TEXTBOOK OF CARDIOVASCULAR MEDICINE

SECOND EDITION

TEXTBOOK OF CARDIOVASCULAR MEDICINE

SECOND EDITION

Editor

ERIC J. TOPOL, M.D.

Provost and Chief Academic Officer
Chairman, Department of Cardiovascular Medicine
The Cleveland Clinic Foundation
Cleveland, Ohio

Associate Editors

ROBERT M. CALIFF, M.D.
Professor of Medicine
Director, Duke Clinical
*   Research Institute*
Durham, North Carolina

JEFFREY M. ISNER, M.D.*
Professor of Medicine and Pathology
Department of Medicine/Vascular
*   Medicine*
Tufts University School of Medicine
Chief of Vascular Medicine and
*   Cardiovascular Research*
St. Elizabeth's Medical Center
Boston, Massachusetts
*Deceased.

ERIC N. PRYSTOWSKY, M.D.
Director, Electrophysiology Laboratory
The CARE Group
Indianapolis, Indiana

JUDITH L. SWAIN, M.D.
Arthur L. Bloomfield Professor of Medicine
Chairman, Department of Medicine
Stanford University School of Medicine
Stanford, California

JAMES D. THOMAS, M.D.
Professor of Medicine and Biomedical Engineering
Director of Cardiovascular Imaging
The Cleveland Clinic Foundation
Cleveland, Ohio

PAUL D. THOMPSON, M.D.
Professor of Medicine
Department of Cardiology
University of Connecticut School
*   of Medicine*
Farmington, Connecticut
Director, Preventive Cardiology
Hartford Hospital
Hartford, Connecticut

JAMES B. YOUNG, M.D.
Professor of Medicine
Medical Director, Kaufman Center
*   for Heart Failure*
The Cleveland Clinic Foundation
Cleveland, Ohio

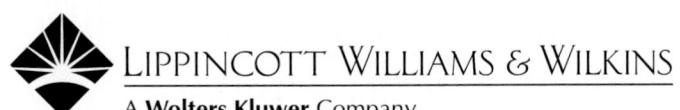

LIPPINCOTT WILLIAMS & WILKINS
A **Wolters Kluwer** Company
Philadelphia · Baltimore · New York · London
Buenos Aires · Hong Kong · Sydney · Tokyo

Executive Editor: Ruth W. Weinberg
Managing Editor: Brian Brown
Developmental Editor: Sonya L. Seigafuse
Supervising Editor: Mary Ann McLaughlin
Production Editors: Alyson Langlois and Holly L. Hoe, Silverchair Science + Communications
Manufacturing Manager: Tim Reynolds
Cover Designer: QT Design
Compositor: Silverchair Science + Communications
Printer: Quebecor World

Library of Congress Cataloging-in-Publication Data

Textbook of cardiovascular medicine / editor, Eric J. Topol ; associate editors, Robert M. Califf ... [et al.].--2nd ed.
   p. ; cm.
  Includes bibliographical references and index.
  ISBN 0-7817-3225-5
  1. Cardiology. 2. Cardiovascular system--Diseases. I. Topol, Eric J., 1954- II. Califf, Robert M.
  [DNLM: 1. Cardiovascular Diseases. 2. Cardiology. WG 100 T3545 2002]
  RC667 .T44 2002
  616.16--dc21

2001038461

10 9 8 7 6 5 4 3 2 1

Dedicated to the memory of
Jeffrey M. Isner, M.D., associate editor for the first and second editions, and one
of the most extraordinary researchers and individuals in the history of cardiovascular medicine

CONTENTS

SECTION III: CARDIOVASCULAR IMAGING
JAMES D. THOMAS

SECTION IV: ELECTROPHYSIOLOGY AND PACING
ERIC N. PRYSTOWSKY

SECTION V: INVASIVE CARDIOLOGY AND SURGICAL TECHNIQUES
ERIC J. TOPOL

CONTRIBUTING AUTHORS

PHILIP A. ADES, M.D.
Professor of Medicine
Division of Cardiology
University of Vermont College
 of Medicine
Burlington, Vermont

KEIKO AIKAWA, M.D.
Fellow in Cardiology
Department of Medicine
Division of Cardiology
University of Washington
 Medical Center
Seattle, Washington

MASOOD AKHTAR, M.D.
Clinical Professor of Medicine
University of Wisconsin Medical School
Milwaukee Clinical Campus
Milwaukee, Wisconsin

HOOMAN ALLAYEE, PH.D.
Postdoctoral Fellow
Department of Human Genetics
University of California, Los Angeles,
 UCLA School of Medicine
Los Angeles, California

JOSEPH S. ALPERT, M.D.
Robert S. and Irene P. Flinn Professor
 of Medicine
Head, Department of Medicine
University of Arizona Health
 Sciences Center
Tucson, Arizona

PETER B. AMSTERDAM, M.D.
Department of Cardiology
Grant Medical Center
Heart Care, Inc.
Columbus, Ohio

RENE A. ARCILLA, M.D.
Professor of Pediatrics
University of Illinois at Chicago College
 of Medicine
Chicago, Illinois
Director of the Heart Institute
 for Children
Hope Children's Hospital
Oak Lawn, Illinois

PAUL W. ARMSTRONG, M.D.
Professor of Medicine
University of Alberta Faculty of Medicine
 and Dentistry
Edmonton, Alberta, Canada

DORON ARONSON, M.D.
Department of Cardiology
Rambam Medical Center
Haifa, Israel

LUIS H. ARROYO, M.D.
Department of Cardiology
Newark Beth Israel
 Medical Center
Newark, New Jersey

CRAIG R. ASHER, M.D.
Assistant Staff
Department of Cardiovascular
 Medicine
The Cleveland Clinic Foundation
Cleveland, Ohio

GARY J. BALADY, M.D.
Professor of Medicine
Section of Cardiology
Boston Medical Center
Boston, Massachusetts

THOMAS M. BASHORE, M.D.
Professor of Medicine
Division of Cardiology
Duke University
 Medical Center
Durham, North Carolina

CRAIG T. BASSON, M.D., PH.D.
Assistant Professor of Medicine
Cardiology Division
Weill Medical College of
 Cornell University
New York Presbyterian Hospital–Cornell
 Medical Center
New York, New York

KENNETH L. BAUGHMAN, M.D.
Professor of Medicine
The Johns Hopkins University School
 of Medicine
Baltimore, Maryland

CHRISTOPHE BAUTERS, M.D.
Professor of Cardiology
CHRU de Lille
Lille, France

ROBERT H. BEEKMAN III, M.D.
Professor of Pediatric Cardiology
Department of Pediatrics
Children's Hospital Medical Center
Cincinnati, Ohio

SUSAN M. BEGELMAN, M.D.
Associate Staff
Department of Cardiovascular Medicine
Section of Vascular Medicine
The Cleveland Clinic Foundation
Cleveland, Ohio

DAVID G. BENDITT, M.D.
Professor of Medicine
Department of Medicine/Cardiology
University of Minnesota Medical
 School—Minneapolis
Minneapolis, Minnesota

DEEPAK L. BHATT, M.D.
Staff Cardiologist
Department of Cardiovascular Medicine
The Cleveland Clinic Foundation
Cleveland, Ohio

LEE A. BIBLO, M.D.
Associate Professor of Medicine
Case Western Reserve University School
 of Medicine
MetroHealth Medical Center
Cleveland, Ohio

J. THOMAS BIGGER, M.D.
Professor of Medicine and Pharmacology
Department of Medicine
Columbia University College of Physicians
 and Surgeons
New York, New York

EUGENE H. BLACKSTONE, M.D.
Professor of Surgery
Department of Thoracic and
 Cardiovascular Surgery
The Cleveland Clinic Foundation
Cleveland, Ohio

MEREDITH BOND, PH.D.
Staff, Department of
    Molecular Cardiology
The Cleveland Clinic Foundation
Cleveland, Ohio

LAWRENCE M. BOXT, M.D.
Professor of Clinical Radiology
Albert Einstein College
    of Medicine of
    Yeshiva University
Bronx, New York
Department of Radiology
Beth Israel Medical Center
New York, New York

ANDREW JAMES BOYLE, M.D.
Clinical Fellow
Department of Heart
    Failure and Cardiac
    Transplantation
The Cleveland Clinic Foundation
Cleveland, Ohio

ROBERT M. CALIFF, M.D.
Professor of Medicine
Director, Duke Clinical
    Research Institute
Durham, North Carolina

BLASE A. CARABELLO, M.D.
Professor of Medicine
Baylor College of Medicine
Houston Veterans Affairs
    Medical Center
Houston, Texas

J. JEFFREY CARR, M.D.
Associate Professor
Department of Public
    Health Sciences
Division of Radiological Sciences
Wake Forest University Baptist
    Medical Center
Winston-Salem, North Carolina

GIULIA L. CEBULLA, M.D.
Fellow in Cardiology
Boston Medical Center
Boston, Massachusetts

KANU CHATTERJEE, M.B.
Professor of Medicine
Lucie Stern Professor
    of Cardiology
University of California, San Francisco,
    School of Medicine
San Francisco, California

MELVIN D. CHEITLIN, M.D.
Emeritus Professor of Medicine
Department of Cardiology
University of California, San Francisco,
    School of Medicine
Former Chief of Cardiology
San Francisco General Hospital
San Francisco, California

PENG-SHENG CHEN, M.D.
Professor of Medicine
Department of Medicine/Cardiology
Cedars-Sinai Medical Center
Los Angeles, California

DEREK P. CHEW, M.B.B.S.
Interventional Fellow
Department of Cardiovascular Medicine
The Cleveland Clinic Foundation
Cleveland, Ohio

MYLAN C. COHEN, M.D., M.P.H.
Clinical Associate Professor of Medicine
Division of Cardiology
University of Vermont College of Medicine
Burlington, Vermont
Maine Medical Center
Portland, Maine

JOSEPH A. COLADONATO, M.D.
Fellow, Department of Nephrology
Duke University Medical Center
Durham, North Carolina

CHRISTOPHER R. COLE, M.D.
Electrophysiology Fellow
Department of Cardiovascular Medicine
The Cleveland Clinic Foundation
Cleveland, Ohio

PIERRE CORVOL, M.D.
Professor of Medicine
Department of Experimental Medicine
College de France
Paris, France

DELOS M. COSGROVE, M.D.
Chairman, Department of Thoracic and
    Cardiovascular Surgery
The Cleveland Clinic Foundation
Cleveland, Ohio

SANJAY S. DESHPANDE, M.D.
Clinical Associate Professor of Medicine
Department of Cardiology
University of Wisconsin-Milwaukee
    Clinical Campus
Sinai Samaritan and St. Luke's
    Medical Centers
Milwaukee, Wisconsin

ROBERT DETRANO, M.D., PH.D.
Professor of Medicine
Department of Cardiology
South Bay Heart Watch
Harbor-UCLA Research and
    Education Institute
Torrance, California

CARLO DI MARIO, M.D., PH.D.
Department of Interventional Cardiology
San Raffaelo Hospital
Milan, Italy

SANDRA A. DISSE-NICODÈME, PH.D.
Department of Gene Identification
Centre National de Genotypage
Cedex, France

JOHN S. DOUGLAS, JR., M.D.
Professor of Medicine
Director, Interventional Cardiology
Emory University Hospital
Atlanta, Georgia

THOMAS A. DRAKE, M.D.
Professor of Pathology and
    Laboratory Medicine
University of California, Los Angeles,
    UCLA School of Medicine
Los Angeles, California

THOMAS J. DRESING, M.D.
Clinical Fellow
Department of Cardiovascular Medicine
The Cleveland Clinic Foundation
Cleveland, Ohio

KIM A. EAGLE, M.D.
Albion Walter Hewlett Professor of
    Internal Medicine
Department of Internal
    Medicine/Cardiology
University of Michigan Medical School
Ann Arbor, Michigan

PERRY M. ELLIOTT, M.B.B.S., M.D.
Senior Lecturer in Cardiology
Department of Cardiological Sciences
St. George's Hospital Medical School
London, United Kingdom

ROBERT C. ELSTON, PH.D.
Professor of Epidemiology
    and Genetics
Department of Epidemiology and
    Biostatistics
Case Western Reserve University School
    of Medicine
MetroHealth Medical Center
Cleveland, Ohio

CHARLES F. EMERY, PH.D.
Associate Professor of Psychology
The Ohio State University
Columbus, Ohio

N. A. MARK ESTES III, M.D.
Professor of Medicine
Tufts University School of Medicine
Boston, Massachusetts

GORDON A. EWY, M.D.
Professor and Chief of Cardiology
Department of Medicine
University of Arizona College
    of Medicine
Arizona Health Sciences Center
Sarver Heart Center
Tucson, Arizona

JOHN D. FISHER, M.D.
Professor of Medicine
Director, Arrhythmia Services
Department of Cardiology
Montefiore Medical Center
Bronx, New York

FRANK A. FLACHSKAMPF, M.D.
Associate Professor of Medicine
Medizinische Klinik II
University Erlangen–Nürnberg
Erlangen, Germany

GARY S. FRANCIS, M.D.
Professor of Medicine
Director, Coronary Intensive
    Care Unit
The Cleveland Clinic Foundation
Cleveland, Ohio

ROBERT M. FREEDOM, M.D.
Chief, Division of Cardiology
The Hospital for Sick Children
Toronto, Ontario, Canada

GOTTLIEB C. FRIESINGER, M.D.
Betty and Jack Bailey Professor of
    Cardiology
Department of Medicine
Vanderbilt University
    Medical Center
Nashville, Tennessee

ANTHONY J. FURLAN, M.D.
Head, Section of Stroke and Neurological
    Intensive Care
Medical Director,
    Cerebrovascular Center
Department of Neurology
The Cleveland Clinic Foundation
Cleveland, Ohio

W. BRUCE FYE, M.D.
Professor of Medicine
Cardiovascular Division
Mayo Medical School
Mayo Clinic
Rochester, Minnesota

MARIO J. GARCIA, M.D.
Staff Cardiologist and Director of
    Echocardiography
Department of Cardiovascular Medicine
The Cleveland Clinic Foundation
Cleveland, Ohio

ARTHUR GARSON, JR., M.D., M.P.H.
Professor of Pediatrics (Cardiology)
Department of Pediatric Cardiology
Baylor College of Medicine
Houston, Texas

BERNARD J. GERSH, M.D., CH.B., D.PHIL.
Professor of Medicine
Division of Cardiovascular Diseases
Mayo Clinic
Rochester, Minnesota

GARY H. GIBBONS, M.D.
Associate Professor of Medicine
Director, Cardiovascular Research Institute
Morehouse School of Medicine
Atlanta, Georgia

A. MARC GILLINOV, M.D.
Heart Surgeon
Department of Thoracic and
    Cardiovascular Surgery
The Cleveland Clinic Foundation
Cleveland, Ohio

**ANNE-PAULE GIMENEZ-ROQUEPLO,
M.D., PH.D.**
Department of Molecular Genetics
Hôpital Européen Georges Pompidou
Paris, France

MICHAEL G. GOLDSTEIN, M.D.
Adjunct Professor
Department of Psychiatry and Human
    Behavior
Brown University School of Medicine
The Miriam Hospital
Providence, Rhode Island
The Bayer Institute for Health Care
    Communication
West Haven, Connecticut

AUGUSTUS O. GRANT, M.B., CH.B., PH.D.
Professor of Medicine
Duke University Medical Center
Durham, North Carolina

BRIAN P. GRIFFIN, M.D.
Director, Cardiovascular
    Training Program
Department of Cardiovascular
    Medicine
The Cleveland Clinic Foundation
Cleveland, Ohio

MADHU GUPTA, PH.D.
Assistant Professor
Department of Physiology
    and Biophysics
University of Illinois
Hope Children's Hospital
Palos Heights, Illinois

MAHESH P. GUPTA, PH.D.
Associate Professor
Department of Surgery (Cardiac
    and Thoracic)
The University of Chicago Pritzker
    School of Medicine
Chicago, Illinois

GARRIE J. HAAS, M.D.
Director, Heart Failure Disease
    Management Program
Mid Ohio Cardiology Consultants
Riverside Methodist Hospital
Columbus, Ohio

DAVID E. HAINES, M.D.
Professor of Medicine
Cardiovascular Division
University of Virginia
    Health System
Charlottesville, Virginia

STEPHEN C. HAMMILL, M.D.
Professor of Medicine
Director, Electrocardiography
    and Electrophysiology
Mayo Clinic
Rochester, Minnesota

DAVID L. HAYES, M.D.
Professor of Medicine
Mayo Medical School
Consultant, Division of
    Cardiovascular Diseases and
    Internal Medicine
Mayo Clinic
Rochester, Minnesota

FREDERICK A. HEUPLER, JR., M.D.
Staff Cardiologist
Department of Cardiovascular
    Medicine
The Cleveland Clinic Foundation
Cleveland, Ohio

L. DAVID HILLIS, M.D.
Professor and Vice Chair
Department of Internal Medicine
University of Texas Southwestern Medical
  Center at Dallas
Dallas, Texas

JUDITH S. HOCHMAN, M.D.
Professor of Medicine
Department of Cardiology
Columbia University College of Physicians
  and Surgeons
St. Luke's-Roosevelt Hospital Center
New York, New York

AMI E. ISKANDRIAN, M.D.
Distinguished Professor of Medicine and
  Radiology
Section Chief, Nuclear Cardiology
Division of Cardiovascular Disease
University of Alabama School
  of Medicine
Birmingham, Alabama

JEFFREY M. ISNER, M.D.*
Professor of Medicine and Pathology
Department of Medicine/Vascular
  Medicine
Tufts University School of Medicine
Chief of Vascular Medicine and
  Cardiovascular Research
St. Elizabeth's Medical Center
Boston, Massachusetts

**XAVIER LAURENT JEUNEMAITRE,
M.D., PH.D.**
Professor of Genetics
Hôpital Européen Georges Pompidou
Paris, France

RONALD J. KANTER, M.D.
Associate Professor of Pediatrics
Department of Pediatric Cardiology
Duke University Medical Center
Durham, North Carolina

SAMIR R. KAPADIA, M.D.
Assistant Professor
Department of Cardiology
University of Washington School
  of Medicine
Seattle, Washington

AMOS KATZ, M.D.
Professor of Medicine
Department of Cardiology
Soroka University Medical Center
Beersheva, Israel

*Deceased.

ARNOLD M. KATZ, M.D.
Professor of Medicine Emeritus
University of Connecticut School
  of Medicine
Farmington, Connecticut
Visiting Professor of Medicine
Dartmouth Medical School
Hanover, New Hampshire

ALLAN L. KLEIN, M.D.
Professor of Medicine
Department of Cardiovascular Medicine
The Cleveland Clinic Foundation
Cleveland, Ohio

ROBERT A. KLONER, M.D., PH.D.
Professor of Medicine
Division of Cardiology
University of Southern California School
  of Medicine
Director of Research
Heart Institute
Good Samaritan Hospital
Los Angeles, California

ROBERT H. KNOPP, M.D.
Professor of Medicine
University of Washington School
  of Medicine
Director, Northwest Lipid
  Research Clinic
Seattle, Washington

RICHARD A. LANGE, M.D.
Professor of Medicine
Department of Internal Medicine
University of Texas Southwestern
  Medical Center at Dallas
Dallas, Texas

DANIEL T. LASKOWITZ, M.D.
Assistant Professor of Medicine
  (Neurology) and Anesthesiology
Department of Medicine
Duke University School
  of Medicine
Duke University Medical Center
Durham, North Carolina

MICHAEL S. LAUER, M.D.
Director of Clinical Research
Department of Cardiovascular
  Medicine
The Cleveland Clinic Foundation
Cleveland, Ohio

DAVID H. LEWIS, M.D.
Cardiologist
Mid America Heart Institute
Kansas City, Missouri

MARK E. LIEB, M.D.
Assistant Professor of Medicine
Mount Sinai School of Medicine of the
  City University of New York
New York, New York

A. MICHAEL LINCOFF, M.D.
Associate Professor of Medicine
Director, Experimental Interventional
  Laboratory
Department of Cardiovascular Medicine
The Cleveland Clinic Foundation
Cleveland, Ohio

FLOYD D. LOOP, M.D.
Chief Executive Officer
The Cleveland Clinic Foundation
Cleveland, Ohio

JOSEPH LOSCALZO, M.D., PH.D.
Wade Professor and Chairman
Department of Medicine
Boston University School of Medicine
Boston Medical Center
Boston, Massachusetts

ALDONS J. LUSIS, PH.D.
Professor
Departments of Medicine and
  Human Genetics
Division of Cardiology
University of California, Los Angeles,
  UCLA School of Medicine
Los Angeles, California

SUZANNE R. LUTTON, M.D.
Diagnostic Cardiology Associates
Youngstown, Ohio

JOHN S. MACGREGOR, M.D., PH.D.
Associate Professor of Medicine
University of California, San Francisco,
  School of Medicine
San Francisco, California

KENNETH W. MAHAFFEY, M.D.
Assistant Professor of Medicine
Department of Cardiology
Duke Clinical Research Institute
Duke University Medical Center
Durham, North Carolina

ARIANE J. MARELLI, M.D.
Assistant Professor of Medicine
McGill University Faculty
  of Medicine
Director, Adult Congenital Heart
  Disease Unit
McGill University Health Center
Montreal, Quebec, Canada

DANIEL B. MARK, M.D., M.P.H.
Professor of Medicine
Department of Cardiology
Duke University Medical Center
Durham, North Carolina

THOMAS H. MARWICK, M.B.B.S., PH.D.
Professor of Medicine
University of Queensland
Princess Alexandra Hospital
Brisbane, Queensland, Australia

WILLIAM J. MCKENNA, M.D., D.SC.
Professor of Molecular
    Cardiovascular Sciences
Department of Cardiological Sciences
St. George's Hospital
    Medical School
London, United Kingdom

DENNIS M. MCNAMARA, M.D.
Associate Professor of Medicine
Cardiovascular Institute
University of Pittsburgh
    Medical Center
Pittsburgh, Pennsylvania

BERNHARD MEIER, M.D.
Professor of Cardiology
    and Chairman
Cardiovascular Department
University Hospital
Bern, Switzerland

ALAN M. MENDELSOHN, M.D.
Associate Director of Cardiovascular
    Medical Affairs
Centocor, Inc.
Malvern, Pennsylvania

DAVID J. MOLITERNO, M.D.
Associate Professor of Medicine
Department of Cardiovascular
    Medicine
The Cleveland Clinic Foundation
Cleveland, Ohio

DOUGLAS S. MOODIE, M.D.
Chairman, Department of
    Pediatrics
Ochsner Clinic Foundation
New Orleans, Louisiana

ELIZABETH G. NABEL, M.D.
Scientific Director
National Heart, Lung, and
    Blood Institute
National Institutes of Health
Bethesda, Maryland

GERALD V. NACCARELLI, M.D.
Professor of Medicine and Chief
Division of Cardiology
Director, Cardiovascular Center
Pennsylvania State University College
    of Medicine
Hershey, Pennsylvania

RAYMOND NIAURA, PH.D.
Professor of Psychiatry
Centers for Behavioral and
    Preventive Medicine
Brown University School of Medicine
The Miriam Hospital
Providence, Rhode Island

STEVEN E. NISSEN, M.D.
Professor of Medicine and
    Vice Chairman
Department of Cardiovascular
    Medicine
The Cleveland Clinic Foundation
Cleveland, Ohio

DAVID G. NYKANEN, M.D.
Division of Cardiology
Miami Children's Hospital
Miami, Florida

CHRISTOPHER M. O'CONNOR, M.D.
Associate Professor of Medicine
Duke University Medical Center
Durham, North Carolina

PETER M. OKIN, M.D.
Professor of Medicine
Division of Cardiology
Weill Medical College of
    Cornell University
New York, New York

JEFFREY W. OLIN, D.O.
Director, The Heart and
    Vascular Institute
Morristown, New Jersey

JOHN N. O'NEIL, PH.D.
Postdoctoral Fellow
Department of Psychology
The Ohio State University
Columbus, Ohio

JOSEPH P. ORNATO, M.D.
Professor and Chairman
Department of Emergency
    Medicine
Virginia Commonwealth University
    School of Medicine
Richmond, Virginia

LARS G. OSTERBERG, M.D.
Clinical Assistant Professor of Medicine
Department of Internal Medicine
Stanford University School of Medicine
Stanford University Medical Center
Stanford, California

DOUGLAS L. PACKER, M.D.
Professor of Medicine
Divisions of Cardiovascular Diseases
    and Electrophysiology
Mayo Clinic
Rochester, Minnesota

**THOMAS A. PEARSON, M.D.,
PH.D., M.P.H.**
Albert D. Kaiser Professor
    and Chair
Department of Community and
    Preventive Medicine
University of Rochester School of
    Medicine and Dentistry
Rochester, New York

MARY ANN PEBERDY, M.D.
Assistant Professor of Medicine and
    Emergency Medicine
Department of Internal Medicine
Virginia Commonwealth University
    School of Medicine
Richmond, Virginia

SERGIO L. PINSKI, M.D.
Associate Professor of Medicine
Section of Cardiology
Rush Medical College of
    Rush University
Rush-Presbyterian-St. Luke's
    Medical Center
Chicago, Illinois

JEFFREY J. POPMA, M.D.
Associate Professor of Medicine
Cardiovascular Division
Brigham and Women's Hospital
Boston, Massachusetts

ERIC N. PRYSTOWSKY, M.D.
Director, Electrophysiology Laboratory
The CARE Group
Indianapolis, Indiana

REED E. PYERITZ, M.D., PH.D.
Professor of Medicine and Genetics
Chief, Division of Medical Genetics
Department of Medicine
University of Pennsylvania School
    of Medicine
Philadelphia, Pennsylvania

MARLENE RABINOVITCH, M.D.
HSFO Research Endowed Chair
Professor of Pediatrics and
    Pathology Medicine
University of Toronto
Director, Cardiovascular Research Program
Hospital for Sick Children
Toronto, Ontario, Canada

DANIEL J. RADER, M.D.
Associate Professor of Medicine
University of Pennsylvania Medical Center
Philadelphia, Pennsylvania

RAVI RASALINGAM, M.B., CH.B.
Department of Medicine
Strong Memorial Hospital
Rochester, New York

NORMAN B. RATLIFF, M.D.
Professor of Pathology
Faculty Director of Cardiovascular
    Pathology and Autopsy Service
Department of Anatomic Pathology
The Cleveland Clinic Foundation
Cleveland, Ohio

ELLIOT J. RAYFIELD, M.D.
Clinical Professor of Medicine
Mount Sinai School of Medicine of the
    City University of New York
New York, New York

DONAL N. REDDAN, M.B., M.H.S.
Associate in Medicine
Department of Medicine/Nephrology
Duke University Medical Center
Durham, North Carolina

TIMOTHY J. REGAN, M.D.*
Professor of Medicine
New Jersey Medical School
Newark, New Jersey

DALE G. RENLUND, M.D.
Professor of Internal Medicine
University of Utah School of Medicine
LDS Hospital
Salt Lake City, Utah

CLARA I. RESTREPO, M.D.
Instructor
Department of Medicine
Division of Pulmonary and Critical
    Care Medicine
National Jewish Medical and Research Center
University of Colorado Health
    Sciences Center
Denver, Colorado

*Deceased.

SHEREIF H. REZKALLA, M.D.
Clinical Professor of Medicine
University of Wisconsin
    Medical School
Madison, Wisconsin
Director, Cardiovascular Research
Department of Cardiology
Marshfield Clinic
Marshfield, Wisconsin

WILLIAM C. ROBERTS, M.D.
Medical Director
Baylor Heart and Vascular Center
Baylor University Medical Center
Dallas, Texas

KILLIAN ROBINSON, M.D.
Associate Professor of Cardiology and
    Internal Medicine
Department of Internal Medicine
Section of Cardiology
Wake Forest University School
    of Medicine
Wake Forest University Baptist
    Medical Center
Winston-Salem, North Carolina

DAN M. RODEN, M.D.
Professor of Medicine and Pharmacology
Vanderbilt University School
    of Medicine
Nashville, Tennessee

MARCO ROFFI, M.D.
Fellow in Interventional Cardiology
Department of Cardiovascular Medicine
The Cleveland Clinic Foundation
Cleveland, Ohio

KENNETH ROSENFIELD, M.D.
Assistant Professor of Medicine
Department of Cardiovascular Medicine
    and Research
Tufts University School of Medicine
St. Elizabeth's Medical Center
Boston, Massachusetts

JAMES H. F. RUDD, M.B.
BHF Clinical Research Fellow and
    Honorary Registrar in Cardiology
Division of Cardiovascular Medicine
University of Cambridge
Addenbrooke's Hospital
Cambridge, United Kingdom

PETER RUDD, M.D.
Professor of Medicine
Department of General
    Internal Medicine
Stanford University School of Medicine
Stanford, California

JOSEPH F. SABIK III, M.D.
Heart Surgeon
Department of Thoracic and
    Cardiovascular Surgery
The Cleveland Clinic Foundation
Cleveland, Ohio

PAULO R. SCHVARTZMAN, M.D.
Fellow in Cardiovascular Imaging
Department of Radiology
The Cleveland Clinic Foundation
Cleveland Ohio

MARKUS SCHWAIGER, M.D.
Professor of Nuclear Medicine
Klinikum Rechts der Isar
Technische Universität München
München, Germany

ROBERT A. SCHWEIKERT, M.D.
Staff Cardiologist
Department of Cardiovascular Medicine
The Cleveland Clinic Foundation
Cleveland, Ohio

CHRISTINE E. SEIDMAN, M.D.
Professor of Medicine and Genetics
Department of Genetics
Harvard Medical School
Boston, Massachusetts

DANIEL J. SEXTON, M.D.
Professor of Medicine
Division of Infectious Diseases
Duke University Medical Center
Durham, North Carolina

ELENA B. SGARBOSSA, M.D.
Assistant Professor of Medicine
Associate Director of Clinical Research
Department of Cardiology
Rush-Presbyterian-St. Luke's
    Medical Center
Chicago, Illinois

SAEED R. SHAIKH, M.D.
Fellow, Cardiovascular Diseases
Department of Cardiology
Maine Medical Center
Portland, Maine

DEBRA L. SHERMAN, M.D.
Staff, Department of Cardiology
Caritas Norwood Hospital
Norwood, Massachusetts

DAVID SHIM, M.D.
Assistant Professor of Pediatrics
Division of Cardiology
Children's Hospital Medical Center
Cincinnati, Ohio

CATHY A. SILA, M.D.
Associate Medical Director
Cerebrovascular Center
Section of Stroke and Neurologic
    Intensive Care
The Cleveland Clinic Foundation
Cleveland, Ohio

NICHOLAS G. SMEDIRA, M.D.
Staff, Department of Thoracic and
    Cardiovascular Surgery
The Cleveland Clinic Foundation
Cleveland, Ohio

REBECCA L. SMITH, M.D.
Fellow in Cardiovascular Imaging
Department of Cardiovascular
    Medicine
The Cleveland Clinic Foundation
Cleveland, Ohio

PETER C. SPITTELL, M.D.
Assistant Professor of Medicine
Mayo Medical School
Consultant, Department of Internal
    Medicine
Division of Cardiovascular
    Diseases
Mayo Medical Center
Rochester, Minnesota

RANDALL C. STARLING, M.D., M.P.H.
Director of Advanced Heart Failure
Department of Cardiovascular
    Medicine
Section of Heart Failure and Cardiac
    Transplant Medicine
The Cleveland Clinic Foundation
Cleveland, Ohio

WILLIAM J. STEWART, M.D.
Associate Professor of Medicine
Department of Cardiovascular Medicine
The Cleveland Clinic Foundation
Cleveland, Ohio

NEIL J. STONE, M.D.
Professor of Clinical Medicine
Department of Cardiology
Northwestern University Medical School
Chicago, Illinois

D. EUGENE STRANDNESS, JR., M.D.*
Professor of Medicine
Department of Surgery
University of Washington
    Medical Center
Seattle, Washington

Deceased.

JUDITH L. SWAIN, M.D.
Arthur L. Bloomfield Professor
    of Medicine
Chairman, Department of Medicine
Stanford University School of Medicine
Stanford, California

LYNDA ANNE SZCZECH, M.D.
Assistant Professor of Medicine
Duke University Medical Center
Durham, North Carolina

VICTOR F. TAPSON, M.D.
Associate Professor of Medicine
Division of Pulmonary and Critical
    Care Medicine
Duke University Medical Center
Durham, North Carolina

MARK B. TAUBMAN, M.D.
Professor of Medicine
The Cardiovascular Institute
Mount Sinai School of Medicine of the
    City University of New York
New York, New York

DAVID O. TAYLOR, M.D.
Professor of Medicine
Division of Cardiology
University of Utah School of Medicine
Salt Lake City, Utah

PATRICK J. TCHOU, M.D.
Head, Cardiac Electrophysiology and Pacing
Department of Cardiovascular Medicine
The Cleveland Clinic Foundation
Cleveland, Ohio

JAMES D. THOMAS, M.D.
Professor of Medicine and Biomedical
    Engineering
Director of Cardiovascular Imaging
The Cleveland Clinic Foundation
Cleveland, Ohio

PAUL D. THOMPSON, M.D.
Professor of Medicine
Department of Cardiology
University of Connecticut School
    of Medicine
Farmington, Connecticut
Director, Preventive Cardiology
Hartford Hospital
Hartford, Connecticut

XIAO-LI TIAN, PH.D.
Department of Molecular Cardiology
Center for Molecular Genetics
The Cleveland Clinic Foundation
Cleveland, Ohio

ERIC J. TOPOL, M.D.
Provost and Chief Academic Officer
Chairman, Department of
    Cardiovascular Medicine
The Cleveland Clinic Foundation
Cleveland, Ohio

E. MURAT TUZCU, M.D.
Professor of Medicine
Department of Cardiovascular Medicine
The Cleveland Clinic Foundation
Cleveland, Ohio

ALEC SYLVAIN VAHANIAN, M.D.
Professor of Medicine
Department of Cardiology
Bichat Hospital
Paris, France

PETER R. VALE, M.D.
Interventional Vascular Physician
    and Cardiologist
Department of Vascular Medicine
University of New South Wales
    School of Medicine
St. Vincent's Hospital
St. Vincent's Clinic
Sydney, Australia

ERIC VAN BELLE, M.D., PH.D.
Professor of Medicine
Department of Cardiology
Hôpital Cardiologique
Lille, France

FRANS J. VAN DE WERF, M.D., PH.D.
Professor and Chairman of Cardiology
Gasthuisberg University Hospital
Leuven, Belgium

MARIO S. VERANI, M.D.
Professor of Medicine and Director
    of Nuclear Cardiology
Department of Medicine (Cardiology)
The Methodist Hospital
Houston, Texas

GALEN S. WAGNER, M.D.
Associate Professor of Medicine
Duke University Medical Center
Durham, North Carolina

ALBERT L. WALDO, M.D.
The Walter H. Pritchard Professor of
    Cardiology and Professor of Medicine
Department of Medicine
Case Western Reserve University School
    of Medicine
University Hospitals of Cleveland
Cleveland, Ohio

QING WANG, PH.D.
Assistant Staff
Assistant Professor of Molecular
 Genetics, Molecular Cardiology,
 and Cardiology
Departments of Molecular Genetics and
 Molecular Cardiology
The Cleveland Clinic Foundation
Cleveland, Ohio

JUDAH WEINBERGER, M.D., PH.D.
Associate Professor of Medicine
New York-Presbyterian Hospital
New York, New York

ARI WEINREB, M.D., PH.D.
Assistant Professor of Medicine
University of California, Los Angeles,
 UCLA School of Medicine
Associate Chief of Rheumatology
VA Greater Los Angeles Healthcare
 System
Los Angeles, California

PETER L. WEISSBERG, M.D.
BHF Professor of Cardiovascular
 Medicine
Division of Cardiovascular
 Medicine
Addenbrooke's Hospital
Cambridge, United Kingdom

HEIN J. WELLENS, M.D.
Professor of Cardiology
 and Director
Interuniversity Cardiology Institute
 of The Netherlands
Utrecht, The Netherlands

**DAVID W. WHALLEY, M.B.B.S.(HON.),
PH.D.**
Senior Lecturer in Cardiology
Royal North Shore Hospital,
 Sydney
University of Sydney
Sydney, Australia

HARVEY D. WHITE, CH.B., D.SC.
Honorary Clinical Professor
 of Medicine
University of Auckland
Director of Coronary Care and
 Cardiovascular Research
Green Lane Hospital
Auckland, New Zealand

RICHARD D. WHITE, M.D.
Professor of Medicine
 and Radiology
Division of Radiology
The Cleveland Clinic
 Foundation
Cleveland, Ohio

DEBORAH L. WOLBRETTE, M.D.
Associate Professor of Medicine
Division of Cardiology
Pennsylvania State University College
 of Medicine
The Milton S. Hershey Medical Center
Hershey, Pennsylvania

RAYMOND L. WOOSLEY, M.D., PH.D.
Vice President for Health Sciences
Dean, College of Medicine
University of Arizona College of Medicine
Tucson, Arizona

DAVID M. YAMADA, M.D.
Consulting Cardiologist
Department of Cardiovascular Medicine
Sarasota Memorial Hospital
Sarasota, Florida

JAMES B. YOUNG, M.D.
Professor of Medicine
Medical Director, Kaufman Center for
 Heart Failure
The Cleveland Clinic Foundation
Cleveland, Ohio

SIBYLLE I. ZIEGLER, PH.D.
Department of Nuclear Medicine
Technische Universität München
München, Germany

PREFACE

Textbook of Cardiovascular Medicine, *2nd Edition*
A Pioneering Concept in the Era of Electronic Textbook Publishing

The success of the first edition of the *Textbook* was largely predicated on fulfilling its mission: "building a new, authoritative reference textbook in the field of cardiovascular medicine . . . based on the radical changes that have taken place in the past decade." These changes not only include coverage of the largest specialty within medicine, but also the fully transformed electronic capabilities that have become both pervasive and prosaic. The CD-ROM version of the first edition of the *Textbook* received significant recognition and acclaim as a single disc that contained the entire expanded, two-volume *Comprehensive Cardiovascular Medicine* and hundreds of digital images and multimedia video clips to bring the text alive. Subsequent to the launch of this project, we were the first to make its entire contents fully available on the Internet at http://www.theheart.org.

In this edition of the *Textbook*, we have developed an entirely new concept of electronic textbook publishing. This takes into account a broad embracing of digital technology, with a CD-ROM fully integrated with the textbook. The book and CD-ROM are a unit, with each component providing invaluable support for the other. The hard copy of the book is intended to capture the core material in our specialty; those sections of each chapter and whole chapters that are critical to providing a comprehensive reference source of the field are incorporated in the CD-ROM. This model of full integration of hard copy and an electronic medium has not been done before in medical textbook publishing. It is intended to cater to the realities of and need for rapidly looking up something in a book, which is simplified and limited in bulk, while at the same time providing in-depth probing of virtually all aspects of cardiovascular medicine, from its molecular areas to health care policy. Only via the electronic medium using the CD-ROM can all the detail be provided along with the extensive graphic support without being too voluminous.

The graphics are extensively hyperlinked to the text in an effort to broaden the presentation to not only words, but also multimedia imagery. The extent of this graphic support in magnitude has not been approached to date by any medical textbook, let alone the full integration concept. Clearly, this has been an ambitious and futuristic project for medical textbooks.

Beyond the book and electronic hybridization, there have been radical updates of nearly every chapter from the first edition (with the exception of such topics as history and physical examination!). New chapters include End-of-Life Care, Athlete's Heart, Clinical Assessment of the Autonomic Nervous System, Percutaneous Coronary Intervention, Surgical Considerations in the Treatment of Heart Failure, Gene Therapy, and Molecular Basis of Heart Development. The updates and new chapters were built on the original framework of the eight sections of the book, which we believe continue to represent the optimal partitioning of the field's major components. The digital anchoring of this project fully supports updates in the field, such as the significant advance in a clinical trial of rapamycin-coated stents that proved highly effective in reducing the incidence of restenosis after percutaneous coronary revascularization.

To execute this prodigious effort, we relied on nearly 200 expert contributing authors from all over the world. One of the most significant contributors to and editors of this project from its inception was Dr. Jeffrey M. Isner, who was a veritable pioneer in this field. His untimely death in late 2001 has sent shock waves throughout the biomedical community. Besides all the leadership he provided in gene therapy, angiogenesis, and translational research, he was deeply committed to this book and the value it would have for our field. Although it is only one dimension of Dr. Isner's rich legacy, the editors and authors hope that this initiative will prove helpful in day-to-day care of patients with cardiovascular disease, serve as a stimulus for future research in basic and clinical science, and provide a utilitarian reference for all health care professionals, trainees, and biomedical researchers active in the field of cardiovascular medicine in the twenty-first century.

Eric J. Topol, M.D.
The Cleveland Clinic Foundation

ACKNOWLEDGMENTS

As in the first edition, this project has been utterly consumptive and, without question, the most challenging and enormous undertaking that I have ever encountered. For it to be accomplished, a huge number of dedicated individuals came together in a highly synergistic fashion. The people behind the project include the superb section editors, nearly 200 contributing authors from all over the world, and two project teams. One, based at The Cleveland Clinic Foundation, included Donna Wasiewicz-Bressan, Managing Editor; Steve Nissen, CD-ROM Producer and Director; Suzanne Turner, Charlene Surace, Mary Ann Citraro, and Marion Tomasko, graphic artists; with extensive CD-ROM contributions from Timothy Crowe, Paula Shalling, Arman Askari, Ron Aviles, Keith Ellis, Murray Estess, Hitinder Gurm, Barbara Hesse, Matt Hook, Chris Jones, David Lee, Tom McRae, Chris Merritt, Adrian Messerli, David Rodriguez, Ravish Sachar, Niranjan Seshadri, Barb Srichai, Mike Yen, and Frank Zidar. Heart sounds were collected by Deb Mukherjee, Steve Lin, Khaldoun Tarakji, and Raymond Migrino. The other group, based at Lippincott Williams & Wilkins and Silverchair Science + Communications, included Ruth Weinberg, Executive Editor, and the editorial and production teams of Sonya Seigafuse, Brian Brown, Mary Ann McLaughlin, Alyson Langlois, Holly Hoe, and Lisa Cunningham. Only with the tight collaboration and dedication of all the editors, authors, and the project teams could such a vast endeavor come together so successfully. My personal appreciation to all of these people runs very deep and cannot be adequately expressed in words.

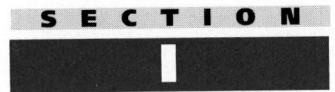

PREVENTIVE CARDIOLOGY

PAUL D. THOMPSON

ATHEROSCLEROTIC BIOLOGY AND EPIDEMIOLOGY OF DISEASE

PETER L. WEISSBERG
JAMES H. F. RUDD

▼▼ *ADDITIONAL ELECTRONIC TOPICS*

Theories of Atherogenesis a01;   Lipid Hypothesis a02;   Thrombogenic Hypothesis a03;   Response to Injury Hypothesis a04;   Modified Response to Injury Hypothesis a05;   Inflammation Theory a06

EPIDEMIOLOGY OF CARDIOVASCULAR DISEASE

Atherosclerosis, with its complications, is the leading cause of mortality and morbidity in the developed world. In the United States, a snapshot of the population would reveal that 60 million adults currently suffer from atherosclerotic cardiovascular disease, which accounts for 42% of all deaths annually, at a cost to the nation of $128 billion. Fortunately, despite this catastrophic burden of disease, much evidence has emerged over the last decade suggesting that the progression of atherosclerosis can be slowed or even reversed in many people with appropriate lifestyle and drug interventions.

The origin of the current epidemic of cardiovascular disease can be traced back to the time of industrialization in the 1700s. The three factors largely responsible for this

---

P. L Weissberg: Division of Cardiovascular Medicine, Addenbrooke's Hospital, Cambridge, United Kingdom
J. H. F. Rudd: Division of Cardiovascular Medicine, University of Cambridge, Addenbrooke's Hospital, Cambridge, United Kingdom

were an increase in the use of tobacco products; reduced physical activity; and the adoption of a diet high in fat, calories, and cholesterol. This rising tide of cardiovascular disease continued into the twentieth century but began to recede when data from the Framingham study identified a number of modifiable risk factors for cardiovascular disease, including cigarette smoking, hypertension, and hypercholesterolemia [1].

The number of deaths per 100,000 attributable to cardiovascular disease peaked in the Western world in 1964 to 1965, since which time there has been a gradual decline in death rates (Fig. 1.1) [2]. The age-adjusted coronary heart disease mortality in the United States dropped by more than 40% and cerebrovascular disease mortality by more than 50%, with the greatest reductions being seen among whites and males. This reduction has occurred despite a quadrupling of the proportion of the population older than 65 years of age and has been due to a number of factors, particularly major health promotion campaigns aimed at reducing the prevalence of Framingham risk factors. Indeed, there has been a substantial change in the prevalence of population cardiovascular risk factors over the last

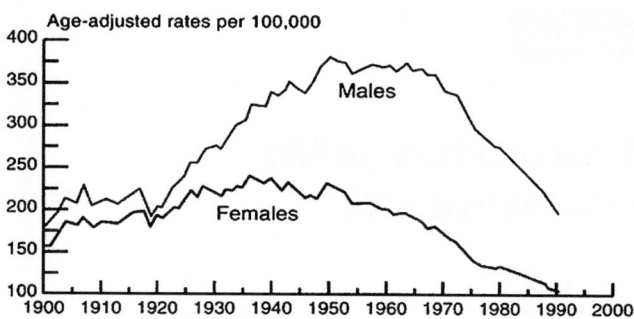

FIGURE 1.1 Trends in death rates for heart diseases: United States, 1900 to 1991. [From Feinleib M. Trends in heart disease in the United States (review). *Am J Med Sci* 1995;310(Suppl 1):S8–S14, with permission.]

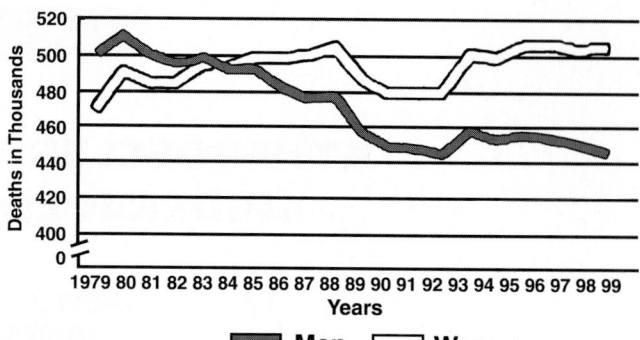

FIGURE 1.2 Cardiovascular disease mortality trends for men and women: United States, 1979 to 1998. (Source: CDC/NCHS and the American Heart Association, with permission.)

30 years (Table 1.1). The war is not won, however, and the decline in the death rate from cardiovascular disease slowed in the 1990s (Fig. 1.2). This is likely due to a large increase in the prevalence of both obesity and type 2 diabetes mellitus, as well as a resurgence of cigarette smoking in some sectors of society (3). Female death rates from cardiovascular disease overtook male death rates in 1984 and have shown a smaller decline over the last 30 years (4). The consequences of atherosclerosis are also beginning to be felt in less well-developed regions of the globe (5), with death from atherosclerotic cardiovascular disease set to replace infection as the leading cause of death in the Third World in the near future.

BIOLOGY OF ATHEROSCLEROSIS

Traditionally, atherosclerosis has been viewed as a degenerative disease, affecting predominantly older people, slowly progressing over many years, and eventually leading to symptoms through mechanical effects on blood flow. The perceived insidious and relentless nature of its development has meant that a somewhat pessimistic view of the potential to

TABLE 1.1 TEMPORAL CHANGES IN CORONARY RISK FACTORS

Cigarette smoking	1960	Men: 55%; Women: 33%
	1990	Men: 30%; Women: 27%
Undiagnosed hypertension	1960	52%
	1980	29%
Mean serum cholesterol	1960	225 mg/dL
	1990	208 mg/dL
Diabetes mellitus	1970	2.6%
	1990	9.1%
Sedentary lifestyle	1970	41%
	1985	27%
Obesity	1960	25%
	1990	38%

From Miller M, Vogel RA. *The practice of coronary disease prevention.* Baltimore: Williams & Wilkins, 1996.

modify its progression by medical therapy has held sway. There has been little emphasis on the diagnosis and treatment of high-risk asymptomatic patients. Disease management has instead been dominated by interventional revascularization approaches, targeting the largest and most visible or symptomatic lesions with coronary angioplasty or bypass surgery.

Recently, for three reasons, this defeatist view of the pathogenesis and progression of atherosclerosis has begun to change. First, careful descriptive studies of the underlying pathology of atherosclerosis have revealed that atherosclerotic plaques differ in their cellular composition and that the cell types predominating in the plaque can determine the risk of fatal clinical events. Second, recent cellular and molecular biologic work has emphasized the importance of inflammatory cells and inflammatory mediators in the pathogenesis of atherosclerosis. The third and most important reason is because several large-scale clinical trials have reported that drugs—in particular, the HMG-CoA reductase inhibitors—are able to reduce the number of clinical events in patients with established atherosclerosis and do so without necessarily affecting the size of atherosclerotic plaques. These three strands of evidence have shown that, rather than being an irreversibly progressive disease, atherosclerosis is a dynamic, inflammatory process that may be amenable to medical therapy. Understanding the cellular and molecular interactions that determine the development and progression of atherosclerosis brings with it opportunities to develop novel therapeutic agents targeting key molecular and cellular interactions in its etiology. In addition, the recognition that the clinical consequences of atherosclerosis depend almost entirely on plaque composition argues for a new approach to diagnosis, with less emphasis placed on the degree of lumen narrowing and more interest in the cellular composition of the plaque.

NORMAL ARTERY

The healthy artery consists of three histologically distinct layers. Innermost and surrounding the lumen is the tunica intima, which comprises a single layer of endothelial cells in close proximity to the internal elastic lamina. The tunica media surrounds the internal elastic lamina, and its composition varies depending on the type of artery. The tunica media of the smallest arterial vessels, arterioles, comprises a single layer of vascular smooth muscle cells (VSMCs). Small arteries have a similar structure but with a thicker layer of medial VSMCs. Arterioles and small arteries are termed *resistance vessels* because they contribute vascular resistance and, hence, directly affect blood pressure. At the opposite end of the spectrum are large elastic or conduit arteries, named for the high proportion of elastin in the tunica media. The tunica media of all arteries is contained within a connective tissue layer that contains blood vessels and nerves and that is known as the *tunica adventitia*. In normal arteries, the vessel lumen diameter can be altered by contraction and relaxation of the medial VSMCs in response to a variety systemic and locally released signals.

ATHEROSCLEROTIC VESSEL

Atherosclerosis is primarily a disease affecting the intimal layer of elastic arteries. For reasons that remain largely unknown, some arterial beds appear more prone than others. Coronary, carotid, cerebral, and renal arteries and the aorta are most often involved. The arteries supplying the lower limb are also vulnerable to disease. Interestingly, the internal mammary artery is almost always spared, making it an invaluable vessel for coronary bypass surgery.

Atherosclerotic lesions develop over many years and pass through several stages. Histologically, the earliest lesion is a subendothelial accumulation of lipid-laden macrophage foam cells and associated T lymphocytes known as a *fatty streak*. Fatty streaks are asymptomatic and nonstenotic. Postmortem examinations have shown that they are present in the aorta at the end of the first decade of life, are present in the coronary arteries by the second, and begin to appear in the cerebral circulation by the third decade. With time, the lesion progresses and the core of the early plaque becomes necrotic, containing cellular debris, crystalline cholesterol, and inflammatory cells, particularly macrophage foam cells. This necrotic core becomes bounded on its luminal aspect by an endothelialized fibrous cap, consisting of VSMCs embedded in an extensive collagenous extracellular matrix. Inflammatory cells are also present in the fibrous cap, concentrated particularly in the "shoulder" regions, where T cells, mast cells, and especially macrophages have a tendency to accumulate. Advanced lesions may become increasingly complex, showing evidence of calcification, ulceration, new vessel formation, and rupture or erosion. Thus, the composition of atherosclerotic plaques is variable and complex, and it is the interaction between the various cell types within a plaque that determines the progression, complications, and outcome of the disease.

CELLULAR ROLES IN ATHEROGENESIS

Endothelial Cells

The endothelium plays a central role in maintaining vascular health by virtue of its vital antiinflammatory and anticoagulant properties. Many of these characteristics are mediated by the nitric oxide molecule (NO). This molecule was discovered in the 1980s, having been isolated from lipopolysaccharide-primed macrophages (13). NO is synthesized by endothelial cells under the control of the enzyme endothelial nitric oxide synthase and has a number of antiatherogenic properties. First, it acts as a powerful inhibitor of platelet aggregation on endothelial cells. Second, it can reduce inflammatory cell recruitment into the intima by abrogating the expression of genes involved in this process, such as those encoding intercellular adhesion molecule-1 (ICAM-1), vascular cell adhesion molecule-1 (VCAM-1), P-selectin, and monocyte chemoattractant protein-1 (MCP-1) (14–16). There is some evidence that NO may also reduce lipid entry into the arterial intima (17). NO is also a potent antiinflammatory molecule and, depending on concentration, may be a scavenger or a producer of potentially destructive oxygen free radicals, such as peroxynitrite (18–20).

The earliest detectable manifestation of atherosclerosis is a decrease in the bioavailability of NO in response to pharmacologic or hemodynamic stimuli (12). This may occur for two reasons. Either there may be decreased manufacture of NO because of endothelial cell dysfunction, or increased NO breakdown may take place. There is evidence that both mechanisms may be important in different situations (21). Many atherosclerosis risk factors can lead to impaired endothelial function and reduced NO bioavailability. For example, hyperlipidemic patients have reduced NO-dependent vasodilatation. This reduction is reversed when patients are treated with lipid-lowering medication (22). Patients with diabetes mellitus also have impaired endothelial function, occurring primarily as a result of impaired NO production. There is, however, some evidence to suggest that increased oxidative stress leading to enhanced NO breakdown may also be a factor (23). Similarly, other risk factors for atherosclerosis, such as hypertension and cigarette smoking, are associated with reduced NO bioavailability (24,25). In cigarette smokers, endothelial impairment is thought to be due to enhanced NO degradation by oxygen-derived free radical agents such as the superoxide ion. There are also other consequences of an increased reactivity between NO and superoxide species. The product of their interaction, ONOO– (peroxynitrite), is a powerful oxidizing agent and can reach high concentrations in atherosclerotic lesions. This may result in cellular oxidative injury.

Another consequence of endothelial cell dysfunction that occurs in early atherosclerosis is the expression of surface-bound selectins and adhesion molecules, including P-selectin, ICAM-1, and VCAM-1. These molecules attract and capture circulating inflammatory cells and facilitate their migration into the subendothelial space (*e*Fig. 1.2.1) (12). Normal endothelial cells do not express these molecules, but their appearance may be induced by abnormal arterial shear stress, subendothelial oxidized lipid, and, in diabetic patients, advanced glycosylation products in the arterial wall. The importance of selectins and adhesion molecules in the development of atherosclerosis is demonstrated by experiments using mice, which lack their expression. These animals develop smaller lesions with a lower lipid content and fewer inflammatory cells than control mice when fed a lipid-rich diet (26). Animal models have reinforced the importance of inflammatory cell recruitment to the pathogenesis of atherosclerosis, but because inflammatory cells are never seen in the intima in the absence of lipid, the results suggest that subendothelial lipid accumulation is also necessary for the development of atherosclerosis.

The tendency for atherosclerosis to occur preferentially in particular sites may be explained by subtle variations in endothelial function. This is probably caused by variations in local blood flow patterns, especially conditions of low flow, which can influence expression of a number of endothelial cell genes, including those encoding ICAM-1 and endothelial nitric oxide synthase (27,28). In addition to flow speed, flow type can have a direct effect on cell morphology. In areas of laminar flow, endothelial cells tend to have an ellipsoid shape, contrasting with the situation found at vessel branch points and curves, where turbulent flow induces a conformational change toward polygonal-shaped cells. Such cells have an increased permeability to low-density lipoprotein (LDL) cholesterol and may promote lesion formation (29).

These data are consistent with the idea that the primary event in atherogenesis is endothelial dysfunction. The endothelium can be damaged by a variety of means, leading to dysfunction and, by unknown mechanisms, subsequent subendothelial lipid accumulation. In this situation, the normal homeostatic features of the endothelium break down; it becomes more adhesive to inflammatory cells and platelets, it loses its anticoagulant properties, and there is reduced bioavailability of NO. Importantly, endothelial function is improved by drugs that have been shown to substantially reduce death from vascular disease, including statins and angiotensin-converting enzyme inhibitors (30,31).

Inflammatory Cells

LDL from the circulation is able to diffuse passively through the tight junctions that bind neighboring endothelial cells.

The rate of passive diffusion is increased when the circulating levels of LDL are elevated. In addition, other lipid fractions may be important in atherosclerosis. Lipoprotein(a) has the same basic molecular structure as LDL, with an additional apolipoprotein(a) element attached by a disulfide bridge. It has been shown to be highly atherogenic (32), to accumulate in the arterial wall in a manner similar to LDL (33), to impair vessel fibrinolysis (34), and to stimulate smooth muscle cell proliferation (35). The accumulation of subendothelial lipids, particularly when at least partly oxidized, is thought to stimulate the local inflammatory reaction that initiates and maintains activation of overlying endothelial cells. The activated cells express a variety of selectins and adhesion molecules and also produce a number of chemokines—in particular, MCP-1, whose expression is upregulated by the presence of oxidized LDL in the subendothelial space (36). Interestingly, the protective effect of HDL against atherosclerotic vascular disease may be partly explained by its ability to block endothelial cell expression of adhesion molecules (37,38). Chemokines are proinflammatory cytokines that are responsible for chemoattraction, migration, and subsequent activation of leukocytes. Mice lacking the MCP-1 gene develop smaller atherosclerotic lesions than normal animals (39). The first stage of inflammatory cell recruitment to the intima is the initiation of "rolling" of monocytes and T cells along the endothelial cell layer. This phenomenon is mediated by the selectin molecules, which selectively bind ligands found on these inflammatory cells. The subsequent firm adhesion to and migration of leukocytes through the endothelial cell layer is dependent on the endothelial expression of adhesion molecules such as ICAM-1 and VCAM-1 and their binding to appropriate receptors on inflammatory cells. Once present in the intima, monocytes differentiate into macrophages under the influence of chemokines such as macrophage colony-stimulating factor. Such molecules also stimulate the expression of the scavenger receptors that allow macrophages to ingest oxidized lipids and to develop into macrophage foam cells, the predominant cell in an early atherosclerotic lesion (*e*Fig. 1.2.2). The formation of scavenger receptors is also regulated by peroxisome proliferator-activated receptor-γ, a nuclear transcription factor expressed at high levels in foam cells (40).

In early atherosclerosis at least, the macrophage can be thought of as performing a predominantly beneficial role as a "neutralizer" of potentially harmful oxidized lipid components in the vessel wall. However, macrophage foam cells also synthesize a variety of proinflammatory cytokines and growth factors that contribute both beneficially and detrimentally to the evolution of the plaque. Some of these factors are chemoattractant (osteopontin) (41,42) and growth-enhancing (platelet-derived growth factor) for VSMCs. Under the influence of these cytokines, VSMC migrate from the media to the intima, where they adopt a synthetic phenotype, well-suited to matrix production and protective fibrous cap formation (*e*Fig. 1.2.3).

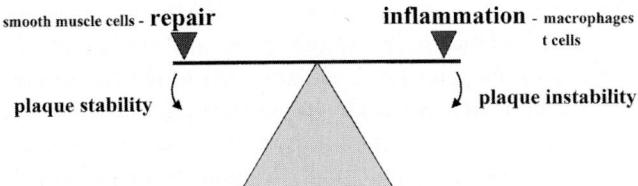

FIGURE 1.3 Factors influencing plaque stability.

However, activated macrophages have a high rate of apoptosis. Once dead, they release their lipid content, which becomes part of the core of the plaque, thereby contributing to its enlargement. The apoptotic cells also contain high concentrations of tissue factor, which may invoke thrombosis if exposed to circulating platelets (43). a07

It is now generally recognized that the pathologic progression and consequences of atherosclerotic lesions are determined by dynamic interactions between inflammatory cells recruited in response to subendothelial lipid accumulation, and the local reparative "wound healing" response of surrounding VSMCs (Fig. 1.3).

Vascular Smooth Muscle Cells

VSMCs reside mostly in the media of healthy adult arteries, where their role is to regulate vascular tone. Thus, medial VSMCs contain large amounts of contractile proteins, including myosin, alpha-actin, and tropomyosin. Continued expression of this "contractile" phenotype is maintained by the influence of extracellular proteins in the media, which act via integrins in the VSMC membrane. In atherosclerosis, however, the cells become influenced by cytokines produced by activated macrophages and endothelial cells. Under these influences, VSMCs migrate to the intima and undergo a phenotypic change characterized by a reduction in content of contractile proteins and a large increase in the number of synthetic organelles (eFig. 1.2.3). This migration of VSMCs from the media to the intima, and the consequent change from a contractile to a "synthetic" phenotype, was previously thought be a crucial step in the development of atherosclerosis in the modified response to injury hypothesis discussed previously. More recently, it has been recognized that intimal VSMCs in atherosclerotic plaques bear a remarkable similarity to VSMCs found in the early developing blood vessels (45), suggesting that intimal VSMCs may be performing a beneficial, reparative role rather than a destructive one in atherosclerosis. VSMCs are well-equipped for this action. First, they can express the proteinases that they require to break free from the medial basement membrane and allow them to migrate to the site of inflammation or injury in response to chemokines. Second, they can produce various growth factors, including vascular endothelial growth factor and platelet-derived growth factor, that act in an autocrine loop to facilitate their proliferation at the site of injury. Finally, and most important, they produce large quantities of

matrix proteins, in particular glycosaminoglycans, elastin, and collagen isoforms 1 and 3, necessary to repair the vessel and form a fibrous cap over the lipid-rich core of the lesion. This fibrous cap separates the highly thrombogenic lipid-rich plaque core from circulating platelets and the proteins of the coagulation cascade and also confers structural stability to the atherosclerotic lesion. And because the VSMC is the only cell capable of synthesizing this cap, it follows that VSMCs play a pivotal role in maintaining plaque stability and protecting against the potentially fatal thrombotic consequences of atherosclerosis (eFigs. 1.3.1 and 1.3.2) (46).

CELLULAR INTERACTIONS AND LESION STABILITY

Generally, early atherosclerosis progresses without symptoms until a lesion declares itself in one of two ways. As discussed previously, macrophage foam cells may undergo apoptosis, especially in the presence of high concentrations of oxidized LDL. Their cellular remnants then become part of an enlarging lipid-rich core. Plaque size thus increases, and there may be a consequent reduction in vessel lumen area. At times of increased demand, such as exercise, this may be sufficient to cause ischemic symptoms such as angina. More hazardous is if the plaque presents with disruption of the fibrous cap, leading to exposure of the thrombogenic lipid core. This is likely to result in subsequent platelet accumulation and activation, fibrin deposition, and intravascular thrombosis. Depending on factors such as collateral blood supply, extent of arterial thrombus and local fibrinolytic activity, the end result may be arterial occlusion and downstream necrosis.

By studying the pathology of ruptured plaques, several characteristics have been identified that seem to be predictive of the risk of rupture in individual lesions (47). Plaques that are vulnerable to rupture tend to have thin fibrous caps with a high ratio of inflammatory cells to VSMCs and contain a lipid core that occupies more than 50% of the volume of the plaque. Of these, the most important is the cellular composition of the fibrous cap. Plaques containing a heavy inflammatory cell infiltrate and relatively few VSMCs have the highest risk of rupture (eFig. 1.3.3) (48).

Inflammatory cells in plaques act to promote plaque rupture by a number of synergistic mechanisms. First, activated T cells produce proinflammatory cytokines, typified by IFN-γ, that directly inhibit VSMC proliferation (49) and almost completely shut down collagen synthesis (50,51). Thus, VSMCs in the vicinity of activated T cells in plaques are poorly able to lay down or repair extracellular matrix. Second, macrophage-derived inflammatory cytokines, in particular interleukin-1β and tumor necrosis factor-α, along with IFN-γ from T cells, are synergistically cytotoxic for VSMCs, causing depletion in cell number by apoptosis (52). These cytokines are found at high levels in vulnerable plaques (53). Third, activated macrophages can induce VSMC apoptosis by direct cell-cell contact (54). Finally, and probably most important, macrophages secrete a variety of matrix metallo-proteinases that degrade the matrix components of the fibrous cap by proteolytic cleavage of its protein components (46). The production of matrix metalloproteinases is upregulated by inflammatory mediators such as tumor necrosis factor-α. As well as being under threat from such an array of insults, VSMCs themselves within the fibrous cap of a mature plaque have a reduced ability to proliferate (55,56) and an enhanced susceptibility to apoptosis (57). Thus, inflammatory cells can destroy the fabric of the fibrous cap, and resident VSMCs are poorly equipped to compensate, particularly in the presence of inhibitory inflammatory cytokines (*e*Figs. 1.3.4 and 1.3.5). It is important to note that all of these features can be present in small, hemodynamically insignificant plaques that are clinically silent and angiographically invisible. Thus, plaque composition is far more important than plaque size in determining outcome.

INFLAMMATORY MARKERS IN ATHEROSCLEROSIS

The cell biology of plaque development and subsequent rupture illustrates that atherosclerosis is fundamentally an inflammatory condition. Confirmation of the inflammatory basis of atherosclerosis has come from several studies that have all demonstrated a correlation between levels of markers of systemic inflammation, principally C-reactive protein (CRP), and risk of a clinical event due to plaque rupture (58–61). However, unlike in other systemic inflammatory conditions, such as rheumatoid arthritis, levels of CRP in atherosclerosis are characteristically not elevated above the conventional normal range, and a correlation between CRP level and coronary events was demonstrated only after development of a highly sensitive assay for CRP that was capable of measuring levels below the lower limit of detection of conventional assays. Similar, although less compelling, correlations with clinical events have also been published for other markers of inflammation, including soluble ICAM-1 (62), VCAM-1 (63,64), P-selectin (65), and interleukin-6 (the primary driver of CRP production) (66). Results of these studies have been interpreted by some as indicating that atherosclerosis arises as a consequence of a systemic inflammatory process, for example chronic infection, and by others that it reflects the inflammatory processes of atherosclerosis itself. However, there is accumulating evidence in favor of the latter interpretation.

TWO FORMS OF PLAQUE DISRUPTION: FIBROUS CAP RUPTURE AND ENDOTHELIAL EROSION

Atherosclerotic plaques become life-threatening when they initiate clot formation in the vessel lumen and disturb blood flow. This can occur in two different ways. Either there can be fibrous cap rupture, with consequent exposure of the thrombogenic extracellular matrix of the cap and the tissue factor–rich lipid core to circulating blood, or less commonly, there is erosion of the endothelial cells covering the fibrous cap, also potentially leading to the buildup of platelet-rich thrombus. Endothelial erosion probably accounts for approximately 30% of acute coronary syndromes overall and seems particularly common in females (67). Both forms of plaque disruption invariably lead to local platelet accumulation and activation. This may result in triggering of the clotting cascade, thrombus formation and, if extensive, complete vessel occlusion. Platelet-rich thrombus contains chemokines and mitogens, in particular platelet-derived growth factor and thrombin that induce migration and proliferation of VSMCs from the arterial media to the plaque and transforming growth factor-β that contributes to healing of the disrupted lesion (68). Platelets also express CD40 on their cell membranes, which causes local endothelial cell activation, resulting in the recruitment of more inflammatory cells to the lesion and perpetuating the cycle of inflammation, rupture, and thrombosis. However, fibrous cap rupture or erosion does not invariably lead to vessel occlusion. Up to 70% of plaques causing high-grade stenosis contain histologic evidence of previous subclinical plaque rupture with subsequent repair (69). This is particularly likely to occur if high blood flow through the vessel prevents the accumulation of a large occlusive thrombus. Thus, nonocclusive plaque rupture induces formation of a new fibrous cap over the organizing thrombus, which restabilizes the lesion but at the expense of increasing its size (*e*Figs. 1.3.6 and 1.3.7). Because this occurs suddenly, there is little opportunity for adaptive remodeling of the artery, and the healed lesion may now impede flow sufficiently to produce ischemic symptoms. This explains why patients who have previously had normal exercise tolerance may suddenly develop symptoms of stable angina pectoris. It also follows that if lesions can grow as a consequence of repeated episodes of silent rupture and repair, a reduction of plaque rupture rate will reduce progression of atherosclerosis. Therefore, atheromatous plaques may become larger by two methods. The first is a gradual increase in size as a consequence of macrophage foam cell apoptosis and the plaques' incorporation into an enlarging necrotic lipid-laden plaque core. The second is a stepwise increase in size because of repeated, often silent episodes of plaque rupture or erosion with subsequent VSMC-driven repair.

BALANCE OF ATHEROSCLEROSIS: THERAPEUTIC IMPLICATIONS

Atherosclerosis is a dynamic process in which the balance between the destructive influence of inflammatory cells and the reactive, stabilizing effects of VSMCs determines out-

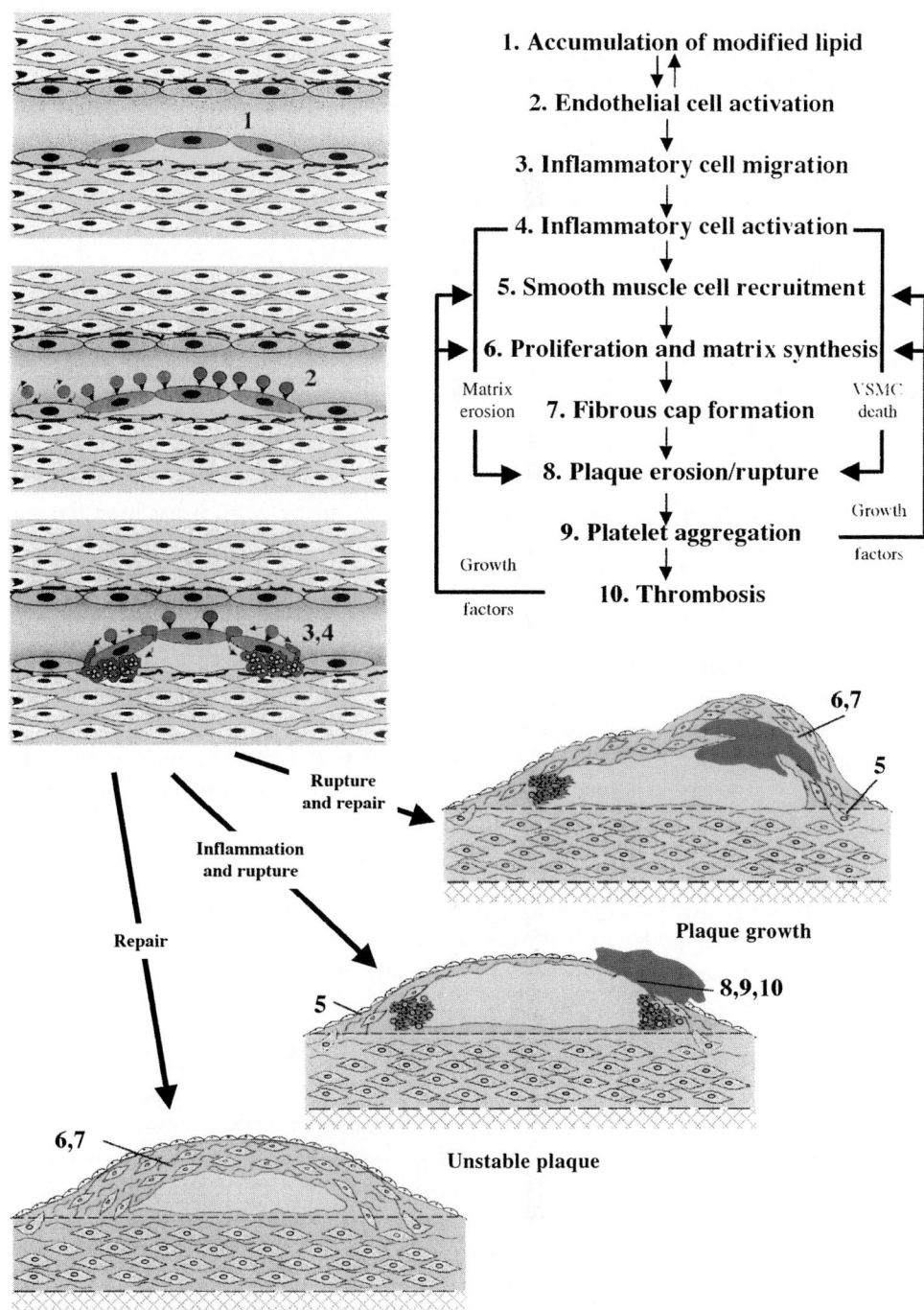

1. Accumulation of modified lipid

2. Endothelial cell activation

3. Inflammatory cell migration

4. Inflammatory cell activation

5. Smooth muscle cell recruitment

6. Proliferation and matrix synthesis

Matrix erosion   VSMC death

7. Fibrous cap formation

8. Plaque erosion/rupture

Growth

9. Platelet aggregation

factors

Growth

factors

10. Thrombosis

Rupture and repair

Inflammation and rupture

Repair

6,7

5

Plaque growth

5

8,9,10

Unstable plaque

6,7

Stable plaque

FIGURE 1.4 Cellular interactions in the development and progression of atherosclerosis. (From Weissberg PL. Atherogenesis: current understanding of the causes of atheroma. *Heart* 2000;83:247–252, with permission.)

come (Fig. 1.4 and *e*Fig. 1.4.1). This balance can be tipped toward plaque rupture by factors such as an atherogenic lipoprotein profile, high levels of lipid oxidation, local free radical generation, and genetic variability in expression and activity of certain central inflammatory molecules. For example, an association between plaque progression and a polymorphism in the stromelysin-1 gene promoter has been described (70). It is also possible that infectious organisms might be involved in atherosclerosis, either as plaque initiators or as having some role in initiating plaque rupture. This

fiercely debated question has still to be resolved. *Chlamydia pneumoniae* remains the most plausible candidate pathogen. It is found in plaques, localizing at high concentrations within macrophages, but is rarely found in normal arteries (71). Although these data imply a pathologic association between the presence of chlamydia infection and atherosclerosis, neither a causative role nor an association between serum markers of infection and ischemic heart disease has been established. Animal work has shown that healthy rabbits that are nasally inoculated with chlamydia develop extensive atherosclerosis (72). The situation appears to be somewhat different in humans. Two large prospective studies and an extensive metaanalysis of previous data failed to show any association between serum markers of infection with chlamydia and incidence of or mortality from ischemic heart disease (73,74). The results of these two studies effectively exclude a strong association but allow the possibility of a weaker link, and several trials of antichlamydial antibiotics for the prevention of ischemic heart disease are in progress (ACES, WIZARD, PROVEIT, MARBLE, STAMINA).

The balance can be tipped toward plaque stability by a reduction in plaque inflammation or an increase in VSMC-driven repair. Lipid reduction, by whatever means, reduces clinical events. Evidence that this may be due to a plaque-stabilizing effect comes from animal studies that showed that statins reduced inflammatory cell and increased VSMC content of plaques (75,76), changes that would be expected to enhance stability. More important, however, evidence from human clinical studies also points to a plaque-stabilizing effect of statins. Angiographic studies have shown that statins produce only a small, hemodynamically insignificant reduction in progression of established stenoses (77–79). They also reduce new lesion formation, and, importantly, the number of new vessel occlusions. These arise after a plaque ruptures, leading to an occlusive thrombus in the context of a well-collateralized myocardial circulation. This seems to imply that statins are stabilizing plaques by reducing rupture rate. This conclusion is supported by the results of all the large primary and secondary prevention studies, which have demonstrated that statins (pravastatin, simvastatin and lovastatin) produce major reductions in events due to plaque rupture, such as myocardial infarction and stroke (30,80–83). Because statins have only a modest effect on plaque size but cause profound reductions in the number of clinical events, these studies highlight the inadequacy of angiography for the prediction of clinical events and suggest that statins have beneficial effects on plaque inflammation in addition to, or as a result of, their lipid-lowering effects. Importantly, this notion is supported by the observation that the reduction in clinical events due to statin therapy is accompanied by a parallel reduction in highly sensitive assay for CRP levels that is unlikely to be due to effects of statins on nonatherosclerotic inflammation (84,85). Also, in the first study of its kind, it has been shown that statins reduce inflammation and increase plaque collagen content in human carotid artery atherosclerosis (86).

Statin drugs may help stabilize plaques in a number of different ways (*e*Fig. 1.4.2). It is known that they can exert direct effects on endothelial cell function, inflammatory cell number and activity, VSMC proliferation, platelet aggregation, and thrombus formation (87–91). Evidence that non–lipid-lowering effects may be important *in vivo* comes from animal studies in which pravastatin caused beneficial changes in plaque composition (but

not size), even when lipid levels were maintained at pretreatment levels (76). Additionally, in mice, simvastatin has direct antiinflammatory effects comparable to those of indomethacin (92). Recently, a newly recognized effect of statins as immune modulators has been described, whereby major histocompatibility complex class II mediated T-cell activation is reduced by a variety of statins (93). These observations point to potentially important effects of statins that are poorly understood and have yet to be fully defined.

RESTENOSIS

Restenosis is the term used for the late loss of gain in lumen diameter achieved immediately after balloon dilatation of an atherosclerotic plaque. For many years, it has been thought of as an undesirable response to vascular injury. However, in effect, it represents an extreme form of plaque stabilization. Whether performed on a stable or unstable plaque, angioplasty causes endothelial disruption and often substantial damage to the full thickness of the vessel wall. The initial thrombotic response that would otherwise lead to early vessel occlusion is prevented by antiplatelet and antithrombotic therapy. There then follows a reparative response driven by medial VSMCs and adventitial myofibroblasts. The former form a matrix-rich neointima over the exposed plaque, whereas the latter produce a collagenous matrix in the adventitia. The net result is that the adventitial reaction "splints" the vessel and prevents the remodeling that would normally allow expansion of the vessel to accommodate the neointima. However, although this phenomenon may lead to angiographic or clinical restenosis, much more important, it renders the lesion stable, making the likelihood of a further plaque rupture at that site extremely remote. In effect, by stimulating a vigorous VSMC repair response, balloon angioplasty tips "the balance of atherosclerosis" in favor of plaque stability (Fig. 1.4 and *e*Fig. 1.4.1). This phenomenon undoubtedly underlies the success of angioplasty in the treatment of acute myocardial infarction. Most of the adverse effects of the response to balloon angioplasty on remodeling can be countered by deployment of a stent. Nevertheless, the neointimal response remains problematic but is probably a worthwhile price for the stability achieved because restenosis is rarely life-threatening.

CONTROVERSIES AND PERSONAL PERSPECTIVES

Many issues concerning the initiation and progression of atherosclerosis remain to be resolved. In particular, controversy persists over the extent to which endothelial dysfunction precedes or is the consequence of intimal lipid accumulation; the relative contributions of endothelial ero-

THE FUTURE

It is almost inconceivable that the combination of these approaches will not lead to the development of new drugs that will act synergistically with statins and angiotensin-converting enzyme inhibitors. Furthermore, we predict that advances in genetics and diagnostics will combine with therapeutic advances to produce substantial reductions in premature cardiovascular deaths. Thus, new gene polymorphisms and mutations will be identified that confer increased likelihood either of developing atheroma or of experiencing its consequences. This will lead, in turn, to better prescription of lifestyle modifications and better targeting of current and new therapies for primary prevention of cardiovascular events. This approach will be aided by new diagnostic tests—based on specific circulating markers of vascular inflammation or imaging of the inflammatory process underlying plaque rupture—that will lead to better preclinical diagnosis of patients at greatest risk of cardiovascular events and better monitoring of plaque-modifying therapies.

---

sion and plaque rupture to clinical events; the specific role, if any, of infective agents such as *C. pneumoniae* in the pathogenesis and progression of atherosclerosis; and the extent to which statins achieve their plaque stabilizing effects directly via lipid lowering or by their so-called pleiotropic effects on the intercellular interactions that lead to plaque rupture. Integral to this latter issue is the outstanding question of what is the optimal level of lipid reduction. In other words, is greater always better?

Despite these controversies, it is certain that drug treatment will become increasingly prominent in the management of patients with, and at high risk of developing, atherosclerosis. Improvements in drug design will come from a number of complementary approaches. First, improvement will come by modifications of existing molecules, based on understanding how currently available drugs such as statins and angiotensin-converting enzyme inhibitors influence plaque progression. This will include evaluation of how other lipid-modifying strategies, such as inhibiting cholesterol absorption in the gut and modifying the balance between pro- and antiatherogenic lipoproteins and triglycerides, might influence the atherosclerotic process. Second, improvements will come by targeting molecular interactions known to be involved in atherogenesis. Likely candidates include endothelial adhesion molecules, matrix metalloproteinases, inflammatory cytokines and their signaling molecules, in particular, nuclear factor-κB and its downstream transcriptional activators. Here the challenge lies in identifying pathways or molecular species that are specific for atherosclerosis whose modification will not compromise the normal inflammatory response to pathogens. This approach will include developing regulators of VSMC behavior, such as modulators of transforming growth factor-β–driven matrix production, that may lead to enhanced maintenance of the fibrous cap. Another important example includes establishing the role of drugs targeting peroxisome proliferator–activated receptors in modifying inflammation and the vascular consequences of the metabolic syndrome that links insulin resistance, diabetes, hypertension, and dyslipidemia with premature atherosclerosis. The potentially beneficial effects of thiazolidinediones (the glitazones) on atherosclerotic events have yet to be determined. The third approach is to use new technologies such as proteomics to design new therapeutic molecules and gene array technologies to identify new molecular targets in vascular disease. In addition, as a consequence of sequencing the human genome, a number of "orphan" receptors have already been identified that might provide vascular specific targets for novel therapies.

REFERENCES

1. Wong ND, Wilson PW, Kannel WB. Serum cholesterol as a prognostic factor after myocardial infarction: the Framingham Study. *Ann Intern Med* 1991;115:687–693.
2. NHLBI. *NHLBI fact book fiscal year 1997*. Bethesda, MD: National Heart, Lung, and Blood Institute, 1998.
3. Cooper R, Cutler J, Desvigne-Nickens P, et al. Trends and disparities in coronary heart disease, stroke, and other cardiovascular diseases in the United States: findings of the national conference on cardiovascular disease prevention. *Circulation* 2000;102:3137–3147.
4. McGovern PG, Pankow JS, Shahar E, et al. Recent trends in acute coronary heart disease—mortality, morbidity, medical care, and risk factors. The Minnesota Heart Survey Investigators. *N Engl J Med* 1996;334:884–890.
5. Reddy KS, Yusuf S. Emerging epidemic of cardiovascular disease in developing countries. *Circulation* 1998;97:596–601.
6. Berliner JA, Navab M, Fogelman AM, et al. Atherosclerosis: basic mechanisms. Oxidation, inflammation, and genetics. *Circulation* 1995;91:2488–2496.
7. Bini A, Fenoglio JJ Jr, Mesa-Tejada R, et al. Identification and distribution of fibrinogen, fibrin, and fibrin(ogen) degradation products in atherosclerosis. Use of monoclonal antibodies. *Arteriosclerosis* 1989;9:109–121.
8. Wilcox JN, Smith KM, Williams LT, et al. Platelet-derived growth factor mRNA detection in human atherosclerotic

plaques by in situ hybridization. *J Clin Invest* 1988;82:1134–1143.

9. Ross R, Glomset JA. Atherosclerosis and the arterial smooth muscle cell: proliferation of smooth muscle is a key event in the genesis of the lesions of atherosclerosis. *Science* 1973;180:1332–1339.

10. Ross R. The pathogenesis of atherosclerosis—an update. *N Engl J Med* 1986;314:488–500.

11. Ross R. The pathogenesis of atherosclerosis: a perspective for the 1990s. *Nature* 1993;362:801–809.

12. Ross R. Atherosclerosis—an inflammatory disease. *N Engl J Med* 1999;340:115–126.

13. Palmer RM, Ferrige AG, Moncada S. Nitric oxide release accounts for the biological activity of endothelium-derived relaxing factor. *Nature* 1987;327:524–526.

14. Tsao PS, Wang B, Buitrago R, et al. Nitric oxide regulates monocyte chemotactic protein-1. *Circulation* 1997;96:934–940.

15. Gauthier TW, Scalia R, Murohara T, et al. Nitric oxide protects against leukocyte-endothelium interactions in the early stages of hypercholesterolemia. *Arterioscler Thromb Vasc Biol* 1995;15:1652–1659.

16. Tsao PS, Buitrago R, Chan JR, Cooke JP. Fluid flow inhibits endothelial adhesiveness. Nitric oxide and transcriptional regulation of VCAM-1. *Circulation* 1996;94:1682–1689.

17. Cardona-Sanclemente LE, Born GV. Effect of inhibition of nitric oxide synthesis on the uptake of LDL and fibrinogen by arterial walls and other organs of the rat. *Br J Pharmacol* 1995;114:1490–1494.

18. Hobbs AJ, Higgs A, Moncada S. Inhibition of nitric oxide synthase as a potential therapeutic target. *Annu Rev Pharmacol Toxicol* 1999;39:191–220.

19. Anggard E. Nitric oxide: mediator, murderer, and medicine. *Lancet* 1994;343:1199–1206.

20. Bhagat K, Vallance P. Nitric oxide 9 years on. *J R Soc Med* 1996;89:667–673.

21. Li H, Forstermann U. Nitric oxide in the pathogenesis of vascular disease. *J Pathol* 2000;190:244–254.

22. Stroes ES, Koomans HA, de Bruin TW, Rabelink TJ. Vascular function in the forearm of hypercholesterolaemic patients off and on lipid-lowering medication. *Lancet* 1995;346:467–471.

23. Williams SB, Cusco JA, Roddy MA, et al. Impaired nitric oxide-mediated vasodilation in patients with non-insulin-dependent diabetes mellitus. *J Am Coll Cardiol* 1996;27:567–574.

24. Panza JA, Garcia CE, Kilcoyne CM, et al. Impaired endothelium-dependent vasodilation in patients with essential hypertension. Evidence that nitric oxide abnormality is not localized to a single signal transduction pathway. *Circulation* 1995;91:1732–1738.

25. Heitzer T, Just H, Munzel T. Antioxidant vitamin C improves endothelial dysfunction in chronic smokers. *Circulation* 1996;94:6–9.

26. Nakashima Y, Plump AS, Raines EW, et al. ApoE-deficient mice develop lesions of all phases of atherosclerosis throughout the arterial tree. *Arterioscler Thromb* 1994;14:133–140.

27. Resnick N, Yahav H, Khachigian LM, et al. Endothelial gene regulation by laminar shear stress. *Adv Exp Med Biol* 1997;430:155–164.

28. Topper JN, Cai J, Falb D, Gimbrone MA Jr. Identification of vascular endothelial genes differentially responsive to fluid mechanical stimuli: cyclooxygenase-2, manganese superoxide dismutase, and endothelial cell nitric oxide synthase are selectively up-regulated by steady laminar shear stress. *Proc Natl Acad Sci U S A* 1996;93:10417–10422.

29. Gimbrone MA Jr. Vascular endothelium, hemodynamic forces, and atherogenesis. *Am J Pathol* 1999;155:1–5.

30. LIPID Study Group. Prevention of cardiovascular events and death with pravastatin in patients with coronary heart disease and a broad range of initial cholesterol levels. The Long-Term Intervention with Pravastatin in Ischaemic Disease (LIPID) Study Group. *N Engl J Med* 1998;339:1349–1357.

31. Yusuf S, Sleight P, Pogue J, et al. Effects of an angiotensin-converting-enzyme inhibitor, ramipril, on cardiovascular events in high-risk patients. The Heart Outcomes Prevention Evaluation Study Investigators [published errata appear in *N Engl J Med* 2000;342:748 and 2000;342:1376]. *N Engl J Med* 2000;342:145–153.

32. Poon M, Zhang X, Dunsky KG, et al. Apolipoprotein(a) induces monocyte chemotactic activity in human vascular endothelial cells. *Circulation* 1997;96:2514–2519.

33. Rath M, Niendorf A, Reblin T, et al. Detection and quantification of lipoprotein(a) in the arterial wall of 107 coronary bypass patients. *Arteriosclerosis* 1989;9:579–592.

34. Loscalzo J, Weinfeld M, Fless GM, Scanu AM. Lipoprotein(a), fibrin binding, and plasminogen activation. *Arteriosclerosis* 1990;10:240–245.

35. Grainger DJ, Kirschenlohr HL, Metcalfe JC, et al. Proliferation of human smooth muscle cells promoted by lipoprotein(a). *Science* 1993;260:1655–1658.

36. Boring L, Gosling J, Cleary M, Charo IF. Decreased lesion formation in CCR2–/– mice reveals a role for chemokines in the initiation of atherosclerosis. *Nature* 1998;394:894–897.

37. Xia P, Vadas MA, Rye KA, et al. High density lipoproteins (HDL) interrupt the sphingosine kinase signaling pathway. A possible mechanism for protection against atherosclerosis by HDL. *J Biol Chem* 1999;274:33143–33147.

38. Calabresi L, Franceschini G, Sirtori CR, et al. Inhibition of VCAM-1 expression in endothelial cells by reconstituted high density lipoproteins. *Biochem Biophys Res Commun* 1997;238:61–65.

39. Gosling J, Slaymaker S, Gu L, et al. MCP-1 deficiency reduces susceptibility to atherosclerosis in mice that overexpress human apolipoprotein B. *J Clin Invest* 1999;103:773–778.

40. Tontonoz P, Nagy L, Alvarez JG, et al. PPARgamma promotes monocyte/macrophage differentiation and uptake of oxidized LDL. *Cell* 1998;93:241–252.

41. Shanahan CM, Cary NR, Metcalfe JC, Weissberg PL. High expression of genes for calcification-regulating proteins in human atherosclerotic plaques. *J Clin Invest* 1994;93:2393–2402.

42. Liaw L, Almeida M, Hart CE, et al. Osteopontin promotes vascular cell adhesion and spreading and is chemotactic for smooth muscle cells in vitro. *Circ Res* 1994;74:214–224.

43. Zaman AG, Helft G, Worthley SG, Badimon JJ. The role of plaque rupture and thrombosis in coronary artery disease. *Atherosclerosis* 2000;149:251–266.

44. de Boer OJ, van der Wal AC, Becker AE. Atherosclerosis, inflammation, and infection. *J Pathol* 2000;190:237–243.

45. Shanahan CM, Weissberg PL. Smooth muscle cell heterogeneity: patterns of gene expression in vascular smooth muscle cells in vitro and in vivo. *Arterioscler Thromb Vasc Biol* 1998;18:333–338.

46. Libby P. Molecular bases of the acute coronary syndromes. *Circulation* 1995;91:2844–2850.

47. Galis ZS, Sukhova GK, Lark MW, Libby P. Increased expression of matrix metalloproteinases and matrix degrading activity in vulnerable regions of human atherosclerotic plaques. *J Clin Invest* 1994;94:2493–2503.

48. Davies MJ. Stability and instability: two faces of coronary atherosclerosis. The Paul Dudley White Lecture 1995. *Circulation* 1996;94:2013–2020.

49. Warner SJ, Friedman GB, Libby P. Immune interferon inhibits proliferation and induces 2'-5'-oligoadenylate synthetase gene expression in human vascular smooth muscle cells. *J Clin Invest* 1989;83:1174–1182.

50. Amento EP, Ehsani N, Palmer H, Libby P. Cytokines and growth factors positively and negatively regulate interstitial collagen gene expression in human vascular smooth muscle cells. *Arterioscler Thromb* 1991;11:1223–1230.

51. Libby P, Sukhova G, Lee RT, Galis ZS. Cytokines regulate vascular functions related to stability of the atherosclerotic plaque. *J Cardiovasc Pharmacol* 1995;25(Suppl 2):S9–S12.

52. Geng YJ, Wu Q, Muszynski M, et al. Apoptosis of vascular smooth muscle cells induced by in vitro stimulation with interferon-gamma, tumor necrosis factor-alpha, and interleukin-1 beta. *Arterioscler Thromb Vasc Biol* 1996;16:19–27.

53. Sukhova GK, Schonbeck U, Rabkin E, et al. Evidence for increased collagenolysis by interstitial collagenases-1 and -3 in vulnerable human atheromatous plaques. *Circulation* 1999;99:2503–2509.

54. Boyle JJ, Bennett MR, Proudfoot D, et al. Human monocyte/macrophages induce human smooth muscle cell apoptosis in culture. *Arterioscler Thromb Vasc Biol* 2001 (*in press*).

55. Ross R, Wight TN, Strandness E, Thiele B. Human atherosclerosis. I. Cell constitution and characteristics of advanced lesions of the superficial femoral artery. *Am J Pathol* 1984;114:79–93.

56. Bennett MR, Macdonald K, Chan SW, et al. Cooperative interactions between RB and p53 regulate cell proliferation, cell senescence, and apoptosis in human vascular smooth muscle cells from atherosclerotic plaques. *Circ Res* 1998;82:704–712.

57. Bennett MR, Littlewood TD, Schwartz SM, Weissberg PL. Increased sensitivity of human vascular smooth muscle cells from atherosclerotic plaques to p53-mediated apoptosis. *Circ Res* 1997;81:591–599.

58. Ridker PM, Hennekens CH, Buring JE, Rifai N. C-reactive protein and other markers of inflammation in the prediction of cardiovascular disease in women. *N Engl J Med* 2000;342:836–843.

59. Sacks FM, Ridker PM. Lipid lowering and beyond: results from the CARE study on lipoproteins and inflammation. Cholesterol and Recurrent Events. *Herz* 1999;24:51–56.

60. Ridker PM, Cushman M, Stampfer MJ, et al. Inflammation, aspirin, and the risk of cardiovascular disease in apparently healthy men [published erratum appears in *N Engl J Med* 1997;337:356]. *N Engl J Med* 1997;336:973–979.

61. Ridker PM. High-sensitivity C-reactive protein: potential adjunct for global risk assessment in the primary prevention of cardiovascular disease. *Circulation* 2001;103:1813–1818.

62. Ridker PM, Hennekens CH, Roitman-Johnson B, et al. Plasma concentration of soluble intercellular adhesion molecule 1 and risks of future myocardial infarction in apparently healthy men. *Lancet* 1998;351:88–92.

63. de Lemos JA, Hennekens CH, Ridker PM. Plasma concentration of soluble vascular cell adhesion molecule-1 and subsequent cardiovascular risk. *J Am Coll Cardiol* 2000;36:423–426.

64. Peter K, Weirich U, Nordt TK, et al. Soluble vascular cell adhesion molecule-1 (VCAM-1) as potential marker of atherosclerosis. *Thromb Haemost* 1999;82(Suppl 1):38–43.

65. Ridker PM, Buring JE, Rifai N. Soluble P-selectin and the risk of future cardiovascular events. *Circulation* 2001;103:491–495.

66. Ridker PM, Rifai N, Stampfer MJ, Hennekens CH. Plasma concentration of interleukin-6 and the risk of future myocardial infarction among apparently healthy men. *Circulation* 2000;101:1767–1772.

67. Farb A, Burke AP, Tang AL, et al. Coronary plaque erosion without rupture into a lipid core. A frequent cause of coronary thrombosis in sudden coronary death. *Circulation* 1996;93:1354–1363.

68. McNamara CA, Sarembock IJ, Bachhuber BG, et al. Thrombin and vascular smooth muscle cell proliferation: implications for atherosclerosis and restenosis. *Semin Thromb Hemost* 1996;22:139–144.

69. Davies MJ. Acute coronary thrombosis—the role of plaque disruption and its initiation and prevention. *Eur Heart J* 1995;16(Suppl L):3–7.

70. Ye S, Eriksson P, Hamsten A, et al. Progression of coronary atherosclerosis is associated with a common genetic variant of the human stromelysin-1 promoter which results in reduced gene expression. *J Biol Chem* 1996;271:13055–13060.

71. Kol A, Sukhova GK, Lichtman AH, Libby P. Chlamydial heat shock protein 60 localizes in human atheroma and regulates macrophage tumor necrosis factor-alpha and matrix metalloproteinase expression. *Circulation* 1998;98:300–307.

72. Muhlestein JB, Anderson JL, Hammond EH, et al. Infection with *Chlamydia pneumoniae* accelerates the development of atherosclerosis and treatment with azithromycin prevents it in a rabbit model. *Circulation* 1998;97:633–636.

73. Danesh J, Whincup P, Walker M, et al. *Chlamydia pneumoniae* IgG titres and coronary heart disease: prospective study and meta-analysis. *BMJ* 2000;321:208–213.

74. Wald NJ, Law MR, Morris JK, et al. *Chlamydia pneumoniae* infection and mortality from ischaemic heart disease: large prospective study. *BMJ* 2000;321:204–207.

75. Shiomi M, Ito T, Tsukada T, et al. Reduction of serum cholesterol levels alters lesional composition of atherosclerotic plaques. Effect of pravastatin sodium on atherosclerosis in mature WHHL rabbits. *Arterioscler Thromb Vasc Biol* 1995;15:1938–1944.

76. Williams JK, Sukhova GK, Herrington DM, Libby P. Pravastatin has cholesterol-lowering independent effects on the artery wall of atherosclerotic monkeys. *J Am Coll Cardiol* 1998;31:684–691.

77. Investigators. Effect of simvastatin on coronary atheroma: the Multicentre Anti-Atheroma Study (MAAS) [published erratum appears in *Lancet* 1994;344:762]. *Lancet* 1994;344:633–638.

78. Pitt B, Mancini GB, Ellis SG, et al. Pravastatin limitation of atherosclerosis in the coronary arteries (PLAC I): reduction in atherosclerosis progression and clinical events. PLAC I investigation. *J Am Coll Cardiol* 1995;26:1133–1139.

79. Jukema JW, Bruschke AV, van Boven AJ, et al. Effects of lipid lowering by pravastatin on progression and regression of coronary artery disease in symptomatic men with normal to moderately elevated serum cholesterol levels. The Regression Growth Evaluation Statin Study (REGRESS). *Circulation* 1995;91:2528–2540.

80. Shepherd J, Cobbe SM, Ford I, et al. Prevention of coronary heart disease with pravastatin in men with hypercholesterolemia. West of Scotland Coronary Prevention Study Group. *N Engl J Med* 1995;333:1301–1307.

81. Sacks FM, Pfeffer MA, Moye LA, et al. The effect of pravastatin on coronary events after myocardial infarction in patients with average cholesterol levels. Cholesterol and Recurrent Events Trial investigators. *N Engl J Med* 1996;335:1001–1009.

82. Randomised trial of cholesterol lowering in 4444 patients with coronary heart disease: the Scandinavian Simvastatin Survival Study (4S). *Lancet* 1994;344:1383–1389.

83. Downs JR, Clearfield M, Weis S, et al. Primary prevention of acute coronary events with lovastatin in men and women with average cholesterol levels: results of AFCAPS/TexCAPS. Air Force/Texas Coronary Atherosclerosis Prevention Study. *JAMA* 1998;279:1615–1622.

84. Ridker PM, Rifai N, Pfeffer MA, et al. Inflammation, pravastatin, and the risk of coronary events after myocardial infarction in patients with average cholesterol levels. Cholesterol and Recurrent Events (CARE) Investigators. *Circulation* 1998;98:839–844.

85. Jialal I, Stein D, Balis D, et al. Effect of hydroxymethyl glutaryl coenzyme a reductase inhibitor therapy on high sensitive C-reactive protein levels. *Circulation* 2001;103:1933–1935.

86. Crisby M, Nordin-Fredriksson G, Shah PK, et al. Pravastatin treatment increases collagen content and decreases lipid content, inflammation, metalloproteinases, and cell death in human carotid plaques: implications for plaque stabilization. *Circulation* 2001;103:926–933.

87. Treasure CB, Klein JL, Weintraub WS, et al. Beneficial effects of cholesterol-lowering therapy on the coronary endothelium in patients with coronary artery disease. *N Engl J Med* 1995;332:481–487.

88. Katznelson S, Wang XM, Chia D, et al. The inhibitory effects of pravastatin on natural killer cell activity in vivo and on cytotoxic T lymphocyte activity in vitro. *J Heart Lung Transplant* 1998;17:335–340.

89. Negre-Aminou P, van Vliet AK, van Erck M, et al. Inhibition of proliferation of human smooth muscle cells by various HMG-CoA reductase inhibitors—comparison with other human cell types. *Biochim Biophys Acta* 1997;1345:259–268.

90. Rosenson RS, Tangney CC. Antiatherothrombotic properties of statins: implications for cardiovascular event reduction. *JAMA* 1998;279:1643–1650.

91. Lacoste L, Lam JY, Hung J, et al. Hyperlipidemia and coronary disease. Correction of the increased thrombogenic potential with cholesterol reduction. *Circulation* 1995;92:3172–3177.

92. Sparrow CP, Burton CA, Hernandez M, et al. Simvastatin has anti-inflammatory and antiatherosclerotic activities independent of plasma cholesterol lowering. *Arterioscler Thromb Vasc Biol* 2001;21:115–121.

93. Kwak B, Mulhaupt F, Myit S, Mach F. Statins as a newly recognized type of immunomodulator. *Nat Med* 2000;6:1399–1402.

DIET, NUTRITIONAL ISSUES, AND OBESITY

NEIL J. STONE

OVERVIEW

Diet plays an important role in the primary and secondary prevention of coronary artery disease (CAD). It has beneficial effects on the lipid profile and is a crucial part of the treatment of individuals who have multiple metabolic risk factors ("the metabolic syndrome"). Moreover, data on the value of diet in reducing oxidant stress, thrombotic tendencies, ischemic ventricular arrhythmia, and sudden death are encouraging.

N. J. Stone: Department of Cardiology, Northwestern University Medical School, Chicago, Illinois

The American Heart Association's (AHA) recommended population or "healthy" diet focuses on healthy eating patterns and foods. It replaces the older AHA Step I diet. It recommends an overall healthy eating pattern with general advice that should help prevent obesity, hypertension, and hypercholesterolemia (Table 2.1). For individuals who have medical problems that necessitate consumption of a therapeutic cardiovascular diet, consultation with a dietitian for medical nutrition therapy is recommended for guidance in making the necessary lifestyle changes. To reduce levels of low-density lipoprotein cholesterol (LDL-C), the earlier AHA Step II diet restricted saturated fatty acids to less than 7% of energy and dietary

TABLE 2.1 REVISION 2000: AMERICAN HEART ASSOCIATION DIETARY GUIDELINES SUMMARIZED

Have a healthy eating pattern	Achieve and maintain a healthy body weight	Achieve a desirable blood cholesterol profile	Achieve and maintain a desirable blood pressure
Variety of fruits, vegetables, grains, low-fat or nonfat dairy products, fish, legumes, poultry, lean meats	Match energy intake to energy expenditures with appropriate changes to achieve weight loss when indicated	Limit foods high in saturated fat and cholesterol; substitute unsaturated fat from vegetables, fish, legumes, and nuts	Limit salt and alcohol; maintain a healthy body weight and a diet with emphasis on vegetables, fruits, and low-fat or nonfat dairy products

Adapted from Krause RM, Eckel RH, Howard B, et al. Revision 2000: AHA dietary guidelines; a statement for healthcare professionals from the Nutrition Committee of the American Heart Association. *Circulation* 2000;102:2296–2311, with permission.

cholesterol to less than 200 mg per day. The current AHA dietary module to reduce LDL-C preserves this recommendation and also suggests a reduction in *trans* fatty acids (TFAs). For individuals with multiple metabolic risk factors and obesity, treatment begins with caloric restriction and increased energy expenditure. For those with elevated blood pressure, a low-salt regimen with increased emphasis on fruits and vegetables, nonfat dairy products, and weight reduction, if needed, is suggested.

The response to diet is variable and probably is genetically based. Therapeutic diets that reduce risk factors must be targeted to the specific characteristics of the individual [high LDL-C level, combined elevation of cholesterol and triglyceride (TG) levels, obesity, hypertension]. These individual characteristics may also underlie individual responsiveness to diet.

Understanding the response of the individual to various dietary components is useful, because some people may use the therapeutic diet to reach their LDL-C goal or reduce their need for medication to reach LDL-C goals. The response of LDL-C to dietary cholesterol is highly variable. People with combined forms of hyperlipidemia may be the most sensitive to diet. Dietary options such as plant sterol and stanol esters taken as margarines reduce cholesterol absorption significantly and can reduce LDL-C by 10% or more. Some saturated fats raise blood cholesterol more than others. Stearic acid is converted to oleic acid and may even lower blood cholesterol. Nonetheless, restriction of saturated fats is the hallmark of the cholesterol-lowering diet. TFAs, when consumed in high amounts, can raise LDL-C and lower high-density lipoprotein cholesterol (HDL-C). Sources high in TFAs, such as stick margarine, cookies, biscuits, and cakes, should be avoided. Butter contains cholesterol and saturated fat and is cholesterol-raising compared with soft margarine. Therapeutic diets should be low in both saturated fatty acids and TFAs.

Diets high in sources of monounsaturated fats such as canola and olive oil do not lower HDL-C as much as do high-carbohydrate diets. Such diets may be preferred for individuals with the metabolic syndrome or for diabetic patients, when weight control is not an issue. Patients need to be reminded, however, that an excess intake of fats—monounsaturated or not—can lead to weight gain. Reducing excess body weight can be a crucial factor in improving the lipid profile. The addition of regular exercise to changes in diet can be particularly beneficial in helping a patient maintain weight loss. Recent data suggest that omega-3 fatty acids, particularly docosahexaenoic acid (DHA) may reduce cardiovascular events by a mechanism other than improvement of lipid profiles. Several trials have shown a reduction in cardiac death among patients consuming DHA-supplemented diets, and animal models of coronary heart disease (CHD) suggest that an increase in the ventricular fibrillation threshold accompanies consumption of DHA.

Mild alcohol consumption, especially among middle-aged and older adults, is associated with decreased rates of CAD compared with rates among teetotalers. Approximately one-half of the benefit of alcohol can be attributed to increased levels of HDL-C. Benefit is not dependent on the kind of beverage consumed. Excess amounts of alcohol can lead to significant cardiovascular problems, including arrhythmias, cardiomyopathy, and left ventricular hypertrophy (LVH). Women are more sensitive to alcohol than men and develop cardiomyopathy and a decrease in left ventricular function at a lower dose.

Large clinical trials have not shown beneficial effects of vitamin E or beta-carotene supplementation either on total mortality or on cardiovascular end points in both primary and secondary prevention trials. These supplements cannot be recommended for reduction of cardiovascular risk. Diets that emphasize sources of antioxidants in fruits, vegetables, nuts, and whole-grain products are recommended.

The prevalence of overweight and obesity is increasing. This is a serious concern; obesity is now considered to be the second leading cause of preventable death in the United States (after cigarette smoking). The use of the body mass index (BMI) to define overweight as a BMI of 25.0 to 29.9 and obesity as a BMI of 30 or higher is useful in clinical practice. Weight gain into the overweight range increases insulin resistance. The clinical presentation of insulin resistance includes multiple metabolic abnormalities such as high TG levels, low HDL-C levels, glucose intolerance, hypertension, and hypercoagulability. Treatment begins with regular physical activity and reduction of excess weight. The importance of prompt recognition and treatment of individuals with the metabolic syndrome is underscored by data showing that weight gain after the age of 18 years is an important precursor of diabetes and CAD. Most therapies for obesity result in benefits in the short term, with disappointingly low rates of success at 5 years. Popular diets can achieve short-term weight loss, but there is no convincing evidence of long-term efficacy. Medications such as fenfluramine and phentermine or dexfenfluramine are no longer used to treat obesity because of the associated occurrence of valvular lesions that resemble those seen with serotonin excess. Newer medical approaches to weight loss include use of sibutramine and orlistat, which may help the obese patient achieve a 5% to 10% weight loss in 1 year. Gastric bypass surgery is particularly useful for those with marked obesity. Lifestyle change is important even for individuals who are being treated with medication and/or surgery. Thus, a comprehensive approach to weight loss is recommended. Prevention of obesity should be a high priority for public policy, and physicians should consider intervention when patients initiate measures strongly associated with weight gain. Examples include smoking cessation, use of steroids, and initiation of certain antidiabetic or antidepressant medications known to promote weight gain.

GLOSSARY

Alpha-linolenic acid: Plant-based omega-3 polyunsaturated fatty acid.

Android or male pattern obesity: Increased waist-to-hip ratio associated with increased CAD risk and with hypertension, visceral obesity, glucose intolerance, and insulin resistance.

BMI: Body mass index. Calculated as weight/height^2. This index minimizes the effect of height on body weight and has become the preferred index for categorizing levels of obesity. It does not provide information, however, on the pattern of obesity.

Cis: Naturally occurring double bonds that produce a bend in the molecule that impairs crystallization.

DART Trial: Diet and Reinfarction Trial.

DASH Trial: Dietary Approaches to Stop Hypertension Trial.

Dietary cholesterol: A crucial waxy substance that is found in animal cells. Response of blood cholesterol to its consumption is highly variable.

Familial dyslipidemic hypertension: Hypertension and dyslipidemia aggregating in family members.

Gynoid or female pattern obesity: Waist to hip ratio is not increased as fat increases in femoral-gluteal regions. Not associated with increased heart risk.

Insulin-resistance syndrome: Increased insulin levels relative to glucose levels. In some studies, this is an indepen-dent predictor of CAD risk. Associated with atherogenic dyslipidemia, hypertension, and visceral obesity.

Linoleic acid: Major human polyunsaturated fatty acid; an essential fatty acid.

Mediterranean diet pyramid: Graphic summary of eating style that excludes all fats but olive oil; recommends fish, poultry, and red meat less frequently, and includes physical activity and consumption of wine in moderation.

Metabolic syndrome: Describes constellation of multiple metabolic risk factors likely due to insulin resistance. These include high TG levels, low HDL-C level, hypertension, glucose intolerance or diabetes, hypercoagulability, and increased inflammatory markers.

Monounsaturated fatty acids: Fatty acids, such as oleic acid, whose carbon chains have one double bond. Foods high in monounsaturated fats include canola and olive oil.

NHANES II, III: National Health and Nutrition Exam Surveys II (1976–1980) and III (1988–1994).

Oleic acid: A monounsaturated fatty acid.

Omega-3 or *n*-3 polyunsaturated fatty acid: Fatty acids whose first double bond is 3 carbon atoms from the methyl end of the fatty-acid chain. Fish oils and alpha-linolenic acid are *n*-3 fatty acids.

Omega-6 or *n*-6 polyunsaturated fatty acid: Polyunsaturated fatty acids whose first double bond is six carbon atoms from the methyl end of the fatty-acid chain. Linoleic acid is an example.

Partial hydrogenation: A process whereby hydrogen atoms are added to fatty acids. Produces TFAs.

Phytoestrogens: Plant compounds that have estrogen-like activity.

Polyunsaturated fatty acids: Fatty acids whose carbon chains have one or more double bonds.

Saturated fatty acids: Fatty acids whose carbon chains have no double bonds.

SCRIP: Stanford Coronary Risk Intervention Project.

STARS: St. Thomas Atherosclerosis Regression Study.

Syndrome X: Also known as the *metabolic syndrome*, with insulin resistance, glucose intolerance, dyslipidemia, and hypertension as its hallmarks. Patients have visceral obesity. The cardiologic syndrome X is microvascular angina. The link between the two syndromes may be insulin resistance.

Trans **fatty acids:** Fatty-acid configuration in which the molecule is straightened out, leading to a more densely packed form. Solid at room temperatures.

USDA: United States Department of Agriculture.

USDA Diet Pyramid: Graphic summary of eating style based on the dietary guidelines of the USDA.

Waist to hip ratio: Measurement of waist or waist to hip ratio used to determine the pattern of obesity. Men with waist greater than 100 cm (approximately 40 in.) or waist to hip ratio greater than 0.9 and women with waist greater than 90 cm (35 in.) or waist to hip ratio greater than 0.8 are believed to have increased adiposity.

DIETARY PRESCRIPTION AND LIFESTYLE CHANGES TO REDUCE CORONARY ARTERY DISEASE

The contemporary practice of preventive cardiology requires an understanding of the use of dietary prescriptions to reduce the risk of CAD. Diets designed to lower cholesterol and improve multiple metabolic risk factors can lower the risk of CAD. A conference on dietary fatty acids and cardiovascular health reviewed in detail the epidemiologic, clinical trial, and nonhuman primate evidence supporting an important relationship between dietary fat and CAD (1). There are real benefits to an emphasis on solid nutritional principles. Cholesterol-lowering diets may allow therapeutic goals for LDL-C to be reached without additional medication (2). For example, a multicenter trial noted that the effects of intensive dietary therapy added to treatment with lovastatin resulted in a very modest gain of approximately 5% additional lowering of LDL-C levels (3). This trial had several design features that may have caused the value of diet to be underestimated. Nonetheless, even this modest lowering may allow LDL-C targets to be attained without the need to resort to an increased statin dose. For many patients, diet can reduce the expense of medication. In addition, for those with high TG, LDL-C, or HDL-C levels and associated features of the metabolic syndrome, diet, exercise, and weight loss may be particularly effective in normalizing lipid profiles or reducing the need for complex medication regimens (3). Finally, the use of dietary therapy alone, often in conjunction with either reduced tobacco intake or regular exercise, has been associated with significant cardiovascular benefit, including reductions in total mortality (4), angiographic progression (5,6), CHD end points [particularly CHD death (7–9)], and symptoms in patients with CAD (10). [See Tables 2.2 and 2.3 for a comprehensive look at clinical and angiographic trials (11).]

For the population as a whole, the implications of a "healthy" diet that shifts the population mean for serum cholesterol are exciting to contemplate. It has been speculated that a shift in the population mean cholesterol level by 10% would prevent 30% of all CAD events, whereas lifelong treatment with cholesterol-lowering drugs of individuals with cholesterol values in the highest 10% would achieve only a 15% to 20% reduction in CAD events (12).

NATIONAL CHOLESTEROL EDUCATION PROGRAM GUIDELINES FOR DIET

Overall Goals

One major goal of the National Cholesterol Education Program (NCEP) guidelines for diet is to use diet and lifestyle to reduce both risk factors and morbidity and mortality from CHD. The NCEP, through its population and adult treatment panels (13,14), believes that adherence to its dietary recommendations could result in a 10% decrease in blood cholesterol levels (Fig. 2.1). Since those reports were published, emerging information on fiber, plant sterol/stanol esters, alcohol, fish oil, and antioxidants indicate continued relevance of dietary considerations in a total program to reduce CHD risk. Moreover, reducing or preventing obesity is a major goal because it not only indirectly affects CHD risk, through its link with risk factors, but also independently predicts CAD (15).

Therapeutic Diets: Step I and II Diets Give Way to Revised Diets for Year 2000

The NCEP Adult Treatment Panel and the AHA previously recommended the Step I and Step II diets to lower cholesterol and to achieve LDL-C goals (13). The Step I diet restricted total fat to less than 30% of energy, saturated fat to less than 10% of energy, and dietary cholesterol to less than 300 mg per day. The Step II diet also restricted total fat to less than 30% of energy but limited saturated fat to less than 7% of energy, and dietary cholesterol to less than 200 mg per day. To put these diets in proper perspective, the Step I diet was really the "population diet," designed to shift the mean cholesterol level of the population to a lower value, and the Step II diet was the therapeutic or "clinical" diet, designed to provide more optimal lowering of total cholesterol and LDL-C levels. For patients with TG levels that exceed 1,000 mg per dL, the Step II diet's focus on LDL-C lowering was inadequate. Dietary control of severe hypertriglyceridemia requires weight loss, marked fat restriction, and possibly omega-3 fatty acids.

In the new AHA Dietary Guidelines known as "Revision 2000," the Step I diet is supplanted by major guidelines for the general population (16) (Table 2.1). These include the following population goals:

1. Achieve an overall healthy eating pattern
2. Achieve and maintain appropriate body weight
3. Achieve a desirable cholesterol profile
4. Achieve a desirable blood pressure

The revised guidelines stress three underlying principles. First, there are dietary patterns that all individuals can follow throughout their life span that promote and encourage cardiovascular health. This includes particular emphasis on patterns that help individuals avoid obesity. Second, the focus should shift to healthy dietary practices over an extended period of time, rather than insisting on "perfection" with each meal. This allows for the inclusion of a wide variety of healthy foods and avoids restricting the diet to repetitious and unsatisfying dietary experi-

TABLE 2.2 SELECTED BLINDED, CONTROLLED DIETARY INTERVENTION TRIALS USING CHD MORBIDITY OR MORTALITY AS END POINTS

	Subjects		Study characteristics			Change in TC[a] from baseline (%)	
Study	No.	Age (yr)	Design	Randomized	Duration (yr)		Comments
Finnish Mental Hospital[b]	5,115, 5,497	>15	Cross-over	No	6	−12 to 18	53%↓ in CHD mortality among men (*p* <.002), and 34%↓ among women (*p* was not significant).
Los Angeles-VA	846	50–89	Double-blinded	Yes	5–8	−13	31%↓ in end points of MI, CHD mortality, CVA, ruptured aneurysm, and ischemic gangrene (*p* <.01); 20%↓ in primary end points of MI and sudden death (*p* was not significant).
Minnesota Mental Hospital	9,057	All	Double-blinded	Yes	<4.5	−14	No significant differences or trends were noted in incidence of MI or sudden death.
DART	2,033 (CHD)	<70	Factorial	Yes	2	−2.8[c]	29%↓ in 2-yr all-cause mortality in subjects advised to eat fish (*p* <.05) resulting from 33%↓ in CHD mortality (*p* <.01)
Lyon Diet Heart	605 (CHD)	<70	Single-blinded	Yes	5	−7.5	65%↓ in CHD mortality in post-MI patients fed a diet rich in alpha-linolenic acid (*p* <.01).
GISSI	11,324 (CHD)	ND	Factorial	Yes	3.5	7 to 9	15%↓ in relative risk for all-cause mortality, nonfatal MI, and non-fatal stroke in the two groups supplemented with 1 g of *n*-3 PUFA. No benefit was seen in the group given vitamin E.
HOPE	9,541 (CHD)	>55	Double-blinded	Yes	4–6	NR	400 IU of vitamin E taken daily had no beneficial effects on cardiovascular outcomes in a high-risk patient population.

CHD, coronary heart disease; CVA, cerebrovascular accident; DART, Diet and Reinfarction Trial; GISSI, Gruppo Italiano per lo Studio della Sopravvivenza nell'Infarto Miocardico Prevenzione Trial; HOPE, Heart Outcomes Prevention Evaluation; MI, myocardial infarction; ND, not defined; NR, not reported; TC, total cholesterol; VA, Veterans Administration; ↓, decrease.
[a]The percentage change in plasma TC, rather than low-density lipoprotein cholesterol, is reported because the latter value is unavailable in the early intervention trials.
[b]Values are for the periods of 1959–1965 and 1965–1971, respectively.
[c]Value represents decrease of TC among subjects given advice about reducing fat consumption only (*p* was not significant). No changes from baseline were noted among patients who received advice about consumption of fiber or fish.
From Brousseau ME, Schaefer EJ. Diet and coronary heart disease: clinical trials. *Curr Atheroscler Rep* 2000;2:487–493, with permission.

ences. Finally, the new guidelines form a framework on which specific recommendations can be made to individuals, based on their health and risk-factor status, and appropriately modified by their dietary preferences and cultural background.

The new NCEP Adult Treatment Panel III guidelines (17) essentially advocate the Step II diet for individuals with raised LDL-C but provide specific nutritional and lifestyle options for those who need more intensive nutritional efforts to lower LDL-C or who require an approach that more specifically targets the metabolic syndrome. Along with the DASH (Dietary Approaches to Stop Hypertension) diet (18) for individuals with high blood pressure and guidelines for obesity to guide those with weight excess, clinicians can individualize the dietary prescription to address not only an abnormal lipid profile, but also associated hypertension, obesity, and risk of sudden death.

Using Diet to Alter Risk for Coronary Artery Disease

There are several principles that must be remembered in treating patients. First, the response of patients to diets is variable, as discussed earlier. Currently, we cannot predict how a given patient will respond to a particular therapeutic diet. Second, adherence to diets that produce an excellent reduction in serum lipids often also results in clinically important weight loss. Third, dietary factors that lower LDL-C levels include restriction of cholesterol-raising fatty acids and dietary cholesterol and inclusion of plant sterol/stanol esters to reduce cholesterol absorption.

TABLE 2.3 SELECTED CONTROLLED DIETARY INTERVENTION TRIALS USING RESULTS OF ANGIOGRAPHY AS AN END POINT

Study	Subjects		Study characteristics			LDL-C reduction[b] (%)	Comments
	No.[a]	Age (yr)	Design	Randomized	Duration (yr)		
Lifestyle Heart Trial	41	35–75	Prospective, controlled	Yes	1	37	Average percentage of diameter of stenosis regressed 1.8% in the experimental group; yet progressed 2.3% in the control group (*p* <.02).
Lifestyle Heart Trial	35	35–75	Prospective, controlled	Yes	5	20	Average percentage of diameter of stenosis regressed 3.1% from baseline in the experimental group and 11.8% in the control group (*p* <.001).
Heidelberg Trial	113	35–68	Prospective, controlled	Yes	1	9	Progression of coronary lesions was noted in 23% of intervention subjects vs. 48% of control subjects (*p* <.05). Regression occurred in 32% of intervention subjects vs. 17% of control subjects (*p* <.05).
CLAS	162	40–59	Placebo, controlled	Yes	2	7[c]	Increased intake of total fat and polyunsaturated fat associated with development of new lesions. Three fatty acids emerged as significant risk factors for new lesions: lauric acid (at >0.22% of calories), oleic acid (at >11.3% of calories), and linoleic acid (at >9.7% of calories).
STARS	74	>66	End-point blinded	Yes	3	16	Overall CHD progression decreased in 15% of intervention subjects (*p* <.02). Overall CHD regression increased in 38% of intervention subjects (*p* <.02).
SCRIP	300	56[d]	Placebo, controlled	Yes	4	23	Intervention group showed a rate of narrowing of diseased coronary segments that was 47% less than that of subjects in the usual care group (*p* <.02).

CHD, coronary heart disease; CLAS, Cholesterol Lowering Atherosclerosis Study; LDL-C, low-density lipoprotein cholesterol; SCRIP, Stanford Coronary Risk Intervention Project; STARS, St. Thomas' Atherosclerosis Regression Study.
[a]Sum of intervention and control groups (all subjects had CHD).
[b]All reductions were statistically significant (*p* <.05).
[c]Represents decrease among subjects who did not develop new lesions. No change was noted in LDL-C in those who developed new lesions.
[d]Mean value.

Other important factors include substituting mono- or polyunsaturated fats or complex carbohydrates for saturated fats, reducing intake of animal protein, and increasing intake of viscous fiber or cereal. Fourth, factors that affect HDL-C or TG levels include changes in body weight and consumption of sugars, alcohol, and omega-3 fatty acids or fish oils. Supplementation of the diet with fish may reduce cardiovascular end points independent of its effects on the lipid profile. Weight loss or restriction of simple sugars, for example, raises HDL-C levels and lowers TG levels. On the other hand, alcohol intake raises both HDL-C and TG levels. Fifth, changes seen in the first few months of a diet often are not sustained over time. This is particularly true for weight loss. The real hurdle for those with excess weight is not beginning a therapeutic program, it's maintaining the dietary habits and resulting weight loss. For weight maintenance, regular physical activity can be invaluable. The goal, of course, is sustained, not temporary, benefit.

EFFECT OF DIETARY FACTORS ON LIPIDS AND CORONARY ARTERY DISEASE

In published landmark studies, Keys (35) and Hegsted (36) quantified the response of serum cholesterol levels in humans to consumption of varying proportions of dietary fat and cholesterol. They demonstrated that saturated fatty acids (C12:0 to C16:0) are approximately twice as potent in raising cholesterol as polyunsaturated fats are in lowering them. Both investigators showed an independent effect of dietary cholesterol on serum cholesterol, although

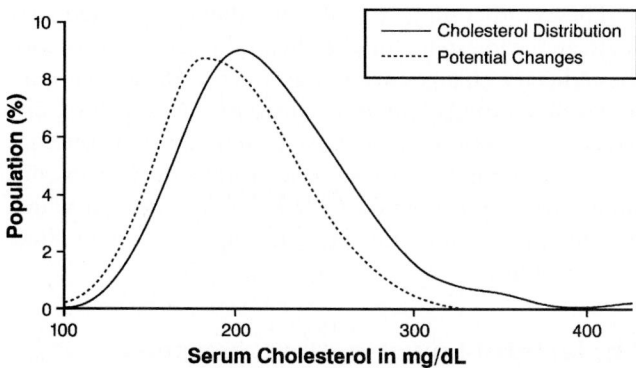

FIGURE 2.1 Cholesterol distribution in the U.S. population from the National Health and Nutrition Exam Survey, showing data from 1976 to 1980 and changes possible (*dotted lines*) if population goals for diet are attained. (Adapted from National Cholesterol Education Program. Report of the expert panel on population strategies for blood cholesterol reduction. Publication NIH 90–3046. Bethesda, MD: National Institutes of Health, US Department of Health and Human Services, 1990, with permission.)

monounsaturated fats (*cis* C18:1) were believed to have no specific independent effect. These equations do not take into account the effects of behenic acid (22:0), caprylic acid (8:0), and capric acid (10:0) that are cholesterol raising as well (37). Moreover, as will be shown later, these equations do not account for the increase in LDL-C levels seen with intake of TFAs and *n*-3 fatty acids that should be considered in any contemporary review of current dietary habits.

Cholesterol-Raising Fatty Acids

Saturated Fats

Saturated Fats and Coronary Artery Disease

Epidemiologic Data. The Seven Countries Study showed a direct relationship between saturated fat intake and rates of CAD (65). In that trial, Finland had the highest rate of CAD mortality, Mediterranean groups were far lower, and the Japanese, who had low intakes of saturated fat, had the lowest rates of CAD. The Ni-Hon-San Trial compared the diets and clinical status of native Japanese men with Japanese men who had migrated to Hawaii or to California. After migration toward the mainland of the United States, the diet increased in calories and saturated fat and the resulting increases in weight and serum cholesterol levels paralleled increases in rates of CAD (66,67). A notable exception to the observation that national diet often predicts risk of CAD is France. Despite similar intakes of saturated fat and dietary cholesterol to those in other Western countries, the rate of CHD in France is lower. The inverse association between wine ethanol and CHD has been one possible explanation for what has become known as the "French paradox" (68). Artaud-Wild and colleagues (69)

reviewed the cholesterol–saturated fat index scores for foods eaten in these countries. They speculated that consumption of milk and butterfat was markedly higher in Finland than in France. They suggested that the lower rates of fatal CAD in France were related to a less thrombogenic diet containing more plant foods and vegetables and small amounts of liquid vegetable oils. Law (70) noted that serum HDL-C levels explained little of the difference and offered a time-lag observation, suggesting that consumption of animal fat increased more recently in France than in Britain and that this accounted for the difference.

Clinical Trial Data. As noted earlier, clinical trials using lipid-lowering drugs with the ability to markedly reduce LDL-C levels have shown more convincing results than have trials involving dietary adjustments alone (71). Nonetheless, the insights gained from the entire range of dietary trials are worth reviewing, even if any single trial is, by itself, not conclusive in proving that dietary reduction of saturated fats prevents CAD.

Interpretation of many of the dietary trials that used clinical end points is hindered by faulty design (Tables 2.2 and 2.3). This is particularly true of early trials that were underpowered, so that achieving a positive result was more difficult. The Minnesota Coronary Survey, for example, did not have sufficient patients on the therapeutic diet for a sufficient length of time to achieve a significant effect—if, in fact, one was possible (72). Other examples of flawed study design that have made interpretation difficult include the Oslo Dietary and Smoking Intervention Trial, which changed smoking habits as well as diet (73), the Los Angeles Veterans Administration Trial, which combined both primary and secondary prevention (74), and the Finnish trial, which suffered from flawed randomization (75). Despite the fact that it was not a "pure" dietary trial, the results of the Oslo trial suggested that dietary reductions in cholesterol may be important in reducing rates of CAD. In this study, participants were randomly assigned to consume a diet low in saturated fat and counseled to reduce smoking. A 47% reduction in the incidence of sudden death and myocardial infarction (MI) was achieved in the intervention group, compared with the control group. The dietary change resulted in a net difference of 10% in serum cholesterol levels between intervention and control groups. The authors used statistical analysis to show that dietary change influenced the reduction in CAD events more than smoking did. At 5 years, the difference between both groups in total mortality became marginally significant, with a 33% lower mortality rate in the intervention group than in the control group.

Three large, multiple–risk factor intervention trials in which dietary change was a component also resulted in a smaller decrease of serum cholesterol values than was anticipated (76–78). When intervention trials (multifactorial or not) that use dietary changes are viewed as a whole, it appears that modest lowering of serum cholesterol by approximately 10% by dietary intervention over a short trial period is unlikely to show significant differences in CHD risk as compared to that seen in a control group.

Clinical trials with angiographic end points have the advantage of providing additional information about the potential beneficial effects of a diet low in total and saturated fat but involve sample sizes that are easier to recruit (Table 2.3). An individual's initial response to a diet can decrease with time, as seen in the Heidelberg trial, in which total fat restriction to less than 20% of calories resulted in initial LDL-C level decrease of 25% in subjects after 3 weeks on a metabolic ward (7). At the end of 1 year, the decrease in LDL-C levels had fallen to 4% as adherence to diet fell sharply. This produced an average lowering of LDL-C levels of 8% over the course of the year. The intervention group also participated in intensive physical exercise. When follow-up angiograms were reviewed, a significant decrease in progression and an increase in regression were seen in the intervention group. In this study, apolipoproteins, lipids, and lipoproteins were measured. Although the exercise component was an important part of this study, the best metabolic predictors of angiographic disease progression were the ratio of total cholesterol to HDL-C and the level of LDL-C (79).

In the St. Thomas Atherosclerosis Trial (STARS), CAD patients were randomly assigned to received treatment with usual care, diet, or diet and cholestyramine resin (6). The diet restricted total fat intake to 27% of total energy and saturated fat intake to 8% to 10% of energy and was high in fiber, chiefly pectin. The primary end point of this angiographic trial was the per-patient change in the mean absolute width of coronary segments. Progression of angiographic CAD correlated significantly with in-trial plasma total cholesterol, LDL-C, apolipoprotein B, and Lp(a) levels. By multiple regression analysis, LDL-C level was the best predictor of change in the diameter of the coronary vessel, appearing to account for 24% of the variance.

Further detailed dietary analysis showed that total fat intake was higher in the usual-care group than in the diet group (97 g vs. 61 g) (80). Patients in whom disease progression occurred consumed 42 g per day of saturated fat, whereas patients who experienced regression consumed only 21 g per day. These distinctions were important, because there were linear correlations between decreased intake of saturated or total fat and increased size of the artery lumen. When multiple regression analysis was used, the associations between change in coronary vessel diameter and total or saturated fat intake persisted, despite adjustment for LDL-C and other clinical descriptors. Thus, in this study of middle-aged British men, progression of CAD was strongly influenced by the intake of saturated fatty acids, possibly mediated in part by mechanisms other than the effect of saturated fat on LDL-C levels.

These studies suggest a role for reducing saturated fatty acids and cholesterol in the diet. The effects seen with these dietary changes are not as great as those seen with 3-hydroxy-3-methylglutaryl coenzyme A (HMG-CoA) reductase inhibitors. Moreover, they do not produce results as dramatic as those seen in individuals who consume diets supplemented with *n*-3 fatty acids, in which benefit appears to be mediated through a nonlipid effect (see Fish Oils).

Cholesterol-Lowering Interventions

Unsaturated Fatty Acids

Unsaturated fatty acids lower LDL-C levels when they are exchanged for saturated fatty acids in the diet. The more unsaturated a fatty acid, the more liquid it tends to be at room temperature. There are important differences, however, in various groups of unsaturated fatty acids that should be considered in the design of therapeutic diets. The two major groups are the polyunsaturated fatty acids (PUFAs) and the monounsaturated fatty acids (MUFAs). A recent metaanalysis found no significant differences in total cholesterol, LDL-C, and HDL-C levels when MUFAs and PUFAs are directly compared (90). Real differences may relate to effects on oxidation and coagulation parameters.

Polyunsaturated Fatty Acids

PUFAs, however, are not a homogenous class but are divided into two groups by the position of the first double bond from the terminal end of the carbon chain. Examples of *n*-6 fatty PUFAs include corn, sunflower, safflower, sesame, and cottonseed oils. The major *n*-6 PUFA, linoleic acid (18:2) is an 18-carbon "essential" fatty acid that cannot be synthesized by the body. Linoleic acid is needed for normal immune response, and essential fatty acid deficiency impairs B and T cell–mediated responses (91). The *n*-3 PUFAs are often referred to as "marine lipids" or "fish oils." Marine *n*-3 PUFAs have a major effect on TG levels, as is discussed later. Alpha-linolenic acid is a plant-based *n*-3 PUFA. Common sources of alpha-linolenic acid are tofu, soybean and canola oil, nuts, and flax seed. These are healthy additions to the diets of vegetarians and those who do not eat seafood; however, alpha-linolenic acid does not appear to lower TG levels as strikingly as do fish oils (92).

Low-Fat, High-Carbohydrate Diets

A diet low in fat and high in complex carbohydrates is typical of an "Asian-style" diet. Often the percentage of energy that comes from carbohydrates is 60% to 65%, allowing total fat calories to be as low as 15% to 20% of total energy.

Thus, intakes of saturated fat and dietary cholesterol are very low.

Low-Fat Diets and Coronary Artery Disease

Some studies have emphasized a total fat content less than 30% of calories and a lowered intake of saturated fat in the diet. The Leiden study was an uncontrolled study of the effects of a vegetarian diet in 39 men who had angina pectoris. The study demonstrated that subjects who improved the ratio of total cholesterol to HDL-C had the least progression of CAD on follow-up angiography (114). Blackenhorn and colleagues (115) noted a striking difference between the 18 men in the placebo group of the Cholesterol Lowering Atherosclerosis Study (CLAS), who developed new atherosclerotic coronary lesions, and the 64 men in the diet group, who did not. Their analysis of the nutritional data suggested that this was related to dietary choices. Subjects who did not show progression had substituted low-fat meats and dairy products for high-fat products. The effect of an increased intake of total, saturated, and polyunsaturated fat was to foster a greater likelihood of new lesion development. These observational results are consistent with, but did not prove, the premise that for individuals at risk, the diet should be low in both total fat and saturated fat to reduce the likelihood of coronary progression.

The value of a low-fat vegetarian-style diet as part of a comprehensive lifestyle intervention that includes exercise was examined in the Lifestyle Heart Trial (10). In this provocative study, a highly motivated group of patients with symptomatic coronary disease consumed a diet in which fewer than 10% of calories came from fat and no cholesterol was allowed. The treatment group lost 22 lb, whereas the control group, who were on what was essentially a Step II diet, did not lose any weight. The intervention subjects showed a decline in LDL-C levels of 37.8%, to 100 mg per dL.

At the end of 1 year, the intensively treated group had decreased progression and/or regression of angiographic CAD compared with the control group. The improvement in angiographic appearance went beyond simple improvements in percentage of stenosis; the treatment group had complex shape-change and stenosis-molding characteristics suggestive of augmented flow reserve (116). At the end of 5 years, improvement was documented by both angiography and decreased size and severity of perfusion abnormalities as seen while the patient was at rest, using dipyridamole positron emission tomography (PET) (117). The small sample size, the difficulties caused when 49% of the subjects refused to participate after randomization, and the fact that multiple interventions were in place, including exercise, stress reduction, and the significant weight reduction seen in the treatment group, preclude any generalizations about the value of the very-low-fat diet to the coronary patient that might be based on the results of this study.

Singh and coworkers (118) performed a randomized, single-blind, controlled clinical trial in patients with acute MI to determine the effect of adding more fruits, vegetables, nuts, and grains to the usual post-MI fat-reduced diet. Both groups consumed a principally vegetarian diet, eating eggs four to five times per week and meat one to two times per week. The treatment group's goal was to eat at least 400 g per day of fruits and vegetables. The results were striking: blood cholesterol and the incidence of cardiac events were significantly lower in the treatment group. Even total mortality was significantly improved. It is important to note that weight fell by 6.3 kg in the treatment group versus 2.4 kg in the usual-care group. As seen in other trials, reduction in LDL-C, particularly when it is accompanied by loss of excess weight, appears to be associated with improvement in rates of CAD events.

The Stanford Coronary Risk Intervention Project was a 4-year multifactor intervention trial. The study used serial, quantitative coronary angiography in 300 men and women to show a significant reduction in new lesion formation in the coronary arteries of those randomly assigned to the risk-reduction group, compared with that in the usual-care group (119). All risk-reduction group subjects were instructed to consume a low-fat, low-cholesterol, and high-carbohydrate diet, with a goal of intake of less than 20% of energy from fat, less than 6% of energy from saturated fat, and less than 75 mg of cholesterol per day. Increased physical activity and a specific endurance exercise-training program were recommended. A staff psychologist supervised a stop-smoking program for smokers. Major goals were to decrease LDL-C levels to fewer than 110 mg per dL and TG levels to fewer than 100 mg per dL, and to increase HDL-C levels to greater than 55 mg per dL, using dietary and pharmacologic interventions. Multiple regression analysis identified in-study dietary fat intake as the best correlate with new lesion formation. Participants randomly assigned to the risk-reduction group preferentially increased complex carbohydrate intake to offset reduction in dietary fat restriction. The authors suggested that the reduction in dietary fat accomplished by subjects in their study, as in the CLAS placebo group, decreased the rate of new lesion formation by mechanisms not limited to LDL reduction.

In addition, a low-fat diet may help relieve symptoms through mechanisms apart from the lipid-lowering effects on atherosclerosis. Several studies that used low-fat diets as part of a multiple intervention approach showed early symptomatic improvements in cardiac status. Ornish (10) reported that patients in the experimental group of his Lifestyle Trial experienced a 91% reduction in frequency of angina, a 42% reduction in duration of angina, and a 28% reduction in severity of angina, whereas angina worsened in the control group. A decrease in angina was also seen in the Heidelberg Trial (7). Both of these studies used intensive exercise regimens. Interestingly, a beneficial effect on angina was seen in the intervention groups in STARS, but not in the control group, even though there was no difference in the exercise advice given to control and to intervention subjects. Gould and colleagues (120) showed that relatively short-term, intensive cholesterol lowering over the course of 90 days resulted in improved myocardial perfusion capacity, as measured noninvasively by dipyridamole PET.

A likely explanation for short-term improvement that occurs with changes in diet is improved endothelial regulation of vasomotion. In both animal and human studies of hypercholesterolemia, abnormal blood-vessel reactivity occurs early and involves both large vessels with overt atherosclerotic change and the microcirculation, where atherosclerosis does not develop (121). Harrison and coworkers demonstrated that dietary treatment of atherosclerosis in monkeys not only produced morphologic improvement of the atherosclerotic lesion, but also restored endothelium-dependent vascular relaxation to normal (122). Later work in rabbits also showed that cholesterol-lowering diets improved endothelium-dependent vascular relaxation (123).

The mechanism by which diet restores endothelium-dependent vascular relaxation to normal most likely involves diet-related reduction of LDL-C levels. Further studies have demonstrated the more potent effects of adding LDL-lowering therapy to diet. Leung and coauthors (124) demonstrated that impairment of endothelium-dependent relaxation in hypercholesterolemic patients with healthy coronary arteries can be reversed by cholesterol-lowering therapy with diet and a lipid-lowering resin that lowered LDL-C levels by 35.7%. In patients with CAD, adherence to a cholesterol-lowering diet and HMG-CoA-reductase therapy for 5.5 months significantly improved endothelium-dependent coronary reactivity in hypercholesterolemic patients, compared with patients whose condition was managed solely by adherence to a Step I diet (125). Anderson and colleagues (126) documented even greater improvement when probucol (which is no longer clinically available, but was used as an antioxidant in this study) was added to treatment with lovastatin. Because the effects of diet may be additive to the effects of drug therapy, these data support the notion that drug therapy should be added to dietary therapy and not given alone.

Dietary Fiber

Fiber, or nondigestible plant-based carbohydrate, is an important part of a balanced diet. Some believe that the ideal diet for both cancer and heart disease prevention is the 25/25 diet (i.e., intake of 25% of calories from fat and 25 g of total fiber per day) (127). However, for the optimal cholesterol-lowering diet, it is useful to think of fiber in terms of its viscous (formerly called "soluble") and nonvis-

cous ("insoluble") forms. Nonviscous fiber aids in the treatment of constipation but is not lipid-lowering.

Fiber and Coronary Artery Disease

The benefits of increased intake of dietary fiber for cardiovascular disease may extend beyond lowering of LDL-C levels. Khaw and Barrett-Connor (136) used 24-h dietary fiber intake by recall in a cohort of men and women in southern California aged 50 to 79 to show a significant inverse relationship between fiber intake and CAD. A 6-g increment in daily fiber intake was associated with a significant 25% reduction in mortality from CAD. A recent report of 43,757 U.S. male health professionals 40 to 75 years of age showed that there was a reduced risk of MI in men in the highest quintile for total dietary fiber intake (137). A 10-g increase in dietary fiber corresponded to a significant 19% reduction in risk. Within the three main dietary contributors to total fiber intake (vegetables, fruits, and cereals), *cereal fiber* was most strongly associated with reduced risk for MI. Finally, fruit and vegetable intake was found to reduce the all-stroke risk, including risk of transient ischemic attack, in men followed in the Framingham Trial, even after adjustment for multiple risk factors, including total fat, ethanol, and total energy intake (138).

Vegetable Protein

Soy protein has been consumed worldwide for centuries, and some Asian populations are known to consume 20 g of soy protein daily in products such as soy milk, tempeh, and tofu (139). This would seem to attest to the long-term safety of a diet enriched with soy protein. The mechanism by which soy lowers cholesterol levels is still unclear (140). The presence of the soybean isoflavone fraction appears to be important to cholesterol-lowering effects (141,142). In addition, high isoflavone intakes in soy breakfast cereals may reduce oxidized LDL levels, even though LDL-C is not significantly lowered (143). The benefit of this on atherosclerosis is not established.

Soy Protein and Coronary Artery Disease

There are no good data from clinical trials that examined the effects of soy protein on CAD end points. Although there are practical concerns regarding intake of sufficient soy protein to improve LDL-C values, products made with soy may prove useful as substitutes for products high in animal fat.

Additional Dietary Factors

Coffee

There has been considerable interest in whether coffee has deleterious effects on the coronary risk profile. A critical analysis must distinguish between filtered coffee and boiled coffee, such as is consumed in Scandinavia, France, or Turkey, which is associated with elevated cholesterol values.

Coffee and Coronary Artery Disease

A prospective cohort analysis from the Health Professionals Study has provided the largest sample to date used to collect data about coffee's effects on cardiovascular disease (150). Although follow-up was only 2 years, they found that increased consumption of caffeinated coffee did not lead to higher risks for cardiovascular disease. They did note that greater consumption of decaffeinated coffee was associated with a marginally significant increase in the risk for CAD. A longer follow-up was used in the Nurses' Health Study, which documented 712 cases of CAD after 10 years of follow-up (151). There was no increase in CAD among women who drank six or more cups of caffeinated coffee, compared with that among women who drank none. The results of a study by La Croix and colleagues (152) that followed 1,130 male medical students for 19 to 35 years supported an independent, dose-responsive association between coffee and overt CAD among coffee drinkers who had more than 5 cups per day. In the absence of a placebo-controlled, clinical trial that would eliminate unknown confounding variables, it would appear that individuals who drink, on average, one to two cups of filtered coffee per day probably incur little change in lipid levels or CAD rates, as long as the coffee consumption is neither associated with the use of dairy creamers nor accompanied by cigarette smoking.

Dietary Factors That Affect High-Density Lipoprotein Cholesterol and Triglyceride Levels

The dietary factors that alter HDL-C and TG levels are not the same as those that alter LDL-C levels. The emphasis shifts to excess dietary energy, high carbohydrate intake, alcohol, and fish oil.

Excess Dietary Energy

Knuiman and colleagues (156) reviewed epidemiologic data on the relationship between diet and HDL-C levels and concluded that three partly opposing dietary factors determine the ratio of total cholesterol to HDL-C in an adult population. They convincingly argued that the proportion of energy from saturated fat raised total cholesterol and LDL-C levels, the proportion of energy from total fat raised HDL-C levels, and an excess in dietary energy, which produces obesity, lowered HDL-C levels. In addition, weight loss markedly affects TG levels and can improve HDL-C levels. A clinical study involving obese men and women quantified the effects of weight loss on the lipid profile as additive to those reducing fat and saturated fat (157). In this 13-week trial, weight loss in and of itself

appeared to explain approximately 50% of the decrease in total cholesterol, 60% of the decrease in LDL-C, and 70% of the decrease in TGs. Moreover, although a low-fat, low–saturated fat diet alone reduced HDL-C by 11.1% and the ratio of HDL-C to LDL-C by 7.7%, weight loss reversed this trend, resulting in an increase in HDL-C of 12.5% and in the ratio of HDL-C to LDL-C of 24%. A metaanalysis of studies on the effects of weight loss on lipid and lipoprotein levels showed a significant negative correlation between weight loss and total cholesterol, LDL-C, and TG levels (158). HDL-C levels decreased during the active weight loss phase but increased by 0.009 mmol per L with every kilogram of weight loss when weight was maintained.

High-Carbohydrate Diets

TG levels have a marked influence on HDL-C levels and are very sensitive to dietary change. Dietary influences on TG levels include high carbohydrate consumption, which, as noted earlier, can both elevate TG levels and lower HDL-C levels. Avoidance of simple sugars is particularly important, because they not only promote dental caries, but also can lead to caloric excess and obesity. The current trend toward fat-free foods has produced many food choices that are high in calories as a result of the addition of corn syrup solids or sucrose. Patients should be cautioned that such fat-free foods cannot be eaten in unlimited quantities. Although limited amounts of these foods can be part of a healthy dietary regimen, a diet that is fat-free is not necessarily nutritious.

Alcohol Intake

Alcohol consumption raises TG levels but, unlike a high-carbohydrate diet, also raises HDL-C levels. The Framingham Offspring Study's analysis of 1,584 middle-aged men and 1,639 middle-aged women showed that TG levels, BMI, and alcohol intake all contributed significantly to fasting HDL-C and apoprotein A-I variability (160).

Alcohol and Coronary Artery Disease

Dietary and alcohol consumption data from 21 countries indicate that alcohol consumption has a strong negative correlation with CAD mortality (68) (Fig. 2.2). Among middle-aged or older British men whose average intake of alcoholic beverages was 1 to 2 U per day, consumption of alcohol was associated with significantly lower all-cause mortality than was consumption of no alcohol or of greater amounts of alcohol (165). A genetic "proof of principle" was seen in a study of individuals with a polymorphism for the gene for alcohol dehydrogenase-3 that alters the rate of alcohol metabolism. Men homozygous for the allele, which is associated with a slow rate of oxidation, who consumed at least one drink per day had the greatest reduction in risk and the highest plasma HDL-C levels (166). This interac-

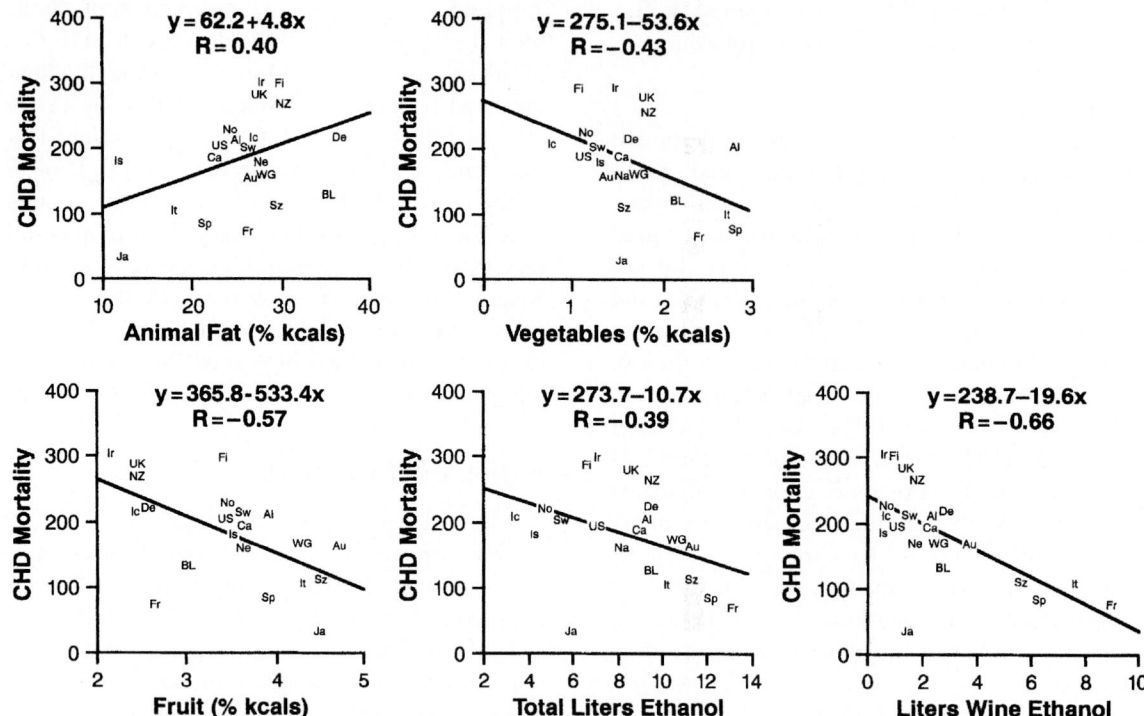

FIGURE 2.2 Graphs showing epidemiologic correlations between intake of fat, vegetables, fruit, alcohol, and wine ethanol. Au, Australia; Ca, Canada; CHD, coronary heart disease; De, Denmark; Fi, Finland; Fr, France; Ic, Iceland; Ir, Ireland; Is, Israel; It, Italy; Ja, Japan; Ne, The Netherlands; No, Norway; NZ, New Zealand; Sp, Spain; Sw, Sweden; Sz, Switzerland; UK, United Kingdom; US, United States; WG, West Germany. (From Criqui MH, Ringel BL. Does diet or alcohol explain the French paradox? *Lancet* 1994;344:1719–1723, with permission.)

tion was confirmed in an independent study of postmenopausal women.

In the MRFIT prospective experience among middle-aged men who were light-to-moderate drinkers, HDL-C levels largely demonstrated the inverse association between alcohol consumption and death from CAD (167). Metaanalysis of 42 experimental studies suggested that 30 g of alcohol per day would cause an estimated reduction of 24.7% in risk of CHD (162). There has been speculation that an effect of alcohol on platelet function could explain the low mortality from CAD that is seen among the population in France despite consumption of a diet that is comparable in intake of saturated fat to those of other nations in which CAD rates are higher (168). Other effects of alcohol on coagulation include a positive association between moderate alcohol intake and plasma levels of endogenous tissue-type plasminogen activator (169).

Various reports indicate that one kind of alcoholic beverage is not preferred over others. A systematic review of 12 ecologic, 3 case-control, and 10 separate prospective cohort studies indicates that *all* alcoholic drinks are linked with lower risk (170). Indeed, a study comparing red and white wine did not show that red wine selectively decreased the susceptibility of LDL to oxidation (171).

Although older men and women may benefit from the effects of mild-to-moderate alcohol intake in reducing rates of CAD, public health considerations argue against an uncritical encouragement of alcohol consumption (172). In men and women younger than 40 years, alcohol consumption has a particularly negative benefit/risk profile; the cardiovascular risk is already low, and the increase in all-cause mortality that accompanies drinking more than offsets any possible health advantage (173). Moreover, individuals who consume five or more drinks per occasion are nearly twice as likely to die from injuries than persons who drink less (174). Cardiac patients, in particular, may suffer from aggravation of hypertension, as well as increased arrhythmia, stroke risk, cardiomyopathy, and LVH, with excess drinking (175).

An important caveat pertains to alcohol intake among women. Women reporting any amount of alcohol consumption in the First National Health and Nutrition Exam Survey had an approximately 20% decrease in risk for CAD compared with women who abstain (176). A recent study that examined asymptomatic alcoholic women and men noted a similar prevalence of cardiomyopathy and myopathy in both groups (177). The threshold dose for the development of cardiomyopathy was significantly lower among women, and the decline in ejection fraction with increasing amounts of alcohol was significantly steeper than among men. These data suggest an increased sensitivity in women to the toxic effects of alcohol on cardiac muscle (Fig. 2.3).

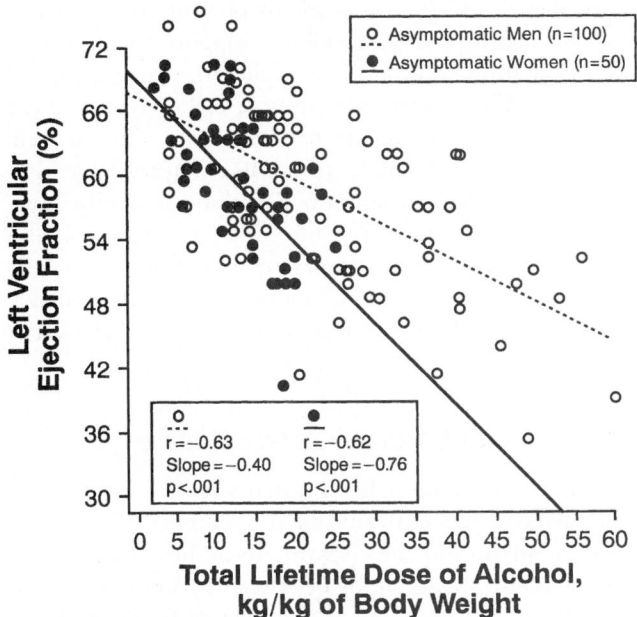

FIGURE 2.3 Lifetime dose of alcohol and left ventricular ejection fraction in men and women.

Fish Oils

The omega-3 PUFAs known as *n-3* fatty acids can be obtained from either plant or marine sources. Alpha-linolenic acid is a plant-based omega-3 PUFA found in tofu, soybean, canola oil, and nuts. Plant-based omega-3 PUFAs do not lower TG levels in a striking fashion in contrast to the marine-based omega-3 fatty acids known as "eicosapentenoic acid" and DHA (92). The sum of these long-chain *n-3* PUFAs in a capsule or fish product determines the amount of omega-3 PUFAs present. Fatty fish such as salmon and mackerel are good sources of *n-3* fatty acids.

Fish Oil and Coronary Artery Disease
Studies using fish or fish oil capsules challenge the traditional diet-lipid-heart paradigm, although fish oil capsules are useful in the control of moderate to severe hypertriglyceridemia. The relationship between fish intake and lowered rates of CHD stemmed from early observational studies comparing Greenland Inuit with their Danish counterparts. The Inuit diet included a strikingly higher intake of *n-3* PUFAs, in which marine sources, such as seal and whale, are rich. The biochemical and hematologic profiles of the Inuit showed lower values for total cholesterol, TG, LDL-C, and VLDL-C, increased values for HDL-C, increased bleeding times, and lower rates of CAD (184). In addition, prospective epidemiologic studies confirmed that men who ate at least some fish every week had a lower mortality from CAD than did men who ate none (185–188). In two studies, however, in which fish intake was high, a beneficial effect was not documented (189,190).

Despite these intriguing results, the results of most primary prevention studies of fish, fish oil, and CAD have been negative. The Health Professionals Follow-up Study, a large-scale prospective cohort study, reported no association between increases in consumption of fish and CAD (191). The authors concluded that increasing fish intake beyond one or two servings per week is not beneficial in the primary prevention of CAD. A nested case-control study among the 14,916 participants of the Physician's Health Study also showed no beneficial effect from consumption of fish oil on CAD (192). No association was found between fish oil levels and the incidence of MI, even when results were adjusted for major cardiovascular risk factors. Fish oil has not always produced beneficial results in trials of secondary CAD prevention. A clinical trial large enough to find a significant effect if one existed showed that 8 g per day of *n-3* PUFA was well-tolerated, but not helpful in preventing clinical restenosis after angioplasty (193). Among normocholesterolemic men with angiographically documented CAD, fish oil treatment (6 g of *n-3* PUFAs for 2 years) did not produce significant changes in the diameter of the coronary arteries (194).

Yet the ability of fish and fish oil capsules to reduce all-cause mortality in two intervention trials and a putative relationship between increased omega-3 fatty acid ingestion and CHD mortality in a third trial are compelling data that must be examined carefully (8,9,195). The Diet and Reinfarction Trial (DART) noted that those men who were instructed to eat fish after they had experienced MI showed a 29% decline in all-cause mortality compared with those in the placebo group (8). The mechanism for this beneficial effect was independent of lipid levels. In this trial, a group of the men (25%) who could not tolerate fish were given 875 mg of fish oil in capsule form. This study raised speculation that the beneficial effect of fish oil in survivors of MI may relate to its effects on thrombosis and/or risk for arrhythmia. The Gruppo Italiano per lo Studio della Sopravvivenza nell'Infarto Miocardio (GISSI)–Prevenzione Trial, a large-scale open-label, randomized, controlled trial involving 11,324 MI survivors, demonstrated that 875-mg fish oil capsules, but not vitamin E, reduced the primary cumulative end point of all-cause mortality, nonfatal MI, and nonfatal stroke (9). Neither intervention significantly reduced the other primary end point, the cumulative rate of cardiovascular death, nonfatal MI, and nonfatal stroke. Analysis of secondary end points suggested that the benefit lay in reduction of mortality and not in reduction of nonfatal MI. It was a safe intervention, although LDL-C levels were slightly increased as TG levels were decreased.

The Lyon Trial, which was mentioned previously in the section on Mediterranean diet, used a diet rich in a vegetable-based omega-3 fatty acid known as *alpha-linolenic acid*

(107). The striking reduction in sudden death, similar to that seen in DART, suggested a beneficial effect on cardiac health from intake of omega-3 fatty acids, independent of any lipid-lowering effect. Viewed critically, the Lyon results seem almost too good to be true: When the major primary and secondary end points are combined, 59 events occurred in control subjects and 14 events occurred in study patients—a risk reduction of 76% (195). Although these data seem to overestimate the true effect of such dietary change, they do suggest that certain components of the Mediterranean-type diet, such as omega-3 fatty acids, oleic acid, and dietary antioxidants, may play important roles in reducing the risk for CAD. Moreover, a cohort questionnaire study involving 43,757 male health professionals aged 40 to 75 years and free of cardiovascular disease or diabetes reported that subjects who consumed diets high in alpha-linolenic acid had a reduced risk of CAD (196).

These provocative findings were followed by a carefully done population-based case-control study from Seattle and King County, Washington (197). Among 334 patients who had experienced primary cardiac arrest, the monthly intake of *n*-3 PUFAs was significantly less than that seen in age- and sex-matched community controls. The equivalent of one fatty-fish meal per week was associated with a 50% reduction in the risk for primary cardiac arrest after adjustment for potential confounding factors. These findings were consistent with experimental evidence suggesting that the *n*-3 PUFAs have an important effect on the vulnerability to ventricular fibrillation in the setting of myocardial ischemia (198).

Recommending consumption of one or two fish-based meals weekly is reasonable, particularly if it substitutes for sources of protein in the diet such as fatty meats, which increase total saturated fat intake. Patients should be cautioned to avoid fish contaminated with mercury and other toxins. Mercury contamination not only could prove an important hazard to susceptible persons (children, pregnant women), but has been shown to attenuate the cardiac benefits of fish (199). The use of fish oil capsules can be considered for MI survivors, based on the GISSI trial, but additional studies and standardized, widely available preparations are needed before this is a routine recommendation (200). The potential benefit of decreasing sudden cardiac death using fish oil therapy is exciting to contemplate. Additional research studies are awaited.

Antioxidants, Vitamins, and Coronary Artery Disease

The available data support the hypothesis that oxidation of LDL by cells in the arterial wall is a pivotal step in the initiation of the early lesions seen in coronary atherosclerosis (201). Thus, there has been a heightened interest in antioxidants, which may work to prevent or retard this process. Several lines of evidence support an important role for vitamin E (or alpha-tocopherol), which is carried on LDL and is a potent lipid-soluble antioxidant. There is also considerable interest in beta-carotene, which is lipid soluble, and in vitamin C, which is a water-soluble vitamin. Food sources of vitamin E include seed oils, nuts, avocados, whole-grain and fortified cereals, eggs, and green vegetables. Food sources of beta-carotene include carrots and boiled broccoli. Vitamin C is widely available in fruits and vegetables, but losses of vitamin C can occur with cooking.

Vitamin E and Coronary Artery Disease

The effects of vitamin E on atherosclerosis and clinical CAD are controversial and do not support enthusiastic recommendation of the vitamin. To be sure, early observational studies suggested a beneficial effect of vitamin E (204–206). Furthermore, a prospective study of postmenopausal women from Iowa showed that the intake of vitamin E from foods is inversely associated with the risk by death from CAD. Importantly, the data suggested that such women might lower their risk without using vitamin supplements (207). These were not randomized clinical trials, and unforeseen bias may have influenced the results.

The Cambridge Heart Antioxidant Study used a randomized, double-blind design in 2,002 patients with angiographic CAD who were assigned to receive 400 IU of alpha-tocopherol daily or placebo. Nonfatal MI decreased significantly at 1 year among subjects who took vitamin E (208). One feature of the study that is worthy of concern was the lack of a significant reduction in either total mortality or cardiovascular deaths in the alpha-tocopherol group. In fact, a slight, nonsignificant increase was seen in these categories in the treatment group. Since publication of the results of this trial, two large randomized trials have shown no benefit from vitamin E on primary end points. In the previously mentioned GISSI trial, vitamin E did not affect either of the two primary combined end points. Although benefit was suggested in a secondary analysis that examined cardiovascular death, the authors speculated that a longer trial would be required to show beneficial effects from vitamin E on cardiovascular end points. The Heart Outcomes Prevention Evaluation Study found no significant effect associated with daily ingestion of 400 U of vitamin E on cardiovascular end points in 9,541 high-risk subjects older than 55 years who were randomly assigned to receive vitamin E or placebo and followed for 4.5 years (209). Moreover, a substudy of this trial showed no differences in atherosclerosis progression rates, as determined by carotid ultrasound, associated with ingestion of vitamin E, whereas a beneficial effect was seen with the angiotensin-converting enzyme inhibitor ramipril (210). Because strong evidence for effects associated with vitamin E on subclinical atherosclerosis as well as clinical rates of CHD is lacking, a routine recommendation for its use is not reasonable at this time.

Vitamin C and Coronary Artery Disease

A large prospective observation of 19,496 men and women in a nine-country study showed that plasma ascorbic acid levels were inversely related to mortality from all causes, from cardiovascular disease, and from ischemic heart disease (211). The authors speculated on the potential benefits of a small increase in intake of fruits and vegetables. The Atherosclerosis Risk in Communities Study examined the relationship between the intake of dietary and supplemental vitamin C, alpha-tocopherol, and provitamin A carotenoids and average carotid artery–wall thickness among 6,318 women and 4,989 men aged 45 to 64 years (212). Among men and women older than 55 years, but not among individuals younger than 55 years, who had not recently begun a special diet, there was a significant inverse relationship between vitamin C intake and average carotid artery wall thickness, adjusted for pertinent variables. In Kuopio, in Eastern Finland, men and postmenopausal women in a double-masked, two-by-two factorial trial were randomly assigned to four strata and received either 136 IU daily of D-alpha-tocopherol, 250 mg of slow-release vitamin C, a combination of these, or placebo for 3 years. Progression of common carotid atherosclerosis was decreased significantly among men who received a combination of D-alpha-tocopherol and slow-release vitamin C (213).

Beta-Carotene and Coronary Artery Disease

The European Community Multicenter Study on Antioxidants, Myocardial Infarction, and Breast Cancer was a controlled study that looked at adipose tissue levels of beta-carotene and alpha-tocopherol in individuals with a history of MI (214). The data suggested that consumption of foods rich in beta-carotene, such as carrots and green leafy vegetables, might reduce the risk for MI.

In contrast, three carefully done trials using beta-carotene supplementation did not show beneficial effects on cancer or cardiovascular disease (215–217). Moreover, the Beta Carotene and Retinol Efficacy Trial showed that the combination of beta-carotene and vitamin A may have led to an adverse effect on lung cancer and the risk of death from lung cancer, from cardiovascular disease, and from all causes in both cigarette smokers and workers exposed to asbestos. Thus, the time and expense necessary to obtain clinical trial data to document or refute contentions derived from observational data was clearly worth it. There is no good evidence to support the endorsement of beta-carotene supplementation to reduce cardiovascular disease end points.

OBESITY, LIPIDS, CORONARY ARTERY DISEASE, AND CARDIOVASCULAR DISEASE

The terminology of the obesity literature can be confusing. Terms useful to the following discussion are summarized in *e*Table 2.3.3. Bray has proposed a classification of obesity that avoids misleading descriptors such as "progressive" or "morbid" (226). Using the BMI, obesity can be classified from Class 1 to Class 4, at the extreme. This system is summarized in *e*Table 2.3.4.

According to recent data, 50% of all adult Americans are overweight or obese (227). This reflects an increasing prevalence over the course of the past decade. This finding is worrisome, because obesity, over the long term, increases the risk for death (228–231). In addition, obesity contributes to at least one-half of the diseases that are chronic in Western societies (232). Although abdominal obesity is cause for particular concern, noncentral obesity is not metabolically benign. A cross-sectional study in Manitoba showed that, in its survey of adults aged 18 to 74 years, the BMI as an overall measure of obesity compared favorably with waist-to-hip ratio in predicting effects of obesity on blood pressure, glucose, and plasma lipids (233).

A review published in 1993 of 13 reports from 11 diverse populations looked at weight changes in subjects aged 17 years or older (234). It concluded that the highest mortality rates occur in adults who either have lost weight or have gained excessive weight. Andres (235) believed that data suggesting that the lowest mortality rates in these studies accompanied modest weight gains in adulthood supported his previously held views. This was disputed by a detailed analysis of U.S. women enrolled in the Nurses' Health Study (236) (*e*Table 2.3.5). The data showed that body weight and all-cause mortality were directly related. Lean women did not show excess mortality, and a weight increase ≥10 kg after the age of 18 was associated with increased mortality in middle adulthood. When the BMI exceeded 27, mortality was substantially elevated. In terms of attributable risk, 53% of deaths among women with a BMI greater than 29 could be attributed to their obesity. Mortality from CAD in this study was more strongly related to waist-hip ratio, which is a measure of abdominal obesity.

The Nurses' Health Study data should be compared with observations from the Honolulu Heart Program, in which men who had a weight loss of 4.5 kg or more, large fluctuations in weight, or both over the course of a 6-year period were in poorer health than those whose weight was more stable (237). Like the Nurses' Health Study, an increase in mortality occurred primarily among subjects with a BMI greater than 27. Subjects whose weight fluctuated the most had a significantly higher risk for death from cardiovascular causes. This relationship was not seen in healthy men who had not smoked. In fact, one of the problems with analyzing "weight cycling" is the inability to distinguish between intentional and unintentional weight loss. Stunkard (238) noted that evidence that weight cycling is a cause of either upper-body obesity with metabolic changes or increased mortality is lacking.

In a prospective cohort study of Dutch men and women aged 30 to 54 years, with an average follow-up of 12 years, all-cause mortality was increased among obese men (BMI greater than 30) and among underweight men, but not among women (239). The Framingham Heart Study looked at the relationship of weight at age 65 among 1,723 nonsmokers who were followed for a mean of 9.5 years (240). The study found that the risk of death was increased twofold over the course of the entire follow-up period for persons with a BMI higher than the 70th percentile at both 55 and 65 years of age. This works out to a BMI greater than or equal to 28.5 that is attained by a 5-ft 9-in. man who weighs at least 193 lb.

Obesity and the Heart

Cardiac output and blood volume increase in obesity to supply the increased adipose stores (*e*Fig. 2.3.1). Systolic function is generally preserved, even in patients with marked obesity. Nonetheless, in a small subgroup who had low left ventricular fractional shortening before surgical therapy for morbid obesity, the mean fractional shortening increased significantly when body weight decreased from 13 to 79 kg of the amount over ideal body weight. Blood pressure and left ventricular internal dimension in diastole also decreased (260). Obesity affects diastolic function and is a strong stimulus for LVH. Messerli (261) noted, among subjects matched for blood pressure values, that LVH was found in more than 50% of all obese subjects and only in less than 20% of nonobese subjects. When heart size is examined, eccentric enlargement is seen in obese patients with hypertension, compared with symmetric LVH in hypertensive patients who were not obese. In addition to magnitude of obesity, the duration of obesity must also be taken into account (262). In the Framingham Heart Study, BMI was strongly associated with echocardiographic LVH, particularly when the BMI was greater than 30 kg per m² (263). Finally, obesity leads to a prolonged QT interval, which may increase the potential for arrhythmias (264).

For the Class 4 obese patient, the situation is especially grim. Cardiovascular disease is the most frequent cause of death (265). Life-table techniques that compare the mortality among Class 4 obese individuals with that among men in the general population demonstrated a 12-fold excess mortality among obese patients aged 25 to 34 years, and a sixfold excess among those aged 35 to 44 years. This ratio

diminished with advancing age. Postmortem examination of 12 Class 4 obese patients aged 12 to 59 years disclosed dilated left ventricular and right ventricular cavities, but only two patients had one or more epicardial coronary arteries that had narrowed at least 75% in cross-sectional diameter (266). Kasper and colleagues (267) looked at patients greater than 35% overweight who presented with congestive heart failure and compared them with patients whose weight was normal. A significantly higher percentage of the obese patients had a dilated cardiomyopathy. Among patients with similar degrees of cardiomyopathy, obese patients had elevated right-heart pressures, cardiac outputs, and pulmonary vascular resistance index. On biopsy, the most common finding in the obese group was mild myocyte hypertrophy.

Importantly, the cardiac dysfunction associated with obesity may occur with weight loss (268). Cardiac studies were repeated in 12 Class 4 obese patients after a 54.8 ± 1.9-kg weight loss. Echocardiography documented a decrease in dilatation (27.3% to 9.1%) and a significant decrease in hypertrophy. After the weight loss, radionuclide and right-heart catheterization studies demonstrated improved cardiac function with reduced filling pressures and increased left ventricular work during fluid and exercise challenges. In addition, the prolonged QT interval seen in obese patients may shorten after weight reduction (269).

The Class 4 obese patient may present with significant noncardiovascular problems as well. The Pickwickian syndrome, involving sleep apnea, pituitary/gonadal dysfunction, acanthosis nigricans, and pronounced osteoarthritis, is well described (226). Weight loss achieved by consumption of a very-low-calorie diet improves lung volumes in morbidly obese patients but may not be enough to improve arterial oxygenation (270). In one study, hypoxemia was not relieved in patients who assumed a supine position but was significantly relieved when patients stood up, both before and after weight loss. Comorbidity seen with significant obesity includes respiratory disease, gout, osteoarthritis, and gallbladder disease (271). The presence of obesity more than doubles the risk for gallstones, because it increases the flux of cholesterol through the biliary tree. In fact, after 8 weeks of dieting, sludge was detected in three subjects and gallstones in 25.5% of subjects, compared with nonfasting control subjects (272). Depression commonly accompanies significant obesity. Individuals more likely to show symptoms of emotional illness include patients with a history of obesity from childhood, those undergoing severe caloric restriction, and those undergoing outpatient treatment (273).

CONCLUSIONS

What diet can cardiologists recommend at present? For those with coronary disease or who are greatly at risk for coronary disease, a healthy AHA diet is inadequate. A therapeutic diet that is nutritionally adequate and contains from 25% to 35% of calories as fat is recommended, but less than 7% of calories should come from saturated fat and intake of dietary cholesterol should be less than 200 mg per day. There should be at least five servings of fruits and vegetables daily, along with nonfat dairy products and salt restriction, if the patient is hypertensive. Whether the patient prefers an Asian regimen with more-complex carbohydrates or a Mediterranean-type regimen with more olive or canola oil is best decided on a case-by-case basis. Two servings of fatty fish per week should be recommended. For individuals who have experienced MI and cannot eat fish, consideration should be given to use of approximately 875 mg of omega-3 fatty acids as a fish oil capsule. Sugar calories are "empty" calories and should be eliminated from the diet. Because weight reduction is given high priority in the overweight heart patient, calories in excess of energy expenditure must be discouraged. An alcoholic drink with dinner is not prohibited, and moderate alcohol consumption may prove to be salutary. Nonetheless, as noted earlier, the negative effects seen in individuals who cannot limit alcohol consumption and in special circumstances (e.g., pregnancy) should make physicians wary about casual, global endorsement of alcoholic drinking to improve risk for CAD.

Although some patients may do well with highly restricted low-fat diets (as recommended by Ornish and Pritikin), there are no available data to show that this is the preferred nutritional choice for the patient with CAD. Nonetheless, these programs have taught us the value of a real commitment to a low-fat diet. As is seen even with drug therapy, individuals who adhere most consistently to a therapeutic regimen often get the best results (10). A possible danger of advising a very-low-fat regimen to patients who do not receive adequate instruction is the adoption of a dietary regimen that is too low in protein and too high in carbohydrates. If detailed individualized instruction is provided and there is a comprehensive approach to lifestyle changes, the dietary and lifestyle changes achieved can be impressive in the short term (302). Certainly, when noninvasive testing such as PET can monitor the efficacy of these regimens, the potential for improvement in coronary status can motivate patients considerably (301,303). Most often, surrogates such as improved risk factors (and possibly markers of subclinical disease) should provide the reassurance that patients often require to continue with these regimens. In addition, we need further studies of the Mediterranean-type diet used in the Lyon Trial (107). We need to understand whether the crucial intervention was the increase in omega-3 fatty acids, MUFAs, or both together with the low–saturated fat, low-cholesterol, low-fiber regimen that produced the striking results.

The growing weight of evidence suggests that lifestyle changes should be recommended to the coronary patient that encourage the avoidance of excess calories and promote regular exercise to reduce the likelihood of excessive weight gain. These are crucial supplements to dietary advice. Also helpful would be the presence of a registered dietitian to help the patient learn how to deal with external cues from the environment and to develop important skills such as label reading, wise restaurant menu selections, and recipe modification. This cannot be emphasized enough; individualized recommendations for lifestyle change and feedback are crucial to obtaining good results. Many excellent books on eating a healthier diet are available. Sources such as the AHA; the National Heart, Lung, and Blood Institute; and the American Dietetic Association should be consulted (by phone or through the Internet) to obtain help.

CONTROVERSIES AND PERSONAL PERSPECTIVES

Several major controversies need to be resolved. The first is whether we should adopt the Mediterranean diet pyramid (*e*Fig. 2.1.2) instead of our current pyramid for primary prevention of CAD. As noted in this chapter, there are aspects of the Mediterranean-type diet that are particularly helpful for certain patients. However, although the potential cardioprotective effects associated with a diet supplemented with omega-3 fatty acids and oleic acid are exciting to contemplate, their efficacy needs to be explored with more data from clinical trials.

Many physicians are under the false impression that basic nutrition principles do not work in clinical practice. Well-meaning but poorly reinforced suggestions about diet are certainly likely to fail. As noted in earlier sections of this chapter, failure is much less likely when individualized counseling and follow-up are provided. Results can occasionally be dramatic. In a recent small study involving healthy, motivated individuals that was designed to determine whether use of the Dietary Guidelines for Americans and the Food Guide Pyramid, combined with exercise training, could result in significant reductions in cardiovascular risk compared with a regimen of exercise therapy alone, subjects randomly assigned to the diet and exercise group fared better than those assigned to exercise alone (302). In the half of the group that received individualized dietary counseling using the Food Guide Pyramid as a primary educational tool, the percentage of energy intake from fat decreased from 39% to 23% (*e*Fig. 2.1.3). This was associated with significant reductions in BMI, total cholesterol levels, and LDL-C levels, whereas no change was observed in the group who used exercise alone.

Another controversial aspect of medical nutritional therapy is whether patients with CAD require a very-low-fat diet. Again, the data supporting this approach are inadequate at present because of the highly selected nature of the patients who have been involved in studies of the effect of

THE FUTURE

As we approach the year 2010, the United States is well on its way to attaining an even lower overall serum cholesterol level through improved diet. The ongoing change in health care delivery toward a system of managed care has the potential to improve the nutritional health of the population through innovative, low-cost nutritional programs. The ability to document improved outcomes associated with such endeavors is an important task that lies ahead. Finally, exciting advances in medical genetics hold the promise of more-targeted nutritional advice, not only for the general population, but particularly for those at high risk for heart disease.

such diets. Although these patients have been able to make the major lifestyle changes required for these regimens, it is not clear that this is feasible for the population at large. In fact, diets with less than 15% fat are not likely to have wide appeal. For those with CAD, a diet markedly restricted in saturated fats is still the primary approach and retains the appropriate focus. Well-motivated patients should be encouraged to learn the basics of a vegetarian lifestyle and supplement their diets with small amounts of lean meat, fish, and skinless fowl. The use of exercise as an adjunct to diet cannot be stressed enough. The best diets will invariably be the ones that promote loss of excessive weight while augmenting the use of drugs to lower LDL-C and TG levels and to raise subnormal levels of HDL-C.

An important controversy that appears to be resolving is whether it is better to have a diet supplemented with fish, vegetables, and fruits as a supply of antioxidants, or to load up on a handful of pills each morning that contain megadoses of minerals and vitamins. The adverse experience with beta-carotene and the lack of data confirming cardiovascular benefit from vitamin E supplementation in large-scale clinical trials should make all cardiologists more cautious about the supplements they recommend for their patients. Physicians should remember that, although tempting, recommendation of interesting but unproved nutritional supplements may not work to a patient's advantage.

A word of caution should be given about "fad diets" that are presented to cardiologists by their patients. Many diets have had glowing testimonials in the short term only to fall short of the mark in the long term. In addition, at the extremes of the life cycle, children and the elderly are likely to do poorly with dietary plans that may not have the proper nutritional balance for their age group. This can lead to unwanted nutritional deficiencies. Many patients look for endorsement because they feel the most important hurdle is getting started on weight loss. Actually, the most formidable hurdle is *maintaining* weight loss. As a general rule, diets that promise dramatic short-term weight loss fail to teach our patients the proper behaviors that are needed for long-term weight maintenance. Should it be surprising that so many regain lost weight and become even heavier?

A final controversy relates to the treatment of obesity. As the prevalence of obesity increases, its impact will be seen in cardiology practices. As noted earlier, the increase in insulin resistance with accompanying dyslipidemia, hypertension, and glucose intolerance (i.e., the metabolic syndrome) greatly increases coronary risk. The risk factors in turn magnify the negative effects of obesity on cardiac status. Moreover, for individuals with CAD, obesity limits or adversely affects the accuracy of diagnostic procedures. Although more vigorous attempts at adhering to dietary recommendations under the watchful eye of a registered dietitian are very useful, they have not proven as productive as might be wished. The current antiobesity drugs may be useful if 5% to 10% weight loss is required to improve risk-factor status. I do not recommend sibutramine in patients with CHD, because of its small but definite effects on blood pressure and heart rate. Further clinical trials of the newer generations of obesity drugs are needed to determine their proper place in both primary and secondary prevention of CAD. More widespread use of surgical techniques by qualified surgeons with appropriate multidisciplinary support may prove most helpful to severely obese patients. Given the high recidivism rate in weight-loss programs, the focus for the obese patient should be on learning new behaviors, such as dietary changes, exercise, and stress management. Increasing social support may be extremely helpful in this regard. Most important, the cardiologist should use every opportunity to endorse prevention of obesity through regular exercise and diet among individuals who are just beginning to increase their weight status as they age. Given the difficulty of successfully treating obesity, prevention of obesity should remain a high priority for public policy. Physicians should play a role as well and try to anticipate the expected weight gain from patients who stop smoking or start medications such as steroids, antidepressants, and antidiabetic drugs. These patients constitute a high-risk group to which heightened attention should be given.

REFERENCES

1. Kris-Etherton P, Daniels SR, Eckel RH, et al. Summary of the Scientific Conference on Dietary Fatty Acids and Cardiovascular Health. Conference summary from the Nutrition Committee of the American Heart Association. *Circulation* 2001;103:1034–1039.
2. Cobb MM, Teitelbaum HS, Breslow JL. Lovastatin efficacy in reducing low-density lipoprotein cholesterol levels on high- vs. low-fat diets. *JAMA* 1991;265:997–1001.
3. Hunninghake DB, Stein EA, Dujovne CA, et al. The efficacy of intensive dietary therapy alone or combined with lovastatin in outpatients with hypercholesterolemia. *N Engl J Med* 1993;328:1213–1219.
4. Grundy SM. Small LDL, atherogenic dyslipidemia, and the metabolic syndrome. *Circulation* 1997;95:1–4.
5. Hjermann I, Holme I, Leren P. Oslo Study Diet and Anti-Smoking Trial: results after 102 months. *Am J Med* 1986;80[Suppl 2A]:7–12.
6. Watts GF, Lewis B, Brunt JNH, et al. Effects of coronary artery disease of lipid lowering diet, or diet plus cholestyramine in the St. Thomas Atherosclerosis Regression Study (STARS). *Lancet* 1992;339:563–569.
7. Schuler G, Hambrecht R, Schlierf G, et al. Regular physical exercise and low-fat diet: effects of progression on coronary artery disease. *Circulation* 1992;86:1–11.
8. Burr ML, Fehily AM, Gilbert JF, et al. Effects of changes in fat, fish, and fibre intakes on death and myocardial reinfarction: Diet and Reinfarction Trial (DART). *Lancet* 1989;2:757–761.
9. Dietary supplementation with *n-3* polyunsaturated fatty acids and vitamin E after myocardial infarction: results of the GISSI-Prevenzione trial. GISSI-Prevenzione Investigators. *Lancet* 1999;354:447–455.
10. Ornish D, Brown SE, Scherwitz LW, et al. Can lifestyle changes reverse coronary heart disease? The Lifestyle Heart Trial. *Lancet* 1990;335:129–133.
11. Brousseau ME, Schaefer EJ. Diet and coronary heart disease: clinical trials. *Curr Atheroscler Rep* 2000;2:487–493.
12. Yusuf S, Anand S. Cost of prevention: the case of lipid lowering. *Circulation* 1996;93:1774–1776.
13. National Cholesterol Education Program. Report of the expert panel on population strategies for blood cholesterol reduction. Publication NIH 90–3046. Bethesda, MD: National Institutes of Health, US Department of Health and Human Services, 1990.
14. National Cholesterol Education Program Expert Panel. Summary of the second report of the National Cholesterol Education Program (NCEP) Expert Panel on detection, evaluation, and treatment of high blood cholesterol in adults (Adult Treatment Panel II). *JAMA* 1993;269:3015–3023.
15. Eckel RH. Obesity and heart disease: a statement for healthcare professionals from the Nutrition Committee, American Heart Association. Nutrition Committee, American Heart Association. *Circulation* 1997;96:3248–3250.
16. Krause RM, Eckel RH, Howard B, et al. Revision 2000: AHA dietary guidelines; a statement for healthcare professionals from the Nutrition Committee of the American Heart Association. *Circulation* 2000;102:2296–2311.
17. National Cholesterol Education Program. Adult Treatment Panel III. May 2001.
18. Appel LJ, Moore TJ, Obarzanek E, et al. A clinical trial of the effects of dietary patterns on blood pressure. DASH Collaborative Research Group. *N Engl J Med* 1997;336:1117–1124.
19. Denke MA. Cholesterol-lowering diets: a review of the evidence. *Arch Intern Med* 1995;155:17–26.
20. Denke MA, Grundy SM. Individual responses to a cholesterol-lowering diet in 50 men with moderate hypercholesterolemia. *Arch Intern Med* 1994;154:317–325.
21. Denke MA. Review of human studies evaluating individual dietary responsiveness in patients with hypercholesterolemia. *Am J Clin Nutr* 1995;62:471S–477S.
22. Hopkins PN, Williams RR, Kuida H, et al. Predictive value of a short dietary questionnaire for changes in serum lipids in high-risk Utah families. *Am J Clin Nutr* 1989;50:292–300.
23. Denke MA, Frantz ID Jr. Response to a cholesterol-lowering diet efficacy is greater in hypercholesterolemic subjects even after adjustment for regression to the mean. *Am J Med* 1993;94:626–631.
24. Denke MA, Sempos CT, Grundy SM. Excess body weight: an under-recognized contributor to dyslipidemia in white American women. *Arch Intern Med* 1994;154:401–410.
25. Denke MA, Sempos CT, Grundy SM. Excess body weight: an underrecognized contributor to high blood cholesterol levels in white American men. *Arch Intern Med* 1993;153:1093–1103.
26. Assouline L, Levy E, Feoli-Fonseca JC, et al. Familial hypercholesterolemia: molecular, biochemical, and clinical characterization of a French-Canadian pediatric population. *Pediatrics* 1995;96[2 Pt 1]:239–246.
27. Kesaniemi YA, Einholm C, Miettinen TA. Intestinal cholesterol absorption efficiency in man is related to apoprotein E phenotype. *J Clin Invest* 1987;80:578–581.
28. Lopez-Miranda J, Ordovas JM, Mata P, et al. Effect of apolipoprotein E phenotype on diet-induced lowering of plasma low density lipoprotein cholesterol. *J Lipid Res* 1994;35:1965–1975.
29. Cobb MM, Teitelbaum H, Risch N, et al. Influence of dietary fat, apolipoprotein E, phenotype and sex on plasma lipoprotein levels. *Circulation* 1992;86:849–857.
30. McCombs RJ, Marcadis DE, Ellis J, et al. Attenuated hypercholesterolemic response to a high cholesterol diet in subjects heterozygous for the apolipoprotein A-IV-2 allele. *N Engl J Med* 1994;331:706–710.
31. Mata P, Ordovas JM, Lopez-Miranda J, et al. ApoA-IV phenotype affects diet-induced plasma LDL cholesterol lowering. *Arterioscler Thromb* 1994;14:884–891.
32. Tikkanen MJ, Xu C-F, Hamalainen T, et al. XbaI polymorphism of the apolipoprotein B gene influences plasma lipid response to dietary intervention. *Clin Genet* 1990;37:327–334.
33. Lopez-Miranda J, Ordovas JM, Espino A, et al. Influence of mutation in human apolipoprotein A-1 gene promoter on plasma LDL cholesterol response to dietary fat. *Lancet* 1994;343:1246–1249.
34. Krauss RM, Dreon DM. Low-density-lipoprotein subclasses and response to a low-fat diet in healthy men. *Am J Clin Nutr* 1995;62:478S–487S.

35. Keys A, Anderson JT, Grande F. Prediction of serum-cholesterol responses of man to changes in fats in the diet. *Lancet* 1957;2:959–966.

36. Hegsted DM, McGandy RB, Myers ML, et al. Quantitative effects of dietary fat on serum cholesterol levels in man. *Am J Clin Nutr* 1995;17:281–295.

37. Cater NB, Denke MA. Behenic acid is a cholesterol-raising saturated fatty acid. *Am J Clin Nutr* 2001;73:41–44.

38. Woolett LA, Spady DK, Dietschy JM. Mechanisms by which saturated triacylglycerols elevate the plasma low density lipoprotein–cholesterol concentration in hamsters: differential effects of fatty acid chain length. *J Clin Invest* 1989;84:119–128.

39. McNamara DJ, Kolb R, Parker TS, et al. Heterogeneity of cholesterol homeostasis in man: response to changes in dietary fat quality and cholesterol quantity. *J Clin Invest* 1987;79:1729–1739.

40. Beynen AC, Katan MB, Van Zutphen LF. Dietary cholesterol and responsiveness hypo- and hyperresponders: individual differences in the response of serum cholesterol concentration to changes in diet. *Adv Lipid Res* 1987;22:115–171.

41. Ginsberg HN, Karmally W, Siddiqui M, et al. A dose-response study of the effects of dietary cholesterol on fasting and postprandial lipid and lipoprotein metabolism in healthy young men. *Arterioscler Thromb* 1994;14:576–586.

42. Ginsberg HN, Karmally W, Siddiqui M, et al. Increases in dietary cholesterol are associated with modest increases in both LDL and HDL cholesterol in healthy women. *Arterioscler Thromb Vasc Biol* 1995;15:169–178.

43. Lichtenstein AH, Ausman LM, Carrasco W, et al. Hydrogenation impairs the hypolipidemic effect of corn oil in humans: hydrogenation, *trans* fatty acids, and plasma lipids. *Arterioscler Thromb* 1993;13(2):154–161.

44. Fielding CJ, Havel RJ, Todd KM, et al. Effects of dietary cholesterol and fat saturation on plasma lipoproteins in an ethnically diverse population of healthy young men. *J Clin Invest* 1995;95:611–618.

45. Retzlaff BM, Walden CE, Dowdy AA, et al. Effects of two eggs per day versus placebo in moderately hypercholesterolemic and combined hyperlipidemic subjects consuming an NCEP Step One Diet. *Circulation* 1995;92:I-350.

46. Tippett KS, Cleveland LE. How current diets stack up: comparison with dietary guidelines. In: Frazao E, ed. *America's eating habits: changes and consequences* (Agricultural Information Bulletin no. 750). Washington, DC: US Department of Agriculture, Economic Research Service, Food and Rural Economics Division, 1999:51–70.

47. Shekelle RB, Shyrock AM, Paul O, et al. Diet, serum cholesterol, and death from coronary heart disease: the Western Electric Study. *N Engl J Med* 1981;304:65–70.

48. Stamler J, Shekelle R. Dietary cholesterol and human coronary heart disease. *Arch Pathol Lab Med* 1988;112:1032–1040.

49. Hu F, Stampfer MJ, Rimm EB, et al. A prospective study of egg consumption and risk of cardiovascular disease in men and women. *JAMA* 1999;281:1387–1394.

50. Law M. Plant sterol and stanol margarines in health. *BMJ* 2000;320:861–864.

51. Miettinen TA, Gylling H. Regulation of cholesterol metabolism by dietary plant sterols. *Curr Opin Lipidol* 1999;10(1):9–14.

52. Jones PJ, MacDougall DE, Ntanios F, et al. Dietary phytosterols as cholesterol-lowering agents in humans. *Can J Physiol Pharmacol* 1997;75(3):217–227.

53. Nguyen TT, Dale LC, von Bergmann K, et al. Cholesterol-lowering effect of stanol ester in a US population of mildly hypercholesterolemic men and women: a randomized controlled trial. *Mayo Clin Proc* 1999;74:1198–1206.

54. Lichtenstein AH, Deckelbaum RJ. Stanol/sterol ester-containing foods and blood cholesterol levels: a statement for healthcare professionals from the Nutrition Committee of the Council on Nutrition, Physical Activity and Metabolism of the American Heart Association. American Heart Association Nutrition Committee. *Circulation* 2001;103:1177–1179.

55. Hallikainen MA, Sarkkinen ES, Gylling H, et al. Comparison of the effects of plant sterol ester and plant stanol ester–enriched margarines in lowering serum cholesterol concentrations in hypercholesterolaemic subjects on a low-fat diet. *Eur J Clin Nutr* 2000;54:715–725.

56. Miettinen TA, Strandberg TE, Gylling H. Noncholesterol sterols and cholesterol lowering by long-term simvastatin treatment in coronary patients: relation to basal serum cholestanol. *Arterioscler Thromb Vasc Biol* 2000;20:1340–1346.

57. Sacks FM, Ornish D, Rosner B, et al. Plasma lipoprotein levels in vegetarians: the effect of ingestion of fats from dairy products. *JAMA* 1985;254:1337–1341.

58. Jousilahti P, Vartianen E, Tuomilehto J, et al. Twenty-year dynamics of serum cholesterol levels in the middle-aged population of eastern Finland. *Ann Intern Med* 1996;125:713–722.

59. Ginsberg HN, Kris-Etherton P, Dennis B. Effects of reducing dietary saturated fatty acids on plasma lipids and lipoproteins in healthy subjects: The Delta Study, Protocol 1. DELTA Research Group. *Arterioscler Thromb Vasc Biol* 1998;18:441–449.

60. Denke MA, Grundy SM. Comparison of effects of lauric acid and palmitic acid on plasma lipids and lipoprotein. *Am J Clin Nutr* 1992;56:895–898.

61. Temme EHM, Mensink RP, Hornstra G. Comparison of the effects of diets enriched in lauric, palmitic, or oleic acids on serum lipids and lipoproteins in healthy women and men. *Am J Clin Nutr* 1996;63:897–903.

62. Grundy SM. Influence of stearic acid on cholesterol metabolism relative to other long-chain fatty acids. *Am J Clin Nutr* 1994;60[Suppl 6]:986S–990S.

63. Zock P, de Vries J, Katam M. Impact of myrisitic acid versus palmitic acid on serum lipid and lipoprotein levels in healthy women and men. *Arterioscler Thromb* 1994;14:567–575.

64. Lichtenstein AH, Ausman LM, Carrasco W, et al. Hypercholesterolemic effect of dietary cholesterol in diets enriched in polyunsaturated and saturated fat: dietary cholesterol, fat saturation, and plasma lipids. *Arterioscler Thromb* 1994;14:168–175.

65. Keys A. *Seven countries: a multivariate analysis of death and coronary heart disease.* Cambridge, MA: Harvard University Press, 1980.

66. Kato H, Tillotson J, Nichaman MZ, et al. Epidemiologic studies of coronary heart disease and stroke in Japanese men living in Japan, Hawaii and California. *Am J Epidemiol* 1973;97:372–385.

67. Robertson TI, Kato H, Rhoads GG, et al. Epidemiology studies of coronary heart disease and stroke in Japanese men living in Japan, Hawaii, and California. *Am J Cardiol* 1977;39:239–243.

68. Criqui MH, Ringel BL. Does diet or alcohol explain the French paradox? *Lancet* 1994;344:1719–1723.

69. Artaud-Wild SM, Connor SL, Sexton G, et al. Differences in coronary mortality can be explained by differences in cholesterol and saturated fat intakes in 40 countries but not in France and England: a paradox. *Circulation* 1993;88:2771–2779.

70. Law M, Wald N. Why heart disease mortality is low in France: the time lag explanation. *BMJ* 1999;318:1471–1480.

71. Holme I. An analysis of randomized trials evaluating the effect of cholesterol reduction on total mortality and coronary heart disease incidence. *Circulation* 1990;82:1916–1924.

72. Frantz ID, Dawson EA, Ashman PL, et al. Test of effect of lipid lowering by diet on cardiovascular risk: The Minnesota Coronary Survey. *Arteriosclerosis* 1989;9:129–135.

73. Hjermann I, Holme I, Velve Byre K, et al. Effect of diet and smoking intervention on the incidence of coronary heart disease. *Lancet* 1981;2:1303–1310.

74. Dayton S, Pearce ML, Hashimoto S, et al. A controlled clinical trial of a diet high in unsaturated fat in preventing complications of atherosclerosis. *Circulation* 1969;39–40[Suppl 20]:1–63.

75. Turpeinen O, Karvonen MJ, Pekkarinen M, et al. Dietary prevention of heart disease: The Finnish Mental Hospital Study. *Int J Epidemiol* 1979;8:99–118.

76. Multifactorial trial in the prevention of coronary heart disease. III. Incidence and mortality results. World Health Organization Collaborative Group. *Eur Heart J* 1983;4:141–147.

77. Wilhelmsen L, Berglund G, Elmfeldt D, et al. The Multifactor Primary Prevention Trial in Goteborg, Sweden. *Eur Heart J* 1986;7:279–288.

78. Multiple Risk Factor Intervention Trial: risk factor changes and mortality results. Multiple Risk Factor Intervention Trial Research Group. *JAMA* 1982;248:1465–1477.

79. Niebauer J, Hambrecht R, Velich T, et al. Predictive value of lipid profile for salutary coronary angiographic changes in patients on a low-fat diet and physical exercise program. *Am J Cardiol* 1996;78:163–167.

80. Watts GF, Jackson P, Mandalia S, et al. Nutrient intake and progression of coronary artery disease. *Am J Cardiol* 1994;73:328–332.

81. Mensink RP, Katan MB. Effect of dietary *trans* fatty acids on high-density and low-density lipoprotein cholesterol levels in healthy subjects. *N Engl J Med* 1990;323:439–445.

82. Zock PL, Katan MB. Hydrogenation alternatives: effects of *trans* fatty acids and stearic acid v linoleic acid on serum lipids and lipoproteins in humans. *J Lipid Res* 1992;33:399–410.

83. Judd JT, Clevidence BA, Muesing RA, et al. Dietary *trans* fatty acids: effects on plasma lipids and lipoproteins of healthy men and women. *Am J Clin Nutr* 1994;59:861–886.

84. Mensink RP, Zock PL, Katan MB, et al. Effect of dietary *cis* and *trans* fatty acids on serum lipoprotein(a) levels in humans. *J Lipid Res* 1992;33:1493–1501.

85. Lichtenstein AH, Ausman LM, Carrasco W, et al. Hydrogenation impairs the hypolipidemic effect of corn oil in humans: hydrogenation, *trans* fatty acids, and plasma lipids. *Arterioscler Thromb* 1993;13:154–161.

86. *Trans fatty acids, plasma lipids and cardiovascular disease risk.* Institute of Shortening and Edible Oils. March 1994:28.

87. van Tol A, Zock PL, van Gent T, et al. Dietary *trans* fatty acids increase serum cholesteryl ester transfer protein activity in man. *Atherosclerosis* 1995;115:129–134.

88. Willett WC, Stampfer MJ, Manson JE, et al. Intake of *trans* fatty acids and risk of coronary heart disease among women. *Lancet* 1993;341:581–585.

89. Lichtenstein AH. *Trans* fatty acids and cardiovascular disease risk. *Curr Opin Lipidol* 2000;11(1):37–42.

90. Gardner CD, Kraemer HC. Monounsaturated versus polyunsaturated dietary fat and serum lipids: a meta-analysis. *Arterioscler Thromb Vasc Biol* 1995;15:1917–1927.

91. Meydani SN, Lichtenstein AH, White PJ, et al. Food use and health effects of soybean and sunflower oils. *J Am Coll Nutr* 1991;10:406–428.

92. Kestin M, Clifton P, Belling GB, et al. n-3 Fatty acids of marine origin lower systolic blood pressure and triglycerides but raise LDL cholesterol compared with n-3 and n-6 fatty acids from plants. *Am J Clin Nutr* 1990;51:1028–1034.

93. Sturdevant RAL, Pearce ML, Dayton S. Increased prevalence of cholelithiasis in men ingesting a serum cholesterol lowering diet. *N Engl J Med* 1973;288:24–27.

94. Dolecek TA. Epidemiological evidence of relationships between dietary polyunsaturated fatty acids and mortality in the multiple risk factor intervention trial. *Proc Soc Exp Biol Med* 1992;200:177–182.

95. Kris-Etherton P. Monounsaturated fats and the risk of cardiovascular disease. *Circulation* 1999;100:1253–1258.

96. Berry EM, Eisenberg S, Friedlander Y, et al. Effects of diets rich in monounsaturated fatty acids on plasma lipoproteins: the Jerusalem Nutrition Study. II. Monounsaturated fatty acids vs. carbohydrates. *Am J Clin Nutr* 1992;56:394–403.

97. Reaven P, Parthasarathy S, Grasse BJ, et al. Effects of oleate-rich and linoleate-rich diets on the susceptibility of low density lipoprotein to oxidative modification in mildly hypercholesterolemic subjects. *J Clin Invest* 1993;91:668–676.

98. Parthasarathy S, Khoo JC, Miller E, et al. Low-density lipoprotein enriched in oleic acid is protected against oxidative modification: implications for dietary prevention of atherosclerosis. *Proc Natl Acad Sci U S A* 1990;87:3894–3898.

99. Reaven PD, Grasse BJ, Tribble DL. Effects of linoleate-enriched and oleate-enriched diets in combination with alpha-tocopherol on the susceptibility of LDL and LDL subfractions to oxidative modification in humans. *Arterioscler Thromb* 1994;14:557–566.

100. Grundy SM. Comparison of monounsaturated fatty acids and carbohydrates for lowering plasma cholesterol. *N Engl J Med* 1986;3143:745–748.

101. Mensink RP, Katan MB. Effect of monounsaturated fatty acids versus complex carbohydrates on high density lipoproteins in healthy men and women. *Lancet* 1987;1:125–129.

102. Ginsberg HN, Barr SL, Gilbert A, et al. Reduction of plasma cholesterol levels in normal men on an American Heart Association Step I diet or a Step I diet with added monounsaturated fat. *N Engl J Med* 1990;322:574–579.

103. Kris-Etherton P, Pearson TA, Wan Y, et al. High-monoun-saturated fatty acid diets lower both cholesterol and triacyl-glycerol concentrations. *Am J Clin Nutr* 1999;70:1009–1015.

104. Willett WC, Sacks F, Trichopoulou A, et al. Mediterranean diet pyramid: a cultural model for healthy eating. *Am J Clin Nutr* 1995;61[Suppl]:1402S–1406S.

105. O'Brien P. Dietary shifts and implications for US agriculture. *Am J Clin Nutr* 1995;61[Suppl 6]:1390S–1396S.

106. Garg A, Grundy SM, Koffler M. Effect of high carbohydrate intake on hyperglycemia, islet function, and plasma lipoproteins in NIDDM. *Diabetes Care* 1992;15:1572–1580.

107. de Lorgeril M, Renaud S, Marnelle N, et al. Mediterranean alpha-linolenic acid rich diet in secondary prevention of coronary heart disease. *Lancet* 1994;343:1454–1459.

108. de Lorgeril M. Mediterranean diet, traditional risk factors, and the rate of cardiovascular complications after myocardial infarction: final report of the Lyon Diet Heart Study. *Circulation* 1999;99:779–785.

109. Ullmann D, Connor WE, Hatcher LF, et al. Will a high-carbohydrate, low-fat diet lower plasma lipids and lipoproteins without producing hypertriglyceridemia? *Arterioscler Thromb* 1991;11:1059–1067.

110. Barnard RJ. Effects of life-style modification on serum lipids. *Arch Intern Med* 1991;151:1389–1394.

111. Grundy S. Critique of short-term lifestyle change. *Arch Intern Med* 1991;151:1275–1276.

112. Lichtenstein AH, Ausman LM, Carrasco W, et al. Short-term consumption of a low-fat diet beneficially affects plasma lipid concentrations only when accompanied by weight loss: hypercholesterolemia, low-fat diet, and plasma lipids. *Arterioscler Thromb* 1994;14:1751–1760.

113. Yu-Poth S, Zhao G, Etherton T, et al. Effects of the National Cholesterol Education Program's Step I and Step II dietary intervention programs on cardiovascular disease risk factors: a meta-analysis. *Am J Clin Nutr* 1999;69:632–646.

114. Arntzenius AC, Kromhout D, Barth JD, et al. Diet, lipoproteins, and the progression of coronary atherosclerosis. The Leiden Intervention Trial. *N Engl J Med* 1985;312:805–811.

115. Blankenhorn DH, Johnson RL, Mack WJ, et al. The influence of diet on the appearance of new lesions in the human coronary arteries. *JAMA* 1990;263:1646–1652.

116. Gould KL, Ornish D, Kirkeeide R, et al. Improved stenosis geometry by quantitative coronary arteriography after vigorous risk factor modification. *Am J Cardiol* 1992;69:845–853.

117. Gould KL, Ornish D, Scherwitz L, et al. Changes in myocardial perfusion abnormalities by positron emission tomography after long-term, intense risk factor modification. *JAMA* 1995;274:894–901.

118. Singh RB, Rastogi SS, Verma R, et al. Randomized controlled trial of cardioprotective diet in patients with recent myocardial infarction: results of one year followup. *BMJ* 1992;304:1015–1019.

119. Quinn TG, Alderman EL, McMillan A, et al. Development of new coronary atherosclerotic lesions during a 4-year multifactor risk reduction program: The Stanford Risk Intervention Project (SCRIP). SCRIP Investigators. *J Am Coll Cardiol* 1994;24:900–908.

120. Gould KL, Martucci JP, Goldberg DI, et al. Short-term cholesterol lowering decreases size and severity of perfusion abnormalities by positron emission tomography after dipyridamole inpatients with coronary artery disease: a potential noninvasive marker of healing coronary endothelium. *Circulation* 1994;89:1530–1538.

121. Harrison DG, Ohara Y. Physiologic consequences of increased vascular oxidant stresses in hypercholesterolemia and atherosclerosis: implications for impaired vasomotion. *Am J Cardiol* 1995;75:75B–81B.

122. Harrison DG, Armstrong ML, Freiman PC, et al. Restoration of endothelium-dependent relation by dietary treatment of atherosclerosis. *J Clin Invest* 1987;80:1808–1811.

123. Ohara Y, Peterson TE, Sayegh HS, et al. Dietary correction of hypercholesterolemia in the rabbit normalizes endothelial superoxide anion production. *Circulation* 1995;92:898–903.

124. Leung WH, Lau CP, Wong CK. Beneficial effect of cholesterol-lowering therapy on coronary endothelium-dependent relaxation in hypercholesterolemic patients. *Lancet* 1993;341:1496–1500.

125. Treasure CB, Klein JL, Weintraub WS, et al. Beneficial effects of cholesterol-lowering therapy on the coronary endothelium in patients with coronary artery disease. *N Engl J Med* 1995;332:481–487.

126. Anderson TJ, Meredith IT, Yeung AC, et al. The effect of cholesterol-lowering and antioxidant therapy on endothelium-dependent coronary vasomotion. *N Engl J Med* 1995;332:488–493.

127. Van Horn L. Fiber, lipids, and coronary heart disease. Nutrition Committee. *Circulation* 1997;95:2701–2704.

128. Lia A, Hallmans G, Sandberg AS, et al. Oat beta-glucan increases bile acid excretion and a fiber-rich barley fraction increases cholesterol excretion in ileostomy subjects. *Am J Clin Nutr* 1995;62:1245–1251.

129. Jenkins DJ, Axelsen M, Kendall CW, et al. Dietary fibre, lente carbohydrates and insulin-resistant diseases. *Br J Nutr* 2000;83[Suppl 1]:S157–S163.

130. Ripsin CM, Keenan JM, Jacobs DR, et al. Oat products and lipid lowering: a meta-analysis. *JAMA* 1992;267:3317–3325.

131. Jenkins DJ, Kendall CW, Vuksan V. Viscous fibers, health claims, and strategies to reduce cardiovascular disease risk. *Am J Clin Nutr* 2000;71:401–402.

132. Davidson MH, Dugan LD, Burns JH, et al. A psyllium-enriched cereal for the treatment of hypercholesterolemia in children: a controlled, double-blind, crossover study. *Am J Clin Nutr* 1996;63:96–102.

133. Sprecher DL, Harris BV, Goldberg AC, et al. Efficacy of psyllium in reducing serum cholesterol levels in hypercholesterolemic patients on high- or low-fat diets. *Ann Intern Med* 1993;119:545–554.

134. Jenkins DJA, Wolever TMS, Venketeshwer R, et al. Effect of blood lipids on very high intakes of fiber in diets low in saturated fat and cholesterol. *N Engl J Med* 1993;329:21–26.

135. Hunninghake DB, Miller VT, LaRosa JC, et al. Long-term treatment of hypercholesterolemia with dietary fiber. *Am J Med* 1994;97:501–503.

136. Khaw KT, Barrett-Connor E. Dietary fiber and reduced ischemic heart disease mortality rates in men and women: a

12-year prospective study. *Am J Epidemiol* 1987;126:1093–1102.

137. Rimm EB, Ascherio A, Giovannucci E, et al. Vegetable, fruit, and cereal fiber intake and risk of coronary heart disease among men. *JAMA* 1996;275:447–451.

138. Gillman MW, Cupples LA, Gagnon D, et al. Protective effect of fruits and vegetables on development of stroke in men. *JAMA* 1995;273:1113–1117.

139. Erdman JW. Control of serum lipids with soy protein. *N Engl J Med* 1995;333:313–315.

140. Potter SM, Potter SM. Soy protein and serum lipids. *Curr Opin Lipidol* 1996;7:260–264.

141. Lichtenstein AH. Soy protein, isoflavones and cardiovascular disease risk. *J Nutr* 1998;128:1589–1592.

142. Crouse JR, Morgan T, Terry JG, et al. A randomized trial comparing the effect of casein with that of soy protein containing varying amounts of isoflavones on plasma concentrations of lipids and lipoproteins. *Arch Intern Med* 1999;159:2070–2076.

143. Jenkins DJ, Kendall CW, Vidgen E, et al. Effect of soy-based breakfast cereal on blood lipids and oxidized low-density lipoprotein. *Metabolism* 2000;49:1496–1500.

144. Anderson JW, Johnstone BM, Cook-Newell ME. Meta-analysis of the effects of soy protein intake on serum lipids. *N Engl J Med* 1995;333:276–282.

145. de Roos B, Caslake MJ, Stalenhoef AFH, et al. The coffee diterpene cafestol increased plasma triacylglycerol by increasing the production rate of large VLDL apolipoprotein in healthy normolipidemic subjects. *Am J Clin Nutr* 2001;73:45–52.

146. Post SM, de Roos B, Vermeulen M, et al. Cafestol increases serum cholesterol in apolipoprotein E*3 Leiden transgenic mice by suppression of bile acid synthesis. *Arterioscler Thromb Vasc Biol* 2000;20;1551–1556.

147. Superko HR, Bortz W, Williams PT, et al. Caffeinated and decaffeinated coffee effects on plasma lipoprotein cholesterol, apolipoproteins, and lipase activity: a controlled, randomized trial. *Am J Clin Nutr* 1991;54:599–605.

148. Wahrburg U, Martin H, Schulte H, et al. Effects of two kinds of decaffeinated coffee on serum lipid profiles in healthy young adults. *Eur J Clin Nutr* 1994;48:172–179.

149. Fried RE, Levine DM, Kwiterovich PO, et al. The effect of filtered-coffee consumption on plasma lipid levels. *JAMA* 1992;267:811–815.

150. Grobbee DE, Rimm EB, Giovannucci E, et al. Coffee, caffeine, and cardiovascular disease in men. *N Engl J Med* 1990;323:1026–1032.

151. Willett W, Stampfer MJ, Manson JE, et al. Coffee consumption and coronary heart disease in women: a ten-year followup. *JAMA* 1996;275:458–462.

152. LaCroix AZ, Mead LA, Liang KY, et al. Coffee consumption and the incidence of coronary heart disease. *N Engl J Med* 1986;315:377–382.

153. Warshafsky S, Kamer RS, Sivak SL. Effect of garlic on total serum cholesterol: a meta-analysis. *Ann Intern Med* 1993;119[7 Pt 1]:599–605.

154. Isaacsohn JL, Moser M, Stein EA, et al. Garlic powder and plasma lipids and lipoproteins: a multicenter, randomized, placebo-controlled trial. *Arch Intern Med* 1998;158:1189–1194.

155. Superko HR, Krauss RM. Garlic powder, effect on plasma lipids, postprandial lipemia, low density lipoprotein particle size, high-density lipoprotein subclass distribution and lipoprotein(a). *J Am Coll Cardiol* 2000;35(2):321–326.

156. Knuiman JT, West CE, Katan MB, et al. Total cholesterol and high density lipoprotein cholesterol levels in populations differing in fat and carbohydrate intake. *Arteriosclerosis* 1987;7:612–619.

157. Leenen R, van der Kooy K, Meyboom S, et al. Relative effects of weight loss and dietary fat modification on serum lipid levels in the dietary treatment of obesity. *J Lipid Res* 1993;34:2183–2191.

158. Dattilo AM, Kris-Etherton PM. Effects of weight reduction on blood lipids and lipoproteins: a meta-analysis. *Am J Clin Nutr* 1992;56:320–328.

159. Brinton EA, Eisenberg S, Breslow JL. A low-fat diet decreases high density lipoprotein (HDL) cholesterol levels by decreasing HDL apolipoprotein transport rates. *J Clin Invest* 1990;85:1.

160. Schaefer EJ, Lamon-Fava S, Ordovas JM, et al. Factors associated with low and elevated plasma high density lipoprotein cholesterol and apolipoprotein A-I levels in the Framingham Offspring Study. *J Lipid Res* 1994;35:871–882.

161. Walsh BW, Sacks FM. Effects of low dose oral contraceptives on very low density and low density lipoprotein metabolism. *J Clin Invest* 1993;91:2126–2132.

162. Rimm EB, Williams P, Fosher K, et al. Moderate alcohol intake and lower risk of coronary heart disease: meta-analysis of effects on lipids and haemostatic factors. *BMJ* 1999;319:1523–1528.

163. Chait A, Mancini M, February AW, et al. Clinical and metabolic study of alcoholic hyperlipidaemia. *Lancet* 1972;2:62–64.

164. Hartung GH, Lawrence SJ, Reeves RS, et al. Effect of alcohol and exercise on postprandial lipemia and triglyceride clearance in men. *Atherosclerosis* 1993;100:33–40.

165. Doll R, Peto R, Hall E, et al. Mortality in relation to consumption of alcohol: 13 years observations on male British doctors. *BMJ* 1994;309:911–918.

166. Hines LM, Stampfer MJ, Ma J, et al. Genetic variation in alcohol dehydrogenase and the beneficial effect of moderate alcohol consumption on myocardial infarction. *N Engl J Med* 2001;344:549–555.

167. Langer RD, Criqui MH, Reed DM. Lipoproteins and blood pressure as biological pathways for effect of moderate alcohol consumption on coronary heart disease. *Circulation* 1992;85:910–915.

168. Renaud S, de Lorgeril M. Wine, alcohol, platelets, and the French paradox for coronary heart disease. *Lancet* 1992;339:1523–1526.

169. Ridker PM, Vaughan DE, Stampfer MJ, et al. Association of moderate alcohol consumption and plasma concentration of endogenous tissue-type plasminogen activator. *JAMA* 1994;272:929–933.

170. Rimm EB, Klatsky A, Grobbee D, et al. Review of moderate alcohol consumption and reduced risk of coronary heart disease: is the effect due to beer, wine, or spirits? *BMJ* 1996;312:731–736.

171. de Rijke YB, Demacker PMN, Assen NA, et al. Red wine

consumption does not affect oxidizability of low-density lipoproteins in volunteers. *Am J Clin Nutr* 1996;63:329–334.

172. Cutler JA, Kuller LH. Alcohol use and mortality from coronary heart disease: the role of high-density lipoprotein cholesterol. The Multiple Risk Factor Intervention Trial Research Group. *Ann Intern Med* 1992;116:881–887.

173. Jackson R, Beaglehole R. Alcohol consumption guidelines: relative safety vs. absolute risks and benefits. *Lancet* 1995;346:716.

174. Anda RF, Williamson DF, Remington PL. Alcohol and fatal injuries among US adults: findings from the NHANES I Epidemiologic Follow-up Study. *JAMA* 1988;260:2529–2532.

175. Manolio TA, Levy D, Garrison RJ, et al. Relation of alcohol intake to left ventricular mass: The Framingham Study. *J Am Coll Cardiol* 1991;17:717–721.

176. Garg R, Wagener DK, Madans JH. Alcohol consumption and risk of ischemic heart disease in women. *Arch Intern Med* 1993;153:1211–1216.

177. Urbano-Marquez A, Estruch R, Fernandez-Sola J, et al. The greater risk of alcoholic cardiomyopathy and myopathy in women compared with men. *JAMA* 1995;274:149–154.

178. Connor WE, DeFrancesco CA, Connor SL. n-3 Fatty acids from fish oil: effects on plasma lipoproteins and hypertriglyceridemic patients. *Ann N Y Acad Sci* 1993;683:16–34.

179. Dyerberg J, Bang HO, Stoffersen E, et al. Eicosapentaenoic acid and prevention of thrombosis and atherosclerosis. *Lancet* 1978;2:117–119.

180. Zambon S, Friday KE, Childs MT, et al. Effect of glyburide and omega 3 fatty acid dietary supplements on glucose and lipid metabolism in patients with non–insulin-dependent diabetes mellitus. *Am J Clin Nutr* 1992;56:447–454.

181. Connor WE, Prince MJ, Ullman D, et al. The hypotriglyceridemic effect of fish oil in adult-onset diabetes without adverse glucose control. *Ann N Y Acad Sci* 1993;683:337–440.

182. Westerveld HT, de Graaf JC, van Breugel HH, et al. Effects of low-dose EPA-E on glycemic control, lipid profile, lipoprotein(a), platelet aggregation, viscosity, and platelet and vessel wall interaction in NIDDM. *Diabetes Care* 1993;16:683–688.

183. Meydani SN, Lichtenstein AH, Cornwall S, et al. Immunologic effects of a National Cholesterol Education Panel Step-2 diet with and without fish-derived n-3 fatty acid enrichment. *J Clin Invest* 1993;92:105–113.

184. Dyerberg J, Bang HO. Haemostatic function and platelet polyunsaturated fatty acids in Eskimos. *Lancet* 1979;2:433–435.

185. Kromhout D, Bosschieter EB, de Lezenne-Coulander C. The inverse relation between fish consumption and 20-year coronary mortality from coronary heart disease. *N Engl J Med* 1985;312:1205–1209.

186. Shekelle RB, Missell L, Paul O, et al. Fish consumption and mortality from coronary heart disease. *N Engl J Med* 1985;313:820.

187. Dolecek TA, Grandits G. Dietary polyunsaturated fatty acids and mortality in the multiple risk factor intervention trial (MRFIT). *World Rev Nutr Diet* 1991;66:205–216.

188. Kromhout D, Feskens EJM, Bowles CH. The protective effect of a small amount of fish on coronary heart disease

189. Vollset SE, Heuch I, Bjelke E. Fish consumption and mortality from coronary heart disease. *N Engl J Med* 1985;313:820–821.

190. Curb JD, Reed DM. Fish consumption and mortality from coronary heart disease. *N Engl J Med* 1985;313:821–822.

191. Ascherio A, Rimm EB, Stampfer MJ, et al. Dietary intake of marine n-3 fatty acids, fish intake and the risk of coronary heart disease among men. *N Engl J Med* 1995;332:977–982.

192. Guallar E, Hennekens CH, Sacks FM, et al. A prospective study of plasma fish oil levels and incidence of myocardial infarction in US male physicians. *J Am Coll Cardiol* 1995;25:387–394.

193. Leaf A, Jorgensen MB, Jacobs AK, et al. Do fish oils prevent restenosis after coronary angioplasty? *Circulation* 1994;90:2248–2257.

194. Sacks FM, Stone PH, Gibson CM, et al. Controlled trial of fish oil for regression of human coronary atherosclerosis. HARP Research Group. *J Am Coll Cardiol* 1995;25:1492–1498.

195. de Lorgeril M, Salen P, Martin JL, et al. Effect of a Mediterranean type of diet on the rate of cardiovascular complications in patients with coronary artery disease: insights into the cardioprotective effect of certain nutrients. *J Am Coll Cardiol* 1996;28:1103–1108.

196. Ascherio A, Rimm EB, Giovannucci EL, et al. Dietary fat and risk of coronary heart disease in men: cohort followup study in the United States. *BMJ* 1996;313:84–90.

197. Siscovick DS, Raghunathan TE, King I, et al. Dietary intake and cell membrane levels of long-chain n-3 polyunsaturated fatty acids and the risk of primary cardiac arrest. *JAMA* 1995;274:1363–1367.

198. Billman GE, Hallaq H, Leaf A. Prevention of ischemia-induced ventricular fibrillation by n-3 fatty acids. *Proc Natl Acad Sci U S A* 1994;91:4427–4430.

199. Rissanen T, Voutilainen S, Nyyssönen K, et al. Fish oil–derived fatty acids, docosahexaenoic acid and docosapentaenoic acid, and the risk of acute coronary events: The Kuopio Ischaemic Heart Disease Risk Factor Study. *Circulation* 2000;102:2677.

200. Stone NJ. The Gruppo Italiano per lo Studio della Sopravvivenza nell'Infarto Miocardio (GISSI)–Prevenzione Trial on fish oil and vitamin E supplementation in myocardial infarction survivors. *Curr Cardiol Rep* 2000;2:445–451.

201. Steinberg D, Parthasarathy S, Carew TE, et al. Beyond cholesterol: modifications of low-density lipoprotein that increase its atherogenicity. *N Engl J Med* 1989;320:915–924.

202. Princen HMG, van Poppel G, Vogelzang C, et al. Supplementation with vitamin E but not beta carotene *in vivo* protects low density lipoprotein from lipid peroxidation *in vitro*. *Arterioscler Thromb* 1992;12:554–562.

203. Levine GN, Frei B, Koulouris SN, et al. Ascorbic acid reverses endothelial vasomotor dysfunction in patients with coronary artery disease. *Circulation* 1996;93:1107–1113.

204. Regnstrom J, Nilsson J, Moldeus P, et al. Inverse relation between the concentration of low-density-lipoprotein vitamin E and severity of coronary artery disease. *Am J Clin Nutr* 1996;63:377–385.

mortality in an elderly population. *Int J Epidemiol* 1995;24:340–345.

205. Rimm EB, Stampfer MJ, Ascherio A, et al. Vitamin E consumption and the risk of coronary heart disease in men. *N Engl J Med* 1993;328:1450–1456.

206. Stampfer MJ, Hennekens CH, Manson JE, et al. Vitamin E consumption and the risk of coronary disease in women. *N Engl J Med* 1993;328:1444–1449.

207. Kushi LH, Folsom AR, Prineas RJ, et al. Dietary antioxidant vitamins and death from coronary heart disease in postmenopausal women. *N Engl J Med* 1996;334:1156–1162.

208. Stephans NG, Parsons A, Schofield PM, et al. Randomized controlled trial of vitamin E in patients with coronary disease: Cambridge Heart Antioxidant Study (CHAOS). *Lancet* 1996;347:781–786.

209. Yusuf S, Dagenais G, Pogue J, et al. Vitamin E supplementation and cardiovascular events in high-risk patients. The Heart Outcomes Prevention Evaluation Study Investigators. *N Engl J Med* 2000;342(3):154–160.

210. Lonn EM, Yusuf S, Dzavik V, et al. Effects of ramipril and vitamin E on atherosclerosis: the Study to Evaluate Carotid Ultrasound Changes in Patients Treated with Ramipril and Vitamin E (SECURE). SECURE Investigators. *Circulation* 2001;103;919–925.

211. Khaw K-T, Bingham S, Welch A, et al. Relation between plasma ascorbic acid and mortality in men and women in EPIC–Norfolk Prospective Study: a prospective population study. *Lancet* 2001;357:657–663.

212. Kritchevsky SB, Shimakawa T, Tell GS, et al. Dietary antioxidants and carotid artery wall thickness: The ARIC Study. Atherosclerosis Risk in Communities Study. *Circulation* 1995;92:2142–2150.

213. Salonen JT, Nyyssonen K, Salonen R, et al. Antioxidant Supplementation in Atherosclerosis Prevention (ASAP) study: a randomized trial of the effect of vitamins E and C on 3-year progression of carotid atherosclerosis. *J Intern Med* 2000;248:377–386.

214. Kardinaal AF, Kok FJ, Ringstad J, et al. Antioxidants in adipose tissue and risk of myocardial infarction: The EURAMIC Study. *Lancet* 1993;342:1379–1384.

215. Hennekens CH, Buring JE, Manson JE, et al. Lack of effect of long-term supplementation with beta carotene on the incidence of malignant neoplasms and cardiovascular disease. *N Engl J Med* 1996;334:1145–1149.

216. Omenn GS, Goodman GE, Thornquist MD, et al. Effects of a combination of beta carotene and vitamin A on lung cancer and cardiovascular disease. *N Engl J Med* 1996;334:1150–1155.

217. The effect of vitamin E and beta carotene on the incidence of lung cancer and other cancers in male smokers. Alpha Tocopherol, Beta Carotene Prevention Study Group. *N Engl J Med* 1994;330:1029–1035.

218. Hertog MG, Hollman PC, Katan MB, et al. Intake of potentially anticarcinogenic flavonoids and their determinants in adults in the Netherlands. *Nutr Cancer* 1993;20:21–29.

219. Hertog MG, Feskens EJ, Hollman PC, et al. Dietary antioxidant flavonoids and risk of coronary heart disease: the Zutphen Elderly Study. *Lancet* 1993;342:1007–1011.

220. Hertog MG, Kromhout D, Aravanis C, et al. Flavonoid intake and long-term risk of coronary heart disease and cancer in the Seven Countries Study. *Arch Intern Med* 1995;155:381–386.

221. Sullivan JL. Iron and the sex difference in heart disease. *Lancet* 1981;1:1293–1294.

222. Meyers DG. The iron hypothesis: does iron cause atherosclerosis? *Clin Cardiol* 1996;19:925–929.

223. Zacharski LR, Chow B, Lavori PW, et al. The Iron (Fe) and Atherosclerosis Study (FeAST): a pilot study of reduction of body iron stores in atherosclerotic peripheral vascular disease. *Am Heart J* 2000;139[2 Pt 1]:337–345.

224. Ascherio A, Willett WC, Rimm EB, et al. Dietary iron intake and risk of coronary disease among men. *Circulation* 1994;89:969–974.

225. Ascherio A, Willett WC. New directions in dietary studies of coronary heart disease. *J Nutr* 1995;125[Suppl 3]:647S–655S.

226. Bray G. Pathophysiology of obesity. *Am J Clin Nutr* 1992;55[Suppl]:488S–494S.

227. Mokdad AH, Serdula MK, Dietz WH, et al. The spread of the obesity epidemic in the United States, 1991–1998. *JAMA* 1999;282:1519–1522.

228. Must A, Spadano J, Coakley EH, et al. The disease burden associated with overweight and obesity. *JAMA* 1999;282:1523–1529.

229. Rabkin SW, Mathewson FA, Hsu PH. Relation of body weight to development of ischemic heart disease in a cohort of young North American men after a 26 year observation period: The Manitoba Study. *Am J Cardiol* 1977;39:452–458.

230. Feinleib M. Epidemiology of obesity in relation to health hazards. *Ann Intern Med* 1985;103:1019–1024.

231. Garrison RJ, Castelli WP. Weight and thirty-year mortality of men in the Framingham Study. *Ann Intern Med* 1985;103:1006–1009.

232. NHLBI Obesity Education Initiative. *Summary report: Strategy development workshop for public education on weight and obesity.* NIH publication 94-3314. Bethesda, MD: National Institutes of Health, 1994:139.

233. Young TK, Gelskey DE. Is noncentral obesity metabolically benign? Implications for prevention from a population survey. *JAMA* 1995;274:1939–1941.

234. Andres R, Muller DC, Sorkin JD. Long-term effects of change in body weight on all-cause mortality. *Ann Intern Med* 1993;119[7 Pt 2]:737–743.

235. Andres R. Mortality and obesity: the rationale for age-specific height-weight tables. In: Andres R, Bierman EL, Hazzard WR, eds. *Principles of geriatric medicine.* New York: McGraw-Hill, 1985:311–318.

236. Mamson JE, Willett WC, Stampfer MJ, et al. Body weight and mortality among women. *N Engl J Med* 1995;333:677–685.

237. Iribarren C, Sharp DS, Burchfield CM, et al. Association of weight loss and weight fluctuation with mortality among Japanese American men. *N Engl J Med* 1995;333:686–692.

238. Stunkard AJ. Current views on obesity. *Am J Med* 1996;100:230–236.

239. Seidell JC, Verschuren WMM, van Leer EM, et al. Overweight, underweight, and mortality: a prospective study of 48,287 men and women. *Arch Intern Med* 1996;156:958–963.

240. Harris T, Cook EF, Garrison R, et al. Body mass index and mortality among nonsmoking older persons: the Framingham Heart Study. *JAMA* 1988;259:1520–1524.

241. Bouchard C, Tremblay A, Despres JP, et al. The response to long-term overfeeding in identical twins. *N Engl J Med* 1990;322:1477–1482.

242. Ravussin E, Valencia ME, Esparza J, et al. Effects of a traditional lifestyle on obesity in Pima Indians. *Diabetes Care* 1994;17:1067–1074.

243. Gibbs WW. Gaining on fat. *Sci Am* 1996;275(2):88–94.

244. Poehlman ET, Toth MJ, Bunyard LB, et al. Physiologic predictors of increasing total and central adiposity in aging men and women. *Arch Intern Med* 1995;155:2443–2448.

245. Grundy SM, Barnett JP. Metabolic and health complications of obesity. *Dis Mon* 1990;36:641–731.

246. Hunt SC, Williams RR, Adams TD. Biochemical and anthropometric characterization of morbid obesity in a large Utah pedigree. *Obes Res* 1995;3[Suppl 2]:165S–172S.

247. Despres J-P, Lemieux I, Prud'homme D. Treatment of obesity: need to focus on high risk abdominally obese patients. *BMJ* 2001;322:716–720.

248. Pouliot MC, Despres J-P, Lemieux S, et al. Waist circumference and abdominal sagittal diameter: best simple anthropometric indexes of abdominal visceral adipose tissue accumulation and related cardiovascular risk in men and women. *Am J Cardiol* 1994;73:460–468.

249. Despres JP, Moorjani S, Lupien PJ, et al. Regional distribution of body fat, plasma lipoproteins, and cardiovascular disease. *Arteriosclerosis* 1990;10:497–511.

250. Donahue RP, Abbott RD, Bloom E, et al. Central obesity and coronary heart disease in men. *Lancet* 1987;1:821–824.

251. Walton C, Lees B, Crook D, et al. Body fat distribution rather than overall adiposity influences serum lipids and lipoproteins in healthy men independently of age. *Am J Med* 1995;99:459–563.

252. Reaven GM. Role of insulin resistance in human disease: Banting Lecture in 1988. *Diabetes* 1988;37:1595–1607.

253. Bao W, Srinivasan SR, Wattigney WA, et al. Persistence of multiple cardiovascular risk clustering related to syndrome X from childhood to young adulthood: The Bogalusa Heart Study. *Arch Intern Med* 1994;154:1842–1847.

254. Grundy SM. Atherogenic dyslipidemia: lipoprotein abnormalities and implications for therapy. *Am J Cardiol* 1995;75:45B–52B.

255. Allemann Y, Horber FF, Colombo M, et al. Insulin sensitivity and body fat distribution in normotensive offspring of hypertensive parents. *Lancet* 1993;341:327–331.

256. Davidson MB. Clinical implications of insulin resistance syndromes. *Am J Med* 1995;99:420–426.

257. Williams RR, Hopkins PN, Hunt SC, et al. Familial dyslipidaemic hypertension and other multiple metabolic syndromes. *Ann Med* 1992;24:469–475.

258. Godsland IF, Crook D, Stevenson JC, et al. Insulin resistance syndrome in postmenopausal women with cardiological syndrome X. *Br Heart J* 1995;74:47–52.

259. Lamarche B, Tchernof A, Mauriège P, et al. Fasting insulin and apolipoprotein B levels and low-density lipoprotein particle size as risk factors for ischemic heart disease. *JAMA* 1998;279:1955–1961.

260. Alpert MA, Terry BE, Kelly DL. Effect of weight loss on cardiac chamber size, wall thickness and left ventricular function in morbid obesity. *Am J Cardiol* 1985;55:783–786.

261. Messerli FH, Sundgaard-Riise K, Reisin ED, et al. Dimorphic cardiac adaption to obesity and arterial hypertension. *Ann Intern Med* 1983;99:757–761.

262. Nakajima T, Fujoka S, Tokunaga K, et al. Noninvasive study of left ventricular performance in obese patients: influence of duration of obesity. *Circulation* 1985;71:481–486.

263. Lauer MS, Anderson KM, Kannel WB, et al. The impact of obesity on left ventricular mass and geometry: the Framingham Heart Study. *JAMA* 1992;266:231–236.

264. Frank S, Colliver JA, Frank A. The electrocardiogram in obesity: statistical analysis of 1,029 patients. *J Am Coll Cardiol* 1986;7:295–299.

265. Drenick EJ, Bale GS, Seltzer F, et al. Excessive mortality and causes of death in morbidly obese men. *JAMA* 1980;243:443–445.

266. Warnes CA, Roberts WC. The heart in massive (more than 300 pounds or 136 kilograms) obesity: analysis of 12 patients studied at necropsy. *Am J Cardiol* 1984;54:1087–1091.

267. Kasper EK, Hruban RH, Baughman KL. Cardiomyopathy of obesity: a clinicopathologic evaluation of 43 obese patients with heart failure. *Am J Cardiol* 1992;70:921–924.

268. Alaud-Din A, Meterissian S, Lisbona R, et al. Assessment of cardiac function in patients who were morbidly obese. *Surgery* 1990;108:809–820.

269. Carella MJ, Mantz SL, Rovner DR, et al. Obesity, adiposity, and lengthening of the QT interval: improvement after weight loss. *Int J Obes* 1996;20:938–942.

270. Hakala K, Mustajoki P, Aittomaki J, et al. Effect of weight loss and body position on pulmonary function and gas exchange abnormalities in morbid obesity. *Int J Obes Rel Metab Disorders* 1995;19:343–346.

271. Pi-Sunyer FX. Medical hazards of obesity. *Ann Intern Med* 1993;119:655–660.

272. Liddle RA, Goldstein RB, Saxton J. Gallstone formation during weight-reduction dieting. *Arch Intern Med* 1989;149:1750–1753.

273. Stunkard AJ, Rush J. Diet and depression reexamined: a critical review of reports of untoward responses during weight reduction for obesity. *Ann Intern Med* 1974;81:526–533.

274. National Institutes of Health, National Heart, Lung, and Blood Institute. Obesity Education Initiative. *Clinical guidelines on the identification, evaluation and treatment of overweight and obesity in adults.* Bethesda, MD: National Institutes of Health, 1998.

275. Grodstein F, Levine R, Trooy L, et al. Three-year follow-up of participants in a commercial weight loss program: can you keep it off? *Arch Intern Med* 1996;156:1302–1306.

276. Freedman MR. *Popular diets: a scientific review; executive summary.* Washington, DC: United States Department of Agriculture, Office of Research, Education and Economics, 2000:20.

277. Tuomilehto J, Lindstrom J, Eriksson JG, et al. Prevention of type 2 diabetes mellitus by changes in lifestyle among subjects with impaired glucose tolerance. *N Engl J Med* 2001;344:1343–1350.

278. Sours HE, Frattali VP, Brand CD, et al. Sudden death associated with very low calorie weight reduction regimens. *Am J Clin Nutr* 1981;34:453–461.

279. Wadden TA, Van Itallie TB, Blackburn GL. Responsible and irresponsible use of very–low calorie diets in the treatment of obesity. *JAMA* 1990;263:83–85.

280. Leibel RL, Rosenbaum M, Hirsch J. Changes in energy expenditure resulting from altered body weight. *N Engl J Med* 1995;332:621–628.

281. St. Jeor ST, Brunner RL, Harrington ME, et al. Who are the weight maintainers? *Obes Res* 1995;3[Suppl 2]:249S–259S.

282. Eckel RH. Insulin resistance: an adaption for weight maintenance. *Lancet* 1992;340:1452–1453.

283. Wing RR. Behavioral treatment of severe obesity. *Am J Clin Nutr* 1992;55[Suppl 2]:545S–551S.

284. Wing RR, Koeske R, Epstein LH, et al. Long-term effects of modest weight loss in type II diabetic patients. *Arch Intern Med* 1987;147:1749–1753.

285. Kayman S, Bruvold W, Stern JS. Maintenance and relapse after weight loss in women: behavioral aspects. *Am J Clin Nutr* 1990;52:800–807.

286. Epstein LH, Valoski AM, Vara LS, et al. Effects of decreasing sedentary behavior and increasing activity on weight change in obese children. *Health Psychol* 1995;14:109–115.

287. Lichtman SW, Pisarska K, Berman ER, et al. Discrepancy between self-reported and actual caloric intake and exercise in obese subjects. *N Engl J Med* 1992;327:1893–1898.

288. Bouchard C, Tremblay A, Nadeau A, et al. Long-term exercise training with constant energy intake. I. Effect on body composition and selected metabolic variables. *Int J Obes* 1990;14:57–73.

289. Foreyt JP, Brunner RL, Goodrick GK, et al. Psychological correlates of reported physical activity in normal-weight and obese adults: The Reno Diet-Heart Study. *Int J Obes Rel Metab Disorders* 1995;1[Suppl 4]:69S–72S.

290. Tremblay A, Despres JP, Maheux J, et al. Normalization of the metabolic profile in obese women by exercise and a low fat diet. *Med Sci Sports Exer* 1991;23:1326–1331.

291. Pate RR, Pratt M, Blair SN, et al. Physical activity and public health: a recommendation from the Centers for Disease Control and Prevention and the American College of Sports Medicine. *JAMA* 1995;273:402–407.

292. Weintraub M, Hasday JD, Mushlin AI, et al. A double blind clinical trial in weight control: use of fenfluramine and phentermine alone and in combination. *Arch Intern Med* 1984;144:1143–1148.

293. Connolly HM, Crary JL, McGoon MD, et al. Valvular heart disease associated with fenfluramine-phentermine. *N Engl J Med* 1997;337:581–588.

294. Devereux RB. Appetite suppressants and valvular heart disease. *N Engl J Med* 1998;339:765–767.

295. Rothman RB, Baumann MH, Savage JE, et al. Evidence for possible involvement of 5-HT(2B) receptors in the cardiac valvulopathy associated with fenfluramine and other serotonergic medications. *Circulation* 2000;102:2836–2841.

296. Abenhaim L, Moride Y, Brenot F, et al. Appetite-suppressant drugs and the risk of primary pulmonary hypertension. *N Engl J Med* 1996;335:609–616.

297. McMahon FG, Fujioka K, Singh BN, et al. Efficacy and safety of sibutramine in obese white and African American patients with hypertension: a 1-year, double-blind, placebo-controlled, multicenter trial. *Arch Intern Med* 2000;160:2185–2191.

298. Finer N, James WP, Kopelman PG, et al. One-year treatment of obesity: a randomized, double-blind, placebo-controlled, multicentre study of orlistat, a gastrointestinal lipase inhibitor. *Int J Obes Relat Metab Disord* 2000;24:306–313.

299. Charatan F. Obesity surgery grows in popularity in the US. *BMJ* 2000;321:980.

300. Baxter J. Obesity surgery: another unmet need. It is effective but prejudice is preventing its use [editorial]. *BMJ* 2000;321:523–524.

301. Gould KL. Reversal of coronary atherosclerosis: clinical promise as the basis for noninvasive management of coronary artery disease. *Circulation* 1994;90:1558–1571.

302. Gambera PJ, Schneeman BO, Davis PA. Use of the Food Guide Pyramid and US dietary guidelines to improve dietary intake and reduce cardiovascular risk in active-duty Air Force members. *J Am Diet Assoc* 1995;95:1268–1273.

303. Czernin J, Barnard RJ, Sun KT, et al. Effect of short-term cardiovascular conditioning and low-fat diet on myocardial blood flow and flow reserve. *Circulation* 1995;92:197–204.

3

LIPID DISORDERS

DANIEL J. RADER

OVERVIEW

Lipid disorders are common and are an important risk factor for coronary heart disease (CHD) and all types of atherosclerotic cardiovascular disease (ASCVD). Intervention with diet

D. J. Rader: Department of Medicine, University of Pennsylvania Medical Center, Philadelphia, Pennsylvania

and drugs to reduce low-density lipoprotein (LDL) cholesterol has been proven to decrease the risk of subsequent cardiovascular events, including the total mortality. In patients who have established ASCVD or are at a high risk for developing it, treatment to reduce LDL cholesterol is effective not only when the LDL cholesterol level is elevated, but also when the cholesterol level is average. On the basis of a wealth of clinical trial data, it is widely agreed that virtually all patients with ASCVD should be treated with lipid-lowering drug therapy to reduce the risk of subsequent cardiovascular events. However, sudden cardiac death at the time of the first myocardial infarction (MI) is common, and, therefore, waiting to reduce cholesterol until symptoms of CHD have developed is not an acceptable strategy. Drug therapy to reduce cholesterol in primary prevention has also been shown to reduce cardiovascular events, even when LDL cholesterol levels are only moderately elevated. Thus, the major challenge in primary prevention is to perform an accurate risk assessment so that high-risk patients can be treated with an appropriate level of aggressive drug therapy, and low-risk patients can avoid drug therapy. Traditional risk factors are useful but do not always permit accurate risk assessment; additional tests to assess cardiovascular risk, such as laboratory tests and noninvasive imaging tests of subclinical atherosclerosis, have a role to play. It is likely that those individuals at highest risk for developing premature CHD will be able to be prospectively identified. Cholesterol reduction is a cornerstone of cardiovascular risk reduction. Strategies to achieve cholesterol reduction must include both broad-based public health measures oriented around diet and lifestyle and highly focused, aggressive intervention targeted toward those at highest risk for developing premature CHD.

GLOSSARY

Apolipoprotein: Major protein component of lipoproteins; apolipoproteins have a variety of functions.

Cholesteryl ester transfer protein (CETP): Protein that transfers lipids among lipoproteins, especially cholesteryl ester from high-density lipoprotein to very low-density lipoprotein, in exchange for triglycerides.

Chylomicron: Intestinal triglyceride-rich lipoprotein; elevated when triglycerides are >1,000 mg per dL.

Hepatic lipase (HL): Endothelial-anchored enzyme in liver that is primarily responsible for hydrolysis of triglycerides and phospholipids in intermediate-density lipoprotein and high-density lipoprotein.

High-density lipoprotein (HDL): Small lipoprotein thought to participate in "reverse cholesterol transport"; levels are inversely associated with risk of coronary artery disease.

3-Hydroxy-3-methylglutaryl coenzyme A (HMG-CoA) reductase: Rate-limiting enzyme in cholesterol biosynthesis; inhibition by statins results in reduction of plasma LDL-cholesterol levels.

Intermediate-density lipoprotein (IDL): Lipoprotein formed by hydrolysis of triglycerides in very low-density lipoprotein; elevated in type III hyperlipoproteinemia.

Lecithin-cholesterol acyltransferase (LCAT): Enzyme that converts free cholesterol to cholesteryl ester on high-density lipoprotein.

Lipoproteins: Complexes responsible for transporting lipids (cholesterol, triglyceride, phospholipids) within the blood.

Lipoprotein lipase (LPL): Endothelial-anchored enzyme primarily responsible for hydrolysis of chylomicron and very-low-density lipoprotein triglycerides, especially in muscle and adipose tissue.

Low-density lipoprotein (LDL): Major cholesterol-containing lipoprotein and major atherogenic lipoprotein.

Primary prevention: Treatment to prevent atherosclerosis and coronary artery disease events in persons who do not have evidence of coronary artery disease.

Secondary prevention: Treatment to prevent recurrent coronary artery disease events in persons who have documented coronary artery disease.

Very-low-density lipoprotein (VLDL): Major triglyceride-containing lipoprotein when fasting triglycerides are <1,000 mg per dL; made by the liver.

HISTORICAL PERSPECTIVE

Cholesterol was first postulated to be related to atherosclerosis when it was found to be a major component of advanced atherosclerotic plaques. The association between elevated serum cholesterol and atherosclerotic disease was first reported in the 1930s. Subsequent large epidemiologic studies such as the Seven Countries Study (1) and the Framingham Heart Study (2) confirmed the strong relationship between serum cholesterol and CHD. In the Multiple Risk Factor Intervention Trial, 356,222 men with no history of MI were screened and followed for the development of CHD over the course of 6 years. The relationship between serum cholesterol level and subsequent CHD was found to be continuous, graded, and strong (3). The Lipid Research Clinics Prevalence Study demonstrated in a 10-year follow-up that cholesterol level at baseline was strongly associated with CHD death in men who did and men who did not have CHD when they entered the study (4). In the Johns Hopkins Precursors Study, cholesterol levels determined in young men in their early twenties were predictive of the risk of developing CHD three to four decades later (5). In the Bogalusa Heart Study, aortic fatty streaks in young individuals (mean age, 18 years) were found to be strongly correlated with serum cholesterol level (6). These and many other epidemiologic and observational studies formed the basis of the "cholesterol hypothesis," which states that the relationship between serum cholesterol and atherosclerosis is causal and that reduction of serum cholesterol reduces atherosclerotic disease.

The subfractionation of serum cholesterol into cholesterol contained within specific lipoproteins, such as LDLs and high-density lipoproteins (HDLs), was a major clinical advance. Risk for CHD was found to be strongly associated with LDL cholesterol levels. The seminal observation that HDL cholesterol levels were inversely associated with cardiovascular risk was made in the 1950s and rediscovered in the 1970s (7). Subsequent studies from many parts of the world have confirmed this observation (8) and have ultimately resulted in the use of

HDL cholesterol levels as a key laboratory marker for the screening of cardiovascular risk in all adults (9).

The relationship between fasting serum triglycerides and cardiovascular risk has been confounded by the inverse association between triglycerides and HDL cholesterol, as well as by the association of triglycerides with other risk factors, such as diabetes mellitus and body mass. Earlier epidemiologic studies demonstrated that fasting triglycerides were not independently associated with cardiovascular risk. However, in the last several years, several prospective studies have indicated that triglyceride levels are an important independent predictor of risk (10). Although formal guidelines have not yet established the use of triglycerides as an independent risk factor, many clinicians now incorporate the fasting triglyceride level into a comprehensive cardiovascular risk assessment (see below).

LIPID-MODIFYING THERAPY AND EFFECTS ON ATHEROSCLEROSIS AND CARDIOVASCULAR EVENTS

Despite the wealth of epidemiologic and pathologic data linking serum cholesterol to atherosclerotic disease, proof of the "cholesterol hypothesis" required demonstration that reduction of cholesterol decreased atherosclerosis and clinical cardiovascular events. Over the past two decades, multiple trials have been reported that were designed to test this hypothesis, and more recent studies have been designed to test whether modification of HDL cholesterol and triglyceride levels would reduce atherosclerosis or cardiovascular risk. Many studies have assessed the impact of lipid-modifying therapy on a quantitative measure of atherosclerotic disease (as assessed by coronary angiography or carotid ultrasound) (*e*Table 3.0.1). Other, larger trials have been focused on the effect of lipid-modifying therapy on clinical cardiovascular events (nonfatal MI, CHD death, and total mortality rate) (Table 3.1). These studies encompass both secondary prevention trials (in patients with clinically established CHD) and primary prevention trials (in patients without established CHD).

Trials Using Clinical Events as the Primary End Point

Early Clinical Trials: Niacin, Bile Acid Sequestrants, and Partial Ileal Bypass

The early clinical trials used niacin, bile acid sequestrants, and even the surgical approach of partial ileal bypass to reduce serum cholesterol levels (Table 3.1). The Coronary Drug Project demonstrated a modest benefit of niacin in reducing nonfatal MI after 6 years of treatment (14) and in reducing the total mortality rate after 15 years of follow-up (15). The Program on the Surgical Control of the Hyperlipidemias trial used partial ileal bypass surgery to reduce LDL cholesterol levels and demonstrated a significant 35% relative reduction in fatal CHD and nonfatal MI, although

TABLE 3.1 CLINICAL TRIALS OF CHOLESTEROL REDUCTION WITH CLINICAL EVENTS AS THE PRIMARY END POINT

Study	Intervention	Event rates (%)			Relative risk	
		End point	Placebo	Active	Reduction (%)	
Secondary prevention						
Coronary Drug Project (14,15)	Niacin	Total mortality	19.4	17.3	11[a]	
POSCH (16)	Ileal bypass	Fatal CHD/nonfatal MI	30.0	19.4	35[a]	
		Total mortality	14.9	11.6	22	
4S (20,22)	Simvastatin	Total mortality	11.5	8.2	30[a]	
		Fatal CHD/nonfatal MI	28.0	19.0	44[a]	
CARE (157)	Pravastatin	Fatal CHD/nonfatal MI	13.2	10.2	24[a]	
LIPID (25)	Pravastatin	CHD mortality	8.3	6.4	24[a]	
Primary prevention						
Oslo Study (158)	Multifactorial	Fatal CHD/nonfatal MI	6.2	3.6	42[a]	
WHO (36)	Clofibrate	Nonfatal MI			25[a]	
Lipid Research Clinics (17)	Cholestyramine	Fatal CHD/nonfatal MI	6.6	5.5	19[a]	
		Total mortality	2.5	2.4	7	
Helsinki Heart Study (38)	Gemfibrozil	Fatal CHD/nonfatal MI	4.1	2.7	34[a]	
		Total mortality	2.1	2.2	(−5.8)	
West of Scotland (32)	Pravastatin	Fatal CHD/nonfatal MI	7.9	5.5	31[a]	
		Total mortality	4.1	3.2	22[a]	
AFCAPS/TexCAPS (33)	Lovastatin	MI/SCD/UA	10.9	6.8	37[a]	

4S, Scandinavian Simvastatin Survival Study; AFCAPS/TexCAPS, Air Force/Texas Coronary Atherosclerosis Prevention Study; CARE, Cholesterol and Recurrent Events Study; CHD, coronary heart disease; LIPID, Long-Term Intervention with Pravastatin in Ischaemic Disease Study; MI, myocardial infarction; POSCH, Program on the Surgical Control of the Hyperlipidemias; SCD, sudden cardiac death; UA, unstable angina; WHO, World Health Organization.
[a]*p* <.05.

no significant reduction was seen in the total mortality rate (the primary end point of the trial) (16). In the Lipid Research Clinics Coronary Primary Prevention Trial, which studied the effect of cholestyramine administration in hypercholesterolemic men (17,18), combined fatal CHD and nonfatal MI (the primary end point) was reduced by 19%, but the total mortality rate was not reduced (68 deaths among patients receiving cholestyramine vs. 71 deaths among patients receiving placebo). A higher noncardiovascular mortality rate was seen in patients who were treated with cholestyramine (36 deaths) than in patients who received placebo (27 deaths), mostly because of a higher number of suicides and violent deaths among patients treated with cholestyramine (11 vs. 4 deaths). Extension of the follow-up period to a total of 13.4 years (19) demonstrated that the total number of deaths in the group of patients receiving cholestyramine (143 deaths) was not significantly different from that in the control group (156 deaths).

3-Hydroxy-3-Methylglutaryl Coenzyme A Reductase Inhibitor (Statin) Trials

Secondary Prevention

Five major clinical outcome trials with 3-hydroxy-3-methylglutaryl coenzyme A (HMG-CoA) reductase inhibitors (statins) performed during the 1990s definitively established that reduction of LDL cholesterol reduced cardiovascular risk in both secondary and primary prevention (Table 3.1). Three of these trials were secondary prevention trials, and two were primary prevention trials. The Scandinavian Simvastatin Survival Study (4S) (20) was designed to address the question of whether cholesterol reduction with simvastatin in persons with CHD and elevated cholesterol would reduce the total mortality rate (the primary end point). A total of 4,444 patients with angina or previous MI whose total cholesterol levels were between 212 and 310 mg per dL were randomized to placebo or simvastatin. The simvastatin dose was titrated to reduce the total cholesterol level to <200 mg per dL. Subjects were followed for a mean of 5.4 years. One hundred and eighty-nine deaths occurred in the group receiving placebo, and 111 deaths occurred in the group receiving simvastatin, resulting in a highly significant 30% relative reduction in the total mortality rate (p <.00001) (eFig 3.0.2A). The relative risk of a major coronary event (the secondary end point) such as CHD death or MI was reduced by 44% (p <.00001) (eFig 3.0.2B). The number of revascularization procedures such as coronary bypass surgery and angioplasty also dropped significantly, by 34%. An economic analysis based on the 4S study concluded that in the United States, the reduction in hospital costs alone as a result of the treatment would virtually offset the cost of the medication (21). Importantly, the reduction in risk was not only seen among subjects who had the highest cholesterol levels; the quartile with the lowest LDL cho-

lesterol levels at baseline had proportionately as much benefit from treatment as the highest quartile (22).

This issue is important, because the majority of patients with CHD do not have particularly elevated cholesterol levels; in fact, approximately 35% of all persons with CHD have total cholesterol levels <200 mg per dL (23). Therefore, another major trial, the Cholesterol and Recurrent Events study (24), addressed the previously unanswered question of whether patients who had experienced MI and who had average cholesterol levels would benefit from further cholesterol reduction with pravastatin. In this study, 4,159 patients who had experienced MI 3 to 20 months before the trial and had total cholesterol levels <240 mg per dL were randomly assigned to receive placebo or pravastatin, 40 mg daily, and followed for an average of 5 years. The mean total cholesterol level was 209 mg per dL in each group, and the mean LDL cholesterol level was only 139 mg per dL (range, 115 to 174 mg per dL). After 5 years, 274 subjects in the placebo group had nonfatal MI or CHD death (the primary end point), compared with 212 subjects in the group of patients treated with pravastatin, resulting in a significant 24% reduction in relative risk (p = .003) (eFig 3.0.3A). Revascularization procedures were reduced by 27% (p <.001) (eFig. 3.0.3B). These results demonstrated that the benefit of cholesterol-lowering therapy extends even to CHD patients who have average cholesterol levels.

The Long-Term Intervention with Pravastatin in Ischaemic Disease Study (LIPID) (25) was the largest secondary prevention study performed to date. It included 9,014 patients aged 31 to 75 years who presented with either acute MI or unstable angina and who had baseline cholesterol levels spanning the wide range of 155 to 271 mg per dL. Subjects were randomly assigned to receive placebo or pravastatin, 40 mg daily, and followed for 6 years. Treatment with pravastatin significantly reduced the CHD mortality rate (the primary end point) by 24% (p <.001) and the total mortality rate by 22% (p <0.001). The study was terminated early by the data and safety monitoring committee because of the highly significant difference in total mortality between the two groups. The occurrence of revascularization was reduced by 20%, and the occurrence of stroke of any type was reduced by 19%.

These three studies definitively established the efficacy of statin therapy in reducing cardiovascular events and the total mortality rate in patients who had established CHD over a very wide range of baseline LDL cholesterol levels. Not only is cholesterol-lowering drug therapy clinically effective in secondary prevention, it is cost-effective as well. Aggressive cholesterol reduction in patients with patients with CHD or other ASCVD is now the standard of care, as agreed on in a joint statement issued by the American Heart Association and the American College of Cardiology (26). The majority of patients with ASCVD should be considered candidates for lipid-lowering drug therapy. Current debate in secondary prevention centers around not whether to treat, but how far to reduce the LDL cholesterol level (27). Studies designed to address this issue are currently under way.

All of the statin trials reviewed earlier excluded patients who were within 3 to 6 months of an acute coronary event. The LIPID trial was, in fact, the only secondary-prevention trial to include patients who had presented with unstable angina. In LIPID, the relative risk reduction for total mortality with pravastatin therapy was 20.6% among patients who had experienced MI and 26.3% among patients who had experienced unstable angina, suggesting a trend for even greater benefit in those patients who presented with unstable angina (28). In patients in LIPID who had previous unstable angina, the CHD mortality rate, the total mortality rate, the incidence of MI, the need for coronary revascularization, the number of admissions to the hospital, and the number of days spent in the hospital were all significantly lower in the group of patients receiving pravastatin. One question of substantial clinical interest is whether patients presenting with acute coronary syndromes would benefit from immediate initiation of statin therapy. In a small study called the Randomized Lipid-Coronary Artery Disease Study, patients were randomly assigned, an average of 6 days after presenting with an acute coronary syndrome, to receive pravastatin, 40 mg daily (combined, when necessary, with cholestyramine and/or nicotinic acid to achieve LDL cholesterol levels <130 mg per dL), or usual care (29). After 2 years, 52% of patients in the group receiving usual care but only 23% of patients in the group being aggressively treated experienced a recurrent cardiovascular event (p = .005). In a larger study called the Myocardial Ischemia Reduction with Aggressive Cholesterol Lowering Study, patients who presented with acute coronary syndromes and did not undergo revascularization were randomly assigned to receive immediate therapy with atorvastatin, 80 mg, or placebo and followed for 4 months (30). A 16% reduction in recurrent coronary events was associated with immediate statin therapy, a difference that barely achieved statistical significance (p = .048). Additional studies that include patients undergoing revascularization are under way that also address the important question of the benefit of immediate initiation of statin therapy.

Primary Prevention

Primary prevention of CHD is also important, because approximately one-fourth to one-third of first MIs result in death (31), precluding the opportunity for secondary prevention. Nevertheless, the use of drug therapy in primary prevention has been controversial; before the mid-1990s, relatively few data were available that demonstrated clinical benefit. The West of Scotland Coronary Prevention Study (32) was a landmark trial in primary prevention of CHD. This study involved 6,595 healthy Scottish men aged 45 to 64 years, with total cholesterol levels >252 mg per dL and LDL cholesterol levels of 174 to 232 mg per dL. Although none of the study subjects had documented CHD, 5% had positive results of a Rose questionnaire indicating probable angina. Subjects were randomly assigned to receive pravastatin, 40 mg per day, or placebo and were followed for an average of 5 years. The primary end point of the study was nonfatal MI or CHD death. Two hundred and forty-eight definite events were reported in the group of patients receiving placebo (7.9% of the subjects) and 174 events in the group receiving pravastatin (5.5% of the subjects), resulting in a 31% reduction in relative risk of nonfatal MI or CHD death (p <.001) (eFig. 3.0.4A). In addition, a significant 32% reduction in CHD death (p <.033) (eFig. 3.0.4B) and a 37% reduction in revascularization procedures (p <.009) were seen. Importantly, no significant difference was found in the noncardiovascular mortality rate (eFig. 3.0.4C), indicating that cholesterol reduction with pravastatin did not increase the risk of death from other causes. In fact, the relative risk of death from any cause (total mortality rate) was reduced by 22% among patients treated with pravastatin (p = .051) during the 5-year period of the trial (eFig. 3.0.4D). This trial clearly established that drug therapy for hypercholesterolemia is an effective method of decreasing risk of cardiovascular events in persons who do not have prior evidence of CHD.

The Air Force/Texas Coronary Atherosclerosis Prevention Study (AFCAPS/TexCAPS) extended these findings to a population with modestly elevated to average cholesterol levels (33). A total of 6,608 men and women with LDL cholesterol levels of 130 to 190 mg per dL and HDL cholesterol levels <45 mg per dL in men and <47 mg per dL in women were randomly assigned to receive lovastatin, 20 mg, or placebo and were followed for an average of 5.2 years. The dose of lovastatin was titrated to 40 mg in an attempt to reduce LDL cholesterol levels to <100 mg per dL. A 37% relative risk reduction was seen in the primary end point of combined cardiovascular events in the group of patients who were treated with lovastatin. Interestingly, only 17% of the subjects in this trial would have met National Cholesterol Education Program Adult Treatment Panel II (NCEP-ATPII) 1993 guidelines for drug therapy. Therefore, the major clinical challenge in the use of drug therapy to reduce cholesterol levels in primary prevention of CHD is the accurate identification of individuals who are likely to develop clinical CHD and who are therefore most likely to benefit from drug therapy.

Fibrate Trials

Fibrates have been used as lipid-lowering drugs for several decades. They are particularly effective in reducing triglyceride levels and have modest effectiveness in reducing cholesterol levels and raising HDL cholesterol levels (35). Relatively few clinical endpoint trials examining the use of fibrates have been published. In the World Health Organization cooperative trial using clofibrate to treat hypercholesterolemic men (36), a 25% reduction was seen in relative risk of nonfatal MI (the primary end point) after 5 years, but a substantial 47% increase in noncardiovascular deaths was also found. Extension of the follow-up period to 13 years did not reveal a persistent effect of the drug on the excess mortality rate (37). The Helsinki Heart Study (38) treated men who had elevated non-HDL cholesterol levels, >200 mg per dL, with gemfibrozil and demonstrated a significant 34% reduction in combined fatal and nonfatal MI (the primary end point) but no difference in the total mortality rate (45 deaths among patients receiving gemfibrozil and 42 deaths in the control group). A small trend toward an increase in the noncardiovascular mortality rate was seen (31 vs. 23 deaths, respectively), which was largely due to a difference in accidental and violent death (10 vs. 4 deaths, respectively). Extension of the follow-up period to 8.5 years (39) demonstrated an increased mortality rate in the group treated with gemfibrozil (101 deaths) compared to the group receiving placebo (83 deaths) that was not statistically significant ($p = .19$) and was due to a small increase in cancer deaths among patients receiving gemfibrozil. Neither of these trials were designed with adequate power to assess the impact of fibrates on the total mortality rate. Nevertheless, the lack of effect on the total mortality rate and the small trends toward an increased noncardiovascular mortality rate resulted in uncertainty about the broad use of fibrates for cardiovascular risk reduction in hypercholesterolemic patients.

Two trials of fibrates in the late 1990s provided more data but also generated more questions. The Veteran Affairs High-Density Lipoprotein Cholesterol Intervention Trial (VA-HIT) tested the benefit of gemfibrozil therapy in patients who had CHD and reasonably well-controlled LDL cholesterol levels but low HDL cholesterol levels (40). Two thousand five hundred and thirty-one patients with CHD, low levels of HDL (mean, 32 mg per dL), low LDL cholesterol levels (mean, 112 mg per dL), and triglyceride levels <300 mg per dL were randomly assigned to receive treatment with a sustained-release gemfibrozil formulation (1,200 mg daily) or placebo and followed for an average of 5.1 years. Gemfibrozil therapy was associated with a significant 22% reduction in the primary end point (nonfatal MI and coronary death) compared with placebo. Gemfibrozil resulted in a 6% increase in HDL cholesterol levels, a 31% decrease in triglyceride levels, and no change in LDL cholesterol levels. This important study suggests that lipid-modifying drug therapy using fibrates in patients with CHD and low LDL and HDL cholesterol levels reduces cardiovascular events.

In contrast, the Bezafibrate Infarction Prevention (BIP) trial involved 3,090 patients with established CHD, total cholesterol levels of 180 to 250 mg per dL, HDL cholesterol levels <45 mg per dL, triglyceride levels <300 mg per dL, and LDL cholesterol levels <180 mg per dL who were randomly assigned to receive either bezafibrate, 400 mg daily, or placebo and followed for a mean of 6.2 years (41). The primary end point was fatal or nonfatal MI or sudden death. Bezafibrate therapy was associated with a reduction in the primary end point of only 7.3%, which was not statistically significant ($p = .24$). A post hoc analysis in the subgroup with high baseline triglyceride levels (>200 mg per dL) suggested a reduction in events of 39% ($p = .02$).

These trials differed in a number of important ways, including the agent used and the mean baseline LDL cholesterol levels, which in BIP were 150 mg per dL and in VA-HIT were only 111 mg per dL. A reasonable conclusion is that fibrates are effective as monotherapy in reducing events in secondary prevention if the LDL cholesterol is low, but not if it is elevated. A number of additional studies are under way that address the role of fibrates in reducing cardiovascular events, both as monotherapy and in combination with statins.

PHYSIOLOGY AND PATHOPHYSIOLOGY OF LIPOPROTEIN METABOLISM AND RELATIONSHIP TO ATHEROSCLEROSIS

Clinical management of patients with lipid disorders requires a general working knowledge of normal lipoprotein metabolism (42). Lipoproteins are large macromolecular complexes that transport cholesterol and triglycerides within the blood. They contain a neutral lipid core consisting of triglycerides and cholesteryl esters that is surrounded by phospholipids and specialized proteins known as *apolipoproteins*. The five major families of lipoproteins are chylomicrons, VLDLs, intermediate-density lipoproteins (IDLs), LDLs, and HDLs. Chylomicrons are the largest and most lipid-rich lipoproteins, whereas HDLs are the smallest lipoproteins and contain the least amount of lipid. The major metabolic pathways of lipoproteins are shown in Figures 3.1 through 3.3 and described in detail in the accompanying legends. ✌ a61

SECONDARY DISORDERS OF LIPOPROTEIN METABOLISM

Lipid disorders can be grouped into primary disorders (genetic or inherited) and secondary disorders (caused by disease or environmental factors). Clinically, it is useful to consider and exclude secondary causes. Some of the most important secondary causes of hyperlipidemia are reviewed here and listed in Table 3.2.

Hypothyroidism

Hypothyroidism causes elevated LDL cholesterol levels primarily because of down-regulation of the LDL receptor (54). Because hypothyroidism can be subtle in its clinical presenta-

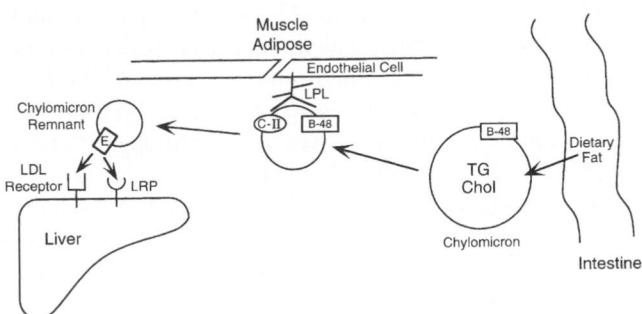

FIGURE 3.1 Exogenous pathway of lipid transport. Dietary fat is absorbed into chylomicrons, which contain the major structural apolipoprotein B-48. Chylomicrons bind to lipoprotein lipase (LPL) on the luminal surface of the capillary endothelium of tissues, especially muscle and adipose tissue. The LPL hydrolyzes the triglycerides [apolipoprotein C-II (C-II) on the chylomicron surface is a required cofactor for LPL]. The free fatty acids enter the tissue to be used for energy (muscle) or storage (adipose), and the triglyceride-depleted chylomicron remnant is released. Chylomicron remnants are taken up by the liver by binding of apolipoprotein E (E) to the low-density lipoprotein (LDL) receptor and the LDL receptor–related protein (LRP). TG Chol, triglyceride cholesterol.

tion, patients presenting with hypercholesterolemia should be screened with a thyroid-stimulating hormone to rule out hypothyroidism. Thyroid replacement therapy usually results in resolution of the hypercholesterolemia. Hypothyroid patients who remain hypercholesterolemic after adequate replacement probably have an underlying lipoprotein disorder and may require lipid-lowering drug therapy.

Diabetes Mellitus

Several forms of hyperlipidemia are recognized clinically in patients with diabetes mellitus (55,56). Patients with type I

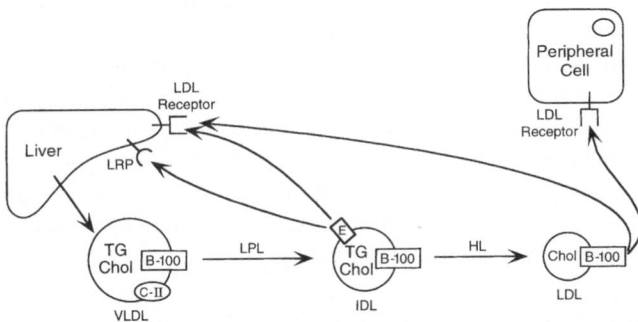

FIGURE 3.2 Endogenous pathway of lipid transport. The liver synthesizes triglycerides and cholesteryl esters and packages them into very-low-density lipoproteins (VLDLs), which contain the major structural apolipoprotein B-100. VLDLs are hydrolyzed by lipoprotein lipase (LPL) to form intermediate-density lipoproteins (IDL). IDLs can be taken up by the liver via binding of apolipoprotein E (E) to the LDL receptor or LDL receptor–related protein (LRP). Alternatively, the triglyceride and phospholipid in IDL can be hydrolyzed by hepatic lipase (HL) within the hepatic sinusoids to form LDL. LDL can be taken up by peripheral cells or by the liver through the binding of apolipoprotein B-100 to the LDL receptor. C-II, apolipoprotein C-II; TG Chol, triglyceride cholesterol.

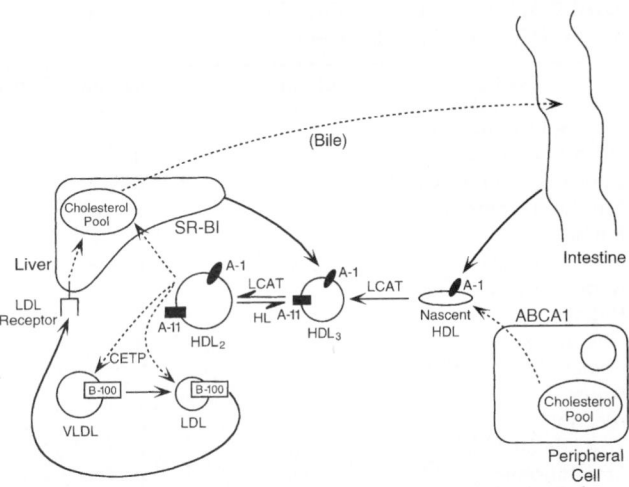

FIGURE 3.3 High-density lipoprotein (HDL) metabolism and reverse cholesterol transport. HDL and its major apolipoprotein, apolipoprotein A-I, are synthesized by both the intestine and the liver. A second major HDL protein, apolipoprotein A-II, is made only by the liver. Nascent HDL interacts with peripheral cells to facilitate the removal of excess free cholesterol through a process that is facilitated by the cellular protein ABCA1. Some of the acquired free cholesterol is esterified to cholesteryl ester on the HDL particle by the action of the enzyme lecithin-cholesterol acyltransferase (LCAT), and the nascent HDL particle becomes the larger HDL3. HDL acquires further cholesteryl ester by continued LCAT action and eventually becomes the even larger HDL2. HDL2 can selectively transfer both cholesteryl ester and free cholesterol to the liver via an HDL receptor in the liver called *scavenger receptor BI*. Cholesteryl esters can also be transferred from HDL2 to apolipoprotein B–containing lipoproteins such as very-low-density lipoproteins (VLDLs) and LDLs via the action of the cholesteryl ester transfer protein (CETP) and then returned to the liver by hepatic uptake of LDL. HDL2 triglycerides and phospholipids can be hydrolyzed by hepatic lipase (HL) to remodel HDL2 to HDL3. Cholesterol derived from HDL contributes to the hepatic cholesterol pool used for bile acid synthesis, and the cholesterol is eventually excreted into the bile and feces as bile acid or free cholesterol. Solid lines indicate the metabolism of the lipoprotein particles, and broken lines indicate the flux of cholesterol independent of lipoprotein particle metabolism.

diabetes mellitus who are under adequate glycemic control do not usually have hyperlipidemia, and the presence of hyperlipidemia in such patients suggests the presence of an underlying genetic lipoprotein abnormality. In contrast, patients with type II diabetes mellitus frequently have associated hyperlipidemia. Insulin resistance results in impaired capacity to catabolize chylomicrons and VLDL, as well as excess hepatic triglyceride and VLDL production (57). Type II diabetes mellitus and even glucose intolerance are often associated with a constellation of lipid abnormalities, including elevated triglyceride and VLDL cholesterol levels, increased small, dense LDL levels, and decreased HDL cholesterol levels. These lipid abnormalities are also common in persons with impaired glucose tolerance and insulin resistance in whom frank diabetes is not present. Occasionally, the triglyceride levels may be extremely elevated (>1,000 mg per dL) and predispose the patient to acute pancreatitis. Significant elevation of LDL cholesterol levels in the diabetic

TABLE 3.2 SELECTED DISORDERS ASSOCIATED WITH SECONDARY HYPERLIPIDEMIA

Disorder	Cholesterol	Triglycerides	HDL
Metabolic/endocrine			
Hypothyroidism	++	N	N
Diabetes mellitus, type II	+	++	–
Cushing's syndrome	+	++	–
Renal			
End-stage renal disease	+	+	–
Nephrotic syndrome	++	++	–
Hepatic			
Obstructive liver disease	++	N	–
Primary biliary cirrhosis	++	N	+
Drugs			
Alcohol	N	++	+
Thiazide diuretics	N	+	–
Beta-blockers	N	+	–
Cyclosporin	++	N	N
Isotretinoin and etretinate	N	++	–
HIV protease inhibitors	+	++	–

–, decreased; +, increased; ++, substantially increased; HDL, high-density lipoprotein; HIV, human immunodeficiency virus; N, not affected.

patient often suggests the presence of an additional lipoprotein abnormality. All patients who present with hyperlipidemia should be screened for diabetes using a fasting glucose test. Aggressive control of diabetes often results in improved control of hyperlipidemia. Furthermore, hyperlipidemia is a major risk factor for diabetic patients, and lipid disorders in patients with diabetes should be aggressively treated to decrease the risk of ASCVD (55).

Renal Diseases

Chronic renal insufficiency and especially end-stage renal disease are often associated with moderate hypertriglyceridemia caused by a defect in triglyceride lipolysis and remnant clearance (54). Nephrotic syndrome is associated with a more pronounced hyperlipidemia involving both elevated triglyceride and cholesterol levels caused by hepatic overproduction of VLDL (58). Both types of renal disease should be considered and excluded when they are suspected in patients who present with hyperlipidemia. Resolution of the nephrotic syndrome improves the lipid profile, but patients with chronic nephrotic syndrome often require lipid-lowering drug therapy. Although the lipid abnormalities in end-stage renal disease are more modest, cardiovascular risk is high, and lipid-modifying drug therapy should be seriously considered. It has been suggested that lipid-lowering therapy could slow the progression of chronic renal insufficiency (59), but clinical trials have not yet been performed to test this hypothesis.

Alcohol Consumption

Alcohol intake often exacerbates hyperlipidemia, but its effects are highly variable (60). The greatest effects of alcohol are on triglyceride levels. Alcohol consumption inhibits oxidation of free fatty acids by the liver, which stimulates hepatic triglyceride synthesis and secretion of VLDL. The usual lipoprotein pattern associated with alcohol consumption is moderate hypertriglyceridemia, although it can raise total and LDL cholesterol levels as well. Regular alcohol use also raises the HDL cholesterol level by a mechanism that is not completely understood. Patients with hyperlipidemia who drink alcohol regularly should be advised to reduce their alcohol intake.

Drug Use

Several drugs are known to influence plasma lipid levels; these are listed in Table 3.2. Retinoids such as isotretinoin and etretinate, used for acne, are known to induce substantial hypertriglyceridemia in susceptible persons. Immunosuppressive therapy used in the posttransplantation setting is well known to cause hypercholesterolemia and hypertriglyceridemia. Finally, since the introduction of the protease inhibitors for therapy for human immunodeficiency virus, it has been recognized that many of these patients develop hyperlipidemia, which appears to result from a complex and poorly understood interaction between the disease and the effect of the drugs.

PRIMARY (INHERITED) DISORDERS OF LIPOPROTEIN METABOLISM

The classification of lipoprotein disorders is useful as a guide to accurate diagnosis and effective treatment. The Frederickson and Levy classification (Table 3.3) is based on the type of lipoprotein that is elevated. This classification system has been used for several decades. It is now gradually being replaced by a classification based on the understanding of the molecular etiology and pathophysiology of the lipoprotein disorders (Table 3.4). In this section, lipoprotein disorders are presented in a way intended to facilitate a practical clinical approach. This approach is based on classifying patients first according to triglyceride levels and can lead to a more rational approach to differential diagnosis and choice of appropriate therapy.

Disorders Associated with Triglyceride Levels >1,000 mg per dL

Severe hypertriglyceridemia (fasting triglyceride levels >1,000 mg per dL) is virtually always an indication of hyperchylomicronemia in the fasting state and points to an underlying genetic predisposition, often exacerbated by another medical condition or a hormonal or environmental factor. The major clinical complication of severe hypertriglyceridemia is acute pancreatitis, and initial treatment is focused on decreasing the triglycerides below 1,000 mg per

TABLE 3.3 FREDERICKSON AND LEVY CLASSIFICATION OF LIPOPROTEIN PHENOTYPES

Phenotype	Lipoprotein	Triglycerides	Cholesterol	Xanthomas	Pancreatitis	Atherosclerosis	Molecular defects
I	CM	+++	+++	Eruptive	+++	0	LPL, apolipoprotein C-II
IIa	LDL	N	++	Tendon	0	+++	LDL receptor, apolipoprotein B-100
IIb	LDL and VLDL	+	+	None	0	+++	Unknown
III	Remnants	+	++	Palmar and tubero-eruptive	0	++	Apolipoprotein E
IV	VLDL	++	+	None	0	±	Unknown
V	CM and VLDL	+++	+++	Eruptive	+++	±	Unknown

+, mildly elevated; ++, moderately elevated; +++, severely elevated; CM, chylomicron; LDL, low-density lipoprotein; LPL, lipoprotein lipase; N, not affected; VLDL, very-low-density lipoprotein; 0, minimal to no risk.

dL to prevent this serious complication. In addition, some but not all patients with severe hypertriglyceridemia are at risk for premature ASCVD and require more aggressive therapy, even after triglyceride levels have been decreased below the 1,000 mg per dL threshold.

Familial Chylomicronemia Syndrome: Lipoprotein Lipase Deficiency and Apolipoprotein C-II Deficiency

The familial chylomicronemia syndrome (61) is characterized by presentation in childhood with acute pancreatitis and triglyceride levels >1,000 mg per dL. Recurrent abdominal pain is a common feature in children with this disorder. On physical examination, eruptive xanthomas (small papu-

lar lesions that occur in showers on the buttocks and back) are often seen. Lipemia retinalis (a pale appearance to the retinal veins) is a clue to the existence of severe hypertriglyceridemia, and hepatosplenomegaly caused by ingestion of chylomicrons by the reticuloendothelial system is often found. Premature ASCVD is not a feature of this disease.

Two different genetic defects can cause the familial chylomicronemia syndrome: LPL deficiency and apoC-II deficiency (Table 3.4). The hydrolysis of triglycerides in chylomicrons requires the action of LPL in tissue capillary beds, and apoC-II is a required cofactor for the activation of LPL (Fig. 3.1). Mutations in either the LPL gene or the apoC-II gene result in functional deficiency of LPL, inability to hydrolyze triglycerides in chylomicrons, and consequent massive hyperchylomicronemia. The disorder is

TABLE 3.4 PRIMARY LIPID DISORDERS

Genetic disorder	Molecular defect	Lipoproteins elevated	Lipoprotein phenotype	Clinical findings	Genetic transmission	Estimated incidence
Familial chylomicronemia syndrome	LPL deficiency, apolipoprotein C-II deficiency	Chylomicrons	Type I	Eruptive xanthomas, hepatosplenomegaly, pancreatitis	Autosomal recessive	Rare
Familial dysbetalipoproteinemia	Abnormal apolipoprotein E (i.e., 2/2)	Chylomicron and VLDL remnants	Type III	Palmar and tubero-eruptive xanthomas, premature atherosclerosis	Autosomal recessive or autosomal codominant	1/5,000
Familial combined hyperlipidemia	Unknown	VLDL and LDL	Type IIb, sometimes IIa or IV, rarely V	Premature atherosclerosis	Autosomal dominant	1/200
Familial hypertriglyceridemia	Unknown	VLDL, occasionally chylomicrons	Type IV, occasionally V	Usually none	Autosomal dominant	1/500
Familial hepatic lipase deficiency	Hepatic lipase	VLDL remnants	Type III deficiency	Premature atherosclerosis	Autosomal recessive	Rare
Familial hypercholesterolemia	LDL receptor	LDL	Type IIa	Tendon xanthomas, premature atherosclerosis	Autosomal codominant	1/500
Familial defective apolipoprotein B-100	Abnormal apolipoprotein B-100 (i.e., $Arg_{3500} \rightarrow Gln$)	LDL	Type IIa	Tendon xanthomas, premature atherosclerosis	Autosomal codominant	1/700

Arg, arginine; Gln, glutamine; LDL, low-density lipoprotein; LPL, lipoprotein lipase; VLDL, very-low-density lipoprotein.

autosomal recessive, meaning that both alleles of the LPL or apoC-II gene must be affected for the disorder to be present. Therefore, the parents of children with this disorder generally have normal or near normal triglyceride levels. Both are rare disorders, but of the two, LPL deficiency is much more common (approximately 1 case in 1 million persons) than apoC-II deficiency.

The diagnosis of the familial hyperchylomicronemia syndrome is usually made based on clinical presentation and some key laboratory features. The plasma is often lactescent, and after overnight refrigeration, a cake of chylomicrons forms on the surface. Triglyceride levels are >1,000 mg per dL and may be 10,000 mg per dL. Total cholesterol levels are also elevated, due to the presence of cholesterol in chylomicrons. Lipoprotein electrophoresis demonstrates markedly elevated chylomicrons at the origin but is not essential for making the diagnosis. The diagnosis of LPL and apoC-II deficiency can be confirmed at specialized centers by the quantitation of LPL activity in the plasma after intravenous heparin injection (postheparin lipolytic activity). Patients with suspected familial chylomicronemia syndrome should be referred to a specialized lipid center for diagnosis and management of the disorder.

The mainstay of therapy for familial chylomicronemia syndrome is restriction of total dietary fat. Consultation with a registered dietitian familiar with this disorder is essential. Caloric supplementation with medium-chain triglycerides, which are absorbed directly into the portal vein and therefore do not promote chylomicron formation, can be useful. If dietary fat restriction alone is not successful, some patients may respond to a cautious trial of fish oils (62). For patients with apoC-II deficiency, an attack of acute pancreatitis can be treated with infusion of fresh-frozen plasma to provide apoC-II in an attempt to clear severe hypertriglyceridemia and promote resolution of the pancreatitis.

Type V Hyperlipoproteinemia

Type V hyperlipoproteinemia (HLP) is a common diagnosis which continues to use the nomenclature of the Frederickson classification system. The label "type V hyperlipoproteinemia" is generally used to describe the disorder of an adult in whom triglyceride levels are >1,000 mg per dL and who does not have known familial chylomicronemia syndrome caused by LPL or apoC-II deficiency (see above). Type V HLP is also associated with risk of acute pancreatitis, which can be the initial presentation of this syndrome and is the major criterion for aggressive treatment of this condition. Type V HLP can also be associated with increased risk of cardiovascular disease, although some patients with type V HLP do not appear to be at significantly increased risk.

Most but not all patients with type V HLP have a family history of hypertriglyceridemia, although specific genetic mutations causing type V HLP have not yet been

identified. Type II diabetes mellitus or glucose intolerance frequently accompanies type V HLP, but type V HLP also occurs in people who have normal glucose tolerance. Some patients with nephrotic syndrome can develop severe hypertriglyceridemia. Estrogen replacement therapy can exacerbate moderate hypertriglyceridemia and lead to a more severe type V HLP, as can heavy alcohol consumption. Finally, treatment with isotretinoin or etretinate sometimes causes severe hypertriglyceridemia. Rarely, patients with familial dysbetalipoproteinemia (type III hyperlipidemia; see below) due to a mutation in apoE can have triglyceride levels >1,000 mg per dL, particularly if another factor is superimposed on the apoE mutation. The diagnostic evaluation of an adult patient presenting with triglyceride levels >1,000 mg per dL should be focused on a search for underlying predisposing factors and an attempt to establish a history of complications (pancreatitis and cardiovascular disease). A comprehensive personal and family history should be obtained, and all medications should be reviewed. On physical examination, lipemia retinalis and tiny eruptive xanthomas on the back or buttocks are the most specific findings for type V HLP. In contrast, larger tuberoeruptive xanthomas on the elbows or knees or palmar xanthomas (orange coloration to the creases of the palms) are more suggestive of familial dysbetalipoproteinemia (see Familial Dysbetalipoproteinemia, later). Diabetes and renal disease should always be excluded as potential contributing factors. No specific laboratory tests are required for the diagnosis of type V HLP except possibly lipoprotein centrifugation to exclude familial dysbetalipoproteinemia.

The management of type V HLP is first targeted at decreasing triglycerides to reduce the risk of pancreatitis, followed by further lipid lowering depending on the presence of CHD or other risk factors for cardiovascular disease. Women who are taking estrogens and patients taking isotretinoin or etretinate should be encouraged to discontinue these medications if triglyceride levels are >1,000 mg per dL. Diabetes mellitus should be controlled as optimally as possible. Metformin is a useful agent in the treatment of type II diabetes mellitus associated with severe hypertriglyceridemia, because it improves control of diabetes and also has a direct effect in lowering triglyceride levels. Patients should be referred to a registered dietitian for dietary counseling. In general, dietary management includes restriction of total fat as well as simple sugars in the diet. Alcohol should be avoided. Regular aerobic exercise can have a significant impact on triglyceride levels and should be actively encouraged. If the patient is overweight, weight loss can help to decrease triglyceride levels as well.

When fasting triglyceride levels remain >1,000 mg per dL despite institution of appropriate dietary and lifestyle measures and control of secondary causes, drug therapy must be considered to decrease the risk of acute pancreatitis. Drug therapy is usually straightforward, although a subset of patients is remarkably resistant to treatment. Three major drug classes should be considered for treatment of very high triglyceride levels: fibrates, nicotinic acid, and fish oils (see below). In practice, fibrates are generally recommended as the first-line agent. Nicotinic acid or fish oils should be considered for patients who fail to respond adequately to fibrates.

Frequently, patients remain significantly hypercholesterolemic after triglyceride levels are adequately controlled. This raises the difficult question of whether a second medication is needed to better control the LDL cholesterol levels. The NCEP guidelines are useful in making decisions about whether to institute further drug therapy in this setting (9). In patients who have CHD or diabetes mellitus or are at high risk for the development of CHD, who continue to have an LDL cholesterol level >130 mg per dL, most specialists recommend consideration of a second drug (usually a statin). Although it is important to recognize that an increased risk of myopathy is associated with this combination, it can be minimized by careful patient selection and by advising the patient to call the physician immediately in the event of generalized muscle pain.

Disorders Associated with Triglyceride Levels of 200 to 1,000 mg per dL

Fasting triglyceride levels <1,000 mg per dL are not generally associated with risk of acute pancreatitis. Therefore, the significance of elevated triglyceride levels of 200 to 1,000 mg per dL is their potential association with risk of ASCVD. There has been increasing recognition of the importance of elevated fasting triglycerides in this range as an independent cardiovascular risk factor (10). The major primary causes of elevated triglycerides of 200 to 1,000 mg per dL are familial hypertriglyceridemia (FHGT), familial dysbetalipoproteinemia (type III hyperlipidemia), and familial combined hyperlipidemia (FCHL). It is important to differentiate among them, because familial dysbetalipoproteinemia and FCHL are both definitely associated with increased risk of premature atherosclerosis, whereas the risk associated with FHGT is variable. The clinical approach to a patient with triglyceride levels of 200 to 1,000 mg per dL generally involves ruling out secondary causes (and, when they are found, treating them), differentiating among major primary causes, assessing the patient for the presence of ASCVD and other cardiovascular risk factors, and managing the lipid disorder based on the clinical assessment of cardiovascular risk. Because no clinical endpoint trials based on treatment of hypertriglyceridemia have been carried out and no formal guidelines for the clinical management of patients with hypertriglyceridemia are available, the clinical approach to reducing cardiovascular risk is focused on decreasing LDL cholesterol levels. However, elevated triglyceride levels can make the determination of the LDL cholesterol level difficult; can be associated with

increased risk, even in the presence of a normal LDL cholesterol level; and can complicate the therapeutic approach.

Familial Hypertriglyceridemia

FHTG is a relatively common disorder characterized by moderately elevated triglyceride levels, usually with an average or only moderately elevated total cholesterol level. FHTG occurs in approximately 1 in 500 persons. It is inherited as an autosomal dominant trait but is not usually expressed until adulthood. The molecular etiology is unknown. In patients with FHTG, the VLDL level is elevated because of increased production, impaired catabolism, or a combination of the two. The LDL cholesterol level is generally not increased in patients with this disorder. Increased intake of simple carbohydrates, a sedentary lifestyle, obesity, insulin resistance, alcohol use, and estrogens can all exacerbate hypertriglyceridemia.

The diagnosis is suggested by elevated triglyceride levels (200 to 1,000 mg per dL) with normal or only mildly increased cholesterol levels (<240 mg per dL) and almost always a low HDL cholesterol level. A history of hypertriglyceridemia in at least one first-degree relative of the patient is useful in making the diagnosis. It is important to consider and rule out secondary causes of hypertriglyceridemia. In the differential diagnosis, both familial dysbetalipoproteinemia (type III HLP) and FCHL should be considered. This is not simply an academic exercise; these two conditions are associated with a significantly increased risk of ASCVD, whereas FHTG often is not. The total cholesterol level relative to the triglyceride level is usually lower in FHTG, compared with that in familial dysbetalipoproteinemia and FCHL, and the plasma apoB level is usually lower in FHTG than in the other two conditions. Determination of lipoprotein particle size using NMR reveals an increase in VLDL as the major lipoprotein abnormality.

Therapy for FHTG should begin with diet and lifestyle changes. Intake of simple carbohydrates should be reduced. Regular aerobic exercise can be very effective in decreasing triglyceride levels, as can weight loss. Alcohol use should be discouraged. Diabetes mellitus should be aggressively controlled. Lipid-lowering drug therapy can often be avoided if appropriate diet and lifestyle changes are made. However, drug therapy should be considered for patients who have triglyceride levels higher than 400 to 600 mg per dL after an adequate trial of diet and exercise changes. A fibrate is a reasonable choice as a first-line drug for FHTG, and niacin can also be considered in this condition.

Familial Dysbetalipoproteinemia (Type III Hyperlipoproteinemia)

Familial dysbetalipoproteinemia is also commonly called *type III hyperlipidemia* (63). It is the best understood of the genetic lipid disorders that cause moderate elevation of triglyceride levels and can usually be definitively diagnosed based on a combination of clinical and laboratory parameters. Patients with familial dysbetalipoproteinemia usually present in adulthood with distinctive xanthomas or premature atherosclerosis, or asymptomatic hyperlipidemia is discovered on routine screening. Two types of xanthomas are seen in patients with familial dysbetalipoproteinemia. Tuberoeruptive xanthomas begin as clusters of small papules on the elbows, knees, or buttocks and can grow to the size of small grapes. Palmar xanthoma, orange-yellow discoloration of the creases of the palms and wrists, may also be present. Either of these xanthomas is highly suggestive of familial dysbetalipoproteinemia. Premature ASCVD is often seen in this disorder. Compared with other lipid disorders, peripheral vascular disease is particularly common in patients with familial dysbetalipoproteinemia.

The pattern of hyperlipidemia can be another clue to the diagnosis of familial dysbetalipoproteinemia. Patients generally have both hypertriglyceridemia and hypercholesterolemia, and in contrast to most other lipid disorders, the cholesterol and triglyceride levels are often elevated to a relatively similar degree. In addition, the HDL cholesterol level is often relatively normal, in contrast to most hypertriglyceridemic conditions, in which the HDL cholesterol level is usually reduced. Hyperlipidemia can be relatively mild or very severe, depending on the presence of other metabolic conditions and unknown factors.

Familial dysbetalipoproteinemia is caused by mutations in the gene for apoE (63,64). ApoE is present on chylomicron and VLDL remnants and mediates their removal from the plasma by binding to receptors in the liver (Figs. 3.1 and 3.2). Defective apoE is impaired in its ability to bind to these receptors, resulting in accumulation of chylomicron and VLDL remnants in the plasma. The most common form of familial dysbetalipoproteinemia is related to a common polymorphism of apoE. The "normal" form of apoE is known as *apoE3*, but another form, called *apoE2*, has an allele frequency of approximately 7%. The apoE2 protein, which differs from apoE3 by a single amino acid, does not bind adequately to lipoprotein receptors, resulting in defective removal of chylomicron and VLDL remnants. Homozygosity for the E2 allele (the E2/E2 genotype) is the most common cause of familial dysbetalipoproteinemia. However, most persons with the apoE2/E2 genotype do not have familial dysbetalipoproteinemia; development of this disorder appears to require an additional factor. Some of these factors include obesity, diabetes mellitus, hypothyroidism, renal disease, and alcohol use, but many patients with familial dysbetalipoproteinemia do not have an obvious predisposing factor other than the E2/E2 genotype. Another common variant of apoE, known as *apoE4*, has an allele frequency of approximately 14%. Although it is associated with elevated LDL cholesterol levels and increased risk of both CHD and Alzheimer's disease (65),

the common apoE4 allele is not associated with familial dysbetalipoproteinemia. ◆ a62

Because familial dysbetalipoproteinemia is associated with increased risk of premature ASCVD, it should be actively treated. General therapeutic measures include decreased intake of dietary fat, regular aerobic exercise, weight loss (if required), and discontinuance of alcohol use. Postmenopausal women who have familial dysbetalipoproteinemia respond very favorably to estrogen replacement therapy. Although estrogens generally elevate triglyceride levels, familial dysbetalipoproteinemia is unusual in that estrogen replacement often decreases the triglyceride levels. Fibrates and niacin are each very effective in the treatment of familial dysbetalipoproteinemia. HMG-CoA reductase inhibitors have also been used with success, but they may be somewhat less effective than in other forms of hyperlipidemia.

Familial Combined Hyperlipidemia

FCHL is the most common primary lipid disorder, occurring in approximately 1 in 200 persons. Approximately 20% of patients with CHD who are younger than 60 years have FCHL (67). FCHL is characterized by a mixed dyslipidemia, usually associated with moderately elevated fasting triglycerides, moderately elevated cholesterol, and reduced HDL cholesterol. In most cases, at least one first-degree relative also has hyperlipidemia, and there is often a family history of premature CHD as well. Xanthomas are not generally seen in patients with this disorder. Visceral obesity, glucose intolerance, insulin resistance, hypertension, and hyperuricemia are sometimes associated with FCHL. Patients with FCHL almost always have a significantly elevated plasma level of apoB that is disproportionate to the LDL cholesterol level (68). This indicates the presence of small, dense LDL particles, which are characteristic of this syndrome and are considered to be highly atherogenic. The term "hyperapobetalipoproteinemia" has been used to describe the syndrome of elevated apoB with normal lipid levels, and that disorder is probably a subset of FCHL. FCHL is inherited as an autosomal dominant trait and can be expressed in childhood, but it sometimes is not fully expressed until adulthood.

The genetic basis of FCHL is not known. Studies of lipoprotein metabolism in carefully selected individuals have indicated that hepatic overproduction of VLDL is a common metabolic basis of this condition (68). It has been suggested that a subset of patients with the FCHL phenotype may be heterozygous for LPL deficiency, but LPL mutations are probably not a common cause of FCHL (69). It is likely that more than one genetic etiology of the FCHL phenotype exists (70).

The diagnosis of FCHL is suggested by the presence of a mixed hyperlipidemia with fasting triglyceride levels of 200 to 800 mg per dL, cholesterol levels of 200 to 400 mg per dL, and decreased HDL cholesterol levels in the absence of secondary causes of hyperlipidemia. A family history of hyperlipidemia and premature coronary disease is often present and supports the diagnosis. The finding of an apoB level that is elevated relative to the LDL cholesterol level suggests increased levels of small, dense LDL. The size and concentration of LDL can be determined using an NMR technique, which helps confirm the diagnosis and assists in decisions regarding therapy.

Because individuals with FCHL are at significantly increased risk of premature CHD, they should be treated aggressively. Decreased dietary intake of saturated fat and simple carbohydrates, regular aerobic exercise, and weight loss can all have beneficial effects on the lipid profile. However, many patients with FCHL require lipid-lowering drug therapy for adequate control. HMG-CoA reductase inhibitors (statins) are effective in lowering LDL cholesterol and apoB levels. Nicotinic acid decreases both LDL cholesterol and triglyceride levels and raises the HDL cholesterol level, and it is often used in combination with statins for this condition (71).

Disorders Associated with Triglyceride Levels <200 mg per dL

Familial Hypercholesterolemia

Familial hypercholesterolemia (FH) is caused by mutations in the gene for the LDL receptor that prevent its appearance on the cell surface or impair its ability to bind and internalize LDL (73). More than 200 different mutations in the LDL receptor have been described in patients with FH (74). FH is an autosomal codominant disorder, meaning that heterozygotes have hypercholesterolemia but homozygotes have even more severe hypercholesterolemia. The presence of one mutant LDL receptor allele results in the production of only approximately one-half the normal number of LDL receptors, whereas the presence of two mutant alleles severely reduces or eliminates functional LDL receptors. The reduction in functional hepatic LDL receptors leads to reduced clearance of plasma LDL by the liver and substantial elevations in LDL cholesterol. Elevated LDL cholesterol levels lead directly to the major complication of this condition, premature ASCVD.

Heterozygous FH occurs in approximately 1 in 500 persons in North America and worldwide, making it one of the most common single gene disorders. It is characterized by elevated LDL cholesterol levels (usually 200 to 400 mg per dL) with normal triglyceride levels and a family history of hypercholesterolemia or premature cardiovascular disease. The finding of tendon xanthomas is virtually diagnostic of FH (although these can also been seen in another disorder, as discussed later). Tendon xanthomas are most easily recognized within the Achilles tendons, where they cause thickening and irregularity. Another common location for tendon xanthomas is the digit extensor tendons of the metacarpophalangeal joints on the dorsa of the hands. Premature arcus corneae is frequently seen in patients with heterozygous FH. There is no definitive diagnostic test for heterozygous FH; the disorder is diagnosed on clinical grounds.

Heterozygous FH is strongly associated with premature ASCVD, especially CHD. Therefore, patients should be aggressively treated to lower the LDL cholesterol level. Most heterozygous FH patients require lipid-lowering drug therapy. Statins are especially effective in treatment of heterozygous FH, inducing up-regulation of the normal LDL receptor allele in the liver. If further lowering of the LDL level is required, the addition of a bile acid sequestrant to the statin is often beneficial. Niacin is also effective in FH and is often used in combination with statins and resins. The combination of all three drug classes (statin, resin, and niacin) is sometimes required to achieve LDL cholesterol level goals. If combination drug therapy is not tolerated or fails to adequately control the cholesterol levels, LDL apheresis should be considered (75) (see below). ⛴ a63

Familial Defective Apolipoprotein B-100

Familial defective apoB-100 (FDB) resembles heterozygous FH clinically. It is characterized by elevated LDL cholesterol levels with normal triglyceride levels, possible tendon xanthomas, and increased risk of premature ASCVD (79). In contrast to FH, FDB is caused by mutations in the receptor-binding region of apoB-100, the ligand for the LDL receptor, which impairs its binding and delays the clearance of LDL from the blood. The most common mutation that causes FDB is a substitution of glutamine for arginine at position 3500 in apoB-100 (79). However, other mutations have been reported that have a similar effect on binding of apoB to the LDL receptor. FDB is a dominantly inherited disorder and occurs in approximately 1 in 700 persons in Europe and North America.

Patients who have FDB clinically resemble those with heterozygous FH, and these disorders cannot be differentiated on purely clinical grounds. The apoB mutation can be detected in specialized laboratories so that a specific diagnosis of FDB can be made. However, there is no compelling reason to make a specific molecular diagnosis, because the clinical management of patients with FDB is similar to that of patients with heterozygous FH. If future therapies are found that are more effective in one condition than in the other, molecular diagnosis could be indicated to guide specific therapy.

Polygenic Hypercholesterolemia

Most forms of hypercholesterolemia are not single-gene disorders, but rather are caused by a complex interaction of several genetic and environmental factors. For example, genetic differences in cholesterol absorption, cholesterol synthesis, or rates of bile acid synthesis may result in very different cholesterol levels in people challenged with a diet rich in fat. Polygenic hypercholesterolemia is characterized by a cholesterol level exceeding the 95th percentile for age and gender, with triglyceride levels that are usually relatively normal. In polygenic hypercholesterolemia, LDL cholesterol levels are usually not as elevated as they are in heterozygous FH and FDB, and tendon xanthomas are not observed. In the differentiation of polygenic hypercholesterolemia from the these single-gene disorders, family studies are useful. Only approximately 7% of first-degree relatives of patients with polygenic hypercholesterolemia are hypercholesterolemic, whereas approximately one-half of the relatives of patients with FCHL, heterozygous FH, and FDB have dyslipidemia. Treatment of polygenic hypercholesterolemia follows the same guidelines as the approach to any patient with hypercholesterolemia.

DISORDERS OF HIGH-DENSITY LIPOPROTEIN METABOLISM

HDL cholesterol levels are inversely associated with CHD, independent of LDL cholesterol levels. The National Cholesterol Education Program recommends that all adults older than 20 years should be screened not only for total cholesterol levels, but also for HDL cholesterol levels. As a result of screening, patients with low HDL cholesterol levels are frequently identified. However, formal guidelines for the approach to the patient with a low HDL cholesterol level have not yet been developed. Many causes of low HDL cholesterol are secondary to other factors. Cigarette smoking, obesity, and physical inactivity contribute to a low HDL cholesterol. Type II diabetes mellitus, end-stage renal disease, and hypertriglyceridemia from any cause are all associated with low HDL. Beta-blockers, thiazide diuretics, androgens, and progestins can all reduce HDL cholesterol levels. Importantly, a low-fat diet often results in a low level of HDL cholesterol; for example, most vegetarians have low levels of HDL cholesterol. In this case, the low HDL is not considered to be associated with an increased risk of CHD, because persons who eat low-fat diets are at substantially reduced risk of premature CHD. However, many persons with low HDL cholesterol levels have a genetic cause for the low HDL cholesterol. Only a few of the genes responsible for inherited syndromes associated with low HDL levels have been identified (*e*Table 3.4.1).

SCREENING AND MANAGEMENT OF PATIENTS WITH LIPID DISORDERS

Screening

A general approach to the screening and management of hyperlipidemia has been developed by an expert panel con-

TABLE 3.5 CLASSIFICATION BASED ON TOTAL, LDL, AND HDL CHOLESTEROL LEVELS

Cholesterol (mg/dL)	Classification
Total	
<200	Desirable
200–239	Borderline high
≥240	High
LDL	
<100	Optimal
100–129	Near or above optimal
130–159	Borderline high
160–189	High
≥190	Very high
HDL	
<40	Low
≥60	High

HDL, high-density lipoprotein; LDL, low-density lipoprotein.

vened by the NCEP of the National Institutes of Health, and the original recommendations (92) underwent one revision in 1993 and another revision in 2001 (9). These guidelines have been widely endorsed by other professional organizations, including the American Heart Association and the American College of Cardiology (26). Alternative screening guidelines issued by the American College of Physicians (93,94) were based on a number of tenuous assumptions and have not been widely accepted.

All adults older than 20 years should be screened through measurement of fasting total, LDL cholesterol, HDL cholesterol, and triglyceride levels. The initial classification according to the NCEP-ATPIII guidelines is described in Table 3.5.

The LDL cholesterol is usually estimated from the other lipid values using the following equation: LDL cholesterol = total cholesterol − (triglycerides/5) − HDL cholesterol. (Because VLDL usually contains triglyceride and cholesterol in a ratio of approximately 5:1, "triglycerides/5" is an estimate of the VLDL cholesterol). This formula is reasonably accurate if test results are obtained from fasting plasma and if the triglyceride level is less than 400 mg per dL. The determination of LDL cholesterol levels in patients who have triglyceride levels >400 mg per dL usually requires application of ultracentrifugal techniques in specialized laboratories, although direct assays for LDL measurement have recently become available. All further evaluation and treatment is based on other cardiovascular risk factors (Table 3.6) and the LDL cholesterol level (Table 3.7).

Diagnosis and Classification of Lipid Disorders

Most patients with hyperlipidemia have a primary or genetic cause for the lipid disorder. However, the clinician should always first consider whether a secondary medical disorder could be causing or contributing to the hyperlipidemia. Treatment of the underlying medical condition can

TABLE 3.6 MAJOR CARDIOVASCULAR RISK FACTORS TO CONSIDER IN THE TREATMENT OF LOW-DENSITY LIPOPROTEIN CHOLESTEROL

Age
  Men ≥45 yr
  Women ≥55 yr
Family history of premature CHD (CHD in male first-degree relative ≤55 yr or female first-degree relative ≤65 yr)
Cigarette smoking
Hypertension
Low high-density lipoprotein cholesterol[a]

CHD, coronary heart disease.
[a]If the high-density lipoprotein cholesterol is ≥60 mg/dL, subtract one risk factor.
Note: Diabetes mellitus is considered a CHD risk equivalent; see Table 3.7.

often result in substantial improvement in the lipid profile and obviate the need for therapy directed at the lipids themselves. Once secondary causes have been considered, the fasting triglyceride level can be used as an initial method of stratifying patients. This approach guides both the initial diagnostic evaluation and the selection of the most effective therapy. It is important to consider the differential diagnosis of hyperlipidemia before treatment is started, because the inherited disorders discussed earlier are associated with different risks of developing CHD, different responses to drug therapy, and differences in family and genetic history.

Although extremely elevated triglyceride levels (>1,000 mg per dL) are associated with a risk of acute pancreatitis, the most important clinical consequence of lipid disorders is ASCVD, including coronary, cerebrovascular, and peripheral vascular disease. The clinical approach to a patient with a lipid disorder is significantly influenced by the presence of established ASCVD and other risk factors. Treatment of hyperlipidemia in patients with ASCVD is called *secondary prevention*, whereas treatment in patients without established ASCVD is known as *primary prevention*.

Management of lipid disorders should be based, whenever possible, on clinical trials that indicate the benefit of treatment in decreasing the risk of cardiovascular morbidity and death, although reasonable extrapolation of these data to specific subgroups is sometimes required (95). LDL cholesterol levels are strongly associated with increased risk of cardiovascular disease, and abundant data exist to show that treatment aimed at lowering LDL levels decreases the risk of clinical cardiovascular events in both secondary and primary prevention (51). Elevated triglyceride levels are also associated with increased risk of cardiovascular disease, but this relationship weakens considerably when statistical corrections are made for LDL and HDL cholesterol levels (96). Furthermore, no trials have been performed specifically to determine whether treatment to decrease triglyceride levels decreases the risk of cardiovascular disease. HDL cholesterol levels are inversely associated with cardiovascular disease, but no clinical trial data exist to date indicating that treatment aimed at elevating HDL levels leads to decreased risk of cardiovascular disease events. However, elevated triglyceride levels, decreased HDL cholesterol levels, or both are important clues to the existence of a lipid disorder and can help to identify individuals who may be at higher risk of cardiovascular disease and therefore are candidates for more aggressive therapy aimed at lowering the LDL cholesterol level. The clinical management of lipid disorders is a major component of an overall strategy directed toward the treatment or prevention of complications related to ASCVD. Some general guidelines for the nonpharmacologic management of patients with lipid disorders are given in the next section.

General Issues in the Nonpharmacologic Management of Lipid Disorders

Identify and Treat Secondary Causes of Hyperlipidemia

Secondary causes of hypercholesterolemia should be considered and excluded with appropriate laboratory testing. Many lipid experts recommend routine screening of all hyperlipidemic patients with a thyroid stimulating hormone to exclude hypothyroidism. Treatment of hypothyroidism usually results in substantial improvement in hypercholesterolemia. A fasting glucose level should always be obtained in the initial workup of a patient with hyperlipidemia. Diabetes mellitus should be controlled as effectively as possible, which often results in substantial improvement in hyperlipidemia. Nephrotic syndrome and chronic renal insufficiency should be excluded if they are clinically suspected. Patients with hyperlipidemia, especially hypertriglyceridemia, who drink alcohol should be encouraged to decrease their intake.

TABLE 3.7 LOW-DENSITY LIPOPROTEIN CHOLESTEROL (LDL-C) GOALS AND CUTPOINTS FOR THERAPY

Risk category	LDL-C Goal (mg/dL)	Lifestyle therapy (mg/dL)	Drug therapy (mg/dL)
CHD or CHD risk equivalent (10-yr risk >20%)	<100	≥100	≥130 (100–130 optional)
2+ risk factors (10-yr risk 10–20%)	<130	≥130	≥130
2+ risk factors (10-yr risk <10%)	<130	≥130	≥160
0–1 risk factors	<160	≥160	≥190 (160–190 optional)

CHD, coronary heart disease.

TABLE 3.8 DIETARY GUIDELINES FOR MANAGING HYPERCHOLESTEROLEMIA

Dietary constituent	Step I diet	Step II diet
Total fat	<30% of total calories	<30% of total calories
Saturated fatty acids	<10% of total calories	<7% of total calories
Polyunsaturated fatty acids	<10% of total calories	<10% of total calories
Monounsaturated fatty acids	10–15% of total calories	10–15% of total calories
Carbohydrates	50–60% of total calories	50–60% of total calories
Protein	10–20% of total calories	10–20% of total calories
Cholesterol	<300 mg/day	<200 mg/day
Total calories	As required to achieve and maintain desired body weight	As required to achieve and maintain desired body weight

Sedentary lifestyle, obesity, and smoking are all associated with low HDL cholesterol levels.

Counsel Patients on an Appropriate Diet

Dietary modification is an important component of the effective management of patients with lipid disorders. It is important for the physician to make a general assessment of the patient's diet, to provide suggestions for improvement, and to recognize whether a patient may benefit from referral to a dietitian for more intensive counseling. The dietary approach depends on the type of hyperlipidemia. For predominant hypercholesterolemia, the major approach is restriction of saturated fat intake. For moderate hypertriglyceridemia, it is also important to restrict intake of simple sugars. For severe hypertriglyceridemia reflecting hyperchylomicronemia, restriction of total fat intake is critical.

To lower the LDL cholesterol level by diet modification, restricting the intake of saturated fats and cholesterol is necessary. The most widely used diet is the "step I diet" developed by the American Heart Association (Table 3.8). If possible, the patient should receive specific instruction in the diet from a dietitian or qualified professional. Periodic review of the diet may be needed to reinforce the need for its continued use. Responses to a step I diet vary widely among individuals, and it can be difficult to predict which persons are most likely to benefit from dietary intervention. However, the majority of patients has relatively modest (<10%) decreases in LDL cholesterol levels on a step I diet. If therapeutic goals for LDL cholesterol are not reached after 3 to 6 months on a step I diet, the patient may be referred to a registered dietitian for more detailed dietary instruction, including the introduction of a step II diet, which is further restricted in total and saturated fat (Table 3.7). Patients with established ASCVD should be instructed on how to maintain a step II diet from the first. Almost all persons experience a decrease in HDL cholesterol levels when they decrease the amount of total and saturated fat in their diets. Patients should be reassured that a low-fat diet is beneficial in terms of reducing overall cardiovascular risk. For patients with hypertriglyceridemia, dietary counseling should also include restriction of simple sugar intake. Treatment of severe hypertriglyceridemia (triglyceride levels >1,000 mg per dL) includes restriction of all fat intake, both saturated and unsaturated.

Certain types of foods and dietary additives can be used to modestly reduce cholesterol levels and in some cases obviate the need for drug therapy. Plant stanol esters were shown to reduce LDL cholesterol levels in randomized controlled trials when the esters are taken three times per day (97); are not absorbed; and are available in a variety of foods, such as spreads, salad dressings, and snack bars under the trade label Benecol. Plant sterol esters also can reduce LDL cholesterol but have not been as extensively studied, and they can be absorbed, so they are not as desirable an option. Chinese red yeast rice has been shown to reduce LDL cholesterol levels and is known to contain small amounts of lovastatin, which probably accounts for its modest cholesterol-lowering properties. Addition of psyllium to the diet can reduce cholesterol levels. Soy protein has been shown to reduce cholesterol levels. Certain types of nuts, such as walnuts, have been shown to reduce cholesterol levels, but this approach requires the daily consumption of a very large amount of nuts and is not practical. Despite some enthusiasm, controlled trials of garlic have not demonstrated a significant cholesterol-lowering effect. Other herbal approaches, such as gugulipid, are interesting but require further study. No controlled studies have been carried out that combined several of these nonpharmacologic options to address their additive or synergistic effects.

Encourage Regular Aerobic Exercise

Regular aerobic exercise can have a positive effect on lipids. Elevated triglyceride levels are especially sensitive to aerobic exercise, and persons with hypertriglyceridemia can substantially lower their triglyceride levels by initiating an exercise program. The effect of exercise on LDL cholesterol levels is more modest. Although aerobic exercise is widely believed to raise HDL cholesterol levels, the effects on HDL are relatively modest in most individuals. Patients should also be reminded that aerobic exercise has cardiovascular benefits that extend well beyond its effect on lipid levels (98).

Encourage the Patient to Achieve and Maintain an Appropriate Weight

Obesity is often associated with dyslipidemia, especially with elevated triglyceride levels, low HDL cholesterol levels, and small, dense LDL levels. In individuals who are overweight, weight loss can have a significant favorable impact on the lipid profile and should be actively encouraged. In addition to providing counseling on other dietary issues, a dietitian should advise patients about the caloric restriction necessary for effective weight loss.

Consider Hormone Replacement Therapy in Postmenopausal Women

The effects of hormone replacement therapy (HRT) on lipid metabolism are complex (99). HRT generally decreases LDL cholesterol levels and modestly increases HDL cholesterol levels. However, HRT raises triglyceride levels, and, in women with underlying triglyceride disorders, can precipitate severe hyperchylomicronemia and acute pancreatitis. Therefore, HRT is relatively contraindicated in women with triglyceride levels >500 mg per dL, until the triglyceride levels are better controlled. When triglyceride levels are between 250 and 500 mg per dL, estrogens can be administered cautiously, but triglyceride levels should be monitored carefully. One exception to this rule is in women with type III HLP, in whom estrogen replacement can substantially improve the lipid profile, including the triglyceride levels. HRT also decreases levels of lipoprotein (a) [Lp(a)] in women (100).

The relationship of HRT to cardiovascular risk has been the topic of substantial debate. On the basis of observational data, HRT was believed to confer substantial cardiovascular benefit associated with an approximately 50% reduction in clinical cardiovascular disease events (101). However, randomized controlled trials with estrogen replacement have not duplicated the positive results seen in observational studies. Both the Heart and Estrogen/Progestin Study clinical outcome trial (102) and an angiographic study (103) have failed to show a benefit of combination estrogen/ progestin HRT in secondary prevention. Therefore, prospective studies do not support a role for HRT in the secondary prevention of cardiovascular disease, at least over the short to medium term. However, many experts feel that estrogen replacement may still have a clinical role, especially in primary prevention. Understanding of the long-term role of HRT and the effect of HRT in primary prevention of cardiovascular disease awaits the results of ongoing studies, including the Women's Health Initiative Study of >50,000 asymptomatic postmenopausal women (104).

Drug Therapy for Lipid Disorders

Deciding to Initiate Drug Therapy for Dyslipidemia

The decision to use drug therapy is highly dependent on whether established CHD is present and, if it is not, on the global cardiovascular risk of the patient. Drug therapy for hypercholesterolemia in patients with established CHD is well supported by clinical trial data. Randomized controlled clinical trials have demonstrated conclusively that lowering LDL cholesterol levels in patients with established CHD reduces not only cardiovascular events and CHD mortality rates but also the total mortality rate after only 5 years. Even patients with CHD who have average LDL cholesterol levels benefit from treatment. Drug treatment to lower LDL cholesterol levels in patients with CHD is also highly cost-effective (21,105). Current guidelines (9) call for drug therapy in all patients who have established CHD and LDL cholesterol levels >130 mg per dL (9,26), with consideration given to treating patients with LDL cholesterol levels 100 to 130 mg per dL (Table 3.7). Based on these guidelines, the majority of patients with established CHD should be treated with cholesterol-lowering drug therapy. Nevertheless, it has been estimated that at least 50% of patients who have CHD are not receiving cholesterol-lowering drug therapy (106).

The decision to initiate lipid-lowering drug therapy in primary prevention is more difficult. However, data now exist that demonstrate a substantial benefit with drug therapy, even in individuals without preexisting CHD. Therefore, persons at high risk for the development of cardiovascular disease are excellent candidates for lipid-modifying drug therapy. For example, patients with diabetes mellitus have a level of absolute cardiovascular risk that is similar to that of patients with established CHD (107). Therefore, lipid disorders in diabetic patients should be treated as aggressively as in patients with established CHD; the NCEP, the American Heart Association, the American College of Cardiology, and the American Diabetes Association all have endorsed this view. Absolute global cardiovascular risk can be quantitated using a simple approach based on the Framingham Heart Study database (108) and used as a guide in the decision about whether to initiate cholesterol-lowering drug therapy. A 10-year risk of less than 20% should be considered a "CHD risk equivalent," and such patients should be treated like those with CHD or diabetes targeting the LDL to <100 mg per dL (Table 3.7). Drug therapy should be used for most individuals who have markedly elevated LDL cholesterol levels (>190 mg per dL), even if the short-term absolute risk is not particularly elevated. However, it is often difficult to decide whether to initiate drug therapy in patients who have LDL cholesterol levels that are in the gray zone between 130 and 190 mg per dL. Although it is desirable to avoid drug treatment in patients who are unlikely to develop CHD, a very high proportion of patients who eventually develop CHD have LDL cholesterol levels in this range (23). Therefore, the use of certain blood and vascular imaging tests may be useful in helping to refine the risk assessment, and therefore the decision about drug therapy (see below). In persons considered to be at low risk, the emphasis should remain primarily on dietary and lifestyle modification.

In certain patients, drug therapy should be targeted initially toward reduction of triglyceride levels rather than the

LDL cholesterol level. For example, when triglyceride levels are >1,000 mg per dL, the patient has a primary triglyceride disorder and should be treated with drug therapy to prevent acute pancreatitis. When triglyceride levels are 400 to 1,000 mg per dL, the decision to use drug therapy depends on the assessment of cardiovascular risk; however, if drug therapy is used, it should usually be targeted first at reducing the triglyceride levels, because cholesterol reduction is difficult in the setting of substantially elevated triglycerides. Importantly, all of the five major clinical endpoint trials with statins have excluded persons with triglyceride levels >350 to 450 mg per dL. Therefore, no data are available regarding the effectiveness of statins in reducing cardiovascular risk in persons with triglyceride levels greater than approximately 400 mg per dL. If the triglyceride levels are <400 mg per dL, the initial emphasis in treatment should be on reduction of the LDL cholesterol level, not the triglyceride levels.

In general, a low level of HDL cholesterol justifies the use of more aggressive therapy to decrease an elevated LDL cholesterol level. In AFCAPS/TexCAPS, subjects were recruited in part on the basis of relatively low HDL cholesterol levels, and individuals with the lowest HDL cholesterol levels at baseline had the highest relative risk reduction with lovastatin therapy (109). Drug therapy targeted primarily toward raising HDL cholesterol is a potentially important strategy for reducing cardiovascular events. The VA-HIT study has provided data to support the initiation of pharmacologic therapy in patients in whom LDL cholesterol levels are con-

trolled but HDL cholesterol levels are low. More data are required before broad recommendations are made about the use of drug therapy targeted specifically toward raising HDL cholesterol levels to prevent cardiovascular events.

Choosing a Lipid-Lowering Drug

Once the decision to initiate drug therapy has been made, the drug must be chosen. A summary of the major drugs for treating dyslipidemia is provided in Table 3.9, and the major classes of drugs are discussed here.

3-Hydroxy-3-Methylglutaryl Coenzyme A Reductase Inhibitors (Statins)

HMG-CoA reductase is the rate-limiting step in cholesterol biosynthesis, and inhibition of this enzyme decreases cholesterol synthesis. There are five HMG-CoA reductase inhibitors currently available: lovastatin (Mevacor), pravastatin (Pravachol), simvastatin (Zocor), fluvastatin (Lescol), and atorvastatin (Lipitor). By inhibiting cholesterol biosynthesis, these drugs lead to increased hepatic LDL receptor expression and in some situations to decreased hepatic production of VLDL as well. Their major effect is reduction of LDL cholesterol, which they do in a dose-dependent fashion. There is wide interindividual variation in the initial response to statins, but once a patient is on a statin, the doubling of the statin dose produces a very predictable 6% further reduction in LDL cholesterol (110). Statins also reduce triglyceride levels in a dose-dependent fashion

TABLE 3.9 MAJOR DRUGS USED FOR THE TREATMENT OF HYPERLIPIDEMIA

Drug	Major indications	Starting dose	Maximal dose	Mechanism	Common side effects
HMG-CoA reductase inhibitors	Elevated LDL			Inhibit cholesterol synthesis and up-regulate LDL receptors in liver	Myositis, arthralgias, GI upset, elevated liver function tests
Lovastatin		20 mg daily	80 mg daily		
Pravastatin		10 mg qhs	40 mg qhs		
Simvastatin		10 mg qhs	40 mg qhs		
Fluvastatin		20 mg qhs	40 mg qhs		
Atorvastatin		20 mg qhs	80 mg qhs		
Cerivastatin		0.2 mg qhs	0.8 mg qhs		
Bile acid sequestrants	Elevated LDL			Promote bile acid excretion and increase LDL receptors in liver	Bloating, constipation, elevated triglycerides
Cholestyramine		4 g daily	As tolerated		
Colestipol		5 g daily	As tolerated		
Colesevelam		3.75 g daily	As tolerated		
Nicotinic acid	Elevated LDL and triglycerides, low HDL			Decrease VLDL synthesis	Cutaneous flushing, GI upset, elevated glucose, uric acid, transaminases
Immediate-release		100 mg t.i.d.	1,000 mg t.i.d.		
Sustained-release (Niaspan)		500 mg qhs	2,000 mg qhs		
Fibric acid derivatives	Elevated triglycerides			Stimulate lipoprotein lipase, may decrease VLDL synthesis	Myositis, GI upset, gallstones
Gemfibrozil		600 mg b.i.d.	600 mg b.i.d.		
Fenofibrate		200 mg qd	200 mg qd		
Fish oils	Elevated triglycerides	3 g daily	12 g daily	Decrease triglyceride synthesis	Diarrhea, GI upset, fishy odor to breath

GI, gastrointestinal; HDL, high-density lipoprotein; HMG-CoA, 3-hydroxy-3-methylglutaryl coenzyme A; LDL, low-density lipoprotein; VLDL, very-low-density lipoprotein.

that is proportional to their effect in decreasing LDL cholesterol levels. Statins have a modest effect in increasing HDL cholesterol levels by 5% to 10% that is not dose dependent. As was reviewed earlier, considerable evidence of efficacy of statins in reducing the risk of clinical cardiovascular events is now available.

Patient acceptance of these drugs is high, because they can be taken in tablet form once a day and are generally well tolerated. Potential side effects include gastrointestinal upset, headaches, sleep disturbance, fatigue, and muscle or joint pains. Severe myopathy and even rhabdomyolysis have been reported with HMG-CoA reductase inhibitors, but these side effects are very rare. The risk of statin-associated myopathy is increased by the administration of drugs that interfere with the cytochrome P450 metabolism of statins, such as erythromycin, and related antibiotics, antifungal agents, immunosuppressive drugs, and fibrates. Severe myopathy can usually be avoided by carefully selecting the patients who will receive treatment with statins, by avoiding interacting drugs, and by informing patients of the potential of severe myopathy and advising immediate discontinuance of the drug in the event of new generalized muscle pain. Serum creatine kinase (CK) levels need not be monitored on a routine basis, because an elevated serum CK level in the absence of symptoms does not predict the development of myopathy and does not suggest the need for discontinuing the drug. The serum CK level can be measured in a patient who is taking a statin and complains of muscle pain, but a normal level does not exclude the possibility that the symptoms are caused by the drug. By convention, liver transaminases (alanine aminotransferase and aspartate aminotransferase) are monitored in patients taking statins (for example, 8 weeks after initiation of the drug and every 6 months thereafter). Other liver function tests, such as those for alkaline phosphatase and gamma glutamyl transpeptidase, are not useful and need not be used to monitor the patient. Substantial elevation (more than three times normal levels) in transaminases is relatively rare, and mild to moderate elevation (one to three times normal levels) in transaminases in the absence of symptoms need not mandate discontinuation of the medication. Severe clinical hepatitis associated with statins is exceedingly rare, if it occurs at all, and the trend is toward less-frequent monitoring of transaminases in patients taking statins.

A careful review of the five major trials with statins indicates a high level of safety (111). These five trials included a total of more than 30,000 subjects, one-half of whom were treated with active statin therapy for an average of 5 to 6 years. A review of this experience demonstrates that the incidence of suicide and fatal trauma did not differ between the patients being treated with statin and those receiving placebo. Likewise, the incidence of cancer did not differ between the two groups.

Bile Acid Sequestrants (Resins)

Bile acid sequestrants include cholestyramine (Questran), colestipol (Colestid), and colesevelam (WelChol). They bind bile acids in the intestine, interrupt their enterohepatic circulation, and accelerate the loss of bile acids in the stool. To maintain an adequate bile acid pool, the liver diverts cholesterol to bile acid synthesis. The decreased intracellular cholesterol content results in up-regulation of the hepatic LDL receptor and enhanced LDL clearance from the plasma. Bile acid sequestrants primarily reduce LDL cholesterol levels and should not be prescribed for patients with triglyceride levels higher than approximately 300 mg per dL, because this exacerbates hypertriglyceridemia. The bile acid sequestrants are very safe drugs that are not systemically absorbed. However, cholestyramine and colestipol are insoluble resins that must be suspended in liquid and are therefore often inconvenient and unpleasant to take. Colestipol is also available in large tablets, but multiple tablets must be taken each day to achieve a substantial effect. The newest bile acid sequestrant, colesevelam, was designed to combat the limitations of the traditional resins by providing a molecule able to bind a larger number of bile acids. Colesevelam is available in smaller tablets than colestipol, and because it binds more bile acids per molecule, fewer tablets are required each day to achieve the desired effect. Most side effects of resins are limited to the gastrointestinal tract; bloating and constipation can occur and are ultimately dose limiting. In addition, bile acid sequestrants may bind some other drugs (e.g., digoxin and warfarin) and interfere with their absorption, so that other medications must be taken 1 hour before or 4 hours after the bile acid sequestrants are taken.

Bile acid sequestrants can be useful in young, highly motivated patients with moderate hypercholesterolemia who wish to avoid systemic drug therapy. These are also the cholesterol-lowering drug of choice in children and in women who are pregnant, could become pregnant, or are lactating. Bile acid sequestrants are especially effective in combination therapy, and their major clinical role has evolved to use in combination with HMG-CoA reductase inhibitors, with which they are synergistic in the reduction of LDL cholesterol.

Nicotinic Acid (Niacin)

Nicotinic acid, or niacin, is a B-complex vitamin that in high doses is a lipid-lowering drug. Niacin reduces triglyceride and LDL cholesterol levels and is the most effective of the available lipid-modifying drugs in raising HDL cholesterol. Niacin is also the only lipid-lowering drug currently available that decreases Lp(a) levels (34–37). Its safety and efficacy were documented in the Coronary Drug Project, which demonstrated a modest benefit to the use of niacin to reduce nonfatal MI after 6 years of treatment (14) and a decrease in the total mortality rate after 15 years of follow-up (15).

The use of immediate-release crystalline niacin has been limited by the occurrence of cutaneous flushing. However, with proper administration and patient education, flushing can be minimized. The starting dose of immediate-release niacin should usually be 100 mg three times per day and always at the end of meals. Food delays the absorption and makes it much easier to tolerate with less flushing. Patients should be told to expect some flushing initially but that it will improve quickly with continued administration. Every 4 to 7 days, the dosage should be increased by 100 mg per dose, eventually reaching 500 mg three times per day. After 1 month of treatment with this dose, lipid and other pertinent levels (e.g., glucose, uric acid, and liver transaminases) should be measured. It is frequently necessary to increase the dose to 3 g per day to achieve a substantial beneficial effect on lipid levels. Rarely, immediate-release niacin is used in doses of up to 4.5 g per day. Despite adherence to the dosing protocol, some patients may continue to have flushing with certain doses (often the morning dose) and may benefit from taking aspirin 30 minutes before the niacin.

Sustained-release forms of niacin are associated with less flushing and therefore are better tolerated. However, the use of over-the-counter sustained-release niacin preparations, which are usually administered twice a day, has been limited because of several cases of severe hepatotoxicity. Niaspan is a prescription sustained-release niacin that is administered once daily at bedtime. Niaspan is better tolerated than immediate-release crystalline niacin and is probably safer than over-the-counter sustained-release niacin because of its pharmacokinetics, the once-a-day dosing, and superior quality control. In one study, Niaspan decreased triglyceride levels by 29% and increased HDL cholesterol levels by 26% at a dose of 2 g (112). Niaspan has also been directly compared to gemfibrozil and had a significantly greater effect on HDL cholesterol levels (increase of 26%), compared with 1,200 mg of gemfibrozil (increase of 13%), although gemfibrozil had a more pronounced effect on triglyceride levels (decrease of 40%) than Niaspan (decrease of 29%) (113).

Use of niacin can be limited by side effects other than flushing. It has been associated with elevation in uric acid and precipitation of gouty attacks and can also exacerbate peptic ulcer disease and symptoms of gastroesophageal reflux. Mild elevations in transaminases occur in as many as 15% of treated patients, but these elevations rarely require cessation of treatment with the medication. Niacin potentiates the effect of warfarin and should be used cautiously for patients taking warfarin. Acanthosis nigricans, a dark-colored, coarse skin lesion, is a rare side effect of niacin that is not dangerous but can be bothersome.

Niacin can elevate fasting glucose in patients with diabetes and therefore has traditionally been avoided in the treatment regimens of these patients. However, the Arterial Disease Multiple Intervention Trial confirmed the benefits of short-acting niacin and extended the safety and efficacy of this therapy to patients with diabetes (114). In this study, niacin given at an average dose of 2,500 mg per day resulted an increase in HDL cholesterol of 29% and a decrease in triglycerides of 25% in patients with and without diabetes. Interestingly, although patients with diabetes who were treated with niacin had a small increase in fasting glucose, their glycosylated hemoglobin levels did not change from baseline but were 0.3% higher than those in patients with diabetes who received placebo. No changes in hypoglycemic agents were required during the 48-week follow-up period.

Successful therapy with niacin requires careful education and motivation on the part of the patient. Its advantages are its low cost, long-term safety, and efficacy in treatment of combined hyperlipidemia and in raising HDL cholesterol levels. It is particularly useful in the secondary prevention of CHD in motivated patients who have combined hyperlipidemia and low HDL levels. Niacin can also be used successfully in combination with bile acid sequestrants and statins. In particular, patients already receiving a statin who require further LDL cholesterol reduction, in whom triglyceride levels remain elevated, or who have low HDL cholesterol levels can benefit substantially from the addition of niacin to treatment regimen (71).

Fibric Acid Derivatives (Fibrates)

Fibric acid derivatives, or fibrates, are agonists of peroxisome proliferator–activated receptor-α, a nuclear hormone receptor involved in metabolic regulation (35). This class includes clofibrate (Atromid-S), gemfibrozil (Lopid), fenofibrate (TriCor), and bezafibrate (not available in the United States). Fibrates work by activating peroxisome proliferator–activated receptor-α to stimulate LPL activity (enhancing triglyceride hydrolysis), reduce apoC-III synthesis (enhancing lipoprotein remnant clearance), and possibly reduce VLDL production. Fibrates decrease triglyceride levels effectively (up to 40%) and generally increase HDL cholesterol levels modestly (up to 15%), but they have less ability to decrease LDL cholesterol levels.

The most straightforward clinical role of fibrates is in the treatment of severe hypertriglyceridemia to prevent acute pancreatitis. They are also highly effective in patients who have type III HLP. Fibrates are first-line agents for individuals with triglyceride levels >400 to 600 mg per dL who need drug therapy. The role of fibrates in the treatment of dyslipidemia for prevention of cardiovascular disease is supported by the Helsinki Heart Study and the more recent VA-HIT trial. Additional clinical endpoint trials with fibrates are under way.

Fibrates are generally well tolerated; the most common side effect is dyspepsia, which occurred in 6% more patients receiving treatment with fibrates than patients receiving placebo in the VA-HIT study. Myopathy has occurred, but in the absence of treatment with other drugs, it is very rare. In both the VA-HIT and BIP studies no statistically different occurrence of muscle complaints was seen between the group of patients receiving fibrates and those receiving placebo. Elevated results of liver function tests can also occur, but the frequency of elevations in transaminases more than three times the upper limit of normal was no different among patients receiving fibrates than those receiving placebo in both the VA-HIT and the BIP trials. Fibrates have also been associated with an increased risk of gallstones, but this was not seen in VA-HIT over the course of 5 years. Fibrates can potentiate the effect of warfarin and interact with certain oral hypoglycemic agents. In the World Health Organization study (37), clofibrate was associated with an increase in gastrointestinal tumors and in the total mortality rate, and therefore clofibrate is rarely used.

Omega-3 Fatty Acids (Fish Oils)

Ω-3 Polyunsaturated fatty acids (Ω-3 PUFAs) are useful tools in the management of severe hypertriglyceridemia. Ω-3 PUFAs are found naturally in high concentrations in fish and in flax seeds, and their use in the form of concentrated fish-oil capsules has been at the center of active investigation. Both epidemiologic and experimental studies have demonstrated the benefit of dietary fish intake and concentrated fish oils in the management of CHD (115). Most of the attention has been focused on the two active molecules in fish oil, eicosapentanoic acid (EPA) and decohexanoic acid (DHA).

Ω-3 PUFAs in doses of 3 to 6 g per day consistently decrease fasting and postprandial triglyceride levels (116). Fish oils are useful as a third-line therapy for patients who have severe hypertriglyceridemia that is resistant to fibrates and niacin or who are intolerant of these drugs. At least 6 g per day is usually required for a substantial effect, and many patients require 9 to 12 g per day. Fish oils should not be used to treat hypercholesterolemia and have been reported to raise LDL cholesterol levels. Interestingly, a large randomized controlled trial demonstrated that one fish-oil capsule daily was associated with a significant reduction in cardiovascular events (117). ▼ a64

Combination Drug Therapy

Some patients with dyslipidemia may require therapy with more than one drug. Patients with FH often have difficulty achieving LDL cholesterol goals with a statin alone but respond very well to the addition of a bile acid sequestrant. In some cases, the addition of niacin to this regimen is required for further decreases in LDL levels (71). Patients with FCHL can often reach their LDL cholesterol goal with a statin alone but frequently have persistent moderate hypertriglyceridemia, low HDL cholesterol levels, or both. In this situation, the addition of niacin to the statin can be highly effective in reducing the triglycerides and increasing the level of HDL cholesterol (71,118). Many patients with triglyceride levels higher than 400 to 600 mg per dL require initial therapy with a fibrate to decrease the triglyceride levels, but once the triglycerides are reduced, the LDL cholesterol often remains elevated. In this situation, the addition of a statin to the fibrate is effective in decreasing the level of LDL cholesterol. Although the risk of myopathy with this combination is a concern, it can be minimized with appropriate patient selection and education (118). Patients should be told of the potential for myopathy and advised to stop the medication and call their physician in the event of unexplained or generalized muscle pain. Practicing physicians are encouraged to consider combination therapy in appropriate high-risk patients or consider referring patients who may benefit from such therapy to a specialized lipid center.

Approaches to Reducing Cholesterol When Drugs Are Not Tolerated or Are Ineffective

Some patients cannot tolerate any of the existing lipid-lowering drugs at the doses required for adequate control of their lipid levels. A larger group of patients, most of whom have genetic lipid disorders, remain significantly hypercholesterolemic despite combination drug therapy. These patients, many of whom already have established CHD, are at high risk for disease progression and clinical events and should be referred to a specialized lipid center. The approaches discussed in the next sections have been used or are being developed for use in such patients.

Partial Ileal Bypass

Partial ileal bypass was developed as a surgical procedure to decrease LDL cholesterol levels in the 1960s (119). Like the mechanism of the bile acid sequestrants, partial ileal bypass interrupts the enterohepatic circulation of bile acids, resulting in up-regulation of the hepatic LDL receptor. One controlled trial of partial ileal bypass in moderately hypercholesterolemic patients who had established CHD demonstrated a 38% decrease in LDL cholesterol and a 35% decrease in the combined end point of nonfatal MI and CHD death (16). The procedure is ineffective in patients with homozygous FH (73), probably because partial ileal bypass works by up-regulating the LDL receptor (which is absent in homozygous FH). Partial ileal bypass has not been proven to be effective in patients with severe hypercholesterolemia who did not respond adequately to HMG-CoA reductase inhibitors. Diarrhea is a common side effect of this procedure, and the incidence of kidney stones, gallstones, and intestinal obstruction increases in patients who have undergone the surgery. The clinical usefulness of partial ileal bypass is limited to treatment of hypercholesterolemic patients who have established CHD, are unable to tolerate standard lipid-lowering medications, and do not wish to undergo LDL apheresis.

Low-Density Lipoprotein Apheresis or Plasma Exchange

The preferred option for management of patients who have refractory or drug-resistant hypercholesterolemia is LDL apheresis (or, if LDL apheresis is not available, plasma exchange). Plasma exchange involves removing a large volume of plasma and replacing it with an albumin/saline solution. It results in acute reduction in plasma cholesterol levels and has been used for decades on a repetitive basis for the management of severe hypercholesterolemia (120). However, plasma exchange also removes all other plasma constituents, such as HDL cholesterol and other plasma proteins, and is often associated with fatigue and other systemic symptoms. In 1996, the FDA approved a device for selective LDL apheresis (Kaneka) as an alternative to plasma exchange. In this approach, the patient's plasma is passed over dextran sulfate columns that selectively remove LDL, and then the LDL-depleted plasma is returned to the patient (121). More recently, another device (Braun) that uses heparin columns was also approved by the FDA. Both methods are in use in many countries around the world. In contrast to plasma exchange, LDL apheresis does not decrease the levels of HDL cholesterol or other plasma constituents and is often better tolerated by patients. Clinical trials have indicated that LDL apheresis can retard progression or cause regression of CHD in patients who have severe drug-resistant hypercholesterolemia (76,77) and have even suggested a decrease in clinical cardiovascular events (77). Patients on maximally tolerated combination drug therapy who have CHD and an LDL cholesterol level >200 mg per dL or no CHD and an LDL cholesterol level >300 mg per dL are considered candidates for LDL apheresis (75). The procedure is usually performed every 2 weeks, although some patients with very severe hypercholesterolemia may benefit from undergoing the procedure every week. LDL apheresis is safe, but it requires a major time commitment on the part of the patient and a substantial expense on the part of the insurer. Nevertheless, it is considered the therapy of choice for patients with severe refractory hypercholesterolemia, and these patients should be referred to a specialized lipid center for management of their condition, including consideration of LDL apheresis.

Future Developments in the Treatment of Dyslipidemia

Small molecules that target new molecular pathways are under development for use in therapy for dyslipidemia. One example is a molecule that inhibits the intestinal bile acid transporter. These molecules inhibit the reuptake of bile acids by the intestine and therefore result in LDL receptor up-regulation and reduction of LDL cholesterol. They are expected to be particularly effective in combination with statins. Somatic gene therapy is a logical treatment of the future for patients with major genetic lipid disorders who cannot be treated adequately with available drugs (122). Homozygous FH due to deficiency of LDL receptors has been a disease model for the development of liver-directed somatic gene therapy, and a pilot clinical trial

involving five patients has been completed (123). However, the development of effective gene therapy for severe genetic dyslipidemias requires advances in the technology of gene delivery and expression.

Approach to the Patient with Low High-Density Lipoprotein Cholesterol

Many individuals are found to have a low HDL cholesterol level during routine lipid screening. The finding of a low HDL cholesterol level can be useful when it is recognized as an independent risk factor in the assessment of CHD risk and in the clinical management of LDL cholesterol levels that are in the gray zone. However, no formal guidelines have been developed specifically for the classification and management of patients with isolated findings of low levels of HDL cholesterol.

Secondary causes of low HDL levels should always be considered. Specifically, the patient should be asked about medications, smoking habits, dietary patterns, and physical activity. Decreased HDL cholesterol levels in patients with substantially elevated triglyceride levels (>500 mg per dL) are common and should not be directly addressed until the triglyceride levels have been reduced. Once secondary causes and hypertriglyceridemia are excluded, the differential diagnosis and management of low HDL cholesterol can be divided into moderately decreased HDL cholesterol levels (20 to 35 mg per dL) and severely decreased HDL levels (<20 mg per dL). Severely decreased HDL cholesterol levels <20 mg per dL accompanied by triglyceride levels <400 mg per dL usually indicate the presence of a specific genetic etiology for the condition, such as mutations in apoA-I, LCAT deficiency, or Tangier disease. A patient in whom one of these diagnoses is suspected should be referred to a specialized lipid center for further evaluation.

No formal clinical practice guidelines are available for the management of the condition of patients with isolated low HDL cholesterol. However, some general guidelines can be proposed. Secondary factors should be sought and corrected when possible. Smoking should be discontinued, obese persons should be encouraged to lose weight, and sedentary persons should be encouraged to exercise. HRT can substantially raise HDL cholesterol and should be considered in postmenopausal women. When possible, medications associated with reduced HDL cholesterol should be discontinued. Diabetes mellitus should be optimally controlled. Isolated low HDL cholesterol levels that are not a result of a secondary factor or a very low-fat diet are often associated with modestly elevated LDL cholesterol levels. In this situation, a finding of decreased HDL cholesterol levels is useful clinically as an additional independent cardiovascular risk factor supporting the use of drug therapy to reduce a slightly increased or even average LDL cholesterol level. If the LDL cholesterol level is well controlled, it can be difficult to decide whether pharmacologic intervention should be used to raise an isolated finding of a low HDL cholesterol level. In individuals with established ASCVD, drug therapy may be a reasonable approach, especially in light of the results of the VA-HIT study. In healthy individuals, no published clinical trials have demonstrated any benefit from treatment targeted specifically at increasing the level of HDL cholesterol. Every effort should be made to assess the risk of future CHD in patients with isolated findings of low HDL cholesterol levels so that appropriate clinical decisions about medical management can be made. In high-risk individuals, drug therapy targeted toward HDL cholesterol could be reasonably considered.

Statins increase HDL cholesterol levels modestly, by approximately 5% to 10%, and are not generally regarded as HDL cholesterol–raising drugs. Fibrates also increase HDL cholesterol modestly, by approximately 5% to 15%, but are most effective when triglyceride levels are elevated. Change in HDL in response to fibrate therapy is relatively slight in many patients who have low HDL cholesterol and normal triglyceride levels. Niacin is the most effective therapy targeted at increasing HDL cholesterol levels that is currently available; increases in HDL cholesterol levels up to approximately 30% have been seen. But some patients who have isolated findings of low HDL cholesterol levels do not even respond significantly to niacin therapy. New molecules designed to raise HDL cholesterol levels or promote reverse cholesterol transport are under active development.

CONTROVERSIES AND PERSONAL PERSPECTIVES

The case for aggressive cholesterol reduction has become much stronger over the past few years as a number of new clinical studies have been published. These studies have contributed to the paradigm shift away from a focus on angiographic disease and degree of luminal stenosis and toward the concept of plaque stabilization in the prevention of acute coronary events. The enthusiasm for using aggressive lipid lowering to markedly reduce the burden of coronary morbidity and death has been apparent in a variety of editorials written by prominent scientists. Nobel laureates Drs. Michael Brown and Joseph Goldstein stated in an editorial in *Science* that "Exploitation of recent breakthroughs—proof of the cholesterol hypothesis, discovery of effective drugs, and better definition of genetic susceptibility factors—may well end coronary disease as a major public health threat early in the next century" (124). Dr. William Roberts, editor of the *American Journal of Cardiology,* has called the statin drugs "miracle drugs" that are to atherosclerosis "what penicillin was to infectious disease" (125). The purpose of this section will be to outline the issues, make practical suggestions based

on current knowledge, and point out needs for future basic and clinical research.

Assessment of Cardiovascular Risk

It is widely agreed that drug therapy to reduce cholesterol is indicated in secondary prevention of clinical events and death in individuals with established CHD (26). Most experts also agree that drug therapy is indicated for primary prevention in certain high-risk individuals (such as diabetics and those with multiple risk factors) who have hypercholesterolemia that cannot be controlled adequately with diet and exercise. Therefore, in primary prevention, the major emphasis has turned to the more precise identification of high-risk individuals who are most likely to benefit from more aggressive therapy. It is now generally recognized that although traditional risk factors are reasonably good at predicting excess risk above the baseline for particular populations, they allow clinicians to predict only approximately 50% to 60% of the variation in absolute risk in individual patients (126). Therefore, factors that enhance predictive ability in an additive fashion over traditional risk factors would have considerable clinical usefulness, allowing better decisions to be made regarding the use of proven preventive therapies. Although traditional risk factors are useful in identifying some high-risk individuals, they identify only approximately one-half of the individuals who are destined to develop premature CHD. Therefore, there is great interest in the use of additional tests to identify high-risk individuals. Such information has immediate implications with regard to decisions about the use and intensity of lipid-lowering drug therapy. Those individuals at the highest risk for future CHD will benefit the most from aggressive lipid-lowering drug therapy (127). This section will briefly review some of the tests that have been proposed and are being used for the purpose of cardiovascular risk assessment.

Low-Density Lipoprotein Particle Concentration and Size

A given level of LDL cholesterol could be caused by a small number of large LDL particles or a large number of small LDL particles. A large body of epidemiologic data indicates that the latter is associated with substantially greater cardiovascular risk than the former. Therefore, determination of LDL particle concentration and size could potentially be used to aid the diagnosis of lipid disorders and to refine the identification of individuals at risk for premature CHD, who therefore deserve more aggressive therapy (128). ApoB is the major protein component of LDL, and each LDL particle has one molecule of apoB per particle. Thus, the apoB concentration is an indirect measure of the number of LDL particles. Although epidemiologic studies have been conflicting, apoB levels are probably predictive of CHD risk independent of LDL cholesterol levels (128,129). Assays to measure apoB have not yet been fully standardized. An NMR imaging–based method has become the gold standard for the quantitation of LDL particle size and LDL particle number (130). Some clinicians choose to use this test, which is FDA-approved and commercially available, to assist them in the treatment of patients with LDL cholesterol levels that are in a borderline range. The finding of an increased concentration of small, dense LDL particles could reasonably lead to the initiation of drug therapy, even if the LDL cholesterol level itself were not significantly elevated.

Lipoprotein(a)

Lp(a) is similar to LDL, but it is characterized by the presence of an additional protein called "apolipoprotein(a)" (131). Lp(a) levels are highly genetically determined, and the gene for apolipoprotein(a) is the major genetic factor controlling the plasma levels of Lp(a). A large number of epidemiologic and observational studies have indicated that Lp(a) levels are associated with premature ASCVD, independent of LDL cholesterol levels (131). A recent prospective study of the Framingham offspring cohort confirmed that the relative risk for premature CHD was increased in the presence of an elevated Lp(a) level (132). The mechanism by which Lp(a) promotes cardiovascular disease is not well understood, although it may inhibit activation of plasminogen to plasmin. Elevated Lp(a) levels may not have the same significance in all ethic groups; in studies of African-Americans, Lp(a) levels have not been associated with CHD. In contrast, elevated levels of Lp(a) are common in Asian Indians who have premature CHD and may play an important role in the early CHD often seen in this population. End-stage renal disease is strongly associated with elevated levels of Lp(a), which may play a role in the cardiovascular disease common in patients with such disease. Lp(a) levels increase in women after menopause and can be reduced with HRT. Some data suggest that an elevated Lp(a) level invites less risk after decrease of an elevated LDL cholesterol level (133). Therefore, an elevated Lp(a) level should be considered in decisions about whether to initiate drug therapy aimed at lowering the LDL cholesterol level. Although there is no proof that reducing levels of Lp(a) reduces the risk of cardiovascular disease, niacin is the only lipid-lowering drug that consistently lowers the Lp(a) level, and it should probably receive extra consideration as a treatment in the hypercholesterolemic patient who has an elevated Lp(a) level. Finally, postmenopausal women with elevated Lp(a) levels should receive special consideration for estrogen replacement therapy. However, the major emphasis in the setting of an elevated Lp(a) should remain on reduction of the LDL cholesterol level.

Homocysteine

Homocysteine levels have a continuous graded relationship with all types of ASCVD (134). This association is independent of known risk factors, and the mechanism has not yet been established. Homocysteine levels are inversely associated with folic acid intake and serum folate levels (135). Therefore, in addition to providing evidence of higher CHD risk, an elevated serum homocysteine level may have therapeutic implications with regard to folic acid supplementation. Randomized controlled clinical trials of the use of folic acid supplementation to lower homocysteine levels in the prevention of CHD are under way, but results have not yet been reported.

Inflammatory Markers

There has been increasing interest in the concept of atherosclerosis as an inflammatory disease (136). This concept has been fueled by the finding that serum markers of inflammation predict future cardiovascular events (137,138). The most-studied marker has been the high-sensitivity C-reactive protein, which has been found to be associated with increased cardiovascular risk in multiple prospective studies. Other inflammatory markers that have also been found to be predictive of risk include interleukin-6, serum amyloid A, and soluble intercellular adhesion molecule 1 (139). In a head-to-head comparison of different serum-based markers, inflammatory markers were clearly additive to lipid markers in predicting future cardiovascular risk (140). The clinical use of certain markers, such as high-sensitivity C-reactive protein, in selected patients for improvement of cardiovascular risk assessment may be reasonable.

Fibrinogen

Fibrinogen levels have been found to have a significant association with premature CHD in several studies (141). The mechanism by which fibrinogen promotes CHD is not well understood but may involve at least in part its effects on plasma viscosity.

Genetic Polymorphisms

Genetic variation plays a role in determining cardiovascular risk. A variety of single-nucleotide polymorphisms in different candidate genes have been reported to be associated with CHD in univariate analyses. In theory, a panel of a large number of single-nucleotide polymorphisms could be used to predict future cardiovascular risk. This type of panel is not yet ready for use in clinical decision-making but is under active study.

Noninvasive Vascular Imaging

In theory, the use of noninvasive tests to examine vascular beds for presence of atherosclerotic plaque before the development of symptoms is an attractive way of identifying high-risk individuals who may be candidates for more aggressive therapy to reduce LDL cholesterol levels (142). Several different modalities are under development and clinical investigation with regard to this concept. Because acute coronary events are frequently caused by lesions that represent <50% stenosis of the vessel, the goal in identifying individuals at high risk for coronary events is not to identify those with significant coronary stenoses (as for exercise testing), but rather to identify individuals who are at higher statistical risk of developing vulnerable coronary lesions and having acute coronary events. Therefore, the most promising methods are likely to be those that sensitively and specifically detect and quantitate atherosclerosis. B-mode carotid ultrasound can be used to quantitate carotid IMT in asymptomatic individuals, and this technique has been used to demonstrate that lowering lipid levels can retard the progression of intimal thickening in comparison with that in control patients (143–145). Prospective studies based on large populations, such as the Atherosclerosis Risk in Communities (ARIC) study and Cardiovascular Health Study (CHS), have shown that carotid IMT is predictive of future coronary events, independent of known cardiovascular risk factors. Another marker for coronary atherosclerotic plaque is coronary calcification (146). Electron-beam tomography can detect and quantitate coronary calcification as a specific marker for atherosclerotic plaque (147). Coronary calcification is highly correlated with the extent of atherosclerotic disease on autopsy (148,149) and with the extent of angiographic coronary disease (147). Several prospective studies have indicated that the extent of coronary calcification is associated with the probability of a future coronary event (150). Therefore, both carotid IMT and coronary calcification could potentially be used as noninvasive methods for stratifying selected asymptomatic persons according to cardiovascular risk, to aid physicians in making more informed decisions regarding drug therapy for cholesterol reduction.

Use of Lipid-Lowering Drug Therapy in Underrepresented Subgroups

Women

Women have been traditionally underrepresented in lipid-lowering trials, although trials such as 4S, Cholesterol and Recurrent Events, LIPID, and AFCAPS/TexCAPS included women. Subgroup analyses have indicated that women are as likely as men to benefit from cholesterol reduction. On the basis of available data, women with CHD or diabetes or who have high cardiovascular risk should receive treatment as aggressive as that in men. Premenopausal women are, on average, at substantially lower risk of developing premature CHD than men of the same age, and therefore the threshold of LDL cholesterol levels for institution of drug therapy should probably be higher for women than for men. Nevertheless, in women at high

risk, such as those with diabetes mellitus or strong family histories of premature CHD, it is appropriate to consider more aggressive therapy. HRT may be considered for postmenopausal women before initiation of lipid-lowering drug therapy, because estrogens can lower LDL cholesterol levels (as well as raise HDL cholesterol). Postmenopausal women who are not receiving estrogen replacement are at similar risk to that in men for developing CHD and therefore should be treated for hypercholesterolemia with a similar degree of intensity.

Elderly Individuals

Some secondary prevention trials have included patients as old as 75 years. Subgroup analyses have indicated that age is not a determinant of benefit from therapy and that patients in older age groups derive benefit similar to that in younger patients. Given the wealth of data demonstrating the benefit of cholesterol reduction in secondary prevention, it is rational to treat elderly persons with CHD as aggressively as younger persons with CHD. However, the decision to use cholesterol-lowering drug therapy should be influenced by the general health of the patient, the need for other medications, and the patient's ability to tolerate the lipid-lowering medication. Primary prevention of CHD using cholesterol-lowering drugs is a more difficult issue in elderly patients. The West of Scotland study included patients as old as 64 years; a subgroup analysis of patients older than 55 years indicated a significant reduction in MI and CHD death, similar to that seen in the group of patients younger than 55 years (32). The approach to hypercholesterolemia in elderly persons without CHD should probably be influenced primarily by the general health and vigor of the patients as well as by their degree of interest in being treated aggressively. For example, a healthy, active 80-year-old with an elevated LDL cholesterol level who wants to do everything possible to prevent his or her first MI should not be denied drug therapy simply on the basis of age.

Role of Antioxidants in Reduction of Risk of Coronary Heart Disease

The Probucol Quantitative Regression Swedish Trial used probucol as an antioxidant to treat patients who had femoral atherosclerosis. No difference was seen between the group of patients who were treated with probucol and the control group with regard to the extent of femoral atherosclerosis (151). Two large trials failed to demonstrate any effect on cardiovascular disease from beta carotene supplementation with relatively low doses of either 50 mg every other day (152) or 30 mg daily (153). The Cambridge Heart Antioxidant Study compared the use of two different doses of vitamin E supplementation (400 and 800 IU per day) to placebo in 2,002 patients with established CHD (154). The analysis was performed by pooling the two different treat-

THE FUTURE

Virtually all experts agree that cholesterol-lowering drugs are underused and that more frequent use will lead to even more impressive reductions in coronary events in the future. Nevertheless, many clinical issues remain unresolved in the treatment of lipid disorders. Although a thorough discussion of all of these issues is beyond the scope of this chapter, several are discussed here: (1) the use of additional diagnostic tests for determining CHD risk as a guide to intensity of lipid-lowering drug therapy in primary prevention, (2) the use of lipid-lowering drug therapy in particular subgroups underrepresented in clinical trials, and (3) the use of antioxidant therapies.

ment groups and comparing them to the placebo group. Combined CHD death and nonfatal MI (the primary end point) was significantly reduced (by 47%; p <.005) in the groups treated with vitamin E. This difference was entirely due to a reduction in nonfatal MI (14 events in the group of patients receiving treatment vs. 41 events in the control group). Although the trial was not powered to address the total mortality rate, the rate was actually increased in the group of patients receiving vitamin E (36 deaths) compared with that in the control group (27 deaths). In the Gruppo Italiano per lo Studio della Sopravvivenza nell'Infarto Miocardico–Prevenzione Trial (117), 11,324 Italian subjects with recent MI (<3 months before enrollment) were randomly assigned to receive 300 mg per day of synthetic vitamin E, 1 g per day of Ω-3 PUFA, or both, or placebo in a 2-by-2 factorial design and followed for 3.5 years. The primary combined efficacy end points were death, nonfatal MI, and stroke. Treatment with Ω-3 PUFAs without vitamin E significantly lowered the risk of the primary end point. The Heart Outcomes Prevention Evaluation study (155) involved 9,541 subjects aged 55 years or older with both symptomatic and asymptomatic cardiovascular disease. Subjects were randomly assigned to receive naturally occurring vitamin E (400 IU) or placebo and followed for 4.5 years. This trial used a two-by-two factorial design that also involved the angiotensin-converting enzyme inhibitor ramipril. No clinical benefit or adverse events were noted in the group of patients treated with vitamin E. The Secondary Prevention with Antioxidants of Cardiovascular Disease in Endstage Renal Disease (SPACE) trial (156) investigated the effect of high-dose vitamin E supplementation on cardiovascular disease outcomes in hemodialysis patients with preexisting heart disease. One hundred and ninety-six hemodialysis patients aged 40 to 75 years were randomly assigned to receive 800 IU per day of vitamin E or placebo in a double-blind design. Patients were followed for approximately 17 months. The primary end points included fatal and nonfatal MI, ischemic stroke, peripheral vascular disease, and unstable angina. Secondary outcomes included cardiovascular mortality and total mortality rates. Results of this study demonstrated a highly significant reduction in the composite primary outcome measure that was chiefly attrib-

utable to a 70% reduction in acute MI. No effect on the total mortality rate or the cardiovascular mortality rate was seen. Therefore, although most of the results of vitamin E supplementation trials have been negative to date, the results of the SPACE trial suggest that patients who have elevated levels of oxidant stress may benefit from therapy with vitamin E. Additional clinical trials are under way that are examining the important question of whether antioxidant therapy will reduce cardiovascular events in both secondary and primary prevention.

REFERENCES

1. Verschuren WMM, Jacobs DR, Bloemberg BPM, et al. Serum total cholesterol and long-term coronary heart disease mortality in different cultures: twenty-five-year follow-up of the seven countries study. *JAMA* 1995;274:131–136.
2. Kannel WB, Castelli WP, Gordon T. Cholesterol in the prediction of atherosclerotic disease: new perspectives based on the Framingham study. *Ann Intern Med* 1979;90:85–91.
3. Stamler J, Wentworth D, Neaton JD. Is relationship between serum cholesterol and risk of premature death from coronary heart disease continuous and graded? Findings in 356,222 primary screenees of the multiple risk factor intervention trial (MRFIT). *JAMA* 1986;256:2823–2828.
4. Pekkanen J, Linn S, Heiss G, et al. Ten-year mortality from cardiovascular disease in relation to cholesterol level among men with and without preexisting cardiovascular disease. *N Engl J Med* 1990;322:1700–1717.
5. Klag MJ, Ford DE, Mead LA, et al. Serum cholesterol in young men and subsequent cardiovascular disease. *N Engl J Med* 1993;328:313–318.
6. Newman III WP, Freedman DS, Voors AW, et al. Relation of serum lipoprotein levels and systolic blood pressure to early atherosclerosis: the Bogalusa Heart Study. *N Engl J Med* 1986;314:138–144.
7. Miller NE, Thelle DS, Forde OH, et al. The Tromso heart-study. High-density lipoprotein and coronary heart-disease: a prospective case-control study. *Lancet* 1977;1:965–968.
8. Gordon DJ, Rifkind BM. High-density lipoproteins: the clinical implications of recent studies. *N Engl J Med* 1989;321:1311–1316.
9. Executive summary of the third report of the National Cholesterol Education Program (NCEP) Expert Panel on Detec-

tion, Evaluation, and Treatment of High Blood Cholesterol in Adults (Adult Treatment Panel III). *JAMA* 2001;285:2486–2497.

10. Austin MA, Hokanson JE, Edwards KL. Hypertriglyceridemia as a cardiovascular risk factor. *Am J Cardiol* 1998;81:7B–12B.

11. Brown BG, Zhoa XQ, Sacco DE, et al. Lipid lowering and plaque regression: new insights into prevention of plaque disruption and clinical events in coronary disease. *Circulation* 1993;87:1781–1791.

12. Pearson TA, Marx HJ. The rapid reduction in cardiac events with lipid-lowering therapy: mechanisms and implications. *Am J Cardiol* 1993;72:1072–1073.

13. Byington RP, Jukema W, Salonen JT, et al. Reduction in cardiovascular events during pravastatin therapy: pooled analysis of clinical events of the pravastatin atherosclerosis intervention program. *Circulation* 1995;92:2419–2425.

14. The Coronary Drug Project Research Group. Clofibrate and niacin in coronary heart disease. *JAMA* 1975;231:360–381.

15. Canner PL, Berge KG, Wenger NK, et al. Fifteen year mortality in Coronary Drug Project patients: long term benefit with niacin. *J Am Coll Cardiol* 1986;8:1245–1255.

16. Buchwald H, Varco RL, Matts JP, et al. Effect of partial ileal bypass surgery on mortality and morbidity from coronary heart disease in patients with hypercholesterolemia: report of the Program on the Surgical Control of the Hyperlipidemias (POSCH). *N Engl J Med* 1990;323:946–955.

17. Lipid Research Clinics Program. The Lipid Research Clinics Coronary Primary Prevention Trial results. 1: Reduction in incidence of coronary heart disease. *JAMA* 1984;251:351–364.

18. Lipid Research Clinics Program. The Lipid Research Clinics Coronary Primary Prevention Trial results. II: The relationship of reduction in incidence of coronary heart disease to cholesterol lowering. *JAMA* 1984;251:365–374.

19. The Lipid Research Clinics Coronary Primary Prevention Trial. *Arch Intern Med* 1992;152:1399–1410.

20. Scandinavian Simvastatin Survival Study Group. Randomized trial of cholesterol lowering in 4444 patients with coronary heart disease: the Scandinavian Simvastatin Survival Study (4S). *Lancet* 1994;344:1383–1389.

21. Pederson TR, Kjekshus J, Berg K, et al. Cholesterol lowering and the use of healthcare resources: results of the Scandinavian Simvastatin Survival Study. *Circulation* 1996;93:1796–1802.

22. Scandinavian Simvastatin Survival Study Group. Baseline serum cholesterol and treatment effect in the Scandinavian Simvastatin Survival Study (4S). *Lancet* 1995;345:1274–1275.

23. Kannel WB. Range of serum cholesterol values in the population developing coronary artery disease. *Am J Cardiol* 1995;76:69C–77C.

24. Sacks FM, Pfeffer MA, Moye L, et al. The effect of pravastatin on coronary events after myocardial infarction in patients with average cholesterol levels. *N Engl J Med* 1996;335:1001–1009.

25. Prevention of cardiovascular events and death with pravastatin in patients with coronary heart disease and a broad range of initial cholesterol levels. The Long-Term Intervention

26. Smith J, Blair SN, Criqui MH, et al. Preventing heart attack and death in patients with coronary disease. *Circulation* 1995;92:2–4.

27. Grundy SM. Statin trials and goals of cholesterol-lowering therapy. *Circulation* 1998;97:1436–1439.

28. Tonkin AM, Colquhoun D, Emberson J, et al. Effects of pravastatin in 3260 patients with unstable angina: results from the LIPID study. *Lancet* 2000;356:1871–1875.

29. Arntz H, Agrawal R, Wunderlich W, et al. Beneficial effects of pravastatin (+/–colestyramine/niacin) initiated immediately after a coronary event (the Randomized Lipid-Coronary Artery Disease [L-CAD] Study). *Am J Cardiol* 2000;86:1293–1298.

30. Schwartz GG, Olsson AG, Ezekowitz MD, et al. Effects of atorvastatin on early recurrent ischemic events in acute coronary syndromes: the MIRACL study, a randomized, controlled trial. *JAMA* 2001;285:1711–1718.

31. Kannel WB, Schatzkin A. Sudden death: lessons from subsets in population studies. *J Am Coll Cardiol* 1985;5:141b–149b.

32. Shepherd J, Cobbe SM, Ford I, et al. Prevention of coronary heart disease with pravastatin in men with hypercholesterolemia. West of Scotland Coronary Prevention Study Group. *N Engl J Med* 1995;333:1301–1307.

33. Downs JR, Clearfield M, Weis S, et al. Primary prevention of acute coronary events with lovastatin in men and women with average cholesterol levels. *JAMA* 1998;279:1615–1622.

34. Sacks FM, Tonkin AM, Shepherd J, et al. Effect of pravastatin on coronary disease events in subgroups defined by coronary risk factors: the Prospective Pravastatin Pooling Project. *Circulation* 2000;102:1893–1900.

35. Rader DJ, Haffner SM. Role of fibrates in the management of hypertriglyceridemia. *Am J Cardiol* 1999;83:30F–35F.

36. Committee of Principal Investigators. A cooperative trial in the prevention of ischaemic heart disease using clofibrate. *Br Heart J* 1978;40:1069–1118.

37. WHO cooperative trial on primary prevention of ischaemic heart disease with clofibrate to lower serum cholesterol: final mortality follow-up. Report of the Committee of Principal Investigators. *Lancet* 1984;2:600–604.

38. Frick MH, Elo O, Haapa K, et al. Helsinki Heart Study: primary-prevention trial with gemfibrozil in middle-aged men with dyslipidemia. Safety of treatment, changes in risk factors, and incidence of coronary heart disease. *N Engl J Med* 1987;317:1237–1245.

39. Huttunen JK, Heinonen O, Manninen V, et al. The Helsinki Heart Study: an 8.5-year safety and mortality follow-up. *J Intern Med* 1994;235:1–4.

40. Rubins HB, Robins SJ, Collins D, et al. Gemfibrozil for the secondary prevention of coronary heart disease in men with low levels of high-density lipoprotein cholesterol. *N Engl J Med* 1999;341:410–418.

41. Secondary prevention by raising HDL cholesterol and reducing triglycerides in patients with coronary artery disease: the Bezafibrate Infarction Prevention (BIP) Study. *Circulation* 2000;102:21–27.

42. Rader DJ, Brewer HB. *Lipids, apolipoproteins and lipoproteins.* Boston: Kluwer Academic Publishers, 1994:83–103.

43. Brown MS, Goldstein JL. A receptor-mediated pathway for cholesterol homeostasis. *Science* 1986;232:34–47.

44. Beisiegel U. Receptors for triglyceride-rich lipoproteins and their role in lipoprotein metabolism. *Curr Opin Lipidol* 1995;6:117–122.

45. Willnow TE, Herz J. Animal models for disorders of hepatic lipoprotein metabolism. *J Mol Med* 1995;73:213–220.

46. Krieger M, Abrams JM, Lux A, et al. Molecular flypaper, atherosclerosis, and host defense: structure and function of the macrophage scavenger receptor. Cold Spring Harbor Symposia on Quantitative Biology. *Circulation* 1992;4:607–615.

47. Rader DJ, Ikewaki K. Unravelling high density lipoprotein-apolipoprotein metabolism in human mutants and animal models. *Curr Opin Lipidol* 1996;7:117–123.

48. Tall AR. Plasma high density lipoproteins: metabolism and relationship to atherogenesis. *J Clin Invest* 1990;86:379–384.

49. Witztum JL, Steinberg D. Role of oxidized low density lipoprotein in atherogenesis. *J Clin Invest* 1991;88:1785–1792.

50. Williams KJ, Tabas I. The response-to-retention hypothesis of early atherogenesis. *Arterioscler Thromb Vasc Biol* 1995;15:551–561.

51. Levine GN, Keaney J, Vita JA. Cholesterol reduction in cardiovascular disease: clinical benefits and possible mechanisms. *N Engl J Med* 1995;332:512–521.

52. Treasure CB, Klein JL, Weintraub WS, et al. Beneficial effects of cholesterol-lowering therapy on the coronary endothelium in patients with coronary artery disease. *N Engl J Med* 1995;332:481–487.

53. Anderson TJ, Meredith IT, Yeung AC, et al. The effect of cholesterol-lowering and antioxidant therapy on endothelium-dependent coronary vasomotion. *N Engl J Med* 1995;332:488–493.

54. Rader DJ, Rosas S. Management of selected lipid abnormalities: hypertriglyceridemia, low HDL cholesterol, lipoprotein(a), in thyroid and renal diseases, and post-transplantation. *Med Clin North Am* 2000;84:43–61.

55. Detection and management of lipid disorders in diabetes. *Diabetes Care* 1993;16:828–834.

56. Abbate SL, Brunzell JD. Pathophysiology of hyperlipidemia in diabetes mellitus. *J Cardiovasc Pharm Ther* 1990;16:S1–S7.

57. Taskinen M. Insulin resistance and lipoprotein metabolism. *Curr Opin Lipidol* 1995;6:153–160.

58. Wanner C, Rader D, Bartens W, et al. Elevated plasma lipoprotein(a) in patients with the nephrotic syndrome. *Ann Intern Med* 1993;119:263–269.

59. Oda H, Keane WF. Lipid abnormalities in end stage renal disease. *Nephrol Dial Transplant* 1998;[13 Suppl 1]:45–49.

60. Gaziano JM, Manson JE. Diet and heart disease: the role of fat, alcohol, and antioxidants. *Cardiol Clin* 1996;14:69–83.

61. Fojo SS, Brewer HB Jr. The familial hyperchylomicronemia syndrome. *JAMA* 1991;265:904–908.

62. Connor WE, DeFrancesco C, Connor SL. N–3 fatty acids from fish oil: effects on plasma lipoproteins and hypertriglyceridemic patients. *Ann N Y Acad Sci* 1993;683:16–34.

63. Brewer HB Jr, Zech LA, Gregg RE, et al. Type III hyperlipoproteinemia: diagnosis, molecular defects, pathology, and treatment. *Ann Intern Med* 1983;98:623–640.

64. Davignon J, Gregg RE, Sing CF. Apolipoprotein E polymorphism and atherosclerosis. *Arteriosclerosis* 1988;8:1–21.

65. Wilson PWF, Myers RH, Larson MG, et al. Apolipoprotein E alleles, dyslipidemia, and coronary heart disease. *JAMA* 1994;272:1666–1671.

66. Rall SC Jr, Mahley RW. The role of apolipoprotein E genetic variants in lipoprotein disorders. *J Intern Med* 1992;231:653–659.

67. Brunzell JD, Austin M, Deeb S, et al. Familial combined hyperlipidemia and genetic risk for atherosclerosis. In: Woodford FP, Davignon J, Sniderman A, eds. *Atherosclerosis X*. New York: Elsevier, 1995:624–627.

68. Grundy SM, Chait A, Brunzell JD. Familial combined hyperlipidemia workshop. *Arteriosclerosis* 1987;7:203–207.

69. Nevin D, Brunzell JD, Deeb SS. The LPL gene in individuals with familial combined hyperlipidemia and decreased LPL activity. *Arterioscler Thromb* 1994;14:869–873.

70. Kwiterovich PO Jr. Genetics and molecular biology of familial combined hyperlipidemia. *Curr Opin Lipidol* 1993;4:133–143.

71. Wolfe ML, Vartanian SF, Ross JL, et al. Safety and effectiveness of Niaspan when added sequentially to a statin for the treatment of dyslipidemia. *Am J Cardiol* 2001;87:476–479.

72. Hegele R, Little JA, Vezina C, et al. Hepatic lipase deficiency: clinical, biochemical, and molecular genetic characteristics. *Arterioscler Thromb* 1993;13:720–728.

73. Goldstein JL, Hobbs HH, Brown MS. Familial hypercholesterolemia. In: Scriver CR, Beaudet AL, Sly WS, et al., eds. *The metabolic basis of inherited disease*. New York: McGraw-Hill, 1995:1981–2030.

74. Hobbs HH, Brown MS, Goldstein JL. Molecular genetics of the LDL receptor gene in familial hypercholesterolemia. *Hum Mutat* 1992;1:445–446.

75. Gordon BR, Stein E, Jones P, et al. Indications for low-density lipoprotein apheresis. *Am J Cardiol* 1994;74:1109–1112.

76. Tatami R, Inoue N, Itoh H, et al. Regression of coronary atherosclerosis by combined LDL-apheresis and lipid-lowering drug therapy in patients with familial hypercholesterolemia: a multicenter study. *Atherosclerosis* 1992;95:1–13.

77. Thompson GR, Maher V, Matthews S, et al. Familial hypercholesterolaemia regression study: a randomised trial of low-density lipoprotein apheresis. *Lancet* 1995;345:811–816.

78. Elam MB, Hunninghake DB, Davis KB. Effect of niacin on lipid and lipoprotein levels and glycemic control in patients with diabetes and peripheral arterial disease. *JAMA* 2000;284:1263–1270.

79. Innerarity TL, Mahley RW, Weisgraber KH, et al. Familial defective apolipoprotein B-100: a mutation of apolipoprotein B that causes hypercholesterolemia. *J Lipid Res* 1990;31:1337–1349.

80. Norum RA, Lakier JB, Goldstein S, et al. Familial deficiency of apolipoproteins A-I and C-III and precocious coronary-artery disease. *N Engl J Med* 1982;306:1513–1519.

81. Schaefer EJ, Heaton WH, Wetzel MG, et al. Plasma apolipoprotein A-1 absence associated with a marked reduction of high density lipoproteins and premature coronary artery disease. *Arteriosclerosis* 1982;2:16–26.

82. Ng D, Leiter L, Vezina C, et al. Apolipoprotein A-I Q[-2]X causing isolated apolipoprotein A-I deficiency in a family

with analphalipoproteinemia. *J Clin Invest* 1994;93:223–229.

83. Breslow JL. Familial disorders of high density lipoprotein metabolism. In: Scriver CR, Beaudet AL, Sly WS, et al., eds. *The metabolic basis of inherited disease.* New York: McGraw-Hill, 1995:2031–2052.

84. Glomset JA, Assmann G, Gjone E, et al. Lecithin:cholesterol acyltransferase deficiency and fish eye disease: In: Scriver CR, Beaudet AL, Sly WS, et al., eds. *The metabolic basis of inherited disease.* New York: McGraw-Hill, 1995:1933–1952.

85. Assmann G, von Eckardstein A, Brewer HB Jr. Familial high density lipoprotein deficiency: Tangier disease. In: Scriver CR, Beaudet AL, Sly WS, et al., eds. *The metabolic basis of inherited disease.* New York: McGraw-Hill, 1995:2053–2072.

86. Young SG, Fielding CJ. The ABCs of cholesterol efflux. *Nat Genet* 1999;22:316–318.

87. Clee SM, Kastelein JJ, van Dam M, et al. Age and residual cholesterol efflux affect HDL cholesterol levels and coronary artery disease in ABCA1 heterozygotes. *J Clin Invest* 2000;106:1263–1270.

88. Third JL, Montag J, Flynn M, et al. Primary and familial hypoalphalipoproteinemia. *Metabolism* 1984;33:136–146.

89. Genest J, Bard JM, Fruchart JC, et al. Familial hypoalphalipoproteinemia in premature coronary artery disease. *Arterioscler Thromb* 1993;13:1728–1737.

90. Breslow JL, Eisenberg S, Brinton EA. Metabolic determinants of low HDL-C levels. *Ann N Y Acad Sci* 1993;676:157–162.

91. Rader DJ, Ikewaki K, Duverger N, et al. Very low high-density lipoproteins without coronary atherosclerosis. *Lancet* 1993;342:1455–1458.

92. Report of the National Cholesterol Education Program Expert Panel on Detection and Treatment of High Blood Cholesterol in Adults. *Arch Intern Med* 1988;148:36–69.

93. American College of Physicians. Guidelines for using serum cholesterol, high-density lipoprotein cholesterol, and triglyceride levels as screening tests for preventing coronary heart disease in adults. *Ann Intern Med* 1996;124:515–517.

94. Garber AM, Browner WS, Hulley SB. Cholesterol screening in asymptomatic adults, revisited. *Ann Intern Med* 1996;124:518–531.

95. Larosa JC. Cholesterol agonistics. *Ann Intern Med* 1996;124:505–508.

96. Austin MA, McKnight B, Edwards KL, et al. Cardiovascular disease mortality in familial forms of hypertriglyceridemia: a 20-year prospective study. *Circulation* 2000;101:2777–2782.

97. Nguyen TT. The cholesterol-lowering action of plant stanol esters. *J Nutr* 1999;129:2109–2112.

98. Fletcher GF. The antiatherosclerotic effect of exercise and development of an exercise prescription. *Cardiol Clin* 1996;14:85–95.

99. The Writing Group for the PEPI Trial. Effects of estrogen or estrogen/progestin regimens on heart disease risk factors in postmenopausal women. *JAMA* 1995;273:199–208.

100. Shlipak MG, Simon JA, Vittinghoff E, et al. Estrogen and progestin, lipoprotein(a), and the risk of recurrent coronary heart disease events after menopause. *JAMA* 2000;283:1845–1852.

101. Kafonek SD. Postmenopausal hormone replacement therapy and cardiovascular risk reduction: a review. *Drugs* 1994;47:16–24.

102. Hulley S, Grady D, Bush T, et al. Randomized trial of estrogen plus progestin for secondary prevention of coronary heart disease in postmenopausal women. Heart and Estrogen/Progestin Replacement Study (HERS) Research Group. *JAMA* 1998;280:605–613.

103. Herrington DM, Reboussin DM, Brosnihan KB, et al. Effects of estrogen replacement on the progression of coronary-artery atherosclerosis. *N Engl J Med* 2000;343:522–529.

104. Design of the Women's Health Initiative clinical trial and observational study. The Women's Health Initiative Study Group. *Control Clin Trials* 1998;19:61–109.

105. Yusuf S, Anand S. Cost of prevention: the case of lipid lowering. *Circulation* 1996;93:1774–1776.

106. Giles WH, Anda RF, Jones DH, et al. Recent trends in the identification and treatment of high blood cholesterol by physicians. *JAMA* 1993;269:1133–1138.

107. Haffner SM, Lehto S, Ronnemaa T, et al. Mortality from coronary heart disease in subjects with type 2 diabetes and in nondiabetic subjects with and without prior myocardial infarction. *N Engl J Med* 1998;339:229–234.

108. Wilson PWF, D'Agostino RB, Levy D, et al. Prediction of coronary heart disease using risk factor categories. *Circulation* 1998;97:1837–1847.

109. Clearfield M, Whitney EJ, Weis S, et al. Air Force/Texas Coronary Atherosclerosis Prevention Study (AFCAPS/Tex-CAPS): baseline characteristics and comparison with USA population. *J Cardiovasc Risk* 2000;7:125–133.

110. Gotto AM. Cholesterol management in theory and practice. *Circulation* 1997;96:4424–4430.

111. Muldoon MF, Manuck SB, Mendelsohn AB, et al. Cholesterol reduction and non-illness mortality: meta-analysis of randomised clinical trials. *BMJ* 2001;322:11–15.

112. Morgan JM, Capuzzi DM, Guyton JR, et al. Treatment effect of Niaspan, a controlled-release niacin, in patients with hypercholesterolemia: a placebo-controlled trial. *J Cardiovasc Pharm Ther* 1996;1:195–202.

113. Guyton JR, Blazing MA, Hagar J, et al. Extended-release niacin vs gemfibrozil for the treatment of low levels of high-density lipoprotein cholesterol. Niaspan-Gemfibrozil Study Group. *Arch Intern Med* 2000;160:1177–1184.

114. Chesney CM, Elam MB, Herd JA, et al. Effect of niacin, warfarin, and antioxidant therapy on coagulation parameters in patients with peripheral arterial disease in the arterial disease multiple intervention trial (ADMIT). *Am Heart J* 2000;140:631–636.

115. Nestel PJ. Fish oil and cardiovascular disease: lipids and arterial function. *Am J Clin Nutr* 2000;71:228S–231S.

116. Weber P, Raederstorff D. Triglyceride-lowering effect of omega-3 LC-polyunsaturated fatty acids: a review. *Nutr Metab Cardiovasc Dis* 2000;10:28–37.

117. Dietary supplementation with Ω-3 polyunsaturated fatty acids and vitamin E after myocardial infarction: results of the GISSI-Prevenzione trial. Gruppo Italiano per lo Studio della Sopravvivenza nell'Infarto Miocardico. *Lancet* 1999;354:447–455.

118. Pasternak RC, Brown LE, Stone PH, et al. Effect of combination therapy with lipid-reducing drugs in patients with

coronary heart disease and "normal" cholesterol levels. *Ann Intern Med* 1996;125:529–540.

119. Buchwald H, Fitch LL, Campos CT. Partial ileal bypass in the treatment of hypercholesterolemia. *J Fam Pract* 1992;35:69–76.

120. King ME, Breslow JL, Lees RS. Plasma-exchange therapy of homozygous familial hypercholesterolemia. *N Engl J Med* 1980;302:1457–1459.

121. Rader DJ, Eder AF. LDL-Apheresis for severe refractory dyslipidemia. *J N Dev Clin Med* 1996;14:165–179.

122. Rader DJ, Wilson JM. Gene therapy for lipid disorders. In: Haber E, ed. *Molecular cardiovascular medicine*, 1st ed. New York: Scientific American, 1995:97–114.

123. Grossman M, Rader DJ, Muller DWM, et al. A pilot study of *ex vivo* gene therapy for homozygous familial hypercholesterolaemia. *Nat Med* 1995;1:1148–1154.

124. Brown MS, Goldstein JL. Heart attacks: gone with the century? *Science* 1996;272:529.

125. Roberts WC. The underused miracle drugs: the statin drugs are to atherosclerosis what penicillin was to infectious disease. *Am J Cardiol* 1996;78:377–378.

126. Greenland P, Abrams J, Aurigemma GP, et al. Prevention Conference V. Beyond secondary prevention: identifying the high-risk patient for primary prevention. Noninvasive tests of atherosclerotic burden. Writing Group III. *Circulation* 2000;101:E16–E22.

127. Pyorala K, DeBacker G, Graham I, et al. Prevention of coronary heart disease in clinical practice. *Eur Heart J* 1994;15:1300–1331.

128. Rader DJ, Hoeg JM, Brewer HB Jr. Quantitation of plasma apolipoproteins in the primary and secondary prevention of coronary artery disease. *Ann Intern Med* 1994;120:1012–1025.

129. Lamarche B, Moorjani S, Lupien PJ, et al. Apolipoprotein A-I and B levels and the risk of ischemic heart disease during a five-year follow-up of men in the Quebec Cardiovascular Study. *Circulation* 1996;94:273–278.

130. Otvos J. Measurement of triglyceride-rich lipoproteins by nuclear magnetic resonance spectroscopy. *Clin Cardiol* 1999;22[Suppl 2]:II-21–II-27.

131. Rader DJ, Brewer HB Jr. Lipoprotein(a): clinical approach to a unique atherogenic lipoprotein. *JAMA* 1992;267:1109–1112.

132. Bostom AG, Cupples LA, Jenner JL, et al. Elevated plasma lipoprotein(a) and coronary heart disease in men aged 55 years and younger. *JAMA* 1996;276:544–548.

133. Maher VMG, Brown BG, Marcovina SM, et al. Effects of lowering elevated LDL cholesterol on the cardiovascular risk of lipoprotein(a). *JAMA* 1995;274:1771–1774.

134. Robinson K, Mayer E, Jacobsen DW. Homocysteine and coronary artery disease. *Cleve Clin J Med* 1994;61:438–450.

135. Morrison HI, Schaubel D, Desmeules M, et al. Serum folate and risk of fatal coronary heart disease. *JAMA* 1996;275:1893–1930.

136. Ross R. Atherosclerosis: an inflammatory disease. *N Engl J Med* 1999;340:115–126.

137. Ridker PM, Cushman M, Stampfer MJ, et al. Inflammation, aspirin, and the risk of cardiovascular disease in apparently healthy men. *N Engl J Med* 1997;336:973–979.

138. Ridker PM, Buring JE, Shih J, et al. Prospective study of C-reactive protein and the risk of future cardiovascular events among apparently healthy women. *Circulation* 1998; 98:731–733.

139. Rader DJ. Inflammatory markers of coronary risk. *N Engl J Med* 2000;343:1179–1182.

140. Ridker PM. Evaluating novel cardiovascular risk factors: can we better predict heart attacks? *Ann Intern Med* 1999;130:933–937.

141. Meade TW. Fibrinogen in ischaemic heart disease. *Eur Heart J* 1995;16:31–35.

142. Rader DJ. Noninvasive procedures for subclinical atherosclerosis risk assessment. *Am J Med* 1999;107:25S–27S.

143. Furberg CD, Adams J, Applegate WB, et al. Effect of lovastatin on early carotid atherosclerosis and cardiovascular events. *Circulation* 1994;90:1679–1687.

144. Crouse JR, Byington RP, Bond MG, et al. Pravastatin, Lipids, and Atherosclerosis in the Carotid Arteries (PLAC-II). *Preventive Cardiology/PLAC-II* 1995;75:455–459.

145. Salonen R, Nyyssonen K, Porkkala E, et al. Kuopio Atherosclerosis Prevention Study (KAPS): a population-based primary preventive trial of the effect of LDL lowering on atherosclerotic progression in carotid and femoral arteries. *Circulation* 1995;92:1758–1764.

146. Demer LL. Lipid hypothesis of cardiovascular calcification. *Circulation* 1997;95:297–298.

147. Rumberger JA, Brundage BH, Rader DJ, et al. Electron beam computed tomographic coronary calcium scanning: a review and guidelines for use in asymptomatic persons. *Mayo Clin Proc* 1999;74:243–252.

148. Rumberger JA, Simons DB, Fitzpatrick LA, et al. Coronary artery calcium areas by electron beam computed tomography and coronary atherosclerotic plaque area: a histopathologic correlative study. *Circulation* 1995;92:2157–2162.

149. Mautner GC, Mautner SL, Froehlich J, et al. Coronary artery calcification: assessment with electron beam CT and histomorphometric correlation. *Radiology* 1994;192:619–623.

150. Arad Y, Spadaro LA, Goodman K, et al. Predictive value of electron beam computed tomography of the coronary arteries: 19-month follow-up of 1173 asymptomatic subjects. *Circulation* 1996;93:1951–1953.

151. Walldius G, Erikson U, Olsson A, et al. The effect of probucol on femoral atherosclerosis: the Probucol Quantitative Regression Swedish Trial (PQRST). *Am J Cardiol* 1994;74:875–883.

152. Hennekens CH, Buring JE, Manson JE, et al. Lack of effect of long-term supplementation with beta carotene on the incidence of malignant neoplasms and cardiovascular disease. *N Engl J Med* 1996;334:1145–1149.

153. Omenn GS, Goodman GE, Thornquist MD, et al. Effects of a combination of beta carotene and vitamin A on lung cancer and cardiovascular disease. *N Engl J Med* 1996;334:1150–1155.

154. Stephens NG, Parsons A, Schofield PM, et al. Randomized controlled trial of vitamin E in patients with coronary disease: Cambridge Heart Antioxidant Study (CHAOS). *Lancet* 1996;347:781–786.

155. Yusuf S, Dagenais G, Pogue J, et al. Vitamin E supplementation and cardiovascular events in high-risk patients. The Heart Outcomes Prevention Evaluation Study Investigators. *N Engl J Med* 2000;342:154–160.

156. Boaz M, Smetana S, Weinstein T, et al. Secondary prevention with antioxidants of cardiovascular disease in endstage renal disease (SPACE): randomised placebo-controlled trial. *Lancet* 2000;356:1213–1218.

157. Pfeffer MA, Sacks FM, Moye LA, et al. Cholesterol and recurrent events: a secondary prevention trial for normolipidemic patients. *Am J Cardiol* 1995;76:98C–106C.

158. Hjermann I, Velve Byre K, Holme I, et al. Effect of diet and smoking intervention on the incidence of coronary heart disease: report from the Oslo Study Group of a randomised trial in healthy men. *Lancet* 1981;2:1303–1310.

159. Brensike JF, Levy RI, Kelsey SF, et al. Effects of therapy with cholestyramine on progression of coronary arteriosclerosis: results of the NHLBI type II coronary intervention study. *Circulation* 1984;69:313–324.

160. Blankenhorn DH, Nessim SA, Johnson RL, et al. Beneficial effects of combined colestipol-niacin therapy on coronary atherosclerosis and coronary venous bypass grafts. *JAMA* 1987;257:3233–3240.

161. Brown G, Albers JJ, Fisher MD, et al. Regression of coronary artery disease as a result of intensive lipid-lowering therapy in men with high levels of apolipoprotein B. *N Engl J Med* 1990;323:1289–1298.

162. Ornish D, Brown SE, Scherwitz LW, et al. Can lifestyle changes reverse coronary heart disease? The Lifestyle Heart Trial. *Lancet* 1990;336:129–133.

163. Kane JP, Malloy MJ, Ports TA, et al. Regression of coronary atherosclerosis during treatment of familial hypercholesterolemia with combined drug regimens. *JAMA* 1990;264:3007–3012.

164. Watts GF, Lewis B, Brunt JNH, et al. Effects on coronary artery disease of lipid-lowering diet, or diet plus cholestyramine, in the St Thomas' Atherosclerosis Regression Study (STARS). *Lancet* 1992;339:563–569.

165. Haskell WL, Alderman E, Fair J, et al. Effects of intensive multiple risk factor reduction on coronary atherosclerosis and clinical cardiac events in men and women with coronary artery disease. The Stanford Coronary Risk Intervention Project (SCRIP). *Circulation* 1994;89:975–990.

166. Blankenhorn DH, Azen SP, Kramsch DM, et al. Coronary angiographic changes with lovastatin therapy: the Monitored Atherosclerosis Regression Study (MARS). *Ann Intern Med* 1993;119:969–976.

167. Waters D, Higginson L, Gladstone P, et al. Effects of monotherapy with an HMG-CoA reductase inhibitor on the progression of coronary atherosclerosis as assessed by serial quantitative arteriography: the Canadian Coronary Atherosclerosis Intervention Trial. *Circulation* 1994;89:959–968.

168. MAAS Investigators. Effect of simvastatin on coronary atheroma: the Multicentre Anti-atheroma Study (MAAS). *Lancet* 1994;344:633–638.

169. Pitt B, Mancini GBJ, Ellis GS, et al. Pravastatin limitation of atherosclerosis in the coronary arteries (PLAC I): reduction in atherosclerosis progression and clinical events. *J Am Coll Cardiol* 1995;26:1133–1139.

170. Jukema JW, Bruschke AVG, Van Boven AJ, et al. Effects of lipid lowering by pravastatin on progression and regression of coronary artery disease in symptomatic men with normal to moderately elevated serum cholesterol levels. The Regression Growth Evaluation Statin Study (REGRESS). *Pravastatin and Coronary Atherosclerosis* 1995;91:2528–2540.

4

EXERCISE AND PHYSICAL ACTIVITY

DEBRA L. SHERMAN
GIULIA L. CEBULLA
GARY J. BALADY

OVERVIEW

Physical activity results in increased exercise capacity and physical fitness, which may lead to many health benefits. Individuals who are more physically active appear to have lower rates of all-cause mortality, probably due to a decrease in chronic diseases, including coronary artery disease (CAD). This low rate may result from an improvement in cardiovascular risk factors, enhanced fibrinolysis, improved endothelial function, decreased sympathetic tone, and other as-yet-undetermined factors.

Regular endurance and resistance exercise leads to favorable alterations in the cardiovascular, musculoskeletal, and neurohumoral systems. These alterations result in a training effect that allows an individual to do increasing amounts of work at a lower heart rate and blood pressure. Such an effect is particularly desirable in patients with CAD, because it allows increased activity with less ischemia.

Current recommendations from the Centers for Disease Control and Prevention (CDC) (8) state that every American should participate in at least moderately intense physical activity for at least 30 minutes on most, if not all, days of the week. Unfortunately, too many Americans are sedentary and perform too little physical activity. This is especially true among racial minorities, low-income groups, the elderly, and women. It is important to educate the public regarding the benefits of physical activity and to help encourage more leisure-time exercise in underactive individuals.

GLOSSARY

Calorie: a unit of energy equal to the amount of heat required to raise the temperature of 1 kg of water 1°C.

D. L. Sherman: Department of Cardiology, Caritas Norwood Hospital, Norwood, Massachusetts

G. L. Cebulla: Section of Cardiology, Boston Medical Center, Boston, Massachusetts

G. J. Balady: Section of Cardiology, Boston Medical Center, Boston, Massachusetts

- 1,000 cal = 1 kcal
- 5 kcal = 1 L oxygen consumed
- 7,000 kcal = 1 kg fat (2.2 lb)

Endurance exercise: Dynamic exercise involving high-repetition movements against low resistance. Endurance exercise also is called *isotonic exercise* because muscle shortening develops predominantly without much muscle tension. Examples include walking, jogging, swimming, and cycling. The term also is referred to as *aerobic exercise*.

Exercise: A form of physical activity; planned physical activity with the goal of achieving or preserving physical fitness.

Maximal oxygen uptake ($\dot{V}O_2$max): Maximal rate of oxygen consumption per minute. $\dot{V}O_2$max is a reliable, reproducible, and objective measure of physical fitness.

Metabolic equivalent (MET): One MET is equal to the amount of oxygen per minute required by the body during resting conditions.

1 MET = 3.5 mL oxygen/kg body weight/minute

Physical activity: Skeletal muscle contraction resulting in bodily movement that requires energy utilization.

Physical fitness: A set of attributes that enables an individual to perform physical activity.

Resistance exercise: Exercise involving low-repetition movements against a high resistance. An example is weightlifting.

Training effect: The ability to achieve a higher peak workrate and $\dot{V}O_2$max with lower heart-rate responses to submaximal levels of exercise compared with pretraining conditions.

Volume of oxygen ($\dot{V}O_2$): Amount of oxygen consumed per minute and expressed as the absolute value or as liters per kilogram of body weight per minute.

$\dot{V}O_2$ = stroke volume × heart rate × arteriovenous oxygen difference

Work: Force × distance.

Workrate: Work per unit of time.

INTRODUCTION

Physical Activity and Public Health

Nearly 60 million (approximately one of every four) persons in the United States have cardiovascular disease (CVD). Of these, 50 million suffer from hypertension, 12 million have CAD, and more than 4 million have suffered a stroke (1). Despite the declining mortality rate observed since 1950 and due to cardiovascular illness, 43% of all deaths are currently attributed to CVD. The morbidity and subsequent disability incurred from cardiovascular illness have far-reaching medical and socioeconomic implications and an estimated total cost of $327 billion in

2000. Thus, continued major efforts in preventing CVD are needed to reduce the overall incidence of atherosclerotic disease and stroke (1).

Physical inactivity is a risk factor for CVD. Regular exercise results in an increase in exercise capacity and lower myocardial oxygen demand, leading to cardiovascular benefits such as lower mortality rates and fewer symptoms of CAD (2–4). Moreover, the long-term cost-effectiveness of an unsupervised exercise training program has been estimated to be less than $12,000 per year of life saved for all individuals (5). The Surgeon General's report on physical activity and health (6) has summarized the findings of five national surveys by the CDC. The results indicate that too many American adults lead sedentary lifestyles, with only 14% of respondents reporting regular vigorous physical activity (i.e., activity performed at 50% of maximum cardiorespiratory capacity for 20 minutes at least three times per week). Approximately 25% of adults report regular moderate physical activity (i.e., activity performed at 3 to 6 METs for 30 minutes on most days of the week), and 25% participate in no leisure-time physical activity (6). More recent data from the National Health Interview Survey (7) estimate that 40% of American adults are sedentary.

Many factors contribute to physical inactivity in adults, but the most-cited reasons are lack of time and risk of injury. Although most Americans are aware that exercise is beneficial for good health, this knowledge does not strongly correlate with physical activity. Other important barriers are lack of companionship or encouragement and the absence of an appropriate environment for exercise (e.g., no available paths for walking or biking, poor weather, or dangerous neighborhood). Regular physical activity is more strongly associated with enjoyment of exercise, confidence in athletic ability, and participation in low to moderate levels of activity (8). ❥ a75

Physical Activity, Exercise, and Fitness

Physical activity, fitness, and exercise are related entities but have different definitions. The definitions described below are as defined in the Surgeon General's report on physical activity and health (6).

Physical Activity

Physical activity is skeletal muscle contraction resulting in bodily movement that requires energy use. Further classification can be based on mechanical and metabolic aspects of contraction. Mechanical properties relate to whether limb movement occurs and includes isometric contraction (i.e., muscle tension without limb movement) and isotonic contraction (i.e., limb movement without change in muscle tension). Metabolic properties of physical activity are divided into categories of aerobic contraction (i.e., energy derived in the presence of oxygen) and anaerobic contrac-

TABLE 4.1   CLASSIFICATION OF PHYSICAL ACTIVITY INTENSITY[a]

	Endurance-type activity					
	Relative intensity		Absolute intensity (METs) in healthy adults (age in yr)			
Intensity	$\dot{V}O_2$max heart-rate reserve (%)	Maximum heart rate (%)	Young (20–39)	Middle-aged (40–64)	Old (65–79)	Very old (80+)
Very light	<25	<30	<3.0	<2.5	<2.0	≤1.25
Light	25–39	30–49	3.0–4.7	2.5–4.4	2.0–3.5	1.26–2.20
Moderate	40–59	50–69	4.8–7.1	4.5–5.9	3.6–4.7	2.30–2.95
Hard	60–84	70–89	7.2–10.1	6.0–8.4	4.8–6.7	3.00–4.25
Very hard	≥85	≥90	≥10.2	≥8.5	≥6.8	≥4.25
Maximum[b]	100	100	12.0	10.0	8.0	5.0

MET, metabolic equivalent; $\dot{V}O_2$max, maximal oxygen uptake.
[a]Based on 8 to 12 repetitions for persons <50 years old and 10 to 15 repetitions for persons ≥50 years old.
[b]Maximum values are mean values achieved during maximum exercise by healthy adults. Absolute intensity (METs) values are approximate mean values for men. Mean values for women are approximately 1 to 2 METs lower than those for men.
Adapted from U.S. Department of Health and Human Services. *Physical activity and health: a report of the surgeon general.* Atlanta: Center for Disease Control and Prevention, National Center for Chronic Disease Prevention and Promotion, 1996.

tion (i.e., energy derived in the absence of oxygen). Most activity involves a combination of the above parameters (6).

The intensity of physical activity can be described as the energy required per unit of time for the performance of an activity and can be obtained by measuring the oxygen uptake required for the activity. This intensity can be expressed in units of oxygen, kilocalories (measure of heat), or kilojoules (measure of energy). In addition, intensity of activity can be expressed by measuring the force of muscle contraction and is expressed in pounds or kilograms. Alternatively, physical activity can be measured in relative terms by relating the amount of activity in relation to the individual's capacity and is usually expressed as a percentage, such as the percentage of $\dot{V}O_2$max or the percentage of maximum heart rate (6) (Table 4.1).

Physical Exercise

Physical exercise is a form of physical activity and is defined as planned physical activity with the goal of achieving or preserving physical fitness. *Exercise training* may be a more accurate term, because similar activity may be viewed as exercise by one person and not by others (6).

Physical Fitness

Physical fitness is a set of attributes that enables an individual to perform physical activity (8). Physical fitness is best assessed by measures of $\dot{V}O_2$max. Many studies estimate fitness levels by measurement of the peak workrate or MET level achieved during graded exercise tests. Numerous exercise training studies have evaluated the frequency, intensity, and duration of the training sessions. Based on these data, it appears that the most consistent benefit on $\dot{V}O_2$max is observed when exercise training is performed at least three to five times per week for 12 or more weeks at an intensity of approximately 60% of the maximum heart rate, or 50% of

$\dot{V}O_2$max, for 20 to 60 minutes (11). Improvements in $\dot{V}O_2$max of 15% to 30% are usually achieved using the above guidelines (11). It also appears that intermittent activity can confer fitness benefits similar to those of continuous activity at similar exercise intensities and total duration (12).

PHYSICAL ACTIVITY AND HEALTH: EPIDEMIOLOGIC OBSERVATIONS AND BIOLOGIC MECHANISMS

All-Cause Mortality

Data accumulated over the past 50 years have confirmed the health benefits of exercise. Epidemiologic studies have shown that active individuals are at lower risk for developing many chronic diseases (8). In addition, all-cause mortality rates are higher in less active people than in those who are more active (16,17). A large-scale epidemiologic study involving 13,375 women and 17,265 men between the ages of 20 and 93 years reported a significant inverse association between leisure-time physical activity and all-cause mortality (18). Approximately 12% of deaths per year in the United States are associated with inactivity (19). The risk for all-cause mortality decreases among inactive individuals who become more physically active (20). Importantly, recent data from an evaluation of 5,209 men and women demonstrate that the performance of recent activity confers a reduction in all-cause mortality, whereas activity performed decades earlier without subsequent maintenance appears to have no long-term benefit (21).

Cardiovascular Disease

Many studies have demonstrated that regular exercise and physical activity prevent primary and secondary cardiac events. In one of the most well-known studies, male Harvard University alumni without a history of CVD were followed for 16 years (16). There was a 39% reduction in cardiovascular morbidity and a 24% reduction in cardiovascular mortality in subjects with exercise energy expenditures of more than 2,000 kcal per week. Oldridge et al. (4) performed a metaanalysis of ten randomized clinical trials that examined the effects of cardiac rehabilitation after myocardial infarction (MI). No differences in nonfatal MI were apparent; however, there was a 24% reduction in all-cause mortality and a 25% reduction in cardiovascular mortality among exercise rehabilitation patients compared with controls. Wannamethee et al. (22) have also demonstrated that in men with established CAD, an increase in leisure-time physical activity was associated with a significant reduction in all-cause mortality.

Several population-based studies show that incremental levels of regular physical activity are inversely proportional to long-term cardiovascular mortality when controlled for the presence of other risk factors in both men and women (2,8,16,20,23) (Fig. 4.1). Among male alumni, the risk of death became progressively lower as physical activity levels increased from 500 to 3,500 kcal per week of energy expended (16). Alumni who were initially inactive and later increased their activity levels demonstrated significantly reduced cardiovascular risk compared with those who remained inactive (20). Moreover, when measured by an exercise tolerance test, higher levels of physical fitness are associated with significantly reduced subsequent cardiovascular mortality among men and women (17,25). In the Nurses' Health Study (24,26), 73,029 women (aged 40 to 65 years) were followed for 4 years. Physical activity in women was inversely related to the risk for stroke and CAD. The largest benefit was seen between the lowest and second-lowest quintile groups, suggesting that the incremental value of exercise is greatest in the least-active subjects compared with the most-active subjects. In a general population of elderly men, the 10-year CVD and all-cause mortality rate was inversely related to increasing levels of physical activity (27).

The relative risk of CAD in physically inactive subjects compared with active individuals is approximately 2.0 (2,8,9). Importantly, the relative risk for cardiovascular mortality in the least-fit or least-active individuals compared with the most-fit or most-active subjects approaches 6.0 (8,9,17). Paffenbarger et al. (20) have reported encouraging data that demonstrate that, when habitual physical activity levels are increased, subsequent mortality is decreased relative to those who remained physically inactive. These data strongly support the need to increase physical activity and fitness levels among both women and men, with the most mortality benefit to be derived by those who are the least fit.

The specific mechanisms by which physical activity reduces CAD mortality are not known. Exercise improves lipid profile, glucose tolerance, obesity, and elevated blood pressure. In a cross-sectional analysis of a large cohort of men and women, increasing levels of physical fitness

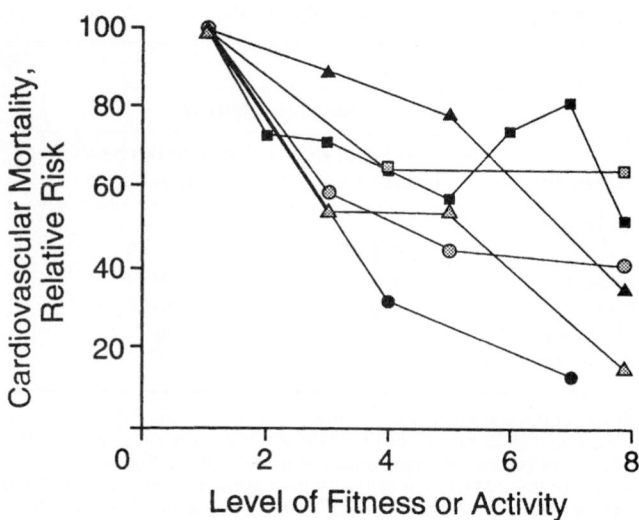

FIGURE 4.1 The relationship between physical activity or fitness and the relative risk for cardiovascular mortality. As fitness improves, the risk for cardiovascular death diminishes. ■, Paffenbarger et al. (1993); ▲, Morris et al. (1990); ●, Blair et al. (1989); ▨, Leon et al. (1987); △, Ekelund et al. (1988); ◉, Sandvik et al. (1993). (From Pate RR, Pratt M, Blair SN, et al. Physical activity and public health: a recommendation from the Centers for Disease Control and Prevention and the American College of Sports Medicine. *JAMA* 1995;273:402–407, with permission.)

assessed by maximal exercise treadmill testing were found to protect against elevations in most coronary heart disease (CHD) risk factors in persons with and without CAD (28). However, modification of atherosclerotic risk factors does not fully explain the benefits that have been observed. Other possible mechanisms—including effects on thrombosis, endothelial function, and autonomic tone—may play an important role (*e*Table 4.1.2).

Cardiovascular Risk Factors

Hypertension

In addition to preventing hypertension, [⛛ a76] regular exercise has also been found to lower blood pressure. In mildly hypertensive men, short-term physical activity decreases blood pressure for 8 to 12 hours after exercise, and average blood pressure is lower on exercise days than on nonexercise days (33). In severely hypertensive black men, moderate physical activity performed for 16 to 32 weeks results in a decrease in diastolic blood pressure that is sustained even after reduction in antihypertensive medications. In addition, a significant decrease in left ventricular (LV) hypertrophy has been reported as early as 16 weeks after the initiation of exercise (34).

Diabetes Mellitus

Physical activity has beneficial effects on glucose metabolism and insulin sensitivity, including increased sensitivity to insulin, decreased production of glucose by the liver, larger numbers of muscle cells that use more glucose than adipose tissue, and reduced obesity (35). In addition, there is evidence that regular exercise may prevent the onset of diabetes mellitus. A study of male alumni from the University of Pennsylvania (36) found that for every 500 calories of energy expended per week participating in leisure-time physical activity, the age-adjusted risk for the development of type 2 diabetes mellitus decreased by 6%. Lynch et al. (37) found that men who participated in moderate physical activity for at least 40 minutes a week were at lower risk for developing type 2 diabetes. This risk reduction was even more pronounced in men at high risk for developing diabetes. In a population-based prospective study, men in the lowest level of cardiorespiratory fitness, as measured by maximal exercise treadmill time, had a 3.7-fold higher risk of developing diabetes compared with men in the highest fitness level (38). In a large prospective cohort study of women, the risk of developing type 2 diabetes was substantially decreased in women who either walked or exercised vigorously, as long as the total energy expenditure was the same (40). Among physically inactive men who already have type 2 diabetes, those with a low fitness level have higher all-cause mortality than those who exercise and are physically fit (39). However, the role of exercise in the prevention and treatment of type 1 diabetes mellitus is unclear.

Overweight and Obesity

The prevalence of obesity has increased over the past 25 years, despite a reduction in fat intake. The most likely explanation for this national trend is an increase in total caloric intake, along with a reduction in physical activity (41). Using a body mass index of 25 or higher as "overweight" and a body mass index of 30 or higher as "obese," nearly 106 million American adults age 20 and older are considered overweight (55 million men and 51 million women), and more than 43 million are considered obese (18 million men and 25 million women). In addition, an estimated 4.9 million children ages 6 to 17 are considered overweight (1).

Exercise training appears to be an important component for weight loss, although the effect of exercise is quite variable. Most controlled exercise training studies show only modest weight loss (approximately 2 to 3 kg) in the treated group versus the control group. When diet is added to exercise programs, the average weight loss is 8.5 kg (42,43). A well-controlled, 1-year randomized trial (44) that included 231 subjects demonstrated a significant 8.7-kg weight loss, most of which was body fat, in the exercise and diet intervention group and a significant 5.1-kg weight loss in the diet-only group. Those in the control group increased their weight by an average of 1.7 kg. Another randomized controlled trial involving 40 obese women demonstrated that moderate-intensity lifestyle activity combined with a low-

fat diet resulted in favorable effects on weight loss, systolic blood pressure, and serum lipoprotein concentrations at 16 weeks and 1 year. Remarkably, the magnitude of benefit was similar to that observed in patients randomized to diet plus a structured program of aerobic exercise (45). These data strongly support the role of both exercise and diet in weight-loss programs.

Body composition and fat distribution are also linked to cardiovascular mortality (43) and are favorably affected by exercise. On average, exercise training programs reduce body fat by approximately 1.6% (42). Physically active men and women have a more favorable waist-hip ratio (p <0.9) than do sedentary individuals (46–49). Although significant, these changes are rather small, even after 1 year of diet and exercise (47). Importantly, physical activity appears to have favorable effects on lipoproteins, glucose metabolism, and blood pressure, even when weight loss is only modest (50).

Lipids

The effect of exercise on lipid levels has been an area of continued research. There is much variability in the results of exercise–lipid-lowering studies, at least in part due to the heterogeneity of the study methods, populations, exercise interventions, and the use of adjunctive interventions such as diet or pharmacologic lipid-lowering agents. A metaanalysis of 95 studies (51), most of which were not randomized controlled trials, concluded that exercise leads to a 6% reduction in total cholesterol, 10% in low-density lipoprotein cholesterol, and 13% in cholesterol/high-density lipoprotein cholesterol (HDL-C), and a 5% increase in HDL-C. The greatest changes in lipids were noted in patients who also lost weight during their exercise program. When body weight increased, lipid levels worsened. Intermediate changes were noted when body weight remained constant. It appears that the training intensities required to yield modest improvements in lipids are not as high as those that lead to improvements in fitness levels, as HDL appears to increase across a broad spectrum of exercise intensities (52,53) (*e*Fig. 4.1.1). Moderate-intensity exercise (i.e., equivalent to briskly walking 10 miles per week), Step 2 AHA diet, and the combination of exercise plus diet were studied in a randomized controlled trial of postmenopausal women and middle-aged men. The most favorable changes in low-density lipoprotein (8% to 12% reduction) occurred among subjects in the diet and exercise group after 1 year. HDL levels decreased by 2% among women in the diet plus exercise groups, but among men there was a favorable increase of 2% (54).

In a study of 82 male and female patients with coronary disease, a 3-month exercise training program in conjunction with diet resulted in an 8% increase in HDL and a 22% decrease in triglycerides in subjects who had baseline triglyceride elevations. However, there was no significant improvement in body weight, low-density lipoprotein cholesterol, glucose level, or insulin level (55). ❦ a77

Thrombosis

Mounting evidence suggests that hemostatic parameters are important cardiovascular risk factors. Hemostasis is a balance between clot formation (thrombosis) and clot dissolution (fibrinolysis). This balance is especially important in CAD, in which the fibrinolytic system plays a protective role. The Framingham Study (60) has shown that elevated fibrinogen levels increase the risk for CAD in men and women between the ages of 47 and 59 years. In fact, patients in the upper tercile of fibrinogen levels had a two- to threefold higher incidence of CVD. Emerging evidence suggests that exercise training favorably affects the fibrinolytic system, which may help to explain the reduction in cardiac events observed in subjects who are more physically active. Strenuous endurance exercise for 6 months in healthy older patients (i.e., aged 60 to 82 years) resulted in a significant improvement in hemostatic parameters, a reduction in plasma fibrinogen levels of 13%, an increase in mean tissue-plasminogen activator (t-PA) of 39%, an increase in active t-PA of 141%, and a reduction of plasminogen activator inhibitor-1 of 58% (61). In contrast, younger patients (i.e., aged 24 to 30 years), whose baseline fibrinolytic variables were lower than the older group, had no significant change in fibrinogen, t-PA, or plasminogen activator inhibitor-1 activity. However, other studies have shown favorable effects of fibrinolytic enzymes after exercise training in younger subjects (62) and in patients after MI (63).

There is also evidence that acute and chronic exercise affect platelet activation. Platelet activation is important in the pathophysiologic mechanisms of unstable coronary syndromes and acute MI. Kestin et al. (64) studied the effects of treadmill exercise on platelet activation in sedentary and physically fit individuals. After acute strenuous exercise of similar duration and intensity, platelet activation and hyperreactivity were increased in sedentary subjects but remained unchanged in physically fit subjects. Rauramaa et al. (65) demonstrated that regular, moderate-intensity physical activity in middle-aged, overweight, mildly hypertensive men results in decreased platelet aggregation. After the 12-week exercise program, the study subjects demonstrated a 52% reduction in secondary platelet aggregation compared with a 17% decrease for the control group. Thus, it appears that, although acute exercise can lead to increased platelet activity, especially in sedentary individuals, regular exercise may abolish or improve this response.

Inflammation

Growing evidence suggests that inflammation plays a role in atherosclerosis. In a recent study, serum levels of cyto-

kines and C-reactive protein levels were measured in 52 volunteers in a 6-month, moderate-intensity exercise program who were at risk for ischemic heart disease. Atherogenic cytokine production fell significantly after the training period, as did levels of C-reactive protein (66).

Endothelial Function

The vascular endothelium plays an important role in the regulation of arterial tone and local platelet aggregation, in part through the release of nitric oxide (NO) (67). NO produces vasodilation and inhibits platelet adhesion and aggregation by a guanylyl cyclase–dependent mechanism in vascular smooth-muscle cells and platelets. These effects are associated with an increase in platelet cyclic–guanosine monophosphate. Release of NO is stimulated by serotonin, thrombin, acetylcholine, and other receptor-dependent agonists (67). NO release is also stimulated by increased shear stress associated with acute and chronic increases in blood flow (68,69). Endothelium-dependent dilation is impaired in patients with coronary atherosclerosis or coronary risk factors, including hypercholesterolemia, diabetes mellitus, cigarette smoking, and hypertension (70–72). Patients with peripheral arterial disease have also been shown to have impaired endothelium-dependent vasodilation in the presence of cardiac risk factors (73). Convincing evidence exists that impaired NO action in atherosclerosis contributes to the pathophysiology of myocardial ischemia in patients with stable and unstable coronary syndromes (71,72,74).

An improvement in endothelial function in such patients has the potential to improve outcome. Growing evidence suggests that exercise improves endothelial function (75). Recent animal studies suggest that an important consequence of chronic exercise is an improvement in vasomotor function. This manifests by increased endothelium-dependent vasodilation in response to increased blood flow and clinically relevant NO agonists (76,77). High-resolution brachial artery ultrasound assessment of flow-mediated dilation has been used and validated as a model to evaluate endothelial function (78,79). Brachial artery diameter is measured at baseline and after reactive hyperemia produced by 5 minutes of cuff occlusion of the upper arm. Relative increases in diameter from baseline are used as measures of endothelium-dependent, flow-mediated dilation. Using this method, Clarkson et al. (80) showed that exercise training improved endothelium-dependent, flow-mediated dilation in young, healthy men. This effect was present in patients with and without CAD risk factors and was not related to lipid levels. Similar effects were demonstrated in patients with heart failure (HF) (81). Aging has been associated with a progressive decline in endothelium-dependent vasodilation, which may partially explain the increased risk of atherosclerosis in the elderly. A cross-sectional study of 68 healthy men demonstrated that regular aerobic exercise prevented this age-associated decline in endothelial function (82). A separate study suggests that the mechanism of the improvement in endothelial function in trained elderly athletes may be an increase in the availability of NO (83).

A seminal study by Hambrecht et al. (84) assessed whether exercise training affects endothelial function in the coronary circulation. In a randomized controlled trial, improvement in coronary endothelial function and coronary flow reserve in men with CAD was demonstrated. After 4 weeks of exercise training, significantly less coronary vasoconstriction in response to acetylcholine was observed.

Autonomic Function

The balance between sympathetic and parasympathetic activity modulates cardiovascular activity. Enhanced sympathetic nervous system activity, which may occur with aging, may be a risk factor for cardiac events. Heart-rate variability (HRV) is a well-accepted noninvasive technique for assessing autonomic tone. HRV increases with higher parasympathetic tone and decreases with sympathetic stimulation. Thus, higher HRV implies augmentation of parasympathetic tone, which may protect against cardiovascular morbidity and mortality. In healthy subjects, HRV appears to be related to exercise training. In a cross-sectional study, Goldsmith et al. (85) evaluated HRV in eight endurance-trained men and eight age-matched controls. Using 24-hour Holter monitors, they found that the standard deviation of the RR intervals, the average RR interval, and the high-frequency power were greater in the trained group, suggesting that exercise training increases parasympathetic tone. In another cross-sectional study, DeMeersman et al. (86) compared HRV in 72 male runners with sedentary age-matched controls. HRV was significantly higher in the physically fit patients, implying higher parasympathetic tone. Whether exercise affects autonomic tone in patients with CVD is unclear. Coats et al. (87,88) found that exercise training increased HRV in 17 patients with chronic HF (*e*Fig. 4.1.2). However, in a recent randomized controlled trial of 25 men with new-onset LV dysfunction after MI, 2 months of high-intensity exercise training did not alter HRV at 1, 2, and 12 months compared with controls (89). ❦ a78

PHYSIOLOGY OF EXERCISE

Types of Exercise

Most types of exercise involve endurance and resistance training. However, usually one type of training predominates. The physiologic responses to exercise lead to specific muscular, neurohumoral, and cardiovascular adaptations that depend, in part, on the type of exercise performed.

Endurance

Endurance (aerobic, dynamic) training consists of dynamic or isotonic exercise, which involves high-repetition movements against low resistance. Examples include walking, jogging, swimming, or cycling. Isotonic exercise implies that muscles shorten but maintain a constant tension, although tension does change to some degree during exercise (11). Endurance exercise involves rhythmic contraction and relaxation of working muscles. This results in increased blood flow to active muscles during relaxation and increased venous return to the heart from the working muscles during contraction. Regular dynamic exercise is referred to as *endurance training*, because it results in improved functional capacity, enabling the individual to exercise for a longer duration or at a higher workrate.

Resistance

Resistance training, also called *static exercise*, involves low-repetition movements against high resistance. This training may also be referred to as *isometric exercise*, because muscle tension develops predominantly without muscle shortening. An example of resistance training is weightlifting. The development of muscle tension during resistance training restricts blood flow during contraction. Regular resistance training leads to increased strength and is commonly referred to as *power* or *strength training*.

Responses to Exercise Training

Regular endurance or resistance training results in specific changes in the muscular, cardiovascular, and neurohumoral systems that lead to improvement in functional capacity and strength. These changes are referred to as the *training effect* and allow an individual to exercise to higher peak workrates with lower heart rates at each submaximal level of exercise.

Muscular Adaptations

Regular endurance training results in changes in skeletal muscle, including increases in mitochondria, myoglobin, capillary density, and metabolic enzymes (107). The increased mitochondrial number is specific to the muscle group exercised. For example, runners have more mitochondria in their lower-extremity muscles than in their arm muscles. Additional capillaries in skeletal muscle serve to aid in the exchange of nutrients and metabolic byproducts during exercise (108). Increased metabolic enzymes enhance a muscle's capacity for converting glycogen and fatty acids to adenosine 6-triphosphate. With endurance training, more energy is derived from fatty-acid metabolism, and glycogen stores are spared (107). As a result, less lactate is produced, and endurance is enhanced. The net effect of the changes in skeletal muscle is to promote aerobic metabolism, which, in turn, improves exercise capacity.

In contrast to endurance training, regular resistance training leads to muscle-cell hypertrophy due to increased synthesis of contractile proteins and connective tissue (109).

Cardiovascular Adaptations

Endurance training results in increased venous return to the heart, which leads to higher LV volumes. Resistance training exposes the patient to chronic increases in afterload due to increased total peripheral resistance and elevated blood pressure, yielding a greater LV wall thickness. These effects result in increased LV mass in both training groups. However, the LV mass–lean body mass ratio is elevated in the endurance trainer, whereas it is normal in the resistance trainer (110). The increase in LV mass in the resistance trainer is proportional to the increase in skeletal muscle mass.

Along with changes in myocardial mass, certain hemodynamic effects are observed from endurance and resistance training. Wall stress at rest in endurance trainers is normal; however, it is lower in resistance trainers due to increased wall thickness without ventricular dilation (111). Systolic function and fractional shortening at rest are normal in both groups. However, compared with nonathletes, stroke volume is increased due to greater end diastolic volumes (111,112). Despite increased LV wall thickening, diastolic function appears to be normal in both groups (113). A cross-sectional study comparing the effects of long-term training among distance runners and wheelchair athletes demonstrated that long-term arm exercise and leg exercise yield increases in LV volume and mass—although to a lesser degree in arm-trained athletes—compared with untrained control subjects (114).

The decline in $\dot{V}O_2$max (exercise capacity) seen with aging has also been shown to be attenuated by habitual exercise. A recent study (115) aimed to explain this observation and noted that, after exercise training, peak leg blood flow increased by 50%, although there was no change in peak cardiac output. This occurrence suggests that exercise yields a reversible deconditioning effect on the distribution of cardiac output to exercising muscle. In patients with CAD, there appears to be less ischemia for a given rate-pressure product after exercise training compared with that before training. Improvements in ischemic threshold manifest as less angina (116), ST-segment depression (117), and thallium defects (118) at the same levels of exercise. These findings suggest that exercise training improves myocardial oxygen supply in patients with CAD. The specific mechanisms responsible are unclear; however, possible explanations include improvement in endothelial function and vasomotor tone, decreased sympathetic tone, and alterations in blood rheology.

Neurohumoral Adaptations

Neurohumoral responses to exercise manifest as lower resting heart rate and reduced heart rate at any level of submaximal exercise. The diminished heart rate at rest and with exercise is due to increased resting parasympathetic tone and decreased sympathetic tone. Lower levels of circulating catecholamines are observed in trained versus untrained individuals (90,91), whereas the number and sensitivity of beta-adrenergic receptors appear unchanged with exercise training (119).

Detraining

Cessation of exercise training for as little as 3 weeks can lead to some loss of the training effect. This may be partially due to the reduction in LV size and stroke volume as a consequence of the absence of increased cardiac filling, which occurs with exercise (120). The lower preload results in less stretching of the myocardium and a lower stroke volume, according to the Frank-Starling mechanism.

PHYSICAL ACTIVITY AND EXERCISE: PRESCRIPTION FOR HEALTH AND FITNESS

Energy Expenditure

Major public health statements have generated recommendations regarding the amount of exercise and physical activity that should be performed each week to generate health benefits. It is important to note that these recommendations are based on studies performed almost exclusively on men, although recent years have witnessed an increasing number of studies performed on women.

Intensity, Frequency, and Duration of Physical Activity

The CDC, ACSM (8), and Surgeon General (6) recommend that adults exercise for 30 minutes at moderate-intensity levels on most, if not all, days of the week to achieve a weekly energy expenditure of at least 1,000 kcal. These statements stem from evidence stating that regular moderate physical activity provides many health benefits. In addition, these recommendations stress that physical activity can be accomplished in multiple short intervals—which may be more feasible for many individuals—rather than continuous 30-minute exercise sessions. Low-intensity exercise should be performed more frequently and for longer duration.

The CDC recommendations are based on data that suggest that the benefits of exercise are related to the total energy expenditure or dose measured in calories or duration of physical activity. Observational studies have shown that cardiovascular mortality decreases when duration of exercise increases from 15 to 47 minutes per day and when caloric expenditure increases from 500 to 2,000 calories per week (16). A recent study of 7,307 Harvard University alumni demonstrated that brief durations of physical activity—as short as 15 minutes—conferred as much of a reduction in CHD risk as longer sessions, as long as the total energy expenditure was equivalent (121). However, an important question remains regarding the intensity of physical activity required to incur a mortality benefit. Intensity can be defined in terms of reflecting the rate of energy expenditure during exercise (expressed in METs or kcal per minute) or the relative percentage of maximum aerobic capacity that is maintained during the exercise or activity (expressed in terms of percentage of maximum heart rate or percentage of $\dot{V}O_2$max achieved on exercise tests) (8). The data regarding exercise intensity are much less clear than those addressing dose. Lee et al. (122) have reported that only energy expended during vigorous activity (>6 METs) yielded a mortality benefit among Harvard University alumni. More recent data from this cohort similarly demonstrate that moderate activities (<6 METs) have no clear association with risk of CHD and that men older than 60 years with coronary risk factors who expended more than 1,000 kcal per week had less CHD risk, as did men without risk factors. The intensity of physical activity was associated with a 20% reduction in CHD risk (29). Conversely, walking also has been shown to reduce the incidence of coronary disease in a large sample of elderly subjects, with a proportionately lower incidence of CVD in men who walked more than 1.5 miles per day (29). One must consider however, that brisk walking in elderly persons may be at moderate-intensity relative to their peak exercise capacity but, in absolute terms, is <6 METs. Similarly, prospective data from the Nurses Health Study suggest that brisk walking (3 to 4 miles per hour; 2.5 to 4.5 METs), as well as vigorous exercise (>6 METs), is associated with a substantial reduction in the risk for CVD (124).

Risks of Exercise

The inherent risks of physical activity must be considered to promote the health benefits of exercise while minimizing injury. Because nearly every activity carries some risk, the risk-benefit ratio must be examined for each individual. Major hazards involve the cardiovascular and musculoskeletal systems.

Cardiovascular Risks

The risks of cardiovascular morbidity and mortality depend on whether one studies the general population or individuals with CAD. Although the risk of death during exercise is low, death in individuals over 35 years of age is usually the result of atherosclerotic CAD, whereas younger individuals are more likely to suffer from congenital cardiac malforma-

tions (128). The incidence of sudden cardiac death during exercise for the population at large is 1 in 565,000 events per hour (129). The risk of sudden death during exercise is much lower for young individuals than for middle-aged and older adults. Among high school and college athletes, the sudden death rate is estimated to be 1 in 133,333 male athletes and 1 in 769,230 female athletes (130). The exertionally related sudden death rate in previously healthy middle-aged men is approximately 6 to 7 in 100,000 events per year (131,132).

For healthy sedentary men, the risk of cardiac arrest is 56 times higher during exercise compared with times of inactivity. In contrast, the risk for active men during exercise is five times the risk during times of inactivity. Despite this transient increased risk during strenuous exercise, regularly active men have a cumulative cardiac arrest risk that is 40% lower than the risk in inactive men (132). In a prospective study of 21,481 male physicians who were reportedly free of CAD, the relative risk of sudden death after an episode of heavy exertion was 1.9. However, the absolute risk of dying was extremely low (1 in 1.5 million episodes of exertion). Furthermore, habitual vigorous exercise was associated with a significant reduction in the incidence of sudden death (133). This and other studies (132,134) demonstrate that the risk of primary cardiac arrest during exertion is reduced among those who are physically active.

There is also evidence that heavy exertion may trigger acute MI. Two studies have found that the relative risk for MI within 1 hour after strenuous physical exertion was increased by two to six times that of patients who were sedentary or less active during that hour (135,136). However, the risk was inversely related to the amount of leisure-time physical activity performed by the subjects. Thus, the more active the individual, the lower the risk for developing acute MI during strenuous exertion. There is also evidence that sexual activity can trigger acute MI; however, the risk is low (137). The relative risk for MI within 2 hours of sexual activity was 2.5 in healthy subjects, 2.1 in those with a history of angina, and 2.9 in those with a history of MI. The absolute risk for MI in all groups was low and was not increased in individuals with CAD. In addition, the risk was reduced in individuals who exercised regularly.

In individuals with known CAD, exercise training is relatively safe. In a study of 167 cardiac rehabilitation programs involving 51,000 patients, the incidence of cardiac arrest was 1 in 112,000 person-hours, with a successful resuscitation rate of 86% (138). The incidence of MI was 1 in 294,000 person-hours, and the incidence of death was 1 in 784,000 person-hours. More recent data from a single cardiac rehabilitation center report the incidence of major cardiovascular complications to be 1 in 60,000 participant-hours, with no deaths occurring (139). Limited data are available regarding home exercise in patients with cardiac disease. Using heart-rate monitors and transtelephonic electrocardiographic transmission, DeBusk and colleagues

(140) found a similar rate of reinfarction and death after 26 weeks in patients randomized to home training versus subjects randomized to group training. Similarly, Ades et al. reported no major cardiac arrest or death during 3,100 hours of home exercise (141).

CONTROVERSIES AND PERSONAL PERSPECTIVES

Promotion of Physical Activity

The message from America's leading scientists is clear, unequivocal, and unified: physical inactivity is a risk factor for CVD. It is highly prevalent and is a matter of public health. This unprecedented focus on physical activity and exercise is the product of copious research, including epidemiologic observational studies, cohort studies, randomized controlled trials, and basic research. It is clear that the promotion of physical activity has reached the forefront of our national public health agenda, as manifested by the publication of the 1996 Surgeon General's report on physical activity and health (6). Much work remains to promulgate this message and implement strategies to achieve the ambitious goals of the Healthy People 2010 objectives (145). Broad-based efforts that affect every level of our social infrastructure are needed ultimately to impact the health status of the United States. Although educational and media campaigns that directly target youth and adults are essential, these efforts must be supported by policy makers, legislators, educators, health care providers and insurers, employers, community leaders, and researchers.

Federal, state, and local governments must adopt policies that foster the promotion of physical activity. Physical education programs in schools throughout our nation are vital for the development of positive attitudes and the acquisition of appropriate knowledge and skills that foster active and healthy lifestyles throughout adult years. All individuals should develop an understanding and appreciation of the benefits that can be derived from the wide range of physical activity options. The nature of these activities range from everyday house chores to organized sports, from walking the dog to running on a treadmill. Physicians, nurses, and allied health care providers play a pivotal role in counseling their patients on physical activity and influencing subsequent behavior. These initiatives by the health care team must, in turn, be supported by government and private health insurance providers, who must realize that appropriate lifestyle interventions can reduce or eliminate a large number of health risks and, ultimately, reduce health care costs. Communities and employers have remarkable opportunities to provide environments and incentives to promote physical activity. Finally, scientists and researchers should be stimulated to answer the many remaining questions regarding physical activity, exercise, and health. Of course, such work cannot be done without the much-needed support of federal and private funding agencies. Funding opportunities and initiatives for clinical, behavioral, and basic research in this area are essential to transform present-day goals into future reality.

Dose and Intensity of Physical Activity

Despite the large body of literature from more than half a century of research in the area of physical activity, large gaps in the knowledge base remain. A prudent conclusion has been drawn from the studies to date: moderate-intensity activity for 30 minutes a day leads to health and, presumably, mortality benefits. Inherent properties in this recommendation are dose (i.e., total energy expanded per week) and intensity (i.e., the energy requirements per unit of time for a given activity). Prospective, randomized controlled trials are needed to evaluate variations of dose versus intensity of activities on specific health outcomes—including definite cardiac events—in any large representative cohort of the population or among any specific subgroup (e.g., youth, elderly, patients with known CVD). Recent studies indicate that exercise training of low to moderate intensity can increase physical fitness and result in improvements in several health variables (e.g., insulin sensitivity, HDL levels, blood pressure). Epidemiologic data support the relation of moderate-intensity activity to lower mortality; however, intensity of activity in these studies is not directly measured, but it is categorized based on estimated energy requirements per unit of time or subjective perception of activity intensity. Indeed, the lowest threshold for dose or intensity to achieve specific cardiovascular benefit is not known, nor is the ideal dose-intensity prescription for specific biologic outcomes or total cardiovascular health.

Considering the high prevalence of physical inactivity among American youth and adults, the existing broad-based public health recommendations are reasonable and scientifically sound. However, it is hoped that customized activity prescriptions tailored to individual needs, risks, and benefits will someday replace the current generic recommendations.

Medical Screening before Exercise

It is anticipated that the public health efforts to promote physical activity will impact all Americans, including the one in four who have some form of CVD. Although regular exercise leads to health benefits, the incidence of cardiovascular events during exercise is estimated to be 10 times greater than that at rest among otherwise healthy persons (129). The CDC (6) and AHA (129) conclude that most persons do not need to see their physician before starting a moderate-intensity physical activity program. However, it is advised that men older than 45 years and women older than 55 years who plan to start a program of vigorous intensity (>60% $\dot{V}O_2$max) or individuals with risk factors, signs, or symptoms of cardiovascular

THE FUTURE

Evidence regarding the health benefits of physical activity is overwhelming; however, there are many unanswered questions, and future research is needed. For example, further study of the specific mechanisms responsible for the decrease in cardiovascular events, as well as total mortality, is needed. In addition, whether specific physiologic and biochemical changes differ among the various types of exercise is undetermined. For instance, what are the effects of chronicity, intensity, and duration of activity on these parameters? The effects of physical activity in persons of different age, gender, race, and ethnicity are unknown (9). Moreover, no prospective, randomized controlled trial has compared the effects that the high-dose versus low-dose range of these exercise recommendations has on fitness levels or modifiable cardiovascular risk factors (including weight, body composition, and lipid profile). Importantly, no study has evaluated the cardiovascular benefits of these recommendations on racial minorities.

The economic effects of physical activity on various diseases need additional investigation. Knowledge of the cost-effectiveness of exercise for the treatment or prevention of atherosclerotic diseases is important (9).

The U.S. Department of Health and Human Services has published recommendations for the promotion of health and prevention of disease in Americans (145). A major objective is to enhance the physical activity of inactive individuals in an attempt to reduce chronic diseases and improve quality of life. Certain special populations have been targeted due to their lack of participation in leisure-time physical activity, including ethnic minorities such as blacks, Hispanics, Native Americans, low-income groups, the elderly, the disabled, and obese individuals. Methods that aid in promoting, implementing, and maintaining physical activity are needed.

---

or chronic disease consult their physician to design an exercise program. These recommendations seem reasonable, yet are they practical? Should asymptomatic men and women, based on their age, undergo a screening exercise test before participation in exercise training programs designed to improve fitness, strength, or both? Indeed, the utility of the exercise test in screening asymptomatic individuals may often result in false-positive tests, which may cause undue concern and lead to further, more expensive and invasive tests. Conversely, are the many individuals with CVD who do not seek regular evaluation by a health care professional placing themselves at significantly increased risk by beginning an unsupervised exercise program at home or at a fitness club? The specific answers to these questions remain unknown, as there are no scientific data that evaluate the benefits, costs, and potential risks of specific medical screening practices—or the lack thereof—for individuals who are about to begin or who are actively participating in moderate- to vigorous-intensity exercise programs. As such, current recommendations must be left to expert consensus opinion until more data are available. General medical screening guidelines (6,127,129) and those directed at cardiovascular screening at fitness facilities (146) must be promulgated to the public and the health care professional in concert with efforts promoting physical activity.

REFERENCES

1. *2000 Heart and stroke statistical supplement*. Dallas: American Heart Association, 2000.

2. Powell KE, Thompson PD, Caspersen CJ, et al. Physical activity and the incidence of coronary heart disease. *Annu Rev Pub Health* 1987;8:253–287.

3. O'Connor GT, Buring JE, Yusuf S, et al. An overview of randomized trials of rehabilitation with exercise after myocardial infarction. *Circulation* 1989;80:234–244.

4. Oldridge NB, Guyatt GH, Fischer ME, et al. Cardiac rehabilitation after myocardial infarction: combined experience of randomized clinical trials. *JAMA* 1988;260:945–950.

5. Lowensteyn I, Coupal L, Zowall H, et al. The cost effectiveness of exercise training for the primary and secondary prevention of cardiovascular disease. *J Cardiopulm Rehabil* 2000;20:147–155.

6. U.S. Department of Health and Human Services. *Physical activity and health: a report of the surgeon general*. Atlanta: Centers for Disease Control and Prevention, National Center for Chronic Disease Prevention and Promotion, 1996.

7. National Health Interview Survey. National Center for Statistics. http://www.cdc.gov/nchs/nhis.htm.

8. Pate RR, Pratt M, Blair SN, et al. Physical activity and public health: a recommendation from the Centers for Disease Control and Prevention and the American College of Sports Medicine. *JAMA* 1995;273:402–407.

9. Fletcher GF, Balady GJ, Blair SN, et al. AHA statement on exercise: benefits and recommendations for physical activity programs for all Americans. *Circulation* 1996;94:857–862.

10. Dunn AL, Marcus BH, Kampert JB, et al. Comparison of lifestyle and structured interventions to increase physical activity and cardiorespiratory fitness. *JAMA* 1999;281:327–334.

11. American College of Sports Medicine. Position stand on the recommended quantity and quality of exercise for developing and maintaining cardiorespiratory and muscular fitness

and flexibility in healthy adults. *Med Sci Sports Exerc* 1998;30:975–991.

12. DeBusk RF, Stenestrand U, Sheehan M, et al. Training effects of long versus short bouts of exercise in healthy subjects. *Am J Cardiol* 1990;65:1010–1013.

13. Hoffman MS, ed. *World almanac*. New York: Pharos Books, 1995.

14. Caplan GA, Keil JB. Socioeconomic factors and cardiovascular disease: a review of the literature. *Circulation* 1993;88:1973–1998.

15. Keil JE, Sutherland SE, Knapp RG, et al. Does equal socioeconomic status in black and white men mean equal risk of mortality? *Am J Pub Health* 1992;82:1133–1136.

16. Paffenbarger RS, Hyde RT, Wing A, et al. Physical activity, all-cause mortality, and longevity of college alumni. *N Engl J Med* 1986;314:605–613.

17. Blair SN, Kohl HW, Paffenbarger RS, et al. Physical fitness and all-cause mortality. *JAMA* 1989;262:2395–2401.

18. Andersen LB, Schnohr P, Schroll M, et al. All-cause mortality associated with physical activity during leisure time, work, sports, and cycling to work. *Arch Intern Med* 2000;160:1621–1628.

19. McGinnis JM, Foege WH. Actual causes of death in the United States. *JAMA* 1993;270:2207–2212.

20. Paffenbarger RS, Hyde RG, Wing AI, et al. The association of changes in physical activity level in other lifestyle characteristics with mortality among men. *N Engl J Med* 1993;328:538–545.

21. Paffenbarger RS, Wing AL, Hyde RD. Physical activity and incidence of hypertension in college alumni. *Am J Epidemiol* 1983;117:245–257.

22. Wannamethee SG, Shaper AG, Walker MA. Physical activity and mortality in older men with diagnosed coronary heart disease. *Circulation* 2000;102:1358–1363.

23. Leon A, Connett J, Jacobs DR, et al. Leisure time physical activity levels and risk of coronary heart disease and death. The Multiple Risk Factor Intervention trial. *JAMA* 1987;258:2388–2395.

24. Manson JE, Stampfer MJ, Colditz GA, et al. A prospective study of exercise and incidence of myocardial infarction in women. *Circulation* 1993;88:1–220.

25. Sandvick L, Erikssen J, Thoulaw WE, et al. Physical fitness as a predictor of mortality among healthy and middle-aged Norwegian men. *N Engl J Med* 1993;328:533–537.

26. Manson JE, Stampfer MJ, Willett WC, et al. Physical activity and incidence of coronary heart disease and stroke in women. *Circulation* 1995;9:927.

27. Bijnen FCH, Caspersen CJ, Feskens EJM, et al. Physical activity and 10-year mortality from cardiovascular diseases and all causes. The Zutphen Elderly Study. *Arch Intern Med* 1998;158:1499–1505.

28. LaMonte MJ, Eisenman PA, Adams TD, et al. Cardiorespiratory fitness and coronary heart disease risk factors. The LDS Hospital Fitness Institute Cohort. *Circulation* 2000;102:1623–1628.

29. Sherman SE, D'Agostino RB, Silbershatz H, et al. Comparison of past versus recent physical activity in the prevention of premature death and coronary artery disease. *Am Heart J* 1999;138:900–907.

30. Blair SN, Goodyear NN, Gibbons LW, et al. Physical fitness and incidence of hypertension in healthy normotensive men and women. *JAMA* 1984;252:487–490.

31. Hayashi T, Tsumura K, Suematsu C, et al. Walking to work and the risk for hypertension in men: the Osaka Health Survey. *Ann Intern Med* 1999;130:21–26.

32. *The sixth report of the Joint National Committee on prevention, detection, evaluation, and treatment of high blood pressure.* NIH Publication #98-4048. Bethesda, MD: National Institutes of Health, 1997.

33. Pescatello LS, Fargo AE, Leach CN, et al. Short term effect of dynamic exercise on arterial blood pressure. *Circulation* 1991;83:1557–1561.

34. Kokkinos PF, Narayan P, Colleran JA, et al. Effects of regular exercise on blood pressure and left ventricular hypertrophy in African-American men with severe hypertension. *N Engl J Med* 1995;333:1462–1467.

35. Wasserman DH, Zinman B. Fuel homeostasis. In: Ruderman N, Devlin JT, eds. *The health professional's guide to diabetes and exercise.* Alexandria, VA: American Diabetes Association, 1995:29–47.

36. Helmrich SP, Ragland DR, Leung RW, et al. Physical activity and reduced occurrence of non–insulin-dependent diabetes mellitus. *N Engl J Med* 1991;325:147–152.

37. Lynch J, Helmrich SP, Lakka TA, et al. Moderately intense physical activities and high levels of cardiorespiratory fitness reduces the risk of non–insulin-dependent diabetes mellitus in middle-aged men. *Ann Intern Med* 1996;156:1307–1314.

38. Wei M, Gibbons LW, Mitchell TD, et al. The association between cardiorespiratory fitness and impaired fasting glucose and type 2 diabetes mellitus in men. *Ann Intern Med* 1999;130:89–96.

39. Wei M, Gibbons LW, Kampert JB, et al. Low cardiorespiratory fitness and physical inactivity as predictors of mortality in men with type 2 diabetes. *Ann Intern Med* 2000;132:605–611.

40. Hu FB, Sigal RJ, Rich-Edwards JW, et al. Walking compared with vigorous physical activity and risk of type 2 diabetes in women. *JAMA* 1999;282:1433–1439.

41. Eckel RH. Obesity and heart disease. A statement for healthcare professionals from the Nutrition Committee, American Heart Association. *Circulation* 1997;96:3248–3250.

42. Wilmore JH. Appetite and body composition consequent to physical activity. *Res Q Exerc Sport* 1983;54:415–425.

43. Blair SN. Evidence for success of exercise in weight loss and control. *Ann Intern Med* 1993;119:702–706.

44. Wood PD, Stefanick ML, Williams PT, et al. The effects on plasma lipoproteins of a prudent weight-reducing diet, with or without exercise, in overweight men and women. *N Engl J Med* 1991;325:461–466.

45. Andersen RE, Wadden TA, Bartlett SJ, et al. Effects of lifestyle activity vs. structured aerobic exercise in obese women. A randomized trial. *JAMA* 1999;281:335–340.

46. Tremblay A, Despres JP, LeBlanc C, et al. Effect of intensity and physical activity on body fatness and fat distribution. *Am J Clin Nutr* 1990;51:153–157.

47. Seidell JC, Cigolini M, Deslypre JP, et al. Body fat distribution in relation to physical activity and smoking habits in 38-year old European men: the European Fat Distribution Study. *Am J Epidemiol* 1991;133:257–265.

48. Troisi RJ, Heinhold JW, Vokonas PS, et al. Cigarette smoking, dietary intake, and physical activity: effects on body fat distribution. The Normative Aging Study. *Am J Clin Nutr* 1991;53:1104–1111.

49. Wing RR, Matthews KA, Kuller LH, et al. Waist to hip ratio in middle aged women: associations with behavioral and psychosocial factors and what changes in cardiovascular risk factors. *Arterioscler Thromb* 1991;11:1250–1257.

50. Krauss RM, Winston M, Fletcher BJ, et al. Obesity. Impact on cardiovascular disease. *Circulation* 1999;98:1472–1476.

51. Tran ZV, Weltman A. Differential effects of exercise on serum lipid and lipoprotein levels seen with changes in body weight. *JAMA* 1985;254:919–924.

52. Laporte RE, Brenes G, Dearwater S. HDL cholesterol across a spectrum of physical activity from a quadriplegia to marathon running. *Lancet* 1983;1:1212–1213.

53. King AC, Haskell WL, Young DR, et al. Long-term effects of varying intensities and formats of physical activity on participation rates, fitness, and lipoproteins in men and women aged 50 to 65 years. *Circulation* 1995;91:2596–2604.

54. Stefanick M, Mackey S, Sheehan M, et al. Effects of diet and exercise in men and postmenopausal women with low levels of HDL cholesterol and high levels of LDL cholesterol. *N Engl J Med* 1998;339:12–20.

55. Brochu M, Poehlman ET, Savage P, et al. Modest effects of exercise training alone on coronary risk factors and body composition in coronary patients. *J Cardiopulm Rehabil* 2000;20:180–188.

56. Moll ME, Williams RS, Lester RM. Cholesterol metabolism in nonobese women: failure of physical conditioning to alter levels of high-dose lipoprotein cholesterol. *Atherosclerosis* 1979;34:159–166.

57. Farrel PA, Barboriak J. The time course of alterations in plasma lipids and lipoprotein concentration during eight weeks of endurance running. *Atherosclerosis* 1980;37:231–238.

58. Tikkanen MJ, Nikkila EA, Kuusi T, et al. Different effects of two progestins on plasma high density lipoprotein (HDL) and postheparin plasma hepatic lipase activity. *Atherosclerosis* 1981;40:365–369.

59. Williams PT. High-density lipoprotein cholesterol and other risk factors for coronary heart disease in female runners. *N Engl J Med* 1996;334:1298–1303.

60. Kannel W, Wolf P, Castelli W, et al. Fibrinogen and risk of cardiovascular disease: the Framingham Heart Study. *JAMA* 1987;258:1183–1186.

61. Stratton JR, Chandler WL, Schwartz RS, et al. Effects of physical conditioning on fibrinolytic variables in young and old healthy adults. *Circulation* 1991;83:1692–1697.

62. de-Geus EJ, Kluft C, de-Bart AC, et al. Effects of exercise training on plasminogen activator inhibitor activity. *Med Sci Sports Exerc* 1992;24:1210–1219.

63. Suzuki T, Yamauchi K, Yamada Y, et al. Blood coagulability and fibrinolytic activity before and after physical training during the recovery phase of acute myocardial infarction. *Clin Cardiol* 1992;15:358–364.

64. Kestin AS, Ellis PA, Barnard MR, et al. Effect of strenuous exercise on platelet activation state and reactivity. *Circulation* 1993;88:1502–1511.

65. Rauramaa R, Salonen JT, Seppanen K, et al. Inhibition of platelet aggregability by moderate-intensity physical exercise: a randomized clinical trial in overweight men. *Circulation* 1986;74:939–944.

66. Smith JK, Dykes R, Douglas JE, et al. Long-term exercise and atherogenic activity of blood mononuclear cells in persons at risk of developing ischemic heart disease. *JAMA* 1999;281:1722–1727.

67. Furchgott R. Role of endothelium in responses of vascular smooth muscle. *Circ Res* 1983;35:557–573.

68. Rubanyi GM, Romero JC, Vanhoutte PM. Flow-induced release of endothelium-derived relaxing factor. *Am J Physiol* 1986;250:H1145–H1149.

69. Miller VM, Vanhoutte PM. Enhanced release of endothelium-derived relaxing factor by chronic increases in blood flow. *Am J Physiol* 1988;255:H446–H451.

70. Cox DA, Vita JA, Treasure CB, et al. Atherosclerosis impairs flow-mediated dilation of coronary arteries in humans. *Circulation* 1989;80:458–465.

71. Okumura K, Yasue H, Matsuyama K, et al. Effect of acetylcholine on the highly stenotic coronary artery. *J Am Coll Cardiol* 1992;19:752–758.

72. Meredith IT, Yeung AC, Weidinger FF, et al. Role of impaired endothelium-dependent vasodilation in ischemic manifestations of coronary artery disease. *Circulation* 1993;87:V56–V66.

73. Yataco AR, Corretti MC, Gardner AW, et al. Endothelial reactivity and cardiac risk factors in older patients with peripheral arterial disease. *Am J Cardiol* 1999;83:754–758.

74. Yeung AC, Vekshstein VI, Krantz TS, et al. The effect of atherosclerosis on the vasomotor response of coronary arteries to mental stress. *N Engl J Med* 1991;325:1551–1556.

75. Charo S, Gokce N, Vita JA. Endothelial dysfunction and coronary risk reduction. *J Cardiopulm Rehabil* 1998;18:60–67.

76. Sessa WC, Pitchard K, Seyedi N, et al. Chronic exercise in dogs increases coronary vascular nitric oxide production and endothelial cell nitric oxide synthase gene expression. *Circ Res* 1994;74:349–353.

77. Muller JM, Meyers PR, Laughlin H. Vasodilator responses of coronary resistance arteries of exercise-trained pigs. *Circulation* 1994;89:2308–2314.

78. Uehata A, Lieberman EH, Meredith I, et al. Noninvasive assessment of flow-mediated dilation in brachial arteries. *Circulation* 1992;86:1–620.

79. Celermajer DS, Sorensen KE, Gooch VM, Deanfield JE. Noninvasive detection of endothelial dysfunction in children and adults at risk of atherosclerosis. *Lancet* 1992;340:1111–1115.

80. Clarkson P, Montgomery HE, Mullen MJ, et al. Exercise training enhances endothelial function in young men. *J Am Coll Cardiol* 1999;33:1379–1385.

81. Hornig B, Maier V, Drexler H. Physical training improves endothelial function in patients with chronic heart failure. *Circulation* 1996;93:210–214.

82. DeSouza CA, Shapiro LF, Clevenger CM, et al. Regular aerobic exercise prevents and restores age-related declines in endothelium-dependent vasodilation in healthy men. *Circulation* 2000;102:1351–1357.

83. Taddei S, Galetta F, Virdis A, et al. Physical activity prevents age-related impairment in nitric oxide availability in elderly athletes. *Circulation* 2000;101:2896–2901.

84. Hambrecht R, Wolf A, Gielen S, et al. Effect of exercise on coronary endothelial function in patients with coronary artery disease. *N Engl J Med* 2000;342:454–460.

85. Goldsmith RL, Bigger JT Jr, Steinman RC, et al. Comparison of 24-hour parasympathetic activity in endurance-trained and untrained young men. *J Am Coll Cardiol* 1992;20:552–558.

86. DeMeersman RE. Heart rate variability and aerobic fitness. *Am Heart J* 1993;125:726–731.

87. Coats AJS, Adamaplous S, Radaelli A, et al. Controlled trial of physical training in chronic heart failure. *Circulation* 1992;85:2119–2131.

88. Coats AJS. Exercise rehabilitation in chronic heart failure. *J Am Coll Cardiol* 1993;22[Suppl A]:172A–177A.

89. Duru F, Candinas R, Dziekan G, et al. Effect of exercise training on heart rate variability in patients with new onset left ventricular dysfunction after myocardial infarction. *Am Heart J* 2000;140:157–161.

90. Blumenthal JA, Fredrikson M, Kuhn CM, et al. Aerobic exercise reduces levels of cardiovascular and sympathoadrenal responses to mental stress in subjects without prior evidence of myocardial ischemia. *Am J Cardiol* 1990;65:93–98.

91. Jennings G, Nelson L, Nestel P, et al. The effects of changes in physical activity on major cardiovascular risk factors, hemodynamics, sympathetic function, and glucose utilization in man: a controlled study of four levels of activity. *Circulation* 1986;73:30–40.

92. Folkins CH, Sime WE. Physical fitness training and mental health. *Am Psychol* 1981;36:373–389.

93. Oldridge N, Guyatt G, Jones N, et al. Effects of quality of life with comprehensive rehabilitation after acute myocardial infarction. *Am J Cardiol* 1991;67:1084–1089.

94. Belardinelli R, Georgiou D, Cianci G, et al. Randomized, controlled trial of long-term moderate exercise training in chronic heart failure. *Circulation* 1999;99:1173–1182.

95. Durstine LJ, Pate RR, Branch JD. Cardiorespiratory responses to acute exercise. In: Durstine JL, King AC, Painter PL, et al., eds. *ACSM resource manual for guidelines for exercise testing and prescription*, 2nd ed. Philadelphia: Lea & Febiger, 1993:66–74.

96. Holloszy JO. Muscle metabolism during exercise. *Arch Phys Med Rehabil* 1982;63:231–234.

97. Durstine JL, Pate RR. Cardiorespiratory responses to acute exercise. In: Durstine JL, Pate RR, eds. *Resource manual for guidelines for exercise testing and prescription. American College of Sports Medicine*. Philadelphia: Lea & Febiger, 1988:48.

98. Clausen JP. Circulatory adjustments to dynamic exercise and effects of physical training in normal subjects and in patients with coronary artery disease. *Prog Cardiovasc Dis* 1976;18:459–495.

99. Francis GS. Hemodynamic and neurohumoral responses to dynamic exercise: normal subjects versus patients with heart disease. *Circulation* 1987;76[Suppl VI]:VI11–VI17.

100. Asmussen E. Similarities and dissimilarities between static and dynamic effort. *Circ Res* 1981;48[Suppl I]:I3–I10.

101. Seals DR, Washborn RA, Hanson PG, et al. Increased cardiovascular response to static contraction of larger muscle groups. *J Appl Physiol* 1983;58:434–437.

102. Miles DS, Cox MH, Bomze JP. Cardiovascular responses to upper body exercise in normals and cardiac patients. *Med Sci Sports Exerc* 1989;21[Suppl 5]:126S–131S.

103. Balady GJ, Weiner DA, Rose L, et al. Physiologic responses to arm ergometry relative to age and gender. *J Am Coll Cardiol* 1990;16:130–135.

104. Cullinane EM, Ribero B, Sady S, et al. Can treadmill exercise capacity be predicted from arm ergometry results? *J Cardiopulm Rehabil* 1992;12:36.

105. Kitamura K, Jorgensen CR, Gobel FL, et al. Hemodynamic correlates of myocardial oxygen consumption during upright exercise. *J Appl Physiol* 1972;32:516–522.

106. Roubin GS, Anderson SD, Shen W, et al. Hemodynamic and metabolic basis of impaired exercise tolerance in patients with severe left ventricular dysfunction. *J Am Coll Cardiol* 1990;15:995–998.

107. Holloszy JO, Coyle EF. Adaptations of skeletal muscle to endurance exercise and their metabolic consequences. *J Appl Physiol* 1984;56:831–838.

108. Terjung RL. Peripheral adaptations in skeletal muscle induced by exercise training. *Heart Failure* 1988;4:93.

109. Sharkey B. Specificity of exercise. In: Durstine JL, Pate RR, eds. *Resource manual for guidelines for exercise testing and prescription. American College of Sports Medicine*. Philadelphia: Lea & Febiger, 1988:55.

110. Longhurst JC, Kelly AR, Gonyea WJ, et al. Echocardiographic left ventricular masses in distance runners and weightlifters. *J Appl Physiol* 1980;48:154–162.

111. Colan SD, Sanders SP, Borow KM. Physiologic hypertrophy: effects on left ventricular systolic mechanics in athletes. *J Am Coll Cardiol* 1987;9:776–783.

112. Fisman E, Frank AG, Ben-Ari E, et al. Altered left ventricular volume and ejection fraction responses to supine dynamic exercise in athletes. *J Am Coll Cardiol* 1990;15:582–588.

113. Colan SD, Sanders SP, MacPherson D, et al. Left ventricular diastolic function in elite athletes with physiologic cardiac hypertrophy. *J Am Coll Cardiol* 1985;6:545–549.

114. Price DT, Davidoff R, Balady GJ. Comparison of cardiovascular adaptations to long term arm and leg exercise in wheelchair athletes vs. long distance runners. *Am J Cardiol* 2000;85:996–1001.

115. Beere PA, Russell SD, Morey MC, et al. Aerobic exercise training can reverse age-related peripheral circulatory changes in healthy older men. *Circulation* 1999;100:1085–1094.

116. Ben-Ari E, Kellerman JJ, Rothbaum DA, et al. Effects of prolonged intensive versus moderate leg training on the untrained arm exercise response in angina pectoris. *Am J Cardiol* 1987;59:231–234.

117. Rogers MA, Yamamoto C, Hagberg JM, et al. The effect of seven years of intense exercise training on patients with coronary artery disease. *J Am Coll Cardiol* 1987;10:321–326.

118. Schuler G, Schierf G, Wirth A, et al. Low fat diet and regular supervised physical exercise in patients with symptomatic coronary artery disease: reduction of stress induced myocardial ischemia. *Circulation* 1988;77:172–188.

119. Williams RS, Eden RS, Moll MG, et al. Autonomic mechanisms of training bradycardia: beta adrenergic receptors in humans. *J Appl Physiol* 1981;51:1232–1237.

120. Martin WH, Coyle EF, Bloomfield SA, et al. Effects of physical deconditioning after intense endurance training on left ventricular dimensions and stroke volume. *J Am Coll Cardiol* 1986;7:982–989.

121. Lee IM, Sesso HD, Paffenbarger RS. Physical activity and coronary heart disease risk in men. Does the duration of exercise episodes predict risk? *Circulation* 2000;102:981–986.

122. Lee IM, Hsieh C, Paffenbarger R. Exercise and intensity and longevity in men. A Harvard Alumni Health Study. *JAMA* 1995;273:1179–1184.

123. Hakim AA, Curb JD, Petrovich H, et al. Effects of walking on coronary heart disease in elderly men. The Honolulu Heart Program. *Circulation* 1999;100:9–13.

124. Manson JE, Hu FB, Rich-Edwards JW, et al. A prospective study of walking as compared with vigorous exercise in the prevention of coronary heart disease in women. *N Engl J Med* 1999;341:650–658.

125. Franklin BA, Gordon S, Timmis GC. Fundamentals of exercise physiology: implications for exercise testing and prescription. In: Franklin BA, Gordon S, Timmis GC, eds. *Exercise in modern medicine.* Baltimore: Williams & Wilkins, 1989:1.

126. Zeni AI, Hoffman MD, Clifford PS. Energy expenditure with indoor exercise machines. *JAMA* 1996;275:1424–1427.

127. Pollock ML, Franklin BA, Balady GJ, et al. Resistance exercise in individuals with and without cardiovascular disease. Benefits, rationale, safety, and prescription. An advisory from the Committee on Exercise, Rehabilitation, and Prevention, Council on Clinical Cardiology, American Heart Association. *Circulation* 2000;101:828–833.

128. Maron BJ, Shirani J, Poliac LC, et al. Sudden death in young competitive athletes: clinical, demographic and pathological profiles. *JAMA* 1996;276:199–204.

129. Fletcher GF, Balady GJ, Froelicher VF, et al. Exercise standards: a statement from the American Heart Association. *Circulation* 1995;91:580–615.

130. Van Camp SP, Bloor CM, Mueller FU, et al. Non-traumatic sports deaths in high school and college athletes. *Med Sci Sports Exerc* 1995;27:641–647.

131. Thompson PD, Funk EJ, Carlton RA, et al. Incidence of death during jogging in Rhode Island from 1975 through 1980. *JAMA* 1982;247:2535–2538.

132. Siscovick DS, Weiss NS, Fletcher RN, et al. The incidence of primary cardiac arrest during vigorous exercise. *N Engl J Med* 1984;311:874–877.

133. Albert CM, Mittelman MA, Chae CU, et al. Triggering of sudden death from cardiac causes by vigorous exertion. *N Engl J Med* 2000;343:1355–1361.

134. Lemaitre RN, Siscovick DS, Raghunathan TE, et al. Leisure-time physical activity and the risk of primary cardiac arrest. *Arch Intern Med* 1999;59:686–690.

135. Mittleman MA, Maclure M, Tofler GH, et al. Triggering of acute myocardial infarction by heavy physical exertion: protection against triggering by regular exertion. *N Engl J Med* 1993;329:1677–1683.

136. Willich SN, Lewis M, Lowel H, et al. Physical exertion as a trigger of acute myocardial infarction. *N Engl J Med* 1993;329:1684–1690.

137. Muller JE, Mittleman MA, Maclure M, et al. Triggering myocardial infarction by sexual activity: low absolute risk and prevention by regular physical exertion. *JAMA* 1996;275:1405–1409.

138. Van Camp SP, Peterson RA. Cardiovascular complications of out-patient cardiac rehabilitation programs. *JAMA* 1986;256:1160–1163.

139. Franklin BA, Bonzheim K, Gordon S, et al. Safety of medically supervised cardiac rehabilitation therapy: a 16 year followup. *Chest* 1998;114:902–906.

140. DeBusk RF, Haskell WL, Miller NH, et al. Medically directed at-home rehabilitation soon after clinically uncomplicated acute myocardial infarction: a new model of patient care. *Am J Cardiol* 1985;55:251–257.

141. Ades P, Pashkow FJ, Fletcher G, et al. A controlled trial of cardiac rehabilitation in the home setting using electrocardiographic and voice transtelephonic monitoring. *Am Heart J* 2000;139:543–548.

142. Bouchard C, Shephard RJ, Stephens T, eds. *Physical activity, fitness, and health: international proceedings and consensus statement.* Champaign, IL: Human Kinetics, 1994.

143. Coplan JP, Powell KE, Sikes RK, et al. An epidemiologic study of the benefits and risks of running. *JAMA* 1982;248:3118–3121.

144. Roy S. Injuries of exercise. *Med Clin North Am* 1985;69:197–209.

145. U.S. Department of Health and Human Services. *Healthy people 2010: Objectives for improving health*, Vol. 2. Publication number (PHS) 017-001-00547-9.

146. Balady GJ, Chaitman B, Driscoll D, et al. American Heart Association/American College of Sports Medicine joint scientific statement. Recommendations for cardiovascular screening, staffing, and emergency policies at health/fitness facilities. *Circulation* 1998;97:2283–2293.

HYPERTENSION: CONTEXT, PATHOPHYSIOLOGY, AND MANAGEMENT

PETER RUDD
LARS G. OSTERBERG

OVERVIEW

Hypertension is a major cardiovascular risk factor that directly contributes to myocardial infarction (MI), cerebrovascular accidents, congestive heart failure (CHF), peripheral arterial insufficiency, and premature mortality. Optimal and cost-effective management of the condition

depends on careful diagnosis, treatment minimization, optimized adherence, parsimonious selection of tests and treatments, and practice efficiency.

Over the natural history of hypertension, early endothelial dysfunction and elevations of cardiac output (CO) usually give way to increased peripheral vascular resistance, reflecting an array of genetic, environmental, and homeostatic factors. Early perturbations may be slight and reversible; subsequent chronic changes tend to be larger, slower, and irreversible.

Successful reduction in blood pressure (BP) and other cardiovascular risk factors can dramatically reduce the inci-

P. Rudd: Department of General Internal Medicine, Stanford University School of Medicine, Stanford, California

L. G. Osterberg: Department of Internal Medicine, Stanford University School of Medicine, Stanford University Medical Center, Stanford, California

dence of cerebrovascular and coronary morbidity and mortality, especially for individuals with the highest elevations of BP, individuals with multiple risk factors, and the elderly. Nondrug therapy is often sufficient for mild or labile elevations of BP. The large number of antihypertensive drug options necessitates individualization for particular patients and a thoughtful balancing of hypotensive efficacy, impact on key vascular beds, patient cost and convenience, and long-term consequences on metabolic and other baseline functions.

Secondary hypertension with curable potential makes up <2% of unselected hypertensive populations and usually produces characteristic clues or refractoriness to therapy. Suboptimal compliance with prescribed medications and suboptimal drug combinations are more common causes of apparent resistance to standard treatment than is secondary hypertension.

Continued controversy surrounds the optimal threshold of treatment and the optimal choice of antihypertensive medications.

INTRODUCTION

Hypertension is a major cardiovascular risk factor that contributes to MI, cerebrovascular accidents, CHF, peripheral arterial insufficiency, and premature mortality (1). Of all the known cardiovascular risk factors, hypertension is the most prevalent: it occurs in up to 30% of the United States population (approximately 80 million Americans), when using a threshold of 140/90 mm Hg (2). Hypertension is the most common reason cited for office visits to American internists (3) and the most common indication for the use of prescription medication in the United States (4). In 1995, direct costs of American antihypertensive management and treatment of its complications totaled $24 billion (2).

Definitions of hypertension continue to evolve as more epidemiologic data and randomized controlled trials clarify the distributions of BPs and the thresholds for net benefit from treatment. Traditional definitions have used systolic BP (SBP) ≥140 mm Hg and/or diastolic BP (DBP) ≥90 mm Hg to delimit the upper bounds of normal. More recently, the recommendation has shifted to defining normal BP as mean daytime SBP <135 mm Hg and DBP as <85 mm Hg (5). ▼ a89

PATHOPHYSIOLOGY

As summarized in *e*Figure 5.0.1, the numerous factors affecting BP control are complex in themselves and their interrelationships. Striking examples of the interdependencies include observations that insulin resistance precedes hypertension in individuals genetically predisposed to it (30) and that hyperinsulinemia, salt sensitivity, obesity, and increased sympathetic drive are covariants (31).

Sodium Intake

Primitive societies have had diets characterized by low salt (10 to 30 mmol per day) and high potassium intakes. In such settings, hypertension is rare. Only a subset of people (20% to 50%) appears to be salt sensitive by showing a pressor response when fed diets of more than 50 mEq sodium per day (~1/2 tsp of salt per day, because 1 tsp of salt = 6 g salt = 2.4 g sodium = 104 mEq sodium = 104 mmol sodium). Most Americans consume substantially more than this level. Proving the unique contribution of excessive salt intake, however, is difficult. Some have argued that the sodium-potassium ratio or the chloride intake may be crucial. Still, most data support a role for dietary sodium excess in producing hypertension in some individuals (40,41).

Despite attractive theories to the contrary, Intersalt—the superbly executed, worldwide study of salt intake and BP (10,079 subjects from 32 countries)—was unable to confirm a consistent relationship between dietary salt intake and BP in diverse settings (42). In other studies, no single marker has predicted salt sensitivity with accuracy. Even the reproducibility of salt loading in such individuals leading to pressor responses has been questioned (40). A recent metaanalysis of 56 published trials could confirm only 3.7/0.9 mm Hg reductions in systolic and diastolic pressures among 1,131 hypertensive subjects who reduced dietary salt intake by 100 mmol per day (41).

Given these small differences, testing for salt sensitivity cannot be justified in routine clinical practice, especially because the standard protocol is difficult to administer: determination of baseline BP after a 4-hour infusion of 2 L of normal saline, and then comparison with BP after 1 day of a 10-mmol sodium diet coupled with three oral doses of furosemide at 10 a.m., 2 p.m., and 6 p.m. in search of ≥10 mm Hg decline in mean BP.

Natriuresis and Renal Function

In healthy individuals, homeostasis prevails. When BP rises, sodium and water excretion via the kidneys increases to return BP to baseline. This process is termed *pressure natriuresis*. Among hypertensives and prehypertensives, renal blood flow appears reduced compared to normotensives. The causative sequence may include preferential constriction of efferent arterioles (perhaps via the renin-angiotensin system), reduction in renal blood flow, and increased filtration fraction. The peritubular capillary blood with less sodium and water develops higher oncotic pressure and facilitates sodium reabsorption, leading to higher blood volume and higher BP. Pressure natriuresis occurs but only to sustain BP at a higher level.

In some individuals, renal function may contribute to elevated BP after reductions in filtration surface area from lower numbers of functioning nephrons. Controversy surrounds whether both the number and the function of nephrons are reduced, either globally or in a patchy distribution (43). Intrarenally, prostaglandin function—especially prostaglandin E_2 influencing natriuresis and prostaglandin I_2 modulating renin release—may serve as intermediary derangements (44). Regardless of the precise mechanism, the kidney acts to return the pressure all the way back to a balance of input and output—the "set point" of the system—even if disease has deranged the set point to pathologic levels (45).

Renin-Angiotensin System

Since its discovery in 1898, renin has assumed growing importance as a pressor hormone and a growth factor. A single-chain polypeptide, renin is secreted from the renal juxtaglomerular apparatus in response to macula densa signals of lowered cytosolic calcium, decreased renal arteriolar pressure, or increased renal alpha- or beta-adrenergic nerve activity. Renin likely has no physiologic effect except for stimulating the activation of angiotensin I from angiotensinogen. Angiotensin I, in turn, undergoes conversion to the four–amino acid angiotensin II (AII, sometimes called *angiotensin 1-8*) in multiple tissues, especially the lung. AII becomes inactivated by angiotensinases that are present in many tissues, especially red blood cells. Complete renin-angiotensin systems operate in the brain, reproductive tract, and heart and play physiologic roles in epithelial, fibroblast, and macrophage cell function (46).

The principal effects of AII consist of the following: (a) vasoconstriction that leads to elevated BP by inhibiting adenylate cyclase mediated through G proteins, particularly for the kidney's efferent arterioles; (b) volume retention via promoting aldosterone secretion by the adrenal and stimulating antidiuretic hormone and thirst; and (c) vascular hypertrophy, especially in the heart, peripheral vessels, and renal vasculature (47,48). Of the two AII receptors, the AT_1 subtype mediates all the known actions of AII on BP control and is widely distributed in the body (49). ▼ a90

Sympathetic Nervous System

In parallel with the renin-angiotensin systems, the sympathetic nervous system (SNS) may couple with high sodium intake to raise BP. Often, stress activates the SNS, especially in patients genetically or environmentally predisposed to respond with increased levels of epinephrine, norepinephrine, and neuropeptide Y (54). Baroreceptor sensitivity—both sinoaortic and cardiopulmonary—rapidly undergoes resetting and decreased sensitivity among hypertensives, predisposing to heightened BP variability (55). Catecholamine-mediated vasoconstriction may con-

tribute to changes in efferent arterioles. In parallel with diurnal cortisol variation, increases in α-sympathetic activity likely play a role in early morning pressor responses. Higher BP, higher pulse rates, and increased risk for cardiovascular events all ensue (56,57). ▼ a91

Vascular Constriction and Vascular Remodeling and Hypertrophy

The simple notion of the circulatory system as a collection of passive pipes attached to a pump is incorrect. *In vivo*, systemic resistance vessels depend on complex interactions among smooth muscle contractility, the vessels' geometric design, vessel wall distensibility, and distending pressure (62). Structural changes increase the ratio between wall thickness and lumen diameter, in turn producing higher wall stress and intraluminal pressure when resistance vessels are sympathetically stimulated.

The vascular tree acts like a Windkessel system, in which there is a distensible component that absorbs energy during systole and releases it during diastole. The net effect is to sustain perfusion to peripheral vascular beds, despite the rhythmic cardiac contractions. In hypertension, vessel wall compliance (i.e., the change in vessel diameter for a given change in pressure) falls. This reduction occurs throughout the arterial side but predominantly among smaller, distal, resistance vessels, rather than large or medium-sized vessels, and increases dramatically with age (63). These changes result from a multitude of vasoactive trophic factors originating within the vessel wall itself (64).

Regardless of the specific initiating events, hypertension is maintained by vascular hypertrophy, which sustains elevated peripheral resistance. In such a pathophysiologic formulation, hypertension proceeds in two steps: (a) an initiating step by which any one of an array of possible small, largely undetectable perturbations occurs, especially in the context of those genetically or environmentally predisposed to derangement; and (b) an amplification step, which is slow, progressive, ultimately large, and likely nonspecific (65).

Hyperinsulinemia and Insulin Resistance

Hyperinsulinemia and insulin resistance commonly coexist with essential hypertension, augmenting the overall cardiovascular risk profile. In contrast, secondary hypertension does not lead to insulin resistance. Prospective follow-up of individuals with elevated fasting insulin demonstrated a high correlation with subsequent development of hypertension at two- to threefold higher rates than controls (82). The association is not perfect; individuals from ethnic groups with high prevalence of diabetes mellitus (e.g., Mexican Americans and Pima Indians) do not display higher incidences of hypertension. Undoubtedly, complex interactions among genetic, environmental, and other factors determine the clinical outcomes (83), because insulin's ability to mediate glucose disposal can differ by as much as tenfold among subjects with normal glucose tolerance (84).

Obese individuals' degree of insulin resistance does not increase if hypertension is present. This lack of additive effect suggests that hypertension, exogenous obesity, and diabetes mellitus may act independently but along a final, common pathway (85). A review of 25 prospective studies correlating plasma insulin levels with heart disease did not support hyperinsulinemia by itself as a major cardiovascular risk factor (86). In contrast, insulin resistance correlates closely with atherosclerosis, thrombogenesis, hypertension, obesity, and diabetes mellitus (87,88).

The vasodilatory effects of insulin appear blunted among hypertensives, compounded by the increased SNS tone of obesity and the insulin resistance all three conditions share (89). Other proposed mechanisms by which insulin resistance and hyperinsulinemia may lead to hypertension include (a) increased sensitivity to dietary salt intake, (b) heightened renal sodium and water reabsorption, (c) augmented pressor and aldosterone responses to AII, (d) increased Na^+-H^+ pump activity and decreased Na^+-K^+ ATPase activity leading to augmented intracellular Na^+, (e) increased intracellular Ca^{2+}, (f) stimulation of vascular smooth muscle growth factors, (g) stimulation of SNS activity, (h) reduced vasodilatory prostaglandins, (i) increased endothelin secretion, and (j) impaired vasodilation (90). Not surprisingly, given the several overlapping effects, hypertension may be clustered with obesity, dyslipidemia, glucose intolerance, and type II diabetes mellitus; sometimes, these conditions are lumped together as "metabolic syndrome X" or "insulin resistance syndrome." Individually and collectively, these conditions lead to accelerated atherosclerosis and cardiovascular disease (91).

CLINICAL PROFILE

Natural History of Hypertension

Whether viewed as a distinct disease or as a cardiovascular risk factor, hypertension commonly produces structural changes in arteries and target organs in a variety of patterns. This sequence appears in *e*Figure 5.0.5.

During the prehypertension phase, repetitive perturbations of cardiovascular homeostasis occur, reflecting an array of hereditary and environmental factors. In time, these small changes accumulate and yield larger changes that are recognizable as early hypertension. If the BP elevations are caught in time and reversed by lifestyle changes, normalization may occur. In the Australian Therapeutic Trial, 13% of screenees with entry DBP >95 mm Hg had spontaneous BP reduction that continued for at least 1 year. An additional 48% of subjects' BPs remained <95 mm Hg while on placebo treatment for 3 years (21).

Patients with sustained elevations may progress to established hypertension. Subsequent events are somewhat difficult to predict in individual patients, because BP on its own provides only the most crude index of prognosis. Observed log-linear associations between BP and risk of coronary heart disease death display approximately constant risk regardless of the specified definition of hypertension (99). A few individuals (<5%) enter a fulminant course with rapid deterioration in cardiac, renal, and neurologic function. Another distinct subset (~20%) undergoes a more subdued course, commonly producing moderate to severe target organ changes with progression over years, rather than over weeks to months. The most common organ systems involved with these destructive processes include (a) the heart itself (diastolic dysfunction, LVH, endocardial scarring, CHF, and coronary insufficiency), (b) the large and medium-sized arteries (accelerated atherosclerosis, aneurysm formation with or without dissection), (c) the brain and intracranial circulation (ischemia, infarction, whether hemorrhagic or thrombotic), and (d) renal circulation (nephrosclerosis, with or without renal failure). These target organ complications reflect a wide array of contributing factors, often inherited, that extend well beyond elevated BP alone. This cluster has been termed *hypertension syndrome* (100). One patient series antedating effective antihypertensive therapy gives a glimpse of the array and progression of events, as summarized in *e*Figure 5.0.6. *e*Figure 5.0.7 displays the cluster of pathophysiologic derangements of the hypertension syndrome. ⌖ a92

Effective treatment that reduces BP dramatically changes the natural history of hypertension-related end points, especially for cerebrovascular events and, somewhat less so, for coronary events. Hypertension carries a high population-attributable risk for subsequent CHF, accounting for 39% of cases in men and 59% in women. The overall RR of CHF in 12 randomized controlled trials between 1967 and 1991 was reduced to 0.48 [95% confidence interval (CI), 0.38–0.59] among treated versus control subjects (106). As in most situations, preventing the end organ damage is more effective than trying to reverse the changes once they are established. There continues to be controversy about the optimal drug therapy for hypertension, especially to prevent major target organ damage, as occurs in stroke, MI, and renal dysfunction (107). The proportions of American hypertensives who are aware of their condition (50% to 82%) and who are treated for it (37% to 72%) have increased dramatically in the last two decades, but the percentage of patients consistently controlled with their medications remains at <30% (108), illustrated by Figure 5.1. The benefits of treatment accrue to both genders (109).

Common Presentations

The vast majority of hypertensive patients (93% to 95%) displays no demonstrable, curable abnormality of anatomy

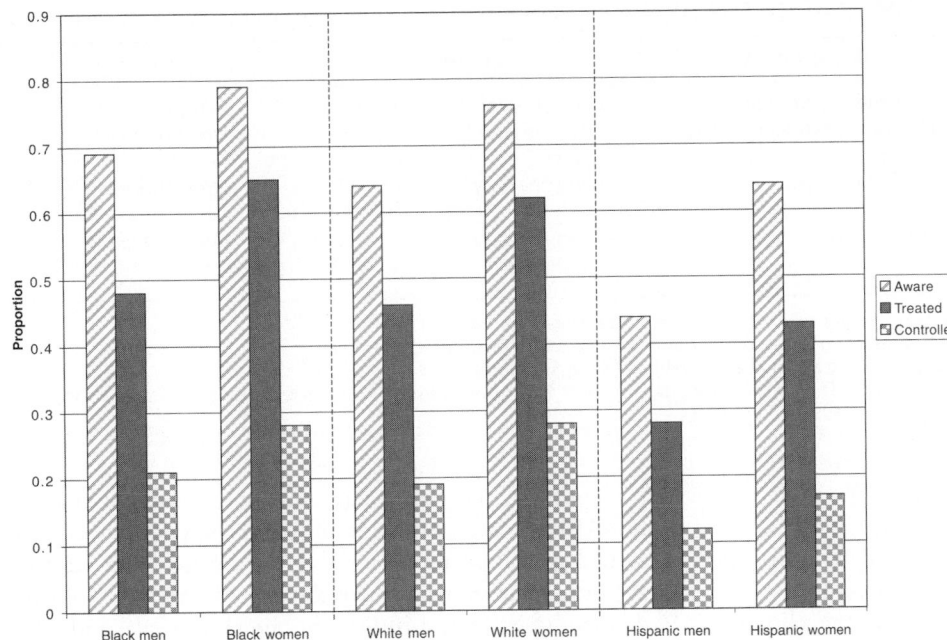

FIGURE 5.1 Data from National Health and Nutrition Examination Survey III (NHANES III) Study classifying American hypertensives by gender, ethnic group, and hypertensive status: Aware of hypertension, under treatment for hypertension, and controlled by treatment. (Adapted from Burt VL, Whelton P, Roccella EJ, et al. Prevalence of hypertension in the U.S. adult population. Results from the Third National Health and Nutrition Examination Survey, 1988–1991. *Hypertension* 1995;25:305–313.)

or physiology (110). Termed *primary hypertension*, the condition carries no consistent hallmark symptoms or signs, except for the elevated BP itself. Most cases are detected incidentally as part of routine examinations and generally in the absence of target organ damage at initial presentation. Reports of headache, dizziness, fatigue, palpitations, and chest discomfort occur commonly among hypertensive and nonhypertensive patients. Because the symptoms prompt clinician attention, hypertension is more likely to be detected among patients with symptoms. For the majority of hypertensives, symptoms and symptom levels do not correlate well with BP level (111).

Even among individuals with proven secondary hypertension, clinical presentations are often nonspecific. Together accounting for 5% to 7% of all hypertensives, secondary causes represent a diverse collection of conditions. Renal parenchymal disease is the most common condition and occurs often in the context of known predisposing illnesses such as diabetes mellitus, connective tissue disease, or drug toxicities. The early (<age 30 years) or late (>age 65 years) onset of hypertension moderately raises the likelihood of secondary causes. The section Evaluation for Secondary Forms of Hypertension explores specific constellations of symptoms and signs by secondary cause (*e*Fig. 5.1.1).

Establishing the Diagnosis and Risk Profile

The Joint National Committee on the Detection, Evaluation, and Treatment of High Blood Pressure has defined hypertension as indirect, sphygmomanometric levels of ≥140 mm Hg systolic, ≥90 mm Hg diastolic, or both (5). Other groups have urged more stringent thresholds for

high-risk populations such as diabetics in special danger of target organ damage, infants, children, and pregnant women. The standard criteria, cardiovascular risk factors, and consequent treatment and risk categories are summarized in Table 5.1, *e*Table 5.1.1, and Table 5.2.

By single BP determinations, nearly one in every four adult Americans have hypertension. Using the somewhat more stringent criteria of intercurrent antihypertensive drug therapy or ≥2 occasions with sustained BP elevations, the prevalence falls to 35 to 45 million Americans. Its prevalence rises with advancing age, from <5% among individuals under age 29 to >50% among those over age 60 (113). On average, black women develop hypertension 10 years before white women do. As the population ages and women tend to outlive men, the number of hypertensive women continues to predominate with higher attributable risk than that of men, even though men and women

TABLE 5.1 BLOOD PRESSURE CLASSIFICATION— ADULTS ≥18 YEARS OLD[a]

Category	Systolic (mm Hg)	Diastolic (mm Hg)
Optimal	<120	<80
Normal	<130	<85
High normal	130–139	85–89
Hypertension		
Stage 1	140–159	90–99
Stage 2	160–179	100–109
Stage 3	≥180	≥110

[a]When systolic and diastolic pressures fall into different categories, the higher category should guide the classification.
Adapted from Joint National Committee. The sixth report of the Joint National Committee on prevention, detection, evaluation, and treatment of high blood pressure. *Arch Intern Med* 1997;157:2413–2446.

TABLE 5.2 DEFINITIONS AND RISK STRATIFICATION FOR HYPERTENSION

Blood pressure stage	Risk group A[a]	Risk group B[b]	Risk group C[c]
High normal (130–139/85–89 mm Hg)	Lifestyle modification	Lifestyle modification	Drug therapy
Stage 1 [140–159/90–99 mm Hg (72% of all hypertensives)]	Lifestyle modification ≤12 mo	Lifestyle modification ≤6 mo	Drug therapy
Stage 2 [160–179/100–109 mm Hg (22% of all hypertensives)]	Drug therapy	Drug therapy	Drug therapy
Stage 3 [≥180/110 mm Hg (6% of all hypertensives)]	Drug therapy	Drug therapy	Drug therapy

[a]Risk group A: *No* cardiovascular (CV) risk factors; *no* clinical CV disease; *no* target organ damage.
[b]Risk group B: *One* CV risk factor; *no* clinical CV disease; *no* target organ damage; *no* diabetes mellitus.
[c]Risk group C: Clinical CV disease *or* target organ damage *or* diabetes mellitus (± CV risk factors).
Adapted from Sheps SG, Black HR, Cohen JD, et al. The sixth report of the Joint National Committee on the Detection, Evaluation, and Treatment of High Blood Pressure. *Am J Mgd Care* 1998;4:366–370.

develop hypertension at comparable rates (3). Each year, approximately 2 million new hypertensive patients are added to the pool of Americans who may benefit from antihypertensive intervention (114).

When assessing a hypertensive patient, the clinician seeks to (a) confirm the existence and magnitude of hypertension, (b) assess the extent of end organ damage, (c) evaluate for contributing comorbidities and risk factors, (d) screen for secondary causes of hypertension, (e) understand any special circumstances that may impact treatment over time, and (f) help create professional trust and the patient's commitment for reducing cardiovascular risk over time. The most important components of initial and follow-up visits in the ambulatory setting are enumerated in Table 5.3.

Not all patients require drug therapy. For individuals with sustained elevations not responding to nondrug treatments over 3 to 6 months, consistent support has emerged for antihypertensive drug therapy as producing net benefit—even among the elderly with isolated systolic hypertension (23–26)—without compromising quality of life (115). The benefit is especially marked in patients with higher pretreatment BPs (116) or multiple risk factors, rather than in patients with hypertension alone (117). ▼ a93

Ambulatory BP monitoring by electronic technology is rarely necessary for the diagnosis of hypertension (136), but it may prove valuable in isolated cases for whom white-coat hypertension (137) needs to be excluded (5).

TABLE 5.3 COMPONENTS OF AMBULATORY ANTIHYPERTENSIVE MANAGEMENT

Initial visit
  Evidence for secondary hypertension?
  Evidence for target organ damage at presentation?
  Clues for optimal future management?
Follow-up visits
  Interim symptoms/signs from hypertension-related pathology?
  Interim symptoms/signs attributable to antihypertensive treatment?
  Obstacles to optimal medication/diet/exercise/other compliance?

No consensus currently exists about the optimal analysis for ABPM data, although the concept of BP load has gained special prominence. The *load* refers to the percentage of readings during which the SBP or DBP exceeds predefined limits (e.g., 140/90 mm Hg while awake and 120/80 mm Hg during sleep). In one study, when the BP load exceeded 40%, the probability of increased LV mass index or decreased LV filling rate was 61%, compared to only 17% when the load was <40% (138). BPs tend to be highest at work, lower at home, and lowest during sleep in most individuals (139).

The remainder of the physical examination should search for target organ damage and evidence of atherosclerotic disease, concentrating on evidence for cardiomegaly, vascular insufficiency, bruits, and possible stigmata of secondary hypertension or comorbidities such as hepatic or renal dysfunction that can complicate therapy. Recent reports indicating increased risk of dementia among the hypertensive elderly (140) and risk of lacunar infarction underscore the importance of a careful baseline neurologic examination.

Hypertension often keeps close company with other cardiovascular risk factors, including diabetes mellitus, dyslipidemia, hyperinsulinemia, and exogenous obesity (82). In the National Health and Nutrition Examination Survey II, the prevalence of hypertension (BP ≥160/95) was 2.9 times higher among patients who were overweight compared to those who were not. Obesity brings a two- to sixfold increase in the probability of developing hypertension (141) and may account for 65% to 78% of its attributable risk (142). Upper-body or android fat patterns (apple-like) are more dangerous cardiovascularly than lower-body or gynoid patterns (pear-like) (143), perhaps more in women than in men (144).

The obese patients were also 2.9 times more likely to have diabetes mellitus and 1.5 times more likely to have hypercholesterolemia, whether mediated through relative insulin resistance (145) or changes in cytosolic calcium (146). Most of the individual factors (e.g., hypercholesterolemia, obesity) exhibit an exponential relation to subsequent rates of adverse outcomes, rising disproportionately as the number of risk factors increases. In combination, these risk factors are multiplicative rather than simply additive (147).

Smoking and alcohol use also contribute to hypertension. Cigarette smoking directly and indirectly leads to endothelial damage and accelerated atherosclerosis. Epidemiologically, smoking is negatively associated with BP, relative body weight, and physical activity during leisure; smoking is positively associated with total cholesterol, psychological stress, and alcohol abuse (148). The use of alcohol itself is associated with higher BP (149). Consuming three or more alcoholic drinks a day (~40 g ethanol per day) increases BP, even when controlling for body mass index, cigarette smoking, and age (150).

PRINCIPLES OF MANAGEMENT

Goal of Antihypertensive Therapy

The overall goal of antihypertensive therapy is to prevent cardiovascular morbidity and mortality. Management generally combines nonpharmacologic and drug therapy to optimize BP control. Table 5.4 summarizes recommendations for nondrug therapy.

Nonpharmacologic Treatment

Most studies confirm that nondrug therapy may be effective for mild or labile hypertension but that combined nondrug and drug therapy is generally more powerful in controlling BP than nondrug treatment alone (151) and more cost-effective for more severe disease (152).

Weight Reduction

Loss of excess weight reduces SBP and DBP. The Trials of Hypertension Prevention (153) produced an average weight loss of 3.8 kg at 18 months, reduction of SBP and DBP by 2.9 mm Hg and 2.3 mm Hg respectively, and a 51% reduction in hypertension incidence among individuals with high normal BP by using caloric restriction and modest physical activity. Similar results have been

TABLE 5.4 RECOMMENDATIONS FOR NONDRUG THERAPY

	Normotensive individuals	Hypertensive patients	Health care professionals
Alcohol	≤2 drinks/d (8 oz wine, 2 oz liquor, 24 oz beer)	≤2 drinks/d (8 oz wine, 2 oz liquor, 24 oz beer); abstinence if BP still uncontrolled	Advise on effects of excess consumption; encourage reduction; refer as appropriate
Obesity	Goal body weight = BMI 20–27 kg/m²	Reduce to acceptable BMI by diet and exercise	Inform patient; use proper BP cuff; refer as appropriate
Saturated fat	Total fat <30% total calories; saturated fat <10% of total calories; cholesterol <100 mg/d	Total fat <30% total calories; saturated fat <10% of total calories; cholesterol <100 mg/d	Provide information on fat content of foods; counsel on methods to reduce fat and cholesterol intake over time
Sodium/salt	Avoid high-salt foods; minimize salt addition; reduce intake to <100 mmol (<2.3 g sodium, <6.0 g salt)/d	Avoid high-salt foods; minimize salt addition; reduce intake to <100 mmol (<2.3 g sodium, <6.0 g salt)/d	Provide information on salt content of foods; counsel on methods to reduce salt intake over time
Smoking	Stop smoking	Stop smoking	Advise on effects of smoking; encourage reduction, then abstinence; refer as appropriate
Exercise	Regular exercise as beneficial for weight regulation and reducing cardiovascular mortality	Regular, progressive exercise as beneficial for weight regulation and reducing cardiovascular mortality; avoid isometric exercise	Encourage regular, appropriate physical activity; refer as appropriate to community resources
Potassium	Eat a potassium-rich diet (high in vegetables, fruits, low-fat dairy products)	Eat a potassium-rich diet (high in vegetables, fruits, low-fat dairy products, especially if on potassium-losing diuretics)	Provide information on potassium-rich diet and optimal preparation (steaming is better than boiling)
Other Calcium Magnesium Stress management	Data at present not sufficient to recommend inclusion	Data at present not sufficient to recommend inclusion	Data at present not sufficient to recommend inclusion

BMI, body mass index; BP, blood pressure.
Adapted from Laidlaw JC, Chockalingam A. Canadian Consensus Conference on Nonpharmacological Approaches to the Management of High Blood Pressure: recommendations. *J Cardiovasc Pharmacol* 1990;16:S48–S50; Cressman MD. Management of hypercholesterolemia in the hypertensive patient. *Cleveland Clin J Med* 1989;56:351–358; and Joint National Committee. The sixth report of the Joint National Committee on prevention, detection, evaluation, and treatment of high blood pressure. *Arch Intern Med* 1997;157:2413–2446.

reported by two other randomized controlled trials of nondrug therapy (154,155) and among patients with morbid obesity (156). None of these trials reported adverse effects from weight loss. Other benefits of weight loss generally include improvement in lipid profile (157) and reduced rates of developing diabetes mellitus, breast cancer, and gout (113).

Most trials confirm that BP reduction is directly related to the weight loss achieved, although less-than-optimal weight loss may still reduce BP to levels below the need for supplemental treatment. If weight gain recurs, hypertension may return, but most trials suggest that the regain is only partial and that long-term benefits of BP reduction persist (153–155,158).

Exercise

Adding physical activity to a weight-loss program accelerates the weight loss and augments BP reduction (159). An addition of even a 20-minute daily walk can reduce the risk of incident hypertension by 29% (160). The precise mechanism likely involves decreases in CO and peripheral resistance, as well as modifications in serum norepinephrine levels, insulin sensitivity, electrolyte balance, neural and baroreflex mechanisms, and vascular structure (161).

After increased physical activity, BP falls as much as 6 to 7 mm Hg for SBP and DBP, independent of any weight changes (113). Escalating daily activity level may be superior to concentrated workouts three times per week (162), and moderate-intensity endurance exercise proves as effective as higher-intensity exercise for reducing BP (163). To plan exercise programs, summaries of energy expenditures for representative activities and lists of contraindications may be helpful (164).

Dietary Adjustment

Some of the most dramatic evidence supporting nondrug therapy has emerged from the Dietary Approaches to Stop Hypertension trial (165). The study evaluated 459 subjects with mild hypertension (<160/80–95) randomized to usual diet or to a diet with increased fruits and vegetables with or without reduced total and saturated fat intake. Despite lasting only 8 weeks, the combined dietary intervention reduced BP by 11.4/5.5 mm versus 7.2/2.8 mm achieved by increasing fruits and vegetables alone (p <.01). Fully 70% of subjects on combination diet—versus only 45% on increased fruits and vegetables alone and 23% on usual diet—were normotensive at the end of 8 weeks (166). The Dietary Approaches to Stop Hypertension combination diet emphasizes fruits, vegetables, and low-fat dairy products; it includes whole grains, poultry, fish, and nuts and decreases fat, red meat, sweets, and sugar-containing beverages. The precise mechanisms

by which such dietary changes can rapidly lower BP remain uncertain.

Sodium Restriction

More than 70 published studies have addressed the impact of reducing sodium intake on BP (40,167). Despite crossover and parallel group comparisons in normotensive and hypertensive trial populations, most trials have been too small to assess definitively the sodium hypothesis of hypertension causation. A metaanalysis of 32 randomized controlled trials of reducing salt intake estimated the net effect of decreasing intake by 100 mmol per day as –6 mm Hg systolic (168). Another review of 56 trials found the BP reduction at –3.7 mm Hg for a mean 95 mmol salt intake reduction (41). A metaanalysis of nine trials of 24-hour urinary sodium excretion suggested that salt intake was an independent determination of LV mass (169).

Pooled estimates suggest that BP reductions are most impressive among older individuals, those with higher baseline levels of BP, and particularly those who are salt-sensitive (167). Most important, sodium restriction often allows reduction in the need for antihypertensive medications, regardless of combination with weight loss (170). In one trial of sodium reduction with or without weight reduction among elderly hypertensives, 34% to 44% of patients were able to remain off their antihypertensives, compared to only 16% who continued on their usual diet (171). The principal hurdles include maintaining such reductions over the long haul and dealing with the high sodium content of most processed foods (36). Despite these data, the optimal guideline for salt use remains controversial (172).

Alcohol Restriction and Smoking Cessation

Restricting habitual consumption to two or fewer alcohol drinks per day can reduce BP in normotensive and hypertensive individuals and may help prevent hypertension (113). Whereas stopping smoking generally does not reduce BP, its cessation dramatically reduces overall cardiovascular risk. An important caution surrounds the weight gain that commonly accompanies the cessation of smoking and creates a major hurdle to individuals otherwise willing to stop.

The impact of alcohol use occurs in both genders, increases with age, combines with obesity, and may be aggravated by cigarette smoking (36). Among individuals consuming four to six standard drinks a day, the pressor effect lasts throughout the 24-hour period (173). There may also be a withdrawal component to patients exhibiting higher pressures after binge intake (36).

Stress Reduction/Relaxation Training

Some benefit of relaxation, meditation, or biofeedback has been reported from workplace and clinical settings (174,175).

One review of 25 published randomized controlled trials enumerated 823 subjects on active treatment, but the studies had many methodologic limitations: small sample sizes (17 of 25 studies had <40 subjects), short duration (average = 3 months), and small effects (176). Only two of five studies with >15 subjects per treatment arm and ≥12 months of treatment duration exhibited significant BP reductions. The one randomized controlled trial testing the value of stress management in preventing the development of hypertension could not demonstrate a clear benefit (153). There is insufficient current evidence to support stress reduction as a principal treatment modality for hypertension. Conflicting data exist as to whether high job stress alone is a powerful predictor of subsequent hypertension or whether the methods for coping with stress are more determinant (36).

Selecting Drug Therapy

If 3 to 6 months of nondrug therapy fail to reduce BP to acceptable levels, the clinician should consider antihypertensive medications. *e*Table 5.4.1 summarizes the objectives for antihypertensive drugs (180).

No single strategy for selecting antihypertensive drug therapy is relevant and helpful for all patients. Four principal approaches have emerged as useful: stepped care, demographic analysis, renin profiling, and individualization.

Stepped Care

Over the past two decades, the concept of progressive, stepped care has evolved from a narrow set of incremental options to a broader set of guidelines by the Joint National Committee VI (JNC VI) (5):

Step 1—Prescribe lifestyle modifications, including weight reduction, moderated alcohol intake, regular physical exercise, reduced sodium intake, and smoking cessation.
Step 2—If response is inadequate, continue the lifestyle modification and add monotherapy for mild to moderate (stage 1–2) hypertension with thiazide diuretics or beta-blockers, unless there is a contraindication. Other agents [e.g., angiotensin-converting enzyme (ACE) inhibitors, calcium antagonists, alpha₁-blockers, and alpha-beta-blockers] are satisfactory substitutes for patients with contraindications, although the long-term net benefit of these drugs is not established.
Step 3—If response to initial treatment is inadequate, increase drug dose, substitute another antihypertensive drug, or add a second agent from a different drug class.
Step 4—If response is still inadequate, add a second or third agent from a different drug class, including an appropriate diuretic (if not already administered).

This approach carries several major advantages: simplicity of understanding and implementation, emphasis on

administration of complementary drug classes for synergism, and titration to minimize toxicities. The JNC VI offers limited sensitivity to three issues: hemodynamic diversity among hypertensives, negative metabolic effects of thiazides and beta-blockers, and the need for direct testing of stepped care versus alternative approaches.

Demographic Analysis

Several investigators have propounded useful, if simplistic, heuristics that summarize relative responsiveness of demographic subgroups to different antihypertensive drug classes. Although helpful as generalizations, these guidelines reflect relative, not absolute, effectiveness.

Younger patients may exhibit high or normal CO, which is often associated with a sympathetically activated, hyperkinetic circulation. Such individuals may be responsive to ACE inhibitors or antiadrenergic agents such as beta-blockers. Older patients more commonly display low or normal plasma renin activity (PRA), volume expansion, and increased peripheral resistance. Such patterns often respond to diuretic or calcium antagonist therapy. A majority of black hypertensive patients shows volume-dependent, low-renin patterns, compared to about 10% of white hypertensives. Whereas diuretic therapy may be especially effective, other drug classes (e.g., beta-blockers, calcium antagonists, and ACE inhibitors) may also control BP among black hypertensives (181). Such differences in demographic responsiveness to medications decrease when more than one class of antihypertensive agents are used. The demographic and hemodynamic differences offer modest support for the principles summarized in *e*Table 5.4.2.

Individualized Approach

Perhaps the most comprehensive strategy for selecting antihypertensive therapy is the individualized approach. It factors in patients' profiles of hemodynamics and pathophysiology, cardiovascular risk analysis, concurrent medical conditions and therapies, demographics, quality-of-life analysis, and cost. In essence, the customized approach corresponds to a type of "mosaic" model of treatment, incorporating a large number of variables that differ for each individual.

The strategy consists of six components. Responding to the projected *pathophysiology and hemodynamics*, the clinician chooses medications to reverse the underlying circulatory dysregulation, lowering the vascular resistance, if elevated, while preserving CO and maintaining perfusion to critical target organs, both at rest and with exercise and over the entire 24 hours.

Reflecting *cardiovascular risk profile analysis*, the clinician should avoid medications that worsen the known risk profile, such as using high-dose thiazides in a patient with elevated low-density lipoprotein cholesterol. In addition, the clinician should prospectively monitor those regimen-affected factors that impact risk and continuously adjust the regimen to minimize overall risk, whether related to atherosclerosis, major arrhythmias, congestive failure, or sudden death (184).

Aware of *concurrent medical conditions and therapies*, the clinician prescribes the fewest antihypertensive drugs to treat the greatest number of concomitant conditions, such as using beta-blockers when angina and hypertension are present in the absence of heart failure, peripheral vascular insufficiency, or bronchospasm. Such therapeutic parsimony facilitates medication adherence by simplifying the overall regimen and minimizes adverse drug reactions and drug-drug interactions. This approach uses the *demographic* patterns previously described but integrates the options related to age and race with the other factors as well (185).

To optimize adherence to the regimen, the clinician seeks to optimize the patient's *quality of life* by considering physical, mental, social, emotional, and sexual functions (186–188).

Finally, the strategy considers cost: the sum of drug acquisition cost, required concomitant treatment (e.g., potassium supplementation for thiazide diuretics) and tests (e.g., monitoring serum potassium and renal function), clinician visits, hospitalizations and emergency evaluations, missed work from disease or side effects, and direct and indirect costs of long-term morbidity and mortality, as well as lost wages and productivity (10,189).

The guidelines for initial drug therapy promulgated by the JNC VI reflect these considerations. They incorporate consideration of patient comorbidities and the use of agents proven to reduce mortality in randomized controlled trials.

The JNC VI suggests three pathways for initiating medical treatment in patients requiring drug therapy for hypertension. First, patients with uncomplicated hypertension should be initiated with a beta-blocker or a diuretic. Second, patients with coexisting conditions and "compelling indications" should be started on medications that have been shown to reduce mortality. The choice of these drugs are "compelling" in that they have been shown by randomized controlled trials to reduce mortality in the specific condition (e.g., use of ACE inhibitors in patients with heart failure) and should be used unless strong contraindications to their use exist. Third, patients with comorbidities should be started on medications that are favorable to other medical conditions present (e.g., use of alpha$_1$-blockers in patients with coexisting prostatism) (*e*Fig. 5.1.2).

One controversial strategy to minimize medication-related cost and toxicity is to attempt cautious "step-down" therapy with progressive reduction and, sometimes, discontinuation of therapy—especially for patients with mild elevations (190) or good control, despite imperfect medication compliance (191,192).

Hemodynamics of Essential Hypertension/Drug Effects

Table 5.5 summarizes the effects of antihypertensive drug therapy on concomitant medical conditions and metabolic disorders, and Table 5.6 lists common drug interactions for antihypertensive therapy. Table 5.7 indicates the dosing guidelines and relative advantages and disadvantages by drug. ❧ a94

TABLE 5.5 EFFECTS OF ANTIHYPERTENSIVE DRUG THERAPY ON CONCOMITANT MEDICAL CONDITIONS AND METABOLIC DISORDERS

Conditions and disorders	Thiazide diuretics	Beta-blockers	Alpha$_1$-blockers	ACE inhibitors or AII receptor antagonists	Calcium antagonists (DHP)	Calcium antagonists (non-DHP)
Angina or acute MI	0	++	0	±	±	++
Atrial tachyarrhythmias	—	++	0	0	0	++
Bronchospasm	0	—	0	0	0	0
Congestive heart failure	++	±; carvedilol, metoprolol	0	++	±	±
Depression	0	±	0	0	0	0
Diabetes mellitus ± proteinuria	±	—	0	++	±	0
Dyslipidemia	—	—	++	0	0	0
Gout	—	0	0	0	0	0
Heart block (second or third degree)	0	—	0	0	±	—
Hypercalcemia	—	0	0	0	0	0
Hypokalemia	—	0	0	±	0	0
Migraine	0	++	0	0	—	0
Osteoporosis	++	0	0	0	0	0
Peripheral arterial disease	0	—	±	0	±	—
Prostatism	±	0	++	0	0	0
Renal insufficiency	±	0	0	±	±	0

AII, angiotensin II; ACE, angiotensin-converting enzyme; DHP, dihydropyridine; MI, myocardial infarction; —, adverse effect; ++, beneficial effect; ±, may be beneficial or adverse; 0, no effect.
Modified from Joint National Committee. The sixth report of the Joint National Committee on prevention, detection, evaluation, and treatment of high blood pressure. *Arch Intern Med* 1997;157:2413–2446.

TABLE 5.6 IMPORTANT DRUG INTERACTIONS IN ANTIHYPERTENSIVE THERAPY

Drug class	Increased antihypertensive efficacy	Decreased antihypertensive efficacy	Effect on other medications
Diuretics	Combine diuretics that act at different nephron sites (e.g., thiazide and furosemide)	NSAIDs Corticosteroids Oral contraceptives Resin-binding agents	↑ Serum lithium levels Cause ↑(K^+) if combining spironolactone or triamterene with ACE inhibitors or AIIRAs May cause ↑ prothrombin time with warfarin therapy
Beta-blockers	Cimetidine and quinidine blunt hepatic metabolism of hepatically metabolized beta-blockers	NSAIDs Drugs inducing hepatic enzymes (e.g., rifampin, phenobarbital)	Propranolol induces hepatic enzymes, increasing clearance of drugs with similar metabolism May mask or prolong insulin-induced hypoglycemia May cause heart block or precipitate CHF with non-DHP calcium antagonists
ACE inhibitors	Chlorpromazine Clozapine	NSAIDs Antacids Food decreases moexipril absorption	↑ Serum lithium levels ↑ Hyperkalemic effect of K^+-sparing diuretics
Calcium antagonists	Cimetidine and ranitidine blunt hepatic metabolism of hepatically metabolized calcium antagonists Grapefruit juice (some DHPs)	Drugs inducing hepatic enzymes (e.g., rifampin, phenobarbital)	↑ Cyclosporine with diltiazem, verapamil, or nicardipine Non-DHPs increase drug levels for drugs using same hepatic metabolism (e.g. digoxin, quinidine, sulfonylureas, theophylline) ↓ Serum lithium levels from verapamil Prazosin may decrease verapamil clearance
Alpha$_1$-blockers Central alpha$_2$-agonists and peripheral neuronal blockers		Tricyclic antidepressants Phenothiazines Monoamine oxidase inhibitors Sympathomimetics (May all lead to paradoxical hypertension)	↑ Serum lithium levels from methyldopa ↑ Clonidine withdrawal from beta-blockers Clonidine potentiates many anesthetics Iron salts reduce methyldopa absorption

ACE, angiotensin-converting enzyme; AIIRAs, angiotensin II receptor antagonists; CHF, congestive heart failure; DHP, dihydropyridine; K^+, potassium; NSAIDs, nonsteroidal antiinflammatory drugs.
Adapted from Joint National Committee. The sixth report of the Joint National Committee on prevention, detection, evaluation, and treatment of high blood pressure. *Arch Intern Med* 1997;157:2413–2446.

EVALUATION FOR SECONDARY FORMS OF HYPERTENSION

Prevalence

Curable secondary hypertension is relatively rare (197). Among unselected patient series, primary hypertension is the ultimate cause in 93% to 94% of cases, renal parenchymal disease in an additional 5% to 6%, and all other causes of presumably reversible secondary hypertension accounting for only 1% to 2% of the total, as summarized in *e*Figure 5.1.1 (197–201). There is little justification for aggressive evaluation of every hypertensive patient for secondary hypertension in the absence of important clues. The diagnostic process may resume if patients later exhibit new clues or refractoriness to treatment. Several important clues from history, physical examination, or baseline testing may indicate a higher-than-usual likelihood of secondary hypertension. The differential for secondary hypertension appears in *e*Table 5.7.2, and the clues are summarized in Table 5.8.

Renal Parenchymal Disease

Renal parenchymal disease constitutes a collection of diverse conditions, and it is the single largest cause of secondary hypertension (202). Most of these conditions may not be reversible.

A large array of clinical situations affect renal parenchyma and produce hypertension. Acute renal failure may result from acute glomerulonephritis (especially postinfectious, crescentic, or focal segmental changes), vasculitis (especially systemic lupus erythematosus, scleroderma, or polyarteritis), or acute obstruction. When the renal dysfunction is more insidious, ultimately destroying ≥80% of the nephrons, chronic renal failure occurs. The most common causes are vasculitis, glomerular disease (especially diabetic nephropathy and crescentic or focal segmental glomerulitis), and polycystic renal disease (203). Two patient clusters predominate. Most patients have a volume-dependent form of hypertension that is indicative of chronic glomerulonephritis and is usually relatively easy to control. A less common subset of patients has nephrosclerosis

TABLE 5.7 ANTIHYPERTENSIVE DRUG THERAPY: A PHARMACOLOGIC SUMMARY

Class	Example(s)	Mechanism(s)	Initial dose	Usual dose	Maximal dose	Usual dose/day	Advantages	Disadvantages	Comments
Diuretics									
Thiazides	Hydrochlorothiazide	Natriuresis	12.5–25.0 mg/d	25–50 mg/d	100 mg/d	1	Potentiates other antihypertensives	Hypokalemia	Especially effective among blacks, obese, elderly
	Chlorothiazide	Vasodilatation	125–250 mg/d	250–500 mg/d	1,000 mg/d			Hyperuricemia	
	Bendroflumethiazide		2.5 mg/d	2.5–5.0 mg/d	10 mg/d		Low cost	Hypercholesterolemia	May increase LVH
	Trichlorothiazide, etc.		1–2 mg/d	1–2 mg/d	4 mg/d		Proven end-organ efficacy	Hyperglycemia	Mediated via low K$^+$
Thiazide-like	Chlorthalidone	Natriuresis	12.5–25.0 mg/d	25–50 mg/d	50 mg/d	1	Lasts 24–48 h	Hypokalemia	Especially effective among blacks, obese, elderly
	Indapamide	Vasodilatation	2.5 mg/d	2.5–5.0 mg/d	5 mg/d		Works even if GFR <50	Hyperuricemia	
	Metolazone		0.5–2.5 mg/d	0.5–5.0 mg/d	5 mg/d		Works even if GFR <50	Hypercholesterolemia	May increase LVH
K$^+$-Sparing	Spironolactone	Natriuresis	25 mg/d	25–50 mg/d	100 mg/d	1–2	Spares K$^+$	Gynecomastia	Higher doses in first-degree hyperaldosteronism
	Triamterene		25–50 mg/d	25–50 mg/d	75 mg/d		No effect on glucose, uric acid, lipid	Little hypotensive effect on its own	Caution in renal dysfunction
	Amiloride	Natriuresis	5 mg/d	5–10 mg/d	10 mg/d	1–2	More potent diuresis	Hypokalemia	Less effective antihypertensive effects despite greater diuresis
Loop	Furosemide		10–20 mg/d	10–40 mg/d	120 mg/d				
	Bumetanide		0.5 mg/d	0.5–1.0 mg/d	5 mg/d			Hyperuricemia Hypercholesterolemia Hyperglycemia	
	Ethacrynic acid		25 mg/d	25–50 mg/d	100 mg/d				
Antiadrenergics									
Beta-blockers Lipophilic	Propranolol	Peripheral beta-blocker (1 vs. 2)	20–40 mg/d	40–160 mg/d	320 mg/d	1–2	Effective for secondary prevention of MIs	Decrease exercise tolerance	All beta-blockers are equally effective antihypertensives
	Timolol		10–20 mg/d	20–40 mg/d	80 mg/d				
	Pindolol (ISA)	Antirenin effect	5–10 mg/d	10–20 mg/d	60 mg/d		Useful when CAD comorbidity is present	May cause bronchospasm	Main differences are convenience of dosing and side-effect profile
	Metoprolol		25–50 mg/d	50–100 mg/d	200 mg/d			Increase TG, decrease HDL except with ISA	
	Labetalol	(Alpha$_1$ + beta)	100 mg/d	100–200 mg/d	1,200 mg/d		May assist for coexistent agitation or tremor		

Class	Drug	Mechanism							
Hydrophilic		Decrease cardiac output						Predispose to CHF	Those with ISA may be less cardioprotective
	Nadolol		20–40 mg/d	40–120 mg/d	320 mg/d			May cause sedation, nightmares, indigestion, vascular insufficiency	
	Atenolol		25–50 mg/d	50–100 mg/d	200 mg/d				
Alpha$_2$-agonists	Acebutolol (ISA) Betaxolol, etc.		200 mg/d	200–400 mg/d	1,200 mg/d				
	Methyldopa	Decrease peripheral catecholamines	5 mg/d 125–250 mg/d	5–10 mg/d 250–500 mg/d	20 mg/d 2,000 mg/d	1–2	Decrease cardiac output when contraindication to beta-blockers	May cause excess sedation, dry mouth, orthostasis, dermatitis from patch	Slow upward titration may minimize unpleasant side effects
	Clonidine		0.1–0.2 mg/d	0.1–0.6 mg/d	1.2 mg/d				
	Clonidine patch	Decrease HR, CO	0.1 mg/d	0.1–0.3 mg/d	0.3 mg/d				
	Guanabenz		2–4 mg/d	2–8 mg/d	64 mg/d		May assist for coexistent agitation or tremor		
	Guanfacine		1 mg/d	1–2 mg/d	3 mg/d				
Alpha$_1$-blockers	Prazosin	Peripheral postganglionic blocker	1 mg/d	1–2 mg/d	10 mg/d	1–2	Lowers LDL	"First-dose" phenomenon	Not yet demonstrated as useful step 1 treatment
	Terazosin	Vasodilatation	1 mg/d	1–2 mg/d	10 mg/d		Raises HDL		Potentiated by diuretics or autonomic dysfunction
	Doxazosin		1 mg/d	1–2 mg/d	8 mg/d				
Peripheral antagonists	Reserpine	Peripheral ganglionic blocker	0.1 mg/d	0.10–0.25 mg/d	0.25 mg/d	1–2	Long half-life (wk)	May cause depression, orthostasis, sedation, peptic exacerbations	(Reserpine) Little used but found effective and safe in low doses
	Guanethidine		10 mg/d	10–50 mg/d	150 mg/d				
	Guanadrel		10 mg/d	10–50 mg/d	100 mg/d				
ACE inhibitors	Captopril	Decrease AII, aldosterone	12.5 mg/d	25–75 mg/d	150 mg/d	2–3	Less side effects	May cause proteinuria, dysgeusia, cough, rash	Useful in context of congestive heart failure, LVH
	Enalapril	Decrease afterload	2.5–5.0 mg/d	10–20 mg/d	40 mg/d	1–2	Useful for diabetic glomerulopathy		
	Lisinopril		5 mg/d	10–20 mg/d	40 mg/d	1		May precipitate renal failure, esp. with stenosis	Use caution in context of renal dysfunction
	Benazepril		5–10 mg/d	20–40 mg/d	80 mg/d	1–2			
	Fosinopril		10 mg/d	20–40 mg/d	80 mg/d	1			
	Moexipril		7.5 mg/d	7.5–30.0 mg/d	30 mg/d	1			
	Perindopril		2–4 mg/d	4–16 mg/d	16 mg/d	1			

(continued)

TABLE 5.7 (Continued)

Class	Example(s)	Mechanism(s)	Initial dose	Usual dose	Maximal dose	Usual dose/day	Advantages	Disadvantages	Comments
	Quinapril		5–10 mg/d	20–80 mg/d	80 mg/d	1–2			Useful for LVH, CHF
	Ramipril		1.25–2.50 mg/d	2.5–20.0 mg/d	20 mg/d	1–2			
	Trandolapril		1–2 mg/d	2–8 mg/d	8 mg/d	1			
All antagonists	Losartan	Block AII, decrease TPR	25 mg/d	25–100 mg/d	100 mg/d	1	May have less side effects than ACE inhibitors	Similar to ACE inhibitors and asthenia	
	Valsartan		80 mg/d	160–320 mg/d	320 mg/d	1			Lowers uric acid
	Irbesartan		100 mg/d	100–200 mg/d	200 mg/d	1			
	Candesartan		8–16 mg/d	4–16 mg/d	32 mg/d	1			
	Eprosartan		400 mg/d	400–800 mg/d	800 mg/d	1–2			
	Telmisartan		20–40 mg/d	20–80 mg/d	80 mg/d	1			
Calcium antagonists Dihydropyridines	Nifedipine	Vasodilatation	30 mg/d	30–90 mg/d	180 mg/d	1–2	Effective in wide array of patients	May cause headache, edema, flushing, weakness, tachycardia	May be useful in context of peripheral insufficiency, angina
	Nicardipine	Reflex sympathetic stimulation	30 mg/d	30–90 mg/d	180 mg/d				
	Nitrendipine		5 mg/d	10–20 mg/d	40 mg/d		May help natriuresis		
	Isradipine	Decrease afterload	5 mg/d	5–15 mg/d	15 mg/d			May predispose to CHF	
	Amlodipine		5 mg/d	5–15 mg/d	15 mg/d	1			
	Felodipine		2.5 mg/d	2.5–10.0 mg/d	20 mg/d				
	Nimodipine		30 mg t.i.d.	60 mg q4h	360 mg/d				Used for subarachnoid hemorrhage
Negative inotropics	Nisoldipine	Decrease HR, CO	10–20 mg/d	20–40 mg/d	60 mg/d	1–2	Useful in context of CAD, arrhythmia	Constipation	Avoid cotreatment with beta-blockers
	Verapamil		80–120 mg/d	120–240 mg/d	480 mg/d				
	Diltiazem		60 mg/d	90–240 mg/d	360 mg/d			May precipitate CHF	
Vasodilators	Hydralazine	Peripheral vasodilatation	25–50 mg/d	50–200 mg/d	300 mg/d	1–2	Useful step 3 agents	May cause angina, edema, pericarditis	Must control HR and fluid retention for good BP control
	Minoxidil		2.5–10.0 mg/d	10–20 mg/d	40 mg/d				

AII, angiotensin II; ACE, angiotensin-converting enzyme; BP, blood pressure; CAD, coronary artery disease; CHF, congestive heart failure; CO, cardiac output; GFR, glomerular filtration rate; HDL, high-density lipoprotein; HR, heart rate; ISA, intrinsic sympathomimetic activity; K+, potassium; LDL, low-density lipoprotein; LVH, left ventricular hypertrophy; MI, myocardial infarction; TG, triglycerides; TPR, total peripheral resistance.

TABLE 5.8 SECONDARY HYPERTENSION: AN OVERVIEW

Condition	Clues from			Diagnostic tests		Comments	Therapy
	History	Physical	Early Lab	Screening	Definitive		
Renal parenchymal disease	Renal disease; urinary tract infections; diabetes mellitus; chronic analgesics	Flank/abdominal mass	Active urinary sediment; elevated creatinine; glycosuria; proteinuria; anemia	24-h urinary protein; creatinine clearance	(Renal biopsy)	False reassurance with "normal" serum creatinine in the elderly	Treat underlying condition; r/o transplant stenosis, immunosuppressive therapy, rejection, volume overload
Renovascular hypertension	Age <30 yr, especially female; age >60 yr, especially male; new onset, rapid course; cardiovascular risk factors; family history of vascular anomalies	Flank bruit; peripheral vascular insufficiency	Proteinuria	Captopril renal scan (MRI)	Renal arteriography	Split vein renins no longer required for diagnosis	Renal angioplasty; renal artery reconstruction
Coarctation of the aorta	—	Asymmetrical pulses and blood pressure; pulse delay (arm or leg); systolic murmur or bruit	Ankle: brachial index; chest radiograph ± notching of ribs	Echocardiogram	Aortography	—	Surgical repair
Cushing's syndrome	Weight gain, acne, fluid retention, bruising	Abdominal mass; moon facies; truncal obesity; striae; plethora; hirsutism; weakness	Hyperglycemia	Overnight dexamethasone suppression test (1 mg); 24-h urinary free cortisol	4–8 mg dexamethasone suppression test; CT or MRI scan; CRH stimulation test	—	Surgical excision vs. drug suppression
Primary hyperaldosteronism	Weakness; paresthesia; polyuria; tetany	—	Hypokalemia, especially after potassium-wasting diuretics (diagnosis excluded by potassium ≥4 mEq/L)	24-h urinary aldosterone; orthostatic test; stimulated plasma renin activity	Abdominal CT or MRI; adrenal vein sampling; response to glucocorticoids	—	Excision for adenoma after spironolactone trial; antialdosterone drugs for hyperplasia (glucocorticoids)
Pheochromocytoma	Paroxysmal hypertension; palpitations; headache; sweating; fainting; weight loss; procedure → attacks; family history of multiple endocrine neoplasm or neurofibromata	Orthostasis, tremor, perspiration; cardiomyopathy	Hyperglycemia; posterior mediastinal mass on chest radiography	Spot urinary metanephrine; 24-h urinary metanephrine, total catecholamines, VMA; clonidine suppression test	CT or MRI scan; 131I-MIBG scan (radiocholesterol scan)	Provocative tests no longer recommended; tumor palpation in operating room	Excision after pretreatment with alpha-blockers, fluid (phenoxybenzamine, labetalol)
Hyperthyroidism	Nervousness; palpitations; dysphagia; weight loss	Tremor; goiter; wide pulse pressure; bruit; exophthalmos	—	Free thyroxine; thyroid stimulating hormone	Thyroid uptake/scan; antithyroid antibodies	—	131I vs. surgery vs. antithyroid medications
Drug response	Vasoconstriction; fluid retainers; nephrotoxins						

CRH, corticotropin-releasing hormone; CT, computed tomography; 131I, iodine-131; MIBG, metaiodobenzylguanidine; MRI, magnetic resonance imaging; r/o, rule out; VMA, vanillylmandelic acid.
Adapted from Rudd P, Dzau VJ. Hypertension: evaluation and management. In: Loscalzo J, Creager MA, Dzau VI, eds. Vascular medicine. Boston: Little, Brown, 1996:609–638.

that is dependent on renin rather than volume and is often more difficult to control. Most patients requiring chronic dialysis display a volume dependency and variable degrees of autonomic dysfunction, whereas those with no functional kidneys or post bilateral nephrectomy usually are volume-dependent.

Other, less common causes of hypertension associated with chronic renal disease include pyelonephritis, membranous and membranoproliferative glomerulonephritis, immunoglobulin A nephropathy, renin-secreting tumors, or drug-induced renal dysfunction (e.g., phenacetin-associated analgesic nephropathy) (204). Even after renal transplantation, hypertension may result from continuation of prior hypertension, excess renin from the native kidney if not removed, posttransplant renal artery stenosis, immunosuppressive therapy [e.g., corticosteroids, cyclosporine, and tacrolimus (205)], chronic rejection, recurrent intrinsic renal disease, or volume overload.

Screening tests usually reveal azotemia, microalbuminuria, proteinuria, or abnormal urinary sediment. The most important management decisions usually revolve around the desirability and timing of dialysis or transplantation, as well as the optimal management of the volume component of the hypertension. The volume component usually responds to diuretics or to dialysis, whereas the renin component may require beta-blockers, ACE inhibitors, AII receptor antagonists, or minoxidil. Several of the standard antihypertensive agents may need dose adjustments in chronic renal failure (204). Optimizing BP control—usually to a lower target pressure (120–130/70–80 mm Hg) than for other hypertensive patients—may slow progression of the renal disease. Proteinuria itself serves as an independent risk factor for renal dysfunction (206), as well as for overall risk of cardiovascular disease (207). Direct comparison of the calcium antagonist nisoldipine versus the ACE inhibitor enalapril revealed that BP control was more important than the specific agent used for preserving creatinine clearance (208). More importantly, the trial demonstrated that renal function can be stabilized in type II diabetes over 5 years before frank albuminuria by achieving BPs no higher than 138/86 mm Hg.

Vascular Causes of Hypertension

Hypertension may result from physiologically significant stenosis of the renal arteries, the aorta, and a variety of other vascular structures.

Renovascular Causes of Hypertension

Activation of the renin-angiotensin-aldosterone system can result from compromise of arterial flow to either or both kidneys. Depending on the status and participation of the contralateral kidney, the ischemic stimulus may elevate renin, promote fluid retention, or both.

Two clinical subgroups comprise the majority of patients with renovascular hypertension: fibromuscular dysplasia and atherosclerotic disease. Fibromuscular dysplasia of the renal arteries accounts for less than 10% of all renovascular hypertension and occurs almost exclusively in younger patients, especially females. Although five pathologic subtypes are described, 70% of affected individuals display medial fibroplasia, and an additional 20% show perimedial fibroplasia. Both of these subtypes exhibit classical beaded appearance on angiography (209). Although the precise pathogenesis is uncertain, the natural history usually consists of slow progression of stenosis without frank occlusion (210).

Atherosclerotic disease, making up about 90% of the total causes, usually involves the proximal third of the renal artery with or without encroachment of the ostium itself. Lesions generally arise bilaterally, although one side may predominate. Atherosclerosis disease may extend for years without signaling its presence with hypertension or even elevated serum creatinine. Left untreated, most lesions progress, including complete occlusion and renal failure (210). If stenosis exceeds 75%, the probability of progression to full occlusion approaches 40% over 1 year (211). As many as 5% to 15% of individuals entering dialysis programs have previously undetected renovascular hypertension (210). ❦ a95

No perfect screening test exists. Baseline testing may demonstrate mild azotemia, proteinuria, or hypokalemia in <20% of individuals with the condition—modestly higher rates than among others with essential hypertension. Proponents exist for elevated peripheral PRA with or without captopril stimulation (213), renal scans, renal digital subtraction angiography (214), intravenous pyelography, and prompt progression to arteriography (215). Although it is an invasive test, arteriography remains the gold standard, searching for critical stenoses of ≥80% (216). Given its poor positive and negative predictive value, the marginal utility of obtaining renal vein renins to confirm unilateral versus bilateral disease has been questioned (217). One alternative to direct angiography is the use of captopril scintigraphy, which combines radionuclide scanning of the kidney (especially with mercaptoacetyltriglycine) with captopril stimulation to enhance differences in renal blood flow (218). The ACE inhibitor produces a fall in glomerular filtration rate on the affected side more than a reduction in renal blood flow. A positive scan correlates with successful angioplasty or surgical intervention in ≥90% of fibromuscular cases, but it may be less definitive in the elderly or in the presence of renal dysfunction (219). Its sensitivity can approach 100%, with specificity of 68% in selected series (220). Doppler ultrasound and magnetic resonance angiography offer promising results, but some consider them not yet cost-effective alternatives (221).

Preserving renal function preferentially involves endarterectomy, stenting, aortorenal bypass with saphenous vein or hypogastric artery, or partial nephrectomy when multiple distal stenoses occur. Rates of overall improvement and rapidity of improved glomerular filtration are superior among patients with fibromuscular dysplasia compared with those with atherosclerosis (222,223). The latter carry a worse prognosis because of progression of the arteriosclerotic process. Higher rates of successful repairs by angioplasty occur for fibromuscular dysplasia than for athero-sclerotic disease. Another advantage of angioplasty is that it may take place at the same time as diagnostic angiography, with or without stenting (224).

The trade-offs for medical management are especially acute for atherosclerotic disease. Progression of arteriosclerosis with occlusion and renal failure may occur even with adequate BP control. There have been no randomized controlled trials directly comparing the two treatment strategies (210). Useful drug classes have included ACE inhibitors or AII receptor antagonists (with cautions about hypotension, dose adjustment with renal dysfunction, and actual deterioration in renal function), beta-blockers, and dihydropyridine calcium channel blockers.

Aortic Coarctation

A variety of congenital and acquired malformations of the aorta may produce hypertension. Although the majority of patients presents during childhood, an important minority may pass into adulthood before definitive diagnosis (225). The variations include a left, right, or double aortic arch, which produces tracheal, bronchial, and esophageal compression. These conditions can be recognized on chest radiographs or esophagrams and confirmed by ultrasound, angiography, computed tomography (CT), or magnetic resonance imaging (MRI). Other congenital lesions of the aortic arch are characterized by aortic obstruction and include supravalvular aortic stenosis, aortic arch interruption or atresia, and coarctation (226).

Angioplasty and surgery remain the treatments of choice, although complications of these procedures include functional impairment, aortic rupture, aneurysmal formation, and restenosis (227). Useful, noninvasive ways to confirm the diagnosis and monitor for complications include Doppler ultrasound with exercise for arm-leg differences (228), transesophageal echocardiography (229), and MRI (227).

Endocrinologic Causes of Hypertension

Cushing's Syndrome

Spontaneous Cushing's syndrome may be classified into (a) corticotropin-dependent forms (e.g., Cushing's disease, ectopic corticotropin syndrome, and the rare ectopic corticotropin-releasing hormone syndrome); and (b) corticotropin-independent forms (e.g., unilateral cortisol-producing

adenomas and carcinomas). Rarely, bilateral adrenal hyperplasia—especially with functioning nodules—may yield the same clinical constellation of hypercortisolism, including hypertension. As the spectrum of conditions causing ectopic adrenocorticotropic hormone (ACTH) hypersecretion has filled in and expanded, even these distinctions have been become blurred (230). Fully 70% to 90% of patients with ACTH-dependent hypercortisolism have a pituitary tumor, but sophisticated special testing and endocrinologic consultation may still be necessary, once the syndrome is confirmed.

In most patients, the physical stigmata are striking: truncal obesity, moon facies, acne, buffalo hump, striae, and ecchymoses are coupled with osteoporosis, hyperglycemia, and hypertension (231). Up to 70% of individuals with the syndrome display hypertension, regardless of the subtype and independent of salt intake. Increased pressor responsiveness has been reported, probably due to local postsynaptic effector mechanisms in the resistance vessels; circadian BP variations have been decreased, absent, or even reversed (232). Initial screening for the diagnosis is best performed by a 1-mg, overnight dexamethasone suppression test or a 24-hour urinary-free cortisol after 2-mg dexamethasone suppression. Further distinctions require repeated plasma ACTH measurements by radioimmune assay, along with the 8-mg dexamethasone suppression test (233) or a corticotropin-releasing hormone stimulation test with inferior petrosal sinus sampling (234). Localization maneuvers include CT, MRI, or scanning using [^{131}I]6β-iodomethyl-19-norcholesterol—a marker of adrenocortical cholesterol uptake that accurately localizes adrenal cortex dysfunction (235).

The majority of individuals with Cushing's disease undergoes transsphenoidal exploration with remission rates of about 80%, especially for localized, relatively small tumors (236). Postoperative courses, particularly for patients undergoing adrenalectomy, may be stormy, in part because of cardiac complications associated with LVH (237). Recently described medical options include metyrapone, bromocriptine, and ketoconazole (238).

Primary Aldosteronism

Whereas Cushing's syndrome reflects glucocorticoid excess, a variety of other conditions exhibit mineralocorticoid excess. These conditions include primary hyperaldosteronism (adenoma, carcinoma, or bilateral hyperplasia), enzymatic deficiencies (11-OH-hydroxylase deficiency, 17-OH-hydroxylase deficiency, and 11-OH-dehydrogenase deficiency syndromes), or chronic licorice ingestion containing glycyrrhetinic acid (239). Although all of these conditions are relatively rare, the most common (60% to 90% of the total) is benign unilateral adenoma of the adrenal [aldosterone-producing adenoma (APA)], which yields inappropriately large and autonomous secretion of aldosterone with predictable metabolic and pathophysiologic consequences. Less common variants include idiopathic hyperaldosteronism (IHA or bilateral hyperplasia), nodular adrenocortical hyperplasia, aldosterone-producing renin-responsive adenoma, and glucocorticoid-suppressible hyperaldosteronism (240).

The autonomous secretion of plasma aldosterone (PA) occurs in distinction to its usual diurnal variation that is linked to plasma cortisol concentrations. Nonhormonal factors, such as increased serum potassium or decreased serum sodium, can stimulate aldosterone synthesis directly. Once secreted, aldosterone increases distal tubular sodium resorption and potassium secretion, increases intravascular volume, and suppresses renin secretion. When secreted in excess, aldosterone produces a volume-dependent hypertension, although there is physiologic escape from incessant sodium retention before frank edema develops.

Patients with primary hyperaldosteronism have no distinguishing symptoms from individuals with hypertension, although they may display nonspecific weakness, fatigue, polyuria, or cramps, presumably reflecting hypokalemia. APA is more common in women than in men, generally presenting in the third to sixth decade (241). An excessive loss of potassium or refractoriness to treatment may prompt further investigation. Hypokalemia may reach panic values (≤2.8 mEq per L), especially after diuretic therapy, but may be in the low normal range (≤4.0 mEq per L) without provocation or after salt restriction in up to 38% of patients (242).

The diagnostic process for primary hyperaldosteronism consists of three components: confirmation of inappropriately high aldosterone secretion, distinction between excisable tumor and nonsurgical glandular hyperplasia, and exclusion of rare variants suitable for medical therapy (other than aldosterone antagonists) (243). Because of many other causes of hypokalemia and low-renin hypertension, the single best screening test for the condition is a 24-hour urinary collection for aldosterone (244). The collection should occur after withdrawing all diuretics and ACE inhibitors for ≥2 weeks and all aldosterone antagonists for ≥6 weeks and repleting fluid status, sodium, and potassium to normal levels, if necessary, with 3 to 5 days of salt loading to ensure 24-hour urinary sodium of ≥200 mEq/L (241). These steps are essential to avoid stimulation of aldosterone secretion by hyperkalemia or its inhibition by hypokalemia. Noninterfering antihypertensive drugs, including alpha$_1$-blockers and ganglionic antagonists such as guanadrel, may be used to control BP before the test. Alternatively, a logistically simpler screening test may be the PA to PRA ratio, if patients can be withdrawn safely from antihypertensive medications for ≥2 weeks. A PA/PRA ratio >30 and a PA >20 ng/mL may yield a sensitivity of 90%, a specificity of 91%, a positive predictive value of 69%, and a negative predictive value of 98%. Some investigators have reported both consistent differentiation from essential hypertension and separation between APA and IHA—the two most common forms of primary hyperaldosteronism (245).

Once the triad of hypertension, high aldosterone, and low renin has been confirmed, the clinician can shift attention to detecting adenomata for which surgical excision is the treatment of choice and curative in 70% of cases (241). The hypertension, hypokalemia, and hyperaldosteronism are generally higher in APA than in IHA, but the distinctions are usually too small to be clinically useful. Imaging studies such as CT scans can detect adenomata of ≥0.7 cm, but ≤8% of the normal population may have nonfunctioning, incidental adrenal adenomata. MRI scanning offers no clear advantage. Dexamethasone and Lugol's solution pretreatment and [^{131}I]6β-iodomethyl-19-norcholesterol scanning may highlight a functioning mass while suppressing surrounding adrenal tissue and protecting the thyroid. Unfortunately, scanning must proceed over 2 to 5 days and carries only a 72% accuracy that is highly dependent on the tumor's size (241). ❧ a96

For the subset of patients with APA, unilateral total adrenalectomy is the treatment of choice in surgical candidates. High-dose spironolactone (200 to 600 mg per day in divided doses) for 2 to 6 weeks preoperatively corrects hypertension and hypokalemia, thereby predicting the surgical result (247). Despite careful workups and uncomplicated perioperative courses, long-term cure rates average <70%, even though most patients display improved BP control and simplified regimens. The BP may require 3 to 6 months postoperatively to fall to normal values (241).

For the remaining patients, no cure is available, although outcomes are often satisfactory (248). Treatment usually consists of a low-sodium diet (≤80 mEq per day), maintenance of near-optimal body weight, and aldosterone antagonist therapy. Spironolactone is the drug of choice in the form of 200 to 600 mg per day in divided doses. Correction of hypokalemia occurs within days, whereas normalization of BP may require 1 to 2 months. Common side effects include painful gynecomastia, impotence, decreased libido, menstrual irregularities, and gastrointestinal discomfort. Alternative therapies include amiloride (10 to 40 mg per day), dihydropyridines (e.g., nifedipine 30 to 180 mg per day), or ACE inhibitors. In patients with the rare syndrome of glucocorticoid-suppressible aldosteronism, spironolactone therapy may be as effective and better tolerated than dexamethasone 2 mg daily (241).

Pheochromocytoma

Pheochromocytomas and other catecholamine-secreting tumors—termed *paragangliomas* when arising outside the adrenal—may prompt some of the most dramatic moments in hypertension. The clinical spectrum is wide, ranging from previously unsuspected tumors, which first gain recognition from hypertensive crisis after a procedure like anesthesia, to incidentally discovered, slow growing, sometimes large, almost metabolically inactive masses. Nearly 80% of the tumors are limited to the adrenal glands, usually unilaterally. The tumors are more likely to be bilateral or multiple in pediatric presentations or in familial forms such as neurofibromatosis, von Hippel-Lindau disease, or multiple endocrine neoplasia type 2a or 2b. An additional 10% to 20% arise in other intraabdominal sites, and <5% appear from intrathoracic sites along the neurosecretory crest or bladder. A small number come from intracranial sites. Up to 20% of tumors are multiple. Less than 10% of all catecholamine-secreting tumors are malignant, although their presentation may be difficult to distinguish from their more benign equivalents. Prompt diagnosis and definitive treatment is essential to avoid cardiomyopathy, CHF, and other potentially lethal outcomes (249).

Disease manifestations reflect the direct and indirect effects of catecholamines, either hypersecreted at random intervals for variable durations or tonically released. The classic triad of episodic headache, palpitations with or without tachycardia, and inappropriate perspiration accompanying the hypertension may suggest pheochromocytoma. The full textbook description, however, occurs less than half of the time. Other findings that may indicate pheochromocytoma include nervousness and anxiety, tremor, nausea, abdominal or chest pain, orthostatic drops in BP, glucose intolerance, weight loss, pallor, and fatigue (249). Usually the most spectacular symptoms accompany the most dramatic BP elevations. Although less likely without one or more of the classical symptoms, the diagnosis of pheochromocytoma should be considered in patients unresponsive to appropriate triple-drug therapy, patients with paroxysmal hypertension associated with clinical procedures, or patients with hypertension developing after phenothiazine, tyramine, or tricyclic medications. Pregnancy may unmask the disease, as the growing uterus applies pressure on the adrenal, or after micturition in the rare presence of bladder wall-based tumors. Tumors that are nearly silent metabolically may grow to large size before detection, whereas metabolically active lesions generate enough early symptoms to be small when first discovered.

Under most circumstances, the diagnosis of catecholamine-secreting tumor receives first confirmation by elevated urinary levels of one or more of the vasoactive hormones. Most tumors secrete norepinephrine and epinephrine, although the former usually predominates. Because any single hormone may or may not be elevated, most published guidelines call for collecting an array, usually consisting of metanephrine, normetanephrine, total catecholamines, vanillylmandelic acid, norepinephrine, and epinephrine. Some have argued that a negative assay for a single catecholamine has a 98% predictive value for ruling out the disease in a primary care population (250). Optimally, the diagnostic procedure consists of a 24-hour collection that includes a catecholamine and creatinine to monitor sufficiency of urine collection. Shorter timed intervals (e.g., 4 to 8 hours) may be useful when full-day collections are impractical or if episodic symptoms are short-lived and potentially diluted by longer collections. Using µg of catecholamine/mg creatinine, the clinician may extrapolate to a full day's collection. Urine collections should occur at times of sustained hypertension. Plasma catecholamines may be equally diagnostic, as long as collection procedures are assiduously followed to minimize false-positives and false-negatives (249). Recent reports suggest that plasma metanephrine is more sensitive (~100%) than serum catecholamines or urinary metanephrines for the diagnosis of pheochromocytoma and retains specificity (~85%) similar to that of serum catecholamine determinations (251). Newer biochemical techniques usually obviate the need for dietary or drug restrictions (252).

The majority of patients with pheochromocytoma has dramatic elevations of catecholamines that are at least twice normal. If the clinical suspicion is high but the urinary concentration is only equivocally elevated, use of an oral clonidine suppression test (plasma catecholamine levels before and after clonidine, 0.3 mg orally) (253) or overnight clonidine suppression test (clonidine, 0.3 mg orally, at 9 p.m. with overnight urine collections) (254) to minimize hypotensive reactions may distinguish clonidine-suppressible versus irrepressible secretion. Clonidine serves to reduce central sympathetic outflow among patients with essential hypertension, but it leaves autonomous secretion unaffected. The provocative tests commonly recommended in prior decades are now relegated only to the small number of individuals with ambiguously mild elevations but strong clinical suspicion.

Definitive diagnosis and full localization usually require biochemical tests for catecholamines and scanning of potential sites by CT or MRI. On occasion, these scans may fail to localize the tumor. Scanning by [^{131}I]-metaiodobenzylguanidine (MIBG) uses a guanethidine analog with affinity for chromaffin tissue to search the entire body, rather than a more focal anatomic study that generally requires a lesion ≥1 cm in diameter for detection. A number of antihypertensive drugs—including labetalol, nifedipine, reserpine, diltiazem, verapamil, and tricyclic medications—may interfere with the test (255).

In most situations, patients with catecholamine-secreting tumors undergo curative resection as definitive therapy. Perioperative management usually includes several weeks of alpha$_1$-blocker therapy, especially phenoxybenzamine, and rehydration to avoid abrupt hypotension from withdrawal of the elevated catecholamines once the tumor pedicle is clamped. Often, the degree of alpha-blockade—using phentolamine or nitroprusside—is only partial to assist the surgeon in localizing the tumor by direct palpation during the exploration and to ensure that BP falls with complete excision. Persistent BP elevations may indicate additional catecholamine-secreting tumors. Beta-blockade can control arrhythmias during the perioperative period but should be administered only in conjunction with alpha-blockers to avoid unopposed alpha-agonist influence. Up to 25% of patients with benign, resected tumors remain hypertensive postoperatively; perhaps this percentage is related to primary hypertension or hypertensive nephropathy (252).

SPECIAL SITUATIONS

Hypertensive Crises

True hypertensive emergencies are unusual. Many reflect mismanagement—sometimes from patient nonadherence, sometimes from medical system failures, sometimes from both factors (263). Rather than a search for secondary causes, the clinical priority should be the safe, prompt, and gradual lowering of BP without major side effects or complications.

Dangers exist from both undertreatment and overtreatment. Diuretic therapy usually is not needed, unless it is applied in the presence of frank fluid overload or with diazoxide or minoxidil therapy to combat fluid retention. Centrally acting antiadrenergic agents (e.g., clonidine) carry the possibility of sedation, confounding the interpretation of altered mental status in hypertensive crisis. Such drugs, therefore, should be avoided in favor of nonsedating alternatives. The principal drug classes useful in hypertensive crisis reduce peripheral resistance. The clinician selects among them by assessing the need for (a) *prompt* (e.g., diazoxide) versus *less prompt* (e.g., minoxidil) treatment, (b) *precisely* controlled (e.g., nitroprusside) versus *less controlled* (e.g., hydralazine) treatment, and (c) *equipment-intensive* (e.g., nitroprusside) versus *uncomplicated* (e.g., fenoldopam) procedures. Most drug-induced complications may be minimized by anticipating which organs will receive pharmacologic effects in the short term and the long term.

Clinical decompensation rather than BP level alone should define the situation as urgent (i.e., no target organ damage) or emergent (i.e., target organ damage present). Others have emphasized the term *malignant hypertension* in reference to the association with encephalopathy or nephropathy (264). Although systolic pressures often exceed 180 to 200 mm Hg and diastolics are ≥110 to 120 mm Hg, the absolute level is less important than the rate of rise and the absolute difference in BP between the patient's usual level and those observed during crisis. The typical patient in hypertensive crisis is a middle-aged male with inconsistent access to medical care. All sociodemographic groups, however, are at risk.

Early pathophysiologic changes reflect arteriolar spasm, whereas later decompensation results from fibrinoid necrosis, release of vasoactive substances, further vasoconstriction, and myointimal proliferation. Target organ damage may affect brain, eye, kidney, heart, and gut, among other tissues. Most patients offer few specific symptoms. Sometimes cardiovascular decompensation produces palpitations, angina, or congestive failure; neurologic manifestations may include headache, nausea, seizures, or obtundation. Clinical examination may demonstrate retinopathy, CHF, arrhythmias, or focal neurologic deficits. Most screening laboratory tests are normal or nonspecific, such as mild azotemia, proteinuria, and hypokalemia.

Several patterns of clinical presentations deserve emphasis. New onset of hypertension in the absence of prior BP elevations is most consistent with acute drug reactions (e.g., cocaine, amphetamines, phencyclidine, monoamine oxidase inhibitor–tyramine reactions) or acute glomerulonephritis. If BP worsening rather than improvement occurs after diuretic therapy, extra stimulation of the renin-angiotensin-aldosterone system from volume depletion may be the cause from prior vasoconstriction.

There is no single recipe for managing hypertensive crises. Each situation should be assessed individually for critical organ involvement, desired time frame for lowering BP (minutes, hours, or days), and available options, including personnel and equipment. A summary of preferred treatments for hypertensive emergencies appears in Table 5.9. Notably, the use of short-acting nifedipine may cause precipitous falls in BP and should be avoided (265).

Accelerated hypertension without major target organ damage is the most common situation. It usually occurs in the context of inadequately treated primary hypertension, but it may also reflect renal parenchymal disease, withdrawal from antiadrenergic agents, vasculitis or renovascular disease. In the absence of significant retinopathic, cardiovascular, or neurologic abnormality, the clinician may elect close follow-up rather than automatic hospitalization (266).

More ominous are central nervous system catastrophes. These may result from hypertensive encephalopathy with failure of autoregulation by cerebral blood flow (CBF). There may be focal neurologic findings. Less commonly, transient hypertension can follow any cerebral insult, such as cerebrovascular accident (thrombotic, embolic, or hemorrhagic), trauma, subdural hematoma, neoplasia, encephalitis, vasculitis, or drug withdrawal. Whereas autoregulation generally maintains CBF within narrow limits over a wide range of BPs, chronic BP elevations shift the curve to higher settings, and abrupt changes in BP carry risks of dangerous rises or falls in CBF (267). Therapeutically, the clinician seeks a 10% to 20% reduction in BP over the first hour, then further, stepped reductions over 12 to 24 hours; this therapy is preferred over prompt and full normalization because more aggressive treatment may impair CBF (268).

Hypertension carries extra hazards for *ischemic heart disease*. Angina, like other acute pain, may briefly elevate BP, but MI usually lowers CO and subsequently BP. If persistent, hypertension may increase periinfarction morbidity and mortality. In pulmonary edema or CHF, the priority

TABLE 5.9 ANTIHYPERTENSIVE THERAPY OF CHOICE FOR HYPERTENSIVE EMERGENCIES

Clinical situation	Agents of choice	Alternatives	Avoid or use cautiously
Malignant hypertension without associated disease	Diazoxide Nitroprusside Minoxidil Fenoldopam	Hydralazine Trimethaphan Clonidine Labetalol Captopril	Nifedipine
Intracerebral or subarachnoid hemorrhage	Nitroprusside Labetalol	Trimethaphan Hydralazine Fenoldopam	Diazoxide Methyldopa Reserpine Clonidine
Ischemic heart disease	Nitrates Nitroprusside Labetalol	Morphine Trimethaphan Calcium antagonists	Diazoxide Hydralazine Minoxidil
Pulmonary edema	Furosemide Morphine Fenoldopam	Other diuretics Nitrates Nitroprusside	Beta-blockers Verapamil Diltiazem
Pregnancy, toxemia	Hydralazine Methyldopa	Nitroprusside Diazoxide Labetalol	Trimethaphan Nitrates Thiazides ACE inhibitors A$_{II}$RAs
Dissecting aortic aneurysm	Nitroprusside + beta-blocker	Trimethaphan + beta-blocker Labetalol	Diazoxide Hydralazine Minoxidil Diuretics
Renal failure or acute nephritis	Diazoxide Nitroprusside Calcium antagonists Fenoldopam	Hydralazine Methyldopa Minoxidil	Trimethaphan Beta-blockers
Pheochromocytoma	Phentolamine or phenoxybenzamine + propranolol	Nitroprusside Prazosin Labetalol Diazoxide	Methyldopa Beta-blockers alone Hydralazine
Postoperative hypertension	Diazoxide Fenoldopam	Nitroprusside Methyldopa Esmolol	Hydralazine Trimethaphan

ACE, angiotensin-converting enzyme; A$_{II}$RAs, angiotensin II receptor antagonists.

should be to ameliorate the LV failure. BP reduction usually follows. Diuretic therapy plays an important role in situations of fluid overload, even though most other hypertensive crises offer little place for diuresis.

Dissecting aortic aneurysms affecting the proximal ascending aorta comprise surgical emergencies and carry poor prognoses. Medical management in that context serves mainly to stabilize the patient as much as possible before transfer to the operating room when surgery is feasible. When localized distal to the left subclavian artery, such aneurysms may be triaged to surgery (good surgical risk) or medical (poor surgical risk) therapy (269). Drug therapy seeks to decrease the rate of pulse wave propagation to limit aneurysmal extension, as well as to lower BP overall.

Less than 5% of pregnant women present with preexisting chronic hypertension (270). During pregnancy, hypertension usually presents among primiparas after the twentieth week. Up to 40% of gestational hypertensives experience sustained hypertension within the subsequent two decades. Preeclampsia, especially when superimposed on chronic hypertension or renal disease, carries substantial risks to mother and fetus, whereas transient hypertension appearing near term is usually mild (271). Pregnancy may unmask previously unrecognized chronic renal disease, renovascular hypertension, and other secondary causes of hypertension. Whereas delivery is the ultimate treatment of choice, interim therapy may include bedrest, methyldopa, or hydralazine. In one study using atenolol, lower birth weights and smaller placentas were observed without demonstrated long-term differences in outcomes (272). ACE inhibitors are specifically contraindicated in pregnancy because of congenital malformations and fetal growth retardation (273).

In the *perioperative period*, hypertension constitutes a relative contraindication to elective surgery. The occurrence of abrupt hypertension during induction may suggest an occult pheochromocytoma. Sudden cessation of beta-blockers, methyldopa, or clonidine in the immediate pre-operative period may precipitate hypertensive crises (274).

Refractory Hypertension

Resistant or *refractory hypertension*—defined as failure to lower BP to <140/90 mm Hg despite a regimen of ≥3 antihypertensive agents—may occur from factors related to the prescribing clinician, the patient, the disease, or combinations of all three (275). Such a definition assumes that careful and appropriate measurement of BP has occurred on several occasions, including adequate patient preparation, elimination of interfering substances, and use of proper instruments and techniques.

The differential diagnosis of refractory hypertension heavily depends on selective factors of primary care versus referral practice. Whereas partial compliance with prescribed regimens may figure prominently in primary care, the most common cause of resistant hypertension is usually inappropriate or inadequate drug regimens in a referral practice (259). Other causes of refractory hypertension are summarized in *e*Table 5.9.1. Even in the context of refractory hypertension, specific, identifiable secondary causes of hypertension comprise only approximately 10% of the total. Although not common, correctable secondary forms of hypertension may first appear more likely after treatment has started. For example, increased BP after starting ACE-inhibitor therapy may suggest occult, bilateral renovascular hypertension, especially in association with drug-induced renal insufficiency.

Once the diagnosis of resistant disease is confirmed, the clinician should review the regimen to confirm its sufficiency. If the dose or dosing frequency of prescribed medications is submaximal, they may be reasonably increased, as long as adverse drug reactions have not occurred. When prescribed as monotherapy, most antihypertensive medications prompt physiologic compensation. These compensatory reactions usually involve reflex tachycardia, fluid retention, or other stimulation of the renin-angiotensin-aldosterone system. Perhaps the most common difficulty surrounds unrecognized "pseudoresistance" from subclinical fluid retention, especially after the use of vasodilators or antiadrenergic agents. BP control usually follows quickly the (re)institution of adequate diuretic therapy, commensurate with the level of renal function. Most thiazide diuretics lose antihypertensive potency as creatinine clearance falls below 40 mL per minute. Inappropriate antihypertensive combinations may also occur. Using more than one drug of the same drug class or creating adverse drug-drug interactions, as summarized in Table 5.6, may blunt BP control.

A patient's failure to adhere to prescribed regimens—sometimes termed *partial compliance* or *adherence*—frequently reflects suboptimal knowledge of the regimen or of the importance of consistent medication taking. When queried nonconfrontationally, many patients acknowledge that a variety of "hassle" factors interfere, such as complex regimens, disruption of daily schedules, side effects, and cost (276).

Other concerns for some patients may include health beliefs discordant from those of the treating clinician, especially about the significance of the "hypertension" diagnosis or the effectiveness of the prescribed treatment (277). ▼ a97

Compliance-enhancing strategies for the clinician include (a) watching for nonattenders and nonresponders, (b) inquiring nonconfrontationally about compliance barriers, (c) encouraging the development and use of the patient's own medication-taking system, (d) providing simple and clear instructions, (e) simplifying the regimen as much as possible, (f) guiding behavioral changes in "small packets," (g) monitoring progress to goal, both in BP and in compliance, (h) reinforcing desirable behaviors and outcomes whenever possible, (i) making explicit the value of the regimen and adherence to it, (j) applying help from all possible sources, (k) emphasizing the importance of dose-timing when appropriate, and (l) customizing the regimen to the patient's needs and preferences (281) (*e*Fig. 5.1.4).

Confronted with a patient demonstrating refractory hypertension, the clinician should review the regimen, goal BP, and past patterns of BP control. Subsequent steps include ruling out confounding conditions such as drug-related side effects, excess salt intake, drug-drug interactions, and secondary hypertension. Inquiring about toxicities should be nonconfrontational and assess potentially embarrassing symptoms such as altered libido, impotence, or incontinence (282). When relevant, the clinician should consider a change in regimen—especially the inclusion of an appropriate diuretic—commensurate with the level of renal function. Adjusting the regimen should permit simplification, tailoring the regimen details to the patient's daily lifestyle, and minimizing side effects. On occasion, powerful additional hypertension agents such as minoxidil may be necessary. Table 5.10 summarizes guidelines for management of refractory hypertension.

CONTROVERSIES AND PERSONAL PERSPECTIVES

In a field as vast and rapidly changing as hypertension, controversies thrive, and new ones emerge just as the old ones appear less compelling. Two of these controversies deserve special attention.

Significance of White-Coat Hypertension

The phenomenon of labile hypertension is familiar, as when patients exhibit a degree of hour-to-hour variability in excess of the usual 15% to 20% variation. Such variation includes physiologic dipping of the BP to lower levels during sleep. In 1983, Mancia et al. (283) proposed the term *white-coat syndrome* to reflect the systolic and diastolic BP increases of 27 mm Hg and 15 mm Hg, respectively, when a physician entered the patient's room during intraarterial

TABLE 5.10 GUIDELINES FOR MANAGEMENT OF REFRACTORY HYPERTENSION

Principle 1	Increase the dose of drug A to the maximal tolerated dose before adding drug B (selected for complementary mechanism of drug action).
Principle 2	Review the fluid/volume/diuretic status for "pseudoresistance." Thiazide diuretics are superior antihypertensive agents than loop diuretics when glomerular filtration rate (GFR $\cong$ C$_{cr}$) >50 mL/min. Longer-acting metolazone or indapamide may be useful when GFR <50.
Principle 3	Simplify the regimen (number of drugs, frequency of dosing).
Principle 4	Decrease out-of-pocket costs (consider using free medication samples as test).
Principle 5	Inquire about side effects (especially awkward symptoms, like decreased libido, impotence, or incontinence) and adjust regimen to reduce them.
Principle 6	Use nonconfrontational phrasing to help detect partial compliance and to explore useful options to reduce it.
Principle 7	Consider formal monitoring of compliance (diary vs. pill count vs. biologic assay vs. electronic dispenser).

C_{cr}, creatinine clearance; GFR, glomerular filtration rate.

BP monitoring. Over time, *white-coat hypertension* has come to mean elevated BP occurring in a medical setting despite normal ambulatory BP monitoring (284). The prevalence of such discrepant BP levels may affect up to 20% of men and 54% of women in reported series (122).

The difficult question then arises: what is the significance of such discrepancies? Unfortunately, the data are murky (284). The original prospective series of Verdecchia et al. (285,286) restricted white-coat hypertension to patients with elevated BP during clinic visits but normal ambulatory BPs (daytime pressures <130/80). Such patients had the same cardiovascular morbidity as patients with normal office BP (<140/90) on at least three visits on different days. Liberalizing the criteria even slightly (≤136/87 for men or ≤131/86 for women) raised CV risks close to those of sustained hypertensive patients. Several additional investigators (287–289) have reported intermediate risk for patients with white-coat hypertension, as reflected in abnormal levels of carotid stiffness and LV relaxation.

Accordingly, some have challenged the assumption that office hypertension among patients with normal ambulatory BP need not be treated. This argument starts with the reminder that office BPs are the basis for most published clinical trials in which treating hypertension appears beneficial (284). Several additional studies suggest that home BPs of ≤135/85 (290) or 137/82 (291) represent the upper limit of normality. Finally, to confound the matter, other investigators report that "white-coat normotension" (i.e., elevated ambulatory pressures despite normal office BP) correlates with augmented LV mass index and relative wall thickness compared to patients with sustained normotension (292). For the moment, there is no simple resolution. Given a curvilinear relation between BP and cardiovascular risk, no simple or universal threshold is likely to emerge.

Best Options for Initial Monotherapy

The JNC VI unambiguously recommended diuretics and beta-blockers as drugs of choice for initial monotherapy in the absence of specific contraindications (5). With the exception of diabetics, for whom the use of ACE inhibitors or AII receptor antagonists are particularly advantageous (147,293), a large number of other primary prevention trials found strong and consistent support for endorsing diuretics and beta-blockers over the alternatives. Diuretics and beta-blockers have been evaluated in 18 long-term randomized trials (294). Compared with placebo, beta-blocker therapy was effective in preventing stroke (RR, 0.71; 95% CI, 0.59–0.86) and CHF (RR, 0.58; 95% CI, 0.40–0.84). The findings were similar for high-dose diuretic therapy (for stroke, RR, 0.49; 95% CI, 0.39–0.62; and for CHF, RR, 0.17; 95% CI, 0.07–0.41). Low-dose diuretic therapy prevented not only stroke (RR, 0.66; 95% CI, 0.55–0.78) and CHF (RR, 0.58; 95% CI, 0.44–0.76), but it also reduced coronary disease (RR, 0.72; 95% CI, 0.61–0.85) and total mortality (RR, 0.90; 95% CI, 0.81–0.99).

Several other randomized controlled trials highlight reduction in stroke risk with the use of the calcium antagonist nitrendipine (295) and reduced rates of stroke, coronary disease, and heart failure among patients receiving the ACE inhibitor ramipril (296), but not in those receiving captopril (297). Concomitantly, the Antihypertensive and Lipid-Lowering Treatment to Prevent Heart Attack Trial (ALLHAT) investigators reported the elimination of the alpha$_1$-blocker doxazosin treatment arm because of unexpectedly higher rates of congestive failure compared to the diuretic chlorthalidone (298). Together, these reports create ambiguities as to whether alternative drug classes offer net benefit versus risk as initial monotherapy for hypertension. At least 2 more years will pass before the final ALLHAT results are published, allowing head-to-head comparisons of the remaining treatment arms among more than 24,000 patients at 625 centers: the calcium antagonist amlodipine, the ACE inhibitor lisinopril, and chlorthalidone. The controversy continues.

Finally, the contention about calcium antagonists and their linkage to higher mortality has greatly softened in recent years. Early reports of higher rates of MI, gas-

THE FUTURE

As one tries to predict the future of hypertension management, there will continue to be exciting developments in three major areas. First, basic scientific advances in molecular and genetic medicine will likely shed light on the initial and initiating events that cause the deranged physiology of hypertension. Second, evolving insights from epidemiology will refine definitions of high-risk groups and clusterings to focus efforts that produce the greatest positive yield for a population, despite resource constraints. Finally, the development of more effective and better tolerated antihypertensive medications will almost certainly combine with more sophisticated behavioral approaches to enhance adherence. In so doing, patients may enjoy the full benefits of risk reduction while maintaining an excellent quality of life.

trointestinal hemorrhage, and breast cancer (299) have not been confirmed in larger trials of nitrendipine (300), nifedipine gastrointestinal therapeutic system, amlodipine (301), or verapamil (302). The risks of shorter-acting dihydropyridines remain debated.

REFERENCES

1. Levy D, Larson MG, Vasan RS, et al. The progression from hypertension to congestive heart failure. *JAMA* 1996;275:1557–1562.
2. Pardell H, Tresserras R, Armario P, et al. Pharmacoeconomic considerations in the management of hypertension. *Drugs* 2000;59:13–20; discussion 39–40.
3. Anastos K, Charney P, Charon RA, et al. Hypertension in women: what is really known? The Women's Caucus, Working Group on Women's Health of the Society of General Internal Medicine. *Ann Intern Med* 1991;115:287–293.
4. Baum D, Kennedy DL, Knapp EE, et al. Prescription drug use in 1984 and changes over time. *Med Care* 1988;26:105–114.
5. Joint National Committee. The sixth report of the Joint National Committee on Prevention, Detection, Evaluation, and Treatment of High Blood Pressure. *Arch Intern Med* 1997;157:2413–2446.
6. Franklin SS. Ageing and hypertension: the assessment of blood pressure indices in predicting coronary heart disease. *J Hypertens* 1999;17:S29–S36.
7. Franklin SS, Khan SA, Wong ND, et al. Is pulse pressure useful in predicting risk for coronary heart disease? The Framingham heart study. *Circulation* 1999;100:354–360.
8. Pearson TA, Fuster V. 27th Bethesda Conference: matching the intensity of risk factor management with the hazard for coronary disease events: executive summary. *J Am Coll Cardiol* 1996;27:961–963.
9. Kannel WB. Blood pressure as a cardiovascular risk factor: prevention and treatment. *JAMA* 1996;275:1571–1576.
10. Stason WB. Opportunities to improve the cost-effectiveness of treatment for hypertension. *Hypertension* 1991;18:I161–I166.
11. O'Rourke MF. What is blood pressure? *Am J Hypertens* 1990;3:803–810.
12. Segall HN. How Korotkoff, the surgeon, discovered the auscultatory method of measuring arterial pressure. *Ann Intern Med* 1975;83:561–562.
13. Janeway TC. A clinical study of hypertensive cardiovascular disease. *Arch Intern Med* 1913;12:755–762.
14. Keith NM, Wagener HP, Barker NW. Some different types of essential hypertension: their course and prognosis. *Am J Med Sci* 1939;197:332–339.
15. Goldblatt H, Lynch J, Hanzal RF, et al. Studies on experimental hypertension. I. The production of persistent elevation of systolic blood pressure by means of renal ischemia. *J Exp Med* 1934;59:347–379.
16. Page IH. The mosaic theory of hypertension. In: Bock KD, Cottier PT, eds. *Essential hypertension*. Berlin: Springer-Verlag, 1960:1–9.
17. Page IH. Some regulatory mechanisms of renovascular and essential arterial hypertension. In: Genest J, Koiw E, Kuchel O, eds. *Hypertension: physiopathology and treatment*. New York: McGraw-Hill, 1979:576–587.
18. Dollery C. Hypertension. *Br Heart J* 1987;58:179–184.
19. Veterans Administration Cooperative Study Group on Antihypertensive Agents. Effects of treatment on morbidity in hypertension: results in patients with diastolic blood pressures averaging 115 through 129 mm Hg. *JAMA* 1967;202:1028–1034.
20. Veterans Administration Cooperative Study Group on Antihypertensive Agents. Effects of treatment on morbidity in hypertension: II. Results in patients with diastolic blood pressures averaging 90 through 114 mm Hg. *JAMA* 1970;213:1143–1152.
21. Australian National Blood Pressure Management Committee. The Australian therapeutic trial in mild hypertension. *Lancet* 1980;1:1261–1267.
22. The Hypertension Detection and Follow-Up Program Cooperative Research Group. The effect of antihypertensive drug treatment on mortality in the presence of resting electrocardiographic abnormalities at baseline: the HDFP experience. *Circulation* 1984;70:996–1003.
23. Dahlof B, Lindholm LH, Hansson L, et al. Morbidity and mortality in the Swedish Trial in Old Patients with Hypertension (STOP-Hypertension). *Lancet* 1991;338:1281–1285.
24. SHEP Cooperative Research Group. Prevention of stroke by antihypertensive drug treatment in older persons with iso-

lated systolic hypertension. Final results of the Systolic Hypertension in the Elderly Program (SHEP). *JAMA* 1991;265:3255–3264.

25. MRC Working Party. Medical Research Council trial of treatment of hypertension in older adults: principal results. *BMJ* 1992;304:405–412.

26. Staessen JA, Gasowski J, Wang JG, et al. Risks of untreated and treated isolated systolic hypertension in the elderly: meta-analysis of outcome trials. *Lancet* 2000;355:865–872.

27. Applegate WB, Pressel S, Wittes J, et al. Impact of the treatment of isolated systolic hypertension on behavioral variables. Results from the systolic hypertension in the elderly program. *Arch Intern Med* 1994;154:2154–2160.

28. Strasser T. Hypertension research related to health care. In: *Hypertension related to health care—research priorities.* Copenhagen: World Health Organization, 1980:24–43.

29. Messerli FH, Garavaglia GE, Schmieder RE, et al. Disparate cardiovascular findings in men and women with essential hypertension. *Ann Intern Med* 1987;107:158–161.

30. Sharma AM, Schorr U, Distler A. Insulin resistance in young salt-sensitive normotensive subjects. *Hypertension* 1993;21:273–279.

31. Hall JE, Brands MW, Zappe DH, et al. Cardiovascular actions of insulin: are they important in long-term blood pressure regulation? *Clin Exp Pharmacol Physiol* 1995;22:689–700.

32. Hamet P, Pausova Z, Adarichev V, et al. Hypertension: genes and environment. *J Hypertens* 1998;16:397–418.

33. Samani NJ. Molecular genetics of susceptibility to the development of hypertension. *Br Med Bull* 1994;50:260–271.

34. Brown MJ. The causes of essential hypertension. *Br J Clin Pharmacol* 1996;42:21–27.

35. Williams RR, Hunt SC, Hopkins PN, et al. Genetic basis of familial dyslipidemia and hypertension: 15-year results from Utah. *Am J Hypertens* 1993;6:319S–327S.

36. Beilin LJ, Puddey IB, Burke V. Lifestyle and hypertension. *Am J Hypertens* 1999;12:934–945.

37. Lifton RP. Genetic determinants of human hypertension. *Proc Natl Acad Sci U S A* 1995;92:8545–8551.

38. Luft FC. Molecular genetics of human hypertension. *J Hypertens* 1998;16:1871–1878.

39. Muldoon MF, Terrell DF, Bunker CH, et al. Family history studies in hypertension research. Review of the literature. *Am J Hypertens* 1993;6:76–88.

40. Muntzel M, Drueke T. A comprehensive review of the salt and blood pressure relationship. *Am J Hypertens* 1992;5:1S–42S.

41. Midgley JP, Matthew AG, Greenwood CMT, et al. Effect of reduced dietary sodium on blood pressure: a meta-analysis of randomized controlled trials. *JAMA* 1996;275:1590–1597.

42. Intersalt Cooperative Research Group. Intersalt: an internationals study of electrolyte excretion and blood pressure. Results for 24-hour urinary sodium and potassium excretion. *BMJ* 1988;297:319–328.

43. Sealey JE, Blumenfeld JD, Bell GM, et al. On the renal basis for essential hypertension: nephron heterogeneity with discordant renin secretion and sodium excretion causing a hypertensive vasoconstriction-volume relationship. *J Hypertens* 1988;6:763–777.

44. Romero JC, Bentley MD, Textor SC, et al. Alterations in blood pressure by derangement of the mechanisms that regulate sodium excretion. *Mayo Clin Proc* 1989;64:1425–1435.

45. Guyton AC. Dominant role of the kidneys and accessory role of whole-body autoregulation in the pathogenesis of hypertension. *Am J Hypertens* 1989;2:575–585.

46. Johnson CJ. Renin-angiotensin system: a dual tissue and hormonal system for cardiovascular control. *J Hypertens* 1992;10:S13–S26.

47. Itoh H, Hukoyama M, Pratt RE, et al. Multiple autocrine growth factors modulate vascular smooth muscle cell growth response to angiotensin II. *J Clin Invest* 1993;91:2268–2274.

48. Weir MR, Dzau VJ. The renin-angiotensin-aldosterone system: a specific target for hypertension management. *Am J Hypertens* 1999;12:205S–213S.

49. Chung O, Unger T. Angiotensin II receptor blockade and end-organ protection. *Am J Hypertens* 1999;12:150S–156S.

50. Williams GH, Dluhy RG, Lifton RP, et al. Non-modulation as an intermediate phenotype in essential hypertension. *Hypertension* 1992;20:788–796.

51. de Leeuw PW. Sensitivity to angiotensin and the risk for hypertension. *Am J Hypertens* 1992;5:251–252.

52. Alderman MH, Madhavan S, Ooi WL, et al. Association of the renin-sodium profile with the risk of myocardial infarction in patients with hypertension. *N Engl J Med* 1991;324:1098–1104.

53. Spence JD. Physiologic tailoring of therapy for resistant hypertension: 20 years' experience with stimulated renin profiling. *Am J Hypertens* 1999;12:1077–1083.

54. Erlinge D, Ekman R, Thulin T, et al. Neuropeptide Y-like immunoreactivity and hypertension. *J Hypertens* 1992;10:1221–1225.

55. Xie P, McDowell TS, Chapleau MW, et al. Rapid baroreceptor resetting in chronic hypertension. Implications for normalization of arterial pressure. *Hypertension* 1991;17:72–79.

56. Muller JE, Tofler GH, Stone PH. Circadian variation and triggers of onset of acute cardiovascular disease. *Circulation* 1989;79:733–743.

57. Brook RD, Julius S. Autonomic imbalance, hypertension, and cardiovascular risk. *Am J Hypertens* 2000;13:112S–122S.

58. Esler M. The sympathetic system and hypertension. *Am J Hypertens* 2000;13:99S–105S.

59. Pickering TG. Does psychological stress contribute to the development of hypertension and coronary heart disease? *Eur J Clin Pharmacol* 1990;39:S1–S7.

60. Widgren BR, Wikstrand J, Berglund G, et al. Increased response to physical and mental stress in men with hypertensive parents. *Hypertension* 1992;20:606–611.

61. Julius S. Changing role of the autonomic nervous system in human hypertension. *J Hypertens* 1990;8:S59–S65.

62. Folkow B. "Structural factor" in primary and secondary hypertension. *Hypertension* 1990;16:89–101.

63. McVeigh GE, Burns DE, Finkelstein SM, et al. Reduced vascular compliance as a marker for essential hypertension. *Am J Hypertens* 1991;4:245–251.

64. Dzau VJ, Gibbons GH, Cooke JP, et al. Vascular biology and medicine in the 1990s: scope, concepts, potentials, and perspectives. *Circulation* 1993;87:705–719.

65. Lever AF. Slow pressor mechanisms in hypertension: a role for hypertrophy of resistance vessels? *J Hypertens* 1986;4:515–524.

66. Bohr DF, Webb RC. Vascular smooth muscle function and its changes in hypertension. *Am J Med* 1984;77:3–16.

67. Swales JD. Is there a cellular abnormality in hypertension? *J Cardiovasc Pharmacol* 1991;18:S39–S44.

68. Swales JD. Membrane transport of ions in hypertension. *Cardiovasc Drug Ther* 1990;4:367–372.

69. Weder AB. Is there a metabolic link between increased red blood cell lithium-sodium countertransport and hypertension? *Nutr Metab Cardiovasc Dis* 1993;3:38–45.

70. Rutherford PA, Thomas TH, Laker MF, et al. Plasma lipids affect maximum velocity not sodium affinity of human sodium-lithium countertransport: distinction from essential hypertension. *Eur J Clin Invest* 1992;22:719–724.

71. Adeoya SA, Norman RI, Bing RF. Erythrocyte membrane calcium adenosine 5'-triphosphate activity in the spontaneously hypertensive rat. *Clin Sci* 1988;77:395–400.

72. Blaustein MP. Sodium/calcium exchange and the control of contractility in cardiac muscle and vascular smooth muscle. *J Cardiovasc Pharmacol* 1988;12:S56–S68.

73. Aviv A. The links between cellular Ca^+ and Na^+/H^+ exchange in the pathophysiology of essential hypertension. *Am J Hypertens* 1996;9:703–707.

74. Berk BC, Vekshtein V, Gordon HM, et al. Angiotensin II-stimulated protein synthesis in cultured vascular smooth muscle cells. *Hypertension* 1989;13:305–314.

75. Naftilan AJ, Pratt RE, Dzau VJ. Induction of platelet-derived growth factor a-chain and c-myc gene expressions by angiotensin II in cultured rat vascular smooth muscle cells. *J Clin Invest* 1989;83:1419–1424.

76. Touyz RM, Schiffrin EL. Signal transduction in hypertension: part II. *Curr Opin Nephrol Hypertens* 1993;2:17–26.

77. Heagerty AM, Bund SJ, Aalkjaer C. Effects of drug treatment on human resistance arteriole morphology in essential hypertension: direct evidence for structural remodeling of resistance vessels. *Lancet* 1988;2:1209–1212.

78. Lüscher TF, Boulanger CM, Yang Z, et al. Interactions between endothelium-derived relaxing and contracting factors in health and cardiovascular disease. *Circulation* 1993;87:V36–V44.

79. Lüscher TF. The endothelium and cardiovascular disease—a complex relation. *N Engl J Med* 1994;330:1081–1083.

80. Panza JA, Quyyumi AA, Callahan TS, et al. Effect of antihypertensive treatment on endothelium-dependent vascular relation in patients with essential hypertension. *J Am Coll Cardiol* 1993;21:1145–1151.

81. Drexler H, Zeiher AM, Meinzer K, et al. Correction of endothelial dysfunction in coronary microcirculation of hypercholesterolemic patients by L-arginine. *Lancet* 1991;338:1546–1550.

82. Haffner SM, Ferrannini E, Hazuda HP, et al. Clustering of cardiovascular risk factors in confirmed prehypertensive individuals. *Hypertension* 1992;20:38–45.

83. Reaven GM. Treatment of hypertension: focus on prevention of coronary heart disease. *J Clin Endocrinol Metab* 1993;76:537–540.

84. Reaven GM, Bfrand RJ, Chen Y-DI, et al. Insulin resistance and insulin secretion are determinants of oral glucose tolerance in normal individuals. *Diabetes* 1993;42:1324–1332.

85. Bonora E, Bonadonna RC, Del Prato S, et al. In vivo glucose metabolism in obese and type II diabetic subjects with or without hypertension. *Diabetes* 1993;42:764–772.

86. Wingard DL, Ferrara A, Barrett-Connor EL. Is insulin really a heart disease risk factor? *Diabetes Care* 1995;18:1299–1304.

87. Genuth S. Exogenous insulin administration and cardiovascular risk in non–insulin-dependent and insulin-dependent diabetes mellitus. *Ann Intern Med* 1996;124:104–109.

88. Howard G, O'Leary DH, Zaccaro D, et al. Insulin sensitivity and atherosclerosis. *Circulation* 1996;93:1809–1817.

89. Baron AD, Brechtel-Hook G, Johnson A, et al. Skeletal muscle blood flow. A possible link between insulin resistance and blood pressure. *Hypertension* 1993;21:129–135.

90. Kaplan NM. Primary hypertension: pathogenesis. In: Kaplan NM, ed. *Clinical hypertension*, 6th ed. Baltimore: Williams & Wilkins, 1994:47–108.

91. Reaven GM, Chen Y-DI. Insulin resistance, its consequences, and coronary heart disease: must we choose one culprit? *Circulation* 1996;93:1780–1783.

92. Laragh JH. Atrial natriuretic hormone, the renin-aldosterone axis, and blood pressure–electrolyte homeostasis. *N Engl J Med* 1985;313:1330–1340.

93. Hollister AS, Inagami T. Atrial natriuretic factor and hypertension: a review and metaanalysis. *Am J Hypertens* 1991;4:850–855.

94. Tan ACI, Russel FGM, Thieu T, et al. Atrial natriuretic peptide. An overview of clinical pharmacology and pharmacokinetics. *Clin Pharmacokinet* 1993;24:28–45.

95. Oates JA, FitzGerald GA, Branch RA, et al. Clinical implications of prostaglandin and thromboxane A_2 formation. *N Engl J Med* 1988;319:761–767.

96. Printz MP, Klett C. Angiotensinogen. In: Izzo JL, Black HR, eds. *Hypertension primer: the essentials of high blood pressure*. Dallas: American Heart Association Council on High Blood Pressure Research, 1993:10–11.

97. Christy IJ, Woods RL, Courneya CA, et al. Evidence for a renomedullary vasodepressor system in rabbits and dogs. *Hypertension* 1991;18:325–333.

98. Klasky AL, Armstrong MA, Friedman GD. Alcohol and mortality. *Ann Intern Med* 1992;117:646–654.

99. MacMahon S. Blood pressure and the risk of cardiovascular disease. *N Engl J Med* 2000;342:50–52.

100. Neutel JM, Smith DH. Hypertension control: multifactorial contributions. *Am J Hypertens* 1999;12:164S–169S.

101. Kuller LH, Shemanski L, Psaty BM, et al. Subclinical disease as an independent risk factor for cardiovascular disease. *Circulation* 1995;92:720–726.

102. Buck C, Baker P, Bass M, et al. The prognosis of hypertension according to age at onset. *Hypertension* 1987;9:204–208.

103. Hall WD, Ferrario CM, Moore MA, et al. Hypertension-related morbidity and mortality in the southeastern United States. *Am J Med Sci* 1997;313:195–209.

104. Kaplan NM. Natural history, special populations, and evaluation. In: Kaplan NM, ed. *Clinical hypertension*, 6th ed. Baltimore: Williams & Wilkins, 1994:109–143.

105. Sutton-Tyrrell K, Alcorn HG, Herzog H, et al. Morbidity, mortality, and antihypertensive treatment effects by extent of atherosclerosis in older adults with isolated systolic hypertension. *Stroke* 1995;26:1319–1324.

106. Moser M. Management of hypertension, part I. *Am Fam Phys* 1996;53:2295–2302.

107. Lasagna L. Diuretics vs. alpha-blockers for treatment of hypertension: lessons from ALLHAT. *JAMA* 2000;283:2013–2014.

108. Burt VL, Whelton P, Roccella EJ, et al. Prevalence of hypertension in the U.S. adult population. Results from the Third National Health and Nutrition Examination Survey, 1988–1991. *Hypertension* 1995;25:305–313.

109. Hayes SN, Taler SJ. Hypertension in women: current understanding of gender differences. *Mayo Clin Proc* 1998;73:157–165.

110. Rudd P, Dzau VJ. Hypertension: evaluation and management. In: Loscalzo J, Creager MA, Dzau VJ, eds. *Vascular medicine.* Boston: Little, Brown, 1996:609–638.

111. Pickering T. Headache and hypertension—something old, something new. *J Clin Hypertens* 2000;2:345–347.

112. Sheps SG, Black HR, Cohen JD, et al. The sixth report of the Joint National Committee on the detection, evaluation, and treatment of high blood pressure. *Am J Mgd Care* 1998;4:366–370.

113. National High Blood Pressure Education Program Working Group. National High Blood Pressure Education Program Working Group report on primary prevention of hypertension. *Arch Intern Med* 1993;153:186–208.

114. Coroni-Huntley J, LaCroix A, Havlik RJ. Race and sex differentials in the impact of hypertension in the United States: the National Health and Nutrition Examination Survey. I. Epidemiologic follow-up study. *Arch Intern Med* 1989;149:780–788.

115. Applegate WB, Pressel S, Wittes J, et al. Impact of the treatment of isolated systolic hypertension on behavioral variables. Results from the Systolic Hypertension in the Elderly Program. *Arch Intern Med* 1994;154:2154–2160.

116. Kawachi I, Malcolm LA. The cost-effectiveness of treating mild-to-moderate hypertension: a reappraisal. *J Hypertens* 1991;9:199–208.

117. Kannel WB. An epidemiological perspective in hypertension problem solving. *Cardiology* 1994;1:71–77.

118. American Society of Hypertension. Recommendations for routine blood pressure measurement by indirect cuff sphygmomanometry. *Am J Hypertens* 1992;5:207–209.

119. Holleman DR, Westman EC, McCrory DC. The effect of sleeved arms on oscillometric blood pressure measurement. *J Gen Intern Med* 1993;8:325–326.

120. McKay DW, Campbell NR, Parab LS, et al. Clinical assessment of blood pressure. *J Hum Hypertens* 1990;4:639–645.

121. Appel LJ, Stason WB. Ambulatory blood pressure monitoring and blood pressure self-measurement in the diagnosis and management of hypertension. *Ann Intern Med* 1993;118:867–882.

122. MacDonald MB, Laing GP, Wilson MP, et al. Prevalence and predictors of the white-coat response in patients with treated hypertension. *Can Med Assoc J* 1999;161:265–269.

123. Sprafka JM, Strickland D, Gomez-Marin O, et al. The effect of cuff size on blood pressure measurement in adults. *Epidemiology* 1991;2:214–217.

124. Askey JM. The auscultatory gap in sphygmomanometry. *Ann Intern Med* 1974;80:94–97.

125. Campbell NR, Chockalingam A, Fodor JG, et al. Accurate, reproducible measurement of blood pressure. *Can Med Assoc J* 1990;143:19–24.

126. Mathieu G, Biron P, Roberge F, et al. Blood pressure determinations during medical examinations: how many? *Can J Pub Health* 1974;65:447–450.

127. Sokolow M, Perloff D, Cowan R. Contribution of ambulatory blood pressure to the assessment of patients with mild to moderate office blood pressure. *Cardiovasc Rev Rep* 1980;1:295–303.

128. Pickering TG, Harshfield GA, Devereux RB, et al. What is the role of ambulatory blood pressure monitoring in the management of hypertensive patients? *Hypertension* 1985;7: 171–177.

129. Asmar RG, Brunel PC, Pannier BM, et al. Arterial distensibility and ambulatory blood pressure monitoring in essential hypertension. *Am J Cardiol* 1988;61:1066–1070.

130. Giaconi S, Levanti C, Fommei E, et al. Microalbuminuria and casual and ambulatory blood pressure monitoring in normotensives and in patients with borderline and mild essential hypertension. *Am J Hypertens* 1989;2:259–261.

131. Julius S. Home blood pressure monitoring: advantages and limitations. *J Hypertens* 1991;9[Suppl]:S41–S46.

132. Soghikian K, Casper SM, Fireman BH, et al. Home blood pressure monitoring. Effect on use of medical services and medical care costs. *Med Care* 1992;30:855–865.

133. Evans CE, Haynes RB, Goldsmith CH, et al. Home blood pressure-measuring devices: a comparative study of accuracy. *J Hypertens* 1989;7:133–142.

134. Mejia A, Julius S. Practical utility of blood pressure readings obtained by self-determination. *J Hypertens* 1989;7[Suppl]:S53–S57.

135. Mejia AD, Egan BM, Schork NJ, et al. Artifacts in measurement of blood pressure and lack of target organ involvement in the assessment of patients with treatment-resistant hypertension. *Ann Intern Med* 1990;112:270–277.

136. Audet AM, Clinical Efficacy Assessment Subcommittee, Health and Public Policy Committee, et al. Automated ambulatory blood pressure and self-measured blood pressure monitoring devices: their role in the diagnosis and management of hypertension. *Ann Intern Med* 1993;118:889–892.

137. Julius S, Mejia A, Jones K, et al. "White coat" versus "sustained" borderline hypertension in Tecumseh, Michigan. *Hypertension* 1990;16:617–623.

138. White WB, Dey HM, Schulman P. Assessment of the daily blood pressure load as a determinant of cardiac function in patients with mild-to-moderate hypertension. *Am Heart J* 1989;118:782–795.

139. Staessen J, Bulpitt CJ, O'Brien E, et al. The diurnal blood pressure profile: a population study. *Am J Hypertens* 1992;5:386–392.

140. Skoog I, Lernfelt B, Landahl S, et al. 15-year longitudinal study of blood pressure and dementia. *Lancet* 1996;347: 1141–1145.

141. Van Itallie TB. Health implications of overweight and obesity in the United States. *Ann Intern Med* 1985;103:983–988.

142. Kannel WB. Framingham study insights into hypertensive risk of cardiovascular disease. *Hypertens Res* 1995;18:181–196.

143. Kaplan NM. The deadly quartet: upper-body obesity, glucose intolerance, hypertriglyceridemia, and hypertension. *JAMA* 1989;149:1514–1520.

144. Haffner SM, Valdez R, Morales PA, et al. Greater effect of glycemia on incidence of hypertension in women than in men. *Diabetes Care* 1992;15:1277–1284.

145. Reaven GM, Lithell H, Landsberg L. Hypertension and associated metabolic abnormalities—the role of insulin resistance and the sympathoadrenal system. *N Engl J Med* 1996;334:374–381.

146. Resnick LM. Cellular calcium and magnesium metabolism in the pathophysiology and treatment of hypertension and related metabolic disorders. *Am J Med* 1992;93:11S–20S.

147. National High Blood Pressure Education Program Working Group. *National High Blood Pressure Education Program Working Group report on hypertension in diabetes.* Bethesda, MD: National Heart, Lung, and Blood Institute, National Institutes of Health, 1995.

148. Wilhelmsen L. Coronary heart disease: epidemiology of smoking and intervention studies of smoking. *Am Heart J* 1988;115:242–249.

149. MacMahon S. Alcohol consumption and hypertension. *Hypertension* 1987;9:111–121.

150. Criqui MH, Mebane I, Wallace RB, et al. Multivariate correlates of adult blood pressures in nine North American populations: the Lipid Research Clinics Prevalence Study. *Prev Med* 1982;11:391–402.

151. Cutler JA. Combinations of lifestyle modification and drug treatment in management of mild-moderate hypertension: a review of randomized clinical trials. *Clin Exp Hypertens* 1993;15:1193–1204.

152. Johannesson M, Fagerberg B. A health-economic comparison of diet and drug treatment in obese men with mild hypertension. *J Hypertens* 1992;10:1063–1070.

153. The Trials of Hypertension Prevention Collaborative Research Group. The effects of nonpharmacologic interventions on blood pressure of persons with high normal levels: results of the Trials of Hypertension Prevention, phase I. *JAMA* 1992;267:1213–1220.

154. Stamler R, Stamler J, Gosch FC, et al. Primary prevention of hypertension by nutritional-hygienic means: final report of a randomized, controlled trial. *JAMA* 1989;262:1801–1807.

155. Hypertension Prevention Trial Research Group. The Hypertension Prevention Trial: three-year effects of dietary changes on blood pressure. *Arch Intern Med* 1990;150:153–162.

156. Ben-Dov I, Grossman E, Stein A, et al. Marked weight reduction lowers resting and exercise blood pressure in morbidly obese subjects. *Am J Hypertens* 2000;13:251–255.

157. Fagerberg B, Berglund A, Andersson OK, et al. Weight reduction versus antihypertensive drug therapy in obese men with high blood pressure: effects upon plasma insulin levels and association with changes in blood pressure and serum lipids. *J Hypertens* 1992;10:1053–1061.

158. Jones DW, Miller ME, Wofford MR, et al. The effect of weight loss intervention on antihypertensive medication requirements in the Hypertension Optimal Treatment (HOT) study. *Am J Hypertens* 1999;12:1175–1180.

159. Blumenthal JA, Sherwood A, Gullette EC, et al. Exercise and weight loss reduce blood pressure in men and women with mild hypertension: effects on cardiovascular, metabolic, and hemodynamic functioning. *Arch Intern Med* 2000;160:1947–1958.

160. Hayashi R, Tsumura K, Suematsu C, et al. Walking to work and the risk for hypertension in men: the Osaka health survey. *Ann Intern Med* 1999;130:21–26.

161. Franklin BA, Gordon S, Timmis GC. Exercise prescription for hypertensive patients. *Ann Med* 1991;23:279–287.

162. NIH Consensus Development Panel on Physical Activity and Cardiovascular Health. Physical activity and cardiovascular health. *JAMA* 1996;276:241–246.

163. Hagberg JM, Montain SJ, Martin WH, et al. Effect of exercise training in 60- to 69-year-old persons with essential hypertension. *Am J Cardiol* 1989;64:348–353.

164. Peterson DM. Exercise and physical activity in the adult population: a general internist's perspective. *J Gen Intern Med* 1993;8:149–159.

165. Appel LJ, Moore TJ, Obarzanek E, et al. A clinical trial of the effects of dietary patterns on blood pressure. DASH Collaborative Research Group. *N Engl J Med* 1997;336:1117–1124.

166. Conlin PR, Chow D, Miller ER, et al. The effect of dietary patterns on blood pressure control in hypertensive patients: results from the Dietary Approaches to Stop Hypertension (DASH) trial. *Am J Hypertens* 2000;13:949–955.

167. Law MR, Frost CD, Wald NJ. By how much does dietary salt reduction lower blood pressure? III. Analysis of data from trials of salt reduction. *BMJ* 1991;302:819–824.

168. Cutler JA, Follman D, Alexander PS. Randomized controlled trials of sodium reduction: an overview. *Am J Clin Nutr* 1997;65:643S–651S.

169. Messerli HF, Schmieder RE, Weir MR. Salt: a perpetrator of hypertensive target organ disease? *Arch Intern Med* 1997;157:2449–2452.

170. Little P, Girling G, Hasler A, et al. A controlled trial of a low sodium, low fat, high fibre diet in treated hypertensive patients: effect on antihypertensive drug requirement in clinical practice. *J Hum Hypertens* 1991;5:175–181.

171. Whelton PK, Appel LJ, Espeland MA, et al. Tone Collaborative Research Group: sodium reduction and weight loss in the treatment of hypertension in older persons. A randomized controlled Trial of Nonpharmacologic interventions in the Elderly (TONE). *JAMA* 1998;279:317–322.

172. MacGregor GA, De Wardener HE. "Salt": a commentary. *Am J Hypertens* 2000;13:313–316.

173. Rakic V, Puddey IB, Burke V, et al. Influence of pattern of alcohol intake on blood pressure in regular drinkers: a controlled trial. *J Hypertens* 1998;16:165–174.

174. Patel C, Marmot MG, Terry DJ, et al. Trial of relaxation in reducing coronary risk: four-year follow-up. *BMJ* 1985;290:1103–1106.

175. Agras WS, Taylor CB, Kraemer HC, et al. Relaxation training for essential hypertension at the worksite. II. The poorly controlled hypertensive. *Psychosom Med* 1987;49:264–273.

176. Johnson DW. The behavioral control of high blood pressure. *Curr Psychol Res Rev* 1987;6:99–114.

177. Whelton PK, He J, Cutler JA, et al. Effects of oral potassium on blood pressure: meta-analysis of randomized controlled trials. *JAMA* 1997;277:1624–1632.

178. Ascherio A, Rimm EG, Giovanucci EL, et al. A prospective study of nutritional factors and hypertension among US men. *Circulation* 1992;86:1475–1484.

179. Appel LJ, Miller ER, Seidler AJ, et al. Does supplementation of diet with "fish oil" reduce blood press? A meta-analy-

sis of controlled clinical trials. *Arch Intern Med* 1993;153: 1429–1438.

180. Houston MC. Hypertension strategies for therapeutic intervention and prevention of end-organ damage. *Prim Care* 1991;18:713–753.

181. Saunders E, Weir MR, Kong BW, et al. A comparison of the efficacy and safety of a beta-blocker, a calcium channel blocker, and a converting enzyme inhibitor in hypertensive blacks. *Arch Intern Med* 1990;150:1707–1713.

182. Dzau VJ. Evolution of the clinical management of hypertension. Emerging role of "specific" vasodilators as initial therapy. *Am J Med* 1987;82:36–43.

183. Dzau VJ. Renin and myocardial infarction in hypertension. *N Engl J Med* 1991;324:1128–1130.

184. Materson BJ, Preston RA. Newer principles of patient profiling for antihypertensive therapy. *Circulation* 1989;80:IV128–IV135.

185. National High Blood Pressure Education Program Working Group. *National High Blood Pressure Education Program Working Group report on hypertension in the elderly.* Bethesda, MD: National Heart, Lung, and Blood Institute, National Institutes of Health, 1994.

186. Beto JA, Bansal VK. Quality of life in treatment of hypertension. A meta-analysis of clinical trials. *Am J Hypertens* 1992;5:125–133.

187. Materson BJ, Reda DJ, Cushman WC, et al. Single-drug therapy for hypertension in men. A comparison of six antihypertensive agents with placebo. The Department of Veterans Affairs Cooperative Study Group on antihypertensive agents. *N Engl J Med* 1993;328:914–921.

188. Neaton JD, Grimm RH, Prineas RJ, et al. Treatment of Mild Hypertension Study. Final results. *JAMA* 1993;270:713–724.

189. Edelson JT, Weinstein MC, Tosteson AN, et al. Long-term cost-effectiveness of various initial monotherapies for mild to moderate hypertension. *JAMA* 1990;263:407–413.

190. Myers MG, Reeves RA, Oh PI, et al. Overtreatment of hypertension in the community? *Am J Hypertens* 1996;9:419–425.

191. Steiner JF, Fihn SD, Blair B, et al. Appropriate reductions in compliance among well-controlled hypertensive patients. *J Clin Epidemiol* 1991;44:1361–1371.

192. Schmieder RE, Rockstroh JK, Messerli FH. Antihypertensive therapy. To stop or not to stop? *JAMA* 1991;265:1566–1571.

193. Magarian GJ. Reserpine: a relic from the past or a neglected drug of the present for achieving cost containment in treating hypertension? *J Gen Intern Med* 1991;6:561–572.

194. van Zwieten PA. An overview of the pharmacodynamic properties and therapeutic potential of combined alpha- and beta-adrenoceptor antagonists. *Drugs* 1993;45:509–517.

195. Packer M, Bristow MR, Cohn JN, et al. The effect of carvedilol on morbidity and mortality in patients with chronic heart failure. U.S. Carvedilol Heart Failure Study Group. *N Engl J Med* 1996;334:1349–1355.

196. Zannad R, Matzzinger A, Larché J. Trough/peak ratios of once daily angiotensin converting enzyme inhibitors and calcium antagonists. *Am J Hypertens* 1996;9:633–643.

197. Lewin A, Blaufox D, Castle H, et al. Apparent prevalence of curable hypertension in the Hypertension Detection and Follow-Up Program. *Arch Intern Med* 1985;145:424–427.

198. Iimura O. Actual incidence of secondary hypertension. *Jpn Circ J* 1973;37:1040–1044.

199. Berglund G, Andersson O, Wilhelmsen L. Prevalence of primary and secondary hypertension: studies in a random population sample. *BMJ* 1976;2:554–556.

200. Rudnick KV, Sackett DL, Hirst S, et al. Hypertension in a family practice. *Can Med Assoc J* 1977;117:492–497.

201. Greminger P, Vetter W, Zimmermann K, et al. Primary and secondary hypertension in polyclinical patients. *Schweiz Med Wochenschr* 1977;107:605–609.

202. National High Blood Pressure Education Program Working Group. *1995 update of the Working Group reports on chronic renal failure and renovascular hypertension.* Bethesda, MD: National Heart, Lung, and Blood Institute, National Institutes of Health, 1995.

203. Gabow PA. Autosomal dominant polycystic kidney disease. *N Engl J Med* 1993;329:332–342.

204. Heyka RJ, Vidt DG. Control of hypertension in patients with chronic renal failure. *Cleveland Clin J Med* 1989;56:65–76.

205. Peters DH, Fitton A, Plosker GL, et al. Tacrolimus. A review of its pharmacology, and therapeutic potential in hepatic and renal transplantation. *Drugs* 1993;46:746–794.

206. Peterson JC, Adler S, Burkart JM, et al. Blood pressure control, proteinuria, and the progression of renal disease: the Modification of Diet in Renal Disease Study. *Ann Intern Med* 1995;123:754–762.

207. Ljungman S, Wikstrand J, Hartford M, et al. Urinary albumin excretion—a predictor of risk of cardiovascular disease: a prospective 10-year follow-up of middle-aged nondiabetic normal and hypertensive men. *Am J Hypertens* 1996;9:770–778.

208. Estacio RO, Jeffers BW, Gifford N, et al. Effect of blood pressure control on diabetic microvascular complications in patients with hypertension and type 2 diabetes. *Diabetes Care* 2000;23:B54–B64.

209. Harrison EG, McCormack LJ. Pathologic classification of renal arterial disease in renovascular hypertension. *Mayo Clin Proc* 1971;46:161–167.

210. Safian RD, Textor SC. Renal-artery stenosis. *N Engl J Med* 2001;344:431–442.

211. Schreiber MJ, Pohl MA, Novick AC. The natural history of atherosclerotic and fibrous renal artery disease. *Urol Clin North Am* 1984;11:383–392.

212. Pickering TG, Herman L, Sotelo JE, et al. Recurrent pulmonary edema in hypertension due to bilateral renal artery stenosis: treatment by renal angioplasty or surgical revascularization. *Lancet* 1988;2:551–552.

213. Muller FB, Sealey JE, Case CB, et al. The captopril test for identifying renovascular disease in hypertensive patients. *Am J Med* 1986;80:633–644.

214. Havey RJ, Krumlovsky F, delGreco F, et al. Screening for renovascular hypertension: is renal digital-subtraction angiography the preferred noninvasive test? *JAMA* 1985;254:388–393.

215. Kumar R, Schreiber MH. The changing indications for excretory urography. *JAMA* 1985;254:403–405.

216. Simon G. What is critical renal artery stenosis? *Am J Hypertens* 2000;13:1189–1193.

217. Sellars L, Shore AC, Wilkinson R. Renal vein renin studies

in renovascular hypertension—do they really help? *J Hypertens* 1985;3:177–181.

218. Nally JV, Black HR. State-of-the-art review: captopril renography—pathophysiological considerations and clinical observations. *Sem Nucl Med* 1992;22(2):85–97.

219. Mann SJ, Pickering TG. Detection of renovascular hypertension. State of the art: 1992. *Ann Intern Med* 1992;117:845–853.

220. Helin KH, Tikkanen I, von Knorring JE, et al. Screening for renovascular hypertension in a population with relatively low prevalence. *J Hypertens* 1998;16:1523–1529.

221. Strotzer M, Fellner CM, Geissler A, et al. Noninvasive assessment of renal artery stenosis. A comparison of MR angiography, color Doppler sonography, and intraarterial angiography. *Acta Radiol* 1995;36:243–247.

222. Novick AC, Ziegelbaum M, Vidt DG, et al. Trends in surgical revascularization for renal artery disease. Ten years' experience. *JAMA* 1987;257:498–501.

223. Airoldi F, Palatresi S, Marana I, et al. Angioplasty of atherosclerotic and fibromuscular renal artery stenosis: time course and predicting factors of the effects on renal function. *Am J Hypertens* 2000;13:1210–1217.

224. Kuhlmann U, Gramminger P, Grüntzig A, et al. Long-term experience in percutaneous transluminal dilatation of renal artery stenosis. *Am J Med* 1985;79:692–698.

225. Jenkins NP, Ward C. Coarctation of the aorta: natural history and outcome after surgical treatment. *Q J Med* 1999;92:365–371.

226. Jaffe RB. Radiographic manifestations of congenital anomalies of the aortic arch. *Radiol Clin North Am* 1991;29:319–334.

227. Kaemmerer H, Theissen P, Konig U, et al. Follow-up using magnetic resonance imaging in adult patients after surgery for aortic coarctation. *Thorac Cardiovasc Surg* 1993;41:107–111.

228. Teien D, Wendel H, Holm S, et al. Estimation of Doppler gradients at rest and during exercise in patients with recoarctation of the aorta. *Br Heart J* 1991;65:155–157.

229. Marelli AJ, Child JS, Perloff JK. Transesophageal echocardiography in congenital heart disease in the adult. *Cardiol Clin* 1993;11:505–520.

230. Findling JW. The Cushing syndromes: an enlarging clinical spectrum. *N Engl J Med* 1989;321:1677–1678.

231. Danese RD, Aron DC. Cushing's syndrome and hypertension. *Endocrinol Metab Clin North Am* 1994;23:299–324.

232. Mantero F, Boscaro M. Glucocorticoid-dependent hypertension. *J Steroid Biochem Mol Biol* 1992;43:409–413.

233. Tyrrell JB, Findling JW, Aron DC, et al. An overnight high-dose dexamethasone suppression test for rapid differential diagnosis of Cushing's syndrome. *Ann Intern Med* 1986;104:180–186.

234. Kaye TB, Crapo L. The Cushing syndrome: an update on diagnostic tests. *Ann Intern Med* 1990;112:434–444.

235. Gross MD, Shapiro B. Scintigraphic studies in adrenal hypertension. *Semin Nucl Med* 1989;19:122–143.

236. Carpenter PC. Cushing's syndrome: update of diagnosis and management. *Mayo Clin Proc* 1986;61:49–58.

237. Sugihara N, Shimizu M, Kita Y, et al. Cardiac characteristics and postoperative courses in Cushing's syndrome. *Am J Cardiol* 1992;69:1475–1480.

238. Miller JW, Crapo L. The medical treatment of Cushing's syndrome. *Endocr Rev* 1993;14:443–458.

239. Stewart PM. Mineralocorticoid hypertension. *Lancet* 1999;353:1341–1347.

240. Irony I, Kater CE, Biglieri EG, et al. Correctable subsets of primary aldosteronism. Primary adrenal hyperplasia and renin responsive adenoma. *Am J Hypertens* 1990;3:576–582.

241. Young WF, Klee GC. Primary aldosteronism: diagnostic evaluation. *Endocr Metab Clin North Am* 1988;17:367–395.

242. Young WF, Hogan MJ, Klee GG, et al. Primary aldosteronism: diagnosis and treatment. *Mayo Clin Proc* 1990;65:96–110.

243. Opocher G, Rocco S, Carpene G, et al. Differential diagnosis in primary aldosteronism. *J Steroid Biochem Mol Biol* 1993;45:49–55.

244. Bravo EL, Tarazi RC, Dustan HP, et al. The changing clinical spectrum of primary aldosteronism. *Am J Med* 1983;74:641–651.

245. Weinberger MH, Fineberg NS. The diagnosis of primary aldosteronism and separation of two major subtypes. *Arch Intern Med* 1993;153:2125–2129.

246. Fontes RG, Kater CE, Biglieri EG, et al. Reassessment of the predictive value of the postural stimulation test in primary aldosteronism. *Am J Hypertens* 1991;4:786–791.

247. Novick AC. Surgery for primary hyperaldosteronism. *Urol Clin North Am* 1989;16:535–545.

248. Ghose RP, Hall PM, Bravo EL. Medical management of aldosterone-producing adenomas (see comments). *Ann Intern Med* 1999;131:105–108.

249. Bravo EL, Gifford RW. Pheochromocytoma: diagnosis, localization and management. *N Engl J Med* 1984;311(20):1298–1303.

250. Young MJ, Dmuchowski C, Wallis JW, et al. Biochemical tests for pheochromocytoma: strategies in hypertensive patients. *J Gen Intern Med* 1989;4:273–276.

251. Lenders JW, Keiser HR, Goldstein DS, et al. Plasma metanephrines in the diagnosis of pheochromocytoma. *Ann Intern Med* 1995;123:101–109.

252. Falterman CJ, Kreisberg R. Pheochromocytoma: clinical diagnosis and management. *South Med J* 1982;75:321–328.

253. Bravo EL, Tarazi RC, Fouad FM, et al. Clonidine-suppression test: a useful aid in the diagnosis of pheochromocytoma. *Med Intell* 1981;305(11):623–626.

254. MacDougall IC, Isles CG, Stewart H, et al. Overnight clonidine suppression test in the diagnosis and exclusion of pheochromocytoma. *Am J Med* 1988;84:993–1000.

255. Khafagi FA, Shapiro B, Fig LM, et al. Labetalol reduces iodine-131 MIBG uptake by pheochromocytoma and normal tissues. *J Nucl Med* 1989;30:481–489.

256. Radack K, Deck C. Do nonsteroidal anti-inflammatory drugs interfere with blood pressure control in hypertensive patients? *J Gen Intern Med* 1987;2:108–112.

257. Palmer FF. Renal complications associated with use of nonsteroidal anti-inflammatory agents. *J Invest Med* 1995;43:516–532.

258. Brook RD, Kramer MB, Blaxall BC, et al. Nonsteroidal anti-inflammatory drugs and hypertension. *J Clin Hypertens* 2000;2:319–323.

259. Setaro JF, Black HR. Refractory hypertension. *N Engl J Med* 1992;327:543–547.

260. Chasan-Tauber L, Willett WC, Manson JE, et al. Prospective study of oral contraceptives and hypertension among women in the United States. *Circulation* 1996;94:483–489.

261. Porter GA, Bennett WM, Sheps SG, et al. Cyclosporine-associated hypertension. *Arch Intern Med* 1990;150:280–283.

262. Bellett M, Cabrol C, Sassano P, et al. Systemic hypertension after cardiac transplantation: effects of cyclosporine on renin-angiotensin-aldosterone system. *Am J Cardiol* 1985;56:927–931.

263. Shea S, Misra D, Ehrlich MH, et al. Predisposing factors for severe, uncontrolled hypertension in an inner-city minority population. *N Engl J Med* 1992;327:776–781.

264. Varon J, Marik PE. The diagnosis and management of hypertensive crisis. *Chest* 2000;118:214–227.

265. Grossman E, Messerli FH, Grodzicki T, et al. Should a moratorium be placed on sublingual nifedipine capsules for hypertensive emergencies and pseudoemergencies? *JAMA* 1996;276:1328–1331.

266. Reuler JB, Magarian GJ. Hypertensive emergencies and urgencies: definition, recognition, and management. *J Gen Intern Med* 1988;3:64–74.

267. Strandgaard S, Paulson OB. Cerebral blood flow and its pathophysiology in hypertension. *Am J Hypertens* 1989;2:486–492.

268. Calhoun DA, Oparil S. Treatment of hypertensive crisis. *N Engl J Med* 1990;323:1177–1183.

269. Cooke JP, Safford RE. Progress in the diagnosis and management of aortic dissection. *Mayo Clin Proc* 1986;61:147–153.

270. Magee LA, Ornstein MP, von Dadelszen P. Management of hypertension in pregnancy. *BMJ* 1999;318:1332–1336.

271. Cunningham FG, Lindheimer MD. Hypertension in pregnancy. *N Engl J Med* 1992;326:927–932.

272. Blake S, McDonald D. The prevention of the maternal manifestations of pre-eclampsia by intensive antihypertensive treatment. *Br J Obstet Gynaecol* 1991;98:244–248.

273. Sibai BM. Treatment of hypertension in pregnant women. *N Engl J Med* 1996;335:257–265.

274. Martin DE, Kammerer WS. The hypertensive surgical patient: controversies in management. *Surg Clin North Am* 1983;63:1017–1033.

275. Schiff RL, Cohen MH, Balson A. What do you do when the blood pressure is up? An approach to the known hypertensive who has an elevated blood pressure (see comments). *J Gen Intern Med* 1991;6:71–76.

276. Rudd P, Marshall G. Antihypertensive medication-taking behavior: outpatient patterns and implications. In: Rosenfeld J, ed. *Hypertension control in the community*. London: John Libbey & Co, 1985:232–236.

277. Huertin-Roberts S, Reisen E. The relation of culturally influenced lay models of hypertension to compliance with treatment. *Am J Hypertens* 1992;5:787–792.

278. Rudd P. Clinicians and patients with hypertension: unsettled issues about compliance. *Am Heart J* 1995;130:572–579.

279. Rudd P, Ramesh J, Bryant-Kosling C, et al. Gaps in cardiovascular medication taking: The tip of the iceberg. *J Gen Intern Med* 1993;8:659–666.

280. Rudd P. Maximizing compliance with antihypertensive therapy. *Drug Ther* 1992;22:25–32.

281. Rudd P. Medication compliance for antihypertensive therapy. In: Oparil S, Weber MA, eds. *Hypertension*. Philadelphia: W.B Saunders, 2000:419–431.

282. Duncan LE, Lewis C, Jenkins P, et al. Does hypertension and its pharmacotherapy affect the quality of sexual function in women? *Am J Hypertens* 2000;13:640–647.

283. Mancia G, Bertinieri G, Grassi G, et al. Effects of blood-pressure measurement by the doctor on patient's blood pressure and heart rate. *Lancet* 1983;2:695–698.

284. Spence JD. Withholding treatment in white-coat hypertension: wishful thinking. *Can Med Assoc J* 1999;161:275–276.

285. Verdecchia P, Schiallaci G, Gorgioni C, et al. Prognostic significance of the white coat effect. *Hypertension* 1997;29:1218–1224.

286. Verdecchia P, Schiallaci G, Gorgioni C, et al. White-coat hypertension: not guilty when correctly defined. *Blood Press Monit* 1998;3:147–152.

287. Weber MA, Neutel JM, Smith DH, et al. Diagnosis of mild hypertension by ambulatory blood pressure monitoring. *Circulation* 1994;90:2291–2298.

288. Cerasola G, Cottone S, Nardi E, et al. White-coat hypertension and cardiovascular risk. *J Cardiovasc Risk* 1995;2:545–549.

289. Glen SK, Elliott HL, Curzio JL, et al. White coat hypertension as a cause of cardiovascular dysfunction. *Lancet* 1996;348:624–630.

290. Mengden T, Uen S, Vetter H. Reference values for office blood pressure measurement cannot be applied to self blood pressure measurement. *Cardiovasc Res Rev* 2000;21:293–301.

291. Stergiou GS, Thomopoulou GC, Skeva II, et al. Home blood pressure normalcy: the Didima study. *Am J Hypertens* 2000;13:678–685.

292. Liu JE, Roman MJ, Pini R, et al. Cardiac and arterial target organ damage in adults with elevated ambulatory and normal office blood pressure. *Ann Intern Med* 1999;131:564–572.

293. Schrier RW. Treating high-risk diabetic hypertensive patients with comorbid conditions. *Am J Kidney Dis* 2000;36:S10–S17.

294. Psaty BM, Smith NL, Siscovick DS, et al. Health outcomes associated with antihypertensive therapies used as first-line agents. A systematic review and meta-analysis. *JAMA* 1997;277:739–745.

295. Staessen JA, Fagard R, Thijs L, et al. Randomised double-blind comparison of placebo and active treatment for older patients with isolated systolic hypertension. The Systolic Hypertension in Europe (Syst-Eur) Trial Investigators (see comments). *Lancet* 1997;350:757–764.

296. Yusuf S, Sleight P, Pogue J, et al. Effects of an angiotensin-converting-enzyme inhibitor, ramipril, on cardiovascular events in high-risk patients. The Heart Outcomes Prevention Evaluation Study Investigators. *N Engl J Med* 2000;342:145–153.

297. Hansson L, Lindholm LH, Niskanen L, et al. Effect of angiotensin-converting-enzyme inhibition compared with conventional therapy on cardiovascular morbidity and mortality in hypertension: the Captopril Prevention Project (CAPPP) randomised trial. *Lancet* 1999;353:611–616.

298. ALLHAT Collaborative Research Group. Major cardiovascular events in hypertensive patients randomized to dox-

azosin vs. chlorthalidone: the antihypertensive and lipid-lowering treatment to prevent heart attack trial (ALLHAT). *JAMA* 2000;283:1967–1975.

299. Straka RJ, Swanson AL, Parra D. Calcium channel antagonists: morbidity and mortality—what's the evidence? Am Fam Phys 1998;57:1551–1560.

300. Tuomilehto J, Rastenyte D, Birkenhager WH, et al. Effects of calcium-channel blockade in older patients with diabetes and systolic hypertension. Systolic Hypertension in Europe Trial Investigators. *N Engl J Med* 1999;340:677–684.

301. Kloner RA, Vetrovec GW, Materson BJ, et al. Safety of long-acting dihydropyridine calcium channel blockers in hypertensive patients. *Am J Cardiol* 1998;81:163–169.

302. Pepine CJ, Faich G, Makuch R. Verapamil use in patients with cardiovascular disease: an overview of randomized trials. *Clin Cardiol* 1998;21:633–641.

303. Laidlaw JC, Chockalingam A. Canadian Consensus Conference on Nonpharmacological Approaches to the Management of High Blood Pressure: recommendations. *J Cardiovasc Pharmacol* 1990;16:S48–S50.

304. Cressman MD. Management of hypercholesterolemia in the hypertensive patient. *Cleveland Clin J Med* 1989;56:351–358.

305. Messerli FH, Garavaglia GE, Schmieder RE, et al. Disparate cardiovascular findings in men and women with essential hypertension. *Ann Intern Med* 1987;107:158–161.

306. Perera GA. Hypertensive vascular disease: description and natural history. *J Chron Dis* 1955;1:33–42.

307. Alderman MH, Cushman WC, Hill MN, et al. International roundtable discussion of national guidelines for the detection, evaluation, and treatment of hypertension. *Am J Hypertens* 1993;6:974–981.

6

SMOKING

RAYMOND NIAURA
MICHAEL G. GOLDSTEIN

▼ ADDITIONAL ELECTRONIC TOPICS

OVERVIEW

Worldwide, there are approximately 1 billion individuals who smoke cigarettes. The overall prevalence of smoking in the United States in 1994 was 25.5%. Cigarette smoking remains the most important preventable contributor to premature death, disability, and unnecessary health expense in this country, and it is a major risk factor for all manifestations of coronary artery disease (CAD), stroke, and peripheral artery disease. Smoking also has been estimated to cause between 17% and 30% of all deaths due to cardiovascular disease.

R. Niaura: Centers for Behavioral and Preventive Medicine, Brown University School of Medicine, The Miriam Hospital, Providence, Rhode Island

M. G. Goldstein: Department of Psychiatry and Human Behavior, Brown University School of Medicine, The Miriam Hospital, Providence, Rhode Island; and The Bayer Institute for Health Care Communication, West Haven, Connecticut

Although the risk of CAD after smoking cessation drops by approximately 50% 1 year after cessation, it approaches that of a person who has never smoked within 3 to 4 years. Smoking contributes to the pathogenesis of CAD and sudden death through a variety of mechanisms, including the promotion of atherosclerosis, the triggering of coronary thrombosis, coronary artery spasm, and cardiac arrhythmias, and through reduced capacity of the blood to deliver oxygen.

Nicotine is a powerful pharmacologic agent with a wide variety of stimulant and depressant effects involving the central and peripheral nervous, cardiovascular, endocrine, and other systems. These effects contribute to nicotine's addictive properties. The characteristics and patterns of chronic nicotine use have much in common with the use of other psychotropic drugs, and nicotine dependence is a recognized psychiatric disorder. Chronic nicotine use associated with smoking produces tolerance and a characteristic withdrawal syndrome that contributes to difficulty in achieving abstinence.

Cardiologists have an especially important role to play in smoking cessation. Because cardiologists frequently encounter patients in the setting of an acute cardiovascular event, they have the opportunity to take advantage of these "teachable moments" when patients may be most receptive to smoking cessation advice or intervention. In 1996, a *Clinical Practice Guideline on Smoking Cessation* was released by the Agency for Health Care Policy and Research based on an extensive review of the scientific literature. The guideline was recently updated and released by the U.S. Department of Health and Human Services, Public Health Service (*Treating Tobacco Use and Dependence: Clinical Practice Guideline*). The guideline recommends that clinicians determine and document the tobacco-use status of every patient treated in a health care setting; provide a minimal intervention to every patient who uses tobacco; offer several first-line pharmacotherapies—including bupropion and nicotine replacement therapy (NRT)—to all patients willing to make a quit attempt; provide a brief intervention designed to increase motivation to quit to all patients unwilling to commit to quitting; and use problem-solving and skills-training strategies, clinician-provided support, and help in securing social support outside of treatment to aid the smoker's quitting efforts. Because most patients seen for routine care are not motivated to make a quit attempt, clinicians should match their counseling interventions to patient's level of readiness for change. Motivational interventions that include personalized feedback and use an empathic style are most likely to be effective for patients not committed to quitting smoking.

NRT (e.g., gum, transdermal nicotine, inhaler, and nasal spray) and bupropion are efficacious smoking cessation treatments. Clonidine and the antidepressant nortriptyline are also efficacious but are considered second-line treatments. Other pharmacotherapies, such as buspirone and the combination of nicotine and mecamylamine, have shown some promise. Among behavioral or psychosocial treatments, problem solving and skills training, clinician-delivered social support, and aversive therapies have the most evidence of efficacy. Multicomponent groups are highly effective, especially when combined with nicotine replacement treatment. Intensive case management for myocardial infarction (MI) patients has produced excellent smoking cessation outcomes. Finally, organizational systems to support office-based smoking interventions are useful for insuring optimal delivery of these interventions in medical care settings.

GLOSSARY

Aversive therapy: A behavioral treatment for smoking cessation that uses aversive experiences to make smoking unpleasant and less reinforcing. Techniques used to produce the aversive experience include rapid smoking, smoke holding, and rapid puffing.

Fagerstrom Tolerance Questionnaire: A scale for measuring the level of nicotine dependence; helpful in determining risk of relapse after attempted cessation and likelihood of benefit from high-dose nicotine gum or nicotine nasal spray.

Nicotine dependence: A well-defined psychiatric disorder characterized by physical dependence on nicotine (i.e., tolerance and withdrawal), as well as a maladaptive pattern of nicotine use.

Nicotine replacement therapy (NRT): Pharmacotherapy that delivers doses of nicotine to help manage nicotine withdrawal and promotes smoking cessation in tobacco users who are attempting to quit. Currently approved forms of NRT are nicotine gum, transdermal nicotine, and nicotine nasal spray.

Nicotine withdrawal: A syndrome of disturbing symptoms that occur in the setting of abstinence from nicotine.

Stimulus control: A behavioral smoking cessation strategy that involves identification of cues associated with smoking and removal or avoidance of these cues during attempts at smoking cessation.

EPIDEMIOLOGY OF SMOKING

Smoking Prevalence and Incidence

There are approximately 1 billion individuals who smoke cigarettes worldwide, with approximately one-third living in China (1). An estimated 48 million adults (25 million men and 23 million women) were current smokers in the United States in 1994 (2); another 46 million adults were former smokers, indicating that almost one-half of all individuals who had ever regularly smoked cigarettes had successfully quit. After a steady decline in the prevalence of cigarette smoking from the late 1960s to the early 1990s, there has been little to no change in these rates from 1990 to 1997 (2) (*e*Fig. 6.0.1). The overall prevalence of current smoking among adults in 1994 was 25.5% (28% of men, 23% of women) (2). In 1997, the prevalence was 24.7% (27.6% for men, 22.1% for women) (3). Because the proportion of "ever-smokers" who are now former smokers is increasing at a yearly rate of less than 1%, smoking prevalence is likely to remain high well beyond the year 2000 (4). In developing countries, prevalence rates of cigarette smoking is actually increasing at an alarming rate; for example, in China, cigarette consumption increased from 700 cigarettes per adult in 1970 to approximately 2,000 per year in 1992 (1).

Several factors contribute to the relatively slow decline in smoking prevalence in the United States. Although approximately 70% of current smokers say they want to quit smoking (2), only approximately 20% are actively attempting to do so (5). Relapse rates for those who do attempt to quit approach 80%, even when smokers use pharmacologic agents or seek assistance from formal treatment programs (6). Moreover, among the 90% of smokers who attempt to quit smoking on their own, only 3% to 5% achieve successful abstinence after 1 year (7). Other factors contributing to the slow decline in smoking prevalence in the United States include tobacco corporations' aggressive marketing and high rates of smoking initiation among youth. In the 1980s, approximately 1 million young persons per year were recruited to regular smoking—the equivalent of about 3,000 new smokers each day (4). Also, as the prevalence of smoking has declined, a greater proportion of smokers are likely to have conditions that make quitting more difficult, such as high levels of physical dependence on nicotine, dependence on other psychoactive substances, depression, and other psychiatric comorbid conditions (8,9). ▼ b09

Morbidity and Mortality Associated with Smoking

Cigarette smoking remains the most important preventable contributor to premature death, disability, and unnecessary medical expense in this country (13). In developed countries as a whole, tobacco was responsible for more than 1.8 million deaths in 1990, representing 24% of all male deaths and 7% of all female deaths (14). Although studies in the 1960s and 1970s reported that overall mortality rates in women were not as high as men at the same age and level of daily consumption, more recent epidemiologic studies show that overall mortality ratios in female smokers are similar to those seen in men (15). In the United States, cigarette smoking accounts for more than 400,000 deaths each year; in 1990, tobacco use accounted for 19% of all deaths (16). Smoking has also been estimated to cause between 17% and 30% of all deaths due to cardiovascular disease (16). The average loss of life for all cigarette smokers is approximately 8 years, whereas loss of life approaches 16 years for those whose deaths are attributed to tobacco (14). Approximately half of all smokers in developed countries die from a smoking-related illness (14). Based on current worldwide smoking patterns, epidemiologists have estimated that approximately half a billion of the world's current population will eventually be killed by tobacco, and approximately half of them will be 35 to 69 years of age when they die (14). ▼ b10

Health Effects of Environmental Tobacco Smoke

Exposure to environmental tobacco smoke (ETS)—also known as *passive smoking*—is associated with an increased risk of death from heart disease, increased risk of lung cancer, and an increased frequency of respiratory infections in children (21).

In ten epidemiologic studies on the risk of death from CAD among nonsmokers living with smokers, the group exposed to tobacco smoke experienced a 20% to 30% increase in risk (21). Individuals with CAD who are exposed to ETS have increases in heart rate, blood pressure, and carboxyhemoglobin; angina patients exposed to ETS experience an approximately 20% to 40% reduction in exercise capacity (22). Moreover, physiologic and biochemical studies have documented deleterious effects of ETS on platelets, the endothelium, and cellular respiration (23).

The risk of lung cancer is increased approximately 30% for nonsmoking spouses of smokers relative to nonsmoking spouses of nonsmokers (21). In 1992, the Environmental Protection Agency reviewed 30 studies of passive smoking and lung cancer and concluded that ETS is a "known human carcinogen" that is responsible for 3,000 lung cancer deaths per year in never-smokers and ex-smokers (24). Among children of parents who smoke, ETS is estimated to produce approximately 300,000 additional cases of bronchitis and pneumonia, as well as up to 1 million exacerbated cases of asthma per year (21).

Smoking and Cardiovascular Disease

Cigarette smoking is a major risk factor for all manifestations of CAD, stroke, and peripheral artery disease (25,26). In ten major cohort studies in several countries, each found a higher incidence of MI and death from coronary heart disease among smokers, averaging 70% higher in cigarette smokers versus nonsmokers (27). The 1990 Surgeon General's report on the health benefits of smoking cessation lists 25 prospective studies that documented the effects of smoking on CAD risk (*e*Table 6.0.1). Pooled data from five large studies demonstrated that middle-aged men (40 to 59 years of age) who smoked 20 or more cigarettes per day have two to three times the risk of experiencing a major coronary event, as compared with nonsmokers (28). An analysis of the 30-year Framingham data found that the relative risk for CAD was almost three times as great in male smokers aged 35 to 44 as nonsmokers, although the relative CAD risk for smokers declined for each succeeding age group (29). The higher relative risk for CAD among younger smokers likely is due to the rather low risk for CAD among nonsmokers in this age group.

The risk for CAD among smokers is dose-related (26) (Fig. 6.1), and smoking as little as one to four cigarettes per day significantly increases risk (30). Women whose smoking patterns are similar to patterns of men have a similar increased risk of CAD morbidity and mortality (15,26). Women in the Nurses' Health Study who smoked more than 25 cigarettes per day had 5.5 times the risk of fatal CAD and 5.8 times the risk of nonfatal CAD than nonsmoking women (30). Women who smoke and use an oral contraceptive have a 13-fold increase in risk of fatal CAD than oral contraceptive users who do not smoke (31).

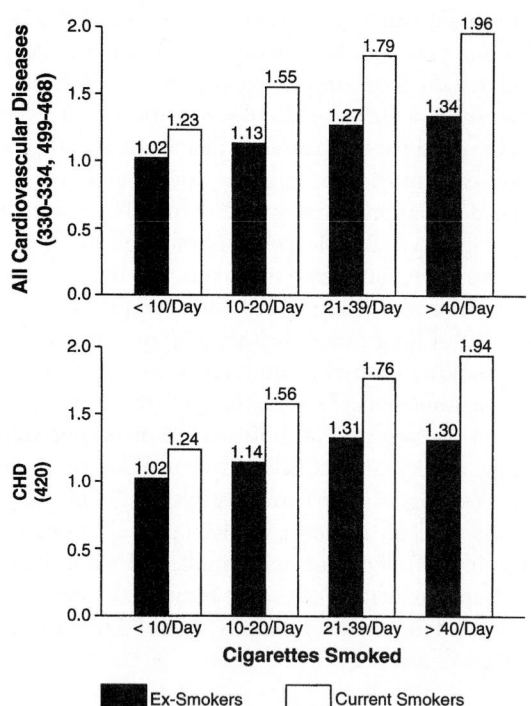

FIGURE 6.1 Mortality ratios for all cardiovascular diseases and congestive heart disease (CHD) by daily cigarette consumption, U.S. Veterans Study, 1954–1969. [From U.S. Department of Health and Human Services. *The health benefits of smoking cessation: a report of the Surgeon General*, DHHS Publication no. (CDC) 90–8416. Rockville, MD: U.S. Department of Health and Human Services, Public Health Service, Centers for Disease Control and Prevention, 1990.]

Smoking in the presence of other coronary risk factors (e.g., hypertension, hypercholesterolemia) appears to have a synergistic effect on cardiovascular disease (CVD) morbidity and mortality (15,26) (Fig. 6.2).

It has been estimated that 15% of the 150,000 stroke deaths that occur annually in the United States are directly related to smoking (15). Male and female cigarette smokers younger than 65 years experience stroke mortality rates that are 3.7 and 4.8 times greater, respectively, than those of nonsmokers (15). There is a clear dose-response relationship between smoking and mortality from stroke (26) (Fig. 6.3). Cigarette smoking is also associated with an increased risk of advanced atherosclerotic vascular disease in peripheral arteries (32). The likelihood of claudication, amputation, abdominal aortic aneurysm, and failure of vascular reconstruction is significantly higher in smokers than nonsmokers (32).

HEALTH EFFECTS OF SMOKING

Cigarette Smoking and Nicotine: Effects on the Cardiovascular System

Smoking contributes to the pathogenesis of CAD and sudden death through a variety of mechanisms, including the promotion of atherosclerosis, the triggering of coronary thrombosis, coronary artery spasm, and cardiac arrhythmias, and reduced capacity of the blood to deliver oxygen (26). Smoking's effects on each of these mechanisms is described in the following sections.

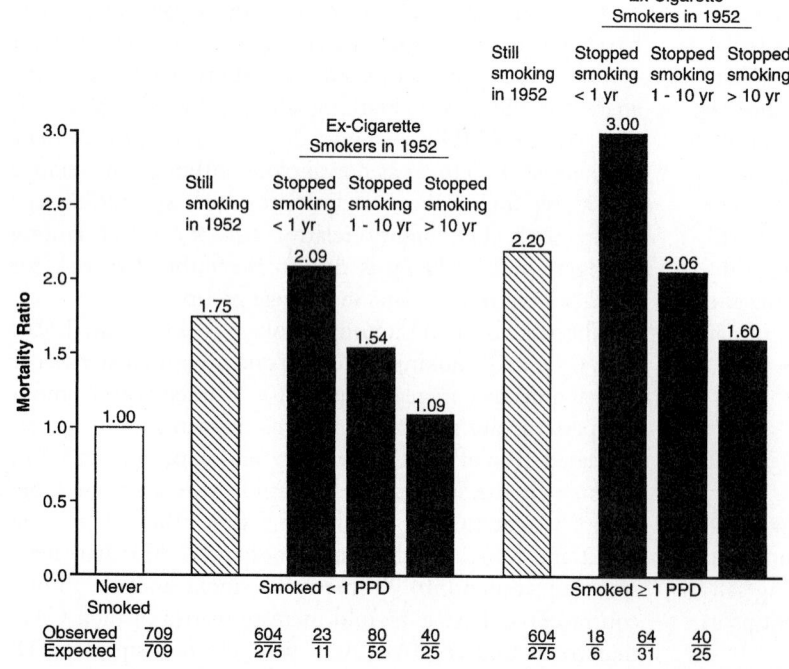

FIGURE 6.2 Mortality ratios due to coronary artery disease. Rates for men who have stopped smoking are compared with rates for men who have never smoked and rates for men still smoking in 1952. PPD, packs per day. [From U.S. Department of Health and Human Services. *The health benefits of smoking cessation: a report of the Surgeon General*, DHHS Publication no. (CDC) 90-8416. Rockville, MD: U.S. Department of Health and Human Services, Public Health Service, Centers for Disease Control and Prevention, 1990.]

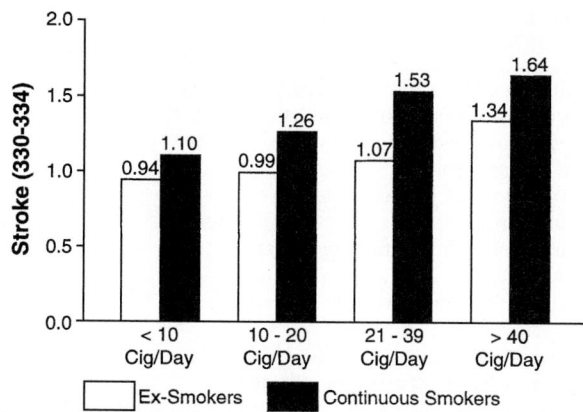

FIGURE 6.3 Mortality ratios for stroke for current smokers and ex-smokers compared with never-smokers by daily cigarette consumption, U.S. Veterans Study, 1954–1969. [From U.S. Department of Health and Human Services. *The health benefits of smoking cessation: a report of the Surgeon General*, DHHS Publication no. (CDC) 90-8416. Rockville, MD: U.S. Department of Health and Human Services, Public Health Service, Centers for Disease Control and Prevention, 1990.]

Thrombosis

In addition to smoking's effects on atherosclerosis, smoking promotes coronary artery thrombosis by increasing platelet adherence to endothelium and platelet aggregation (26,46). Tobacco smoke appears to increase platelet aggregation by inhibiting endothelial cell prostacyclin production and increasing thromboxane (26). Recent research has demonstrated that platelet-derived nitric oxide release, which inhibits platelet aggregation, is significantly impaired in long-term smokers (55). Smoking also appears to decrease platelet monoamine oxidase, which may promote platelet aggregation by increasing catecholamine levels (55). Smoking also may promote thrombosis by increasing fibrinogen levels, increasing plasma viscosity, and decreasing red cell deformity (26). Short-term increases in arterial wall stiffness induced by cigarette smoking may increase the risk for plaque rupture, thereby triggering an acute ischemic event (56). Impairment of endothelium-dependent coronary vasodilation has also been shown in long-term smokers, which may also promote the development of atherosclerosis and thrombosis (57). This finding is likely due to reduced endothelial nitric oxide release (55). Although smoking promotes thrombosis, transdermal delivery of nicotine does not appear to do so (58). ❧ b11

Coronary Artery Spasm

Both chronic and acute cigarette smoking have a vasoconstrictor effect on coronary vasculature (26). Current smokers have 20 times the risk of vasospastic angina compared to never-smokers (65). Smoking even a single cigarette has been demonstrated to produce coronary artery spasm during angiography (66). Smoking-associated vasoconstriction is mediated by an alpha-adrenergic increase in arterial tone and

by smoking-associated increases in platelet and plasma vasopressin, vasopressin carrier protein, and oxytocin (26). In some cases of variant or Prinzmetal's angina, smoking induced a profound vasospastic effect; unless cessation is assured, this may be refractory to medical management (67,68).

Arrhythmias and Reduced Oxygen-Carrying Capacity

Nicotine-induced release of catecholamines increases blood pressure and heart rate and may produce a lowered threshold for ventricular arrhythmias (26). In animal studies, cigarette smoke lowers the threshold for ventricular fibrillation (69). In a study of more than 10,000 men, smoking was associated with a 21% increase in ventricular premature beats on electrocardiographic rhythm strips (70). Moreover, nicotine's sympathetic effects increase myocardial oxygen demand, which is also accompanied by a reduction in oxygen carrying capacity due to the presence of 3% to 6% carbon monoxide in cigarette smoke (26). Carbon monoxide's high affinity for hemoglobin elevates levels of carboxyhemoglobin, interfering with oxygen exchange. The combination of increased myocardial oxygen demand and impaired oxygen exchange can produce or exacerbate myocardial ischemia. These effects on oxygen delivery may also lower the threshold for ventricular arrhythmias (26).

Nicotine as a Psychoactive Drug

Nicotine rapidly accumulates in the brain after cigarette smoking. Maximum brain concentrations are reached within 1 minute (13). This rapid accumulation of nicotine in combination with nicotine's effects on brain activity and function provide optimal conditions for the development of drug dependence (13). Acute and chronic tolerance to many effects of nicotine contribute to an increase in cigarette consumption, as individuals smoke more to obtain desired effects of nicotine (13,74).

Actions of Nicotine

Nicotine is a powerful pharmacologic agent with a wide variety of stimulant and depressant effects involving the central and peripheral nervous, cardiovascular, and endocrine systems, as well as other systems (13,74). These effects contribute to nicotine self-administration. Central effects include electrocortical activation (as noted on an electroencephalogram) and increases in brain serotonin, endogenous opioid peptides, pituitary hormones, catecholamines, and vasopressin (13,74). The rewarding properties of nicotine may be related to nicotine's stimulatory effects on dopaminergic pathways in the mesolimbic system (75). Nicotine has been shown to increase attention, memory, and learning in smokers—especially in the setting of low environmental demand, when stimulation is most desirable (26).

Nicotine also has anxiolytic and antinociceptive effects, and there is evidence that smokers are more apt to use cigarettes during stressful situations or in situations involving negative mood (26). Recently, research has demonstrated an association between a history of clinical depression, depressive symptoms, and difficulty in quitting smoking (76–78). Nicotine's effects on negative mood states in some smokers may help to explain the relationship between smoking, depression, and other psychiatric disorders (77). There is considerable variability in nicotine's effects between and within individuals over time. This variability results from a number of factors including dose, biphasic pharmacologic effects of stimulation and blockade, the influence of setting, the current state of the individual, and individual differences in dependence, genetics, and learning history (79).

Nicotine as an Addicting Drug

The characteristics and patterns of chronic nicotine use have much in common with the use of other psychotropic drugs: Humans self-administer nicotine in the laboratory to reproduce desired effects, patterns of relapse to smoking after smoking cessation are quite similar to the patterns noted after treatment for other forms of drug abuse and dependence, chronic nicotine use produces tolerance, and a withdrawal state is noted with abstinence (13,74).

Nicotine recently has been included among the drugs that may produce psychoactive substance dependence in the American Psychiatric Association's *Diagnostic and Statistical Manual of Mental Disorders, 4th edition* (*DSM-IV*) (80). The diagnosis of nicotine dependence by these criteria require evidence for any three of nine criteria. The criteria are listed in *e*Table 6.0.3. Among older adult smokers, 87% are estimated to meet *DSM-IV* criteria for nicotine dependence (81).

The nicotine withdrawal syndrome is well characterized (Table 6.1 lists the *DSM-IV* criteria for nicotine withdrawal) and experienced by approximately 50% of the smokers who make a serious attempt to quit smoking (80,82). In addition, a craving for sweets and impaired performance on vigilance tasks can occur (82,83). The signs and symptoms of the nicotine withdrawal syndrome can appear within 2 hours after the last use of tobacco, usually peak between 24 and 48 hours after cessation, and usually last from a few days to 4 weeks, although craving and hunger can persist for months (82). The mean decrease in heart rate is eight beats per minute, and the mean weight gain is 2 to 3 kg (82). ▼▼ b12

Effects of Cigarette Smoking and Nicotine on Drug Metabolism

Smoking is known to accelerate the metabolism of many drugs (100,101), including several drugs used regularly in treating cardiovascular disease (e.g., propranolol, lidocaine, and theophylline). The blood levels of these medications may increase significantly when individuals stop smoking. ▼▼ b13

TABLE 6.1 DIAGNOSTIC CRITERIA FOR NICOTINE WITHDRAWAL

1. Daily use of nicotine for at least several weeks
2. Abrupt cessation of nicotine use, or reduction in the amount of nicotine used, followed within 24 h by four (or more) of the following signs:
   a. Dysphoric or depressed mood
   b. Insomnia
   c. Irritability, frustration, or anger
   d. Anxiety
   e. Difficulty concentrating
   f. Restlessness
   g. Decreased heart rate
   h. Increased appetite or weight gain
3. The symptoms in criterion 2 cause clinically significant distress or impairment in social, occupational, or other important areas of functioning.
4. The symptoms are not due to a general medical condition and are not better accounted for by another mental disorder.

Reprinted from American Psychiatric Association. *Diagnostic and statistical manual of mental disorders, 4th edition (DSM-IV)*. Washington, DC: American Psychiatric Press, 1994:489.

Smoking also appears to have an important independent effect on anticoagulation in response to intravenously administered heparin (103). Granger and colleagues (103) monitored the activated partial thromboplastin time in response to intravenous heparin in more than 29,000 patients participating in the Global Utilization of Streptokinase and t-PA for Occluded Coronary Arteries (GUSTO-I) trial. Current smokers had significantly lower activated partial thromboplastin times than nonsmokers, even after adjustment for weight, age, and gender (103). This finding is consistent with previous studies of the pharmacokinetics of heparin, which have demonstrated that heparin is eliminated more rapidly among smokers (104). Therefore, when smokers are treated with heparin, anticoagulation parameters should be followed closely to ensure an adequate response.

SMOKING CESSATION

Role of the Cardiologist and Other Health Care Providers in Smoking Cessation

All physicians can play a central role in reducing the morbidity and mortality associated with cigarette smoking. Cardiologists have an especially important role in smoking cessation, for several reasons. Many cardiologists serve as primary care physicians for many of their patients. Because primary care providers have multiple opportunities over several years to intervene with their patients who smoke, they are in a unique position to provide smoking cessation advice and treatment. Moreover, because cardiologists frequently encounter patients in the setting of an acute cardiovascular event, they have the opportunity to take advantage of these "teachable moments," when patients may be most receptive to smoking cessation advice or intervention (39). *The Clinical Practice Guideline on Cardiac Rehabilitation*, published by the Agency for Health Care Policy and Research and the National Heart, Lung, and Blood Institute, recommends the inclusion of smoking cessation interventions as an essential component of cardiac rehabilitation programs (105). Even if the patient is asymptomatic, health care providers can link the patient's smoking to increased risk for disease in the future (e.g., heart disease, if the patient has a family history of early CAD). Finally, the widespread adoption of smoke-free policies in hospitals and other health care institutions provides additional new opportunities for health care provider intervention.

Although physicians recognize the importance of smoking cessation as a disease-preventive measure, few physicians are confident in their ability to help patients stop smoking (106,107). Moreover, less than half of smokers report that they have ever been advised to quit smoking by their physician (108–110).

Smoking Cessation: Effectiveness of Brief Interventions

Perhaps the most compelling reason to focus on physician-delivered smoking cessation interventions is that they are effective (111–113). In April 1996, after a comprehensive and exhaustive review and analysis of the existing scientific literature, the Agency for Health Care Policy and Research Smoking Cessation Guideline Panel released the *Clinical Practice Guideline on Smoking Cessation* (113,114). The Panel was reconvened recently, and the Guideline was updated and reissued by the Department of Health and Human Services, Public Health Service (114). Table 6.2 outlines the principal recommendations of the Guideline.

The Panel's recommendations were based on evidence that was derived primarily from metaanalyses of published randomized controlled trials (113,114). Highlights of the evidence is summarized in the following paragraphs. First, several studies have demonstrated that systems that identify and document smoking status result in significantly higher rates of smoking cessation interventions by clinicians (113,114). Further, the presence of these screening systems appears to result in higher quit rates among patients who smoke (113,114).

Second, even brief advice (e.g., less than 3 minutes) by a clinician significantly increases quit rates compared to the absence of such advice (113,114). The magnitude of the increase in quit rates with brief clinician advice is approximately 25% (113,114).

Third, smoking cessation interventions delivered by any type of health care provider increase cessation rates with no

---

TABLE 6.2 RECOMMENDATIONS OF THE AGENCY FOR HEALTHCARE AND RESEARCH QUALITY TREATING TOBACCO USE AND DEPENDENCE CLINICAL PRACTICE GUIDELINE

Tobacco dependence is a chronic condition that often requires repeated intervention. However, effective treatments exist that can produce long-term or even permanent abstinence.

Because effective tobacco dependence treatments are available, every patient who uses tobacco should be offered at least one of these treatments: Patients willing to try to quit tobacco use should be provided with treatments identified as effective in the Guideline; patients unwilling to try to quit tobacco use should be provided with a brief intervention designed to increase their motivation to quit.

It is essential that clinicians and health care delivery systems institutionalize the consistent identification, documentation, and treatment of every tobacco user seen in a health care setting.

Brief tobacco dependence treatment is effective, and every patient who uses tobacco should be offered at least brief treatment.

There is a strong dose-response relation between the intensity of tobacco dependence counseling and its effectiveness. Treatments involving person-to-person contact are consistently effective, and their effectiveness increases with treatment intensity.

Three types of counseling and behavioral therapies were found to be especially effective and should be used with all patients attempting tobacco cessation: provision of practical counseling (problem solving or skills training), provision of social support as part of treatment, and help in securing social support outside of treatment.

Numerous effective pharmacotherapies for smoking cessation now exist. Except in the presence of contraindications, these should be used with all patients attempting to quit smoking. Five first-line pharmacotherapies were identified that reliably increase long-term smoking abstinence rates: bupropion SR, nicotine gum, nicotine inhaler, nicotine nasal spray, nicotine patch. Two second-line pharmacotherapies were identified as efficacious and may be considered by clinicians if first-line pharmacotherapies are not effective: clonidine and nortriptyline.

Over-the-counter nicotine patches are effective relative to placebo, and their use should be encouraged. Tobacco-dependence treatments are both clinically effective and cost-effective relative to other medical and disease prevention interventions.

Adapted from Fiore M, Bailey W, Cohen S, et al. *Treating tobacco use and dependence: clinical practice guideline*. Rockville, MD: U.S. Department of Health and Human Services, Public Health Services, 2000.

TABLE 6.3 SMOKING CESSATION RATES FOR VARIOUS INTENSITY LEVELS OF PERSON-TO-PERSON CONTACT

Level of contact	Estimated odds ratio (95% CI)	Estimated abstinence rate (95% CI)
No contact (reference group)	1.0	10.9
Minimal contact (≤3 min)	1.3 (1.1–1.6)	13.4 (10.9–16.1)
Brief counseling (>3 min to ≤10 min)	1.6 (1.2–2.0)	16.0 (12.8–19.2)
Counseling (>10 min)	2.3 (2.0–2.7)	22.1 (19.4–24.7)

CI, confidence interval.
From Fiore M, Bailey W, Cohen S, et al. *Treating tobacco use and dependence: clinical practice guideline.* Rockville, MD: U.S. Department of Health and Human Services, Public Health Services, 2000.

clear advantage to any single provider type (e.g., physician, nurse, psychologist, health counselor) (113,114). Moreover, interventions delivered by multiple types of providers more than double the likelihood of smoking cessation, suggesting that smoking cessation interventions should be delivered by as many clinicians and types of clinicians as feasible (113,114). This finding has implications for specialized inpatient cardiac units and cardiac rehabilitation programs, which provide unique opportunities to deliver interventions from multiple providers.

Fourth, there is a strong dose-response relationship between the intensity of person-to-person contact and a successful smoking cessation outcome (113,114). In Table 6.3, the results of a metaanalysis are presented that examine the relationship between smoking cessation outcome and level of intensity of contact across 43 randomized controlled trials. As noted above, even brief counseling significantly increases quit rates. However, more counseling is clearly even better, with rates exceeding 20.0% (compared with 10.9% for the no-contact reference group) for more than 10 minutes of counseling during a single clinical contact. ▼✔ b14

Smoking Cessation: Matching Interventions to the Patient's Readiness for Change

Although health care provider–mediated smoking cessation interventions are effective, only a small minority of patients who receive interventions from physicians are successful in achieving long-term abstinence. Frustration and feelings of ineffectiveness that result from these low rates of success are important barriers to provider intervention with smokers. The Transtheoretical Model of Change—developed by psychologists James Prochaska and Carlo DiClemente at the University of Rhode Island (118)—can help physicians and other health care providers to intervene more effectively with their smoking patients by offering strategies for the majority of smokers who are not ready to quit smoking when they visit a physician's office.

The Transtheoretical Model of Change identifies five discrete stages of smoking cessation: precontemplation, contemplation, preparation, action, and maintenance

(118,119) (Fig. 6.4). Individuals at the precontemplation stage—representing as many as 40% of current smokers seen in a typical medical practice (5)—are not considering stopping smoking in the immediate future. These patients may be uninformed or underinformed, demoralized about their ability to change, or defensive and resistant to change (118). *Contemplation* is a stage of ambivalence that characterizes another 40% of smokers (5). Although individuals at this stage have given serious thought to giving up smoking, they are not yet ready to commit to quitting (118). Only approximately 20% of smokers who seek medical care are in the preparation stage and are intending to quit smoking in the next month. Many of these patients have attempted to quit in the past year or have taken small steps toward quitting, such as delaying their first cigarette in the morning or cutting down on the number of cigarettes that they smoke (118).

When individuals finally reach the action stage, they have overtly tried to quit smoking. Relapse is the rule dur-

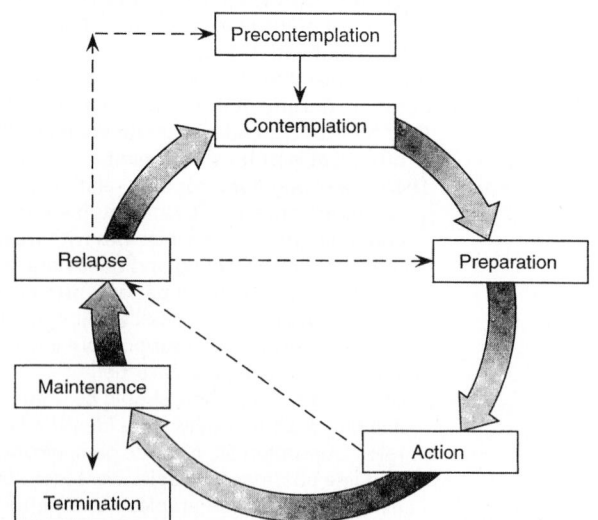

FIGURE 6.4 The Stages of Change (Prochaska and DiClemente). (From Prochaska JO, DiClemente CC. Towards a comprehensive model of change. In: Miller WR, Heather N, eds. *Treating addictive disorders: processes of change.* New York: Plenum Press, 1986.)

ing this stage, rather than the exception, especially during the first few days and weeks after quitting. *Maintenance*, defined as the stage reached 6 months after quitting, is characterized by continued use of processes to help individuals to change or modify their experience to prevent slips or relapse. The average smoker takes three or four cycles through the stages of change over several years before finally reaching a stable period of maintenance (119). ▼ b15

Five A's: A Strategy for Brief Provider Intervention

The Guideline (114) provides clinicians with a brief five-step strategy for smoking cessation intervention in medical care settings that includes the important step of assessing patients' readiness for making a quit attempt. This approach builds upon the "Four A's" of smoking cessation counseling that were developed for the National Cancer Institute's Physician-Delivered Smoking Cessation Program (122). The five steps are as follows:

1. **Ask:** Systematically identify all tobacco users at every visit.
2. **Advise:** Strongly advise all smokers to quit and identify smokers willing to make a quit attempt (provide a motivational intervention if they are not willing to quit).
3. **Assess** willingness to make a quit attempt.
4. **Assist:** Aid the patient in quitting (set a quit date, encourage nicotine replacement, provide advice on successful quitting, refer to formal treatment if desired, and provide supplementary materials).
5. **Arrange:** Schedule follow-up contact. ▼ b16

Smoking Cessation: Pharmacotherapy

Nicotine Replacement Therapy

NRT has been approved by the U.S. Food and Drug Administration (FDA) for use as an aid to smoking cessation. The four approved forms are nicotine gum, transdermal nicotine, nicotine inhaler, and nicotine nasal spray. As noted above, the Panel's review of the scientific literature found that nicotine gum and transdermal nicotine were efficacious as smoking cessation interventions across a variety of diverse settings and populations and regardless of the intensity of adjuvant behavioral and psychosocial interventions (113,114). This conclusion was based on the results of several published metaanalyses on the efficacy of transdermal nicotine (123–127) and nicotine gum (126–129). The American Psychiatric Association's *Practice Guideline for the Treatment of Patients with Nicotine Dependence* also endorsed the use of nicotine gum and patches as effective therapies (121). Moreover, the efficacy of the patch, gum, nasal spray, and inhaler were found to be statistically indistinguishable in the Guideline Panel

metaanalyses and in a recent head-to-head clinical trial comparison (130). ▼ b17

Nicotine nasal spray was approved by the FDA in 1996 as a smoking cessation treatment. Nasal spray provides a more rapid rise in nicotine levels than transdermal or gum products, with peak levels of nicotine occurring within 10 minutes (121). Three published studies of nicotine nasal spray that meet the requirements for the Guideline metaanalyses have documented its efficacy when combined with adjunctive psychosocial treatment (121,114), and one study documented the efficacy of nicotine nasal spray in a minimal contact setting (137). Nicotine nasal spray has considerably more side effects than other forms of NRT and appears to have greater dependence liability (121). Side effects include nasal and throat irritation, rhinitis, sneezing, coughing, and watering eyes (121). However, tolerance to these side effects often develops within several days. At present, nicotine nasal spray seems best suited for individuals who have failed other forms of NRT. In a metaanalysis of four studies, nicotine inhalers—which produce a nicotine vapor when air is drawn through a tube into the mouth and throat—were found to be efficacious when combined with adjunctive behavioral therapy (114). In addition to its pharmacologic benefits in terms of nicotine replacement, the inhaler provides the user with an oral-handling substitute for cigarettes, which may confer additional therapeutic benefit. The inhaler is FDA-approved for use in the United States as a prescription product (121).

Bupropion and Other Pharmacotherapy

Bupropion recently received FDA approval for smoking cessation. Bupropion is a unique antidepressant with noradrenergic and dopaminergic activity. Clinical trials have demonstrated the efficacy of bupropion SR (a delayed release preparation) for smoking cessation with or without concomitant transdermal nicotine (121,138–140). The recommended dose of bupropion SR for smoking cessation is 150 mg twice daily. In clinical trials, medication was started 1 to 2 weeks before patients' quit days and was continued for 7 to 12 weeks. Because bupropion may lower the seizure threshold, it is contraindicated in patients with a seizure disorder and should be avoided when a patient has a condition predisposed to seizures (e.g., head injury, alcohol abuse or dependence) (Table 6.4). Common side effects include headache, insomnia, nausea, and restlessness. If sleep difficulty occurs, move the p.m. dose to the late afternoon or early evening. Bupropion has little or no adverse effects on the cardiovascular system (i.e., no significant alpha-adrenergic blockade, anticholinergic activity, or effects on cardiac conduction) (141–143), although elevations in blood pressure have been noted on occasion.

Clonidine is an alpha$_2$-agonist that dampens sympathetic activity and attenuates withdrawal symptoms associated with alcohol, opiate, and nicotine abstinence

TABLE 6.4   SUGGESTIONS FOR USE OF BUPROPION SR

Selection of patients: Avoid during pregnancy and breast feeding unless increased likelihood of smoking abstinence, with its potential benefits, outweighs the risk of bupropion SR treatment and potential concomitant smoking. There is a small risk of hypertension. Contraindicated in patients with a history of seizure disorder, eating disorder, use of another form of bupropion (e.g., Wellbutrin), or use of a monoamine oxidase inhibitor in the past 14 days.

Dosage and duration: Begin with a dose of 150 mg q.a.m. for 3 days, increasing to 150 mg b.i.d. and continuing for 7–12 weeks after quit date. Patients should begin treatment 1–2 weeks before quitting. Use alcohol in moderation.

Adapted from Fiore M, Bailey W, Cohen S, et al. *Treating tobacco use and dependence: clinical practice guideline.* Rockville, MD: U.S. Department of Health and Human Services, Public Health Services, 2000.

(121,144). Recent metaanalytic reviews (114,145) concluded that clonidine was more effective than placebo in promoting abstinence from smoking (144). Doses used for smoking cessation are 0.1 to 0.4 mg per day for 2 to 6 weeks in oral or transdermal formulations (121). The most common side effects are sedation, dry mouth, constipation, lightheadedness, and postural hypotension (144). Although it is uncommon, rebound hypertension after discontinuation is also a concern, especially in patients with cardiac disease. Clonidine is recommended as a second-line treatment for smokers who have failed NRT or bupropion (114,121) or as an alternative for smokers who prefer not to receive nicotine. b18

Intensive Case Management for Myocardial Infarction Patients

As noted in the section Smoking Cessation and Reduction of Cardiovascular Disease Risk, cessation rates after the diagnosis of clinical CAD range from 35% to 75%. Using an intensive case-management system, DeBusk and colleagues (40) produced a 1-year smoking cessation rate of 70% compared to a rate of 53% for usual care for patients hospitalized with acute MI ($p = .03$). The case-management system included the following components: in-hospital counseling (by a physician) lasting approximately 2 minutes, an in-hospital comprehensive assessment and counseling session conducted by a nurse trained in behavioral problem-solving skills, provision of a self-help manual focusing on relapse prevention and a relaxation audiotape, and telephone calls by the nurse 48 hours and 1 week after hospital discharge and monthly for 6 months. Patients who relapsed after discharge also were offered one additional visit with the nurse for further counseling, as well as nicotine gum or transdermal nicotine. The usual-care condition included physician counseling on smoking cessation, nutritionist counseling on dietary change during hospitalization, and physician-managed, lipid-lowering drug therapy after hospital discharge. Patients in the usual-care group also had access to a group smoking cessation program and group exercise rehabilitation at a number of community facilities.

CONTROVERSIES AND PERSONAL PERSPECTIVES

Harm Reduction

Proponents of a harm-reduction approach maintain that any decrease in smoking rate, even short of complete abstinence, is desirable. On the surface, this makes sense, given the clear dose-dependent relationship between the amount of tobacco smoked or consumed and the risk of cardiovascular diseases. However, this approach has several drawbacks. It is unlikely that most smokers can maintain a decrease in the amount that they smoke. Somewhere between 5% to 10% of all smokers smoke five or fewer cigarettes per day, but these "chippers" are more likely to have maintained this level of smoking for most of their smoking careers than to have decreased the amount that they smoked (154). Very few intervention studies have adopted decreases in smoking as a goal, largely because it is ineffective and because this strikes most smokers as unacceptable. Moreover, even though disease risk is reduced when smoking rate decreases, it is not eliminated. Smoking even one to four cigarettes a day increases risk of cardiovascular disease (30). Therefore, unlike with problem drinking—in which there is some evidence that a harm-reduction approach is feasible and that drinking moderate quantities of alcohol may be salubrious—complete abstinence from smoking should remain the desired outcome.

Another approach to harm reduction, ironically championed by the tobacco industry, is the low-tar and low-nicotine cigarette. However, considerable evidence now suggests that smokers compensate for decreased nicotine yield by smoking more effectively (e.g., more frequent and deeper puffing) and by blocking cigarette ventilation holes. Often, such compensation occurs outside of conscious awareness. In some cases, smokers even overcompensate by increasing their overall nicotine intake (i.e., smoking more cigarettes) after switching to a low-tar, low-nicotine brand. A study of women who smoked "low-yield" cigarettes produced a similar increase in the risk of having a first MI to those who smoked a higher-yield cigarette (155). Thus, there does not appear to be such a thing as a safe or even a safer cigarette, and this approach to harm reduction cannot be condoned because it is false.

Still another variation on harm reduction is the position that all nicotine replacement products should be sold as OTC medications. This includes not only slow-release formulations such as the nicotine patch and gum, but also the faster-release formulations such as nicotine nasal spray and inhaler, although abuse liability appears to be increased with the faster-release formulations. The argument in favor of this approach is simply that it is better to ingest pure nicotine rather than to be exposed simultaneously to carcinogens, carbon monoxide, and the other toxic components of tobacco during the combustion process, thereby increasing the risk of disease. However, because nicotine alone appears to increase the risk for cardiovascular disease by increasing adrenergic tone and by its effect on lipids, one has to question the wisdom of this suggestion. Moreover, an unknown number of non- and former smokers might use OTC nicotine delivery devices to boost memory and cognitive performance, to control weight, or for other "benefits," thereby risking addiction. Our perspective is that, although harm reduction appears laudable, it seems impossible to implement. Therefore, complete abstinence from smoking and nicotine should remain the treatment goal.

Policy, Regulation, and Advocacy

Should the sale of tobacco products be illegal? Can the sale of tobacco products be made illegal? The answer to the former question is a tentative yes; the answer to the latter is very probably no. A ban on tobacco products is extremely unlikely because (a) historically, they have been manufactured and sold legally, (b) a substantial number of Americans smoke, and (c) tobacco is very big business. Can tobacco products be regulated? Possibly. By calling nicotine an addictive drug, the FDA may be able to regulate aspects of tobacco manufacture and sales. However, governmental regulatory efforts face the challenge of the tobacco industry, its lobbyists, and politicians who are friendly toward the tobacco industry. The future of increased government regulation remains uncertain, given the vicissitudes of the political process. In our opinion, only "grass roots" reform will permit more effective regulation; unfortunately, there is as yet no evidence of an antitobacco groundswell.

Economic regulation (e.g., increasing taxes on tobacco products) is probably effective, to some degree, in motivating smokers to quit. However, this type of regulation has its limits. For example, recently the Canadian government substantially increased taxes on cigarettes, which increased the price of a pack of cigarettes two- to threefold. This resulted in a small decrease in smoking prevalence and a substantial increase in the cigarette black market, which is reminiscent of the effects of prohibition on alcohol use in the United States. The Canadian government repealed the high taxes on cigarettes when it was realized that tax revenues were decreasing. As a result, black market activity decreased. This scenario illustrates another reason why banning tobacco would be nearly impossible.

Another approach to regulation that has been debated is the application of a special tax on cigarette sales, which would then be used to offset the cost of smokers' disproportionately high use of health care resources as they become ill as a result of their smoking. In fact, variations on this theme are already in place (e.g., higher life insurance premiums for smokers). It is unclear to what degree such a tax would serve as a disincentive to smoke. There probably would be some effect, but we are not likely to see this form of regulation adopted anytime soon.

Should physicians advocate the control of tobacco? The answer is a resounding "yes!" Indeed, several physician organizations, including the American Medical Association (AMA) and the American Psychiatric Association, have drafted policy papers on this topic. Effective advocacy starts with education. Physicians are urged to learn about tobacco control by reading about the work of the AMA and established advocacy groups such as Doctors Oughta Care and the Action on Smoking and Health. The American Academy of Family Physicians has developed a model tobacco control program called Tar Wars. The principal goal of Tar Wars is to educate youth regarding tobacco-free lifestyles by developing partnerships between physicians, schools, and community agencies supporting tobacco control. The program supports physicians and other health care clinicians to deliver lessons to fifth- and sixth-graders on the effects of tobacco use on health and strategies for countering the advertising images that tobacco companies use to market their products. Physician-teachers also judge "counter-advertising" posters developed by the children as a follow-up activity. As enthusiastic participants in the Tar Wars program in our own communities, we strongly encourage cardiologists and other clinicians treating patients with cardiac disease to get involved in similar community-based tobacco control programs. It is a wonderful way to promote tobacco control, teach children about prevention, and have fun!

We also encourage physicians who are members of clinical and scientific societies to develop position papers similar to the AMA documents and to disseminate these papers to their membership. The AMA has also recommended divestiture of tobacco and tobacco-related stock. Does the American College of Cardiology or other similar societies own stock in tobacco and related industries? Do your employer-related retirement plans invest in tobacco-related stock? Recently, the Teacher's Insurance Annuity Association–College Retirement Equities Fund—the largest retirement fund for employees of educational institutions—was prompted by its membership to hold a vote on whether to divest all of its tobacco-related holdings. The motion was voted down.

An important but neglected topic is reimbursement for smoking cessation treatment provided by health care providers. The *Treating Tobacco Use and Dependence Guideline* recommends that those smoking cessation treatments found to be effective be included as paid services for all subscribers of health insurance programs (113,114). Lack of reimbursement is an important barrier, preventing the busy physician from spending more time motivating and assisting their patients to quit smoking. Physicians and other health care providers should push hard for third-party reimbursement. Voluntary agencies can provide more information on this issue (Table 6.5).

THE FUTURE

This is a time for considerable optimism. New behavioral and pharmacologic treatments for nicotine dependence are currently being developed to add to the many known effective treatments (58,156–158). Research is helping us to understand the biobehavioral mechanisms responsible for nicotine dependence and how to target these mechanisms for treatment. A few areas, however, stand out as especially important in terms of furthering our ability to help smokers to quit; one has to do with increased understanding of the biologic and psychological substrates of nicotine dependence. For example, symptoms of depression are associated with nicotine dependence and difficulty quitting, and promising new treatments for smoking cessation include antidepressant medications and psychosocial treatments that target depressive symptoms. Research on nicotine receptors in the mesolimbic areas associated with addiction suggest that more specific antagonists can be developed to block the reinforcing effects of nicotine, thereby helping smokers quit.

Another area of importance that dovetails with the study of biobehavioral mechanisms is patient–treatment matching. No single treatment proves effective for every smoker; there are many reasons why people smoke and become addicted. However, smokers with certain characteristics may respond more favorably to certain treatments. For example, smokers with symptoms of depression achieve better outcomes when treated with an antidepressant than smokers with no symptoms of depression. Better matching of treatment to patient will increase the chances of successful treatment.

Finally, if we are to truly have a significant impact on smoking, subpopulations in whom smoking prevalence has stabilized—or is even increasing—must be targeted for treatment (9). In particular, there is an epidemic of adolescent smoking in the United States. The adolescent smokers of today are the addicted smokers of tomorrow who will suffer from smoking-related cardiovascular and other diseases. Efforts to prevent the initiation of smoking are of paramount importance (the Tar Wars program described above is one such effort), but so is treatment of the adolescent smoker. Many of the same treatments that have proven effective among adult smokers, (e.g., nicotine replacement and bupropion) should be evaluated for efficacy among adolescent smokers. In addition, new innovative strategies for adolescent smokers need to be evaluated and tested.

Finally, health care providers should not turn a blind eye to tobacco consumption on a worldwide scale. The United States enjoys one of the lowest smoking prevalence rates in the world, due in large part to increasing public awareness about the health risks of smoking and to considerable research on developing and disseminating effective smoking cessation treatments. Other countries, especially underdeveloped or newly developing ones, fare much worse in terms of smoking prevalence and efforts to educate and treat smokers. The American tobacco industry is one of the world's largest suppliers of tobacco. We should question American export practices, which actively promote the sale and distribution of tobacco products to developing countries, thereby directly contributing to a worldwide pandemic in tobacco-related diseases.

REFERENCES

1. Wald N, Hackshaw A. Cigarette smoking: an epidemiological overview. *Br Med Bull* 1996;52(1):3–11.
2. Centers for Disease Control. Cigarette smoking among adults—United States, 1994. *MMWR Morb Mortal Wkly Rep* 1996;45:588–589.
3. Centers for Disease Control & Prevention. Cigarette smoking among adults, United States, 1997. *MMWR Morb Mortal Wkly Rep* 1999;48(93):993–996.
4. Pierce JP, Fiore MC, Novotny TE, et al. Trends in cigarette smoking in the United States. Projections to the year 2000. *JAMA* 1989;261(1):61–65.
5. Velicer WF, Fava JL, Prochaska JO, et al. Distribution of smokers by stage in three representative samples. *Prev Med* 1995;24(4):401–411.
6. Schwartz JL. Methods of smoking cessation. *Med Clin North Am* 1992;76(2):451–476.
7. Lichtenstein E, Glasgow R. Smoking cessation: what have we learned over the past decade? *J Consult Clin Psychol* 1992;60(4):518–527.
8. Brown RA, Goldstein MG, Niaura R, et al. Nicotine dependence: assessment and management. In: Stoudemire A, Fogel BS, eds. *Principles of medical psychiatry*. New York: Oxford University Press, 1993.
9. Lasser K, Boyd JW, Woolhandler S, et al. Smoking and mental illness. A population-based prevalence study. *JAMA* 2000;284:2606–2610.
10. Ockene J. Smoking among women across the life span: prevalence, interventions, and implications for cessation research. *Ann Behav Med* 1993;15:135–148.
11. Solomon L, Flynn B. Women who smoke. In: Orleans CT, Slade J, eds. *Nicotine addiction: principles and management.* New York: Oxford University Press, 1993.
12. Fisher E, Lichtenstein E, Haire-Joshu E. Multiple determi-

nants of tobacco use and cessation. In: Orleans CT, Slade J, eds. *Nicotine addiction: principles and management.* New York: Oxford University Press, 1993.

13. U.S. Department of Health and Human Services. *The health consequences of smoking: nicotine addiction. A report of the Surgeon General,* DHHS Publication No. (CDC) 88–8406. Rockville, MD: U.S. Department of Health and Human Services, Public Health Service, Centers for Disease Control and Prevention, 1988.

14. Peto P, Lopez A, Boreham J, et al. Mortality from smoking worldwide. *Br Med Bull* 1996;52(1):12–21.

15. Shopland D, Burns D. Medical and public health implications of tobacco addiction. In: Orleans CT, Slade J, eds. *Nicotine addiction: principles and management.* New York: Oxford University Press, 1993.

16. McGinnis J, Foege W. Actual causes of death in the United States. *JAMA* 1993;270(18):2207–2212.

17. Wannamethee SG, Shaper AG, Whincup PH, et al. Smoking cessation and the risk of stroke in middle-aged men. *JAMA* 1995;274(2):155–160.

18. Herling S, Kozlowski L. The importance of direct questions about inhalation and daily intake in the evaluation of pipe and cigar smokers. *Prev Med* 1988;17:73–78.

19. Henningfield J, Hariharan M, Kozlowski L. Nicotine content and health risks of cigars. *JAMA* 1996;276(23):1857–1858.

20. National Cancer Institute. *Cigars: health effects and trends. Smoking and tobacco control monograph,* no. 9. Rockville, MD: U.S. Department of Health and Human Services, National Institutes of Health, National Cancer Institute, 1998.

21. Repace J. Tobacco smoke pollution. In: Orleans CT, Slade J, eds. *Nicotine addiction: principles and management.* New York: Oxford University Press, 1993.

22. Aronow W. Effect of passive smoking on angina pectoris. *N Engl J Med* 1978;299:21–24.

23. Glantz S, Parmley W. Passive smoking and heart disease: epidemiology, physiology, and biochemistry. *Circulation* 1991;83:1–12.

24. U.S. Environmental Protection Agency. *Respiratory health effects of passive smoking: lung cancer and other disorders.* Washington, DC: Office of Health and Environmental Assessment, Office of Research and Development, U.S. Environmental Protection Agency, 1992.

25. U.S. Department of Health and Human Services. *The health consequences of smoking: cardiovascular disease. A report of the Surgeon General.* Rockville, MD: U.S. Department of Health and Human Services, 1983.

26. U.S. Department of Health and Human Services. *The health benefits of smoking cessation: a report of the Surgeon General,* DHHS Publication no. (CDC) 90–8416. Rockville, MD: U.S. Department of Health and Human Services, Public Health Service, Centers for Disease Control and Prevention, 1990.

27. Fielding J. Smoking: health effects and control (first of two parts). *N Engl J Med* 1985;313(8):491–498.

28. Pooling Project Research Group. Relationship of blood pressure, serum cholesterol, smoking habit, relative weight, and ECG abnormalities to incidence of major coronary events: final report of the Pooling Project. *J Chronic Dis* 1978;31:201–306.

29. Kannel W, McGee D, Castelli W. Latest perspectives on cigarette smoking and cardiovascular disease: the Framingham Study. *J Card Rehabil* 1984;4:267–277.

30. Willett WC, Green A, Stampfer MJ, et al. Relative and absolute excess risks of coronary heart disease among women who smoke cigarettes. *N Engl J Med* 1987;317(21):1303–1309.

31. Hennekens C, Evans D, Peto R. Oral contraceptive use, cigarette smoking and myocardial infarction. *Br J Fam Plann* 1989;5:66–67.

32. Krupski WC. The peripheral vascular consequences of smoking. *Ann Vasc Surg* 1991;5(3):291–304.

33. Vlietstra R, Kronmal R, Oberman A, et al. Effect of cigarette smoking on survival of patients with angiographically documented coronary artery disease: report from the CASS Registry. *JAMA* 1986;255(8):1023–1027.

34. Hallstrom A, Cobb L, Ray R. Smoking as a risk factor for recurrence of sudden cardiac arrest. *N Engl J Med* 1986;314(5):271–275.

35. Galan K, Deligonul U, Kern M, et al. Increased frequency of restenosis in patients continuing to smoke cigarettes after percutaneous transluminal coronary angioplasty. *Am J Cardiol* 1989;61:260–263.

36. Solymoss B, Nadeau P, Millette D, et al. Late thrombosis of saphenous vein coronary bypass grafts related to risk factors. *Circulation* 1988;78[Suppl I]:I140–I143.

37. Hu FB, Stampfer MJ, Manson JE, et al. Trends in the incidence of coronary heart disease and changes in diet and lifestyle in women. *N Engl J Med* 2000;343:530–537.

38. Frid D, Ockene I, Ockene J, et al. Severity of angiographically proven coronary artery disease predicts smoking cessation. *Am J Prev Med* 1991;7(3):131–135.

39. Ockene J, Kristeller J, Goldberg R, et al. Smoking cessation and severity of disease: the Coronary Artery Smoking Intervention Study. *Health Psychol* 1992;11:119–126.

40. DeBusk R, Miller N, Superko H, et al. A case-management system for coronary risk factor modification after acute myocardial infarction. *Ann Intern Med* 1994;120(9):721–729.

41. Hughes G, Hymowitz N, Ockene J, et al. The Multiple Risk Factor Intervention Trial (MRFIT): V. Intervention on smoking. *Prev Med* 1981;10:476–500.

42. Farquhar J, Wood P, Brietrose H, et al. Community education for cardiovascular health. *Lancet* 1977;1:1192–1195.

43. Zimmerman M, McGeachie J. The effect of nicotine on aortic endothelium. A quantitative ultrastructural study. *Atherosclerosis* 1987;63:33–41.

44. Krupski W, Olive G, Weber CA, et al. Comparative effects of hypertension and nicotine on injury-induced myointimal thickening. *Surgery* 1987;102(2):409–415.

45. Davis J, Shelton L, Hartman C, et al. Smoking-induced changes in endothelium and platelets are not affected by hydroxyethylrutosides. *Br J Exp Pathol* 1986;67(5):765–771.

46. Davis J, Shelton L, Eigenberg D, et al. Effects of tobacco and non-tobacco cigarettes smoking on endothelium and platelets. *Clin Pharmacol Ther* 1985;37(5):529–533.

47. Asmussen I, Kjeldsen K. Intimal ultrastructure of human umbilical arteries. Observations on arteries from newborn children of smoking and nonsmoking mothers. *Circ Res* 1984;22(6):397–402.

48. Morrow JD, Frei B, Longmire AW, et al. Increase in circulating products of lipid peroxidation (F2-isoprostanes) in smokers. Smoking as a cause of oxidative damage. *N Engl J Med* 1995;332(18):1198–1203.

49. Pettilo R, Clarke J, Harris D, et al. Cigarette smoking and platelet adhesion. *Br J Haematol* 1984;58(4):627–632.

50. Rival J, Riddle J, Stein P. Effects of chronic smoking on platelet function. *Thromb Res* 1987;45(1):75–85.

51. Marshall M. Ultrastructural findings on platelet depositions in initial atherogenesis. *Wien Klin Wochenschr* 1986;98(7):212–214.

52. Steinberg D, Parthasarathy S, Carew T, et al. Beyond cholesterol: modifications of low-density lipoprotein that increase its atherogenicity. *N Engl J Med* 1989;320(14):915–924.

53. Nadiger H, Mathew C, Sadasivudu B. Serum malondialdehyde (TBA reactive substance) levels in cigarette smokers. *Atherosclerosis* 1987;64(1):71–73.

54. De Parscau L, Fielding C. Abnormal plasma cholesterol metabolism in cigarette smokers. *Metabolism* 1986;35:1070–1073.

55. Ichiki K, Ikeda H, Haramaki N, et al. Long-term smoking impairs platelet-derived nitric oxide release. *Circulation* 1996;94:3109–3114.

56. Kool MJ, Hoeks AP, Struijker Boudier HA, et al. Short- and long-term effects of smoking on arterial wall properties in habitual smokers. *J Am Coll Cardiol* 1993;22(7):1881–1886.

57. Zeiher A, Schachinger V, Minners J. Long-term cigarette smoking impairs endothelium-dependent coronary arterial vasodilator function. *Circulation* 1995;92:1094–1100.

58. Benowitz NL, Gourlay SG. Cardiovascular toxicity of nicotine: implications for nicotine replacement therapy. *J Am Coll Cardiol* 1997;29(7):1422–1431.

59. Molstad P. First myocardial infarction in smokers. *Eur Heart J* 1991;12:753–759.

60. Barbash G, White H, Modan M, et al. For the Investigators of the International Tissue Plasminogen Activator/Streptokinase Mortality Trial. Significance of smoking in patients receiving thrombolytic therapy for acute myocardial infarction. *Circulation* 1993;87:53–58.

61. Barbash G, Reiner J, White H, et al. Evaluation of paradoxic beneficial effects of smoking in patients receiving thrombolytic therapy for acute myocardial infarction: mechanism of the "smoker's paradox" from the GUSTO-I Trial, with angiographic insights. *J Am Coll Cardiol* 1995;26(5):1222–1229.

62. The TIMI Study Group. Comparison of invasive and conservative strategies after treatment with intravenous tissue plasminogen activator in acute myocardial infarction: results of the Thrombolysis in Myocardial Infarction (TIMI) Phase II Trial. *N Engl J Med* 1989;320:618–627.

63. GISSI-2: a factorial randomised trial of alteplase versus streptokinase and heparin versus no heparin among 12,490 patients with acute myocardial infarction. Gruppo Italiano per lo Studio della Sopravvivenza nell'Infarto Miocardico. *Lancet* 1990;336:65–71.

64. Grines C, Topol E, O'Neil W, et al. Effect of cigarette smoking on outcome after thrombolytic therapy for myocardial infarction. *Circulation* 1995;91:298–303.

65. Scholl J, Benacerraf A, Ducimetiere P, et al. Comparison of risk factors in vasospastic angina without significant fixed coronary narrowing to significant fixed coronary narrowing and no vasospastic angina. *Am J Cardiol* 1986;57:199–202.

66. Maouad J, Fernandez F, Barrillon A, et al. Diffuse or segmental narrowing (spasm) if the coronary arteries during smoking demonstrated on angiography. *Am J Cardiol* 1984;53(2):354–355.

67. Tashiro H, Shimokawa H, Koyanagi S, et al. Clinical characteristics of patients with spontaneous remission of variant angina. *Jpn Circ J* 1993;57(2):117–122.

68. Miwa K, Fujita M, Miyagi Y. Beneficial effects of smoking cessation on the short-term prognosis for variant angina—validation of the smoking status by urinary cotinine measurements. *Int J Cardiol* 1994;44(2):151–156.

69. Downey H, Bashour C, Boutros I, et al. Regional myocardial blood flow during nicotine infusion: effects of beta adrenergic blockade and acute coronary artery occlusion. *J Pharmacol Exper Ther* 1977;202(1):55–68.

70. Hennekens C, Lown B, Rosner B, et al. Ventricular premature beats and coronary risk factors. *Am J Epidemiol* 1980;112(1):93–99.

71. Benowitz NL. Nicotine replacement therapy during pregnancy [see comments]. *JAMA* 1991;266(22):3174–3177.

72. Baron JA, La Vecchia C, Levi F. The antiestrogenic effect of cigarette smoking in women. *Am J Obstet Gynecol* 1990;162(2):502–514.

73. Vingerling J, Hofman A, Grobbee D, et al. Age-related macular degeneration and smoking: the Rotterdam Study. *Arch Ophthalmol* 1996;114:1193–1196.

74. Henningfield J, Cohen C, Pickworth W. Psychopharmacology of nicotine. In: Orleans CT, Slade J, eds. *Nicotine addiction: principles and management.* New York: Oxford University Press, 1993.

75. Clarke P. Nicotine dependence—mechanisms and therapeutic strategies. *Biochem Soc Symp* 1994;59:83–85.

76. Hall SM, Munoz R, Reus V. Smoking cessation, depression and dysphoria. *NIDA Res Monogr* 1991;105(312):312–313.

77. Glassman AH. Cigarette smoking: implications for psychiatric illness. *Am J Psychiatry* 1993;150(4):546–553.

78. Niaura R, Britt DM, Shadel WG, et al. Symptoms of depression and survival experience among three samples of smokers trying to quit. *Psychol Addict Behav* 2001;15(1):13–17.

79. Pomerleau O, Pomerleau C. Neuroregulators and the reinforcement of smoking: towards a biobehavioral explanation. *Neurosci Biobehav Rev* 1984;8:503–513.

80. American Psychiatric Association. *Diagnostic and statistical manual of mental disorders, 4th edition (DSM-IV).* Washington, DC: American Psychiatric Press, 1994.

81. Hale K, Hughes J, Oliverto A, et al. Nicotine dependence in a population-based sample. *Problems of drug dependence, 1992. NIDA Research Monograph 132.* Rockville, MD: National Institute on Drug Abuse, 1993.

82. Hughes J, Hatsukami D. The nicotine withdrawal syndrome: a brief review and update. *Int J Smoking Cessation* 1992;1:21–26.

83. Hughes J, Higgins S, Hatsukami D. Effects of abstinence from tobacco: a critical review. In: Kozlowski L, Annis H, Cappell H, et al., eds. *Recent advances in alcohol and drug problems.* New York: Plenum Press, 1990.

84. Williamson D, Madans J, Anda R, et al. Smoking cessation and severity of weight gain in a national cohort. *N Engl J Med* 1991;324:739–745.

85. Hall S, Ginsberg D, Jones R. Smoking cessation and weight gain. *J Consult Clin Psychol* 1986;57:81–86.

86. Kawachi I, Troisi R, Rotnitzky A, et al. A prospective study of smoking cessation and weight change in women. *J Smoking Rel Disord* 1994;5[Suppl 1]:91–100.

87. Moffat R, Owens S. Cessation from cigarette smoking: changes in body weight, body composition, resting metabolism, and energy consumption. *Metabolism* 1991;40:465–470.

88. Klesges R, Somes G, Pascale R, et al. Knowledge and beliefs regarding the consequences of cigarette smoking and their relationships to smoking status in a biracial sample. *Health Psychol* 1988;7:387–401.

89. Pomerleau C, Kurth C. Willingness of female smokers to tolerate postcessation weight gain. *J Subst Abuse Treat* 1996;8:371–378.

90. Klesges R, Klesges L. Cigarette smoking as a dieting strategy in a university population. *Int J Eat Disord* 1988;7:413–419.

91. French S, Jeffrey R. Weight concerns and smoking: a literature review. *Ann Behav Med* 1995;17:234–244.

92. Borrelli B, Mermelstein R, Shadel W. The role of weight concern and self-efficacy in smoking cessation and weight gain. *Ann Behav Med* 1995;17:S096.

93. Swan G, Ward M, Carmelli D, et al. Differential rates of relapse in subgroups of male and female smokers. *J Clin Epidemiol* 1993;46:1041–1053.

94. Pirie P, McBride CM, Hellerstedt W, et al. Smoking cessation in women concerned about weight. *Am J Public Health* 1992;2:1238–1243.

95. Hall S, Tunstall C, Vila K, et al. Weight gain prevention and smoking cessation: cautionary findings. *Am J Public Health* 1992;82:799–805.

96. Gross J, Stitzer M, Maldonadok J. Nicotine replacement: effects on postcessation weight gain. *J Consult Clin Psychol* 1989;37:87–92.

97. Marcus B, Pinto B, Audrain J, et al. Exercise enhances the maintenance of smoking cessation in women. *Addict Behav* 1994;20:87–92.

98. Spring B, Wurtman J, Gleason R, et al. Efficacies of dexfenfluramine and fluoxetine in preventing weight gain after smoking cessation. *Am J Clin Nutr* 1995;62(6):1181–1187.

99. Fagerstrom K, Schneider N. Measuring nicotine dependence: a review of the Fagerstrom Tolerance Questionnaire. *J Behav Med* 1989;12:159–182.

100. Benowitz N. Pharmacologic aspects of cigarette smoking and nicotine addiction. *N Engl J Med* 1988;319:1318–1330.

101. Zevin S, Benowitz NL. Drug interactions with tobacco smoking. An update. *Clin Pharmacokinet* 1999;36(6):425–438.

102. Walle T, Byington R, Furberg C, et al. Biologic determinants of propranolol disposition: results from 1308 patients the Beta-Blocker Heart Attack Trial. *Clin Pharmacol Ther* 1985;38:509–518.

103. Granger C, Hirsh J, Califf R, et al. Activated partial thromboplastin time and outcome after thrombolytic therapy for acute myocardial infarction: results from the GUSTO-I Trial. *Circulation* 1996;93(5):870–878.

104. Cipolle R, Seifert R, Neilan B, et al. Heparin kinetics: variables related to disposition and dosage. *Clin Pharmacol Ther* 1981;29:387–393.

105. Wenger N, Froelicher E, Smith L, et al. *Cardiac rehabilitation: clinical practice guideline no. 17.* Rockville, MD: Agency for Health Care Policy and Research and the National Heart, Lung, and Blood Institute, Public Health Service, U.S. Department of Health and Human Services, 1995.

106. Ockene JK, Aney J, Goldberg RJ, et al. A survey of Massachusetts physicians' smoking intervention practices. *Am J Prev Med* 1988;4(1):14–20.

107. Orleans CT, George LK, Houpt JL, et al. Health promotion in primary care: a survey of U.S. family practitioners. *Prevent Med* 1985;14:636–637.

108. Goldstein MG, Niaura R, Willey-Lessne C, et al. Physicians counseling smokers. A population-based survey of patients' perceptions of health care provider-delivered smoking cessation interventions. *Arch Intern Med* 1997;157(12):1313–1319.

109. Frank E, Winkleby MA, Altman DG, et al. Predictors of physician's smoking cessation advice [see comments]. *JAMA* 1991;266(22):3139–3144.

110. Anda RF, Remington PL, Sienko DG, Davis RM. Are physicians advising smokers to quit? The patient's perspective. *JAMA* 1987;257(14):1916–1919.

111. Ockene JK. Physician-delivered interventions for smoking cessation: strategies for increasing effectiveness. *Prev Med* 1987;16(5):723–737.

112. Kottke TE, Battista RN, DeFriese GH, et al. Attributes of successful smoking cessation interventions in medical practice. A meta-analysis of 39 controlled trials. *JAMA* 1988;259(19):2883–2889.

113. Fiore M, Bailey W, Cohen S, et al. *Smoking cessation: clinical practice guideline no. 18.* Rockville, MD: Agency for Health Care Policy and Research, Public Health Service, U.S. Department of Health and Human Services, 1996.

114. Fiore M, Bailey W, Cohen S, et al. *Treating tobacco use and dependence: clinical practice guideline.* Rockville, MD: U.S. Department of Health and Human Services, Public Health Services, 2000.

115. Hollis JF, Lichtenstein E, Vogt TM, et al. Nurse-assisted counseling for smokers in primary care. *Ann Intern Med* 1993;118(7):521–525.

116. Cummings SR, Rubin SM, Oster G. The cost-effectiveness of counseling smokers to quit. *JAMA* 1989;261(1):75–79.

117. British Thoracic Society. Smoking cessation guidelines and their cost-effectiveness. *Thorax* 1998;53[Suppl 5, Pt 1]:S1–S38.

118. Prochaska JO, Goldstein MG. Process of smoking cessation. Implications for clinicians. *Clin Chest Med* 1991;12(4):727–735.

119. Prochaska JO, DiClemente CC. Towards a comprehensive model of change. In: Miller WR, Heather N, eds. *Treating addictive disorders: processes of change.* New York: Plenum Press, 1986.

120. Miller WR, Rolnick S. *Motivational interviewing: preparing people to change addictive behavior.* New York: Guilford, 1991.

121. American Psychiatric Association. Practice guideline for the treatment of patients with nicotine dependence. *Am J Psychiatry* 1996;153[Suppl]:1–31.

122. Glynn TJ, Manley MW. *How to help your patients stop smoking. A national cancer institute manual for physicians,* NIH

Publication 89–3064. Bethesda, MD: Smoking, Tobacco and Cancer Program, Division of Cancer Prevention and Control, National Cancer Institute, 1989.

123. Fiore MC, Smith SS, Jorenby DE, et al. The effectiveness of the nicotine patch for smoking cessation. A meta-analysis [see comments]. *JAMA* 1994;271(24):1940–1947.

124. Gourlay S. The pros and cons of transdermal nicotine therapy. *Med J Austr* 1994;160:152–159.

125. Po A. Transdermal nicotine in smoking cessation: a meta-analysis. *Eur J Clin Pharmacol* 1993;24:519–528.

126. Silagy C, Mant D, Fowler G, et al. Meta-analysis on efficacy of nicotine replacement therapies in smoking cessation. *Lancet* 1994;343:139–142.

127. Tang J, Law M, Wald N. How effective is nicotine replacement therapy in helping people to stop smoking? *BMJ* 1994;308:21–26.

128. Cepeda-Benito A. A meta-analytic review of the efficacy of nicotine chewing gum in smoking treatment programs. *J Consult Clin Psychol* 1993;61:822–830.

129. Lam W, Sze PC, Sacks HS, et al. Meta-analysis of randomized controlled trials of nicotine chewing-gum. *Lancet* 1987;2:27–30.

130. Hajek P, West R, Foulds J, et al. Randomized comparative trial of nicotine polacrilex, a transdermal patch, nasal spray, and an inhaler. *Arch Intern Med* 1999;159(17):2033–2038.

131. Joseph A, Norman S, Ferry LH, et al. The safety of transdermal nicotine as an aid to smoking cessation in patients with cardiac disease. *N Engl J Med* 1996;335:1792–1798.

132. Tzivoni D, Keren A, Meyler S, et al. Cardiovascular safety of transdermal nicotine patches in patients with coronary artery disease who try to quit smoking. *Cardiovasc Drugs Ther* 1998;12(3):239–244.

133. Gourlay SG, Benowitz NL, Forbes A, et al. Determinants of plasma concentrations of nicotine and cotinine during cigarette smoking and transdermal nicotine treatment. *Eur J Clin Pharmacol* 1997;51(5):407–414.

134. Working Group for the Study of Transdermal Nicotine in Patients with Coronary Artery Disease. Nicotine replacement therapy for patients with coronary artery disease. *Arch Intern Med* 1994;154(9):989–995.

135. Murray RP, Bailey WC, Daniels K, et al. Safety of nicotine polacrilex gum used by 3,094 participants in the Lung Health Study. Lung Health Study Research Group. *Chest* 1996;109(2):438–445.

136. Shiffman S, Mason KM, Henningfield JE. Tobacco dependence treatments: review and prospectus. *Annu Rev Public Health* 1998;19:335–358.

137. Schneider N, Olmstead R, Mody F, et al. Efficacy of a nicotine nasal spray in smoking cessation: a placebo-controlled, double-blind trial. *Addiction* 1995;90:1671–1682.

138. Niaura R, Bock B, Goldstein M, et al. Nicotine dependence: assessment and management. In: Rommelspacher H, Schuckit M, eds. *Drugs of abuse: Bailliere's clinical psychiatry: international practice and research.* London: Bailliere-Tindall, 1996.

139. Hurt RD, Sachs DP, Glover ED, et al. A comparison of sustained-release bupropion and placebo for smoking cessation. *N Engl J Med* 1997;337(17):1195–1202.

140. Jorenby DE, Leischow SJ, Nides MA, et al. A controlled trial of sustained-release bupropion, a nicotine patch, or both for smoking cessation. *N Engl J Med* 1999;340(9):685–691.

141. Spiller HA, Ramoska EA, Krenzelok EP, et al. Bupropion overdose: a 3-year multi-center retrospective analysis. *Am J Emerg Med* 1994;12(1):43–45.

142. Roose SP, Dalack GW, Glassman AH, et al. Cardiovascular effects of bupropion in depressed patients with heart disease. *Am J Psychiatry* 1991;148(4):512–516.

143. Kiev A, Masco HL, Wenger TL, et al. The cardiovascular effects of bupropion and nortriptyline in depressed outpatients. *Ann Clin Psychiatry* 1994;6(2):107–115.

144. Gourlay S, Benowitz N. Is clonidine an effective smoking cessation therapy? *Drugs* 1995;50:197–207.

145. Gourlay SG, Stead LF, Benowitz NL. Clonidine for smoking cessation (Cochrane Review). In: *The Cochrane library,* issue 1. Oxford: Update Software, 2000.

146. Hall SM, Reus VI, Munoz RF, et al. Nortriptyline and cognitive-behavioral therapy in the treatment of cigarette smoking. *Arch Gen Psychiatry* 1998;55(8):683–690.

147. Prochazka AV, Weaver MJ, Keller RT, et al. A randomized trial of nortriptyline for smoking cessation. *Arch Intern Med* 1998;158(18):2035–2039.

148. Rose JE, Behm FM, Westman EC, et al. Mecamylamine combined with nicotine skin patch facilitates smoking cessation beyond nicotine patch treatment alone. *Clin Pharmacol Ther* 1994;56(1):86–99.

149. Rose JE, Behm FM, Westman EC. Nicotine-mecamylamine treatment for smoking cessation: the role of pre-cessation therapy. *Exp Clin Psychopharmacol* 1998;6(3):331–343.

150. Lando H. Formal quit smoking treatments. In: Orleans CT, Slade J, eds. *Nicotine addiction: principles and management.* New York: Oxford University Press, 1993.

151. Abbot N, Stead L, White ABJ, et al. Hypnotherapy for smoking cessation (Cochrane Review). In: *The Cochrane library,* issue 1. Oxford: Update Software, 1999.

152. Kottke TE, Solberg LI, Brekke ML. Beyond efficacy testing: introducing preventive cardiology into primary care. *Am J Prev Med* 1990;6[Suppl 1]:77–83.

153. Kottke TE, Solberg LI, Brekke ML, et al. Smoking cessation strategies and evaluation. *J Am Coll Cardiol* 1988;12(4):1105–1110.

154. Kassel JD, Shiffman S, Gnys M, et al. Psychosocial and personality differences in chippers and regular smokers. *Addict Behav* 1994;19(5):565–575.

155. Palmer J, Rosenberg L, Shapiro S. "Low-yield" cigarettes and the risk of nonfatal myocardial infarction in women. *N Engl J Med* 1989;320:1569–1573.

156. Mahmarian J, Moyce L, Nasser G, et al. Nicotine patch therapy in smoking cessation reduces the extent of exercise-induced myocardial ischemia. *J Am Coll Cardiol* 1997;30:125–130.

157. Kottke TE. Editorial comment. Managing nicotine dependence. *J Am Coll Cardiol* 1997;30:131–132.

158. Hughes JR, Goldstein MG, Hurt RD, et al. Recent advances in the pharmacotherapy of smoking. *JAMA* 1999;281(1):72–76.

7

DIABETES

DORON ARONSON
ELLIOT J. RAYFIELD

▼▼ **ADDITIONAL ELECTRONIC TOPICS**

D. Aronson: Department of Cardiology, Rambam Medical Center, Haifa, Israel
E. J. Rayfield: Department of Medicine, Mount Sinai School of Medicine of the City University of New York, New York, New York

OVERVIEW

Both type 1 and type 2 diabetes are powerful and independent risk factors for coronary artery disease (CAD), stroke, and peripheral arterial disease (1,2). Atherosclerosis accounts for virtually 80% of all deaths among North American diabetic patients, compared with one-third of all deaths in the general North American population (3). More than 75% of all hospitalizations for diabetic complications are attributable to cardiovascular disease (3). Sixteen million people in the United States are estimated to have diabetes, and more than 90% of these patients have type 2 diabetes (4). In addition, it is estimated that up to one-half of type 2 diabetic patients have not been diagnosed. The World Health Organization estimates that the number of diabetic adults will more than double globally, from 143 million in 1997 to 300 million in 2025, largely because of dietary and other lifestyle factors.

Whereas other major multifactorial diseases (e.g., heart disease, stroke, and many cancers) have declined or remained stable, the age-adjusted death rate for diabetes in the United States has increased 30% since 1980 (5) (*e*Fig. 7.0.1). The decline in heart disease mortality in the general U.S. population has been attributed to the reduction in cardiovascular risk factors and improvement in treatment of heart disease. However, patients with diabetes have not experienced the reduction in age-adjusted heart disease mortality that has been observed in nondiabetic people, and an increase in age-adjusted heart disease mortality has been reported in diabetic women (6). ▼ b56

CORONARY ARTERY DISEASE IN TYPE 1 DIABETES

In contrast to type 2 diabetes, cardiovascular risk in type 1 diabetes can be examined in relation to hyperglycemia *per se*. Long-term follow-up of patients with type 1 diabetes from the Joslin Diabetes Center has shown that an excess of cardiovascular mortality can only be observed after the age of 30 (14). The first cases of clinically manifest CAD occur late in the third decade or in the fourth decade of life, regardless of whether diabetes developed early in childhood or in late adolescence, suggesting that diabetes mainly accelerates the progression of early atherosclerotic lesions that occur at a young age in the general population (14). CAD risk increases rapidly after the age of 40; by the age of 55 years, 35% of men and women with type 1 diabetes die of CAD. This rate of CAD mortality far exceeded that observed in an age-matched nondiabetic cohort from the Framingham Heart Study (8% for nondiabetic men and 4% for nondiabetic women) (14). Similar to women with type 2 diabetes, the protection from CAD observed in nondiabetic women is lost in women with type 1 diabetes (14,15).

Diabetic nephropathy occurs only in a subset of 30% to 40% of type 1 diabetic patients and increases dramatically

the prevalence of CAD. Data from the Steno Memorial Hospital showed that in patients with persistent proteinuria the relative mortality from cardiovascular disease was 37 times that in the general population, whereas in patients without proteinuria cardiovascular mortality was only 4.2 times higher (16). In a case-control study of type 1 diabetes patients who were followed from the onset of microalbuminuria (a urinary albumin excretion rate of greater than 20 μg per min but less than 200 μg per min or 30 to 300 mg per 24 hours), coronary heart disease (CHD) developed eight times more frequently than in a diabetic population of similar age, sex, and diabetes duration (17). In the Joslin clinic cohort, the risk of developing CAD in patients with persistent proteinuria was 15 times higher than in those without this renal complication (14). Microalbuminuria in type 1 diabetes is, therefore, not only a marker for renal disease, but it is also a potent risk marker of CAD.

Prospective studies demonstrated that in type 2 diabetes patients, microalbuminuria is also an independent predictor of increased cardiovascular mortality (18). Proteinuria in a patient with type 2 diabetes increases the risk of fatal CAD by a factor of only two to four.

When nephropathy is superimposed on diabetes, some of the atherogenic mechanisms present in diabetes are accentuated. An aggregation of cardiovascular risk factors for cardiovascular disease, including hypertension, lipid abnormalities, and a hypercoagulable state, are detectable in the early stages of diabetic nephropathy, when renal function is still normal (19). Hypertension is frequently present in diabetic nephropathy even when the creatinine concentrations remain normal and can intensify CAD in type 1 diabetes patients. In the World Health Organization Multinational Study on Vascular Disease in Diabetes, patients with both hypertension and proteinuria experienced 11-fold and 18-fold increased mortality for men and women, respectively (20). Microalbuminuria is associated with an atherogenic lipoprotein profile that includes elevated low-density lipoprotein (LDL) and chylomicron remnants levels, decreased high-density lipoprotein (HDL) levels, and elevated lipoprotein(a) levels (21,22). In addition, plasminogen activator inhibitor-1 (PAI-1) activity, factor VII, and plasma fibrinogen are significantly higher in microalbuminuric type 1 diabetes patients (23). Finally, nephropathy results in accelerated accumulation of advanced glycosylation end products (AGEs) in the circulation and tissue that parallels the severity of renal functional impairment (24). The accumulation of AGEs improves markedly with successful renal transplantation (25). ▼ b57

CORONARY ARTERY DISEASE IN TYPE 2 DIABETES

CHD is the leading cause of death among patients with type 2 diabetes, regardless of duration of diabetes. Several population-based studies have consistently shown that the relative risk ratio of cardiovascular disease in type 2 diabetes compared with the general population is increased twofold to fourfold (2,15,35). Patients with type 2 diabetes without previous myocardial infarction have CAD mortality as high as nondiabetic patients with a previous infarction (36).

The increased cardiovascular risk is particularly striking in women. A number of studies reported a disproportionate effect of CAD on diabetic women compared with diabetic men (37). Indeed, the usual protection that premenopausal women have against atherosclerosis is almost completely lost when diabetes is present (38).

Although the degree and duration of hyperglycemia are the principal risk factors for microvascular complications (39), in type 2 diabetes, there is no obvious association between the extent or severity of macrovascular complications and the duration or severity of the diabetes. An increased prevalence of CAD is apparent in newly diagnosed type 2 diabetes subjects (40). In fact, even impaired glucose tolerance carries an increased cardiovascular risk despite minimal hyperglycemia (41).

In individuals who are genetically prone to develop type 2 diabetes, insulin resistance is the earliest detectable metabolic defect and can occur 15 to 25 years or more before the clinical onset of overt diabetes (42). Although there is some uncertainty regarding the primary lesion and the relative importance of the different tissues, metabolic defects in the liver and peripheral tissues such as fat, muscle, and pancreatic beta cells all contribute to the syndrome.

The term *insulin resistance* usually connotes resistance to the effects of insulin on glucose uptake and metabolism in adipocytes and skeletal muscle and impaired suppression of hepatic glucose output (43). Insulin resistance is a common condition, associated with genetic predisposition, sedentary

TABLE 7.1 CARDIOVASCULAR RISK FACTORS ASSOCIATED WITH INSULIN RESISTANCE

Hypertension (45,46)
Abdominal obesity (47)
Dyslipidemia
  Increased very-low-density lipoprotein triglyceride (52,71,72)
  Decreased high-density lipoprotein (52,71,72)
  Small dense atherogenic low-density lipoprotein particles (91,92)
  Postprandial lipemia (82,87)
Prothrombotic state
  Elevated plasminogen activator inhibitor-1 activity (158)
  Fibrinogen (155)
  von Willebrand factor (154)
Endothelial dysfunction (136)
Chronic subclinical inflammation (?) (51)

lifestyle, and aging. It is exacerbated and produced by obesity. Even in the absence of diabetes, insulin resistance is a major risk factor for CAD (44) because impaired insulin action coupled with compensatory hyperinsulinemia leads to a number of proatherogenic abnormalities referred to as the *insulin resistance syndrome* (Table 7.1). The association of insulin resistance with several established atherogenic risk factors (45–47) (Table 7.1) promotes atherosclerosis many years before overt hyperglycemia ensues (48) (Fig. 7. 1).

The dyslipidemia associated with insulin resistance entails elevated very-low-density lipoprotein (VLDL)–triglyceride levels, low HDL levels, delayed postprandial clearance of triglyceride-rich lipoprotein remnants, and the presence of the very atherogenic, small, dense LDL particles (49) (Table 7.1). This atherogenic lipoprotein phenotype is the most common lipoprotein abnormality seen in patients with CAD and imparts a risk for CAD at least

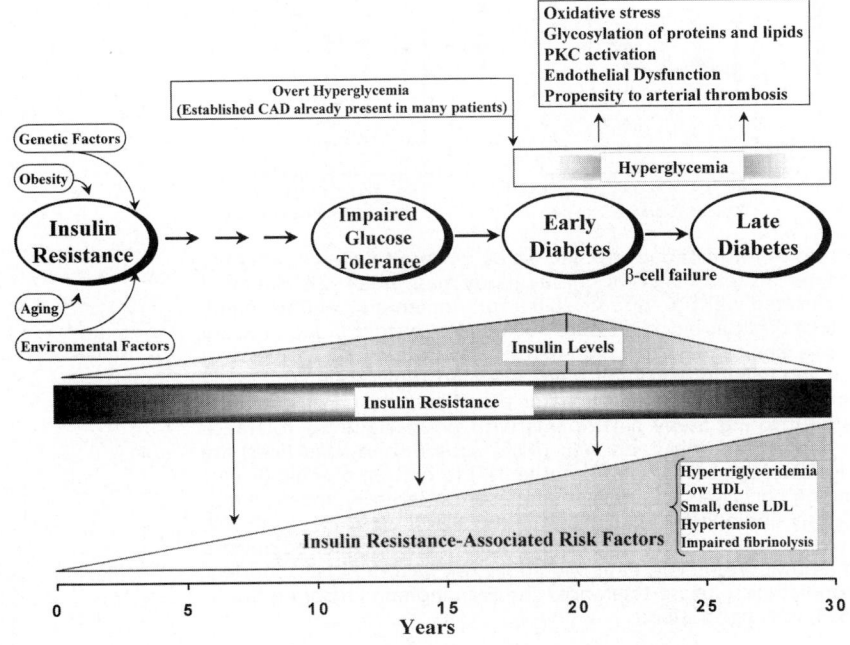

FIGURE 7.1 Schema of cardiovascular risk factors in patients with type 2 diabetes. Patients are exposed to the proatherogenic effects of the insulin resistance many years before the development of frank hyperglycemia. Therefore, macrovascular complications are commonly found when diabetes is diagnosed. When overt hyperglycemia ensues, it promotes atherosclerosis through several other mechanisms. CAD, coronary artery disease; HDL, high-density lipoprotein; LDL, low-density lipoprotein; PKC, protein kinase C.

equal to that of isolated moderate to severe hypercholesterolemia (50) (see Lipoprotein Disorders in Diabetes).

Insulin-resistant subjects also exhibit endothelial dysfunction (see Vascular Endothelial Dysfunction in Diabetes) and a hypercoagulable state (see Diabetes as a Prothrombotic State). Chronic subclinical inflammation has emerged as part of the insulin-resistance syndrome. C-reactive protein, a sensitive marker of inflammation associated with cardiovascular events, is independently related to insulin sensitivity (51).

The proatherogenic metabolic risk factors in insulin-resistance subjects worsen continuously across the spectrum of glucose tolerance (52). In the Framingham Offspring Study, the deterioration of insulin resistance (and glucose tolerance) over time was associated with a continuous increasing gradient of metabolic atherogenic risk factors (Fig. 7.2).

Whether compensatory hyperinsulinemia promotes atherosclerosis in insulin-resistant subjects is still unclear. Several prospective studies reported the association between fasting or postprandial hyperinsulinemia and future CAD (53,54). Other studies reported inverse correlations between insulin sensitivity and atherosclerosis (55,56). In addition, it has been suggested that chronic hyperinsulinemia exerts a deleterious effect on the arterial wall (57) based on the ability of insulin at high concentrations to stimulate the insulin growth factor-1 receptor. However, the association between hyperinsulinemia and atherosclerosis has been demonstrated only in healthy male middle-aged white cohorts (53,54) but not in women (44,58), or in other ethnic groups such as Pima Indians (59) or Hispanic Americans (60).

The inconsistent association between plasma insulin levels and CAD may stem from the fact that hyperinsulinemia

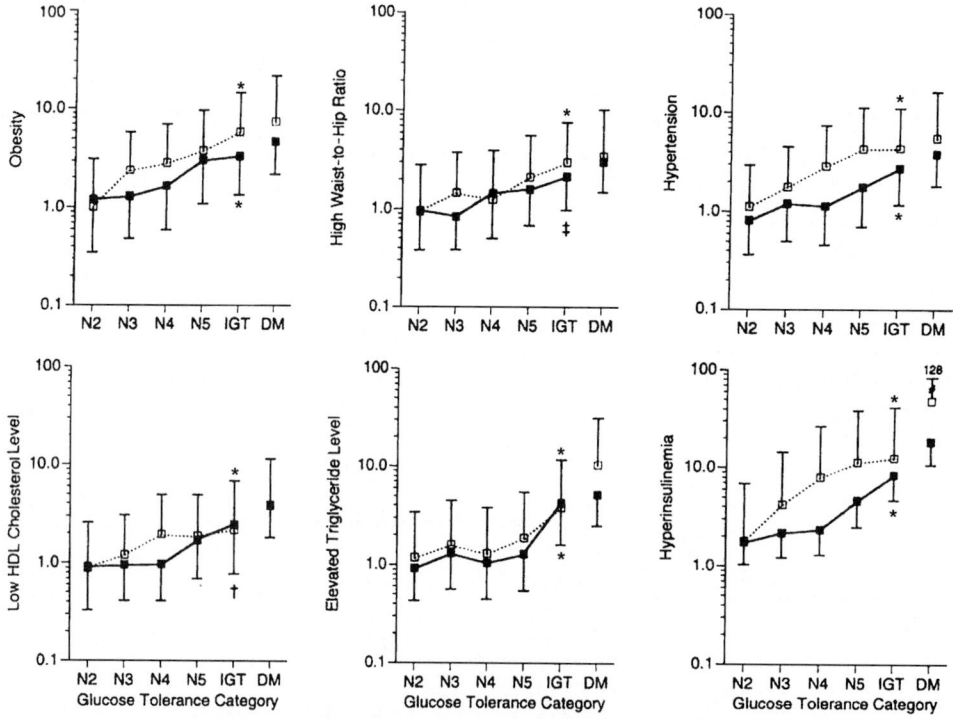

FIGURE 7.2 Multivariable odds ratios for metabolic risk factors by glucose tolerance category: odd ratios and 95% confidence intervals (*error bars*) of obesity (body mass index ≥27.3 kg/m² in women or ≥27.8 kg/m² in men, elevated waist-to-hip ratio (>0.9 for women and >1.0 for men), hypertension (two measurements of diastolic blood pressure >90 mm Hg, systolic blood pressure >140 mm Hg, or use of hypertensive medications), low high-density lipoprotein (HDL) cholesterol level (<45 mg per dL for women and <35 mg per dL for men), elevated triglyceride level (>200 mg per dL), and hyperinsulinemia (fasting insulin level greater than ninetieth percentile of its distribution among Framingham Offspring Study participants with normal glucose tolerance among women (*white squares* and *dotted lines*) and men (*black squares* and *solid lines*) are shown for each glucose tolerance category from lowest quintile (N1) to highest quintile (N5) of fasting plasma glucose level among participants with normal glucose tolerance, impaired glucose tolerance (IGT), and previously undiagnosed diabetes mellitus (DM). *p <.001; †p = .002; ‡p = .008 for trend from the lowest quintile of normal fasting glucose level to impaired glucose tolerance. (From Meigs JB, Nathan DM, Wilson PW, et al. Metabolic risk factors worsen continuously across the spectrum of nondiabetic glucose tolerance. The Framingham Offspring Study. *Ann Intern Med* 1998;128:524–533, with permission.)

TABLE 7.2 LIPOPROTEIN ABNORMALITIES IN DIABETES

Lipoprotein	Type 1 diabetes		Type 2 diabetes		Atherogenic modifications
	Conventional therapy	Intensive therapy	Poor control	Good control	
VLDL	Normal or increased	Decreased	Increased	Normal or increased	Cholesteryl ester–rich VLDL
LDL	Normal or increased	Normal or decreased	Normal	Normal	Glycosylation of LDL apolipoprotein B; LDL susceptible to oxidative modification; high proportion of small, dense LDL
HDL	Normal	Increased	Decreased	Normal or decreased	Decreased HDL; increased cholesteryl ester transfer protein activity; low paraoxonase activity (?)

HDL, high-density lipoprotein; LDL, low-density lipoprotein; VLDL, very-low-density lipoprotein.

is only a compensatory response of pancreatic beta cells to the peripheral insulin resistance. Prospective studies have shown that type 2 diabetes progresses over a continuum of worsening insulin action, beginning with peripheral insulin resistance and ending with a loss of insulin secretion. Thus, plasma insulin levels reflect not only the degree of insulin resistance but also the ability of beta cells to compensate. In fact, the natural course of type 2 diabetes is characterized by gradual loss of insulin secretion. Whereas hyperinsulinemia is characteristic in patients with impaired glucose tolerance and mild type 2 diabetes, increased glucose levels seen in patients with moderate-to-severe type 2 diabetes are associated with a progressive decline in both fasting and postprandial insulin concentrations as a result of pancreatic beta cell failure (43). Cross-sectional (52) and prospective (61) studies have shown that fasting and glucose-stimulated insulin concentrations have an inverted U-shaped curve when plotted against plasma glucose concentrations. This pattern has been termed the *Starling curve of the pancreas* (43). Thus, the insulin-resistance state itself—not the accompanying compensatory hyperinsulinemia—is more important than hyperinsulinemia as a risk factor for atherosclerosis (55).

Insulin-resistant individuals who go on to develop type 2 diabetes become exposed also to the atherogenic effects of hyperglycemia (Fig. 7.1). Indeed, the atherogenic risk factor profile observed in insulin-resistance patients accounts for only a portion of the excess risk for CAD in patients with type 2 diabetes (15,62), indicating that hyperglycemia itself plays a central role in accelerating atherosclerosis in these patients. Because many years of asymptomatic hyperglycemia may precede the clinical diagnosis of type 2 diabetes, the duration of diabetes is frequently underestimated. Furthermore, the threshold above which hyperglycemia becomes atherogenic is unknown but may be in the range defined as impaired glucose tolerance (63). Despite these confounding factors, many population-based studies in patients with type 2 diabetes have shown a positive association between the degree of glycemic control and CAD morbidity and mortality in middle-aged and elderly type 2 diabetic subjects (64–66).

LIPOPROTEIN DISORDERS IN DIABETES

The metabolic abnormalities associated with types 1 and 2 diabetes result in profound changes in the transport, composition, and metabolism of lipoproteins. Lipoprotein metabolism is influenced by several factors including type of diabetes, glycemic control, obesity, insulin resistance, the presence of diabetic nephropathy, and genetic background (67). Abnormalities in plasma lipoprotein concentrations are commonly observed in diabetic individuals and contribute to the atherosclerotic process.

Lipoprotein Profile in Type 2 Diabetes

In contrast to type 1 diabetes, the pathophysiology of dyslipidemia in type 2 diabetes results from a complex relationship between hyperglycemia and the insulin-resistance state (67). An atherogenic pattern of lipoprotein changes (Table 7.1) is often present for years before the development of fasting hyperglycemia and the diagnosis of type 2 diabetes (70).

The typical lipoprotein profile associated with type 2 diabetes includes high triglycerides, low HDL levels, and normal LDL levels (Table 7.2). The most consistent change is an increase in VLDL-triglyceride levels (71,72). Population studies, including studies of the Pima Indians who have virtually no forms of genetic hyperlipidemia, indicate that type 2 diabetes generally produces only a 50% to 100% elevation of VLDL or total triglycerides (73). Thus, type 2 diabetic subjects with total triglycerides greater than 350 to 400 mg per dL probably have other genetic disorders in lipoprotein metabolism that may be exacerbated by diabetes. HDL levels are typically approximately 25% to 30% lower than in nondiabetic subjects and are commonly associated with other lipid and lipoprotein abnormalities, particularly high triglyceride levels.

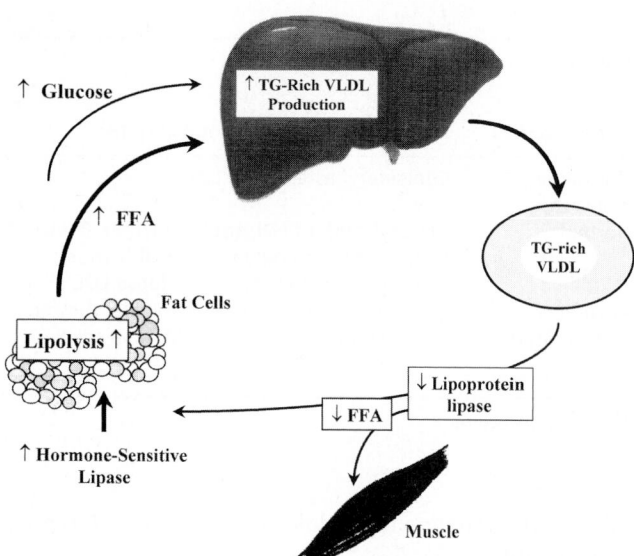

FIGURE 7.3 Mechanism of increased very-low-density lipoprotein (VLDL) triglyceride (TG) in diabetes. In the setting of insulin deficiency or insulin resistance, higher rates of glucose and free fatty acids (FFAs) flux to the liver lead to enhanced VLDL production and secretion. Decreased lipoprotein lipase activity contributes to the accumulation of these particles in the plasma.

Very-Low-Density Lipoprotein Metabolism in Diabetes

Hypertriglyceridemia in type 2 diabetes results from high fasting and postprandial triglyceride-rich lipoproteins, especially VLDL (71). Type 2 diabetic subjects with hypertriglyceridemia have both overproduction and impaired catabolism of VLDL (67,72). Increased VLDL production is almost uniformly present in patients with type 2 diabetes and hypertriglyceridemia (72). Increased VLDL production in diabetes is a consequence of an increase in free fatty acid mobilization (because maintenance of stored fat in adipose tissue depends on the suppression of hormone-sensitive lipase by insulin) and high glucose levels (74) (Fig. 7.3). Because free fatty acid availability is a major determinant of VLDL production by the liver, VLDL overproduction and hypertriglyceridemia occur (72).

The rest of the dyslipidemic phenotype that characterizes insulin resistance and type 2 diabetes (low HDL and small, dense LDL)—which has been termed *atherogenic lipoprotein phenotype* (50)—follows once VLDL secretion increases, mainly through the action of cholesteryl ester transfer protein and lipoprotein compositional changes that occur in plasma (75).

Increased fatty acid flux to the liver also results in the production of large triglyceride-rich VLDL particles because the size of VLDL is also mainly determined by the amount of triglyceride available. VLDL size is an important determinant of its metabolic fate. Large triglyceride-rich VLDL particles may be less efficiently converted to LDL (76), thereby increasing direct removal from the circulation

by non-LDL pathways. In addition, overproduction of large triglyceride-rich VLDL is associated with the atherogenic small, dense LDL subclass (50).

In type 2 diabetic subjects with more severe hypertriglyceridemia, VLDL clearance by lipoprotein lipase (LPL)—the rate-limiting enzyme responsible for the removal of plasma triglyceride-rich lipoproteins—is also impaired (71). LPL requires insulin for maintenance of normal tissue levels (77), and its activity is low in patients with poorly controlled type 2 diabetes (71). The result is enzymatic activity insufficient to match the overproduction rate, with further accumulation of VLDL triglyceride. ⬥ b58

High-Density Lipoprotein Metabolism in Diabetes

As in nondiabetic subjects, low HDL levels are powerful indicators of CHD in diabetic patients (50,78). Decreased HDL levels in diabetes result from decreased production and increased catabolism of HDL and are closely related to the abnormal metabolism of triglyceride-rich lipoproteins (71,72) (Fig. 7.4).

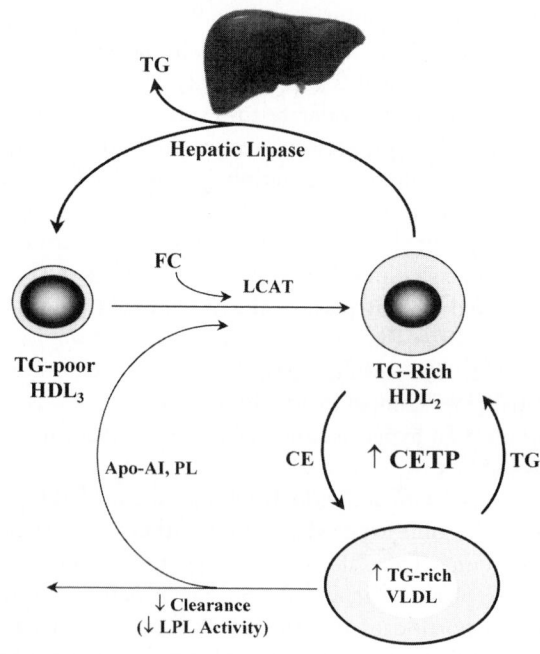

FIGURE 7.4 Mechanism of decreased high-density lipoprotein (HDL) in diabetes. The rate of HDL_2 formation is dependent on the rate of flux of surface components from lipolysis of triglyceride (TG)-rich lipoproteins. Inefficient low-density lipoprotein–mediated TG-rich lipoprotein catabolism reduces the rate of HDL_2 formation. Excess of TG-rich lipoproteins enhances cholesteryl ester transfer protein (CETP), resulting in the formation of HDL_2, which is a TG-rich particle that efficiently interacts with hepatic lipase. The result is the predominance of the small and dense HDL_3 in diabetic patients. A similar mechanism governs the predominance of small, dense species of low-density lipoprotein. Apo-AI, apolipoprotein AI; CE, cholesteryl ester; FC, free cholesterol; LCAT, lecithin-cholesterol acyltransferase; LPL, lipoprotein lipase.

During lipolysis of chylomicrons and VLDL, surface components (free cholesterol, redundant phospholipids, and apolipoproteins) are transferred into the HDL fraction. These components may enter nascent discoid HDL particles secreted by the liver. The free cholesterol is esterified by lecithin-cholesterol acyltransferase to generate mature spherical HDL. Alternatively, these surface components may be incorporated into preexisting HDL particles (see Chapter 3). The latter process results in an increase in size and decrease in density of HDL particles, leading to the conversion of preexisting HDL_3 (triglyceride depleted) to HDL_2.

Decreased HDL synthesis is related to the decreased LPL activity. Both genetic and acquired LPL (89) deficiencies are associated with low HDL because the rate of HDL_2 formation is dependent on the rate of flux of surface components from lipolysis of triglyceride-rich lipoprotein (Fig. 7.4). When LPL-mediated VLDL catabolism is inefficient, less surface material is transferred to HDL, impairing HDL formation.

Increased catabolism of HDL in diabetes can occur because increased secretion of VLDL into plasma promotes the transfer of triglycerides from these lipoproteins to HDL in exchange for cholesteryl ester. This exchange occurs in plasma and is facilitated by cholesteryl ester transfer protein, generating a triglyceride-enriched (and cholesteryl ester–depleted) HDL_2. This particle is highly susceptible to catabolism by hepatic triglyceride lipase (HTGL), an enzyme found primarily on endothelial cells of hepatic sinusoids (72,90). Hepatic triglyceride lipase has both triglyceride hydrolase and phospholipase activity and generates smaller HDL_3 particles that are depleted in triglycerides and phospholipids (Fig. 7.4).

Low-Density Lipoprotein Metabolism in Diabetes

As discussed, patients with types 1 and 2 diabetes in reasonable metabolic control have normal LDL cholesterol levels. However, although the absolute number of LDL particles is normal, alterations in LDL clearance and susceptibility to oxidative modification result in an increase in LDL atherogenic potential.

Low-Density Lipoprotein Composition and Insulin Resistance

In insulin-resistant patients with or without overt type 2 diabetes, the composition of LDL particles is altered, resulting in a preponderance of small, triglyceride-enriched and cholesterol-depleted particles (phenotype B). A preponderance of small, dense LDL particles is related to many characteristics of the insulin-resistance syndrome. In nondiabetic subjects, LDL subclass phenotype B is associated with other components of the insulin-resistance syndrome, including central obesity, hypertension, glucose intolerance, and hyperinsulinemia (91–93).

The formation of small, dense LDL in diabetes occurs in a similar fashion to the increased formation of small and dense HDL_3, as described previously. Cholesteryl ester transfer protein mediates the exchange of triglyceride from VLDL for cholesteryl ester in LDL. If sufficient LDL cholesteryl ester is replaced by triglyceride from VLDL, then when the particle comes into contact with hepatic lipase hydrolysis of newly acquired triglyceride in LDL and HDL by HTGL in turn decreases the size of LDL particles (94). The symmetry of the mechanisms for the formation of small, dense species of LDL and HDL (Fig. 7.4) helps to explain why low HDL levels and a preponderance of small dense LDL are both components of the insulin-resistance syndrome and why HDL cholesterol level is strongly correlated with LDL size (94).

Small, dense LDL has been associated with CAD risk independently of the absolute concentrations of LDL cholesterol or other CAD risk factors (50). Small, dense LDL particles are more susceptible to oxidative modification (95) and are particularly prone to induce endothelial dysfunction (96). In addition, there is enhanced arterial wall penetration by the small LDL particles (97).

Management of Dyslipidemia in Diabetic Patients

The American Diabetes Association recommendations for the management of hyperlipidemia in patients with diabetes generally follow the guidelines of the National Cholesterol Education Program (see Chapter 3) with several differences (106).

Nonpharmacologic strategies to treat dyslipidemia in diabetics include dietary modification (similar to those recommended by the National Cholesterol Education Program), weight loss, physical exercise, and improved glycemic control (106). In patients with type 1 diabetes, optimal glycemic control should result in normal or below normal lipoprotein levels (68) and prevent the atherogenic state associated with lipoprotein glycosylation. Improved diabetic control in type 2 diabetes is beneficial but not always associated with reversal of lipoprotein abnormalities (Table 7.3). Improved glycemic control using sulfonylurea, insulin (21), metformin (107), or thiazolidinediones (e.g., pioglitazone, rosiglitazone) (108) therapy often causes a substantial reduction (20% to 50%) in VLDL triglyceride levels. The magnitude of improvement in triglycerides generally correlates with the change in glucose levels rather than the mode of therapy. However, agents that improve insulin sensitivity such as metformin (107) and thiazolidinediones (108) lead to greater lowering of triglyceride compared with sulfonylurea. The effect of improved glycemic control on HDL is more variable and often

TABLE 7.3 ANTIHYPERLIPIDEMIC DRUG THERAPY IN DIABETIC PATIENTS

Drug	Therapeutic effect				Main indication	Special considerations
	Triglyceride level	LDL level	LDL size	HDL level		
Nicotinic acid	↓45%	↓15%	↑	↑15–30%	Generally not indicated	Adverse effect on glycemic control May be used in refractory dyslipidemias No adverse effect on glucose metabolism Increased risk for cholesterol gallstones
Fibric acid derivatives[a]	↓25–40%[b]	↓ or ↑[c]	↑	↑5–15%	Probably the drugs of choice for the treatment of hypertriglyceridemia	
3-Hydroxy-3-methyl-glutaryl-coenzyme A reductase inhibitors	↓10–25%[c]	↓25–30%	↑→[d]	↑5%	Drugs of choice for the treatment of hypercholesterolemia	
Bile acid resins	↑–↑↑	↓25%	→	→	Mixed dyslipidemias, in combination with fibric acid derivatives	Extreme elevations in triglyceride level occur mainly in patients who already had marked hypertriglyceridemia The only drug therapy recommended for children and adolescents Impaired absorption of several drugs, including glipizide

↑, Increased; ↑↑, markedly increased; ↓, decreased; →, no change.
[a]Studies using 600-mg twice per day gemfibrozil.
[b]Greatest reductions in patients with higher baseline levels.
[c]Depending on initial triglyceride concentrations (see text).
[d]Generally in relation to the magnitude of reduction in plasma triglyceride and very-low-density lipoprotein levels.

results in only a small increase (3 to 4 mg per dL) in HDL levels (21). ▼ b59

Drug Therapy

Antihyperlipidemic drug therapy in diabetic patients is similar to that in nondiabetic subjects (see Chapter 3) with several specific considerations (Table 7.3). 3-Hydroxy-3-methyl-glutaryl-coenzyme A (HMG-CoA) reductase inhibitors are highly effective in lowering cholesterol levels in type 2 diabetic patients in whom the principal finding is elevated LDL cholesterol level. They do not adversely affect glycemic control (21,109).

The fibric acid derivatives are effective in the treatment of hypertriglyceridemia in diabetic patients (110) (Table 7.3). These agents decrease VLDL levels, increase HDL, and can increase LDL particle size in hypertriglyceridemic patients with small, dense LDL particles (110). In the Helsinki Heart Study, gemfibrozil reduced the incidence of cardiovascular events in patients with type 2 diabetes (111). The Veterans Affairs High-Density Lipoprotein Cholesterol Intervention Trial randomized 2,531 patients with CHD (25% of whom had diabetes) with low HDL

cholesterol to gemfibrozil or placebo (112). Treatment with gemfibrozil over 5 years increased HDL 6% and reduced 22% of major coronary artery events, without lowering LDL cholesterol.

Fibric acid derivatives do not adversely affect glucose metabolism. In patients with normal triglyceride levels, these drugs lower LDL cholesterol by 5% to 15%. However, in hypertriglyceridemic patients, the decrease in triglyceride levels is frequently accompanied by an increase in LDL cholesterol levels (110). This increase probably reflects the elimination of small, dense LDL particles characteristic of the hypertriglyceridemic patients, resulting in less atherogenic LDL cholesterol (113).

Cholestyramine is efficacious in decreasing LDL cholesterol levels in diabetic patients (114). However, bile acid resins can increase VLDL triglycerides significantly, particularly if they are already elevated above 250 to 300 mg per dL or in patients with poorly controlled diabetes.

Nicotinic acid is the most effective drug in raising HDL levels in patients with hypertriglyceridemia and can increase particle size in patients with small, dense LDL particles (115). The use of nicotinic acid has been discouraged in patients with diabetes because of possible deterioration

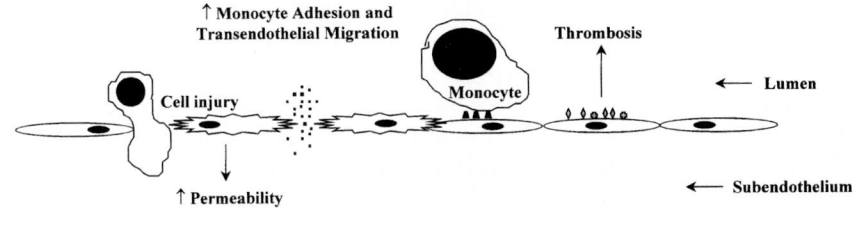

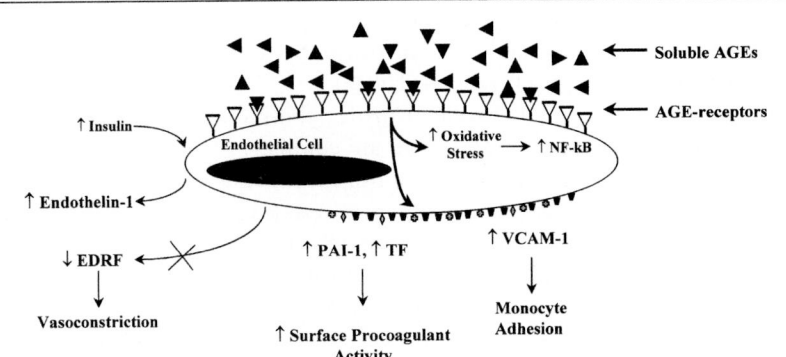

FIGURE 7.5 Generation of a dysfunctional endothelium in diabetes. See text for details. AGE, advanced glycosylation end product; EDRF, endothelium-derived relaxing factor; PAI-1, plasminogen activator inhibitor-1; TF, tissue factor; VCAM-1, vascular cell adhesion molecule-1.

in glycemic control (21,116) secondary to the induction of insulin resistance. In one study of patients with type 2 diabetes, a niacin dose of 4.5 g per day reduced plasma cholesterol levels by 24% and triglyceride levels by 45% and raised HDL cholesterol by 34%. However, the glycosylated hemoglobin level increased by 21% (116). In another study, niacin at a lower dose (3 g per day) produced a 8% reduction in LDL, a 23% reduction in triglycerides, and a 29% increase in HDL level, whereas HbA_{1c} increased by only 0.3% (117).

Niacin therapy may be considered as an alternative to statin drugs or fibrates in patients with diabetes in whom these agents are not tolerated, or in whom they fail to sufficiently correct hypertriglyceridemia or low HDL (117). Glycemic status should be carefully monitored during niacin therapy and the dose modified or discontinued if glycemic control deteriorates.

VASCULAR ENDOTHELIAL DYSFUNCTION IN DIABETES

Endothelial cells situated at the vessel wall–blood interface participate in a number of important homeostatic and cellular functions that protect from atherosclerosis and intraluminal thrombosis (*e*Table 7.3.1). Endothelial dysfunction can promote both the formation of atherosclerotic plaques and the occurrence of acute events. Endothelial *injury*, which results in endothelial *dysfunction*, has a critical role in the pathogenesis of atherosclerosis.

Endothelial dysfunction in diabetes entails profound perturbations in several critical functions of the endothelium (*e*Table 7.3.1, Fig. 7.5) that contribute to the initia-

tion and progression of the atherosclerotic process, as well as to the occurrence of clinical events.

Endothelial Permeability

The endothelial lining of the large arteries is of the continuous type characterized by tight junctions in the lateral borders, which restrict the movement of macromolecules from reaching the subendothelial space. Human vascular endothelial cells cultured in glucose concentrations comparable with those of uncontrolled diabetes exhibit delay in reaching confluence and in the rate of replication (118). Endothelial cell regeneration following deendothelialization (e.g., after balloon angioplasty) is slower (119). Endothelial cells in diabetic animals also exhibit morphologic abnormalities that include the presence of craters resulting from weakened intercellular junctions (120). Furthermore, AGEs, with their specific receptor, diminish endothelial barrier function (121,122). These abnormalities may explain the increased vascular permeability and transendothelial macromolecular transport (118).

DIABETES AS A PROTHROMBOTIC STATE

The coagulation and fibrinolytic systems are especially important in atherosclerosis because of the substantial contribution that mural thrombosis may make to the later stages of plaque progression, and because thrombotic occlusion plays a vital role in the development of clinical events. In the vast majority of cases, the fundamental mechanism in the development of potentially life-threatening events such as unstable angina or myocardial infarction is thrombosis arising at sites of plaque disruption. Not all disruptions of atherosclerotic plaques result in clinically apparent or symptomatic events. Thus, both local and systemic thrombogenic risk factors at the time of plaque disruption may determine the degree of thrombus formation; hence, the clinical outcome. Indeed, several hemostatic variables are powerful predictors of acute events in patients with established CAD (144–146).

Diabetes is characterized by a variety of individual alterations in the coagulation and fibrinolytic systems that combine to produce a prothrombotic state. These alterations include increased platelet functional behavior, increased levels of several coagulation components, and impaired fibrinolysis (*e*Table 7.3.2).

Platelet Aggregation

Platelet hyperaggregability, including the presence of spontaneous platelet aggregation (144) and increased platelet aggregability induced by conventional stimuli (145), increases the risk for cardiovascular events.

Platelets from diabetic subjects exhibit enhanced adhesiveness and hyperaggregability in response to both strong [e.g., thrombin, thromboxane A_2 (TxA_2)] and weak (e.g., adenosine diphosphate, epinephrine, collagen) agonists (147,148). Shear-induced platelet adhesion and aggregation are increased in diabetic patients (149). Platelet hypersensitivity is more evident in diabetic patients with vascular complications. However, it is also observed in newly diagnosed diabetic patients, suggesting that altered platelet function may be a consequence of metabolic changes secondary to the diabetic state (147,150). Elevated fractions of $CD62^+/CD63^+$ (activated) platelets circulate in diabetic patients in the absence of clinically detectable vascular lesions (148,151). Enhanced activity of the arachidonic acid pathway with increased TxA_2 formation occurs in diabetic individuals (152). There is a significant correlation between TxA_2 production and fasting plasma glucose or HbA_{1c}, and TxA_2 production can be restored by strict glycemic control with continuous subcutaneous insulin infusion.

Altered Fibrinolysis in Diabetes

The intensity of endogenous fibrinolysis depends on a dynamic equilibrium involving plasminogen activators, primarily tissue-type plasminogen activator, and inhibitors. The principal physiologic inhibitor of tissue-type plasminogen activator is plasminogen activator inhibitor-1 (PAI-1). Attenuated fibrinolysis caused by an increase of PAI-1 activity has been associated with increased risk for myocardial infarction in patients with established CAD (144,157).

Reduced plasma fibrinolytic activity caused by increased PAI-1 levels is a characteristic feature of insulin resistance

and hyperinsulinemia. Elevated concentrations of PAI-1 have been recognized consistently in the plasma of hyperinsulinemic type 2 diabetics (158) but occur also in normoglycemic insulin-resistant subjects (157,158). Increased plasma PAI-1 strongly correlates with parameters that define the insulin-resistance syndrome—in particular, body mass index and visceral accumulation of body fat, rather than with diabetes *per se* (158,159). Furthermore, interventions that lower insulin resistance, such as weight loss, are invariably accompanied by a reduction in plasma PAI-1 concentrations (160).

The mechanisms for the increased expression of PAI-1 in type 2 diabetes are complex. Insulin and especially proinsulin, a precursor of insulin, augment PAI-1 gene expression in hepatocytes resulting in an increased PAI-1 synthesis by the liver, which is the primary source of PAI-1 in plasma (161). Proinsulin levels are elevated in insulin-resistant subjects because of stimulation of pancreatic beta cells and in part because of the impaired processing of proinsulin to insulin that is typical of the condition. Exogenous insulin administration is accompanied by a decline in plasma PAI-1 levels, as stimulation of the pancreatic beta cells by hyperglycemia decreases. The production of PAI-1 by adipose tissue has been demonstrated and could be an important contributor to the elevated plasma PAI-1 levels observed in insulin-resistant patients (159). Hyperglycemia can also increase PAI-1 levels because it stimulates transcription of the PAI-1 gene through an effect on its promoter region (162).

HYPERGLYCEMIA AS AN ATHEROGENIC FACTOR

Hyperglycemia induces a large number of alterations in vascular tissue that potentially promote accelerated atherosclerosis. Currently, three major mechanisms have emerged that encompass most of the pathologic alterations observed in the vasculature of diabetic animals and humans: (a) nonenzymatic glycosylation of proteins and lipids; (b) oxidative stress; and (c) PKC activation. Importantly, these mechanisms are not independent. For example, hyperglycemia-induced oxidative stress promotes the formation of AGEs and PKC activation (166).

Role of Advanced Glycosylation End Products in Diabetic Atherosclerosis

One of the important mechanisms responsible for the accelerated atherosclerosis in diabetes is the nonenzymatic reaction between glucose and proteins or lipoproteins in arterial walls, collectively known as *Maillard's* or *browning reaction* (167). Glucose forms chemically reversible early glycosylation products with reactive amino groups of circulating or vessel wall proteins (Schiff's bases), which subse-

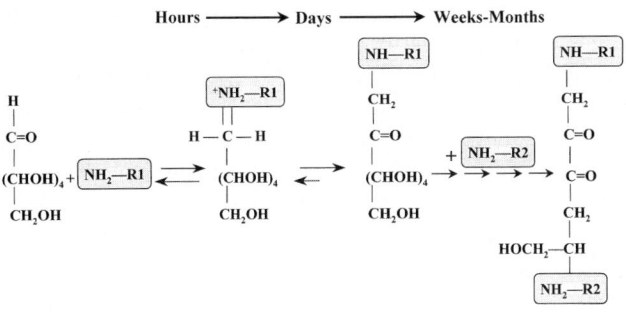

Hours ⟶ Days ⟶ Weeks-Months

| Glucose | Protein | Schiff Base | Amadori Product | Crosslinked AGE |

FIGURE 7.6 The formation of advanced glycosylation end product (AGE).

quently rearrange to form the more stable Amadori-type early glycosylation products. Equilibrium levels of Schiff-base and Amadori products (the best known of which is hemoglobin A_{1c}) are reached in hours and weeks, respectively (168) (Fig. 7.6). Some of the early glycosylation products on long-lived proteins (e.g., vessel wall collagen) continue to undergo complex series of chemical rearrangements to form AGEs (168). Once formed, AGE-protein adducts are stable and virtually irreversible. Although AGEs comprise a large number of chemical structures, carboxy-methyl-lysine-protein adducts are the predominant AGEs present *in vivo* (169).

AGEs accumulate continuously on long-lived vessel wall proteins with aging and at an accelerated rate in diabetes (168). The degree of nonenzymatic glycation is determined mainly by the glucose concentration and time of exposure (168). However, another critical factor to the formation of AGEs is the tissue microenvironment redox potential. Thus, AGEs formation increases substantially in situations in which the local redox potential has been shifted to favor oxidant stress (166,170–174).

TABLE 7.4 ATHEROSCLEROSIS PROMOTING EFFECTS OF ADVANCED GLYCOSYLATION END PRODUCTS: NON–RECEPTOR-MEDIATED MECHANISMS

Extracellular matrix
  Collagen cross-linking (176)
  Enhanced synthesis of extracellular matrix components (168)
  Trapping of LDL in the subendothelium (405)
  Glycosylated subendothelial matrix quenches nitric oxide (406)
Functional alterations of regulatory proteins
  Basic fibroblast growth factor glycosylation reduces its heparin binding capacity and its mitogenic activity on endothelial cells (407)
  Inactivation of the complement regulatory protein CD59 (175)
Lipoprotein modifications
  Glycosylated LDL (99,100)
  Reduced LDL recognition by cellular LDL receptors (98)
  Increased susceptibility of LDL to oxidative modification (99)

LDL, low-density lipoprotein.

TABLE 7.5 ATHEROSCLEROSIS PROMOTING EFFECTS OF ADVANCED GLYCOSYLATION END PRODUCTS: RECEPTOR-MEDIATED MECHANISMS

Promoting inflammation
  Secretion of cytokines such as tumor necrosis factor-α, interleukin-1 (176)
  Chemotactic stimulus for monocyte-macrophages (178,408)
Induction of cellular proliferation
  Stimulation of platelet-derived growth factor (408) and insulin-like growth factor I secretion from monocytes and possibly smooth muscle cells
Endothelial dysfunction
  Increased permeability of endothelial cell monolayers (121,409)
  Increased procoagulant activity (409)
  Increased expression of adhesion molecules (122)
  Increased intracellular oxidative stress (121,124)

AGEs can accelerate the atherosclerotic process by diverse mechanisms that can be classified as non–receptor dependent (Table 7.4) and receptor mediated (Table 7.5).

Non–Receptor-Mediated Mechanisms

Glycosylation-modified proteins and lipoproteins can interfere with their normal function (Table 7.4). Examples are the proatherogenic effect LDL glycosylation described previously (see Low-Density Lipoprotein Metabolism in Diabetes) and glycation of the complement regulatory protein. Deposition of the membrane attack complex of complement (MAC) in blood vessels stimulates proliferation of fibroblasts and smooth muscle cells, in part by releasing growth factors such as fibroblast growth factor and platelet-derived growth factor from MAC-targeted endothelium. MAC deposition is normally restricted because cells express the regulatory membrane protein CD59, which limits complement activation and MAC formation. Glycation of the complement regulatory protein CD59 results in its inactivation (175) and may increase the sensitivity of the diabetic endothelium to MAC-induced release of growth factors and cytokines.

Another important consequence of AGEs formation is the ability to cross-link adjacent proteins. For example, collagen can become cross-linked because AGEs form covalent heat-stable intermolecular bonds (176) (*e*Fig. 7.6.1). The amount of cross-linked collagen peptides formed increases as a function of both time and glucose concentration (176). In contrast to normal cross-links within normal collagen, which occur only at two discrete sites at the N-terminal and C-terminal ends of the molecule, AGEs form cross-links throughout the collagen molecule (168). Collagen cross-linking plays an important role in changing the mechanical properties of tissues, leading to the increased vascular rigidity and the reduced left ventricular compliance in diabetic patients (see Diabetic Cardiomyopathy).

Glycosylation of matrix components such as collagen VI, laminin, and vitronectin decreased binding of anionic heparan sulfate, leading to greater turnover of heparan sulfate (168). The absence of heparan sulfate is thought to stimulate a compensatory overproduction of other matrix components through altered partitioning of growth regulatory factors between matrix-bound proteoglycans and cells (168). AGEs on matrix also alter the normal interactions of transmembrane integrin receptors with three specific matrix ligands. For example, modification of the cell-binding domains of type IV collagen causes decreased endothelial cell adhesion (168).

OXIDATIVE STRESS

Oxidative stress is widely invoked as a pathogenic mechanism for atherosclerosis. Among the sequelae of hyperglycemia, oxidative stress has been suggested as a potential mechanism for accelerated atherosclerosis (166,187,195). Importantly, there appears to be a strong pathogenic link between hyperglycemia-induced oxidant stress and other hyperglycemia-dependent mechanisms of vascular damage, namely AGEs formation and PKC activation (Fig. 7.7).

Hyperglycemia can increase oxidative stress through several pathways. A major mechanism appears to be the hyperglycemia-induced intracellular reactive oxygen species, produced by the proton electromechanical gradient generated by the mitochondrial electron transport chain and resulting in increased production of superoxide (166).

Two other mechanisms have been proposed that may explain how hyperglycemia causes increased reactive oxygen species formation. One mechanism involves the transition metal-catalyzed autoxidation of free glucose, as described in cell-free systems. Through this mechanism, glucose itself initiates an autoxidative reaction and free radical production yielding superoxide anion (O_2^-) and hydrogen peroxide (H_2O_2) (196). The other mechanism involves the transition metal-catalyzed autoxidation of protein-bound Amadori products, which yields superoxide and hydroxyl radicals and highly reactive dicarbonyl compounds (195) (see Glycoxidation).

There is also evidence that hyperglycemia may compromise natural antioxidant defenses. Under normal circumstances, free radicals are rapidly eliminated by antioxidants such as reduced glutathione, vitamin C, and vitamin E. Reduced glutathione content (197), as well as reduced vitamin E (198), have been reported in diabetic patients. Plasma and tissue levels of vitamin C are 40% to 50% lower in diabetic patients compared with nondiabetic subjects (199).

Glycoxidation

Some of the individual advanced glycosylation products such as Nε-(carboxymethyl)lysine and pentosidine are formed in reactions of protein with glucose only under oxidative conditions (172,200,201). Thus, some AGEs are produced by combined processes of glycation and oxidation and have been termed *glycoxidation products* (187). Each AGE structure has its own formation mechanism and thus its own dependence on oxidative stress. However, because glycoxidation products on proteins are irreversible, it has been suggested that they may be an integrative biomarker for the accumulated oxidative stress to which the respective tissue has been exposed (171,195).

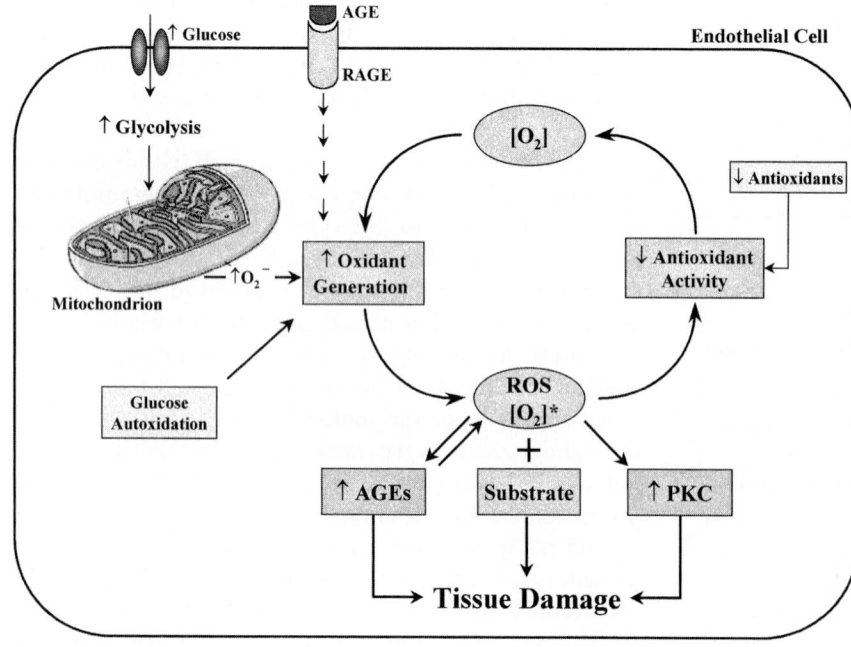

FIGURE 7.7 Relationship between rates of oxidant generation, antioxidant activity, oxidative stress, and oxidative damage in diabetes. *[O₂]** represents various forms of reactive oxygen species (ROS). The overall rate of formation of oxidative products leading to oxidative tissue damage is dependent on ambient levels of both *[O₂]** and substrate. Increased generation of *[O₂]** depends on several sources, including glucose autoxidation, increased mitochondrial superoxide production, and as a result of the receptor for advanced glycosylation end products activation. *[O₂]** deactivation is reduced because antioxidant defenses are compromised in diabetes. Note that oxidative stress also promotes other hyperglycemia-induced mechanisms of tissue damage. Oxidative stress activates protein kinase C (PKC) and accelerates the formation of advanced glycosylation end products (AGEs).

As previously discussed, the interaction between AGE epitopes and the cell surface AGE receptor upregulate oxidative stress response genes (124) and release oxygen radicals (202). Thus, hyperglycemia simultaneously enhances both AGEs formation and oxidative stress, and the mutual facilitatory interactions between glycation and oxidation chemistry can contribute synergistically to the formation of AGEs, oxidative stress, and diabetic complications (Fig. 7.7). Indeed, there are strong correlations between levels of glycoxidation products in skin collagen and the severity of diabetic retinal, renal, and vascular disease (203).

EFFECT OF OTHER CARDIOVASCULAR RISK FACTORS ON CORONARY ARTERY DISEASE RISK IN DIABETIC PATIENTS

Prospective studies indicate that all of the major cardiovascular risk factors continue to act as independent contributors to CAD in diabetic patients (2,206,207). Standard cardiovascular risk factors account for at least two-thirds of the excess risk from cardiovascular disease in diabetic subjects. In general, for any given degree of abnormality, individuals with diabetes have two to four times greater risk of developing CAD than individuals without diabetes (2).

Hypercholesterolemia

The U.K. Prospective Diabetes Study (UKPDS), including 2,693 patients with newly diagnosed type 2 diabetes, evaluated the significance of all major cardiovascular risk factors for CAD by stepwise multivariate Cox analysis (64). The most important risk factor for CAD—fatal and nonfatal myocardial infarction, angina pectoris—was high LDL cholesterol, followed by low HDL cholesterol, and HbA_{1c}. These results emphasize the contribution of concomitant classic risk factors for CAD in diabetic patients.

Hypertension

Hypertension occurs approximately twice as frequently in patients with diabetes as in the general population (208,209). Isolated systolic hypertension is considerably more common in diabetics. Type 1 diabetes mellitus is associated with hypertension only when albuminuria and early nephropathy develop, but type 2 diabetes mellitus may be associated with hypertension at or even preceding diagnosis (208,209).

The combined presence of hypertension and diabetes considerably accelerates the development of both macrovascular and microvascular diabetic complications. However, the most significant manifestation of this combination of diseases is that they confer a greater risk of ischemic heart disease, stroke, and peripheral vascular disease in affected individuals (208–211). The high cardiovascular risk associated with the coexistence of hypertension and diabetes led the Joint National Committee on Prevention, Detection, Evaluation, and Treatment of High Blood Pressure to include hypertensive patients with diabetes in the same risk group as hypertensive patients who have clinically manifest cardiovascular disease (212). These patients should be considered for prompt pharmacologic therapy, even if they have high-normal blood pressure (212).

Pharmacologic Therapy of Hypertension in Diabetic Patients

Current evidence suggests that for the prevention of cardiovascular events, ACE inhibitors (213,214), low-dose diuretics (215), or beta-adrenergic blockers (216) are the preferred first-line agents for hypertensive patients with diabetes, whereas a controversy exists with regard to the efficacy of calcium antagonists in preventing cardiovascular complications (217). In the Appropriate Blood Pressure Control in Diabetes trial, patients in the nisoldipine group had a fivefold higher risk of fatal and nonfatal acute myocardial infarction than did the enalapril group (213). The Swedish Trial in Old Patients with Hypertension 2 reported that ACE inhibitors were superior to calcium channel blockers in preventing myocardial infarction and congestive heart failure (CHF) in the subgroup of elderly patients with diabetes (218).

In the Fosinopril versus Amlodipine Cardiovascular Events Randomized Trial patients receiving fosinopril had half the risk of the combined outcome of acute myocardial infarction, stroke, or hospitalized angina than those receiving amlodipine (214). However, the combined therapy resulted in a lower incidence of cardiovascular events than either treatment alone and could be interpreted as evidence that combination therapy is a safe strategy (219). These results are important because hypertension control is not achieved by monotherapy in many diabetic patients, as demonstrated in Appropriate Blood Pressure Control in Diabetes trial (213) and UKPDS (216).

The Systolic Hypertension in Europe study compared outcomes of treatments with nitrendipine versus placebo in patients with isolated systolic hypertension. Endpoint reduction achieved by active treatment was significantly larger in the diabetic subgroup (–69% vs. –26% cardiovascular events), indicating a remarkable benefit from first-line treatment with a calcium antagonist (220). Similarly, the results of the Hypertension Optimal Treatment trial showed a reduction of myocardial infarction event rates in diabetic patients (n = 1,501, representing the largest calcium antagonist trial in diabetic patients) using the long-acting dihydropyridine calcium antagonist felodipine (221).

In the UKPDS, no difference was found between atenolol and captopril (216). In the Captopril Prevention Project study, no difference in outcomes was noted between subjects receiving a combination of diuretic and beta-blockers and those receiving captopril. By contrast, in the subgroup of patients with diabetes, captopril was associated with an approximately 40% decrease in the primary end point, fatal and nonfatal myocardial infarction, stroke, and cardiovascular deaths (222).

The evidence for aggressive antihypertensive treatment in patients with diabetes, hypertension, and nephropathy is now overwhelming (223,224). ACE inhibitors are particularly useful in this population, with clear evidence that these agents reduced the progression of kidney dysfunction and the number of patients who will develop end-stage renal failure (225–227). Furthermore, the UKPDS indicated that among patients with hypertension and type 2 diabetes, aggressive lowering of blood pressure (mean, 144/82 mm Hg vs. 154/87 mm Hg), either with ACE inhibitors or a beta-blocker, provides greater protection against death from cardiovascular causes and major nonfatal events than did less aggressive therapy (228) (*e*Fig. 7.7.1). A similar benefit was observed in the Hypertension Optimal Treatment study among hypertensive patients with diabetes, who were randomly assigned to intensive therapy with calcium channel blockers (221). In summary, ACE inhibitors appear to be the preferred antihypertensive therapy in diabetic patients, but other antihypertensive agents are also effective in reducing cardiovascular mortality and morbidity. In addition, aggressive blood pressure reduction may be more important than the specific agent being used.

The sixth report of the Joint National Committee on Prevention, Detection, Evaluation, and Treatment of High Blood Pressure has incorporated these principles for the treatment of hypertension in the presence of diabetes and has included a more aggressive program of blood pressure reduction, aiming for a target of less than 130/85 mm Hg in both type 1 and type 2 diabetic patients (212,229). In addition, the guidelines included a target of 125/75 mm Hg in patients with greater than 1 g per day proteinuria (212,223,224).

DIABETIC PATIENT WITH AN ACUTE ISCHEMIC EVENT

Acute ischemic events represent a major cause of death in the diabetic population (281). Diabetics who suffer myocardial infarction have a higher mortality than nondiabetic subjects both in the acute phase and on long-term follow-up (105).

Acute Myocardial Infarction

Numerous studies have shown that in-hospital mortality from myocardial infarction in diabetic patients is 1.5- to 2.0-fold higher than in nondiabetic patients (9,256,282,283). Diabetic women have a particularly poor prognosis, with an almost twofold increase in mortality compared with diabetic men (9,256,282,283).

Diabetes mellitus remains an independent predictor for a poor prognosis in the thrombolytic era. In the Thrombolysis and Angioplasty in Myocardial Infarction trials, the in-hospital mortality was nearly twice as high in patients with diabetes, with more CHF and twice the rate of clinically recognized reinfarction (9). In the GUSTO-I trial, mortality at 30 days was highest among diabetic patients treated with insulin (12.5%) compared with non–insulin-treated diabetic (9.7%) and nondiabetic (6.2%) patients (284). Similar results have been reported from the other large studies (285,286). Diabetes is also a risk factor for cardiogenic shock in the setting of acute ischemic syndromes (287). Despite the overall improvement in survival from an acute myocardial infarction with thrombolysis, the in-hospital mortality in diabetics remains 1.5 to 2.0 times higher than in nondiabetic subjects (9,284,286). Primary angioplasty appears to be an effective alternative to thrombolysis in diabetic patients (288,289).

The excess in-hospital mortality in diabetics correlates primarily with an increased incidence of CHF (105,256,282,283), although increased reinfarction, infarct extension, and recurrent ischemia also contribute (256,290,291).

CHF and cardiogenic shock are more common and more severe in diabetic subjects than would be predicted from the size of the index infarction (282,283,286). Indeed, studies using serial determinations of total creatine kinase activity, radionuclide ventriculography, or echocardiography have shown no evidence that diabetic patients sustain more extensive infarctions than their nondiabetic counterparts (105). However, a reduction in both left ventricular ejection fraction (256) and the regional ejection fraction of the noninfarcted myocardium occurs in diabetic patients following myocardial infarction compared with nondiabetic subjects. For example, early angiography in the Thrombolysis and Angioplasty in Myocardial Infarction trials has demonstrated worse noninfarct zone ventricular function in diabetics (9). These findings can be ascribed to several additional pathogenic processes that reduce the ability of the noninfarcted myocardium to compensate (Fig. 7.8). The observation that clinical manifestations of heart failure occur in diabetic patients despite a modest decrease in left ventricular ejection fraction led to the suggestion that preexisting diastolic dysfunction is a major culprit of the congestive symptoms (256). Subclinical diabetic cardiomyopathy, in which the salient finding is diastolic dysfunction (see Diabetic Cardiomyopathy) is likely to be an important factor in this setting.

The performance of the left ventricle following myocardial infarction is largely determined by the extent of coronary disease and the quality of collateral circulation. Thus, the diffuse nature of coronary atherosclerosis in diabetes may contribute to systolic dysfunction of the noninfarcted myocardium. Moreover, diabetic patients have a reduced ability to develop collateral blood vessels in the presence of

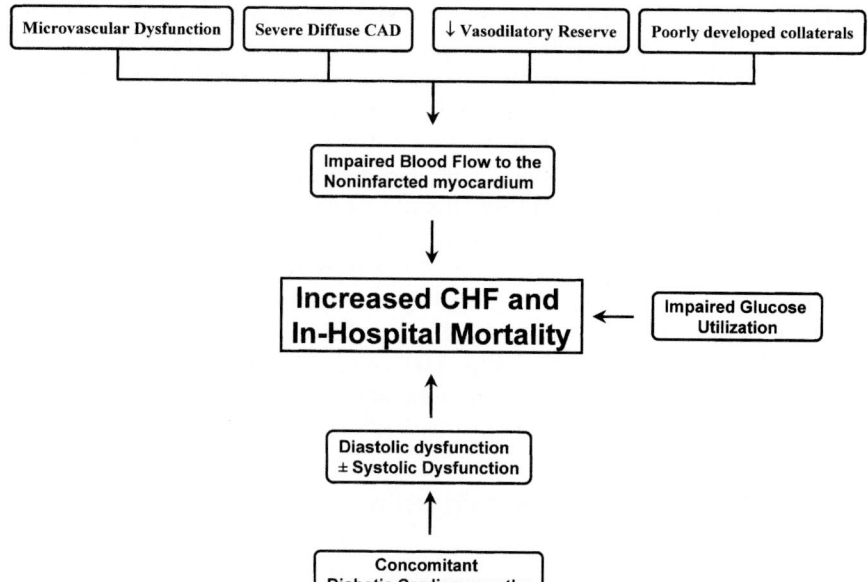

FIGURE 7.8 Factors promoting in-hospital and long-term mortality of diabetic patients following myocardial infarction. CAD, coronary artery disease; CHF, congestive heart failure.

CAD (292), a finding that may also explain the more frequent occurrence of postinfarction angina and infarct extension (105,256,291). Finally, an altered pattern of exogenous substrate use during ischemia and in the postreperfusion period may result in increased oxygen consumption by the myocardium and reduced contractility and may prevent myocardial preservation (see Abnormal Myocardial Substrate Metabolism).

Long-Term Outcome of Diabetic Patients after Myocardial Infarction

Diabetic patients surviving myocardial infarction suffer from higher late mortality than do their nondiabetic counterparts (256,291,293). Late mortality is mainly related to recurrent myocardial infarction and the development of new CHF (104,286).

Survival and recurrent cardiovascular events in diabetic patients after myocardial infarction are closely related to the following categories of risk: (a) extent of global pump dysfunction following the infarct; (b) multivessel CAD; (c) the diabetic hematologic milieu (see Diabetes as a Prothrombotic State); and (d) diabetic autonomic neuropathy, which may predispose to sudden death, especially in postinfarct patients (see Diabetic Autonomic Neuropathy and the Heart).

Medical Therapy in Diabetic Patients with Myocardial Infarction

Diabetic patients treated with fibrinolytic agents benefit by the same mortality reduction as nondiabetic patients (9,105,294). In an overview of fibrinolytic trials in patients with myocardial infarction, the proportion reduction in 35-day mortality was slightly, but not significantly, greater in

diabetic patients than in nondiabetic patients (21.7% vs. 14.3%) (294). Importantly, no increase in serious bleeding complications or stroke has been observed in diabetics (9,285,294). Retinal bleeding is an extremely uncommon complication of thrombolytic therapy in diabetic patients. In the GUSTO-I study, 300 of 6,011 diabetic patients had proliferative retinopathy, but none developed intraocular hemorrhage (295). It is unlikely that thrombolytic therapy would increase vitreous hemorrhage, which is caused by vitreous detachment in patients with diabetic retinopathy. Thus, the concern that many clinicians have with regard to thrombolytic therapy in patients with diabetic retinopathy is not supported by the results of large clinical trials. It is probably unjustified to deny these patients the proven life-saving benefit of thrombolysis.

Beta-blockers are effective in reducing reinfarction and sudden death in diabetic patients, perhaps to a greater extent than in nondiabetic subjects (296–298). Early treatment of myocardial infarction with beta-blockers resulted in a 37% mortality reduction in diabetics compared with a 13% mortality reduction in all patients, whereas long-term mortality reduction was 48% and 33% in diabetics and all patients, respectively (296). Deterioration in glycemic control or blunted counterregulatory response to hypoglycemia are seldom a serious clinical problem, especially when cardioselective beta$_1$-blockers are used (296).

ACE inhibition is unequivocally associated with a substantial mortality reduction in patients surviving myocardial infarction with left ventricular dysfunction (ejection fraction less than 40%) (299). The GISSI-3 investigators compared the effect of early administration (within 24 hours of admission) of lisinopril in patients with and without diabetes presenting with myocardial infarction (300). Compared with placebo, lisinopril dramatically reduced both 6-week (30%

vs. 5%) and 6-month (20% vs. 0%) mortality in diabetics versus nondiabetic subjects. These findings are corroborated by a retrospective analysis using data from the Trandolapril Cardiac Evaluation study, a randomized, double-blind, placebo-controlled trial evaluating trandolapril in patients after acute myocardial infarction with an ejection fraction less than or equal to 35%; it showed a 36% reduction of death from any cause and a 62% reduction in the risk of progression to severe heart failure (301). ACE inhibitors do not adversely affect glycemic control and lipid profile (3,208). In fact, ACE inhibitors may actually enhance insulin sensitivity in type 2 diabetic patients (302).

The Antiplatelet Trialists' Collaboration metaanalysis quantified the benefit of aspirin in diabetic patients who have had a previous cardiovascular event (303). The relative benefit on vascular events was 17% in the diabetic patients and 22% in those without diabetes. Although the number was lower for diabetic patients than for nondiabetic patients in terms of percentage benefit, the absolute number of events prevented was similar in the two groups (38 ± 12 per thousand compared with 36 ± 3 per thousand, respectively), probably because of the higher event rates in diabetic patients.

Unstable Angina in Diabetic Patients

Of all patients presenting with unstable angina, 20% to 25% have diabetes (163,304). Diabetes is an important risk factor for an adverse outcome (e.g., death, infarction, or readmission with unstable angina at 1 year; relative risk, 4.9) (164). Hospitalization for unstable angina or non–Q-wave myocardial infarction predicts a high 2-year morbidity and mortality in patients with diabetes. Diabetic patients with no previous cardiovascular disease have the same long-term morbidity and mortality as nondiabetic patients with established cardiovascular disease after hospitalization for unstable CAD (163).

These observations may be related to the higher proportion of ulcerated plaque (94% vs. 60%) and intracoronary thrombi (94% vs. 55%) observed by angioscopy in diabetic patients presenting with unstable angina (13). Coronary tissue obtained from culprit lesions of diabetic patients with unstable angina or myocardial infarction exhibit a larger content of lipid-rich atheroma, macrophage infiltration, and a higher incidence of coronary thrombus, which occupies a larger area (305).

CORONARY REVASCULARIZATION IN DIABETIC PATIENTS

Because CAD is a major health problem in patients with diabetes, the need for revascularization procedures arises frequently. An increasing proportion of patients undergoing angioplasty are diabetics. In the 1977 to 1981 National Heart, Lung, and Blood Institute registry, 9% of patients undergoing angioplasty were diabetics (318). More recent large trials indicate that the prevalence of diabetes in patients undergoing angioplasty has increased to 17% to 26% (319).

Studies performed in the last decade have evaluated the relative efficacy of revascularization methods in diabetic patients. These studies reveal unique problems in diabetic patients, including higher periprocedural complication rates, a greater incidence of restenosis following successful angioplasty, and adverse long-term outcome after percutaneous and surgical revascularization, especially in the presence of multivessel disease, and suggest that the determination of optimal revascularization in these patients requires special attention.

Coronary Angioplasty

Procedural Outcomes and Complication Rates

In general, procedural success rates and completeness of revascularization do not significantly differ between diabetics and nondiabetic subjects (10,320–323). In-hospital complication (of death, infarction, and need for emergency surgery) rates have been reported to be higher in diabetic patients undergoing balloon angioplasty (10,320) and stenting (323). With stenting, a trend toward higher rates of subacute stent thrombosis was reported (323,324).

These differences are small and have not been confirmed in all studies. Based on data from the EPILOG study, Kleiman et al. concluded that with current angioplasty techniques, the in-hospital event rates for diabetic patients are comparable with those for nondiabetic patients (325). However, when acute ischemic complications occur during angioplasty, they may be poorly tolerated by diabetic patients, leading to a higher rate of periprocedural death (326).

Long-Term Results: Restenosis

Long-term outcomes have been disappointing because of the greater incidence of restenosis following successful angioplasty and adverse long-term outcome, especially in the presence of multivessel disease. The importance of diabetes as a consistent clinical predictor for restenosis after percutaneous transluminal coronary angioplasty (PTCA) has been demonstrated in multiple studies. The initial report from the National Heart, Lung, and Blood Institute Angioplasty Registry (327) that the angiographic restenosis rate in diabetic patients was 47%, as compared with 32% in nondiabetic patients, was subsequently confirmed by many other studies that reported restenosis rates of 49% to 68% among diabetic patients undergoing balloon angioplasty (328–330). Diabetes is also a clinical predictor for restenosis with other percutaneous revascularization techniques, such as excimer laser angioplasty (331) and coronary atherectomy (321).

Intracoronary stents decrease restenosis compared with balloon angioplasty. However, even with stent use, the majority of studies has shown higher restenosis rates, compared with nondiabetic patients (324,332–335).

The full impact of the higher postangioplasty restenosis rates on the cardiovascular morbidity of diabetic patients is significant. Numerous studies have shown that diabetic patients experience a greater need than their nondiabetic counterparts for repeat revascularization [angioplasty or coronary artery bypass graft (CABG)], a high cardiac event rate, and lower overall survival rates after either balloon angioplasty (10,320,321,336) or stenting (333–335).

Whereas restenosis may explain the higher repeat angioplasty and CABG rates among diabetics, the exact relationship between restenosis and recurrent events or increased mortality is more complex. The majority of ischemic events outside the time frame of restenosis appears to be disease progression at other coronary sites rather than late restenosis at the original treatment site. Notwithstanding, percutaneous interventions may affect long-term prognosis through other mechanisms, including increased incidence of heart failure (330) and distal embolization (337). In a study of 485 consecutive patients with diabetes undergoing balloon angioplasty without stenting, at least one vessel with restenosis was found in 68% of patients (330). Many of these occlusions were clinically silent, with no angina in 36% and stable angina in 33% of patients. Occlusions were associated with a significant decrease in left ventricular function.

Because of the diffuse atherosclerotic process, poor collateralization, and preexisting microvascular dysfunction, diabetic patients may have reduced adaptive capacity for embolization during percutaneous interventions (337). Studies suggest that the combination of abciximab and stent placement reduces periprocedural myocardial infarction and short-term mortality (338,339). The beneficial effect of abciximab may be related to the reduction of distal embolization at the time of stenting (338,339). Target vessel revascularization rates were not different, suggesting that the risk for restenosis is not affected (338).

Mechanism of Coronary Artery Bypass Graft Protection

Two major mechanisms have been suggested to explain the apparent superiority of CABG over multivessel balloon angioplasty in diabetic patients: (a) high restenosis rates after angioplasty with incomplete revascularization of ischemic territories (336,361); and (b) accelerated progression of atherosclerosis of native arteries or SVGs (362).

Restenosis with Incomplete Revascularization

Previous CABG studies have shown that complete revascularization, which is accomplished almost exclusively through CABG surgery, is essential for obtaining survival benefit in

patients with multivessel disease (363). The superiority of CABG over angioplasty in providing complete revascularization is exemplified in the BARI study itself. In the BARI population, 3.1 grafts were placed per patient undergoing CABG (364), whereas the mean number of successfully treated lesions in the PTCA group was 2.0 (322). Similar numbers are reported by other studies comparing multivessel angioplasty and CABG (336,357,365). In the Emory cohort, revascularization was achieved in 16% of patients undergoing PTCA, and 80% in the CABG group (365). In the study by Gum et al., complete revascularization was accomplished in 79% of patients undergoing CABG and in 42% of the angioplasty group (*p* <.001) (336).

Given the suboptimal revascularization with multivessel angioplasty compared with CABG, successful application of multivessel angioplasty—which entails a selective high-priority lesion-targeting strategy—requires that a comparable proportion of myocardium supplied through high-priority lesions be revascularized by each of the two strategies. Given the high restenosis rates in diabetic patients, and because when multivessel angiography is preformed, multiple treatment sites can become restenosed independently, it is likely that this goal is frequently not achieved in diabetic patients. Thus, the worse outcome of diabetic patients undergoing PTCA may be mediated in part by the frequent occurrence of incomplete revascularization (336,361). The effect of incomplete revascularization may be even more severe in view of the more diffuse and distal CAD (9–11,320,322), poor collateral development (292), and microcirculatory dysfunction in diabetic patients (see Vascular Endothelial Dysfunction in Diabetes).

The BARI investigators have analyzed the outcome of BARI-eligible patients, a larger group that included randomized patients and 2,010 additional eligible patients who declined randomization (361). This report identified two mechanisms for the protective effect of CABG in diabetes: (a) a strong protective effect with respect to survival in a small group of patients who sustained a Q-wave myocardial infarction, accounting for approximately 50% of the overall reduction in mortality attributable to the procedure; and (b) a moderate constant reduction in mortality throughout follow-up that occurred in the majority of diabetic patients who remained free of myocardial infarction during follow-up (*e*Fig. 7.8.1). A steadily increasing advantage of CABG compared with PTCA was also apparent at 7-year follow-up (366). These protective effects were not present in nondiabetic patients (361).

Accelerated Atherosclerosis Progression

It has been suggested that accelerated progression of atherosclerosis leading to new plaque ruptures located within the native coronary arteries or vein grafts of diabetic patients accounts for the poor long-term prognosis after multivessel angioplasty (362). Bypass surgery offers some protection from atherosclerosis progression in native arteries by providing a bypass conduit beyond the epicardial coronary segment most vulnerable to future plaque development (usually within the proximal 6 cm of epicardial coronary arteries) (362). However, progression of native CAD in postbypass patients is mainly related to dyslipidemia (352). Currently, there is no evidence that in the group of patients who already have an advanced atherosclerotic process (multivessel disease) continued progression is more rapid in the presence of diabetes. Likewise, progression of vein graft atherosclerosis is mainly related to hypercholesterolemia, and aggressive lipid-lowering therapy reduces the progression of atherosclerosis in vein grafts (367), whereas the effect of diabetes on the accelerated atherosclerotic process that characterizes vein grafts is still unclear (see Vein Grafts). Indeed, in the BARI trial, the type of revascularization had no influence on the incidence of Q-wave myocardial infarction during follow-up (361). In a large study comparing the outcomes of 9,920 patients without diabetes and 2,278 diabetic patients after CABG surgery, there was no difference in myocardial infarction rates at 5 and 10 years (347). Of note is the fact that in post-CABG patients with evolving infarction, approximately two-thirds of culprit lesions are located within vein grafts (368).

Although the incidence of plaque disruption leading to a clinical acute coronary event is probably not affected, a greater proportion of the myocardium may become ischemic because of incomplete revascularization with PTCA. This is particularly important given the high long-term incidence of both fatal and nonfatal events among diabetic patients (10,320,322,361,365). For example, in the BARI study, although CABG offered no protection from myocardial infarction, patients with diabetes were 1.9 times as likely as those without diabetes to have a spontaneous (non–procedure-related) Q-wave myocardial infarction at 5 years (361).

DIABETIC AUTONOMIC NEUROPATHY AND THE HEART

Although clinically apparent autonomic neuropathy (e.g., orthostatic hypotension and gastroparesis) generally occurs only in patients with diabetes of long duration, it has become evident that subclinical diabetic autonomic neuropathy, mainly in the form of cardiac autonomic neuropathy (CAN), evolves early in the course of diabetes (376) and in the absence of other microvascular complications (377). CAN is extremely common in both type 1 and type 2 diabetes, affecting up to 60% of unselected populations (376,378).

CAN involves parasympathetic dysfunction (379) as well as derangements of adrenergic cardiac innervation as assessed by myocardial meta-[^{123}I]iodobenzylguanidine

scintigraphy (380). The presence of CAN in diabetic patients has been linked to increased risk of arrhythmias, cardiovascular events, and a high prevalence of silent ischemia and infarction (*e*Fig. 7.8.3).

Silent Ischemia

The propensity of diabetic patients to present with silent or unrecognized myocardial infarction is well established (394). In the Framingham Study, a higher proportion of myocardial infarctions in diabetic patients was silent and unrecognized (395). Atypical symptoms such as confusion, dyspnea, fatigue, or nausea and vomiting were the presenting complaint in 32% to 42% of diabetic patients with myocardial infarction compared with 6% to 15% of nondiabetic patients. More recently, failure to use reperfusion therapy was observed in diabetic patients (396), which may be attributable, in part, to an atypical presentation.

Although silent ischemia frequently can be demonstrated in nondiabetic patients, several studies have shown that, whether assessed by treadmill exercise testing (377), ambulatory Holter monitoring, or exercise thallium scintigraphy (397,398), silent ischemia is more common in diabetic than in nondiabetic subjects. This finding, however, is not supported by all studies (399). For example, in the Asymptomatic Cardiac Ischemia Pilot study, there was a similar prevalence of asymptomatic ischemia during exercise treadmill testing and 48-hour ambulatory electrocardiographic monitoring (399).

Autonomic neuropathy with involvement of the sensory supply to the heart is a plausible explanation for painless infarction and ischemia episodes in diabetic subjects. In autopsies of diabetic patients who died of silent myocardial infarction, typical diabetic neuropathic changes were found in the intracardiac sympathetic and parasympathetic fibers (400), and several studies correlated abnormalities in autonomic function in patients with silent ischemia (377,401). The anginal perceptual threshold—the time from the onset of myocardial ischemia (assessed by ST-segment depression) to the onset of chest pain during exercise testing—is prolonged in diabetic patients compared with nondiabetic subjects. This delay in the perception of pain is related to the impairment of autonomic nervous function (401).

CONTROVERSIES AND PERSONAL PERSPECTIVES

In the last two decades, the advent of effective therapies of hypertension and hypercholesterolemia resulted in a substantial reduction in mortality and morbidity associated with these risk factors for CAD. Diabetes remains a major risk factor for which the optimal therapy has not been established and is increasingly becoming a research focus in the field of preventive and clinical cardiology.

THE FUTURE

Basic and clinical research should be directed to elucidate the unique mechanisms causing accelerated atherosclerosis in insulin-resistant and diabetic individuals. Diabetes promotes initiation of atherosclerosis, progression of lesions, and thrombotic complications by multiple mechanisms. Current lines of investigation focus on the following interactions of diabetes and mechanisms of atherosclerosis: (a) the role of endothelial dysfunction in the pathogenesis of atherosclerosis and propensity to thrombosis; (b) the mechanisms involved in the abnormal hemostatic and fibrinolytic function observed in the diabetic setting; and (c) the role of AGEs and the receptor for AGEs in the pathogenesis of vascular disease in diabetes and the use of specific inhibitors of various steps in the glycosylation process (e.g., aminoguanidine or "AGE breakers") as a potential therapy; (d) diabetes-induced augmentation of oxidative stress; (e) understanding the relationship between the components of the insulin-resistance syndrome and its importance as a cardiovascular risk factor for both diabetic and nondiabetic subjects; and (f) understanding the relation between inflammation and diabetes. Defining the molecular mechanisms responsible for insulin resistance may lead to the development of new "insulin-sensitizing" agents that can improve insulin action, resulting in a wide spectrum of beneficial metabolic effects and a reduced cardiovascular risk.

The pathogenesis, natural history, and clinical significance of diabetic cardiomyopathy remain to be determined. Likewise, the role of autonomic neuropathy in the cardiovascular complications of diabetes should be explored. More research is also needed with regard to the specific mechanisms involved in the pathogenesis of restenosis in diabetic patients and potential therapeutic approaches that will improve the results of angioplasty in diabetic patients.

Finally, the prevention of type 1 and type 2 diabetes is a major focus of basic and clinical investigations. Screening of the human genome can identify regions of genetic susceptibility, after which the final localization of disease genes can be carried out, followed by sequencing of candidate genes to identify the specific mutations. Multiple molecular defects can lead to type 2 diabetes, and the molecular details of several rare forms of type 1 diabetes have already been identified (e.g., pancreatic glucose "sensor" mechanism).

Diabetes prevention trials based on immunologic toleration to prevent type 1 diabetes, lifestyle changes, and pharmacologic interventions to prevent or delay type 2 diabetes are now being carried out.

A central issue in the treatment of diabetic patients is whether tight glycemic control will reduce CAD morbidity and mortality. Whereas randomized primary prevention trials have clearly shown that glycemic control reduces the incidence of microvascular complications in both type 1 and type 2 diabetes, the effect on macrovascular complications was small. Indeed, lipid lowering and aggressive blood pressure reduction appear to be more efficacious as primary prevention in diabetic patients.

There are two key questions with regard to the expected benefit of intensive glycemic control as part of the primary prevention of macrovascular disease. First, the threshold above which hyperglycemia becomes atherogenic is unknown and may be below the range defined as diabetes. It is also unknown whether a continuous relative risk reduction relationship over the range of hemoglobin A_{1c} exists for diabetic macrovascular complications. Second, the time necessary for the reversal of established hyperglycemia-induced vascular damage is not known. For example, in diabetic patients with functioning pancreatic transplants, renal pathology continues to progress for at least 5 years after diabetes has been cured

(402). The mechanism for these observations is unclear but may be related to a slow replacement of glycosylated molecules or because phenotypic alterations in vascular cells may persist despite the return of normoglycemia (the so-called memory effect). Notwithstanding, intensive glycemic control as secondary prevention seems to be effective in reducing short-term mortality (317), suggesting that glycemic control may be valuable even in diabetics with established CAD.

The diffuse nature of the atherosclerotic process in diabetic patients is often emphasized. It is commonly accepted that angiographically severe CAD increases the propensity to develop acute coronary syndromes because the presence of the severe stenoses serves as a marker for the presence of angiographically modest or even inapparent noncritically stenotic plaques that are more prone to disruption. However, the striking excess of coronary events in diabetic patients with or without established CAD appears to be out of proportion to the severity of atherosclerosis. These observations raise the possibility that unique pathogenic mechanisms in diabetes operate to weaken plaque stability.

REFERENCES

1. Schwartz CJ, Valente AJ, Sprague EA, et al. Pathogenesis of the atherosclerotic lesion. Implications for diabetes mellitus. *Diabetes Care* 1992;15:1156–1167.
2. Stamler J, Vaccaro O, Neaton JD, et al. Diabetes, other risk factors, and 12-yr cardiovascular mortality for men screened in the Multiple Risk Factor Intervention Trial. *Diabetes Care* 1993;16:434–444.
3. American Diabetes Association. Consensus statement: role of cardiovascular risk factors in prevention and treatment of macrovascular disease in diabetes. *Diabetes Care* 1993;16:72–78.
4. National Center for Health Statistics. *Health United Stats.* Washington, DC: Government Printing Office, 1998.
5. McKinlay J, Marceau L. US public health and the 21st century: diabetes mellitus. *Lancet* 2000;356:757–761.
6. Gu K, Cowie CC, Harris MI. Diabetes and decline in heart disease mortality in US adults. *JAMA* 1999;281:1291–1297.
7. Robertson WB, Strong JP. Atherosclerosis in persons with hypertension and diabetes mellitus. *Lab Invest* 1968;18:538–551.
8. Waller BF, Palumbo PJ, Lie JT, et al. Status of the coronary arteries at necropsy in diabetes mellitus with onset after age 30 years. Analysis of 229 diabetic patients with and without clinical evidence of coronary heart disease and comparison to 183 control subjects. *Am J Med* 1980;69:498–506.
9. Granger CB, Califf RM, Young S, et al. Outcome of patients with diabetes mellitus and acute myocardial infarction treated with thrombolytic agents. The Thrombolysis and Angioplasty in Myocardial Infarction (TAMI) Study Group. *J Am Coll Cardiol* 1993;21:920–925.
10. Stein B, Weintraub W, Gebhart S, et al. Influence of diabetes mellitus on early and late outcome after percutaneous transluminal coronary angioplasty. *Circulation* 1995;91:979–989.
11. Barzilay JI, Kronmal RA, Bittner V, et al. Coronary artery disease and coronary artery bypass grafting in diabetic patients aged > or = 65 years [report from the Coronary Artery Surgery Study (CASS) Registry]. *Am J Cardiol* 1994;74:334–339.
12. Davies MJ, Bland JM, Hangartner JR, et al. Factors influencing the presence or absence of acute coronary artery thrombi in sudden ischaemic death. *Eur Heart J* 1989;10:203–208.
13. Silva JA, Escobar A, Collins TJ, et al. Unstable angina. A comparison of angioscopic findings between diabetic and nondiabetic patients. *Circulation* 1995;92:1731–1736.
14. Krolewski AS, Kosinski EJ, Warram JH, et al. Magnitude and determinants of coronary artery disease in juvenile-onset, insulin-dependent diabetes mellitus. *Am J Cardiol* 1987;59:750–755.
15. Donahue RP, Orchard TJ. Diabetes mellitus and macrovascular complications. An epidemiological perspective. *Diabetes Care* 1992;15:1141–1155.
16. Borch-Johnsen K, Kreiner S. Proteinuria: value as predictor of cardiovascular mortality in insulin dependent diabetes mellitus. *BMJ* 1987;294:1651–1654.
17. Jensen T, Borch-Johnsen K, Kofoed-Enevoldsen A, et al. Coronary heart disease in young type 1 (insulin-dependent) diabetic patients with and without diabetic nephropathy: incidence and risk factors. *Diabetologia* 1987;30:144–148.
18. Mattock MB, Morrish NJ, Viberti G, et al. Prospective study of microalbuminuria as predictor of mortality in NIDDM. *Diabetes* 1992;41:736–741.
19. Deckert T, Kofoed-Enevoldsen A, Norgaard K, et al. Microalbuminuria. Implications for micro- and macrovascular disease. *Diabetes Care* 1992;15:1181–1191.
20. Wang SL, Head J, Stevens L, et al. Excess mortality and its relation to hypertension and proteinuria in diabetic patients. The World Health Organization multinational study of vascular disease in diabetes. *Diabetes Care* 1996;19:305–312.
21. Haffner SM. Management of dyslipidemia in adults with diabetes. *Diabetes Care* 1998;21:160–178.
22. Winocour PH, Durrington PN, Bhatnagar D, et al. Influence of early diabetic nephropathy on very low density lipoprotein (VLDL), intermediate density lipoprotein (IDL), and low density lipoprotein (LDL) composition. *Atherosclerosis* 1991;89:49–57.
23. Stehouwer CD, Nauta JJ, Zeldenrust GC, et al. Urinary albumin excretion, cardiovascular disease, and endothelial dysfunction in non-insulin-dependent diabetes mellitus. *Lancet* 1992;340:319–323.
24. Makita Z, Radoff S, Rayfield EJ, et al. Advanced glycosylation end products in patients with diabetic nephropathy. *N Engl J Med* 1991;325:836–842.
25. Makita Z, Bucala R, Rayfield EJ, et al. Reactive glycosylation endproducts in diabetic uraemia and treatment of renal failure. *Lancet* 1994;343:1519–1522.
26. Seaquist ER, Goetz FC, Rich S, et al. Familial clustering of diabetic kidney disease. Evidence for genetic susceptibility to diabetic nephropathy. *N Engl J Med* 1989;320:1161–1165.
27. Marre M, Jeunemaitre X, Gallois Y, et al. Contribution of genetic polymorphism in the renin-angiotensin system to the development of renal complications in insulin-dependent diabetes: Genetique de la Nephropathie Diabetique (GENEDIAB) study group. *J Clin Invest* 1997;99:1585–1595.
28. Earle K, Walker J, Hill C, et al. Familial clustering of cardiovascular disease in patients with insulin-dependent diabetes and nephropathy. *N Engl J Med* 1992;326:673–677.
29. Krolewski AS, Canessa M, Warram JH, et al. Predisposition to hypertension and susceptibility to renal disease in insulin-dependent diabetes mellitus. *N Engl J Med* 1988;318:140–145.
30. Geerlings W, Tufveson G, Brunner FP, et al. Combined report on regular dialysis and transplantation in Europe, XXI, 1990. *Nephrol Dial Transplant* 1991;6[Suppl 4]:5–29.
31. Renal failure in diabetics in the UK: deficient provision of care in 1985. Joint Working Party on Diabetic Renal Failure of the British Diabetic Association, the Renal Association, and the Research Unit of the Royal College of Physicians. *Diabet Med* 1988;5:79–84.
32. Lemmers MJ, Barry JM. Major role for arterial disease in morbidity and mortality after kidney transplantation in diabetic recipients. *Diabetes Care* 1991;14:295–301.
33. Manske CL, Thomas W, Wang Y, et al. Screening diabetic transplant candidates for coronary artery disease: identification of a low risk subgroup. *Kidney Int* 1993;44:617–621.

34. Manske CL, Wang Y, Rector T, et al. Coronary revascularisation in insulin-dependent diabetic patients with chronic renal failure. *Lancet* 1992;340:998–1002.

35. Fontbonne A, Eschwege E, Cambien F, et al. Hypertriglyceridaemia as a risk factor of coronary heart disease mortality in subjects with impaired glucose tolerance or diabetes. Results from the 11-year follow-up of the Paris Prospective Study. *Diabetologia* 1989;32:300–304.

36. Haffner SM, Lehto S, Ronnemaa T, et al. Mortality from coronary heart disease in subjects with type 2 diabetes and in nondiabetic subjects with and without prior myocardial infarction. *N Engl J Med* 1998;339:229–234.

37. Barrett-Connor EL, Cohn BA, Wingard DL, et al. Why is diabetes mellitus a stronger risk factor for fatal ischemic heart disease in women than in men? The Rancho Bernardo Study. *JAMA* 1991;265:627–631.

38. Barrett-Connor E, Wingard DL. Sex differential in ischemic heart disease mortality in diabetics: a prospective population-based study. *Am J Epidemiol* 1983;118:489–496.

39. The Diabetes Control and Complications Trial Research Group. The effect of intensive treatment of diabetes on the development and progression of long-term complications in insulin-dependent diabetes mellitus. *N Engl J Med* 1993;329:977–986.

40. Uusitupa M, Siitonen O, Aro A, et al. Prevalence of coronary heart disease, left ventricular failure and hypertension in middle-aged, newly diagnosed type 2 (non-insulin-dependent) diabetic subjects. *Diabetologia* 1985;28:22–27.

41. Fuller JH, Shipley MJ, Rose G, et al. Coronary-heart-disease risk and impaired glucose tolerance. The Whitehall study. *Lancet* 1980;1:1373–1376.

42. Kahn CR. Banting lecture. Insulin action, diabetogenes, and the cause of type II diabetes. *Diabetes* 1994;43:1066–1084.

43. DeFronzo RA. Lilly lecture 1987. The triumvirate: beta-cell, muscle, liver. A collusion responsible for NIDDM. *Diabetes* 1988;37:667–687.

44. Lempiainen P, Mykkanen L, Pyorala K, et al. Insulin resistance syndrome predicts coronary heart disease events in elderly nondiabetic men. *Circulation* 1999;100:123–128.

45. Ferrannini E, Buzzigoli G, Bonadonna R, et al. Insulin resistance in essential hypertension. *N Engl J Med* 1987;317:350–357.

46. Zavaroni I, Bonora E, Pagliara M, et al. Risk factors for coronary artery disease in healthy persons with hyperinsulinemia and normal glucose tolerance. *N Engl J Med* 1989;320:702–706.

47. Peiris AN, Sothmann MS, Hoffmann RG, et al. Adiposity, fat distribution, and cardiovascular risk. *Ann Intern Med* 1989;110:867–872.

48. Reaven GM. Role of insulin resistance in human disease (syndrome X): an expanded definition. *Annu Rev Med* 1993;44:121–131.

49. Grundy SM. Hypertriglyceridemia, atherogenic dyslipidemia, and the metabolic syndrome. *Am J Cardiol* 1998;81:18B–25B.

50. Austin MA, King MC, Vranizan KM, et al. Atherogenic lipoprotein phenotype. A proposed genetic marker for coronary heart disease risk. *Circulation* 1990;82:495–506.

51. Festa A, D'Agostino R Jr, Howard G, et al. Chronic subclinical inflammation as part of the insulin resistance syndrome: the Insulin Resistance Atherosclerosis Study (IRAS). *Circulation* 2000;102:42–47.

52. Meigs JB, Nathan DM, Wilson PW, et al. Metabolic risk factors worsen continuously across the spectrum of nondiabetic glucose tolerance. The Framingham Offspring Study. *Ann Intern Med* 1998;128:524–533.

53. Despres JP, Lamarche B, Mauriege P, et al. Hyperinsulinemia as an independent risk factor for ischemic heart disease. *N Engl J Med* 1996;334:952–957.

54. Fontbonne A, Charles MA, Thibult N, et al. Hyperinsulinaemia as a predictor of coronary heart disease mortality in a healthy population: the Paris Prospective Study, 15-year follow-up. *Diabetologia* 1991;34:356–361.

55. Howard G, O'Leary DH, Zaccaro D, et al. Insulin sensitivity and atherosclerosis. The Insulin Resistance Atherosclerosis Study (IRAS) Investigators. *Circulation* 1996;93:1809–1817.

56. Laakso M, Sarlund H, Salonen R, et al. Asymptomatic atherosclerosis and insulin resistance. *Arterioscler Thromb* 1991;11:1068–1076.

57. Stout RW. Insulin and atheroma. 20-yr perspective. *Diabetes Care* 1990;13:631–654.

58. Modan M, Or J, Karasik A, et al. Hyperinsulinemia, sex, and risk of atherosclerotic cardiovascular disease. *Circulation* 1991;84:1165–1175.

59. Liu QZ, Knowler WC, Nelson RG, et al. Insulin treatment, endogenous insulin concentration, and ECG abnormalities in diabetic Pima Indians. Cross-sectional and prospective analyses. *Diabetes* 1992;41:1141–1150.

60. Ferrara A, Barrett-Connor EL, Edelstein SL. Hyperinsulinemia does not increase the risk of fatal cardiovascular disease in elderly men or women without diabetes: the Rancho Bernardo Study, 1984–1991. *Am J Epidemiol* 1994;140:857–869.

61. Saad MF, Knowler WC, Pettitt DJ, et al. Sequential changes in serum insulin concentration during development of non-insulin-dependent diabetes. *Lancet* 1989;1:1356–1359.

62. Pyorala K, Laakso M, Uusitupa M. Diabetes and atherosclerosis: an epidemiologic view. *Diabetes Metab Rev* 1987;3:463–524.

63. Gerstein HC, Yusuf S. Dysglycaemia and risk of cardiovascular disease. *Lancet* 1996;347:949–950.

64. Turner RC, Millins H, Neil HA, et al. Risk factors for coronary artery disease in non-insulin dependent diabetes mellitus: United Kingdom Prospective Diabetes Study (UKPDS: 23). *BMJ* 1998;316:823–828.

65. Kuusisto J, Mykkanen L, Pyorala K, et al. NIDDM and its metabolic control predict coronary heart disease in elderly subjects. *Diabetes* 1994;43:960–967.

66. Laakso M. Hyperglycemia and cardiovascular disease in type 2 diabetes. *Diabetes* 1999;48:937–942.

67. Ginsberg HN. Lipoprotein physiology in nondiabetic and diabetic states. Relationship to atherogenesis. *Diabetes Care* 1991;14:839–855.

68. Garg A. Management of dyslipidemia in IDDM patients. *Diabetes Care* 1994;17:224–234.

69. Sosenko JM, Breslow JL, Miettinen OS, et al. Hyperglycemia and plasma lipid levels: a prospective study of young insulin-dependent diabetic patients. *N Engl J Med* 1980;302:650–654.

70. Haffner SM, Stern MP, Hazuda HP, et al. Cardiovascular risk factors in confirmed prediabetic individuals. Does the clock for coronary heart disease start ticking before the onset of clinical diabetes? *JAMA* 1990;263:2893–2898.

71. Syvanne M, Taskinen MR. Lipids and lipoproteins as coronary risk factors in non-insulin-dependent diabetes mellitus. *Lancet* 1997;350:SI20–SI23.

72. Ginsberg HN. Diabetic dyslipidemia: basic mechanisms underlying the common hypertriglyceridemia and low HDL cholesterol levels. *Diabetes* 1996;45[Suppl 3]:S27–S30.

73. Howard BV, Knowler WC, Vasquez B, et al. Plasma and lipoprotein cholesterol and triglyceride in the Pima Indian population. Comparison of diabetics and nondiabetics. *Arteriosclerosis* 1984;4:462–471.

74. Chen YD, Coulston AM, Zhou MY, et al. Why do low-fat high-carbohydrate diets accentuate postprandial lipemia in patients with NIDDM? *Diabetes Care* 1995;18:10–16.

75. Ginsberg HN. Insulin resistance and cardiovascular disease. *J Clin Invest* 2000;106:453–458.

76. Packard CJ, Munro A, Lorimer AR, et al. Metabolism of apolipoprotein B in large triglyceride-rich very low density lipoproteins of normal and hypertriglyceridemic subjects. *J Clin Invest* 1984;74:2178–2192.

77. Eckel RH. Lipoprotein lipase. A multifunctional enzyme relevant to common metabolic diseases. *N Engl J Med* 1989;320:1060–1068.

78. Havel RJ, Rapaport E. Management of primary hyperlipidemia. *N Engl J Med* 1995;332:1491–1498.

79. Hodis HN. Myocardial ischemia and lipoprotein lipase activity. *Circulation* 2000;102:1600–1601.

80. Laakso M, Lehto S, Penttila I, et al. Lipids and lipoproteins predicting coronary heart disease mortality and morbidity in patients with non-insulin-dependent diabetes. *Circulation* 1993;88:1421–1430.

81. Goldschmid MG, Barrett-Connor E, Edelstein SL, et al. Dyslipidemia and ischemic heart disease mortality among men and women with diabetes. *Circulation* 1994;89:991–997.

82. Karpe F. Postprandial lipoprotein metabolism and atherosclerosis. *J Intern Med* 1999;246:341–355.

83. Zilversmit DB. Atherogenesis: a postprandial phenomenon. *Circulation* 1979;60:473–485.

84. Patsch JR, Miesenbock G, Hopferwieser T, et al. Relation of triglyceride metabolism and coronary artery disease. Studies in the postprandial state. *Arterioscler Thromb* 1992;12:1336–1345.

85. Plotnick GD, Corretti MC, Vogel RA. Effect of antioxidant vitamins on the transient impairment of endothelium-dependent brachial artery vasoactivity following a single high-fat meal. *JAMA* 1997;278:1682–1686.

86. Syvanne M, Hilden H, Taskinen MR. Abnormal metabolism of postprandial lipoproteins in patients with non-insulin-dependent diabetes mellitus is not related to coronary artery disease. *J Lipid Res* 1994;35:15–26.

87. Jeppesen J, Hollenbeck CB, Zhou MY, et al. Relation between insulin resistance, hyperinsulinemia, postheparin plasma lipoprotein lipase activity, and postprandial lipemia. *Arterioscler Thromb Vasc Biol* 1995;15:320–324.

88. Herz J, Qiu SQ, Oesterle A, et al. Initial hepatic removal of chylomicron remnants is unaffected but endocytosis is delayed in mice lacking the low density lipoprotein receptor. *Proc Natl Acad Sci U S A* 1995;92:4611–4615.

89. Goldberg IJ, Blaner WS, Vanni TM, et al. Role of lipoprotein lipase in the regulation of high density lipoprotein apolipoprotein metabolism. Studies in normal and lipoprotein lipase-inhibited monkeys. *J Clin Invest* 1990;86:463–473.

90. Patsch JR, Prasad S, Gotto AM Jr, et al. Postprandial lipemia. A key for the conversion of high density lipoprotein 2 into high density lipoprotein 3 by hepatic lipase. *J Clin Invest* 1984;74:2017–2023.

91. Selby JV, Austin MA, Newman B, et al. LDL subclass phenotypes and the insulin resistance syndrome in women. *Circulation* 1993;88:381–387.

92. Reaven GM, Chen YD, Jeppesen J, et al. Insulin resistance and hyperinsulinemia in individuals with small, dense low density lipoprotein particles. *J Clin Invest* 1993;92:141–146.

93. Haffner SM, D'Agostino R Jr, Goff D, et al. LDL size in African Americans, Hispanics, and non-Hispanic whites: the insulin resistance atherosclerosis study. *Arterioscler Thromb Vasc Biol* 1999;19:2234–2240.

94. Packard CJ, Shepherd J. Lipoprotein heterogeneity and apolipoprotein B metabolism. *Arterioscler Thromb Vasc Biol* 1997;17:3542–3556.

95. Tribble DL, van den Berg JJ, Motchnik PA, et al. Oxidative susceptibility of low density lipoprotein subfractions is related to their ubiquinol-10 and alpha-tocopherol content. *Proc Natl Acad Sci U S A* 1994;91:1183–1187.

96. Anderson TJ, Meredith IT, Charbonneau F, et al. Endothelium-dependent coronary vasomotion relates to the susceptibility of LDL to oxidation in humans. *Circulation* 1996;93:1647–1650.

97. Nielsen LB. Transfer of low density lipoprotein into the arterial wall and risk of atherosclerosis. *Atherosclerosis* 1996;123:1–15.

98. Bucala R, Mitchell R, Arnold K, et al. Identification of the major site of apolipoprotein B modification by advanced glycosylation end products blocking uptake by the low density lipoprotein receptor. *J Biol Chem* 1995;270:10828–10832.

99. Bucala R, Makita Z, Koschinsky T, et al. Lipid advanced glycosylation: pathway for lipid oxidation in vivo. *Proc Natl Acad Sci U S A* 1993;90:6434–6438.

100. Bucala R, Makita Z, Vega G, et al. Modification of low density lipoprotein by advanced glycation end products contributes to the dyslipidemia of diabetes and renal insufficiency. *Proc Natl Acad Sci U S A* 1994;91:9441–9445.

101. Lyons TJ. Glycation and oxidation: a role in the pathogenesis of atherosclerosis. *Am J Cardiol* 1993;71:26B–31B.

102. Bowie A, Owens D, Collins P, et al. Glycosylated low density lipoprotein is more sensitive to oxidation: implications for the diabetic patient? *Atherosclerosis* 1993;102:63–67.

103. Pyorala K, Pedersen TR, Kjekshus J, et al. Cholesterol lowering with simvastatin improves prognosis of diabetic patients with coronary heart disease. A subgroup analysis of the Scandinavian Simvastatin Survival Study (4S). *Diabetes Care* 1997;20:614–620.

104. Goldberg RB, Mellies MJ, Sacks FM, et al. Cardiovascular events and their reduction with pravastatin in diabetic and glucose-intolerant myocardial infarction survivors with

average cholesterol levels: subgroup analyses in the Cholesterol and Recurrent Events (CARE) trial. The Care Investigators. *Circulation* 1998;98:2513–2519.

105. Aronson D, Rayfield EJ, Chesebro JH. Mechanisms determining course and outcome of diabetic patients who have had acute myocardial infarction. *Ann Intern Med* 1997;126:296–306.

106. American Diabetes Association. Position statement. Management of dyslipidemia in adults with diabetes. *Diabetes Care* 1998;21:179–182.

107. DeFronzo RA, Goodman AM. Efficacy of metformin in patients with non-insulin-dependent diabetes mellitus. The Multicenter Metformin Study Group. *N Engl J Med* 1995;333:541–549.

108. Ghazzi MN, Perez JE, Antonucci TK, et al. Cardiac and glycemic benefits of troglitazone treatment in NIDDM. The Troglitazone Study Group. *Diabetes* 1997;46:433–439.

109. Garg A, Grundy SM. Lovastatin for lowering cholesterol levels in non-insulin-dependent diabetes mellitus. *N Engl J Med* 1988;318:81–86.

110. Vega GL, Grundy SM. Gemfibrozil therapy in primary hypertriglyceridemia associated with coronary heart disease. Effects on metabolism of low-density lipoproteins. *JAMA* 1985;253:2398–2403.

111. Koskinen P, Manttari M, Manninen V, et al. Coronary heart disease incidence in NIDDM patients in the Helsinki Heart Study. *Diabetes Care* 1992;15:820–825.

112. Rubins HB, Robins SJ, Collins D, et al. Gemfibrozil for the secondary prevention of coronary heart disease in men with low levels of high-density lipoprotein cholesterol. Veterans Affairs High-Density Lipoprotein Cholesterol Intervention Trial Study Group. *N Engl J Med* 1999;341:410–418.

113. Lahdenpera S, Tilly-Kiesi M, Vuorinen-Markkola H, et al. Effects of gemfibrozil on low-density lipoprotein particle size, density distribution, and composition in patients with type II diabetes. *Diabetes Care* 1993;16:584–592.

114. Garg A, Grundy SM. Cholestyramine therapy for dyslipidemia in non-insulin-dependent diabetes mellitus. A short-term, double-blind, crossover trial. *Ann Intern Med* 1994;121:416–422.

115. Superko HR, Krauss RM. Differential effects of nicotinic acid in subjects with different LDL subclass patterns. *Atherosclerosis* 1992;95:69–76.

116. Garg A, Grundy SM. Nicotinic acid as therapy for dyslipidemia in non-insulin-dependent diabetes mellitus. *JAMA* 1990;264:723–726.

117. Elam MB, Hunninghake DB, Davis KB, et al. Effect of niacin on lipid and lipoprotein levels and glycemic control in patients with diabetes and peripheral arterial disease: the ADMIT study: A randomized trial. Arterial Disease Multiple Intervention Trial. *JAMA* 2000;284:1263–1270.

118. Lin SJ, Hong CY, Chang MS, et al. Increased aortic endothelial death and enhanced transendothelial macromolecular transport in streptozotocin-diabetic rats. *Diabetologia* 1993;36:926–930.

119. Winocour PD, Richardson M, Kinlough-Rathbone RL. Continued platelet interaction with de-endothelialized aortae associated with slower re-endothelialization and more extensive intimal hyperplasia in spontaneously diabetic BB Wistar rats. *Int J Exp Pathol* 1993;74:603–613.

120. Dolgov VV, Zaikina OE, Bondarenko MF, et al. Aortic endothelium of alloxan diabetic rabbits: a quantitative study using scanning electron microscopy. *Diabetologia* 1982;22:338–343.

121. Wautier JL, Zoukourian C, Chappey O, et al. Receptor-mediated endothelial cell dysfunction in diabetic vasculopathy. Soluble receptor for advanced glycation end products blocks hyperpermeability in diabetic rats. *J Clin Invest* 1996;97:238–243.

122. Schmidt AM, Hori O, Chen JX, et al. Advanced glycation endproducts interacting with their endothelial receptor induce expression of vascular cell adhesion molecule-1 (VCAM-1) in cultured human endothelial cells and in mice. A potential mechanism for the accelerated vasculopathy of diabetes. *J Clin Invest* 1995;96:1395–1403.

123. Richardson M, Hadcock SJ, DeReske M, et al. Increased expression in vivo of VCAM-1 and E-selectin by the aortic endothelium of normolipemic and hyperlipemic diabetic rabbits. *Arterioscler Thromb* 1994;14:760–769.

124. Yan SD, Schmidt AM, Anderson GM, et al. Enhanced cellular oxidant stress by the interaction of advanced glycation end products with their receptors/binding proteins. *J Biol Chem* 1994;269:9889–9897.

125. Wautier JL, Wautier MP, Schmidt AM, et al. Advanced glycation end products (AGEs) on the surface of diabetic erythrocytes bind to the vessel wall via a specific receptor inducing oxidant stress in the vasculature: a link between surface-associated AGEs and diabetic complications. *Proc Natl Acad Sci U S A* 1994;91:7742–7746.

126. Kim JA, Berliner JA, Natarajan RD, et al. Evidence that glucose increases monocyte binding to human aortic endothelial cells. *Diabetes* 1994;43:1103–1107.

127. Hadcock S, Richardson M, Winocour PD, et al. Intimal alterations in rabbit aortas during the first 6 months of alloxan-induced diabetes. *Arterioscler Thromb* 1991;11:517–529.

128. Johnstone MT, Creager SJ, Scales KM, et al. Impaired endothelium-dependent vasodilation in patients with insulin-dependent diabetes mellitus. *Circulation* 1993;88:2510–2516.

129. De Vriese AS, Verbeuren TJ, Van de Voorde J, et al. Endothelial dysfunction in diabetes. *Br J Pharmacol* 2000;130:963–974.

130. Williams SB, Goldfine AB, Timimi FK, et al. Acute hyperglycemia attenuates endothelium-dependent vasodilation in humans in vivo. *Circulation* 1998;97:1695–1701.

131. Ting HH, Timimi FK, Boles KS, et al. Vitamin C improves endothelium-dependent vasodilation in patients with non-insulin-dependent diabetes mellitus. *J Clin Invest* 1996;97:22–28.

132. Tesfamariam B, Cohen RA. Free radicals mediate endothelial cell dysfunction caused by elevated glucose. *Am J Physiol* 1992;263:H321–H326.

133. O'Driscoll G, Green D, Rankin J, et al. Improvement in endothelial function by angiotensin converting enzyme inhibition in insulin-dependent diabetes mellitus. *J Clin Invest* 1997;100:678–684.

134. Scherrer U, Randin D, Vollenweider P, et al. Nitric oxide release accounts for insulin's vascular effects in humans. *J Clin Invest* 1994;94:2511–2515.

135. Steinberg HO, Brechtel G, Johnson A, et al. Insulin-mediated skeletal muscle vasodilation is nitric oxide dependent.

A novel action of insulin to increase nitric oxide release. *J Clin Invest* 1994;94:1172–1179.

136. Steinberg HO, Chaker H, Leaming R, et al. Obesity/insulin resistance is associated with endothelial dysfunction. Implications for the syndrome of insulin resistance. *J Clin Invest* 1996;97:2601–2610.

137. Balletshofer BM, Rittig K, Enderle MD, et al. Endothelial dysfunction is detectable in young normotensive first-degree relatives of subjects with type 2 diabetes in association with insulin resistance. *Circulation* 2000;101:1780–1784.

138. Petrie JR, Ueda S, Webb DJ, et al. Endothelial nitric oxide production and insulin sensitivity. A physiological link with implications for pathogenesis of cardiovascular disease. *Circulation* 1996;93:1331–1333.

139. Steinberg HO, Tarshoby M, Monestel R, et al. Elevated circulating free fatty acid levels impair endothelium-dependent vasodilation. *J Clin Invest* 1997;100:1230–1239.

140. Hopfner RL, Gopalakrishnan V. Endothelin: emerging role in diabetic vascular complications. *Diabetologia* 1999;42:1383–1394.

141. Oliver FJ, de la Rubia G, Feener EP, et al. Stimulation of endothelin-1 gene expression by insulin in endothelial cells. *J Biol Chem* 1991;266:23251–23256.

142. Takahashi K, Ghatei MA, Lam HC, et al. Elevated plasma endothelin in patients with diabetes mellitus. *Diabetologia* 1990;33:306–310.

143. Park JY, Takahara N, Gabriele A, et al. Induction of endothelin-1 expression by glucose: an effect of protein kinase C activation. *Diabetes* 2000;49:1239–1248.

144. Thompson SG, Kienast J, Pyke SD, et al. Hemostatic factors and the risk of myocardial infarction or sudden death in patients with angina pectoris. European Concerted Action on Thrombosis and Disabilities Angina Pectoris Study Group. *N Engl J Med* 1995;332:635–641.

145. Meade TW, Mellows S, Brozovic M, et al. Haemostatic function and ischaemic heart disease: principal results of the Northwick Park Heart Study. *Lancet* 1986;2:533–537.

146. Trip MD, Cats VM, van Capelle FJ, et al. Platelet hyperreactivity and prognosis in survivors of myocardial infarction. *N Engl J Med* 1990;322:1549–1554.

147. Winocour PD. Platelet abnormalities in diabetes mellitus. *Diabetes* 1992;41[Suppl 2]:26–31.

148. Tschoepe D, Roesen P, Schwippert B, et al. Platelets in diabetes: the role in the hemostatic regulation in atherosclerosis. *Semin Thromb Hemost* 1993;19:122–128.

149. Knobler H, Savion N, Shenkman B, et al. Shear-induced platelet adhesion and aggregation on subendothelium are increased in diabetic patients. *Thromb Res* 1998;90:181–190.

150. Davi G, Gresele P, Violi F, et al. Diabetes mellitus, hypercholesterolemia, and hypertension but not vascular disease per se are associated with persistent platelet activation in vivo. Evidence derived from the study of peripheral arterial disease. *Circulation* 1997;96:69–75.

151. Tschoepe D, Driesch E, Schwippert B, et al. Exposure of adhesion molecules on activated platelets in patients with newly diagnosed IDDM is not normalized by near-normoglycemia. *Diabetes* 1995;44:890–894.

152. Davi G, Catalano I, Averna M, et al. Thromboxane biosynthesis and platelet function in type II diabetes mellitus. *N Engl J Med* 1990;322:1769–1774.

153. Nichols TC, Bellinger DA, Reddick RL, et al. Role of von Willebrand factor in arterial thrombosis. Studies in normal and von Willebrand disease pigs. *Circulation* 1991;83:IV56–IV64.

154. Conlan MG, Folsom AR, Finch A, et al. Associations of factor VIII and von Willebrand factor with age, race, sex, and risk factors for atherosclerosis. The Atherosclerosis Risk in Communities (ARIC) Study. *Thromb Haemost* 1993;70:380–385.

155. Kannel WB, Agostino RB, Wilson PW, et al. Diabetes, fibrinogen, and risk of cardiovascular disease: the Framingham experience. *Am Heart J* 1990;120:672–676.

156. Paisey RB, Harkness J, Hartog M, et al. The effect of improvement in diabetic control on plasma and whole blood viscosity. *Diabetologia* 1980;19:345–349.

157. Kohler HP, Grant PJ. Plasminogen-activator inhibitor type 1 and coronary artery disease. *N Engl J Med* 2000;342:1792–1801.

158. Juhan-Vague I, Alessi MC. PAI-1, obesity, insulin resistance and risk of cardiovascular events. *Thromb Haemost* 1997;78:656–660.

159. Alessi MC, Peiretti F, Morange P, et al. Production of plasminogen activator inhibitor 1 by human adipose tissue: possible link between visceral fat accumulation and vascular disease. *Diabetes* 1997;46:860–867.

160. Svendsen OL, Hassager C, Christiansen C, et al. Plasminogen activator inhibitor-1, tissue-type plasminogen activator, and fibrinogen: effect of dieting with or without exercise in overweight postmenopausal women. *Arterioscler Thromb Vasc Biol* 1996;16:381–385.

161. Nordt TK, Sawa H, Fujii S, et al. Induction of plasminogen activator inhibitor type-1 (PAI-1) by proinsulin and insulin in vivo. *Circulation* 1995;91:764–770.

162. Chen YQ, Su M, Walia RR, et al. Sp1 sites mediate activation of the plasminogen activator inhibitor-1 promoter by glucose in vascular smooth muscle cells. *J Biol Chem* 1998;273:8225–8231.

163. Malmberg K, Yusuf S, Gerstein HC, et al. Impact of diabetes on long-term prognosis in patients with unstable angina and non-Q-wave myocardial infarction: results of the OASIS (Organization to Assess Strategies for Ischemic Syndromes) Registry. *Circulation* 2000;102:1014–1019.

164. Calvin JE, Klein LW, Vandenberg BJ, et al. Risk stratification in unstable angina. Prospective validation of the Braunwald classification. *JAMA* 1995;273:136–141.

165. Kurnik PB. Circadian variation in the efficacy of tissue-type plasminogen activator. *Circulation* 1995;91:1341–1346.

166. Nishikawa T, Edelstein D, Du XL, et al. Normalizing mitochondrial superoxide production blocks three pathways of hyperglycaemic damage. *Nature* 2000;404:787–790.

167. Maillard L. Action des acides amines sur les sucres: formation des melanoidines par voie methodique. *C R Hebd Seances Acad Sci* 1912;154:66–68.

168. Brownlee M, Cerami A, Vlassara H. Advanced glycosylation end products in tissue and the biochemical basis of diabetic complications. *N Engl J Med* 1988;318:1315–1321.

169. Ikeda K, Higashi T, Sano H, et al. N (epsilon)-(carboxymethyl)lysine protein adduct is a major immunological epitope in proteins modified with advanced glycation end products of the Maillard reaction. *Biochemistry* 1996;35:8075–8083.

170. Giardino I, Edelstein D, Brownlee M. BCL-2 expression or antioxidants prevent hyperglycemia-induced formation of intracellular advanced glycation endproducts in bovine endothelial cells. *J Clin Invest* 1996;97:1422–1428.

171. Fu MX, Knecht KJ, Thorpe SR, et al. Role of oxygen in cross-linking and chemical modification of collagen by glucose. *Diabetes* 1992;41[Suppl 2]:42–48.

172. Dunn JA, Ahmed MU, Murtiashaw MH, et al. Reaction of ascorbate with lysine and protein under autoxidizing conditions: formation of N epsilon-(carboxymethyl)lysine by reaction between lysine and products of autoxidation of ascorbate. *Biochemistry* 1990;29:10964–10970.

173. Schmidt AM, Hori O, Brett J, et al. Cellular receptors for advanced glycation end products. Implications for induction of oxidant stress and cellular dysfunction in the pathogenesis of vascular lesions. *Arterioscler Thromb* 1994;14:1521–1528.

174. Schmidt AM, Yan SD, Wautier JL, et al. Activation of receptor for advanced glycation end products: a mechanism for chronic vascular dysfunction in diabetic vasculopathy and atherosclerosis. *Circ Res* 1999;84:489–497.

175. Acosta J, Hettinga J, Fluckiger R, et al. Molecular basis for a link between complement and the vascular complications of diabetes. *Proc Natl Acad Sci U S A* 2000;97:5450–5455.

176. Brownlee M, Vlassara H, Kooney A, et al. Aminoguanidine prevents diabetes-induced arterial wall protein cross-linking. *Science* 1986;232:1629–1632.

177. Schmidt AM, Yan SD, Brett J, et al. Regulation of human mononuclear phagocyte migration by cell surface-binding proteins for advanced glycation end products. *J Clin Invest* 1993;91:2155–2168.

178. Vlassara H, Fuh H, Makita Z, et al. Exogenous advanced glycosylation end products induce complex vascular dysfunction in normal animals: a model for diabetic and aging complications. *Proc Natl Acad Sci U S A* 1992;89:12043–12047.

179. Vlassara H, Brownlee M, Manogue KR, et al. Cachectin/TNF and IL-1 induced by glucose-modified proteins: role in normal tissue remodeling. *Science* 1988;240:1546–1548.

180. Kirstein M, Aston C, Hintz R, et al. Receptor-specific induction of insulin-like growth factor I in human monocytes by advanced glycosylation end product-modified proteins. *J Clin Invest* 1992;90:439–446.

181. Park L, Raman KG, Lee KJ, et al. Suppression of accelerated diabetic atherosclerosis by the soluble receptor for advanced glycation endproducts. *Nat Med* 1998;4:1025–1031.

182. Makita Z, Vlassara H, Rayfield E, et al. Hemoglobin-AGE: a circulating marker of advanced glycosylation. *Science* 1992;258:651–653.

183. Onorato JM, Jenkins AJ, Thorpe SR, et al. Pyridoxamine, an inhibitor of advanced glycation reactions, also inhibits advanced lipoxidation reactions. Mechanism of action of pyridoxamine. *J Biol Chem* 2000;275:21177–21184.

184. Vasan S, Zhang X, Zhang X, et al. An agent cleaving glucose-derived protein crosslinks in vitro and in vivo. *Nature* 1996;382:275–278.

185. Wolffenbuttel BH, Boulanger CM, Crijns FR, et al. Breakers of advanced glycation end products restore large artery properties in experimental diabetes. *Proc Natl Acad Sci U S A* 1998;95:4630–4634.

186. Asif M, Egan J, Vasan S, et al. An advanced glycation end-product cross-link breaker can reverse age-related increases

187. in myocardial stiffness. *Proc Natl Acad Sci U S A* 2000;97:2809–2813.

187. Baynes JW. Role of oxidative stress in development of complications in diabetes. *Diabetes* 1991;40:405–412.

188. Ishii H, Jirousek MR, Koya D, et al. Amelioration of vascular dysfunctions in diabetic rats by an oral PKC beta inhibitor. *Science* 1996;272:728–731.

189. Koya D, King GL. Protein kinase C activation and the development of diabetic complications. *Diabetes* 1998;47:859–866.

190. Xia P, Inoguchi T, Kern TS, et al. Characterization of the mechanism for the chronic activation of diacylglycerol-protein kinase C pathway in diabetes and hypergalactosemia. *Diabetes* 1994;43:1122–1129.

191. Inoguchi T, Battan R, Handler E, et al. Preferential elevation of protein kinase C isoform beta II and diacylglycerol levels in the aorta and heart of diabetic rats: differential reversibility to glycemic control by islet cell transplantation. *Proc Natl Acad Sci U S A* 1992;89:11059–11063.

192. Koya D, Jirousek MR, Lin YW, et al. Characterization of protein kinase C beta isoform activation on the gene expression of transforming growth factor-beta, extracellular matrix components, and prostanoids in the glomeruli of diabetic rats. *J Clin Invest* 1997;100:115–126.

193. Koya D, Haneda M, Nakagawa H, et al. Amelioration of accelerated diabetic mesangial expansion by treatment with a PKC beta inhibitor in diabetic db/db mice, a rodent model for type 2 diabetes. *FASEB J* 2000;14:439–447.

194. Inaba T, Ishibashi S, Gotoda T, et al. Enhanced expression of platelet-derived growth factor-beta receptor by high glucose. Involvement of platelet-derived growth factor in diabetic angiopathy. *Diabetes* 1996;45:507–512.

195. Baynes JW, Thorpe SR. Role of oxidative stress in diabetic complications: a new perspective on an old paradigm. *Diabetes* 1999;48:1–9.

196. Wolff SP. Diabetes mellitus and free radicals. Free radicals, transition metals and oxidative stress in the aetiology of diabetes mellitus and complications. *Br Med Bull* 1993;49:642–652.

197. Yoshida K, Hirokawa J, Tagami S, et al. Weakened cellular scavenging activity against oxidative stress in diabetes mellitus: regulation of glutathione synthesis and efflux. *Diabetologia* 1995;38:201–210.

198. Karpen CW, Cataland S, O'Dorisio TM, et al. Production of 12-hydroxyeicosatetraenoic acid and vitamin E status in platelets from type I human diabetic subjects. *Diabetes* 1985;34:526–531.

199. Chen MS, Hutchinson ML, Pecoraro RE, et al. Hyperglycemia-induced intracellular depletion of ascorbic acid in human mononuclear leukocytes. *Diabetes* 1983;32:1078–1081.

200. Dyer DG, Blackledge JA, Thorpe SR, et al. Formation of pentosidine during nonenzymatic browning of proteins by glucose. Identification of glucose and other carbohydrates as possible precursors of pentosidine in vivo. *J Biol Chem* 1991;266:11654–11660.

201. Wells-Knecht MC, Thorpe SR, Baynes JW. Pathways of formation of glycoxidation products during glycation of collagen. *Biochemistry* 1995;34:15134–15141.

202. Yan SD, Chen X, Schmidt AM, et al. Glycated tau protein in Alzheimer disease: a mechanism for induction of oxidant stress. *Proc Natl Acad Sci U S A* 1994;91:7787–7791.

203. Beisswenger PJ, Moore LL, Brinck-Johnsen T, et al. Increased collagen-linked pentosidine levels and advanced glycosylation end products in early diabetic nephropathy. *J Clin Invest* 1993;92:212–217.

204. Konishi H, Tanaka M, Takemura Y, et al. Activation of protein kinase C by tyrosine phosphorylation in response to H_2O_2. *Proc Natl Acad Sci U S A* 1997;94:11233–11237.

205. Kunisaki M, Fumio U, Nawata H, et al. Vitamin E normalizes diacylglycerol-protein kinase C activation induced by hyperglycemia in rat vascular tissues. *Diabetes* 1996;45[Suppl 3]:S117–S119.

206. UK Prospective Diabetes Study (UKPDS) Group. Intensive blood-glucose control with sulphonylureas or insulin compared with conventional treatment and risk of complications in patients with type 2 diabetes (UKPDS 33). *Lancet* 1998;352:837–853.

207. Grundy SM, Benjamin IJ, Burke GL, et al. Diabetes and cardiovascular disease: a statement for healthcare professionals from the American Heart Association. *Circulation* 1999;100:1134–1146.

208. National High Blood Pressure Education Program Working group report on hypertension and diabetes. *Hypertension* 1994;23:145–158.

209. American Diabetes Association. Consensus statement on the treatment of hypertension in diabetes. *Diabetes Care* 1993;16:1394–1401.

210. Alderman MH, Cohen H, Madhavan S. Diabetes and cardiovascular events in hypertensive patients. *Hypertension* 1999;33:1130–1134.

211. Hypertension in Diabetes Study Group. HDS II. Increased risk of cardiovascular complications in hypertensive type 2 diabetic patients. *J Hypertens* 1993;11:319–325.

212. The sixth report of the Joint National Committee on prevention, evaluation, and treatment of high blood pressure. *Arch Intern Med* 1997;157:2413–2446.

213. Estacio RO, Jeffers BW, Hiatt WR, et al. The effect of nisoldipine as compared with enalapril on cardiovascular outcomes in patients with non-insulin-dependent diabetes and hypertension. *N Engl J Med* 1998;338:645–652.

214. Tatti P, Pahor M, Byington RP, et al. Outcome results of the Fosinopril Versus Amlodipine Cardiovascular Events Randomized Trial (FACET) in patients with hypertension and NIDDM. *Diabetes Care* 1998;21:597–603.

215. Curb JD, Pressel SL, Cutler JA, et al. Effect of diuretic-based antihypertensive treatment on cardiovascular disease risk in older diabetic patients with isolated systolic hypertension. Systolic Hypertension in the Elderly Program Cooperative Research Group. *JAMA* 1996;276:1886–1892.

216. Efficacy of atenolol and captopril in reducing risk of macrovascular and microvascular complications in type 2 diabetes: UKPDS 39. *BMJ* 1998;317:713–720.

217. Pahor M, Psaty BM, Furberg CD. Treatment of hypertensive patients with diabetes. *Lancet* 1998;351:689–690.

218. Hansson L, Lindholm LH, Ekbom T, et al. Randomised trial of old and new antihypertensive drugs in elderly patients: cardiovascular mortality and morbidity the Swedish Trial in Old Patients with Hypertension-2 study. *Lancet* 1999;354:1751–1756.

219. Sowers JR. Comorbidity of hypertension and diabetes: the

fosinopril versus amlodipine cardiovascular events trial (FACET). *Am J Cardiol* 1998;82:15R–19R.

220. Tuomilehto J, Rastenyte D, Birkenhager WH, et al. Effects of calcium-channel blockade in older patients with diabetes and systolic hypertension. Systolic Hypertension in Europe Trial Investigators. *N Engl J Med* 1999;340:677–684.

221. Hansson L, Zanchetti A, Carruthers SG, et al. Effects of intensive blood-pressure lowering and low-dose aspirin in patients with hypertension: principal results of the Hypertension Optimal Treatment (HOT) randomised trial. HOT Study Group. *Lancet* 1998;351:1755–1762.

222. Hansson L, Lindholm LH, Niskanen L, et al. Effect of angiotensin-converting-enzyme inhibition compared with conventional therapy on cardiovascular morbidity and mortality in hypertension: the Captopril Prevention Project (CAPPP) randomised trial. *Lancet* 1999;353:611–616.

223. Cooper ME. Pathogenesis, prevention, and treatment of diabetic nephropathy. *Lancet* 1998;352:213–219.

224. Parving HH. Renoprotection in diabetes: genetic and non-genetic risk factors and treatment. *Diabetologia* 1998;41:745–759.

225. Ravid M, Brosh D, Levi Z, et al. Use of enalapril to attenuate decline in renal function in normotensive, normoalbuminuric patients with type 2 diabetes mellitus. A randomized, controlled trial. *Ann Intern Med* 1998;128:982–988.

226. Ravid M, Savin H, Jutrin I, et al. Long-term stabilizing effect of angiotensin-converting enzyme inhibition on plasma creatinine and on proteinuria in normotensive type II diabetic patients. *Ann Intern Med* 1993;118:577–581.

227. Lewis EJ, Hunsicker LG, Bain RP, et al. The effect of angiotensin-converting-enzyme inhibition on diabetic nephropathy. The Collaborative Study Group. *N Engl J Med* 1993;329:1456–1462.

228. Tight blood pressure control and risk of macrovascular and microvascular complications in type 2 diabetes: UKPDS 38. *BMJ* 1998;317:703–713.

229. 1999 World Health Organization-International Society of Hypertension Guidelines for the Management of Hypertension Guidelines Subcommittee. *J Hypertens* 1999;17:151–183.

230. Moy CS, LaPorte RE, Dorman JS, et al. Insulin-dependent diabetes mellitus mortality. The risk of cigarette smoking. *Circulation* 1990;82:37–43.

231. Hanefeld M, Fischer S, Julius U, et al. Risk factors for myocardial infarction and death in newly detected NIDDM: the Diabetes Intervention Study, 11-year follow-up. *Diabetologia* 1996;39:1577–1583.

232. Haire-Joshu D, Glasgow RE, Tibbs TL. Smoking and diabetes. *Diabetes Care* 1999;22:1887–1898.

233. Nakanishi N, Nakamura K, Matsuo Y, et al. Cigarette smoking and risk for impaired fasting glucose and type 2 diabetes in middle-aged Japanese men. *Ann Intern Med* 2000;133:183–191.

234. Rimm EB, Chan J, Stampfer MJ, et al. Prospective study of cigarette smoking, alcohol use, and the risk of diabetes in men. *BMJ* 1995;310:555–559.

235. Facchini FS, Hollenbeck CB, Jeppesen J, et al. Insulin resistance and cigarette smoking. *Lancet* 1992;339:1128–1130.

236. Cryer PE, Haymond MW, Santiago JV, et al. Norepinephrine and epinephrine release and adrenergic mediation of

smoking-associated hemodynamic and metabolic events. *N Engl J Med* 1976;295:573–577.

237. Cerami C, Founds H, Nicholl I, et al. Tobacco smoke is a source of toxic reactive glycation products. *Proc Natl Acad Sci U S A* 1997;94:13915–13920.

238. Hoogeveen EK, Kostense PJ, Jakobs C, et al. Hyperhomocysteinemia increases risk of death, especially in type 2 diabetes: 5-year follow-up of the Hoorn Study. *Circulation* 2000;101:1506–1511.

239. Hoogeveen EK, Kostense PJ, Beks PJ, et al. Hyperhomocysteinemia is associated with an increased risk of cardiovascular disease, especially in non-insulin-dependent diabetes mellitus: a population-based study. *Arterioscler Thromb Vasc Biol* 1998;18:133–138.

240. Welch GN, Loscalzo J. Homocysteine and atherothrombosis. *N Engl J Med* 1998;338:1042–1050.

241. Tarnow L, Cambien F, Rossing P, et al. Insertion/deletion polymorphism in the angiotensin-I-converting enzyme gene is associated with coronary heart disease in IDDM patients with diabetic nephropathy. *Diabetologia* 1995;38:798–803.

242. Ruiz J, Blanche H, Cohen N, et al. Insertion/deletion polymorphism of the angiotensin-converting enzyme gene is strongly associated with coronary heart disease in non-insulin-dependent diabetes mellitus. *Proc Natl Acad Sci U S A* 1994;91:3662–3665.

243. Keavney BD, Dudley CR, Stratton IM, et al. UK prospective diabetes study (UKPDS) 14: association of angiotensin-converting enzyme insertion/deletion polymorphism with myocardial infraction in NIDDM. *Diabetologia* 1995;38:948–952.

244. Ruiz J, Blanche H, James RW, et al. Gln-Arg192 polymorphism of paraoxonase and coronary heart disease in type 2 diabetes. *Lancet* 1995;346:869–872.

245. Shih DM, Gu L, Xia YR, et al. Mice lacking serum paraoxonase are susceptible to organophosphate toxicity and atherosclerosis. *Nature* 1998;394:284–287.

246. Kannel WB, Hjortland M, Castelli WP. Role of diabetes in congestive heart failure: the Framingham study. *Am J Cardiol* 1974;34:29–34.

247. Shindler DM, Kostis JB, Yusuf S, et al. Diabetes mellitus, a predictor of morbidity and mortality in the Studies of Left Ventricular Dysfunction (SOLVD) Trials and Registry. *Am J Cardiol* 1996;77:1017–1020.

248. Ho KK, Pinsky JL, Kannel WB, et al. The epidemiology of heart failure: the Framingham Study. *J Am Coll Cardiol* 1993;22:6A–13A.

249. Ho KK, Anderson KM, Kannel WB, et al. Survival after the onset of congestive heart failure in Framingham Heart Study subjects. *Circulation* 1993;88:107–115.

250. Zarich SW, Arbuckle BE, Cohen LR, et al. Diastolic abnormalities in young asymptomatic diabetic patients assessed by pulsed Doppler echocardiography. *J Am Coll Cardiol* 1988;12:114–120.

251. Paillole C, Dahan M, Paycha F, et al. Prevalence and significance of left ventricular filling abnormalities determined by Doppler echocardiography in young type I (insulin-dependent) diabetic patients. *Am J Cardiol* 1989;64:1010–1016.

252. Mildenberger RR, Bar-Shlomo B, Druck MN, et al. Clinically unrecognized ventricular dysfunction in young diabetic patients. *J Am Coll Cardiol* 1984;4:234–238.

253. Shapiro LM, Leatherdale BA, Mackinnon J, et al. Left ventricular function in diabetes mellitus. II: Relation between clinical features and left ventricular function. *Br Heart J* 1981;45:129–132.

254. Mustonen JN, Uusitupa MI, Laakso M, et al. Left ventricular systolic function in middle-aged patients with diabetes mellitus. *Am J Cardiol* 1994;73:1202–1208.

255. Raev DC. Which left ventricular function is impaired earlier in the evolution of diabetic cardiomyopathy? An echocardiographic study of young type I diabetic patients. *Diabetes Care* 1994;17:633–639.

256. Stone PH, Muller JE, Hartwell T, et al. The effect of diabetes mellitus on prognosis and serial left ventricular function after acute myocardial infarction: contribution of both coronary disease and diastolic left ventricular dysfunction to the adverse prognosis. The MILIS Study Group. *J Am Coll Cardiol* 1989;14:49–57.

257. Grossman E, Messerli FH. Diabetic and hypertensive heart disease. *Ann Intern Med* 1996;125:304–310.

258. Levy D, Larson MG, Vasan RS, et al. The progression from hypertension to congestive heart failure. *JAMA* 1996;275:1557–1562.

259. Grossman E, Shemesh J, Shamiss A, et al. Left ventricular mass in diabetes-hypertension. *Arch Intern Med* 1992;152:1001–1004.

260. D'Ercole AJ, Underwood LE, Groelke J, et al. Leprechaunism: studies of the relationship among hyperinsulinism, insulin resistance, and growth retardation. *J Clin Endocrinol Metab* 1979;48:495–502.

261. Rheuban KS, Blizzard RM, Parker MA, et al. Hypertrophic cardiomyopathy in total lipodystrophy. *J Pediatr* 1986;109:301–302.

262. Breitweser JA, Meyer RA, Sperling MA, et al. Cardiac septal hypertrophy in hyperinsulinemic infants. *J Pediatr* 1980;96:535–539.

263. Lauer MS, Anderson KM, Kannel WB, et al. The impact of obesity on left ventricular mass and geometry. The Framingham Heart Study. *JAMA* 1991;266:231–236.

264. Sasson Z, Rasooly Y, Bhesania T, et al. Insulin resistance is an important determinant of left ventricular mass in the obese. *Circulation* 1993;88:1431–1436.

265. Liebson PR, Grandits GA, Dianzumba S, et al. Comparison of five antihypertensive monotherapies and placebo for change in left ventricular mass in patients receiving nutritional-hygienic therapy in the Treatment of Mild Hypertension Study (TOMHS). *Circulation* 1995;91:698–706.

266. MacMahon SW, Wilcken DE, Macdonald GJ. The effect of weight reduction on left ventricular mass. A randomized controlled trial in young, overweight hypertensive patients. *N Engl J Med* 1986;314:334–339.

267. Ohya Y, Abe I, Fujii K, et al. Hyperinsulinemia and left ventricular geometry in a work-site population in Japan. *Hypertension* 1996;27:729–734.

268. Verdecchia P, Reboldi G, Schillaci G, et al. Circulating insulin and insulin growth factor-1 are independent determinants of left ventricular mass and geometry in essential hypertension. *Circulation* 1999;100:1802–1807.

269. Marcus R, Krause L, Weder AB, et al. Sex-specific determinants of increased left ventricular mass in the Tecumseh Blood Pressure Study. *Circulation* 1994;90:928–936.

270. Reaven GM, Laws A. Insulin resistance, compensatory hyperinsulinaemia, and coronary heart disease. *Diabetologia* 1994;37:948–952.

271. Agewall S, Fagerberg B, Attvall S, et al. Carotid artery wall intima-media thickness is associated with insulin-mediated glucose disposal in men at high and low coronary risk. *Stroke* 1995;26:956–960.

272. Koren MJ, Devereux RB, Casale PN, et al. Relation of left ventricular mass and geometry to morbidity and mortality in uncomplicated essential hypertension. *Ann Intern Med* 1991;114:345–352.

273. Wakasaki H, Koya D, Schoen FJ, et al. Targeted overexpression of protein kinase C beta2 isoform in myocardium causes cardiomyopathy. *Proc Natl Acad Sci U S A* 1997;94:9320–9325.

274. Takeishi Y, Chu G, Kirkpatrick DM, et al. In vivo phosphorylation of cardiac troponin I by protein kinase C beta2 decreases cardiomyocyte calcium responsiveness and contractility in transgenic mouse hearts. *J Clin Invest* 1998;102:72–78.

275. Salomaa V, Riley W, Kark JD, et al. Non–insulin-dependent diabetes mellitus and fasting glucose and insulin concentrations are associated with arterial stiffness indexes. The ARIC Study. Atherosclerosis Risk in Communities Study. *Circulation* 1995;91:1432–1443.

276. Airaksinen KE, Salmela PI, Linnaluoto MK, et al. Diminished arterial elasticity in diabetes: association with fluorescent advanced glycosylation end products in collagen. *Cardiovasc Res* 1993;27:942–945.

277. Monnier VM, Kohn RR, Cerami A. Accelerated age-related browning of human collagen in diabetes mellitus. *Proc Natl Acad Sci U S A* 1984;81:583–587.

278. Monnier VM, Cerami A. Nonenzymatic browning in vivo: possible process for aging of long-lived proteins. *Science* 1981;211:491–493.

279. Norton GR, Candy G, Woodiwiss AJ. Aminoguanidine prevents the decreased myocardial compliance produced by streptozotocin-induced diabetes mellitus in rats. *Circulation* 1996;93:1905–1912.

280. Huijberts MS, Wolffenbuttel BH, Boudier HA, et al. Aminoguanidine treatment increases elasticity and decreases fluid filtration of large arteries from diabetic rats. *J Clin Invest* 1993;92:1407–1411.

281. Morrish NJ, Stevens LK, Head J, et al. A prospective study of mortality among middle-aged diabetic patients (the London Cohort of the WHO Multinational Study of Vascular Disease in Diabetics). I: Causes and death rates. *Diabetologia* 1990;33:538–541.

282. Jaffe AS, Spadaro JJ, Schechtman K, et al. Increased congestive heart failure after myocardial infarction of modest extent in patients with diabetes mellitus. *Am Heart J* 1984;108:31–37.

283. Savage MP, Krolewski AS, Kenien GG, et al. Acute myocardial infarction in diabetes mellitus and significance of congestive heart failure as a prognostic factor. *Am J Cardiol* 1988;62:665–669.

284. Mak KH, Moliterno DJ, Granger CB, et al. Influence of diabetes mellitus on clinical outcome in the thrombolytic era of acute myocardial infarction. GUSTO-I Investigators. Global utilization of streptokinase and tissue plasminogen activator for occluded coronary arteries. *J Am Coll Cardiol* 1997;30:171–179.

285. Barbash GI, White HD, Modan M, et al. Significance of diabetes mellitus in patients with acute myocardial infarction receiving thrombolytic therapy. Investigators of the International Tissue Plasminogen Activator/Streptokinase Mortality Trial. *J Am Coll Cardiol* 1993;22:707–713.

286. Zuanetti G, Latini R, Maggioni AP, et al. Influence of diabetes on mortality in acute myocardial infarction: data from the GISSI-2 study. *J Am Coll Cardiol* 1993;22:1788–1794.

287. Holmes DR Jr, Berger PB, Hochman JS, et al. Cardiogenic shock in patients with acute ischemic syndromes with and without ST-segment elevation. *Circulation* 1999;100:2067–2073.

288. Hasdai D, Granger CB, Srivatsa SS, et al. Diabetes mellitus and outcome after primary coronary angioplasty for acute myocardial infarction: lessons from the GUSTO-IIb Angioplasty Substudy. Global use of strategies to open occluded arteries in acute coronary syndromes. *J Am Coll Cardiol* 2000;35:1502–1512.

289. Shindler DM, Palmeri ST, Antonelli TA, et al. Diabetes mellitus in cardiogenic shock complicating acute myocardial infarction: a report from the SHOCK Trial Registry. Should we emergently revascularize occluded coronaries for cardiogenic shock? *J Am Coll Cardiol* 2000;36:1097–1103.

290. Malmberg K, Ryden L. Myocardial infarction in patients with diabetes mellitus. *Eur Heart J* 1988;9:259–264.

291. Ulvenstam G, Aberg A, Bergstrand R, et al. Long-term prognosis after myocardial infarction in men with diabetes. *Diabetes* 1985;34:787–792.

292. Abaci A, Oguzhan A, Kahraman S, et al. Effect of diabetes mellitus on formation of coronary collateral vessels. *Circulation* 1999;99:2239–2242.

293. Herlitz J, Malmberg K, Karlson BW, et al. Mortality and morbidity during a five-year follow-up of diabetics with myocardial infarction. *Acta Med Scand* 1988;224:31–38.

294. Fibrinolytic Therapy Trialists' (FTT) Collaborative Group. Indications for fibrinolytic therapy in suspected acute myocardial infarction: collaborative overview of early mortality and major morbidity results from all randomized trials of more than 1000 patients. *Lancet* 1994;343:311–322.

295. Mahaffey KW, Granger CB, Toth CA, et al. Diabetic retinopathy should not be a contraindication to thrombolytic therapy. *J Am Coll Cardiol* 1997;30:1606–1610.

296. Kendall MJ, Lynch KP, Hjalmarson A, et al. Beta-blockers and sudden cardiac death. *Ann Intern Med* 1995;123:358–367.

297. Gundersen T, Kjekshus J. Timolol treatment after myocardial infarction in diabetic patients. *Diabetes Care* 1983;6:285–290.

298. Kjekshus J, Gilpin E, Cali G, et al. Diabetic patients and beta-blockers after acute myocardial infarction. *Eur Heart J* 1990;11:43–50.

299. Pfeffer MA. ACE inhibitors in acute myocardial infarction: patient selection and timing. *Circulation* 1998;97:2192–2194.

300. Zuanetti G, Latini R, Maggioni AP, et al. Effect of the ACE inhibitor lisinopril on mortality in diabetic patients with acute myocardial infarction: data from the GISSI-3 study. *Circulation* 1997;96:4239–4245.

301. Gustafsson I, Torp-Pedersen C, Kober L, et al. Effect of the angiotensin-converting enzyme inhibitor trandolapril on mortality and morbidity in diabetic patients with left ventricular dysfunction after acute myocardial infarction. Trace Study Group. *J Am Coll Cardiol* 1999;34:83–89.

302. Torlone E, Rambotti AM, Perriello G, et al. ACE-inhibition increases hepatic and extrahepatic sensitivity to insulin in patients with type 2 (non–insulin-dependent) diabetes mellitus and arterial hypertension. *Diabetologia* 1991;34:119–125.

303. Antiplatelet Trialists' Collaboration. Collaborative overview of randomized trials of antiplatelet therapy. I. Prevention of death, myocardial infarction, and stroke by prolonged antiplatelet therapy in various categories of patients. *BMJ* 1994;308:81–106.

304. Braunwald E, Antman EM, Beasley JW, et al. ACC/AHA guidelines for the management of patients with unstable angina and non-ST-segment elevation myocardial infarction: executive summary and recommendations. A report of the American College of Cardiology/American Heart Association task force on practice guidelines (Committee on the Management of Patients with Unstable Angina). *Circulation* 2000;102:1193–1209.

305. Moreno PR, Murcia AM, Palacios IF, et al. Coronary composition and macrophage infiltration in atherectomy specimens from patients with diabetes mellitus. *Circulation* 2000;102:2180–2184.

306. Lopaschuk GD, Stanley WC. Glucose metabolism in the ischemic heart. *Circulation* 1997;95:313–315.

307. Depre C, Vanoverschelde JL, Taegtmeyer H. Glucose for the heart. *Circulation* 1999;99:578–588.

308. Russell RR 3rd, Yin R, Caplan MJ, et al. Additive effects of hyperinsulinemia and ischemia on myocardial GLUT1 and GLUT4 translocation in vivo. *Circulation* 1998;98:2180–2186.

309. Katz EB, Stenbit AE, Hatton K, et al. Cardiac and adipose tissue abnormalities but not diabetes in mice deficient in GLUT4. *Nature* 1995;377:151–155.

310. Eberli FR, Weinberg EO, Grice WN, et al. Protective effect of increased glycolytic substrate against systolic and diastolic dysfunction and increased coronary resistance from prolonged global underperfusion and reperfusion in isolated rabbit hearts perfused with erythrocyte suspensions. *Circ Res* 1991;68:466–481.

311. Kurien VA, Yates PA, Oliver MF. Free fatty acids, heparin, and arrhythmias during experimental myocardial infarction. *Lancet* 1969;2:185–187.

312. Apstein CS. Glucose-insulin-potassium for acute myocardial infarction: remarkable results from a new prospective, randomized trial. *Circulation* 1998;98:2223–2226.

313. Oliver MF, Opie LH. Effects of glucose and fatty acids on myocardial ischaemia and arrhythmias. *Lancet* 1994;343:155–158.

314. Runnman EM, Lamp ST, Weiss JN. Enhanced utilization of exogenous glucose improves cardiac function in hypoxic rabbit ventricle without increasing total glycolytic flux. *J Clin Invest* 1990;86:1222–1233.

315. von Dahl J, Herman WH, Hicks RJ, et al. Myocardial glucose uptake in patients with insulin-dependent diabetes mellitus assessed quantitatively by dynamic positron emission tomography. *Circulation* 1993;88:395–404.

316. Gorge G, Chatelain P, Schaper J, et al. Effect of increasing degrees of ischemic injury on myocardial oxidative metabolism early after reperfusion in isolated rat hearts. *Circ Res* 1991;68:1681–1692.

317. Malmberg K, Ryden L, Efendic S, et al. Randomized trial of insulin-glucose infusion followed by subcutaneous insulin treatment in diabetic patients with acute myocardial infarction (DIGAMI study): effects on mortality at 1 year. *J Am Coll Cardiol* 1995;26:57–65.

318. Detre K, Holubkov R, Kelsey S, et al. Percutaneous transluminal coronary angioplasty in 1985–1986 and 1977–1981. The National Heart, Lung, and Blood Institute Registry. *N Engl J Med* 1988;318:265–270.

319. Lincoff A. Dose stenting prevent diabetic arterial shrinkage after percutaneous coronary revascularization. *Circulation* 1997;96:1134–1137.

320. Kip KE, Faxon DP, Detre KM, et al. Coronary angioplasty in diabetic patients. The National Heart, Lung, and Blood Institute Percutaneous Transluminal Coronary Angioplasty Registry. *Circulation* 1996;94:1818–1825.

321. Levine GN, Jacobs AK, Keeler GP, et al. Impact of diabetes mellitus on percutaneous revascularization (CAVEAT-I). CAVEAT-I Investigators. Coronary Angioplasty Versus Excisional Atherectomy Trial. *Am J Cardiol* 1997;79:748–755.

322. The Bypass Angioplasty Revascularization Investigation (BARI). Influence of diabetes on 5-year mortality and morbidity in a randomized trial comparing CABG and PTCA in patients with multivessel disease. *Circulation* 1997;96:1761–1769.

323. Abizaid A, Mintz GS, Pichard AD, et al. Clinical, intravascular ultrasound, and quantitative angiographic determinants of the coronary flow reserve before and after percutaneous transluminal coronary angioplasty. *Am J Cardiol* 1998;82:423–428.

324. Elezi S, Kastrati A, Neumann F, et al. Vessel size and long-term outcome after coronary stent placement. *Circulation* 1998;98:1875–1880.

325. Kleiman NS, Lincoff AM, Kereiakes DJ, et al. Diabetes mellitus, glycoprotein IIb/IIIa blockade, and heparin: evidence for a complex interaction in a multicenter trial. EPILOG Investigators. *Circulation* 1998;97:1912–1920.

326. Goldberg S, Savage MP, Fischman DL. The interventional cardiologist and the diabetic patient. Have we pushed the envelope too far or not far enough? *Circulation* 1996;94:1804–1806.

327. Holmes DJ, Vietstra R, Smith H, et al. Restenosis after percutaneous transluminal coronary angioplasty (PTCA): a report from the PTCA Registry of the National Heart, Lung, and Blood Institute. *Am J Cardiol* 1984;53:77C–81C.

328. Weintraub W, Kosinski A, Brown C, et al. Can restenosis after coronary angioplasty be predicted from clinical variables? *J Am Coll Cardiol* 1993;21:6–14.

329. Vandormael MG, Deligonul U, Kern MJ, et al. Multilesion coronary angioplasty: clinical and angiographic follow-up. *J Am Coll Cardiol* 1987;10:246–252.

330. Van Belle E, Abolmaali K, Bauters C, et al. Restenosis, late vessel occlusion and left ventricular function six months after balloon angioplasty in diabetic patients. *J Am Coll Cardiol* 1999;34:476–485.

331. Rabbani L, Edelman E, Ganz P, et al. Relation of restenosis after excimer laser angioplasty to fasting insulin levels. *Am J Cardiol* 1994;73:323–327.

332. Kastrati A, Schomig A, Elezi S, et al. Predictive factors of restenosis after coronary stent placement. *J Am Coll Cardiol* 1997;30:1428–1436.

333. Abizaid A, Kornowski R, Mintz GS, et al. The influence of diabetes mellitus on acute and late clinical outcomes following coronary stent implantation. *J Am Coll Cardiol* 1998;32:584–589.

334. Carrozza JP Jr, Kuntz RE, Fishman RF, et al. Restenosis after arterial injury caused by coronary stenting in patients with diabetes mellitus. *Ann Intern Med* 1993;118:344–349.

335. Elezi S, Kastrati A, Pache J, et al. Diabetes mellitus and the clinical and angiographic outcome after coronary stent placement. *J Am Coll Cardiol* 1998;32:1866–1873.

336. Gum P, O'Keefe JJ, Borkon A, et al. Bypass surgery versus coronary angioplasty for revascularization of treated diabetic patients. *Circulation* 1997;96:II-7–II-10.

337. Topol EJ, Yadav JS. Recognition of the importance of embolization in atherosclerotic vascular disease. *Circulation* 2000;101:570–580.

338. Bhatt DL, Marso SP, Lincoff AM, et al. Abciximab reduces mortality in diabetics following percutaneous coronary intervention. *J Am Coll Cardiol* 2000;35:922–928.

339. Theroux P, Alexander J Jr, Pharand C, et al. Glycoprotein IIb/IIIa receptor blockade improves outcomes in diabetic patients presenting with unstable angina/non-ST-elevation myocardial infarction: results from the platelet receptor inhibition in ischemic syndrome management in patients limited by unstable signs and symptoms (PRISM-PLUS) study. *Circulation* 2000;102:2466–2472.

340. Kornowski R, Mintz GS, Kent KM, et al. Increased restenosis in diabetes mellitus after coronary interventions is due to exaggerated intimal hyperplasia. A serial intravascular ultrasound study. *Circulation* 1997;95:1366–1369.

341. Aronson D, Bloomgarden Z, Rayfield EJ. Potential mechanisms promoting restenosis in diabetic patients. *J Am Coll Cardiol* 1996;27:528–535.

342. Nishimoto Y, Miyazaki Y, Toki Y, et al. Enhanced secretion of insulin plays a role in the development of atherosclerosis and restenosis of coronary arteries: elective percutaneous transluminal coronary angioplasty in patients with effort angina. *J Am Coll Cardiol* 1998;32:1624–1649.

343. Marso SP, Ellis SG, Tuzcu M, et al. The importance of proteinuria as a determinant of mortality following percutaneous coronary revascularization in diabetics. *J Am Coll Cardiol* 1999;33:1269–1277.

344. Kennedy J, Kaiser G, Fisher L, et al. Multivariate discriminate analysis of clinical and angiographic predictors of operative mortality from the Collaborative Study in Coronary Artery Surgery (CASS). *J Thorac Cardiovasc Surg* 1980;80:876–887.

345. Salomon NW, Page US, Okies JE, et al. Diabetes mellitus and coronary artery bypass. Short-term risk and long-term prognosis. *J Thorac Cardiovasc Surg* 1983;85:264–271.

346. Johnson WD, Pedraza PM, Kayser KL. Coronary artery surgery in diabetics: 261 consecutive patients followed four to seven years. *Am Heart J* 1982;104:823–827.

347. Thourani VH, Weintraub WS, Stein B, et al. Influence of diabetes mellitus on early and late outcome after coronary artery bypass grafting. *Ann Thorac Surg* 1999;67:1045–1052.

348. Loop FD, Lytle BW, Cosgrove DM, et al. J. Maxwell Chamberlain memorial paper. Sternal wound complications after isolated coronary artery bypass grafting: early and late mortality, morbidity, and cost of care. *Ann Thorac Surg* 1990;49:179–186; discussion 186–187.

349. Zerr KJ, Furnary AP, Grunkemeier GL, et al. Glucose control lowers the risk of wound infection in diabetics after open heart operations. *Ann Thorac Surg* 1997;63:356–361.

350. Davies M, Kim J, Klyachkin M, et al. Diabetes mellitus and experimental vein graft structure and function. *J Vasc Surg* 1994;19:1031–1043.

351. Lytle BW, Loop FD, Cosgrove DM, et al. Long-term (5 to 12 years) serial studies of internal mammary artery and saphenous vein coronary bypass grafts. *J Thorac Cardiovasc Surg* 1985;89:248–258.

352. Campeau L, Enjalbert M, Lesperance J, et al. The relation of risk factors to the development of atherosclerosis in saphenous-vein bypass grafts and the progression of disease in the native circulation. A study 10 years after aortocoronary bypass surgery. *N Engl J Med* 1984;311:1329–1332.

353. Hoogwerf BJ, Waness A, Cressman M, et al. Effects of aggressive cholesterol lowering and low-dose anticoagulation on clinical and angiographic outcomes in patients with diabetes: the Post Coronary Artery Bypass Graft Trial. *Diabetes* 1999;48:1289–1294.

354. Loop F. Internal-thoracic-artery grafts—biologically better coronary arteries. *N Engl J Med* 1996;334:263.

355. Morris JJ, Smith LR, Jones RH, et al. Influence of diabetes and mammary artery grafting on survival after coronary bypass. *Circulation* 1991;84:III-275–III-284.

356. Chaitman B, Rosen A, Williams D, et al. Myocardial infarction and cardiac mortality in the Bypass Angioplasty Revascularization Investigation (BARI) randomized trial. *Circulation* 1997;96:2162–2170.

357. Barsness GW, Peterson ED, Ohman EM, et al. Relationship between diabetes mellitus and long-term survival after coronary bypass and angioplasty. *Circulation* 1997;96:2551–2556.

358. The Bypass Angioplasty Revascularization Investigation (BARI) Investigators. Comparison of coronary bypass surgery with angioplasty in patients with multivessel disease. *N Engl J Med* 1996;335:217–225.

359. King SB 3rd, Kosinski AS, Guyton RA, et al. Eight-year mortality in the Emory Angioplasty versus Surgery Trial (EAST). *J Am Coll Cardiol* 2000;35:1116–1121.

360. Bertran M. Long-term follow-up of European revascularization trials. Presented at the 68th Scientific Sessions XII of the American Heart Association. Anaheim, CA, November 16, 1995.

361. Detre KM, Lombardero MS, Brooks MM, et al. The effect of previous coronary-artery bypass surgery on the prognosis of patients with diabetes who have acute myocardial infarction. Bypass Angioplasty Revascularization Investigation Investigators. *N Engl J Med* 2000;342:989–997.

362. Kuntz RE. Importance of considering atherosclerosis progression when choosing a coronary revascularization strategy: the diabetes-percutaneous transluminal coronary angioplasty dilemma. *Circulation* 1999;99:847–851.

363. Bell MR, Gersh BJ, Schaff HV, et al. Effect of completeness of revascularization on long-term outcome of patients with three-vessel disease undergoing coronary artery bypass surgery. A report from the Coronary Artery Surgery Study (CASS) Registry. *Circulation* 1992;86:446–457.

364. Schaff HV, Rosen AD, Shemin RJ, et al. Clinical and operative characteristics of patients randomized to coronary artery bypass surgery in the Bypass Angioplasty Revascularization Investigation (BARI). *Am J Cardiol* 1995;75:18C–26C.

365. Weintraub W, Stein B, Kosinski A, et al. Outcome of coronary bypass surgery versus coronary angioplasty in diabetic patients with multivessel coronary artery disease. *J Am Coll Cardiol* 1998;31:10–19.

366. The BARI Investigators. Seven-year outcome in the Bypass Angioplasty Revascularization Investigation (BARI) by treatment and diabetic status. *J Am Coll Cardiol* 2000;35:1122–1129.

367. The Post Coronary Artery Bypass Graft Trial Investigators. The effect of aggressive lowering of low-density lipoprotein cholesterol levels and low-dose anticoagulation on obstructive changes in saphenous-vein coronary-artery bypass grafts. *N Engl J Med* 1997;336:153–162.

368. Grines CL, Booth DC, Nissen SE, et al. Mechanism of acute myocardial infarction in patients with prior coronary artery bypass grafting and therapeutic implications. *Am J Cardiol* 1990;65:1292–1296.

369. Engler RL, Yellon DM. Sulfonylurea KATP blockade in type II diabetes and preconditioning in cardiovascular disease. Time for reconsideration. *Circulation* 1996;94:2297–2301.

370. Brady PA, Terzic A. The sulfonylurea controversy: more questions from the heart. *J Am Coll Cardiol* 1998;31:950–956.

371. Aguilar-Bryan L, Nichols CG, Wechsler SW, et al. Cloning of the beta cell high-affinity sulfonylurea receptor: a regulator of insulin secretion. *Science* 1995;268:423–426.

372. Cleveland JC Jr, Meldrum DR, Cain BS, et al. Oral sulfonylurea hypoglycemic agents prevent ischemic preconditioning in human myocardium. Two paradoxes revisited. *Circulation* 1997;96:29–32.

373. Meinert CL, Knatterud GL, Prout TE, et al. A study of the effects of hypoglycemic agents on vascular complications in patients with adult-onset diabetes. II. Mortality results. *Diabetes* 1970;19:789–830.

374. Garratt KN, Brady PA, Hassinger NL, et al. Sulfonylurea drugs increase early mortality in patients with diabetes mellitus after direct angioplasty for acute myocardial infarction. *J Am Coll Cardiol* 1999;33:119–124.

375. Klamann A, Sarfert P, Launhardt V, et al. Myocardial infarction in diabetic vs. non-diabetic subjects. Survival and infarct size following therapy with sulfonylureas (glibenclamide). *Eur Heart J* 2000;21:220–229.

376. Rollins MD, Jenkins JG, Carson DJ, et al. Power spectral analysis of the electrocardiogram in diabetic children. *Diabetologia* 1992;35:452–455.

377. Marchant B, Umachandran V, Stevenson R, et al. Silent myocardial ischemia: role of subclinical neuropathy in patients with and without diabetes. *J Am Coll Cardiol* 1993;22:1433–1437.

378. Toyry JP, Niskanen LK, Mantysaari MJ, et al. Occurrence, predictors, and clinical significance of autonomic neuropathy in NIDDM. Ten-year follow-up from the diagnosis. *Diabetes* 1996;45:308–315.

379. Ziegler D. Diabetic cardiovascular autonomic neuropathy: prognosis, diagnosis and treatment. *Diabetes Metab Rev* 1994;10:339–383.

380. Kreiner G, Wolzt M, Fasching P, et al. Myocardial m-[123I]iodobenzylguanidine scintigraphy for the assessment of adrenergic cardiac innervation in patients with IDDM. Comparison with cardiovascular reflex tests and relationship to left ventricular function. *Diabetes* 1995;44:543–549.

381. Schwartz PJ, La Rovere MT, Vanoli E. Autonomic nervous system and sudden cardiac death. Experimental basis and clinical observations for post-myocardial infarction risk stratification. *Circulation* 1992;85:177–191.

382. La Rovere MT, Bigger JT Jr, Marcus FI, et al. Baroreflex sensitivity and heart-rate variability in prediction of total cardiac mortality after myocardial infarction. ATRAMI (Autonomic Tone and Reflexes after Myocardial Infarction) Investigators. *Lancet* 1998;351:478–484.

383. Ewing DJ, Boland O, Neilson JM, et al. Autonomic neuropathy, QT interval lengthening, and unexpected deaths in male diabetic patients. *Diabetologia* 1991;34:182–185.

384. Wei K, Dorian P, Newman D, et al. Association between QT dispersion and autonomic dysfunction in patients with diabetes mellitus. *J Am Coll Cardiol* 1995;26:859–863.

385. Muller JE, Tofler GH, Stone PH. Circadian variation and triggers of onset of acute cardiovascular disease. *Circulation* 1989;79:733–743.

386. ISIS-2 (Second International Study of Infarct Survival) Collaborative Group. Morning peak in the incidence of myocardial infarction: experience in the ISIS-2 trial. *Eur Heart J* 1992;13:594–598.

387. Hjalmarson A, Gilpin EA, Nicod P, et al. Differing circadian patterns of symptom onset in subgroups of patients with acute myocardial infarction. *Circulation* 1989;80:267–275.

388. Bernardi L, Ricordi L, Lazzari P, et al. Impaired circadian modulation of sympathovagal activity in diabetes. A possible explanation for altered temporal onset of cardiovascular disease. *Circulation* 1992;86:1443–1452.

389. O'Brien E, Sheridan J, O'Malley K. Dippers and non-dippers [letter]. *Lancet* 1988;2:397.

390. Verdecchia P, Schillaci G, Guerrieri M, et al. Circadian blood pressure changes and left ventricular hypertrophy in essential hypertension. *Circulation* 1990;81:528–536.

391. Mann S, Altman DG, Raftery EB, et al. Circadian variation of blood pressure in autonomic failure. *Circulation* 1983;68:477–483.

392. Spallone V, Bernardi L, Ricordi L, et al. Relationship between the circadian rhythms of blood pressure and sympathovagal balance in diabetic autonomic neuropathy. *Diabetes* 1993;42:1745–1752.

393. Nielsen FS, Rossing P, Bang LE, et al. On the mechanisms of blunted nocturnal decline in arterial blood pressure in NIDDM patients with diabetic nephropathy. *Diabetes* 1995;44:783–789.

394. Bradley RF, Schonfeld A. Diminished pain in diabetic patients with acute myocardial infarction. *Geriatrics* 1962;17:322–326.

395. Kannel WB, Abbott RD. Incidence and prognosis of unrecognized myocardial infarction. An update on the Framingham study. *N Engl J Med* 1984;311:1144–1147.

396. Barron HV, Bowlby LJ, Breen T, et al. Use of reperfusion therapy for acute myocardial infarction in the United States: data from the National Registry of Myocardial Infarction 2. *Circulation* 1998;97:1150–1156.

397. Nesto RW, Phillips RT, Kett KG, et al. Angina and exertional myocardial ischemia in diabetic and nondiabetic patients: assessment by exercise thallium scintigraphy. *Ann Intern Med* 1988;108:170–175.

398. Milan Study on Atherosclerosis and Diabetes (MiSAD) Group. Prevalence of unrecognized silent myocardial ischemia and its association with atherosclerotic risk factors in noninsulin-dependent diabetes mellitus. *Am J Cardiol* 1997;79:134–139.

399. Caracciolo EA, Chaitman BR, Forman SA, et al. Diabetics with coronary disease have a prevalence of asymptomatic ischemia during exercise treadmill testing and ambulatory ischemia monitoring similar to that of nondiabetic patients. An ACIP database study. ACIP Investigators. Asymptomatic Cardiac Ischemia Pilot Investigators. *Circulation* 1996;93:2097–2105.

400. Faerman I, Faccio E, Milei J, et al. Autonomic neuropathy and painless myocardial infarction in diabetic patients. Histologic evidence of their relationship. *Diabetes* 1977;26:1147–1158.

401. Ambepityia G, Kopelman PG, Ingram D, et al. Exertional myocardial ischemia in diabetes: a quantitative analysis of anginal perceptual threshold and the influence of autonomic function. *J Am Coll Cardiol* 1990;15:72–77.

402. Fioretto P, Steffes MW, Sutherland DE, et al. Reversal of lesions of diabetic nephropathy after pancreas transplantation. *N Engl J Med* 1998;339:69–75.

403. Haffner SM, Alexander CM, Cook TJ, et al. Reduced coronary events in simvastatin-treated patients with coronary heart disease and diabetes or impaired fasting glucose levels: subgroup analyses in the Scandinavian Simvastatin Survival Study. *Arch Intern Med* 1999;159:2661–2667.

404. Prevention of cardiovascular events and death with pravastatin in patients with coronary heart disease and a broad range of initial cholesterol levels. The Long-Term Intervention with Pravastatin in Ischaemic Disease (LIPID) Study Group. *N Engl J Med* 1998;339:1349–1357.

405. Brownlee M, Vlassara H, Cerami A. Nonenzymatic glycosylation products on collagen covalently trap low-density lipoprotein. *Diabetes* 1985;34:938–941.

406. Bucala R, Tracey KJ, Cerami A. Advanced glycosylation products quench nitric oxide and mediate defective endothelium-dependent vasodilatation in experimental diabetes. *J Clin Invest* 1991;87:432–438.

407. Giardino I, Edelstein D, Brownlee M. Nonenzymatic glycosylation in vitro and in bovine endothelial cells alters basic fibroblast growth factor activity. A model for intracellular glycosylation in diabetes. *J Clin Invest* 1994;94:110–117.

408. Kirstein M, Brett J, Radoff S, et al. Advanced protein glycosylation induces transendothelial human monocyte chemotaxis and secretion of platelet-derived growth factor: role in vascular disease of diabetes and aging. *Proc Natl Acad Sci U S A* 1990;87:9010–9014.

409. Esposito C, Gerlach H, Brett J, et al. Endothelial receptor-mediated binding of glucose-modified albumin is associated with increased monolayer permeability and modulation of cell surface coagulant properties. *J Exp Med* 1989;170:1387–1407.

410. Downs JR, Clearfield M, Weis S, et al. Primary prevention of acute coronary events with lovastatin in men and women with average cholesterol levels: results of AFCAPS/TexCAPS. Air Force/Texas Coronary Atherosclerosis Prevention Study. *JAMA* 1998;279:1615–1622.

8

ESTROGEN, FEMALE GENDER, AND HEART DISEASE

ROBERT H. KNOPP
KEIKO AIKAWA

▼▼ ADDITIONAL ELECTRONIC TOPICS

Plasma Triglyceride Elevations b60; Remnant Lipoprotein Metabolism b61; Low-Density Lipoprotein Metabolism b62; Lipoprotein(a) Metabolism b63; High-Density Lipoprotein Metabolism b64; Oral Contraceptive Steroid Effects on Lipoprotein Metabolism and Atherogenesis b65; Dehydroepiandrosterone b66; Diet b67; Drug Therapy Efficacy b68; Arteriosclerosis Prevention and Regression b69; Lipid Screening Guidelines for Hyperlipidemic Women b70; Gender Differences in Drug Treatment b71; Bile Acid–Binding Resin b72; Niacin b73; Fibric Acid Derivatives b74; Reductase Inhibitors b75; Reductase and Fibrate Combination Therapy b76

OVERVIEW

Cardiovascular disease (CVD) across the entire lifetime is slightly more common as a cause of mortality in women than

R. H. Knopp: Department of Medicine, University of Washington School of Medicine, Northwest Lipid Reseach Clinic, Seattle, Washington
K. Aikawa: Department of Medicine, Division of Cardiology, University of Washington Medical Center, Seattle, Washington

in men. In addition, CVD in women is a formidable problem because of difficulties in diagnosis and increased morbidity and mortality associated with CVD events at all ages. In the middle years, CVD is associated with multiple risk factors, generally more in women than in men of the same age. Diabetes appears to be a particularly more severe risk factor in women than in men, but smoking is still probably the worst CVD risk factor in any gender. Specific lipid management guidelines are available for the treatment of elevated low-density lipoprotein cholesterol (LDL-C) in women, but the management of combined hyperlipidemia is a more common condition and more important. Postmenopausal hormone replacement therapy, unfortunately, has not been beneficial in preventing progression of established coronary disease in prospective double-blind randomized studies. The evidence of benefit from experimental models may relate to the early rather than the late use of estrogen in the atherogenic process; this is analogous to the lower rates of heart disease in premenopausal women. There are many examples of interaction of sex steroids with lipid disorders that require care and thought and have long-term implications for the cardiovascular health of both men and women.

GLOSSARY

Combined hyperlipidemia: The concomitant elevation of total triglyceride level above 200 mg per dL and LDL-C level above 100, 130, or 160 mg per dL, depending on National Cholesterol Education Program risk factors.

Lipid transfer protein: Also known as *cholesterol ester transport protein*, lipid transfer protein facilitates the transfer of triglyceride from very-low-density lipoprotein (VLDL) to high-density lipoprotein (HDL) and cholesterol from HDL to VLDL and LDL, thereby maintaining a cycle of transport of cholesterol in the body.

Lipoprotein(a) [Lp(a)]: A nonfibrinolytic plasminogen analog that is attached to low-density lipoprotein (LDL) apoprotein B and plasminogen binding sites, inhibiting fibrinolysis and enhancing LDL trapping in the arterial wall.

Polycystic ovary syndrome (PCOS): Syndrome associated with the metabolic syndrome, obesity, and hyperandrogenemia in young women.

Remnant lipoprotein: A lipoprotein particle that is intermediate between VLDL and LDL (also known as *intermediate-density lipoprotein*) and has powerful atherogenic potential.

Syndrome X: The metabolic syndrome that is caused by insulin resistance. Syndrome X is associated with combined hyperlipidemia, obesity, hypertension, diabetes, and PCOS.

INTRODUCTION

The main points of this chapter are raised in the following true case. A 25-year-old woman who used oral contraceptives (OCs) and smoked one pack of cigarettes per day was having vague chest pains for a year, which were variously diagnosed as anxiety and acid reflux. On July 4, 2000, she was seen at an emergency room and sent away. Twelve hours later at the same emergency room, the possibility of a myocardial infarction (MI) was entertained as she went into shock. An emergency two-vessel angioplasty procedure was performed, saving the patient's life. Several other angioplasties and three-vessel bypass surgery have been done

since, complicated by bilateral iliac vessel stenosis. She is now somewhat intellectually impaired. On presentation to clinic, the cholesterol was 182 mg per dL, triglyceride was 175 mg per dL, and high-density lipoprotein cholesterol (HDL-C) was 24 mg per dL on 40 mg atorvastatin. The Lp(a) was 19.2 (seventy-fifth percentile). Why did this patient have an MI? Why was it so severe? Why was the MI not recognized during the first emergency room visit? Is this case as rare as it might seem? Is the constellation of symptoms unique to this case or to women in general? What is the approach to managing this patient's lipid disorder? This chapter addresses these and other questions.

INCIDENCE OF CORONARY ARTERY DISEASE IN WOMEN VERSUS MEN

The perception persists that coronary artery disease is a rare occurrence in women, especially in young women, leading to the view that arteriosclerotic disease of the vascular tree is less important in women overall. Both perceptions are incorrect. CVD is an equal-opportunity killer in men and women over their lifetimes. In Washington State in 1991, the incidence of CVD death was 42% in women and 39% in men (1). Nationwide, these numbers approach 50%. The slightly higher percentage of female cardiovascular deaths can be attributed to the greater longevity of women, which is an extremely powerful risk factor in its own right and allows female CVD mortality rates to "catch up" in old age.

A lower rate of CVD mortality in women is certainly observed in young women, especially premenopausally; still, the rates of CVD in women are not negligible and have defined relationships to cardiovascular risk factors. In fact, as shown in Figure 8.1, the increase in CVD with age in the Framingham study (2) lags behind the male age-associated increase by only 10 to 15 years. A similar pattern is seen even in high-risk conditions such as heterozygous familial hypercholesterolemia, again with a delay of 10 years in women compared to men. The delay in onset in women versus men is attributed to the premenopausal exposure to endogenous ovarian estrogen, but, even premenopausally, this effect diminishes with advancing age (Fig. 8.1). The most important point is that the rise in female CVD is highly parallel to the rise of CVD in men. A major inflection in the female risk curve around the time of menopause is not seen (Fig. 8.1). ❧ b77

The early lesions of arteriosclerosis—the fatty streak and the fibrous arteriosclerotic plaque—are seen in young women and men. In teenagers and young adults who died traumatic deaths in Bogalusa (7), half of the men and one-fourth of the women were so affected. In blacks, half of men and women were affected and were equal in extent. In both genders, the fatty streak lesions were proportional in extent to the plasma LDL-C. However, the plasma level of VLDL-C (7), which is closely related to the plasma trigly-

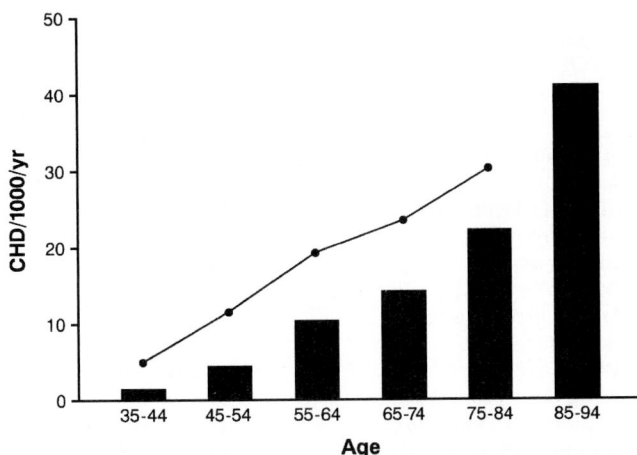

FIGURE 8.1 Annual rate of coronary heart disease (CHD) in men (*line*) and women (*bars*), from the Framingham Heart Study. (From Castelli WP. Cardiovascular disease in women. *Am J Obstet Gynecol* 1988;158:1553–1560, with permission.)

ceride level, was associated with lesions only in women (see the discussion of triglyceride as a CVD risk factor in women in the section Plasma Triglyceride Elevations). When coronary lesions are examined, female lesions are more lipid filled, rich in macrophages, and less densely fibrous (8). Thus, lesions in women could be more unstable under certain circumstances, as well as more readily reversed (9). Likewise, coronary calcification is half that of men on ultrafast computed tomography until age 60 years, when the difference between the genders narrows (10).

An excess in female acute MI susceptibility among young blacks is seen in the Bogalusa data (7). This trend is borne out by national mortality data, in which black women have consistently had a 50% to 75% greater risk of death from diseases of the heart since 1950 (11) and into the 1990s (3). The approximate rates (adjusted for age) for white and black women were 110 per 100,000 and 190 per 100,000, respectively, in 1988 (11). The reasons for this greater risk are unclear but could relate to higher blood pressure and Lp(a) levels in blacks.

DIFFERENCES IN CARDIOVASCULAR DISEASE PRESENTATION, MANAGEMENT, AND OUTCOME IN WOMEN VERSUS MEN

The tendency to overlook CVD in women because of its lesser frequency in youth and middle age is compounded by less classical presentation, which is more frequently angina in women and MI in men (*e*Table 8.0.1). In the Framingham study, the annual incidence of angina pectoris in women exceeded that of MI by a ratio of more than 2:1 in the age ranges of 45 to 54 years and 55 to 64 years. In men, frank MI exceeded angina for all four age groups examined, ranging from 1.5:1.0 between ages 45 and 64

years, 2.4:1.0 between ages 65 and 74 years, and 6.5:1.0 between ages 75 and 84 years (12,13). In a recent study, women presenting for stenting had fewer MIs than men (14). These data are consistent with the clinical impression that angina pectoris is an earlier and more common presentation of the arteriosclerotic process in women.

Recognition of cardiovascular chest pain is difficult in women because (a) it is not expected, (b) it is often atypical, and (c) noncardiac chest pain seems to be more common in women than in men. As a result of atypical symptoms, misdiagnosis as chronic fatigue or a psychiatric disorder is not uncommon. The reason for the lack of classical anginal symptoms in many women—despite having validated myocardial ischemia—is unknown. The greater incidence of silent MI in women (13) may also be related to the atypicality of chest pain presentation. One of our patients had fatigue with exercise without ischemic electrocardiogram changes on treadmill testing that did not resolve until she developed overt angina and had bypass surgery. A tip-off to performing anatomic studies earlier might have been recognition of her severe combined hyperlipidemia.

As this case suggests, the exercise tolerance test is not as useful in clarifying atypical chest pain in women as in men because it is too susceptible to false-positive and false-negative results. In general, radionuclide or echocardiographic imaging are recommended if an exercise test is to be done (15,16). On the other hand, a female patient with chest pain with a positive exercise test and a negative angiogram might have arteriosclerotic vasospasm with a normal lumen. In this instance, estrogen may be beneficial and even diagnostic if it eliminates the vasospasticity and the chest pain syndrome. In such cases, the long-term prognosis is favorable, and angina in women is collectively associated with approximately one-half the rate of subsequent MI as that in men (16).

Frank MI in women has more unfavorable consequences than in men. Sudden death is more frequent, and early post-MI mortality is greater in women than in men. In the Thrombolysis in Myocardial Infarction (TIMI)-II trial, the 6-week mortality rate was 9% in women versus 4% in men, and post-MI mortality was 1.54 times more likely in women compared to men when adjusting for age and other baseline inequalities (17). The Global Utilization of Streptokinase and Tissue Plasminogen Activator for Occluded Coronary Arteries (GUSTO)-I trial demonstrated a similar twofold excess that decreased to a relative risk of 1.4 when adjusted for age and 1.06 when adjusting predictors of 30-day mortality (18). In keeping with this observation, recent Scandinavian data (19) and experience from a Cleveland clinic (18) indicate that nearly all of the excess mortality in women is concentrated within the first 4 weeks post-MI (Fig. 8.2); these data influence all subsequent statistics. After 1 year, a mortality rate of 32% in women versus 16% in men has been observed in the Framingham study (20,21). Thus, postevent nonadjusted mortality is approximately 50% greater in women than in men for various

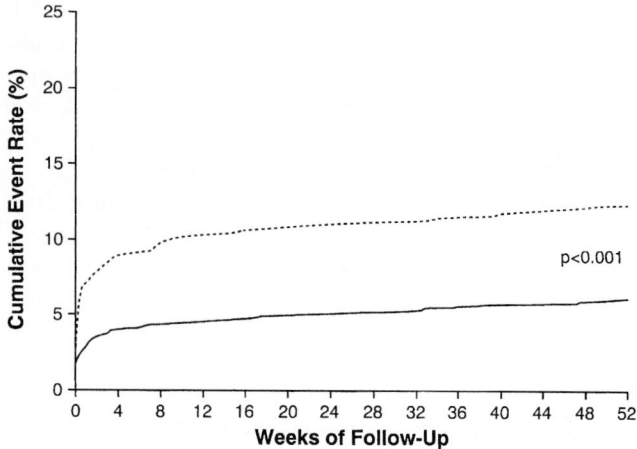

FIGURE 8.2 One-year Kaplan-Meier mortality curves for women and men. The solid line represents men; the dashed line represents women. (From Becker RC, Terrin M, Ross R, et al. Comparison of clinical outcomes for women and men after acute myocardial infarction. *Ann Intern Med* 1994;120:635–645, with permission.)

TABLE 8.1 DIFFERENCES IN CARDIOVASCULAR DISEASE PRESENTATION AND OUTCOME IN WOMEN (W) VERSUS MEN (M)

	Comparison of W and M
Presentation	
Angina	W > M
Atypical chest pain	W > M
Death from MI	W > M
Sudden death	W > M
Exercise test false-positive	W > M
Angina prognosis for MI	W < M
Consequences	
MI morbidity	W > M
MI morbidity (unadjusted)	W > M
MI mortality (adjusted)	W = to slightly > M
Coronary artery bypass graft mortality	W = to > M
Angioplasty mortality (adjusted and unadjusted)	W > M
Stenting	W ≥ M[a]

MI, myocardial infarction.
[a]W > M at 30 days, W = M at 1 year.

intervals. These trends have been confirmed recently and extended (22) with a higher risk for death relative to younger men (23). ⌖ b78

Operative procedures also show greater short- and long-term morbidity and mortality in women than in men, though the probability of benefit remains high in both genders. At the Mayo Clinic, percutaneous transluminal coronary angioplasty was successful in 85% of women and 86% of men, but age-adjusted in-hospital mortality was 4.2% in women and 2.7% in men—a significant difference that persisted with multivariate analysis (38). In the case of bypass surgery, in-hospital mortality at Cedars-Sinai Medical Center was 4.6% and 2.6% in women and men, respectively, despite a difference in age of only 4 years (68.2 vs. 64.0) (39). However, more of the women had unstable angina and CHF, whereas more men were referred for abnormal exercise-test results. In this instance, the later stage of disease at the time of operation or the greater inherent severity accounted for the greater mortality in women (39). A recent analysis of stent experience from Germany found rates of death and MI greater in women at 30 days, (3.1% vs. 1.8% in men) but equal after 1 year (6.0 vs. 5.8%) (14) (*e*Fig. 8.2.3). Male-female differences in clinical presentation and prognosis are summarized in Table 8.1.

The most important message from the greater morbidity and mortality associated with coronary disease in women is that high priority should be given to early recognition and treatment of risk factors and early ischemic symptoms in women, as well as in men. The other point is that obscure symptoms of fatigue or atypical chest pain should be worked up aggressively for potential coronary ischemia with exercise and performance imaging, particularly when risk factors for coronary artery disease are present and especially when present in combination.

CARDIOVASCULAR DISEASE RISK FACTORS IN WOMEN COMPARED TO MEN

Similarities in risk factor relationships to arteriosclerotic vascular disease in women and men include hypertension and smoking (12). In the Framingham study, smoking was the worst of any single risk factor among male subjects (40) but had less impact among females. However, in a study of 119,404 female nurses, the cardiovascular risk of smoking is clear (41) and may be increasing in severity in recent birth cohorts (42). The interaction of smoking with OC use is also strong (see the section Oral Contraceptive Use and Cardiovascular Disease Risk). Lp(a), fibrinogen, and homocystine all function as risk factors in women, as well as in men (43–45). Abdominal obesity, weight gain since age 18, and increments in body weight—even at body mass indexes less than 27—are all associated with increased CVD incidence in women (46). Recently, highly sensitive C-reactive protein (CRP) was found to be a stronger single risk factor than any other, including lipids and apoproteins (47). Marital stress (48) and being early in the menstrual cycle (49) are two other risk factors.

Differences between men and women have been identified for the impact of diabetes, plasma triglyceride, and HDL-C on female vascular health. Diabetes confers a greater increment of susceptibility to atherosclerosis in women than men, resulting in diabetic women having an absolute coronary disease rate equalling or approaching that of men (50,51). The exaggerated diabetic effect on CVD in women is most marked in middle-aged women and attenuates with age (*e*Table 8.1.1), as does the cholesterol effect due to the increased incidence of coronary disease from other causes, especially age (25).

The greater impact of diabetes on CVD in women compared to men is not well understood but may be due to more greatly disturbed lipoprotein levels in the female diabetic than in the male diabetic (50). Specifically, the change experienced by diabetic versus nondiabetic women exceeds that for diabetic versus nondiabetic men for increases in total plasma triglyceride, cholesterol, and LDL-C and reductions in HDL-C (50,52), although insulin deficiency may affect lipoprotein metabolism equally in men and women (*e*Fig. 8.2.4). Whether other effects of gender bear on the atherogenic effects of lipoprotein oxidation and glycoxidation in diabetes requires further study. ✨ b79

The cluster of risk factors associated with CVD in middle age also differs between men and women. Because women tend to be protected compared to men and have a 10- to 15-year delay in the curve describing the rise in CVD (Fig. 8.1), it follows that for a woman to have coronary disease in middle age, she must have more risk factors or a greater risk burden than a man to experience coronary artery disease, as seen in many studies (14,54). The leading condition embodying multiple risk factors is the metabolic syndrome, also known as the *insulin resistance syndrome* or *syndrome X* (55–58). Along with insulin resistance, abdominal obesity, a propensity to hypertension, overt diabetes, and combined hyperlipidemia characterize this syndrome. Combined hyperlipidemia consists of elevated plasma triglyceride, VLDL-C, intermediate-density lipoprotein cholesterol, LDL-C, small dense LDL, and low HDL-C (56,57). Clotting factor abnormalities are also associated, including elevated factor VII and plasminogen activator inhibitor-1 levels. Thus, in a single entity, four to eight risk factors can be present, affecting approximately 25% of the population.

It is not known if the metabolic syndrome has a greater association with women versus men, but the presence of coronary disease in middle-aged women is highly associated with the metabolic syndrome. For instance, diabetes and hypertension are overrepresented three- and fivefold, respectively, in women with coronary disease compared to women without. In addition, diabetes, hypertension, and hyperlipidemia are present in more women than men with acute MI in virtually every study (14,17–19,28,29,33,36,37,59,60). In other words, for women to have "premature" coronary disease, they must have a greater number of risk factors; therefore, it is not surprising that the metabolic syndrome is so overrepresented.

The predilection of the metabolic syndrome for coronary disease in women contributes to plasma triglyceride being a stronger risk factor in women than in men—1.8-fold versus 1.2-fold, or even higher (61). Conversely, a reduction in HDL-C is more strongly associated with CVD risk in women than in men, such that a 1-mg-per-dL drop in HDL-C in women is associated with a 3% to 4% increase in coronary artery disease, whereas a 1-mg-per-dL

decrease in HDL-C in men is associated with a 2% increment in coronary disease (62) (*e*Fig. 8.2.5). When coronary arteriosclerosis in men and women is graded according to angiographic severity, lipoprotein abnormalities correlating with disease severity in men are total cholesterol, LDL-C, and apoprotein B; in women, the abnormalities are VLDL-C, intermediate-density lipoprotein cholesterol, LDL triglyceride, and low HDL apoprotein (also termed *apoprotein A-I*) (63). Again, it is the combined hyperlipidemia phenotype that seems to predominate as the lipoprotein risk factor in women. The case presented in the introduction to this chapter is a striking and unfortunate example of this association.

Triglyceride should not be rejected as a CVD risk factor because it is overtaken by HDL-C in some multivariate analyses (61). At the very least, triglyceride is a major and easily measured marker for CVD risk in the metabolic syndrome. Second, triglyceride-rich lipoproteins can be found as intact particles in the arterial wall (64). A third point is that regardless of which lipoprotein abnormality one may believe to be important, triglyceride and HDL are highly inversely associated, and treatment of one with lipid-lowering agents helps correct both abnormalities.

PCOS is the earliest manifestation of the metabolic syndrome in the young woman. Such individuals have the plasma lipid profile of combined hyperlipidemia, as described above. Conversely, women with coronary artery disease more frequently have PCOS (65). CVD risk is further aggravated by the excessive secretion of androgen, which attenuates the effect of endogenous estrogen, as discussed in the section Postmenopausal Sex Steroid Hormone Effects on Lipoproteins, Carbohydrate Metabolism, and Clotting.

Two treatments of the insulin resistance syndrome are at hand. Metformin (500 mg b.i.d. for the first week and 1 g b.i.d. thereafter) and the thiazolidinediones rosiglitazone (2 to 8 mg q.d.) and pioglitazone (15 to 45 mg q.d.) are associated with improved insulin sensitivity (even in normoglycemic individuals), a fall in plasma insulin, and a reduction in plasma free testosterone levels in PCOS (66,67). Weight loss is also important in obese individuals with serious CVD risk. The diet and lipid-lowering approach to the management of combined hyperlipidemia in women is discussed in the section Cholesterol-Lowering Interventions and Reductions in Coronary Artery Disease in Women. ✨ b80

In summary, the metabolic syndrome and combined hyperlipidemia are more prevalent in women than in men with arteriosclerosis in middle age. The clinical management point is that treatment should be directed holistically toward the entire metabolic disorder (e.g., insulin resistance, obesity, hypertension, hyperglycemia, dyslipidemia) and not toward a single factor such as elevated LDL, as important as it is (69). Important risk factors in women are listed in Table 8.2.

TABLE 8.2 RISK FACTORS FOR CARDIOVASCULAR DISEASE IN WOMEN

The metabolic syndrome (syndrome X)
Insulin resistance
Obesity
Hypertension[a]
Diabetes[a]
Combined hyperlipidemias
Low high-density lipoprotein cholesterol (<40 mg/dL)[a]
Polycystic ovary syndrome (amenorrhea, hirsutism, infertility)
Smoking[a]
Inactivity
Age ≥55 yr[a]
Familial or polygenic hypercholesterolemia
Homocystine elevations
Family history of premature coronary disease: younger than 55 yr in men and 65 yr in women (first-degree relatives)[a]
Oral contraceptive use in the presence of other risk factors
Lipoprotein(a)

[a]Denotes official National Cholesterol Education Program risk factors. See Executive Summary of The Third Report of the National Cholesterol Education Program (NCEP) Expert Panel on Detection, Evaluation, and Treatment of High Blood Cholesterol in Adults (Adult Treatment Panel III). *JAMA* 2001;285:2486–2497.

DIETARY RESPONSE AND CARDIOVASCULAR DISEASE

Some small-scale diet studies suggest that women are less responsive to diet than men. However, a large study from our own clinic indicates that the National Cholesterol Education Program (NCEP) Step II Diet lowers LDL-C equally in men and women, with LDL-C levels above approximately 160 mg per dL (70). On the other hand, HDL-C declined with Step II Diet to a greater extent in women—5% to 6% as compared to 1% to 3% in men after 6 and 12 months of diet—with the greatest reduction in HDL(2), the estrogen-exercise–sensitive portion of HDL (71).

This study indicates that chronic differences exist in the HDL-C response to diet between men and women. The mechanism and significance of the greater HDL-C decrease in women for CVD risk are not known. At this point, the recommendation for dietary intervention in men and women is not different. Nonetheless, in a woman with coronary disease needing dietary and drug management of hyperlipidemia, the greater propensity to HDL-C lowering with diet further reinforces the point that triglyceride and HDL—as well as LDL—be aggressively managed in the at-risk woman. The NCEP Adult Treatment Panel III (ATP-III) guidelines advocate a diet containing 35% of fat as calories rather than <30%, which is less likely to decrease HDL-C (71a).

EFFECTS OF GONADAL STEROIDS ON LIPOPROTEIN METABOLISM AND THEIR CLINICAL SIGNIFICANCE

The effects of estrogens and progestins on lipoprotein metabolism are shown in Figure 8.3. The main point from the illustration is that estrogen enhances the metabolic traffic of cholesterol transport in virtually every pathway except one, raising triglyceride, lowering LDL, and raising HDL, whereas progestins and androgens have the opposite effect (1,72,73). Details of the pathway effects are presented in the online version of this textbook and in the accompanying CD-ROM.

ENDOTHELIAL AND VASCULAR BIOLOGY EFFECTS OF ESTROGENS, PROGESTINS, AND ANDROGENS

Some animal studies of estrogen effects on lipoprotein levels in plasma show little impact on the extent of atherogenesis and suggest that direct arterial wall effects of estrogen are more

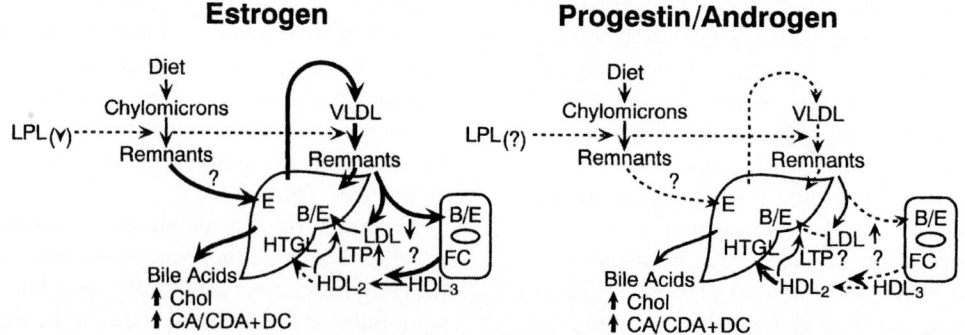

FIGURE 8.3 Effects of sex steroids on lipoprotein metabolism. Width of the lines indicates the rate of cholesterol traffic under the influence of estrogen or progestin/androgen. Question marks indicate effects for which documentation is uncertain or unclear. B/E, low-density lipoprotein receptor; CA, cholic acid; CDA, chenodeoxycholic acid; Chol, cholesterol; DC, deoxycholate; FC, free cholesterol; HDL, high-density lipoprotein; HTGL, hepatic triglyceride lipase; LDL, low-density lipoprotein; LPL, lipoprotein lipase; LTP, leukocyte thromboplastin; VLDL, very-low-density lipoprotein.

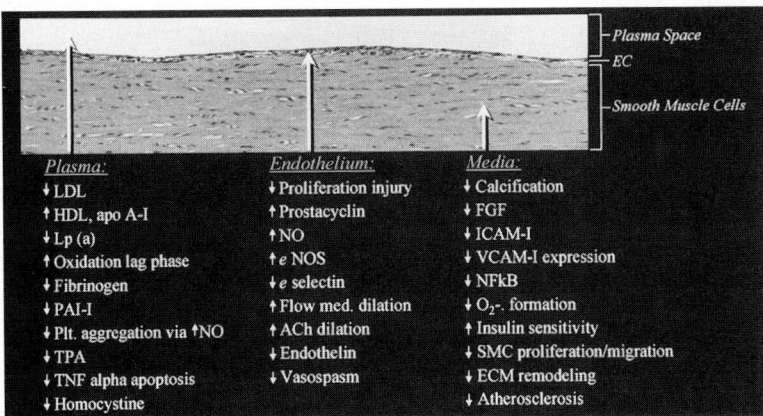

FIGURE 8.4 Beneficial effects of estrogen on arterial wall biology. In this scenario, estrogen-mediated events in plasma, endothelium, and intima-media are beneficial to the arterial wall. ACh, acetylcholine; apo, apoprotein; EC, epidermal cell; ECM, extracellular matrix; eNOS, endothelial nitric oxide synthase; FGF, fibroblast growth factor; HDL, high-density lipoprotein; ICAM-1, intercellular adhesion molecule-1; LDL, low-density lipoprotein; Lp(a), lipoprotein(a); NFκB, nuclear factor kappa B; NO, nitrous oxide; PAI-1, plasminogen activator inhibitor-1; Plt, platelet; SMC, smooth muscle cell; TNF, tumor necrosis factor; TPA, tissue plasminogen activator; VCAM-1, vascular cell adhesion molecule-1.

important (80). Whether this observation applies to humans is doubtful, but it is clear that estrogen has direct arterial wall effects. These effects include diminished penetration of arterial wall by LDL (80), diminished arterial wall LDL retention (81), and diminished inflammatory response (82) involving a diminished cytokine release and generation of inflammatory response molecules in arterial endothelium and intima-media (see reference 83 for review and Figure 8.4).

Some of these effects may be related to the antioxidant effect of estrogen, a non–receptor-mediated effect of estrogen believed to inhibit atherogenesis (83). Alternatively, estrogen effects may be mediated via genomic or nongenomic effects on estrogen receptors or macrophages and arterial walls (84,85). Importantly, estrogen receptors are found in diminished amounts or are absent in areas of atherosclerosis, which may explain the lack of vascular benefit from estrogen in recent clinical trials (86) (see the section Effects of Postmenopausal Hormone Use on Coronary Disease).

A moment-to-moment effect of estrogen increases endothelial nitric oxide synthase activity, nitric oxide generation, and vasodilation. This effect can reverse the paradoxical vasoconstrictor response to acetylcholine in arteriosclerotic arteries (87) (*e*Table 8.2.3 and Fig. 8.5). In fact, estrogen administration can reverse clinical vasospasm within minutes and may be a useful treatment in cardiologic syndrome X (88,89). Some of this benefit may also be due to the antioxidant effect of estrogen, which may slow the rate of oxidative destruction of endothelial nitric oxide (1,72,88–90). In addition, estrogen is associated with lower plasma levels of the vasoconstrictor endothelin (91). Surprisingly, testosterone and other androgens also have a vasodilatory effect in healthy arteries that is mediated directly and by an acetylcholine mechanism (92,93).

Most recently, vasoconstrictive effects of progestins on arterial vasomotion have been reported (94), and medroxyprogesterone acetate (MPA) has been reported to abolish the antiatherosclerotic effect of estrogen in cholesterol-fed monkeys and rats (95,96). Testosterone and one androgenic progestin also promote atherogenesis in cholesterol-fed monkeys (97). We have found that progestins and andro-

gens also have a weak prooxidant effect and oppose the antioxidant effect of estrogen (98).

Another way in which sex hormones affect arterial wall physiology is through the arterial wall–prostaglandin system, which can favor vasoconstriction and platelet aggregation if thromboxane formation is dominant and vasodilation and diminished platelet aggregation if prostacyclin is dominant. Consistent with its effects on nitric oxide metabolism and probably arterial wall redox state, estrogen favors prostacyclin dominance, whereas testosterone favors thromboxane formation, diminishes prostacyclin formation, and enhances platelet thromboxane receptor binding on platelets (see reference 93 for review). Again, the estrogen-androgen antagonism is borne out in another physiologic system.

In summary, ample evidence exists for the presence of estrogen receptors in healthy arterial walls and direct, almost moment-to-moment regulation of endothelial nitric oxide

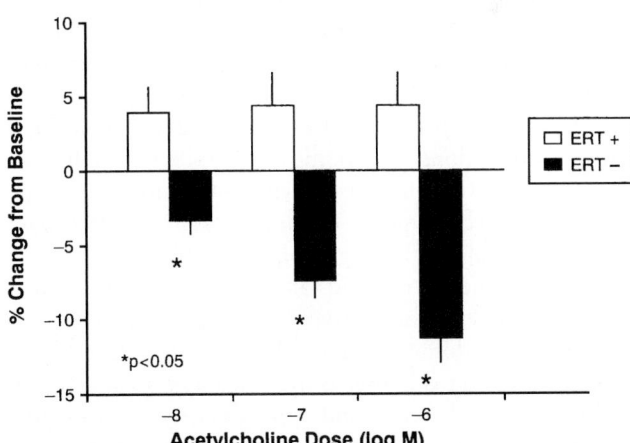

FIGURE 8.5 Mean percent change in coronary diameter after graded doses of acetylcholine. Vertical lines indicate standard error of the mean. Actual *p* values for comparison of estrogen replacement therapy (ERT)+ versus ERT– for each dose of acetylcholine are .03, .001, and .0004, respectively. (From Herrington DM, Braden GA, Williams JK, et al. Endothelial-dependent coronary vasomotor responsiveness in postmenopausal women with and without estrogen replacement therapy. *Am J Cardiol* 1994; 73:951–952, with permission.)

generation, vasomotion, arterial wall LDL penetration and metabolism, and underlying inflammatory response. Whether these effects are all estrogen receptor–mediated is unknown, but the fact that progestin and androgen can oppose some of the effects suggests receptor-mediated mechanisms.

ORAL CONTRACEPTIVE USE AND CARDIOVASCULAR DISEASE RISK

Shortly after the introduction of oral contraception in the early 1960s, a flurry of reports appeared of venous thrombosis and stroke among OC users. In light of today's experience, the occurrence of venous thrombosis is not surprising because the earliest OCs contained between 100 and 150 μg of ethinyl estradiol, which is approximately 20 to 30 times the postmenopausal replacement amount! Reports of an excess of coronary artery disease among OC users appeared in 1975, in which British epidemiologists found an approximately threefold excess of coronary disease among OC users (102,103). Most importantly, these researchers found that a basic tenet of the risk factor theory of arteriosclerosis applied to women and OC users, with single risk factors increasing coronary disease risk approximately threefold and combinations of risk factors increasing risk geometrically (102,103).

The doses of OC estrogen have declined over the ensuing decades to 20 to 35 μg daily of ethinyl estradiol, which is approximately 1.3 to 2.0 times postmenopausal replacement levels. Even at these doses, venous thrombosis still occurs (100) and may actually be somewhat promoted by the reduced androgenicity of certain third-generation OCs; this androgenicity allows the formulation to be more estrogenic, even though the estrogen dose is unchanged (101). The preferred initial formulations contain 35 μg of ethinyl estradiol and 0.250 mg of norgestimate (Ortho-Cyclen) or 0.250 mg of desogestrel and 30 μg of ethinyl estradiol (Ortho-Cept). The triphasic form of Ortho-Cyclen contains less progestin (0.180, 0.215, and 0.250 mg weekly). Other formulations containing less ethinyl estradiol or stronger progestin can be used—depending on gynecologic symptoms or requirements—such as Alesse 21 or 28 (20 μg ethinyl estradiol and 100 μg levonorgestrel).

Several studies in the mid- and late 1980s have verified the earlier epidemiologic surveys that show that, even with lower estrogen–dose OCs, the risk of coronary disease in a cigarette-smoking OC user is increased approximately 20- to 30-fold from baseline and approximately six- to eightfold above the risk of cigarette smoking alone for coronary disease (104,105). The data of Croft and Hannaford in *e*Table 8.2.4 (105) and Rosenberg et al. in Figure 8.6 are representative of the danger of combinations of risk factors for MI, even in young women (104).

The pathophysiologic mechanism for the increased risk for CVD with high- and mid-dose estrogen pills, especially with smoking, probably reflects the propensity for thrombosis at a

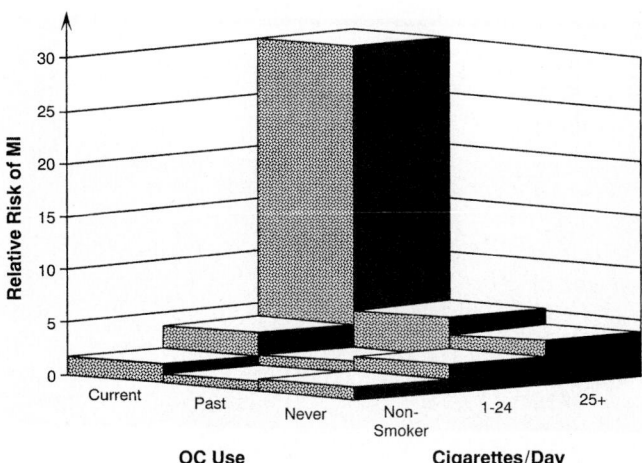

FIGURE 8.6 The effect of smoking and oral contraceptives (OCs) on the risk of myocardial infarction (MI) in women younger than 50 years. (Adapted from Rosenberg L, Kaufman DW, Helmrich S, et al. Myocardial infarction and cigarette smoking in women younger than 50 years of age. *JAMA* 1985;253:2965.)

site of arterial wall injury such as an endothelial erosion. Such erosion might arise from a toxic effect of cigarette smoke, smoke-induced depletion of antioxidant defenses, or enhanced LDL oxidation in the absence of major atherosclerosis. On the other hand, arteriosclerotic plaque rupture and thrombosis (106) and advanced arteriosclerotic disease (107) have been reported among OC users; this seems to be the situation in the case presented in the introduction to this chapter.

Young women with high degrees of CVD risk should avoid the use of OCs, especially after the age of 35 years, unless the risk factors can be modified. It is the standard of clinical practice that OCs not be prescribed to cigarette-smoking women who are older than 35 years. A schema that takes this and other risk factors into account as a function of initial LDL-C is presented in *e*Table 8.2.5, which is modeled on the NCEP guidelines (108). The important message is that CVD risk factors must be considered seriously when prescribing OCs and that every woman should have her lipid profile checked when OC use is contemplated and then instituted. CVD risk factors in women are summarized in Table 8.2. Obviously, venous thrombosis due to an estrogen-containing OC is a separate contraindication to continued use of the drug. In the case mentioned in the introduction, the combination of cigarette smoking, OC use, and severe combined hyperlipidemia was nearly lethal, even at age 25 years. Had the patient's lipids been checked before OC use, her high-risk status might have been appreciated.

POSTMENOPAUSAL SEX STEROID HORMONE EFFECTS ON LIPOPROTEINS, CARBOHYDRATE METABOLISM, AND CLOTTING

LDL-C levels are higher in postmenopausal women than in younger women—a condition likely due in part to the absence of endogenous estrogen (1,72,73) (*e*Fig. 8.6.1). When women have been studied through menopause and estrogen deficiency develops, the LDL-C level increases by 12.0 mg per dL (0.31 mmol), and HDL-C decreases by 3.5 mg per dL (0.09 mmol) (109). These differences reflect the absence of endogenous ovarian estrogen secretion into the systemic circulation. It is also noteworthy that plasma insulin, glucose, and body weight all increase more in women becoming menopausal than in those not becoming menopausal; this is consistent with a loss of insulin efficacy (discussed earlier).

When hormone users are compared to nonhormone users, estrogen treatment raises the HDL-C level as much as 8 mg per dL (0.2 mmol). Compared to the smaller difference associated with menopause, the greater difference with hormone replacement may be due to higher doses of estrogen or to the oral route of administration. The Postmenopausal Estrogen-Progestin Intervention trial showed a 6-mg-per-dL (0.16-mmol) HDL-C increase above control in women given 0.625 mg of Premarin daily, as shown in *e*Table 8.2.6 (110). Premarin given with MPA (10.0 mg given cyclically or 2.5 mg given continuously) resulted in HDL-C increases to 1.6 and 1.2 mg (0.04 and 0.03 mmol) above baseline, respectively. Most interestingly, when micronized natural progesterone was given cyclically with Premarin, the Premarin effect on HDL-C was almost entirely preserved (5 mg per dL or 0.13 mmol increase above baseline). On the other hand, all of the postmenopausal hormonal formulations examined were associated with reductions in LDL-C concentrations of approximately 14.5 to 17.5 mg per dL (0.37 to 0.45 mmol) without any distinctions among the groups. Finally, the triglyceride elevations were minor, ranging from 11.4 to 13.7 mg per dL (0.13 to 0.15 mmol), and less than the triglyceride elevations associated with oral contraception.

In the Postmenopausal Estrogen-Progestin Intervention study (*e*Table 8.2.6), plasma glucose and insulin levels were lowest with estrogen alone and highest with high-dose progestin plus estrogen (110). Thus, the antagonism of estrogen and progestin on carbohydrate metabolism is seen with postmenopausal hormone replacement, as with OC steroids of varied composition.

The estrogen-progestin antagonism is also seen in the levels of clotting factors. Fibrinogen concentration is diminished among postmenopausal estrogen users, as with OC users (101), despite lower doses. Addition of natural progesterone or increasing doses of Provera (MPA) oppose these effects. Although the range of these effects is small, the data indicate that progestins can oppose the effect of estrogen on the clotting system. Recent work from our own laboratory indicates that progestins are prooxidants, opposing the antioxidant and anticytotoxic effects of estrogen (83,98).

An unexpected effect of estrogen—increased CRP levels—has been seen in several studies (111). This increase is said to drive an increase in activity in the complement pathway and favor inflammatory processes (112), and it may explain the strong predictive effect of CRP on atherosclerosis in women (47).

EFFECTS OF POSTMENOPAUSAL HORMONE USE ON CORONARY DISEASE

More than 30 case-controlled and prospective cohort studies have been performed over the last 20 years comparing arteriosclerotic vascular disease in estrogen users versus nonusers (1,72,73,113–115). These studies indicate that the incidence of coronary artery disease among estrogen users is approximately one-half of that among nonusers. Even before the recent negative clinical trials of estrogen efficacy on heart disease, it was postulated that the putative estrogen benefit was due in part to a "healthy user effect" (i.e., healthier women use estrogen). Barrett-Connor and associates (113) estimated that 50% of the lower rate of coronary artery disease among estrogen users might be ascribed to this selection bias.

Nonetheless, it was a great surprise that the Heart and Estrogen/Progestin Replacement Study (HERS) showed no benefit of equine estrogen (Premarin) 0.625 mg plus MPA (Provera, Cycrin) 2.50 mg continuously versus placebo (116). The results showed a hazard ratio of 0.99 with 95% confidence interval (CI) of 0.80–1.22, p = .91. Various CVD subgroups showed no significant differences with hormone replacement, but the number of subjects with unstable angina tended to be fewer with estrogen, whereas the number of individuals with CHF or cardiac death tended to be greater with estrogen (*e*Table 8.2.7). Because unstable angina involves plaque rupture and nonocclusive thrombus formation, it is hard to argue that the lack of overall benefit from estrogen was due to an enhanced susceptibility to thrombosis. It seems that the sicker or more vulnerable persons were at slightly greater risk from estrogen plus progestin therapy.

Contrary to popularly held view, equine estrogen plus MPA was without benefit over the entire course of the study, particularly concerning CHD death (Fig. 8.7). Only in a secondary hypothesis-generating analysis was a downward trend detected in nonfatal coronary events, but this analysis included an adverse trend of excess nonfatal CHD events in the first year (116). The results of a HERS follow-up study will be reported in late 2001 and will address the questions of whether the downward trend in CHD events among hormone users continued after the conclusion of the main trial. At present, the conclusion is that coronary disease is not prevented by estrogen among older women (average age, 67 years) with established heart disease (116).

A similar negative result was observed on angiographically quantified coronary atherosclerosis after 3.2 years in 309 women randomized to placebo, 0.625 mg equine estrogen

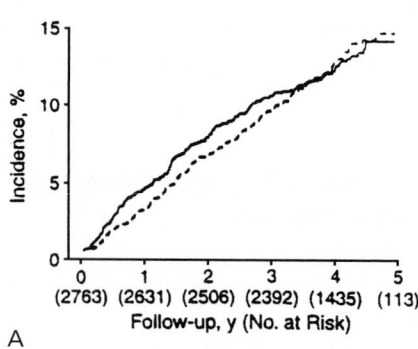
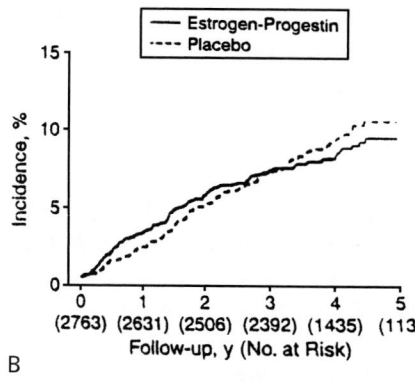
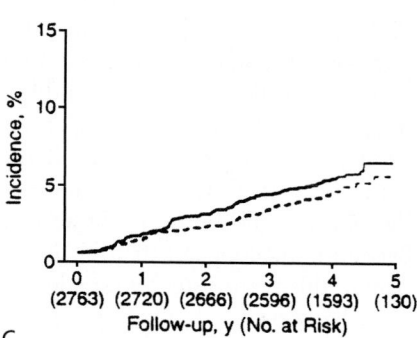

FIGURE 8.7 Heart and Estrogen/Progestin Replacement Study Kaplan-Meier curve estimates of the cumulative incidence of primary coronary heart disease and its constituents. **A:** All events. **B:** Nonfatal events. **C:** Fatal events. Numbers in parentheses are subjects followed to each time-point. Curves are fainter where the sample size falls to less than one-half of the original cohort. (From Hulley S, Grady D, Bush T, et al. Randomized trial of estrogen plus progesterone for secondary prevention of coronary heart disease in postmenopausal women. *JAMA* 1998;280:605–613, with permission.)

alone, or with 2.5 mg medroxyprogesterone acetate daily in the Estrogen Replacement Atherosclerosis trial (117). Again, these were women with established coronary disease, with mean ages ranging from 65.6, 66.3, and 65.5 years, respectively, in the three groups. Minimum coronary diameter change and change in percent stenosis were indistinguishable in the equine estrogen and placebo groups and slightly worse with the equine estrogen plus MPA group (Table 8.3).

Possible reasons why neither the HERS nor the Estrogen Replacement Atherosclerosis studies were successful are listed in Table 8.4. These reasons range from too high an estrogen dose in older, estrogen-naïve women to an inflammatory effect of CRP. Not listed among these possibilities is an enhanced sensitivity to arterial thrombosis, because unstable coronary syndromes that are thrombotic in nature tended to be *less* frequent in the HERS hormone-treated group. Other possibilities include an adverse effect of progestin. In animal models, MPA completely blocks the cardioprotective effect of estrogen (95,96), and estrogen seems to be without benefit in animals who have been fed cholesterol and have established atherosclerosis (118,119).

Another argument against arterial thrombosis being a factor in the negative HERS trial results is the rather low occurrence of venous thrombosis in the hormone-treated groups: 25 versus 8 cases in the placebo group and pulmonary embolism in 11 cases in the hormone-treated group versus 4 in the placebo group for totals of 34 and 12, respectively. These totals are well below the 172 and 176 primary CHD events in the two groups, respectively. Whereas these totals are low relative to coronary disease events, the approximately threefold increased rate of venous thrombosis is similar to that reported recently in a number of observational studies of postmenopausal estrogen use (120–123).

Notwithstanding the above data, Psaty et al. have reported association between a prothrombin polymorphism (20210 G→A) and first MI in hormone-treated postmenopausal women who are hypertensive (124). However, the patients are relatively few. Factor V Leiden was not a predictive factor.

A much longer-term prospective randomized trial of estrogen and estrogen plus progestin replacement therapy is being conducted by the Women's Health Initiative in at least 40 centers nationwide. The larger number of 40,000 to 50,000 subjects is required because of the lower incidence of coronary disease in a primary prevention setting. This study will be reported in approximately 2004.

TABLE 8.3 EFFECTS OF POSTMENOPAUSAL HORMONE REPLACEMENT ON CORONARY LUMEN DIAMETER[a]

	Placebo	Equine estrogen (E)	E + MPA	E vs. placebo	E + MPA vs. placebo
				p values	
Minimal coronary diameters adjusted change (mm)	−0.09 ± 0.02	−0.12 ± 0.02	−0.09 ± 0.02	.97	.38
% stenosis adjusted change	4.01 ± 0.92	4.75 ± 0.92	4.11 ± 4.93	.93	.56

MPA, medroxyprogesterone acetate.
[a]Data include all subjects with adjustments for baseline inequalities.
From Herrington DM, Reboussin DM, Brosnihan KB, et al. Effects of estrogen replacement on the progression of coronary-artery atherosclerosis. *N Engl J Med* 2000;343:522–529, with permission.

TABLE 8.4 REASONS WHY ESTROGEN MAY NOT PREVENT CORONARY DISEASE IN RANDOMIZED CLINICAL TRIALS

The observational case-control and cohort studies are wrong and do not control for the "healthy user" effect (i.e., there may be no real benefit).

C-reactive protein is increased with estrogen and may activate complement and inflammatory response.

Estrogen receptors are reduced or absent in arteriosclerotic tissue.

Estrogen prevents atherosclerosis only in early animal models of atherosclerosis and not established disease.

The progestin opposes diverse effects of estrogen, possibly those that may benefit the arterial wall.

Too high an equine estrogen dose was given too late in secondary prevention studies in menopausal women (late 60s).

Estrogen appears to aggravate cardiovascular risk factor effects, whereas "statins" as an example yield extra benefit in women with high risk.

The oral estrogen route induces first pass effects on hepatic protein synthesis, including lipid and clotting effects; this route is not the systemic ovarian route and may actually diminish effective systemic estrogen delivery.

Clinical Advice

In the meantime, what do we tell patients? It does not seem possible dogmatically to recommend estrogen replacement therapy to prevent existing coronary disease, given the negative results of two prospective randomized trials. On the other hand, many reasons can be given for offering or suggesting estrogen replacement therapy, including sense of well-being, prevention of osteoporosis, preservation of skin turgor, prevention of senility and even Alzheimer's disease (1,72,73), preservation of vaginal mucosa, metabolic benefits (see below), and higher intellectual function (1,72,73). Most women come to this decision aware of at least some of these benefits and some of the side effects and often have their own well-established viewpoint about whether to take estrogen.

As to androgen effects on human atherosclerosis, more than 20 case reports of coronary artery disease have been documented among athletes taking androgen (125). This clinical experience and the atherogenic effects of androgens in animal models provide evidence against the use of excessive or pharmacologic amounts of androgen in young athletes and provides evidence for minimizing the exposure to androgenic progestins in hormone replacement and OC therapy.

The most frequently prescribed dose of postmenopausal estrogen replacement therapy is equine estrogen (Premarin) 0.625 mg daily. Whether generic equine estrogen is equivalent in the 8 to 10 estrogenic steroids of pregnant mares' urine is hotly debated. Occasionally, 0.9 or 1.2 mg daily of equine estrogens is necessary to control hot flashes in women entering menopause. Doses of 2.5 mg daily of equine estrogens have little or no use and may be associated with MI excess, especially in association with cigarette smoking, as found in the Framingham study—one of the

few observational studies in which postmenopausal estrogen replacement was associated with an increased rate of coronary artery disease (126). This effect resembles the increase in coronary disease among men given 2.5 or 5.0 mg of equine estrogen in the Coronary Drug Project (127). These data are compatible with the idea that coronary disease is *worse* with high-dose estrogen and major CVD risk factors, as in the OC experience. Thus, one might predict diminished estrogen benefit or even harm with increasing estrogen dose, older age, and multiple CVD risk factors (*e*Fig. 8.7.1).

Alternatives to equine estrogens are pure 17β-estradiol (Estrace), which is given in 1- to 2-mg-per-day doses, or estropipate (Ogen), which is estrone sulfate given in doses ranging from 0.75, 1.50, or 3.00 mg daily (Ogen: 0.625, 1.250, or 2.50 mg). Ogen does not appear to be quite equivalent to equine estrogen, and doses higher than 0.75 mg daily may be needed to relieve flushing symptoms.

When women have oral intolerance to estrogens or have a metabolic contraindication (chiefly hypertriglyceridemia), then systemically administered estrogen is indicated by one of three routes: patch, injection, or sublingual. There are 3-day patches in the form of 50- or 100-μg doses of Estraderm or Vivelle or 7-day patches of Climara in 50 or 100 μg delivered daily. Most women prefer the longer duration patch, but, often, use is dictated by sensitivity to the patch adhesive. In this respect, Vivelle may be better tolerated. When no patch can be tolerated, sublingual estrogen in the form of Estrace (1 mg) is a viable alternative or 17β-estradiol valerate in oil (10 to 20 mg intramuscularly), although injectable preparations do not yield an even blood level over a month's time. Side effects of estrogen are most typically breast tenderness and, possibly, pelvic fullness. In postmenopausal women, and especially in elderly women, lower doses of estrogen are advisable to start (e.g., 0.3 mg of equine estrogen daily or every other day) to avoid these symptoms. Another advantage of patch estrogen is that a higher systemic dose can be obtained with better control of symptoms than the oral route, in which hepatic inactivation can limit symptom control.

Estrogen can be used without a progestin only in women without uteri. All other women require progestin in some form. The most popular form is 2.5 mg of MPA (Provera, Cycrin, or the combination formulation Prempro) given continually. This regimen is associated with vaginal spotting and bleeding in more than 50% of users during the first months of treatment and does not decline to a few percent until after 24 to 36 months of use. The unpredictability of this bleeding is the most troublesome aspect for older women. Cyclic progestin given 12 days out of each month can produce vaginal bleeding on a predictable basis in approximately 50% of the women who resume bleeding, but most women do not want this regimen, and the higher MPA doses of 5 and 10 mg daily have deleterious metabolic effects, as described above. Micronized natural progesterone taken cyclically in doses of 100 to 200 mg daily is an alternative form, as are 1 mg micronized 17β-estradiol with norgestimate (Ortho-Prefest) and 5 mg ethinyl estradiol with 1 mg norethindrone acetate (Femhrt)—a more androgenic progestin.

Side effects of progestins are not negligible and include weight gain, fluid retention, headache, and symptoms resembling premenstrual tension. Fortunately, most women are not bothered by these symptoms, but they can be virtually incapacitating when these symptoms are present. Oral progestin can be given with estrogen by any route. An alternative to oral progestin is Depo-Provera administered intramuscularly.

CHOLESTEROL-LOWERING INTERVENTIONS AND REDUCTIONS IN CORONARY ARTERY DISEASE IN WOMEN

Lipid-Lowering Treatment Guidelines

The NCEP guidelines for lipid lowering specify that risk factors apply equally for men and women—except for family history, in which, in contrast to men younger than 55 years, CVD under age 65 in a female relative is considered to be premature and a risk factor (71a). Likewise, age as a risk factor is later in women (age 55 years) than in men (age 45 years). Formerly, male gender was a risk factor at any age, but this guideline no longer applies. Finally, an unwritten difference exists in the application of the HDL-C <40 mg per dL rule as a risk factor. Because women have a mean HDL-C of approximately 55 mg per dL and men have a mean HDL-C of 45 mg per dL, fewer women qualify for low HDL-C as a risk factor than men. Similarly, more women qualify for subtracting one risk factor on the basis of HDL-C >60 mg per dL, yielding a significant number of women in population surveys (especially premenopausally) having a risk factor total of –1. Otherwise, the less than 160-, 130-, and 100-mg-per-dL LDL-C target values apply equally to men and women, with the gender differences in risk being embodied in the risk factor assessments.

CONTROVERSIES AND PERSONAL PERSPECTIVES

Postmenopausal Hormone Replacement Therapy

The view is still held by some that all women should be placed on sex hormone replacement therapy postmenopausally and, conceivably, supplemental estrogen premenopausally. Those who hold this view argue that the lipoprotein effects, the direct arterial wall effects, the antioxidant effects, the benefit on vasomotion, and the epidemiologic surveys are sufficient information and that the proposed cardiologic benefit is so great that side effects, some of which could be fatal, such as pulmonary embolism, can be ignored. This line of reasoning is flawed because, according to epidemiologic surveys, the benefit of estrogen may be overestimated by 50% due to the healthy user effect (113), side effects may possibly be underestimated, and clinical trials in women with advanced coronary disease do not show benefit. Younger women may benefit. The take-home message is that estrogen currently cannot be prescribed for CVD prevention with any assurance, especially in women with coronary disease. Nonetheless, I certainly prescribe hormone replacement to women for specific noncardiovascular indications, which are many.

When counseling patients, I tell them what I know, but I also listen to their concerns, fears, and family history, especially when it involves ovarian and breast cancer, venous thrombosis, and heart disease. If a patient declines to use postmenopausal hormone replacement therapy, she may be making the right decision for her! If hormone replacement therapy is initiated, it must be in conjunction with annual gynecologic evaluation, breast examination, and mammography.

Oral Contraceptives and Vascular Health

Over the years, the argument has raged over whether "undesirable" lipoprotein effects of androgenic progestin-dominant OCs have any material effect on the arterial wall. Given the absence of any arteriosclerotic carryover effect of prior OC use on subsequent risk for arteriosclerotic vascular disease, the possible deleterious effects of the progestin have been dismissed, especially in light of animal studies that show no arteriosclerotic effect in conjunction with estrogen administration (72). The reservations about this point of view are as follows: the monkey studies may not apply to humans, and the older, high-estrogen–dose OCs may have been sufficiently estrogen dominant to overcome any arterial wall progestogenic effect. We must recognize that our understanding of the interaction between estrogen and progestin in OCs and metabolic and vascular physiology is developing, as is our understanding of postmenopausal hormone replacement effects. For now, the clinical message is to minimize the estrogen exposure, the androgenicity of the progestin, and the presence of concomitant risk factors. In this context, not measuring a young woman's cholesterol because CVD mortality is not high enough to justify the expense (132,133) overlooks a vast area of biology and pharmacology that is pertinent to women's health. Greater refinement of our knowledge of new third-generation OC effects on vascular health is needed to secure the possibil-

THE FUTURE

The following statements are as much hopes as predictions. First, physicians and caregivers will remember that coronary disease and arteriosclerotic vascular disease are the most prevalent causes of death in women as well as in men but that the symptomatologies and presentations are likely to differ. Second, physicians and caregivers will have the patience to let patients tell us the story as they see it, so that we can better appreciate and describe the male-female difference and treat appropriately. The third expectation is that ongoing clinical trials will further refine the nature and extent of the heightened vulnerability of women for certain morbidities associated with coronary disease. The fourth expectation is that we will learn the reasons for these excessive morbidities and find better ways to prevent and treat them. The fifth hope is that caregivers will recognize that treatable CVD risk factors—especially hypertension, diabetes, and, in all probability, syndrome X with its associated dyslipidemia—are consistently more common among women with CVD than among men. The sixth expectation is that we will learn to use metabolic treatments more effectively and in combination to treat these risk factors. These treatments will include use of antihypertensives without adverse metabolic effect, agents to minimize insulin resistance, cautious use of existing and forthcoming appetite suppressants, and more informed, target-oriented treatment of diabetes and dyslipidemia. Treatments will also include management of female hyperandrogenic states premenopausally and hormone replacement postmenopausally, avoiding or minimizing the androgenic side effects of certain progestational agents. The future of hormone therapy of arteriosclerotic vascular disease may include the use of chimeric agents combining estrogenic and progestogenic effects and estrogens that are selective for specific tissues and organs. Seventh, women and men should be treated aggressively with lipid-lowering agents to target (while awaiting resolution of) the estrogen–heart disease enigma.

ity that these OCs may be noninjurious and even beneficial to the arterial wall.

Future Directions

Clinical trials currently under way will better define the effects of postmenopausal hormone replacement therapy on cardiovascular health in healthy postmenopausal women without heart disease. We can also expect future development of estrogenic compounds that have hybrid or chimeric effects of estrogen and progestin or that only act on certain, but not all, estrogen-sensitive systems (e.g., the selective estrogen receptor modulators). A heart disease prevention study of one of these agents, raloxifene (Evista; 60 mg q.d.), is under way in high-risk women. These specific therapies may eventually be directed to the arterial wall or bone, for instance, without effects on clotting, hepatic lipoprotein production, or breast metaplasia. Knowledge is also developing rapidly in understanding the postreceptor signaling system of the estrogen receptor (137) and the specificities it entails that may eventually be used for pharmacologic benefit.

Female-Male Cardiovascular Disease Issues

As is apparent from the foregoing text, the epidemiology, management, risk predictors, and subsequent morbidities of CVD are incompletely distinguished in women compared to men. Although better descriptions are constantly appearing (17,36–38), we will never discover a better way to treat CVD in females without listening to and looking for the ways that early CVD presents differently in women than in men. In this regard, the basic skills of the practitioner must be joined with those of the epidemiologist, the clinical trialist, and the clinical and basic researchers to carry this field forward.

CONCLUSIONS

CVD can occur in women of all ages, depending on risk factor burden. The insulin resistance syndrome (syndrome X) appears to be more important as a risk factor in women than in men. Triglyceride and HDL levels are more important in women than in men until late in life, when the relationships are reversed. Because almost every category of CVD carries worse morbidity and mortality in women compared to men, it seems very important to use every means at hand to prevent its occurrence. The interplay of estrogen and progestin bears on this issue in all stages of life and has to be considered, along with all other cardiovascular therapies.

In general, estrogen at replacement hormone–dose levels is associated with a favorable effect on lipoprotein metabolism, arterial wall penetration of LDL, insulin sensitivity, and plasma glucose concentrations; some clotting factors and progestins oppose these effects (138–141). The best available information from clinical trials is that estrogen is without cardiovascular benefit in women with established heart disease. It remains to be seen if estrogen or its selective estrogen receptor modulator relatives will have benefit in a primary prevention setting in younger women or those without heart disease.

Caution is also advised for clinicians giving estrogen in any case in which the patient has underlying hypertriglyceridemia or a history of thrombosis. Should hypertriglyceridemia result from estrogen administration or if the patient has a baseline plasma triglyceride level >300 mg per dL (3.38 mmol), an estrogen-patch regimen should be used as an alternative.

With the recent growth in understanding of the effects of sex steroid hormones on many body functions and of the many differences between the genders in arterial physiology and pathophysiology, there is an excellent prospect that this knowledge can be used to minimize coronary disease in both men and women if the undesirable side effects can be avoided.

REFERENCES

1. Knopp RH, Zhu X, Bonet B. Effects of estrogens on lipoprotein metabolism and cardiovascular disease in women. *Atherosclerosis* 1994;110[Suppl]:S83–S91.
2. Castelli WP. Cardiovascular disease in women. *Am J Obstet Gynecol* 1988;158:1553–1560, 1566–1567.
3. Rosamond WD, Chambless LE, Folsom AR, et al. Trends in the incidence of myocardial infarction and in mortality due to coronary heart disease, 1987 to 1994. *N Engl J Med* 1998;339:861–867.
4. Centers for Disease Control and Prevention. Update: mortality attributable to HIV infection among persons aged 25–44 years in the United States, 1994. *MMWR Morb Mortal Wkly Rep* 1996;45:121–125.
5. Raymond JR, van den Berg EK Jr, Knapp MJ. Nontraumatic prehospital sudden death in young adults. *Arch Intern Med* 1988;148:303–308.
6. Negus BH, Willard JE, Glamann DB, et al. Coronary anatomy and prognosis of young, asymptomatic survivors of myocardial infarction. *Am J Med* 1994;96:354–358.
7. Berenson GS, Wattigney WA, Tracy RE, et al. Atherosclerosis of the aorta and coronary arteries and cardiovascular risk factors in persons aged 6 to 30 years and studied at necropsy (The Bogalusa Heart Study). *Am J Cardiol* 1992;70:851–858.
8. Mautner SL, Lin F, Mautner GC, et al. Comparison in women versus men of composition of atherosclerotic plaques in native coronary arteries and in saphenous veins used as aortocoronary conduits. *J Am Coll Cardiol* 1993;21:1312–1318.
9. Kane JP, Malloy MJ, Ports TA, et al. Regression of coronary atherosclerosis during treatment of familial hypercholesterolemia with combined drug regimens. *JAMA* 1990;264:3007–3012.
10. Janowitz WR, Agatston AS, Kaplan G, et al. Differences in prevalence and extent of coronary artery calcium detected by ultrafast computed tomography in asymptomatic men and women. *Am J Cardiol* 1993;72:247–254.
11. U. S. Public Health Service. National Center for Health Statistics. *Health, United States, 1988.* Vol. PHS Publication 1988. Washington, DC: U.S. Government Printing Office, 1988:89–1232.
12. Dustan HP. Coronary artery disease in women. *Can J Cardiol* 1990;6(Suppl B):19B–21B.
13. Lerner DJ, Kannel WB. Patterns of coronary heart disease morbidity and mortality in the sexes: a 26-year follow-up of the Framingham population. *Am Heart J* 1986;111:383–390.
14. Mehilli J, Kastrati A, Dirschinger J, et al. Differences in prognostic factors and outcomes between women and men undergoing coronary artery stenting. *JAMA* 2000;284:1799–1805.
15. Wenger NK, Speroff L, Packard B. Cardiovascular health and disease in women. *N Engl J Med* 1993;329:247–256.
16. Wenger N. Coronary heart disease in women: an overview (myths, misperceptions and missed opportunities). In: Wenger N, Speroff L, Packard B, eds. *Cardiovascular disease and health in women.* Greenwich, CT: LeJacq Communications, 1993:21–29.
17. Becker RC, Terrin M, Ross R, et al. Comparison of clinical outcomes for women and men after acute myocardial infarction. The Thrombolysis in Myocardial Infarction Investigators. *Ann Intern Med* 1994;120:638–645.
18. Moen EK, Asher CR, Miller DP, et al. Long-term follow-up of gender-specific outcomes after thrombolytic therapy for acute myocardial infarction from the GUSTO-I trial. Global Utilization of Streptokinase and Tissue Plasminogen Activator for Occluded Coronary Arteries. *J Womens Health* 1997;6:285–293.
19. Kober L, Torp-Pedersen C, Ottesen M, et al. Influence of gender on short- and long-term mortality after acute myocardial infarction. TRACE study group. *Am J Cardiol* 1996;77:1052–1056.
20. Higgins M, Thom T. Cardiovascular disease in women as a public health problem. In: Wenger N, Speroff L, Packard B, eds. *Cardiovascular disease and health in women.* Greenwich, CT: LeJacq Communications, 1993:15–19.
21. Cupples L, D'Agostino R. Some risk factors related to the annual incidence of cardiovascular disease and death using pooled repeated biennial measurements: Framingham Heart Study, 30-year follow-up. In: Kannel W, Wolf P, Garrison R, eds. *The Framingham Heart Study: an epidemiological investigation of heart disease.* Vol. NIH Publication 87-2703, Section 34. Rockville, MD: National Heart, Lung and Blood Institute, 1987.
22. Hochman JS, Tamis JE, Thompson TD, et al. Sex, clinical presentation, and outcome in patients with acute coronary syndromes. Global Use of Strategies to Open Occluded Coronary Arteries in Acute Coronary Syndromes IIb Investigators. *N Engl J Med* 1999;341:226–232.
23. Vaccarino V, Parsons L, Every NR, et al. Sex-based differences in early mortality after myocardial infarction. National Registry of Myocardial Infarction 2 participants. *N Engl J Med* 1999;341:217–225.
24. Vaccarino V, Krumholz HM, Berkman LF, et al. Sex differences in mortality after myocardial infarction. Is there evidence for an increased risk for women? *Circulation* 1995;91:1861–1871.

25. Bueno H, Vidan MT, Almazan A, et al. Influence of sex on the short-term outcome of elderly patients with a first acute myocardial infarction. *Circulation* 1995;92:1133–1140.

26. Krumholz HM, Douglas PS, Lauer MS, et al. Selection of patients for coronary angiography and coronary revascularization early after myocardial infarction: is there evidence for a gender bias? *Ann Intern Med* 1992;116:785–790.

27. Chiriboga DE, Yarzebski J, Goldberg RJ, et al. A community-wide perspective of gender differences and temporal trends in the use of diagnostic and revascularization procedures for acute myocardial infarction. *Am J Cardiol* 1993;71:268–273.

28. Maynard C, Litwin PE, Martin JS, et al. Gender differences in the treatment and outcome of acute myocardial infarction. Results from the Myocardial Infarction Triage and Intervention Registry. *Arch Intern Med* 1992;152:972–976.

29. Bickell NA, Pieper KS, Lee KL, et al. Referral patterns for coronary artery disease treatment: gender bias or good clinical judgment? *Ann Intern Med* 1992;116:791–797.

30. Mark DB, Shaw LK, DeLong ER, et al. Absence of sex bias in the referral of patients for cardiac catheterization. *N Engl J Med* 1994;330:1101–1106.

31. Maynard C, Beshansky JR, Griffith JL, et al. Influence of sex on the use of cardiac procedures in patients presenting to the emergency department. A prospective multicenter study. *Circulation* 1996;94:II93–II98.

32. Gan SC, Beaver SK, Houck PM, et al. Treatment of acute myocardial infarction and 30-day mortality among women and men. *N Engl J Med* 2000;343:8–15.

33. Healy B. The Yentl syndrome [editorial; comment]. *N Engl J Med* 1991;325:274–276.

34. Vacek JL, Handlin LR, Rosamond TL, et al. Gender-related differences in reperfusion treatment allocation and outcome for acute myocardial infarction. *Am J Cardiol* 1995;76:226–229.

35. Kudenchuk PJ, Maynard C, Martin JS, et al. Comparison of presentation, treatment, and outcome of acute myocardial infarction in men versus women (the Myocardial Infarction Triage and Intervention Registry). *Am J Cardiol* 1996;78:9–14.

36. Weaver WD, White HD, Wilcox RG, et al. Comparisons of characteristics and outcomes among women and men with acute myocardial infarction treated with thrombolytic therapy. GUSTO-I investigators. *JAMA* 1996;275:777–782.

37. Lincoff AM, Califf RM, Ellis SG, et al. Thrombolytic therapy for women with myocardial infarction: is there a gender gap? Thrombolysis and Angioplasty in Myocardial Infarction Study Group. *J Am Coll Cardiol* 1993;22:1780–1787.

38. Bell MR, Holmes DR Jr, Berger PB, et al. The changing in-hospital mortality of women undergoing percutaneous trans-luminal coronary angioplasty. *JAMA* 1993;269:2091–2095.

39. Khan SS, Nessim S, Gray R, et al. Increased mortality of women in coronary artery bypass surgery: evidence for referral bias. *Ann Intern Med* 1990;112:561–567.

40. Bostom AG, Cupples LA, Jenner JL, et al. Elevated plasma lipoprotein(a) and coronary heart disease in men aged 55 years and younger. A prospective study. *JAMA* 1996;276:544–548.

41. Willett WC, Green A, Stampfer MJ, et al. Relative and absolute excess risks of coronary heart disease among women who smoke cigarettes. *N Engl J Med* 1987;317:1303–1309.

42. Thun MJ, Day-Lally CA, Calle EE, et al. Excess mortality among cigarette smokers: changes in a 20-year interval. *Am J Public Health* 1995;85:1223–1230.

43. Guyton JR, Dahlen GH, Patsch W, et al. Relationship of plasma lipoprotein Lp(a) levels to race and to apolipoprotein B. *Arteriosclerosis* 1985;5:265–272.

44. Kannel WB, Wolf PA, Castelli WP, et al. Fibrinogen and risk of cardiovascular disease. The Framingham Study. *JAMA* 1987;258:1183–1186.

45. Kang SS, Wong PW, Glickman PB, et al. Protein-bound homocyst(e)ine in patients with rheumatoid arthritis undergoing D-penicillamine treatment. *J Clin Pharmacol* 1986;26:712–715.

46. Willett WC, Manson JE, Stampfer MJ, et al. Weight, weight change, and coronary heart disease in women. Risk within the 'normal' weight range. *JAMA* 1995;273:461–465.

47. Ridker PM, Hennekens CH, Buring JE, et al. C-reactive protein and other markers of inflammation in the prediction of cardiovascular disease in women. *N Engl J Med* 2000;342:836–843.

48. Orth-Gomer K, Wamala SP, Horsten M, et al. Marital stress worsens prognosis in women with coronary heart disease: the Stockholm Female Coronary Risk Study. *JAMA* 2000;284:3008–3014.

49. Methot J, Bogaty P, Poirier P, et al. The relationship of the occurrence of acute coronary events in women to the timing of their menstrual cycle. *Circulation* 2000;102[Suppl II]:II–613.

50. Knopp R, Broyles F, Bonet B, et al. Exaggerated lipoprotein abnormalities in diabetic women as compared with diabetic men: possible significance for atherosclerosis. In: Wenger N, Speroff L, Packard B, eds. *Cardiovascular health and disease in women.* Greenwich, CT: LeJacq Communications, 1993:131–138.

51. Kannel W. Cardiovascular sequelae in diabetes. In: Moskowitz J, ed. *Diabetes and atherosclerosis connection.* Rockville, MD: National Heart, Lung and Blood Institute, 1981:5–15.

52. Walden CE, Knopp RH, Wahl PW, et al. Sex differences in the effect of diabetes mellitus on lipoprotein triglyceride and cholesterol concentrations. *N Engl J Med* 1984;311:953–959.

53. Corti MC, Guralnik JM, Salive ME, et al. HDL cholesterol predicts coronary heart disease mortality in older persons. *JAMA* 1995;274:539–544.

54. Arnold AM, Mick MJ, Piedmonte MR, et al. Gender differences for coronary angioplasty. *Am J Cardiol* 1994;74:18–21.

55. Reaven GM. Banting lecture 1988. Role of insulin resistance in human disease. *Diabetes* 1988;37:1595–1607.

56. Kwiterovich PO Jr, Motevalli M, Miller M, et al. Further insights into the pathophysiology of hyperapobetalipoproteinemia: role of basic proteins I, II, III. *Clin Chem* 1991;37:317–326.

57. Brunzell JD, Albers JJ, Chait A, et al. Plasma lipoproteins in familial combined hyperlipidemia and monogenic familial hypertriglyceridemia. *J Lipid Res* 1983;24:147–155.

58. Kahn SE, Prigeon RL, McCulloch DK, et al. Quantification of the relationship between insulin sensitivity and beta-cell function in human subjects. Evidence for a hyperbolic function. *Diabetes* 1993;42:1663–1672.

59. Kostis JB, Wilson AC, O'Dowd K, et al. Sex differences in the management and long-term outcome of acute myocardial infarction. A statewide study. MIDAS Study Group.

Myocardial Infarction Data Acquisition System. *Circulation* 1994;90:1715–1730.

60. Yarzebski J, Col N, Pagley P, et al. Gender differences and factors associated with the receipt of thrombolytic therapy in patients with acute myocardial infarction: a community-wide perspective. *Am Heart J* 1996;131:43–50.

61. Hokanson JE, Austin MA. Plasma triglyceride level is a risk factor for cardiovascular disease independent of high-density lipoprotein cholesterol level: a meta-analysis of population-based prospective studies. *J Cardiovasc Risk* 1996;3:213–219.

62. Gordon DJ, Probstfield JL, Garrison RJ, et al. High-density lipoprotein cholesterol and cardiovascular disease. Four prospective American studies. *Circulation* 1989;79:8–15.

63. Reardon MF, Nestel PJ, Craig IH, et al. Lipoprotein predictors of the severity of coronary artery disease in men and women. *Circulation* 1985;71:881–888.

64. Rapp JH, Lespine A, Hamilton RL, et al. Triglyceride-rich lipoproteins isolated by selected-affinity anti-apolipoprotein B immunoabsorption from human atherosclerotic plaque. *Arterioscler Thromb* 1994;14:1767–1774.

65. Birdsall MA, Farquhar CM, White HD. Association between polycystic ovaries and extent of coronary artery disease in women having cardiac catheterization. *Ann Intern Med* 1997;126:32–35.

66. Nestler JE, Jakubowicz DJ. Decreases in ovarian cytochrome P450c17 alpha activity and serum free testosterone after reduction of insulin secretion in polycystic ovary syndrome. *N Engl J Med* 1996;335:617–623.

67. Gasic S, Bodenburg Y, Nagamani M, et al. Troglitazone inhibits progesterone production in porcine granulosa cells. Endocrinology 1998;139:4962–4966.

68. Blankenhorn DH, Hodis HN. George Lyman Duff Memorial Lecture. Arterial imaging and atherosclerosis reversal. *Arterioscler Thromb* 1994;14:177–192.

69. Kannel WB, Wilson PW. Risk factors that attenuate the female coronary disease advantage. *Arch Intern Med* 1995;155:57–61.

70. Walden CE, Retzlaff BM, Buck BL, et al. Lipoprotein lipid response to the National Cholesterol Education Program step II diet by hypercholesterolemic and combined hyperlipidemic women and men. *Arterioscler Thromb Vasc Biol* 1997;17:375–382.

71. Walden CE, Retzlaff BM, Buck BL, et al. Differential effect of National Cholesterol Education Program (NCEP) step II diet on HDL cholesterol, its subfractions, and apoprotein A-I levels in hypercholesterolemic women and men after 1 year: the beFIT Study. *Arterioscler Thromb Vasc Biol* 2000;20:1580–1587.

72. Knopp R, Zhu X-D, Lau J, et al. Sex hormones and lipid interactions: implications for cardiovascular disease in women. *Endocrinologist* 1994;4:285–301.

73. Knopp RH, Zhu X, Bonet B, et al. Effects of sex steroid hormones on lipoproteins, clotting, and the arterial wall. *Semin Reprod Endocrinol* 1996;14:15–27.

74. Applebaum-Bowden D, McLean P, Steinmetz A, et al. Lipoprotein, apolipoprotein, and lipolytic enzyme changes following estrogen administration in postmenopausal women. *J Lipid Res* 1989;30:1895–1906.

75. Knopp RH, Bergelin RO, Wahl PW, et al. Population-based lipoprotein lipid reference values for pregnant women compared to nonpregnant women classified by sex hormone usage. *Am J Obstet Gynecol* 1982;143:626–637.

76. Knopp R, Bonet B, Zhu X-D. Lipid metabolism in pregnancy. In: Cowett R, ed. *Principles of perinatal-neonatal metabolism*. New York: Springer-Verlag, 1998:221–258.

77. Knopp R, Wheeler B, Brunzell J, et al. Effect of raloxifene hydrochloride on serum triglycerides in postmenopausal women with a history of enhanced hypertriglyceridemia in response to oral estrogen therapy [manuscript submitted]. *J Clin Endocrinol Metab* 2001.

78. Olsson AG, Oro L, Rossner S. Effects of oxandrolone on plasma lipoproteins and the intravenous fat tolerance in man. *Atherosclerosis* 1974;19:337–346.

79. Zambon A, Brown B, Deeb S, et al. Hepatic lipase as a focal point for the development and treatment of coronary artery disease. *J Invest Med* 2001;49:112–118.

80. Wagner JD, Clarkson TB, St Clair RW, et al. Estrogen and progesterone replacement therapy reduces low density lipoprotein accumulation in the coronary arteries of surgically postmenopausal cynomolgus monkeys. *J Clin Invest* 1991;88:1995–2002.

81. Haarbo J, Nielsen LB, Stender S, et al. Aortic permeability to LDL during estrogen therapy. A study in normocholesterolemic rabbits. *Arterioscler Thromb* 1994;14:243–247.

82. Chen SJ, Li H, Durand J, et al. Estrogen reduces myointimal proliferation after balloon injury of rat carotid artery. *Circulation* 1996;93:577–584.

83. Zhu X, Bonet B, Gillenwater H, et al. Opposing effects of estrogen and progestins on LDL oxidation and vascular wall cytotoxicity: implications for atherogenesis. *Proc Soc Exp Biol Med* 1999;222:214–221.

84. Kovacs EJ, Faunce DE, Ramer-Quinn DS, et al. Estrogen regulation of JE/MCP-1 mRNA expression in fibroblasts. *J Leuk Biol* 1996;59:562–568.

85. Mendelsohn ME, Karas RH. The protective effects of estrogen on the cardiovascular system. *N Engl J Med* 1999;340:1801–1811.

86. Losordo DW, Kearney M, Kim EA, et al. Variable expression of the estrogen receptor in normal and atherosclerotic coronary arteries of premenopausal women. *Circulation* 1994;89:1501–1510.

87. Herrington DM, Braden GA, Williams JK, et al. Endothelial-dependent coronary vasomotor responsiveness in postmenopausal women with and without estrogen replacement therapy. *Am J Cardiol* 1994;73:951–952.

88. Gerhard M, Ganz P. How do we explain the clinical benefits of estrogen? From bedside to bench [editorial; comment]. *Circulation* 1995;92:5–8.

89. Guetta V, Cannon RO III. Cardiovascular effects of estrogen and lipid-lowering therapies in postmenopausal women. *Circulation* 1996;93:1928–1937.

90. Rosselli M, Imthurn B, Keller PJ, et al. Circulating nitric oxide (nitrite/nitrate) levels in postmenopausal women substituted with 17 beta-estradiol and norethisterone acetate. A two-year follow-up study. *Hypertension* 1995;25:848–853.

91. Polderman KH, Stehouwer CD, van Kamp GJ, et al. Influence of sex hormones on plasma endothelin levels. *Ann Intern Med* 1993;118:429–432.

92. Yue P, Chatterjee K, Beale C, et al. Testosterone relaxes rabbit coronary arteries and aorta. *Circulation* 1995;91:1154–1160.

93. Practico D, FitzGerald GA. Testosterone and thromboxane. Of muscles, mice, and men. *Circulation* 1995;91:2694–2698.

94. Miller VM, Vanhoutte PM. Progesterone and modulation of endothelium-dependent responses in canine coronary arteries. *Am J Physiol* 1991;261:R1022–R1027.

95. Adams MR, Register TC, Golden DL, et al. Medroxyprogesterone acetate antagonizes inhibitory effects of conjugated equine estrogens on coronary artery atherosclerosis. *Arterioscler Thromb Vasc Biol* 1997;17:217–221.

96. Levine RL, Chen SJ, Durand J, et al. Medroxyprogesterone attenuates estrogen-mediated inhibition of neointima formation after balloon injury of the rat carotid artery. *Circulation* 1996;94:2221–2227.

97. Adams MR, Williams JK, Kaplan JR. Effects of androgens on coronary artery atherosclerosis and atherosclerosis-related impairment of vascular responsiveness. *Arterioscler Thromb Vasc Biol* 1995;15:562–570.

98. Zhu X, Bonet B, Knopp RH. Estradiol 17beta inhibition of LDL oxidation and endothelial cell cytotoxicity is opposed by progestins to different degrees. *Atherosclerosis* 2000;148:31–41.

99. Bloemenkamp KW, Rosendaal FR, Helmerhorst FM, et al. Enhancement by factor V Leiden mutation of risk of deep-vein thrombosis associated with oral contraceptives containing a third-generation progestogen. *Lancet* 1995;346:1593–1596.

100. Lewis MA, Spitzer WO, Heinemann LA, et al. Third generation oral contraceptives and risk of myocardial infarction: an international case-control study. Transnational Research Group on Oral Contraceptives and the Health of Young Women. *BMJ* 1996;312:88–90.

101. Knopp RH, Broyles FE, Cheung M, et al. Comparison of the lipoprotein, carbohydrate, and hemostatic effects of phasic oral contraceptives containing desogestrel or levonorgestrel. *Contraception* 2001;63:1–11.

102. Mann JI, Vessey MP, Thorogood M, et al. Myocardial infarction in young women with special reference to oral contraceptive practice. *BMJ* 1975;2:241–245.

103. Mann JI, Inman WH. Oral contraceptives and death from myocardial infarction. *BMJ* 1975;2:245–248.

104. Rosenberg L, Kaufman DW, Helmrich SP, et al. Myocardial infarction and cigarette smoking in women younger than 50 years of age. *JAMA* 1985;253:2965–2969.

105. Croft P, Hannaford PC. Risk factors for acute myocardial infarction in women: evidence from the Royal College of General Practitioners' oral contraception study. *BMJ* 1989;298:165–168.

106. Spain D. Concerning the pathology of acute coronary heart disease in young women. In: Olver M, ed. Coronary heart disease in young women. Edinburgh: Churchill Livingstone, 1978:61–70.

107. Holden J. Clinicopathologic conference: sudden death in a 29-year old woman. *Am J Med* 1988;84:265–272.

108. Knopp RH, LaRosa JC, Burkman RT Jr. Contraception and dyslipidemia. *Am J Obstet Gynecol* 1993;168:1994–2005.

109. Matthews KA, Meilahn E, Kuller LH, et al. Menopause and risk factors for coronary heart disease. *N Engl J Med* 1989;321:641–646.

110. The Writing Group for the PEPI Trial. Effects of estrogen or estrogen/progestin regimens on heart disease risk factors in postmenopausal women. The Postmenopausal Estrogen/Progestin Interventions (PEPI) Trial. *JAMA* 1995;273:199–208.

111. Cushman M, Legault C, Barrett-Connor E, et al. Effect of postmenopausal hormones on inflammation-sensitive proteins: the Postmenopausal Estrogen/Progestin Interventions (PEPI) Study. *Circulation* 1999;100:717–722.

112. Pasceri V, Willerson JT, Yeh ET. Direct proinflammatory effect of C-reactive protein on human endothelial cells. *Circulation* 2000;102:2165–2168.

113. Barrett-Connor E. Postmenopausal estrogen and prevention bias. *Ann Intern Med* 1991;115:455–456.

114. Grodstein F, Stampfer MJ, Manson JE, et al. Postmenopausal estrogen and progestin use and the risk of cardiovascular disease. *N Engl J Med* 1996;335:453–461.

115. Psaty BM, Heckbert SR, Atkins D, et al. The risk of myocardial infarction associated with the combined use of estrogens and progestins in postmenopausal women. *Arch Intern Med* 1994;154:1333–1339.

116. Hulley S, Grady D, Bush T, et al. Randomized trial of estrogen plus progestin for secondary prevention of coronary heart disease in postmenopausal women. Heart and Estrogen/progestin Replacement Study (HERS) Research Group. *JAMA* 1998;280:605–613.

117. Herrington DM, Reboussin DM, Brosnihan KB, et al. Effects of estrogen replacement on the progression of coronary-artery atherosclerosis. *N Engl J Med* 2000;343:522–529.

118. Hanke H, Kamenz J, Hanke S, et al. Effect of 17-beta estradiol on pre-existing atherosclerotic lesions: role of the endothelium. *Atherosclerosis* 1999;147:123–132.

119. Williams JK, Anthony MS, Honore EK, et al. Regression of atherosclerosis in female monkeys. *Arterioscler Thromb Vasc Biol* 1995;15:827–836.

120. Daly E, Vessey MP, Hawkins MM, et al. Risk of venous thromboembolism in users of hormone replacement therapy. *Lancet* 1996;348:977–980.

121. Jick H, Derby LE, Myers MW, et al. Risk of hospital admission for idiopathic venous thromboembolism among users of postmenopausal estrogens. *Lancet* 1996;348:981–983.

122. Grodstein F, Stampfer MJ, Goldhaber SZ, et al. Prospective study of exogenous hormones and risk of pulmonary embolism in women. *Lancet* 1996;348:983–987.

123. Grady D, Wenger NK, Herrington D, et al. Postmenopausal hormone therapy increases risk for venous thromboembolic disease. The Heart and Estrogen/Progestin Replacement Study. *Ann Intern Med* 2000;132:689–696.

124. Psaty B, Smith N, Lemaitre R, et al. Hormone replacement therapy, prothrombotic mutations and the risk of incident nonfatal myocardial infarction in postmenopausal women. *JAMA* 2001;285:906–913.

125. Glazer G. Atherogenic effects of anabolic steroids on serum lipid levels. A literature review. *Arch Intern Med* 1991;151:1925–1933.

126. Wilson PW, Garrison RJ, Castelli WP. Postmenopausal estrogen use, cigarette smoking, and cardiovascular morbidity in women over 50. The Framingham Study. *N Engl J Med* 1985;313:1038–1043.

127. The Coronary Drug Project. Initial findings leading to modifications of its research protocol. *JAMA* 1970;214:1303–1313.

128. Barrett-Connor E, Khaw KT, Yen SS. A prospective study of dehydroepiandrosterone sulfate, mortality, and cardiovascular disease. *N Engl J Med* 1986;315:1519–1524.

129. Derman RJ. Effects of sex steroids on women's health: implications for practitioners. *Am J Med* 1995;98:137S–143S.

130. Sacks FM, Pfeffer MA, Moye LA, et al. The effect of pravastatin on coronary events after myocardial infarction in patients with average cholesterol levels. Cholesterol and Recurrent Events Trial investigators. *N Engl J Med* 1996;335:1001–1009.

131. Dollar AL, Kragel AH, Fernicola DJ, et al. Composition of atherosclerotic plaques in coronary arteries in women less than 40 years of age with fatal coronary artery disease and implications for plaque reversibility. *Am J Cardiol* 1991;67:1223–1227.

132. Jacobs D, Blackburn H, Higgins M, et al. Report of the Conference on Low Blood Cholesterol: mortality associations. *Circulation* 1992;86:1046–1060.

133. Hulley SB, Walsh JM, Newman TB. Health policy on blood cholesterol. Time to change directions. *Circulation* 1992;86:1026–1029.

134. Knopp RH. Drug Treatment of lipid disorders. *N Engl J Med* 1999;341:498–511.

135. Shear CL, Franklin FA, Stinnett S, et al. Expanded Clinical Evaluation of Lovastatin (EXCEL) study results. Effect of patient characteristics on lovastatin-induced changes in plasma concentrations of lipids and lipoproteins. *Circulation* 1992;85:1293–1303.

136. Pierce LR, Wysowski DK, Gross TP. Myopathy and rhabdomyolysis associated with lovastatin-gemfibrozil combination therapy. *JAMA* 1990;264:71–75.

137. Kato S, Endoh H, Masuhiro Y, et al. Activation of the estrogen receptor through phosphorylation by mitogen-activated protein kinase. *Science* 1995;270:1491–1494.

138. Barrett-Connor E. Sex differences in coronary heart disease. Why are women so superior? The 1995 Ancel Keys Lecture. *Circulation* 1997;95:252–264.

139. Woodfield SL, Lundergan CF, Reiner JS, et al. Gender and acute myocardial infarction: is there a different response to thrombolysis? *J Am Coll Cardiol* 1997;29:35–42.

140. Koh KK, Mincemoyer R, Bui MN, et al. Effects of hormone-replacement therapy on fibrinolysis in postmenopausal women. *N Engl J Med* 1997;336:683–690.

141. Miyagawa K, Rosch J, Stanczyk F, et al. Medroxyprogesterone interferes with ovarian steroid protection against coronary vasospasm. *Nat Med* 1997;3:324–327.

142. Rosenfeld ME, Polinsky P, Virmani R, et al. Advanced atherosclerotic lesions in the innominate artery of the ApoE knockout mouse. *Arterioscler Thromb Vasc Biol* 2000;20:2587–2592.

ETHANOL AND THE HEART

LUIS H. ARROYO
TIMOTHY J. REGAN

▼▼ *ADDITIONAL ELECTRONIC TOPICS*

Subclinical Cardiomyopathy b81;   Hypertension b82

OVERVIEW

The influence of ethanol on the cardiovascular system generally has been attributed to its toxic action rather than to malnutrition. Whereas many individuals addicted to ethanol have subclinical diastolic dysfunction presumably related to interstitial fibrosis of the myocardium, a minority goes on to develop symptomatic cardiac problems such as heart failure and arrhythmias. In addition to supraventricular arrhythmias that often normalize spontaneously, there is an increased incidence of sudden death that apparently peaks at approximately 50 years of age in the alcoholic population. The combined use of tobacco and alcohol increases the risk of many of these clinical abnormalities. A significant degree of blood pressure elevation occurs in individuals who abuse alcohol. This tends to be transient and is normalized in most individuals during abstinence from alcohol. In addition to these risks, there is also a preventive effect of mild to moderate drinking on coronary heart disease.

GLOSSARY

Alcoholism: a disorder characterized by a pathologic pattern of alcohol use and resulting in serious impairment of social and occupational functioning.

Holiday heart: an acute arrhythmic process that appears after an episode of heavy drinking.

Light alcohol consumption: one to two drinks per day in women, two to three drinks per day in men.

PERSONAL PERSPECTIVES

Recent decades have seen a growing public awareness of the multiple negative consequences associated with excess intake of ethyl alcohol. Moreover, there has been some progress in the long-term management of this addiction. At the other end of the spectrum is the realization from multiple studies that low-dose alcohol intake can have positive

L. H. Arroyo: Department of Cardiology, Newark Beth Israel Medical Center, Newark, New Jersey

T. J. Regan: Department of Medicine, New Jersey Medical School, Newark, New Jersey (Deceased)

effects in terms of prevention of cardiovascular disease in middle age and beyond.

HISTORICAL PERSPECTIVE

During the 1860s, controversy existed among members of the British medical profession on the therapeutic effects of alcohol, which had a prominent place in medical practice at the time. The debate focused mainly on the scientific basis that would support this practice (1). During the same period, new investigations called attention to the potential toxic effect of alcohol on the heart. Early studies in the nineteenth century demonstrated a relationship between excessive consumption of beer and the presence of cardiomegaly at autopsy (2). Clinical heart disease related to ethanol abuse was later described in the British medical literature (3). Since then, ethanol has been recognized as a toxic agent affecting different organ functions, both acutely and chronically.

The discovery of the beriberi heart syndrome drew attention to the role of thiamine deficiency as an underlying factor in alcoholic heart disease. Diminished thiamine intake was common among alcoholics in a period when vitamin supplementation was uncommon. Since the middle part of the twentieth century, this confusion between the direct effects of alcohol and the effects of nutritional deficiency has been reduced by evidence of the direct deleterious effects of alcohol on the heart. Numerous studies performed during the late 1960s and early 1970s have confirmed the role of ethanol in the genesis of low-output heart failure, as opposed to the high cardiac output of wet beriberi (4,5). There is persistent controversy, however, about the roles that concomitant risk factors (e.g., tobacco) and lack of trace elements have in the development of cardiac abnormalities.

Recently, epidemiologic studies have reported beneficial effects of light to moderate alcohol consumption on cardiovascular risk. However, further evidence is required to recommend the use of alcohol as a general health policy.

ANATOMY

Specimens from autopsies and biopsies of alcoholic hearts have shown varying degrees of morphologic abnormalities, depending on the stage and progression of the disease. During the preclinical phase, left ventricular mass may be normal or moderately enhanced due to increased wall thickness. With progression of the disease, varying degrees of cardiomegaly reflecting chamber dilatation are seen, particularly when there is concomitant mitral insufficiency as part of the cardiomyopathic picture. On gross observation, the heart appears flabby, large, and pale. ▾ b83

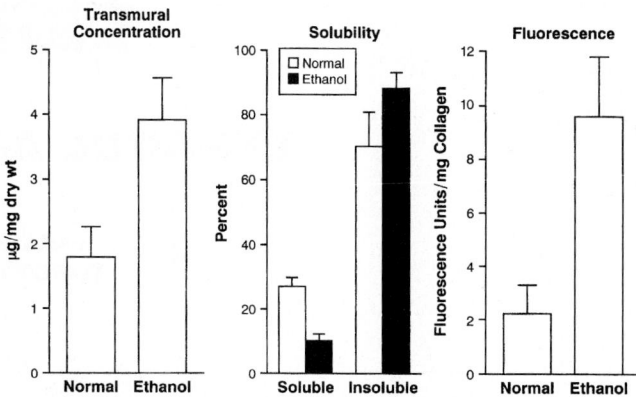

FIGURE 9.1 Differences in the concentration and solubility of collagen found in left ventricular muscle in comparison of healthy and ethanol-fed animals.

PATHOPHYSIOLOGY

Acute ingestion of ethanol is responsible for a direct negative inotropic effect due to diminished ventricular contractile force. A modest increase in heart rate is commonly observed secondary to increased autonomic activity (8). Because these actions of ethanol tend to have opposing effects, evidence of direct acute damage from alcohol can be minimal in healthy individuals or asymptomatic alcoholics. However, clear demonstration of diminished contractility secondary to acute ingestion of alcohol has been shown in human and animal models under conditions of autonomic blockade (8–10).

The hemodynamic changes that alcohol produces are of greater clinical significance in the chronic user, especially in those with underlying cardiac disease. A potential morphologic basis for the increased diastolic stiffness observed early in the alcoholic heart is related to the accumulation of myocardial collagen in the extracellular matrix. Collagen accumulation has been associated with greater intermolecular cross-links, translating into an increased diastolic stiffness of the ventricle. Staining with Alcian blue shows the deposition of glycoprotein-like material in the interstitium of the ventricular wall (Fig. 9.1). The role of ethanol in the accumulation of collagen can be enhanced by the use of tobacco (11), which is commonly a coaddiction. ▾ b84

EPIDEMIOLOGY

Two-thirds of the population of the United States consume alcohol, and approximately 10% of these are considered heavy users. Among the identifiable etiologies of nonischemic dilated cardiomyopathy, alcohol is the most common in industrialized countries, accounting for almost half of those diagnosed at autopsy. Prevalence of alcohol consumption differs between genders; however, the risk of alcoholic cardiomyopathy is greater in women than in men.

CLINICAL PRESENTATION

Congestive Heart Failure

With continuing ethanol abuse, the initial subclinical process eventually deteriorates in many patients with the development of heart failure (Fig. 9.2). Continuation of alcohol consumption at this stage produces a marked decrease of left ventricular function compared to normals (*e*Fig. 9.2.1). Abstinence still plays a role during this period, resulting in evidence of partial improvement in ventricular function and reduced mortality. Cardiac decompensation commonly affects patients in the age range from 30 years to the mid-50s. Intake history averages 80 g of alcohol per day (approximately 8 oz of 86-proof whiskey or 1 L of wine) for a minimum of 10 years. Occasionally, an episode of intense drinking is reported before the development of symptoms, but a particular pattern of drinking has not been found to be associated with the onset of heart failure. ▼ b85

Thiamine Deficiency (Wet Beriberi)

Thiamine deficiency should be considered as a factor contributing to alcoholic cardiomyopathy. Approximately 15% of asymptomatic alcoholics are moderately deficient in thiamine, as determined by dietary history and excretion of

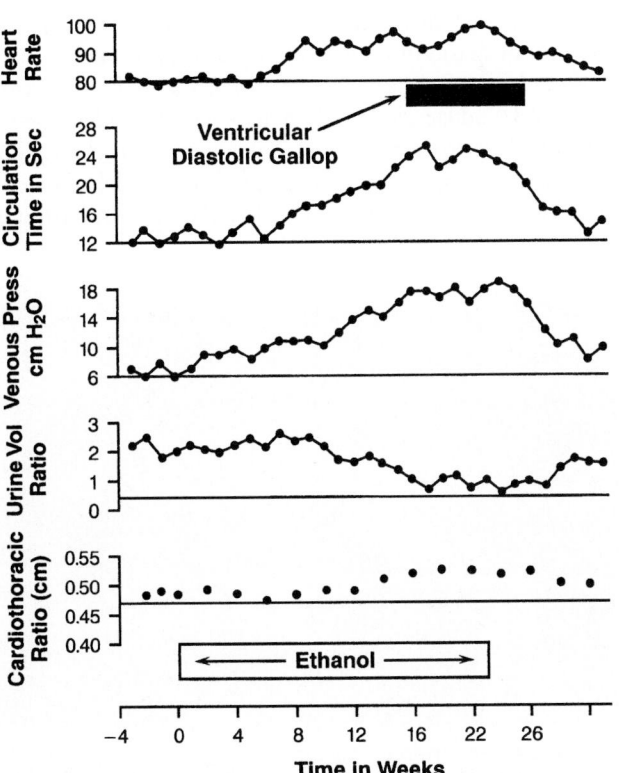

FIGURE 9.2 Evidence of cardiac depression developing as a result of chronic ethanol abuse. The various parameters became progressively abnormal after 8 weeks of alcohol ingestion. The abnormalities disappeared with abstinence.

vitamin metabolites (27). There has been no survey of patients with clinical heart disease. The physiologic derangements observed in beriberi heart disease are different from those seen in alcoholic cardiomyopathy; the hallmark is the existence of a hyperkinetic state affecting the cardiovascular system, characterized by decreased peripheral resistance, increased cardiac output, tachycardia, and biventricular failure. In addition to the findings of congestion, on physical examination, there is a wide pulse pressure with a bounding arterial pulse. Frequently, an early diastolic gallop and a systolic murmur can be heard in the apical area. A machinery-type murmur is heard in the peripheral arteries as a manifestation of the arteriovenous shunts that are common in this disorder. The electrocardiogram may show low voltage with an increased QT interval and nonspecific T-wave abnormalities. Cardiomegaly is the common finding in chest radiography.

For the diagnosis of beriberi heart disease, several criteria are required, including a history of thiamine deficiency for more than 3 months, absence of another etiology of heart failure, evidence of peripheral neuropathy, and a therapeutic response to thiamine (28).

Arrhythmias

Dysrhythmias in the heart are associated with underlying changes in myocardial composition and electrophysiology as a consequence of chronic alcohol ingestion. Healthy subjects do not appear to be affected after mild to moderate intake. Arrhythmias tend to appear in the late stages of an episode of excessive drinking or in the subsequent hours. These episodes of intense drinking are particularly more prevalent among the middle-aged population, as compared to older individuals. A seasonal variability has been described, but similar episodes may not appear in the same individual, despite a similar drinking pattern. Frequent clinical presentations of alcoholics are dizziness and syncope, which are usually attributed to the individual's inebriated state. However, the arrhythmia is detected by electrocardiography.

The most common arrhythmia is atrial fibrillation. This condition can revert spontaneously to normal sinus rhythm, but, on occasion, electrical or pharmacologic cardioversion is required. With sustained abuse of alcohol, chronic atrial fibrillation can develop. *Holiday heart* describes the development of an acute arrhythmic process, generally atrial fibrillation, after an episode of heavy alcohol consumption (Fig. 9.3). These episodes frequently occur during long weekends or annual holidays, during which there is a rise in the consumption of spirits—thus the name *holiday heart* (29).

An increased incidence of sudden death has been found among the alcoholic population. It has been postulated that this increased incidence might be due to rapid degeneration of ventricular tachycardias into ventricular fibrillation,

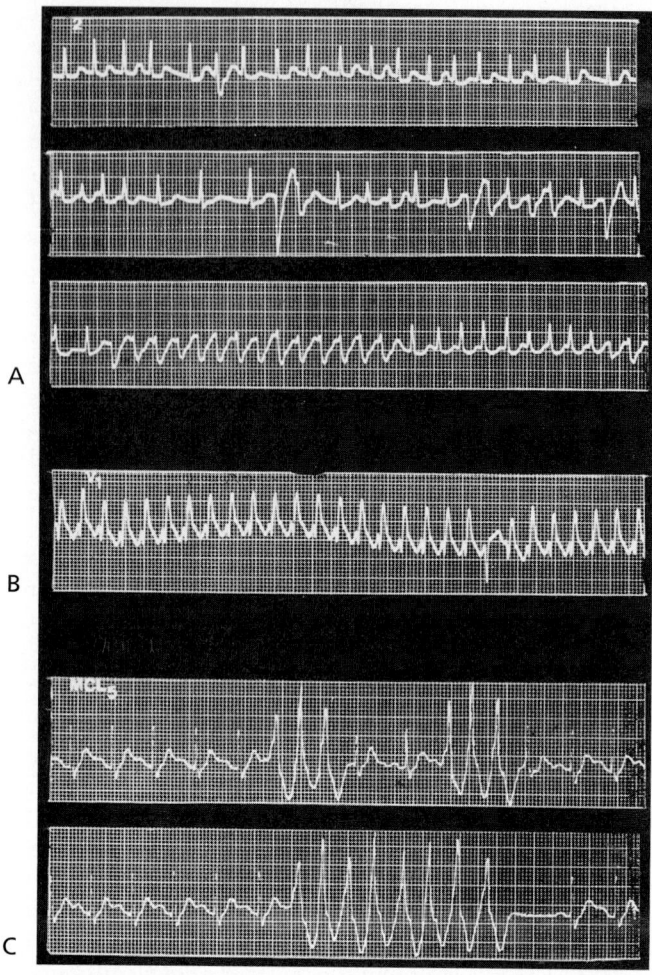

A

B

C

FIGURE 9.3 Electrocardiographic manifestations in alcoholic patients. **A:** The first strip demonstrates rapid atrial fibrillation with one aberrant beat (Ashman phenomenon); the following two strips show increased rate in the same patient with wide complex tachycardia (rate of 240 beats/min). **B:** Atrial flutter with 1:1 conduction (verified after carotid massage) at a rate of 250 beats/min with right bundle branch block aberration. **C:** Nonsustained ventricular tachycardia.

TABLE 9.1 AMOUNT OF ALCOHOL IN DIFFERENT BEVERAGES[a]

Beer (360 mL)	18 g
Wine (1 L)	100 g
Whiskey (90 mL)	36 g

[a]1 oz = 30 mL.

Dose is an important factor in determining the relationship of alcohol to the development of sudden death (Table 9.1). No effect on mortality was found with doses of <80 g of ethanol per day in an epidemiologic study (32). The mortality rate rose threefold with increased intake compared to that of those taking less alcohol. This finding was confirmed in an analysis of the Framingham population. Individuals consuming more than 2,500 g of alcohol per month had an increased risk of sudden death without evidence of CAD (33). b86

Chest Pain

Underlying cardiac or gastrointestinal processes are often the cause of chest pain in alcoholics. Minimal CAD typically is found among these patients. However, transmural myocardial infarction associated with perivascular fibrosis of subepicardial vessels has been described (40). This fibrosis may limit the coronary blood flow during a period of high myocardial diastolic and systolic tension (Fig. 9.4). No evidence of spasm or embolization has been found.

Elevations of creatine kinase (CK), CK-MB isoenzyme, troponin I, and lactate dehydrogenase have been described in individuals with alcoholic heart disease, both in clinical and in subclinical stages. Whereas its significance is debatable, the elevation of creatine kinase and CK-MB has been attributed

because the former are rarely described in clinical practice. Two European studies have confirmed these observations. Cases of witnessed cardiac arrest were evaluated at the Pathology Institute of Moscow, showing that 17% of the deaths were related to alcohol abuse (30). The majority of the cases were in men younger than the age of 50 years and with alcoholemia. Autopsy revealed no significant coronary artery disease (CAD), but there was evidence of subclinical cardiomyopathy on light and electron microscopy. A large prospective study using a registration system established by the Swedish social authorities for alcoholism examined the role of alcohol as a general and specific cause of mortality (31). In a period of 11 years, the incidence of sudden death between the group registered for alcoholism was double that of the nonregistered group. This association was observed in men with and without coronary disease.

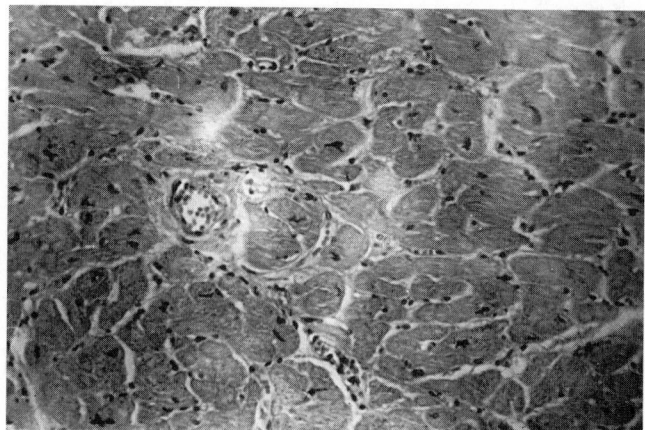

FIGURE 9.4 Periarterial interstitial collagen accumulation with distribution between myofibers (Alcian blue staining), graded as 2 to 3+, indicating increased deposition of glycoprotein material in the extracellular matrix. (From Regan TJ, Wu CF, Weisse AB, et al. Acute myocardial infarction in toxic cardiomyopathy without coronary obstruction. *Circulation* 1975;51:453, with permission.)

to the existence of skeletal muscle myopathy that is common in alcoholics. Despite the absence of electrocardiographic changes, a cardiac origin is still possible because myocardial enzyme release is induced by acute alcohol administration (41–43). To make the diagnosis of coronary ischemia related to alcohol, physicians cannot rely entirely on enzyme levels but must consider the entire clinical picture.

DIAGNOSIS AND MANAGEMENT

Identification of the alcoholic patient can often represent a challenge, because denial of the underlying problem is a common characteristic. It is estimated that approximately 60% to 80% of cases of alcoholism are undiagnosed. Physicians rarely use any screening method to identify the addiction. Screening tests have a sensitivity and specificity of 70% to 90%. Clinician specialists use the criteria established by the *Diagnostic and Statistical Manual of Mental Disorders (DSM-IV)* (44). These criteria require a maladaptive pattern of alcohol use associated with other typical characteristics (*e*Table 9.1.1).

In clinical practice, there are clues that aid in the diagnosis: unexplained hepatic dysfunction, parotid enlargement, hypertension, seizures, anxiety, depression, tremors, and alcohol on the breath. Laboratory data have a low sensitivity and specificity, but they provide a hint of the existence of an alcoholic disorder when used in combination with the history and physical findings. Abnormal laboratory values include a high or slightly elevated mean corpuscular volume, aspartate aminotransferase, γ-glutamyl transferase, serum uric acid, triglycerides, and high-density lipoprotein (HDL). ▾ᵧ b87

The therapy of heart failure in alcoholic patients is guided by the same principles as other forms of cardiomyopathy. Initial management with diuretics and bed rest may be the only treatment required in patients with minimal clinical symptomatology. Although no clinical investigation has evaluated the efficacy of angiotensin-converting enzyme inhibitors or beta-blockade in the alcoholic heart, these medications' beneficial effect on heart failure patients in general should encourage their use. ▾ᵧ b88

Reduction in the amount of alcohol consumed lowers blood pressure in the hypertensive alcoholic. A period of 2 to 4 weeks of abstinence should be allowed before considering antihypertensive medications in this population. In the absence of any specific data demonstrating the efficacy of any particular drug in the treatment of alcohol-induced hypertension, angiotensin-converting enzyme inhibitors could be considered the drugs of first choice due to the possibility of concomitant cardiomyopathy. It is important to note that a substantial portion of these patients may experience some degree of autonomic dysfunction secondary to alcohol, resulting in the development of orthostatic hypotension and making alpha-adrenergic blockers the least desirable drug in this population.

There are two objectives in managing patients who present with arrhythmias secondary to ethanol: control of the ventricular response and alcohol cessation. Control of the ventricular response in rapid atrial fibrillation or flutter is best achieved with medications that block atrioventricular nodal conduction, such as beta-blockers and calcium-channel antagonists. Atrial fibrillation in holiday heart tends to revert to sinus rhythm spontaneously, but chemical or electrical cardioversion should be considered if the arrhythmia persists. Ventricular tachycardia or fibrillation require aggressive management with electrical cardioversion or defibrillation. Individuals who are unresponsive to drug therapy or have experienced an episode of sudden cardiac death need to be considered for an implantable defibrillator. Correction of electrolyte abnormalities—especially potassium and magnesium—should ideally be done via intravenous infusion, because many patients present with clouded sensorium or gastrointestinal symptoms that limit oral therapy.

CONTROVERSIES AND PERSONAL PERSPECTIVES

Light to Moderate Alcohol Consumption and the Prevention of Cardiovascular Diseases

A series of epidemiologic studies have suggested that one to two drinks a day of any alcoholic beverage helps protect against CAD (46–49,54). The low incidence of CAD seen in France (French paradox) (50,51) compared to other countries with similar dietary habits has been well publicized. This difference was initially attributed to red wine and its antioxidant components (e.g., tannins, anthocyanins, and flavonoids) (51). However, similar findings have been reported with the use of other alcoholic beverages (52,53).

This beneficial effect of moderate drinking also appears to have a secondary prevention effect by reducing total and cardiovascular mortality in individuals with a history of previous myocardial infarction (55). In this regard, a study of the myocardial response to ischemia in guinea pigs is of interest (56). Low-dose ethanol feeding for several weeks was followed by 45 minutes of no-flow ischemia in the isolated heart with a similar period of reflow. Compared to controls, the ethanol-fed group had lower ventricular diastolic pressure and decreased myocardial damage measured as the level of creatinine-kinase. Adenosine A_1 receptors were required for this effect.

A biologically plausible basis for the effect of ethanol in reducing CAD is the rise of circulating HDL2 and HDL3 with moderate use. Both subfractions have been associated with a decreased incidence of CAD (57). Complementing this effect may be the increased incidence in thrombolytic activity secondary to enhanced endogenous tissue plasminogen activator (58,62), downregulation of plasminogen activator inhibitor-1 (59), prevention of mononuclear-macrophage activation (60), decreased platelet activity (61), and reduced fibrinogen levels after ethanol ingestion (62). A study by McConnell et al. demonstrated only increasing levels of HDL and its subfractions but no effect on hemostatic parameters in individuals exposed to light drinking over a period of 6 weeks (63).

Prospective studies on the relationship of ethanol consumption and incidence of CAD have demonstrated, in general, a U-shaped or J-shaped pattern with a lower risk among light to moderate drinkers. The increased incidence of cardiac mortality observed in heavy drinkers may be secondary to alcohol-related arrhythmias, hypertension, or cardiomyopathy. The benefit of moderate drinking compared to abstaining has been challenged on the basis that these studies did not separate true abstainers from ex-drinkers.

Major contributions to this field have been made by the Physicians' Health Study, which showed cardiovascular benefits of light ethanol consumption in men. These researchers have recently indicated that no further benefit was achieved above two drinks per day in men. Of greater interest is recent evidence showing no difference in benefit between the consumption of one drink per week and intake of one to two drinks per day. This evidence applies to cardiac events (64), stroke (65), and total mortality.

These findings have prompted others to evaluate the relationship of ethanol use and other cardiovascular diseases. A recent examination of carotid atherosclerosis by ultrasound did not find a significant difference in the wall thickness between patients with moderate drinking habits and the control group (66). In contrast, a recent prospective study on the relationship between alcohol use and peripheral artery disease among American physicians demonstrated that moderate ethanol intake appears to decrease the risk of peripheral artery disease in men (67). This inverse relationship is not affected by other known cardiovascular risk factors, except for smoking. Similarly, in a retrospective analysis of patients with mainly ischemic cardiomyopathy, light to moderate alcohol consumption was not associated with an adverse prognosis and decreased the risk of fatal myocardial infarction. However, a trend towards increasing hospitalization was seen with light to moderate alcohol intake among patients with nonischemic heart failure (68). In a large prospective study of apparently healthy males, a decrease in the incidence of sudden cardiac death was observed in those who reported a light consumption of ethanol. The nadir in risk occurred in those individuals who consumed two to six drinks per week (69).

An association between stroke and alcohol consumption has also been analyzed. In a study by Berger et al., approximately half of those individuals consuming alcohol were also using aspirin, making the absolute effect of ethanol *per se* unclear (65). The association with total stroke incidence showed a risk reduction of 20% after adjusting for impor-

TABLE 9.2 FACTORS THAT CONTRIBUTE TO THE DEVELOPMENT OF ALCOHOLIC CARDIOMYOPATHY

Quantity
Frequency
Duration
Ill-defined variables: nutrition, gender, cigarette use, age of onset

tant confounders. Benefit was observed among those consuming only one drink per week, and the degree of protection did not increase with higher doses.

The question of who may benefit from moderate alcohol consumption revolves around determinants such as age, gender, the influence of risk factors for disease, and the concomitant use of other drugs (70) (Table 9.2). Young adults have minimal risk for CAD but are at risk for vehicular accidents, which are commonly related to ethanol use. Individuals older than 50 years with coexisting cardiovascular risk factors may benefit from moderate ethanol intake (49). In fact, a major study in the United States indicated that a significant preventive effect was present only in subjects older than 60 years (48). Analysis of population subsets among women has revealed that only those with coronary risk factors experience a significant benefit from low-dose ethanol consumption (71,72) (*e*Table 9.2.1). Recent data also have shown a significant decrease in the risk of coronary disease among diabetics consuming one drink per week. The apparent lack of influence of light to moderate drinking on the regulation of blood glucose is especially important. In contrast to results of the Physicians' Health Study, these diabetics obtained apparent benefit with only one drink per day.

At issue in the prevention of CAD by alcohol is the question of increased premature mortality rates from other alcohol-related causes, even at moderate doses. The risk-benefit ratio concept has been used to indicate the public health utility of a recommendation for light ethanol use. In a prospective study of 276,000 men aged 40 to 59 years, there was a benefit for reduction of coronary heart disease, but this was only at low dose (i.e., two to three drinks per day) (73). No additional benefit was achieved at higher levels of alcohol intake. Over the 12 years of follow-up, beginning at two drinks per day, there was a progressive increase in the risk of cancer (colon and breast), stroke, accidents, violence, and overall mortality with increasing use of alcohol (Fig. 9.5). Thus, the benefit was limited to low-dose consumption of alcohol. Particularly relevant is a French report that included a prospective cohort study of middle-aged men for nearly a decade and national mortality data from a single year. Whereas consumption of >60 g per day of ethanol correlated with an increase in mortality, lower levels of 26 to 60 mL per day (i.e., two to five drinks) were not associated with reduced total mortality (74).

In the context of the positive epidemiologic message for moderate ethanol use, the statement of Castelli (75) pro-

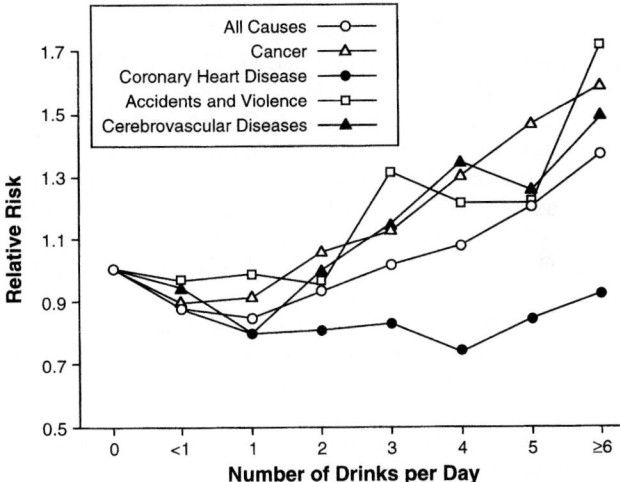

FIGURE 9.5 Alcohol consumption and relative risk of death over 12 years in an American Cancer Society prospective study of 276,802 men, ages 40 to 59 years. Mortality ratios are adjusted for age, smoking habits, the four most common causes of death, and death from all causes. (From Boffetta P, Garfinkel L. Alcohol drinking and mortality among men enrolled in an American Cancer Society prospective study. *Epidemiology* 1990;1:342–348, with permission.)

vides a sobering perspective: "With 17 million alcoholics in this country, we perhaps have a message for which this country is not yet ready." Moreover, the use of alcohol for cardioprotective purposes has been discouraged by some as a general public health measure, because alcohol abuse appears to correlate with overall ethanol consumption in the general population (76). Although the body of evidence supporting the cardiovascular benefits of light to moderate alcohol drinking appears to be reassuring, hazards of moderate intake must be weighed on an individual basis; even modest doses of two drinks per day are associated with an increase in blood pressure. Because of age-related body changes, the National Institute on Alcohol Abuse and Alcoholism recommends that individuals older than 65 years

consume no more than one drink per day (77). Extrapolation of these epidemiologic findings to the general population has to take into account several issues: the potential beneficial effect of ethanol is likely to occur over several years; these reports are based on self-reporting habits, which tend to be inaccurate; consumption of ethanol varies among different cultures and societies, which, in turn, reflect different types of diet and lifestyles. Until the precise mechanisms by which ethanol affects cardiovascular diseases are determined, no public health recommendations should be established.

Cardiotoxicity of Alcohol in Women

A gender difference in the left ventricular function has been found among alcoholics (78), suggesting that there may be a varied prevalence of alcoholic cardiomyopathy between men and women, especially during the subclinical period. A lower prevalence of alcoholism among women may be responsible for the lower incidence of cardiac involvement. It is estimated that, currently, one-third of the alcoholics in the United States are women. Alcoholic heart failure is observed in postmenopausal women, but statistical data are lacking in terms of younger women.

However, a similar or slightly greater propensity for developing cardiomyopathy was seen in women, despite their consumption of lesser amounts of alcohol (79,80). In the study conducted by Urbano-Marquez et al. (80) in ethnically homogeneous and adequately nourished women, a decrease in the mean left ventricular ejection fraction was present, compared to that in a control group (men). However, the group was small (n = 4), and the women were at an age approximating menopausal years. Kupari et al. (79) found that the development of subclinical cardiomyopathy, as established by echocardiographic findings, was similar in alcoholics of both genders. The caveat to this study is the lack of data indicating whether the younger women ever developed clinical heart failure.

THE FUTURE

In the next decade, further diagnostic refinement should be developed for identification of cardiac patients who abuse alcohol. These developments include biochemical alterations in blood and specific histochemical changes identified on cardiac biopsy. Progress is needed in promoting abstinence in such patients. Pharmacologic interventions to reverse or impede progression of the

pathophysiology in myocytes and extracellular matrix are likely to be forthcoming.

Although the research to demonstrate ethanol's beneficial effect at low to moderate doses has been provocative (81), further extensive study is required to define the mechanisms involved and the precise subgroups of patients who may benefit.

REFERENCES

1. Warner JH. Physiological theory and therapeutic explanation in the 1860s: the British debate on the medical use of alcohol. *Br Hist Med* 1980;59:235–237.

2. Bollinger, O. Über die Häufigkeit und Ursachen der idiopathischen Herzhypertrophie in München. *Deutsche Med Wchnschr* 1884;10:180–181.

3. Steel G. Heart failure as a result of alcoholism. *Med Chron* 1893;18:1.

4. Burch GE, DePasquale NP. Alcoholic cardiomyopathy. *Am J Cardiol* 1969;23:723.

5. Demakis JG, Proskey A, Rahimtoola SH, et al. The natural course of alcoholic cardiomyopathy. *Ann Intern Med* 1974;80:293–297.

6. Urbano-Marquez A, Estruch R, Navarro-Lopez F, et al. The effects of alcoholism on skeletal and cardiac muscle. *N Engl J Med* 1989;320:409–415.

7. Factor SM. Intramyocardial small-vessel disease in chronic alcoholism. *Am Heart J* 1976;92:561–575.

8. Thomas AP, Rozansli DJ, Renard DC, Rubin E. Effects of ethanol on contractile function of the heart. *Alcohol Clin Exp Res* 1994;18:121–131.

9. Kupari M, Heikkila J, Tolppanen EM, et al.: Acute effects of alcohol, beta-blockade, and their combination on left ventricular function and hemodynamics in normal man. *Eur Heart J* 1983;7:463–471.

10. Regan TJ, Koroxenidis G, Moschos CB, et al. The acute metabolic and hemodynamic responses of the left ventricle to alcohol. *J Clin Invest* 1966;45:270–280.

11. Rayiyah G, Agarwal R, Avendano G, et al. Influence of nicotine on myocardial stiffness and fibrosis during chronic ethanol use. *Alcohol Clin Exp Res* 1996;20:985–989.

12. Sarma JSM, Ikeda S, Fisher R, et al. Biochemical and contractile properties of heart muscle after prolonged alcohol administration. *J Mol Cell Cardiol* 1976;8:951–972.

13. Burch GE, Giles TD. The importance of magnesium deficiency in cardiovascular disease. *Am Heart J* 1977;94(5):649–657.

14. Heggtviet HA, Herman L, Mishra RK. Cardiac necrosis and calcification in experimental magnesium deficiency: a light and electron microscopic study. *Am J Pathol* 1964;45:757.

15. Rotruck JT, Pope AL, Ganther HE, et al. Selenium: biochemical role as a component of glutathione peroxidase. *Science* 1973;179:588–590.

16. Morin Y, Daniel P. Quebec beer-drinkers cardiomyopathy: etiological considerations. *Can Med Assoc J* 1967;97:926.

17. Sullivan J, Parker M, Carson SB. Tissue cobalt content in beer drinkers myocardiopathy. *J Lab Clin Med* 1968;71:893.

18. Wilberg GS. Factors affecting the cardiotoxic potential of cobalt. *Clin Toxicol* 1969;2:257.

19. Asokan SK. Experimental lead cardiomyopathy: myocardial structural changes in rats given small amounts of lead. *J Lab Clin Med* 1974;84:20.

20. Regan TJ, Levinson GE, Oldewurtel HA, et al. Ventricular function in noncardiacs with alcoholic fatty liver disease: Role of ethanol in the production of cardiomyopathy. *J Clin Invest* 1969;48:397.

21. Lazarevic AM, Nakatani S, Neskovic AN, et al. Early changes in left ventricular function in chronic asymptom-atic alcoholics: relation to the duration of heavy drinking. *J Am Coll Cardiol* 2000;35:1599–1607.

22. Mathews EC, Gardin JM, Henry WL, et al. Echocardiographic abnormalities of chronic alcoholics with and without overt congestive heart failure. *Am J Cardiol* 1981;47:570–578.

23. Kupari M, Koskinen P, Suokas A. Left ventricular size, mass and function in relation to the duration and quantity of heavy drinking in alcoholics. *Am J Cardiol* 1991;67:274–279.

24. Read R, Bell J, Batey R. Cardiac function assessed by gated heart pool studies in an alcohol clinic population: A preliminary study. *Alcohol Clin Exp Res* 1984;8:467–469.

25. Reeves WC, Nanda NC, Gramiak R. Echocardiography in chronic alcoholics following prolonged periods of abstinence. *Am Heart J* 1978;95:578–583.

26. Urbano-Marquez A, Estruch R, Navarro-Lopez F, et al. The effects of alcoholism on skeletal and cardiac muscle. *N Engl J Med* 1989;320:409–415.

27. Neville JN, Eagles JA, Sampson G, et al. The nutritional status of alcoholics. *Am J Clin Nutr* 1968;21:1329–1340.

28. Blakenhorn MA. Effects of vitamin deficiency on the heart and circulation. *Circulation* 1955;11:288–291.

29. Ettinger PO, Wu CF, De la Cruz C. Arrhythmias and the holiday heart: Alcohol associated cardiac rhythm disorders. *Am Heart J* 1978;95:555–562.

30. Vikhert AM, Tsiplenkova VG, Cherpachenka NM. Alcoholic cardiomyopathy and sudden death. *J Am Coll Cardiol* 1986;8:3A–11A.

31. Rosengren A, Wilhelmsen L, Wedel H. Separate and combined effects of smoking and alcohol abuse in middle aged men. *Acta Med Scand* 1988;223:111–118.

32. Dwyer AR, Stamler J, Paul O, et al. Alcohol consumption and 17 year mortality in the Chicago Western Electric company study. *Prev Med* 1980;9:78–90.

33. Gordon T, Kannel WB. Drinking habits and cardiovascular disease: the Framingham Study. *Am Heart J* 1983;105:667–673.

34. Carpentier RG, Gallardo-Carpentier A. Effect of ethanol on guinea pig ventricular action potential. *J Electrocardiogr* 1981;14:333–334.

35. Walsh MJ, Hollander PB, Truit EB, et al. Sympathomimetic effects of acetaldehyde on the electrical and contractile characteristics of isolated left atria of guinea pigs. *J Pharmacol Exp Ther* 1969;167:173–186.

36. Patel R, McArdle JJ, Regan TJ. Increased ventricular vulnerability in chronic ethanol model despite reduced electrophysiologic responses to catecholamines. *Alcohol Clin Exp Res* 1991;15:785–789.

37. Abdel-Rahman AA, Wooles WR. Ethanol induced hypertension involves impairment of baroreceptors. *Hypertension* 1987;10:67–73.

38. Grassi GM, Somers VK, Renk WS, et al. Effects of alcohol intake on blood pressure and sympathetic nerve activity in normotensive humans: a preliminary report. *J Hypertens* 1989;7[Suppl 6]:S20–S21.

39. Altura BM, Altura BT. Microvascular and vascular smooth muscle actions of ethanol, acetaldehyde, and acetate. *Fed Proc* 1982;41:2447–2451.

40. Regan TJ, Wu CF, Weisse AB, et al. Acute myocardial infarction in toxic cardiomyopathy without coronary obstruction. *Circulation* 1975;51:453–461.

41. Siegel RJ, Kligerman M, Haywood LJ, et al. Increased MB-creatinine kinase isoenzymes in an alcoholic population. *J Natl Med Assoc* 1985;77(6):459–464.

42. Fink R, Marjot DH, Rosalki SB. Detection of alcoholic cardiomyopathy by serum enzyme and isoenzyme determination. *Ann Clin Biochem* 1979;16:165–166.

43. Siegel AJ, Dawson DM. Peripheral source of MB band of creatinine kinase in alcoholic rhabdomyolysis: non-specificity of MB isoenzyme for myocardial injury in undiluted serum samples. *JAMA* 1980;244:580–582.

44. American Psychiatric Association. *Diagnostic and Statistical Manual of Mental Disorders (DSM-IV)*, 4th ed. Washington, DC: American Psychiatric Association, 1994.

45. Adams ML, Sewing BN, Chen J, et al. Nitric oxide-related agents alter alcohol withdrawal in male rats. *Alcohol Clin Exp Res* 1995;19:195–199.

46. Jackson R, Scragg R, Beaglehole R. Alcohol consumption and risk of coronary heart disease. *BMJ* 1991;303:211–216.

47. Stampfer MJ, Colditz GA, Willett WC, et al. Prospective study of moderate alcohol consumption and the risk of coronary artery disease and stroke in women. *N Engl J Med* 1988;319:267–273.

48. Klatzky AL, Armstrong MA, Friedman GD. Alcohol and mortality. *Ann Intern Med* 1992;117:646–654.

49. Ajani UA, Gaziano JM, Lotufo PA, et al. Alcohol consumption and the risk of coronary heart disease by diabetes status. *Circulation* 2000;102:500–505.

50. Criqui MH, Ringel BL. Does diet or alcohol explain the French paradox? *Lancet* 1994;344:1719–1723.

51. Renaud S, de Lorgeril M. Wine, alcohol, platelets, and the French paradox for coronary heart disease. *Lancet* 1992;339:1523–1526.

52. Rimm EC, Giovannucci EL, Willett WC, et al. Prospective study for alcohol consumption and coronary disease in men. *Lancet* 1991;338:464–468.

53. Yano K, Reed DM, McGee DL. Ten year incidence of coronary heart disease in the Honolulu Heart Program. *Am J Epidemiol* 1984;119:653–664.

54. Stampfer MJ, Colditz GA, Willett WC, et al. A prospective study of moderate alcohol consumption and the risk of coronary disease and stroke in women. *N Engl J Med* 1988;319:267–273.

55. Muntwyler J, Hennekens CH, Buring JE, et al. Mortality and light to moderate alcohol consumption after myocardial infarction. *Lancet* 1998;352:1882–1885.

56. Miyamae M, Diamond I, Weiner MW, et al. Regular alcohol consumption mimics cardiac preconditioning by protecting against ischemia-reperfusion injury. *Proc Natl Acad Sci U S A* 1997;94:3235–3239.

57. Gardner CD, Tribble DL, Young DR, et al. Associations of HDL, HDL2, HDL3 cholesterol and apolipoproteins A-I and B with lifestyle factors in healthy women and men: Stanford five city project. *Prev Med* 2000;31:346–356.

58. Ridker PM, Vaughan DE, Stampfer MJ, et al. Association of moderate alcohol consumption and plasma concentration of endogenous tissue-type plasminogen activator. *JAMA* 1994;272:929–933.

59. Grenett HE, Aikens ML, Tabengwa EM, et al. Ethanol downregulates transcription of PAI-1 gene in cultured human endothelial cells. *Thromb Res* 2000;97:247–255.

60. Blanco-Colio LM, Valderrama M, Alvare-Sala LA, et al. Red wine intake prevents nuclear factor-kappaB activation in peripheral blood mononuclear cells of healthy volunteers during postprandial lipemia. *Circulation* 2000;102: 1020–1026.

61. Haut MJ, Cowan DH. The effect of ethanol in hemostatic properties of human blood platelets. *Am J Med* 1974;56:22–33.

62. Margaglione M, Cappucci G, Colaizzo D, et al. Fibrinogen plasma levels in apparently healthy general population: relation to environmental and genetic determinants. *Thromb Haemost* 1998;80:805–810.

63. McConnell MV, Vavouranakis I, Wu LL, et al. Effect of a single, daily alcoholic beverage on lipid and hemostatic markers of cardiovascular risk. *Am J Cardiol* 1997;80:1226–1228.

64. Gaziano JM, Gaziano TA, Glynn RJ, et al. Light-to-moderate alcohol consumption and mortality in the Physician's Health Study enrollment cohort. *J Am Coll Cardiol* 2000; 35:96–105.

65. Berger K, Ajani UA, Kase CS, et al. Light-to-moderate alcohol consumption and the risk of stroke among US male physicians. *N Engl J Med* 1999;341:1557–1564.

66. Demirovic J, Nabulsi A, Folsom AR, et al. Alcohol consumption and ultrasonographically assessed carotid artery wall thickness and distensibility: the Atherosclerosis Risk in Communities (ARIC) Study Investigators. *Circulation* 1993; 88(6):2787–2793.

67. Camargo CA, Stamfer MJ, Glynn RJ, et al. Prospective study of moderate alcohol consumption and risk of peripheral arterial disease in US male physicians. *Circulation* 1997;95:577–580.

68. Cooper HA, Exner DV, Domanski MJ. Light to moderate alcohol consumption and prognosis in patients with left ventricular systolic dysfunction. *J Am Coll Cardiol* 2000; 35:1753–1759.

69. Albert CM, Manson JE, Cook NR, et al. Moderate alcohol consumption and the risk of sudden cardiac death among US male physicians. *Circulation* 1999;100:944–950.

70. Criqui MH. Moderate drinking: benefits and risks. In: Zakhari S, Wassef M, eds. *Alcohol and the cardiovascular system*. Bethesda, MD: National Institutes of Health, 1996:4133.

71. Solomon CG, Hu FB, Stampfer MJ, et al. Moderate alcohol consumption and risk of coronary heart disease among women with type 2 diabetes mellitus. *Circulation* 2000; 102:494–499.

72. Fuchs CS, Stampfer MJ, Golditz GA, et al. Alcohol consumption and mortality among women. *N Engl J Med* 1995;332:1245–1255.

73. Boffetta P, Garfinkel L. Alcohol drinking and mortality among men enrolled in an American Cancer Society prospective study. *Epidemiology* 1990;1:342–348.

74. Zureik M, Ducimetiere P. High alcohol related premature mortality in France: concordant estimates from a prospective cohort study and national mortality statistics. *Alcohol Clin Exp Res* 1996;20(3):428–433.

75. Castelli WP. How many drinks a day? *JAMA* 1979; 242:2000.

76. Haskel WL, Camargo C, Williams PT, et al. The effect of cessation and resumption of moderate alcohol intake on serum high-density lipoprotein subfractions. *N Engl J Med* 1984;310:805–810.

77. Archer L, Gordi E. Alcohol and the elderly. *Clin Geriatr Med* 1992;8:127–141.

78. Wu CF, Sudhakar M, Jaferi G, et al. Preclinical cardiomyopathy in chronic alcoholics: a sex difference. *Am Heart J* 1976;91:281–286.

79. Kupari M, Koskinen P. Comparison of the cardiotoxicity of ethanol in women versus men. *Am J Cardiol* 1992;70:645–649.

80. Urbano-Marquez A, Estruch E, Fernandez-Sola J, et al. The greater risk of alcoholic cardiomyopathy and myopathy in women compared with men. *JAMA* 1995; 274:149–154.

81. Booyse FM, Parks DA. Moderate wine and alcohol consumption: beneficial effects on cardiovascular disease. *Thromb Haemost* 2001;86:517–528.

OTHER RISK FACTORS FOR CORONARY ARTERY DISEASE: HOMOCYSTEINE, LIPOPROTEIN(a), FIBRINOGEN, AND PLASMINOGEN ACTIVATOR INHIBITOR

KILLIAN ROBINSON
JOSEPH LOSCALZO

KEY CONCEPTS

1. Nontraditional risk factors are now recognized as important determinants of coronary heart disease.

2. Hyperhomocysteinemia confers an independent risk for coronary heart disease, probably by imparting oxidative stress-induced endothelial dysfunction and inducing atherothrombosis.

3. Many patients with elevated homocysteine concentrations in plasma are relatively deficient in folate or pyridoxine; the possible benefits of treating patients with vascular diseases using vitamins is now being evaluated in clinical trials.

4. Lipoprotein(a) [Lp(a)] confers an independent risk for coronary heart disease in selected populations and may do so by impairing fibrinolysis, promoting thrombosis, or stimulating vascular smooth muscle cell proliferation.

5. Fibrinogen and other prothrombotic risk factors, including plasminogen activator inhibitor-1 (PAI-1) excess and factor VII, confer independent risk for coronary heart disease.

K. Robinson: Department of Internal Medicine, Wake Forest University School of Medicine, Wake Forest University Baptist Medical Center, Winston-Salem, North Carolina

J. Loscalzo: Department of Medicine, Boston University School of Medicine, Boston University Medical Center, Boston, Massachusetts

6. Thrombosis is a major determinant of atherogenesis; thrombin stimulates smooth muscle cell proliferation, activates platelets, and promotes plaque growth. In addition, a prothrombotic state in the vasculature supports thrombus propagation at sites of vascular injury.

OVERVIEW

Traditional risk factors are commonplace in patients with coronary artery disease. Their absence in many patients with vascular disorders provides a stimulus to search for other abnormalities that may also confer an increased risk of atherosclerosis. Several such abnormalities have received more widespread attention recently as their possible roles in the genesis of atherosclerosis and thrombosis become more evident. A high plasma homocysteine concentration has been proposed as a risk factor in most case-control studies and some prospective studies. Elevated levels of this sulfur-containing amino acid may cause vascular damage, perhaps by increasing intracellular oxidative stress in endothelial cells. High concentrations may be readily reduced by folic acid, either alone or combined with vitamin B_6 or vitamin B_{12}. The effects of such treatment on prognosis are being evaluated by a number of secondary prevention studies in patients with vascular diseases. An elevated Lp(a) level is also a recognized risk factor for atherosclerosis. The mechanism of vascular damage is unclear but may be related to enhancement of the toxicity of low-density lipoprotein (LDL) cholesterol or, because of structural homology to plasminogen, interference with normal thrombolysis. Although high Lp(a) levels may be reduced by certain drugs and LDL apheresis, such measures are not always successful, and no prognostic benefit has been demonstrated. High fibrinogen and factor VII concentrations are also independently linked with coronary artery disease by mechanisms that remain obscure. Prospective studies are needed to clarify the precise role of the elevated concentrations of PAI in patients with atherosclerosis and thrombosis. Levels of fibrinogen may be lowered by exercise and modest alcohol intake, but a specific fibrinogen-lowering agent is not yet available. The effect of reducing the levels of these prothrombotic clotting factors on prognosis is unknown. This chapter outlines the relationship between these risk factors and coronary artery disease.

HOMOCYSTEINE

Homocysteine, a sulfhydryl-containing amino acid, was first discovered as a product of demethylation of methionine (1), which is essential as a methyl donor (2). Excessive quantities of homocysteine were noted to accumulate in the blood of patients with homocystinuria—a rare disease characterized by skeletal, neurologic, and vascular abnormalities

(3). From this initial observation, a link has been established between more moderate elevations of plasma homocysteine concentrations and atherosclerosis (4–19), even in patients without any apparent defined genetic trait for homocystinuria.

Nomenclature

The term *total homocysteine* refers to all species of this amino acid circulating in the blood (4,5,20) and may be abbreviated to *tHcy*. Approximately 80% of homocysteine is protein bound, principally to albumin. The sulfhydryl group of free, unbound homocysteine reacts readily with other sulfhydryl groups to form disulfides. Thus, homocysteine may combine with itself (forming homocystine) or with cysteine to form the mixed disulfide homocysteine-cysteine. Approximately 1% of all circulating homocysteine exists in the free, reduced state. The range of fasting homocysteine currently reported as normal is 5 to 15 µmol per L and includes all free, disulfide-linked and protein-bound species (4,5). Some evidence exists that this range may be too high, because concentrations as low as 12 µmol per L have been associated with atherosclerosis (4,5) and thrombosis in many of the studies of patients with vascular disease (4,5,11–16). A concentration above this range defines hyperhomocysteinemia; this is sometimes written as *hyperhomocyst(e)inemia* to emphasize the inclusion of all disulfide-linked bound and free species of the amino acid. ☜ c01

Homocysteine Metabolism

Following ingestion, methionine is converted to *S*-adenosylmethionine and then to *S*-adenosylhomocysteine, from which homocysteine is formed (Fig. 10.1). Methionine may be regenerated by the recycling of homocysteine via two remethylation pathways (2). One pathway uses vitamin B_{12}–dependent methionine synthase, using 5-methyltetrahydrofolate as a methyl donor; the presence of 5,10-methylenetetrahydrofolate reductase is also required. An additional pathway exists for methionine remethylation involving the enzyme betaine-methionine methyltransferase (2). This route is independent of folate and vitamin B_{12}, but it requires trimethylglycine (betaine) as a methyl donor. When methionine stores are adequate, homocysteine enters the transsulfuration pathway, where it is converted to cystathionine by vitamin B_6–dependent cystathionine β-synthase. Cystathionine, in turn, serves as a source for the generation of cysteine, which is required for the synthesis of many major biologic compounds, including glutathione—the most important and abundant intracellular thiol (Fig. 10.2). Ultimately, sulfur-containing amino acids are metabolized to water and sulphate and are excreted in the urine. Activity of cystathionine β-synthase is low or absent in classical homocystinuria. From a review of this metabolic pathway, it can be seen that plasma

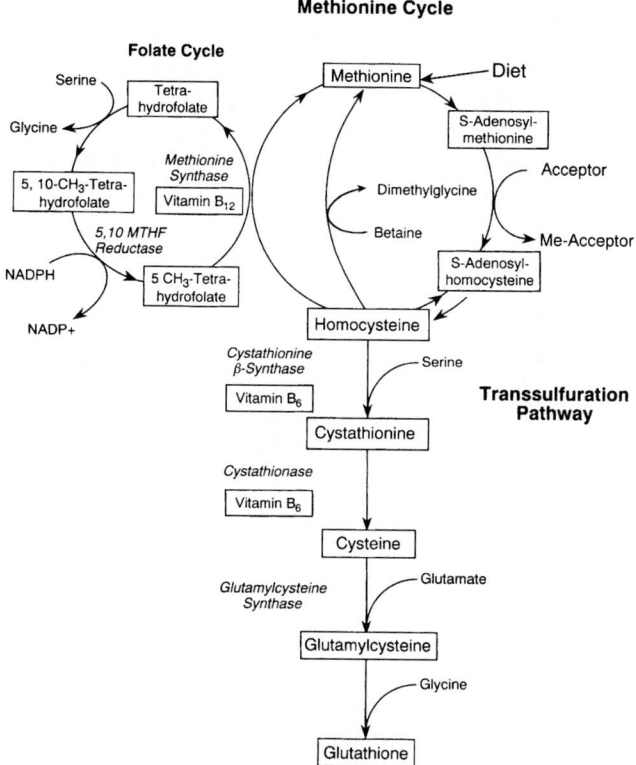

FIGURE 10.1 The metabolic pathway for the metabolism of methionine and homocysteine (see text for discussion). Me, methyl; MTHF, methylenetetrahydrofolate; NADP+, oxidized form of nicotinamide adenine dinucleotide phosphate; NADPH, reduced nicotinamide adenine dinucleotide phosphate.

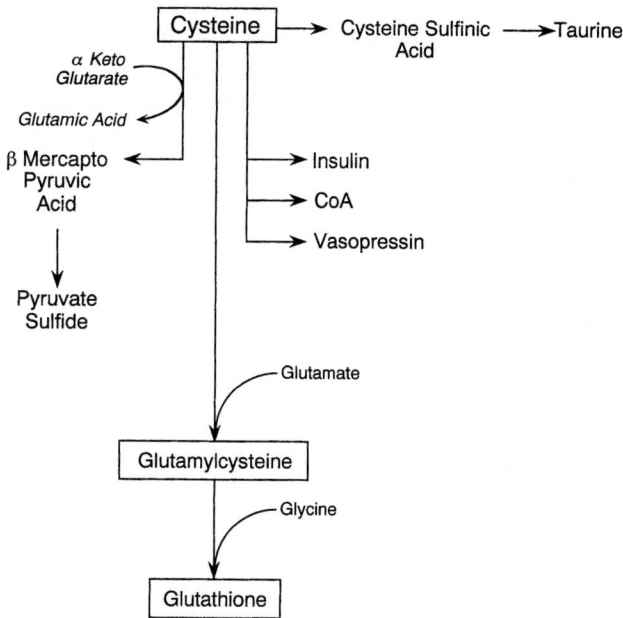

FIGURE 10.2 Pathways showing the fate of cysteine and its central role in the synthesis of essential metabolic compounds, including insulin, coenzyme A (CoA), and glutathione.

homocysteine concentrations may increase, owing to decreased activity of certain enzymes, reduced vitamin cofactor availability, or both.

Causes of Altered Homocysteine Concentrations

See Table 10.1 for the causes of hyperhomocysteinemia.

Genetic Factors

Classical homozygous homocystinuria is associated with low or absent activity of cystathionine β-synthase and leads to extremely high (>250 µmol per L) plasma concentrations of homocysteine (3). The heterozygous state is also associated with higher levels of the amino acid. Rare mutations in the remethylation enzyme methylenetetrahydrofolate reductase—which may be associated with excessively high homocysteine concentrations and early death—have also been reported (22). A more common abnormality yielding a temperature-sensitive enzyme (C677T mutation) is also associated with high homocysteine levels (23–25). Importantly, this abnormality leads to a requirement for high concentration of folate for optimal enzyme activity,

TABLE 10.1 CAUSES OF HYPERHOMOCYSTEINEMIA

Inherited causes
  Disorders of transsulfuration
    Cystathionine β-synthase deficiency
  Disorders of remethylation
    Defective vitamin B_{12} transport
    Defective vitamin B_{12} coenzyme synthesis
    Defective methionine synthase
    5,10-methylenetetrahydrofolate reductase deficiency or
    defects
Acquired causes
  Diseases
    Chronic renal failure
    Hypothyroidism
    Chronic inflammatory bowel disease
    Some malignant disorders
    Systemic lupus erythematosus
    Psoriasis
  Vitamin deficiencies
    Vitamin B_{12}
    Folate
    Vitamin B_6
  Drugs
    Cholestyramine, colestipol, and metformin (affect folate
      and cobalamin absorption)
    Methotrexate (inhibits dihydrofolate reductase)
    L-Dopa (increases transmethylation)
    Niacin and theophylline (induce vitamin B_6 deficiency)
    Androgens
    Cyclosporine (reduces renal function)
    Fibric acid derivatives (possibly alter renal function)
    Phenytoin and carbamazepine (antagonize folate)
    Nitrous oxide (inactivates of methionine synthase)

and folate supplementation can correct the hyperhomocysteinemia observed in these individuals (26). Uncommon inherited abnormalities of cobalamin metabolism may produce similar clinical disorders (4,5). A genetic influence on plasma concentration has been observed in healthy subjects (27) and in patients with vascular disease (28).

Age

Plasma homocysteine levels rise with age in both men and women (4,5). This age-dependent increase may be secondary to decreases in vitamin cofactor levels or coexisting renal impairment; both are common in this age group. An age-related reduction in the activity of cystathionine β-synthase has also been reported (29).

Gender

Homocysteine concentrations are higher in men than women (4,5), which may be due to differences in muscle mass, renal function, essential vitamin cofactors, or even protein intake. Homocysteine levels are also higher in postmenopausal women than premenopausal women. Sex steroids play an important role in modulating homocysteine concentrations, as illustrated by one study of transsexual males and females in which homocysteine concentrations rose in the subjects treated with androgens but fell in the subjects treated with estrogens (30).

Lifestyle

Lifestyle is also an important determinant of plasma total homocysteine concentrations. In the Hordaland Homocysteine Study, gender, age, folate intake, smoking status, and coffee consumption were the strongest determinants of homocysteine concentration in apparently healthy subjects. A lifestyle of low folate intake, smoking, and higher coffee consumption was associated with a higher homocysteine concentration. Conversely, a high folate intake, nonsmoking status, and low coffee consumption were associated with a median homocysteine concentration that was 3.0 to 4.8 μmol per L lower (31).

Vitamin Deficiencies

Folate and vitamin B_{12} are required for remethylation of homocysteine to methionine. Concentrations of homocysteine rise with decreasing levels of these vitamins (4,5). Frank deficiency can give rise to a markedly increased homocysteine concentration (32). Levels also rise with a decreasing concentration of vitamin B_6 (4,5).

Drugs

Total plasma homocysteine concentrations may also be increased by drugs that affect the metabolism of folate or vitamin B_{12}, including methotrexate, phenytoin, carbamazepine, and nitrous oxide (4,5). Several preparations commonly used in patients with vascular disease—including the cholesterol-lowering agents cholestyramine and colestipol, niacin, and fibric acid derivatives—have also been shown to be associated with an increased homocysteine concentration (4,5). Metformin, theophylline, and L-dopa may have similar effects. A lower homocysteine concentration may be seen in patients taking hormone replacement therapy or penicillamine (4,5).

Renal Dysfunction and Other Disease States

Total plasma homocysteine concentration rises with declining renal function (4,5,33–35). c02

Homocysteine and Vascular Disease

Homocystinuria

Homocystinuria has been the paradigm of homocysteine-related atherosclerosis since the early work of Mudd and coworkers (20). The classical disorder—characterized by complete, or almost complete, absence of cystathionine β-synthase—is rare and occurs in the United States once in every 400,000 births (20). The condition is transmitted in autosomal recessive fashion. Reduced enzyme activity is observed in heterozygotes for the disorder and may be demonstrated by administering a methionine challenge. A markedly elevated plasma homocysteine concentration is typical and is accompanied by an increase in urinary homocystine. The clinical manifestations include skeletal abnormalities, ocular lens dislocation, and mental retardation. The other major complications of early atherosclerosis and a tendency to thromboembolic events soon became evident after the disorder was first described in a survey of mentally retarded children from Ireland (40). The plasma homocysteine concentration can be reduced by dietary methionine restriction or by the administration of vitamin B_6, which may protect against vascular complications (20).

Major Clinical Studies of Homocysteine and Vascular Disease

In 1976, Wilcken and colleagues undertook the first studies of patients younger than 50 years with angiographically proven coronary disease (6) and found higher homocysteine concentrations in patients than in controls. In a later study, the same investigators were unable to confirm these results (68). However, many other studies have since been performed (7–19) that have reached conclusions similar to the initial investigation. In the study by Malinow and coworkers (8), after controlling for conventional risk factors, the odds ratio for vascular disease in patients with hyperhomocysteinemia was 3.3, which was higher than the ratio associated

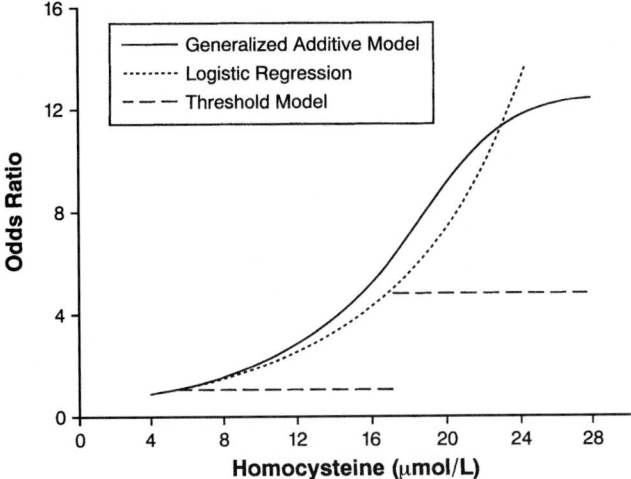

FIGURE 10.3 The relationship of rising plasma homocysteine concentrations to the risk of coronary heart disease. A higher risk is noted with higher concentrations. When homocysteine values are analyzed across the range of plasma concentrations, no threshold effect is evident. (From Robinson K, Mayer EL, Miller D, et al. Hyperhomocysteinemia and low pyridoxal phosphate: common and independent reversible risk factors for coronary artery disease. *Circulation* 1995;92:2825–2830, with permission.)

with smoking or hypercholesterolemia. In addition, the increased risk does not have a threshold and is present over much of the range of plasma homocysteine concentrations (Fig. 10.3). A European multicenter case-control study using an internationally accepted methodology and definitions of vascular disease has confirmed other case-control studies (14). Although some prospective studies have confirmed these findings (18,19), a number of major investigations have not (69,70), raising the question of whether an elevated homocysteine level may be causally related to the development of vascular disease or may simply be an epiphenomenon. There are a number of useful recent reviews of studies in this area to which we refer the interested reader (4,5).

Effect of Homocysteine on Prognosis in Patients with Atherosclerosis

An elevated homocysteine concentration is associated with an adverse prognosis in patients with established coronary artery disease. In patients with angiographically confirmed coronary artery disease, Nygard and colleagues found a graded relation between plasma homocysteine levels and overall mortality. After 4 years, 3.8% of patients with homocysteine levels below 9 μmol per L had died, as compared with 24.7% of patients with homocysteine levels of 15 μmol per L or higher (75). Stubbs and coworkers evaluated the relationship between plasma homocysteine and short-term (28 days) and long-term (median 2.5 years) prognosis in patients with acute coronary syndromes. Although the event rate within the first 28 days was unre-

lated to the homocysteine concentration, an apparent threshold effect was noted on long-term follow-up, with a 2.6-fold increase in the risk of cardiac events for patients in the upper two quintiles compared with the lowest three quintiles (76).

Renal Failure

High homocysteine concentrations occur frequently in patients with renal failure (89). Case-control studies have shown that higher levels of homocysteine are associated with an increased risk of atherosclerosis independent of traditional risk factors in dialyzed patients with end-stage renal disease (35). In addition, high homocysteine levels are closely related to B-vitamin metabolism in these patients. Prospective studies have also demonstrated a relationship between vascular complications of end-stage renal disease and elevated homocysteine concentrations (89,90). Recently, Suliman and colleagues (91) have shown that elevated homocysteine concentrations are a predictor of adverse outcomes in patients with end-stage renal disease and that nutritional status may also be an important determining factor of homocysteine concentrations.

Cardiac Transplantation

After cardiac transplantation, homocysteine concentrations rise (92–94) and are associated with abnormalities of B vitamins and renal function, suggesting a multifactorial etiology. Follow-up of these patients, however, has shown that low vitamin B_6—but not high homocysteine concentrations—predicted cardiovascular morbidity and mortality in this patient group (95).

Therapeutic Implications

Metabolism of homocysteine requires vitamin B_6, vitamin B_{12}, folate, and betaine. Vitamin B_6 and folate reduce homocysteine concentrations in homocystinuria, and vitamin B_6 may reduce the incidence of vascular complications in patients with atherosclerosis (20). The treatment of homocystinuria is reviewed extensively elsewhere (96).

In healthy subjects and in patients with atherosclerotic vascular disease, homocysteine concentrations may be reduced by folic acid alone or in combination with vitamins B_6 or B_{12} (4,5,97,98). The effect is greatest with folic acid, which, in doses of only 0.5 mg per day, may reduce homocysteine concentrations by approximately 30% (98). Vitamin B_{12} may produce a more modest 10% reduction. Vitamin B_6 is most effective in reducing homocysteine concentrations after a methionine challenge. Other agents that may reduce homocysteine include betaine, choline (13), estrogen (99), and *N*-acetylcysteine (100). The use of penicillamine has also been associated with a reduction in homocysteine concentrations. A number of clinical trials are ongoing in patients with coronary artery disease and stroke using folic acid, vitamin B_6, and vitamin B_{12}. In addition, other studies are in progress using high-dose folic acid in patients with end-stage renal disease. These studies may help provide more definitive answers concerning the contribution of homocysteine to the development of atherosclerosis and whether the routine use of B-vitamin supplements is justified in these patients.

At the current time, measurement of homocysteine concentrations and use of these vitamins in patients with vascular disease remains speculative, although the American Heart Association has suggested that the measurement of homocysteine concentrations in high-risk individuals—such as those with a positive family history or the development of early atherosclerosis—may be reasonable. Until the ongoing treatment trials have been concluded, the benefit of routine use of vitamin supplements in these patients remains unproven (101).

LIPOPROTEIN(a)

Genetics

The gene for the apoprotein(a) is located on the long arm of chromosome 6 and is closely linked to the gene for plasminogen (106,107). There is a high degree of homology between these two genes. Utermann and colleagues (103) reported six size isoforms of Lp(a) that were inherited, but more than 30 isoforms have now been reported (106,108).

Effects of Age, Gender, and Race on Lipoprotein(a) Levels

Plasma levels of Lp(a) do not bear any clear relationship to age or gender, although levels are higher after menopause (109). Concentrations also increase with the levels of LDL cholesterol (109). A weak correlation with age in men and women was reported by the Northern Sweden World Health Organization (WHO) MONICA project investigators (110). Lp(a) levels vary substantially among ethnic groups and are higher in American and African blacks than in whites; levels are normally distributed rather than skewed in blacks. Despite the higher levels, the risk of coronary artery disease may not be increased in blacks compared with whites (110). In Asian populations, Lp(a) has also been associated with an increased incidence of coronary artery disease (111). Recent studies have shown that dietary fat content may increase Lp(a) concentrations, perhaps by modulating apoprotein(a) mRNA levels (106). Levels are higher in patients with nephrotic syndrome and chronic renal failure and may be three times higher than normal controls in patients undergoing dialysis (112). Higher levels have also been noted in patients with diabetes mellitus and immediately after MI (113,114). Lp(a) concentrations are higher in patients who have undergone renal transplantation treated with cyclosporin than in patients taking azathioprine or prednisone (115).

Mechanism of Thrombosis and Atherosclerosis

The mechanism of thrombosis and atherosclerosis is unknown (*e*Table 10.1.2), but the structural similarity of apoprotein(a) to plasminogen suggests that high levels of Lp(a) may inhibit endogenous fibrinolytic activity (129). Unlike plasminogen, apoprotein(a) cannot be converted to a plasmin-like molecule. Indeed, it inhibits plasminogen activation by streptokinase and competitively inhibits plasminogen activation by t-PA. In addition, owing to its kringle-like domains, apoprotein(a) binds and displaces plasminogen from sites on fibrin and fibrinogen (130). Lp(a) may increase the endothelial release of PAI and downregulate plasmin generation (131). In one study, the rate of plasmin generation was most effectively inhibited by low-molecular-weight isoforms of Lp(a). However, it is important to point out that there is extraordinary polymorphism in apoprotein(a) with respect to kringle number and sequence heterogeneity within kringles—both of which can affect fibrin(ogen) binding properties (132). Alternatively, Lp(a) may affect the delivery of LDL cholesterol to the vessel wall, favoring atherogenesis by binding to plaque elements and enhancing cholesterol deposition (133). Recently, additional potential proatherothrombotic actions have been identified, including induction of monocyte chemotaxis by endothelial cells (134) and, possibly, control of angiogenesis (135).

Treatment

Niacin and neomycin (136) may lower Lp(a) levels, as may stanozolol (137) and *N*-acetylcysteine (138). In one study, the angiotensin-converting enzyme inhibitor fosinopril lowered Lp(a) levels in patients with mild to moderate renal impairment, including blacks and diabetics (139). In a study of 31 postmenopausal women given conjugated equine estrogen for 3 months, Lp(a) concentrations fell by approximately 15% (140). In men with prostatic cancer, large doses of estrogen reduced Lp(a) concentrations by approximately 50% (141); androgens and androgenic progestins have similar effects (141,142). The effects of estrogen may be mediated by accelerated LDL-receptor–mediated clearance (140), as may the effects of the fibric acid derivative bezafibrate (143). Despite the potential for lowering Lp(a) levels, there are no data showing the clinical benefit of this treatment approach (144). In patients with a borderline LDL cholesterol level, an elevated Lp(a) level may provide a rationale for more aggressive LDL-lowering therapy (144). In one study (145), higher levels of Lp(a) did not confer greater cardiovascular risk if LDL had been lowered (Fig. 10.4).

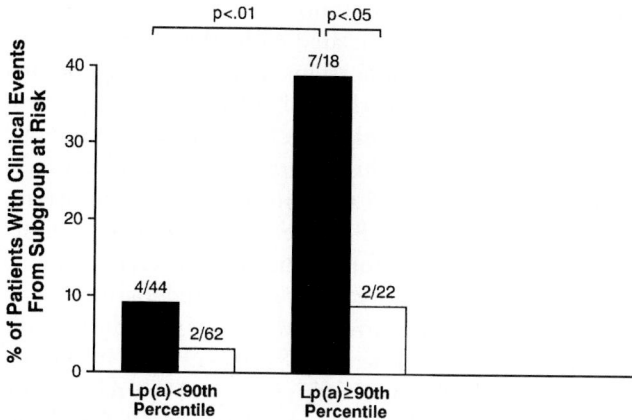

FIGURE 10.4 Relationship of in-treatment lipoprotein(a) [Lp(a)] level and low-density lipoprotein cholesterol (LDL-C) response to occurrence of clinical events. Dark bars indicate LDL-C reductions of ≤10% (i.e., minimal); light bars indicate LDL-C reductions of >10% (i.e., substantial). The number of clinical events divided by the number of patients at risk in subgroup is listed above each bar. It is assumed that patients dropping out of the study (n = 26) had LDL-C reductions ≤10%. [From Maher V, Brown BG, Marcovina SM, et al. Effects of lowering LDL cholesterol on the cardiovascular risk of lipoprotein(a). *JAMA* 1995;274;1771–1774, with permission.]

COAGULATION AND FIBRINOLYTIC ABNORMALITIES

Fibrinogen

As long ago as 1954, levels of fibrinogen were noted to be high in patients with acute MI (146). A large body of evidence has now accumulated that links fibrinogen independently to cardiovascular disease.

Structure

Fibrinogen is a glycoprotein synthesized in the liver and has a molecular mass of 340,000 d. The circulating concentration ranges from 200 to 400 mg per dL. Levels are higher in women than in men and increase with age, after menopause, and with increasing body fat. Elevated fibrinogen concentrations occur as a consequence of increased hepatic production or reduced clearance from the circulation. The fibrinogen molecule consists of three pairs of polypeptide chains (α, β, and γ) linked by disulfide bonds (147).

Genetics

The three polypeptide chains are encoded by three separate genes on chromosome 4 band 4q32 (148). Genotype may be associated with significant differences in fibrinogen levels (149).

Function

Formation of a fibrin clot and support of platelet-platelet associations are the principal functions of fibrinogen. The proteolytic fragments of fibrinogen have several other functions, including stimulating hematopoiesis, promoting smooth muscle proliferation, and having a possible role in containing bacterial infection.

Mechanism of Thrombosis and Atherosclerosis

The mechanism of thrombosis and atherosclerosis is unknown and reflects the complex interactions among plaque development, lipid abnormalities, and derangements of endothelium and the coagulation system (167) (*e*Table 10.1.4). Fibrinogen is the major determinant of plasma viscosity and binds to platelet glycoprotein IIb/IIIa receptors, which is a necessary prerequisite for platelet aggregation (168). In patients with type II hyperlipoproteinemia and familial hypercholesterolemia, fibrinogen binding to platelets is increased (169). In addition, fibrinogen is incorporated into arteriosclerotic plaques and stimulates smooth muscle cell proliferation and growth (151,170,171).

Treatment

Several drugs lower plasma fibrinogen concentrations, including some beta-adrenergic blocking agents, platelet inhibitors (172), and fibric acid derivatives (especially bezafibrate) (167), but lifestyle interventions such as increased exercise and modest alcohol intake may be the most satisfactory initial treatment choice (172). A specific fibrinogen-lowering agent is not yet available.

Plasminogen Activator Inhibitor-1

Plasminogen activator inhibitors (PAIs) are specific inhibitors of t-PA and urokinase-type plasminogen activator. There are several PAIs: PAI-1, PAI-2, and PAI-3; the most extensively investigated in relation to atherosclerosis is PAI-1.

Structure

PAI-1 is a glycoprotein that belongs to the α_1-protease inhibitor class of serine protease inhibitors (i.e., serpins) (173). The gene for PAI-1 is located on chromosome 7 (174). PAI-1 has a molecular mass of 52 kd and consists of 379 amino acids. It is found in plasma, platelets, and extracellular fluid. The relatively high circulating levels of PAI-1 activity in pregnancy may be explained by the high concentrations in the placenta (173).

Synthesis

Synthesis and secretion of PAI-1 can be modulated by various substances that may exert their effects at the level of gene transcription (173,175). Some substances, such as insulin, may have a posttranscriptional effect by modification of mRNA stability (176). When synthesized in endothelium, PAI-1 is rapidly secreted, although it may also be stored in the alpha-granules of platelets and is released on activation (173).

Function

Under normal circumstances, fibrinolysis is tightly regulated by the balance between activation of plasminogen and inhibition of plasmin—the active serine protease derived from plasminogen. Inhibition of fibrinolysis may occur through inhibition of plasminogen activation. Plasma PAI-1 circulates bound to vitronectin (176); its plasma levels exhibit a circadian variation reaching a peak in the morning and a trough in the evening. Importantly, this variation is opposite that for t-PA (173).

Age

Levels of PAI-1 increase with age (177,178) but are not related to smoking or cholesterol levels (179). Levels rise with increasing systolic blood pressure and are higher in patients with higher triglyceride and insulin concentrations and with higher body-mass indices (180). There is a correlation of PAI-1 with insulin resistance and with the components of this syndrome (181). Endothelial synthesis of PAI-1 may also be enhanced by Lp(a) (131), although plasma levels of these substances do not correlate with one another (182). The clinical value of measurement of PAI concentrations may be enhanced by drawing blood samples before and after venous occlusion for 10 minutes, using a blood pressure cuff inflated to 100 mm Hg (137). This maneuver should produce an increase in fibrinolysis expressed as increased plasminogen activator level and a fall in the concentrations of PAI-1. The test requires further evaluation, as it conceivably could be a better marker for vascular disease than the fasting value alone; the test has already been applied in therapeutic studies in which the fibrinolytic properties of drugs are being evaluated (137).

Epidemiologic Links with Coronary Artery Disease

Increased levels of PAI-1 have been reported in several thrombotic disorders, including venous thrombosis, coronary artery disease, and especially MI (*e*Fig. 10.4.2), although the mechanism remains unclear (*e*Table 10.1.5). ▾❦ c03

INFLAMMATORY MARKERS

Inflammatory responses within coronary atheromata are important determinants of plaque activation and subsequent acute atherothrombotic events (203). Systemic inflammation is also associated with atherogenesis and its acute thrombotic complications. Recent data suggest that circulating systemic markers of inflammation can identify subjects at high risk for clinical atherothrombotic events (204,205). In this regard, the acute phase reactants serum amyloid A protein and, more important, C-reactive protein (CRP) have been identified as independent risk factors for cardiovascular events among both apparently healthy individuals and patients with unstable angina pectoris (206,207). In addition, the increase in CRP after acute MI (208–210) or in the setting of unstable angina pectoris (211,212) correlates with adverse outcome. The association between CRP and cardiovascular disease is believed to be indirect, because circulating CRP reflects the extent of acute phase response to nonspecific stimuli that induce acute inflammation, including ischemia, plaque rupture, vascular injury, and necrosis. Nevertheless, CRP has been demonstrated to be an independent risk factor for atherothrombotic events (207) and may, therefore, be a direct mechanistic determinant of outcome by as yet poorly defined molecular processes. Importantly, aspirin suppresses CRP levels, and this effect may account, in part, for the benefits of aspirin in prevention (207).

CONTROVERSIES AND PERSONAL PERSPECTIVES

Research into the relationship between homocysteine and vascular disorders has uncovered important links between folic acid and atherosclerosis. Although folate is important, it is not the sole determinant of plasma homocysteine levels. It is essential to realize that high homocysteine concentrations may reflect reduced activities of a number of enzyme systems and several B vitamins. By extension, the relationship between vitamin B_6 and atherosclerosis—although proposed almost 50 years ago by Rinehart and Greenberg (78) and since developed by others (79,80,216)—is largely unknown by clinicians and requires greater recognition. Controversy also surrounds the relationship of mutations in methylenetetrahydrofolate reductase and cystathionine β-synthase to hyperhomocysteinemia and vascular disease. Treatment of high homocysteine levels by the routine use of multivitamins in patients with atherosclerosis remains entirely speculative, although trials are now ongoing. Indeed, even the routine measurement of homocysteine, Lp(a), or the concentrations of fibrinogen, factor VII, or PAI-1 in patients with atherosclerosis cannot be recommended until controlled intervention studies have demonstrated a clinical benefit of therapy.

THE FUTURE

Whereas the elevated concentrations of homocysteine, Lp(a), and prothrombotic clotting factors may confer increased risk of atherosclerosis and thrombosis, much additional investigation is required before their role in these disorders can be fully understood. For example, the underlying abnormalities that lead to high homocysteine levels in patients with vascular disease are complex and involve nutritional and genetic factors (25,26,203–211). The cellular mechanism, if any, leading to vascular damage in patients with high homocysteine levels is also unclear. Interactions with traditional risk factors (e.g., smoking, hypercholesterolemia, and hypertension) may predispose to a greater likelihood of vascular disease (14,72), but attention should also focus on interactions with nontraditional risk factors. The increased risk of thrombosis in patients with homocystinuria possessing the R506Q (Leiden) mutation of factor V (212) highlights the possibility of multiple coexisting genetic abnormalities predisposing to atherosclerosis and emphasizes the evolving concept of disease-modifying genes as an explanation for the diverse manifestation of complex phenotypes. Perhaps the most important issue is whether reduction is associated with an improved prognosis in primary or secondary prevention studies, and these issues should now be tested by clinically appropriate trials.

The role of Lp(a) in atherosclerosis and thrombosis remains unclear, but complex interactions with nontraditional risk factors are evident. There is increased binding of Lp(a) to fibrin by homocysteine (73). In addition, Lp(a) regulates PAI-1 expression in endothelial cells (131) and accumulates with fibrinogen in atherosclerotic plaque (127). It is also possible that Lp(a) may be more atherogenic in the presence of specific cholesterol subfractions and that certain Lp(a) phenotypes may be more atherogenic than others. Different populations may be at varying risk; this also requires further study. Reduction of high Lp(a) levels is possible, but, at present, this may not confer any benefit if LDL is maximally reduced. Future development of more specific and effective treatment may alter this perspective.

High circulating levels of fibrinogen and PAI are frequently seen in patients with atherothrombotic disorders, but their origin is obscure. Genetic determinants and their relationship to environmental factors require further study. Newer genetic polymorphisms in platelet glycoproteins (213,214) and procoagulants (215) and other prothrombotic determinants are likely to gain importance as we unravel the complexities of gene-gene interactions in atherothrombotic risk. Therapeutic studies are also needed but are made more complex, as in the case of fibrinogen, by the lack of a specific agent that selectively reduces levels of this clotting factor. As with other heritable abnormalities, the atherosclerotic and thrombotic tendency associated with specific phenotypic abnormalities—alone or combined with other risk factors—requires further evaluation. Additional prospective study is required to define the specific role of high levels PAI in atherosclerosis and thrombosis.

REFERENCES

1. du Vigneaud V, Ressler C, Rachele JR. The biological synthesis of "labile methyl groups." *Science* 1959;112:267–271.
2. Finkelstein JD. Methionine metabolism in mammals. *J Nutr Biochem* 1990;1:228–237.
3. Mudd SH, Levy HL, Skovby F. Disorders of transsulfuration. In: Scriver CR, Beaudet AL, Sly WS, et al., eds. *The metabolic basis of inherited disease*, 7th ed. New York: McGraw-Hill, 1995:1279–1327.
4. Refsum H, Ueland PM, Nygard O, et al. Homocysteine and cardiovascular disease. *Annu Rev Med* 1998;49:31–62.
5. Seshadri N, Robinson K. Homocysteine, B vitamins, and coronary artery disease. *Med Clin North Am* 2000;84:215–237.
6. Wilcken DEL, Wilcken B. The pathogenesis of coronary artery disease. A possible role for methionine metabolism. *J Clin Invest* 1976;57:1079–1082.
7. Boers GH, Smals AG, Trijbels FJ, et al. Heterozygosity for homocystinuria in premature peripheral and cerebral occlusive arterial disease. *N Engl J Med* 1985;313:709–715.
8. Malinow MR, Kang SS, Taylor LM, et al. Prevalence of hyperhomocyst(e)inemia in patients with peripheral arterial occlusive disease. *Circulation* 1989;79:1180–1188.
9. Clarke R, Daly L, Robinson K, et al. Hyperhomocysteinemia: an independent risk factor for vascular disease. *N Engl J Med* 1991;324:1149–1155.
10. Brattström L, Israelsson B, Norrving B, et al. Impaired homocysteine metabolism in early-onset cerebral and peripheral occlusive arterial disease. Effects of pyridoxine and folic acid treatment. *Atherosclerosis* 1990;81:51–60.
11. Wu LL, Wu J, Hunt SC, et al. Plasma homocyst(e)ine as a risk factor for early familial coronary artery disease. *Clin Chem* 1994;40:552–561.
12. Pancharuniti N, Lewis CA, Sauberlich HE, et al. Plasma homocyst(e)ine, folate, and vitamin B-12 concentrations and risk for early-onset coronary artery disease. *Am J Clin Nutr* 1994;59:940–948.
13. Dudman NP, Wilcken DE, Wang J, et al. Disordered methionine/homocysteine metabolism in premature vascular disease. Its occurrence, cofactor therapy, and enzymology. *Arterioscler Thromb* 1993;13:1253–1260.

14. Graham IM, Daly LE, Refsum HM, et al. Plasma homocysteine as a risk factor for vascular disease: the European Concerted Action Project. *JAMA* 1997;277:1775–1781.
15. Selhub J, Jacques PF, Bostom AG, et al. Association between plasma homocysteine concentrations and extracranial carotid artery stenosis. *N Engl J Med* 1995;332:286–291.
16. Robinson K, Mayer EL, Miller D, et al. Hyperhomocysteinemia and low pyridoxal phosphate: common and independent reversible risk factors for coronary artery disease. *Circulation* 1995;92:2825–2830.
17. Stampfer MJ, Malinow MR, Willett WC, et al. A prospective study of plasma homocyst(e)ine and risk of myocardial infarction in US physicians. *JAMA* 1992;268:877–881.
18. Arnesen E, Refsum H, Bonaa KH, et al. Serum total homocysteine and coronary heart disease. *Int J Epidemiol* 1995;24:704–709.
19. Perry IJ, Refsum H, Morris RW, et al. Prospective study of serum total homocysteine concentration and risk of stroke in middle-aged British men. *Lancet* 1995;346:1395–1398.
20. Mudd SH, Levy HL. Plasma homocyst(e)ine or homocysteine? *N Engl J Med* 1995;333:325.
21. Malinow MR, Axthelm MK, Meredith MJ, et al. Synthesis and transsulfuration of homocysteine in blood. *J Lab Clin Med* 1994;123:421–429.
22. Rosenblatt DS. Inherited disorders of folate transport and metabolism. In: Scriver CR, Beaudet AL, Sly WS, et al., eds. *The metabolic basis of inherited disease*, 7th ed. New York: McGraw-Hill, 1995.
23. Kang S-S, Wong PWK, Susmano A, et al. Thermolabile methylenetetrahydrofolate reductase: an inherited risk factor for coronary artery disease. *Am J Hum Genet* 1991;48:536–545.
24. Frosst P, Blom HJ, Milos R, et al. A candidate genetic risk factor for vascular disease: a common mutation in methylenetetrahydrofolate reductase. *Nat Genet* 1995;10:111–113.
25. Kluijtmans LA, van den Heuvel LP, Boers GH, et al. Molecular genetic analysis in mild hyperhomocysteinemia: a common mutation in the methylenetetrahydrofolate reductase gene is a genetic risk factor for cardiovascular disease. *Am J Hum Genet* 1996;58:35–41.
26. Jacques PF, Bostom AG, Williams RR, et al. Relation between folate status, a common mutation in methylenetetrahydrofolate reductase and plasma homocysteine concentrations. *Circulation* 1996;93:7–9.
27. Reed T, Malinow MR, Christian JC, et al. Estimates of heritability of plasma homocyst(e)ine levels in aging adult male twins. *Clin Genet* 1991;39:425–428.
28. Genest JJ, McNamara JR, Upson B, et al. Prevalence of familial hyperhomocyst(e)inemia in men with premature coronary artery disease. *Arterioscler Thromb* 1991;11:1129–1136.
29. Nordström M, Kjellström T. Age dependency of cystathione beta-synthase activity in human fibroblasts in homocyst(e)inemia and atherosclerotic vascular disease. *Atherosclerosis* 1992;94:213–221.
30. Giltay EJ, Hoogeveen EK, Elbers JM, et al. Effects of sex steroids on plasma total homocysteine levels: a study in transsexual males and females. *J Clin Endocrinol Metab* 1998;83:550–553.
31. Nygard O, Refsum H, Ueland PM, et al. Major lifestyle determinants of plasma total homocysteine distribution: the Hordaland Homocysteine Study. *Am J Clin Nutr* 1998;67:263–270.
32. Brattström L, Israelsson B, Lindgärde F, et al. Higher total plasma homocysteine in vitamin B12 deficiency than in heterozygosity for homocystinuria due to cystathionine β-synthase deficiency. *Metabolism* 1988;37:175–178.
33. Wilcken DEL, Gupta VJ. Sulfur containing amino acids in chronic renal failure with particular reference to homocystine and cysteine-homocysteine mixed disulfide. *Eur J Clin Invest* 1979;9:301–307.
34. Chauveau P, Chadefaux B, Coude M, et al. Hyperhomocysteinemia, a risk factor for atherosclerosis in chronic uremic patients. *Kidney Int* 1993;41[Suppl 41]:S72–S77.
35. van Guldener C, Robinson K. Homocysteine and renal disease. *Semin Thromb Hemost* 2000;26:313–324.
36. van Guldener C, Donker AJ, Jakobs C, et al. No net renal extraction of homocysteine in fasting humans. *Kidney Int* 1998;54:166–169.
37. Refsum H, Helland S, Ueland PM. Radioenzymic determination of homocysteine in plasma and urine. *Clin Chem* 1985;31:624–628.
38. Guttormsen AB, Ueland PM, Svarstad E, et al. Kinetic basis of hyperhomocysteinemia in patients with chronic renal failure. *Kidney Int* 1997;52:495–502.
39. Bostom AG, Gohh RY, Tsai MY, et al. Excess prevalence of fasting and postmethiomime-loading hyperhomocysteinemia in stable renal transplant recipients. *Arterioscler Thromb Biol* 1997:17:1894–1900.
40. Carson NAJ, Neill DW. Metabolic abnormalities detected in a summary of mentally backward individuals in Northern Ireland. *Arch Dis Children* 1962;37:505–513.
41. McCully KS. Vascular pathology of homocysteinemia: implications for the pathogenesis of arteriosclerosis. *Am J Pathol* 1969;56:111–128.
42. deGroot PG, Willems C, Boers GHJ, et al. Endothelial cell dysfunction in homocystinuria. *Eur J Clin Invest* 1983;13:405–410.
43. Landefeld CS, Rosenblatt MW, Goldman L. Bleeding in patients treated with warfarin: relation to the prothrombin time and important remedial lesions. *Am J Med* 1989;87:153–159.
44. Jacobsen DW, Savon SR, Stewart RW, et al. Limited capacity for homocysteine catabolism in vascular cells and tissues: a pathophysiologic mechanism for arterial damage in hyperhomocysteinemia? *Circulation* 1995;92(Suppl I):104.
45. Mudd SH, Matorin AI, Levy HL. Homocysteine thiolactone: failure to detect in human serum or plasma. *Res Commun Chem Pathol Pharmacol* 1989;63:297–300.
46. Harker LA, Slichter SJ, Scott CR, et al. Homocystinemia. Vascular injury and arterial thrombosis. *N Engl J Med* 1974;291:537–543.
47. Harker LA, Ross R, Slichter SJ, et al. Homocystine-induced arteriosclerosis. The role of endothelial cell injury and platelet response in its genesis. *J Clin Invest* 1976;58:731–741.
48. Loscalzo J. The oxidant stress of hyperhomocyst(e)inemia. *J Clin Invest* 1996;98:5–7.
49. Eberhardt RT, Forgione MA, Cap A, et al. Endothelial dys-

function in a murine model of mild hyperhomocsyt(e)inemia. *J Clin Invest* 2000;106:483–491.

50. Welch GN, Upchurch GR Jr, Keaney KF Jr, et al. Homocyst(e)ine decreases cell redox potential in vascular smooth muscle cells (abstract). *J Am Coll Cardiol* 1996;27:164A.

51. Stamler JS, Osborne JA, Jaraki O, et al. Adverse vascular effects of homocysteine are modulated by endothelium-derived relaxing factor and related oxides of nitrogen. *J Clin Invest* 1993;91:308–318.

52. Upchurch GR Jr, Welch GN, Fabian AJ, et al. Homocyst(e)ine decreases bioavailable nitric oxide by a mechanism involving glutathione peroxidase. *J Biol Chem* 1997;272:17012–17017.

53. Lentz SR, Sobey CG, Piegors DJ, et al. Vascular dysfunction in monkeys with diet-induced hyperhomocyst(e)inemia. *J Clin Invest* 1996;98:24–29.

54. Woo KS, Chook P, Lolin Y, et al. Hyperhomocyst(e)inemia is a risk factor for arterial endothelial dysfunction in humans. *Circulation* 1997;96:2542–2544.

55. Wang J, Dudman NP, Wilcken DE. Effects of homocysteine and related compounds on prostacyclin production by cultured human vascular endothelial cells. *Thromb Haemost* 1993;70:1047–1052.

56. Panganamala RV, Karpen CW, Merola AJ. Peroxide mediated effects of homocysteine on arterial prostacyclin synthesis. *Prostaglandins Leukot Med* 1986;22:349–356.

57. Rodgers GM, Conn MT. Homocysteine, an atherogenic stimulus, reduces protein C activation by arterial and venous endothelial cells. *Blood* 1990;75:895–901.

58. Rodgers GM, Kane WH. Activation of endogenous factor V by a homocysteine-induced vascular endothelial cell activator. *J Clin Invest* 1986;77:1909–1916.

59. Fryer RH, Wilson BD, Gubler DB, et al. Homocyst(e)ine, a risk factor for premature vascular disease and thrombosis, induces tissue factor activity in endothelial cells. *Arterioscler Thromb* 1993;13:1327–1333.

60. Undas A, Williams EB, Butenas S, et al. Homocysteine inhibits inactivation of factor Va by activated protein C. *J Biol Chem* 2000 Nov 16 [epub ahead of print].

61. Hayashi T, Honda G, Suzuki K. An atherogenic stimulus homocysteine inhibits cofactor activity of thrombomodulin and enhances thrombomodulin expression in human umbilical vein endothelial cells. *Blood* 1992;79:2930–2936.

62. Nishinaga M, Ozawa T, Shimada K. Homocysteine, a thrombogenic agent, suppresses anticoagulant heparan sulfate expression in cultured porcine aortic endothelial cells. *J Clin Invest* 1993;92:1381–1386.

63. Hajjar KA. Homocysteine-induced modulation of tissue plasminogen activator binding to its endothelial cell membrane receptor. *J Clin Invest* 1993;91:2873–2879.

64. von Eckardstein A, Malinow MR, Upson B. Effects of age, lipoproteins, and hemostatic parameters on the role of homocyst(e)inemia as a cardiovascular risk factor in men. *Arterioscler Thromb* 1994;14:960–964.

65. Tsai JC, Perrella MA, Yoshizumi M, et al. Promotion of vascular smooth muscle cell growth by homocysteine: a link to atherosclerosis. *Proc Natl Acad Sci U S A* 1994;91:6369–6373.

66. Dudman NP, Temple SE, Gu XW. Homocysteine enhances neutrophil-endothelial interactions in both cultured human cells and rats in vivo. *Circ Res* 1999;84:409–416.

67. Welch GN, Upchurch G, Loscalzo J. Hyperhomocyst(e)inemia and atherothrombosis. *Ann N Y Acad Sci* 1997;811:48–59.

68. Wilcken EL, Reddy SG, Gupta VJ. Homocysteinemia, ischemic heart disease, and the carrier state for homocystinuria. *Metabolism* 1993;32:363–370.

69. Alfthan G, Pekkanen J, Jauhiainen M, et al. Relation of serum homocysteine and lipoprotein (a) concentrations to atherosclerotic disease in a prospective Finnish population based study. *Atherosclerosis* 1994;106:9–19.

70. Folsom AR, Nieto FJ, McGovern PG, et al. Prospective study of coronary heart disease incidence in relation to fasting total homocysteine, related genetic polymorphisms, and B vitamins: the Atherosclerosis Risk in Communities (ARIC) study. *Circulation* 1998;98:204–210.

71. Nygard O, Vollset SE, Refsum H, et al. Total plasma homocysteine and cardiovascular risk profile. *JAMA* 1995;274:1526–1533.

72. Hirano K, Ogihara T, Miki M, et al. Homocysteine induces iron-catalyzed lipid peroxidation of low-density lipoprotein that is prevented by alpha-tocopherol. *Free Rad Res* 1994;21:267–276.

73. Glueck CJ, Shaw P, Lang J, et al. Evidence that homocysteine is an independent risk factor for atherosclerosis in hyperlipidemic patients. *Am J Cardiol* 1995;75:132–136.

74. Harpel PC, Chang VT, Borth W. Homocysteine and other sulfhydryl compounds enhance the binding of lipoprotein(a) to fibrin: a potential biochemical link between thrombosis, atherogenesis, and sulfhydryl compound metabolism. *Proc Natl Acad Sci U S A* 1992;89:10193–10197.

75. Nygard O, Nordrehaug JE, Refsum H, et al. Plasma homocysteine levels and mortality in patients with coronary artery disease. *N Engl J Med* 1997;337:230–236.

76. Stubbs PJ, Al-Obaidi MK, Conroy RM, et al. Effect of plasma homocysteine concentration on early and late events in patients with acute syndromes. *Circulation* 2000;102:605–610.

77. Brattstrom L, Wilcken D, Ohrvick J, et al. Common methylenetetrahydrofolate reductase gene mutation leads to hyperhomocysteinemia but not to vascular disease: the results of a meta-analysis. *Circulation* 1998;98:2520–2526.

78. Robinson K, Arheart K, Refsum H, et al. Low circulating folate and vitamin B_6 concentrations: risk factors for stroke, peripheral vascular disease and coronary artery disease. *Circulation* 1998;97:437–443.

79. Rinehart JF, Greenberg LD. Arteriosclerotic lesions in pyridoxine-deficient monkeys. *Am J Pathol* 1949;25:481–491.

80. Vermaak WJH, Barnard HC, Potgieter GM, et al. Vitamin B6 and coronary artery disease. Epidemiological observations and case studies. *Atherosclerosis* 1987;63:235–238.

81. Kok FJ, Schrijver J, Hofman A, et al. Low vitamin B_6 status in patients with acute myocardial infarction. *Am J Cardiol* 1989;63:513–516.

82. den Heijer M, Blom HJ, Gerrits WBJ, et al. Is hyperhomocyst(e)inaemia a risk factor for recurrent venous thrombosis? *Lancet* 1995;345:882–885.

83. Bienvenu T, Ankri A, Chadefaux B, et al. Elevated total plasma homocysteine, a risk factor for thrombosis. Relation

to coagulation and fibrinolytic parameters. *Thromb Res* 1993;70:123–129.

84. Brattström L, Tengborn L, Lagerstedt C, et al. Plasma homocysteine in venous thromboembolism. *Haemostasis* 1991;21:51–57.

85. Kottke-Marchant K, Green R, Jacobsen DW, et al. High plasma homocysteine: a risk factor for arterial and venous thrombosis in patients with normal hypercoagulation profiles. *Clin Appl Thromb Hemost* 1997;3:239–244.

86. Falcon CR, Cattaneo M, Panzeri D, et al. High prevalence of hyperhomocyst(e)inemia in patients with juvenile venous thrombosis. *Arterioscler Thromb* 1994;14:1080–1083.

87. den Heijer M, Rosendaal FR, Blom HJ, et al. Hyperhomocysteinemia and venous thrombosis: a meta-analysis. *Thromb Haemost* 1998;80:874–877.

88. Ray JG. Meta-analysis of hyperhomocysteinemia as a risk factor for venous thromboembolic disease. *Arch Intern Med* 1998;158:2101–2106.

89. Moustapha A, Naso A, Nahlawi M, et al. Prospective study of hyperhomocysteinemia as an adverse cardiovascular risk factor in end-stage renal disease. *Circulation* 1998;97:138–141.

90. Bostom AG, Lathrop L. Hyperhomocysteinemia in end-stage renal disease: prevalence, etiology, and potential relationship to arteriosclerotic outcomes. *Kidney Int* 1997;52:10–20.

91. Suliman ME, Qureshi AR, Barany P, et al. Hyperhomocysteinemia, nutritional status, and cardiovascular disease in hemodialysis patients. *Kidney Int* 2000;57:1727–1735.

92. Ambrosi P, Barlatier A, Habib G, et al. Hyperhomocysteinaemia in heart transplant recipients. *Eur Heart J* 1994;15:1191–1195.

93. Berger PB, Jones JD, Olson LJ, et al. Increase in total plasma homocysteine concentration after cardiac transplantation. *Mayo Clin Proc* 1995;70:125–131.

94. Gupta A, Moustapha A, Jacobsen DW, et al. High homocysteine, low folate and low vitamin B_6 concentrations: prevalent risk factors for vascular disease in heart transplant recipients. *Transplantation* 1998;65:544–550.

95. Nahlawi M, Naso A, Boparai N. Low vitamin B6: an independent predictor of cardiovascular morbidity and mortality in heart transplant recipients. *Circulation* 1998;98(Suppl I):690.

96. Boers GHJ, Yap S, Naughten E, et al. Treatment of high homocysteine concentrations in homocysteinuria. In: Robinson K, ed. *Homocysteine and vascular disease*. Dordrecht: Kluwer Academic Publishers, 2000:389–411.

97. Brattström L. Vitamins as homocysteine-lowering agents. *J Nutr* 1996;126(4 Suppl):1276S–1280S.

98. Homocysteine Lowering Trialists' Collaboration. Lowering blood homocysteine with folic acid based supplements: meta-analysis of randomised trials. *BMJ* 1998;316:894–898.

99. van der Mooren MJ, Wouters MG, Blom HJ, et al. Hormone replacement therapy may reduce high serum homocysteine in postmenopausal women. *Eur J Clin Invest* 1994;24:733–736.

100. Wiklund O, Fager G, Andersson A, et al. N-acetylcysteine treatment lowers plasma homocysteine levels but not serum lipoprotein(a) levels. *Atherosclerosis* 1996;119:99–106.

101. Malinow MR, Bostom AG, Krauss RM. Homocyst(e)ine, diet, and cardiovascular diseases: a statement for healthcare professionals from the Nutrition Committee, American Heart Association. *Circulation* 1999;99:178–182.

102. Berg K. A new serum system type in man—the Lp system. *Acta Pathol Microbiol Scand* 1963;59:369–382.

103. Utermann G. The mysteries of lipoprotein(a). *Science* 1989;246:904–910.

104. Mann AW, Kraft HG, Rader DJ, et al. Human in vivo catabolism of lipoprotein(a). *Circulation* 1989;890:II–181.

105. Rader DJ, Cain W, Ikewaki K, et al. The inverse association of plasma lipoprotein(a) concentrations with apolipoprotein(a) isoform size is not due to differences in LP(a) catabolism but to differences in production rate. *J Clin Invest* 1994;93:2758–2763.

106. White AL, Lanford RE. Biosynthesis and metabolism of lipoprotein (a). *Curr Opin Lipidol* 1995;6:75–80.

107. Fortmann SP, Marcovina SM. Lipoprotein(a), a clinically elusive lipoprotein particle. *Circulation* 1997;95:295–296.

108. Gaw A, Hobbs HH. Molecular genetics of lipoprotein(a): new pieces to the puzzle. *Curr Opin Lipidol* 1994;5:149–155.

109. Heinrich J, Sandkamp M, Kokott R, et al. Relationship of lipoprotein(a) to variables of coagulation and fibrinolysis in a healthy population. *Clin Chem* 1991;37:1950–1954.

110. Moliterno DJ, Leffert CC, Lange RA, et al. Plasma lipoprotein(a) is not a risk factor for atherosclerosis in blacks. *Circulation* 1992;86:I–337.

111. Sandholzer CH, Boerwinkle E, Soha N, et al. Apolipoprotein(a) phenotypes, LP(a) concentration and plasma lipid levels in relation to coronary heart disease in a Chinese population: evidence for role of the apo(a) gene in coronary heart disease. *J Clin Invest* 1992;89:1040–1046.

112. Parra HJ, Mezdour H, Cachera C, et al. Lp(a) lipoprotein in patients with chronic renal failure treated by hemodialysis. *Clin Chem* 1987;33:721.

113. Maeda S, Abe A, Seishima M, et al. Transient changes of serum lipoprotein(a) as an acute phase protein. *Atherosclerosis* 1989;78:145–150.

114. Mbewu AD, Durrington PN. Lipoprotein(a): structure properties and possible involvement in thrombogenesis and atherogenesis. *Atherosclerosis* 1990;85:1–14.

115. Webb AT, Reaveley DA, O'Donnell M, et al. Does cyclosporin increase lipoprotein(a) concentrations in renal transplant recipients? *Lancet* 1993;341:268–270.

116. Seed M, Hoppichler F, Reavely D, et al. Relation of serum lipoprotein(a) concentration and apolipoprotein(a) phenotype to coronary heart disease in patients with familial hypercholesterolemia. *N Engl J Med* 1990;322:1494–1499.

117. Rosengren A, Wilhelmsen L, Eriksson E, et al. Lipoprotein(a) and coronary heart disease: a prospective case-control study in a general population sample of middle aged men. *BMJ* 1990;301:1248–1251.

118. Dahlen GH, Guyton JR, Attar M, et al. Association of levels of lipoprotein Lp(a), plasma lipids, and other lipoproteins with coronary artery disease documented by angiography. *Circulation* 1986;74:758–765.

119. Sigurdsson G, Baldursdottir A, Sigvaldason H, et al. Predictive value of apolipoproteins in a prospective survey of coronary artery disease in men. *Am J Cardiol* 1992;69:1251–1254.

120. Jauhiainen M, Koskinen P, Ehnholm C, et al. Lipoprotein (a) and coronary heart disease risk: a nested case-control study of the Helsinki Heart Study participants. *Atherosclerosis* 1991;89:59–67.

121. Ridker PM, Hennekens CH, Stampfer MJ. A prospective study of lipoprotein(a) and the risk of myocardial infarction. *JAMA* 1993;270:2195–2199.

122. Hoff HF, Beck GJ, Skibinski CI, et al. Serum Lp(a) level as a predictor of vein graft stenosis after coronary artery bypass surgery in patients. *Circulation* 1988;77:1238–1244.

123. Eritsland J, Arnesen H, Seljeflot I, et al. Influence of serum lipoprotein(a) and homocyst(e)ine levels on graft patency after coronary artery bypass grafting. *Am J Cardiol* 1994;74:1099–1102.

124. Milionis HJ, Winder AF, Mikhailidis DP. Lipoprotein(a) and stroke. *J Clin Pathol* 2000;53:487–496.

125. Rath M, Niendorf A, Reblin T, et al. Detection and quantification of lipoprotein(a) in the arterial wall of 107 coronary bypass patients. *Arteriosclerosis* 1989;9:579–592.

126. Smith EB, Cochran S. Factors influencing the accumulation in fibrous plaques of lipid derived from low density lipoprotein. II. Preferential immobilization of lipoprotein(a). *Atherosclerosis* 1990;84:173–181.

127. Simon DA, Schoen FJ, Fless GM, et al. Lipoprotein(a) accumulates intracellularly in coronary atherectomy specimens obtained from primary and restenotic lesions after PTCA. *J Am Coll Cardiol* 1991;17:299.

128. Berg K, Dahlen G, Borresen AL. Lp(a) phenotypes, other lipoprotein parameters and a family history of coronary heart disease in middle-aged males. *Clin Genet* 1979;16:347–352.

129. Hervio L, Chapman MJ, Thillet J, et al. Does apolipoprotein(a) heterogeneity influence lipoprotein(a) effects on fibrinolysis? *Blood* 1993;82:392–397.

130. Loscalzo J, Weinfeld M, Fless GM, et al. Lipoprotein(a), fibrin binding, and plasminogen activation. *Arteriosclerosis* 1990;10:240–245.

131. Etingin OR, Hajjar DP, Hajjar KA, et al. Lipoprotein (a) regulates plasminogen activator inhibitor-1 expression in endothelial cells. A potential mechanism in thrombogenesis. *J Biol Chem* 1991;266:2459–2465.

132. Soulat T, Loyau S, Baudouin V, et al. Effect of individual plasma lipoprotein(a) variations in vivo on its competition with plasminogen for fibrin and cell binding. *Arterioscler Thromb Vasc Biol* 2000;20:575–584.

133. Bihari-Varga M, Gruber E, Rothenender M, et al. Interaction of lipoprotein Lp(a) and low density lipoprotein with glycosaminoglycans from human aorta. *Arteriosclerosis* 1988;8:851–857.

134. Poon M, Zhang X, Dunoky KG, et al. Apolipoprotein(a) induces monocyte chemotactic activity in human vascular endothelial cells. *Circulation* 1997;96:2574–2579.

135. Nachman RL. Lipoprotein(a): molecular mischief in the microvasculature. *Circulation* 1997;96:2485–2487.

136. Gurakar A, Hoeg JM, Kostner G, et al. Levels of lipoprotein Lp(a) decline with neomycin and niacin treatment. *Atherosclerosis* 1985;57:293–301.

137. Glueck CJ, Freiberg R, Glueck HI, et al. Idiopathic osteonecrosis, hypofibrinolysis, high plasminogen activator inhibitor, high lipoprotein(a), and therapy with stanozolol. *Am J Hematol* 1995;48:213–220.

138. Gavish D, Breslow JL. Lipoprotein(a) reduction by (N)-acetylcysteine. *Lancet* 1991;337:203–204.

139. Schlueter W, Keilani T, Batlle DC. Metabolic effects of converting enzyme inhibitors: focus on the reduction of cholesterol and lipoprotein(a) by fosinopril. *Am J Cardiol* 1993;72:37H–44H.

140. Sachs FM, McPherson R, Walsh BW. Effects of postmenopausal estrogen replacement on plasma Lp(a) lipoprotein concentrations. *Arch Intern Med* 1994;154(10):1106–1110.

141. Henriksson P, Angelin B, Berglund L. Hormonal regulation of serum Lp(a) levels: opposite effects after estrogen treatment and orchidectomy in males with prostatic carcinoma. *J Clin Invest* 1992;89:1166–1171.

142. Farish E, Rolton HA, Barnes JF, et al. Lipoprotein (a) concentrations in postmenopausal women taking norethisterone. *BMJ* 1991;303:694.

143. Perez-Jimenez F, Hidalgo L, Zambrana JL, et al. Comparison of lovastatin and bezafibrate on lipoprotein(a) plasma levels in cardiac transplant recipients. *Am J Cardiol* 1995;75:648–650.

144. Rader DJ, Rosas S. Management of selected lipid abnormalities. *Med Clin North Am* 2000;84:43–61.

145. Maher V, Brown BG, Marcovina SM, et al. Effects of lowering LDL cholesterol on the cardiovascular risk of lipoprotein(a). *JAMA* 1995;274;1771–1774.

146. Losner S, Volk BW, Wilensky ND. Fibrinogen concentration in acute myocardial infarction. *Arch Intern Med* 1954;93:231–238.

147. Henschen A, McDonagh J. Fibrinogen, fibrin and factor XIII. In: Zwaal RFA, Henker HC, eds. *Blood coagulation.* Amsterdam: Elsevier, 1986:171–242.

148. Kant JA, Fornace AJ, Saxe D, et al. Evolution and organization of the fibrinogen locus on chromosome 4: gene duplication accompanied by transposition and inversion. *Proc Natl Acad Sci U S A* 1985;82:2344–2348.

149. Thomas AE, Green FR, Kelleher C, et al. Variation in the promoter region of the β-fibrinogen gene is associated with plasma fibrinogen levels in smokers and non-smokers. *Thromb Haemost* 1991;65:487–490.

150. Folsom AR, Wu KK, Conlan MG. Fibrinogen and cardiovascular risk in the Atherosclerosis Risk in Communities (ARIC) Study. In: Ernst E, ed. *Fibrinogen, a "new" cardiovascular risk factor.* Oxford: Blackwell, 1992:124–129.

151. Folsom AR. Epidemiology of fibrinogen. *Eur Heart J* 1995;16:21–24.

152. Thompson WD, Smith EB. Atherosclerosis and the coagulation system. *J Pathol* 1989;159:97–106.

153. Ernst E, Matrai A, Scholzl C, et al. Dose-effect relationship between smoking and blood rheology. *Br J Haematol* 1987;65:485–487.

154. Yarnell JW, Sweetnam PM, Rogers S, et al. Some long-term effects of smoking on the haemostatic system: a report from the Caerphilly and Speedwell Collaborative Surveys. *J Clin Pathol* 1987;40:909–913.

155. Green F, Hamsten A, Blombäck M, et al. The role of β-fibrinogen genotype in determining plasma fibrinogen levels in young survivors of myocardial infarction and healthy controls from Sweden. *Thromb Haemost* 1993;70:915–920.

156. Kannel WB, Wolf PA, Castelli WP, et al. Fibrinogen and risk of cardiovascular disease. The Framingham Study. *JAMA* 1987;258:1183–1186.

157. Letcher RI, Chien S, Pickering TG, et al. Direct relationship between blood pressure and blood viscosity in normal and hypertensive subjects. Role of fibrinogen concentration. *Am J Med* 1981;70:1195–1202.

158. Kannel WB, D'Agostino RB, Wilson PW, et al. Diabetes, fibrinogen, and risk of cardiovascular disease: the Framingham experience. *Am Heart J* 1990;120:672–676.

159. Eisenberg S. Blood viscosity and fibrinogen concentration following cerebral infarction. *Circulation* 1966;33:10–14.

160. Ernst E, Krauth U, Resch KL, et al. Does blood rheology revert to normal after myocardial infarction? *Br Heart J* 1990;64:248–250.

161. Vaziri ND, Gonzales EC, Wang J, et al. Blood coagulation, fibrinolytic, and inhibitory proteins in end-stage renal disease: effect of hemodialysis. *Am J Kidney Dis* 1994;23:828–835.

162. Cavagna R, Schiavon R, Tessarin C, et al. Risk factors of ischemic cardiac disease in patients on continuous ambulatory peritoneal dialysis. *Perit Dial Int* 1993;13:S402–S405.

163. de Maat MP, Kastelein JJ, Jukema JW, et al. –455G/A polymorphism of the beta-fibrinogen gene is associated with the progression of coronary atherosclerosis in symptomatic men: proposed role for an acute-phase reaction pattern of fibrinogen. *Arterioscler Thromb Vasc Biol* 1998;18:265–271.

164. Meade TW, Mellows S, Brozovic M, et al. Haemostatic function and ischemic heart disease: principal results of the Northwick Park Heart Study. *Lancet* 1986;2:533–537.

165. Wilhelmsen L, Svardsudd K, Korsan-Bengtsen K, et al. Fibrinogen as a risk factor for stroke and myocardial infarction. *N Engl J Med* 1984;311:501–505.

166. Barasch E, Benderly M, Graff E, et al. Plasma fibrinogen levels and their correlates in 6457 coronary heart disease patients. The Bezafibrate Infarction Prevention (BIP) Study. *J Clin Epidemiol* 1995;48:757–765.

167. Ernst E, Resch KL. Fibrinogen as a cardiovascular risk factor: a meta-analysis and review of the literature. *Ann Intern Med* 1993;118:956–963.

168. Cook NS, Ubben D. Fibrinogen as a major cardiovascular risk factor in cardiovascular disease. *Trends Pharmacol Sci* 1990;11:444–451.

169. DiMinno G, Silver MJ, Cerbone AM, et al. Increased fibrinogen binding to platelets from patients with familial hypercholesterolemia. *Arteriosclerosis* 1986;6:203–211.

170. Smith EB, Keen GA, Grant A, et al. Fate of fibrinogen in human arterial intima. *Arteriosclerosis* 1990;10:263–275.

171. Rabbani LE, Loscalzo J. Recent observations on the role of hemostatic determinants in the development of atherothrombotic plaque. *Atherosclerosis* 1994;105:1–7.

172. Ernst E, Resch KL. Therapeutic interventions to lower fibrinogen concentration. *Eur Heart J* 1995;16:47–53.

173. Lijnen HR, Bachmann F, Collen D, et al. Mechanisms of plasminogen activation. *J Intern Med* 1994;236:415–424.

174. Klinger KW, Winqvist R, Riccio A, et al. Plasminogen activator inhibitor type 1 gene is located at region q21.3-q22 of chromosome 7 and genetically linked with cystic fibrosis. *Proc Natl Acad Sci U S A* 1987;84:8548–8552.

175. Loskutoff DJ. Regulation of PAI-1 gene expression. *Fibrinolysis* 1991;5:197–206.

176. Green F, Humphries S. Genetic determinants of arterial thrombosis. *Ballieres Clin Haematol* 1994;7:675–692.

177. Aillaud MF, Pignol F, Alessi MC, et al. Increase in plasma concentration of plasminogen activator inhibitor, fibrinogen, von Willebrand factor, F VIII:c and in erythrocyte sedimentation rate with age. *Thromb Haemost* 1986;35:250–253.

178. Hashimoto Y, Kobayashi A, Yamazaki N, et al. Relationship between age and plasma t-PA, PA-inhibitor, and PA activity. *Thromb Res* 1987;46:625–633.

179. Wiman B, Hamsten A. The fibrinolytic enzyme system and its role in the etiology of thromboembolic disease. *Semin Thromb Haemost* 1990;16:207–216.

180. Juhan-Vague I, Vague P, Alessi MC, et al. Relationships between plasma insulin, triglyceride, body mass index and plasminogen activator inhibitor 1. *Diabetes Metab* 1987;13:331–336.

181. Juhan-Vague I, Alessi MC, Vague P. Increased plasma plasminogen activator inhibitor-1 levels. A possible link between insulin resistance and atherothrombosis. *Diabetologia* 1991;34:457–462.

182. Alessi MC, Parra HJ, Joly P, et al. Increased plasma Lp(a): B lipoprotein particle concentration in angina pectoris is not associated with hypofibrinolysis. *Clin Chim Acta* 1990;188:119–128.

183. Korninger C, Lechner K, Niessner H, et al. Impaired fibrinolytic capacity predisposes for recurrence of venous thrombosis. *Thromb Haemost* 1984;52:127–130.

184. Grimaudo V, Bachman F, Hauert J, et al. Hypofibrinolysis in patients with a history of idiopathic deep vein thrombosis and/or pulmonary embolism. *Thromb Haemost* 1992;67:397–401.

185. Prins MH, Hirsh J. A critical review of the evidence supporting a relationship between impaired fibrinolytic activity and venous thromboembolism. *Arch Intern Med* 1991;151:1721–1731.

186. Fay WP, Shapiro AD, Shih JL, et al. Complete deficiency of plasminogen activator inhibitor type 1 due to a frameshift mutation. *N Engl J Med* 1992;327:1729–1733.

187. Hamsten A, Wiman B, De Faire U, et al. Increased plasma levels of a rapid inhibitor of tissue plasminogen activator in young survivors of myocardial infarction. *N Engl J Med* 1985;313:1557–1563.

188. Johnson O, Mellbring G, Nilsson T. Defective fibrinolysis in survivors of myocardial infarction. *Int J Cardiol* 1984;6:380–382.

189. Paramo JA, Colucci M, Collen D, et al. Plasminogen activator inhibitor in the blood of patients with coronary artery disease. *BMJ* 1985;291:575–576.

190. Aznar J, Estelles A, Tormo G, et al. Plasminogen activator inhibitor activity and other fibrinolytic variables in patients with coronary artery disease. *Br Heart J* 1988;59:535–541.

191. Hamsten A, Blomback M, Wiman B, et al. Haemostatic function in myocardial infarction. *Br Heart J* 1986;55:58–66.

192. Francis RB, Kawasnishi D, Baruchi T, et al. Impaired fibrinolysis in coronary artery disease. *Am Heart J* 1988;115:776–780.

193. Olofsson BO, Dahlen G, Nilsson TK. Evidence for increased levels of plasminogen activator in plasma of patients with angiographically verified coronary artery disease. *Eur Heart J* 1989;10:77–82.

194. Zalewski A, Shi Y, Nardone D, et al. Evidence for reduced fibrinolytic activity in unstable angina at rest. Clinical, biochemical and angiographic correlates. *Circulation* 1991;83:1685–1691.

195. Jansson JJ, Nilsson TK, Johnson O. Von Willebrand factor in plasma: a novel risk factor for recurrent myocardial infarction and death. *BMJ* 1991;66:351–355.

196. Hamsten A, Walldius G, Szamosi A, et al. Plasminogen activator inhibitor in plasma: risk factor for recurrent myocardial infarction. *Lancet* 1987;2:3–9.

197. Margaglione M, Capucci G. Colaizzo D, et al. The PAI-1 gene locus 4G/5G polymorphism is associated with a family history of coronary artery disease. *Arterioscler Thromb Vasc Biol* 1998;18:152–156.

198. Anderson JL, Muhlestein JB, Habashi J, et al. Lack of association of a common polymorphism of the plasminogen activator inhibitor-1 gene with coronary artery disease and myocardial infarction. *J Am Coll Cardiol* 1999;34:1778–1783.

199. Jansson JJ, Nilsson TK, Olofsson BO. Tissue plasminogen activator and other risk factors as predictors of cardiovascular events in patients with severe angina pectoris. *Eur Heart J* 1991;12:157–161.

200. Huber K, Jorg M, Probst P, et al. A decrease in plasminogen activator inhibitor 1 activity after successful percutaneous transluminal coronary angioplasty is associated with a significantly reduced risk for coronary restenosis. *Thromb Haemost* 1992;67:209–213.

201. Schneiderman J, Sawdey MS, Keeton MR, et al. Increased type 1 plasminogen activator inhibitor gene expression in atherosclerotic human arteries. *Proc Natl Acad Sci U S A* 1989;86:6998–7002.

202. Ridker PM, Hennekens CH, Stampfer MJ, et al. Prospective study of endogenous tissue plasminogen activator and risk of stroke. *Lancet* 1994;343:940–943.

203. Ross R. The pathogenesis of atherosclerosis: a perspective for the 1990's. *Nature* 1993;362:801–809.

204. Ridker PM. C-reactive protein and risks of future myocardial infarction and thrombotic stroke. *Eur Heart J* 1998;19:1–3.

205. Thompson SG, Kienast J, Pyke SD, et al. Hemostatic factors and the risk of myocardial infarction or sudden death in patients with angina pectoris. *N Engl J Med* 1995;332:635–641.

206. Mendall MA, Patel P, Ballam L, et al. C-reactive protein and its relation to cardiovascular risk factors: a population based cross-sectional study. *BMJ* 1996;312:1061–1065.

207. Ridker PM, Cushman M, Stampfer MJ, et al. Inflammation, aspirin, and risk of cardiovascular disease in apparently healthy men. *N Engl J Med* 1997;336:973–979.

208. deBeer FC, Hind CRK, Fox KM, et al. Measurement of serum C-reactive protein concentration in myocardial ischaemia and infarction. *Br Heart J* 1982;46:239–243.

209. Pietila KO, Harmoinen AP, Jokiniitty J, et al. Serum C-reactive protein concentration in acute myocardial infarction and its relationship to mortality during 24 months of follow-up in patients under thrombolytic treatment. *Eur Heart J* 1996;17:1345–1349.

210. Casl MT, Surina B, Glojnaric-Spasic I, et al. Serum amyloid A protein in patients with acute myocardial infarction. *Ann Clin Biochem* 1995;32:196–200.

211. Berk BC, Weintraub WS, Alexander RW. Elevation of C-reactive protein in "active" coronary artery disease. *Am J Cardiol* 1990;65:168–172.

212. Liuzzo G, Biasucci LM, Gallimore JR, et al. The prognostic value of C-reactive protein and serum amyloid A protein in severe unstable angina. *N Engl J Med* 1994;331:417–424.

213. Schmitz C, Lindpaintner K, Verhoef P, et al. Genetic polymorphism of methylenetetrahydrofolate reductase and myocardial infarction. *Circulation* 1996;94:1812–1814.

214. Narang R, Callaghan G, Haider AW, et al. Methylenetetrahydrofolate reductase mutation and coronary artery disease. *Circulation* 1996;94:2322–2323.

215. Adams M, Smith PD, Martin D, et al. Genetic analysis of thermolabile methylenetetrahydrofolate reductase as a risk factor for myocardial infarction. *QJM* 1996;89:437–444.

216. de Franchis R, Mancini FP, D'Angelo AD, et al. Elevated total plasma homocysteine and 677C→T mutation of the 5,10-methylenetetrahydrofolate reductase gene in thrombotic vascular disease. *Am J Hum Genet* 1996;59:252–264.

217. Gallagher PM, Meleady R, Shields DC, et al. Homocysteine and risk of premature coronary heart disease: evidence for a common gene mutation. *Circulation* 1996;94:2154–2158.

218. Izumi M, Iwai N, Ohmichi N, et al. Molecular variant of 5,10-methylenetetrahydrofolate reductase is a risk factor of ischemic heart disease in the Japanese population. *Atherosclerosis* 1996;121:293–294.

219. Harmon DL, Woodside JV, Yarnell JWG, et al. The common "thermolabile" variant of methylene tetrahydrofolate reductase is a major determinant of mild hyperhomocysteinaemia. *QJM* 1996;89:571–577.

220. Bostom AG, Shemin D, Lapane KL, et al. Folate status is the major determinant of fasting total plasma homocysteine levels in maintenance dialysis patients. *Atherosclerosis* 1996;123:193–202.

221. Wilcken DEL, Wang XL, Sim AS, et al. Distribution in healthy and coronary populations of the methylenetetrahydrofolate reductase (MTHFR) $C_{677}T$ mutation. *Arterioscler Thromb Vasc Biol* 1996;16:878–882.

222. Mandel H, Brenner B, Berant M, et al. Coexistence of hereditary homocystinuria and factor V Leiden–effect on thrombosis. *N Engl J Med* 1996;334:763–768.

223. Murata M, Kawano K, Matsubara Y, et al. Genetic polymorphisms and risk of coronary artery disease. *Semin Thromb Hemost* 1998;24:245–250.

224. Anderson JL, King GJ, Bair TL, et al. Associations between a polymorphism in the gene encoding glycoprotein IIIa and myocardial infarction or coronary artery disease. *J Am Coll Cardiol* 1999;33:727–733.

225. Rosendaal FR, Siscovick DS, Schwartz SM, et al. A common prothrombin variant (20210 G to A) increases the risk of myocardial infarction in young women. *Blood* 1997;90:1747–1750.

226. Robinson K, Gupta A, Dennis V, et al. Homocysteinemia confers an independent increased risk of atherosclerosis in end-stage renal disease and is closely linked to plasma folate and pyridoxine concentrations. *Circulation* 1996;94:2743–2748.

BEHAVIORAL MEDICINE AND HEART DISEASE

CHARLES F. EMERY
JOHN N. O'NEIL

▼▽ ADDITIONAL ELECTRONIC TOPICS
Additional Psychological Factors c04;   Social Support c05;   Behavioral Counseling and Therapy c06

OVERVIEW

Behavioral medicine integrates behavioral sciences with the science of medicine. Thus, the behavioral medicine approach to cardiac disease includes evaluation of behavioral, psychological, and social functioning in relation to the etiology and treatment of disease. Behavioral and psychological factors associated with coronary artery disease (CAD) include personality [e.g., Type A behavior pattern (TABP)], affective state (e.g., depression, anxiety), and social or work environment.

Although global Type A (TA) behavior previously was found to be strongly associated with the development of CAD, refinements of the TA construct have indicated that hostility and cynicism may be the most toxic components of the TABP. In addition, negative emotions other than

C. F. Emery: Department of Psychology, The Ohio State University, Columbus, Ohio
J. N. O'Neil: Department of Psychology, The Ohio State University, Columbus, Ohio

hostility, especially depression, and environmental factors such as work strain (high demand, low control) have been associated with the development of CAD. Social support, on the other hand, appears to mitigate the negative effects of stress and environment on CAD.

Comprehensive evaluation of stress usually includes a subjective appraisal of stress, as well as physiologic indicators of stress as measured in laboratory studies of cardiovascular (CV) function. Stress-related hemodynamic alterations are important to evaluate because CV reactivity of the sympathoadrenal and pituitary adrenal-cortical systems is thought to be a pathophysiologic mechanism linking stress with development of CAD. Recent data also reveal stress-related changes in neuroendocrine function and blood lipids, which may contribute to CAD.

Intervention studies suggest that relaxation training may have beneficial effects on CV reactivity to laboratory stressors and that stress-management training may be beneficial for reducing components of the TABP. Stress-management interventions can minimize the impact of depression on future cardiac events among post–myocardial infarction (MI) patients, and stress management is a central component of multimodal treatments for patients with CAD. Studies have not yet demonstrated the optimal components or dosage of stress-management interventions among patients with CAD, but ongoing research is documenting various aspects of stress-management interventions that may be important in the treatment of cardiac patients.

GLOSSARY

Appraisal: The mechanism by which social support is thought to mitigate the effects of stress on health. *Primary appraisal* refers to support that helps to prevent the individual from viewing an event as stressful. *Secondary appraisal* refers to social support facilitating reappraisal (in a less stressful way) after an event that was viewed as stressful.

Biofeedback-assisted relaxation training: The use of auditory and visual feedback from electromyographic sensors to enhance individual awareness and control of muscle tension.

Cognitive-behavioral counseling: An approach to stress management that includes increasing the patient's awareness of negative and stressful ways of thinking that are likely to result in unhealthy behavior and negative social interactions. Cognitive counseling is directed toward increasing the frequency of positive, rational thinking.

Health behavior model: A theoretical model linking hostility with CAD and suggesting that hostile individuals are less likely to engage in good health habits.

Progressive muscle relaxation (PMR): A technique for reducing muscle tension and subjective stress by means of focused, systematic relaxation of muscle groups throughout the body.

Psychophysiologic (CV) reactivity model: A theoretical model linking hostility with CAD and suggesting that individuals high in hostility manifest larger increases in heart rate, blood pressure, and stress hormones than individuals with low hostility.

Psychosocial vulnerability model: A theoretical model linking hostility with CAD and suggesting that hostile individuals experience a more conflict-laden environment with less available social support.

Self-efficacy: The individual judgment of one's ability to achieve a goal. This is a widely studied concept in health psychology literature that has been proved to be an important psychological factor in behavioral change (e.g., exercise, smoking cessation, diet).

Structured Interview: An interview assessment of TABP and related characteristics (e.g., potential for hostility) that is widely regarded as the best assessment tool for evaluating TA characteristics.

Thought stopping: A stress-management technique in which patients are trained to stop the rapid succession of negative thoughts and feelings associated with stressful circumstances and to substitute alternative behaviors (e.g., relaxation) or thoughts.

Type A behavior pattern (TABP): Also described as *coronary-prone behavior*, TABP includes a constellation of behaviors and personality traits (e.g., excessive competitiveness, chronic feelings of time pressure and urgency, chronic feelings of anger and hostility) associated with increased rates of CAD.

HISTORICAL PERSPECTIVE

This chapter elaborates on the historical perspective [▼ c07] by delineating the contribution of each area of research toward understanding behavioral and psychological factors in CAD. Subsequent sections of the chapter address biobehavioral factors in the etiology of CAD, behavioral and psychological interventions, and select issues and controversies relevant to future behavioral medicine research.

Stress

Stress has been broadly defined as an experience in which the demands of a situation exceed the perceived ability to cope with the situation (9), most often resulting from a person-environment transaction and leading to overarousal or underarousal of the organism (10). Much research has been directed toward elucidating the nature of the *stress response*, first described by Cannon (11) and characterized as an innate "fight-or-flight" response in animals when confronted by a threatening situation of a physical or social nature. Although this fight-or-flight response is an adaptive response to physical threats, it is not adaptive in most modern social circumstances and often is suppressed. In human beings, the stress response is marked by a cognitive appraisal of a situation as threatening, followed by physiologic changes such as increases in blood pressure, heart rate, respiratory rate, output of stress hormones, blood homocysteine levels (12), and blood platelet activity. It has been hypothesized that stress-associated physiologic arousal may contribute to chronic elevations in blood pressure and increased risk of cardiac disease (6). Thus, the stress response is a function of personality and individual differences that may affect the appraisal of the situation, as well as influence person-environment interactions.

An expanded view of the stress response was proposed in a recent review (13), in which it was observed that the majority of studies describing the fight-or-flight phenomenon has included only men. After extensive review of animal and human research, Taylor and colleagues (13) have postulated that women respond to stress with a "tend-and-befriend" pattern of behavior. *Tending* is described as nurturing activities that enhance safety and alleviate distress to protect the self and offspring; *befriending* involves the development and maintenance of social relationships that facilitate tending.

The tend-and-befriend pattern is thought to be a product of the biobehavioral attachment-caregiving system involving oxytocin, estrogen, and endogenous opioid mechanisms, which, in turn, down-regulate sympathetic nervous system responses. Taylor and colleagues suggest an evolutionary basis for this behavioral pattern, speculating that the tend-and-befriend stress response may help to explain gender differences in CV reactivity and life span. At a minimum, this view of the stress response indicates the importance of evaluating responses to stressful circumstances in the context of gender.

Several studies provide data suggestive of the importance of stress—physical or mental—in the onset of cardiac symptoms. Stressful, frustrating interpersonal relations may elicit anger and general excitement among CAD-prone individuals (14). In addition, epidemiologic research suggests that the onset of symptoms of acute MI are triggered by external factors (e.g., heavy physical work, violent quarrel, unusual mental stress) in a substantial minority of cases (10%) (15).

Work environment has become one of the most commonly studied environmental precipitants of stress-related cardiac disease, and it has been argued that work environment is more important to evaluate than individual factors (16). Johnson and Hall (17) found that job strain (high demand and low control) was associated with increased rates of CVD prevalence and that workers with the lowest level of social support had higher prevalence rates, regardless of level of job strain. Figure 11.1 provides a schematic of relative job strain associated with various common professions.

This research shows promise in providing evidence of the complex interaction of factors (e.g., work stress and social support) associated with CAD. Longitudinal data from a 14-year follow-up study revealed that working Swedish men with low control in their jobs had a significantly elevated risk for CVD mortality compared to men with high-control jobs (5). CV risk factors may also be affected by work stress. A study of 715 male shipyard workers found that the threat of job loss was associated with increased serum cholesterol, especially among those men reporting sleep disturbance (18). Thus, data suggest that work and related environmental stressors may have a significant influence on the development of CAD. However, individual differences in the frequency and magnitude of the stress response also suggest the importance of personality variables such as the TABP.

Type A Behavior Pattern

The TABP was first described in the late 1950s by cardiologists Meyer Friedman and Ray Rosenman, who observed in

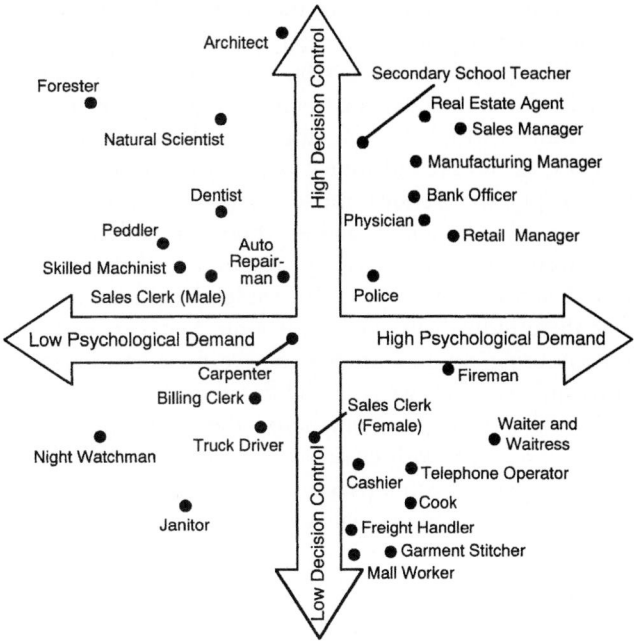

FIGURE 11.1 Illustration of the Karasek job strain model. Based on a job characteristics scoring system, occupations are characterized according to level of job demand and control. Workers with high demand and low control are at greater risk for cardiovascular disease. (Adapted from *The New York Times*, 3 April 1983.)

their patients a number of common behavioral characteristics and personality traits, including excessive competitiveness, extreme desire for recognition and achievement, chronic feelings of time pressure and urgency, as well as chronic feelings of anger and hostility (1). Although early research suggested a strong association of TABP with development of CAD (19), more recent data suggest that global TABP may not be associated with CAD (20,21). Thus, there remains controversy regarding the prognostic importance of TABP in primary and secondary prevention settings. Data from a recent metaanalysis indicate that global TABP may not be as relevant as more specific aspects of TABP, especially hostility (2).

Hostility and Heart Disease

Epidemiologic data evaluating personality traits associated with CAD suggest that chronic hostility and cynicism are the most pathogenic components of the coronary-prone personality (22). Smith has reviewed evidence for several models to explain the association (23). The psychophysiologic reactivity model is founded on the notion that individuals high in hostility are more likely to manifest larger increases in heart rate, blood pressure, and stress hormones in response to stressors than individuals with low hostility (22). However, the nature of the stressor may be important, as demonstrated by studies finding no association of hostility with reactivity in the context of nonsocial stressors (24) but significant associations in the context of interpersonal stressors (25). Other theoretical models linking hostility with disease include the psychosocial vulnerability model (i.e., hostile individuals experience a more conflict-laden environment with less social support) and a health behavior model (e.g., hostile individuals may engage in poor health habits). The transactional model—representing a synthesis of the psychophysiologic and psychosocial models—posits that hostile individuals tend to respond to daily stressors with heightened CV and neuroendocrine reactivity and that these individuals experience more frequent, extreme, and enduring episodes of stress due to their hostile cognitions and overt behavior (23). Thus, all of the models linking hostility with CAD emphasize the interaction of the hostile individual with environmental stressors; this interaction supports the importance of individual constitutional variation and environmental factors.

Gender

Several studies suggest that gender differences may mediate the relationship between hostility and psychophysiologic reactivity. Davidson et al. (26) examined correlations between hostility scores from a Structured Interview assessment (27), scores on antagonism and neuroticism scales, and resting blood pressure among 193 undergraduate women and men. Whereas hostility was related to antagonism and higher resting blood pressure in men, hostility was related to neuroticism and lower resting blood pressure in women. ☜ c08

Blood Serum

Recent studies have explored the relationship between hostility and lipid reactivity. In a study of 77 healthy women, Suarez et al. (30) observed significant elevations in total serum cholesterol and low-density lipoprotein cholesterol among women assessed as high in cynical and antagonistic hostility. Among healthy men (n = 98), Richards et al. (31) found significant associations between angry reactions (i.e., the tendency to experience and express anger in response to criticism or unfair treatment) and elevated total serum cholesterol and low-density lipoprotein cholesterol levels. Data also indicate that healthy women and men with high levels of hostility and men with inhibited anger expression may have higher levels of blood homocysteine (32). One hypothesized mechanism for this effect may be increased hemoconcentration associated with stress (33).

Depression and Anxiety

Although much early research was devoted to the relationship of CAD to TABP and its components, more recent data have suggested additional important psychological factors associated with CAD, especially anxiety and depression. In a

metaanalysis of studies evaluating psychological functioning and CAD, it was found that the effect size for depression was as great as that of TABP or other known risk factors for CAD (2). Although anxiety was related to CAD, it was not as strongly related as depression. Thus, the traditional image of the coronary-prone individual as time pressured, impatient, and work oriented is not consistent with the data. Instead, a more appropriate image is that of someone harboring negative emotions, such as depression, anxiety, hostility, or aggression. Thus, hostility or anger would be supported as the most important component of TABP, but depression and anxiety also may be important predictors of CAD (2).

Depression has been implicated as an important factor in the initial onset of CAD (34), as well as among patients with previously diagnosed CAD. Frasure-Smith and colleagues (35) confirmed the importance of negative emotions, including depression, anxiety, and history of depression, for prognosis of post-MI patients. Results from their longitudinal study, included in Figure 11.2, suggested that post-MI depression was more strongly associated with arrhythmic deaths (3), whereas anxiety was more strongly associated with acute coronary syndromes (30). ☜ c09

Adherence and Risk-Factor Reduction

As awareness of risk factors for CAD has become more widespread through community education efforts, the need has grown for programs to support health behavior change. Most of the risk factors for CAD are behaviorally mediated and, thus, may be readily influenced and modified. For example, smoking, diet, and exercise activity all involve

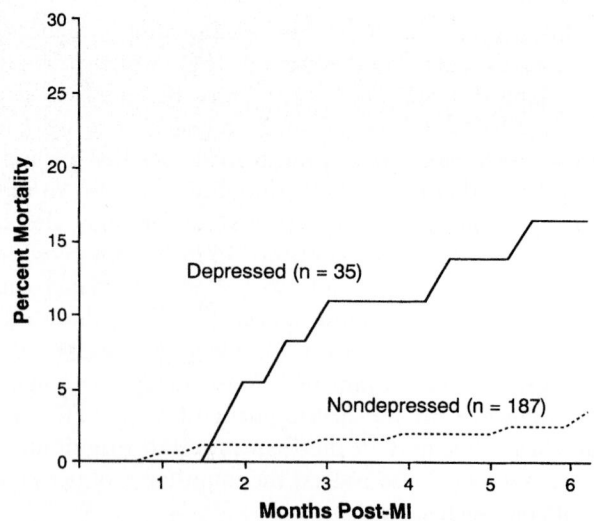

FIGURE 11.2 Cumulative 6-month mortality for depressed and nondepressed post–myocardial infarction (MI) patients. Depression was assessed with structured interviews during inpatient hospitalization (approximately 7 days post-MI). (Adapted from Frasure-Smith N, Lesperance F, Talajic M. Depression following myocardial infarction. Impact on 6-month survival. *JAMA* 1993;270:1821.)

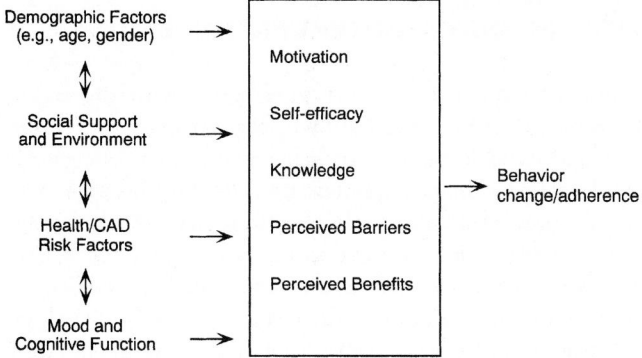

FIGURE 11.3 Hypothesized model of factors associated with adherence and behavior change. CAD, coronary artery disease.

modifiable behaviors. However, it may be difficult to reach high-risk individuals in primary prevention, because it has been found that high-risk CAD groups (e.g., men, older adults, and individuals with less education) are less likely to make use of educational materials regarding CVD risk (57).

As shown in Figure 11.3, adherence to a behavioral program may be influenced by a number of factors, both individual and environmental. Among the most clearly identified individual factors affecting adherence are self-efficacy (i.e., the patient's belief that he or she will be able to achieve the behavioral goal) and self-motivation (58). ⚐ c10

BIOBEHAVIORAL FACTORS IN THE PATHOPHYSIOLOGY OF HEART DISEASE

As theoretical advances have been made in evaluating physiologic mechanisms of behavioral and psychological effects in CAD, the major thrust of research has been directed toward studies of CV reactivity.

Cardiovascular Reactivity

Studies suggest that stress may contribute to the development of CAD via stress-associated, chronic, exaggerated reactivity of the sympathoadrenal-medullary and pituitary adrenal-cortical systems, triggering hemodynamic changes or biochemical alterations that lead to damage of artery walls (6). The impact of CV reactivity is thought to be cumulative, contributing to injury of the endothelium and to deposition of cholesterol on the artery wall. Among patients with CAD, CV reactivity may also contribute to myocardial ischemia and arrhythmias (23). Studies generally confirm an association of elevated CV reactivity in individuals with symptoms of CAD or hypertension (6). ⚐ c11

Health-Damaging Behavior

The health behavior model described by Smith (23) suggests that the association between hostility and CAD is the result of poor health behavior among hostile individuals. In support of this model, Smith summarizes studies that have demonstrated associations between hostility and low physical exercise, low self-care, higher alcohol consumption, higher body mass index, and more cigarette smoking. However, the interrelationship of hostility, health behavior, and CAD has not been evaluated. Frasure-Smith et al. (3) suggest that health behavior change among cardiac patients also may be impaired by affective distress (e.g., depression and anxiety). Although social support may serve to moderate somewhat the negative effects of emotional state and personality on health behavior change, the effect of personality and emotions on adherence to preventive and rehabilitative health behaviors has not been investigated.

Cognitive functioning also may affect an individual's ability to conduct adequate self-care and follow prescribed health care regimens. Although several studies have documented cognitive deficits among cardiac patients (67,68), only one study has evaluated the association of cognitive functioning with health behavior in cardiac patients. In a sample of clinically stable cardiac rehabilitation patients, Barclay and colleagues (69) found that 35% were so cognitively impaired that they were unable to self-administer medications appropriately. The evaluation of interactions of cognitive performance with health and health behavior is especially important among older adults with or at risk for CAD.

Relationship among Areas of Behavioral Medicine

As the research data indicate, it is difficult to define psychosocial functioning by addressing only one of the many psychosocial factors in CAD because these factors are likely to be interrelated. For example, social support may mitigate the association of TABP with CAD, as well as minimize CV reactivity to laboratory stress. Figure 11.4 provides an illustration of the relationships among various behavioral factors suggested by the research data thus far.

CLINICAL PROFILE AND ASSESSMENT

The historical research data suggest that the typical CAD patient is likely to manifest one or more components of TABP—most likely hostility or cynicism, as well as other negative emotions such as depression or anxiety. In addition, the patient's work and home environments may present obvious or subtle stressors of a chronic nature, and social support may be limited. Although not all CAD patients present with psychosocial problems, the clinician addressing behavioral issues among CAD patients must use adequate assessment techniques to facilitate appropriate treatment strategies.

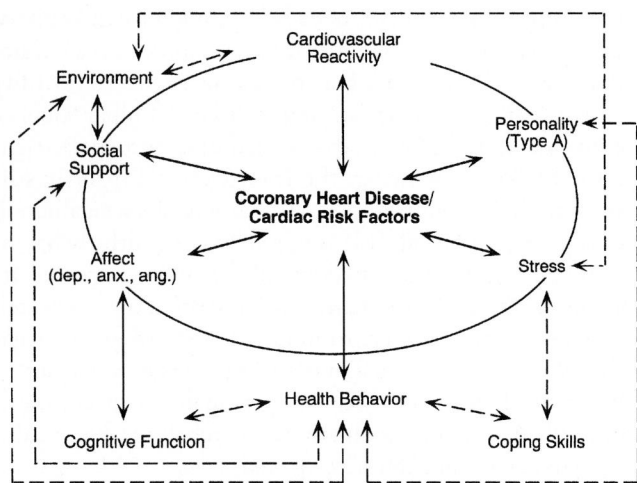

FIGURE 11.4 Psychosocial factors associated with coronary heart disease and cardiac risk factors. Stronger associations are depicted with solid arrows; less strong associations are depicted with hatched arrows. ang., anger; anx., anxiety; dep., depression.

Several assessment instruments have been used by researchers to measure psychiatric symptoms, physical symptoms, psychological functioning, social support, and stress. A listing of common assessment instruments is included in Table 11.1. ⚑ c12

TABLE 11.1 PSYCHOSOCIAL ASSESSMENT INSTRUMENTS COMMONLY USED IN CARDIOVASCULAR MEDICINE

Stress and coping
  Hopkins Symptom Checklist-90-R (SCL-90-R)
  Millon Behavioral Health Inventory (MBHI)
  General Health Questionnaire (GHQ)
  Sickness Impact Profile (SIP)
  Schedule of Recent Life Events (SRLE)
  Life Experiences Survey (LES)
  Perceived Stress Scale (PSS)
Personality/type A
  Structured Interview (SI)
  Jenkins Activity Survey (JAS)
  Cook-Medley Hostility Scale (Ho)
  Buss Durkee Hostility Inventory (BDHI)
  Minnesota Multiphasic Personality Inventory (MMPI)
  Eysenck Personality Questionnaire (EPQ)
Social support
  Social Support Questionnaire (SSQ)
  Perceived Social Support Scale (PSSS)
  Dyadic Adjustment Scale (DAS)
Work
  Job Content Questionnaire (JCQ)
Psychiatric comorbidity
  NIMH Interview Schedule (DIS)
  Beck Depression Inventory (BDI)
  Center for Epidemiological Studies Depression Inventory (CES-D)
  Profile of Mood States (POMS)
  State Trait Anxiety Inventory (STAI)

NIMH, National Institute of Mental Health.

BEHAVIORAL AND PSYCHOLOGICAL INTERVENTIONS

Most cardiac risk factors are modifiable, with the exceptions of age, gender, and family history. Primary prevention strategies tend to target at-risk behaviors, such as cigarette smoking, poor dietary habits, and sedentary lifestyle. Secondary prevention efforts also aim to reduce health-damaging behaviors and improve compliance with physicians' recommendations; these efforts often include additional therapeutic techniques to reduce the impact of psychological distress and other psychosocial risks that can interfere with a positive prognosis. Among the intervention strategies commonly used are stress reduction techniques, relaxation training, biofeedback, and other psychotherapeutic interventions. However, none of these techniques is mutually exclusive. Most studies of psychosocial interventions among cardiac patients have evaluated the effects of stress-management interventions encompassing relaxation training and selected other techniques, such as cognitive counseling (e.g., identifying and challenging irrational, stress-producing thought patterns) or behavioral counseling (e.g., modifying contingencies for desired behavior). Relaxation techniques typically include breathing exercises and PMR—a process of systematic tensing and relaxing of major muscle groups throughout the body. Cognitive and behavioral components of stress management have included specific skills training, such as public speaking training, stress-inoculation training emphasizing positive self-statements, biofeedback-assisted relaxation training with electromyography and heart-rate feedback, and affect regulation, including appropriate expression of anger and hostility. Few studies have been conducted to compare the relative efficacy of the stress-management components. The only study contrasting components of stress management among cardiac patients found no significant differences between a relaxation condition and a no-relaxation stress-management condition (i.e., monitoring negative self-statements) with regard to psychological functioning (i.e., decreases in social anxiety) (77).

Stress Management

The effects of stress management on cardiac outcomes have been studied mainly in secondary prevention. The Ischemic Heart Disease Life Stress Monitoring Program (35) examined the impact of stress monitoring and intervention in 543 male post-MI patients randomly assigned to a treatment condition or no-treatment control. Subjects in the treatment condition received monthly telephone calls from nurses who assessed stress levels. If the subject's monthly stress level was above the standard criterion (i.e., above 4 on the General Health Questionnaire; 78), he would receive individual counseling and advice designed to alleviate stress. Results indicated that the monitored group showed a

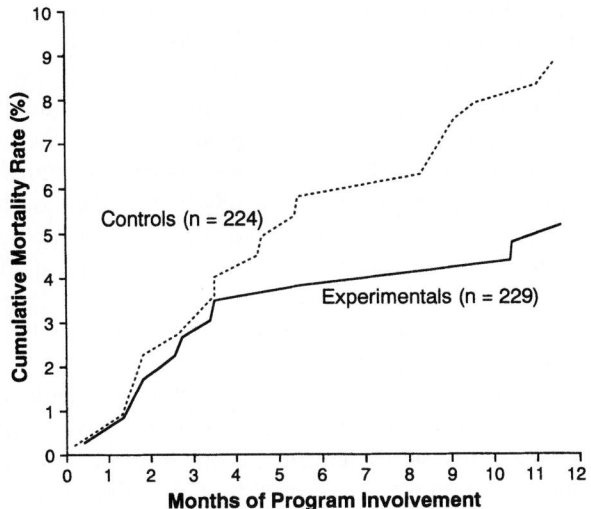

FIGURE 11.5 Life-table cumulative mortality rates for post–myocardial infarction patients randomly assigned to experimental group (stress monitoring) or no-treatment control group. (From Frasure-Smith N, Prince R. The ischemic heart disease life stress monitoring program: impact on mortality. *Psychosom Med* 1985;47:438, with permission.)

greater decline in stress levels compared to no-treatment controls. Although the monitored group did not differ from the controls in the incidence and length of hospital readmissions, the rate of mortality for that group was significantly lower. Data from this study are depicted in Figure 11.5. The authors suggest that stress reduction interventions may play a greater role in lowering cardiac mortality than in preventing future nonlethal cardiac episodes. Unfortunately, the investigators did not control for the type of counseling offered to each subject; indeed, they suggested that the phone call itself might have been responsible for lowering stress levels.

Among post-MI subjects, stress-management interventions (e.g., coping skills training, PMR, deep breathing exercises, biofeedback) have been found to provide greater cardiac benefit (i.e., significantly fewer arrhythmias, less chest pain, and better overall cardiac status) than cardiac education alone (79), and the effect of stress management on psychophysiologic reactivity has been found to be comparable to that of drug treatment (e.g., propranolol) (80). Stress management also has been evaluated as an adjunct to exercise rehabilitation in a study of 45 post–coronary artery bypass graft patients randomly assigned to (a) conventional medical therapy and exercise rehabilitation or (b) conventional therapy, exercise rehabilitation, and stress-management intervention (81). Exercise rehabilitation included three 1-hour workouts per week for 18 weeks. Stress-management intervention included eight 90-minute sessions that provided education about TABP, expression of anger and hostility, use of humor, and autogenic training—a form of relaxation training. Subjects received a booster session 1 month after the end of the program. Results indi-

cated that subjects in the stress-management intervention experienced reduced blood pressure reactivity, as well as improved perceived health status and decreased triglyceride levels. The conventional treatment showed a decrease in high-density lipoprotein. Blumenthal et al. (82) compared the effects of stress management or exercise on myocardial ischemia and risk for cardiac events among 107 CAD patients exhibiting ischemia during mental stress tasks or ambulatory monitoring. Patients were randomized to stress management (i.e., psychoeducational group sessions, monitoring and modifying irrational thoughts, PMR, and biofeedback) or an exercise intervention (i.e., riding on a stationary bicycle, walking, and jogging three times per week) for 4 months. Patients residing at a distance from the study site comprised a nonrandom, usual-care control group. Patients were contacted at 4 months, 10 months, and at yearly intervals up to 5 years to assess cardiac morbidity and mortality. Compared to patients in the usual-care control group, patients in the stress-management group had significantly lower relative risk for cardiac events throughout the 5-year follow-up period. In addition, subjects in the stress-management condition experienced reductions in ischemia during mental stress and ambulatory monitoring. ❦ c13

In a primary prevention study, Patel and colleagues (84) examined the effects of relaxation training—including breathing exercises and meditation techniques—among 192 men and women with two or more coronary risk factors (e.g., high blood pressure, high cholesterol, or cigarette smoking). Subjects were randomly assigned to a treatment group that received health-education leaflets and 8 weeks of relaxation training or to a control group that received only the educational leaflets. In the relaxation group, systolic and diastolic blood pressure were significantly reduced after 8 weeks, as well as at 4-year follow-up. No significant blood pressure changes were observed in the control group; at 4-year follow-up, the control group had a significantly higher incidence of ischemic heart disease, fatal MI, or electrocardiographic evidence of ischemia. ❦ c14

Multidisciplinary Interventions

Recent cardiac intervention studies have incorporated several behavioral strategies into multidisciplinary efforts. Ornish and colleagues (100) conducted a randomized controlled clinical study of an intensive multidisciplinary intervention on patients with CAD. Twenty-eight subjects participated in the treatment group, and 20 subjects participated in the usual-care control group. Treatment subjects were provided an intensive 1-week retreat at which they were instructed in numerous areas of lifestyle change, including initiating a low-fat vegetarian diet (i.e., <10% calories from fat), practicing stress management for at least 1 hour per day (e.g., stretching and breathing exercises, meditation, progressive relaxation, and imagery), and exercising regularly (i.e., minimum of 3 hours per week with 30 minutes at target heart rate). After the retreat, intervention subjects participated in group support meetings for 4 hours twice a week. At 12-month follow-up, experimental subjects had reduced cholesterol, fewer angina episodes, and significant regression of coronary atherosclerosis, but control subjects were unchanged. Better adherence to the experimental regime was associated with greater decreases in stenosis of the arteries, as shown in Figure 11.6. Experimental subjects continued to exhibit regression of coronary atherosclerosis at 5-year follow-up; control subjects showed progressive coronary atherosclerosis and had twice as many cardiac events (101). Although the results are impressive, the study has been criticized for several reasons. The intensive nature of the treatment raises questions as to its viability, cost-effectiveness, and generalizability to larger samples. Only half of the 94 original subjects randomized to treatment and control conditions agreed to participate in the study, raising the possibility of selection bias. In addition, the study did not discriminate between the effects of individual components of the multidisciplinary treatment program.

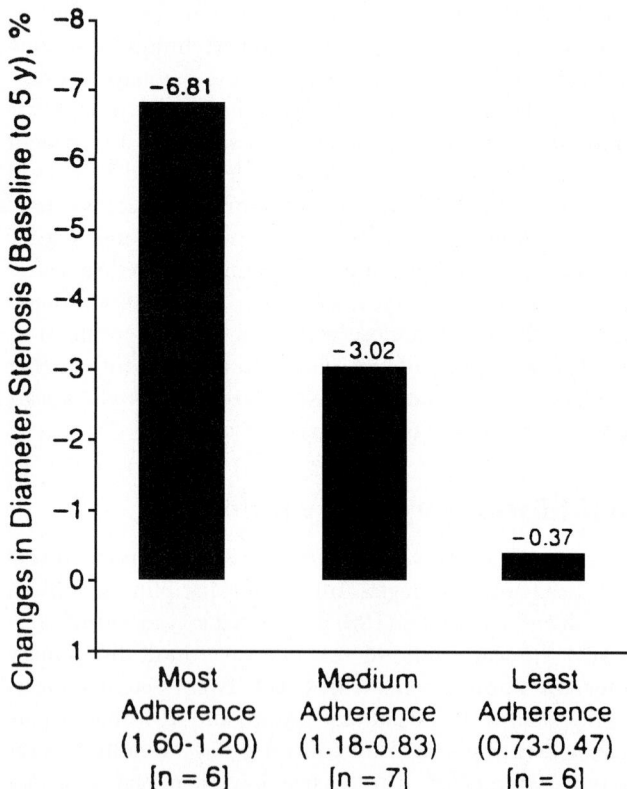

FIGURE 11.6 Percentage change in coronary arterial diameter stenosis over 5 years by adherence tertiles for coronary heart disease patients assigned to intensive lifestyle (exercise, diet, stress management) intervention. (Adapted from Ornish D, Scherwitz LW, Billings JH, et al. Intensive lifestyle changes for reversal of coronary heart disease. *JAMA* 1998;280:2005.)

The Women's Lifestyle Heart Trial (102) used the methodology developed by Ornish et al. (100) in a study of 25 postmenopausal women with CAD. Fourteen women were randomized to the treatment group, and 11 were randomized to the usual-care control group. Results at 4-, 12-, and 24-month follow-up showed significantly greater improvement for the treatment group, as reflected by decreases in body mass, angina symptoms, and hypertension medications, as well as increases in self-reported quality of life. There were also trends toward lower lipids and blood pressure in the treatment group, as well as reductions in lipid-lowering medications.

Spoth et al. (103) assessed a minimal multidisciplinary intervention in 47 patients undergoing coronary angioplasty. Patients were randomized to one of three treatment conditions: minimal intervention (1-day risk-reduction educational workshop plus individual consultation on behavior change), minimal intervention plus biofeedback training (six 1-hour sessions), or waiting-list control. Both intervention groups showed greater increases in knowledge about CVD risk reduction strategies, but the group in the combined program had a greater benefit in self-reported lifestyle behavior change.

Several community-wide primary intervention trials aimed at reducing behavioral and psychosocial risk factors have been studied [e.g., Purdue Stepped Approach Model (104); Stanford Five-Cities Project (105)]. Although clinical interventions are more intensive and responsive to individual cognitive, behavioral, and psychological needs, community interventions have the advantage of reaching a much larger audience (104). The majority of these interventions is based on health-education and health-promotion strategies; the results are generally encouraging, revealing improved use of educational resources and compliance with health-promotion programs.

The intervention strategies reviewed show promising results, but they suffer from methodologic shortcomings. Most strategies are lacking randomized control groups; many have high dropout rates, small samples, and unbalanced sample sizes in treatment conditions and lack assessment of long-term cardiac outcomes. Ethical concerns may contribute to the methodologic problems, such as reluctance to include a no-treatment control group in clinical settings. There may also be a bias toward publishing only positive results. Despite these shortcomings, the findings are encouraging and suggest that stress-management approaches can be an effective component of primary and secondary efforts to minimize the impact of CAD. Specifically, the data suggest that clinical behavioral and psychological management of cardiac patients should include (a) relaxation training, (b) education regarding cardiac risk factors, (c) identification of social and environmental stressors, (d) facilitation of social support mechanisms, and (e) focused cognitive approaches to stressful interactions (e.g., positive self-talk, thought stopping, distraction).

The data suggest that such interventions provide additional benefit to cardiac patients beyond the benefits of exercise per se. Although the efficacy of stress management and relaxation has been demonstrated, no studies have evaluated the appropriate "dose" required.

CONTROVERSIES AND PERSONAL PERSPECTIVES

Psychological Influences in Heart Disease

Decades of research have helped to refine the TABP construct and delimit its components (e.g., hostility and cynicism), which appear to be associated with the etiology of CAD. Recent data suggest that depression also may be an extremely important psychological factor in the etiology of CAD, as well as in mortality post-MI. There is acknowledgment of the importance of environmental or interpersonal factors in the manifestation of coronary-prone behavior, as well as the importance of situational appraisal as a hypothesized modifiable link between stimulus and physiologic response. The transactional model described by Smith (23) posits that the hostile individual creates situations that are challenging and stressful. Although no studies have directly tested this model, it deserves further scrutiny to evaluate the full extent to which the hostile or coronary-prone individual exerts control over physiologic responses and cognitive or emotional responses. In the treatment literature, it is assumed that individuals exert a considerable amount of influence over select aspects of physiology and cognition. However, the parameters of control must be explicated further to help direct future psychosocial interventions among patients at risk for cardiac disease.

Environmental influences also may affect the individual's health-promoting behavior, thereby having an indirect influence on the development or progression of CAD. Although the research literature has addressed various psychosocial components related to CAD, studies have not addressed more complex models integrating psychophysiologic, social, environmental, and personality variables. Thus, despite data suggesting the relevance of several psychosocial variables, there is minimal documentation of the way in which the variables interact or the relative importance of psychosocial variables. For example, O'Neil and Emery (99) found a positive relationship between anger expression and quality of social support among college undergraduates with a family history of CAD. This counterintuitive result of a higher quality of social support for people who express anger may reflect the positive aspects of a greater willingness to discuss problems and emotions with close friends. In addition, the presence of a curvilinear relationship between hostility and quantity of social support in this study suggested the possibility that social relationships may increase with a moderate degree of cynicism but not

with a high degree of cynicism (99). Thus, it is important to recognize that factors associated with CAD may interact in unexpected ways.

Brummett et al. (106) found a directly inverse relationship between CAD patients' perceived social support during hospitalization and depressive symptoms 1 month after discharge; hostility was indirectly predictive of postdischarge depressive symptomatology due to its negative association with social support. In a comparative population study of Lithuanian and Swedish men (107), a four-fold higher CAD mortality rate for Lithuanian men was associated with poor social support, low self-esteem and quality of life, depression, vital exhaustion, and poor expectations for health and well-being. Data suggest that social support may have less impact than negative emotions on cardiac events among post-MI patients (3), but further research will help to clarify models describing the relative impact of psychological and social factors in CAD.

In clinical practice, data suggest the importance of teaching relaxation skills, addressing psychological distress, especially depression and anger, and working with patients in identifying social and environmental sources of stress and support. Although none of these areas is easily addressed by the practicing cardiologist, recent data suggest that cardiac patients' satisfaction with health care providers' support is associated with enhanced recovery times (108). Thus, it is important for the cardiologist to attend to the patient's concerns and provide support directed at those concerns while encouraging the patient to make positive steps forward in recovery and health-behavior change. The cardiologist may help the patient view the illness as an opportunity to reevaluate priorities and set new goals, thereby encouraging the patient to remain oriented toward the future instead of dwelling on perceived past mistakes. Perhaps the most important role for the cardiologist is to help the patient identify specific individuals (e.g., spouse, child, friend) who will be supportive of the patient and future behavioral changes. Toward that end, cardiac rehabilitation programs provide an excellent environment for the patient to receive emotional and physical support from staff members and fellow patients, in addition to learning further strategies for exercise, nutrition, and stress management.

Measurement and Data Analysis

Despite the availability of a wide range of psychosocial assessment procedures, implementation of the assessments may be restricted. For example, metaanalysis has indicated that self-report measures of TABP are not adequate and that the Structured Interview is a preferable assessment technique for TABP (2). However, the Structured Interview is a more cumbersome and expensive assessment because it requires a face-to-face interview conducted by trained interviewers and scoring of videotaped interviews. Thus, the Structured Interview may be impractical in many settings, and clinical investigations of TABP and related factors (e.g., potential for hostility) may be constrained by inadequate measurement. Studies of more specific psychological and personality factors (e.g., depression or neuroticism) are likely to be easier because of the availability of valid and reliable self-report measures.

Technological advances have enhanced the reliability of CV reactivity measurement, and CV reactivity may have utility as an outcome for the clinician to document changes over time in physiologic response to laboratory or environmental stress. However, analysis of reactivity data remains controversial due to conflicting methodologies for analysis of the complex data resulting from reactivity studies. In addition, measurement of CV parameters, especially determination of baseline values, may be subject to experimental bias or neglect (66). Although data indicate the importance of the cardiac patient's home and work environment as potential sources of interpersonal conflict and work stress, there is a lack of reliable measurement of environmental factors and a lack of agreement regarding choice of environmental factors to measure. Because the analysis of psychological-environmental interactions in the pathogenesis of CAD remains a critical area for further study, it is important for clinicians working with cardiac patients to help elucidate relevant environmental factors to consider for evaluation.

Implementation of Behavioral and Psychological Interventions

Evidence exists for the importance of psychological factors (e.g., depression, hostility) in the pathogenesis of CAD, as well as for the effectiveness of behavioral and psychological interventions in modifying psychosocial risk factors (109). Although behavioral and psychological approaches are increasingly embraced in the practice of CV medicine, there remains a bias against directly addressing psychological issues. This bias may stem from several sources, including (a) patients and family members who are reluctant to acknowledge that psychological or social factors may play a role in the patient's health and heart condition and (b) inadequate resources available for behavioral assessment and treatment. The result of this bias is that, often, only patients who are most distressed, most difficult to manage, or unresponsive to traditional medical care are referred for behavioral and psychological evaluation. Such patients may be angry at the health care system and less

willing to address psychological issues, thereby undermining the efficacy of the intervention. However, data from randomized clinical studies support the utility of behavioral and psychological interventions for the average patient. Thus, the most efficacious approach for addressing behavioral and psychological issues among cardiac patients is to provide all patients with psychological evaluation, group support, and individual follow-up intervention as needed. The accumulated evidence supporting the relevance of behavioral and psychological factors in CAD indicates that a behavioral and psychological assessment and treatment model would be appropriate in primary care settings, as well as in rehabilitation settings. By making behavioral evaluation a routine part of practice, all patients would benefit without fear of being stigmatized.

Factors limiting the ability to implement a behavioral and psychological evaluation and treatment program among cardiac patients are the reluctance of third-party payers to reimburse for behavioral services and the difficulty that most patients have paying for medical costs out-of-pocket. This problem can be addressed, in part, by health care providers who are sensitive and responsive to behavioral issues. More important, systematic collection of behavioral and psychological outcome data can help to clarify the utility of behavioral and psychological assessment and treatment among cardiac patients and patients at risk for CAD. In addition, further clinical studies are needed that compare the effects of established behavioral interventions (e.g. relaxation training, cognitive therapy) and lifestyle interventions on the incidence and progression of CAD and that evaluate psychological factors associated with long-term adherence and behavior change among patients with CV risk factors and CAD. The accumulated evidence to date suggests that behavioral and psychological factors are of critical importance in the etiology and treatment of CAD and cardiac risk factors. By implementing and evaluating behavioral interventions, it is possible to refine intervention techniques and develop symptom- and illness-specific behavioral and psychological assessment and treatment protocols.

ACKNOWLEDGMENT

This work was supported, in part, by a grant from the National Heart, Lung, and Blood Institute.

THE FUTURE

Empirical studies have documented the potent effects of negative emotions on the development and course of CAD, and studies support the importance of CV reactivity and related neuroendocrine changes as pathophysiologic mechanisms by which stressful events may contribute to the development of CAD. Future clinical research will be dedicated to the task of evaluating the complicated interactions of social, psychophysiologic, and health behavior factors in the development of CAD and the mechanisms explaining interactions of these factors with emotions and coping skills. In addition, future research will further explore the mechanisms by which gender may interact with behavioral, psychological, and physiologic factors in the etiology of CAD. Studies will also address treatment outcomes among cardiac patients to determine the most effective strategies for minimizing the influence of negative psychosocial factors in the epidemiology of CAD.

REFERENCES

1. Friedman M, Rosenman RH. Association of specific overt behavior pattern with blood and cardiovascular findings. *JAMA* 1959;169:1286–1296.
2. Booth-Kewley S, Friedman HS. Psychological predictors of heart disease: a quantitative review. *Psychol Bull* 1987;101:343–362.
3. Frasure-Smith N, Lesperance F, Talajic M. Depression and 18-month prognosis after myocardial infarction. *Circulation* 1995;91:999–1005.
4. Orth-Gomer K, Johnson JV. Social network interaction and mortality. *J Chron Dis* 1987;40:949–957.
5. Johnson JV, Stewart W, Hall EM, et al. Long-term psychosocial work environment and cardiovascular mortality among Swedish males. *Am J Pub Health* 1996;86:324–331.
6. Krantz DS, Manuck SB. Acute physiological reactivity and risk of cardiovascular disease: a review and methodologic critique. *Psychol Bull* 1984;96:435–464.
7. Manuck SB, Olsson G, Hjemdahl P, et al. Does cardiovascular reactivity to mental stress have prognostic value in postinfarction patients? A pilot study. *Psychosom Med* 1992;54:102–108.
8. Matarazzo JD. Behavioral health and behavioral medicine: frontiers for a new health psychology. *Am Psychol* 1980;37:1–14.
9. Lazarus RS, Folkman S. *Stress, appraisal, and coping.* New York: Springer, 1984:331.
10. Aldwin CM. *Stress, coping, and development.* New York: Guilford, 1994.
11. Cannon WB. *The wisdom of the body.* New York: Norton, 1939.
12. Stoney CM. Plasma homocysteine levels increase in women during psychological stress. *Life Sci* 1999;64:2359–2365.
13. Taylor SE, Klein LC, Lewis BP, et al. Biobehavioral responses to stress in females: tend-and-befriend, not fight-or-flight. *Psychol Rev* 2000;107:411–429.
14. Eysenck HJ. Personality as a risk factor in coronary heart disease. *Eur J Pers* 1991;5:81–92.
15. Behar S, Halabi M, Reicher-Reiss H, et al. Circadian variation and possible external triggers of onset of myocardial infarction. *Am J Med* 1993;94:395–400.
16. Marmot M. Work and other factors influencing coronary health and sickness absence. *Work Stress* 1994;8:191–201.
17. Johnson JV, Hall EM. Job strain, work place social support, and cardiovascular disease: a cross-sectional study of a random sample of the Swedish working population. *Am J Pub Health* 1988;78:1336–1342.
18. Mattiasson I, Lindgarde F, Nilsson JA, et al. Threat of unemployment and cardiovascular risk factors: longitudinal study of quality of sleep and serum cholesterol concentrations in men threatened with redundancy. *BMJ* 1990;301:461–466.
19. Rosenman RH, Brand RJ, Jenkins D, et al. Coronary heart disease in Western Collaborative Group Study: final follow-up experience of 8.5 years. *JAMA* 1975;233:872–877.
20. Ragland DR, Brand RJ. Type A behavior and mortality from coronary heart disease. *N Engl J Med* 1988;318:65–69.
21. Matthews KA. Coronary heart disease and type A behaviors: update on and alternative to the Booth-Kewley and Friedman (1987) quantitative review. *Psychol Bull* 1988;104:373–380.
22. Williams RB. Refining the Type A hypothesis: emergence of the hostility complex. *Am J Cardiol* 1987;60:27J–32J.
23. Smith TW, Leon AS. *Coronary heart disease: a behavioral perspective.* Champaign, IL: Research Press, 1992:187.
24. Kamarck TW, Manuck SB, Jennings JR. Social support reduces cardiovascular reactivity to psychological challenge: a laboratory model. *Psychosom Med* 1990;52:42–58.
25. Suarez EC, Williams RB. Situational determinants of cardiovascular and emotional reactivity in high and low hostile men. *Psychosom Med* 1989;51:404–418.
26. Davidson K, Hall P, MacGregor M. Gender differences in the relation between interview-derived hostility scores and resting blood pressure. *J Behav Med* 1996;19:185–201.
27. Rosenman RH. The interview method of assessment of the coronary-prone behavior pattern. In: Dembroski TM, Weiss SM, Shields JL, et al., eds. *Coronary-prone behavior.* New York: Springer-Verlag, 1978:55–70.
28. Siegman AW, Townsend ST, Civelek AC, et al. Antagonistic behavior, dominance, hostility, and coronary heart disease. *Psychosom Med* 2000;62:248–257.
29. Lahad A, Heckbert SR, Koepsell TD, et al. Hostility, aggression and the risk of nonfatal myocardial infarction in postmenopausal women. *J Psychosom Res* 1997;43:183–195.
30. Suarez EC, Bates MP, Harralson TL. The relation of hostility to lipids and lipoproteins in women: evidence for the

role of antagonistic hostility. *Ann Behav Med* 1998;20:59–63.

31. Richards JC, Hof A, Marlies A. Serum lipids and their relationships with hostility and angry affect and behaviors in men. *Health Psychol* 2000;19:393–398.

32. Stoney CM, Engebretson TO. Plasma homocysteine concentrations are positively associated with hostility and anger. *Life Sci* 2000;66:2267–2275.

33. Muldoon MF, Herbert TB, Patterson SM, et al. Effects of acute psychological stress on serum lipid levels, hemoconcentration, and blood viscosity. *Arch Intern Med* 1995;155:615–620.

34. Barefoot JC, Schroll M. Symptoms of depression, acute myocardial infarction, and total mortality in a community sample. *Circulation* 1996;93:1976–1980.

35. Frasure-Smith N, Prince R. The ischemic heart disease life stress monitoring program: impact on mortality. *Psychosom Med* 1985;47:431–445.

36. Carney RM, Rich MW, Freedland KE, et al. Major depressive disorder predicts cardiac events in patients with coronary artery disease. *Psychosom Med* 1988;50:627–633.

37. Dalack GW, Roose SP. Perspectives on the relationship between cardiovascular disease and affective disorder. *J Clin Psychiatr* 1990;51:4–9.

38. Stein PK, Carney RM, Freedland KE, et al. Severe depression is associated with markedly reduced heart rate variability in patients with stable coronary heart disease. *J Psychosom Res* 2000;48:493–500.

39. Carney RM, Freedland KE, Veith RC, et al. Major depression, heart rate, and plasma norepinephrine in patients with coronary heart disease. *Biol Psychiatr* 1999;45:458–463.

40. Blumenthal JA, Babyak M, Moore KA, et al. Effects of exercise training on older adults with major depression. *Arch Intern Med* 2000;159:2349–2356.

41. Babyak M, Blumenthal JA, Herman S, et al. Exercise treatment for major depression: maintenance of therapeutic benefit at 10 months. *Psychosom Med* 2000;62:633–638.

42. Travella JI, Forrester AW, Schultz SK, et al. Depression following myocardial infarction: a one year longitudinal study. *Int J Psychiatr Med* 1994;24:357–369.

43. Denollet J, Sys SU, Brutsaert DL. Personality and mortality after myocardial infarction. *Psychosom Med* 1995;57:582–591.

44. Powell LH, Thoresen CE. Behavioral and physiologic determinants of long-term prognosis after myocardial infarction. *J Chron Dis* 1985;38:253–263.

45. Shekelle RB, Vernon SW, Ostfeld AM. Personality and coronary heart disease. *Psychosom Med* 1991;53:176–184.

46. Cohen S, Wills TA. Stress, social support, and the buffering hypothesis. *Psychol Bull* 1985;98:310–357.

47. Olsen RB, Olsen J, Gunner-Svensson F, et al. Social networks and longevity. A 14 year follow-up study among elderly in Denmark. *Soc Sci Med* 1991;33:1189–1195.

48. Welin L, Larsson B, Svardsudd K, et al. Social network an activities in relation to mortality from cardiovascular diseases, cancer other causes: a 12 year follow up of the study of men born in 1913 and 1923. *J Epidemiol Commun Health* 1992;46:127–132.

49. O'Reilly P, Thomas HE. Role of support networks in maintenance of improved cardiovascular health status. *Soc Sci Med* 1989;28:249–260.

50. Olsen O. Impact of social network on cardiovascular mortality in middle aged Danish men. *J Epidemiol Commun Health* 1993;47:176–180.

51. Blumenthal JA, Burg MM, Barefoot J, et al. Social support, Type A behavior, and coronary artery disease. *Psychosom Med* 1987;49:331–340.

52. Gorkin L, Follick MJ, Wilkin DL, et al. Social support and the progression and treatment of cardiovascular disease. In: Shumaker SA, Czajkowski SM, eds. *Social support and cardiovascular disease*. New York: Plenum, 1994:281–300.

53. Gliksman MD, Lazarus R, Wilson A, et al. Social support, marital status and living arrangement correlates of cardiovascular disease risk factors in the elderly. *Soc Sci Med* 1995;40:811–814.

54. Venters M, Jacobs DR, Pirie P, et al. Marital status and the cardiovascular risk: the Minnesota Heart Survey and the Minnesota Heart Health Program. *Prev Med* 1986;15:591–605.

55. Carmelli D, Swan GE, Rosenman RH. The relationship between wives' social and psychologic status and their husbands' coronary heart disease. A case-control family study from the Western Collaborative Group Study. *Am J Epidemiol* 1985;122:90–100.

56. Kamarck TW, Annunziato B, Amateau LM. Affiliation moderates the effects of social threat on stress-related cardiovascular responses: boundary conditions for a laboratory model of social support. *Psychosom Med* 1995;57:183–194.

57. Jackson C, Winkleby MA, Flora JA, et al. Use of educational resources for cardiovascular risk reduction in the Stanford Five-City Project. *Am J Prev Med* 1991;7:82–88.

58. Ewart CK. A social problem-solving approach to behavior change in coronary heart disease. In: Shumaker SA, Schron EB, Ockene JK, eds. *The handbook of health behavior change*. New York: Springer, 1990:153–190.

59. Hellman EA. Use of the stages of change in exercise adherence model among older adults with a cardiac diagnosis. *J Cardiopulm Rehabil* 1997;17:145–155.

60. Prochaska JO, DiClemente CC. Stages and processes of self-change in smoking: toward an integrative model of change. *J Consult Clin Psychol* 1983;51:390–395.

61. Bock BC, Albrecht AE, Traficante RM, et al. Predictors of exercise adherence following participation in a cardiac rehabilitation program. *Int J Behav Med* 1997;4:60–75.

62. Hershberger PJ, Robertson KB, Markert RJ. Personality and appointment-keeping adherence in cardiac rehabilitation. *J Cardiopulm Rehabil* 1999;19:106–111.

63. Naslund GK, Fredrikson M, Hellenius ML, et al. Determinants of compliance in men enrolled in a diet and exercise intervention trial: a randomized, controlled study. *Patient Educ Couns* 1996;29:247–256.

64. Burker EJ, Fredrikson M, Rifai N, et al. Serum lipids, neuroendocrine, and cardiovascular responses to stress in men and women with mild hypertension. *Behav Med* 1994;19:155–161.

65. Manuck SB, Kaplan JR, Clarkson TB. Behaviorally-induced heart rate reactivity and atherosclerosis in cynomolgus monkeys. *Psychosom Med* 1983;45:95–108.

66. Krantz DS, Falconer JJ. Measurement of cardiovascular responses. In: Cohen S, Kessler RC, Underwood GL, eds. *Measuring stress: a guide for health and social scientists*. New York: Oxford University Press, 1995:193–212.

67. Garcia CA, Tweedy JR, Blass JP. Underdiagnosis of cognitive impairment in a rehabilitation setting. *J Am Geriatr Soc* 1984;32:339–342.

68. Reich P, Regestein QR, Murawski BJ, et al. Unrecognized organic mental disorders in survivors of cardiac arrest. *Am J Psychiatr* 1983;140:1194–1197.

69. Barclay LL, Weiss EM, Mattis S, et al. Unrecognized cognitive impairment in cardiac rehabilitation patients. *J Am Geriatr Soc* 1988;36:22–28.

70. Byrne DG, Rosenman RH, Schiller E, et al. Consistency and variation among instruments purporting to measure the Type A behavior pattern. *Psychosom Med* 1985;47:242–261.

71. Dembroski TM, Costa PT Jr. Coronary-prone behavior: components of the Type A pattern and hostility. *J Pers* 1987;55:211–235.

72. Cook WW, Medley DM. Proposed hostility and pharisaic-virtue scales for the MMPI. *J Appl Psychol* 1954;38:414–418.

73. Hathaway SR, McKinley JC. *The Minnesota multiphasic personality inventory manual.* Minneapolis: University of Minnesota Press, 1943.

74. Beck AT, Steer RA. *Beck depression inventory manual.* San Antonio: The Psychological Corporation, Harcourt Brace Jovanovich, 1987.

75. Sarason IG, Levine HM, Basham RB, et al. Assessing social support: the Social Support Questionnaire. *J Pers Soc Psychol* 1983;44:127–139.

76. Schnall PL, Pieper C, Schwartz JE, et al. The relationship between "job strain," workplace diastolic blood pressure, and left ventricular mass index. Results of a case-control study. *JAMA* 1990;263:1929–1935.

77. Langosch W, Seer P, Grodner G, et al. Behavior therapy with coronary heart disease patients: results of a comparative study. *J Psychosom Res* 1982;26:475–484.

78. Goldberg DP. *The detection of psychiatric illness by questionnaire.* London: Oxford University Press, 1972.

79. Nelson DV, Baer PE, Cleveland SE, et al. Six-month follow-up of stress management training versus cardiac education during hospitalization for acute myocardial infarction. *J Cardiopulm Rehabil* 1994;14:384–390.

80. Gatchel RJ, Gaffney FA, Smith JE. Comparative efficacy of behavioral stress management versus propranolol in reducing psychophysiological reactivity in post-myocardial infarction patients. *J Behav Med* 1986;9:503–513.

81. Turner L, Linden W, van der Wal R, et al. Stress management for patients with heart disease: a pilot study. *Heart Lung* 1995;24:145–153.

82. Blumenthal JA, Jiang W, Babyak MA, et al. Stress management and exercise training in cardiac patients with myocardial ischemia. Effects on prognosis and evaluation of mechanisms. *Arch Intern Med* 1997;157:2213–2223.

83. Dusseldorp E, van Elderen T, Maes S, et al. A meta-analysis of psychoeducational programs for coronary heart disease patients. *Health Psychol* 1999;18:506–519.

84. Patel C, Marmot MG, Terry DJ, et al. Trial of relaxation in reducing coronary risk: four year follow up. *BMJ* 1985;290:1103–1106.

85. Trzcieniecka-Green A, Steptoe A. Stress management in cardiac patients: a preliminary study of the predictors of improvement in quality of life. *J Psychosom Res* 1994;38:267–280.

86. Bohachick P. Progressive relaxation training in cardiac rehabilitation: effect on psychologic variables. *Nurs Res* 1984;33:283–287.

87. Munro BH, Creamer AM, Haggerty MR, et al. Effect of relaxation therapy on post-myocardial infarction patients' rehabilitation. *Nurs Res* 1988;37:231–235.

88. van Dixhoorn J, Duivenvoorden HJ, Staal HA, et al. Physical training and relaxation therapy in cardiac rehabilitation assessed through a composite criterion for training outcome. *Am Heart J* 1989;118:545–552.

89. van Dixhoorn J, Duivenvoorden HJ, Staal JA, et al. Cardiac events after myocardial infarction: possible effect of relaxation therapy. *Eur Heart J* 1987;8:1210–1214.

90. van Dixhoorn J, Duivenvoorden HJ, Pool J, et al. Psychic effects of physical training and relaxation therapy after myocardial infarction. *J Psychosom Res* 1990;34:327–337.

91. Conn VS, Taylor SG, Wiman P. Anxiety, depression, quality of life, and self-care among survivors of myocardial infarction. *Issues Ment Health Nurs* 1991;12:321–331.

92. Adsett CA, Bruhn JG. Short-term group psychotherapy for post-myocardial infarction patients and their wives. *Can Med Assoc J* 1968;99:577–584.

93. Oldenburg B, Perkins RJ, Andrews G. Controlled trial of psychological intervention in myocardial infarction. *J Consult Clin Psychol* 1985;53:852–859.

94. Friedman M, Thoresen CE, Gill JJ, et al. Alteration of Type A behavior and its effect on cardiac recurrences in post myocardial infarction patients: summary results of the recurrent coronary prevention project. *Am Heart J* 1986;112:653–665.

95. Bennet P, Carroll D. Cognitive-behavioural interventions in cardiac rehabilitation. *J Psychosom Res* 1994;38:169–182.

96. Gidron Y, Davidson K, Bata I. The short-term effects of a hostility-reduction intervention on male coronary heart disease patients. *Health Psychol* 1999;18:416–420.

97. Davidson K, MacGregor W, Stuhr J, et al. Increasing constructive anger verbal behavior decreases resting blood pressure: a secondary analysis of a randomized controlled hostility intervention. *Int J Behav Med* 1999;6:268–278.

98. Stoney CM, Engebretson TO. Anger and hostility: potential mediators of the gender difference in coronary heart disease. In: Siegman AW, Smith TW, eds. *Anger, hostility, and the heart.* New Jersey: Erlbaum, 1994:215–237.

99. O'Neil JN, Emery CF. Family history of coronary heart disease, psychosocial vulnerability, and hostility among male and female college students. Manuscript under review, 2001.

100. Ornish D, Brown SE, Scherwitz LW, et al. Can lifestyle changes reverse coronary heart disease? *Lancet* 1990;336:129–133.

101. Ornish D, Scherwitz LW, Billings JH, et al. Intensive lifestyle changes for reversal of coronary heart disease. *JAMA* 1998;280:2001–2007.

102. Toobert DJ, Glasgow RE, Radcliffe JL. Physiologic and related behavioral outcomes from the Women's Lifestyle Heart Trial. *Ann Behav Med* 2000;22:1–16.

103. Spoth RL, Dush DM, Conley M. Evaluating minimal intervention health promotion in a clinical context. *Int Q Commun Health Educ* 1992;12:203–216.

104. Black DR, Hultsman JT. The Purdue Stepped Approach Model: sequencing community and clinical interventions to

reduce cardiovascular risk factors. *Int Q Commun Health Educ* 1989–90;10:19–37.

105. Winkleby MA, Flora JA, Kraemer HC. A community-based heart disease intervention: predictors of change. *Am J Pub Health* 1994;84:767–772.

106. Brummett BH, Babyak MA, Barefoot JC, et al. Social support and hostility as predictors of depressive symptoms in cardiac patients one month after hospitalization: a prospective study. *Psychosom Med* 1998;60:707–713.

107. Kristenson M, Kucinskiene Z, Bergdahl B, et al. Increased psychosocial strain in Lithuanian versus Swedish men: the LiVicordia study. *Psychosom Med* 1998;60:277–282.

108. Yates BC. The relationships among social support and short- and long-term recovery outcomes in men with coronary heart disease. *Res Nurs Health* 1995;18:193–203.

109. Kawachi I, Sparrow D, Spiro A III, et al. A prospective study of anger and coronary heart disease: the normative aging study. *Circulation* 1996;94:2090–2095.

CARDIAC REHABILITATION AND SECONDARY PREVENTION

PHILIP A. ADES

▼▼ ADDITIONAL ELECTRONIC TOPICS

Adaptations to Exercise Conditioning in Patients with Coronary Heart Disease c15;   Psychological Factors c16;   Exercise Prescription c17;   Organizational Issues c18;   Cost-Effectiveness Analysis c19

Cardiac rehabilitation is a well-defined process that has changed over the years from a narrowly focused, closely monitored exercise program for coronary patients to a widely applied secondary prevention process, available to a broad range of patients with cardiovascular disease. Risk reduction outcomes are closely tied to specific individualized patient goals, often delivered in a case-management format. The greatest benefits are often manifest in the highest-risk patients and extend to women, elderly patients, and patients with chronic heart failure (CHF). The best determinant of patient participation in cardiac rehabilitation is the strength of the primary physician's recommendations, and these physicians should be actively recruited into the rehabilitation process from acute coronary event to participation in long-term preventive care.

Cardiac rehabilitation is highly cost-effective and is associated with a decrease in cardiac hospitalizations. The cardiac rehabilitation facility should be viewed as the clinical site at which systematic secondary prevention services are delivered in an outpatient setting in collaboration with the primary physician. The maintenance of physical functioning, the prevention of coronary disability, and the

prevention of recurrent coronary events are the primary outcome goals.

BACKGROUND

Cardiovascular disease is the leading cause of death and premature disability in the United States for both men and women (1). It is also a major cause of disability in the rapidly growing elderly population (2,3). Coronary artery disease (CAD) usually presents clinically as angina pectoris or acute myocardial infarction and affects more than 13 million Americans, with many more cases remaining undiagnosed. More than 1 million individuals survive a myocardial infarction yearly in the United States, and another 750,000 undergo coronary revascularization procedures (4,5). The maintenance of physical functioning and the prevention of second coronary events and rehospitalizations in these populations are major preventive health challenges and require a systematic approach.

The current perspective of cardiac rehabilitation is that of a structured "secondary prevention" center, with on-site and home-based exercise programs, lipid clinics, weight loss programs, and other risk-factor modification components aimed at preventing second coronary events, cardiac rehos-

P. A. Ades: Division of Cardiology, University of Vermont College of Medicine, Burlington, Vermont

pitalizations, and cardiac disability in patients with established CAD (6,7). Cardiac rehabilitation services include medical evaluation; prescribed exercise; and cardiac risk-factor modification, education, and counseling. Services are tied to a series of short-term and longer-term outcomes, which include return to work and measures of physical functioning, cardiac symptoms, psychological well-being, risk factors, progression of coronary atherosclerosis, recurrence of cardiac events, and number of rehospitalizations. Cardiac rehabilitation is prescribed for patients with myocardial infarction, coronary bypass surgery or percutaneous angioplasty, chronic angina pectoris, CHF, or heart transplantation and for selected patients who have had valvular heart surgery or exertional arrhythmias (8,9). Debate is ongoing as to whether early outpatient exercise training requires direct supervision or whether it could effectively be more widely applied, for low- and moderate-risk patients, in the home setting (10–13).

HISTORICAL PERSPECTIVE

Cardiac rehabilitation was conceived in an era when post–myocardial infarction activity prescriptions were evolving from 6 weeks of bed rest in the 1930s, to "chair" therapy in the 1940s, to 3 to 5 minutes of walking per day at 4 weeks in the 1950s (14–16). By the early 1960s, clinicians recognized that early ambulation helped patients avoid many of the complications of bed rest, such as pulmonary embolism and deconditioning, and in-hospital ambulation gradually displaced long-term bed rest as the standard of care (17–19). As the ambulation process extended beyond hospital discharge, concerns about the safety of unsupervised exercise resulted in the development of highly structured, physician-supervised, electrocardiographically monitored exercise programs in the 1970s. The focus was almost exclusively on exercise. By the 1990s, hospitalizations for acute myocardial infarction had shortened and are now as brief as 3 to 4 days (20), so that deconditioning is minimal. However, so is the opportunity to counsel patients about risk-factor modification. Smoking-relapse prevention programs, initiated in-hospital, have proven effective (21), but therapy and education for other modifiable risk factors are largely left for the postdischarge period.

With the development of a body of literature supporting the benefits of risk-factor modification in coronary patients (called *secondary prevention*), the cardiac rehabilitation center has evolved to become a clinical site for the systematic delivery of secondary prevention services. Recently demonstrated benefits of cardiac rehabilitation and secondary prevention in coronary patients are broad and compelling. Metaanalyses of exercise rehabilitation after acute myocardial infarction have demonstrated a 20% to 25% decrease in the overall mortality rate and in sudden cardiac death in the 3 years after infarction (22,23). Complementary trials

of exercise and low-fat diets have demonstrated a slowing of the atherosclerotic process (24,25), and studies that incorporated multiple risk-factor interventions (10), pharmacologic lipid-lowering, or both, demonstrated a decrease in coronary events and a retardation of atherosclerosis (26). Despite these well-described advantages, fewer than 15% of patients who might benefit currently participate in formal cardiac rehabilitation (27). ⌖ c20

SCIENTIFIC FOUNDATION OF CARDIAC REHABILITATION AND SECONDARY PREVENTION

Determinants of Exercise Capacity and Physical Functioning in Coronary Patients

The cardinal symptoms of coronary heart disease (CHD), angina, and exertional dyspnea depend on a complex interplay of vascular biologic abnormalities and cardiac hemodynamics, compounded by deconditioning and psychological factors. [⌖ c21] Angina pectoris and ischemic left ventricular (LV) dysfunction result from an imbalance of myocardial oxygen supply and demand. In the presence of coronary atherosclerosis, exercise-induced increases in blood flow are limited both by the presence of atheroma and by an abnormal vascular endothelial response that paradoxically results in exertional vasoconstriction (31,32).

In the presence of chronic exertional angina, supervised aerobic exercise training programs have clearly been shown to increase the anginal threshold, and at a given workload, myocardial oxygen demand is lower (33) (Fig. 12.1). In one study, after 3 months of aerobic training, 7 of 18 patients who had exertional angina before conditioning could no longer reach their angina threshold after conditioning (34). In the 1-year study by Ornish and associates, a combination of aerobic exercise, a very low-fat diet, and meditation led to a 91% decrease in angina frequency and a 28% decrease in angina severity (25).

Many patients with CAD are limited by coronary ischemia in the absence of angina, often manifested as dyspnea or fatigue. Furthermore, LV diastolic abnormalities, which are particularly common in older coronary patients, lead to exertional dyspnea, which may be exercise limiting (35,36). A smaller number of patients are limited by exertional arrhythmias, peripheral vascular disease, and comorbidities independent of their CAD.

More than 25% of patients with CAD appear to terminate exercise at treadmill testing before the attainment of a true physiologic maximal effort in the absence of coronary ischemia, heart failure, and arrhythmias (37,38). This effect is particularly notable in the older coronary population, in which as many as one-third of patients terminate exercise prematurely, before significant anaerobic metabolism has

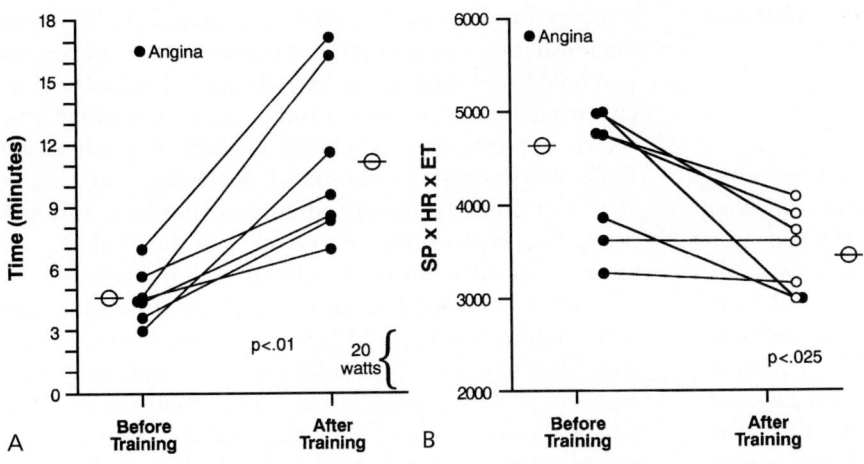

FIGURE 12.1 Effect of 6 weeks of training on exercise capacity **(A)** and triple product **(B)** in patients who have exertional angina. ET, ejection time; HR, heart rate; SP, systolic pressure. (From Redwood DR, Rosing DR, Epstein SE. Circulatory and symptomatic effects of physical training in patients with coronary-artery disease and angina pectoris. *N Engl J Med* 1972;286:959–965, with permission.)

been measured, in the absence of angina or ischemia (37). These findings are supported by a study on cardiac disability in which many patients describe limiting their daily activities because of a fear of adverse cardiac consequences, based on advice or misinformation, rather than on account of specific symptoms, such as angina or dyspnea (38) (Fig. 12.2). Rehabilitation programs that counsel patients about the safety of specific employment-related and daily living activities and that reproduce these activities in a monitored setting are designed to facilitate return to premorbid activities (39,40). This is supported by improvements in patient-reported physical function scores after cardiac rehabilitation (11,13,41). ⚓ c22

Clinical Effects of Exercise Conditioning in Coronary Patients

Exercise Tolerance

The effect of supervised exercise conditioning programs on exercise tolerance in populations of patients with

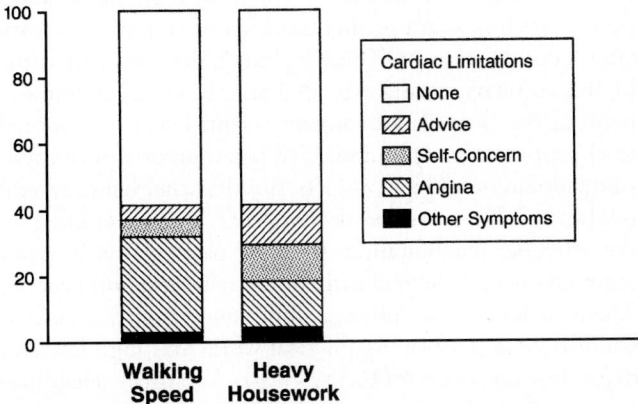

FIGURE 12.2 Patients' perception of reasons why heart disease limited them in walking speed and in heavy housework. (From Neill WA, Branch LG, De Jong GD, et al. Cardiac disability. The impact of coronary heart disease on patient's daily activities. *Arch Intern Med* 1985;145:1642–1647, with permission.)

CAD has been extensively studied. The Federal Clinical Practice Guideline on cardiac rehabilitation describes a total of 35 randomized, controlled trials of cardiac rehabilitation exercise training on measures of exercise tolerance, and the vast majority documents a clear benefit of exercise training on the outcome measure of exercise tolerance (8) (*e*Fig. 12.2.2). These exercise conditioning studies consisted of uncomplicated patients after myocardial infarction who began their exercise program 4 to 52 weeks after the coronary event (22–24,66,67). After 3 months of aerobic conditioning three times weekly, at an intensity of 70% to 85% of maximal heart rate, exercise tolerance on the treadmill increased by 30% to 50%, and peak oxygen consumption increased by 15% to 20%. ⚓ c23

Morbidity and Mortality Rate

The effect of cardiac rehabilitation programs on long-term morbidity and mortality rates, particularly in patients who have experienced myocardial infarction, has been extensively studied. These studies, however, took place in the 1970s and 1980s, before the widespread use of thrombolytic therapy, coronary angioplasty, stents, and angiotensin-converting enzyme inhibitors. Although several individual randomized, controlled trials documented significant decreases in the long-term mortality rate (66,80–82), metaanalyses have provided the best data on the effect of cardiac rehabilitation on the mortality rate in patients who have experienced myocardial infarction. In the metaanalyses of Oldridge, O'Connor, and their coworkers, which included more than 4,000 patients in 21 randomized, controlled trials, cardiac rehabilitation was associated with a 25% reduction in the mortality rate compared with the rate among control subjects at an average follow-up of 3 years (22,23) (*e*Fig. 12.2.3). More than 80% of the patients in these studies were male, and they were primarily younger than 65 years. Studies in which the intervention involved exercise and risk-factor modification showed a greater benefit than studies in which the intervention was exercise only (23). ❦ c24

Effects on Lipid Levels and Obesity

Studies of cardiac rehabilitation exercise programs on serum lipid levels in the absence of focused nutritional counseling document modest, though favorable, effects. Although exercise has no consistent effect on low-density lipoprotein (LDL) cholesterol levels, a consistent favorable increase of high-density lipoprotein (HDL) cholesterol of 8% to 23% has been demonstrated (89–91). Decreases of 3% to 21% in serum triglyceride levels after 1 to 2 years of exercise have also been demonstrated (92–94). Numerous studies that combined exercise with behavioral counseling and dietary instruction have documented consistent beneficial effects on serum lipid levels that include decreases in LDL cholesterol and serum triglyceride levels and maintenance or slight increase in HDL cholesterol (10,11,24,25,95). For example, in the diet-exercise studies of Schuler and Ornish, reductions in LDL cholesterol of 11% and 37%, respectively, were attained (24,25). In some patients, lipid-lowering medications are required to meet treatment goals (29), and the benefits of aggressive therapy include a retardation of the atherosclerotic process and a decrease in long-term coronary events (10,26).

Studies on the effect of cardiac rehabilitation exercise without intensive nutritional counseling on measures of obesity have documented only modest benefits (82,90, 96,97). This may be because of the surprisingly low exercise-related caloric expenditure noted with cardiac rehabilitation exercise programs, particularly in female and older participants (98,99). A promising intervention that merits further study is the modification of cardiac rehabilitation exercise protocols to maximize caloric expenditure. This involves increasing the frequency and duration of exercise, at slightly lower intensities, and using non–weight-supported exercise such as walking (100). In studies that incorporated a very low-fat dietary intervention in addition to the exercise intervention, consistent improvements in body mass index [(weight in kg)/(height in m)^2] have been demonstrated (10,24,25). Although obesity is an independent risk factor for the development of CAD (101,102), in the setting of established CAD, reduction of obesity, particularly abdominal obesity, acts as a multifactorial intervention with associated improvements in lipid profiles and measures of insulin resistance and a lowering of blood pressure (96,103–105). Aerobic exercise training alone is associated with a reduction in abdominal obesity, even in the absence of major changes of weight in healthy elderly individuals and in CHD patients (90,106).

Psychological Effects

Many patients state that psychological effects of cardiac rehabilitation programs play a major role in their successful recovery from a cardiac event. In practice, the objective demonstration of measurable improvements in markers of psychological function has been difficult. Studies of exercise rehabilitation without psychological counseling have shown improvements in selected markers of psychological functioning, such as measures of depression and tension (107,108), although these findings have not been universal (109). Group psychological counseling in the rehabilitation setting has demonstrated objective improvements in selected psychological measures, such as depression and social adjustment (110–112). In addition, a metaanalytic study has noted that the addition of psychosocial treatments to standard cardiac rehabilitation regimens results in a reduction in mortality rates and morbidity over a 2-year period, along with a reduction in psychological distress (113). A randomized, controlled trial of relaxation training in cardiac rehabilitation resulted in a significant decrease in total cardiac events (114).

The magnitude of improvement in dysfunctional behavior in CHD patients is a function of the intensity of the counseling component of a multifactorial rehabilitation intervention. This generally includes group counseling on stress management, relaxation training, and guidance on social adjustment and recovery. Another important role of the group sessions is to identify patients who require more intensive counseling or pharmacologic therapy to avoid psychological symptoms and psychological disability. Depression, in particular, has been demonstrated not only to be a quality-of-life issue, but to predict 6-month mortality rates after myocardial infarction and rate of cardiac rehospitalizations, independent of the severity of cardiac disease (115,116).

Employment

A return to prior employment status is an important integrated measure of successful recovery from a coronary event. Numerous factors independent of the rehabilitation process are important predictors of failure to return to work after a coronary event. These include older age at the time of the coronary event, extended sick leave or unemployment at the time of the coronary event, lower educational level, employment in an unskilled position, or a prior myocardial infarction (86,117–119). On the other hand, several predictors of return to work may be favorably modified by the exercise rehabilitation process, particularly if work requirements are defined early in the rehabilitation process. These include a low physical function capacity, a lack of confidence in performing physical work, and high levels of depression or anxiety (86,117–119). A cardiac rehabilitation program that simulates elements of work during the training process has proven to be more effective at returning cardiac patients to work than standard cardiac rehabilitation without job simulation (39,40,117). Studies that have applied a generic exercise training routine to all participants have had little success in enhancing return-to-work rates (67,81,82,85,109,119). ❦ c25

Older Patients

More than one-half of the patients who are eligible for cardiac rehabilitation services are older than 65 years. According to the Framingham Disability Study, which defined disability by work and mobility limitations, disability rates in older coronary patients are extremely high (2). In patients older than 70 years, 79% of women and 49% of men with CAD were found to be disabled (Table 12.1). The direct causes of disability in older coronary patients have received little study, although preliminary work suggests that the best predictors of poor physical function in older coronary patients are a low aerobic fitness capacity and the presence of mental depression, both of which are treatable (121). Despite this, older coronary patients are far less likely to participate in cardiac rehabilitation than younger patients (122,123). The rate of participation for patients older than 62 years is less than one-half that seen in younger patients (122). The primary reason for nonparticipation is a low rate of physician referral (122). ❦ c26

Women

After menopause, the incidence of CAD rises steadily; by age 65 years, the prevalence of CAD in women approaches that in men (126,127). Despite this, women are a definite minority among cardiac rehabilitation participants (122). The primary reason for this appears to be lower referral rates by primary physicians rather than clinical differences between male and female patients (122). Relatively little study has been made of the relative benefits and special needs of women in cardiac rehabilitation, although women and men improve exercise capacity with training to a similar degree (122,128). Women, however, appear to experience less weight loss, and risk factors improve to a lesser degree, probably owing to a significantly lower exercise-related energy expenditure during cardiac rehabilitation sessions (90,99).

TABLE 12.1 FRAMINGHAM DISABILITY STUDY DISABILITY RATES: AGES 70–88 YEARS

	Men (%)	Women (%)
No CAD or CHF	27	49
CAD	39	61
Angina	56	84
CHF	57	88

CAD, coronary artery disease; CHF, congestive heart failure.
Adapted from Pinsky JL, Jette AM, Branch LG, et al. The Framingham Disability Study: relationship of various coronary heart disease manifestations to disability in older persons living in the community. *Am J Public Health* 1990;80:1363–1368.

The current model of cardiac rehabilitation was developed primarily for middle-aged male coronary patients in the 1960s and 1970s. Early after myocardial infarction, women have a lower functional capacity than men, they are generally older, they are more likely to have residual angina, and they have more prominent risk-factor profiles; therefore, rehabilitation needs may differ from those of male participants (122,126,129,130). ❦ c27

Chronic Heart Failure

Patients with CHF are the most highly symptomatic group of patients with cardiovascular disease, and their activities are often limited by low-threshold exertional dyspnea and fatigue. Because of the progressive aging of the population and the improved prognosis of patients with CHF who receive pharmacologic therapy with angiotensin-converting enzyme inhibitors (133,134), the absolute size of the American population with CHF is gradually increasing. At present, more than 2 million Americans experience CHF, with 400,000 new cases diagnosed yearly (135). The mortality rate is high, at a 5-year mortality rate of roughly 50% (135).

Recent studies show that patients with CHF can safely undergo exercise conditioning and that regular exercise improves functional status and decreases symptoms (47,136–138) (Fig. 12.3). Furthermore, in a randomized, controlled trial, 1 year of moderately intense aerobic exercise improved patient-reported measures of quality of life and decreased overall mortality and hospital readmission rates (139)

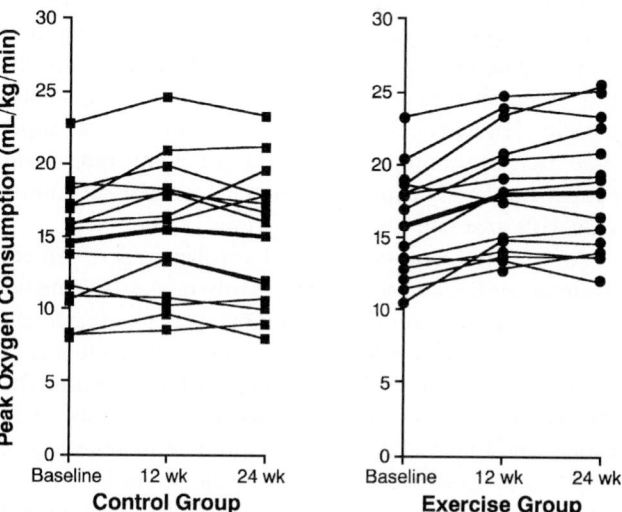

FIGURE 12.3 Peak oxygen consumption in patients with compensated heart failure who do not have exercise training (control group, n = 14) and who did have exercise training (exercise group, n = 15). The heavy line represents the mean value across time, with a significant difference between groups (*p* <.05). (From Keteyian SJ, Levine AD, Brawner CA, et al. Exercise training in patients with heart failure: a randomized, controlled trial. *Ann Intern Med* 1996;124:1051–1057, with permission.)

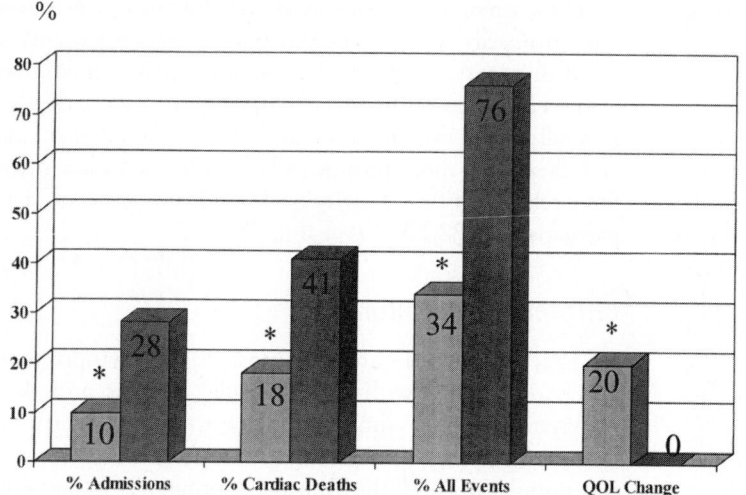

FIGURE 12.4 Randomized, controlled trial of exercise training in patients with chronic heart failure (n = 99; mean follow-up, 3.3 ± 0.15 years). *$p < .05$ compared with control group. QOL, quality of life. (Adapted from Belardinelli R, Georgiou D, Cianci G, et al. Randomized, controlled trial of long-term moderate exercise training in chronic heart failure: effects on functional capacity, quality of life, and clinical outcome. *Circulation* 1999;99:1173–1182.)

(Fig. 12.4). Neurohormonal activation and lactate production during submaximal exercise is also diminished by a regular, supervised, home-based exercise program (136), and exercise training augments the symptomatic and functional benefits of angiotensin-converting enzyme inhibitors (137). Peripheral (skeletal muscle) adaptations appear to mediate the improvement in exercise tolerance (47). In addition to improving the peripheral extraction of oxygen, aerobic conditioning in CHF is associated with an increase in cardiac output both during submaximal and maximal exercise (136).

There is insufficient evidence to recommend a specific type of training program for patients with CHF, although existing studies have focused primarily on aerobic exercises such as cycling or treadmill walking rather than resistance training (47,136–138). Effects of combined strength and aerobic training in patients with CHF is a promising intervention that improves muscular strength, aerobic capacity, and endothelial-dependent and -independent vasodilator capacity (140,141). In addition to the benefits of supervised exercise training, rehabilitation programs can provide patient and family counseling and facilitate patient compliance with treatment recommendations (135).

An exercise conditioning trial involving CHF patients awaiting cardiac transplantation involved maximal medical therapy and a prescribed walking program. Patients gradually worked up to walking 20 to 30 minutes or 2 miles four times per week at a moderate exercise intensity for 6 months. Peak exercise tolerance improved in 38 of 68 clinically stable patients, and after an average of 6 months of follow-up, 31 of those 38 patients had improved sufficiently to be removed from the transplant list (142). After transplantation, exercise tolerance improves with aerobic exercise training, using perceived exertion as a guide to exercise intensity (143–145).

Resistance Training

Resistance- or weight-training protocols have long been discouraged in coronary patients because of fears of cardiac complications that can be caused by blood pressure elevations during the lifting phase of such exercise (146). However, carefully screened subsets of CAD patients younger than 65 years have safely participated in resistance-training programs, with impressive increases in strength and no adverse cardiac effects (146–149). Recent data also confirm increases in strength measures after 3 months of resistance training in older coronary patients of approximately 19% to 24% (124). It is important to note that when strength is low, it is a limiting factor in endurance activities, such as walking (150). Thus, in elderly patients, walking endurance improves with resistance training in the absence of aerobic training (151).

Resistance training is of particular importance in women, elderly patients, and coronary patients who plan to return to physically demanding employment (132,148). In healthy individuals, the conditioning response to resistance training includes fiber hypertrophy and an increase in oxidative enzyme activity without an increase in peak aerobic capacity (152). An important functional result is a decreased heart-rate response to a given resistive workload (147,151,152). c28

From a practical point of view, the onset of upper body resistance training should be delayed until 3 months after coronary bypass grafting surgery to allow full sternal healing to occur, whereas it can commence as early as 1 month after myocardial infarction or 1 to 2 weeks after a successful percutaneous coronary intervention, after performance of a satisfactory baseline exercise tolerance test. The resistance-training program should include training of the leg extensor muscles to assist with walking and stair climbing and upper body training to aid in the lifting and pushing required for the performance of daily household activities. A report on the results of resistance training in disabled older women with CHD documented increased strength, endurance, balance, coordination, and measures of physical performance during practical activities such as stair climbing and grocery carrying (125).

Secondary Prevention

Lipids

It is now well established that lowering blood lipid levels reduces clinical events and mortality rates in patients known to have CHD. Numerous controlled clinical trials [✌ c29], most with quantitative coronary angiography, have demonstrated the efficacy of pharmacologic and diet-induced lipid lowering on slowing the progression of angiographic measures of atherosclerosis and on reducing clinical coronary events (10,24,25,84,162–164). Low-fat diets, without accompanying drug treatment, have been effective in reducing the prevalence of angiographic progression of CAD when combined with exercise (24,25) and stress management (25), which strengthens the case for widespread institution of lipid-lowering dietary therapy. The reduction in clinical coronary events was most conclusively demonstrated in the Scandinavian Simvastatin Survival Study, which reported a 30% to 35% reduction in deaths and major coronary events (84). Data from these studies suggest that even patients who have mild to moderate lipid abnormalities benefit from therapy in a manner similar to that in patients who have more severe abnormalities. The National Cholesterol Education Program recommends setting an LDL cholesterol level of <100 mg per dL as a goal of therapy for all coronary patients (165).

The cardiac rehabilitation program is an optimal site for systematic screening and treatment of hyperlipidemia. This includes dietary counseling and active participation by the patient in pharmacologic therapy. A rehabilitation-based screening and treatment program has been documented to triple the likelihood that, with the collaboration of the referring physician, patients for whom such treatment is appropriate receive lipid-lowering therapy (166). Affiliation with a clinician who is expert in lipid management is necessary, and in many cases a lipid clinic can be organized at the rehabilitation facility itself.

Smoking Cessation

Cigarette smoking cessation is associated with a marked decrease in coronary event rates in coronary patients (167,168). In the study of Wilhelmsson and associates, patients who quit smoking after experiencing myocardial infarction reduced their 1-year mortality rate from 10% to 5% and their 1-year reinfarction rate from 18% to 9% (168). Exercise training in and of itself has minimal, if any, effect on smoking cessation rates in coronary patients (82). The best results with smoking cessation after a coronary event have been obtained using a physician-recommended, nurse-managed intervention that takes place during hospitalization for an acute coronary event (while patients are unable to smoke) and is aimed at relapse prevention (11,21). These interventions include teaching skills to deal with high-risk situations, relaxation training, provision of nicotine or bupropion when necessary, and long-term telephone contact. At the end of 6 months (21), and 1 year (11), cessation rates were significantly increased, from 32% to 61%.

Weight Reduction

Although no study has addressed the effect of weight reduction on second coronary events, its well-defined role in the treatment of hyperlipidemia, hypertension, and insulin resistance makes it an important multifactorial risk-factor intervention (97). In the studies of Haskell, Schuler, and Ornish that incorporated a low-fat dietary intervention and exercise, reductions in body mass index were demonstrated in coronary populations (10,24,25). For example, in the Stanford Coronary Risk Intervention Project, a sustained 4% decrease in body mass index was attained with a combination of nutritional counseling and home-based exercise (10). On the other hand, studies of exercise rehabilitation alone have generally not been associated with substantial weight change (82,90). When weight loss is accomplished in the rehabilitation setting, it is generally associated with improvements in lipid profiles, insulin resistance, and blood pressure (96). Nutrition education combined with behavioral interventions and prescribed exercise can achieve modest and sustained weight loss in the rehabilitation setting (169). However, the accomplishment of weight loss in cardiac rehabilitation is not a passive process, and it requires the development of a weight loss module for selected patients, staffed by appropriately trained professionals, with clear definitions of goals and desired outcomes and long-term follow-up. A well-established and effective behavior-based weight reduction program has been adapted to the cardiac rehabilitation setting (170,171). The intervention includes behavioral concepts of stimulus control, self-monitoring, problem-solving, and social support; a daily caloric goal; and a daily calorie count. The weight loss goal is not to reach ideal body weight, but rather to achieve improvements in obesity-related risk factors. In many cases, a relatively modest but sustained weight loss of 5% to 10% of body weight significantly improves risk factors such as lipid measures and insulin resistance. An advantage of cardiac rehabilitation–based weight reduction programs is that patients are already performing the exercise component needed to prevent them from regaining lost weight (172).

Diabetes

No clinical trials involving patients with established CAD have been carried out to determine whether tight control of diabetes, in patients with either type I or type II diabetes, prevents cardiac complications or slows the course of macrovascular disease. Results of a recent multicenter clinical trial of tight glucose control in patients with type I (insulin-dependent) diabetes who did not have CAD demonstrated improved lipid profiles, an increase in body weight, a decrease in microvascular complications (retinal and renal), and a trend toward decreased macrovascular events, with such events (cardiac and cerebrovascular) reduced by almost 50% (173). In patients with type II diabetes, exercise and weight reduction resulted in improved measures of insulin resistance and associated coronary risk factors, such as lipid abnormalities and hypertension (174,175). Poor glycemic control predicts an increased likelihood of cardiac events in type II diabetes (176,177). An important role of the cardiac rehabilitation program, beyond encouraging exercise and proper nutrition, is to assist primary physicians with monitoring and treatment of diabetes. Patients are taught self-monitoring techniques, and medications are adjusted as needed (6,178).

Hypertension

Rehabilitation programs assist primary physicians with the treatment and follow-up of coronary patients with hypertension. Although weight reduction, exercise, and salt restriction have all been associated with modest reductions in systemic blood pressure, definite benefits in the cardiac rehabilitation setting have not been demonstrated. Frequent surveillance of blood pressure, teaching of self-monitoring techniques, nutritional instruction, and adjustment of medications are all useful (6,179).

PRINCIPLES OF MANAGEMENT, PROGRAM STRUCTURE, AND ORGANIZATIONAL ISSUES

Inpatient Rehabilitation

In-hospital rehabilitation, or phase I rehabilitation, has necessarily evolved in recent years in response to ever-shortening hospitalizations for acute myocardial infarction and coronary revascularizations. With many infarction patients hospitalized for only 4 to 6 days (20), and much of this period occupied by acute care and recovery from interventional techniques, it is no longer realistic to expect patients to participate in a comprehensive course providing information about coronary risk factors and cardiac diets, and a graded in-hospital exercise program. However, in addition to the economic benefits of a shorter hospitalization, less deconditioning occurs, and patients are more capable of resuming premorbid physical activities. Many patients report that in the current environment, the most important aspect of phase I rehabilitation is to be directed to the phase II outpatient program (185).

Nonetheless, several important interventions take place during this brief hospitalization. Most important is smoking-relapse prevention. Because essentially all American hospitals now prohibit smoking, the issue is no longer smoking cessation, but planning for continued cessation on hospital discharge. Well-designed studies demonstrate that in the setting of acute myocardial infarction, 32% of patients stop smoking without a program, which can be increased to 61% with a nurse-managed smoking-relapse prevention program, as demonstrated by Taylor and colleagues (21).

It is also important during this brief index admission to define coronary risk factors and to set up an outpatient plan for long-term therapy. Defining lipid profiles early on is of particular importance; studies of aggressive lipid lowering in coronary patients document decreasing secondary event rates beginning 6 months to 1 year after therapy is begun (84,164). Serum lipid values are accurate when measured within 24 hours of myocardial infarction. When they are measured later in a hospitalization for myocardial infarction, they are inaccurate, with total, LDL, and HDL cholesterol levels lower and triglyceride levels higher (186–189). For 1 month after coronary bypass surgery, serum cholesterol levels measure falsely low, and therefore baseline measures should be determined preoperatively, with follow-up measures performed after 1 month (190). ⚐ c30

Outpatient Rehabilitation

Intake Evaluation

The cardiac rehabilitation intake evaluation is the optimal opportunity to stratify patients into risk categories and to systematically define secondary risk factors for the progression of CAD (Fig. 12.5). Therefore, as part of this evaluation, a fasting lipid profile and a glucose measure should be obtained for all patients. Other risk factors, such as smoking status, blood pressure, obesity, and diabetes-related measures, should also be assessed.

An exercise tolerance test needs to be performed so that an exercise prescription can be developed and the risk associated with exercise can be assessed. Patients in whom high-risk characteristics are identified at risk-stratification (Table 12.2) should participate in a supervised program in which electrocardiographic monitoring is available. Patients who are stratified to low- or intermediate-risk groups can be considered for a home-based exercise program. Although the requirements for electrocardiographic monitoring remain poorly defined, the American College of Cardiology, in its "Report on Cardiac Rehabilitation," recommends electrocardiographic monitoring for high-risk patients (*e*Table 12.2.1) (191).

Only 15% of eligible patients in the United States receive cardiac rehabilitation services. In many cases, cardiac rehabilitation programs are not geographically available, whereas in other cases, formal rehabilitation is not recommended by the primary physician. For some patients, insurance coverage is incomplete or unavailable. Whereas cardiac rehabilitation services have classically been delivered on-site at a well-defined exercise training facility, the need to expand preventive cardiology services to include the

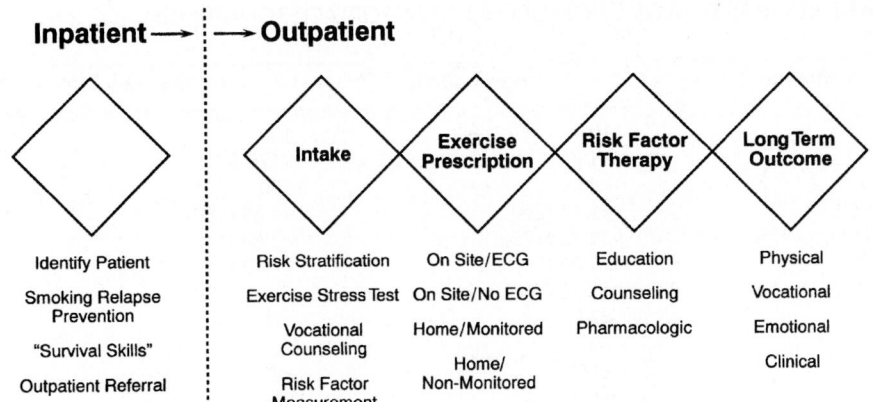

FIGURE 12.5 Elements of cardiac rehabilitation. ECG, electrocardiogram.

TABLE 12.2 GUIDELINES FOR RISK-STRATIFICATION

Risk level	Characteristics
Low	No significant left ventricular dysfunction (i.e., ejection fraction, ≥50%)
	No resting or exercise-induced myocardial ischemia manifested as angina and/or ST segment displacement
	No resting or exercise-induced complex arrhythmias
	Uncomplicated myocardial infarction, coronary artery bypass surgery, angioplasty, or atherectomy
	Functional capacity ≥6 METs on graded exercise test ≥3 weeks after clinical event
Intermediate	Mildly to moderately depressed left ventricular function (ejection fraction, 31–49%)
	Functional capacity <5–6 METs on graded exercise test ≥3 wk after clinical event
	Failure to comply with exercise intensity prescription
	Exercise-induced myocardial ischemia (1–2 mm ST segment depression) or reversible ischemic defects (see on echocardiography or nuclear radiography)
High	Severely depressed left ventricular function (ejection fraction, ≤30%)
	Complex ventricular arrhythmias while patient is at rest or appearing or increasing with exercise
	Decrease in systolic blood pressure of >15 mm Hg during exercise or failure to rise with increasing exercise workloads
	Patient is survivor of sudden cardiac death
	Myocardial infarction complicated by congestive heart failure, cardiogenic shock, and/or complex ventricular arrhythmias
	Severe coronary artery disease and marked exercise-induced myocardial ischemia (>2 mm ST segment depression)

METs, multiple of resting energy expenditure.
From American Association of Cardiovascular and Pulmonary Rehabilitation. *Guidelines for cardiac rehabilitation programs.* Champaign, IL: Human Kinetics Books, 1995, with permission.

majority of eligible patients necessitates a redefinition of this model.

The development of alternate approaches to delivery of cardiac rehabilitation services is an ongoing process, aimed at a goal of expanding the base of patients who receive services, at the lowest possible health care cost. Numerous investigators have documented the safety of home-based exercise programs for individuals who are at low to medium risk by use of varying degrees of transtelephonic monitoring (12,13,28,192). Case management (i.e., evaluation and management of risk factors for the individual patient) complements exercise conditioning and allows the individualization of preventive care in health care delivery systems that focus on efficiency and outcomes. Case management, whether delivered in an office practice or in a structured rehabilitation program, should focus on attainment of risk-factor goals (Table 12.3) and identification of highest risk patients (Table 12.2) (10,11). Exercise programs can be individualized for moderate- and higher-risk patients, and patients at highest risk of disability should be referred to a rehabilitation program for closer supervision and monitoring.

Compliance with Exercise and Long-Term Follow-Up

Long-term adherence to cardiac rehabilitation exercise is approximately 50% at 1 year (197,198). This compares to 1-year adherence rates of 64% for antihypertensive medication regimens (199) and 82% for treatment with lipid-lowering agents (200). Several interventions have been shown to optimize compliance with cardiac rehabilitation exercises. A gradual transition to home-based exercise sessions with self-monitoring while the patient was still in the rehabilitation program increased 6-month compliance rates from 76% to 92% (201). The use of lower-intensity exercise (202), participation of nurse case-managers (10,11), and the signing of a written agreement (203) have all been

TABLE 12.3 RISK-FACTOR GOALS FOR PATIENTS IN RISK REDUCTION GROUP: STANFORD CORONARY RISK INTERVENTION PROJECT MODEL

Variable	Minimum	Intermediate	Maximum
Body weight, % ideal	110	105	100
Systolic BP, mm Hg	<140	<130	≤120
Diastolic BP, mm Hg	<90	<85	≤80
Plasma cholesterol, mmol/L (mg/dL)	<5.69 (220)	<5.17 (200)	<4.65 (180)
LDL cholesterol, mmol/L (mg/dL)	<3.62 (140)	<3.23 (125)	<2.84 (110)
HDL cholesterol, mmol/L (mg/dL)	>1.16 (45)	>1.29 (50)	>1.42 (55)
Plasma triglycerides, mmol/L (mg/dL)	<1.81 (160)	<1.58 (140)	<1.13 (100)
Dietary fat, % calories	<30	<25	<20
Saturated fat, % calories	<10	<8	<6
Dietary cholesterol, mg/d	<250	<150	<75
P:S ratio[a]	≥1.0	≥1.0	≥1.0
Sodium, mg/d[b]	3,000	3,000	2,500
Cigarette smoking, no./d	<10	<5	0
Exercise capacity (METs)			
Men	>8	>10	>12
Women	>7	>8.5	>10
Fasting glucose, mg/dL	<110	<100	<90
1-h glucose, mg/dL	<200	<180	<160
Physical activity			
Routine aerobic, calories/d	+200	+300	+400
Training session, % MHR	50–75	60–75	70–85
	15- to 30-min sessions every other day	20- to 30-min sessions every other day	30- to 45-min sessions every other day

BP, blood pressure; HDL, high-density lipoprotein; LDL, low-density lipoprotein; METs, multiple of resting energy expenditure; MHR, maximal heart rate; P:S, polyunsaturated:saturated fat.
[a]Emphasis was placed on achieving the desired percentage of calories from saturated fat, with P:S ratio approximately 1.0.
[b]Hypertensive participants were encouraged to reduce sodium further, with attention also given to other aspects of their diet.
From Haskell WL, Alderman EL, Fair JM, et al. Effects of intensive multiple risk factor reduction on coronary atherosclerosis and clinical cardiac events in men and women with coronary artery disease: the Stanford Coronary Risk Intervention Project (SCRIP). *Circulation* 1994;89:975–990, with permission.

associated with increased long-term compliance with the exercise component of cardiac rehabilitation.

Provisions for the long-term continuation of risk-factor modification also need to be specified. The long-term surveillance and treatment of coronary risk factors is generally transferred to the primary physician, in a case-management format, whereas the long-term surveillance and maintenance of the exercise component is often delegated to the rehabilitation program. Although long-term, institutional phase III programs successfully maintain patients in a supervised exercise program and are particularly useful for older patients because they provide supervision and social interactions, a fully "rehabilitated" patient exercises independently at home.

Strategies to improve participation in cardiac rehabilitation programs are of major importance in view of the relationship between adherence with preventive cardiology recommendations and better clinical outcomes (204–206). The most important determinant of early post–coronary event cardiac rehabilitation participation, studied in a population of patients ≥62 years old, is the strength of the primary physician's recommendation for participation (207). When the recommendation was graded as moderate to strong (4 to 5, on a scale of 1 to 5), participation was 70%; when the recommendation was weak (1 to 3), participation

rate was 2% (Fig. 12.6). Other predictors of poor participation rates included older age; presence of comorbidities, especially arthritis; and the presence of mental depression (207). c31

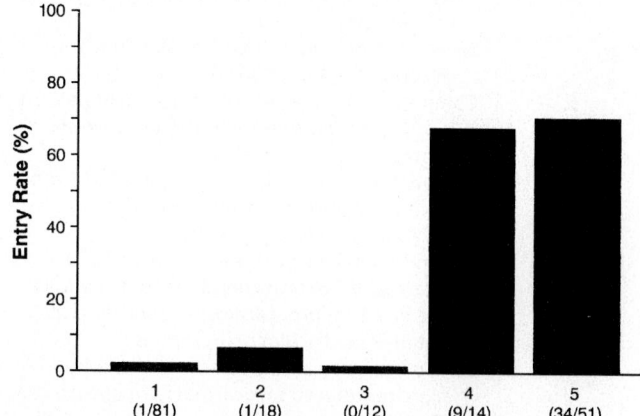

FIGURE 12.6 Cardiac rehabilitation participation by physician's recommendation. The physician's recommendation score was graded from 1 (not recommended, or recommended against) to 5 (strongly recommended). (From Ades PA, Waldmann ML, McCann W, et al. Predictors of cardiac rehabilitation participation in older coronary patients. *Arch Intern Med* 1992;152:1033–1035, with permission.)

Home-Based Cardiac Rehabilitation

So that cardiac rehabilitation services can be extended to increasing numbers of patients, the development of home-based programs is essential. The same principles of management described for facility-based rehabilitation apply. Specifically, an on-site intake evaluation is required, with risk-stratification, development of an exercise prescription, and delineation of long-term preventive cardiology goals (*e*Table 12.3.1). The Stanford Coronary Risk Intervention Project describes a model of health care delivery that has been successfully incorporated into a community setting (10). It is a physician-directed, nurse case-managed, multiple risk-factor modification program with well-defined short-term and longer-term individualized goals for specific risk factors (Fig. 12.3). It incorporates personal instruction, home-based programs, and periodic phone and office follow-up and requires no specialized exercise facilities. It has been successfully adapted for use in community programs (208). ⚑ c32

All but the highest-risk cardiac patients, such as those with exertional arrhythmias or low-threshold angina, may participate in home-based rehabilitation, although patients in the moderate-risk category, such as older individuals, those with exertional angina, or those with stable CHF, require more frequent periodic checks and a slower progression of exercise. New technologies include commercially available heart-rate monitors and transtelephonic monitoring and online nurse supervision for selected patients (13). Patients should be encouraged to keep records of their exercise sessions and to perform home monitoring of other individualized risk factors, such as body weight, dietary intake, and blood pressure measures. Short- and longer-term risk-factor goals should be realistic and individualized based on the current status of the patient, the patient's readiness for change, and the available resources. The use of community resources should be maximized to provide climate-controlled exercise spaces, assistance in measurements such as weight or blood pressure, and support groups. Appropriate consultations in the medical environment, such as nutritional instruction or physical therapy, should be available for selected patients to aid them in meeting risk-factor goals. The nurse case-manager should be capable of providing the majority of the necessary education about risk factors related to diet, exercise, and smoking cessation. Patients should be referred as needed to the physician director or the primary health care physician for medical therapy for lipid abnormalities, diabetes, and other risk factors.

CONTROVERSIES AND PERSONAL PERSPECTIVES

In a health care environment that is rapidly incorporating the precepts of managed care and other delivery models, cardiovascular services are undergoing a consolidation designed to maximize efficiency and minimize the use of expensive technologies. Advances in knowledge about the development of coronary atherosclerosis and the prevention of acute coronary events will drive continued interest in the delivery of efficient preventive cardiology services well into the new century. Furthermore, the patient population is aging, and the prevention of coronary disability and second coronary events in elderly patients is a major priority. In patients of all ages, costly cardiac rehospitalizations can be prevented, clinical event rates can be reduced, and coronary disability can be treated and prevented by the systematic application of secondary prevention services.

Many physicians question the need for distinct cardiac rehabilitation facilities, arguing that they can effectively measure and treat cardiac risk factors and recommend home-based exercise in the office setting. In reality, it is the rare physician whose practice is sufficiently regimented, who possesses sufficient expertise in preventive cardiology, and who has sufficient time available to meet the multidisciplinary medical, psychosocial, and vocational needs of the complex cardiac patient. Cardiac rehabilitation is a comprehensive process, and the complex patient benefits greatly from the expertise that is concentrated in the rehabilitation program, including specialists in preventive cardiology, exercise physiology, physical therapy, psychology, nutrition, and vocational counseling. The rehabilitation program has methods in place to maximize the likelihood of attaining outcome goals, and patients describe receiving great psychological support from the peer-group exercise and counseling sessions. Well-defined rehabilitation algorithms have been demonstrated to attain risk-factor goals more successfully than "usual care" in several clinical trials (10,11,24).

Successful modification of coronary risk is not a passive process. Care-management systems need to be established so that patients who would benefit from treatment are referred for care. Risk factors need not only to be identified and measured, but also to be actively treated according to systematic algorithms, with transition to primary health care providers for long-term care and follow-up.

Overall, only 15% of eligible patients participate in cardiac rehabilitation programs, whereas more than 30% of patients at academic medical centers participate (8). Alternative modes of delivery of cardiac rehabilitation services need to be developed to increase the availability of programs. These include home-based programs, with and without transtelephonic monitoring, and case-management systems coordinated through rehabilitation programs or physicians' offices (208). Exercise programs and risk modification need to be individualized, with an emphasis on clinical outcomes.

In summary, the scientific foundations of cardiac rehabilitation and secondary prevention are on firm ground, supported by recent authoritative clinical practice guidelines and clinical trials (8,6,215,216). As is true of many other preventive interventions, we need not await a "magic bullet." If currently available therapies can be systematically applied to targeted populations, recurrent coronary event rates will plummet, and coronary disability will be minimized.

THE FUTURE

An established body of scientific knowledge exists that supports the foundations of cardiac rehabilitation and secondary prevention for coronary patients. Systems of delivery need to be established so that patients are systematically involved in the prevention process. The future of cardiac rehabilitation will be defined by the medical care delivery system within which it operates and by the aging of the cardiac population. Prevention of costly rehospitalizations will be a high priority, as will preventing coronary disability in elderly patients. Ever-shortening lengths of stay for acute coronary events and interventional procedures will increase the need for prevention in the outpatient setting.

REFERENCES

1. *Heart and stroke facts.* Dallas: American Heart Association, 1990.
2. Pinsky JL, Jette AM, Branch LG, et al. The Framingham Disability Study: relationship of various coronary heart disease manifestations to disability in older persons living in the community. *Am J Public Health* 1990;80:1363–1368.
3. LaPlante MP. *Data on disability from the National Health Interview Survey, 1983–1985.* Washington, DC: National Institute on Disability and Rehabilitation Research, 1989.
4. Ellis SG, Miller DP, Brown KJ, et al. In-hospital cost of percutaneous coronary revascularization. *Circulation* 1995;92:741–747.
5. American Heart Association. *Heart and stroke facts: 1995 statistical supplement.* Dallas: American Heart Association, 1995.
6. Balady GJ, Ades PA, Comoss P, et al. Core components of cardiac rehabilitation/secondary prevention programs: a statement for healthcare professionals from the American Heart Association and the American Association of Cardiovascular and Pulmonary Rehabilitation Writing Group. *Circulation* 2000;102:1069–1073.
7. Ades PA. Cardiac rehabilitation and the secondary prevention of coronary heart disease. *N Engl J Med* 2001 (*in press*).
8. Wenger NK, Froehlicher ES, Smith LK, et al. *Cardiac rehabilitation: clinical practice guidelines.* AHCPR publication no. 96-0672. Rockville, MD: U.S. Department of Health and Human Services, Public Health Service, Agency for Health Care Policy and Research, and the National Heart, Lung, and Blood Institute, 1995.
9. Feigenbaum E, Carter E. *Health technology assessment report, 1987, no. 6.* Rockville, MD: U.S. Department of Health and Human Services, Public Health Service, National Center for Health Services Research and Health Care Technology Assessment, 1988.
10. Haskell WL, Alderman EL, Fair JM, et al. Effects of intensive multiple risk factor reduction on coronary atherosclerosis and clinical cardiac events in men and women with coronary artery disease: the Stanford Coronary Risk Intervention Project (SCRIP). *Circulation* 1994;89:975–990.
11. DeBusk RF, Houston-Miller N, Superko HR, et al. A case-management system for coronary risk factor modification after acute myocardial infarction. *Ann Intern Med* 1994;120:721–729.
12. DeBusk RF, Haskell WL, Miller NH, et al. Medically directed at-home rehabilitation soon after uncomplicated acute myocardial infarction: a new model for patient care. *Am J Cardiol* 1985;55:251–257.
13. Ades PA, Pashkow F, Fletcher G, et al. A controlled trial of cardiac rehabilitation in the home setting using electrocardiographic and voice transtelephonic monitoring. *Am Heart J* 2000;139:543–548.
14. Mallory G, Shite P, Salcedo-Salgar J. The speed of healing of myocardial infarction: a study of the pathological anatomy in seventy-two cases. *Am Heart J* 1939;18:647–671.
15. Levine S, Lown B. "Armchair" treatment of acute coronary thrombosis. *JAMA* 1952;148:1365–1369.
16. Newman L, Andrews M, Koblish M. Physical medicine and rehabilitation in acute myocardial infarction. *Arch Intern Med* 1952;89:552–561.
17. Cain HD, Frasher WG, Stivelman R. Graded activity program for safe return to self-care after myocardial infarction. *JAMA* 1961;177:111–115.
18. Berra K. Cardiac and pulmonary rehabilitation: historical perspectives and future needs. *J Cardiopulm Rehabil* 1991;11:8–15.
19. Pashkow FJ. Issues in contemporary cardiac rehabilitation: a historical perspective. *J Am Coll Cardiol* 1993;21:822–834.
20. Newby LK, Eisenstein EL, Califf RM, et al. Cost effectiveness of early discharge after uncomplicated acute myocardial infarction. *N Engl J Med* 2000;342:749–755.
21. Taylor CB, Houston-Miller N, Killen JD, et al. Smoking cessation after acute myocardial infarction: effects of a nurse-managed intervention. *Ann Intern Med* 1990;113:118–123.
22. Oldridge NB, Guyatt GH, Fischer ME, et al. Cardiac rehabilitation after myocardial infarction: combined experience of randomized clinical trials. *JAMA* 1988;260:945–950.
23. O'Connor GT, Buring JE, Yusuf S, et al. An overview of randomized trials of rehabilitation with exercise after myocardial infarction. *Circulation* 1989;80:234–244.
24. Schuler G, Hambrecht R, Schlierf G, et al. Regular physical exercise and low-fat diets: effects on progression of coronary artery disease. *Circulation* 1992;86:1–11.
25. Ornish D, Brown SE, Scherwitz LW, et al. Can lifestyle changes reverse coronary heart disease? The Lifestyle Heart Trial. *Lancet* 1990;336:129–133.
26. Brown BG, Zhao XQ, Sacco DE, et al. Lipid lowering and plaque regression: new insights into prevention of plaque disruption and clinical events in coronary disease. *Circulation* 1993;87:1781–1791.

27. Leon AS, Certo C, Comoss P, et al. Scientific evidence of the value of cardiac rehabilitation services with emphasis on patients following myocardial infarction. Section I: Exercise conditioning component. *J Cardiopulm Rehabil* 1990;10:79–87.

28. Miller NH, Haskell WL, Berra K, et al. Home vs. group exercise training for increasing functional capacity after myocardial infarction. *Circulation* 1984;70:645–649.

29. Smith SC, Blair SN, Criqui MH, et al. Preventing heart attack and death in patients with coronary disease. *Circulation* 1995;92:2–4.

30. Pashkow P, Ades PA, Emery CF, et al. Outcome measurement in cardiac and pulmonary rehabilitation. *J Cardiopulm Rehabil* 1995;15:394–405.

31. Hambrecht R, Wolf A, Gielen S, et al. Effect of exercise on coronary endothelial function in patients with coronary artery disease. *N Engl J Med* 2000;342:454–460.

32. Kaufmann P, Mandinov L, Hess OM. Coronary stenosis vasoconstriction: impact on myocardial ischaemia. *Eur Heart J* 1997;12:1853–1859.

33. Redwood DR, Rosing DR, Epstein SE. Circulatory and symptomatic effects of physical training in patients with coronary-artery disease and angina pectoris. *N Engl J Med* 1972;286:959–965.

34. Ades PA, Grunvald MH, Weiss RM, et al. Usefulness of myocardial ischemia as predictor of training effect in cardiac rehabilitation after acute myocardial infarction or coronary artery bypass grafting. *Am J Cardiol* 1989;63:1032–1036.

35. Rockman HA, Lew W. Left ventricular remodeling and diastolic dysfunction in chronic ischemic heart disease. In: Gaasch WH, LeWinter MM, eds. *Left ventricular diastolic dysfunction and heart failure.* Philadelphia: Lea and Febiger, 1994.

36. Levy W, Cerqueira M, Abrass IB, et al. Endurance exercise training augments diastolic filling abnormalities at rest and during exercise in healthy young and older men. *Circulation* 1993;88:116–126.

37. Ades PA, Grunvald MH. Cardiopulmonary exercise testing before and after conditioning in older coronary patients. *Am Heart J* 1990;120:585–589.

38. Neill WA, Branch LG, DeJong G. Cardiac disability. The impact of coronary disease on patients' daily activities. *Arch Intern Med* 1985;145:1642–1647.

39. Mital A, Shrey DE, Govindaraju M, et al. Accelerating the return to work (RTW) chances of coronary heart disease (CHD) patients. Part 1: Development and validation of a training programme. *Disabil Rehabil* 2000;22:604–620.

40. Shrey DE, Mital A. Accelerating the return to work (RTW) chances of coronary heart disease (CHD) patients. Part 2: Development and validation of a vocational rehabilitation programme. *Disabil Rehabil* 2000;22:621–626.

41. Ades PA, Maloney AE, Savage P, et al. Determinants of physical function in coronary patients: response to cardiac rehabilitation. *Arch Intern Med* 1999;159:2357–2360.

42. Zelis R, Nellis SH, Longhurst J, et al. Abnormalities in the regional circulations accompanying congestive heart failure. *Prog Cardiovasc Dis* 1975;18:181–199.

43. Cowley AJ, Stainer K, Rowley JM, et al. Abnormalities of the peripheral circulation and respiratory function in patients with severe heart failure. *Br Heart J* 1986;55:75–80.

44. Minotti J, Christoph I, Oka R, et al. Impaired skeletal muscle function in patients with congestive heart failure: relationship to systemic exercise performance. *J Clin Invest* 1991;88:2077–2082.

45. Franciosa JA, Park M, Levine B. Lack of correlation between exercise capacity and indexes of resting left ventricular performance in heart failure. *Am J Cardiol* 1981;47:3–39.

46. Captopril Multicenter Study Group. A placebo controlled trial of captopril in refractory chronic congestive heart failure. *J Am Coll Cardiol* 1983;2:755–763.

47. Sullivan MJ, Higginbotham MB, Cobb FR. Exercise training in patients with severe left ventricular dysfunction: hemodynamic and metabolic effects. *Circulation* 1988;78:506–515.

48. Minotti JR, Johnson EC, Hudson TL, et al. Skeletal muscle response to exercise training in congestive heart failure. *J Clin Invest* 1990;86:751–758.

49. Detry JMR, Rousseau M, Vandenbroecke O, et al. Increased arteriovenous oxygen difference after physical training in coronary heart disease. *Circulation* 1971;44:109–118.

50. Clausen JP. Circulatory adjustments to dynamic exercise and effect of physical training in normal subjects and in patients with coronary artery disease. *Prog Cardiovasc Dis* 1976;18:459–495.

51. Ferguson RJ, Taylor AW, Cote P, et al. Skeletal muscle and cardiac changes with training in patients with angina pectoris. *Am J Physiol* 1982;12:H830–H836.

52. Ehsani A, Martin WH, Heath GW, et al. Cardiac effects of prolonged intense exercise training in patients with coronary artery disease. *Am J Cardiol* 1982;50:246–254.

53. Hagberg JM, Ehsani AA, Holloszy JO. Effects of 12 months of intense exercise training on stroke volume in patients with coronary artery disease. *Circulation* 1983;67:1194–1199.

54. Ehsani AA, Biello DR, Schultz J, et al. Improvement of left ventricular contractile function by exercise training in patients with coronary artery disease. *Circulation* 1986;74:350–358.

55. Hagberg JM. Physiologic adaptations to prolonged high-intensity exercise training in patients with coronary artery disease. *Med Sci Sports* 1991;23:661–667.

56. Snell PG, Martin WH, Buckey JC, et al. Maximal vascular leg conductance in trained and untrained men. *J Appl Physiol* 1987;62:606–610.

57. Gobel FL. Rate pressure product as an index of myocardial oxygen consumption during exercise in patients with angina. *Circulation* 1978;57:549–556.

58. Ades P, Waldmann ML, Meyer WL, et al. Skeletal muscle and cardiovascular adaptations to exercise conditioning in older coronary patients. *Circulation* 1996;94:323–330.

59. Froelicher V, Jensen D, Genter F, et al. A randomized trial of exercise training in patients with coronary heart disease. *JAMA* 1984;252:1291–1297.

60. Schuler G, Hambrecht R, Schlierf G, et al. Myocardial perfusion and regression of coronary artery disease in patients on a regimen of intensive physical exercise and low fat diet. *J Am Coll Cardiol* 1992;19:34–42.

61. Haskell WL, Sims C, Myll J, et al. Coronary artery size and dilating capacity in ultradistance runners. *Circulation* 1993;87:1076–1082.

62. Schachinger V, Britten MB, Zeiher AM. Prognostic impact of coronary vasodilator dysfunction on adverse long-term outcome of coronary heart disease. *Circulation* 2000;101:1899–1906.

63. Wang J, Wolin MS, Hintze TH. Chronic exercise enhances endothelium-mediated dilation of epicardial coronary artery in conscious dogs. *Circ Res* 1993;73:829–838.

64. Sessa WC, Pritchard K, Seyedi N, et al. Chronic exercise in dogs increases coronary vascular nitric oxide production and endothelial cell nitric oxide synthase gene expression. *Circ Res* 1994;74:349–353.

65. Loscalzo J, Vita JA. Ischemia, hyperemia, exercise and nitric oxide: complex physiology and complex molecular adaptations. *Circulation* 1994;90:2556–2559.

66. Kallio V, Hamalainen H, Hakkila J, et al. Reduction in sudden deaths by a multifactorial intervention programme after acute myocardial infarction. *Lancet* 1979;2:1091–1094.

67. DeBusk RF, Houston N, Haskell W, et al. Exercise training soon after myocardial infarction. *Am J Cardiol* 1979;44:1223–1229.

68. Williams MA, Maresh CM, Esterbrooks DJ, et al. Early exercise training in patients older than age 65 years compared with that in younger patients after acute myocardial infarction of coronary bypass grafting. *Am J Cardiol* 1985;55:263–266.

69. Ades PA, Hanson JS, Gunther PG, et al. Exercise conditioning in the elderly coronary patient. *J Am Geriatr Soc* 1987;35:121–124.

70. Lavie CJ, Milani RV, Littman AB. Benefits of cardiac rehabilitation and exercise training in secondary coronary prevention in the elderly. *J Am Coll Cardiol* 1993;22:678–683.

71. Williams MA, Thalken LJ, Esterbrooks DJ, et al. Effects of short-term and long-term exercise training in older-elderly cardiac patients. *Circulation* 1992;86:I-670(abst).

72. Ades PA, Waldmann ML, Gillespie C. A controlled trial of exercise training in older coronary patients. *J Gerontol* 1995;50:M7–M11.

73. Arvan S. Exercise performance of the high risk acute myocardial infarction patient after cardiac rehabilitation. *Am J Cardiol* 1988;62:197–201.

74. Hammond HK, Kelly TL, Froelicher VF, et al. Use of clinical data in predicting improvement in exercise capacity after cardiac rehabilitation. *J Am Coll Cardiol* 1985;6:19–26.

75. Ades PA, Waldmann ML, Poehlman ET, et al. Exercise conditioning in older coronary patients: submaximal lactate response and endurance capacity. *Circulation* 1993;88:572–577.

76. Ades PA. Coronary disability in the elderly. *Cardiovasc Rev Rep* 1994;15:32–36.

77. Pratt CM, Welton DE, Squires WJ, et al. Demonstration of training effect during chronic α-adrenergic blockade in patients with coronary artery disease. *Circulation* 1981;64:1125–1129.

78. Sable DL, Brammell HL, Sheehan MW, et al. Attenuation of exercise conditioning by beta-adrenergic blockade. *Circulation* 1982;65:679–684.

79. Marsh RC, Hiatt WR, Brammell HL, et al. Attenuation of exercise conditioning by low dose beta-adrenergic receptor blockade. *J Am Coll Cardiol* 1983;2:551–556.

80. Hamalainen H, Luurila OJ, Kallio V, et al. Long-term reduction in sudden deaths after a multifactorial intervention programme in patients with myocardial infarction: 10 year results of a controlled investigation. *Eur Heart J* 1989;10:55–62.

81. Lamm G, Denolin H, Dorossiev D, et al. Rehabilitation and secondary prevention of patients after acute myocardial infarction. WHO collaborative study. *Adv Cardiol* 1982;31:107–111.

82. Carson P, Phillips R, Lloyd M, et al. Exercise after myocardial infarction: a controlled trial. *J R Coll Physicians Lond* 1982;16:147–151.

83. Vanhees L, Fagard R, Thijs L, et al. Prognostic value of training-induced change in peak exercise capacity in patients with myocardial infarcts and patients with coronary bypass surgery. *Am J Cardiol* 1995;76:1014–1019.

84. Scandinavian Simvastatin Survival Study Group. Randomized trial of cholesterol lowering in 4444 patients with coronary heart disease. *Lancet* 1994;345:1383–1389.

85. Hedback B, Perk J. 5 Year results of a comprehensive rehabilitation programme after myocardial infarction. *Eur Heart J* 1987;8:234–242.

86. Hedback B, Perk J, Wodlin P. Long-term reduction of cardiac mortality after myocardial infarction: 10-year results of a comprehensive rehabilitation programme. *Eur Heart J* 1993;14:831–835.

87. Van Camp SP, Peterson RA. Cardiovascular complications of outpatient cardiac rehabilitation programs. *JAMA* 1986;256:1160–1163.

88. Franklin BA, Bonzheim K, Gordon S, et al. Safety of medically supervised outpatient cardiac rehabilitation exercise therapy: a 16-year follow-up. *Chest* 1998;114:902–906.

89. Warner JG Jr, Brubaker PH, Zhu Y, et al., Long-term (5-year) changes in HDL cholesterol in cardiac rehabilitation patients: do sex differences exist? *Circulation* 1995;92:772–777.

90. Brochu M, Poehlman ET, Savage P, et al. Modest effects of exercise training alone on coronary risk factors and body composition in coronary patients. *J Cardiopulm Rehabil* 2000;20:180–188.

91. Mendoza SG, Carrasco H, Zerpa A, et al. Effect of physical training on lipids, lipoproteins, apolipoproteins, lipases, and endogenous sex hormones in men with premature myocardial infarction. *Metabolism* 1991;40:368–377.

92. Wilhelmsen L, Sanne H, Elmfeldt D, et al. A controlled trial of physical training after myocardial infarction: effects of risk factors, nonfatal reinfarction, and death. *Prev Med* 1975;4:491–508.

93. Oberman A, Cleary P, Larosa JC, et al. Changes in risk factors among participants in a long-term exercise rehabilitation program. *Adv Cardiol* 1982;31:168–175.

94. Engblom E, Hietanen EK, Hamalainen H, et al. Exercise habits and physical performance during comprehensive rehabilitation after coronary bypass surgery. *Eur Heart J* 1992;13:1053–1059.

95. Hambrecht R, Niebauer J, Marburger C, et al. Various intensities of leisure time physical activity in patients with coronary artery disease: effects on cardiorespiratory fitness and progression of coronary atherosclerotic lesions. *J Am Coll Cardiol* 1993;22:468–477.

96. Lavie CJ, Milani RV. Effects of cardiac rehabilitation and exercise training in obese patients with coronary artery disease. *Chest* 1996;109:52–56.

97. Brochu M, Poehlman ET, Ades PA. Obesity, body fat distribution and coronary artery disease. *J Cardiopulm Rehabil* 2000;20:96–108.

98. Schairer JR, Kostelnik T, Proffitt SM, et al. Caloric expenditure during cardiac rehabilitation. *J Cardiopulm Rehabil* 1998;18:290–294.

99. Savage PD, Brochu M, Scott P, et al. Low caloric expenditure in cardiac rehabilitation. *Am Heart J* 2000;140:527–533.

100. Mertens DJ, Kavanagh T, Campbell RB, et al. Exercise without dietary restriction as a means to long-term fat loss in the obese cardiac patient. *J Sports Med Phys Fitness* 1998;38:310–316.

101. Hubert HB, Feinleib M, McNamara PM, et al. Obesity as an independent risk factor for cardiovascular disease: a 26-year follow-up of participants in the Framingham Heart Study. *Circulation* 1983;67:968–977.

102. Manson SE, Colditz GA, Stampfer MJ, et al. A prospective study of obesity and risk of coronary heart disease in women. *N Engl J Med* 1990;322:882–889.

103. Wood PD, Stephanick ML, Dreon D, et al. Changes in plasma lipids and lipoproteins in overweight men during weight loss through dieting as compared with exercise. *N Engl J Med* 1988;319:1173–1179.

104. Schotte DE, Stunkard AJ. The effects of weight reduction on blood pressure in 201 obese patients. *Arch Intern Med* 1990;150:1701–1704.

105. Consensus development conference. Diet and exercise in non-insulin dependent diabetes mellitus. *Diabetes Care* 1987;10:639–644.

106. Kohrt WM, Obert KA, Holloszy JO. Exercise training improves fat distribution patterns in 60–70-year old men and women. *J Gerontol* 1992;47:M99–M105.

107. Taylor CB, Houston-Miller N, Ahn DK, et al. The effects of exercise training programs on psychosocial improvement in uncomplicated postmyocardial infarction patients. *J Psychosom Res* 1986;30:581–587.

108. Newton M, Mutrie N, McArthur JD. The effects of exercise in a coronary rehabilitation programme. *Scott Med J* 1991;60:38–41.

109. Erdman RA, Duivenvoorden HJ, Verhage F, et al. Predictability of beneficial effects in cardiac rehabilitation: a randomized clinical trial of psychosocial variables. *J Cardiopulm Rehabil* 1986;6:206–213.

110. Ott CR, Sivarajan ES, Newton KM, et al. A controlled randomized study of early cardiac rehabilitation: the Sickness Impact Profile as an assessment tool. *Heart Lung* 1983;9:846–853.

111. Oldridge NB, Guyatt G, Jones N, et al. Effects on quality of life with comprehensive rehabilitation after acute myocardial infarction. *Am J Cardiol* 1991;67:1084–1089.

112. Stern MJ, Gorman PA, Kaslow P. The group counseling vs. exercise therapy study: a controlled intervention with subjects following myocardial infarction. *Arch Intern Med* 1983;143:1719–1725.

113. Linden W, Stossel C, Maurice J. Psychosocial interventions for patients with coronary artery disease: a meta-analysis. *Arch Intern Med* 1996;156:745–752.

114. van Dixhoorn J, Duivenvoorden HJ. Effect of relaxation therapy on cardiac events after myocardial infarction: a five-year follow-up study. *J Cardiopulm Rehabil* 1999;19:178–185.

115. Frasure-Smith N, Lesperance F, Talajic M. Depression following myocardial infarction: impact on 6-month survival. *JAMA* 1993;270:1819–1825.

116. Levine JB, Covino NA, Slack WV, et al. Psychologic predictors of subsequent medical care among patients hospitalized with cardiac disease. *J Cardiopulm Rehabil* 1996;16:109–116.

117. Schiller E, Baker J. Return to work after a myocardial infarction: evaluation of planned rehabilitation and of a predictive rating scale. *Med J Aust* 1976;1:859–862.

118. Bar FW, Hoppener P, Diederiks J, et al. Cardiac rehabilitation contributes to the restoration of leisure and social activities after myocardial infarction. *J Cardiopulm Rehabil* 1992;12:1117–1125.

119. Hedback B, Perk J, Engvall J. Predictive factors for return to work after coronary artery bypass grafting: the role of cardiac rehabilitation. *Int J Rehabil Res* 1992;15:148–153.

120. Dennis C, Houston-Miller N, Schwartz RG, et al. Early return to work after uncomplicated myocardial infarction: results of a randomized trial. *JAMA* 1988;260:214–220.

121. Ades P, Tischler MD, Savage PD, et al. Determinants of disability in older coronary patients. *Circulation* 1996;94;I-497(abst).

122. Ades PA, Waldmann ML, Polk D, et al. Referral patterns and exercise response in the rehabilitation of female coronary patients aged ≥62 years. *Am J Cardiol* 1992;69:1422–1425.

123. Evenson KR, Rosamond WD, Leupker RV. Predictors of outpatient cardiac rehabilitation utilization: the Minnesota Heart Survey Registry. *J Cardiopulm Rehabil* 1998;18:192–198.

124. Fragnoli-Munn K, Savage PD, Ades PA. Combined resistive-aerobic training in older coronary patients early after myocardial infarction. *J Cardiopulm Rehabil* 1998;18:416–420.

125. Ades PA, Savage P, Brochu M, et al. Resistance training on physical function in older women with coronary heart disease. *Circulation* 2000:18;II-679(abst).

126. Bueno H. Influence of sex on the short-term outcome of elderly patients with a first acute myocardial infarction. *Circulation* 1995;92:1133–1140.

127. Greenland P. In-hospital and 1-year mortality in 1524 women after myocardial infarction: comparison with 4315 men. *Circulation* 1991;83:484–491.

128. Balady GJ, Jette D, Scheer J, et al. Changes in exercise capacity following cardiac rehabilitation in patients stratified according to age and gender. *J Cardiopulm Rehabil* 1996;16:38–46.

129. Cannistra LB, Balady GJ, O'Malley CJ, et al. Comparison of the clinical profile and outcome of women and men in cardiac rehabilitation. *Am J Cardiol* 1992;69:1274–1279.

130. Rich MW, Bosner MS, Chung MK, et al. Is age an independent predictor of early and late mortality in patients with acute myocardial infarction? *Am J Med* 1992;92:7–13.

131. Moore SM, Kramer FM. Women's and men's preferences for cardiac rehabilitation program features. *J Cardiopulm Rehabil* 1996;16:163–168.

132. Ades PA. Cardiac rehabilitation in older coronary patients. *J Am Geriatr Society* 1999;47:98–105.

133. Pfeffer MA, Braunwald E, Moye LA, et al. Effect of captopril on mortality and morbidity in patients with left ventricular dysfunction after myocardial infarction: results of the survival and ventricular enlargement trial. *N Engl J Med* 1992;327:669–677.

134. SOLVD Investigators. Effect of enalapril on survival in patients with reduced left ventricular ejection fractions and congestive heart failure. *N Engl J Med* 1991;325:293–302.

135. Konstam M, Dracup K, Baker D, et al. *Heart failure: evaluation and care of patients with left-ventricular systolic dysfunction.* Clinical practice guideline no. 11. AHCPR publication no. 94-0612. Rockville, MD: Agency for Health Care Policy and Research, Public Health Service, U.S. Department of Health and Human Services, 1994.

136. Coats AJ, Adamopoulos S, Radaelli A, et al. Controlled trial of physical training in chronic heart failure: exercise performance, hemodynamics, ventilation, and autonomic function. *Circulation* 1992;85:2119–2131.

137. Meyer TR, Casadei B, Coats AJ. Angiotensin-converting enzyme inhibition and physical training in heart failure. *J Intern Med* 1991;230:407–413.

138. Keteyian SJ, Levine AD, Brawner CA, et al. Exercise training in patients with heart failure: a randomized, controlled trial. *Ann Intern Med* 1996;124:1051–1057.

139. Belardinelli R, Georgiou D, Cianci G, et al. Randomized, controlled trial of long-term moderate exercise training in chronic heart failure: effects on functional capacity, quality of life, and clinical outcome. *Circulation* 1999;99:1173–1182.

140. Maiorana A, O'Driscoll G, Dembo L, et al. Effect of aerobic and resistance exercise training on vascular function in heart failure. *Am J Physiol* 2000;279:H1999–H2005.

141. Maiorana A, O'Driscoll G, Cheetham C, et al. Combined aerobic and resistance exercise training improves functional capacity and strength in CHF. *J Appl Physiol* 2000;88:1565–1570.

142. Stevenson LW, Steimle AE, Fonarow G, et al. Improvement in exercise capacity of candidates awaiting heart transplantation. *J Am Coll Cardiol* 1995;25:163–170.

143. Kobashigawa JA, Leaf DA, Lee N, et al. A controlled trial of exercise rehabilitation after heart transplantation. *N Engl J Med* 1999;340:272–277.

144. Kavanagh T, Yacoub MH, Mertens DJ, et al. Cardiorespiratory responses to exercise training after orthotopic cardiac transplantation. *Circulation* 1988;77:162–171.

145. Squires RW. Rehabilitation after cardiac transplantation: 1980 to 1990. *J Cardiopulm Rehabil* 1991;11:84–92.

146. Weicek EM, McCartney N, McKelvie RS. Comparison of direct and indirect measures of systemic arterial pressure during weightlifting in coronary artery disease. *Am J Cardiol* 1990;66:1065–1068.

147. McCartney N, McKelvie RS, Haslam DR, et al. Usefulness of weight-lifting training in improving strength and maximal power in coronary artery disease. *Am J Cardiol* 1991;67:939–945.

148. Franklin BA, Bonzheim K, Gordon S, et al. Resistance training in cardiac rehabilitation. *J Cardiopulm Rehabil* 1991;11:99–107.

149. Squires RW, Muri AJ, Anderson LJ, et al. Weight training during phase II (early outpatient) cardiac rehabilitation: heart rate and blood pressure responses. *J Cardiopulm Rehabil* 1991;11:360–364.

150. Buchner DM, deLateur BJ. The importance of skeletal muscle strength to physical function in older adults. *Ann Behav Med* 1991;13:91–98.

151. Ades PA, Ballor DL, Ashikaga T, et al. Weight training improves walking endurance in the healthy elderly. *Ann Intern Med* 1996;124:568–572.

152. Frontera WR, Meridith CN, O'Reilly KP, et al. Strength training and determinants of VO$_2$ max. *J Appl Physiol* 1990;68:329–333.

153. Effron MB. Effects of resistance training on left ventricular function. *Med Sci Sports* 1989;21:694–697.

154. Pearson AC, Schiff M, Mrosek D, et al. Left ventricular diastolic function in weight lifters. *Am J Cardiol* 1986;58:1254–1259.

155. Longhurst JC, Kelly AR, Gonyea WJ, et al. Echocardiographic left ventricular masses in distance runners and weight lifters. *J Appl Physiol* 1980;48:154–162.

156. Snoeckx LHEH, Abeling HRM, Lambregts JAC, et al. Echocardiographic dimensions in athletes in relation to their training program. *Med Sci Sports* 1982;14:428–434.

157. Featherstone JF, Holly RG, Amsterdam EA. Physiologic response to weight training in coronary artery disease. *Am J Cardiol* 1993;71:287–292.

158. DeBusk R, Pitts W, Haskell W, Houston N. Comparison of cardiovascular responses to static-dynamic effort and dynamic effort alone in patients with chronic coronary heart disease. *Circulation* 1979;59:977–984.

159. Kerber RE, Miller RA, Najjar SM. Myocardial ischemic effects of isometric, dynamic and combined exercise in coronary artery disease. *Chest* 1975;67:388–394.

160. Bertagnoli K, Hanson P, Ward A. Attenuation of exercise-induced ST depression during combined isometric and dynamic exercise in coronary artery disease. *Am J Cardiol* 1990;65:314–317.

161. Roussow JE, Lewis B, Rifkind BM. The value of lowering cholesterol after myocardial infarction. *N Engl J Med* 1990;323:1112–1116.

162. Blankenhorn DH, Nessim SA, Johnson RL, et al. Beneficial effects of combined colestipol-niacin therapy on coronary atherosclerosis and coronary venous bypass grafts. *JAMA* 1987;257:3233–3240.

163. Brown G, Alvers JJ, Fisher LD, et al. Regression of coronary artery disease as a result of intensive lipid-lowering therapy in men with high levels of apolipoprotein B. *N Engl J Med* 1990;323:1289–1298.

164. Sacks FM, Pfeffer MA, Moye LA, et al. The effect of pravastatin on coronary events after myocardial infarction in patients with average cholesterol levels. Cholesterol and Recurrent Events Trial investigators. *N Engl J Med* 1996;335:1001–1009.

165. National Cholesterol Education Program. *Detection, evaluation, and treatment of high blood cholesterol in adults (Adult Treatment Panel II).* Bethesda, MD: National Institutes of Health, National Heart, Lung, and Blood Institute, 1993.

166. Ades PA, Savage PD, Poehlman ET, et al. Lipid lowering in the cardiac rehabilitation setting. *J Cardiopulm Rehabil* 1999;19:255–260.

167. Hermanson B, Omenn GS, Kronmal RA, et al. Beneficial

six-year outcome of smoking cessation in older men and women with coronary artery disease. *N Engl J Med* 1988;319:1365–1369.

168. Wilhelmsson C, Vedin JA, Elmfeldt D, et al. Smoking and myocardial infarction. *Lancet* 1975;1:415–419.

169. Dracup K, Meleis AI, Clark S, et al. Group counseling in cardiac rehabilitation: effect on patient compliance. *Patient Educ Couns* 1984;6:169–177.

170. Brownell KD. *The LEARN program for weight control,* 6th ed. Dallas: American Health Publishing Company, 1994.

171. Harvey-Berino J. Weight loss in the clinical setting: applications for cardiac rehabilitation. *Coron Artery Dis* 1998;9:795–798.

172. Perry MG, McAdoo WG, McAllister DA, et al. Enhancing the efficacy of behavior therapy for obesity: effects of aerobic exercise and a multicomponent maintenance program. *J Consult Clin Psychol* 1986;54:670–675.

173. Diabetes Control and Complications Trial (DCCT) Research Group. Effect of intensive diabetes management on macrovascular events and risk factors in the Diabetes Control and Complications Trial. *Am J Cardiol* 1995;75:894–903.

174. Horton ES. Role and management of exercise in diabetes mellitus. *Diabetes Care* 1988;11:201–211.

175. Dylewicz P, Bienkowska S, Szczesniak L, et al. Beneficial effect of short-term endurance training on glucose metabolism during rehabilitation after coronary bypass surgery. *Chest* 2000;117:47–51.

176. Lehto S, Ronnemaa T, Haffner SM, et al. Dyslipidemia and hyperglycemia predict coronary heart disease events in middle-aged patients with NIDDM. *Diabetes* 1997;46:1354–1359.

177. Haffner SM. Epidemiological studies on the effects of hyperglycemia and improvement of glycemic control on macrovascular events in type 2 diabetes [review]. *Diabetes Care* 1999;22[Suppl 3]:C54–C56.

178. Ruderman N, Devlin JT, eds. *The health professional's guide to diabetes and exercise.* Alexandria, VA: American Diabetes Association, 1995.

179. Vongvanich P, Bairey Merz CN. Supervised exercise and electrocardiographic monitoring during cardiac rehabilitation: impact on patient care. *J Cardiopulm Rehabil* 1996;16:233–238.

180. Rosenman RH, Brand RJ, Jenkins D, et al. Coronary heart disease in Western Collaborative Group Study: final follow-up experience of 8 1/2 years. *JAMA* 1975;233:872–877.

181. Case RB, Heller SS, Case NB, et al. Type A behavior and survival after acute myocardial infarction. *N Engl J Med* 1985;312:737–741.

182. Friedman M, Thoresen CE, Gill JJ, et al. Alteration of type A behavior and its effect on cardiac recurrences in post myocardial infarction patients: summary results of the Recurrent Coronary Prevention Project. *Am Heart J* 1986;112:663–665.

183. Schleifer SJ, Macari-Hinson MM, Coyle DA, et al. The nature and course of depression following myocardial infarction. *Arch Intern Med* 1989;149:1785–1789.

184. Ruberman W, Weinblatt E, Goldberg JD, et al. Psychosocial influences on mortality after myocardial infarction. *N Engl J Med* 1984;311:552–559.

185. Piscatella JC. *Don't eat your heart out cookbook.* New York: Workman Publishing, 1994:662.

186. Watson WC, Buchanan KD, Dickson C. Serum cholesterol levels after myocardial infarction. *Br Med J* 1963;2:709–712.

187. Ronnemaa T, Viikari J, Irjala K, et al. Marked decrease in serum HDL cholesterol level during acute myocardial infarction. *Acta Med Scand* 1980;207:161–166.

188. Ryder REJ, Hayes TM, Mulligan IP, et al. How soon after myocardial infarction should plasma lipid values be assessed? *Br Med J* 1984;289:1651–1653.

189. Rosenson R. Myocardial injury: the acute phase response and lipoprotein metabolism. *J Am Coll Cardiol* 1993;22:933–940.

190. Cunningham MJ, Boucher TM, McCabe CH, et al. Changes in total cholesterol and high-density lipoprotein cholesterol in men after coronary bypass grafting. *Am J Cardiol* 1987;60:1393–1394.

191. Parmley WW. Position report on cardiac rehabilitation: recommendations of the American College of Cardiology on cardiovascular rehabilitation. *J Am Coll Cardiol* 1986;7:451–453.

192. Fletcher GF, Chiaramida AJ, LeMay MR, et al. Telephonically-monitored home exercise early after coronary bypass surgery. *Chest* 1984;86:198–202.

193. Borg GA. Perceived exertion: a note on history and methods. *Med Sci Sports* 1973;5:90–93.

194. Blumenthal JA, Rejeski WJ, Walsh-Riddle M, et al. Comparison of high- and low-intensity exercise training early after acute myocardial infarction. *Am J Cardiol* 1988;61:26–30.

195. Goble AJ, Hare DL, Macdonald PS, et al. Effect of early programmes of high and low intensity exercise on physical performance after transmural acute myocardial infarction. *Br Heart J* 1991;65:126–131.

196. Stewart AL, Hays RD, Ware JE. The MOS short-form general health survey: reliability and validity in a patient population. *Med Care* 1988;26:724–735.

197. Oldridge NB. Compliance and dropout in cardiac rehabilitation. *J Cardiac Rehabil* 1984;4:166–177.

198. Burke L, Dunbar-Jacob J, Hill M. Compliance with cardiovascular disease prevention strategies: a review of the research. *Ann Behav Med* 1997;19:239–263.

199. Dunbar-Jacob J, Dwyer K, Dunning E. Compliance with antihypertensive regimen: a review of the research in the 1980's. *Ann Behav Med* 1991;13:31–39.

200. Kruse W. Compliance with treatment of hyperlipoproteinemia in medical practice and clinical trials. In: Kramer J, Spilker B, eds. *Patient compliance in medical practice and clinical trials.* New York: Raven Press, 1991:175–186.

201. Carlson JJ, Johnson JA, Franklin BA, et al. Program participation, exercise adherence, cardiovascular outcomes, and program cost of traditional versus modified cardiac rehabilitation. *Am J Cardiol* 2000;86:17–23.

202. Lee JY, Jensen BE, Oberman A, et al. Adherence in the training levels comparison trial. *Med Sci Sports Exerc* 1996;28:47–52.

203. Oldridge N, Jones N. Improving patient compliance in cardiac exercise rehabilitation: effects of a written agreement and self-monitoring. *J Cardiopulm Rehabil* 1983;3:257–262.

204. Mulcahy R. Influence of cigarette smoking on morbidity and mortality after myocardial infarction. *Br Heart J* 1983;49:410–415.

205. Singh RB, Rostogi S, Verma R, et al. Randomized controlled trial of cardioprotective diet in patients with recent acute myocardial infarction: results of one year follow up. *Br Med J* 1992;304:1015–1019.

206. Hypertension Detection and Follow-up Program Cooperative Group. Persistence of reduction in blood pressure and mortality of participants in the Hypertension Detection and Follow-up Program. *JAMA* 1988;259:2113–2122.

207. Ades PA, Waldmann ML, McCann W, et al. Predictors of cardiac rehabilitation participation in older coronary patients. *Arch Intern Med* 1992;152:1033–1035.

208. Gordon NF, Haskell WL. Comprehensive cardiovascular disease risk reduction in a cardiac rehabilitation setting. *Am J Cardiol* 1997;80:69H–73H.

209. Connolly D, Fernhall B, McHugh M. Reliability of the rating of perceived exertion scale in a population with coronary heart disease. *Sports Med Training Rehab* 1996;7:7–16.

210. Oldridge N, Furlong W, Feeny D, et al. Economic evaluation of cardiac rehabilitation soon after acute myocardial infarction. *Am J Cardiol* 1993;72:154–161.

211. Ades P, Huang D, Weaver S. Cardiac rehabilitation participation predicts lower rehospitalization costs. *Am Heart J* 1992;123:916–921.

212. Levin LA, Perk J, Hedback B. Cardiac rehabilitation: a cost analysis. *J Intern Med* 1991;230:427–434.

213. Ades PA, Pashkow F, Nestor J. Cost-effectiveness of cardiac rehabilitation after myocardial infarction. *J Cardiopulm Rehabil* 1997;17:222–231.

214. Bondestam E, Breikss A, Hartford M. Effects of early rehabilitation on consumption of medical care during the first year after acute myocardial infarction in patients >65 years of age. *Am J Cardiol* 1995;75:767–771.

215. American Association of Cardiovascular and Pulmonary Rehabilitation. *Guidelines for cardiac rehabilitation programs.* Champaign, IL: Human Kinetics, 1995;155.

216. Fuster V, Pearson TA. 27th Bethesda Conference: matching the intensity of risk factor management with the hazard for coronary disease events. *J Am Coll Cardiol* 1996;27:957–1047.

217. Pedersen TR, Kjekshus J, Berg K, et al. Cholesterol lowering and the use of healthcare resources: results of the Scandinavian Simvastatin Survival Study. *Circulation* 1996;93:1796–1802.

218. Mark DB, Hlatky MA, Califf RM, et al. Cost effectiveness of thrombolytic therapy following acute myocardial infarction. *N Engl J Med* 1995;332:1418–1424.

219. Kupersmith J, Holmes-Rovner M, Hogan A, et al. Cost effectiveness analysis in heart disease. *Prog Cardiovasc Dis* 1995;37:243–271.

13

AN INTEGRATED APPROACH TO RISK-FACTOR MODIFICATION

RAVI RASALINGAM
THOMAS A. PEARSON

NEED FOR A SYSTEMATIC APPROACH
TO PREVENTIVE CARDIOLOGY

The evidence base supportive of preventive cardiology has
steadily become more comprehensive. Studies of vascular
biology, natural history studies, and multicenter clinical trials have clearly delineated the role of factors in the atherosclerotic process and the effectiveness of practices to reduce
the morbidity and mortality resulting from coronary artery
disease. This evidence base has been used by the scientific
community and the medical profession to develop a number of comprehensive clinical guidelines and scientific statements, which have been endorsed by the major
cardiovascular associations (4–13) (eFig. 13.0.1). But
guidelines are not enough. The next step to realize these
potential benefits are critical. Evaluations of the performance of health care providers and health care systems to

implement prevention and rehabilitation from coronary
artery disease have shown continuing deficiencies. ▼ c44

Rationale for a Comprehensive Risk
Reduction Approach

What form should risk-factor modification take in the
management of the high-risk patient? Several scenarios
might be entertained, including intervention by a specialty
clinic, for example, lipid management or preventive cardiology clinics, referral of this responsibility back to the primary care provider, or integration of modification efforts as
part of the overall care of the high-risk patient. Table 13.1
identifies several of the many reasons to support the latter
approach for all patients with symptomatic or high risk for
atherosclerotic disease.

   One important consideration deals with which disease is
actually being targeted for intervention. Although acute
syndromes of myocardial ischemia and their sequelae
demand acute intervention to reduce the risk of death and
disability over the short-term, long-term prognosis is dictated by the extent of the atherosclerotic disease in the cor-

   R. Rasalingam: Department of Medicine, Strong Memorial Hospital,
Rochester, New York
   T. A. Pearson: Department of Community and Preventive Medicine, Uni-
versity of Rochester School of Medicine and Dentistry, Rochester, New York

TABLE 13.1 RATIONALE FOR COMPREHENSIVE RISK-FACTOR MODIFICATION INTEGRATED INTO THE OVERALL MANAGEMENT OF THE PATIENT WITH CORONARY ARTERY DISEASE

Treatment of the primary disease process (atherosclerosis) rather than the symptomatic complications of the disease
    Long-term efficacy in reducing risk of events
    Reduced risk of symptoms from disease in other vascular beds (e.g., cerebral, peripheral)
Improved effectiveness of acute coronary care
    Risk-factor interventions efficacious over very short intervals
    Risk-factor modifications may be more successful in the acute phases of coronary disease
    Benefits additive to those of other cardiologic procedures
Improved safety of interventions
    Reduce potentially deleterious interactions between risk-factor modifications
    Reduce deleterious interactions between risk-factor modifications and other cardiologic therapies
Improve follow-up care and compliance by considering risk-factor modification as a cornerstone of cardiologic care worthy of initiation early in clinical course

onary vasculature and the factors related to it. Perhaps a better concept is that risk-factor modification constitutes the *medical management of atherosclerosis* (14). After alleviation of the acute manifestations of ischemia, the focus of the physician should then turn to those pathophysiologic processes within the arterial wall that allowed the ischemic event to develop. Although invasive or surgical approaches to atherosclerosis have their place in cardiac care, a considerable array of interventions, both behavioral and pharmacologic, are now available. These focus on reestablishing normal endothelial function, inhibiting the initiation and growth of atherosclerotic plaques, stabilizing these plaques to prevent ulceration and rupture, and reducing thrombogenicity of the blood. This represents the management of the atherosclerotic arterial system, in conjunction with the correction of myocardial ischemia, left ventricular dysfunction, ventricular arrhythmias, and other pathophysiologic processes. Clinical trials have proven the long-term benefits of this approach (*e*Table 13.0.1).

Second, limiting intervention to atherosclerotic disease that is symptomatic in one vascular bed ignores the fact that atherosclerosis is a systemic disease. Although the relief of symptoms through revascularization is important to the patient, without intervention on recurrence of the systemic atherosclerotic process itself, symptomatic disease in the coronary arteries or in other vascular beds is highly likely. It is well known that the leading cause of death in patients with atherosclerotic abdominal aneurysm or peripheral arterial disease is MI and sudden cardiac death (24). Moreover, reductions in risk factors in patients with symptomatic coronary disease have been shown to reduce events elsewhere in the vasculature. A metaanalysis of clinical trials observed that LDL cholesterol reduction with 3-hydroxy-3-methylglutaryl coenzyme A (HMG-CoA)

reductase inhibitors in patients with coronary disease not only reduced MI and cardiac death but also reduced the occurrence of fatal and nonfatal stroke by approximately 30% (27). Clearly, the management of the atherosclerotic disease process must occur concomitantly with the management of its symptoms.

Third, the traditional approach has been to consider risk-factor modification as adjunctive therapy, to be provided only after the completion of diagnostic and therapeutic steps in the acutely ill patient. This is based on the old notion that risk-factor management acts on the slowly progressive atherosclerotic process, thereby taking months or years to benefit the patient. More recent evidence, suggesting that a number of modifiable risk factors affects endothelial function, plaque stability, and hemostasis, establishes the biologic plausibility for rapid benefits of risk-factor modification in the acute care of a coronary patient (28). Clinical studies corroborate the acute benefits of risk-factor modification. It has long been recognized that smoking cessation reduces the risk of reinfarction and death after MI in a matter of weeks or months (29,30). More recent randomized trials of lipid-lowering agents have demonstrated substantial reduction of myocardial ischemia on ambulatory electrocardiograms within months of MI (31). There is now agreement that these effective behavioral and pharmacologic measures should be instituted before hospital discharge for maximal benefit (32). Studies using HMG-CoA reductase inhibitors suggest that sizable reductions in clinical coronary events can be realized in a matter of weeks or months. The Pravastatin Multinational study showed a 95% reduction in coronary events with pravastatin after only 6 months, with sizable differences discernible at 8 weeks (33). In a prospective cohort study evaluating early statin use post-MI, a relative risk reduction of 25% in 1-year mortality was noted (Fig. 13.1) (34). Likewise, the preliminary results of a randomized trial of a high-dose statin within the first 48 hours after symptom onset showed a significant 16% reduction in events over the next 6 months (35). Several randomized double-blind placebo trials of early initiation of statins are currently being completed to further delineate the best time to introduce statin use. The Diabetes Mellitus Insulin Glucose Infusion in Acute Myocardial Infarction trial showed a mortality reduction in those patients who had more aggressive management of their blood sugars post-MI, again highlighting short-term benefits of effective risk-factor management (36). The magnitude of these benefits is similar to that expected with angiotensin-converting enzyme (ACE) inhibitors or beta-blocker therapies. This shift in preference toward early risk-factor modification again highlights the need for an effective, structured risk reduction strategy to be in place.

Next, there are a number of psychosocial benefits of integrating risk-factor modification into the overall management of acute and chronic ischemic heart disease. Dur-

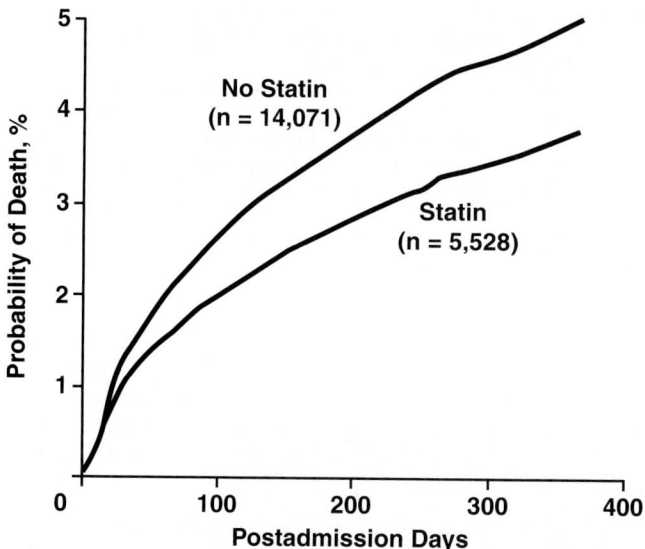

FIGURE 13.1 Statin treatment initiated early in the postinfarction period for patients with acute myocardial infarction. Data were calculated using multiple Cox regression analysis (relative risk, 0.75; 95% confidence interval, 0.63–0.89; p = .001). (From Stenestrand U, Wallentin L. Early statin treatment following acute myocardial infarction and 1-year survival. *JAMA* 2001;285:430–436, with permission.)

ing acute phases of illness, the patient and his or her family members may be especially receptive to behavioral interventions. This is the concept of the *teachable moment*. For example, during hospitalization for acute ischemia, the coronary disease patient is prohibited from smoking. This may be a propitious time to initiate a program of behavior modification that can extend to the outpatient phases of the patient's treatment.

Another erroneous notion is that traditional cardiac interventions such as revascularization or beta-blocker therapies may somehow negate the need for risk-factor management. Risk factors and clinical factors both strongly influence the natural history of coronary disease (37,38). Although prevention of ischemia, congestive heart failure, and arrhythmia is an important goal in caring for the atherosclerotic patient, stabilization of the atherosclerotic process, slowing its progression, and prevention of thrombosis are discrete benefits of risk-factor management. Subanalyses in large clinical trials such as the Scandinavian Simvastatin Survival Study, for example, were able to examine the benefits of LDL cholesterol lowering in patients who were undergoing a variety of secondary preventive interventions such as treatment with aspirin, beta-blockers, ACE inhibitors, as well as those who were not (39). Consistently, cholesterol lowering was found to have benefits additive to other interventions. Another example is the prevention of saphenous vein bypass graft atherosclerosis. Both the Cholesterol Lowering Atherosclerosis Study (40) and the Post Coronary Artery Bypass Graft Study (41) have shown that the lowering of LDL cholesterol can prevent the initiation

and progression of lesions in bypass grafts, preventing the need for repeated surgical revascularization. These observations point to the need to integrate risk-factor modification into the initial stages of therapy, with the expectation of short- and long-term benefits additive to those of traditional cardiac interventions.

On the other hand, another reason for coordination of efforts in comprehensive risk reduction is the potential deleterious interactions between risk-factor modifications and other therapies. Bile acid–binding resins, useful agents for reducing LDL cholesterol, can bind up coumadin, beta-blockers, and digoxin. Similarly, smoking cessation, a major means of reducing risk, can nonetheless lead to postcessation weight gain and deleterious effects on lipids and glucose. A diet that reduces saturated fat and cholesterol may also reduce HDL cholesterol. Proven antihypertensive therapies, namely, thiazide diuretics and beta-blockers, can also reduce HDL cholesterol and raise serum triglycerides in some patients. Clearly, when considering overall risk, a patient's entire risk-factor profile must be considered, especially because most patients with coronary disease have two or more risk factors (39). Intervention on one risk factor should take others into consideration, with the goal being maximal reduction of overall risk. ❦ *c45*

Evidence for the Underutilization of Interventions to Reduce Risk

The American Heart Association (AHA), American College of Cardiology (ACC), and other organizations have released a number of consensus statements addressing prevention of coronary artery disease (4–13), based on basic epidemiologic and clinical trial evidence (14) (*e*Fig. 13.0.1). Despite the increasing evidence supporting effective preventive therapies, their application has been disappointing. An example is the National Cholesterol Education Program (NCEP) Adult Treatment panel II guidelines for LDL cholesterol management (10). As an evidence-based document, these guidelines established LDL cholesterol thresholds for treatment and LDL cholesterol goals that should be attained for low-risk, high-risk, and coronary heart disease patients. A review of office visits from the National Ambulatory Medical Care Surveys showed that cholesterol screening, both for primary and secondary prevention, was much lower than predicted by NCEP guidelines (42). Cholesterol testing occurred in only 22.9% of office visits and counseling was infrequent (34%) in known hyperlipidemic patients. The Heart and Estrogen/Progestin Study trial enrolled women with coronary artery disease, identifying 91% of participants who had not achieved the NCEP LDL cholesterol goal of less than 100 mg per dL. (43). The Lipid Treatment Assessment Project, a survey to evaluate the proportion of 4,888 dyslipidemic patients receiving lipid-lowering therapy, also provided evidence of a low success rate, especially in high-risk, noncoronary, and coronary heart disease groups (44). Only 18% of patients with established coronary heart disease met the NCEP goal for LDL cholesterol. This was despite surveying 618 physicians who were among the most frequent prescribers of lipid-lowering drugs. The lack of use of medications, an inappropriate choice or dose of medication, or the infrequent use of combination therapy appeared to be the cause of the low success rates. The majority (80%) of participants did not receive dietary counseling.

This treatment gap does not appear to be limited to lipid management. Further review analyzed medication use and showed disappointing rates of use of well-established medications such as beta-blockers (45), ACE inhibitors (46), and aspirin (47), even when clearly indicated. Smoking cessation counseling is addressed in less than one-half of smokers with coronary disease (48,49). A multicenter study conducted in Europe looked retrospectively at hospital records and conducted prospective interviews of patients to determine whether major coronary risk factors had been addressed (50). There was a striking twofold difference between countries' use of proven beneficial therapies such as beta-blockers post-MI. There was also a threefold variation in ACE inhibitor use in those patients with symptoms of heart failure that could not be explained. Reduced assessment and inappropriate modification of risk factors have also been documented in the elderly (aged 65 years and older) despite their high burden of disease and proven significant risk reduction with these therapies (51,52). An outpatient survey of predominately cardiology practices documented a reluctance to titrate the dose of ACE inhibitors for patients with congestive heart failure and of HMG-CoA reductase inhibitors in patients with lipid disorders (53). Only 26% of patients achieved the recommended target dose as described by a number of studies clearly showing mortality benefit (54). Finally, the majority of patients with premature coronary heart disease were not encouraged to have first-degree relatives screened for cardiac risk. This was further emphasized in a study using the ACC Evaluation of Preventative Therapeutics data, in which less than 1% of inpatient medical records contained a discharge plan detailing recommended screening of family members of patients younger than 55 years (55). Only 17.8% of these patients had their families screened within 6 months of their cardiovascular event, despite NCEP guideline recommendations to screen all patients with a recognized history of premature coronary artery disease (10).

Thus, the gap between the goals of treatment and the actual levels of risk-factor control appears large, and it must translate into considerable numbers of preventable cases of recurrence and death caused by atherosclerotic disease. Table 13.2 illustrates this gap by showing the numbers of lives potentially saved each year if proven preventions were optimally implemented, suggesting that tens of thousands of deaths might be averted merely by following guidelines (56).

TABLE 13.2 ESTIMATION OF ADDITIONAL LIVES SAVED EACH YEAR BY IMPLEMENTATION OF PREVENTIVE CARDIOLOGY INTERVENTIONS

Therapy	Ideal–actual use (%)	Relative risk reduction (%)	No. of additional lives saved/yr
Antiplatelet	15	15	13,500
Beta-blockers	10	21	12,600
Angiotensin-converting enzyme 1	30	17	30,600
Statins	20	23	27,600
Total			**84,300**

From Bahit MC, Granger CB, Alexander KP, et al. Applying the evidence: opportunity in US for 80,000 additional lives saved per year. *Circulation* 2000;102:11–874, with permission.

STRATEGIES FOR INTEGRATION OF COMPREHENSIVE RISK REDUCTION INTO CARDIOLOGIC PRACTICE

Opportunities in the Inpatient Care Setting

Role of the Hospital

An inpatient cardiology service can be organized to efficiently and reliably assess the levels of risk factors prevalent in patients admitted with acute coronary syndromes or for revascularization procedures. A convenient tool is the joint AHA–American Association of Cardiovascular Preventive Health statement regarding core components for secondary prevention (26), which includes strategies for optimal risk-factor management. These guidelines include the goals for each risk-factor intervention and have been modified to provide a form to comprehensively document the initial status of the risk factor as well as plans for intervention and follow-up (Fig.13.2). The checklist format has been used successfully to improve levels of preventive care (81,82). In one study, computer-generated preventive-care reminders, individualized to the patient, increased preventive services provided by 126 physicians by 20% (83). Such a form could be filled out by physicians, nurses, or other health professionals. The AHA has provided a number of Web-based tools to quickly and efficiently document risk-factor assessments and interventions for individual patients (http://www.american-heart.org/CAP, "Get with the Guidelines Program"). These tools track compliance of risk-factor modifications and can even generate letters clearly outlining proposed programs. This provides a time-efficient, vital communication between physicians participating in care. Nurse-generated checklists also have been successful in increasing preventive services (84,85). Similar reminder messages and forms have also been used to implement a variety of acute care guidelines, suggesting their feasibility and desirability even in acute care settings (86). The Cardiac Hospitalization Atherosclerosis

Primary and Secondary CVD Patient Tracking Form

American Heart Association.

Fighting Heart Disease and Stroke

Patient Name _____

Patient Age _____   Patient Sex _____

Pre-existing ❑ CVD conditions ❑ Diabetes ❑ Other _____

Indicate acceptable range in grey areas.

Risk Interventions	Initial Status		Patient Goal	Date	Date	Date	Date
Smoking Complete Cessation	Smoker Nonsmoker			Smoking Not Smoking	Smoking Not Smoking	Smoking Not Smoking	Smoking Not Smoking
Blood Pressure • ≤140/90 mm Hg or • <130/85 mm Hg if heart failure, renal insufficiency, or diabetes	mm Hg mm Hg						
Cholesterol Primary • LDL <160 mg/dL (If ≤1 risk factor) or • LDL <130 mg/dL (If ≥2 risk factors) Secondary • LDL <100 mg/dL Primary & Secondary • HDL >35 mg/dL • TG <200 mg/dL	❑ Test sent out	Total	mg/dL mg/dL				
		LDL	mg/dL mg/dL				
		HDL	mg/dL mg/dL				
		TG	mg/dL mg/dL				
Physical Activity Duration P1: 30–60 min P2: 30 min Frequency 3–4 times/week	DUR.		min min				
	FRQ.		times/wk times/wk				
Weight Management BMI: 21–25 kg/m² Height:	Weight		lbs lbs				
	BMI		kg/m²kg/m²				
Diabetes Management Near Normal: • Glucose • HbA1c (<7)	Glucose		mg/dL mg/dL				
	HbA1c		% %				
Estrogens *Primary*- Consider ERT in all postmenopausal women *Secondary*- Estrogen Replacement	Yes / No		Compliant? Rx	Y / N Rx	Y / N Rx	Y / N Rx	Y / N Rx
Antiplatelet Agents/ Anticoagulants	Yes / No		Compliant? Rx	Y / N Rx	Y / N Rx	Y / N Rx	Y / N Rx
ACE Inhibitors Post-MI	Yes / No		Compliant? Rx	Y / N Rx	Y / N Rx	Y / N Rx	Y / N Rx
Beta Blockers Post-MI	Yes / No		Compliant? Rx	Y / N Rx	Y / N Rx	Y / N Rx	Y / N Rx

©1999 American Heart Association 8/6/99

FIGURE 13.2 American Heart Association form to track risk-factor modification and secondary preventive intervention. ACE, angiotensin-converting enzyme; BMI, body mass index; CVD, cardiovascular disease; DUR, duration; ERT, estrogen replacement therapy; FRQ, frequency; HDL, high-density lipoprotein; LDL, low-density lipoprotein; MI, myocardial infarction; Rx, prescription; TG, triglyceride.

Management Program at the University of California Los Angeles has implemented such a system of early risk-factor intervention and has shown increasing rates of use of known effective interventions during long-term follow-up (Table 13.3) (87). Another approach is the development of more elaborate care protocols, or *critical pathways*, that comprehensively define care of a specific problem. The joint AHA-ACC guidelines for management of patients with acute myocardial infarction is an example of this, defining multiple dimensions of acute myocardial infarction management but including risk-factor assessment and management as part of the initial intervention (13).

Hospitals can also provide a variety of other opportunities to identify risk factors. One example is the chemistry laboratory. The AHA-ACC guidelines for management of acute myocardial infarction suggest a lipid profile at the time of admission to the hospital (13). This can be made automatic, so that serum collected for cardiac enzymes such as troponin and creatinine phosphokinase might also be analyzed for serum lipids. The importance of this lies in the observation that serum cholesterol levels (and most lipoprotein cholesterol levels) decrease 24 hours after an MI (88). The routine measurement of a lipid profile in the patient with the presumptive diagnosis of MI would ensure a baseline assessment of lipids and lipoproteins. Furthermore, laboratory reports can include various messages identifying abnormal levels and the steps needed to correct those levels. Cholesterol levels identified as abnormal serve as cues to change physician behavior and are more likely to lead to further diagnosis and treatment of a lipid abnormality than those values not identified as normal (89). This has taken on even more importance with increasing evidence of the benefits of in-hospital preventive interventions.

TABLE 13.3 RATES OF APPROPRIATE AND INAPPROPRIATE CARDIOLOGIC MEDICATION USE BEFORE AND AFTER AN INPATIENT PROGRAM TO IMPROVE ATHEROSCLEROSIS: THE CARDIAC HOSPITALIZATION ATHEROSCLEROSIS MANAGEMENT PROGRAM (CHAMP) STUDY

Discharge therapy	Pre-CHAMP (1992–1993) (n = 256; %)	Post-CHAMP (1994–1995) (n = 302; %)
Aspirin	78	92
Beta-blocker	12	61
Nitrate	62	34
Calcium antagonists	68	12
Angiotensin-converting enzyme inhibitors	4	56
3-Hydroxy-3-methylglutaryl coenzyme A reductase inhibitor	6	86

From Fonarow GC, Gawlinski A. Rationale and design of the cardiac hospitalization atherosclerosis management program at the University of California Los Angeles. *Am J Cardiol* 2000;85:10A–17A, with permission.

Another important reason for encouraging early assessment and treatment of risk factors is that hospitalization for an acute ischemic episode often represents an opportunity to change patient attitude and behavior. Patients are unable to smoke in the hospital and are subject to dietary restrictions. This provides as ideal opportunity to begin the discussion of what permanent changes need to be made in their lifestyles (49,60,61).

Role of the Cardiovascular Specialist

The usual role of the physician admitting the patients acutely ill with vascular disease, or the cardiovascular consultant asked for advice, is to make and confirm the diagnosis, to set goals for treatment, and to formulate the optimal plan to achieve these goals. The same should be true for the modification of risk factors. In this way, the cardiovascular specialist plays a leadership role in the integration of risk reduction strategies into the overall plan. Those patients admitted with symptomatic coronary artery disease already fall into the high-risk group of patients likely to experience further cardiac events. Therefore, risk-factor modulation should aim to meet recommended goals over the next few months after the onset of symptoms and the diagnosis of a risk factor.

After the plan is constructed, the physician may or may not be the person implementing it. However, the physician does need to communicate the overall treatment plan to the patient, including the importance of risk-factor control in the prognosis of disease. Other supporting team members charged with counseling or other behavior-modifying activities need to emphasize the importance of nonpharmacologic life-style changes as well as pharmacologic interventions and revascularization procedures.

The duration of hospital stays is continuing to decrease, with many diagnostic and nonsurgical revascularization procedures being performed on a same-day basis. Much of the care plan, especially that dealing with long-term issues, is carried out by the specialist or by the primary care provider on an outpatient basis. This does not alter the need to integrate risk-factor management into the overall treatment plan of the patient. Rather, it emphasizes the importance of communicating to the ambulatory care provider the need for risk-factor management and the appropriate strategies to achieve specified goals. Frequently, discharge summaries describe findings of diagnostic or therapeutic procedures in great detail, only to ignore altogether the presence of risk factors and any plan to control them. The ambulatory care provider is then led to believe that risk-factor management is not an essential part of the patient's care. Discharge plans and letters to the referring physician should identify risk factors on the patient's problem list, including diagnostic tests performed (e.g., fasting lipid profiles at the time of admission for MI). Furthermore, steps taken, including counseling by members of the multidisciplinary team, should be recorded. Finally, additional interventions and the goals of these interventions, which still need to be completed, should be provided. Again, the emphasis is on communicating the optimal care plan for the patient with vascular disease and this includes risk-factor management.

Opportunities in the Ambulatory Care Setting

Role of the Primary Care Provider

The primary care provider plays a variety of important roles in risk-factor management. It is hoped that detailed notes on the recommendations and progress to date will be available from the specialist after discharge from an inpatient unit. Construction of this plan requires the ability to accurately assess an individual patient's risk factors and place them in a category of appropriate risk-factor intervention. Currently, many discharge forms are poorly organized. There are a number of easily accessible forms that provide more comprehensive communication and prompt the physician to consider a number of key issues (Fig. 13.2, http://www.americanheart.org/CAP). The primary care provider needs to integrate these new plans with the overall care plan. Monitoring and feedback of patients' progress are often best carried out by the primary care provider, who has more frequent and regular access to the patient. The primary care provider may also wish to organize his or her practice to provide preventive care more efficiently. The office nurse frequently serves as a counselor on smoking cessation, diet, exercise, medication compliance, and other risk factors. Additional training of nonphysician professionals can expand considerably the services provided by an ambulatory care practice.

In terms of preventive strategies in the patient without symptomatic coronary artery disease, the physician must be able to assess multiple risk factors and estimate an overall risk of future coronary artery disease events. In this instance, the calculation of a global risk-scoring equation using multiple risk-factor variables gives an overall estimate of absolute risk of developing coronary artery disease over a 10-year period (24,25). A variety of risk assessment instruments are available, including wall charts, slide rules, handheld risk calculators, and software programs. With use of this risk-stratification, the physician is able to provide the appropriate level of risk-factor modification based on accepted guidelines, including the identification of the *coronary heart disease risk equivalent* patient who deserves aggressive risk-factor management.

Role of Specialty Clinics and Cardiac Rehabilitation Units

Larger ambulatory practices, especially those tied to inpatient units, may have the opportunity to develop specialized programs for risk-factor management. The key element is the focus of risk-factor management expertise and resources in a person or team of people to whom problems can be referred. Clearly, most patients with vascular disease should be provided with risk-factor counseling and appropriate pharmacologic therapy as part of optimal cardiology care. However, there will continue to be a subgroup of patients in whom specialized expertise will likely be needed. These include patients who are resistant, recalcitrant, rare, or risky (the four Rs). Patients not responding to usual interventions for dyslipidemia or hypertension may benefit from an additional opinion. Patients who are recalcitrant may benefit from physicians, nurses, nutritionists, and exercise specialists skilled in behavior modification and counseling. Patients with rare risk-factor abnormalities, such as genetic hyperlipidemias, coronary disease without obvious risk factors, or coexisting medical diagnoses, may also require specialist expertise. Finally, patients at extreme risk of bad outcomes may have aggressive risk-factor management programs more successfully implemented by a multidisciplinary team (e.g., the patient with symptomatic vascular disease in the fourth or fifth decade of life and those patients with coronary heart disease and type 2 diabetes mellitus).

These specialized programs may take several forms. A preventive cardiology clinic is likely preferable over a clinic emphasizing a single risk factor, as most patients have several risk factors (90). In general, the staff includes one or more physicians with specialized training and expertise in risk-factor management, a coordinator, a nurse skilled in risk-factor counseling, a nutritionist knowledgeable about lipid-lowering diets, and an exercise physiologist who can develop an exercise prescription. The team may be supported by a variety of data collection tools, including computerized databases, patient education materials, and follow-up protocols.

Cardiac rehabilitation programs are often underused as sites for risk-factor management (see Chapter 12). Their efficacy in reducing total and cardiovascular mortality has been well documented in metaanalyses (91), especially when they include comprehensive risk-factor management services (92,93). Again, a team approach is optimal. Cardiac rehabilitation programs have the added advantage of providing considerable psychosocial support from other patients and their family members.

Nurse case managers are being used widely as a cost-effective means to provide comprehensive risk reduction with excellent continuity between inpatient and ambulatory care settings. Nurse-managed programs have been shown to be effective in the management of single risk factors, including smoking cessation (94), diabetes (95), hypertension (96), and lipid lowering (97). Specially trained nurses have implemented comprehensive risk-factor reduction programs targeting multiple risk factors. An example of such a program, the Stanford Cardiac Risk Intervention Program, is illustrated in *e*Figure 13.2.1 (98,99). During a 1-year

TABLE 13.4 LEVELS OF RISK-FACTOR MODIFICATION IN PATIENTS AFTER MYOCARDIAL INFARCTION: A TRIAL OF NURSE CASE MANAGER–BASED PROGRAMS VERSUS USUAL CARE

	Intervention	
Risk-factor modification	Nurse case manager (n = 293)	Usual care (n = 292)
Smoking cessation at 12 mo (%)	70.0	53.0
Low-density lipoprotein cholesterol <100 mg/dL at 12 mo (%)	42.0	15.0
Functional capacity	9.3	8.4

From DeBusk RF, Houston-Miller N, Superko HR, et al. A case-management system for coronary risk factor modification after acute myocardial infarction. *Ann Intern Med* 1994;120:721–729, with permission.

period, patients received a combination of visits, telephone calls, and mailing reminders. Nurses formed the central point of contact, interacting with patients and other health professionals and laboratories. There was a clear delineation of professionals' responsibilities. The system successfully enhanced pharmacologic and dietary therapy and improved patient symptomatology and use of health services. DeBusk et al. (98) demonstrated a significantly higher rate of smoking cessation, a tripling of the proportion of patients reaching the LDL cholesterol goal of less than 100 mg per dL, and an improved exercise capacity among those patients managed by nurses trained in multiple risk-factor management (Table 13.4). Nurse case managers appear to be particularly effective in increasing patients' adherence to diet and drugs; in implementing a program of self-monitoring of weight, blood pressure, symptoms, and smoking cessation; and in teaching patients to recognize and respond to changes in their symptoms (100,101). Among the numerous advantages of such nurse case manager programs is the opportunity to initiate contact with the patient while he or she is still in the hospital (98,99), thereby integrating the inpatient and outpatient risk-factor management into a single, continuous program. Furthermore, patient satisfaction has been high, and significant cost savings, even over the short-term, can be realized (101).

Opportunities for the Patient

Patient Compliance and Adherence to Interventions

A detailed discussion of patient compliance and adherence with behavioral and therapeutic regimens is beyond the scope of this review. It is an issue of enormous importance (69). First, the prevalence of noncompliance is exceptionally high, with estimates suggesting that only one-third of patients are fully compliant, another one-third are somewhat compliant, and one-third are fully noncompliant (102). This results in approximately 50% of the 2 billion prescriptions written in the United States annually being taken incorrectly (69). Compliance with behavioral interventions is even lower, with the maintenance of smoking cessation, weight-control diets, and low–saturated fat diets estimated at 10% to 20% over a 1-year period (103). The costs resulting from this noncompliance are staggering, with approximately 10% of hospitalization caused by patients' inability to follow therapeutic regimens (69). In the Beta Blocker Heart Attack Trial, both men and women taking fewer than 75% of their prescribed beta-blocker medication had 2.5- to 3.0-fold higher mortality than those who took their medications more than 75% of the time (104,105). The problem of noncompliance encompasses all diseases, risk factors, and therapies (70). Improving patient compliance and adherence is clearly a major challenge and opportunity for improving the outcome of any intervention program.

The determinants of noncompliance and nonadherence are multiple and complex (106). For example, patient factors (knowledge, beliefs, attitudes, and values), their families, the health care setting, the provider–patient relationship, characteristics of the disease, and nature of the treatment all play important roles (69,107). A 2-year study of patients with hypertension, diabetes, or cardiac disease showed that characteristics of health care providers (physician specialty, number of patients seen per week, willingness to answer patients' questions), the health care facility itself (scheduling a follow-up appointment, number of tests ordered), the seriousness of the illness, and the level of patient distress all have an effect on compliance (70).

Because of the complexity of this issue, no single intervention has been shown to be effective in solving the problem. Although a variety of strategies of varying sophistication have been proposed (102), some rather simple steps can be emphasized (Table 13.5) (107). These include clear communication of goals, simplification of the intervention, and monitoring with feedback to the patient. Special programs, such as those with nurse case managers, may succeed because of their abilities to carry out these compliance-enhancing steps. Increasingly, programs in the electronic media have been developed to ensure compliance. The AHA has also provided several Web-based tools that have a wide variety of applications for physicians, patients, and hospital staff. The *one-of-a-kind* program allows patients to enter data regarding their cardiac risk factors and track their progress as well as compare their values with a composite mean of the database (http://www.onelife.americanheart.org). This compliance-enhancing, Web-based tool is versatile. Physicians and staff in busy practices can provide their patients with access to cardiovascular services by a brief but strong recommendation to enroll in this program, which prompts a wide range of risk-factor management issues based on current guidelines.

TABLE 13.5 RECOMMENDATIONS TO IMPROVE PATIENT ADHERENCE TO TREATMENT

Initiation of treatment
  Convey the importance of the recommendations
  Emphasize required behaviors to provide the rationale for them
  Simplify the regimen
  Discuss costs
Record keeping
  Use a systematic and consistent tracking form
  Send reminders of follow-up appointments
  Monitor effects
Follow-up
  Reinforce treatment message
  Probe about side effects, problems, and adherence

From Luepker RV. Patient adherence: a "risk factor" for cardiovascular disease. *Heart Dis Stroke* 1993;2:418–421, with permission.

Opportunities by Health Care Organizations, Professional Societies, and Third-Party Payers

Clinical Guidelines

Fortunately, the AHA, ACC, and other bodies have issued joint guidelines on risk-factor management in patients with vascular disease (4) and without vascular disease (8), as well as for women (7) and diabetic patients (6). These guidelines are consistent with statements addressing individual risk-factor modification such as hypertension (9), hypercholesterolemia (10), sedentary lifestyle, smoking (11), and obesity (12). The essence of these guidelines has also been incorporated into recommendations for acute cardiac care (13).

Despite good consensus on risk-factor management, the efficacy of guidelines is mixed. It appears that they are least likely to succeed if no incentives (or removal of disincentives) are provided for the practicing physician (114). Guidelines need to be actively disseminated and implemented. They are most effective when coupled with evaluation of physician performance (115). As databases evaluating patient risk-factor modification become increasingly available, this may provide such an opportunity in the future.

Quality Assurance Standards

Some of the components of a quality assurance program are already in place, including substantial evidence from basic science, epidemiology clinical trials, cost-effectiveness analyses (14), and guidelines reflecting broad consensus on criteria for optimal risk-factor management (4). The next component in a quality assurance program is the feedback loop, in which levels of performance toward accepted criteria are linked to incentives, including credentialing, remuneration, or competitiveness (*e*Fig. 13.2.2) (116,117). One performance report has been the Health Plan Employer

Data and Information Set (HEDIS), which employers use in contracting for care with managed care organizations (118). Risk-factor management indices have become especially well represented, probably because of the presence of consensus statements and the evidence of nearly universal benefits of many of the interventions. HEDIS 3.0, for example, used a number of risk-factor levels and management practices as end points for the next *report card* (Table 13.6) (119). The National Committee for Quality Assurance is routinely developing new performance guidelines as part of the HEDIS process (118). This now requires a mandatory report from health maintenance organizations, quantifying the percentage of cardiac patients who have met HEDIS criteria. The National Committee for Quality Assurance have defined a difference between clinical and performance goals. Although they endorse the NCEP guidelines, they have stipulated a goal LDL of less than 130 mg per dL, rather than less than 100 mg per dL, in patients with coronary heart disease. The reason for this difference is to provide a realistic, attainable goal that allows physicians room for clinical judgment in individual cases. The important point to note, however, is the change in focus for health maintenance organizations and consequently physician practice in terms of evaluation of efficacy of risk-factor modification (120).

Relatively recent medical-legal actions may be another example of use of quality assurance standards. One settled suit, successfully charging a wrongful death caused in part by the lack of treatment of hyperlipidemia, illustrates the use of guidelines in medical malpractice claims (121).

Reimbursement Policies

The lack of reimbursement can serve as a powerful disincentive to risk-factor management for practicing physicians (122). Statements, guidelines, and accreditation by professional societies and the acceptance of risk-factor manage-

TABLE 13.6 MEASURES RELEVANT TO THE COMPREHENSIVE RISK REDUCTION OF PATIENTS WITH VASCULAR DISEASE PROPOSED FOR REPORTING IN HEALTH PLAN EMPLOYER DATA AND INFORMATION SET

Beta-blocker treatment after myocardial infarction
Advising smokers to quit
Controlling high blood pressure[a]
Aspirin treatment after myocardial infarction[a]
Prevention of stroke in patients with atrial fibrillation[a]
Angiotensin-converting enzyme inhibitors in patients hospitalized with congestive heart failure[a]
Cholesterol management in patients hospitalized with coronary disease[a]

[a]Being evaluated for inclusion in future Health Plan Employer Data and Information Set.
From Committee on Performance Measurement of the National Center for Quality Assurance. Health plan employer data and information set. HEDIS 3.0 Draft, 1996, with permission.

ment as quality indicators are powerful motivators for third-party payers to reimburse for preventive services. Such motivation will be needed for physicians, clinics, and hospitals to allocate personnel, space, and funds for risk-factor management programs.

CONTROVERSIES AND PERSONAL PERSPECTIVES

The demand for risk modification is likely to continue to expand because of several irreversible trends. First, the prevalence of coronary heart disease and other vascular diseases will continue to expand for at least the next 30 years (123). Currently, among U.S. adults aged 45 years and older, 12% of men and 8% of women carry the diagnosis of coronary disease. Second, cardiovascular specialists are likely to be consulted in the management of a new cohort of patients in whom asymptomatic atherosclerotic disease has been identified by noninvasive means. Third, current guidelines are now identifying, on the basis of a global risk score, a potentially large group of patients who have a coronary heart disease risk equivalent. Thus, the demand for preventive services will only expand, necessitating efficacious, effective, and efficient methods to reduce risk. This chapter has identified gaps in the successful implementation of risk-factor modification. How might we do better? The controversy is not why, whether, or how to do it, but who should do it.

This author's personal impression is that this responsibility is a shared one. Although additional research is needed to identify specific barriers to preventive care and to test strategies to remove them, it is clear that we can organize ourselves to be more effective. For every coronary disease patient admitted to an inpatient service, we recommend an organized, comprehensive assessment of risk factors, which then triggers the development of a plan to manage the patient. Next, a nurse case manager either follows up on the patient from the inpatient to the outpatient setting or clearly communicates the plan to the referring generalist. The plan is then carried out by a coordinated, multidisciplinary team of physicians, nurses, nutritionists, and exercise physiologists either in the inpatient service or in the outpatient clinic. In general, the patient is cared for until risk-factor goals have been met.

Cardiovascular specialists often cite their lack of responsibility in this area. This position is increasingly untenable, because most or all of the goals of revascularization or cardiac pharmacotherapy are the same as those for risk-factor management. Risk-factor management alleviates chest pain, reduces the risk of MI, prevents disability caused by stroke and heart disease, prolongs survival, and, in many instances, reduces health care costs. Few invasive procedure and high-technology interventions can boast of such an effect. The cardiovascular specialist who does not integrate risk-factor management into his or her patient care then has the simple goal of performing procedures, rather than optimizing clinical outcomes.

The bedrock, which is unmoved by contemporary deficiencies in medical education, health care economics, and practice disorganization, will remain the scientific evidence defining the role of risk-factor management in beneficially altering the natural history of atherosclerotic disease. This is likely only to strengthen. In addition to studies of basic mechanisms and randomized clinical trials of new interventions, research on the implementation and maintenance of optimal care practices is needed to ensure the appropriate application of all that we have learned.

This would then require us to reform our research agenda. The World Health Organization perspective on disease control is illustrated in *e*Figure 13.2.2 (1). The WHO identified three areas for improvement. The first is to reduce disease currently unavoidable with existing interventions through biomedical research and the development of new interventions. Clearly, there are many opportunities to elucidate new disease mechanisms amenable to intervention, to identify new risk factors, and to test new drugs and technologies with randomized trials. Indeed, the vast majority of our research and development resources go into this activity. A controversial position may be that, as biomedical science advances, further development of interventions will result in only a modicum of disease reduction unless there is attention to two other causes of the disease burden, namely, disease that would be averted with improved efficiency and disease that would be averted if existing interventions were more cost effective. These two areas currently receive a small fraction of research and development funds. To really affect this disease, these sources of avoidable coronary heart disease must likewise be reduced.

TABLE 13.7 PREVENTIVE CARE OF THE CORONARY DISEASE PATIENT: USUAL, OPTIMAL, AND FUTURE

Phase of disease	Usual, contemporary care	Optimal contemporary care	Future care
Early (1–5 d)	Risk-stratification with echocardiogram/angiogram; acetylsalicylic acid; beta-blockers with or without angiotensin-converting enzyme inhibitors	Usual care, plus lipid, glucose screening; smoking cessation counseling; nutrition intervention; aggressive glucose management; lipid-lowering drugs (statins); diagnosis and treatment of depression	Usual and optimal care plus risk-stratification by noninvasive tests, including inflammatory markers; risk-factor assessment, including phenotyping and genotyping; initiation of diet and exercise regimens targeted at risk; selection of drugs to reduce risk with greatest cost-effectiveness
Postdischarge (6–8 wk)	Smoking cessation; lipid profile; physical activity advise; diabetes screening	Nurse case-managed care; standard cardiac rehabilitation; titration of lipid management; titration of glucose management; titration of blood pressure medication; risk-factor screening of first-degree relatives	Risk management program via electronic media; titration of LDL, HDL, glucose, and blood pressure to optimal levels; genotyping and phenotyping of first-degree relatives
Long-term	Risk-factor monitoring; lipid management; diabetes therapy	Treatment to goals of LDL, HDL, blood pressure and blood glucose; compliance with dietary recommendations; compliance with exercise recommendations; monitoring for evidence of recurrence	Titration of LDL, HDL, glucose and blood pressure to optimal levels, based on noninvasive markers; compliance enhancers for diet; compliance enhancers for exercise

HDL, high-density lipoprotein; LDL, low-density lipoprotein.

THE FUTURE

Applications of the principles of vascular biology to the practice of cardiology will likely be of such priority that the two fields will become one. The concepts of *metabolic revascularization* and *risk-based intervention* will be cornerstones for care.

eTable 13.0.1 provides a view of contemporary interventions as well as those likely to evolve in the near future to become established modes of care. Improved intervention and studies to establish their efficiency will be forthcoming in the next decade for diabetes, low HDL and high triglycerides, and obesity. Improvements in compliance with physical activity and diet will also take place, it is hoped.

Table 13.7 furthers this vision, starting with current care using known strategies, expanded to optimal evidence-based care projected into the future. Several trends clearly stand out. First, risk-stratification will improve through the use of noninvasive imaging and biochemical or genetic markers, such as inflammatory markers. Likewise, risk-factor assessment in early and postdischarge periods will be sharpened by use of genetic markers and improved phenotypic indicators, for both probands and their relatives. Selection of nonpharmacologic and pharmacologic interventions will be more precise, with clusters of interventions chosen to optimize prognosis and cost effectiveness. These interventions will

be guided by knowledge of disease processes and by empirical data from clinical trials. Compliance will be strongly emphasized, with the use of multidisciplinary teams led by risk-factor managers supported by a variety of electronic media. Titration of drugs and lifestyle interventions may rely less on metabolic or behavioral end points and more on noninvasive measures of altered pathophysiology, such as endothelial dysfunction or disease progression.

This explosion of knowledge and technology should not lull us into a false sense that cardiovascular disease will be conquered without the continued reliance on interpersonal skills. Preventive cardiology will still need to rely on the ability of the preventive cardiology team to modify the patient's behaviors that led to the disease in the first place. It is difficult to conceive of pharmacologic or surgical interventions that will even partially displace the need for effective smoking cessation counseling, the alteration of ingestion of dietary fats and cholesterol, and the increase in physical activity. Although patients will benefit from the skills of a variety of health professionals, the cardiovascular specialist will still need to ensure optimal care through his or her implementation. Thus, the integration of risk-factor modification will undoubtedly cease to be adjunctive therapy and take its rightful place as the cornerstone of cardiac care.

REFERENCES

1. Ad Hoc Committee on Health Research to Future Intervention Options: investing in health research development. Geneva: World Health Organization, 1996:1–18.
2. Byers T, Anda R, McQueen D, et al. The correspondence between coronary heart disease mortality and risk factor prevalence among states in the United States, 1991–1992. *Prev Med* 1998;27:311–316.
3. Stampfer MJ, Hu FB, Monson JE, et al. Primary prevention of coronary heart disease in women through diet and lifestyle. *N Engl J Med* 2000;343:16–22.
4. Smith SC Jr, Blair SN, Criqui MH, et al. Preventing heart attack and death in patients with coronary disease. *Circulation* 1995;92:2–4.
5. Grundy SM, Balady JG, Criqui MH, et al. Guide to primary prevention of cardiovascular disease. *Circulation* 1997;95:2329–2331.
6. American Diabetes Association. Standards of medical care for patients with diabetes mellitus. *Diabetes Care* 1999;22:S32–S41.
7. Mosca L, Grundy SM, Judelson D, et al. AHA/ACC Scientific Statement Consensus Panel: guide to preventive cardiology for women. *Circulation* 1999;99:2480–2484.
8. Agency for Health Care Policy and Research. Treating tobacco use and dependence. US Department of Health and Human Services. Public Health Services Report, June 2000.
9. The Sixth Report of the Joint National Committee on Prevention, Detection, Evaluation, and Treatment of High Blood Pressure. Bethesda, MD: National Institutes of Health, National Heart, Lung, and Blood Institute, 1998, NIH Publication 98-4080.
10. Expert Panel on Detection, Evaluation, and Treatment of High Blood Cholesterol in Adults. National Cholesterol Education Program: second report of the expert panel on detection, evaluation, and treatment of high blood cholesterol (Adult Treatment Panel II). Bethesda, MD: National Institutes of Health, National Heart, Lung and Blood Institute, 1993, NIH Publication 93-3095.
11. Fletcher GF, Balady G, Blair SN, et al. Statement on exercise: benefits and recommendations for physical activity programs for all Americans: a statement for health professionals by the Committee on Exercise and Cardiac Rehabilitation of the Council on Clinical Cardiology. American Heart Association. *Circulation* 1996;94:857–862.
12. NHLBI Obesity Education Initiative Expert Panel. Clinical guidelines on identification, evaluation, and treatment of overweight and obesity in adults: the evidence report. *Obesity Research* 1998;6[Suppl]:51S–209S.
13. Ryan TJ, Antman EM, Brooks NH, et al. 1999 update: ACC/AHA guidelines for the management of patients with acute myocardial infarction: executive summary and recommendations: a report of the American College of Cardiology/American Heart Association Task Force on Practice Guidelines. *Circulation* 1999;100:1016–1030.
14. Pearson TA, Fuster V. Executive summary of the 27th Bethesda Conference: matching the intensity of risk factor management with the hazard for coronary disease events. *J Am Coll Cardiol* 1996;27:961–963.
15. DeLorgeril M, Salen P, Martin JL, et al. Mediterranean diet, traditional risk factors, and the rate of cardiovascular complications after MI: final report of the Lyon Diet Heart Study. *Circulation* 1999;99:779–785.
16. Pearson TA, Boden WE. The imperative to raise low levels of high density lipoprotein cholesterol: a better clinical strategy in the prevention and treatment of coronary artery diseases. *Am J Cardiol* 2000;86[Suppl]:1L–65L.
17. Robins HB, Robins SJ, Collins D, et al. VA-HIT study group. Gemfibrozil for the secondary prevention of coronary heart disease in men with low levels of high-density lipoprotein cholesterol. Veteran Affairs High Density Lipoprotein Cholesterol Intervention Study for Group. *N Engl J Med* 1999;341:410–418.
18. HOPE investigators. Vitamin E supplementation and cardiovascular events in high-risk patients: the Heart Outcomes Prevention Evaluation Study Investigation. *N Engl J Med* 2000;342:154–160.
19. Ridker PM, Hennekens CH, Buring JE, et al. C-reactive protein and other markers of inflammation in the prediction of cardiovascular disease in women. *N Engl J Med* 2000;342:836–843.
20. Danesh J, Collins R, Appleby P, et al. Association of fibrinogen, C-reactive protein, or leukocyte count with coronary heart disease: meta-analyses of prospective studies. *JAMA* 1998;279:1477–1482.
21. Hulley S, Grady D, Bush T, et al. Randomized trial of estrogen plus progestin for secondary prevention of coronary heart disease in postmenopausal women: Heart and Estrogen/Progestin Study (HERS) Research Group. *JAMA* 1998;280:605–613.
22. Herrington DM, Reboussin DM, Klein KP, et al. The estrogen replacement and atherosclerosis (ERA) study: study design and baseline characteristics of the cohort. *Control Clin Trials* 2000;21:257–285.
23. Petitti D. Hormone replacement therapy and heart disease prevention. experimentation trumps observation. *JAMA* 1998;280:650–652.
24. Wilson PW, D'Agostino RB, Levy D, et al. Prediction of coronary heart disease using risk factor categories. *Circulation* 1998;97:1837–1847.
25. Grundy SM, Pasternak R, Greenland P, et al. Assessment of cardiovascular risk by use of multiple risk factor assessment equations. *Circulation* 1999;100:1481–1492.
26. Wood DA, DeBacker G, Faergeman O, et al. Prevention of coronary heart disease in clinical practice. Recommendations of the second joint task force of the European Society of Cardiology, European Atherosclerosis Society, and European Society of Hypertension. *Eur Heart J* 1998;19:1434–1503.
27. Crouse JR 3rd, Byington RP, Furberg CD. HMG-CoA reductase inhibitor therapy and stroke risk reduction: an analysis of clinical trials data. *Atherosclerosis.* 1998;138:11–24.
28. Fuster V, Gotto AM, Libby P, et al. Pathogenesis of coronary disease: the biologic role of risk factors. *J Am Coll Cardiol* 1996;27:964–976.
29. Wilhelmsson C, Elmsfeldt D, Vedin JA, et al. Smoking and myocardial infarction. *Lancet* 1975;1:415–419.
30. US Department of Health and Human Services. The Health Benefits of Smoking Cessation, A Report of the Sur-

geon General. Centers for Disease Control, Office of Smoking and Health, 1990, Department of Health and Human Services Publication CDC 909–8416.

31. Andrews TC, Raby K, Barry J, et al. The effect of LDL cholesterol reduction on myocardial ischemia in patients with coronary disease. *Circulation* 1997;95:324–328.

32. Grundy SM, Balady GJ, Criqui MH, et al. When to start cholesterol-lowering therapy in patients with coronary heart disease. A statement for healthcare professionals from the American Heart Association Task Force on Risk Reduction. *Circulation* 1997;95:1683–1685.

33. The Pravastatin Multinational Study Group of Cardiac Risk Patients. Effects of pravastatin in patients with serum total cholesterol levels from 5.2 to 7.8 mmol/liter (200 to 300 mg/dl) plus two additional atherosclerotic risk factors. *Am J Cardiol* 1993;72:1031–1037.

34. Stenestrand U, Wallentin L. Early statin treatment following acute myocardial infarction and 1-year survival. *JAMA* 2001;285:430–436.

35. Schwartz GG, Oliver MF, Ezekowitz MD, et al. Rationale and design of the myocardial ischemia reduction with aggressive cholesterol lowering (MIRACL) study that evaluates atorvastatin in unstable angina pectoris and in non-Q-wave acute myocardial infarction. *Am J Cardiol* 1998;81:578–581.

36. Malmberg K, Ryden L, Efendic S, et al. Randomized trial of insulin-glucose infusion followed by subcutaneous insulin treatment in diabetic patients with acute myocardial infarction (DIGAMI study): effects on mortality at 1 year. *J Am Coll Cardiol* 1995;26:57–65

37. Mathew J, Pearson TA. Clinical and epidemiologic predictors of recurrent coronary artery disease. *Coronary Artery Dis* 1995;6:447–456.

38. Califf RM, Armstrong PW, Carver JR, et al. Stratification of patients into high, medium, and low risk subgroups for purposes of risk factor management. *J Am Coll Cardiol* 1996;27:1007–1019.

39. Scandinavian Simvastatin Study Group. Randomized trial of cholesterol lowering in 4444 patients with coronary heart disease: the Scandinavian Simvastatin Survival Study (4S). *Lancet* 1994;344:1385–1389.

40. Blankenhorn DH, Nessim SA, Johnson RL, et al. Beneficial effects of combined colestipol-niacin therapy on coronary atherosclerosis and coronary venous bypass grafts. *JAMA* 1987;257:3233–3240.

41. Post Coronary Artery Bypass Graft Trial Investigators. The effect of aggressive lowering of low-density lipoprotein cholesterol levels and low-dose anticoagulation on obstructive changes in saphenous-vein coronary-artery bypass grafts. *N Engl J Med* 1997;336:153–162.

42. Stafford RS, Blumenthal D, Pasternak RC. Variations in cholesterol management practices of U.S. physicians. *J Am Coll Cardiol* 1997;29:139–146.

43. Schrott HG, Bittner V, Vittinghoff E, et al. Adherence to national cholesterol education program treatment goals in postmenopausal women with heart disease. The Heart and Estrogen/Progestin Replacement Study (HERS). *JAMA* 1997;277:1281–1286.

44. Pearson TA, Laurora I, Chu H, et al. The Lipid Treatment Assessment Project (L-TAP). A multicenter survey to evaluate the percentage of dyslipidemic patients receiving lipid-lowering drugs. *Arch Intern Med* 2000;160:459–467.

45. Wang TJ, Stafford RS. National patterns and predictors of beta-blocker use in patients with coronary artery disease. *Arch Intern Med* 1998;158:1901–1906.

46. Stafford RS, Saglam D, Blumenthal D. National patterns of angiotensin-converting enzyme inhibitor use in congestive heart failure. *Arch Intern Med* 1997;157:2460–2464.

47. Stafford RS. Aspirin use is low among United States outpatients with coronary artery disease. *Circulation* 2000;101:1097–1101.

48. Thorndike AN, Rigotti NA, Stafford RS, et al. National patterns in the treatment of smokers by physicians. *JAMA* 1998;279:604–608.

49. Rigotti NA, Singer DE, Mulley AG, et al. Smoking cessation following admission to a coronary care unit. *J Gen Intern Med* 1991;6:305–311.

50. Anonymous. A European Society of Cardiology survey of secondary prevention of coronary heart disease: principal results, EUROSPIRE Study Group. *Eur Heart J* 1998;18:1569–1582.

51. Grundy SM, Cleeman JI, Rifkind BM, et al. Cholesterol lowering in the elderly population. *Arch Intern Med* 1999;159:1670–1678.

52. McAlister F. The treatment and prevention of coronary heart disease in Canada: do older patients receive efficacious therapies? The Clinical Quality Improvement Network (CQIN) Investigators. *J Am Geriatr Soc* 1999;47:811–818.

53. Sueta C, Chowdury M, Boccuzzi SJ. Analysis of the degree of undertreatment of hyperlipidemia and congestive heart failure secondary to coronary artery disease. *Am J Cardiol* 1999;83:1303–1307.

54. Bourassa MG, Gurne O, Bangdiwala SI. Natural history and patterns of current practice in heart failure, The Studies of Left Ventricular Dysfunction (SOLUD) Investigations. *J Am Coll Cardiol* 1993;22[4 Suppl A]:14A–19A.

55. Swanson J, Pearson TA. Screening family members at high risk for coronary disease—why isn't it done? *Am J Prev Med* 2001;20:50–55.

56. Bahit MC, Granger CB, Alexander KP, et al. Applying the evidence: opportunity in US for 80,000 additional lives saved per year. *Circulation* 2000;102:11–874.

57. Pearson TA, McBride PE, Houston Miller N, et al. 27th Bethesda Conference: matching the intensity of risk factor management with the hazard for coronary disease events. Task Force 8. Organization of preventive cardiology service. *J Am Coll Cardiol* 1996;27:1039–1047.

58. Solberg LI, Boyle RG, Davidson G, et al. Patient satisfaction and discussion of smoking cessation during clinical visits. *Mayo Clin Proc* 2001;76:138–143.

59. Kottke TE, Brekke ML, Solberg LI. Making time for preventative services. *Mayo Clin Proc* 1993;68:785–791.

60. Miller NH, Smith PM, DeBusk RF, et al. Smoking cessation in hospitalized patients. Results of a randomized trial. *Arch Intern Med* 1997;157:409–415.

61. Taylor CB, Houston-Miller N, Killen JD, et al. Smoking cessation after acute myocardial infarction: effects of a nurse managed intervention. *Ann Intern Med* 1990;113:118–123.

62. Cohen MC, Stafford RS, Misra B. Stress testing: national patterns and predictors of test ordering. *Am Heart J* 1999;138:1019–1024.

63. Ayanian JZ, Epstein AM. Differences in the use of procedures between women and men hospitalized for coronary heart disease. *N Engl J Med* 1991;325:221–225.

64. Steingart RM, Packer M, Hamm P, et al. Sex differences in the management of coronary artery disease. *N Engl J Med* 1991;325:226–230.

65. Williams RB, Barefoot JC, Califf RM, et al. Prognostic importance of social and economic resources among medically treated patients with angiographically defined coronary heart disease. *JAMA* 1992;267:520–524.

66. Lenfant C. Conference on socioeconomic status and cardiovascular health and disease. *Circulation* 1996;94:2041–2044.

67. Castaner A, Simmons BE, Mar M, et al. Myocardial infarction in black patients: poor prognosis after hospital discharge. *Ann Intern Med* 1988;109:33–35.

68. Tofler GH, Stone PH, Muller JE, et al. Effects of gender and race on prognosis after myocardial infarction: adverse prognosis in women, particularly black women. *J Am Coll Cardiol* 1987;9:473–482.

69. Berg JS, Dischler J, Wagner DJ, et al. Medication compliance: a health care problem. *Ann Pharmacother* 1993;27[Suppl]:S2–S22.

70. Morris LS, Schultz RM. Patient compliance—a review. *J Clin Pharmacol Ther* 1992;17:283–295.

71. Simons LA. Apparent discontinuation rates in patients prescribed lipid-lowering drugs. *Med J Aust* 1996;164:208–211.

72. Harlan WR, Sandler SA, Lee KL, et al. Importance of baseline functional and socioeconomic factors for participation in cardiac rehabilitation. *Am J Cardiol* 1995;76:36–39.

73. Mark DB, Clapp-Channing N, Lam LC, et al. Medical care: access, utilization, and cost. In: *Report of the Conference on Socioeconomic Status and Cardiovascular Health and Disease.* Public Health Service, National Institutes of Health, National Heart, Lung, and Blood Institute, 1996;133–138.

74. Sullivan JM, Frohlich ED, Lewis RP, et al. Guidelines for training in adult cardiovascular medicine. Core Cardiology Training Symposium(CO-CATS). Task Force 10: training in preventive cardiovascular medicine. *J Am Coll Cardiol* 1995;25:33–34.

75. AVERT study group. Efficacy and safety of aggressive lipid lowering therapy with atorvastatin to catheter based revascularization followed by conventional care in patients with stable angina pectoris and documented coronary artery disease. *Am J Cardiol* 1997;80:1130–1133.

76. Balady GJ, Ades PA, Comoss P, et al. Core components of cardiac rehabilitation/prevention programs: a statement for healthcare professionals from the American Heart Association and the American Association of Cardiovascular and Pulmonary Rehabilitation Writing Group. *Circulation* 2000;102:1069–1073.

77. Shea S, Gemson DH, Mossel P. Management of high blood cholesterol by primary care physicians: diffusion of the National Cholesterol Education Program Adult Treatment Panel guidelines. *J Gen Intern Med* 1990;5:327–334.

78. Roberts WC. Getting cardiologists interested in lipids. *Am J Cardiol* 1993;72:744–745.

79. Swan HJC. Why cardiologists must be interested in lipids. *Am J Cardiol* 1995;76:1067–1068.

80. Pearson TA, Rapaport E, Criqui M, et al. Optimal risk factor management in the patient after coronary revascularization: a statement for health professionals from an American Heart Association Writing Group. *Circulation* 1994;90:3125–3133.

81. Williams BJ. Efficiency of a checklist to promote a preventive medicine approach. *J Tenn Med Assoc* 1981;74:489–491.

82. Cohen DI, Littenburg B, Wetzel C, et al. Improving physician compliance with preventive medicine guidelines. *Med Care* 1982;20:1040–1045.

83. McDonald CJ. Protocol-based computer reminders, the quality of care and the non-perfectibility of man. *N Engl J Med* 1976;295:1351–1355.

84. Davidson RA, Fletcher SW, Retchin S, et al. A nurse-initiated reminder system for the periodic health examination: implementation and evaluation. *Arch Intern Med* 1984;144:2167–2170.

85. Harris RP, O'Malley MS, Fletcher SW, et al. Prompting physicians for preventive procedures: a five year study of manual and computer reminders. *Am J Prev Med* 1990;6:145–152.

86. Weingarten SR, Reidinger MS, Connor L, et al. Practice guidelines and reminders to reduce duration of hospital stay for patients with chest pain: an interventional trial. *Ann Intern Med* 1994;120:257–263.

87. Fonarow GC, Gawlinski A. Rationale and design of the cardiac hospitalization atherosclerosis management program at the University of California Los Angeles. *Am J Cardiol* 2000;85:10A–17A.

88. Rosenson RS. Myocardial injury: the acute phase response and lipoprotein metabolism. *J Am Coll Cardiol* 1993;22:933–940.

89. Reed RG, Jenkins PL, Pearson TA. Laboratory's manner of reporting serum cholesterol affects clinical care. *Clin Chem* 1994;40:847–848.

90. Genest J. Prevalence of risk factors in men with premature coronary artery disease. *Am J Cardiol* 1991;67:1185–1190.

91. Oldridge NB, Guyatt GH, Fisher ME, et al. Cardiac rehabilitation after myocardial infarction: combined experience of randomized clinical trials. *JAMA* 1988;260:945–950.

92. Kallio V, Hamalainen H, Hakkila J, et al. Reduction in sudden deaths by a multifactorial intervention program after acute myocardial infarction. *Lancet* 1979;2:1091–1094.

93. Hedback B, Perk J. Five-year results of a comprehensive rehabilitation program after myocardial infarction. *Eur Heart J* 1987;8:234–242.

94. Taylor CB, Houston-Miller N, Killen JD, et al. Smoking cessation after acute myocardial infarction: effects of a nurse managed intervention. *Ann Intern Med* 1990;113:118–123.

95. Weinberger M, Kirkman MS, Samson GP, et al. A nurse coordinated intervention for primary care patients with non-insulin dependent diabetes mellitus: impact on glycemic control and health-related quality of life. *J Gen Intern Med* 1995;10:59–66.

96. Rechgott MJ, Pearson S, Hill MN. The nurse practitioner's role in complex patient management: hypertension. *J Natl Med Assoc* 1983;75:1197–1204.

97. Blair TP, Bryant FJ, Bocuzzi S. Treatment of hypercholesterolemia by a clinical nurse using a stepped-care protocol in an nonvolunteer population. *Arch Intern Med* 1988;148:1046–1048.

98. DeBusk RF, Houston-Miller N, Superko HR, et al. A case-management system for coronary risk factor modification after acute myocardial infarction. *Ann Intern Med* 1994;120:721–729.

99. Hammer L. Kaiser Permanente Northern California Region MULTIFIT program provides alternative approach to cardiac rehabilitation. *Nurse Week* February 1995;26–27.

100. Allison TG, Squires RW, Johnson BD, et al. Achieving national cholesterol education program goals for low-density lipoprotein cholesterol in cardiac patients: importance of diet, exercise, weight control and drug therapy. *Mayo Clin Proc* 1999;74:466–473.

101. Miller NH, Warren D, Myers D. Home-based cardiac rehabilitation and lifestyle modification: the MULTIFIT model. *J Cardiovasc Nurs* 1996;11:76–87.

102. Wright EL. Noncompliance—or how many aunts has Matilda? *Lancet* 1993;342:909–913.

103. Levine DM. Behavioral and psychosocial factors, processes and strategies. In: Pearson TA, Criqui MH, Luepker RV, et al., eds. *Primer in preventive cardiology.* Dallas: American Heart Association, 1994;217–226.

104. Horwitz RI, Viscoli CM, Berkman L, et al. Treatment adherence and risk of death after a myocardial infarction. *Lancet* 1990;336:542–545.

105. Gallagher EJ, Viscoli CM, Horwitz RI. The relationship of treatment adherence to the risk of death after myocardial infarction in women. *JAMA* 1993;270:742–744.

106. Eraker SA, Knight JP, Becker MH. Understanding and improving patient compliance. *Ann Intern Med* 1984;100:258–268.

107. Luepker RV. Patient adherence: A "risk factor" for cardiovascular disease. *Heart Dis Stroke* 1993;2:418–421.

108. Stein LS. The effectiveness of continuing medical education: eight research reports. *J Med Educ* 1981;56:103–110.

109. Davis AA, Thompson MA, Oxman AA, et al. Changing physician performance: a systematic review of the effect of continuing medical education strategies. *JAMA* 1995;274:700–705.

110. Hill MH, Levine DM, Whelton PK. Awareness, use and impact of the 1984 Joint National Committee consensus report on high blood pressure. *Am J Public Health* 1988;78:1190–1194.

111. Cope DW, Linn LS, Leake BD, et al. Modification of resident's behavior by preceptor feedback of patient satisfaction. *J Gen Intern Med* 1986;1:394–398.

112. Hershey CO, Porter DK, Breslau D, et al. Influence of simple computerized feedback on prescription charges in an ambulatory clinic: a randomized clinical trial. *Med Care* 1986;24:472–481.

113. Boekeloo BO. *Evaluation of strategies for increasing intern cholesterol management in inpatients.* Baltimore: Johns Hopkins University, 1988, dissertation.

114. Lomas J, Enkin M, Anderson GM, et al. Opinion leaders vs audit and feedback to implement practice guidelines: delivery after previous cesarean section. *JAMA* 1995;265:2022–2207.

115. Grimshaw JM, Russell IT. Effect of clinical guidelines on medical practice: a systematic review of rigorous evaluations. *Lancet* 1993;342:1317–1322.

116. Palmer RH, Nesson HR. A review of methods for ambulatory medical care evaluations. *Med Care* 1982;20:758–781.

117. Epstein A. Performance reports on quality—prototypes, problems, and prospects. *N Engl J Med* 1993;333:57–61.

118. Lee TA, Cleeman JI, Grundy SM, et al. Clinical goals and performance measures for cholesterol management in secondary prevention of coronary heart disease. *JAMA* 2000;283:94–98.

119. Committee on Performance Measurement of the National Center for Quality Assurance. *Health plan employer data and information set.* HEDIS 3.0 Draft, 1996.

120. Eisenberg JM. Physician utilization: the state of research about physicians' practice patterns. *Med Care* 1985;23:461–483.

121. Woman's death leads to award by jurors. *Oregonian.* May 1, 1996.

122. Taylor RB. Health promotion: can it succeed in the office? *Prev Med* 1981;10:258–262.

123. Cooper R, Cutler J, Desvigne-Nickens P, et al. Trends and disparities in coronary heart disease, stroke and other cardiovascular diseases in the United States: findings of the national conference on cardiovascular disease prevention. *Circulation* 2000;102:3137–3147.

CLINICAL CARDIOLOGY

ROBERT M. CALIFF

14

THE HISTORY

ERIC J. TOPOL

OVERVIEW

The history is the most essential part of the diagnostic evaluation. A careful interview with the patient not only lays the foundation for an appropriate further workup, but it also serves as the framework for a bond between patient and physician, thereby promoting mutual respect, trust, and understanding. Listening to the patient cannot be adequately emphasized, and this goes beyond what is verbally communicated through gestures and nonverbal language. The major symptoms to review with each patient include chest discomfort or pain, dyspnea or cough, and syncope or palpitations—each of which are discussed in more depth. It is hoped that directly obtaining a meticulous history will become more routine and prioritized in the years ahead.

GENERAL PERSPECTIVE

Obtaining a careful, detailed history is fundamental to the proper evaluation of the patient. This takes time, as it requires listening to the patient and, ideally, his or her family members without interruption. Beyond listening, it is vital to cue in to the patient's nonverbal communication, such as affect and gestures. The time spent with the patient and the attitude displayed set the tone for the whole relationship and, therefore, represent a critical investment for the long-term bond and mutual trust that need to be nurtured. It is important for the patient to understand that the physician is a compassionate person

who frankly cares about his or her condition and who genuinely wants to help. The relationship that is built on strong communication with attention to details during the interview leads to a "full disclosure" history that often preempts the need for expensive, potentially hazardous, and certainly inconvenient diagnostic testing (1,2). History taking is a true art that yields unique and valuable information.

Before zooming in on the chief complaint, it is helpful to establish the patient's noncardiovascular history and medications and to query the risk factors for atherosclerosis. Pertinent conditions such as thyroid disease, anemia or gastrointestinal bleeding, asthma or chronic bronchitis, recent upper respiratory or viral illness, prostatitis, or arthritis frequently interrelate to the chief complaint and need to be fully characterized. Similarly, trauma or recent procedures such as oral surgery need to be surveyed. The entire list of medications with corresponding dosages must be known, given the preponderance of symptoms that can arise from side effects of drug therapy. Furthermore, the list of medications often serves as a checkpoint that all relevant medical conditions have been reviewed. Known allergies should be ascertained, and if coronary angiography is even a remote possibility, direct questioning about exposure to contrast dye or shellfish is imperative.

The risk factors for atherosclerosis must be carefully examined. As reviewed in detail in the first section of this textbook, each of the "big five"—hypertension, smoking, diabetes, hypercholesterolemia, and family history—is discussed. In this era of recognition of the primacy of genetics for influencing diseases, it is especially essential to obtain a detailed family history to consider for precocious atherosclerotic coronary disease (presenting at younger than 40 years for men or 45 years for women), any history of coro-

E. J. Topol: Department of Cardiovascular Medicine, The Cleveland Clinic Foundation, Cleveland, Ohio

nary artery disease, and other heart disease such as hypertrophic cardiomyopathy, arrhythmias, or other conditions (see Chapters 97 and 100). As recently noted, a family history of myocardial infarction may not be accurate (3,4).

The patient's weight at the time of graduation from high school and over the next few years (with any significant fluctuations) is helpful information. For women, determination of menstrual status and, if postmenopausal, of whether hormone replacement therapy has been recommended are important to resolve but are too frequently overlooked. The patient's diet and nutritional status are worthy of full review, providing some insight into a patient's level of commitment to a healthy lifestyle. Similarly, the level of physical activity and whether regular exercise is part of the patient's weekly routine frame the symptomatic assessment and corroborate the previous commitment to cardiovascular health. The pattern of alcohol use is a particularly worthwhile item about which to question the patient. Similarly, the potential for drug abuse should be explored in particular circumstances. Considerable revelation about the psychosocial makeup of the patient becomes evident, provided the physician is cueing in to the intensity level and manner in which the words and responses are being conveyed.

EVALUATION OF CARDIOVASCULAR SYMPTOMS

For each patient, a review of cardiovascular symptoms beyond the primary symptom is useful. The major symptoms are chest discomfort, dyspnea, syncope, edema, and fatigue. Other symptoms such as cough, palpitations, orthopnea, and dizziness or light-headedness are supportive and need to be ascertained in relation to the primary complaint. Often, a patient is not in touch with the symptoms or is in such fear or denial that he or she is unlikely to volunteer the information. For this reason, it is imperative to perform detailed questioning about chest discomfort or dyspnea in patients with a clustering of risk factors for atherosclerosis irrespective of the lack of a complaint. Symptoms of atherosclerosis of other arterial beds are systematically surveyed. For the cerebrovasculature, a check on symptoms such as transient loss of speech or motor function (suggesting a transient ischemic attack) or, for the peripheral blood vessels, calf discomfort on exertion that is promptly relieved by rest (suggesting intermittent claudication) help resolve the diffuseness of the atherosclerotic process, if present.

A functional classification of the patient's symptoms should be obtained (5,6). For angina, the Canadian Cardiovascular Society Functional Classification System is usually used (Table 14.1), whereas for dyspnea and other symptoms of heart failure, the New York Heart Association Functional Classification is relied on (Table 14.2).

Chest Discomfort, Pain, and Related Symptoms

One of the most frequent, yet difficult, symptoms to assess is chest discomfort or pain (7–23). Because this can be so frightening to patients, these symptoms may precipitate emergency evaluation. A variety of cardiac and noncardiac conditions can produce chest discomfort or pain, as summarized in Table 14.3. The key to determining whether the discomfort is cardiac is to review its character, location, and

TABLE 14.1   ASSESSING CARDIOVASCULAR DISABILITY

Canadian Cardiovascular Society Functional Classification	Specific activity scale
Ordinary physical activity, such as walking and climbing stairs, does not cause angina. Angina with strenuous, rapid, or prolonged exertion at work or recreation.	Patients can perform to completion any activity requiring ≤7 metabolic equivalents [e.g., can carry 24 lb up eight steps, carry objects that weigh 80 lb, do outdoor work (shovel snow, spade soil), and do recreational activities (skiing, basketball, squash, handball, jog/walk 5 mph)].
Slight limitation of ordinary activity. Walking or climbing stairs rapidly, walking uphill, walking or stair climbing after meals, in cold, in wind, or when under emotional stress, or only during the few hours after awakening. Walking more than two blocks on the level and climbing more than one flight of ordinary stairs at a normal pace and in normal conditions.	Patients can perform to completion any activity requiring ≤5 metabolic equivalents (e.g., have sexual intercourse without stopping, garden, rake, weed, roller skate, dance fox trot, walk at 4 mph on level ground), but cannot and do not perform to completion activities requiring ≤7 metabolic equivalents.
Marked limitation of ordinary physical activity. Walking one to two blocks on the level and climbing more than one flight in normal conditions.	Patients can perform to completion any activity requiring ≤2 metabolic equivalents (e.g., shower without stopping, strip and make bed, clean windows, walk 2.5 mph, bowl, play golf, dress without stopping), but cannot and do not perform to completion any activities requiring ≤5 metabolic equivalents.
Inability to perform any physical activity without discomfort—anginal syndrome may be present at rest.	Patients cannot or do not perform to completion activities requiring ≤2 metabolic equivalents.

Adapted from Criteria Committee, New York Heart Association. *Diseases of the heart and blood vessels: nomenclature and criteria for diagnosis*, 6th ed. Boston: Little, Brown, 1964:114; and Goldman L, Hashimoto B, Cook EF, et al. Comparative reproducibility and validity of systems for assessing cardiovascular functional class: advantages of a new specific activity scale. *Circulation* 1981;64:1227–1234.

TABLE 14.2 FUNCTIONAL CLASSIFICATION

Class	New York Heart Association functional classification
I	Patients with cardiac disease but without resulting limitations of physical activity. Ordinary physical activity does not cause undue fatigue, palpitations, dyspnea, or anginal pain.
II	Patients with cardiac disease resulting in slight limitation of physical activity. They are comfortable at rest. Ordinary physical activity results in fatigue, palpitation, dyspnea, or anginal pain.
III	Patients with cardiac disease resulting in marked limitation of physical activities. They are comfortable at rest. Less than ordinary physical activity causes fatigue, palpitation, dyspnea, or anginal pain.
IV	Patients with cardiac disease resulting in inability to perform any physical activity without discomfort.

Goldman L, Hashimoto B, Cook EF, et al. Comparative reproducibility and validity of systems for assessing cardiovascular functional class: advantages of a new specific activity scale. *Circulation* 1981;64:1227–1234.

precipitating factors. Because conditions such as esophageal reflux and musculoskeletal abnormalities are quite common, it is not unusual for a given patient to have two or more different types of chest discomfort (22,23). In such instances, a careful assessment of each of the symptom complexes is necessary to determine the underlying condition(s).

Character and Location

Although *angina* literally means "choking," most patients with true angina do not use this term to describe their sensation. Despite Herberden's early description in 1768 of a "painful and most disagreeable sensation in the breast" (24), the unpleasant sensation is more typically characterized as a pressure, tightness, heaviness, or burning. The pressure is not perceived by the patient as "pain," such that the interviewer who specifically asks about pain may be misled. On the other hand, "pain" is much more apt to be

TABLE 14.3 CAUSES OF CHEST DISCOMFORT AND PAIN

Cardiac	Noncardiac
Angina	Esophagitis, esophageal spasm, or reflex
Acute myocardial infarction	Peptic ulcer
Aortic dissection	Gallbladder disease
Pericarditis	Musculoskeletal causes, including osteochondritis or cervical disk, thoracic outlet syndrome
Myocarditis	Hyperventilation
	Anxiety
	Psychogenic causes
Mitral valve prolapse	Pneumonia
	Pulmonary embolus
	Pneumothorax
	Pulmonary hypertension

used by the patient to describe a heart attack; on occasion, the patient may clench the fist while describing the discomfort—the so-called Levine sign. The discomfort of angina is usually easy to differentiate from the pain of acute myocardial infarction by the duration, radiation, and lack of precipitating or alleviating factors. As opposed to angina, which usually lasts for 1 to 3 minutes, heart attack pain lasts for longer than 10 minutes; rather than having one focus (usually the retrosternal region), there is commonly radiation of the pain, such as down the arm. Heart attack pain is described in more depth in Chapter 18. Angina most commonly is felt in the midline of the chest, but it can manifest exclusively in the jaw or neck, the left shoulder or arm, and, when present in the arm, particularly on the ulnar aspect of the forearm and hand (Table 14.4). Rather than in the chest, the principal pressure or burning can be perceived in the epigastrium, causing the patient to believe the problem is simple indigestion. More rarely, the back interscapular region or the right side of the chest, shoulder, arm, or forearm is involved. Unlike the chest discomfort of angina, severe pain that radiates to the back is a classic indication of aortic dissection. However, patients with aortic dissection or expanding aortic aneurysm can have predominant anterior chest pain that may be mistaken for acute myocardial infarction. In the course of evaluating patients with chest pain, it is helpful to adopt the philosophy of "aortic dissection until proven otherwise" so that this diagnosis is never missed, even though it is a relatively uncommon entity in the current era of improved control of hypertension.

Chest pain or discomfort in women is more difficult to assess, and there have been studies to address the issue of whether there is gender bias resulting in inappropriate underinvestigation or undertreatment in women (25,26). A careful history and assessment of risk is especially critical among women, as the correct diagnosis is more elusive—even with noninvasive testing—and pivotal.

Acute pericarditis is a precordial pain that is typically left sided; it is usually worse with inspiration and described as sharp, often referred to the neck. Unlike angina or myocardial infarction pain, this pain is often positional in character such that if the patient sits up and leans forward, the pain may be relieved. Congenital absence of the pericardium is exceedingly rare, but the telltale symptom is chest pain produced by lying on the left side lasting only a few seconds or minutes (27). On occasion, patients with acute

TABLE 14.4 ANGINAL "EQUIVALENTS"

Dyspnea
Jaw or neck discomfort
Shoulder, elbow, or arm discomfort, particularly along the side of the left forearm and hand
Epigastric discomfort
Back (interscapular) discomfort

myocarditis may present with chest pain, which may be attributed to pericardial involvement or the actual inflammation of cardiac muscle. Mitral valve prolapse often is accompanied by atypical chest discomfort because it is sharp, stabbing, protracted in duration, and associated with a constellation of symptoms (see Chapter 21).

A long list of noncardiac causes of chest pain or discomfort (Table 14.3) is capped by the esophageal disorders of reflux, esophagitis, or spasm—all of which may coexist in certain patients with myocardial ischemia. Esophageal discomfort can fully mimic the character and location of myocardial ischemic symptoms, but, more commonly, the retrosternal burning or epigastric heaviness is brought on by food ingestion and recumbency, with relief by antacids and H$_2$-blockers. When there is a sour taste in the mouth (so-called water brash) as a result of the acid reflux, this is helpful in differentiating esophageal-induced symptoms from other etiologies. Other gastrointestinal disorders such as peptic ulcer disease, gall bladder disease, and pancreatitis can produce epigastric discomfort and need to be considered in the differential diagnosis.

The symptoms of chest discomfort may be the presenting feature for a host of musculoskeletal conditions. Costal chondritis, or Tietze's syndrome (11), is characterized by a chest-wall pain that includes point tenderness and, frequently, is exacerbated by movement or coughing. Chest wall syndromes are particularly common among cigarette smokers and seem to be responsive to cessation of smoking; the etiology remains unclear. A thoracic outlet syndrome is associated with ulnar distribution paresthesias in the arm and forearm that are worsened by arm abduction or lifting. Herpes zoster of the chest wall displays a specific dermatome pattern of the pain with exquisite sensitivity of the skin to touch and, ultimately, the development of characteristic skin vesicles.

In the continuum of musculoskeletal chest discomfort, terms frequently used for discharge diagnosis in emergency departments when the cause is uncertain are *hyperventilation*, *anxiety*, and the *Da Costa's syndromes* (also known as *neurocirculatory asthenia*) (10). Emotional stress precipitates pain characterized by a dull, persistent ache and may be accompanied by point or even diffuse chest-wall tenderness (28–32). This pain may last for hours or even days and may be quite localized (e.g., below the left nipple) with a "stabbing" quality. A component of hyperventilation may be diagnosed by eliciting the symptoms of circumoral or fingertip paresthesias with occasional carpal-pedal spasm and the response of the symptoms to breathing into a paper bag. Pulmonary causes of chest discomfort include pneumonia, pneumothorax, pulmonary hypertension, and pulmonary embolus. On occasion, pneumonia can present simultaneously with acute myocardial infarction such that the "either/or" process of ruling out one diagnosis should be considered carefully. Pulmonary hypertension may simulate angina, likely due to right ventricular ischemia. A pneumothorax presents with sudden onset of chest pain in the lateral chest with acute shortness of breath. Pulmonary embolism is also sudden, occurring at rest, and is usually associated with pleuritic chest pain exacerbated by coughing.

Exacerbating and Alleviating Factors

The most helpful aspect of angina is the classic precipitation by exercise or emotional stress. Interestingly, some patients never have angina with peak levels of robust exercise but, rather, experience the tightness or burning during a high-pressure business meeting or a stressful emotional incident. Cold weather, rushing to do an activity, and heavy meals are all common precipitants of angina. When angina occurs nocturnally or in the early morning hours on a cyclic basis, or when it occurs at rest, the possibility of coronary artery spasm or Prinzmetal's angina should be considered. This "variant" angina may be associated with a history of migraine headaches, Raynaud's phenomenon, or both, signifying a vasospastic tendency of multiple arterial beds. Coronary artery spasm, expressed as rest pain or discomfort, can occur concomitantly with classic exertional angina.

Alleviating factors that help in the diagnosis are relief by cessation of the activity or by sublingual nitroglycerin. Getting out of the cold or completing the uphill walk are excellent examples of ways that angina is usually relieved. Interestingly, lying down may not relieve angina and, at times, may precipitate it by the increase in venous return. The response to nitroglycerin is not specific, because esophageal spasm also is alleviated by nitroglycerin. However, the rapidity of relief for angina is quite impressive. The freshness of the nitroglycerin tablets needs to be ascertained in the context of whether the discomfort was responsive; if the tablets are old and did not induce mucosal tingling or a headache, it remains unclear whether a true effect was tested.

Precipitating Factors

There are several key subgroups of patients that deserve particular emphasis. Diabetes mellitus frequently leads to significant atherosclerotic coronary disease, but the symptoms are much less apt to be present and probably are related to a sensory neuropathy (13). Silent ischemia must, therefore, be considered in these patients, but careful interrogation for anginal equivalent symptoms (Table 14.4) is especially worthwhile. Of course, many diabetics have classic angina, but missing the underlying coronary disease in patients who are not fortunate enough to have an intact "alarm system" can have serious or even fatal consequences. Compared with men, women with documented coronary artery disease more often do not have the characteristic symptoms of angina, for unclear reasons. Whereas an exertional or emotional stress component is frequently elicited, the quality of the discomfort can be misleading and seem atypical. A full diagnostic evaluation and extra time to delineate fully the symptoms, precipitants, and risk factors are imperative.

After cardiac transplantation, patients cannot expect to experience chest pain or discomfort due to denervation, except in rare situations in which apparent reinnervation occurs (33,34). Systematic screening for coronary atherosclerosis has to be set up (see Chapter 94). For patients presenting with the chest pain of acute myocardial infarction, women, the elderly, and minority patients (particularly African-American and Hispanic) tend to present later in the course of the event and are more apt to have atypical or nonclassic features (15–17).

Dyspnea and Cough

Difficulty breathing is one of the cardinal symptoms of cardiac and pulmonary disease. Strictly, *dyspnea* denotes an abnormally uncomfortable awareness of breathing that is easily differentiated from normal, quiet, unnoticed breathing. The history can be particularly important in pinpointing the cause of dyspnea because there are a number of potential etiologies (35,36), including heart failure, pulmonary edema, obstructive airway disease, and pulmonary embolism.

Sudden dyspnea occurs not only with acute pulmonary edema but also with a pneumothorax, pulmonary embolism, or airway obstruction. In congestive heart failure, the onset of dyspnea is insidious and frequently precipitated by exertion. Conditions that simulate the chronic development of dyspnea are chronic obstructive pulmonary disease, pleural effusions, pregnancy, and obesity. Asthma or obstructive airway disease is suggested by inspiratory dyspnea, wheezing, and prior episodes responsive to bronchodilators. Although it is a rare symptom, sudden dyspnea while sitting rather than recumbent suggests the possibility of atrial myxoma, whereas dyspnea relieved by squatting is a classic indication for the congenital lesion of tetralogy of Fallot.

Paroxysmal nocturnal dyspnea is a classic sign of interstitial pulmonary edema and is most commonly due to heart failure. It usually begins 2 to 4 hours after going to sleep; is associated with sweating, cough, and, at times, wheezing; and can gradually improve (over 10 to 20 minutes) by getting out of bed or sitting on the side of the bed. The cough follows the dyspnea in heart failure but occurs in the opposite order in patients with chronic obstructive pulmonary disease. Of lesser severity is orthopnea due to pulmonary venous hypertension, and it occurs in the recumbent position with relief by sitting upright or standing. The number of pillows used by the patient is a good way to semiquantify orthopnea, because patients learn to use one or more extra pillows to combat their sense of breathlessness. Symptoms of heart failure that also cluster with dyspnea and orthopnea are nocturia, edema, and, more rarely, upper abdominal discomfort due to hepatosplenomegaly.

Dyspnea on exertion as a sole symptom may signify an anginal equivalent (Table 14.4); if it occurs with angina, there is an increased likelihood of a large myocardium in jeopardy, compared with angina and no symptoms of breathlessness.

Two alterations of breathing, both with a component of apnea, deserve mention. *Cheyne-Stokes respiration* refers to periods of hyperpnea followed by apnea. The pattern is a feature of the elderly who have heart failure, often with concomitant cerebrovascular disease. Sleep apnea has emerged as an important trigger of pulmonary hypertension and is characterized by episodes of snoring with prolonged periods of apnea due to upper airway obstruction. It typically occurs in patients who are overweight or mildly obese and can be responsive to measures that counter the upper airway obstruction. The diagnosis, however, can only be supported by obtaining a history from the patient's spouse or significant other.

Cough as a symptom is considerably more frequent but equally less specific (37). Perhaps the most common cause of cough today results from the side effect of angiotensin-converting enzyme inhibitors—popularly used for the treatment of hypertension and heart failure—that occurs as a result of activating bradykinin. The dry cough from this class of medications can be difficult to differentiate from that of pulmonary hypertension or mitral stenosis. Both types of cough are irritating and spasmodic, although the heart failure or mitral stenosis cough is more likely to be nocturnal, despite considerable overlap. Cough associated with hoarseness in the absence of upper respiratory disease may suggest a very enlarged left atrium with compression of the recurrent laryngeal nerve. Hoarseness without obvious upper respiratory infection in such patients is known as *Ortner's syndrome*, in which the large left atrium exerts pressure on an enlarged pulmonary artery and peribronchial lymph nodes to compress the recurrent laryngeal nerve. Dysphagia and right posterior chest pain occur only if left atrial enlargement is extreme due to severe chronic mitral regurgitation.

Sputum production and, particularly, hemoptysis are symptoms that tend to localize the disorder in the lungs, except for hemoptysis that is associated with severe mitral stenosis and is characterized by sudden increases in left atrial pressure and rupture of small bronchopulmonary veins. Frank hemoptysis that occurs with pulmonary arterial hypertension due to congenital left-to-right shunts may not share this pathophysiology, as bronchial arterioles rupture, in this case, to cause massive hemorrhage.

In patients with dyspnea and suspect valvular disease, determining whether there is a history of rheumatic fever is customary but can be misleading. Determination of whether there was scarlet fever with a rash, joint pains, chorea (St. Vitus' dance) with twitches or clumsiness, frequent sore throats, prolonged bed rest, or a family history of rheumatic fever are all in this line of questioning. However, frequently, the absence of these symptoms does not rule out rheumatic fever; a positive history can also be inaccurate (38).

Syncope and Palpitations

Syncope is a loss of consciousness due to inadequate perfusion of the brain. The history is fundamental for narrowing down a wide differential diagnosis (see Chapter 71). Sudden loss of consciousness without an aura or warning characterizes cardiac syncope. This condition can result from an arrhythmia such as ventricular fibrillation, ventricular tachycardia, advanced atrioventricular block, or asystole (38,39). A family history of syncope raises the possibility of a long QT syndrome (see Chapter 97). Beyond arrhythmic causes of syncope, the hemodynamically significant lesions of aortic stenosis, hypertrophic cardiomyopathy, or primary pulmonary hypertension are important causes of cardiac syncope. With these disorders, syncope classically occurs just after exertion, and although hemodynamic lesions are present that can account for the loss of consciousness, serious arrhythmias should not be discounted as the primary trigger. Hypertrophic cardiomyopathy is usually familial such that the family history is important to raise or support this possibility. Besides the postexertional syncope, fainting during prolonged standing, posttussive, or even during exertion can occur with this condition.

The most common cause of cardiac syncope is known as *vasodepressor* and is mediated through the autonomic nervous system, with unconsciousness developing a bit more gradually and lasting for a few seconds; this condition can be induced by emotional stress or pain. It can be preceded by dim vision, sweating, nausea, light-headedness, giddiness, or yawning, reflecting autonomic nervous system hyperactivity, and can be fully alleviated by lying down. After the spell, it is common for the patient to be quite pale and to have a slow heart rate. Closely related in underlying pathophysiology is the syncope due to direct stimulation of the carotid sinus in patients who are "hypersensitive"; this syncope is manifested by fainting spells after sudden head motion or wearing of a tight collar. Hypovolemia in patients experiencing fainting while standing and orthostatic hypotension-related syncope are other possible and related etiologies of cardiac syncope.

Compared with cardiac syncope, neurologic causes often have an aura, as in the case of epilepsy (which, in some cases, is familial and in others posttraumatic) or associated neurologic deficits of transient cerebrovascular ischemia (e.g., vision loss, speech impairment, or motor weakness). Furthermore, after some neurologic causes of syncope such as a grand mal seizure, there is postictal confusion. Importantly, vasodepressor syncope is not typically linked with trauma, but patients with seizures or other forms of sudden cardiac syncope can sustain physical injury with a fainting spell. Near syncope, which is described by the patients as "nearly" losing consciousness or "graying" out, is similar in its differential to actual syncope but, overall, is less likely to be associated with serious pathologic conditions compared with true loss of consciousness.

Calkins and colleagues (39) studied the differentiating symptoms of the history to resolve the etiology of syncope. Features of the history predictive of syncope not due to ventricular tachycardia or atrioventricular block were palpitation, blurred vision, nausea, warmth, diaphoresis, and lightheadedness before syncope and nausea, warmth, diaphoresis, and fatigue after the syncopal event (40).

Palpitations represent an unpleasant awareness of the heartbeat and frequently are described as "skipping," "jumping," "pounding," or "racing." The skipping is often attributed to the postextrasystolic pause, whereas the pounding or forceful beat is accounted for by the postextrasystolic potentiation of contractility. A variety of rhythm disturbances may be considered, with the full spectrum from bradyarrhythmias to supraventricular or ventricular tachycardias being potential triggers. Palpitations are remarkably common and can simply occur with anxiety (e.g., palpitations occurring with the syndrome of hyperventilation previously described), with tingling around the mouth and in the hands, although the underlying rhythm is sinus tachycardia. Similarly, other benign forms occur with postural hypotension due to the reflex heart acceleration or in response to medications (e.g., amphetamines), cocaine, alcohol, tobacco, and caffeine. With physical exertion, a sense of the heart "pounding" may certainly be anticipated.

However, when the complaint occurs despite lack of exertion or with only minimal effort, other causes need to be surveyed, such as heart failure, anemia, thyrotoxicosis, and atrial fibrillation. A pulse rate of approximately 150 beats per minute suggests atrial flutter, whereas faster rates suggest paroxysmal supraventricular tachycardia. Rates slower than 140 beats per minute (as low as 100 beats per minute) are more suggestive of sinus tachycardia and, therefore, are more likely to be benign.

Edema, Fatigue, and Other Symptoms

Swollen legs manifesting at the end of the day are characteristic of heart failure or chronic venous insufficiency. Early on, this can sometimes be associated only with difficulty in getting one's shoes on but can also be linked to appreciable weight gain due to fluid retention. Usually, the edema is symmetric and progresses "from the ground up." In patients with prior bypass surgery who have had saphenous vein grafts harvested, the edema may begin unilaterally on the side of decreased venous competence. In patients confined to bed with heart failure, presacral edema is common. In the presence of hyperpigmentation of the legs, ulcers, and other changes suggesting venous stasis, chronic venous insufficiency may be the likely explanation, but, frequently, the coincident finding of heart failure and chronic venous

THE FUTURE

Although the history has been deemphasized in the past decade, it will become increasingly relied on in the future because of its relatively low cost and pivotal importance in guiding more diagnostic and therapeutic decision making. With the reduced sense of patient satisfaction and bonding with the physician, spending more time with the patient to relay information and develop mutual understanding and trust hopefully will override the forces that have deprioritized such a core component of high-quality cardiovascular medicine.

insufficiency is present. This is especially true in patients who have had long-standing heart failure and other reasons for venous insufficiency (e.g., marked obesity). Generalized edema, known as *anasarca*, can occur with severe heart failure but also with cirrhosis and the nephrotic syndrome. Periorbital edema occurs with hypoproteinemia, myxedema, hereditary angioneurotic edema, and acute glomerulonephritis. Edema localized to the upper body, involving the face, arms, and neck, raises the possibility of a superior vena cava syndrome, which may herald carcinoma of the lung. Edema of cardiac origin that is not associated with dyspnea or orthopnea suggests a right-sided heart lesion such as constrictive pericarditis, tricuspid stenosis, or, for example, a tumor that has invaded the inferior vena cava or right atrium.

Fatigue is a nonspecific and common symptom that may not have cardiovascular basis. However, it may signal poor cardiac output or result from overdiuresis or from the use of beta-blocker drugs. In some cases, episodic fatigue from physical exertion or emotional stress disproportionate to the amount of effort expended may represent an anginal equivalent.

Nausea and vomiting can occur with acute myocardial infarction (see Chapter 18). Fever and chills, along with other constitutional signs, may be associated with infectious endocarditis (see Chapter 25).

CONTROVERSIES AND PERSONAL PERSPECTIVES

It is clear that taking a thorough history has become less of a priority for a few pivotal reasons. First, there is less time available for physician-patient direct contact as a result of the demands placed on a physician's time. Frequently, a physician extender or nurse obtains part or all of the history to reduce the time burden on the doctor. Under the putative heading of "efficiency," the priority of the detailed, thorough interview has been markedly reduced. Second, with advances in technology, the history and physical examination have been partially supplanted by rapid use of bedside tools such as the two-dimensional echocardiogram, a treadmill or dobutamine thallium test, a Holter recording, or even diagnostic angiography or electrophysiologic study—all instead of the meticulous history.

These two forces are unfortunate. The history is the most important way to create a physician-patient bond and is precious and irreplaceable. Ideally, the task should not be delegated to a physician extender, except for such perfunctory aspects as the medications and doses, risk factors, and minor details. It is absolutely essential to query the patient directly and in depth for the principal symptoms (e.g., chest discomfort, loss of consciousness, or dyspnea). Only in this way can there be the optimal accuracy and relationship building that are critical. Also, the use of advanced diagnostic technology easily can be imprudent with respect to cost and can uncover findings that, although accurate, have no bearing on the patient's symptoms. The detailed history preempts or properly guides the use of more refined diagnostic tests. Intuitively, the history is the most cost-effective tool that one can use to lay soundly the foundation of the patient's evaluation.

REFERENCES

1. Belkin BM, Neelon FA. The art of observation: William Osler and the method of Zadig. *Ann Intern Med* 1992;116:863–866.
2. Sandler G. The importance of the history in the medical clinic and the cost of unnecessary tests. *Am Heart J* 1980;100:928.
3. Kee F, Tiret L, Robo JY, et al. Reliability of reported family history of myocardial infarction. *BMJ* 1993;307:1528–1530.
4. Hunt K, Emslie C, Watt G. Lay constructions of a family history of heart disease: potential for misunderstandings in the clinical encounter? *Lancet* 2001;357:1168–1171.
5. Goldman L, Hashimoto B, Cook EF, et al. Comparative reproducibility and validity of systems for assessing cardiovascular functional class: advantages of a new specific activity scale. *Circulation* 1981;64:1227–1234.
6. Criteria Committee, New York Heart Association. *Diseases of the heart and blood vessels: nomenclature and criteria for diagnosis*, 6th ed. Boston: Little, Brown, 1964:114.
7. Serlie AW, Erdman RA, Passchier J, et al. Psychological aspects of non-cardiac chest pain [review]. *Psychother Psychosom* 1995;64:62–73.

8. Pryor DB, Shaw L, McCants CB, et al. Value of the history and physical in identifying patients at increased risk for coronary artery disease. *Ann Intern Med* 1993;118:81–90.

9. Tatum JL, Jesse RL, Kontos MC, et al. Comprehensive strategy for the evaluation and triage of the chest pain patient. *Ann Emerg Med* 1997;29:116–125.

10. Jarcho S. Functional heart disease in the Civil War (Da Costa, 1871). *Am J Cardiol* 1959;4:809–817.

11. Levey GS, Calabro JJ. Tietze's syndrome: report of two cases and review of the literature. *Arthritis Rheum* 1962;5:261.

12. Epstein SE, Gerber LN, Boren JS. Chest wall syndrome: a common cause of unexpected pain. *JAMA* 1979;241:279.

13. Chiariello M, Indolfi C. Silent myocardial ischemia in patients with diabetes mellitus. *Circulation* 1996;93:2089–2091.

14. Gregor RD, Bata IR, Eastwood BJ, et al. Gender differences in the presentation, treatment, and short-term mortality of acute chest pain. *Clin Invest Med* 1994;17:551–562.

15. Ell K, Haywood LJ, Sobel E, et al. Acute chest pain in African Americans: factors in the delay in seeking emergency care. *Am J Public Health* 1994;84:965–970.

16. Haywood LJ, Ell K, deGuman M, et al. Chest pain admissions: characteristics of black, Latino, and white patients in low- and mid-socioeconomic strata. *J Natl Med Assoc* 1993;85:749–757.

17. Johnson PA, Goldman L, Orav EJ, et al. Comparison of the medical outcomes study short-form 36-item health survey in black patients and white patients with acute chest pain. *Med Care* 1995;33:145–160.

18. Lehmann JB, Wehner PS, Lehmann CU, et al. Gender bias in the evaluation of chest pain in the emergency department. *Am J Cardiol* 1996;77:641–644.

19. Chang RA, Rossi NF. Intermittent cocaine use associated with recurrent dissection of the thoracic and abdominal aorta. *Chest* 1995;108:1758–1762.

20. Hollander JE, Todd KH, Green G, et al. Chest pain associated with cocaine: an assessment of prevalence in suburban and urban emergency departments. *Ann Emerg Med* 1995;26:671–676.

21. Hollander JE. The management of cocaine-associated myocardial ischemia. *N Engl J Med* 1995;333:1267–1272.

22. Chauhan A, Petch MC, Schofield PM. Cardioesophageal reflex in humans as a mechanism for "linked angina." *Eur Heart J* 1996;17:407–413.

23. Saltissi S. Cardio-esophageal reflex and "linked angina"—is the way to a man's (or woman's) heart through the stomach? *Eur Heart J* 1996;17:329–331.

24. Eslick GD. Chest pain: a historical perspective. *Int J Cardiol* 2001;77:5–11.

25. Wong Y, Rodwell A, Livesey SA, et al. Sex differences in investigation results and treatment in subjects referred for investigation of chest pain. *Heart* 2001;85:149–152.

26. Sharaf BL, Pepine CJ, Kerensky RA, et al. Detailed angiographic analysis of women with suspected ischemic chest pain (pilot phase data from the NHLBI-sponsored Women's Ischemia Syndrome Evaluation [WISE] study angiographic core laboratory). *Am J Cardiol* 2001;87:937–941.

27. Constant J, ed. *Bedside cardiology*, 2nd ed. Boston: Little, Brown, 1976.

28. Bradley LA, Richter JE, Scarinci IC, et al. Psychosocial and psychophysical assessments of patients with unexplained chest pain. *Am J Med* 1992;92:65S–73S.

29. Yingling KW, Wulsin LR, Arnold LM, et al. Estimated prevalences of panic disorder and depression among consecutive patients seen in an emergency department with acute chest pain. *J Gen Intern Med* 1993;8:231–235.

30. Tew R, Guthrie EA, Creed FH, et al. A long-term follow-up study of patients with ischemic heart disease versus patients with nonspecific chest pain. *J Psychosom Res* 1995;39:977–985.

31. Mayou R, Bryant B, Forfar C, et al. Non-cardiac chest pain and benign palpitations in the cardiac clinic. *Br Heart J* 1994;72:548–553.

32. Cannon RO III, Quyyumi AA, Mincemoyer R, et al. Imipramine in patients with chest pain despite normal coronary angiograms. *N Engl J Med* 1994;330:1411–1417.

33. Schroeder JS, Hunt SA. Chest pain in heart-transplant recipients. *N Engl J Med* 1986;324:1805–1807.

34. Stark RP, McGinn AL, Wilson RF. Chest pain in cardiac-transplant recipients: Evidence of sensory reinnervation after cardiac transplantation. *N Engl J Med* 1991;324:1791–1794.

35. Duncan AK, Vittone J, Fleming KC, et al. Cardiovascular disease in elderly patients. *Mayo Clin Proc* 1996;71:184–196.

36. Valacio R, Lye M. Heart failure in the elderly patient. *Br J Clin Pract* 1995;49:200–204.

37. Irwin RS, Curley FJ, French CL, et al. Chronic cough: the spectrum and frequency of causes, key components of the diagnostic evaluation, and outcome of specific therapy. *Am Rev Respir Dis* 1990;141:640–647.

38. Reichek N, Shelburne JC, Perloff JK. Clinical aspects of rheumatic valvular disease. *Prog Cardiovasc Dis* 1973;15:491–537.

39. Calkins H, Shyr Y, Frumin H, et al. The value of the clinical history in the differentiation of syncope due to ventricular tachycardia, atrioventricular block, and neurocardiogenic syncope. *Am J Med* 1995;98:365–373.

40. Sutton R, Nathan A, Perrins J, et al. Syncope: a good history is not enough. *BMJ* 1994;309:474.

PHYSICAL EXAMINATION

KANU CHATTERJEE

OVERVIEW

A systematic approach to the bedside examination of a patient is essential in determining the significance of an abnormal physical finding, such as decreased or increased intensity of the first heart sound (S_1), a pathologic third heart sound (S_3), or a systolic or diastolic murmur. Assessment of the abnormalities of the systemic venous pressure and pulse, arterial pulse, precordial impulse, heart sound, and murmurs provides clues not only for the diagnosis of the anatomic abnormalities, but also for the determination

K. Chatterjee: Department of Cardiology, University of California, San Francisco, School of Medicine, San Francisco, California of the severity of the hemodynamic abnormalities. It should be emphasized that appropriate investigations (e.g., echocardiography, radionuclide ventriculography and scintigraphy, and cardiac catheterization) should be considered to establish the diagnosis.

In the present era of technological advances, particularly in the various imaging modalities, there is a growing conception among practicing physicians in cardiovascular medicine that bedside physical examination is unnecessary. It should be emphasized, however, that for proper application and interpretation of various new and old tests that are available for cardiovascular evaluation in a given patient, a careful physical examination is essential. Furthermore, a careful, systematic, and methodical bedside clinical evaluation—including analysis of clinical history—can provide enough information to decide whether further investigations are necessary and, if necessary, which investigations are appropriate. Bedside clinical examination should be performed and practiced in the same way after similar sequences and usually begins with *general inspection* of the patient.

INSPECTION

During general inspection (1,2), the stature, body habitus, approximate weight, and presence or absence of obesity are noted. An unusually short stature is seen in patients with osteogenesis imperfecta, which is associated with aortic and mitral regurgitation and calcification of the arterial system. Congenital heart disease, such as Noonan's syndrome, also occurs in association with short stature due to dwarfism. In Noonan's syndrome, short stature is associated with web-neck, dental malocclusion, antimongoloid slanting of the eyes, mental retardation, and hypogonadism. Pulmonary valve stenosis and obstructive and nonobstructive cardiomyopathy are also observed. Dwarfism is an essential phenotypic feature of the various types of mucopolysaccharidosis, which can be associated with various valvular and myocardial dysfunctions due to mucopolysaccharide deposition. An unusually tall stature, however, is seen in patients with Marfan's syndrome, which is frequently associated with aortic aneurysm, aortic regurgitation, and mitral regurgitation. When severe chest pain or back pain is the presenting symptom in a patient with Marfan's syndrome, acute aortic dissection should always be suspected. A tall stature, long extremities, and eunuchoid appearance is observed in patients with Klinefelter's syndrome, which can be associated with congenital heart diseases such as ventricular septal defects, patent ductus arteriosus, and tetralogy of Fallot. During initial cardiac evaluation, it is customary to notice any obvious musculoskeletal deformity, such as kyphoscoliosis, straight back, and pectus deformity of the chest. A higher incidence of mitral valve prolapse is observed in the presence of such musculoskeletal deformities. An increased incidence of mitral valve prolapse is also observed in females with smaller breasts. Muscular dystrophies such as pseudohypertrophic, fascioscapular humoral, or limb-girdles varieties can be suspected during general inspection. These muscular dystrophies may be associated with various cardiovascular abnormalities, including myocardial disease, mitral valve prolapse, ventricular septal defect, and dysrhythmias.

Gait

Abnormalities of gait are also noted during inspection. Neurologic deficits resulting from cardioembolic strokes or hypertensive cerebrovascular disease may be associated with abnormalities of gait. A parkinsonian gait may indicate Shy-Drager syndrome, which may be associated with orthostatic hypotension (3). Certain metabolic disorders (e.g., hyperthyroidism, hypothyroidism, Cushing's syndrome, and acromegaly) can be suspected during inspection, and these metabolic diseases may be associated with various cardiovascular abnormalities, including systemic and pulmonary hypertension and myocardial and pericardial diseases.

Body Habitus

During inspection, the general nutritional status of the patient is also noted. Although marked weight loss, wasting, and cachexia occur more frequently from metabolic and neoplastic diseases, they can be manifestations of severe congestive heart failure. Cardiac cachexia (4) does not correlate to cardiac output as usually perceived, but to a marked neuroendocrine abnormality characterized by an activated renin angiotensin system as well as increased levels of cytokines, including tumor necrosis factor and interleukins. The presence and severity of obesity should be noted, as various cardiovascular abnormalities can be associated with obesity. Obesity, particularly abdominal and truncal types, is one of the components of the metabolic syndrome X, which comprises hypertension, hyperlipidemia, and insulin resistance (5,6). In patients with metabolic syndrome, there is increased risk of developing atherosclerotic macrovascular disease, including coronary artery disease. Furthermore, in markedly obese patients, there is increased incidence of sleep apnea, hypertension, and dilated cardiomyopathy. Truncal obesity, if associated with buffalo hump or moon facies, should raise the suspicion of Cushing's syndrome, which may be complicated by hypertension and hypertensive heart disease. In African-Americans, severe obesity and marked increase in body mass index and diabetes are more important predictors of primary diastolic heart failure than hypertension or coronary artery disease.

Respiration

During inspection, presence of respiratory distress and types of altered respiration should be observed. Labored and uncomfortable breathing, however, may be of cardiac or noncardiac origin. Inability to lie down or a dry, irritating cough with dyspnea when in the supine position usually indicates pulmonary venous congestion. Sleep-disordered breathing is common in chronic congestive heart failure (7). Typical Cheyne-Stokes respiration with central sleep apnea is observed in 20% to 30% of patients with moderate or severe congestive heart failure with reduced left ventricular ejection fraction and, usually, elevated pulmonary capillary wedge pressure and lower cardiac output. Cheyne-Stokes respiration with central sleep apnea should be distinguished from obstructive sleep apnea, which is associated with inspiratory efforts during apneic phase, because central sleep apnea is a risk factor for increased mortality (7a). Also, patients with only central sleep apnea are likely to benefit from continuous positive airway pressure therapy (7b). Frequent sighing respirations and a restless, anxious look are more frequently encountered in patients with anxiety and neurocirculatory asthenia. The "blue bloater" and "pink puffer" appearances, which can be detected during inspection, usually indicate chronic obstructive pulmonary disease. During inspection, it is desirable to note any obvious changes in the color of the skin. A bluish discoloration of the skin usually indicates cyanosis, which can be either peripheral or central. Peripheral cyanosis is detected in exposed skin (e.g., lips, nose, and earlobes, and in extremities) and indicates impaired peripheral perfusion. A bluish discoloration of the tongue, uvula, and buccal mucus membrane suggests central cyanosis, which results from intrapulmonary or intracardiac right-to-left shunt. When differential cyanosis (i.e., cyanosis in the inferior extremities without cyanosis in the superior extremity) is observed along with differential clubbing, Eisenmenger's syndrome associated with patent ductus arteriosus should be suspected.

Edema

Generalized edema is easily detected during inspection, usually results from nephrotic syndrome and sepsis, and rarely results from severe heart failure. Dependent edema, on the other hand, is associated with right heart failure. When dependent edema is discovered, careful evaluation of systemic venous pressure and pulse is essential for the diagnosis of right heart failure. The presence of ascites, which also may be a manifestation of right heart failure, can be suspected from the protuberant abdomen. Ascites in the absence of edema of the lower extremities is more frequently a manifestation of liver disease, such as cirrhosis, rather than heart failure. However, in patients with constrictive pericarditis and restrictive cardiomyopathy, disproportionately large ascites with little or no edema of the lower extremities can be observed (8). Again, careful examination for the presence of systemic venous hypertension, pulmonary arterial hypertension, and physical findings suggestive of restrictive physiology is essential for the differential diagnosis between liver disease and cardiac failure.

Skin

Slate or bronze pigmentation of the skin may suggest hemochromatosis, which may be associated with various cardiac complications (e.g., restrictive or dilated cardiomyopathy, arrhythmias, and conduction disturbances). It also should be appreciated that patients on chronic amiodarone therapy also develop similar discoloration of the skin with exposure to sunlight (9). Discoloration of the skin similar to marked suntan is also seen in patients with carcinoid syndrome. Mild jaundice may be observed in patients with heart failure with congestive hepatopathy and with pulmonary embolism. Prosthetic valve malfunction should be suspected if jaundice is detected in a patient with artificial heart valves. The livido reticulares with cyanosis of the toes and preserved peripheral pulses (blue toes syndrome) suggest cholesterol emboli (10). Acrosclerosis with taut, thickened, or edematous skin bound tightly to subcutaneous tissue in the hands and fingers suggests systemic sclerosis, which may be associated with pulmonary hypertension, pericarditis, right heart failure, systemic hypertension, restrictive cardiomyopathy, and dilated cardiomyopathy. If malar flush is detected, mitral stenosis with pulmonary hypertension should be suspected. Malar flush, however, can also occur in patients with severe precapillary pulmonary hypertension and may be confused with butterfly rash of lupus erythematosus. The presence of transverse or diagonal earlobe creases in a relatively young person (i.e., under 45 years of age), may suggest the presence of premature atherosclerotic coronary artery disease. The presence of arcus—a circumferential light ream around the iris that begins inferiorly—further increases the risk of premature atherosclerotic coronary artery disease. Arcus is also frequently associated with hypercholesterolemia and xanthelasma (i.e., deposits of cholesterol on the eyelids). When telangiectasia of the lips, tongue, and buccal mucosa are detected, Osler-Weber-Rendu disease, which is associated with pulmonary arteriovenous fistulae, should be suspected. Exfoliative dermatitis, purpura, and petechial rashes usually indicate drug reactions. Although an erythema marginatum is characteristic of acute rheumatic fever, erythema nodosum is a nonspecific finding and occurs in many systemic diseases. In patients with suspected bacterial endocarditis, searches should be made for conjunctival hemorrhages, skin purpuric, and petechial lesions, as well as for splinter hemorrhages. It should be realized that splinter hemorrhages in the nail beds may occur in normal patients after mild trauma and in patients with trichinosis or hemorrhagic disorders.

During examination of the skin, it is customary to check for the presence of cutaneous and subcutaneous nodular lesions, which may suggest some systemic and metabolic diseases that may also involve the cardiovascular system. The rheumatic nodules associated with acute rheumatic fever are small, nontender, and most frequently seen on the knuckles, extensor surface of the elbows, and suboccipital regions. Rheumatoid nodules, on the other hand, are large, nontender, and characteristically localized over points of pressure or friction—most commonly the extensor surfaces of the proximal forearms. If rheumatoid nodules are detected, attention should be directed to detect the cardiovascular complications of rheumatoid arthritis (e.g., pericarditis, aortic and mitral valvular disease, conduction disturbances, and, rarely, cardiomyopathy). Xanthomas, the cholesterol-filled nodules, occur in different types of abnormalities of lipoprotein metabolism, and recognition of the distribution of xanthomas aids in the diagnosis of these disorders. Tendon xanthomas, xanthomas occurring on digital extensors, and tuberous xanthomas occur in familial hypercholesterolemia (11). Eruptive xanthomas are small yellow papules in the skin that are surrounded by an erythematous halo. They occur in patients with primary familial hypertriglyceridemia that results from lipoprotein lipase deficiency and is associated with recurrent episodes of pancreatitis, but not with premature coronary artery disease. Eruptive xanthomas also occur in patients with endogenous and mixed hypertriglyceridemia, which can be associated with ischemic vascular disease. In patients with suspected bacterial endocarditis, it is desirable to search for Osler's nodes and Janeway's lesions. Osler's nodes are most frequently observed on the palms, soles of the feet, and pads of the fingers or toes. These nodes are tender, nodular, erythematous skin lesions and result from emboli. Janeway's lesions are nontender, raised, hemorrhagic nodules that usually occur on the palms of the hands and soles of the feet. These lesions were initially thought to be due to vasculitis, but they also appear to be of embolic origin. Café au lait spots—sometimes detected only in the axilla—occur in neurofibromatosis, which occasionally is associated with hypertrophic cardiomyopathy.

Funduscopy

In patients with established or suspected systemic hypertension, funduscopic examination should be performed. Based on the degree of narrowing or irregularities of retinal artery, the presence or absence of arteriovenous nicking or nipping, hemorrhages, exudates, and papilledema, four grades are recognized (12). Grade 1 consists of minimal irregularity of the arterial lumen and narrowing with increased light reflex. Grade 2 changes consist of arteriovenous nicking, more marked narrowing and irregularity of the arterioles, and distention of the veins. Grade 3 changes are characterized by the presence of flame-shaped hemorrhages and fluffy "cotton wool" exudates in addition to arterial changes. Hard exudates may also be present. Grade 4 funduscopic changes are characterized by the presence of papilledema and any other changes in grades 1 through 3. Generally, grade 1 and 2 changes are present in benign hypertension, whereas grade 3 or 4 changes are seen in accelerated or malignant hypertension. Funduscopic examination should also be per-

formed in patients with suspected bacterial endocarditis and may reveal vascular occlusions and hemorrhagic areas with white centers (Roth's spots), which result from emboli in the nerve fiber retinal layer. Roth's spots, however, are not diagnostic of bacterial endocarditis and can be seen in hemorrhagic disorders, including leukemia. Mycotic aneurysms resulting from large emboli occasionally may be discovered in retinal vessels during funduscopic examination. Identification of such lesions should lead to further evaluation for the source of emboli, and appropriate investigations—including transthoracic and, occasionally, transesophageal echocardiography—must be undertaken. Occasionally, funduscopic examination may reveal unusual findings that may provide clues for the diagnosis of the underlying pathophysiology. Beading of the retinal artery may suggest hypercholesterolemia. Microinfarction in the peripheral retina is seen in sickle cell disease, which may also involve the cardiovascular system. Angioid streaks may suggest pseudoxanthoma elasticum, which may be associated with coronary artery calcification, systemic hypertension, intermittent claudication, and arrhythmias. A wreath-like arteriovenous anastomosis around the optic disk is a characteristic of Takayasu's syndrome. In adult cardiology practice, the abnormal findings that are often detected during inspection, along with their significance, are summarized in Table 15.1.

TABLE 15.1 INSPECTION

Cyanosis
Peripheral cyanosis only—suspect low cardiac output and impaired peripheral perfusion
Central cyanosis—suspect intrapulmonary or intracardiac right-to-left shunt
Differential cyanosis—suspect Eisenmenger's syndrome with patent ductus arteriosus

Respiratory distress
Cheyne-Stokes respiration with central sleep apnea—suspect heart failure
Blue bloater and pink puffer—suspect pulmonary disease
Frequent sighing respiration—suspect anxiety syndromes

Nutritional status
Cachexia—suspect severe heart failure with abnormal neuroendocrine profile
Obesity—suspect metabolic syndrome X, sleep apnea, cardiomyopathy
Ascites and peripheral edema—suspect severe heart failure, constrictive pericarditis

Musculoskeletal deformity, kyphoscoliosis, straight back, pectus excavatum
Suspect mitral valve prolapse, aortic and mitral valve regurgitation, congenital heart disease such as atrial septal defect

Abnormal movement of the head and neck
Bobbing of the head, coincident with each heart beat—suspect severe aortic regurgitation
Lateral movements of the earlobes with each cardiac cycle—suspect severe tricuspid regurgitation

Slate or bronze discoloration of the skin
Suspect chronic amiodarone therapy, hemochromatosis, carcinoid syndrome

EXAMINATION OF THE ARTERIAL PULSE

During initial evaluation, all accessible arterial pulses should be examined; in the inferior extremities, dorsales pedes, posterior tibials, and femoral pulses should be examined bilaterally. In the upper extremities, both brachial and radial pulses should be examined, and, in special circumstances, the ulnar pulses and axillary arterial pulses should also be examined. Temporal arteries are examined when temporal arteritis is suspected in patients with headache and jaw claudication. Carotid arteries should be examined sequentially in all patients. Diminished or absent pulses may result from atherosclerotic peripheral vascular disease, which is associated with increased incidence of atherosclerotic coronary artery disease. Loss of or decreased femoral pulse unilaterally or bilaterally most frequently suggests local obstructive lesions due to atherosclerotic disease. However, diminished amplitudes of the lower extremity pulses, including femoral, popliteals, posterior tibials, and dorsales pedes arterial pulsations, also occur from isolated aortoiliac diseases, such as Leriche's syndrome (13), postsubclavian coarctation of the aorta, aortic dissection, descending thoracic and abdominal aortic aneurysms, and abdominal aortic disease such as giant cell arteritis. When coarctation of the aorta is suspected, it is desirable to examine the radial and femoral pulses simultaneously to assess radial/femoral delay. In a normal adult, the pulse transmission time from aorta to the radial artery is approximately 75 ms and to the femoral artery is approximately 70 ms. Thus, in the presence of coarctation, delay in the onset of femoral pulse compared to that of radial pulse can be detected. The radial/femoral delay is rarely observed in patients with Leriche's syndrome and abdominal coarctation. Also in pseudocoarctation, the degree of obstruction is not severe enough to decrease the amplitude of the femoral pulse or to cause delay in the onset of femoral pulse compared with that of radial pulse (14). In patients with radial/femoral delay and suspected coarctation, blood pressure should be recorded in the upper and lower extremities. In the supine position, the inferior extremity pressure is normally slightly higher than that of the upper extremity arterial pressure. In coarctation, inferior extremity pressure is lower than upper extremity pressure. While examining the peripheral arterial pulses, it is desirable to assess the rigidity and elasticity of the arteries. The rigidity of the arterial pulses are best appreciated by examining the femoral, radial, brachial, and carotid pulses. In clinical practice, the thickness and firmness of the arterial walls are examined by rolling the vessel, usually the radial artery, against underlying tissue. The more rigid the artery, the less it is compressible. The appreciation of nonelastic, rigid peripheral arteries may indicate the presence of systolic hypertension. If the significant rigidity of the peripheral arteries is observed, it is desirable to perform Osler's maneuver. Osler's maneuver is performed by elevating the cuff pressure to obliterate the radial pulse; if, after obliteration of the pulse, the radial artery is easily palpable and appears rigid (i.e., a positive Osler's sign), then there might be a significant difference between indirect measurement of arterial pressure by cuff method and directly determined intraarterial pressure.

The peripheral arterial pulses are also examined at the bedside for detection of arrhythmias. If the pulse rate is regular but slow, sinus bradycardia, junctional rhythm, or complete atrioventricular block is suspected. Occasionally, bigeminy may produce an irregular slow pulse because of the nonconducted pulse associated with the ectopic beat. Careful examination of the venous pulse and simultaneous auscultation may be helpful for the differential diagnosis of slow regular pulse. If regular cannon waves with each cardiac cycle are recognized, junctional rhythm is suspected. In the presence of a slow regular pulse, if irregular cannon waves and changing intensity of the S_1 are observed, atrioventricular dissociation due to complete atrioventricular block is the most likely diagnosis. Bigeminy can be diagnosed easily by auscultation, which demonstrates the postectopic compensatory pause. Atrial fibrillation can be suspected if irregularly irregular pulses are appreciated. However, frequent premature beats or multifocal atrial tachycardia can also produce an irregularly irregular pulse similar to that of atrial fibrillation. If atrial fibrillation is suspected, it is desirable to determine the ventricular rate by simultaneous auscultation to assess the degree of pulse deficit. The difference between the heart rate by auscultation and the pulse rate is the pulse deficit. The rapid ventricular responses are the cause of the hemodynamic abnormalities of atrial fibrillation. A fast and regular pulse rate (150 beats or more) should raise the possibility of supraventricular or ventricular tachycardia. It is mandatory to do electrocardiographic evaluation of every patient with suspected arrhythmia.

Peripheral arterial pulses are also examined to detect any alteration of the character of the pulse, which can provide important diagnostic clues. Pulsus alternans is suspected when strong and weak amplitude pulses are appreciated with alternate beats in the presence of a regular pulse. Pulsus alternans can be confirmed by measuring blood pressure by sphygmomanometer. When the cuff pressure is slowly released, phase I Korotkoff's sound is heard initially only during the alternate strong beats; with further release of cuff pressure, the softer sounds of the weak beat also appear. The most important cause of pulsus alternans is left ventricular systolic failure. Pulsus alternans is rarely encountered in patients with cardiac tamponade. In patients with tamponade with pulsus paradoxus, if the respiratory rate is half of the heart rate, pulsus alternans may occur. However, in these patients, when respiration is held transiently, the pulsus alternans is resolved. Pulsus alternans (mechanical alternans) can also occur occasionally in aortic stenosis, in hypertrophic obstructive cardiomyopathy, with sudden increase of afterload, with ischemia, with abrupt fall of preload, and with the onset of a tachyarrhythmia. Rapid atrial pacing may induce pulsus alternans in the presence of normal left ventricular systolic function. However, clinically detectable sustained pulsus alternans almost always indicates left ventricular systolic dysfunction.

In experimental and clinical studies, alternating changes in preload, afterload, and contractility have been suggested as potential mechanisms for mechanical alternans (15); ventricular dyssynchrony with alternating contraction of the interventricular septum, incomplete relaxation in the alternate beats, partial asystole of the left ventricle, alternating changes in action potential duration, and alternating amounts of Ca^{2+} sparks from the sarcoplasmic reticulum are the other proposed mechanisms (15a). The failing heart is sensitive to altered afterload and resistance to left ventricular ejection. The increased arterial pressure associated with a strong beat increases the resistance to left ventricular ejection for the following beat, which is thus associated with decreased forward stroke volume and decreased arterial pressure. This reduction in arterial pressure lowers the resistance to left ventricular ejection, which allows increase in forward stroke volume and, therefore, increase in arterial pressure. These changes in arterial pressure, reflecting changes in the ejection impedance with alternate beats, can perpetuate pulsus alternans (Fig. 15.1). It should be emphasized, however, that the absence of pulsus alternans does not exclude left ventricular systolic dysfunction. Nevertheless, the pulsus alternans is a reliable and helpful physical finding for the diagnosis of left ventricular systolic dysfunction.

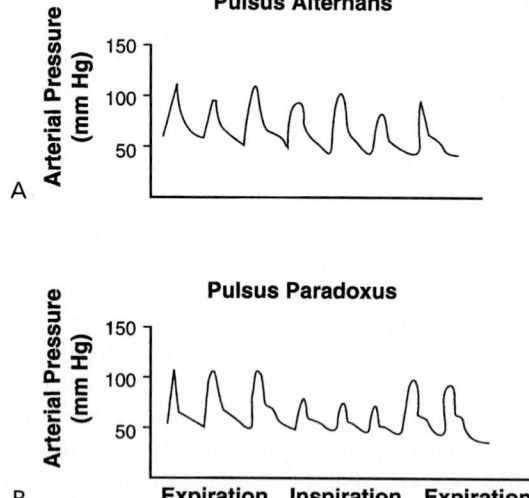

FIGURE 15.1 Schematic illustrations of pulsus alternans **(A)** and pulsus paradoxus **(B)**. In clinical practice, pulsus alternans usually indicates systolic ventricular failure and occurs in patients with chronic ischemic or nonischemic dilated cardiomyopathy, aortic stenosis, and acute myocardial infarction. Pulsus paradoxus, however, is observed in pericardial tamponade, constrictive pericarditis (rare), emphysema, asthma, marked obesity, and severe congestive heart failure (rare).

During examination of the peripheral arterial pulses, if there is a substantial reduction in the amplitude of the arterial pulse during inspiration, pulsus paradoxus should be suspected, and determination of arterial pressure by sphygmomanometry during inspiration and expiration should be performed. Systolic arterial pressure normally falls during inspiration; however, the magnitude of fall in arterial pressure during inspiration usually does not exceed 8 to 12 mm Hg. A more marked inspiratory decrease in arterial pressure exceeding 12 to 15 mm Hg is regarded as pulsus paradoxus and usually is detectable by palpation of the peripheral pulses. However, the magnitude of pulsus paradoxus should be measured by sphygmomanometry. When the cuff pressure is slowly released, the systolic pressure at expiration is noted. With further slow deflation of the cuff, the systolic pressure during inspiration can also be detected. The difference between the pressure during expiration and inspiration is the magnitude of the pulsus paradoxus. The abnormal pulsus paradoxus is an important physical finding of cardiac tamponade (16). The marked inspiratory decrease in arterial pressure in tamponade results from the marked inspiratory decline of left ventricular stroke volume due to a decreased end diastolic volume. In cardiac tamponade during inspiration, there is an increase in venous return to the right atrium and the right ventricle. Due to increased intrapericardial pressure, the intraventricular septum shifts toward the left ventricle during inspiration, which decreases left ventricular preload. There is also an expected decrease in venous return to the left ventricle during inspiration because of increased pulmonary venous reservoir capacity during inspiration. In clinical practice, besides cardiac tamponade, pulsus paradoxus is observed in patients with chronic obstructive pulmonary disease. It should be emphasized that pulsus paradoxus is a rare finding in patients with constrictive pericarditis. Pulsus paradoxus is rarely observed in pulmonary embolism, pregnancy, marked obesity, and partial obstruction of the superior vena cava. In hypertrophic obstructive cardiomyopathy, arterial pressure occasionally increases during inspiration (i.e., reversed pulsus paradoxus) (17). The precise mechanism for this phenomenon is not clear.

The amplitude of the peripheral arterial pulse may provide some information about stroke volume, systemic vascular resistance, and compliance of the arteries. A small-amplitude, rapid pulse usually indicates hypotension, reduced stroke volume, and increased systemic vascular resistance. A large-amplitude, arterial pulse suggests large stroke volume or decreased compliance. A large-volume, bounding pulse is noted after exercise; in high-output states such as chronic anemia, hyperthyroidism, and aortic regurgitation; and in patients with bradycardia (e.g., complete heart block). Decreased compliance and increased rigidity of the peripheral arteries may also increase the amplitude of the arterial pulse, as seen in elderly patients with systolic hypertension. In elderly patients, when the carotid pulse amplitude is decreased, local carotid disease or aortic stenosis should be suspected. Decreased amplitudes of the carotid pulse in elderly subjects should prompt further evaluation, such as echocardiography, to exclude aortic stenosis.

Changes in the contour of the arterial pulses (Fig. 15.2) should also be noted. In patients with significant aortic valve stenosis, a delayed upstroke of the ascending limb of the carotid pulse (so-called pulsus tardus), an anacrotic character of the carotid pulse, delayed peak, and small amplitude (pulsus parvus) of the carotid pulse are frequently appreciated. In patients with aortic stenosis, a thrill over the carotid pulse, which usually is termed a shudder, may also be detected. These abnormalities are best appreciated in the central pulse. In the central aortic ascending pressure pulse, normally there is a notch on the ascending limb: the anacrotic notch. On the upstroke of the carotid pulse, however, the anacrotic notch is not normally appreciated. An anacrotic carotid pulse gives the impression of interruption of the ascending limb or the upstroke of the carotid pulse. When the anacrotic notch is felt immediately after the onset of the upstroke, aortic stenosis is likely to be hemodynamically significant. An anacrotic radial pulse also suggests moderate to severe aortic stenosis. At the bedside, the delayed peak of the carotid pulse is appreciated by simultaneous auscultation of the duration of the systole. Normally, the peak of the carotid pulse is closer to the S_1. In the presence of significant aortic stenosis, the peak of the carotic pulse is delayed and is closer to the second heart

sound (S_2). With increasing severity of aortic stenosis, the peak of the carotid pulse is not only further delayed and closer to the S_2, but the amplitude of the carotid pulse is also substantially reduced. It needs to be emphasized, however, that these changes in the contour of the carotid pulse may not be present in elderly patients with aortic stenosis with decreased and noncompliant carotid arteries. When aortic stenosis is suspected, whether in young or older patients, an echocardiographic evaluation is highly desirable.

Pulsus bisferiens is appreciated by the presence of two positive impulses near the peak of the arterial pulse. These two positive impulses represent accentuated percussion and tidal waves, which can be recorded in the carotid arterial pulse tracing and the central aortic pulse waveform, even in normal subjects. The percussion wave results from the rapid left ventricular ejection, and a second, usually smaller peak represents the tidal wave that results from a reflected wave from the periphery. Normally, radial and femoral pulse tracings demonstrate a single sharp peak. In pulsus bisferiens, percussion and tidal waves are accentuated. At the bedside, it is often difficult to distinguish between anacrotic, pulsus bisferiens and dicrotic pulse. The anacrotic pulse, however, is characterized by a positive palpable wave during the ascending limb of the arterial pulse. Thus, it should be easily distinguished from pulsus bisferiens or the dicrotic pulse. However, if the two positive waves are felt near where the maximum amplitude of the pulse wave occurs, it is difficult to distinguish between pulsus bisferiens and dicrotic pulse. In these circumstances, one has to rely on detection of the etiologic conditions that can be associated with pulsus bisferiens or dicrotic pulse (18). The most frequent conditions associated with pulsus bisferiens are isolated hemodynamically significant aortic regurgitation, mixed aortic stenosis and regurgitation with predominant aortic regurgitation, and obstructive hypertrophic cardiomyopathy. Pulsus bisferiens is rarely appreciated in patients with large patent ductus arteriosus with large left-to-right shunt, multiple arteriovenous fistulas, and, rarely, complete heart block. If these etiologies are excluded at the bedside, then one should consider dicrotic pulse if double-picked arterial pulse is appreciated. The arterial pressure waveform, when recorded, reveals a single percussion wave and a prominent, accentuated dicrotic wave. At the bedside, however, it is difficult to differentiate between dicrotic pulse and pulsus bisferiens. The dicrotic pulse is appreciated in some patients with severe heart failure, for example, due to dilated cardiomyopathy, low cardiac output, and increased systemic vascular resistance. On the other hand, dicrotic pulse is also appreciated in patients with septic shock with high cardiac output and low systemic vascular resistance. However, in clinical practice, a dicrotic pulse is appreciated frequently in patients after aortic valve replacement and usually indicates impaired left ventricular systolic function. In patients with aortic valve replacement, if a double-picked carotid pulse with sharp initial upstroke is

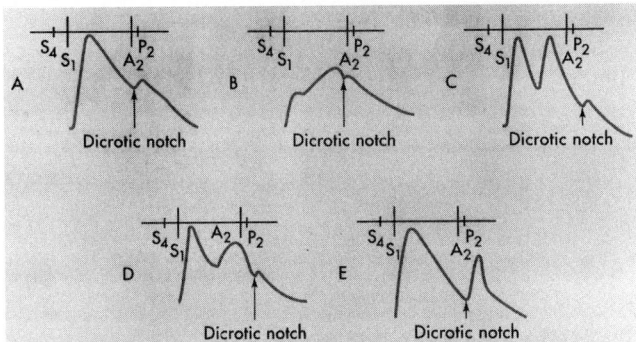

FIGURE 15.2 Schematic illustration of the configurational changes in the carotid pulse and their differential diagnoses. Heart sounds are also illustrated. **A:** Normal. **B:** Anacrotic pulse with slow initial upstroke and delayed peak, which is close to the aortic component of the second heart sound (A_2), indicate fixed aortic stenosis. **C:** Pulsus bisferiens with increased amplitude of percussion and tidal waves occurs during systole. This type of pulsus bisferiens carotid pulse is most frequently observed in patients with significant aortic regurgitation. **D:** Pulsus bisferiens in hypertrophic obstructive cardiomyopathy is rarely appreciated at the bedside. **E:** Dicrotic pulse results from an accentuated dicrotic wave and tends to occur in severe heart failure, hypovolemic shock, cardiac tamponade, sepsis, and after aortic valve replacement. P_2, pulmonary component of the second heart sound; S_1, first heart sound; S_4, atrial sound. (From Chatterjee K. Bedside evaluation of the heart: the physical examination. In: Parmley W, Chatterjee K, eds. *Cardiology.* Philadelphia: JB Lippincott Co, 1997;1:13, with permission.)

TABLE 15.2 ALTERED CHARACTERS OF THE ARTERIAL PULSE AND THEIR CLINICAL SIGNIFICANCE

Pulsus alternans—suspect acute or chronic reduction in left ventricular ejection fraction

Anacrotic pulse, delayed upstroke, palpable thrill, delayed peak—suspect fixed left ventricular outflow tract obstruction such as aortic valve stenosis

Pulsus biferiens—suspect aortic regurgitation, aortic stenosis with dominant aortic regurgitation, dynamic left ventricular outflow tract obstruction (obstructive hypertrophic cardiomyopathy), large patent ductus arteriosus with left-to-right shunt, complete heart block, hyperkinetic heart syndrome (e.g., in hyperthyroidism)

Dicrotic pulse—suspect "low output syndrome" with increased systemic vascular resistance, "high output" with low systemic resistance (e.g., in septic shock), postaortic valve replacement with depressed left ventricular ejection fraction

Pulsus paradoxus—suspect tamponade, emphysema

appreciated, it is desirable to evaluate prosthetic valve and left ventricular function by echocardiography to exclude paraprosthetic leak, which usually is associated with pulsus bisferiens, or depressed left ventricular ejection fraction, which is associated with dicrotic pulse. The significance of altered character of the arterial pulse that is sometimes encountered at the bedside in adult patients is summarized in Table 15.2.

EXAMINATION OF JUGULAR VENOUS PULSE AND PRESSURE

Examination of jugular venous pulse and pressure (1,2) is essential to assess hemodynamic changes in the right side of the heart. Jugular venous pressure and pulses usually are examined with the patient in a 45-degree, semirecumbent position. However, if, in this position, the venous pulsations are not recognized, the examination of venous pressure and pulse should be done with the patient in a supine position or even with the head and neck tilted below the level of the chest. Occasionally, if the venous pressure is normal or low, the legs need to be raised to increase the venous return and increase right-sided venous pressure. When the venous pressure is extremely elevated and the veins appear to be distended, it is preferable to examine the jugular venous pulses with the patient in an upright position or even in a standing position. It is preferable to examine the internal jugular venous pressure and pulse. In adults, particularly in elderly patients, the external jugular venous pressure may be elevated due to partial obstruction at the level of the external jugular venous bulb due to partial thrombosis or even obstruction by the platysma muscle. The internal jugular venous pulse usually is located medial to the mandibular portion of the sternomastoid muscle. The proximal internal jugular venous pulse is located in the supraclavicular area between the two proximal heads of the sternomastoid muscle. Both right and left jugular venous pulsations need to be examined, because sometimes, disparity between left and right internal jugular venous pressures can be recognized. Occasionally in elderly patients, the left internal jugular venous pressure is higher than the right internal jugular venous pressure because of the partial obstruction of the left innominate vein by unfolded aorta. In these circumstances, with inspiration and descent of the diaphragm, partial obstruction of the left innominate vein is relieved, and the pressures in the right and left internal jugular veins become equal.

At the bedside, venous pulsation needs to be differentiated from carotid artery pulsation. By inspection, the venous pulse is characterized by a sharp inward movement, whereas the arterial pulse is characterized by a sharp outward movement. During inspection, the venous pulse is also recognized by its double undulation character in sinus rhythm. In the presence of atrial fibrillation, the double undulation character of the venous pulse is lost due to the absence of an 'a' wave associated with atrial systole. The venous pressure and the amplitude of the venous pulse can be decreased or increased by appropriate maneuvers. The pressure and amplitude can be decreased by raising the level of the head and trunk above the level of the right atrium (in a sitting or standing position), or they can be increased by enhancing the venous return to the right side of the heart by raising the legs or by abdominal compression. In the presence of low systemic venous pressure, when a patient is examined in a head-down position, it is possible to recognize the venous pulsation in the neck. When a pulsation in the neck is recognized, a gentle to moderate compression—by the fingers or stethoscope tubes—at the root of the neck obliterates the venous pulse, but the arterial pulse remains visible. This maneuver is extremely useful for differentiating between arterial and venous pulsations. Normally during inspection, the jugular venous pulse amplitude decreases during inspiration, whereas the arterial pulse amplitude does not change during respiration.

After recognizing the venous pulse, the venous pressure is estimated by noting the height of the oscillating top of the venous pulse above the sternal angle. Right atrial pressure is approximated by adding 5 cm to the height of the venous column, as it is assumed that the right atrium is located about 5 cm below the sternal angle. The normal right atrial pressure is <9 cm of water. If the jugular venous pressure is increased in the absence of obvious pulsation, it is desirable to exclude superior vena cava obstruction, which does not permit transmission of right atrial pulsation to the internal jugular veins. If pulsation of the neck veins can be recognized, the estimated venous pressure can be used to estimate right atrial pressure. It should be recognized that although jugular venous pressure reflects right atrial pressure, the cause of elevated right atrial pressure cannot be determined by simply noting the height of the jugular venous pulse. The character of the venous pulse and

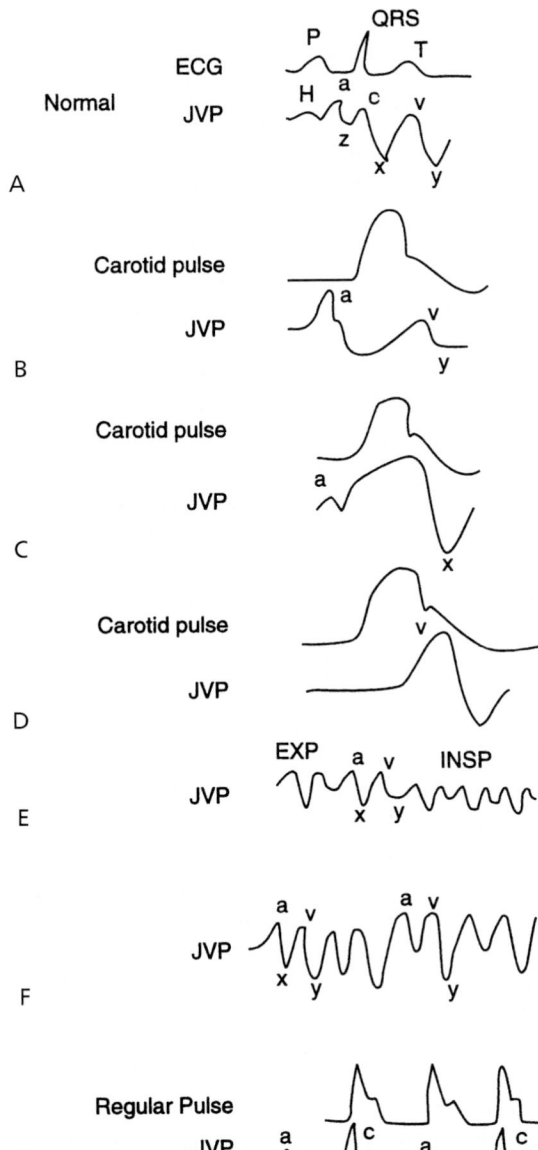

FIGURE 15.3 Schematic illustrations of a normal jugular venous pulse (JVP) and a few commonly encountered abnormalities of the JVP. **A:** Normal venous pulse along with electrocardiogram (ECG). The 'a' wave associated with right atrial systole occurs after the P wave and just before the upstroke of the carotid pulse. Normally, 'a' wave is dominant and appears more obvious during inspiration. During simultaneous palpitation of the carotid pulse at the bedside, an impression of "out of phase" between the 'a' wave and the carotid pulse upstroke is appreciated. During right atrial relaxation, the venous pulse descends and may continue up to a plateau interval (z) or can be interrupted by the 'c' wave, which is produced by the bulging of the tricuspid valve into the right atrium at the onset of the isovolumic systole and also transmitted from the carotid pulse when observed in the neck. After the 'c' wave, the venous pulse descends (x), which results from atrial relaxation. The 'v' wave occurs during right atrial filling with closed tricuspid valve and during right ventricular ejection. After the peak of the 'v' wave, which corresponds to the T wave of the ECG, right atrial pressure exceeds right ventricular diastolic pressure, which causes opening of the tricuspid valve, rapid filling of the right ventricle, and subsequent 'y' descent. When diastole is long (e.g., with a slow heart rate), the 'y' descent may be followed by a brief positive wave (H) or a plateau. It should be recognized that, at the bedside, it is difficult to appreciate the 'x' descent, H wave, and 'z' wave; usually only 'a' and 'v' waves and 'y' descents are appreciated. **B:** A prominent 'a' wave precedes the carotid pulse upstroke; when jugular venous pulse is inspected during simultaneous palpitation of the carotid pulse upstroke, an impression of "out of phase" between pulses is appreciated at the bedside. Once a prominent 'a' wave is recognized, an increased resistance to right ventricular filling during atrial systole (e.g., tricuspid stenosis) and right ventricular hypertrophy from right ventricular outflow obstruction should be suspected. In adults, however, pulmonary hypertension is the most frequent cause. **C:** Prominent 'v' wave (regurgitant wave) followed by a sharp 'y' descent and coincident with the carotid pulse. At the bedside, venous pulse appears in phase with carotid pulse, and tricuspid regurgitation is the most common cause. **D:** In atrial fibrillation, a prominent 'v' in the JVP and even pulsatile liver in the absence of tricuspid regurgitation can be recognized in the absence of tricuspid regurgitation. **E:** In cardiac tamponade, mean jugular venous pressure (JVP) is elevated, and a lack of a sharp 'x' or 'y' descent is appreciated at the bedside. A quiet precordium and significant pulsus paradoxus are also usually appreciated. EXP, expiration; INSP, inspiration. **F:** Jugular venous pulsation in constrictive pericarditis usually reveals a marked elevation of the mean venous pressure and sharp 'y' descent. During inspiration, the venous pressure may not decrease and may even increase (Kussmaul's sign). These altered characteristics of the JVP, however, are nondiagnostic of constrictive pericarditis and can be present in patients with right ventricular infarction, pulmonary embolism, restrictive cardiomyopathy, and severe tricuspid regurgitation. **G:** In a patient with a slow regular pulse, appreciation of irregular cannon waves ('c') in the jugular venous pulse suggests complete atrioventricular block.

other physical findings need to be incorporated to assess the cause of elevation of systemic venous and right atrial pressures. The normal jugular venous pulse wave or right atrial pressure wave recordings usually consist of three positive waves ('a,' 'c,' and 'v') and two negative waves ('x' and 'y' descents) (Fig. 15.3). The 'a' wave is caused by transmitted right atrial pressure to the jugular veins during right atrial systole. The 'a' wave in the jugular venous pulse is appreciated by its occurrence just prior to the left ventricular ejection, which is recognized by simultaneous palpation of the carotid pulse upstroke. At the bedside, simultaneous palpation of the carotid pulse upstroke and inspection of the venous pulse give the impression that the 'a' wave of the venous pulse and the carotid pulse upstroke occur out of phase. On the other hand, the prominent 'v' wave in the venous pulse occurs more or less simultaneously with the

carotid pulse upstroke. Atrial relaxation initiates the descent of the 'a' wave. Rarely, when the PR interval is markedly prolonged, the descent may continue until a plateau is reached: the 'z' point, which occurs just prior to the ventricular systole. The descent after atrial systole usually is interrupted by the 'c' wave. In the right atrial pressure pulse, the 'c' wave is recognized with the onset of right ventricular systole and occurs from bulging of the tricuspid valve into the right atrium. It should be emphasized, however, that the 'c' wave in the jugular venous pulse probably results from transmission of the carotid artery pulsation and not from the transmission of the right atrial 'c' wave. The 'v' wave is caused by the rise in right atrial and jugular venous pressure due to continued inflow of blood to the venous system during right ventricular systole when the tricuspid valve is still closed. Although in right atrial and jugular venous pressure tracings, the peak of the normal 'v' wave occurs immediately after ventricular systole; at the bedside, the normal or abnormal 'v' wave coincides with the carotid pulse upstroke and downstroke. Although the regurgitant wave of tricuspid regurgitation (a prominent 'v' wave) occurs earlier and coincides with the beginning of left ventricular ejection, at the bedside the tricuspid regurgitant wave is appreciated simultaneously with the carotid pulse upstroke (Fig. 15.3).

The descending limb of the 'v' wave—the 'y' descent—is caused by the opening of the tricuspid valve and the rapid inflow of blood to the right ventricle from the right atrium. The 'y' descent is almost always recognized in the jugular venous pulse, and it follows the 'v' wave.

During examination of the jugular venous pulse at the bedside, if a prominent 'a' wave is appreciated, the conditions that are associated with increased resistance to right atrial emptying during atrial systole should be considered. The 'a' waves need to be distinguished from regular cannon waves, which occur in junctional rhythm or ventricular tachycardia with retrograde ventriculoatrial conduction. Cannon waves occur during atrial systole with closed tricuspid valve. Cannon waves, therefore, occur concurrently with the onset of ventricular systole (i.e., concurrently with carotid pulse upstroke). Cannon waves are distinguished from 'v' waves by lack of obvious 'y' descents that follow 'v' waves or regurgitant waves. In the presence of a regular pulse, if irregular cannon waves are recognized by a sudden appearance of a large positive wave coincident with ventricular systole (with carotid upstroke), atrioventricular dissociation should be suspected. Regular cannon waves also occur in patients with a prolonged PR interval when atrial systole occurs during the preceding ventricular systole. However, more frequent causes of regular cannon waves are junctional rhythm and ventricular tachycardia with retrograde conduction.

In an adult cardiac patient, when a prominent 'a' wave with large amplitude is appreciated, it is desirable to exclude tricuspid valve obstruction; this can be done by noting absence of a mid-diastolic rumble along the lower left sternal border, which increases in intensity during inspiration. Although in severe tricuspid stenosis the 'y' descent is abbreviated and presystolic hepatic pulsations can be observed, such degree of tricuspid stenosis is rarely encountered in adult patients. It should also be emphasized that isolated tricuspid stenosis is almost never encountered in rheumatic heart disease, and rheumatic tricuspid stenosis occurs almost always in the presence of mitral or aortic valve disease and in patients who are usually in atrial fibrillation. Thus, in rheumatic tricuspid stenosis, it is uncommon to appreciate a prominent 'a' wave. In adult cardiac patients, if isolated tricuspid stenosis is recognized with a prominent 'a' wave (in sinus rhythm) with a mid-diastolic rumble along the lower left sternal border that increases in intensity during inspiration (Carvello's sign), right atrial

myxoma or carcinoid heart disease should be considered in the differential diagnosis. However, the most common cause of a prominent 'a' wave in adults is right ventricular hypertrophy, which offers increased resistance to right atrial emptying during right atrial systole. Right ventricular hypertrophy may result from a right ventricular outflow tract obstruction, such as pulmonary valve stenosis or precapillary or postcapillary pulmonary hypertension. Significant pulmonary valve stenosis can be easily diagnosed by noting a long ejection systolic murmur, which is heard best over the left second intercostal space, a pulmonary ejection sound, and a widely split S_2 with reduced intensity of the pulmonary component of the S_2. Pulmonary stenosis is an infrequent cause of right ventricular hypertrophy in adult patients, and the most common cause of right ventricular hypertrophy is chronic pulmonary arterial hypertension. Pulmonary hypertension is also easily recognized at the bedside by noting the increased intensity of the pulmonic component of the S_2 and its transmission to the cardiac apex (mitral area).

If a prominent 'v' wave in the jugular venous pulse is recognized at the bedside, tricuspid regurgitation should be suspected, and physical findings that will confirm the diagnosis should be sought. In tricuspid regurgitation, jugular venous pulse always reveals a sharp 'y' descent after a prominent 'v' wave. In severe tricuspid regurgitation, lateral pulsatile motions of the earlobes coincident with each cardiac cycle are observed in many patients. There usually is a systolic murmur either early or pansystolic in duration, which is heard best over the left third and fourth intercostal space, along the left sternal border. Tricuspid regurgitation murmur frequently radiates to the epigastrium and the right side of the sternum. The tricuspid regurgitation murmur also increases in intensity after inspiration. When the diagnosis of tricuspid regurgitation is confirmed, it is desirable to assess carefully the intensity of the pulmonic component of the S_2 to distinguish between primary and secondary tricuspid regurgitation. Secondary tricuspid regurgitation is defined when tricuspid regurgitation occurs due to right ventricular dilatation and failure secondary to pulmonary hypertension.

Occasionally, a prominent 'v' wave is detected in patients with atrial septal defect in the absence of pulmonary arterial hypertension and tricuspid regurgitation (19). The mechanism of the prominent 'v' wave in atrial septal defect is not clear; however, a concomitant increase in systemic venous return and left-to-right shunt during ventricular systole may cause a rapid increase in right atrial pressure—hence, a prominent 'v' wave. It should be emphasized that a prominent 'v' wave in patients with atrial septal defect is not followed by a sharp 'y' descent.

Although a sharp 'y' descent most frequently occurs in tricuspid regurgitation, it can be observed in constrictive pericarditis and restrictive cardiomyopathy. In constrictive pericarditis and restrictive cardiomyopathy, systemic venous pressure is elevated, and inspection of the jugular venous pulse may reveal a sharp 'y' descent of brief duration. In the presence of sinus rhythm, the amplitudes of the 'a' and 'v' waves are similar. In patients with atrial fibrillation, because there is no 'a' wave present in the venous pulse, changes in the venous pulse character may seem similar to those in tricuspid regurgitation (i.e., a 'v' wave followed by a 'y' descent). In such circumstances, it is difficult to distinguish between constrictive pericarditis, restrictive cardiomyopathy, or primary or secondary tricuspid regurgitation. However, it is easy to recognize tricuspid regurgitation by other physical findings. In constrictive pericarditis or restrictive cardiomyopathy, the jugular venous pressure does not fall appropriately or even increase during inspiration (Kussmaul's sign) (20) (Fig. 15.3). It should be recognized that Kussmaul's sign is not diagnostic of constrictive pericarditis or restrictive cardiomyopathy. Kussmaul's sign can be observed in patients with right ventricular infarction (21), primary severe right ventricular failure resulting from any cause, primary or secondary severe tricuspid regurgitation, partial obstruction of the vena cava, or right atrial and right ventricular tumors; in some patients with severe congestive heart failure without tricuspid regurgitation; and, occasionally, in patients with tricuspid stenosis. It should also be emphasized that Kussmaul's sign is uncommon and seldom noted in cardiac tamponade. The mechanism of Kussmaul's sign has not been adequately studied; however, increased resistance to right atrial filling during inspiration seems to be a common contributory factor. For practical purposes, in patients with chronic congestive heart failure, a presence of Kussmaul's sign should raise the possibility of constrictive pericarditis or restrictive cardiomyopathy, and appropriate evaluations should be considered. The presence of physical findings of pulmonary hypertension (e.g., a sustained systolic left parasternal lift, a loud pulmonic component of the S_2, and severe tricuspid regurgitation with pulsatile hepatic impulse) favor the diagnosis of restrictive cardiomyopathy. In contrast, lack of findings suggestive of pulmonary hypertension, a quiet precordium or presence of a prominent diastolic left parasternal impulse, and absence of hepatic pulsation favor the diagnosis of constrictive pericarditis. In constrictive pericarditis, a pericardial "knock" (similar to right-sided S_3 gallop) and, rarely, a mid-diastolic murmur are heard. It should be emphasized that when constrictive pericarditis or restrictive cardiomyopathy are suspected, appropriate investigations—particularly cardiac catheterization—should be undertaken. After confirming the presence of constrictive or restrictive hemodynamics by cardiac catheterization, magnetic resonance imaging or computed tomography are appropriate noninvasive investigations to distinguish between constrictive pericarditis and restrictive cardiomyopathy (see Chapter 54).

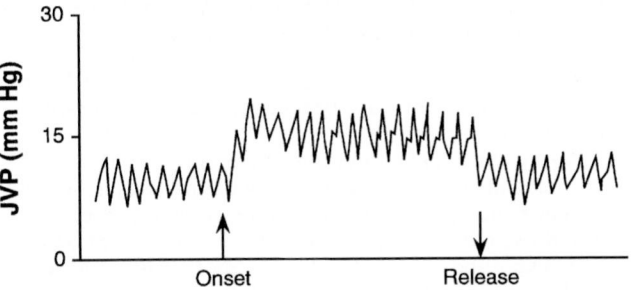

FIGURE 15.4 An example of a positive hepatojugular reflux (abdominojugular maneuver). Jugular venous pressure (JVP) increases with the onset of abdominal compression (↑) and remains elevated until it is released (↓). In adults, the most common cause of positive hepatojugular reflux is left heart failure due to dilated cardiomyopathy. However, positive hepatojugular reflux also is observed in tricuspid stenosis and isolated right ventricular failure due to pulmonary hypertension and right ventricular infarction.

In patients with suspected congestive heart failure but with normal resting venous pressure, it is desirable to perform the hepatojugular reflux test (22,23). With the patient breathing normally and in the semirecumbent position, a firm pressure is applied with the palm of the hand to the upper right quadrant of the abdomen for at least 10 seconds. In normal patients, there may be a transient increase in jugular venous pressure with rapid return to or near baseline in <10 seconds. The abnormal hepatojugular reflux is defined when there is a rapid increase in jugular venous pressure that remains elevated by 4 cm or more until abdominal compression is released. During abdominal compression with increased intraabdominal pressure, there is an increase in venous return to the right atrium and right ventricle. Concurrently, there is an increase in right ventricular afterload due to upward movement of the diaphragm, which reduces the intrathoracic volume capacity. The normally functioning right ventricle handles this increase in preload and afterload, and systemic venous pressure remains normal. The dysfunctioning right ventricle, however, fails to accept this increase in preload and afterload; therefore, there is a persistent elevation of systemic venous pressure. A positive hepatojugular reflux is most frequently associated with congestive heart failure resulting from left heart failure (24). In these circumstances, an abnormal sustained elevation of right atrial pressure during hepatojugular reflux indicates incipient right heart failure or abnormal compliance of the right ventricle in the presence of intact pericardium (Fig. 15.4). It should be emphasized that a positive hepatojugular reflux is noted in patients with isolated right heart failure due to precapillary pulmonary hypertension or right ventricular infarction. The abnormalities of the venous pressure and pulse and associated suspected cardiovascular disorders are summarized in Table 15.3.

TABLE 15.3 ABNORMALITIES OF THE VENOUS PRESSURE AND PULSE AND THEIR CLINICAL SIGNIFICANCE

Positive hepatojugular reflux—suspect congestive heart failure, particularly left ventricular systolic dysfunction (echocardiography recommended)

Elevated systemic venous pressure without obvious 'x' or 'y' descent and quiet precordium and pulsus paradoxus—suspect cardiac tamponade (echocardiography recommended)

Elevated systemic venous pressure with sharp 'y' descent, Kussmaul's sign, and quiet precordium—suspect constrictive pericarditis (cardiac catheterization and MRI or CT recommended)

Elevated systemic venous pressure with a sharp, brief 'y' descent, Kussmaul's sign, and evidence of pulmonary hypertension and tricuspid regurgitation—suspect restrictive cardiomyopathy (cardiac catheterization and MRI or CT recommended)

A prominent 'a' wave with or without elevation of mean systemic venous pressure—exclude tricuspid stenosis, right ventricular hypertrophy due to pulmonary stenosis, and pulmonary hypertension (echo-Doppler study recommended)

A prominent 'v' wave with a sharp 'y' descent—suspect tricuspid regurgitation (echo-Doppler study or cardiac catheterization recommended to determine the etiology)

CT, computed tomography; MRI, magnetic resonance imaging.

EXAMINATION OF THE PRECORDIAL PULSATIONS

Inspection and palpation of precordial pulsation during bedside cardiac evaluation may provide important diagnostic clues (1,2). Normally, a slight, abrupt, inward pulsation can be seen occasionally over the lower left parasternal area, particularly in children and thin-chested patients. Epigastric and subxyphoid pulsations are usually abnormal, although they can be seen in the absence of right heart failure in patients with chronic obstructive pulmonary disease. A pronounced epigastric or subxyphoid pulsation should raise the possibility of right ventricular failure or abdominal aortic aneurysm, and appropriate evaluations should be undertaken. A visible pulsation over the right second intercostal space or right sternoclavicular joint may indicate aneurysm of the ascending aorta. Aneurysm of the arch of the aorta may also cause suprasternal pulsation. The most common cause of right supraclavicular pulsation is a kinked, tortuous right carotid artery. A visible pulsation over the left second or third interspace may be due to dilated pulmonary artery, which may result from increased flow, such as with atrial septal defect or increased pressure, as in patients with precapillary or postcapillary pulmonary hypertension. Systolic outward parasternal and left ventricular outward movements are better appreciated by palpation. However, in many patients, an abnormal left ventricular apical impulse is visible and may result from a pronounced, sustained, outward movement or hyperdynamic left ventricular apical impulse. When cardiac pulsations are visible lateral to the left mid-clavicular line, cardiac enlargement should be suspected. Leftward dis-

placement of the cardiac apex may occur due to fibrosis of the left lung, right-sided tension pneumothorax, or massive left pleural effusion. Absent left pericardium (a congenital anomaly) and thoracic deformity may also cause visible pulsations beyond the mid-clavicular line. Occasionally in patients with adhesive pericarditis, retraction of the ribs in the left axilla (Broadbent's sign) are recognized. In patients with severe dilated congestive cardiomyopathy, a double or triple impulse over the left ventricular apex can be recognized and represents a sustained left ventricular outward movement, a prominent atrial filling wave, and early diastolic filling impulse.

Although conventional teaching recommends palpation of the precordium to detect any abnormal impulse in the apical, mid-precordial, lower left and right parasternal, pulmonary, aortic, suprasternal, and epigastric areas, palpation of left ventricular impulse and left parasternal impulse provide the most useful information to assess changes in cardiac dynamics and function. The left ventricular apical impulse is best palpated when the patient lies in a partial left lateral decubitus position. The outward movement of the left ventricular apical impulse is normally brief and localized and does not extend significantly into the left ventricular ejection phase (Fig. 15.5). The beginning of left ventricular ejection at the bedside is appreciated by the onset of the carotid pulse upstroke. The normal outward movement of the left ventricular apical impulse recedes from the chest wall and becomes impalpable with the onset of ejection after the upstroke of the carotid pulse and during the downstroke of the carotid pulse (25). Thus, at the bedside, when carotid pulse and left ventricular apical impulse are examined concurrently, these two impulses appear out of phase or asynchronous. The sustained apical impulse is characterized by a prolonged duration of the outward movement extending into the ejection phase of the left ventricle. Usually, this outward movement is diffuse and occupies more than one intercostal space. When the carotid pulse upstroke and duration are evaluated simultaneously with the left ventricular outward movement, the sustained apical impulse appears in phase with the carotid pulse upstroke and remains palpable during the downstroke of the carotid pulse.

With a hyperdynamic apical impulse, the amplitude of the outward movement is increased, but the sequence between the onset of the carotid pulse and the outward movement remains normal. The hyperdynamic apical impulse is appreciated as a thrust of large amplitude that immediately disappears from the palpating fingers. When the duration of the ejection phase is estimated from the carotid pulse upstroke and downstroke or from the interval between the S_1 and S_2, the hyperdynamic apical impulse does not extend throughout systole. The sustained outward movement usually is felt as a heave. The duration of the outward movement of the apical impulse when it is sustained extends throughout the ejection phase. A sustained apical

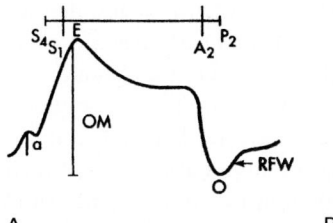
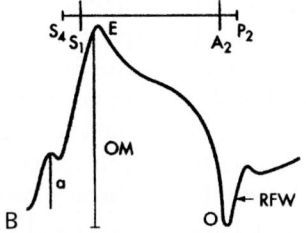
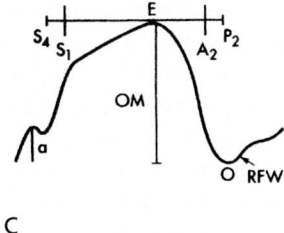

FIGURE 15.5 Schematic diagrams of normal, hyperdynamic, and sustained left ventricular impulse. Heart sounds are also illustrated. **A:** Normal apical impulse. The 'a' wave related to ventricular filling during atrial systole usually is not palpable. Similarly, the rapid filling wave (RFW) in early diastole is also not palpable. The E point, which coincides with the beginning of the left ventricular ejection, is brief in normal individuals. Normal apical impulse usually is associated with normal left ventricular ejection fraction. **B:** Hyperdynamic left ventricular impulse usually is seen in left ventricular volume overloaded conditions such as primary mitral regurgitation and aortic regurgitation. Left ventricular ejection fraction usually is normal. A palpable 'a' wave or presystolic wave indicates increased left ventricular end diastolic pressure. **C:** Sustained left ventricular impulse, which extends into the ejection phase, usually is seen in the presence of decreased left ventricular ejection fraction or when there is marked left ventricular hypertrophy. A palpable 'a' wave or early rapid filling spike is associated with increased diastolic pressure. A_2, aortic component of the second heart sound; P_2, pulmonary component of the second heart sound; S_1, first heart sound; S_4, fourth heart sound.

impulse usually is found when there is significant impairment of left ventricular systolic function (i.e., reduced ejection fraction) (26,27). Another cause of sustained apical impulse is marked left ventricular hypertrophy resulting from systemic hypertension or left ventricular outflow tract obstruction. If, at the bedside, these conditions are excluded, a sustained apical impulse should be regarded as an indication of depressed left ventricular ejection fraction. In patients with known coronary artery disease or previous myocardial infarction, a sustained apical impulse almost invariably indicates reduced left ventricular ejection fraction. Similar hemodynamic correlates should be suspected in patients with known nonischemic dilated cardiomyopathy. In patients with angina pectoris, early systolic, late systolic, or combined early and late systolic bulges occasionally can be appreciated at the bedside when left ventricular apical impulse is analyzed carefully. These abnormal systolic motions are more frequently appreciated in patients with previous myocardial infarction. Systolic bulges occasionally may be appreciated in the absence of previous myocardial infarction and probably result from myocardial ischemia. If these abnormal apical impulses are transient and appreciated during anginal pain, reversible myocardial ischemia should be considered. At the bedside, however, these transient abnormal systolic motions are difficult to appreciate. Occasionally in patients with mitral valve prolapse, a deep notch in the systolic portion of the left ventricular apical impulse, which coincides with the mid-systolic click, is recorded in the apex cardiogram, but it is difficult to recognize at the bedside. The hyperdynamic apical impulse occurs in conditions associated with an increased stroke volume or volume overload. Hyperdynamic impulse is found in patients with hypermetabolic state, such as hyperthyroidism, anemia, primary mitral regurgitation, and aortic regurgitation, and in some patients with a patent ductus arteriosus and ventricular septal defect with a large left-to-right shunt. A hyperdynamic impulse, in general, suggests preserved left ventricular ejection fraction.

While examining the left ventricular apical impulse, particularly in the left lateral decubitus, a double impulse is felt and almost always represents a palpable 'a' wave (presystolic wave) and a prominent outward movement. The palpable 'a' wave is related to an accentuated atrial filling wave and is most frequently observed in patients with noncompliant left ventricle, such as in patients with aortic stenosis, hypertensive heart disease, or ischemic heart disease. The hemodynamic correlate of palpable 'a' wave is increased left ventricular end diastolic pressure. Occasionally, a palpable, rapid filling spike, which coincides with a prominent S_3 gallop, is appreciated during palpation of left ventricular apical impulse. At the bedside, this palpable early diastolic rapid filling spike is appreciated after the outward movement. The hemodynamic correlate of palpable S_3 gallop is also increased left ventricular diastolic pressure. The characteristics of the left ventricular outward movement, along with changes in the filling waves, are illustrated in Fig. 15.5.

Right ventricular impulse is appreciated by palpation of the lower left parasternal area. In children and in some adults with thin chest walls, a brief, gentle impulse may be palpable over the left third and fourth interspaces. This impulse usually is in diastole. A prolonged left parasternal impulse extending during the ejection phase (i.e., throughout the carotid pulse upstroke and downstroke or between S_1 and S_2) is distinctly abnormal and reflects right ventricular failure or right ventricular hypertrophy. It should be realized, however, that in the presence of significant mitral regurgitation, left atrial expansion during left ventricular systole may also produce a sustained systolic left parasternal impulse. Thus, at the bedside, before the diagnosis of right ventricular failure or right ventricular hypertrophy is suspected, it is necessary to exclude significant mitral regurgitation. In patients with right ventricular hypertrophy and failure, a sustained epigastric impulse is also appreciated. An inward systolic movement and an outward diastolic movement are sometimes appreciated in some patients with constrictive pericarditis. (28) The diastolic movement usually coincides in timing with the pericardial knock. The precise explanation for these unusual precordial impulses in constrictive pericarditis has not been clarified. It has been suggested that this unusual outward movement during isovolumic systole is inhibited by the constriction, and the outward movement during early diastole becomes accentuated. In patients with severe chronic constrictive pericarditis, however, the precordium usually is quiet, and no obvious precordial impulses are appreciated at the bedside. In patients with Ebstein's anomaly, the precordium may also be quiet. In some patients with Ebstein's anomaly, a right parasternal systolic outward movement resulting from a large, ventricularized right atrium is appreciated.

A left ventricular aneurysm can be associated with a systolic impulse in unusual locations, such as over the midprecordium. Pulsation in the left second interspace usually reflects an enlarged pulmonary artery resulting from chronic severe pulmonary arterial hypertension or from increased pulmonary flow, as in atrial septal defect. Occasionally, a higher-frequency impulse is appreciated coincident with the downstroke of the carotid pulse in the left second interspace and usually reflects an accentuated pulmonary component of the S_2, as in patients with severe chronic pulmonary hypertension. A pulsatile mass in the suprasternal notch may indicate aneurysm of the ascending aorta. Aneurysm of the ascending aorta is sometimes associated with the tracheal tug, which is appreciated when the trachea is slightly pulled upward and the pulsation in the trachea is recognized with each cardiac cycle. A pulsatile mass in the right supraclavicular area is most frequently caused by a kinked right carotid artery. Such an abnormal impulse may indicate the presence of atherosclerotic peripheral vascular disease.

AUSCULTATION

A systematic and careful cardiac auscultation (1,29) is essential for the diagnosis of a cardiovascular abnormality. Auscultation should be performed whenever possible with the patient in the left lateral decubitus, supine, and sitting positions. However, in many clinical circumstances, particularly with patients with critical illness in intensive-care units, such approaches are not practical. Auscultation can begin over the cardiac apex—the so-called mitral area—and one can proceed counterclockwise to the left fourth interspace (tricuspid area), left third interspace, left second interspace, pulmonic area and right second interspace (aortic area), sometimes, over the right fourth interspace adjacent to the sternal borders, and, finally, over the epigastrium. It is customary to assess the intensity and splitting of the S_1 and S_2 and the presence of S_3 and the

fourth heart sound (S_4). It is also desirable to listen for the presence of abnormal early systolic, mid-systolic, early diastolic, and late diastolic heart sounds. After the analysis of the normal and abnormal heart sounds, heart murmurs, if present, are analyzed. When certain diagnoses are suspected, areas of auscultation should include the left axilla, thoracic and lumber spine, vortex (mitral regurgitation), axilla and back (pulmonary artery branch stenosis), posterior chest (coarctation of aorta), left infraclavicular area (patent ductus arteriosus), and sternoclavicular joints (venous hum).

First Heart Sound

For the analysis of the S_1, the diaphragm is used, and auscultation is performed over the mitral and tricuspid areas. The intensity of the S_1 is determined primarily by the intensity of mitral component (M_1) of the S_1. Several factors contribute to the intensity of M_1 (30,31). The position of the mitral valve at the onset of systole, the rate of mitral valve closure, the mobility of the mitral valve, the PR interval, and the dP/dT of the left ventricle—all are important factors that influence the intensity of M_1. Of all these contributing factors, the position of the atrioventricular valves at the beginning of the ventricular systole, and the velocity of closure seem to be the major determinants of the intensity of the S_1. When the mitral valve remains fully open until the very end of diastole and then closes rapidly, the intensity of M_1 is increased. The greater the distance that the mitral valve leaflets have to travel from the open to closed positions and the greater the velocity of closure of the mitral valve, the louder the S_1. In clinical practice, if a substantial increase in the intensity of the S_1 is recognized at the bedside, an increase in transmitral valvular pressure gradient (e.g., in mitral stenosis), increased transvalvular flow (e.g., in the presence of large left-to-right shunt due to ventricular septal defect or a patent ductus arteriosus), a very short PR interval (e.g., in preexcitation syndrome), or markedly shortened left ventricular diastole (e.g., in tachycardia) should be suspected. When mitral valve obstruction and short PR interval are excluded, increased intensity of the S_1 may reflect an increased left ventricular dP/dT, as during adrenergic stimulation. The increased intensity of the tricuspid valve closure sound (T_1), which is appreciated over the left third and fourth interspaces along the lower sternal border, usually occurs when the transtricuspid valve pressure gradient is increased, as in patients with tricuspid stenosis or right atrial myxoma. A substantial increase in diastolic flow across the tricuspid valve, as in large atrial septal defect, may also increase the intensity of the T_1. Intermittent increased intensity of the S_1 in the presence of regular pulse and heart rhythms indicates atrioventricular dissociation, results from varying PR intervals, and is associated with variable rates of closure of atrioventricular valves. An increase in intensity of the S_1 has been observed in some patients with mitral valve prolapse, despite mitral regurgitation, and probably reflects increased adrenergic activity (32).

Intensity of the First Heart Sound

A decrease in intensity of the S_1 can result from a substantial loss of the tissue mass of the atrioventricular valves, as occurs in severe rheumatic tricuspid and mitral valve diseases and bacterial endocarditis. This decrease can also result from the marked restriction of the movement of the atrioventricular valves due to calcification or sclerosis of the valve leaflets, which occasionally occurs in patients with rheumatic mitral valve stenosis and may be associated with decreased—rather than increased—intensity of the S_1. When the PR interval is prolonged (i.e., exceeding 200 ms), the intensity of the S_1 decreases because semiclosure of the mitral valve occurs after atrial systole and before ventricular systole begins. In severe aortic regurgitation, premature closure of the mitral valve may occur due to a rapid rise in left ventricular diastolic pressure, and the mitral valve may be virtually closed at the onset of ventricular systole, resulting in a markedly decreased intensity of the S_1. In patients with acute severe aortic regurgitation associated with marked increase in left ventricular diastolic pressure, the S_1 may be inaudible and should be regarded as an indication for surgical intervention (33). A substantial increase in left ventricular diastolic pressure and a reduction in transmitral valve pressure gradient are important mechanisms for decreased intensity of the S_1 in the absence of prolonged PR interval and restricted mitral valve mobility. Impaired pump and contractile function, as in dilated cardiomyopathy, is an important cause of reduced intensity of the S_1. In these patients, left ventricular diastolic pressure is also frequently elevated. In clinical practice, decreased intensity of the S_1 in the absence of prolonged PR interval should be regarded as indicative of increased left ventricular diastolic pressure with or without impairment of contractile function. Occasionally, decreased intensity of S_1 is observed in isolated left bundle branch block, probably reflecting impaired left ventricular function (34).

A variable intensity of the S_1 is common in atrial fibrillation. However, atrial fibrillation can be suspected at the bedside from analysis of the arterial pulse, which is irregularly irregular. Auscultatory alternans—in which the S_1 is soft and loud in intensity with alternate beats—is a rare finding of severe cardiac tamponade and is almost always associated with electrical alternans and pulsus paradoxus. Auscultatory alternans also has been observed in patients with pulsus alternans, in whom beat-to-beat alteration in the left ventricular dP/dT occurs (35).

Decreased conduction of sounds through the chest wall reduces the intensity of the S_1 in patients with chronic obstructive pulmonary disease, obesity, and pericardial effusion. In these circumstances, all heart sounds appear soft and distant. One of the practical difficulties in assessing the intensity of the S_1 at the bedside is the lack of any objective method to standardize its intensity. The S_1 normally is loudest at the apex and along the lower left sternal border. In the tricuspid and mitral areas, the intensity of the S_1 is louder than the intensity of the S_2. If the S_1 is softer than the S_2 over the mitral or tricuspid area, it can be assumed that the intensity of the S_1 is reduced. On the other hand, if the S_1 is much louder than the S_2 over the left or right second interspace, the intensity of the S_1 is likely to be increased.

Splitting of the First Heart Sound

The splitting of the S_1 (36) is best appreciated along the left parasternal areas and is most frequently observed in the presence of complete or incomplete right bundle branch block. In right bundle branch block, the S_2 is also widely split, and the A_2-P_2 interval widens during inspiration. Delayed closure of T_1 due to increased flow across the tricuspid valve (atrial septal defect) or increased transtricuspid valve pressure gradient (tricuspid stenosis) causes wide splitting of S_1 without splitting of the S_2. The widely split S_1 is recognized in patients with Ebstein's anomaly, not only because of right ventricular conduction disturbances but also from the delayed closure of the tricuspid valve due to atrialization of the right ventricle. In Ebstein's anomaly, the S_2 is also widely split, and, frequently, systolic and diastolic, scratchy, superficial sounds—so-called "sail sounds"—are present (37). In adult cardiac patients, however, Ebstein's anomalies are encountered infrequently. The diagnosis of Ebstein's anomaly can only be suspected at the bedside and needs to be confirmed by other investigations, including echocardiography. The reversed splitting of the S_1 is extremely rare and difficult to recognize at the bedside. Reversed splitting of the S_1 can result from severe mitral stenosis and is rarely due to left bundle branch block. However, in left bundle branch block, it is easier to appreciate the reversed splitting of the S_2 than that of the S_1. In patients with severe mitral stenosis, delayed closure of the mitral valve contributes to the reversed splitting of the S_1. However, earlier closure of the tricuspid valve resulting from secondary tricuspid regurgitation is also necessary for the reversed splitting of the S_1 in mitral stenosis. The severity of mitral stenosis at the bedside also is not diagnosed based on the presence or absence of reversed splitting of the S_2. The duration of the diastolic murmur, associated pulmonary hypertension, and the A_2–opening snap interval are assessed to determine the severity of mitral stenosis at the bedside. Furthermore, in all patients with suspected mitral valve obstruction, echocardiographic evaluation is mandatory.

Sounds Mimicking the First Heart Sound

At the bedside, it is necessary to distinguish between splitting of the S_1 and the presence of a loud atrial sound preceding the S_1 (Fig. 15.6). The left ventricular atrial sound (S_4) usually is localized over the cardiac apex and is heard best with the bell of the stethoscope. When auscultation is

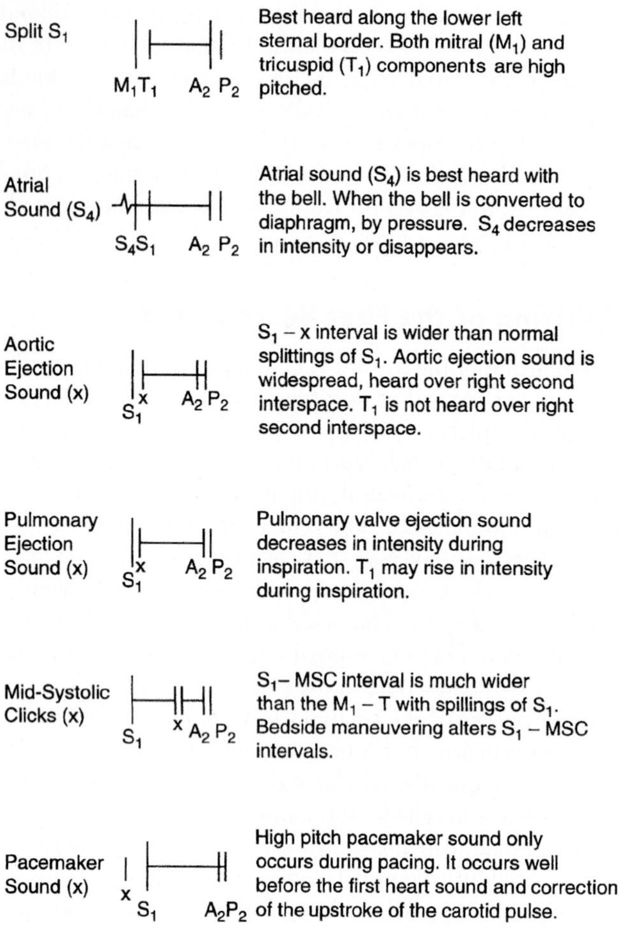

Split S₁ — Best heard along the lower left sternal border. Both mitral (M₁) and tricuspid (T₁) components are high pitched.

M₁T₁   A₂ P₂

Atrial Sound (S₄) — Atrial sound (S₄) is best heard with the bell. When the bell is converted to diaphragm, by pressure. S₄ decreases in intensity or disappears.

S₄S₁   A₂ P₂

Aortic Ejection Sound (x) — S₁ – x interval is wider than normal splittings of S₁. Aortic ejection sound is widespread, heard over right second interspace. T₁ is not heard over right second interspace.

S₁ ˣ   A₂ P₂

Pulmonary Ejection Sound (x) — Pulmonary valve ejection sound decreases in intensity during inspiration. T₁ may rise in intensity during inspiration.

S₁ ˣ   A₂ P₂

Mid-Systolic Clicks (x) — S₁ – MSC interval is much wider than the M₁ – T with spillings of S₁. Bedside maneuvering alters S₁ – MSC intervals.

S₁   ˣ A₂ P₂

Pacemaker Sound (x) — High pitch pacemaker sound only occurs during pacing. It occurs well before the first heart sound and correction of the upstroke of the carotid pulse.

ˣ S₁   A₂P₂

FIGURE 15.6 The causes and differential diagnosis of the first heart sound (S₁). A₂, aortic component of the second heart sound; P₂, pulmonary component of the second heart sound.

started with the use of the bell over the cardiac apex, S₁ and S₄ are heard easily. When the bell is converted to the diaphragm by applying firm pressure over the underlying skin, the S₄ decreases in intensity or disappears, whereas the splitting of the S₁ becomes more obvious.

The combination of a systolic ejection sound and S₁ may also appear as split S₁. The S₁ and the ejection sound interval usually is greater than the normal M₁-T₁ interval. The aortic ejection sound is widely transmitted and, therefore, can be heard easily over the aortic area, along the left sternal border, and over the cardiac apex. On the other hand, the split S₁ is best appreciated along the lower left sternal border, over the left third and fourth interspaces. Pulmonary valvular ejection sounds can be easily distinguished from T₁. Pulmonary ejection sounds are usually localized and heard best over the left second interspace. Pulmonary valvular ejection sounds decrease in intensity during inspiration, whereas the intensity of T₁ remains unchanged or increases after inspiration.

A combination of S₁ and a mid-systolic click due to mitral valve prolapse is rarely confused with a split S₁. The interval between S₁ and a mid-systolic click is much greater than the

interval between M₁ and T₁. Furthermore, the S₁ to mid-systolic click interval can be changed by maneuvers such as standing and squatting. These maneuvers, however, usually do not alter the interval between M₁ and T₁ significantly enough to be appreciated at the bedside. The presence of a pacemaker sound preceding S₁ may seem like a widely split S₁. The pacemaker sound results from the stimulation of the intercostal muscles during pacing, precedes S₁, and occurs well before the upstroke of the carotid pulse (38). Furthermore, the pacemaker sound disappears with discontinuation of pacing. The causes and the differential diagnosis of the abnormalities of the S₁ are summarized in Table 15.4.

TABLE 15.4 USUAL CAUSES OF THE ABNORMALITIES OF THE FIRST HEART SOUND

Increased intensity
Mitral or tricuspid valve obstruction—mitral stenosis, left atrial myxoma, tricuspid stenosis, and right atrial myxoma. These conditions are also associated with other findings of atrioventricular valvular obstruction such as mid-diastolic rumble.
Increased transatrioventricular valve flow—patent ductus arteriosus, ventricular septal defect, atrial septal defect. These conditions are also associated with characteristic findings such as continuous murmur, pansystolic murmur, or widely split second heart sound, respectively.
Increased dP/dT—hyperkinetic heart syndrome, tachycardia, mitral valve prolapse. These conditions are also associated with additional physical findings such as mid-systolic click in mitral valve prolapse.
Short PR interval—preexcitation syndrome, which is confirmed by the electrocardiographic findings.

Decreased intensity
Restrictive mitral valve movement—calcific mitral stenosis. This condition is also associated with other auscultatory findings such as mid-diastolic rumble and findings suggestive of pulmonary hypertension.
Lack of apposition of the mitral valve leaflets—rheumatic mitral regurgitation, which is associated with a pansystolic murmur over the cardiac apex.
Presystolic semiclosure of the mitral valves due to increase in left ventricular diastolic pressure—noncompliant left ventricle, acute aortic regurgitation, dilated cardiomyopathy.
Conduction anomaly, left bundle branch block, prolonged PR interval. These conditions are confirmed by electrocardiography.

Wide splitting of the first heart sound
Conduction abnormalities—complete right bundle branch block, left ventricular pacing, preexcitation syndrome with left ventricular connection. These conditions are confirmed by other associated findings, as well as by electrocardiography.
Ebstein's anomaly—also associated with widely split second heart sound, sail sounds, and tricuspid regurgitation murmur.
Mechanical—tricuspid stenosis, atrial septal defect. These conditions are also associated with characteristic physical findings such as mid-diastolic rumble and wide fixed splitting of the second heart sound, respectively.

Reversed splitting of the first heart sound
Arrhythmias—premature beats of right ventricular origin.
Conduction disturbances—left bundle branch block, right ventricular pacing. These conditions are confirmed by electrocardiography.
Mechanical—severe mitral stenosis and left atrial myxoma.

dP/dT, upstroke pattern.

SECOND HEART SOUND

The genesis of the S_2 appears to be related to closure of the aortic and pulmonary valves; thus, the S_2 traditionally is regarded to consist of two components designated as A_2 (associated with aortic valve closure) and P_2 (associated with pulmonary valve closure). The first high-frequency component of A_2 and P_2 is coincident with completion of closure of these semilunar valves (39). It should be appreciated that A_2 and P_2 are not produced by the clapping together of the valve leaflets but by the sudden deceleration of retrograde flow of the blood column in the aorta and pulmonary artery when the maximum tensing of these valve leaflets occurs. The abrupt deceleration of flow produces the vibration of the cardiohemic system, and the lower frequency vibrations are coincident with the incisura of the great vessels, whereas the higher frequency components cause A_2 and P_2. It should be recognized that left and right ventricular ejection ceases before the closure of the aortic and pulmonary valves.

Aortic Component

The amplitude and intensity of A_2 and P_2 are directly proportional to the rate of change of the diastolic pressure gradient that develops across the semilunar valves—that is, the driving force that accelerates the blood mass retrograde into the base of the great vessels (40). The rate of pressure decline in the ventricle and the level of the diastolic pressure in the great vessels determine the pressure gradient in the root of the great vessels. Normally, the diastolic pressure gradient in the aorta is significantly greater than that in the pulmonary artery, which explains the normal increased intensity of A_2 compared with that of P_2. The most common cause of the increased intensity of A_2 is systemic hypertension. Occasionally, in addition to the increased intensity, a tambour quality of A_2 is recognized in systemic hypertension. Such altered quality of A_2 also is appreciated in some patients with aneurysm of the ascending aorta without aortic insufficiency. The decreased intensity of A_2 most frequently occurs from immobility of calcified, sclerosed aortic valves in calcific aortic stenosis. It should be appreciated, however, that the degree of intensity of A_2 does not correlate well with the severity of aortic stenosis. In aortic regurgitation resulting from fibrosed and retracted aortic valve leaflets, as in syphilitic aortic regurgitation, the aortic component of the S_2 also is decreased in intensity. Normally, A_2 is widely transmitted and well heard at the cardiac apex. However, in patients with significant mitral regurgitation, A_2 may be drowned at the cardiac apex by the regurgitant murmur that frequently extends beyond the aortic valve closure. However, in these circumstances, the intensity of A_2 can be appreciated by listening over other areas of the precordium.

Pulmonic Component

The pulmonic component of the S_2—that is, P_2—is softer than A_2 and is rarely audible at the apex. Increase in the intensity of P_2 indicates pulmonary hypertension, irrespective of its etiology. When there is a substantial increase in its intensity, P_2 is also heard at the cardiac apex. Without pulmonary hypertension, it is uncommon for the P_2 to be transmitted to the cardiac apex. In only approximately 5% of healthy subjects, and only when they are young (i.e., under 20 years old), can P_2 be recorded by phonocardiography over the cardiac apex (41). Although an increased intensity of P_2 is the most important physical finding for the diagnosis of pulmonary arterial hypertension, other physical findings that support the diagnosis should be searched for at the bedside. A prominent 'a' wave in the jugular venous pulse, a sustained left parasternal outward impulse, epigastric pulsation, a palpable P_2 over the left second interspace, and auscultatory features of tricuspid regurgitation and secondary pulmonary insufficiency all support the diagnosis of significant pulmonary arterial hypertension. These secondary findings, however, result from severe pulmonary hypertension and are not present in all patients.

When the cardiac apex is occupied by the right ventricle—as in patients with large atrial septal defects—P_2 can be heard at the apex, even when the pulmonary artery pressure is not increased. Similarly, in patients with primary tricuspid regurgitation without pulmonary hypertension, P_2 occasionally is heard at the apex. In patients with a widely split S_2 due to right bundle branch block, P_2 rarely can be heard at the apex in the absence of pulmonary hypertension.

Decreased intensity of P_2 results from a reduction in the pulmonary artery diastolic pressure, as in patients with pulmonary valve stenosis. Decreased intensity of P_2 or absence of P_2 may also occur from the loss of the pulmonary valve leaflets or from the congenital absence of the pulmonary valves. In these clinical conditions, however, a loud pulmonary insufficiency murmur is appreciated over the precordium.

Splitting of the Second Heart Sound

The sequence of closure of the aortic and pulmonary valves (i.e., the splitting of A_2 and P_2 during respiratory phases) should be analyzed whenever feasible. Normally, A_2 precedes P_2 during expiration and inspiration. The A_2-P_2 interval also increases considerably during normal inspiration.

In adults, the splitting of the S_2 during the expiratory phase of respiration usually is not appreciated at the bedside, because the degree of splitting usually does not exceed 30 ms. However, during inspiration, the splitting is easily appreciated, particularly in the semirecumbent position and even in elderly patients. The splitting of the S_2 should be assessed during normal respiration with the diaphragm of the stethoscope over the left second and third interspaces close to the sternal border. Normally, the aortic component of the S_2 (A_2) precedes the pulmonic component (P_2). The normal splitting of the S_2 primarily results from the differences between pulmonary artery and aortic "hangout" times (42). The left ventricular ejection starts a few milliseconds before the onset of right ventricular ejection because of the earlier onset of left ventricular depolarization. The earlier onset of left ventricular ejection certainly contributes to the earlier completion of left ventricular ejection. However, this earlier completion of left ventricular ejection only accounts for 10 to 15 ms of the degree of splitting of the S_2. The hangout time is the interval between the end of ventricular ejection and the closure of the semilunar valves. The hangout time in the aorta is considerably shorter than that of the pulmonary artery. The hangout time in the pulmonary artery may be as long as 60 to 70 ms; the hangout time in the aorta may be as short as 15 to 30 ms. The difference between the pulmonary artery and aortic hangout times primarily determines the degree of splitting of the S_2, both in physiologic situations and in many pathologic conditions (Fig. 15.7). The hangout time also is determined by the compliance of the aorta and the pulmonary artery. Normally, the aorta is much stiffer than the pulmonary artery—a characteristic that accounts for the shorter hangout time in the aorta than in the pulmonary artery. When the pulmonary artery compliance decreases, as in chronic pulmonary hypertension, the hang-

out time also decreases; thus, the degree of splitting of the S_2 may actually be shorter in the presence of significant chronic pulmonary arterial hypertension. The normal inspiratory splitting of the S_2 is explained by an increase in the pulmonary hangout time during inspiration that results from an increase in right ventricular stroke volume. An increase in the right ventricular ejection time after inspiration also contributes, to some extent, to the inspiratory splitting of the S_2. More negative intrathoracic pressure during inspiration is associated with an increased venous return to the right ventricle and an increased right ventricular stroke volume, which increases the ejection time and delays the P_2. During inspiration, A_2 occurs slightly earlier due to slight reduction of left ventricular ejection time associated with a transient, slight reduction of left ventricular stroke volume. After one to three cardiac cycles, the increase in right ventricular stroke volume with inspiration is followed by a similar increase in stroke volume of the left ventricle associated with a slight increase in left ventricular ejection time. During normal respiration, prolongation of left ventricular ejection time and a delayed A_2 usually occur during the expiratory phase, whereas lengthening of the right ventricular ejection time and delay in P_2 coincide with the inspiratory phase.

Wide Splitting of the Second Heart Sound

When splitting of the S_2 is appreciated during expiration, abnormal wide splitting of the S_2 should be suspected. The longer the A_2-P_2 interval during expiration, the more abnormal is the splitting of the S_2. The inspiratory increase in the degree of splitting of the S_2 indicates the presence of physiologic delay in the pulmonary valve closure sound. The widely split S_2 during expiration (with further increase in splitting during inspiration) most frequently occurs in right bundle branch block. In right bundle branch block, the S_1 also is frequently split. A widely split S_2 may be present in Wolff-Parkinson-White syndrome with left ventricular preexcitation. Left ventricular pacing also produces right bundle branch block–types of conduction disturbances and is associated with widely split S_2. Premature beats and an idioventricular rhythm of left ventricular origin with QRS complex of right bundle branch block morphology are also associated with wide splitting of the S_2. The wide splitting of the S_2 in conduction disturbances occurs from delayed activation of the right ventricle and consequently delayed completion of right ventricular ejection.

The wide splitting of the S_2 may also result from increased resistance of right ventricular ejection, as in patients with pulmonary valve stenosis, infundibular stenosis, supravalvular stenosis, and pulmonary branch stenosis. In pulmonary valve stenosis, the intensity of the P_2 is substantially decreased, and pulmonary valve stenosis can be easily recognized from the presence of a long ejection systolic murmur. In pulmonary valve stenosis, the degree of

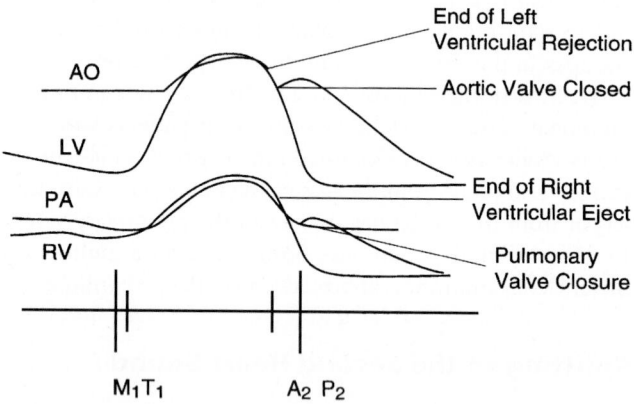

FIGURE 15.7 Schematic illustrations of "hangout" times, which are the time intervals between the end of ventricular ejection and closure of the aortic valve (A_2) and closure of the pulmonary valve (P_2). The hangout time is primarily determined by the compliance of the great vessels and the stroke volume ejected into the great vessels. The aortic hangout time is much shorter (aorta is less compliant than the pulmonary artery) than that of the pulmonary artery. The differences between the pulmonary and aortic hangout time may explain physiologic or pathologic splitting of the second heart sound. The mitral component (M_1) and the tricuspid component (T_1) of the first heart sound and left ventricular (LV), right ventricular (RV), aortic (AO), and pulmonary artery (PA) pressure waveforms are also illustrated.

expiratory splitting of the S_2 is directly related to the severity of stenosis and right ventricular systolic hypertension (43). If the expiratory splitting of the S_2 is approximately 40 to 50 ms, right ventricular systolic pressure is also 40 to 50 mm Hg. When the degree of splitting of the S_2 exceeds 70 to 80 ms, the right ventricular systolic pressure is extremely high and may exceed 80 mm Hg. In patients with pulmonary branch stenosis, the intensity of P_2 is increased, and, frequently, unilateral or bilateral continuous murmurs are appreciated. In adults, the most common cause of obvious expiratory splitting of the S_2 with increased intensity of P_2 is precapillary or postcapillary pulmonary arterial hypertension. In pulmonary hypertension, although the expiratory splitting is obvious, the degree of splitting is less than that expected from the degree of pulmonary hypertension. The relatively shorter splitting of the S_2—even in patients with severe pulmonary hypertension—is related to the substantial reduction in pulmonary hangout time due to decreased pulmonary arterial compliance. For the same reason, in patients with severe pulmonary hypertension, the magnitude of inspiratory widening of the interval between A_2 and P_2 is smaller. Wide expiratory splitting of the S_2 may also result from isolated reduction of the left ventricular ejection time, as in patients with hemodynamically significant mitral regurgitation (44). In patients with severe mitral regurgitation with relatively preserved left ventricular ejection fraction, as in patients with primary mitral regurgitation, left ventricular forward stroke volume may decrease with a substantial shortening of left ventricular ejection time and an earlier occurrence of A_2 (45). In patients with unrestricted ventricular septal defect with increased pulmonary flow and decreased pulmonary vascular resistance, a widely split S_2 is appreciated due to a decrease in left ventricular ejection time and an increase in pulmonary artery hangout time (46). In constrictive pericarditis, a wide inspiratory splitting of the S_2 occasionally is observed, and it results from marked reduction in left ventricular ejection time during inspiration (47). Decreased impedence of the pulmonary vascular bed resulting in an increase in pulmonary hangout time may also cause a wide splitting of the S_2 (29). In patients with idiopathic dilatation of the pulmonary artery, mild pulmonary valve stenosis, atrial septal defect with normal pulmonary artery pressure, and postoperative atrial septal defect, the increase in pulmonary hangout time is the principal mechanism for the wide splitting of the S_2. In patients with a primum or secondary type of atrial septal defect and also with common atrium, the interval between A_2 and P_2 during expiration and inspiration may not change significantly (widely split fixed S_2). The mechanism of wide expiratory splitting of the S_2 appears to be due to isolated shortening of the ejection time of the left ventricle, whereas the right ventricular ejection time remains normal. There is also an increase in the pulmonary hangout time, which results from the decreased pulmonary vascular impedence. During inspira-

tion, P_2 is delayed, as in healthy patients, due to prolongation of the right ventricular ejection time. However, in atrial septal defect, A_2 does not occur earlier, suggesting the absence of inspiratory shortening of left ventricular ejection time (48). This lack of shortening of left ventricular ejection time may result from the transient increase in the venous return to the left ventricle due to a reduction in the magnitude in the left-to-right shunt. Thus, the A_2-P_2 interval may remain relatively constant during normal expiration and inspiration.

In adults, the most frequent cause of fixed splitting of the S_2 is the occurrence of severe right ventricular failure when there is little or no increase in right ventricular stroke volume after inspiration. The degree of splitting of the S_2 during expiration, however, usually is normal in the absence of right bundle branch block. In patients with severe right ventricular failure and right bundle branch block, a wide fixed splitting of the S_2 frequently is appreciated at the bedside.

Paradoxical Split of the Second Heart Sound

Reversed or paradoxical splitting of the S_2 is recognized when splitting of the S_2 during expiration is appreciated. However, during inspiration, the A_2-P_2 interval shortens, and the S_2 may appear single (48). The reversed splitting of the S_2 almost always occurs due to a delay in A_2. The sequence of these closure sounds is reversed, with P_2 preceding A_2 during expiration. During inspiration, P_2 moves toward A_2, and the splitting of the interval narrows. The reversed splitting of the S_2 may occur due to a delay in the electrical activation of the left ventricle, which results in a delay in the onset and completion of left ventricular ejection. The most common cause of reversed splitting of the S_2 in adults is left bundle branch block, which is associated with a prolonged electromechanical interval. Right ventricular ectopic beats and right ventricular pacing produce a delay in the onset of left ventricular contraction and result in reversed splitting of the S_2. The Wolff-Parkinson-White syndrome with right ventricular preexcitation is associated with reversed splitting of the S_2. In all of these conditions, conduction disturbance resulting in delayed activation of the left ventricle causes a delay in the onset and completion of left ventricular ejection and, thus, results in reversed splitting of the S_2. It should be appreciated that left ventricular systolic function may also be impaired and can accompany conduction disturbances (49). In these circumstances, the degree of expiratory reversed splitting may be significantly greater than when the conduction disturbances are present without myocardial dysfunction.

Reversed splitting of the S_2 may occur due to prolongation of the left ventricular ejection time, which is due to a selective increase in the left ventricular forward stroke volume or a marked increase in resistance to left ventricular ejection. A selective increase in left ventricular forward stroke volume can occur in patients with significant aortic regurgitation or with patent ductus arteriosus with a large left-to-right shunt. Increased resistance to left ventricular ejection producing a reversed splitting of the S_2 occurs in patients with significant aortic stenosis and obstructive hypertrophic cardiomyopathy. In patients with aortic stenosis, reversed splitting in the absence of left bundle branch block indicates hemodynamically significant aortic stenosis. In patients with hypertrophic cardiomyopathy with left ventricular outflow tract obstruction, reversed splitting occurs despite significant mitral regurgitation (50). The systolic murmur associated with primary mitral regurgitation, ventricular septal defect, and hypertrophic obstructive cardiomyopathy may appear similar in character and duration at the bedside. The behavior of the S_2 may be useful in the differential diagnosis of these conditions. If the S_2 is paradoxically split in the absence of left bundle branch block, the diagnosis of hypertrophic cardiomyopathy is most likely. The presence of widely split S_2 favors the diagnosis of primary mitral regurgitation or ventricular septal defect. The reversed splitting also occurs in patients with severe chronic systemic hypertension with a marked increase in systemic vascular resistance, which increases resistance to left ventricular ejection. However, a compensatory increase in adrenergic activity and left ventricular wall thickness, which reduces left ventricular wall stress, may normalize left ventricular ejection time; therefore, S_2 may be normal. In systemic hypertension, the intensity of A_2 is always increased. If there is dilatation of the aortic root, a tambour quality of the A_2 frequently can be recognized. Acute elevation of systemic arterial pressure (e.g., during administration of methoxamine) has been shown to produce reversed splitting of the S_2, even in normal subjects, suggesting that acute increase in left ventricular afterload may cause a substantial prolongation of the left ventricular ejection time (51). Reversed splitting of the S_2 also has been recognized in patients with ischemic heart disease and during episodes of angina. These findings, however, are rarely encountered in clinical practice in patients with ischemic heart disease. Furthermore, the mechanism of reversed splitting in these patients remains unclear, but it may be related to a prolonged isovolumic systole of the ischemic left ventricle and an increase in left ventricular afterload. This mechanism may also be related to transient left bundle branch block. Poststenotic aortic root dilatation is associated with a decrease in the impedance in the systemic vascular bed; delayed A_2 can occur, which may contribute to the reversed splitting of the S_2 (52). Such mechanisms have also been entertained in explaining the reversed splitting of the S_2 in patients with chronic aortic regurgitation and patent ductus arteriosus. In clinical practice, however, when reversed splitting of the S_2 is clearly recognized at the bedside, it is desirable first to exclude left bundle branch block or any other conduction anomaly that can be associated with paradoxical splitting of the S_2. After

exclusion of these conduction abnormalities, covert left ventricular systolic dysfunction should be suspected in the absence of left ventricular outflow tract obstruction or aortic regurgitation, which can be diagnosed easily at the bedside.

WIDELY SPLIT SECOND HEART SOUND

A marked increase in the intensity of the pulmonic component of the S_2 (P_2) with narrow expiratory splitting of the S_2 is a common and almost universally present physical finding in severe pulmonary hypertension. The degree of expiratory splitting (i.e., the A_2-P_2 interval) may even be <30 ms in patients with pulmonary hypertension, but the splitting is still clearly appreciated because of the marked increase in the intensity of P_2 (53). In some patients with pulmonary hypertension, a wide splitting with an increased amplitude of P_2 is present in the absence of right bundle branch block (54). It has been suggested that, in these circumstances, wide splitting may represent impairment of right ventricular systolic function. In some patients with severe pulmonary hypertension, fixed splitting of the S_2 has been observed, and it has been suggested that this fixed splitting occurs due to concomitant right ventricular failure secondary to pulmonary hypertension. In these patients, the altered pulmonary vascular impedance associated with severe pulmonary hypertension may also be contributory in the diminished inspiratory splitting of the S_2.

At the bedside, when pulmonary hypertension is suspected from the presence of the increased intensity of the P_2, it is desirable to search for other findings that may be associated with or result from chronic severe pulmonary hypertension. These findings include the pulmonary ejection sound, left parasternal systolic lift associated with right ventricular failure, pulmonary insufficiency murmur, right ventricular S_4, S_3 gallops, and tricuspid regurgitation. It is also desirable to investigate at the bedside the potential etiology of pulmonary hypertension. In adult patients, Eisenmenger's syndrome is suspected from the presence of cyanosis and clubbing and the characteristic changes in the S_2. In Eisenmenger's syndrome, central cyanosis occurs due to intracardiac right-to-left shunt. In Eisenmenger's syndrome associated with atrial and ventricular septal defects, peripheral cyanosis and clubbing involve fingers and toes bilaterally. In Eisenmenger's syndrome associated with patent ductus arteriosus, however, the cyanosis and clubbing are usually recognized in the toes, and the fingers are spared. Differential cyanosis and clubbing in adult patients almost always indicate patent ductus arteriosus and reversal of shunt due to marked increase in pulmonary artery pressure and pulmonary vascular resistance, which allows shunting of the desaturated blood from the pulmonary artery to the descending thoracic aorta. The S_2 in Eisenmenger's syndrome associated with atrial septal defect remains widely split, and the degree of splitting during expiration and inspiration usually does not change significantly (wide fixed splitting of S_2). In Eisenmenger's syndrome associated with a ventricular septal defect, the duration of right and left ventricular systole is essentially equal; therefore, a loud, single S_2 is appreciated because of simultaneous closure of the aortic and pulmonary valves (41). In Eisenmenger's syndrome associated with patent ductus arteriosus, the S_2 behaves like that in precapillary primary pulmonary hypertension.

It should be appreciated that pulmonary hypertension and central and peripheral cyanosis and clubbing can also occur from primary pulmonary disease, such as severe pulmonary fibrosis.

In adults, postcapillary pulmonary hypertension is much more frequent than precapillary pulmonary hypertension, including Eisenmenger's syndrome. Postcapillary pulmonary hypertension can be caused by mitral valve obstruction, such as rheumatic mitral stenosis, mitral regurgitation, aortic stenosis, and aortic regurgitation. These valvular abnormalities can be suspected at the bedside and subsequently confirmed by further investigations, such as echocardiography. If valvular heart disease is excluded, an increase in left ventricular diastolic pressure resulting from left ventricular myocardial dysfunction should be suspected. Systolic ventricular failure due to ischemic and nonischemic dilated cardiomyopathy, diastolic ventricular failure resulting from hypertrophic cardiomyopathy, hypertensive heart disease, and restrictive cardiomyopathy all can be associated with a substantial increase in left ventricular diastolic pressure, a passive increase in left atrial and pulmonary venous pressure, and an obligatory rise in pulmonary artery pressure. If a left ventricular S_3 gallop is appreciated in patients with suspected dilated cardiomyopathy or aortic valve disease, an abnormally elevated left ventricular diastolic pressure and, thus, postcapillary pulmonary hypertension, should be suspected. Careful analysis of the characters of the cardiac apex, diastolic and systolic murmurs, and gallop sounds is essential for exclusion of postcapillary pulmonary hypertension. The causes of precapillary pulmonary hypertension in adults include primary pulmonary diseases, such as chronic obstructive pulmonary disease, chronic thromboembolic pulmonary hypertension, and unexplained or primary pulmonary hypertension. When precapillary pulmonary hypertension is suspected at the bedside, it is desirable to look for conditions such as systemic lupus erythematosus, scleroderma, or CREST syndrome, which can also be associated with precapillary pulmonary hypertension.

Single S_2 may result from the absence of either of the two components of the S_2 or from the fusion of A_2 and P_2 without the inspiratory splitting. The most common cause of an apparently single S_2 is the inability to hear the faint pulmonic component because of chronic obstructive lung disease, obesity, or even normal but accentuated respiratory noise. Another common cause of single S_2 is advanced age and most likely occurs due to a decreased inspiratory delay in P_2, rather than a delayed A_2. Decreased inspiratory delay of P_2 probably results from a decreased right-sided hangout interval related to aging changes in the pulmonary artery compliance. However, all conditions that can delay A_2 may produce a single S_2 when the splitting interval becomes <30 ms. In conditions in which one component of the S_2 is absent or inaudible (e.g., in patients with severe tetralogy of Fallot, severe pulmonary valve stenosis, severe aortic stenosis, pulmonary atresia, and most cases of tricuspid atresia), S_2 is single. The abnormalities of the S_2 and their potential mechanisms and associated causes are summarized in Table 15.5.

EJECTION SOUNDS

The ejection sounds are relatively high-pitched sounds occurring with the onset of ejection or soon after ventricular ejection starts. The ejection sounds are classified as valvular (i.e., arising from deformed aortic or pulmonic valves) or vascular (i.e., caused by a forceful ejection of blood into the great vessels).

Aortic Sounds

Aortic valvular ejection sounds are recognized in bicuspid aortic valve and valvular aortic stenosis. The aortic valvular ejection sounds occur 20 to 40 ms after the onset of pressure rises in the central aorta, and they coincide with the sharp anacrotic notch on the upstroke of the aortic pressure curve. The aortic valvular ejection sounds also are coincident with the maximal excursion of the domed valve. When the aortic valve is immobile due to severe calcification, no excursion or pistol-like ascent of the deformed valve is present; therefore, in severe calcific aortic stenosis, ejection sound is frequently absent. The intensity of the aortic valvular ejection sound also correlates directly with the mobility of the valve. Thus, if the ejection sound is present in patients with aortic valvular stenosis, it indicates the presence of a mobile stenotic valve. In bicuspid aortic valve, the ejection sound usually is loud and is followed by a short ejection systolic murmur, normal S_2, and trivial aortic regurgitation. The aortic valvular ejection sound is widely transmitted and often heard best at the apex. Aortic vascular ejection sounds originate from the aortic root and are common in systemic hypertension, aortic aneurysm, and, sometimes, with aortic root dilatation resulting from hemodynamically significant aortic regurgitation. Aortic vascular ejection sounds occur later than aortic valvular ejection sounds and frequently are localized and poorly transmitted. Aortic vascular ejection sounds are sometimes confused with the tricuspid valve closure sounds. The differential diagnosis between tricuspid valve closure sounds and aortic vascular ejection sounds depends

TABLE 15.5 ABNORMALITIES OF THE SECOND HEART SOUND

Single S$_2$

If there is no evidence of left ventricular outflow tract obstruction, hypertensive heart disease, Eisenmenger's syndrome with ventricular septal defect, and right ventricular outflow obstruction (e.g., tetralogy of Fallot), a clinically relevant pathology can be excluded.

Wide splitting of S$_2$ with inspiratory delay of P$_2$

No other abnormal finding except widely split S$_1$—suspect right ventricular conduction delay such as right bundle branch block.

Pulmonary ejection sound, ejection systolic murmur, a short early diastolic murmur in the left second interspace—suspect idiopathic dilatation of the pulmonary artery or mild pulmonary valve stenosis. Chest x-ray and echo-Doppler study are appropriate ancillary investigations.

Longer ejection systolic murmur with or without pulmonary ejection sound and decreased intensity of the P$_2$—suspect pulmonary valve stenosis or right ventricular infundibular stenosis and consider echo-Doppler study. The increased intensity of P$_2$ with or without a short ejection systolic murmur along left sternal border; with or without evidence of right ventricular hypertrophy, tricuspid regurgitation, and right heart failure; and unilateral or bilateral continuous murmur—suspect peripheral pulmonary artery branch stenosis. MRI and transesophageal echocardiography are appropriate noninvasive investigations.

Increased intensity of the P$_2$ with or without ejection systolic murmur and evidence of right ventricular hypertrophy or failure—suspect precapillary pulmonary hypertension with right ventricular dysfunction. Transthoracic and transesophageal echo-Doppler studies are appropriate noninvasive investigations to assess the etiology of pulmonary hypertension and right ventricular function.

Widely split fixed S$_2$—suspect primum or secundum atrial septal defect

In the presence of cyanosis or pulmonary hypertension—suspect Eisenmenger's syndrome with atrial septal defect or complete atrioventricular canal or common atrium. Electrocardiogram, chest x-ray, and echocardiographic evaluations are appropriate.

Increased intensity of P$_2$ with P$_2$ transmitted to the cardiac apex suggesting pulmonary hypertension

Search for evidence for right ventricular hypertrophy, right ventricular failure, and secondary tricuspid regurgitation.

Cyanosis and clubbing—suspect Eisenmenger's syndrome. Differential cyanosis and clubbing—suspect patent ductus arteriosus. Widely split S$_2$—suspect atrial septal defect. Single S$_2$—suspect ventricular septal defect. In the absence of Eisenmenger's syndrome—suspect primary pulmonary disease.

Mid-diastolic rumble in left lateral decubitus—suspect mitral valve obstruction. Early systolic or pansystolic regurgitant murmur over the cardiac apex—suspect mitral regurgitation. An ejection systolic murmur with a small-volume, delayed upstroke and peaked carotid pulse—suspect aortic stenosis. An ejection systolic murmur along the left sternal border with or without a regurgitant murmur and a normal carotid pulse upstroke—suspect obstructive hypertrophic cardiomyopathy. An early diastolic murmur with displaced hyperdynamic or sustained left ventricular apical impulse—suspect aortic regurgitation. In the absence of evidence for valvular heart disease, a sustained left ventricular apical impulse with a left ventricular S$_3$ gallop—suspect nonischemic or ischemic dilated cardiomyopathy. Elevated systemic venous pressure with sharp 'y' descent and positive Kussmaul's sign—suspect restrictive cardiomyopathy. In all patients with suspected postcapillary pulmonary hypertension, further investigations, including echocardiography, should be entertained.

After exclusion of the causes of postcapillary pulmonary hypertension—suspect precapillary pulmonary hypertension such as thromboembolic pulmonary hypertension, collagen vascular disease, primary pulmonary disease, and primary pulmonary hypertension. Appropriate radiologic, echocardiographic, and laboratory investigations should be considered in patients with suspected precapillary pulmonary hypertension.

Paradoxical splitting of the S$_2$

Suspect conduction disturbances such as left bundle branch block, preexcitation syndrome, arrhythmias, right ventricular pacing—electrocardiogram is indicated. Ejection systolic murmur—suspect aortic stenosis, obstructive hypertrophic cardiomyopathy. Early diastolic murmur—suspect aortic regurgitation. Loud A$_2$—suspect hypertension.

A$_2$, aortic component of the second heart sound; MRI, magnetic resonance imaging; P$_2$, pulmonary component of the second heart sound; S$_1$, first heart sound; S$_2$, second heart sound; S$_3$, third heart sound.

on the clinical circumstances when these sounds are expected to be present.

Pulmonic Sounds

Pulmonary valvular ejection sounds are observed in mild to moderate pulmonary valve stenosis and idiopathic dilatation of the pulmonary artery. Pulmonary valvular ejection sounds occur at the maximal excursion of the stenotic pulmonary valve. In contrast to the aortic valvular ejection sounds and to most right-sided sounds and murmurs, a pulmonary ejection sound or click decreases in intensity—or even disappears—with inspiration (55). The pulmonary valvular ejection sounds coincide with the movement of the domed pulmonary valve. During expiration, a pressure gradient between the pulmonary artery end diastolic pressure and right ventricular end diastolic pressure exists, allowing the deformed domed pulmonary valve excursion and, therefore, the presence of the ejection sounds. During inspiration, the pressure gradient between the pulmonary artery and the right ventricle in end diastole substantially decreases, and there is preopening of the pulmonary valve; there is no further excursion of the domed pulmonary valve, which explains the absence of pulmonary ejection sounds during inspiration. In severe pulmonary stenosis, the pulmonary valvular ejection sounds appear fused with the S_1, which may explain the lack of pulmonary valvular ejection sounds in these patients. Pulmonary vascular ejection sounds arise from the pulmonary artery and are associated with dilatation of the pulmonary artery. The dilated pulmonary artery can be seen in patients with idiopathic dilatation of the pulmonary artery or secondary to severe pulmonary hypertension. Vascular pulmonary ejection sounds are louder in the second and third left intercostal spaces. Echocardiographic studies have suggested that pulmonary vascular ejection sounds coincide with the complete opening of the pulmonary valve and occur during the upstroke of the pulmonary artery pressure recordings (56). It should be recognized that the intensity of pulmonary vascular ejection sounds may not vary substantially during the phases of respiration. In patients with pulmonary hypertension with vascular pulmonary ejection sounds, the intensity of P_2 is markedly accentuated. In idiopathic dilatation of the pulmonary artery, the S_2 intensity is normal and may or may not be associated with a short ejection systolic murmur and a short early diastolic murmur. In pulmonary valve stenosis with pulmonary valvular ejection sounds, there is a long ejection systolic murmur. The S_2 is widely split, and the intensity of P_2 is decreased.

NONEJECTION SOUNDS

Clicks

Systolic nonejection sounds (mid-systolic clicks) occur most frequently in mitral valve prolapse syndrome. Mid-systolic clicks also occur in prolapse of the tricuspid valve.

The mechanism of the mid-systolic click is the tensing of the atrioventricular valves during systole.

At the bedside, when a nonejection or a mid-systolic click is recognized, the initial diagnosis, until proved otherwise, should be mitral valve prolapse. The sound has a sharp, high-frequency, clicking quality, and, although it is heard best over the cardiac apex, it can be transmitted widely. It may be an isolated finding occurring in mid- to late systole, or there may be multiple clicks resulting from prolapsing of the different areas of the large, redundant, scalloped mitral leaflets at different times. Echocardiographic studies have shown the presence of the mid- to late systolic prolapse, as well as pansystolic prolapse, in patients with mid-systolic clicks. All of these different types of prolapse of the mitral valve can occur in patients with only systolic clicks, with clicks and late systolic murmur, or with late systolic murmur alone (57–59). Mid-systolic clicks usually occur at the time of maximum prolapse. Valvuloventricular disproportion (i.e., a valve too big for the ventricle) has been thought to be the principal cause of mitral valve prolapse. It has been suggested that the ventricular volume or dimension associated with prolapse of the mitral valve (click dimension) is relatively fixed in a given patient. After the onset of ejection, the mitral valve prolapse occurs whenever this click dimension is reached (60). Thus, the S_1-click interval and the relative proportion of systole occupied by the regurgitant murmur vary with maneuvers (Fig. 15.8). When the patient maintains an upright posture and the ventricular volume is reduced, the S_1-click interval is shorter, and the duration of the murmur is longer. When the patient is supine and the ventricular volume is increased, the S_1-click interval is longer, and the duration of the murmur is shorter. With the postectopic beat—even though the ventricular volume is increased—the postectopic potentiation causes a rapid ejection; therefore, the S_1-click interval gets shorter, and the duration of the murmur gets longer (60). These bedside maneuvers are helpful for the differential diagnosis between nonejection click and early ejection sound, a split S_2, and an S_3.

Although mitral valve prolapse and tricuspid valve prolapse are the most frequent causes of mid-systolic clicks, nonejection sounds also have been observed in patients with left-sided pneumothorax, adhesive pericarditis, atrial myxomas, left ventricular aneurysm, and aneurysm associated with ventricular septal defects (61–64). These nonejection clicks vary in their timing, and the maneuvers that influence the mid-systolic click associated with mitral valve prolapse and the S_1 interval are not recognized in these patients. In some patients with hypertrophic cardiomyopathy, a nonejection sound has been observed to occur with systolic anterior motion of the anterior mitral leaflet. This sound, termed *pseudoejection sound*, begins considerably after the upstroke of the carotid pulse (65). The precise mechanism of this pseudoejection sound in hypertrophic cardiomyopathy remains unclear. It may result from the contact of the anterior leaflet with the septum or from the deceleration of blood flow in the left ventricular outflow tract. The S_1–pseudoejec-

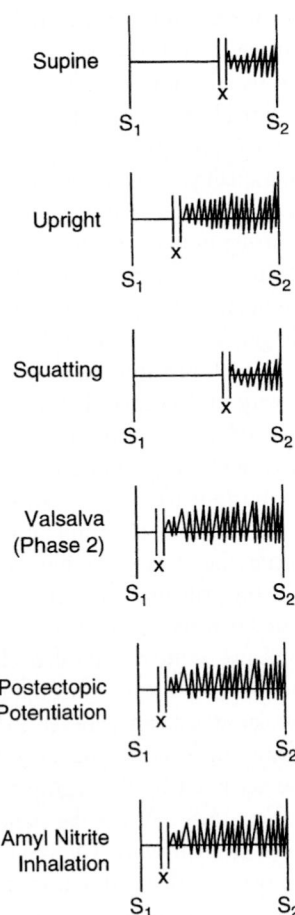

FIGURE 15.8 The influences of various bedside maneuvers on the first heart sound (S₁) and mid-systolic click (x) intervals and the duration of the late systolic murmur, which usually extends to the second heart sound (S₂). With an increase in left ventricular volumes (supine and squatting), S₁-x intervals are longer and the duration of the late systolic murmur is shorter. With a smaller left ventricular diastolic volume (upright, Valsalva phase 2, amyl nitrite inhalation), S₁-x intervals are shorter and the duration of the late systolic murmur is relatively longer.

tion sound interval also does not change with maneuvers. The effects of different maneuvers on the S₁–mid-systolic click interval and mitral regurgitation murmur associated with mitral valve prolapse are summarized in Figure 15.8.

Opening Snap

The opening snap is a high-pitched (high-frequency), early diastolic sound associated with mitral or tricuspid valve opening. These opening sounds of the atrioventricular valves are normally silent, but they become audible in the presence of mitral or tricuspid stenosis. The most common cause of opening snap is mitral stenosis, and the snap is heard best with the diaphragm of the stethoscope just medial to the cardiac apex. The opening snap associated with mitral stenosis usually is widely transmitted and frequently heard along the left sternal border and even over the left second interspace.

Thus, the transmitted opening snap can be confused with the pulmonic component of the S₂. However, during the inspiratory phase of respiration, three high-frequency sounds can be recognized: The initial two sounds are the two components of the S₂, and the third is the opening snap. The opening snap coincides with the full opening of the mitral valve and usually occurs 40 to 100 ms after the S₂. The opening snap results from rapid opening of the mitral valve to its maximal open position; thus, the mobility of the valve contributes to its genesis. When the mitral valve is heavily calcified and immobile, the opening snap may be absent. A careful analysis of the interval between A₂ and the opening snap can provide information regarding the severity of mitral stenosis. The shorter the A₂–opening snap interval is, the more severe is the mitral stenosis. The A₂–opening snap interval is related to the difference in pressures at the time of the aortic valve closure and the opening of the mitral valve. When mitral stenosis is severe, left atrial pressure is higher, and the pressure crossover point between the left ventricle and the left atrium is closer to A₂, which reduces the A₂–opening snap interval. At the bedside, if the A₂–opening snap interval appears like widely split S₂, the A₂–opening snap interval is short and suggests severe mitral stenosis. On the other hand, if the opening snap seems to occur at the time when the S₃ gallop is expected, the A₂–opening snap interval is wide and indicates mild mitral stenosis. It needs to be emphasized that the A₂–opening snap interval should be assessed when the heart rate is relatively normal. When the heart rate is fast, the A₂–opening snap interval is shorter, even when the mitral stenosis is not severe. Similarly, in the presence of aortic stenosis, mitral regurgitation, or aortic regurgitation, it is difficult to assess the severity of mitral stenosis based on the A₂–opening snap interval (66) (Fig. 15.9). However, in the presence of significant mitral regurgitation or aortic stenosis, if the A₂–opening snap interval is wide, it is unlikely that significant mitral stenosis is present.

Although an opening snap is most frequently encountered in mitral stenosis, it also can occur in patients with tricuspid stenosis. Left atrial and right atrial myxomas may cause an early diastolic sound (tumor plop) and seem to occur when tumors move into the ventricle and come to a sudden halt. In patients with hypertrophic cardiomyopathy with a decreased left ventricular cavity, high-frequency, early diastolic sounds are heard in some patients; these sounds coincide with the time of contact of the anterior leaflet of the mitral valve to the interventricular septum (67). The tricuspid opening snap also can be heard in patients with atrial septal defect with a large left-to-right shunt. Rarely, a high-pitched diastolic sound can be heard in patients with mitral valve prolapse. This high-frequency sound seems to be related to the rapid, inward movement of the prolapsed mitral valve toward the left ventricular cavity before the opening of the mitral valve. Also, rarely in patients with severe mitral regurgitation due to ruptured chordae, a high-pitched, early diastolic sound similar to the

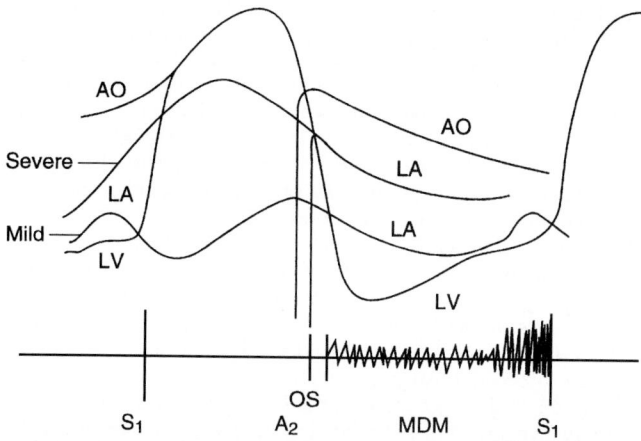

FIGURE 15.9 Schematic illustrations of left ventricular (LV), aortic (AO), and left atrial (LA) pressures to explain the relationship between the severity of mitral stenosis and the interval between the closure of the aortic valve sound (A_2) and the opening snap (OS). Compared to mild mitral stenosis, left atrial pressure is higher in severe mitral stenosis; thus, LA-LV pressures cross over at the end of isovolumic relaxation phase occur closer to A_2; thus, the A_2-OS interval is shorter with more severe mitral stenosis. The mid-diastolic murmur (MDM) is longer in more severe mitral stenosis and may extend to a loud first heart sound (S_1). The A_2-OS interval, however, is related to aortic pressure at the time of aortic valve closure; the interval is related to left ventricular pressure at the time of the opening of the mitral valve, which is also related to arterial pressure, ventricular relaxation, associated mitral regurgitation, aortic stenosis, and aortic regurgitation, as well as heart rate, which influences the duration of diastole. Thus, a relatively poor correlation exists between A_2-OS intervals and the mitral valve areas.

opening snap can be heard (44). If a high-frequency, early diastolic sound is heard in clinical practice, one should exclude mitral valve stenosis by echocardiography.

Bioprosthesis and mechanical prosthesis also produce systolic and diastolic high-pitched sounds. The relative intensity of the opening and closing sounds vary according to the type and design of the prosthetic valve. With the ball-and-cage type of valve, the opening and closing sounds are loud and clicking in character. With the disc valve, however, the closing sound is louder and clickier than the opening sound. The artificial valve sounds are of high frequency and are much louder than normal valve sounds. The opening or closing sounds may consist of multiple clicks, which do not necessarily indicate valve malfunction. The absence of an opening click has been observed with normally functioning mitral valve prosthesis. Obstruction of a prosthetic valve in the mitral position may be associated with a markedly decreased A_2–opening click interval. For the diagnosis of the malfunction of prosthetic valve, however, one should not rely on the physical findings.

THIRD AND FOURTH HEART SOUNDS

S_3 and S_4 are of relatively low frequency, are lower-pitched sounds, and are related to early and late diastole filling of the ventricles (68). When these sounds are recognized in the pathologic states, they are termed *gallop sounds*. In certain pathologic conditions, the presence of gallop sounds provides useful information about the hemodynamic and functional abnormalities. The S_3 is commonly heard in children, adolescents, and young adults in the absence of any pathologic condition or hemodynamic abnormality and is termed *physiologic S_3*. The physiologic or pathologic S_3 is a low-frequency sound that follows A_2 by 120 to 200 ms and occurs during the ventricular early rapid filling phase.

The mechanisms for the production of physiologic and pathologic S_3 have not been precisely determined. The opening and tensing of the atrioventricular valves in early diastole, the tensing of the ventricular wall, and the impact of the ventricular wall with the chest wall at the end of the rapid filling phase had been proposed to explain physiologic and pathologic S_3. The fast cineangiographic, echocardiographic, and Doppler studies have indicated that the S_3 is most likely related to the rapid deceleration of flow in early diastole. During the early filling phase—when there is an abrupt deceleration of the column of blood entering the ventricle after the opening of the atrioventricular valves—the cardiohemic system is set into vibration, which contributes to the genesis of the S_3 (69). It also has been suggested that the dynamic impact of the heart with the chest wall at the end of the rapid filling phase may contribute to the genesis of the S_3 that is recognized at the bedside (70).

At the bedside, S_3 is best recognized when the bell of the stethoscope is pressed very lightly over the skin in the left lateral decubitus position. When the bell of the stethoscope is pressed harder and converted to a diaphragm, the intensity of the S_3 decreases and may even disappear. In a number of pathologic conditions, an S_3 gallop indicates an increase in left ventricular diastolic pressure (71). In patients with dilated cardiomyopathy, coronary artery disease, and aortic valve disease, a relatively crisper and sharper S_3 gallop indicates abnormally elevated left ventricular diastolic pressure. In patients with chronic aortic regurgitation, the presence of an S_3 gallop has been reported to reflect reduced left ventricular ejection fraction (72). An S_3 gallop is very common in aortic regurgitation and usually is followed by a mid-diastolic rumble of the Austin Flint murmur.

An S_3 is frequently appreciated in patients with hemodynamically significant atrioventricular valvular regurgitation (mitral and tricuspid regurgitation) and in hyperkinetic states. In these conditions, there is an excessive early diastolic filling of the left ventricle that may not be associated with any impairment of ventricular systolic function or elevation of left ventricular diastolic pressure. An S_3 gallop also is heard in patients with a large left-to-right shunt due to high flow across the mitral valve with ventricular septal defect or patent ductus arteriosus and to high flow across the tricuspid valve with atrial septal defects. The presence of S_3 in these conditions does not imply abnormal ventricular function or congestive heart failure.

A pathologic S_3 is almost invariably recognized in patients with restrictive cardiomyopathy. The pathologic S_3 in constrictive pericarditis is termed the *pericardial knock*. However, the frequency of the pericardial knock is somewhat higher than the physiologic or other pathologic S_3. The pericardial knock or S_3 associated with restrictive cardiomyopathy may occur earlier and soon after A_2 and may be confused with opening snap; it usually increases in intensity with inspiration and occurs coincident with the 'y' descent of the jugular venous pulse.

The S_4 is related to ventricular filling during atrial systole and, therefore, is absent in patients with atrial fibrillation. The S_4 follows the onset of the P wave of the electrocardiogram and precedes the S_1; thus, it is frequently termed the *atrial diastolic gallop* or the *presystolic gallop*. The S_4 is heard best at the cardiac apex with the patient in the left lateral decubitus position. The right ventricular S_4 gallop, however, is heard best along the lower left sternal border over the third or fourth intercostal space. The intensity of the right-sided S_4 increases after inspiration. In contrast, the left-sided S_4 is heard best during expiration. Occasionally, a loud, audible S_4 is accompanied by a palpable presystolic apical impulse—the so-called palpable S_4. The precise mechanism for the genesis of the S_4 has not been identified; however, both the ventricular origin due to the abrupt deceleration of the incoming blood column during atrial contraction and the impact theory have been proposed (70,73). Regardless of the mechanism of genesis of S_4, its presence—particularly when associated with a palpable, presystolic, apical impulse—indicates abnormal hemodynamics and ventricular diastolic dysfunction. The common pathologic conditions in which a prominent left-sided S_4 is recognized are systemic hypertension, aortic valvular stenosis, and hypertrophic cardiomyopathy—the conditions that produce significant left ventricular hypertrophy. Similarly, pulmonary hypertension and pulmonary valvular stenosis, which produce right ventricular hypertrophy, are associated with right-sided S_4. Although it initially was thought that the presence of S_4 in a patient with aortic stenosis indicated hemodynamically significant aortic valvular stenosis with a gradient of 70 mm Hg or greater and a left ventricular end diastolic pressure of 13 mm Hg or greater, recent studies have suggested that S_4 is good evidence of significant aortic stenosis only in patients younger than age 40 (74).

An audible S_4 with or without a palpable presystolic impulse is common in patients during angina associated with ischemic heart disease. In the absence of acute ischemia, S_4 is uncommon, except in patients with ischemic dilated cardiomyopathy with elevated left ventricular diastolic pressure. In patients with left ventricular aneurysm or idiopathic or ischemic cardiomyopathy, the S_4 is often associated with a pathologic S_3, producing a quadruple rhythm. If there is also tachycardia or a markedly prolonged PR interval, S_3 and S_4 can be fused and give rise to a loud summation gallop. A gallop rhythm, which usu-

TABLE 15.6 PATHOPHYSIOLOGIC MECHANISMS AND CLINICAL SIGNIFICANCE AFTER GALLOP SOUND

S_3 is common in children and young adults (physiologic), but it is uncommon in normal subjects older than 40 years.

S_3 usually indicates an increase in left or right ventricular diastolic pressure in the presence of impaired ejection fraction.

Chronic aortic regurgitation—the presence of S_3 indicates impaired left ventricular ejection fraction.

Right ventricular failure resulting from congenital heart disease and pulmonary hypertension or primary right ventricular failure—S_3 gallop indicates an increase in right ventricular diastolic pressure and reduced right ventricular ejection fraction.

In hyperkinetic states, hyperthyroidism, anemia, arteriovenous fistulae, left-to-right shunts, and chronic tricuspid or mitral regurgitation, S_3 does not indicate hemodynamic abnormalities.

Primary myocardial or pericardial disease (constrictive pericarditis)—S_3 and S_4 gallops indicate increased ventricular diastolic pressures.

In the presence of first-degree atrioventricular block, S_4 can be audible without any associated hemodynamic abnormality.

S_3, third heart sound; S_4, fourth heart sound.

ally is associated with tachycardia and results from the fusion of S_3 and S_4 gallops, is most frequently observed in patients with dilated cardiomyopathy with clinical overt heart failure. With improvement in ventricular function and reduction in heart rate, as well as improved hemodynamics, gallop rhythm is no longer observed in these patients. Thus, clinical evaluation to assess the presence or absence of an S_3 gallop or gallop rhythm can provide information regarding response to therapy. In acute atrioventricular valve regurgitation, as in patients with mitral regurgitation due to ruptured chordae, an S_4 associated with a presystolic apical impulse is frequently present and results from vigorous atrial contraction into an acutely volume-loaded ventricle. In chronic mitral regurgitation, it should be appreciated that an S_4 is uncommon, whereas an S_3 is frequently present. In patients with first degree atrioventricular block, S_4 is more easily heard because of its separation of the S_1. In complete atrioventricular block, intermittent S_4 is recognized frequently. It is of interest that S_4 occasionally is recognized in patients with complete atrioventricular block with atrial contraction during ventricular systole with closed atrioventricular valves. These sounds associated with atrial contraction, therefore, cannot be due to ventricular filling, and different mechanisms need to be postulated for the genesis of these sounds (70). The pathophysiologic mechanisms and clinical significance of the gallop sounds are summarized in Table 15.6.

PERICARDIAL FRICTION RUB

Pericardial friction sounds are high pitched, leathery, and scratchy in quality and heard best with the patient leaning forward or in the knee/chest position during held, forced expiration. The pericardial rub may have three components: (a) during atrial systole, (b) during ventricular systole, and (c) during rapid ventricular filling. Frequently, the pericardial rub consists of two components; occasionally, it consists of only one component. Three-component pericardial rubs are more frequently observed in patients with acute primary pericarditis, uremic pericarditis, postoperative pericarditis, and traumatic pericarditis. In episternal pericarditis after acute myocardial infarction, it is more common to recognize one or two components of the pericardial rub. Episternal pericarditis, however, is transient, and persistent pericardial rub in acute myocardial infarction may indicate Dressler's syndrome or subacute rupture of the ventricular free wall.

A one-component pericardial rub occurring during ventricular systole can be confused with certain mid-systolic ejection murmurs with a scratchy quality, as recognized in some patients with hyperthyroidism (Means-Lerman sign) (75). Superficial, scratchy ejection systolic murmurs also are recognized in patients with Ebstein's anomaly.

Mediastinal crunch (Hamman's sign) is a series of scratchy sounds that occur with cardiac cycles and result from the presence of air in the pericardium and mediastinum (76). These sounds occur most frequently during ventricular systole. The mediastinal crunch sounds also are influenced by respiratory excursion. The pleuropericardial rubs are accentuated during inspiration. However, the character of the pleuropericardial rub is different from that of the mediastinal crunch. Mediastinal crunch is observed in patients with mediastinal emphysema, which may also be associated with chest pain syndrome similar to angina. Mediastinal emphysema is associated with crepitations in the neck, secondary to subcutaneous air. The most common cause of mediastinal crunch is the presence of air and blood in the open pericardial sac after cardiac surgery. In the postoperative patient, mediastinal crunch does not indicate any significant hemodynamic abnormality.

Pacemaker sounds are also high-frequency sounds of brief duration and are produced by the contraction of the intercostal muscles resulting from stimulation of the intercostal nerves by the transvenous pacemakers located in the right ventricular apex (38). The pacemaker sounds coincide with the pacemaker stimuli and are abolished when the pacing is discontinued. The stimulation of pectoral muscles and the diaphragm during epicardial or endocardial pacing may also produce extracardiac sounds.

EVALUATION OF HEART MURMURS

During bedside evaluation of a cardiovascular murmur, it is customary to assess the location of the maximum intensity, radiation, timing (systolic, diastolic, or continuous), intensity (loudness), and frequency (pitch) of the murmur, as well as its configuration (shape, quality, and duration).

Although the exact mechanisms for the production of murmurs are not clear, it is generally agreed that turbulence is the principle determinant for the genesis of most murmurs. In clinical practice, six grades are used to assess the intensity of a murmur at the bedside. Grade 1 is the faintest murmur and can be heard only with special effort or maneuvers. A grade 2 murmur is faint but can be heard easily. A grade 3 murmur is moderately loud. A grade 4 murmur is very loud, and a grade 5 murmur is extremely loud and can be heard with a light touch of the stethoscope. A grade 6 murmur is exceptionally loud and can be heard with the stethoscope just removed from contact with the chest. Systolic murmurs of grade 4 or more usually are associated with a palpable thrill. The intensity or loudness of the murmur can vary depending on the hemodynamic determinants that govern the production of a given murmur. The frequency of the murmur determines its pitch, which may be high or low. During auscultation, a mental image is formed to recognize the shape of a murmur and its configuration. A crescendo murmur is recognized when there is increasing intensity; a decrescendo murmur is defined when the intensity of the murmur is diminishing. A crescendo/decrescendo murmur is defined when there is initial increasing intensity followed by decreasing intensity, and a plateau murmur is recognized when there is no change in intensity of the murmur. The quality of a murmur that is recognized during auscultation can be harsh, rumbling, scratchy, grunting, blowing, squeaky, and musical. The duration of a murmur is assessed by determining the length of systole or diastole that the murmur occupies. The murmur can be long or brief. The direction of radiation of a murmur follows the direction of blood flow and can provide information regarding the origin of the murmur. At the bedside, initially, it is essential to determine the timing of the murmur in relation to the cardiac cycle. A murmur can be systolic, diastolic, or continuous. Systolic and diastolic murmurs can be left-sided or right-sided. At the bedside, there usually is little difficulty in distinguishing between systolic and diastolic murmurs, because at normal heart rate, systole is much shorter in duration than diastole. However, when the heart rate is fast, the duration of systole and diastole may become equal; in these circumstances, the timing of the murmur can be determined by simultaneous palpation of the carotid pulse. In rare circumstances, a high-pitched, pandiastolic murmur can be confused with a pansystolic murmur. Whenever there is any doubt about the timing of a given murmur, it is desirable to auscultate with simultaneous palpation of the carotid pulse. After recognizing a systolic murmur at the bedside, it is desirable to determine whether the systolic murmur is of ejection type (mid-systolic) or regurgitant type (Fig. 15.10). The ejection systolic murmur starts after the S_1 and does not extend to the S_2. A left-sided ejection systolic murmur ends before A_2, and a right-sided ejection systolic murmur ends before P_2. The ejection, or mid-systolic, murmur is related to flow

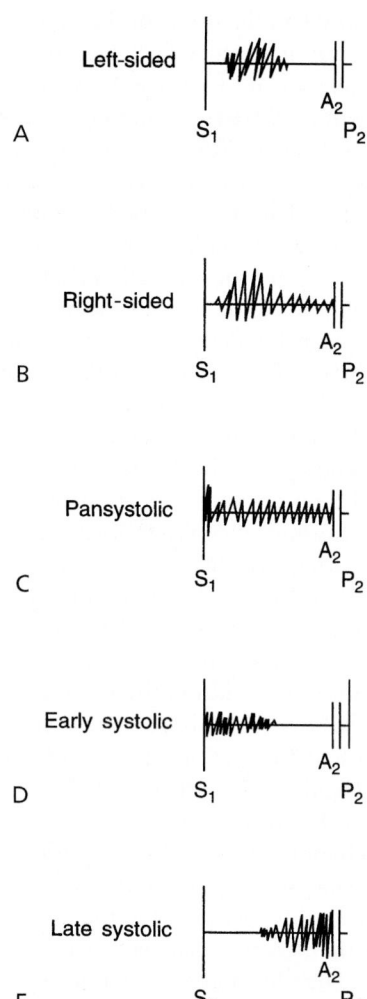

FIGURE 15.10 A left-sided ejection systolic murmur starts after the first heart sound (S₁) and terminates before the aortic component of the second heart sound (A₂). A right-sided ejection systolic murmur starts after S₁ and terminates before the pulmonary component of the second heart sound (P₂). A pansystolic murmur starts with S₁ and extends to the second heart sound. An early systolic murmur starts with the S₁ and terminates before the second heart sound. A late systolic murmur starts after the S₁ and extends up to second heart sound. **A:** Aortic stenosis, aortic sclerosis, flow murmur, innocent murmur, hypertrophic cardiomyopathy, and bicuspid aortic valve. **B:** Pulmonary stenosis, infundibular stenosis, flow murmur (ASD), idiopathic dilatation of the pulmonary artery, and innocent murmurs. **C:** Mitral regurgitation, tricuspid regurgitation, and ventricular septal defect. **D:** Mitral regurgitation, tricuspid regurgitation, and ventricular septal defect. **E:** Mitral regurgitation and tricuspid regurgitation.

across the semilunar valves. Onset of the murmur coincides with the beginning of the ejection, and termination of the murmur coincides with the cessation of forward flow. The S₁ occurs at the onset of isovolumic systole, and the beginning of ejection occurs at the end of the isovolumic systole, explaining why ejection systolic murmur starts after the S₁. The ventricular ejection ends before closure of the semilunar valves; thus, an ejection systolic murmur cannot extend to the semilunar valve closure sounds. The configuration or

shape of most ejection systolic murmurs is crescendo/decrescendo. The crescendo part of the ejection systolic murmur is related to the initial rapid ejection phase, and the decrescendo part of the ejection systolic murmur is related to the slower ejection phase.

Ejection Systolic versus Regurgitant Murmur

When the S₁ and S₂ are decreased in intensity, it is often difficult to distinguish between an ejection systolic murmur and a regurgitant murmur. There are a number of distinguishing features, however, that can be appreciated at the bedside (76). If A₂ is clearly audible over the cardiac apex, the murmur is likely to be ejection or mid-systolic (77). If A₂ is heard over the right and left second interspaces but not over the apex, it is likely that A₂ is drowned out by the holosystolic murmur of mitral regurgitation. If the patient is in atrial fibrillation, and if the intensity of the murmur substantially increases with longer RR cycle length, the murmur is likely to be an ejection murmur. Similarly, if the intensity of the murmur increases during the postectopic beat after a postectopic pause, the murmur is likely to be of ejection variety. At the bedside, a response to hand grip can be used to distinguish between left-sided ejection and regurgitant murmurs. In response to sustained hand grip, the intensity of a mitral regurgitation murmur increases, whereas the intensity of murmur associated with aortic stenosis usually decreases. The physiologic responses to hand grip are complex. In addition to an increase in systemic vascular resistance and arterial pressure, a reflex increase in contractility may also occur, which can increase the intensity of the stenotic murmur. Amyl nitrite inhalation is also a helpful bedside pharmacologic maneuver to distinguish between an ejection systolic murmur and a holosystolic regurgitant murmur of left ventricular origin. The intensity of the ejection systolic murmur increases, whereas the intensity of the regurgitant holosystolic murmur decreases. Amyl nitrite inhalation is associated with decreased systemic vascular resistance and arterial pressure, which decreases the severity of the regurgitation—hence, the intensity of the regurgitation murmur. In aortic stenosis, the intensity of the systolic murmur increases because of the increased flow across the stenotic aortic valve. In obstructive hypertrophic cardiomyopathy, the intensity of the murmur in response to amyl nitrite inhalation increases due to an accentuated left ventricular outflow obstruction. The intensity of an ejection systolic murmur is markedly influenced by the changes in stroke volume. With increased stroke volume—such as during exercise, anxiety, or fever; after volume loading or passive leg elevation; or with a long diastolic filling period—the intensity of the ejection systolic murmur increases. Likewise, conditions that decrease cardiac output and stroke volume (e.g., congestive heart failure, beta blockade, or other negative inotropic agents)

TABLE 15.7 EFFECTS OF MANEUVERS ON THE INTENSITY OF THE SYSTOLIC MURMURS AND CAROTID PULSE IN AORTIC STENOSIS, HYPERTROPHIC OBSTRUCTIVE CARDIOMYOPATHY, AND MITRAL REGURGITATION

Maneuvers	Aortic stenosis		Hypertrophic obstructive cardiomyopathy		Mitral regurgitation	
	ESM	CAR AMP	ESM	CAR AMP	PSM	CAR AMP
Leg raising	Increased	Increased	Decreased	Increased No change	Increased	Decreased No change
Standing	Decreased	Decreased No change	Increased	Decreased No change	Decreased	Increased No change
Squatting	Decreased No change	No change	Decreased	Increased No change	Increased	Decreased No change
Hand grip	Decreased Increased	Increased No change	Decreased	No change	Increased	No change
Supine position	No change	No change	Decreased	No change	No change	No change
Postectopic beat	Increased	Increased	Increased	Decreased No change	No change	No change
Valsalva (phase 2)	Decreased	Decreased	Increased	Decreased	Decreased	Decreased
Amyl nitrite	Increased	Increased	Increased	Decreased No change	Decreased	Increased No change

CAR AMP, carotid pulse amplitude; ESM, ejection systolic murmur; PSM, pansystolic murmur.

decrease the intensity of the ejection murmur. The effects of different pharmacologic and nonpharmacologic interventions on systolic murmurs of fixed and dynamic left ventricular outflow obstruction and of mitral regurgitation are summarized in Table 15.7.

Once the presence of an ejection systolic murmur is established, a systematic evaluation to establish its etiology should be undertaken (Table 15.8). In adults, it is desirable to search for the findings that might indicate fixed or dynamic left ventricular outflow obstruction. The conditions of congenital aortic, valvular, subvalvular, or supravalvular stenosis, acquired aortic stenosis, and hypertrophic obstructive cardiomyopathy are all associated with an ejection systolic murmur. The murmur of fixed stenosis of the left ventricular outflow tract is crescendo/decrescendo in configuration and usually is heard best at the right second and left second and third interspaces near the sternal border. This murmur usually radiates widely into the neck and along the great vessels. The murmur of aortic stenosis is of lower pitch and has a harsh quality. With calcific aortic stenosis, particularly in the elderly, the murmur may radiate to the apex. Also in calcific aortic stenosis in the elderly, the high-frequency components of the murmur may predominate, and the apical murmur may have a high pitch and, often, a musical quality (78). This murmur has been frequently confused with the mitral regurgitation murmur. However, it should be emphasized that the murmur associated with aortic stenosis is an ejection murmur and not a regurgitant murmur. An aortic ejection sound is frequently appreciated in congenital and acquired valvular aortic stenosis. With increasing severity of aortic stenosis and with calcification of the aortic valves, however, the aortic ejection sound may not occur. In congenital aortic stenosis—whether valvular, subvalvular, or supravalvular—the S_2 split-

ting usually is normal or single. In acquired aortic stenosis, the S_2 usually is single, or it may be reversed with severe outflow obstruction. The intensity of A_2 in congenital valvular aortic stenosis usually is normal but may decrease with calcification. The intensity of A_2 in subvalvular and supravalvular aortic stenosis is normal or decreased. In acquired aortic stenosis, the intensity of A_2 is decreased, or it may be absent with calcification of the aortic valve. The murmur of aortic regurgitation frequently is present in congenital valvular and subvalvular aortic stenosis, as well as in acquired aortic valvular stenosis. A murmur of aortic regurgitation is uncommon in supravalvular congenital aortic stenosis. In supravalvular congenital aortic stenosis (William's syndrome), elf-like facial appearance, mental retardation, and hypercalcemia are common (79). The carotid artery upstroke is slow rising, the peak is delayed, and the amplitude is decreased in congenital valvular and subvalvular aortic stenosis, as well as in acquired aortic stenosis. In congenital supravalvular aortic stenosis, the right brachial and carotid pulsations have greater amplitudes than those of left brachial and left carotid pulsations. Left ventricular hypertrophy can occur in response to valvular, subvalvular, supravalvular, and acquired aortic stenosis; thus, it can be associated with a sustained left ventricular apical impulse. A significant hypertrophy and noncompliant ventricle may also be associated with a palpable presystolic impulse (S_4).

Severity of Aortic Stenosis

After establishing the diagnosis of aortic stenosis, attempts should be made to assess its severity (Fig. 15.11). The physical finding that indicates that hemodynamically significant aortic stenosis is a substantial increase in left ventricular ejection time. A palpable anacrotic character of radial pulse,

TABLE 15.8 DIFFERENTIAL DIAGNOSIS OF SYSTOLIC MURMURS—BEDSIDE EVALUATION

Determine the timing of the systolic murmur; the murmur starts after the S$_1$ and does not extend up to the S$_2$—ejection systolic murmur

Consider conditions associated with left or right ventricular outflow tract obstruction such as aortic stenosis, pulmonary stenosis, or hypertrophic cardiomyopathy.

The flow murmurs in systole are ejection systolic murmurs and can be observed in hyperkinetic states such as hyperthyroidism and after exercise.

The murmur associated with aortic sclerosis (grunting quality) is an ejection systolic murmur.

The innocent murmur in children (Still's murmur) is an ejection systolic murmur.

In patients with suspected aortic stenosis, careful analysis of the changes in the carotid pulse upstroke, volume, and presence or absence of left ventricular hypertrophy, behavior of the S$_2$, and intensity of the S$_1$ to assess the severity of aortic stenosis.

Hypertrophic cardiomyopathy is suspected from the presence of an ejection systolic murmur and normal or sharp carotid pulse upstroke. Auscultation and simultaneous palpations of the carotid pulse volume during Valsalva's maneuvers (standing and squatting) are used to confirm the diagnosis.

Bicuspid aortic valve suspected from the presence of an aortic ejection sound, normal S$_2$, and a brief, early diastolic murmur of aortic regurgitation.

Superficial, scratchy ejection systolic murmur—suspect Means-Lerman scratch of hyperthyroidism, Ebstein's anomaly, one-component pericardial friction rub. Appropriate noninvasive investigations are recommended to confirm diagnosis.

A long ejection systolic murmur with widely split S$_2$ and reduced intensity of P$_2$—suspect pulmonary stenosis. Presence of a pulmonary valve ejection sound suggests pulmonary valve stenosis; absence of a pulmonary valve ejection sound suggests infundibular stenosis.

Presence of a pulmonary valve ejection sound short ejection systolic murmur, normal physiologic splitting of the S$_2$ with or without short early diastolic murmur—suspect idiopathic dilatation of the pulmonary artery.

Pulmonary vascular ejection sound, a short ejection systolic murmur, and increased intensity of the P$_2$—suspect pulmonary hypertension; the presence of a left parasternal systolic lift, secondary tricuspid, and pulmonary regurgitation suggests severe pulmonary hypertension. Once pulmonary hypertension is suspected, causes for postcapillary pulmonary hypertension should be excluded before the diagnosis of precapillary pulmonary hypertension is entertained.

When an ejection systolic murmur is recognized without any evidence of left or right ventricular outflow obstruction, hyperkinetic states and innocent ejection systolic murmur are diagnosed.

Murmurs start with the S$_1$ and extend up to the S$_2$ or beyond—pansystolic or holosystolic murmur

These murmurs can be associated with mitral regurgitation, tricuspid regurgitation, or ventricular septal defect (VSD). Mitral regurgitation is suspected from the radiation of murmur to the axilla or to the base and changes in the intensity and duration with maneuvers such as hand grip and amyl nitrite inhalation.

Tricuspid regurgitation murmur is suspected when there is an increase in intensity of the murmur during inspiration. Associated findings of tricuspid regurgitation are a prominent 'v' wave and 'y' descent in jugular venous pulse and hepatic pulsation. Secondary tricuspid regurgitation is associated with increased intensity of P$_2$.

The pansystolic murmur of VSD is associated with a palpable thrill and does not change in intensity with inspiration and does not radiate to the axilla. Once the VSD is suspected, appropriate noninvasive investigations, such as echocardiography and echo-Doppler evaluation, are recommended.

Murmurs start with the S$_1$ and do not extend up to the S$_2$—early systolic murmur

The early systolic murmur can be due to either mild or severe mitral regurgitation. Acute severe mitral regurgitation is associated with a crescendo/decrescendo, early systolic murmur and pulmonary hypertension. If left ventricular ejection fraction is normal, suspect primary acute severe mitral regurgitation such as ruptured chordae. If left ventricular ejection fraction is depressed, suspect papillary muscle dysfunction and coronary artery disease.

Early systolic murmur can also result from mild mitral regurgitation associated with ventricular dilatation, as in patients with ischemic or nonischemic dilated cardiomyopathy or annular calcification of the mitral valve.

Early systolic murmur may also result from tricuspid regurgitation. At the bedside, if the murmur increases in intensity during inspiration, tricuspid regurgitation should be considered. Early systolic murmur associated with tricuspid regurgitation most frequently results from secondary severe tricuspid regurgitation associated with pulmonary hypertension. A prominent 'v' wave with a sharp 'y' descent and systolic hepatic pulsation confirm the diagnosis of severe tricuspid regurgitation. If the intensity of P$_2$ is increased, it suggests that tricuspid regurgitation is secondary. Primary tricuspid regurgitation in the absence of evidence of pulmonary hypertension occurs in patients with carcinoid heart disease, right ventricular infarct, and traumatic rupture of the chordae of the tricuspid valve.

Murmurs start after the S$_1$ and extend up to the S$_2$—late systolic murmur

The most common cause of late systolic murmurs is mitral valve prolapse, which is frequently associated with mid-systolic clicks. The S$_1$–mid-systolic click interval and the onset of late systolic murmur in mitral valve prolapse are influenced by left ventricular volume and inotropic state. Maneuvers such as sitting, the supine, squatting, and standing positions, and amyl nitrite inhalation can confirm the diagnosis of mitral valve prolapse at the bedside.

Tricuspid regurgitation due to tricuspid valve prolapse can also produce a late systolic murmur and mid-systolic clicks. The late systolic murmur associated with tricuspid valve prolapse increases in intensity during inspiration.

P$_2$, pulmonary component of the second heart sound; S$_1$, first heart sound; S$_2$, second heart sound.

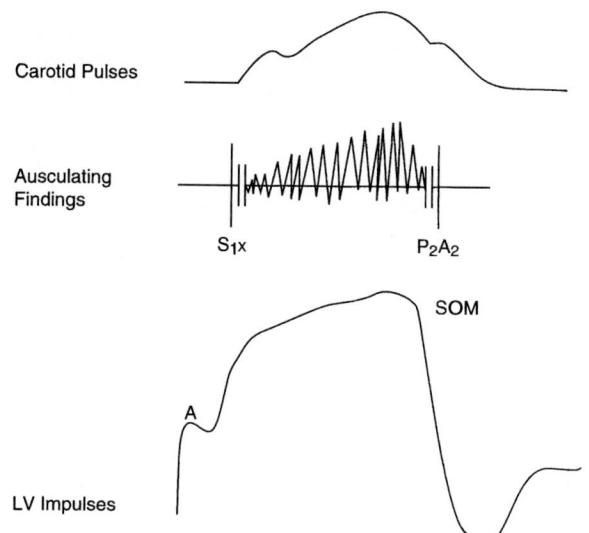

Carotid Pulses

Ausculating Findings

S_1x P_2A_2

SOM

A

LV Impulses

FIGURE 15.11 Schematic illustration of the physical findings of aortic stenosis at the bedside, which suggest hemodynamically significant aortic stenosis, are slow-rising, delayed-peaking anacrotic pulse (carotid pulse), palpable presystolic (A) and sustained outward movement (SOM) in left ventricular (LV) impulse and delayed-peaking ejection systolic murmur, reversed splitting of the second heart sound in the absence of left bundle branch block, and reduced intensity of the first heart sound (S_1) (see text). A_2, aortic component of the second heart sound; P_2, pulmonary component of the second heart sound; x, aortic ejection sound.

slow-rising carotid pulse, and reduced amplitude and delayed peak of the carotid pulse indicate significant aortic stenosis. The decrease in intensity of the S_1 in the absence of prolonged PR interval (first degree atrioventricular block) indicates an increase in left ventricular end diastolic pressure, which indirectly suggests hemodynamically significant aortic stenosis. The intensity of the aortic valve closure sound (A_2) does not correlate with the severity of aortic stenosis. A longer and delayed peaking ejection systolic murmur suggests significant aortic stenosis. However, in the presence of heart failure and reduced stroke volume, the duration and intensity of the ejection murmur is decreased, and it may even be absent (silent aortic stenosis). Hemodynamically significant aortic stenosis usually is associated with left ventricular hypertrophy, which can be appreciated at the bedside by the presence of a sustained left ventricular apical impulse. The presence of an ejection systolic murmur with a musical quality along the left sternal border or over the cardiac apex strongly suggests calcification of the aortic valves. In elderly patients, diagnosis of hemodynamically significant aortic valve stenosis may be difficult (80). The ejection murmur is often of low intensity due to decreased stroke volume associated with impaired left ventricular ejection fraction. The murmur is often loudest at the apex, may have a high-frequency component, and may be difficult to define as ejection in nature because of decreased S_1 and S_2. In the elderly, the rate of rise of the carotid pulse may be normal or near normal because of the sclerotic changes in the carotid

arteries. The carotid pulse amplitude may also be normal—even in the presence of significant aortic stenosis—because of the rigid, noncompliant carotid vessels. In elderly patients with aortic stenosis, hypertension may coexist and cause further difficulties in the diagnosis.

Hypertrophic Cardiomyopathy

In adult patients, when aortic stenosis for the cause of the ejection systolic murmur is excluded, dynamic left ventricular outflow tract obstruction (obstructive hypertrophic cardiomyopathy) should be considered. It is generally believed that the systolic anterior motion of the mitral valve apparatus, impinging on the thickened interventricular septum and producing high-velocity flow and obstruction during mid-systole, causes the mid-systolic ejection murmur in hypertrophic cardiomyopathy. The maximum intensity of this ejection murmur is appreciated over the left second or third interspace along the sternal edge. In many patients with obstructive hypertrophic cardiomyopathy, the systolic murmur along the left sternal edge is longer in duration and may appear regurgitant in nature. In fact, in many patients with obstructive hypertrophic cardiomyopathy, mitral regurgitation occurs after the onset of left ventricular outflow tract obstruction. The sequence of dynamic events in these patients is rapid, high-velocity ejection in mid-systole followed by obstruction in the left ventricular outflow tract due to systolic anterior motion, which also produces incompetence of the mitral valve associated with mitral regurgitation (ejection, obstruction, regurgitation). The initial part of the systolic murmur seems to be related to left ventricular outflow tract obstruction, and the latter part is related to mitral regurgitation (81). The ejection murmur that is appreciated at the bedside is the summation of both murmurs as transmitted to the chest wall. In patients with obstructive hypertrophic cardiomyopathy, the intensity of the ejection systolic murmur resulting from outflow tract obstruction and the intensity of the systolic murmur resulting from mitral regurgitation vary directly with the degree of left ventricular outflow tract obstruction and pressure gradient and, therefore, the orifice size of the left ventricular outflow tract (82). The larger the size of the left ventricular outflow tract, the lower the pressure gradient and the lesser the intensity of the murmur. The narrower the left ventricular outflow tract, the higher the pressure gradient and the louder the murmur. The size of the left ventricular outflow tract is directly related to left ventricular volume and intraventricular pressure during systole, and it is inversely related to muscle tension and contractile state. The higher the distending pressure (i.e., the arterial pressure), the larger the left ventricular outflow tract and, therefore, the softer the murmur. Similarly, the larger the left ventricular volume, the larger the size of the left ventricular outflow tract and the softer the murmur. With increased inotropic state, such as during postectopic potentiation or

TABLE 15.9 DIAGNOSIS OF OBSTRUCTIVE HYPERTROPHIC CARDIOMYOPATHY

Manuevers	Hemodynamic changes	LV outflow tract size	LV outflow pressure gradient	Intensity of the murmur
Standing	↓ LV volume ↑ Heart rate	↓	↑	↑
Squatting	↑ LV volume ↑ SVR, ART pressure	↑	↓	↓
Valsalva phase 2	↑ Heart rate ↓↓ LV volume	↓↓	↑↑	↑↑
Hand grip	↓ Heart rate ↑ ART pressure	↑	↓	↓
Post-PVC	↑↑ Contractility ↑ LV volume	↓↓	↑↑	↑↑
Amyl nitrite inhalation	↑ Heart rate ↓ LV volume ↓ ART pressure	↓↓	↑↑	↑↑

ART, arterial; LV, left ventricular; PVC, premature ventricular contraction; SVR, systemic vascular resistance; ↑, mild increase; ↓, mild decrease; ↑↑, marked increase; ↓↓, marked decrease.

during the challenge with positive inotropic drugs, the size of the left ventricular outflow tract decreases with an increase in the pressure gradient and intensity of the ejection systolic murmur. At the bedside, when obstructive hypertrophic cardiomyopathy is suspected from the presence of a loud ejection systolic murmur along the left sternal border, it is desirable to perform certain maneuvers that may confirm the diagnosis (Table 15.9). Auscultation for the changes in the intensity of the murmur during supine, sitting, standing, and squatting positions can demonstrate characteristic changes. The ejection systolic murmur in obstructive hypertrophic cardiomyopathy increases in intensity while standing and decreases in intensity in the supine and squatting positions. When the patient is standing, there is a reduction of intracardiac volume due to decreased systemic venous return associated with transient fall in blood pressure and an increase in heart rate. These hemodynamic changes decrease the size of the left ventricular outflow tract and increase the pressure gradient and intensity of the murmur. The supine and squatting positions, on the other hand, increase intracardiac volume by increasing venous return and left ventricular outflow resistance. The size of the left ventricular outflow tract, therefore, increases with a decrease in pressure gradient and intensity of the murmur. Valsalva's maneuver is another intervention that can be applied at the bedside to establish the diagnosis of obstructive hypertrophic cardiomyopathy. During phase 2 of Valsalva's maneuver, there is a decrease in venous return, which reduces left ventricular volume; a decrease in arterial pressure, which results from decreased stroke volume; and a reflex increase in heart rate. All of these hemodynamic changes enhance left ventricular outflow obstruction and increase the intensity of the murmur. Furthermore, there is a simultaneous reduction in the carotid pulse volume. In patients with aortic stenosis during phase 2 of Valsalva's maneuver, the carotid pulse volume decreases, but there is also a reduction in the intensity of the ejection systolic murmur. Similarly, during phase 2 of Valsalva's maneuver in patients with chronic primary mitral regurgitation, there is a reduction in the carotid pulse volume and the intensity of the regurgitant murmur (Table 15.7). If premature beats occur during clinical evaluation, it is desirable to assess the intensity of the ejection systolic murmur and the amplitude of the carotid pulse simultaneously during the postectopic beat. In obstructive hypertrophic cardiomyopathy, postectopic potentiation increases the left ventricular outflow pressure gradient; therefore, the intensity of the murmur is increased. However, the carotid pulse volume is either decreased or remains unchanged. In patients with aortic stenosis, the intensity of the murmur increases during the postectopic beat, but there is also a substantial increase in the carotid pulse volume. The most useful pharmacologic intervention that can be applied easily at the bedside is the use of amyl nitrite inhalation. After inhalation of amyl nitrite, the intensity of the ejection systolic murmur in obstructive hypertrophic cardiomyopathy increases along with decreased or unchanged carotid pulse volume. The murmur of mitral regurgitation, however, decreases with amyl nitrite inhalation as a decreased systemic vascular resistance, and arterial pressure decreases the severity of mitral regurgitation. In aortic stenosis, the intensity of the murmur tends to increase after amyl nitrite inhalation. The pharmacologic agents that increase the contractile state (e.g., isoprenaline, dobutamine, or dopamine) increase the intensity of the murmur; agents that decrease the inotropic state (e.g., intravenous beta blocker, or disopyramide) decrease the intensity of the murmur. Similarly, pharmacologic agents that increase left ventricular outflow resistance (e.g., methoxamine or phenylephrine) decrease the intensity of the murmur as the left ventricular outflow tract obstruction decreases (83). In clinical practice, however, these pharmacologic agents are rarely used or necessary for the differential diagnosis of obstructive hypertrophic cardiomyopathy, aortic stenosis, or mitral regurgitation. In patients with suspected or confirmed obstructive hypertrophic cardiomyopathy, careful analysis of the carotid pulse and left ventricular apical impulse may provide additional information about the severity of hypertrophic cardiomyopathy. In patients with significant left ventricular outflow tract obstruction, the carotid pulse usually has a sharp initial upstroke, a large volume, and, occasionally, a bisferiens quality. The left ventricular apical impulse frequently is sustained due to significant increase in left ventricular mass. A presystolic wave (a palpable S_4) also is frequently appreciated. The outward movement of the left ventricular apical impulse may occasionally have bifid character. If the left ventricular outward movement is associated with a presystolic wave, three distinct impulses can be appreciated in rare patients (triple ripple). It should also be realized that in patients with known obstructive hypertrophic cardiomyopathy, the carotid pulse character may be normal, and ejection systolic murmur may be absent. The only indication of hypertrophic cardiomyopathy may be a palpable S_4 or a sustained left ventricular apical impulse. In apical hypertrophic cardiomyopathy, the electrocardiogram may provide some clues for the diagnosis. The electrocardiogram in apical hypertrophic cardiomyopathy frequently reveals a giant T-wave inversion in the lateral precordial leads, along with large QRS voltages due to left ventricular hypertrophy (84). The absence of electrocardiographic changes, however, does not exclude nonobstructive hypertrophic cardiomyopathy. In all patients with suspected hypertrophic cardiomyopathy, echocardiographic evaluation is essential.

Other Left-Sided Ejection Systolic Murmurs

When aortic stenosis or obstructive hypertrophic cardiomyopathy is excluded as the cause of an ejection systolic murmur, other potential causes of left-sided ejection systolic murmur should be considered. Hemodynamically significant isolated aortic regurgitation can also be associated with an ejection systolic murmur, which usually reflects increased flow during systole. Predominant aortic regurgitation can be diagnosed at the bedside from the presence of characteristic physical findings of significant chronic aortic regurgitation, such as pulsus bisferiens, hyperdynamic left ventricular apical impulse, and a high-pitched, early diastolic murmur along the left sternal border. A bicuspid aortic valve may be associated with an ejection systolic murmur. The bicuspid aortic valve at the bedside is suspected from the presence of an aortic ejection sound, normal carotid pulse upstroke, a short early diastolic murmur, and no evidence of hemodynamically significant aortic stenosis. Once suspected, the bicuspid aortic valve should be confirmed by two-dimensional transthoracic echocardiography. A left-sided ejection systolic murmur is also recognized in the presence of normal valves when the flow across the aortic valve is significantly increased, as in anemia in pregnancy or thyrotoxicosis. In these clinical conditions, however, the findings suggestive of fixed or dynamic left ventricular outflow tract obstruction

are absent. The murmur of so-called aortic sclerosis is also a mid-systolic ejection murmur. It is benign because it is not associated with hemodynamic abnormalities. In aortic sclerosis, the physical findings of left ventricular outflow tract obstruction are absent. The benign aortic systolic murmur results from the stiffening and degenerative fibrous thickening of the roots of the aortic cusps at the site of their insertions. These morphologic changes do not cause any impairment of mobility of the valve and, thus, no obstruction. The murmur of aortic sclerosis usually is heard best over the right second interspace, and the murmur usually does not radiate to the carotid arteries. In some patients, a musical, high-frequency murmur of brief duration can be heard along the lower left sternal border and cardiac apex. The S_1 and S_2 are normal, and there is no evidence of aortic regurgitation. Clinical recognition of aortic sclerosis is relevant, as it is an adverse risk factor for long-term prognosis probably due to increased atherothrombotic complications. When diagnosis of aortic sclerosis is suspected, echocardiography for confirmation should be considered.

Right-Sided Ejection Systolic Murmurs

In the adult cardiac patient, it is infrequent to encounter pathophysiologic conditions that produce right-sided ejection systolic murmurs. Right-sided systolic murmurs can result from obstructions to right ventricular outflow, such as pulmonary valvular stenosis, subvalvular right ventricular outflow obstruction, or supravalvular pulmonary stenosis. Isolated infundibular pulmonary stenosis without ventricular septal defect is rare. Infundibular pulmonary stenosis usually is associated with ventricular septal defect, as in patients with tetralogy of Fallot. Pulmonary valvular stenosis, however, may be present in the absence of ventricular septal defect. One finding at the bedside that suggests the presence of pulmonary valvular stenosis is a long ejection systolic murmur that starts after the S_1 and terminates before the P_2 and which can be markedly decreased in intensity. Frequently, a pulmonic valvular ejection sound is also present, and, characteristically, the pulmonary valvular ejection sound decreases in intensity during inspiration. There may or may not be an associated early diastolic murmur due to pulmonary insufficiency. Depending on the severity of pulmonary valvular stenosis, evidence of right ventricular hypertrophy may be recognized at the bedside. Significant pulmonary valvular stenosis causing right ventricular hypertrophy frequently is associated with a prominent 'a' wave in the jugular venous pulse, which reflects increased resistance to right ventricular filling during right atrial systole. In severe pulmonary valvular stenosis, the pulmonary ejection sound may fuse with the S_1 and cannot be recognized at the bedside. Typically, in pulmonary valvular stenosis and isolated subvalvular right ventricular outflow obstruction, the S_2 is widely split. The degree of splitting of the S_2 roughly correlates to the severity of the pressure gradient across the pulmonary valve or the right ventricular outflow tract. In patients with valvular pulmonary stenosis or subvalvular infundibular fixed stenosis, the intensity of the P_2 is decreased substantially, as the pulmonary artery diastolic pressure in these circumstances is low. In patients with supravalvular pulmonary stenosis, however, the intensity of P_2 is not decreased. Supravalvular pulmonary stenosis, or pulmonary artery branch stenosis, is frequently associated with a continuous murmur. Pulmonary valve stenosis, or obstruction in the right ventricular outflow tract, and supravalvular pulmonary stenosis can be associated with significant right ventricular hypertrophy. Occasionally, the long, harsh ejection systolic murmur of pulmonary stenosis is confused with the holosystolic murmur of a ventricular septal defect. This confusion is more likely to occur with infundibular stenosis because of the lower location of the murmur. In ventricular septal defect the splitting of the S_2 and the intensity of the P_2 are normal. In infundibular pulmonary stenosis, the S_2 is widely split, and the intensity of P_2 is significantly reduced. Amyl nitrite inhalation—which usually decreases the intensity of the murmur associated with ventricular septal defect, whereas the intensity of the murmur due to right ventricular outflow obstruction remains unchanged—is sometimes helpful.

The idiopathic dilatation of the pulmonary artery may be associated with a right-sided ejection systolic murmur. The usual findings of idiopathic dilatation of the pulmonary artery are a pulmonary ejection sound, a short ejection systolic murmur, a relatively widely split S_2 with normal intensity of P_2, and, occasionally, a short pulmonary insufficiency murmur. There is no hemodynamic abnormality. It should be noted that the auscultatory findings associated with idiopathic dilatation of the pulmonary artery are similar to those observed in patients with precapillary or postcapillary pulmonary hypertension—except that the S_2 is narrowly split, with P_2 markedly accentuated in intensity, and the pulmonary ejection sound is late due to vascular origin. Evidence of pulmonary insufficiency, right ventricular hypertrophy, and tricuspid regurgitation also is present in patients with significant pulmonary hypertension, but is absent in patients with idiopathic dilatation of the pulmonary artery. A right-sided ejection systolic murmur also is heard in atrial septal defect with relatively large left-to-right shunt. This ejection murmur occurs because of increased flow across the pulmonary valve, and it is not related to any pulmonary valve stenosis. Atrial septal defect can be suspected from the presence of wide fixed splitting of the S_2 and the evidence for right ventricular volume overload. Increased flow across the pulmonary valve associated with increased flow due to hyperthyroidism may also be associated with an ejection systolic murmur. The ejection systolic murmur due to hyperthyroidism may have a scratchy quality (Means-Lerman scratch), and, frequently, the intensity of P_2 is increased due to mild to moderate pulmonary hypertension (75). The right-sided flow murmurs, however, usually are not associated with evidence of any hemodynamic compromise, such as right ventricular hypertrophy or right heart failure.

Innocent Murmurs

Innocent murmurs are, by and large, ejection in type and mid-systolic in timing. In adults, innocent ejection systolic murmurs are diagnosed when there is no evidence for right or left ventricular outflow tract obstruction. The short ejection systolic murmur associated with aortic sclerosis is often regarded as an innocent murmur. In children, a short, vibrating murmur can be heard over the mid-precordium, and it is not accompanied by any other abnormality. The precise mechanism of this murmur, termed *Still's murmur*, is not known (85,86). Another type of innocent systolic ejection murmur most frequently heard in children has a blowing quality and is heard best over the left second interspace. This murmur is thought to originate from the flow across the pulmonary artery. With increasing age, these innocent murmurs tend to decrease in intensity and, ultimately, disappear. In patients with straight back syndrome with a decreased anteroposterior diameter of the chest, a superficial ejection systolic murmur is heard over the left second interspace. The mechanism of this murmur remains unclear. It should be emphasized that whether an ejection systolic murmur is innocent should not depend on the duration or intensity of the murmur but on whether any other abnormal finding is present. If any abnormal finding coexists, such as an abnormality of S_2, even a short and sharp ejection systolic murmur should not be considered benign or innocent.

Regurgitant Systolic Murmurs

Regurgitant systolic murmurs can be pansystolic (holosystolic), early systolic, or late systolic in nature. A pansystolic murmur starts with the S_1 and lasts throughout the systole; the murmur extends to A_2 when it is left sided or to P_2 when it is right sided. In clinical practice, when a pansystolic or holosystolic murmur is recognized at the bedside, mitral regurgitation, tricuspid regurgitation, or ventricular septal defect should be considered in the differential diagnosis. The pansystolic mitral regurgitation murmur usually is of higher pitch and has a blowing character. The murmur frequently extends beyond the left ventricular systole, and A_2 is frequently drowned by the murmur. In patients with hemodynamically significant primary mitral regurgitation, the left ventricular pressure remains higher than the left atrial pressure throughout the systole and during the isovolumic relaxation phase. This hemodynamic abnormality explains the onset of pansystolic murmur with S_1 and extension of the murmur beyond A_2. Primary mitral regurgitation is defined when mitral regurgitation occurs due to the abnormalities of the components of the mitral valve apparatus, particularly of the mitral valve leaflets. Rheumatic mitral valve disease, bacterial endocarditis, and ruptured chordae due to idiopathic degenerations that produce pansystolic mitral valve prolapse are examples of primary mitral regurgitation. Hemodynamically significant chronic mitral regurgitation usually is associated with an S_3 gallop and left ventricular dilatation with preserved left ventricular ejection fraction. When mitral regurgitation results from mitral valve prolapse, particularly of the posterior leaflet, the radiation of the murmur occurs toward the base and occasionally radiates to the neck. Thus, this murmur can be confused with an ejection systolic murmur due to aortic stenosis. The murmur resulting from aortic stenosis is ejection in nature, and other findings for left ventricular outflow tract obstruction, such as delayed upstroke of the carotid pulse, are evident. The pansystolic murmur due to mitral valve prolapse occasionally can be confused with the ejection systolic murmur resulting from left ventricular outflow obstruction in hypertrophic cardiomyopathy. Bedside maneuvers (e.g., Valsalva's, hand grip, squatting, and standing) usually can differentiate between obstructive hypertrophic cardiomyopathy and primary mitral regurgitation. Posterior radiation of the mitral regurgitation murmur can be detected when auscultation is done over the thoracic spine or on the vortex. When the regurgitant murmur is heard over the lower back (i.e., on the lumbar spine), a substantial increase in left atrial size should be suspected. The S_2 in hemodynamically significant primary mitral regurgitation usually is widely split—a condition that results from decreased left ventricular ejection time. The intensity of P_2 remains normal until pulmonary hypertension develops, when its intensity is increased. Chronic primary hemodynamically significant mitral regurgitation is associated not only with an increase in left ventricular diastolic volume but also with normal ejection fraction. A displaced and hyperdynamic left ventricular apical impulse indicates normal ejection fraction and, therefore, primary mitral regurgitation. A displaced and sustained left ventricular apical impulse usually is associated with a decreased left ventricular ejection fraction, which, of course, can result from long-standing, severe mitral regurgitation, or it may indicate secondary mitral regurgitation due to dilated cardiomyopathy. Thus, normal left ventricular ejection fraction is helpful in establishing the diagnosis of primary mitral regurgitation. When the left ventricular ejection fraction seems to be decreased, further evaluation by echocardiography or cardiac catheterization is required to establish the mechanism of mitral regurgitation.

Tricuspid Regurgitation

The pansystolic murmur of tricuspid regurgitation usually is heard best at the lower left sternal border. Occasionally, the murmur is heard best near the cardiac apex because of significant right ventricular dilatation. The tricuspid regurgitation murmur, however, does not radiate to the left axilla. Frequently, the murmur of tricuspid regurgitation is heard along the right sternal border, over the epigastrium, and over the right subcostal region. The intensity of the murmur, as expected, increases during inspiration due to the increased venous return and right ventricular filling. Occasionally, a severe tricuspid regurgitation is associated with a diastolic flow murmur that is characterized as a short diastolic rumble along the lower left sternal border. When present, this murmur also increases in intensity during inspiration. Hemodynamically significant tricuspid regurgitation frequently is associated with right ventricular S_3 gallop, which also increases in intensity during inspiration. Tricuspid regurgitation is diagnosed at the bedside from the presence of a prominent 'v' wave followed by a sharp 'y' descent in the jugular venous pulse and systolic hepatic pulsation. Tricuspid regurgitation is most often secondary to pulmonary arterial hypertension; thus, a prominent left parasternal impulse and narrow splitting of S_2 with an accentuated P_2 suggest secondary tricuspid regurgitation. Although severe tricuspid regurgitation can be associated with reversed splitting of the S_2 due to a marked reduction in right ventricular ejection time, this finding is rarely observed at the bedside. Tricuspid regurgitation not accompanied by pulmonary hypertension (primary tricuspid regurgitation) can occur after right-sided bacterial endocarditis, right ventricular infarction, Ebstein's anomaly, carcinoid heart disease, right ventricular papillary muscle dysfunction or infarction, and traumatic rupture of the chordae of the tricuspid valve. Predominant tricuspid regurgitation also can occur in rheumatic heart disease; however, rheumatic tricuspid regurgitation is almost always accompanied by aortic or mitral valvular disease. The diagnosis of primary tricuspid regurgitation depends on the demonstration of normal pulmonary artery pressure; thus, echo-Doppler evaluation is recommended.

Ventricular Septal Defect

Ventricular septal defect is associated with a pansystolic murmur, because the pressure in the right ventricle is lower than the pressure in the left ventricle throughout systole (87). This hemodynamic profile usually is observed in unrestricted ventricular septal defect with normal pulmonary vascular resistance. Thus, the S_2 in these patients usually is normal. The murmur is loud and may be accompanied by a thrill (46). The murmur is heard best over the left third or fourth interspace along the left sternal border. In supracristal ventricular septal defect, the maximum intensity of the murmur may be located over the left second interspace, and it can be confused with the murmur of pulmonary valve stenosis. The changes in the splitting of the S_2 may help in the differential diagnosis. A wide splitting of the S_2 with reduced intensity of P_2 is present in pulmonary stenosis, and a normal S_2 favors ventricular septal defect. The murmur of ventricular septal defect does not radiate to the axilla, as with mitral regurgitation, and does not increase in intensity with inspiration, as with tricuspid regurgitation. When the magnitude of the left-to-right shunt is large, wide physiologic splitting of the S_2 with normal intensity of P_2 is recognized. Furthermore, left ventricular S_3 gallop with or without a mid-diastolic rumble suggesting increased flow across the mitral valve can be heard at the cardiac apex. It should be appreciated that the intensity of the murmur correlates poorly with the degree of left-to-right shunt. A grade 5 murmur usually is associated with a high-velocity flow through a small hemodynamically insignificant ventricular septal defect (88). When the septal defect is large and the right and left ventricular pressures are equal, no murmur may be produced across the defect (89). Pansystolic murmur of mitral regurgitation and the murmur of ventricular septal defect decrease in intensity in response to amyl nitrite. Amyl nitrite inhalation reduces systemic vascular resistance and left ventricular/right ventricular pressure gradient associated with decreased left-to-right shunt. However, with certain vasodilators, which have the potential to decrease pulmonary vascular resistance by greater magnitude than systemic vascular resistance, the intensity of the murmur may increase. Nitroglycerin and sodium nitroprusside can cause a greater reduction of pulmonary vascular resistance than of systemic resistance and, therefore, may cause an increase in the magnitude of left-to-right shunt and the intensity of the murmur.

Early systolic regurgitant murmurs can occur in mitral and tricuspid valvular regurgitation and in certain types of ventricular septal defects. Early systolic regurgitant murmurs begin with the S_1 but do not extend to S_2 and generally have a decrescendo configuration. The early systolic murmur associated with mitral regurgitation is heard best at the cardiac apex, but it may have limited radiation. The early systolic murmur usually suggests relatively mild mitral regurgitation and results most frequently from left ventricular dilatation with or without annular dilatation. In some patients with mitral stenosis, an early systolic murmur is heard and probably represents mild mitral regurgitation. Mitral annular calcification may also be associated with an early systolic murmur, indicating mild mitral regurgitation. Mitral annular calcification is associated with lack of a reduction of the circumference of the annulus at the beginning of the systole, thus inducing mild mitral regurgitation.

Acute Severe Mitral Regurgitation

Early systolic murmur may also be associated with acute severe mitral regurgitation (90). The conditions producing acute severe mitral regurgitation include spontaneous rupture of the chordae, acute or subacute bacterial endocarditis of the mitral valve, papillary muscle rupture or infarction secondary to acute myocardial infarction, and disruption of the mitral valve apparatus due to chest trauma. In acute severe mitral regurgitation, there is regurgitation of a relatively large volume of blood into a normal-sized left atrium. As a result, there is a rapid increase in the magnitude of 'v' wave, and, during mid- or late systole, 'v' wave pressure may be similar to

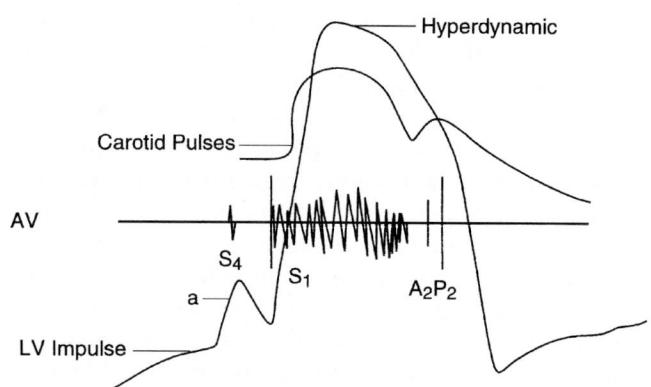

FIGURE 15.12 Schematic illustrations of the physical findings suggestive of acute or subacute severe primary mitral regurgitation (e.g., due to ruptured chordae). Examination of the carotid pulse reveals a sharp upstroke, but the amplitude is small. Palpation of the left ventricular (LV) impulse usually reveals a palpable 'a' wave and a hyperdynamic outward movement, indicating increased LV diastolic pressure and normal LV ejection fraction, respectively. Auscultation usually reveals a fourth heart sound (S_4), an early systolic murmur, and a relatively widely split second heart sound. The pulmonary component of the second heart sound (P_2) usually is accentuated, indicating pulmonary hypertension. A_2, aortic component of the second heart sound; AV, atrioventricular; S_1, first heart sound.

sure gradient between the left ventricle and left atrium during mid-systole stops the regurgitation, and, therefore, the murmur terminates before the A_2 (Fig. 15.12). In patients with ruptured chordae, left ventricular apical impulse usually is normal in character, indicating normal ejection fraction. In contrast, when mitral regurgitation occurs after acute myocardial infarction, left ventricular ejection fraction usually is depressed. In acute mitral regurgitation, a palpable S_4 and audible S_4 are commonly recognized. In contrast to chronic mitral regurgitation, an S_3 gallop may be absent. Acute severe mitral regurgitation almost always is associated with a substantial increase in the left atrial and pulmonary capillary wedge pressure and with postcapillary pulmonary hypertension. The S_2 is widely split, and the intensity of P_2 is increased (Fig. 15.12). The systolic murmur of acute mitral regurgitation may radiate to the axilla and back, especially if it is due to prolapse of the anterior leaflet of the mitral valve. When the murmur is loud, it may be conducted to the top of the head and to the lower back along the spinal column. Occasionally, the murmur is conducted to the base of the heart and over the neck vessels and can be confused with the murmur of aortic stenosis. However, the sharp initial upstroke of the carotid pulse and the wide physiologic splitting of the S_2 allow differentiation from aortic stenosis. The systolic murmur associated with primary tricuspid regurgitation is often early systolic and ends well before the S_2 (91). Early systolic murmur may also represent severe tricuspid regurgitation. When the right ventricular pressure is near normal and there is minimal gradient between right ventricular systolic pressure and right atrial pressure, the flow velocity is low and there is minimal turbulence, producing an abbreviated systolic murmur. In these patients, a large 'v' wave with a sharp 'y' descent frequently is encountered, indicating severe tricuspid regurgitation. There may also be a short mid-diastolic rumble (flow murmur) along the left sternal border, which increases in intensity during inspiration. Frequently, a right-sided S_3 gallop is appreciated. The early systolic murmur associated with severe tricuspid regurgitation also increases in intensity during inspiration. A right-sided S_4 with a prominent diastolic tricuspid flow rumble is appreciated when the tricuspid regurgitation is acute and severe, as occurs in endocarditis of the tricuspid valve. After total excision of the tricuspid valve, severe tricuspid regurgitation may not be associated with any systolic murmur, although there is a prominent 'v' wave in the jugular venous pulse, and systolic hepatic pulsations are easily appreciated. Palpable venous thrills and a murmur at the base of the neck are due to rapid retrograde flow to the jugular venous system (92).

Other Systolic Murmurs

An early systolic murmur may occur in certain types of ventricular septal defects. The ventricular septal defects causing early systolic murmur usually are small and located in the muscular septa, which are sealed because of systolic thickening of the ventricular septa (93). This early systolic murmur associated with ventricular septal defect may indicate that the defect may eventually close spontaneously. The small ventricular septal defect causing early systolic murmur is not associated with any other hemodynamic compromise, such as right ventricular failure or pulmonary hypertension.

Late systolic murmurs are most frequently recognized in mitral regurgitation due to papillary muscle dysfunction or mitral valve prolapse. The late systolic murmur resulting from papillary muscle dysfunction in patients with ischemic heart disease may or may not be associated with mid-systolic clicks. The late systolic murmur due to papillary muscle dysfunction can be intermittent or constant and may occur only during myocardial ischemia. Late systolic murmur with or without mid-systolic clicks may occur due to fibrosis of the posterior left ventricular wall, as seen in patients with pseudohypertrophic muscular dystrophy. In these patients, the electrocardiogram always reveals evidence of posterior wall infarction (i.e., a tall R wave in the leads V_1 and V_2). Mitral valve prolapse associated with myxomatous disease of the mitral valve is the most common cause of late systolic murmur. The murmur is heard best at the apex and often has a late systolic crescendo character. Single or multiple mid-systolic clicks frequently accompany late systolic murmur associated with mitral valve prolapse.

Precordial whoop or honk also is associated with mitral valve prolapse. These murmurs are loud, high pitched, musical, sonorous, and vibratory. These murmurs are heard best at the apex in late systole and can be intermittent. The unusual quality of this precordial whoop or honk is secondary to the high-frequency vibrations of the mitral apparatus.

Late systolic murmur with or without mid-systolic clicks can be observed in tricuspid regurgitation due to prolapse of the tricuspid valve. Isolated prolapse of the tricuspid valve is extremely unusual and almost always accompanies mitral valve prolapse. However, isolated tricuspid valve prolapse can be observed in patients with Ebstein's anomaly. Tricuspid valve prolapse may also produce precordial whoop or honk, as with mitral valve prolapse.

DIASTOLIC MURMURS

Early Diastolic Murmurs (Aortic Regurgitation)

Early diastolic murmurs typically start at the time of closure of the semilunar valves, and their onset coincides with S_2 (Table 15.10; Fig. 15.13). The aortic regurgitation murmur begins with the A_2, whereas the pulmonary regurgitation murmur begins with the P_2. The configuration of the aortic regurgitation murmur usually is decrescendo. The aortic regurgitation diastolic murmurs are high pitched and have a blowing character. Occasionally, these murmurs have a musical quality (diastolic whoop) and can be heard best with the diaphragm of the stethoscope. The musical quality of the aortic regurgitation murmur has been attributed to everted aortic cusps or perforated aortic cusps (94). The duration of the murmur is variable but usually terminates before the S_1. The low-intensity, high-pitched murmur of aortic regurgitation may not be heard easily until the patient sits and leans forward with the breath held during expiration and firm pressure with the diaphragm of the stethoscope is applied along the left sternal border or over the right second interspace. The radiation of an aortic regurgitation murmur is toward the cardiac apex. In some patients, the murmur can be heard best over the mid-precordium, along the lower left sternal border, or even over the cardiac apex. Radiation of the murmur along the right sternal border is more frequent in aortic regurgitation caused by aortic root abnormalities (95). After the diagnosis of aortic regurgitation is suspected at the bedside, it is desirable to assess the severity of aortic regurgitation (Fig. 15.14). In hemodynamically significant chronic aortic regurgitation, the carotid pulse upstroke is sharp, and the volume is increased. Frequently, a pulsus bisferiens quality of the carotid arterial pulse is appreciated. In patients with hemodynamically significant chronic aortic regurgitation, arterial diastolic pressure usually is <60 mm Hg. The pulse pressure is increased substantially in severe aortic regurgitation. The presence of water-hammer pulse or Corrigan's pulse is also suggestive of hemodynamically significant chronic aortic regurgitation. The various peripheral signs of chronic aortic regurgitation should also be determined at the bedside. Hemodynamically significant chronic aortic regurgitation is almost always associated with a consider-

TABLE 15.10 DIFFERENTIAL DIAGNOSIS OF THE DIASTOLIC MURMUR

Murmurs start with S₂ and have a decrescendo quality—suspect aortic regurgitation or pulmonary regurgitation

Chronic aortic regurgitation signs of hemodynamically significant aortic regurgitation are large pulse pressure, low arterial diastolic pressure, sharp carotid pulse upstroke, pulsus bisferiens quality of the carotid pulse, water-hammer pulse, Corrigan's sign, left ventricular enlargement. Reduced intensity of S₁ indicates increased left ventricular diastolic pressure. Presence of S₃ gallop indicates increased left ventricular end diastolic pressures and reduced left ventricular ejection fraction.

If aortic regurgitation is associated with increased intensity of A₂, suspect hypertensive aortic regurgitation.

Aortic regurgitation due to bicuspid aortic valve is associated with an aortic ejection sound, short ejection systolic murmur, and normal S₂.

If early diastolic murmur increases in intensity during inspiration, suspect pulmonary insufficiency. Once pulmonary insufficiency is suspected, a careful analysis of the intensity of the P₂ should be performed to assess whether pulmonary insufficiency is secondary to pulmonary hypertension. If the intensity of P₂ is increased, one should suspect secondary pulmonary insufficiency. This can occur in patients with precapillary or postcapillary pulmonary hypertension. Once secondary pulmonary hypertension is suspected, conditions that can be associated with postcapillary pulmonary hypertension—such as mitral stenosis and mitral regurgitation, aortic stenosis and aortic regurgitation, and primary left ventricular myocardial dysfunction (dilated, hypertrophic, and restrictive cardiomyopathy)—should be excluded before the diagnosis of precapillary pulmonary hypertension causing pulmonary regurgitation can be entertained.

When the intensity of P₂ is normal or decreased, consider primary pulmonary regurgitation. Primary pulmonary regurgitation can occur from bacterial endocarditis, congenital absence of the pulmonary valve, or after pulmonary valvulotomy.

The murmur starts after S₂ and extends to S₁ (mid-diastolic rumble with or without presystolic accentuation); consider organic or functional mitral or tricuspid valve stenosis

The presence of an opening snap indicates organic mitral or tricuspid stenosis.

Left or right atrial myxomas are associated with similar auscultatory findings of mitral and tricuspid stenosis of rheumatic origin.

Once the organic mitral and tricuspid valve obstruction is excluded, increased flow across the atrioventricular valves should be suspected as the cause of the mid-diastolic flow murmur. In these circumstances, one is obliged to exclude atrial septal defect, ventricular septal defect, hyperkinetic heart syndromes, and aortic regurgitation.

A₂, aortic component of the second heart sound; P₂, pulmonary component of the second heart sound; S₁, first heart sound; S₂, second heart sound; S₃, third heart sound.

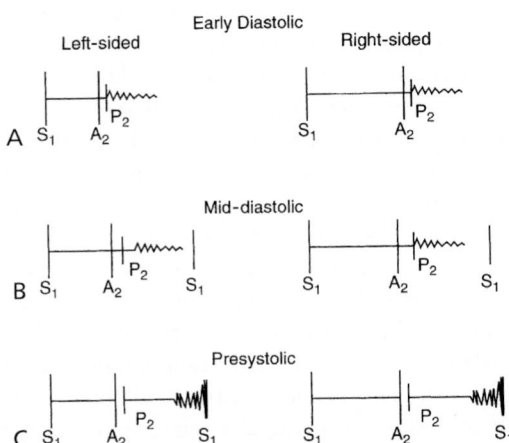

FIGURE 15.13 A: An early diastolic murmur, when the left-sided murmur starts with the aortic component of the second heart sound (A₂) and when the right-sided murmur starts with the pulmonary component of the second heart sound (P₂) or soon after P₂. **B:** A mid-diastolic murmur starts after A₂ when left sided and after P₂ when right sided and does not extend up to the first heart sound (S₁). **C:** A presystolic murmur starts before S₁ and terminates at S₁.

to selective increase in the left ventricular stroke volume, which increases its ejection time. Frequently, it is difficult to appreciate A₂, which may be decreased in intensity or absent because of the lack of coaptation of the valve cusp (96). Left ventricular apical impulse usually is displaced downward and laterally and maintains the normal asynchronous sequence with the carotid pulse upstroke, indicating normal left ventricular ejection fraction. In severe chronic aortic regurgitation, there may be a substantial increase in left ventricular mass due to eccentric hypertrophy that may be associated with a sustained left ventricular apical impulse. In these circumstances, it is desirable to assess ventricular function by echocardiography or radionuclide ventriculography. The presence of S₃ gallop in patients with hemodynamically significant chronic aortic regurgitation usually indicates reduced left ventricular ejection fraction. The presence of S₃ may also indicate increased left ventricular diastolic pressure. A soft S₁ in the absence of a prolonged PR interval in chronic aortic regurgitation indicates elevated left ventricular diastolic pressure. The duration of the aortic regurgitant murmur does not correlate well with the severity of aortic regurgitation. The presence of a pandiastolic murmur is more likely to be associated with significant aortic regurgitation. The Austin Flint murmur is a mid-diastolic rumble with late systolic accentuation; it is heard best at the cardiac apex and results from relative functional mitral stenosis. Evidence of pulmonary venous congestion and pulmonary hypertension should also be considered indicative of hemodynamically significant aortic regurgitation if these hemodynamic abnormalities are related to aortic regurgitation.

The hemodynamic consequences of acute severe aortic regurgitation are characterized by a sudden, severe volume

able increase in left ventricular size, which should be determined at the bedside and by chest x-ray. The lack of cardiac enlargement usually suggests hemodynamically insignificant chronic aortic regurgitation. In severe aortic regurgitation, ejection systolic murmur along the left sternal border and over the aortic area indicates increased stroke volume rather than aortic stenosis. S₂ can be paradoxically split due

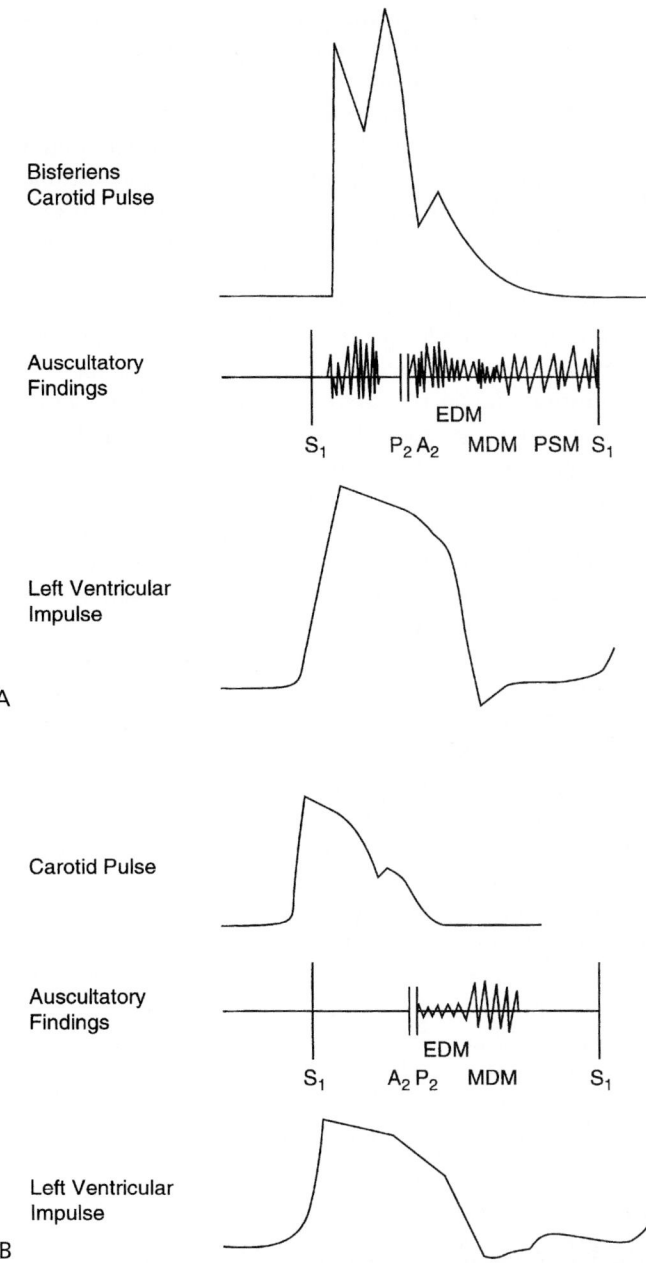

FIGURE 15.14 A: Schematic illustrations of the physical findings that can indicate hemodynamically significant chronic aortic regurgitation and can be appreciated at the bedside. The carotid pulse upstroke is sharp or may have bisferiens quality. The amplitude is increased. Left ventricular apical impulse reveals a hyperdynamic quality that suggests increased left ventricular volume with normal ejection fraction. Auscultation usually reveals an early diastolic murmur (EDM), and an Austin Flint murmur with both mid-diastolic (MDM) and presystolic (PSM) components are usually appreciated. The second heart sound can be paradoxically split (P_2-A_2), and the first heart sound (S_1) may be soft if left ventricular diastolic pressure is elevated. **B:** Schematic illustrations of the physical findings that may indicate hemodynamically significant acute aortic regurgitation. The carotid pulse usually is normal. Left ventricular apical impulse is also normal. The EDM of aortic regurgitation usually is brief. Austin Flint murmur only consists of an MDM component. The S_1 is soft or absent as the second heart sound is physiologically split (A_2-P_2), but the pulmonary component of the second heart sound (P_2) may be increased in intensity, indicating pulmonary hypertension. A_2, aortic component of the second heart sound.

overload to a nondilated left ventricle, which is associated with a rapid increase in left ventricular diastolic pressure and, often, equalization of left ventricular and aortic pressures in mid-diastole. The regurgitant murmur, therefore, can be brief (97). Because of a noncompliant ventricle and a substantial increase in left ventricular diastolic pressure, pulmonary venous pressure and pulmonary artery pressure may increase considerably—a condition that can be suspected from the increased intensity of P_2 as left ventricular wall stress increases due to the lack of compensatory eccentric hypertrophy—and forward stroke volume may decrease, which may cause a decrease in carotid pulse amplitude and arterial pulse pressures. Displacement of the left ventricular apical impulse is not appreciated. The apical impulse maintains the normal character, indicating normal ejection fraction. Decreased intensity of the S_1 or absent S_1 indicates acute severe aortic regurgitation and results from premature closure of the mitral valve due to a marked and rapid increase in left ventricular diastolic pressure (Fig. 15.14). A marked increase in left ventricular end diastolic pressure may also prevent effective left ventricular filling during left atrial systole; thus, an S_4 gallop may be absent in acute aortic regurgitation.

Mild aortic regurgitation without any hemodynamic compromise can occur in association with bicuspid aortic valve or systemic hypertension. The bicuspid aortic valve can be suspected at the bedside from the presence of an aortic ejection sound, a short ejection systolic murmur, and a normal S_2. Aortic regurgitation resulting from systemic hypertension usually is associated with an accentuated A_2, and the duration of the regurgitation is brief. However, the duration of the murmur varies with the degree of systemic hypertension. The higher the diastolic blood pressure, the longer the duration of the murmur.

Dock's Murmur

Diastolic murmur similar to murmurs of aortic regurgitation can be heard in some patients with stenosis of the left anterior descending coronary artery (Dock's murmur) (98). The murmur of left anterior descending coronary artery stenosis, however, is not transmitted widely and usually is heard best over the left second or third interspace, a little lateral to the left sternal border. This murmur is caused by turbulent flow across the coronary artery stenosis, and its duration may be short or long. After successful angioplasty or coronary artery bypass surgery, this murmur is abolished.

Pulmonary Regurgitation (Graham Steell's Murmur)

An early diastolic murmur also results from pulmonary regurgitation. In adult patients, pulmonary regurgitation occurs most frequently due to pulmonary artery hypertension (Graham Steell's murmur) (99,100). The early diastolic murmur associated with pulmonary hypertension is a high-pitched, blowing murmur that starts with an accentuated P_2 and can be of variable duration. In Eisenmenger's syndromes associated with atrial septal defect or patent ductus arteriosus, when right ventricular diastolic pressure may remain normal, the pulmonary regurgitant murmur may be pandiastolic. On the other hand, in the presence of modest precapillary or postcapillary pulmonary hypertension, the duration of the murmur may be brief. The pulmonary regurgitant murmur has a decrescendo configuration like that of aortic regurgitation. The murmur may increase in intensity during inspiration and may be very localized. It is heard best over the left second and third interspaces. Pulmonary regurgitation is suspected when other findings of pulmonary hypertension are present and peripheral signs of aortic regurgitation are absent.

Pulmonary regurgitation can occur in the absence of pulmonary hypertension, as in patients with idiopathic dilatation of the pulmonary artery. Pulmonary regurgitation is also frequently observed after pulmonary valvulotomy. It may occur as a complication of right-sided endocarditis and with the congenital absence of the pulmonary valve. In these conditions, the pulmonary artery diastolic pressure is normal or low, and the pulmonary regurgitant murmur is of lower pitch. The murmur usually begins after the onset of P_2 (101). The degree of pulmonary regurgitation associated with idiopathic dilatation of the pulmonary artery or after pulmonary valvulotomy usually does not produce any hemodynamic compromise. Congenital absence of the pulmonary valve may be associated with severe pulmonary regurgitation, and a loud "to and fro" murmur and absent pulmonary component of the S_2 should raise the suspicion of absent pulmonary valve.

Mid-Diastolic Murmurs

The mid-diastolic murmurs result from turbulent flow across the atrioventricular valves during ventricular diastole. These murmurs result from either functional or organic mitral or tricuspid valve stenosis.

Mitral Stenosis

The mid-diastolic murmur of mitral stenosis has a rumbling character and is heard best with the bell of the stethoscope and over the left ventricular impulse and with the patient in the left lateral decubitus position. If the stenotic mitral valve is mobile, an opening snap and a loud S_1 are present. The mid-diastolic rumble starts with the opening snap and may extend to the S_1 with presystolic accentuation (Fig. 15.9). The presystolic component of the mid-diastolic murmur of mitral stenosis may be present in sinus rhythm and atrial fibrillation (102). The mechanism of the presystolic accentuation of the mid-diastolic murmur is not entirely clear. It was initially thought to be related to atrial systole. However, it may occur in the presence of atrial fibrillation. Doppler-echocardiographic studies have suggested that the presys-

tolic murmur is related to antegrade flow through a progressively narrowing mitral orifice during the end of the ventricular diastole. It should be recognized that the onset of mitral valve closure starts approximately 60 ms before the valves close and produce S_1. With an obstructed mitral valve, the presence of a pressure gradient at end diastole allows antegrade flow across the closing mitral valve before the mitral valves close completely, explaining the presystolic murmur—even in patients with atrial fibrillation. The duration of the murmur correlates well with the severity of mitral stenosis. The longer the mid-diastolic murmur, the more severe the mitral stenosis. However, the duration of the murmur should be assessed during normal or slower heart rate. In the presence of sinus tachycardia or rapid ventricular response with atrial fibrillation, a pandiastolic rumble may not necessarily indicate severe mitral stenosis. Although duration of the mid-diastolic murmur correlates reasonably well with the severity of mitral stenosis, there is a poor correlation between the intensity of the murmur and the severity of mitral stenosis. The intensity of the murmur is related not only to the severity of the mitral valve obstruction but also to the flow across the valve. When there is a marked reduction in cardiac output resulting from severe mitral valve obstruction, the flow across the valve also is markedly reduced and may be associated with a soft murmur or absent murmur (silent mitral stenosis). At the bedside, the severity of mitral stenosis also can be assessed by noting the A_2–opening snap interval. The shorter the A_2–opening snap interval, the higher the left atrial pressure and the higher the pressure gradient across the mitral valve. In patients with severe postcapillary pulmonary hypertension associated with low cardiac output and calcified immobile mitral valve, the auscultatory findings of mitral stenosis may not be recognized at the bedside. The severity of mitral stenosis also should be suspected from the associated findings, such as evidence of pulmonary hypertension.

Left Atrial Myxoma and Tumor Plop

Although rheumatic mitral stenosis is the most common cause of mitral valve obstruction, left atrial myxoma, left atrial ball valve thrombus, cor triatriatum, and congenital mitral stenosis all can be associated with findings of mitral valve obstruction. Left atrial myxoma may cause intermittent obstruction of the mitral valve and, therefore, may be associated with a mid-diastolic murmur. Indeed, the auscultatory findings may be identical to those of rheumatic mitral stenosis (103). A loud tumor plop sound at the beginning of the mid-diastolic rumble may be similar to opening snap. The presystolic component of the mid-diastolic murmur may occur when the tumor is ejected into the left atrium at the beginning of the systole. A systolic murmur of mitral regurgitation may also be present. The auscultatory findings of left atrial myxoma may vary from examination to examination and even with changes in the body position. Patients with left atrial myxoma may also present with positional syncope and intermittent pulmonary edema.

OTHER DIASTOLIC MURMURS

Tricuspid valve stenosis is associated with a mid-diastolic rumbling murmur, which usually is heard best in the xyphoid area or over the lower left third and fourth interspaces along the sternal border. The diastolic murmur resulting from tricuspid valve obstruction increases in intensity during inspiration (Carvello's sign). The mid-diastolic murmur of tricuspid valve stenosis may be preceded by tricuspid opening snap. As right atrial systole occurs before the left atrial systole, the diastolic murmur of tricuspid stenosis may have a crescendo/decrescendo configuration without presystolic accentuation (104). Isolated tricuspid stenosis is infrequently encountered in clinical practice. Systemic lupus erythematosus and carcinoid heart disease may produce tricuspid stenosis. Rarely, constrictive pericarditis may cause functional tricuspid stenosis and may be associated with a mid-diastolic murmur. Tricuspid stenosis most frequently occurs in association with rheumatic mitral valve disease. Right atrial myxoma is an infrequent cause of tricuspid valve obstruction and may be associated with mid-diastolic murmur with presystolic accentuation preceded by a tumor plop sound. Both tumor plop sound and mid-diastolic murmur resulting from tricuspid valve obstruction due to right atrial myxoma increase in intensity during inspiration.

Diastolic rumbles may occur due to high flow across the atrioventricular valves. Diastolic murmurs at the cardiac apex are appreciated in patients with severe isolated mitral regurgitation or ventricular septal defect and patent ductus arteriosus with a large left-to-right shunt. Similarly, a large left-to-right shunt associated with atrial septal defect may cause a mid-diastolic murmur along the left sternal border due to increased flow across the tricuspid valve. Similar low-pitched, rumbling murmurs may be present in hyperkinetic states such as hyperthyroidism, chronic severe anemia, and arteriovenous fistulae. These flow murmurs occur not due to anatomic obstruction of the atrioventricular valves but due to functional stenosis.

Carey-Coombs Murmur

Mitral valvulitis associated with acute rheumatic fever may cause a short diastolic rumble (Carey-Coombs murmur) (105). This rumble usually is preceded by an S_3 gallop and most often is recognized in children in the presence of fever and anemia. These physical findings do not indicate mitral valve obstruction, but they do indicate rheumatic carditis.

Austin Flint Murmur

The mid-diastolic murmur associated with aortic regurgitation in the absence of organic mitral stenosis is called the *Austin Flint murmur*, after the man who first described this murmur in 1862 (106). It is heard best at the apex and can be mid-diastolic or presystolic in timing. In some patients, however, a long mid-diastolic rumble with presystolic accentuation is appreciated. Unlike organic mitral stenosis, the Austin Flint murmur is preceded by an S_3 gallop rather than opening snap. The S_1 in patients with aortic regurgitation and the Austin Flint murmur is normal or decreased in amplitude, but in mitral stenosis, S_1 usually is increased in amplitude. The duration and intensity of the Austin Flint murmur is directly related to the severity of aortic regurgitation. With amyl nitrite inhalation and when aortic regurgitation is decreased, the Austin Flint murmur is decreased in duration and intensity. The mid-diastolic murmur of organic mitral stenosis, however, increases in intensity and duration after amyl nitrite inhalation. In most cases of severe aortic regurgitation—particularly when there is a marked increase in left ventricular end diastolic pressure, as in acute severe aortic regurgitation—the presystolic component of the Austin Flint murmur is not appreciated. In this situation, there is reversal of the pressure gradient between the left ventricle and the left atrium in mid-diastole, which causes premature closure of the mitral valve and loss of the presystolic component of the Austin Flint murmur.

The mechanisms of the genesis of the Austin Flint murmur are incompletely understood and likely to be multifactorial (107). Although late diastolic mitral regurgitation has been excluded as one of the mechanisms, antegrade flow across the mitral valve with closing mitral orifice and incomplete mitral valve opening because of the regurgitant jet impinging on the anterior leaflet of the mitral valve may be contributory to the genesis of the Austin Flint murmur. In clinical practice, an easily appreciated Austin Flint murmur usually indicates hemodynamically significant aortic regurgitation.

Rytand's Murmur

Occasionally in patients with complete atrioventricular heart block, a mid-diastolic murmur is heard at the apex (Rytand's murmur) and may be confused with mitral stenosis. The slow heart rate, variable duration of the murmur, changing intensity of the S_1, and lack of opening snap are helpful findings for the differential diagnosis. The mechanism of Rytand's murmur is not clear, but increased flow due to slow heart rate and increased antegrade flow with atrial contraction, which occurs randomly, may be contributory (108).

CONTINUOUS MURMURS

Continuous murmurs (109) begin in systole and extend up to diastole without interruption. Continuous murmurs do not necessarily occupy the total duration of systole and diastole. These murmurs may result from blood flow from a higher-pressure chamber or vessel to a lower-pressure system associated with the persistent pressure gradient between the structures during systole and diastole. Patent ductus arteriosus is one relatively common cause of a continuous murmur that is occasionally encountered in adult patients. Descending thoracic, aortic pressure is higher than pulmonary artery pressure during both systole and diastole, and the blood flow from the high-pressure descending thoracic aorta to the low-pressure pulmonary artery causes the continuous machinery murmur (Gibson murmur) (110). The maximum intensity of the murmur usually occurs at the S_2, and the duration of the murmur is variable and depends on the pressure difference between aorta and the pulmonary artery. When pulmonary hypertension develops, pulmonary diastolic pressure increases, and the diastolic portion of the continuous murmur becomes shorter. When the diastolic pressure in the pulmonary artery is equal to the aortic pressure, the diastolic component of the continuous murmur is absent. With more severe pulmonary hypertension, the pulmonary artery systolic pressure may be similar to the aortic systolic pressure, and the systolic component of the murmur may be absent (silent patent ductus arteriosus). In patients with severe pulmonary hypertension with reversal of shunt across the patent ductus arteriosus (Eisenmenger's syndrome), differential cyanosis and clubbing may provide clues for diagnosis.

Continuous murmurs may be present in patients with aorticopulmonary window or Lutembacher's syndrome, which consists of a small atrial septal defect and mitral valve obstruction (111), total anomalous pulmonary venous drainage, and mitral stenosis with a persistent left superior vena cava. These conditions, however, are rarely encountered in clinical practice. A communication between the sinus of Valsalva and the right atrium or right ventricle is associated with a continuous murmur. Systemic and pulmonary arteriovenous fistulae also produce continuous murmurs. Systemic arteriovenous communications usually produce loud continuous murmurs. The murmurs of pulmonary arteriovenous fistulae are softer and may be primarily systolic. Coronary arteriovenous fistulae are occasionally encountered in adult cardiac patients. The location, duration, and character of the continuous murmur due to a coronary atriovenous communication depend on the anatomic type of coronary arteriovenous fistulae. The right coronary and right atrial or coronary sinus communication produce continuous murmurs that usually are located along the parasternal areas. The circumflex coronary artery–coronary sinus communication, however, produces continuous murmurs in the left axilla (112).

Constriction in the systemic or pulmonary arteries can be associated with a continuous murmur due to a pressure gradient across the narrow segment during both systole and diastole. In coarctation of the aorta, a continuous murmur can be heard in the back overlying the areas of constriction. Continuous murmurs in coarctation of the aorta may also originate from the tortuous collateral arteries, which are heard in the back over the interscapular regions. Sometimes, large, tortuous intercostal vessels are visible when the

TABLE 15.11 CAUSES OF CONTINUOUS MURMUR

Continuous murmur due to flow from high- to low-pressure systems

    Systemic artery to pulmonary artery connection—patent ductus arteriosus, aortopulmonary window, truncus arteriosus, pulmonary atresia, and coronary arteriovenous fistulae

    Systemic artery to right heart connection—rupture of sinus of Valsalva coronary artery fistulae

    Left-to-right atrial shunting—Lutembacher's syndrome

    Venovenous shunts—anomalous pulmonary veins, portosystemic shunts

    Arteriovenous fistulae—systemic or pulmonic

Continuous murmur secondary to localized arterial obstruction

    Coarctation of the aorta, pulmonary artery branch stenosis, carotid stenosis

Continuous murmur due to rapid blood flow

    Venous hum, mammary shuffle

shoulders are rotated and separated (Suzman's sign) (113). Pulmonary artery branch stenosis may also be associated with continuous murmur. Chronic obstruction of the pulmonary artery from pulmonary embolism has been shown to produce continuous murmur on rare occasions. Bronchial arterial collateral vessels develop in certain types of cyanotic congenital heart disease, as in tricuspid atresia and pulmonary atresia with ventricular septal defect; these collateral vessels can produce continuous murmur. An example of innocent continuous murmur is venous hum (114). The venous hum is heard with the patient in the sitting position and usually in the supraclavicular areas; it disappears when the patient is in the supine position. A loud, left-sided venous hum transmitted below the clavicle should not be mistaken for the patent ductus arteriosus. A venous hum is not heard in the supine position, and pressure on the internal jugular vein abolishes the venous hum. The mammary shuffle associated with pregnancy is another example of an innocent continuous murmur. These innocent murmurs are usually of higher frequency (i.e., high-pitched) and louder in systole. The causes of continuous murmurs and the mechanisms of their geneses are summarized in Table 15.11.

CONTROVERSIES AND PERSONAL PERSPECTIVES

Often in today's clinical practice, bedside examination is considered unnecessary and a waste of time. Indeed, the investigative tools available today are far superior to the bedside examination in establishing the diagnosis of the anatomic abnormality and severity of the pathophysiologic consequences. However, only bedside examination allows you to know the patient, understand the patient's sufferings and expectations, and establish rapport with the patient. Thus, I believe that we should practice more—not less—bedside physical examination.

THE FUTURE

The future of the physical examination as an investigation tool is likely to be compromised with the increasing availability of sonocardiographic and other allied imaging techniques. It should be remembered, however, that the bedside physical examination is still the cheapest and, in certain circumstances, most informative investigation.

CONCLUSION

Bedside clinical examination of the cardiovascular system provides useful information about the potential etiology of valvular, myocardial, and pericardial diseases, which can be confirmed by further noninvasive and invasive investigations. Physical examination also is helpful in deciding the appropriate investigations to establish the diagnosis. Furthermore, appropriate clinical evaluations are helpful to assess the therapeutic response and prognosis of patients with cardiovascular disorders. There is no cost-effective substitute for the information and insight derived from a careful bedside examination.

REFERENCES

1. Chatterjee K. Bedside evaluation of the heart: the physical examination. In: Parmley W, Chatterjee K, eds. *Cardiology,* 1st ed. Philadelphia: JB Lippincott Co, 1997.
2. O'Rourke RA, Silverman ME, Schlant RC. General examination of the patient. In: Schlant RC, Alexander RW, eds. *Hurst's the heart,* 8th ed. New York: McGraw-Hill, 1994:10217.
3. Shy GM, Drager GA. A neurologic syndrome associated with orthostatic hypotension: a clinical-pathologic study. *Arch Neurol* 1960;2:511.
4. Anker SD, Coats AJS. Syndrome of cardiac cachexia. In: Poole-Wilson PA, Colucci WS, Massie BM, et al., eds. *Heart failure,* 1st ed. New York: Churchill Livingstone, 1997:18261.
5. Kaplan NM. The deadly quartet. Upper-body obesity, glucose intolerance, hypertriglyceridemia, and hypertension. *Arch Intern Med* 1989;149:1514.
6. Solymoss BC, Marcil M, Chadur M, et al. Fasting hyperinsulinism, insulin resistance syndrome, and coronary artery disease in men and women. *Am J Cardiol* 1995;76:1152.
7. Javaheri S, Parker TJ, Liming JD, et al. Sleep apnea in 81 ambulatory male patients with stable heart failure: types and their prevalences. *Circulation* 1998;97:1254.
7a. Lanfranchi PA, Braghiroli A, Bosmini E, et al. Prognostic value of nocturnal Cheyne-Stokes respiration in chronic heart failure. *Circulation* 1999;99:1435.
7b. Sin D, Logan A, Fitzgerald F, et al. Effects of continuous positive airway pressure on cardiovascular outcomes in heart failure patients with and without Cheyne-Stokes respiration. *Circulation* 2000;102:61.
8. Benotti JR, Grossman W, Cohn EF. Clinical profile of restrictive cardiomyopathy. *Circulation* 1980;61:1206.
9. Zachary CB, Slater DN, Holt DW, et al. The pathogenesis of amiodarone-induced pigmentation and photosensitivity. *Br J Dermatol* 1984;110:451.
10. Richards AM, Eliot RS, Kanjuh VI, et al. Cholesterol embolism: a multiple-system disease masquerading as polyarteritis nodosa. *Am J Cardiol* 1965;15:696.
11. Malloy MJ, Kane JP, Kunitake ST, et al. Complementarity of colestipol, niacin, and lovastatin in treatment of severe familial hypercholesterolemia. *Ann Intern Med* 1987;107:616.
12. Keith NM, Wagener HP, Barker ND. Some different types of essential hypertension: their course and prognosis. *Am J Med Sci* 1939;197:332.
13. Leriche R, Morel A. The syndrome of thrombotic obliteration of the aortic bifurcation. *Ann Surg* 1948;127:193.
14. Smyth PT, Edwards JE. Pseudocoarctation, kinking, or buckling of the aorta. *Circulation* 1972;46:1027.
15. McGaughey MD, Maughan L, Sunagawa K, et al. Alternating contractility in pulsus alternans studied in the isolated canine heart. *Circulation* 1985;71:357.
15a. Narayan P, McCune SA, Robitaille PML, et al. Mechanical alternans and the force-frequency relationship in failing rat hearts. *J Moll Cell Cardiol* 1995;27:523.
16. Chabetai R, Fowler NO, Guntheroth WG. The hemodynamics of cardiac tamponade and constrictive pericarditis. *Am J Cardiol* 1970;26:480.
17. Massumi RA, Mason DT, Zakuddin V, et al. Reserved pulsus paradoxus. *N Engl J Med* 1973;289:1272.
18. Robinson B. The carotid pulse: 1. Diagnosis of aortic stenosis by external recordings. *Br Heart J* 1963;25:51.
19. Dexter L. Atrial septal defect. *Br Heart J* 1956;18:209.
20. Kussmaul A. User schwielige Mediastino-pericarditis und den parodoxen pulse. *Berl Klin Wochenschr* 1873;10:433.
21. Dell'Italia L, Starling MR, O'Rourke RA. Physical examination for exclusion of hemodynamically important right ventricular infarction. *Ann Intern Med* 1983;99:608.
22. Ducas J, Magder S, McGregor M. Validity of the hepatojugular reflux as a clinical test for congestive heart failure. *Am J Cardiol* 1983;52(10):1299.
23. Ewy GA. The abdominojugular test: technique and hemodynamic correlates. *Ann Intern Med* 1989;108:456.
24. Cohn J, Hamosh P. Experimental observations on pulsus paradoxus and hepatojugular reflux. In: Reddy PS, ed. *Pericardial disease.* New York: Raven Press, 1982:249.
25. Sutton GC, Craige E. Quantitation of precordial movement: I. Normal subjects. *Circulation* 1967;35:476.
26. Sutton GC, Prewitt TA, Craige E. Relationship between quantitated precordial movement and left ventricular function. *Circulation* 1970;31:179.

27. Manttleman SJ, Hakki AH, Iskandrian AS, et al. Reliability of bedside evaluation in determining left ventricular function: correlation with left ventricular ejection fraction determined by radionuclide ventriculography. *J Am Coll Cardiol* 1983;1:417.

28. El-Sherif A, El-said G. Jugular, hepatic and precordial pulsations in constrictive pericarditis. *Br Heart J* 1971;33:305.

29. Shaver JA, Salerni R. Auscultation of the heart. In: Schlant RC, Alexander RW, eds. *Hurst's the heart,* 8th ed. New York: McGraw-Hill, 1994:253.

30. Leech G, Brooks N, Green-Wilkinson A, Leatham A. Mechanisms of influence of P-R interval on loudness of first heart sound. *Br Heart J* 1980;43:138.

31. Shah PM. Hemodynamic determinants of the first heart sound. In: Leon DF, Shaver JA, eds. *Physiologic principles of heart sounds and murmurs. Monograph 46.* New York: American Heart Association, 1975:2.

32. Tei C, Shah PM, Cherian G, et al. The correlates of an abnormal first heart sound in mitral valve prolapse syndromes. *N Engl J Med* 1982;307:334.

33. Mann T, McLaurin L, Grossman W, et al. Acute aortic regurgitation due to infective endocarditis. *N Engl J Med* 1975;293:108.

34. Shaver JA, Rahko PS, Grines CL, et al. Effect of left bundle branch block on the events of the cardiac cycle. *Acta Cardiol* 1988;4:459.

35. Sakamoto T, Kusukawa R, MacCanon DM, Luisada AA. First heart sound amplitude in experimentally induced alternans. *Dis Chest* 1966;50:470.

36. Leatham A. Splitting of the first and second heart sounds. *Lancet* 1954;267:607.

37. Crews TL, Pridie RB, Benham R, et al. Auscultatory and phonocardiographic findings in Ebstein's anomaly: correlation of first heart sound with ultrasonic records of tricuspid valve movement. *Br Heart J* 1972;34:681.

38. Harris A. Pacemaker "heart sound." *Br Heart J* 1967;29:608.

39. Hirschfeld S, Liebman J, Borkat G, Bormuth C. Intracardiac pressure-sound correlates of echocardiographic aortic valve closure. *Circulation* 1977;55:602.

40. Stein PD, Sabbah HN, Anbe DT, Khaja F. Hemodynamic and anatomic determinants of relative differences in amplitude of the aortic and pulmonary components of the second heart sound. *Am J Cardiol* 1978;42:539.

41. Harris A, Leatham A, Sutton G. The second heart sound in pulmonary hypertension. *Br Heart J* 1968;30:743.

42. Shaver JA, Nadolny RA, O'Toole JD, et al. Sound pressure correlates of the second heart sound: an intracardiac sound study. *Circulation* 1974;49:316.

43. Leatham A, Weitzman DW. Auscultatory and phonocardiographic signs of pulmonary stenosis. *Br Heart J* 1957;19:303.

44. Sutton GC, Chatterjee K, Caves PK. Diagnosis of severe mitral regurgitation due to nonrheumatic chordal abnormalities. *Br Heart J* 1973;35:877.

45. Adolph RJ. Second heart sound: role of altered electromechanical events. In: Leon DF, Shaver JA, eds. *Physiologic principles of heart sounds and murmurs. Monograph 46.* New York: American Heart Association, 1975:45.

46. Leatham, Segal B. Auscultatory and phonocardiographic signs of ventricular septal defect with left to right shunt. *Circulation* 1962;25:318.

47. Beck W, Schrire V, Vogelpoel L. Splitting of the second heart sound in constrictive pericarditis with observations on the mechanism of pulsus paradoxus. *Am Heart J* 1962;64:765.

48. Gray I. Paradoxical splitting of the second heart sound. *Br Heart J* 1956;18:21.

48a. Leatham A, Gray I. Auscultatory and phonocardiographic signs of atrial septal defect. *Br Heart J* 1956;18:193.

49. Luisada AA, Kumar S, Pouget MJ. On the causes of the changes of the second heart sound in left bundle branch block. *Jpn Heart J* 1972;13:281.

50. Alvares RF, Shaver JA, Gamble WH, Goodwin JF. The isovolumic relaxation period in hypertrophic cardiomyopathy. *J Am Coll Cardiol* 1984;3:71.

51. Shaver JA, Kroetz FW, Leonard JJ, Paley HW. Effect of study state increase in systemic arterial pressure on the duration of left ventricular ejection time. *J Clin Invest* 1968;47:217.

52. Shaver JA, O'Toole JD. The second heart sound: newer concepts, part 2. Paradoxical splitting and narrow physiologic splitting. *Mod Concepts Cardiovasc Dis* 1977;46:13.

53. Perloff JK. Auscultatory and phonocardiographic manifestations of pulmonary hypertension. *Prog Cardiovasc Dis* 1967;9:303.

54. Shapiro S, Clark TJH, Goodwin JF. Delayed closure of the pulmonary valve in obliterative pulmonary hypertension. *Lancet* 1965;2:1207.

55. Hultgren HN, Reeve R, Cohn K, McLeod R. The ejection click of valvular pulmonic stenosis. *Circulation* 1969;40:631.

56. Sakamoto T, Matsuhisa M, Hayashi T, Ichiyasu H. Echocardiogram and phonocardiogram related to the movement of the pulmonary valve. *Jpn Heart J* 1975;16:107.

57. Barlow JB, Pocock WA, Marchand P, Denny M. The significance of late systolic murmurs. *Am Heart J* 1963;66:443.

58. Criley JM, Lewis KB, Humphries JO, Ross RS. Prolapse of the mitral valve: clinical and cine-angiographic findings. *Br Heart J* 1966;28:488.

59. Popp RL, Brown OR, Silverman JF, Harrison D. Echocardiographic abnormalities in the mitral valve prolapse syndrome. *Circulation* 1974;49:428.

60. Mathey DG, Decodt PR, Allen HN, Swan HJC. The determinants of onset of mitral valve prolapse in the systolic click-late systolic murmur syndrome. *Circulation* 1976;53:872.

61. Roelandt J, Willems J, Van der Hauwaert LG, deGreest H. Clicks and sounds (whoops) in left-sided pneumothorax: clinical and phonocardiographic study. *Dis Chest* 1969;56:31.

62. Martin CE, Hufnagel CA, deLeon AC Jr. Calcified atrial myxoma: diagnostic significance of the "systolic tumor sound" in a case presenting as tricuspid insufficiency. *Am Heart J* 1969;78:245.

63. Pickering D, Keith JD. Systolic clicks, with ventricular septal defects: a sign of aneurysm of ventricular septum? *Br Heart J* 1971;22:538.

64. Killebrew E, Cohn K. Observations on murmurs originating from incompetent heterograft mitral valves. *Am Heart J* 1971;81:490.

65. Sze KC, Shah PM. Pseudoejection sound in hypertrophic subaortic stenosis: an echocardiographic correlative study. *Circulation* 1976;54:504.

66. Ranko PS, Shaver JA, Salerni R, et al. Echo-phonocardiographic estimates of pulmonary artery wedge pressure in mitral stenosis. *Am J Cardiol* 1985;55:462.

67. Spodick DH. Hypertrophic obstructive cardiomyopathy of the left ventricular (idiopathic hypertrophic subaortic stenosis). In: Burch GE, Brest AN, eds. *Cardiovascular clinics.* Philadelphia: FA Davis, 1972:156.

68. Abrams J. The third and fourth heart sounds. *Primary Cardiol* 1982;8:47.

69. Vancheri F, Gibson D. Relation of third and fourth heart sounds to blood velocity during left ventricular filling. *Br Heart J* 1989;61:144.

70. Reddy PS, Salerni R, Shaver JA. Normal and abnormal heart sounds in cardiac diagnosis: part II. Diastolic sounds. *Current Probl Cardiol* 1985;April:10.

71. Shah PM, Jackson D. Third heart sound and summation gallop. In: Leon DF, Shaver JA, eds. *Physiologic principles of heart sounds and murmurs. Monograph 46.* New York: American Heart Association, 1975:79.

72. Abdulla AM, Frank MJ, Erdin RA Jr, et al. Clinical significance and hemodynamic correlates of the third heart sound gallop in aortic regurgitation: a guide to optimal timing of cardiac catheterization. *Circulation* 1981;64:463.

73. Vandewerf F, Minten J, Carmeliet P, et al. The genesis of the third and fourth heart sounds: a pressure-flow study in dogs. *J Clin Invest* 1984;73:1400.

74. Caulfield WH, deLeon AC, Perloff JK, Steelman RB. The clinical significance of the fourth heart sound in aortic stenosis. *Am J Cardiol* 1971;28:179.

75. Lerman J, Means JH. Cardiovascular symptomatology in exophthalmic goiter. *Am Heart J* 1932;8:55.

76. Hamman L. Spontaneous mediastinal emphysema. *Bull Johns Hopkins Hosp* 1939;64:1.

77. Lembo NJ, Dell'Italia LJ, Crawford MH, O'Rourke RA. Bedside diagnosis of systolic murmurs. *N Engl J Med* 1988; 318:1572.

78. Gallavardin L, Ravault P. Le souffle du retre'cissem-ent aortique puce changer de timbre et devenir musical dans sa propagation apexienne. *Lyon Med* 1925;135:523.

79. Pagon RA, Bennett FC, La Veek B, et al. Williams syndrome. *J Pediatr* 1987;80:85.

80. Thompson ME, Shaver JA. Aortic stenosis in the elderly. *Geriatrics* 1983;38:50.

81. Shaver JA, Alvares RF, Reddy PS, Salerni R. Phonoechocardiography and intracardiac phonocardiography in hypertrophic cardiomyopathy. *Postgrad Med J* 1986;62:527.

82. Shah PM. Controversies in hypertrophic cardiomyopathy. *Curr Probl Cardiol* 1986;11(10):563.

83. Braunwald E, Lambrew CT, Rockoff SD, et al. Idiopathic hypertrophic subaortic stenosis: I. A description of the disease based upon analysis of 64 patients. *Circulation* 1964;30[Suppl 4]:3.

84. Yamaguchi H, Ishimura T, Nishiyama S, et al. Hypertrophic non-obstructive cardiomyopathy with giant negative T-waves (apical hypertrophy): ventriculographic and echocardiographic features in 30 patients. *Am J Cardiol* 1979;44:401.

85. Darazs B, Hesdorfer CS, Butterworth AM, Ziady F. The possible etiology of the vibratory systolic murmur. *Clin Cardiol* 1987;10:341.

86. Schwartz ML, Goldberg SJ, Wilson N, et al. Relation of Still's murmur, small aortic diameter, and high aortic velocity. *Am J Cardiol* 1986;57:1344.

87. Craig E. Phonocardiography in interventricular septal defects. *Am Heart J* 1960;60:51.

88. Roger H. Recherches cliniques sur la communication congenitale. Des deux coeurs par inocclusion du septum interventriculaire. *Bull Acad Med (Paris)* 1879;8:1074.

89. Wood P. The Eisenmenger syndrome or pulmonary hypertension with reversed central shunt. *BMJ* 1958; Sept:701.

90. Sutton GC, Craig E. Clinical signs of severe acute mitral regurgitation. *Am J Cardiol* 1967;20:141.

91. Rios JC, Massumi RA, Breesmen WT, Sarin RK. Auscultatory features of acute tricuspid regurgitation. *Am J Cardiol* 1969;23:4.

92. Amidi M, Irwin JM, Salerni R, et al. Venous systolic thrill and murmur in the neck: a consequence of severe tricuspid insufficiency. *J Am Coll Cardiol* 1986;7:942.

93. Vogelpoel L, Schrire V, Beck W, et al. A typical systolic murmur of minute ventricular septal defect and its recognition by amyl nitrite and phenylephrine. *Am Heart J* 1961; 62:101.

94. Gelfand D, Bellet S. The musical murmur of aortic insufficiency: clinical manifestations based on study of 18 cases. *Am J Med Sci* 1951;221:644.

95. Harvey WP, Corrado MA, Perloff JK. Right sided murmurs of aortic insufficiency. *Am J Med Sci* 1963;245:533.

96. Sabbah HN, Khaja F, Anbe DT, Stein PD. The aortic closure sound in pure aortic insufficiency. *Circulation* 1977; 56:859.

97. Reddy PS, Leon DF, Krishnaswami V, et al. Syndrome of acute regurgitation. In: Leon DF, Shaver JA, eds. *Physiologic principles of heart sounds and murmurs. Monograph 46.* New York: American Heart Association, 1975:166.

98. Dock W, Zoneraich S. A diastolic murmur arising in a stenosed coronary artery. *Am J Med* 1967;742:617.

99. Steell G. The murmur of high pressure in the pulmonary artery. *Med Chron* 1888;9:182.

100. Runco V, Molnar W, Meckstroth CV, Ryan JM. The Graham Steell murmur versus aortic regurgitation in rheumatic heart disease. *Am J Med* 1961;31:71.

101. Runco V, Levin HS. The spectrum of pulmonic regurgitation. In: Leon DF, Shaver JA, eds. *Physiologic principles and heart sounds and murmurs. Monograph 46.* New York: American Heart Association, 1975:175.

102. Criley JM, Hermer AJ. The crescendo presystolic murmur of mitral stenosis with atrial fibrillation. *N Engl J Med* 1971;285:1284.

103. Nasser WK, Davis RH, Dillon JC, et al. Atrial myxoma: II. Phonocardiographic, echocardiographic, hemodynamic and angiographic features in nine cases. *Am Heart J* 1972; 83:810.

104. Wooley CF, Fontana ME, Kilman JW, Ryan JM. Tricuspid sounds: atrial systolic murmur, tricuspid opening snap, and right atrial pressure pulse. *Am J Med* 1985;78:375.

105. Coombs CF. *Rheumatic Heart Disease.* New York: William Wood, 1924:190.

106. Flint A. On cardiac murmurs. *Am J Med Sci* 1862;44:29.

107. Reddy PS, Curtiss EI, Salerni R, et al. Sound pressure correlates of the Austin Flint murmur: An intracardiac sound study. *Circulation* 1976;53:210.

108. Panidis IP, Ross J, Munley B, et al. Diastolic mitral regurgi-

tation in patients with atrioventricular conduction abnormalities: a common finding by Doppler echocardiography. *J Am Coll Cardiol* 1986;7:768.

109. Craige E, Milward DK. Diastolic and continuous murmurs. *Prog Cardiovasc Dis* 1971;14:38.
110. Gibson GA. Lecture on patent ductus arteriosus. *Edinburgh Med J* 1900;8:1.
111. Steinbrunn W, Cohn KE, Selzer A. Atrial septal defect associated with mitral stenosis: the Lutembacher syndrome revisited. *Am J Med* 1970;48:295.
112. Harris A, Jefferson K, Chatterjee K. Coronary arteriovenous fistula with aneurysm of coronary sinus. *Br Heart J* 1969;31:400.
113. Campbell M, Suzman SS. Coarctation of the aorta. *Br Heart J* 1947;9:185.
114. Fowler NO, Gause R. The cervical venous hum. *Am Heart J* 1964;67:135.

STABLE ISCHEMIC SYNDROMES

PAUL W. ARMSTRONG

▼▼ ADDITIONAL ELECTRONIC TOPICS

OVERVIEW

The phenomenon of coronary atherosclerosis mediates the development of myocardial ischemia through a complex interaction of fixed atherosclerotic plaque, impaired coronary vasomotion, and diffuse disease underestimated by conventional coronary angiography.

The frequency of angina grossly underestimates the frequency of ischemia; it is the composite impact of the latter that has an important impact on prognosis. Attention to the particular diagnostic and therapeutic strategies most appropriate to individual patient needs is warranted. Exercise testing remains the pivotal diagnostic test for assessment of patients with stable angina pectoris. Perfusion imaging and dobutamine echocardiography (ECHO) can complement exercise testing, especially in patients with inconclusive results or of intermediate risk. Although not routinely indicated, ambulatory ST-segment monitoring may be helpful in establishing the relationship between symptoms and objective manifestations of ischemia, quantifying the total ischemic burden and confirming the presence of Prinzmetal's variant angina.

Matching the intensity of risk-reduction strategies to an accurate assessment of individual patient risk is a fundamental responsibility of the practitioner. Intelligent medical (both pharmacologic and nonpharmacologic) management offers genuine benefits in controlling symptoms and ischemia. Revascularization is a valuable alternative in high-risk subsets and in those in whom symptoms and/or ischemia persist on effective medical management. Future opportunities of exciting potential that harness the results of ongoing research into the pathogenesis, diagnosis, and treatment of coronary disease offer exciting prospects for patients and physicians alike.

HISTORY AND BACKGROUND

But there is a disorder of the breast marked with strong and peculiar symptoms, considerable for the kind of danger belonging to it, and not extremely rare, which deserves to be mentioned more at length. The seat of it, and the sense of strangling and anxiety with which it is attended, may make it not improperly be called angina pectoris.

Those who are afflicted with it are seized while they are walking (more especially if it be uphill, and soon after eating), with a painful and most disagreeable sensation in the breast,

---

P. W. Armstrong: Department of Medicine, University of Alberta Faculty of Medicine and Dentistry, Edmonton, Alberta, Canada

which seems as if it would extinguish life, if it were to increase or to continue; but the moment they stand still, all this uneasiness vanishes.

This elegant description by William Heberden first published 225 years ago eloquently captures the symptomatic characteristics of angina pectoris (1). It is a common and important symptom affecting many patients with coronary artery disease. Recent estimates indicate that there are 6.75 million Americans with angina pectoris, and an additional 350,000 new cases occur each year (2). These figures, however, are likely very conservative: Current estimates reveal that between 3.0% and 3.5% of patients with angina experience an acute myocardial infarction each year (3,4). Back-calculating from the observed rates of patients with acute myocardial infarction who survive to hospital admission suggests a more realistic prevalence for stable angina of at least 16.5 million individuals (5). The prevalence of angina pectoris in elderly men varies from 21.1% (aged 65 to 69 years) to 27.3% (aged 80 to 84 years), whereas in women the comparable figures are 13.7% (aged 65 to 69 years) and 24.7% (aged 85 years and older) (6). The socioeconomic implications of angina pectoris are staggering and in the United States alone likely extend to tens of billions of dollars. A comprehensive approach to diagnostic assessment, risk stratification, medical treatment, revascularization, and prevention of other cardiac complications through secondary prevention is a key priority and responsibility of the physician.

PATHOPHYSIOLOGY

Stable Angina

Cardiac ischemic pain is thought to arise from sensory afferents located in the coronary vessels and myocardium (7). These afferents were reasoned to be sensitive to both stretch and irritation promoted by local expression of noxious chemical stimuli. The latter theory has gained credence through the work of Crea and colleagues (8), who demonstrated that intracoronary adenosine reproduced typical cardiac ischemic pain in patients with stable angina pectoris yet did not promote electrocardiographic (ECG) signs of ischemia. Furthermore, in some of these same patients, prior treatment with aminophylline, an antagonist of adenosine P_1 receptors, attenuated exercise-induced angina without nullifying the ST-segment depression associated with the symptoms. Maseri and colleagues (7) have categorized cardiac ischemic pain into three components: (a) a diffuse visceral component, (b) a better-defined somatic component conforming to a distribution by dermatomes, and (c) an interpretive component modulated by psychological factors. Pain-producing stimuli traveling through afferent nerve endings converge with others from the same dermatome on the same dorsal horn spinal neu-

rons. Cardiac afferents distributed from the first to the fourth thoracic spinal neurons interact with other afferents and descending signals from supraspinal sources, then ascend to the thalamus and from thence to the cortex, where the decoding is processed by a complex collage of physical, emotional, and other factors.

The symptomatic discomfort that represents angina pectoris is usually associated with inadequate oxygenation of the myocardium. Most often this reflects underlying coronary atherosclerosis that involves at least a 50% diameter stenosis sufficient to reduce maximal blood flow during exercise (9). Whereas fixed segmental coronary stenosis may preclude adequate myocardial blood flow to meet the increased oxygen requirements imposed by physical exercise, it is important to realize that coronary atherosclerosis is a diffuse vascular disease associated with deficient endothelial-dependent relaxation (10). It is this deficiency that may mediate exercise-induced coronary vasoconstriction of a narrowed coronary artery, with resultant imbalance between oxygen supply and demand culminating in angina. ⟁ c48

Mental as well as physical stress is known to precipitate angina pectoris and ischemia; mental stress is mediated by sympathetic activation, with a commensurate increase in myocardial oxygen requirements resulting from tachycardia, hypertension, and increased contractility (18). This exerts a double jeopardy on the ischemic myocardium by also reducing regional coronary flow (19). Although failure of endothelial-dependent epicardial coronary vasodilatation is evident during mental stress in patients with stable angina, it seems likely that this is, by itself, inadequate to explain the genesis of ischemia (19). Hence, vasoconstriction of coronary resistance vessels is likely operational. Several neurohumoral factors may be at work to produce this, including serotonin, neuropeptide Y, norepinephrine, angiotensin II, thromboxane A_2, endothelin, and arginine vasopressin (20). Moreover, as many as one of five stable angina patients has been shown to have features of recent injury and/or repair in their culprit coronary lesions; hence, the stage is obviously set in such patients for both aggregation and activation of platelets (21). The demonstration of increased levels of both serotonin and thromboxane A_2 in the coronary sinus of patients with angina pectoris, coupled with the capacity of ketanserin, a selective serotonin II receptor antagonist, to blunt coronary vasoconstriction is further support for this reasoning (22).

Silent Ischemia

Ambulatory ECG monitoring of patients with established coronary disease and stable angina has revolutionized our understanding of myocardial ischemia in these individuals. In patients with established or a high likelihood of coronary disease, transient ST-segment depression of at least 1 mm persisting for at least 1 minute has been well validated as a marker of myocardial ischemia through concomitant studies involving positron emission tomography, radionuclide and echocardiographic assessment of ventricular function, and myocardial perfusion imaging (18,23–25). At least 75% of the ischemia occurring in patients with stable angina is clinically silent, and effective symptomatic control of angina notwithstanding, a substantial proportion (i.e., 40% of patients with stable angina) continue to demonstrate ischemia on ambulatory monitoring (26). On reflection, it is perhaps not surprising that evidence of ischemia occurs so frequently in the absence of symptomatic complaints, given prior pathophysiologic studies of myocardial ischemia in patients with stable coronary disease. Ample evidence in the literature predating the concept of silent ischemia clearly documents a chronologic sequence of events during ischemia that begins with diminished myocardial perfusion and is followed by diminished diastolic and systolic left ventricular function, abnormal myocardial lactate metabolism, ECG changes, and then finally symptoms of angina pectoris (26,27). Moreover, impairment of contractile function may persist for a surprisingly extended period of time—that is, 60 to 120 minutes after exercise-induced angina despite abrupt normalization of hemodynamic and ECG parameters. This temporal dissociation has been elegantly delineated by Ambrosio and colleagues (eFig. 16.0.1) (28), who have demonstrated delay in return of contractile performance despite normal perfusion after the development and relief of exertional angina—that is, myocardial stunning—which is thought to represent severe coronary artery disease.

According to the classification of Cohn (29), ischemia detected on ambulatory monitoring in the absence of symptoms (i.e., silent ischemia) may be categorized into three types: Type 1 patients are totally asymptomatic, type 2 are those who are symptomatic after a prior documented myocardial infarction, and type 3 patients manifest silent ischemia but also have symptomatic ischemia (29). It is patients in the type 3 category who are further discussed here. In a series of insightful studies, Krantz et al. and Gabbay et al. (30,31) examined the relationship between symptomatic and silent ischemia during daily life activities, the role of triggers of myocardial ischemia, and the response and significance of mental stress testing. In a study of 63 patients, they found that 85% of episodes of ST depression were asymptomatic. Importantly, however, only one-third of 90 symptomatic reports of anginal symptoms was associated with ST-segment depression, yet the majority of these was associated with significant heart-rate increments (30). This bidirectional uncoupling of symptoms and ECG evidence of ischemia highlights the difficulties in developing a treatment program aimed solely at the modification of symptoms in patients with stable angina. Whereas some of these symptoms may have reasonably been attributable to noncardiac causes, ischemia can clearly occur, as documented by evidence of left ventricular functional abnor-

malities without ST-segment shift (i.e., so-called super-silent ischemia) (24). After adjusting for duration of time spent, intense physical activity was found far more likely to be associated with ambulatory symptomatic ischemia, most particularly walking, stair climbing, and related activities (31). Similar temporal adjustments associated with the evaluation of mental activity revealed that ischemia was evident approximately 5% of the time during intense mental activity such as anger or anxiety and only 0.2% of the time when low-intensity mental activities were occurring. A significant relationship existed between elevated heart rate at the onset of ischemic activities associated with physically and mentally intense activities. Finally, ischemia was fivefold more prominent when cigarette consumers smoked than when they did not. Mental stress induced in a laboratory setting, especially when it involves personally relevant speech, may induce abnormalities in regional and global left ventricular function at lower heart rates but comparable elevations in blood pressure to exercise (32). This has led to the suggestion that a decrease in myocardial oxygen supply may be as important or more important than an increase in myocardial oxygen demand and lends credence to the notion that a dynamic decrease in coronary flow mediates this phenomenon. Interestingly, the ability to demonstrate mental stress–induced ischemia has been found to be associated with a significantly higher prevalence, longer duration, and greater frequency of ambulatory ischemia during everyday activity (33). Gabbay and colleagues (31) have also demonstrated a relationship between ambulatory ischemia and intense mental activity unaccompanied by physical activity, as well as a similar proportion of ischemia during marked physical activity (accounting for roughly one-half of all ischemia). ▼ c49

Rosen and colleagues conducted a landmark study (47) of patients with symptomatic and silent ischemia in which they evaluated regional cerebral blood flow via positron emission tomography [ironically the same imaging technique that Deanfield and coworkers (17) used in 1983 to validate ambulatory ST monitoring as the surrogate for myocardial ischemia] during dobutamine-induced myocardial ischemia. Ischemia was confirmed both electrocardiographically and echocardiographically in those without chest pain, whereas symptomatic patients experienced angina that in all cases was associated with ischemic ECG changes. The hemodynamic response to dobutamine was similar in both symptomatic and silent patients, but the cerebral blood flow findings were significantly different. Whereas in symptomatic patients both thalami were activated, in patients with silent ischemia, cortical activation was limited to the right frontal region. The absence of activation of basal frontal, anterior, and ventral cingulate cortices and the left temporal pole suggested that gating of the afferent signals at the thalamic level is a possible mechanism for silent ischemia (eFig. 16.0.3). These findings open up new avenues of investigation aimed at evaluating, as suggested by Pepine (48), whether silent ischemia could be considered a conditioned autonomic response to environmental and psychosocial stressors (48). Hence, repeated ischemia could attenuate painful stimuli associated with ischemia, possibly through involvement of endogenous neurochemical analgesia.

Syndrome X

Fully 25% of patients with stable angina have coronary lesions on angiography that are inadequate to alter exercise-induced coronary flow (59,60). It is appreciated that abnormalities of coronary vasomotor tone in arteries that are by angiography apparently normal may also mediate angina. Most commonly, angina, or angina-like chest pain in the presence of normal coronary arteries, has been related to so-called syndrome X, a term coined by Kemp in 1973 (61). Despite a host of investigative studies in these patients over the past quarter century, uncertainty remains regarding the exact etiology. Most likely, cardiac syndrome X represents a heterogeneous group of disorders best characterized by a reduced capacity of the coronary circulation to augment flow in the face of an increase in oxygen demand. Although some have argued that a positive exercise test should constitute part of the definition of syndrome X, it seems clear that this should not be a mandatory requirement given the demonstration of abnormal myocardial lactate production with isoproterenol stress in some symptomatic patients who do not have ischemic ECG changes during exercise (62). Evidence for myocardial ischemia in such patients has also been evident through the demonstration of reversible perfusion defects with thallium scintigraphy and transient impairment of global and regional left ventricular function by radionuclide ventriculography (63).   c50

Prinzmetal's Variant Angina

Originally described in 1959 by Prinzmetal and colleagues (74) in association with resting angina and ST-segment elevation, these workers noted organic obstruction of the proximal portion of the coronary artery supplying the territory of ST elevation. Subsequently, this uncommon but well-recognized syndrome, evident in approximately 2% to 3% of patients presenting with chest pain undergoing invasive study at large referral centers, is known to be usually associated with underlying fixed coronary obstruction, although a substantial cohort may have either normal coronary arteries or minimally evident disease angiographically (75). The evidence for focal coronary spasm as the mechanism for variant angina is clear, based on the association of transient ST elevation concurrent with symptoms and localized myocardial perfusion and function abnormalities (76). Although usually confined to a single epicardial vessel, multivessel spasm is well documented, as is the occurrence of spasm at different levels within the same vessel (77). Based on an exaggerated vasodilator response to nitroglycerin, it is evident that the resting tone of the coronary vessels is not only augmented in patients afflicted with variant angina, but also indeed is supersensitive to intracoronary acetylcholine, which reliably provokes spasm (78).   c51

CLINICAL PROFILE

Perhaps more than any other cardiac symptom, descriptions of angina are rich with history and a delicate mix of elegant clinical observation buttressed by an interesting and still-unfolding pathophysiologic foundation. A glossary of the terminology associated with the term *angina* is provided in *e*Table 16.0.1. Most patients with stable angina describe retrosternal chest discomfort or distress, not pain, that occupies a physical area of clenched-fist proportion or more. Anginal discomfort is sometimes characterized as a burning, tightness, choking, heaviness, and occasionally a hot or cold sensation. It may be exclusively located outside the chest, however, and reside in the epigastrium, neck, shoulders, back or arms, and, occasionally, the jaw or head. Patterns of anginal radiation from the chest typically spread to the neck, shoulders, arms (usually left), and jaw. Anginal equivalents characterized by dyspnea, profound fatigue, weakness, or syncope may occur in the absence of any discomfort whatsoever. Ischemic symptoms during stable angina are usually of brief duration, persisting for 3 to 5 minutes, and are typically relieved by rest, dissipation of emotional distress, or the administration of nitroglycerin. Typically the symptoms are produced by vigorous physical activity or emotional distress, and the threshold at which they occur may be lowered by exposure to cold weather, by smoking a cigarette, or after ingestion of a meal. Some patients experience walk-through angina such that they can characteristically maintain the same or a slightly lesser degree of physical activity while the symptoms disappear within a few minutes. Thereafter, they are able to continue for a sustained time at the same or even an accelerated pace. A variation on this theme is the warm-up, or so-called second-wind angina, which is evident in approximately 20% of patients; hence, the second exertional effort is predictably better than the first if there is separation of at least 2 to 5 minutes between them (91). However, if the second effort is initiated later than 30 to 60 minutes after the first, the improvement disappears. If the interval between symptom-limited exercise in chronic stable angina is separated by 30, 60, or 240 minutes, the impact on both exercise performance and left ventricular dysfunction presumed secondary to stunning diverges (92). Hence, after 30 minutes, exercise time is extended, and comparable depression in contractile and diastolic function recovers more quickly. When the interval is separated by 60 minutes, total exercise time remains unchanged, but left ventricular performance is more severely depressed than initially and recovers more slowly, whereas if the interval is 240 minutes, both exercise time and cardiac performance behave in a fashion similar to controls. These data provide further physiologic underpinning for the warm-up phenomenon in patients with stable angina during exercise. Marber and colleagues (91), along with others (93,94), have suggested a pathophysiologic link triggered by favorable adaptive myocardial metabolic changes that result in less of a decline in high-energy phosphate and less lactate production despite recurrent ischemia. Experimental and clinical insights into the phenomenon of ischemic preconditioning suggest that enhanced ischemic adenosine production is a likely putative mechanism for warm-up angina, leading to reduced requirement for oxygenated substrate and attendant reduction in myocardial oxygen consumption and coronary flow (94,95).

Another clinical feature is angina pectoris when first reclining in bed at night that is thought to be related to blood volume redistribution centrally and an increase in preload. Nocturnal angina may be provoked by an emotionally charged dream and is known to be exacerbated by sleep apnea in patients with severe disabling angina (96).

Angina is traditionally categorized into four grades based on the Canadian Cardiovascular Society grading scale (97). Hence, patients in class I experience angina only with strenuous or protracted physical activity; those in class II experience only slight limitation with vigorous physical activity such as walking up a hill briskly. Patients in class III have marked limitation, with symptoms during the activities of everyday living, and those in class IV have the inability to perform the activities of daily living because of symptoms as well as angina that may occur at rest. Although this classification has some virtue, it also has limitations; hence, it does not address changes in the pattern or frequency of angina or take into account the warm-up effect or the self-imposed alteration in activities of daily living that may subtly modify symptomatic status (98).

New-onset angina, defined as occurring within 2 to 3 months of presentation, has been found to be associated with at least a doubling of the risk of nonfatal myocardial infarction within the first year after onset (99). This accentuated risk over patients with chronic coronary disease appears in spite of a lesser extent of triple-vessel disease and a greater frequency of single-vessel disease than in patients with chronic stable angina (100). Within the broad rubric of patients with new-onset angina, a story of progressive symptoms with more frequent and more readily provoked pain, nocturnal pain, and sustained resting discomfort with an abnormal baseline electrocardiogram are indicators of increased risk and a need to investigate promptly. Noninvasive stratification (see the section Diagnostic Tests) is usually helpful and feasible, but direct interrogation of the coronary anatomy may also be desirable.

Evaluation of a general outpatient population of 5,125 patients with stable angina enrolled by 1,266 primary care physicians in the United States provides a basis for reevaluating the common notion that this is a disorder that largely occurs in middle-aged men (101). This population was nearly evenly split between men and women, with the mean age of women of 71 years and that of men of 67 years. Most patients had more than one cardiovascular-related illness, usually systemic hypertension, hypercholesterolemia, prior infarction, heart failure, or diabetes. The majority perceived their health to be either poor or fair and had experienced at least two episodes of angina per week, and although more than 90% had angina with activity, nearly half also experienced angina at rest, highlighting the commonality of mixed angina. One-third had mental stress–induced angina, and one-fourth reported sleep-related symptoms. Accordingly, the traditional requirement that stable angina conform to a pattern of exercise-induced symptoms is no longer tenable given the aforementioned new insights into its pathophysiology, as well as surveillance data from both ambulatory monitoring and symptomatic surveys.

The approach to women with angina has undergone careful scrutiny in recent years, especially as it relates to the vigor with which diagnostic studies and hospital admission are undertaken. Atypical pain is more common in women than in men and may be related to a higher prevalence of less common causes of ischemia such as vasospasm and microvascular and microcirculatory disturbances as well as causes of nonischemic chest pain such as mitral valve prolapse (102). In the Coronary Artery Surgery Study, 62% of women with definite angina had coronary disease compared with a much higher proportion (89%) in men (103). Women with chronic stable angina are more likely to have chest pain at rest, during sleep, or at times of emotional stress. Paradoxically, analysis of cardiovascular risk factors alone more correctly predicts the existence and extent of coronary disease in women than in men, especially in young women. ❦ c52

Blacks, especially those born in the southern United States, have an excess of cardiovascular mortality compared with American whites (105). Less aggressive use of diagnostic procedures in blacks is known to occur. It has been suggested that, in addition to racial bias, blacks are less likely to request major procedures and have more of a tendency to decline them when offered (106,107). Asian Indians living outside of India have an excess risk of myocardial infarction (range of 2.5 to 5.0) and mortality for coronary artery disease (range of 1.5 to 3.0) compared with indigenous populations (108). Their disease is characterized by premature onset and a severe and diffuse nature such that it is less amenable to coronary artery bypass graft (CABG) and more likely to lead to permanent disability. Factors promoting this more malignant course include increased triglycerides and lipoprotein(a) levels, low HDL cholesterol levels, insulin resistance, and more prevalent diabetes occurring earlier in life (108). A consistent inverse relationship exists between indicators of socioeconomic status and coronary artery disease (109). Although socioeconomic status is strongly linked to conventional risk factors such as cigarette smoking, hypertension, cholesterol, and obesity, it is likely to be an independent risk factor for cardiovascular disease.

PRINCIPLES OF MANAGEMENT

The clinical assessment of patients with angina pectoris should involve a systematic review of cardiac and extracardiac factors that might contribute to the genesis of symptoms. Hence, cardiovascular factors such as hypertension, left ventricular hypertrophy, aortic and other valvular disease, aortitis, and arteritis must be considered. Important associated confounding systemic illnesses such as anemia, thyrotoxicosis, renal disease, chronic volume overload, and high output states from other causes such as arteriovenous fistula need identification. Homocysteinuria (estimated prevalence of 1% to 2% of the population in a heterozygous state) has been found to be a relatively common and correctable factor associated with symptomatic coronary artery disease (110). In the U.S. Physician Health Study, the adjusted relative risk for disease in the highest 5% versus the lowest 90% of homocysteine levels was 3.4 (95% confidence interval, 1.3% to 8.8%, $p = .01$) compared with matched-paired controls (111). The impact of correcting this risk factor is under study and is as yet unknown.

In addition to identifying cardiac and systemic factors on clinical examination that might support the clinical suspicion of coronary disease, a survey for systemic hyperlipidemia; hypertension with associated signs of target organ damage; and concomitant vascular disease in the extracranial neck vessels, abdominal aorta, and peripheral vascular tree should be undertaken. Evidence of left ventricular dysfunction and elevated left ventricular filling pressure are commonly accompanied by a presystolic fourth heart sound gallop, cardiomegaly, mitral regurgitation, and paradoxical splitting of the second sound. If the clinician is presented with the opportunity to assess a patient during a typical attack of angina, physical examination may be rewarded by detection of transient signs of left ventricular dysfunction and pulmonary congestion.

Diagnostic Tests

Whereas the ECG at rest may commonly be normal in patients with angina pectoris, it is useful to seek evidence of prior infarction and persisting ST-segment depression, which are both factors portending an unfavorable prognosis. T-wave change, intraventricular conduction defects, and atrial abnormalities may also be evident. ECG observations captured during an episode of angina permit evaluation of the location and extent of ECG changes. When the total amount of ST-segment change is extensive (i.e., more than

12 mm), there is a high positive predictive accuracy for the detection of three-vessel or left main coronary disease (121).

In the Rochester, Minnesota, area, 59% of 1,154 individuals presenting with chest pain were found to have normal resting electrocardiograms (122). In these individuals, assessment of clinical variables such as age, gender, and presence of diabetes, coupled with the results of an exercise electrocardiogram, can achieve a predictive value comparable with that of exercise thallium-201 scintigraphy in the estimation of three-vessel or left main coronary disease (123). It has been suggested that conventional exercise testing can readily triage patients into three major groups: (a) those who have normal or near-normal responses, comprising approximately 30% to 40% of patients with resultant mortality of less than 1% per year; (b) those with markedly abnormal tests, comprising 10% to 15% of the population who have a high risk of mortality (5% or more per year), and (c) the remaining population of approximately half the patients who are in an intermediate-risk area (124).

The graded exercise stress test forms the cornerstone of diagnostic testing in patients with known or suspected stable angina pectoris. It should be performed in all such patients before moving toward more detailed, costly, or invasive procedures. At least four important potential objectives may be achieved by conducting this test:

1. Correlation of patient symptoms with the presence of ischemia. When angina occurs with ischemic ECG changes, the prediction of coronary disease is more reliable (125).
2. Definition of risk of future events. Hence, those patients who are unable to exercise for more than 6 minutes on the Bruce protocol or demonstrate significant ischemia within this temporal window are at increased risk and deserving of further investigation (126). A summary of high-risk variables associated with unfavorable prognosis during exercise testing is shown in Table 16.1. A recent addition to this profile is the observation that a delay in the decrease in heart rate during the first minute after a graded exercise test was strongly predictive of mortality at 6 years (19% vs. 5%; relative risk of –4.0). This finding occurred in 26% of 639 patients and was associated with 56% of the deaths (127).
3. To provide the patient with an "exercise prescription" based on the level of activity and heart rate–blood pressure product at which ischemia develops.
4. To evaluate the efficacy of pharmacologic and revascularization therapy directed toward the subjective and objective manifestations of ischemia.

Deriving an index or score from information relating to the duration of exercise, the extent of ST-segment deviation, and the reproduction of limiting or nonlimiting angina has been shown to provide a more precise estima-

TABLE 16.1 HIGH-RISK EXERCISE TEST

Inability to complete 6 min (Bruce protocol)
Early positive test (i.e., 3 min)
Strongly positive test (i.e., 2-min ST depression)
Sustained ST depression 3 min after cessation of exercise
Delayed decrease in heart rate during first minute after cessation of exercise
Downsloping ST depression
Ischemia developed at a low heart rate (i.e., 120 beats/min)
Flat or lowered blood pressure response
Serious ventricular arrhythmia at a heart rate of 120 beats/min

---

tion of prognosis. Using such an approach (as depicted in Fig. 16.1), Mark and colleagues (128) in a series of 613 consecutively evaluated outpatients with suspected coronary disease found that two-thirds of patients had low risk, with a 4-year survival of 99%, whereas 4% had high risk, with a 4-year survival of 79%. In general, the location of

ST depression during exercise testing is an unreliable guide to the location of coronary narrowing. ▼ c53

There are a variety of circumstances where more specialized noninvasive assessment of the coronary circulation beyond that provided by conventional exercise testing may be warranted (*e*Table 16.1.1). If an adequate exercise test is feasible, it remains a highly effective, diagnostically accurate test when coupled with either myocardial nuclear imaging or two-dimensional echocardiography. Both exercise and the infusion of dobutamine induce ischemia through an increase in myocardial oxygen consumption mediated by augmented heart rate, systolic blood pressure, and contractility. However, exercise results in a 50% greater increment in heart-rate systolic blood pressure product versus dobutamine in direct comparisons, probably accounting for its greater sensitivity in detecting coronary artery disease in some series (143). The findings of lower end systolic volume and higher ratio of systolic blood pressure to end systolic

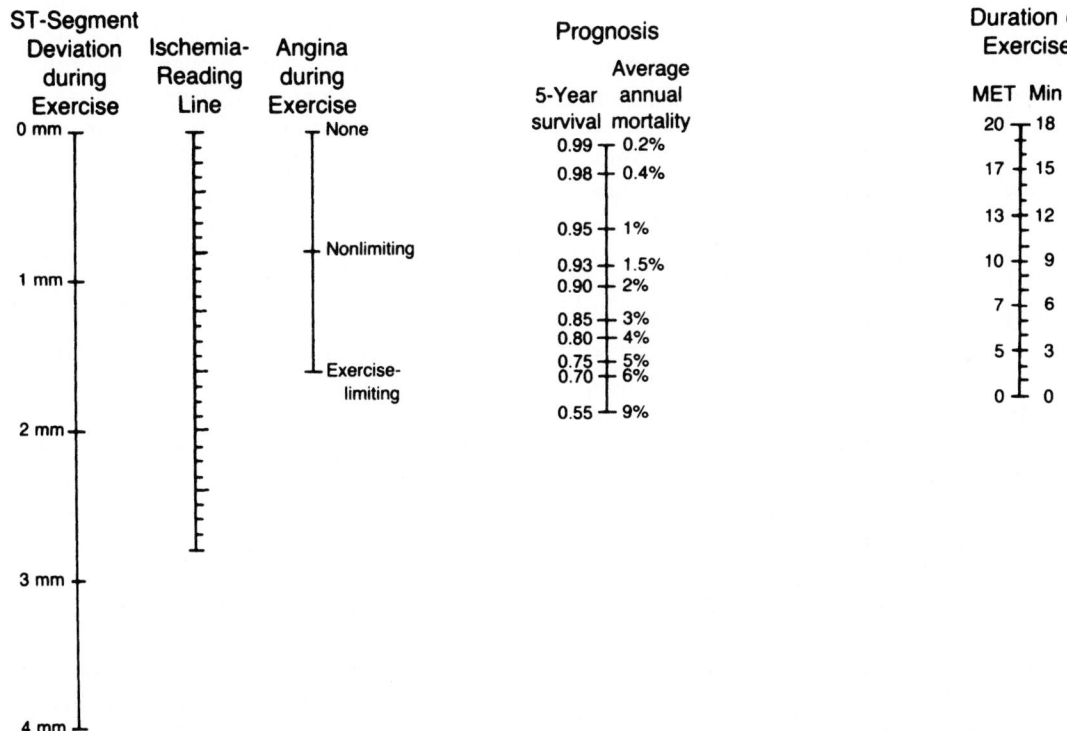

FIGURE 16.1 Nomogram of the prognosis relations embodied in the treadmill score. Determination of prognosis proceeds in five steps. First, the observed amount of exercise-induced ST-segment deviation (the largest elevation or depression after resting changes have been subtracted) is marked on the line for ST-segment deviation during exercise. Second, the observed degree of angina during exercise is marked on the line for angina. Third, the marks for ST-segment deviation and degree of angina are connected with a straight edge. The point where this line intersects the ischemia-reading line is noted. Fourth, the total number of minutes of exercise in treadmill testing according to the Bruce protocol [or the equivalent in multiples of resting oxygen consumption (METs) from an alternative protocol] is marked on the exercise duration line. Fifth, the mark for ischemia is connected with that for exercise duration. The point at which the line intersects the line for prognosis indicates the 5-year survival rate and average annual mortality for patients with these characteristics. (From Mark DB, Shaw L, Harrell FE, et al. Prognostic value of a treadmill exercise score in outpatients with suspected coronary artery disease. *N Engl J Med* 1991;325:850, with permission.)

volume index at the ischemic threshold during dobutamine echocardiography (compared with exercise) support the notion that there is greater augmentation of contractility as a contributor to the increase in myocardial oxygen consumption with dobutamine versus exercise (143).

Given that a high proportion of patients with stable angina have prior infarction and/or wall motion abnormalities at rest detected by two-dimensional echocardiography or resting perfusion defects, the question of whether such wall motion abnormalities possess residual myocardial perfusion and viability becomes highly relevant in therapeutic planning. Dobutamine enhancement of left ventricular dysfunction or inotropic stimulation evident after a ventricular premature beat is predictive of improvement in function with revascularization of the affected segment (144). Delayed imaging—that is, 18 to 24 hours after thallium exercise scintigraphy—reveals that 50% or more of segments (with apparently irreversible thallium defects on delayed imaging, i.e., at 3 to 4 hours) demonstrate isotope redistribution thought to be indicative of severe ischemia and predictive of favorable response to revascularization (145). Thallium reinjection at rest, 3 to 4 hours after stress imaging, has been demonstrated to provide similar information to delayed imaging in a more time-efficient and practical fashion (146). The use of thallium in this fashion to detect myocardial viability has been validated by concomitant metabolic imaging using positron emission tomography with oxygen-15–labeled water and exogenous glucose use with fluorine-18–labeled fluorodeoxyglucose (146).

By contrast, dipyridamole- and adenosine-induced hyperemia resulting in maldistribution of coronary flow occurs by maximally dilating normal vascular segments, whereas those with fixed coronary stenosis already have near-maximal dilatation, and hence, a resulting uneven flow pattern emerges. Adenosine's rapid onset of action and extremely short half-life, as opposed to that of dipyridamole, circumvents the need for theophylline reversal of troublesome side effects such as bronchial constriction (147). Two-dimensional echocardiography performed before and immediately after exercise testing and continuously before, during, and after dobutamine infusion is used to detect new or worsening preexisting wall motion abnormalities (24,148). These findings bear excellent concordance with the territory of the affected coronary vessel (143). Dobutamine stress echocardiography has been demonstrated to be of value in determining prognosis in patients with known or suspected coronary artery disease (149). In 108 medically treated patients with left ventricular dysfunction and known or suspected coronary disease observed for 16 months, Williams and coworkers (150) noted a significant relationship between cardiac events (death, myocardial infarction, and unstable angina requiring revascularization) and the development of ischemia or demonstration of viability—that is, enhanced myocardial thickening of a dysfunctional left ventricular segment.

Marcovitz et al. (151) found an increased likelihood of death or myocardial infarction in 291 patients observed for a mean of 15 months who had a combination of fixed and inducible wall motion abnormalities with dobutamine stress echocardiography. Perfusion imaging with thallium-201– or technetium-99m–labeled radiopharmaceuticals [either sestamibi (MIBI) or tetrofosmin] provides visualization of myocardial blood flow. Injected immediately before cessation of exercise or pharmacologic stress, these agents can delineate relative differences in myocardial blood flow conforming to areas of myocardial ischemia. With thallium-201, a late image associated with redistribution of blood flow 3 to 4 hours after exercise is commonly obtained to assess reversibility of defects observed during exercise (152). By contrast, with the technetium-99m–labeled MIBI, myocardial distribution is relatively fixed without significant redistribution; hence, imaging can be conducted for a few hours after the time of injection during pharmacologic or exercise stress (153). A second injection is necessary to characterize blood flow at rest. In addition to the value of perfusion scintigraphy in depicting coronary artery disease, it is useful in assessing ischemia in specific vascular segments when coronary disease has been established. In a study evaluating the prediction of cardiac events in patients without prior infarction presenting with suspicion of coronary artery disease, Ladenheim and coworkers (154) found that the frequency of cardiac events bore an exponential relationship to the number of reversible perfusion defects (*e*Fig. 16.1.3). Thus, substantial data are now available to support the role of myocardial perfusion imaging in more precisely defining prognosis; in this regard a high-risk scan may be especially useful, and the characteristics of this finding are depicted in Table 16.2 (155–159). c54

Although coronary calcification has long been recognized as a marker of atherosclerosis, its clinical utility has been limited by the low sensitivity of cardiac fluoroscopy for detection. The availability of electron beam (ultrafast) tomography has dramatically increased the sensitivity of coronary calcium detection. Notwithstanding evidence supporting electron beam tomography's ability to predict both the presence and severity of coronary disease, other data indicate marked intrapatient variability on repeat testing. Its ultimate role remains both uncertain and controversial (5). Recently an American College of Cardiology/

TABLE 16.2 HIGH-RISK NUCLEAR SCAN

More than 15% of left ventricle involved
Multiple defects (two or more)
Both fixed and reversible defects
"Left main pattern" (i.e., mid/upper septum and upper posterolateral wall involvement)
Left involvement dilatation after exercise
Lung uptake after exercise

American Heart Association consensus document concluded that "the test has proven to have a predictive accuracy approximately equivalent to alternative methods for diagnosing coronary artery disease but has not been found to be superior to alternative non-invasive tests" (160).

Selective coronary angiography remains the most definitive diagnostic investigation to define the anatomic extent and severity of intrinsic coronary narrowing. In general, it should be performed in patients (a) when the diagnosis of coronary disease is important to establish yet remains in doubt after noninvasive assessment, (b) when high-risk coronary disease is suspected based on the results of clinical and noninvasive evaluation, and (c) when significant symptoms persist despite adequate medical therapy (or, alternatively, when compliance with medical therapy is problematic). Although angiography was originally considered to be an unequivocal gold standard, it is now evident (not surprisingly) that some tarnish has emerged on this valuable diagnostic tool. Hence, the physiologic importance of moderate apparently similar stenoses has been demonstrated to be markedly different (161). Advances in technology using miniaturized wires that permit measurement of coronary velocity and pressure change across a stenosis allow evaluation of coronary flow reserve in living humans (162). Coupling the physiologic importance of a lesion with its anatomic definition is a key step toward appropriate revascularization therapy (161). Provocative testing with ergonovine maleate in patients with known or suspected Prinzmetal's variant angina may be useful during coronary angiography to identify the location and extent of provokable coronary spasm (90). In patients without major anatomic narrowing and in the absence of Prinzmetal's variant angina, vasoreactivity of lesions may be provoked by intravenous ergonovine; in this regard, Harding and coworkers (90) identified a subset of patients with a 10% likelihood of provokable spasm; this occurred in 17% of their study group and was identified by a history of smoking and the presence of 50% or less coronary stenosis. Building on the insights provided by coronary angioscopy, intravascular ultrasound provides precise definition of not only the contents of the coronary lumen and the extent of its narrowing, but also the thickness and characteristics of the coronary arterial wall, thereby portraying coronary anatomy in an entirely new fashion (Fig. 16.2) (163,164).

Therapy

The traditional approach to therapy of angina is aimed at the relief of symptoms and the reduction of risk to future untoward events known to develop (i.e., unstable angina, myocardial infarction, and death). Early observations suggest that obliteration of silent as well as symptomatic ischemia may well be a desirable long-term objective. It is also now evident that merely retarding or halting the progression of underlying atherosclerosis is too modest a goal; hence, reversal of atherosclerosis is a feasible aim. Accordingly, this section deals first with medical therapy, then the approach to revascularization, and finally the natural history and potential for modifying it. Comprehensive recommendations for the management of stable angina have been developed both by task forces of the European Society of Cardiology (165) and the American College of Cardiology/American Heart Association (5). In approaching therapy of patients with stable angina, it is useful to develop an overall strategy that emerges from the individual patient profile (166). Developing this profile involves several issues:

1. A risk assessment (i.e., What is the natural history of this individual?).
2. What factors are modifiable that will favorably alter the likelihood of future adverse events?
3. A comprehensive review of the following:
   a. Systemic factors that may aggravate ischemia (i.e., intercurrent disease such as anemia, thyrotoxicosis, renal failure, and infection).
   b. Cardiac-specific issues (e.g., hypertension, heart failure, valvular disease, and arrhythmia).
4. What patient-specific characteristics need special consideration as one chooses a medical treatment program (i.e., the presence of peptic ulcer and gastrointestinal hemorrhage such that aspirin may be relatively contraindicated; advanced left ventricular failure, brittle insulin-dependent diabetes that would make the use of beta-blockers problematic; marked sinus bradycardia or atrioventricular conduction delay where beta-blockers and certain negative chronotropic calcium antagonists could be deleterious)?
5. What characteristics of the anginal pattern suggest typical exercise-induced angina in which attention to favorably modifying the determinants of oxygen consumption will result in treatment benefit versus mental stress–induced angina where coronary vasoconstriction may be operative? Is mixed angina present where both of the above may exist? Is nocturnal angina present?

All patients with stable angina should receive 80 to 325 mg per day of regular or enteric-coated aspirin unless contraindicated (167). Aspirin produces a sustained functional defect in the platelet associated with prolongation of the bleeding time (168). This is induced by cyclooxygenase inhibition and subsequent suppression of thromboxane A_2, the key modulator of irreversible platelet aggregation. The Swedish Angina Pectoris Aspirin Trial, a prospective study of 2,035 patients with stable angina, revealed that 75 mg of aspirin added to sotalol produced a 34% decrease in primary outcome events of myocardial infarction and sudden death (95% confidence interval of 24% to 49%, $p = .003$) and a 32% reduction in secondary vascular events (169). Although 325 mg of coated aspirin is a common daily dose,

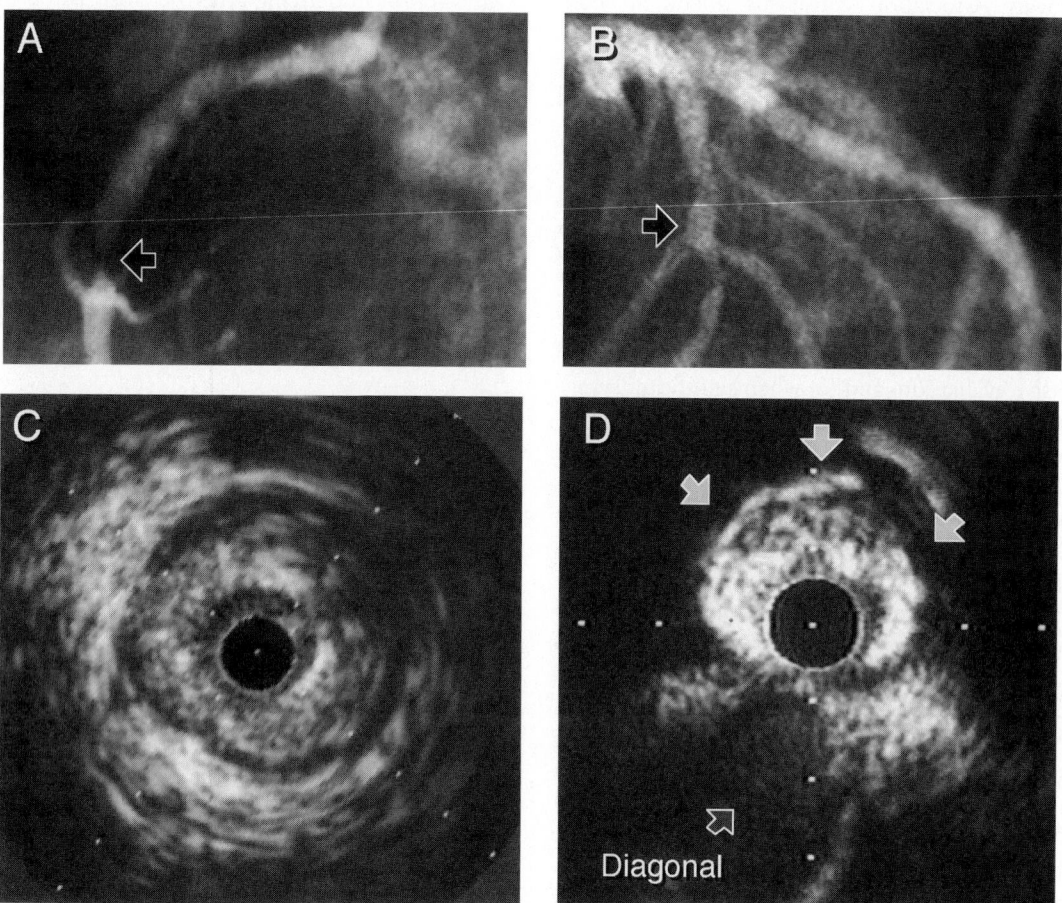

FIGURE 16.2 Angiographic and intravascular ultrasound patterns in stable angina. Stable lesions are often concentric **(A)** and have an echodense appearance and distinct fibrous cap **(C)**. In this example of a bifurcation lesion **(B)**, intravascular ultrasound examination reveals a significant and calcified plaque (*closed arrows*) at the mid left anterior descending artery opposite the origin of a large diagonal branch that was not angiographically apparent **(D)**.

this amount is in excess of what has been shown to be efficacious. Given the dose-related increase in gastrointestinal bleeding with aspirin, this dose could be administered on alternate days, or a daily dose of 75 to 100 mg would suffice. When aspirin cannot be used because of genuine allergy or gastrointestinal complications, ticlopidine or clopidogrel should be considered. These agents, which inhibit platelet aggregation induced by adenosine diphosphate collagen, arachidonic acid thrombin, and platelet aggregating factor, are known to reduce blood viscosity probably as a result of a reduction in plasma fibrinogen and an increase in red cell deformability. A number of trials have shown a consistent positive reduction with ticlopidine in a dose of 250 mg twice a day in nonfatal and fatal vascular events in peripheral, cerebral, and coronary vascular disease (170). Because hematologic changes including neutropenia, thrombocytopenia, and pancytopenia may occur (usually within 3 months of commencement of ticlopidine therapy), this therapy requires careful monitoring and is usually but not always reversible. Added to these concerns with

ticlopidine have been a series of cases demonstrating a small but genuine increase in the risk of thrombotic thrombocytopenic purpura (171). Accordingly, an agent structurally similar to ticlopidine—that is, clopidogrel in a dose of 75 mg daily—is the preferred agent in this class because it does not have the hematologic problems associated with ticlopidine and has been demonstrated to have a favorable effect on vascular complications that is slightly superior to that of aspirin (relative risk reduction, 8.7%; $p = .043$) (172).

There are three main classes of drugs with demonstrated efficacy on the relief of the symptoms of stable angina. It is important to recognize the presence of a strong placebo effect associated with any new therapy: This was well typified by a 76% improvement in the placebo arm of an internal mammary ligation study conducted in 1958 (173,174).

Nitrates have a multitude of effects on the cardiovascular system that promote the relief of ischemia and angina (Fig. 16.3). They reduce left ventricular preload and afterload through effects on the venous and arterial circulation, thereby reducing the oxygen consumption of the heart;

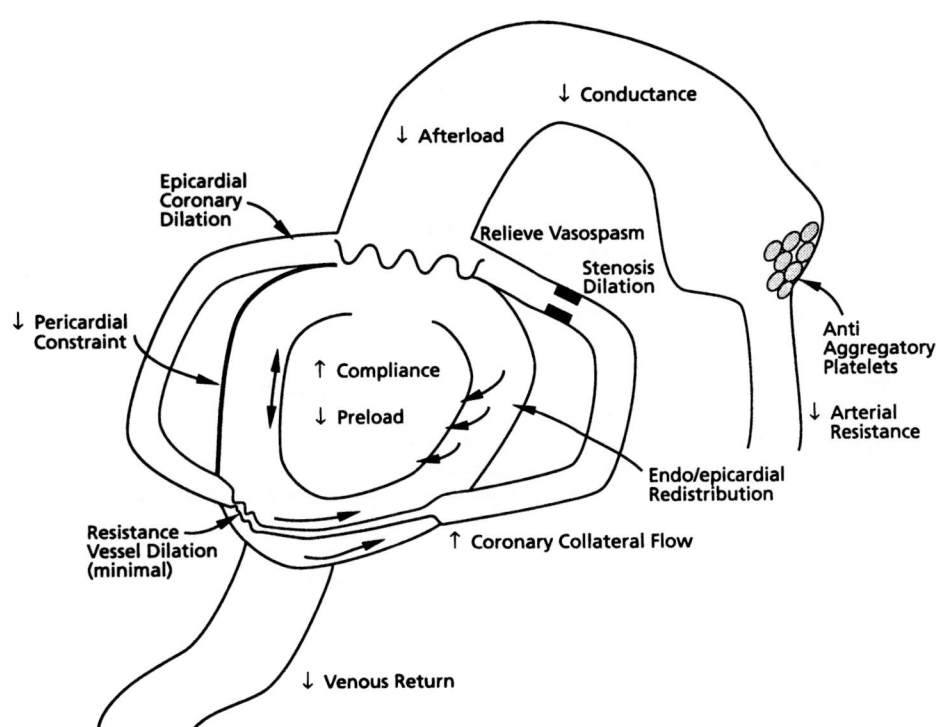

↓ Conductance

↓ Afterload

Epicardial
Coronary
Dilation

Relieve Vasospasm

Stenosis
Dilation

↓ Pericardial
Constraint

↑ Compliance

↓ Preload

Anti
Aggregatory
Platelets

↓ Arterial
Resistance

Resistance
Vessel Dilation
(minimal)

Endo/epicardial
Redistribution

↑ Coronary Collateral Flow

↓ Venous Return

FIGURE 16.3 Mechanism of nitrates.

they also dilate epicardial coronary vessels through their smooth muscle relaxant effect and in selected circumstances may enhance intracoronary collateral flow, relieve epicardial vasoconstriction and spasm, and produce a favorable redistribution of transmural coronary flow from epicardial to endocardial layers. Finally, they have a direct effect on the compliance of the left ventricle, producing a downward shift in the pressure-volume relationship (175). This increase in compliance is thought secondary to a reduction in pericardial restraint. Nitrates are metabolized through a common intermediary and after reaction with a sulfhydryl moiety are converted to an S-nitrosothiol. This in turn stimulates guanylate cyclase, which catalyzes the conversion of guanosine triphosphate to guanosine monophosphate, resulting in a decrease in intracellular calcium (176). When this develops in smooth muscle, it results in relaxation; a similar biochemical reaction seems to mediate the antiaggregatory effects on platelets that nitrates have been demonstrated to possess (177). It is thought that the nitric oxide produced by nitrate metabolism is similar or identical to that endogenously produced by the vascular endothelium—that is, endothelium-derived relaxing factor. Initial enthusiasm for sustained nitrate therapy as effective prophylaxis against angina has abated in the face of evidence that this strategy produces tolerance to its hemodynamic and antianginal effects (178). Tolerance can appear rapidly within days of commencement of sustained nitrate therapy, and three major mechanisms have been implicated: (a) the depletion of sulfhydryl groups necessary to promote metabolism of nitrates to nitric oxide, (b) expansion of blood volume leading to attenuation of the hemodynamic effects of

nitrates, and (c) activation of counterregulatory vasoconstrictor neurohumoral influences that would again attenuate the peripheral circulatory effects of nitrates (179,180). It is unlikely that a single unifying explanation can satisfactorily explain the phenomenon of tolerance, and controversy exists about the relative importance of the aforementioned hypotheses. Hence, the addition of a sulfhydryl donor, *N*-acetyl cysteine, to patients made tolerant to the antianginal effects of oral isosorbide was not successful in reversing the effect (181). Whereas chronic nitrate therapy is associated with an expanded intravascular volume and diuretic therapy was associated with improvement in exercise tolerance, it seems that this benefit is independent of any direct effect on nitrate tolerance (182). The addition of an angiotensin-converting enzyme inhibitor in patients with chronic stable angina receiving sustained nitrate therapy seems to restore short-term efficacy of nitrate effect (183,184). The long-term implications of this strategy are unclear.

In Table 16.3, a summary of the variety of nitrate dosing preparations and strategies is demonstrated. Nitroglycerin, either sublingual or as an oral spray, remains the most effective remedy for relief of individual attacks. Nitroglycerin may also provide good short-term (i.e., 20-minute) prophylaxis when activities known to predictively produce symptoms are about to be commenced (e.g., physical exercise or sexual intercourse). Oral or buccal nitrates administered twice or three times a day can produce sustained and effective symptomatic relief, as can topical preparations (185,186). Care should be taken to avoid the tolerance associated with sustained use by ensuring a nitrate-free

TABLE 16.3 NITRATE DOSING

Formulation	Dose	Frequency	Onset/action duration
Sublingual tablet GTN	0.3–0.6 mg	As required	2 min/20–30 min
Sublingual tablet ISDN	2.5–10 mg	As required	5–10 min/1–2 h
Oral spray GTN	0.4-mg metered dose	As required	2 min/20–30 min
Oral GTN SR	2.6 mg	Three times a day	2–5 min/3–5 h
Buccal tablet GTN	1, 2, 3, and 5 mg	Two or three times a day	2–5 min/3–5 h
Oral ISDN	10–30 mg	Two or three times a day	15 min/4–6 h
Oral ISDN SR	80–120 mg	Daily	Approximately 60 min/10–12 h
Oral IS-5-MN	20 mg	Twice a day	30 min/5–7 h
Oral IS-5-MN SR	60–240 mg	Daily	Approximately 60 min/10–14 h
GTN ointment 2%	0.5–2.0 in.	Twice a day	15 min/8 h
Transdermal GTN patch	0.2–0.8 mg/h[a]	Daily	30 min/12–24 h

GTN, nitroglycerin; ISDN, isosorbide mononitrate; IS-5-MN, isosorbide-5-mononitrate; SR, sustained release.
[a]A nitrate-free interval of at least 8 hours per 24-hour period should be provided to avoid tolerance.
Adapted from Abrams J. Therapy of angina pectoris with long-acting nitrates: which agent and when? *Can J Cardiol* 1996;12[Suppl C]:9C–16C.

interval of at least 8 hours; this can be achieved by once-daily topical or asymmetric oral dosing in patients in whom nocturnal angina is especially problematic (187). Using a bedtime application of nitrate may be especially useful for patients with nocturnal angina. In addition, care should be taken to use the smallest effective dose of nitrate required to minimize tolerance development (187). The best approach to long-acting nitrate therapy is to begin with the minimally effective and tolerated dose and be prepared to individualize the timing of administration in accordance with the pattern of symptoms and/or ischemia one is aiming to relieve. Gradual upward adjustment to maximally tolerated doses should be undertaken within 6 to 12 weeks. Nitrates are the most venerable of the medical therapies for angina pectoris and, despite challenge, have stood the test of time very well.

The principal side effects associated with the use of nitrates are headache, flushing, and lightheadedness. Occasionally, nitrate syncope can occur with a rapid decline in systolic blood pressure in the upright position, associated with arterial dilatation and venous pooling. Patients who experience lightheadedness while taking sublingual or oral short-acting nitrates should be cautioned to sit or adopt a semirecumbent position when taking short-acting nitrates. Generally, concomitant analgesia for headache for the first several days or weeks is successful in circumventing this side effect, but approximately 30% of patients are unable to take sustained long-acting nitrate therapy because of troublesome side effects. Oral isosorbide should be taken with milk or meals to avoid the heartburn sometimes associated with its use.

The role of nitrate therapy in stable angina has recently undergone reexamination in conjunction with the availability of sildenafil (Viagra), a selective phosphodiesterase inhibitor indicated for the enhancement of sexual performance. The commonality of erectile dysfunction in males with stable angina presents a significant therapeutic challenge to the practitioner. Many men so afflicted have asso-

ciated diabetes, have peripheral vascular disease, and/or are receiving beta-blockers, all or none of which may contribute to this symptomatic complaint. Because sildenafil releases endothelium-bound nitric oxide, concomitant use of nitrates (which also function as nitric oxide donors) may result in a synergistic decline in blood pressure (188). Accordingly, a recent American College of Cardiology/American Heart Association consensus document (189) advises that sildenafil is contraindicated in patients receiving long-acting nitrates and should be used with substantial caution if patients require short-acting nitrates for symptoms that develop during mild or moderate exercise.

The introduction of beta-blockers more than 25 years ago has markedly improved the medical therapy of patients with stable angina. These agents have a variety of cardiovascular effects that ameliorate ischemia (Fig. 16.4) (190). Occasionally, unfavorable effects on the cardiovascular system occur—that is, (a) patients with impaired left ventricular function may develop cardiac dilatation with an increase in myocardial oxygen consumption and aggravation of angina and/or left ventricular failure and (b) the blockade of beta$_2$-adrenergic effects in the coronary circulation may lead to vasoconstriction in patients with coronary vasospasm (191). This tendency becomes unmasked by the unopposed impact of alpha-adrenergic–mediated vasoconstriction. ☞ c55

Both propranolol and metoprolol, two first-generation beta-blockers, have relatively short pharmacologic half-lives, are metabolized by the liver, and are lipid soluble. Lipid solubility tends to be associated with enhanced central nervous system concentration of beta-blockers and has been linked to the side effects of lethargy, depression, sleep disruption with vivid dreaming, and hallucinations (190). By contrast, atenolol and nadolol are water-soluble agents that are excreted unchanged by the kidney, have relatively long half-lives, and can be administered once daily. It has been suggested that these agents may be associated with fewer central nervous system effects given their water solu-

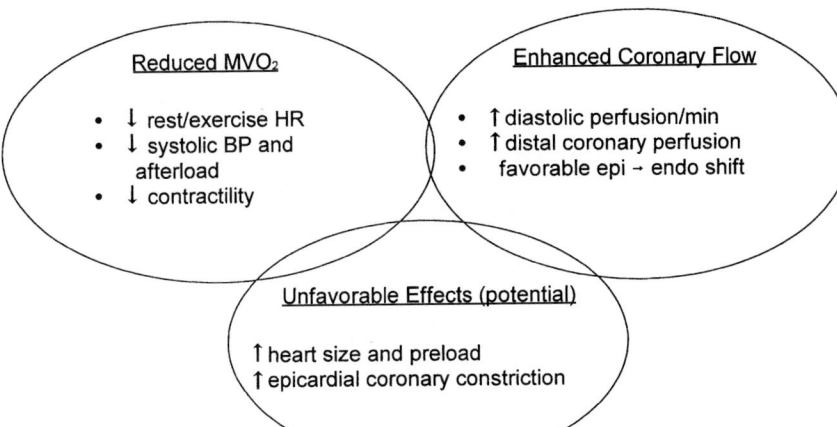

Reduced MVO$_2$

- ↓ rest/exercise HR
- ↓ systolic BP and afterload
- ↓ contractility

Enhanced Coronary Flow

- ↑ diastolic perfusion/min
- ↑ distal coronary perfusion
- favorable epi → endo shift

Unfavorable Effects (potential)

↑ heart size and preload
↑ epicardial coronary constriction

FIGURE 16.4 Mechanism of action—beta-blockers. BP, blood pressure; endo, endocardial; epi, epicardial; HR, heart rate; MVO$_2$, myocardial oxygen consumption. ↓, decreased; ↑, increased.

bility. This proposition has recently been buttressed by evidence from a randomized double-blind study of propranolol and nadolol in normal volunteers whose memory for emotional events was tested by observation of both a neutral and an arousal version of a slide show. The study confirmed that propranolol significantly impaired memory for an emotionally arousing but not a neutral story, whereas an equipotent beta-blocking dose of nadolol did not impair either type of memory and was comparable to placebo (193). Agents with beta$_1$-selective action, such as metoprolol and atenolol, may circumvent the undesirable consequences of nonselective beta-blockade (Table 16.4). Other side effects of beta-blockers include lightheadedness and postural hypotension, cold extremities and Raynaud's phenomenon, gastric upset with heartburn and diarrhea, decreased libido, impotence, and reversible alopecia. Selective beta$_1$-blocker effects, however, are only relatively selective, and at increased doses these agents produce beta$_2$-blockade. Beta-blocking agents with partial agonist activity such as pindolol and acebutolol do not lower resting heart rate or slow atrioventricular conduction and may obviate the untoward effects of beta-blockers on plasma lipids and the central nervous system (194).

Unless contraindicated or limited by unacceptable side effects, all patients should be considered as candidates for beta-blockers, given their demonstrated antianginal efficacy and favorable effect on long-term survival in patients after myocardial infarction (195,196). A variety of beta-blocker

TABLE 16.4 UNTOWARD EFFECTS OF NONSELECTIVE BETA-BLOCKADE

Coronary vasoconstriction
Peripheral circulatory vasoconstriction
Bronchial constriction
Response to hypoglycemia
Impaired hepatic gluconeogenesis
Impaired general awareness
Triglycerides/high-density lipoprotein cholesterol

preparations are available for clinical use in angina, and an inventory of their characteristics, dosages, and frequency of administration is depicted in Table 16.5. Despite initial suggestions that four daily dosages were required, most beta-blockers can now be given either twice a day or once daily, both of which are well received by patients and therefore conducive to good compliance. Although those agents characterized as beta$_1$-selective lose their selectivity at the higher dose ranges, at more modest doses they may be advantageous in patients in whom nonselective beta-blockade is undesirable—those with chronic obstructive lung disease or brittle insulin-dependent diabetes. In general, beta-blockers with significant intrinsic sympathomimetic activity, such as pindolol, have fewer cardioprotective effects and seem to be less effective in control of symptoms and ischemia (194). Although sotalol may be useful in some patients because of its additional antiarrhythmic effects, its propensity to prolong the QT interval and be proarrhythmic limits its broad applicability (197). Whereas heart failure can occasionally be precipitated, there is now unequivocal evidence that the use of beta$_1$-selective beta-blockers—that is, metoprolol (sustained action) (198) and bisoprolol (199)—ameliorate the symptoms, morbidity, and mortality of heart failure. The introduction of carvedilol (200), a third-generation beta-blocker with alpha$_1$-adrenergic blocking activity (which produces vasodilatation), as well as antioxidant and antiproliferative properties, has shown an impressive reduction in cardiac mortality and morbid events in patients with chronic heart failure (201); this has recently been extended to include those with class IV symptoms (202). Recent data support the efficacy of carvedilol, as superior to placebo and comparable to metoprolol, as it relates to antianginal efficacy, exercise time, and time to 1-mm ST-segment depression (203,204).

In a study of 306 patients with mildly symptomatic or asymptomatic ischemia and well-documented coronary disease, Pepine and coworkers (141) examined the effects of atenolol, 100 mg daily, versus placebo on event-free sur-

TABLE 16.5 BETA RECEPTOR ANTAGONISTS FOR ANGINA PECTORIS

Name (proprietary)	Property	Frequency	Daily dose (mg)
Propranolol (Inderal)	Nonselective	Twice a day	80–320
(Inderal LA)		Daily	60–320
Nadolol (Corgard)	Nonselective	Daily	80–240
Timolol (Blocadren)	Nonselective	Twice a day	15–45
Metoprolol (Lopressor)	Beta$_1$-selective	Twice a day	100–400
(Lopressor SR)		Daily	100–400
Atenolol (Tenormin)	Beta$_1$-selective	Daily	50–200
Bisoprolol (Zebeta)	Beta$_1$-selective	Daily	5–10
Acebutolol (Sectral)	Beta$_1$-selective partial ISA	Twice a day	200–600
Pindolol (Visken)	Nonselective ISA	Twice a day	15–45
		Three times a day (>30 mg total)	
Sotalol (Sotacor)[a]	Nonselective with type 3 antiarrhythmic effect	Twice a day	160–480
Carvedilol (Coreg)	Nonselective with vasodilator effects	Twice a day	50–100

ISA, intrinsic sympathomimetic activity; LA, long acting; SR, sustained release.
[a]Sotalol is not approved for angina pectoris use.

vival at 1 year. Because of a significant reduction in risk of adverse events with atenolol versus placebo [relative risk, 0.44; 95% confidence interval, 0.26 to 0.75 (p = .001)], this study was terminated earlier than planned. Importantly, these events were a composite of hard and soft outcomes—that is, death, resuscitation from ventricular arrhythmia, nonfatal myocardial infarction, hospitalization for unstable angina, aggravation of angina requiring known antianginal therapy, and the need for revascularization. Atenolol also significantly reduced heart rate, the number of ischemic episodes on ambulatory monitoring, and the average total duration of ischemia over 48 hours of monitoring. As in other studies, the frequency of ischemia on ambulatory monitoring was predictive of the long-term cardiac risk. Although this study was relatively small in size and underpowered to detect a significant change in death and myocardial infarction, the linkage in treatment response to silent ischemia and the clinical outcome was suggestive.

To ensure patient compliance and minimize adverse side effects, the use of once-daily atenolol or metoprolol twice a day (or a once-daily long-acting preparation) is usually an effective strategy. Titrating the dose to symptomatic relief and assessing the adequacy of beta-blockade based on the response of exercise (not resting) heart rate is a useful approach. Initial unfavorable adverse effects can sometimes be circumvented by dropping the dose to one-half the initial maintenance dose and building gradually over weeks such that full-dose therapy or maximally tolerated amounts can be reached within 6 to 12 weeks.

When symptoms persist or side effects limit treatment with beta-blockers and/or nitrates, the use of calcium antagonists may provide significant additional relief. It has been suggested that a special niche for calcium antagonists resides with Prinzmetal's variant angina patients and those in whom hyperventilation precipitates angina with ST depression during the recovery phase of this form of pro-

vocative stress (205). Although often considered as a single class of therapeutic agents for angina, calcium antagonists, like nitrates and beta-blockers, have substantial heterogeneity (206).

Calcium channel blockers inhibit intracellular entry of calcium ions primarily through the voltage-dependent L-type slow- or long-acting calcium channel. The subsequent reduction in intracellular calcium availability is critical to an activation process that binds actin to myosin, resulting in contraction of cardiac, skeletal, and smooth muscle. Each of these agents possesses significant smooth muscle relaxing effects, resulting in peripheral arterial vasodilatation and afterload reduction, as well as coronary vasodilatation with reduced potential for coronary vasospasm. In the intact circulation, each agent possesses negative inotropic effects; this is most marked with verapamil, least evident with nifedipine, and represents the composite impact of the latter agent's more prominent arterial unloading influence of the direct cardiodepressive effect.

In September 1995, a special announcement from the National Heart, Lung, and Blood Institute on the safety of calcium channel blockers proved a focus for major scientific debate on the safety of these agents. This announcement was fueled in part by a retrospective case control study of patients with hypertension, suggesting an increased risk of myocardial infarction for nifedipine, diltiazem, and verapamil (31%, 63%, and 61%, respectively) (207). Shortly thereafter, a metaanalysis by Furberg of 16 trials using short-acting nifedipine in patients with clinical coronary disease, primarily those with acute ischemic syndromes, revealed a dose-related influence on excess mortality (208). This analysis has been the subject of substantial scientific debate, and the weight of this and other evidence suggests that nifedipine's use as a short-acting preparation without concomitant beta-blocker therapy should be avoided (209). The resulting reflex tachycardia, increased cardiac output, and untoward precipitation of angina and ischemic events that are associated with its use all support this posture. Observational clinical evidence suggests increased ischemic activity during nifedipine therapy in patients who have well-developed coronary collaterals on angiography, implying a possible coronary steal phenomenon as an explanation for this observation (210).

Significant differences also exist between the electrophysiologic effects of dihydropyridines and the verapamil and diltiazem classes; these are absent with nifedipine, but both verapamil and diltiazem slow the resting and exercise heart rate and delay atrioventricular conduction (206). Verapamil and diltiazem also are effective in controlling the ventricular response to atrial fibrillation and in intravenous form are effective in converting reentry paroxysmal supraventricular tachycardia to sinus rhythm. Oral verapamil is effective as prophylaxis against paroxysmal supraventricular tachycardia as well. Sustained-release nifedipine preparations and newer longer-acting dihydropyridine agents such as felodipine and amlodipine have circumvented some of the untoward effects of dihydropyridines and, along with sustained-release formulations of verapamil and diltiazem, have facilitated patient use and compliance through once-daily dosing regimens (211,212). Although initial animal studies suggested calcium antagonists might have a role in retarding or reversing atherosclerosis, clinical studies of nifedipine and nicardipine have failed to show benefit on either lesion progression or regression (213,214). The dosing schedule and effects on heart, atrioventricular conduction, and blood pressure of the various calcium channel blockers available for angina are depicted in Table 16.6. Side effects of headache, dizziness, and flushing along with peripheral edema are most prominent with the dihydropyridines, whereas they are much less frequent with verapamil and diltiazem. Overall, diltiazem is the best tolerated of the first-generation calcium antagonists; constipation, which may be especially troubling in the elderly, is a significant side effect of verapamil. However, each of these first-generation calcium antagonists has negative inotropic effects. This is most pronounced with

verapamil and least with nifedipine, and they are relatively contraindicated in patients with significant left ventricular dysfunction. Special note should be made of the propensity for bepridil to prolong the QT interval and promote proarrhythmic effects in a small proportion of patients; accordingly, the QT interval should be monitored during the initiation of therapy with this agent and the drug discontinued or dosage reduced if there is a more than 25% increment. Accordingly, bepridil should be reserved for patients with refractory angina. The newer-generation dihydropyridines exhibit less net negative inotropic effects, presumably attributable to their greater vascular selectivity. Opie has suggested that amlodipine has a more favorable side effect profile than beta-blocker therapy in angina based on overview of a number of small studies (215). Amlodipine has also been demonstrated to reduce the extent of postexercise ischemic-induced myocardial stunning as compared with isosorbide mononitrate: In 24 patients with chronic stable angina and normal resting left ventricular function, exercise was undertaken until limited by chest pain (216).

Despite similar extent of radionuclide-confirmed perfusion abnormalities, comparable exercise duration, hemodynamic parameters, and ST-segment depression, postexercise stunning defined as a new wall motion abnormality in the area of a perfusion defect occurred less frequently and was less marked while receiving amlodipine than isosorbide mononitrate. These data support prior experimental work demonstrating a direct antistunning effect of calcium antagonists thought to be secondary to inhibition of calcium overload.

In summary, all three classes of antiischemic agents have been demonstrated to relieve symptoms, improve exercise tolerance, and reduce the frequency of silent ischemia. On balance, beta-blockers and, more specifically, the two beta$_1$-antagonists atenolol and metoprolol, seem to be most effective in the relief of ischemia. Ardissino and colleagues (217) studied 280 patients with mild stable angina and compared long-acting metoprolol, 200 mg daily, versus nifedipine in a sustained formulation, 20 mg twice a day. Whereas both

TABLE 16.6 CALCIUM CHANNEL BLOCKERS: DOSING AND PROPERTIES

Blocker	Dose (mg/frequency)	Heart rate	Atrioventricular conduction	Blood pressure
Nifedipine	30–120 three times a day	↑	→	↓↓
Nifedipine GITS	30–180 daily	→	→	↓↓
Diltiazem	30–90 three or four times a day	↓↓	↓	↓
Diltiazem SR	60–120 twice a day	↓↓	↓	↓
Verapamil	80–120 three or four times a day	↓	↓↓	↓
Verapamil SR	120–240 daily or twice a day	↓	↓↓	↓
Amlodipine	2.5–10.0 daily	↑	→	↓↓
Felodipine	5–20 daily	↑	→	↓↓
Nicardipine	10–20 three times a day	↑	→	↓↓
Isradipine	2.5–10.0 twice daily	↑	→	↓↓
Bepridil	200–400 daily	↓	→↓	↓

GITS, gastrointestinal system; SR, sustained release.

agents improved exercise tolerance, there was a greater effect for metoprolol, which seemed most prominent in patients with low exercise tolerance and high-rate pressure products either at rest or during exercise (*e*Fig. 16.4.1). Interestingly, the same investigators (the International Multicentre Angina Exercise Study group) found that the benefit of combination metoprolol and nifedipine seemed to be mainly related to an enhanced response to one versus another agent in nonresponders and not a function of the additive effects of the two agents (218). (The total nifedipine dose in both these studies was somewhat modest, at 40 mg, compared with full 200-mg doses of metoprolol.) The Tibet study of patients with mild stable angina compared 100-mg atenolol to 40-mg nifedipine, and then the combination on exercise testing, ambulatory ECG monitoring, symptoms, and cardiac events (219). Both therapies were equally effective in reducing evidence of ischemia, and combination therapy did not further improve these measures. However, cardiac events at 2 years consisting of mortality, myocardial infarction, unstable angina, and the need for revascularization and further treatment showed a trend for benefit with combination therapy (8.5%) over that observed with atenolol and nifedipine alone (12.8% and 11.2%, respectively, *p* = .14). Hence, it would seem that once symptoms are adequately controlled, reassessment of the patient for continuing objective evidence of ischemia while on treatment may be warranted because such patients seem to be at high risk and potentially deserving of more aggressive intervention (220). This question is under active continuing clinical investigation.

Other Medical Therapy

Despite some initial enthusiasm, angiotensin-converting enzyme inhibitors have proved to be disappointing in ameliorating symptoms or evidence of myocardial ischemia in patients with chronic stable angina (221). However, their role in enhancing survival among patients with left ventricular dysfunction after myocardial infarction is well established. Importantly, angiotensin-converting enzyme inhibitors have been found in both the Survival and Ventricular Enlargement studies and Studies of Left Ventricular Dysfunction to reduce the long-term risk of developing unstable angina and myocardial infarction (222). These studies have now been confirmed and their implications broadened by the Heart Outcomes Prevention Evaluation study, which studied more than 9,000 patients with a history of coronary disease, stroke, peripheral vascular disease, or diabetes in conjunction with at least one additional cardiovascular risk factor and no evidence of heart failure or depressed ejection fraction. More than one-half of the patients had stable angina, and more than one-third had diabetes with coexisting hypertension and prior infarction also common. The treatment group received 10 mg of ramipril for a mean of 5 years, with a significant reduction in all-

cause mortality, cardiovascular death, myocardial infarction, stroke, coronary revascularization, cardiac arrest, heart failure and, not only complications related to diabetes, but also the appearance of new-onset diabetes (223). Interestingly, the Heart Outcomes Prevention Evaluation study, which was a two-by-two design also studying vitamin E, found no difference for this therapy as compared with placebo on cardiovascular outcomes (224). It seems clear that angiotensin-converting enzyme inhibitors exert a multiplicity of effects on the vasculature at diverse sites that extend beyond any of their well-documented hemodynamic effects. These include a potential antiproliferative effect that may retard atherosclerotic plaque growth, an inhibitory effect on the endothelium that may attenuate both vasoconstriction and plaque rupture, and modulation of collagen deposition and left ventricular remodeling. ➤ c56

The role of postmenopausal hormone replacement therapy (HRT) is thought to have been important in secondary prevention among women with coronary disease based on impressive observational data. This thesis has finally been subjected to a randomized study in 2,763 women younger than 80 years of age with established coronary disease who were postmenopausal but possessed an intact uterus (227). HRT was provided by 0.625 mg of conjugated estrogen coupled with 2.500 mg of medroxyprogesterone acetate, and an evaluation of the primary outcome was evaluated over a mean of 4.1 years. Although no significant differences in the primary outcome were found, there was a statistically significant time trend for excess coronary events in the HRT group during the first year and less in years 4 and 5. This was largely modulated by an increase in nonfatal myocardial infarction and overall coronary deaths remained nonsignificantly higher for the HRT group compared with placebo throughout the study despite an 11% lower LDL cholesterol and 10% higher HDL cholesterol in the HRT group. Importantly, there was also an excess of venous thromboembolic events and gallbladder disease in the HRT group. As suggested in an accompanying editorial, "these findings are a sobering reminder of the limitations of observational research, the incompleteness of current understanding of the mechanisms of vascular disease, and the dangers of extrapolation" (228). Whereas there is now clearly no indication for commencing HRT for secondary prevention, sustaining such therapy in women who have received it for longer than a year may be reasonable. HRT in women with prior hysterectomy and as a strategy for primary prevention is the subject of ongoing study.

Hormone therapy in the form of supplemental testosterone in men has recently been demonstrated in a pilot study using low-dose supplemental testosterone (5 mg daily by transdermal patch) to improve exercise-induced ischemia in chronic stable angina (229). These findings were accompanied by a twofold increase in androgen levels, and the magnitude of the response was somewhat greater in those with lower baseline testosterone levels. As the coronary circulation appears more sensitive to the vasodilatory effects of testosterone in larger blood vessels and age-related decrements in androgens are common in elderly men, this interesting initial work deserves confirmation and wider study.

In patients with syndrome X and systemic hypertension, enalapril therapy has been shown to reduce left ventricular hypertrophy, normalize thallium perfusion defects, and increase exercise capacity (230). In a randomized double-blind study, Cannon and coworkers (231) demonstrated that imipramine, 50 mg every night, reduced chest pain frequency by half among patients with syndrome X; the mechanism is unknown but was speculated to relate to a visceral analgesic effect.

In Prinzmetal's variant angina, when symptoms do not respond to nitrates and calcium antagonists, a variety of options have been suggested. Conflicting data exist regarding serotonin antagonism; hence, short-term intravenous ketanserin (232), a specific serotonin blocker, did not attenuate ischemic episodes, whereas chronic therapy with cyproheptadine, a nonselective serotonergic antagonist, has been reported to be of benefit in two case reports (233). Supplementary vitamin E therapy (vitamin acetate, 300 mg per day) added to calcium antagonist in patients with persisting attacks of variant angina significantly inhibited recurrent symptoms (81).

Nonpharmacologic Therapy

Factors associated with mental and physical stress are often underestimated in the therapeutic approach to stable angina. Similarly, the increased physical demands associated with obesity, an increasingly common and correctable risk factor, provide both patient and physician a significant opportunity for reducing cardiac work and enhancing a general sense of well-being. Diet, environmental manipulation, exercise conditioning, stress relaxation, and behavior modification applied appropriately and judiciously (in conjunction with patient and family counseling), may yield significant symptomatic benefit. A recent review of exercise as cardiovascular therapy outlines the physiologic effects of regular exercise and suggests an approach to a rationale for exercise prescription and how this may improve cardiac performance, quality of life, and secondary prevention (234). These considerations are too often neglected, yet they commonly comprise powerful opportunities for enhancing short- and long-term quality of life in stable angina (5).

Revascularization Therapy

Angiography plays a pivotal role in modulating the advisability and need for revascularization. Confirmation of significant epicardial coronary stenosis—that is, 50% or more diameter narrowing—helps to define patient risk and guide therapeutic decision making. If the patient falls into a high-

risk anatomic subset where surgical revascularization is known to improve prognosis, the course of action is relatively clear. Hence, those patients with left main coronary stenosis or a triple-vessel coronary disease are best managed with coronary bypass surgery (234,235). This strategy may also be reasonably applied to patients with two-vessel disease involving the proximal left anterior descending coronary artery, given the recent report of the Coronary Artery Bypass Surgery Trialists Collaboration (236). In the first large-scale prospective observational assessment of angioplasty versus CABG for patients with coronary disease, Mark and colleagues (237) described the 5-year survival experience of patients in the Duke data bank evaluated between 1984 and 1990. As is evident from *e*Figure 16.4.2, a survival advantage was evident for coronary bypass grafting over angioplasty in patients with three-vessel disease and those with two-vessel disease that involved the proximal left anterior descending coronary artery. In 1995, Pocock and colleagues (238) conducted a metaanalysis of 3,371 patients from eight randomized trials comparing angioplasty with coronary bypass surgery for patients with angina observed for a mean of 2.7 years. Three of the trials and 22% of the patients had single-vessel disease and the remaining had multivessel disease. Those with high-risk proximal three-vessel disease and left main stenosis were excluded (*e*Fig. 16.4.3). As is evident in Table 16.7, there was no difference in cardiac death and myocardial infarction at 1 year; however, patients receiving angioplasty had a substantially greater requirement for repeat revascularization and less complete relief of symptoms, which required more antianginal medical therapy. Examples of anatomic subsets well suited for surgical revascularization are depicted in *e*Figure 16.4.3.

The Bypass Angioplasty Revascularization Investigation trial compared the results of coronary bypass surgery with percutaneous transluminal coronary angioplasty (PTCA) in 1,829 patients with multivessel coronary disease and demonstrated superior survival with CABG in the 25% of the patients with diabetes mellitus (239). Hence, the 5-year survival with CABG versus PTCA (80.6% vs. 65.5%, respectively; *p* = .003) was substantially better. Summary results for the major 5-year outcomes of the Bypass Angioplasty Revascularization Investigation trial are depicted in Table 16.7. Subsequently, investigators in the Bypass Angioplasty Revascularization Investigation analyzed a subgroup of 353 patients (19% of the overall sample) who were diabetic with multivessel disease and found a substantial reduction in 5-year all-cause and cardiac mortality in those receiving CABG (especially with internal mammary artery grafts) as compared with PTCA; thus, for CABG, these mortalities were 19.1% and 5.8% and for PTCA 34.7% and 20.6%, respectively. Some, but not universal, support from post hoc analysis of this issue has merged from other trials; accordingly, caution should be exercised in applying PTCA to diabetic patients in the setting of

TABLE 16.7 RANDOMIZED TRIALS COMPARING PTCA AND CABG[a]

	Metaanalysis (n = 3,371; mean follow-up duration 2.7 yr)		Bypass Angioplasty Revascularization Investigation (n = 1,829; mean follow-up duration 5 yr)	
	PTCA	CABG	PTCA	CABG
Mortality (%)	4.6	4.4	13.7	10.7
Myocardial infarction (%)	4.2	5.4	10.9	11.7
Need for PTCA/CABG (%)	33.7	3.3	54.0	8.0
Need for CABG (%)	21.2	1.5	31.0[b]	1.0

CABG, coronary artery bypass graft; PTCA, percutaneous transluminal coronary angioplasty.
[a]Data are percentages and represent mean follow-up of 2.7 years for metaanalysis (218) and 5 years for the Bypass Angioplasty Revascularization Investigation) (239), except for Q-wave myocardial infarction (and need for PTCA/CABG), which is 1 year, in metaanalysis.
[b]11.0% of the PTCA group underwent both PTCA and CABG.

multivessel or multilesion disease (240,241). A summary of the pros and cons of PTCA versus CABG for patients with multivessel disease who fit the criteria of the randomized trials to date is outlined in Figure 16.5 (242). Multivessel disease accounts for approximately 12% of all candidates for revascularization. It is conceptually useful to consider revascularization as a strategy rather than a choice of single procedure (243,244). Hence, in a young patient, angioplasty may be useful in avoiding early surgical procedure and the use of grafts that are of finite number, with the expectation that they will ultimately be required. Angioplasty may be extremely useful in dealing with the problem of graft stenosis that markedly accelerates in venous conduits after the first 6 years. Superior long-term patency with internal mammary as opposed to saphenous vein grafts unequivocally points to using this conduit wherever possible, especially when the left anterior descending coronary artery is being surgically revascularized (241). When revascularization is planned and the prognosis judged to be equal, irrespective of the procedure, the decision regarding the type of revascularization depends on a host of factors that are best left to an informed discussion between patient and physician, taking into account local expertise and experience. Such a discussion will involve the risk and morbidity of the initial procedure, the time for recovery, cost-benefit issues, acceptance of the need for follow-up, and the likelihood of need for ongoing medical therapy and repeat procedures as well as the completeness of revascularization.

The evidence base for these revascularization decisions is now somewhat dated, and major changes in the content and application of medical therapy PTCA and CABG have occurred since its acquisition. These include the use of angiotensin-converting enzyme inhibitors and statins as part of a broad secondary prevention strategy. For percutaneous interventions they are composed of the use of intravenous glycoprotein IIb/IIIa inhibitors, which reduce acute complications, the use of coronary stenting to reduce the recurrence rate of restenosis, and the application of intracoronary radiation to reduce the risk of restenosis after coronary stenting (245–247). For CABG surgery, significant attempts have been made to diminish the morbidity of the operation by using smaller incisions and obviating the use of cardiopulmonary bypass. In particular, minimally invasive direct coronary artery bypass ("MID-CAB" operation)

PRO	CON
PTCA	**PTCA**
• Avoids or defers major surgery • Rapid recovery • Shorter initial hospitalization • Less early morbidity and MI • 80% less costly @ 2 yrs	• Incomplete revascularization • More angina • More medical therapy • More subsequent hospitalization • More subsequent revascularization • Possibly less long-term survival in MVD
CABG	**CABG**
• More complete revascularization • Excellent symptom relief • Less anti-anginal meds • Less subsequent hospitalization • Less subsequent revascularization • Possibly better survival in multivessel CAD	• More early morbidity/MI • Longer recovery • Longer initial hospital stay

FIGURE 16.5 Weighing the balance for revascularization. CABG, coronary artery bypass graft surgery; CAD, coronary artery disease; MI, myocardial infarction; MVD, multivessel disease; PTCA, percutaneous transluminal coronary angioplasty. [Adapted from Simoons ML. Myocardial revascularization—bypass surgery or angioplasty? (editorial). *N Engl J Med* 1996;335:275–277, with permission.]

through a small left thoracotomy incision with a thoraco-scope permits surgery on the left anterior descending coronary artery and its diagonal branches, whereas a right-sided incision allows access to the right coronary artery. Early results in appropriately selected patients are encouraging, with reduced morbidity and hospital stay and rapid return to normal activity (241).

In patients with single-vessel coronary disease, exclusive of the proximal left anterior descending and at low risk—that is, with normal left ventricular function, preserved exercise tolerance, and nondisabling angina—the evidence from two randomized trials supports contemporary medical therapy to be at least as effective as PTCA (248) with regard to the outcomes of death and myocardial infarction (249). In a third study, where the medical group received aggressive lipid-lowering therapy with 80 mg of atorvastatin (250), medically treated patients tended to have a lower frequency of ischemic events as well as a delay to their first occurrence. Relief of angina was superior with PTCA in all three trials, but the majority of this benefit attenuated over time. It should be emphasized that none of these trials used state-of-the-art interventional procedures with systematic concurrent intravenous glycoprotein IIb/IIIa platelet inhibition or intracoronary stenting (245,246). This composite approach has been shown to have a substantial effect on reducing the risk of 30-day myocardial infarction and death (246).

Three novel alternatives to conventional PTCA and CABG have recently been introduced: percutaneous transmyocardial laser revascularization (PTMR), enhanced external counterpulsation, and spinal cord stimulation (SCS). These are discussed in detail in the CD-ROM and online version of this chapter. ❦ c57

NATURAL HISTORY, RISK ASSESSMENT, AND REDUCTION

Substantial progress has been made in the evaluation of the risk of fatal events in patients with coronary artery disease. A remarkable spectrum of risk exists within patients depending on the interaction of a variety of information that can be acquired from the history, clinical examination, electrocardiogram, and laboratory findings.

Whereas a 60-year-old patient with stable angina and no comorbid conditions may have a 98.7% 1-year survival, the presence of prior infarction, diabetes, heart failure, and a high-risk exercise treadmill can markedly reduce the 1-year survival (261). Nomograms developed during the twenty-seventh Bethesda, Maryland, conference, "Matching the Intensity of Risk Factor Management with the Hazard for Coronary Events," exist to assimilate the variety of factors known to predict outcome and permit the physician to practically apply such information for purposes of the assessment of an individual patient (*e*Fig. 16.5.1) (261). A defining principle of this strategy is the application of com-

prehensive risk management in direct proportion to the level of risk identified, giving both physician and patient the requisite knowledge and enthusiasm to initiate and sustain a risk-reduction program (262). This strategy is particularly important given the dramatic new developments in risk reduction.

A rigorous effort to address correctable risk factors is a fundamental component of the overall management of the patient with stable angina. Smoking cessation is the single most powerful contribution patients can make to their own well-being and destiny. A variety of approaches including behavior modification and pharmacologic assistance have been used. Nicotine-replacement therapy using transdermal patches has had modest success without adversely affecting angina frequency (263). Achieving an ideal body weight through dietary modification, which also reduces cholesterol and saturated fat, controlling elevated blood pressure and blood sugar, along with incorporating regular physical activity into a patient's daily routine, can lead to enhanced quality of life with a higher threshold of physical activity before symptom development and improved prognosis (264). Improved cardiovascular conditioning such that the same degree of effort can be achieved at a lower rate pressure product may account in part for this phenomenon (265). The most important development in risk modification is the introduction of inhibitors of hydroxymethylglutaryl coenzyme A reductase, which have been substantially more successful in reducing LDL cholesterol than diet or prior drug interventions. Appreciation that reduction in total and LDL cholesterol of the order of 25% and 35%, respectively, can achieve a similar dramatic reduction in total and coronary mortality, myocardial infarction, and the need for coronary revascularization has provided the physician with important new opportunities and responsibilities (266). Sequential angiographic studies have demonstrated both a reduction in the frequency of progression and an increase in the frequency of regression of coronary atherosclerotic lesions in conjunction with clinical improvement (267). Because the extent of coronary arterial regression by sequential angiography seems too modest to explain the dramatic clinical benefit, it is presumed that this benefit relates to stabilization of coronary plaque and extraluminal remodeling with a commensurate reduction in the frequency of plaque fissuring and the coronary vascular accidents that ensue. It has been speculated that the interaction between hypercholesterolemia, lipid peroxidation, and platelet activation provides the statin drugs with an opportunity to favorably modulate the attendant prothrombotic state (268). The documentation of an antiaggregatory effect on platelets in patients with coronary artery disease after only 2 to 3 months of pravastatin therapy, coupled with evidence that statins can reduce fibrinogen levels, demonstrates their potential to behave as antithrombotic agents (269,270). This effect could be expressed temporally in advance of their effect on plaque stabilization and regression. Emerging data from two clinical studies have confirmed the ability of the statins to reduce ischemia detected by ambulatory monitoring. Andrews and coworkers (271) have shown in 96 patients with known stable coronary disease that lovastatin reduced the number of ischemic episodes by 65% in the control group versus 10% in placebo patients ($p <.001$) within only 4 to 6 months of commencing therapy. Van Boven and colleagues (272) assessed the efficacy of 40 mg of pravastatin in 768 male patients with stable angina and found a reduction in the duration and number of ischemic episodes coupled with a decline in ischemic-related clinical events. They observed changes from baseline in the duration of ischemia (60 ± 13 mm per minute and 80 ± 12 mm per minute) and ischemic burden (34 ± 6 and 41 ± 5 mm per minute) for placebo and pravastatin, respectively (*e*Fig. 16.5.2). Restoration toward normal coronary vasomotion as a result of lipid-lowering strategies with lovastatin has been unequivocally demonstrated after 6 months of therapy, and this improvement in endothelium-dependent vasomotion seems to be accentuated by combining cholesterol-lowering therapy produced by lovastatin with antioxidant therapy achieved with the use of probucol (273). Given that the majority of lesions responsible for acute myocardial infarction develops from noncritically stenosed coronary lesions, these observations from lipid-lowering trials acquire additional credibility and coherence (274). Targeting a reduction of total cholesterol to the range of 3.0 to 5.2 mmol per L as identified in the Scandinavian Simvastatin Survival Study of secondary prevention seems a legitimate goal (266). It is likely, however, that the risk associated with elevated total and LDL cholesterol is continuous. Hence, when other risk factors for coronary disease are present, more aggressive lipid lowering may be sensible. Pharmacologic management of serum cholesterol in patients older than 75 years remains of uncertain value and requires individualization of therapy. However, the benefit seen in the Scandinavian Simvastatin Survival Study was evident among all age groups up to the exclusion cutpoint of 70 years of age and, importantly, was also seen in both genders. A variety of endogenous factors known to play either a thrombogenic or coagulation inhibitory role have been identified as markers of increased risk (275). Serum fibrinogen is the most powerful and independent of these and has a particularly potent impact when present in association with increased cholesterol (276). Increased platelet aggregability, thrombin activity and generation, factor VII, and tissue-type plasminogen activator antigen have all been associated with increased risk of coronary events. The benefit of aspirin and warfarin and the interest in the development of oral antithrombin compounds relate to these risks. Continuing epidemiologic evidence provides considerable but not uniform weight to the role of homocysteine

as a risk factor for cardiovascular disease. A recent American Heart Association Science Advisory cautions that there is as yet still no indication for population-wide screening or therapy (277). However, in high-risk patients, a strategy associated with dietary incorporation of a diet fortified with the recommendations of the Food and Nutrition Board of the Academy of Sciences Institute of Medicine that includes folic acid, vitamin B_6, and vitamin B_{12} of 400 µg, 1.7 mg, and 2.4 µg, respectively, is appropriate. In the event that this is unsuccessful in reducing basal homocysteine less than 10 µmol per L, supplementation with a multivitamin of 400 µg of folic acid, 2 mg of vitamin B_6, and 6 µg of vitamin B_{12} is suggested (277). The potential benefit of vitamin supplementation to reduce oxidation of LDL cholesterol is currently under investigation (262).

CONTROVERSIES AND PERSONAL PERSPECTIVES

Using symptoms as the solitary guide for appropriate therapy of stable angina is no longer an acceptable treatment strategy. Most ischemia is clinically silent, and its total extent bears a prognostic relationship to outcome. Hence, consideration should be given to assessing provocable or ambulatory ischemia as part of overall management. Validation that effective medical treatment of silent ischemia improves long-term outcome remains a promising and plausible hypothesis that is currently under study and requires confirmation.

Pharmacologic interventions such as the use of angiotensin-converting enzyme inhibitors and hydroxymethylglutaryl coenzyme A reductase inhibitors that reduce morbid events and the progression of coronary vascular disease have broad implications for huge populations. Movement of the gains achieved through secondary prevention toward primary prevention among patients at risk is one of the most fundamental and major future challenges. Realization of this goal requires incorporation of a collaborative approach with a variety of nonphysician health care providers, who are often better equipped to provide the necessary advice and follow-up (278).

Now that regression of disease and enhanced prognosis as a result of angiotensin-converting enzyme inhibitors and lipid-lowering strategies is a clinical reality, the time is ripe for new prospective studies comparing this strategy with revascularization in selected anatomic subsets.

The growing epidemic of obesity and diabetes will place new emphasis not only on understanding the multiplicity of the effects of insulin resistance but also on how to modify this especially unhappy synergism between environmental factors and genetics. Further insights into the triggers of myocardial ischemia and their relationship to behavior and mental stress will lead to nonpharmacologic strategies aimed at stress relaxation and behavior modification with avoidance of ischemia (279).

Angiography with a view to revascularization of all lesions more than 50% diameter narrowing in patients with stable coronary disease irrespective of prognostic stratification is unwarranted. An appropriate profile of risk, including noninvasive documentation of left ventricular function, reversible ischemia, exercise tolerance, and the response to pharmacologic therapy, is sensible, cost-effective, and responsible stewardship of resources.

The promise of transmyocardial and percutaneous laser revascularization appears more elusive than 5 years ago given the attendant morbidity and mortality of the procedure(s) and uncertainty about long-term efficacy. Rigorous phase IV surveillance of this technique, now that it has been U.S. Food and Drug Administration–approved, will be necessary to establish its ultimate role.

Finally, care of the patient with chronic stable angina is a lifelong proposition. It takes time and patience to provide a comprehensive treatment plan, especially in non–high-risk patients. Issues associated with lifestyle, occupation, age, quality of life, the ability and motivation to comply with a complex medical program, and lifestyle preferences all require consideration. Active participation of the patient as a full partner in this collaborative venture is most likely to lead to a successful long-term strategy that couples symptom control, prevention of morbid events, improved survival, and retardation or reversal of the underlying disease based on targeting correctable risk factors.

FUTURE DIRECTIONS

The frequency of thrombus and complex plaque formation including inflammation within culprit lesions in patients with stable angina suggests a continuum between stable and unstable syndromes mediated by platelet activation, oxidative stress, dysfunctional endothelium, vasoconstriction, thrombus formation, and the potential for rapid acceleration in growth of atherosclerotic plaque (275). Endothelial injury and its interaction with inflammation, monocytes and mediators extruded from inflammatory cells, platelets, and other sources are an intense focus of investigation. It now appears that the proinflammatory milieu associated with unstable angina can also be demonstrated in some patients with stable angina as demonstrated by elevations in C-reactive protein, macrophage colony-stimulating factor, interleukin-6, and leukocyte elastase (280–283). There appears to be at least a modest relationship between serologic evidence of inflammation, the extent of coronary disease and ischemia, and the likelihood

of future unfavorable cardiovascular events. Explosive developments in cell biology associated with better understanding of adhesion molecules and their role of the growth of the atherosclerotic plaque are likely to lead to entirely new classes of efficacious drugs (275). Despite its limitations, aspirin's venerability is likely to survive, possibly related, in part, to its antiinflammatory as well as its relatively weak antiplatelet effect (284). Notwithstanding the clinical disappointment associated with the introduction of oral glycoprotein IIb/IIIa antagonists during the convalescence of acute coronary syndromes (285), the identification and cloning of the P2Y subset 1,2 receptor and its demonstration of abundant expression on the surface of human platelets provides new opportunities for more rational drug design (286). So too is the future development of specific oral antithrombin agents likely to add usefully to our therapeutic armamentarium.

Further advances in the assessment of the coronary arterial tree will enhance our on-line assessment of coronary arterial plaque burden as well as its composition and stability (164,287). These will use novel ultrasonic measures, thermal detection interrogating temperature heterogeneity, and magnetic resonance imaging (288,289). These techniques will underscore the diffuse nature of coronary atherosclerosis and highlight the need for an appropriately broad strategy directed toward the total endothelial lining and what modulates its health and disease.

Major advances within the next 5 years are likely to be seen in association with the conduct of percutaneous coronary intervention (290). Further refinement in the development of intravascular stents that are biologically degradable and pharmacologically active may well additionally reduce the frequency of restenosis. The long-term effects of intracoronary radiation will establish whether enthusiasm concerning its short-term impact on restenosis after stent implantation is warranted. Advances in molecular biology coupled with the introduction of vascular endothelial growth factor provide creative new opportunities for revascularization in the face of inoperable diffuse disease and obstructed vessels (291). This will be especially applicable to the increasing cohort of patients who present with recurrent symptoms after prior revascularization. Less traumatic, minimally invasive coronary bypass surgery will become one component of an overall revascularization strategy: This will include percutaneous delivery of a melange of options such as mechanical dilation, stenting, radiation, and molecular modulation of both vascular and tissue growth. A central challenge for the practicing clinician and the majority of patients with stable angina will be how to apply and integrate a sensible, cost-effective solution from such a dazzling array of medical advances.

THE FUTURE

One of the most extraordinary features of stable ischemic syndromes is that our knowledge and approach are anything but stable! Since the publication of the first edition of this text, major new clinical trials and evidence have emerged to influence our thinking about pharmacologic therapy and approaches to revascularization. The sequencing of the human genome and the exploitation of the potential of molecular biology have begun to dramatically alter our thinking and, in some instances, management. This will accelerate progress toward closing the gap on the 50% of coronary atherosclerotic cases where known risk factors fail to account for its development. Polymorphisms of a variety of genes regulating the immune system, vascular tone, coagulation, and lipid metabolism are or will be uncovered (292). These discoveries will in turn spawn pharmacogenetic developments that provide "boutique" solutions for specific defects.

The future seems both challenging and filled with opportunity given the tremendous advances in cell biology that are enhancing our ability to comprehend the pathophysiology of coronary disease, better assess its long-term risk, and construct novel therapies (293). The therapeutic success of the past decade with its attendant prolongation of life will further accelerate the number of elderly patients seeking relief from symptomatic coronary disease. Further diagnostic advances will help discern the risk of future events and thereby guide the application of multiple therapeutic choices. Better strategies will be required to ensure practitioners apply evidence-based medicine to the broad population at risk; the emergence of two major guidelines concerning chronic stable angina management and the application of coronary artery bypass surgery are required reading for the clinical practitioner.

Engagement of the broad public in a response to the evidence supporting the promotion of healthy lifestyles and the adoption of behavior that reduces morbidity and mortality from atherosclerosis must surely constitute the centerpiece of our ongoing efforts.

REFERENCES

1. Heberden W. Commentaries on the history and cure of diseases. In: Wilius FA, Keys TE, eds. *Classics of cardiology*. New York: Henry Schuman, Dover Publications, 1941:I–221.
2. *2000 Heart and stroke statistical update [report]*. Dallas: American Heart Association, 2001.
3. Kannel WB, Feinleib M. Natural history of angina pectoris in the Framingham study. Prognosis and survival. *Am J Cardiol* 1972;29:154–163.
4. Elveback LR, Connolly DC. Prognosis of patients with coronary heart disease based on initial manifestation. *Mayo Clin Proc* 1985;60:305–311.
5. Gibbons RJ, Chatterjee K, Daley J, et al. ACC/AHA/ACP-ASIM guidelines for the management of patients with chronic stable angina: a report of the American College of Cardiology/American Heart Association Task Force on Practice Guidelines (Committee on the Management of Patients with Chronic Stable Angina). *J Am Coll Cardiol* 1999;33:2092–2197.
6. *Heart and stroke facts: 1996 statistical supplement [report]*. Dallas: American Heart Association, 1997.
7. Maseri A, Crea F, Kaski JC, Davies G. Mechanisms and significance of cardiac ischemic pain. *Prog Cardiovasc Dis* 1992;35:1–18.
8. Crea F, Pupita G, Galassi AR, et al. Role of adenosine in pathogenesis of anginal pain. *Circulation* 1990;81:164–172.
9. Gould KL, Lipscomb K, Hamilton GW. Physiologic basis for assessing critical coronary stenosis: instantaneous flow response and regional distribution during coronary hyperemia as measures of coronary flow reserve. *Am J Cardiol* 1974;33:87–94.
10. Treasure CB, Klein JL, Weintraub WS, et al. Beneficial effects of cholesterol-lowering therapy on the coronary endothelium in patients with coronary artery disease. *N Engl J Med* 1995;332:481–487.
11. Uren NG, Crake T, Lefroy DC, et al. Reduced coronary vasodilator function in infarcted and normal myocardium after myocardial infarction. *N Engl J Med* 1994;331:222–227.
12. Uren NG, Marraccini P, Gistri R, et al. Altered coronary vasodilator reserve and metabolism in myocardium subtended by normal arteries in patients with coronary artery disease. *J Am Coll Cardiol* 1993;22:650–658.
13. Smith KS, Papp C. Episodic, postural and linked angina. *BMJ* 1962;(Dec):1425–1430.
14. Juneau M, Johnstone M, Dempsey E, Waters DD. Exercise-induced myocardial ischemia in a cold environment. *Circulation* 1989;79:1015–1020.
15. Adams KF, Koch G, Chatterjee B, et al. Acute elevation of blood carboxyhemoglobin to 6% impairs exercise performance and aggravates symptoms in patients with ischemic heart disease. *J Am Coll Cardiol* 1988;12:900–909.
16. Winniford MD, Wheelan KR, Kremers MS. Smoking-induced coronary vasoconstriction in patients with atherosclerotic coronary artery disease: evidence for adrenergically mediated alterations in coronary artery tone. *Circulation* 1986;73:662–667.
17. Deanfield J, Wright C, Krikler S, et al. Cigarette smoking

and the treatment of angina with propranolol, atenolol, and nifedipine. *N Engl J Med* 1984;310:951–954.

18. Deanfield JE, Selwyn AP, Chierchia S, et al. Myocardial ischaemia during daily life in patients with stable angina: its relation to symptoms and heart rate changes. *Lancet* 1983;2:753–758.

19. Yeung AC, Vekshtein VI, Krantz DS, et al. The effect of atherosclerosis on the vasomotor response of coronary arteries to mental stress. *N Engl J Med* 1991;325:1551–1556.

20. Rubanyi GM, Frye R, Holmes DR, Vanhoutte PM. Vasoconstrictor activity of coronary sinus plasma from patients with coronary artery disease. *J Am Coll Cardiol* 1987;9:1243–1249.

21. van der Wal AC, Becker AE, Koch KT, et al. Clinically stable angina pectoris is not necessarily associated with histologically stable atherosclerotic plaques. *Heart* 1996;76:312–316.

22. Golino P, Piscione F, Benedict CR, et al. Local effect of serotonin released during coronary angioplasty. *N Engl J Med* 1994;330:523–528.

23. Freeman MR, de Yang L, Langer A, et al. Frequency of transient reductions in left ventricular ejection fraction at rest in coronary artery disease. *Am J Cardiol* 1994;74:137–143.

24. Beleslin BD, Ostojic M, Stepanovic J, et al. Stress echocardiography in the detection of myocardial ischemia. *Circulation* 1994;90:1168–1176.

25. Langer A, Freeman MR, Josse RG, et al. Detection of silent myocardial ischemia in diabetes mellitus. *Am J Cardiol* 1991;67:1073–1078.

26. Parker JO, Chiong MA, West RO, Case RB. Sequential alterations in myocardial lactate metabolism, S-T segments, and left ventricular function during angina induced by atrial pacing. *Circulation* 1969;XL:113–131.

27. Upton MT, Rerych SK, Newman GE, et al. Detecting abnormalities in left ventricular function during exercise before angina and ST-segment depression. *Circulation* 1980;62:341–349.

28. Ambrosio G, Betocchi S, Pace L, et al. Prolonged impairment of regional contractile function after resolution of exercise-induced angina. *Circulation* 1996;94:2455–2464.

29. Cohn PF. *Silent myocardial ischemia: present status modern concepts cardiovascular disease.* New York: Marcel Dekker, 1987:1–5.

30. Krantz DS, Hedges SM, Gabbay FH, et al. Triggers of angina and ST-segment depression in ambulatory patients with coronary artery disease: evidence for an uncoupling of angina and ischemia. *Am Heart J* 1994;128:703–712.

31. Gabbay FH, Krantz DS, Kop WJ, et al. Triggers of myocardial ischemia during daily life in patients with coronary artery disease: physical and mental activities, anger and smoking. *J Am Coll Cardiol* 1996;27:585–592.

32. Rozanski A, Bairey CN, Krantz DS, et al. Mental stress and the induction of silent myocardial ischemia in patients with coronary artery disease. *N Engl J Med* 1988;318:1005–1012.

33. Legault SE, Langer A, Armstrong PW, Freeman MR. Usefulness of ischemic response to mental stress in predicting silent myocardial ischemia during ambulatory monitoring. *Am J Cardiol* 1995;75:1007–1011.

34. Mulcahy D, Keegan J, Cunningham D, et al. Circadian variation of total ischaemic burden and its alteration with anti-anginal agents. *Lancet* 1988;2:755–758.

35. Sheps DS, Heiss G. Sudden death and silent myocardial ischemia. *Am Heart J* 1989;117:177–184.

36. Rocco MB, Barry J, Campbell S, et al. Circadian variation of transient myocardial ischemia in patients with coronary artery disease. *Circulation* 1987;75:395–400.

37. Benhorin J, Banai S, Moriel M, et al. Circadian variations in ischemic threshold and their relation to the occurrence of ischemic episodes. *Circulation* 1993;87:808–814.

38. Andrews TC, Fenton T, Toyosaki N, et al. Subsets of ambulatory myocardial ischemia based on heart rate activity: circadian distribution and response to anti-ischemic medication. *Circulation* 1993;88:92–100.

39. Parker JD, Testa MA, Jimenez AH, et al. Morning increase in ambulatory ischemia in patients with stable coronary artery disease. *Circulation* 1994;89:604–614.

40. Stone PH. Unravelling the mechanisms of ambulatory ischemia. *Circulation* 1990;82:1528–1530.

41. Sheps DS, Maixner W, Hinderliter AL. Mechanisms of pain perception in patients with silent myocardial ischemia. *Am Heart J* 1990;119:983–987.

42. Falcone C, Auguadro C, Sconocchia R, et al. Susceptibility to pain during coronary angioplasty: usefulness of pulpal test. *J Am Coll Cardiol* 1996;28:903–909.

43. Falcone C, Specchia G, Rondanelli R, et al. Correlation between beta-endorphin plasma levels and anginal symptoms in patients with coronary artery disease. *J Am Coll Cardiol* 1988;11:719–723.

44. Miller PF, Sheps DS, Bragdon EE, et al. Aging and pain perception in ischemic heart disease. *Am Heart J* 1990;120:22–30.

45. Levine SA. Carotid sinus massage: a new diagnostic test for angina pectoris. *JAMA* 1962;182:1332–1334.

46. Langer A, Freeman MR, Josse RG, Armstrong PW. Metaiodobenzylguanidine imaging in diabetes mellitus: assessment of cardiac sympathetic denervation and its relation to autonomic dysfunction and silent myocardial ischemia. *J Am Coll Cardiol* 1995;25:610–618.

47. Rosen SD, Paulesu E, Nihoyannopoulos P, et al. Silent ischemia as a central problem: regional brain activation compared in silent and painful myocardial ischemia. *Ann Intern Med* 1996;124:939–949.

48. Pepine CJ. Does the brain know when the heart is ischemic? [editorial]. *Ann Intern Med* 1996;124:1006–1007.

49. Kramer JR, Kitazume H, Proudfit WL, Sones FM. Clinical significance of isolated coronary bridges: benign and frequent condition involving the left anterior descending artery. *Am Heart J* 1982;103:283–288.

50. Angelini P, Trivellato M, Donis J, Leachman RD. Myocardial bridges: a review. *Prog Cardiovasc Dis* 1983;26:75–88.

51. Ge J, Erbel R, Rupprecht HJ, et al. Comparison of intravascular ultrasound and angiography in the assessment of myocardial bridging. *Circulation* 1994;89:1725–1732.

52. Schwarz ER, Klues HG, vom Dahl J, et al. Functional, angiographic and intracoronary Doppler flow characteristics in symptomatic patients with myocardial bridging: effect of short-term intravenous beta blocker medication. *J Am Coll Cardiol* 1996;27:1637–1645.

53. Hartnell GG, Parnell BM, Pridie RB. Coronary artery ectasia. *Br Heart J* 1985;54:392–395.

54. Swanton RH, Thomas ML, Coltart DJ, et al. Coronary artery ectasia: a variant of occlusive coronary arteriosclerosis. *Br Heart J* 1978;40:393–400.

55. Markis JE, Joffe CD, Cohn PF, et al. Clinical significance of coronary arterial ectasia. *Am J Cardiol* 1976;37:217–222.

56. Sorrell VL, Davis MJ, Bove AA. Origins of coronary artery ectasia. *Lancet* 1996;347:136–137.

57. Om A, Ellahham S, Vetrovec GW. Radiation-induced coronary artery disease. *Am Heart J* 1992;124:1598–1602.

58. Tuzcu EM, De Franco A, Goormastic M, et al. Dichotomous pattern of coronary atherosclerosis 1 to 9 years after transplantation: insights from systematic intravascular ultrasound imaging. *J Am Coll Cardiol* 1996;27:839–846.

59. Likoff W, Segal BL, Kasparian H. Paradox of normal selective coronary arteriograms in patients considered to have unmistakable coronary heart disease. *N Engl J Med* 1967;276:1063–1066.

60. Kemp HG, Elliott WC, Gorlin R. The anginal syndrome with normal coronary arteriography. *Trans Assoc Am Physicians* 1967;80:59–70.

61. Kemp HG, Vokonas PS, Cohn PF, Gorlin R. The anginal syndrome associated with normal coronary arteriograms: report of a six year experience. *Am J Med* 1973;54:735–742.

62. Cannon RO. Chest pain with normal coronary angiograms [editorial]. *N Engl J Med* 1993;328:1706–1708.

63. Cannon RO, Camici PG, Epstein SE. Pathophysiological dilemma of syndrome X. *Circulation* 1992;85:883–892.

64. Cannon RO, Dilsizian V, Correa R, et al. Chronic deterioration in left ventricular function in patients with microvascular angina [abstract]. *J Am Coll Cardiol* 1991;17:28A.

65. Cannon RO, Cattau EL, Yakshe PN, et al. Coronary flow reserve, esophageal motility, and chest pain in patients with angiographically normal coronary arteries. *Am J Med* 1990;88:217–222.

66. Egashira K, Inou T, Hirooka Y, et al. Evidence of impaired endothelium-dependent coronary vasodilatation in patients with angina pectoris and normal coronary angiograms. *N Engl J Med* 1993;328:1659–1664.

67. Cannon RO, Peden DB, Berkebile C, et al. Airway hyperresponsiveness in patients with microvascular angina: evidence for a diffuse disorder of smooth muscle responsiveness. *Circulation* 1990;82:2011–2017.

68. Sax FL, Cannon RO, Hanson C, Epstein SE. Impaired forearm vasodilator reserve in patients with microvascular angina: evidence of a generalized disorder of vascular function? *N Engl J Med* 1987;317:1366–1370.

69. Inobe Y, Kugiyama K, Morita E, et al. Role of adenosine in pathogenesis of syndrome X: assessment with coronary hemodynamic measurements and thallium-201 myocardial single-photon emission computed tomography. *J Am Coll Cardiol* 1996;28:890–896.

69a. Gibbons RJ, Chatterjee K, Daley J, et al. ACC/AHA/ACP-ASIM guidelines for the management of patients with chronic stable angina: a report of the American College of Cardiology/American Heart Association Task Force on Practice Guidelines (Committee on the Management of Patients with Chronic Stable Angina). *J Am Coll Cardiol* 1999;33:2092–2197.

70. Iriarte MM, Caso R, Murga N, et al. Microvascular angina pectoris in hypertensive patients with left ventricular hypertrophy and diagnostic value of exercise thallium-201 scintigraphy. *Am J Cardiol* 1995;75:335–339.

71. Reaven GM. Role of insulin resistance in human disease: Banting lecture 1988. *Diabetes* 1988;37:1595–1607.

72. Godsland IF, Stevenson JC. Insulin resistance: syndrome or tendency? *Lancet* 1995;346:100–103.

73. Goodfellow J, Owens D, Henderson A. Cardiovascular syndromes X, endothelial dysfunction and insulin resistance. *Diabetes Res Clin Pract* 1996;31[Suppl]:S163–S171.

74. Prinzmetal M, Kennamer R, Merliss R, et al. Angina pectoris: I. A variant form of angina pectoris. *Am J Med* 1959;27:375–388.

75. Mark DB, Califf RM, Morris KG, et al. Clinical characteristics and long-term survival of patients with variant angina. *Circulation* 1984;69:880–888.

76. Maseri A, Parodi O, Severi S, Pesola A. Transient transmural reduction of myocardial blood flow, demonstrated by thallium-201 scintigraphy, as a cause of variant angina. *Circulation* 1976;54:280–288.

77. Onaka H, Hirota Y, Shimada S, et al. Clinical observation of spontaneous anginal attacks and multivessel spasm in variant angina pectoris with normal coronary arteries: evaluation by 24-hour 12-lead electrocardiography with computer analysis. *J Am Coll Cardiol* 1996;27:38–44.

78. Morita E, Ohmori K, Matsuyama T, et al. A new noninvasive method of diagnosing vasospastic angina based on dilation response of the left main coronary artery to nitroglycerin as measured by echocardiography. *J Am Coll Cardiol* 1996;27:1450–1457.

79. Kugiyama K, Yasue H, Okumura K, et al. Nitric oxide activity is deficient in spasm arteries of patients with coronary spastic angina. *Circulation* 1996;94:266–272.

80. Satake K, Lee JD, Shimizu H, et al. Relation between severity of magnesium deficiency and frequency of anginal attacks in men with variant angina. *J Am Coll Cardiol* 1996;28:897–902.

81. Miwa K, Miyaga Y, Igawa A, et al. Vitamin E deficiency in variant angina. *Circulation* 1996;94:14–18.

82. Lanza GA, Pedrotti P, Pasceri V, et al. Autonomic changes associated with spontaneous coronary spasm in patients with variant angina. *J Am Coll Cardiol* 1996;28:1249–1256.

83. Ogawa H, Yasue H, Oshima S, et al. Circadian variation of plasma fibrinopeptide A level in patients with variant angina. *Circulation* 1989;80:1617–1626.

84. Previtali M, Ardissino D, Barberis P, et al. Hyperventilation and ergonovine tests in Prinzmetal's variant angina pectoris in men. *Am J Cardiol* 1989;63:17–20.

85. Sugiishi M, Takatsu F. Cigarette smoking is a major risk factor for coronary spasm. *Circulation* 1993;87:76–79.

86. Nademanee K, Gorelick DA, Josephson MA, et al. Myocardial ischemia during cocaine withdrawal. *Ann Intern Med* 1989;111:876–880.

87. Yasue H, Takizawa A, Nagao M, et al. Long-term prognosis for patients with variant angina and influential factors. *Circulation* 1988;78:1–9.

88. Yasue H, Omote S, Takizawa A, et al. Circadian variation

of exercise capacity in patients with Prinzmetal's variant angina: role of exercise-induced coronary arterial spasm. *Circulation* 1979;59:938–948.

89. Crea F, Chierchia S, Kaski JC, et al. Provocation of coronary spasm by dopamine in patients with active variant angina pectoris. *Circulation* 1986;74:262–269.

90. Harding MB, Leithe ME, Mark DB, et al. Ergonovine maleate testing during cardiac catheterization: a 10 year perspective in 3,447 patients without significant coronary artery disease or Prinzmetal's variant angina. *J Am Coll Cardiol* 1992;20:107–111.

91. Marber MS, Joy MD, Yellon DM. Is warm-up in angina ischaemic preconditioning? *Br Heart J* 1994;72:213–215.

92. Rinaldi CA, Masani ND, Linka AZ, Hall RJ. Effect of repetitive episodes of exercise induced myocardial ischaemia on left ventricular function in patients with chronic stable angina: evidence for cumulative stunning or ischaemic preconditioning? *Heart* 1999;81:404–411.

93. Stewart RAH, Simmonds MB, Williams MJA. Time course of "warm up" in stable angina. *Am J Cardiol* 1995;76:70–73.

94. Williams DO, Bass TA, Gewirtz H, Most AS. Adaptation to the stress of tachycardia in patients with coronary artery disease: insight into the mechanism of the warm-up phenomenon. *Circulation* 1985;71:687–692.

95. Okazaki Y, Kodama K, Sato H, et al. Attenuation of increased regional myocardial oxygen consumption during exercise as a major cause of warm-up phenomenon. *J Am Coll Cardiol* 1993;21:1597–1604.

96. Franklin KA, Nilsson JB, Sahlin C. Sleep apnea and nocturnal angina. *Lancet* 1995;345:1085–1087.

97. Campeau L. Grading of angina pectoris. *Circulation* 1976;54:522–523.

98. Cox J, Naylor CD. The Canadian Cardiovascular Society grading scale for angina pectoris: is it time for refinements? *Ann Intern Med* 1992;117:677–683.

99. Roberts KB, Califf RM, Harrell FE Jr, et al. The prognosis for patients with new-onset angina who have undergone cardiac catheterization. *Circulation* 1983;68:970–978.

100. Castaner A, Roig E, Serra A, et al. Risk stratification and prognosis of patients with recent onset angina. *Eur Heart J* 1990;11:868–875.

101. Pepine CJ, Abrams J, Mark RG, et al. Characteristics of a contemporary population with angina pectoris. *Am J Cardiol* 1994;74:226–231.

102. Douglas PS, Ginsberg GS. The evaluation of chest pain in women. *N Engl J Med* 1996;334:1311–1315.

103. Weiner DA, Ryan TJ, McCabe CH, et al. Exercise stress testing: correlations among history of angina, ST-segment response and prevalence of coronary-artery disease in the Coronary Artery Surgery Study (CASS). *N Engl J Med* 1979;301:230–235.

104. Birdsall MA, Farquhar CM, White HD. Association between polycystic ovaries and extent of coronary artery disease in women having cardiac catheterization. *Ann Intern Med* 1997;126:32–35.

105. Fang J, Madhavan S, Alderman MH. The association between birthplace and mortality from cardiovascular causes among black and white residents of New York City. *N Engl J Med* 1996;335:1545–1551.

106. Peterson ED, Shaw LK, DeLong ER, et al. Racial variation in the use of coronary-revascularization procedures. *N Engl J Med* 1997;336:480–486.

107. Whittle J, Conigliaro J, Good CB, Lofgren RP. Racial differences in the use of invasive cardiovascular procedures in the Department of Veterans Affairs medical system. *N Engl J Med* 1993;329:621–627.

108. Enas EA, Yusuf S, Mehta JL. Prevalence of coronary artery disease in Asian Indians. *Am J Cardiol* 1992;70:945–949.

109. Kaplan GA, Keil JE. Socioeconomic factors and cardiovascular disease: a review of the literature [AHA Medical/Scientific Statement-Special Report]. *Circulation* 1993;88[4 Pt 1]:1973–1998.

110. Clarke R, Daly L, Robinson K, et al. Hyperhomocysteinemia: an independent risk factor for vascular disease. *N Engl J Med* 1991;324:1149–1155.

111. Stampfer MJ, Malinow MR, Willett WC, et al. A prospective study of plasma homocyst(e)ine and risk of myocardial infarction in US physicians. *JAMA* 1992;268:877–881.

112. Birdwell BG, Herbers JE, Kroenke K. Evaluating chest pain: the patient's presentation style alters the physician's diagnostic approach. *Arch Intern Med* 1993;153:1991–1995.

113. Constant J. The clinical diagnosis of nonanginal chest pain: the differentiation of angina from nonanginal chest pain by history. *Clin Cardiol* 1983;6:11–16.

114. Dry TJ. Thoracic pain in cardiovascular disease. *Proc Staff Mayo Clin* 1956;31:10–15.

115. Babu SC, Shah PM. Celiac territory ischemic syndrome in visceral artery occlusion. *Am J Surg* 1993;166:227–230.

116. Davies HA, Jones DB, Rhodes J, Newcombe RG. Angina-like esophageal pain: differentiation from cardiac pain by history. *J Clin Gastroenterol* 1985;7:477–481.

117. Chauhan A, Mullins PA, Taylor G, et al. Cardioesophageal reflex: a mechanism for "linked angina" in patients with angiographically proven coronary artery disease. *J Am Coll Cardiol* 1996;27:1621–1628.

118. Rao SS, Gregersen H, Hayek B, et al. Unexplained chest pain: The hypersensitive, hyperreactive, and poorly compliant esophagus. *Ann Intern Med* 1996;124:950–958.

119. Frøbert O, Funch-Jensen P, Bagger JP. Diagnostic value of esophageal studies in patients with angina-like chest pain and normal coronary angiograms. *Ann Intern Med* 1996;124:959–968.

120. Goyal RK. Changing focus on unexplained esophageal chest pain. *Ann Intern Med* 1996;124:1008–1010.

121. Gorgels APM, Vos MA, Mulleneers R, et al. Value of the electrocardiogram in diagnosing the number of severely narrowed coronary arteries in rest angina pectoris. *Am J Cardiol* 1993;72:999–1003.

122. Connolly DC, Elveback LR, Oxman HA. Coronary heart disease in residents of Rochester, Minnesota: IV. Prognostic value of the resting electrocardiogram at the time of initial diagnosis of angina pectoris. *Mayo Clin Proc* 1984;59:247–250.

123. Christian TF, Miller TD, Bailey KR, Gibbons RJ. Exercise tomographic thallium-201 imaging in patients with severe coronary artery disease and normal electrocardiograms. *Ann Intern Med* 1994;121:825–832.

124. Chaitman BR. What has happened to risk stratification with noninvasive testing? *ACC Curr J Rev* 1996;33–35.

125. Weiner DA, McCabe C, Hueter DC, et al. The predictive value of anginal chest pain as an indicator of coronary disease during exercise testing. *Am Heart J* 1978;96:458–462.

126. Goldschlager N, Sox HC Jr. The diagnostic and prognostic value of the treadmill exercise test in the evaluation of chest pain, in patients with recent myocardial infarction, and in asymptomatic individuals. *Am Heart J* 1988;116:523–535.

127. Cole CR, Blackstone EH, Pashkow FJ, et al. Heart rate recovery immediately after exercise as a predictor of mortality. *N Engl J Med* 1999;341:1351–1357.

128. Mark DB, Shaw L, Harrell FE, et al. Prognostic value of a treadmill exercise score in outpatients with suspected coronary artery disease. *N Engl J Med* 1991;325:849–853.

129. Mark DB, Hlatky MA, Lee KL, et al. Localizing coronary artery obstructions with the exercise treadmill test. *Ann Intern Med* 1987;106:53–55.

130. Rocco MB, Nabel EG, Campbell S, et al. Prognostic importance of myocardial ischemia detected by ambulatory monitoring in patients with stable coronary artery disease. *Circulation* 1988;78:877–884.

131. Deedwania PC, Carbajal EV. Silent ischemia during daily life is an independent predictor of mortality in stable angina. *Circulation* 1990;81:748–756.

132. Pepine CJ, Sharaf B, Andrews TC, et al. Relation between clinical, angiographic and ischemic findings at baseline and ischemic-related adverse outcomes at 1 year in the asymptomatic cardiac ischemia pilot study. *J Am Coll Cardiol* 1997;29:1483–1489.

133. Mulcahy D, Husain S, Zalos G, et al. Ischemia during ambulatory monitoring as a prognostic indicator in patients with stable coronary artery disease. *JAMA* 1997;277:318–324.

134. Reis SE, Gottlieb SO. Prognostic implications of transient asymptomatic myocardial ischemia as detected by ambulatory electrocardiographic monitoring. *Prog Cardiovasc Dis* 1992;35:77–96.

135. Stone PH, Chaitman BR, McMahon RP, et al. Asymptomatic cardiac ischemia pilot (ACIP) Study. Relationship between exercise-induced and ambulatory ischemia in patients with stable coronary disease. *Circulation* 1996;94:1537–1544.

136. Campbell S, Barry J, Rocco MB, et al. Features of the exercise test that reflect the activity of ischemic heart disease out of hospital. *Circulation* 1986;74:72–80.

137. Goodman SG, Freeman MR, Armstrong PW, Langer A. Does ambulatory monitoring contribute to exercise testing and myocardial perfusion scintigraphy in the prediction of the extent of coronary artery disease in stable angina? *Am J Cardiol* 1994;73:747–752.

138. Sharaf B, Williams DO, Miele NJ, et al. A detailed angiographic analysis of patients with ambulatory electrocardiographic ischemia: results from the Asymptomatic Cardiac Ischemia Pilot (ACIP) Study Angiographic Core Laboratory. *J Am Coll Cardiol* 1997;29:78–84.

139. Langer A, Freeman MR, Armstrong PW. Relation of angiographic detected intracoronary thrombosis and silent myocardial ischemia in unstable angina pectoris. *Am J Cardiol* 1990;66:1381–1382.

140. Lim R, Dyke L, Dymond DS. Effect on prognosis of abolition of exercise-induced painless myocardial ischemia by medical therapy. *Am J Cardiol* 1992;69:733–735.

141. Pepine CJ, Cohn PF, Deedwania PC, et al. Effects of treatment on outcome in mildly symptomatic patients with ischemia during daily life: the Atenolol Silent Ischemia Study (ASIST). *Circulation* 1994;90:762–768.

142. Davies RF, Goldberg AD, Forman S, et al. Asymptomatic Cardiac Ischemia Pilot (ACIP) Study two-year follow-up: outcomes of patients randomized to initial strategies of medical therapy versus revascularization. *Circulation* 1997;95:2037–2043.

143. Dagianti A, Penco M, Agati L, et al. Stress echocardiography: comparison of exercise, dipyridamole and dobutamine in detecting and predicting the extent of coronary artery disease. *J Am Coll Cardiol* 1995;26:18–25.

144. Nesto RW, Cohn LH, Collins JJ Jr, et al. Inotropic contractile reserve: a useful predictor of increased 5 year survival and improved postoperative left ventricular function in patients with coronary artery disease and reduced ejection fraction. *Am J Cardiol* 1982;50:39–44.

145. Bonow RO, Dilsizian V, Cuocolo A, Bacharach SL. Identification of viable myocardium in patients with chronic coronary artery disease and left ventricular dysfunction. *Circulation* 1991;83:26–37.

146. Dilsizian V, Smeltzer WR, Freedman NMT, et al. Thallium reinjection after stress re-distribution imaging. Does 24-hour delayed imaging after reinjection enhance detection of viable myocardium? *Circulation* 1991;83:1247–1255.

147. Marwick T, Willemart B, D'Hondt AM, et al. Selection of the optimal nonexercise stress for the evaluation of ischemic regional myocardial dysfunction and malperfusion. *Circulation* 1993;87:345–354.

148. Ling LH, Pellikka PA, Mahoney DW, et al. Atropine augmentation in dobutamine stress echocardiography: role and incremental value in a clinical practice setting. *J Am Coll Cardiol* 1996;28:551–557.

149. Kamaran M, Teague SM, Finkelhor RS, et al. Prognostic value of dobutamine stress echocardiography in patients referred because of suspected coronary artery disease. *Am J Cardiol* 1995;76:887–889.

150. Williams MJ, Odabashian J, Lauer MS, et al. Prognostic value of dobutamine echocardiography in patients with left ventricular dysfunction. *J Am Coll Cardiol* 1996;27:132–139.

151. Marcovitz PA, Shayna V, Horn RA, et al. Value of dobutamine stress echocardiography in determining the prognosis of patients with known or suspected coronary artery disease. *Am J Cardiol* 1996;78:404–408.

152. Kaul S, Lilly DR, Gascho JA, et al. Prognostic utility of the exercise thallium-201 test in ambulatory patients with chest pain: comparison with cardiac catheterization. *Circulation* 1988;77:745–758.

153. Berman DS, Hachamovitch R, Kiat H, et al. Incremental value of prognostic testing in patients with known or suspected ischemic heart disease: a basis for optimal utilization of exercise technetium-99m sestamibi myocardial

perfusion single-photon emission computed tomography. *J Am Coll Cardiol* 1995;26:639–647.

154. Ladenheim ML, Pollock BH, Rozanski A, et al. Extent and severity of myocardial hypoperfusion as predictors of prognosis in patients with suspected coronary artery disease. *J Am Coll Cardiol* 1986;7:464–471.

155. Brown KA. Prognostic value of thallium-201 myocardial perfusion imaging: a diagnostic tool comes of age. *Circulation* 1991;83:363–381.

156. Shaw L, Chaitman BR, Hilton TC, et al. Prognostic value of dipyridamole thallium-201 imaging in elderly patients. *J Am Coll Cardiol* 1992;19:1390–1398.

157. Zabel KM, Califf RM. The value of exercise thallium imaging [editorial]. *Ann Intern Med* 1994;121:891–893.

158. Nygaard TW, Gibson RS, Ryan JM, et al. Prevalence of high-risk thallium-201 scintigraphic findings in left main coronary artery stenosis: Comparison with patients with multiple- and single-vessel coronary artery disease. *Am J Cardiol* 1984;53:462–469.

159. Dash H, Massie BM, Botvinick EH, Brundage BH. The noninvasive identification of left main and three vessel coronary artery disease by myocardial stress perfusion scintigraphy and treadmill exercise electrocardiography. *Circulation* 1979;60:276–284.

160. O'Rourke RA, Brundage BH, Froelicher VF, et al. American College of Cardiology/American Heart Association Expert Consensus document on electron-beam computed tomography for the diagnosis and prognosis of coronary artery disease. *Circulation* 2000;102:126–140.

161. Wilson RF. Assessing the severity of coronary-artery stenoses [editorial]. *N Engl J Med* 1996;334:1735–1737.

162. Pijls NHJ, De Bruyne B, Peels K, et al. Measurement of fractional flow reserve to assess the functional severity of coronary-artery stenoses. *N Engl J Med* 1996;334:1703–1708.

163. Forrester JS, Litvack F, Grundfest W, Hickey A. A perspective of coronary disease seen through the arteries of living man. *Circulation* 1987;75:505–513.

164. Nissen SE, Yock P. Intravascular ultrasound: novel pathophysiologic insights and current clinical applications. *Circulation* 2001;103:604–616.

165. Task Force of the European Society of Cardiology. Guidelines on management of stable angina pectoris: recommendations from the Task Force of the ESC. *Eur Heart J* 1997;18:394–413.

166. Thadani U, Chohan A. Chronic stable angina pectoris: strategies for effective drug therapy. *Postgrad Med* 1995;98:175–188.

167. Ridker PM, Manson JE, Gaziano M, et al. Low-dose aspirin therapy for chronic stable angina: a randomized, placebo-controlled clinical trial. *Ann Intern Med* 1991;114:835–839.

168. Patrono C. Aspirin as an antiplatelet drug. *N Engl J Med* 1994;330:1287–1294.

169. Juul-Moller S, Edvardsson N, Jahnmatz B, et al. Double-blind trial of aspirin in primary prevention of myocardial infarction in patients with stable chronic angina pectoris. *Lancet* 1992;340:1421–1425.

170. Anonymous. Ticlopidine [editorial]. *Lancet* 1991;337:459–460.

171. Bennett CL, Weinberg PD, Rozenberg-Ben-Dror K, et al. Thrombotic thrombocytopenic purpura associated with ticlopidine: a review of 60 cases. *Ann Intern Med* 1998;128:541–544.

172. CAPRIE Steering Committee. A randomized, blinded, trial of clopidogrel versus aspirin in patients at risk of ischaemic events (CAPRIE). *Lancet* 1996;348:1329–1339.

173. Benson H, McCallie DP. Angina pectoris and the placebo effect. *N Engl J Med* 1979;300:1424–1429.

174. Diamond EG, Kittle CF, Crockett JE. Evaluation of internal mammary artery ligation and sham procedure in angina pectoris. *Circulation* 1958;18:712–713.

175. Smith ER, Smiseth OA, Kingma I, et al. Mechanism of action of nitrates: role of changes in venous capacitance and in the left ventricular diastolic pressure-volume relation. *Am J Med* 1984;76(6A):14–21.

176. Armstrong PW, Moffat JA. Tolerance of organic nitrates: clinical and experimental perspectives. *Am J Med* 1983;74(6B):73–84.

177. Diodata JG, Cannon RO, Hussain N, Quyyumi AA. Inhibitory effect of nitroglycerin and sodium nitroprusside on platelet activation across the coronary circulation in stable angina pectoris. *Am J Cardiol* 1995;75:443–448.

178. Parker JO. Drug therapy: nitrate therapy in stable angina pectoris. *N Engl J Med* 1987;316:1635–1642.

179. Packer M. What causes tolerance to nitroglycerin? The 100 year old mystery continues [editorial]. *J Am Coll Cardiol* 1990;16:932–935.

180. Thadani U. Role of nitrates in angina pectoris. *Am J Cardiol* 1992;70:43B–53B.

181. Parker JD, Farrell B, Lahey KA, Rose BF. Nitrate tolerance: the lack of effect of *N*-acetylcysteine. *Circulation* 1987;76:572–576.

182. Parker JD, Parker AB, Farrell B, Parker JO. Effects of diuretic therapy on the development of tolerance to nitroglycerin and exercise capacity in patients with chronic stable angina. *Circulation* 1996;93:691–696.

183. Katz RJ, Levy WS, Buff L, Wasserman AG. Prevention of nitrate tolerance with angiotensin converting enzyme inhibitors. *Circulation* 1991;83:1271–1277.

184. Muiesan ML, Boni E, Castellano M, et al. Effects of transdermal nitroglycerin in combination with an ACE inhibitor in patients with chronic stable angina pectoris. *Eur Heart J* 1993;14:1701–1708.

185. Thadani U, Maranda CR, Amsterdam E, et al. Lack of pharmacologic tolerance and rebound angina pectoris during twice-daily therapy with isosorbide-5-mononitrate. *Ann Intern Med* 1994;120:353–359.

186. Abrams J. Therapy of angina pectoris with long-acting nitrates: which agent and when? *Can J Cardiol* 1996; 12[Suppl C]:9C–16C.

187. Abrams J. Interval therapy to avoid nitrate tolerance: paradise regained? *Am J Cardiol* 1989;64:931–934.

188. Webb DJ, Muirhead GJ, Wulff M, et al. Sildenafil citrate potentiates the hypotensive effects of nitric oxide donor drugs in male patients with stable angina. *J Am Coll Cardiol* 2000;36:25–31.

189. Cheitlin MD, Hutter AM, Brindis RG, et al. ACC/AHA expert consensus document: use of sildenafil (Viagra) in

patients with cardiovascular disease. *J Am Coll Cardiol* 1999;33:273–282.

190. Frishman WH. Beta-adrenergic blockers. *Med Clin North Am* 1988;72:37–81.

191. Robertson RM, Wood AJJ, Vaughn WK, et al. Exacerbation of vasotonic angina pectoris by propranolol. *Circulation* 1982;65:281–285.

192. Frishman WH. Drug therapy: beta-adrenoceptor antagonists: new drugs and new indications. *N Engl J Med* 1981;305:500–506.

193. van Stegeren AH, Everaerd W, Cahill L, et al. Memory for emotional events: differential effects of centrally versus peripherally acting beta-blocking agents. *Psychopharmacology* 1998;138:305–310.

194. Quyyumi AA, Wright C, Mockus L, Fox KM. Effect of partial agonist activity in beta-blockers in severe angina pectoris: a double blind comparison of pindolol and atenolol. *BMJ* 1984;289:951–953.

195. NHLBI Beta-Blocker Heart Attack Trial Research Group. A randomized trial of propranolol in patients with acute myocardial infarction: I. Mortality results. *JAMA* 1982;247:1707–1714.

196. Yusuf S, Peto R, Lewis J, et al. Beta blockade during and after myocardial infarction: an overview of the randomized trials. *Prog Cardiovasc Dis* 1985;27:335–371.

197. Hohnloser SH, Woosley RL. Sotalol. *N Engl J Med* 1994;331:31–38.

198. MERIT-HF Study Group. Effect of metoprolol CR/XL in chronic heart failure: metoprolol CR/XL Randomized Intervention Trial In Congestive Heart Failure (MERIT-HF). *Lancet* 1999;353:2001–2007.

199. CIBIS-II Investigators and Committees. The Cardiac Insufficiency Bisoprolol Study II (CIBIS-II): a randomized trial. *Lancet* 1999;353:9–13.

200. Rodrigues EA, Lahira A, Hughes LO, et al. Antianginal efficacy of carvedilol: a beta-blocking drug with vasodilating activity. *Am J Cardiol* 1986;58:916–921.

201. Packer M, Bristow MR, Cohn JN, et al. The effect of carvedilol on morbidity and mortality in patients with chronic heart failure. *N Engl J Med* 1996;334:1349–1355.

202. Packer M. COPERNICUS (Carvedilol Prospective Randomized Cumulative Survival): evaluates the effects of carvedilol top-of-ACE on major cardiac events in patients with heart failure NYHAA II-IV. Presented at the XXII Congress of the European Society of Cardiology, 2000.

203. Weiss R, Ferry D, Pickering E, Smith LK, et al., on behalf of the Carvedilol-Angina Study Group. Effectiveness of three different doses of carvedilol for exertional angina. *Am J Cardiol* 1998;82:927–931.

204. van der Does R, Hauf-Zachariou U, Pfarr E, et al. Comparison of safety and efficacy of carvedilol and metoprolol in stable angina pectoris. *Am J Cardiol* 1999;83:643–649.

205. Ardissino D, Barberis P, De Servi S, et al. Usefulness of the hyperventilation test in stable exertional angina pectoris in selecting medical therapy. *Am J Cardiol* 1990;65:417–421.

206. Weiner DA. Calcium antagonists in the treatment of ischemic heart disease: angina pectoris. *Coron Artery Dis* 1994;5:14–20.

207. Psaty BM, Heckbert SR, Koepsell MD, et al. The risk of myocardial infarction associated with antihypertensive drug therapies. *JAMA* 1995;274:620–625.

208. Furberg CD, Psaty BM, Meyer JV. Nifedipine: dose-related increase in mortality in patients with coronary heart disease. *Circulation* 1995;92:1326–1331.

209. Opie LH, Messerli FH. Nifedipine and mortality: grave defects in the dossier. *Circulation* 1995;92:1068–1073.

210. Egstrup K, Andersen PE Jr. Transient myocardial ischemia during nifedipine therapy in stable angina pectoris, and its relation to coronary collateral flow and comparison with metoprolol. *Am J Cardiol* 1993;71:177–183.

211. de Vries RJM, Dunselman PH, van Veldhuisen DJ, et al. Comparison between felodipine and isosorbide mononitrate as adjunct to beta blockade in patients > 65 years of age with angina pectoris. *Am J Cardiol* 1994;74:1201–1206.

212. Ezekowitz MD, Hossack K, Mehta JL, et al. Amlodipine in chronic stable angina: results of a multicenter, double-blind crossover trial. *Am Heart J* 1995;129:527–535.

213. Lichtlen PR, Hugenholtz PG, Rafflenbeul W, et al. Retardation of angiography progression of coronary artery disease by nifedipine: results of the International Nifedipine Trial on Antiatherosclerotic Therapy (INTACT). *Lancet* 1990;335:1109–1113.

214. Waters D, Lesperance J, Francetich M, et al. A controlled trial to assess the effect of a calcium channel blocker on the progression of coronary atherosclerosis. *Circulation* 1990;82:1940–1953.

215. Opie LH. First line drugs in chronic stable effort angina—the case for newer, longer-acting calcium channel blocking agents. *J Am Coll Cardiol* 2000;36:1967–1971.

216. Rinaldi CA, Linka AZ, Navroz D, et al. Randomized, double-blind crossover study to investigate the effects of amlodipine and isosorbide mononitrate on the time course and severity of exercise-induced myocardial stunning. *Circulation* 1998;98:749–756.

217. Ardissino D, Savonitto S, Egstrup K, et al. Selection of medical treatment in stable angina pectoris: results of the International Multicenter Angina Exercise (IMAGE) Study. *J Am Coll Cardiol* 1995;25:1516–1521.

218. Savonitto S, Ardissino D, Egstrup K, et al. Combination therapy with metoprolol and nifedipine versus monotherapy in patients with stable angina pectoris. *J Am Coll Cardiol* 1996;27:311–316.

219. Fox KM, Mulcahy D, Findlay I, et al. The Total Ischaemic Burden European Trial (TIBET): effects of atenolol, nifedipine SR and their combination on the exercise test and the total ischaemic burden in 608 patients with stable angina. *Eur Heart J* 1996;17:96–103.

220. Bertolet BD, Hill JA, Pepine CJ. Treatment strategies for daily life silent myocardial ischemia: a correlation with potential pathogenic mechanisms. *Prog Cardiovasc Dis* 1992;35:97–118.

221. Davies MK. Effects of ACE inhibitors on coronary hemodynamics and angina pectoris. *Br Heart J* 1994;72[Suppl]:52–56.

222. Lonn EM, Yusuf S, Jha P, et al. Emerging role of angiotensin-converting enzyme inhibitors in cardiac and vascular protection. *Circulation* 1994;90:2056–2069.

223. Heart Outcomes Prevention Evaluation Study Investigators. Effects of an angiotensin-converting-enzyme inhibi-

tor, ramipril, on cardiovascular events in high risk patients. *N Engl J Med* 2000;342:145–153.

224. Heart Outcomes Prevention Evaluation Study Investigators. Vitamin E supplementation and cardiovascular events in high-risk patients. *N Engl J Med* 2000;342:154–160.

225. Doval HC, Nul DR, Grancelli HO, et al. Randomized trial of low dose amiodarone in severe congestive heart failure. *Lancet* 1994;344:493–498.

226. Meyer BJ, Amann FW. Additional antianginal efficacy of amiodarone in patients with limiting angina pectoris. *Am Heart J* 1993;125:996–1001.

227. Hulley S, Grady D, Bush T, et al., for the Heart and Estrogen/progestin Replacement Study (HERS) Research Group. Randomized trial of estrogen plus progestin for secondary prevention of coronary heart disease in postmenopausal women. *JAMA* 1998;280:605–613.

228. Petitti DB. Hormone replacement therapy and heart disease prevention: experimentation trumps observation. *JAMA* 1998;280:650–651.

229. English KM, Steeds RP, Jones TH, et al. Low-dose transdermal testosterone therapy improves angina threshold in men with chronic stable angina: a randomized, double-blind, placebo-controlled study. *Circulation* 2000;102:1911.

230. Iriarte MM, Caso R, Murga N, et al. Microvascular angina in systemic hypertension: diagnosis and treatment with enalapril. *Am J Cardiol* 1995;76:31D–34D.

231. Cannon RO, Quyyumi AA, Mincemoyer R, et al. Imipramine in patients with chest pain despite normal coronary angiograms. *N Engl J Med* 1994;330:1411–1417.

232. De Caterina R, Carpeggiani C, L'Abbate A. A double-blind, placebo-controlled study of ketanserin in patients with Prinzmetal's angina. *Circulation* 1984;69:889–894.

233. Schecter AD, Chesebro JH, Fuster V. Refractory Prinzmetal angina treated with cyproheptadine. *Ann Intern Med* 1994;121:113–114.

234. Passamani E, Davis KB, Gillespie MJ, et al. A randomized trial of coronary artery bypass surgery. *N Engl J Med* 1985;312:1665–1671.

235. European Coronary Surgery Study Group. Coronary artery bypass surgery and stable angina pectoris: survival at two years. *Lancet* 1979;1:889–893.

236. Yusuf S, Zucker D, Peduzzi P, et al. Effect of coronary artery bypass graft surgery on survival: overview of 10-year results from randomized trials by the Coronary Artery Bypass Graft Surgery Trialists Collaboration. *Lancet* 1994;334:563–570.

237. Mark DB, Nelson CL, Califf RM, et al. Continuing evolution of therapy for coronary artery disease. *Circulation* 1994;89:2015–2025.

238. Pocock SJ, Henderson RA, Rickards AF, et al. Meta-analysis of randomized trials comparing coronary angioplasty with bypass surgery. *Lancet* 1995;346:1184–1189.

239. Bypass Angioplasty Revascularization Investigation (BARI) Investigators. Comparison of coronary bypass surgery with angioplasty in patients with multivessel disease. *N Engl J Med* 1996;335:217–225.

240. BARI Investigators. Influence of diabetes on five year mortality and morbidity in a randomized trial comparing CABG and PTCA in patients with multivessel disease: the

Bypass Angioplasty Revascularization Investigation (BARI). *Circulation* 1997;96:1761–1769.

241. Eagle KA, Guyton RA, Davidoff R, et al. ACC/AHA guidelines for coronary artery bypass graft surgery: a report of the American College of Cardiology/American Heart Association Task Force on Practice Guidelines (Committee to Revise the 1991 Guidelines for CABG Surgery). *J Am Coll Cardiol* 1999;34:1262–1346.

242. Simoons ML. Myocardial revascularization—bypass surgery or angioplasty? [editorial]. *N Engl J Med* 1996;335:275–277.

243. Baim DS. Angioplasty as a treatment for coronary artery disease. *N Engl J Med* 1992;326:56–58.

244. Hillis LD, Rutherford JD. Coronary angioplasty compared with bypass grafting. *N Engl J Med* 1994;331:1086–1087.

245. EPILOG Investigators. Platelet glycoprotein IIb/IIIa receptor blockade and low-dose heparin during percutaneous coronary revascularization. *N Engl J Med* 1997;336:1689–1696.

246. EPISTENT Investigators. Randomized placebo-controlled and balloon-angioplasty-controlled trial to assess safety of coronary stenting with use of platelet glycoprotein IIb/IIIa blockade. *Lancet* 1998;352:87–92.

247. Sapirstein W, Zuckerman B, Dillard J. FDA approval of coronary-artery brachytherapy [editorial]. *N Engl J Med* 2001;344:297–299.

248. Pocock SJ, Henderson RA, Clayton T, et al., for the RITA-2 Trial Participants. Quality of life after coronary angioplasty or continued medical treatment for angina: three year follow-up in the RITA-2 trial. *J Am Coll Cardiol* 2000;35:907–914.

249. Parisi AF, Folland ED, Hartigan P, on behalf of the Veterans Affairs ACME Investigators. A comparison of angioplasty with medical therapy in the treatment of single-vessel coronary artery disease. *N Engl J Med* 1992;326:10–16.

250. Pitt B, Waters D, Brown WV, et al., for the Atorvastatin versus Revascularization Treatment Investigators. Aggressive lipid-lowering therapy compared with angioplasty in stable coronary artery disease. *N Engl J Med* 1999;341:70–76.

251. Horvath KA, Cohn LH, Cooley DA, et al. Transmyocardial laser revascularization: results of a multicenter trial with transmyocardial laser revascularization used as sole therapy for end-stage coronary artery disease. *J Thorac Cardiovasc Surg* 1997;113:645–654.

252. Aaberge L, Nordstrand K, Dragsund M, et al. Transmyocardial revascularization with CO_2 laser in patients with refractory angina pectoris. Clinical results from the Norwegian Randomized Trial. *J Am Coll Cardiol* 2000;35:1170–1177.

253. Allen KB, Dowling RD, Fudge TL, et al. Comparison of transmyocardial revascularization with medical therapy in patients with refractory angina. *N Engl J Med* 1999;341:1029–1036.

254. Burkhoff D, Schmidt S, Schulman SP, et al., for the ATLANTIC investigators. Transmyocardial laser revascularization compared with continued medical therapy for treatment of refractory angina pectoris: a prospective randomized trial. *Lancet* 1999;354:885–890.

255. Frazier OH, March RJ, Horvath KA, for the Transmyocardial Carbon Dioxide Laser Revasularization Study Group. Transmyocardial revascularization with a carbon dioxide laser in patients with end-stage coronary artery disease. *N Engl J Med* 1999;341:1021–1028.

256. Jones JW, Schmidt SE, Richman BW, et al. Holmium: YAG laser transmyocardial revascularization relieves angina and improves functional status. *Ann Thorac Surg* 1999;67:1596–1602.

257. Schofield PM, Sharples LD, Caine N, et al. Transmyocardial laser revascularization in patients with refractory angina: a randomized controlled trial. *Lancet* 1999;353:519–524.

258. Oesterle SN, Sanborn TA, Ali N, et al. Percutaneous transmyocardial laser revascularization for severe angina: the PACIFIC randomised trial. *Lancet* 2000;356:1705–1710.

259. Arora RR, Chou TM, Jain D, et al. The multicenter study of enhanced external counterpulsation (MUST-EECP): effect of EECP on exercise-induced myocardial ischemia and anginal episodes. *J Am Coll Cardiol* 1999;33:1833–1840.

260. Mannheimer C, Eliasson T, Augustinsson L-E, et al. Electrical stimulation versus coronary artery bypass surgery in severe angina pectoris. The ESBY Study. *Circulation* 1998;97:1157–1163.

261. Califf RM, Armstrong PW, Carver JR, et al. Task Force 5: stratification of patients into high, medium and low risk subgroups for purposes of risk factor management. *J Am Coll Cardiol* 1996;27:1007–1019.

262. Forrester JS, Merz NB, Bush TL, et al. Task Force 4: efficacy of risk factor management. *J Am Coll Cardiol* 1996;27:991–1006.

263. Anonymous. Nicotine replacement therapy for patients with coronary artery disease. Working Group for the Study of Transdermal Nicotine in Patients with Coronary Artery Disease. *Arch Intern Med* 1994;154:989–995.

264. Schuler G, Hambrecht R, Schlierf G, et al. Myocardial perfusion and regression of coronary artery disease in patients on a regimen of intensive physical exercise and low fat diet. *J Am Coll Cardiol* 1992;19:34–42.

265. Hambrecht R, Niebauer J, Marburger C, et al. Various intensities of leisure time physical activity in patients with coronary artery disease: effects on cardiorespiratory fitness and progression of coronary atherosclerotic lesions. *J Am Coll Cardiol* 1993;22:468–477.

266. The Scandinavian Simvastatin Survival Study Group. Randomized trial of cholesterol lowering in 4,444 patients with coronary heart disease: the Scandinavian Simvastatin Survival Study (4S). *Lancet* 1994;344:1383–1389.

267. Brown G, Albers JJ, Fisher LD, et al. Regression of coronary artery disease as a result of intensive lipid-lowering therapy in men with high levels of apolipoprotein B. *N Engl J Med* 1990;323:1289–1298.

268. Vaughan CJ, Murphy MB, Buckley BM. Statins do more than just lower cholesterol. *Lancet* 1996;348:1079–1082.

269. Lacoste L, Lam JYT, Hung J, et al. Hyperlipidemia and coronary disease: correction of the increased thrombogenic potential with cholesterol reduction. *Circulation* 1995;92:3172–3177.

270. Mayer J, Eller T, Brauer P, et al. Effects of long term treatment with lovastatin on the clotting system and blood platelets. *Ann Hematol* 1992;64:196–201.

271. Andrews TC, Raby K, Barry J, et al. Effect of cholesterol reduction on myocardial ischemia in patients with coronary disease. *Circulation* 1997;95:324–328.

272. Van Boven AJ, Jukema W, Zwinderman AH. Reduction of transient myocardial ischemia with pravastatin in addition to the conventional treatment in patients with angina pectoris. *Circulation* 1996;94:1503–1505.

273. Anderson TJ, Meredith IT, Yeung AC, et al. The effect of cholesterol-lowering and antioxidant therapy on endothelium-dependent coronary vasomotion. *N Engl J Med* 1995;332:488–493.

274. Little WC, Constantinescu M, Applegate RJ, et al. Can coronary angiography predict the site of a subsequent myocardial infarction in patients with mild-to-moderate coronary artery disease? *Circulation* 1988;78:1157–1166.

275. Fuster V, Gotto AM, Libby P, et al. Task Force 1: pathogenesis of coronary disease: the biologic role of risk factors. *J Am Coll Cardiol* 1996;27:964–975.

276. Grady D, Rubin SM, Petitti DB, et al. Hormone therapy to prevent disease and prolong life in postmenopausal women. *Ann Intern Med* 1992;117:1016–1037.

277. Malinow MR, Bostom AJ, Krauss RM. Homocysteine diet in cardiovascular diseases. A statement for healthcare professionals from the Nutrition Committee for the American Heart Association. *Circulation* 1999;99:178–182.

278. Pearson TA, McBride PE, Miller NH, Smith SC. Task Force 8: organization of preventive cardiology service. *J Am Coll Cardiol* 1996;27:1039–1047.

279. Rozanski A, Blumenthal JA, Kaplan J. Impact of psychological factors on the pathogenesis of cardiovascular disease and implications for therapy. *Circulation* 1999;99:2192–2217.

280. Garcia-Moll X, Zouridakis E, Cole D, Kaski JC. C-reactive protein in patients with chronic stable angina: differences in baseline serum concentration between women and men. *Eur Heart J* 2000;21:1598–1606.

281. Saitoh T, Kishida H, Tsukada Y, et al. Clinical significance of increased plasma concentration of macrophage colony-stimulating factor in patients with angina pectoris. *J Am Coll Cardiol* 2000;35:655–665.

282. Ikonomidis I, Andreotti F, Economou E, et al. Increased proinflammatory cytokines in patients with chronic stable angina and their reduction by aspirin. *Circulation* 1999;100:793–798.

283. Smith FB, Fowkes FGR, Rumley A, et al. Tissue plasminogen activator and leucocyte elastase as predictors of cardiovascular events in subjects with angina pectoris: Edinburgh Artery Study. *Eur Heart J* 2000;21:1607–1613.

284. Ridker PM. Inflammation: aspirin and the risk of cardiovascular disease in apparently healthy men. *N Engl J Med* 1997;336:973–979.

285. Chew DP, Bhatt DL, Sapp S, Topol EJ. Increased mortality with oral platelet glycoprotein IIb/IIIa antagonists: a meta-analysis of phase III multicenter randomized trials. *Circulation* 2001;103:201–206.

286. Hollopeter G, Jantzen H-M, Vincent D, et al. Identification of the platelet ADP receptor targeted by antithrombotic drugs. *Nature* 2001;409:202–207.

287. Violaris AG, Linnemeier TJ, Campbell S, et al. Intravascular ultrasound imaging combined with coronary angioplasty. *Lancet* 1992;339:1571–1572.

288. Casscells W, Hathorn B, David M, et al. Thermal detection of cellular infiltrates in living atherosclerotic plaques: possible implications for plaque rupture and thrombosis. *Lancet* 1996;347:1447–1451.

289. Fayad ZA, Fuster V, Fallon JT, et al. Noninvasive in vivo human coronary artery lumen and wall imaging using black-blood magnetic resonance imaging. *Circulation* 2000;102:506–510.

290. Topol EJ, Serruys PW. Frontiers in Interventional Cardiology. *Circulation* 1998;98:1802–1820.

291. Hendel RC, Henry TD, Rocha-Singh K, et al. Effect of intracoronary recombinant human vascular endothelial growth factor on myocardial perfusion. *Circulation* 2000;101:118–121.

292. Lefkowitz RJ, Willerson JT. Prospects for cardiovascular research. *JAMA* 2001;285:581–587.

293. Theroux P, Willerson JT, Armstrong PW. Progress in the treatment of acute coronary syndromes: a 50 year perspective (1950–2000). *Circulation* 2000;102:IV-2–IV-13.

17

NON–ST-ELEVATION ACUTE CORONARY SYNDROMES: UNSTABLE ANGINA AND NON–ST-ELEVATION MYOCARDIAL INFARCTION

HARVEY D. WHITE

H. D. White: University of Auckland, Coronary Care and Cardiovascular Research, Green Lane Hospital, Auckland, New Zealand

---

▼ **ADDITIONAL ELECTRONIC TOPICS**

Upstream Treatment with IIb/IIIa Antagonists: Guidelines c58;   Agents in Development c59;   Direct Antithrombins c60;   Hirudin c61;   Bivalirudin c62;   Argatroban, Inogatran, and Efegatran c63;   Other Agents c64

OVERVIEW

The major pathophysiologic mechanism of acute ischemic syndromes is plaque rupture or fissuring with superimposed thrombus. Patients with non–ST-elevation acute coronary syndromes should be risk profiled at admission, and therapy should be tailored to individual patient characteristics and risk. Many low- and intermediate-risk patients can be managed without the need for interventions.

The goals of a conservative treatment strategy should be to risk-stratify all patients at admission, revascularize those at high risk, and "passivate" (i.e., inactivate) the platelet-active surface of the ruptured or fissured plaque in patients at intermediate risk. Patients at low risk should be discharged early.

Combination therapy with aspirin, a platelet glycoprotein IIb/IIIa receptor antagonist, and unfractionated heparin is effective for preventing myocardial infarction (MI) and death. The combination of aspirin and clopidogrel also reduces the risk of death/MI. Low-molecular-weight heparins are more convenient to use than unfractionated heparin, and the combined results of two trials showed that one low-molecular-weight heparin reduced the risk of death/MI compared with unfractionated heparin. Beta-blockers, nitrates, and calcium channel antagonists relieve angina but have no significant effect on intracoronary thrombus and do not necessarily reduce the risks of MI and death.

In high-risk patients, a revascularization strategy combined with a IIb/IIIa antagonist or an antithrombotic agent such as low-molecular-weight heparin prevents death/MI more effectively than a conservative medical strategy. The patient has less need for antianginal medications, a shorter hospital stay, and less need for readmission. This approach is cost effective in many health-care settings.

Better treatments and new therapeutic strategies are needed to improve the outcomes of patients with non–ST-elevation acute coronary syndromes. It is important that primary and secondary preventative measures are instituted to reduce the community burden of acute coronary syndromes.

GLOSSARY

Conservative management: Risk-stratification and medical therapy with selective use of angiography and revascularization procedures according to the patient's risk status.

Invasive management: Medical therapy plus early coronary arteriography and revascularization, irrespective of the patient's risk status.

Plaque instability: Propensity for atheromatous plaque to rupture or fissure.

Plaque passivation: Inactivation of the platelet-active surface of a ruptured or fissured plaque.

Rebound ischemia: Increase in ischemic events when heparin therapy is stopped.

Risk profiling: Estimation of the risk of coronary events—usually death or MI—by studying patient characteristics and the results of investigations.

INTRODUCTION

The first documented description of a patient with an acute ischemic syndrome is in the Ebers papyrus from 2600 BCE, which states, "If you find a man with heart discomfort, with pain in his arms, at the side of his heart, death is near." The description is still apt, but the prognosis has changed over the centuries. Today unstable angina is one of the most frequent causes of hospitalization (1), and the number of patients admitted with this condition is on the increase.

The syndromes of unstable angina, non–ST-elevation MI and ST-elevation MI are a continuum, and the pathophysiology is heterogeneous and dynamic. The clinical presentation depends on the severity of the arterial injury, the size and type of thrombus formed, the extent and duration of ischemia, and the amount of previous myocardial necrosis. The extent of ischemia depends on the myocardial distribution of the ischemia-producing artery, the severity of the ischemia-producing stenosis, the absence or presence of collateral circulation, factors that affect the supply of oxygenated blood, and increased myocardial demands, including the heart rate, blood pressure, and contractility. Patients may die, have an MI, require revascularization for refractory angina, or be readmitted with recurrent symptoms, and management continues to pose a major clinical challenge (1).

DEFINITIONS

The term *acute coronary syndromes* describes a spectrum of clinical syndromes that ranges from unstable angina to non–ST-elevation MI and ST-elevation MI. Patients who present with acute coronary syndromes are divided into those with ST elevation or new left bundle branch block and those with non–ST-elevation acute coronary syndromes including unstable angina and non–ST-elevation MI (2) (Fig. 17.1).

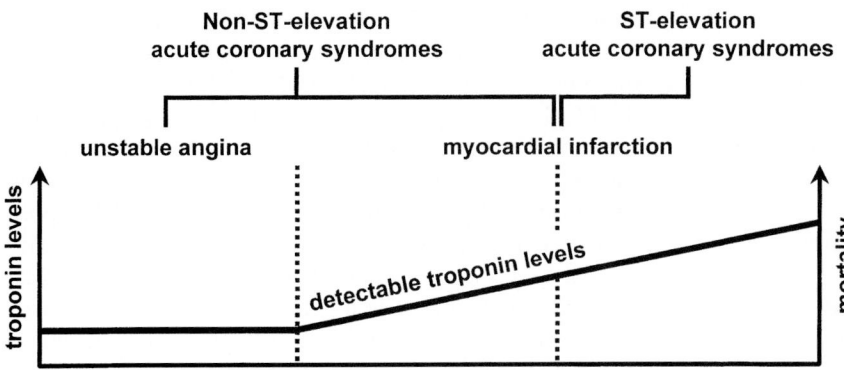

FIGURE 17.1 New terminology for coronary syndromes. [Adapted from Aroney C, Boyden AN, Jelinek MV, et al. Management of unstable angina: guidelines 2000. *Med J Aust* 2000;173(Suppl):S65–S88, with permission.]

The term *unstable angina* describes a syndrome that is intermediate between chronic stable angina and MI. It is a clinical diagnosis based on a history of chest pain and exclusion of the diagnosis of MI by electrocardiography (ECG) or cardiac enzyme testing. The chest pain may be prolonged at rest or of new onset, or it may represent accelerating symptoms of previously stable angina. It can also occur after MI. Patients who present without ST elevation are diagnosed as having either unstable angina or non–ST-elevation MI based on whether or not an elevation in myocardial protein levels, such as the troponins (3) or creatine kinase (CK)–MB, is detected. In 2% to 15% of patients, Q-wave MI subsequently develops. Braunwald (4) developed an unstable angina classification in 1989, which has proved to be clinically useful (5) and has been found to correlate with the underlying coronary angiographic findings in patients with unstable angina (6) (Table 17.1). This classification is based on the severity of symptoms, the clinical circumstances in which the unstable angina occurs, and the intensity of medical treatment. It has been updated to include troponin levels (7). Prinzmetal's angina (8) (i.e., recurrent rest angina accompanied by ST elevation on the ECG) is considered as a separate entity.

PATHOPHYSIOLOGY

The five major causes of acute coronary syndromes are thrombus, mechanical obstruction, dynamic obstruction, inflammation, and increased organ demand (9). c65

CORONARY ARTERY SPASM

In 1959, Prinzmetal et al. (8) described a variant form of angina characterized by chest pain predominantly at rest and usually associated with ST elevation on the ECG. Rarely, variant angina is associated with other vasospastic disorders, such as migraine or Raynaud's syndrome, in patients with angiographically normal coronary arteries. c66

PATHOPHYSIOLOGIC IMPLICATIONS FOR CLINICAL MANAGEMENT

The management of patients with non–ST-elevation acute coronary syndromes should focus on etiology (9). The pri-

TABLE 17.1 CLASSIFICATION OF UNSTABLE ANGINA[a]

| Severity | Clinical circumstances | | |
	A: Develops in presence of extracardiac condition that intensifies myocardial ischemia (secondary unstable angina)	B: Develops in absence of extracardiac condition (primary unstable angina)	C: Develops within 2 wk after acute myocardial infarction (postinfarction unstable angina)
I: New onset of severe angina or accelerated angina; no rest pain	IA	IB	IC
II: Rest angina within past month but not within preceding 48 h (rest angina, subacute)	IIA	IIB	IIC
III: Rest angina within 48 h (rest angina, acute)	IIIA	IIIB (troponin negative) IIIB (troponin positive)	IIIC

[a]Patients with unstable angina can also be divided into three groups, depending on whether unstable angina occurs (a) in the absence of treatment for chronic stable angina, (b) during treatment for chronic stable angina, or (c) despite maximal antiischemic drug therapy. These three groups can be designated by subscripts 1, 2, or 3, respectively. Patients with unstable angina can be further divided into those with and those without transient ST-T–wave changes during pain.
Modified from Hamm CW, Braunwald E. A classification of unstable angina revisited. *Circulation* 2000;102:118–122, with permission.

mary aims of treatment are to reduce initial symptoms and to prevent death or MI.

In individual patients, the mechanisms of plaque fissuring, platelet aggregation, thrombus formation, and increased vasomotor tone may play different roles at different times. A variety of therapeutic approaches are needed to modify these processes.

Platelet activation and aggregation and thrombus formation are central to the pathophysiology of unstable angina, and greater understanding of these mechanisms has led to improvements in treatment. The main emphases of medical management are antithrombotic therapy with aspirin and heparin (67) and antiplatelet therapy with IIb/IIIa antagonists or clopidogrel to reduce the risks of MI and death. Beta-blockers, nitrates, and calcium channel antagonists should be used for relief of symptoms.

Patients with an increased oxygen demand or a decreased oxygen supply (e.g., those with anemia or thyrotoxicosis) need to be managed differently from those with a severe coronary artery stenosis that is causing mechanical obstruction. Patients with vasospasm require therapies such as nitrates and calcium channel antagonists, whereas those with evidence of inflammation may be best treated with aspirin and statins (68). The choice of medical therapies also depends on whether an invasive or a conservative treatment strategy is planned. Risk-stratification is pivotal to triage, and the results determine whether patients should be discharged early, admitted and monitored closely, or undergo early angiography and revascularization (*e*Fig. 17.1.3). Revascularization reduces the likelihood of death, MI, and readmission (69,70).

CLINICAL PROFILE

History and Physical Examination

The site, character and radiation of the discomfort, and physical findings are similar to those in patients with MI, except that unstable angina may occur at rest with an unclear relationship to exercise or stress, and there may be little or no response to nitroglycerin therapy.

Electrocardiography

The ECG is a very important investigation and should be performed at admission and during episodes of ischemia. Patients with recurrent episodes of pain should have ECGs recorded while the pain is present. If there is sustained ST elevation or left bundle branch block (either new or old with evidence of troponin or myoglobin elevation), administration of thrombolytic therapy or transfer to a catheterization laboratory for primary percutaneous coronary intervention (PCI) should be considered. A normal ECG does not exclude the possibility of unstable angina. Tran-

sient ST depression (or, less frequently, elevation) and T-wave inversion occur commonly only during ischemia, and the prognosis and management are critically dependent on the ECG (71–74). ST depression of 0.5 mm or greater has been shown to be a significant risk factor for the composite end point of death/MI at 1 year (73), and 4-year follow-up has shown that patients with 0.5 mm or greater ST depression have a significantly higher mortality than those with normal ECGs or T-wave inversion (19% vs. 4% at 1 year and 18% vs. 6% at 4 years) (74) (*e*Fig. 17.1.4). Patients with isolated T-wave inversion usually have a benign course (72). The presence of inverted T waves in five or more leads has been shown to be associated with higher risk (75). Little information is available regarding the outcome of patients with deep T-wave inversion (0.2 mV), who are usually classified as being at intermediate risk.

Continuous Electrocardiographic Monitoring

Ischemic ST-segment changes are detected in 85% to 90% of patients with unstable angina who are undergoing continuous ECG monitoring, but these changes are often silent (76,77). Silent ischemia on Holter monitoring has been shown to correlate with reduced myocardial perfusion and ventricular function (77), and patients with this feature are more likely to die, develop MI, or require revascularization (77–79). The European guidelines for the management of acute coronary syndromes without persistent ST elevation (80) recommend that patients with suspected acute ischemic heart disease should have multilead continuous ST-segment monitoring if it is available or, failing that, frequent ECGs.

Troponins

The cardiac troponins are sensitive and specific markers of myocyte necrosis (81). Troponin levels are useful prognosticators, with a clear gradient of risk as levels increase (82,83), but because of their release pattern, patients who present within 6 hours of symptom onset may have a normal troponin test result despite being at high risk. For this reason, it is important that troponin tests be done at admission and repeated 6 to 8 hours later.

Only one troponin T assay is available. A number of different troponin I assays are available with a wide variety of cutoff values, and discrepancies have been found between the results obtained using different assays (84). The prognostic value of third-generation assays for troponin T (cutoff point, 0.03 mg per L) and troponin I (cutoff point, 1.0 mg per L) was confirmed in the Fragmin and Fast Revascularization during Instability in Coronary Artery Disease (FRISC II) study (85).

It is important to measure troponin levels because they correlate with the pathophysiology of acute coronary syndromes (i.e., the presence of thrombus in the coronary

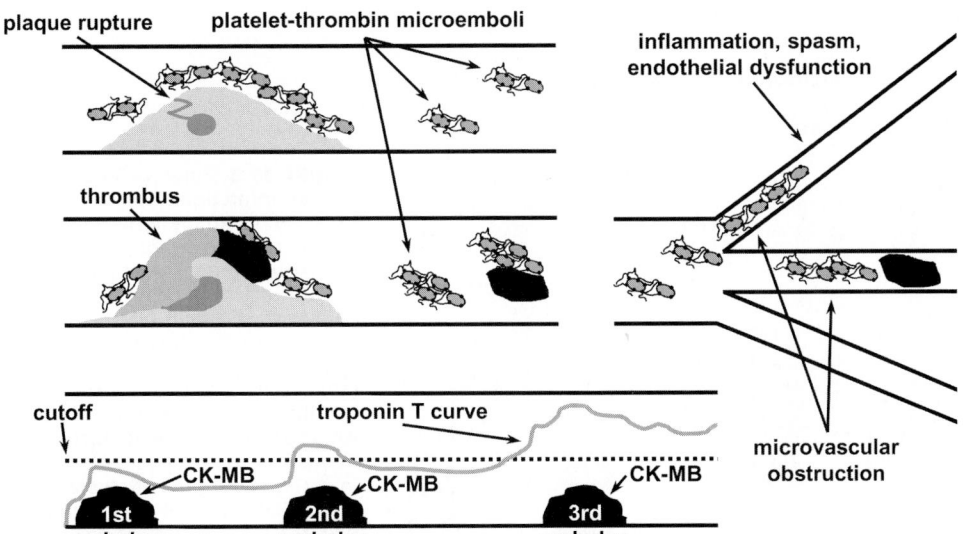

FIGURE 17.2 Microvascular obstruction after plaque rupture. CK-MB, creatine kinase-MB. (Adapted from Goldmann BU, Christenson RH, Hamm CW, et al. Implications of troponin testing in clinical medicine. *Curr Control Trials Cardiovasc Med* 2001;2:75–84, with permission.)

artery) (86) and may reflect the thrombogenic activity of ruptured or fissured plaques (86,87). The prognostic value of the troponins is greater than would be expected from the extent of myocyte necrosis and impairment of left ventricular function, perhaps reflecting preceding episodes of micromyocyte necrosis following embolization of platelets from ruptured or fissured plaques (Fig. 17.2). Several angiographic studies have reported that evidence of thrombus, complex lesions, and impairment of TIMI flow were more common in patients with elevated troponin levels than in those with normal levels (86,87).

Troponin levels identify patients at short- and long-term risk (83,88–94), enabling therapies such as low-molecular-weight heparins (95), IIb/IIIa antagonists (83,91,96), and interventions (69,70) to be targeted toward those who are most likely to benefit. Troponin testing is thus a valuable addition to the history, examination, and ECG, and troponin levels have been added as a subclassification to the Braunwald definition of unstable angina (7) (Table 17.1). Thirty percent of patients who present with non–ST-elevation acute coronary syndromes and normal CK-MB levels have elevated troponin levels (82,95,97), and these patients have poor outcomes (95,98). ❦ c67

The combination of troponin T testing and exercise testing further defines patients at low, intermediate, and high risk (99) (*e*Fig. 17.2.2).

Figure 17.3 shows the risk of death/MI at various time points in trials of the IIb/IIIa antagonists, abciximab (88,93), tirofiban (89,90), and lamifiban (91), and the low-molecular-weight heparins, dalteparin (92) and enoxaparin (94). In all seven trials there was a clear association between elevated troponin levels and risk. However, a normal troponin test does not ensure a good clinical outcome, as shown by the event rates in these trials.

A metaanalysis of trials, totaling more than 5,000 patients, reported odds ratios of 4.19 [95% confidence interval (CI), 2.01 to 4.20] for the short-term risk of an event (i.e., inhospital or within 30 days) and 2.05 (95% CI, 1.98 to 4.11) for longer-term risk (up to 150 days). Troponins T and I were found to have equivalent prognostic values (100). An urgent troponin test should therefore be incorporated into the initial risk assessment, along with the clinical features, ECG changes, measures of left ventricular function, and extent of coronary disease. If the initial troponin test is negative, it should be repeated at 6 to 8 hours (3).

Cardiac Enzymes

Because troponin levels may remain elevated for 2 weeks, other measures of myocyte necrosis are required to diagnose reinfarction, such as CK levels (or preferably CK-MB, which is more cardiac specific). A myoglobin test may be helpful if troponin levels are not elevated, as this enzyme is the first to become elevated following ischemia. Baseline point-of-care testing with a multimarker strategy including myoglobin has been shown to be a more effective means of risk-stratification than a single-marker laboratory-based strategy (101). Other tests such as myosin light-chain assays (102) are not currently recommended as standard practice.

Chest X-Ray

Unless MI has occurred previously, the heart size is normal. Transient pulmonary edema may occur with global ischemia and should raise suspicions of left main coronary artery stenosis or mitral papillary muscle dysfunction.

C-Reactive Protein

C-reactive protein is an acute-phase protein produced by the liver when there is tissue injury, infection, or inflamma-

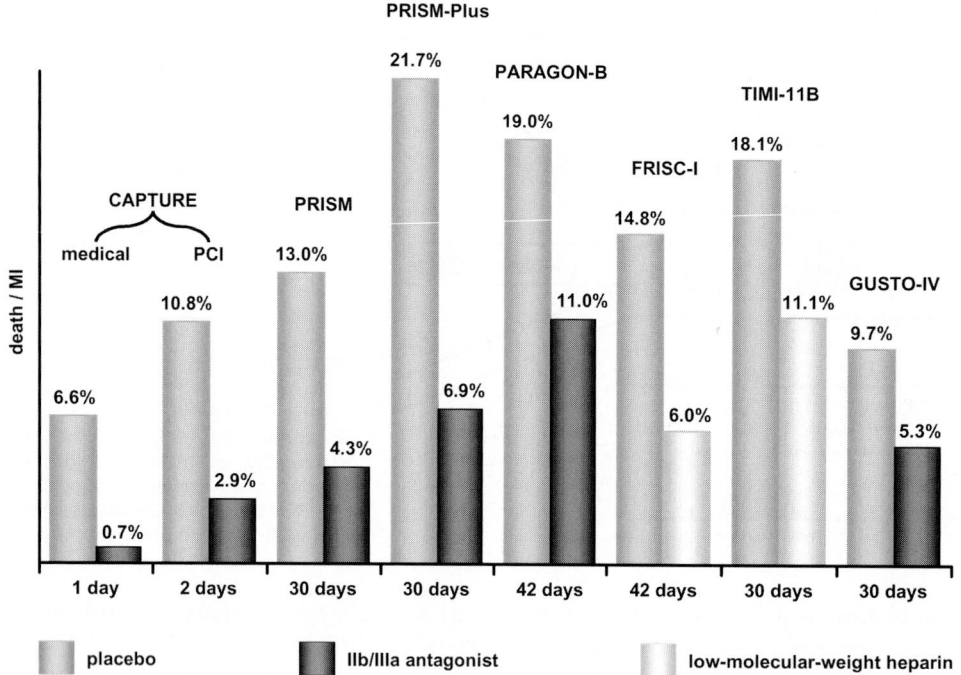

FIGURE 17.3 Rates of death/myocardial infarction (MI) at various time points in patients with elevated troponin levels in the c7E3 Fab Antiplatelet Therapy in Unstable Refractory Angina (CAPTURE) study of abciximab (88), the Platelet Receptor Inhibition in Ischemic Syndrome Management (PRISM) (89) and PRISM-PLUS (90) studies of tirofiban, the Platelet IIb/IIIa Antagonism for the Reduction of Acute Coronary Syndrome Events in a Global Organization Network (PARAGON-B) trial of lamifiban (88), the FRISC I study of dalteparin (92), the TIMI 11B trial of enoxaparin (94), and the Global Utilization of Streptokinase and t-PA for Occluded Coronary Arteries (GUSTO) IV trial (93) of abciximab. PCI, percutaneous coronary intervention.

tion. High-sensitivity C-reactive protein levels have been shown to correlate with future risks of MI, stroke, and peripheral vascular occlusion in apparently healthy people (103), and elevated levels have been noted in studies of patients with unstable angina (31). C-reactive protein levels are elevated in 50% to 70% of patients with Braunwald class IIIB angina (31).

Patients with elevated C-reactive protein levels at admission have been shown to have worse inhospital and 1-year outcomes, and elevated levels at discharge have been linked to recurrent instability long term (32). The major application of C-reactive protein testing appears to be in determining the long-term strategy after hospital discharge. Reduced C-reactive protein levels have been observed with aspirin (104) and statin therapy (105).

Amyloid A

Amyloid A is an acute-phase protein that is produced by the liver. Its predictive value appears to be similar to that of C-reactive protein (31).

Fibrinopeptide A

Fibrinopeptide A is a polypeptide cleaved from fibrinogen by thrombin. It is a sensitive marker of thrombin activity and fibrin generation. Elevated urinary fibrinopeptide A levels have been shown to correlate with the presence of intracoronary thrombus (106) and are an individual predictor of death/MI/revascularization within 1 week (odds ratio, 4.8) and within 6 months (odds ratio, 9.6). Persistently elevated levels signify an increased risk of coronary events (46). A

number of other markers that are currently under investigation include interleukin-6, intercellular adhesion molecule-1, lipoprotein-associated phospholipase A_2, and infectious seropositivity for *Chlamydia* (eTable 17.1.1).

Other Laboratory Tests

The white cell count is normal unless myocardial necrosis has occurred or there is underlying infection. Primary risk factors should be assessed at admission, including cholesterol and glucose intolerance, and possible secondary causes of unstable angina should be investigated if appropriate to the clinical circumstances, for example, hemoglobin, thyroid function, oxygen saturation, and so forth.

Risk-Stratification

Risk-stratification is critically important because it determines the choice of treatment strategy and provides prognostic information for the patient and relatives. Risk-stratification should take into account clinical factors, ECG and serum markers, evidence of spontaneous or inducible ischemia, measures of left ventricular function, and coronary anatomy. Patients at low risk can be discharged early. They should be asked to report any changes in their symptoms (e.g., recurring discomfort at rest or at night) and be reviewed subsequently at an outpatient clinic. Patients at intermediate risk may either receive initial medical therapy and be closely monitored for high-risk features or undergo early angiography with a view to revascularization. Patients at high risk should undergo early angiography and revascularization if their anatomy is suitable.

TABLE 17.2 AMERICAN COLLEGE OF CARDIOLOGY/AMERICAN HEART ASSOCIATION GUIDELINES FOR RISK-STRATIFICATION IN PATIENTS PRESENTING WITH NON–ST-ELEVATION ACUTE CORONARY SYNDROMES

	High risk: At least one of the following features must be present	Intermediate risk: No high-risk features but must have one of the following features	Low risk: No high- or intermediate-risk features but may have any of the following features
History	Accelerating tempo of ischemic symptoms in preceding 48 h	Previous MI, peripheral vascular disease or cerebrovascular disease, CABG, or prior aspirin use	
Character of pain	Prolonged and ongoing (>20 min) rest angina	Prolonged (>20 min) rest angina now resolved, rest angina (<20 min) or angina relieved by rest or sublingual nitroglycerin	New-onset Canadian Cardiovascular Society class III or IV angina in the previous 2 wk without prolonged (>20 min) rest pain
Clinical features	Pulmonary edema (most likely due to ischemia), new/worse murmur of mitral regurgitation, third heart sound or new/worsening rales, hypotension, bradycardia, tachycardia, age >75 yr	Age >70 yr	
ECG features	Rest angina with transient ST-segment changes (>0.05 mV), new bundle branch block, sustained ventricular tachycardia	T-wave inversion (>0.2 mV), pathologic Q waves	Normal or unchanged ECG during an episode of angina
Cardiac markers	Markedly elevated troponin T or I (>0.1 mg/L)	Slightly elevated troponin T (>0.01 mg/L but <0.1 mg/L)	Normal

CABG, coronary artery bypass grafting; ECG, electrocardiography; MI, myocardial infarction.
Adapted from Braunwald E, Jones RH, Mark DB, et al. Unstable angina: diagnosis and management. AHCPR Publication No. 94-0602 (204). Rockville, MD: Agency for Health Care Policy and Research and the National Heart, Lung, and Blood Institute. US Public Health Service, US Department of Health and Human Services, 1994, with permission.

A variety of risk factors have been identified, and various models for risk-stratification have been developed. Table 17.2 summarizes the guidelines for risk-stratification that were published by the American College of Cardiology (ACC) and American Heart Association (AHA) (1). Special emphasis is given to the tempo and momentum of ischemia, the patient's age (the most powerful determinant of risk), troponin levels, and ECG features, based on the TIMI IIIB study (73), which showed that ST depression of 0.5 mm or greater was a significant risk factor for the composite end point of death/MI at 1 year, and a study from Auckland (74), which showed that patients who presented with 0.5 mm or greater ST depression had a significantly higher mortality than those with normal ECGs or T-wave inversion (10% vs. 4% at 1 year and 18% vs. 6% at 4 years) (eFig. 17.1.4). Certain clinical features are not included in risk-stratification models, and the clinical assessment should always be regarded as paramount; for example, a patient who is gray, sweating, and anxious is at higher risk than one who is relaxed and appears well.

Different markers have been shown to have different prognostic values for acute risk and long-term risk, and the European Society of Cardiology guidelines (80) divide patients into these two categories (eTable 17.2.1). Patients should be assessed fully when first seen and then reviewed at 6 to 8 hours for recurrence of ischemia, response to treatment, and results of cardiac marker investigations, particularly the troponins. Further assessments should be done at 24 hours and again before discharge (eTable 17.2.2). Patients who have new-onset or accelerated angina without severe pain or pain at rest within 2 weeks and who have normal troponin levels and a normal ECG or an ECG that shows new T-wave changes are considered to be low risk and can be treated as outpatients (1,2) or in chest pain units (107). ▼ c68

NONINVASIVE TESTING

Stress Testing

Exercise or pharmacologic testing with or without imaging can be performed when patients have been asymptomatic for 24 to 48 hours. Exercise stress testing on a treadmill or bicycle, with ECG monitoring for ischemia and arrhythmias, is adequate in most patients. Ischemia occurring at a low workload (<6 metabolic equivalents) is associated with a poor prognosis (112), and coronary angiography is recommended. When exercise testing for ischemia is negative in patients with a normal baseline ECG, the 5-year survival rate is 95% (112).

Exercise thallium imaging can predict the severity of coronary artery disease and the risk of subsequent cardiac events in patients with unstable angina (113). ▼ c69

A number of patients are unable to undergo exercise testing because of physical limitations, and others have ECG changes that are difficult to interpret because of baseline abnormalities such as left ventricular hypertrophy, left bundle branch block, preexcitation, or the effects of digoxin. Pharmacologic stress testing is of particular value in these patients (115). Dipyridamole can be administered intravenously to cause coronary artery vasodilatation and flow discrepancies on perfusion scintigraphy (116), or echocardiography may reveal wall motion abnormalities in myocardial segments that are supplied by stenosed coronary arteries. By increasing myocardial contractility and, to a lesser extent, the heart rate, dobutamine stress testing can also detect areas of ischemia (113,117,118).

Early noninvasive testing is an important part of risk-stratification and should be performed soon after stabilization. If it is performed 1 month later, events that occur during this time—which may amount to 50% of all events in the first year—cannot be predicted. Sensitivity is not lost if exercise tests are performed before discharge. Stress testing can determine whether severe coronary artery stenoses are present (119) and indicate the likelihood of multivessel disease but does not show whether there is instability of coronary artery plaque with ongoing thrombosis.

Echocardiography

Two-dimensional echocardiography can provide anatomic and functional information, which is helpful in determining the diagnosis and prognosis. Transient abnormalities of wall motion and changes in ventricular volumes can be detected during ischemia (120). These findings may be helpful if the symptoms are atypical or if the ECG findings are nondiagnostic. Echocardiographic changes may precede pain or ischemic ST-segment changes. Transesophageal echocardiography is particularly useful for evaluating the possibility of aortic dissection.

Coronary Arteriography

The findings at coronary arteriography depend on the population studied. Single-vessel disease has been demonstrated in 43% of those with new-onset angina (55), and angiographically normal coronary arteries are found in 10% of patients (121). However, angiography outlines only the arterial lumen, and there may be large plaques within the arterial wall. Intravascular ultrasound may show that some of these patients have ruptured plaques with probable thrombus. In others, even intravascular ultrasound and angiography are normal, and the likely pathophysiology is coronary spasm. Alternatively, there may have been a misleading history of false-positive ECG features.

In a selected group of patients from the Coronary Artery Surgery Study Registry who had CABG for unstable angina, 14% had left main coronary artery stenoses and 50% had triple-vessel coronary artery disease. In the TIMI IIIB trial, 19% of patients had no coronary artery stenoses of greater than 60% narrowing. Single-vessel disease was found in 38%, double-vessel disease in 29%, and triple-vessel disease in 15%. A left main coronary artery stenosis of greater than 50% narrowing was found in 4% (122).

Eccentric plaques and complex plaques (*e*Fig. 17.3.4) are more commonly found in patients with unstable angina than in those with chronic stable angina (6). Coronary artery thrombi may be seen in 40% of patients if arteriography is performed soon after an episode of rest pain (48).

Left Ventriculography

Abnormalities of regional wall motion may be detected, caused by previous MI or "hibernation" due to prolonged or recurrent ischemia. Wall motion abnormalities and changes in ventricular volumes may also occur during episodes of acute ischemia (123).

PROGNOSIS

The prognosis of patients who present with unstable angina depends on their risk factors. Within 1 month, 2% to 5% die and 5% to 16% experience an MI (70,90,124). Within 1 year, 26% to 35% require readmission to the hospital for recurrent symptoms (125) and 4% to 15% die (122,125–129). Patients with unstable angina and a normal coronary arteriogram have good short-term (130) and long-term prognoses (131).

CLINICAL VARIABLES

The most important variables are age (110), left ventricular function (110), coronary anatomy (132), diabetes, and comorbid conditions such as chronic obstructive pulmonary disease, renal failure, cerebrovascular disease, and malignancy. Diabetics with non–ST-elevation acute coronary syndromes are at higher risk of death/MI than are nondiabetics (70,90,124). ♥ c70

Rest pain at admission and recurrent episodes of ischemia are high-risk features (71,122,135–137). Patients with recurrent rest pain within 48 hours after admission have a 20% lower survival rate (135).

The incidence of MI is approximately 3% in patients with accelerating angina without ECG changes and about 18% in those with rest pain and ECG changes (136). Ischemic ST changes on the admission ECG are high-risk features (71,109,135). The presence of myocardial ischemia on continuous ST-segment monitoring increases the risk of death/MI significantly (79) (*e*Fig. 17.3.5). Mortality at 1 year can be predicted by the extent of ST depression on the admission ECG (*e*Table 17.2.7). ECG changes of greater than 1 mm of ST depression after admission have an 89% sensitivity for predicting MI, further angina, or the need for revascularization (71). The number of ischemic episodes is related to outcomes (109). ♥ c71

ST-segment shifts increase the risk of death/MI (71). Patients with rebound ischemia during continuous ST-segment monitoring have an increased risk of death/MI at 1 year (18.4% vs. 8.3%, p = .02) (139).

The medicines that patients are taking when angina develops can be an important indicator of risk. In the TIMI IIIB trial, patients in whom unstable angina developed while they were receiving beta-blockers did worse, whereas those on angiotensin-converting enzyme (ACE) inhibitors at the time did better (122).

PRINCIPLES OF MANAGEMENT

Aims of Treatment

The immediate aims of treatment are to relieve pain with morphine and antianginal therapy and to prevent MI and death by stabilizing the thrombotic process with antithrombotic therapy (*e*Table 17.2.8). If MI develops, treatments to preserve the myocardium should be used, such as thrombolytic therapy or primary PCI in the event of ST elevation or left bundle branch block that is not preexisting. Revascularization is recommended for high-risk patients and can also be performed as primary treatment in intermediate-risk patients or reserved for use in those who are refractory to medical therapy.

Longer-term goals involve identification and treatment of cardiac risk factors such as hypertension, dyslipidemia, and smoking. Patients should also be enrolled in a cardiac rehabilitation program (*e*Table 17.2.8). It is incumbent on physicians to use the most cost-effective strategy that is available to them.

General Measures

Patients with rest pain or ECG changes, or both, within the previous 48 hours should be admitted to the hospital. Antithrombotic and antiischemic therapy should be commenced without delay when the patient is first seen in the emergency department, chest pain unit (107), or coronary care unit. Patients should be placed on bed rest, ideally with continuous ECG monitoring for arrhythmias and ischemia, or, failing that, 12-lead ECGs should be performed at baseline, 30 minutes, and 1 hour and repeated if further pain occurs.

Oxygen

Oxygen is commonly administered to all patients with acute chest pain. The Agency for Health Care Policy and Research guidelines recommend more selective use of oxygen in patients with obvious cyanosis, respiratory distress, or high-risk features (1) (Table 17.2).

Morphine

Morphine is very effective for relieving pain and anxiety. It may also reduce the cardiac workload and oxygen con-

sumption by causing venodilation and slightly decreasing the heart rate and blood pressure. Morphine should be administered in intravenous (i.v.) doses of 2 to 5 mg if angina has not been relieved by nitroglycerin tablets or spray (see Nitrates), provided that there are no contraindications. The dose can be repeated every 5 to 30 minutes.

Antiplatelet Agents

Aspirin

Aspirin potently inhibits thromboxane A_2-dependent platelet aggregation by irreversibly inhibiting the platelet enzyme, cyclooxygenase, which reduces platelet synthesis of thromboxane A_2. ☛ c72

In a metaanalysis of five studies, aspirin or ticlopidine reduced mortality by 59 ± 8% (67,126,127,154,155) (*e*Fig. 17.3.6). The dosages used varied from 75 mg per day (154) to 325 mg four times a day (127). The effect of aspirin is rapid. In normal volunteers, 162.5 mg aspirin inhibited 91% of arachidonic acid–induced platelet aggregation *ex vivo* within 15 minutes (156).

All patients with a diagnosis of unstable angina should receive aspirin as soon as possible unless there is active bleeding or documented hypersensitivity. The initial dose should be 150 to 325 mg because of the possibility of reduced intestinal blood flow during ischemia and to ensure complete inhibition of thromboxane A_2 production. ☛ c73

Ticlopidine and Clopidogrel

Ticlopidine and clopidogrel are thienopyridine derivatives, and both are prodrugs. They are selective antagonists of ADP-induced aggregation and also reduce responses to other agonists that require ADP.

Because of its side effects and delayed onset of action (2 to 3 days for maximal antiplatelet effect), ticlopidine is not recommended as initial therapy for patients with unstable angina.

Clopidogrel (75 mg per day) was compared with aspirin (325 mg per day) in the Clopidogrel versus Aspirin in Patients at Risk of Ischaemic Events (CAPRIE) trial of 19,000 patients with symptomatic peripheral vascular disease, recurrent MI, or a recent ischemic stroke. A modest reduction in vascular death/MI/ischemic stroke occurred with clopidogrel (5.32% vs. 5.83% with aspirin, p = .04; relative risk reduction, 8.7%; 95% CI, 0.3 to 16.5). The safety profile was similar to that of aspirin (158). Thrombotic thrombocytopenic purpura can occur when clopidogrel is commenced, but this is rare and tends to manifest within the first 2 weeks of therapy (159).

The Clopidogrel in Unstable Angina to Prevent Recurrent Events (CURE) trial randomized 12,562 patients with acute coronary syndromes to receive either aspirin (75 to 325 mg per day) or aspirin plus clopidogrel, given as a 300-

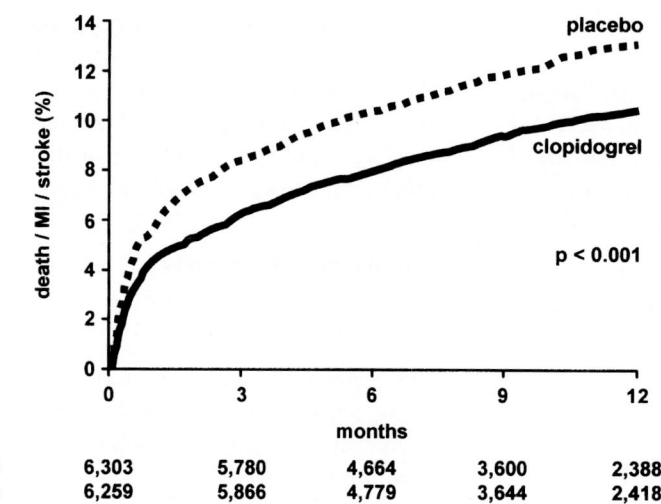

FIGURE 17.4 Rates of cardiovascular death/myocardial infarction (MI)/stroke within 9 months in patients given either aspirin alone or aspirin plus clopidogrel in the CURE trial. (Redrawn from The Clopidogrel in Unstable Angina to Prevent Recurrent Events Trial Investigators. Effects of clopidogrel in addition to aspirin in patients with acute coronary syndromes without ST-segment elevation. *N Engl J Med* 2001;345:494–502. Copyright © 2001, Massachusetts Medical Society. All rights reserved, with permission.)

mg loading dose followed by 75 mg per day. At 9 months, the incidence of cardiovascular death/MI/stroke was reduced by 20% from 11.47% to 9.28% in the patients who had received aspirin plus clopidogrel (p <.01) (Fig. 17.4). The major component of this reduction was a 23% decrease in MI (Table 17.3). A 31% reduction in refractory ischemia (defined as ischemic ECG changes leading to intervention while receiving at least one antianginal and one antithrombotic agent) also occurred. The reduction in death/MI/stroke beyond 30 days was similar to that observed within 30 days, and the benefits of clopidogrel were seen across many subgroups. The effect was similar in patients with and patients without elevated markers. A 1% absolute increase in major bleeding occurred among patients who were given aspirin plus clopidogrel (3.6% vs. 2.7% in patients given aspirin alone, p <.01) (160).

Clopidogrel is thus indicated for acute and long-term use in addition to aspirin in intermediate-risk patients. It is not known whether it is superior to small-molecule IIb/IIIa antagonists in high-risk patients. In high-risk patients, its use should be considered in addition to IIb/IIIa antagonists. The use of clopidogrel should also be considered in patients in whom emergency surgery is

likely, such as those with hemodynamic instability or widespread ST-segment changes. It is also recommended for adjunctive use with a IIb/IIIa antagonist in the setting of PCI (161,162). Approximately 1,500 patients undergoing CABG in the CURE trial received clopidogrel, with no increase in the relative bleeding excess (160). However, there is concern among surgeons about the possibility of increased bleeding in patients who have received clopidogrel, and there was a trend in the CURE trial toward increased bleeding in patients who received clopidogrel within 5 days of their surgery.

Platelet Glycoprotein IIb/IIIa Receptor Antagonists

The final common pathway to platelet aggregation is the binding of fibrinogen to the IIb/IIIa receptors on the surface of platelets, with cross-linking and formation of a platelet thrombus. On the surface of each platelet are 50,000 to 80,000 of these receptors, but they are usually unreceptive unless activated by the conformational changes associated with disruption of endothelium. Inhibition of these receptors blocks the final common pathway to plate-

TABLE 17.3 RESULTS OF THE CURE TRIAL

End point	Aspirin (n = 6,303)	Aspirin + clopidogrel (n = 6,259)	Risk ratio
Cardiovascular death/MI/stroke[a]	11.40%	9.30%	0.80
Cardiovascular death	5.50%	5.10%	0.93
MI	6.70%	5.20%	0.77
Stroke	1.40%	1.20%	0.86
Noncardiovascular end point	0.70%	0.70%	0.91

CURE, Clopidogrel in Unstable Angina to Prevent Recurrent Events; MI, myocardial infarction.
[a]Primary end point.
From The Clopidogrel in Unstable Angina to Prevent Recurrent Events Trial Investigators. Effects of clopidogrel in addition to aspirin in patients with acute coronary syndromes without ST-segment elevation. *N Engl J Med* 2001;345:494–502. Copyright © 2001, Massachusetts Medical Society. All rights reserved, with permission.

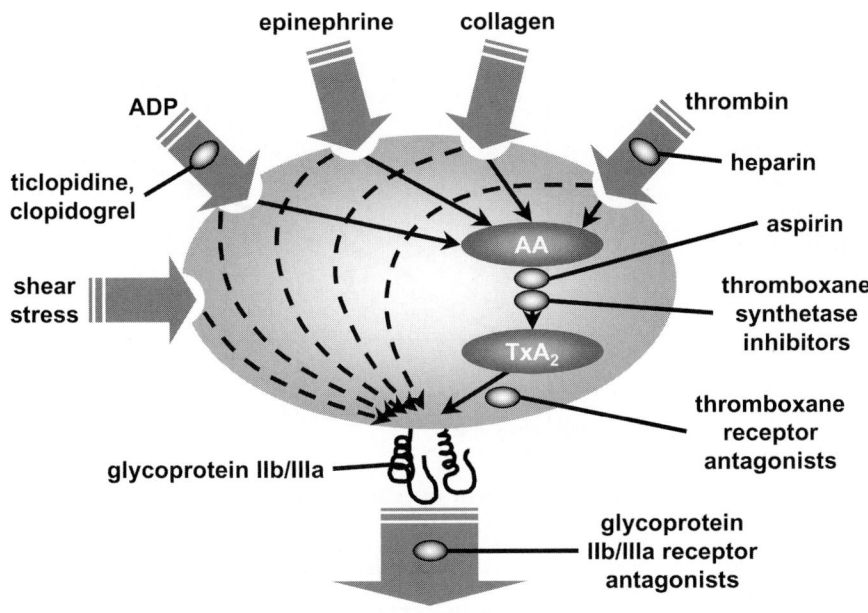

FIGURE 17.5 Stimuli that increase the affinity of the glycoprotein IIb/IIIa receptor for fibrinogen. AA, arachidonic acid; ADP, adenosine diphosphate; TxA$_2$, thromboxane A$_2$.

let aggregation (Fig. 17.5). The effects of thrombin, thromboxane A$_2$, collagen, ADP, catecholamine, and shear-induced platelet aggregation can be prevented by specific blockers of these receptors. Dose-dependent inhibition of platelet aggregation can be achieved, and the effect of the nonantibody agents is reversible within a few hours of stopping the infusion. With the monoclonal antibody, abciximab, there is a gradual decline in the antithrombotic effect, with 50% recovery of ADP-induced aggregation at 24 to 48 hours.

Glycoprotein IIb/IIIa antagonists can limit platelet aggregation at the site of plaque rupture, erosion, or fissuring and reduce the amount of platelet thrombus and embolization causing myocyte necrosis. Abciximab was shown in the CAPTURE study to reduce the amount of thrombus present at coronary arteriography (96), and the Platelet Receptor Inhibition in Ischemic Syndrome Management in Patients Limited by Unstable Signs and Symptoms (PRISM-PLUS) study found that tirofiban reduced peak troponin levels (163). In 16 trials of IIb/IIIa antagonists in acute coronary syndromes, totaling more than 32,000 patients, mortality was reduced by 30% at 48 to 96 hours (p <.03), but the mortality reductions at 30 days and 6 months were not significant. The incidence of death/MI was significantly reduced by 24% at 30 days and at 6 months (164). Seven trials have shown that IIb/IIIa antagonists reduce the incidence of death/MI by approximately 35% at 30 days in patients who are undergoing PCI (162).

Abciximab

The efficacy of abciximab, a monoclonal antibody to the IIb/IIIa receptor, has been evaluated in several trials. ⚐ c74

In the GUSTO IV trial (93), 7,800 patients who presented within 24 hours of the onset of chest pain that lasted at least 5 minutes and who had either 0.5 mm or greater ST depression or elevated troponin I or T levels were randomized to receive a placebo infusion, abciximab for 24 hours, or abciximab for 48 hours. The aim of the trial was to test an intensive medical regimen, and only 1.6% of patients underwent PCI in the first 48 hours. Abciximab was found to have no effect on the incidence of death/MI within 30 days (MI being defined as a CK-MB level of three times normal), with rates of 8.0% in the placebo group, 8.2% in the 24-hour abciximab group, and 9.1% in the 48-hour abciximab group. In patients with elevated troponin levels, the event rates were 10.0%, 10.0%, and 11.6%, respectively. Abciximab also had no effect in patients with ST depression, with event rates of 8.4%, 8.5%, and 9.9%, respectively, or in patients with both elevated troponins and ST depression. ⚐ c75

Tirofiban

Tirofiban is a small nonpeptide antagonist of the IIb/IIIa receptor that mimics the tripeptide arginine-glycine-aspartate sequence in fibrinogen. It is nonimmunogenic and has a high degree of selectivity for the platelet fibrinogen receptor, producing an acute effect within 5 minutes of administration. The effects are reversible in 4 to 6 hours. ⚐ c76

The PRISM and PRISM-PLUS studies showed that tirofiban is effective at reducing acute ischemic events during the infusion of the drug. Tirofiban was more effective than heparin in the PRISM study (89) and added to the effects of heparin in the PRISM-PLUS study (90). Because of the mortality increase observed with tirofiban in the dropped arm of PRISM-PLUS, which enrolled higher-risk patients than PRISM, it is recommended that adjunctive heparin be given with tirofiban.

In the Do Tirofiban and ReoPro Give Similar Efficacy (TARGET) trial (161), tirofiban was compared with abciximab in patients who were undergoing stenting. At 30 days, there was a 20% reduction in death/MI/rescue revascularization in the patients treated with abciximab (6.0% vs. 7.5% with tirofiban, $p = .037$). The difference was greater in the subgroup of patients with acute coronary syndromes (6.3% with abciximab vs. 9.3% with tirofiban). No difference was found in death/MI in patients undergoing elective PCI (5.6% with abciximab vs. 4.5% with tirofiban).

Eptifibatide

Eptifibatide is a cyclic peptide inhibitor of the IIb/IIIa receptor that exerts rapid platelet inhibition. It has a short half-life, with platelet aggregation returning to baseline within 2 to 4 hours. ▼ c77

The PURSUIT trial compared eptifibatide with a placebo in 9,461 patients with ischemic chest pain and 1 mm or greater ST depression and reported that it reduced the incidence of death/MI from 15.7% to 14.2% at 30 days ($p = .03$).

Lamifiban

Lamifiban is a synthetic, nonpeptide, highly selective IIb/IIIa antagonist. It has been tested in several clinical trials (91,170) but is not yet available for clinical use. Its pharmacodynamic half-life is approximately 4 hours (179). ▼ c78

Time to Treatment

The longer the delay before commencement of IIb/IIIa antagonist therapy, the longer patients are exposed to the risk of MI. In the PURSUIT trial, patients were randomized to receive eptifibatide either within 6 hours, between 6 and 12 hours, or more than 12 hours after symptom onset. A larger absolute reduction in death/MI occurred within 30 days in patients who received eptifibatide earlier (2.8%, 2.5%, and 1.4%, respectively) (124,180) (*e*Fig. 17.5.1).

Upstream Treatment with IIb/IIIa Antagonists

IIb/IIIa antagonists may be beneficial in three situations: during PCI, before PCI ("upstream" treatment), and in patients who are treated with medical therapy alone. Upstream treatment was assessed in the CAPTURE (88), PRISM-PLUS (90), and PURSUIT (124) trials, totaling more than 12,000 patients, and the combined results demonstrated a substantial reduction in death/MI in the period before intervention (from 4.3% to 2.9%, equating to 14 fewer events per 1,000 patients treated) (181) (Fig. 17.6).

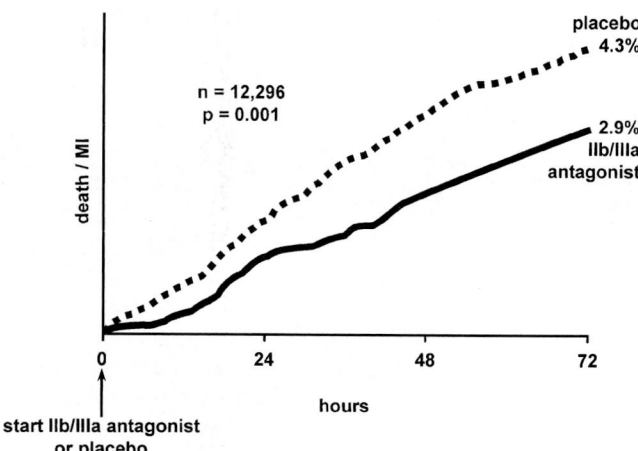

FIGURE 17.6 Event rates before intervention in the CAPTURE (88), PRISM-PLUS (90), and PURSUIT (124) trials of IIb/IIIa antagonists in patients with non–ST-elevation acute coronary syndromes. MI, myocardial infarction. (Redrawn from Boersma E, Akkerhuis M, Théroux P, et al. Platelet glycoprotein IIb/IIIa receptor inhibition in non-ST-elevation acute coronary syndromes: early benefit during medical treatment only, with additional protection during percutaneous coronary intervention. *Circulation* 1999;100:2045–2048, with permission.)

Most of this reduction was in MI rather than death. From the time of the intervention up until 48 hours afterward, the effect was greater, but after that time there was no effect.

Upstream treatment with a IIb/IIIa antagonist also reduces the incidence of MI before CABG (90) and may reduce the risk of perioperative events. Cardiopulmonary bypass activates platelets, leading to thromboembolism. Paradoxically, it may also lead to thrombocytopenia and increased bleeding via binding of platelets through the IIb/IIIa receptors. In the PURSUIT trial, 1,558 patients underwent CABG. Eptifibatide reduced the rate of death/MI within 30 days from 30.8% to 26.1%, and the effect was maintained at 6-month follow-up (*e*Fig. 17.6.1). The reduction in events was greatest among patients who received eptifibatide within 72 hours of CABG (23.8% vs. 33.6%, $p = .002$). The incidence of major bleeding was not increased, occurring in 58.2% of the eptifibatide group and 56.6% of the placebo group ($p = .7$) (182). In the PRISM-PLUS study, tirofiban reduced the 30-day incidence of death/MI in patients who were undergoing CABG from 16.8% to 12.2% (90). Given the logistical difficulties in many hospitals of performing procedures at night and during the weekend, upstream use of a IIb/IIIa antagonist before procedures is very practical.

Use of IIb/IIIa Antagonists in Patients Treated without Interventions

In the PARAGON-A (170), PRISM (89), PRISM-PLUS (90), PURSUIT (124) PARAGON-B (91), and GUSTO IV (93) trials, intervention was not recommended to be performed routinely, and only approximately 11% of patients underwent intervention while on randomized IIb/IIIa antagonist or placebo therapy. These trials were thus trials of medical therapy with intervention performed at the discretion of the treating physician, and so conclusions cannot be drawn from analysis of the medically managed patients alone. These trials showed that IIb/IIIa antagonists reduced the incidence of death/MI by 8% at 30 days (see Fig. 17.7). In the PURSUIT trial, in which PCI was performed at the discretion of the treating physician, an analysis with censoring for PCI across the 30-day follow-up period showed that eptifibatide accounted for a 31% reduction in the incidence of death/MI (from 16.8% to 15.1%, $p = .035$) (183). Correction of the event rates using a PCI propensity score produced no evidence that the eptifibatide treatment effect differed between the two groups.

Which Patients Should Receive IIb/IIIa Antagonists?

IIb/IIIa antagonists should be targeted at patients who are undergoing PCI (184), patients at high risk, and, in particular, those with ST depression or elevated troponin levels (1,80,89,91,96) (Table 17.4). In the PRISM study (89), tirofiban reduced the risk of death/MI in patients with elevated troponins to a level similar to that of patients without elevated troponins (83) (Fig. 17.6.2). In the PARAGON-B trial, lamifiban had no beneficial effect overall, but in patients with troponin levels it reduced the incidence of death/MI/recurrent ischemia from 19.4% to 11.0% at 30 days ($p = .01$) (91). Diabetic patients are at high risk, and in PRISM-PLUS tirofiban reduced their incidence of death/MI from 19.2% to 11.2% at 30 days (90).

Patients who are already receiving aspirin therapy at admission are at particularly high risk (111,185) because the

TABLE 17.4 INDICATIONS FOR INTRAVENOUS IIB/IIIA ANTAGONISTS

Elevated troponin levels
≥ 0.5-mm ST depression
Elevated cardiac enzyme levels
Patients undergoing PCI
Patients with high-risk features
    Age >65 yr
    Ejection fraction <50%
    Hemodynamic instability
    Angiographic evidence of thrombus
    PCI within the previous 6 mo
    Previous CABG
    Previous myocardial infarction
    Pulmonary edema
Diabetes
Patients already receiving aspirin at admission
Recurrent ischemia
Inpatients awaiting CABG

CABG, coronary artery bypass grafting; PCI, percutaneous coronary intervention.

aspirin has usually been prescribed for secondary prevention due to a previous coronary event or known coronary artery disease or for primary prevention; for example, they are considered at high risk because of a strong family history of coronary disease (186). When such patients present with an acute coronary syndrome, it signifies that they have broken through the antiplatelet and antiinflammatory effects of the aspirin (103), and it could mean either that they are unresponsive to aspirin or that they have a large thrombus load associated with plaque rupture or fissuring. In patients who are already receiving aspirin, the rates of death/MI were reduced from 17.3% to 14.9% at 30 days with eptifibatide in PURSUIT (185) and from 21.8% to 14.8% at 7 days with tirofiban in PRISM-PLUS (90).

Patients with intracoronary thrombus detected at angiography are also at high risk. In PRISM-PLUS (187) the presence of thrombus was shown to increase the 30-day incidence of death from 2% to 5%, MI from 4% to 9%, and recurrent ischemia from 5% to 9%. IIb/IIIa antagonists have been shown to reduce the amount of thrombus detected at angiography (96), and their use may be indicated in patients with angiographic thrombus unsuitable for PCI who are awaiting CABG over the next few days.

More than 30,000 patients have been randomized into IIb/IIIa antagonist studies in which they received medical treatment primarily and underwent revascularization procedures only at the discretion of the treating physician. If all of the results are combined (including GUSTO IV), there was a significant 8% reduction in death/MI at 30 days in patients who were given IIb/IIIa antagonists, down from 11.8% to 10.6% ($p <.02$) (89–91,93,124,170) (Fig. 17.7). In the subgroup of patients with elevated troponin levels, analysis using a similar definition of MI in all of the trials (namely, a CK-MB level of twice normal) shows that the incidence of death/MI was reduced by 22% (83,90,91,93) (Fig. 17.8). A few studies have evaluated the cost effectiveness of IIb/IIIa antagonists and found it to be similar to that of other therapies (188).

Combination Therapy with IIb/IIIa Antagonists and Clopidogrel

There have been no randomized trials of combination therapy with IIb/IIIa antagonists and clopidogrel, but retrospective analysis of several studies has suggested that this combination is both beneficial and safe. In the EPISTENT Trial, ticlopidine was found to be beneficial when given prior to stenting in patients who also received abciximab in the catheterization laboratory (188a). In the TARGET trial (161), patients who received clopidogrel prior to either abciximab or tirofiban had lower event rates. In the CURE trial (188b), there was less usage of IIb/IIIa antagonists in the clopidogrel treatment group, and no increase in major bleeding was observed in patients who did receive a IIb/IIIa antagonist. Upstream treatment with both clopidogrel and

Trial	N	Death / MI IIb/IIIa antagonist	Control	Reduction ± SD	Odds ratio and 95% CI
PARAGON-A*	1,513	10.6%	11.7%	11 ± 15%	
PARAGON-A†	1,526	12.0%	11.7%	−2 ± 16%	
PRISM	3,232	5.8%	7.1%	19 ± 13%	
PRISM-Plus‡	1,570	8.7%	11.9%	30 ± 14%	
PRISM-Plus§	695	13.6%	11.7%	−19 ± 25%	
PURSUIT	9,461	14.2%	15.7%	11 ± 5%	
PARAGON-B	5,169	10.5%	11.5%	9 ± 8%	
GUSTO-IV	7,800	8.7%	8.0%	−8 ± 9%	
Total	30,966	10.6%	11.8%	8 ± 4%	

Treatment effect: 2p = 0.027
χ^2 test for heterogeneity = 9.07

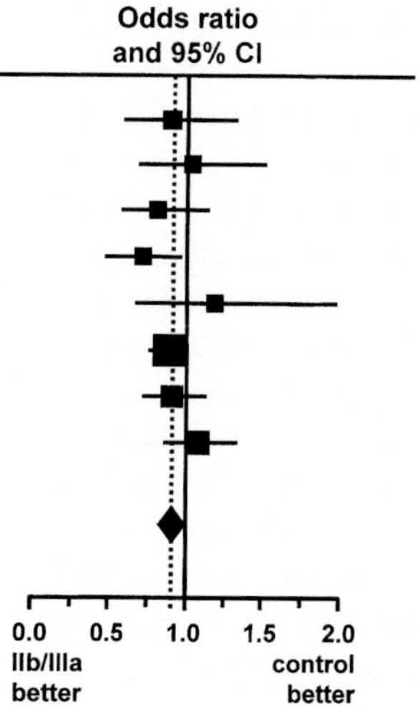

0.0 0.5 1.0 1.5 2.0
IIb/IIIa   control
better   better

FIGURE 17.7 Metaanalysis of death/ myocardial infarction (MI) at 30 days in trials (89–91,93,124,170) comparing IIb/IIIa antagonists with control treatment in patients with non–ST-elevation acute coronary syndromes who were also receiving aspirin therapy and in whom immediate percutaneous coronary intervention was not planned. *Low-dose lamifiban; †high-dose lamifiban; ‡tirofiban plus heparin versus heparin alone; §tirofiban alone versus heparin alone; CI, confidence interval; SD, standard deviation.

a IIb/IIIa antagonist prior to PCI should be considered in high-risk patients but avoided in those likely to require urgent CABG.

Heparin

A pooled analysis of heparin trials is shown in Figure 17.9. [✍ c79] Overall, unfractionated heparin had no effect on the incidence of death/MI within 30 days (197).

Duration and Monitoring of Heparin Therapy

Limited data are available regarding the optimal duration and intensity of heparin therapy. When administered for 6 to 7 days, heparin has been shown to reduce the incidence of death/MI (67,189,194). However, in two studies, 2 days of heparin therapy had no effect on myocardial ischemia or on the incidence of death/MI (79).

Low-Molecular-Weight Heparins

Although unfractionated heparin is standard therapy in acute coronary syndromes, the data for its use are not compelling (194). Its bioavailability varies because it binds to

plasma proteins and to the endothelium, and this makes it difficult to use, necessitating precise dosage adjustment to maximize therapeutic efficacy while minimizing the risk of bleeding.

Low-molecular-weight heparins have a mean molecular mass of only 46 kd and lack the minimum 18 saccharides that are required for simultaneous binding of thrombin and antithrombin III, although they bind to and inhibit factor X_a more effectively than does unfractionated heparin. Because the different low-molecular-weight heparins have different chemical structures and different molecular weights, they have different biologic properties, antifactor X_a to antifactor II_a ratios, and effects on the release of tissue factor pathway inhibitor. The antifactor X_a effects of low-molecular-weight heparins can be partially reversed (by approximately 60%) by administration of protamine sulfate (198).

Low-molecular-weight heparins have a number of practical advantages over unfractionated heparin, including greater bioavailability and a more predictable dose response due to minimal protein binding, and higher antifactor X_a to antifactor II_a ratios with an enhanced ability to inhibit thrombin generation, inhibition of von Willebrand's factor release, resistance to inactivation by platelet factor 4, no

Trial	N	Death / MI IIb/IIIa antagonist	Control	Reduction ± SD	Odds ratio and 95% CI
PRISM	629	4.3%	13.0%	66 ± 17%	
PRISM-Plus	105	5.7%	17.3%	68 ± 36%	
PARAGON-B	464	11.0%	19.0%	46 ± 19%	
GUSTO-IV	3,259	12.9%	13.0%	2 ± 11%	
Total	4,457	11.6%	14.0%	22 ± 8%	

Treatment effect: 2p < 0.01
χ^2 test for heterogeneity = 17.49

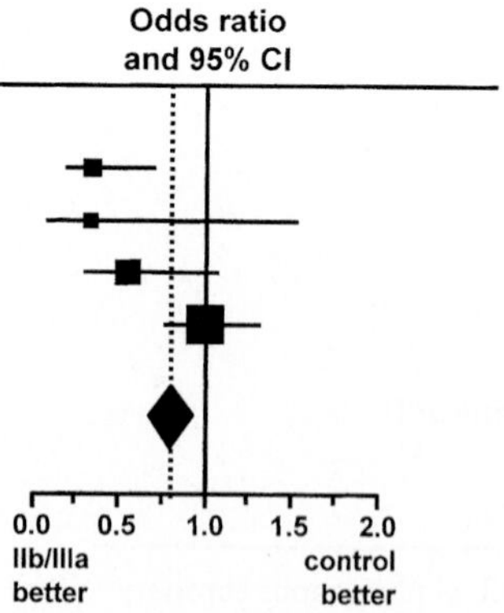

0.0 0.5 1.0 1.5 2.0
IIb/IIIa   control
better   better

FIGURE 17.8 Metaanalysis of death/ myocardial infarction (MI) at 30 days in patients with elevated troponin levels in the PRISM (83), PRISM-PLUS (90), PARAGON-B (91), and GUSTO IV (93) trials. In GUSTO IV, MI was defined as a creatine kinase (CK)–MB level of three times normal. Here, MI is defined as a CK-MB level of twice normal. CI, confidence interval; SD, standard deviation.

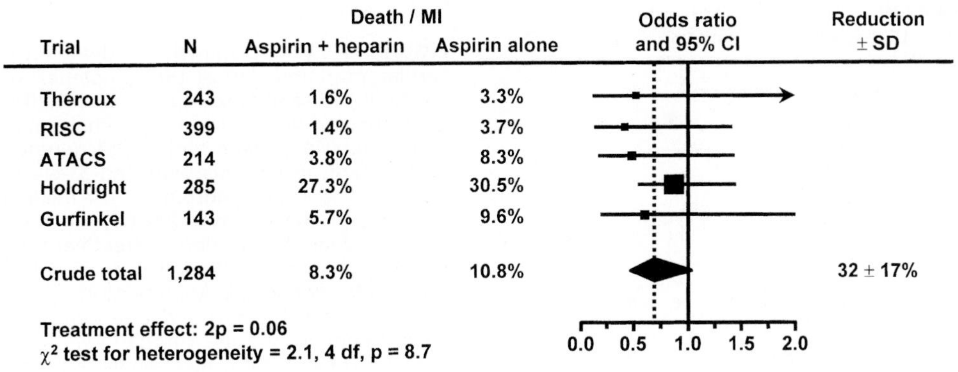

Trial	N	Death / MI Aspirin + heparin	Aspirin alone	Odds ratio and 95% CI	Reduction ± SD
Théroux	243	1.6%	3.3%		
RISC	399	1.4%	3.7%		
ATACS	214	3.8%	8.3%		
Holdright	285	27.3%	30.5%		
Gurfinkel	143	5.7%	9.6%		
Crude total	1,284	8.3%	10.8%		32 ± 17%

Treatment effect: 2p = 0.06
χ^2 test for heterogeneity = 2.1, 4 df, p = 8.7

0.0 0.5 1.0 1.5 2.0

FIGURE 17.9 Metaanalysis of death/myocardial infarction (MI) in trials (79,154,190,192,193) comparing aspirin plus unfractionated heparin with aspirin alone in patients with unstable angina. Low-molecular-weight heparin was used in the trial by Gurfinkel et al. (192). CI, confidence interval; df, degrees of freedom; SD, standard deviation.

heparin resistance, and no activation of platelets. They are more convenient to use because they require no monitoring of the APTT and no i.v. lines, and their use has been shown to save money in some health-care systems (199). The associated rates of thrombocytopenia and osteoporosis are lower (200), and rebound ischemia may be less common after cessation than it is with unfractionated heparin (139). The patients who benefit most are those older than 65 years (92,94,201); those who are currently receiving aspirin; those with elevated troponins, ST depression, or previous or current MI; and those waiting for interventions (69).

As of yet, there is no compelling evidence that the low-molecular-weight heparins as a group are superior to unfractionated heparin in the management of patients with acute coronary syndromes. The five trials that compared enoxaparin (94,201), dalteparin (202), and Fraxiparine (192,203) with unfractionated heparin yielded mixed results.

The TIMI 11B trial (94) compared enoxaparin (30-mg i.v. bolus followed by 1.0 mg per kg subcutaneously twice a day) with unfractionated heparin (70-IU-per-kg i.v. bolus followed by 15-IU-per-kg-per-hour i.v. infusion). c80

In the ESSENCE trial (201), 3,171 patients with unstable angina or non–Q-wave MI were randomized to receive either i.v. dose-adjusted unfractionated heparin or subcutaneous enoxaparin (1 mg per kg 12-hourly). [c81] A prospective metaanalysis of the TIMI 11B and ESSENCE trials (204) showed that enoxaparin reduced the incidence of death/MI by 18% at 43 days (*p* = .02) (Fig. 17.10). c82

A metaanalysis of these five trials (94,192,201–203) concluded that there was no significant overall reduction in death/MI during short-term follow-up (odds ratio, 0.88; 95% CI, 0.69 to 1.12; *p* = NS) (197) (Fig. 17.11). The combined event rates in these trials—2.2% in patients given low-molecular-weight heparin and 2.3% in those given unfractionated heparin—were much lower than the event rates in the IIb/IIIa antagonist trials.

The disparate findings of these trials using various low-molecular-weight heparins may be partly due to differences in the trial methodologies and patient selection. Firm conclusions regarding the relative efficacy of the low-molecular-weight heparins will only be possible once directly comparative trials have been performed.

A number of differences between the agents, such as the doses of the drugs used, rates of clearance, amount of nonspecific binding, and effects on von Willebrand's factor (205) or tissue factor pathway inhibitor, could produce dif-

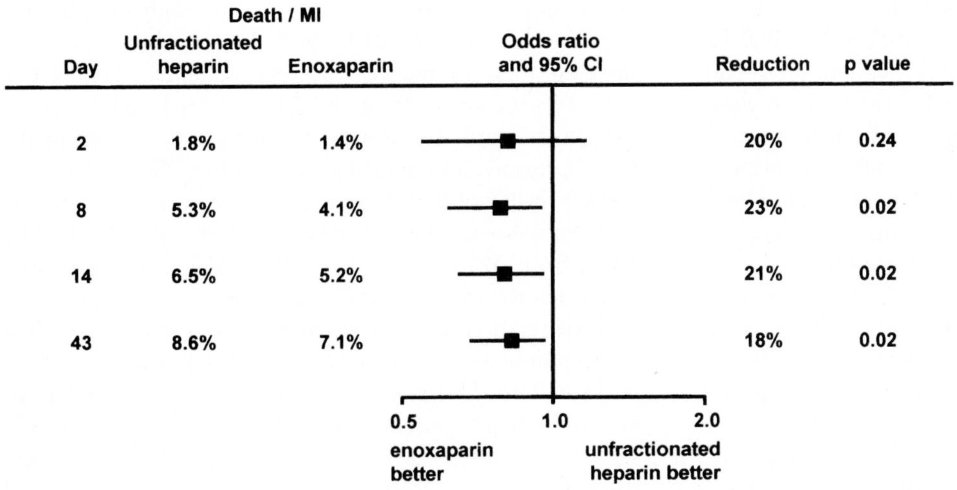

Day	Death / MI Unfractionated heparin	Enoxaparin	Odds ratio and 95% CI	Reduction	p value
2	1.8%	1.4%		20%	0.24
8	5.3%	4.1%		23%	0.02
14	6.5%	5.2%		21%	0.02
43	8.6%	7.1%		18%	0.02

0.5 1.0 2.0
enoxaparin better   unfractionated heparin better

FIGURE 17.10 Metaanalysis of death/myocardial infarction (MI) at days 2, 8, 14, and 43 in the TIMI IIB (94) and ESSENCE (201) trials comparing enoxaparin with unfractionated heparin. CI, confidence interval. (Redrawn from Antman EM, Cohen M, Radley D, et al. Assessment of the treatment effect of enoxaparin for unstable angina/non-Q-wave myocardial infarction: TIMI 11B-ESSENCE meta-analysis. *Circulation* 1999;100: 1602–1608, with permission.)

Trial	N	Death / MI		Odds ratio and 95% CI
		LMW heparin	UF heparin	
Gurfinkel	138	0.0%	4.2%	
FRIC	1,482	3.9%	3.6%	
ESSENCE*	3,171	1.1%	1.3%	
TIMI-11B†	3,912	1.7%	2.1%	
FRAXIS	3,468	3.0%	3.1%	
Pooled results (276 events)	12,171	2.2%	2.3%	

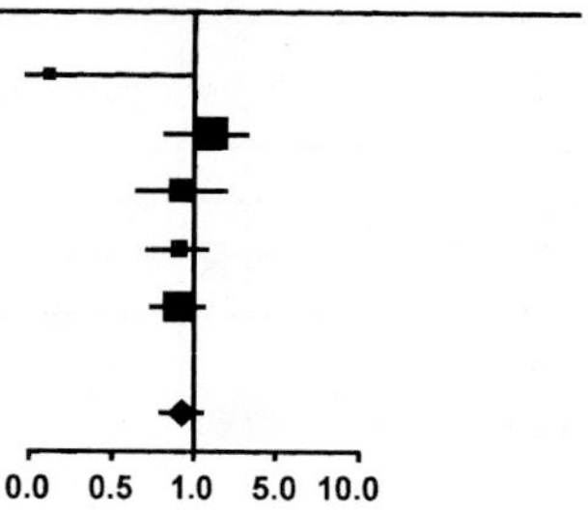

0.0 0.5 1.0 5.0 10.0

Pooled results for death: odds ratio 1.35 (95% CI 0.87 - 2.10)
χ^2 test for heterogeneity = 4.49, p = 0.49

FIGURE 17.11 Metaanalysis of death/myocardial infarction (MI) at the completion of treatment in randomized trials (94,192,201–203) comparing short-term low-molecular-weight (LMW) heparin with unfractionated (UF) heparin in patients with non–ST-elevation acute coronary syndromes. *The median duration of therapy was 2.6 days in both groups. †Unequal duration of treatment. CI, confidence interval. (Redrawn from Eikelboom JW, Anand SS, Malmberg K, et al. Unfractionated heparin and low-molecular-weight heparin in acute coronary syndrome without ST elevation: a meta-analysis. *Lancet* 2000;355:1936–1942, with permission.)

ferent clinical outcomes (206). A low-molecular-weight pentasaccharide with anticoagulant activity has been found to persist for several days after the administration of enoxaparin, but this has not been demonstrated with dalteparin or unfractionated heparin (207). More prolonged treatment with low-molecular-weight heparins has not been found to be beneficial (92,94,202,203). ❧ c83

Rebound Ischemia

Following the cessation of heparin therapy, there may be a rebound increase in ischemic events. In the first of the two Montreal Heart Institute trials that compared heparin with aspirin (209), there was a recurrence of angina at a median of 9.5 hours after stopping heparin in patients who were not taking aspirin. ❧ c84

Rebound ischemia was also noted with unfractionated heparin in the GUSTO IIB study despite concomitant aspirin therapy (133). ❧ c85

Recommendations for Heparin Use

Patients with intermediate- or high-risk non–ST-elevation acute coronary syndromes (Table 17.2) should receive either low-molecular-weight heparin or weight-adjusted i.v. unfractionated heparin immediately, provided that they have no contraindications (1). The initial dose should be a 5,000-IU bolus followed by an infusion of 1,000 IU per hour in patients who weigh 80 kg or greater or 800 IU per hour in those weighing less than 80 kg to maintain the APTT between 50 and 70 seconds (210,211). The infusion should be continued for 2 to 5 days or until revascularization (1). The APTT should be measured 6 hours after any change in dosage, and the heparin dose should be readjusted if necessary.

If recurrent ischemia develops, the APTT should be measured immediately. A validated bedside APTT measurement can be used to expedite management. If the APTT is subtherapeutic, an appropriate weight-adjusted bolus of heparin should be administered. Urgent cardiac catheterization should be considered with a view to revascularization if the ischemic episode is prolonged or associated with ECG changes despite a therapeutic APTT. When i.v. heparin is stopped, patients should be monitored closely for ischemic events over the next 12 hours.

Low-molecular-weight heparin should be considered as an alternative to unfractionated heparin. The European Society of Cardiology and American College of Chest Physicians guidelines (212) recommend low-molecular-weight heparin as the antithrombotic agent of choice. However, patients with heparin-induced thrombocytopenia should not be given low-molecular-weight heparins, which have a high degree of *in vitro* cross-reactivity with the antibody that causes this disorder (213), and can cause heparin-induced thrombocytopenia in patients with a history of this condition (214–216).

Combination of IIb/IIIa Antagonists and Low-Molecular-Weight Heparins

No large clinical trials to date have compared aspirin plus low-molecular-weight heparin with aspirin plus unfractionated heparin plus a IIb/IIIa antagonist. However, several small trials have suggested that the combination of tirofiban and enoxaparin is safe. ❧ c86

Beta-Adrenoreceptor Blockers

Beta-blockers are effective when used singly in unstable angina (128,129,189,219) and in combination with nitrates (220) to reduce recurrent ischemia. They block beta-receptors on all cell membranes and reduce myocardial oxygen demands by slowing the heart rate, lowering the blood pressure, and reducing contractility. ❧ c87

In a review of 4,700 randomized patients, beta-blockers reduced the percentage of those in whom MI developed by 13%, from 32% to 29% (p <.05) (219). It has not been clearly shown whether beta-blockers reduce mortality.

Patients should be started on a beta-blocker or have their existing dose adjusted to keep the resting heart rate at 50 to 60 beats/min. Intravenous beta-blockers should be considered in high-risk patients with rest pain and widespread ST-segment changes or tachycardia. The choice of beta-blocker should take into account the patient's characteristics and the pharmacologic profile and side effects of the particular agent. Esmolol (50 to 250 µg per kg per minute intravenously), which has an effect that lasts for only 20 to 30 minutes after discontinuation, can be considered for patients with relative contraindications. Standard contraindications include marked first- (>0.24 seconds), second-, or third-degree atrioventricular block, asthma, and severe left ventricular dysfunction. The degree of left ventricular dysfunction at which beta-blockers become contraindicated is not clearly defined, and they can and should be used in stable patients with heart failure provided that doses are carefully titrated. Therapy should be continued long term.

Nitrates

No large randomized trials of nitrates in unstable angina have been done, and there is no compelling evidence that these agents reduce the incidence of death/MI. They do, however, relieve angina.

Nitrates dilate normal and atherosclerotic epicardial coronary arteries and inhibit platelet-mediated thrombus formation. Their vasodilatory effect plays an important role in reducing the preload and afterload of the heart, and they are of particular value in patients with vasospasm or a physiologic increase in coronary artery tone. They reduce ischemia very effectively, but tolerance can develop within 24 hours.

Small doses or concomitant administration of the sulfhydryl donor, *N*-acetylcysteine, may augment the effect of nitroglycerin and decrease tolerance (221). Nitroglycerin should be given immediately, either as a sublingual tablet or spray, to relieve angina. If symptoms are not relieved, i.v. nitroglycerin can be infused to relieve pain and to optimize hemodynamics, commencing at an infusion rate of 5 to 10 µg per minute, with increases every 5 to 10 minutes depending on symptoms and side effects such as headache or hypotension. It is usually recommended that the infusion be decreased slowly, as abrupt cessation can precipitate ischemia. However, a study of 200 patients reported savings in nursing time and patient transfer time, with no compromise in safety, when i.v. nitroglycerin was discontinued abruptly as opposed to being tapered off with concurrent use of topical nitrates. To avoid tolerance, nitrate patches or oral therapy may be preferred, with nitrate-free periods of 6 to 10 hours.

Calcium Channel Antagonists

Calcium channel antagonists act as coronary artery dilators by reducing the cellular membrane influx of calcium. They have variable vasodilatory effects in peripheral arteries and negative inotropic, chronotropic, and atrioventricular conduction-slowing effects. They may also enhance diastolic relaxation and left ventricular compliance. Agents that increase the heart rate (e.g., short-acting nifedipine) may be associated with worse outcomes than those that reduce the heart rate (e.g., verapamil or diltiazem) (222,223). c88

Nicorandil, which has nitrate and potassium channel-opening effects, was compared with a placebo in 188 patients with unstable angina and found to reduce the incidence of recurrent ischemia but not death or MI (226).

Because there is a risk of excessive bradycardia or atrioventricular block when drugs such as verapamil or diltiazem are added to a beta-blocker, it may be appropriate to use dihydropyridines (e.g., nifedipine, amlodipine, or nicardipine) as combination therapy. If the patient cannot tolerate a beta-blocker, a non-dihydropyridine calcium channel antagonist with sinus node-slowing effects, such as diltiazem or verapamil, should be used.

Calcium channel antagonists should be used as needed in patients with ongoing ischemia despite beta-blocker and nitrate therapy or in combination with a beta-blocker if hypertension is present. Calcium channel antagonists should be avoided in patients with pulmonary edema or left ventricular dysfunction (222) but are the agents of choice in individuals with variant angina. The choice of agent should be based on the clinical profile of the patient and also depends on whether concomitant beta-blocker therapy is prescribed. Few published data are available evaluating the effects of newer agents on hard clinical end points.

Oral Anticoagulants

Because of their delayed onset of action, oral anticoagulants are not appropriate for acute treatment but can be considered for long-term use if aspirin is contraindicated. c89

Thrombolytic Therapy

Thrombolytic therapy is not recommended for routine use in patients with unstable angina because it has been shown to increase the rate of MI (231). c90

Intraaortic Balloon Counterpulsation

Intraaortic balloon pump counterpulsation (IABP) stabilizes patients and relieves symptoms very effectively (253). By increasing aortic diastolic pressure, coronary blood flow is improved distal to critical stenoses, and there is a decrease in myocardial oxygen demands due to reduction of afterload. No randomized trials of IABP have been done in patients with unstable angina. c91

IABP should be considered in patients with refractory symptoms or hemodynamic instability to stabilize the patient on the way to the cardiac catheterization room or operating room (1).

Indications for Angiography

Coronary angiography determines the extent and severity of coronary artery disease and may detect thrombus. Assessment of valvular and left ventricular function can be performed at the same time. The information obtained is a useful indicator of prognosis and determines the choice of revascularization strategy. Patients who are more likely to have severe coronary artery stenoses, multivessel disease, or left main stenosis can be identified by ECG changes (71) or a recent history of rest angina (135,136). Angiography is not normally performed if revascularization is contraindicated due to comorbidity. ☜ c92

Revascularization

Despite the effectiveness of aspirin, heparin, and beta-blockers, refractory angina that requires an intervention commonly develops in patients with unstable angina (122,154,190,193). The FRISC II study (69) and the Treat Angina with Aggrastat and Determine Cost of Therapy with an Invasive or Conservative Strategy—Thrombolysis in Myocardial Infarction 18 (TACTICS-TIMI 18) trial (70) have shown that patients at high risk should undergo interventions (1,80). ☜ c93

Percutaneous Coronary Intervention

PCI techniques have evolved rapidly over the past several years, particularly with the advent of stenting and the use of adjunctive therapies such as IIb/IIIa antagonists and thienopyridines. ☜ c94

Although PCI improves coronary flow by reducing the coronary artery stenosis, it is associated with periprocedural MI (*e*Fig. 17.11.3) due to obstruction of branch vessels or distal embolization of plaque material and microvascular injury, or both. Acute thrombotic closure and MI associated with PCI are more common in patients with non–ST-

elevation acute coronary syndromes than in those who are undergoing elective interventions (287,288). Furthermore, PCI may not treat the unstable plaques that cause the clinical syndrome, which may be non-flow limiting (289) and multiple (290). Revascularization is not recommended unless the benefits are likely to outweigh the risks. ☜ c95

Six trials have compared an invasive treatment strategy with a conservative treatment strategy in which patients underwent revascularization procedures only if recurrent or inducible ischemia developed (Fig. 17.12). Four of these trials were conducted exclusively in patients with non–ST-elevation acute coronary syndromes (69,70,122,292), one was conducted in patients with postinfarction ischemia (293), and one was conducted in patients with ST elevation or depression (294). In one of these trials, early PCI did not reduce the incidence of death/MI at 1 year (122). In two trials a conservative strategy was better (292,294), and three trials favored an invasive strategy (69,122). Both approaches are therefore supported by clinical trial evidence, but the weight of evidence, including recent trials that are relevant to contemporary practice, suggests that patients at higher risk do better with an invasive strategy.

The percentage of patients in these trials who were randomized to receive conservative treatment but then underwent revascularization procedures varied from 2% (293) to 40% (294) (Fig. 17.12). In some of the trials, there was little difference in revascularization rates between the invasive and conservative treatment groups; for example, in the Veterans Affairs Non–Q-Wave Infarction Strategies in Hospital (VANQWISH) trial, revascularization was performed in 33% of the conservative treatment group and 44% of the invasive treatment group. In the TIMI IIIB trial, the rates were 40% and 60%, respectively. In contrast, only 9% of

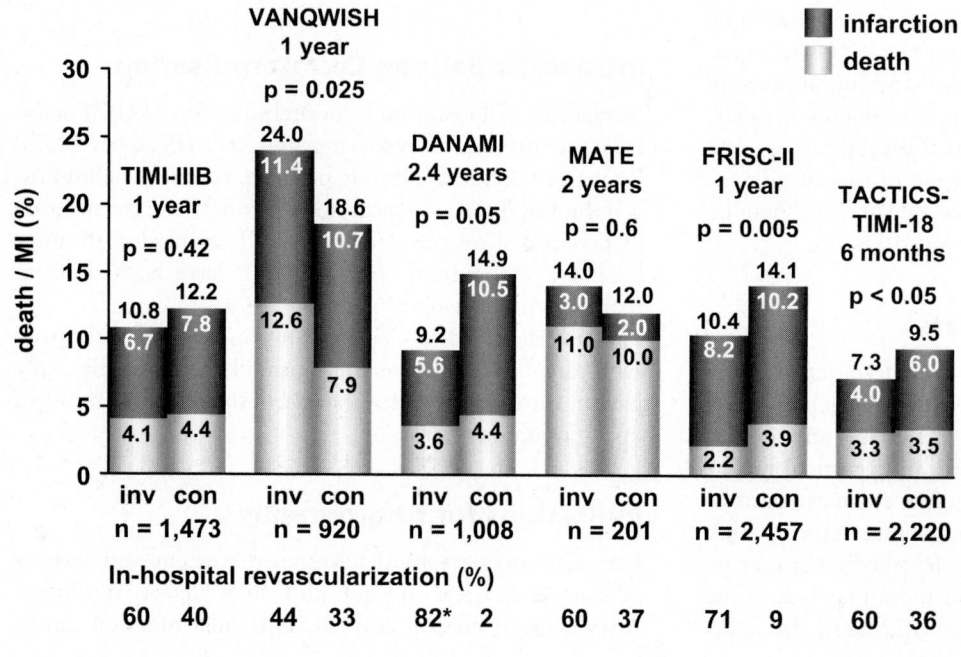

FIGURE 17.12 Rates of death/myocardial infarction (MI) at various time points in six trials comparing invasive (inv) with conservative (con) medical management in patients with acute coronary syndromes. Four of these trials were conducted in patients with non–ST-elevation acute coronary syndromes (69,70,122,292), one was conducted in patients with postinfarction angina (293), and one was conducted in patients with either ST elevation or ST depression who were ineligible for thrombolytic therapy (294). *At 2 months. DANAMI, Danish Trial in Acute Myocardial Infarction; MATE, Medicine versus Angiography in Thrombolytic Exclusion; VANQWISH, Veterans Affairs Non–Q-Wave Infarction Strategies in Hospital.

the conservative treatment group in the FRISC II study underwent revascularization, as opposed to 71% of the invasive treatment group. ❦ c96

In the VANQWISH trial, most of the mortality excess among patients who underwent early CABG was perioperative (11.6%). This may have been due to the urgency of the operation, as acuity is known to be one of the most powerful predictors of a poor outcome after CABG (295). The operative mortality among patients whose CABG was not performed acutely was 3.4%. At 23-month follow-up, there was no difference between the groups.

The FRISC II study (296) showed that intervention was beneficial after an initial period of dalteparin treatment (4 days in patients undergoing PCI and 7 days in those undergoing CABG). As noted above, the rate of inhospital revascularization in the conservative group (9%) was very low. The invasive group had a higher incidence of MI than the conservative group during the first month because of periprocedural events (*e*Fig. 17.12.1) but a lower incidence from then on. At 6 months, the incidence of angina was reduced from 39% to 22% and hospital readmission rates from 49% to 31% (both *p* <.001). At 1 year, the mortality was reduced from 3.9% to 2.2% (*p* <.02), MI from 11.6% to 8.6% (*p* = .02), and readmissions from 57% to 37% (*p* <.001). The patients in FRISC II were at high risk, with 57.5% having elevated troponin T levels and 45.5% having ST depression. In addition, the angiograms of patients with ST depression showed that 13% of the invasive treatment group had left main coronary artery disease and 33% had triple-vessel disease—both of which are better treated with revascularization (297). The patients who benefited most from revascularization were those (n = 756) with ST depression and elevated troponin T levels (more than 0.03 mg per L) (87). No significant benefit was found in patients who had ST depression with normal troponin T levels (n = 301) or in patients who had elevated troponin T levels without ST depression (n = 800). ❦ c97

The TACTICS-TIMI 18 trial (70) enrolled 2,220 patients who presented with unstable or minimal-effort angina and ECG changes, elevated troponins, or a history of prior MI, PCI, or CABG, that is, largely intermediate/high-risk patients according to the ACC/AHA guidelines (1). The patients received heparin, aspirin, and tirofiban for 48 to 108 hours and were randomized to undergo either conservative or invasive treatment. Patients in the invasive treatment group underwent catheterization between 4 and 48 hours and were revascularized if their anatomy was suitable, whereas those in the conservative treatment group did not undergo revascularization procedures unless they had refractory angina (more than 10 minutes of rest pain with ECG changes), hemodynamic instability, a positive exercise test or stress echocardiogram, new MI, hospitalization with unstable angina, or class III or IV angina. The study prospectively evaluated the TIMI risk score (111) and the use of troponin levels in determining the optimal treatment

strategy. The primary end point was a composite of death/MI/rehospitalization for an acute coronary syndrome during 6 months of follow-up.

During the initial hospital admission, 97% of the invasive group and 51% of the conservative group underwent cardiac catheterization. In the invasive group, the mean duration of the tirofiban infusion before catheterization was 24 hours, and 41% of patients underwent PCI, 19% had CABG, and 40% had no intervention. The 30-day mortality in patients who underwent CABG was 3.5%. In the conservative group, 36% of patients underwent revascularization procedures during the initial hospital admission. Although there was no difference in mortality at 6 months between the two groups, the incidence of death/MI/rehospitalization was reduced from 19.4% in the conservative group to 15.9% in the invasive group (odds ratio, 0.78; *p* = .025) (Fig. 17.13). Periprocedural MI was not increased among patients who were pretreated with tirofiban (*e*Fig. 17.12.1), unlike the FRISC II findings with dalteparin (69). The length of hospital stay was 1 day shorter in the invasive group (mean 7.4 days).

Invasive treatment was beneficial in patients with elevated troponin levels and in those with ST depression, reducing their rates of death/MI/rehospitalization from 24.2% to 14.3% (*e*Fig. 17.13.1) and from 26.3% to 16.4%, respectively—but not in patients with a low TIMI risk score of 0 to 2, who represented 25% of the study cohort. The odds ratios for death/MI/rehospitalization were 0.76 (95% CI, 0.57 to 1.00) in patients at intermediate risk and 0.56 (95% CI, 0.33 to 0.95) in those at high risk.

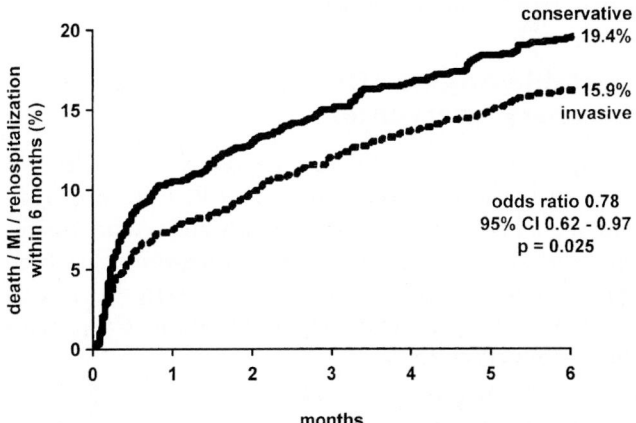

FIGURE 17.13 Cumulative incidence of death/myocardial infarction (MI)/rehospitalization for an acute coronary syndrome within 6 months in patients who were managed either conservatively or invasively in the TACTICS–TIMI 18 trial. CI, confidence interval. (Redrawn from Cannon CP, Weintraub WS, Demopoulos LA, et al. Comparison of early invasive and conservative strategies in patients with unstable coronary syndromes treated with the glycoprotein IIb/IIIa inhibitor tirofiban. *N Engl J Med* 2001;344:1879–1887. Copyright © 2001, Massachusetts Medical Society. All rights reserved, with permission.)

In view of the TACTICS-TIMI 18 findings, early invasive treatment should be considered in high-risk patients after treatment with aspirin, unfractionated heparin, and a small-molecule IIb/IIIa antagonist for 4 to 48 hours. If catheterization facilities are not available, high-risk patients should be started on aspirin, unfractionated heparin, and a IIb/IIIa antagonist and then transferred to an appropriate center. An alternative approach for high-risk patients would be to transfer them promptly to a catheterization facility (preferably within 4 hours) (1) and to administer abciximab or eptifibatide if PCI is performed. The superiority of either approach is yet to be determined in clinical trials.

A powerful motivation for an early revascularization strategy is the evidence showing that patients can be discharged earlier and that readmissions are reduced (122,298). Hospital beds can thus be used more efficiently. In TACTICS-TIMI 18, inhospital costs were higher in patients who were treated invasively, but follow-up costs were higher in those treated conservatively; consequently, at 6 months there was no difference in cost between the invasive and conservative strategies (298). Intervention was most cost effective in patients with elevated troponin levels, ST depression, or diabetes. Angina scores, as measured by the Seattle Angina Questionnaire, improved in both treatment groups and were no different at 6 months.

Coronary Artery Bypass Grafting

CABG is an excellent therapy for relieving angina and was an important component of the FRISC II and TACTICS-TIMI 18 trials, being performed in 35% of the invasive group in FRISC II (69) and in 20% of the invasive group in TACTICS-TIMI 18 (70). Both trials reported that revascularization was beneficial. ❦ c98

Unstable Angina after Percutaneous Coronary Intervention

If angina develops in the first 6 months after PCI, it is likely that restenosis has occurred at the PCI site. Angiography should be performed expeditiously and repeat revascularization if indicated. Intravenous nitroglycerin has been shown to be superior to antithrombotic therapy in preventing recurrent or refractory angina in nonstented patients without restenosis (308).

Unstable Angina after Coronary Artery Bypass Grafting

Patients with unstable angina and subtotally occluded bypass grafts have a high risk of thrombotic occlusion, which is very difficult to treat. [❦ c99] If important symptoms of angina develop, particularly with ischemic ST-segment changes in the distribution of a vein graft, the patient should undergo expeditious angiography to define

the anatomy and to determine appropriate treatment. PCI with stenting may prevent occlusion of a vein graft with a severe stenosis, thereby avoiding reoperation and its associated risks. Unfortunately, progressive disease frequently occurs in nonstented segments of the vein graft within 2 years (312).

The Case for Conservative Management in Low- and Intermediate-Risk Patients

The good prognosis of many patients with unstable angina may justify a conservative treatment strategy provided that troponin levels are not elevated, symptoms settle, and left ventricular function is normal. Many patients can be managed with antithrombotic and antianginal therapy without the need for revascularization. For example, 40% of patients in TACTICS-TIMI 18 (70) and 46.5% of those in PRISM-PLUS (90), which encouraged angiography in everyone, were managed without the need for revascularization.

The aim of medical management is to passivate the plaque. Subsequent management can be based on the amount of inducible ischemia rather than the presenting clinical features and coronary arteriographic findings. If the symptoms settle, exercise testing, stress echocardiography, or dipyridamole sestamibi imaging can be performed to assess the hemodynamic significance of the residual coronary artery stenosis. Testing should be delayed until 24 to 48 hours after the last episode of angina. However, noninvasive stress testing does not predict plaque instability or the risk of future MI, and therefore it is important that patients are seen for review and instructed to report any continuing symptoms.

Early Lipid Lowering

The European (313), U.S. (314), and British guidelines (315) for the management of dyslipidemia in patients with ischemic heart disease recommend the use of lipid-lowering drugs only after diet and lifestyle modifications have been attempted. They do not recommend early drug treatment when patients are admitted with an acute coronary syndrome. ❦ d01

In the LIPID study, 9,014 patients with an acute MI or a hospital discharge diagnosis of unstable angina 3 to 36 months previously and total cholesterol levels of 4.0 to 7.0 mmol per L were randomized to receive either pravastatin (40 mg per day) or a placebo for 6 years. Approximately one-third of the cohort (3,260 patients) were included in the unstable angina stratum, and pravastatin reduced their relative risk of mortality by 26.3% (332) (*e*Fig. 17.13.3). Overall, the patients who received pravastatin also had significantly lower rates of coronary heart disease mortality, MI, need for revascularization, admission to the hospital, and number of drugs received in hospital. In absolute terms, pravastatin prevented 33 deaths, 24 nonfatal MIs, and 26 revascularization procedures per 1,000 patients treated for 6 years.

In the Myocardial Ischemia Reduction with Aggressive Cholesterol Lowering (MIRACL) trial (333), 3,086 patients were randomized to receive either 80 mg atorvastatin or a placebo 1 to 4 days after presenting with an acute coronary syndrome. On average, atorvastatin increased high-density lipoprotein cholesterol levels by 4% and reduced total cholesterol by 27%, low-density lipoprotein cholesterol by 40%, and triglycerides by 16%. At 16 weeks, the incidence of death/MI/resuscitated cardiac arrest/worsening angina/urgent rehospitalization was reduced from 17.4% to 14.8% (p = .048), but there was no reduction in the need for revascularization. Early atorvastatin therapy was confirmed as being safe, with no episodes of myositis, although 2.5% of patients who were given atorvastatin developed elevated liver transaminases (three times the upper limit of normal) as opposed to 0.6% of patients given the placebo. ❦ d02

A major rationale for beginning lipid lowering early is that it emphasizes to the patient that therapy is important and needs to be continued long term. A low-fat diet alone is usually inadequate to achieve the recommended cholesterol targets in patients with coronary artery disease (334). Compliance and achievement of target levels may be improved if therapy is begun in conjunction with dietary advice while the patient is still in hospital.

Antiinflammatory Agents

Some survivors of MI have been shown to have elevated levels of *Chlamydia pneumoniae* antibodies, and these patients have worse outcomes (335). A pilot trial of roxithromycin in patients with unstable angina reported reductions in ischemic events at 30 days and at 6 months (336).

A small randomized trial compared 48 hours of methylprednisolone therapy with a placebo in 166 patients with unstable angina and reported a reduction in C-reactive protein levels, but no effect on short-term outcomes (337). Large-scale trials are currently under way to establish whether antibiotics or antiinflammatory agents will improve outcomes.

Secondary Prevention

Smoking cessation and treatment of dyslipidemia and hypertension are important secondary preventative measures in all patients with coronary artery disease. The risk of dying is five times greater if patients with unstable angina continue to smoke than if they quit.

Other measures that should be instituted after presentation with a non–ST-elevation acute coronary syndrome include achievement of ideal weight, a regular exercise program, an appropriate low-cardiovascular-risk diet, and achievement of optimal diabetic control where necessary. If

facilities are available, patients should be referred to a cardiac rehabilitation program (338). Appropriate education should also be undertaken.

Pharmacologic measures are also indicated, such as aspirin, beta-blockers, lipid-modifying agents (see above), and ACE inhibitors in patients with decreased ejection fractions or another risk factor. The Heart Outcome Prevention Evaluation (HOPE) study (339), which excluded patients who had experienced MI within the previous 30 days, showed that the ACE inhibitor, ramipril, reduced the rate of cardiovascular death/MI/stroke from 17.8% to 14.0% (p <.001) over 5 years in patients older than 55 years with a history of vascular disease or diabetes with one other risk factor.

Strong evidence has now been found that better outcomes are achieved with higher usage rates of proven therapies (340). Compliance with published guidelines has been shown to reduce mortality in patients with acute MI (341) and also offers the potential to improve outcomes in patients with non–ST-elevation acute coronary syndromes if physicians adhere to their recommendations (1,2,80).

CONTROVERSIES AND PERSONAL PERSPECTIVES

Upstream versus In-Laboratory Use of IIb/IIIa Antagonists

Revascularization by PCI or CABG is the preferred option in patients at high risk (219,292). Patients with non–ST-elevation MI are often treated by PCI, although in TACTICS-TIMI 18 only 41% of patients had PCI, 19% had CABG, and 40% had no intervention (70). When used appropriately, IIb/IIIa antagonists have been shown to improve outcomes in patients who are treated with revascularization procedures (70,162,165,168,177,182), but the optimal timing of therapy has not yet been established. A distinct advantage of starting IIb/IIIa antagonist therapy in advance of the procedure (upstream treatment) is that it allows even those patients who are not undergoing interventions to benefit from the drug. As seen in the TACTICS-TIMI 18 trial (70), upstream treatment with a small-molecule IIb/IIIa antagonist such as tirofiban reduces the risk of preprocedural MI and periprocedural events (69,88) in patients who are undergoing PCI, thereby allowing hospitals greater freedom in planning the timing of interventions in patients presenting at night or during the weekend.

In a metaanalysis of upstream IIb/IIIa antagonist therapy in more than 12,000 patients in the CAPTURE, PRISM-PLUS, and PURSUIT trials (181), the incidence of death/MI was reduced from 4.3% to 2.3% (p = .001). This equates to 14 fewer events (predominantly MIs) per 1,000 all-comers randomized in these trials. The risk reduction is far greater in patients at high risk (e.g., those with

THE FUTURE

Patient outcomes may well be improved by new combinations of current therapies such as clopidogrel with IIb/IIIa antagonists and low-molecular-weight heparin (*e*Fig. 17.13.5). Predictors of plaque instability are needed so that patients at high risk can be targeted. The new biomarkers for risk assessment, ischemia, inflammation, thrombosis, necrosis, heart failure, and plaque instability will enable targeting of therapies for efficacy and safety, as will advances in pharmacogenomics.

High-resolution three-dimensional magnetic resonance imaging is able to distinguish intact thick fibrous plaque caps from intact thin and disrupted caps in human carotid arteries (360). This technology may allow the relationship between fibrous cap changes and clinical outcomes to be examined, enabling the development of therapies to stabilize plaques. Innovative work is also being done with noninvasive assessment of plaque temperature (361). Plaques with higher temperatures have increased numbers of macrophages and a greater propensity for rupture (362).

Further developments in noninvasive imaging may enable detection of coronary thrombi composed mostly of platelets, at which agents such as IIb/IIIa antagonists could be targeted. If imaging showed that a thrombus was composed mostly of red blood cells, a direct anti-thrombin might be more effective, whereas if the thrombus were a mixture of platelets and red blood cells, combination therapy might be more suitable. If imaging were able to show that there was an elevated plaque with little thrombus, PCI without adjunctive drug therapy might be the most appropriate first-line treatment.

Our knowledge of the mechanisms that lead to plaque instability will expand. Treatments that reduce the vulnerability of plaques to rupture include matrix metalloproteinase inhibitors and locally delivered growth factor inhibitors. Modulation of the ability of the myocardium to survive ischemia, including angiogenesis and metabolic manipulation, will be an area of active research. It may be possible to develop rapid bedside tests to obtain the genomic profile of patients so that therapies can be targeted to those who are most likely to benefit and least likely to experience side effects. Safer, more effective, cost-effective, and easily administered agents, including oral compounds, are needed. In the long term, however, greater emphasis must be placed on primary prevention.

elevated troponins)—on the order of 100 fewer events per 1,000 patients, as seen in the PRISM study (83).

An alternative to upstream treatment with a small-molecule IIb/IIIa antagonist is to wait and give abciximab in the catheterization laboratory. This approach is based on the TARGET trial (161), which found that abciximab was superior to tirofiban for in-laboratory use, producing a greater reduction in the incidence of periprocedural MI. Dosing is critical when using small-molecule agents such as tirofiban, because there may be a dip in the level of platelet inhibition between the bolus dose and the infusion (359), unless a double bolus is administered or upstream treatment is continued for several hours before the procedure. No large randomized trials to date have addressed the issue of whether patients benefit more if catheterization is performed within 4 hours. In TACTICS-TIMI 18, patients underwent revascularization between 4 and 48 hours (70). It may well be appropriate to perform revascularization as expeditiously as possible and administer abciximab in the catheterization laboratory, but this approach has yet to be evaluated in comparison with upstream IIb/IIIa antagonist therapy before intervention.

ACKNOWLEDGMENT

The author gratefully acknowledges the assistance of Anna Breckon, who edited the manuscript and prepared the artwork.

REFERENCES

1. Braunwald E, Antman EM, Beasley JW, et al. ACC/AHA guidelines for the management of patients with unstable angina and non–ST-segment elevation myocardial infarction: a report of the American College of Cardiology/American Heart Association Task Force on Practice Guidelines (Committee on the Management of Patients with Unstable Angina). *J Am Coll Cardiol* 2000;36:970–1062.

2. Aroney C, Boyden AN, Jelinek MV, et al. Management of unstable angina: guidelines—2000. *Med J Aust* 2000;173[Suppl]:S65–S88.

3. Joint European Society of Cardiology/American College of Cardiology Committee. Myocardial infarction redefined—a consensus document of the Joint European Society of Cardiology/American College of Cardiology Committee for the Redefinition of Myocardial Infarction. *J Am Coll Cardiol* 2000;36:959–969.

4. Braunwald E. Unstable angina: a classification. *Circulation* 1989;80:410–414.

5. Cannon CP, McCabe CH, Stone PH, et al. Prospective validation of the Braunwald classification of unstable angina: results from the Thrombolysis in Myocardial Ischemia (TIMI) III registry. *Circulation* 1995;92[Suppl I]:I-19(abst).

6. Ahmed WH, Bittl JA, Braunwald E. Relation between clinical presentation and angiographic findings in unstable angina pectoris, and comparison with that in stable angina. *Am J Cardiol* 1993;72:544–550.

7. Hamm CW, Braunwald E. A classification of unstable angina revisited. *Circulation* 2000;102:118–122.

8. Prinzmetal M, et al. A variant form of angina pectoris. *Am J Med* 1959;27:375–388.

9. Braunwald E. Unstable angina: an etiologic approach to management [Editorial]. *Circulation* 1998;98:2219–2222.

10. Falk E. Plaque rupture with severe pre-existing stenosis precipitating coronary thrombosis. Characteristics of coronary atherosclerotic plaques underlying fatal occlusive thrombi. *Br Heart J* 1983;50:127–134.

11. Davies MJ, Thomas AC. Plaque fissuring: the cause of acute myocardial infarction, sudden ischemic death, and crescendo angina. *Br Heart J* 1985;53:363–373.

12. Fuster V, Badimon L, Badimon JJ, et al. The pathogenesis of coronary artery disease and the acute coronary syndromes (Pt 1). *N Engl J Med* 1992;326:242–250.

13. Fuster V, Badimon L, Badimon JJ, et al. The pathogenesis of coronary artery disease and the acute coronary syndromes (Pt 2). *N Engl J Med* 1992;326:310–318.

14. Mizuno K, Satomura K, Miyamoto A, et al. Angioscopic evaluation of coronary-artery thrombi in acute coronary syndromes. *N Engl J Med* 1992;326:287–291.

15. Ross R. Atherosclerosis—an inflammatory disease. *N Engl J Med* 1999;340:115–126.

16. Libby P. Molecular bases of the acute coronary syndromes. *Circulation* 1995;91:2844–2850.

17. Little WC, Constantinescu M, Applegate RJ, et al. Can coronary angiography predict the site of a subsequent myocardial infarction in patients with mild-to-moderate coronary artery disease? *Circulation* 1988;78:1157–1166.

18. Haft JI, Haik BJ, Goldstein JE, et al. Development of significant coronary artery lesions in areas of minimal disease: a common mechanism for coronary disease progression. *Chest* 1988;94:731–736.

19. Ambrose JA, Tannenbaum MA, Alexopoulos D, et al. Angiographic progression of coronary artery disease and the development of myocardial infarction. *J Am Coll Cardiol* 1988;12:56–62.

20. Hackett D, Verwilghen J, Davies G, et al. Coronary stenoses before and after acute myocardial infarction. *Am J Cardiol* 1989;63:1517–1518.

21. Giroud D, Li JM, Urban P, et al. Relation of the site of acute myocardial infarction to the most severe coronary arterial stenosis at prior angiography. *Am J Cardiol* 1992;69:729–732.

22. Pétursson MK, Jónmundsson EH, Brekkan A, et al. Angiographic predictors of new coronary occlusions. *Am Heart J* 1995;129:515–520.

23. Yamagishi M, Terashima M, Awano K, et al. Morphology of vulnerable coronary plaque: insights from follow-up of patients examined by intravascular ultrasound before an acute coronary syndrome. *J Am Coll Cardiol* 2000;35:106–111.

24. Davies MJ, Richardson PD, Woolf N, et al. Risk of thrombosis in human atherosclerotic plaques: role of extracellular lipid, macrophage, and smooth muscle cell content. *Br Heart J* 1993;69:377–381.

25. Moreno PR, Falk E, Palacios IF, et al. Macrophage infiltration in acute coronary syndromes. Implications for plaque rupture. *Circulation* 1994;90:775–778.

26. van der Wal AC, Becker AE, van der Loos CM, et al. Site of intimal rupture or erosion of thrombosed coronary atherosclerotic plaques is characterized by an inflammatory process irrespective of the dominant plaque morphology. *Circulation* 1994;89:36–44.

27. van der Wal AC, Piek JJ, de Boer OJ, et al. Recent activation of the plaque immune response in coronary lesions underlying acute coronary syndromes. *Heart* 1998;80:14–18.

28. Kaartinen M, Penttila A, Kovanen PT. Accumulation of activated mast cells in the shoulder region of human coronary atheroma, the predilection site of atheromatous rupture. *Circulation* 1994;90:1669–1678.

29. Adams JEI, Sicard GA, Allen BT, et al. Diagnosis of perioperative myocardial infarction with measurement of cardiac troponin I. *N Engl J Med* 1994;330:670–674.

30. Biasucci LM, Liuzzo G, Fantuzzi G, et al. Increasing levels of interleukin (IL)-1Ra and IL-6 during the first 2 days of hospitalization in unstable angina are associated with increased risk of in-hospital coronary events. *Circulation* 1999;99:2079–2084.

31. Liuzzo G, Biasucci LM, Gallimore JR, et al. The prognostic value of C-reactive protein and serum amyloid A protein in severe unstable angina. *N Engl J Med* 1994;331:417–424.

32. Biasucci LM, Liuzzo G, Grillo RL, et al. Elevated levels of C-reactive protein at discharge in patients with unstable angina predict recurrent instability. *Circulation* 1999;99:855–860.

33. Milazzo D, Biasucci LM, Luciani N, et al. Elevated levels of C-reactive protein before coronary artery bypass grafting predict recurrence of ischemic events. *Am J Cardiol* 1999;84:459–461.

34. Mulvihill NT, Foley JB, Murphy R, et al. Evidence of prolonged inflammation in unstable angina and non–Q wave myocardial infarction. *J Am Coll Cardiol* 2000;36:1210–1216.

35. Liuzzo G, Kopecky SL, Frye RL, et al. Perturbation of the T-cell repertoire in patients with unstable angina. *Circulation* 1999;100:2135–2139.

36. Kuo CC, Shor A, Campbell LA, et al. Demonstration of *Chlamydia pneumoniae* in atherosclerotic lesions of coronary arteries. *J Infect Dis* 1993;167:841–849.

37. Mendall MA, Goggin PM, Molineaux N, et al. Relation of *Helicobacter pylori* infection and coronary heart disease. *Br Heart J* 1994;71:437–439.

38. Mendall MA, Patel P, Ballam L, et al. C-reactive protein and its relation to cardiovascular risk factors; a population based cross-sectional study. *BMJ* 1996;312:1061–1065.

39. Caligiuri G, Paulsson G, Nicoletti A, et al. Evidence for antigen-driven T-cell response in unstable angina. *Circulation* 2000;102:1114–1119.

40. Kol A, Sperti G, Shani J, et al. Cytomegalovirus replication is not a cause of instability in unstable angina. *Circulation* 1995;91:1910–1913.

41. Folts JD, Crowell EB, Rowe GG. Platelet aggregation in partially obstructed vessels and its elimination with aspirin. *Circulation* 1976;54:365–370.

42. Davies MJ, Thomas AC, Knapman PA, et al. Intramyocardial platelet aggregation in patients with unstable angina suffering sudden ischemic cardiac death. *Circulation* 1986;73:418–427.

43. Fitzgerald DJ, Roy L, Catella F, et al. Platelet activation in unstable coronary disease. *N Engl J Med* 1986;315:983–989.

44. Buja LM, Willerson JT. Role of inflammation in coronary plaque disruption [Editorial]. *Circulation* 1994;89:503–505.

45. Hoffmeister HM, Jur M, Wendel HP, et al. Alterations of coagulation and fibrinolytic and kallikrein-kinin systems in the acute and postacute phases in patients with unstable angina pectoris. *Circulation* 1995;91:2520–2527.

46. Merlini PA, Bauer KA, Oltrona L, et al. Persistent activation of coagulation mechanism in unstable angina and myocardial infarction. *Circulation* 1994;90:61–68.

47. Ault KA, Cannon CP, Mitchell J, et al. Platelet activation in patients after an acute coronary syndrome: results from the TIMI-12 trial. *J Am Coll Cardiol* 1999;33:634–639.

48. Freeman MR, Williams AE, Chisholm RJ, et al. Intracoronary thrombus and complex morphology in unstable angina: relation to timing of angiography and in-hospital cardiac events. *Circulation* 1989;80:17–23.

49. Ambrose JA, Winters SL, Stern A, et al. Angiographic morphology and the pathogenesis of unstable angina pectoris. *J Am Coll Cardiol* 1985;5:609–616.

50. Gotoh K, Minamino T, Katoh O, et al. The role of intracoronary thrombus in unstable angina: angiographic assessment and thrombolytic therapy during ongoing angina attacks. *Circulation* 1988;77:526–534.

51. Sherman CT, Litvak F, Grundfest W, et al. Coronary angioscopy in patients with unstable angina pectoris. *N Engl J Med* 1986;315:913–919.

52. Mizuno K. Angioscopy in acute coronary syndromes. *Cardiology Today* 1992;20:1–2.

53. De Feyter PJ, Ozaki Y, Baptista J, et al. Ischemia-related lesion characteristics in patients with stable or unstable angina: a study with intracoronary angioscopy and ultrasound. *Circulation* 1995;92:1408–1413.

54. Moise A, Theroux P, Taeymans Y, et al. Unstable angina and progression of coronary atherosclerosis. *N Engl J Med* 1983;309:685–689.

55. Victor MF, Likoff MJ, Mintz GS, et al. Unstable angina pectoris of new onset: a prospective clinical and arteriographic study of 75 patients. *Am J Cardiol* 1981;47:228–232.

56. Kloner RA, Hale S, Alker K, et al. The effects of acute and chronic cocaine use on the heart. *Circulation* 1992;85:407–419.

57. Muller JE, Stone PH, Turi ZG, et al. Circadian variation in the frequency of onset of acute myocardial infarction. *N Engl J Med* 1985;313:1315–1322.

58. Tofler GH, Brezinski D, Schafer AI, et al. Concurrent morning increase in platelet aggregability and the risk of myocardial infarction and sudden cardiac death. *N Engl J Med* 1987;316:1514–1518.

59. Mittleman MA, Maclure M, Tofler GH, et al. Triggering of acute myocardial infarction by heavy physical exertion. Protection against triggering by regular exertion. *N Engl J Med* 1993;329:1677–1683.

60. Baroldi G. Coronary thrombosis: facts and beliefs. *Am Heart J* 1976;91:683–688.

61. Yasue H, Horio Y, Nakamura N, et al. Induction of coronary artery spasm by acetylcholine in patients with variant angina: possible role of the parasympathetic nervous system in the pathogenesis of coronary artery spasm. *Circulation* 1986;74:955–963.

62. McFadden EP, Clarke JG, Davies GJ, et al. Effect of intracoronary serotonin on coronary vessels in patients with stable angina and patients with variant angina. *N Engl J Med* 1991;324:648–654.

63. Toyo-Oka T, Aizawa T, Suzuki N, et al. Increased plasma level of endothelin-1 and coronary spasm induction in patients with vasospastic angina pectoris. *Circulation* 1991;83:476–483.

64. Brown BG, Bolson EL, Dodge HT. Dynamic mechanisms in human coronary stenosis. *Circulation* 1984;70:917–922.

65. Ludmer PL, Selwyn AP, Shook TL, et al. Paradoxical vasoconstriction induced by acetylcholine in atherosclerotic coronary arteries. *N Engl J Med* 1986;315:1046–1051.

66. Bogaty P, Hackett D, Davies G, et al. Vasoreactivity of the culprit lesion in unstable angina. *Circulation* 1994;90:5–11.

67. Théroux P, Ouimet H, McCans J, et al. Aspirin, heparin, or both to treat acute unstable angina. *N Engl J Med* 1988;319:1105–1111.

68. Ridker PM, Rifai N, Pfeffer MA, et al. Inflammation, pravastatin, and the risk of coronary events after myocardial infarction in patients with average cholesterol levels. *Circulation* 1998;98:839–844.

69. Fragmin and Fast Revascularisation during Instability in Coronary Artery Disease (FRISC II) investigators. Invasive compared with non-invasive treatment in unstable coronary-artery disease: FRISC II Prospective Randomised Multicentre study. *Lancet* 1999;354:708–715.

70. Cannon CP, Weintraub WS, Demopoulos LA, et al. Comparison of early invasive and conservative strategies in patients with unstable coronary syndromes treated with the glycoprotein IIb/IIIa inhibitor tirofiban. *N Engl J Med* 2001;344:1879–1887.

71. Langer A, Freeman MR, Armstrong PW. ST segment shift in unstable angina: pathophysiology and association with coronary anatomy and hospital outcome. *J Am Coll Cardiol* 1989;13:1495–1502.

72. Savonitto S, Ardissino D, Granger CB, et al. Prognostic value of the admission electrocardiogram in acute coronary syndromes. *JAMA* 1999;281:707–713.

73. Cannon CP, McCabe CH, Stone PH, et al. The electrocardiogram predicts one-year outcome of patients with unstable angina and non–Q wave myocardial infarction: results of the TIMI III Registry ECG Ancillary study. *J Am Coll Cardiol* 1997;30:133–140.

74. Hyde TA, French JK, Wong C-K, et al. Four-year survival of patients with acute coronary syndromes without ST-segment elevation and prognostic significance of 0.5-mm ST-segment depression. *Am J Cardiol* 1999;84:379–385.

75. Holmvang L, Luscher MS, Clemmensen P, et al. Very early risk stratification using combined ECG and biochemical assessment in patients with unstable coronary artery disease [a Thrombin Inhibition in Myocardial Ischemia (TRIM) substudy]. *Circulation* 1998;98:2004–2009.

76. Deanfield JE, Maseri A, Selwyn AP, et al. Myocardial ischaemia during daily life in patients with stable angina:

its relation to symptoms and heart rate changes. *Lancet* 1983;2:753–758.

77. Chierchia S, Lazzari M, Freedman B, et al. Impairment of myocardial perfusion and function during painless myocardial ischemia. *J Am Coll Cardiol* 1983;1:924–930.

78. Gottlieb SO, Weisfeldt ML, Ouyang P, et al. Silent ischemia as a marker for early unfavorable outcomes in patients with unstable angina. *N Engl J Med* 1986;314:1214–1219.

79. Holdright D, Patel D, Cunningham D, et al. Comparison of the effect of heparin and aspirin versus aspirin alone on transient myocardial ischemia and in-hospital prognosis in patients with unstable angina. *J Am Coll Cardiol* 1994;24:39–45.

80. Bertrand ME, Simoons ML, Fox KAA, et al. Management of acute coronary syndromes: acute coronary syndromes without persistent ST segment elevation: recommendations of the Task Force of the European Society of Cardiology. *Eur Heart J* 2000;21:1406–1432.

81. Jaffe AS, Ravkilde J, Roberts R, et al. It's time for a change to a troponin standard. *Circulation* 2000;102:1216–1220.

82. Antman EM, Tanasijevic MJ, Thompson B, et al. Cardiac-specific troponin I levels to predict the risk of mortality in patients with acute coronary syndromes. *N Engl J Med* 1996;335:1342–1349.

83. Heeschen C, Hamm CW, Goldmann B, et al. Troponin concentrations for stratification of patients with acute coronary syndromes in relation to therapeutic efficacy of tirofiban. *Lancet* 1999;354:1757–1762.

84. Apple FS. Clinical and analytical standardization issues confronting cardiac troponin I. *Clin Chem* 1999;45:18–20.

85. Lindahl B, Diderholm E, Lagerqvist B, et al. Troponin I and T are comparable for risk stratification in unstable coronary artery disease. *Eur Heart J* 2000;21[Abstract Suppl]:521(abst).

86. Heeschen C, van den Brand MJ, Hamm CW, et al. Angiographic findings in patients with refractory unstable angina according to troponin T status. *Circulation* 1999;104:1509–1514.

87. Lindahl B, Diderholm E, Lagerqvist B, et al. Invasive vs noninvasive strategy in relation to troponin T level and ECG findings—a FRISC-2 substudy. *Eur Heart J* 2000;21[Abstract Suppl]:469(abst).

88. The CAPTURE investigators. Randomised placebo-controlled trial of abciximab before and during coronary intervention in refractory unstable angina: the CAPTURE study. *Lancet* 1997;349:1429–1435.

89. The Platelet Receptor Inhibition in Ischemic Syndrome Management (PRISM) study investigators. A comparison of aspirin plus tirofiban with aspirin plus heparin for unstable angina. *N Engl J Med* 1998;338:1498–1505.

90. The Platelet Receptor Inhibition in Ischemic Syndrome Management in Patients Limited by Unstable Signs and Symptoms (PRISM-PLUS) study investigators. Inhibition of the platelet glycoprotein IIb/IIIa receptor with tirofiban in unstable angina and non–Q-wave myocardial infarction. *N Engl J Med* 1998;338:1488–1497.

91. Harrington RA, on behalf of the PARAGON-B Investigators. The PARAGON-B study. Proceedings of the Late Breaking Clinical Trials II Session. Anaheim: 49th Annual Scientific Sessions of the American College of Cardiology, March 14, 2000.

92. Fragmin during Instability in Coronary Artery Disease (FRISC) study group. Low-molecular-weight heparin during instability in coronary artery disease. *Lancet* 1996;347:561–568.

93. The GUSTO IV–ACS investigators. Effects of glycoprotein IIb/IIIa receptor blocker abciximab on outcome in patients with acute coronary syndromes without early coronary revascularisation: the GUSTO IV–ACS randomized trial. *Lancet* 2001;357:1915–1924.

94. Antman EM, McCabe CH, Gurfinkel EP, et al. Enoxaparin prevents death and cardiac ischemic events in unstable angina/non–Q-wave myocardial infarction: results of the Thrombolysis in Myocardial Infarction (TIMI) 11B trial. *Circulation* 1999;100:1593–1601.

95. Lindahl B, Venge P, Wallentin L, et al. Relation between troponin T and the risk of subsequent cardiac events in unstable coronary artery disease. *Circulation* 1996;93:1651–1657.

96. Hamm CW, Heeschen C, Goldmann B, et al. Benefit of abciximab in patients with refractory unstable angina in relation to serum troponin T levels. *N Engl J Med* 1999;340:1623–1629.

97. Ohman EM, Armstrong PW, Christenson RH, et al. Cardiac troponin T levels for risk stratification in acute myocardial ischemia. *N Engl J Med* 1996;335:1333–1341.

98. Hamm CW, Ravkilde J, Gerhardt W, et al. The prognostic value of serum troponin T in unstable angina. *N Engl J Med* 1992;327:146–150.

99. Lindahl B, Andrén B, Ohlsson J, et al. Risk stratification in unstable coronary artery disease: additive value of troponin T determinations and pre-discharge exercise tests. *Eur Heart J* 1997;18:762–770.

100. Ottani F, Galvani M, Nicolini FA, et al. Elevated cardiac troponin levels predict the risk of adverse outcome in patients with acute coronary syndromes. *Am Heart J* 2000;140:917–927.

101. Newby LK, Storrow AB, Gibler WB, et al. Bedside multimarker testing for risk stratification in chest pain units: the Chest Pain Evaluation by Creatine Kinase-MB, Myoglobin, and Troponin I (CHECKMATE) study. *Circulation* 2001;103:1832–1837.

102. Sonel A, Sasseen BM, Fineberg N, et al. Prospective study correlating fibrinopeptide A, troponin I, myoglobin, and myosin light chain levels with early and late ischemic events in consecutive patients presenting to the emergency department with chest pain. *Circulation* 2000;102:1107–1113.

103. Ridker PM, Cushman M, Stampfer MJ, et al. Inflammation, aspirin, and the risk of cardiovascular disease in apparently healthy men. *N Engl J Med* 1997;336:973–979.

104. Ikonomidis I, Andreotti F, Economou E, et al. Increased proinflammatory cytokines in patients with chronic stable angina and their reduction by aspirin. *Circulation* 1999;100:793–798.

105. Ridker PM, Rifai N, Pfeffer MA, et al. Long-term effects of pravastatin on plasma concentration of C-reactive protein. *Circulation* 1999;100:230–235.

106. Wilensky RL, Bourdillon PD, Vix VA, et al. Intracoronary artery thrombus formation in unstable angina: a clinical, biochemical and angiographic correlation. *J Am Coll Cardiol* 1993;21:692–699.

107. Farkouh ME, Smars PA, Reeder GS, et al. A clinical trial of a chest-pain observation unit for patients with unstable angina. *N Engl J Med* 1998;339:1882–1888.

108. Savonitto S, Granger CB, Ardissino D, et al. Even minor elevations of creatine kinase predict increased risk of cardiac events in acute coronary syndromes without ST-segment elevation. *J Am Coll Cardiol* 1999;33[Suppl A]:346A(abst).

109. Armstrong PW, Fu Y, Chang W-C, et al. Acute coronary syndromes in the GUSTO-IIb trial: prognostic insights and impact of recurrent ischemia. *Circulation* 1998;98:1860–1868.

110. Boersma E, Pieper KS, Steyerberg EW, et al. Predictors of outcome in patients with acute coronary syndromes without persistent ST-segment elevation: results from an international trial of 9461 patients. *Circulation* 2000;101:2557–2567.

111. Antman EM, Cohen M, Bernink PJ, et al. The TIMI risk score for unstable angina/non–ST elevation MI: a method for prognostication and therapeutic decision making. *JAMA* 2000;284:835–842.

112. Severi S, Orsini E, Marraccini P, et al. The basal electrocardiogram and the exercise stress test in assessing prognosis in patients with unstable angina. *Eur Heart J* 1988;9:441–446.

113. Brown KA. Prognostic value of thallium-201 myocardial perfusion imaging in patients with unstable angina who respond to medical treatment [published erratum appears in *J Am Coll Cardiol* 1991;18:889]. *J Am Coll Cardiol* 1991;17:1053–1057.

114. Hilton TC, Thompson RC, Williams HJ, et al. Technetium-99m sestamibi myocardial perfusion imaging in the emergency room evaluation of chest pain. *J Am Coll Cardiol* 1994;23:1016–1022.

115. Zhu YY, Chung WS, Botvinick EH, et al. Dipyridamole perfusion scintigraphy: the experience with its application in one hundred seventy patients with known or suspected unstable angina. *Am Heart J* 1991;121:33–43.

116. Younis LT, Byers S, Shaw L, et al. Prognostic value of intravenous dipyridamole thallium scintigraphy after an acute myocardial ischemic event. *Am J Cardiol* 1989;64:161–166.

117. Stratmann HG, Tamesis BR, Younis LT, et al. Prognostic value of predischarge dipyridamole technetium 99m sestamibi myocardial tomography in medically treated patients with unstable angina. *Am Heart J* 1995;130:734–740.

118. Stratmann HG, Younis LT, Wittry MD, et al. Exercise technetium-99m myocardial tomography for the risk stratification of men with medically treated unstable angina pectoris. *Am J Cardiol* 1995;76:236–240.

119. Wilson RF, Marcus ML, Christensen BV, et al. Accuracy of exercise electrocardiography in detecting physiologically significant coronary arterial lesions. *Circulation* 1991;83:412–421.

120. Nixon JV, Brown CN, Smitherman TC. Identification of transient and persistent segmental wall motion abnormalities in patients with unstable angina by two-dimensional echocardiography. *Circulation* 1982;65:1497–1503.

121. Bugiardini R, Pozzati A, Borghi A, et al. Angiographic morphology in unstable angina and its relation to transient myocardial ischemia and hospital outcome. *Am J Cardiol* 1991;67:460–464.

122. The TIMI IIIB investigators. Effects of tissue plasminogen activator and a comparison of early invasive and conservative strategies in unstable angina and non–Q-wave myocardial infarction: results of the TIMI IIIB trial. *Circulation* 1994;89:1545–1556.

123. Davies GJ, Bencivelli W, Fragasso G, et al. Sequence and magnitude of ventricular volume changes in painful and painless myocardial ischemia. *Circulation* 1988;78:310–319.

124. The PURSUIT trial investigators. Inhibition of platelet glycoprotein IIb/IIIa with eptifibatide in patients with acute coronary syndromes. *N Engl J Med* 1998;339:436–443.

125. Anderson HV, Cannon CP, Stone PH, et al. One-year results of the Thrombolysis in Myocardial Infarction (TIMI) IIIB clinical trial: a randomized comparison of tissue-type plasminogen activator versus placebo and early invasive versus early conservative strategies in unstable angina and non–Q wave myocardial infarction. *J Am Coll Cardiol* 1995;26:1643–1650.

126. Lewis HD, Davis JW, Archibald DG, et al. Protective effects of aspirin against acute myocardial infarction and death in men with unstable angina: results of a Veterans Administration cooperative study. *N Engl J Med* 1983;309:396–403.

127. Cairns JA, Gent M, Singer J, et al. Aspirin, sulfinpyrazone, or both in unstable angina: results of a Canadian multicenter trial. *N Engl J Med* 1985;313:1369–1375.

128. Lubsen J, Tijssen JGP, Kerkkamp HJJ. Early treatment of unstable angina in the coronary care unit: a randomised, double blind, placebo controlled comparison of recurrent ischaemia in patients treated with nifedipine or metoprolol or both: report of the Holland Interuniversity Nifedipine/Metoprolol trial (HINT) research group. *Br Heart J* 1986;56:400–413.

129. Gottlieb SO, Weisfeldt ML, Ouyang P, et al. Effect of the addition of propranolol to therapy with nifedipine for unstable angina pectoris: a randomized, double-blind, placebo-controlled trial. *Circulation* 1986;73:331–337.

130. Diver DJ, Bier JD, Ferreira PE, et al. Clinical and arteriographic characterization of patients with unstable angina without critical coronary arterial narrowing (from the TIMI-IIIA trial). *Am J Cardiol* 1994;74:531–537.

131. Yasue H, Takizawa A, Nagao M, et al. Long-term prognosis for patients with variant angina and influential factors. *Circulation* 1988;78:1–9.

132. McCormick JR, Schick EC Jr, McCabe CH, et al. Determinants of operative mortality and long-term survival in patients with unstable angina: the CASS experience. *J Thorac Cardiovasc Surg* 1985;89:683–688.

133. The Global Use of Strategies to Open Occluded Coronary Arteries (GUSTO) IIB investigators. A comparison of recombinant hirudin with heparin for the treatment of acute coronary syndromes. *N Engl J Med* 1996;335:775–782.

134. Schuster EH, Bulkley BH. Early post-infarction angina. Ischemia at a distance and ischemia in the infarct zone. *N Engl J Med* 1981;305:1101–1105.

135. Betriu A, Heras M, Cohen M, et al. Unstable angina: outcome according to clinical presentation. *J Am Coll Cardiol* 1992;19:1659–1663.

136. Rizik DG, Healy S, Margulis A, et al. A new clinical classification for hospital prognosis of unstable angina pectoris. *Am J Cardiol* 1995;75:993–997.

137. Bazzino O, Díaz R, Tajer C, et al. Clinical predictors of in-hospital prognosis in unstable angina: ECLA 3. *Am Heart J* 1999;137:322–331.

138. Akkerhuis M, Klootwijk PAJ, Lindeboom WK, et al. The risk of adverse outcome in patients with acute coronary syndromes is directly proportional to the number of episodes of recurrent ischemia detected by multilead ST-segment monitoring: meta-analysis of three studies involving 995 patients. *Circulation* 2000;102[Suppl II]:II-589.

139. Goodman SG, Barr A, Sobtchouk A, et al. Low molecular weight heparin decreases rebound ischemia in unstable angina or non–Q-wave myocardial infarction: the Canadian ESSENCE ST Segment Monitoring substudy. *J Am Coll Cardiol* 2000;36:1507–1513.

140. Tschopp TB. Aspirin inhibits platelet aggregation on, but not adhesion to, collagen fibrils: an assessment of platelet adhesion and deposited platelet mass by morphometry and ^{51}Cr-labeling. *Thromb Res* 1977;11:619–632.

141. Oates JA, Fitzgerald GA, Branch RA, et al. Clinical implications of prostaglandin and thromboxane A2 formation (Pt 1). *N Engl J Med* 1988;319:689–698.

142. Cooke GE, Bray PF, Hamlington JD, et al. PIA$_2$ polymorphism and efficacy of aspirin [Letter]. *Lancet* 1998;351:1253.

143. Pappas JM, Westengard JC, Bull BS. Population variability in the effect of aspirin on platelet function: implications for clinical trials and therapy. *Arch Pathol Lab Med* 1994;118:801–804.

144. Buchanan MR, Brister SJ. Individual variation in the effects of ASA on platelet function: implications for the use of ASA clinically. *Can J Cardiol* 1995;11:221–227.

145. Patrono C, Coller B, Dalen JE, et al. Platelet-active drugs: the relationships among dose, effectiveness, and side effects. *Chest* 1998;114:470S–488S.

146. Roderick PJ, Wilkes HC, Meade TW. The gastrointestinal toxicity of aspirin: an overview of randomised controlled trials. *Br J Clin Pharmacol* 1993;35:219–226.

147. Derry S, Loke YK. Risk of gastrointestinal haemorrhage with long term use of aspirin: meta-analysis. *BMJ* 2000;321:1183–1187.

148. White HD. Unstable angina: ischemic syndromes. In: Topol EJ, ed. *Comprehensive cardiovascular medicine.* Philadelphia: Lippincott–Raven Publishers, 1998:395–423.

149. Antiplatelet Trialists' Collaboration. Collaborative overview of randomised trials of antiplatelet therapy—I: prevention of death, myocardial infarction, and stroke by prolonged antiplatelet therapy in various categories of patients. *BMJ* 1994;308:81–106.

150. Komatsu H, Yaju H, Chiba K, et al. Inhibition by cyclo-oxygenase inhibitors of interleukin-6 production by human peripheral blood mononuclear cells. *Int J Immunopharmacol* 1991;13:1137–1146.

151. Rosenblum WI, Nishimura H, Nelson GH. L-NMMA in brain microcirculation of mice is inhibited by blockade of cyclooxygenase and by superoxide dismutase. *Am J Physiol* 1992;262:H1343–H1349.

152. Mehta P, Mehta JL. Effects of aspirin in arterial thrombosis: why don't animals behave the way humans do? [Editorial]. *J Am Coll Cardiol* 1993;21:511–513.

153. Kyrle PA, Eichler HG, Jager U, et al. Inhibition of prostacyclin and thromboxane A2 generation by low-dose aspirin at the site of plug formation in man in vivo. *Circulation* 1987;75:1025–1029.

154. The RISC group. Risk of myocardial infarction and death during treatment with low dose aspirin and intravenous heparin in men with unstable coronary artery disease. *Lancet* 1990;336:827–830.

155. Balsano F, Rizzon P, Violi F, et al. Antiplatelet treatment with ticlopidine in unstable angina: a controlled multicenter clinical trial. The Studio della Ticlopidina nell'Angina Instabile group. *Circulation* 1990;82:17–26.

156. Dabaghi SF, Kamat SG, Payne J, et al. Effects of low-dose aspirin on in vitro platelet aggregation in the early minutes after ingestion in normal subjects. *Am J Cardiol* 1994;74:720–723.

157. Coumadin Aspirin Reinfarction study (CARS) investigators. Randomised double-blind trial of fixed low-dose warfarin with aspirin after myocardial infarction. *Lancet* 1997;350:389–396.

158. CAPRIE Steering Committee. A randomised, blinded, trial of clopidogrel versus aspirin in patients at risk of ischaemic events (CAPRIE). *Lancet* 1996;348:1329–1339.

159. Bennett CL, Connors JM, Carwile JM, et al. Thrombotic thrombocytopenic purpura associated with clopidogrel. *N Engl J Med* 2000;342:1773–1777.

160. The Clopidogrel in Unstable Angina to Prevent Recurrent Events Trial Investigators. Effects of clopidogrel in addition to aspirin in patients with acute coronary syndromes without ST-segment elevation. *N Engl J Med* 2001;345:494–502.

161. Topol EJ, Moliterno DJ, Herrmann HC, et al. Comparison of two platelet glycoprotein IIb/IIIa inhibitors, tirofiban and abciximab, for the prevention of ischemic events with percutaneous coronary revascularization. *N Engl J Med* 2001;344:1888–1894.

162. The ESPRIT investigators. Novel dosing regimen of eptifibatide in planned coronary stent implantation (ESPRIT): a randomised, placebo-controlled trial. *Lancet* 2000;356:2037–2044.

163. Januzzi JL, Hahn SS, Chae CU, et al. Effects of tirofiban plus heparin versus heparin alone on troponin I levels in patients with acute coronary syndromes. *Am J Cardiol* 2000;86:713–717.

164. Kong DF, Califf RM, Miller DP, et al. Clinical outcomes of therapeutic agents that block the platelet glycoprotein IIb/IIIa integrin in ischemic heart disease. *Circulation* 1998;98:2829–2835.

165. The EPIC investigators. Use of a monoclonal antibody directed against the platelet glycoprotein IIb/IIIa receptor in high-risk coronary angioplasty. *N Engl J Med* 1994;330:956–961.

166. Holmes DR Jr, Hartzler GO, Smith HC, et al. Coronary artery thrombosis in patients with unstable angina. *Br Heart J* 1981;45:411–416.

167. Topol EJ, Califf RM, Weisman HF, et al. Randomised trial of coronary intervention with antibody against platelet IIb/IIIa integrin for reduction of clinical restenosis: results at six months. *Lancet* 1994;343:881–886.

168. The EPILOG investigators. Platelet glycoprotein IIb/IIIa receptor blockade and low-dose heparin during percutaneous coronary revascularization. *N Engl J Med* 1997;336:1689–1696.

169. The EPISTENT investigators. Randomised placebo-controlled and balloon-angioplasty–controlled trial to assess safety of coronary stenting with use of platelet glycoprotein-IIb/IIIa blockade. *Lancet* 1998;352:87–92.

170. The PARAGON investigators. International, randomized, controlled trial of lamifiban (a platelet glycoprotein IIb/IIIa inhibitor), heparin, or both in unstable angina. *Circulation* 1998;97:2386–2395.

171. Wu AH. Biochemical markers of cardiac damage: from traditional enzymes to cardiac-specific proteins. IFCC Subcommittee on Standardization of Cardiac Markers (S-SCM). *Scand J Clin Lab Invest* 1999;230[Suppl]:74–82.

172. Peter K, Schwarz M, Ylänne J, et al. Induction of fibrinogen binding and platelet aggregation as a potential intrinsic property of various glycoprotein IIb/IIIa ($\alpha_{IIb}\beta_3$) inhibitors. *Blood* 1998;92:3240–3249.

173. Simon DI, Chen Z, Xu H, et al. Platelet glycoprotein Ibα is a counterreceptor for the leukocyte integrin Mac-1 (CD11b/CD18). *J Exp Med* 2000;192:193–204.

174. Mascelli MA, Lance ET, Damaraju L, et al. Pharmacodynamic profile of short-term abciximab treatment demonstrates prolonged platelet inhibition with gradual recovery from GP IIb/IIIa receptor blockade. *Circulation* 1998;97:1680–1688.

175. Kereiakes DJ, Broderick TM, Roth EM, et al. Time course, magnitude, and consistency of platelet inhibition by abciximab, tirofiban, or eptifibatide in patients with unstable angina pectoris undergoing percutaneous coronary intervention. *Am J Cardiol* 1999;84:391–395.

176. Murphy RT, Quinn M, Dooley M, et al. Abciximab fails to fully inhibit internal pool of GP IIb/IIIa receptors in patients undergoing coronary angioplasty. *Circulation* 2000;102[Suppl II]:II-428(abst).

177. The RESTORE investigators. Effects of platelet glycoprotein IIb/IIIa blockade with tirofiban on adverse cardiac events in patients with unstable angina or acute myocardial infarction undergoing coronary angioplasty. *Circulation* 1997;96:1445–1453.

178. Horrigan MCG, Tcheng JE, Califf RM, et al. Maximal benefit of integrelin platelet IIb/IIIa blockade 6–12 hours after therapy: results of the IMPACT-II trial. *J Am Coll Cardiol* 1996;27:55A(abst).

179. Kouns WC, Kirchhofer D, Hadvary P, et al. Reversible conformational changes induced in glycoprotein IIb–IIIa by a potent and selective peptidomimetic inhibitor. *Blood* 1992;80:2539–2547.

180. Bhatt DL, Marso SP, Houghtaling P, et al. Does earlier administration of eptifibatide reduce death and MI in patients with acute coronary syndromes? *Circulation* 1998;98[Suppl I]:I-560–I-561.

181. Boersma E, Akkerhuis M, Théroux P, et al. Platelet glycoprotein IIb/IIIa receptor inhibition in non–ST-elevation acute coronary syndromes: early benefit during medical treatment only, with additional protection during percutaneous coronary intervention. *Circulation* 1999;100:2045–2048.

182. Marso SP, Bhatt DL, Roe MT, et al. Enhanced efficacy of eptifibatide administration in patients with acute coronary syndrome requiring in-hospital coronary artery bypass grafting. *Circulation* 2000;102:2952–2958.

183. Kleiman NS, Lincoff AM, Flaker GC, et al. Early percutaneous coronary intervention, platelet inhibition with eptifibatide, and clinical outcomes in patients with acute coronary syndromes. *Circulation* 2000;101:751–757.

184. The IMPACT-II investigators. Randomised placebo-controlled trial of effect of eptifibatide on complications of percutaneous coronary intervention: IMPACT-II. *Lancet* 1997;349:1422–1428.

185. Alexander JH, Harrington RA, Tuttle RH, et al. Prior aspirin use predicts worse outcomes in patients with non–ST-elevation acute coronary syndromes. *Am J Cardiol* 1999;83:1147–1151.

186. Hebert PR, Hennekens CH. An overview of the 4 randomized trials of aspirin therapy in the primary prevention of vascular disease. *Arch Intern Med* 2000;160:3123–3127.

187. Zhao X-Q, Théroux P, Snapinn SM, et al. Intracoronary thrombus and platelet glycoprotein IIb/IIIa receptor blockade with tirofiban in unstable angina or non–Q-wave myocardial infarction: angiographic results from the PRISM-PLUS trial (Platelet Receptor Inhibition for Ischemic Syndrome Management in Patients Limited by Unstable Signs and Symptoms). *Circulation* 1999;100:1609–1615.

188. Szucs TD, Meyer BJ, Kiowski W. Economic assessment of tirofiban in the management of acute coronary syndromes in the hospital setting: an analysis based on the PRISM PLUS trial. *Eur Heart J* 1999;20:1253–1260.

188a. Steinhubl SR, Ellis SG, Wolski K, et al. Ticlopidine pretreatment before coronary stenting is associated with sustained decrease in adverse cardiac events: data from the Evaluation of Platelet IIb/IIIa Inhibitor for Stenting (EPISTENT) trial. *Circulation* 2001;103:1403–1409.

188b. Mehta SR, Yusuf S, Peters RJG, et al. Effects of pretreatment with clopidogrel and aspirin followed by long-term therapy in patients undergoing percutaneous coronary intervention: the PCI-CURE study. Lancet 2001;358:527–533.

189. Telford AM, Wilson C. Trial of heparin versus atenolol in prevention of myocardial infarction in intermediate coronary syndrome. *Lancet* 1981;1:1225–1228.

190. Théroux P, Waters D, Qiu S, et al. Aspirin versus heparin to prevent myocardial infarction during the acute phase of unstable angina. *Circulation* 1993;88:2045–2048.

191. Cohen M, Adams PC, Hawkins L, et al. Usefulness of antithrombotic therapy in resting angina pectoris or non–Q-wave myocardial infarction in preventing death and myocardial infarction (a pilot study from the Antithrombotic Therapy in Acute Coronary Syndromes study group). *Am J Cardiol* 1990;66:1287–1292.

192. Gurfinkel EP, Manos EJ, Mejaíl RI, et al. Low molecular weight heparin versus regular heparin or aspirin in the treatment of unstable angina and silent ischemia. *J Am Coll Cardiol* 1995;26:313–318.

193. Cohen M, Adams PC, Parry G, et al. Combination antithrombotic therapy in unstable rest angina and non–Q-wave infarction in nonprior aspirin users: primary end points analysis from the ATACS trial. Antithrombotic Therapy in Acute Coronary Syndromes research group. *Circulation* 1994;89:81–88.

194. Neri Serneri GG, Gensini GF, Poggesi L, et al. Effect of heparin, aspirin, or alteplase in reduction of myocardial ischaemia in refractory unstable angina. *Lancet* 1990;335:615–618.

195. Neri Serneri GG, Modesti PA, Gensini GF, et al. Randomised comparison of subcutaneous heparin, intravenous heparin, and aspirin in unstable angina [published erratum appears in *Lancet* 1995;346:130]. *Lancet* 1995;345:1201–1204.

196. Becker RC, Spencer FA, Li Y, et al. Thrombin generation after the abrupt cessation of intravenous unfractionated heparin among patients with acute coronary syndromes: potential mechanisms for heightened prothrombotic potential. *J Am Coll Cardiol* 1999;34:1020–1027.

197. Eikelboom JW, Anand SS, Malmberg K, et al. Unfractionated heparin and low-molecular-weight heparin in acute coronary syndrome without ST elevation: a meta-analysis. *Lancet* 2000;355:1936–1942.

198. Massonnet-Castel S, Pelissier E, Bara L, et al. Partial reversal of low molecular weight heparin (PK 10169) anti-Xa activity by protamine sulfate: in vitro and in vivo study during cardiac surgery with extracorporeal circulation. *Haemostasis* 1986;16:139–146.

199. Mark DB, Cowper PA, Berkowitz SD, et al. Economic assessment of low-molecular-weight heparin (enoxaparin) versus unfractionated heparin in acute coronary syndrome patients: results from the ESSENCE randomized trial. *Circulation* 1998;97:1702–1707.

200. Warkentin TE, Levine MN, Hirsh J, et al. Heparin-induced thrombocytopenia in patients treated with low-molecular-weight heparin or unfractionated heparin. *N Engl J Med* 1995;332:1330–1335.

201. Cohen M, Demers C, Gurfinkel EP, et al. A comparison of low-molecular-weight heparin with unfractionated heparin for unstable coronary artery disease. *N Engl J Med* 1997;337:447–452.

202. Klein W, Buchwald A, Hillis SE, et al. Comparison of low-molecular-weight heparin with unfractionated heparin acutely and with placebo for 6 weeks in the management of unstable coronary artery disease: Fragmin in Unstable Coronary Artery Disease study (FRIC). *Circulation* 1997;96:61–68.

203. The FRAXIS study group. Comparison of two treatment durations (6 days and 14 days) of a low molecular weight heparin with a 6-day treatment of unfractionated heparin in the initial management of unstable angina or non–Q wave myocardial infarction: FRAXIS (Fraxiparine in Ischaemic Syndrome). *Eur Heart J* 1999;20:1553–1562.

204. Antman EM, Cohen M, Radley D, et al. Assessment of the treatment effect of enoxaparin for unstable angina/non–Q-wave myocardial infarction: TIMI 11B-ESSENCE meta-analysis. *Circulation* 1999;100:1602–1608.

205. Montalescot G, Philippe F, Ankri A, et al. Early increase of von Willebrand factor predicts adverse outcome in unstable coronary artery disease: beneficial effects of enoxaparin. *Circulation* 1998;98:294–299.

206. Hansen J-B, Sandset PM. Differential effects of low molecular weight heparin and unfractionated heparin on circulating levels of antithrombin and tissue factor pathway inhibitor (TFPI): a possible mechanism for the difference in therapeutic efficacy. *Thromb Res* 1998;91:177–181.

207. Brieger D, Dawes J. Characterisation of persistent anti-Xa activity following administration of the low molecular weight heparin enoxaparin sodium (Clexane). *Thromb Haemost* 1994;72:275–280.

208. Fragmin and Fast Revascularisation during Instability in Coronary Artery Disease (FRISC II) investigators. Long-term low-molecular-mass heparin in unstable coronary-artery disease: FRISC II Prospective Randomised Multicentre study [published erratum appears in *Lancet* 1999;354:1478]. *Lancet* 1999;354:701–707.

209. Théroux P, Waters D, Lam J, et al. Reactivation of unstable angina after the discontinuation of heparin. *N Engl J Med* 1992;327:141–145.

210. Granger CB, Califf RM, Van de Werf F, et al. Activated partial thromboplastin time and clinical outcome among patients with unstable angina or non–Q-wave MI treated with intravenous heparin. *Circulation* 1995;92[Suppl I]:I-416–I-417(abst).

211. Granger CB, Hirsh J, Califf RM, et al. Activated partial thromboplastin time and outcome after thrombolytic therapy for acute myocardial infarction: results from the GUSTO-I trial. *Circulation* 1996;93:870–878.

212. Hirsh J, Dalen JE, Guyatt G. The Sixth (2000) ACCP Guidelines for Antithrombotic Therapy for Prevention and Treatment of Thrombosis. *Chest* 2001;119[Suppl 1]:1S–2S.

213. Chong BH, Ismail F, Cade J, et al. Heparin-induced thrombocytopenia: studies with a new low molecular weight heparinoid, Org 10172. *Blood* 1989;73:1592–1596.

214. Horellou MH, Conard J, Lecrubier C, et al. Persistent heparin induced thrombocytopenia despite therapy with low molecular weight heparin [Letter]. *Thromb Haemost* 1984;51:134.

215. Leroy J, Leclerc MH, Delahousse B, et al. Treatment of heparin-associated thrombocytopenia and thrombosis with low molecular weight heparin (CY 216). *Semin Thromb Hemost* 1985;11:326–329.

216. Vitoux JF, Mathieu JF, Roncato M, et al. Heparin-associated thrombocytopenia treatment with low molecular weight heparin. *Thromb Haemost* 1986;55:37–39.

217. Cohen M, Théroux P, Weber S, et al. Combination therapy with tirofiban and enoxaparin in acute coronary syndromes. *Int J Cardiol* 1999;71:273–281.

218. Cohen M, Théroux P, Frey MJ, et al. Anti-thrombotic combination using tirofiban and enoxaparin: the ACUTE II study. *Circulation* 2000;102[Suppl II]:II-826(abst).

219. Yusuf S, Wittes J, Friedman L. Overview of results of randomized clinical trials in heart disease. II. Unstable angina, heart failure, primary prevention with aspirin, and risk factor modification. *JAMA* 1988;260:2259–2263.

220. Muller JE, Turi ZG, Pearle DL, et al. Nifedipine and conventional therapy for unstable angina pectoris: a random-

ized, double-blind comparison. *Circulation* 1984;69:728–739.

221. Horowitz JD, Henry CA, Syrjanen ML, et al. Combined use of nitroglycerin and *N*-acetylcysteine in the management of unstable angina pectoris. *Circulation* 1988;77:787–794.

222. Gibson RS, Boden WE, Théroux P, et al. Diltiazem and reinfarction in patients with non–Q-wave myocardial infarction. Results of a double-blind, randomized, multicenter trial. *N Engl J Med* 1986;315:423–429.

223. Hansen JF, Hagerup L, Sigurd B, et al. Cardiac event rates after acute myocardial infarction in patients treated with verapamil and trandolapril versus trandolapril alone. Danish Verapamil Infarction Trial (DAVIT) study group. *Am J Cardiol* 1997;79:738–741.

224. Muller JE, Morrison J, Stone PH, et al. Nifedipine therapy for patients with threatened and acute myocardial infarction: a randomized, double-blind, placebo-controlled comparison. *Circulation* 1984;69:740–747.

225. Gerstenblith G, Ouyang P, Achuff SC, et al. Nifedipine in unstable angina: a double-blind, randomized trial. *N Engl J Med* 1982;306:885–889.

226. Patel DJ, Purcell HJ, Fox KM, et al. Cardioprotection by opening of the K_{ATP} channel in unstable angina: is this a clinical manifestation of myocardial preconditioning? Results of a randomized study with nicorandil. *Eur Heart J* 1999;20:51–57.

227. Anticoagulants in the Secondary Prevention of Events in Coronary Thrombosis (ASPECT) research group. Effect of long-term oral anticoagulant treatment on mortality and cardiovascular morbidity after myocardial infarction. *Lancet* 1994;343:499–503.

228. Hoogwerf BJ, Waness A, Cressman M, et al. Effects of aggressive cholesterol lowering and low-dose anticoagulation on clinical and angiographic outcomes in patients with diabetes: the Post Coronary Artery Bypass Graft trial. *Diabetes* 1999;48:1289–1294.

229. Stroke Prevention in Atrial Fibrillation investigators. Adjusted-dose warfarin versus low-intensity, fixed-dose warfarin plus aspirin for high-risk patients with atrial fibrillation: Stroke Prevention in Atrial Fibrillation III randomised clinical trial. *Lancet* 1996;348:633–638.

230. Anand SS, Yusuf S, Pogue J, et al. Long-term oral anticoagulant therapy in patients with unstable angina or suspected non–Q-wave myocardial infarction: Organization to Assess Strategies for Ischemic Syndromes (OASIS) pilot study results. *Circulation* 1998;98:1064–1070.

231. Waters D, Lam JYT. Is thrombolytic therapy striking out in unstable angina? *Circulation* 1992;86:1642–1644.

232. Fibrinolytic Therapy Trialists' (FTT) collaborative group. Indications for fibrinolytic therapy in suspected acute myocardial infarction: collaborative overview of early mortality and major morbidity results from all randomised trials of more than 1000 patients. *Lancet* 1994;343:311–322.

233. DeWood MA, Stifter WF, Simpson CS, et al. Coronary arteriographic findings soon after non–Q-wave myocardial infarction. *N Engl J Med* 1986;315:417–423.

234. The TIMI IIIA investigators. Early effects of tissue-type plasminogen activator added to conventional therapy on the culprit coronary lesion in patients presenting with ischemic cardiac pain at rest: results of the Thrombolysis in Myocardial Ischemia (TIMI IIIA) trial. *Circulation* 1993;87:38–52.

235. Karlsson J-E, Berglund U, Björkholm A, et al. Thrombolysis with recombinant human tissue-type plasminogen activator during instability in coronary artery disease: effect on myocardial ischemia and need for coronary revascularization. *Am Heart J* 1992;124:1419–1426.

236. Ambrose JA, Almeida OD, Sharma SK, et al. Adjunctive thrombolytic therapy during angioplasty for ischemic rest angina: results of the TAUSA trial. *Circulation* 1994;90:69–77.

237. Bär FW, Verheugt FW, Col J, et al. Thrombolysis in patients with unstable angina improves the angiographic but not the clinical outcome: results of UNASEM, a multicenter, randomized, placebo-controlled, clinical trial with anistreplase. *Circulation* 1992;86:131–137.

238. Schreiber TL, Rizik D, White C, et al. Randomized trial of thrombolysis versus heparin in unstable angina. *Circulation* 1992;86:1407–1414.

239. Oltrona L, Merlini PA, Spinola A, et al. Prolonged streptokinase infusion in patients with unstable angina: results of a randomized, placebo-controlled clinical trial. *Coronary Artery Disease* 1996;7:377–382.

240. Shabani F, Théroux P, de Guise P, et al. A randomized, double-blind trial of streptokinase versus placebo for the management of unstable angina and non–Q wave myocardial infarction in patients with previous coronary artery bypass surgery. *J Am Coll Cardiol* 1995;25[Suppl A]:421A(abst).

241. Romeo F, Rosano GMC, Martuscelli E, et al. Effectiveness of prolonged low dose recombinant tissue-type plasminogen activator for refractory unstable angina. *J Am Coll Cardiol* 1995;25:1295–1299.

242. ISIS-2 (Second International Study of Infarct Survival) collaborative group. Randomised trial of intravenous streptokinase, oral aspirin, both, or neither among 17,187 cases of suspected acute myocardial infarction: ISIS-2. *Lancet* 1988;2:349–360.

243. ISIS-3 (Third International Study of Infarct Survival) collaborative group. ISIS-3: a randomised comparison of streptokinase vs tissue plasminogen activator vs anistreplase and of aspirin plus heparin vs aspirin alone among 41,299 cases of suspected acute myocardial infarction. *Lancet* 1992;339:753–770.

244. Gruppo Italiano per lo Studio della Streptochinasi nell'Infarto Miocardico (GISSI). Effectiveness of intravenous thrombolytic treatment in acute myocardial infarction. *Lancet* 1986;1:397–402.

245. LATE study group. Late Assessment of Thrombolytic Efficacy (LATE) study with alteplase 6–24 hours after onset of acute myocardial infarction. *Lancet* 1993;342:759–766.

246. Kornreich F, Montague TJ, Rautaharju PM. Body surface potential mapping of ST segment changes in acute myocardial infarction: implications for ECG enrollment criteria for thrombolytic therapy. *Circulation* 1993;87:773–782.

247. O'Keefe JH Jr, Sayed-Taha K, Gibson W, et al. Do patients with left circumflex coronary artery–related acute myocardial infarction without ST-segment elevation bene-

fit from reperfusion therapy? *Am J Cardiol* 1995;75:718–720.

248. Huey BL, Beller GA, Kaiser DL, et al. A comprehensive analysis of myocardial infarction due to left circumflex artery occlusion: comparison with infarction due to right coronary artery and left anterior descending artery occlusion. *J Am Coll Cardiol* 1988;12:1156–1166.

249. French JK, Williams BF, Hart HH, et al. Prospective evaluation of eligibility for thrombolytic therapy in acute myocardial infarction. *BMJ* 1996;312:1637–1641.

250. Fitzgerald DJ, Catella F, Roy L, et al. Marked platelet activation in vivo after intravenous streptokinase in patients with acute myocardial infarction. *Circulation* 1988;77:142–150.

251. Kroll MH, Schafer AI. Biochemical mechanisms of platelet activation. *Blood* 1989;74:1181–1195.

252. Langer A, Goodman SG, Topol EJ, et al. Late Assessment of Thrombolytic Efficacy (LATE) study: prognosis in patients with non–Q wave myocardial infarction. *J Am Coll Cardiol* 1996;27:1327–1332.

253. Szatmary LJ, Marco J, Fajadet J, et al. The combined use of diastolic counterpulsation and coronary dilation in unstable angina due to multivessel disease under unstable hemodynamic conditions. *Int J Cardiol* 1988;19:59–66.

254. Ohman EM, George BS, White CJ, et al. Use of aortic counterpulsation to improve sustained coronary artery patency during acute myocardial infarction: results of a randomized trial. *Circulation* 1994;90:792–799.

255. Stone GW, Marsalese D, Brodie BR, et al. A prospective, randomized evaluation of prophylactic intraaortic balloon counterpulsation in high risk patients with acute myocardial infarction treated with primary angioplasty. *J Am Coll Cardiol* 1997;29:1459–1467.

256. Mark DB, Nelson CL, Califf RM, et al. Continuing evolution of therapy for coronary artery disease: initial results from the era of coronary angioplasty. *Circulation* 1994;89:2015–2025.

257. White HD. Angioplasty versus bypass surgery [Commentary]. *Lancet* 1995;346:1174–1175.

258. Pocock SJ, Henderson RA, Rickards AF, et al. Meta-analysis of randomised trials comparing coronary angioplasty with bypass surgery. *Lancet* 1995;346:1184–1189.

259. The Bypass Angioplasty Revascularization Investigation (BARI) investigators. Comparison of coronary bypass surgery with angioplasty in patients with multivessel disease. *N Engl J Med* 1996;335:217–225.

260. De Feyter PJ, Serruys PW. Percutaneous transluminal coronary angioplasty for unstable angina. In: Topol EJ, ed. *Textbook of interventional cardiology*, 2nd ed. Philadelphia: WB Saunders, 1994:274–291.

261. Bentivoglio LG, Detre K, Yeh W, et al. Outcome of percutaneous transluminal coronary angioplasty in subsets of unstable angina pectoris. A report of the 1985–1986 National Heart, Lung, and Blood Institute Percutaneous Transluminal Coronary Angioplasty Registry. *J Am Coll Cardiol* 1994;24:1195–1206.

262. Myler RK, Shaw RE, Stertzer SH, et al. Unstable angina and coronary angioplasty. *Circulation* 1990;82:II-88–II-95.

263. De Feyter PJ, Suryapranata H, Serruys PW, et al. Coronary angioplasty for unstable angina: immediate and late

results in 200 consecutive patients with identification of risk factors for unfavorable early and late outcome. *J Am Coll Cardiol* 1988;12:324–333.

264. Sugrue DD, Holmes DR Jr, Smith HC, et al. Coronary artery thrombus as a risk factor for acute vessel occlusion during percutaneous transluminal coronary angioplasty: improving results. *Br Heart J* 1986;56:62–66.

265. Deligonul U, Gabliani GI, Caralis DG, et al. Percutaneous transluminal coronary angioplasty in patients with intracoronary thrombus. *Am J Cardiol* 1988;62:474–476.

266. Grines CL, Cox DA, Stone GW, et al. Coronary angioplasty with or without stent implantation for acute myocardial infarction. *N Engl J Med* 1999;341:1949–1956.

267. Mehran R, Ambrose JA, Bongu RM, et al. Angioplasty of complex lesions in ischemic rest angina: results of the Thrombolysis and Angioplasty in Unstable Angina (TAUSA) trial. *J Am Coll Cardiol* 1995;26:961–966.

268. Mabin TA, Holmes DR Jr, Smith HC, et al. Intracoronary thrombus: role in coronary occlusion complicating percutaneous transluminal coronary angioplasty. *J Am Coll Cardiol* 1985;5:198–202.

269. Arora RR, Platko WP, Bhadwar K, et al. Role of intracoronary thrombus in acute complications during percutaneous transluminal coronary angioplasty. *Cathet Cardiovasc Diagn* 1989;16:226–229.

270. Ryan TJ, Faxon DP, Gunnar RM, et al. Guidelines for percutaneous transluminal coronary angioplasty: a report of the American College of Cardiology/American Heart Association Task Force on Assessment of Diagnostic and Therapeutic Cardiovascular Procedures (Subcommittee on Percutaneous Transluminal Coronary Angioplasty). *Circulation* 1988;78:486–502.

271. Ellis SG, Vandormael MG, Cowley MJ, et al. Coronary morphologic and clinical determinants of procedural outcome with angioplasty for multivessel coronary disease: implications for patient selection. *Circulation* 1990;82:1193–1202.

272. Goudreau E, DiSciascio G, Vetrovec GW, et al. Intracoronary urokinase as an adjunct to percutaneous transluminal coronary angioplasty in patients with complex coronary narrowings or angioplasty-induced complications. *Am J Cardiol* 1992;69:57–62.

273. Gulba DC, Daniel WG, Simon R, et al. Role of thrombolysis and thrombin in patients with acute coronary occlusion during percutaneous transluminal coronary angioplasty. *J Am Coll Cardiol* 1990;16:563–568.

274. Schieman G, Cohen BM, Kozina J, et al. Intracoronary urokinase for intracoronary thrombus accumulation complicating percutaneous transluminal coronary angioplasty in acute ischemic syndromes. *Circulation* 1990;82:2052–2060.

275. Verna E, Repetto S, Boscarini M, et al. Management of complicated coronary angioplasty by intracoronary urokinase and immediate re-angioplasty. *Cathet Cardiovasc Diagn* 1990;19:116–122.

276. Laskey MA, Deutsch E, Barnathan E, et al. Influence of heparin therapy on percutaneous transluminal coronary angioplasty outcome in unstable angina pectoris. *Am J Cardiol* 1990;65:1425–1429.

277. Laskey MA, Deutsch E, Hirshfeld JW Jr, et al. Influence of heparin therapy on percutaneous transluminal coronary

angioplasty outcome in patients with coronary arterial thrombus. *Am J Cardiol* 1990;65:179–182.

278. Antoniucci D, Santoro GM, Bolognese L, et al. Early coronary angioplasty as compared with delayed angioplasty in patients with high-risk unstable angina. *Coronary Artery Disease* 1996;7:75–80.

279. Serruys PW, de Jaegere P, Kiemeneij F, et al. A comparison of balloon-expandable-stent implantation with balloon angioplasty in patients with coronary artery disease. *N Engl J Med* 1994;331:489–495.

280. Fischman DL, Leon MB, Baim DS, et al. A randomized comparison of coronary-stent placement and balloon angioplasty in the treatment of coronary artery disease. *N Engl J Med* 1994;331:496–501.

281. Hong MK, Wong C, Kent KM, et al. An aggressive stent strategy improves procedure success and reduces major in-hospital ischemic complications. *Circulation* 1995;92[Suppl I]:I-535–I-536(abst).

282. Schömig A, Neumann F-J, Kastrati A, et al. A randomized comparison of antiplatelet and anticoagulant therapy after the placement of coronary-artery stents. *N Engl J Med* 1996;334:1084–1089.

283. Colombo A, Hall P, Nakamura S, et al. Intracoronary stenting without anticoagulation accomplished with intravascular ultrasound guidance. *Circulation* 1995;91:1676–1688.

284. Moussa I, Di Mario C, Reimers B, et al. Subacute stent thrombosis in the era of intravascular ultrasound-guided coronary stenting without anticoagulation: frequency, predictors and clinical outcome. *J Am Coll Cardiol* 1997;29:6–12.

285. Malosky SA, Hirshfeld JW Jr, Herrmann HC. Comparison of results of intracoronary stenting in patients with unstable vs. stable angina. *Cathet Cardiovasc Diagn* 1994;31:95–101.

286. Kussmaul WGI, Krol J, Laskey WK, et al. One-year follow-up results of "culprit" versus multivessel coronary angioplasty trial. *Am J Cardiol* 1993;71:1431–1433.

287. De Feyter PJ, Suryapranata H, Serruys PW, et al. Coronary angioplasty for unstable angina: immediate and late results in 200 consecutive patients with identification of risk factors for unfavorable early and late outcome. *J Am Coll Cardiol* 1988;12:324–333.

288. Ellis SG, Roubin GS, King SBI, et al. Angiographic and clinical predictors of acute closure after native vessel coronary angioplasty. *Circulation* 1988;77:372–379.

289. Little WC, Applegate RJ. Role of plaque size and degree of stenosis in acute myocardial infarction. *Cardiol Clin* 1996;14:221–228.

290. Goldstein JA, Demetriou D, Grines CL, et al. Multiple complex coronary plaques in patients with acute myocardial infarction. *N Engl J Med* 2000;343:915–922.

291. Fu Y, Chang W-C, Mark D, et al. Canadian-American differences in the management of acute coronary syndromes in the GUSTO IIb trial: one-year follow-up of patients without ST-segment elevation. *Circulation* 2000;102:1375–1381.

292. Boden WE, O'Rourke RA, Crawford MH, et al. Outcomes in patients with acute non–Q-wave myocardial infarction randomly assigned to an invasive as compared with a conservative management strategy. *N Engl J Med* 1998;338:1785–1792.

293. Madsen JK, Grande P, Saunamäki K, et al. Danish multicenter randomized study of invasive versus conservative treatment in patients with inducible ischemia after thrombolysis in acute myocardial infarction (DANAMI). *Circulation* 1997;96:748–755.

294. McCullough PA, O'Neill WW, Graham M, et al. A prospective randomized trial of triage angiography in acute coronary syndromes ineligible for thrombolytic therapy: results of the Medicine Versus Angiography in Thrombolytic Exclusion (MATE) trial. *J Am Coll Cardiol* 1998;32:596–605.

295. Jones RH, Hannan EL, Hammermeister KE, et al. Identification of preoperative variables needed for risk adjustment of short-term mortality after coronary artery bypass graft surgery. The Working Group Panel on the Cooperative CABG Database Project. *J Am Coll Cardiol* 1996;28:1478–1487.

296. Wallentin L, Lagerqvist B, Husted S, et al. Outcome at 1 year after an invasive compared with a non-invasive strategy in unstable coronary-artery disease: the FRISC II invasive randomised trial. *Lancet* 2000;356:9–16.

297. Yusuf S, Zucker D, Peduzzi P, et al. Effect of coronary artery bypass graft surgery on survival: overview of 10-year results from randomised trials by the Coronary Artery Bypass Graft Surgery Trialists' Collaboration. *Lancet* 1994;344:563–570.

298. Mahoney EM, Jurkovitz CT, Chu H, et al. Hospital costs for acute coronary syndromes in the TACTICS-TIMI 18 trial. *J Am Coll Cardiol* 2001;37[Suppl A]:510A(abst).

299. Bertolasi CA, Tronge JE, Riccitelli MA, et al. Natural history of unstable angina with medical or surgical therapy. *Chest* 1976;70:596–605.

300. Neutze JM, White HD. What contribution has cardiac surgery made to the decline in mortality from coronary heart disease? *Br Med J Clin Res Ed* 1987;294:405–409.

301. Russell RO, Moraski RE, Kouchoukos N, et al. Unstable angina pectoris: National Cooperative Study Group to compare surgical and medical therapy: II. In-hospital experience and initial follow-up results in patients with one, two and three vessel disease. *Am J Cardiol* 1978;42:838–848.

302. Scott SM, Luchi RJ, Deupree RH. Veterans Administration Cooperative Study for treatment of patients with unstable angina: results in patients with abnormal left ventricular function. *Circulation* 1988;78:I-113–I-121.

303. Sharma GVRK, Lapsley D, Vita JA, et al. Usefulness and tolerability of hirulog, a direct thrombin-inhibitor, in unstable angina pectoris. *Am J Cardiol* 1993;72:1357–1360.

304. Scott SM, Deupree RH, Sharma GVRK, et al. VA Study of Unstable Angina: 10-year results show duration of surgical advantage for patients with impaired ejection fraction. *Circulation* 1994;90:II-120–II-123.

305. Luchi RJ, Scott SM, Deupree RH, et al. Comparison of medical and surgical treatment for unstable angina pectoris: results of a Veterans Administration cooperative study. *N Engl J Med* 1987;316:977–984.

306. Parisi AF, Khuri S, Deupree RH, et al. Medical compared with surgical management of unstable angina 5 year mortality and morbidity in the Veterans Administration study. *Circulation* 1989;80:1176–1189.

307. Cannon CP, Weintraub WS, Demopoulos LA, et al. Invasive versus conservative strategies in unstable angina and

non–Q-wave myocardial infarction following treatment with tirofiban: rationale and study design of the international TACTICS–TIMI 18 trial. *Am J Cardiol* 1998;82:731–736.

308. Doucet S, Malekianpour M, Théroux P, et al. Randomized trial comparing intravenous nitroglycerin and heparin for treatment of unstable angina secondary to restenosis after coronary artery angioplasty. *Circulation* 2000;101:955–961.

309. FitzGibbon GM, Leach AJ, Keon WJ, et al. Coronary bypass graft fate. Angiographic study of 1,179 vein grafts early, one year, and five years after operation. *J Thorac Cardiovasc Surg* 1986;91:773–778.

310. Galbut DL, Traad EA, Dorman MJ, et al. Seventeen-year experience with bilateral internal mammary artery grafts. *Ann Thorac Surg* 1990;49:195–201.

311. Campeau L, Enjalbert M, Lesperance J, et al. Atherosclerosis and late closure of aortocoronary saphenous vein grafts: sequential angiographic studies at 2 weeks, 1 year, 5 to 7 years, and 10 to 12 years after surgery. *Circulation* 1983;68[Suppl II]:II-1–II-7.

312. Piana RN, Moscucci M, Cohen DJ, et al. Palmaz-Schatz stenting for treatment of focal vein graft stenosis: immediate results and long-term outcome. *J Am Coll Cardiol* 1994;23:1296–1304.

313. Prevention of coronary heart disease in clinical practice: recommendations of the Second Joint Task Force of European and other Societies on Coronary Prevention. *Eur Heart J* 1998;19:1434–1503.

314. Executive Summary of the Third Report of the National Cholesterol Education Program (NCEP) Expert Panel on Detection, Evaluation, and Treatment of High Blood Cholesterol in Adults (Adult Treatment Panel III). *JAMA* 2001;285:2486–2497.

315. British Cardiac Society, British Hyperlipidemia Association, British Hypertension Society, British Diabetic Association. Joint British recommendations on primary prevention of coronary heart disease in clinical practice: summary. *BMJ* 2000;320:705–708.

316. Brown G, Albers JJ, Fisher LD, et al. Regression of coronary artery disease as a result of intensive lipid-lowering therapy in men with high levels of apolipoprotein B. *N Engl J Med* 1990;323:1289–1298.

317. Loscalzo J. Regression of coronary atherosclerosis [Editorial]. *N Engl J Med* 1990;323:1337–1339.

318. Scandinavian Simvastatin Survival Study Group. Randomised trial of cholesterol lowering in 4444 patients with coronary heart disease: the Scandinavian Simvastatin Survival Study (4S). *Lancet* 1994;344:1383–1389.

319. Long-Term Intervention with Pravastatin in Ischaemic Disease (LIPID) study group. Prevention of cardiovascular events and death with pravastatin in patients with coronary heart disease and a broad range of initial cholesterol levels. *N Engl J Med* 1998;339:1349–1357.

320. Dupuis J, Tardif J-C, Cernacek P, et al. Cholesterol reduction rapidly improves endothelial function after acute coronary syndromes: the RECIFE (Reduction of Cholesterol in Ischemia and Function of the Endothelium) trial. *Circulation* 1999;99:3227–3233.

321. Treasure CB, Klein JL, Weintraub WS, et al. Beneficial effects of cholesterol-lowering therapy on the coronary endothelium in patients with coronary artery disease. *N Engl J Med* 1995;332:481–487.

322. Anderson TJ, Meredith IT, Yeung AC, et al. The effect of cholesterol-lowering and antioxidant therapy on endothelium-dependent coronary vasomotion. *N Engl J Med* 1995;332:488–493.

323. Andrews TC, Raby K, Barry J, et al. Effect of cholesterol reduction on myocardial ischemia in patients with coronary disease. *Circulation* 1997;95:324–328.

324. Guethlin M, Kasel AM, Coppenrath K, et al. Delayed response of myocardial flow reserve to lipid-lowering therapy with fluvastatin. *Circulation* 1999;99:475–481.

325. Huggins GS, Pasternak RC, Alpert NM, et al. Effects of short-term treatment of hyperlipidemia on coronary vasodilator function and myocardial perfusion in regions having substantial impairment of baseline dilator reverse. *Circulation* 1998;98:1291–1296.

326. Baller D, Notohamiprodjo G, Gleichmann U, et al. Improvement in coronary flow reserve determined by positron emission tomography after 6 months of cholesterol-lowering therapy in patients with early stages of coronary atherosclerosis. *Circulation* 1999;99:2871–2875.

327. Liem A, van Boven AJ, Withagen AP, et al. Fluvastatin in acute myocardial infarction: effects on early and late ischemia and events (the FLORIDA trial). Proceedings of the Special Session VIII: clinical trials results. New Orleans: American Heart Association Scientific Sessions 2000, November 15, 2000.

328. Weber C, Erl W, Weber KS, et al. HMG-CoA reductase inhibitors decrease CD11b expression and CD11b-dependent adhesion of monocytes to endothelium and reduce increased adhesiveness of monocytes isolated from patients with hypercholesterolemia. *J Am Coll Cardiol* 1997;30:1212–1217.

329. Lacoste L, Lam JY, Hung J, et al. Hyperlipidemia and coronary disease. Correction of the increased thrombogenic potential with cholesterol reduction. *Circulation* 1995;92:3172–3177.

330. Aronow HD, Topol EJ, Roe MT, et al. Effect of lipid-lowering therapy on early mortality after acute coronary syndromes: an observational study. *Lancet* 2001;357:1063–1068.

331. Hamm CW, Heeschen C, Boehm M, et al. Role of statins in patients with acute coronary syndromes. *Circulation* 2000;102[Suppl II]:II-435(abst).

332. Tonkin AM, Colquhoun D, Emberson J, et al. Effect of pravastatin in 3260 patients with unstable angina: results from the LIPID study. *Lancet* 2000;356:1871–1875.

333. Schwartz GG, Olsson AG, Ezekowitz MD, et al. Effects of atorvastatin on early recurrent ischemic events in acute coronary syndromes: the MIRACL study: a randomized controlled trial. *JAMA* 2001;285:1711–1718.

334. Aquilani R, Tramarin R, Pedretti RF, et al. Despite good compliance, very low fat diet alone does not achieve recommended cholesterol goals in outpatients with coronary heart disease. *Eur Heart J* 1999;20:1020–1029.

335. Gupta S, Leatham EW, Carrington D, et al. Elevated *Chlamydia pneumoniae* antibodies, cardiovascular events, and azithromycin in male survivors of myocardial infarction. *Circulation* 1997;96:404–407.

336. Gurfinkel E, Bozovich G, Beck E, et al. Treatment with the antibiotic roxithromycin in patients with acute non–

Q-wave coronary syndromes: the final report of the ROXIS study. *Eur Heart J* 1999;20:121–127.

337. Azar RR, Rinfret S, Théroux P, et al. A randomized placebo-controlled trial to assess the efficacy of antiinflammatory therapy with methylprednisolone in unstable angina (MUNA trial). *Eur Heart J* 2000;21:2026–2032.

338. O'Connor GT, Buring JE, Yusuf S, et al. An overview of randomized trials of rehabilitation with exercise after myocardial infarction. *Circulation* 1989;80:234–244.

339. Heart Outcome Prevention Evaluation study investigators. Effects of ramipril on cardiovascular and microvascular outcomes in people with diabetes mellitus: results of the HOPE study and MICRO-HOPE substudy. *Lancet* 2000;355:253–259.

340. Thiemann DR, Coresh J, Oetgen WJ, et al. The association between hospital volume and survival after acute myocardial infarction in elderly patients. *N Engl J Med* 1999;340:1640–1648.

341. Chen J, Radford MJ, Wang Y, et al. Do "America's best hospitals" perform better for acute myocardial infarction? *N Engl J Med* 1999;340:286–292.

342. Weitz JI, Hudoba M, Massel D, et al. Clot-bound thrombin is protected from inhibition by heparin-antithrombin III but is susceptible to inactivation by antithrombin III-independent inhibitors. *J Clin Invest* 1990;86:385–391.

343. Lefkovits J, Topol EJ. Direct thrombin inhibitors in cardiovascular medicine. *Circulation* 1994;90:1522–1536.

344. Topol EJ, Fuster V, Harrington RA, et al. Recombinant hirudin for unstable angina pectoris: a multicenter, randomized angiographic trial. *Circulation* 1994;89:1557–1566.

345. Organisation to Assess Strategies for Ischemic Syndromes (OASIS-2) investigators. Effects of recombinant hirudin (lepirudin) compared with heparin on death, myocardial infarction, refractory angina, and revascularisation procedures in patients with acute myocardial ischaemia without ST elevation: a randomised trial. *Lancet* 1999;353:429–438.

346. Direct Thrombin Inhibitor Trialists' Collaborative Group. Direct thrombin inhibitors in acute coronary syndromes: principal results of a meta-analysis based on individual patient data. *Lancet* 2001 (*in press*).

347. Bates SM, Weitz MD. Direct thrombin inhibitors for treatment of arterial thrombosis: potential differences between bivalirudin and hirudin. *Am J Cardiol* 1998;82:12P–18P.

348. Lidon RM, Théroux P, Juneau M, et al. Initial experience with a direct antithrombin, Hirulog, in unstable angina: anticoagulant, antithrombotic, and clinical effects. *Circulation* 1993;88:1495–1501.

349. Fuchs J, Cannon CP, and the TIMI 7 investigators. Hirulog in the treatment of unstable angina: results of the Thrombin Inhibition in Myocardial Ischemia (TIMI) 7 trial. *Circulation* 1995;92:727–733.

350. Organization to Assess Strategies for Ischemic Syndromes (OASIS) Investigators. Comparison of the effects of two doses of recombinant hirudin compared with heparin in patients with acute myocardial ischemia without ST elevation: a pilot study. *Circulation* 1997;96:769–777.

351. Bittl JA, Strony J, Brinker JA, et al. Treatment with bivalirudin (Hirulog) as compared with heparin during coronary angioplasty for unstable or postinfarction angina. *N Engl J Med* 1995;333:764–769.

352. Gold HK, Torres FW, Garabedian HD, et al. Evidence for a rebound coagulation phenomenon after cessation of a 4-hour infusion of a specific thrombin inhibitor in patients with unstable angina pectoris. *J Am Coll Cardiol* 1993;21:1039–1047.

353. Thrombin Inhibition in Myocardial Ischaemia (TRIM) study group. A low molecular weight, selective thrombin inhibitor, inogatran, vs heparin, in unstable coronary artery disease in 1209 patients: a double-blind, randomized, dose-finding study. *Eur Heart J* 1997;18:1416–1425.

354. Klootwijk P, Lenderink T, Meij S, et al. Anticoagulant properties, clinical efficacy and safety of efegatran, a direct thrombin inhibitor, in patients with unstable angina. *Eur Heart J* 1999;20:1101–1111.

355. Abendschein DR, Meng YY, Torr-Brown S, et al. Maintenance of coronary patency after fibrinolysis with tissue factor pathway inhibitor. *Circulation* 1995;92:944–949.

356. Scholz W, Albus U. Na$^+$/H$^+$ exchange and its inhibition in cardiac ischemia and reperfusion. *Basic Res Cardiol* 1993;88:443–455.

357. Théroux P, Chaitman BR, Erhardt L, et al. Design of a trial evaluating myocardial cell protection with cariporide, an inhibitor of the transmembrane sodium-hydrogen exchanger: the Guard during Ischemia against Necrosis (GUARDIAN) trial. *Current Controlled Trials in Cardiovascular Medicine* 2000;1:59–67.

358. Théroux P, Chaitman BR, Danchin N, et al. Inhibition of the sodium-hydrogen exchanger with cariporide to prevent myocardial infarction in high-risk ischemic situations: main results of the GUARDIAN trial. *Circulation* 2000;102:3032–3038.

359. Kereiakes D, Kleiman NS, Ambrose J, et al. Randomized, double-blind, placebo-controlled dose-ranging study of tirofiban (MK-383) platelet IIb/IIIa blockade in high risk patients undergoing coronary angioplasty. *J Am Coll Cardiol* 1996;27:536–542.

360. Hatsukami TS, Ross R, Polissar NL, et al. Visualization of fibrous cap thickness and rupture in human atherosclerotic carotid plaque in vivo with high-resolution magnetic resonance imaging. *Circulation* 2000;102:959–964.

361. Casscells W, Hathorn B, David M, et al. Thermal detection of cellular infiltrates in living atherosclerotic plaques: possible implications for plaque rupture and thrombosis. *Lancet* 1996;347:1447–1451.

362. Stefanadis C, Diamantopoulos L, Vlachopoulos C, et al. Thermal heterogeneity within human atherosclerotic coronary arteries detected in vivo: a new method of detection by application of a special thermography catheter. *Circulation* 1999;99:1965–1971.

363. Campeau L. Grading of angina pectoris [Letter]. *Circulation* 1976;54:522–523.

364. Antman EM, for the TIMI 9B investigators. Hirudin in acute myocardial infarction: Thrombolysis and Thrombin Inhibition in Myocardial Infarction (TIMI) 9B trial. *Circulation* 1996;94:911–921.

365. Metz BK, White HD, Granger CB, et al. Randomized comparison of direct thrombin inhibition versus heparin in conjunction with fibrinolytic therapy for acute myocardial infarction: results from the GUSTO-IIb trial. *J Am Coll Cardiol* 1998;31:1493–1498.

ACUTE MYOCARDIAL INFARCTION: EARLY DIAGNOSIS AND MANAGEMENT

ERIC J. TOPOL
FRANS J. VAN DE WERF

▼▼ **ADDITIONAL ELECTRONIC TOPICS**

Historical Perspective d03; Prehospital Therapy d04; Antiarrhythmics, Cardioversion, and Pacemaker Use d05; Magnesium d06; Inotropic Support, Vasodilators, Intraaortic Balloon Counterpulsation, and Hemodynamic Monitoring d07; Left Ventricular Assist Devices and Emergency Transplantation d08; Functional Testing d09

E. J. Topol: Department of Cardiovascular Medicine, The Cleveland Clinic Foundation, Cleveland, Ohio
F. J. Van de Werf: Department of Cardiology, Gathuisberg University Hospital, Leuven, Belgium

OVERVIEW

Not only has our approach to the patient with acute myocardial infarction (MI) radically changed since the 1980s, but there continues to be steady refinement. The cardinal goal is to consider reperfusion therapy, either fibrinolytic or catheter-based, and to initiate such therapy as quickly as possible. Patients who present within the first 12 hours of symptom onset who have no contraindications for fibrinolytics are considered appropriate candidates, but the maximum benefit is achieved in patients treated within the first hour or two. The admission electrocardiogram (ECG), which provides the location and approximate size of the infarct, is remarkably important for prognosis, and combined with the main clinical parameters of age (the single most important parameter), heart rate, blood pressure, and Killip class, more than 90% of prognostic information is quickly assembled.

Patients without ST-segment elevation have non–Q-wave MI or unstable angina and are generally treated the same way, except without the use of fibrinolytic agents. Therapy with aspirin, anticoagulation, and beta-blockade is appropriate in most patients. Consideration for coronary angiography, either on an urgent or elective basis, and coronary revascularization, are key decisions that need to be made as a function of the patient's risk profile, the occurrence of recurrent ischemia, and resource availability.

Although there has been considerable progress in recent years, our current armamentarium leaves many patients with suboptimal reperfusion at the tissue level. This problem is currently being addressed with the assessment of platelet glycoprotein IIb/IIIa inhibitors and other antiplatelets, better anticoagulants, antiinflammatory agents, and emboli capture devices for catheter-based reperfusion. Undoubtedly, we will have more effective restoration of epicardial and tissue-level perfusion.

GLOSSARY

Myocardial reperfusion: Restoration of coronary blood flow through the infarct-related artery.

Primary angioplasty: Use of balloon angioplasty to achieve myocardial reperfusion.

Rescue angioplasty: For patients who fail thrombolytic therapy, the use of catheter-based reperfusion as a fall-back approach in the early hours of the event.

TIMI-3 flow: Brisk, complete flow as assessed by the Thrombolysis in Myocardial Infarction semiquantitative scoring system.

PATHOPHYSIOLOGY

Coronary atherosclerotic disease is the underlying substrate in nearly all patients with acute MI. The initiating event is a crack or fissure in the diseased arterial wall, which occurs as a result of loss of integrity of the plaque cap, which is the fibrous tissue overlying the plaque and partitioning the atheroma from the arterial lumen (*e*Fig. 18.0.2) (15). The fissure or even frank plaque rupture leads to exposure of subendothelial matrix elements such as collagen, stimulating platelet activation, and thrombus formation. Furthermore, tissue factor is released with the arterial injury, which directly activates the extrinsic coagulation cascade and promotes the formation of fibrin (16). If an occlusive thrombus forms, patients may develop an acute ST-segment elevation MI unless the subtended myocardium is richly collateralized. On the other hand, the thrombus formed may not be occlusive, but rather mural, and the patient may develop unstable angina or non–ST-segment elevation changes on the ECG (ST-depression or T-wave changes), which denote the lack of a "current of injury" or full-thickness (subendocardial to epicardial) myocardial ischemia (Fig. 18.1).

Understanding the reasons why plaques crack may provide a better means of preventing acute MI, rather than intervening at the late phase after the event has been initiated. Plaques that rupture or fissure tend to have a thin fibrous cap, a high lipid content, few smooth muscle cells, and a high proportion of macrophages and monocytes (17,18). These mononuclear cells are conceived as a major trigger in plaque rupture by their release of such proteases as monocyte chemotactic protein (MCP-1) and matrix metalloproteinases (examples are collagenases, stromelysin, elastases), which chemically digest the plaque cap. Of note, the 3-hydroxy-3-methylglutaryl coenzyme A (HMG-CoA) reductase inhibitors have been shown to reduce the incidence of MI, and this is likely related to reduction in lipid content, as well as a favorable antiinflammatory effect on the cellular plaque constituents and chemokines (19–22). Loss of integrity of the arterial wall and platelet thrombus, with cessation of coronary blood flow through the infarct-related artery, thus drives myocardial ischemia and injury. As elegantly described by Reimer and Jennings, the *wavefront* of necrosis extends from the subendocardium to the subepicardium (23), and the extent of necrosis varies as a function of collateral flow, the length of time that coronary blood flow has halted, and the extent of diminution of coronary blood flow. In many patients, there is a stuttering quality of MI with severe pain often denoting the cutoff of blood supply, and less chest pain, with partial, albeit insufficient, reflow. This dynamic quality of the infarct vessel blood flow pattern in acute MI (altered vasomotor tone or spasm) is likely related to the release of vasoactive amines from the activated platelets and loss of endothelial function.

The thrombus that occludes the coronary artery is a mixture of white (platelet-rich) and red (fibrin- and erythrocyte-rich) clot. In some patients, there is a more dominant role of platelets, whereas in others predominantly fibrin-rich thrombus at the arterial injury site is found. Stagnation thrombosis results from the lack of blood flow through the infarct vessel, thus leading to calumniation of red thrombus proximal to the original occlusion site (24).

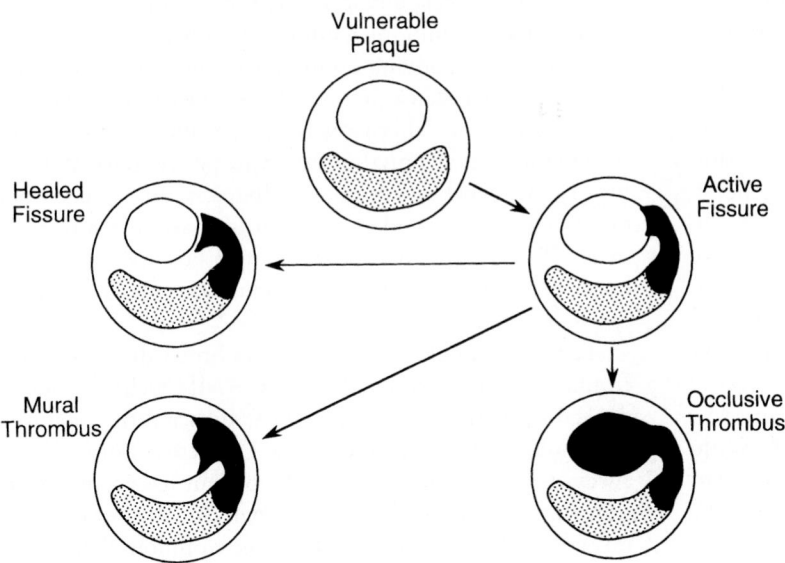

FIGURE 18.1 Different types of acute coronary syndromes as a function of mural versus occlusive thrombus. The vulnerable plaque develops a fissure, which can heal or result in a mural or occlusive thrombus. The fate of the plaque fissure depends, in part, on the extent of vessel wall disruption.

There is rarely frank herniation of the plaque occluding the lumen, which is known as *plaque disaster* (24,25).

On the other hand, the mural thrombus in patients without ST-segment elevation MI is more apt to be platelet rich and not accompanied by stagnation as there is not sustained cutoff of coronary blood flow. Depending on the extent and duration of ischemia, the patient may not experience any myocardial necrosis (unstable angina) or develop myocardial damage (non–ST-elevation or non–Q-wave infarction). Beyond what is occurring at the arterial injury site and proximal to it, there is the potential for embolization of atheroma constituents or platelet thrombus distally. This is not typically found at postmortem but requires careful histologic inspection (26). When this occurs, a further explanation to cessation of myocardial blood flow is provided.

Although there is considerable variability in time of presentation, the plaque fissure events are more likely to happen in the early morning hours, especially on awakening, owing to the circadian rhythm, with its temporal cyclic-enhanced platelet aggregation, and reduced fibrinolytic potential related to higher plasminogen activator inhibitor levels (27). Surges of epinephrine may also have a role, as evidenced by a considerably higher rate of MIs during Scud missile attacks in the Gulf War and during the Los Angeles earthquake (28,29). Beyond catecholamine excess, there are several factors that ultimately may precipitate plaque fissure, including infection or inflammation of the diseased coronary artery segment.

INCIDENCE AND SIGNIFICANCE

The true incidence of acute MI is unknown. Beyond the significant proportion of patients who die before reaching the hospital, estimated at 200,000 to 300,000 patients in the United States per year (30), it is estimated that approximately 1 million patients present to a hospital each year with some type of MI as the principal diagnosis (31). Of these, we know that roughly 200,000 patients receive reperfusion therapy in the United States per year, and that this represents only 20% to 30% of the patients who are assessed for eligibility for aggressive management (32,33). The breakdown of infarctions is also unclear, with a split between the classic ST-segment elevation and the non–ST-segment elevation (also known as *non–Q wave*). The latter group is difficult to differentiate from unstable angina on presentation, but it is estimated that approximately one-half of patients present with either significant ST-segment elevation (greater than 1 mm) or fall into the latter category with abnormal ST-segment depression or T-wave inversion.

The incidence and mortality resulting from MI is on the decline. Not only has the fatality rate been reduced as better therapies have evolved (*e*Fig. 18.1.1), but the absolute number of MI events has continued to decrease since the 1970s. This is likely attributable to the many advances in preventive cardiology, including treatment of hypertension, avoidance of smoking, management of hypercholesterolemia, improved diet and exercise, and the use of prophylactic aspirin. It may also be an outgrowth of the high rates of surgical and percutaneous coronary revascularization in the United States, where the treatment of angina is more apt to be bypass surgery or angioplasty, rather than medical management. Although prevention of MI is not a prominent effect of coronary revascularization, intervening early in the course of atherosclerotic coronary disease may change its natural history. The most pronounced effect on reducing the incidence of MI appears to have resulted from the use of HMG-CoA reductase inhibitors (19–22), which has led to the concept that acute MI may even be "extinct" someday (34). Clearly, the most important initiatives for the condition of MI are in its prevention, because once the process of plaque rupture is unleashed, it is much more difficult to interrupt.

Although the incidence is declining, acute MI remains the principal cause of death in Western society (35). With the many rapid advances that have occurred in this field, the serious and potentially catastrophic outcome of an MI event has been taken for granted in more recent years. Although reperfusion has made important progress in lowering mortality, most patients with acute MI are not eligible for this therapy and face in-hospital death rates of 10% to 20% (36–38). With the increasing proportion of our population being represented by the elderly, who have a high incidence of fatality even with reperfusion therapy, MI remains as the most critical single event in medicine. With the global burden of atherosclerotic disease, Beaglehole has predicted even greater prevalence and pervasiveness of MI by 2020 (38a).

DIAGNOSIS

Acute MI is a clinical syndrome for which a constellation of subjective and objective parameters need to be assessed. The diagnosis must be obtained rapidly and accurately, and misdiagnosis can have catastrophic sequelae. The individual components of making the diagnosis are discussed separately, but it is the integration of all of them that facilitates the accuracy and speed of the clinical syndrome recognition.

History

The classic symptoms of MI are intense, oppressive, excruciating chest pressure, with an impending sense of doom and radiation of the pain to the left arm. However, the other symptoms of chest heaviness or burning, radiation to the jaw, neck, shoulder, back, or both arms may be encountered. Indigestion is common, especially with inferior wall MI. Nausea and vomiting, particularly the former, are typical. Profuse diaphoresis is also a frequent characteristic. Taken together, the patient with a clear-cut presentation is experiencing a unique, discrete, painful event that has induced fear. However, the subtleties of the history are more common and challenging. It is important to ask whether there were premonitory signs of chest discomfort (not necessarily pain) in the preceding week or two. Pain or discomfort may be completely localized to the arm or shoulder. Quite commonly, only the symptoms of indigestion and nausea prevail, such that the patient attributes the episode to heartburn and resorts to taking antacids.

The identification of risk factors, such as smoking, known cholesterol elevation, diabetes, hypertension, and family history, is a supportive piece that helps to put the acute history into context. The chest discomfort that causes the patient to seek medical attention is usually sustained (greater than 20 minutes), but can be stuttering.

Other accompanying symptoms include dyspnea, which is of concern because it may denote incipient congestive heart failure or, alternatively, is an outgrowth of the patient's anxiety. Palpitations or syncope are unusual, but a history of lightheadedness or dizziness and presyncope often reflects the underlying vagotonia or bradyarrhythmias. When syncope, or an out-of-hospital arrest has occurred, there is a high likelihood of ventricular tachycardia as an explanation.

The differential diagnosis is quite broad (because many conditions can masquerade as acute MI) including aortic dissection, pericarditis, esophagitis, myocarditis, pneumonia, cholecystitis, and pancreatitis. Of these conditions, it is always worth considering that the patient has aortic dissection until proven otherwise, so that this diagnosis is not missed. Although considerably less common than acute MI, the therapies for the two conditions are entirely different and, for example, the use of fibrinolytic therapy for aortic dissection could be disastrous.

Physical Examination

The patient appears to be in distress and may even be writhing in pain. Pallor is common. The pulse is usually regular, although ventricular extrasystoles may be present. Bradycardia or tachycardia is helpful in understanding the infarct location, the effect on the conduction system, the vagal tone, and the extent of myocardium at jeopardy. Significant tachycardia (pulse greater than 120) is worrisome and usually denotes an extensive MI, although a "hyperdynamic" subset of patients who have relatively small infarcts, but are hyperadrenergic, may be encountered. The blood pressure is typically elevated owing to the body's response to pain. Hypotension is either due to vagotonia, dehydration, a right ventricular infarction, or impending power failure.

Major examination findings to be aware of include whether there is elevation of jugular venous pressure, the character and location of the apical impulse, the splitting of the second heart sound, the presence of a third or fourth heart sound, a mitral regurgitant murmur, and whether there are rales. Examination of the peripheral pulses and the extremities is important. Collectively, this information provides a sense of the size of the myocardial infarct. If a third heart sound is present, along with rales halfway up the posterior chest fields, a large anterior wall MI is likely present. On the other hand, a normal examination suggests either a small infarction or that more extensive myocardial damage has not yet occurred.

Electrocardiography

It is imperative to obtain the 12-lead ECG as quickly as possible to secure the diagnosis. The presence of a true normal ECG rules out the occlusion of a major epicardial vessel at the moment the tracing was obtained. Hyperacute, tall T-wave changes are the first manifestations of acute coronary occlusion, but are frequently not present when the patient reaches the hospital for medical attention. The presence of ST-segment elevation (*e*Fig. 18.1.2) is the principal feature that denotes "current of injury" and should be associated with reciprocal depression in contralateral leads. If only minimal (1 to 2 mm) ST elevation is present, then either the patient has collaterals to the infarct territory or the vessel is not fully occluded, or there has already been evolution of the ECG changes. If only ST-segment depression or T-wave inversion or both are manifest, this may denote either unstable angina or a non–ST-elevation (non–Q-wave) MI. This usually is not associated with an occluded infarct vessel, but rather one that is stenotic with myocardial ischemia. If a patient has a normal ECG, but the history is suggestive or even compelling, it is vital to observe the patient over an extended period (6 to 24 hours) to get additional ECG tracings and to determine if the chest discomfort or other symptoms recur. Certainly transient but marked ischemia can resolve before the patient has an ECG and a normal ECG can be recorded. It is worthwhile to give sublingual nitroglycerin (0.4 mg) to a patient with marked ST-segment elevation to see if this represents coronary artery spasm, while more definitive therapy (vide infra) is being initiated. If the patient's chest pain and ECG quickly revert to normal after nitroglycerin, this strongly suggests vasospasm as the principal trigger.

In patients with ST-segment elevation largely confined to the right precordial leads (V_1 to V_2), it is important to differentiate ST-segment elevation due to current of injury and fast (early) repolarization, which is a normal variant, especially common in young African-American men. Early repolarization is diminished or undetectable when the heart rate is increased, so that if the ECG remains equivocal it may be helpful to have the patient do some sit-ups to increase the heart rate, and then repeat the ECG.

Creatine Phosphokinase

The creatine phosphokinase (CPK) is unhelpful to make the initial diagnosis. It takes at least 6 hours for there to be an enzyme "leak," which denotes myocardial cell necrosis. Enzymes should be assessed every 8 hours for the first 24 hours, and longer if the peak is not firmly established. The peak CPK occurs earlier when there has been successful reperfusion (*e*Fig. 18.1.3) (39). This enzyme is much more helpful in gauging the size of the MI than in making the diagnosis.

Troponin T and I

More sensitive measures of myocardial necrosis have become available, which have a similar obligatory lag in appearing in the blood (as CPK) but appear to detect cell damage more readily (40–44). The troponins are part of the tropomyosin-binding protein of the contractile apparatus of cardiac myocytes and therefore are highly specific for cardiac origin. A rapid, bedside assay for troponin is available and is a practical, rapid way to assess patients with ischemic symptoms and non–ST-segment elevation. The off-line quantitative assays of both troponin T and I have been particularly helpful in differentiating risk, better than CPK, in patients with unstable angina and non–ST-elevation MI (Fig. 18.2). Both are extremely promising for offering a more sensitive means of not only diagnosing whether infarction has occurred, but also discriminating the risk. However, the real utility of tests such as troponin goes beyond the determination of risk level to favorably alter the prognosis of the patient by knowledge of whether the test result is abnormal or not. Indeed, responses of patients to either IIb/IIIa inhibitors or low-molecular-weight heparins are predicted by abnormal troponin. These sensitive markers should be applied routinely for patients without ST-segment elevation. Troponins offer little incremental value in classic ST-elevation MI.

Echocardiography

The diagnosis of acute MI cannot be made by echocardiography, as it is based on the combination of symptoms, the ECG findings, and the enzyme abnormalities. However, there are several findings that may be considered ancillary from a two-dimensional echo, including a segmental wall abnormality and hyperkinesis of the contralateral wall. If a segment is akinetic, dyskinetic, or severely hypokinetic, it is not possible to know whether there was ischemia, with attendant dysfunction or stunning, or irrevocable damage due to necrosis. This can only be differentiated by serial echocardiographic examination. However, the finding of lack of hyperkinesis of the contralateral territory (e.g., the anterolateral wall in an inferior MI) in the acute setting suggests that the infarct vessel has recanalized or that there is multivessel coronary disease. This finding may be especially valuable in assessing a patient with congestive heart failure or cardiogenic shock, as the main compensation of the ventricle to preserve its global ejection fraction is preempted if there is a significant stenosis of a major epicardial vessel supplying the noninfarct territory. In patients with inferior MI, the echocardiogram of the right ventricle is helpful in demonstrating dilation or hypocontractility and is more sensitive than the ECG (45). A significant prior MI is also diagnosed by scarring and thinning of a specific territory and can easily be differentiated from an acute MI by its echocardiographic appearance.

Angiography

On occasion, even with all of the tools outlined, the diagnosis is uncertain. This may be the result of atypical

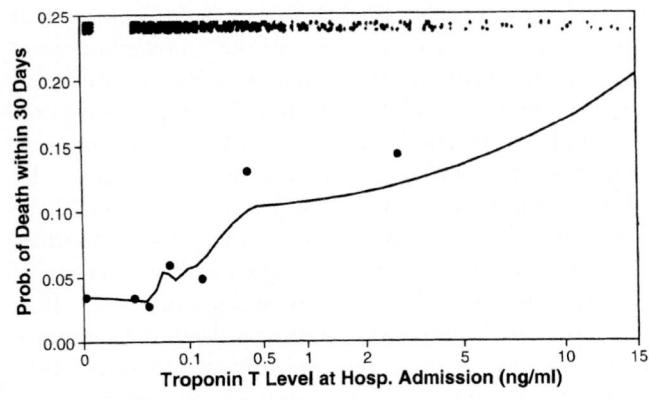

A

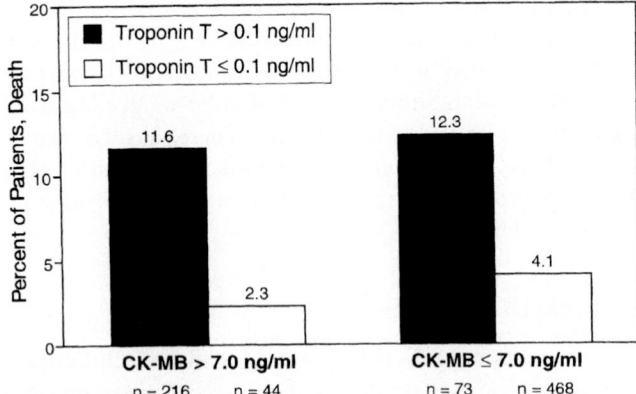

B

FIGURE 18.2 A: Probability of death within 30 days according to the troponin T level at hospital admission. Smoothed nonparametric estimates are shown. The troponin T levels are plotted on a cube-root scale. The density of the data is indicated at the top, with each mark representing one patient. The dots represent simple estimates of mortality derived from ranges of the troponin T level that contained at least 70 patients. (From Ohman EM, Armstrong PW, Christenson RH, et al. for the GUSTO-IIa Investigators. Risk stratification with admission cardiac troponin T levels in acute myocardial ischemia. *N Engl J Med* 1996;335:1333–1341, with permission.) **B:** Sensitivity of troponin compared with creatine kinase-myocardial band (CK-MB). Even in patients with a low CK-MB (less than 7.0 ng per mL), the troponin T–positive patients (greater than 0.1 ng per mL) had a worse outcome with respect to mortality. (Data from Ohman EM, Armstrong PW, Christenson RH, et al. for the GUSTO-IIa Investigators. Risk stratification with admission cardiac troponin T levels in acute myocardial ischemia. *N Engl J Med* 1996;335:1333–1341.)

symptoms and an ECG that is difficult to interpret. In a patient in whom reperfusion therapy is contemplated, an approach that can rapidly establish the diagnosis is emergency coronary angiography. By demonstrating an acutely occluded infarct vessel, with the characteristic appearance of thrombus or a cutoff sign at the point of occlusion, coupled with left ventriculography to ascertain the segmental wall motion profile, angiography can at times be helpful for a difficult diagnosis. Examples of patients who may present with ambiguity are those with an acute myocarditis with diffuse ECG changes, or patients with prior bypass surgery and previous MI, or those without a characteristic pattern on ECG. Furthermore, angiography can

serve as the foundation for primary balloon angioplasty to achieve reperfusion.

MAJOR SUBGROUPS AT PRESENTATION

By Electrocardiography

In Table 18.1, the five types of ST-segment elevation MI are presented. These represent specific patterns of ECG abnormalities that correlate with a clinical presentation, the underlying coronary anatomy, and prognosis. The most worrisome type is the proximal left anterior descending (LAD) MI, often referred to as the *widow-maker* infarction, which carries a high mortality and is attributed to an occlusion of the LAD before or at the first septal perforator. All of the precordial leads and I and aVL show ST-segment elevation (*e*Fig. 18.2.1). The proximal location of occlusion is associated with compromised perfusion to the His-Purkinje conduction tissue owing to loss of septal supply and often accompanied by a new bundle branch block. Usually, left anterior hemiblock or right bundle branch block is present, but bifascicular blocks, left bundle branch block, or Mobitz II atrioventricular block are all possible. Cardiogenic shock or power failure is not unexpected in this subgroup, unless there has been effective reperfusion established.

In contrast, occlusion of the LAD just distal to the first septal perforator is an anterior MI, which is less serious and called the *mid-LAD infarction* (*e*Fig. 18.2.2). Although the ECG may be indistinguishable from that of the proximal anterior MI patient with respect to the leads with ST elevation, there is no conduction disturbance. Cardiogenic shock in these patients is considerably less frequent, as restriction of the damage to the anterolateral and anteroapical segments spares the proximal interventricular septum. If shock is present, one should be concerned about prior myocardial damage or other noncardiac causes such as massive hemorrhage. Heart failure can occur, and the complications of ventricular aneurysm with potential of apical thrombus are common, especially if reperfusion has been delayed or is unsuccessful.

One segment distal in the LAD, sparing a large diagonal, represents the distal LAD infarction, which is less common. Only leads V_1 to V_4 are affected, but still there is the potential for apical hypokinesis, thrombus formation, and a milder form of the mid-LAD infarct clinical syndrome. Importantly, cardiogenic shock cannot result from this type of infarction per se.

Two types of infarcts that are relatively small are due to less significant territory affected. These are the LAD diagonal branch "lateral" MI, involving only leads I, aVL, V_5, and V_6 (*e*Fig. 18.2.3), also classified in the distal LAD tensitory MI, and the small inferior MI, with ECG ST elevation confined to leads II, III, and aVF (*e*Fig. 18.2.4). The latter is usually attributed to a distal right coronary artery

TABLE 18.1 A NEW CLASSIFICATION OF ACUTE MYOCARDIAL INFARCTION BASED ON ELECTROCARDIOGRAPHIC ENTRY CRITERIA WITH ANGIOGRAPHIC CORRELATION

Categories	Anatomy of occlusion	Electrocardiographic entry	30-day mortality (%)[a]	1-year mortality (%)[a]
1. Proximal left anterior descending	Proximal to first septal perforator	ST↑ V_{1-6}, I, aVL and fascicular or bundle branch block	19.6	25.6
2. Mid-left anterior descending	Proximal to large diagonal, but distal to first septal perforator	ST↑ V_{1-6}, I, aVL	9.2	12.4
3. Distal left anterior descending or diagonal	Distal to large diagonal or of diagonal itself	ST↑ V_{1-4} or ST↑ I, aVL, V_{5-6}	6.8	10.2
4. Moderate to large inferior (posterior, lateral, right ventricular)	Proximal RCA or left circumflex	ST↑ II, III, aVF and any or all of the following: a. V_1, V_{3R}, V_{4R} or b. $V_5 V_6$ or c. R > S in V_1, V_2	6.4	8.4
5. Small inferior	Distal RCA or left circumflex, branch occlusion	ST↑ II, III, aVF only	4.5	6.7

RCA, right coronary artery.
[a]Based on Global Use of Streptokinase and t-PA for Occluded Coronary Arteries (GUSTO-I) cohort population in each of the 5-year categories, all receiving reperfusion therapy.

lesion or branch (posterolateral or posterior descending), but in patients with a dominant left circumflex, it may be a branch from this vessel. Both of these types of MIs are usually uncomplicated and rarely associated with serious outcomes such as congestive heart failure or significant arrhythmias.

Patients with moderate or large inferior MIs are a key subgroup, which is heterogeneous, representing a spectrum of involvement of the inferior, posterior, lateral, and right ventricular myocardial involvement. The proximal, dominant right coronary artery is responsible for supplying all of these territories and can result in a large and potentially catastrophic event. The ECG leads involved include II, III, aVF, and additional changes in the V_5, V_6 lateral leads, right ventricular leads (V_1 or V_{3R}, V_{4R}), or posterior leads (R/S ratio greater than 1 in V_1, V_2, with or without ST depression, ST elevation in aVR). The largest inferior MI involves the composite of all of these territories (*e*Fig. 18.2.5). Dreaded complications, such as power failure or cardiogenic shock due to a large right ventricular infarct, or the development of a ventricular septal defect due to extensive distal septal necrosis, are possible. In all patients with inferior MI, a systematic approach to obtaining the right precordial ECG must be incorporated. Although right ventricular lead ST elevation of 1 to 2 mm in V_{3R} or V_{4R} is highly specific for right ventricular infarct, the sensitivity is still suboptimal, and one should carefully examine the patient for elevated jugular venous pressure, a right-sided S_3 gallop, and, in cases in which there is uncertainty, perform either or both echocardiography or right-sided heart catheterization. Inferior MI is characterized by hypervagotonia, with bradycardia and hypotension that is responsive to atropine (0.6 to 1.0 mg intravenously). Type I atrioventricular block (Wenckebach) is exceedingly common with inferior MI, particularly if continuous ECG monitoring is

reviewed. The conduction disturbances and bradyarrhythmias of inferior MI are usually benign, most often not requiring specific therapy except occasional atropine.

Diagnosis of a true posterior infarction is rare, but the posterior wall is the least well expressed on the 12-lead ECG, such that occlusion of the left circumflex branches, which are usually responsible for the true posterior myocardial territory, can be missed. When the findings of ST depression in V_1 to V_4 are present, especially when accompanied by an R greater than S wave in V_1 or V_2 (or both), the ECG is highly supportive of a posterior MI. The ST depression follows the "mirror rule" as the reflection of the tracing would fit the conventional ST-elevation pattern that one would expect in other MI locations. Posterior wall MIs are usually well tolerated, but it is imperative to interrogate the possibility of concomitant involvement of the right ventricle and free wall of the left ventricle.

All of the patterns described have associated reciprocal ECG changes, which are important to confirm the diagnosis. For example, most patients with inferior MI have ST depression in either leads I, aVL, or precordial leads V_1 to V_4, and the prognostic significance of this latter finding has been debated for many years (46). The extent of reciprocal changes is usually similar to the primary current of injury, such that if there is 5 mm of ST elevation, there is more pronounced evidence of contralateral, reciprocal ECG changes. For the most part, this finding is useful for confirming the diagnosis and represents an ECG contrecoup expression, which does not carry vital clinical prognostic information. In most series, however, there is some incremental risk of adverse outcomes as a function of the extent and severity of reciprocal ST-segment depression (46).

Repeat 12-lead ECGs are vital 60 to 90 minutes after administration of fibrinolytic therapy to detect whether tissue-level reperfusion has occurred. As shown in Table 18.2

TABLE 18.2 MYOCARDIAL REPERFUSION:
ST RESOLUTION VERSUS MORTALITY (30 DAY)

Study (reference)	Time (min)	Complete	Partial	No.
ISAM (47)	180	2.8	4.3	9.2
INJECT (48)	180	2.5	4.3	17.5
HIT 4 (49)	180	2.8	6.0	14.3
GUSTO-III (50)	90	4.0	5.4	10.7
TIMI 14 (51)	90	1.0	4.2	5.9
InTIME (52)	60	1.7	4.5	7.7

with the early repeat ECG in many large-scale trials (47–52), the prognosis of patients is greatly differentiated by whether there has been greater than or equal to 70% resolution of ST-segment elevation. This has come to serve as the "lie detector" or "truth serum" as an inexpensive, readily available means of assessing tissue-level reperfusion. It is also worthwhile to recheck the ECG after catheter-based reperfusion because approximately 20% to 30% of patients do not achieve ST-segment resolution and carry an unfavorable prognosis (53).

Non–ST-Segment Elevation

Patients with acute ECG changes but without ST-segment elevation fit into the non–ST-elevation category. This was formerly known as *subendocardial, non–Q-wave MI,* but the reperfusion era has provided ample evidence that many patients with initial ST elevation do not go on to evolve a Q-wave MI (54). Giant T-wave inversion, characteristic of a proximal LAD lesion if occurring throughout the precordial leads, is an example of a non–ST-elevation MI with a discrete ECG pattern. However, many of the ECGs in this patient group do not fit a particular pattern of myocardial

necrosis or ischemia, and at the time of evaluation, one is uncertain whether the changes are fixed or transient. Clearly, ST-segment depression is more ominous than T-wave inversion for 30-day mortality or nonfatal reinfarction (55). In a large-scale trial, the death rates were 6.8% versus 1.4%, and the composite event rates were 12.4% and 6.8%, respectively (55). Especially worrisome is the finding of global ischemia, when there is an ST depression in virtually every lead except aVR (where there is elevation); this frequently denotes a left main or equivalent non–ST-elevation MI.

By Hemodynamic (Killip) Class

Besides the ECG, which establishes the location of the infarct and often the precise location of the affected coronary artery, it is important to establish the patient's hemodynamic class. The Killip categories are most useful and validated for this purpose (56). Killip class I is the most common presenting class, occurring in 85% of patients with MI, and, by definition, with no evidence of heart failure. Early heart failure, as manifested by bibasilar rales and at times an S_3 gallop, is present in Killip II, the category that approximately 10% of patients present with. Pulmonary edema, as denoted by Killip III, and cardiogenic shock, classified as Killip IV, are uncommon, collectively accounting for 5% of patients in large-scale trials. In evaluating the patient's risk, five simple baseline parameters have been demonstrated, explaining more than 90% of the prognostic information for 30-day mortality. As shown in the pyramid (Fig. 18.3), the key five characteristics are age, systolic blood pressure, Killip class, heart rate, and location of the MI (57). Thus, evaluation of the patient's age, ECG, and hemodynamics provides crucial information that stratifies risk and may be helpful in guiding therapy.

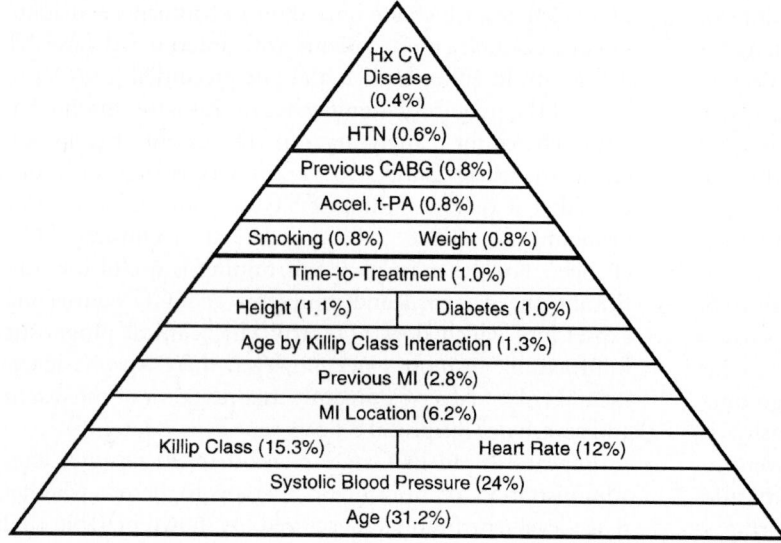

FIGURE 18.3 A multivariate model of mortality at 30 days in the Global Utilization of Streptokinase and t-PA for Occluded Coronary Arteries (GUSTO-I) trial. The factors in the pyramid provide the relative importance in affecting mortality among the 41,021 patients studied. CABG, coronary artery bypass grafting; HTN, hypertension; Hx CV, history of cardiovascular disease; MI, myocardial infarction; t-PA, tissue plasminogen activator. (Data adapted from Lee KL, Woodlief L, Topol EJ, et al. Predictors of 30-day mortality in the era of reperfusion for acute myocardial infarction: results from an international trial of 41,021 patients. *Circulation* 1995;91:1659–1668.)

TREATMENT

Analgesia and Supportive Measures

The first step in treating the patient, while more definitive therapy is being prepared (such as fibrinolytics or transfer to a cardiac catheterization laboratory), is to make the patient comfortable via supplemental oxygen (usually nasal cannula at 2 L per minute) and morphine (2 to 4 mg intravenously and repeat as necessary). Before using morphine, it is helpful to have quickly tried sublingual nitroglycerin to determine whether there is a reversible component of the ischemia, pain, and ECG changes. Furthermore, if the patient is Killip class I or II and has no bradycardia or hypotension (systolic pressure less than 110 mm Hg), then use of intravenous beta-blockade can be considered as a means of reducing the extent of ischemia and lessening the need for narcotic analgesia (58).

Aspirin

The use of aspirin is a cornerstone of therapy for patients with acute coronary syndromes. It should be initiated as quickly as possible when the diagnosis is made, at a dose of 160 mg by chewable administration (2 × 80 mg "baby" aspirin) or a 325-mg orally administered tablet. No enteric coated formulation of aspirin should be used. The validation for the importance of aspirin in this setting is derived from the landmark International Studies of Infarct Survival (ISIS-2) trial (Fig. 18.4), which showed it is lifesaving (59). Since this trial, aspirin has been used in all patients with acute MI, and other trials have provided strong evidence for its use in unstable angina and non–ST-elevation MI (60–62). The dose that has been routinely recommended is 325 mg per day, and it is continued indefinitely.

Clopidogrel

The Clopidogrel in Unstable Angina to Prevent Recurrent Events trial (63) assessed the combination of aspirin plus clopidogrel compared with aspirin in patients without ST-segment elevation MI. With a 20% reduction of ischemic events, particularly MI (or reinfarction), there are supportive data to use this second antiplatelet (see Chapter 17). However, this has not been assessed in patients with ST-elevation MI.

Thrombolytics or Primary Mechanical Reperfusion

Patient Selection

All patients with ST-segment elevation MI who present within 12 hours from the onset of symptoms should be considered for myocardial reperfusion therapy (64,65). The list of absolute and relative contraindications is provided in

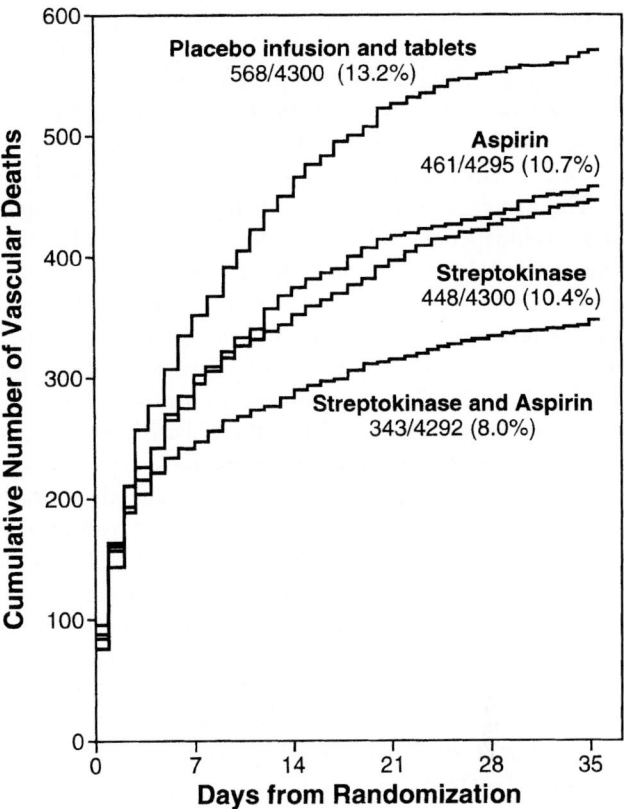

FIGURE 18.4 Second International Study of Infarct Survival (ISIS-2) showing significant reduction of mortality at 35 days for aspirin or streptokinase, and an additive effect for the two combined. [From ISIS-2 (Second international study of infarct survival) Collaborative Group. Randomized trial of intravenous streptokinase, oral aspirin, both, or neither among 17,187 cases of suspected acute myocardial infarction. *Lancet* 1988;11:349–360, with permission.]

eTable 18.2.1 and is quite straightforward in most respects. The only definite contraindications for thrombolytic therapy are active bleeding and recent stroke, trauma, or major surgery. Relative contraindications include severe or uncontrolled hypertension (systolic blood pressure greater than 180/110 mm Hg), any previous cerebrovascular history, prior gastrointestinal hemorrhage, active menstruation, pregnancy, prolonged cardiopulmonary resuscitation (CPR) (greater than 10 minutes), noncompressible vascular punctures, and coumadin therapy with an international normalized ratio of greater than 2 to 3. For patients with relative contraindications to thrombolytic therapy, consideration for primary angioplasty can be made.

Patients with new bundle branch block are also considered suitable candidates for reperfusion on the basis of the collaborative overview of the large-scale controlled trials of thrombolytic therapy (65). However, right bundle branch block does not obscure ST elevation, and as pointed out by Sgarbossa et al., ST-segment elevation MI can frequently be diagnosed in the presence of left bundle branch block (see Chapter 59) (66). Thus, for the most part, ST-segment elevation is the hallmark ECG feature guiding the use of thrombolytic therapy along with symptoms, appropriate timing, and consideration of the clinical profile. Occasionally, left bundle branch block is present and the ST-segment elevation or ECG signs of acute MI are lacking. In these cases, a search for the old ECG is warranted; alternatively, or concomitantly, echocardiography may be considered.

The benefit of thrombolytic therapy or primary angioplasty is independent of age, gender, and most of the baseline characteristics. However, the patients who derive the most benefit are patients treated earliest, the elderly, those with anterior MI, and, in general, those with the highest risk. The critical dogma is to restore myocardial perfusion as quickly as possible. Accordingly, in a hospital with an experienced team for acute MI catheter-based intervention with an open laboratory, it may be the most rapid strategy to perform primary percutaneous transluminal coronary angioplasty (PTCA). Patient selection criteria will also be extended by the availability of primary PTCA owing to some relative exclusions of systemic fibrinolytic administration, which do not pose an incremental risk to mechanical reperfusion. Owing to the relative lack of efficacy of fibrinolytic intervention in specific settings, patients with cardiogenic shock and those with prior bypass surgery may be especially well suited for mechanical reperfusion, instead of fibrinolytic therapy.

Review of Clinical Trials

After the GISSI-1 (13) and ISIS-2 (59) trials, other placebo-controlled trials of 1,000 or more patients were pooled in the Fibrinolytic Therapy Trialists collaborative project (65,67–70). Collectively, the pooled data of more than 60,000 patients treated with different fibrinolytics (SK, t-PA, urokinase, or anistreplase) demonstrated an 18% reduction of mortality from 11.5% to 9.6% (13,59,65,67–72). Survival benefit was confirmed across a variety of subgroups, including the patients with ST elevation or bundle branch block, patients receiving therapy within 12 hours from symptom onset, diabetics, and patients with prior MI. Although patients with a systolic blood pressure less than 100 mg Hg had particular benefit, the GISSI-1 trial showed poor efficacy of thrombolytic therapy in patients with cardiogenic shock (13,65). Subsequent trials have confirmed minimal evidence for benefit of fibrinolytic therapy alone for cardiogenic shock (73,74). As discussed in the chapter by Hochman and Gersh (see Chapter 19), catheter-based reperfusion is preferred if it is available.

Time to Treatment

The time to treatment is a pivotal parameter in reperfusion. Patients treated in the first hour have the highest absolute and relative mortality benefit (75,76). This observation has led to the first 60 minutes to be referred to as the *golden hour* of reperfusion. The dominant explanation for the

exaggerated benefit appears to be related to prevention of myocardial damage, as thallium studies have indicated the ability to prevent an MI in up to 40% of such patients (77). However, as judged from the high placebo group mortality of patients treated in the first hour, it may be that patients who present early (e.g., in less than 30 minutes from their onset of symptoms) have a larger MI and are therefore preselected to derive pronounced benefit. Certainly all of the trials convey an inverse relationship between treatment onset and survival benefit with little to no beneficial effect for patients treated at 12 hours or beyond. Two large-scale trials have been dedicated to the issue of late therapy (78,79), and both suggested that treatment benefit is restricted to the first 12 hours.

Selection of Fibrinolytic Agents

There have been three large trials that studied the differences in effects on mortality for t-PA and SK (73,74,88,89). In the GISSI-2/International trial (73,74) 20,749 patients were randomly assigned to t-PA or SK, with a factorial design also randomized to subcutaneous heparin started after 12 hours or no heparin. The t-PA was alteplase given over 3 hours. Mortality at 30 days was 8.9% and 8.5%, respectively (74). The ISIS-3 trial evaluated 41,299 patients with three different thrombolytic agents: the duteplase form of t-PA, which has not been commercially developed; SK; and anistreplase. A factorial design for evaluating subcutaneous heparin started after 4 hours versus placebo was also used. There were no differences in mortality (10.3%, 10.5%, and 10.6%, respectively) (88). Subsequently, the Global Use of Streptokinase and t-PA for Occluded Coronary Arteries (GUSTO-I) trial evaluated 41,021 patients randomly assigned to one of four thrombolytic strategies (89). Accelerated alteplase t-PA over 90 minutes, administered with intravenous heparin, was shown to significantly reduce 30-day mortality by 15% as compared with SK with intravenous or with subcutaneous heparin, or the combination of t-PA and SK with intravenous heparin (Fig. 18.5). The benefit was highly consistent across virtually all subcategories, including age, location of MI, and the time from symptom onset (*e*Fig. 18.5.1). Although the superiority of t-PA was contested because of the eight- to tenfold increase in its cost compared with SK ($2,200 vs. $300), the differences were highly significant, consistent, and durable at 1 year of follow-up (89–92). The mechanism for the benefit, with earlier complete infarct vessel patency, as discussed later in this chapter (see Importance of Early and Complete Reperfusion), was also fully characterized (83) (*e*Fig. 18.5.2 and Fig. 18.6). As would be expected, the patients with the higher risk derived the most substantial benefit of t-PA compared with SK (91). Formal cost-effectiveness analysis has shown that accelerated t-PA saved 14 additional years of life per 1,000 patients treated, which translates to a cost of $32,678 per year of life saved

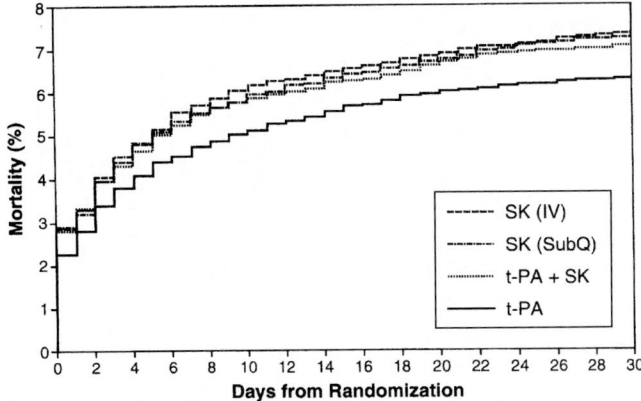

FIGURE 18.5 Thirty-day mortality in four treatment groups. The group receiving accelerated treatment with tissue plasminogen activator (t-PA) had lower mortality than both the two streptokinase (SK) groups (p = .001) and each individual treatment group: streptokinase and subcutaneous (SubQ) heparin (p = .009), streptokinase and intravenous (IV) heparin (p = .003), and tissue plasminogen activator and streptokinase combined with IV heparin (p = .04). (From The GUSTO Investigators. An international randomized trial comparing four thrombolytic strategies for acute myocardial infarction. *N Engl J Med* 1993;329:1615–1622, with permission.)

(90). This compares favorably with such benchmarks as the cost of hypertension treatment ($20,000 per year of life saved) or the cost-effectiveness ratio of hemodialysis for chronic renal failure ($35,000 per year of life saved), but still represents a significant toll on an individual patient basis and on a societal level.

New Plasminogen Activators

As shown in Figure 18.7, many new thrombolytic agents are being developed and these have been termed *third-gen-*

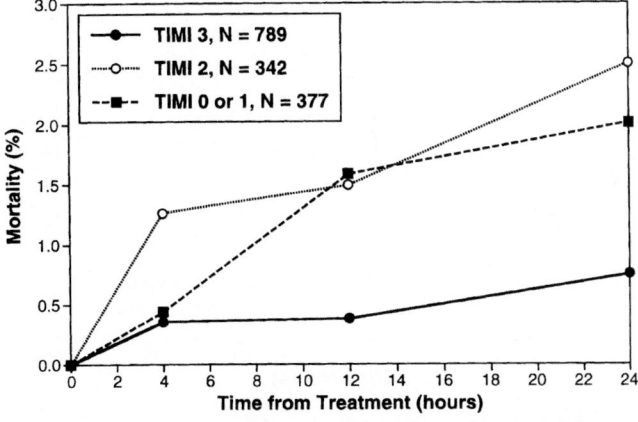

FIGURE 18.6 Plot of mortality according to Thrombolysis in Myocardial Infarction (TIMI) flow grade on the angiogram performed at 90 minutes in the angiographic study. Data are taken according to flow grade regardless of treatment arm. (Adapted from Kleiman NS, White, Ohman EM, et al. Mortality within 24 hours of thrombolysis for myocardial infarction: the importance of early reperfusion. *Circulation* 1994;90:2658–2665.)

eration plasminogen activators (91–102). The mutants of native t-PA include reteplase (r-PA, Retevase, Roche/Centocor), lanoteplase (n-PA, Bristol-Myers Squibb), and TNK (a triple mutant Genentech; see Fig. 18.7). Other agents that are being developed include recombinant staphylokinase and vampire bat plasminogen activator.

The common theme for many of these agents is their prolonged half-life and the ability to use a bolus-type administration. Three of the agents have remarkable fibrin specificity: TNK, staphylokinase, and bat PA, which affords almost no fibrinogenolysis. All have the theoretical potential to be more potent in lysing coronary thrombi and therefore are being pursued for acute MI as a chief indication. Each of the agents is briefly addressed.

Reteplase

r-PA was approved for use in the United States in 1996 and represents the first of the third-generation thrombolytics to become commercially available. As shown in Figure 18.7, it is a deletion mutant of t-PA and is given as two 10-MU boluses, 30 minutes apart. Like t-PA, intravenous heparin is used in conjunction with r-PA, and the results of two angiographic trials (103,104) indicate the potential of superiority for speed and extent of coronary thrombolysis for r-PA compared with conventional or accelerated t-PA. The International Joint Evaluation of Coronary Thrombolysis trial compared r-PA with SK in over 6,000 patients and demonstrated a small, but not statistically meaningful benefit for r-PA (105). The GUSTO-III trial compared r-PA and accelerated t-PA in 15,072 patients. No benefit for r-PA over t-PA was demonstrated (50) (Fig. 18.8). There was a higher mortality and hemorrhagic stroke rate in GUSTO-III compared with previous trials, probably owing to a more aged population enrolled. Both t-PA and r-PA cost approximately $2,200 per dose. The major benefit of r-PA over t-PA is the ease of use. Equivalence has not been established at 30 days or 1 year with respect to mortality point estimates, although the findings in GUSTO-III were supportive of a minimal gap.

Tenecteplase

An outgrowth of the Assessment of the Safety and Efficacy of a New Thrombolytic (ASSENT-2) trial (106) was the validation of TNK as equivalent (or not inferior) to accelerated t-PA. As shown in Figure 18.9, the mortality at 30 days was remarkably similar with this single-bolus agent compared with the more complicated accelerated t-PA regimen. Furthermore, there was superiority established for patients presenting late (receiving therapy after 4 hours) and a significant reduction in noncerebral bleeding complications. Taken together, the profile of TNK is particularly favorable, and this is the most fibrin-specific agent currently available. Its cost, however, is similar to alteplase and r-PA.

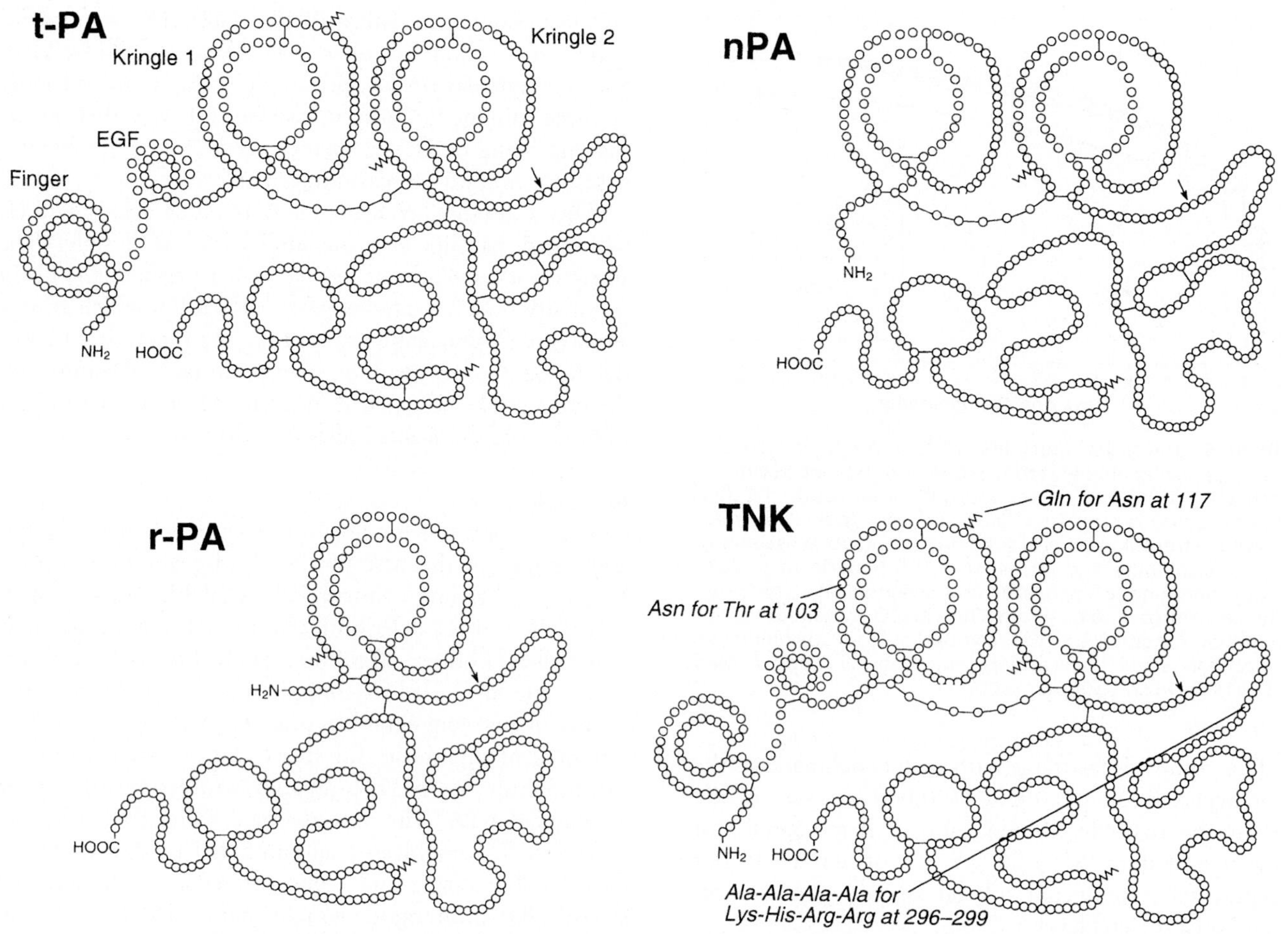

t-PA

Kringle 1   Kringle 2

EGF

Finger

NH₂   HOOC

nPA

NH₂

HOOC

r-PA

H₂N—

HOOC

TNK

Gln for Asn at 117

Asn for Thr at 103

NH₂   HOOC

Ala-Ala-Ala-Ala for Lys-His-Arg-Arg at 296–299

FIGURE 18.7 Structure of wild-type tissue plasminogen activator (t-PA) and three mutants. Reteplase (r-PA) is missing the finger, epidermal growth factor (EGF), and Kringle-1 domain. Lanoteplase (nPA) is similar to r-PA but maintains the Kringle-1. TNK is a triple site-directed mutagenic plasminogen activator with changes at three sites, as shown.

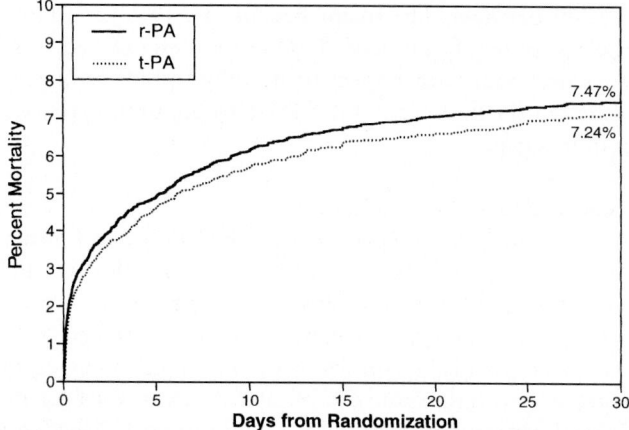

FIGURE 18.8 Primary results of Global Utilization of Streptokinase and t-PA for Occluded Coronary Arteries (GUSTO-III) trial for 30-day mortality. r-PA, reteplase; t-PA, tissue plasminogen activator.

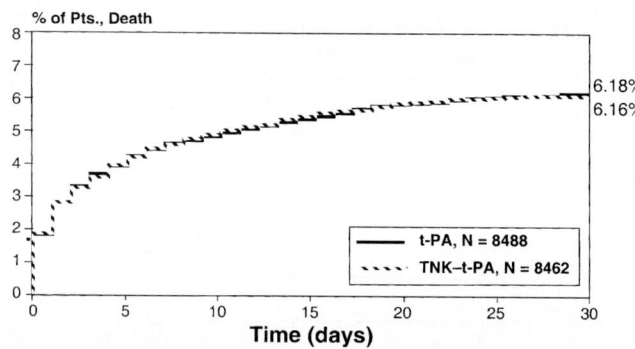

FIGURE 18.9 Mortality at 30 days for TNK as compared with accelerated tissue plasminogen activator (t-PA) in the Assessment of the Safety and Efficacy of a New Thrombolytic (ASSENT-2) trial.

Other Agents

n-PA was studied in the *I*ntravenous *n*PA for *T*reatment of *I*nfartcting *M*yocardium *E*arly (InTIME)-2 trial and did not fare particularly well against accelerated t-PA (52). Although the mortality at 30 days was within 0.3% absolute, possibly fulfilling noninferiority criteria, there was a significant excess in intracerebral hemorrhage with this single-bolus mutant t-PA. Thus far, n-PA has not become commercially available.

Staphylokinase has had promising phase II angiographic trial data and is a fibrin-specific agent such as TNK (107–109). However, it has yet to go forward with a mortality reduction trial and, despite efforts to reduce immunogenicity, has some intrinsic homology to SK. Saruplase, recombinant single-chain urokinase-type plasminogen activator, has been shown to provide better angiographic results than SK (110), but is not available on a commercial basis.

Importance of Early and Complete Reperfusion

The mechanism of benefit of accelerated t-PA in the GUSTO-I trial was clearly demonstrated to be the improvement in timely and complete restoration of coronary blood flow (111). As shown in *e*Figure 18.5.2, the proportion of patients in the angiographic trial who had TIMI-3 flow at 90 minutes after therapy was initiated, reflecting brisk infarct vessel blood flow, was considerably higher for the patients receiving t-PA compared with the other three strategies assessed. Nonetheless, even for accelerated t-PA, the rate of TIMI-3 flow was only 54%, leaving room for improvement in future pharmacologic reperfusion strategies (111). The patency status at 90 minutes was a critical index of outcomes, including survival at 24 hours, 30 days, and 1 and 2 years (Figs. 18.5, 18.6, and 18.10; *e*Fig. 18.10.1) (89,111–114). Beside the salutary effects on improving survival, the TIMI-3 flow status was closely associated with global left ventricular function, cavity dilatation, and regional wall motion of the infarct zone (111,115) (*e*Fig. 18.10.2). In *e*Figure 18.10.3, the linkage of early (90- to 180-minute) end systolic volume and 1-year mortality is shown (114). ⚑ d10

Primary Mechanical Reperfusion

Although thrombolytic therapy is a strategy that can be applied in virtually all hospitals, the 54% plateau of TIMI-3 flow (at 90 minutes) for even the most effective plasminogen activator available is a major shortcoming. The technique of mechanical reperfusion using balloon angioplasty that was introduced by Hartzler et al. in the mid-1980s (9) has been convincingly superior to thrombolytic therapy for establishing TIMI-3 flow in a greater proportion of patients. As assessed in the GUSTO-IIb substudy that directly compared accelerated t-PA and primary angioplasty, the rate of infarct vessel TIMI-3 flow was 80%

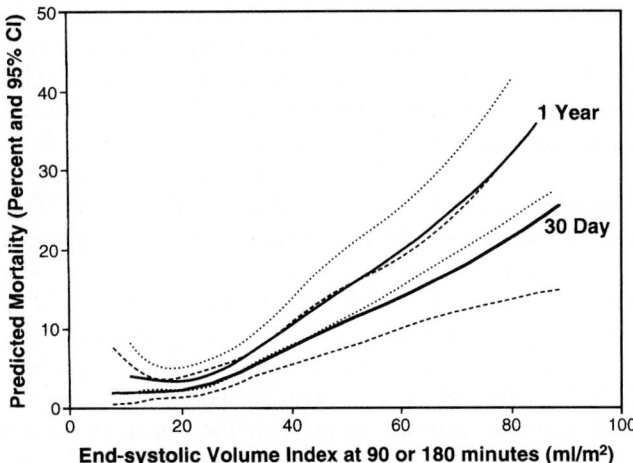

FIGURE 18.10 Model of the relationship between end systolic volume index and 30-day and 1-year mortality. Dashed lines represent 95% confidence interval (CI) for 1-year mortality, and dotted lines represent 95% CI for 30-day mortality. (From Migrino RQ, Young JB, Ellis SG, et al. End-systolic volume index at 90–180 minutes into reperfusion therapy for acute myocardial infarction is a strong predictor of early and late mortality. *Circulation* 1997;96:116–121, with permission.)

(119), representing a near 50% proportionate improvement over accelerated t-PA. In *e*Table 18.2.1, the major features of the nine randomized trials of thrombolytics and primary angioplasty are summarized (119–127). In aggregate, approximately 2,500 patients have been incorporated in these trials, with two different thrombolytic agents, and, in the case of t-PA, both the 3-hour and accelerated dosing strategies. The number of patients assessed is thus two orders of magnitude less than the thrombolytic trial experience, and the scientific rigor of the trials, most of which had no central adjudication of clinical events or core angiographic laboratories, is suboptimal. The primary end point in these trials could not be mortality, owing to the small sample size, but pooling the studies affords a look into whether mortality is significantly affected. The pooled results of the trials are presented in *e*Figure 18.10.5, which shows a strong trend toward mortality reduction, and a significant reduction of the composite of death and reinfarction. Another benefit of major outcomes that has been unraveled in these trials has been the reduced incidence of intracerebral hemorrhage with balloon angioplasty as compared with thrombolytic therapy.

The early benefit of angioplasty over thrombolytic therapy is attenuated during more extended follow-up. As shown in *e*Figure 18.10.6, at 6 months' follow-up in the largest trial, GUSTO-IIb, there was near equivalence of the death and nonfatal reinfarction end point (119). In parallel, there was little difference in the actual cumulative costs associated with the two strategies ($18,643 vs. $19,395 for PTCA and t-PA, respectively, *p* = .19) (128).

A number of trials have compared balloon angioplasty with stenting for acute MI reperfusion (129–136), and the mortality data for eight of these trials are summarized in *e*Figure 18.10.7. Overall, the in-hospital or 30-day mortality did not favor stenting. On the other hand, all of these trials showed less need for repeat target vessel revascularization, and overall the rate of reinfarction was reduced from 2.5% to 0.9% (137). The *S*tent versus *T*hrombolysis for *O*ccluded Coronary Arteries in *P*atients with *A*cute *My*ocardial *I*nfarction (STOP AMI) trial trial compared alteplase with stenting and abciximab and demonstrated a substantial reduction of infarct size along with a trend of improved survival (138). The Controlled Abciximab and Device Investigation to Lower Late Angioplasty Complications (CADILLAC) trial compared balloon and stenting in a two-by-two factorial design with abciximab or control (not blinded) and showed an advantage for stenting for the primary end point (139). Overall, the mortality of stenting compared with balloon angioplasty has not been shown to be significantly reduced in the aggregate of all of the trials. Nevertheless, the overriding benefits of lessened reinfarction and the need for repeat revascularization have made stenting the standard for catheter-based reperfusion. As discussed subsequently (see Rescue Percutaneous Transluminal Coronary Angioplasty), more recent trials have incorporated IIb/IIIa inhibition, which may further ameliorate the results of stenting in acute MI.

One major criticism that has been raised regarding primary PTCA is that the clinical trial experience may not be mirrored or replicated in community hospitals (140–143). It is clear that critical factors, such as the time from patient arrival ("door") to successful angioplasty-mediated reperfusion ("balloon") must be minimized and has been less than 60 minutes in the trials in which the most extensive advantage over thrombolysis was demonstrated. Many studies have shown that the average door-to-balloon time is approximately 2 hours for many hospitals, which may serve as the principal explanation for the failure to achieve excellent results (140–143). Furthermore, operator experience probably plays a meaningful role as the technical aspects of the procedure are important (140). Infarct vessels, as compared with diseased arteries in patients without acute coronary syndromes, are particularly prone to intimal dissection, vasospasm, and thrombosis. Furthermore, the complexity of the patient, with respect to hemodynamic management and arrhythmias, is heightened. Specific expertise in performing rapid, high-volume, high-quality (superior risk-adjusted outcomes) mechanical reperfusion probably accounts for some of the discrepancies between clinical trials and the community at large.

As far as recommendations for the use of mechanical reperfusion, it is clear that if a patient is in the right time and the right place with an evolving acute MI, then primary PTCA would be preferred. This is an infrequent phenomenon, however, as only a limited number of hospitals have the facilities, operators and teams, their timely availability, and the expertise. Nevertheless, if a patient presents

to an appropriate center with these features, primary PTCA should be considered the superior strategy. In most cases, even in centers in which primary PTCA is used but the catheterization laboratory or personnel are not quickly available, thrombolytic fibrinolytic therapy is more easily implemented. It is worth bearing in mind, however, that for thrombolytic fibrinolytic therapy to actually dissolve the coronary thrombus and reestablish coronary blood flow it takes approximately 45 to 60 minutes. Therefore, in a situation in which the door-to-balloon time is anticipated to be 60 minutes, there is still legitimacy in using primary PTCA for more rapid and reliable reperfusion. This important triage decision must be made on an individual patient basis, but should not be accompanied by any delay.

Other patients who specifically benefit from primary PTCA are those with an absolute or relative contraindication to thrombolytic therapy (*e*Table 18.2.2), owing to safety concerns, and in patients with prior bypass surgery or cardiogenic shock, attributed to the markedly reduced efficacy of thrombolytic therapy in both of these settings (13,73,74,144–147). The reasons for poor efficacy are different. In cardiogenic shock, t-PA fibrinolytics have a high failure rate because their effect relies on adequate perfusion (148), whereas the failure rate of thrombolytics in saphenous vein grafts is attributed to the extensive clot burden and slow runoff (145). Furthermore, patients with a large MI (especially the proximal LAD; Table 18.1) should be considered for primary mechanical reperfusion because the risk profile is so high if successful reperfusion is not achieved.

Clinical Detection of Reperfusion

Apart from administering thrombolytic therapy or performing PTCA as rapidly as possible after the diagnosis is established, it is important to emphasize that in most patients one cannot rely on bedside signs to reliably detect whether pharmacologic reperfusion has been successful (114–117). First, it is not possible to use the patient's chest pain as a guide to whether the therapy is effective. The reasons for this are multiple, including the confounding effects of narcotic analgesics, the partial denervation that occurs at some point after coronary thrombosis in some patients with MI (118), the stuttering pattern of infarct vessel blood flow in the early hours of infarction, and the natural evolution of the necrosis with eventual attenuation or relief from chest pain. Second, so-called reperfusion arrhythmias are a misnomer, such as ventricular tachycardia, as they more commonly occur in patients who either do not receive reperfusion therapy or fail to achieve successful reperfusion (119–121). One arrhythmia that has been correlated with restoration of infarct vessel patency is accelerated idioventricular rhythm (114,115). Third, resolution of the ST-segment elevation is an unreliable means of establishing reperfusion success. There may be partial resolution from natural, evolutionary features of the event or the dynamic blood flow pattern so characteristic of the first 12 hours of acute MI. If a patient develops sudden and near complete relief of chest pain, full resolution of the ECG abnormalities, and has a run of accelerated idioventricular rhythm, this is highly specific for successful reperfusion, but this only occurs in less than 10% of patients receiving thrombolytic therapy (example in Fig. 18.5) (114,115).

Accordingly, we do not have a sensitive bedside, clinical means of detecting reperfusion. A variety of enzymatic tests have been advocated, including myoglobin, creatine kinase isoforms, and troponin, but these have not yet been proven to be clinically useful (122–131). Continuous recording of the 12-lead ECG or serial assessment of the 12-lead ECG at baseline and 60 minutes into therapy may be more useful methods for the diagnosis of successful or unsuccessful reperfusion (132–134), but there is a suboptimal relationship between the extent of ST-segment resolution and the completeness of coronary blood flow. This may be related to the temporal instability of coronary blood flow in the early hours of acute MI, and that many of the studies that evaluated the correlation did not have simultaneous assessment of the ECG and angiographic indices. Alternatively, because up to one-third of patients with TIMI-3 flow on the angiogram do not have flow at the tissue level as evaluated with contrast echo perfusion imaging or positron emission tomography (135), it is possible that the ECG parameters are more indicative or authentically reflect the true myocardial perfusion status. Noninvasive markers continue to be intensely investigated, with more recent studies of cine magnetic resonance angiography (136,137), echocardiography (138), high-frequency QRS monitoring (139), and continuous vector ECG (140). Although in clinical practice there is frequent use of the term *clinical reperfusion*, it is essential to point out that this is usually based on quite soft criteria that may be misleading.

Heparin

Even though heparin was administered as early as 1916, it has only been in relatively recent years that we have generated data to study the appropriate ways of its use. A critical advance came with the analysis of the GUSTO-I trial in which more than 30,000 patients had intravenous heparin, serial measurements of the activated partial thromboplastin time (aPTT), and assessment of clinical outcomes (149). As shown in Figure 18.11, there is a relationship between aPTT and 30-day mortality, with the optimal range between 50 and 70 seconds. The same preferred range of 50 to 70 seconds proved to be associated with lower bleeding complications, and particularly intracerebral hemorrhage, than more aggressive heparin effects. These data, importantly, are not from a randomized trial of conserva-

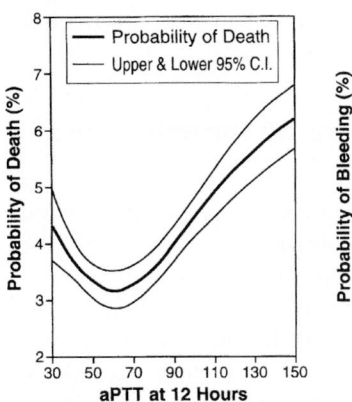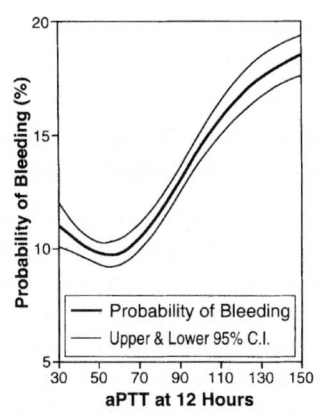

FIGURE 18.11 Activated partial thromboplastin time (aPTT) versus probability of death (30 days) or of severe or moderate bleeding. C.I., confidence interval. (Adapted from Granger CB, Hirsh J, Califf RM, et al. Activated partial thromboplastin time and outcome after thrombolytic therapy for acute myocardial infarction. *Circulation* 1996;93:870–878.)

tive or aggressive heparin dosing strategies, but represent the largest data set that compares heparin effects and clinical outcomes.

When used in conjunction with thrombolytic therapy, heparin should be administered on a weight-adjusted basis at 60 U per kg bolus (maximum, 4,000 U) and followed by 12 U per kg per hour (maximum, 1,000 U per hour initially) (149a). Consideration for a lower bolus should be given in patients who are aged, lightweight (less than 50 kg), and female, as these are the major determinants of the aPTT after heparin administration (149). The use of intravenous heparin is essential with t-PA, as verified in a number of controlled angiographic trials (150–153), but less documented with SK (73,88,89,154–156). SK has considerably more fibrinogenolytic action, such that it will intrinsically elevate the aPTT to a higher extent than t-PA. In the GISSI-2 International and ISIS-3 controlled trials of high-dose subcutaneous heparin after SK, there was little evidence of mortality reduction and more bleeding complications (73,74,88). In GUSTO-I comparing SK with intravenous versus subcutaneous heparin, there were no significant differences for mortality even though predischarge infarct vessel patency favored intravenous heparin in the angiographic trial (88). There is considerable debate as to whether any heparin should be routinely conjunctively administered with SK (155–157), but more recent trials of direct thrombin inhibitors strongly suggest the potential for better adjunctive therapy with this plasminogen activator (158,159). Heparin is used for the first 48 hours, with serial assessment of the aPTT at 6, 12, and 24 hours and active titration of the aPTT to the 50- to 70-second value. After 24 hours, in the uncomplicated patients, heparin can be discontinued. In patients with recurrent ischemia, however, atrial fibrillation, or those with an antero-apical MI who may require oral anticoagulation to prevent stroke (see Chapters 19 and 20), heparin should be continued until hospital discharge or the oral anticoagulation effect is fully established.

Bleeding Complications of Thrombolytics and Anticoagulation

With the judicious use of heparin, the potential for bleeding complications of thrombolytics is reduced. Nevertheless, the most feared complication of intracerebral hemorrhage occurs in approximately 1 of 200 patients (0.5%) treated with thrombolytic therapy. The incidence is definitely higher with t-PA (0.7%) than SK (0.4%) (73,74,88,89,160,161). Prompt recognition of this catastrophe can be helpful because there are case reports of successful neurosurgical evacuation of the hemorrhage or hematoma, and in many patients, the location of the event is one that will not incur long-term disability (162,163). Presentation can be heralded by the complaint of a headache, an acute confusional state, a seizure, visual disturbance, or any new, focal neurologic sign. Still, even with rapid recognition and immediate computed tomography or magnetic resonance brain imaging, approximately two-thirds of patients with an intracerebral hemorrhage will die or sustain fixed neurologic disability (89,161). In patients older than 75 years of age, the rate of fatality exceeds 90% (160,164). In the clinical trials that have evaluated thrombolytics, the mortality incorporates all causes, and the end point of death plus nonfatal, disabling stroke is important to consider (89,165) to understand the net clinical benefit of a particular reperfusion strategy. Other sites of serious bleeding, such as gastrointestinal or retroperitoneal, are unusual (less than 5%), but can be life threatening if not quickly diagnosed and treated. The most common cause of bleeding, periaccess site, is usually self-limiting (89,166).

Beta-Blockade

Nearly all of the data available for the use of beta-blockers in acute MI are derived from the prereperfusion era. There is extensive support for the usefulness of beta-blockade to reduce recurrent ischemia and arrhythmias and improve survival (167–173). The largest trial of intravenous beta-blockade, ISIS-1, suggested that the predominant benefit was mediated via the reduction of cardiac rupture events (167). Only two placebo-controlled trials in the contemporary era of reperfusion therapy have been conducted, and one of these showed reduction in recurrent ischemia with the use of early intravenous followed by oral metoprolol (174). The trial was relatively small, however, and the primary end point of preserving cardiac function was not significantly affected. Likewise, a trial of intravenous metoprolol conducted by Van de Werf et al. was negative (175). In the GUSTO-I trial, the use of intravenous beta-blockade was associated with an adverse profile of clinical outcomes including worse mortality and congestive heart failure (175a). In this trial, the use of intrave-

nous beta-blockade in 44% of patients was higher than many other large-scale thrombolytic studies, and it remains possible that the ill effects were related to administering therapy to patients with a large infarction or with marginal left ventricular function (73,88,89,175a). Current recommendations are to use beta-blockers orally in patients with a preserved left ventricular ejection fraction (estimated at >40%), and to initiate this on the first or second day after presentation. Intravenous beta-blockade is particularly useful in patients who are hyperdynamic and hyperadrenergic, representing the unusual subset of relatively young patients who have tachycardia and hypertension disproportionate to the smallness of their MI territory. But the potential for reducing intracerebral hemorrhage, as demonstrated in the TIMI-2 trial, has not been confirmed in subsequent large-scale efforts (174,175a).

Nitrates

Intravenous nitroglycerin is frequently used (89), but the data to support its use do not originate from trials conducted in the era of myocardial reperfusion. A review of trials that were conducted with nitrates in the period that antedated thrombolytic therapy suggested a significant 35% mortality benefit (176,177). The benefit is believed to be related to reduction of infarct size, improvement of regional myocardial function, along with reduction in right and left ventricular preload. More recent large-scale trials that have assessed either intravenous nitrates or long-acting oral nitrate preparations have failed to demonstrate benefit (178,179). However, in these trials there was extensive use of nitrates in the first few hospital days in the control group patients, confounding the assessment of the effect.

Often, intravenous nitroglycerin is inadequately administered, as the correct dose to achieve the desired hemodynamic benefit is to titrate the infusion to achieve at least a 10% to 15% reduction in the systolic blood pressure for normotensive patients and a 30% reduction in hypertensive patients, not to exceed a systolic blood pressure less than 90 mm Hg. Appropriate administration is to use a bolus dose of 12.5 to 20.0 μg, followed by an infusion of 10 to 20 μg per minute with an increase in this infusion level by 5 to 10 μg every 5 to 10 minutes, along with careful surveillance of blood pressure, heart rate, and hemodynamic and clinical signs. In appropriate patients who do not have a large MI and are not at risk for congestive heart failure, it is especially helpful to combine beta-blocker therapy with the intravenous nitroglycerin to avoid the undesired tachycardia. Intravenous nitroglycerin is continued for the first 24 to 48 hours and replaced by oral or topical nitroglycerin preparations in patients with heart failure and recurrent ischemia.

Angiotensin-Converting Enzyme Inhibitors

One of the most important advances in cardiovascular medicine in the last decade has been the demonstration of survival benefit for angiotensin-converting enzyme (ACE) inhibitors in patients with left ventricular dysfunction. In several trials of acute MI (178–182) various ACE inhibitors have been tested and shown, in aggregate, to promote survival, reduce the incidence of heart failure, and, in selected trials, reduce the incidence of reinfarction and the need for revascularization. The details of these trials and the rationale are reviewed in Chapters 19 and 20. ACE inhibitors can be recommended in the first 24 hours of an anterior MI (proximal or mid-LAD, Table 18.1) or an MI complicated by either heart failure or ejection fraction less than 40%, or both. A graded dose schedule is used to avoid hypotension, especially with the first dose, with initiation of therapy on the first hospital day once the blood pressure is stabilized. The Heart Outcomes Preventions Evaluation (HOPE) trial findings of ramipril compared with placebo in a broad population of patients with coronary disease supports a greater than or equal to 20% reduction of death, recurrent MI, stroke, or need for revascularization (183). The combination of ACE inhibitors and beta-blockers with asymptomatic left ventricular dysfunction was studied in post-MI patients and appears to provide additive benefit (184).

Calcium Channel Blockade

Unlike ACE inhibitors, which have almost uniformly been shown to have salutary effects, the calcium channel blockers have limited data to support their use in this setting and, more recently, there has been heightened awareness of their potential for toxicity and risk of mortality (171,185–190). Nifedipine is contraindicated because of its intrinsic negative inotropic effects, reflex sympathetic activation, tachycardia, and hypotension. The excess of adverse outcomes in four placebo-controlled post-MI trials of nifedipine (none with reperfusion) (185–190) raised the possibility that coronary steal was occurring, referring to an imbalance in vasodilatation and reduction in coronary perfusion pressure. Other calcium channel beta-blockers, such as verapamil or diltiazem, may be used for specific indications, such as treatment of supraventricular tachyarrhythmia or relief of postinfarction angina, if nitrates and beta-blockers are ineffective or not adequately tolerated. All calcium channel blockers should otherwise be avoided, especially in patients who develop heart failure.

Management of Lipids

With the marked salutary effects on long-term survival, prevention of reinfarction, and subsequent coronary revascularization of HMG-CoA reductase drugs (19–22,191–194), it is important that a cholesterol panel (total, low-density lipoprotein, high-density lipoprotein) be obtained on admission and no later than the first 24 hours. This will

be useful for predischarge planning, and the use of lipid-lowering drugs is discussed fully in Chapter 20.

EMERGENCY ANGIOGRAPHY AND REVASCULARIZATION

Emergency Angiography

The role of emergency angiography remains controversial, apart from its obligatory role in primary mechanical reperfusion. If a patient has received thrombolytic therapy, emergency angiography should be considered if there is recurrent chest pain or ECG changes, if there is new-onset hypotension or heart failure, or in an uncomplicated, large MI for which the success of pharmacologic reperfusion is unknown, but critical to the patient's outcome. As reviewed in the clinical assessment of reperfusion, in the vast majority of patients it remains unclear whether thrombolytic therapy has been effective.

The advantages of emergency angiography are that the coronary anatomy is fully defined, and a more precise assessment of the patient's status is determined regarding the presence of multivessel disease, which carries key independent prognostic information (213), and the patency status of the infarct vessel, which as reviewed is the most important treatment determinant of clinical outcome. On the other hand, disadvantages are the need for an emergency on-call team, as for primary PTCA, the cost, and potential for bleeding complications, which are usually in a periaccess site. Just as is the case with primary mechanical reperfusion, most hospitals do not have the potential to perform this procedure. However, transfer to a referral center may be appropriate for the categories of patients for whom this strategy has the most potential benefit.

Rescue Percutaneous Transluminal Coronary Angioplasty

Rescue PTCA refers to using a mechanical strategy of balloon angioplasty as a fallback if thrombolytic therapy is unsuccessful (214). The decision to perform emergency angiography should be made promptly, as it sets up the foundation to achieve reperfusion mechanically even if thrombolytic therapy has proven ineffective. Ideally, the decision is made before a waiting period in a patient with a large MI (e.g., proximal LAD infarct) who is at considerable risk for adverse sequelae. If a waiting period of 60 to 120 minutes is interposed before making a decision, then the patient's potential gain from the rescue PTCA is substantially reduced.

The primary data supportive of the use of rescue PTCA are derived from a randomized trial of 150 patients with LAD artery occlusion after thrombolytic therapy (215). In this trial, the incidence of death at 30 days was 5.2% with

PTCA as compared with 9.9% without PTCA. The composite of death or heart failure occurred in 6.5% versus 16.4%, respectively (*p* = .05). Although this trial was small, it was extremely difficult to do because it meant leaving half the patients with a known occluded LAD without reperfusion. These data, combined with many observational studies that provide a favorable clinical and left ventricular function profile, including long-term follow-up, for patients with successful rescue PTCA (216–224), support the application of rescue PTCA in select patients. The overall reocclusion rate in the studies with more than 560 patients in aggregate was 18%, and it should be noted that the reasons for failure of thrombolytic therapy are frequently more extensive intimal disruption, a large thrombus burden unresponsive to the plasminogen activator, or platelet-rich clot that is intrinsically resistant to current therapies. In right coronary artery occlusion, a higher incidence of periprocedural complications has been reported, as compared with the left coronary (225). But these complications of bradyarrhythmias, sustained hypotension, ventricular tachycardia, and fibrillation were responsive to therapy and do not represent a contraindication to rescue PTCA for patients with an inferior MI. However, the rationale for rescue PTCA in a patient with an uncomplicated inferior wall MI remains unclear, because this carries a low risk of fatality. It should also be pointed out that virtually all of the studies and the trial of rescue PTCA were performed in an era of suboptimal anticoagulation, one in which stents for intimal dissection were not available, and there was lack of antiplatelet coverage (215–225). With contemporary pharmacologic therapy, including platelet glycoprotein IIb/IIIa inhibitors, along with stents and in-laboratory monitoring of the activated clotting time, it is likely that the results of rescue PTCA will be improved. The safety, however, of combining full doses of fibrinolytic agents with IIb/IIIa inhibitors is unknown and will require careful study. The use of reduced lytic doses, judicious heparin, and IIb/IIIa inhibitors may be especially useful in maximizing benefit-risk ratio in these patients.

Immediate Angioplasty

The strategy of performing PTCA immediately after successful thrombolysis was essentially abandoned as a result of three randomized trials (218,226–228) that demonstrated a higher incidence of adverse events, including mortality and the need for emergency bypass surgery, and no improvement in left ventricular function. These trials were performed in the mid-1980s, and again the improvement in pharmacologic and catheter-based alternatives may lead to different results. However, the predominant benefit to the patient is restoration of TIMI-3 flow, such that alleviation of the underlying infarct vessel stenosis on an immediate basis provides little added benefit but certainly poses a risk. For these reasons, the practice of angioplasty after success-

ful thrombolytic therapy in an uncomplicated patient has largely become unnecessary and obsolete.

Emergency Bypass Surgery

Still an essential part of reperfusion strategies today, although infrequently reported on, is the use of emergency bypass surgery for patients who undergo early coronary angiography, with or without thrombolytic therapy. In patients who are intended to undergo primary mechanical reperfusion, but an unsuspected critical left main stem lesion is detected, or there is the equivalent scenario with advanced, diffuse, three-vessel coronary artery disease that is not approachable by percutaneous revascularization, emergency bypass surgery should be contemplated. In 1% to 2% of primary PTCA cases, emergency surgery proves to be necessary (119–126) and for this reason having a facility with rapid, in-house surgical capabilities is quite important. The results for emergency bypass surgery as a reperfusion treatment for acute MI are particularly encouraging, despite the lack of a randomized controlled design and the fact that these studies were reported in the 1980s before pharmacologic and catheter-based reperfusion was popularized (229–233).

PREDISCHARGE ASSESSMENT AND ELECTIVE REVASCULARIZATION

Elective Coronary Angiography and Revascularization

In the GUSTO-I trial of 21,722 patients in the United States with acute MI, 71% underwent coronary angiography (246), and most of this was elective, predischarge. The major determinants of angiography were the patient's age, hospital availability, and recurrent ischemia. The age characteristic is particularly troubling, as there was a pronounced reduction for use of angiography patients older than 73 years, and it is precisely these patients who have the highest risk of major events (164). Other studies have confirmed that hospital availability of the procedure is a key predictive factor of its use (247,248), which is also a sobering realization. Of note, recurrent ischemia, which could have been conceived as the most salient driving feature for performing coronary angiography, was third in importance (246). There is marked variability in the use of coronary angiography in the eight different regions of the United States, ranging from 52% to 81%, and reflective of the uncertainty of how this procedure should be applied (248).

When angiography is performed, patients can be categorized into five groups. An interesting group is the 15% of patients who have "minimal lesion syndrome" (249). These patients are usually young, quite often smokers, and of the male sex, who at the time of predischarge angiography have less than 30% residual stenosis. The underlying pathophysiology is likely to involve coronary vasospasm, or fissure, with subsequent thrombus formation overlying a minimally encroaching atherosclerotic plaque. Of course, revascularization is not necessary, but it is vital for smoking cessation to be achieved. The prognosis for these patients is excellent, but in 2% despite the use of nitrates, calcium channel blockers, or both, there is recurrence. The other angiographic subsets include patients with occluded infarct vessels and single-vessel disease, patients with single-vessel disease of the infarct-related artery, those with two- or three-vessel disease, and the small subgroup of patients with left main stem lesions.

Coronary angiography is advocated for all patients who have recurrent ischemia. For the reasons discussed for using emergency angiography, as far as establishing infarct vessel patency, extent of multivessel disease, and suitability for revascularization, angiography can be considered an integral part of the early post-MI assessment. Of note, if a patient has provocable ischemia, angiography is fully justified with the results of the Danish Multicenter Study of Acute MI trial (241).

A major question remains as to patients who do not have provocable ischemia or do not undergo functional testing but, by clinical criteria, have evidence of viable myocardium of the infarct zone. These criteria may include a lower peak CPK than expected, hypokinesia but not akinesia of the infarct zone by echocardiography, early thrombolytic therapy in the first 2 hours of symptom onset with rapid relief of chest pain and ECG findings, or the lack of development of Q waves on the ECG. These patients, on an empiric basis, may be suitable for coronary angiography because of the clinical judgment that they have sustained an "incomplete" infarct and will likely have a significant residual stenosis of the infarct vessel. On the other hand, patients with a complicated MI, with such features as congestive heart failure or ventricular tachycardia, are at high risk for subsequent events and deserve consideration for angiography. The groups of patients who do not need angiography are those in whom revascularization, be it percutaneous or surgical, could not be considered or those patients with a small inferior or lateral infarct who do not have provocable ischemia. This analysis suggests that a substantial portion of patients probably deserve consideration for predischarge angiography, but this must be considered an unsettled controversy as there has not been a clinical trial to address this issue per se.

Coronary Angioplasty or Bypass Surgery

Revascularization is used commonly in hospitals in the United States, as evidenced by the GUSTO-I data of 30% use of PTCA and 13% use of CABG. The coronary anatomy strongly predicts which procedure is performed, with single-vessel disease resulting in PTCA for 86% of patients undergoing any revascularization, whereas CABG was used in 79% of patients with three-vessel disease who had some form of revascularization (246). Even though the use of coronary angiography and revascularization was much lower outside the United States in this large trial, the proportionate use of angioplasty and bypass surgery among patients undergoing angioplasty was similar (250). Bypass surgery carries a risk of mortality that is independent of the acute MI event and, even risk adjusted, in the first year after surgery there is a small excess of deaths (not statistically meaningful) compared with patients not undergoing surgery (251). However, the benefit of complete revascularization in these patients with advanced, multivessel disease is much more likely to be manifest over a more prolonged follow-up (251). One of the controversies in surgical revascularization in this setting is whether bypass surgery to the infarct-related vessel, especially if it was not successfully rendered patent from reperfusion therapy, is worthwhile. This dilemma is usually resolved by grafting the infarct-related territory, but determination of viability (see Chapters 50 and 55) may be helpful. In patients with spontaneous or provokable ischemia who have extensive and diffuse atherosclerotic involvement, bypass surgery should be strongly considered as the revascularization procedure of choice, provided that the distal vessels are suitable for grafting. It would be anticipated that the patients with compromised left ventricular function would stand the most to benefit from the standpoint of survival (251).

SPECIAL SUBGROUPS

The Aged

The highest risk group of patients with acute MI are clearly the elderly, as they account for more than one-half of the deaths of patients hospitalized (252), and age represents the single most important risk factor (57). In GUSTO-I, the 30-day mortality for patients between 75 and 85 years of age was 19.1% and for those older than 85 it was 27.9% (164). The risk of death in the aged was coupled with a higher risk of hemorrhagic stroke and bleeding complications. Overall, intracranial hemorrhage occurred in 3.3% of patients older than the age of 75 years and moderate or severe bleeding, as reflected by need for transfusion or significant blood loss, affected more than 20% of these patients. Of note, the elderly have more comorbidities and many have relative contraindications to thrombolytic therapy; they present later to the hospital by approximately 30 minutes and paradoxically have smaller infarcts based on creatine kinase measurements. The discrepancy between lower creatine kinase and higher mortality was explained on the basis of less muscle mass in the elderly (164,253). Some evidence suggests that the myocardial band fraction release is higher among elderly patients (164). These patients are much more apt to have multivessel disease, prior MI, diminished ejection fraction, and an increased risk of cardiac rupture (254,255). It has also been pointed out that advanced age is a major factor associated with the "early hazard" of thrombolytic therapy, such that in the first 24 hours after treatment, compared with placebo, there are actually more deaths in the elderly (65,115,164). Age is the single factor that most predicts whether a patient will undergo coronary angiography after acute MI, and it is the elderly, who by and large have the most to gain, who are at highest risk of not undergoing the procedure (246,256).

The most important issue is that reperfusion therapy should be used more aggressively in the elderly. The net benefit of reduction of death and disabling stroke is pronounced in the aged. In the ISIS-2 trial, the number of lives saved for SK was 16 per 1,000 in patients less than 65 years, but 36 lives per 1,000 in the older patients (59). For accelerated t-PA as compared with SK, the net clinical benefit of reducing the number of deaths or disabling strokes was 5 per 1,000 patients for those aged younger than 65 years as compared with 17 events per 1,000 patients for patients aged 75 to 85 years (164). The main explanations for this large amplification of net benefit include the considerably higher risk of the aged, and the fact that when hemorrhagic stroke occurs, it is much more likely to be a fatal event. Despite these findings, in several registries (257–259) the proportion of patients aged older than 75 years who do not receive therapy is one-half or more. It appears that there is more use of thrombolytic therapy in the elderly as based on the proportion of patients older than age 75 enrolled from the GUSTO-I to the GUSTO-III trials (an increase from 12% to 16%). Even patients up to the age of 110 years have been successfully treated (260), according to one of the most instructive case reports that have been published. After deciding on reperfusion for an elderly patient, the next choice is whether to use thrombolytic therapy or primary angioplasty. In GUSTO-I, for patients younger than 85 years, there is benefit of accelerated t-PA over SK (253). For patients older than age 85, the experience is limited and there are no cogent, statistically robust data to draw on. But in the 412 patients in GUSTO-I, the best regimen appeared to be SK and subcutaneous heparin (164). When fibrinolytic therapy is used in this subgroup, it is essential to lower the dose of heparin as age is a critical determinant to aPTT elevation (149), and SK with intravenous heparin (associated with the highest aPTTs) had a hemorrhagic stroke rate of 3.0% compared with 0.9% for accelerated t-PA and intravenous heparin (164). Alternatively, primary angioplasty can be used and is associated with a lesser risk of hemorrhagic strokes. Although early studies suggested that the risk of primary PTCA in the elderly might be excessive, more recent trials have pointed out the potential for heightened benefit over fibrinolytic therapy (261–263). The use of primary angioplasty is preferred in the appropriate settings as previously

discussed and should be strongly considered if there is marked concern about hemorrhagic stroke or major bleeding, particularly in patients with absolute or relative contraindications to thrombolytic therapy.

More recently, there has been considerable debate about the use of fibrinolytic therapy in the elderly (264–269). This resulted, in part, from a report by Thiemann and colleagues of a large registry, which called into question whether the elderly were being harmed by fibrinolytic therapy. It is difficult to make a judgment from data in registries, although certainly important to reconsider the value and risk of the therapy in a population with a known high risk of intracerebral hemorrhage. The classic Fibrinolytic Therapy Trialists' analysis of the data was originally hampered by inclusion of patients without certain criteria for reperfusion therapy. An update of the data from all of the large-scale fibrinolytic trials is shown in Figure 18.12. Among patients 75 years or older, there was an important 15% reduction of mortality (from 29.4% to 26.0%), and this translated to 34 deaths avoided per 1,000 elderly patients treated. This is an absolute benefit that compares favorably with the other age groups (Fig. 18.12). Furthermore, Krumholz and colleagues have demonstrated that at 1-year follow-up there is clear-cut advantage of therapy in the elderly (267). The issue is not completely settled, however, because of relatively limited data from the randomized trials. Overall, if catheter-based reperfusion were immediately available it would be considered preferable with the relative avoidance of intracerebral hemorrhage. Nonetheless, this is frequently not available on a timely basis and fibrinolytic therapy should still be considered as an established and important treatment for the aged with acute MI.

Women

The subgroup of women with acute MI has been a controversial one, and particularly the issue of whether gender differences were responsible for worse outcomes, including more than doubling of mortality (261–263). Beginning

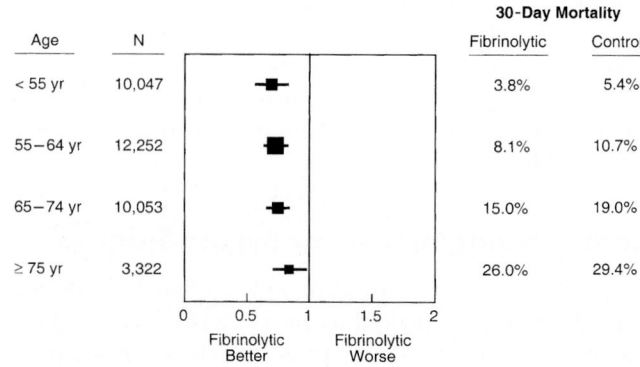

FIGURE 18.12 Revised Fibrinolytic Therapy Trialists' data. [From Estess JM, Topol EJ. *Heart* 2001 (*in press*).]

from presentation, it is clear that women are less apt to receive reperfusion therapy, even though their presenting symptoms and ECG manifestations are similar (261). The reasons for this appears to be that women are considerably older at presentation than men, on average 7 to 10 years, and as a result have more risk factors, including hypertension, smoking, and diabetes. They present later for medical attention, a median of 18 minutes, and have a longer time to treatment than men (263). Of note, by creatine kinase peak, women typically evolve a smaller MI (median, 1,223 U per L vs. 1,491 U per L for women vs. men, respectively, in GUSTO-I), even adjusted for weight, which is dissociated from their higher propensity for fatal and nonfatal complications, especially the more frequent but unexplained risk of heart failure (262).

The death rate for women in GUSTO-I, as shown in *e*Figure 18.12.1, at 30 days was 11.3% versus 5.5%, which seems like a major gender-specific adverse effect. However, by adjusting for the important differences in baseline characteristics (262), and especially age, these differences tended to disappear. After adjustment, the mortality at 30 days was 15% higher in women, which was of marginal statistical significance. After 1-year follow-up, the differences were completely absent (*e*Fig. 18.12.1) (263). Similarly, the excess in stroke of 2.1% versus 1.2% (*p* = .02) is canceled out by adjusting for the baseline feature differences, particularly age and weight.

The use of the GUSTO-I trial to evaluate the gender differences is helpful because this trial enrolled almost five-fold the number of women as previous trials and registries (262). Importantly, there was no imbalance in the use of coronary angiography and only small differences in the use of revascularization (angioplasty in 35% vs. 32%, bypass surgery in 9% vs. 7%, for women compared with men, respectively). Accordingly, despite the marked controversy over the existence of a gender gap for acute MI patients in their diagnosis or treatment, more recent evidence suggests that this is not the case when adequate sized sample populations and differences in baseline features are appropriately analyzed.

Prior Myocardial Infarction

The patients with prior MIs denote a high-risk subgroup who have largely been understudied to date. The proportion of patients with prior MIs is at least 16% in thrombolytic trials (270), and the mortality for these patients is at least doubled (*e*Fig. 18.12.2). Like the women subgroup, these patients are older (median increase of approximately 3 years) and have a greater preponderance of risk factors. In contrast to the elderly or women, they tend to present to the hospital earlier, probably owing to their familiarity with the symptoms. The chance for their presentation to be in Killip class III or IV is doubled (3.7% vs. 1.8%), as is the incidence of shock during the hospitalization (8.8% vs.

5.4%). Heart failure occurs much more commonly (22.6% vs. 14.9%), and ejection fraction is much lower (52% vs. 60%). As would be expected, the incidence of multivessel coronary disease is substantially increased (71.5% vs. 35.0%), but the response to coronary thrombolysis similar compared with the patients having de novo MI. As in the overall GUSTO-I and in this high-risk subgroup, the benefit of accelerated t-PA over SK for reducing mortality at 30 days and 1 year was significant (270). There is a gradient of prior MI with respect to risk, with the patients having an old inferior and new inferior MI having the lowest risk, and those with a prior inferior and new anterior MI demonstrating the highest risk of mortality (271).

This subgroup deserves emphasis because the risks are so exaggerated compared with the patients presenting with their first MI. Many of the patients have had prior CABG (17% of patients with prior MI) and already have the potential for a conduit that is resistant to thrombolytics owing to such an extensive clot burden (144,145). But even the patients with prior MI who have not had bypass surgery deserve special consideration for aggressive therapy. In the TIMI-2 trial comparing an invasive and conservative strategy of angiography and revascularization after thrombolysis, the subgroup of prior MI patients emerged as one with distinct benefit of the invasive approach (272). The group of patients with prior MI, like those who have Killip III or IV on presentation, or prior CABG, deserves careful consideration for emergency coronary angiography with an eye toward revascularization. If thrombolytic therapy is used, it should be thought of as only a temporizing measure because one cannot rely on either the success of the therapy (which leaves one-half of patients without early TIMI-3 flow) or our ability to clinically differentiate whether reperfusion has been achieved.

Cardiopulmonary Resuscitation

Administering fibrinolytics to patients with CPR (particularly when unsuccessful), has been quite controversial. A prospective study by Böttiger et al. (273) showed safety and supported efficacy in patients with initially unsuccessful out-of-hospital CPR. The odds ratio of return of spontaneous circulation was 2.7 for t-PA compared with controls. In patients with successful CPR, especially if brief (less than 5 minutes), fibrinolytics should not be considered contraindicated. This is an important area that has not been sufficiently studied (274).

Non–ST-Elevation Myocardial Infarction

A considerable part of this chapter has been dedicated to ST elevation because of the pressing need to establish reperfusion therapy. Patients without ST elevation, unless they have true posterior MI (*e*Table 18.2.1), do not usually have an occluded infarct-related artery and have not been shown to benefit from thrombolytic therapy. In fact, the aggregate data suggest that these patients may be put at risk of reinfarction if thrombolytic therapy is used (275). The reasons for this include the presence of a mural thrombus, rather than an occlusive one, with the potential for a plasminogen activator to engender free thrombin and facilitate platelet aggregation and the autocatalytic formation of thrombin. Essentially, the prothrombotic effects of thrombolytic therapy pose a risk in this setting, and this class of agents should be avoided. One more recent study (276), which raised the potential salutary effects of t-PA in this setting, is difficult to interpret because it represents a post hoc analysis from a trial dedicated to testing reperfusion in patients presenting later after symptom onset (6 to 24 hours). More data would be necessary to condone the use of empiric thrombolytic therapy in this subgroup.

As we learned from the GUSTO-IIb trial (277), which enrolled more than 12,140 patients without ST elevation, they are clearly older and more frequently female, diabetic, and hypertensive than their ST-elevation counterparts. In many respects, their characteristics pull together the features of the three previous subgroups of the aged, women, and prior MI. They are twice as likely to have had a prior MI (32% vs. 17%) and have more than twice the frequency of prior CABG (12% vs. 5%). The outcomes for these patients are still indicative of the need for improved therapies, as the incidence of death and nonfatal MI in the first 30 days was 9.4% and quite similar to the patients with ST-segment elevation. Of this composite, the non–ST-elevation patients have more reinfarction than death as compared with the ST-elevation patients (277). The therapy for non–ST-elevation MI is the same as that delineated for the ST-elevation MI patients, with emphasis on the use of aspirin, heparin, nitrates, and beta-blockade. The use of calcium channel blockers in this setting is supported by the results of one trial, albeit with marginal statistical significance (278).

With the pivotal importance of thrombin in these patients, it was thought that a direct inhibitor rather than heparin, which is effective on both circulating and clot-bound thrombin, would be associated with improved clinical outcomes. This was the focus of the GUSTO-IIb trial, which demonstrated a small but statistically insignificant benefit of hirudin over heparin (eFig. 18.12.3) (277). Although hirudin provided important benefits in the first few days of therapy while the infusion was being maintained, the lack of a robust effect at 30 days likely reflects the inability of hirudin or any direct thrombin inhibitor to block thrombin generation. Future trials directed at both antagonizing thrombin generation and activity might well build on the early phase, encouraging data on hirudin in the non–ST-elevation subgroup. Low-molecular-weight heparin (enoxaparin), given subcutaneously, has been shown to reduce death and nonfatal MI in patients with unstable angina or non–ST-elevation MI in the Efficacy

Safety Subcutaneous Enoxaparin in Non-Q Wave Coronary Events study and TIMI-11 without an ill effect on major bleeding complications (279). Platelet glycoprotein IIb/IIIa inhibition is being actively studied in large-scale trials for reducing death and MI in this subgroup, and initial trials, as reviewed in Chapter 19, are encouraging. Patients without ST-segment elevation constitute a group with appreciable risk despite our current armamentarium. The use of troponin to differentiate risk among these patients may prove to be helpful for the purposes of triage to early coronary angiography, and when suitable, revascularization. While new therapies and diagnostics are being assessed, it is important to bear in mind that the absence of ST elevation does not, in any way, convey lower risk.

Direct Thrombin Inhibitors and New Anticoagulants

The GUSTO-IIb trial was, in actuality, testing the thrombin activity hypothesis, rather than whether thrombin plays a pivotal role in acute coronary syndromes. Because it has been shown that hirudin does nothing to block thrombin generation, the beneficial effects that have been demonstrated in the trial, namely, an 11% reduction in death or reinfarction (eFig. 18.12.3), may be built on in the future.

The more substantial benefit realized in the first 24 hours and 3 days of therapy, while therapy was being administered, suggests that even directly blocking thrombin activity would be advantageous compared with our standard approach.

Several pilot studies have shown beneficial effects of low-molecular-weight heparins given in conjunction with fibrinolytics. In the ASSENT-3 trial, 2,040 patients were treated with full-dose TNK–t-PA and enoxaparin (30 mg intravenous bolus immediately followed by a subcutaneous dose of 1 mg per kg repeated every 12 hours until revascularization or discharge, with a maximum of 7 days). Enoxaparin cotherapy was associated with a significant 27% reduction in the composite of 30-day mortality, in-hospital reinfarction, or refractory ischemia when compared with unfractionated heparin. No excess of major bleeding complications or intracranial hemorrhage was observed, and a benefit was also present in patients above 75 years of age. These results suggest that prolonged administration of enoxaparin should be the anticoagulant treatment of choice in conjunction with TNK–t-PA. Whether it can replace unfractionated heparin with other less fibrin-specific agents needs to be determined (280).

Many agents work higher in the coagulation cascade and would be potentially more effective than hirudin. These include tissue factor pathway inhibitor, factor VII mimetics, factor X_a inhibitors, activated protein C, mutant thrombins that facilitate thrombomodulin or the protein C system, nematode anticoagulant protein (nAPc2), and factor IX inhibitors (281–284). Beyond the action of hirudin,

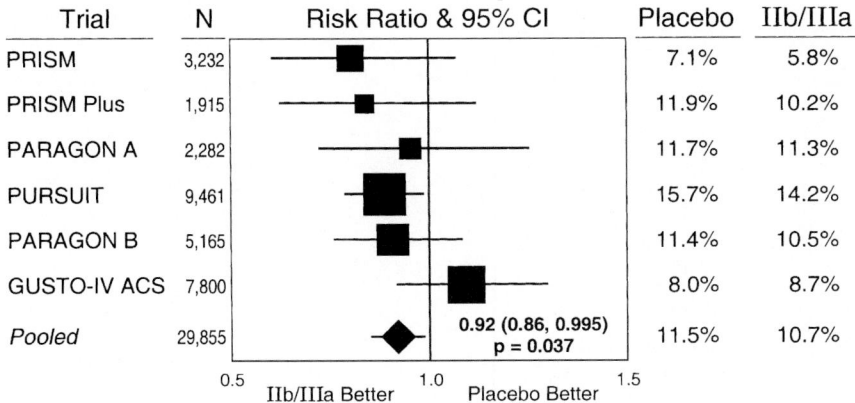

Trial	N	Risk Ratio & 95% CI	Placebo	IIb/IIIa
PRISM	3,232		7.1%	5.8%
PRISM Plus	1,915		11.9%	10.2%
PARAGON A	2,282		11.7%	11.3%
PURSUIT	9,461		15.7%	14.2%
PARAGON B	5,165		11.4%	10.5%
GUSTO-IV ACS	7,800		8.0%	8.7%
Pooled	29,855	0.92 (0.86, 0.995) p = 0.037	11.5%	10.7%

0.5   IIb/IIIa Better   1.0   Placebo Better   1.5

p = 0.339 Breslow-Day homogeneity

FIGURE 18.13 IIb/IIIa inhibition for acute coronary syndromes. Death or nonfatal myocardial infarction end point at 30 days. CI, confidence interval.

these agents have the potential to be fully effective in blocking thrombin generation, and future clinical investigation will be devoted to extending the "thrombin hypothesis" and building on the encouraging GUSTO-IIb results. The better results obtained in the Efficacy Safety Subcutaneous Enoxaparin in Non-Q Wave Coronary Events study with the low-molecular-weight heparin (enoxaparin), which exerts a higher anti-X_a activity than standard heparin, seems to support the thrombin generation hypothesis.

Platelet Glycoprotein IIb/IIIa Inhibitors

There has been intensive clinical trial assessment of IIb/IIIa inhibitors in patients with acute MI. For the intravenous IIb/IIIa inhibitors, there are six trials of 29,855 patients (285–290) focusing on acute coronary syndromes: unstable angina and non–ST-segment elevation MI. The results of these six trials are summarized in Figure 18.13. Overall, there was only an 8% reduction of death or MI at 30 days. However, the benefit for patients with an abnormal troponin at entry (or the subsequent sample at 6 to 8 hours) and diabetics was striking, especially in the PRISM trials (troponin was not assessed in PURSUIT). Furthermore, the overall positive results for eptifibatide in *P*latelet IIb/IIIa in *U*nstable Angina: *R*eceptor *S*uppression *U*sing *I*ntegrilin *T*herapy (PURSUIT) and tirofiban in the *P*latelet *R*eceptor *I*nhibition for *I*schemic *S*yndrome *M*anagement (PRISM) trials were offset by the single trial with a trend of worsened outcome: In the GUSTO-IV study of abciximab an interesting paradox has arisen. Abciximab was associated with worse outcomes in the GUSTO-IV trial, while being regarded as the reference standard for superior outcomes in percutaneous coronary revascularization trials (291–294). This is likely due to the long (24- and 48-hour) infusions of abciximab in GUSTO-IV, given without percutaneous revascularization. The likely explanation involves subthreshold platelet inhibition (below 80% inhibition of platelet aggregation) and the link with proinflammatory

expression of P-selectin and shedding of platelet CD40 ligand. This also probably explains the disappointing results of the oral IIb/IIIa inhibitors, which are subthreshold with respect to their IIb/IIIa receptor inhibition. Overall, these agents have induced a 35% excess of mortality for patients with acute coronary syndromes (295).

In acute MI, the GUSTO-V trial tested, for the first time in a large-scale definitive trial, low-dose fibrinolytic and IIb/IIIa inhibition. With enrollment of more than 16,000 patients comparing r-PA with r-PA at half-dose and abciximab, there was little difference in mortality (5.9% vs. 5.6%) (Fig. 18.14) (296). Noninferiority was established for the new strategy of combined therapy with respect to 30-day mortality, but superiority with respect to significantly less reinfarction and almost all MI complications (Table 18.3) was demonstrated. On the other hand, there was an excess of bleeding complications (5.6% vs. 3.9%). Of note, no increase in intracerebral hemorrhage was encountered (0.6% in both groups). Overall, the GUSTO-V trial validated combined fibrinolytics (at reduced doses) with IIb/IIIa inhibition as an alternative therapy to traditional fibrinolytic monotherapy. This may be particularly well suited for younger patients, those with high-risk MIs such as anterior location, and patients who are being considered for acute transfer to a cardiac catheterization laboratory.

The overall effect of abciximab given with half-dose TNK–t-PA in ASSENT-3 was similar to that in GUSTO-V. Significant reduction in in-hospital reinfarction and refractory ischemia rates as well as in the need for urgent intervention was observed, at the cost of a significant increase in major bleedings. Like GUSTO-V, there was no excess in intracranial hemorrhage with this combination. In the elderly no beneficial effects were seen. Major bleeding complications in this age category more than doubled as compared with full-dose TNK and unfractionated heparin (280).

This brings up the findings of IIb/IIIa used in conjunction with angioplasty or stenting in acute MI. Thus far, all of the five trials have tested abciximab, and the mortality

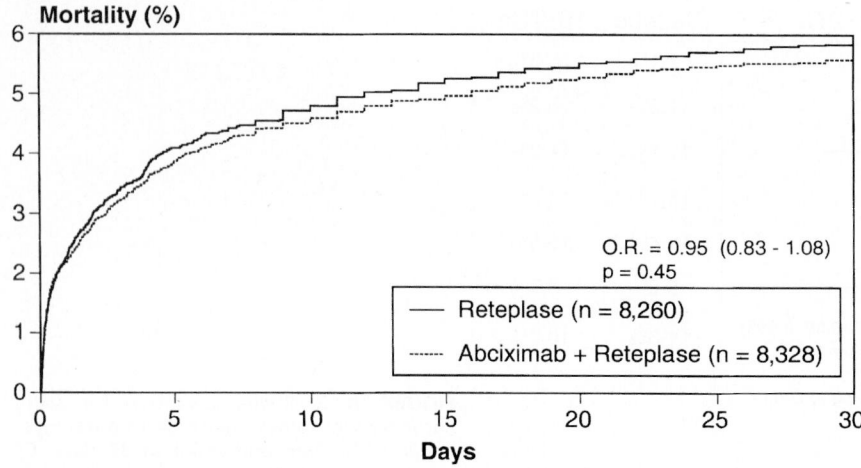

FIGURE 18.14 Kaplan-Meier mortality curves. O.R., odds ratio.

results are summarized in Table 18.4. There is an overall reduction of mortality seen with all trials in aggregate, even though the open-labeled CADILLAC trial did not show an advantage of abciximab in the stent arm (297). Besides mortality as an end point, there was a significant reduction in reinfarction, recurrent ischemia, and stent thrombosis in these trials. The data from the various trials and the way in which clinical practice has evolved suggest that IIb/IIIa inhibition has evolved as an important adjunct for catheter-based reperfusion.

The next phase of IIb/IIIa inhibition in clinical trials will take place with catheter-based reperfusion. A major issue is the time delay (from presentation to effective reperfusion) termed *door-to-balloon time*, which still averages almost 2 hours in most centers. Use of the combined strategy of half-dose fibrinolytic and full-dose IIb/IIIa inhibi-

tion may be a useful bridge to catheter-based reperfusion. Furthermore, the use of the IIb/IIIa inhibitor will likely be incorporated subsequently to deal with the microvascular embolization of platelet-thrombus and microscopic atheromatous debris.

CONTROVERSIES AND PERSONAL PERSPECTIVES

The field of acute MI therapy has been characterized by a long-standing debate of pharmacologic versus catheter-based reperfusion. If a patient presents to a hospital with an experienced team and can be mobilized to the catheterization laboratory quickly, catheter-based reperfusion has emerged as a preferred strategy. It is hoped that there will

TABLE 18.3 COMPLICATIONS OF MYOCARDIAL INFARCTION (THROUGH DAY 7)

Complication	Reteplase (n = 8,260) (%)	Reteplase + abciximab (n = 8,328) (%)	Odds ratio	p Value
Reinfarction	3.5	2.3	0.67 (0.55, 0.80)	<.001
Recurrent ischemia	12.8	11.3	0.87 (0.79, 0.96)	.004
Sustained ventricular tachycardia	2.8	2.2	0.79 (0.65, 0.96)	<.02
Ventricular fibrillation	3.5	2.7	0.79 (0.66, 0.94)	<.008
Second- or third-degree atrioventricular block	3.3	2.7	0.80 (0.67, 0.96)	.018
Cardiogenic shock	0.2	0.2	0.76 (0.37, 1.56)	.45
Pulmonary embolism	0.04	0.06	1.65 (0.39, 6.92)	.49
Pericardial effusion	1.0	1.2	1.19 (0.89, 1.59)	.23
New, severe congestive heart failure	4.8	4.6	0.95 (0.83, 1.10)	.51
Tamponade	0.4	0.4	0.96 (0.59, 1.58)	.88
Asystole	2.2	2.1	0.95 (0.77, 1.17)	.66
Ventricular septal defect	0.3	0.2	0.52 (0.26, 1.00)	.049
Papillary muscle rupture	0.07	0.059	0.66 (0.19, 2.34)	.52
Hypotension requiring therapy	9.4	9.1	0.96 (0.82, 1.07)	.49
Atrial fibrillation/flutter	4.4	4.2	0.95 (0.82, 1.11)	.52
Electromechanical dissociation	1.8	1.5	0.83 (0.65, 1.05)	.12
Myocardial rupture	0.6	0.4	0.67 (0.44, 1.03)	.065

TABLE 18.4 MORTALITY IN ALL ABCIXIMAB MYOCARDIAL INFARCTION TRIALS

	Placebo		Abciximab		Hazard ratio	95% Confidence interval	*p* Value
	No.	Death (%)	No.	Death (%)			
RAPPORT, 6 mo	242	4.6	241	4.2	0.91	(0.38, 2.13)	0.821
ISAR-2, 1 yr	200	8.5	201	6.0	0.69	(0.33, 1.45)	0.331
ADMIRAL, 6 mo	151	7.3	149	3.4	0.45	(0.16, 1.31)	0.144
CADILLAC, Balloon 6 mo	515	4.3	529	2.3	0.53	(0.26, 1.06)	0.073
CADILLAC, Stent 6 mo	513	2.8	525	3.8	1.38	(0.70, 2.74)	0.350
STOP AMI, 6 mo	69	13	71	4.2	0.31	(0.08, 1.16)	—

be convergence established with the ability to have a strategy that facilitates mechanical coronary intervention and promotes early patency of the infarct vessel and the microvasculature. For this reason, the combination of IIb/IIIa inhibition and a low-dose fibrinolytic is an attractive foundation. This still remains to be demonstrated, but the hope is that one day there will be no "confusional" delays, deciding on whether to use drugs or the catheterization laboratory. The use of the 60-minute ECG after pharmacologic therapy is attractive in ferreting out the patients who do not yet have tissue-level reperfusion established, and who may indeed have considerable benefit from early catheterization laboratory transfer with consideration for rescue catheter reperfusion.

A considerable challenge exists in avoidance of microvascular obstruction with either pharmacologic or catheter-based reperfusion. To this end, emboli protection devices offer considerable promise to prevent the atheromatous and platelet-thrombus material from getting downstream at the time of the balloon or stenting procedure. Their use will probably become routine over the next few years as the devices go through iterative refinement and the results of the first vein-graft trial (298) become extrapolated to catheter-based reperfusion.

THE FUTURE

Patients with acute ST-segment elevation MI continue to have a compromised prognosis with a relatively constant rate of death or reinfarction by 30 days at 9% to 10%. Today MI remains as the number-one killer in Western society. The intrinsic delays of approximately 2.7 hours from onset of symptoms to initiation of therapy appear to have been immutable since the 1990s. Prehospital administration of pharmacologic reperfusion is frequently used in Europe, but has not been incorporated in practice at most centers in the United States. Once extensive damage has occurred, it is particularly hard to change the natural history. The *Sh*ould We Emergently Revascularize *O*ccluded Coronaries for *C*ardiogenic Shoc*k*? (SHOCK) trial shows benefit for aggressive therapy, but a persistent poor prognosis for those patients with extensive myocardial necrosis.

On the encouraging side, the incidence of classic MI appears to be decreasing, and this trend will likely continue with the use of statins, aspirin, clopidogrel, and ACE inhibitors. But even with improved preventive therapies, we will still need to improve the outcomes of patients with acute MI.

For therapeutic advances, the use of emboli protection devices is attractive and will likely become commonplace. Likewise, the early results of coated stents to control the local inflammatory response will likely become standard. Better antiinflammatory agents, such as selectin or complement inhibitors, may also afford improved outcomes of acute MI, and a focus on lessening heart failure and survival over a longer-term window (1 year rather than 30 days) is likely. For this reason, the early work with stem cells (CD34 positive) is very exciting (299–303) and may ultimately restore human heart tissue. It will be a challenge to perform autologous bone marrow transplantation in the early hours of acute MI, but it is nevertheless intriguing for patient with extensive necrosis.

A big change in the future is likely to be affected by the unraveling of the human genome. Although this is unlikely to affect the actual care provided on an emergency basis for acute MI, the ability to provide better primary and secondary prevention will be greatly enhanced. Tailored therapy according to the specific genotypic variant will likely markedly amplify the efficacy and safety of our preventive therapies.

REFERENCES

1. Herrick JB. Clinical features of sudden obstruction of the coronary arteries. *JAMA* 1912;59:2015–2020.
2. Fye WB. A historical perspective on atherosclerosis and coronary artery disease. In: Fuster VRR, Topol EJ, ed. *Atherosclerosis and coronary artery disease.* Philadelphia: Lippincott–Raven, 1996:1–12.
3. Levine SA, ed. *Coronary thrombosis: its various clinical features.* Baltimore: Williams & Wilkins, 1929.
4. Fletcher AP, Alkjaersig N, Smyrniotis F, et al. The treatment of patients suffering from early myocardial infarction with massive and prolonged streptokinase therapy. *Trans Assoc Am Physicians* 1958;71:287–296.
5. Boucek RJ, Murphy WP. Segmental perfusion of the coronary arteries with fibrinolysis in man following a myocardial infarction. *Am J Cardiol* 1960;6:525–533.
6. Chazov EI, Mateeva LS, Mazaev AV, et al. Intracoronary administration of fibrinolysis in acute myocardial infarction. *Ter Arkh* 1976;48:8–19.
7. Rentrop P, Blanke H, Karsch KR, et al. Selective intracoronary thrombolysis in acute myocardial infarction and unstable angina pectoris. *Circulation* 1981;63:307–317.
8. DeWood MA, Spores J, Notske R, et al. Prevalence of total coronary occlusion during the early hours of transmural myocardial infarction. *N Engl J Med* 1980;303:897–902.
9. Hartzler GO, Rutherford BD, McConahay DR. Percutaneous transluminal coronary angioplasty: application for acute myocardial infarction. *Am J Cardiol* 1984;53:117C–121C.
10. Collen D, Topol EJ, Tiefenbrunn AJ, et al. Coronary thrombolysis with recombinant human tissue-type plasminogen activator: a prospective, randomized, placebo-controlled trial. *Circulation* 1984;68:1012–1017.
11. Schroder R, Biamino G, Leitner E-RV, et al. Intravenous short-term infusion of streptokinase in acute myocardial infarction. *Circulation* 1983;67:536–548.
12. Ganz W, Geft I, Shah PK, et al. Intravenous streptokinase in evolving acute myocardial infarction. *Am J Cardiol* 1984;53:1209–1216.
13. Gruppo Italiano per lo Studio della Streptochinasi nell'Infarto Miocardico (GISSI). Effectiveness of intravenous thrombolytic treatment in acute myocardial infarction. *Lancet* 1986;1:397–401.
14. Topol E. Which thrombolytic agent should one choose? *Prog Cardiovasc Dis* 1991;34:165–178.
15. Davies MJ, Treasure T, Richardson PD. The pathogenesis of spontaneous arterial dissection. *Heart* 1996;75:434–435.
16. Moreno PR, Bernardi VH, Lopez-Cuellar J, et al. Macrophages, smooth muscle cells, and tissue factor in unstable angina: implications for cell-mediated thrombogenicity in acute coronary syndromes. *Circulation* 1996;94:3090–3097.
17. Moreno PR, Falk E, Palacios IF, et al. Macrophage infiltration in acute coronary syndromes: implications for plaque rupture. *Circulation* 1994;90:775–778.
18. Libby P. Molecular basis of the acute coronary syndromes. *Circulation* 1995;91:2844–2850.
19. Scandinavian Simvastatin Survival Study Group. Randomized trial of cholesterol lowering in 4444 patients with coronary heart disease: the Scandinavian Simvastatin Survival Study (4S). *Lancet* 1994;344:1383–1389.
20. West of Scotland Coronary Prevention Group. Identification of high-risk groups and comparison with other cardiovascular interventional trials. *Lancet* 1996;348:1339–1342.
21. Sacks FM, Pfeffer MA, Moye LA, et al. The effect of pravastatin on coronary events after myocardial infarction in patients with average cholesterol levels. *N Engl J Med* 1996;335:1001–1009.
22. Vaughan CJ, Murphy MB, Buckley BM. Statins do more than just lower cholesterol. *Lancet* 1996;348:1079–1082.
23. Reimer KA, Jennings RB. The "wavefront phenomenon" of myocardial ischemic cell death. II. Transmural progression of necrosis within the framework of ischemic bed size (myocardium at risk) and collateral flow. *Lab Invest* 1979;40:633–644.
24. Falk E, Shah PK, Fuster V. Coronary plaque disruption. *Circulation* 1995;92:657–671.
25. Fuster V, Badimon L, Badimon JJ, et al. The pathogenesis of coronary artery disease and the acute coronary syndromes. *N Engl J Med* 1992;326:242–250, 310–318.
26. Falk E. Morphologic features of unstable atherothrombotic plaques underlying acute coronary syndromes. *Am J Cardiol* 1989;63:114E–120E.
27. Kono T, Morita H, Nishina T, et al. Circadian variations of onset of acute myocardial infarction and efficacy of thrombolytic therapy. *J Am Coll Cardiol* 1996;27:774–778.
28. Leor J, Poole WK, Kloner RA. Sudden cardiac death triggered by an earthquake. *N Engl J Med* 1996;334:413–419.
29. Meisel SR, Kutz I, Dayan KI, et al. Effect of Iraqi missile war on incidence of acute myocardial infarction and sudden death in Israeli civilians. *Lancet* 1991;338:660–661.
30. American Heart Association. Heart and stroke facts. *AHA 1996 Supplement.* Dallas, 1996:1–23.
31. Hunink MG, Goldman L, Tosteson ANA, et al. The recent decline in mortality from coronary heart disease, 1980–1990. *JAMA* 1997;277:535–542.
32. European Secondary Prevention Study Group. Translation of clinical trials into practice: a European population-based study of the use of thrombolysis for acute myocardial infarction. *Lancet* 1996;347:1203–1207.
33. Jha P, Deboer D, Sykora K, et al. Characteristics and mortality outcomes of thrombolysis trial participants and non-participants: a population-based comparison. *J Am Coll Cardiol* 1996;27:1335–1342.
34. Brown MS, Goldstein JL. Heart attacks: gone with the century. *Science* 1996;272:629.
35. McGovern PG, Pankow JS, Shahar E, et al. Recent trends in acute coronary heart disease: mortality, morbidity, medical care, and risk factors. *N Engl J Med* 1996;334:884–890.
36. Paul SD, O'Gara PT, Mahjoub ZA, et al. Geriatric patients with acute myocardial infarction: cardiac risk factor profiles, presentation, thrombolysis, coronary interventions, and prognosis. *Am Heart J* 1996;131:710–715.
37. Cragg DR, Friedman HZ, Bonema JD, et al. Outcome of patients with acute myocardial infarction who are ineligible for thrombolytic therapy. *Ann Intern Med* 1991;115:173–177.

38. Pfeffer MA, Moye LA, Braunwald E, et al. Selection bias in the use of thrombolytic therapy in acute myocardial infarction. *JAMA* 1991;266:528–532.

38a. Beaglehole R. Global cardiovascular disease prevention: time to get serious. *Lancet* 2001;358:661–663.

39. Puleo PR, Meyer D, Wathen C, et al. Use of a rapid assay of subforms of creatine kinase MB to diagnose or rule out acute myocardial infarction. *N Engl J Med* 1994;331:561–566.

40. Antman EM, Grudzien C, Sacks DB. Evaluation of a rapid bedside assay for detection of serum cardiac troponin T. *JAMA* 1995;273:1279–1282.

41. Ravkilde J, Nissen H, Horder M, et al. Independent prognostic value of serum creatinine kinase isoenzyme MB mass, cardiac troponin T and myosin light chain levels in suspected acute myocardial infarction. *J Am Coll Cardiol* 1995;25:574–581.

42. Antman EM, Tanasijevic MJ, Thompson B, et al. Cardiac-specific troponin levels to predict the risk of mortality in patients with acute coronary syndromes. *N Engl J Med* 1996;335:1342–1349.

43. Ohman EM, Armstrong PW, Christenson RH, et al. for the GUSTO-IIa Investigators. Risk stratification with admission cardiac troponin T levels in acute myocardial ischemia. *N Engl J Med* 1996;335:1333–1341.

44. Christensen RH, Ohman EM, Topol EJ, et al. Assessment of coronary reperfusion after thrombolysis with a model containing myoglobin, creatine kinase-MB, and clinical variables. *Circulation* 1997;96:1776-1782.

45. Bairey CN, Shah PK, Lew AS, et al. Electrocardiographic differentiation of occlusion of the left circumflex versus the right coronary artery as a cause of inferior acute myocardial infarction. *Am J Cardiol* 1987;60:456–459.

46. Peterson ED, Hathaway WR, Zabel KM, et al. Prognostic significance of precordial ST segment depression during inferior myocardial infarction in the thrombolytic era: results in 16,521 patients. *J Am Coll Cardiol* 1996;28:305–312.

47. Schroder R, Dissmann R, Bruggemann T, et al. Extent of early ST segment elevation resolution: a simple but strong predictor of outcome in patients with acute myocardial infarction. *J Am Coll Cardiol* 1994;24:384–391.

48. Schroder R, Wegscheider K, Schroeder K, et al. For the INJECT Trial Group. Extent of early ST-segment elevation resolution: a simple but strong predictor of outcome in patients with acute myocardial infarction and a sensitive measure to compare thrombolytic regimens. A substudy of the International Joint Efficacy Comparison of Thrombolytics (INJECT) Trial. *J Am Coll Cardiol* 1995;26:1657–1664.

49. Zeymer U, Schroder R, Tebbe U, et al. Non-invasive detection of early infarct vessel patency by resolution of ST-segment elevation in patients with thrombolysis for acute myocardial infarction. *Eur Heart J* 2001;22:769–775.

50. The GUSTO-III Investigators. An international, multicenter, randomized comparison of reteplase with alteplase for acute myocardial infarction. *N Engl J Med* 1997;337:1118–1123.

51. de Lemos JA, Antman EM, Giugliana RP, et al. for the TIMI 14 Investigators. ST segment resolution and infarct-related artery patency and flow after thrombolytic therapy. *Am J Cardiol* 2000;85:299–304.

52. de Lemos JA, Antman EM, Giugliano RP, et al., for the InTIME-II Investigators. Very early risk stratification after thrombolytic therapy with a bedside myoglobin assay and the 12-lead electrocardiogram. *Am Heart J* 2000;140:373–378.

53. Claeys MJ, Bosmans J, Veenstra L, et al. Determinants and prognostic implications of persistent ST-segment elevation after primary angioplasty for acute myocardial infarction: importance of microvascular injury on clinical outcome. *Circulation* 1999;99:1972–1977.

54. Schechtman KB, Capone RJ, Kleiger RE, et al. Risk stratification of patients with non-Q wave myocardial infarction. *Circulation* 1989;80:1148–1158.

55. Moliterno DJ, Sgarbossa EB, Armstrong PW, et al. A major dichotomy in unstable angina outcome: ST depression versus T-wave inversion: GUSTO II results. *J Am Coll Cardiology* 1996;27:182A(abstr).

56. Killip T, Kimball JT. Treatment of myocardial infarction in a coronary unit: a two-year experience with 250 patients. *Am J Cardiol* 1967;20:457–464.

57. Lee KL, Woodlief L, Topol EJ, et al. Predictors of 30-day mortality in the era of reperfusion for acute myocardial infarction: results from an international trial of 41,021 patients. *Circulation* 1995;91:1659–1668.

58. Roberts R, Rogers WJ, Mueller HS, et al. Immediate versus deferred β-blockade following thrombolytic therapy in patients with acute myocardial infarction. Results of the Thrombolysis in Myocardial Infarction (TIMI) II-B Study. *Circulation* 1991;83:422–437.

59. ISIS-2 (Second international study of infarct survival) Collaborative Group. Randomized trial of intravenous streptokinase, oral aspirin, both, or neither among 17,187 cases of suspected acute myocardial infarction. *Lancet* 1988;11:349–360.

60. Cairns JA, Gent M, Singer J, et al. Aspirin, sulfinpyrazone, or both in unstable angina: results of a Canadian multicenter trial. *N Engl J Med* 1985;313:1369–1375.

61. Lewis HDJ, Davis JW, Archibald DG, et al. Protective effects of aspirin against acute myocardial infarction and death in men with unstable angina: results of a Veterans Administration Cooperative Study. *N Engl J Med* 1983;309:396–403.

62. Theroux P, Ouimet H, McCans J, et al. Aspirin, heparin, or both to treat acute unstable angina. *N Engl J Med* 1988;319:1105–1111.

63. CURE Trial Investigators. Effects of clopidogrel in addition to aspirin in preventing major vascular events in patients with non-ST elevation acute coronary syndromes. *N Engl J Med* 2001 (*in press*).

64. Muller DWM, Topol EJ. Selection of patients with acute myocardial infarction for thrombolytic therapy. *Ann Intern Med* 1990;113:949–960.

65. Fibrinolytic therapy trialists' (FTT) collaborative group. Indications for fibrinolytic therapy in suspected acute myocardial infarction: collaborative overview of early mortality and major morbidity results from all randomized trials of more than 1000 patients. *Lancet* 1994;343:311–322.

66. Sgarbossa E, Pinski SL, Barbagelata A, et al. Electrocardiographic diagnosis of acute myocardial infarction in the presence of left bundle branch block. *N Engl J Med* 1996;334:481–487.

67. AIMS Trial Study Group. Effect of intravenous APSAC on mortality after acute myocardial infarction: preliminary report of a placebo-controlled clinical trial. *Lancet* 1988;1:545–549.

68. Wilcox RG, von der Lippe G, Olsson CG, et al. Trial of tissue plasminogen activator for mortality reduction in acute myocardial infarction (ASSET). *Lancet* 1988;2:525–530.

69. The ISAM Study Group. A prospective trial of intravenous streptokinase in acute myocardial infarction (ISAM). Mortality, morbidity, and infarct size at 21 days. *N Engl J Med* 1986;314:1465–1471.

70. Rossi P, Bolognese L, on behalf of Urochinasi per via Sistemica nell'Infarto Miocardio (USIM) Collaborative Group. Comparison of intravenous urokinase plus heparin versus heparin alone in acute myocardial infarction. *Am J Cardiol* 1991;68:585–592.

71. ISIS (International Studies of Infarct Survival) Pilot Study Investigators. Randomized factorial trial of high-dose intravenous streptokinase, of oral aspirin and of intravenous heparin in acute myocardial infarction. *Eur Heart J* 1987;8:634–642.

72. Granger CB, Califf RM, Topol EJ. Thrombolytic therapy for acute myocardial infarction, a review. *Drugs* 1992;44:293–325.

73. The International Study Group. In-hospital mortality and clinical course of 20,891 patients with suspected acute myocardial infarction randomized between alteplase and streptokinase with or without heparin. *Lancet* 1990;336:71–75.

74. Gruppo Italiano Per Lo Studio Della Sopravvivenza Nell'Infarto Miocardico. GISSI-2: a factorial randomized trial of alteplase versus streptokinase and heparin versus no heparin among 12,490 patients with acute myocardial infarction. *Lancet* 1990;336:65–71.

75. Lincoff AM, Topol EJ. The illusion of reperfusion. Does anyone achieve optimal myocardial reperfusion? *Circulation* 1993;87:1792–1805, and 88:1361–1374.

76. Boersma E, Maas AC, Deckers JW, et al. Early thrombolytic treatment in acute myocardial infarction: reappraisal of the golden hour. *Lancet* 1996;348:771–775.

77. Weaver WD, Cerqueira M, Hallstrom AP, et al. Prehospital-initiated vs hospital-initiated thrombolytic therapy. *JAMA* 1993;270:1211–1216.

78. LATE Study Group. Late assessment of thrombolytic efficacy (LATE) study with alteplase 6–24 hours after onset of acute myocardial infarction. *Lancet* 1993;342:759–766.

79. Estudio Multicentrico Estreptoquinasa Republicas de Americas del Sur (EMERAS). Randomized trial of late thrombolysis in patients with suspected acute myocardial infarction. *Lancet* 1993;342:767–772.

80. The European Myocardial Infarction Project Group. Prehospital thrombolytic therapy in patients with suspected acute myocardial infarction. *N Engl J Med* 1993;329:383–389.

81. Trent R, Adams J, Rawles J, on behalf of the GREAT Group. Electrocardiographic evidence of reperfusion occurring before hospital admission. A Grampian Region Early Anistreplase Trial (GREAT) sub-study. *Eur Heart J* 1994;15:895–897.

82. Rawles J. Halving of mortality at 1 year by domiciliary thrombolysis in the Grampian region early anistreplase trial (GREAT). *J Am Coll Cardiol* 1994;23:1–5.

83. Rawles J. Magnitude of benefit from earlier thrombolytic treatment in acute myocardial infarction: new evidence of Grampian region early anistreplase trial (GREAT). *BMJ* 1996;312:212–215.

84. (Belgian Eminase Prehospital Study) BEPS Collaborative Group. Prehospital thrombolysis in acute myocardial infarction: the Belgian Eminase Prehospital Study. *Eur Heart J* 1991;12:965–967.

85. Brouwer MA, Martin JS, Maynard C, et al. Influence of early prehospital thrombolysis on mortality and event-free survival (The Myocardial Infarction Triage and Intervention—MITI—Randomized Trial). *Am J Cardiol* 1996;78:497–502.

86. Every NR, Weaver WD. Prehospital treatment of myocardial infarction. *Curr Probl Cardiol* 1995;20:1–52.

87. Rogers WJ, Bowlby LJ, Chandra NC, et al. Treatment of myocardial infarction in the United States (1990 to 1993). Observations from the National Registry of Myocardial Infarction. *Circulation* 1994;90:2103–2114.

88. ISIS-3 (Third International Study of Infarct Survival) Collaborative Group. ISIS-3: a randomized comparison of streptokinase vs tissue plasminogen activator vs anistreplase and of aspirin plus heparin vs aspirin among 41,299 cases of suspected acute myocardial infarction. *Lancet* 1992;339:753–770.

89. The GUSTO Investigators. An international randomized trial comparing four thrombolytic strategies for acute myocardial infarction. *N Engl J Med* 1993;329:1615–1622.

90. Mark DB, Hlatky MA, Califf RM, et al. Cost effectiveness of thrombolytic therapy with tissue plasminogen activator as compared with streptokinase for acute myocardial infarction. *N Engl J Med* 1995;332:1418–1424.

91. Collen D. Synergism of thrombolytic agents: investigational procedures and clinical potential. *Circulation* 1988;77:731–735.

92. Larsen GR, Henson K, Blue Y. Variants of human tissue-type plasminogen activator. *J Biol Chem* 1988;263:1023–1029.

93. Gheysen D, Lijnen HR, Pierard L, et al. Characterization of a recombinant fusion protein of the finger domain of tissue-type plasminogen activator with a truncated single chain urokinase-type plasminogen activator. *J Biol Chem* 1987;262:11779–11784.

94. Pannekoek H, de Vries C, van Zonneveld A. Mutants of human tissue-type plasminogen activator (t-PA): structural aspects and functional properties. *Fibrinolysis* 1988;2:123–132.

95. Jackson CV, Crowe VG, Craft TJ, et al. Thrombolytic activity of a novel plasminogen activator, LY210825, compared with recombinant tissue-type plasminogen activator in a canine model of coronary artery thrombosis. *Circulation* 1990;82:930–940.

96. Martin U, Sponer G, Strein K. Evaluation of thrombolytic and systemic effects of the novel recombinant plasminogen

activator BM 06.022 compared with alteplase, anistreplase, streptokinase and urokinase in a canine model of coronary artery thrombosis. *J Am Coll Cardiol* 1992;19:433–440.

97. Neuhaus K-L, von Essen R, Vogt A, et al. Dose finding with a novel recombinant plasminogen activator (BM 06.022) in patients with acute myocardial infarction: results of the German recombinant plasminogen activator study. *J Am Coll Cardiol* 1994;24:55–60.

98. Witt W, Maass B, Baldus B, et al. Coronary thrombolysis with Desmodus salivary plasminogen activator in dogs. *Circulation* 1994;90:421–426.

99. Rijken DC, Groeneveld E, Barrett-Bergshoeff MM. In vitro stability of a tissue-type plasminogen activator mutant, BM 06.022, in human plasma. *Thromb Haemost* 1994;72:906–911.

100. Mellott MJ, Ramjit DR, Stabilito II, et al. Vampire bat salivary plasminogen activator evokes minimal bleeding relative to tissue-type plasminogen activator as assessed by a rabbit cuticle bleeding time model. *Thromb Haemost* 1995;73:478–483.

101. Verstraete M, Lijnen HR, Collen D. Thrombolytic agents in development. *Drugs* 1995;50:29–42.

102. Benedict CR, Refino CJ, Keyt BA, et al. New variant of human tissue plasminogen activator (TPA) with enhanced efficacy and lower incidence of bleeding compared with recombinant human TPA. *Circulation* 1995;92:3032–3040.

103. Smalling RW, Bode C, Kalbfleisch J, et al. More rapid, complete, and stable coronary thrombolysis with bolus administration of reteplase compared with alteplase infusion in acute myocardial infarction. *Circulation* 1995;91:2725–2732.

104. Bode C, Smalling RW, Berg G, et al. Randomized comparison of coronary thrombolysis achieved with double-bolus reteplase (recombinant plasminogen activator) and front-loaded, accelerated alteplase (recombinant tissue plasminogen activator) in patients with acute myocardial infarction. *Circulation* 1996;94:891–898.

105. International Joint Efficacy Comparison of Thrombolytics. Randomised, double-blind comparison of reteplase double-bolus administration with streptokinase in acute myocardial infarction (INJECT): trial to investigate equivalence. *Lancet* 1995;346:329–336.

106. ASSENT-2 Investigators (Assessment of the Safety and Efficacy of a New Thrombolytic). Single-bolus tenecteplase compared with front-loaded alteplase in acute myocardial infarction: the ASSENT-2 double-blind randomized trial. *Lancet* 1999;354:716–722.

107. Vanderschueren S, Barrios L, Kerdsinchai P, et al. A randomized trial of recombinant staphylokinase versus alteplase for coronary artery patency in acute myocardial infarction. *Circulation* 1995;92:2044–2049.

108. Collen D, Lijnen HR. Staphylokinase, a fibrin-specific plasminogen activator with therapeutic potential. *Blood* 1994;84:680–686.

109. Collen D, Bernaerts R, Declerck P, et al. Recombinant staphylokinase variants with altered immunoreactivity: I: construction and characterization. *Circulation* 1996;94:197–206.

110. The PRIMI study group. Randomized double-blind trial of recombinant prourokinase against streptokinase in acute myocardial infarction. *Lancet* 1989;1:863–869.

111. The GUSTO Angiographic Investigators. The effects of tissue plasminogen activator, streptokinase, or both on coronary-artery patency, ventricular function, and survival after acute myocardial infarction. *N Engl J Med* 1993;329:1615–1622.

112. Califf RM, White HD, Van de Werf F, et al. One-year results from the Global Utilization of Streptokinase and TPA for Occluded Coronary Arteries (GUSTO-I) Trial. *Circulation* 1996;94:1233–1238.

113. Genentech Activase growth slowed by shrinking thrombolytics market, firm says: Pfizer Zithromax sales up 75% on severe flu season, new indications. *F-D-C Reports— "The Pink Sheet"* 1997:9–10.

114. Migrino RQ, Young JB, Ellis SG, et al. End-systolic volume index at 90–180 minutes into reperfusion therapy for acute myocardial infarction is a strong predictor of early and late mortality. *Circulation* 1997;96:116–121.

115. Kleiman NS, White, Ohman EM, et al. Mortality within 24 hours of thrombolysis for myocardial infarction: the importance of early reperfusion. *Circulation* 1994;90:2658–2666.

116. White HD, Norris RM, Brown MA, et al. Left ventricular end-systolic volume as the major determinant of survival after recovery from myocardial infarction. *Circulation* 1987;76:44–51.

117. Jeremy RW, Hackworthy RA, Bautovich G, et al. Infarct artery perfusion and changes in left ventricular volume in the month after acute myocardial infarction. *J Am Coll Cardiol* 1987;9:989–995.

118. Simes RJ, Topol EJ, Holmes DR, et al. The link between the angiographic substudy and mortality outcomes in a large randomized trial of myocardial reperfusion: the importance of early and complete infarct artery reperfusion. *Circulation* 1995;91:1923–1928.

119. GUSTO II Angioplasty Substudy Investigators. An international randomized trial of 1138 patients comparing primary coronary angioplasty versus tissue plasminogen activator for acute myocardial infarction. *N Engl J Med* 1997;336:1621–1628.

120. Grines CL, Browne KF, Marco J, et al. A comparison of immediate angioplasty with thrombolytic therapy for acute myocardial infarction. *N Engl J Med* 1993;328:673–679.

121. Zijlstra F, Jan De Boer M, Hoorntje CA, et al. A comparison of immediate coronary angioplasty with intravenous streptokinase in acute myocardial infarction. *N Engl J Med* 1993;328:680–684.

122. Gibbons RJ, Holmes DR, Reeder GS, et al. Immediate angioplasty compared with the administration of a thrombolytic agent followed by conservative treatment for myocardial infarction. *N Engl J Med* 1993;328:685–691.

123. Ribeiro EE, Silva LA, Carneiro R, et al. Randomized trial of direct coronary angioplasty versus intravenous streptokinase in acute myocardial infarction. *J Am Coll Cardiol* 1993;22:376–380.

124. Elizaga J, Garcia EJ, Bueno H, et al. Primary coronary angioplasty versus systemic thrombolysis in acute anterior

myocardial infarction: in-hospital results from a prospective randomized trial. *Eur Heart J* 1993;14:118(abstr).

125. Dewood MA. Direct PTCA vs. intravenous t-PA in acute myocardial infarction: results from a prospective randomized trial. Thrombolysis and Interventional Therapy in Acute Myocardial Infarction Symposium IV, George Washington University, 1990.

126. Grinfeld L, Berrocal D, Belardi J, et al. Fibrinolytics vs. primary angioplasty in acute myocardial infarction (FAP): randomized trial in a community in Argentina. *J Am Coll Cardiol* 1996;27:222A(abstr).

127. Ribichini F, Steffenino G, Dellavalle A, et al. Primary angioplasty versus thrombolysis in inferior acute myocardial infarction with anterior ST-segment depression: a single-center randomized study. *J Am Coll Cardiol* 1996;27:221A(abstr).

128. Mark D, for the GUSTO-IIb Investigators. Costs of PTCA versus thrombolysis in the GUSTO IIb trial. Presented at the American Heart Association (AHA), New Orleans, November 1996.

129. Saito S, Hosokawa G. Primary Palmaz-Schatz stent implantation for acute myocardial infarction: the final results of the Japanese PASTA (Primary Angioplasty vs Stent Implantation in AMI in Japan) trial. *Circulation* 1997;96:I-595(abstr).

130. Suryapranata H, van't Hof AWJ, Hoorntje JCA, et al. Randomized comparison of coronary stenting with balloon angioplasty in selected patients with acute myocardial infarction. *Circulation* 1998;97:2502–2505.

131. Grines CL, Cox DA, Stone GW, et al., for the Stent Primary Angioplasty in Myocardial Infarction Study Group. Coronary angioplasty with or without stent implantation for acute myocardial infarction. *N Engl J Med* 1999;341:1949–1956.

132. Maillard L, Hamon M, Monassier J-P, et al., Investigators STENTIM 2. Six months angiographic results. Elective Wiktor stent implantation in acute myocardial infarction compared with balloon angioplasty. *Circulation* 1998;98:I-21.

133. Kawashima A, Ueda K, Nishida Y, et al. Quantitative angiographic analysis of restenosis of primary stenting using Wiktor stent for acute myocardial infarction: results from a multicenter randomized PRISM Study. *Circulation* 1998;98:I-153.

134. Rodriguez A, Bernardi V, Fernandez M, et al., on behalf of the GRAMI Investigators. In-hospital and late results of coronary stents versus conventional balloon angioplasty in acute myocardial infarction (GRAMI trial). *Am J Cardiol* 1998;81:1286–1291.

135. Antoniucci D, Santoro GM, Bolognese L, et al. A clinical trial comparing primary stenting of the infarct-related artery with optimal primary angioplasty for acute myocardial infarction. Results from the Florence Randomized Elective Stenting in Acute Coronary Occlusions (FRESCO) trial. *J Am Coll Cardiol* 1998;31:1234–1239.

136. Jacksch R, Niehues R, Knobloch W. PTCA versus stenting in acute myocardial infarction: single centre prospective randomized trial. *Eur Heart J* 1998;19:239(abstr).

137. Steinhubl S, Topol EJ. Primary angioplasty and stenting in acute MI. In: Topol EJ, ed. *Acute coronary syndromes*, 2nd ed. New York: Marcel Dekker, 2001:373–390.

138. Schomig A, Kastrati A, Dirschinger J, et al. Coronary stenting plus platelet glycoprotein IIb/IIIa blockade compared with tissue plasminogen activator in acute myocardial infarction. *N Engl J Med* 2000;343:385–391.

139. Stone GW. Stenting and IIb/IIIa receptor blockade in acute myocardial infarction: final results of the CADILLAC Trial. American Heart Association (AHA), November 2000.

140. Every NR, Parsons LS, Hlatky M, et al. For the Myocardial Infarction Triage and Intervention Investigators: a comparison of thrombolytic therapy with primary coronary angioplasty for acute myocardial infarction. *N Engl J Med* 1996;335:1253–1260.

141. Rogers WJ, Dean LS, Moore PB, et al. Comparison of primary angioplasty versus thrombolytic therapy for acute myocardial infarction. *Am J Cardiol* 1994;74:111–118.

142. Tiefenbrunn AJ, Chandra NC, French WJ, et al. Clinical experience with primary PTCA compared with alteplase (recombinant tissue-type plasminogen activator) in patients with acute myocardial infarction. A report from the Second National Registry of Myocardial Infarction (NRMI 2). *J Am Coll Cardiol* 1998;31:1240-1245.

143. Cannon CP, Braunwald E. Time to reperfusion: the critical modulator in thrombolysis and primary angioplasty. *J Thromb Thrombol* 1996;3:117–125.

144. Topol EJ. Mechanical interventions for acute myocardial infarction. In: Topol EJ, ed. *Textbook of interventional cardiology.* Vol 1. Philadelphia: WB Saunders, 1994:292–317.

145. DeFranco A, Abramowitz B, Krichbaum D, et al., for the GUSTO Investigators. Substantial (three-fold) benefit of accelerated t-PA over standard thrombolytic therapy in patients with prior bypass surgery and acute MI: results of the GUSTO trial. *J Am Coll Cardiol* 1994;23:355A(abstr).

146. Holmes DR, Bates ER, Kleiman NS, et al. Contemporary reperfusion therapy for cardiogenic shock: the GUSTO I trial experience. *J Am Coll Cardiol* 1995;26:668–674.

147. Holmes DR, Califf RM, Van de Werf F, et al. Difference in countries use of resources and clinical outcome in patients with cardiogenic shock after myocardial infarction: results from the GUSTO trial. *Lancet* 1997;349:75–78.

148. Prewitt RM, Downes AMT, Gu S, et al. Effects of hydralazine and increased cardiac output on recombinant tissue plasminogen activator-induced thrombolysis in canine pulmonary embolism. *Chest* 1991;99:708–714.

149. Granger CB, Hirsh J, Califf RM, et al. Activated partial thromboplastin time and outcome after thrombolytic therapy for acute myocardial infarction. *Circulation* 1996;93:870–878.

149a. Ryan TJ, Antman EM, Brooks NH, et al. 1999 update: ACC/AHA guidelines for the management of patients with acute myocardial infarction: executive summary and recommendations: a report of the American College of Cardiology/American Heart Association Task Force on Practice Guidelines (Committee on Management of Acute Myocardial Infarction). *Circulation* 1999;100:1016–1030.

150. Hsia J, Hamilton WP, Kleiman N, et al. A comparison between heparin and low-dose aspirin as adjunctive therapy with tissue plasminogen activator for acute myocardial infarction. *N Engl J Med* 1990;323:1433–1437.

151. Thompson PL, Aylward PE, Federman J, et al. A randomized comparison of intravenous heparin with oral aspirin and dipyridamole 24 hours after recombinant tissue-type plasminogen activator for acute myocardial infarction. *Circulation* 1991;83:1534–1542.

152. de Bono DP, Simoons JL, Tijssen J, et al. Effect of early intravenous heparin on coronary patency, infarct size, and bleeding complications after alteplase thrombolysis: results of a randomized double blind European Cooperative Study Group trial. *Br Heart J* 1992;67:122–128.

153. Bleich SD, Nichols TC, Schumacher RR, et al. Effect of heparin on coronary arterial patency after thrombolysis with tissue plasminogen activator in acute myocardial infarction. *Am J Cardiol* 1990;66:1412–1417.

154. O'Connor CM, Meese R, Carney R, et al. A randomized trial of intravenous heparin in conjunction with anistreplase (anisoylated plasminogen streptokinase activator complex) in acute myocardial infarction: the Duke University clinical cardiology study (DUCCS) 1. *J Am Coll Cardiol* 1994;23:11–18.

155. White HD, Yusuf S. Issues regarding the use of heparin following streptokinase therapy. *J Thromb Thrombol* 1995;2:5–10.

156. Mahaffey KW, Granger CB, Collins R, et al. Overview of randomized trials of intravenous heparin in patients with acute myocardial infarction treated with thrombolytic therapy. *Am J Cardiol* 1996;77:551–556.

157. Collins R, MacMahon S, Flather M, et al. Clinical effects of anticoagulant therapy in suspected acute myocardial infarction: systematic overview of randomised trials. *BMJ* 1996;313:652–659.

158. Metz BK, Granger CB, White HD, et al. Streptokinase and hirudin reduces death and reinfarction in acute myocardial infarction compared with streptokinase and heparin: results from GUSTO IIb. *Circulation* 1996;94:I430.

159. Ellis CJ, French JK, Williams BF, et al. Thrombolytic therapy can be given to half of hospitalized patients with acute myocardial infarction. *J Am Coll Cardiol* 1996;27:249A.

160. Gore JM, Granger CB, Simoons ML, et al. Stroke after thrombolysis: mortality and functional outcomes in the GUSTO-I trial. *Circulation* 1995;92:2811–2818.

161. Neuhaus KL. More on thrombolysis and hemorrhagic stroke. *Circulation* 1995;92:2794–2795.

162. Mahaffey KW, Granger CB, Sloan MA, et al. Risk factors for in-hospital nonhemorrhagic stroke in patients with acute myocardial infarction treated with thrombolysis: results from GUSTO-I. *Circulation* 1998;97:7575–7576.

163. Illingworth RD. Burr holes, trephine, and craniotomy. In: Dudley H, Carter D, Russell RCG, eds. *Operative surgery: neurosurgery.* London: Butterworth, 1989:12–29.

164. White H, Barbash GI, Califf RM, et al. Age and outcome with contemporary thrombolytic therapy: results from the GUSTO trial. *Circulation* 1996;94:1826–1833.

165. Topol EJ, Califf RM. Thrombolytic therapy for elderly patients. *N Engl J Med* 1992;327:45–46.

166. Califf RM, Topol EJ, George BS, et al. Hemorrhagic complications associated with the use of intravenous tissue plasminogen activator in treatment of acute myocardial infarction. *Am J Med* 1988;85:353–359.

167. ISIS-1 (First International Study of Infarct Survival) Collaborative Study. Randomized trial of intravenous atenolol among 16,027 cases of suspected acute myocardial infarction: ISIS-1. *Lancet* 1986;2:57–65.

168. ISIS-1 (First International Study of Infarct Survival) Collaborative Group. Mechanisms for the early mortality reduction produced by beta-blockade started early in acute myocardial infarction: ISIS-1. *Lancet* 1988;1:823–921.

169. Jang I, van de Werf F, Vanhaecke J, et al. Coronary reperfusion by thrombolysis and early beta-adrenergic blockade in acute experimental myocardial infarction. *J Am Coll Cardiol* 1989;14:1816–1823.

170. Viskin S, Barron HV. Beta blockers prevent cardiac death following a myocardial infarction: so why are so many infarct survivors discharged without beta blockers? *Am J Cardiol* 1996;78:821–822.

171. Yusuf S, Peto R, Lewis J, et al. Beta blockade during and after myocardial infarction: an overview of the randomized trials. *Prog Cardiovasc Dis* 1985;27:335–371.

172. The MIAMI Trial Research Group. Metoprolol in acute myocardial infarction: patient population. *Am J Cardiol* 1985;56:1G–57G.

173. Conti CR. Beta-adrenergic blockade and acute myocardial infarction. *J Am Coll Cardiol* 1989;14:1824–1825.

174. Soumerai SB, McLaughlin TJ, Spiegelman D, et al. Adverse outcomes of underuse of β-blockers in elderly survivors of acute myocardial infarction. *JAMA* 1997;277:115–121.

175. Van de Werf F, Janssens L, Brzostek T, et al. Short-term effects of early intravenous treatment with a beta-adrenergic blocking agent or a specific bradycardiac agent in patients with acute myocardial infarction receiving thrombolytic therapy. *J Am Coll Cardiol* 1993;22:407–416.

175a. Brener SJ, Cox JL, Pfisterer ME, Armstrong PW, et al., for the GUSTO Investigators. The potential for unexpected hazard of intravenous beta-blockade for acute myocardial infarction: results from the GUSTO trial. *J Am Coll Cardiol* 1995;25:5A(abstr).

176. Yusuf S, Collins R, MacMahon S, et al. Effect of intravenous nitrates on mortality in acute myocardial infarction: an overview of the randomized trials. *Lancet* 1988;1:1088–1092.

177. Yusuf S, Wittes J, Friedman L. Overview of results of randomized clinical trials in heart disease. Treatments following myocardial infarction. *JAMA* 1988;260:2088–2093.

178. ISIS-4 (Fourth International Study of Infarct Survival) Collaborative Group. ISIS-4: a randomised factorial trial assessing early oral captopril, oral mononitrate, and intravenous magnesium sulphate in 58,050 patients with suspected acute myocardial infarction. *Lancet* 1995;345:669–685.

179. Gruppo Italiano per lo Studio della Sopravvivenza nell'Infarto Miocardico. GISSI-3: effects of lisinopril and transdermal glyceryl trinitrate singly and together on 6-week mortality and ventricular function after acute myocardial infarction. *Lancet* 1994;343:1115–1122.

180. Kober L, Torp-Pedersen C, Carlsen JE, et al. A clinical trial of the angiotensin-converting enzyme inhibitor trandolapril in patients with left ventricular dysfunction after myocardial infarction. *N Engl J Med* 1995;333:1670–1676.

181. Ambrosioni E, Borghi C, Magnani B. The effect of the angiotensin-converting enzyme inhibitor zofenopril on

mortality and morbidity after anterior myocardial infarction. *N Engl J Med* 1995;332:80–85.

182. Chinese cardiac study collaborative group. Oral captopril versus placebo among 13,634 patients with suspected acute myocardial infarction: interim report from the Chinese Cardiac Study (CCS-1). *Lancet* 1995;345:686–687.

183. The HOPE Study Investigators. Effects of an angiotensin-converting-enzyme inhibitor, ramipril, on cardiovascular events in high-risk patients. *N Engl J Med* 2000;342:145–153.

184. Vantrimpont P, Rouleau JL, Chuan-Chuan W, et al. Additive beneficial effects of beta-blockers to angiotensin-converting enzyme inhibitors in the survival and ventricular enlargement (SAVE) study. *J Am Coll Cardiol* 1997;29:229–236.

185. Goldbourt U, Behar S, Reicher-Reiss H, et al. Early administration of nifedipine in suspected acute myocardial infarction: the Secondary Prevention Reinfarction Israel Nifedipine Trial 2 Study. *Arch Intern Med* 1993;153:345–353.

186. Wilcox RG, Hampton JR, Banks DC, et al. Trial of early nifedipine in acute myocardial infarction: the TRENT study. *BMJ* 1986;293:1204–1208.

187. Furberg CD, Psaty BM, Mayer JV. Nifedipine: dose-related increase in mortality in patients with coronary heart disease. *Circulation* 1995;92:1326–1331.

188. The Israeli Sprint Study Group. Secondary Prevention Reinfarction Israeli Nifedipine Trial (SPRINT): a randomized intervention trial of nifedipine in patients with acute myocardial infarction. *Eur Heart J* 1988;9:354–364.

189. Muller JE, Morrison J, Stone PH, et al. Nifedipine therapy for patients with threatened and acute myocardial infarction: a randomized, double-blind, placebo-controlled comparison. *Circulation* 1984;69:740–747.

190. Sirnes PA, Overskeid K, Pedersen TR, et al. Evolution of infarct size during the early use of nifedipine in patients with acute myocardial infarction: the Norwegian Nifedipine Multicenter Trial. *Circulation* 1984;70:638–644.

191. Roberts WC. The underused miracle drugs: the statin drugs are to atherosclerosis what penicillin was to infectious disease. *Am J Cardiol* 1996;78:377–378.

192. Anderson TJ, Meredith IT, Yeung AC, et al. The effect of cholesterol-lowering and antioxidant therapy on endothelium-dependent coronary vasomotion. *N Engl J Med* 1995;332:488–493.

193. Treasure CB, Klein JL, Weintraub WS, et al. Beneficial effects of cholesterol-lowering therapy on the coronary endothelium in patients with coronary artery disease. *N Engl J Med* 1995;332:481–487.

194. Levine GN, Keaney JF, Vita JA. Cholesterol reduction in cardiovascular disease. *N Engl J Med* 1995;332:512–521.

195. MacMahon S, Collins R, Peto R, et al. Effects of prophylactic lidocaine in suspected acute myocardial infarction. An overview of results from the randomized, controlled trials. *JAMA* 1988;260:1910–1916.

196. Alexander JH, Granger CB, Sadowski Z, et al., for the GUSTO-I and GUSTO IIb Investigators. Prophylactic lidocaine in acute myocardial infarction: incidence and outcomes from two international acute myocardial infarction trials. *Circulation* 1996;94[Suppl 1]:I-197(abstr).

197. Ward SR, Crenshaw BS, Stebbins AL, for the GUSTO Trial Investigators. Atrial fibrillation after thrombolysis denotes more extensive coronary artery disease and increased likelihood of reperfusion failure. *Circulation* 1995;92:I-777(abstr).

198. Crenshaw BS, Ward SR, Stebbins AL, et al. Risk factors and outcomes in patients with atrial fibrillation following acute myocardial infarction. *Circulation* 1995;92:I-177(abstr).

199. Goldberg RJ, Seeley D, Becker RC, et al. Impact of atrial fibrillation on the in-hospital and long-term survival of patients with acute myocardial infarction: a community-wide perspective. *Am Heart J* 1990;119:996–1001.

200. Behar S, Zahavi Z, Goldbourt U, et al. Long-term prognosis of patients with paroxysmal atrial fibrillation complicating acute myocardial infarction: SPRINT Study Group. *Eur Heart J* 1992;13:45–50.

201. Ryan TJ, Anderson JL, Antman EM, et al. ACC/AHA guidelines for the management of patients with acute myocardial infarction. *J Am Coll Cardiol* 1996;28:1328–1428.

202. Wood MA. Temporary transvenous pacing. In: Ellenbogen KA, Kay GN, Wilkoff BL, eds. *Clinical cardiac pacing.* Philadelphia: WB Saunders, 1995:687–700.

203. Horner S. Efficacy of intravenous magnesium in acute myocardial infarction in reducing arrhythmias and mortality: meta-analysis of magnesium in acute myocardial infarction. *Circulation* 1992;86:774–779.

204. Woods KL, Fletcher S, Roffee C, et al. Intravenous magnesium sulphate in suspected acute myocardial infarction: results of the second Leicester Intravenous Magnesium Intervention Trial (LIMIT-2). *Lancet* 1992;339:1553–1558.

205. Antman EM. Randomized trials of magnesium in acute myocardial infarction: big numbers do not tell the whole story. *Am J Cardiol* 1995;75:391–393.

206. Antman EM. Magnesium in acute MI: timing is critical. *Circulation* 1995;92:2367–2372.

207. Topol EJ, Lerman BB. Hypomagnesemic torsades de pointes. *Am J Cardiol* 1983;52:1367–1368.

208. Gheorghiade M. A symposium: management of heart failure in the 1990s: a reassessment of the role of digoxin therapy. *Am J Cardiol* 1992;69:1G–154G.

209. Gorlin R, Garg R. The effect of digitalis on mortality and hospitalizations in patients with heart failure, American College of Cardiology Annual Scientific Session, Orlando, FL, March 1996.

210. Ohman EM, George BS, White CJ, et al. Use of aortic counterpulsation to improve sustained coronary artery patency during acute myocardial infarction. Results of a randomized trial. *Circulation* 1994;90:792–799.

211. Champagnac D, Claudel JP, Chevalier P, et al. Primary cardiogenic shock during acute myocardial infarction: results of emergency cardiac transplantation. *Eur Heart J* 1993;14:925–929.

212. Smalling RW. The use of mechanical assist devices in the management of cardiogenic shock: secondary to acute myocardial infarction. *Texas Heart Inst J* 1991;18:275–281.

213. Topol EJ, Holmes DR, Rogers WJ. Coronary angiography after thrombolytic therapy for acute myocardial infarction. *Ann Intern Med* 1991;114:877–885.

214. Topol EJ. Coronary angioplasty for acute myocardial infarction. *Ann Intern Med* 1988;109:970–980.

215. Ellis SG, Ribeiro da Silva E, Heyndrickx G, et al. Randomized comparison of rescue angioplasty with conservative management of patients with early failure of thrombolysis for acute anterior myocardial infarction. *Circulation* 1994;90:2280–2284.

216. Abbottsmith CW, Topol EJ, George BS, et al. Fate of patients with acute myocardial infarction with patency of the infarct-related vessel achieved with successful thrombolysis versus rescue angioplasty. *J Am Coll Cardiol* 1990;16:770–778.

217. Ellis SG, Van de Werf F, Riberior-daSilva E, et al. Present status of rescue coronary angioplasty: current polarization of opinion and randomized trials. *J Am Coll Cardiol* 1992;19:681–686.

218. Topol EJ, Califf RM, George BS, et al. A randomized trial of immediate versus delayed elective angioplasty after intravenous tissue plasminogen activator in acute myocardial infarction. *N Engl J Med* 1987;317:581–588.

219. Califf RM, Topol EJ, Stack RS, et al. The TAMI Study Group: evaluation of combination thrombolytic therapy and timing of cardiac catheterization in acute myocardial infarction. *Circulation* 1991;83:1543–1556.

220. Belenkie I, Knudston ML, Roth DL, et al. Relation between flow grade after thrombolytic therapy and the effect of angioplasty on left ventricular function: a prospective randomized trial. *Am Heart J* 1991;121:407–416.

221. Fung AY, Lai P, Topol EJ, et al. Value of percutaneous transluminal coronary angioplasty after unsuccessful intravenous streptokinase therapy in acute myocardial infarction. *Am J Cardiol* 1986;58:686–691.

222. O'Connor CM, Mark DB, Hinohara T, et al. Rescue coronary angioplasty after failure of intravenous streptokinase in acute myocardial infarction: in-hospital and long-term outcomes. *J Invest Cardiol* 1989;1:85–95.

223. Ellis SG, Van de Werf F, Ribeiro-daSilva E, et al. Present status of rescue coronary angioplasty: current polarization of opinion and randomized trials. *J Am Coll Cardiol* 1992;19:681–686.

224. Grines CL, Nissen SE, Booth DC, et al. Kentucky Acute Myocardial Infarction Trial (KAMIT) group: a prospective, randomized trial comparing combination half-dose tissue-type plasminogen activator and streptokinase with full-dose tissue-type plasminogen activator. *Circulation* 1991;84:540–549.

225. McKendall GR, Forman S, Sopko G, et al. Value of rescue percutaneous transluminal coronary angioplasty following unsuccessful thrombolytic therapy in patients with acute myocardial infarction. *Am J Cardiol* 1995;76:1108–1111.

226. Gacioch GM, Topol EJ. Sudden paradoxic clinical deterioration during angioplasty of the occluded right coronary artery in acute myocardial infarction. *J Am Coll Cardiol* 1989;14:1202–1209.

227. Simoons ML, Arnold AER, Betriu A, et al. Thrombolysis with tissue plasminogen activator in acute myocardial infarction: no additional benefit from immediate percutaneous transluminal coronary angioplasty. *Lancet* 1988;1:197–203.

228. TIMI Research Group. Immediate vs delayed catheterization and angioplasty following thrombolytic therapy for acute myocardial infarction. TIMI II A results. *JAMA* 1988;260:2849–2858.

229. Cheitlin MD. The aggressive war on acute myocardial infarction: is the Blitzkrieg strategy changing (editorial)? *JAMA* 1988;260:2894–2896.

230. DeWood MA, Notske RN, Hensley GR, et al. Intraaortic balloon counterpulsation with and without reperfusion for myocardial infarction shock. *Circulation* 1980;61:1105–1112.

231. Phillips SJ, Zeff RH, Skinner JR, et al. Reperfusion protocol and results in 738 patients with evolving myocardial infarction. *Ann Thorac Surg* 1986;41:119–125.

232. Flameng W, Sargeant P, Vanhaecke J, et al. Emergency coronary bypass grafting for evolving myocardial infarction. *Cardiovasc Surg* 1987;94:124–131.

233. DeWood MA, Notske RN, Berg RJ, et al. Medical and surgical management of early Q wave myocardial infarction. I. Effects of surgical reperfusion on survival, recurrent myocardial infarction, sudden death and functional class at 10 or more years of follow-up. *J Am Coll Cardiol* 1989;14:65–77.

234. Kennedy JW, Ivey TD, Misbach G, et al. Coronary artery bypass graft surgery early after acute myocardial infarction. *Circulation* 1989;79:173–178.

235. Topol EJ, Ellis SG, Cosgrove DM, et al. Analysis of coronary angioplasty practice in the United States using a private insurance database. *Circulation* 1993;87:1489–1497.

236. Guetta V, Topol EJ. Pacifying the infarct vessel. *Circulation* 1997;96:713–715.

237. Topol EJ, Nissen S. Our preoccupation with coronary luminology: the dissociation between clinical and angiographic findings in ischemic heart disease. *Circulation* 1995;92:2333–2342.

238. Northridge DB, Hall RJC. Post myocardial-infarction exercise testing in the thrombolytic era. *Lancet* 1994;343:1175–1176.

239. Detrano R, Froelicher VF. Exercise testing: uses and limitations considering recent studies. *Prog Cardiovasc Dis* 1988;31:173–204.

240. Lavie CJ, Gibbons RJ, Zinsmeister AR, et al. Interpreting results of exercise studies after acute myocardial infarction altered by thrombolytic therapy, coronary angioplasty or bypass. *Am J Cardiol* 1991;67:116–120.

241. Haber HL, Beller GA, Watson DD, et al. Exercise thallium-201 scintigraphy after thrombolytic therapy with or without angioplasty for acute myocardial infarction. *Am J Cardiol* 1993;71:1257–1261.

242. Madsen JK, Grand P, Saunamaki K, et al. The Danish multicentre randomized study of invasive vs conservative treatment in patients with inducible ischemia following thrombolysis in acute myocardial infarction (DANAMI). *Circulation* 1997;96:748–755.

243. TIMI Study Group. Comparison of invasive and conservative strategies after treatment with intravenous tissue plasminogen activator in acute myocardial infarction. Results of the Thrombolysis in Myocardial Infarction (TIMI) phase II trial. *N Engl J Med* 1989;320:618–627.

244. SWIFT Trial Study Group. SWIFT trial of delayed elective intervention v conservative treatment after thrombolysis with anistreplase in acute myocardial infarction. *BMJ* 1991;302:555–560.

245. Barbash GI, Roth A, Hod H, et al. Randomized controlled trial of late in-hospital angiography and angioplasty versus conservative management after treatment with recombinant tissue-type plasminogen activator in acute myocardial infarction. *Am J Cardiol* 1990;66:538–545.

246. van den Brand MJ, Betriu A, Bescos LL, et al. Randomized trial of deferred angioplasty after thrombolysis for acute myocardial infarction. *Coron Artery Dis* 1992;3:393–401.

247. Pilote L, Miller DP, Califf RM, et al. Determinants of the use of coronary angiography and revascularization after thrombolysis for acute myocardial infarction in the United States. *N Engl J Med* 1996;335:1198–1205.

248. Every NR, Larson EB, Litwin PE, et al. The association between onsite cardiac catheterization facilities and the use of coronary angiography after acute myocardial infarction. *N Engl J Med* 1993;329:546–551.

249. Pilote L, Califf RM, Sapp S, et al. Regional variability in the United States for the management of acute myocardial infarction: insights from the GUSTO trial. *N Engl J Med* 1995;333:565–572.

250. Kereiakes DJ, Topol EJ, George BS, et al. The Thrombolysis and Angioplasty in Myocardial Infarction (TAMI) Study Group: myocardial infarction with minimal coronary atherosclerosis in the era of myocardial reperfusion. *J Am Coll Cardiol* 1991;17:304–312.

251. Van de Werf F, Topol EJ, Lee KL, et al. Variations in patient management and outcomes for acute myocardial infarction in the United States and other countries. *JAMA* 1995;273:1586–1591.

252. Tardiff BE, Califf RM, Morris D, et al. Coronary revascularization surgery following myocardial infarction: the effect of bypass surgery on survival following thrombolysis. *J Am Coll Cardiol* 1997;29:240–249.

253. Stason WB, Sanders CA. Cardiovascular care of the elderly: economic consideration. *J Am Coll Cardiol* 1987;10:18A–21A.

254. Maggioni AP, Maseri A, Fresco C, et al. Age related increase in mortality among patients with first myocardial infarctions treated with thrombolysis. *N Engl J Med* 1993;329:1442–1448.

255. De Franco AC, Topol EJ. Invasive strategies for acute myocardial infarction in the elderly. *Cardiology in the Elderly* 1994;2:274–289.

256. Gurwitz JH, Goldberg RJ, Gore JM. Coronary thrombolysis for the elderly. *JAMA* 1991;265:1720–1723.

257. Krumholz HM, Forman DE, Kuntz RE, et al. Coronary revascularization after myocardial infarction in the very elderly: outcomes and long-term follow up. *Ann Intern Med* 1993;119:1084–1090.

258. Udvarhelyi IS, Gatsonis C, Epstein AM, et al. Acute myocardial infarction in the Medicare population: process of care and clinical outcomes. *JAMA* 1992;268:2530–2536.

259. Ketley D, Woods KL. Selection factors for the use of thrombolytic treatment in acute myocardial infarction: a population based study of current practice in the United Kingdom. *Br Heart J* 1995;74:224–228.

260. Gurwitz JH, Gore JM, Goldberg RJ, et al. Recent age-related trends in the use of thrombolytic therapy in patients who have had acute myocardial infarction. *Ann Intern Med* 1996;124:283–291.

261. Katz A, Cohn G, Mashal A, et al. Thrombolytic therapy for acute myocardial infarction in a 110-year-old man. *Am J Cardiol* 1993;71:1122–1123.

262. Paul SD, Eagle KA, Guidry U, et al. Do gender-based differences in presentation and management influence predictors of hospitalization costs and length of stay after an acute myocardial infarction. *Am J Cardiol* 1995;76:1122–1125.

263. Weaver WD, White HD, Wilcox RG, et al. Comparisons of characteristics and outcomes among women and men with acute myocardial infarction treated with thrombolytic therapy. *JAMA* 1996;275:777–782.

264. Moen EK, Miller DP, Asher CR, et al. Long-term follow-up of gender specific outcomes after thrombolytic therapy for acute myocardial infarction from the GUSTO-I trial. *J Women's Health* 1997;6:285–293.

265. Thiemann DR, Coresh J, Schulman SP, et al. Thrombolytic therapy and mortality. *Lancet* 2001;357:1367.

266. White HD. Thrombolytic therapy in the elderly. *Lancet* 2001;356:2028–2030.

267. Thiemann DR, Coresh J, Schulman SP, et al. Lack of benefit for intravenous thrombolysis in patients with myocardial infarction who are older than 75 years. *Circulation* 2000;101:2239–2246.

268. Berger AK, Radford MJ, Wang Y, et al. Thrombolytic therapy in older patients. *J Am Coll Cardiol* 2000;36:366–374.

269. White HD. Thrombolytic therapy and mortality—reply. *Lancet* 2001;357:1367–1368.

270. Stenestrand U, Wallentin L. Thrombolysis is beneficial in elderly acute myocardial infarction patients. *J Am Coll Cardiol*, 2001 (*in press*).

271. Brieger DB, Mak K-H, White HD, et al. The benefit of early sustained reperfusion in patients with acute myocardial infarction superimposed on prior infarction. Insights from the GUSTO-I trial. *Am J Cardiol* 1998;81:282–287.

272. Brieger DB, Mak K-H, Miller DP, for the GUSTO-I Investigators. Second MI patients derive particular benefit from aggressive establishment of infarct artery patency. Insights from GUSTO-I. *Circulation* 1996;94:I-441(abstr).

273. Mueller HS, Cohen LS, Braunwald E, et al. Predictors of early morbidity and mortality after thrombolytic therapy of acute myocardial infarction. Analyses of patient subgroups in the Thrombolysis in Myocardial Infarction (TIMI) Trial, phase II. *Circulation* 1992;85:1254–1264.

274. Bottiger BW, Bode C, Kern S, et al. Efficacy and safety of thrombolytic therapy after initially unsuccessful cardiopulmonary resuscitation: a prospective clinical trial. *Lancet* 2001;357:1583–1585.

275. Kern KB. Thrombolytic therapy during cardiopulmonary resuscitation. *Lancet* 2001;357:1549–1550.

276. The TIMI IIIB Investigators. Effects of tissue plasminogen activator and a comparison of early invasive and conservative strategies in unstable angina and non-Q-wave myocardial infarction: results of the TIMI IIIB trial. *Circulation* 1994;89:1545–1556.

277. Langer A, Goodman SG, Topol EJ, et al. Late Assessment of Thrombolytic Efficacy (LATE) Study: prognosis in

patients with non-Q-wave myocardial infarction. *J Am Coll Cardiol* 1996;27:1327–1332.

278. The Global Use of Strategies to Open Occluded Coronary Arteries (GUSTO) IIb Investigators. A comparison of recombinant hirudin with heparin for the treatment of acute coronary syndromes. *N Engl J Med* 1996;335:775–782.

279. Gibson RS, Boden WE, Theroux P, et al. Diltiazem and reinfarction in patients with non-Q-wave myocardial infarction: results of a double-blind, randomized, multicenter trial. *N Engl J Med* 1986;315:423–429.

280. Cohen M, Demers C, Gurfinkel E, et al. Primary end point analysis from the ESSENCE trial: enoxaparin vs unfractionated heparin in unstable angina and non-Q-wave infarction. *Circulation* 1996;94:I-554(abstr).

281. ASSENT-3 Investigators. Efficacy and safety of tenecteplase in combination with enoxaparin abciximab or unfractionated heparin: the ASSENT-3 randomized trial in acute myocardial infarction. *Lancet* 2001;358:605–613.

282. Lefkovits J, Malycky JL, Rao JS, et al. Selective inhibition of factor Xa is more efficient than factor VIIa-tissue factor complex blockade at facilitating coronary thrombolysis in the canine model. *J Am Coll Cardiol* 1996;28:1858–1865.

283. Maraganore JM, Adelman BA. Hirulog: a direct thrombin inhibitor for management of acute coronary syndromes. *Coron Artery Dis* 1996;7:438–448.

284. Ragni M, Cirillo P, Pascucci I, et al. Monoclonal antibody against tissue factor shortens tissue plasminogen activator lysis time and prevents reocclusion in a rabbit model of carotid artery thrombosis. *Circulation* 1996;93:1913–1918.

285. Stanssens P, Bergum PW, Gansemans Y, et al. Anticoagulant repertoire of the hookworm *Ancylostoma caninum*. *Proc Natl Acad Sci U S A* 1996;93:2149–2154.

286. PURSUIT Trial Investigators. Inhibition of platelet glycoprotein IIb/IIIa with eptifibatide in patients with acute coronary syndromes. *N Engl J Med* 1998;339:436–443.

287. PRISM PLUS Study Investigators. Inhibition of the platelet glycoprotein IIb/IIIa receptor with tirofiban in unstable angina and non-Q-wave myocardial infarction. *N Engl J Med* 1998;338:1488–1497.

288. PARAGON Investigators. International, randomized controlled trial of lamifiban (a platelet glycoprotein IIb/IIIa inhibitor), heparin or both in unstable angina. *Circulation* 1998;97:2386–2395.

289. PRISM Study Investigators. A comparison of aspirin plus tirofiban with aspirin plus heparin for unstable angina. *N Engl J Med* 1998;338:1498–1505.

290. Mukherjee D, Mahaffey KW, Moliterno DJ, et al. The promise of combined low-molecular-weight heparin and platelet glycoprotein IIb/IIIa inhibition—results from PARAGON-B. *Circulation* 2001 (*submitted*).

291. The GUSTO IV-ACS Investigators. Glycoprotein IIb/IIIa receptor blocker abciximab does not improve outcome in patients with acute coronary syndromes without early coronary revascularization. *Lancet* 2001;357:1915–1924.

292. The EPIC Investigators. Use of a monoclonal antibody directed against the platelet glycoprotein IIb/IIIa receptor in high-risk coronary angioplasty. *N Engl J Med* 1994;330:956–961.

293. EPILOG Investigators. Platelet glycoprotein IIb/IIIa receptor blockade and low-dose heparin during percutaneous coronary revascularization. *N Engl J Med* 1997;336:1689–1696.

294. The EPISTENT Investigators. Randomised, placebo-controlled and balloon-angioplasty controlled trial to assess safety of coronary stenting with use of platelet glycoprotein IIb/IIIa blockade. *Lancet* 1998;352:87–92.

295. Topol EJ, Moliterno DJ, Herrmann HC, et al., for the TARGET Investigators. Comparison of two platelet glycoprotein IIb/IIIa inhibitors, tirofiban and abciximab, for the prevention of ischemic events with percutaneous coronary revascularization. *N Engl J Med* 2001;344:1888–1894.

296. Chew DP, Bhatt DL, Sapp S, et al. Increased mortality with oral platelet glycoprotein IIb/IIIa antagonists: a meta-analysis of the phase III multi-center randomized trials. *Circulation* 2001;103:201–206.

297. The GUSTO V Investigators. Reperfusion therapy for acute myocardial infarction with fibrinolytic therapy or combination low dose fibrinolytic therapy and platelet glycoprotein IIb/IIIa inhibition: the GUSTO 5 trial. *Lancet* 2001;357:1905–1914.

298. Khot UN, Neumann F-J, Brener SJ, et al. Is IIb/IIIa blockade state-of-the-art for catheter-based reperfusion? A meta-analysis of five randomized trials in acute myocardial infarction. *JACC* 2001;37:368A(abstr).

299. Baim D. Saphenous vein graft Angioplasty Free of Emboli Randomized trial (SAFER). Presented at the Transcatheter Cardiovascular Therapeutics Twelfth Annual Symposium, Washington Hospital Center, Washington, DC, September, 2000.

300. Jackson KA, Majka SM, Wang H, et al. Regeneration of ischemic cardiac muscle and vascular endothelium by adult stem cells. *J Clin Invest* 2001;107:1395–1402.

301. Shintani S, Murohara T, Ikeda H, et al. Mobilization of endothelial progenitor cells in patients with acute myocardial infarction. *Circulation* 2001;103:2776–2779.

302. Orlic D, Kajstura J, Chimenti S, et al. Bone marrow cells regenerate infarcted myocardium. *Nature* 2001;410:701–705.

303. Kocher AA, Schuster MD, Szabolcs MJ, et al. Neovascularization of ischemic myocardium by human bone-marrow-derived angioblasts prevents cardiomyocyte apoptosis, reduces remodeling and improves cardiac function. *Nat Med* 2001;4:430–436.

ACUTE MYOCARDIAL INFARCTION: COMPLICATIONS

JUDITH S. HOCHMAN
BERNARD J. GERSH

J. S. Hochman: Department of Cardiology, Columbia University College of Physicians and Surgeons, St. Luke's-Roosevelt Hospital Center, New
York, New York
B. J. Gersh: Division of Cardiovascular Diseases, Mayo Clinic, Rochester, Minnesota

OVERVIEW

Complications of myocardial infarction (MI) are related to
myocardial factors including infarct size, transmural extent,
and location and to coronary factors including extent and

severity of coronary artery disease (CAD), as well as the status of the infarct-related artery (IRA) (i.e., patent or occluded). Arrhythmic complications, such as atrial tachyarrhythmias and ventricular tachycardia after the first day, are also largely related to infarct size and left ventricular (LV) function. Major complications include (a) pump failure [LV or right ventricular (RV)], which is the leading cause of death in hospitalized MI patients; (b) LV aneurysm; (c) systemic emboli; (d) reinfarction (infarct extension); (e) ischemia; (f) myocardial rupture (free wall, ventricular septal and papillary muscle); (g) pericardial effusion; and (h) pericarditis. Except for reinfarction and hemorrhagic complications, reperfusion therapy reduces the incidence of most complications.

Echocardiography with color flow Doppler is an excellent tool for rapidly assessing all complications and for evaluating hypotension, congestive heart failure (CHF), and cardiogenic shock. Mimics of shock complicating acute MI, such as aortic dissection, can be readily detected. Management of each complication must be related to its pathophysiology. Mechanical problems, such as ventricular septal rupture (VSR) and mitral regurgitation (MR), should be surgically corrected. A randomized trial of patients in cardiogenic shock demonstrated improved 6- and 12-month survival for those assigned to early angiography and revascularization compared with initial intensive medical therapy and delayed revascularization as indicated. After 20 years of unchanging high in-hospital mortality for shock, the Worcester community reported improved in-hospital survival in 1995 and 1997. Aspirin (ASA) therapy reduces the incidence of early reinfarction, which may be managed with percutaneous transluminal coronary angioplasty (PTCA) or thrombolysis when ST elevations occur. Future efforts must focus on preventing complications because mortalities are high once complications develop.

GENERAL PATHOPHYSIOLOGY

The spectrum of complications of myocardial necrosis from CHF to arrhythmias to post-MI angina is illustrated in Figure 19.1 (12). Complications of MI tend to occur when infarcts are large and extensively transmural (i.e., when they involve the full thickness of the myocardium). A large, transmural infarct is more prone to expansion (i.e., thinning and dilation) with its attendant increased risk for myocardial rupture, LV aneurysm, LV thrombus, pump failure, and pericarditis (Fig. 19.1) (12). Refractory, sustained ventricular tachycardia develops after MI most frequently in relation to large transmural infarcts that result in LV dilation. Although infarct size is a major determinant of complications, certain strategic locations of small, extensively transmural infarcts can result in devastating complications, such as LV free-wall rupture or rupture of the posteromedial papillary muscle, even when expansion does

not occur (Fig. 19.1) (12). Indeed, in an autopsy study of patients dying of an acute MI, infarct size was substantially smaller in patients with cardiac rupture than in patients dying of primary pump function or arrhythmias (*e*Fig. 19.1.1). An anteroapical location of MI increases the likelihood of acute infarct expansion and mural thrombosis. Massive acute myocardial necrosis, multiple small infarcts (acute and prior), and recurrent ischemia or reinfarction may each lead to cardiogenic shock (Fig. 19.1) (12). New myocardial necrosis or infarct extension (i.e., reinfarction) may occur after the initial MI and result in a larger total area of infarction. In contrast, infarct expansion involves no additional myocardial necrosis but results in a larger functional infarct size with a greater percentage of the LV being composed of necrotic myocardium or scar (13). These two complications are compared in Figure 19.1 (12). Extent and severity of disease in noninfarct-related coronary arteries and important characteristics of the patient—including age, gender, and comorbidities (e.g., diabetes mellitus and prior hypertension)—also contribute significantly to the development of acute MI complications. These complications are not entirely independent, and each can lead to other complications (Fig. 19.2).

INFARCT EXPANSION, LEFT VENTRICULAR REMODELING, AND LEFT VENTRICULAR ANEURYSM

Pathophysiology

LV remodeling after MI refers to topographic and functional changes in the infarct zone and in remote, uninfarcted myocardium that begin minutes after MI and may continue for months or years later. These changes include (a) infarct expansion (i.e., thinning and dilation of the infarct zone) (*e*Fig. 19.2.1); (b) subsequent dilation of the remote, uninfarcted myocardium with hypertrophy; (c) interstitial fibrosis and impairment of contraction; and (d) global change from a normal LV, elongated ellipse to a more spherical shape (26–31). LV aneurysm, a discrete bulge of the LV composed of fibrotic tissue, results when severe infarct expansion persists and scar is laid down on the topographic substrate.

Infarct Expansion and Left Ventricular Remodeling

Infarct expansion occurs soon after onset of coronary occlusion (26,32). It is reversible if coronary flow is reestablished rapidly; however, it may progress in a time-dependent manner if flow is not reestablished or is reestablished late (33). Infarct size is a major determinant, with large infarcts expanding more frequently and more severely than small ones (27,30). Anterior infarcts and those involving the apex

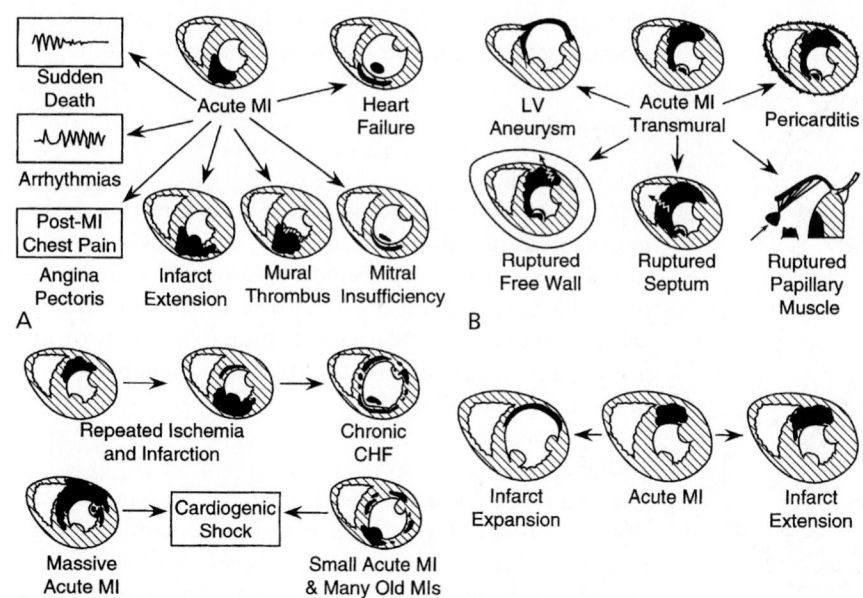

FIGURE 19.1 Complications of myocardial infarction (MI) (schematic). **A:** General complications. **B:** Complications of transmural infarctions. **C:** Cardiogenic shock as a result of either a massive acute infarction or a small acute process in a heart already involved by multiple old infarctions. **D:** Comparison of infarct expansion (aneurysm formation) and infarct extension (reinfarction). CHF, congestive heart failure; LV, left ventricle. (From Edwards WD. Pathology of myocardial infarction and reperfusion. In: Gersh BJ, Rahimtoola SH, eds. *Acute myocardial infarction.* Boston: Chapman & Hall, 1996:16–50, with permission.)

are at greatest risk for infarct expansion (13,26,34), probably as a result of a thinner LV wall and greater radius of curvature at the apex, which increase stress on the LV wall per Laplace's equation. Inferior, posterior, or lateral infarcts without apical necrosis less frequently expand. Transmural infarcts are more likely to expand; nontransmural infarcts are largely protected from expansion (27,33). The greater the extent of transmural infarct, the more likely it is to expand, even though a thin rim of noninfarcted subepicardial myofibrils helps to limit infarct expansion. Infarct expansion is the pathologic substrate for type III cardiac rupture. Disruption of the intercellular collagen matrix may lead to slippage of sheets of myofibrils and expansion of the affected area (31,35).

Infarct expansion results in early LV dilation (26–28). It is associated with CHF and LV intracavitary thrombosis (29,36,37). Long-term global remodeling with dilation and long-term impairment of uninfarcted, myocardial segment

contraction begins soon after a large infarction and progresses for months to years (28,30,31,38). LV volume strongly correlates with long-term mortality (39,40).

Left Ventricular Aneurysm

Regional expansion of the infarct zone that results in a discrete diastolic and systolic bulge and that is not reversed by reperfusion or other measures produces chronic, true LV aneurysm. LV aneurysm pathologically is composed of scar that is laid down by fibroblasts on the topographic substrate formed early by infarct expansion (41). Scar laid down soon after infarction does not subsequently dilate to form aneurysms. Early LV aneurysms may be referred to as *functional aneurysms* (42) because they may be reversible. In fact, LV aneurysms resected years after MI sometimes contain viable and presumably hibernating myocardium (43). In contrast to true LV aneurysm, pseudoaneurysm or false LV aneurysm represents localized rupture of the myocardium and is discussed later in this chapter (Fig. 19.3) (44).

Left Ventricular Thrombus

Inflammation of the endocardium resulting from myocardial necrosis in any location may produce layered, mural thrombus; however, thrombus most frequently develops in anterior infarcts (37,54) with expansion or aneurysmal dilation that involves the apex, caused by the combination of endocardial inflammation and stasis. More extensive thrombi with a protruding appearance are at increased risk for systemic embolization (37,55), and they typically occur in the apex. Mural thrombi are more frequently found in recently formed LV aneurysms than in older aneurysms (56).

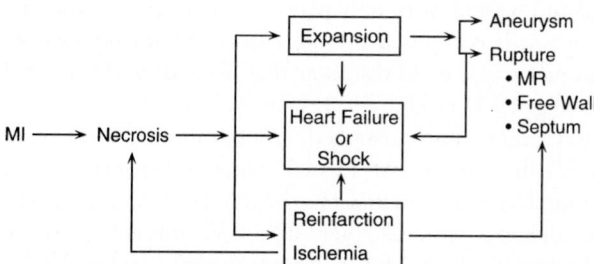

FIGURE 19.2 Overview of the interrelated nature of many complications of myocardial infarction (MI). One complication is often the substrate for another (e.g., expansion is the substrate for left ventricular aneurysms and myocardial rupture, or directly leads to another complication; reinfarction results in pump failure). MR, mitral regurgitation.

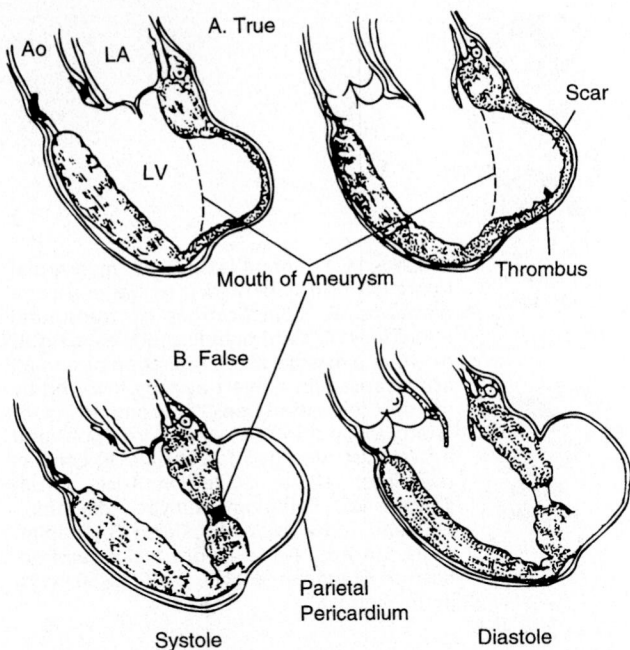

FIGURE 19.3 Hearts in systole and diastole with true and false anatomic left ventricular (LV) aneurysms and healed myocardial infarction. The true anatomic LV aneurysm protrudes during both systole and diastole, has a mouth that is as wide as or wider than the maximal diameter, has a wall that was formerly the wall of the left ventricle, and is composed of fibrous tissue with or without residual myocardial fibers. A true aneurysm may or may not contain thrombus and almost never ruptures once the wall is healed. The false anatomic LV aneurysm protrudes during both systole and diastole, has a mouth that is considerably smaller than the maximal diameter of the aneurysm and represents a myocardial rupture site, has a wall made up of parietal pericardium, virtually always contains thrombus, and often ruptures. Ao, aorta; LA, left atrium. (Adapted from Cabin HS, Roberts WC. Left ventricular aneurysm, intraaneurysmal thrombus, and systemic embolus in coronary heart disease. *Chest* 1980;77:586, with permission.)

Clinical Profile

Risk Factors

Patients with myocardial infarcts that involve the apex of the left ventricle, particularly those with anteroapical, Q-wave (i.e., transmural) infarcts are at greatest risk for infarct expansion and aneurysm formation (34). A discrete, posterobasal aneurysm may less frequently develop following inferoposterior MI. Patients who do not receive reperfusion therapy or in whom reperfusion therapy fails are at greater risk for aneurysm formation.

High ventricular afterload states, such as hypertension during acute MI and elevated plasma angiotensin-converting enzyme (ACE) activity levels, are associated with infarct expansion (36,57,58). Administration of corticosteroids after acute MI is associated with delayed infarct healing and development of LV aneurysms (59). Both corticosteroids and nonsteroidal antiinflammatory drugs have been dem-

onstrated experimentally to induce infarct expansion when administered acutely after coronary occlusion (60–62).

Diagnosis

Clinical Findings

The classic physical finding of LV aneurysm is a dyskinetic apical impulse on palpation. The ECG typically shows an extensive, anteroapical Q-wave MI with persistent ST-segment elevation. Persistent T-wave inversion is also a marker of progressive LV dilation (63). Chest roentgenography is insensitive but typically demonstrates a bulge in the LV silhouette.

Imaging

On imaging, LV aneurysm is defined as a discrete bulge in the LV contour during both diastole and systole, which typically exhibits dyskinetic (i.e., paradoxical) expansion during systole. Echocardiography with color flow Doppler is the imaging modality of choice and can be used to distinguish discrete, LV aneurysms from false aneurysms. Other techniques to assess an aneurysm include biplane left ventriculography, which is the traditional gold standard, radionuclide ventriculography, computed tomography (CT), and magnetic resonance imaging (MRI).

Clinical Consequences

Cardiac Rupture, Congestive Heart Failure, and Arrhythmias

Rupture of the myocardium may result from acute infarct expansion, but it does not occur in chronic LV aneurysms with scar. Acute CHF complicating MI more frequently occurs when infarct expansion is demonstrated (29,36). Infarct expansion and acute aneurysmal dilation may result in CHF caused by paradoxic systolic bulging with reduced mechanical efficiency of the left ventricle (i.e., wasted work) (43) and elevated wall stress in the remote, uninfarcted myocardium, causing global ischemia. Chronic LV aneurysms are associated with chronic CHF. In this context, the extent of systolic bulging with chronic scar is minimal and wasted work only plays a significant role when the aneurysm is composed of viable myocardium interspersed with scar tissue or of thin scar that expands with each systole (Fig. 19.3) (44).

Recurrent and sustained, monomorphic ventricular tachycardia may occur in acute infarct expansion or in chronic LV aneurysm and may be refractory to antiarrhythmic therapy (see Chapter 67). LV volume correlates strongly with short- and long-term mortality (*e*Fig. 19.3.1) (39,40), with sudden cardiac death occurring at least as frequently as death from progressive pump failure. Early LV dilation results in late progressive LV enlargement with associated CHF and malignant ventricular arrhythmias late post-MI (64).

Left Ventricular Thrombi and Systemic Emboli

Layered mural and protruding thrombi typically develop within the first week following acute anterior Q-wave MIs with expanded or aneurysmal akinetic or dyskinetic segments, especially those involving the LV apex. The estimated incidence in an echocardiographic study in 1986 was approximately 33% for anterior MI and less than 5% to 10% for other locations (65). Because LV thrombi more frequently occur with large infarctions, they have become less common in the reperfusion era. Of 8,326 patients in the Gruppo Italiano Per lo Studio Della Streptokinase nell'Infarto Miocardio (GISSI)-3 study who had a predischarge echocardiogram, the overall LV thrombus incidence was 5.1% of anterior MIs and 2.3% of nonanterior MIs. These rates were higher when the ejection fraction (EF) was less than 40%. Independent risk factors for LV thrombus are Killip class greater than I and early intravenous beta-blocker use (54). LV thrombi are associated with increased risk for systemic embolization (55), particularly when they have a protruding appearance (37). Stroke is the primary manifestation of cardiac emboli (occurring in 85% of cases); however, the overall incidence of arterial embolism is low (65–69), whether LV thrombus is visualized or not. The reported incidence (69) of systemic emboli associated with anterior MI in the prereperfusion era was 2% to 6%. Patients with atrial fibrillation (AF) after MI are at increased risk for systemic emboli from left atrial thrombi. Patients with chronic LV aneurysm are at low risk for systemic embolization (70), perhaps because the aneurysmal area containing thrombus is noncontractile and there is no longer endocardial inflammation. However, when global LVEF is reduced after MI (less than 40%), the rate of stroke is 1.5% per year even when CHF is not present. The risk increases with decreasing EF and older age (71). Patients with LVEF less than 28.0% have a 5-year stroke rate of 8.9%. These strokes, however, are undoubtedly caused by cerebrovascular disease, as well as cardiac emboli.

Management

Medical Therapy

Angiotensin-Converting Enzyme Inhibitors

ACE inhibitors have been shown in experimental models and in clinical investigations (64,72,73) to reduce acute infarct expansion and progressive LV remodeling. When successful reperfusion has inhibited infarct expansion and aneurysm formation, ACE inhibitors have not been clearly shown to limit expansion further (74). A detailed discussion of the use of ACE inhibitors in MI can be found elsewhere in this textbook (see Chapter 20). Because infarct expansion begins early, therapy should be instituted within the first 24 hours of onset of MI in patients at risk for expansion and aneurysms (i.e., those with nonreperfused or large anteroapical Q-wave MIs, particularly with associated hypertension). A short-acting ACE inhibitor is recommended for initial therapy (e.g., captopril), so that it can be discontinued if hypotension develops, dissipating its effect more rapidly. The initial dose should be 6.25 mg followed by 12.5 mg, then 25 to 50 mg every 8 hours as tolerated. After several days, the patient may be switched to a long-acting ACE inhibitor. The use of ACE inhibitors in patients presenting with pulmonary congestion is discussed in Acute Left Ventricular Failure, later in this chapter.

Anticoagulation: Therapy for Left Ventricular Thrombus

Full oral anticoagulation for 3 months significantly accelerated the resolution of LV thrombus in a small randomized trial (82) of acenocoumarol versus sulfinpyrazone versus placebo. Full-dose warfarin is recommended when LV thrombus is visualized, although there are no data from randomized trials of this subset demonstrating decreased events.

Anticoagulation: Prevention of Systemic Emboli

In the prethrombolytic era, the effect of anticoagulant therapy on systemic and pulmonary embolism (PE) was assessed in two major randomized trials. Patients assigned to heparin followed by high-dose pheninidione had significantly lower rates of systemic and PE compared with those assigned to low-dose pheninidione (4.8% vs. 11%; *p* = .01) (83). In the Veterans Administration Cooperative Trial (84), heparin followed by warfarin significantly reduced the rate of systemic embolism, including stroke (5.6% vs. 0.8%; *p* = .001). In the thrombolytic era, the GISSI (85) showed that the rate of pulmonary and systemic thromboembolism was significantly reduced by streptokinase (SK) alone compared with placebo (0.4% vs. 1.1%, respectively; *p* = .05).

The Survival and Ventricular Enlargement investigators (71) reported that long-term use of warfarin in patients with EF less than 40% after MI was strongly associated with a reduced 5-year stroke rate (relative risk, 0.19; range, 0.13 to 0.27; *p* <.001). Of note, ASA was also associated with a reduced risk (relative risk, 0.49; range, 0.29 to 0.65; *p* <.001) (71). In the Anticoagulants in the Secondary Prevention of Events in Coronary Thrombosis-2 (ASPECT 2) randomized trial, warfarin alone or in combination with ASA was superior to ASA alone post-MI in preventing stroke (0% versus 0.3% versus 1.5%) as well as MI and death (86). However, stroke, MI, and death were not reduced by warfarin (Coumadin) plus ASA compared with ASA alone in the Combined Hemotherapy and Mortality Prevention (CHAMP) trial (87). Larger trials comparing Coumadin with ASA and their combination are ongoing.

Anticoagulant Regimens

Warfarin Dosing. Warfarin therapy with a target international normalized ratio (INR) of 2.0 to 3.0 is recommended following infarction in patients with anterior Q-wave MI (69) and, in particular, in those with akinetic or dyskinetic apical wall motion, or in the presence of ECG-documented LV thrombus. Warfarin is also recommended in patients with large, nonanterior infarcts complicated by depressed LVEF and CHF and in those with AF (65,69). Perhaps a higher target INR of 2.5 to 3.5 is appropriate for at least 6 months in patients with LV thrombi who have had systemic emboli. It is unclear whether patients with these high-risk characteristics should be treated with Coumadin indefinitely or 3 months of therapy followed by ASA. The former approach is supported by the ASPECT 2 study, which demonstrated reduction of vascular events, stroke, death, and MI with Coumadin plus ASA compared to ASA alone (86). However, the larger CHAMP study, which achieved lower INRs than ASPECT 2, showed similar event rates for Coumadin plus ASA compared with ASA alone (87). Long-term warfarin therapy should be strongly considered in asymptomatic patients with depressed EFs after MI, particularly EFs less than 30% (71). Until larger trials are completed, it is reasonable to continue warfarin indefinitely for the higher risk group patients who are suitable candidates.

Lower intensity warfarin (1 or 3 mg) combined with ASA (80 mg) in survivors of acute MI of any location (patients with LV thrombi are largely excluded) was associated with similar long-term outcomes when compared with ASA (160 mg) alone in the Coumadin Aspirin Reinfarction Study (92), except for a small excess of stroke in the two low-dose Coumadin with ASA (80 mg) arms.

REINFARCTION AND ISCHEMIA

Pathophysiology

Importance of Coronary Perfusion Pressure

It is critical to maintain coronary perfusion pressure during acute MI to facilitate reperfusion and sustain patency of the IRA. Recurrent MI and ischemia may result from a decrease in coronary perfusion pressure in patients with a preexisting coronary stenosis. Reocclusion following reperfusion with PTCA may result from hypotension. Hypotension during thrombolytic therapy substantially reduces the rate of lysis of thrombi (117,118), as well as the overall reperfusion rate (119,120), and may predispose patients to reocclusion. There is also evidence of worse outcomes and larger MIs when hypotension occurs with use of nitrates and ACE inhibitors early in acute MI (74,121).

Clinical Profile

Diagnosis

The diagnosis and incidence of reinfarction or infarct extension vary widely depending on the clinical definition

and the diligence with which it is sought. ECG changes alone are the least specific method of diagnosing infarct extension and they markedly overestimate its occurrence (13,122). ST-segment elevation that progresses days after MI may represent pericarditis or infarct expansion. Evolution of deepening T waves is typical after MI and does not usually represent ischemia or infarct extension. Recurrent chest pain is also nonspecific, with angina or pericarditis pain as other causes of post-MI chest pain. Recurrent elevations in creatine kinase with muscle and brain subunits (CK-MB) after its disappearance or to >50% of the prior value are regarded as the standard for reinfarction (89). Because troponin I and T may remain elevated for up to 2 weeks, they are not used to diagnose reinfarction (123). The full constellation of recurrent chest discomfort and recurrent elevation in ST segments followed by recurrent elevation in CK-MB infrequently occurs but constitutes the typical diagnosis, both in large clinical trials and in clinical practice. We recommend obtaining daily CK-MB measurements for 2 days after MI as well as 8-hour samplings for 24 hours if a recurrent event develops (e.g., chest pain, worsening ST elevations or depressions).

Incidence, Risk Factors, and Prognosis

The incidence of short-term reinfarction in the prereperfusion era in studies (124–126) in which it was carefully assessed by repeated CK-MB measurements is shown in Table 19.1 and is compared with rates reported in large clinical trials (84,85,124–140). The rates reported in clinical trials are all relatively low probably because of (a) reporting of only those reinfarctions with the full clinical constellation of pain, ECG changes, and cardiac marker elevations in the same trials; (b) lack of adequate data collected; and (c) lower risk patients enrolled in clinical trials (141).

Risk factors for recurrent MI in patients not receiving reperfusion therapy include diabetes, female gender, obesity, and non–Q-wave MI (125). In the thrombolytic era, recurrent ischemia after MI is associated with an increased risk for in-hospital reinfarction as demonstrated by a substudy of GISSI-2 (142) (28% vs. 2% reinfarction; *p* <.001). Among these 453 patients, aged 70 years or younger, there were no baseline or MI characteristics that predicted early recurrent ischemia. Recurrent ischemia and reinfarction increase the risk of death after MI (143,144).

Prevention

Recurrent MI is, in part, related to the early therapy used in treating the initial MI. Although there was originally some concern that thrombolytic therapy may increase the rate of reinfarction, with the residual active culprit lesion supplying an incomplete or aborted infarct zone, the large body of data does not support such concern (Table 19.1) (130–134) provided ASA is used adjunctively (130). Randomized

TABLE 19.1 REINFARCTION (INFARCT EXTENSION) RATES ≤6 MONTHS POST–MYOCARDIAL INFARCTION

Prethrombolysis	Reference	Number	Reinfarction (%)
Clinical (pooled)	122,124–126	761	16

Clinical trial reinfarction rates					
			Reinfarction (%)		
Beta-blockers	**Reference**	**Number**	**Beta-blocker**	**Control**	***p* value[a]**
No thrombolysis Pooled (ISIS-1, MIAMI, 26 other studies)	127,128	>27,000	2.8	3.4	<.02
			Immediate i.v. beta-blockade	Deferred oral beta-blockade	
Thrombolysis TIMI 2	129	1,390	2.6	4.5	.06

			Reinfarction (%)			
Anticoagulation and antiplatelet therapy	**Reference**	**Number**	**Heparin/ Coumadin**	**Control**	**ASA**	***p* value**
Veterans Cooperative (no thrombolysis)	84	999	3.4	4.8	N/A	.28
APRICOT 1 (after thrombolysis)	109	248	8	11	3	
ISIS 2 (with and without SK)	130	16,981	N/A	3.3	1.8	≤.0001
			ASA + Coumadin	Coumadin	ASA	
ASPECT 2	86		3.3	4.0	3.3	

			Reinfarction (%)		
Thrombolysis	**Reference**	**Number**	**Thrombolysis**	**Control**	
GISSI-1 (no ASA)	85	11,712	4.1	2.1	[b]
ISIS 2 (SK vs. no SK)	130	16,981	2.8	2.4	
ISIS 2					
(SK no ASA vs. placebo)		8,489	3.8	2.9	[b]
(SK and ASA vs. ASA)		8,492	1.8	1.9	
AIMS, ECSG, ISAM, ASSET	131–134	8,725	3.95	3.86	

Thrombolytic agent	**Reference**	**Number**	**t-PA**	**SK/APSAC**	**Reteplase**	**Tenecteplase**
International	135	20,768	2.65	3.0	—	—
ISIS 3	136	40,775	2.92	3.50	—	—
GUSTO 1	137	27,164	4.0	3.7	—	—
GISSI-2	138	12,381	1.9	2.3	—	—
GUSTO 3	407	15,059	4.2	—	4.2	—
ASSENT-II	408	16,949	4.1	—	—	3.8

Adjunctive heparin (full dose, s.c.)	**Reference**	**Number**	**Heparin**	**Control**
GISSI-2[c]	138	12,381	1.9	2.3
International	135	20,768	2.8	2.9
ISIS 3	136	40,775	3.2	3.5

		Reinfarction (%)		
Glycoprotein IIb/IIIa antagonists[d]	**Reference**	**Lytic**	**Lytic + glycoprotein IIb/IIIa**	***p* value**
TIMI 14A[c]	409	3.0	3.0	
SPEED	410	2.8	0.9	
Intro-AMI	411	3.8	1.8	
GUSTO V	147a	3.5	2.3	<.0001

(continued)

TABLE 19.1 *(Continued)*

Primary PTCA	Reference	Number	Reinfarction (%)	
			Primary PTCA	Thrombolysis
MITRA/MIR Registry (in-hospital)	412	1,625	1.0	5.4
NRMI	413	28,757	2.6	2.9
PAMI (in-hospital)	203	195	2.6	6.5
GUSTO IIB-PTCA substudy	291	1,138	4.4	6.5

Other therapy	Reference	Number	Reinfarction (%)	
			Nitrates	Control
Nitrates				
ISIS 4	139	57,061	4.0	3.9
GISSI-3	140	18,895	3.1	3.2

ACE inhibitors[e]	Reference	Number	ACE	Control
SIS 4	139	57,061	4.1	3.9
GISSI-3	140	18,895	3.2	3.1
ACE Collaborative Group		98,483	3.9	3.8

ACE, angiotensin-converting enzyme; APSAC, anisoylated plasminogen streptokinase activator complex; ASA, acetylsalicylic acid; N/A, not available; PTCA, percutaneous transluminal coronary angioplasty; SK, streptokinase; t-PA, tissue plasminogen activator.
[a]p values are listed when reported in the published report.
[b]Reports of GISSI and ISIS 2 note significant increases in reinfarction with SK if no ASA is used (no p values reported).
[c]GISSI-2 is also included in International Study.
[d]For non–ST-elevation myocardial infarction, see Chapter 17. Different reduced doses of lytics combined with glycoprotein IIb/IIIa antagonists are pooled.
[e]Long-term reduction in reinfarction, see Chapter 20.

trials (135–138) report slightly lower short-term reinfarction rates following tissue-type plasminogen activator (t-PA) compared with SK. After t-PA therapy, reocclusion is significantly reduced by full-dose i.v. heparin (145). However, there are no data demonstrating that heparin per se reduces the rate of reinfarction (146). Delayed, full-dose s.c. heparin after thrombolysis does not reduce reinfarction nor does i.v. heparin compared with full-dose s.c. heparin after administration of SK (135–138,146). ▼ d43

For patients with ST-elevation MI who do not receive thrombolysis, full-dose heparin followed by warfarin has not been shown to reduce rates of reinfarction occurring over 6 weeks after the initial MI (84). ASA significantly reduced the rate of reinfarction in the International Study of Infarct Survival (ISIS) 2 (130). Beta-blockers in patients not receiving thrombolytic therapy did not reduce reinfarction in the large ISIS 1 or in the Metoprolol in Acute Myocardial Infarction trial (127,128). However, when patients in these trials were pooled with those in 26 small studies (127) of i.v. beta-blockade (greater than 27,000 patients), an 18% reduction in reinfarction was demonstrated (2.8% versus 3.4%; $p <.02$). In conjunction with thrombolysis, early i.v. beta-blockade followed by oral beta-blockade reduced reinfarction and recurrent ischemia compared with oral, deferred beta-blockade (129), particularly when administered less than or at 2 hours of symptom onset. In large-scale trials (139,140), neither nitrates nor ACE inhibitors reduced early reinfarction (Table 19.1). Long-term

reinfarction is reduced with ACE inhibitors (150,151). Routine revascularization using PTCA or CABG following thrombolysis to prevent reinfarction at 6 weeks proved disappointing in several major randomized trials (129,152–154). Direct PTCA as an initial treatment for acute MI appears to result in lower early reinfarction rates compared with thrombolytic therapy (Table 19.1) (see Chapter 18).

Management

Reinfarction is managed using the same treatment modalities as those used for the initial MI, including ASA, heparin, and beta-blockers, but with the caveat that patients with recurrent ischemia are a high-risk group who merit early cardiac catheterization. Readministration of thrombolytics for recurrent MI with recurrent ST-segment elevations on ECG has been used (155,156), with high successful response rates. If SK is used previously, t-PA or recombinant plasminogen activator or tenecteplase should be administered because antibodies to SK may develop. Direct PTCA should be performed, if available for recurrent coronary artery occlusion.

GP IIb/IIIa antagonists and low-molecular-weight or unfractionated heparin are efficacious in reducing death and reinfarction when used in patients with non–ST-elevation acute coronary syndromes, which include patients with post-MI angina (see Chapters 17 and 18). Recurrent ischemia is initially managed with beta-blockers and nitrates. Calcium channel blockers may be added if recurrent angina occurs on maximal doses of beta-blockers and nitrates. IABP counterpulsation should be used for patients with ischemia and hemodynamic instability (i.e., hypotension, hypoperfusion, or low cardiac output) and for refractory ischemia if revascularization facilities are not immediately available. Recurrent ischemia postinfarction and reinfarction identifies a high-risk subgroup of patients in whom urgent cardiac catheterization is indicated to prompt revascularization with PTCA or CABG, depending on the coronary anatomy, LV function, and the extent of myocardial jeopardy. The Danish Trial in Acute Myocardial Infarction (DANAMI) trial demonstrated reduced long-term events for post-MI patients with spontaneous or stress-induced significant ischemia who underwent revascularization (157).

ACUTE LEFT VENTRICULAR FAILURE

Pathophysiologic Principles

General

LV failure in acute MI varies widely in terms of pathophysiology and severity. Mild-to-severe pulmonary congestion may occur alone or in association with depressed stroke volume (SV) and cardiac output. Diastolic or systolic dysfunction may predominate. At the severe end of the spectrum of pump failure, cardiogenic shock is a state of severe tissue hypoperfusion caused by cardiac dysfunction.

Congestive Heart Failure

After acute coronary occlusion, LV systolic and diastolic functions change over minutes, hours, and weeks. Superimposed fixed or transient MR, recurrent ischemia, or reinfarction may have a major effect. Compliance of the infarct zone evolves over time (158–160), and stunned myocardium may recover function (161–163). Furthermore, elevations in LV filling pressures resulting from systolic or diastolic dysfunction may reduce the pressure gradient that maintains coronary blood flow (*e*Fig. 19.3.3) (164) and thereby initiate a cycle of hypoperfusion and worsening LV dysfunction (Fig. 19.4) (165,166).

Systolic Dysfunction

The composite number of dysfunctional myocardial segments—including hypokinetic, akinetic, and dyskinetic regions, as well as the hyperkinetic or normokinetic motion of the uninfarcted myocardium—determines global LV function. These abnormalities may be old (e.g., caused by prior infarctions) or new and may be reversible or irreversible. Global LV function is the strongest determinant of pump failure and death caused by MI (167–170). Lack of compensatory hyperkinesis of uninfarcted zones correlates with the development of pump failure (114). The LV typically dilates when significant systolic dysfunction is present, caused by early infarct expansion and the effect of the resultant increased wall stress on the remote myocardium. LV dilation plays an acute compensatory role by allowing the high end diastolic volume (EDV) to maintain SV when EF is significantly depressed.

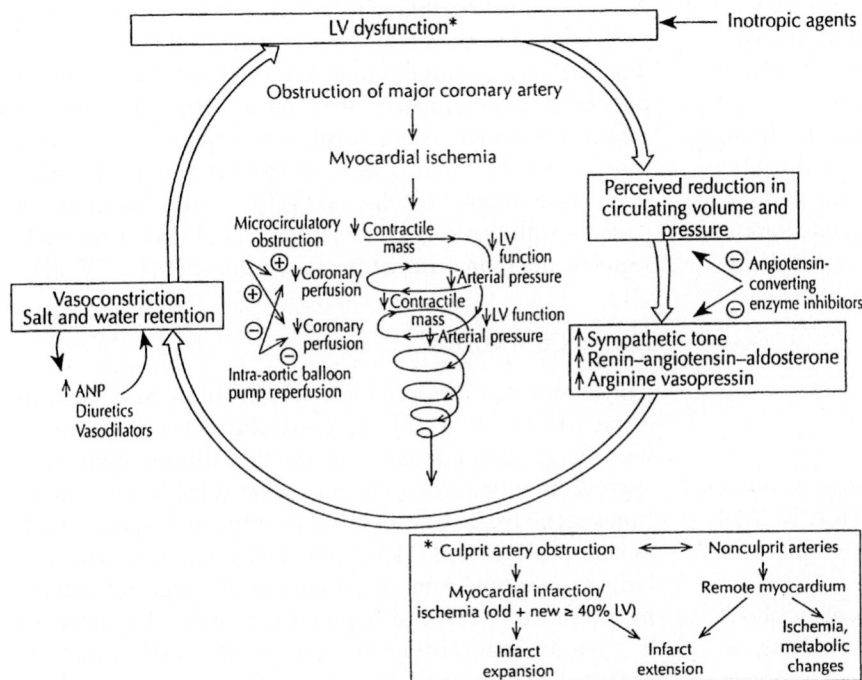

FIGURE 19.4 Pathophysiology of cardiogenic shock caused by primary left ventricular (LV) failure. The complex interplay of LV dysfunction, neurohormonal activation, and the vicious cycle of progressively worsening ventricular function that characterizes cardiogenic shock is illustrated. LV dysfunction results from dysfunction of the infarct zone and remote myocardium, as illustrated in the inset in the lower, right-hand corner. For discussion, see text. ANP, atrial natriuretic peptide. (Adapted from Califf RM, Bengtson JR. Cardiogenic shock. *N Engl J Med* 1994;330:1724–1730; and Hochman JS, Palazzo A. Cardiogenic shock complicating acute myocardial infarction. In: Braunwald E, ed. *Atlas of heart diseases.* Boston: Current Medicine, 1996;8:12.1–12.23, with permission.)

$$EF = SV/EDV$$

The acute adaptive role of LV dilation is counterbalanced by deleterious long-term effects of LV dilation including increased wall stress, hypertrophy, and dilation, followed by failure of the remote myocardium.

The clinical manifestations of CHF when LV systolic function is depressed vary. Neurohormonal activation (171–173) (Fig. 19.4) and hydration status may explain why some patients with low EFs have pulmonary congestion and others do not (174). Varying degrees of diastolic dysfunction associated with infarction contribute substantially to alterations in LV compliance and filling pressure. Furthermore, alterations in peripheral circulation and in end organs, particularly those with prior LV damage, may influence the symptomatic response to the acute insult.

Recovery of contractile function in akinetic and even dyskinetic segments following acute MI is well documented and is caused by resolution of myocardial stunning and hibernation. Stunning may take weeks to months to resolve, and function of hibernating myocardium is only restored when coronary flow is normalized. Even late reperfusion may improve wall motion and global EF.

Diastolic Dysfunction

Diastolic dysfunction with reduced LV compliance is a relatively common cause of pulmonary congestion in acute MI. Ischemia causes impaired myocardial relaxation and diastolic dysfunction (175). Severe pulmonary edema may result from global subendocardial ischemia caused by three-vessel or left main CAD with a normal heart size. Additionally, the infarct zone undergoes alterations in compliance that result in varying LV distensibility over time following coronary occlusion (158–160). Reperfusion into areas of irreversible necrosis leads to contraction band necrosis, hemorrhage, and edema, resulting in acutely stiff infarcts (48,176) and, therefore, reduced LV compliance.

Diastolic abnormalities of the LV that impede LV filling may result in both an increase in LV filling pressures and a decrease in SV in the absence of global LV systolic dysfunction. Preexisting conditions that may cause reductions in ventricular compliance, such as hypertension and diabetes, result in an even greater shift of the pressure-volume curve when ischemia or infarction is superimposed.

Cardiogenic Shock Caused by Primary Left Ventricular Failure

LV failure is the most common cause of cardiogenic shock complicating acute MI. The prospective SHOCK Trial Registry identified LV failure as the etiology of shock in 78.5% of patients (Fig. 19.5) (177).

Patients with acute MI who develop cardiogenic shock typically have severe atherosclerotic disease involving all three major coronary arteries and often a severe stenosis in

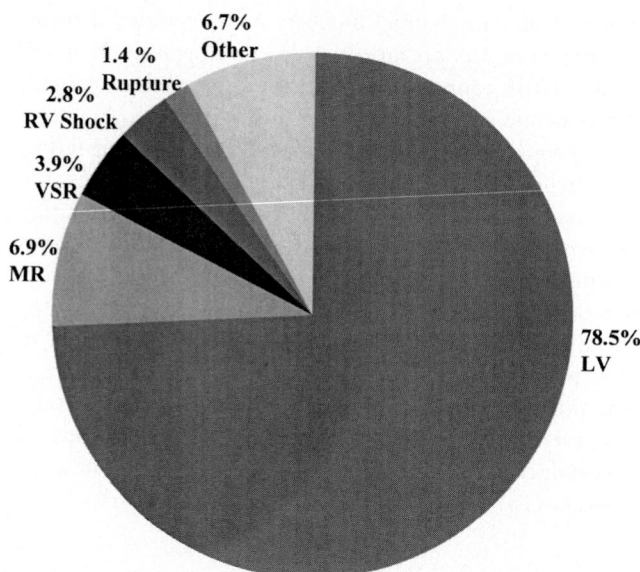

FIGURE 19.5 Etiologies of cardiogenic shock complicating acute myocardial infarction in the SHOCK Trial Registry (n = 1,190) and patients enrolled concurrently in the SHOCK Trial Registry (n = 232). The other category includes all other etiologies not noted (i.e., prior severe valvular heart disease, cardiomyopathy, or sustained arrhythmias). LV, left ventricular; MR, mitral regurgitation; RV, right ventricular; VSR, ventricular septal rupture. (Data from Hochman JS, Buller CE, Sleeper LA, et al. Cardiogenic shock complicating acute myocardial infarction—etiologies, management and outcome; overall findings of the SHOCK Trial Registry. *J Am Coll Cardiol* 2000;36:1063–1070.)

the LAD coronary artery. Significant stenosis in the left main coronary artery is seen in 16% to 21% of patients and single-vessel disease in approximately 13% to 22% of patients (178–180), with the LAD most often the IRA. Autopsy studies traditionally have demonstrated that at least 40% of the LV mass is affected in patients dying from cardiogenic shock complicating MI (179,181). Prior MI is present in approximately 40% of patients; when an old infarct is extensive, even a small, new infarction may lead to shock. Global ischemia, with or without minor infarction, may cause shock. In the GUSTO 2 trial one-third of patients with cardiogenic shock presented with a non–ST-segment elevation acute coronary syndrome (182). ▼ d44

Other Conditions

Conditions that result in high-output failure may occur in acute MI (Table 19.2). In particular, fever is common with large infarctions, and in the thrombolytic and aggressive anticoagulation era, acute anemia was sometimes seen. Excess use of negative inotropic agents, such as beta-blockers and calcium channel antagonists, particularly in combination, in patients with large infarctions may result in CHF and hypotension. When hypotension is present, noncardiogenic causes of shock must be excluded. These include volume depletion, particularly

TABLE 19.2 CARDIOGENIC SHOCK: DIFFERENTIAL DIAGNOSIS

Complications of acute myocardial infarction
    Extensive left ventricular infarction and ischemia
    Extensive right ventricular infarction and ischemia
    Ventricular septal rupture
    Acute, severe mitral regurgitation
    Tamponade
        With free wall rupture
        Without free wall rupture
Other conditions
    Aortic dissection
    Myocarditis
    Pulmonary embolism
    Critical aortic or mitral stenosis
    Acute aortic or mitral regurgitation
    Pericarditis with tamponade
    Metabolic/toxic
        Calcium channel or beta-blocker overdose
        Acidosis, hyperkalemia, hypoxemia
        Thyroid storm, myxedema coma
    Acute myocardial infarction with
        Ischemic/infarcted bowel
        Ruptured abdominal aortic aneurysm
        Sepsis
        Hemorrhage
        Anaphylaxis
        Excessive beta- or calcium channel blockade

common in the elderly with or without hemorrhage, sepsis, and PE. Even when shock results from primary LV failure, MR caused by papillary muscle dysfunction (191,192) often contributes to shock. Each of the mechanical causes of cardiogenic shock discussed later in this chapter—including VSR, acute severe MR, pericardial tamponade, and PE—must be excluded. Aortic dissection with acute aortic regurgitation, tamponade, or both may mimic acute MI with cardiogenic shock (*e*Fig. 19.5.1, Table 19.2). An acute MI may occur in association with another catastrophic event (e.g., ruptured aortic aneurysm, ischemic bowel, and so forth), and the diagnosis may be difficult in an obtunded patient in shock.

Clinical Profile: Congestive Heart Failure and Cardiogenic Shock

The Killip clinical classification system (5) stratifies patients at risk based on severity of CHF and the presence of cardiogenic shock and provides a useful approach with continued applicability in the reperfusion era. In a classic study at a single center of 250 consecutive patients with acute MI, Killip et al. (5) defined criteria for risk-stratification based on clinical evidence of LV failure:

1. Killip class I is defined as no evidence of CHF.
2. Killip class II is defined as presence of a third heart sound gallop, basilar rales, or both.
3. Killip class III is defined as pulmonary edema.

4. Killip class IV is defined as cardiogenic shock (*e*Tables 19.2.1 and 19.2.2).

The worst Killip class may be present on hospital admission or may develop at any point during hospitalization.

Incidence of Congestive Heart Failure and Cardiogenic Shock

The incidence of CHF by Killip class in the original description in 1967 is shown in *e*Table 19.2.2. The rates of CHF by Killip class reported 20 to 30 years later in large thrombolytic trials and two registries are shown in *e*Table 19.2.1. These data suggest that the incidence of CHF may be decreasing over time. However, this cannot be firmly established, as more complicated patients have been excluded from clinical trials (141), and the definition and diagnosis of CHF varies. Furthermore, the original description by Killip et al. (5) involved only 250 patients in a single, university hospital center. Data from placebo-controlled, randomized trials assessing the effect of thrombolysis on the occurrence of CHF after hospital admission demonstrate variable results (Table 19.3) (131,133,134,193–198). Overall, however, the short-term incidence of CHF is 20% for the placebo group and is slightly lower (17%) for the thrombolytic group. The 7-month to 1-year follow-up pooled data also appear to show a slight reduction in the incidence of CHF (Table 19.3).

From 1975 to 1988, which antedates the widespread use of reperfusion therapy, the incidence of cardiogenic shock in the Worcester community was relatively constant at 7.5%, with a consistently high mortality of 78% (199). This incidence is similar to that reported in more recent large thrombolytic trials (137). The Worcester community studied 7 additional years (up to 1997) and reported no change in the incidence of cardiogenic shock (200). The U.S. National Registry of Myocardial Infarction (NRMI) data since 1989 demonstrate that 4.1% of patients not treated with thrombolysis (n = 228,512) died of cardiogenic shock, which represented 32.0% of deaths (201). Of those receiving thrombolysis (n = 91,218), 2.3% died of cardiogenic shock, which represented 39.0% of deaths. These data are consistent with a decrease in the incidence of cardiogenic shock in more recent years and a decrease in the incidence of shock associated with reperfusion therapy. Randomized trials (134,196) of thrombolysis versus heparin alone have demonstrated a significantly lower incidence of cardiogenic shock with thrombolysis, particularly of shock that develops 24 or more hours after MI.

Direct PTCA has not been compared with placebo in terms of its effect on pump failure or on the frequency of cardiogenic shock; however, by extrapolating from comparisons with thrombolysis, the incidence of shock is reduced compared with that following no reperfusion (202–204).

TABLE 19.3 INCIDENCE OF CONGESTIVE HEART FAILURE

Study	Reference	Thrombolysis		Placebo	
		Number	Percent	Number	Percent
In-hospital					
ASSET	134	2,512	17.7	2,493	18.4
Guerci et al.	193	72	14.0	66	33.0
NHF	194	73	27.4	71	36.6
Simoons et al.	195	269	13.8	264	20.1
Meinertz et al.	196	162	20.0	151	29.0
Bassand et al.	197	112	6.7	119	13.4
Follow-up					
ISAM (7 mo)	133	859	6.6	882	9.1
AIMS (1 yr)	131	624	21.0	634	24.0

Study	Reference	Thrombolysis		Primary PTCA	
		Number	Percent	Number	Percent
GUSTO IIB PTCA substudy (30 days)	291	573	4.9	565	4.3

PTCA, percutaneous transluminal coronary angioplasty.
Modified from Bates ER, Topol EJ. Limitations of thrombolytic therapy for acute myocardial infarction complicated by congestive heart failure and cardiogenic shock. *J Am Coll Cardiol* 1991;18:1077–1084, with permission.

Nevertheless, pump failure remains the leading cause of death in patients hospitalized with acute MI in the reperfusion era (201).

Congestive Heart Failure and Cardiogenic Shock: Risk Factors

Patient Profile
Risk factors for the development of shock have been studied extensively in the prereperfusion and postreperfusion eras and in ST-elevation and non–ST-elevation MI patients. Age, female sex, prior MI, and diabetes are consistently associated with risk of pump failure (184,185,199), as is anterior MI location (182,200,205). The characteristics of 1,190 patients with suspected cardiogenic shock in the prospective SHOCK Trial Registry, which includes all etiologies, infarct types, and therapies, were age 68.7, 40% women, history of MI in 37%, hypertension in 53%, and diabetes in 33% (177). Systolic BP, HR, and Killip class II or III on admission make up approximately 90% of the predictive information in thrombolytic-treated patients (205) (Fig. 19.5.2). Other factors associated with the development of cardiogenic shock include EF less than or equal to 35%, persistent occlusion of the IRA, and the absence of hyperkinesis of the uninfarcted LV segments (114,168,184).

Non–ST-Elevation Myocardial Infarction.
Cardiogenic shock complicates non–ST-elevation MI approximately half as often as it does ST-elevation MI (182). In the SHOCK Trial Registry, 17% of patients with predominant LV failure had non–ST-elevation MI (206). These patients are older and have more prior MI, CHF, CABG, and peripheral vascular disease than patients with ST-elevation MI. They more often have severe three-vessel and left main CAD. Importantly, in 35% the circumflex artery was the culprit vessel, reflecting the difficulty in diagnosing posterior ST-elevation infarction.

Congestive Heart Failure and Cardiogenic Shock: Timing

As noted, patients often develop CHF and cardiogenic shock after hospital admission. In the SHOCK Trial Registry, patients with cardiogenic shock caused by primary LV failure demonstrated a predominance of early shock: 47% within the first 6 hours and 72% within 24 hours of MI onset (209). Nevertheless, only 9% of those with cardiogenic shock presented to the hospital in shock. The large GUSTO 1 (185) thrombolytic trial reported that 0.8% of enrolled patients presented with cardiogenic shock, and an additional 6.5% developed shock after hospital admission.

Clinical Assessment

Overview
Patients who develop pump failure must be assessed for other complicating conditions (Table 19.2; *e*Fig. 19.5.1) (see Pathophysiologic Principles).

A history should be obtained and a physical examination should be performed rapidly as well as ECG, arterial blood gas analysis, and hematology and chemistry profiles. Chest roentgenography should be promptly performed.

Clinical Findings: Congestive Heart Failure

Pump failure most frequently manifests as pulmonary congestion with pulmonary rales on examination, and pulmonary vascular redistribution with interstitial edema on chest roentgenography, initially with a normal heart size. Patients with mild CHF (Killip class II) may or may not report dyspnea. Tachypnea is usually present, but the respiratory rate may be only mildly elevated. Tachycardia and hypertension may or may not be present. Pulmonary edema (Killip class III) with acute interstitial and alveolar edema is associated with tachypnea, tachycardia, and hypertension caused by sympathetic stimulation. Lack of hypertension suggests profound LV failure and impending cardiogenic shock.

Electrocardiographic Findings: Congestive Heart Failure

There are large variations in the ECG findings in patients with pulmonary congestion, although most patients have changes consistent with a large infarction. Extensive ST-segment depressions are not uncommon and may represent extensive subendocardial infarction or small infarcts with extensive ischemia.

Clinical Findings: Cardiogenic Shock

The patient with classic cardiogenic shock complicating acute MI has severe systemic hypotension, end-organ hypoperfusion with cool extremities and oliguria, and respiratory distress caused by pulmonary congestion. This syndrome may develop either as a sudden event or slowly *after* hospital admission. There is a wide range in the clinical manifestations and severity of cardiogenic shock, and all components for classic cardiogenic shock may not be present. Clinical pulmonary edema need not be present to diagnose or suspect cardiogenic shock. An adequate or elevated PCWP must be documented by right-sided heart catheterization in the setting of systemic hypotension to confirm the diagnosis when pulmonary edema is not present (unless RV cardiogenic shock is diagnosed) (see Right Ventricular Infarction). In the SHOCK Trial Registry, 29% of patients diagnosed with cardiogenic shock caused by predominant LV failure had no pulmonary congestion on physical or radiographic examination, despite having mean PCWP of 22 mm Hg and LVEF of 30% (210) (*e*Fig. 19.5.3).

Preshock. Categorization of patients is not absolute, and gray zones exist. Patients who develop delayed cardiogenic shock following MI often slowly slip into shock, with evidence of a low cardiac output clinically before the onset of hypotension. Sympathetic stimulation may result in maintenance of normal BP in patients with high systemic vascular resistance and low cardiac output. This preshock or nonhypotensive shock state is associated with predominately anterior MI and a 46% in-hospital mortality in the SHOCK Trial Registry (211). Sinus tachycardia and low urine output are clinical findings of reduced SV and cardiac output. It must be appreciated that these signs reflect severe depression of cardiac output and necessitate rapid evaluation of patients before the onset of frank hypotension.

Electrocardiographic Findings: Cardiogenic Shock

Most patients have ECG findings consistent with a transmural acute MI; however, 15% to 30% of patients who develop cardiogenic shock may have nonspecific ECG findings consistent with non–Q-wave MI (177,199,206) including widespread ST-segment depression. Anterior ST depression with upright T waves that improve across the precordium suggests acute posterior MI. More than one-half of all infarcts (55%) in the SHOCK Trial Registry (177) were anterior, 46% inferior, 19% posterior, and 32% lateral. Patients often have multiple infarct locations (50%) on ECG that are a composite of old and new MIs. Of note, ischemia in an old infarct zone may result in recurrent ST-segment elevations.

Patients with cardiogenic shock caused by *LV failure* should have extensive ECG abnormalities consistent with massive, acute infarct, severe and diffuse acute ischemia, or evidence of prior substantial damage (e.g., extensive pathologic Q waves or left bundle branch block). A relative lack of ECG abnormalities in contrast to the severity of the hemodynamic status should alert one to another cause of cardiogenic shock such as aortic dissection or rupture of the myocardium (i.e., free wall, ventricular septum, papillary muscle, or chordae) or hemorrhage (Table 19.2; *e*Fig. 19.5.1).

Patients with first inferior or posterior or lateral MI do not develop cardiogenic shock caused by LV failure, and one should suspect acute severe MR. In patients with cardiogenic shock and mild ECG abnormalities, such as only limited ST-segment elevations, aortic dissection should be ruled out (Table 19.2).

Echocardiography with Color Flow Doppler

Echocardiography with color flow Doppler is an extremely valuable diagnostic tool and should be obtained as rapidly as possible once CHF or cardiogenic shock is suspected. LV and RV function can be visualized, and tamponade can be diagnosed (212–214). Color flow Doppler mapping can diagnose severe MR and VSR (214). Proximal aortic dissection with aortic insufficiency, pericardial tamponade, or both can also be visualized. In critically ill patients, who are often supported by mechanical ventilation, it may be difficult to obtain adequate images with transthoracic echocardiography, and transesophageal echocardiography may reveal a flail mitral leaflet with severe MR (215). Even adequate transthoracic echocardiography may miss localized MR caused by a flail mitral leaflet (212).

Management: Pharmacologic Therapy, Mechanical Support, and Revascularization

General Measures

Hypoxemia caused by pulmonary congestion must be corrected rapidly with mechanical ventilatory support to reduce the work of breathing and improve oxygenation, as necessary. In the presence of cardiogenic shock, lactic acidosis is common; this leads to further myocardial depression and renders patients resistant to the vasopressor effects of dopamine and norepinephrine. Rapid correction of acidosis is extremely important and empiric hyperventilation is appropriate until arterial blood gas results can be obtained. Ventilator settings can then be guided by arterial blood gas values. Hyperventilation is preferred to administration of sodium bicarbonate for correction of acidosis, because the buffering capacity of sodium bicarbonate is limited and short-lived, requiring a large sodium load.

Bradycardia and atrioventricular (AV) block must be corrected. If pacing is indicated, preservation of atrial contraction is an important goal; thus, AV pacing is preferred. New onset of AF should be rapidly cardioverted. An antiarrhythmic agent, such as amiodarone, may be required to maintain sinus rhythm. When severe LV dysfunction leads to reduction in SV, high HRs are necessary to maintain cardiac output. This needs to be taken into account when setting the HR for patients with hemodynamically significant bradycardia who require pacing. In general, HRs of approximately 90 to 100 beats/min are advisable.

Volume Status

Pulmonary Congestion. Pulmonary congestion with acute MI is caused by a transient or sustained increase in the PCWP. Patients who present with pulmonary edema who have no prior history of myocardial dysfunction and have not received fluid administration have a normal total body sodium and fluid status. There is acute redistribution of fluid into the lungs, and with diaphoresis and no oral intake, this results in *relative* intravascular depletion in the early phase. Diuretics can cause further intravascular depletion and hypotension and can precipitate cardiogenic shock. It must also be appreciated that there is a lag between normalization of the PCWP and resolution of interstitial and alveolar edema (224). Patients with findings on examination or on chest roentgenography suggesting congestion (e.g., basilar rales or interstitial fluid) for 24 hours do not necessarily require continued diuretic therapy provided dyspnea is resolving and respiratory status is improving. Excessive diuresis may result in severe intravascular depletion in patients who present with pulmonary edema, which initiates a vicious cycle of hypotension, hypoperfusion, infarct extension and ischemia, additional LV dysfunction, and so forth (Fig. 19.4). The best means of assessing volume status is careful measurement of the intake and output record including the prehospital and emergency department phases as well as the patient's weight. Measurement of PCWP is useful but reflects ventricular compliance as well as volume status. An elevated blood urea nitrogen to creatinine ratio may reflect intravascular depletion or poor renal perfusion caused by a low CI. However, a low blood urea nitrogen level in a patient with severely depressed LVEF and persistent pulmonary congestion reflects underdiuresis.

The volume status of patients with prior myocardial dysfunction and prior use of diuretics is more variable. These patients may be volume overloaded because of chronic CHF, or those on chronic diuretics may be intravascularly depleted at the time of onset of their acute MI, with a sudden increase in PCWP caused by acute infarction.

Hypotension. Hypotension complicating acute MI may be caused by hypovolemia as a result of vomiting, diaphoresis, use of diuretics, or associated hemorrhage. In addition, many of the medications (e.g., nitrates and morphine) administered during acute MI cause venodilation and preload reduction, which, in turn, causes hypotension. Placing the patient in Trendelenburg's position is appropriate for treatment of these causes of hypotension. For patients who do not have evidence on examination or on chest roentgenography of pulmonary congestion and who are not in respiratory distress, an empiric i.v. volume challenge of 250 mL of normal saline can be given. Repeated empiric fluid challenges may be used before PA catheterization, but caution must be exercised for those at increased risk for precipitation of CHF with volume infusion (e.g., older patients, patients with prior MI, prior CHF or impaired LV function, hypertensive heart disease, diabetes, and a small body size). Transcutaneous continuous oximetric monitoring of systemic oxygen saturation is advised. In some patients, hypotension and bradycardia are manifestations of Bezold-Jarisch reflex (225) or a vasovagal response to volume depletion. Although atropine may be helpful, the key to management is fluid administration. This is particularly true in patients with a first inferior MI and in association with the administration of nitrates, which accentuates preload reduction in an already volume-depleted patient. PA catheterization is needed only in refractory patients. Overly vigorous fluid challenges in patients with extensive LV infarction result in pulmonary edema and should be avoided. Elderly patients, in particular, are sensitive to excessive administration of fluids caused by reduced LV compliance.

Pulmonary Congestion and Hypotension—Cardiogenic Shock. When pulmonary congestion and hypotension are both present, cardiogenic shock is diagnosed; these patients should not have a fluid challenge. Diuretics have a limited role in the acute management of these patients because they can cause further hypotension and are ineffective when marked reduction in renal blood flow and glomerular filtration are present. The circulation must be first supported by pharmacologic and mechanical interventions discussed in the following sections, followed by i.v. diuretics.

Medications

General

Agents with negative inotropic properties should be avoided in patients with acute large infarctions and pump failure. These agents include both beta-blockers and calcium channel antagonists. This does *not* preclude the use of beta-blockers as secondary prevention at a later time in the clinical course once hemodynamics are stabilized. Beta-blockers, initiated in low doses, are indicated in these patients before hospital discharge (226). Amiodarone is the agent of choice for ventricular tachycardia or fibrillation that occurs in patients with severe pump failure. Medications that are primarily cleared by the kidneys or liver must be used in reduced doses in patients with hepatic or renal dysfunction and end-organ hypoperfusion. In particular, lidocaine doses must be reduced when this agent is used to treat ventricular arrhythmias.

Morphine sulfate reduces preload and therefore improves pulmonary congestion. It also provides analgesia and lessens anxiety. To avoid hypotension, small incremental doses (2 to 4 mg) should be administered.

Medications that are used in acute MI patients with or without pump failure are discussed in the CD-ROM and online versions of this text and Chapter 18.

Specific Medications

Diuretics. Furosemide, 20 mg i.v., should be the initial dose for patients who have not been given diuretics and who have normal creatinine levels; higher and repeated doses should be given as needed. Other loop diuretics, such as torsemide, bumetanide, or ethacrynic acid, are alternatives. After the early phase of acute MI with pulmonary congestion, continued doses of diuretics are necessary for patients with significantly impaired LV systolic function and persistent CHF. Potent loop diuretics also activate the renin-angiotensin-aldosterone system, thereby leading to an increase in cardiac afterload and promoting sodium retention once their short-term effects resolve. For refractory patients, a combination of a loop and a thiazide diuretic, such as hydrochlorothiazide or metolazone, produces additive effects. Diuretics should be withheld or the dosage reduced when ACE inhibitors are initiated to avoid hypotension and transient renal insufficiency.

Angiotensin-Converting Enzyme Inhibitors. ACE inhibitors, by reducing cardiac preload and afterload in patients with heart failure and acute MI, improve LV performance. The renin-angiotensin-aldosterone system is frequently activated in patients with acute MI (172) and further activated in patients with CHF. In addition to directly blocking the renin-angiotensin-aldosterone system, ACE inhibitors vasodilate by increasing circulating bradykinins (240–242). Other beneficial effects on atherogenesis and plaque rupture may occur at a cellular level and the long-term vascular event rate is reduced (151). ACE inhibitors produce a dilating effect on the cerebral, coronary, and renal circulation, decreasing blood flow in the hepatic and splanchnic circulations (243,244). ACE inhibitors should be instituted early in patients with pulmonary congestion and particularly in those with hypertension. They should be administered orally and initiated in low doses with rapid upward titration provided hypotension is not induced. ACE inhibitors should not be used acutely in patients who are hypotensive.

The only study that evaluated the effect of ACE inhibitors on morbidity and mortality in patients presenting with acute CHF complicating MI was the Acute Infarction Ramipril Efficacy study (227). Ramipril or placebo was instituted in 2,006 patients between days 3 and 10, and mortality was significantly reduced at 30 days (relative hazard, 0.73; 95% confidence interval: 0.602, 0.89; $p <.002$) (eFig. 19.5.4) (227). This beneficial effect was seen in all subgroups analyzed, including those patients with or without thrombolytic and ASA therapy. Therefore, all patients with pump failure complicating acute MI, including those whose cardiogenic shock has resolved, should be treated with ACE inhibitors. The timing of initiation depends on the stability of the BP, with hypertensive or normotensive patients tolerating early initiation. Based on the excellent tolerance of early oral captopril and lisinopril in ISIS 4 and GISSI-3 and on the benefits on infarct expansion, we recommend early (≤12 hours) oral initiation of captopril, 6.25 mg, for patients presenting with pulmonary congestion. The dosage may be doubled with each subsequent dosage, as tolerated up to 25 to 50 mg every 8 hours. Hypotension should be avoided, particularly during reperfusion, and we therefore recommend initiating oral ACE inhibitors after direct PTCA or thrombolysis has established reperfusion. If reperfusion fails or is not attempted, early administration of ACE inhibitors plays an important role. Long-acting ACE inhibitors (e.g., enalapril, lisinopril, ramipril, trandolapril) can be given after the acute phase.

Cardiac Glycosides. Digoxin increases myocardial contractility to a lesser extent compared with dobutamine or phosphodiesterase inhibitors (245). Acute administration is associated with alpha adrenergically mediated coronary and systemic vasoconstriction (246). However, in patients with CHF, the positive inotropic effects may result in reflex sympathetic withdrawal and vasodilation. Digoxin is associated with an increased risk for ventricular arrhythmias during the first 24 hours of acute MI. Therefore, digoxin has no clear role in acute pulmonary congestion or cardiogenic shock complicating MI. For patients with AF with a rapid ventricular response, digoxin has limited efficacy, but it is a good agent for rate control because it does not have the negative inotropic properties of beta-blockers or verapamil and diltiazem. The recommended dose for digoxin is 0.5 mg i.v., followed by 0.25 mg i.v. 4 to 6 hours later, until a 1-mg total loading dose has been administered or the target HR has been achieved (maximum dose, 1 mg). Of note, the target ventricular rate for a patient with pump failure is 90 to 110 beats/min to compensate for a depressed SV.

Pharmacologic Circulatory Support

General. The choice of a sympathomimetic agent for patients with pump failure depends on the patient's hemodynamics and, specifically, whether hypotension is present (*e*Table 19.3.2). Patients with pulmonary congestion without significantly depressed cardiac output should be treated with vasodilators alone. Patients in ACC/AHA hemodynamic subset 1 of pump failure (89) with an elevated PCWP and a CI ≤2.5 L per minute per m^2 and with systolic BP ≥100 mm Hg can be treated with combined inotropic and vasodilating agents, such as dobutamine or milrinone if needed for hypoperfusion. Beta-adrenergic agents have been demonstrated to enhance contractility of stunned myocardium and therefore can provide temporary support for pump failure until stunned myocardium recovers (247). Patients with cardiogenic shock and profound hypoperfusion need initial vasopressor support with alpha-dose dopamine or norepinephrine.

The lowest doses of sympathomimetic amines needed to maintain adequate cardiac output and adequate systemic perfusion should be used. For patients in cardiogenic shock, therapy should be guided with a PA catheter. Because each patient's response to different doses varies, systemic vascular resistance should be calculated, and the relationship between PCWP and CI should be defined repeatedly for patients as they remain on support. All sympathomimetic agents may cause atrial and ventricular tachyarrhythmias.

Dobutamine. This synthetic catecholamine increases myocardial contractility through preferential stimulation of myocardial beta$_1$-adrenergic receptors. Beta$_2$-peripheral vasodilator receptors and myocardial alpha$_1$-adrenergic receptors are also stimulated but to a lesser extent (248–250). Dobutamine has less chronotropic effect than does dopamine and typically does not cause significant changes in HR when the dose is less than 15 µg per kg per minute. The initial dosage of dobutamine is 2 µg per kg per minute followed by a gradual increase in dosage to 15 µg per kg per minute as needed. The lowest dosage required should be used for maintenance. Cardiac output should increase, and PCWP should decrease. Systemic vascular resistance decreases somewhat, and the balance of the increase in cardiac output and the decrease in systemic vascular resistance results in an unchanged BP. Dobutamine therefore is not the drug of choice for hypotension. Its short half-life, approximately 2 minutes, is highly desirable because it can be discontinued if ventricular tachycardia develops or it can be titrated down for excess increases in HR.

A concern with use of any inotropic agent is the risk for increase in myocardial oxygen requirements by increased myocardial contractility, tachycardia, and exacerbation of myocardial ischemia. However, when LV dilation and elevated diastolic filling pressures are present, wall tension decreases because EDV and pressure are reduced by dobutamine (251,252). Dobutamine can be combined with i.v. nitroglycerin when significant elevation in PCWP persists. Although dobutamine improves the patient's immediate hemodynamic status, there are no randomized trials assessing its effect on outcome.

Dopamine. The hemodynamic effects of dopamine are dose-dependent and vary from patient to patient. Low doses (i.e., 1 to 3 µg per kg per minute) result in renal vasodilation caused by dopamine receptor stimulation. Intermediate doses of 5 to 10 µg per kg per minute result in beta$_1$-adrenergic stimulation and increased myocardial contractility. High doses (i.e., ≥15 µg per kg per minute) result in alpha$_1$-receptor stimulation and arterial vasoconstriction. High-dose dopamine increases pulmonary vascular pressures, including PCWP, as well as systemic arterial pressure. High-dose dopamine is required for cardiogenic shock with profound hypotension to support perfusion of the vital organs. Hypotension must be aggressively corrected during attempted reperfusion with thrombolytic therapy. As other support measures are instituted (e.g., IABP), dopamine should be titrated down to the minimum dosage required.

Norepinephrine and Epinephrine. Norepinephrine is a powerful alpha$_1$ stimulant that results in arterial vasoconstriction and is a beta$_1$-stimulant that increases inotropy (259). It is used primarily as a last resort if dopamine proves inadequate to maintain systemic and coronary perfusion pressures. Epinephrine also acts on the beta$_1$ myocardial receptors and on both alpha$_2$- and beta$_2$-receptors in peripheral blood vessels. Small amounts may constrict renal as well as cutaneous vessels while dilating skeletal and mesenteric vessels, which may result in a decrease in BP. At larger doses, epinephrine primarily acts as a vasoconstrictor. It causes tachycardia and arrhythmias, which limits its use in acute MI with cardiogenic shock, except in resuscitating patients in cardiac arrest.

Mechanical Circulatory Support

Mechanical circulatory support plays an extremely important role in providing temporary support for patients in cardiogenic shock. Support devices are superior to pharmacologic support for cardiogenic shock in that perfusion is supported without increasing myocardial work and V̇O$_2$. It must be noted, however, that mechanical circulatory support alone has never been demonstrated in randomized trials to improve outcome in patients with cardiogenic shock.

Intraaortic Balloon Counterpulsation

The IABP is placed in the descending thoracic aorta distal to the left subclavian artery and above the renal arteries through the femoral artery, with balloon inflations and deflations synchronized with the cardiac cycle. This augments diastolic blood flow in the coronary and systemic circulation, and reduces afterload and aortic impedance. Both mechanisms increase CI and systemic and coronary diastolic pressures and improve myocardial metabolism (9,263–266). It is not clear, however, whether coronary flow distal to a critical stenosis increases with IABP. There are conflicting results with Doppler flow wire measurements of coronary blood flow versus great cardiac vein thermodilution flow measurements (267–269). However, in hypotensive states an increase in aortic pressure by IABP should improve coronary blood flow (270), particularly when combined with PTCA. ▼ d45

IABP remains extremely effective in supporting patients undergoing coronary angiography, PTCA, and CABG in cardiogenic shock. It also provides bridging support until an LV assistance device can be implanted or cardiac transplantation can be performed.

A randomized trial (274) has demonstrated that IABP improves angiographic patency following PTCA of the IRA in patients not in cardiogenic shock. Reports have suggested that IABP may be combined with thrombolytic therapy to improve reperfusion rates when cardiogenic shock is present (see Thrombolysis). The GUSTO 1 thrombolytic trial investigators (275) reported that patients in the United States were more frequently treated with invasive therapy including IABP than patients not in the United States, and that use of IABP correlated with lower mortality in an adjusted model. The SHOCK Trial Registry also reported improved survival associated with IABP use (276). However, most of these patients were revascularized, which was the strongest determinant of survival. Use of IABP allows for rapid stabilization of cardiogenic shock patients so that they can survive long enough to undergo urgent revascularization. Rapid IABP insertion and transfer of patients from primary to tertiary care hospitals is associated with improved survival (277). ACC/AHA guideline indications for use of IABP include preparation for angiography and revascularization in cardiogenic shock that has not quickly reversed, acute MR or VSR, refractory post-MI angina (89), and refractory ventricular arrhythmias with hemodynamic instability. Less firm indications include hemodynamic instability without shock, poor LV function, or persistent ischemia with large regions at risk (89). Risks associated with IABP include (a) leg ischemia possibly necessitating thrombectomy, vascular surgery, or amputation; (b) dissection, perforation, or damage to the aorta with insertion; (c) hemorrhage; and (d) infection and thrombocytopenia. Full-dose i.v. heparin is required. IABP is contraindicated when significant aortic insufficiency is present or when peripheral vascular disease is severe or aortic pathology (e.g., aortic aneurysm) precludes it. IABP is not effective when there is no spontaneous circulation, and the timing of IABP inflation is difficult when there are uncontrolled tachyarrhythmias.

Coronary Artery Reperfusion and Revascularization

Therapy that rapidly reestablishes blood flow in a totally occluded IRA is the single most important treatment of acute MI. This is true for patients with pump failure, in whom the absolute gain is large based on the high event rates (11,177,287–289). Observational data (287) demonstrate that an open IRA in patients with cardiogenic shock complicating MI correlates strongly with survival. Randomized trial results confirm that early revascularization, with either PTCA or CABG, improves 1-year survival compared with initial aggressive medical stabilization, including thrombolysis and IABP (11).

Congestive Heart Failure

The mortality among patients with CHF complicating acute MI (Killip classes II and III) has been only modestly reduced by thrombolytic therapy (Table 19.4) (5,85,135,156). However, GISSI-1 (85) provides the only randomized data available from patients with CHF on presentation that tested SK without ASA and included MIs with non–ST-segment elevations. Few patients with CHF have been enrolled in PTCA versus thrombolytic trials (202–204,290). One small trial (290) suggested benefit of PTCA over SK. In the GUSTO 2b PTCA substudy (291), patients who presented in Killip class II to III had similar relative reductions in mortality at 30 days from PTCA compared with front-loaded t-PA as was demonstrated in the overall study (292). Based on the higher event rates, the absolute reduction in events with direct PTCA was larger than for Killip class I patients. Unfortunately, the mortality remained high even with direct PTCA. It is likely that prior and acute *irreversible* myocardial damage in many of these patients will continue to result in mortality that is significantly higher than those among patients who present without CHF. Nevertheless, *early* successful reperfusion is the goal. We recommend direct PTCA when available; if direct PTCA is not available, thrombolytic therapy should be administered with rescue PTCA for failure of reperfusion. Based on the high event rate among patients with CHF complicating MI if early PTCA was not performed (Table 19.4), subsequent revascularization is indicated based on the anatomy. If CABG is indicated for multivessel disease, its timing must be individualized based on whether the IRA is patent and on the patient's degree of pulmonary congestion and clinical stability.

Cardiogenic Shock

Thrombolysis

Early Shock. There is limited efficacy of thrombolysis in patients who present in shock. This appears to be the result

TABLE 19.4 MORTALITY BY KILLIP CLASS

| | | Thrombolytic trials (30 days) | | | |
| | Killip and Kimball (in-hospital) | GISSI-1 | | International: thrombolytic | ASSENT-II: thrombolytic |
Killip class		Placebo	Thrombolytic		
I	6	7	6	5	5
II	17	20	16	18	13
III	38	39	33	32	26
IV	81	70	70	72	56

Data from references 5, 85, 133, and 408.

of failure to reperfuse thrombosed arteries in the setting of low coronary perfusion pressure. Experimentally, the rate of dissolution of coronary artery thrombus is markedly depressed when hypotension is present (117,118). If BP is augmented (to a systolic pressure of 130 mm Hg as demonstrated in the canine model) by aggressive use of vasopressors (118) or by IABP (117) during reperfusion, the rate of thrombus dissolution can be restored to more normal values. ⚐ d46

Mechanical Revascularization

Percutaneous Transluminal Coronary Angioplasty. The in-hospital mortality in mostly retrospective studies of patients undergoing PTCA for cardiogenic shock is 45% (10,177,178,287,288,297,298), which is lower than the historic mortality of 80% in controls (5,199). When PTCA is successful, mortality is significantly lower than when it is not (36% vs. 83%, respectively). The overall success rate for PTCA in shock is lower (75%), than for primary PTCA for acute myocardial infarction. GUSTO 1 investigators (185,275) also reported the association of revascularization (using PTCA or CABG) with lower mortality. Nonetheless, as shown in the SHOCK Trial Registry, selection bias plays a major role in improved outcomes following PTCA and CABG (177,299).

The randomized SHOCK Trial Registry compared a direct invasive strategy of emergency early revascularization to initial medical stabilization including thrombolysis and IABP, followed by delayed revascularization as clinically determined. Patients with shock (n = 302) caused by predominant LV failure that developed less than or equal to 36 hours after an ST elevation or Q wave or new left bundle branch block MI were enrolled (289). Angiography and early revascularization were performed in 97% and 87% of the invasive strategy group, respectively, and delayed revascularization was performed in 25% of the medical stabilization group. Both groups were supported with IABP (86%) and thrombolytic agents were used in 63% of the medical stabilization group and 49% of the invasive group. Although the difference in 30-day mortality of 9.3 percentage points between the groups (17% relative risk reduction, 46.7% vs. 56.0%) in favor of early revascularization did not

reach statistical significance (p = .109), the difference increased over time. At 6 and 12 months, 13 lives were saved for every 100 patients treated with early revascularization compared with intensive medical therapy, including IABP, thrombolysis, and delayed revascularization (53% vs. 66%; p = .025 at 12 months) (11) (Fig. 19.6). This benefit is comparable with that seen at 1 year with CABG surgery for left main disease (300,301). The improved survival was seen for patients with early and late shock and regardless of infarct location or the presence of comorbidities (e.g., diabetes, prior hypertension, or MI) (Fig. 19.7). The small subgroup of those older than 75 years (n = 56) did not appear to benefit. However, the small sample size precludes firm conclusions. The larger nonrandomized Registry suggested a markedly lower in-hospital mortality for elderly patients who were carefully clinically selected for early revascularization, even after adjustment for their lower risk profile (302). In the SHOCK Trial Registry, more than 80% of 1-year survivors were in New York Heart Association CHF class I to II.

PTCA should be performed with IABP support. Although there are insufficient data in shock, we recom-

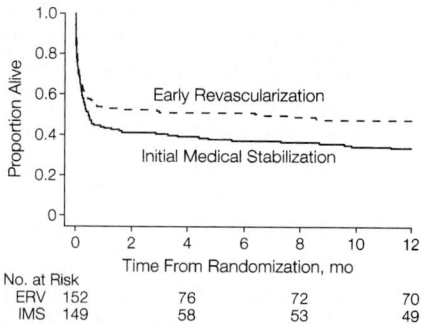

FIGURE 19.6 Kaplan-Meier survival curve 1-year postrandomization: 1-year survival of patients with acute myocardial infarction complicated by cardiogenic shock caused by predominant left ventricular failure. Patients were randomized to early revascularization (ERV) or initial medical stabilization (IMS) in the SHOCK Trial Registry (log rank, p = .043). (From Hochman JS, Sleeper LA, White HD, et al. One year survival following early revascularization for acute myocardial infarction complicated by cardiogenic shock. *JAMA* 2001;285:190–192, with permission.)

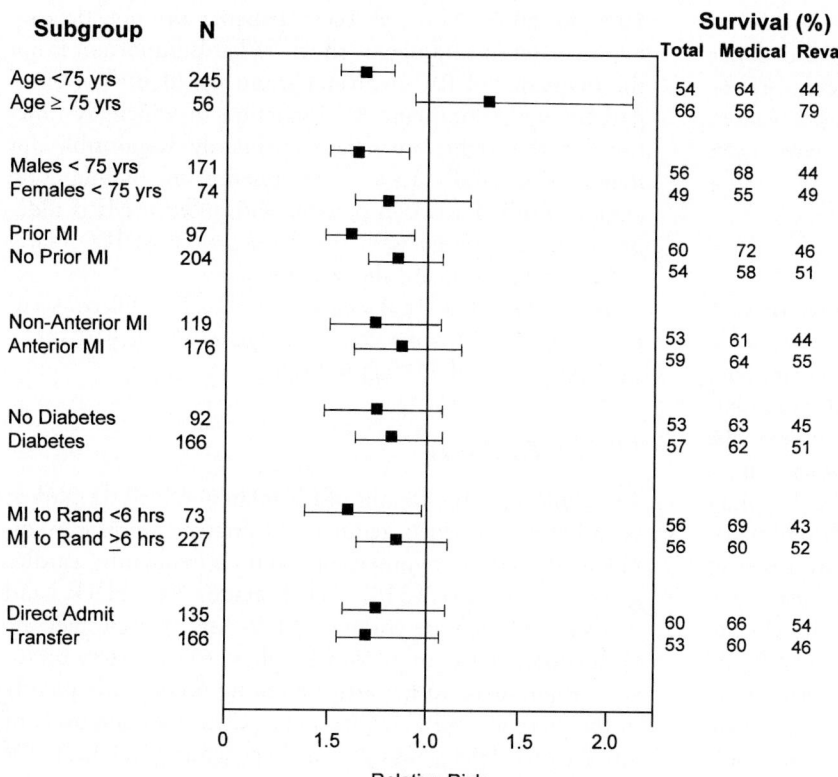

Subgroup	N		Survival (%)		
			Total	Medical	Revasc.
Age <75 yrs	245		54	64	44
Age ≥ 75 yrs	56		66	56	79
Males < 75 yrs	171		56	68	44
Females < 75 yrs	74		49	55	49
Prior MI	97		60	72	46
No Prior MI	204		54	58	51
Non-Anterior MI	119		53	61	44
Anterior MI	176		59	64	55
No Diabetes	92		53	63	45
Diabetes	166		57	62	51
MI to Rand <6 hrs	73		56	69	43
MI to Rand ≥6 hrs	227		56	60	52
Direct Admit	135		60	66	54
Transfer	166		53	60	46

Relative Risk

Early Revascularization Benefit   Medical Therapy Benefit

FIGURE 19.7 Relative risk of 6-month death with early revascularization compared with initial medical stabilization (medical therapy) for selected subgroups of patients with cardiogenic shock in the SHOCK Trial Registry. MI, myocardial infarction.

mend use of stents and GP IIb/IIIa antagonists. The outcome of patients who underwent PTCA after thrombolysis was similar to those who underwent direct PTCA in the SHOCK Trial Registry (297). Most patients have triple-vessel disease (65%) and the options for revascularization include (a) PTCA of the IRA followed by complete revascularization by multivessel PTCA; (b) initial multivessel PTCA; (c) initial CABG; and (d) PTCA of the IRA followed by CABG. These strategies have not been directly compared. We recommend PTCA for patients with one-, two-, or moderate three-vessel disease and CABG for those with severe three-vessel or left main disease. Continuous, noninvasive monitoring of the systemic oxygen saturation is required. Most patients with cardiogenic shock have required prior intubation; for others, intubation is recommended before injecting angiographic dye. Low osmolality, ionic contrast dye is recommended. Despite these measures, relatively low PTCA success rates and no reflow remain challenges. Some patients improve rapidly and dramatically after PTCA, whereas others show no immediate hemodynamic improvement. Patients may deteriorate hemodynamically after reperfusion is established, particularly if they are reperfused late. It is not uncommon for significant arrhythmias, including profound bradycardia and ventricular fibrillation, to develop during reperfusion in these patients. Immediate therapy must be available.

Coronary Artery Bypass Graft. In patients with shock, severe triple-vessel disease is present in most (65%), and left main disease is present in 20% (180,289). Such patients are often unsuitable for PTCA; hence, CABG is the preferred alternative. The in-hospital mortality among patients who underwent CABG at some time during their hospitalization for cardiogenic shock complicating acute MI was 35%. This constitutes the lowest mortality reported for cardiogenic shock in acute MI (9,177,287,298,299,303). In the SHOCK Trial Registry, early CABG surgery was performed in 40% of those who underwent emergency revascularization at a median of 2.7 hours after randomization. Despite significantly higher rates of left main (40% vs. 14%; *p* = .001) and triple-vessel CAD (79% vs. 59%; *p* = .007), the 30-day and 1-year mortality for those who underwent emergency CABG was the same as for those who underwent emergency PTCA (42% vs. 46% at 30 days; 52% vs. 55% at 1 year) (289,304).

We recommend emergency early CABG with IABP support for patients with cardiogenic shock and severe triple-vessel or left main disease. Although some surgeons prefer a period of medical stabilization, there is a high risk of death on the first day (almost 50% of all deaths). The SHOCK Trial Registry demonstrated that an initial intensive medical stabilization approach was associated with poorer 1-year survival than early revascularization (11).

Optimization of cardioprotection is most critical in patients with severe LV dysfunction and shock, and newer cardioprotective techniques including antegrade and retrograde cardioplegia, warm induction, prolonged vented bypass, and use of substrate-enriched blood have been advocated (303).

Summary

Rapid support of the circulation and restoration of IRA blood flow is the goal for managing patients with acute LV failure complicating acute MI. We strongly recommend rapid IABP support, coronary angiography, and revascularization, particularly for those aged less than 75 years. The choice of PTCA or CABG is based on the coronary anatomy and the experience of the personnel. For hospitals without the facilities for PTCA or CABG, thrombolytic agents should be administered with aggressive measures to augment BP, including IABP, followed rapidly by transfer to tertiary care facilities. For young patients who do not respond to available measures, LV assistance devices should be considered as a bridge to urgent cardiac transplantation. Despite the marked reduction in mortality and the good functional class of survivors, overall 30-day survival is only 45% with aggressive care. Patients, especially the elderly, and their families must be involved in the decisions regarding their care, which should be individualized.

RIGHT VENTRICULAR INFARCTION

Pathology

RV infarction is typically associated with an inferior MI involving the interventricular septum and with occlusion of the proximal, right coronary artery. The extent of infarction varies greatly depending on whether occlusion occurs before the RV free wall and RV marginal branches, whether collateral flow from the LAD is present, and on the extent of blood flow through the thebesian veins (311). Because the right ventricle is a thin-walled chamber that functions at low-oxygen demands and low pressure with coronary perfusion throughout systole and diastole, extensive irreversible infarction is unusual. Transient, ischemic dysfunction and stunning are more typical, with long-term recovery of function being the rule (312,313). RV infarction is typically seen in association with LV infarction, with isolated RV infarction reported in less than 5% of autopsies (314).

Clinical Profile

Incidence

Depending on the diagnostic criteria used, the incidence of RV infarction in patients with inferior MI ranges from 10% to 50%. Most of these patients do not develop hypotension or cardiogenic shock. What is important is not the frequency of RV involvement but the identification of patients with dominant RV infarction in which dysfunction of the right ventricle is primarily responsible for hypotension and shock. The absence of preinfarction angina within 1 week in patients with inferior MI is independently associated with the development of RV infarction, hypotension, and shock (315).

In the SHOCK Trial Registry, 2.8% of 1,190 consecutive patients with suspected cardiogenic shock had shock caused by isolated RV failure (316).

Clinical Findings

The clinical manifestations of RV infarction include marked sensitivity to preload reduction (nitrates, morphine sulphate, diuretics), hypotension, and, infrequently, cardiogenic shock (317–319). High-grade AV block and bradyarrhythmias are common (320–322) because they are both consequences of proximal, right coronary artery occlusion. Right atrial to left atrial shunting occurs infrequently in the presence of RV failure and a patent foramen ovale or atrial septal defect, resulting in hypoxemia (323,324). RV free wall rupture and tamponade are rare, but patients with extensive RV necrosis are at risk for RV catheter- (i.e., pacemaker lead or PA catheter) related perforation.

Diagnosis

The classic, clinical constellation of hypotension, elevated jugular venous pressure with clear lung fields, and no dyspnea (316) is highly specific but insensitive for RV infarction (325).

When performed early after onset of symptoms, ECG can be highly sensitive and specific. Right precordial (RV) leads should be obtained in patients with inferior MI. An ST elevation of greater than or equal to 0.5 mm in lead V_{4R} is highly sensitive (326,327) and correlates with major clinical complications (328). The added criteria of ST elevations greater than 0.5 mm in lead V_{4R} compared with leads V_1 to V_3 has higher specificity but lower sensitivity than does ST-segment elevation in lead V_{4R} alone (327). Technetium 99m pyrophosphate myocardial scintigraphy can diagnose RV infarction; however, at present, it is infrequently performed. Echocardiography and gated blood pool scintigraphy have proven to be efficacious (329) in diagnosing clinically significant RV infarction by assessing RV size and wall motion. Echocardiography is typically preferred because it can be performed at the bedside and simultaneously offers assessment of pericardial effusion and tamponade, which is the chief differential diagnosis when predominant RV infarction and hypotension are present. When this syndrome is found on acute presentation before cardiac marker confirmation, acute PE is part of the differential diagnosis as well. Echocardiography may also be useful because Doppler estimation of PA pressures may be obtained.

Accepted hemodynamic criteria for dominant RV infarction include a right atrial (RA) pressure >10 mm Hg, an RA/PCWP ratio ≥0.8, or an RA pressure that is no less than 5 mm Hg below the PCWP. These values may only be demonstrated after volume infusion (330). Equalization of RA pressure and PCWP is often seen, necessitating exclusion of cardiac tamponade. The CI will be ≤2.2 L per minute per m² in patients with severe RV dysfunction.

Prognosis

The prognosis for RV infarction is largely determined by the degree of associated LV infarction (321,331). Overall, RV infarction is an independent risk factor for death in patients with inferior MI, and this risk increases substantially with increasing age (328,332,333). Patients with isolated RV infarction and normal or near normal LV function infrequently have severe hemodynamic compromise leading to death. For the small subset with shock, the in-hospital mortality is 53% (316). This poor prognosis is despite the predominance of single-vessel disease (65%). For survivors of acute RV infarction, the long-term prognosis is excellent, with improved RVEF seen over time (312,334).

Hemodynamics and Management

Although RV cauterization in animal models with normal pulmonary vascular resistance and an open pericardium has not resulted in significant hemodynamic abnormalities, the clinical syndrome of hemodynamic compromise with RV infarction has been well described (335,336). A subsequent dog model (337) confirmed this hemodynamic profile and a favorable response of the systemic arterial pressure and cardiac output to volume administration. The difference between the animal model of isolated RV infarction and clinical isolated RV infarction is that in the latter, the inferior wall of the LV and the interventricular septum are almost invariably involved. This, in turn, may result in relatively elevated LV filling pressures and RV afterload, which further compromise RV SV. Contraction of the interventricular septum also contributes to normal RV function (338). The role of the pericardium and ventricular interdependence is important to the understanding of the pathophysiology of RV failure. As the size of the RV cavity increases because of extensive infarction and volume administration, flattening of the interventricular septum or bowing of the septum into the left ventricle develops, resulting in restriction of LV filling (339,340) (Fig. 19.8). This resolves when the pericardium is removed (339).

Volume infusion became standard treatment for hypotension and low cardiac output in RV infarction based on the experimental data and early clinical series (317,337).

In those patients who demonstrated the typical hemodynamic finding of an RA/PCWP ratio ≥0.8, the goal was to increase RV output and LV filling pressure. However, patients in these studies may have been receiving inappropriate preload-reducing therapy because RV infarction perhaps was not recognized initially. Dell'Italia et al. (341) demonstrated that despite progressive volume infusion with RA pressure rising from 11 to 15 mm Hg (*p* ≤.001) and PCWP increasing from 10 to 15 mm Hg (*p* ≤.001), the CI did not significantly increase (1.9 ± 0.5 L per minute per m² to 2.1 ± 0.4 L per minute per m²). This was confirmed in patients. PCWP increased with i.v. volume infusion, but CI was unchanged (342) and RVEF decreased (343). This more contemporary experience probably reflects a patient population with more severely compromised RV function in contrast to earlier series of patients with milder RV infarction complicated by inappropriate diuresis in whom one would expect fluid administration to be beneficial. Radionuclide angiography demonstrated an increase in RVEDV, whereas LVEDV remained unchanged. The thin wall infarcted RV markedly dilates and, because of pericardial restraint, the interventricular septum shifts into the LV. This important finding demonstrates that PCWP may not accurately reflect LVEDV but, rather, impaired LV filling caused by the interventricular septal shift (Fig. 19.8). Therefore, echocardiographic imaging is critical for the diagnosis and management of patients with hemodynamic compromise caused by RV infarction, because the PCWP may be misleading. Nonetheless, an elevated PCWP is detrimental as a component of RV afterload. Hemodynamic monitoring is advisable. In patients with low output caused by dominant RV infarction, the RA should be maintained at 10 to 15 mm Hg and the PCWP should be maintained at less than or equal to 15 mm Hg. The finding of ventricular interaction and limitation of LV filling by RV dilation has important therapeutic implications for the efficacy of volume infusion. Patients may deteriorate with excess volume administration. In addition, excess volume administration precipitates pulmonary edema when LV infarction is present in association with RV infarction.

The crucial management issue is not whether there is anatomic involvement of the right ventricle, but rather the pathophysiologic consequences of dominant RV infarction. If the jugular venous pressure is elevated in a patient with an inferior MI and hypotension, all that is necessary is to avoid preload reduction. For patients with hypotension and RV and first inferior MI, emergency empiric volume administration is indicated. These patients require variable amounts of fluid (200 mL to 1 L of fluid over the first several hours) depending on the estimated or measured RA pressure. If hypotension or evidence of low cardiac output persists, an emergency echocardiogram should be obtained, and subsequent management should be guided by PA catheter monitoring of cardiac output. As noted, additional fluid administration may be detrimental. Patients who are

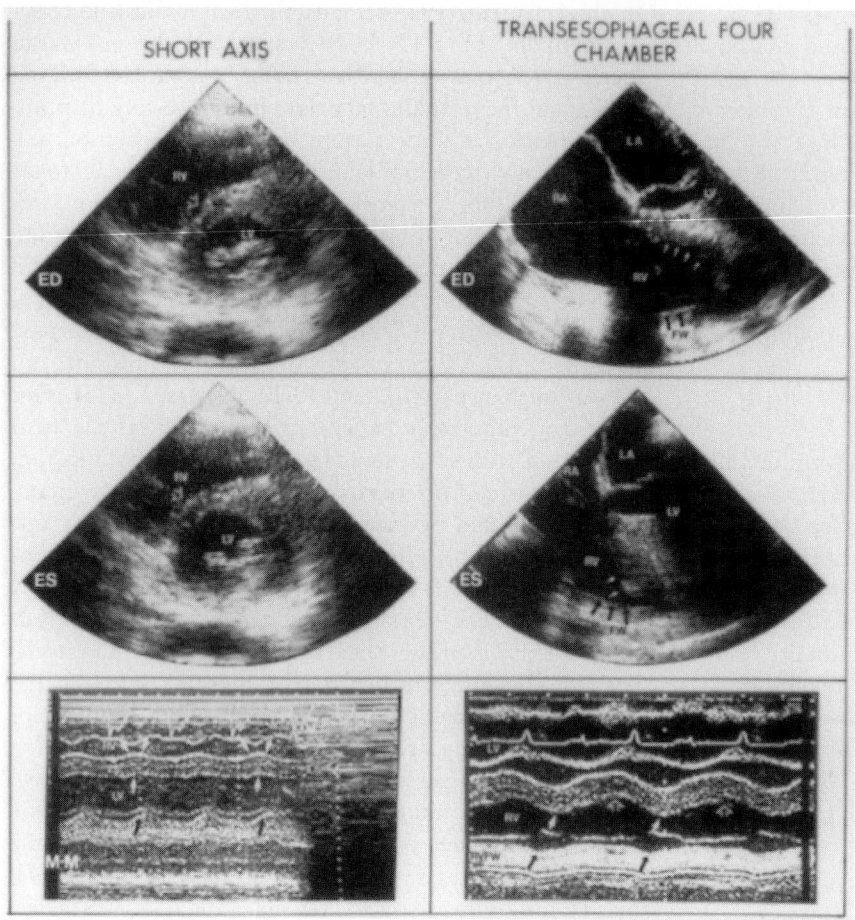

FIGURE 19.8 Transthoracic, transesophageal, and M-mode echocardiograms from a patient with right ventricular infarction, refractory shock, and right atrial infarction. In short axis at end diastole (ED), the right ventricle (RV) is markedly dilatated, and the interventricular septal curvature is reversed (*open arrow*) with a shift into the left ventricle (LV). The four-chamber view demonstrates marked right atrial (RA) enlargement as well as severe RV dilation and bowing of the septum into the LV (*white arrows*). At end systole (ES), the septum bulges paradoxically into the RV in both short-axis (*open arrow*) and four-chamber views (*white arrows*). RV free wall (FW, *dark arrows*) was dyskinetic in four-chamber view. These findings are confirmed in the M-mode views from the transthoracic and transesophageal images. Excess volume administration can cause RV dilatation, septal shift into the LV with impairment of LV filling, and paradoxic decrease in cardiac output despite an increase of pulmonary capillary wedge pressure. (From Goldstein JA, Barzilai B, Rosamound TL, et al. Determinants of hemodynamic compromise with severe right ventricular infarction. *Circulation* 1990;82:359–368, with permission. Original figure courtesy of Dr. J. Goldstein.)

at risk for pulmonary edema should not receive this degree of rapid volume administration. These patients include those with (a) prior MIs; (b) acute, extensive LV infarction; (c) associated MR or other valvular lesions; (d) acute anterior MI; and (e) advanced age. If pulmonary congestion is not present, these patients may receive 200 to 250 mL of fluid, and an emergency echocardiogram should be obtained. If hypotension, evidence of a low cardiac output, or both persist, PA monitoring is required with further volume infusion.

The positive inotropic effects of dobutamine play an important role in managing patients with RV infarction and low cardiac output. Dobutamine significantly increases the CI and RVEF and is superior to afterload reduction therapy with nitroprusside (341). Patients in whom the initial central venous pressure or RA pressure are greater than 10 mm Hg or in whom an initial volume infusion fails and leads to an increase in RA and PCWP but a persistently low CI should be treated with dobutamine. When pacing is indicated for sinus bradycardia or complete heart block, it should be dual-chamber, AV sequential. Of note, there is an increased incidence of ventricular fibrillation with RV pacing caused by RV ischemia (344). IABP and PA counterpulsation have been used for RV shock (345–347). In rare cases of refractory

shock caused by RV infarction, pericardiectomy should be considered (339).

Reperfusion Therapy

Rapid reperfusion with either thrombolytics or direct PTCA should be the initial treatment for RV infarction. RVEF improved in patients with successful intracoronary thrombolysis compared with no improvement in those in whom thrombolysis failed (348). Similarly, patients who received intracoronary SK had higher RVEFs than did those who did not receive intracoronary SK. Occluded IRAs at angiography correlated with evidence of RV infarction in contrast to a lower incidence of RV infarction in those with a patent IRA in Thrombolysis in Myocardial Infarction (TIMI) II (349). RV infarction is associated with low rates of reperfusion by thrombolysis, possibly caused by prolonged hypotension (120). Systemic arterial pressure should be augmented during thrombolytic administration for RV infarction with hypotension (117,118). Observational studies (350,351) of PTCA report marked improvement in hemodynamics and RV function after successful PTCA. In the SHOCK Trial Registry, 65% of those with RV shock had single-vessel disease with proximal right coronary artery occlusion (316). Based on extrapolation of the SHOCK Trial Registry results and the poor outcome if shock complicates RV infarction, we recommend direct (or rescue) PTCA for these patients.

MECHANICAL COMPLICATIONS OF ACUTE MYOCARDIAL INFARCTION

Cardiac Rupture: Overview

Rupture may occur through a zone of necrosis in the LV free wall, interventricular septum, papillary muscle, or the contiguous chordae tendineae. Spontaneous RV free wall rupture rarely occurs. When one of these types of rupture occurs, it is typically referred to as a *mechanical complication* of acute MI; when shock results, this is termed a *mechanical cause* of shock. The relative infrequency of the often lethal mechanical complications of acute MI such as acute MR caused by papillary muscle rupture, VSR, or rupture of the free wall should not detract from their importance, because they are amenable to surgical repair. Moreover, these potentially catastrophic complications are, in turn, compatible with an excellent long-term prognosis among perioperative survivors. In a series (177) of 1,493 patients in 36 centers, acute septal rupture or MR accounted for only 11% of patients with cardiogenic shock. Acute MR without papillary muscle rupture can cause severe hemodynamic compromise and is discussed in this section as a mechanical complication. It is the etiology of MR in a substantial number of patients, although its exact frequency remains undetermined. Reperfusion therapy has reduced the overall incidence of cardiac rupture and shifted its occurrence to earlier after MI onset. Distinct clinical syndromes result, depending on the location and extent (i.e., partial or complete) of the rupture.

Left Ventricular Free Wall Rupture

Rupture of the LV free wall is not a uniformly fatal event, and early recognition of rupture with subacute tamponade may result in successful intervention.

Pathology

Pseudoaneurysm

Rupture that is sealed by the pericardium and then develops into a discrete aneurysmal outpouching with a narrow neck is referred to as a *pseudoaneurysm* or *false aneurysm* (Fig. 19.3) (44). The wall of a pseudoaneurysm is composed of pericardium and not infarcted myocardium or scar tissue, in contrast to a true LV aneurysm. The neck of a pseudoaneurysm is narrower than that of a true aneurysm.

Clinical Profile

Subacute Ventricular Wall Rupture and Subacute Tamponade
Rupture with a period of temporary pericardial sealing (less stable than pseudoaneurysm) and subacute tamponade has

been characterized in the prospective, large series by Lopez-Sendon et al. (360). Of 1,457 consecutive patients with acute MI, 6.2% were diagnosed with free wall rupture; approximately one-third of these patients had a subacute presentation. Thirty-nine patients went to surgery and a myocardial rupture site was confirmed in 33. The clinical constellation in these patients may include transient hypotension, syncope, transient EMD, chest pain (360), and transient bradycardia, repetitive emesis, and restlessness (358). These clinical findings are sensitive but nonspecific. The ECG findings of pericarditis may be seen and include persistent or new ST-segment elevations, persistently positive T waves, or inverted T waves becoming positive. However, these findings are insensitive and nonspecific (360). Subacute rupture can often be identified on echocardiography and successfully repaired (*e*Table 19.4.1) (360,361). This is in contrast to the classic constellation of sudden chest pain and cardiovascular collapse with EMD seen in uncontained free wall rupture with tamponade. A right-sided heart catheterization can be performed to confirm tamponade hemodynamics with equalization of diastolic pressures, if the echocardiogram is not diagnostic.

Management

Early recognition of subacute rupture with echocardiography is critical for early intervention before uncontained intrapericardial hemorrhage and acute tamponade. Pericardiocentesis has been used to confirm that effusion is hemorrhagic and to relieve tamponade. However, we recommend emergency open drainage and repair, when possible, for subacute rupture with subacute tamponade. A stabilized patient with temporary sealing of the rupture site by thrombus on the epicardial surface is at risk for dislocation of the thrombus and precipitation of acute tamponade. Surgical repair is often successful and is accepted therapy (360,361). That subacute rupture is accessible to surgical repair is not in dispute. Unfortunately, the diagnostic criteria are not specific, and the decision to undergo surgical exploration frequently has to be made on the basis of a high index of clinical suspicion without definitive documentation of a site of rupture. Echocardiography may be helpful with the demonstration of an effusion, RV and RA compression, and shaggy, intrapericardial echo densities consistent with thrombus, at times visualized as a thrombus on the epicardial surface of the heart. ▼ d47

Acute Mitral Regurgitation

Pathophysiology

An autopsy study (362) in the precardiac surgical era established that among patients dying of papillary muscle rupture, the extent of LV infarction was relatively small; approximately one-half of patients had single-vessel disease, the annulus was usually not involved, and there was a marked predominance of inferior infarcts.

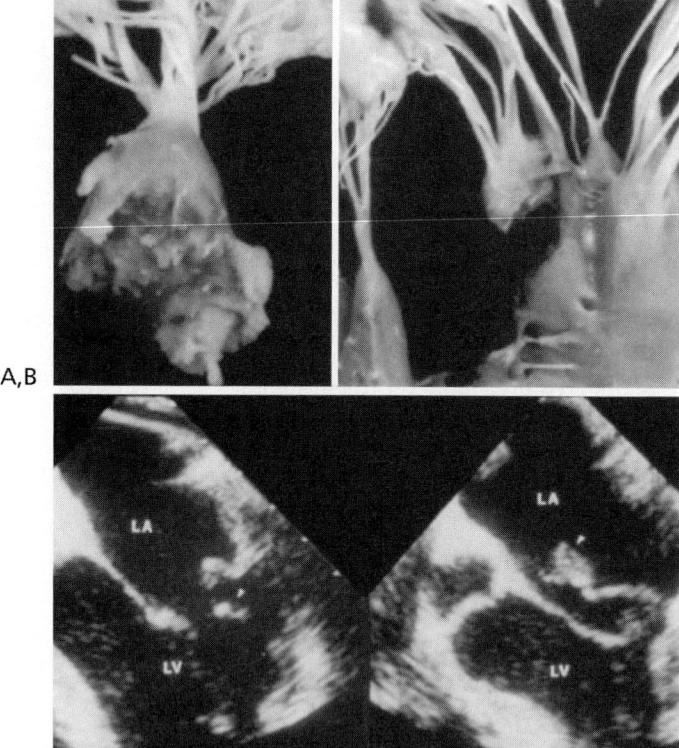

FIGURE 19.9 **A, B:** Examples of a ruptured belly of a papillary muscle **(A)** and a partial rupture **(B)** following acute myocardial infarction. **C:** The utility of transesophageal echocardiography. The ruptured belly of the papillary muscle can be seen prolapsing into the left atrium (LA) during systole and in the left ventricle (LV) during diastole. (Pathology specimens courtesy of Dr. W. D. Edwards.)

The conclusions that were drawn had major potential implications for surgical repair; patients dying of papillary muscle rupture died from MR and not from primary pump failure. The striking predominance of inferior infarcts in this autopsy study and in other studies (363) underscores the consequence of the vulnerability of the posteromedial papillary muscle because of its single blood supply from the posterior descending coronary artery, which is in contrast to the dual blood supply from both the LAD and left circumflex arteries to the anterolateral papillary muscle. Rupture of the papillary muscle may be partial or complete, but either condition results in severe MR (Fig. 19.9). These pathophysiologic features and, in particular, the limited extent of LV necrosis, highlight the potential for excellent long-term results from surgical correction and for the inefficacy of medical therapy (362,364). ▼ d48

Clinical Profile

Incidence, Patient Characteristics, and Prognosis
Acute MR often develops during the course of MI, and the frequency of a murmur during hospitalization has been reported to be 20% to 55% (367). Transient MR is common during the early phase of acute MI and is not usually the cause of hemodynamic compromise. Angiographic studies (368,369) reported incidences of MR of 13% and 18% within hours of MI, respectively; 13% of patients entering phase I of the TIMI trial (368) had MR documented on left ventriculography, and it was clinically silent in nearly all patients. When sought by Doppler echocardiography, a frequency of 39% has been reported (367). ▼ d49

Acute severe MR was the cause of shock in 7% of patients with cardiogenic shock complicating MI in the SHOCK Trial Registry (177,371) (Fig. 19.5). Compared with those with LV failure, MR patients were more often female and had inferior and posterior infarcts. Although the EF was higher in patients with MR, the mean EF for those in shock was only 37%. The in-hospital mortality (55%) was similar to those with shock caused by LV failure (59%) (177).

Clinical Presentation and Diagnosis
The clinical picture of acute papillary muscle rupture is characterized by the sudden onset of LV failure, hypotension, or both. Although older studies reported the onset approximately 2 to 7 days post-MI (362), the median time in the SHOCK Trial Registry is 22 hours (25%, 75%: 2, 36 hours) (371). As with other locations of myocardial rupture, thrombolytic therapy is associated with a shift in the time course to earlier occurrence, with an overall reduced incidence. Other clinical findings and physical examination are nonspecific. The apex beat may be dyskinetic, and heart sounds are usually soft, muffled, or masked by the auscultatory features of severe pulmonary edema. Accentuated pulmonary component of the second heart sound caused by pulmonary hypertension is often not appreciable. A harsh, but relatively short, systolic murmur typically is heard at the apex and left sternal edge; a thrill is uncommon. It should be strongly emphasized that the murmur may be soft or even absent as a result of the early pressure equalization between the left ventricle and left atrium caused by severe regurgitation into a nondilated atrial chamber and low-flow state. The key to the diagnosis is a heightened index of clinical suspicion, which should always be entertained in any patient with an inferior MI, particularly a first MI, who is hemodynamically compromised, particularly in the absence of any identifiable cause (e.g., an arrhythmia, PE, or tamponade) (Table 19.5).

Two-dimensional, and often transesophageal, echocardiography is a pivotal noninvasive diagnostic tool (372,373) (Fig. 19.9). Identification of the freely mobile head of the papillary muscle either in the left atrium or the left ventricle or of a flail mitral leaflet is diagnostic (373). The addition of color flow imaging, with the aim of semiquantitation of the severity of MR is frequently helpful, and, in one series, it correctly identified MR in all patients. Transesophageal echocardiography may be particularly advantageous in patients on mechanical ventilation because transthoracic echocardiography may not provide adequate images. An

TABLE 19.5 DIAGNOSTIC CONSIDERATIONS IN PATIENTS WITH INFERIOR MYOCARDIAL INFARCTION AND CONGESTIVE HEART FAILURE OR CARDIOGENIC SHOCK

Prior myocardial infarction
High-grade atrioventricular block/bradyarrhythmias
Acute severe mitral regurgitation
Right ventricular infarction (characterized by an absence of pulmonary edema)
Left ventricular pseudorupture/subacute rupture
Pulmonary embolism
Acute interventricular septal rupture

extremely helpful clinical feature, particularly when the mitral valve apparatus is not well visualized, is the demonstration of reasonably well-preserved or even hyperdynamic LV function in the face of pulmonary edema, cardiogenic shock, or both. This constellation of clinical and echocardiographic features should point toward a mechanical complication as the putative cause of pulmonary edema or shock and is an indication for further diagnostic or confirmatory tests (e.g., left ventriculography). Those in shock often have depressed LV function (371). Documentation of tall V waves on PCWP tracing catheterization is a helpful finding but has limitations (374), and the role of PA catheterization as a diagnostic modality has been superseded by advances in echocardiography. Nonetheless, the former may be useful in monitoring the effects of pharmacologic therapy. Ventriculography may be required to confirm the severity of the MR in patients for whom surgery is being considered.

Management

The cornerstone of management is prompt diagnosis and aggressive medical therapy with a view to emergency cardiac surgery. The natural history of medically treated chordal or papillary muscle rupture, whether partial or complete, is poor and characterized by a volatile, unpredictable clinical course even when medical therapy results in initial stabilization (362). Sudden hemodynamic deterioration is frequent, and the consequences are usually catastrophic. ☞ d50

Papillary muscle rupture remains a potentially catastrophic and fatal complication of acute MI; however, there is a window of opportunity for emergency surgical correction with the encouraging prospect of excellent long-term survival and a return to an active life.

In contrast, patients with moderate or severe MR in the face of severely compromised LV function (i.e., EF <30% to 35%), in whom clear evidence of papillary muscle or chordal rupture is not documented by echocardiography, pose a particularly difficult problem in diagnosis and management. The mechanism of MR in these patients may be underlying LV failure with dilation of the annulus or malalignment of the mitral valve apparatus caused by a severe regional wall motion abnormality adjacent to a papillary

muscle or multiple areas by dyssynergy (366). A more prudent approach in these patients is aggressive medical therapy, including high-dose vasodilators and perhaps IABP. This may give time for LV function to improve and for additional diagnostic testing to help avoid the dilemma of a surgical procedure in the absence of a clearly delineated correctable cause of CHF. Factors to be addressed before performing surgery are the extent and reversibility of LV dysfunction, the potential for revascularization to improve LV size and function, the degree of MR, and the extent of structural abnormalities of the mitral valve apparatus.

Acute Interventricular Septal Rupture

Incidence, Timing, Clinical Profile, and Prognosis

Acute rupture of the interventricular septum occurs in approximately 1% to 3% of all infarcts (377). In the GUSTO 1 trial in which all patients received thrombolytic therapy, the incidence was 0.2% (378). In the SHOCK Trial Registry, VSR was the etiology of shock in 3.9% of those with shock complicating MI (Fig. 19.5). Patients with VSR are more often older, female, with less prior MI and comorbidity compared with those without mechanical complications of MI (379) and with those with shock caused by LV failure. Older reports suggested that rupture occurred several days post-MI. However, in GUSTO 1 the median time was 1 day (378). When VSR causes shock, it occurs early after MI onset. The median time was 16 hours (25%, 75%: 2, 45 hours) for patients in the SHOCK Trial Registry. Once shock has developed, the prognosis is grim (87% mortality) (379).

Pathophysiology

Interventricular septal rupture is nearly always a complication of a transmural MI, particularly a first MI; however, in contrast to papillary muscle rupture, anterior or anterolateral infarcts are slightly more frequent than are inferior infarcts (378–382). A history of prior angina is uncommon, and hypertension may be a predisposing factor (378,382). Concomitant involvement of other structures including the papillary muscles and free wall of the left and right ventricles has been well described (381). Septal rupture may occur in patients with single-vessel disease, but multivessel disease is common. Two- or three-vessel CAD was present in 43% and 31%, respectively, in the SHOCK Trial Registry (379) and in 51% in GUSTO (378).

Interventricular septal rupture has been categorized morphologically into simple and complex forms (Fig. 19.10). The former is a discrete defect with a direct through-and-through communication across the septum, usually the apical septum. The ventricular openings are therefore at the same level on both sides of the septum. Complex ruptures are characterized by extensive hemor-

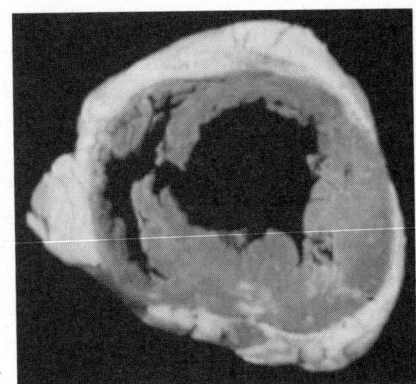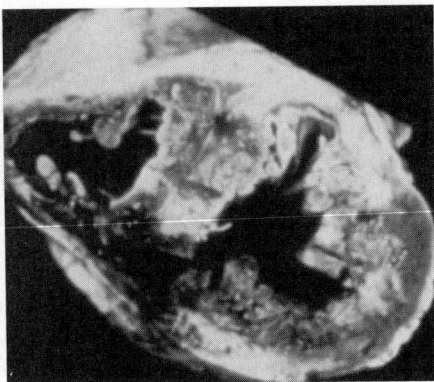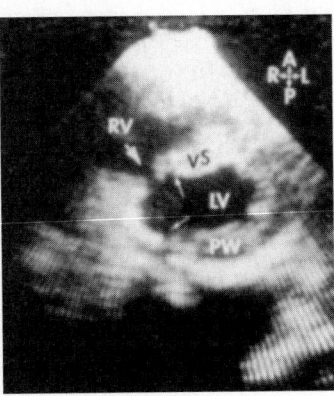

A–C

FIGURE 19.10 Ventricular septal rupture complicating acute myocardial infarction. This illustrates two types of rupture of the ventricular septum, which in 53 autopsied hearts were simple (in 28 patients) or complex (in 25 patients). **A:** Simple rupture is a direct through-and-through defect. **B:** Complex ruptures are associated with serpiginous dissection tracts, which are remote from the primary site of tear of the ventricular septum. Complex ruptures are more frequent with inferior infarcts involving the inferobasal portion of the septum and may be associated with rupture of a second structure, such as the free wall of the right ventricle (RV) in this patient. **C:** The marked utility of two-dimensional echocardiography in the diagnosis, illustrating a parasternal short-access view using transthoracic echocardiography. The echocardiogram illustrates a complex ventricular septal rupture. LV, left ventricle; PW, posterior wall; VS, ventricular septum. (From Edwards BS, Edwards WD, Edwards JE. Ventricular septal rupture complicating acute myocardial infarction: identification of simple and complex types in 53 autopsied hearts. *Am J Cardiol* 1984;54:1201–1205, with permission.)

rhage around irregular, serpiginous tracts that extend in different directions within extensive necrotic tissue; they more frequently involve the inferobasal septum as a complication of inferior MIs. Complex ruptures are more likely to involve associated structures including extensive areas of the right ventricle (381).

Clinical Presentation and Diagnosis

The typical presentation is the acute development of shock and pulmonary edema in the face of severe right-sided heart failure and a new systolic murmur. The murmur is usually loud and pansystolic and is accompanied by a thrill in 50% of patients. The distinction between papillary muscle rupture and acute interventricular septal rupture can be made clinically on the basis of the intensity and characteristics of the murmur and the presence of a thrill and right-sided heart failure in most patients with septal rupture. Nonetheless, physical findings may be unreliable, particularly in a low-output state. ☞ d51

Among patients with acute septal rupture, left-sided heart catheterization and left ventriculography confirm the diagnosis, but the decision to employ these diagnostic modalities depends on the patient's hemodynamic stability and the need to identify the coronary anatomy in the event that concomitant coronary artery bypass surgery is being considered.

Management

The key to management is prompt diagnosis, an aggressive approach to stabilization, rapid angiography, and surgery.

Medical therapy consists of diuretics, vasodilators, and frequently inotropes in addition to intermittent positive-pressure ventilation and IABP in patients with severe CHF or cardiogenic shock. As is the case with papillary muscle rupture, initial stabilization on medical therapy may provide only a temporary respite.

A small, asymptomatic VSR may be managed without surgery. For most patients with VSR who are severely symptomatic, the need for surgical repair has never been questioned, but its timing has been an issue of debate (383). ☞ d52

The current approach, therefore, is to advocate early or emergency surgery in all patients, preferably before decompensation (90). It must be accepted that an aggressive approach may be associated with a high perioperative mortality but may have the potential for an overall reduction in mortality (379,382). This is particularly relevant in patients with cardiogenic shock as opposed to pulmonary edema alone in whom short-term survival with medical therapy is extremely poor and among whom apparent stabilization is usually transient (380,386–390).

There is little consensus in the literature (391) regarding the need for concomitant coronary revascularization during surgical repair of postinfarction VSR. Theoretically, revascularization of residual and viable but ischemic myocardium should facilitate weaning the patient off cardiopulmonary bypass and should accelerate recovery during the perioperative period as well as provide a beneficial effect on long-term outcome. There are, however, no prospective studies documenting the merits of such an approach. On balance, preoperative coronary angiography with a view to concomitant CABG appears reasonable and may be indicated, provided the patient is sufficiently stable as to tolerate the procedure. ▼ d53

In summary, the approach to patients with acute septal rupture and hemodynamic decompensation is rapid stabilization and prompt surgery. Rarely, patients with small shunts and without CHF who remain hemodynamically stable may be managed medically over the long term.

MISCELLANEOUS COMPLICATIONS OF ACUTE MYOCARDIAL INFARCTION

Pericarditis

Inflammation of the pericardium may occur acutely during acute MI and may be largely localized to the pericardium adjacent to the infarction, or it may occur as a delayed, more generalized inflammatory syndrome (i.e., Dressler's syndrome). Pericarditis associated with acute infarction results from the infarction extending to the epicardial surface of the heart, with an associated inflammatory response.

Diagnosis

The diagnosis is made clinically by history, physical examination, and ECG. Pericarditic chest pain is typically sharp, severe, substernal pain that may radiate to the neck, shoulders, and back, increasing with inspiration and on reclining. Patients with pericarditis are often severely distressed and uncomfortable. A typical three-component pericardial friction rub may be heard but may be absent when effusion develops. The typical ECG changes of pericarditis are uncommon when the pericarditis is localized to the infarct zone (396). Nonetheless, persistent or new ST-segment elevations in multiple leads may be seen when pericarditis is more generalized. Pericarditis should heighten the index of suspicion for subacute rupture and warrants echocardiography. Atypical T-wave evolution, either with T waves remaining consistently positive for 48 hours or longer after onset of acute MI or with initially inverted T waves gradually becoming positive deflections, has been described in postinfarction pericarditis (358,397). An effusion may or may not be present on echocardiography; presence of effusion is more common than is clinical pericarditis (398). Most cases of acute pericarditis are diagnosed within 3 days of acute MI (399) but may occur as early as day 1.

Incidence

Clinical studies (399) report a higher incidence of pericarditis in patients with Q-wave MI than in patients with non–Q-wave MI; it is more common with large infarcts. Its clinical incidence varies depending on the diagnostic criteria. Most studies require a pericardial friction rub to be present. Large clinical trials such as GISSI-1 (85) define pericarditis as either a friction rub or as typical pericarditis chest pain. The incidence of postinfarction pericarditis has decreased by approximately 50% in patients treated with thrombolytic therapy (85,131,195,396,399,400) (Table 19.6).

TABLE 19.6 PERICARDITIS IN ACUTE MYOCARDIAL INFARCTION (MI): INCIDENCE

Prethrombolytic era	Reference	Number	Incidence (%)		
Kranin	396	423	7.3		
MILIS	399	703	20.0		
			Q wave MI	Non–Q wave MI	*p* value
			25.0%	9.0%	<.001
			Incidence (%)		
Thrombolytic era	**Reference**	**Number**	**Control**	**Thrombolysis**	*p* value
Simoons	152	533	17.4	7.0	0.0004
GISSI-1	85	11,483	12.0	6.7	<.001
ECSG	400	721	11.0	6.3	<.005
AIMS	131	1,258	15.5	6.9	<.001
ASSENT-II	408	16,949	—	3.0	
			Incidence (%)		
Primary PTCA			**PTCA**	**Thrombolysis**	*p* value
PAMI	203	395	1.5	1.5	0.31

PTCA, percutaneous transluminal coronary angiography.

Reperfusion therapy results in smaller infarcts that less often extend to the epicardial surface, resulting in less localized pericarditis.

Pericardial Effusion

Pericardial effusions occur relatively frequently after acute MI (incidence, up to 45%) (398). They are more common with large, anterior, or both large and anterior infarcts and when CHF is present. They are typically asymptomatic. If tamponade develops, it is usually caused by free wall rupture or hemorrhage into the pericardium. Effusions most frequently occur without clinical pericarditis. Conversely, patients with clinical pericarditis frequently do not have associated effusion.

CONTROVERSIES AND PERSONAL PERSPECTIVES

Pump Failure

We now have randomized trial evidence that a direct invasive strategy, with IABP-supported rapid angiography, PTCA, or CABG markedly improves 1-year survival when post-MI shock develops caused by predominant LV failure. The treatment benefit is derived despite comorbidities such as diabetes and despite profound hemodynamic abnormalities. Although the long-term survival is improved by intervention, even successful procedures are associated with high in-hospital mortality, and operators may be reluctant to intervene. Quality improvement measures must track not only procedural death rates but the rate of refusals for interventions based on the high-risk profile. However, when the outcome is grim even with intervention, such as surgery for VSR with inferior MI once shock is present, treatment may be deemed futile.

Reperfusing Occluded Infarct-Related Arteries in Asymptomatic Patients: Any Benefits?

Despite the wealth of data implicating a beneficial effect of an open artery independent of myocardial salvage, the late open artery concept remains a tantalizing but unproven hypothesis. The implications for clinical practice, however, are far reaching. If it could be demonstrated that reperfusion of a closed IRA in asymptomatic patients without stress-induced ischemia reduces mortality or improves LV function, routine angiography in all MI survivors might then be recommended to identify those with an occluded IRA. To accomplish this, a randomized trial is ongoing.

Reinfarction

In contrast to the efficacy of heparin (low-molecular-weight heparin or unfractionated) and GP IIb/IIIa antagonists demonstrated in non–ST-elevation acute coronary syndrome, their role after ST-elevation MI is less clear. Full anticoagulation is recommended for patients treated with t-PA and for those with large anterior MIs and other MI locations complicated by pump failure. Based on beneficial trends and the knowledge that the ulcerated plaque is thrombogenic, for other patients we recommend full-dose i.v. unfractionated or s.c. low-molecular-weight heparin for 48 hours in addition to ASA, 160 mg every day. However, patients at risk for intracranial or other hemorrhagic events should not be fully anticoagulated in an attempt to prevent reinfarction.

GP IIb/IIIa receptor antagonists and low-molecular-weight heparin are superior to i.v. unfractionated heparin in preventing reinfarction in the non–ST-elevation acute coronary syndromes. Their role in ST elevation MI is still being defined. Other antiplatelet agents, such as clopidogrel, have been reported to reduce long-term death rates compared with ASA in patients with vascular disease (149). The efficacy of clopidogrel in reducing short-term reinfarction rates after unstable angina and non–ST elevation has recently been demonstrated (416). The role of these antiplatelet agents in acute ST elevation MI is being evaluated.

When recurrent chest pain with ST reelevation develops after MI, the efficacy of readministering thrombolytic agents versus performing emergency PTCA remains an issue of debate. We recommend emergency PTCA when immediately available. When there is inherent delay, however (e.g., at hospitals that do not perform PTCA), we recommend thrombolytic administration (t-PA, tenecteplase, or recombinant plasminogen activator if SK has been used previously) followed by transfer for coronary angiography and PTCA or CABG.

ACKNOWLEDGMENTS

We gratefully acknowledge the following persons for their help in the preparation of this chapter: Venu Menon, MD, for his assistance with review of the literature and preparation of tables; Maziar Azadapour, MD, for assistance with review of the literature; Richard M. Fuchs, MD, for editing the manuscript; and Ashley McDonell for assistance with all aspects of the manuscript preparation.

THE FUTURE

Pump Failure

Prevention of Pump Failure

Strategies to prevent pump failure in patients at high risk need to be further investigated. Such strategies should include (a) agents that inhibit reperfusion injury (e.g., leukocyte inhibitors, free radical scavengers, and magnesium); (b) metabolic support solutions (e.g., glucose, insulin, and potassium; carnitine; dichloroacetate; sodium-proton pump exchange inhibitors); (c) early coronary angiography and revascularization with and without circulatory support (e.g., IABP); and (d) other strategies to reduce reinfarction, such as newer antiplatelet and antithrombotic agents.

Treatment of Pump Failure

Use of magnesium, metabolic support for the remote, ischemic, and reperfused myocardium, and agents that inhibit reperfusion injury need further evaluation. The role of alternative vasopressors such as the nitric oxide synthase inhibitor L-NMMA and vasopressin should be investigated.

The role of newer LV support devices compared with IABP and criteria for selecting appropriate patients for newer LV support devices need to be defined.

Cardiac Rupture and Left Ventricular Remodeling: Basic Mechanisms

Measures to prevent cardiac rupture in patients at increased risk need to be evaluated. The role of interstitial matrix degradation by metalloproteinases in myocardial rupture should be explored further and metalloproteinase inhibitor evaluated in high-risk patients. Similarly, the effects of disruption of the intercellular collagen struts that link myofibrils with potential slippage of myocytes, infarct expansion, and LV remodeling and the role metalloproteinase inhibitors for patients at risk need to be investigated. Aging and female gender are associated with an increased incidence of rupture and pump failure. The basic myocyte and interstitial myocardial changes that may be associated with such increased incidence need to be elucidated. The development of improved techniques for the noninvasive diagnosis of subacute cardiac rupture is a priority.

In summary, despite the dramatic advances in the treatment of acute MI, reinfarction, pump failure, and myocardial rupture remain major challenges for the future and their basic mechanisms, prevention, and management must be explored and elucidated.

REFERENCES

1. Day HW. A cardiac resuscitation program. *Lancet* 1962;82:153–156.
2. Julian DG. The history of coronary care units. *Br Heart J* 1987;57:497–502.
3. Zoll PM, Linenthal AJ, Gibson W, et al. Termination of ventricular fibrillation in man by externally applied electric countershock. *N Engl J Med* 1956;254:727–732.
4. Zoll PM. Resuscitation of the heart in ventricular standstill by external electric stimulation. *N Engl J Med* 1952;247:768–771.
5. Killip T, Kimball JT. Treatment of myocardial infarction in a coronary care unit: a two-year experience with 250 patients. *Am J Cardiol* 1967;20:457–464.
6. Monlopoulos SD, Tiopez S, Kolff WJ. Diastolic balloon pumping in the aorta: a mechanical assistance to the failing circulation. *Am Heart J* 1962;63:669–675.
7. Kantrowitz A, Phillips SJ, Butner AN, et al. Technique of femoral artery cannulation for phase-shift balloon pumping. *J Thorac Cardiovasc Surg* 1968;56:219–220.
8. Swan HJ, Ganz W, Forrester J, et al. Catheterization of the heart in man with the use of a flow-directed balloon-tipped catheter. *N Engl J Med* 1970;283:447–451.
9. Dunkman WB, Leinbach RC, Buckley MJ, et al. Clinical and hemodynamic results of intraaortic balloon pumping and surgery for cardiogenic shock. *Circulation* 1972;46:465–477.
10. O'Neill W, Erbel R, Laufer N, et al. Coronary angioplasty therapy of cardiogenic shock complicating acute myocardial infarction. *Circulation* 1985;72[Suppl II]:309.
11. Hochman JS, Sleeper LA, White HD, et al. One year survival following early revascularization for acute myocardial infarction complicated by cardiogenic shock. *JAMA* 2001;285:190–192.
12. Edwards WD. Pathology of myocardial infarction and reperfusion. In: Gersh BJ, Rahimtoola SH, eds. *Acute myocardial infarction.* Boston: Chapman & Hall, 1996:16–50.
13. Hutchins GM, Bulkley BH. Infarct expansion versus extension: two different complications of acute myocardial infarction. *Am J Cardiol* 1978;41:1127.
14. Reimer KA, Lowe JE, Rasmussen MM, Jennings RB. The wavefront phenomenon of ischemic cell death. 1. Myocardial infarct size versus duration of coronary occlusion in dogs. *Circulation* 1977;56:786–794.
15. Blumgart HL, Schlesinger MJ, Zoll PM. Angina pectoris, coronary failure and acute myocardial infarction: the role of coronary occlusions and collateral circulation. *JAMA* 1941;116:91.
16. Topol EJ, Ellis SG. Coronary collaterals revisited: Accessory pathway to myocardial preservation during infarction. *Circulation* 1991;83:1084.

17. Yellon DM, Baxter GF, Garcia-Dorado D, et al. Ischaemic preconditioning: present position and future directions. *Cardiovascular Research* 1998;37:21–33.

18. Ito H, Maruyama A, Iwakura K, et al. Clinical implications of the "no reflow" phenomenon: a predictor of complications and left ventricular remodeling in reperfused anterior wall myocardial infarction. *Circulation* 1996;93:223–228.

19. Kenner MD, Zajac EJ, Kondos GT, et al. Ability of the no-reflow phenomenon during an acute myocardial infarction to predict left ventricular dysfunction at one-month follow-up. *Am J Cardiol* 1995;76:861–868.

20. de Lemos JA, Antman EM, Gibson CM, et al. Abciximab improves both epicardial flow and myocardial reperfusion in ST-elevation myocardial infarction. Observation from the TIMI 14 trial. *Circulation* 2000;101:239–243.

21. Gibson CM, Cannon CP, Murphy SA, et al. Relationship of TIMI myocardial perfusion grade to mortality after administration of thrombolytic drugs. *Circulation* 2000;101:125–130.

22. Wu KC, Zerhouni EA, Judd RN, et al. Prognostic significance of microvascular obstruction by magnetic resonance imaging in patients with acute myocardial infarction. *Circulation* 1998;97:765–772.

23. Braunwald E, Kloner RA. The stunned myocardium: prolonged, postischemic ventricular dysfunction. *Circulation* 1982;66:1146.

24. Rahimtoola SH. The hibernating myocardium. *Am Heart J* 1989;117:211.

25. Braunwald E, Rutherford JD. Reversible ischemic left ventricular dysfunction: evidence for the hibernating myocardium. *J Am Coll Cardiol* 1986;8:1467.

26. Picard MH, Wilkins GT, Gillam LD, et al. Immediate regional endocardial surface expansion following coronary occlusion in the canine left ventricle: disproportionate effects of anterior versus inferior ischemia. *Am Heart J* 1991;121:753–762.

27. Hochman JS, Bulkley BH. Expansion of acute myocardial infarction: an experimental study. *Circulation* 1982;65:1446–1450.

28. Erlebacher JA, Weiss JL, Eaton LW, et al. Late effects of acute infarct dilation on heart size: a two dimensional echocardiographic study. *Am J Cardiol* 1982;49:1120–1126.

29. Eaton LW, Weiss JL, Bulkley BH, et al. Regional cardiac dilatation after acute myocardial infarction: recognition by two-dimensional echocardiography. *N Engl J Med* 1979;300:57–62.

30. Pfeffer JM, Pfeffer MA, Fletcher PJ, et al. Progressive ventricular remodeling in rats with myocardial infarction. *Am J Physiol* 1991;260:H1406–H1414.

31. Olivetti G, Capasso JM, Sonnenblick EH, et al. Side-to-side slippage of myocytes participates in ventricular wall remodeling acutely after myocardial infarction in rats. *Circ Res* 1990;67:23–34.

32. Tennant R, Wiggers CJ. The effect of coronary occlusion on myocardial contraction. *Am J Physiol* 1935;112:351–361.

33. Hochman JS, Choo H. Limitation of myocardial infarct expansion by reperfusion independent of myocardial salvage. *Circulation* 1987;75:299–306.

34. Bulkley BH. Site and sequelae of myocardial infarction. *N Engl J Med* 1981;305:337–338.

35. Herzog E, Gu A, Kohmoto T, et al. Early activation of metalloproteinases after experimental myocardial infarction occurs in infarct and non-infarct zones. *Cardiovasc Pathol* 1998;7:307–312.

36. Pierard LA, Albert A, Gilis F, et al. Hemodynamic profile of patients with acute myocardial infarction at risk of infarct expansion. *Am J Cardiol* 1987;60:5–9.

37. Meltzer RS, Visser CA, Kan G, et al. Two-dimensional echocardiographic appearance of left ventricular thrombi with systemic emboli after myocardial infarction. *Am J Cardiol* 1984;53:1511–1513.

38. Neubauer S, Horn M, Naumann A, et al. Impairment of energy metabolism in intact residual myocardium of rat hearts with chronic myocardial infarction. *J Clin Invest* 1995;95:1092–1100.

39. White HD, Norris RM, Brown MA, et al. Left ventricular end-systolic volume as the major determinant of survival after recovery from myocardial infarction. *Circulation* 1987;76:44–51.

40. Migrino RQ, Young JB, Ellis SG, et al. End-systolic volume index at 90 to 180 minutes into reperfusion therapy for acute myocardial infarction is a strong predictor of early and late mortality. The Global Utilization of Streptokinase and t-PA for Occluded Coronary Arteries (GUSTO)-I Angiographic Investigators. *Circulation* 1997;96:116–121.

41. Hochman JS, Bulkley BH. Pathogenesis of left ventricular aneurysms: an experimental study in the rat model. *Am J Cardiol* 1982;50:83–88.

42. Visser CA, Kan G, Meltzer RS, et al. Incidence, timing, and prognostic value of left ventricular aneurysm formation after myocardial infarction: a prospective serial echocardiographic study of 158 patients. *Am J Cardiol* 1986;57:729.

43. Gorlin R, Klein MD, Sullivan JM. Prospective correlative study of ventricular aneurysm: mechanistic concept and clinical recognition. *Am J Med* 1967;42:512–531.

44. Cabin HS, Roberts WC. Left ventricular aneurysm, intraaneurysmal thrombus, and systemic embolus in coronary heart disease. *Chest* 1980;77:586.

45. Jeremy RW, Hackworthy RA, Bautovich G, et al. Infarct artery perfusion and changes in left ventricular volume in the month after acute myocardial infarction. *J Am Coll Cardiol* 1987;9:989–995.

46. Popovic A, Neskovic A, Babic R, et al. Independent impact of thrombolytic therapy and vessel patency on left ventricular dilation after myocardial infarction. *Circulation* 1994;90:800–807.

47. Dzavik V, Beanlands DS, Davies RF, et al. Effects of late percutaneous transluminal coronary angioplasty of an occluded infarct-related coronary artery on left ventricular function in patients with a recent (<6-week) Q wave acute myocardial infarction (Total Occlusion Post-Myocardial Infarction Intervention Study [TOMIIS]—a pilot study). *Am J Cardiol* 1994;73:856–861.

48. Force T, Kemper A, Leavitt M, et al. Acute reduction in functional infarct expansion with late coronary reperfusion: assessment with quantitative two-dimensional echocardiography. *J Am Coll Cardiol* 1988;11:192–200.

49. Marino P, Destro G, Barbieri E, et al. Reperfusion of the infarct-related coronary artery limits left ventricular expansion beyond myocardial salvage. *Am Heart J* 1992;123:1157–1165.

50. Garot J, Scherrer-Crosbie M, Monin JL, et al. Effect of delayed percutaneous transluminal coronary angioplasty of occluded coronary arteries after acute myocardial infarction. *Am J Cardiol* 1996;77:915–921.

51. Galli M, Marcassa C, Bolli R, et al. Spontaneous delayed recovery of perfusion and contraction after the first 5 weeks after anterior infarction: evidence for the presence of hibernating myocardium in the infarcted area. *Circulation* 1994;90:1386–1397.

52. Meijer A, Verheugt FWA, van Eenige MJ, et al. Left ventricular function at 3 months after successful thrombolysis. Impact of reocclusion without reinfarction on ejection fraction, regional function, and remodeling. *Circulation* 1994;90:1706–1714.

53. Sabia PJ, Powers ER, Ragosta M, et al. An association between collateral blood flow and myocardial viability in patients with recent myocardial infarction. *N Engl J Med* 1992;327:1825–1834.

54. Chiarella F, Santoro E, Domenicucci S, et al. Predischarge two-dimensional echocardiographic evaluation of left ventricular thrombosis after acute myocardial infarction in the GISSI-3 study. *Am J Cardiol* 1998;8:822–827.

55. Stratton JR, Resnick AD. Increased embolic risk in patients with left ventricular thrombi. *Circulation* 1987;75:1004–1011.

56. Hochman JS, Platia EV, Bulkley BH. Endocardial abnormalities in left ventricular aneurysms: a clinicopathologic study. *Ann Intern Med* 1984;100:29.

57. Nolan SE, Mannisi JA, Bush DE, et al. Increased afterload aggravates infarct expansion after acute myocardial infarction. *J Am Coll Cardiol* 1988;12:1318–1325.

58. Oosterga M, Voors AA, de Kam PJ, et al. Plasma angiotensin-converting enzyme activity and left ventricular dilation after myocardial infarction. *Circulation* 1997;95:2607–2609.

59. Bulkley BH, Roberts WC. Steroid therapy during acute myocardial infarction: a cause of delayed healing and of ventricular aneurysm. *Am J Med* 1974;56:244–250.

60. Jugdutt BI, Basualdo CA. Myocardial infarct expansion during indomethacin or ibuprofen therapy for symptomatic post infarction pericarditis: influence of other pharmacologic agents during remodeling. *Can J Cardiol* 1989;5:211–221.

61. Hammerman H, Kloner RA, Schoen FJ, et al. Indomethacin-induced scar thinning after experimental myocardial infarction. *Circulation* 1983;67:1290–1295.

62. Hammerman H, Kloner RA, Hale S, et al. Dose-dependent effects of short-term methylprednisolone on myocardial infarct extent, scar formation, and ventricular function. *Circulation* 1983;68:446–452.

63. Bosimini E, Giannuzzi P, Temporelli PL, et al. Electrocardiographic evolutionary changes and left ventricular remodeling after acute myocardial infarction: results of the GISSI-3 Echo substudy. *J Am Coll Cardiol* 2000;35:135–137.

64. St. John Sutton M, Pfeffer MA, Plappert T, et al. Quantitative two-dimensional echocardiographic measurements are major predictors of adverse cardiovascular events after acute myocardial infarction. The protective effects of captopril. *Circulation* 1994;89:68–75.

65. Meltzer RS, Visser CA, Fuster V. Intracardiac thrombi and systemic embolization. *Ann Intern Med* 1986;104:689–698.

66. Lupi G, Domenicucci S, Chiarella F, et al. Influence of thrombolytic treatment followed by full dose anticoagulation on the frequency of left ventricular thrombi in acute myocardial infarction. *Am J Cardiol* 1989;64:588–590.

67. Kontny F, Dale J, Hegrerves L, et al. Left ventricular thrombosis and arterial embolism after thrombolysis in acute anterior myocardial infarction: predictors and effects of adjunctive antithrombotic therapy. *Eur Heart J* 1993;14:1489–1492.

68. Mooe T, Teien D, Karp K, et al. Left ventricular thrombosis after anterior myocardial infarction with and without thrombolytic treatment. *J Intern Med* 1995;237:563–569.

69. Hirsh J, Fuster V. Guide to anticoagulant therapy. Part 2: oral anticoagulants. *Circulation* 1994;89:1469–1480.

70. Lapeyre AC III, Steele PM, Kazmier FJ, et al. Systemic embolism in chronic left ventricular aneurysm: incidence and the role of anticoagulation. *J Am Coll Cardiol* 1985;6:534–538.

71. Loh E, St. John Sutton M, Wun CCC, et al. Ventricular dysfunction and the risk of stroke after myocardial infarction. *N Engl J Med* 1997;336:251–257.

72. Pfeffer MA, Lamas GA, Vaughan DE, et al. Effect of captopril on progressive ventricular dilatation after anterior myocardial infarction. *N Engl J Med* 1988;319:80–86.

73. Carstensen S, Bonarjee VVS, Berning J, et al. Effects of early enalapril treatment on global and regional wall motion in acute myocardial infarction. *Am Heart J* 1995;129:1101–1107.

74. de Kam PJ, Voors AA, van der Berg MP, et al. Effect of very early angiotensin-converting enzyme inhibition on left ventricular dilation after myocardial infarction in patients receiving thrombolysis: results of a meta-analysis of 845 patients. *J Am Coll Cardiol* 2000;36:2047–2053.

75. Spinar J, Vitovec J, Spinarova L, et al. A comparison of intervention with losartan or captopril in acute myocardial infarction. *Eur J Heart Failure* 2000;2:91–100.

76. Di Pasquale P, Bucca V, Scalzo S, et al. Does the addition of losartan improve the beneficial effects of ACE inhibitors in patients with anterior myocardial infarction? A pilot study. *Heart* 1999;81:606–611.

77. Jugdutt BI, Warnica JW. Intravenous nitroglycerin therapy to limit myocardial infarct size, expansion, and complications: Effect of timing, dosage, and infarct location. *Circulation* 1988;78:906–919.

78. Jugdutt BI, Khan MI. Effect of prolonged nitrate therapy on left ventricular remodeling after canine acute myocardial infarction. *Circulation* 1994;89:2297–2307.

79. Mahmarian JJ, Moye LA, Chinoy DA, et al. Transdermal nitroglycerin patch therapy improves left ventricular function and prevents remodeling after acute myocardial infarction: results of a multicenter prospective randomized, double-blind, placebo-controlled trial. *Circulation* 1998;97:2017–2024.

80. Pipilis A, Flather M, Collins R, et al. Hemodynamic effects of captopril and isosorbide mononitrate started

early in acute myocardial infarction: a randomized placebo-controlled study. *J Am Coll Cardiol* 1993;22:73–79.

81. Turpie AG, Robinson JG, Doyle DJ et al. Comparison of high-dose with low-dose subcutaneous heparin to prevent left ventricular mural thrombosis in patients with acute transmural anterior myocardial infarction. *N Engl J Med* 1989;320:352–357.

82. Tramarin R, Pozzoli M, Febo O, et al. Echocardiographic assessment of therapy efficacy in left ventricular thrombosis post myocardial infarction. *Circulation* 1983;68(Suppl 3):331.

83. Medical Research Council. Assessment of short-anticoagulant administration after cardiac infarction: report of the Working Party on Anticoagulant Therapy in Coronary Thrombosis to the Medical Research Council. *BMJ* 1969;1:335–342.

84. Veterans Administration Hospital Investigators. Anticoagulants in acute myocardial infarction: results of a cooperative clinical trial. *JAMA* 1973;225:724–729.

85. Gruppo Italiano Per Lo Studio Della Streptochinasi nell'Infarto Miocardico (GISSI). Effectiveness of intravenous thrombolytic treatment in acute myocardial infarction. *Lancet* 1986;2:397–401.

86. ASPECT 2 Trial. Presented at European Society of Cardiology, 2000.

87. CHAMP Trial. Presented at the American Heart Association 72nd Scientific Sessions, November 1999.

88. Granger CB, Hirsch J, Califf RM, et al. Activated partial thromboplastin time and outcome after thrombolytic therapy for acute myocardial infarction. Results from the GUSTO-1 trials. *Circulation* 1996;93:870–878.

89. Ryan TJ, for ACC/AHA. Guidelines for the management of patients with acute myocardial infarction. *J Am Coll Cardiol* 1996;28:1328–1419.

90. Ryan TJ, for ACC/AHA. Guidelines for the management of patients with acute myocardial infarction. *J Am Coll Cardiol* 1999;34:890–911.

91. Cohen M, Demers C, Gurfinkel EP, et al. for the ESSENCE Study Group. A comparison of low-molecular weight heparin with unfractionated heparin for unstable coronary artery disease. *N Engl J Med* 1997;14:447–452.

92. Coumadin Aspirin Reinfarction Study (CARS) Investigators. Randomized double-blind trial of fixed low-dose warfarin with aspirin after myocardial infarction. *Lancet* 1997;350:389–396.

93. Komeda M, David TE, Malik A, et al. Operative risks and long-term results of operation for left ventricular aneurysm. *Ann Thorac Surg* 1992;53:22.

94. Lamas GA, Flaker GC, Mitchell G, et al. Effect of infarct artery patency on prognosis after acute myocardial infarction. *Circulation* 1995;92:1101–1109.

95. Galvani M, Ottani F, Ferrini D, et al. Patency of the infarct-related artery and left ventricular function as the major determinants of survival after Q-wave acute myocardial infarction. *Am J Cardiol* 1993;71:1–7.

96. White HD, Cross DB, Elliott JM, et al. Long-term prognostic importance of patency of the infarct-related coronary artery after thrombolytic therapy for acute myocardial infarction. *Circulation* 1994;89:61–67.

97. Steinberg JS, Hochman JS, Morgan CD, et al. The effect of thrombolytic therapy given 6 to 24 hours after myocar-

dial infarction on the signal averaged electrocardiogram: results of a randomized placebo controlled trial. *Circulation* 1994;90:746–752.

98. Chandrasekaran S, Hochman JS, Slater J, et al. Relations between infarct artery patency at late angiography after acute myocardial infarction and signal-averaged electrocardiogram. *Am J Cardiol* 1999;86:734–736.

99. Puma JA, Sketch MH Jr, Thompson TD, et al. Support for the open-artery hypothesis in survivors of acute myocardial infarction: analysis of 11,228 patients treated with thrombolytic therapy. *Am J Cardiol* 1999;83:482–487.

100. Topol EJ, Califf RM, Vandormael M, et al. A randomized trial of late reperfusion therapy for acute myocardial infarction. Thrombolysis and angioplasty in myocardial infarction-6 study group. *Circulation* 1992;85:2090–2099.

101. Buller CE, Dzavik V, Carere RG, et al. Primary stenting versus balloon angioplasty in occluded coronary arteries: the Total Occlusion Study of Canada (TOSCA). *Circulation* 1999;100:236–242.

102. Moliterno DJ, Lange RA, Meidell RS, et al. Relation of plasma lipoprotein (a) to infarct artery patency in survivors of myocardial infarction. *Circulation* 1993;88:935–940.

103. Dakik HA, Mahmarian JJ, Verani MS, et al. Association of angiotensin I converting enzyme gene polymorphism with myocardial ischemia and patency of infarct related artery in patients with acute myocardial infarction. *J Am Coll Cardiol* 1997;29:1468–1473.

104. Yousef ZR, Redwood SR, Bucknall C, et al. A randomized trial of delayed intervention after myocardial infarction: clinical endpoint and echocardiographic data from The Open Artery Trial (TOAT- study). *Circulation* 2000;102[Suppl]:II-755(abst).

105. Horie H, Takahashi M, Minai K, et al. Long-term beneficial effect of late reperfusion for acute anterior myocardial infarction with percutaneous transluminal coronary angioplasty. *Circulation* 1998;98:2377–2382.

105a. Sadanandan S, Buller C, Menon V, et al. The late open artery hypothesis—a decade later. *Am Heart J* 2001;142:411–421.

106. Hochman JS. Has the time come to seek and open all occluded infarct-related arteries after myocardial infarction? *J Am Coll Cardiol* 1996;28:846–848.

107. Schuster EH, Bulkley BH. Early post-infarction angina: ischemia at a distance and ischemia in the infarct zone. *N Engl J Med* 1981;305:1101.

108. Schuster EH, Bulkley BH. Ischemia at a distance after acute myocardial infarction: a cause of early post-infarction angina. *Circulation* 1980;62:509.

109. Meijer A, Verheugt FW, Werter CJ, et al. Aspirin versus Coumadin in the prevention of reocclusion and recurrent ischemia after successful thrombolysis: a prospective placebo-controlled angiographic study. Results of the APRICOT study. *Circulation* 1993;87:1524–1530.

110. Ohman ME, Califf RM, Topol EJ, et al. Consequences of reocclusion after successful reperfusion therapy in acute myocardial infarction. *Circulation* 1990;82:781–791.

111. Roberts WC, Potkin BN, Solus DE, et al. Mode of death, frequency of healed and acute myocardial infarction, number of major epicardial coronary arteries severely narrowed

by atherosclerotic plaque, and heart weight in fatal athero-sclerotic coronary artery disease: analysis of 889 patients studied at necropsy. *J Am Coll Cardiol* 1990;15:196.

112. Betriu A, Castaner A, Sanz GA, et al. Angiographic findings 1 month after myocardial infarction: a prospective study of 259 survivors. *Circulation* 1982;65:1099–1105.

113. Goldstein JA, Demetriov D, Grenes DL, et al. Multiple complex coronary plaques in patients with acute myocardial infarction. *N Engl J Med* 2000;343:915–922.

114. Widimsky P, Gregor P, Cervenka V, et al. Severe diffuse hypokinesis of the remote myocardium: the main cause of cardiogenic shock? An echocardiographic study of 75 patients with extremely large myocardial infarctions. *Cor Vasa* 1988;30:27–34.

115. Uren NG, Crake T, Lefroy DC, et al. Reduced coronary vasodilator function in infarcted and normal myocardium after myocardial infarction. *N Engl J Med* 1994;331:222–227.

116. Gibson CM, Ryan KA, Murphy SA, et al. Impaired coronary blood flow in nonculprit arteries in the setting of acute myocardial infarction. The TIMI Study Group. Thrombolysis in myocardial infarction. *J Am Coll Cardiol* 1999;34:974–982.

117. Prewitt RM, Gu S, Schick U, et al. Intraaortic balloon counterpulsation enhances coronary thrombolysis induced by intravenous administration of a thrombolytic agent. *J Am Coll Cardiol* 1994;23:794–798.

118. Prewitt RM, Gu S, Garger PJ, et al. Marked systemic hypotension depresses coronary thrombolysis induced by intracoronary administration of recombinant tissue-type plasminogen activator. *J Am Coll Cardiol* 1992;20:1626–1633.

119. Kennedy JW, Gensini GG, Timmis GC, et al. Acute myocardial infarction treated with intracoronary streptokinase: a report of the Society for Cardiac Angiography. *Am J Cardiol* 1985;55:871–877.

120. Giannitsis E, Potratz J, Schmuecker G, et al. Impact of right ventricular infarction on in-hospital patency after early thrombolysis with an accelerated dose regimen of 100 mg tPA. *Circulation* 1996;94[Suppl]:I-733.

121. Swedberg K, Held P, Kjekshus J, et al. Effects of the early administration of enalapril on mortality in patients with acute myocardial infarction: results of the Cooperative New Scandinavian Enalapril Survival Study II (CONSENSUS II). *N Engl J Med* 1992;327:678–684.

122. Reid PR, Taylor DR, Kelly DT, et al. Myocardial infarct extension detected by precordial ST segment mapping. *N Engl J Med* 1974;290:123.

123. The Joint European Society of Cardiology/American College of Cardiology Committee. Myocardial infarction redefined—a consensus document of the Joint European Society of Cardiology/American College of Cardiology Committee for the redefinition of myocardial infarction. The Joint ESC/ACC Committee. *J Am Coll Cardiol* 2000;36:959–969.

124. Fraker TD Jr, Wagner GS, Rosati RA. Extension of myocardial infarction: incidence and prognosis. *Circulation* 1979;60:126–129.

125. Marmor A, Sobel BE, Roberts R. Factors presaging early recurrent myocardial infarction (extension). *Am J Cardiol* 1981;48:603–610.

126. Buda AJ, Macdonald IL, Dubbin JD, et al. Myocardial infarct extension: prevalence, clinical significance and problems in diagnosis. *Am Heart J* 1983;105:744–749.

127. ISIS-1 (First International Study of Infarct Survival) Collaborative Group. Randomized trial of intravenous atenolol among 16,027 cases of suspected acute myocardial infarction: ISIS-1. *Lancet* 1986;1:57–66.

128. The Miami Trial Research Group. Metoprolol in Acute Myocardial Infarction (MIAMI). A randomized, placebo-controlled international trial. *Eur Heart J* 1985;6:199–226.

129. The TIMI Study Group. Comparison of invasive and conservative strategies after treatment with intravenous tissue plasminogen activator in acute myocardial infarction. Results of the Thrombolysis in Myocardial Infarction (TIMI) phase II trial. *N Engl J Med* 1989;320:618–627.

130. ISIS-2 (Second International Study of Infarct Survival) Collaborative Group. Randomized trial of intravenous streptokinase, oral aspirin, both, or neither among 17,187 cases of suspected acute myocardial infarction. ISIS-2. *Lancet* 1988;2:349–360.

131. AIMS Trial Study Group. Long-term effects of intravenous anistreplase in acute myocardial infarction: final report of the AIMS study. *Lancet* 1990;335:427–431.

132. Arnold AE, Simoons ML, Van de Werf F, et al. Recombinant tissue-type plasminogen activator and immediate angioplasty in acute myocardial infarction. *Circulation* 1992;86:111–120.

133. Schroder R, Neuhaus KL, Leizorovicz A, et al. A prospective placebo-controlled double-blind multicenter trial of intravenous streptokinase in acute myocardial infarction (ISAM): long-term mortality and morbidity. *J Am Coll Cardiol* 1987;9:197–203.

134. Wilcox RG, Von der Lippe G, Olsson CG, et al. Trial of tissue plasminogen activator for mortality reduction in acute myocardial infarction. Anglo-Scandinavian study of early thrombolysis (ASSET). *Lancet* 1988;2:525–530.

135. The International Study Group. In-hospital mortality and clinical course of 20,891 patients with suspected acute myocardial infarction randomized between alteplase and streptokinase with or without heparin. *Lancet* 1990;336:71–75.

136. ISIS-3 (Third International Study of Infarct Survival) Collaborative Group. ISIS-3: a randomized comparison of streptokinase versus tissue plasminogen activator versus anistreplase and of aspirin plus heparin versus aspirin alone among 41,299 cases of suspected acute myocardial infarction. *Lancet* 1992;339:753–770.

137. The GUSTO Investigators. An international randomized trial comparing four thrombolytic strategies for acute myocardial infarction. *N Engl J Med* 1993;329:673–682.

138. Gruppo Italiano per lo Studio della Sopravvivenza Nell'Infarto Miocardico. GISSI-2: a factorial randomized trial of alteplase versus streptokinase and heparin versus no heparin among 12,490 patients with acute myocardial infarction. *Lancet* 1990;336:65–71.

139. ISIS-4 (Fourth International Study of Infarct Survival) Collaborative Group. ISIS-4: a randomized factorial trial assessing early oral captopril, oral mononitrate, and intravenous magnesium sulphate in 58,050 patients with sus-

pected acute myocardial infarction. *Lancet* 1995;345:669–685.

140. Gruppo Italiano per lo Studio della Sopravvivenza Nell'Infarto Miocardico. GISSI-3: effects of lisinopril and transdermal glyceryl trinitrate singly and together on 6-week mortality and ventricular function after acute myocardial infarction. *Lancet* 1994;343:1115–1122.

141. Jha P, Deboer D, Sykora K, et al. Characteristics and mortality outcomes of thrombolysis trial participants and nonparticipants: a population-based comparison. *J Am Coll Cardiol* 1996;27:1335–1342.

142. Silva P, Galli M, Campolo L, for the IRES (Ischemia Residual) Study Group. Prognostic significance of early ischemia after acute myocardial infarction in low-risk patients. *Am J Cardiol* 1993;71:1142–1147.

143. Armstrong PW, Fu Y, Chang WC, et al. Acute coronary syndromes in the GUSTO-IIb trial: prognostic insights and impact of recurrent ischemia. The GUSTO-IIb Investigators. *Circulation* 1998;98:1860–1868.

144. Mueller HS, Forman SA, Menegus MA, et al. Prognostic significance of nonfatal reinfarction during 3-year follow-up: results of the Thrombolysis in Myocardial Infarction (TIMI) phase II clinical trial. *J Am Coll Cardiol* 1995;26:900–907.

145. Hsia J, Hamilton WP, Kleiman N, et al. A comparison between heparin and low-dose aspirin as adjunctive therapy with tissue plasminogen activator for acute myocardial infarction. *N Engl J Med* 1990;323:1433–1437.

146. Mahaffey KW, Granger CB, Collins R, et al. Overview of randomized trials of intravenous heparin in patients with acute myocardial infarction treated with thrombolytic therapy. *Am J Cardiol* 1996;77:551–556.

147. The Global Use of Strategies to Open Occluded Coronary Arteries (GUSTO) IIb Investigators. A comparison of recombinant hirudin with heparin for the treatment of acute coronary syndromes. *N Engl J Med* 1996;335:775–785.

147a. The GUSTO V Investigators. Reperfusion therapy for acute myocardial infarction with fibrinolytic therapy or combination reduced fibrinolytic therapy and platelet glycoprotein IIb/IIIa inhibition: the GUSTO V randomized trial. *Lancet* 2001;357:1905–1914.

148. Moliterno DJ. A critical appraisal of platelet glycoprotein IIb/IIa inhibitors. *J Am Coll Cardiol* 2000;36:2028–2035.

149. CAPRIE Steering Committee. A randomized, blinded, trial of clopidogrel versus aspirin in patients at risk of ischaemic events (CAPRIE). *Lancet* 1996;348:1329–1339.

150. Rutherford JD, Pfeffer MA, Moye LA, et al. Effects of captopril on ischemic events after myocardial infarction. Results of the Survival and Ventricular Enlargement Trial. SAVE Investigators. *Circulation* 1994;90:1731–1738.

151. Yusuf S, Sleight P, Pogue J, et al. Effects of an angiotensin-converting-enzyme inhibitor, ramipril, on cardiovascular events in high-risk patients. The Heart Outcomes Prevention Evaluation Study Investigators. *N Engl J Med* 2000;342:145–153.

152. Simoons ML, Arnold AE, Betriu A, et al. Thrombolysis with tissue plasminogen activator in acute myocardial infarction: no additional benefit from immediate percutaneous coronary angioplasty. *Lancet* 1988;1:197–203.

153. SWIFT (Should We Intervene Following Thrombolysis?) Trial Study Group. SWIFT trial of delayed elective intervention versus conservative treatment after thrombolysis with anistreplase in acute myocardial infarction. *BMJ* 1991;302:555–560.

154. Barbash GI, Roth A, Hod H, et al. Randomized controlled trial of late in-hospital angiography and angioplasty versus conservative management after treatment with recombinant tissue-type plasminogen in acute myocardial infarction. *Am J Cardiol* 1990;66:538–545.

155. White HD, Cross DB, Williams BF, et al. Safety and efficacy of repeat thrombolytic treatment after acute myocardial infarction. *Br Heart J* 1990;64:177–181.

156. Hudson MP, Barbash GI, Granger CB, et al. Temporal and regional differences in therapy for reinfarction following thrombolysis: results from GUSTO I and ASSENT II. *J Am Coll Cardiol* 2000;76:386A.

157. Madsen JK, Grande P, Saunamäki K. Danish multicenter randomized study of invasive versus conservative treatment in patients with inducible ischemia after thrombolysis in acute myocardial infarction (DANAMI). *Circulation* 1997;96:748–755.

158. Hood WB Jr, Bianco JA, Kumar R, et al. Experimental myocardial infarction. IV. Reduction of left ventricular compliance in the healing phase. *J Clin Invest* 1970;49:1316–1323.

159. Forrester JS, Diamond G, Parmley WW, et al. Early increase in left ventricular compliance after myocardial infarction. *J Clin Invest* 1972;51:598–603.

160. Vokonas PS, Pirzada F, Hood WB Jr. Experimental myocardial infarction. XII. Dynamic changes in segmental mechanical behavior of infarcted and noninfarcted myocardium. *Am J Cardiol* 1976;37:853–859.

161. Becker LC, Levine JH, DiPaula AF, et al. Reversal of dysfunction in postischemic stunned myocardium by epinephrine and postextrasystolic potentiation. *J Am Coll Cardiol* 1986;7:580–589.

162. Matsuzaki M, Gallagher KP, Kemper WS, et al. Sustained regional dysfunction produced by prolonged coronary stenosis: gradual recovery after reperfusion. *Circulation* 1983;68:170–182.

163. Ross J Jr. Myocardial perfusion-contraction matching: implications for coronary heart disease and hibernation. *Circulation* 1991;83:1076–1083.

164. McGhie AI, Goldstein RA. Pathogenesis and management of acute heart failure and cardiogenic shock: role of inotropic therapy. *Chest* 1992;102:626S–632S.

165. Califf RM, Bengtson JR. Cardiogenic shock. *N Engl J Med* 1994;330:1724–1730.

166. Hochman JS, Palazzo A. Cardiogenic shock complicating acute myocardial infarction. In: Braunwald E, ed. *Atlas of heart diseases*. Boston: Current Medicine, 1996;8:12.1–12.23.

167. Shah PK, Maddahi J, Staniloff HM, et al. Variable spectrum and prognostic implications of left and right ventricular ejection fractions in patients with and without clinical heart failure after acute myocardial infarction. *Am J Cardiol* 1986;58:387–393.

168. Berning J, Steensgaard-Hansen F. Early estimation of risk by echocardiographic determination of wall motion index

in an unselected population with acute myocardial infarction. *Am J Cardiol* 1990;65:567–576.

169. Nishimura RA, Tajik AJ, Shub C, et al. Role of two-dimensional echocardiography in the prediction of in-hospital complications after acute myocardial infarction. *J Am Coll Cardiol* 1984;4:1080–1087.

170. Volpi A, De Vita C, Franzosi MG, et al. Determinants of 6-month mortality in survivors of myocardial infarction after thrombolysis: results of the GISSI-2 data base. *Circulation* 1993;88:416–429.

171. Remme WJ, Look MP, Bootsma M, et al. Neurohumoral activation during acute myocardial ischaemia: effects of ACE inhibition. *Eur Heart J* 1990;[Suppl B]:162–171.

172. Dargie HJ, McAlpine HM, Morton JJ. Neuroendocrine activation in acute myocardial infarction. *J Cardiovasc Pharmacol* 1987;9[Suppl 2]:21S–24S.

173. Omland T. Natriuretic peptides as markers of ventricular dysfunction. *Hypertension* 1997;30:305–306.

174. Sanford CF, Corbett J, Nicod P, et al. Value of radionuclide ventriculography in the immediate characterization of patients with acute myocardial infarction. *Am J Cardiol* 1982;49:637–644.

175. Oh JK, Ding ZP, Gersh BJ, et al. Restrictive left ventricular diastolic filling identifies the patients with heart failure after acute myocardial infarction. *J Am Soc Echocardiol* 1992;5:497–503.

176. Brown EJ, Swinford RD, Gadde P, et al. Acute effects of delayed reperfusion on myocardial infarct shape and left ventricular volume: a potential mechanism of additional benefits from thrombolytic therapy. *J Am Coll Cardiol* 1991;17:1641–1650.

177. Hochman JS, Buller CE, Sleeper LA, et al. Cardiogenic shock complicating acute myocardial infarction—etiologies, management and outcome; overall findings of the SHOCK Trial Registry. *J Am Coll Cardiol* 2000;36:1063–1070.

178. Himbert D, Juliard JM, Steg PG, et al. Limits of reperfusion therapy for immediate cardiogenic shock complicating acute myocardial infarction. *Am J Cardiol* 1994;74:492–494.

179. Alonso DR, Scheidt S, Post M, et al. Pathophysiology of cardiogenic shock: quantification of myocardial necrosis, clinical, pathologic, and electrocardiographic correlations. *Circulation* 1973;48:588–596.

180. Wong SC, Antonelli T, Sleeper LA, et al. Angiographic findings and clinical correlates in patients with cardiogenic shock complicating acute myocardial infarction in the SHOCK Registry. *J Am Coll Cardiol* 2000;36:1077–1083.

181. Page DL, Caulfield JB, Kastor JA, et al. Myocardial changes associated with cardiogenic shock. *N Engl J Med* 1971;285:133–137.

182. Holmes DR Jr, Berger PB, Granger CB, et al. Cardiogenic shock in patients with acute ischemic syndromes with and without ST-segment elevation. *Circulation* 1999;100:2067–2073.

183. Gutovitz AL, Sobel BE, Roberts R. Progressive nature of myocardial injury in selected patients with cardiogenic shock. *Am J Coll Cardiol* 1978;41:469–475.

184. Hands ME, Rutherford JD, Muller JE. The in-hospital development of cardiogenic shock after myocardial infarction: incidence, predictors of occurrence, outcome, and prognostic factors. The MILIS Study Group. *Am J Coll Cardiol* 1989;14:40–46.

185. Holmes DR Jr, Bates ER, Kleiman NS, et al. for the GUSTO-I Investigators. Contemporary reperfusion therapy for cardiogenic shock: the GUSTO-I trial experience. Global utilization of streptokinase and tissue plasminogen activator for occluded coronary arteries. *J Am Coll Cardiol* 1995;26:668–674.

186. de Villalobos DH, Taegtmeyer H. Metabolic support for the postischaemic heart. *Lancet* 1995;345:1552–1555.

187. Opie LH. Glucose and the metabolism of ischaemic myocardium. *Lancet* 1995;345:1520–1521.

188. Beyersdorf F, Acar C, Buckberg GD, et al. Studies on prolonged acute regional ischemia. III. Early natural history of simulated single and multivessel disease with emphasis on remote myocardium. *J Thorac Cardiovasc Surg* 1989;98:368–380.

189. Beyersdorf F, Acar C, Buckberg GD, et al. Studies on prolonged acute regional ischemia. V. Metabolic support of remote myocardium during left ventricular power failure. *J Thorac Cardiovasc Surg* 1989;98:567–579.

190. Coven DL, Suter TM, Eberli FR, Apstein CS. Dobutamine and glucose-insulin-potassium (GIK) improve cardiac function and survival in a randomized trial of experimental cardiogenic shock. *Circulation* 1994;90:I–480.

191. Ballester M, Tasca R, Marin L. Different mechanisms of mitral regurgitation in acute and chronic forms of coronary heart disease. *Eur Heart J* 1983;4:557–565.

192. Forrester JS, Diamond G, Freedman S, et al. Silent mitral insufficiency in acute myocardial infarction. *Circulation* 1971;44:877–883.

193. Guerci AD, Gerstenblith G, Brinker JA, et al. A randomized trial of intravenous tissue plasminogen activator for acute myocardial infarction with subsequent randomization to elective coronary angioplasty. *N Engl J Med* 1987;317:1613–1618.

194. National Heart Foundation of Australia Coronary Thrombolysis Group. Coronary thrombolysis and myocardial salvage by tissue plasminogen activator given up to 4 hours after onset of myocardial infarction. *Lancet* 1988;1:203–208.

195. Simoons ML, Serruys PW, van den Brand M, et al. Early thrombolysis in acute myocardial infarction: limitation of infarct size and improved survival. *J Am Coll Cardiol* 1986;7:717–728.

196. Meinertz T, Kasper W, Schumacher M, et al., for the APSAC Multicenter Trial Group. The German multicenter trial of anisoylated plasminogen streptokinase activator complex versus heparin for acute myocardial infarction. *Am J Cardiol* 1988;62:347–351.

197. Bassand JP, Machecourt J, Cassagnes J, et al. Multicenter trial of intravenous anisoylated plasminogen streptokinase activator complex (APSAC) in acute myocardial infarction: effects on infarct size and left ventricular function. *J Am Coll Cardiol* 1989;13:988–997.

198. Bates ER, Topol EJ. Limitations of thrombolytic therapy for acute myocardial infarction complicated by congestive heart failure and cardiogenic shock. *J Am Coll Cardiol* 1991;18:1077–1084.

199. Goldberg RJ, Gore JM, Alpert JS, et al. Cardiogenic shock after acute myocardial infarction: incidence and mortality from a community-wide perspective, 1975 to 1988. *N Engl J Med* 1991;325:1117–1122.

200. Goldberg RJ, Samad NA, Yarzebski J, et al. Temporal trends in cardiogenic shock complicating acute myocardial infarction. *N Engl J Med* 1999;340:1162–1168.

201. Rogers WJ, Bowlby LJ, Chandra NC, et al. Treatment of myocardial infarction in the United States (1990 to 1993). Observations from the national registry of myocardial infarction. *Circulation* 1994;90:2103–2114.

202. Gibbons RJ, Holmes DR, Reeder GS, et al. for the Mayo Coronary Care Unit and Catheterization Laboratory Groups. Immediate angioplasty compared with the administration of a thrombolytic agent followed by conservative treatment for myocardial infarction. *N Engl J Med* 1993;328:685–691.

203. Grines CL, Browne KF, Marco J, et al. for the Primary Angioplasty in Myocardial Infarction Study Group. A comparison of immediate angioplasty with thrombolytic therapy for acute myocardial infarction. *N Engl J Med* 1993;328:673–679.

204. Zijlstra F, de Boer MJ, Hoorntje JC, et al. A comparison of immediate coronary angioplasty with intravenous streptokinase in acute myocardial infarction. *N Engl J Med* 1993;328:680–684.

205. Hasdai D, Califf RM, Thompson TD, et al. Predictors of cardiogenic shock after thrombolytic therapy for acute myocardial infarction. *J Am Coll Cardiol* 1999;35:136–143.

206. Jacobs AK, French J, Col J, et al. Cardiogenic shock without ST segment elevation myocardial infarction. A report from the SHOCK Registry. *J Am Coll Cardiol* 2000;36;1091–1096.

207. Hasdai D, Holmes D Jr, Califf RM, et al. for the GUSTO-1 Investigators. Cardiogenic shock complicating acute myocardial infarction: predictors of death. *Am Heart J* 1999;138:21–31.

208. Sleeper LA, Jacobs AK, LeJemtel TH, et al. A mortality model and severity scoring system for cardiogenic shock complicating acute myocardial infarction. *Circulation* 2000;102:II-795(abst).

209. Webb JG, Buller CE, Thompson CR, et al. Implications of the timing of onset of cardiogenic shock after acute myocardial infarction: a report from the SHOCK Registry. *J Am Coll Cardiol* 2000;36;1084–1090.

210. Menon V, White H, LeJemtel T, et al. The clinical profile of patients with suspected cardiogenic shock due to predominant left ventricular failure. *J Am Coll Cardiol* 2000;36:1071–1076.

211. Menon V, Slater JN, White HD, et al. Acute myocardial infarction complicated by systemic hypoperfusion: report of the SHOCK Registry. *Am J Med* 2000;108:374–380.

212. Chirillo F, Cavarzerani A, Ius P, et al. Role of transthoracic, transesophageal, and transgastric two-dimensional and color Doppler echocardiography in the evaluation of mechanical complications of acute myocardial infarction. *Am J Cardiol* 1995;76:833–836.

213. Heidenreich PA, Stainback RF, Redberg RF, et al. Transesophageal echocardiography predicts mortality in critically ill patients with unexplained hypotension. *J Am Coll Cardiol* 1995;26:152–158.

214. Smyllie JH, Sutherland GR, Geuskens R, et al. Doppler color flow mapping in the diagnosis of ventricular septal rupture and acute mitral regurgitation after myocardial infarction. *J Am Coll Cardiol* 1990;15:1449–1455.

215. Oh JK, Seward JB, Khandheria BK, et al. Transesophageal echocardiography in critically ill patients. *Am J Cardiol* 1990;66:1492–1495.

216. Forrester JS, Diamond G, Chatterjee K, et al. Medical therapy of acute myocardial infarction by application of hemodynamic subsets (first of two parts). *N Engl J Med* 1976;295:1356–1362.

217. Forrester JS, Diamond GC, Chatterjee K, et al. Medical therapy of acute myocardial infarction by application of hemodynamic subsets (second of two parts). *N Engl J Med* 1976;295:1404–1413.

218. Scheinman M, Brown MA, Rapaport E. Critical assessment of use of central venous oxygen saturation as a mirror of mixed venous oxygen in severely ill cardiac patients. *Circulation* 1969;40:165–172.

219. Kasnitz P, Druger GL, Yorra F, Simmons DH. Mixed venous oxygen tension and hyperlactatemia: Survival in severe cardiopulmonary disease. *JAMA* 1976;236:570–574.

220. da Luz PL, Cavanilles JM, Michaels S, et al. Oxygen delivery, anoxic metabolism, and hemoglobin-oxygen affinity (P_{50}) in patients with acute myocardial infarction and shock. *Am J Cardiol* 1975;36:148–154.

221. Yang SC, Puri VK, Raheja R. Oxygen delivery and consumption and P_{50} in patients with acute myocardial infarction. *Circulation* 1986;73:1183–1185.

222. Connors AF, Speroff T, Dawson NV, et al. The effectiveness of right-heart catheterization in the initial care of critically ill patients. *JAMA* 1996;276:889–897.

223. Rackley CE, Satler LF, Pearle DL, et al. Use of hemodynamic measurements for management of acute myocardial infarction. *Cardiovasc Clin* 1986;16:3–15.

224. Biddle TL, Yu PN. Effect of furosemide on hemodynamics and lung water in acute pulmonary edema secondary to myocardial infarction. *Am J Cardiol* 1979;43:86–90.

225. Mark AL. The Bezold-Jarisch reflex revisited: clinical implications of inhibitory reflexes originating in the heart. *J Am Coll Cardiol* 1983;1:90–102.

226. Rochon TA, Tu JV, Anderson GM, et al. Rate of heart failure and 1-year survival for older patients receiving low-dose beta-blocker therapy after myocardial infarction. *Lancet* 2000;356:639–644.

227. The Acute Infarction Ramipril Efficacy (AIRE) Study Investigators. Effect of ramipril on mortality and morbidity of survivors of acute myocardial infarction with clinical evidence of heart failure. *Lancet* 1993;342:821–828.

228. The EPIC Investigators. Use of a monoclonal antibody directed against the platelet glycoprotein IIb/IIIa receptor in high-risk coronary angioplasty. *N Engl J Med* 1994;330:956–961.

229. The EPILOG Investigators. Platelet glycoprotein IIb/IIIa receptor blockade and low-dose heparin during percutaneous coronary revascularization. *N Engl J Med* 1997;336:1689–1696.

230. The ESPRIT Investigators. Novel dosing regimen of eptifibatide in planned coronary stent implantation (ESPRIT): a randomized placebo-controlled trial. *Lancet* 2000;356:2037–2044.

231. Hasdai D, Harrington RA, Hochman JS. Platelet glycoprotein IIb/IIIa blockade and outcome of cardiogenic shock complicating acute coronary syndromes without persistent ST-segment elevation. *J Am Coll Cardiol* 2000;36:685–692.

232. Nelson GI, Silke B, Ahuja RC, et al. Hemodynamic advantages of isosorbide dinitrate over furosemide in acute heart failure following myocardial infarction. *Lancet* 1983;1:730–733.

233. Chiche P, Derrida JP, Baligadoo S, et al. The treatment of recent myocardial infarction by prolonged infusion of trinitrin. *Nouv Presse Med* 1977;6:4119–4122.

234. Chiariello M, Gold HK, Leinbach RC, et al. Comparison between the effects of nitroprusside and nitroglycerin on ischemic injury during acute myocardial infarction. *Circulation* 1976;54:766–773.

235. Armstrong PW, Walker DC, Burton JR, Parker JO. Vasodilator therapy in acute myocardial infarction. A comparison of sodium nitroprusside and nitroglycerin. *Circulation* 1975;52:1118.

236. Keren G, Bier A, LeJemtel TH. Improvement in forward cardiac output without a change in ejection fraction during nitroglycerin therapy in patients with functional mitral regurgitation. *Can J Cardiol* 1986;2:206–211.

237. Gold HK, Chiariello M, Leinbach RC. Deleterious effects of nitroprusside on myocardial injury during acute myocardial infarction. *Herz* 1976;1:161–166.

238. Franciosa JA, Limas CJ, Guiha NH. Improved left ventricular function during nitroprusside infusion in acute myocardial infarction. *Lancet* 1972;1:650–657.

239. Ivankovich AD, Miletich DJ, Albrecht RF, Zahed B. Sodium nitroprusside and cerebral blood flow in the anesthetized and unanesthetized goat. *Anesthesiology* 1976;44:21.

240. Farhy RD, Carretero OA, Ho KL, Scicli AG. Role of kinins and nitric oxide in the effects of angiotensin converting enzyme inhibitors on neointima formation. *Circ Res* 1993;72:1202–1210.

241. Cody RJ. Renin system inhibition: beginning the fourth epoch [editorial]. *Circulation* 1992;85:362–364.

242. McCaa RE, Hall JE, McCaa CS. The effects of angiotensin I-converting enzyme inhibitors on arterial blood pressure and urinary sodium excretion: role for the renal-serum-angiotensin and kallikrein-kinin systems. *Circ Res* 1978;43:I-32–I-39.

243. Kugler J, Maskin C, Frishman WH, et al. Regional and systemic metabolic effects of angiotensin converting enzyme inhibition during exercise in patients with severe heart failure. *Circulation* 1982;66:1256–1261.

244. Foult JM, Tavolaro O, Antony I, et al. Direct myocardial and coronary effects of enalaprilat in patients with dilated cardiomyopathy: Assessment by a bilateral intracoronary infusion technique. *Circulation* 1988;77:337–344.

245. Goldstein RA, Passamani ER, Roberts R. A comparison of digoxin and dobutamine in patients with acute infarction and cardiac failure. *N Engl J Med* 1980;303:846–850.

246. Hamlin NP, Willerson JT, Garan H, et al. The neurogenic vasoconstrictor effect of digitalis on coronary vascular resistance. *J Clin Invest* 1974;53:288–296.

247. Arnold JM, Braunwald E, Sandor T, et al. Inotropic stimulation of reperfused myocardium with dopamine: effects on infarct size and myocardial function. *J Am Coll Cardiol* 1985;6:1026–1034.

248. Sonnenblick EH, Frishman WH, LeJemtel TH. Dobutamine: a new synthetic cardioactive sympathetic amine. *N Engl J Med* 1979;300:17–22.

249. Tuttle RR, Hillmann CC, Toomey RE. Differential β-adrenergic sensitivity of atrial and ventricular tissue assessed by chronotropic, inotropic, and cyclic AMP responses to isoprenaline and dobutamine. *Cardiovasc Res* 1976;10:452–458.

250. Tuttle RR, Mills J. Dobutamine: development of a new catecholamine to selectively increase cardiac contractility. *Circ Res* 1975;36:185–196.

251. Kirk ES, LeJemtel TH, Nelson GR, et al. Mechanisms of beneficial effects of vasodilators and inotropic stimulation in the experimental failing ischemic heart. *Am J Med* 1978;65:189–196.

252. Tuttle RR, Pollock GD, Todd G, et al. The effect of dobutamine on cardiac oxygen balance, regional blood flow, and infarction severity after coronary artery narrowing in dogs. *Circ Res* 1977;41:357–364.

253. Karlsberg RP, DeWood MA, DeMaria AN, et al. Comparative efficacy of short-term intravenous infusions of milrinone and dobutamine in acute congestive heart failure following acute myocardial infarction. Milrinone-Dobutamine Study Group. *Clin Cardiol* 1996;19:21–30.

254. Gage J, Rutman H, Lucido D, et al. Additive effects of dobutamine and amrinone on myocardial contractility and ventricular performance in patients with severe heart failure. *Circulation* 1986;74:367–373.

255. Guimond JG, Matuschak GM, Meyers F, et al. Augmentation of cardiac function in end-stage heart failure by combined use of dobutamine and amrinone. *Chest* 1986;90:302–304.

256. Verma SP, Silke B, Taylor SH. Haemodynamic dose-response effects of amrinone in left ventricular failure complicating myocardial infarction. *Br J Clin Pharmacol* 1992;19:540P.

257. Taylor SH, Verma SP, Hussain M, et al. Intravenous amrinone in left ventricular failure complicated by acute myocardial infarction. *Am J Cardiol* 1985;56:29B–32B.

258. Gold J, Culinane S, Chen J, et al. Treatment of milrinone induced hypotension in severe heart failure. *Am J Cardiol* 2000;85:506–508.

259. Mueller HS, Ayres SM, Gregory JJ, et al. Hemodynamics, coronary blood flow, and myocardial metabolism in coronary shock: response of l-norepinephrine and isoproterenol. *J Clin Invest* 1970;49:1885–1902.

260. Advanced cardiac life support—algorithmic life exercises art 6. *Circulation* 2000;102:136–166.

261. Morales DL, Gregg DG, Helman DN, et al. Arginine vasopressin in the treatment of 50 patients with postcardiotomy vasodilatory shock. *Ann Thorac Surg* 2000;69:102–106.

262. Cotter G, Kaluski E, Blatt A, et al. L-NMMA (a nitric oxide synthase inhibitor) is effective in the treatment of cardiogenic shock. *Circulation* 2000;101:1358–1361.

263. Nanas JN, Moulopoulos SD. Counterpulsation: historical background, technical improvements, hemodynamic and metabolic effects. *Cardiology* 1994;84:156–167.

264. Mueller H, Ayres SM, Conklin EF, et al. The effects of intra-aortic counterpulsation on cardiac performance and metabolism in shock associated with acute myocardial infarction. *J Clin Invest* 1971;50:1885–1900.

265. Leinbach RC, Dinsmore RE, Mundth ED, et al. Selective coronary and left ventricular cineangiography during intraaortic balloon pumping for cardiogenic shock. *Circulation* 1972;45:845–852.

266. Mueller H, Ayres SM, Giannelli S, et al. Effect of isoproterenol, 1-norepinephrine and intraaortic counterpulsation on hemodynamics and myocardial metabolism in shock following acute myocardial infarction. *Circulation* 1972;45:335–351.

267. Kern MJ, Aguirre FV, Tatrineni S, et al. Enhanced coronary blood flow velocity during intraaortic balloon counterpulsation in critically ill patients. *J Am Coll Cardiol* 1993;21:359–368.

268. Kimura A, Toyota E, Songfang L, et al. Effects of intraaortic balloon pumping on the septal arterial blood flow velocity waveform during severe left main coronary artery stenosis. *J Am Coll Cardiol* 1996;27:810–816.

269. Fuchs RM, Brin KP, Brinker JA, et al. Augmentation of regional coronary blood flow by intraaortic balloon counterpulsation in patients with unstable angina. *Circulation* 1983;68:117–123.

270. Williams DO. Intra-aortic balloon counterpulsation: deciphering its effects on coronary flow. *J Am Coll Cardiol* 1996;27:817–818.

271. Scheidt S, Wilner G, Mueller H, et al. Intra-aortic balloon counterpulsation in cardiogenic shock: report of a cooperative clinical trial. *N Engl J Med* 1973;288:979–984.

272. O'Rourke MF, Norris RM, Campbell TJ, et al. Randomized controlled trial of intra-aortic balloon counterpulsation in early myocardial infarction with acute heart failure. *Am J Cardiol* 1981;47:815–820.

273. Waksman R, Weiss AT, Gotsman MS, et al. Intra-aortic balloon counterpulsation improves survival in cardiogenic shock complicating acute myocardial infarction. *Eur Heart J* 1993;14:71–74.

274. Ohman EM, George BS, White CJ, et al. for the Randomized IABP Study Group. Use of aortic counterpulsation to improve sustained coronary artery patency during acute myocardial infarction: results of a randomized trial. *Circulation* 1994;90:792–799.

275. Holmes DR, Califf RM, Van de Werf F, et al. Difference in countries' use of resources and clinical outcome for patients with cardiogenic shock after myocardial infarction: results from the GUSTO trial. *Lancet* 1997;349:75–78.

276. Sanborn TA, Sleeper LA, Bates E, et al. Impact of thrombolysis, aortic counterpulsation, and their combination in cardiogenic shock complicating acute myocardial infarction. *J Am Coll Cardiol* 2000;36:1123–1129.

277. Barron HV, Every NR, Parsons LS, et al. The use of intra-aortic balloon counterpulsation in patients with cardiogenic shock complicating acute myocardial infarction: data from the National Registry of Myocardial Infarction 2. *Am Heart J* 2001;141:933–939.

278. Farrar DJ, Lawson JH, Litwak P, et al. Thoratec VAD system as a bridge to heart transplantation. *J Heart Transplant* 1990;9:415–422.

279. Miller CA, Pae WE, Pierce WS. Combined registry for the clinical use of mechanical ventricular assist devices: postcardiotomy cardiogenic shock. *Trans Am Soc Artif Intern Organs* 1990;36:43–46.

280. Moritz A, Wolner E. Circulatory support with shock due to acute myocardial infarction. *Ann Thorac Surg* 1993;55:238–244.

281. Shawl F, Domanski MA, Hernandez TJ, et al. Emergency percutaneous cardiopulmonary bypass support in cardiogenic shock from acute myocardial infarction. *Am J Cardiol* 1989;64:967.

282. Vogel RA, Shawl F, Tommaso C, et al. Initial report of the national registry of elective cardiopulmonary bypass supported coronary angioplasty. *J Am Coll Cardiol* 1990;15:23–29.

283. Hill JG, Bruhn PS, Cohen SE, et al. Emergent applications of cardiopulmonary support: a multi-institutional experience. *Ann Thorac Surg* 1992;54:699–704.

284. Grambow DW, Deeb GM, Pavlides GS, et al. Emergent percutaneous cardiopulmonary bypass in patients having cardiovascular collapse in the cardiac catheterization laboratory. *Am J Cardiol* 1994;73:872–875.

285. Overlie PA, Walter PD, Hurd HP II, et al. Emergency cardiopulmonary support with circulatory support devices. *Cardiology* 1994;84:231–237.

286. Thiele H, Lauer B, Hambrecht R, et al. Reversal of cardiogenic shock by percutaneous left atrial-to-femoral arterial bypass assistance. (Personal communication with Dr. Schuler.)

287. Bengtson JR, Kaplan AJ, Pieper KS, et al. Prognosis in cardiogenic shock after acute myocardial infarction in the interventional era. *J Am Coll Cardiol* 1992;20:1482–1489.

288. Lee L, Erbel R, Brown TM, et al. Multicenter registry of angioplasty therapy of cardiogenic shock: initial and long-term survival. *J Am Coll Cardiol* 1991;17:599–603.

289. Hochman JS, Sleeper LA, White HD, et al. Early revascularization in acute myocardial infarction complicated by cardiogenic shock. *N Engl J Med* 1999;341:625–634.

290. de Boer MJ, Suryapranata H, Hoorntje JC, et al. Limitation of infarct size and preservation of left ventricular function after primary coronary angioplasty compared with intravenous streptokinase in acute myocardial infarction. *Circulation* 1994;90:753–761.

291. The GUSTO IIb Angioplasty Substudy Investigators. A clinical trial comparing primary coronary angioplasty with tissue plasminogen activator for acute myocardial infarction. *N Engl J Med* 1997;23:1621–1628.

292. Hochman JS, Jaber W, Bates ER, et al. Angioplasty versus thrombolytics for patients presenting with congestive heart failure: GUSTO IIb substudy findings. *J Am Coll Cardiol* 1998;31:856–864.

293. Fibrinolytic Therapy Trialists' (FTT) Collaborative Group. Indications for fibrinolytic therapy in suspected acute myocardial infarction: collaborative overview of early mortality and major morbidity results from all randomised trials of more than 1000 patients. *Lancet* 1994;343:311–322.

294. Stomel RJ, Rasak M, Bates ER. Treatment strategies for acute myocardial infarction complicated by cardiogenic shock in a community hospital. *Chest* 1994;105:997–1002.

295. Ohman ME, Nannas J, Stomel RJ. Thrombolysis and counterpulsation to improve cardiogenic shock survival (TACTICS): results of a prospective randomized trial. *Circulation* 2000;102[Suppl]:II-600.

296. Bates ER, Kleiman NS, Morris DC, Holmes DR, for the GUSTO Investigators. Influence on Killip class on mortality in the international trial and the GUSTO Trial. *J Am Coll Cardiol* 1994;23:313A.

297. Webb JG, Sanborn TA, Sleeper TA, et al. Percutaneous coronary intervention in the management of cardiogenic shock in the SHOCK Registry. *Am Heart J* 2001;1441:964–970.

298. Hochman JS. Cardiogenic shock: can we save the patient? *Am Coll Cardiol* 1996;12:1–5.

299. Hochman JS, Boland J, Sleeper LA. Current spectrum of cardiogenic shock and effect of early revascularization on mortality: results of an international registry. *Circulation* 1995;91:873–881.

300. Varnauskas E, and the European Coronary Surgery Study Group. Twelve-year follow-up of survival in the randomized European coronary surgery study. *N Engl J Med* 1988;319:332–337.

301. Takaro T, Hultgren HN, Lipton MJ, Detre KM, and participants in the study group. The VA Cooperative randomized study of surgery for coronary artery occlusive disease. Subgroup with significant left main lesions. *Circulation* 1976;54[Suppl 3]:III-107–III-117.

302. Dzavik V, Sleeper LA, Cocke JR, et al. Effect of age on treatment and outcome in patients with acute myocardial infarction complicated by cardiogenic shock: a report for the SHOCK Trial Registry. (Personal communication with Dr. Dzavik.)

303. Allen BS, Buckberg GD, Fontan FM, et al. Superiority of controlled surgical reperfusion versus percutaneous transluminal coronary angioplasty in acute coronary occlusion. *J Thorac Cardiovasc Surg* 1993;105:864.

304. White HD, Stewart JT, Aylward PEG, et al. Angioplasty versus surgery for cardiogenic shock: results from the SHOCK trial. *Circulation* 1999;18:370.

305. Lazar HL, Philippides G, Fitzgerald C, et al. Glucose-insulin-potassium solutions enhance recovery after urgent coronary artery bypass grafting. *J Thorac Cardiovasc Surg* 1997;113:354–360.

306. Gradinac S, Coleman GM, Taegtmeyer H, et al. Improved cardiac function with glucose-insulin-potassium after aorto-coronary bypass grafting. *Ann Thorac Surg* 1998;48:2227–2234.

307. Malmberg K, Ryden L, Efendic S, et al. Randomized trial of insulin-glucose infusion followed by subcutaneous insulin treatment in diabetic patients with acute myocardial infarction (DIGAMI study): effect on mortality at 1 year. *J Am Coll Cardiol* 1995;26:57–65.

308. Corbucci GG, Loche F. L-carnitine in cardiogenic shock therapy: pharmacodynamic aspects and clinical data. *Int J Clin Pharmacol Res* 1993;13:87–91.

309. Woods KL, Fletcher S, Roffe C, et al. Intravenous magnesium sulphate in suspected acute myocardial infarction: results of the second Leicester Intravenous Magnesium Intervention Trial (LIMIT-2). *Lancet* 1992;339:1553–1558.

310. Kloner RA. Does reperfusion injury exist in humans? *J Am Coll Cardiol* 1993;21:537–545.

311. Farrer-Brown G. Vascular pattern of myocardium or right ventricle of human heart. *Br Heart J* 1968;30:679–686.

312. Dell'Italia LJ, Lembo NJ, Starling MR, et al. Hemodynamically important right ventricular infarction: follow-up evaluation of right ventricular systolic function at rest and during exercise with radionuclide ventriculography and respiratory gas exchange. *Circulation* 1987;75:996.

313. Steele P, Kirch D, Ellis J, et al. Prompt return to normal of depressed right ventricular ejection fraction in acute inferior infarction. *Br Heart J* 1977;39:1319.

314. Setaro JF, Cabin HS. Right ventricular infarction. *Cardiol Clin* 1992;10:69–90.

315. Shiraki H, Yoshikawa T, Anzai T, et al. Association between preinfarction angina and a lower risk of right ventricular infarction. *N Engl J Med* 1998;338:941–947.

316. Jacobs AK, Leopold JA, Modur S, et al. Right ventricular infarction complicated by cardiogenic shock: observations and implications. The NHLBI SHOCK Registry. *J Am Coll Cardiol* 2000;873:385A.

317. Cohn JN, Guiha NH, Broder MI, et al. Right ventricular infarction. Clinical and hemodynamic features. *Am J Cardiol* 1974;33:209.

318. Cintron GB, Hernandez E, Linares E, et al. Bedside recognition, incidence, and clinical course of right ventricular infarction. *Am J Cardiol* 1981;47:224.

319. Baigre RS, Hag A, Morgan CD, et al. The spectrum of right ventricular involvement in inferior wall myocardial infarction: a clinical, hemodynamic, and noninvasive study. *J Am Coll Cardiol* 1983;1:1396.

320. Braat SH, de Zwann C, Brugada P, et al. Right ventricular involvement with acute inferior wall myocardial infarction identifies high risk of developing atrioventricular nodal conduction disturbances. *Am Heart J* 1984;107:1183–1187.

321. Kulbertus HE, Rigo P, Legrand V. Right ventricular infarction: pathophysiology, diagnosis, clinical course, and treatment. *Mod Concepts Cardiovasc Dis* 1985;54:1–5.

322. Love JC, Haffajee CI, Gore JM, et al. Reversibility of hypotension and shock by atrial or atrioventricular sequential pacing in patients with right ventricular infarction. *Am Heart J* 1984;108:5–13.

323. Rietveld AP, Merrman L, Essed CE, et al. Right-to-left shunt with severe hypoxemia at the atrial level in a patient with hemodynamically important right ventricular infarction. *J Am Coll Cardiol* 1983;2:776.

324. Manno BV, Bemis CE, Carver J, et al. Right ventricular infarction complicated by right-to-left shunt. *J Am Coll Cardiol* 1983;2:554.

325. Dell'Italia LJ, Starling MR, O'Rourke RA. Physical examination for exclusion of hemodynamically important right ventricular infarction. *Ann Intern Med* 1983;99:608.

326. Klein HO, Tordjman T, Ninio R, et al. The early recognition of right ventricular infarction: diagnostic accuracy of the electrocardiographic V4R lead. *Circulation* 1983;67:558.

327. Lopez-Sendon J, Coma-Canella I, Alcasena S, et al. Electrocardiographic findings in acute right ventricular infarc-

tion: sensitivity and specificity of electrocardiographic alterations in right precordial leads V4R, V3R, V1, V2 and V3. *J Am Coll Cardiol* 1984;6:1273.

328. Zehender M, Kasper W, Kauder E, et al. Right ventricular infarction as an independent predictor of prognosis after acute inferior myocardial infarction. *N Engl J Med* 1993;328:981–988.

329. Sharpe DN, Botvinick EH, Shames DM, et al. The noninvasive diagnosis of right ventricular infarction. *Circulation* 1978;57:483.

330. Dell'Italia LJ, Starling MR, Crawford MH, et al. Right ventricular infarction: Identification by hemodynamic measurements before and after volume loading and correlation with noninvasive techniques. *J Am Coll Cardiol* 1984;4:931–939.

331. Lloyd EA, Gersh BJ, Kennelly BM. Hemodynamic spectrum of "dominant" right ventricular infarction in 19 patients. *Am J Cardiol* 1981;48:1016.

332. Mehta SR, Eikelboom JW, Natarajan MK, et al. Impact of right ventricular involvement on mortality and morbidity in patients with inferior myocardial infarction. *J Am Coll Cardiol* 2001;27:37–43.

333. Bueno H, Lopez-Palop R, Perez-David E, et al. Combined effect of age and right ventricular involvement on acute inferior myocardial infarction prognosis. *Circulation* 1998;27:1714–1720.

334. Haines DE, Beller GA, Watson DD, et al. A prospective clinical, scintigraphic, angiographic, and functional evaluation of patients after inferior myocardial infarction with and without right ventricular dysfunction. *J Am Coll Cardiol* 1985;6:995.

335. Kagan A. Dynamic responses of the right ventricle following extensive damage by cauterization. *Circulation* 1952;5:816.

336. Donald DE, Essex HE. Pressure studies after inactivation of the major portion of the canine right ventricle. *Am J Physiol* 1954;176:155.

337. Guiha NH, Limas CJ, Cohn JN. Predominant right ventricular dysfunction after right ventricular destruction in the dog. *Am J Cardiol* 1974;33:254.

338. Goldstein JA, Tweddell JS, Barzilai B, et al. Importance of left ventricular function and systolic ventricular interaction to right ventricular performance during acute right heart ischemia. *J Am Coll Cardiol* 1992;19:704–711.

339. Goldstein JA, Vlahakes GJ, Verrier ED, et al. The role of right ventricular systolic dysfunction and elevated intrapericardiac pressure in the genesis of low output in experimental right ventricular infarction. *Circulation* 1982;65:513.

340. Sharkey SW, Shelley W, Carlyle PF, et al. M-mode and two-dimensional echocardiographic analysis of the septum in experimental right ventricular infarction: correlation with hemodynamic alterations. *Am Heart J* 1985;110:1210.

341. Dell'Italia LJ, Starling MR, Blumhardt R, et al. Comparative effects of volume loading, dobutamine, and nitroprusside in patients with predominant right ventricular infarction. *Circulation* 1985;72:1327.

342. Ferrario M, Poli A, Prvitali M, et al. Hemodynamics of volume loading compared with dobutamine in severe right ventricular infarction. *Am J Cardiol* 1994;74:329–333.

343. Siniorakis EE, Nikolaou NI, Sarantopoulos CD, et al. Volume loading in predominant right ventricular infarc-

tion: bedside haemodynamics using rapid response thermistors. *Eur Heart J* 1994;15:1340–1347.

344. Sclarovsky S, Zafrir N, Strasberg B, et al. Ventricular fibrillation complicating temporary ventricular pacing in acute myocardial infarction: significance of right ventricular infarction. *Am J Cardiol* 1981;48:1160–1166.

345. Iqbal MZ, Liebson PR. Counterpulsation and dobutamine: their use in treatment of cardiogenic shock due to right ventricular infarct. *Arch Intern Med* 1981;141:247–249.

346. Miller DC, Moreno-Cabral RJ, Stinson EB, et al. Pulmonary artery balloon counterpulsation for acute right ventricular failure. *J Thorac Cardiovasc Surg* 1980;80:760–763.

347. Moran JM, Opravil M, Gorman AF. Pulmonary artery balloon counterpulsation for right ventricular failure. II. Clinical experience. *Ann Thorac Surg* 1984;38:254.

348. Schuler G, Hofmann M, Schwarz F, et al. Effect of successful thrombolytic therapy on right ventricular function in acute inferior wall myocardial infarction. *Am J Cardiol* 1984;54:951–957.

349. Berger PB, Ruocco NA, Timm TC. The impact of thrombolytic therapy on right ventricular infarction complicating inferior myocardial infarction. Results from thrombolysis in myocardial infarction. II. *Circulation* 1989;80:II-313.

350. Moreyra AE, Suh C, Porway MN, et al. Rapid hemodynamic improvement in right ventricular infarction after coronary angioplasty. *Chest* 1988;94:197–199.

351. Bowers TR, O'Neill WW, Grene C, et al. Effect of reperfusion on ventricular function and survival after right ventricular infarction. *N Engl J Med* 1998;338:933–940.

352. Saffitz JE, Fredrickson RC, Roberts WC. Relation of size of transmural acute myocardial infarct to mode of death: interval between infarction and death in frequency of coronary arterial thrombus. *Am J Cardiol* 1986;112:1088–1090.

353. Becker AE, van Mantgem JP. Cardiac tamponade: a study of 50 hearts. *Eur J Cardiol* 1975;15:349–358.

354. Becker R, Charlesworth A, Wilcox R, et al. Cardiac rupture associated with thrombolytic therapy: impact of time to treatment in the Late Assessment of Thrombolytic Efficacy (LATE) study. *J Am Coll Cardiol* 1995;25:1063–1068.

355. Peuhkurinen KJ, Risteli L, Melkko JT, et al. Thrombolytic therapy with streptokinase stimulates collagen breakdown. *Circulation* 1991;83:1969–1975.

356. Schuster EH, Bulkley BH. Expansion of transmural myocardial infarction: a pathophysiologic factor in cardiac rupture. *Circulation* 1979;60:1532–1538.

357. Becker RC, Gore JM, Lambrew C, et al. A composite view of cardiac rupture in the United States National Registry of Myocardial Infarction. *J Am Coll Cardiol* 1996;27:1321–1326.

358. Oliva PB, Hammill SC, Edwards WD. Cardiac rupture, a clinically predictable complication of acute myocardial infarction: report of 70 cases with clinicopathological correlations. *J Am Coll Cardiol* 1993;22:720–726.

359. Becker RC, Hochman JS, Cannon CP, et al. Fatal cardiac rupture among patients treated with thrombolytic agents and adjunctive thrombin antagonists: observations from

the Thrombolysis and Thrombin Inhibitions in Myocardial Infarction 9 Study. *J Am Coll Cardiol* 1999;2:479–487.

360. Lopez-Sendon J, Gonzales A, Lopez de Sa E, et al. Diagnosis of subacute ventricular wall rupture after acute myocardial infarction: sensitivity and specificity of clinical, hemodynamic, and echocardiographic criteria. *J Am Coll Cardiol* 1992;19:1145–1153.

361. Park WM, Connery CP, Hochman JS, et al. Successful repair of myocardial free wall rupture after thrombolytic therapy for acute infarction. *Ann Thorac Surg* 2000;70:1345–1349.

362. Wei JY, Hutchins GM, Bulkley BH. Papillary muscle rupture in fatal acute myocardial infarction: a potentially treatable form of cardiogenic shock. *Ann Intern Med* 1979;90:149–152.

363. Voci P, Bilotta F, Caretta Q, et al. Papillary muscle perfusion pattern: a hypothesis for ischemic papillary muscle dysfunction. *Circulation* 1995;91:1714–1718.

364. Nishimura RA, Scaff HV, Gersh BJ, et al. Early repair of mechanical complications after acute myocardial infarction. *JAMA* 1986;256:47–50.

365. Burch GE, DePasquale NP, Phillips SH. The syndrome of papillary muscle dysfunction. *Am Heart J* 1968;75:399–415.

366. Kono T, Sabbah HN, Stein PD, et al. Left ventricular shape as a determinant of functional mitral regurgitation in patients with severe heart failure secondary to either coronary artery disease or idiopathic dilated cardiomyopathy. *Am J Cardiol* 1991;68:355–359.

367. Barzilai B, Gessler C, Perez JE, et al. Significance of Doppler-detected mitral regurgitation in acute myocardial infarction. *Am J Cardiol* 1988;61:220–223.

368. Lehmann KG, Francis CK, Dodge HT, et al. Mitral regurgitation in early myocardial infarction: incidence, clinical detection, and prognostic implications. TIMI Study Group. *Ann Intern Med* 1992;117:10–17.

369. Tcheng JE, Jackman JD, Nelson CL, et al. Outcome of patients sustaining acute ischemic mitral regurgitation during myocardial infarction. *Ann Intern Med* 1992;117:18–24.

370. Perloff JK, Roberts WC. The mitral apparatus. *Circulation* 1997;46:227–239.

371. Thompson CR, Christopher BE, Sleeper LA, et al. Cardiogenic shock due to acute severe mitral regurgitation complicating acute myocardial infarction: a report for the SHOCK Trial Registry. *J Am Coll Cardiol* 2000;36:1104–1109.

372. Nishimura RA, Shub C, Tajik AJ. Two-dimensional echocardiographic diagnosis of partial papillary muscle rupture. *Br Heart J* 1982;48:598–600.

373. Moursi MH, Bhatnagar SK, Vilacosta I, et al. Transesophageal echocardiographic assessment of papillary muscle rupture. *Circulation* 1996;94:1003–1009.

374. Fuchs RM, Heuser RR, Yin FCP, et al. Limitations of pulmonary wedge V waves in diagnosing mitral regurgitation. *Am J Cardiol* 1982;49:849–854.

375. Giuliani ER, Danielson GK, Pluth JR, et al. Postinfarction ventricular septal rupture: surgical considerations and results. *Circulation* 1974;49:455–459.

376. Kishon Y, Oh JK, Schaff HV, et al. Mitral valve operation in post infarction rupture of a papillary muscle: immediate results and long-term follow-up of 22 patients. *Mayo Clin Proc* 1992;67:1023–1030.

377. Hutchins GM. Rupture of the interventricular septum complicating myocardial infarction: pathological analysis of 10 patients with clinically diagnosed perforations. *Am Heart J* 1979;97:165–173.

378. Gershaw BS, Granger CB, Bunbaum Y, et al. Risk factors, angiographic patterns and outcomes in patients with ventricular septal defect complicating acute myocardial infarction. GUSTO I Investigators. *Circulation* 2000;101:27–32.

379. Menon V, Webb JG, Hillis D, et al. Outcome and profile of ventricular septal rupture with cardiogenic shock after myocardial infarction: a report from the SHOCK Registry. *J Am Coll Cardiol* 2000;36:1110–1117.

380. Radford MJ, Johnson RA, Daggett WM Jr, et al. Ventricular septal rupture: a review of clinical and physiological features and an analysis of survival. *Circulation* 1981;64:545–553.

381. Edwards BS, Edwards WD, Edwards JE. Ventricular septal rupture complicating acute myocardial infarction: identification of simple and complex types in 53 autopsied hearts. *Am J Cardiol* 1984;54:1201–1205.

382. Parry G, Goudevenos J, Adams PC, et al. Septal rupture after myocardial infarction: Is very early surgery really worthwhile? *Eur Heart J* 1992;13:373–382.

383. Daggett WM, Guyton RA, Mundth ED. Surgery for postmyocardial infarct ventricular septal defect. *Ann Surg* 1977;186:260–271.

384. Cummings RG, Reimer KA, Califf R, et al. Quantitative analysis of right and left ventricular infarction in the presence of postinfarction ventricular septal defect. *Circulation* 1988;77:33–42.

385. Giuliani ER, Danielson GK, Pluth JR, et al. Postinfarction ventricular septal rupture. Surgical considerations and results. *Circulation* 1974;49:455–459.

386. Gaudiani VA, Miller DG, Stinson EB, et al. Postinfarction ventricular septal defect: an argument for early operation. *Surgery* 1981;89:43–55.

387. Moore CA, Nygard TW, Kaser DI, et al. Postinfarction ventricular septal rupture: the importance of location of infarction and right ventricular function in determining survival. *Circulation* 1986;74:45–55.

388. Davies RH, Dawkins KD, Skillington PD, et al. Late functional results after surgical closure of acquired ventricular septal defect. *J Thorac Cardiovasc Surg* 1993;106:592–598.

389. Muehrcke DD, Blank S, Daggett WM. Survival after repair of postinfarction ventricular septal defects in patients over the age of 70. *J Cardiac Surg* 1992;7:290–300.

390. Held AC, Cole PL, Lipton B, et al. Rupture of the interventricular septum complicating acute myocardial infarction: a multicenter analysis of clinical findings and outcome. *Am Heart J* 1988;116:1330–1336.

391. Cox FF, Plokker HWM, Morshuis WJ, et al. Importance of coronary revascularization for late survival after postinfarction ventricular septal rupture. *Eur Heart J* 1996;17:1841–1845.

392. David TE, Dale L, Sun Z. Postinfarction ventricular septal rupture. Repair by endocardial patch with infarct exclusion. *J Thorac Cardiovasc Surg* 1995;110:1315–1322.

393. Lemery R, Smith HC, Giuliani ER, et al. Prognosis in rupture of the ventricular septum after acute myocardial infarction and role of early surgical intervention. *Am J Cardiol* 1992;70:147–151.

394. Fananapazir L, Bray CL, Dark JF, et al. Right ventricular dysfunction and surgical outcome in postinfarction ventricular septal defect. *Eur Heart J* 1983;4:155–167.

395. Keenan DJ, Monro JL, Ross JK, et al. Acquired ventricular septal defect. *J Thorac Cardiovasc Surg* 1983;85:116–119.

396. Krainin FM, Flessas AP, Spodick DH. Infarction-associated pericarditis: rarity of diagnostic electrocardiogram. *N Engl J Med* 1984;311:1211–1214.

397. Oliva PB, Hammill SC, Talano JV. Effect of definition on incidence of postinfarction pericarditis: is it time to redefine postinfarction pericarditis? *Circulation* 1994;90:1537–1541.

398. Widimsky P, Gregor P. Pericardial involvement during the course of myocardial infarction: a long-term clinical and echocardiographic study. *Chest* 1995;108:89–93.

399. Tofler GH, Muller JE, Stone PH, et al. Pericarditis in acute myocardial infarction: characterization and clinical significance. *Am Heart J* 1989;117:86–92.

400. Van de Werf F, for the investigators of the European Cooperative Study Group for recombinant tissue-type plasminogen activation. Lessons from the European Cooperative Recombinant Tissue-Type Plasminogen Activator (rt-PA) versus Placebo Trial. *J Am Coll Cardiol* 1988;12:14A–19A.

401. Wall TC, Califf RM, Harrelson-Woodlief L, et al. Usefulness of a pericardial friction rub after thrombolytic therapy during acute myocardial infarction in predicting amount of myocardial damage. *Am J Cardiol* 1990;66:1418–1421.

402. Musselman DR, Dehmer GJ, Hoffman BJ Jr, et al. Localized right atrial tamponade and right-to-left shunting as a complication of pericarditis after myocardial infarction. *Am Heart J* 1993;125:241–242.

403. Renkin J, DeBruyne B, Benit E, et al. Cardiac tamponade early after thrombolysis for acute myocardial infarction: a rare but not reported hemorrhagic complication. *J Am Coll Cardiol* 1991;17:280–285.

404. Khan AH. The postcardiac injury syndromes. *Clin Cardiol* 1992;15:67–72.

405. Shahar A, Hod H, Barabash GM, et al. Disappearance of a syndrome: Dressler's syndrome in the era of thrombolysis. *Cardiology* 1994;85:255–258.

406. Berman J, Haffajee CI, Alpert JS. Therapy of symptomatic pericarditis after myocardial infarction: retrospective and prospective studies of aspirin, indomethacin, prednisone, and spontaneous resolution. *Am Heart J* 1981;101:750–753.

407. The Global Use of Strategies to Open Occluded Coronary Arteries (GUSTO III) Investigators. A comparison of reteplase with alteplase for acute myocardial infarction. *N Engl J Med* 1997;337:1118–1123.

408. Single-bolus tenecteplase compared with front-loaded alteplase in acute myocardial infarction: the ASSENT-2 double-blind randomized trial. *Lancet* 1999;354:716–722.

409. Antman EM, Guigliano RP, Gibson CM, et al. for the TIMI 14 Investigators. Abciximab facilitates the rate and extent of thrombolysis. Results of the Thrombolysis in Myocardial Infarction (TIMI) 14 trial. *Circulation* 1999;99:2720–2732.

410. Strategies for Patency Enhancement in the Emergency Department (SPEED) Group. Trial of abciximab with and without low-dose reteplase for acute myocardial infarction. *Circulation* 2000;101:2988–2994.

411. Brener SJ, Adgey JA, Zeymer U, et al. Combination low-dose T-PA and eptifibatide for acute myocardial infarction—final results of the INTRO-AMI Study. *Circulation* 2000;102:II-599.

412. Zahn R, Schiele R, Schneider S, et al. Pooled data of the Maximal Individual Therapy in Acute myocardial infarction (MITRA) Registry and the Myocardial Infarction Registry (MIR). *J Am Coll Cardiol* 2000;36:2064–2071.

413. Tiefenbrunn AJ, Chandra NC, French WJ, et al. Clinical experience with primary percutaneous transluminal coronary angioplasty compared with alteplase (Recombinant tissue-type plasminogen activator) in patients with acute myocardial infarction. A report from the second National Registry of Myocardial Infarction (NRMI-2). *J Am Coll Cardiol* 1998;31:1240–1245.

414. Rogers WJ, Canto JG, Lambrew CT, et al. Temporal trends in the treatment of over 1.5 million patients with myocardial infarction in the U.S. from 1990 through 1999: The National Registry of Myocardial Infarction. *J Am Coll Cardiol* 2000;36:2056–2063.

415. Gottlieb S, Harpaz D, Shotan A, et al. Sex differences in management and outcome after acute myocardial infarction in the 1990's—a prospective observational community based study. *Circulation* 2000;102:2484–2490.

416. Yusuf S, Zhao F, Mehta SR, et al. Effects of clopidogrel in addition to aspirin in patients with acute coronary syndromes without ST-segment elevation. *N Engl J Med* 2001;345:494–502.

20

POST–MYOCARDIAL INFARCTION MANAGEMENT

DEEPAK L. BHATT
ERIC J. TOPOL

OVERVIEW

The management of acute ST-segment elevation myocardial infarction (MI) has been revolutionized in the past decade. Advances in pharmacologic and mechanical reperfusion therapy have improved the survival of patients who experience MI. As more patients survive the initial myocardial insult, subsequent medical care has increased in importance. An appreciation of pathologic left ventricular

remodeling after MI has permitted the study of medications that preserve left ventricular function. The role of plaque stabilization with lipid-lowering therapy has been established. The use of antiplatelet therapy to prevent recurrent atherothrombotic events continues to grow. Appropriate control of risk factors such as diabetes and hypertension remains prominent. Additionally, inflammation has been identified as having a significant role in the pathogenesis of ischemic events. Controversy over noninvasive risk-stratification versus the need for invasive assessment continues, although the pendulum seems to be swinging toward aggressive management. Despite impressive technological advances, lifestyle modification remains a key component of secondary prevention after MI.

D. L. Bhatt: Department of Cardiovascular Medicine, The Cleveland Clinic Foundation, Cleveland, Ohio
E. J. Topol: Department of Cardiovascular Medicine, The Cleveland Clinic Foundation, Cleveland, Ohio

GLOSSARY

Acute coronary syndrome: Plaque rupture leading to various degrees of coronary artery thrombosis. Most often refers to unstable angina and non–Q-wave myocardial infarction, although sometimes meant also to include ST-segment elevation myocardial infarction.

Non–Q-wave myocardial infarction: Older nomenclature for myocardial infarction believed to be caused by nonocclusive coronary arterial thrombus. Now often referred to as *non–ST-segment elevation myocardial infarction.*

Q-wave myocardial infarction: Older term for myocardial infarction meant to imply transmural myocardial necrosis.

Remodeling: The process of left ventricular cellular and geometric adaptation to compensate for damage sustained during myocardial infarction.

ST-segment elevation myocardial infarction: Myocardial infarction resulting from coronary arterial occlusion by thrombus, manifested on the surface electrocardiogram as ST-segment elevation.

GENERAL PRINCIPLES

Historical Perspective

Because of the use of fibrinolytic therapy and, in communities where it is available, primary percutaneous intervention, the past decade has seen dramatic decreases in deaths resulting from MI. However, in the recent Global Utilization of Streptokinase and t-PA for Occluded Coronary Arteries III (GUSTO III) trial of acute MI, in which two different fibrinolytic regimens were tested, the 1-year mortality rate was still 11% (1). In fact, the additional 4% mortality rate observed in GUSTO III between 30 days and 1 year was quite high, illustrating the importance of initiating secondary preventive efforts during a patient's hospitalization for acute MI. Outside the context of clinical trials, mortality rates are even higher, with a 9.4% in-hospital mortality rate seen in the National Registry of Myocardial Infarction (NRMI) in 1999 (2). Therefore, despite improved therapies for acute MI, risk-stratification and secondary prevention are still critically important in improving the outcomes of patients with acute MI by decreasing the likelihood of recurrent ischemic events, in both the short term and the long term.

Pathophysiology

An appreciation of the pathophysiology of acute MI is necessary to understand how specific therapies may be used to target different components of the cascade of events that lead to acute MI. Plaque rupture, arterial thrombosis, myocardial necrosis, and adverse left ventricular remodeling are part of the continuum that leads to symptomatic manifestations and long-term sequelae of acute MI.

Plaque Rupture and Thrombosis

The inciting event of acute MI is plaque rupture. Numerous factors, which are only partially understood, determine the occurrence of plaque rupture in a susceptible individual. Production of matrix metalloproteinases leads to degradation of the shoulder of a coronary plaque, leading to exposure of its lipid-rich core to flowing blood (3–5). This triggers formation of platelet-rich thrombus. When the degree of thrombus is flow-occlusive, ischemia occurs, and myocardial stunning and necrosis follow.

The 3-hydroxy-3-methylglutaryl coenzyme A (HMG-CoA) reductase inhibitors (statins) may exert part of their benefit by decreasing the lipid content of plaques, making them less prone to rupture (6,7). Antithrombotic therapy decreases the tendency for occlusive thrombus formation. Antiplatelet therapy, in particular, decreases platelet aggregation at the site of ruptured plaque. Thus, in concert, statin therapy and antiplatelet therapy decrease the chance of MI occurring.

Left Ventricular Remodeling

When occlusive thrombus has developed and caused ischemia for several hours, myocardium is damaged. When this necrosis is transmural, the left ventricle may undergo a process of remodeling. This adaptation occurs at both the cellular level and the whole-organ level (8). Angiotensin-converting enzyme (ACE) inhibitors greatly decrease this process of adverse remodeling. This explains, at least in part, the marked benefits ACE inhibition has on patients who have ventricular dysfunction after MI.

Arrhythmogenic Substrate

The zone of myocardium surrounding the infarcted area is particularly prone to electrical instability. This often manifests as premature ventricular contractions (PVCs) and predisposes the patient to ventricular arrhythmia. Beta-blockers are useful in reducing the electrical irritability of the damaged myocardium, as is amiodarone. Implantable cardioverter-defibrillators (ICDs) are the last line of defense in treating electrical excitability that causes potentially lethal arrhythmia.

Open-Artery Hypothesis

Even if the left ventricular muscle supplied by an occluded artery is dead, revascularization may still favorably effect ventricular remodeling and promote electrical stability. Depending on the duration of ischemia, among other factors, the myocardial cells either die or go into a state of hibernation. In this latter stage, revascularization can restore contractile functionality to what otherwise appears to be dead myocardium. Thus, there are a number of reasons, both established and theoretical, why vessel patency can improve prognosis (Fig. 20.1) (9).

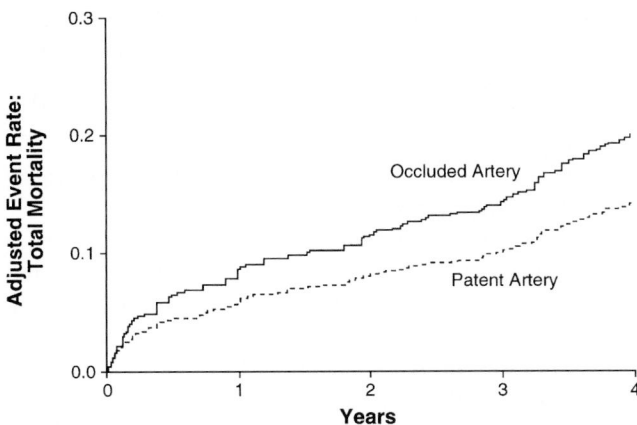

FIGURE 20.1 An occluded coronary artery is associated with a much lower survival rate, as illustrated by these data from the Survival and Ventricular Enlargement (SAVE) Trial, which provides indirect evidence supporting the "open-artery hypothesis." (From Lamas GA, Flaker GC, Mitchell G, et al. Effect of infarct artery patency on prognosis after acute myocardial infarction. The Survival and Ventricular Enlargement Investigators. *Circulation* 1995;92:1101–1109, with permission.)

CLINICAL MANAGEMENT

Exercise stress testing, noninvasive imaging, and coronary angiography are all used to risk-stratify patients and determine their subsequent management. Risk-stratification models may help determine the most appropriate in-hospital and long-term management of patients with acute MI (10).

Assessment of Left Ventricular Function and Reperfusion

Echocardiography has assumed a large role in the management of the condition of patients who have experienced an acute MI. In addition to its role in determining the presence of mechanical complications of MI, echocardiography is able to provide an estimate of left ventricular systolic and diastolic function. Indeed, at least on a population level, the left ventricular ejection fraction has been shown to be a powerful predictor of outcome (Fig. 20.2) (11).

Contrast echocardiography may, additionally, allow an assessment of whether successful tissue-level reperfusion has occurred (12,13). In conjunction with ST-segment resolution, important insights may be gained by gauging reperfusion with contrast echocardiography (14). Magnetic resonance imaging appears to be even more sensitive than contrast echocardiography in detection of microvascular obstruction (15). The *in vivo* study of microvascular function is not an arcane exercise in physiology, but rather adds important prognostic ability to more conventional determinants of infarct size (16). These newer modalities will refine assessment of left ventricular function so that an evaluation of microvascular integrity will become part of analyzing the

state of the infarcted myocardium, at both a whole-organ and a cellular level.

Stress Testing

The role of stress testing in the management of patients after MI has been extensively studied. The value of exercise stress testing depends greatly on whether the patient has undergone revascularization (17). Guidelines have been developed to aid in the appropriate use of stress testing (18). As a practical point, based on data from the NRMI, predischarge stress testing currently is performed in fewer than 10% of American patients, with the majority undergoing in-hospital revascularization or outpatient stress testing (2).

Certain features on a stress test identify patients at high risk of recurrent ischemic events. Left ventricular dilatation, pulmonary uptake of thallium-201, ejection fraction less than 40%, and reversible defects in the territory of the infarction are all markers of high risk on postexercise nuclear imaging scans. Additionally, large fixed defects and multivessel disease considerably raise the risk profile of the patient. Normal or low-risk results of a dipyridamole stress test predict an annual rate of death, MI, or urgent revascularization of less than 2%.

The Danish Trial in Acute Myocardial Infarction (DAN-AMI) randomly assigned 1,008 patients who had received fibrinolysis for MI and had inducible ischemia on stress testing to receive either invasive or conservative treatment (19). Those patients assigned to the invasive arm had a statistically significant reduction in the primary end points of death, MI, or readmission for unstable angina. The authors

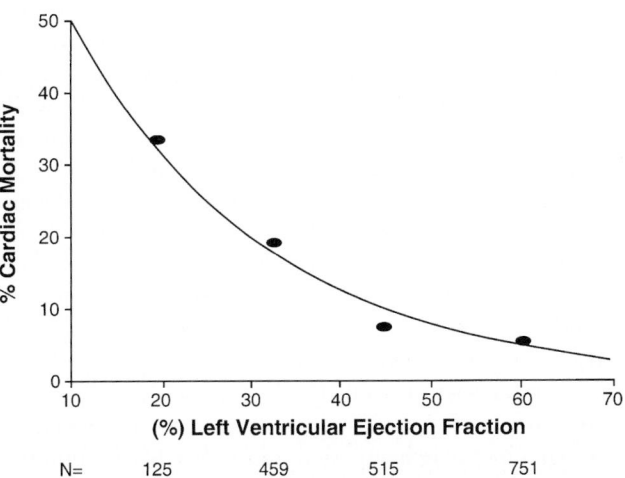

FIGURE 20.2 Diminished left ventricular ejection fraction after myocardial infarction is a powerful predictor of death after myocardial infarction. (From Gottlieb S, Moss AJ, McDermott M, et al. Interrelation of left ventricular ejection fraction, pulmonary congestion and outcome in acute myocardial infarction. *Am J Cardiol* 1992;69:977–984, with permission.)

appropriately concluded that patients who have inducible ischemia detected before discharge should undergo coronary angiography.

Exercise stress testing can provide valuable information, primarily because the inability to exercise confers a poor prognosis (20,21). Although rare, myocardial rupture is possible during exercise stress testing or dobutamine stress testing in the post-MI period (22). As an alternative to submaximal exercise stress testing before hospital discharge, pharmacologic stress testing with dipyridamole 2 to 4 days after MI may be performed safely (23). In fact, dipyridamole stress testing outperformed submaximal exercise testing with nuclear imaging in its ability to predict postdischarge cardiac events (23). Therefore, if predischarge stress testing instead of invasive evaluation is the approach, dipyridamole stress testing may be the noninvasive test of choice.

Coronary Angiography

As noted, the DANAMI study showed that patients with inducible ischemia after acute MI had better outcomes if they were treated with an invasive strategy as opposed to a conservative one (19). Revascularization, either percutaneously or surgically, was found to be beneficial. An analysis of the patients from the DANAMI study who underwent coronary artery bypass grafting (CABG) was performed (24). The median time to CABG after acute MI was approximately 6 weeks. Patients who had inducible ischemia, including silent ischemia, after acute MI benefited from CABG.

Similarly, spontaneous ischemia in the form of post-infarction angina is a serious development that warrants invasive investigation. The Gruppo Italiano per lo Studio della Sopravvivenza nell'Infarto Miocardico 3 (GISSI-3) trial prospectively analyzed patients with early angina after MI who were managed conservatively (25). Patients with post-MI angina suffered a higher rate of in-hospital reinfarction. Although the condition of many patients who developed post-MI angina was successfully controlled medically while the patient was in the hospital, these patients nevertheless had a higher rate of death or reinfarction at 6 months. In fact, the presence of early post-MI angina was an independent predictor of the 6-month rate of reinfarction or death. In patients with early angina, the rate of reinfarction was 12%, versus 5% in patients without early angina (*p* <.0001). The rate of death was also higher in patients with early angina than in those without early angina (13% vs. 7%, respectively; *p* <.0001). The presence of post-MI angina is a strong indication for coronary arteriography. Angiography for ischemic symptoms after MI is appropriately given a class I indication in the American College of Cardiology/American Heart Association guidelines for coronary arteriography (26).

Indirect evidence from comparative studies favors an invasive approach to treatment of MI. Compared with Canadian patients, American patients are more likely to undergo catheterization and angioplasty. This difference in approach appears to lead to better outcomes in American patients (27). A study comparing outcomes after MI in areas in France and Spain with different rates of angiography reached a similar conclusion regarding the superiority of an invasive approach (28).

However, older, randomized studies such as the Treatment of Post-Thrombolytic Stenoses (TOPS) trial do not favor routine angiography after successful fibrinolysis, even when angiography demonstrates a "significant" stenosis (29). The Should We Intervene following Thrombolysis (SWIFT) trial did not find a benefit for routine angiography after fibrinolysis either (30). Likewise, the Thrombolysis in Myocardial Infarction (TIMI) II-B and European Cooperative Study Group (ECSG) trials were unable to demonstrate an advantage to a routine invasive approach (31,32). The Thrombolysis and Angioplasty in Myocardial Infarction (TAMI) study found no advantage to immediate angioplasty after fibrinolysis in comparison with delayed angioplasty 5 to 10 days later (33). Perhaps the prothrombotic effects at the site of ruptured plaque that systemic fibrinolysis can create, coupled with further arterial trauma from balloon angioplasty, led to lack of favorable outcomes with invasive therapy (34). Therefore, the results of these trials may no longer apply in an era marked by greater use of stents and intravenous glycoprotein IIb/IIIa inhibition, but this issue needs to be examined prospectively (35). Nevertheless, in patients who appear to have successfully reperfused after fibrinolysis, or those who have received no reperfusion therapy acutely, it is still reasonable to use noninvasive risk-stratification before invasive therapy, with its attendant risk. An algorithm for risk-stratification is shown in Figure 20.3. ☛ d70

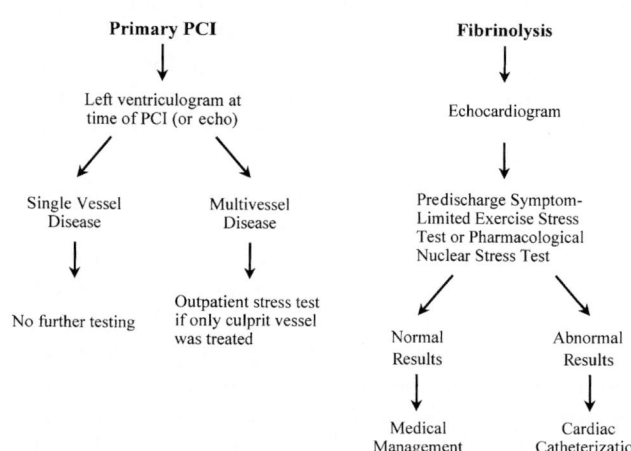

FIGURE 20.3 Risk assessment algorithm for the post–myocardial infarction patient, depending on the primary mode of reperfusion. echo, echocardiogram; PCI, percutaneous coronary intervention.

Assessment of Inflammatory Activity

Although an assessment of myocardial necrosis and microvascular obstruction is useful, measures of heightened inflammation, such as an elevated C-reactive protein (CRP) level, may provide additional ability to risk-stratify patients. The value of CRP levels was examined in a study of 64 patients with an uncomplicated MI (39). All patients had normal left ventricular function with no evidence of ischemia on a predischarge ergometer test. Interestingly, with each successive increase in quartile of CRP, the risk of cardiac death, recurrent MI, or new-onset angina in the ensuing year increased (Fig. 20.4). Even cruder indices of inflammation, such as the white blood cell (WBC) count, appear to help risk-stratify patients (40). A study of 975 patients with acute MI found that those who had angiographic thrombus were more likely to have an elevated WBC count, perhaps illustrating the interplay between inflammation and thrombosis (40). Furthermore, increasing elevation in levels of WBCs were associated with higher rates of death.

Beyond their role in risk-stratification, markers of inflammation may help gauge the incremental benefit of invasive therapy, in a manner complementary to troponin elevation. This paradigm has been shown to be true for non–ST-segment elevation acute coronary syndromes in two separate analyses, the results of which may apply to the acute MI setting also. In an analysis of almost 12,000 patients with acute coronary syndromes, an elevated WBC count correlated with 6-month mortality (177). However, in those patients undergoing in-hospital revascularization, the deleterious effect of an elevated WBC count were substantially lessened (177). Similarly, in FRISC-II, an invasive strategy (compared with a conservative approach) was seen

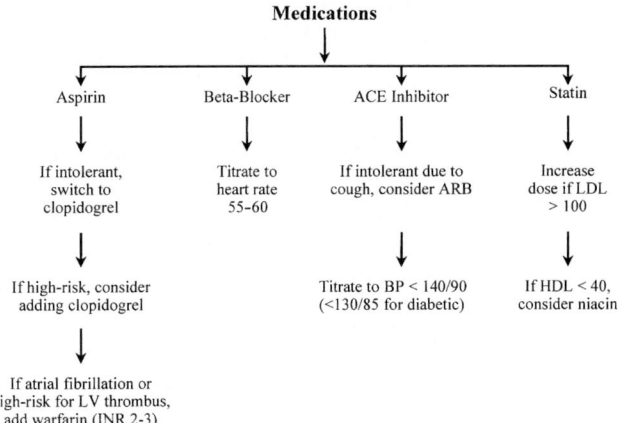

FIGURE 20.5 Flow chart for appropriate medications in patients after myocardial infarction. If left ventricular (LV) dysfunction is not present, it is not clear whether both beta-blockers and angiotensin-converting enzyme (ACE) inhibitors are necessary. ARB, angiotensin-receptor blocker; BP, blood pressure; HDL, high-density lipoprotein; INR, international normalized ratio; LDL, low-density lipoprotein.

to be of particular benefit in patients with elevated CRP, troponin T, or interleukin-6 levels (41).

MEDICAL THERAPY

Several classes of medications designed to improve outcomes after acute MI have undergone rigorous evaluation in large, randomized, controlled trials. It is imperative that physicians screen post-MI patients for criteria that indicate that specific medications should be prescribed (Fig. 20.5).

Afterload Reduction

Angiotensin-Converting Enzyme Inhibitors

Use of ACE inhibitors after acute MI is supported by a vast amount of evidence (Table 20.1) (54–56). The Acute Infarction Ramipril Efficacy study found that ramipril decreased mortality rates after MI among patients with heart failure (57). The Survival and Ventricular Enlargement trial demonstrated the significant benefit, with regard to mortality rates, of administration of captopril after MI among patients with asymptomatic left ventricular dysfunction as well (58). The Trandolapril Cardiac Evaluation study showed that the benefit of ACE inhibition persisted through 2 years of therapy, suggesting that ACE inhibition should be continued indefinitely (59). In fact, the results of the Heart Outcomes Prevention Evaluation (HOPE) study suggest that ACE inhibitors may be indicated in all patients who have had an MI (60).

Early initiation of oral ACE inhibitors is recommended for these patients, unless hypotension is present (61–63). However, the data do not support the early administration

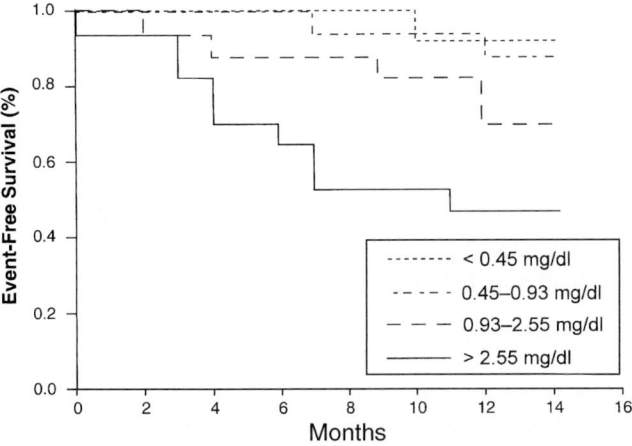

FIGURE 20.4 Even in patients who have an uncomplicated myocardial infarction, the risk of subsequent cardiac events increases with each successive quartile elevation of the C-reactive protein level. (From Tommasi S, Carluccio E, Bentivoglio M, et al. C-reactive protein as a marker for cardiac ischemic events in the year after a first, uncomplicated myocardial infarction. *Am J Cardiol* 1999;83:1595–1599, with permission.)

TABLE 20.1 LARGE TRIALS OF THE USE OF ANGIOTENSIN-CONVERTING ENZYME (ACE) INHIBITORS AFTER ACUTE MYOCARDIAL INFARCTION, DEMONSTRATING MORTALITY RATES FOR PLACEBO AND ACE INHIBITOR ARMS

Study	ACE inhibitor	No. of patients	Length of follow-up	Mortality rates (%)	
				Placebo	ACE inhibitor
AIRE (57)	Ramipril	2,006	15 mo	22.4	16.8
CCS-1 (61)	Captopril	13,634	4 wk	9.6	9.1
CONSENSUS II (64)	Enalapril	6,090	6 mo	10.2	11.0
GISSI-3 (54)	Lisinopril	18,895	6 wk	7.1	6.3
ISIS-4 (55)	Captopril	58,050	5 wk	7.7	7.2
SAVE (58)	Captopril	2,231	42 mo	24.6	20.4
SMILE (293)	Zofenopril	1,556	1 yr	14.1	10.0
TRACE (294)	Trandolapril	1,749	24–50 mo	42.3	34.7

AIRE, Acute Infarction Ramipril Efficacy Study; CCS-1, Chinese Cardiac Study; CONSENSUS II, Cooperative New Scandinavian Enalapril Survival Study II; GISSI-3, Gruppo Italiano per lo Studio della Sopravvivenza nell'Infarto Miocardico 3; ISIS-4, Fourth International Study of Infarct Survival; SAVE, Survival and Ventricular Enlargement Trial; SMILE, Survival of Myocardial Infarction Long-Term Evaluation Study; TRACE, Trandolapril Cardiac Evaluation Study.

of intravenous ACE inhibitors (64). The early benefit of ACE inhibition on minimizing left ventricular dilatation is most marked when reperfusion has not occurred, but other beneficial effects of ACE inhibitors likely apply to all patients (65). Despite all these favorable data, ACE inhibitors are underprescribed after acute MI (66). Unless systolic blood pressure is <100 mm Hg, ACE inhibition should generally be initiated within 24 hours of acute MI (63).

Beta-Blockers

The role of beta-blockers in patients who have experienced MI is well established (Table 20.2) (68). Beneficial effects result from decreases in heart rate, blood pressure, myocardial oxygen demand, and arrhythmogenesis (69). Newer evidence suggests a favorable influence on left ventricular remodeling as well (70). The Beta-Blocker Heart Attack Trial (BHAT) demonstrated that propranolol safely decreased cardiac mortality, sudden death, and all-cause mortality rates (71). Furthermore, side effects caused by propranolol that prompted drug discontinuation were relatively infrequent. The BHAT investigators recommended continuation of therapy for at least 3 years. In aggregate, the data suggest that beta-blockade reduces nonfatal MI by approximately 25%, which is paralleled by a 25% reduction in the mortality rate (72). Although these data were gathered largely before the fibrinolytic era, TIMI II-B found that even in patients who have received fibrinolysis, compared with later administration of beta-blockers, early beta-blockade reduced recurrent chest pain and reinfarction (73). Furthermore, early beta-blockade appears to reduce the incidence of intracranial hemorrhage after fibrinolysis, as well as the incidence of reinfarction (74).

Beta-blockers remain underused after MI, sometimes because of unfounded concerns regarding relative contraindications such as diabetes or chronic obstructive pulmonary disease (75–77). Beta-blockers have a similar relative benefit

in the presence and in the absence of heart failure, although the absolute benefit is magnified in those with heart failure (78). Underuse is a problem particularly among elderly patients (79,80). Numerous studies have confirmed that use of beta-blockade is safe in elderly patients and in diabetic patients (81). The optimal dose of beta-blockade, particularly in elderly patients, is not known, but doses lower than those that were used in several of the early randomized trials may be just as effective (82,83). If all eligible patients received beta-blockers after MI, thousands of recurrent MIs and deaths could be averted.

The limited available evidence suggests that beta-blockade and ACE inhibition are complementary (84–89). In patients who experience congestive heart failure after MI, both classes of medication seem to be indicated. At the other end of the spectrum, in patients with normal left ventricular function, perhaps only one of these classes of medication is needed. Without prospective data examining the incremental value of combination therapy, other patient factors, such as history of arrhythmia or diabetes, should also be considered in deciding which of these agents to use.

3-Hydroxy-3-Methylglutaryl Coenzyme A Reductase Inhibitors

Statins are strongly indicated for use as secondary prevention after acute MI. The Cholesterol and Recurrent Events (CARE) trial demonstrated that pravastatin, compared with placebo, reduced the rate of death or MI in patients with previous MI (107). In addition to beneficial effects on reinfarction, the CARE study showed that statin use decreases the risk of stroke in survivors of acute MI (108,109). Several other trials have validated the role of statins in secondary, and even primary, prevention (110). Whether there are benefits specific to one statin or whether

TABLE 20.2 EVENT RATES FOR SELECTED LARGE TRIALS OF THE USE OF BETA-BLOCKERS VERSUS PLACEBO AFTER ACUTE MYOCARDIAL INFARCTION

Study	Beta-blocker	No. of patients	Length of follow-up	End point	Event rate (%) Placebo	Event rate (%) Beta-blocker
BHAT (295)	Propranolol	3,837	24 mo	Death	9.8	7.2
Goteborg Trial (296)	Metoprolol	1,395	3 mo	Death	8.9	5.7
ISIS-1 (297)	Atenolol	16,027	7 d	Vascular death	4.6	3.9
MIAMI (298)	Metoprolol	5,778	15 d	Death	4.9	4.3
Norwegian Multicenter Study (69,299)	Timolol	1,884	7 yr	Death	32.3	26.4
TIMI II-B (73)	Metoprolol	1,434	6 d	Reinfarction	5.1[a]	2.7

BHAT, Beta-Blocker Heart Attack Trial; ISIS-1, First International Study of Infarct Survival; MIAMI, Metoprolol in Acute Myocardial Infarction Trial; TIMI II-B, Thrombolysis in Myocardial Infarction II-B Study.
[a]The placebo was delayed administration of metoprolol on day 6 after myocardial infarction versus immediate intravenous administration followed by oral dosing on day 1.

the protective attributes result from a class effect remains to be elucidated.

Antithrombotic Therapy

Because of the important role that thrombosis plays in acute MI, much research has been done on the use of antithrombotic therapy for the secondary prevention of MI (126).

Antiplatelet Therapy

Aspirin

With its metaanalysis of 174 randomized trials of antiplatelet therapy for cardiovascular disease, the Antiplatelet Trialists' Collaboration conclusively demonstrated the value of aspirin use after MI (127). Approximately 20,000 patients with acute MI were included in this metaanalysis; aspirin reduced the rate of recurrent ischemic events from 14% to 10%. Because the majority of trials included in this metaanalysis lasted an average of 2 years and a significant benefit of aspirin therapy was found between years 1 and 3, aspirin should be continued for at least several years after MI, and, in the absence of bleeding complications, should be continued indefinitely. The Second International Study of Infarct Survival found that aspirin therapy given for 1 month after acute MI was beneficial (128). The benefit was on the same order of magnitude as the benefit of administration of fibrinolysis with streptokinase. The dose of aspirin should be no greater than 325 mg per day, although it is unclear whether more than 81 mg per day is actually necessary for chronic therapy. Thus, aspirin is a simple, highly cost-effective intervention in MI patients. Nevertheless, aspirin remains underused after MI (129).

Clopidogrel

Clopidogrel is an antiplatelet agent that works by blocking the adenosine diphosphate receptor. In the Clopidogrel versus Aspirin in Patients at Risk of Ischaemic Events (CAPRIE) study, 19,185 patients with established atherosclerosis

of the coronary, cerebral, or peripheral circulation were randomly assigned to undergo secondary prevention with either aspirin or clopidogrel (130). After a mean follow-up period of 1.9 years, this trial found an overall 8.7% relative risk reduction in the primary end point of vascular death, MI, or ischemic stroke ($p = .043$). Interestingly, the CAPRIE study found a 19.2% relative risk reduction in fatal or nonfatal MI ($p = .008$) (131). Thus, compared with aspirin, clopidogrel's ability to reduce the incidence of MI in patients with previous ischemic events is particularly notable. The Clopidogrel and Metoprolol in Myocardial Infarction Trial (COMMIT) is currently enrolling approximately 30,000 patients within 6 hours of acute ST-elevation MI in China and randomly assigning them to therapy with either clopidogrel or placebo, in addition to aspirin, for 4 weeks. Whereas CAPRIE showed that clopidogrel was more effective than aspirin in secondary prevention of MI, COMMIT will help determine whether clopidogrel should be used in the acute setting in combination with aspirin.

In a subgroup analysis from CAPRIE, patients who were on statin therapy and were randomly assigned to clopidogrel had a lower rate of recurrent ischemic events than patients who were randomly assigned to aspirin (132). Furthermore, the relative risk reduction for MI was slightly greater than 50% with this combination. Thus, the benefits of statin therapy and clopidogrel appear to be complementary. In patients who have had an MI while taking aspirin or who are intolerant to aspirin, it is therefore reasonable to consider long-term therapy with clopidogrel, in addition to statin therapy (133). Whether aspirin plus clopidogrel plus a statin should be standard care after an acute MI will be determined in part by the results of the COMMIT trial. The results from the recently presented Clopidogrel in Unstable Angina to Prevent Recurrent Ischemic Events (CURE) trial demonstrate that clopidogrel plus aspirin was superior to aspirin alone in patients presenting with non–ST-elevation acute coronary syndromes (134). After an average of 9 months, the rate of cardiovascular death, MI, or stroke was reduced from 11.5% in the aspirin-only group to 9.3% in the group assigned to receive both aspirin and clopidogrel (p = .00005). Furthermore, the rate of life-threatening bleeding was low: 2.1% in the dual antiplatelet therapy group versus 1.8% in the aspirin group. These findings from CURE are likely applicable to the ST-segment elevation MI population as well.

RISK FACTORS

Inflammation

The role of inflammation in MI is being investigated, with identification of several markers that appear to correlate with adverse outcome after episodes of coronary instability (40,41,177,178). The possibility of using agents to treat inflammation to decrease the risk of recurrent ischemic events is appealing. Potential targets include tumor necrosis factor-α, CD 40, and peroxisome proliferator–activated receptor alpha and gamma (178–180). Additionally, agents already in use may have beneficial effects on inflammatory pathways. Statins may possess clinically relevant antiinflammatory properties (181). Antiplatelet agents such as clopidogrel and low-dose aspirin may have secondary antiinflammatory actions mediated through their ability to interfere with platelet activation and subsequent triggering of inflammatory processes. Ultimately, revascularization may prove to be the best "antiinflammatory" therapy (41,177).

LIFESTYLE MODIFICATION

The post-MI patient must incorporate several elements of lifestyle modification into daily practice (Fig. 20.6). Physician involvement in this process is crucial. Although counseling a patient and family can be time-consuming for the busy clinician, the likelihood of effecting change is highest during the first few days after MI, and this opportunity must not be lost.

Smoking Cessation

It is critical for patients who smoke to stop. The physician must always counsel the patient about the importance of this step, the message should be repeated often during the hospitalization and subsequent outpatient visits, and smoking status should be documented on follow-up (183). The patient is particularly receptive to such messages while in the cardiac care unit (184). The risk of recurrent MI is greatly increased if smoking is continued. However, if the post-MI patient ceases smoking, the risk of death is decreased by almost one-half (185,186). The deleterious effects of smoking include elevation of fibrinogen, which is particularly undesirable in someone who is recovering from an MI (187). ▼ d71

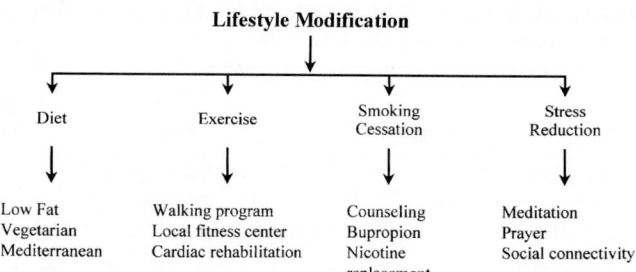

FIGURE 20.6 Lifestyle modification should consist of a multi-pronged effort to eliminate behaviors that are likely to contribute to adverse cardiac events. Although a comprehensive approach is mandatory, substantial latitude exists in specific recommendations, which allows therapy to be tailored to individual patients.

Exercise

Ambulation in the hallways should begin as soon as the patient is hemodynamically stable and shows no evidence of ischemia. Prolonged bed rest is undesirable and leads to deconditioning and an increase in the risk of deep vein thrombosis. Simple measures, such as a daily walking program, may lead to weight loss (203). Exercise can trigger acute MI, which is something patients fear, but this occurs most often from sudden bursts of exercise, rather than from a gradual increase in the intensity of an exercise program. If a patient has been revascularized, the decision to proceed with an exercise program is simplified. Some have asserted that a preentrance exercise test may not be absolutely necessary in an appropriately monitored cardiac rehabilitation program (204). However, if no invasive investigation has occurred, standard practice consists of use of an exercise stress test to guide the decision about beginning an exercise program. Even a structured weight-training program appears safe when it is started 6 or more weeks after acute MI in low-risk patients, with a rate of complications lower than that for aerobic exercise (205). The importance of exercise training is most pronounced in post-MI patients who have left ventricular dysfunction. Exercise training improves exercise capacity without causing left ventricular dilatation or increasing left ventricular wall thickness, which were concerns raised by older studies (206). Beta-blockade does not attenuate the benefits of exercise training (207). ▼ d72

Diet

Diet is an important part of realigning the patient's lifestyle after MI. Ideally, nutritional change should be implemented in the cardiac unit setting to emphasize the importance of this component of the patient's care. Consultation with a nutritionist can help the patient make practical changes and can ensure that the person who is most involved with food preparation in the household also understands the changes that must take place. ➼ d73

Psychosocial Aspects

Patients who have completed high school education fare better after MI than those who have not graduated from high school (257). Higher rates of smoking only partially accounted for this difference in outcome between patients who graduated from high school and those who did not. Thus, a patient's socioeconomic background does influence the outcome after MI.

Whether mental stress has a role in MI has been debated, and data are available that support both sides of the argument. Psychological distress does appear to increase the risk of rehospitalization, MI, cardiac death, and sudden death in patients who have had acute coronary events (258,259). In fact, psychological distress may have more to do with the failure to return to previous levels of functioning than the extent of myocardial damage (260). Patients' self-perception of their level of functioning after MI contributes to actual levels of function (261). ➼ d74

Depression appears to increase the risk of MI. Similarly, MI can lead to depression. Therefore, the physician must be vigilant for signs of depression and not merely assume that it is "normal" for a patient to be depressed after a heart attack. The options for treating depression pharmacologically include the use of selective serotonin reuptake inhibitors (270). Although concerns exist over the cardiac side effects of tricyclic antidepressants, use of selective serotonin reuptake inhibitors after acute MI appears safe (271). Additionally, the social support provided by a spouse can have substantial effects on recovery after MI. Interestingly, the social support provided by a pet can have a tremendous positive influence on survival after MI as well (272).

Ideally, all the aforementioned aspects of lifestyle modification can be incorporated into a comprehensive cardiac rehabilitation program. Whether this will be a formal or informal program depends largely on patient preference and local availability of resources, but in either case, the commitment to change on the part of the patient and physician is most critical.

CONTROVERSIES AND PERSONAL PERSPECTIVES

In the patient who appears to have experienced clinical reperfusion after fibrinolysis, the value of routine angiography remains controversial. Newer methods to assess microvascular reperfusion, such as electrocardiographic ST-segment resolution, contrast echocardiography, and magnetic resonance imaging, may help further clarify which patients will benefit from early angiography. Patients with recurrent spontaneous ischemia or abnormal results of a stress test should definitely undergo cardiac catheterization, with the goal of performing revascularization. After initial treatment, much of the distinction between therapy for ST-segment elevation MI and non–ST-segment elevation acute coronary syndromes will continue to be blurred as an early invasive approach becomes the standard treatment for chest pain syndromes associated with electrocardiographic deviation or elevated markers of myocardial necrosis and inflammation.

Efforts to increase the use of beta-blockers and ACE inhibitors should continue, given the widespread availability of these proven medications, and, unless new data emerge, calcium channel blockers should not be used as first-line agents for secondary prevention in patients with MI. Whether both beta-blockers *and* ACE inhibitors are necessary in every patient requires clarification from clinical trials. Because beta-blockade has been shown to decrease adverse ventricular remodeling and ACE inhibition has been shown to decrease sudden death, the two classes of drugs may have overlapping protective effects, and both may not be necessary in the patient who has normal left ventricular function after MI. The role of warfarin in acute MI should be limited to specific indications, such as atrial fibrillation or left ventricular thrombus. Instead, oral antiplatelet therapy should be continued after acute MI. Aggressive identification and treatment of hypertension, hypercholesterolemia, and diabetes should occur, with medical therapy begun in the hospital phase.

Quality improvement initiatives directed at the physician and the patient can increase the use of appropriate medications and lifestyle measures (273). Measures to improve quality do appear to be able to affect "hard" end points such as mortality rates (274). Communication between the hospital-based specialist and the outpatient physician is necessary to ensure a smooth transition of care for the patient. Effective methods to enhance such communication need to be developed and integrated into health care delivery systems (275). The availability of guidelines to aid the practitioner in management of MI should be welcomed (276,277). In fact, one of the few measurable differences between treatment of patients with MI in "top" hospitals and mediocre hospitals appears to be a difference in the use of medications such as aspirin and beta-blockers, and this appears to translate into better outcomes, including reduced mortality rates (278). Although physician resistance to implementation of guidelines is often the result of a perceived intrusion into the "art" of medicine, in reality, much of the variation in physician practice stems from a failure to incorporate new data (279). For example, a large degree of geographic variation exists in the prescription of medications that have been proven to be effective in multiple, randomized clinical trials (280,281). Payer status also appears to influence management after acute MI (282). A comprehensive approach that integrates care at multiple levels in the health care system will help standardize and optimize the care of patients after MI.

THE FUTURE

Early revascularization will become the favored strategy throughout Western health care systems. Optimal medical management begun early in the hospital course after MI will include statin therapy, beta-blockade, ACE inhibition, and antiplatelet therapy. The coupling of early revascularization with aggressive medical therapy will lead to dramatically improved outcomes after MI. Efforts targeting thrombus formation will continue to be an important part of secondary prevention and will consist of antiplatelet therapy with aspirin, clopidogrel, or possibly a combination. Inflammatory markers will help stratify risk beyond current measures, and therapies directed specifically at inflammatory pathways will be developed. A more refined understanding of the role of inflammation will complement efforts directed at treating thrombosis. The relative effectiveness, cost-effectiveness, incremental benefit, and potential for interaction of all these different medications in combination remain to be determined, although industry is unlikely to fund this type of research (283,284). Potentially, pharmacogenomics will allow targeting of patients most likely to benefit from therapy. Initially, based on the knowledge of the human genome, efforts will be directed toward the development of pharmaceuticals tailored to specific genotypes. For example, factor VII, glycoprotein IIIa (PlA2 allele), and thrombospondin genes have all been demonstrated to have clinically relevant single-nucleotide polymorphisms that could guide the use of different antithrombotic cocktails (285–291). Eventually, therapies designed to modify or enhance an individual's genetic structure will be created. Lifestyle modification will remain an important part of secondary preventive efforts, although pharmaceutical adjuncts to aid in smoking cessation and weight loss will continue to be tested. The appreciation of psychosocial factors in the well-being of post-MI patients will grow. The aging of the population will continue to challenge the health care system. The mortality rate among aged patients with acute MI remains extremely high, and a shift toward more aggressive management in both the acute and chronic phases of therapy will be necessary (292). Use of practice guidelines and critical care pathways, aided by developments in medical informatics, will play an even larger role in reducing variability in physician management and improving the care of the post-MI patient.

REFERENCES

1. Topol EJ, Ohman EM, Armstrong PW, et al. Survival outcomes 1 year after reperfusion therapy with either alteplase or reteplase for acute myocardial infarction: results from the Global Utilization of Streptokinase and t-PA for Occluded Coronary Arteries (GUSTO) III Trial. *Circulation* 2000;102:1761–1765.

2. Rogers WJ, Canto JG, Lambrew CT, et al. Temporal trends in the treatment of over 1.5 million patients with myocardial infarction in the US from 1990 through 1999: the National Registry of Myocardial Infarction 1, 2 and 3. *J Am Coll Cardiol* 2000;36:2056–2063.

3. Nikkari ST, O'Brien KD, Ferguson M, et al. Interstitial collagenase (MMP-1) expression in human carotid atherosclerosis. *Circulation* 1995;92:1393–1398.

4. Ikeda U, Shimpo M, Ohki R, et al. Fluvastatin inhibits matrix metalloproteinase-1 expression in human vascular endothelial cells. *Hypertension* 2000;36:325–329.

5. Loftus IM, Naylor AR, Goodall S, et al. Increased matrix metalloproteinase-9 activity in unstable carotid plaques. A potential role in acute plaque disruption. *Stroke* 2000;31:40–47.

6. Huang Y, Mironova M, Lopes-Virella MF. Oxidized LDL stimulates matrix metalloproteinase-1 expression in human vascular endothelial cells. *Arterioscler Thromb Vasc Biol* 1999;19:2640–2647.

7. Rabbani R, Topol EJ. Strategies to achieve coronary arterial plaque stabilization. *Cardiovasc Res* 1999;41:402–417.

8. Dietz R, Osterziel KJ, Willenbrock R, et al. Ventricular remodeling after acute myocardial infarction. *Thromb Haemost* 1999;82[Suppl 1]:73–75.

9. Lamas GA, Flaker GC, Mitchell G, et al. Effect of infarct artery patency on prognosis after acute myocardial infarction. The Survival and Ventricular Enlargement Investigators. *Circulation* 1995;92:1101–1109.

10. Newby LK, Califf RM. Identifying patient risk: the basis for rational discharge planning after acute myocardial infarction. *J Thromb Thrombolysis* 1996;3:107–115.

11. Gottlieb S, Moss AJ, McDermott M, et al. Interrelation of left ventricular ejection fraction, pulmonary congestion and outcome in acute myocardial infarction. *Am J Cardiol* 1992;69:977–984.

12. Brochet E, Czitrom D, Karila-Cohen D, et al. Early changes in myocardial perfusion patterns after myocardial infarction: relation with contractile reserve and functional recovery. *J Am Coll Cardiol* 1998;32:2011–2017.

13. Sakuma T, Hayashi Y, Sumii K, et al. Prediction of short- and intermediate-term prognoses of patients with acute myocardial infarction using myocardial contrast echocardiography one day after recanalization. *J Am Coll Cardiol* 1998;32:890–897.

14. Santoro GM, Valenti R, Buonamici P, et al. Relation between ST-segment changes and myocardial perfusion

evaluated by myocardial contrast echocardiography in patients with acute myocardial infarction treated with direct angioplasty. *Am J Cardiol* 1998;82:932–937.

15. Wu KC, Kim RJ, Bluemke DA, et al. Quantification and time course of microvascular obstruction by contrast-enhanced echocardiography and magnetic resonance imaging following acute myocardial infarction and reperfusion. *J Am Coll Cardiol* 1998;32:1756–1764.

16. Wu KC, Zerhouni EA, Judd RM, et al. Prognostic significance of microvascular obstruction by magnetic resonance imaging in patients with acute myocardial infarction. *Circulation* 1998;97:765–772.

17. Abboud L, Hir J, Eisen I, et al. Long-term value of exercise testing after acute myocardial infarction: influence of thrombolytic therapy. *Chest* 2000;117:556–561.

18. Gibbons RJ, Balady GJ, Beasley JW, et al. ACC/AHA Guidelines for Exercise Testing: a report of the American College of Cardiology/American Heart Association Task Force on Practice Guidelines (Committee on Exercise Testing). *J Am Coll Cardiol* 1997;30:260–311.

19. Madsen JK, Grande P, Saunamaki K, et al. Danish multicenter randomized study of invasive versus conservative treatment in patients with inducible ischemia after thrombolysis in acute myocardial infarction (DANAMI). Danish Trial in Acute Myocardial Infarction. *Circulation* 1997;96:748–755.

20. Chaitman BR, McMahon RP, Terrin M, et al. Impact of treatment strategy on predischarge exercise test in the Thrombolysis in Myocardial Infarction (TIMI) II Trial. *Am J Cardiol* 1993;71:131–138.

21. Zaret BL, Wackers FJ, Terrin ML, et al. Value of radionuclide rest and exercise left ventricular ejection fraction in assessing survival of patients after thrombolytic therapy for acute myocardial infarction: results of Thrombolysis in Myocardial Infarction (TIMI) phase II study. The TIMI Study Group. *J Am Coll Cardiol* 1995;26:73–79.

22. Joao I, Cotrim C, Duarte JA, et al. Cardiac rupture during exercise stress echocardiography: a case report. *J Am Soc Echocardiogr* 2000;13:785–787.

23. Brown KA, Heller GV, Landin RS, et al. Early dipyridamole (99m)Tc-sestamibi single photon emission computed tomographic imaging 2 to 4 days after acute myocardial infarction predicts in-hospital and postdischarge cardiac events: comparison with submaximal exercise imaging. *Circulation* 1999;100:2060–2066.

24. Hjelms E, Alstrup P, Paulsen PK, et al. CABG shortly after AMI treated with thrombolysis: an analysis of the surgical group and a comparison with PTCA in the DANAMI study. Danish Multicenter Randomized Study of Invasive Versus Conservative Treatment in Patients with Inducible Ischemia after Thrombolysis in Acute Myocardial Infarction. *Eur J Cardiothorac Surg* 1998;13:555–558.

25. Early and six-month outcome in patients with angina pectoris early after acute myocardial infarction (the GISSI-3 APPI [angina precoce post-infarto] study). The GISSI-3 APPI Study Group. *Am J Cardiol* 1996;78:1191–1197.

26. Scanlon PJ, Faxon DP, Audet AM, et al. ACC/AHA guidelines for coronary angiography: a report of the American College of Cardiology/American Heart Association Task Force on practice guidelines (Committee on Coronary Angiography).

Developed in collaboration with the Society for Cardiac Angiography and Interventions. *J Am Coll Cardiol* 1999;33:1756–1824.

27. Langer A, Fisher M, Califf RM, et al. Higher rates of coronary angiography and revascularization following myocardial infarction may be associated with greater survival in the United States than in Canada. The CARS Investigators (Coumadin/Aspirin Reinfarction Study). *Can J Cardiol* 1999;15:1095–1102.

28. Marrugat J, Ferrieres J, Masia R, et al. Differences in use of coronary angiography and outcome of myocardial infarction in Toulouse (France) and Gerona (Spain). The MONICA-Toulouse and REGICOR Investigators. *Eur Heart J* 2000;21:740–746.

29. Ellis SG, Mooney MR, George BS, et al. Randomized trial of late elective angioplasty versus conservative management for patients with residual stenoses after thrombolytic treatment of myocardial infarction. Treatment of Post-Thrombolytic Stenoses (TOPS) Study Group. *Circulation* 1992;86:1400–1406.

30. SWIFT trial of delayed elective intervention v conservative treatment after thrombolysis with anistreplase in acute myocardial infarction. The Should We Intervene following Thrombolysis Group. *BMJ* 1991;302:555–560.

31. Terrin ML, Williams DO, Kleiman NS, et al. Two- and three-year results of the Thrombolysis in Myocardial Infarction (TIMI) Phase II clinical trial. *J Am Coll Cardiol* 1993;22:1763–1772.

32. de Bono DP. The European Cooperative Study Group trial of intravenous recombinant tissue-type plasminogen activator (rt-PA) and conservative therapy versus rt-PA and immediate coronary angioplasty. *J Am Coll Cardiol* 1988;12:20A–23A.

33. Topol EJ, Califf RM, George BS, et al. A randomized trial of immediate versus delayed elective angioplasty after intravenous tissue plasminogen activator in acute myocardial infarction. *N Engl J Med* 1987;317:581–588.

34. Duber C, Jungbluth A, Rumpelt HJ, et al. Morphology of the coronary arteries after combined thrombolysis and percutaneous transluminal coronary angioplasty for acute myocardial infarction. *Am J Cardiol* 1986;58:698–703.

35. Miller JM, Smalling R, Ohman EM, et al. Effectiveness of early coronary angioplasty and abciximab for failed thrombolysis (reteplase or alteplase) during acute myocardial infarction (results from the GUSTO-III trial). Global Use of Strategies to Open Occluded Coronary Arteries. *Am J Cardiol* 1999;84:779–784.

36. Fragmin and Fast Revascularisation during Instability in Coronary Artery Disease Investigators. Invasive compared with non-invasive treatment in unstable coronary-artery disease: FRISC II prospective randomised multicentre study. *Lancet* 1999;354:708–715.

37. Cannon CP, Weintraub WS, Demopoulos LA, et al. Invasive versus conservative strategies in unstable angina and non–Q-wave myocardial infarction following treatment with tirofiban: rationale and study design of the international TACTICS-TIMI 18 Trial. Treat Angina with Aggrastat and Determine Cost of Therapy with an Invasive or Conservative Strategy. Thrombolysis in Myocardial Infarction. *Am J Cardiol* 1998;82:731–736.

38. Cannon CP. TACTICS-TIMI 18. Presented at the American Heart Association Annual Meeting, New Orleans, LA, 2000.

39. Tommasi S, Carluccio E, Bentivoglio M, et al. C-reactive protein as a marker for cardiac ischemic events in the year after a first, uncomplicated myocardial infarction. *Am J Cardiol* 1999;83:1595–1599.

40. Barron HV, Cannon CP, Murphy SA, et al. Association between white blood cell count, epicardial blood flow, myocardial perfusion, and clinical outcomes in the setting of acute myocardial infarction: a thrombolysis in myocardial infarction 10 substudy. *Circulation* 2000;102:2329–2334.

41. Lagerqvist B, Siegbahn A, Diderholm E, et al. Raised mortality at inflammatory activity or myocardial damage in unstable CAD is reduced by an invasive strategy. *Circulation* 2000;102:II-390.

42. Kober L, Bloch Thomsen PE, Moller M, et al. Effect of dofetilide in patients with recent myocardial infarction and left-ventricular dysfunction: a randomised trial. Danish Investigations of Arrhythmia and Mortality on Dofetilide (DIAMOND) Study Group. *Lancet* 2000;356:2052–2058.

43. Bigger JT, Fleiss JL, Kleiger R, et al. The relationships among ventricular arrhythmias, left ventricular dysfunction, and mortality in the 2 years after myocardial infarction. *Circulation* 1984;69:250–258.

44. Preliminary report: effect of encainide and flecainide on mortality in a randomized trial of arrhythmia suppression after myocardial infarction. The Cardiac Arrhythmia Suppression Trial (CAST) Investigators. *N Engl J Med* 1989;321:406–412.

45. Echt DS, Liebson PR, Mitchell LB, et al. Mortality and morbidity in patients receiving encainide, flecainide, or placebo. The Cardiac Arrhythmia Suppression Trial. *N Engl J Med* 1991;324:781–788.

46. Effect of the antiarrhythmic agent moricizine on survival after myocardial infarction. The Cardiac Arrhythmia Suppression Trial II Investigators. *N Engl J Med* 1992;327:227–233.

47. Denes P, el-Sherif N, Katz R, et al. Prognostic significance of signal-averaged electrocardiogram after thrombolytic therapy and/or angioplasty during acute myocardial infarction (CAST substudy). Cardiac Arrhythmia Suppression Trial (CAST) SAECG Substudy Investigators. *Am J Cardiol* 1994;74:216–220.

48. Pedretti RF, Migliori GB, Mapelli V, et al. Cost-effectiveness analysis of invasive and noninvasive tests in high risk patients treated with amiodarone after acute myocardial infarction. *J Am Coll Cardiol* 1998;31:1481–1489.

49. A comparison of antiarrhythmic-drug therapy with implantable defibrillators in patients resuscitated from near-fatal ventricular arrhythmias. The Antiarrhythmics Versus Implantable Defibrillators (AVID) Investigators. *N Engl J Med* 1997;337:1576–1583.

50. Moss AJ, Hall WJ, Cannom DS, et al. Improved survival with an implanted defibrillator in patients with coronary disease at high risk for ventricular arrhythmia. Multicenter Automatic Defibrillator Implantation Trial Investigators. *N Engl J Med* 1996;335:1933–1940.

51. Buxton AE, Lee KL, DiCarlo L, et al. Electrophysiologic testing to identify patients with coronary artery disease who are at risk for sudden death. Multicenter Unsustained Tachycardia Trial Investigators. *N Engl J Med* 2000;342:1937–1945.

52. Buxton AE, Lee KL, Fisher JD, et al. A randomized study of the prevention of sudden death in patients with coronary artery disease. Multicenter Unsustained Tachycardia Trial Investigators. *N Engl J Med* 1999;341:1882–1890.

53. Prystowsky EN. Screening and therapy for patients with nonsustained ventricular tachycardia. *Am J Cardiol* 2000;86:K34–K39.

54. GISSI-3: effects of lisinopril and transdermal glyceryl trinitrate singly and together on 6-week mortality and ventricular function after acute myocardial infarction. Gruppo Italiano per lo Studio della Sopravvivenza nell'Infarto Miocardico. *Lancet* 1994;343:1115–1122.

55. ISIS-4: a randomised factorial trial assessing early oral captopril, oral mononitrate, and intravenous magnesium sulphate in 58,050 patients with suspected acute myocardial infarction. ISIS-4 (Fourth International Study of Infarct Survival) Collaborative Group. *Lancet* 1995;345:669–685.

56. Young JB. Angiotensin-converting enzyme inhibitors post-myocardial infarction. *Cardiol Clin* 1995;13:379–390.

57. Effect of ramipril on mortality and morbidity of survivors of acute myocardial infarction with clinical evidence of heart failure. The Acute Infarction Ramipril Efficacy (AIRE) Study Investigators. *Lancet* 1993;342:821–828.

58. Pfeffer MA, Braunwald E, Moye LA, et al. Effect of captopril on mortality and morbidity in patients with left ventricular dysfunction after myocardial infarction: results of the survival and ventricular enlargement trial. The SAVE Investigators. *N Engl J Med* 1992;327:669–677.

59. Torp-Pedersen C, Kober L. Effect of ACE inhibitor trandolapril on life expectancy of patients with reduced left-ventricular function after acute myocardial infarction. TRACE Study Group. Trandolapril Cardiac Evaluation. *Lancet* 1999;354:9–12.

60. Yusuf S, Sleight P, Pogue J, et al. Effects of an angiotensin-converting-enzyme inhibitor, ramipril, on cardiovascular events in high-risk patients. The Heart Outcomes Prevention Evaluation Study Investigators. *N Engl J Med* 2000;342:145–153.

61. Oral captopril versus placebo among 13,634 patients with suspected acute myocardial infarction: interim report from the Chinese Cardiac Study (CCS-1). *Lancet* 1995;345:686–687.

62. Flather MD, Lonn EM, Yusuf S. Effects of ACE inhibitors on mortality when started in the early phase of myocardial infarction: evidence from the larger randomized controlled trials. *J Cardiovasc Risk* 1995;2:423–428.

63. Indications for ACE inhibitors in the early treatment of acute myocardial infarction: systematic overview of individual data from 100,000 patients in randomized trials. ACE Inhibitor Myocardial Infarction Collaborative Group. *Circulation* 1998;97:2202–2212.

64. Swedberg K, Held P, Kjekshus J, et al. Effects of the early administration of enalapril on mortality in patients with acute myocardial infarction: results of the Cooperative New Scandinavian Enalapril Survival Study II (CONSENSUS II). *N Engl J Med* 1992;327:678–684.

65. de Kam PJ, Voors AA, van den Berg MP, et al. Effect of very early angiotensin-converting enzyme inhibition on left ven-

tricular dilation after myocardial infarction in patients receiving thrombolysis: results of a meta-analysis of 845 patients. FAMIS, CAPTIN and CATS Investigators. *J Am Coll Cardiol* 2000;36:2047–2053.

66. Barron HV, Michaels AD, Maynard C, et al. Use of angiotensin-converting enzyme inhibitors at discharge in patients with acute myocardial infarction in the United States: data from the National Registry of Myocardial Infarction 2. *J Am Coll Cardiol* 1998;32:360–367.

67. Pfeffer MA. Enhancing cardiac protection after myocardial infarction: rationale for newer clinical trials of angiotensin receptor blockers. *Am Heart J* 2000;139:S23–S28.

68. Yusuf S, Peto R, Lewis J, et al. Beta blockade during and after myocardial infarction: an overview of the randomized trials. *Prog Cardiovasc Dis* 1985;27:335–371.

69. Timolol-induced reduction in mortality and reinfarction in patients surviving acute myocardial infarction. *N Engl J Med* 1981;304:801–807.

70. Groenning BA, Nilsson JC, Sondergaard L, et al. Antiremodeling effects on the left ventricle during beta-blockade with metoprolol in the treatment of chronic heart failure. *J Am Coll Cardiol* 2000;36:2072–2080.

71. Goldstein S. Propranolol therapy in patients with acute myocardial infarction: the Beta-Blocker Heart Attack Trial. *Circulation* 1983;67:I53–I57.

72. Furberg CD, Bell RL. Effect of beta-blocker therapy on recurrent nonfatal myocardial infarction. *Circulation* 1983;67:I83–I85.

73. Roberts R, Rogers WJ, Mueller HS, et al. Immediate versus deferred beta-blockade following thrombolytic therapy in patients with acute myocardial infarction: results of the Thrombolysis in Myocardial Infarction (TIMI) II-B Study. *Circulation* 1991;83:422–437.

74. Barron HV, Rundle AC, Gore JM, et al. Intracranial hemorrhage rates and effect of immediate beta-blocker use in patients with acute myocardial infarction treated with tissue plasminogen activator. Participants in the National Registry of Myocardial Infarction-2. *Am J Cardiol* 2000;85:294–298.

75. Woods KL, Ketley D, Lowy A, et al. Beta-blockers and antithrombotic treatment for secondary prevention after acute myocardial infarction: towards an understanding of factors influencing clinical practice. The European Secondary Prevention Study Group. *Eur Heart J* 1998;19:74–79.

76. Gottlieb SS, McCarter RJ, Vogel RA. Effect of beta-blockade on mortality among high-risk and low-risk patients after myocardial infarction. *N Engl J Med* 1998;339:489–497.

77. Phillips KA, Shlipak MG, Coxson P, et al. Health and economic benefits of increased beta-blocker use following myocardial infarction. *JAMA* 2000;284:2748–2754.

78. Houghton T, Freemantle N, Cleland JG. Are beta-blockers effective in patients who develop heart failure soon after myocardial infarction? A meta-regression analysis of randomised trials. *Eur J Heart Fail* 2000;2:333–340.

79. Gurwitz JH, Goldberg RJ, Chen Z, et al. Beta-blocker therapy in acute myocardial infarction: evidence for underutilization in the elderly. *Am J Med* 1992;93:605–610.

80. Krumholz HM, Radford MJ, Wang Y, et al. Early beta-blocker therapy for acute myocardial infarction in elderly patients. *Ann Intern Med* 1999;131:648–654.

81. Chen J, Marciniak TA, Radford MJ, et al. Beta-blocker therapy for secondary prevention of myocardial infarction in elderly diabetic patients: results from the National Cooperative Cardiovascular Project. *J Am Coll Cardiol* 1999;34:1388–1394.

82. Barron HV, Viskin S, Lundstrom RJ, et al. Beta-blocker dosages and mortality after myocardial infarction: data from a large health maintenance organization. *Arch Intern Med* 1998;158:449–453.

83. Rochon PA, Tu JV, Anderson GM, et al. Rate of heart failure and 1-year survival for older people receiving low-dose beta-blocker therapy after myocardial infarction. *Lancet* 2000;356:639–644.

84. Flather MD, Yusuf S, Kober L, et al. Long-term ACE-inhibitor therapy in patients with heart failure or left-ventricular dysfunction: a systematic overview of data from individual patients. ACE-Inhibitor Myocardial Infarction Collaborative Group. *Lancet* 2000;355:1575–1581.

85. Vaur L, Danchin N, Genes N, et al. Epidemiology of myocardial infarction in France: therapeutic and prognostic implications of heart failure during the acute phase. *Am Heart J* 1999;137:49–58.

86. McAlister FA. Trial is needed of ACE inhibitors plus beta blockers in survivors of myocardial infarction. *BMJ* 1998;317:751.

87. Anthonio RL, van Veldhuisen DJ, van Gilst WH. Left ventricular dilatation after myocardial infarction: ACE inhibitors, beta-blockers, or both? *J Cardiovasc Pharmacol* 1998;32:S1–S8.

88. Coletta C, Ricci R, Ceci V, et al. Effects of early treatment with captopril and metoprolol singly or together on six-month mortality and morbidity after acute myocardial infarction: results of the RIMA (Rimodellamento Infarto Miocardico Acuto) study. The RIMA researchers. *G Ital Cardiol* 1999;29:115–124; discussion 125–129.

89. Frishman WH, Cheng A. Secondary prevention of myocardial infarction: role of beta-adrenergic blockers and angiotensin-converting enzyme inhibitors. *Am Heart J* 1999;137:S25–S34.

90. Skolnick AE, Frishman WH. Calcium channel blockers in myocardial infarction. *Arch Intern Med* 1989;149:1669–1677.

91. Held PH, Yusuf S. Effects of beta-blockers and calcium channel blockers in acute myocardial infarction. *Eur Heart J* 1993;14[Suppl F]:18–25.

92. Aronow WS. Prevalence of use of beta blockers and of calcium channel blockers in older patients with prior myocardial infarction at the time of admission to a nursing home. *J Am Geriatr Soc* 1996;44:1075–1077.

93. The effect of diltiazem on mortality and reinfarction after myocardial infarction. The Multicenter Diltiazem Postinfarction Trial Research Group. *N Engl J Med* 1988;319:385–392.

94. Hager WD, Davis BR, Riba A, et al. Absence of a deleterious effect of calcium channel blockers in patients with left ventricular dysfunction after myocardial infarction: the SAVE Study experience. SAVE Investigators. Survival and Ventricular Enlargement. *Am Heart J* 1998;135:406–413.

95. Secondary prevention with verapamil after myocardial infarction. The Danish Study Group on Verapamil in Myocardial Infarction. *Am J Cardiol* 1990;66:33I–40I.

96. Effect of verapamil on mortality and major events after

acute myocardial infarction (the Danish Verapamil Infarction Trial II—DAVIT II). *Am J Cardiol* 1990;66:779–785.

97. Muller JE, Morrison J, Stone PH, et al. Nifedipine therapy for patients with threatened and acute myocardial infarction: a randomized, double-blind, placebo-controlled comparison. *Circulation* 1984;69:740–747.

98. The Danish studies on verapamil in acute myocardial infarction. The Danish Study Group on Verapamil in Myocardial Infarction. *Br J Clin Pharmacol* 1986;21:197S–204S.

99. Goldbourt U, Behar S, Reicher-Reiss H, et al. Early administration of nifedipine in suspected acute myocardial infarction. The Secondary Prevention Reinfarction Israel Nifedipine Trial 2 Study. *Arch Intern Med* 1993;153:345–353.

100. Ishikawa K, Nakai S, Takenaka T, et al. Short-acting nifedipine and diltiazem do not reduce the incidence of cardiac events in patients with healed myocardial infarction. Secondary Prevention Group. *Circulation* 1997;95:2368–2373.

101. Reicher-Reiss H, Behar S, Boyko V, et al. Long-term mortality follow-up of hospital survivors of a myocardial infarction randomized to nifedipine in the SPRINT study. Secondary Prevention Reinfarction Israeli Nifedipine Trial. *Cardiovasc Drugs Ther* 1998;12:171–176.

102. Rengo F, Carbonin P, Pahor M, et al. A controlled trial of verapamil in patients after acute myocardial infarction: results of the calcium antagonist reinfarction Italian study (CRIS). *Am J Cardiol* 1996;77:365–369.

103. Jespersen CM. Verapamil in acute myocardial infarction: the rationales of the VAMI and DAVIT III trials. *Cardiovasc Drugs Ther* 2000;14:99–105.

104. Hansen JF, Hagerup L, Sigurd B, et al. Cardiac event rates after acute myocardial infarction in patients treated with verapamil and trandolapril versus trandolapril alone. Danish Verapamil Infarction Trial (DAVIT) Study Group. *Am J Cardiol* 1997;79:738–741.

105. Boden WE, van Gilst WH, Scheldewaert RG, et al. Diltiazem in acute myocardial infarction treated with thrombolytic agents: a randomised placebo-controlled trial. Incomplete Infarction Trial of European Research Collaborators Evaluating Prognosis Post-Thrombolysis (INTERCEPT). *Lancet* 2000;355:1751–1756.

106. Psaty BM, Heckbert SR, Koepsell TD, et al. The risk of myocardial infarction associated with antihypertensive drug therapies. *JAMA* 1995;274:620–625.

107. Sacks FM, Pfeffer MA, Moye LA, et al. The effect of pravastatin on coronary events after myocardial infarction in patients with average cholesterol levels. Cholesterol and Recurrent Events Trial investigators. *N Engl J Med* 1996;335:1001–1009.

108. Plehn JF, Davis BR, Sacks FM, et al. Reduction of stroke incidence after myocardial infarction with pravastatin: the Cholesterol and Recurrent Events (CARE) study. The CARE Investigators. *Circulation* 1999;99:216–223.

109. White HD, Simes RJ, Anderson NE, et al. Pravastatin therapy and the risk of stroke. *N Engl J Med* 2000;343:317–326.

110. LaRosa JC, He J, Vupputuri S. Effect of statins on risk of coronary disease: a meta-analysis of randomized controlled trials. *JAMA* 1999;282:2340–2346.

111. Gaziano JM, Hennekens CH, Satterfield S, et al. Clinical utility of lipid and lipoprotein levels during hospitalization for acute myocardial infarction. *Vasc Med* 1999;4:227–231.

112. Shepherd J. From best evidence to best practice: what are the obstacles? *Atherosclerosis* 1999;147[Suppl 1]:S45–S51.

113. Stenestrand U, Wallentin L. Early statin treatment following acute myocardial infarction and 1-year survival. *JAMA* 2001;285:430–435.

114. Schwartz GG, Oliver MF, Ezekowitz MD, et al. Rationale and design of the Myocardial Ischemia Reduction with Aggressive Cholesterol Lowering (MIRACL) study that evaluates atorvastatin in unstable angina pectoris and in non-Q-wave acute myocardial infarction. *Am J Cardiol* 1998;81:578–581.

115. Schwartz GG, Olsson AG. The myocardial ischemia reduction with aggressive cholesterol lowering (MIRACL) trial: effects of intensive atorvastatin treatment on early recurrent events after an acute coronary syndrome. American Heart Association Annual Meeting 2000.

116. van Boven AJ, Liem A. Effects of fluvastatin administered immediately after an acute MI on myocardial ischemia (FLORIDA). American Heart Association Annual Meeting 2000.

117. Ganz DA, Kuntz KM, Jacobson GA, et al. Cost-effectiveness of 3-hydroxy-3-methylglutaryl coenzyme A reductase inhibitor therapy in older patients with myocardial infarction. *Ann Intern Med* 2000;132:780–787.

118. Schiele R, Gitt AK, Schneider S, et al. Early statin use in acute myocardial infarction is associated with a reduced hospital mortality: results of MITRA-2. *Eur Heart J* 2000;21:155.

119. Gylling H, Radhakrishnan R, Miettinen TA. Reduction of serum cholesterol in postmenopausal women with previous myocardial infarction and cholesterol malabsorption induced by dietary sitostanol ester margarine: women and dietary sitostanol. *Circulation* 1997;96:4226–4231.

120. de Faire U, Ericsson CG, Grip L, et al. Secondary preventive potential of lipid-lowering drugs. The Bezafibrate Coronary Atherosclerosis Intervention Trial (BECAIT). *Eur Heart J* 1996;17[Suppl F]:37–42.

121. Secondary prevention by raising HDL cholesterol and reducing triglycerides in patients with coronary artery disease: the Bezafibrate Infarction Prevention (BIP) study. *Circulation* 2000;102:21–27.

122. Rubins HB, Robins SJ, Collins D, et al. Gemfibrozil for the secondary prevention of coronary heart disease in men with low levels of high-density lipoprotein cholesterol. Veterans Affairs High-Density Lipoprotein Cholesterol Intervention Trial Study Group. *N Engl J Med* 1999;341:410–418.

123. Krakoff J, Vela BS, Brinton EA. The role of fibric acid derivatives in the secondary prevention of coronary heart disease. *Curr Cardiol Rep* 2000;2:452–458.

124. Guyton JR, Blazing MA, Hagar J, et al. Extended-release niacin vs gemfibrozil for the treatment of low levels of high-density lipoprotein cholesterol. Niaspan-Gemfibrozil Study Group. *Arch Intern Med* 2000;160:1177–1184.

125. Belalcazar LM, Ballantyne CM. Defining specific goals of therapy in treating dyslipidemia in the patient with low high-density lipoprotein cholesterol. *Prog Cardiovasc Dis* 1998;41:151–174.

126. Bhatt DL, Topol EJ. Antiplatelet and anticoagulant therapy in the secondary prevention of ischemic heart disease. *Med Clin North Am* 2000;84:163–179, ix.

127. Antiplatelet Trialists' Collaboration. Collaborative overview of randomised trials of antiplatelet therapy: I. Prevention of death, myocardial infarction, and stroke by prolonged antiplatelet therapy in various categories of patients. *BMJ* 1994;308:81–106.

128. Randomised trial of intravenous streptokinase, oral aspirin, both, or neither among 17,187 cases of suspected acute myocardial infarction: ISIS-2. ISIS-2 (Second International Study of Infarct Survival) Collaborative Group. *Lancet* 1988;2:349–360.

129. Aronow WS. Underutilization of aspirin in older patients with prior myocardial infarction at the time of admission to a nursing home. *J Am Geriatr Soc* 1998;46:615–616.

130. CAPRIE Steering Committee. A randomised, blinded, trial of clopidogrel versus aspirin in patients at risk of ischaemic events (CAPRIE). *Lancet* 1996;348:1329–1339.

131. Gent M. Benefit of clopidogrel in patients with coronary disease. *Circulation* 1997;96:I-467.

132. Bhatt DL, Foody JM, Hirsch AT, et al. Complementary, additive benefit of clopidogrel and lipid-lowering therapy in patients with atherosclerosis. *J Am Coll Cardiol* 2000;35[Suppl A]:326.

133. Bhatt DL, Hirsch AT, Ringleb PA, et al. Reduction in the need for hospitalization for recurrent ischemic events and bleeding with clopidogrel instead of aspirin. CAPRIE investigators. *Am Heart J* 2000;140:67–73.

134. Yusuf S. Clopidogrel in unstable angina to prevent recurrent ischemic events (CURE). Presented at the Annual Meeting of the American College of Cardiology 2001.

135. Hart RG, Benavente O, McBride R, et al. Antithrombotic therapy to prevent stroke in patients with atrial fibrillation: a meta-analysis. *Ann Intern Med* 1999;131:492–501.

136. A double-blind trial to assess long-term oral anticoagulant therapy in elderly patients after myocardial infarction. Sixty Plus Reinfarction Study Research Group. *Lancet* 1980;2:989–994.

137. Smith P. Long-term anticoagulant treatment after acute myocardial infarction. The Warfarin Re-Infarction Study. *Ann Epidemiol* 1992;2:549–552.

138. Effect of long-term oral anticoagulant treatment on mortality and cardiovascular morbidity after myocardial infarction. Anticoagulants in the Secondary Prevention of Events in Coronary Thrombosis (ASPECT) Research Group. *Lancet* 1994;343:499–503.

139. Azar AJ, Cannegieter SC, Deckers JW, et al. Optimal intensity of oral anticoagulant therapy after myocardial infarction. *J Am Coll Cardiol* 1996;27:1349–1355.

140. Meijer A, Verheugt FW, Werter CJ, et al. Aspirin versus coumadin in the prevention of reocclusion and recurrent ischemia after successful thrombolysis: a prospective placebo-controlled angiographic study. Results of the APRICOT Study. *Circulation* 1993;87:1524–1530.

141. Randomised double-blind trial of fixed low-dose warfarin with aspirin after myocardial infarction. Coumadin Aspirin Reinfarction Study (CARS) Investigators. *Lancet* 1997;350:389–396.

142. Fiore L, Brophy M, Peduzzi P, et al. Combination Hemotherapy and Mortality Prevention (CHAMP) Study rationale and design. *J Thromb Thrombolysis* 1998;6:133–140.

143. Brower MA. Antithrombotics in the Prevention of Reocclu-sion in Coronary Thrombolysis-2 (APRICOT-2). European Society of Cardiology Annual Meeting 2000.

144. Hurlen M, Smith P, Arnesen H. Effects of warfarin, aspirin and the two combined, on mortality and thromboembolic morbidity after myocardial infarction: the WARIS-II (Warfarin-Aspirin Reinfarction Study) design. *Scand Cardiovasc J* 2000;34:168–171.

145. Leon MB, Baim DS, Popma JJ, et al. A clinical trial comparing three antithrombotic-drug regimens after coronary-artery stenting. Stent Anticoagulation Restenosis Study Investigators. *N Engl J Med* 1998;339:1665–1671.

146. Bhatt DL, Topol EJ. Clopidogrel reduces major adverse cardiac events after stenting compared with ticlopidine. *Eur Heart J* 2000;21:381.

147. The Writing Group for the PEPI Trial. Effects of estrogen or estrogen/progestin regimens on heart disease risk factors in postmenopausal women. The Postmenopausal Estrogen/Progestin Interventions (PEPI) Trial. *JAMA* 1995;273:199–208.

148. Herrington DM, Reboussin DM, Brosnihan KB, et al. Effects of estrogen replacement on the progression of coronary-artery atherosclerosis. *N Engl J Med* 2000;343:522–529.

149. Grady D, Wenger NK, Herrington D, et al. Postmenopausal hormone therapy increases risk for venous thromboembolic disease. The Heart and Estrogen/Progestin Replacement Study. *Ann Intern Med* 2000;132:689–696.

150. Cushman M, Legault C, Barrett-Connor E, et al. Effect of postmenopausal hormones on inflammation-sensitive proteins: the Postmenopausal Estrogen/Progestin Interventions (PEPI) Study. *Circulation* 1999;100:717–722.

151. Herrington DM. The HERS trial results: paradigms lost? Heart and Estrogen/Progestin Replacement Study. *Ann Intern Med* 1999;131:463–466.

152. Herrington D. Role of estrogens, selective estrogen receptor modulators and phytoestrogens in cardiovascular protection. *Can J Cardiol* 2000;16[Suppl E]:5E–9E.

153. Cairns JA, Connolly SJ, Gent M, et al. Post-myocardial infarction mortality in patients with ventricular premature depolarizations. Canadian Amiodarone Myocardial Infarction Arrhythmia Trial Pilot Study. *Circulation* 1991;84:550–557.

154. Burkart F, Pfisterer M, Kiowski W, et al. Effect of antiarrhythmic therapy on mortality in survivors of myocardial infarction with asymptomatic complex ventricular arrhythmias: Basel Antiarrhythmic Study of Infarct Survival (BASIS). *J Am Coll Cardiol* 1990;16:1711–1718.

155. Pfisterer ME, Kiowski W, Brunner H, et al. Long-term benefit of 1-year amiodarone treatment for persistent complex ventricular arrhythmias after myocardial infarction. *Circulation* 1993;87:309–311.

156. Ceremuzynski L, Kleczar E, Krzeminska-Pakula M, et al. Effect of amiodarone on mortality after myocardial infarction: a double-blind, placebo-controlled, pilot study. *J Am Coll Cardiol* 1992;20:1056–1062.

157. Cairns JA, Connolly SJ, Roberts R, et al. Randomised trial of outcome after myocardial infarction in patients with frequent or repetitive ventricular premature depolarisations: CAMIAT. Canadian Amiodarone Myocardial Infarction Arrhythmia Trial Investigators. *Lancet* 1997;349:675–682.

158. Julian DG, Camm AJ, Frangin G, et al. Randomised trial of effect of amiodarone on mortality in patients with left-ventricular dysfunction after recent myocardial infarction: EMIAT. European Myocardial Infarct Amiodarone Trial Investigators. *Lancet* 1997;349:667–674.

159. Sim I, McDonald KM, Lavori PW, et al. Quantitative overview of randomized trials of amiodarone to prevent sudden cardiac death. *Circulation* 1997;96:2823–2829.

160. Jafri SM, Borzak S, Goldberger J, et al. Role of antiarrhythmic agents after myocardial infarction with special reference to the EMIAT and CAMIAT trials of amiodarone. European Myocardial Infarct Amiodarone Trial. Canadian Amiodarone Myocardial Infarction Trial. *Prog Cardiovasc Dis* 1998;41:65–70.

161. Elizari MV, Martinez JM, Belziti C, et al. Morbidity and mortality following early administration of amiodarone in acute myocardial infarction. GEMICA study investigators, GEMA Group, Buenos Aires, Argentina. Grupo de Estudios Multicentricos en Argentina. *Eur Heart J* 2000;21:198–205.

162. Janse MJ, Malik M, Camm AJ, et al. Identification of post acute myocardial infarction patients with potential benefit from prophylactic treatment with amiodarone: a substudy of EMIAT (the European Myocardial Infarct Amiodarone Trial). *Eur Heart J* 1998;19:85–95.

163. Effect of prophylactic amiodarone on mortality after acute myocardial infarction and in congestive heart failure: meta-analysis of individual data from 6500 patients in randomised trials. Amiodarone Trials Meta-Analysis Investigators. *Lancet* 1997;350:1417–1424.

164. Boutitie F, Boissel JP, Connolly SJ, et al. Amiodarone interaction with beta-blockers: analysis of the merged EMIAT (European Myocardial Infarct Amiodarone Trial) and CAMIAT (Canadian Amiodarone Myocardial Infarction Trial) databases. The EMIAT and CAMIAT Investigators. *Circulation* 1999;99:2268–2275.

165. Rakugi H, Yu H, Kamitani A, et al. Links between hypertension and myocardial infarction. *Am Heart J* 1996;132:213–221.

166. Gustafsson F, Kober L, Torp-Pedersen C, et al. Long-term prognosis after acute myocardial infarction in patients with a history of arterial hypertension. TRACE study group. *Eur Heart J* 1998;19:588–594.

167. Haider AW, Chen L, Larson MG, et al. Antecedent hypertension confers increased risk for adverse outcomes after initial myocardial infarction. *Hypertension* 1997;30:1020–1024.

168. Fresco C, Avanzini F, Bosi S, et al. Prognostic value of a history of hypertension in 11,483 patients with acute myocardial infarction treated with thrombolysis. GISSI-2 Investigators. Gruppo Italiano per lo Studio della, Sopravvivena nell'Infarto Miocardico. *J Hypertens* 1996;14:743–750.

169. Gustafsson F, Torp-Pedersen C, Kober L, et al. Effect of angiotensin converting enzyme inhibition after acute myocardial infarction in patients with arterial hypertension. TRACE Study Group, Trandolapril Cardiac Event. *J Hypertens* 1997;15:793–798.

170. Aylward PE, Wilcox RG, Horgan JH, et al. Relation of increased arterial blood pressure to mortality and stroke in the context of contemporary thrombolytic therapy for acute myocardial infarction: a randomized trial. GUSTO-I Investigators. *Ann Intern Med* 1996;125:891–900.

171. Chowdhury TA, Lasker SS, Dyer PH. Comparison of secondary prevention measures after myocardial infarction in subjects with and without diabetes mellitus. *J Intern Med* 1999;245:565–570.

172. Tenenbaum A, Fisman EZ, Boyko V, et al. Prevalence and prognostic significance of unrecognized systemic hypertension in patients with diabetes mellitus and healed myocardial infarction and/or stable angina pectoris. *Am J Cardiol* 1999;84:294–298.

173. Zuanetti G, Latini R, Maggioni AP, et al. Effect of the ACE inhibitor lisinopril on mortality in diabetic patients with acute myocardial infarction: data from the GISSI-3 study. *Circulation* 1997;96:4239–4245.

174. MacDonald TM, Butler R, Newton RW, et al. Which drugs benefit diabetic patients for secondary prevention of myocardial infarction? DARTS/MEMO Collaboration. *Diabet Med* 1998;15:282–289.

175. Zuanetti G, Latini R. Impact of pharmacological treatment on mortality after myocardial infarction in diabetic patients. *J Diabetes Complications* 1997;11:131–136.

176. Bhatt DL, Marso SP, Hirsch AT, et al. Superiority of clopidogrel versus aspirin in patients with a history of diabetes mellitus. *J Am Coll Cardiol* 2000;35[Suppl A]:409.

177. Bhatt DL, Chew DP, Simoons ML, et al. An elevated white blood cell count is an independent predictor of mortality in patients with acute coronary syndromes. *Circulation* 2000;102:II-776.

178. Ridker PM, Rifai N, Pfeffer M, et al. Elevation of tumor necrosis factor-alpha and increased risk of recurrent coronary events after myocardial infarction. *Circulation* 2000;101:2149–2153.

179. Phipps RP. Atherosclerosis: the emerging role of inflammation and the CD40-CD40 ligand system. *Proc Natl Acad Sci U S A* 2000;97:6930–6932.

180. Takano H, Nagai T, Asakawa M, et al. Peroxisome proliferator–activated receptor activators inhibit lipopolysaccharide-induced tumor necrosis factor-alpha expression in neonatal rat cardiac myocytes. *Circ Res* 2000;87:596–602.

181. Ferro D, Parrotto S, Basili S, et al. Simvastatin inhibits the monocyte expression of proinflammatory cytokines in patients with hypercholesterolemia. *J Am Coll Cardiol* 2000;36:427–431.

182. Naghavi M, Barlas Z, Siadaty S, et al. Association of influenza vaccination and reduced risk of recurrent myocardial infarction. *Circulation* 2000;102:3039–3045.

183. van Berkel TF, Boersma H, De Baquer D, et al. Registration and management of smoking behaviour in patients with coronary heart disease. The EUROASPIRE survey. *Eur Heart J* 1999;20:1630–1637.

184. Rigotti NA, Singer DE, Mulley AG Jr, et al. Smoking cessation following admission to a coronary care unit. *J Gen Intern Med* 1991;6:305–311.

185. Wilson K, Gibson N, Willan A, et al. Effect of smoking cessation on mortality after myocardial infarction: meta-analysis of cohort studies. *Arch Intern Med* 2000;160:939–944.

186. Greenwood DC, Muir KR, Packham CJ, et al. Stress, social support, and stopping smoking after myocardial infarction in England. *J Epidemiol Community Health* 1995;49:583–587.

187. Fisher SD, Zareba W, Moss AJ, et al. Effect of smoking on lipid and thrombogenic factors two months after acute myocardial infarction. *Am J Cardiol* 2000;86:813–818.

188. Dobson AJ, Alexander HM, Heller RF, et al. How soon after quitting smoking does risk of heart attack decline? *J Clin Epidemiol* 1991;44:1247–1253.

189. McElduff P, Dobson A, Beaglehole R, et al. Rapid reduction in coronary risk for those who quit cigarette smoking. *Aust N Z J Public Health* 1998;22:787–791.

190. Rosenberg L, Palmer JR, Shapiro S. Decline in the risk of myocardial infarction among women who stop smoking. *N Engl J Med* 1990;322:213–217.

191. Negri E, La Vecchia C, D'Avanzo B, et al. Acute myocardial infarction: association with time since stopping smoking in Italy. GISSI-EFRIM Investigators. Gruppo Italiano per lo Studio della Sopravvivenza nell'Infarto. Epidemiologia dei Fattori di Rischio dell'Infarto Miocardico. *J Epidemiol Community Health* 1994;48:129–133.

192. Kawachi I, Colditz GA, Stampfer MJ, et al. Smoking cessation and time course of decreased risks of coronary heart disease in middle-aged women. *Arch Intern Med* 1994;154:169–175.

193. Lightwood JM, Glantz SA. Short-term economic and health benefits of smoking cessation: myocardial infarction and stroke. *Circulation* 1997;96:1089–1096.

194. Glantz SA, Parmley WW. Passive smoking and heart disease: epidemiology, physiology, and biochemistry. *Circulation* 1991;83:1–12.

195. Dornelas EA, Sampson RA, Gray JF, et al. A randomized controlled trial of smoking cessation counseling after myocardial infarction. *Prev Med* 2000;30:261–268.

196. Krumholz HM, Cohen BJ, Tsevat J, et al. Cost-effectiveness of a smoking cessation program after myocardial infarction. *J Am Coll Cardiol* 1993;22:1697–1702.

197. Goldstein MG, Niaura R. Methods to enhance smoking cessation after myocardial infarction. *Med Clin North Am* 2000;84:63–80, viii.

198. Joseph AM, Norman SM, Ferry LH, et al. The safety of transdermal nicotine as an aid to smoking cessation in patients with cardiac disease. *N Engl J Med* 1996;335:1792–1798.

199. Dacosta A, Guy JM, Tardy B, et al. Myocardial infarction and nicotine patch: a contributing or causative factor? *Eur Heart J* 1993;14:1709–1711.

200. Hurt RD, Sachs DP, Glover ED, et al. A comparison of sustained-release bupropion and placebo for smoking cessation. *N Engl J Med* 1997;337:1195–1202.

201. Jorenby DE, Leischow SJ, Nides MA, et al. A controlled trial of sustained-release bupropion, a nicotine patch, or both for smoking cessation. *N Engl J Med* 1999;340:685–691.

202. Huijbrechts IP, Duivenvoorden HJ, Deckers JW, et al. Modification of smoking habits five months after myocardial infarction: relationship with personality characteristics. *J Psychosom Res* 1996;40:369–378.

203. Mertens DJ, Kavanagh T, Campbell RB, et al. Exercise without dietary restriction as a means to long-term fat loss in the obese cardiac patient. *J Sports Med Phys Fitness* 1998;38:310–316.

204. McConnell TR, Klinger TA, Gardner JK, et al. Cardiac rehabilitation without exercise tests for post-myocardial infarction and post-bypass surgery patients. *J Cardiopulm Rehabil* 1998;18:458–463.

205. Daub WD, Knapik GP, Black WR. Strength training early after myocardial infarction. *J Cardiopulm Rehabil* 1996;16:100–108.

206. Dubach P, Myers J, Dziekan G, et al. Effect of exercise training on myocardial remodeling in patients with reduced left ventricular function after myocardial infarction: application of magnetic resonance imaging. *Circulation* 1997;95:2060–2067.

207. Pavia L, Orlando G, Myers J, et al. The effect of beta-blockade therapy on the response to exercise training in postmyocardial infarction patients. *Clin Cardiol* 1995;18:716–720.

208. Jolliffe JA, Rees K, Taylor RS, et al. Exercise-based rehabilitation for coronary heart disease (Cochrane Review). *Cochrane Database Syst Rev* 2000;(4):CD001800.

209. Oldridge NB, Guyatt GH, Fischer ME, et al. Cardiac rehabilitation after myocardial infarction: combined experience of randomized clinical trials. *JAMA* 1988;260:945–950.

210. O'Connor GT, Buring JE, Yusuf S, et al. An overview of randomized trials of rehabilitation with exercise after myocardial infarction. *Circulation* 1989;80:234–244.

211. van Dixhoorn J, Duivenvoorden HJ, Staal JA, et al. Cardiac events after myocardial infarction: possible effect of relaxation therapy. *Eur Heart J* 1987;8:1210–1214.

212. Miller TD, Balady GJ, Fletcher GF. Exercise and its role in the prevention and rehabilitation of cardiovascular disease. *Ann Behav Med* 1997;19:220–229.

213. Pashkow FJ. Rehabilitation in the patient after myocardial infarction with or without surgical management. *Semin Thorac Cardiovasc Surg* 1995;7:240–247.

214. Hedback B, Perk J, Wodlin P. Long-term reduction of cardiac mortality after myocardial infarction: 10-year results of a comprehensive rehabilitation programme. *Eur Heart J* 1993;14:831–835.

215. Hamalainen H, Luurila OJ, Kallio V, et al. Reduction in sudden deaths and coronary mortality in myocardial infarction patients after rehabilitation: 15 year follow-up study. *Eur Heart J* 1995;16:1839–1844.

216. Stahle A, Mattsson E, Ryden L, et al. Improved physical fitness and quality of life following training of elderly patients after acute coronary events: a 1 year follow-up randomized controlled study. *Eur Heart J* 1999;20:1475–1484.

217. Melville MR, Packham C, Brown N, et al. Cardiac rehabilitation: socially deprived patients are less likely to attend but patients ineligible for thrombolysis are less likely to be invited. *Heart* 1999;82:373–377.

218. Ades PA, Pashkow FJ, Nestor JR. Cost-effectiveness of cardiac rehabilitation after myocardial infarction. *J Cardiopulm Rehabil* 1997;17:222–231.

219. Oldridge N, Furlong W, Feeny D, et al. Economic evaluation of cardiac rehabilitation soon after acute myocardial infarction. *Am J Cardiol* 1993;72:154–161.

220. Muller JE. Sexual activity as a trigger for cardiovascular events: what is the risk? *Am J Cardiol* 1999;84:2N–5N.

221. Papadopoulos C, Larrimore P, Cardin S, et al. Sexual concerns and needs of the postcoronary patient's wife. *Arch Intern Med* 1980;140:38–41.

222. Papadopoulos C, Beaumont C, Shelley SI, et al. Myocardial infarction and sexual activity of the female patient. *Arch Intern Med* 1983;143:1528–1530.

223. DeBusk R, Drory Y, Goldstein I, et al. Management of sexual dysfunction in patients with cardiovascular disease: recommendations of The Princeton Consensus Panel. *Am J Cardiol* 2000;86:175–181.

224. DeBusk RF. Evaluating the cardiovascular tolerance for sex. *Am J Cardiol* 2000;86:51F–56F.

225. Porter A, Mager A, Birnbaum Y, et al. Acute myocardial infarction following sildenafil citrate (Viagra) intake in a nitrate-free patient. *Clin Cardiol* 1999;22:762–763.

226. Kloner RA. Cardiovascular risk and sildenafil. *Am J Cardiol* 2000;86:57F–61F.

227. Johnston BL, Cantwell JD, Watt EW, et al. Sexual activity in exercising patients after myocardial infarction and revascularization. *Heart Lung* 1978;7:1026–1031.

228. Muller JE, Mittleman A, Maclure M, et al. Triggering myocardial infarction by sexual activity: low absolute risk and prevention by regular physical exertion. Determinants of Myocardial Infarction Onset Study Investigators. *JAMA* 1996;275:1405–1409.

229. Kimmel SE. Sex and myocardial infarction: an epidemiologic perspective. *Am J Cardiol* 2000;86:10F–13F.

230. Hebert PR, Buring JE, O'Connor GT, et al. Occupation and risk of nonfatal myocardial infarction. *Arch Intern Med* 1992;152:2253–2257.

231. Petrie KJ, Weinman J, Sharpe N, et al. Role of patients' view of their illness in predicting return to work and functioning after myocardial infarction: longitudinal study. *BMJ* 1996;312:1191–1194.

232. Boudrez H, De Backer G, Comhaire B. Return to work after myocardial infarction: results of a longitudinal population based study. *Eur Heart J* 1994;15:32–36.

233. Zahger D, Leibowitz D, Tabb IK, et al. Long-distance air travel soon after an acute coronary syndrome: a prospective evaluation of a triage protocol. *Am Heart J* 2000;140:241–242.

234. Muntwyler J, Hennekens CH, Buring JE, et al. Mortality and light to moderate alcohol consumption after myocardial infarction. *Lancet* 1998;352:1882–1885.

235. Gaziano JM, Hennekens CH, Godfried SL, et al. Type of alcoholic beverage and risk of myocardial infarction. *Am J Cardiol* 1999;83:52–57.

236. Shaper AG, Wannamethee SG. Alcohol intake and mortality in middle aged men with diagnosed coronary heart disease. *Heart* 2000;83:394–399.

237. Kaufman DW, Rosenberg L, Helmrich SP, et al. Alcoholic beverages and myocardial infarction in young men. *Am J Epidemiol* 1985;121:548–554.

238. Cleophas TJ, Tuinenberg E, van der Meulen J, et al. Wine consumption and other dietary variables in males under 60 before and after acute myocardial infarction. *Angiology* 1996;47:789–796.

239. La Vecchia C, Decarli A, Franceschi S, et al. Prevalence of chronic diseases in alcohol abstainers. *Epidemiology* 1995;6:436–438.

240. Ridker PM, Vaughan DE, Stampfer MJ, et al. Association of moderate alcohol consumption and plasma concentration of endogenous tissue-type plasminogen activator. *JAMA* 1994;272:929–933.

241. Serebruany VL, Lowry DR, Fuzailov SY, et al. Moderate alcohol consumption is associated with decreased platelet activity in patients presenting with acute myocardial infarction. *J Thromb Thrombolysis* 2000;9:229–234.

242. Numminen H, Syrjala M, Benthin G, et al. The effect of acute ingestion of a large dose of alcohol on the hemostatic system and its circadian variation. *Stroke* 2000;31:1269–1273.

243. Moreyra AE, Kostis JB, Passannante AJ, et al. Acute myocardial infarction in patients with normal coronary arteries after acute ethanol intoxication. *Clin Cardiol* 1982;5:425–430.

244. Fraser GE, Upsdell M. Alcohol and other discriminants between cases of sudden death and myocardial infarction. *Am J Epidemiol* 1981;114:462–476.

245. Bergstrand R, Vedin A, Wilhelmsson C, et al. Characteristics of males with myocardial infarction below age 40. *J Chronic Dis* 1983;36:289–296.

246. Wannamethee SG, Shaper AG. Patterns of alcohol intake and risk of stroke in middle-aged British men. *Stroke* 1996;27:1033–1039.

247. Bianchi C, Negri E, La Vecchia C, et al. Alcohol consumption and the risk of acute myocardial infarction in women. *J Epidemiol Community Health* 1993;47:308–311.

248. Gould L, Gopalaswamy C, Yang D, et al. Effect of oral alcohol on left ventricular ejection fraction, volumes, and segmental wall motion in normals and in patients with recent myocardial infarction. *Clin Cardiol* 1985;8:576–582.

249. Yano K, Rhoads GG, Kagan A. Coffee, alcohol and risk of coronary heart disease among Japanese men living in Hawaii. *N Engl J Med* 1977;297:405–409.

250. D'Avanzo B, La Vecchia C, Tognoni G, et al. Coffee consumption and risk of acute myocardial infarction in Italian males. GISSI-EFRIM. Gruppo Italiano per lo Studio della Sopravvivenza nell'Infarto, Epidemiologia dei Fattori di Rischio dell'Infarto Miocardico. *Ann Epidemiol* 1993;3:595–604.

251. Kleemola P, Jousilahti P, Pietinen P, et al. Coffee consumption and the risk of coronary heart disease and death. *Arch Intern Med* 2000;160:3393–3400.

252. La Vecchia C, Gentile A, Negri E, et al. Coffee consumption and myocardial infarction in women. *Am J Epidemiol* 1989;130:481–485.

253. Klatsky AL, Friedman GD, Armstrong MA. Coffee use prior to myocardial infarction restudied: heavier intake may increase the risk. *Am J Epidemiol* 1990;132:479–488.

254. Singh RB, Rastogi SS, Verma R, et al. Randomised controlled trial of cardioprotective diet in patients with recent acute myocardial infarction: results of one year follow up. *BMJ* 1992;304:1015–1019.

255. Morris MC, Manson JE, Rosner B, et al. Fish consumption and cardiovascular disease in the physicians' health study: a prospective study. *Am J Epidemiol* 1995;142:166–175.

256. Pais P, Pogue J, Gerstein H, et al. Risk factors for acute myocardial infarction in Indians: a case-control study. *Lancet* 1996;348:358–363.

257. Tofler GH, Muller JE, Stone PH, et al. Comparison of long-term outcome after acute myocardial infarction in patients never graduated from high school with that in more educated patients. Multicenter Investigation of the Limitation of Infarct Size (MILIS). *Am J Cardiol* 1993;71:1031–1035.

258. Allison TG, Williams DE, Miller TD, et al. Medical and economic costs of psychologic distress in patients with coronary artery disease. *Mayo Clin Proc* 1995;70:734–742.

259. Hoffmann A, Pfiffner D, Hornung R, et al. Psychosocial factors predict medical outcome following a first myocardial infarction. Working Group on Cardiac Rehabilitation of the Swiss Society of Cardiology. *Coron Artery Dis* 1995;6:147–152.

260. Friedman S. Cardiac disease, anxiety, and sexual functioning. *Am J Cardiol* 2000;86:46F–50F.

261. Bar-On D, Gilutz H, Maymon T, et al. Long-term prognosis of low-risk, post-MI patients: the importance of subjective perception of disease. *Eur Heart J* 1994;15:1611–1615.

262. Trzcieniecka-Green A, Steptoe A. The effects of stress management on the quality of life of patients following acute myocardial infarction or coronary bypass surgery. *Eur Heart J* 1996;17:1663–1670.

263. Shekelle RB, Gale M, Ostfeld AM, et al. Hostility, risk of coronary heart disease, and mortality. *Psychosom Med* 1983;45:109–114.

264. Everson SA, Kauhanen J, Kaplan GA, et al. Hostility and increased risk of mortality and acute myocardial infarction: the mediating role of behavioral risk factors. *Am J Epidemiol* 1997;146:142–152.

265. Welin CL, Rosengren A, Wilhelmsen LW. Behavioural characteristics in patients with myocardial infarction: a case-control study. *J Cardiovasc Risk* 1995;2:247–254.

266. Eaker ED, Abbott RD, Kannel WB. Frequency of uncomplicated angina pectoris in type A compared with type B persons (the Framingham Study). *Am J Cardiol* 1989;63:1042–1045.

267. Gallacher JE, Yarnell JW, Butland BK. Type A behaviour and prevalent heart disease in the Caerphilly study: increase in risk or symptom reporting? *J Epidemiol Community Health* 1988;42:226–231.

268. O'Connor NJ, Manson JE, O'Connor GT, et al. Psychosocial risk factors and nonfatal myocardial infarction. *Circulation* 1995;92:1458–1464.

269. Denollet J, Sys SU, Stroobant N, et al. Personality as independent predictor of long-term mortality in patients with coronary heart disease. *Lancet* 1996;347:417–421.

270. Shores MM, Pascualy M, Veith RC. Major Depression and Heart Disease: Treatment Trials. *Semin Clin Neuropsychiatry* 1998;3:87–101.

271. Roose SP, Spatz E. Treating depression in patients with ischaemic heart disease: which agents are best to use and to avoid? *Drug Saf* 1999;20:459–465.

272. Friedmann E, Thomas SA. Pet ownership, social support, and one-year survival after acute myocardial infarction in the Cardiac Arrhythmia Suppression Trial (CAST). *Am J Cardiol* 1995;76:1213–1217.

273. Mehta RH, Das S, Tsai TT, et al. Quality improvement initiative and its impact on the management of patients with acute myocardial infarction. *Arch Intern Med* 2000;160:3057–3062.

274. Marciniak TA, Ellerbeck EF, Radford MJ, et al. Improving the quality of care for Medicare patients with acute myocardial infarction: results from the Cooperative Cardiovascular Project. *JAMA* 1998;279:1351–1357.

275. Jolly K, Bradley F, Sharp S, et al. Randomised controlled trial of follow up care in general practice of patients with myocar-

dial infarction and angina: final results of the Southampton heart integrated care project (SHIP). The SHIP Collaborative Group. *BMJ* 1999;318:706–711.

276. Ryan TJ, Anderson JL, Antman EM, et al. ACC/AHA guidelines for the management of patients with acute myocardial infarction: a report of the American College of Cardiology/American Heart Association Task Force on Practice Guidelines (Committee on Management of Acute Myocardial Infarction). *J Am Coll Cardiol* 1996;28:1328–1428.

277. Ryan TJ, Antman EM, Brooks NH, et al. 1999 update: ACC/AHA guidelines for the management of patients with acute myocardial infarction. A report of the American College of Cardiology/American Heart Association Task Force on Practice Guidelines (Committee on Management of Acute Myocardial Infarction). *J Am Coll Cardiol* 1999;34:890–911.

278. Chen J, Radford MJ, Wang Y, et al. Do "America's Best Hospitals" perform better for acute myocardial infarction? *N Engl J Med* 1999;340:286–292.

279. Ellerbeck EF, Jencks SF, Radford MJ, et al. Quality of care for Medicare patients with acute myocardial infarction: a four-state pilot study from the Cooperative Cardiovascular Project. *JAMA* 1995;273:1509–1514.

280. Pilote L, Califf RM, Sapp S, et al. Regional variation across the United States in the management of acute myocardial infarction. GUSTO-1 Investigators. Global Utilization of Streptokinase and Tissue Plasminogen Activator for Occluded Coronary Arteries. *N Engl J Med* 1995;333:565–572.

281. O'Connor GT, Quinton HB, Traven ND, et al. Geographic variation in the treatment of acute myocardial infarction: the Cooperative Cardiovascular Project. *JAMA* 1999;281:627–633.

282. Canto JG, Rogers WJ, French WJ, et al. Payer status and the utilization of hospital resources in acute myocardial infarction: a report from the National Registry of Myocardial Infarction 2. *Arch Intern Med* 2000;160:817–823.

283. Hall D, Zeitler H, Rudolph W. Counteraction of the vasodilator effects of enalapril by aspirin in severe heart failure. *J Am Coll Cardiol* 1992;20:1549–1555.

284. Peterson JG, Topol EJ, Sapp SK, et al. Evaluation of the effects of aspirin combined with angiotensin-converting enzyme inhibitors in patients with coronary artery disease. *Am J Med* 2000;109:371–377.

285. Beer JH, Pederiva S, Pontiggia L. Genetics of platelet receptor single-nucleotide polymorphisms: clinical implications in thrombosis. *Ann Med* 2000;32[Suppl 1]:10–14.

286. Mrozikiewicz PM, Cascorbi I, Ziemer S, et al. Reduced procedural risk for coronary catheter interventions in carriers of the coagulation factor VII-Gln353 gene. *J Am Coll Cardiol* 2000;36:1520–1525.

287. Vijayan KV, Goldschmidt-Clermont PJ, Roos C, et al. The Pl(A2) polymorphism of integrin beta(3) enhances outside-in signaling and adhesive functions. *J Clin Invest* 2000;105:793–802.

288. Undas A, Sanak M, Musial J, et al. Platelet glycoprotein IIIa polymorphism, aspirin, and thrombin generation. *Lancet* 1999;353:982–983.

289. Walter DH, Schachinger V, Elsner M, et al. Platelet glycoprotein IIIa polymorphisms and risk of coronary stent thrombosis. *Lancet* 1997;350:1217–1219.

290. Nurden AT. Platelet glycoprotein IIIa polymorphism and coronary thrombosis. *Lancet* 1997;350:1189–1191.

291. Topol EJ, Bolk S, Moliterno D, et al. Genetic basis of premature coronary atherosclerosis and myocardial infarction: role of the thrombospondin genes. *Circulation* 2000;102:II-31.

292. Haase KK, Schiele R, Wagner S, et al. In-hospital mortality of elderly patients with acute myocardial infarction: data from the MITRA (Maximal Individual Therapy in Acute Myocardial Infarction) registry. *Clin Cardiol* 2000;23:831–836.

293. Ambrosioni E, Borghi C, Magnani B. The effect of the angiotensin-converting-enzyme inhibitor zofenopril on mortality and morbidity after anterior myocardial infarction. The Survival of Myocardial Infarction Long-Term Evaluation (SMILE) Study Investigators. *N Engl J Med* 1995;332:80–85.

294. Kober L, Torp-Pedersen C, Carlsen JE, et al. A clinical trial of the angiotensin-converting-enzyme inhibitor trandolapril in patients with left ventricular dysfunction after myocardial infarction. Trandolapril Cardiac Evaluation (TRACE) Study Group. *N Engl J Med* 1995;333:1670–1676.

295. A randomized trial of propranolol in patients with acute myocardial infarction: I. Mortality results. *JAMA* 1982;247:1707–1714.

296. Hjalmarson A, Elmfeldt D, Herlitz J, et al. Effect on mortality of metoprolol in acute myocardial infarction: a double-blind randomised trial. *Lancet* 1981;2:823–827.

297. Randomised trial of intravenous atenolol among 16,027 cases of suspected acute myocardial infarction: ISIS-1. First International Study of Infarct Survival Collaborative Group. *Lancet* 1986;2:57–66.

298. Metoprolol in acute myocardial infarction (MIAMI): a randomised placebo-controlled international trial. The MIAMI Trial Research Group. *Eur Heart J* 1985;6:199–226.

299. Pedersen TR. Six-year follow-up of the Norwegian Multicenter Study on Timolol after Acute Myocardial Infarction. *N Engl J Med* 1985;313:1055–1058.

MITRAL VALVE DISEASE

JOSEPH S. ALPERT
JOSEPH F. SABIK III
DELOS M. COSGROVE

▼▼ ADDITIONAL ELECTRONIC TOPICS

Differential Diagnosis d75; Nonrheumatic Mitral Stenosis d76; Results of Valve Repair for Rheumatic Mitral Stenosis d77; Magnetic Resonance Imaging d78; Cardiac Catheterization d79; Mitral Valve Repair for Mitral Insufficiency d80

OVERVIEW

Mitral stenosis is almost invariably the result of chronic rheumatic heart disease secondary to one or more prior episodes of acute rheumatic fever. The beginning of modern cardiology is defined by the earliest clinical studies of mitral stenosis [1,2]. The disease can be recognized and its severity appreciated from a careful history and physical examination [3]. In more recent years, it has become possible to obtain a highly accurate assessment of the pathologic status of the mitral valve by means of a Doppler-echocardiographic examination. ▼▼ d81

NATURAL HISTORY OF MITRAL STENOSIS

The natural history of untreated mitral stenosis was carefully studied before the advent of cardiac surgical tech-

niques for relieving mitral stenosis [1,9]. Children who developed acute rheumatic fever had a 30% chance of dying over the subsequent 20 years, with more than 90% of these deaths attributed to heart disease [1]. Forty-five percent of survivors had clinical evidence of rheumatic heart disease; almost invariably, mitral stenosis was present in these latter patients.

Prospective clinical studies of patients with known mitral stenosis have shown that approximately one-half of these individuals are asymptomatic at the time of diagnosis if a young population (mean age, 28 years) is examined [9]. An additional 47% of patients had mild or moderate symptoms. Mortality was 39% at 10 years and 78% at 20 years. Most of the deaths were the result of heart failure or arterial embolism. If an older population (mean age, 42 years) is followed, more of the patients are symptomatic at the time of diagnosis (86%), and the 10-year mortality is higher (70%) [10]. The mortality at 20 years was only slightly higher (83%) than in the younger population, however. The 10-year mortality in a more recent observational study was 60% [11].

The average patient with mitral stenosis develops acute rheumatic fever for the first time at age 12. In general, the murmur of mitral stenosis is heard approximately 20 years

J. S. Alpert: Department of Medicine, University of Arizona Health Sciences Center, Tucson, Arizona

J. F. Sabik III: Department of Thoracic and Cardiovascular Surgery, The Cleveland Clinic Foundation, Cleveland, Ohio

D. M. Cosgrove: Department of Thoracic and Cardiovascular Surgery, The Cleveland Clinic Foundation, Cleveland, Ohio

later (2). Cardiac symptoms usually appear in the fourth or fifth decade in patients who live in industrialized nations. In developing countries, particularly tropical areas, the disease progresses more rapidly. This may be the result of prolonged or repetitive episodes of untreated acute rheumatic fever. In developing countries, one commonly observes teenagers or young adults with severe mitral stenosis. Symptoms develop gradually in approximately one-half of the patients; sudden development of symptoms is often the result of new onset atrial fibrillation.

The progression of mitral stenosis is generally slow, although wide variation in clinical progression exists among different patients. In Rowe's series, 40% of patients were clinically unaltered after 10 years (9). Grant followed 238 British servicemen with mitral stenosis for 10 years and noted that disease in one-third had progressed, one-third were unchanged, and one-third had died (12). More recent serial hemodynamic and Doppler-echocardiographic studies have demonstrated annual mitral valve area loss ranging from 0.09 to 0.32 cm² (13,14). The rate of progression of mitral valve narrowing was variable among individuals, however. Patients with the most stenotic valves and the largest mitral valve gradients tended to progress the most rapidly (14).

Anatomic Considerations

As already noted, stenotic mitral valves are the result of relatively few conditions, with rheumatic heart disease as the etiology in all but a rare patient. With respect to operatively excised rheumatic mitral valves, 83% were stenotic with or without accompanying mitral regurgitation; 17% were purely regurgitant (4,15). Because of a decreasing incidence of acute rheumatic fever in the United States, the percentage of operatively excised valves that are stenotic is declining in comparison with valves that are purely regurgitant.

The anatomic features of rheumatic mitral stenosis are listed in Table 21.1. The initial valvular pathologic lesion in acute rheumatic fever consists of valvulitis manifesting as a series of translucent nodules along the line of closure of the mitral valve. With chronic mitral stenosis, the mitral valve is thickened, fibrotic, and often calcified. Aschoff bodies in the myocardium demonstrate that an attack of rheumatic fever has occurred in the past. ◥ d82

TABLE 21.1 ANATOMIC FEATURES OF RHEUMATIC MITRAL STENOSIS

Diffuse fibrous thickening of the margins of closure
Fibrous thickening involving the entire anterior and posterior leaflets, producing leaflet rigidity
One or both valve commissures fuse, reducing the size of the mitral orifice
Shortened, thickened, and fused chordae tendineae leading to subvalvular stenosis
Calcific deposits in one or both leaflets
Presence of Aschoff's nodules (bodies) in the myocardium

Pathophysiology

It has been suggested that the mitral valvulitis associated with an episode of acute rheumatic fever leads to abnormal flow patterns across the valve. These altered flow patterns place increased tension on an already damaged valve. Furthermore, valve inflammation can lead to fibrin deposition on the valve surface, thereby further increasing abnormality of flow patterns across the valve. The eventual outcome from years of abnormal tension and stress placed on the mitral valve is fibrosis and thickening. It is also possible that smoldering rheumatic immunologic activity continues to damage the valve, leading to progressive fibrosis (3).

In adults, the normal mitral valve area is approximately 4 to 6 cm². As mitral stenosis progressively narrows the valve orifice, a gradient develops between the left atrium and the left ventricle. This gradient is usually small and clinically unimportant until the mitral valve area is narrowed to less than 2.0 cm². Cardiac output and heart rate also affect the mitral valve gradient: The greater the cardiac output, the larger the gradient; faster heart rates are associated with shortened diastolic filling times and hence larger mitral valve gradients. Atrial fibrillation with fast ventricular response markedly shortens the diastolic filling time, thereby leading to a large increase in the mitral valve gradient. Of course, the larger the mitral valve gradient, the higher the left atrial, pulmonary venous, and pulmonary capillary pressures.

Exercise augments cardiac output and heart rate simultaneously. This can lead to marked increases in left atrial pressure with resulting pulmonary congestion and dyspnea on exertion. When the mitral orifice is reduced to 1.0 cm² or less, severe mitral stenosis is said to be present: Left atrial pressure is elevated at rest. At this point in the natural history of mitral stenosis, the gradient across the valve is approximately 20 mm Hg, depending, of course, on the magnitude of the cardiac output. Because normal left ventricular mean diastolic pressure is usually 5 mm Hg, left atrial and pulmonary capillary wedge pressure in these patients is approximately 25 mm Hg (3). Pulmonary capillary wedge pressure in this range leads to marked transudation of fluid into the pulmonary interstitium. ◥ d83

The etiology of a number of complications of mitral stenosis can be explained by examining the abnormal hemodynamic state produced by severe mitral stenosis (Table 21.2). Thus, pulmonary edema develops when the pulmonary capillary pressure exceeds 25 mm Hg, thereby favoring transudation of fluid from the capillary lumen into the pulmonary interstitium and alveoli. Atrial fibrillation is the result of left atrial dilatation and hypertrophy. Systemic embolism occurs as a result of left atrial thrombosis, which, in turn, is the result of sluggish flow in the dilated, fibrillating left atrium. Factors that increase the risk of systemic embolism for patients still in sinus rhythm include advanced age, the presence of left atrial thrombus, decreasing mitral valve area, and the presence of significant aortic regurgitation. For individuals in atrial fibrillation, the risk

TABLE 21.2 PATHOPHYSIOLOGY OF SYMPTOMS AND COMPLICATIONS OF MITRAL STENOSIS

Elevated left atrial, pulmonary venous, and pulmonary capillary pressure leads to dyspnea, pulmonary edema, hemoptysis

Dilated left atrium leads to atrial fibrillation, systemic embolism, dysphagia (rare)

Pulmonary hypertension leads to right ventricular failure (fatigue, peripheral edema, ascites, cyanosis, venous thromboembolism), vocal cord paralysis secondary to left recurrent laryngeal nerve compression

Abnormal valvular structure with roughened surface leads to infective endocarditis

---

TABLE 21.3 FINDINGS ON PHYSICAL EXAMINATION IN PATIENTS WITH MITRAL STENOSIS

Inspection
  Malar flush
  Peripheral cyanosis (severe mitral stenosis)
  Jugular venous distension (right ventricular failure)
Palpation
  Parasternal right ventricular impulse
  Palpable pulmonary arterial impulse
  Palpable first heart sound, pulmonary component of the second heart sound, and occasionally, the diastolic rumble
Auscultation
  Increased intensity of the first heart sound
  Opening snap
  Low-pitched diastolic rumbling murmur

---

of arterial embolism increases if there is a history of a previous embolic episode. Mitral commissurotomy decreases the risk for arterial embolism (20a). Hemoptysis results from the rupture of small venules secondary to sudden increases in pulmonary venous pressure, such as might occur in a patient with moderate to severe mitral stenosis who performs strenuous exercise. In industrialized countries, progression of the mitral stenotic process is slow as is the development of pulmonary hypertension. Pulmonary venules gradually thicken in response to increased pulmonary venous pressure. Thus, rupture of venules secondary to sudden accentuation of pulmonary venous hypertension (e.g., in response to exercise) is uncommon, as is hemoptysis. As noted earlier, the pathophysiologic sequence of mitral stenosis occurs at an accelerated pace in patients living in developing nations where the symptom of hemoptysis is more common. An unusual complication of mitral stenosis is hoarseness that develops secondary to compression of the left recurrent laryngeal nerve by a dilated left pulmonary artery, thereby leading to vocal cord paralysis. Rarely, patients report dysphagia, which is the result of esophageal compression by a dilated left atrium. ▼ d84

Clinical Profile

History

Fifty percent or more of patients with mitral stenosis do not recall having had acute rheumatic fever. In midlife, these patients report dyspnea on exertion. Younger female patients may report an unusual degree of dyspnea during pregnancy. The onset of atrial fibrillation with a rapid ventricular response may also produce marked dyspnea and even pulmonary edema. This is the result of a marked decrease in diastolic filling period, resulting in a concomitant increase in left atrial pressure. Cardiac output may also decrease, producing the sensation of fatigue. ▼ d85

Physical Examination

Patients with mitral stenosis have a number of characteristic physical findings (Table 21.3). The malar flush may be observed in patients with fair complexions. Jugular venous

distension is the result of right ventricular failure. Prominent cardiovascular waves are noted in patients with concomitant tricuspid regurgitation. Peripheral cyanosis is a late finding resulting from low cardiac output. The dilated hypertrophied right ventricle may be palpated during systole along the left sternal border. A systolic impulse from the dilated pulmonary artery can occasionally be felt in the second or third left intercostal space.

The low-pitched, diastolic rumble of mitral stenosis is best heard at the apex with the patient in the left lateral decubitus position. It is usually accompanied by an accentuated first heart sound (S_1), which is the result of rapid closure of a thickened but pliable valve. The more severe the mitral stenosis, the shorter the interval between the second heart sound (S_2) and the opening snap (OS). As the stenotic valve becomes progressively fibrotic, calcified, and "fixed" (i.e., minimal to no valve mobility), the intensity of the S_1 diminishes and the OS may become inaudible. This is the result of ever-decreasing cardiac output and excursion of the mitral valve leaflets at the time of valve closure. The rumbling diastolic murmur may also be extremely difficult to hear in patients with severe "end-stage" mitral stenosis accompanied by low cardiac output and right ventricular failure.

The OS is the most characteristic feature of mitral stenosis. It occurs when the mitral valve reaches its maximum opening excursion into the left ventricular cavity. The OS may occur between 0.03 and 0.13 seconds after the S_2. An S_2-OS interval (time from the S_2 to the OS) of less than 0.08 seconds implies a markedly elevated left atrial pressure and severe mitral stenosis (24,25). The OS is unfortunately not pathognomonic for mitral stenosis. It can also be heard in patients with mitral regurgitation, ventricular septal defect, second- and third-degree heart block, tricuspid atresia with a large atrial septal defect, and tetralogy of Fallot treated with a Blalock-Taussig shunt (26,27). The OS of mitral stenosis is best heard using the diaphragm of the stethoscope and searching between the left sternal border and the apex. The OS can be differentiated from the pulmonic component of the S_2 because the latter occurs earlier.

The mitral stenotic diastolic rumble may be difficult to hear, particularly in a thick-chested or obese individual. A brief period of exercise may accentuate the murmur. In the early stages of mitral stenosis, the murmur is confined to mid-diastole; as the stenotic valve worsens, the murmur becomes holodiastolic with presystolic accentuation (25). The intensity of the murmur does not correlate with the severity of mitral stenosis, but the duration of the murmur does; patients with severe mitral stenosis often display a holodiastolic murmur (25). The murmur of mitral stenosis is best heard with the bell of the stethoscope held lightly against the shin over the apex impulse with the patient in the left lateral decubitus position. The murmur can be accentuated by exercise, deeply held expiration, or inhalation of amyl nitrite. Presystolic accentuation of the murmur is normally heard when the patient is in sinus rhythm. However, presystolic accentuation is occasionally observed in patients with moderately regular atrial fibrillation (28,29). ☜ d86

Diastolic rumbles can be the result of other conditions besides mitral stenosis, including left atrial myxoma, atrial or ventricular septal defect, patent ductus arteriosus, cor triatriatum, severe aortic regurgitation (the Austin Flint murmur), or tricuspid stenosis. Mitral stenosis may go unsuspected in patients who are elderly, obese, emphysematous, or have other complicating pulmonary, cardiovascular, or chest wall diseases (31).

Electrocardiography

Many patients with mitral stenosis are in atrial fibrillation. Those in sinus rhythm usually demonstrate left atrial enlargement on electrocardiography (ECG) (Table 21.4). Left atrial enlargement by ECG correlates more closely with atrial volume than with atrial pressure (32). ECG signs of left atrial enlargement often regress following successful valvulotomy (2). Left ventricular hypertrophy is notably absent. When pulmonary hypertension leads to right ventricular hypertrophy and dilatation, the pattern of right ventricular hypertrophy may be seen in the ECG (Table 21.4). The sensitivity of the ECG diagnosis of right ventricular hypertrophy is not high. However, right ventric-

TABLE 21.4 ELECTROCARDIOGRAPHY IN MITRAL STENOSIS

Atrial fibrillation is common
In sinus rhythm, P mitrale is present
   Prolonged M-shaped P wave (duration >0.12 sec in lead II)
   Marked terminal negative component to the P wave in lead V_1
     (1.0 mm wide and 1.0 mm deep)
   P wave axis between +45 and −30 degrees
Severe mitral stenosis is often accompanied by findings of right
    ventricular hypertrophy
   Right axis deviation (QRS axis >80 degrees)
   R wave >S wave in lead V_1

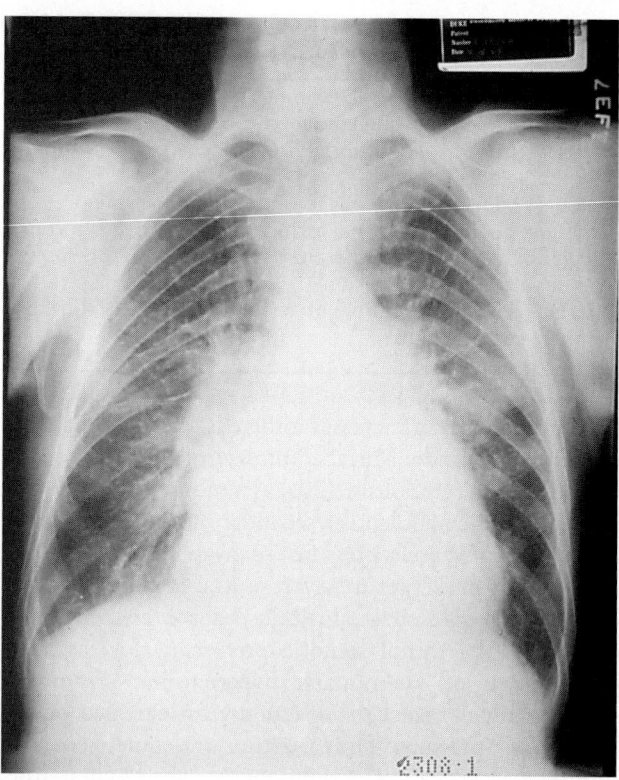

FIGURE 21.1 Chest roentgenogram from a 50-year-old woman with severe, long-standing mitral stenosis complicated by pulmonary hypertension. The overall cardiac silhouette is enlarged secondary to right atrial, right ventricular, left atrial, and pulmonary arterial dilatation. The left ventricle was found to be normal in size during an echocardiographic examination. Marked pulmonary congestion is present.

ular hypertrophy by ECG is almost always present if right ventricular systolic pressure exceeds 100 mm Hg.

Chest Roentgenography

Chest roentgenographic findings in mitral stenosis include left atrial enlargement, redistribution of pulmonary vascular flow to the upper lung fields, calcification of the mitral valve, an enlarged pulmonary artery, and an enlarged right ventricle (3). Other signs of elevated pulmonary venous pressure may be present, such as Kerley A and B lines and interstitial pulmonary edema (Fig. 21.1). ☜ d87

Echocardiography

A modern two-dimensional Doppler-echocardiographic examination of the heart can accurately characterize the severity and extent of the pathologic process in patients with mitral stenosis. A variety of M-mode and two-dimensional findings have been shown to correlate quite well with the hemodynamic determination of mitral valve area (33–37). Severe mitral valvular calcification, fibrosis, and limited leaflet excursion can also be identified. The anatomic abnormalities of the stenotic mitral valve (i.e., thickening, diastolic doming, and restriction of leaflet motion) are usually well defined by transthoracic echocardiography. The size of the stenotic mitral valvular orifice is often clearly visualized and quantitated. Doppler-echocardiographic analysis identifies the presence and severity of regurgitation of the aortic, mitral, and tricuspid valves. Two-dimensional echocardiography is more accurate than M-mode echocardiography in defining the severity of mitral stenosis (38). This is especially true when Doppler studies are added to the two-dimensional echocardiographic analysis. An occasional patient requires a transesophageal study to visualize the stenotic mitral valve. Transthoracic echocardiography is sufficient for diagnosis in the vast majority of patients with mitral stenosis. Valvular vegetations can almost invariably be seen with the aid of transthoracic or transesophageal echocardiography in mitral stenosis patients whose course has been complicated by infectious endocarditis.

Echocardiographic study also yields important information concerning left and right ventricular systolic and diastolic function and size, left atrial size, and the presence of other valvular lesions. Transesophageal echocardiography is quite accurate in identifying thrombus in the left atrium and the left atrial appendage, as well as spontaneous echoes in the left atrial cavity that can predict thrombus formation in the future (39,40). Factors that correlate with spontaneous left atrial echoes and hence an increased risk for thrombus formation and eventual arterial embolism include decreasing degrees of mitral regurgitation, absence of left atrial appendage blood flow, and decreasing mitral valve area (40a). Finally, an accurate measure of mean pulmonary arterial pressure can be obtained from a Doppler examination of a tricuspid valve regurgitant jet. Only a small regurgitant jet is required for this analysis. Many patients do not require invasive study once a thorough Doppler-echocardiographic examination is completed. Coronary arteriography may be the only form of diagnostic catheterization performed in the patient with severe mitral stenosis. ❦ d88

Cardiac Catheterization

Cardiac catheterization was formerly the gold standard for determining the severity of mitral stenosis. The accuracy of Doppler-echocardiographic techniques has resulted in only selective use of cardiac catheterization in patients with mitral stenosis, however. As noted in Table 21.5, cardiac catheterization is most useful in identifying concomitant coronary artery disease and quantifying the degree of mitral regurgitation that is present. Assessing the level of pulmonary hypertension is also of considerable importance. Less important is the evaluation of left and right ventricular function, because this information is often obtained with considerable accuracy from the echocardiographic study. Quantifying the amount of aortic regurgitation that is present can also be of value, because the Doppler-echocardiographic study may underestimate the aortic regurgitant volume. Most centers accept the echocardiographic assessment of severity of aortic regurgitation, and only an occasional patient requires aortic root cineangiography. ❦ d89

TABLE 21.5 INFORMATION THAT MAY BE OBTAINED FROM CARDIAC CATHETERIZATION IN PATIENTS WITH MITRAL STENOSIS THAT MAY NOT BE ALREADY AVAILABLE FROM A DOPPLER-ECHOCARDIOGRAPHIC STUDY

Important
  Assessment of coronary artery disease
  Quantification of mitral regurgitation
  Confirmation of presence or absence of pulmonary hypertension (pulmonary vascular disease)
Moderately important
  Assessment of right ventricular and right atrial pressures: presence of right ventricular failure
  Assessment of aortic valve function: presence and quantity of aortic regurgitation
Modestly important
  Confirmation and quantification of the degree of mitral valve obstruction

Therapy

Medical Therapy of Mitral Stenosis

Medical therapy of mitral stenosis seeks to prevent and treat complications associated with the disease (Table 21.6). In general, symptomatic mitral stenosis is best treated by relieving the mitral valvular obstruction either by means of balloon valvuloplasty or surgical intervention (valvuloplasty, valve replacement). However, prevention or treatment of a variety of complications associated with mitral stenosis is often necessary (Table 21.6).

Symptomatic dyspnea can be ameliorated with diuretics, as well as short- or long-acting nitrate preparations, but these agents are usually only of temporary benefit. Patients with dyspnea associated with bronchospasm may respond to inhaled corticosteroids (45a). Mitral valvuloplasty or replacement is indicated in symptomatic patients with mitral stenosis. Cerebral embolism is often a devastating complication of mitral stenosis, accounting for 60% to 70%

TABLE 21.6 THERAPEUTIC GOALS IN PATIENTS WITH MITRAL STENOSIS

Reduce symptoms of pulmonary congestion (dyspnea on exertion, paroxysmal nocturnal dyspnea, pulmonary edema): diuretics, nitrates
Prevent arterial embolism (cerebral or peripheral arterial embolism): anticoagulation
Prevent infectious endocarditis: prophylactic antibiotics
Treat bacterial endocarditis: antibiotics
Prevent/treat atrial fibrillation: digoxin, beta-blockers, antiarrhythmic agents, anticoagulants

of episodes of systemic embolism (46). Episodes of systemic embolism can occur in patients with moderate, severe, and even mild mitral stenosis; the risk for this complication increases markedly when atrial fibrillation develops. Embolism can be fatal. In the series of patients with mitral stenosis followed by Rowe et al., 19% of the deaths were attributed to arterial embolism (9). Increasing age and left atrial size both augment the risk of systemic embolism (47,48).

Prophylactic antibiotics are administered to patients with mitral stenosis before dental work, as well as a variety of other interventions (see Chapter 25), to minimize the risk of developing infectious endocarditis. Prolonged courses of intravenous antibiotics are given to patients who develop infectious endocarditis, which is more likely to develop in patients with concomitant mitral or aortic regurgitation (46). Mitral regurgitation usually develops or worsens in patients with mitral stenosis who develop infectious endocarditis.

Atrial fibrillation is a commonly occurring complication in patients with mitral stenosis. Initially, it develops as transient paroxysms; later in the course of the illness, atrial fibrillation is sustained. Often the ventricular response is rapid (>140 beats/min), resulting in a shortened diastolic filling period with concomitant pulmonary venous hypertension. Many of these patients complain of dyspnea at rest, and pulmonary edema may develop.

The loss of atrial contraction has little effect on mitral valve flow in the patient with mitral stenosis in whom left atrial pressure is already quite elevated (49). The size of the fibrillatory waves in the ECG are unrelated to left atrial size (50). In most series of patients with mitral stenosis, approximately 40% of patients have sustained atrial fibrillation with the incidence of the arrhythmia increasing with age and left atrial size (51,52). Patients with mitral stenosis and atrial fibrillation, paroxysmal or sustained, should receive prophylactic anticoagulation with warfarin unless a strong contraindication exists. Some authorities favor prophylactic anticoagulation for all patients with mitral stenosis—even those in sinus rhythm—once they are older than 35 to 40 years, because cerebral or peripheral arterial embolism can occur at any time in the course of the illness (50). Patients who are candidates for warfarin anticoagulation should receive 5 mg per day for 3 days. Thereafter, the daily dose of warfarin is determined by the measured prothrombin time (52). An international normalized ratio between 2.0 and 3.0 should be maintained long-term (52).

Attempts to maintain sinus rhythm with antiarrhythmic medication are often unrewarding and carry the risk of proarrhythmia, syncope, and even sudden death. Many clinicians favor controlling the ventricular response with digoxin combined with beta-blockers or diltiazem. Verapamil may also be employed for this purpose. Chronic anticoagulation with warfarin is also employed. Patients who develop pulmonary edema secondary to a rapid ventricular response are candidates for urgent electrical cardioversion. In less urgent circumstances, reversion to sinus rhythm can often be achieved by administering 1,000 mg of intravenous procainamide over 30 to 60 minutes. Once sinus rhythm is reestablished, it can usually be maintained with intravenous procainamide, 2 mg per minute. Blood pressure and QRS duration should be followed closely during procainamide infusion. The dosage should be decreased if arterial blood pressure falls below 100 mm Hg systolic or if QRS duration exceeds 0.10 seconds. If the clinical decision is in favor of elective cardioversion, patients who have been in atrial fibrillation for 48 hours or more should be anticoagulated with warfarin for 3 to 4 weeks before and for 4 weeks after cardioversion.

Beta-blocker therapy has occasionally been used to slow the heart rate in patients still in sinus rhythm. Because the size of the mitral valvular gradient is directly proportional to heart rate, interventions that lower the heart rate, such as beta-blockade, lead to a reduction in the valvular gradient and hence to a lower pulmonary capillary wedge pressure.

Interventional Therapy: Percutaneous Balloon Mitral Commissurotomy

Percutaneous transvenous valvotomy is usually performed with specially designed balloon catheters that are advanced across the stenotic mitral valve from the left atrial side. The catheter is placed in the left atrium using a venous transseptal technique. The balloon is inflated, thereby separating the stenotic leaflets (55–57). However, the procedure can also be performed by placing the balloon catheter across the mitral valve using a retrograde, transaortic, arterial route. Early results with this retrograde technique have been good, although local arterial complications were more common than with the transvenous technique (57a,57b). A new percutaneous technique, employing a metallic valvulotome attached to a catheter, has given excellent short-term results. Multiple uses are possible with this device, thereby reducing the cost for percutaneous mitral commissurotomy. Comparison with the traditional balloon technique and long-term results are not available as yet (58c). The procedure resembles surgical, closed mitral valvuloplasty. In some patients, leaflet calcification may also fracture.

Patients should be carefully selected for this procedure by means of two-dimensional echocardiography. Individuals with symptomatic mitral stenosis and pliable, mobile, relatively thin, and minimally calcified valves are the best candidates for balloon valvuloplasty. Some clinicians favor studying the patient with transesophageal echocardiography before balloon valvuloplasty to ensure that no thrombus is present in the left atrium. Short-term and intermediate-term results are quite good when compared with surgical valvuloplasty (55–57). Long-term results are excellent as well (58,59). In one study, two-thirds of patients treated with percutaneous balloon mitral commissurotomy were in good clinical condition and free of any major event 7 years after the procedure. However, the mitral valve area decreased progressively with time, although mitral regurgitation did not progress (58a). Similar good long-term results have also been observed by other investigators (58a,58b,58d). However, Hildick-Smith and coworkers reported more modest but still acceptable long-term results in a western European population with unfavorable characteristics (58e). In addition to the usual adult population of patients with mitral stenosis, balloon valvulotomy has been successfully employed in children and pregnant women (58e–58g).

Mitral valve area usually increases to 2.0 cm² or more following balloon valvuloplasty, whereas left atrial pressure declines and cardiac output increases (60,61). Symptoms of pulmonary congestion are relieved. A small residual atrial septal defect can be identified in a small number of patients. It is of considerable interest that relief of mitral stenosis is associated with improvement in both systolic and diastolic measures of left ventricular performance (62–64). Repeat balloon valvuloplasty can be performed successfully in patients who develop restenosis (64b). ⚐ d90

Surgery for Rheumatic Mitral Stenosis

The pioneering work of Souttar, Cutler, Harken, and Bailey (68–71) began the era of the surgical treatment of mitral valve disease. Their early operations were closed mitral commissurotomies for rheumatic mitral stenosis. Today, with the assistance of cardiopulmonary bypass and myocardial protection, surgeons are no longer blinded to the valve pathology but can directly inspect the mitral valve and repair or replace the valve. Techniques for mitral valve repair have evolved to such a degree that severely regurgitant or stenotic mitral valves may be repaired with excellent long-term results. For mitral valves unsuitable for repair, both bioprosthetic and prosthetic valves are available.

The standard approach to mitral valve surgery is through a median sternotomy. Cardiopulmonary bypass is performed with direct aortic cannulation for arterial return and bicaudal cannulation for venous drainage. During the cross-clamp period, the heart may be protected with either antegrade cardioplegia or a combination of both antegrade and retrograde cardioplegia. Exposure for the mitral valve may be through a standard left atriotomy or through a transseptal approach, as advocated by Guirdon.

Mitral Valve Replacement

Two types of valves may be used to replace the mitral valve: prosthetic or bioprosthetic valves. The prosthetic valves are the mechanical valves and come in three main types: tilting single disk valves, bileaflet valves, and ball valves (see Chapter 24). Although excellent durability has been reported with the mechanical valves, the major drawback of these valves is that patients with mechanical valves must be anticoagulated with coumadin for life to prevent thromboembolic events. The bioprosthetic valves are stented, glutalderhyde-treated por-

cine valves (see Chapter 24) or trileaflet, glutalderhyde-treated bovine pericardial valves. Although the bioprosthetic valves lack the durability of the mechanical valves, patients in sinus rhythm with bioprosthetic valves do not need to be systemically anticoagulated with coumadin to prevent thrombosis or embolism. The major drawback of bioprosthetic porcine valves is that 20% to 40% fail over 10 years secondary to structural deterioration and require reoperation (72). In patients over the age of 70, however, structural deterioration is rare (73,74). Results of bovine pericardial mitral valve use suggest better long-term durability compared with porcine valves. In one study, actuarial freedom from structural valve deterioration at 10 years in patients with bovine pericardial mitral valves was 95% in patients 61 to 70 years old and 100% in patients greater than 71 years old (74a).

Although attempts have been made at establishing guidelines to assist surgeons as to which type of valve is best for certain patients, valve selection must be individualized for each patient. The selection of which type of valve to insert in which patient is based on weighing the disadvantages of anticoagulation-related complications associated with mechanical valves against the disadvantages of decreased longevity of the bioprosthetic valves. Mechanical valves are usually inserted in younger patients (<70) who have no contraindications to anticoagulation or in any patient who is already systemically anticoagulated for another reason, such as atrial fibrillation. Bioprosthetic valves are usually placed in older patients (>70) or in any patient who has a contraindication to systemic anticoagulation, such as a history of gastrointestinal hemorrhage. ⚐ d91

Results of Mitral Valve Replacement

Operative mortality correlates directly with the preoperative functional class of the patients undergoing mitral valve replacement. Patients in functional class three or less have a reported operative mortality of ≤2% (85–87). However, patients in functional class four have an operative mortality of 25% (85).

Five-year survival rates of 80% to 85% have been reported for patients undergoing mitral valve replacement (88–91). Surprisingly, long-term survival is independent of the type of valve inserted, but it is directly related to preoperative myocardial function (88–91). This emphasizes that patients with significant mitral valvular lesions should undergo mitral valve surgery before a significant decrease in their left ventricular function.

Thromboembolic complications occur in 2% to 4% of patients with mechanical valves per year who are adequately anticoagulated with coumadin (72). Of these thromboembolic events, however, 50% are minor, without any residual deficit or complication. Patients with porcine mitral valves who are not anticoagulated have a yearly thromboembolic rate of 1% to 3% (72,89,92). In patients in sinus rhythm with bioprosthetic valves and no anticoagulation, however, Cohn et al. observed no embolic events in patients followed for a mean of 3 years (89). For patients anticoagulated with warfarin, the risk of a major hemorrhage is 1.5% per year, and the risk of a fatal hemorrhage is 0.5% per year (93,94).

Structural valve deterioration is rare in mechanical valves, except for the 70-degree Björk-Shiley convexo-concave valve. This valve had structural failure of the welded outflow strut, and this mechanical valve has been removed from the market.

Mitral Valve Repair

Unlike mitral valve replacement, mitral valve repair surgical techniques are individualized to the specific mitral valve pathology. Both stenotic and regurgitant valves may be successfully repaired with excellent long-term results. The ability to successfully repair the valve depends not only on the severity of the valve pathology, but also on the experience and ability of the surgeon.

Mitral Repair for Rheumatic Mitral Stenosis

The first operations performed on the mitral valve were closed mitral valve commissurotomies to relieve mitral valve stenosis secondary to rheumatic mitral valve disease (68–71). Today, mitral valve repairs for rheumatic mitral stenosis not only correct commissural fusion, but also restore leaflet mobility and pliability and relieve subvalvular chordal and papillary muscle fusion. ▼▶ d92

Comparison of Mitral Valve Repair and Percutaneous Balloon Mitral Commissurotomy

In recent years, percutaneous balloon commissurotomy has largely replaced surgical repair of the stenotic mitral valve. Farhat et al. performed a randomized controlled trial comparing percutaneous balloon mitral commissurotomy with surgical closed and open commissurotomy in 90 patients with mitral stenosis and pliable valves (103a). The best long-term results were obtained with balloon and open surgical commissurotomy, with only a 6.6% restenosis rate after 7 years as compared with a 37% restenosis rate for closed mitral commissurotomy. Moreover, larger initial mitral valve areas were obtained with the percutaneous and open surgical techniques as compared with the closed surgical procedure. The authors concluded that the procedure of first choice was the percutaneous balloon technique because of the lower costs and the elimination of the need for thoracotomy and cardiopulmonary bypass. Ommen et al. observed no difference in long-term, event-free survival between patients with mitral stenosis treated by percutaneous balloon versus closed surgical mitral commissurotomy (103b).

MITRAL REGURGITATION

During the first half of the twentieth century, textbooks of cardiovascular disease emphasized mitral stenosis over mitral regurgitation. Moreover, during the 1950s and

TABLE 21.7   CAUSES OF MITRAL REGURGITATION

Chronic
  Inflammatory
    Rheumatic heart disease
    Systemic lupus erythematosus
    Progressive systemic sclerosis
    Methysergide therapy
  Degenerative
    Myxomatous degeneration of the valve
    Calcification of the mitral valve annulus
    Marfan's syndrome
    Ehlers-Danlos syndrome
    Pseudoxanthoma elasticum
    Ankylosing spondylitis
    Infiltrative amyloidosis
  Infectious
    Infectious endocarditis
  Structural
    Ruptured chordae tendineae (acute mitral regurgitation that can become chronic)
    Dysfunction of a papillary muscle: ischemia (acute mitral regurgitation that can become chronic)
    Dilatation of mitral valve annulus secondary to left ventricular dilatation (cardiomyopathy)
    Hypertrophic cardiomyopathy
    Paravalvular prosthetic valve leak
  Congenital
    Cleft mitral valve [associated with other congenital heart diseases (e.g., primum atrial septal defect)]
    Parachute mitral valve [associated with other congenital heart diseases (e.g., endocardial cushion defect, endocardial fibroelastosis, transposition of the great arteries)]
Acute
  Structural
    Trauma
    Dysfunction or rupture of a papillary muscle (ischemic heart disease)
    Prosthetic valve malfunction with paravalvular leak or leaflet malfunction or disruption
  Infectious
    Infectious endocarditis
    Acute rheumatic fever
  Degenerative
    Myxomatous degeneration with chordal rupture

1960s, some clinicians stated that mitral regurgitation was a relatively unimportant valvular lesion rarely requiring therapy. As rheumatic fever has waned in the United States and the understanding of the multiple etiologies of mitral regurgitation has increased, the latter lesion has assumed greater importance than the former. Current thinking distinguishes the various causes of mitral regurgitation and the difference between acute and chronic forms of this pathophysiologic entity (Table 21.7).

During the last 25 years, the incidence of rheumatic mitral regurgitation has declined steadily. Conversely, degenerative and structural etiologies (Table 21.7) have increased in number. Mitral valve prolapse is the most common form of valvular heart disease in the United States. Consequently, in addition to material cited throughout the section on mitral regurgitation, a separate section is dedicated to mitral valve prolapse.

Anatomic Considerations

Anatomic changes in patients with mitral regurgitation vary according to the underlying etiology. Thus, patients with rheumatic mitral regurgitation develop progressive fibrosis, contracture, and calcification of the mitral valve and the chordae tendineae, which can lead to predominant mitral stenosis, predominant mitral regurgitation, or mixed stenosis and regurgitation.

Patients with floppy or prolapsing mitral valves demonstrate redundant myxomatous tissue with excess deposits of proteoglycans within the spongiosa layer of the valve (104,105). This excess tissue impinges on the supporting fibrosa layer of the valve, resulting in the laxity and redundancy of the leaflets. There is associated mitral annular dilation. Moreover, all major components of mitral valvular connective tissue are abnormal in patients with floppy mitral valves. ▼ d93

Calcification of the mitral annulus interferes with the normal closure of the valve leaflets. Moreover, the sphincter-like action of the annulus, which occurs during ventricular systole, is lost. Mitral annular calcification is commonly seen in patients with Marfan's syndrome and in elderly women. In the latter group, mitral annular calcification often parallels the presence of coronary arterial and aortic atherosclerosis. On occasion, mitral annular calcification spreads into the conduction system, leading to varying degrees of heart block (116,117). Mitral annular calcification is accelerated in patients with diabetes, arterial hypertension, calcific aortic stenosis, and Marfan's and Hurler's syndromes. Mitral annular calcification is also common in patients with chronic renal failure and secondary hyperparathyroidism. Calcified protrusions may extend from the heavily calcified annulus into the adjacent myocardium, with resulting conduction system abnormalities (118). In most patients, calcification is modest as is the degree of mitral regurgitation.

Infectious endocarditis involving the mitral valve can cause mitral regurgitation secondary to leaflet destruction, perforation, or chordal rupture (119). Acute mitral regurgitation may gradually give way to subacute and chronic valvular insufficiency. Large vegetations can prevent appropriate leaflet coaptation, whereas healed vegetations may lead to valvular fibrosis and deformity (119a).

A variety of uncommon congenital abnormalities can lead to chronic mitral incompetence. For example, clefts of the anterior leaflet are often associated with partial or total AV canal or anomalous mitral arcade (120). Other congenital malformations associated with mitral regurgitation include endocardial fibroelastosis, transposition of the great arteries, and anomalous origin of the left coronary artery from the pulmonary artery.

Trauma may lead to acute, severe mitral regurgitation as a result of disruption of a chordae tendineae or a mitral valve leaflet. Ischemia or infarction is commonly associated with acute as well as chronic mitral regurgitation. Abnormal papillary muscle contractile function is often accompanied by hypokinesis or akinesis of the adjacent left ventricular wall. If papillary muscle ischemic necrosis is present, partial or total papillary muscle rupture may occur (119). The latter almost invariably leads to cardiogenic shock secondary to severe, acute mitral regurgitation with the subsequent demise of the patient. The former may be associated with mild, moderate, or severe mitral regurgitation (119). Papillary muscle rupture usually occurs during the first week after infarction (see Chapter 19). Healing and fibrosis of an infarcted papillary muscle can lead to chronic mitral insufficiency. ▼ d94

Mitral regurgitation can be expected in approximately 30% of patients who are undergoing evaluation for coronary bypass surgery (121). In most of these individuals, mitral regurgitation is mild. The presence of severe mitral regurgitation is associated with reduced left ventricular function and a worsened prognosis (122). However, even milder degrees of mitral regurgitation that develop following acute myocardial infarction are associated with a worsened 1- and 4-year prognosis (122a,122b).

Left ventricular dilatation, such as that which occurs in patients with dilated cardiomyopathy, can cause mitral regurgitation by altering the position and axis of the papillary muscles. Moreover, ventricular dilatation causes dilation of the mitral annulus with resulting incomplete coaptation of the mitral leaflets. Mitral regurgitation leads to left atrial dilatation and thereby results in retraction of the posterior mitral leaflet by the dilated left atrium. In this manner, mitral regurgitation amplifies itself (i.e., "mitral regurgitation begets more mitral regurgitation") (119). Abnormal position of the papillary muscle, combined with altered hydraulic forces in the left ventricular outflow tract, results in mitral regurgitation in patients with hypertrophic cardiomyopathy. The presence and degree of this type of mitral regurgitation (often termed *functional*) is unrelated to the severity of left ventricular dysfunction. Rather, local left ventricular remodeling with apical and posterior displacement of the papillary muscles leads to valvular tenting. This, combined with decreased or absent mitral annular contraction, results in mitral insufficiency that may be mild, moderate, or severe (119a).

Pathophysiology

Chronic mitral regurgitation is a form of volume overload that affects the left ventricle and the left atrium. The lesion is well tolerated for years but eventually leads to failure of the left ventricle. In patients with mitral incompetence, a portion of each systolic stroke volume is ejected retrograde into the left atrium. This results in abnormal left atrial expansion with resulting left atrial dilation (123). Left ventricular eccentric (dilated as opposed to concentric) hypertrophy develops as new myocardial sarcomeres are added end to end (i.e., in series). Total left ventricular volume increases progressively (124). Increased left ventricular dilatation changes the spatial relationship between the papillary muscles and the mitral valve annulus (124a). These spatial changes lead to increases in the volume of mitral regurgitant flow. Thus, mitral regurgitation worsens over time as a result of left ventricular remodeling.

Enlargement of the left ventricle increases that chamber's diastolic compliance, allowing it to fill to a greater volume at a lower filling pressure than would otherwise be allowed. Mitral regurgitant volume is delivered into the low-pressure left atrium during the earliest phase of systole, before aortic ejection commences. As much as 50% of the regurgitant volume can be ejected into the left atrium *before* aortic valve opening. This may represent as much as 20% of the total left ventricular stroke volume in patients with severe mitral incompetence (125). Preload is increased in patients with severe mitral regurgitation as a result of left ventricular dilatation and the addition of new sarcomeres in series. Afterload is maintained in the normal range by the addition of these new left ventricular sarcomeres. Left ventricular contractile function remains within the normal range for many years despite the presence of severe mitral insufficiency (124). Late in the course of the disease, interstitial fibrosis of the left ventricle, which accompanies long-standing pathologic hypertrophy, results in a decline in left ventricular contractile function. At this point in the natural history of mitral regurgitation, left ventricular ejection fraction declines (124). ❦ d95

Acute Mitral Regurgitation

The pathophysiologic consequences of acute, severe mitral incompetence—such as that observed in patients following rupture of a chorda tendineae—differ from those of chronic mitral insufficiency. With acute mitral regurgitation, a sudden volume overload is imposed on an unprepared, nondilated, nonhypertrophied left ventricle and left atrium. Preload is increased, whereas afterload decreases as a result of the newly developed low-pressure runoff to the left atrium during systole (132). In the absence of coronary artery disease or myocardial infarction, left ventricular contractile function can be normal or even supranormal secondary to augmented sympathetic nervous stimulation of the myocardium (132,133).

Despite increased left ventricular preload and contractility and decreased afterload, overall left ventricular pump function declines in acute mitral regurgitation. This decline is considerably greater if recent or previous myocardial infarction is present. Total left ventricular stroke volume increases, but a large amount of this flow is directed into the left atrium rather than the aorta. Forward cardiac output declines. Pressures in the noncompliant, nondilated left atrium and left ventricle increase, often dramatically. Pulmonary congestion results with the development of dyspnea at rest or with minimal exertion. At times, acute pulmonary edema may be observed. Large, regurgitant CV waves are observed in the pulmonary capillary wedge pressure tracing secondary to the arrival of a large bolus of regurgitant blood flow in the small noncompliant left atrium. In most patients with chronic mitral regurgitation, the left atrium dilates progressively so that left atrial and pulmonary capillary wedge pressures remain normal or only modestly elevated.

Major complications in patients with long-standing mitral regurgitation include left ventricular failure, atrial fibrillation, arterial embolism, and infectious endocarditis. Left ventricular failure usually develops when mitral regurgitation has been present for decades and marked left ventricular and left atrial dilatation are present. At that time, left ventricular systolic and diastolic function are almost always abnormal (137).

Clinical Profile

Natural History

Chronic Mitral Regurgitation

The clinical course of patients with chronic mitral regurgitation is determined by the severity of the regurgitant lesion and its etiology. Many patients with mild to moderate amounts of mitral regurgitation remain asymptomatic for their entire lives. Patients with moderate to severe mitral regurgitation are usually without symptoms for decades. During this time period, the left ventricle and left atrium slowly dilate and hypertrophy, thereby maintaining left ventricular filling pressures at or near the normal range. Mitral regurgitation tends to increase with time, although considerable individual variation occurs from patient to patient. Independent predictors of progression include flail leaflet, progression of the underlying cardiac disease (e.g., arteriosclerotic coronary artery disease), and increase in mitral valve annulus diameter (137a). Depending on the severity of the regurgitant lesion, the state of left ventricular and left atrial function, and the disease entity producing mitral regurgitation, symptoms of left ventricular failure begin to develop usually during the fourth through the sixth decade of life. This course is quite different from that observed in patients with mitral stenosis, who often become symptomatic in their 30s.

The prognosis is often worse for patients whose mitral regurgitation is the result of ischemic heart disease. In patients with connective tissue disease, the severity of mitral regurgitation tends to increase with time. Patients with coronary artery disease may suffer complications

TABLE 21.8 COMPARISON OF ACUTE AND CHRONIC MITRAL REGURGITATION

	Chronic	Acute
Time to symptoms	Decades	Immediate
Symptoms	Often asymptomatic	Highly symptomatic
Left ventricular size	Enlarged	Normal
Left atrial size	Enlarged	Normal
Left ventricular filling pressure	Normal to increased	Invariably increased
Left atrial pressure	Normal to increased	Invariably increased
Cardiac output	Normal to decreased	Invariably decreased
Ability of the cardiovascular system to compensate	Usually compensated	Usually not compensated
Electrocardiography	Left ventricular hypertrophy	No left ventricular hypertrophy
Chest roentgenography	Left ventricular, left atrial enlargement	No cardiac enlargement, pulmonary edema
Therapy	Medical-surgical	Usually urgent surgical

related to the latter entity (e.g., myocardial infarction), thereby worsening mitral regurgitation or left ventricular function; hence the prognosis. ☜ d96

Acute Mitral Regurgitation

As noted earlier, the clinical course of patients with acute forms of mitral regurgitation differs greatly from that of individuals with chronic mitral regurgitation. The acute form of the illness is usually associated with the sudden development of severe left ventricular failure. Patients are often in pulmonary edema when initially seen, and cardiogenic shock may ensue. The "unprepared" left ventricle and atrium cannot accept the large quantity of mitral regurgitant blood flow and maintain low or modestly elevated filling pressures as in patients with chronic mitral incompetence. Patients with acute mitral regurgitation have marked elevations in left ventricular filling pressures and decreased cardiac output (Table 21.8). Their clinical course is marked by the development of sudden disability; they are almost invariably hospitalized and undergo urgent mitral valve repair or replacement.

History

Chronic Mitral Regurgitation

Patients with symptomatic chronic mitral regurgitation develop dyspnea on exertion as their initial complaint. Later, these individuals report orthopnea and paroxysmal nocturnal dyspnea. Dyspnea at rest and even pulmonary edema may develop if medical therapy is not instituted or if atrial fibrillation with a rapid ventricular response occurs. These symptoms are the result of increased left ventricular diastolic and left atrial pressures. Decreased cardiac output produces fatigue and generalized weakness. Pulmonary hypertension develops late in the course of the illness and can lead to right ventricular failure with associated peripheral edema and even ascites.

Acute Mitral Regurgitation

Acute mitral regurgitation is associated with the rapid development of symptoms resulting from markedly increased left ventricular filling pressures: severe dyspnea at rest and anxiety.

Physical Examination

Chronic Mitral Regurgitation

Patients with chronic mild mitral regurgitation may have a normal physical examination except for the characteristic murmur. At the other end of the spectrum are patients with chronic, severe, or acute mitral regurgitation who often manifest signs of left ventricular failure (i.e., pulmonary rales and pleural effusion). Patients with long-standing left ventricular failure and associated pulmonary hypertension may have signs of right ventricular failure: distended neck veins, hepatomegaly, ascites, and peripheral edema.

The typical patient with chronic, severe, compensated mitral regurgitation often displays many of the physical findings listed in Table 21.9. The characteristic murmur of chronic mitral regurgitation begins with the S_1 and ceases at or slightly after the aortic component of the S_2 (140). The intensity of the murmur of mitral regurgitation is usually constant throughout systole. Patients with mitral valve prolapse are an exception to this rule: The murmur commences in mid- to late systole and has a brief ejection quality. It is often associated with one or more early systolic clicks.

Patients with long-standing mitral regurgitation often have an easily palpable, enlarged, and laterally displaced apical impulse resulting from left ventricular dilatation. Right ventricular dilatation may be inferred if a left parasternal impulse is felt. An occasional patient demonstrates a modest systolic left parasternal lift secondary to anterior displacement of the heart by a markedly enlarged left atrium. It is often difficult to distinguish this left atrial impulse from a right ventricular lift (140). ☜ d97

Acute Mitral Regurgitation

In individuals with acute mitral regurgitation, the physical examination is dominated by findings associated with left ventricular failure. The heart size is usually normal by palpation; tachycardia and tachypnea are common. The murmur is usually loud if normal left ventricular function is

TABLE 21.9 FINDINGS ON PHYSICAL EXAMINATION IN PATIENTS WITH CHRONIC SEVERE MITRAL REGURGITATION

Head, eyes, ears, nose, throat	Anxious facies; diaphoresis secondary to left ventricular failure
Jugular venous pulse	Distended in patients with right ventricular failure
Carotids	Small or normal volume; brisk upstroke with more rapid than normal falloff
Chest	Rales; dullness and decreased breath sounds at lung bases and e to a change resulting from pleural effusions
Cardiac	Apex impulse laterally displaced, enlarged apical impulse; ↓ intensity of first heart sound; holosystolic murmur loudest at apex with radiation to the axilla, ± third/fourth heart sound; ↑P_2 if pulmonary hypertension is present
Abdomen	Hepatomegaly, ascites if right ventricular failure is present
Extremities	Peripheral edema if right ventricular failure is present

↓, decreased; ↑, increased.

present. The murmur may be soft if left ventricular function is markedly reduced (e.g., with mitral regurgitation secondary to papillary muscle dysfunction following an extensive myocardial infarction). The murmur of acute mitral regurgitation may be harsh and even ejection in quality with wide radiation (142). The S_2 is often widely split secondary to early aortic valve closure. Both the S_3 and the fourth heart sound are also frequently present.

Electrocardiography

Long-standing mitral regurgitation with associated left atrial and left ventricular dilatation alters the morphology of the P waves and the QRS complex: The patterns of left atrial dilatation and left ventricular hypertrophy are usually observed. Atrial fibrillation is often present in patients with chronic mitral regurgitation. Other ECG findings may relate to the pathologic entity producing mitral regurgitation (e.g., myocardial infarction with associated papillary muscle dysfunction). Patients with mitral valve prolapse often manifest nonspecific ST-T changes on the ECG. Individuals with acute mitral regurgitation demonstrate neither left atrial enlargement nor left ventricular hypertrophy.

Chest Roentgenography

Chest roentgenography in patients with chronic mitral insufficiency is usually characterized by left ventricular and left atrial enlargement. Cardiac chamber enlargement is rarely noted in patients with acute mitral regurgitation. Left atrial size is a reasonable gauge to the duration and severity of mitral regurgitation. The larger the atrium, the more severe and chronic is the regurgitation. An occasional

patient with very severe and long-standing mitral incompetence is noted to have a giant left atrium.

The pulmonary vasculature is usually normal in patients with chronic mitral regurgitation reflecting normal or only minimally elevated pulmonary venous pressure. Pulmonary vascular redistribution and interstitial pulmonary edema are observed late in the course of the illness or in patients with acute mitral regurgitation. Cardiac fluoroscopy may reveal mitral leaflet or annular calcification. These findings may often be inferred from the postero-anterior chest roentgenogram as well. Patients with mitral valve prolapse usually demonstrate a normal cardiac silhouette, clear lungs, and an abnormal chest configuration (i.e., narrow anteroposterior diameter or pectus excavatum). Patients with acute mitral regurgitation usually have a normal cardiac silhouette as well as signs of left ventricular failure (e.g., interstitial edema and Kerley A and B lines).

Echocardiography

Chronic Mitral Regurgitation

A Doppler-echocardiographic study is useful in patients with chronic mitral regurgitation (143–146b). Such examinations reveal (a) abnormalities of valvular architecture, (b) left atrial size, (c) left ventricular size and function, (d) a semiquantitative estimate of the severity of mitral regurgitation, (e) size and function of the right ventricle, (f) a rather accurate estimate of pulmonary arterial systolic pressure, and (g) associated valvular lesions (e.g., mitral stenosis, tricuspid regurgitation) (Table 21.10). This information can be obtained from a transthoracic Doppler-echocardiographic study in the overwhelming majority of patients. A number of individuals require a transesophageal echocardiographic examination (e.g., patients with prosthetic mitral valves and paravalvular leaks or individuals in whom mitral valve repair is being contemplated). Transesophageal Doppler-echocardiographic studies provide more accurate anatomic assessment of all types of mitral regurgitant lesions as well as prosthetic valves than can be obtained with transthoracic examinations (see Chapter 52) (146a). As noted earlier, end systolic volume is an excellent discriminator of prognosis in patients with chronic mitral regurgitation. Serial determination of this variable is of considerable value in determining the timing of mitral valve surgery (127–130). ▼ d98

Acute Mitral Regurgitation

In patients with acute mitral regurgitation, Doppler-echocardiographic studies frequently demonstrate the etiology of the acute regurgitant lesion (e.g., vegetations in patients with infectious endocarditis or ruptured chordae in individuals with mitral valve prolapse). Transesophageal echocardiographic examination is more sensitive than transthoracic study for revealing pathologic entities associated with acute mitral regurgitation. Other subtle findings may also be observed in patients with acute mitral incompetence:

TABLE 21.10 SPECTRUM OF ECHOCARDIOGRAPHIC FINDINGS IN PATIENTS WITH MITRAL REGURGITATION

Mitral valve	Prolapse; myxomatous thickened valve; fibrotic or calcified valve (rheumatic); valvar vegetations; ruptured chordae; mild, moderate or severe mitral regurgitation (Doppler)
Left atrium	Dilatation; thrombus
Left ventricle	Dilatation; hypertrophy; normal or reduced contractile function
Right ventricle	Dilatation; hypertrophy; normal or reduced contractile function
Pulmonary artery	Dilatation, estimated pulmonary arterial systolic pressure (Doppler analysis of tricuspid regurgitant jet)
Right atrium	Dilatation
Tricuspid valve	Mild, moderate, or severe tricuspid regurgitation (Doppler)
Pulmonary veins	Reduced systolic and diastolic flow ratios and reversed systolic flow (Doppler)

decreased pulmonary venous systolic and diastolic flow ratios and reversed pulmonary venous systolic flow (143).

Differential Diagnosis

Patients with mitral regurgitation must be distinguished from individuals with other entities that produce systolic murmurs. The murmur of aortic stenosis is usually loudest at the base and radiates to the carotid arteries. It increases following longer cycle lengths (e.g., in patients with atrial fibrillation or extra systoles with compensatory pauses). Echocardiography usually defines the presence or absence of aortic stenosis. Hypertrophic cardiomyopathy can produce two systolic murmurs: a left ventricular outflow tract murmur and a mitral regurgitant murmur. It may be difficult to distinguish these two murmurs during an auscultatory examination. Echocardiography reveals the correct diagnosis and helps to define the severity of mitral regurgitation.

In patients with acute myocardial infarction, a loud systolic murmur of recent onset may be the result of acute mitral regurgitation, or it may result from an acute ventricular septal rupture. The murmur of an acute septal rupture is often more localized than that of mitral regurgitation; the former murmur has its greatest intensity along the lower left sternal border. A systolic thrill is often palpable in patients with septal rupture. Echocardiographic study or right-sided heart catheterization with blood-oxygen content determination in the right atrium, right ventricle, and pulmonary artery defines the cause of the systolic murmur in these patients.

Therapy

Medical Therapy of Mitral Regurgitation

Chronic Mitral Regurgitation

Medical therapy for the patient with chronic mitral regurgitation involves a number of different strategies: antibiotic prophy-

laxis with various interventions in order to prevent infectious endocarditis; antiarrhythmic therapy to maintain sinus rhythm in the patient who develops atrial fibrillation (see Medical Therapy of Mitral Stenosis); anticoagulation for the patient with sustained atrial fibrillation; and vasodilators, digoxin, and diuretics for the patient with left ventricular failure.

From an understanding of the pathophysiology of mitral regurgitation, it seems reasonable that chronic therapy with a vasodilator, particularly an angiotensin-converting enzyme (ACE) inhibitor, or hydralazine, would reduce left ventricular wall stress and thereby delay or obviate entirely the need for mitral valve surgery (152,153). Studies in patients with chronic aortic regurgitation have demonstrated such an effect (see Chapter 22). Unfortunately, minimal long-term outcome data are currently available involving patients with chronic mitral incompetence. Tischler et al. observed significant reduction in left ventricular end diastolic and end systolic volumes and mass following 6 months of ACE inhibitor therapy (153a). Levine et al. noted improvement in severe functional mitral regurgitation following 1 year of ACE inhibitor and nitrate therapy in 19 patients with chronic heart failure and severe mitral regurgitation (153b). Despite the modest volume of evidence, the rationale for such therapy seems compelling and can be recommended for patients with chronic, asymptomatic mitral regurgitation of moderate or greater severity. Such therapy is particularly rational if some degree of left ventricular dilatation is present (152–160). We favor ACE inhibition for this indication. ☙ d99

Acute Mitral Regurgitation

In patients with acute mitral regurgitation, left ventricular failure is almost invariably present. Intravenous vasodilator therapy with nitroprusside can produce dramatic benefit with subsequent reduction in ventricular cavity dilatation, diastolic filling pressures, and mitral regurgitant orifice (154,155). The nitroprusside infusion is continued until the patient is stabilized by either surgical intervention (e.g., mitral valvuloplasty or replacement) or long-term oral medical therapy (e.g., ACE inhibitors, digoxin, and diuretics). Intravenous nitroglycerin is often effective in reducing pulmonary vascular congestion in these patients, particularly if the underlying etiology for mitral regurgitation is ischemic heart disease. Surgical therapy is almost always required.

It is essential that the clinician serially monitor left ventricular function and cavity size by echocardiography when following patients with chronic mitral regurgitation of moderate severity or greater. Declining left ventricular function or progressive left ventricular dilatation should prompt the clinician to consider mitral valve surgery seriously.

MITRAL VALVE PROLAPSE

The syndrome known as *mitral valve prolapse* has been characterized and studied for more than 30 years. It has been given a variety of names including the floppy valve syndrome, Barlow's syndrome, the click-murmur syndrome, and myxomatous mitral valve, among others (106,161–166). There is great variability in the expression of this syndrome, with some patients demonstrating severely involved valves that often require surgical intervention. The overwhelming majority of individuals with this entity, however, has only a minor derangement of mitral valvular structure, which is usually clinically insignificant. The syndrome in any of its manifestations is quite common, with 3% to 5% of the adult U.S. population affected (164,167). Female subjects are affected twice as commonly as male subjects. The Framingham Heart Study employed strict echocardiographic criteria to determine the prevalence of mitral valve prolapse. They noted a prevalence of 2.4% in their population; 60% of the patients with mitral valve prolapse were women (167a). ⚑ e01

Myxomatous changes may not be restricted to the mitral valve. Indeed, the tricuspid, aortic, and pulmonic valves can also be affected. The myxomatous valve syndrome has a strong genetic transmission; in some cases, familial inheritance is by an autosomal dominant mechanism (161,171). An occasional patient demonstrates mitral valve prolapse as well as rheumatic mitral valve disease or ischemic heart disease. It is still unclear whether prolapse in this setting is the result of rheumatic or ischemic heart disease or merely the simultaneous occurrence of two common entities (172–174).

Patients with mitral valve prolapse may have absent, mild, moderate, or severe mitral regurgitation. The majority of patients have mild or no mitral regurgitant blood flow. These individuals are at risk for bacterial endocarditis but will almost certainly not require mitral valve surgery unless chordal rupture develops with attendant acute mitral regurgitation. In patients with minimal or absent mitral regurgitation, left ventricular size and function should remain normal because there is no, or only the most minimal, increase in left ventricular volume work and wall stress. In patients with moderate or severe mitral regurgitation, left ventricular dilatation and dysfunction may develop as described for other individuals with chronic mitral regurgitation.

Clinical Profile

Natural History

Mitral valve prolapse can be recognized in children, adolescents, and adults. The outlook in children is excellent, with the overwhelming majority remaining asymptomatic and without complications for many years (138,161,175). Increasingly severe mitral regurgitation is the result of progressive mitral valvular degeneration. This complication occurs in 10% to 15% of patients and can require mitral valvular surgery if symptoms of left ventricular dysfunction develop (138,176,177). Correlates with severe mitral

regurgitation and the need for mitral valve surgery include male gender, older age, and the presence of obesity and hypertension (177a). Patients with posterior mitral valve leaflet prolapse have a worse prognosis than patients with anterior leaflet prolapse (177b). As already noted, chordal rupture with the development of acute, severe, mitral regurgitation is also a feared complication. Severe regurgitation requiring consideration of mitral valve repair or replacement is more common in men over age 50 than in any other group (177). Mitral valve prolapse is the most common underlying etiology in patients who undergo mitral valve surgery for mitral regurgitation. When chordal rupture occurs, the affected leaflet begins to flail with marked systolic prolapse into the left atrium, leading to severe mitral regurgitation. This complication is associated with a poor prognosis if medical therapy alone is employed. Indeed, sudden death is relatively common in these patients. Surgical intervention with valve repair or replacement should be strongly considered for these patients early in the course of their illness (178–178b). All patients with mitral valve prolapse are at risk for developing infectious endocarditis; however, patients with isolated systolic clicks appear to have a low risk for this complication. Endocarditis is more common in men and in patients older than age 50 (179,180). As might be expected, endocarditis exacerbates the degree of mitral regurgitation present and can lead to chordal rupture.

Cerebral embolism occasionally occurs in patients with mitral valve prolapse. It is manifested as either a transient ischemic attack or a permanent neurologic deficit (181,182). ⚑ e02

Arrhythmias are also quite common in patients with mitral valve prolapse. Both supraventricular and ventricular arrhythmias have been reported. Because arrhythmias occur quite commonly in the general population, it remains unclear to what degree mitral valve prolapse is the actual cause of these rhythm disturbances. It is quite possible that arrhythmias in patients with mitral valve prolapse are merely the result of two common events occurring simultaneously (184,185). An occasional patient with mitral valve prolapse suffers sudden death. Because this event can occur in the absence of obvious structural heart disease, it is unclear what role mitral valve prolapse plays in the etiology of such sudden deaths. Evaluating the relationship between mitral valve prolapse and sudden death, Kligfield et al. have concluded that patients with mitral valve prolapse and significant mitral regurgitation, complex ventricular arrhythmias, prolongation of the QT interval, and a history of syncope were at increased risk for sudden death (184,185). ⚑ e03

History

The overwhelming majority of patients with mitral valve prolapse are asymptomatic (138,164,177). Many patients have symptoms that seem unrelated to the cardiac manifestations of the syndrome. For example, anxiety, easy fatigue, palpitations, and orthostatic hypotension have all been ascribed to this syndrome. Some authorities ascribe these symptoms to dysfunction of the autonomic nervous system with inappropriately increased sympathetic nervous activity at rest and with mild exertion (134–136,180,187).

A relationship to neurocirculatory asthenia, commonly diagnosed in an earlier era, has been postulated (163,166). The exact relationship of these autonomic abnormalities to mitral valve prolapse is unclear. It is possible that abnormally heightened sympathetic tone leads to a decrease in left ventricular volume with resulting mitral valve prolapse. In this scenario, mitral valve prolapse is merely an epiphenomenon related to the abnormality in sympathetic nervous function. It is also possible that some of the symptoms reported by patients with mitral valve prolapse are psychosomatic in origin, resulting from anxiety generated when the patient was informed that he or she had heart disease. Some patients report chest discomfort that, at times, is obviously musculoskeletal in origin and at other times seems anginal in nature. Some authorities have suggested that anginal chest discomfort is cardiac in origin, resulting from abnormal tension and traction on papillary muscles (174).

Physical Examination

Patients with mitral valve prolapse are often asthenic in habitus with low body weights. Arterial blood pressure is often low and orthostatic hypotension may be present. Straight-back syndrome, pectus excavatum, scoliosis, and a narrow thoracic anteroposterior diameter may be present. If severe mitral regurgitation is present, the carotid pulse may be brisk in upstroke with a hint of rapid falloff. Palpation of the precordium may reveal a brief inward movement of the apex impulse in mid-systole coinciding with the occurrence of the mid-systolic click.

Auscultation of these patients is best performed using the diaphragm of the stethoscope with the patient lying and standing. The left lateral decubitus position while lying and movement from standing to squatting may assist the examiner in clarifying the relationship between the ausculted clicks and murmurs. The usual finding is a sharp, systolic click heard 0.14 seconds or more after the S_1. This click differs from the ejection click of aortic valve disease because it occurs well after the onset of the carotid arterial upstroke. At times, more than one click is heard. The click(s) is best heard along the lower left sternal border. It is thought that they are generated by tensing of the chordae tendineae and billowing of the mitral valve leaflets. The click(s) is usually, but not always, followed by a mid- to late systolic crescendo murmur heard best at the apex. The duration of the murmur correlates directly with the severity of mitral regurgitation: The earlier and more prolonged the murmur, the more severe the regurgitation. ⚓ e04

Electrocardiography

Most patients with mitral valve prolapse have normal ECG results. In a small number of patients, and particularly in those with symptoms, the ECG demonstrates nonspecific ST-T changes in the inferior leads (II, III, augmented voltage unipolar left foot lead) and rarely in the anterolateral leads (V_4–V_6) (163,166,174). It has been suggested that these findings are the result of increased papillary muscle tension with resulting ischemia (151). Few data support this supposition, however, and it is just as reasonable to believe that these ECG findings are the result of altered autonomic tone in some patients or ventricular dilatation in individuals with more marked degrees of mitral regurgitation. Some investigators report that arrhythmias and even sudden death are more common in patients with mitral valve prolapse.

Chest Roentgenography

Chest roentgenography is usually normal in patients with mitral valve prolapse unless severe, chronic, or acute mitral regurgitation is present. If chronic severe mitral regurgitation is present, cardiomegaly secondary to left ventricular enlargement, left atrial enlargement, and pulmonary congestion are often noted. If severe acute mitral regurgitation secondary to chordal rupture is present, heart size is usually normal, but severe pulmonary congestion with or without frank pulmonary edema is often observed.

Echocardiography

As already noted, echocardiography yields important diagnostic and prognostic information in patients with mitral valve prolapse. Echocardiography confirms the diagnosis of mitral valve prolapse by demonstrating systolic posterior displacement of one or both leaflets into the left atrium (168,169). The mitral leaflets are usually thickened. Indeed, risk for complications in this syndrome is correlated with thickened leaflets. Patients with mitral valve prolapse but without leaflet thickening have a benign prognosis (147,168,169). Patients with thickened leaflets and dilated mitral valve annuli are at highest risk for complications such as infectious endocarditis and progressive mitral regurgitation. The echocardiographic findings in patients with mitral valve prolapse are quite variable, with individuals at one end of the spectrum demonstrating only mild prolapse, whereas patients at the other end of spectrum manifest thickened valves, dilated mitral valve annuli, and left atrial and left ventricular dilatation. ⚓ e05

Most patients with this syndrome have mild mitral valve prolapse and, in the absence of any change in their physical examination results, only a single echocardiographic examination is necessary. For screening purposes, often an abbreviated, single-view echocardiographic study is all that is required (163a). Individuals with moderate to severe mitral regurgitation require more careful monitoring, and serial echocardiographic examinations should be undertaken. Asymptomatic patients with severe mitral regurgitation should have a yearly echocardiographic study. Individuals with more moderate degrees of mitral regurgitation can be studied less frequently.

Radionuclear Imaging

Patients with mitral valve prolapse and angina-like chest discomfort may benefit from a thallium or sestamibi exercise or pharmacologic stress test. The resulting normal study result reassures the clinician and the patient that the chest discomfort is the result of the mitral valve prolapse syndrome and not coronary artery disease.

Cardiac Catheterization

Invasive hemodynamic and angiography study is usually not necessary in patients with mitral valve prolapse because all manifestations of this syndrome can be exquisitely defined by echocardiography. When angiography is performed, mitral valve prolapse is clearly seen in the right anterior oblique left ventriculogram. Mitral valve redundancy is also often observed in this projection. If severe acute mitral regurgitation secondary to chordal rupture is present, the pulmonary capillary wedge and left ventricular diastolic pressures are markedly elevated. ❦ e06

Therapy

Most patients with mitral valve prolapse have an excellent prognosis. Therefore, they should receive strong reassurance concerning the usually benign nature of their condition. The importance of such reassurance cannot be overemphasized because cardiac neurosis is common in these patients, often as a result of inadequate time spent by the physician when the diagnosis was initially explained to the patient. Individuals with mitral valve prolapse should be carefully instructed concerning antibiotic endocarditis prophylaxis for dental work or surgical procedures. Some physicians believe that patients with isolated clicks without a late systolic murmur or without a thickened valve by echocardiography do not need endocarditis prophylaxis (179,179a). Opinion is divided in this regard, however, and many physicians still provide prophylaxis to the latter group of patients.

Patients with severe mitral regurgitation, particularly if a flail leaflet is present, should be considered for mitral valve surgery (see Results of Mitral Valve Repair for Mitral Insufficiency) (178–178b). If left ventricular size and function are normal or nearly so, the patient can be observed with careful

and frequent follow-up, including at least yearly echocardiographic study. Mitral valve prolapse is now the most common underlying etiology observed in patients who undergo mitral valve surgery for mitral regurgitation. Most patients with mitral valve prolapse who require surgery can have their valves repaired rather than replaced with a prosthetic valve. Older individuals should have coronary arteriography before surgery so that clinically significant coronary arterial obstructions can be bypassed at the time of mitral valve surgery.

Individuals with a history of palpitations, particularly if syncope or presyncope has occurred, should undergo evaluation for arrhythmia, including ambulatory monitoring and routine ECG. If a prolonged QT interval, or repetitive ventricular ectopy such as ventricular tachycardia is detected, further evaluation is indicated, including signal-averaged ECG and possibly an invasive electrophysiologic arrhythmia evaluation to assess the risk for sudden death (184,185). Beta-adrenergic–blocking agents in modest dose are often effective in abolishing these arrhythmias as well as episodes of supraventricular tachycardia. Patients who are resuscitated from sudden death or whose electrophysiologic study demonstrates sustained ventricular tachycardia should be considered for aggressive antiarrhythmic therapy (i.e., amiodarone and an implantable defibrillator) (see Chapter 75). If paroxysms of atrial fibrillation or if an episode of arterial embolism have occurred (e.g., a transient or permanent neurologic deficit), life-long anticoagulation with warfarin should be strongly considered.

Results of Mitral Valve Repair for Mitral Insufficiency

The ability to perform mitral valve repair for mitral insufficiency successfully depends on the valve pathology and the experience of the surgical team (197). Degenerative or myxomatous mitral valves are the most likely to be repaired, followed by mitral insufficiency secondary to ischemia (186). In 1995, at The Cleveland Clinic Foundation, 86% (247 of 286) of patients with mitral insufficiency secondary to degenerative mitral valve disease were successfully repaired, whereas 76% (29 of 38) of patients with ischemic mitral regurgitation underwent successful repair, 59% (10 of 17) of patients with mitral insufficiency secondary to endocarditis underwent successful mitral valve repair, and 42% (13 of 31) of patients with mitral insufficiency secondary to rheumatic disease underwent successful valve repair. In addition, the ability to perform mitral valve repair for mitral insufficiency successfully depends also on the experience of the surgical team. At The Cleveland Clinic Foundation, the percentage of patients with mitral valve disease undergoing mitral valve repair increased from 20% in 1980 to 71% in 1995 (186). Others have reported a similar trend (187).

The operative mortality of mitral valve repair has been documented to be low, with reported rates of 0% to 6.3% (80,198–216). Although it had been speculated that the operative mortality for mitral valve repair would be greater than that for mitral valve replacement secondary to the increased operative time required for mitral valve repair and greater incidence of patients undergoing mitral valve repair with mitral insufficiency, this concern has not been substantiated. The literature demonstrates an overall decreased operative mortality in patients undergoing mitral valve repair versus mitral valve replacement (Table 21.1) (200–203,205,206,208–210). ⚐ e07

The long-term results for mitral valve repair for mitral insufficiency have been encouraging. Five-year survival rates of 86% to 91% have been reported, and rates of freedom from reoperation for structural valve failure at 5 years have been reported at 83% to 95% (186,213,214). Cohn et al. noted an increased rate of valve failure in patients undergoing mitral valve repair who did not undergo a ring annuloplasty at the time of surgery (54). This finding has been confirmed by Marwick et al. (217). Cohn reported a 5-year rate of freedom from reoperation of 88% in patients who underwent an annuloplasty as compared with 67% for patients who did not undergo an annuloplasty ring at the time of mitral valve repair (213). In a multivariate analysis, David et al. noted an increased risk of valve failure in patients with advanced myxomatous changes (214).

Complication rates after mitral valve repair have also been low, with a 93% to 94% rate of freedom from thromboembolic complications after 5 years (213,214). Freedom from endocarditis at 5 years has also been low with reported rates of 97% to 100%.

Minimally Invasive Mitral Valve Surgery

To decrease the morbidity associated with cardiac surgery, minimally invasive procedures for coronary artery bypass surgery, aortic valve surgery, and mitral valve replacement and repair are being developed. In minimally invasive mitral valve operations, the median sternotomy is avoided, and the operations are performed through an 8-cm hemisternotomy or right lateral thoracotomy. These incisions are associated with less morbidity than the median sternotomy, and the hope is that the decreased morbidity associated with the minimally invasive approaches will result in less postoperative pain, decreased need for postoperative ventilatory support, shorter intensive care unit stays, shorter hospitalizations, decreased hospital costs, and quicker functional patient recovery. ⚐ e08

CONTROVERSIES AND PERSONAL PERSPECTIVES

Mitral Stenosis

Although clinicians have been quite successful in managing mitral stenosis for the last 50 years, a number of controver-

sial aspects remain. As already noted, some clinicians favor prophylactic warfarin anticoagulation for all but the most mild forms of mitral stenosis. Others prefer to await the onset of atrial fibrillation, the development of marked left atrial dilatation, or age 35 to 40 before instituting anticoagulant therapy. The recommendations of the Sixth American College of Chest Physicians Consensus Conference on Antithrombotic Therapy are reasonable and favor this course of action (52). Patients are anticoagulated when the following criteria are met: Individuals with rheumatic mitral valve disease with a history of either systemic embolism or paroxysmal or sustained atrial fibrillation should receive chronic warfarin anticoagulation with an international normalized ratio maintained between 2.0 and 3.0. Individuals with rheumatic mitral valve disease in normal sinus rhythm but with a left atrial size exceeding 5.5 cm in diameter should also receive chronic warfarin therapy as previously mentioned. Other patients with rheumatic mitral valve disease may be considered candidates for chronic warfarin anticoagulation if they are older than 65 to 70 years and have more modest but nonetheless definite left atrial dilatation. This is particularly the case if moderately severe or severe mitral stenosis is present. If recurrent systemic embolism occurs, the international normalized ratio range should be increased to 2.5 to 3.5, or 81 to 100 mg of aspirin daily should be added to long-term warfarin therapy. Patients with nonrheumatic mitral disease and paroxysmal or sustained atrial fibrillation should also be anticoagulated with warfarin (see Chapter 64).

A number of randomized trials are currently evaluating the role of transesophageal two-dimensional echocardiography in the management of patients with atrial fibrillation (see Chapters 52 and 64). One school of thought favors immediate cardioversion if left atrial thrombus is not identified during a transesophageal study. Other investigators point out that an occasional patient has an episode of arterial embolism following cardioversion despite a negative transesophageal study. The correct strategy will evolve from the results of ongoing trials. The traditional approach is 3 to 4 weeks of warfarin anticoagulation before and 4 weeks following elective cardioversion. Routine transesophageal echocardiographic studies are not obtained in these patients.

The long-term results of balloon valvuloplasty are still not available. Some patients are now 10 years from this procedure; but the numbers are small, and definitive long-term comparisons between balloon and surgical valvotomy await further follow-up results. Essop and coworkers anticipate that the long-term results of these two procedures will be similar, and it seems reasonable to concur with their arguments (222). Whether surgical repair of the mitral stenotic valve will largely displace prosthetic valve replacement also awaits the results of further clinical trials. Surgical advances, including minithoracotomies and endoscopic techniques are currently being developed and evaluated.

THE FUTURE

Further research, in the form of clinical trials, is needed to determine the appropriate role of vasodilator therapy in delaying or completely removing the need for mitral valve surgery. Continuing clinical and pathologic studies will provide data for improving therapy in patients with mitral valve prolapse as well as mitral regurgitation.

What role, if any, these procedures will play in the future remains to be seen.

Mitral Regurgitation

The most controversial decision for patients with chronic mitral regurgitation involves the timing of surgical intervention. At one time, it was commonly taught that mitral regurgitation was a benign lesion rarely, if ever, requiring mitral valve replacement. Subsequently, a number of clinician investigators argued for relatively early mitral valve replacement before insidious, irreversible left ventricular dysfunction developed. At the present time, most authorities favor serial, noninvasive follow-up for patients with chronic mitral regurgitation. Mitral valve repair or replacement is advised when early left ventricular dysfunction (left ventricular ejection fraction ≤50%) or dilatation (left ventricular end systolic volume index ≥55 mL per m²; end diastolic dimension between 65 and 68 mm; end systolic dimension between 44 and 45 mm) develops (160). Patients may be symptomatic or asymptomatic when significant left ventricular dysfunction or dilatation is observed. Controversy remains, however, concerning the level of left ventricular dysfunction or dilatation that should trigger an evaluation leading to mitral valve surgery (223). Long-term data from the Mayo Clinic suggest that patients with a flail mitral leaflet should be considered for surgery early in the course (224). As data accumulate, it is possible that evaluation of left ventricular function or size during and after a stress echocardiographic study will yield discriminating information, thereby making it easier to select patients for mitral valve repair.

Another controversy involves the decision for medical or surgical therapy in patients with mitral regurgitation and an already dilated hypokinetic left ventricle. Is this entity the result of a congestive cardiomyopathy with mitral regurgitation secondary to ventricular and mitral annular dilatation, or did this patient once have normal left ventricular function with severe, chronic mitral regurgitation leading to marked left ventricular dysfunction? Patients in the latter group may still be surgical candidates, whereas individuals in the former category are rarely offered surgical intervention. Moreover, to what degree, if any, is left ventricular dysfunction or dilatation reversible following surgery? Most of these patients are better served by aggressive vasodilator therapy with ACE inhibitors than with mitral valve surgery unless severe mitral regurgitation is present.

Yet another controversial topic is the role of vasodilator therapy (e.g., ACE inhibition) in delaying or entirely obviating the need for mitral valve surgery. Should prophylactic ACE inhibitor therapy be given to all patients with moderate to severe chronic mitral regurgitation? The answer to this question awaits an appropriately designed randomized clinical trial.

Finally, a number of arguments surround the entity of mitral valve prolapse: How many of the myriad individuals with echocardiographic prolapse actually have myxomatous degeneration of the valve? What intensity of follow-up is required for these individuals? How should they be counseled and what therapy should they receive? Is their exercise intolerance and orthostatic hypotension the result or the cause of their mitral valve prolapse? These and many other questions await the results of further clinical and pathologic studies (225).

REFERENCES

1. Bland EF, Jones TD. Rheumatic fever and rheumatic heart disease. *Circulation* 1951;4:836.
2. Wood P. An appreciation of mitral stenosis. Part I. Clinical features. *BMJ* 1954;1:1051.
3. Dalen JE, Fenster PE. Mitral stenosis. In: Alpert JS, Dalen JE, Rahimtoola SH, eds. *Valvular heart disease.* Philadelphia: Lippincott Williams & Wilkins, 2000.
4. Waller BF, Howard J, Fass S. Pathology of mitral stenosis and pure mitral regurgitation. Part I. *Clin Cardiol* 1994;17:330.
5. Bortolotti U, Valente M, Agozzino L, et al. Rheumatoid mitral stenosis requiring valve replacement. *Am Heart J* 1984;107:1049.
6. Misch KA. Development of heart valve lesions during methysergide therapy. *BMJ* 1974;2:365.
7. Ladefoged C, Rohr N. Amyloid deposits in aortic and mitral valves. *Virchow Arch* 1984;404:301.
8. Wrisley D, Giambartolomei A, Lee L, et al. Left atrial ball thrombus: review of clinical and echocardiographic manifestations with suggestions for management. *Am Heart J* 1991;121:1784.
9. Rowe JC, Bland EF, Sprague HB, et al. The course of mitral stenosis without surgery: ten- and twenty-year perspectives. *Ann Intern Med* 1960;52:741.
10. Olesen KH. The natural history of 271 patients with

mitral stenosis under medical treatment. *Br Heart J* 1962;24:349.

11. Rapaport E. Natural history of aortic and mitral value disease. *Am J Cardiol* 1975;35:221.

12. Grant RT. After histories for 10 years of 1000 men suffering from heart disease: a study in prognosis. *Heart* 1933;16:275.

13. Dubin AA, March HW, Cohn K, et al. Longitudinal hemodynamic and clinical study of mitral stenosis. *Circulation* 1971;44:381.

14. Gordon SPF, Douglas PS, Come PC, et al. Two-dimensional and Doppler echocardiographic determinants of the natural history of mitral valve narrowing in patients with rheumatic mitral stenosis: implications for follow-up. *J Am Coll Cardiol* 1992;19:968.

15. Waller BF, Howard J, Fess S. General concepts in the morphologic assessment of operatively excised cardiac valves. Part I. *Clin Cardiol* 1994;17:41.

16. Lachman AS, Roberts WC. Calcific deposits in stenotic mitral valves: extent and relation to age, sex, degree of stenosis, cardiac rhythm, previous commissurotomy and left atrial body thrombus. From a study of 164 operatively excised valves. *Circulation* 1978;57:808.

17. Alpert JS. Pulmonary hypertension. In: Goldman L, Bennett JC, eds. *Cecil textbook of medicine,* 21st ed. Philadelphia: WB Saunders, 2000:273.

17a. Schwammenthal E, Vered Z, Agranat O, et al. Impact of atrioventricular compliance on pulmonary artery pressure in mitral stenosis—an exercise echocardiographic study. *Circulation* 2000;102:2378.

18. Gash AK, Carabello BA, Cepin D, et al. Left ventricular ejection performance and systolic muscle function in patients with mitral stenosis. *Circulation* 1983;67:148.

19. Colle JP, Rahal S, Ohayon J, et al. Global left ventricular function and regional wall motion in pure mitral stenosis. *Clin Cardiol* 1984;7:573.

20. Mohan JC, Khalilullah M, Arora R. Left ventricular intrinsic contractility in pure rheumatic mitral stenosis. *Am J Cardiol* 1989;64:240.

20a. Chiang CW, Lo SK, Ko YS, et al. Predictors of systemic embolism in patients with mitral stenosis—a prospective study. *Ann Intern Med* 1998;128:885.

21. Keren G, Etzion T, Sherez J, et al. Atrial fibrillation and atrial enlargement in patients with mitral stenosis. *Am Heart J* 1987;114:1146.

22. Nielson GH, Galea EG, Houssack KF. Thromboembolic complications of mitral valve disease. *Aust N Z J Med* 1978;8:372.

23. Lie JT, Entmann ML. "Hole-in-one" sudden death: mitral stenosis and left atrial thrombus. *Am Heart J* 1976;91:798.

24. Legler JR, Benchimol A, Dimond EG. The apex cardiogram in the study of the 2-05 interval. *Br Heart J* 1963;25:246.

25. Craige E. Phonocardiographic studies in mitral stenosis. *N Engl J Med* 1957;257:650.

26. Nixon PG, Wooler GH, Radigan LR. The opening snap in mitral incompetence. *Br Heart J* 1960;22:395.

27. Millward DK, Laurin LP, Craige E. Echocardiographic studies to explain opening snaps in the presence of nonstenotic mitral valves. *Am J Cardiol* 1973;31:64.

28. Bonner AJ Jr, Stewart J, Tavel ME. "Presystolic" augmentation of diastolic heart sounds in atrial fibrillation. *Am J Cardiol* 1976;37:427.

29. Criley JM, Herman AJ. The crescendo presystolic murmur of mitral stenosis with atrial fibrillation. *N Engl J Med* 1971;285:1284.

30. Perloff JK. Auscultatory and phonocardiographic manifestations of pulmonary hypertension. *Prog Cardiovasc Dis* 1967;9:303.

31. Sherrid M, Goyal A, Delia E, et al. Unsuspected mitral stenosis. *Am J Med* 1991;90:189.

32. Cooksey JD, Dunn M, Massie E. *Clinical vectorcardiography and electrocardiography,* 2nd ed. Chicago: Year Book Medical, 1977:272.

33. Lutas EM, Deveraux RB, Borer JS, et al. Echocardiographic evaluation of mitral stenosis: a critical appraisal of its clinical value in detection of severe stenosis and valvular calcification. *J Cardiovasc Ultrasound* 1983;2:131.

34. Yang SS, Goldberg H. Simplified Doppler estimate of mitral valve area. *Am J Cardiol* 1985;56:488.

35. Smith MD, Handshoe R, Handshoe W, et al. Comparative accuracy of two-dimensional echocardiography and Doppler pressure half-time methods in assessing severity of mitral stenosis in patients with and without prior commissurotomy. *Circulation* 1986;73:100.

36. Pearlman JD, Gibson RS. Doppler measurement of left atrial depressurization and mitral valve area in patients with suspected mitral stenosis: validation of a new method. *Am Heart J* 1987;113:868.

37. Stoddard MF, Prince CR, Ammash NM, et al. Two-dimensional transesophageal echocardiographic determination of mitral valve area in adults with mitral stenosis. *Am Heart J* 1994;127:1348.

38. Shapiro LM. Echocardiography of the mitral valve. In: Wells FC, Shapiro LM, eds. *Mitral valve disease,* 2nd ed. London: Butterworth, 1996:47.

39. Daniel WG, Nellessen U, Schroeder E, et al. Left atrial spontaneous echo contrast in mitral valve disease: an indicator for an increased thromboembolic risk. *J Am Coll Cardiol* 1988;11:1204.

40. Leung DYC, Black IW, Cranney GB, et al. Resolution of left atrial spontaneous echocardiographic contrast after percutaneous mitral valvuloplasty: implications for thromboembolic risk. *Am Heart J* 1995;129:65.

40a. Gonzalez-Torrecilla E, Garcia-Fernandez MA, Perez-David E, et al. Predictors of left atrial spontaneous echo contrast and thrombi in patients with mitral stenosis and atrial fibrillation. *Am J Cardiol* 2000;86:529.

41. Sagie A, Freitas N, Padial LR, et al. Doppler echocardiographic assessment of long-term progression of mitral stenosis in 103 patients: valve area and right heart disease. *J Am Coll Cardiol* 1996;28:472.

41a. Binder TM, Rosenhek R, Porenta G, et al. Improved assessment of mitral valve stenosis by volumetric real-time three-dimensional echocardiography. *J Am Coll Cardiol* 2000;36:1355.

42. Gorlin R, Gorlin SG. Hydraulic formula for calculations of the area of the stenotic mitral valve, other cardiac valves, and central circulatory shunts. *Am Heart J* 1951;41:1.

43. Bulkley BH, Hutchins GM. Atrial myxomas: a fifty-year review. *Am Heart J* 1979;97:639.

44. Lappe DL, Buckley BH, Weiss JL. Two dimensional echocardiographic diagnosis of left atrial myxoma. *Chest* 1978;74:55.

45. Ehrich DA, Vieweg WVR, Alpert JS, et al. Cor triatriatum: report of a case in a young adult with special reference to the echocardiographic features and etiology of the systolic murmur. *Am Heart J* 1977;94:217.

45a. Cieslewicz G, Juszczyk G, Foremny J, et al. Inhaled corticosteroid improves bronchial reactivity and decreases symptoms in patients with mitral stenosis. *Chest* 1998;114:1070.

46. Selzer A, Cohn KE. Natural history of mitral stenosis: a review. *Circulation* 1972;45:878.

47. Sherrid MV, Clark RD, Cohn K. Echocardiographic analysis of left atrial size before and after operation in mitral valve disease. *Am J Cardiol* 1979;43:171.

48. Coulshed N, Epstein EJ, McKendrick CS, et al. Systemic embolism in mitral valve disease. *Br Heart J* 1970;32:26.

49. Meisner JS, Keran G, Pajaro OE, et al. Atrial contribution to ventricular filling in mitral stenosis. *Circulation* 1991;84:1469.

50. Morganroth J. Relationship of atrial fibrillatory wave amplitude to left atrial size and etiology of heart disease. *Am Heart J* 1979;97:184.

51. Deverall PB, Olley PM, Smith DR, et al. The incidence of systemic embolism before and after mitral valvotomy. *Thorax* 1968;23:530.

52. Dalen JE, Hirsh J, eds. Sixth ACCP Consensus Conference on Antithrombotic Therapy. *Chest* 2001;119[Suppl]:194S and 207S.

53. Husband EM, Lannigan R. Unusual giant cell lesions in biopsy specimens of left atrial appendages in mitral stenosis. *Br Heart J* 1965;27:269.

54. Coffman JD, Sommers SC. Familial pseudoxanthoma elasticum and valvular heart disease. *Circulation* 1959;19:242.

55. Patel JJ, Sharma D, Mitha A, et al. Percutaneous balloon valvuloplasty versus closed commissurotomy for pliable mitral stenosis: a prospective hemodynamic study. *J Am Coll Cardiol* 1991;18:1318.

56. Turi ZG, Reyes VP, Raju BS, et al. Percutaneous balloon versus surgical closed commissurotomy for mitral stenosis: a prospective randomized trial. *Circulation* 1991;83:1179.

57. Reyes VP, Raju S, Wynne J, et al. Percutaneous balloon valvuloplasty compared with open surgical commissurotomy for mitral stenosis. *N Engl J Med* 1994;331:951.

57a. Stefanadis CI, Stratos CG, Lambrou SG, et al. Retrograde non-transseptal balloon mitral valvuloplasty: immediate results and intermediate long-term outcome in 441 cases—a multicenter experience. *J Am Coll Cardiol* 1998;32:1009.

57b. Bahl VK, Chandra S, Jhamb DK, et al. Balloon mitral valvotomy: comparison between antegrade Inoue and retrograde non-transseptal techniques. *Eur Heart J* 1997;18:1765.

58. Iung B, Cormier B, Ducimatiere P, et al. Functional results 5 years after successful percutaneous mitral commissurotomy in a series of 528 patients and analysis of prediction factors. *J Am Coll Cardiol* 1996;27:407.

58a. Hernandez R, Banuelos C, Alfonso F, et al. Long-term clinical and echocardiographic follow-up after percutaneous mitral valvuloplasty with the Inoue balloon. *Circulation* 1999;99:1580.

58b. Ommen SR, Nishimura RA, Grill DE, et al. Comparison of long-term results of percutaneous mitral balloon valvotomy with closed transventricular mitral commissurotomy at a single North American institution. *Am J Cardiol* 1999;84:575.

58c. Cribier A, Eltchaninoff H, Koning R, et al. Percutaneous mechanical mitral commissurotomy with a newly designed metallic valvulotome. Immediate results of the initial experience in 153 patients. *Circulation* 1999;99:793.

58d. Iung B, Garbarz E, Michaud P, et al. Late results of percutaneous mitral commissurotomy in a series of 1024 patients. Analysis of late clinical deterioration: frequency, anatomic findings, and predictive factors. *Circulation* 1999;99:3272.

58e. Hildick-Smith DJR, Taylor GJ, Shapiro LM. Inoue balloon mitral valvuloplasty: Long-term clinical and echocardiographic follow-up of a predominantly unfavorable population. *Eur Heart J* 2000;21:1690.

58f. Zaki A, Salama M, El Masry M, et al. Five-year follow-up after percutaneous balloon mitral valvuloplasty in children and adolescents. *Am J Cardiol* 1999;83:735.

58g. Martinez-Reding J, Cordero A, Kuri J, et al. Treatment of severe mitral stenosis with percutaneous balloon valvotomy in pregnant patients. *Clin Cardiol* 1998;21:659.

59. Arora R, Nair M, Kalra GS, et al. Immediate and long-term results of balloon and surgical closed mitral valvotomy: a randomized comparative study. *Am Heart J* 1993;125:1091.

60. Ribeiro PA, Zaibag MA, Abdullah M. Pulmonary artery pressure and pulmonary vascular resistance before and after mitral balloon valvotomy in 100 patients with severe mitral stenosis. *Am Heart J* 1993;125:1110.

61. Chen CR, Chen TO. Percutaneous balloon mitral valvuloplasty by the Inoue technique: a multi center study of 4832 patients in China. *Am Heart J* 1995;129:1197.

62. Goto S, Hand S, Akaishi M, et al. Left ventricular ejection performance in mitral stenosis, and effects of successful percutaneous transvenous mitral commissurotomy. *Am J Cardiol* 1992;69:233.

62a. Stefanadis CI, Dernellis J, Stratos C, et al. Effects of balloon mitral valvuloplasty on left atrial function in mitral stenosis as assessed by pressure-area relation. *J Am Coll Cardiol* 1998;32:159.

63. Tischler MD, St. John Sutton M, Bittl JA, et al. Effects of percutaneous mitral valvuloplasty on left ventricular mass and volume. *Am J Cardiol* 1991;68:940.

64. Liu CP, Ting CT, Yang TM, et al. Reduced left ventricular compliance in human mitral stenosis: role of reversible internal constraint. *Circulation* 1992;85:1447.

64a. Ashino K, Gotoh E, Sumita S, et al. Percutaneous transluminal mitral valvuloplasty normalizes baroreflex sensitivity and sympathetic activity in patients with mitral stenosis. *Circulation* 1997;96:3443.

64b. Pathan AZ, Mahdi NA, Leon MA, et al. Is redo percutaneous mitral balloon valvuloplasty (PMV) indicated in patients with post-PMV mitral restenosis. *J Am Coll Cardiol* 1999;34:49.

65. Vahanian A. Percutaneous mitral commissurotomy. *Eur Heart J* 1996;17:1465.

66. Gupta S, Vora A, Lokhandwalla Y, et al. Percutaneous balloon mitral valvotomy in mitral restenosis. *Eur Heart J* 1996;17:1560.

67. Dean LS, Mickel M, Bonan R, et al. Four-year follow-up of patients undergoing percutaneous balloon mitral commissurotomy: a report from the NHLBI Balloon Valvuloplasty Registry. *J Am Coll Cardiol* 1996;28:1452.

67a. Pavlides GS, Nahhas GT, London J, et al. Predictors of long-term event-free survival after percutaneous balloon mitral valvuloplasty. *Am J Cardiol* 1997;79:1370.

67b. Zhang HP, Yen GSH, Allen JW, et al. Comparison of late results of balloon valvotomy in mitral stenosis with versus without mitral regurgitation. *Am J Cardiol* 1998;81:51.

67c. Langerveld J, Plokker HWT, Ernst SMPG, et al. Predictors of clinical events or restenosis during follow-up after percutaneous mitral balloon valvotomy. *Eur Heart J* 1999;20:519.

68. Souttar HS. The surgical treatment of mitral stenosis. *BMJ* 1925;2:603.

69. Cutler EC, Levine SA. Cardiotomy and valvulotomy for mitral stenosis: experimental observations and clinical notes concerning an operated case with recovery. *Boston Med Surg J* 1923;188:1023.

70. Harken DE, Ellis LB, Ware PF, et al. The surgical treatment of mitral stenosis: I. valve repair. *N Engl J Med* 1948;239:804.

71. Bailey CP. The surgical treatment of mitral stenosis (mitral commissurotomy). *Dis Chest* 1949;15:377.

72. Grunkemeier GL, Starr A, Rahimtoola S. Prosthetic heart valve performance: long-term follow-up. *Curr Probl Cardiol* 1992;17:333.

73. Jamieson WRE, Burr LH, Munro I, et al. Cardiac valve replacement in the elderly: clinical performance of biological prosthesis. *Ann Thorac Surg* 1989;48:173.

74. Lougie Y, Noirhomme P, Aranguis E, et al. Use of the Carpentier-Edwards porcine bioprosthesis: assessment of patient selection policy. *J Thorac Cardiovasc Surg* 1992;104:1013.

74a. Jamieson WRE, Marchand MA, Pelletier CL, et al. Structural valve deterioration in mitral replacement surgery: comparison of Carpentier-Edwards supre-annular porcine and Perimount pericardial bioprosthesis. *J Thorac Cardiovasc Surg* 1999;118:297.

75. Lillihei CW, Levy MJ, Bonnabeau RC Jr. Mitral valve replacement with preservation of papillary muscles and chordae tendineae. *J Thorac Cardiovasc Surg* 1964;47:532.

76. Peter CA, Austin EH, Jones RH. Effect of valve replacement for chronic mitral insufficiency on left ventricular function during rest and exercise. *J Thorac Cardiovasc Surg* 1981;82:127.

77. Goldman ME, Mora F, Guarino T, et al. Mitral valve repair is superior to valve replacement for preservation of left ventricular function: an intraoperative two-dimensional echocardiographic study. *J Am Coll Cardiol* 1987;10:568.

78. Bonchek LI, Olinger GN, Siegel R, et al. Left ventricular performance after mitral reconstruction for mitral regurgitation. *J Thorac Cardiovasc Surg* 1984;88:122.

79. David TE, Uden DE, Strauss HD. The importance of the mitral apparatus in left ventricular function after correction of mitral regurgitation. *Circulation* 1983;68(Suppl II):II-76.

80. Hetzer R, Bougioukas G, Frenz M, et al. Mitral valve replacement with preservation of papillary muscles and chordae tendineae—revival of a seemingly forgotten concept. *Thorac Cardiovasc Surg* 1983;31:291.

81. Craver JM, Jones EL, Guyton RA, et al. Avoidance of transverse midventricular disruption following mitral valve replacement. *Ann Thorac Surg* 1985;40:163.

82. Karlson KJ, Ashraf MM, Berger RL. Rupture of left ventricle following mitral valve replacement. *Ann Thorac Surg* 1988;46:590.

83. Spencer FC, Galloway AC, Colvin SB. A clinical evaluation of the hypothesis that rupture of the left ventricle following mitral valve replacement can be prevented by preservation of the chordae of the mural leaflet. *Ann Surg* 1985;202:673.

84. Goor DA, Mohr R, Lavee J, et al. Preservation of the posterior leaflet during mechanical valve replacement for ischemic mitral regurgitation and complete myocardial revascularization. *J Thorac Cardiovasc Surg* 1988;96:253.

85. Appelbaun A, Kouchoukos NT, Blackstone EH, et al. Early risks of open heart surgery for mitral valve disease. *Am J Cardiol* 1976;37:201.

86. Bonchek LI, Anderson RP, Starr A. Mitral valve replacement with cloth-covered composite-seat prosthesis. *J Thorac Cardiovasc Surg* 1974;67:93.

87. Junrod FI, Harlan BJ, Payne J, et al. Preoperative risk assessment in cardiac surgery: comparison of predicted and observed results. *Ann Thorac Surg* 1987;43:59.

88. Arom KV, Nicoloff DM, Kersten TE, et al. Ten years' experience with the St. Jude medical valve prosthesis. *Ann Thorac Surg* 1989;47:831.

89. Cohn LH, Koster JK, Mee RBB, et al. Long-term follow-up of the Hancock bioprosthetic heart valve: a 6-year review. *Circulation* 1979;60:[Suppl I]:I-87.

90. Lytle BW, Cosgrove DM, Gill GC, et al. Mitral valve replacement combined with myocardial revascularization: early and late results for 300 patient, 1970 to 1983. *Circulation* 1985;71:1179.

91. Starr A, Grunkemeier G, Lambert L, et al. Mitral valve replacement: a 10-year follow-up of noncloth-covered vs. cloth-covered caged-ball prosthesis. *Circulation* 1976;54(Suppl III):III-47.

92. Oyer PE, Stinson EB, Reitz BA, et al. Long-term evaluation of the porcine xenograft bioprosthesis. *J Thorac Cardiovasc Surg* 1979;78:343.

93. Allen WB, Karp RB, Kouchoukos NT. Mitral valve replacement: Starr-Edwards cloth-covered composite seat prosthesis. *Arch Surg* 1975;109:642.

94. Isom OW, Spencer FC, Glassman E, et al. Long term results in 1375 patients undergoing valve replacement with the Starr-Edwards cloth-covered composite-seat prosthesis: a six year appraisal. *Ann Surg* 1989;48:173.

95. Kumar AS, Rao PN. Restoration of pliability to the mitral leaflets during reconstruction. *J Heart Valve Dis* 1995;4:251.

96. Bernal JM, Rabasa JM, Olalla JJ, et al. Repair of chordae tendineae for rheumatic mitral valve disease. *J Thorac Cardiovasc Surg* 1996;111:211.

97. Cohn LH, Allred EN, Cohn LA, et al. Long-term results of open mitral valve reconstruction for mitral stenosis. *Am J Cardiol* 1985;55:731.

98. Antunes MJ, Magalhaes MP, Colsen PR, et al. Valve repair for rheumatic mitral valve disease: a surgical challenge. *J Thorac Cardiovasc Surg* 1987;94:44.

99. Eguaras MG, Jimenez MAG, Calleja F, et al. Early open mitral commissurotomy: long-term results. *J Thorac Cardiovasc Surg* 1993;106:421.

100. Laschinger JC, Cunningham JN Jr, Baumann FG, et al. Early open radical commissurotomy: surgical treatment of choice for mitral stenosis. *Ann Thorac Surg* 1982;34:287.

101. Vega JL, Fleitas M, Martinez R, et al. Open mitral commissurotomy. *J Thorac Cardiovasc Surg* 1977;73:742.

102. Herrera JM, Vega JL, Bernal JM, et al. Open mitral commissurotomy: fourteen- to eighteen-year follow-up clinical study. *Ann Thorac Surg* 1993;55:641.

103. Duran CMG, Gometza B, Saad E. Valve repair in rheumatic mitral disease: an unsolved problem. *J Cardiovasc Surg* 1994;9(Suppl):282.

103a. Farhat MB, Ayari M, Maatouk F, et al. Percutaneous balloon versus surgical closed and open mitral commissurotomy—seven year follow-up results of a randomized trial. *Circulation* 1998;97:245.

103b. Ommen SR, Nishimura RA, Grill DE, et al. Comparison of long-term results of percutaneous mitral balloon valvotomy with closed transventricular mitral commissurotomy at single North American institution. *Am J Cardiol* 1999;84:575.

104. Pini R, Devereux RB, Grappi B, et al. Comparison of mitral valve dimensions and motion in mitral valve prolapse with severe mitral regurgitation to uncomplicated mitral valve prolapse and to mitral regurgitation without prolapse. *Am J Cardiol* 1988;62:257.

105. Tamura K, Fukuda Y, Ishizaki M, et al. Abnormalities in elastic fibers and other connective-tissue components of floppy mitral valve. *Am Heart J* 1995;129:1149.

106. Barlow JB, Pocock WA. Mitral valve prolapse: the specific billowing mitral leaflet syndrome, or an insignificant non-ejection click systolic click. *Am Heart J* 1979;97:277.

107. Leier CV, Call TD, Fulkerson PK, et al. The spectrum of cardiac defects in the Ehlers-Danlos syndrome, types I and II. *Ann Intern Med* 1980;92:171.

108. Udoshi MB, Shah A, Fisher VJ, et al. Incidence of mitral valve prolapse in subjects with thoracic skeletal abnormalities—a prospective study. *Am Heart J* 1979;97:303.

109. Rippe JM, Sloss LJ, Angoff G, et al. Mitral valve prolapse in adults with congenital heart disease. *Am Heart J* 1979;97:561.

110. O'Rourke RA, Crawford MH. The systolic click-murmur syndrome: clinical recognition and management. *Curr Probl Cardiol* 1976;1:1.

111. Lebwohl MG, Distefano D, Prioleau PG, et al. Pseudoxanthoma elasticum and mitral valve prolapse. *N Engl J Med* 1982;307:228.

112. Zema MJ, Chiaramida S, DeFilipp GJ, et al. Somatotype and idiopathic mitral valve prolapse. *Cathet Cardiovasc Diagn* 1982;8:105.

113. Froom P, Margulis T, Grenadier E, et al. Von Willebrand factor and mitral valve prolapse. *Thromb Haemostasis* 1988;60:230.

114. Noah MS, Sulimani RA, Famuyiwa FO, et al. Prolapse of the mitral valve in hyperthyroid patients in Saudi Arabia. *Int J Cardiol* 1988;19:217.

115. Devereux RB, Kramer-Fox R, Kligfield P. Mitral valve prolapse: etiology, clinical manifestations and management. *Ann Intern Med* 1989;111:305.

115a. Zhou L, Lu K. Inflammatory valvular prolapse produced by acute rheumatic carditis: echocardiographic analysis of 66 cases of acute rheumatic carditis. *Int J Cardiol* 1997;58:175.

115b. Raggi P, Callister TQ, Lippolis NJ, et al. Is mitral valve prolapse due to cardiac entrapment in the chest cavity? A CT view. *Chest* 2000;117:636.

115c. Trochu JN, Kyndt F, Schott JJ, et al. Clinical characteristics of a familial inherited myxomatous valvular dystrophy mapped to Xq28. *J Am Coll Cardiol* 2000;35:1890.

116. D'Cruz IA, Colien HC, Prabhu R, et al. Clinical manifestations of mitral annulus calcification with emphasis on its echocardiographic features. *Am Heart J* 1977;94:367.

117. Leibovitch ER. Cardiac value disorders: growing significance in the elderly. *Geriatrics* 1989;44:91.

118. Mellino M, Salcedo EE, Lever HM, et al. Echographic-quantified severity of mitral annulus calcification: prognostic correlation to related hemodynamic, valvular, rhythm, and conduction abnormalities. *Am Heart J* 1982;103:222.

119. Roberts WC. Morphologic features of the normal and abnormal mitral valve. *Am J Cardiol* 1983;51:1005.

119a. Yiu SF, Enriquez-Sarano M, Tribouilloy C, et al. Determinants of the degree of functional mitral regurgitation in patients with systolic left ventricular dysfunction. A quantitative clinical study. *Circulation* 2000;102:1400.

120. Layman TE, Edwards JE. Anomalous mitral arcade: a type of congenital mitral insufficiency. *Circulation* 1969;35:389.

121. Izumi S, Miyatake K, Beppu S, et al. Mechanism of mitral regurgitation in patients with myocardial infarction: a study using real-time two-dimensional Doppler flow imaging and echocardiography. *Circulation* 1987;76:777.

121a. Komeda M, Glasson JR, Bolger AF, et al. Geometric determinants of ischemic mitral regurgitation. *Circulation* 1997;96(Suppl II):II-128.

121b. Gorman JH, Jackson BM, Gorman RC, et al. Papillary muscle discoordination rather than increased area facilitates mitral regurgitation after acute posterior myocardial infarction. *Circulation* 1997;96(Suppl II):II-124.

122. Hickey MS, Smith LR, Muhlbaier LH, et al. Current prognosis of ischemic mitral regurgitation: implications for future management. *Circulation* 1988;78[Suppl I]:I51.

122a. Feinberg MS, Schwammenthal E, Shlizerman L, et al. Prognostic significance of mild mitral regurgitation by color Doppler echocardiography in acute myocardial infarction. *Am J Cardiol* 2000;86:903.

122b. Lamas GA, Mitchell GF, Flaker GC, et al. Clinical significance of mitral regurgitation after acute myocardial infarction. *Circulation* 1997;96:827.

123. Gehl LG, Mintz GS, Kotler MN, et al. Left atrial volume overload in mitral regurgitation: a two-dimensional echocardiographic study. *Am J Cardiol* 1982;49:33.

124. Carabello BA. Mitral regurgitation: Part 1. Basic pathophysiological principles. *Mod Conc Cardiovasc Dis* 1988;57:53.

124a. Otsuji Y, Handschumacher MD, Schwammenthal E, et al. Insights from three-dimensional echocardiography into the mechanism of functional mitral regurgitation. Direct in vivo demonstration of altered leaflet tethering geometry. *Circulation* 1997;96:1999.

125. Eckberg DL, Gault JH, Bouchard RL, et al. Mechanics of left ventricular contraction in chronic severe mitral regurgitation. *Circulation* 1973;47:1252.

126. Starling MR, Kirsh MM, Montgomery DG, et al. Impaired left ventricular contractile function in patients with long-term mitral regurgitation and normal ejection fraction. *J Am Coll Cardiol* 1993;22:239.

127. Ramanthan KB, Knowles J, Connor MJ, et al. Natural history of chronic mitral insufficiency: relation of peak systolic pressure/end-systolic volume ratio to morbidity and mortality. *J Am Coll Cardiol* 1984;3:1412.

128. Borow K, Green LH, Mann T, et al. End-systolic volume as a predictor of postoperative left ventricular performance in volume overload from valvular regurgitation. *Am J Med* 1980;68:655.

129. Mudge GH. Asymptomatic mitral regurgitation. *J Cardiovasc Surg* 1994;9(Suppl):248.

130. Wisenbaugh T, Spann JF, Carabello BA. Differences in myocardial performance and load between patients with similar amounts of chronic aortic versus mitral regurgitation. *J Am Coll Cardiol* 1984;3:916.

131. Carabello BA, Usher BW, Hendrix GH, et al. Predictors of outcome for aortic valve replacement in patients with aortic regurgitation and left ventricular dysfunction: a change in the measuring stick. *J Am Coll Cardiol* 1987;10:991.

131a. Tse HF, Lau CP, Cheng G. Relation between mitral regurgitation and platelet activation. *J Am Coll Cardiol* 1997;30:1813.

132. Ross J Jr. Afterload mismatch and preload reserve: a conceptual framework for the analysis of ventricular function. *Prog Cardiovasc Dis* 1985;18:255.

133. Kass DA, Maughan WL, Guo ZM, et al. Comparative influence of load versus inotropic states on indexes of ventricular contractility: experimental and theoretical analysis based on pressure-volume relationships. *Circulation* 1987;76:1422.

134. Gaffney FA, Karlson ES, Campbell W, et al. Autonomic dysfunction in women with mitral valve prolapse syndrome. *Circulation* 1979;59:894.

135. Coghlan HC, Phares P, Cowley M, et al. Dysautonomia in mitral valve prolapse. *Am J Med* 1979;67:236.

136. Maraugoni S, Scalvini S, Mai R, et al. Heart rate variability assessment in patients with mitral valve prolapse syndrome. *Am J Noninvas Cardiol* 1993;7:210.

137. Corin WJ, Murakami T, Monrad S, et al. Left ventricular passive diastolic properties in chronic mitral regurgitation. *Circulation* 1991;83:797.

137a. Enriquez-Sarano M, Basmadjian AJ, Rossi A, et al. Progression of mitral regurgitation—a prospective doppler echocardiographic study. *J Am Coll Cardiol* 1999;34:1137.

138. Zuppiroli A, Rinaldi M, Kramer-Fox R, et al. Natural history of mitral valve prolapse. *Am J Cardiol* 1995;75:1028.

139. Stoddard MF, Prince CR, Dillon S, et al. Exercise-induced mitral regurgitation is a predictor of morbid events in subjects with mitral valve prolapse. *J Am Coll Cardiol* 1995;25:693.

140. Enriquez-Sarano M, Schaff HV, Tajik AJ, et al. Chronic mitral regurgitation. In: Alpert JS, Dalen JE, Rahimtoola SH, eds. *Valvular heart disease.* Philadelphia: Lippincott Williams & Wilkins, 2000.

141. Porter CM, Baxley WA, Eddleman EF Jr, et al. Left ventricular dimensions and dynamics of filling in patients with gallop sounds. *Am J Med* 1971;50:721.

142. Carabello BA. Acute mitral regurgitation. In: Alpert JS, Dalen JE, Rahimtoola SH, eds. *Valvular heart disease*, 3rd ed. Philadelphia: Lippincott Williams & Wilkins, 2000.

143. Klein AL, Stewart WJ, Bartlett J, et al. Effects of mitral regurgitation on pulmonary venous flow and left atrial pressure: an intraoperative transesophageal echocardiographic study. *J Am Coll Cardiol* 1992;20:1345.

144. Hellemans IM, Pieper EG, Ravelli ACJ, et al. Comparison of transthoracic and transesophageal echocardiography with surgical findings in mitral regurgitation. *Am J Cardiol* 1996;77:728.

145. Tribouilly C, Shen WF, Quere JP, et al. Assessment of severity of mitral regurgitation by measuring regurgitant jet width at its origin in the transesophageal Doppler color flow imaging. *Circulation* 1992;85:1248.

146. Castello R, Lenzen P, Aguirre F, et al. Quantitation of mitral regurgitation by transesophageal echocardiography with Doppler color flow mapping: correlation with cardiac catheterization. *J Am Coll Cardiol* 1992;19:1516.

146a. Enriquez-Sarano M, Freeman WK, Tribouilloy CM, et al. Functional anatomy of mitral regurgitation—accuracy and outcome implications of transesophageal echocardiography. *J Am Coll Cardiol* 1999;34:1129.

146b. Thomas L, Foster E, Hoffman JIE, et al. The mitral regurgitation index: an echocardiographic guide to severity. *J Am Coll Cardiol* 1999;33:2016.

147. Marks AR, Choong CY, Sanfillipos AJ, et al. Identification of high-risk and low-risk subgroups of patients with mitral valve prolapse. *N Engl J Med* 1989;320:1031.

147a. Kimura BJ, Scott R, Willis CL, et al. Accuracy and cost-effectiveness of single-view echocardiographic screening for suspected mitral valve prolapse. *Am J Med* 2000;108:331.

148. Hundley WG, Li HF, Willard JE, et al. Magnetic resonance imaging assessment of the severity of mitral regurgitation: comparison with invasive techniques. *Circulation* 1995;92:1151.

149. Carabello BA, Spann JF. The uses and limitations of end-systolic indexes of left ventricular function. *Circulation* 1984;69:1058.

150. Wisenbaugh T. Does normal pump function relieve muscle dysfunction in patients with chronic severe mitral regurgitation? *Circulation* 1988;77:515.

151. Pape LA, Price JM, Alpert JS, et al. Relation of left atrial size to pulmonary capillary wedge pressure in severe mitral regurgitation. *Cardiology* 1991;78:297.

152. Greenberg BH, Masic BM, Brundage BH, et al. Beneficial effects of hydralazine in severe mitral regurgitation. *Circulation* 1978;58:273.

153. Hoit BD. Medical treatment of valvular disease. *Curr Opin Cardiol* 1991;6:207.

153a. Tischler MD, Rowan M, LeWinter MM. Effect of enalapril therapy on left ventricular mass and volumes in asymptomatic chronic, severe mitral regurgitation secondary to mitral valve prolapse. *Am J Cardiol* 1998;82:242.

153b. Levine AB, Muller C, Levine TB. Effects of high-dose lisinopril-isosorbide dinitrate on severe mitral regurgitation and heart failure remodeling. *Am J Cardiol* 1998;82:1299.

154. Chatterjee K, Parmley WW, Swan HJC, et al. Beneficial effects of vasodilator agents in severe mitral regurgitation due to dysfunction of the subvalvular apparatus. *Circulation* 1973;48:684.

155. Goodman DJ, Rossen RM, Holloway EL, et al. Effect of nitroprusside on left ventricular dynamics in mitral regurgitation. *Circulation* 1974;50:1025.

156. Greenberg BH, DeMots H, Murphy E, et al. Arterial vasodilators in mitral regurgitation: effects on rest and exercise hemodynamics and long-term clinical follow-up. *Circulation* 1982;65:181.

157. Keren G, Katz S, Strom J. Dynamic mitral regurgitation: an important determinant of the hemodynamic response to load alterations and inotropic therapy in severe heart failure. *Circulation* 1989;80:306.

158. Schon HR, Schroter G, Barthal P, et al. Quinapril therapy in patients with chronic mitral regurgitation. *J Heart Valve Dis* 1994;3:303.

159. Wisenbaugh T, Sinovich V, Dullabh A, et al. Six-month pilot study of captopril for mildly symptomatic severe isolated mitral and isolated aortic regurgitation. *J Heart Valve Dis* 1994;3:197.

160. Gaasch WH, John RM, Aurigemma GP. Managing asymptomatic patients with chronic mitral regurgitation. *Chest* 1995;108:842.

161. Devereux RB. Recent developments in the diagnosis and management of mitral valve prolapse. *Curr Opin Cardiol* 1995;10:107.

162. Perloff JK, Child JS, Edwards JE. New guidelines for clinical diagnosis of mitral valve prolapse. *Am J Cardiol* 1986;57:1124.

163. Fontana ME, Sparks EA, Boudoulas H, et al. Mitral valve prolapse and the mitral valve prolapse syndrome. *Curr Probl Cardiol* 1991;16:311.

163a. Kimura BJ, Scott R, Willis CL, et al. Accuracy and cost-effectiveness of single-view echocardiographic screening for suspected mitral valve prolapse. *Am J Med* 2000;108:331.

164. Levy D, Savage DD. Prevalence and clinical features of mitral valve prolapse. *Am Heart J* 1987;113:1281.

165. Barlow JB, Pocock WA, Marchand P, et al. The significance of the late systolic murmurs. *Am Heart J* 1963;66:443.

166. Wooley CF. From irritable heart to mitral valve prolapse: the Osler connection. *Am J Cardiol* 1984;53:870.

167. Devereux RB, Hawkins I, Kramer-Fox R, et al. Complications of mitral valve prolapse: disproportionate occurrence in men and older patients. *Am J Med* 1986;81:751.

167a. Freed LA, Levy D, Levine RA, et al. Prevalence and clinical outcome of mitral valve prolapse. *N Engl J Med* 1999;341:1.

168. Levine RA, Handschumacher MD, Sanfilippo AJ, et al. Three-dimensional echocardiographic reconstruction of the mitral valve, with implications for the diagnosis of mitral valve prolapse. *Circulation* 1989;80:589.

169. Levine RA, Stathogiannis E, Newell JB, et al. Reconsideration of echocardiographic standards for mitral valve prolapse: lack of association between leaflet displacement isolated to the apical four chamber view and independent echocardiographic evidence of abnormality. *J Am Coll Cardiol* 1988;11:1010.

169a. Trochu JN, Kyndt F, Schott JJ, et al. Clinical characteristics of a familial inherited myxomatous valvular dystrophy mapped to Xq28. *J Am Coll Cardiol* 2000;35:1890.

170. Stein PD, Wang G-H, Riddle JM, et al. Scanning electron microscopy of operatively excised severely regurgitant floppy mitral valves. *Am J Cardiol* 1989;64:392.

171. Malcolm AD. Mitral valve prolapse associated with other disorders: causal coincidence, common link, or fundamental genetic disturbance? *Br Heart J* 1985;53:353.

172. Zuppiroli A, Roman MJ, O'Gardy M, et al. Lack of association between mitral valve prolapse and history of rheumatic fever. *Am Heart J* 1996;131:525.

173. Tomaru T, Uchida Y, Mohri N, et al. Postinflammatory mitral and aortic valve prolapse: a clinical and pathological study. *Circulation* 1987;76:68.

174. Sanfilippo AJ, Harrigan P, Popovic AD, et al. Papillary muscle traction in mitral valve prolapse: quantitation by two-dimensional echocardiography. *J Am Coll Cardiol* 1993;19:564.

175. Mills P, Rose J, Hollingsworth J, et al. Long-term prognosis of mitral valve prolapse. *N Engl J Med* 1977;297:13.

176. Olson LJ, Subramanian R, Ackermann DM, et al. Surgical pathology of the mitral valve: a study of 712 cases spanning 21 years. *Mayo Clin Proc* 1987;62:22.

177. Wilcken DE, Hickey AJ. Lifetime risk for patients with mitral prolapse of developing severe valve regurgitation requiring surgery. *Circulation* 1988;78:10.

177a. Singh RG, Cappucci R, Kramer-Fox R, et al. Severe mitral regurgitation due to mitral valve prolapse: risk factors for development, progression, and need for mitral valve surgery. *Am J Cardiol* 2000;85:193.

177b. Kamei F, Nakahara N, Yuda S, et al. Long-term site related differences in the progression and regression of the idiopathic mitral valve prolapse syndrome. *Cardiology* 1999;91:161.

178. Ling LH, Enriquez-Sarano M, Seward JB, et al. Clinical outcome of mitral regurgitation due to flail leaflet. *N Engl J Med* 1996;335:1417.

178a. Grigioni F, Enriquez-Sarano M, Ling LH, et al. Sudden death in mitral regurgitation due to flail leaflet. *J Am Coll Cardiol* 1999;34:802.

178b. Ling LH, Enriquez-Sarano M, Seward JB, et al. Early surgery in patients with mitral regurgitation due to flail leaflets—a long-term outcome study. *Circulation* 1997;96:1819.

179. Hickey AJ, MacMahon SW, Wilcken DEL. Mitral valve prolapse and bacterial endocarditis: when is antibiotic prophylaxis necessary? *Am Heart J* 1985;109:431.

179a. Stefanadis CI, Toutouzas P. Mitral valve prolapse: *The Merchant of Venice* or *Much Ado about Nothing*? *Eur Heart J* 2000;21:255.

180. Danchin N, Briancon S, Mathieu P, et al. Mitral valve prolapse as a risk factor for infective endocarditis. *Lancet* 1989;1:743.

181. Barletta GA, Gagliardi R, Benvenuti L, et al. Cerebral

ischemic attacks as a complication of aortic and mitral valve prolapse. *Stroke* 1985;16:218.

182. Schnee MA, Bucal AA. Fatal embolism in mitral valve prolapse. *Chest* 1983;83:825.

183. Makino H, Al-Sadir J. Myocardial infarction in patients with mitral valve prolapse and normal coronary arteries. *J Am Coll Cardiol* 1983;1:661.

183a. Gilon D, Buonanno FS, Joffe MM, et al. Lack of evidence of an association between mitral valve prolapse and stroke in young patients. *N Engl J Med* 1999;341:8.

184. Kligfield P, Devereux RB. Arrhythmia in mitral valve prolapse. In: Podrid PR, Kowey PR, eds. *Cardiac arrhythmia: mechanisms, diagnosis and management.* Baltimore: Williams & Wilkins, 1995:1253.

185. Kligfield P, Hochreiter C, Niles N, et al. Relation of sudden death in pure mitral regurgitation with and without mitral valve prolapse, to repetitive ventricular arrhythmias and right and left ventricular ejection fraction. *Am J Cardiol* 1987;60:397.

186. Cosgrove DM, Stewart WJ. Mitral valve repair. *Curr Probl Cardiol* 1989;10:359.

187. Smedira NG, Selman R, Cosgrove DM, et al. Repair of anterior leaflet prolapse: chordal transfer is superior to chordal shortening. *J Thorac Cardiovasc Surg* 1996;112(2):287.

188. Salati M, Scrofani R, Fundaro P, et al. Correction of anterior mitral prolapse: results of chordal transposition. *J Thorac Cardiovasc Surg* 1992;104:1268.

189. Sousa Uva M, Grare P, Jebara V, et al. Transposition of chordae in mitral valve repair: mid-term results. *Circulation* 1993;88[Pt 2]:35.

190. Lee KS, Stewart WJ, Savage RM, et al. Systolic anterior motion of mitral valve after the posterior leaflet sliding advancement procedure. *Ann Thorac Surg* 1994;57:1338.

191. Perier P, Clausnizer B, Mistarz K, et al. A "sliding leaflet" technique for repair of the mitral valve: early results. *Ann Thorac Surg* 1994;57:383.

192. Jebara VA, Mihaileanu S, Acar C, et al. Left ventricular outflow tract obstruction after mitral valve repair. Results of the sliding leaflet technique. *Circulation* 1993;88(Pt 2):30.

193. Lee KS, Stewart WJ, Lever HM, et al. Mechanism of outflow tract obstruction causing failed mitral valve repair: anterior displacement of leaflet coaptation. *Circulation* 1993;88[Pt 2]:24.

194. Heikkila J. Mitral incompetence as a complication of acute myocardial infarction. *Acta Med Scand* 1967; 182[Suppl]:1.

195. Roberts WC, Cohen LS. Left ventricular papillary muscles. Description of the normal and a survey of conditions causing them to be abnormal. *Circulation* 1972;46:138.

196. Roberts WC. Morphologic features of the normal and abnormal mitral valve. *Am J Cardiol* 1983;51:1005.

197. Antunes MJ, Colsen PR, Kinsley RH. Mitral valve repair: a learning curve. *Circulation* 1983;68(Suppl II):II70.

198. Carpentier A. Cardiac valve surgery—the "French correction." *J Thorac Cardiovasc Surg* 1983;86:323.

199. Spencer FFC, Colvin SB, Sulliford AT, et al. Experiences with the Carpentier techniques of mitral valve reconstruction in 103 patients (1980–1985). *J Thorac Cardiovasc Surg* 1985;90:341.

200. Yacoub M, Halim M, Radley-Smith R, et al. Surgical treatment of mitral regurgitation caused by floppy valves. Repair versus replacement. *Circulation* 1981;64(Suppl II):II210.

201. Oury JH, Peterson KL, Folkerth TL, et al. Mitral valve replacement versus reconstruction: an analysis of indications and results of mitral valve procedures in a consecutive series of 80 patients. *J Thorac Cardiovasc Surg* 1977;73:825.

202. Oliveira DBG, Dawkins KD, Kay PH, et al. Chordal rupture: comparison between repair and replacement. *Br Heart J* 1980;50:318.

203. Orszulak TA, Schaff HV, Danielson GK, et al. Mitral regurgitation due to ruptured chordae tendineae: early and late results of valve repair. *J Thorac Cardiovasc Surg* 1985;89:491.

204. Lessana A, Romano M, Lutfalla G, et al. Treatment of ruptured or elongated anterior mitral valve chordae by partial transposition of the posterior leaflet: experience with 29 patients. *Ann Thorac Surg* 1988;45:404.

205. Adebo OA, Ross JK. Surgical treatment of ruptured mitral valve chordae: a comparison between valve replacement and valve repair. *Thorac Cardiovasc Surg* 1984;32:139.

206. Duran CG, Pomar JL, Revuelta JM. Conservative operation for mitral insufficiency—critical analysis supported by postoperative hemodynamic studies in 72 patients. *J Thorac Cardiovasc Surg* 1980;79:326.

207. Antunes MJ, Magalhaes MP, Colsen PR, et al. *Valve repair for rheumatic mitral valve disease: a surgical challenge.* Thesis. University of the Witwatersrand, Witwatersrand and Johannesburg Group of Teaching Hospitals, South Africa, 1985.

208. Cohn LH. Mitral valve surgery: reconstruction versus replacement. Presented at the International Symposium: Advance in cardiology—controversial views. Berlin, West Germany, December 2–4, 1984.

209. Sand ME, Naftel DC, Blackstone EH, et al. A comparison of repair and replacement for mitral valve incompetence. *J Thorac Cardiovasc Surg* 1987;94:208.

210. Angell WW, Oury JH, Shah P. A comparison of replacement and reconstruction in patients with mitral regurgitation. *J Thorac Cardiovasc Surg* 1987;93:665.

210a. Tribouilloy CM, Enriquez-Sarano M, Schaff HV, et al. Impact of preoperative symptoms on survival after surgical correction of organic mitral regurgitation—rationale for optimizing surgical indications. *Circulation* 1999;99:400.

210b. Wencker D, Borer JS, Hochreiter C, et al. Preoperative predictors of late postoperative outcome among patients with nonischemic mitral regurgitation with "high risk" descriptors and comparison with unoperated patients. *Cardiology* 2000;93:37.

211. Nunley DL, Starr A. The evolution of reparative techniques for the mitral valve. *Ann Thorac Surg* 1984;37:393.

212. Cosgrove DM, Chavez AM, Lytle BW, et al. Results of mitral valve reconstruction. *Circulation* 1986;74[Suppl I]:I-82.

213. Cohn LH, Couper GS, Aranki SF, et al. Long-term results of mitral valve reconstruction for regurgitation of the myxomatous mitral valve. *J Thorac Cardiovasc Surg* 1994;107:143.

214. David TE, Armstrong S, Sun Z, et al. Late results of mitral valve repair for mitral regurgitation due to degenerative disease. *Ann Thorac Surg* 1993;56:7.

215. Carpentier A, Chauvaud S, Fabiana JN, et al. Reconstructive surgery of mitral valve incompetence: ten-year appraisal. *J Thorac Cardiovasc Surg* 1980;79:338.

216. Deloche A, Jebara VA, Relland JYM, et al. Valve repair with Carpentier techniques. *J Thorac Cardiovasc Surg* 1990;99:990.

217. Marwick T, Currie PJ, Stewart WS, et al. Echo evaluation of immediate and late failed mitral valve repair [abstract]. *J Am Coll Cardiol* 1989;13:114A.

218. Navia JL, Cosgrove DM. Minimally invasive mitral valve surgery: a new method. *Ann Thorac Surg* 1996;62:1542.

219. Pompili MF, Stevens JH, Burdon TA, et al. Port-access mitral valve replacement in dogs. *J Thorac Cardiovasc Surg* 1996;112:1268.

220. Pompili MF, Yakub AZ, Siegel LC, et al. Port-access mitral valve replacement: initial clinical experience. *Circulation* 1996;94:I131.

220a. Chitwood WR Jr, Elbeery JR, Moran P. Minimally invasive mitral valve repair using transthoracic aortic occlusion. *Ann Thorac Surg* 1997;63:1477.

221. Cosgrove DM, Sabik JF, Navia J. Minimally invasive valve surgery. *Ann Thorac Surg* 1998;65:1535.

221a. Galloway AC, Shemin RJ, Glower DD, et al. First Report of the Port Access International Registry. *Ann Thorac Surg* 1999;67:51.

222. Essop R, Rothlisberger C, Dullabh A, et al. Can the long-term outcomes of percutaneous balloon mitral valvotomy and surgical commissurotomy be expected to be similar? *J Heart Valve Dis* 1995;4:446.

223. Stewart WJ: Choosing the "golden moment" for mitral valve replacement. *J Am Coll Cardiol* 1994;24:1544.

224. Ling LH, Enriquez-Sarano M, Seward JB, et al. Clinical outcome of mitral regurgitation due to flail leaflet. *N Engl J Med* 1997;335:1417.

225. O'Rourke RA. Syndrome of mitral valve prolapse. In: Alpert, JS, Dalen JE, Rahimtoola SH, eds. *Valvular heart disease*, 3rd ed. Philadelphia: Lippincott Williams & Wilkins, 2000.

AORTIC VALVE DISEASE

WILLIAM J. STEWART
BLASE A. CARABELLO

▼▼ ADDITIONAL ELECTRONIC TOPICS

Historical Perspective e09;   Rheumatic Disease e10;   Congenital Aortic Stenosis e11;   Syncope e12;   Congestive Heart Failure e13; Electrocardiogram e14;   Chest X-Ray e15;   Differential Diagnosis of Aortic Stenosis versus Hypertrophic Cardiomyopathy e16;   Balloon Valvotomy (Valvuloplasty) e17;   Aortic Valve Replacement with Homograft (Allograft) e18;   Aortic Valve Replacement with Pulmonary Autograft (Ross Procedure) e19;   Thromboembolism e20;   Heart Block e21;   Hemolysis e22;   Infection e23;   Choice of Valve e24;   Mechanical Valves e25;   Porcine Bioprostheses e26;   Bovine Pericardial Bioprostheses e27;   Stentless Porcine Bioprostheses e28;   Cryopreserved Homograft Valves e29;   Pulmonary Autograft e30;   Management of Aortic Stenosis in Patients with a Small Hyperdynamic Ventricle e31;   Aortic Valve Surgery: Minimally Invasive Procedures e32;   Angina and Aortic Regurgitation e33;   Use of Exercise Ejection Fraction e34;   Aortic Valve Replacement and Repair e35

AORTIC STENOSIS

Etiology

Valvular Degeneration and Calcification

Several etiologies of valvular AS have been described, including senile calcific, bicuspid, rheumatic, and congenital varieties. In developed countries, the most common cause of adult-acquired AS at present is idiopathic degeneration and calcification of the aortic valve (16), a process that can occur

W. J. Stewart: Department of Cardiovascular Medicine, The Cleveland Clinic Foundation, Cleveland, Ohio
B. A. Carabello: Department of Medicine, Baylor College of Medicine, Houston Veterans Affairs Medical Center, Houston, Texas

on a bileaflet or a trileaflet valve. Among the 1% of Americans born with a bicuspid aortic valve, the valve opens well at birth, but gradual and progressive degeneration leads to stenosis in approximately one-third (17,18). Because bicuspid aortic valves occur more frequently in men, AS also has a male predominance. When it occurs, clinically significant stenosis of a bicuspid valve usually develops in the fifth and sixth decades of life. Presumably, the flow characteristics of the valve increase the process of degenerative changes. In contrast, rheumatic AS, on average, becomes symptomatic in the fourth decade, and congenital AS becomes symptomatic in the first to third decades (Fig. 22.1) (19).

Although the exact incidence of AS in patients born with tricuspid aortic valves is unknown, it is probably less than 1%. In patients with a previously normal tricuspid aortic valve who

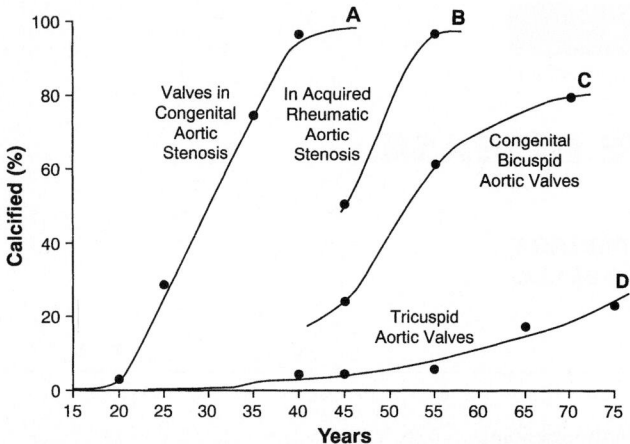

FIGURE 22.1 This figure shows the timing of onset of symptoms and significantly calcified and stenotic valves versus the major etiologies of aortic stenosis, including (A) congenital, (B) bicuspid, (C) rheumatic, and (D) senile. (From Campbell M. Calcific aortic stenosis and congenital bicuspid aortic valves. *Br Heart J* 1968;30:606–616, with permission.)

eventually develop AS, the same process of degeneration and calcification leads to symptoms of critical disease in the seventh and eighth decades (19). Why some patients with previously normal trileaflet valves develop AS whereas others do not remains a mystery. Otto and colleagues (20) have noted that the early lesion of AS is characterized by subendothelial thickening on the aortic side of the leaflet. Thickening occurs as the elastic lamina is displaced by the accumulation of cellular lipid infiltration and extracellular mineralization. There is proliferation of smooth muscle cells and lipid-laden foam cells resembling the plaque of coronary atherosclerosis (17).

An association has been discovered between the standard risk factors for coronary disease and development of AS, suggesting that thickening of the aortic valve as aortic sclerosis, eventually leading to AS, is often a manifestation of an atherosclerotic process on the aortic valve (21–21c). Cholesterol, lipoprotein disorders, smoking, male gender, and age may accelerate the age-related degenerative effects (21d). Duration of exposure to high cholesterol concentrations correlates with development of AS in patients with familial hypercholesterolemia (21e). In fact, even mild degrees of fibrosis, termed *aortic sclerosis*, have a major impact on prognosis, probably due to its link to atherosclerosis in all parts of the cardiovascular system (21c).

The same histologic changes occur in bicuspid valves at an earlier age, and there is no evidence to suggest that the valve pathology differs in bicuspid versus tricuspid disease or that the ultimate outcome of these two types of acquired AS differs.

Clinical Presentation

Natural History

The natural history of acquired AS determines management of the disease. Depicted by Ross and Braunwald in

Figure 22.2 and confirmed by recent studies (25a,26–28), the patient with asymptomatic AS has a nearly normal survival for a long latency period. During this time, the valve is slowly developing fibrosis and calcification, but the patient remains well. Once the symptoms of angina, syncope, or CHF develop, however, survival is dramatically shortened. Approximately 35% of patients who become symptomatic present with angina (29). In this group, 50% survive for only 5 years unless AVR is performed. In the 15% of patients who present with syncope, 50% survive for only 3 years; for the 50% with AS who present with symptoms of CHF, mean survival is less than 2 years unless the aortic valve is replaced. The risk of sudden cardiac death in asymptomatic or minimally symptomatic patients is rare, being less than 2% (28). Because this risk is less than that associated with AVR in many centers, there is usually no indication for surgery before the development of symptoms.

The progression of AS is more rapid, and prognosis with medical therapy is worse in patients who have moderate or severe valvular calcification and in those who have a rapid increase in their Doppler-derived gradient compared with previous studies (29a–29c). Similarly, smoking, hypercholesterolemia, and elevated serum creatinine and calcium levels have been associated with a more rapid rate of progression of AS (29d).

Pathophysiology of Aortic Stenosis and Its Relation to Symptoms

Understanding the pathophysiology of the symptoms of AS is key to understanding the disease. As stenosis worsens and the gradient increases, a progressive pressure overload is placed on the left ventricle. Pressure overload and increased

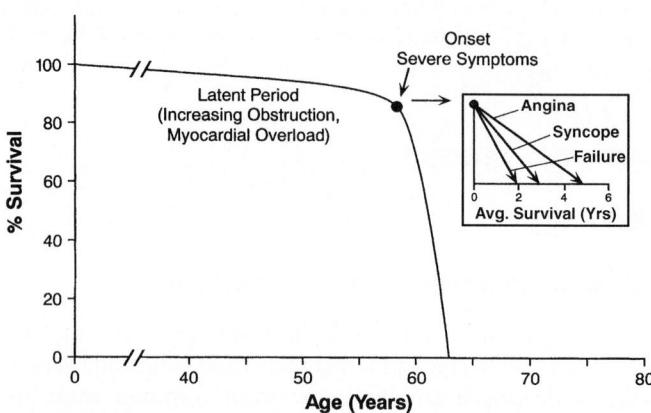

FIGURE 22.2 The natural history of aortic stenosis. A long latent period with a nearly normal survival rate is present until the symptoms of angina, syncope, or congestive heart failure develop. At that time, a precipitous decline in survival occurs unless the problem is surgically corrected. **Inset:** The prognosis is worst with presenting symptoms of congestive heart failure, second worst with syncope. [From Ross J Jr, Braunwald E. Aortic stenosis. *Circulation* 1968;38(Suppl 5):V-61, with permission.]

systolic wall stress are thought to signal the development of concentric LV hypertrophy (LVH) (30). The mechanism is not apparently dependent solely on the renin-angiotensin system (30a,30b). Rather, the signaling cascade is complex, and hypertrophy can develop by activation of a variety of pathways. The pressure overload appears to selectively influence myocardial matrix metalloproteinase activity and expression and therefore the LV myocardial remodeling process (30c). The increased muscle mass that develops allows the ventricle to generate increased pressure while maintaining normal wall stress; thus, the hypertrophy compensates for the increased pressure load. The Laplace equation for wall stress is the following:

$$\text{stress} = \frac{\text{pressure} \times \text{radius}}{2 \times \text{thickness}}$$

This equation is used to approximate afterload on a given area of myocardium. As pressure in the numerator increases, increased thickness in the denominator offsets the pressure overload, and wall stress remains normal. However, as the pressure overload progresses, the hypertrophy that develops takes on pathologic characteristics, becomes involved in the pathogenesis of symptoms (e.g., subendocardial ischemia and arrhythmias), and thus is associated with a worsened outcome.

Angina

Angina, which stems from myocardial ischemia, occurs when myocardial oxygen supply is outstripped by demand either because demand increases or supply decreases. In AS, both factors probably play a role. With the development of concentric hypertrophy, coronary blood flow reserve becomes reduced from its normal five- to eightfold increase above baseline to just a two- to threefold increase (eFig. 22.2.1) (31). Reduced flow reserve may derive from the endocardial compression caused by increased diastolic filling pressure, or it may be due to a relative lack of capillary ingrowth to compensate for the increased muscle mass (32,33). In either case, limited flow reserve helps to precipitate ischemia during exertion. On the other side of the equation, myocardial oxygen demand is determined by heart rate (HR), contractile state, and wall stress. Patients with AS and angina have lower LV mass, increased peak systolic pressure, and increased wall stress than do patients without angina (34). Although hypertrophy initially helps to normalize wall stress in AS, in many patients the hypertrophy is inadequate to offset the increase in pressure, and stress and myocardial oxygen demand increase, precipitating ischemia and angina during exercise (35).

Hemodynamics

The best measurements for assessing the severity of AS are the mean systolic gradient and AVA, which are obtained accurately both by catheterization and Doppler methods.

The invasive and noninvasive techniques for establishing the severity of stenosis are derived from similar principles. The Gorlin formula uses direct pressure measurements from a catheter and pressure manometer. The continuity equation uses direct velocity measurements from Doppler echocardiographic instruments (8). Both methods derive AVA from Torricelli's equation:

$$F = A \times V, \text{ or } A = F/V$$

where A is orifice area, F is flow, and V is velocity.

Using Doppler methods, velocity is measured directly (by determining the amount of shift in the frequency of reflected ultrasound), both in the valve orifice (by continuous wave Doppler) and in the LV outflow tract (by pulsed Doppler). The area is calculated by measuring a diameter of the LV outflow tract directly from a two-dimensional echo image and assuming circular symmetry. Outflow tract area and velocity are multiplied and divided by valvular velocity to obtain the valve area using the continuity equation.

Using catheter methods, cardiac output is measured using the Fick or indicator dilution (thermodilution) technique. Pressure gradient is measured and converted to velocity:

$$V = \sqrt{gh}$$

where g is acceleration due to gravity, and h is mean gradient. These are combined in the Gorlin formula for calculating AVA (45), which is the following:

$$AVA = \frac{Q}{K\sqrt{h}}$$

where Q is cardiac output, and h is the mean valve gradient.

An alternative, third method for determining AVA is transesophageal echocardiography (TEE). Using careful planimetry of the multiplane systolic TEE short-axis views of the aortic valve, the accuracy approaches that of the above-mentioned methods (46a). In addition, TEE from deep transgastric views can accurately determine transvalvular pressure gradients, a method that may be useful in patients with technically difficult transthoracic echo studies or when the data from transthoracic echo do not correlate with other information such as the physical examination.

To obtain pressure gradient, the catheter-derived pressures on both sides of the valve are compared. For Doppler methods, velocity is converted to gradient using the simplified Bernoulli equation (Fig. 22.3) (6,7,46).

$$\text{Gradient} = 4 \times V^2$$

Both methods can accurately derive the mean systolic gradient. Instantaneous gradient measured by Doppler has

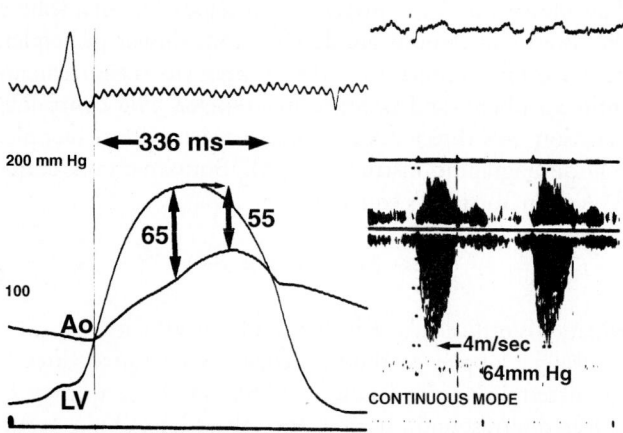

FIGURE 22.3 Micromanometer recordings of left ventricular and ascending aortic pressure tracing (*left*) and continuous-wave Doppler velocity envelope (*right*) demonstrate correspondence of Doppler-derived peak instantaneous gradient (64 mm Hg) with peak instantaneous gradient determined by catheter measurements (65 mm Hg), which differs from the peak-to-peak gradient (55 mm Hg). The catheter- and Doppler-derived mean gradients matched perfectly (42 mm Hg). (From Assey ME, Usher BW, Carabello BA, Spann JF Jr. The patient with valvular heart disease. In: Pepine CJ, Hill JA, Lambert CR, eds. *Diagnostic and therapeutic cardiac catheterization*, 2nd ed. Baltimore: Williams & Wilkins, 1994:692, with permission.)

no convenient direct-pressure measurement counterpart and specifically is not the same as peak-to-peak gradient.

Progression of Aortic Stenosis

As shown in Table 22.1, reduction in aortic orifice area from its normal 3.0 cm² by 50% to approximately 1.5 cm² results in only a small gradient. However, from that degree of stenosis, small additional increments in the reduction of orifice area lead to progressively more dramatic increases in gradient. The average increase in gradient is 7 to 10 mm Hg per year across a wide group of patients (47). However, there is a large and unpredictable individual variation.

Although it is not uncommon for some patients to advance from mild AS with a small gradient of 10 mm Hg to severe AS with a gradient of 70 mm Hg in 3 or 4 years, in other patients the rate of progression is considerably less. Occasionally, the transvalvular gradient increases by as

TABLE 22.1 MEAN SYSTOLIC PRESSURE GRADIENT AND ORIFICE AREA IN AORTIC STENOSIS

Cardiac output (L/min)	Aortic valve area (cm²)	Gradient[a] (mm Hg)
5.0	1.5	14.0
5.0	1.0	21.0
5.0	0.7	42.0
5.0	0.5	82.0

[a]Calculated at a heart rate of 76 beats/min and a systolic ejection period of 330 ms.

much as 25 mm Hg in 1 year, depending, in part, on the amount of stenosis already present (48). A rapid rate of progression of stenosis, as reflected by an increase in aortic-jet maximum velocity of more than 0.3 m per second in the course of a year, is significantly higher in patients who have clinical cardiac events (29a).

The unpredictable rate of progression of stenosis mandates careful follow-up by the physician and education of the patient who should be counseled to inform the physician of the onset of symptoms as soon as they occur. Although most patients with critical AS who require surgery have an AVA of less than 0.7 cm² and a mean systolic gradient of more than 50 mm Hg, patients may develop symptoms and therefore require surgery before or after reaching those thresholds.

Diagnosis

Physical Examination

The presence of AS is frequently first suspected when a systolic ejection murmur that radiates to the neck is heard during physical examination. Early in the disease when cardiac output is high, the murmur may be quite loud, typically peaking in early to mid-systole and is associated with a systolic thrill. The murmur often has a harsh quality and is lower in pitch than the higher-frequency blowing sound of mitral regurgitation. As the disease progresses, the murmur peaks progressively later until it becomes loudest during the later half of systole. The murmur may become softer as cardiac output through the stenotic valve decreases. The murmur is frequently well heard in the aortic area, disappears over the sternum, and becomes louder again over the apex, thus mimicking coexisting mitral regurgitation (Gallivardin's phenomenon). In some cases, the murmur is actually louder at the apex than it is in the aortic area. In congenital AS, the murmur is usually preceded by an early ejection sound.

The severity of AS is best estimated at the bedside by palpation of the carotid arteries. As ejection begins, work is lost at the stenotic valve, and the carotid upstroke becomes reduced in amplitude and delayed in timing (*parvus et tardus*) (Fig. 22.3). In one controlled study, the only predictor of outcome based on physical examination was carotid upstroke amplitude (48a). Occasionally in elderly patients, inelasticity of the carotid arteries causes the carotid contour to maintain a more brisk upstroke, causing the examiner to underestimate the severity of the disease.

The intensity of the second heart sound may also be helpful in assessing the severity of AS. The aortic component typically becomes diminished in intensity (because leaflet mobility is reduced). The second heart sound may also be single, when the aortic component is absent, and only the soft pulmonic component of the second heart sound (S_2) is heard. In some cases, prolongation of LV ejection time, caused by severe outlet obstruction in conjunction with LV dysfunction, leads to a paradoxically split S_2. In severe congenital AS, the valve is still quite mobile, so both components of the S_2 are preserved. ⚓ e36

Echo-Doppler Studies

Ultrasonic examination of the heart in AS is the most important diagnostic modality in confirming the diagnosis and for quantifying disease severity. Two-dimensional echocardiography demonstrates thickened and calcified aortic valve leaflets with reduced leaflet motion. The aortic annulus and sometimes the surrounding aortic walls are echodense and often calcified. Distinction between bicuspid and tricuspid anatomy is often possible (eFig. 22.3.3) when the amount of calcification is small but is difficult in many patients with severe fibrosis and calcification. In addition, the extent of concentric LVH can be quantitated by calculating LV mass (48b). LV ejection performance can be evaluated and the ejection fraction (EF) measured. Doppler studies (6,7,32,46,49) can accurately quantify the transvalvular pressure gradient (Fig. 22.4) and the valve area, using the formulas listed above. Doppler assessment of diastolic dysfunction is also useful, often defining the presence of abnormal LV relaxation (49a).

In practice, an initial Doppler echocardiographic study should be performed when AS is first suspected to confirm the diagnosis and assess the hemodynamics. Clinical follow-up should be frequent enough to ascertain development of symptoms. Echo follow-up should be frequent enough to detect the development or worsening of problems such as LV dysfunction, LVH, or mitral regurgitation (47). Repeat echo studies do not need to be performed every year because quantifying the progression of the disease in the absence of symptoms does not normally influence management. A case can be made for periodic echo examination of asymptomatic patients: yearly in patients with severe AS, every 2 years or so in patients with moderate AS, and every 5 years or so in patients with mild AS (49b). Once symptoms develop, a repeat echo-Doppler helps confirm worsening of disease severity.

Stress Testing

Stress testing has traditionally been avoided in AS for fear of complications (50). Indeed, stress testing *should be avoided* in obviously symptomatic patients. However, stress testing can be performed safely in patients with AS and equivocal symptoms to more clearly establish symptom status and to evaluate exercise tolerance (51,52). Nuclear imaging has also been used to evaluate the presence of coronary disease, which may coexist with AS; one study of perfusion imaging (53) suggests a sensitivity and specificity of approximately 80% for concomitant coronary disease. Stress echo can be done safely in stable patients with AS. Dobutamine echo is often a useful way to redefine valve area and gradient at a higher cardiac output, especially useful in patients with moderate to severe AS with a low gradient and depressed LV function (134).

Cardiac Catheterization

Because all of the information needed to quantify the extent and severity of AS can usually be obtained by physical examination combined with echo-Doppler studies, the need to perform invasive hemodynamics in this population has declined to a small number of patients for whom the data are conflictive (53a,53b). However, most patients with AS fall into the age range in which coronary disease is likely. Unfortunately, the presence or absence of angina pectoris is a poor indicator of the presence or absence of coronary disease. Coronary disease may be present in as many as 25% of AS patients who do not complain of angina, and it is present in 40% to 80% of AS patients who complain of angina (54–56). Although coronary revascularization at the time of AVR does not improve prognosis compared to that of patients who have isolated AS without coronary disease, coronary revascularization of severe coronary stenoses is conventionally performed at the time of AVR and is probably beneficial (57–59). Thus, coronary arteriography is performed in most adult patients with AS to assess coronary anatomy. If the severity of AS is in doubt, the transvalvular gradient should be measured at the time of cardiac catheterization and a right-heart catheterization

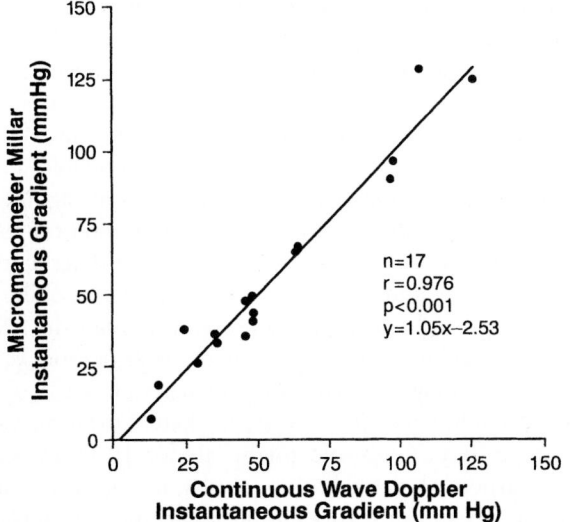

n=17
r=0.976
p<0.001
y=1.05x−2.53

FIGURE 22.4 This figure shows correlation of peak instantaneous aortic valve gradient determined at cardiac catheterization using a micromanometer catheter technique with Doppler-derived estimated peak instantaneous gradient. (Data from the Medical University of South Carolina.) (From Assey ME, Usher BW, Carabello BA, Spann JF Jr. The patient with valvular heart disease. In: Pepine CJ, Hill JA, Lambert CR, eds. *Diagnostic and therapeutic cardiac catheterization*, 2nd ed. Baltimore: Williams & Wilkins, 1994:693, with permission.)

should be performed to measure cardiac output for the AVA calculation.

Management

Medical Therapy

There is no effective medical treatment for AS. Most patients who are asymptomatic do not require therapy. The onset of symptoms should prompt a recommendation for performing AVR (59a). In some patients who are deemed not to be surgical candidates, digitalis and diuretics may transiently improve CHF, and nitrates may be used cautiously to treat angina pectoris. However, these therapies provide no long-term benefit. Although vasodilators, especially angiotensin I–converting enzyme inhibitors, are widely used in treating most forms of CHF, they are relatively contraindicated in patients with AS. In patients with AS, vasodilators lower peripheral pressure without increasing cardiac output. In addition, adequate cardiac output may depend on a high LV filling pressure; thus, vasodilators that reduce preload may cause potentially dangerous hypotension. Like other types of valvular heart diseases, prophylactic antibiotics are indicated as pretreatment for dental or surgical procedures that have a moderate likelihood of causing bacteremia.

Aortic Valve Replacement: Surgical Procedures

AVR is the definitive therapy for symptomatic AS. It is mandatory for all symptomatic patients. Very few patients with symptomatic severe AS should defer aortic valve surgery unless there are compelling contraindications for operation. Surgery for acquired aortic valvular disease usually requires AVR because the thickened aortic valve is difficult to repair (62a). Aortic valve débridement for calcific AS enjoyed a brief period of popularity in the mid-1980s but has since been abandoned because of early and progressive postoperative regurgitation from leaflet fibrosis and retraction (63). Aortic repair for true aortic regurgitation (64) is discussed later in this chapter (see Aortic Valve Replacement and Repair).

Aortic valve surgery is usually a mechanical or bioprosthetic valve, performed through a median sternotomy incision, although recently less invasive techniques have been carried out through smaller hemisternotomy incisions or anterior thoracotomies in the right second or third intercostal space (65) (see the section Aortic Valve Surgery: Minimally Invasive Procedures) ▼▼ e37

Results of Surgery

Surgical Mortality

Operative mortality after aortic valve surgery should be less than 3% to 5%, depending on a variety of factors, includ-

ing the individual surgeon's skill. The risk of operative mortality is higher in elderly or debilitated patients; in the presence of significantly impaired LV function; and in patients with extensive coronary artery disease or other valvular disease, infective endocarditis, or other associated diseases (e.g., renal failure). Operative mortality is slightly higher in patients with aortic regurgitation compared with that in patients with AS, but it is not influenced by the type of prosthesis used.

After surgery there is an improvement in symptoms, a drop in LV mass, and an increase in EF, although not necessarily an increase in exercise capacity (65a). Long-term survival is affected by many of the same variables that affect operative mortality. In general, actuarial survival is approximately 80% to 85% at 5 years and 70% at 10 years postoperatively. As noted, coronary artery disease that is not treated at the time of AVR adversely affects long-term survival.

Postoperative Valve-Related Complications

Postoperative valve-related complications include (a) structural deterioration of the valve; (b) hemodynamic valvular dysfunction; (c) valve thrombosis; (d) thromboembolism; (e) anticoagulant-related bleeding; (f) infection; (g) prosthetic valve endocarditis; (h) hemolysis; and (i) heart block.

Unlike earlier valves, such as some models of the Björk-Shiley prosthesis, structural deterioration of currently available mechanical prostheses is extremely unusual (66–69). In contrast, virtually all tissue valves are prone to progressive, gradual deterioration, usually due to leaflet calcification. For the porcine bioprosthesis, the first primary valve failures usually occur at 7 to 8 years postoperatively and occur at a rate of approximately 2% per year thereafter (69a); freedom from hemodynamically significant structural tissue valve deterioration in the aortic position has been reported to be 80% to 85% at 10 years and 54% to 58% at 15 years (70–72). For currently available aortic pericardial valve bioprostheses, freedom from significant structural tissue valve deterioration has been reported to be 91% to 96% at 10 years (73–75). Structural deterioration of both porcine and pericardial valves in infants, children, and young adults occurs more rapidly than in older patients. Even in adults, the rate of deterioration varies indirectly with age so that a bioprosthesis placed in a 50-year-old might fail in 5 to 10 years, whereas the same valve implanted in a 70-year-old might last for 10 to 15 years. When structural deterioration results in significant and recurrent AS and/or regurgitation, reoperation for replacement of the deteriorated prosthesis may become necessary.

Structural deterioration with the development of aortic regurgitation also occurs after AVR with homograft valves. Its incidence varies widely in different reports depending on different techniques of homograft valve procurement, preservation, and implantation (76,77). The exact incidence of structural valve deterioration with homograft valves remains unknown because little long-term follow-up is available. In some reports (78) the rate of reoperation at 10 years is as low as 10%. Nevertheless, progressive degeneration of the homograft tissue does occur, and it may be more accentuated in younger patients (79) in whom homografts are otherwise an attractive alternative. Ross (80) has estimated that the useful life of a homograft valve is approximately 15 years.

Being native tissue, the pulmonary autograft has less calcific degeneration; however, it is not without some risk of functional deterioration, and the patient is susceptible to postoperative problems with valve replacements in both the pulmonic and the aortic position. Therefore, long-term follow-up of a large series of patients who have undergone the Ross procedure is necessary to determine how long these valves remain functional (81,82).

All standard prosthetic valves (mechanical valves as well as standard stented tissue valves) are stenotic compared with the native aortic valve because part of the potential orifice area of prosthetic valves is occupied by struts, stents, hinge mechanisms, sewing rings, and valve leaflets. Accordingly, all of these valves have a measurable gradient, which is inversely proportional to prosthesis size. Small-sized standard porcine bioprostheses (i.e., sizes 19 and 21) may be associated with gradients that are unacceptable in adult patients. Bioprosthetic valve gradients would be even higher, except for the substitution in manufactured processing of the right coronary valve leaflet (which contains a muscle bar in pigs) with the noncoronary leaflet from another pig. This so-called modified orifice porcine valve appears to have improved hemodynamic function and no increase in structural dysfunction compared with the standard porcine valve prosthesis (71,72). Tissue valves manufactured from glutaraldehyde-preserved bovine pericardium have improved hemodynamic function and may be adequate even in smaller sizes (73–75).

In general, modern bileaflet mechanical valves are also relatively stenotic but have better hemodynamic function than that of porcine bioprostheses and similar function compared with that of pericardial bioprostheses. Accordingly, smaller sizes of these valves are adequate in most adults, especially those who are elderly and those with smaller body surface area. Relatively little hemodynamic data are available from direct postoperative catheterization in patients with current mechanical prostheses because of the difficulties and dangers associated with crossing these delicate valves with stiff catheters. The echo-Doppler technique remains the best way to follow the function of an AVR noninvasively but provides a numerically higher gradient compared with a catheter-derived gradient due to pressure recovery, the "airplane wing" effect (83,83a). This discrepancy between catheter- and Doppler-derived gradients is most substantial in small aortic mechanical prosthetic valves such as bileaflet valves, where there is a localized area of low pressure at the mouth of the orifice between the two open prosthetic leaflets, creating higher velocity recordings.

The aortic valve homograft and the pulmonary autograft are natural valves and their hemodynamic function is excellent. Excellent hemodynamic function may be obtained from the stentless porcine valve because of the absence of sewing ring and stent (84,85). However, there is less experience with its implantation. ▼ e38

Management of Aortic Stenosis Patients with Low Cardiac Output, Low Ejection Fraction, and Low Transvalvular Gradient

In most patients with even far-advanced AS that has resulted in reduced LV EF and severe CHF, outcome after surgery is remarkably good (129). Surgical intervention relieves the afterload excess on the left ventricle, allowing an increase in LV performance (*e*Fig. 22.4.4), which results in a stable postoperative course and rapid improvement in the symptoms of CHF. Unfortunately, this positive outlook frequently does not extend to patients with reduced EF who also have a small transvalvular gradient (125,130). Only about 50% of these patients improve after surgery; the other 50% suffer perioperative death or have persistent symptoms of CHF (131).

Connolly et al. published a paper on 154 patients with severe AS and LV systolic dysfunction, finding a perioperative mortality of 9% and a high incidence of postoperative death, with 50 patients dying in follow-up. Coronary artery disease and a reduced preoperative cardiac output were primarily correlated with adverse outcome (131a). However, a subsequent study of valve replacement in 52 patients with a low gradient found a 21% operative and a 50% 4-year mortality (131b). Pereira et al. found a better prognosis in a series of somewhat different patients, including a perioperative mortality of 5.9%, compared with 4.0% in patients with similarly severe AS without bad LV function (131c). Serum creatinine level and RV systolic function may be more important predictors of outcome after AVR than LV systolic function and valve gradient.

The obvious challenge is to distinguish preoperatively between those patients who may benefit from AVR while avoiding surgery in patients for whom the outcome will be poor. Although at present there is no universally accepted means of distinguishing these patients, surgical candidates can be selected by making the distinction between AS and aortic "pseudostenosis" (132,132a). In true AS, severe valve disease has led to progressive LV dysfunction. Accordingly, correcting the valve lesion, the primary etiologic agent, may be expected to improve the patient's condition. Alternatively, an AVA may be calculated either during echocardiography or cardiac catheterization, which suggests that the valve is severely stenotic when, in fact, it is not (pseudostenosis). Underestimation of the AVA made by hemodynamic calculations occurs at low cardiac output because the Gorlin formula and continuity equation are flow-dependent and will therefore overestimate severity, obtaining an artificially low calculated AVA in low output states (133). ⚐ e39

Prophylactic Valve Replacement in Patients with Coronary Disease

As noted in this chapter, AS frequently coexists with coronary disease. In many cases severe coronary disease requiring revascularization is present at a time when the patient has only mild or moderate AS or regurgitation. Although isolated AVR would not be considered in such a patient in the absence of coronary disease, the question arises as to the proper management of the aortic valve during bypass surgery. Prophylactic valve replacement has been considered because in some patients the severity of their AS may progress very rapidly and reoperation with a very high mortality rate [as high as 20% (137)] may be required just a few years after bypass surgery. These reoperations also have more chance of damage to bypass grafts implanted during the first surgery. On the other hand, in patients whose severity of AS does not progress rapidly, prophylactic surgery results in the presence of an unneeded valve prosthesis with all of its attendant risks and limited durability. Unfortunately, it is impossible to know preoperatively in which patients the severity of AS will progress rapidly and in which patients it will not. Although prophylactic valve replacement would probably be considered appropriate in most patients in whom the mean transvalvular gradient exceeds 40 mm and inappropriate if it were less than 10 mm, this leaves a broad middle range where clinical judgment must hold sway because there are few data for guidance. In general, aortic valve surgery should probably be done with the initial operation if the AS is at least moderate in severity. It also seems more reasonable in patients with higher transvalvular gradients and calcified valves (137a).

A preliminary report suggested that patients with mild to moderate AS actually have a better outcome with prophylactic valve replacement (137b). However, we make this decision on a case-by-case basis, considering the age of the patient and the morphology of the valve. An older patient is less likely to undergo a prophylactic valve operation as is a patient with a more structurally normal valve as determined by echocardiography, surgical inspection, or both. Long-term studies are needed to resolve these issues.

CHRONIC AORTIC REGURGITATION

Etiology

Aortic regurgitation results from failure of leaflet coaptation either due to diseased valve cusps or a diseased aortic root, which distorts cusp suspension (Fig. 22.5) (101). Common causes of cusp disease include bicuspid aortic valve, rheumatic heart disease, infective endocarditis, or calcification of the leaflets, which often causes mixed AS and aortic regurgitation (AR). Although a congenitally bicuspid aortic valve frequently leads to AS in adulthood, approximately 10% of bicuspid valve patients who require surgery present with pure aortic regurgitation without stenosis; these patients are usually younger, averaging approximately 40 years of age. Aortic regurgitation from a bicuspid aortic valve often results from leaflet prolapse, especially when one cusp is larger than the other (102). Although rheumatic heart disease primarily attacks the mitral valve, leading to mitral stenosis, many patients with rheumatic involvement also have some degree of aortic regurgitation, and in some patients aortic regurgitation is the predominant lesion. As mentioned earlier, the presence of rheumatic mitral valve findings is the hallmark of diagnosing rheumatic aortic valve involvement. Infective endocarditis is the most common cause of acute aortic regurgitation. If infection is tolerated acutely without requiring surgery, it becomes a cause of chronic aortic regurgitation.

Diseases of the aortic root leading to aortic regurgitation include atherosclerosis, Marfan's syndrome, aortic dissection, hypertension with associated annuloaortic ectasia, syphilitic aortitis, ankylosing spondylitis, osteogenesis imperfecta, and systemic lupus. In Marfan's syndrome and in annuloaortic ectasia, dilation of the proximal root increases the aortic diameter at the level of the sinotubular ridge, which lifts the cusp suspension superiorly, causing cusp separation and lack of central coaptation (103). Although annuloaortic ectasia is often associated with hypertension, its presence usually correlates better with age than with elevated blood pressure. In Marfan's syndrome, in hypertension, and in some patients with bicuspid aortic valves, cystic medial necrosis of the aorta occurs, and in some patients, it arises in isolation. Whether an aneurysm is caused by atherosclerosis or cystic medial necrosis, an intimal tear can occur, producing aortic dissection. Proximal dissection may undermine aortic valve cusp support if the aortic dissection affects the commissural ridge. Ankylosing spondylitis and syphilis also cause ascending aortic dilation, but they also produce aortic wall thickening, which, in turn, distorts the commissures and prevents leaflet coaptation.

Pathophysiology

The pathophysiologic stages of acute and chronic aortic regurgitation are shown in Figure 22.6 (104). At the time of severe acute aortic regurgitation, there is a small increase in end-diastolic volume as the volume overload of aortic regurgitation increases LV preload. Increased filling volume allows only a modest increase in total stroke volume (SV), which is not enough to compensate for the volume that is regurgitated. Because pulse pressure is proportional to SV, which is only slightly increased, there is usually no percepti-

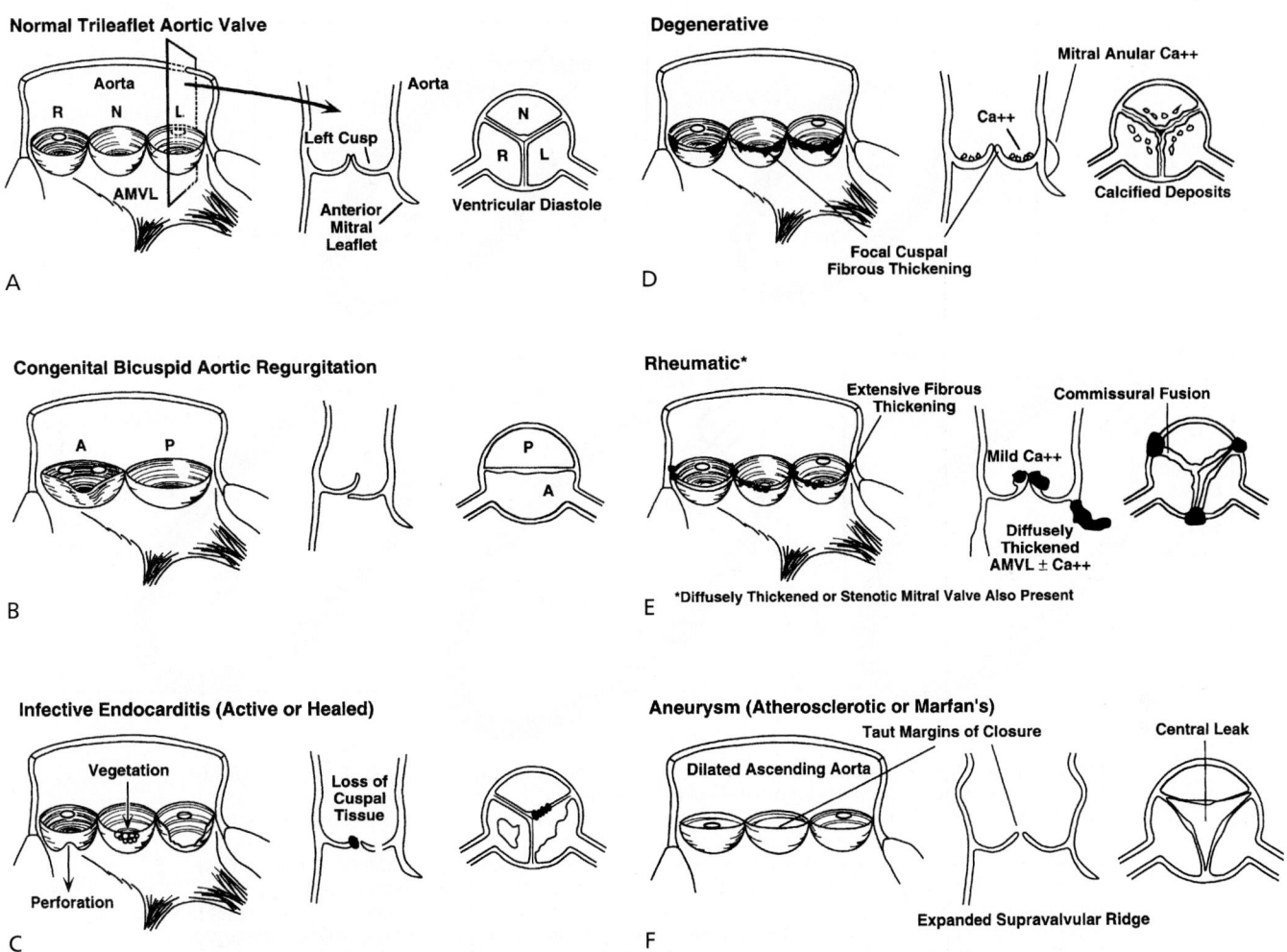

FIGURE 22.5 Diagrams showing various etiologies of aortic regurgitation (AR). Each of the six panels shows a long axis of the aortic root opened up to show all the leaflets (*left*), a schematic of the long axis of the sinus of Valsalva (*middle*), and a schematic of the short axis of the aortic valve (*right*). **A:** Normal trileaflet aortic valve. **B:** Congenital bicuspid valve with a raphe between what would be the right and left coronary cusps in an anterior cusp that is larger than the posterior cusp, causing prolapse and AR. **C:** Endocarditis causes AR through disruption of valve suspension or leaflet perforation. **D:** Degenerative changes cause AR by restricting leaflet motion and coaptation. **E:** Rheumatic valvulitis causes AR with postinflammatory leaflet fusion and fibrosis. **F:** Aneurysms from atherosclerosis or cystic medial necrosis (Marfan's type) cause AR by outward displacement of the leaflet suspension, with central noncoaptation, or by dissection causing failure of leaflet support. (A, anterior; AMVL, anterior mitral valve leaflet coronary cusp; Ca++, calcification; L, left; N, noncoronary cusp; P, posterior; R, right coronary cusp.) (Modified from Frankl WS, Brest AN, eds. Valvular heart disease: comprehensive evaluation and management. *Cardiovasc Clin* 1986;30–31, with permission.)

ble increase in pulse pressure at this stage of the disease. The large regurgitant volume entering the relatively small LV chamber greatly increases LV and left atrial diastolic pressure, leading to pulmonary congestion.

If aortic regurgitation develops more slowly or if the patient can be managed successfully through the acute episode without surgery, the patient enters the chronic compensated phase. In this phase, eccentric cardiac hypertrophy in addition to increased preload allows a large increase in LV end-diastolic volume. Because muscle function remains normal in this phase, normal performance of an enlarged ventri-

cle permits ejection of a very large total SV. The large total SV allows forward SV to be normal despite a large regurgitant volume. The enlarged left ventricle accommodates filling at a lower pressure, more normal than in acute AR. In this stage, the patient may be entirely asymptomatic even during fairly strenuous activity. The large total SV interacts with the aorta to produce a wide pulse pressure causing systolic hypertension. The wide pulse pressure produces most of the physical signs of aortic regurgitation. ❦ e40

The combined pressure and volume overload stimulates the development of both concentric and eccentric hypertrophy

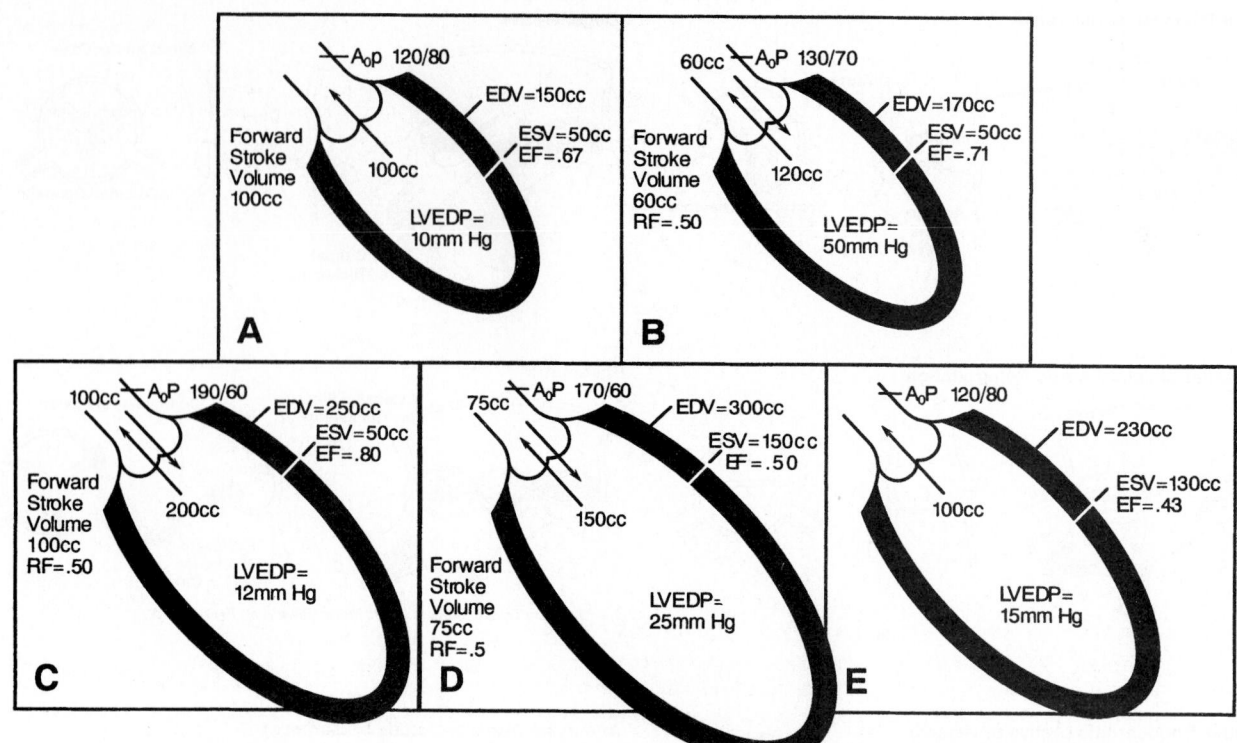

FIGURE 22.6 Hemodynamics of the clinical stages of aortic regurgitation (AR). **A:** Normal conditions. **B:** Severe acute AR, although total stroke volume (SV) is increased, forward SV is reduced. Left ventricular end-diastolic pressure (LVEDP) rises dramatically. **C:** Chronic, compensated AR. Eccentric hypertrophy produces increased end-diastolic volume (EDV), which permits an increase in total as well as forward SV. The volume overload is accommodated, and LVEDP is normalized. Ventricular emptying and end-systolic volume (ESV) remain normal. **D:** Chronic, decompensated AR. Impaired LV emptying produces an increase in ESV and a decrease in ejection fraction (EF), total SV, and forward SV. There is further cardiac dilation and recurrence of moderately elevated LVEDP. **E:** Immediately after aortic valve replacement, preload estimated by EDV decreases, as does LVEDP. ESV is also decreased but to a lesser extent, resulting in an initial decrease in EF. Despite these changes, elimination of AR leads to an increase in forward SV. (A_oP, aortic pressure; RF, regurgitant fraction.) (Modified from Carabello BA. Aortic regurgitation: hemodynamic determinants of prognosis. In: Cohn LH, DiSesa VJ, eds. *Aortic regurgitation: medical and surgical management.* New York: Marcel Dekker, 1986, with permission.)

(*e*Table 22.1.3). In this regard, aortic regurgitation differs markedly from mitral regurgitation, which is a pure volume overload (105) without pressure overload and without an increase in LV wall thickness. AR also differs from AS, which is a pure pressure overload without volume overload. The hypertrophy that occurs in both appears to be related to changes in LV myocardial matrix metalloproteinase activity and inhibitory control, but with some differences—for example, in interstitial collagenase activity and stromelysin levels (30c).

Although the patient may remain in the compensated phase for many years, LV dysfunction eventually develops. In this stage, LV dilation increases further, LV filling pressure becomes elevated, and EF decreases, reducing both total and forward SV. Although most patients develop symptoms at this time, some still may enter this decompensated phase without complaints.

The final panel of Figure 22.6 depicts the patient after AVR has been performed. Shortly after AVR, there is a fall in both end-diastolic volume and end-systolic volume (ESV), with a greater decrease in the former. This results in a temporary reduction in ejection performance. However, if AVR has been performed before LV dysfunction has become permanent, additional remodeling occurs, resulting in an additional fall in ESV, with a return of ejection performance toward normal (106).

To summarize, in chronic aortic regurgitation, there is a large increase in total SV ejected into the aorta, which produces a widened pulse pressure and systolic hypertension accounting for the physical signs of the disorder; the widened pulse pressure and systolic hypertension are responsible for adding a pressure overload to this volume-overloaded state. Although initially compensated by cardiac dilation to increase total SV, eventually afterload mismatch and contractile dysfunction lead to reduced ejection performance and cardiac decompensation (107). If the aortic regurgitation is recognized and corrected surgically in a

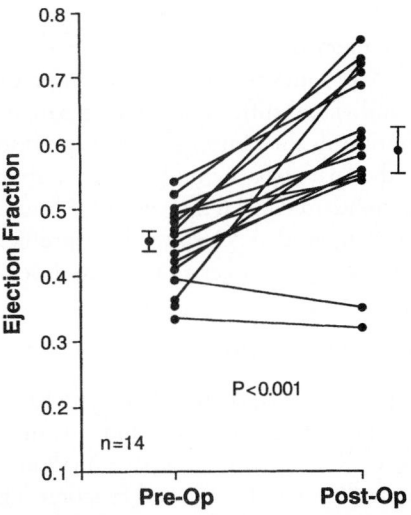

FIGURE 22.7 Shown here is preoperative and postoperative ejection fraction from 14 patients with aortic regurgitation. (From Carabello BA, Usher BW, Hendrix GH, et al. Predictors of outcome for aortic valve replacement in patients with aortic regurgitation and left ventricular dysfunction: a change in the measuring stick. *J Am Coll Cardiol* 1987;10:991–997, with permission.)

TABLE 22.2   SIGNS OF AORTIC INSUFFICIENCY

Sign	Finding
Corrigan's pulse	Rapid forceful carotid upstroke followed by rapid decline
Quincke's pulse	Systolic plethora and diastolic blanching in nail bed when nail is slightly compressed
de Musset's sign	Bobbing of head
Duroziez's sign	Systolic and diastolic bruit heard over femoral artery when compressed by bell of stethoscope
Hill's sign	Augmentation of systolic blood pressure in leg by ≥30 mm Hg compared with that in arm

timely fashion, decompensation is reversed after AVR, afterload is reduced, and EF returns to normal (Fig. 22.7).

Clinical Profile: Symptoms

Congestive Heart Failure

Patients with aortic regurgitation in the chronic compensated phase are often entirely asymptomatic and can remain so for many years, even after myocardial dysfunction develops. As LV decompensation proceeds, in many patients symptoms occur, typically including dyspnea on exertion, orthopnea, and in advanced cases, paroxysmal nocturnal dyspnea and peripheral edema.

Physical Examination

Chronic and severe aortic regurgitation results in a dramatic physical examination. Cardiac dilation and large total SV produce a hyperdynamic circulation. The point of maximum impulse is forceful, enlarged, sustained, and displaced downward and to the left. The typical murmur of aortic regurgitation is a diastolic, blowing, decrescendo murmur heard best at the left sternal border with the patient sitting upright. The length of the murmur is in part related to the severity of the aortic regurgitation. In mild disease a short, early diastolic murmur is the rule. As the degree of valvular regurgitation worsens, the murmur may become pandiastolic. With the late onset of LV dysfunction and in acute, severe aortic regurgitation, high LV diastolic pressure causes earlier equilibration of the aortic and LV diastolic pressures in mid-diastole, reshortening the length

of the diastolic murmur. Many patients with aortic regurgitation also have a systolic murmur even if they do not have AS because of the increase in antegrade flow. A second diastolic murmur, an apical mitral rumble (Austin Flint murmur), usually indicates that the aortic regurgitation is severe. Although still debated, the Austin Flint murmur is probably the result of the aortic jet impinging on the mitral valve, causing it to vibrate or causing diastolic turbulence without true LV inflow obstruction.

The large forward SV and wide aortic pulse pressure affect the process of taking the patient's blood pressure with a sphygmomanometer, during which Korotkoff's sounds are often heard almost down to a pressure of zero. The widened pulse pressure is also responsible for a myriad of signs, listed in Table 22.2, resulting from the hyperdynamic pulse contour. Among them, Hill's sign and Duroziez's sign seem to be the most useful as a bedside gauge of the presence of severe aortic regurgitation. However, when LV decompensation occurs, the pulse pressure may narrow and become pseudonormalized by a reduction in the systolic hypertension. This accrues from reduced total SV by the weakened left ventricle. Elevated LV diastolic pressures often cause an early diastolic apical filling sound [third heart sound (S_3) or gallop].

Electrocardiogram

The ECG in chronic aortic regurgitation is nonspecific, but it almost always demonstrates LVH.

Echocardiography and Doppler Examination

At present, echocardiography with Doppler interrogation of the aortic valve is the most important test to diagnose this disease. Two-dimensional echocardiography is able to visualize the structure, thickness, and mobility of the aortic valve leaflets and the size of the aortic annulus and ascending aorta. ▼ e41

With each etiology of aortic regurgitation, there are typical structural changes that are definable by echo. In the patients with bicuspid aortic valve, rheumatic heart disease, infective endocarditis, or calcific degeneration of the leaflets, typical imaging features of the aortic cusps have become well recognized. Aortic dilation can also be easily detected when it is a cause of valvular regurgitation.

Echo also gauges LV performance, chamber dimensions, and the extent of LVH, which are used with clinical data to time aortic valve surgery (see Aortic Valve Replacement and Repair). Doppler interrogation is used to gauge the degree of aortic regurgitation in several ways. First, the spatial extent of the color Doppler aliasing in the outflow tract is used as a rough guide to the severity of aortic regurgitation (109). A semiquantitative scale of mild, moderate, moderately severe, and severe regurgitation is predicated primarily on the width (in long axis) and the area (in short axis) of the proximal portion of the jet of disturbed flow in the outflow tract. To a lesser extent, the depth to which the jet penetrates toward the apex of the left ventricle is also important. ❦ e42

Cardiac Catheterization

In patients with severe aortic regurgitation in whom the diagnosis is obvious from the physical examination and the noninvasive results, cardiac catheterization need not be performed before AVR. In general, valve surgery without catheterization is more reasonable in men younger than 40 years or in women younger than 50 years, but atherosclerotic risk factors and symptoms should also be considered in this decision. In patients in whom severity of aortic regurgitation is in question or for the purposes of defining concomitant coronary disease, catheterization should be performed. During cardiac catheterization, additional assessment of the severity of aortic regurgitation is made using aortography. Unlike echocardiography, which visualizes the velocity of flow, aortography visualizes regurgitant flow by opacifying the left ventricle with contrast injected into the aorta. The denser the opacification, the worse the aortic regurgitation (111). At least 60 mL of contrast should be injected to opacify both the enlarged left ventricle and aortic root.

Management

Timing of Surgery

Although severe chronic aortic regurgitation may be tolerated for years in many patients, the combined LV pressure and volume overload eventually leads to muscle damage and LV dysfunction. Aortic valve surgery should be performed when symptoms develop, but before muscle dysfunction becomes irreversible. If the patient with aortic regurgitation develops New York Heart Association class II symptoms of CHF, surgery should be performed to help improve the quality of the patient's life and functional status. However, surgery should be performed even in the asymptomatic patient if there is evidence that contractile dysfunction has begun to develop (112–114a). Contractil-

ity is the ability of the myocardium to develop force independent of preload. Unfortunately, there is no easily applied device or index to measure this property. Moreover, because of individual differences among patients with aortic regurgitation in the abnormalities of preload and afterload and the patient's hemodynamic response to the disease, the standard clinical indices of LV function, such as EF, may be confounded. Despite these problems, reliable guides to the timing of surgery have been developed.

Use of Echocardiography

During the past 15 years, echocardiography has become preeminent in predicting outcome and in timing surgery because it provides a safe, noninvasive method for frequent periodic interrogation of LV size and function. The two indices that have demonstrated efficacy in predicting outcome in patients with chronic asymptomatic or minimally symptomatic aortic regurgitation are echocardiographic shortening fraction or EF and end-systolic cavity size (either LV diameter or volume) (112–114a). Shortening fraction and systolic diameter are the minor axis one-dimensional equivalents of EF and ESV, respectively. A patient with a shortening fraction of less than 27% or a resting EF of less than 55% has presumed LV dysfunction. Aortic valve surgery should be considered even in the asymptomatic patient before systolic function declines further. End-systolic diameter, a more preload-independent index than EF, has also proved helpful in timing surgery (112–114). When the combination of eccentric hypertrophy and LV dysfunction has developed so that the left ventricle has an end-systolic diameter of 55 mm or larger, postoperative survival is significantly decreased. To avoid the prospects of a higher risk of perioperative mortality, surgery should be strongly considered when the end-systolic diameter reaches or exceeds 50 mm. It should be noted that there is a window of time of approximately 18 months after either of these thresholds is crossed during which surgery can be performed and systolic function will likely still return to normal (115). Although echocardiographic and clinical follow-up must be tailored to the needs of individual patients, Bonow et al. (113) have recommended that frequency of echo studies be gauged by the end-systolic diameter. When this dimension is less than 40 mm, it is very unlikely that dysfunction will develop within the next 2 years, and thus echocardiography should be performed biannually. When echocardiographic end-systolic diameter ranges from 40 to 50 mm, yearly follow-up is recommended. If end-systolic diameter is more than 50 mm, the patient should also be given the option of surgery, but if delay is chosen, echocardiography should be performed every 6 months.

Medical Therapy

Use of vasodilators in treating patients with asymptomatic aortic regurgitation has been found to forestall the development of LV dysfunction. The premise in their use is that arteriolar vasodilation reduces regurgitant flow and diminishes the severity of the lesion. Hydralazine, nifedipine, and angiotensin-converting enzyme inhibitors have been investigated for this purpose. The most compelling data point to nifedipine, although it is likely that angiotensin-converting enzyme inhibitors and other dihydropyridine calcium blockers would also be effective. In a randomized 2-year study of hydralazine (117), asymptomatic patients given hydralazine had less ventricular dilation and better ejection performance than did a placebo group. Similar results have been reported with angiotensin-converting enzyme inhibitors (118). A large controlled study of nifedipine versus digoxin (119) recently found that nifedipine substantially delayed the time when surgery was required and reduced the number of patients requiring surgery. Thus, there is evidence supporting long-term use of vasodilators in asymptomatic patients with severe, chronic aortic regurgitation who do not yet have LV dysfunction or other clear indications for surgery.

ACUTE AORTIC REGURGITATION

Background

Severe, acute aortic regurgitation frequently constitutes a surgical emergency. Mortality may be as high as 75% in medically treated patients but only 25% after surgery. Thus, recognition of acute aortic regurgitation and its proper management are crucial in ensuring good patient outcome (120).

Etiology

Infective Endocarditis

Infective endocarditis is the most common cause of acute aortic regurgitation. Frequently occurring in younger patients, especially those that practice illicit intravenous drug use, acute endocarditis may develop on a previously bicuspid valve or a normal valve, especially if aggressive organisms, such as *Staphylococcus aureus* or enterococcus, are the etiologic agents. Often mistaken for influenza, the sudden development of a high fever, malaise, and the early symptoms of CHF should be given immediate attention, especially in the patient with a previously known abnormal aortic valve or a valve prosthesis. Cutaneous manifestations of endocarditis, systemic emboli, a new or changing murmur of aortic regurgitation, positive blood cultures, and echocardiographic demonstration of aortic valve vegetations all help to make the diagnosis (see Chapter 25) (120a).

Aortic Dissection

Acute proximal aortic dissection is the other major cause of acute aortic regurgitation. However, unlike endocardi-

tis, other hemodynamic manifestations of proximal dissection, such as hemopericardium with tamponade, myocardial infarction from coronary dissection, or progression to aortic rupture, are usually more problematic than aortic regurgitation.

Pathophysiology

In chronic aortic regurgitation, the development of eccentric LVH permits compensation of the left ventricle by allowing it to generate a large total SV. Apart from being compensatory, this large SV causes a wide pulse pressure, the source of most of the signs of chronic aortic regurgitation. However, in acute regurgitation, eccentric LVH and compensatory LV dilation have not yet developed. Thus, most of the signs of chronic aortic regurgitation, such as a widened pulse pressure, Quincke's pulse, and so forth, are absent. Indeed, the new murmur of aortic regurgitation may be the only clue that this deadly disease is present (121). However, the murmur may be quite short or heard only in very early diastole because of the rapid equilibration of LV and aortic pressures.

At the bedside, considerable attention should be paid to the first heart sound (S_1). In severe, acute aortic regurgitation the high LV diastolic pressure closes the mitral valve before the onset of LV systole (preclosure). Preclosure of the mitral valve is an ominous sign, almost always indicating the need for urgent surgery.

Management

Echocardiography

Once the diagnosis of acute aortic regurgitation is suspected, echocardiography should be performed immediately. In either bacterial endocarditis or in aortic dissection, the echocardiogram is invaluable in helping to define the etiology and severity of the valve dysfunction. Aortic valve vegetations are key to the diagnosis in endocarditis. In aortic dissection, enlargement of the aorta, the intimal flap, and distinguishing true from false lumen velocities by color flow Doppler are keys to diagnosis, which may require TEE (see Chapter 52).

In either etiology, M-mode echo is useful in demonstrating premature mitral valve closure as a sign of high LV diastolic pressure (122). Occurring for the same reason, diastolic mitral regurgitation by Doppler and other signs of elevated LV pressure can be recorded in some cases. Endocarditis patients with severe AR may be followed medically if they have no heart block, mitral valve preclosure, or evidence of CHF on physical examination or chest x-ray. However, a repeat echocardiogram should be performed to look for an increase in vegetation size, especially if new evidence suggests that aortic regurgitation has worsened. Echocardiography, and particularly TEE, is helpful in diag-

THE FUTURE

In the future, improvements in our understanding of the contributing factors of the "atherosclerosis-like" process of AS will fuel prevention strategies. Innovations in cardiac surgery and perioperative medical management will promote the ongoing trend for surgical techniques for AS and AR to become safer, with less perioperative mortality and morbidity. No longer should surgery be put off until the patient's symptoms cannot be managed medically, late in the course of the disease. New valvular replacement options will become more physiologic, with less prosthetic valve "penalty" in terms of persistent gradients, postoperative hypertrophy, and limited durability. Reoperations for a second, third, or even sixth time will continue to become more frequent and with acceptable operative risk. In addition, our abilities to monitor hemodynamics of surgery patients noninvasively and repeatedly and to study groups of patients to understand the disease processes will improve. These factors will further improve the prognosis for patients with aortic valve disease. The progress continues.

nosing endocarditis, perivalvular abscesses, and aortic dissection (120a,120b).

Medical Therapy

In the case of endocarditis, multiple blood cultures should be drawn before antibiotics are started. Thereafter, broadspectrum antibiotics are begun empirically and are adjusted later when blood cultures identify the least toxic antibiotic regimen to which the organism is sensitive. In the absence of CHF or mitral valve preclosure, careful daily assessment for progression of the disease is mandatory. This should include a careful history and physical examination, looking for symptoms and signs of even mild CHF, as well as an ECG rhythm strip looking for prolongation of the PR interval, which might indicate the development of an aortic ring abscess. In some patients, aggressive management with vasodilators may temporarily allow for improvement; however, this therapy should be used to better prepare the patient for surgery rather than as an attempt to delay surgery.

Surgical Therapy

If CHF or mitral preclosure develops, immediate AVR should be contemplated. Although there is always a concern that implantation of a prosthesis in an infected patient may lead to prosthetic endocarditis, reinfection of a prosthetic valve has an incidence of approximately 10%, even if surgery is performed within 48 hours of the last positive blood culture (123). In patients with aortic valve endocarditis, particularly those with extension of the infection into heart tissue (i.e., annular ring abscess), valve replacement with an aortic homograft may be advantageous because it entails implantation of less foreign body and reduced early postoperative valve infection (124).

CONTROVERSIES AND PERSONAL PERSPECTIVES

Aortic Valve Replacement in Asymptomatic Aortic Stenosis Patients

Some change has occurred recently in our understanding of the optimum time for surgery in patients with AS (59a). With the mortality and morbidity risks of valve surgery declining due to improved technology and methods, the question has arisen whether patients with no symptoms should be considered candidates for surgery. In AS, there is a widely recognized risk of sudden death. Although most patients have antecedent symptoms before their event, in many patients the symptoms are not significant enough to bring them in for medical attention before their death and are therefore just as bad as the less common collapse and immediate death. As mentioned above, some factors have been associated with worse prognosis, including the presence of moderate or severe valvular calcification and a rapid increase in aortic jet velocity between two echocardiographic studies (29a). In addition, the flow-dependent rate of change in AVA measured during the ejection phase of a cardiac cycle predicts the rate of hemodynamic progression in patients with asymptomatic AS (25a). Exercise testing may also reveal latent symptoms or hemodynamic instability. If further studies confirm these findings, consideration for early valve replacement in some asymptomatic patients may be appropriate, rather than delaying surgery until symptoms develop.

ACKNOWLEDGMENT

We are indebted to Fred A. Crawford, Jr., M.D., who contributed to the first edition of this chapter, published in the first edition of this book in 1998. His wisdom and experience are still an integral part of this manuscript.

REFERENCES

1. Lindblom D, Lindblom U, Qvist J, Lundstrom H. Long-term relative survival rates after heart valve replacement. *J Am Coll Cardiol* 1990;15:566.

2. Facquet L, Lemoine JM, Alhomme P, et al. La mesure de la pression auriculaire gauche par voie transbronchique. *Arch Mal Coeur* 1952;45:741.

3. Bjork VO, Malmstrom G, Uggla LG. Left auricular pressure measurements in man. *Ann Surg* 1953;138:718.

4. Cope C. Technique for transseptal catheterization of the left atrium: preliminary report. *J Thorac Surg* 1959;37:482.

5. Dodge HT, Sandler H, Ballew DW. The use of biplane angiocardiography for the measurement of left ventricular volume in man. *Am Heart J* 1960;60:762.

6. Hatle L. Noninvasive assessment and differentiation of left ventricular outflow obstruction with Doppler ultrasound. *Circulation* 1981;64:381–387.

7. Hegrenaes L, Hatle L. Aortic stenosis in adults: noninvasive estimation of pressure differences by continuous wave Doppler echocardiography. *Br Heart J* 1985;54:396–404.

8. Skjaerpe T, Hegrenaes L, Hatle L. Noninvasive estimation of valve area in patients with aortic stenosis by Doppler ultrasound and two-dimensional echocardiography. *Circulation* 1985;72:810–881.

9. Huffnagel CA, Harvey WP. The surgical correction of aortic insufficiency. *Bull Georgetown Univ Med Ctr* 1953;6:30.

10. Harken DE, Soroff HS, Taylor WJ, et al. Partial and complete prostheses in aortic insufficiency. *J Thorac Cardiovasc Surg* 1960;40:744.

11. Murray G. Homologous aortic-valve-segment transplants as surgical treatment for aortic and mitral insufficiency. *Angiology* 1956;7:466.

12. Ross DN. Homograft replacement of the aortic valve. *Lancet* 1962;2:487.

13. Ross DN. Replacement of aortic and mitral valves with a pulmonary autograft. *Lancet* 1967;2:956.

14. Carpentier A, Lemaigre G, Robert L, et al. Biologic factors affecting long-term results of valvular heterografts. *J Thorac Cardiovasc Surg* 1969;58:467.

15. Ionescu MI, Pakrashi BC, Holden MP, et al. Results of aortic valve replacement with frame-supported fascia lata and pericardial grafts. *J Thorac Cardiovasc Surg* 1972;64:340.

16. Passik CS, Ackermann DM, Pluth JR, Edwards WD. Temporal changes in the causes of aortic stenosis: a surgical pathologic study of 646 cases. *Mayo Clin Proc* 1987;62:119.

17. Fenoglio JJ Jr, McAllister HA Jr, DeCastro CM, et al. Congenital bicuspid aortic valve after age 20. *Am J Cardiol* 1977;39:164.

18. Roberts WC. The congenitally bicuspid aortic valve: a study of 85 autopsy cases. *Am J Cardiol* 1970;26:72.

18a. Kim YM, Yoo SJ, Choi JY, et al. Natural course of supravalvar aortic stenosis and peripheral pulmonary arterial stenosis in Williams' syndrome. *Cardiol Young* 1999;9:37–41.

19. Campbell M. Calcific aortic stenosis and congenital bicuspid aortic valves. *Br Heart J* 1968;30:606–616.

20. Otto CM, Kuusisto J, Reichenbach DD, et al. Characterization of the early lesion of "degenerative" valvular aortic stenosis: histological and immunohistochemical studies. *Circulation* 1994;90:844.

21. Juvonen J, Laurila A, Juvonen T, et al. Detection of *Chlamydia pneumoniae* in human nonrheumatic stenotic aortic valves. *J Am Coll Cardiol* 1997;29:1054–1059.

21a. Wierzbicki A, Shetty C. Aortic stenosis: an atherosclerotic disease? *J Heart Valve Dis* 1999;8:416–423.

21b. Carabello BA. Aortic sclerosis—a window to the coronary arteries? *N Engl J Med* 1999;341:193–195.

21c. Otto CM, Lind BK, Kitzman DW, et al. Association of aortic-valve sclerosis with cardiovascular mortality and morbidity in the elderly. *N Engl J Med* 1999;341:142–147.

21d. Stewart BF, Siscovick D, Lind BK, et al. Clinical factors associated with calcific aortic valve disease. Cardiovascular Health Study. *J Am Coll Cardiol* 1997;29:630–634.

21e. Rallidis L, Naoumova RP, Thompson GR, Nihoyannopoulos P. Extent and severity of atherosclerotic involvement of the aortic valve and root in familial hypercholesterolaemia. *Heart* 1998;80:583–590.

22. Donner RM, Carabello BA, Black I, Spann JF. Left ventricular wall stress in compensated aortic stenosis in children. *Am J Cardiol* 1983;51:946.

23. Assey ME, Wisenbaugh T, Spann JF Jr, et al. Unexpected persistence into adulthood of low wall-stress in patients with congenital aortic stenosis: is there a fundamental difference in the hypertrophic response to a pressure overload present from birth? *Circulation* 1987;75:973.

24. Keane JF, Driscoll DJ, Gersony WM, et al. Second natural history study of congenital heart defects: results of treatment of patients with aortic valvular stenosis. *Circulation* 1993;87[Suppl 2]:116.

25. Witsenburg M, Cromme-Dijkhuis AH, Frohn-Mulder IM, Hess J. Short- and midterm results of balloon valvuloplasty for valvular aortic stenosis in children. *Am J Cardiol* 1992;69:945.

25a. Lester SJ, Heilbron B, Gin K, et al. The natural history and rate of progression of aortic stenosis. *Chest* 1998;113:1109–1114.

26. Ross J Jr, Braunwald E. Aortic stenosis. *Circulation* 1968;38[Suppl 5]:61–67.

27. Kelly TA, Rothbart RM, Cooper CM, et al. Comparison of outcome of asymptomatic to symptomatic patients older than 20 years of age with valvular aortic stenosis. *Am J Cardiol* 1988;61:123.

28. Pellikka PA, Nishimura RA, Bailey KR, Tajik AJ. The natural history of adults with asymptomatic, hemodynamically significant aortic stenosis. *J Am Coll Cardiol* 1990;15:1012.

29. Lombard JT, Selzer A. Valvular aortic stenosis: a clinical and hemodynamic profile of patients. *Ann Intern Med* 1987;106:292.

29a. Rosenhek R, Binder T, Porenta G, et al. Predictors of outcome in severe, asymptomatic aortic stenosis. *N Engl J Med* 2000;343:611–617.

29b. Bahler RC, Desser DR, Finkelhor RS, et al. Factors leading to progression of valvular aortic stenosis. *Am J Cardiol* 1999;84:1044–1048.

29c. Otto CM, Burwash IG, Legget ME, et al. Prospective study of asymptomatic valvular aortic stenosis. *Circulation* 1997;95:2262–2270.

29d. Palta S, Pai AM, Gill KS, Pai RG. New insights into the progression of aortic stenosis: implications for secondary prevention. *Circulation* 2000;101:2497–2502.

30. Grossman W, Jones D, McLaurin LP. Wall stress and patterns of hypertrophy in the human left ventricle. *J Clin Invest* 1975;56:56.

30a. Hamawaki M, Coffman TM, Lashus A, et al. Pressure-overload hypertrophy is unabated in mice devoid of AT1A receptors. *Am J Physiol* 1998;274[3 Pt 2]:H868–H873.

30b. Koide M, Carabello BA, Conrad CC, et al. Hypertrophic response to hemodynamic overload: role of load vs. renin-angiotensin system activation. *Am J Physiol* 1999;276[2 Pt 2]:H350–H358.

30c. Nagatomo Y, Carabello BA, Coker ML, et al. Differential effects of pressure or volume overload on myocardial MMP levels and inhibitory control. *Am J Physiol Heart Circ Physiol* 2000;278:H151–H161.

31. Marcus ML, Doty DB, Hiratzka LF, et al. Decreased coronary reserve: a mechanism for angina pectoris in patients with aortic stenosis and normal coronary arteries. *N Engl J Med* 1982;307:1362–1367.

32. Dunn RB, Griggs DM. Ventricular filling pressure as a determinant of coronary blood flow during ischemia. *Am J Physiol* 1983;244:H429.

33. Breisch EA, Houser SR, Carey RA, et al. Myocardial blood flow and capillary density in chronic pressure overload of the feline left ventricle. *Cardiovasc Res* 1980;14:469.

34. Julius BK, Spillman M, Vassali G, et al. Angina pectoris in patients with aortic stenosis and normal coronary arteries: mechanisms and pathophysiologic concepts. *Circulation* 1997;95:892–898.

35. Strauer BE. Ventricular function and coronary hemodynamics in hypertensive heart disease. *Am J Cardiol* 1979;44:999.

36. Schwartz LS, Goldfischer J, Sprague GJ, Schwartz SP. Syncope and sudden death in aortic stenosis. *Am J Cardiol* 1969;23:647.

37. Richards AM, Nicholls MG, Ikram A, et al. Syncope in aortic valvular stenosis. *Lancet* 1984;2:1113.

38. Peterson KL, Tsuji J, Johnson A, et al. Diastolic left ventricular pressure-volume and stress-strain relations in patients with valvular aortic stenosis and left ventricular hypertrophy. *Circulation* 1978;58:77.

39. Hess OM, Ritter M, Schneider J, et al. Diastolic stiffness and myocardial structure in aortic valve disease before and after valve replacement. *Circulation* 1984;69:855.

40. Huber D, Grimm J, Koch R, Krayenbuehl HP. Determinants of ejection performance in aortic stenosis. *Circulation* 1981;64:126.

40a. Lorell BH, Carabello BA. Left ventricular hypertrophy: pathogenesis, detection, and prognosis. *Circulation* 2000;102:470–479.

41. Koide M, Nagatsu M, Zile MR, et al. Premorbid determinants of left ventricular dysfunction in a novel model of gradually induced pressure overload in the adult canine. *Circulation* 1997;95:1601–1610.

42. Herzig JW, Ruegg JC, Solaro RJ. Myocardial excitation contraction coupling as influenced through modulation of the calcium sensitivity of the contractile proteins. *Heart Failure* 1991;6:244.

43. Nakano K, Corin WJ, Spann JF Jr, et al. Abnormal subendocardial blood flow in pressure overload hypertrophy is associated with pacing-induced subendocardial dysfunction. *Circ Res* 1989;65:1555.

44. Tsutsui H, Ishihara K, Cooper G IV. Cytoskeletal role in the contractile dysfunction of hypertrophied myocardium. *Science* 1993;260:682.

44a. Tagawa H, Koide M, Sato H, et al. Cytoskeletal role in the transition from compensated to decompensated hypertrophy during adult canine left ventricular pressure overloading. *Circ Res* 1998;82:751–761.

44b. Koide M, Hamawaki M, Narishige T, et al. Microtubule depolymerization normalizes in vivo myocardial contractile function in dogs with pressure-overload left ventricular hypertrophy. *Circulation* 2000;102:1045–1052.

45. Gorlin R, Gorlin SG. Hydraulic formula for calculation of the area of the stenotic mitral valve, other cardiac valves, and central circulatory shunts. *Am Heart J* 1951;41:1.

46. Assey ME, Usher BW, Carabello BA, Spann JF Jr. The patient with valvular heart disease. In: Pepine CJ, Hill JA, Lambert CR, eds. *Diagnostic and therapeutic cardiac catheterization*, 2nd ed. Baltimore: Williams & Wilkins, 1989:471–507.

46a. Blumberg FC, Pfeifer M, Holmer SR, et al. Quantification of aortic stenosis in mechanically ventilated patients using multiplane transesophageal Doppler echocardiography. *Chest* 1998;114:94–97.

47. Brener SJ, Duffy CI, Thomas JD, Stewart WJ. Progression of aortic stenosis in 394 patients. Relation to changes in myocardial and mitral valve dysfunction. *J Am Coll Cardiol* 1995;25:305–310.

48. Otto CM, Pearlman AS, Gardner CL. Hemodynamic progression of aortic stenosis in adults assessed by Doppler echocardiography. *J Am Coll Cardiol* 1989;13:545.

48a. Munt B, Legget ME, Kraft CD, et al. Physical examination in valvular aortic stenosis: correlation with stenosis severity and prediction of clinical outcome. *Am Heart J* 1999;137:298–306.

48b. Wyatt H, Heng MK, Meerbaum S, et al. Cross-sectional echocardiography: I. Analysis of mathematic models for quantifying mass of the left ventricle in dogs. *Circulation* 1977;60:1104–1110.

49. Currie PJ, Seward JB, Reeder GS, et al. Continuous-wave Doppler echocardiographic assessment of severity of calcific aortic stenosis: a simultaneous Doppler-catheter correlative study in 100 adult patients. *Circulation* 1985;71:1162.

49a. Vanoverschelde JL, Essamri B, Michel X, et al. Hemodynamic and volume correlates of left ventricular diastolic relaxation and filling in patients with aortic stenosis. *J Am Coll Cardiol* 1992;20:813–821.

49b. ACC/AHA guidelines for the management of patients with valvular heart disease. A report of the American College of Cardiology/American Heart Association. Task Force on Practice Guidelines (Committee on Management of Patients with Valvular Heart Disease). *J Am Coll Cardiol* 1998;32:1486–1588.

50. Schlant RC, Friesinger GC II, Leonard JJ. Clinical competence in exercise testing: a statement for physicians from the ACP/ACC/AHA Task Force on Clinical Privileges in Cardiology. *J Am Coll Cardiol* 1990;16:1061.

51. Areskog NH. Exercise testing in the evaluation of patients with valvular aortic stenosis. *Clin Physiol* 1984;4:201.

52. Linderholm H, Osterman G, Teien D. Detection of coronary artery disease by means of exercise ECG in patients with aortic stenosis. *Acta Med Scand* 1985;218:181.

53. Samuels B, Kiat H, Friedman JD, Berman DS. Adenosine pharmacological stress myocardial perfusion tomographic imaging in patients with significant aortic stenosis: diagnostic efficacy and comparison of clinical, hemodynamic, and electrocardiographic variables with 100 age-matched control subjects. *J Am Coll Cardiol* 1995;25:99.

53a. Popovic AD, Thomas JD, Neskovic AN, et al. Time-related trends in the preoperative evaluation of patients with valvular stenosis. *Am J Cardiol* 1997;80:1464–1468.

53b. Roger V, Tajik AJ, Reeder GS, et al. Effect of Doppler echocardiography on utilization of hemodynamic cardiac catheterization in the preoperative evaluation of aortic stenosis. *Mayo Clin Proc* 1996;71:141–149.

54. Vandeplas A, Willems JL, Piessens J, De Geest H. Frequency of angina pectoris and coronary artery disease in severe isolated valvular aortic stenosis. *Am J Cardiol* 1988;62:117.

55. Garcia-Rubira JC, Lopez V, Cubero J. Coronary arterial disease in patients with severe isolated aortic stenosis. *Int J Cardiol* 1992;35:121.

56. Alexopoulos D, Kolovou G, Kyriakidis M, et al. Angina and coronary artery disease in patients with aortic valve disease. *Angiology* 1993;44:707.

57. Lytle BW. Impact of coronary artery disease on valvular heart surgery. *Cardiol Clin* 1991;9:301.

58. Czer LS, Gray RJ, Stewart ME, et al. Reduction in sudden late death by concomitant revascularization with aortic valve replacement. *J Thorac Cardiovasc Surg* 1988;95:390.

59. Di Lello F, Flemma RJ, Anderson AJ, et al. Improved early results after aortic valve replacement analysis by surgical time frame. *Ann Thorac Surg* 1989;47:51.

59a. Carabello BA. Timing of valve replacement in aortic stenosis. Moving closer to perfection. *Circulation* 1997;95:2241–2243.

60. Safian RD, Berman AD, Diver DJ, et al. Balloon aortic valvuloplasty in 170 consecutive patients. *N Engl J Med* 1988;319:125.

61. Litvack F, Jakubowski AT, Buchbinder NA, Eigler N. Lack of sustained clinical improvement in an elderly population after percutaneous aortic valvuloplasty. *Am J Cardiol* 1988;62:270.

62. Otto CM, Mickel MC, Kennedy JW, et al. Three-year outcome after balloon aortic valvuloplasty: insights into prognosis of valvular aortic stenosis. *Circulation* 1994;89:642–650.

62a. Carabello BA. Timing of valve replacement in aortic stenosis. *Circulation* 1997;95:2241–2242.

63. Craver JM. Aortic valve debridement by ultrasonic surgical aspirator: a word of caution. *Ann Thorac Surg* 1990;49:746.

64. Cosgrove DM, Rosenkranz ER, Hendren WG, et al. Valvuloplasty for aortic insufficiency. *J Thorac Cardiovasc Surg* 1991;102:571–576.

65. Cosgrove DM, Sabik JF. Minimally invasive approach for aortic valve operations. *Ann Thorac Surg* 1996;62:596–597.

65a. Munt BI, Legget ME, Healy NL, et al. Effects of aortic valve replacement on exercise duration and functional status in adults with valvular aortic stenosis. *Can J Cardiol* 1997;13:346–350.

66. Akins CW. Results with mechanical cardiac valvular prostheses. *Ann Thorac Surg* 1995;60:1836.

67. Emery RW, Arom KV, Nicoloff DM. Utilization of the St. Jude medical prosthesis in the aortic position. *Semin Thorac Cardiovasc Surg* 1996;8:231.

68. Copeland JG. The Carbo-Medics prosthetic heart valve: a second generation bileaflet prosthesis. *Semin Thorac Cardiovasc Surg* 1996;8:237.

69. Akins CW. Medtronic-Hall prosthetic aortic valve. *Semin Thorac Cardiovasc Surg* 1996;8:242.

69a. Hammermeister K, Sethi GK, Henderson WG, et al. Outcomes 15 years after valve replacement with a mechanical versus a bioprosthetic valve: final report of the veterans affairs randomized trial. *J Am Coll Cardiol* 2000;36:1152–1158.

70. Jamieson WR, Munro IA, Miyagishima RT, et al. Carpentier-Edwards standard porcine bioprosthesis: clinical performance to seventeen years. *Ann Thorac Surg* 1995;60:999.

71. Yun KL, Miller DC, Moore KA, et al. Durability of the Hancock MO bioprosthesis compared with standard aortic valve bioprostheses. *Ann Thorac Surg* 1995;60:S221.

72. Fann JI, Miller DC. Porcine valves: Hancock and Carpentier-Edwards aortic prostheses. *Semin Thorac Cardiovasc Surg* 1996;8:259.

73. Cosgrove DM, Lytle BW, Taylor PC, et al. The Carpentier-Edwards pericardial aortic valve: ten-year results. *J Thorac Cardiovasc Surg* 1995;110:653.

74. Aupart MR, Sirinelli AL, Diemont FF, et al. The last generation of pericardial valves in the aortic position: ten-year follow-up in 589 patients. *Ann Thorac Surg* 1996;61:615.

75. Cosgrove DM. Carpentier pericardial valve. *Semin Thorac Cardiovasc Surg* 1996;8:269.

76. Jones EL, Shah VB, Shanewise JS, et al. Should the freehand allograft be abandoned as a reliable alternative for aortic valve replacement? *Ann Thorac Surg* 1995;59:1397.

77. Doty DB. Aortic valve replacement with homograft and autograft. *Semin Thorac Cardiovasc Surg* 1996;8:249.

78. Barratt-Boyes BG, Roche AHG, Subramanyan R, et al. Long-term follow-up of patients with antibiotic-sterilized aortic homograft inserted freehand in the aortic position. *Circulation* 1987;75:768–777.

79. Clarke DR, Campbell DN, Hayward AR, Bishop DA. Degeneration of aortic valve allografts in young recipients. *J Thorac Cardiovasc Surg* 1993;105:934.

80. Ross DN. Evolution of the homograft valve. *Am Thorac Surg* 1995;59:565.

81. Gerosa G, Ross DN, Brucke PE, et al. Aortic valve replacement with pulmonary homografts: early experience. *J Thorac Cardiovasc Surg* 1994;107:424.

82. Elkins RC. Congenital aortic valve disease: evolving management. *Ann Thorac Surg* 1995;59:269.

83. Niederberger J, Schima H, Maurer G, Baumgartner H. Importance of pressure recovery for the assessment of aortic stenosis by Doppler ultrasound: role of aortic size, aortic valve area, and direction of the stenotic jet in vitro. *Circulation* 1996;94:1934–1940.

83a. Baumgartner H, Stefenelli T, Niederberger J, et al. "Over-estimation" of catheter gradients by Doppler ultrasound in patients with aortic stenosis: a predictable manifestation of pressure recovery. *J Am Coll Cardiol* 1999;33:1655–1661.

84. David TE, Feindel CM, Bos J, et al. Aortic valve replacement with a stentless porcine aortic valve: a six-year experience. *J Thorac Cardiovasc Surg* 1994;108:1030.

85. Kon ND, Westaby S, Amarasena N, et al. Comparison of implantation techniques using freestyle stentless porcine aortic valve. *Ann Thorac Surg* 1995;59:857.

85a. Thomson HL, O'Brien MF, Almeida AA, et al. Haemodynamics and left ventricular mass regression: a comparison of the stentless, stented and mechanical aortic valve replacement. *Eur J Cardiothorac Surg* 1998;13:572–575.

85b. Maselli D, Pizio R, Bruno LP, et al. Left ventricular mass reduction after aortic valve replacement: homografts, stentless and stented valves. *Ann Thorac Surg* 1999;67:966–971.

85c. Basarir S, Islamoglu F, Ozkisacik E, et al. Comparative analysis of left ventricular hemodynamics and hypertrophy after aortic valve replacement with homografts or mechanical valves. *J Heart Valve Dis* 2000;9:45–52.

86. Kratz JM, Sade RM, Crawford FA Jr, et al. The risk of small St. Jude aortic valve prostheses. *Ann Thorac Surg* 1994;59:1114.

87. Carrel T, Zingg U, Jeni R, et al. Early in vivo experience with the Hemodynamic Plus St. Jude medical heart valves in patients with narrowed aortic annulus. *Ann Thorac Surg* 1996;61:1418.

88. Nicks R, Cartmill T, Bernstein L. Hypoplasia of the aortic root: the problem of aortic valve replacement. *Thorax* 1970;25:339.

89. Manouguian S, Seybold-Epting W. Patch enlargement of the aortic valve ring by extending the aortic incision into the anterior mitral leaflet. *J Thorac Cardiovasc Surg* 1979;78:402.

90. Konno S, Imai Y, Iida Y, et al. A new method for prosthetic valve replacement in congenital aortic stenosis associated with hypoplasia of the aortic valve ring. *J Thorac Cardiovasc Surg* 1975;70:909.

91. Horstkotte D, Burckhardt D. Prosthetic valve thrombosis. *J Heart Valve Dis* 1995;4:141.

92. Birdi I, Angelini GD, Bryan AJ. Thrombolytic therapy for left-sided prosthetic heart valve thrombosis. *J Heart Valve Dis* 1995;4:154.

93. Horstkotte D, Schulte HD, Bircks W, Strauer BE. Lower intensity anticoagulation therapy results in lower complication rates with the St. Jude medical prosthesis. *J Thorac Cardiovasc Surg* 1994;107:1136.

94. Agnihotri AK, McGriffin DC, Galbraith AJ, O'Brien MF. The prevalence of infective endocarditis after aortic valve replacement. *J Thorac Cardiovasc Surg* 1995;110:1708.

95. Fraser CD Jr, Wang N, Mee RBB, et al. Repair of insufficient bicuspid aortic valves. *Ann Thorac Surg* 1994;58:386.

96. Khan S, Chaux A, Matloff J, et al. The St. Jude medical valve: experience with 1000 cases. *J Thorac Cardiovasc Surg* 1994;108:1010.

97. Baudet EM, Puel V, McBride JT, et al. Long-term results of valve replacement with the St. Jude medical prosthesis. *J Thorac Cardiovasc Surg* 1995;109:858.

98. Masters RG, Pipe AL, Walley VM, Keon WJ. Comparative

99. Akins CW. Long-term results with the Medtronic-Hall valvular prosthesis. *Ann Thorac Surg* 1996;61:806.

100. Fiane AE, Saatvedt K, Svennevig JL, et al. The CarboMedics valve: midterm follow-up with analysis of risk factors. *Ann Thorac Surg* 1995;60:1053.

101. Waller BF, Howard J, Fess S. Pathology of aortic valve stenosis and pure aortic regurgitation: II: a clinical morphologic assessment. *Clin Cardiol* 1994;17:150.

102. Stewart WJ, King ME, Weyman AE. Prevalence of aortic valve prolapse with bicuspid aortic valve and its relation to aortic regurgitation: a cross-sectional echocardiographic study. *Am J Cardiol* 1984;54:1277–1282.

103. Roberts WC, Dangel JC, Bulkley BH. Nonrheumatic valvular cardiac disease: a clinicopathological survey of 27 different conditions causing valvular dysfunction. *Cardiovasc Clin* 1973;5:334.

104. Carabello BA. Aortic regurgitation: hemodynamic determinants of prognosis. In: Cohn LH, DiSesa VJ, eds. *Aortic regurgitation: medical and surgical management.* New York: Marcel Dekker, 1986.

105. Wisenbaugh T, Spann JF, Carabello BA. Differences in myocardial performance and load between patients with similar amounts of chronic aortic versus chronic mitral regurgitation. *J Am Coll Cardiol* 1984;3:916.

106. Bonow RO, Dodd JT, Maron BJ, et al. Long-term serial changes in left ventricular function and reversal of ventricular dilatation after valve replacement for chronic aortic regurgitation. *Circulation* 1988;78:1108.

107. St. John-Sutton M, Plappert T, Spiegel A, et al. Early postoperative changes in left ventricular chamber size, architecture, and function in aortic stenosis and aortic regurgitation and their relation to intraoperative changes in afterload: a prospective two-dimensional echocardiographic study. *Circulation* 1987;76:77.

108. Timmermans P, Willems JL, Piessens J, De Geest H. Angina pectoris and coronary artery disease in severe aortic regurgitation. *Am J Cardiol* 1988;61:826.

109. Perry GJ, Helmcke F, Nanda NC, et al. Evaluation of aortic insufficiency by Doppler color flow mapping. *J Am Coll Cardiol* 1987;9:952.

110. Teague SM, Heinsimer JA, Anderson JL, et al. Quantification of aortic regurgitation utilizing continuous wave Doppler ultrasound. *J Am Coll Cardiol* 1986;8:592.

111. Sellers RD, Levy MJ, Amplatz K. Left retrograde cardioangiography in acquired cardiac disease: technique, indications, and interpretations in 700 cases. *Am J Cardiol* 1964;14:437.

112. Henry WL, Bonow RO, Borer JS, et al. Observations on the optimum time for operative intervention for aortic regurgitation: I. Evaluation of the results of aortic valve replacement in symptomatic patients. *Circulation* 1980;61:471.

113. Bonow RO, Lakatos E, Maron BJ, Epstein SE. Serial long-term assessment of the natural history of asymptomatic patients with chronic aortic regurgitation and normal left ventricular systolic function. *Circulation* 1991;84:1625.

114. Carabello BA, Usher BW, Hendrix GH, et al. Predictors of outcome for aortic valve replacement in patients with aor-

tic regurgitation and left ventricular dysfunction: a change in the measuring stick. *J Am Coll Cardiol* 1987;10:991.

114a. Carabello BA, Crawford FA Jr. Valvular heart disease (review). *N Engl J Med* 1997;337:32–41.

115. Bonow RO, Rosing DR, Maron BJ, et al. Reversal of left ventricular dysfunction after aortic valve replacement for chronic regurgitation: influence of duration of preoperative left ventricular dysfunction. *Circulation* 1984;70:570.

116. Borer JS, Herrold EM, Hochreiter C, et al. Natural history of left ventricular performance at rest and during exercise after aortic valve replacement for aortic regurgitation. *Circulation* 1991;84[Suppl III]:III133–III139.

116a. Movsowitz HD, Levine RA, Hilgenberg AD, Isselbacher EM. Transesophageal description of the mechanisms of aortic regurgitation in acute type A aortic dissection—implications for aortic valve repair. *J Am Coll Cardiol* 2000;3:884–890.

116b. David TE, Feindel CM, Bos J. Repair of the aortic valve in patients with aortic insufficiency and aortic root aneurysm. *J Thorac Cardiovasc Surg* 1995;109:345–351.

117. Greenberg BH, DeMots H, Murphy E, Rahimtoola S. Beneficial effects of hydralazine on rest and exercise hemodynamics in patients with chronic severe aortic insufficiency. *Circulation* 1980;62:49.

118. Schon HR. Hemodynamic and morphologic changes after long-term angiotensin-converting enzyme inhibition in patients with chronic valvular regurgitation. *J Hypertension* 1994;12[Suppl 4]:S95.

119. Scognamiglio R, Rahimtoola SH, Fasoli G, et al. Nifedipine in asymptomatic patients with severe aortic regurgitation and normal left ventricular function. *N Engl J Med* 1994;331:689.

120. Cohn LH, Birjiniuk V. Therapy of acute aortic regurgitation. *Cardiol Clin* 1991;9:339.

120a. Roe MT, Abramson MA, Li J, et al. Clinical information determines the impact of transesophageal echocardiography on the diagnosis of infective endocarditis by the Duke criteria. *Am Heart J* 2000;139:945–951.

120b. Habib G, Derumeaux G, Avierinos JF, et al. Value and limitations of the Duke criteria for the diagnosis of infective endocarditis. *J Am Coll Cardiol* 1999;33:2023–2029.

121. Mann T, McLaurin L, Grossman W, Craige E. Assessing the hemodynamic severity of acute aortic regurgitation due to infective endocarditis. *N Engl J Med* 1975;293:108.

122. Sareli P, Klein HO, Schamroth CL, et al. Contribution of echocardiography and immediate surgery to the management of severe aortic regurgitation from active infective endocarditis. *Am J Cardiol* 1986;57:413.

123. al Jubair K, al Fagih MR, Ashmeg A, et al. Cardiac operations during active endocarditis. *J Thorac Cardiovasc Surg* 1992;104:487.

124. Glazier JJ. Treatment of complicated prosthetic aortic valve endocarditis with annular abscess formation by homograft aortic root replacement. *J Am Coll Cardiol* 1991;17:1177–1182.

125. Carabello BA, Green LH, Grossman W, et al. Hemodynamic determinants of prognosis of aortic valve replacement in critical aortic stenosis and advanced congestive heart failure. *Circulation* 1980;62:42.

126. Carroll JD, Carroll EP, Feldman T, et al. Sex-associated differences in left ventricular function in aortic stenosis of the elderly. *Circulation* 1992;86:1099.

127. Aurigemma GP, Silver KH, McLaughlin M, et al. Impact of chamber geometry and gender on left ventricular systolic function in patients >60 years of age with aortic stenosis. *Am J Cardiol* 1994;74:794.

128. Morris JJ, Schaff HV, Mullany CJ, et al. Gender differences in left ventricular functional response to aortic valve replacement. *Circulation* 1994;90[5 Pt 2]:II183–II189.

129. Smith N, McAnulty JH, Rahimtoola SH. Severe aortic stenosis with impaired left ventricular function and clinical heart failure: results of valve replacement. *Circulation* 1978;58:255.

130. Lund O. Preoperative risk evaluation and stratification of long-term survival after valve replacement for aortic stenosis: reasons for earlier operative intervention. *Circulation* 1990;82:124.

131. Brogan WC III, Grayburn PA, Lange RA, Hillis LD. Prognosis after valve replacement in patients with severe aortic stenosis and a low transvalvular pressure gradient. *J Am Coll Cardiol* 1993;21:1657.

131a. Connolly HM, Oh JK, Orszulak TA, et al. Aortic valve replacement for aortic stenosis with severe left ventricular dysfunction. *Circulation* 1999;795:2395–2400.

131b. Connolly HM, Oh JK, Schaff HV, et al. Severe aortic stenosis with low transvalvular gradient and severe left ventricular dysfunction, result of aortic valve replacement in 52 patients. *Circulation* 2000;101:1940–1946.

131c. Pereira J, Afridi I, Lauer MS, et al. Survival after aortic valve replacement for severe aortic stenosis with low transvalvular gradients and severe left ventricular dysfunction. (manuscript submitted).

132. Carabello BA, Ballard WL, Gazes PC. Patient #65. In: Sahn SA, Heffner JE, eds. *Cardiology pearls*. Philadelphia: Hanley & Belfus, 1994:142.

132a. Carbello BA, Crawford FA. Valvular heart disease. *N Engl J Med* 1997;337:32–41.

133. Marcus R, Bednarz J, Abruzzo J, et al. Mechanism underlying flow-dependency of valve orifice area determined by the Gorlin formula in patients with aortic valve obstruction. *Circulation* 1993;88:I-103.

134. deFilippi CR, Willett DL, Brickner E, et al. Usefulness of dobutamine echocardiography in distinguishing severe from nonsevere valvular aortic stenosis in patients with depressed left ventricular function and low transvalvular gradients. *Am J Cardiol* 1995;75:191.

134a. Pop C, Metz D, Tassan-Mangina S, et al. Dobutamine Doppler echocardiography in severe aortic stenosis with left ventricular dysfunction. Comparison with postoperative examination. *Arch Mal Coeur Vaiss* 1999;92:1487–1493.

135. Ford LE, Feldman T, Chiu YC, Carroll JD. Hemodynamic resistance as a measure of functional impairment in aortic valvular stenosis. *Circ Res* 1990;66:1.

136. Cannon JD Jr, Zile MR, Crawford FA Jr, Carabello BA. Aortic valve resistance as an adjunct to the Gorlin formula in assessing the severity of aortic stenosis in symptomatic patients. *J Am Coll Cardiol* 1992;20:1517–1523.

136a. Faggiano P, Gualeni A, Antonini-Canterin F, et al. Doppler echocardiographic assessment of hemodynamic progression of valvular aortic stenosis over time: comparison between aortic valve resistance and valve area. *G Ital Cardiol* 1999;29:1131–1136.

137. Odell JA, Mullany CJ, Schaff HV, et al. Aortic valve replacement after previous coronary artery bypass grafting. *Ann Thorac Surg* 1996;62:1424–1430.

137a. Tam JW, Masters RG, Burwash IG, et al. Management of patients with mild aortic stenosis undergoing coronary artery bypass grafting. *Ann Thorac Surg* 1998;65:1215–1219.

137b. Balaban KW, Pereira JJ, Bashir M, et al. Aortic valve replacement improves survival in patients undergoing coronary bypass surgery with mild to moderate aortic valve stenosis (abstract). *Circulation* 2000;102:I-371(abst).

23

ACQUIRED TRICUSPID AND PULMONARY VALVE DISEASE

MELVIN D. CHEITLIN
JOHN S. MACGREGOR

▼⁄ ADDITIONAL ELECTRONIC TOPICS

OVERVIEW

Acquired disease of the tricuspid and pulmonary valves is uncommon. Tricuspid valve (TV) disease can be due to intrinsic disease of the valve or to functional tricuspid regurgitation (TR) secondary to right ventricular dysfunction. This condition, in turn, is due to intrinsic disease of the right ventricle (e.g., cardiomyopathy or coronary disease) or to pulmonary hypertension and right ventricular dilatation. Tricuspid stenosis is rare; when seen, it is often due to carcinoid heart disease rather than to rheumatic heart disease. Rarely, infective endocarditis—especially with fungal etiology—can result in tricuspid stenosis. Pulmonary steno-

sis is overwhelmingly congenital in etiology. Pulmonary regurgitation is rarely due to acquired organic disease of the valve, but when it occurs, it is most often iatrogenic due to surgery on a congenitally stenotic valve. Carcinoid can involve the pulmonary valve, causing pulmonary stenosis, regurgitation, or both. Most frequently, pulmonary regurgitation is secondary to pulmonary hypertension.

TR can result in right ventricular systolic and diastolic dysfunction and right heart failure. When cardiac output falls, with a rise in systemic venous pressure, hepatic congestion, ascites, and edema can result, requiring TV surgery, either annuloplasty or replacement. Long-term results of replacement of the TV are not as favorable as with left-sided valve replacement. With tricuspid stenosis, balloon valvotomy, surgical commissurotomy, or valve replacement can be beneficial. With pulmonary stenosis, almost always congenital in etiology, balloon valvotomy has replaced surgical commissurotomy and is probably as successful in the long term. With pulmonary regurgitation, usually due to

M. D. Cheitlin: Department of Cardiology, University of California, San Francisco, School of Medicine, San Francisco General Hospital, San Francisco, California

J. S. MacGregor: Department of Medicine, University of California, San Francisco, School of Medicine, San Francisco General Hospital, San Francisco, California

pulmonary hypertension, it is rarely necessary to consider pulmonary valve surgery; treatment of the pulmonary hypertension is the most beneficial approach. With medically or surgically created pulmonary regurgitation with systolic dysfunction of the right ventricle, pulmonary valve replacement is indicated.

ANATOMY

The right ventricle lies anterior to the left ventricle and leftward of the right atrium. It consists of an inflow tract (including the annulus, TV, and chordal and papillary muscles) and an outflow tract (including the infundibulum of the right ventricle and the pulmonary valve). The outflow and the inflow tracts are separated by four muscle bands: the infundibular septum, the parietal and septal bands of the crista ventricularis, and the moderator band. The blood supply of the right ventricle is mainly from the acute marginal branch of the right coronary artery, with small bands of right ventricle adjacent to the septum receiving blood from the posterior descending and the left anterior descending coronary arteries. In approximately 10% of hearts, the posterolateral branches of the circumflex supply portions of the posterior right ventricle. The moderator band is supplied by a branch of the first septal perforator of the left anterior descending coronary, and the conus artery from the right coronary artery supplies the anterior wall of the right ventricle.

The TV arises from a fibrous annulus and has the largest circumference of all the valves: 10.0 to 12.5 cm, with an estimated valve area of approximately 7 cm². The TV has three leaflets separated by commissures: anterior, posterior, and septal leaflets. The chordae tendineae from the anterior and posterior leaflets arise from a large anterior papillary muscle, which itself arises from the anterior wall of the right ventricle. The posterior papillary muscles are variable in number, arising from the posterior wall of the right ventricle and contributing chordae that insert on the posterior and septal leaflets. There is a conal papillary muscle arising from the septum, its chordae inserted on the anterior and septal leaflets. Frequently, these chordae arise from the septum itself, without a defined papillary muscle. The valve cusps are thin and consist of a dense collagen layer facing the right ventricle (the fibrosa) and a loose matrix composed of mucopolysaccharides (the spongiosa). The TV on the atrial surface has a variable, sparse layer of fibroelastic fibers adjacent to the annulus (1).

By Doppler echocardiography, it is possible to see a jet of TR in approximately 75% of healthy people (2), because the valve ring is so large and the leaflets are relatively narrow. Because the volume of regurgitant blood is so small and the regurgitant pressure gradients are so low, there is normally no murmur of TR. Because the tricuspid annulus forms the orifice of the right ventricular inflow tract, dilation of the right ventricle, for any reason, worsens the failure of coaptation of the tricuspid leaflets and increases the volume of TR. Any disease affecting connective tissue can be associated with TR, because the TV and chordae are composed of connective tissue.

The pulmonary valve is a semilunar valve with three cusps of equal arc similar to the aortic valve; these cusps align approximately 1.5 cm superior, anterior, and leftward of the aortic valve. The cusps have similar histologic structure to the TV, with a dense fibrosa facing the pulmonary artery and the spongiosa facing the right ventricle. Because the stress sustained by the valve is far less than that of the aortic valve, the pulmonary leaflets are thinner and more delicate. Because the pulmonary annulus acts as the root of the pulmonary artery, anything enlarging the root or increasing the diastolic pulmonary arterial pressure causes commissural separation and pulmonary valve insufficiency. Obviously, any disease altering the structure of the pulmonary leaflets also results in pulmonary valve insufficiency.

ETIOLOGY OF ACQUIRED TRICUSPID STENOSIS

Because the tricuspid ring is so large, there are very few diseases that can cause enough obstruction to the opening of the leaflets—either by commissural fusion, fibrosis, and calcification or by vegetative mass—to result in tricuspid stenosis. Etiologies of tricuspid stenosis are presented in Table 23.1.

In more than 90% of cases, TV stenosis is caused by rheumatic heart disease. In 92 excisions of the TV for tricuspid stenosis reported by Hauck and colleagues (3), 85 (93%) were due to rheumatic heart disease.

Rheumatic tricuspid stenosis occurs almost always in association with mitral stenosis and is rare as an isolated finding (4). With rheumatic heart disease, the TV is

TABLE 23.1 DISEASES CAUSING ACQUIRED TRICUSPID STENOSIS

Rheumatic heart disease
Carcinoid heart disease
Metabolic abnormalities
  Fabry's disease
  Whipple's disease
  Methysergide
Eosinophilic myocarditis (Loeffler's myocarditis)
Prosthetic valve thrombosis
Infective endocarditis
Prosthetic valve degeneration and/or calcification
Trauma produced by pacemaker leads or indwelling right-sided
   transvenous catheters
Tumors (differential diagnosis)
  Right atrial tumors
  Extracardiac tumors
  Constrictive pericarditis

involved pathologically in up to 67% of patients with MV disease (5). Functionally important TR occurs in 56%, combined TR/tricuspid stenosis occurs in 41%, and isolated tricuspid stenosis occurs in only 3% (3). ⛟ e46

Carcinoid heart disease is the second most common etiology for tricuspid stenosis. It is almost always accompanied by TR. Carcinoid heart involvement occurs in 10% to 50% of patients with carcinoid syndrome (1,8–9a), depending on whether the patients with isolated carcinoid tumors are included or only those with a diagnosis of metastatic carcinoid tumors. Thus, the incidence of carcinoid heart disease depends on the method of diagnosis, either by physical examination or by Doppler echocardiography.

The primary site of origin for malignant carcinoid tumor is the gastrointestinal tract, including the appendix, ileum, small intestine, colon, and stomach. The tumor secretes vasoactive amines, including bradykinin, 5-hydroxytryptamine (serotonin), and histamine, which are responsible for the systemic manifestations of flushing, diarrhea, and bronchospasm. These substances are largely detoxified in the liver and, therefore, reach the right heart in low concentration. However, when the carcinoid tumor metastasizes to the liver, these substances are released directly into the hepatic venous system and reach the right heart in massive concentration; there, they cause endocardial injury, resulting in the development of fibrous plaques on the endocardium and on the surfaces of the TV and pulmonary valve. ⛟ e47

Pathophysiology

When the TV becomes stenotic by fibrosis, disease, or commissural fusion, the blood flow from systemic veins and the right atrium into the right ventricle is obstructed; with atrial contraction against this stenotic valve, a large 'a' wave is seen. A pressure gradient develops between the right atrium and right ventricle in diastole. This results in a low-pitched diastolic rumbling murmur that is generated by the entire stroke volume crossing the obstructive valve under a low-pressure gradient. The gradient can be accentuated in inspiration, when there is an increase in systemic venous return to the right atrium and a drop in right ventricular filling pressure, and decreased in expiration; therefore, the murmur may become louder during inspiration and decrease in expiration. If the valve is flexible, a high-pitched tricuspid opening snap may be generated at the time of the opening of the TV (21). With severe tricuspid stenosis, there is a drop in cardiac output. With the elevation of pressure in the right atrium, right atrial dilatation occurs. With increasing right atrial pressure, systemic venous pressure, and systemic capillary pressure, edema develops, first in the dependent areas (e.g., the ankles) and then progressively advancing to the thighs, abdomen, and thorax. Finally, edema advances to the face, a condition known as

anasarca. There is also the development of ascites and pericardial effusions (4,22).

History and Physical Examination

In patients with tricuspid stenosis, the history depends on the severity of the tricuspid stenosis and the symptoms associated with the etiology and concomitant cardiac lesions. Therefore, patients with rheumatic heart disease almost always have concomitant MV disease, usually mitral stenosis. The symptoms of shortness of breath, orthopnea, and paroxysmal nocturnal dyspnea due to the mitral stenosis may dominate the patient's symptomatology (22). Decrease in cardiac output in the patient with severe mitral stenosis results in a lower-than-expected left atrial pressure and protects against pulmonary congestion (23).

In metastatic carcinoid tumors, the symptoms of flushing and diarrhea may be the most impressive symptoms. In the patient with mitral stenosis, atrial fibrillation and its concomitant palpitations may occur.

From the tricuspid stenosis alone, the symptoms alone are increased fatigability due to a decreased cardiac output and the effects of fluid retention and elevated systemic venous pressure. Edema—in the most severe cases, anasarca—may be the patient's major complaint. Ascites and abdominal enlargement, hepatic distention, and right upper quadrant discomfort may dominate the history.

The physical findings due to tricuspid stenosis are an abnormally large 'a' wave in the jugular venous pulse. The 'a' wave occurs at the time of the first heart sound and is rapid-rising, resembling a carotid arterial pulse. The difference is that the 'a' wave can be eliminated by firm pressure on the jugular vein, whereas an arterial pulse cannot. The 'v' wave, without accompanying TR, is inconspicuous, and the 'y' descent is slow or absent (24).

The classic finding is that of a low-pitched diastolic murmur, usually along the left sternal border in the third and fourth intercostal spaces (25,25a). In sinus rhythm, it is most prominent at end diastole, whereas in atrial fibrillation, it is usually more prominent in early and mid-diastole. If the valve is flexible, an opening snap can be heard along the lower left sternal border, although this is more unusual than the opening snap heard with mitral stenosis. If the right atrium is very large, an impulse can be felt in diastole along the lower right sternal border. With pure tricuspid stenosis, there is no right ventricular lift.

Because mitral stenosis is almost always present when tricuspid stenosis is due to rheumatic heart disease, the physical findings of mitral stenosis (the diastolic murmur, the loud first heart sound, and opening snap at the apex) are more conspicuous than the findings of tricuspid stenosis. However, tricuspid stenosis should be suspected when mitral stenosis is present when the elevation in the jugular venous pressure is greater than the signs of pulmonary congestion and the patient complaints of dyspnea, orthopnea, and paroxysmal nocturnal dyspnea. The accentuation with inspiration of a diastolic murmur along the lower left sternal border is known as the *Rivero-Carvallo sign*; it is characteristic of tricuspid stenosis (26), even in the presence of mitral stenosis, in which inspiration does not affect the loudness of the murmur. Also, the presence of a large 'a' wave in the jugular venous pulse in the presence of mitral stenosis should raise suspicion of concomitant tricuspid stenosis. Because of the elevation in systemic venous pressure, there may be hepatomegaly, edema, or ascites. If the tricuspid stenosis is due to a metastatic carcinoid tumor, then a large nodular liver is frequently present, and a ruddy cyanotic flush of the face may be seen periodically.

Laboratory Findings

Chest X-Ray

Cardiomegaly due to right atrial enlargement is frequent. The superior vena cava and azygous vein may be prominent. With pure tricuspid stenosis, the left atrium and right ventricle are not enlarged, and the pulmonary vascular markings are normal or decreased (23). With concomitant mitral stenosis, there is left atrial enlargement, although signs of pulmonary congestion are less prominent and without tricuspid stenosis.

Electrocardiogram

A large, peaked P wave in lead II is consistent with right atrial abnormality. A peaked, broad, notched, or biphasic P wave with terminal negative potential in the V_1 lead is consistent with left atrial abnormality and may be present, especially if there is concomitant mitral stenosis. Atrial arrhythmias, especially atrial fibrillation, are often present with severe tricuspid or mitral stenosis.

Doppler and Two-Dimensional Echocardiography

The findings on Doppler echocardiography depend on the etiology of the tricuspid stenosis. With rheumatic heart disease, the TV is domed in diastole. The leaflets are often thickened, with decreased mobility due to fusion along the commissures by the inflammatory process. The chordae tendineae may appear shortened and thickened. There is increased flow velocity across the TV in diastole; from this, by the modified Bernoulli equation, the diastolic gradient can usually be accurately estimated. With M-mode echocardiography, the E-F slope of the anterior leaflet is reduced, and there is increased reflectance from the valve. If rheumatic mitral stenosis or mitral regurgitation is present, the characteristic echocardiographic findings of these diseases can also be seen.

With carcinoid involvement, the valve is thickened and rigid, frequently fixed in the open position and acting like a washer, neither opening nor closing. Most often, TR is the predominant finding, along with an increase in diastolic velocity across the valve, with a reduced E-F slope that is consistent with tricuspid stenosis (8,27). ▼▼ 48

Cardiac Catheterization

At the present time, the diagnosis and estimation of severity of tricuspid stenosis are made by physical examination and confirmed by Doppler echocardiography. Cardiac catheterization is usually not necessary. When catheterization is done, the right atrial pressure is characterized by a large 'a' wave with an inconspicuous 'v' wave and a slow 'y' descent. The cardiac output is low, and the right ventricular and pulmonary artery pressures are normal or low. The TV area is decreased, and clinical tricuspid stenosis does not occur until the valve area is reduced to approximately 1.5 cm^2. Depending on the cardiac output, the diastolic gradient can be quite low (3 to 5 mm Hg) and should be measured with simultaneous catheters in the right atrium and right ventricle (21). An example of right atrial and right ventricular pressure tracings in a patient with carcinoid heart disease and tricuspid stenosis is shown in *e*Figure 23.0.11. The gradient is accentuated by increasing the cardiac output and decreasing the diastolic filling period by exercising, lifting the legs, and increasing the heart rate with atropine. Because the gradient is so low, gradients estimated by pullback of the catheter across the TV from the right ventricle to the right atrium can miss significant tricuspid stenosis.

DIFFERENTIAL DIAGNOSIS OF TRICUSPID STENOSIS

Any disease that delays emptying of the right atrium in diastole can simulate tricuspid stenosis; this includes right atrial myxoma, which can prolapse into the tricuspid orifice in diastole and obstruct diastolic flow across the valve. In this situation, an early diastolic sound, or "tumor plop," may simulate the opening snap of tricuspid stenosis. A tumor growing up from the inferior vena cava (e.g., renal cell carcinoma) can involve the TV and simulate tricuspid stenosis. Other intracardiac tumors, including lymphoma and sarcoma, can obstruct TV flow and mimic tricuspid stenosis. Constrictive pericarditis can involve primarily the right ventricle and stimulate tricuspid stenosis (27a).

Etiology of Tricuspid Regurgitation

In contrast to tricuspid stenosis, TR can be due to a number of different etiologies. Diseases affecting any part of the tricuspid apparatus can result in TR, including pathology of the annulus, leaflets, chordae, and papillary muscles of the right ventricular wall.

The etiologies of TR can be classified as (a) diseases causing pulmonary hypertension and right ventricular failure with tricuspid annular dilatation, or (b) primary diseases of the tricuspid apparatus (28). Table 23.2 lists diseases under each group. The most common etiology for TR is failure of the right ventricle due to pulmonary hypertension caused by left heart failure. Common causes of left heart failure are hypertension, coronary artery disease, mitral and aortic valve disease, and cardiomyopathy. Diseases causing an increase in pulmonary vascular resistance and pulmonary hypertension are listed in Table 23.2. The latest additions to this list have been acquired immunodeficiency syndrome (28a,28b) and anorexic drugs (e.g., fenfluramine or phentermine) (28c).

The pathologic changes of the TV seen in rheumatic heart disease, carcinoid heart disease, and eosinophilic myocarditis have been described. Endomyocardial fibrosis is a rare disease that is found mainly in women. It is charac-

TABLE 23.2 DISEASES CAUSING TRICUSPID REGURGITATION

Diseases causing pulmonary hypertension
  All left ventricular disease with left ventricular failure followed by right ventricular failure (coronary heart disease, cardiomyopathy, aortic stenosis and insufficiency, hypertension, mitral regurgitation)
  Mitral stenosis
  Pulmonary venous obstruction
  Diseases causing an increase in pulmonary vascular resistance
  Anorexic agents (e.g., fenfluramine or phentermine)
  Acquired immunodeficiency syndrome
  Primary pulmonary hypertension
  Congenital heart disease with increased pulmonary vascular resistance (atrial septal defect, ventricular septal defect, patent ductus arteriosus)
  Intrinsic pulmonary diseases (chronic obstructive pulmonary disease, pulmonary fibrosis, pulmonary resection)
  Collagen vascular disease (systemic sclerosis)
  Sleep apnea and hypoventilation syndromes
  Pulmonary emboli, acute and chronic
Diseases of the tricuspid apparatus
  Rheumatic heart disease
  Carcinoid heart disease
  Trauma, penetrating and nonpenetrating
  Infective endocarditis
  Right atrial myxoma
  Connective tissue disorders (Marfan and Ehlers-Danlos syndromes)
  Eosinophilic myocarditis
  Right ventricular endomyocardial fibrosis
  Prosthetic and bioprosthetic valve malfunction, both thrombolytic and degenerative
  Right ventricular myocardial infarction
  Radiation therapy
  Right ventricular cardiomyopathy (right ventricular dysplasia, Uhl's disease)
  Myxomatous tricuspid valve (tricuspid valve prolapse)
  Congenital diseases (Ebstein's anomaly, non-Ebstein's tricuspid regurgitation, cleft tricuspid leaflet, endometrial cardiac defects)

terized by endocardial fibrosis that affects mainly the left ventricle (but also the right ventricle) and may involve the atrioventricular valves, causing mitral regurgitation or TR. It is also characterized by mural thrombus, which can obliterate the ventricular apices (28d). With TR, there is thickening, shortening, and increased stiffness of the valve without significant commissural fusion (29). With pulmonary hypertension, the tricuspid leaflets and chordae tendineae are normal. There is right ventricular hypertrophy, dilatation of the right ventricle and tricuspid annulus, and TR. Malalignment and decreased force of contraction of the papillary muscles are also factors (30). With right ventricular infarction—which is almost always associated with diaphragmatic wall infarction because the acute marginal artery from the right coronary artery is the major source of blood supply to the anterior wall of the right ventricle—there is infarction and, later, fibrosis of the right ventricular papillary muscles and dilatation of the right ventricle (31,32). With right ventricular cardiomyopathy or dysplasia and Uhl's disease, which may be the most severe form of right ventricular dysplasia, the patient can present right ventricular failure and TR (33,34). Myxomatous changes in the TV are similar to changes seen in the MV, with thickening of the spongiosa and undermining support of the chordae tendineae insertions (3). The floppy TV is seen almost exclusively in the presence of a myxomatous prolapsing MV. The incidence of floppy TV in an autopsy population is as high as 3.2% of consecutive autopsies (35,36). An example of a myxomatous TV is shown in Figure 23.1. With connective tissue diseases like Marfan syndrome, there can be dilation of the tricuspid annulus, prolapsing valve leaflets, and elongated chordae (37).

Penetrating trauma can puncture the leaflets, rupture the chordae, or sever the papillary muscles (38). With blunt trauma (most frequently due to motor vehicle accidents), the right ventricle is the most common site of myocardial contusion. If right ventricular myocardial contusion is extensive, right ventricular failure and dilatation occur. With nonpenetrating injury (usually compressive injury or deceleration injury), complete fracture of the papillary muscles is not uncommon (39). A right ventriculogram from a patient with traumatic rupture of a tricuspid papillary muscle with resultant TR is shown in *e*Figure 23.1.1.

Infective endocarditis is seen almost exclusively in intravenous drug users and, occasionally, in patients who have trauma to the TV from the jet of a ventricular septal defect or an indwelling catheter across the TV (Fig. 23.2). Chronic alcoholism and hereditary immunodeficiency disease are also associated with an increased incidence of tricuspid endocarditis (40,41). *Staphylococcus aureus* is the most common organism seen. Hecht and colleagues reported *S. aureus* to be responsible for tricuspid endocarditis in 82% of 132 cases seen in intravenous drug users (40). An autopsy specimen demonstrating a large vegetation on the TV is shown in *e*Figure 23.2.1.

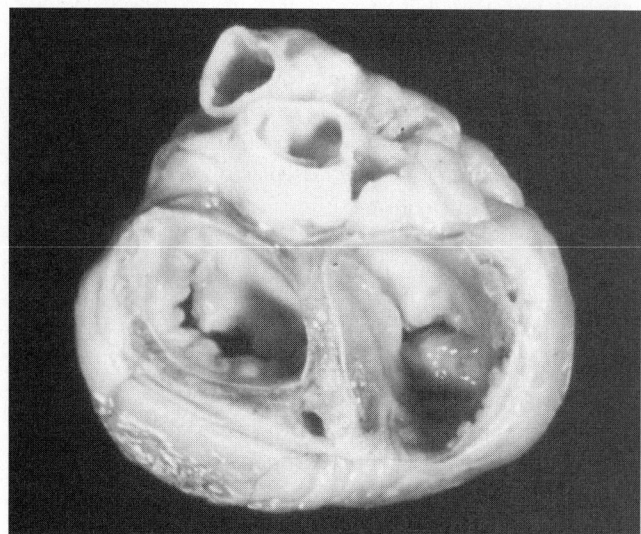

FIGURE 23.1 Autopsy specimen demonstrating the tricuspid valve (*right*) with three myxomatous prolapsed leaflets and the mitral valve (*left*) with both the anterior and the posterior leaflets myxomatous and prolapsed. (Courtesy of William Nelson, M.D.; from Cheitlin MD, MacGregor JS. Acquired tricuspid and pulmonic valve disease. In: Rahimtoola SH, Braunwald E, eds. *Atlas of heart diseases, vol. 11. Valvular heart disease.* St. Louis: Mosby, 1997, with permission.)

Congenital heart lesions (e.g., Ebstein's anomaly, primary TR, and cleft leaflets with endocardial cushion defects) are developmental defects due to malformation of the TV with displacement of the attachment of septal and posterior leaflets into the body of the right ventricle (e.g., Ebstein's anomaly) (28), tethering of the tricuspid leaflets (e.g., congenital non-Ebstein primary TR), or abnormal formation of the leaflets and clefting (e.g., endocardial cushion defects). Congenital lesions of the TV are not discussed further in this chapter.

There are other etiologies of TR that are unusual, such as mediastinal radiation (42,43), systemic lupus erythematosus (44), and methysergide-induced valvular fibrosis (45).

Pathophysiology of Tricuspid Regurgitation

The primary problem in TR is the presence of a regurgitant orifice during systole, resulting in a jet of regurgitant blood from the right ventricle to the right atrium. This is the cause of the systolic murmur. When TR is secondary to pulmonary hypertension, the initial response to increased afterload on the right ventricle depends on the acuteness of the development of the pulmonary hypertension. If it is acute and sudden, as is the case with acute pulmonary embolism, the right ventricle suddenly dilates, and there is increased right ventricular wall stress and a marked increase in right ventricular filling pressure. The right ventricular annulus dilates, TR occurs, there is a marked drop in cardiac output, and there is no time for compensatory right ventricular hypertrophy to occur. In addition, with a sudden increase in right ventricular diastolic volume, there is a shift in diastole of the septum so that it bulges toward the center of the left ventricle. With an intact, stiff pericardium, the sudden increase in right ventricular volume occupies more space within the pericardial sac and, thus, interferes with the filling of the left ventricle. This leads to a decrease in stretch of the left ventricle and possibly a decrease in diastolic volume, thus decreasing left ventricular stroke volume (46–49).

When the pulmonary vascular resistance is gradually increased, and, therefore, pulmonary hypertension gradually

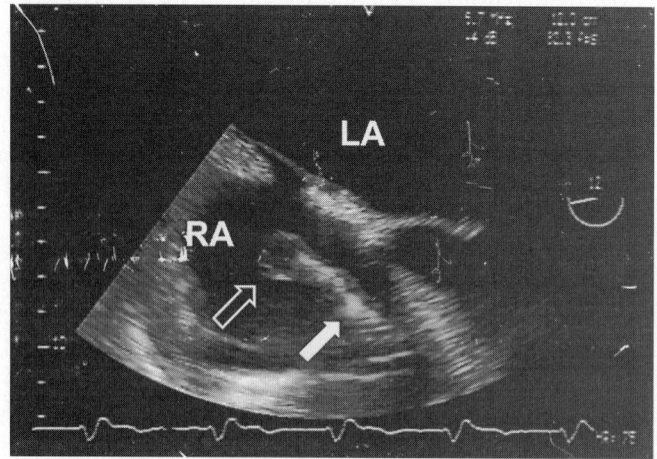
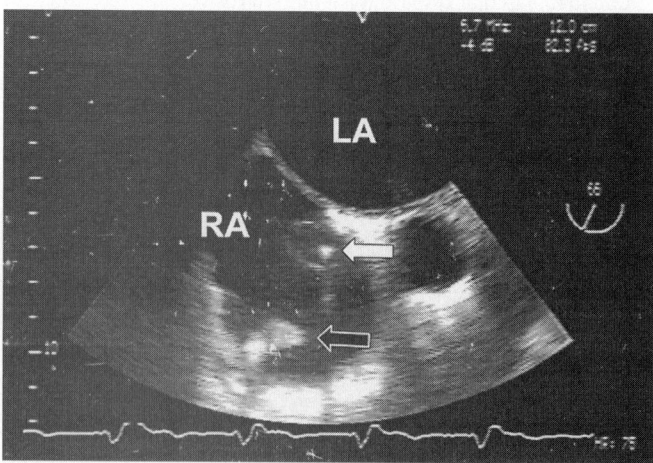

FIGURE 23.2 A: Transesophageal echocardiogram of a patient with right ventricular pacemaker wire and tricuspid valve endocarditis. The white arrow points to the pacemaker wire on tricuspid leaflet. The open arrow indicates vegetation/thickening on wire. **B:** Transesophageal echocardiogram of the same patient. The white arrow indicates the pacemaker on end with halo of thrombus, or vegetation, around it. The open arrow points to vegetation on tricuspid leaflet. LA, left atrium; RA, right atrium.

develops, compensatory right ventricular hypertrophy occurs; without right ventricular dilatation, there may be little or no TR until right ventricular systolic dysfunction and right ventricular failure occur. With right ventricular dilatation, as the tricuspid annulus enlarges, there is reduction of the narrowing of the tricuspid os in systole and failure of coaptation of the TV leaflets (30,50). Displacement of the papillary muscles and alteration in direction of the chordal tension on the valve may also contribute to TR. With treatment and decrease in the volume of the right ventricle, the degree of TR can diminish or completely disappear.

With primary disease of the TV, chordae, or papillary muscles, the primary event is the development of a systolic tricuspid regurgitant jet into the right atrium, which causes a prominent 'v' wave, the height of which is related to the volume of the blood and compliance of the right atrial–systemic venous system. In diastole, the regurgitant volume is added to the systemic venous return, thereby increasing the diastolic right ventricular volume. The larger right ventricular volume causes the right ventricle to contract more forcefully, increasing the right ventricular stroke volume sufficiently to accommodate the regurgitant volume and maintain the effective stroke volume ejected into the pulmonary artery; therefore the cardiac output remains normal. With increased diastolic volume, there is increase in the diastolic wall stress, which is compensated for by eccentric right ventricular hypertrophy, finally resulting in a larger diastolic right ventricle with normal filling pressure. Eventually, right ventricular systolic dysfunction occurs, with failure of the right ventricle. With this, the diastolic filling pressure of the right ventricle increases, increasing the mean pressure in the right atrium and systemic veins and resulting in the clinical picture of right ventricular failure.

History and Physical Examination in Tricuspid Regurgitation

The patient with primary valve regurgitation can do very well for prolonged periods without significant symptomatology until right ventricular dysfunction occurs. Occasionally, the patient may notice active neck vein pulsations due to the marked 'v' wave in the jugular venous pulse (51). Even pulsating eyeballs have been reported by the patient (52). In the presence of pulmonary hypertension with right ventricular dilatation and TR, there is a marked decrease in the cardiac output and an increase in the mean right ventricular and right atrial filling pressures. This results in the signs of right ventricular failure: increased central venous pressure, hepatomegaly, edema, and ascites.

The clinical picture may be dominated by the symptoms related to the various etiologies of TR. If the patient has MV disease, the symptoms of pulmonary congestion may dominate the clinical picture. With severe TR and decreased cardiac output, there is reduction in left atrial pressure in a patient with mitral stenosis and, therefore,

reduction in the symptoms of pulmonary congestion with a concomitant increase in easy fatigability and malaise. In patients with carcinoid syndrome, the systemic symptoms of facial flushing, diarrhea, and bronchospasm may predominate. In intravenous drug users with infective endocarditis, fever is the usual symptom that brings the patient to medical attention.

The physical examination is dominated by evidence of the regurgitant systolic jet and its effects. On palpation of the precordium, there is a precordial lift due to the increased diastolic right ventricular filling and increased right ventricular stroke volume. Depending on the severity of the TR and compliance of the right atrial–systemic venous system, there may be a large 'v' wave seen in the jugular venous pulse, with maximal height at the time of the second heart sound. It can be distinguished from a carotid pulse by pressure over the lower neck, which eliminates the 'v' wave but cannot change the carotid pulse. The descent of the 'v' wave, the 'y' descent, is rapid. With inspiration, the 'y' descent becomes more prominent due to a decrease in right ventricular pressure (53). With failure of the right ventricle, the mean central venous pressure is elevated, and the large 'v' wave occurs over and above the elevated mean venous pressure. Frequently, the external jugular vein is also distended when right ventricular failure occurs; this is not true when right ventricular function is normal, because the valves in the external jugular vein prevent the regurgitant blood from distending the vein. Because the systolic jet of regurgitant blood is directed mostly into the right innominate vein, there may be a peculiar right-to-left pulsation of the head that is different from the to-and-fro bobbing of the head seen in severe aortic regurgitation. Also, due to systolic distention of the cranial veins, pulsation of all veins—and even pulsation of the eyeballs—can be present (52). With auscultation over the jugular veins, a transmitted systolic murmur may be audible (54).

A pansystolic murmur is often present, usually in the third and fourth interspaces at the left sternal border and, occasionally, loudest to the right of the sternum or in the subxyphoid region. If the right ventricle is dilated, or if Ebstein's anomaly is present, the murmur may be heard best toward the apex and may be confused with the murmur of mitral regurgitation. The murmur may be increased with deep inspiration as a result of increased venous return and diastolic right ventricular filling with a more forceful contraction (the Rivero-Carvallo sign) (51). Other maneuvers, such as lifting of the legs or application of abdominal pressure (hepatojugular reflux), also increase venous return and increase the murmur (55). When the right ventricle can no longer respond with increased contraction to the increased venous return, the murmur does not augment. There may be a right-sided third and fourth heart sound gallop along the left sternal border, increasing in loudness with inspiration. Because of the increased diastolic flow across the TV, there may be a short, low-pitched, early diastolic rumble along the

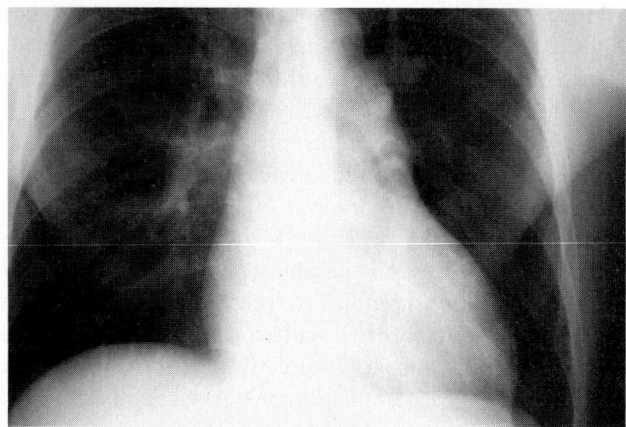
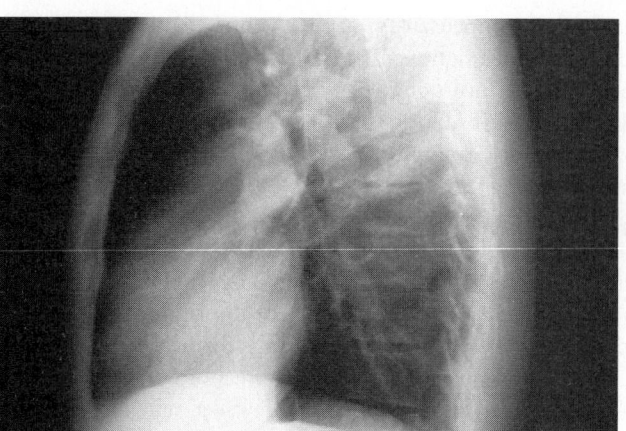

A   B

FIGURE 23.3 Posteroanterior **(A)** and lateral **(B)** chest x-rays of a patient with pulmonary hypertension and severe tricuspid regurgitation. The pulmonary arteries and right heart are markedly enlarged.

lower left sternal border. In patients with minimal TR, the systolic murmur may be short or inaudible. In patients with massive TR, because there is little pressure gradient between the right ventricle and right atrium in systole (the so-called ventricularization of the right atrium), the systolic murmur may be minimal or absent. Occasionally with TV prolapse, one or more nonejection clicks may be present at the beginning of the murmur; at times, the murmur may be vibratory, loud, and "honking" in quality.

If the TR is secondary to mitral or aortic valve disease, the auscultatory and other signs of mitral stenosis, mitral regurgitation, or aortic valve disease may be heard. With cardiomyopathy, there is frequently a left-sided third and fourth heart sound gallop, as well as mitral regurgitation. With pulmonary hypertension, a loud second heart sound, occasionally with a high-pitched diastolic murmur of pulmonary regurgitation, can be heard. With carcinoid heart disease, a large multinodular liver is commonly present. Atrial fibrillation is especially common with MV disease. Signs of right heart failure—with dependent edema, hepatomegaly, and, frequently, a pulsatile liver and ascites—may be present. With severe pulmonary hypertension and terminal right ventricular failure, cachexia and stasis cyanosis frequently are seen.

Laboratory Findings

Chest X-Ray

The effect on the cardiac silhouette depends on the severity of the TR. With severe pulmonary hypertension, there is frequently enlargement of the main pulmonary artery and primary branches. With further increases in pulmonary vascular resistance, the lung fields in the lateral third are diminished, and that part of the lung field is clear (pruning). The right ventricle is enlarged both anteriorly and to the left so that the retrosternal space is encroached upon.

With dilatation of the right ventricle, the cardiothoracic ratio is increased, and the apex of the heart is formed by the dilated right ventricle. The right atrium may be enlarged to the right; with right ventricular failure, the azygos vein may be prominent as it enters the superior vena cava. A chest x-ray of a patient with severe TR and pulmonary hypertension is shown in Figure 23.3. With TR due to infective endocarditis, multiple infiltrations and densities in both lung fields due to septic embolic pulmonary infarction may be present. The appearance of the chest x-ray in patients with septic pulmonary emboli changes over time. Initially, multiple, peripherally based discrete nodules may be present. Depending on the identity of the infecting organism, these nodules may cavitate or become confluent diffuse infiltrates. An example of this process is shown in Figure 23.4. Hecht and Berger reported infiltrates compatible with septic pulmonary emboli in 72 (55%) of 132 patients with right-sided endocarditis (40).

Electrocardiogram

In isolated mild-to-moderate TR, the electrocardiogram may be normal. With moderate-to-severe TR and dilation of the right ventricle, an rSR' in the V$_1$ lead consistent with incomplete right bundle branch block and delayed activation of the right ventricle is seen. In normal sinus rhythm, a peaked P wave consistent with right atrial abnormality can be seen, but it is most common with TR due to pulmonary hypertension in which right ventricular hypertrophy is present. If mitral stenosis is the underlying etiology, biatrial abnormality or atrial fibrillation is present, as well as right ventricular hypertrophy.

Doppler Echocardiography

The findings on Doppler echocardiography depend on the severity of the TR, the presence of pulmonary hypertension, and the etiology of the disease producing the TR.

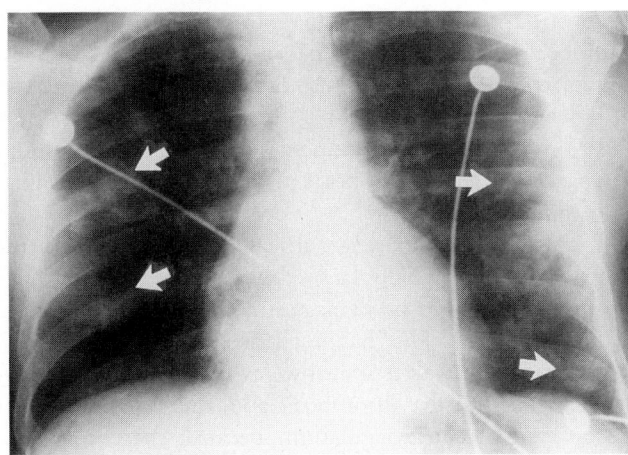
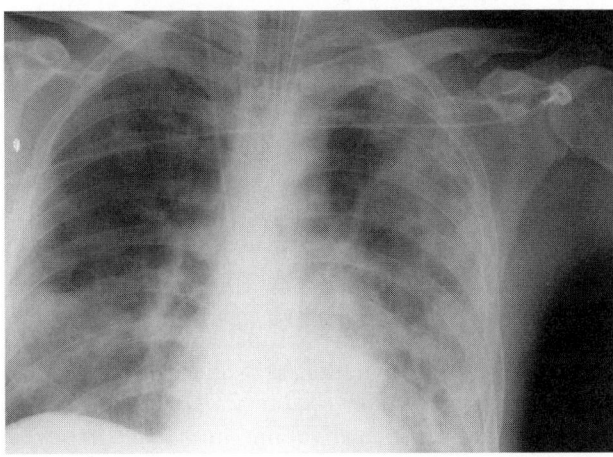

FIGURE 23.4 A: Chest x-ray (posteroanterior view) of a patient with infective endocarditis involving the tricuspid valve with septic emboli. Multiple, somewhat nodular, peripheral infiltrates are indicated by arrows. **B:** Chest x-ray of the same patient 2 days later (posteroanterior view). The relatively discrete nodules have now formed more confluent, diffuse infiltrates.

With minimal TR, the two-dimensional echocardiogram can be entirely normal. Pulsed-wave Doppler or color imaging shows the presence and direction of the regurgitant jet. An estimation of severity can be made by measuring the size of the regurgitant orifice, as outlined by the jet at the valve, and the area of the right atrium occupied by the turbulent and increased regurgitant jet velocities (56,57). Also, the detection of reverse blood-flow velocity in the inferior vena cava and hepatic veins is a measure of the severity of the TR (58). In severe TR, the shape of the velocity-time jet envelope is characteristically that of a dagger, with a high initial velocity and rapid dropoff due to rapid equalization of right atrial and right ventricular pressures in systole.

To quantify the regurgitant-jet velocities precisely, continuous-wave Doppler is needed. The peak pressure gradient from right ventricle to right atrium in systole can be estimated accurately by the modified Bernoulli equation (pressure gradient = $4 \times$ velocity^2) (59,60). When added to the estimated jugular venous pressure (which equals the right atrial pressure), this formula gives an accurate estimate of right ventricular and pulmonary artery systolic pressure (PASP) in the absence of pulmonary stenosis. ⚑ e49

The echocardiogram can show dilatation of the TV annulus. In diseases affecting the TV itself, an echocardiogram can show thickening and increased reflectance caused by fibrosis, retraction and lack of coaptation of the leaflets, prolapse of the tricuspid leaflets and myxomatous changes (62), vegetations with infective endocarditis, and flail cusps due to ruptured chordae or papillary muscles. The thickened, immobile valve and fused chordae characteristic of carcinoid syndrome can also be detected (8,9a). With isolated right-sided infective endocarditis, the size of the vegetation is predictive of the development of a complication. In one study, vegetations >1.0 cm were present in 80% of tricuspid endocarditis in intravenous drug users. Vegetations >2.0 cm were associated with a significantly higher mortality than those ≤2.0 cm (33.3% vs. 1.3%; p <.001) (40). Furthermore, in right-sided infective endocarditis, the association of fever that persists for 3 weeks in the presence of a vegetation ≥1.0 cm identifies those patients who require surgical intervention (62a). A two-dimensional echocardiogram demonstrating a large vegetation on the TV is shown in *e*Figure 23.4.2. Right atrial myxoma or thrombus can also be detected. With pulmonary hypertension, there is enlargement of the right ventricular outflow tract, right ventricular hypertrophy, and characteristic **W**-shaped motion of the pulmonary valve on M-mode echocardiography. There may also be pulmonary regurgitation.

Cardiac Catheterization

Invasive studies are not needed to make the diagnosis of TR or to estimate its severity. In the presence of a tricuspid regurgitant jet on echocardiography, the right ventricular and PASPs can be estimated accurately from the modified Bernoulli equation. With severe TR, there is a dominant 'v' wave in the right atrial pressure curve. With increasing severity of TR, the right atrial pressure becomes ventricularized and resembles the right ventricular pressure curve. An increase in right atrial pressure occurs on deep inspiration in patients with severe TR, especially with right ventricular systolic dysfunction (63). Right ventricular end diastolic pressure is elevated; with right ventricular failure, the mean filling pressures in the right ventricle and right atrium are elevated. Right ventricular and pulmonary artery pressures are normal or low in isolated TV regurgitation, but they may be elevated with septic emboli to the lungs. With diseases causing pulmonary hypertension, the pulmonary artery pressure and pulmonary vascular resistance can be accurately measured at catheterization. Usually the forward, or effective, cardiac output is normal or low, especially with severe TR.

With angiocardiography, injection of contrast is made in the right ventricle, films are taken in the right anterior oblique projection, and the tricuspid regurgitant jet can be seen and semiquantitatively estimated. However, because the catheter is across the TV and the injection produces premature ventricular complexes, there is the possibility of spurious TR (64). A right ventricular angiogram demonstrating severe TV regurgitation in a patient with carcinoid heart disease is shown in eFigure 23.4.3. Because calculation of right ventricular volume from angiography is unreliable (unlike left ventricular volume in mitral regurgitation), it is difficult to make an accurate estimate of regurgitant volume.

TREATMENT OF TRICUSPID VALVE DISEASE

Because most patients with tricuspid stenosis have rheumatic heart disease as the etiology, almost all have concomitant MV disease—mostly mitral stenosis. In these patients, indications for surgery or balloon valvotomy are mainly determined by the severity of the MV disease; however, tricuspid stenosis, when severe, can markedly reduce the cardiac output and cause severe limitation of physical activity, as well as eventually result in right-sided heart failure. Diuretics can be helpful, but, eventually, the valvular obstruction must be relieved. Until recently, with organic involvement of the TV, TV surgery, either commissurotomy or valve replacement, was necessary. Recently, there have been case reports (65) of balloon valvuloplasty in patients with tricuspid stenosis with encouraging results: The right atrial–right ventricular gradient has fallen, and the calculated TV area has increased. When mitral stenosis and tricuspid stenosis are both present, the valvotomy can be done with the same balloon (66,67). With the few cases and in the relatively short time the procedure has been available, it is not known whether balloon valvotomy will have long-term results equal to or better than those of open commissurotomy or TV replacement.

With tricuspid stenosis due to carcinoid syndrome, there have been reports of valve replacement (68,69); with tricuspid stenosis, there have even been attempts at balloon valvuloplasty (70). Connolly and colleagues (69) reported valve replacement in 26 patients with carcinoid TV disease. There were nine (35%) perioperative deaths, primarily from bleeding and right ventricular failure. Of the 17 survivors, eight were alive at a mean follow-up of 25 months, with substantial improvement in functional class. Late deaths were due to hepatic dysfunction due to metastatic disease. Compared to 40 patients with TV disease medically treated, the surgical group displayed a trend toward increased survival (69). In a review of the literature, Robiolio et al. described 47 carcinoid patients with valve replacement. The 30-day mortality was 56% in patients older than 60 years and 0% for those 60 years or younger (p <.001). Valve replacement in carcinoid syndrome has appreciable mortality but can afford prolonged palliation of symptoms (68).

With carcinoid heart disease, mechanical prosthetic valves were originally favored because of the fear that tissue valves would be damaged by the vasoactive carcinoid peptides (71). This has not proved to be the case (72). Bioprosthetic valves are now favored because of reduced incidence of valve thrombosis and, therefore, lack of need for systemic anticoagulation, because these patients are more prone to bleeding because of hepatic dysfunction (69). With the introduction of somatostatin and its derivatives—which inhibit the release of numerous peptides and improve symptoms and survival of patients with metastatic carcinoid tumors (73)—it is possible that the biologic tissue valves would be protected (69). Because of the small number of patients available, it is difficult to know what additional survival advantage there will be with surgery, together with debulking of the tumor by hepatic artery embolization (74), in these patients with carcinoid heart disease.

Bioprosthetic valve degeneration with fibrosis and calcification, with or without thrombus, has been an indication for reoperation to replace the valve with a new prosthetic valve. However, there have been case reports of successful balloon valvuloplasty in patients with bioprosthetic TVs developing stenosis, with reduced right atrial pressure, increased cardiac output, and improved symptomatology (75–77).

Finally, in patients with thrombosed mechanical valves, there has been success in using fibrinolysis (78,79). The largest number of these studies has been of patients with mechanical left-sided valves, with a few patients with thrombosed mechanical TVs. Initial success rates of 75% have been reported, with a 15% to 20% incidence of rethrombosis (80). The danger with thrombolysis in left-sided valves is systemic embolization with serious consequences, such as stroke. The incidence quoted in the literature of systemic embolization occurring with thrombolysis in left-sided thrombosed valves is 15% (81,82). With the TV, there is probably also embolization to the lung, but so far, there have been no reports of clinically significant embolization, probably because the emboli have been small enough not to cause hemodynamic problems. At the present time, Silber and colleagues (81) suggest that thrombolysis is the treatment of choice for a thrombosed mechanical valve, even a thrombosed left-sided mechanical valve.

With TR due to organic involvement of the TV, it is generally agreed that surgical repair or replacement of the TV is necessary. Unfortunately, it is not always possible to tell preoperatively, even with two-dimensional Doppler echocardiography, that the TV regurgitation is due to organic TV disease. In a study of 306 patients requiring TV surgery, Duran (83) stated that only 42% were preoperatively diagnosed by Doppler echocardiography as having organic involvement of the valve, with the rest diagnosed only at the time of surgery. Similar findings were reported by Georgeson and colleagues (84).

In patients who have had surgery for MV stenosis, regression of pulmonary hypertension and a decrease in functional TR have been described (85). Patients with mild TR due to pulmonary hypertension usually do not need a surgical procedure (85,86). Eventually, numerous patients with mitral stenosis potentially have a reduction in pulmonary hypertension (87); however, whether moderate-to-severe TR in these patients will be reduced is not predictable (88). ♈ e50

The long-term results of TV replacement reported in the past were not as good as with MVR. At least in part, this finding is related to the fact that patients with TV replacement are operated on at a later stage of their MV disease. Other reported reasons for poorer results are increased thrombosis seen in tricuspid mechanical valves and degenerative calcification seen in biologic valves (91). Van Nooten and colleagues (92) studied 146 consecutive patients undergoing TV replacement from 1969 to 1987, 69 of whom had bioprosthetic valves and 77 of whom had mechanical ball, disc, or bileaflet valves. Ninety-seven percent were NYHA functional class III or IV, and 40% had previous cardiac surgery. Hospital mortality was 16.1%. In a follow-up of 92 months, there were 70 late deaths, for an actuarial survival of 74% at 5 years and less than 25% at 14 years. Mortality was affected by the type of valve (mechanical worse than biologic), preoperative functional classification, and type of operative myocardial protection. The recommendation was that a large bioprosthetic valve was preferable to a mechanical valve (92).

McGrath and colleagues (91) studied 154 patients with bioprosthetic valve replacement in the tricuspid position. Ninety percent had TR, and 10% had tricuspid stenosis or regurgitation; 54% had Carpentier-Edwards prostheses, and 35% had Ionescu-Shiley valves. Concomitant procedures were performed in 95% of cases. Preoperatively, 90% were NYHA class III or IV. There were 20 in-hospital deaths (13%). All survivors were followed for a mean of 66 months. There were 70 late deaths (52%), and the deaths were related to earlier date of surgery, more complex repairs requiring prolonged aortic occlusion, and signs of increased right heart failure. Valve-related events were thrombosis (1%) and endocarditis (2%). Seventeen patients (12.7%) had structural degeneration of the bioprosthetic valves, with 15 having a second operation at a mean of 74 months after the first operation. Actuarial freedom from TV replacement was 70% at 10 years. McGrath and colleagues concluded that patients

with bioprostheses in the tricuspid position are at a relatively low risk for valve-related events but are at considerable risk for decreased overall survival from their underlying heart disease. ♈ e51

Tricuspid Regurgitation Due to Infective Endocarditis

TR caused by endocarditis is almost always seen in intravenous drug users; the etiologic organism most commonly is *S. aureus*, which readily responds to appropriate antibiotic therapy. TR can be severe, and if the pulmonary vascular resistance is normal, hemodynamically severe TR can be present with few or no symptoms. This condition is best seen in those patients who have resistant organisms such as *Serratia marcescens* or fungal endocarditis, in which removal of the infected valve without valve replacement allows for bacteriologic cure (96,97). Months or years later, a tricuspid prosthesis can be safely placed. As previously mentioned, in patients with TV endocarditis, persistent fever on antibiotics for more than 3 weeks and a vegetation ≥1.0 cm identifies those patients requiring surgical intervention (62a).

If pulmonary hypertension is present, as could be the situation with multiple septic emboli and hypoxia, then cardiac output decreases, exercise intolerance occurs, and right ventricular failure can occur rapidly. A less common problem is the development of a right-to-left shunt through a blown-open foramen ovale with arterial desaturation and even cyanosis. There is also the possibility of systemic embolization.

Most patients with infective endocarditis of the TV are treatable with appropriate antibiotics and do not need TV replacement (40). Hecht and Berger (40), in their report of 132 episodes of right-sided endocarditis in intravenous drug users, had only one patient with an infected porcine TV who underwent surgery. There were ten deaths due to multiorgan failure, adult respiratory distress syndrome, pulmonary embolism, or persistent sepsis (40). If right ventricular failure occurs with severe TR, diuretics, preload reduction, digoxin, and afterload reduction can be initiated. In these patients, valvuloplasty or valve replacement is indicated (97a).

Treatment of Traumatic Tricuspid Regurgitation

TR can occur as a result of penetrating or nonpenetrating trauma to the valve, chordae, or papillary muscles. Right ventricular myocardial contusion can also occur, leading to right ventricular dilatation and TR. Because the pulmonary vascular resistance is usually normal, acute TR may be present without symptoms (98). Surgery to repair or replace the valve is indicated if progressive right ventricular dilatation and systolic dysfunction occur or if the patient develops right ventricular failure or exercise intolerance (39,98a).

Etiology of Acquired Pulmonary Valve Stenosis

With few exceptions, pulmonary valve stenosis is congenital in etiology (*e*Table 23.2.1). Of 116 excised pulmonary valves, 95% were congenital or associated with congenital heart disease, as reported by Altrichter (99). There are reported instances, however, of pulmonary valve stenosis due to rheumatic heart disease, but this is the rarest of all the rheumatic valve diseases. Carcinoid heart disease can cause pulmonary valve stenosis: of the 74 patients with carcinoid heart disease studied by Pellikka and colleagues (8), a murmur of pulmonary stenosis was noted in 24 patients (32%). Echocardiography showed valvular thickening and retraction or stenosis with narrowing of the pulmonary annulus in 36 patients (49%). The pulmonary valve was diminutive to where it could not be visualized in 29 of the patients (39%). In the 47 patients with carcinoid heart disease who underwent Doppler echocardiography of the pulmonary valve, regurgitation was seen in 81% and stenosis in 53% (8). The pathology is similar to that seen in carcinoid involvement of the TV, leaving the valve thickened, retracted, and immobile. A gross anatomic specimen from a patient with carcinoid heart disease and pulmonary stenosis and regurgitation is shown in *e*Figure 23.4.4.

Most acquired pulmonary stenosis is not valvular but the result of obstruction to the right ventricular outflow tract (100,101) or compression of the main pulmonary artery by mediastinal masses (100,102). Marshall and Trump (103) reviewed the literature reporting mediastinal masses causing acquired extrinsic pulmonary stenosis. Teratomas and Hodgkin's disease were responsible for more than 50% of the cases, although carcinoma of the lung, thymoma, pericardial sarcoma, and non-Hodgkin's lymphoma have all been reported.

Pathophysiology of Pulmonary Stenosis

With obstruction of the pulmonary outflow tract, there is increased afterload on the right ventricle, resulting in right ventricular hypertrophy. The degree of right ventricular hypertrophy depends on the severity and the duration of the pulmonary stenosis. In congenital pulmonary valve stenosis, infundibular stenosis, and even double right ventricle with anomalous pulmonary band obstructing the outflow tract, the obstruction is present from birth; therefore, with severe obstruction, right ventricular hypertrophy is almost always present.

With acquired pulmonary stenosis, the obstruction occurs gradually and is frequently not severe; thus, right ventricular hypertrophy is frequently not present. In carcinoid heart disease, for example, in 36 patients with pulmonary valve involvement (53% of whom had pulmonary stenosis), the gradients were 7 to 37 mm Hg (mean, 14 ± 9 mm Hg), and none of the patients had right ventricular hypertrophy (8). The same is true for external compression of the right ventricular outflow tract or pulmonary artery, causing pulmonary stenosis (100–102). Although large systolic pressure gradients across the right ventricular outflow tract can be generated (100), most of the patients had only a mildly dilated right ventricle on two-dimensional echocardiography. ⚐ e52

Pathophysiology of Pulmonary Valve Regurgitation

Isolated pulmonary valve regurgitation is rare; the most common form occurs after pulmonary valve surgery. In pulmonary valve regurgitation, there is a volume overload of the right ventricle, resulting in dilatation of the right ventricle and, eventually, eccentric right ventricular hypertrophy. With the increased right ventricular stroke volume, there is dilatation of the proximal pulmonary arteries. The regurgitant volume depends on the size of the regurgitant orifice, the diastolic filling period, and the pressure gradient driving the regurgitant volume from the pulmonary artery to the right ventricle. Other important factors are pulmonary artery distensibility and right ventricular compliance (105,106). With the large right ventricular stroke volume, a small systolic gradient can be generated, even without pulmonary stenosis (106). With severe pulmonary regurgitation, there is equalization of the pulmonary artery pressure and the right ventricular pressure in diastole. In the absence of pulmonary hypertension, even severe volume overload of the right ventricle is well tolerated for many years (108); however, the prognosis is not entirely benign, because right ventricular dysfunction and right heart failure can occur (109).

With pulmonary hypertension, the patient has right ventricular hypertrophy, and pulmonary regurgitation occurs with dilatation of the pulmonary valve annulus. The degree of the pulmonary regurgitation is usually not severe and is rarely hemodynamically significant. Right ventricular dilatation and dysfunction leading to right ventricular failure are more frequent in these patients as a result of the right ventricular systolic overload rather than as a result of the pulmonary regurgitation.

History and Physical Examination of the Patient with Pulmonary Regurgitation

The symptomatology that the patient develops is dependent on the cause of the pulmonary regurgitation. Patients with pulmonary hypertension have symptoms related to the cause of the pulmonary hypertension; that is, with pulmonary disease or primary pulmonary hypertension, the patient with pulmonary hypertension can have syncope, dyspnea, hemoptysis, and right heart failure. The patient with mitral stenosis can have a history of orthopnea and paroxysmal nocturnal dyspnea. Patients with pulmonary regurgitation due to endocarditis have symptoms related to the infection such as fever, left heart failure if the mitral or aortic valve is infected, or septic pulmonary emboli with an infected TV. When the patient has pulmonary regurgitation due to carcinoid tumor, the symptoms are dominated by those seen with metastatic carcinoid tumor.

The patient with isolated pulmonary regurgitation has no symptoms if the regurgitant volume is small. With a large regurgitant volume, the majority of patients remains asymptomatic. Only 40% of patients with isolated pulmonary regurgitation present with exertional dyspnea, easy fatigability, and intermittent nonexertional left upper chest pain, possibly due to pounding of the enlarged main pulmonary artery and right ventricle against the chest wall (106).

The physical findings in isolated pulmonary regurgitation are those of a prominent right ventricular anterior precordial lift, frequently with a lift in the second left interspace that is caused by the dilated pulmonary artery and its exaggerated expansion due to the increased right ventricular stroke volume. There is also a diastolic murmur along the left sternal border in the second and third interspaces. With isolated pulmonary valve regurgitation, this murmur starts 0.04 to 0.06 seconds after the aortic second sound and is characteristically short and low-pitched (25a). The pulmonary second sound may be audible before the diastolic murmur. If the pulmonary valve cusp is fibrotic and retracted, the pulmonary second sound may be absent.

If pulmonary hypertension is present, the second heart sound is single and accentuated, and the diastolic murmur is high-pitched and decrescendo and cannot be distinguished from aortic regurgitation. This is called the *Graham-Steell murmur*.

If the pulmonary regurgitant volume is large, an early-peaking systolic ejection murmur ending before the second heart sound may be heard and can be grade III to IV/VI in loudness. Such a systolic murmur was heard in 84% of isolated pulmonary valve regurgitation patients, accompanied by a systolic thrill in 10% (106). The murmur can be loud and late-peaking, sounding much like that in pulmonary stenosis. On rare occasions, a low-frequency late presystolic rumbling murmur (110) has been described, analogous to a right-sided Austin-Flint murmur. This murmur is said to increase with inspiration (110).

Laboratory Findings

Electrocardiogram

With pulmonary valve stenosis, the electrocardiogram reflects the hemodynamic severity of the lesion. With severe pulmonary stenosis, the electrocardiogram shows right axis deviation and right ventricular hypertrophy with a qR wave in the V_1 lead. With moderately severe pulmonary stenosis, there is an rSR' in the V_1 lead. With severe right ventricular hypertrophy, peaked P waves in the II, III, and augmented voltage unipolar left foot leads reflect right atrial abnormality (111). With acquired pulmonary stenosis, the obstruction is usually not severe, and the obstruction is present for a shorter period; therefore, severe right ventricular hypertrophy is less frequently present.

With TR with pulmonary hypertension, right ventricular hypertrophy is usually present. If the pulmonary regurgitation is an isolated lesion (which is very uncommon), and if the regurgitant volume is small, the electrocardiogram remains normal. With a large regurgitant volume, an rSR' may be seen in the V_1 lead.

Chest X-Ray

The chest x-ray with pulmonary valve stenosis shows poststenotic dilatation of the main pulmonary artery and, frequently, the proximal left pulmonary artery. With severe pulmonary stenosis, right ventricular hypertrophy manifested by lifting of the apex off the left hemidiaphragm and filling in of the retrosternal space in the lateral chest x-ray can be seen. With right ventricular failure, dilatation of the right ventricle results in an increased size of the cardiac silhouette in the posteroanterior film and encroachment of the retrosternal space. The chest x-ray of a patient with combined valvular and subpulmonary stenosis is shown in *e*Figure 23.4.5. With pulmonary regurgitation, dilatation of the main pulmonary artery with clear lung fields can be seen, together with right ventricular dilatation.

Doppler Echocardiography

With pulmonary stenosis, the two-dimensional echocardiogram, in the parasternal long-axis view and in the four-chamber view, can show right ventricular hypertrophy. Dilatation of the right atrium can be present, and the main pulmonary artery may be dilated in a short-axis view at the level of the aortic ring. At times, doming of the pulmonary valve can be seen. With carcinoid involvement of the pulmonary valve, thickening and lack of flexibility can be seen (8,10,27). With pulsed-wave and color Doppler echocardiography, the exact location of the obstruction to the right ventricular outflow tract can be seen, and obstruction can be seen locally at the valvular, subvalvular, or supravalvular level. Also, if there are masses, either intrinsic to the myocardium or extrinsic to the heart, these can be localized. With intrinsic masses causing obstruction to the right ventricular outflow tract, computed tomography and nuclear magnetic resonance imaging are extremely useful (112,113). With right ventricular failure, right ventricular dilatation and decreased contractility of the right ventricle can be seen. With continuous-wave Doppler echocardiography, the systolic gradient across the right ventricular outflow tract can be determined accurately by the modified Bernoulli equation (114).

With pulmonary regurgitation due to pulmonary hypertension, right ventricular hypertrophy can be seen with dilatation of the main pulmonary artery. With pure pulmonary regurgitation, the right ventricle and the main pulmonary artery are dilated. With pulsed-wave and color Doppler echocardiography, the presence and magnitude of the pulmonary incompetence can be estimated both by the extent of the turbulence of the regurgitant jet in the right ventricle and by the width of the jet under the valve (115). Caution must be exercised because it is possible to detect minimal jets of pulmonary regurgitation in the majority of healthy people (116). With pathologic pulmonary regurgitation, the depth of the jet into the right ventricle is usually 1 to 2 cm below the pulmonary valve, and the duration of the jet usually occupies 75% or more of the entire duration of diastole (117). A Doppler echocardiographic examination demonstrating pulmonary regurgitation is shown in *e*Figure 23.4.6. Two-dimensional echocardiography is also useful in demonstrating vegetations on the pulmonary valve in patients with infective endocarditis (*e*Fig. 23.4.7).

Catheterization and Angiocardiography

Catheterization and angiocardiography are usually not necessary in the diagnosis or estimation of severity of pulmonary stenosis or pulmonary regurgitation. However, in planning surgery (especially for an extrinsic mass), angiocardiography and coronary arteriography used to see the position of the coronary arteries in relationship to the extrinsic mass can be valuable. Cineangiography may be useful in localizing the level of pulmonary stenosis. A cineradiograph showing congenital pulmonary valve stenosis is shown in Figure 23.5. The domed appearance is characteristic of pulmonary valve stenosis, and the right ventricular outflow tract shows no infundibular stenosis. In *e*Figure 23.5.1, the pulmonary valves are normal, and the pressure gradient of 160 mm Hg between the right ventricle and pulmonary artery is due to infundibular stenosis. With pulmonary stenosis, the exact position of the obstruction can be seen; with pullback across the right ventricular outflow tract, the gradient can be accurately calculated. With pulmonary hypertension, pulmonary vascular resistance can be accurately measured. With angiocardiography and an injection into the right ventricle in the posteroanterior and left lateral views, the outflow tract, pulmonary valve, and main pulmonary artery can be seen, and the flexibility of the pulmonary valve can be judged.

With pulmonary valve regurgitation, if the regurgitation is severe, the pulmonary artery pressure curve becomes ventricularized and takes on the configuration seen in the right ventricle, with end diastolic pulmonary artery pressure and right ventricular end diastolic pressure equilibrating. Evalu-

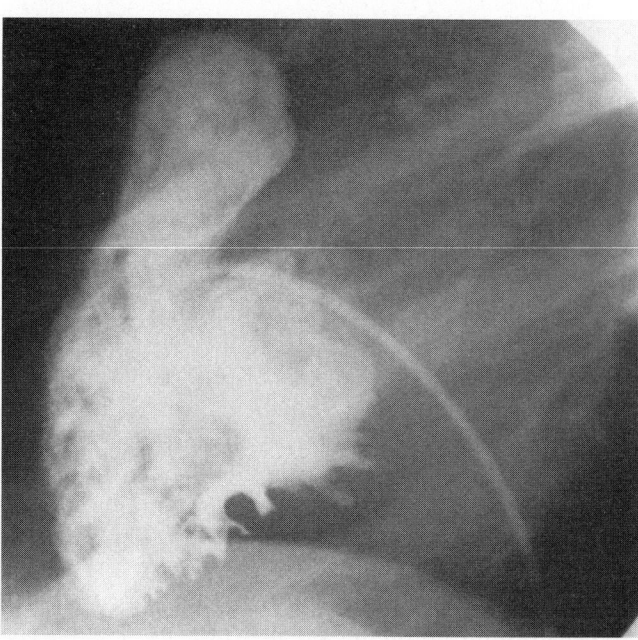

FIGURE 23.5 Right ventricular angiogram (left lateral projection) of a patient with congenital pulmonary stenosis. The doming pulmonary valve (*top*) is characteristic of congenital pulmonary valve stenosis. The right ventricular outflow tract shows no infundibular stenosis. (From MacGregor JS, Ports TA. Catheter balloon valvuloplasty. In: Parmley WW, Chatterjee K, eds. *Cardiology: physiology, pharmacology, diagnosis.* Philadelphia: Lippincott, 1993:1–24, with permission.)

ation of pulmonary regurgitation by angiocardiography is more difficult because the catheter is across the pulmonary valve; with injection into the pulmonary artery, any regurgitation into the right ventricle may be artifactual. Here, Doppler echocardiography is more reliable.

It is also possible to quantify the magnitude of pulmonary regurgitation by radionuclide angiography with the inversion of the left ventricular stroke volume–right ventricular stroke volume ratio, called the *radionuclide regurgitation index.* In patients with pulmonary valve regurgitation, this index is usually 0.59 ± 0.23, which is significantly different from that seen in control subjects (1.49 ± 0.32) (118).

Treatment

With pulmonary stenosis, the prognosis depends on the etiology. With pulmonary valve stenosis that is mild or moderate, the patient does well without surgery. In the minority of cases, the degree of stenosis increases in severity with growth of the patient (119). With severe unrepaired pulmonary stenosis, right ventricular failure most commonly occurs after the fourth decade (107). With severe pulmonary valve stenosis, surgical repair in the past has given good long-term results, usually with residual moderate pulmonary regurgitation. If the operation occurs in childhood, the patient's long-term survival is similar to that of age- and sex-matched controls (120). In adults, long-term prognosis is not as good after surgery because right ventricular dysfunction can still lead to late-life right ventricular failure and death.

At present, balloon valvotomy is the treatment of choice, even in the adult with congenital pulmonary valve stenosis. Immediate and intermediate results are similar to those of surgery (121). Simultaneous right ventricular and pulmonary artery pressure tracings are shown in Figure 23.6 for a patient with congenital pulmonary stenosis. The pressure tracing on the left was obtained before pulmonary valvuloplasty, and the tracing on the right was obtained immediately after balloon valvuloplasty. The peak gradient after the procedure had decreased by 162 mm Hg. The sequence of balloon inflation is demonstrated in *e*Figure 23.6.1.

With carcinoid heart disease, the prognosis is very poor (27). In the report by Pellikka and colleagues (8), in 74 patients with carcinoid heart disease, the median survival was 1.6 years. Balloon valvuloplasty has been reported in carcinoid pulmonary stenosis (68,70), but with the thickened, immobile valve, it is frequently unsuccessful, and valve replacement (rather than valvuloplasty) has been recommended (122). With extrinsic or intrinsic compression, surgical removal of the mass—or radiation therapy, if the neoplasm is sensitive—is indicated.

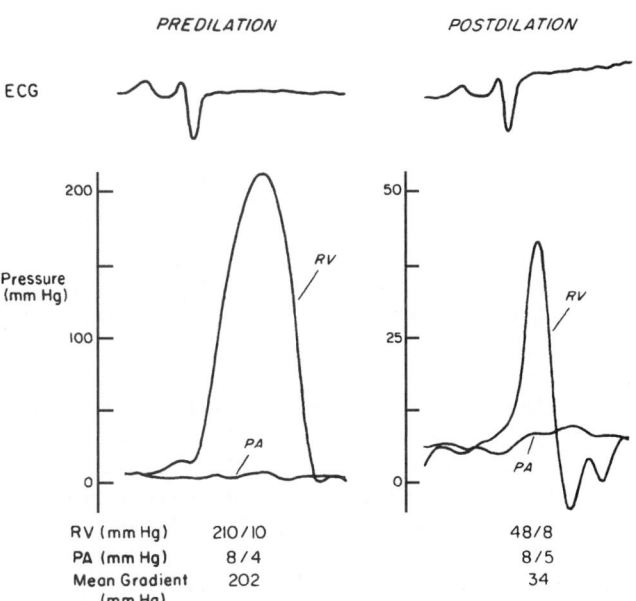

FIGURE 23.6 Simultaneous right ventricular (RV) and pulmonary artery (PA) pressure tracings in a patient with congenital pulmonary stenosis before (*left*) and immediately after (*right*) percutaneous balloon valvuloplasty. The mean pressure gradient across the pulmonary valve fell by 168 mm Hg after the procedure. ECG, electrocardiogram. (From MacGregor JS, Ports TA. Catheter balloon valvuloplasty. In: Parmley WW, Chatterjee K, eds. *Cardiology: physiology, pharmacology, diagnosis.* Philadelphia: Lippincott, 1993:1–24, with permission.)

With pulmonary regurgitation, surgery is rarely necessary (106). Treatment of the primary condition is indicated; for instance, with pulmonary regurgitation due to pulmonary hypertension from mitral stenosis, valvuloplasty of the MV is needed. With endocarditis, treatment of the infection is necessary. If the pulmonary valve regurgitation is severe and right ventricular systolic dysfunction or failure is present, diuretics and digitalis are helpful, and pulmonary valve replacement is indicated (106a).

CONTROVERSIES AND PERSONAL PERSPECTIVES

As with left-sided valve replacement, a durable nonthrombotic prosthetic valve to be used in the pulmonary or tricuspid position would be a major advance in the treatment of severe TR or pulmonary regurgitation. TR secondary to pulmonary hypertension due to mitral stenosis or some other left-sided lesion may diminish or disappear after treatment of the left-sided lesion. An annuloplasty that would spontaneously reverse after a period of time, as suggested by Duran, could avoid the problems of a permanent annuloplasty ring, which can create relative tricuspid stenosis, especially if placed in children or adolescents. With the increased popularity of the Ross procedure (123), in which the patient's pulmonary valve is used to replace a diseased aortic valve and a bioprosthetic valve is placed in the pulmonary area, the question of how long the tissue valve will function in the pulmonary position will become increasingly important with continued investigation. Recent research of growing the patient's fibrocytes in cell culture on a biodegradable scaffold shaped in the form of a semilunar valve promises, one day, to lead to a bioprosthetic valve of the patient's own tissue, which could be as free of complications and as durable as the patient's original valve. Continued investigations of medications that reverse the vasoactive effects of amines produced in the patient with metastatic carcinoid tumor and of whether this approach will prevent tissue valves placed in the tricuspid or pulmonary regions from becoming diseased are important in the treatment of carcinoid heart disease. Continued investigation into possible vasoactive drugs that can reduce pulmonary resistance in patients who have severe pulmonary hypertension, as well as the development of successful lung transplantation, will be important in the control of severe functional TR. Finally, the most important advance to decrease the incidence of TR from infective endocarditis is in the control and eradication of intravenous drug use, which may be the most intractable problem of all.

THE FUTURE

The development of a durable nonthrombotic prosthetic valve would be a major advance in the treatment of severe tricuspid and pulmonary regurgitation. Research into developing a bioprosthetic valve of the patient's own tissues is promising a valve as durable and free of complications as the patient's own valve. Continued investigation into medical therapies for disease processes such as metastatic carcinoid tumor and pulmonary hypertension, as well as the successful development of lung transplantation, will be important in the treatment of tricuspid and pulmonary valve disease. The control and eradication of intravenous drug use would be the most important step toward decreasing the incidence of TR from infective endocarditis.

REFERENCES

1. Farb A, Burke AP, Virmani R. Anatomy and pathology of the right ventricle (including acquired tricuspid and pulmonic valve disease). *Cardiol Clin* 1992;10:1–21.
2. Torres F, Tye T, Gibbons R, et al. Echocardiographic contrast increases the yield for right ventricular pressure measurement by Doppler echocardiography. *J Am Soc Echocardiogr* 1989;2:419–424.
3. Hauck AJ, Freeman DP, Ackermann DM, et al. Surgical pathology of the tricuspid valve: a study of 363 cases spanning 25 years. *Mayo Clin Proc* 1988;63:851–863.
4. Waller BF, Howard J, Fess S. Pathology of tricuspid valve stenosis and pure tricuspid regurgitation. Part I. *Clin Cardiol* 1995;18:97–102.
5. Waller BF, Block T, Eble JN, et al. Etiology of tricuspid stenosis and pure tricuspid regurgitation. In: Waller BF, ed. *Pathology of the heart and the great vessels*. New York: Churchill Livingstone, 1988:149.
6. Hollman A. The anatomical appearance in rheumatic tricuspid valve disease. *Br Heart J* 1957;19:211–216.
7. Datta BN, Nagrani B, Khattri HN, et al. Rheumatic heart disease at autopsy: an analysis of 260 cases in Chandigarh. *Ind Heart J* 1978;30:39–46.
8. Pellikka PA, Tajik AJ, Khandheria BK, et al. Carcinoid heart disease. Clinical and echocardiographic spectrum in 74 patients. *Circulation* 1993;87:1188–1196.
9. Lundin L, Norheim I, Landelius J, et al. Carcinoid heart disease: relationship of circulating vasoactive substances to ultrasound-detectable cardiac abnormalities. *Circulation* 1988;77:264–269.
9a. Moyssakis IE, Rallidis LS, Guida GF, et al. Incidence and evolution of carcinoid syndrome in the heart. *J Heart Valve Dis* 1997;6:625–630.
9b. Lundin L, Funa K, Hansson HE, et al. Histochemical and immunohistochemical morphology of carcinoid heart disease. *Path Res Pract* 1991;187:73–77.
10. Robiolio PA, Rigolin VH, Wilson JS, et al. Carcinoid heart disease. Correlation of high serotonin levels with valvular abnormalities detected by cardiac catheterization and echocardiography. *Circulation* 1995;92:790–795.
11. Olsen EGJ, Spry CJ. Relationship between eosinophilia and endomyocardial disease. *Prog Cardiovasc Dis* 1985;27:241–254.
12. Arnold M, McGuire L, Lee JC. Loeffler's fibroplastic endocarditis. *Pathology* 1988;20:79–82.
12a. Spodick DH. Eosinophilic myocarditis [letter; comment]. *Mayo Clin Proc* 1997;72:996.
13. Sasano H, Virmani R, Patterson RH, et al. Eosinophilic products lead to myocardial damage. *Hum Pathol* 1989;20:850–857.
13a. Borczuk AC, van Hoeven KH, Factor SM. The eosinophil and peripartum heart disease (myocarditis and coronary artery dissection)—coincidence or pathogenetic significance? Review and hypothesis. *Cardiovasc Res* 1997;33:527–532.
14. Frustaci A, Abdulla AK, Possati G, et al. Persisting hypereosinophilia and myocardial activity in the fibrotic stage of endomyocardial disease. *Chest* 1989;96:674–675.
15. Jegaden O, Perinetti M, Barthelet M, et al. Long-term results of porcine bioprostheses in the tricuspid position. *Eur J Cardio-Thorac Surg* 1992;6:256–260.
16. Pai RG, Pai SM. Severe bioprosthetic tricuspid valve stenosis with systolic antegrade flow across the tricuspid valve. *J Heart Valve Dis* 1996;5:436–438.
17. Glotzer TV, Tunick PA, Kloth H, et al. Thrombosis of a Starr-Edwards tricuspid prosthesis: diagnosis by Doppler echocardiography and treatment with thrombolysis. *Am Heart J* 1994;127:705–708.
17a. Saito T, Horimi H, Hasegawa T, et al. Isolated tricuspid valve stenosis caused by infective endocarditis in an adult: report of a case. *Surg Today* 1993;23:1081–1084.
18. Vargas-Barron J, Buenfil-Medina C, Sanchez-Ugarte T, et al. Ventriculoatrial shunts for hydrocephalus and cardiac valvuloplasty: an echocardiographic evaluation. *Am Heart J* 1991;121:1498–1501.
19. Foster-Smith K, Edwards WD, O'Murchu B, et al. Severe tricuspid stenosis: an unusual and unique cause. *Am Heart J* 1995;130:621–624.
20. Old WD, Paulsen W, Lewis SA, et al. Pacemaker lead-induced tricuspid stenosis: diagnosis by Doppler echocardiography. *Am Heart J* 1989;117:1165–1167.
21. Killip T III, Lukas DS. Tricuspid stenosis: physiologic criteria for diagnosis and hemodynamic abnormalities. *Circulation* 1957;16:3–13.
22. el-Sherif N. Rheumatic tricuspid stenosis: a haemodynamic correlation. *Br Heart J* 1971;33:16–31.
23. Perloff JK, Harvey WP. Clinical recognition of tricuspid stenosis. *Circulation* 1960;22:346–364.

24. Kitchin A, Turner R. Diagnosis and treatment of tricuspid stenosis. *Br Heart J* 1964;26:354–379.

25. Killip T, Lukas DS. Tricuspid stenosis: clinical features in twelve cases. *Am J Med* 1958;24:836–852.

25a. Shaver JA. Cardiac auscultation: a cost-effective diagnostic skill. *Curr Probl Cardiol* 1995;20:441–530.

26. Rivero-Carvallo JM. El diagnostico de la estenosis tricuspidea. *Arch Inst Cardiol Mex* 1950;20:1–11.

27. Himelman RB, Schiller NB. Clinical and echocardiographic comparison of patients with the carcinoid syndrome with and without carcinoid heart disease. *Am J Cardiol* 1989;63:347–352.

27a. Vogt PR, Bauer EP, Carrel T, et al. Pericarditis constrictiva after aortic valve replacement simulating tricuspid stenosis. *Eur J Cardio-Thorac Surg* 1992;6:108–110.

28. Waller BF, Howard J, Fess S. Pathology of tricuspid valve stenosis and pure tricuspid regurgitation—Part II. *Clin Cardiol* 1995;18:167–174.

28a. Michaels AD, Lederman RJ, MacGregor JS, et al. Cardiovascular involvement in AIDS. *Curr Probl Cardiol* 1997;22:109–148.

28b. Mesa RA, Edell ES, Dunn WF, et al. Human immunodeficiency virus infection and pulmonary hypertension: two new cases and a review of 86 reported cases. *Mayo Clin Proc* 1998;73:37–45.

28c. Rich S, Rubin L, Walker AM, et al. Anorexigens and pulmonary hypertension in the United States: results from the Surveillance of North American Pulmonary Hypertension [SNAP]. *Chest* 2000;117:870–874.

28d. Schneider U, Jenni R, Turina J, et al. Long-term follow-up of patients with endomyocardial fibrosis: effects of surgery. *Heart* 1998;79:362–367.

29. Waller BF, Moriarty AT, Eble JN, et al. Etiology of pure tricuspid regurgitation based on annular circumference and leaflet area: analysis of 45 necropsy patients with clinical and morphologic evidence of pure tricuspid regurgitation. *J Am Coll Cardiol* 1986;7:1063–1074.

30. Mikami T, Kudo T, Sakurai N, et al. Mechanisms for development of functional tricuspid regurgitation determined by pulsed Doppler and two-dimensional echocardiography. *Am J Cardiol* 1984;53:160–163.

31. Vatterott PJ, Nishimura RA, Gersh BJ, et al. Severe isolated tricuspid insufficiency in coronary heart disease. *Int J Cardiol* 1987;14:295–301.

32. McAllister RG Jr, Friesinger GC, Sinclair-Smith BC. Tricuspid regurgitation following inferior myocardial infarction. *Arch Intern Med* 1976;136:95–99.

33. Mohan JC, Chutani SK, Sethi KK, et al. Dominant right ventricular dilated cardiomyopathy: clinical, echocardiographic and haemodynamic profile. *Ind Heart J* 1989;41:177–181.

34. Blomstrom-Lundqvist C, Sabel KG, Olsson SB. A long term follow up of 15 patients with arrhythmogenic right ventricular dysplasia. *Br Heart J* 1987;58:477–488.

35. Davies MJ, Moore BP, Braimbridge MV. The floppy mitral valve. Study of incidence, pathology and complications in surgical, necropsy and forensic material. *Br Heart J* 1978;40:468–481.

36. Lucas RV Jr, Edwards JE. The floppy mitral valve. *Curr Prob Cardiol* 1982;7(4):1–48.

37. Roberts WC, Honig HS. The spectrum of cardiovascular disease in the Marfan syndrome: a clinico-morphologic study of 18 necropsy patients and comparison to 151 previously reported necropsy patients. *Am Heart J* 1982;104:115–135.

38. Parmley LF, Mattingly TW, Manion WC. Penetrating wounds of the heart and aorta. *Circulation* 1958;17:953–973.

39. Holper KM, Hahnel C, Augustin N, Meisner H. Operative correction of traumatic tricuspid insufficiency. *Herz* 1996;21:172–178.

40. Hecht SR, Berger M. Right-sided endocarditis in intravenous drug users. Prognostic features in 102 episodes. *Ann Intern Med* 1992;117:560–566.

41. Arnett EN, Roberts WC. Active infective endocarditis: a clinicopathologic analysis of 137 necropsy patients. *Curr Prob Cardiol* 1976;1(7):2–76.

42. Brosius FC III, Waller BF, Roberts WC. Radiation heart disease. Analysis of 16 young (aged 15 to 33 years) necropsy patients who received over 3,500 rads to the heart. *Am J Med* 1981;70:519–530.

43. Raviprasad GS, Salem BI, Gowda S, et al. Radiation-induced mitral and tricuspid regurgitation with severe ostial coronary artery disease: a case report with successful surgical treatment. *Cathet Cardiovasc Diagn* 1995;35:146–148.

44. Gabrielli F, Alcini E, Di Prima MA, et al. Cardiac valve involvement in systemic lupus erythematosus and primary antiphospholipid syndrome: lack of correlation with antiphospholipid antibodies. *Int J Cardiol* 1995;51:117–126.

45. Mason JW, Billingham ME, Friedman JP. Methysergide-induced heart disease: a case of multivalvular and myocardial fibrosis. *Circulation* 1977;56:889–890.

46. Louie EK, Lin SS, Reynertson SI, et al. Pressure and volume loading of the right ventricle has opposite effects on left ventricular ejection fraction. *Circulation* 1995;92:819–824.

47. Goldstein JA, Vlahakes GJ, Verrier ED, et al. The role of right ventricular systolic dysfunction and elevated intrapericardial pressure in the genesis of low output in experimental right ventricular infarction. *Circulation* 1982;65:513–522.

48. Goldstein JA, Barzilai B, Rosamond TL, et al. Determinants of hemodynamic compromise with severe right ventricular infarction. *Circulation* 1990;82:359–368.

49. Kingma I, Tyberg JV, Smith ER. Effects of diastolic transseptal pressure gradient on ventricular septal position and motion. *Circulation* 1983;68:1304–1314.

50. Come PC, Riley MF. Tricuspid annular dilatation and failure of tricuspid leaflet coaptation in tricuspid regurgitation. *Am J Cardiol* 1985;55:599–601.

51. Reichek N, Shelburne JC, Perloff JK. Clinical aspects of rheumatic valvular disease. *Prog Cardiovasc Dis* 1973;15:491–537.

52. Allen SJ, Naylor D. Pulsation of the eyeballs in tricuspid regurgitation. *Can Med Assoc J* 1985;133:119–120.

53. Cha SD, Gooch AS. Diagnosis of tricuspid regurgitation. Current status. *Arch Intern Med* 1983;143:1763–1768.

54. Amidi M, Irwin JM, Salerni R, et al. Venous systolic thrill and murmur in the neck: a consequence of severe tricuspid insufficiency. *J Am Coll Cardiol* 1986;7:942–945.

55. Maisel AS, Atwood JE, Goldberger AL. Hepatojugular reflux: useful in the bedside diagnosis of tricuspid regurgitation. *Ann Intern Med* 1984;101:781–782.

56. Curtius JM, Thyssen M, Breuer HW, et al. Doppler versus contrast echocardiography for diagnosis of tricuspid regurgitation. *Am J Cardiol* 1985;56:333–336.

57. Suzuki Y, Kambara H, Kadota K, et al. Detection and evaluation of tricuspid regurgitation using a real-time, two-dimensional, color-coded Doppler flow imaging system: comparison with contrast two-dimensional echocardiography and right ventriculography. *Am J Cardiol* 1986;57:811–815.

58. Diebold B, Touati R, Blanchard D, et al. Quantitative assessment of tricuspid regurgitation using pulsed Doppler echocardiography. *Br Heart J* 1983;50:443–449.

59. Yock PG, Popp RL. Noninvasive estimation of right ventricular systolic pressure by Doppler ultrasound in patients with tricuspid regurgitation. *Circulation* 1984;70:657–662.

60. Skjaerpe T, Hatle L. Noninvasive estimation of systolic pressure in the right ventricle in patients with tricuspid regurgitation. *Eur Heart J* 1986;7:704–710.

60a. Borgeson DD, Seward JB, Miller FA Jr, et al. Frequency of Doppler measurable pulmonary artery pressures. *J Am Soc Echocardiogr* 1996;9:832–837.

61. Meltzer RS, van Hoogenhuyze D, Serruys PW, et al. Diagnosis of tricuspid regurgitation by contrast echocardiography. *Circulation* 1981;63:1093–1099.

62. Schlamowitz RA, Gross S, Keating E, et al. Tricuspid valve prolapse: a common occurrence in the click-murmur syndrome. *J Clin Ultrasound* 1982;10:435–439.

62a. Robbins MJ, Frater RW, Soeiro R, et al. Influence of vegetation size on clinical outcome of right-sided infective endocarditis. *Am J Med* 1986;80:165–171.

63. Lingamneni R, Cha SD, Maranhao V, et al. Tricuspid regurgitation: clinical and angiographic assessment. *Cathet Cardiovasc Diagn* 1979;5:7–17.

64. Ubago JL, Figueroa A, Colman T, et al. Right ventriculography as a valid method for the diagnosis of tricuspid insufficiency. *Cathet Cardiovasc Diagn* 1981;7:433–441.

65. Orbe LC, Sobrino N, Arcas R, et al. Initial outcome of percutaneous balloon valvuloplasty in rheumatic tricuspid valve stenosis. *Am J Cardiol* 1993;71:333–354.

66. Bahl VK, Chandra S, Sharma S. Combined dilatation of rheumatic mitral and tricuspid stenosis with Inoue balloon catheter. *Int J Cardiol* 1993;42:178–181.

67. Goel SI, Desai DM, Shah LS. Concurrent balloon dilatation of rheumatic trivalvular stenosis. *Cathet Cardiovasc Diagn* 1995;36:283–286.

68. Robiolio PA, Rigolin VH, Harrison JK, et al. Predictors of outcome of tricuspid valve replacement in carcinoid heart disease. *Am J Cardiol* 1995;75:485–488.

69. Connolly HM, Nishimura RA, Smith HC, et al. Outcome of cardiac surgery for carcinoid heart disease. *J Am Coll Cardiol* 1995;25:410–416.

70. Onate A, Alcibar J, Inguanzo R, et al. Balloon dilation of tricuspid and pulmonary valves in carcinoid heart disease. *Tex Heart Inst J* 1993;20:115–119.

71. Strickman NE, Hall RJ. Carcinoid heart disease. In: Kapoor AS, Reynolds RD, eds. *Cancer and the heart.* New York: Springer-Verlag, 1986:135–161.

72. DiSesa VJ, Mills RM Jr, Collins JJ Jr. Surgical management of carcinoid heart disease. *Chest* 1985;88:789–791.

73. Kvols LK, Moertel CG, O'Connell MJ, et al. Treatment of the malignant carcinoid syndrome. Evaluation of a long-acting somatostatin analogue. *N Engl J Med* 1986;315:663–666.

74. Mitty HA, Warner RR, Newman LH, et al. Control of carcinoid syndrome with hepatic artery embolization. *Radiology* 1985;155:623–626.

75. MacGregor JS, Cavero PG, McCluskey ER, et al. Percutaneous valvuloplasty to relieve stenosis of a bioprosthetic tricuspid valve in a patient with bacterial endocarditis. *Am Heart J* 1994;128:199–202.

76. Block PC, Smalling R, Owings RM. Percutaneous double balloon valvotomy for bioprosthetic tricuspid stenosis. *Cathet Cardiovasc Diagn* 1994;33:342–344.

77. Slama MS, Drieu LH, Malergue MC, et al. Percutaneous double balloon valvuloplasty for stenosis of porcine bioprostheses in the tricuspid valve position: a report of 2 cases. *Cathet Cardiovasc Diagn* 1993;28:142–148.

78. Hurrell DG, Schaff HV, Tajik AJ. Thrombolytic therapy for obstruction of mechanical prosthetic valves. *Mayo Clin Proc* 1996;71:605–613.

79. Roudaut R, Labbe T, Lorient-Roudaut MF, et al. Mechanical cardiac valve thrombosis. Is fibrinolysis justified? *Circulation* 1992;86[Suppl]:II-8–II-15.

80. Edmunds HL. Thrombotic and bleeding complications of prosthetic heart valve. *Ann Thorac Surg* 1987;44:430–435.

81. Silber H, Khan SS, Matloff JM, et al. The St. Jude valve. Thrombolysis as the first line of therapy for cardiac valve thrombosis. *Circulation* 1993;87:30–37.

82. Ledain LD, Ohayon JP, Colle JP, et al. Acute thrombotic obstruction with disc valve prostheses: diagnostic considerations and fibrinolytic treatment. *J Am Coll Cardiol* 1986;7:743–751.

83. Duran CMG. Tricuspid valve surgery revisited. *J Card Surg* 1994;9[Suppl 2]:242–247.

84. Georgeson S, Panidis IP, Kleaveland JP, et al. Effect of percutaneous balloon valvuloplasty on pulmonary hypertension in mitral stenosis. *Am Heart J* 1993;125:1374–1379.

85. Foltz BD, Hessel EA Jr, Ivey TD. The early course of pulmonary artery hypertension in patients undergoing mitral valve replacement with cardioplegic arrest. *J Thorac Cardiovasc Surg* 1984;88:238–247.

86. Minale C, Lambertz H, Nikol S, et al. Selective annuloplasty of the tricuspid valve. Two-year experience. *J Thorac Cardiovasc Surg* 1990;99:846–851.

87. Camara ML, Aris A, Padro JM, et al. Long-term results of mitral valve surgery in patients with severe pulmonary hypertension. *Ann Thorac Surg* 1988;45:133–136.

88. Porter A, Shapira Y, Wurzel M, et al. Tricuspid regurgitation late after mitral valve replacement: clinical and echocardiographic evaluation. *J Heart Valve Dis* 1999;8:57–62.

88a. Kaul TK, Ramsdale DR, Mercer JL. Functional tricuspid regurgitation following replacement of the mitral valve. *Int J Cardiol* 1991;33:305–313.

89. Sagie A, Schwammenthal E, Palacios IF, et al. Significant tricuspid regurgitation does not resolve after percutaneous balloon mitral valvotomy. *J Thorac Cardiovasc Surg* 1994;108:727–735.

90. Pellegrini A, Colombo T, Donatelli F, et al. Evaluation and treatment of secondary tricuspid insufficiency. *Eur J Cardio-Thorac Surg* 1992;6:288–296.

90a. Bajzer CT, Stewart WJ, Cosgrove DM, et al. Tricuspid valve surgery and intraoperative echocardiography: factors affecting survival, clinical outcome and echocardiographic success. *J Am Coll Cardiol* 1998;32:1023–1031.

91. McGrath LB, Chen C, Bailey BM, et al. Early and late phase events following bioprosthetic tricuspid valve replacement. *J Card Surg* 1992;7:245–253.

92. Van Nooten GJ, Caes FL, Francois KJ, et al. The valve choice in tricuspid valve replacement: 25 years of experience. *Eur J Cardio-Thorac Surg* 1995;9:441–446.

93. Scully HE, Armstrong CS. Tricuspid valve replacement. Fifteen years of experience with mechanical prostheses and bioprostheses. *J Thorac Cardiovasc Surg* 1995;109:1035–1041.

93a. Ratnatunga CP, Edwards MB, Dore CJ, et al. Tricuspid valve replacement: UK Heart Valve Registry mid-term results comparing mechanical and biological prostheses. *Ann Thorac Surg* 1998;66:1940–1947.

94. Jegaden O, Perinetti M, Barthelet M, et al. Long-term results of porcine bioprostheses in the tricuspid position. *Eur J Cardio-Thorac Surg* 1992;6:256–260.

94a. Glower DD, White WD, Smith LR, et al. In-hospital and long-term outcome after porcine tricuspid valve replacement. *J Thorac Cardiovasc Surg* 1995;109:877–883; discussion 883–884.

95. Duran CM, Balasundaram SG, Bianchi S, et al. The vanishing tricuspid annuloplasty. A new concept. *J Thorac Cardiovasc Surg* 1992;104:796–801.

96. Barbour DJ, Roberts WC. Valve excision only versus valve excision plus replacement for active infective endocarditis involving the tricuspid valve. *Am J Cardiol* 1986;57:475–478.

97. Arbulu A, Holmes RJ, Asfaw I. Surgical treatment of intractable right-sided infective endocarditis in drug addicts. 25 years' experience. *J Heart Valve Dis* 1993;2:129–137; discussion 138–139.

97a. Renzulli A, Foe DM, Carozza A, et al. Surgery for tricuspid valve endocarditis: a selective approach. *Heart Vessels* 1999;14:163–169.

98. Gayet C, Pierre B, Delahaye JP, et al. Traumatic tricuspid insufficiency. An underdiagnosed disease. *Chest* 1987;92:429–432.

98a. Sugita T, Watarida S, Katsuyama K, et al. Valve repair with chordal replacement for traumatic tricuspid regurgitation. *J Heart Valve Dis* 1997;6:651–652.

99. Altrichter PM, Olson LJ, Edwards WD, et al. Surgical pathology of the pulmonary valve: a study of 116 cases spanning 15 years. *Mayo Clin Proc* 1989;64:1352–1360.

100. Putterman C, Gilon D, Uretzki G, et al. Right ventricular outflow tract obstruction due to extrinsic compression by non-Hodgkin's lymphoma: importance of echocardiographic diagnosis and follow-up. *Leuk Lymphoma* 1992;7:211–215.

101. Viseur P, Unger P. Doppler echocardiographic diagnosis and follow-up of acquired pulmonary stenosis due to external cardiac compression. *Cardiology* 1995;86:80–82.

102. Lynch M, Blevins LS, Martin RP. Acquired supravalvular pulmonary stenosis due to extrinsic compression by a metastatic thymic carcinoid tumor. *Int J Card Imag* 1996;12:61–63.

103. Marshall ME, Trump DL. Acquired extrinsic pulmonic stenosis caused by mediastinal tumors. *Cancer* 1982;49:1496–1499.

104. Llosa JC, Gosalbez F, Cofina JL, et al. Pulmonary valve endocarditis: mid-term follow-up of pulmonary valvulectomies. *J Heart Valve Dis* 2000;9:359–363.

105. Roistacher N, Kronzon I, Winer HE. Unusual clinical and echocardiographic features of severe isolated pulmonic insufficiency. *Chest* 1983;84:227–229.

106. Ansari A. Isolated pulmonary valvular regurgitation: current perspectives. *Prog Cardiovasc Dis* 1991;33:329–344.

106a. Vrandecic M, Filho BG, Fantini F, et al. The use of bovine pericardium for pulmonary valve reconstruction or conduit replacement: long-term clinical follow-up. *J Heart Valve Dis* 1998;7:54–61.

106b. Nishimura RA, Pieroni DR, Bierman FZ, et al. Second natural history study of congenital heart defects. Pulmonary stenosis: echocardiography. *Circulation* 1993;87[Suppl]:I-73–I-79.

107. Kaplan S, Adolph RJ. Pulmonic valve stenosis in adults. *Cardiovasc Clin* 1979;10(1):327–339.

108. Ellison RG, Brown WJ Jr, Hague EE Jr, et al. Physiologic observations in experimental pulmonary insufficiency. *J Thorac Surg* 1955;30:633–640.

109. Price BO. Isolated incompetence of the pulmonic valve. *Circulation* 1961;23:591–602.

109a. Richardson TR, Moody JM Jr. Bedside cardiac examination: constancy in a sea of change. *Curr Prob Cardiol* 2000;25:785–825.

110. Green EW, Agruss NS, Adolph RJ. Right-sided Austin-Flint murmur. Documentation by intracardiac phonocardiography, echocardiography and postmortem findings. *Am J Cardiol* 1973;32:370–374.

111. Ellison RC, Miettinen OS. Interpretation of RSR' in pulmonic stenosis. *Am Heart J* 1974;88:7–10.

112. Barakos JA, Brown JJ, Higgins CB. MR imaging of secondary cardiac and paracardiac lesions. *AJR: Am J Roentgenol* 1989;153:47–50.

113. Cho CS, Blank N, Castellino RA. Computerized tomography evaluation of chest wall involvement in lymphoma. *Cancer* 1985;55:1892–1894.

114. Aldousany AW, DiSessa TG, Dubois R, et al. Doppler estimation of pressure gradient in pulmonary stenosis: maximal instantaneous vs. peak-to-peak, vs. mean catheter gradient. *Pediatr Cardiol* 1989;10:145–149.

115. Switzer DF, Nanda WC. Color Doppler evaluation of valvular regurgitation. *Echocardiography* 1985;2:533–543.

116. Kostucki W, Vandenbossche JL, Friart A, et al. Pulsed Doppler regurgitant flow patterns of normal valves. *Am J Cardiol* 1986;58:309–313.

117. Miyatake K, Okamoto M, Kinoshita N, et al. Pulmonary regurgitation studied with the ultrasonic pulsed Doppler technique. *Circulation* 1982;65:969–976.

118. Novack H, Machac J, Horowitz SF. Inversion of the radio-

nuclide regurgitant index in right-sided valvular regurgitation. *Eur J Nucl Med* 1985;11:205–209.

119. Danilowicz D, Hoffman JI, Rudolph AM. Serial studies of pulmonary stenosis in infancy and childhood. *Br Heart J* 1975;37:808–818.

120. Perloff JK, Child JS. *Congenital heart disease in adults.* Philadelphia: Saunders, 1991.

121. Stanger P, Cassidy SC, Girod DA, et al. Balloon pulmonary valvuloplasty: results of the Valvuloplasty and Angio-

plasty of Congenital Anomalies Registry. *Am J Cardiol* 1990;65:775–783.

122. Grant SC, Scarffe JH, Levy RD, Brooks NH. Failure of balloon dilatation of the pulmonary valve in carcinoid pulmonary stenosis. *Br Heart J* 1992;67:450–453.

123. Schmidtke C, Bechtel JFM, Noetzold A, et al. Up to seven years of experience with the Ross procedure in patients >60 years of age. *J Am Coll Cardiol* 2000;36:1173–1177.

24

PROSTHETIC VALVE DISEASE

MARIO J. GARCIA

HISTORICAL PERSPECTIVE

After a decade of research, in 1952 (1) Charles Hufnagel successfully inserted the first prosthetic valve in the descending aorta of a patient with aortic regurgitation. Since then, more than 80 different types of heart valve prostheses have been developed. Valve replacement surgery today represents the primary treatment modality for most types of valvular heart disease and is performed in 60,000 Americans each year.

Shortly after the introduction of the pump oxygenator in cardiac surgery, the first aortic valve replacement was performed by Harken (2) in 1953, and the first mitral valve replacement was performed by Starr (3) in 1960. The bare-strut ball valves that were initially used underwent further refinement for the next several years, leading to the development of the Starr-Edwards ball-and-cage valve. The first nontilting-disc valves were introduced shortly afterward, in an attempt to improve the profile of the ball-and-cage valve in the mitral and tricuspid positions. Although these are no longer implanted, nontilting-disc valves such as the Kay-Suzuki, Kay-Shiley, and Beall valves are occasionally found in a patient (4). The tilting-disc valves developed in the late 1960s represented a significant advance, demonstrating a hemodynamic performance far superior to that of the ball-and-cage and nontilting-disc valves. The Björk-Shiley (5) and Lillehei-Kaster (6) hingeless tilting-disc valves had a basic design similar to that of the Medtronic-Hall prosthesis that is commonly used today (7). Double-leaflet hingeless tilting-disc valves were developed in the early 1970s, and in 1977 the first St. Jude Medical bileaflet mechanical prosthesis (8) was made available for clinical use, becoming the most popular mechanical heart valve over the last two decades.

The undesirable thromboembolic complications of the mechanical valves raised interest in the development of tissue valves. The first tissue valve was an aortic homograft inserted by Ross in 1962 (9). The limited availability of fresh homografts made their use impractical until the devel-

M. J. Garcia: Department of Cardiovascular Medicine, The Cleveland Clinic Foundation, Cleveland, Ohio

opment of cryopreservation in 1987. Advances in methods of preservation led to the development of the stented porcine valve xenografts, first implanted in 1965 by Carpentier (10) and later marketed as the Hancock and the Carpentier-Edwards valves. Although these valves eliminated the need for anticoagulation, they were limited to suboptimal hemodynamic performance at smaller sizes because of the bulk and position of their supporting stents. The Ionescu-Shiley (11) and the Carpentier-Edwards bovine valve, which were fashioned from bovine pericardium, were later developed to improve the hemodynamic profile of the tissue heterografts. Aortic homografts, aortic pulmonary autografts (12), and, more recently, stentless porcine valves are capable of providing hemodynamic performance comparable to that of native valves, although these are mostly available for use in the aortic position and have less durability than mechanical valves. A few institutions have limited experience with the use of a mitral valve homograft (13). The long-term results of this operation still need to be determined. Thus, efforts to improve the design and performance of prosthetic valves continue, because none of the options currently available can match the hemodynamic performance, durability, low risk of infection, and low thrombogenicity of native human valves.

ANATOMIC AND PHYSIOLOGIC CONSIDERATIONS

General Principles

Magnetic resonance imaging can be performed safely in most patients with prosthetic valves (14). [▼Ⓨ e68] This test may be of clinical advantage in patients in whom valvular regurgitation is suspected when the results of Doppler echocardiographic studies are inconclusive (15,16). Uncommonly, invasively obtained catheter gradients are needed to determine prosthetic valve dysfunction. Retrograde catheter crossing of tissue prostheses and ball-and-cage prostheses may be performed safely to determine transvalvular gradients. Tilting-disc prostheses should not be crossed with these catheters because of the risk of catheter entrapment (17). Direct left ventricular puncture using a percutaneous approach may be performed in some cases to measure pressure gradients. Fortunately, in most instances, transvalvular gradients can be determined by Doppler echocardiography, obviating the need for catheterization.

When evaluating the function of prosthetic valves, the following general principles should be taken into consideration:

1. With the exception of the aortic homograft and stentless porcine valves, all currently available tissue and mechanical prosthesis have a smaller effective orifice than a native valve in the same position. This reduction in effective orifice is caused by the profile of the suture ring and the supporting

stents in tissue valves or the occluders in mechanical valves. Thus, most tissue and mechanical prostheses in a semilunar position generate a systolic flow murmur. Diastolic murmurs in atrioventricular prosthetic valves are uncommonly heard unless prosthetic stenosis, high forward flow caused by severe valvular regurgitation, or patient-prosthesis mismatch is present (18). The normal auscultatory findings of prosthetic valves may be altered by factors such as chest wall thickness, emphysema, stroke volume, heart rate and rhythm, and the presence of other prostheses.

2. Transvalvular gradients may be estimated from continuous-wave Doppler velocities by means of the modified Bernoulli equation ($\Delta P = 4V^2$), where P represents pressure and V represents velocity. Transvalvular gradients are determined by several factors: the effective orifice of the prosthesis, the stroke volume, and the presence of intravalvular obstruction. Thus, the published normal ranges of transvalvular gradients are only general guidelines that are applicable to normally functioning prostheses at average resting cardiac outputs. Transvalvular gradients are often higher in patients in high output states, such as in patients with anemia, hyperthyroidism, or pregnancy. Forward transvalvular flow may be increased also in the presence of large paravalvular regurgitant leaks. Doppler-derived and catheter-derived peak and mean gradients are comparable, with perhaps the single exception of small ball-and-cage and bileaflet tilting-disc valves that are in the aortic position, in which Doppler gradients have been shown to exceed transcatheter gradients by as much as 44 mm Hg (19). This discrepancy between catheter-derived gradients and Doppler gradients is the result of pressure recovery upstream from the prosthesis.

3. The ratio of Doppler velocity across the valve and velocity proximal to the valve orifice, or "dimensionless index," is independent of flow and should remain relatively constant over time; thus, it is useful in detecting changes in effective valvular orifice (20). The continuity equation of flow (21) provides accurate estimates of the effective valve orifice in single-leaflet tilting-disc mechanical valves and in bioprostheses but underestimates the orifice of the bileaflet tilting-disc valves by approximately 0.5 cm^2 (20). A decrease in effective valve orifice is often seen in bioprosthetic valves at low flow rates, suggesting that bioprosthetic leaflets do not open fully in these cases because of the increased resistance (22).

4. All normally functioning mechanical prosthetic valves have a certain amount of intravalvular regurgitation. This regurgitation is generated by the closure flow backwash and by built-in mechanisms that prevent the deposition of thrombogenic material. Small paravalvular leaks are commonly detected intraoperatively by transesophageal echocardiography immediately after surgical implantation, most of which improve after reversal of anticoagulation (23).

5. Prosthetic valve suture rings, cages, discs, and stents may produce echocardiographic shielding or make it impos-

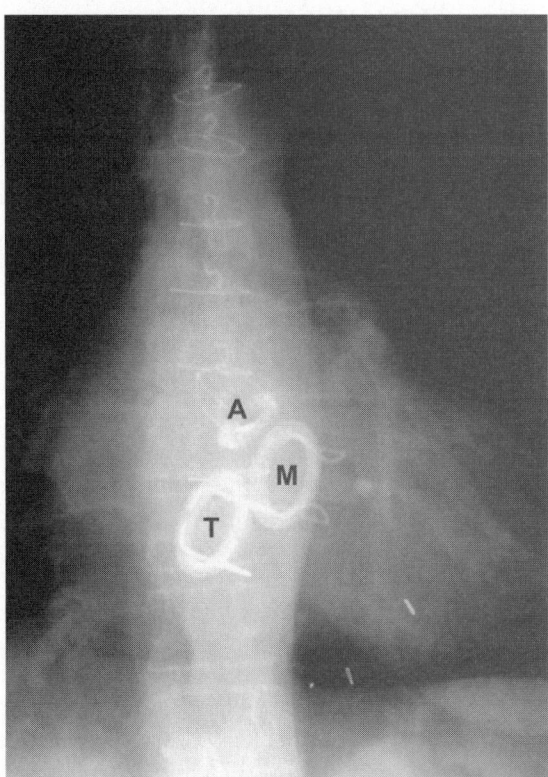

FIGURE 24.1 Radiographic appearance in the anteroposterior projection of mechanical valves in the aortic (A), mitral (M), and tricuspid (T) positions.

sible to visualize structures or flow beyond the location of the ultrasound reflecting surface. This limits the ability to detect transvalvular or paravalvular regurgitation, thrombi, or vegetations of infective endocarditis in some prostheses by transthoracic echocardiography, particularly in prostheses that are in the mitral position (24). In those cases, transesophageal echocardiography offers a superior visualization.

6. Certain types of prosthetic valves and their locations may be identified using plain chest radiography (Fig. 24.1, *e*Figs. 24.1.1 and 24.1.2). Suture rings are always radiopaque, as are prosthetic cages and some tissue valve supporting stents. Tilting discs may or may not be seen in a plain film, depending on the angle of the prosthesis, the construction material, and the radiographic penetration. Cinefluoroscopy may be useful in evaluating the mobility of the occluder of mechanical valves in patients in whom obstruction is suspected. This technique, however, may not necessarily detect subvalvular obstruction by pannus and cannot be used to assess valvular regurgitation.

Mechanical Valves

Tilting-Disc Valves

Tilting-disc prostheses [✌ e69] are available in diameters from 19 to 33 mm for implantation in the mitral or aortic

positions. Their mean transvalvular gradient is significantly lower than that of equally sized Starr-Edwards ball-and-cage valves, from 6 to 15 mm Hg in the aortic position and from 2 to 7 mm Hg in the mitral position. The estimated effective orifices range from 2.1 to 3.9 cm^2 for mitral prostheses and from 1.3 to 2.5 cm^2 for aortic prostheses. The Carbomedics "Top-Hat" valve is mechanically designed to increase the effective orifice in relation to the annular size, due to the supraannular location of the occluder (47). The auscultatory findings of tilting-disc prostheses include a loud single or double closing click and a soft mid-systolic ejection murmur in the aortic position or a low-frequency diastolic rumble in the mitral position. Tilting-disc prostheses also produce a softer opening click. The radiographic appearance of these valves differs according to the number and position of the struts and the tilting discs. In some valves, such as the Björk-Shiley valve and the Wada-Cutter valve, the discs may be radiolucent. The two half discs of bileaflet valves can be observed from a tangential plane. The motion of the valve ring and the opening angle of the discs can be evaluated under fluoroscopic guidance. The movement of the tilting discs also can be detected by two-dimensional echocardiography. Two-dimensional echocardiography frequently demonstrates microcavitations in the left ventricular cavity of patients with mechanical tilting valves in the mitral position (48). These microcavitations appear to be gaseous and do not cause any clinical symptoms. However, transcranial Doppler often detects these microembolic signals, and some cases have been reported in which this phenomenon appeared to be related to episodes of amaurosis fugax (49).

Color Doppler imaging may help to identify the type of prosthesis. The Medtronic-Hall tilting-disc valve has a characteristic regurgitant flow jet through its central orifice. The St. Jude's Medical valve has two central divergent and multiple peripheral convergent regurgitant jets that may be visualized depending on the imaging angle. The amount of intravalvular regurgitation may vary according to heart rate and cardiac output. The regurgitant fraction of single tilting-disc valves averages approximately 12% under normal hemodynamic conditions, but it may be as high as 37% at high heart rates and low cardiac output (50). Continuous-wave Doppler imaging is useful for estimating transvalvular gradients using the modified Bernoulli equation. Mean pressure gradients obtained by Doppler imaging generally have a good correlation with catheter-derived gradients (51). Doppler imaging may overestimate the gradient, however, in small prostheses in the aortic position, particularly in those with bileaflet valves. The mean Doppler gradient may be 10 mm Hg higher than the catheter gradient in these circumstances (52). This apparent overestimation is caused by the effect of pressure recovery, which determines that part of the kinetic energy present at the valve level is converted back to pressure distal to the valve if the geometry of the valve prevents turbulence (53). Thus, discrepancy exists because the Doppler imaging method measures the highest gradient at the intravalvular level, whereas the catheter method measures the gradient distal to the valve. Extended M-mode and Doppler recordings are important in excluding intermittent entrapment of the discs.

Tissue Valves

Heterografts

Advances in tissue valve preservation are expected to increase the longevity of these valves. [▼ e70] Intermediate follow-up of the Hancock II porcine bioprostheses suggests that their durability will be superior to that of their predecessors. Freedom from reoperation has been reported to be 100%, 97%, and 89% after aortic, mitral, and combined valve replacement, respectively, after 7 years of follow-up (66).

Bioprosthetic valves are available in diameters of 19 to 31 mm. The effective orifice area for bioprostheses ranges from 1.4 to 2.5 cm² in the mitral position and from 0.9 to 1.8 cm² in the aortic position. The auscultatory findings of bioprosthetic valves include a systolic ejection murmur in the aortic position and an opening sound in the mitral position. Frequently, a systolic murmur is heard in patients who have mitral bioprostheses, which is caused by turbulent flow in the left ventricular outflow track. The bioprosthetic valve sewing ring is radiopaque in radiographic films. In some models, wire-framed stents may also be seen. The three equidistant stents seen on two-dimensional echocardiography are the hallmark of bioprostheses. The three leaflets can also be imaged, although they are less echogenic than the native aortic valve. Normal bioprostheses showed no or minimal intravalvular regurgitation on color Doppler imaging.

Stentless heterograft prostheses consist of a tubular segment of a porcine proximal ascending aorta containing its *in situ* aortic valve, which is sutured proximally to the aortic annulus and distally to the mid-ascending aorta (eFig. 24.1.4). Although surgical implantation of these valves is technically more demanding, studies have failed to show higher in-hospital morbidity or mortality rates (67). Short and intermediate follow-up of stentless valves have, thus far, demonstrated better hemodynamics with smaller resting and exercise gradients and greater regression of left ventricular hypertrophy than stented tissue valves of similar size (68,69). One study suggested that patients with severe aortic stenosis and left ventricular dysfunction who receive a stentless valve demonstrate a greater early improvement in left ventricular systolic function than patients who receive a stented valve (70). Stentless aortic root bioprostheses can be used safely to replace the aortic root for aortic valve and aortic root pathology (71). Freedom from structural valve degeneration has been reported to be approximately 85% at 9 years (72).

Selection of Prosthetic Valve Type

Age

Children who require valve replacement benefit most from mechanical prostheses (86). [▼ e71] Tilting-disc mechanical valves provide better hemodynamic performance than bioprostheses, particularly at smaller sizes, thus delaying the need for reoperation. Structural valve deterioration of bioprosthetic valves also occurs more rapidly in children and young adults (eFig. 24.1.7) (61,82–87). The main cause of dysfunction of porcine valves appears to be calcification of the leaflets. Premature calcification of porcine valves in children is thought to be caused by the patients' accelerated metabolism of calcium, reduced mobility of the leaflets due to lower cardiac output, and stronger immune reactivity to porcine valve tissue. The life expectancy of bioprostheses increases linearly with the patient's age at the time of implantation, from a mean of 6 years at age 20 years to 12 years at age 80 years. Approximately 60% to 80% of patients who are younger than 40 years at the time of bioprosthetic valve replacement will experience structural valve deterioration, versus 5% to 40% of patients older than 60 years (87,88). Therefore, as a general rule, mechanical valves are preferred in younger patients, and bioprosthetic valves are recommended in older patients, in whom the risk of anticoagulation therapy is higher. In young adults who may want to avoid the risks associated with long-term anticoagulation therapy, valve repair and homograft replacement may offer longer durability than replacement with heterograft prostheses.

Calcium Metabolism

Accelerated calcium turnover is associated with rapid degeneration of bioprosthetic valves. This is frequently seen in patients with chronic renal failure, Paget's disease, and other chronic illnesses associated with hypercalcemia. Mechanical valves offer an advantage to those patients who have no contraindications for anticoagulation and do not have a short life expectancy. Although mechanical valve replacement traditionally has been recommended for patients who require hemodialysis, most of these patients have a limited survival, and few live long enough to develop bioprosthetic valve degeneration (98). Thus, in this patient population, the choice of valve prosthesis should be individualized according to life expectancy and the relative risk of thrombotic and hemorrhagic complications.

PATHOPHYSIOLOGY AND PRINCIPLES OF THERAPY

Complications related to prosthetic heart valves can occur as early as in the immediate postoperative period. Their relative frequency and timing vary with each type of prosthesis and determine the manner in which patients with prosthetic valves should be clinically followed.

Antithrombotic Therapy in Patients with Prosthetic Valves

Thromboembolism represents one of the most important causes of morbidity and death in patients with prosthetic valves. In one of the largest follow-up series of patients with Starr-Edwards ball-and-cage valves, 44% of patients had experienced a thromboembolic episode within 10 years after implantation (103). Of these episodes, 50% resulted in permanent neurologic sequelae and 10% resulted in death. The incidence of thromboembolic events is significantly higher in patients with mechanical prosthesis who are not receiving anticoagulation therapy, ranging from 7% to 34% per year (104–106). Several mechanisms are involved in the pathogenesis of prosthetic valve–mediated thromboembolism, including platelet activation by the synthetic surfaces of the sewing ring, sutures and mechanical occluders, flow stagnation, increased shear stress, and activation of intrinsic clotting factors by the prosthetic material or the damaged endothelium (107). Patient-related contributing risk factors include older age, atrial fibrillation, and left ventricular dysfunction (108). The risk of thromboembolism is higher with both mechanical valves and bioprostheses in the early postoperative period and declines after the first 3 months for bioprosthetic valves. The risk also varies with the type, size, position, and synthetic components of the valve.

Mechanical Valves

The first generation of Starr-Edwards ball-and-cage valves demonstrated a very high incidence of thromboembolic complications in the absence of anticoagulation therapy (104,105,109). In an attempt to reduce this risk by promoting endothelialization of the prosthetic surface, cloth-covered strut models (models 2300 and 6300) were introduced in the late 1960s. However, rapid destruction of cloth fragments resulted in a much higher embolization rate (110), requiring the discontinuation of these models. Oral anticoagulation therapy with warfarin significantly reduces the risk of thromboembolism in patients who have mechanical heart valves. Improved prosthetic design and anticoagulation therapy reduced the rate of embolism to 2.5% to 4.0% per patient-year in patients receiving anticoagulation therapy who had Starr-Edwards valves that were implanted after 1970 (111). The incidence of thromboembolic complications with Björk-Shiley tilting-disc valves is approximately 4% per year for valves in the mitral position and 2.5% per year for valves in the aortic position, and an average of 1% to 3% with Medtronic-Hall valves in patients receiving anticoagulation therapy (112). Bileaflet mechanical valves have a risk of approximately 2.5% per

year in the mitral position and 1% per year in the aortic position (113–115).

Whether the small difference in these rates is associated with intrinsic properties of the prostheses or merely represents differences in patient characteristics, level of anticoagulation therapy, or study design is unclear. For example, Horstkotte and associates (116) reported a lower rate of embolism with the St. Jude's Medical valve, but their study did not include transient ischemic attacks as an outcome. On the other hand, another study, which involved a large group of patients in atrial fibrillation, showed a rate of 3.9 events per 100 patient-years with the same valve (117). Regardless of the type of mechanical prosthesis, the incidence of thromboembolism is lower than 1% in patients who maintain therapeutic anticoagulation (116–118). Studies have shown that the majority of patients with mechanical valves who experience thromboembolic complications has a subtherapeutic INR (international normalized ratio) at the time of the event (103). However, chronic anticoagulation therapy increases the long-term incidence of hemorrhagic complications. Pooled data from 46 studies that observed more than 13,000 patients with mechanical heart valves for more than 50,000 patient-years have shown an incidence of major bleeding complications of approximately 1.4 per 100 patient-years (119). Cannegieter and coworkers (120) reported a risk of intracranial and spinal hemorrhage of approximately 0.6% per 100 patient-years. In their study, 72% of hemorrhagic strokes resulted in permanent neurologic damage and 44% in death, compared to 21% and 5% of ischemic strokes, respectively (Table 24.1). Other common sites of bleeding are the gastrointestinal and genitourinary tracts and the retroperitoneal, intramuscular, subcutaneous, nasopharyngeal, and joint spaces.

In the absence of a predisposing factor, hemorrhagic complications occur significantly more frequently in patients with an INR higher than the therapeutic range (121). In the study by Cannegieter and associates (120), in which 1,608 patients with mechanical valves were observed during 6,475 patient-years, the incidence of adverse events (hemorrhagic and thromboembolic) increased from 2 per 100 patient-years among patients with INRs of 2.5 to 4.9, to 7.5 per 100 patient-years among patients with INRs of 2.0 to 2.4, and to 27 per 100 patient-years among patients with INRs of 1.0 to 1.4 (Fig. 24.2). Similarly, adverse events increased to 4.8 per 100 patient-years among patients with INRs of 5.0 to 5.5 and to 75 per 100 patient-years among patients with INRs >6.5. Predisposing conditions such as trauma or underlying illness were identified in one-half of the patients who experienced hemorrhagic events, regardless of the INR level. Both hemorrhagic and thromboembolic complications are more frequent in older patients (120). Patients younger than 50 years had an incidence of thromboembolism of 0.1 per 100 patient-years and an incidence of hemorrhage of 2.5 per 100 patient-

TABLE 24.1 INCIDENCE OF ADVERSE EVENTS (THROMBOEMBOLISM, MAJOR BLEEDING, AND STROKE) IN PATIENTS WITH MECHANICAL VALVES RECEIVING CHRONIC ANTICOAGULATION

Event	No.	Incidence (per 100 patient-yr)[a]
Thromboembolism		
Cerebral infarction	43	0.68
Peripheral embolism	2	0.03
Valve thrombosis	0	—
Any thromboembolism	45	0.71
Fatal thromboembolism	2	0.03
Bleeding episode		
Intracranial and spinal bleeding	36	0.57
Extracranial bleeding	128	2.11
Any bleeding	64	2.68
Fatal bleeding	20	0.30
Unclassified stroke	14	0.23
First events	210	3.50

[a]Because follow-up ended when the event of interest occurred, the denominators differ for the various end points.
Adapted from Cannegieter SC, Rosendaal RF, Wintzen AR, et al. Optimal oral anticoagulant therapy in patients with mechanical heart valves. *N Engl J Med* 1995;333:14.

years, compared with incidences of 1.1 and 5.6, respectively, among patients older than 70 years.

Accomplishing optimal anticoagulation requires not only achievement of a target INR but also maintenance of that level through careful patient education and rigorous monitoring. Monitoring anticoagulation by means of the INR eliminates uncertainty about the intensity of anticoagulation therapy that is caused by variability in the results of different commercial thromboplastins. The intensity of anticoagulation therapy should vary according to the type of mechanical device and to the presence of other predisposing factors (*e*Fig. 24.1.6). In patients with ball-and-cage prostheses, the incidence of thromboembolic events is low-

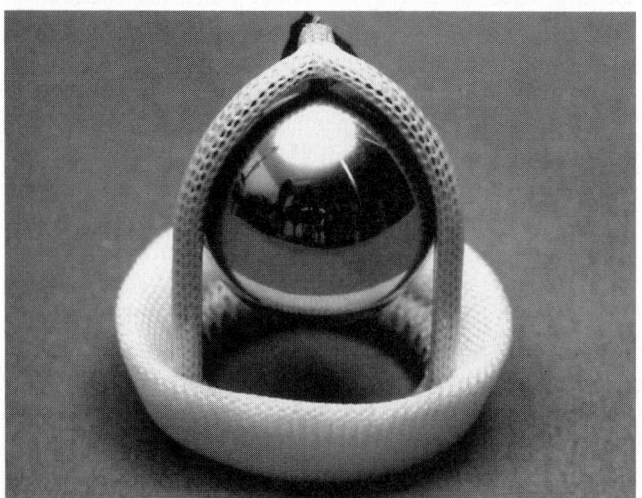

FIGURE 24.2 Cloth-covered Starr-Edwards ball-and-cage valve. This mechanical prosthesis was discontinued due to the high incidence of hemolysis and embolization of cloth fragments.

est when the INR is maintained between 4.0 and 4.9 (121). This higher INR also appears to reduce the rate of embolic events in patients who have multiple mechanical prostheses. An INR of 3.0 to 3.9 is associated with a very low incidence of thromboembolic events in patients with Medtronic-Hall or Björk-Shiley valves, whereas an INR of 2.0 to 2.9 appears to be sufficient in patients with St. Jude's Medical valves. Because the risk of thromboembolic events is higher for patients with any mechanical prostheses in the mitral position and for patients who have chronic atrial fibrillation, efforts should be made to maintain a higher anticoagulation level in these patients. Most hemorrhagic and thromboembolic complications can be avoided by maintaining a stable level of anticoagulation (*e*Fig. 24.2.1).

Studies have shown that patients with prosthetic valves who receive chronic anticoagulation therapy that is monitored in a specialized clinic experienced a lower incidence of thromboembolic and hemorrhagic complications compared with patients who are followed sporadically by primary care physicians (122). Recently, studies have shown that weekly self-testing and self-dosing leads to a better control of anticoagulation therapy than standard treatment in an anticoagulation clinic (123). Whether the widespread use of home-monitoring anticoagulation kits will result in a reduction of thromboembolic complications, bleeding complications, or both remains to be determined.

Antiplatelet therapy may be used in combination with warfarin in patients who have mechanical heart valves. Aspirin may have a beneficial effect by reducing the platelet-mediated activation of the coagulation cascade. Turpie and colleagues (124) demonstrated that low-dose aspirin (100 mg per day) in patients with a target INR of 3.0 to 4.5 has been shown to reduce the annualized risk of death and major systemic thromboembolic events from 11.7% to

4.2% (*e*Fig. 24.2.2). Although the risk of all hemorrhage increased in the group of patients receiving aspirin in this study from 22% to 35%, the risk of major hemorrhagic events (cerebrovascular bleeding, gastrointestinal bleeding, and major bleeding requiring transfusion) appeared to be similar in both groups (13% vs. 10%; 95% confidence interval, −30% to 132%; *p* = .43). The additive benefit of aspirin appeared to be greater in patients who had experienced previous embolic events and were at higher risk for thromboembolism. The reduction in death rate in the group of patients receiving aspirin may also be associated with the prevention of myocardial infarction in patients with coronary artery disease, which present in at least 35% of the patients in this study. Another study has demonstrated that patients randomly assigned to receive oral anticoagulation therapy with a target INR of 2.5 to 3.5 and 200 mg per day of aspirin after mechanical mitral valve replacement had a lower risk of visualization of periprosthetic thrombi by transesophageal echocardiography 9 days after surgery (5% vs. 13%), compared with patients who received standard anticoagulation therapy without aspirin (125). The risk of thromboembolic events was also lower after 1 year of follow-up (9% vs. 25%). Nevertheless, these results have to be interpreted with caution; the incidence of thromboembolism with anticoagulation therapy alone in this study was considerably higher that previously reported. In addition, with the combination treatment, the rate of gastrointestinal hemorrhage was significantly increased (7% vs. 0%). High-dose aspirin (500 mg per day) may reduce the risk of thromboembolism in patients with a low INR (1.8 to 2.3), but it results in a higher incidence of gastrointestinal bleeding (126,127). There is no apparent benefit, but certainly a higher risk of hemorrhage, with the use of high-dose aspirin in patients who have high-intensity INR.

The use of other antiplatelet agents alone or in combination with warfarin in patients with prosthetic valves has been studied. The value of dipyridamole in preventing thromboembolism in patients with mechanical valves is controversial (128,129). A study by Hayashi and coauthors suggested that both dipyridamole and ticlopidine have beneficial effects similar to those of low-dose aspirin in combination with warfarin therapy (130). Because of the high cost and significant side effects of these drugs, their use should be reserved for high-risk patients who are intolerant to aspirin.

Special Situations

Anticoagulation Therapy during Pregnancy

Because pregnancy causes relative hypercoagulability (134), rigorous anticoagulation therapy is required throughout gestation (89,92) in patients with mechanical valve prostheses. Anticoagulant therapy is associated, however, with higher fetal morbidity and mortality rates, especially if the drugs are administered during the first trimester (135).

Warfarin has teratogenic effects in the embryo and may result in fetal death when the embryo is exposed between the sixth and ninth week of gestation (90). Pregnant women with mechanical valves who receive warfarin during this period carry a risk of embryopathy as high as 30% (136) and a risk of spontaneous abortion of 25% to 30% (136). Therapeutic abortion should be considered if advanced gestation is discovered accidentally while the patient is receiving this drug. Anticoagulation should be maintained during pregnancy with either continuous intravenous or subcutaneous heparin, administered twice daily starting at 17,500 to 20,000 units and adjusted to a target activated partial thromboplastin time greater than two times control 6 hours after administration (137). Subtherapeutic doses of heparin are associated with a significant risk of thromboembolism. Large doses of heparin are commonly required because of the relatively hypercoagulable state during pregnancy (138). The risk of major hemorrhagic complications in pregnant patients treated with heparin is approximately 2% (139). Substituting heparin from the sixth week until the twelfth week of gestation eliminates the risk of embryopathy in pregnant women with mechanical valves (90). Larrea and coworkers (140) also found a reduction in the risk of spontaneous abortion from 34.6% in patients receiving warfarin to 9.5% in those receiving intravenous heparin. Warfarin appears to be safe during the second trimester and the first half of the third trimester, and it reduces the risk of thromboembolism that is associated with inadequate anticoagulation with heparin. Heparin should be substituted for warfarin again after the thirty-eighth week and until delivery, because warfarin crosses the placenta and may cause fetal intracranial hemorrhage in the peripartum period (92,141). Heparin should be discontinued 24 hours before elective induction of labor. Both heparin and warfarin can be used safely by nursing mothers, because they do not appear to be secreted into breast milk (139).

Low-molecular-weight heparins have been shown to be safe and effective for the prevention and treatment of deep venous thrombosis in pregnant women (142). Because they have a longer plasma half-life, they provide steady levels of anticoagulation and a more predictable dose response than unfractionated heparin. Low-molecular-weight heparins do not cross the placenta, and they carry lower risks of heparin-induced thrombocytopenia, but they are considerably more expensive. Studies are needed, however, to determine whether low-molecular-weight heparins are safe and effective during pregnancy in patients who have mechanical valves. Low-dose aspirin has been shown to be safe when used in combination with heparin or warfarin in pregnant patients who have a high risk of thromboembolism (143).

Anticoagulation in Patients with Prosthetic Endocarditis

The risk of thromboembolism in patients with mechanical valve endocarditis who are not receiving anticoagulation therapy has been reported to be as high as 50% in different studies (148,149). These studies suggest that anticoagulation may reduce this risk to less than 10%, although such therapy may be associated with a 14% risk of cerebral hemorrhage. The risk of hemorrhage is particularly high in patients who have clinical or radiographic evidence of cerebral embolization. In these patients, anticoagulation therapy should be discontinued for 48 to 72 hours, until resumption is considered safe. Because patients with prosthetic valve endocarditis are hospitalized, oral anticoagulation therapy should be replaced by intravenous heparin, which can be quickly discontinued if necessary. Low-molecular-weight heparins should be used in patients developing heparin-induced thrombocytopenia.

Prosthetic Valve Thrombosis

Prosthetic valve thrombosis is a serious complication associated with both mechanical and bioprosthetic valves (Fig. 24.3). The incidence is higher, approximately 6% per year, for patients with mechanical prostheses who are receiving suboptimal anticoagulation therapy (150,151). Thrombosis occurs more frequently in patients with older models of Björk-Shiley (150,151) and Omniscience (152) single-tilting-disc valves than with Starr-Edwards ball-and-cage, Medtronic Hall single-tilting-disc, and St. Jude's Medical bileaflet valves. Patients with mechanical prostheses who are receiving adequate anticoagulation therapy, regardless of the type of valve, have a lower risk, 0.1% to 2.0% per 100 patient-years, similar to the risk among patients with bioprosthetic valves who are not receiving anticoagulation therapy (25). Valve thrombosis occurs more commonly among patients with prostheses in the mitral position than among patients with prostheses in the aortic position. The incidence of thrombosis appears to be much higher (4% per year) among patients with prostheses in the tricuspid valve position (153).

The thrombus may directly obstruct the valve orifice, cause entrapment of the pivoting mechanism of tilting-disc prostheses, or interfere with the occluding mechanism, causing valvular stenosis, regurgitation, or both. Many patients who have prosthetic thrombosis also have redundant endocardial tissue growth (pannus) that partially obstructs the prosthesis. In the series by Deviri and coworkers (154), thrombus alone was seen in 54% of 106 patients undergoing reoperation for prosthetic valve obstruction. A combination of thrombus and pannus was present in 39%, and pannus alone was found in 6% of the patients. Pannus may be detected as early as 6 weeks and may cause prosthetic valve obstruction as early as 6 months after valve replacement (154). Patients with prosthetic valve thrombosis manifest systemic or pulmonary embolization and symptoms of congestive heart failure and cardiovascular collapse. The onset of symptoms may be insidious, occurring over a period of several weeks, or, more commonly,

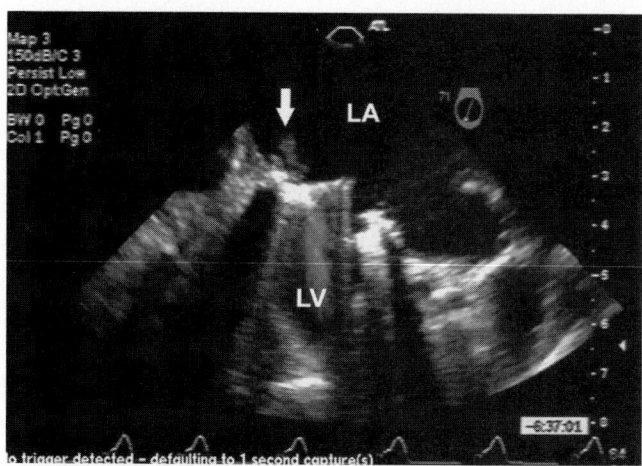

FIGURE 24.3 Thrombosis of a bileaflet mechanical valve in the mitral position. There is partial opening of one of the hemidiscs to a 45-degree angle while the other is stuck in the closed position. The arrow demonstrates the presence of a predunculated thrombus. LA, left atrium; LV, left ventricle.

abrupt, presenting as cardiovascular collapse (155). Acute pulmonary edema appears to be more frequent with single-tilting-disc than with dual-tilting-disc thrombosed prostheses. A murmur of prosthetic stenosis, regurgitation, or both and decreased or absent opening and closing sounds are found on auscultation.

The diagnosis is easily established by two-dimensional and Doppler echocardiography; transesophageal imaging is frequently required. Single or multiple echo densities representing thrombus are often visualized within the valve. Incomplete or intermittent opening and closing of the occluder mechanism may be detected by two-dimensional or M-mode imaging (156). Thorough examination should be performed from different examining positions and angles. Thrombosis of a bileaflet mechanical valve may only affect the excursion of one of the discs. In these cases, careful identification and imaging of both discs should be performed to avoid false-negative results. M-mode images should be recorded for a reasonably long interval, because the valve mechanism may be impaired only intermittently. Continuous-wave Doppler examination is useful, demonstrating elevated transvalvular gradients, and color Doppler imaging may demonstrate abnormal regurgitant flow if there is incomplete closure of the prosthesis. ▼ e72

Structural Degeneration

Mechanical Valves

Malfunction of a mechanical valve prosthesis is relatively uncommon during the first decade after implantation. Prosthetic failure of a mechanical valve resulting in stenosis, regurgitation, or both may occur as a result of ball degeneration, strut fracture, or impaired mechanical function due to thrombus, pannus formation, or infection. The Starr-

Edwards ball-and-cage prosthesis has a very low incidence of mechanical failure (170). Degeneration of the silastic valve as a result of lipid infiltration or abrasion injury was common in models manufactured before 1965 (Fig. 24.4) (27). The incidence of ball degeneration, also called "ball variance," is very low with the more recent models 1260 and 6120, but it may be a concern with valves that have been in use for 20 years or more. Auscultatory findings that suggest malfunction of a ball-and-cage valve include decreased intensity or absence of the opening or closing clicks; new diastolic murmurs, indicating incomplete closure and regurgitation with valves in the aortic position; or new diastolic rumbling murmurs or systolic regurgitant murmurs with valves in the mitral position. Two-dimensional and M-mode echocardiography may show diminished mobility of the ball. It is of paramount importance to register extended Doppler recordings, M-mode recordings, or both of the prosthesis, because obstruction may occur intermittently. Color M-mode Doppler imaging may indicate abnormal intravalvular regurgitant jets.

Degeneration of the occluding disc of nontilting-disc valves is common. Abrasion of the edges of the disc results in incomplete occlusion and regurgitation. Entrapment of the disc by thrombus occurs also more commonly than in ball-and-cage prostheses. Tilting-disc valves may fail for a variety of reasons because of their complex structure. Immobilization of a disc can result from entrapment of the pivoting mechanism by free-floating sutures or chordae tendineae (171), resulting in valvular stenosis or regurgitation. Intermittent closure of the disc and a reduced opening angle are diagnostic features that may be found on echocardiographic and cinefluoroscopic examinations. Abnormal intravalvular regurgitation may be observed by color Doppler imaging. Although dislodgment and embolization of a disc has been reported with the Harken (172), the Duromedics (173), and the Omnicarbon (174) tilting-disc valves, most instances of disc escape due to strut fracture have been associated primarily with the Björk-Shiley convexo-concave tilting-disc valve.

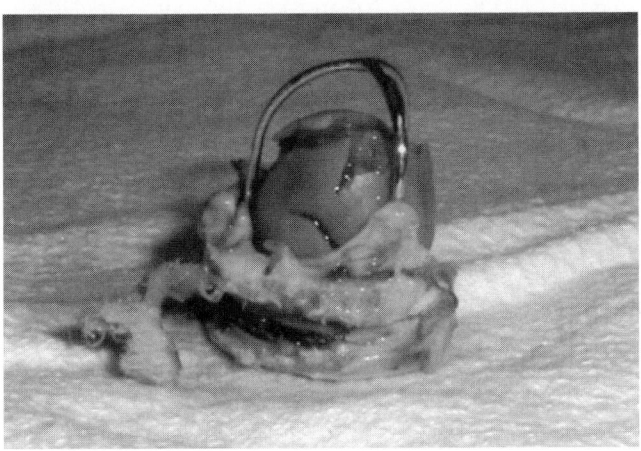

FIGURE 24.4 Structural degeneration of a Silastic ball in a Starr-Edwards valve.

Björk-Shiley Valve and Risk of Strut Fracture

The risk of fracture is estimated according to the size of the prosthesis, position, specific welder group and shop order fracture rates, and the patient's current age and gender. [◆ e73] Risk factor multipliers for 60-degree models are listed in *e*Table 24.1.4. These guidelines must be applied, however, after the characteristics of the individual patient have been considered, which may determine different risk or normal life expectancy.

Strut fracture and disc embolization of an aortic prosthesis is usually fatal. Patients with strut fracture of a mitral prosthesis often survive (179). Acute pulmonary edema, syncope, shock, and acute neurological deficits are often the presenting signs and symptoms. Absence of the opening and closing clicks on auscultation, absence of the disc on radiographic or echocardiographic examination, and severe regurgitation found on color Doppler imaging help establish the diagnosis. Emergency valve replacement is required in these patients.

Incomplete fracture of the strut may be detected by high-resolution cineradiography (180) and also is an indication for valve replacement. This method appears to be very specific when specimens that have been explanted are analyzed. However, its sensitivity is unknown. Of 315 patients with mitral convexo-concave valves who were examined cineradiographically every 6 months after implantation, 11 who showed probable or definite single-leg separations underwent prophylactic explantation. In ten of these, the fracture was confirmed. The mortality rate was slightly lower than the expected mortality rate for this group, for which the fracture rate is estimated to be 0.46% per year or higher. However, two complete outlet-strut fractures occurred 3 and 7 months after radiographic examination yielded apparently normal results, which indicates that some cases were not detected or that complete outlet-strut fracture may not necessarily be preceded by incomplete fracture for a significant period of time. Thus, further studies are necessary to establish specific guidelines about the use of this method as an effective screening procedure. Acoustic analysis has been more recently proposed as a cost-effective method for detecting strut fracture (181).

Prosthetic Valve Endocarditis

Early Prosthetic Valve Endocarditis

By definition, early endocarditis occurs during the first 60 days after valve implantation. It carries a higher mortality rate, ranging between 20% and 70% (195–197). [◆ e74] The classic signs of endocarditis may be masked by the signs of extracardiac sites of infection, such as sternal osteomyelitis and indwelling catheter infections. Symptoms are usually less typical in early prosthetic valve endocarditis. Fever is the most common symptom, occurring in 97% of patients with this condition, followed by diaphoresis and back pain. Anemia is found in 74% of patients, although most of these patients are anemic because of recent blood loss during surgery. Elevated sedimentation rate is uncommonly found in early prosthetic valve endocarditis. Peripheral findings occur in approximately 10% of the cases. The clinical course tends to be more fulminant, with congestive heart failure observed in 60% and shock in 33% of patients (195). Cerebral thromboembolism is more frequent among patients with mechanical valves who are receiving inadequate anticoagulation (38% to 71%), compared to 10% among patients with therapeutic INR. The severity of neurologic deficits is higher, however, in patients receiving anticoagulant therapy, because of the increased risk of hemorrhagic complications. The differential diagnosis of early prosthetic valve endocarditis includes sternal wound, indwelling line infection, and pneumonia. Endocarditis is more frequently associated with sustained bacteremia, which is usually transient with extracardiac infections. Other features of endocarditis include (a) a longer interval between the time of surgery and the onset of symptoms (>25 days), (b) the presence of a new murmur, (c) identification of a microorganism known to be causative, and (d) the absence of an obvious extracardiac source of infection. Gram-negative organisms are not frequently associated with prosthetic valve endocarditis and most likely indicate an extracardiac source.

The incidence of early prosthetic valve endocarditis decreased steadily during the last two decades. This decrease has been attributed to the administration of prophylactic antibiotics in the perioperative period. However, no randomized study has been done to prove this belief. Studies have shown, however, that a shorter course of antibiotics (1 to 2 days) is not associated with a significant increase in risk compared to a longer course (5 to 6 days) (198). The risk of early prosthetic valve endocarditis in prostheses in the aortic position is similar to that of prostheses in the mitral position and is higher in multiple-valve recipients (193–195). Early prosthetic valve endocarditis is more common in men, perhaps as a result of skin infections related to shaving of chest hair during surgery.

Staphylococcus epidermidis is the most common causative organism of early prosthetic endocarditis, accounting for approximately 40% of the cases (199). These organisms have a particularly high affinity for implanted or indwelling synthetic surfaces. They are also the most common organisms causing infection throughout the first year after surgery. The majority of infections caused by *S. epidermidis* during the first year (80%) is resistant to methicillin. In contrast, methicillin resistance is low (20% to 30%) among these organisms after 1 year, suggesting that most infections occurring during the first year after surgery are nosocomial in origin. *Staphylococcus aureus* is the second most common causative organism of both early and late prosthetic valve endocarditis, accounting for 20% of the cases. Gram-negative organisms, diphtheroids, and fungi may also be caus-

ative organisms during the first 2 months after surgery. *Mycoplasma, Legionella* pneumonia, and atypical mycobacteria and enterococci are less frequent causative organisms during this period. Culture-negative endocarditis most commonly occurs as a result of antibiotic therapy. However, *Mycoplasma, Legionella,* fungi, *Coxiella burnetii,* and mycobacteria may cause prosthetic valve endocarditis with negative blood cultures.

Treatment of Prosthetic Valve Endocarditis

Medical treatment of prosthetic valve endocarditis requires longer courses of antibiotics than are used for treatment of native valve endocarditis. The presence of large vegetations usually requires a longer course of antibiotics to achieve sterilization. Regardless of the size of vegetation, however, medical cure is unlikely if there is extensive tissue invasion or if the organism is relatively insensitive to the antibiotic of choice (minimum bactericidal concentration, >4 µg per mL). Treatment of prosthetic valve endocarditis frequently requires surgical replacement of the prosthesis. Streptococcal prosthetic endocarditis is perhaps the only exception; this condition responds to medical treatment alone in 50% of the cases. Medical cure of prosthetic valve endocarditis caused by *Staphylococcus,* gram-negative organisms, or fungi is rare. In patients who are receiving antibiotics and are hemodynamically stable at the time of diagnosis, antibiotics should be withheld briefly to attempt the isolation of an organism from blood cultures. The duration, dosage, and choice of antibiotics is similar to those used in treatment of native valve endocarditis caused by the same organisms, with the following exceptions: (a) treatment of prosthetic valve endocarditis caused by *S. aureus* should include rifampin (300 mg three times per day) and either a semisynthetic penicillin or vancomycin and an aminoglycoside, and (b) in patients who have culture-negative endocarditis associated with a prosthetic valve, vancomycin should be added to ampicillin and gentamycin (209). In cases of penicillin allergy, vancomycin should be used as a second choice.

Surgical replacement should be promptly performed if (a) bacteremia persists after 5 days of intravenous antibiotic therapy; (b) infection recurs after discontinuation of antibiotic therapy; (c) there is evidence of tissue invasion or fistulous tracks; (d) recurrent embolization occurs on antibiotic therapy; (e) infection is caused by a fungal organism; or (f) prosthetic obstruction, dehiscence, heart block, or congestive heart failure develops (210,211). Patients with vegetations that are larger than 10 mm in diameter carry a high risk of embolization, and treatment is less likely to be successful. In these patients, early surgical replacement should be performed. Patients with prosthetic valve endocarditis who have experienced an embolic event while receiving antibiotics and who have residual vegetations carry a significant risk of recurrent embolization and should be considered candidates for early surgical replacement. Patients in whom bacteremia persists for more than 2 days despite effective antibiotic therapy have a better prognosis with early surgical intervention (199). The overall mortality rate of patients treated with antibiotics alone is 61%, compared with 38% among patients who undergo valve replacement (212). In earlier surgical series, however, the mortality rate was high because of delayed operations in patients in whom medical therapy failed. Surgery should not be delayed in any of these circumstances, with perhaps one exception: Patients with cerebral embolization have a significant risk of intracranial hemorrhage during surgery, particularly if they have large neurologic deficits, large abnormalities on a cranial CT scan, or evidence of mycotic aneurysms on a cerebral angiogram. Aggressive removal of all infected tissue should be performed to avoid recurrence of the infection. Occasionally, the annular tissue needs to be reconstructed with autologous pericardium. The stentless aortic homograft is an excellent choice for replacement of infected aortic prostheses. The risk of recurrent endocarditis in aortic homografts is very low (213). Antibiotic treatment should be administered for 6 weeks after surgery. If the organism is methicillin-sensitive *Staphylococcus,* gentamycin should be also administered for 2 weeks. Vancomycin should be used to treat infections caused by methicillin-resistant strains.

Prosthetic valve endocarditis remains a serious complication of valve replacement, but the in-hospital mortality rate associated with reoperations for prosthetic valve endocarditis has declined. In experienced centers, most patients in whom prosthetic valve endocarditis is surgically treated have a favorable outcome. Of 146 patients reoperated for the treatment of prosthetic valve endocarditis by Lytle and colleagues (214) from 1975 through 1992, only 13% died in-hospital (*e*Table 24.1.5). In this study, the surgical mortality rate decreased from 20% between 1975 and 1984 to 10% between 1984 and 1992. The improvement in the prognosis of patients with prosthetic valve endocarditis during the last decade was probably caused by advancements in surgical techniques, including extensive débridement of infected tissue, use of homografts, and improved antibiotic therapy, as well as earlier surgical intervention and patient selection. Both homograft (215) and allograft (216) replacement are associated with a low risk of recurrence in aortic valve endocarditis. Recent efforts have aimed at reducing the incidence of early prosthetic valve endocarditis, such as coating the suture ring with silver (217). However, a higher than expected incidence of paravalvular regurgitation and dehiscence lead to the withdrawal of silver nitrate–impregnated mechanical valves from the market (218).

Hemolysis

Several mechanisms may contribute to the development of hemolysis in normal and malfunctioning prosthetic valves, including shear stress, turbulence, pressure fluctuations, interaction with foreign surfaces, and intrinsic abnormalities of the erythrocyte membrane (221). With the first class of ball-and-cage prosthesis that was implanted, the observed incidence of hemolysis was between 6% and 15% in different series (222–224). The improved hemodynamic performance and surface materials of the newer mechanical and bioprosthetic valves have resulted in a significant reduction of this risk (225,226). Subclinical hemolysis (increased reticulocyte count and lactate dehydrogenase, decreased haptoglobin) is found in most patients who have mechanical valves, but it rarely results in significant anemia. However, hemolytic anemia still represents a relatively common complication among patients with malfunctioning prostheses. Hemolysis is commonly found in association with paravalvular regurgitant leaks. In a series published by Kastor and coauthors (222), 40% of patients with prosthetic valves and paravalvular regurgitation had significant hemolysis that required surgical repair or resulted in death.

Shear stress that causes morphologic alterations in the erythrocyte membrane and results in hemolysis has been well documented. By means of transesophageal echocardiography and fluid dynamic simulation, it has been demonstrated that flow acceleration, deceleration, and fragmentation may be important causes of increased shear stress associated with periprosthetic leaks (227). Patients with clinical hemolysis demonstrate patterns of flow that are associated with peak shear stresses of 4,500 to 6,000 dynes per cm². Direct collision with cardiac structures, such as the limbus of the left atrial appendage, that caused rapid flow deceleration was the most common flow pattern associated with hemolysis in this study. Regurgitation through several small orifices or orifices of irregular shape is associated with greater hemolysis than regurgitation through large, round orifices, perhaps because of the higher acceleration required for passage through the small orifice.

Other factors are also important in the development of hemolytic anemia with prosthetic valves. The surface area and the type of prosthetic material are important factors in the genesis of hemolysis. This phenomenon was noted with the introduction of the completely cloth-covered ball-and-cage prosthesis (Starr-Edwards, series 2300, 2310; Fig. 24.2) (110). These valves, which were developed in an attempt to decrease the incidence of thromboembolism, were associated with a 15% incidence of severe hemolytic anemia. The foreign surface effect is of greater importance when considering the probability of a patient developing hemolysis with malfunctioning prostheses. Teflon and other prosthetic materials that are used to construct the sewing ring and to partially cover the struts in some contemporary valve models become rapidly endothelialized within several weeks after implantation. However, regurgitant jets from paravalvular leaks may denude this endothelium, revealing the prosthetic surface and increasing the propensity to develop hemolysis.

Abnormal flow through a partially thrombosed prosthetic valve may cause hemolytic anemia. Hemolytic anemia is also a common finding in patients who have prosthetic valve endocarditis (228) and in patients who have bioprosthetic valves with structural failure (229). The presence of multiple prosthetic valves or unusually small mechanical prostheses is also associated with higher incidence and severity of hemolysis (230). Mild hemolytic anemia may be treated medically with erythropoietin, iron and folic acid supplementation, and blood transfusions. Control of hypertension with beta-blockers may reduce the severity of hemolysis, probably by reducing the velocity of regurgitant flows and thus the shear stress (231). Closure of paravalvular regurgitant leaks or valve replacement is indicated in patients with severe hemolysis that requires repeated blood transfusions or in patients with congestive heart failure.

Conduction Abnormalities

Heart block may occur after replacement of aortic valves that have become severely calcified, as a result of trauma to the bundle of His that occurs during removal of calcium from the region of the right trigone, beneath the commissure between the noncoronary and the right coronary cusp. Fortunately, complete heart block is uncommon and is usually transient and caused by postoperative edema of the periannular tissue.

Myocardial Infarction

Embolization of air through the right coronary artery is a relatively common cause of perioperative infarction of the inferior wall myocardium, but it rarely results in permanent systolic dysfunction. Myocardial infarction due to obstruction or dissection of the coronary ostia after reimplantation of the coronary trunks in stentless aortic homografts or prosthetic valve conduits may rarely occur. Intraoperative echocardiography is useful demonstrating the presence of postoperative wall motion abnormalities and the patency of flow in the coronary arteries of such patients (236). Myocardial infarction may also be caused by coronary embolization of thrombotic material or infective and aseptic vegetations of endocarditis (237). Coexisting coronary artery disease represents, however, the most common cause of myocardial infarction in patients with prosthetic heart valves.

Ventricular Pseudoaneurysm

Perforation of the posterior mitral annular region may occur after mitral valve replacement, particularly when severe calcification of the mitral annulus is present (238). The posterior pericardium may initially contain the rupture, preventing cardiac tamponade and death. The diagnosis of this infrequent complication is often incidentally made on the basis of a routine echocardiogram. Pseudoaneurysms detected early after mitral valve prosthetic implantation require prompt surgical repair.

Left Ventricular Outflow Obstruction

Some patients with aortic valvular stenosis have significant hypertrophy of the basal muscular septum, either as a result of long-standing pressure overload or as a separate, coexisting condition. In these patients, left ventricular outflow tract obstruction may be subtle before valve replacement because of the high afterload imposed by the stenotic valve. After replacement, the decrease in afterload may result in significant obstruction of the left ventricular outflow tract caused by systolic anterior motion of the anterior mitral valve leaflet. Intraoperative transesophageal echocardiography is useful in diagnosing this complication and should be considered in patients undergoing aortic valve replacement who have severe septal hypertrophy and a small left ventricular outflow tract. Septal myectomy is usually successful correcting this problem when the obstruction is severe. Patients with mitral stenosis and small left ventricular cavities may also develop left ventricular outflow tract obstruction that is caused by one of the supporting struts of a bioprostheses. In these patients, replacement with a mechanical valve is preferred.

CONTROVERSIES AND PERSONAL PERSPECTIVES

Selecting a Prosthetic Valve

The choice between mechanical and bioprosthetic valves should be an early point of discussion between the cardiologist, the cardiac surgeon, and the patient. Multiple factors need to be considered in the decision-making process, including the age of the patient; the probability of future pregnancy in young women; and the patient's occupation, lifestyle, and life expectancy. The risk of a future reoperation should also be considered and may be greater after more extensive surgery such as stentless valve or allograft replacements. When feasible, valve repair should be considered. Otherwise, with very few exceptions, such as a patient who is already receiving chronic anticoagulation therapy or whose anticipated life expectancy is short, no absolute advantages are associated with a specific valve type. Mechanical valve prostheses have a longer durability but require a lifelong commitment to chronic anticoagulation therapy. They should be chosen for younger patients who do not have contraindications and are expected to be medically compliant. The relative benefit-to-risk ratio shifts earlier toward bioprosthetic valves in the aortic position. We recommend bioprosthetic valves for aortic replacement in patients older than 65 years and for mitral valve replacement in patients who are

THE FUTURE

The development and refinement of prosthetic valves during the last three decades have resulted in a remarkable improvement in survival and quality of life for millions of patients who have valvular heart disease. Replacement of a malfunctioning native valve with a prosthesis, however, substitutes one disease for another. None of the available mechanical or biologic valves has the performance and durability of the native human semilunar and atrioventricular valves. Stentless valves appear to have better hemodynamic performance than mechanical valves and stented heterografts, but their long-term durability is still unknown. Refinement of the mitral valve homograft will likely occur in the near future. Mitral homografts may become the procedure of choice for young patients and women of childbearing age who have mitral stenosis that is not amenable to commissurotomy or mitral insufficiency that is not amenable to surgical repair. Future improvements in prosthetic valve design are likely to provide less thrombogenic mechanical materials and better hemodynamic profiles. Future generations of mechanical valves may not require chronic anticoagulation therapy with warfarin. At the same time, chemical and biologic preservation techniques will continue to improve the longevity of bioprostheses. Newer advances in surgical techniques may reduce the morbidity and mortality rates associated with valve surgery. Improved surgical instruments, limited incision surgical techniques, and robotic surgery are now available in many specialized centers and likely will reduce the morbidity associated with heart valve surgery.

70 to 75 years old. Middle-aged or younger patients who wish to avoid long-term anticoagulation therapy and who require aortic valve replacement are good candidates for homograft or allograft replacement, because the durability of theses valves appears to be greater than that of bioprostheses. It remains to be determined whether the durability of stentless porcine valves is comparable.

Prosthetic Valves and Pregnancy

The risk of complications to the mother and to the fetus is significant with both mechanical and bioprosthetic valves. Anticoagulation therapy carries a risk to the fetus even when heparin is substituted for warfarin in the first and third trimesters. Bioprosthetic valves undergo rapid structural degenerative changes in young patients and still carry a higher than expected fetal mortality rate. Women of childbearing age who have mild or regurgitant valvular heart disease should carry their pregnancies earlier in their childbearing years and undergo tubal ligation before prosthetic valve replacement with a mechanical valve. Valve repair should be performed whenever feasible. If valve replacement cannot be avoided, bioprosthetic valves should be used, because they carry a smaller risk of fetal and maternal complications.

Medical versus Surgical Treatment of Prosthetic Valve Complications

Most hemorrhagic and embolic complications seen in patients who have mechanical valves are managed medically, although a few patients with mechanical valves who experience recurrent embolic or hemorrhagic events may benefit from replacement with a bioprosthetic valve. With rare exceptions, other prosthetic valve complications, such as prosthetic valve degeneration, dehiscence, severe hemolysis, and most cases of endocarditis are best treated surgically. No adequate treatment for prosthetic valve degeneration is available. Balloon valvuloplasty of bioprosthetic valve stenosis has been attempted but carries an unacceptably high risk of systemic embolization, acute severe regurgitation, and early restenosis. Thrombolytic therapy of left heart prosthetic valve thrombosis carries a significant risk of stroke. In our opinion, thrombolytic therapy should be reserved for patients who have right-heart prostheses, who are otherwise at high risk for surgery, or for whom skilled surgical treatment is not readily available. Medical cure of prosthetic valve endocarditis occasionally may be accomplished, depending on the valve type and the infecting organism. *Streptococcus viridans* endocarditis in patients with bioprosthetic valves usually responds well to antibiotic therapy. In our experience, these patients should be followed closely; they frequently require valve replacement because of recurrence of infection, incomplete cure, or premature structural degeneration. Valve-induced hemolysis is frequently insidious in onset and may be managed medically, often for several years. The rate of hemolysis and thus requirements for blood transfusion tend to increase steadily over time. Often, the diagnosis of hemolysis is missed in these patients; because of chronic iron losses in urine, they present with predominant signs of iron-deficiency anemia. Because of the risks associated with repeated blood transfusions, valve replacement should be considered early in these patients.

REFERENCES

1. Hufnagel CA, Harvey WP. The surgical correction of aortic regurgitation: preliminary report. *Bull Georgetown Univ Med Cent* 1953;6:60–61.

2. Harken DE, Soroff HS, Taylor WJ, et al. Partial and complete prostheses in aortic insufficiency. *J Thorac Cardiovasc Surg* 1960;40:744–762.

3. Starr A, Edwars ML. Mitral replacement: clinical experience with a ball valve prosthesis. *Ann Surg* 1961;154:726.

4. Kay JH, Tsuji HK, Redington JV, et al. Clinical use of a new mitral disc valve. *Calif Med* 1967;106:165–169.

5. Björk VO. A new tilting disc valve prosthesis. *Scand J Thorac Cardiovasc Surg* 1969;3:1–10.

6. Kaster RL, Lillehei CW, Starek PJ. The Lillehei-Kaster pivoting disc aortic prosthesis and a comparative study of its pulsatile flow characteristics with four other prostheses. *Trans Am Soc Artif Intern Organs* 1970;16:233–243.

7. Hall KV. The Medtronic Hall heart valve: background, latest results, and future work. *Ann Thorac Surg* 1989;48[Suppl 3]:S47–S48.

8. Gott VL, Daggett RL, Young WP. Development of a carbon-coated, central-hinging, bileaflet valve. *Ann Thorac Surg* 1989:48[Suppl 3]:S28–S30.

9. Ross DN. Homograft replacement of the aortic valve. *Lancet* 1967;2:487.

10. Carpentier A, Chanard JC, Laurens P, et al. Use of aortic heterografts in treatment of mitral valvulopathy: experimental basis and first clinical case. *Mem Acad Chir (Paris)* 1967;93:617–622.

11. Ionescu MI, Pakrashi BC, Mary DA, et al. Replacement of heart valves with frame-mounted tissue grafts. *Thorax* 1974;29:56–67.

12. Ross D, Jackson M, Davies J. The pulmonary autograft: a permanent aortic valve. *Eur J Cardiothorac Surg* 1992;6:113–116.

13. Doty DB, Acar C. Mitral valve replacement with homograft. *Ann Thorac Surg* 1998;66:2127–2131.

14. Shellock FG, Curtis JS. MR imaging and biomedical implants, materials, and devices: an updated review. *Radiology* 1991;180:541–550.

15. Deutsch HJ, Bachmann R, Sechtem U, et al. Regurgitant flow in cardiac valve prostheses: diagnostic value of gradient echo nuclear magnetic resonance imaging in reference to transesophageal two-dimensional color Doppler echocardiography. *J Am Coll Cardiol* 1992;119:1500–1507.

16. Botnar R, Nagel E, Scheidegger MB, et al. Assessment of prosthetic aortic valve performance by magnetic resonance velocity imaging. *MAGMA* 2000;10:18–26.

17. Grossman W. Profiles in valvular heart disease. In: Bain DS, Grossman W. *Cardiac catheterization, angiography and intervention*, 5th ed. Baltimore: Williams & Wilkins, 1996:735–756.

18. Morton MJ, Rahimtoola SH. How to follow patients with prosthetic heart valves. *J Cardiovasc Med* 1980;5:475–495.

19. Baumgartner H, Khan S, DeRobertis M, et al. Effect of prosthetic aortic valve design on the Doppler-catheter gradient correlation: an in vitro study of normal St. Jude, Medtronic-Hall, Starr-Edwards and Hancock valves. *J Am Coll Cardiol* 1992;19:324–332.

20. Baumgartner H, Schima H, Kuhn P. Effect of prosthetic valve malfunction on the Doppler-catheter gradient relation for bileaflet aortic valve prostheses. *Circulation* 1993;87:1320–1327.

21. Weyman AE. Principles of flow. In: Weyman AE. *Principles and practice of echocardiography*. 2nd ed. Philadelphia: Lea & Febiger, 1994:184–200.

22. Baumgartner H, Khan SS, DeRobertis M, et al. Doppler assessment of prosthetic valve orifice area: an in vitro study. *Circulation* 1992;85:2275–2283.

23. Morehead AJ, Firstenberg MS, Shiota T 3d, et al. Intraoperative echocardiographic detection of regurgitant jets after valve replacement. *Ann Thorac Surg* 2000;69:135–139.

24. van den Brink RB, Visser CA, Basart DC, et al. Comparison of transthoracic and transesophageal color Doppler flow imaging in patients with mechanical prostheses in the mitral valve position. *Am J Cardiol* 1989;63:1471–1474.

25. Fuster V, Pumphrey CW, McGoon MD, et al. Systemic thromboembolism in mitral and aortic Starr-Edwards prostheses: a 10–19 year follow-up. *Circulation* 1982;66[2 Part 2]:I157–I161.

26. Hammermeister KE, Sethi GK, Henderson WG, et al. A comparison of outcomes in men 11 years after heart-valve replacement with a mechanical valve or bioprosthesis. Veterans Affairs Cooperative Study on Valvular Heart Disease. *N Engl J Med* 1993;328:1289–1296.

27. Krosnick A. Death due to migration of the ball from an aortic valve prosthesis. *JAMA* 1965;191:1083–1094.

28. Currie PJ, Seward JB, Lam JB, et al. Left ventricular outflow tract obstruction related to a valve prosthesis: case caused by a low-profile mitral prosthesis. *Mayo Clin Proc* 1985;60:184–187.

29. Gabbay S, McQueen DM, Yellin EL, et al. In vitro hydrodynamic comparison of mitral valve prostheses at high flow rates. *J Thorac Cardiovasc Surg* 1978;76:771–787.

30. Horstkotte D, Haerten K, Herzer JA, et al. Five-year results after randomized mitral valve replacement with Björk-Shiley, Lillehei-Kaster, and Starr-Edwards prostheses. *Thorac Cardiovasc Surg* 1983;31:206–214.

31. Sala A, Schoevaerdts JC, Jaumin P, et al. Review of 387 isolated mitral valve replacements by the Model 6120 Starr-Edwards prosthesis. *J Thorac Cardiovasc Surg* 1982;84:744–750.

32. Walker DK, Scotten LN, Modi VJ, et al. In vitro assessment of mitral valve prostheses. *J Thorac Cardiovasc Surg* 1980;79:680–688.

33. Schaff HV, Chesebro JH. Experience with the Starr-Edwards silastic ball valve. *Cardiol Clin* 1985;3:405–416.

34. Pyle RB, Mayer JE Jr, Lindsay WG, et al. Hemodynamic evaluation of Lillehei-Kaiser and Starr-Edwards prosthesis. *Ann Thorac Surg* 1978;26:336–343.

35. Winter TQ, Reis RL, Glancy DL, et al. Current status of the Starr-Edwards cloth-covered prosthetic cardiac valves. *Circulation* 1972;45[5 Suppl 1]:14–24.

36. Williams GA, Labovitz AJ. Doppler hemodynamic evaluation of prosthetic (Starr-Edwards and Björk-Shiley) and bioprosthetic (Hancock and Carpentier-Edwards) cardiac valves. *Am J Cardiol* 1985;56:325–332.

37. Dellsperger KC, Wieting DW, Baehr DA, et al. Regurgitation of prosthetic heart valves: dependence on heart rate and cardiac output. *Am J Cardiol* 1983;51:321–328.

38. Cartwright RS, Smeloff EA, Davey TB, et al. Development of a titanium double-caged full-orifice ball valve. *Trans Am Soc Artif Intern Organs* 1964;10:231–236.

39. Magovern GJ, Cromie HW. Sutureless prosthetic heart valves. *J Thorac Cardiovasc Surg* 1963;46:726–736.

40. Braunwald NS, Tatooles C, Turina M, et al. New developments in the design of fabric-covered prosthetic heart valves. *J Thorac Cardiovasc Surg* 1971;62:673–682.

41. Thulin LI, Bain WH, Huysmans HH, et al. Heart valve replacement with the Björk-Shiley Monostrut valve: early results of a multicenter clinical investigation. *Ann Thorac Surg* 1988;45:164–170.

42. Reif TH, Huffstutler MC Jr. Design considerations for the omniscience pivoting disc cardiac valve prosthesis. *Int J Artif Organs* 1983;6:131–138.

43. Scotten LN, Racca RG, Nugent AH, et al. New tilting disc cardiac valve prostheses: in vitro comparison of their hydrodynamic performance in the mitral position. *J Thorac Cardiovasc Surg* 1981;82:136–146.

44. Emery RW, Mettler E, Nicoloff DM. A new cardiac prosthesis: the St. Jude Medical cardiac valve: in vivo results. *Circulation* 1979;60[2 Part 2]:48–54.

45. Subotic S, Petrovic P, Boskovic D, et al. Clinical and functional evaluation of the CarboMedics Prosthetic Heart Valve in the mitral position: preliminary results. *J Cardiovasc Surg* 1990;31:509–511.

46. Wang JH. The design simplicity and clinical elegance of the St. Jude Medical heart valve. *Ann Thorac Surg* 1989;48[3 Suppl]:S55–S56.

47. Bernal JM, Martin-Duran R, Rabasa J, et al. The CarboMedics "Top-Hat" supraannular prosthesis. *Ann Thorac Surg* 1999;67:1299–1303.

48. Kaps M, Hansen J, Weiher M, et al. Clinically silent microemboli in patients with artificial prosthetic aortic valves are predominantly gaseous and not solid. *Stroke* 1997;28:322–325.

49. Muller HR, Pfister M, Gradel E, et al. Simultaneous bilateral transcranial Doppler sonography for the detection of middle cerebral artery microemboli from mechanical prosthetic valves. *Cerebrovasc Dis* 1994;4:393–397.

50. Yoganathan AP, Chaux A, Gray RJ, et al. Bileaflet, tilting disc and porcine aortic valve substitutes: in vitro hydrodynamic characteristics. *J Am Coll Cardiol* 1984;3[2 Part 1]:313–320.

51. Holen J, Aaslid R, Landmark K, et al. Determination of pressure gradient in mitral stenosis with a non-invasive ultrasound Doppler technique. *Acta Med Scand* 1976;199:455–460.

52. Wilkins GT, Gillam LD, Kritzer GL, et al. Validation of continuous-wave Doppler echocardiographic measurements of mitral and tricuspid prosthetic valve gradients: a simultaneous Doppler-catheter study. *Circulation* 1986;74:786–795.

53. Baumgartner H, Khan S, DeRobertis M, et al. Discrepancies between Doppler and catheter gradients in aortic prosthetic valves in vitro: a manifestation of localized gradients and pressure recovery. *Circulation* 1990;82:1467–1475.

54. Carpentier A, Lemaigre G, Robert L, et al. Biological factors affecting long-term results of valvular heterografts. *J Thorac Cardiovasc Surg* 1969;58:467–483.

55. Logeais Y, Langanay T, Leguerrier A, et al. Aortic Carpentier-Edwards supraannular porcine bioprosthesis: a 12-year experience. *Ann Thorac Surg* 1999;68:421–425.

56. Wong SP, Legget ME, Greaves SC, et al. Early experience with the mosaic bioprosthesis: a new generation porcine valve. *Ann Thorac Surg* 2000;69:1846–1850.

57. Lurie AJ, Miller RR, Maxwell KS, et al. Hemodynamic assessment of the glutaraldehyde-preserved porcine heterograft in the aortic and mitral positions. *Circulation* 1977;56[3 Suppl]:II104–II110.

58. Stinson EB, Griepp RB, Oyer PE, et al. Long-term experience with porcine aortic valve xenografts. *J Thorac Cardiovasc Surg* 1977;73:54–63.

59. Cohn LH, Collins JJ Jr, Rizzo RJ, et al. Twenty-year follow-up of the Hancock modified orifice porcine aortic valve. *Ann Thorac Surg* 1998;66[6 Suppl]:S30–S34.

60. Jamieson WR, Tyers GF, Janusz MT, et al. Age as a determinant for selection of porcine bioprostheses for cardiac valve replacement: experience with Carpentier-Edwards standard bioprosthesis. *Can J Cardiol* 1991;7:181–188.

61. Jamieson WR, Rosado LJ, Munro AI, et al. Carpentier-Edwards standard porcine bioprosthesis: primary tissue failure (structural valve deterioration) by age groups. *Ann Thorac Surg* 1988;46:155–162.

62. Ionescu MI, Tandon AP, Mary DA, et al. Heart valve replacement with the Ionescu-Shiley pericardial xenograft. *Thorac Cardiovasc Surg* 1977;3:31–42.

63. Bove EL, Marvasti MA, Potts JL, et al. Rest and exercise hemodynamics following aortic valve replacement: a comparison between 19 and 21 mm Ionescu-Shiley pericardial and Carpentier-Edwards porcine valves. *J Thorac Cardiovasc Surg* 1985;90:750–755.

64. Pelletier LC, Carrier M, Leclerc Y, et al. Porcine versus pericardial bioprostheses: a comparison of late results in 1,593 patients. *Ann Thorac Surg* 1989;47:352–361.

65. Cosgrove DM, Lytle BW, Williams GW. Hemodynamic performance of the Carpentier-Edwards pericardial valve in the aortic position in vivo. *Circulation* 1985;72[3 Part 2]:II146–II152.

66. Bortolotti U, Milano A, Mazzaro E, et al. Hancock II porcine bioprosthesis: excellent durability at intermediate-term follow-up. *J Am Coll Cardiol* 1994;24:676–682.

67. Van Nooten G, Caes F, Francois K, et al. Stentless or stented aortic valve implants in elderly patients? *Eur J Cardiothorac Surg* 1999;15:31–36.

68. Williams RJ, Muir DF, Pathi V, et al. Randomized controlled trial of stented and stentless aortic bioprostheses: hemodynamic performance at 3 years. *Semin Thorac Cardiovasc Surg* 1999;11[4 Suppl 1]:93–97.

69. Pibarot P, Dumesnil JG, Jobin J, et al. Hemodynamic and physical performance during maximal exercise in patients with an aortic bioprosthetic valve: comparison of stentless versus stented bioprostheses. *J Am Coll Cardiol* 1999;34:1609–1617.

70. Collinson J, Henein M, Flather M, et al. Valve replacement for aortic stenosis in patients with poor left ventricular function: comparison of early changes with stented and stentless valves. *Circulation* 1999;100[19 Suppl]:II1–II5.

71. Kon ND, Cordell AR, Adair SM, et al. Aortic root replacement with the freestyle stentless porcine aortic root bioprosthesis. *Ann Thorac Surg* 1999;67:1609–1615.

72. David TE, Feindel CM, Scully HE, et al. Aortic valve replacement with stentless porcine aortic valves: a ten-year experience. *J Heart Valve Dis* 1998;7(3):250–254.

73. Doty DB, Michielon G, Wang ND, et al. Replacement of the aortic valve with cryopreserved aortic allograft. *Ann Thorac Surg* 1993;56:228–235.

74. Heslop BF, Wilson SE, Hardy BE. Antigenicity of aortic valve allografts. *Ann Surg* 1973;177:301–306.

75. Angell WW, Angell JD, Oury JH, et al. Long-term follow-up of viable frozen aortic homografts: a viable homograft valve bank. *J Thorac Cardiovasc Surg* 1987;93:815–822.

76. Langley SM, McGuirk SP, Chaudhry MA, et al. Twenty-year follow-up of aortic valve replacement with antibiotic sterilized homografts in 200 patients. *Semin Thorac Cardiovasc Surg* 1999;11[4 Suppl 1]:28–34.

77. Barratt-Boyes BG, Roche AH, Subramanyan R, et al. Long-term follow-up of patients with the antibiotic-sterilized aortic homograft valve inserted freehand in the aortic position. *Circulation* 1987;75(4):768–777.

78. Grenadier E, Sahn DJ, Roche AH, et al. Detection of deterioration or infection of homograft and porcine xenograft bioprosthetic valves in mitral and aortic positions by two-dimensional echocardiographic examination. *J Am Coll Cardiol* 1983;2:452–459.

79. O'Brien MF, Stafford EG, Gardner MA, et al. A comparison of aortic valve replacement with viable cryopreserved and fresh allograft valves, with a note on chromosomal studies. *J Thorac Cardiovasc Surg* 1987;94:812–823.

80. Chan KC, Fyfe DA, McKay CA, et al. Right ventricular outflow reconstruction with cryopreserved homografts in pediatric patients: intermediate-term follow-up with serial echocardiographic assessment. *J Am Coll Cardiol* 1994;24:483–489.

81. Petrou M, Wong K, Albertucci M, et al. Evaluation of unstented aortic homografts for the treatment of prosthetic aortic valve endocarditis. *Circulation* 1994;90[5 Part 2]:II198–II204.

82. Bloomfield P, Wheatley DJ, Prescott RJ, et al. Twelve-year comparison of a Björk-Shiley mechanical heart valve with porcine bioprostheses. *N Engl J Med* 1991;324:573–579.

83. Pansini S, Ottino G, Forsennati PG, et al. Reoperations on heart valve prostheses: an analysis of operative risks and late results. *Ann Thorac Surg* 1990;50:590–596.

84. Bortolotti U, Milano A, Mossuto E, et al. The risk of reoperation in patients with bioprosthetic valves. *J Card Surg* 1991;6[4 Suppl]:638–643.

85. Jones EL, Weintraub WS, Craver JM, et al. Ten-year experience with the porcine bioprosthetic valve: interrelationship of valve survival and patient survival in 1,050 valve replacements. *Ann Thorac Surg* 1990;49:370–383.

86. Ibrahim M, Cleland J, O'Kane H, et al. St. Jude Medical prosthesis in children. *J Thorac Cardiovasc Surg* 1994;108:52–56.

87. Bernal JM, Rabasa JM, Cagigas JC, et al. Valve-related complications with the Hancock I porcine bioprosthesis: a twelve- to fourteen-year follow-up study. *J Thorac Cardiovasc Surg* 1991;101:871–880.

88. Grunkemeier GL, Jamieson WR, Miller DC, et al. Actuarial versus actual risk of porcine structural valve deterioration. *J Thorac Cardiovasc Surg* 1994;108:709–718.

89. Sareli P, England MJ, Berk MR, et al. Maternal and fetal sequelae of anticoagulation during pregnancy in patients with mechanical heart valve prostheses. *Am J Cardiol* 1989;63:1462–1465.

90. Iturbe-Alessio I, Fonseca MC, Mutchinik O, et al. Risks of anticoagulant therapy in pregnant women with artificial heart valves. *N Engl J Med* 1986;315:1390–1393.

91. Hammond GL, Geha AS, Kopf GS, et al. Biological versus mechanical valves: analysis of 1,116 valves inserted in 1,012 adult patients with a 4,818 patient-year and a 5,327 valve-year follow-up. *J Thorac Cardiovasc Surg* 1987;93:182–198.

92. Hanania G, Thomas D, Michel PL, et al. Pregnancy and prosthetic heart valves: a French cooperative retrospective study of 155 cases. *Eur Heart J* 1994;15:1651–1658.

93. Salazar E, Espinola N, Roman L, et al. Effect of pregnancy on the duration of bovine pericardial bioprosthesis. *Am Heart J* 1999;137[4 Part 1]:714–720.

94. Clark SL. Cardiac disease in pregnancy. *Obst Gyn Clin North Am* 1991;18:237–256.

95. Cohn LH. Surgery for mitral regurgitation. *JAMA* 1988;260:2883–2887.

96. Strauss B, Marquis JF. Percutaneous valvuloplasty as a treatment for aortic and mitral valve disease. *Am Heart J* 1990;119:1184–1192.

97. Kouchoukos NT, Davila-Roman VG, Spray TL, et al. Replacement of the aortic root with a pulmonary autograft in children and young adults with aortic-valve disease. *N Engl J Med* 1994;330:1–6.

98. Kaplon RJ, Cosgrove DM 3d, Gillinov AM, et al. Cardiac valve replacement in patients on dialysis: influence of prosthesis on survival. *Ann Thorac Surg* 2000;70:438–441.

99. Bolooki H, Mallon S, Kaiser GA, et al. Failure of Hancock xenograft valve: importance of valve position (4- to 9-year follow-up). *Ann Thorac Surg* 1983;36:246–252.

100. Magilligan DJ Jr, Kemp SR, Stein PD, et al. Asynchronous primary valve failure in patients with porcine bioprosthetic aortic and mitral valves. *Circulation* 1987;76[3 Part 2]:III141–III145.

101. Chen CR, Cheng TO, Huang T, et al. Percutaneous balloon valvuloplasty for pulmonic stenosis in adolescents and adults. *N Engl J Med* 1996;335:21–25.

102. Ohri SK, Schofield JB, Hodgson H, et al. Carcinoid heart disease: early failure of an allograft valve replacement. *Ann Thorac Surg* 1994;58:1161–1163.

103. Pumphrey CW, Fuster V, Chesebro JH. Systemic thromboembolism in valvular heart disease and prosthetic heart valves. *Mod Concepts Cardiovasc Dis* 1982;51(12):131–136.

104. Moggio RA, Hammond GL, Stansel HC Jr, et al. Incidence of emboli with cloth-covered Starr-Edwards valve without anticoagulation and with varying forms of anticoagulation: analysis of 183 patients followed for 3 1/2 years. *J Thorac Cardiovasc Surg* 1978;75:296–299.

105. Akbarian M, Austen G, Yurchak PM, et al. Thromboembolic complications of prosthetic cardiac valves. *Circulation* 1968;37:826–831.

106. Chaux A, Gray RJ, Matloff JM, et al. An appreciation of the new St. Jude valvular prosthesis. *J Thorac Cardiovasc Surg* 1981;81:202–211.

107. Dewanjee MK, Trastek VF, Tago M, et al. Noninvasive radioisotopic technique for detection of platelet deposition on bovine pericardial mitral-valve prosthesis and in vitro quantification of visceral microembolism in dogs. *Trans Am Soc Artif Intern Organs* 1983;29:188–193.

108. Burchfiel CM, Hammermeister KE, Krause-Steinrauf H, et al. Left atrial dimension and risk of systemic embolism in patients with a prosthetic heart valve. Department of Veterans Affairs Cooperative Study on Valvular Heart Disease. *J Am Coll Cardiol* 1990;15:32–41.

109. Yeh TJ, Anabtawi IN, Cornett VE, et al. Influence of rhythm and anticoagulation upon the incidence of embolization associated with Starr-Edwards prostheses. *Circulation* 1967;35[4 Suppl]:I77–I81.

110. Boruchow IB, Ramsey HW, Wheat MW Jr. Complications following destruction of the cloth covering of a Starr-Edwards aortic valve prosthesis. *J Thorac Cardiovasc Surg* 1971;62:290–293.

111. Miller DC, Oyer PE, Stinson EB, et al. Ten to fifteen year reassessment of the performance characteristics of the Starr-Edwards Model 6120 mitral valve prosthesis. *J Thorac Cardiovasc Surg* 1983;85:1–20.

112. Antunes MJ, Wessels A, Sadowski RG, et al. Medtronic Hall valve replacement in a third-world population group: a review of the performance of 1000 prostheses. *J Thorac Cardiovasc Surg* 1988;95:980–993.

113. Arom KV, Nicoloff DM, Kersten TE, et al. St. Jude Medical prosthesis: valve-related deaths and complications. *Ann Thorac Surg* 1987;43:591–598.

114. Czer LS, Matloff JM, Chaux A, et al. The St. Jude valve: analysis of thromboembolism, warfarin-related hemorrhage, and survival. *Am Heart J* 1987;114:389–397.

115. Duncan JM, Cooley DA, Reul GJ, et al. Durability and low thrombogenicity of the St. Jude Medical valve at 5-year follow-up. *Ann Thorac Surg* 1986;42:500–505.

116. Horstkotte D, Korfer R, Seipel L, et al. Late complications in patients with Björk-Shiley and St. Jude Medical heart valve replacement. *Circulation* 1983;68[3 Part 2]:II175–II184.

117. LeClerc JL, Wellens P, Douvaert FE, et al. Long-term results with the St. Jude Medical valvular prosthesis. In: DeBakey ME, ed. *Advances in cardiac valves, clinical perspectives.* New York: Yorke Medical Books, 1983:33–41.

118. Murphy DA, Levine FH, Buckley MJ, et al. Mechanical valves: a comparative analysis of the Starr-Edwards and Björk-Shiley prostheses. *J Thorac Cardiovasc Surg* 1983;86:746–752.

119. Cannegieter SC, Rosendaal FR, Briet E. Thromboembolic and bleeding complications in patients with mechanical heart valve prostheses. *Circulation* 1994;89:635–641.

120. Cannegieter SC, Rosendaal FR, Wintzen AR, et al. Optimal oral anticoagulant therapy in patients with mechanical heart valves. *N Engl J Med* 1995;333:11–17.

121. Saour JN, Sieck JO, Mamo LA, et al. Trial of different intensities of anticoagulation in patients with prosthetic heart valves. *N Engl J Med* 1990;322:428–432.

122. Patrassi GM, Cardin G, Schiavinato ML, et al. Decreased thrombotic mortality and morbidity after valvular cardiac surgery as a consequence of adequate coumarin anticoagulation: a retrospective study in 516 patients. *Folia Haematol Int Mag Klin Morphol Blutforsch* 1978;105:690–699.

123. Watzke HH, Forberg E, Svolba G, et al. A prospective controlled trial comparing weekly self-testing and self-dosing with the standard management of patients on stable oral anticoagulation. *Thromb Haemost* 2000;83:661–665.

124. Turpie AG, Gent M, Laupacis A, et al. A comparison of aspirin with placebo in patients treated with warfarin after heart-valve replacement. *N Engl J Med* 1993;329:524–529.

125. Laffort P, Roudaut R, Roques X, et al. Early and long-term (one-year) effects of the association of aspirin and oral anticoagulant on thrombi and morbidity after replacement of the mitral valve with the St. Jude medical prosthesis: a clinical and transesophageal echocardiographic study. *J Am Coll Cardiol* 2000;35:739–746.

126. Altman R, Boullon F, Rouvier J, et al. Aspirin and prophylaxis of thromboembolic complications in patients with substitute heart valves. *J Thorac Cardiovasc Surg* 1976;72:127–129.

127. Dale J, Myhre E, Storstein O, et al. Prevention of arterial thromboembolism with acetylsalicylic acid: a controlled clinical study in patients with aortic ball valves. *Am Heart J* 1977;94:101–111.

128. Sullivan JM, Harken DE, Gorlin R. Effect of dipyridamole on the incidence of arterial emboli after cardiac valve replacement. *Circulation* 1969;39[5 Suppl]:I149–I153.

129. Israel DH, Sharma SK, Fuster V. Antithrombotic therapy in prosthetic heart valve replacement. *Am Heart J* 1994;127:400–411.

130. Hayashi J, Nakazawa S, Oguma F, et al. Combined warfarin and antiplatelet therapy after St. Jude Medical valve replacement for mitral valve disease. *J Am Coll Cardiol* 1994;23:672–677.

131. Heras M, Chesebro JH, Fuster V, et al. High risk of thromboemboli early after bioprosthetic cardiac valve replacement. *J Am Coll Cardiol* 1995;25:1111–1119.

132. Turpie AG, Gunstensen J, Hirsh J, et al. Randomised comparison of two intensities of oral anticoagulant therapy after tissue heart valve replacement. *Lancet* 1988;1:1242–1245.

133. Nunez L, Gil Aguado M, Larrea JL, et al. Prevention of thromboembolism using aspirin after mitral valve replacement with porcine bioprosthesis. *Ann Thorac Surg* 1984;37:84–87.

134. Laros RK Jr, Alger LS. Thromboembolism and pregnancy. *Clin Obstet Gynecol* 1979;22:871–878.

135. Stevenson RE, Burton OM, Ferlauto GJ, et al. Hazards of oral anticoagulants during pregnancy. *JAMA* 1980;243:1549–1551.

136. Lutz DJ, Noller KL, Spittell JA Jr, et al. Pregnancy and its complications following cardiac valve prostheses. *Am J Obstet Gynecol* 1978;131:460–468.

137. Ginsberg JS, Hirsh J. Use of antithrombotic agents during pregnancy. *Chest* 1995;108[4 Suppl]:305S–311S.

138. Whitfield LR, Lele AS, Levy G. Effect of pregnancy on the relationship between concentration and anticoagulant action of heparin. *Clin Pharmacol Ther* 1983;34:23–28.

139. Ginsberg JS, Kowalchuk G, Hirsh J, et al. Heparin therapy during pregnancy. *Arch Intern Med* 1989;149:2233–2236.

140. Larrea JL, Nunez L, Reque JA, et al. Pregnancy and mechanical valve prostheses: a high-risk situation for the mother and the fetus. *Ann Thorac Surg* 1983;36:459–463.

141. Hirsh J, Cade JF, Gallus AS. Anticoagulants in pregnancy: a review of indications and complications. *Am Heart J* 1972;83:301–305.

142. Rasmussen C, Wadt J, Jacobsen B. Thromboembolic prophylaxis with low molecular weight heparin during pregnancy. *Int J Gynaecol Obst* 1994;47:121–125.

143. CLASP (Collaborative Low-Dose Aspirin Study in Pregnancy): a randomised trial of low-dose aspirin for the prevention and treatment of pre-eclampsia among 9364 pregnant women. *Lancet* 1994;343:619–629.

144. Tinker JH, Tarhan S. Discontinuing anticoagulant therapy in surgical patients with cardiac valve prostheses: observations in 180 operations. *JAMA* 1978;239:738–739.

145. Sherman DG, Dyken ML Jr, Gent M, et al. Antithrombotic therapy for cerebrovascular disorders: an update. *Chest* 1995;108[4 Suppl]:444S–456S.

146. Cerebral Embolism Study Group. Immediate anticoagulation of embolic stroke: a randomized trial. *Stroke* 1983;14:668–676.

147. Cerebral Embolism Study Group. Immediate anticoagulation of embolic stroke: brain hemorrhage and management option. *Stroke* 1984;15:779–789.

148. Wilson WR, Geraci JE, Danielson GK, et al. Anticoagulant therapy and central nervous system complications in patients with prosthetic valve endocarditis. *Circulation* 1978;57:1004–1007.

149. Block PC, DeSanctis RW, Weinberg AN, et al. Prosthetic valve endocarditis. *J Thorac Cardiovasc Surg* 1970;60:540–548.

150. Copans H, Lakier JB, Kinsley RH, et al. Thrombosed Björk-Shiley mitral prostheses. *Circulation* 1980;61:169–174.

151. Edmunds LH Jr. Thromboembolic complications of current cardiac valvular prostheses. *Ann Thorac Surg* 1982;34:96–106.

152. Cortina JM, Martinell J, Artiz V, et al. Comparative clinical results with Omniscience (STM1), Medtronic-Hall, and Björk-Shiley convexo-concave (70 degrees) prostheses in mitral valve replacement. *J Thorac Cardiovasc Surg* 1986;91:174–183.

153. Thorburn CW, Morgan JJ, Shanahan MX, et al. Long-term results of tricuspid valve replacement and the problem of prosthetic valve thrombosis. *Am J Cardiol* 1983;51:1128–1132.

154. Deviri E, Sareli P, Wisenbaugh T, et al. Obstruction of mechanical heart valve prostheses: clinical aspects and surgical management. *J Am Coll Cardiol* 1991;17:646–650.

155. Kontos GJ Jr, Schaff HV, Orszulak TA, et al. Thrombotic obstruction of disc valves: clinical recognition and surgical management. *Ann Thorac Surg* 1989;48:60–65.

156. Ledain LD, Ohayon JP, Colle JP, et al. Acute thrombotic obstruction with disc valve prostheses: diagnostic considerations and fibrinolytic treatment. *J Am Coll Cardiol* 1986;7:743–751.

157. Gueret P, Vignon P, Fournier P, et al. Transesophageal echocardiography for the diagnosis and management of nonobstructive thrombosis of mechanical mitral valve prosthesis. *Circulation* 1995;91:103–110.

158. Vasan RS, Kaul U, Sanghvi S, et al. Thrombolytic therapy for prosthetic valve thrombosis: a study based on serial Doppler echocardiographic evaluation. *Am Heart J* 1992;123:1575–1580.

159. Kurzrok S, Singh AK, Most AS, et al. Thrombolytic therapy for prosthetic cardiac valve thrombosis. *J Am Coll Cardiol* 1987;9:592–598.

160. Reddy NK, Padmanabhan TN, Singh S, et al. Thrombolysis in left-sided prosthetic valve occlusion: immediate and follow-up results. *Ann Thorac Surg* 1994;58:462–470.

161. Roudaut R, Labbe T, Lorient-Roudaut MF, et al. Mechanical cardiac valve thrombosis: is fibrinolysis justified? *Circulation* 1992;86[5 Suppl]:II8–II15.

162. Jost CM, Yancy CW Jr, Ring WS. Combined thrombolytic therapy for prosthetic mitral valve thrombosis. *Ann Thorac Surg* 1993;55:159–161.

163. Hurrell DG, Schaff HV, Tajik AJ. Thrombolytic therapy for obstruction of mechanical prosthetic valves. *Mayo Clin Proc* 1996;71:605–613.

164. Guerrero Lopez F, Vazquez Mata G, Reina Toral A, et al. Thrombolytic treatment for massive thrombosis of prosthetic cardiac valves. *Intensive Care Med* 1993;19:145–150.

165. Vitale N, Renzulli A, Cerasuolo F, et al. Prosthetic valve obstruction: thrombolysis versus operation. *Ann Thorac Surg* 1994;57:365–370.

166. Puleo JA, Fontanet HL, Schocken DD. The role of prolonged thrombolytic infusions and transesophageal echocardiography in thrombosed prosthetic heart valves: case report and review of the literature. *Clin Cardiol* 1995;18:679–684.

167. Ozkan M, Kaymaz C, Kirma C, et al. Intravenous thrombolytic treatment of mechanical prosthetic valve thrombosis: a study using serial transesophageal echocardiography. *J Am Coll Cardiol* 2000;35:1881–1889.

168. Shapira Y, Herz I, Vaturi M, et al. Thrombolysis is an effective and safe therapy in stuck bileaflet mitral valves in the absence of high-risk thrombi. *J Am Coll Cardiol* 2000;35:1874–1880.

169. Husebye DG, Pluth JR, Piehler JM, et al. Reoperation on prosthetic heart valves: an analysis of risk factors in 552 patients. *J Thorac Cardiovasc Surg* 1983;86:543–552.

170. Grunkemeier GL, Starr A. Twenty-five year experience with Starr-Edwards heart valves: follow-up methods and results. *Can J Cardiol* 1988;4:381–385.

171. Williams DB, Pluth JR, Orszulak TA. Extrinsic obstruction of the Björk-Shiley valve in the mitral position. *Ann Thorac Surg* 1981;32:58–62.

172. Berger RL. Retrograde disc escape in a Harken mitral valve prosthesis. *Ann Thorac Surg* 1992;54:394–395.

173. Dimitri WR, Williams BT. Fracture of the Duromedics mitral valve housing with leaflet escape. *J Cardiovasc Surg* 1990;31:41–46.

174. Kornberg A, Wildhirt SM, Schulze C, et al. Leaflet escape in Omnicarbon monoleaflet valve. *Eur J Cardiothorac Surg* 1999;15:867–869.

175. Björk VO. The improved Björk-Shiley tilting disc valve prosthesis. *Scand J Thorac Cardiovasc Surg* 1978;12:81–84.

176. Hiratzka LF, Kouchoukos NT, Grunkemeier GL, et al. Outlet strut fracture of the Björk-Shiley 60 degrees Convexo-Concave valve: current information and recommendations for patient care. *J Am Coll Cardiol* 1988;11:1130–1137.

177. Birkmeyer JD, Marrin CA, O'Connor GT. Should patients with Björk-Shiley valves undergo prophylactic replacement? *Lancet* 1992;340:520–523.

178. van der Meulen JH, Steyerberg EW, van der Graaf Y, et al. Age thresholds for prophylactic replacement of Björk-Shiley convexo-concave heart valves: a clinical and economic evaluation. *Circulation* 1993;88:156–164.

179. Lindblom D, Rodriguez L, Björk VO. Mechanical failure of the Björk-Shiley valve: updated follow-up and considerations on prophylactic rereplacement. *J Thorac Cardiovasc Surg* 1989;97:95–97.

180. O'Neill WW, Chandler JG, Gordon RE, et al. Radiographic detection of strut separations in Björk-Shiley convexo-concave mitral valves. *N Engl J Med* 1995;333:414–419.

181. Dow JJ, Plemons TD, Scarbrough K, et al. Acoustic assessment of the physical integrity of Björk-Shiley convexo-concave heart valves. *Circulation* 1997;95:905–909.

182. Schoen FJ, Levy RJ. Bioprosthetic heart valve failure: pathology and pathogenesis. *Cardiol Clin* 1984;2:717–739.

183. Ferrans VJ, Spray TL, Billingham ME, et al. Structural changes in glutaraldehyde-treated porcine heterografts used as substitute cardiac valves: transmission and scanning electron microscopic observations in 12 patients. *Am J Cardiol* 1978;41:1159–1184.

184. Alam M, Lakier JB, Pickard SD, et al. Echocardiographic evaluation of porcine bioprosthetic valves: experience with 309 normal and 59 dysfunctioning valves. *Am J Cardiol* 1983;52:309–315.

185. O'Brien MF, Stafford EG, Gardner MA, et al. Allograft aortic valve replacement: long-term follow-up. *Ann Thorac Surg* 1995;60[2 Suppl]:S65–S70.

186. Yacoub M, Rasmi NR, Sundt TM, et al. Fourteen-year experience with homovital homografts for aortic valve replacement. *J Thorac Cardiovasc Surg* 1995;110:186–193, discussion 193–194.

187. Oyer PE, Stinson EB, Reitz BA, et al. Long-term evaluation of the porcine xenograft bioprosthesis. *J Thorac Cardiovasc Surg* 1979;78:343–350.

188. Cohn LH, Mudge GH, Pratter F, et al. Five to eight-year follow-up of patients undergoing porcine heart-valve replacement. *N Engl J Med* 1981;304:258–262.

189. Jamieson WR, Marchand MA, Pelletier CL, et al. Structural valve deterioration in mitral replacement surgery: comparison of Carpentier-Edwards supra-annular porcine and perimount pericardial bioprostheses. *J Thorac Cardiovasc Surg* 1999;118:297–304.

190. Tansley PD, Sheppard MN, Pepper J. Symptomatic calcific stenosis of a Toronto stentless porcine valve. *Eur J Cardiothorac Surg* 2000;17:763–765.

191. Bansal RC, Morrison DL, Jacobson JG. Echocardiography of porcine aortic prosthesis with flail leaflets due to degeneration and calcification. *Am Heart J* 1984;107:591–593.

192. Akiyama K, Sawatani O, Imamura E, et al. Stent creep of porcine bioprosthesis in the mitral position. *Ann Thorac Surg* 1988;46:73–78.

193. Calderwood SB, Swinski LA, Waternaux CM, et al. Risk factors for the development of prosthetic valve endocarditis. *Circulation* 1985;72:31–37.

194. Wilson WR, Danielson GK, Giuliani ER, et al. Prosthetic valve endocarditis. *Mayo Clin Proc* 1982;57:155–161.

195. Ivert TS, Dismukes WE, Cobbs CG, et al. Prosthetic valve endocarditis. *Circulation* 1984;69:223–232.

196. Horstkotte D, Piper C, Niehues R, et al. Late prosthetic valve endocarditis. *Eur Heart J* 1995;16[Suppl B]:39–47.

197. Chastre J, Trouillet JL. Early infective endocarditis on prosthetic valves. *Eur Heart J* 1995;16[Suppl B]:32–38.

198. Goldmann DA, Hopkins CC, Karchmer AW, et al. Cephalothin prophylaxis in cardiac valve surgery: a prospective, double-blind comparison of two-day and six-day regimens. *J Thorac Cardiovasc Surg* 1977;73:470–479.

199. Conte JE Jr, Cohen SN, Roe BB, et al. Antibiotic prophylaxis and cardiac surgery: a prospective double-blind comparison of single-dose versus multiple-dose regimens. *Ann Intern Med* 1972;76:943–949.

200. Kloster FE. Diagnosis and management of complications of prosthetic heart valves. *Am J Cardiol* 1975;35:872–885.

201. Arnett EN, Roberts WC. Prosthetic valve endocarditis: clinicopathologic analysis of 22 necropsy patients with comparison observations in 74 necropsy patients with active infective endocarditis involving natural left-sided cardiac valves. *Am J Cardiol* 1976;38(3):281–292.

202. Effron MK, Popp RL. Two-dimensional echocardiographic assessment of bioprosthetic valve dysfunction and infective endocarditis. *J Am Coll Cardiol* 1983;2:597–606.

203. Erbel R, Rohmann S, Drexler M, et al. Improved diagnostic value of echocardiography in patients with infective endocarditis by transoesophageal approach: a prospective study. *Eur Heart J* 1988;9:43–53.

204. Daniel WG, Mugge A, Grote J, et al. Comparison of transthoracic and transesophageal echocardiography for detection of abnormalities of prosthetic and bioprosthetic valves in the mitral and aortic positions. *Am J Cardiol* 1993;71:210–215.

205. Daniel WG, Mugge A, Martin RP, et al. Improvement in the diagnosis of abscesses associated with endocarditis by transesophageal echocardiography. *N Engl J Med* 1991;324:795–800.

206. Sochowski RA, Chan KL. Implication of negative results on a monoplane transesophageal echocardiographic study in patients with suspected infective endocarditis. *J Am Coll Cardiol* 1993;21:216–221.

207. Yu VL, Fang GD, Keys TF, et al. Prosthetic valve endocarditis: superiority of surgical valve replacement versus medical therapy only. *Ann Thorac Surg* 1994;58:1073–1077.

208. Wolff M, Witchitz S, Chastang C, et al. Prosthetic valve endocarditis in the ICU: prognostic factors of overall survival in a series of 122 cases and consequences for treatment decision. *Chest* 1995;108:688–694.

209. Tunkel AR, Kaye D. Endocarditis with negative blood cultures. *N Engl J Med* 1992;326:1215–1217.

210. Threlkeld MG, Cobbs CG. Infectious disorders of prosthetic valves and intravascular devices. In: Mandell GL, Bennett JE, Dolin R, eds. *Mandell, Douglas and Bennett's principles and practice of infectious diseases,* 4th ed, vol 1. New York: Churchill Livingstone, 1995:783–793.

211. Baumgartner WA, Miller DC, Reitz BA, et al. Surgical treatment of prosthetic valve endocarditis. *Ann Thorac Surg* 1983;35:87–104.

212. Cowgill LD, Addonizio VP, Hopeman AR, et al. A practical approach to prosthetic valve endocarditis. *Ann Thorac Surg* 1987;43:450–457.

213. Kirklin JK, Kirklin JW, Pacifico AD. Aortic valve endocarditis with aortic root abscess cavity: surgical treatment with aortic valve homograft. *Ann Thorac Surg* 1988;45:674–677.

214. Lytle BW, Priest BP, Taylor PC, et al. Surgical treatment of prosthetic valve endocarditis. *J Thorac Cardiovasc Surg* 1996;111:198–207.

215. Dossche KM, Defauw JJ, Ernst SM, et al. Allograft aortic root replacement in prosthetic aortic valve endocarditis: a review of 32 patients. *Ann Thorac Surg* 1997;63:1644–1649.

216. Pettersson G, Tingleff J, Joyce FS. Treatment of aortic valve endocarditis with the Ross operation. *Eur J Cardiothorac Surg* 1998;13:678–684.

217. Bertrand S, Houel R, Vermes E, et al. Preliminary experi-

ence with Silzone-coated St. Jude Medical valves in acute infective endocarditis. *J Heart Valve Dis* 2000;9:131–134.

218. Herold U, Van De Wal H, Piotrowski J, et al. Disruption of the silver and non-silver coated sewing cuff of a new generation bileaflet valve prosthesis during aortic valve replacement: report on four cases. *Eur J Cardiothorac Surg* 2000;18:225–227.

219. Fang G, Keys TF, Gentry LO, et al. Prosthetic valve endocarditis resulting from nosocomial bacteremia: a prospective, multicenter study. *Ann Intern Med* 1993;119[7 Part 1]:560–567.

220. Dajani AS, Taubert KA, Wilson W, et al. Prevention of bacterial endocarditis: recommendations by the American Heart Association. *JAMA* 1997;277:1794–1801.

221. Weed RI, Reed CF. Membrane alterations leading to red cell destruction. *Am J Med* 1966;41:681–698.

222. Kastor JA, Akbarian M, Buckley MJ, et al. Paravalvular leaks and hemolytic anemia following insertion of Starr-Edwards aortic and mitral valves. *J Thorac Cardiovasc Surg* 1968;56:279–288.

223. Rodgers BM, Sabiston DC. Hemolytic anemia following prosthetic valve replacement. *Circulation* 1969;39:I-155–I-161.

224. Clark RE, Grubbs FL, McKnight RC, et al. Late clinical problems with Beall model 103 and 104 mitral valve prostheses: hemolysis and valve wear. *Ann Thorac Surg* 1976:21:475–482.

225. Emery RW, Anderson RW, Lindsay WG, et al. Clinical and hemodynamic results with the St. Jude Medical aortic valve prosthesis. *Surg Forum* 1979;30:235–238.

226. Rao KM, Learoyd PA, Rao RS, et al. Chronic haemolysis after Lillehei-Kaster valve replacement: comparison with the findings after Björk-Shiley and Starr-Edwards mitral valve replacement. *Thorax* 1980;35:290–293.

227. Garcia MJ, Vandervoort P, Stewart W, et al. Mechanisms of hemolysis with mitral prosthetic regurgitation: a study using transesophageal echo and fluid dynamic simulation. *J Am Coll Cardiol* 1996;27:399–406.

228. Gradon JD, Hirschbein M, Milligan J. Fragmentation hemolysis: an unusual indication for valve replacement in native valve infective endocarditis. *South Med J* 1996;89:818–820.

229. Enzenauer RJ, Berenberg JL, Cassell PF Jr. Microangiopathic hemolytic anemia as the initial manifestation of porcine valve failure. *South Med J* 1990;83:912–917.

230. Skoularigis J, Essop MR, Skudicky D, et al. Frequency and severity of intravascular hemolysis after left-sided cardiac valve replacement with Medtronic Hall and St. Jude Medical prostheses, and influence of prosthetic type, position, size and number. *Am J Cardiol* 1993;71:587–591.

231. Okita Y, Miki S, Kusuhara K, et al. Propranolol for intractable hemolysis after open heart operation. *Ann Thorac Surg* 1991;52:1158–1160.

232. Dhasmana JP, Blackstone EH, Kirklin JW, et al. Factors associated with periprosthetic leakage following primary mitral valve replacement: with special consideration of the suture technique. *Ann Thorac Surg* 1983;35:170–178.

233. Schapira JN, Martin RP, Fowles RE, et al. Two dimensional echocardiographic assessment of patients with bioprosthetic valves. *Am J Cardiol* 1979;43:510–519.

234. Kotler MN, Goldman A, Parry WR. Noninvasive evaluation of cardiac valve prostheses. *Cardiovasc Clin* 1986;17:201–241.

235. Hourihan M, Perry SB, Mandell VS, et al. Transcatheter umbrella closure of valvular and paravalvular leaks. *J Am Coll Cardiol* 1992;20:1371–1377.

236. Redberg RF, Schiller NB. Use of transesophageal echocardiography in evaluating coronary arteries. *Cardiol Clin* 1993;11:521–528.

237. Herzog CA, Henry TD, Zimmer SD. Bacterial endocarditis presenting as acute myocardial infarction: a cautionary note for the era of reperfusion. *Am J Med* 1991;90:392–397.

238. Waller BF, Taliercio CP, Clark M, et al. Rupture of the left ventricular free wall following mitral valve replacement for mitral stenosis: a cause of complete (fatal) or contained (false aneurysm) cardiac rupture. *Clin Cardiol* 1991;14:341–345.

239. Zabalgoitia M, Kopec K, Abochamh DA, et al. Usefulness of dobutamine echocardiography in the hemodynamic assessment of mechanical prostheses in the aortic valve position. *Am J Cardiol* 1997;80:523–526.

240. Becassis P, Hayot M, Frapier JM, et al. Postoperative exercise tolerance after aortic valve replacement by small-size prosthesis: functional consequence of small-size aortic prosthesis. *J Am Coll Cardiol* 2000;36:871–877.

241. David TE, Uden DE. Aortic valve replacement in adult patients with small aortic annuli. *Ann Thorac Surg* 1983;36:577–583.

242. Piehler JM, Danielson GK, Pluth JR, et al. Enlargement of the aortic root or anulus with autogenous pericardial patch during aortic valve replacement: long-term follow-up. *J Thorac Cardiovasc Surg* 1983;86:350–358.

243. Jaffe WM, Coverdale HA, Roche AH, et al. Rest and exercise hemodynamics of 20 to 23 mm allograft, Medtronic Intact (porcine), and St. Jude Medical valves in the aortic position. *J Thorac Cardiovasc Surg* 1990;100:167–174.

244. Foster AH, Tracy CM, Greenberg GJ, et al. Valve replacement in narrow aortic roots: serial hemodynamics and long-term clinical outcome. *Ann Thorac Surg* 1986;42:506–516.

INFECTIVE ENDOCARDITIS

DANIEL J. SEXTON
THOMAS M. BASHORE

GLOSSARY

Actinobacillus: A nonmotile, fastidious, gram-negative rod that can cause endocarditis in humans.

Actinobacillus actinomycetemcomitans: A species of *Actinobacillus*.

Adenovirus: A family of double-stranded DNA viruses.

Aminoglycosides: A group of antibiotics made from species of *Streptomyces* or *Micromonosporum*. Effective against many gram-negative bacilli and *Mycobacterium tuberculosis*.

Amoxicillin: A semisynthetic penicillin with an antimicrobial spectrum similar to ampicillin.

Ampicillin: A semisynthetic penicillin that has a broader spectrum of antimicrobial activity than penicillin G.

Bacillus: A genus of anaerobic, spore-forming gram positive rods found in the soil.

Bartonella: A genus of bacteria that is difficult to grow in the laboratory. These bacteria cause infection in cats and can be transmitted to humans by scratches or louse bites.

Blalock-Taussig shunt: A shunt created by routing the left or right subclavian artery to the pulmonary artery.

Brucella: A genus of encapsulated, gram-negative bacteria that are pathogens of humans and a variety of animals.

Candida: A genus of fungi found on the skin and in feces, vaginal, pharyngeal, and gastrointestinal tracts.

Cefazolin: A broad-spectrum cephalosporin.

Ceftriaxone: A semisynthetic parenteral cephalosporin antibiotic.

Cephalosporin: One of several antibiotic substances obtained from *Cephalosporium* species of fungi. Effective against many gram-positive and gram-negative organisms.

Chlamydia: A genus that includes all the agents of the psittacosis, lymphogranuloma, trachoma group.

Clindamycin: A class of antibiotics with broad activity against anaerobic bacteria and many gram-positive cocci.

Corynebacterium: A genus of gram-positive rods found widely in nature; can be found in oropharynx.

Coxiella burnetii: The bacteria that causes Q fever in humans.

Coxsackie B: A picornavirus responsible for a variety of diseases in humans.

Eikenella: A nonmotile, gram-negative, anaerobic rod part of normal oral cavity.

Endarteritis: Inflammation of the intima of an artery.

Enterococcus: A genus of gram-positive cocci that inhabits the intestinal tract of humans.

D. J. Sexton: Division of Infectious Diseases, Duke University Medical Center, Durham, North Carolina

T. M. Bashore: Division of Cardiology, Duke University Medical Center, Durham, North Carolina

Escherichia coli: A gram-negative rod widely found in nature; inhabits the intestines and causes infections of the urogenital and gastrointestinal tract.

Fibronectin: A fibrous-linking glycoprotein found in connective tissue, basement membranes, and cell surfaces; acts as an adhesive.

Gentamicin: An aminoglycoside antibiotic that inhibits growth of gram-negative and some gram-positive bacteria.

Haemophilus: A gram-negative rod in the respiratory tract.

Histoplasma: A dimorphic fungus normally found in soil; it causes pulmonary infections.

Janeway lesion: Erythematous, nontender lesions on fingers, palm, or sole.

Keyhole surgery: Surgery performed through a small thoracotomy rather than large median sternotomy or large lateral thoracotomy.

Laminin: A large polypeptide glycoprotein component of basement membrane.

Legionella: An aerobic gram-negative bacillus that is found in fresh water. It can cause pulmonary wound or renal infections.

Listeria: A genus of motile bacteria containing small gram-positive rods; can cause meningitis, encephalitis, septicemia, endocarditis, abortion, and abscesses.

MacCallum's patch: Vegetations found along the mural surface of a cardiac chamber.

Mycoplasma: A genus of gram-negative organism that lack a true cell wall; may cause pulmonary or genitourinary and postpartum infections.

Mycotic aneurysms: Aneurysmal dilatation of a vessel caused by invasion of the vascular wall from infective endocarditis.

Nafcillin: A semisynthetic penicillin resistant to penicillinase and effective against some strains of *Staphylococcus aureus*.

Osler's nodes: Small, tender, purple erythematous subcutaneous nodules visibly found on the pulp of digits.

Penicillin G: An antibiotic produced from cultures of the molds' *Penicillium* species.

Propionibacterium: A genus of nonmotile, non–spore-forming gram-positive rods found on the skin and in the intestinal tract.

Proteus: A genus of gram-negative bacteria that can cause genitourinary and nosocomial infections.

Pseudomonas aeruginosa: A species of gram-negative, aerobic bacteria found in soil, water, and clinical specimens.

Rickettsia: A genus of intracellular gram-negative bacteria that causes a variety of diseases such as spotted fever and typhus.

Roth's spots: Retinal hemorrhages with a clear center.

Salmonella: A genus of gram-negative bacilli that can cause gastrointestinal and bacteremic illnesses.

Serratia marcescens: Gram-negative rods that may produce infection in immunocompromised and hospitalized patients.

Splinter hemorrhage: An embolic subungual hemorrhage located proximally in the nailbed.

Staphylococcus aureus: Gram-positive bacteria that may colonize the nasal mucous membranes and skin (hair follicles) and cause serious skin, soft tissue, blood, and endocardial infections.

Streptococcus bovis: Gram-positive bacteria found in the gastrointestinal tract.

Streptococcus milleri: A gram-positive coccus found in human throat, mouth, and nasopharynx.

Streptococcus pneumoniae: A gram-positive, lancet-shaped diplococcus frequently occurring in chains; normal inhabitant of the respiratory tract.

Streptococcus sanginosus: A gram-positive coccus found on oral and nasopharyngeal mucous membranes.

Streptococcus sanguis: A gram-positive coccus found normally in oral and nasopharyngeal mucous membranes.

Streptococcus viridans: Name applied to a group of alpha-hemolytic streptococci describing organisms isolated from the mouth and intestines.

Streptomycin: An antibiotic agent from *Streptomycesgriseus* active against *Mycobacterium tuberculosis* bacillus and a large number of gram-negative bacteria.

Type 4 collagen: A protein with a less distinct fibrillar form, characteristic of basement membranes.

Vancomycin: An antibiotic with activity against most gram-positive organisms.

Vegectomies: Surgical removal of endocarditis vegetations from a valvular surface.

Vegetations: Growth consisting of fused platelets, fibrin, and other bacteria adherent to a heart valve or other vascular structure.

ANATOMIC CONSIDERATIONS

Vegetations in patients with preexisting valvular lesions are usually located on the atrial surface of incompetent atrioventricular valves or the ventricular surfaces of incompetent semilunar valves. This is likely because of the fact that these surfaces are subjected to injury from regurgitant jets. In patients with ventricular septal defects, vegetations tend to occur on the orifice of the defect, on the right ventricular side of the opening, and secondarily on the tricuspid and pulmonic valves (10). Vegetations may occasionally localize on the chordae tendineae of the anterior leaflet of the mitral valve in patients with aortic insufficiency. Patients with mitral regurgitation may also develop a vegetation (MacCallum's patch) on the wall of the left atrium where the regurgitant jet strikes the atrial wall and results in endocardial thickening (Fig. 25.1).

The source of infection in some patients with endocarditis may be clinically evident (e.g., an infected vascular catheter, a dental abscess, or an infected skin lesion), but in many patients, there is no history of an antecedent localized

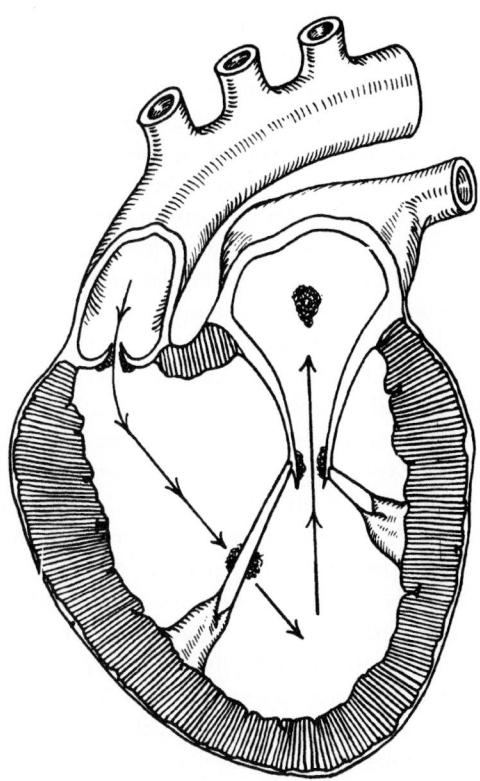

FIGURE 25.1 Sites of high-velocity streams where endocardial injury occurs in mitral and aortic insufficiency. (From Robard S. Blood velocity and endocarditis. *Circulation* 1963;27:24, with permission.)

infection. In most such instances, the source is presumed to be from minor trauma to the oropharyngeal, gastrointestinal, or genitourinary mucosa.

Endocarditis in injection drug users is dominated by one pathogen: *S. aureus*. *S. aureus* is known to have a predilection for normal as well as abnormal cardiac valves (11). This phenomenon may explain why the majority of injection drug–using patients with endocarditis has no known prior valvular disease (12). Endocarditis in injection drug users is presumed to result as a consequence of the trauma to heart valves from contaminating inorganic debris and bacteria injected along with the illicit drugs, from the paraphernalia used for drug injection, or via bacteria on the skin surface at the site of injection. Tricuspid valve involvement has been noted in 78%, mitral in 24%, and aortic in 8% of drug addicts with endocarditis (12). Simultaneous involvement of more than one valve may occur in approximately 20% of drug-abusing patients (13), and some of these infections are polymicrobial (14).

Approximately three-fourths of all patients with endocarditis have a preexisting structural cardiac abnormality at the time that endocarditis begins (15,16). During the period from 1938 to 1967, rheumatic heart disease was the underlying cardiac lesion in 39% of patients hospitalized with endocarditis at the Presbyterian Hospital in New York

(17). In contrast, the authors of a large case series from Tennessee reported that only 6% of patients with endocarditis had underlying rheumatic cardiac lesions (16). Simultaneously, preexisting degenerative valvular lesions such as mitral valve prolapse (usually with coexistent mitral regurgitation) have become relatively more important as a predisposing cause for endocarditis. For example, preexisting mitral valve prolapse was the underlying cardiac lesion in 22% and 29% of cases of endocarditis in two case series (16,18). The estimated risk of endocarditis in patients with mitral valve prolapse and regurgitation has been estimated to be five to eight times higher than the normal population (19,20). However, mitral valve prolapse is a common abnormality and the overall risk of endocarditis in an individual with this lesion is quite small. Aortic valve disease (with stenosis, regurgitation, or both) is a predisposing cause for endocarditis in 12% to 30% of cases (21).

Congenital heart disease is now the underlying lesion in 10% to 20% of cases of endocarditis (10). The most common congenital heart lesions predisposing to endocarditis include bicuspid aortic valves, patent ductus arteriosus, ventricular septal defects, coarctation of the aorta, and tetralogy of Fallot. Unlike most other congenital defects, secundum atrial septal defects are not associated with an increased risk (21).

A succession of new surgical techniques for correction of congenital and acquired valvular lesions has affected the distribution of cardiac abnormalities now seen in patients with infective endocarditis (IE). The risk of endocarditis in patients with mechanical or bioprosthetic valves is similar. In a multicenter follow-up study of over 1,000 patients who were randomized to receive mechanical or bioprosthetic cardiac valves, the overall rate of prosthetic valve endocarditis was similar in both groups (0.8 cases per year of follow-up) (22). Duration of follow-up averaged 7.7 years; the cumulative percentage of patients who developed prosthetic valve endocarditis was 5.8% (22). However, other authors have suggested that mechanical prosthetic valves are more susceptible to endocarditis initially, whereas after 1 year, bioprosthetic valves are more likely to develop endocarditis (23,23a). In another study, endocarditis was more common after 11 years in patients with mechanical valves than in patients with bioprosthetic valves (23b). ❦ e79

A history of endocarditis is an additional important predisposing cause for endocarditis. Recurrent endocarditis occurred in 4.5% of patients in a follow-up study of a large cohort of patients who survived their initial episode of endocarditis (26). Other studies have reported rates of recurrence of endocarditis ranging from 2.5% to 9.0% (27). Also, not surprisingly, prosthetic valve endocarditis occurs more frequently when the original indication for the valve replacement was active endocarditis (28).

Other uncommon but notable predisposing causes for endocarditis include pregnancy (10), arteriovenous fistulas used for hemodialysis (29), the use of central venous and pulmonary artery catheters (30), the presence of peritoneovenous (LeVeen) shunts for the control of intractable ascites (31), and the use of ventriculoatrial shunts for the management of hydrocephalus (32). In addition, patients with ulcerative lesions of the colon caused by carcinoma or inflammatory bowel disease have a poorly understood predilection to develop endocarditis caused by *S. bovis* (33,34). Infective endocarditis has also been reported in patients undergoing liver, heart, and heart–lung transplantation (35).

A number of cases of endocarditis in patients with human immunodeficiency virus (HIV) have also been reported (36). Some patients with HIV and endocarditis have had infection with unusual organisms such as *Salmonella* and *Listeria* (37,38). Although one study suggested that HIV infection was an independent risk factor for IE in injection drug abusers (39), the results of another study of a large cohort of injection drug users found no evidence that supported this concept (37). Cocaine use may be an additional risk factor for IE in injection drug users. In a study of a large number of injection drug users with fever, those who used cocaine were significantly more likely to have endocarditis (40).

PATHOPHYSIOLOGY

The endothelial lining of the heart and its valves is normally resistant to infection with bacteria and fungi. Experiments in animal models have demonstrated that a sequence of interrelated events must occur before microbes can establish an infective nidus or vegetation on the endocardium. Although a few highly virulent organisms such as *S. aureus* are capable of infecting normal human heart valves, the initial step in the establishment of a vegetation is injury to the endocardium followed by focal adherence of platelets and fibrin. This sterile platelet–fibrin nidus, in turn, becomes infected by microorganisms circulating in the bloodstream from a distant source of focal infection or as a result of a transient bacteremia from a mucosal or skin source (41,42).

Following colonization of the platelet–fibrin aggregate, microbial growth results in the secondary accumulation of more platelets and fibrin until a macroscopic excrescence or vegetation is present. The culmination of this process is mature vegetation consisting of an amorphous collection of fibrin, platelets, leukocytes, red blood cell debris, and dense clusters of bacteria. The surface of most vegetations consists of fibrin and scant numbers of leukocytes. Clumps of bacteria, histiocytes, and monocytes are usually found deep within the vegetation. Giant cells containing phagocytic bacteria may be found in some vegetations. Extremely high concentrations of bacteria (e.g., 10^9 to 10^{11} bacteria per g of tissue) may accumulate deep within vegetations. Some of these bacteria exist in a state of reduced metabolic activity.

Following therapy and during the process of healing, capillaries and fibroblasts appear within vegetations, but without treatment, vegetations are avascular structures.

Vegetations often prevent proper valvular leaflet or cusp coaptation, resulting in worsening valvular incompetence and congestive heart failure (43). Vegetation growth may result in leaflet perforation that can manifest as acute congestive heart failure (44). Patients with mitral or tricuspid valve vegetations may develop chordal rupture when infection progresses beyond the valve orifice. Extension of infection may also occur into surrounding structures such as the valve ring, the adjacent myocardium, the cardiac conduction system, or the mitral-aortic intravalvular fibrosa (45). Rarely, cavitation of periaortic abscesses may occur into the adjacent aortic wall, resulting in the formation of a diverticulum or aneurysm. Even more rarely such aneurysms may perforate into surrounding structures resulting in aortic-atrial or aortic-pericardial fistulae (44).

Endocarditis on prosthetic valve tissue differs from native valve endocarditis in that infection commonly extends outside the actual valvular apparatus, resulting in valvular dehiscence, abscess formation, and myocardial invasion (46) (Fig. 25.2). Endothelial cell proliferation overgrowing the valvular cuff of the bioprosthesis may provide a nidus that explains this propensity for valvular ring involvement (28). In addition, bioprosthetic valves are vulnerable to infection of the leaflets themselves (47). ⦿ e80

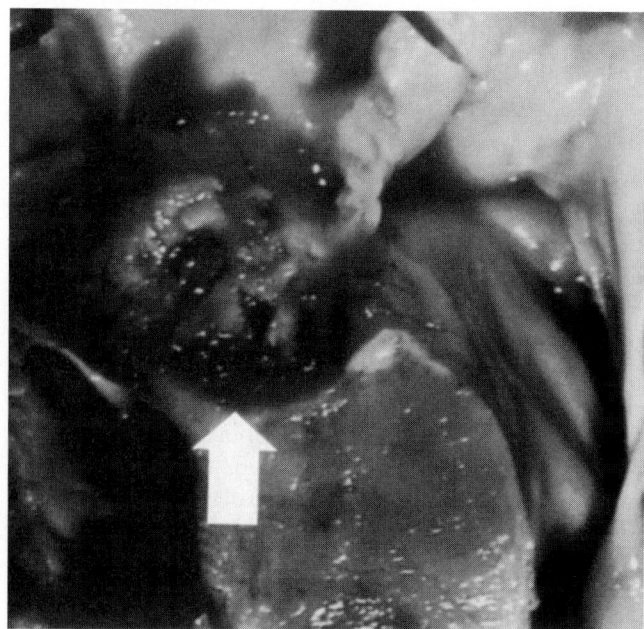

FIGURE 25.2 Pathology of a staphylococcal abscess (*arrow*) involving the annulus of the mitral valve. (From Kissane JM. Staphylococcal infections. In: Connor DH, et al., eds. *Pathology of infectious diseases*. Vol 1. Stamford, CT: Appleton & Lange, 1997:811, with permission.)

Vegetations tend to occur when blood travels from an area of high pressure through a narrow orifice into an area of lower pressure. The explanation for this phenomenon can be deduced from *in vitro* experiments that demonstrate the physics of turbulent flow. If nebulized *Serratia marcescens* are injected into an air stream passing through an agar-coated Venturi tube, the highest concentration of bacteria is found in the low-pressure area immediately distal to the narrowing (55). A similar phenomenon is presumed to occur when bacteria circulate in the blood. The propensity for vegetations to form at specific sites may also relate to a decrease in lateral pressure downstream from the regurgitant flow, which causes a decrease in the perfusion of the intimal lining at these sites (49).

CLINICAL PROFILE

Classification of Infective Endocarditis

Various terms have been used to describe the many forms of endocarditis encountered by clinicians. The term *IE* should now replace the older terms *subacute* and *acute bacterial endocarditis* for several reasons. First, not all cases are caused by gram-positive and gram-negative bacteria; fungi, rickettsia, and *Chlamydia* may also cause endocarditis. Second, presentation and duration of endocarditis are not easily categorized. Although rapidly progressing (acute) endocarditis is usually due to *S. aureus*, the clinical utility of separating cases on the basis of the activity of the presentation is limited because pathogens such as *S. aureus* and streptococci can cause either fulminant or indolent disease in different patients. However, there is clinical utility in separating cases as to whether there is involvement of native or prosthetic valves; for in the latter group, the causative organisms vary if the infection occurs early (during the first 60 days after surgery) or late. In addition, right-sided endocarditis in intravenous drug users results in such a characteristic illness that it is useful to separate it from infection solely involving the left-sided structures of the heart. Although heart valves are the usual sites of infection, vegetations may also appear on pacemaker leads (56), in the mural endocardium (57), in arteriovenous shunts or fistulae (58), in vascular structures such as a patent ductus or a Blalock-Taussig shunt (59), or in coarctation of the aorta, or even in intracardiac masses such as myxomas (60).

Infective endocarditis is a highly variable disease. Its clinical course is dependent on numerous factors, including the causative pathogen, the age and underlying health of the patient, and the nature and extent of the underlying valvular disease. Decisions concerning clinical management are directly related to an accurate diagnosis. Underdiagnosis can lead to catastrophe. Overdiagnosis can lead to weeks of unnecessary therapy at great cost and risk of drug-related toxicity. Distinguishing between IE and an alternate focus of infection in a bacteremic patient with underlying heart disease can be extremely difficult. To help distinguish endocarditis from other bacteremic syndromes, consistent definitions are important. Clinical research concerning the natural history, complications, epidemiology, and treatment outcomes of endocarditis all depend on the accurate identification of patients with this disease. Definitions that are specific but not sensitive may lead to biased conclusions, as can definitions that are sensitive but not specific.

Petersdorf and Pelletier (61) developed the first diagnostic criteria for IE. Their schema classified cases as definite, possible, and probable. Surgical or autopsy confirmation was required to classify a case as definite. Designation of a case as probable or possible was based on the presence of one or more of the following criteria: predisposing valvular disease, bacteremia, the presence of emboli, and the presence of indirect evidence of an active endocardial disease process such as a new regurgitant murmur. In practice, many patients with presumed endocarditis did not meet these criteria. Thus, although this classification was reasonably specific, it lacked sensitivity.

In 1981, the Beth Israel criteria were proposed by von Reyn and colleagues (62). Four diagnostic categories were created: definite, probable, possible, and rejected. As in the Petersdorf and Pelletier schema, histologic or microbiologic confirmation either at autopsy or at surgery were required to categorize a case as definite. Other criteria included the presence of (a) persistent bacteremia, (b) predisposing valvular heart disease, (c) vascular phenomena such as emboli or splinter hemorrhages, and (d) evidence of active endocardial pathology such as a new regurgitant murmur. Echocardiography was not used as a diagnostic criterion nor was the use of illicit intravenous drugs considered to be a predisposing risk factor for endocarditis. The Beth Israel criteria were widely used during the following decade, but despite modifications by various investigators, this classification system still lacked sufficient sensitivity.

In 1994, investigators at Duke University developed a new diagnostic schema that addressed weaknesses in the Beth Israel classification: The Duke criteria used echocardiography as a major criteria for diagnosis, expanded the list of predisposing heart conditions to include intravenous drug use, and devised a system by which cases could be classified as definite using purely clinical criteria (63). The pathologic criteria used in the Duke classification were virtually identical to those proposed by Pelleteir, Petersdorf, and von Reyn. Cases were classified as definite in the Duke schema using major and minor criteria in a manner analogous to the Jones criteria for rheumatic fever (Tables 25.1 and 25.2). In 2000, investigators from the Duke Endocarditis Service further modified the Duke criteria.

Several studies have compared the clinical utility and validity of the Duke criteria with those of von Reyn et al. (63–67). In each of these studies, a substantial number of cases that were considered as rejected when the Beth Israel

TABLE 25.1 DUKE CRITERIA FOR THE DIAGNOSIS OF INFECTIVE ENDOCARDITIS

Definite
  Pathologic criteria
    Microorganism: demonstrated by culture, in a vegetation at surgery, from an embolized vegetation, or from an intra-cardiac abscess
    Pathologic lesions: vegetations or intracardiac abscess present and confirmed by histology showing active endocarditis
  Clinical criteria, using specific definitions listed in Table 25.2
    Two major criteria, or
    One major and three minor criteria, or
    Five minor criteria
Possible
  Findings consistent with infective endocarditis that fall short of *definite*, but not *rejected*
Rejected
  Firm alternate diagnosis for manifestations of endocarditis, or
  Resolution of manifestations of endocarditis, with antibiotic therapy for 4 d or less, or
  No pathologic evidence of infective endocarditis at surgery or autopsy, after antibiotic therapy for 4 d or less

TABLE 25.2 DEFINITIONS OF TERMINOLOGY USED IN THE DUKE CRITERIA FOR INFECTIVE ENDOCARDITIS

Major criteria
  Positive blood culture[a] for infective endocarditis
    Typical microorganism for infective endocarditis from two separate blood cultures: *Streptococcus viridans,*[b] *Streptococcus bovis,* HACEK group, or community-acquired *Staphylococcus aureus* or enterococci, in the absence of a primary focus, *or*
    Persistently positive blood culture, defined as recovery of a microorganism consistent with infective endocarditis from:
      (i) Blood cultures drawn more than 12 h apart, *or*
      (ii) All of three or a majority of four or more separate blood cultures, with first and last drawn at least 1 h apart
  Evidence of endocardial involvement
    Positive echocardiogram for infective endocarditis
      (i) Oscillating intracardiac mass on valve or supporting structures, or in the path of regurgitant jets, or on implanted material, in the absence of an alternative anatomic explanation, *or*
      (ii) Abscess, *or*
      (iii) New partial dehiscence of prosthetic valve, *or*
    New valvular regurgitation (increases or changes in preexisting murmur not sufficient)
Minor criteria
  Predisposition: predisposing heart condition or intravenous drug use
  Fever ≥38.0°C (100.4°F)
  Vascular phenomena: major arterial emboli, septic pulmonary infarcts, mycotic aneurysm, intracranial hemorrhage, conjunctival hemorrhages, and Janeway lesions
  Immunologic phenomena: glomerulonephritis, Osler's nodes, Roth's spots, rheumatoid factor
  Microbiologic evidence: positive blood culture result but not meeting major criterion as noted previously or serologic evidence of active infection with organism consistent with infective endocarditis
  Echocardiogram: consistent with infective endocarditis but not meeting major criterion noted previously

HACEK, *Haemophilus* species, *Actinobacillus actinomycetemcomitans, Cardiobacterium hominis, Eikenella* species, and *Kingella kingae.*
[a]Excluding single positive culture results for coagulase-negative staphylococci and organisms that do not cause endocarditis.
[b]Including nutritional variant strains.

criteria were applied prospectively were simultaneously classified as clinically definite by the Duke criteria (67). The negative predictive value of the Duke criteria was subsequently assessed in a follow-up study of patients considered to be rejected for a diagnosis of IE. None of 52 patients who had been considered as rejected by the Duke criteria had proven IE in follow-up (68). In another study of 100 cases of acute fever or fever of unknown origin, the specificity of the Duke criteria was found to be 99% (69).

The utility of the Duke criteria was subsequently assessed in patients with prosthetic valve endocarditis, pediatric patients, and hospitalized patients. Modifications (such as the use of serologic criteria for diagnosing endocarditis caused by *Coxiella burnetii*) have been adopted (70), and it is likely that further modifications will occur in the future (67). However, the Duke schema is currently the most sensitive and specific diagnostic criteria available and is particularly useful in diagnosing endocarditis in patients with *S. aureus* bacteremia, those with right-sided endocarditis, and those with negative blood culture results (67).

Laboratory Diagnosis

Infective endocarditis is usually a "syndrome diagnosis" based on the presence of multiple findings rather than on a single definitive test result. The diagnosis of IE is usually obvious when a patient has numerous positive blood culture results in the presence of a well-recognized predisposing cardiac lesion and the absence of infection elsewhere.

The bacteriologic diagnosis of IE is facilitated by the relative constancy of bacteremia originating from vegetations. Bacteria are discharged from vegetations at a relatively constant rate rather than haphazardly (85). A minimum of

three blood cultures should be obtained. If the tempo of illness is subacute, and the patient is not critically ill, it is reasonable and often preferable to delay therapy for 1 to 3 days awaiting the results of blood cultures and other diagnostic tests. If the patient is acutely ill, three blood cultures should be obtained at least 1 hour apart before beginning empiric therapy. The constancy of bacteremia in patients with endocarditis makes it unnecessary to await the arrival of a fever spike or chills to obtain blood cultures; in addition, prior studies may have shown that venous blood culture results give approximately the same yield as arterial blood cultures.

Many patients with bacterial endocarditis have low-grade bacteremia (i.e., 1 to 10 colony-forming units per mL of blood) (86); thus, a minimum of 10 mL, and preferably

20 mL, should be obtained from adults and 0.5 to 5.0 mL from infants and children. Blood cultures inoculated with at least 5 mL of blood have a significantly higher detection rate for bacteremia than bottles inoculated with less than 5 mL of blood (92% vs. 69%; *p* <.001). The estimated yield of blood cultures in bacteremic adults increases approximately 3% per mL of blood cultured (87).

Not all microorganisms have the same propensity to cause endocarditis. For example, organisms such as viridans streptococci and *S. aureus* are more likely to cause endocarditis than are gram-negative rods such as *E. coli* and *Proteus*. This distinction has clinical importance. For instance, the Duke Criteria distinguishes among the type of organism isolated from blood cultures. The following organisms are considered to be *likely causes* of IE when isolated from two or more blood cultures: *S. aureus*, viridans streptococci, and enterococci (if the infection was acquired in the community and not nosocomially).

The setting in which bacteremia occurs also has an effect on the probability that an individual patient will have endocarditis. For example, patients who present with community-acquired enterococcal bacteremia are significantly more likely to have endocarditis than are patients who develop enterococcal bacteremia while hospitalized for another cause. ⍄ e81

Although unusual or fastidious organisms are an important consideration when patients with clinical findings of endocarditis are found to have negative routine blood culture results, the most common cause for negative blood culture results in patients with IE is prior antimicrobial therapy. Thus, it may be necessary to delay the institution of therapy for several days for such patients while additional blood cultures are obtained.

A total of three blood cultures is usually adequate to diagnose IE in most cases. In a study of 206 cases of endocarditis, all blood culture results were positive in 91% of the patients. In patients with streptococcal endocarditis, the first blood culture result was positive in 96% of cases and one of two culture results was positive in 98% of patients. In endocarditis, with organisms other than streptococci, the first blood culture obtained was positive in 82% of cases and one of two was positive in 100% of patients (86).

The white blood cell count is rarely helpful in making a diagnosis of endocarditis. Some patients with streptococcal endocarditis may have normal white blood cell counts when they seek medical attention. In contrast, most patients with staphylococcal endocarditis have leukocytosis (90).

The utility of other laboratory tests in the diagnosis of endocarditis is limited. An elevated erythrocyte sedimentation rate, an elevated level of C-reactive protein, or both are usually present, but these findings alone have little specific diagnostic or monitoring value. Most patients with endocarditis quickly develop a normochromic normocytic anemia, but this finding is equally nonspecific. Elevated

levels of serum globulins, the presence of cryoglobulins and circulating immune complexes, hypocomplementemia, and false-positive serologic test results for syphilis may also occur in some patients with IE, but none of these findings is diagnostic or particularly helpful by itself. However, an elevated level of rheumatoid factor may occasionally be useful in diagnosis, particularly when the duration of illness is greater than 6 weeks (91). When present in individuals without a known prior rheumatologic disorder, this finding is considered to be one of the six minor criteria in the Duke Endocarditis Service diagnostic schema (63).

Most patients with endocarditis have an abnormal urinalysis result. Urinary sediment examination may disclose microscopic or gross hematuria, proteinuria, or pyuria. Microscopic hematuria and mild proteinuria occur in many cases and are often found in the absence of other renal complications (48). Like the erythrocyte sedimentation rate, all of these urinary findings lack specificity. However, the presence of red blood cell casts and a low serum complement level may be an indicator of immune-mediated glomerular disease. When present, this uncommon finding is an important minor diagnostic criterion (63).

Electrocardiography should be part of the initial evaluation of all patients with suspected endocarditis, even though this test rarely shows diagnostic findings. Besides the presence of changes suggestive of ischemia or infarction, the electrocardiogram may also reveal the presence or new appearance of heart block, an important clue to extension of infection to the valve annulus and adjacent conduction system. The presence of new prolongation of the PR interval in a patient with endocarditis, if unrelated to drug therapy or recent surgery, is virtually diagnostic of the presence of a ring abscess.

Chest radiography occasionally reveals important diagnostic clues. For example, patients with tricuspid valve endocarditis often present with radiographic evidence of septic pulmonary emboli. In such cases, there may be a few or multiple focal lung infiltrates. Some of these infiltrates may reveal central cavitation. Rarely, chest radiography discloses calcification in a *native* cardiac valve that may in turn raise the suspicion of endocarditis in a febrile patient.

Since its introduction in 1973, echocardiography has greatly simplified the process of diagnosing IE (44). Echocardiography is often of crucial importance in detecting a vegetation that is usually defined as a mass of echoes of distinct echogenicity from the adjacent valve >5 mm in its largest dimension with independent motion from the valve itself (92) (Fig. 25.3). Echocardiography should be obtained in all patients suspected of having endocarditis. Echocardiography not only may confirm the presence of vegetations in the setting of bacteremia, but it may also provide important physiologic information regarding right and left ventricular function and an estimate of valvular obstruction or regurgitation severity. Mitral valve preclosure in the setting of acute aortic insufficiency implies a marked increase in left ventricu-

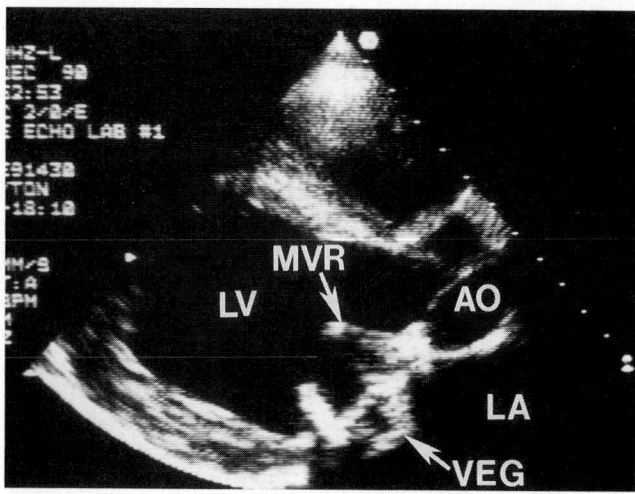

FIGURE 25.3 A vegetation (VEG) is shown on a prosthetic porcine mitral valve. The large mobile vegetation is noted to prolapse into the left atrium (LA). AO, aorta; LV, left ventricle; MVR, mitral valve replacement. (Courtesy of Dr. Thomas Ryan, Duke Medical Center.)

lar diastolic pressure and the likely need for more urgent intervention (93) (*e*Fig. 25.3.1).

Three major incremental advances have occurred in echocardiographic technology in the past 25 years: (a) the advent of two-dimensional echocardiography, (b) the institution of color flow Doppler technology, and (c) the introduction of TEE. M-mode echocardiography has now largely been replaced by two-dimensional echocardiographic methods. M-mode methods detect vegetations in approximately one-half of patients with IE. Although transthoracic two-dimensional echocardiography provides a remarkable improvement in visualizing spatial anatomic relationships compared with M-mode methods, the sensitivity of transthoracic two-dimensional echocardiography is still only approximately 60% (94,95). Furthermore, two-dimensional echocardiography is often of limited utility in the detection of vegetation in patients with obesity, emphysema, and chest wall deformities.

TEE, especially when biplane probes are used, has improved the rate of detection of vegetations on native valves to 90% to 95% (95–100) (*e*Fig. 25.3.2). TEE is particularly useful in visualizing right-sided heart structures and masses on pacemaker leads or intravenous lines and in visualizing abnormalities on the pulmonic valve (101,102). The superiority of TEE over transthoracic imaging methods is particularly important in the detection of small vegetations. However, the sensitivity of both methods is approximately equal when vegetations are ≥5 mm in size (35). In a study of 112 patients with 114 episodes of endocarditis, all of whom underwent transthoracic and TEE, Roe and colleagues reported that the findings on TEE resulted in reclassification of 22 patients from possible to definite endocarditis. Three patients were reclassified from rejected to possible (102a).

Transthoracic echocardiography in patients with prosthetic valve endocarditis often produces poor images, as shadowing of the echo beam may prevent adjacent structures from being adequately visualized and the mass effect from the prosthetic valve can obscure the identification of vegetations. As a result, transthoracic echocardiography has a sensitivity of only 35% for detecting vegetations in patients with prosthetic valve endocarditis.

TEE improves the sensitivity of detecting vegetations on prosthetic valves to up to 96% (103,104). TEE is especially useful in detecting ring abscesses or intracardiac fistulae (105–109). In one study of 44 patients with endocarditis complicated by perivalvular abscesses, transthoracic echocardiography identified only 28% of the abscesses, whereas TEE detected 87% (Fig. 25.4). Most such perivalvular abscesses communicate with the intravascular space (as evidenced by color flow turbulence observable within the lesion). These may be referred to as *pseudoaneurysms* by some. This phenomenon is not always evident, however. TEE is a particularly sensitive method for the detection of mitral regurgitation in the presence of mitral annular calcification or when a prosthetic mitral valve is present (110,111) (Fig. 25.5). The presence of spontaneous echo contrast in the atria of patients with endocarditis may imply a higher risk for systemic emboli in such patients (112). ⬦ e82

The role of cardiac catheterization in the evaluation of patients with endocarditis remains controversial. Traditionalists have argued that intracardiac vegetations should not be crossed with intracardiac catheters; this view makes good sense, even though there are no data to confirm the danger of such maneuvers. Echocardiographic color flow Doppler methods that define the severity of regurgitation are helpful. However, it has been our experience that aortic regurgita-

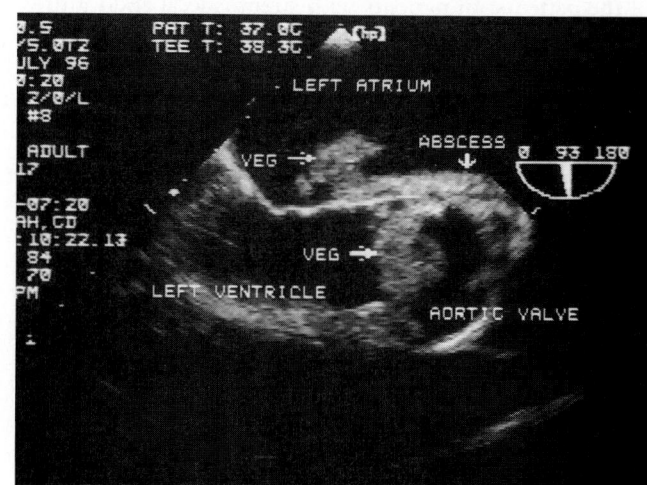

FIGURE 25.4 Transesophageal echocardiogram of a large aortic valve vegetation (VEG) with erosion through the aortic wall into the left atrium. Associated with this is an abscess. (Courtesy of Dr. Carolyn Donovan, Duke Medical Center.)

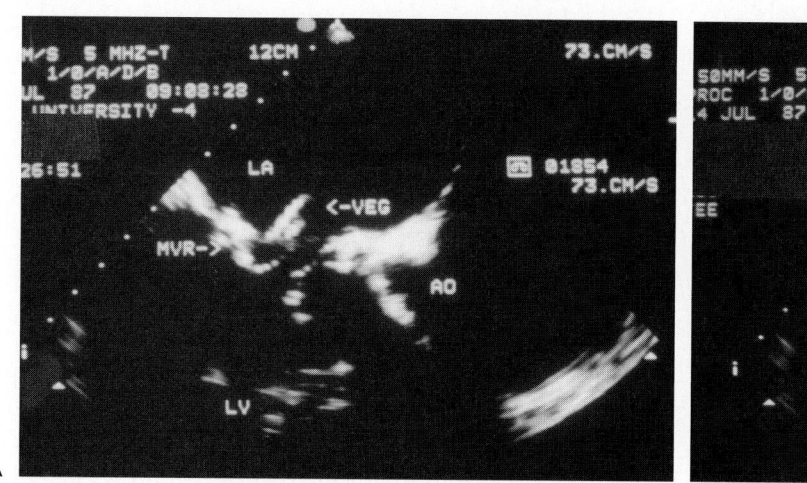
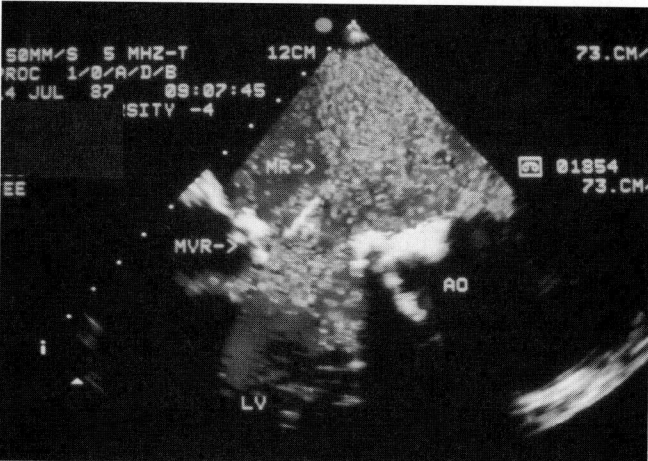

FIGURE 25.5 A: A linear vegetation (VEG) is shown on the St. Jude mitral valve. This was not visible by chest wall echocardiogram. **B:** Same view with color flow Doppler revealing marked mitral insufficiency. AO, aorta; LA, left atrium; LV, left ventricle; MVR, mitral valve replacement. (Courtesy of Dr. Joseph Kisslo, Duke Medical Center.)

tion and mitral regurgitation often appear more severe using color flow Doppler methods than the estimates using contrast angiography. Thus, if the severity of aortic insufficiency or mitral regurgitation observed by Doppler methods is inconsistent with the clinical findings, then catheterization should be undertaken to clarify the degree of valvular competence. In addition, cardiac catheterization may occasionally be a useful tool to visual abnormal intracardiac anatomy or flow if these features are ambiguous or uncertain after use of routine clinical assessment and echocardiography (132). Aortography may reveal the presence and extent of a perivalvular abscess (*e*Fig. 25.5.1) or fully outline fistulous channels in patients before surgical intervention.

As endocarditis has progressively become a disease of the elderly, concomitant coronary artery disease is often present. It has become our practice to perform coronary angiography routinely in all patients over age 55 before surgery for endocarditis or in those at high risk for coronary artery disease based on their coronary risk factors. Coronary angiography may also be important to delineate coronary emboli from vegetations, if the clinical syndrome is suspected. In younger patients, the anatomic information provided by both transthoracic echocardiography and TEE usually provides adequate information to safely proceed to surgical repair or valve replacement without the need for invasive studies.

Clinical Manifestations

The clinical presentation of IE ranges from an illness characterized by subtle, chronic fatigue with low-grade fevers, weight loss, and malaise to one of abrupt fulminant acute pulmonary edema brought on by massive acute aortic regurgitation. The virulence of the infecting organism generally determines the acuteness of the presentation. However, the interval from onset of infection to onset of symptoms is usually short. Most patients with endocarditis

develop symptoms within 2 weeks of the inciting bacteremia (133). Symptoms in staphylococcal endocarditis may even begin within a few days of the onset of infection.

A variety of nonspecific constitutional complaints may dominate the clinical presentation in individual cases (*e*Table 25.2.1) (133a,133b). Fever is the most common constitutional complaint. Fevers are usually low grade. Fever may be absent in the elderly and those with congestive heart failure, uremia, severe debility, and infection with coagulase-negative *Staphylococcus* (10,134). Chills, night sweats, and weight loss are also commonly present, as are a variety of neurologic and musculoskeletal complaints.

Heart murmurs are frequently noted but may be difficult to hear under certain conditions. As many as 15% or more of patients may not have a murmur at the time of initial evaluation (76,135). In acute staphylococcal endocarditis, it is even rarer to recognize a new or changing murmur in the first few days of illness (133c). Right-sided endocarditis, for instance, may be associated with inaudible tricuspid regurgitation. **⚑** e83

Neurologic symptoms occur in 30% to 40% of patients with endocarditis in most series. Headache is the most common of these neurologic complaints. Cerebral embolic events occur in one-fourth of patients and may be the cause of the presenting symptoms in an important number of patients (139). In a review of 218 episodes of IE from one center, 55 of 218 episodes (25%) had a neurologic complication. An embolic event was responsible for 25 of 55 (42%) of the events. In 45% of the 55 neurologic events, the neurologic manifestations were present before antimicrobial therapy had begun (139a). **⚑** e84

Clinical Complications

Surprisingly, the overall incidence of complications related to IE may not have changed significantly in the past three or four decades despite improvements in diagnostic techniques and in medical and surgical therapy (152). However, the types of complications seen in modern practice have changed substantially since the preantibiotic era. Patients now rarely die of sepsis. As a result of medical therapy, patients with IE often live longer and, thus, develop complications such as emboli, mycotic aneurysms, and heart failure more frequently. Estimates of the incidence of complications in the modern antibiotic era are presented in *e*Table 25.2.1.

Patients with endocarditis who undergo surgery are susceptible to a wide array of complications that were largely unknown 30 years ago (43). In a study of 287 patients treated for 300 episodes of IE in a tertiary cardiology referral center, a total of 386 complications occurred in 223 episodes. Most patients had either one (57%) or two (26%) complications, but 8% of patients had four or more complications (153). The most important and frequent cardiac complication of endocarditis is congestive heart failure. Heart failure in patients with endocarditis may be insidious or rapid in onset, but in both instances its primary cause usually is valvular insufficiency, rather than myocardial dysfunction. Patients with prosthetic valve endocarditis or endocarditis caused by fungal infection occasionally develop large bulky vegetations that may functionally occlude a valve orifice and secondarily cause heart failure. Regardless of the mechanism, the development of heart failure in patients with IE is an ominous sign. Unless valve replacement or valve repair is undertaken, most patients with this complication die, even if effective antimicrobial therapy is administered. Congestive heart failure may occur as a result of infection of any cardiac valve, but is most common in patients with aortic valve endocarditis and is least common in patients with tricuspid valve endocarditis (154).

Most other cardiac complications in IE are related directly or indirectly to extension of infection from the valve leaflets or other areas of initial endocardial injury to surrounding cardiac structures such as the valve annulus, the adjacent cardiac conduction system, the sinus of Valsalva, or the mitral aortic intervalvular fibrosa. Rarely, vegetations on the aortic valve enlarge to the point that they occlude the left main coronary ostium (155).

Abscess in or adjacent to the valve annulus is often heralded by the appearance of first or second degree heart block, fever that persists despite appropriate therapy, or both. Rarely, patients with annular abscesses develop purulent pericarditis (89,156,157). Annular abscesses are more common in patients with aortic valvular infection than in those with mitral valve endocarditis (43). If infection extends beyond the valve ring, erosion may occur into the ventricular septum and secondarily into the cardiac conduction system. If the abscess extends into the lower portion of the septum, varying degrees of heart block may ensue. Extension of infection into the upper portion of the septum is less likely to produce electrocardiographic abnor-

malities (43). The new onset of atrioventricular or bundle branch block in a patient with endocarditis has a specificity of greater than 80% for the presence of an abscess (158). Furthermore, patients with perivalvular abscesses have higher rates of embolization and a higher risk of death than patients with endocarditis without abscess formation (116). ☞ e85

The most feared and most common extracardiac complication of endocarditis is embolism. Although valvular vegetations are the source of cerebral and systemic emboli in patients with endocarditis, rarely septic pulmonary arteriovenous fistulae may also provide a conduit for left-sided emboli (160). Cerebral infarction in patients with IE is usually caused by embolism that is later complicated by cerebral hemorrhage. Approximately three-fourths of all cerebral emboli involve the distribution of the middle cerebral artery. Cerebral infarction, caused by emboli or mycotic aneurysm, is the presenting sign of endocarditis in 4.5% to 14.0% of all cases of IE (161). Patients with endocarditis who develop cerebral emboli have clinically apparent evidence of systemic emboli in approximately one-half of cases; in contrast, only 2% of patients with other causes of stroke have associated systemic emboli (162).

The risk of symptomatic embolism decreases rapidly after effective therapy for endocarditis is initiated. In a study that used transthoracic echocardiography to detect vegetations, the overall risk of embolism was 6.2 per 1,000 patient-days. The rate of embolism fell from 13 per 1,000 patient-days during the first week of therapy to less than 1.2 per 1,000 patient-days at the completion of therapy (163). ☞ e86

Metastatic abscesses develop in the kidneys, spleen, or soft tissues (e.g., the psoas muscle) of some patients with IE. Surprisingly, patients with splenic abscesses often do not have marked abdominal pain or splenomegaly. Splenic abscesses usually require splenectomy for cure (43). In contrast, splenic infarcts, which are far more common than splenic abscesses in left-sided endocarditis, usually resolve spontaneously. Splenic infarct, on occasion, may be the presenting manifestation of endocarditis. Most metastatic abscesses in other locations require open or percutaneous drainage procedures.

Patients with tricuspid valve endocarditis may develop septic pulmonary emboli that later cavitate and produce hemoptysis. Such patients may also develop sterile or purulent, bloody or nonbloody pleural effusions (169). Septic pulmonary emboli may also result in the occurrence of a pneumothorax (170).

Clinical Course and Prognosis

Most patients with IE become afebrile within a few days after the institution of antimicrobial therapy. However, a small number of patients, particularly those with endocarditis caused by *S. aureus*, may remain febrile for 7 to 10 days and occasionally even longer. Drug fever, a secondary nosocomial infection, or intracardiac or extracardiac abscess formation should all be considered in such patients.

Congestive heart failure may first appear after an initial positive clinical response to medical therapy. Similarly, emboli to the CNS, coronary arterial, and systemic circulation may all occur after an initial response to antimicrobial therapy.

The prognosis in IE is related to the virulence of the infecting microorganism, the general health of the host, the valvular structures that are involved, the duration of the infection, and the presence or absence of congestive heart failure. *S. aureus* endocarditis is still fatal in 20% to 40% of cases, despite the best available medical and surgical therapies. In contrast, the prognosis of streptococcal endocarditis is substantially better. Between 90% and 95% of patients with endocarditis caused by viridans streptococci are now cured with medical or combined medical and surgical therapy. A similarly good prognosis exists for patients with endocarditis caused by other species of streptococci. Fungal endocarditis is virtually impossible to cure with medical therapy; only a small minority of such patients is currently cured with combined antifungal and surgical therapy (171). Some of these patients remain on antifungal treatment for extended periods of time on the assumption that sterilization of the infection is otherwise impossible.

The prognosis of patients with right-sided endocarditis, even those with infections caused by *S. aureus*, is remarkably good. In an analysis of 11 studies involving 362 cases of right-sided endocarditis, Chambers was able to document only two treatment failures (0.6%) and seven deaths (2.0%) in the same series (40).

Despite early surgical intervention, the prognosis of late-onset prosthetic valve endocarditis is better than for patients who acquire infection within 60 days of their replacement valve surgery. For example, in a review of 56 cases of prosthetic valve endocarditis that occurred among 3,200 recipients of bioprosthetic valves, the mortality for cases that occurred within 2 months of surgery was 75%, whereas only 25% of cases with late-onset prosthetic valve endocarditis were fatal (172). ▼ e87

PRINCIPLES OF MANAGEMENT

Prevention of Infective Endocarditis

Antimicrobial prophylaxis before selected dental and invasive surgical and diagnostic procedures has become standard and routine in most countries, despite the fact that no prospective study has been performed that proves that such therapy is clearly beneficial. Only one-half of all patients who develop endocarditis have a cardiac disorder that would have prompted endocarditis prophylaxis in the first place (176). Furthermore, follow-up incidence of endocarditis is low even if patients with predisposing valvular

lesions do not receive prophylactic antibiotics: One in five untreated patients develops endocarditis after having had an invasive procedure. Thus, perhaps only one in ten endocarditis episodes can be prevented by the appropriate use of antibiotic prophylaxis before an invasive procedure.

It is our view that maintenance of meticulous dental hygiene is of equal importance to antibiotic prophylaxis in the prevention of IE. It has been our experience that some patients with valvular and congenital heart disease actually visit their dentist less often, rather than more often, when the infectious risks of dental procedures are explained to them. Vigorous brushing of teeth or even chewing gum may result in transient bacteremia in patients with periodontal disease; it is important to emphasize to the patient that maintenance of good dental hygiene is vital. In addition, it is advisable to instruct all patients to avoid gingival trauma with toothpicks and high-pressure water irrigation devices (177).

The guidelines for antimicrobial prophylaxis for endocarditis formulated by an expert committee of the American Heart Association (178) are the regimens most widely used by clinicians in the United States. Expert groups in Europe (45) have published similar guidelines. Both guidelines are based on results of *in vitro* studies, clinical experience, data from experimental animal models, and clinical assumptions concerning the bacteria most likely to produce bacteremia and cause endocarditis. These recommendations should not be assumed to be the standard of care in all clinical situations. Clinicians can reasonably deviate from these guidelines in individual cases. ▼ e88

Three studies have been published in an attempt to measure the efficacy of prophylactic antibiotic therapy in the prevention of endocarditis. Two of these studies (8,181) produced results that suggested a benefit of prophylactic antibiotics; the third (182) found no benefit of such therapy. However, all three studies had serious limitations in their design or lacked appropriate numbers of patients to achieve necessary statistical power (180).

*e*Table 25.2.2 outlines the current clinical situations wherein antibiotic prophylaxis is recommended based on the risk involved. The precise risk of endocarditis following invasive dental or surgical procedures in patients with any of the listed conditions cannot be precisely measured; in fact, differences in opinions continue to exist as to whether even patients with each of the listed predisposing conditions should receive antibiotic therapy before an invasive procedure. There is general agreement, however, that those patients with a prior history of endocarditis and those with prosthetic heart valves are at higher risk than patients with acquired congenital and valvular lesions.

In general, risk of IE is considered to be highest for oral or dental procedures in which the oral mucosa is penetrated and in which gingival or mucosal bleeding is likely to occur. Invasive dental procedures in which the risk of transient bacteremia is above 50% include tooth extractions, periodontal surgery, and cleaning of teeth with removal of tartar. The risk of bacteremia is substantially lower for invasive genitourinary procedures such as dilation of strictures, insertion of endoscopes and catheters, and prostatectomy. The risk of bacteremia following invasive gastrointestinal procedures such as colonoscopy with biopsy and endoscopic retrograde cholangiopancreatography is generally less than 5% to 10%. The American Heart Association has listed those invasive procedures in which endocarditis prophylaxis is and is not recommended (*e*Table 25.2.2). Clinicians may choose to use antimicrobial prophylaxis in some patients with a high risk for endocarditis who undergo a procedure with a low or intermediate risk of bacteremia, yet reasonably forego antimicrobial prophylaxis in patients with a very low risk of endocarditis (e.g., those with a history of drug allergy) who undergo a procedure with an intermediate or high risk of bacteremia (*e*Table 25.2.3).

The antimicrobial regimens suggested by the American Heart Association for endocarditis prophylaxis are listed in Table 25.3. Although the evidence supporting the routine use of antibiotic prophylaxis is spotty, failure to adhere to these guidelines in the current medicolegal climate may invite litigation. Other expert groups such as the British Society for Antimicrobial Chemotherapy proposed guidelines that differ only slightly. For example, the American Heart Association guidelines recommend that the primary antibiotic regimen for patients undergoing dental, oral, or upper respiratory procedures should be amoxicillin, 2 g orally, 1 hour before the procedure, whereas the British Society for Antimicrobial Chemotherapy recommends a single 3-g oral dose of amoxicillin (183). Some authors (184) have suggested that prophylaxis in patients with prosthetic heart valves should always be parenteral (184), but such recommendations are certainly not a consensus opinion, and we do not routinely use parenteral therapy in such patients.

Medical Therapy during the Course of Infective Endocarditis

General Principles

Individuals with IE often present with unique issues that must be addressed while treating the disease. For that reason, cases of endocarditis caused by the same organism may not be treated in precisely the same manner. On the other hand, common medical and social issues often arise while treating individuals with endocarditis caused by dissimilar pathogens. Table 25.4 outlines a typical approach that might be used for the patient without complications.

After establishing the initial diagnosis, as previously described, a search should be undertaken for the source of the valvular infection. This extent and nature of this search is dependent on the infecting organism. For instance, a dental abnormality is often associated with *S. viridans* endocarditis; a skin infection, deep abscess, or infected vas-

TABLE 25.3   RECOMMENDED BACTERIAL ENDOCARDITIS PROPHYLAXIS REGIMENS

Standard regimen for dental/oral/upper respiratory tract procedures
    Standard regimen in patients at risk (includes those with prosthetic heart valves and other high-risk patients): amoxicillin, 2.0 g, orally 1 h before procedure
    For amoxicillin/penicillin-allergic patients: clindamycin (600 mg orally), cephalexin or cefadroxil (2 g orally), or azithromycin (500 mg orally) taken 1 h before procedure
Alternate standard regimens for dental/oral/upper respiratory tract procedures
    For patients unable to take oral medications: ampicillin, 2.0 g i.v. (or i.m.) 30 minutes before procedure; then ampicillin, 1.0 g i.v. (or i.m.) 6 h after initial dose
    For ampicillin/amoxicillin/penicillin-allergic patients unable to take oral medications: clindamycin, 600 mg i.v., or cefazolin, 1 g i.v., 30 min before procedure
Standard regimen for genitourinary/gastrointestinal procedures
    Standard regimen in patients at high risk: ampicillin, 2.0 g i.v. (or i.m.), plus gentamicin, 1.5 mg/kg i.v. (or i.m.) (not to exceed 120 mg) 30 min before procedure; then amoxicillin, 1 g orally, i.m. or i.v. 6 h after initial dose
    For amoxicillin/ampicillin/penicillin-allergic patients: vancomycin, 1.0 g i.v. administered over 1 h, plus gentamicin, 1.5 mg/kg i.v. (or i.m.) (not to exceed 120 mg) 1 h before procedure
    Alternate oral regimen for genitourinary/gastrointestinal patients at moderate risk: amoxicillin, 3.0 g orally; ampicillin, 2 g i.v.; or vancomycin, 1 g i.v. to be completed 30 min before the procedure

Adapted from Prevention of bacterial endocarditis: recommendations by the American Heart Association. *JAMA* 1997;277:1794–1801.

cular catheter may be the origin if the organism is *Staphylococcus*, whereas a gastrointestinal source, such as colon cancer, may be the source of *S. bovis* endocarditis. If a source for the endocarditis can be found, then its treatment or eradication should be undertaken before cardiac valve repair or replacement is undertaken. For example, if an infected catheter or foreign body is the source of *S. aureus* endocarditis, this source should be removed before proceeding to valve replacement.

In the 1990s, it became acceptable and often necessary to reduce the length of hospitalization by use of a home health agency to administer home intravenous therapy. The patient's home situation should to be evaluated and the suitability for home intravenous therapy should be assessed soon after the diagnosis of IE is established. For most native valve endocarditis, at least 5 to 7 days of in-hospital intravenous therapy is given, followed typically by several more weeks of intravenous antibiotics that, in selected patients, may be completed at home. Criteria for outpatient treatment of endocarditis include the following: (a) unequivocal clinical response to initial therapy, (b) stable hemodynamic status, (c) absence of metastatic or intracardiac complications, and (d) ability to comply with the mechanics and scheduling of outpatient antibiotic therapy. For some patients home therapy is simply not an option because of their social situations.

TABLE 25.4 REPRESENTATIVE THERAPEUTIC APPROACH FOR UNCOMPLICATED NATIVE VALVE INFECTIVE ENDOCARDITIS

Initial evaluation

    Establish diagnosis (including history, physical, blood cultures, echocardiogram, supportive laboratory studies).

    Initiate appropriate antibiotic therapy using minimum inhibitory concentration levels as guide.

    Obtain other baseline studies (electrocardiography, sedimentation rate, complete blood cell counts, electrolytes, chest roentgenography).

    Continue chronic medications except warfarin.

    If on warfarin, discontinue and let international normalized ratio drift down to 2.0, then begin therapeutic heparin.

    Begin search for source of valvular infection.

    If significant valvular regurgitation present, begin angiotensin-converting enzyme inhibitor.

    Cardiovascular surgical consult in most instances, particularly if resistant organism, prosthetic valve endocarditis, evidence of hemodynamic instability, or perivalvular abscess is present.

    Evaluate home situation and lifestyle regarding potential for home therapy.

Once therapy has begun

    Daily vital signs, physical examination; telemetry at least the first week.

    Insert percutaneous indwelling central venous catheter line (or Hickman's) for intravenous antibiotic use.

    Continue search for source of valvular infection if appropriate.

    Repeat blood cultures after 72 h of therapy and repeat if fever persists.

    Obtain trough and peak antibiotic drug levels initially, and if dosage altered.

    Ongoing laboratory studies: Every 3 d, complete blood cell counts, electrolytes. Weekly, electrocardiography, chest roentgenography.

    Continue i.v. antibiotic therapy 5 to 14 d in-hospital, then arrange for completion of course (usually 4 wk) as outpatient.

    If patient on chronic warfarin, may resume after first week of therapy if surgery not apparently required.

    As outpatient on therapy, continue daily vital signs and weekly complete blood cell counts and electrolytes.

    Once therapy complete, follow-up echocardiography.

In patients with those home environments, completing the entire antibiotic course as an inpatient or in a convalescent care facility is preferred. Six weeks of therapy is used for most prosthetic valve endocarditis or when a relatively resistant organism causes native valve endocarditis. At times, more than 6 weeks of therapy may be needed, especially when a virulent or relatively resistant organism such as a gentamicin-resistant enterococcus is present.

Once the diagnosis of endocarditis is established, a baseline electrocardiogram, complete blood count with differential, sedimentation rate, electrolytes, and chest roentgenography should be obtained. A chest wall echocardiogram should be obtained in all patients. TEE should be employed in accordance with the guidelines noted previously. After the initial blood cultures, repeat blood cultures should be obtained in most patients after 3 days of treatment to ensure that bacteremia has resolved. Persistent bacteremia on surveillance cultures should raise concern that the antibiotic therapy is less than adequate. After that, blood cultures are usually only obtained again if fever resumes or if other signs of active infection, such as recurrent leukocytosis, occur.

Persistent fevers in the face of seemingly appropriate therapy are an occasional clinical dilemma. When fever is accompanied by mental confusion or congestive heart failure, therapy with antipyretics such as acetaminophen is warranted, but in general it is preferable to avoid antipyretics in order to monitor the clinical response to therapy. The blood counts and electrolytes are repeated every 3 days until the results are stable or normal. Patients are usually monitored with telemetry for the first week of therapy; electrocardiography and chest roentgenography are repeated weekly. Prolongation of the PR interval on electrocardiography (unrelated to drug usage) or radiographic or clinical signs of congestive heart failure may in turn lead to other studies and more careful clinical assessment. When aminoglycosides or vancomycin are used as therapy, antibiotic drug levels should be monitored at least once during therapy. Specialized microbiologic testing of the etiologic agent should be assessed with certain organisms such as viridans staphylococci and enterococci. Repeat echocardiography may be necessary if there is confusion regarding the clinical status of the patient, but, in most instances, serial echocardiograms are not necessary while therapy is ongoing. ⚛ e89

Antimicrobial Therapy

Before the availability of antimicrobial therapy, IE was invariably fatal. Even today a substantial percentage of patients with IE die because of highly virulent organisms such as *S. aureus*, despite having received appropriate antimicrobial therapy in a timely manner and despite the skillful use of modern diagnostic techniques, surgical methods, and supportive care. However, the majority of patients with endocarditis now survives infections.

Following the establishment of a diagnosis using clinical deduction and microbiologic and echocardiographic methods, antimicrobial therapy should be administered in a dose designed to give sustained bactericidal serum concentrations throughout much of or the entire dosing interval. The duration of this therapy has to be long enough to eradicate microorganisms growing in the valvular vegetations. ⚛ e90

The need for prolonged therapy in treating endocarditis and the problem of reduced *in vitro* sensitivity to commonly used antimicrobial agents has stimulated interest in using combination therapy to treat endocarditis. Combination therapy using a beta-lactam agent such as penicillin with an aminoglycoside has been shown to be highly effective in streptococcal endocarditis and somewhat effective in a small subset of patients with staphylococcal endocarditis. Combination therapy with penicillin or ceftriaxone and an aminoglycoside for 2 weeks is highly effective in viridans streptococcal endocarditis (188–190).

Combination therapy with nafcillin and an aminoglycoside for 2 weeks has been shown to be effective in patients with right-sided endocarditis caused by *S. aureus* (191). One study suggests that aminoglycoside therapy is not critical to the success of these short-course regimens. In a randomized trial, cloxacillin therapy alone for 2 weeks was as effective as the combination of cloxacillin and gentamicin (192). However, combined therapy with vancomycin and an aminoglycoside administered for 2 weeks does not appear to be effective. Also, combined therapy with nafcillin and an aminoglycoside is not effective in left-sided endocarditis if treatment is given for only 2 weeks.

Several reports have described the successful use of oral regimens for selected patients with IE (193). Despite reports of success with such regimens, oral regimens should not be used as initial therapy for endocarditis. Nonconventional regimens should only be used in highly selected cases in which the causative organism is known, in which the antimicrobial susceptibility has been carefully studied, and in which *in vitro* studies show high levels of susceptibility. Generally, there should be a compelling reason to use oral therapy over conventional intravenous therapy now that home health agencies allow for home antibiotic infusions. We do not believe there are adequate data to support a preference for oral antibiotic usage.

Until more recently, most patients with endocarditis received the entire duration of their antimicrobial therapy while in the hospital. However, the development of systems and equipment that allows for prolonged and safe administration of intravenous therapy to outpatients has made it acceptable and appropriate to treat selected patients with endocarditis as outpatients during much or even all of their therapy (190). Patients selected for outpatient therapy should have responded clinically to inpatient therapy and without evidence of metastatic or intracardiac complications. In addition, they should be hemodynamically stable, compliant, and capable of managing the technical aspects of intravenous therapy (188). Such patients still require careful and regular monitoring and must have ready access to full medical care should complications such as drug allergy, emboli, or cardiac failure occur.

Endocarditis Caused by Streptococcus Viridans and Streptococcus bovis

The various species of streptococci that make up the viridans group and *S. bovis* account for approximately 40% to 50% of all cases of native valve endocarditis in community practice. Endocarditis caused by these organisms can usually be microbiologically cured if one of four different regimens is used (*e*Table 25.4.1). Most of these organisms are highly penicillin-susceptible [i.e., have a minimum inhibitory concentration (MIC) ≤0.1 μg per mL].

Endocarditis caused by highly penicillin-susceptible streptococci can be reliably cured using aqueous crystalline penicillin G at a dose of 12 to 18 million units daily for 4 weeks. This regimen or an equally effective regimen consisting of ceftriaxone, given as a 2-g daily dose for 1 month, remains the preferred treatment for elderly patients or in other patients in whom aminoglycoside therapy is considered risky or contraindicated.

Selected patients with native valve endocarditis without evidence of intracardiac or extracardiac complications or preexisting renal or otic disease can be treated with shorter courses of combination therapy consisting of either aqueous crystalline penicillin G or ceftriaxone with gentamicin. The latter agent should be given at a dose (usually 1 mg per kg) designed to give a peak gentamicin serum level of 3 μg per mL. Although streptomycin can also be used with either of the previously mentioned beta-lactam antibiotics to achieve the same effect, gentamicin is currently more widely used in clinical practice. Furthermore, determinations of gentamicin serum levels are more widely available and dosing regimens are more familiar to clinicians than streptomycin.

Patients with histories of penicillin allergy can usually be treated with other beta-lactam antibiotics, such as cefazolin, if their prior history of penicillin allergy consists of skin rash without other signs of immediate-type hypersensitivity. Patients with histories of immediate-type hypersensitivity may be treated either with vancomycin for 4 weeks or desensitized to penicillin and treated with a standard regimen.

Patients with endocarditis caused by viridans streptococci and MICs >0.1 μg per mL and patients with endocarditis caused by streptococci with nutritional deficiencies that hinder their growth in routine laboratory culture media should receive aqueous penicillin G for a total of 4 weeks. Gentamicin should be added to this regimen for the first 2 weeks. As for other patients with streptococcal endocarditis with immediate-type hypersensitivity reactions to beta-lactams, vancomycin is an acceptable alternative (*e*Table 25.4.2).

Other streptococcal species (e.g., groups A, B, C, and G and *Streptococcus pneumoniae*) are occasional causes of endocarditis. Therapy should always be based on the results of susceptibility tests. As most such organisms are highly sensitive to penicillin, regimens used to treat endocarditis caused by viridans streptococci are usually effective. However, increasing numbers of isolates of *S. pneumoniae* have become relatively or highly penicillin resistant. Such organisms may be simultaneously resistant to other beta-lactams as well as to other antimicrobial agents. Therapy in such cases usually requires the input of an infectious disease specialist or a microbiologist. A few strains of *S. pneumoniae* only respond to vancomycin therapy.

Endocarditis Caused by Enterococci

Unlike streptococci, members of the genus *Enterococcus* are uniformly resistant to low concentrations of penicillin.

Enterococci are also relatively resistant to expanded spectrum penicillins and vancomycin. Furthermore, they are uniformly highly resistant to all cephalosporins and typically resistant to aminoglycosides at concentrations achieved after standard dosing regimens. However, if penicillin, ampicillin, or vancomycin is given in synergistic combination with aminoglycosides such as gentamicin, most strains of enterococci are killed both *in vitro* and *in vivo* (*e*Table 25.4.3).

During the past 10 to 15 years, a number of new trends in the resistance pattern of enterococci have appeared. Some strains (particularly strains of *Enterococcus faecalis*) have acquired genetic material that allows them to produce beta-lactamase. Other strains, particularly strains of *E. faecium*, have acquired high-level resistance to streptomycin, gentamicin, or both. In addition, intrinsic high-level resistance to penicillin and ampicillin has appeared in some strains of enterococci. Finally, increasing numbers of enterococci have acquired high-level resistance to vancomycin. Some, but not all, of these highly resistant strains are also resistant to the investigational glycopeptide antibiotic, teicoplanin.

The previously mentioned microbiologic characteristics have a direct effect on the guidelines for treatment of enterococcal endocarditis. Standard therapy for enterococci with "typical" low-level penicillin resistance consists of a combination of intravenous aqueous penicillin G or ampicillin combined with gentamicin for 4 to 6 weeks. Patients with symptoms for less than 3 months can usually be treated successfully with 4 weeks of therapy. Patients with symptoms of more than 3 months' duration before the initiation of treatment, those with a relapsed infections, and those patients with prosthetic valve infection should receive a 6-week course of therapy. Gentamicin therapy should be given at doses designed to achieve peak serum levels of approximately 3 µg per mL and trough serum concentrations <1 µg per mL. Patients with a history of penicillin allergy should be treated with a combination of vancomycin and gentamicin for 4 to 6 weeks.

Enterococcal endocarditis caused by strains with intrinsic high-level penicillin resistance (MIC >16 µg per mL) should be treated with a combination of vancomycin and gentamicin. Organisms that are resistant to penicillin via the production of beta-lactamase can be treated with either ampicillin-sulbactam, gentamicin, or vancomycin and gentamicin (188). ▼ e91

Staphylococcal Endocarditis

The success of therapy for staphylococcal endocarditis is dependent on numerous factors. These include whether the right- or left-sided valvular structures are involved, whether the staphylococcus is coagulase-negative or -positive, whether the infection occurs on a native or prosthetic valve, and whether there is favorable antimicrobial susceptibility to the staphylococcal isolate (*e*Tables 25.4.4 and 25.4.5).

Native valve endocarditis caused by *S. aureus* is best treated with a semisynthetic penicillin such as nafcillin or oxacillin for 4 to 6 weeks. As methicillin-susceptible strains of *S. aureus* are more rapidly killed both *in vitro* and *in vivo* in a rabbit experimental model of endocarditis, many authorities recommend the addition of gentamicin for the first 3 to 5 days of therapy.

The combination of nafcillin and gentamicin given for the first 2 weeks of therapy in a multicenter collaborative study of native valve endocarditis caused by methicillin-susceptible strains of staphylococcal endocarditis was associated with more rapid clearing of the bacteremia than in patients randomized to receive monotherapy with nafcillin, but such combination therapy did not improve cure rates. Furthermore, combination nafcillin and gentamicin therapy was associated with a higher incidence of renal dysfunction.

Patients with native valve endocarditis caused by *S. aureus* who have histories of penicillin allergy can be treated with either first-generation cephalosporins such as cefazolin (if there is history of penicillin reaction that is not typical of an immediate-type allergy) or vancomycin. Vancomycin should not be used on the basis of convenience related to its pharmacokinetics in patients without a history of penicillin allergy, as clinical experience and *in vitro* studies have suggested that vancomycin is a less effective antistaphylococcal antibiotic than either nafcillin or oxacillin (188,194).

Selected patients with native valve endocarditis caused by *S. aureus* that involves the right-sided heart valves can be successfully treated with a 2-week treatment regimen using the combination therapy of nafcillin and gentamicin (191). Regimens that substitute vancomycin or cefazolin for nafcillin are not considered to be reliably effective in such patients if only 2 weeks of therapy are given (195). It is important to realize that short-course regimens using combination therapy are not suitable for patients with simultaneous infection of both left-sided heart valves, in patients with isolates that demonstrate high-level gentamicin resistance (MIC >500 µg per mL), or in patients with metastatic infection outside of the lungs.

Patients with prosthetic valve endocarditis caused by methicillin-susceptible *S. aureus* should be treated with nafcillin or an equivalent beta-lactamase–resistant beta-lactam antibiotic for at least 6 weeks. Because such infections are notoriously difficult to cure with medical therapy, most authorities recommend simultaneously treating with oral rifampin. In addition, many experts advise the addition of gentamicin for the first 2 weeks of therapy. A first-generation cephalosporin or vancomycin can be substituted for nafcillin in patients with a history of penicillin allergy.

The only effective therapy for patients with endocarditis caused by methicillin-resistant staphylococci is vancomycin. Monotherapy with vancomycin for 4 to 6 weeks is usually adequate for therapy with endocarditis caused by methicillin-resistant native valve endocarditis caused by

TABLE 25.5 THERAPY FOR ENDOCARDITIS CAUSED BY HACEK MICROORGANISMS (*HAEMOPHILUS PARAINFLUENZAE, HAEMOPHILUS APHROPHILUS, ACTINOBACILLUS ACTINOMYCETEMCOMITANS, CARDIOBACTERIUM HOMINIS, EIKENELLA CORRODENS,* AND *KINGELLA KINGAE*)

Antibiotic	Dosage and route	Duration (wk)	Comments
Ceftriaxone sodium	2 g once daily i.v. or i.m.	4	Cefotaxime sodium or other third-generation cephalosporins may be substituted
Ampicillin sodium	12 g/24 h i.v. either continuously or in six equally divided doses	4	
With gentamicin sulfate	1 mg/kg i.m. or i.v. every 8 h		

either *S. aureus* or coagulase-negative staphylococci. However, when methicillin-resistant staphylococci cause infection in patients with prosthetic valves or other prosthetic material, combination therapy is generally used. Such patients can be treated with intravenous vancomycin and oral rifampin therapy for 6 to 8 weeks. The addition of gentamicin is recommended for the first 2 weeks of this therapeutic regimen. The appearance of strains of *S. aureus* that have intermediate- or high-level resistance to vancomycin has raised the possibility that such organisms could cause endocarditis for which all currently available therapy is ineffective. At present, there is little *in vivo* information available on the optimal treatment of human infection with such organisms.

Endocarditis Caused by HACEK Organisms

A number of fastidious gram-negative bacilli, collectively grouped by the acronym *HACEK*, accounts for 5% to 10% of all cases of native valve endocarditis in individuals who do not use illicit intravenous drugs. Organisms in this category include the following: *Haemophilus parainfluenzae, Haemophilus aphrophilus, Actinobacillus actinomycetemcomitans, Cardiobacterium hominis, Eikenella corrodens,* and *Kingella kingae*. All of these organisms grow slowly in blood culture media, and incubation for 7 to 14 days may be required to detect their growth. This delayed growth makes standard antibiotic susceptibility testing difficult. Although in the past most HACEK organisms were ampicillin-sensitive, this is no longer true, as many species in this group have acquired the ability to produce beta-lactamase. However, virtually all of these organisms are highly susceptible to third-generation cephalosporins such as ceftriaxone and cefotaxime (Table 25.5). Either agent is usually effective when given for 3 to 4 weeks to patients with native valve endocarditis; patients with prosthetic valve endocarditis should be treated for 6 weeks (188).

Serum Bactericidal Levels

A commonly asked question in clinical practice relates to serum bactericidal levels. In general, serum bactericidal levels are of little clinical benefit since there is a relatively poor correlation between bactericidal levels and outcome and

because results obtained when performing serum bactericidal levels may vary depending on laboratory technique.

Surgical Therapy

The classic indications for cardiac surgery in patients with IE have remained relatively constant for the past two decades. [✔ e92] Surgery is recommended for patients who develop congestive heart failure, who exhibit recurrent emboli during the course of therapy, and who fail to achieve an adequate bactericidal response to therapy. Most clinicians, including the authors, believe that abscess formation or the presence of a fungal endocarditis is a relative indication for surgical intervention. There is now a general consensus that the indication for surgery in active endocarditis differs little between native valve (Table 25.6) and prosthetic valve infection (Table 25.7). Large bulky vegetations—especially if they represent infections with organisms with a propensity to embolize, such as HACEK—may be an indication for surgical intervention, although no adequately controlled prospective study has examined this question. Congestive heart failure is the most common indication for surgery in patients with left-sided endocarditis, whereas refractory infection is the most frequent indication for surgery in right-sided endocarditis. There is widespread consensus that surgical intervention has been shown to improve patient survival in virtually every instance in which congestive heart failure complicates endocarditis. Before the rou-

TABLE 25.6 INDICATIONS FOR CARDIAC SURGERY IN NATIVE VALVE ENDOCARDITIS

Major indications
  Congestive heart failure (New York Heart Association Functional Classification III or IV) caused by valve dysfunction
  Persistent sepsis while receiving antimicrobial therapy
  Recurrent embolism
Minor indications
  Intracardiac abscess or fistula formation
  Rupture of sinus of Valsalva aneurysm
  Pathogen not susceptible to antimicrobial therapy
  Fungal endocarditis
  Acute *Staphylococcus aureus* endocarditis on left-sided heart valves with congestive failure
  Relapse after an adequate course of antimicrobial therapy
  Culture-negative endocarditis with persistent (>10 d) fever

TABLE 25.7 INDICATIONS FOR CARDIAC SURGERY IN PROSTHETIC VALVE ENDOCARDITIS

Major indications
  Congestive heart failure caused by unstable prosthesis
  Fungal endocarditis
  Significant perivalvular dehiscence
  Recurrent septic emboli
  Evidence for intracardiac abscess or fistula formation
  Persistent sepsis (>3 d on antimicrobial therapy)
  Interference with valve function caused by vegetation
  Pathogen not susceptible to antimicrobial therapy
Minor indications
  Nonstreptococcal pathogen
  Relapse after adequate course of antibiotic therapy
  Culture-negative endocarditis with persistent (>10 d) fever

tine use of surgery in patients with complicated endocarditis, congestive heart failure caused over 90% of all deaths. At times, congestive heart failure may be subtle, clinically evident only by a persistent tachycardia for no other reason. Thus, careful daily assessment by experienced clinicians is necessary for patients with hemodynamic instability or unexplained tachycardia or dyspnea.

It is important to realize that the severity of cardiac and extracardiac manifestations of heart failure and the degree of hemodynamic stability of the individual patient are the major determinants of the optimal timing for surgery (198). In most case series, congestive heart failure caused by endocarditis-induced aortic insufficiency has a worse prognosis than endocarditis-induced mitral insufficiency. However, regardless of the valve involved, valve replacement should be undertaken in most patients as soon as signs and symptoms of congestive heart failure appear. It has been our experience that clinical signs of heart failure are more important than the echocardiographic assessment of left ventricular function. However, when aortic insufficiency is severe enough to result in preclosure of the mitral valve as detected by echocardiography, then operative intervention is likely to be required (137).

Recurrent emboli are a difficult criterion on which to base the need for surgical intervention. Some patients who experience episodes of peripheral embolism after the institution of antimicrobial therapy can be successfully managed without surgery. Furthermore, there is no precise threshold for the number of embolic events that mandate surgery. However, the authors share the opinion of Weinstein that surgery is usually indicated when a second episode of embolization occurs, especially in patients with endocarditis caused by *S. aureus*, any fungal pathogen, or *Haemophilus* species (43). The optimal timing of surgery for recurrent cerebral embolism is often problematic, because full heparinization during bypass surgery may exacerbate the clinical course of a recent cerebral infarct regardless of whether it is hemorrhagic or ischemic. However, it is our experience, and that of others, that surgery can usually be safely undertaken in such patients (199).

Despite the availability of an array of antimicrobial agents, failure to control infection is still a problem in the treatment of endocarditis. Such failure remains an indication for surgical intervention as one is removing the source of the bacteremia. The definition of bacteriological failure though is not clear-cut. Some organisms, such as *S. aureus*, may persist in the bloodstream for up to 5 days after initiation of therapy that will ultimately be curative. However, in general, persistently positive blood culture results after 5 to 7 days of therapy are an indication of the need for surgical intervention. Fungal endocarditis is notoriously difficult to cure with medical therapy alone. A few cases of endocarditis caused by *Candida* species have been cured without surgery (200–202), but most patients with *Candida* endocarditis, and virtually all patients with endocarditis caused by *Aspergillus*, require surgery to control their infections. Even combined surgical and medical therapy often leads to a poor outcome in patients with fungal endocarditis. For example, in a review of the outcome of 108 cases of fungal endocarditis, 97 of 108 (90%) died (35).

Bacteriological cure may be particularly difficult to achieve in patients with prosthetic valve endocarditis. The authors agree with others that prosthetic valve endocarditis caused by organisms other than viridans streptococci and that the HACEK group is difficult to cure with medical therapy. Most such patients eventually require surgery to achieve cure (203). In addition, when prosthetic valve endocarditis relapses after a course of medical therapy, a perivalvular infection is usually present. Such patients almost always require surgery. Certain organisms such as vancomycin-resistant enterococci cannot be effectively treated with any currently available agent. Patients with endocarditis caused by this organism should undergo early surgery whenever this is feasible. ▼ e93

CONTROVERSIES AND PERSONAL PERSPECTIVES

Controversies revolving around the diagnosis and treatment of IE include the duration of therapy needed, the use of outpatient therapy, the use of expensive diagnostic tests such as TEE, the risks and benefits and indications for prophylactic antibiotic therapy (especially in the mitral valve prolapse syndrome), the timing of surgical intervention (including when surgical colleagues should be consulted), and the ethical issues that arise when recurrent endocarditis results from destructive or erratic patient behavior such as often seen among illicit drug users.

All but the ethical issues have been addressed in detail in this chapter. It is our belief that endocarditis requires intravenous therapy. Until conclusive data showing efficacy of oral therapy are published or presented, we do not advocate therapy with any currently available oral antibiotic agent. We also advocate inpatient therapy for at least 5 to 7 days

THE FUTURE

Despite advances in echocardiography and surgery, IE remains a serious and fatal disease. Our basic understanding of the disease process remains incomplete. More research is needed to better understand vegetation propagation and the role of anticoagulant therapy. Refinements in antibiotic prophylaxis and treatment as well as surgical techniques are also important areas of research currently being pursued.

before considering outpatient intravenous therapy. The use of once-a-day administration of drugs with a long half-life, such as ceftriaxone, greatly assists in the administration of outpatient therapy. If there is any question regarding the suitability of the patient and family regarding home therapy though, we favor completing the entire antibiotic course as an inpatient or in a convalescent facility or infusion center.

We believe that TEE provides a substantial and clinically important identification of vegetations on leaflets and involvement of contiguous structures so that its routine use makes some sense even though the chest wall echo may be adequate for diagnosis alone. This is particularly true for aortic valve endocarditis in which annular abscess may be discovered. The presence of abscess by TEE has prompted us to recommend surgery when other indications may not have been present.

Despite few data supporting prophylactic antibiotic usage to prevent endocarditis, our practice is to be quite liberal in its use. As prevention potentially protects from a serious disease that is seemingly much easier to potentially prevent than treat, the risk-benefit ratio of antibiotic usage, especially with dental procedures, seems in favor of antibiotic usage. Antimicrobial prophylaxis for mitral valve prolapse often presents a true therapeutic dilemma given the high prevalence in the population. Because the presence of mitral regurgitation in this disease is dependent on the relationship between the valve apparatus and left ventricular volume, mitral regurgitation may be audible at one time but not another. Given the reduction in emphasis on the physical examination in the majority of training programs in this country, the ability to properly auscultate also is troublesome if the criteria for use of antibiotic prophylaxis in patients with mitral valve prolapse require careful auscultation for murmur detection. For that reason, we are quite liberal in the use of antibiotic prophylaxis in patients with mitral valve prolapse.

We also believe that a close relationship with cardiovascular surgery is mandatory to ensure proper care of these often complex patients. We have formed an endocarditis team that includes cardiologists with an interest in valvular and congenital heart disease, specialists in infectious disease and bacteriology, and cardiovascular surgeons. We believe that consultation with cardiovascular surgeons should be done in almost all patients, regardless of their current clinical status. As mentioned in this chapter, this is particularly important in prosthetic valve endocarditis or when a potential complication, such as ring abscess, fungal valvular infection, or mycotic aneurysm, is present. Issues surrounding the surgical options can be complex, especially if there has been CNS bleeding or significant comorbid disease.

Finally, the debate on the treatment of recurrent endocarditis in patients who chronically use illicit intravenous drugs should be openly discussed and resolved. Ethical dilemmas and controversies often arise in patients with endocarditis who clearly indicate that their illicit drug use will continue. Our current policy is to replace or repair the infected heart valve in intravenous drug abusers only once; the ethical and financial issues that such an approach raise need to be resolved. We believe that every effort should be made to provide medical care for all intravenous drug abusers with special emphasis on efforts at rehabilitation. However, in an era of managed care and reduced resources, it is critical that personal responsibility for health become the accepted norm. Our policy at this time is to involve the ethics committee to provide a forum to understand the specifics for each individual who abused intravenous drugs and also has recurrent infective endocarditis.

REFERENCES

1. Major RH. Notes on the history of endocarditis. *Bull Hist Med* 1945;17:351–359.
2. Contrepois A. Notes on the early history of infective endocarditis and the development of an experimental model. *Clin Infect Dis* 1995;20:461–466.
3. Rosenow EC. Experimental infectious endocarditis. *J Infect Dis* 1912;11:210–218.
4. Luschka H. Das endocardium inad die endocarditis. *Arch Pathol Anat Physiol* 1852;4:171.
5. Gross L. Significance of blood vessels in human heart valves. *Am Heart J* 1937;13:275–280.
6. Thayer WS. Bacterial or infective endocarditis. *Edinburgh Med J* 1931;38:237, 334.
7. Osler W. Chronic infective endocarditis. *QJM* 1901;2:219.
8. Kerr AJ. *Subacute bacterial endocarditis.* Springfield, IL: Thomas, 1955.
9. Weiss S. Self-observations and psychologic reactions of medical student A.S.R. to the onset and symptoms of sub-

acute bacterial endocarditis. *J Mount Sinai Hosp* 1941;42:79–94.

10. Bansal RC. Infective endocarditis [review]. *Med Clin North Am* 1995;79:1205–1240.

11. Clifford CP, Eykyn SJ, Oakley CM. Staphylococcal tricuspid valve endocarditis in patients with structurally normal hearts and no evidence of narcotic abuse. *QJM* 1994;87:755–757.

12. Levine DP, Crane LR, Zervos MJ. Bacteremia in narcotic addicts at the Detroit Medical Center. II. Infectious endocarditis: a prospective comparative study. *Rev Infect Dis* 1986;8:374–396.

13. Mathew J, Addai T, Anand A, et al. Clinical features, site of involvement, bacteriologic findings, and outcome of infective endocarditis in intravenous drug users. *Arch Intern Med* 1995;155:1641–1648.

14. Saravolatz LP, Burch KH, Quinn EL. Polymicrobial infective endocarditis: an increasing clinical entity. *Am Heart J* 1978;95:163.

15. Griffin MR, Wilson WR, Edwards WD, et al. Infective endocarditis, Olmsted County, Minnesota, 1950 through 1981. *JAMA* 1985;254:1199–1202.

16. McKinsey DS, Ratts TE, Bisno AL. Underlying cardiac lesions in adults with infective endocarditis. The changing spectrum. *Am J Med* 1987;82:681–688.

17. Cherubin CE, Neu HC. Infective endocarditis at the Presbyterian Hospital in New York from 1938–1967. *Am J Med* 1971;51:83.

18. Weinberger I, Rotenberg Z, Zacharovitch D, et al. Native valve infective endocarditis in the 1970s versus the 1980s: underlying cardiac lesions and infecting organisms. *Clin Cardiol* 1990;13:94–98.

19. Clemens JD, Horwitz RI, Jaffe CC, et al. A controlled evaluation of the risk of bacterial endocarditis in persons with mitral-valve prolapse. *N Engl J Med* 1982;307:776–781.

20. Beton DC, Brear SG, Edwards JD, et al. Mitral valve prolapse: an assessment of clinical features, associated conditions, and prognosis. *QJM* 1983;52:150–164.

21. Michel PL, Acar J. Native cardiac disease predisposing to infective endocarditis [review]. *Eur Heart J* 1995;16[Suppl B]:2–6.

22. Grover FL, Cohen DJ, Oprian C, et al. Determinants of the occurrence of and survival from prosthetic valve endocarditis. Experience of the Veterans Affairs Cooperative Study on Valvular Heart Disease. *J Thorac Cardiovasc Surg* 1994;108:207–214.

23. Calderwood SB, Swinski LA, Waternaux CM, et al. Risk factors for the development of prosthetic valve endocarditis. *Circulation* 1985;72:31–37.

23a. Gordon SM, Serkey JM, Longworth DL, et al. Each onset prosthetic valve endocarditis: the Cleveland Clinic experience 1992–1997. *Ann Thorac Surg* 2000;69:1388–1392.

23b. Kassai B, Gueyffier F, Cucherat M, et al. Comparison of bioprosthesis and mechanical valves; meta-analysis of randomized clinical trials. *Cardiovasc Surg* 2000;8:477–483.

24. Gersony WM, Hayes CJ, Driscoll DJ, et al. Bacterial endocarditis in patients with aortic stenosis, pulmonary stenosis, or ventricular septal defect. *Circulation* 1993;87:1121–1126.

25. Horstkotte D. Prosthetic valve endocarditis. In: Horstkotte D, Bodnar E, eds. *Infective endocarditis*. London: IRC Publishers, 1991:229–261.

26. Tornos MP, Permanyer-Miralda G, Olona M, et al. Long-term complications of native valve infective endocarditis in non-addicts. A 15-year follow-up study [see comments]. *Ann Intern Med* 1992;117:567–572.

27. Delahaye F, Ecochard R, De Gevigney G, et al. The long term prognosis of infective endocarditis [review]. *Eur Heart J* 1995;16[Suppl B]:48–53.

28. Karchmer AW, Dismukes WE, Buckley MG, et al. Late prosthetic valve endocarditis. Clinical features influencing therapy. *Am J Med* 1978;64:199–207.

29. King LHJ, Bradley KP, Shire DLJ, et al. Bacterial endocarditis in chronic hemodialysis patients: a complication more common than previously reported. *Surgery* 1971;69:554.

30. Martino P, Micozzi A, Venditti M, et al. Catheter-related right-sided endocarditis in bone marrow transplant recipients. *Rev Infect Dis* 1990;12:250–257.

31. Valla D, Pariente E, Degott C, et al. Right-sided endocarditis complicating peritoneovenous shunting for ascites. *Arch Intern Med* 1983;143:1801.

32. Daly JS, Worthington MG, Brenner DJ, et al. *Rochalimaea elizabethae* sp. *nov.* isolated from a patient with endocarditis. *J Clin Microbiol* 1993;31:872–881.

33. Klein RS, Recco RA, Catalono MT, et al. Association of streptococcus bovis with carcinoma of the colon. *N Engl J Med* 1961;264:257.

34. Kreuzpaintner G, Horstkotte D, Heyll A, et al. Increased risk of bacterial endocarditis in inflammatory bowel disease [see comments]. *Am J Med* 1992;92:391–395.

35. Fowler VG, Durack DT. Infective endocarditis [review]. *Curr Opin Cardiol* 1994;9:389–400.

36. Horstkotte D, Piper C, Niehues R, et al. Late prosthetic valve endocarditis [review]. *Eur Heart J* 1995;16[Suppl B]:39–47.

37. Bestetti RB, Figueiredo JF, Da Costa JC. Salmonella tricuspid endocarditis in an intravenous drug abuser with human immunodeficiency virus infection. *Int J Cardiol* 1991;30:361–362.

38. Riancho JA, Echevarria S, Napal J, et al. Endocarditis due to *Listeria monocytogenes* and human immunodeficiency virus infection [published erratum appears in *Am J Med* 1989; March 1986:366]. *Am J Med* 1988;85:737.

39. Nahass RG, Weinstein MP, Bartels J, et al. Infective endocarditis in intravenous drug users: a comparison of human immunodeficiency virus type 1-negative and -positive patients. *J Infect Dis* 1990;162:967–970.

40. Chambers HF, Morris DL, Tauber MG, et al. Cocaine use and the risk for endocarditis in intravenous drug users. *Ann Intern Med* 1987;106:833–836.

41. Garrison PK, Freedman LR. Experimental endocarditis. I. Staphylococcal endocarditis in rabbits resulting from placement of a polyethylene catheter in the right side of the heart. *Yale J Biol Med* 1970;42:394–410.

42. Durack DT, Beeson PB. Experimental bacterial endocarditis. I. Colonization of a sterile vegetation. *Br J Exp Pathol* 1972;53:44–49.

43. Weinstein L. Life-threatening complications of infective

endocarditis and their management. *Arch Intern Med* 1986;146:953–957.

44. Yvorchuk KJ, Chan KL. Application of transthoracic and transesophageal echocardiography in the diagnosis and management of infective endocarditis. *J Am Soc Echocardiogr* 1994;7:294–308.

45. Karalis DG, Bansal RC, Hauck AJ, et al. Transesophageal echocardiographic recognition of subaortic complications in aortic valve endocarditis. Clinical and surgical implications. *Circulation* 1992;86:353–362.

46. Arnett EN, Roberts WC. Prosthetic valve endocarditis: clinicopathologic analysis of 22 necropsy patients with comparison observations in 74 necropsy patients with active infective endocarditis involving natural left-sided cardiac valves. *Am J Cardiol* 1976;38:281–292.

47. Zussa C, Galloni MR, Zattera GF, et al. Endocarditis in patients with bioprostheses: pathology and clinical correlations. *Int J Cardiol* 1984;6:719–735.

48. Weinstein L, Rubin RH. Infective endocarditis—1973. *Prog Cardiovasc Dis* 1973;16:239.

49. Gould K, Ramerez-Ronda CH, Holmes RK, et al. Adherence of bacteria to heart valves in vitro. *J Clin Invest* 1975;56:1314.

50. Freedman LR, Valvone JJ. Experimental infective endocarditis. *Prog Cardiovasc Dis* 1979;22:169.

51. Scheld WM, Valvone JA, Sande MA. Bacterial adherence in the pathogenesis of endocarditis. Interaction of bacterial dextran, platelets, and fibrin. *J Clin Invest* 1978;61:1394.

52. Kuypers JM, Proctor RA. Reduced adherence to traumatized rat heart valves by a low-fibronectin-binding mutant of *Staphylococcus aureus*. *Infect Immunol* 1989;57:2306–2312.

53. Mair W. Pneumococcal endocarditis in rabbits. *J Pathol Bacteriol* 1923;26:426.

54. Durack DT, Gilliland BC, Petersdorf RG. Effect of performed antibody on experimental *Streptococcus mutans* and *Streptococcus sanguis* endocarditis. *Infect Immunol* 1978;22:52.

55. Robbard S. Blood velocity and endocarditis. *Circulation* 1963;27:18–28.

56. Arber N, Pras E, Copperman Y, et al. Pacemaker endocarditis. Report of 44 cases and review of the literature. *Medicine* 1994;73:299–305.

57. Mohamed M, Habte-Gabr E, Mueller W. Infected arteriovenous hemodialysis graft presenting as left and right infective endocarditis. *Am J Nephrol* 1995;15:521–523.

58. Zijlstra F, Fioretti P, Roelandt JR. Echocardiographic demonstration of free wall vegetative endocarditis complicated by a pulmonary embolism in a patient with ventricular septal defect. *Br Heart J* 1986;55:497–499.

59. Turner SW, Wyllie JP, Hamilton JR, et al. Diagnosis of infected modified Blalock-Taussig shunt by computed tomography. *Ann Thorac Surg* 1995;59:1216–1217.

60. Graham HV, vonHartitzsch B, Medina JR. Infected atrial myxoma. *Am J Cardiol* 1976;38:658–661.

61. Pelletier LLJ, Petersdorf RG. Infective endocarditis: a review of 125 cases from the University of Washington Hospitals, 1963–72. *Medicine (Baltimore)* 1977;56:287–313.

62. von Reyn CF, Levy BS, Arbeit RD, et al. Infective endocarditis: an analysis based on strict definitions. *Ann Intern Med* 1981;94:505–518.

63. Durack DT, Lukes AS, Bright DK. New criteria for diagnosis of infective endocarditis: utilization of specific echocardiographic findings. Duke Endocarditis Service [see comments]. *Am J Med* 1994;96:200–209.

64. Bayer AS, Ward JI, Ginzton LE, et al. Evaluation of new clinical criteria for the diagnosis of infective endocarditis [see comments]. *Am J Med* 1994;96:211–219.

65. Hoen B, Selton-Suty C, Danchin N, et al. Evaluation of the Duke Criteria versus the Beth Israel criteria for the diagnosis of infective endocarditis. *Clin Infect Dis* 1995;21:905–909.

66. Del Pont JM, De Cicco LT, Vartalitis C, et al. Infective endocarditis in children: clinical analysis and evaluation of two diagnostic criteria. *Pediatr Infect Dis J* 1995;14:1079–1086.

67. Bayer AS. Editorial: diagnostic criteria for identifying cases of endocarditis–revisiting the Duke criteria two years later. *Clin Infect Dis* 1996;23:303–304.

68. Dodds GA, Sexton DJ, Durack DT. Negative predictive value of the Duke criteria for infective endocarditis. *Am J Cardiol* 1996;77:403–407.

69. Hoen B, Beguinot I, Rabaud C, et al. The Duke criteria for diagnosing infective endocarditis are specific: analysis of 100 patients with acute fever or fever of unknown origin. *Clin Infect Dis* 1996;23:298–302.

70. Fourneir PE, Casalta JP, Habib G, et al. Modification of the diagnostic criteria proposed by the Duke endocarditis service to permit improved diagnosis of Q fever endocarditis. *Am J Med* 1996;100:629–633.

71. Bayer AS. Infective endocarditis [see comments]. *Clin Infect Dis* 1993;17:313–322.

72. Berlin JA, Abrutyn E, Strom BL, et al. Incidence of infective endocarditis in the Delaware Valley, 1988–1990. *Am J Cardiol* 1995;76:933–936.

73. Smith RH, Radford DJ, Clark RA, et al. Infective endocarditis: a survey of cases in the South-East region of Scotland, 1968–1972. *Thorax* 1976;31:373–379.

74. Hickey AJ, MacMahon SW, Wilken DEL. Mitral valve prolapse and bacterial endocarditis: when is antibiotic prophylaxis necessary? *Am Heart J* 1985;109:431–435.

75. Alestig K, Hogevik H, Olaison L. Infective endocarditis. A diagnostic and therapeutic challenge for the new millennium. *Scand Infect Dis* 2000;32:343–356.

76. Lerner PI, Weinstein L. Infective endocarditis in the antibiotic era. *N Engl J Med* 1966;274:199–266.

77. Watanakunakorn C. Changing epidemiology and newer aspects of infective endocarditis. *Adv Intern Med* 1977;22:21.

78. Johnson CM, Rhodes KH. Pediatric endocarditis. *Mayo Clin Proc* 1982;57:86–94.

79. Cantrell M, Yoshikawa TT. Infective endocarditis in the aged patient. *Gerodontology* 1984;30:316.

80. Cerubin CE, Baden M, Favaler F, et al. Infectious endocarditis in narcotic addicts. *Ann Intern Med* 1968;69:1091.

81. Terpenning MS, Buggy BP, Kauffman CA. Infective endocarditis: clinical features in young and elderly patients. *Am J Med* 1987;83:626–634.

82. Larenby D, Gold JP. Prevention and management of prosthetic valve endocarditis. *Infect Med* 1991;8:42–45.

83. Millaire A, Belle EV, de Groote P, et al. Obstruction of the left main coronary ostium due to an aortic vegetation: survival after early surgery. *Clin Infect Dis* 1996;22:192–193.

84. Fang G, Keys TF, Gentry LO, et al. Prosthetic valve endocarditis resulting from nosocomial bacteremia. A prospective, multicenter study. *Ann Intern Med* 1993;119:560–567.

84a. Gouella JP, Asfar P, Brenet O, et al. Nosocomial endocarditis in the intensive care unit: analysis of 22 cases. *Crit Care Med* 2000;28:377–382.

85. Beeson PB, Brannon ES, Warren JS. Observations on the sites of removal of bacteria from the blood of patients with bacterial endocarditis. *J Exp Med* 1945;81:9–23.

86. Werner AS, Cobbs CG, Kaye D, et al. Studies on the bacteremia of bacterial endocarditis. *JAMA* 1967;202:127–131.

87. Mermel LA, Maki D. Detection of bacteremia in adults: consequences of culturing an inadequate volume of blood. *Ann Intern Med* 1993;119:270.

88. Parker MT, Ball LC. Streptococci and aerococci associated with systemic infection in man. *J Med Microbiol* 1976;9:275–302.

89. Molavi A. Endocarditis: recognition, management, and prophylaxis. *Cardiovasc Clin* 1993;23:139–174.

90. Whitby M, Fenech A. Infective endocarditis in adults in Glasgow, 1976–1981. *Int J Cardiol* 1985;7:391–403.

91. Williams RCJ. Subacute bacterial endocarditis as an immune disease. *Hosp Pract* 1971;3:111–122.

92. Vuille C, Nidorf M, Weyman AE, et al. Natural history of vegetations during successful medical treatment of endocarditis. *Am Heart J* 1994;128:1200–1209.

93. Starkebaum M, Durack D, Beeson PB. The "incubation period" of subacute bacterial endocarditis. *Yale J Biol Med* 1977;50:49–58.

94. Stagaman DJ, Presti C, Rees C, et al. Septic pulmonary arteriovenous fistula. An unusual conduit for systemic embolization in right-sided valvular endocarditis. *Chest* 1990;97:1484–1486.

95. Stewart JA, Silimperi D, Harris P, et al. Echocardiographic documentation of vegetative lesions in infective endocarditis: clinical implications. *Circulation* 1980;61:274–280.

96. Mugge A, Daniel WG, Frank G, et al. Echocardiography in infective endocarditis: reassessment of prognostic implications of vegetation size determined by the transthoracic and the transesophageal approach. *J Am Coll Cardiol* 1989;14:631–638.

97. Shively BK, Gurule FT, Roldan CA, et al. Diagnostic value of transesophageal compared with transthoracic echocardiography in infective endocarditis. *J Am Coll Cardiol* 1991;18:391–397.

98. Mugge A. Echocardiographic detection of cardiac valve vegetations and prognostic implications. *Infect Dis Clin North Am* 1993;7:877–898.

99. Sochowski RA, Chan KL. Implication of negative results on a monoplane transesophageal echocardiographic study in patients with suspected infective endocarditis [see comments]. *J Am Coll Cardiol* 1993;21:216–221.

100. Lowry RW, Zoghbi WA, Baker WB, et al. Clinical impact of transesophageal echocardiography in the diagnosis and management of infective endocarditis. *Am J Cardiol* 1994;73:1089–1091.

101. Shapiro SM, Young E, Ginzton LE, et al. Pulmonic valve endocarditis as an underdiagnosed disease: role of transesophageal echocardiography. *J Am Soc Echocardiogr* 1992;5:48–51.

102. Essop R. Transesophageal echocardiography in infective endocarditis: the standard for the 1990s? [editorial]. *Am Heart J* 1995;130:402–404.

102a. Roe MT, Abramson MA, Li J, et al. Clinical information determines the impact of transesophageal echocardiography on the diagnosis of infective endocarditis by the Duke criteria. *Am Heart J* 2000;139:945–951.

103. Daniel WG, Mugge A, Grote J, et al. Comparison of transthoracic and transesophageal echocardiography for detection of abnormalities of prosthetic and bioprosthetic valves in the mitral and aortic positions. *Am J Cardiol* 1993;71:210–215.

104. Vered Z, Mossinson D, Peleg E, et al. Echocardiographic assessment of prosthetic valve endocarditis. *Eur Heart J* 1995;16[Suppl B]:63–67.

105. Daniel WG, Mugge A, Martin RP, et al. Improvement in the diagnosis of abscesses associated with endocarditis by transesophageal echocardiography. *N Engl J Med* 1991;324:795–800.

106. Currier JS, Feinberg J. Bacterial infections in HIV disease. *AIDS Clin Rev* 1995;3:131–152.

107. Karalis DG, Chandrasekaran K, Wahl JM, et al. Transesophageal echocardiographic recognition of mitral valve abnormalities associated with aortic valve endocarditis. *Am Heart J* 1990;119:1209–1211.

108. Leung DY, Cranney GB, Hopkins AP, et al. Role of transesophageal echocardiography in the diagnosis and management of aortic root abscess. *Br Heart J* 1994;72:175–181.

109. Bansal RC, Graham BM, Jutzy KR, et al. Left ventricular outflow tract to left atrial communication secondary to rupture of mitral-aortic intervalvular fibrosa in infective endocarditis: diagnosis by transesophageal echocardiography and color flow imaging. *J Am Coll Cardiol* 1990;15:499–504.

110. Groundstroem K, Rittoo D, Hoffman P, et al. Additional value of biplane transesophageal imaging in assessment of mitral valve prostheses. *Br Heart J* 1993;70:259–265.

111. Job FP, Franke S, Lethen H, et al. Incremental value of biplane and multiplane transesophageal echocardiography for the assessment of active infective endocarditis. *Am J Cardiol* 1995;75:1033–1037.

112. Rohmann S, Erbel R, Darius H, et al. Spontaneous echo contrast imaging in infective endocarditis: a predictor of complications? *Int J Card Imaging* 1992;8:197–207.

113. Hojnik M, George J, Ziporen L, et al. Heart valve involvement (Libman-Sacks endocarditis) in the antiphospholipid syndrome. *Circulation* 1996;93:1579–1587.

114. Gleason CB, Stoddard MF, Wagner SG, et al. A comparison of cardiac valvular involvement in the primary antiphospholipid syndrome versus anticardiolipin-negative systemic lupus erythematosus. *Am Heart J* 1993;125:1123–1129.

115. Ozkutlu S, Saraclar M, Atalay S, et al. Two-dimensional echocardiographic diagnosis of tricuspid valve noninfective endocarditis due to protein C deficiency (lesion mimicking tricuspid valve myxoma). *Jpn Heart J* 1991;32:139–145.

115a. Tak T, Matthews S, Ulene R, et al. Active vegetations can be differentiated from chronic vegetations by visual inspection of standardized two-dimensional echocardiograms. *Echocardiography* 2000;17:109–114.

116. Heinle SK, Kisslo J. The clinical utility of transesophageal echocardiography in patients with left-sided infective endocarditis. *Am J Card Imaging* 1995;9:199–202.

117. Lutas EM, Roberts RB, Devereux RB, et al. Relation between the presence of echocardiographic vegetations and the complication rate in infective endocarditis. *Am Heart J* 1986;112:107–113.

118. Wann LS, Dillon JC, Weyman AE, et al. Echocardiography in bacterial endocarditis. *N Engl J Med* 1976;295:135–139.

119. Heinle S, Wilderman N, Harrison JK, et al. Value of transthoracic echocardiography in predicting embolic events in active infective endocarditis. Duke Endocarditis Service. *Am J Cardiol* 1994;74:799–801.

120. Steckleberg JM, Murphy JG, Ballard D, et al. Emboli in infective endocarditis: the prognostic value of echocardiography. *Ann Intern Med* 1991;114:635–640.

121. Desai SP, Yuille DL. The unsuspected complications of bacterial endocarditis imaged by gallium-67 scanning. *J Nucl Med* 1993;34:955–957.

122. Wiseman J, Rouleau J, Rigo P, et al. Gallium-67 myocardial imaging for the detection of bacterial endocarditis. *Radiology* 1976;120:135–138.

123. Sty JR, Chusid MJ. 99mTc-pyrophosphate imaging: bacterial endocarditis. *Pediatr Radiol* 1979;8:223–224.

124. Morguet AJ, Munz DL, Ivancevic V, et al. Immunoscintigraphy using technetium-99m-labeled anti-NCA-95 antigranulocyte antibodies as an adjunct to echocardiography in subacute infective endocarditis. *J Am Coll Cardiol* 1994;23:1171–1178.

125. Ramackers JM, Kotzki PO, Couret I, et al. The use of technetium-99m hexamethylpropylene amine oxime labeled granulocytes with single-photon emission tomography imaging in the detection and follow-up of recurrence of infective endocarditis complicating transvenous endocardial pacemaker. *Eur J Nucl Med* 1995;22:1351–1354.

126. Morguet AJ, Munz DL, Kreuzer H, et al. Scintigraphic detection of inflammatory heart disease. *Eur J Nucl Med* 1994;21:666–674.

127. Oates E, Sarno RC. Detection of bacterial endocarditis with indium-111 labeled leukocytes. *Clin Nucl Med* 1988;13:691–693.

128. Cowan JC, Patrick D, Reid DS. Aortic root abscess complicating bacterial endocarditis. Demonstration by computed tomography. *Br Heart J* 1984;52:591–593.

129. Akins EW, Slone RM, Wiechmann BN, et al. Perivalvular pseudoaneurysm complicating bacterial endocarditis: MR detection in five cases. *AJR Am J Roentgenol* 1991;31:1155–1158.

130. Miller SW, Palmer EL, Dinsmore RE, et al. Gallium-67 and magnetic resonance imaging in aortic root abscess. *J Nucl Med* 1987;28:1616–1619.

131. Bertorini TE, Laster RE Jr, Thompson BF, et al. Magnetic resonance imaging of the brain in bacterial endocarditis. *Arch Intern Med* 1989;149:815–817.

132. Hosenpud JD, Greenberg BH. The preoperative evaluation in patients with endocarditis. Is cardiac catheterization necessary? *Chest* 1983;84:690–694.

133. Tzukert AA, Leviner E, Sela M. Prevention of infective endocarditis: not by antibiotics alone. A 7-year follow-up of 90 dental patients. *Oral Surg Oral Med Oral Pathol* 1986;62:385–388.

133a. Weinstein L, Brusch JL, eds. *Infective endocarditis*. New York: Oxford University Press, 1996.

133b. Cecchi E, Parrini I, Chinaglea A, et al. New diagnostic criteria for infective endocarditis. *Eur Heart J* 1997;18:1149–1156.

133c. Fowler VG Jr, Sanders LL, Sexton DJ. Infective endocarditis due to *Staphylococcus aureus*. 59 prospectively identified cases with follow-up. *Clin Infect Dis* 1999;28:106–114.

134. Weinstein L, Brusch JL, eds. Prophylaxis. In: *Infective Endocarditis*. New York: Oxford University Press, 1996;333.

135. Kaye D. Changes in the spectrum, diagnosis, and management of bacterial and fungal endocarditis. *Med Clin North Am* 1973;57:941.

136. Weinstein L, Schlesinger JJ. Pathoanatomic, pathophysiologic and clinical correlations in endocarditis. *N Engl J Med* 1974;291:1122–1126.

136a. Lamas CC, Eykyn SJ. Suggested modification to the Duke criteria for the clinical diagnosis of native valve and prosthetic valve endocarditis: analysis of 118 pathologically proven cases. *Clin Infect Dis* 1997;25:713–719.

137. Mann T, McLaurin L, Grossman W, et al. Assessing the hemodynamic severity of acute aortic regurgitation due to infective endocarditis. *N Engl J Med* 1975;293:108–113.

138. Sapico FL, Liquete JA, Sarma RJ. Bone and joint infections in patients with infective endocarditis: review of a 4-year experience. *Clin Infect Dis* 1996;22:783–787.

139. Libman E, Celler HL. The etiology of subacute infectious endocarditis. *Am J Med Sci* 1910;140:516–521.

139a. Heiro M, Nikoskelainen J, Engblom E, et al. Neurologic manifestations of infective endocarditis. A 17-year experience in a teaching hospital in Finland. *Arch Intern Med* 2000;160:2781–2787.

140. Kilpatrick ZM, Greenberg PA, Sanford JP. Splinter hemorrhages—their clinical significance. *Arch Intern Med* 115:730.

141. Dickinson CJ. The aetiology of clubbing and hypertrophic osteoarthropathy. *Eur J Clin Invest* 1993;23:330–338.

142. Salgado AV, Furlan AJ, Keys TF, et al. Neurologic complications of endocarditis: a 12-year experience. *Neurology* 1989;39:173–178.

143. Blumer G. The digital manifestations of subacute bacterial endocarditis. *Am Heart J* 1926;1:256–259.

144. Alpert JS, Krous HF, Dalen JE, et al. Pathogenesis of Osler's nodes. *Ann Intern Med* 1976;85:471–473.

145. Yee J, McAllister CK. Osler's nodes and the recognition of infective endocarditis: a lesion of diagnostic importance. *South Med J* 1987;80:753–757.

146. Maisch B. Autoreactive mechanisms in infective endocarditis. *Springer Seminars in Immunopathology* 1989;11:439–456.

147. Farrior JBI, Silverman ME. A consideration of the differences between a Janeway lesion and Osler's node in infective endocarditis. *Chest* 1974;70:239.

148. Alport JS, Krous HF, Dalen JE, et al. Pathogenesis of Osler's nodes. *Ann Intern Med* 1976;85:471.

149. Janeway EG. Certain clinical observations upon heart disease. *Med News* 1899;75:257–260.

150. Khawly JA, Pollock SC. Litten's sign (Roth's spots) in bacterial endocarditis. *Arch Ophthalmol* 1994;112:683–684.

151. Kerr AJ, Tan JS. Biopsies of the Janeway lesion of infective endocarditis. *J Cutan Pathol* 1979;6:124–129.

152. Hollanders G, De Scheerder I, De Buyzere M, et al. A six years review on 53 cases of infective endocarditis: clinical, microbiological and therapeutical features. *Acta Cardiol* 1988;43:121–132.

153. Mansur AJ, Grinberg M, da Luz PL, et al. The complications of infective endocarditis. A reappraisal in the 1980s [see comments]. *Arch Intern Med* 1992;152:2428–2432.

154. Mills J, Utley J, Abbott J. Heart failure in infective endocarditis: predisposing factors, course, and treatment. *Chest* 1974;66:151–159.

155. Model A, Craig CP. Isolated tricuspid valve endocarditis due to *Streptococcus bovis*. *Clin Infect Dis* 1996;22:178–179.

156. Douglas A, Moore-Gillon J, Eykyn S. Fever during treatment of infective endocarditis. *Lancet* 1986;1:1341–1343.

157. DiNubile MJ, Calderwood SB, Steinhaus DM, et al. Cardiac conduction abnormalities complicating native valve active infective endocarditis. *Am J Cardiol* 1986;58:1213–1217.

158. Aguado JM, Gonzalez-Vilchez F, Martin-Duran R, et al. Perivalvular abscesses associated with endocarditis. Clinical features and diagnostic accuracy of two-dimensional echocardiography [see comments]. *Chest* 1993;104:88–93.

159. Falcone PM, Larrison WI. Roth spots seen on ophthalmoscopy: diseases with which they may be associated. *Conn Med* 1995;59:271–273.

160. Blankenhorn MA, Gall EA. Myocarditis and myocardiosis: clinicopathological appraisal. *Circulation* 1956;13:217–222.

161. Jones HR Jr, Siekert RG. Neurological manifestations of infective endocarditis. Review of clinical and therapeutic challenges. *Brain* 1989;112:1295–1315.

162. Mohr JP, Caplan LR, Melski JW, et al. The Harvard cooperative stroke registry: a prospective registry. *Neurology* 1978;28:754–762.

163. Steckelberg JM, Murphy JG, Ballard D, et al. Emboli in infective endocarditis: the prognostic value of echocardiography. *Ann Intern Med* 1991;114:635–640.

164. Corr P, Wright M, Handler LC. Endocarditis-related cerebral aneurysms: radiologic changes with treatment. *Am J Neuroradiol* 1995;16:745–748.

165. Ziment I. Nervous system complications in bacterial endocarditis. *Am J Med* 1969;47:593.

166. Garvey GJ, Neu HC. Infective endocarditis—an evolving disease. A review of endocarditis at the Columbia-Presbyterian Medical Center 1968–1973. *Medicine (Baltimore)* 1978;57:105–126.

167. Harrison MJG, Hampton JR. Neurological presentation of bacterial endocarditis. *BMJ* 1967;2:148–151.

168. Orfila C, Lepert JC, Modesto A, et al. Rapidly progressive glomerulonephritis associated with bacterial endocarditis: efficacy of antibiotic therapy alone. *Am J Nephrol* 1993;13:218–222.

168a. Colon PJ, Jefferies F, Korigman HR, et al. Predictors of prognosis and risk of renal insufficiency in bacterial endocarditis. *Clin Nephrol* 1998;49:96–101.

169. Sexauer WP, Quezado Z, Lippmann ML, et al. Pleural effusions in right-sided endocarditis: characteristics and pathophysiology. *South Med J* 1992;85:1176–1180.

170. Corzo JE, Lozano de Leon F, Gomez-Mateos J, et al. Pneumothorax secondary to septic pulmonary emboli in tricuspid endocarditis. *Thorax* 1992;47:1080–1081.

171. Gilbert HM, Peters ED, Lang SJ, et al. Successful treatment of fungal prosthetic valve endocarditis: case report and review. *Clin Infect Dis* 1996;22:348–354.

172. Sett SS, Hudon MP, Jamieson WR, et al. Prosthetic valve endocarditis. Experience with porcine bioprostheses. *J Thorac Cardiovasc Surg* 1993;105:428–434.

173. Cortina JM, Martinell J, Artiz V, et al. Surgical treatment of active prosthetic valve endocarditis. Results in 66 patients. *Thorac Cardiovasc Surg* 1987;35:209–214.

174. Horstkotte D, Korfer R, Loogen F, et al. Prosthetic valve endocarditis: clinical findings and management. *Eur Heart J* 1984;5[Suppl C]:117–122.

175. Kay PH, Oldenshaw PJ, Lincoln JCR, et al. The management of prosthetic valve endocarditis. *J Cardiovasc Surg* 1983;24:127–131.

175a. Traninger K, Jost K, Ahenhofer CH, et al. Long term follow-up of prosthetic valve endocarditis: what characteristics identify patients who were treated successfully with antibiotics above? *Heart* 1999;82:714–720.

176. Baddour LM. Twelve-year review of recurrent native-valve infective endocarditis: a disease of the modern antibiotic era. *Rev Infect Dis* 1988;10:1163–1170.

177. Kaye D, Abrutyn E. Prevention of bacterial endocarditis: 1991. *Ann Intern Med* 1991;114:803–804.

178. Dajani AS, Taubert KA, Watson W, et al. Prevention of bacterial endocarditis. Recommendations by the American Heart Association. *JAMA* 1997;277:1794–1801.

179. Glauser MP, Francioli P. Relevance of animal models to the prophylaxis of infective endocarditis. *J Antimicrob Chemother* 1987;20[Suppl A]:87–98.

180. Durack DT. Prevention of infective endocarditis. *N Engl J Med* 1995;332:38–44.

181. Imperiale TF, Horwitz RI. Does prophylaxis prevent post-dental infective endocarditis? A controlled evaluation of protective efficacy. *Am J Med* 1990;88:131–136.

182. van der Meer JT, van Wijk W, Thompson J, et al. Efficacy of antibiotic prophylaxis for prevention of native-valve endocarditis [see comments]. *Lancet* 1992;339:135–139.

183. Anonymous. Antibiotic prophylaxis of infective endocarditis. Recommendations from the Endocarditis Working Party of the British Society for Antimicrobial Chemotherapy [review]. *Lancet* 1990;335:88–89.

184. Everett E, Hirschmann J. Transient bacteremia and endocarditis prophylaxis. A review. *Medicine (Baltimore)* 1977;56:61–67.

185. Claristie RV. Penicillin in subacute bacterial endocarditis. Report of the medical research council on 269 patients

treated in 14 centres appointed by the penicillin clinical trials committee. *BMJ* 1948;1:1–7.

186. Hamburger M, Stein L. *Streptococcus viridans* subacute bacterial endocarditis. Two-week therapy schedule with penicillin. *JAMA* 1952;149:542–545.

187. Durack DT, Beeson PB. Experimental bacterial endocarditis. II Survival of bacteria in endocardial vegetations. *Br J Exp Pathol* 1972;53:50.

188. Wilson WR, Karchmer AW, Dajani AS, et al. Antibiotic treatment of adults with infective endocarditis due to streptococci, enterococci, staphylococci, and HACEK microorganisms. American Heart Association. *JAMA* 1995;274:1706–1713.

188a. Chien JW, Kucia ML, Salata RA. Use of linezolid, an oxazolidinone in the treatment of multidrug-resistant gram-positive bacterial infections. *Clin Infect Dis* 2000;30:146–151.

189. Stamboulian D. Outpatient treatment of endocarditis in a clinic-based program in Argentina. *Eur J Clin Microbiol Infect Dis* 1995;14:648–654.

190. Francioli P, Stamboulian D, and the International Infective Endocarditis Study Group. Treatment of streptococcal endocarditis with a single daily dose of ceftriaxone and netilmicin for 14 days: a prospective multicenter study. *Clin Infect Dis* 1995;21:1406–1410.

191. Chambers HF, Miller RT, Newman MD. Right-sided *Staphylococcus aureus* endocarditis in intravenous drug abusers: two-week combination therapy. *Ann Intern Med* 1988;109:619–624.

192. Ribera E, Gomez-Jimenez J, Cortes E, et al. Effectiveness of cloxacillin with and without gentamicin in short-term therapy for right-sided *Staphylococcus aureus* endocarditis. A randomized, controlled trial. *Ann Intern Med* 1996;125:969–974.

193. Heldman AW, Hartert TV, Ray SC, et al. Oral antibiotic treatment of right-sided staphylococcal endocarditis in injection drug users: prospective randomized comparison with parenteral therapy. *Am J Med* 1996;101:68–76.

194. Levine DP, Fromm BS, Reddy BR. Slow response to vancomycin or vancomycin plus rifampin in methicillin-resistant *Staphylococcus aureus* endocarditis. *Ann Intern Med* 1991;115:674–680.

195. DiNubile MJ. Short-course antibiotic therapy for right-sided endocarditis caused by *Staphylococcus aureus* in injection drug users. *Ann Intern Med* 1994;121:873–876.

196. Yeh TJ, Hall D, Ellison RG. Surgical treatment of aortic valve perforation due to bacterial endocarditis. *Am J Med* 1964;30:766–769.

197. Wallace AG, Young WG, Osterhout S. Treatment of acute bacterial endocarditis by valve excision and replacement. *Circulation* 1965;31:450–453.

198. Aranki SF, Adams DH, Rizzo RJ, et al. Determinants of early mortality and late survival in mitral valve endocarditis. *Circulation* 1995;92:II143–II149.

199. Ting W, Silverman N, Levitsky S. Valve replacement in patients with endocarditis and cerebral septic emboli. *Ann Thorac Surg* 1991;51:18–21; discussion 22.

200. Kanawaty DS, Stalker MJ, Munt PW. Nonsurgical treatment of histoplasma endocarditis involving a bioprosthetic valve. *Chest* 1991;99:253–256.

201. Faix RG, Feick HJ, Frommelt P, et al. Successful medical treatment of *Candida parapsilosis* endocarditis in a premature infant. *Am J Perinatol* 1990;7:272–275.

202. Mayrer AR, Brown A, Weintraub RA, et al. Successful medical therapy for endocarditis due to *Candida parapsilosis*. *Chest* 1978;73:546.

203. Lupinetti FM, Lemmer JH Jr. Comparison of allografts and prosthetic valves when used for emergency aortic valve replacement for active infective endocarditis. *Am J Cardiol* 1991;68:637–641.

204. Mullany CJ, Chau YL, Schaff HV, et al. Early and late survival after surgical treatment of culture-positive active endocarditis. *Mayo Clin Proc* 1995;70:517–525.

204a. Knosalla C, Weng Y, Yankal AC, et al. Surgical treatment of active infective aortic valve endocarditis with associated periannular abscesses with 11 year results. *Eur Heart J* 2000;21:490–497.

205. David TE, Bos J, Christakis GT, et al. Heart valve operations in patients with active infective endocarditis. *Ann Thorac Surg* 1990;49:701–705; discussion 712–713.

206. Middlemost S, Wisenbaugh T, Meyerowitz C, et al. A case for early surgery in native left-sided endocarditis complicated by heart failure: results in 203 patients. *J Am Coll Cardiol* 1991;18:663–667.

207. Haydock D, Barratt-Boyes B, Macedo T, et al. Aortic valve replacement for active infectious endocarditis in 108 patients. A comparison of freehand allograft valves with mechanical prostheses and bioprostheses. *J Thorac Cardiovasc Surg* 1992;103:130–139.

208. Glazier JJ, Verwilghen J, Donaldson RM, et al. Treatment of complicated prosthetic aortic valve endocarditis with annular abscess formation by homograft aortic root replacement. *J Am Coll Cardiol* 1991;17:1177–1182.

209. Dreyfus G, Serraf A, Jebara VA, et al. Valve repair in acute endocarditis. *Ann Thorac Surg* 1990;49:706–711.

210. Hendren WG, Morris AS, Rosenkranz ER, et al. Mitral valve repair for bacterial endocarditis. *J Thorac Cardiovasc Surg* 1992;103:124–128.

211. Tuna IC, Orszulak TA, Schaff HV, et al. Results of homograft aortic valve replacement for active endocarditis. *Ann Thorac Surg* 1990;49:619–624.

212. Danielson GR, Titus JL, DuShane JW. Successful treatment of aortic valve endocarditis and aortic root abscesses by insertion of prosthetic valves in the ascending aorta and placement of bypass grafts to coronary arteries. *J Thorac Cardiovasc Surg* 1974;67:443–449.

213. Franz PT, Murray GF, Wilcox BR. Surgical management of left ventricular-aortic discontinuity complicating bacterial endocarditis. *Ann Thorac Surg* 1980;29:1–6.

214. Fiore A, Ivey T, McKeown P. Patch closure of aortic annulus mycotic aneurysm. *Ann Thorac Surg* 1986;42:372–379.

215. Arvay A, Lengyel M. Incidence and risk factors of prosthetic valve endocarditis. *Eur J Cardiothorac Surg* 1988;2:340–346.

216. Weinstein L, Schlesinger J. Pathoanatomic, pathophysiologic and clinical correlations in endocarditis. *N Engl J Med* 1974;291:832.

216a. Dhewan VK, Yeaman MR, Cheung AL, et al. Phenotypic resistance to thrombin-induced platelet microbicidal protein in vitro is correlated with enhanced virulence in experimental endocarditis due to *Staphylococcus aureus.* *Infect Immunol* 1997;65:3293–3299.

216b. Fowler VG Jr, McIntyre LM, Yeamen MR, et al. In vitro resistance to thrombin-induced platelet microbicidal protein in isolates of *Staphylococcus aureus* from endocarditis patients correlates with an intravascular device source. *J Infect Dis* 2000;182:1251–1254.

217. Macdonell RA, Robbins S. The significance of nonbacterial thrombotic endocarditis: an autopsy and clerical study of 78 cases. *Ann Intern Med* 1957;46:255.

218. Loewe L, Rosenblatt P, Green HJ, et al. Combined penicillin and hepatitis therapy of subacute bacterial endocarditis. Report of severe consecutive successfully treated patients. *JAMA* 1944;124:14.

219. Francis C. Cardiac involvement in AIDS. *Curr Publ Cardiol* 1990;15:571.

220. Burch G, Tsai C. Evaluation of coxsackie viral valvular and mural endocarditis in mice. *Br J Exp Pathol* 1971;52:360.

221. Loulmet D, Carpenter A, LeBret E. Minimally invasive surgery for complex mitral valve repair. *Circulation* 1996;94[Suppl 1]:1–314.

222. Kaji S, Yoshida K, Takagi T, et al. Mitral valve repair for native valve endocarditis. *Circulation* 1996;94[Suppl 1]:1–195.

26

DISEASES OF THE PERICARDIUM, RESTRICTIVE CARDIOMYOPATHY, AND DIASTOLIC DYSFUNCTION

ALLAN L. KLEIN
CRAIG R. ASHER

▼◢ ADDITIONAL ELECTRONIC TOPICS

Historical Perspective e94; Pathophysiology of Diastolic Function e95; Phases of Diastole e96; Isovolumic Relaxation e97; Rapid Filling e98; Diastasis (Slow Filling) e99; Atrial Filling (Contraction) f01; Determinants of Diastolic Function f02; Acoustic Quantification and Color Kinesis f03; TEI Index f04; Exercise Capacity and Diastolic Function f05; Cardiac Catheterization f06; Radionuclide Angiography f07; Magnetic Resonance Imaging f08; Transmitral Flow Assessment in Health and Diastolic Dysfunction f09; Physics of Mitral Inflow f10; Right-Sided Doppler Flows f11; Color M-Mode Doppler f12; Tissue Doppler Echocardiography f13; Idiopathic Restrictive Cardiomyopathy: Pathophysiology f14; Endomyocardial Disease f15; Löffler's Endocarditis: Pathology f16; Cardiac Amyloidosis: Etiology and Classification of Amyloidosis f17; Cardiac Amyloidosis: Pathology f18; Left Ventricular Diastolic Dysfunction f19; Right Ventricular Diastolic Function f20; Prognostic Stratification f21; Differentiation from Hypertrophic Cardiomyopathy f22; Magnetic Resonance Imaging f23; Cardiac Sarcoidosis: Pathology f24; Gaucher's Disease f25; Hurler's Syndrome f26; Metastatic Malignancies f27; Hemochromatosis: Pathology f28; Glycogen Storage Disease f29; Fabry's Disease f30; Carcinoid Heart Disease: Pathology f31; Radiation Heart Disease f32; Anthracycline Cardiomyopathy f33; Scleroderma f34; Pericardial Disease: Anatomic Considerations f35; Normal Physiology of Pericardium f36; Pericardial Tamponade: Pathophysiology f37; Magnetic Resonance Imaging for Pericardial Disease f38; Idiopathic and Viral Pericarditis: Pathology f39; Purulent Pericarditis: Epidemiology and Etiology f40; Fungal Pericarditis f41; Tuberculous Pericarditis f42; Tuberculous Pericarditis: Pathology f43; Tuberculous Pericarditis: Clinical Presentation f44; Tuberculous Pericarditis: Investigations f45; Tuberculous Pericarditis: Management f46; Human Immunodeficiency Virus–Associated Pericardial Effusion f47; Uremic Pericarditis f48; Uremic Pericarditis: Pathophysiology f49; Uremic Pericarditis: Clinical Presentation f50; Uremic Pericarditis: Management f51; Early Acute Pericarditis: Pathophysiology f52; Trauma and the Postpericardiotomy Syndrome f53; Radiation Pericarditis f54; Radiation Pericarditis: Pathology f55; Radiation Pericarditis: Clinical Presentation f56; Radiation Pericarditis: Diagnosis and Management f57; Pericardial Involvement in Autoimmune Diseases f58; Rheumatoid Arthritis f59; Rheumatoid Arthritis: Clinical Presentation f60; Systemic Lupus Erythematosus f61; Systemic Lupus Erythematosus: Clinical Presentation f62; Systemic Lupus Erythematosus: Management f63; Scleroderma f64; Myxedema f65; Malignant Pericarditis f66; Malignant Pericarditis: Clinical Presentation f67; Malignant Pericarditis: Prognosis f68; Congenital Abnormalities of the Pericardium f69; Drugs f70

A. L. Klein: Department of Cardiovascular Medicine, The Cleveland Clinic Foundation, Cleveland, Ohio
C. R. Asher: Department of Cardiovascular Medicine, The Cleveland Clinic Foundation, Cleveland, Ohio

OVERVIEW

Diseases of the pericardium and restrictive cardiomyopathies cause impairment of diastolic function of the heart. Myriad underlying etiologies, via several mechanisms, result in final common clinical presentations, making specific diagnosis difficult. Historically, in the realm of invasive cardiac investigation (1,2), these disorders have become illuminated by several evolving noninvasive techniques including echocardiography (3,4) and magnetic resonance imaging (MRI) (5). This chapter discusses the general principles of diastolic heart failure including the biology and physiology, clinical presentation, epidemiology, investigation, and treatment. Specific diseases of the myocardium and pericardium that may cause diastolic dysfunction are reviewed.

GENERAL PRINCIPLES OF DIASTOLIC HEART DISEASE

Definition of Diastolic Dysfunction

Clinical congestive heart failure is most often secondary to impairment of left ventricular (LV) systolic function (22). Diastolic impairment, although less common, is associated with significant morbidity and mortality (23). Clinically, it is important to distinguish isolated diastolic heart failure (normal ejection fraction) from systolic heart failure; although combined, systolic and diastolic heart failure will be more commonly observed (24,25). Several pathophysiologic definitions of diastolic heart failure have been proposed: (a) impaired capacity of the ventricles to fill without a compensatory increase in left atrial pressure (26); (b) abnormal ventricular filling that would produce inadequate cardiac output with a mean pulmonary venous pressure of less than 12 mm Hg (27); and (c) resistance to filling of one or both ventricles with an inappropriate upward shift of the pressure-volume loop, especially with exercise (28). These definitions have in common an abnormal resistance to filling causing elevated left-sided filling pressures and congestion. Diastolic dysfunction impairs filling of the ventricle by impairing relaxation (early diastole), reducing compliance (early to late diastole), or by external constraint from the pericardium (28,29). Numerous pathologic processes and disease states may produce the clinical constellation of diastolic dysfunction (Table 26.1).

As a framework to design and implement treatment trials, diagnostic criteria for patients with diastolic heart failure have been proposed. The 1998 European Study Group on Diastolic Heart Failure required (a) clinical evidence of congestive heart failure, (b) normal or mild LV dysfunction, and (c) the presence of impaired relaxation, filling, or compliance to diagnose diastolic heart failure (30) (*e*Table 26.1.1). All three components as assessed by noninvasive testing or cardiac catheterization were necessary for a diagnosis. Vasan and Levy subsequently proposed a less rigid criteria using similar inclusions but defining diastolic heart failure as definite, probable, or possible depending on the number of elements present (31). It has been suggested that the incorporation of exclusionary criteria will be required before using these standards for selection of patients for drug therapies to understand the specific effects on various pathologic conditions (32).

Diagnostic Approach to Diastolic Function

Clinical heart failure with normal systolic function (usually by echocardiography or nuclear techniques) would suggest

TABLE 26.1   CONDITIONS INVOLVING DIASTOLIC HEART FAILURE

Condition	Mechanism of diastolic dysfunction
Restrictive cardiomyopathy (idiopathic restrictive cardiomyopathy, cardiac amyloidosis)	Increased resistance to ventricular inflow
Constrictive pericarditis	Increased resistance to ventricular inflow, with decreased ventricular diastolic capacity
Ischemic heart disease	
Flash pulmonary edema, dyspnea during angina	Impaired myocardial relaxation
	Diastolic calcium overload
Postinfarction scarring and hypertrophy (remodeling)	Increased resistance to ventricular inflow
Hypertrophic heart disease (hypertrophic cardiomyopathy, chronic hypertension, aortic stenosis)	Impaired myocardial relaxation
	Diastolic calcium overload
	Increased resistance to ventricular inflow due to thick chamber walls, altered collagen matrix
	Activation of renin-angiotensin system
Volume overload (aortic or mitral regurgitation, arteriovenous fistula)	Increased diastolic volume relative to ventricular capacity
	Myocardial hypertrophy, fibrosis
Dilated cardiomyopathy	Impaired myocardial relaxation
	Diastolic calcium overload
	Myocardial fibrosis or scar
Mitral or tricuspid stenosis	Increased resistance to atrial emptying

Adapted from Grossman W. Diastolic dysfunction in congestive heart failure. *N Engl J Med* 1991;325:1557–1564, with permission.

diastolic dysfunction. The goals of investigation should include identification and quantification of diastolic dysfunction using the LV filling patterns (92–94) and newer Doppler techniques (16); semiquantitation of mean left atrial and end diastolic filling pressures (17,95–98); determination of underlying pathophysiologic mechanisms (constriction vs. restriction) (99–102); and stratification and prognostication and monitoring and guidance of therapy (103,104). Cardiac catheterization, echocardiography, radionuclide angiography techniques, and MRI are discussed in the following sections (24,105).

Echocardiography

Echocardiography has emerged as the main technique in the evaluation of patients with diastolic dysfunction and can be used as an alternative to cardiac catheterization (4,15). This modality encompasses M-mode, two-dimensional echocardiography, and Doppler echocardiography. This noninvasive modality quickly and safely assesses systolic ventricular function, atrial size, and function and valvular function; indirectly infers filling pressures and inflow patterns; and offers information to identify specific pathologies such as constrictive pericarditis, pericardial effusion, cardiac amyloidosis, and sarcoidosis (15,51).

With its enhanced spatial and temporal resolution, M-mode echocardiography has been used to time cardiac events such as the period of LV contraction and relaxation and the timing of valve opening and closing. Digitized M-mode echocardiography of the endocardium has been used to characterize diastolic filling in various diseases (106–108). M-mode echocardiography has been used to demonstrate abnormal RV diastolic collapse in cardiac tamponade (109), the abnormal septal bounce in constrictive pericarditis (110), and decreased annular motion in coronary artery disease (111). Ultrasound systems with high frame rate imaging now have the ability to generate anatomic M-mode tracings in any plane from digitally acquired two-dimensional images (112).

A complete two-dimensional echocardiogram is part of the diastolic function evaluation. It allows for assessment of global and regional systolic evaluation, LV mass and volumes, atrial dimensions, and pericardial thickness. Two-dimensional echocardiography helps exclude other causes of heart failure such as valvular heart disease (15,16). Diastolic dysfunction is unlikely with no organic heart disease, as documented by echocardiography. Similarly, there is a significant relationship with increasing left atrial size and stage of diastolic dysfunction (113). Inferior vena cava (IVC) plethora by echocardiography is closely associated with elevated right atrial (RA) pressure (114).

An integrated approach to the Doppler evaluation of diastolic function includes an evaluation of filling of both the left and right ventricles. The phase of respiration can be assessed simultaneously with Doppler flow velocities using a nasal thermistor to measure the change in temperature between inspiration, expiration, and apnea. Respiratory variations are crucial in differentiating constrictive pericarditis from restrictive cardiomyopathy (4). Transmitral flow is assessed in the apical four-chamber view with the pulsed Doppler sample volume (1 to 2 mm) at the leaflet tips along a laminar flow stream into the LV cavity. Optimal recordings depend on many technical features including sample volume placement, transducer alignment, and machine settings (115). Peak velocities of E and A, E/A ratio, and deceleration times are obtained and can be compared with age- and gender-matched subjects (84). Isovolumic relaxation time can be measured by placing a continuous wave Doppler beam between the LV outflow tract and the LV inflow to measure the time from the aortic valve closure to mitral valve opening. An alternative approach to measuring isovolumic relaxation time is to use pulsed wave Doppler (116).

Pulmonary venous flow can be assessed by transthoracic echocardiography by placing the sample volume (3 to 4 mm) into the right upper pulmonary vein from the apical four-chamber view. Adequate recordings can be achieved in up to 80% to 90% of patients, especially with the use of contrast echocardiography (15,117,118). Failure to obtain this information, critical to some cases, is an indication to proceed to transesophageal echocardiography (119).

RV inflow is assessed by placing the sample volume (1 to 2 mm) at the leaflet tips of the tricuspid inflow from the apical four-chamber view or the RV inflow view (120). The inferior vena cava diameter can be measured from the subcostal view and its respiratory variation calculated using M-mode echocardiography. Also from the subcostal position, hepatic venous flow sample volume (3 to 4 mm) can be recorded by placing the sample volume 1 to 2 cm into the right superior hepatic vein. The patient may have to control his or her depth of respiration to maintain the sample volume in a stable position. Finally, superior vena cava flow can be measured by placing the sample volume (3 to 4 mm) at a depth of 5 to 7 cm into the vein from the supraclavicular position (4). The diastolic filling variables that are typically measured are shown in Table 26.2.

Color M-mode Doppler is increasingly performed as a routine component of the diastolic function assessment. Pulsed wave Doppler records flow at a single spatial location in time. In contrast, color M-mode Doppler provides a map of LV filling velocities across a scan line with enhanced spatial and temporal resolution. In the apical four-chamber view with a standard depth, the M-mode cursor is aligned with the mitral inflow color Doppler flow, with the color Doppler sector size covering only the left ventricle and mitral valve. The positioning of the image should be adjusted to align the scan line parallel to the direction of flow. The color Doppler Nyquist limit is set below the mitral E wave peak velocity to allow for color Doppler aliasing of flow. The scan line from the mitral leaflet tips to

TABLE 26.2 DIASTOLIC FILLING VARIABLES

Left ventricular filling	Right ventricular filling
Left ventricular inflow	Right ventricular inflow
E-wave velocity (cm/sec)	E-wave velocity (cm/sec)
A-wave velocity (cm/sec)	A-wave velocity (cm/sec)
E/A ratio	E/A ratio
Deceleration time (ms)	Deceleration time (ms)
Isovolumic relaxation time (ms)	Superior vena cava and hepatic vein
Pulmonary vein flow	Forward flow
Forward flow	S-wave velocity (cm/sec)
S-wave velocity (cm/sec)	D-wave velocity (cm/sec)
D-wave velocity (cm/sec)	Reverse flow
Reverse flow	V-wave reversal (cm/sec)
Atrial reversal wave velocity (cm/sec)	Atrial reversal wave velocity (cm/sec)
Atrial reversal wave duration (ms)	Tissue Doppler echocardiography (cm/sec)
Tissue Doppler echocardiography (cm/sec) of	of tricuspid annulus
mitral annulus	
Color M-mode flow propagation velocity (cm/sec)	

the LV apex is obtained. LV filling is measured from the slope of the early propagation velocity (Vp) at the mitral valve plane to 4 cm into the LV cavity. Measurements are made at a sweep speed of 100 mm per second using the slope of the first aliasing velocity (17,121). Care must be taken to avoid measuring intracavitary flow starting before the onset of the mitral inflow. This may be prominent in some patients with hypertrophic cardiomyopathy or restrictive cardiomyopathy. It may be difficult to obtain accurate recordings in patients with sinus tachycardia as well as first-degree heart block because of fusion of the E and A waves (similar to mitral inflow).

TDE allows for evaluation of myocardial performance by evaluating myocardial rather than blood flow velocities. By means of a filter and amplification method, low-velocity and high-amplitude signals of tissue are preferentially displayed. A pulsed wave or color-encoded M-mode or two-dimensional map can be displayed and is superimposed over the two-dimensional image (122). TDE is able to provide myocardial velocities at different locations of the myocardium from different acoustic windows. Both systolic and diastolic patterns are displayed. For the assessment of diastolic function, Doppler velocities are obtained from the apical four-chamber view where the myocardium is near parallel with the transducer. The sample volume is approximately of 10-mm length, and the filter is set at 100 Hz or lower with a sweep speed of 100 mm per second. Sampling can be done at the lateral and septal annulus as well as the anterior and inferior annulus in the two-chamber view (16,123). TDE has the same limitations as the standard Doppler techniques. There are several limitations of TDE, including the effect of translation motion, Doppler angle of incidence, sample volume size, and inability to interrogate the apical segment (16,21).

Transesophageal echocardiography can complement transthoracic echocardiography in the comprehensive assessment of diastolic filling, providing both a physiologic assessment using Doppler echocardiography and excellent anatomic delineation. Optimal pulmonary venous flow recordings can be obtained by pulsed Doppler in virtually all patients from both the left and right upper veins from multiple planes. Isovolumic relaxation time, using continuous wave Doppler, is difficult to record using the transesophageal approach, but sometimes can be recorded from the apical five-chamber view from the deep transgastric approach. The pericardium can be visualized and measured when it is thickened by constrictive pericarditis (124). This is especially obvious over the RA and ventricular free walls, which are often seen to be "tethered" (101,119).

Diastolic Filling Patterns

Extensive literature exists regarding the empirically observed patterns of transmitral flow observed in normal individuals and patients with diastolic dysfunction. These patterns are the end result of the complex events only briefly described previously and are nonspecific for any particular physiologic perturbation. Diastolic filling patterns may be influenced by technical (sample volume placement) and hemodynamic factors (heart rate, volume status, conduction disorders) and not always be concordant with diastolic function (115).

Most simply, investigators have measured the peak velocity of the E wave and A wave by transmitral pulsed wave Doppler and their relationship, the *E/A ratio* (168). These basic parameters vary with age and within the spectrum of diastolic filling (Fig. 26.1) (84,92). Taken alone, the normal situation (E/A ratio greater than 1) passes through a delay relaxation phase (E/A ratio less than 1), then through a "pseudonormal" pattern (E/A ratio greater than 1) to the most abnormal "restrictive" pattern (E/A ratio greater than or equal to 1). Thus, the E/A ratio demonstrates a **U**-shaped curve, making it impossible to tell from this single parameter where in the spectrum a given

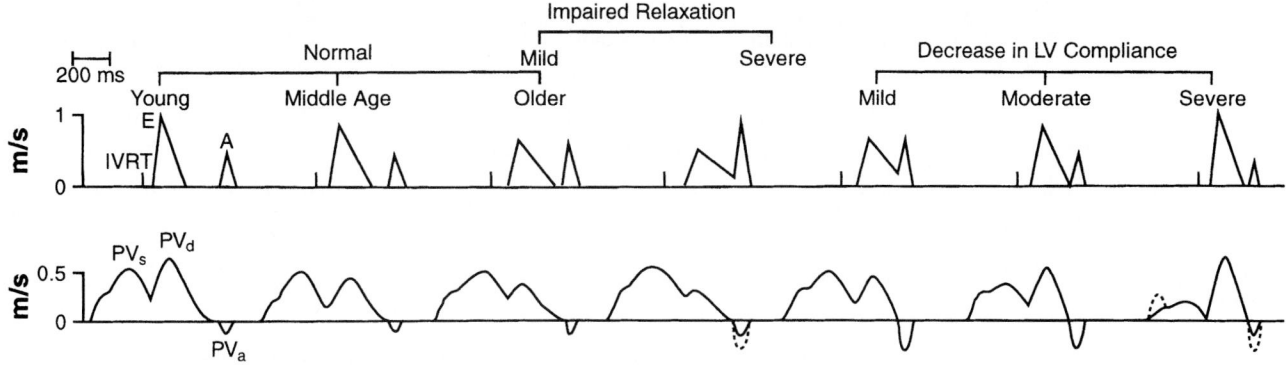

FIGURE 26.1 Natural history of left ventricular (LV) filling. Schematic representation of transmitral and pulmonary venous Doppler profiles, demonstrating the progression of the patterns with the normal aging process, and with diseases of diastolic function showing impaired relaxation and decrease in LV compliance. Isovolumic relaxation time (IVRT), E wave (E), A-wave (A) filling, pulmonary venous systolic (PV$_s$), diastolic (PV$_d$), and atrial reversal (PV$_a$) waves are shown. *Left*: In young healthy subjects, the E/A is greater than 1, the deceleration time and IVRT are short, and there is mild blunting of pulmonary venous systolic flow. With age, ventricular relaxation becomes impaired and the E/A ratio reverses, the A wave increases, the mitral deceleration time and IVRT lengthen, and the pulmonary venous systolic flow increases. *Middle*: With diseases showing impaired relaxation, there may be similar findings with a further decrease in E/A ratio. *Right*: With more severe derangements of diastolic function, as chamber compliance decreases, left-atrial pressure rises, the deceleration time decreases, the E/A ratio increases, and IVRT becomes shorter (restrictive physiology). PV$_s$ flow becomes progressively blunted as mean left atrial pressure and the PV$_a$ increases, helping to differentiate the "pseudonormal" pattern from normal. (From Appleton CP, Hatle LK. The natural history of left ventricular filling abnormalities: assessment by 2-D and Doppler echocardiography. *Echocardiography* 1992;9:453, with permission.)

patient lies (16). The pulmonary venous pattern is an important source of added information (43) that may overcome the limitations of the E/A ratio for determining diastolic function in many patients. An increased pulmonary atrial reversal (AR) flow, reversal velocity, or width, as well as Valsalva maneuver, may aid to differentiate "pseudonormal" from normal diastolic function, corresponding to elevation of mean left atrial or LV diastolic pressures, respectively (113,169,170).

Still, exceptions and limitations to the utility of pulmonary venous flow diminish the capability of distinguishing diastolic flow patterns in all individuals. Some patients may not have adequate pulmonary venous flow profiles, particularly the AR wave may not be well delineated. Blunting of pulmonary venous systolic waves may be present in young individuals due to rapid diastolic "suction," and AR may be absent in advanced diastolic dysfunction due to the loss of atrial function with amyloid infiltration (169,171). Therefore, newer modalities for assessment of diastolic function including color M-mode Doppler and TDE have evolved that provide important adjunct information to determine diastolic function and LV filling pressures (16) (Fig. 26.2).

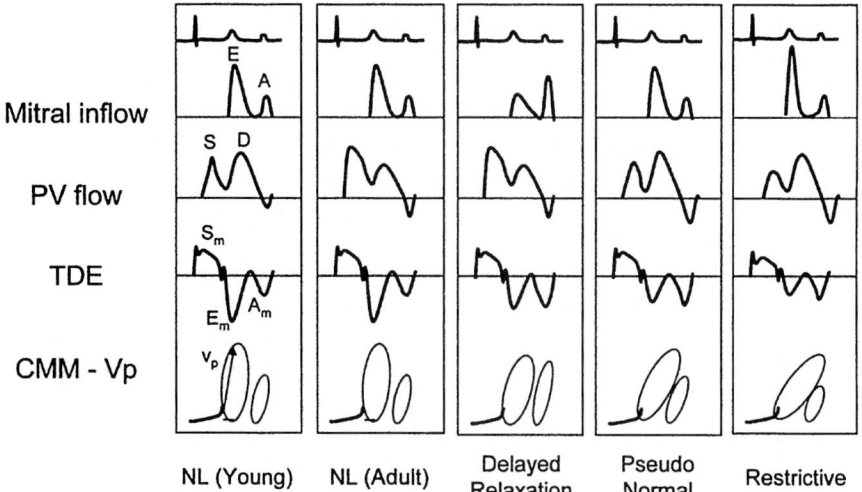

Mitral inflow

PV flow

TDE

CMM - Vp

NL (Young)   NL (Adult)   Delayed Relaxation   Pseudo Normal   Restrictive

FIGURE 26.2 Stages of diastolic function. Schematic representation of the typical patterns seen with mitral inflow, pulmonary venous flow, tissue Doppler echocardiography (TDE), and color M-mode (CMM) – propagation velocity (Vp) for normal (NL, young and adult), impaired relaxation, pseudonormal, and restrictive diastolic function. Using an integrated approach with these four different modalities for assessment of diastolic flow pattern the stages of diastolic dysfunction can be determined. A, late mitral filling; A$_m$, diastolic filling during atrial contraction; D, diastolic filling; E, early mitral filling; E$_m$, early diastolic; S, systolic filling; S$_m$, systolic. (Adapted from Garcia MJ, Thomas JD, Klein AL. New Doppler echocardiographic applications for the study of diastolic function. *J Am Coll Cardiol* 1998;32:865–875.)

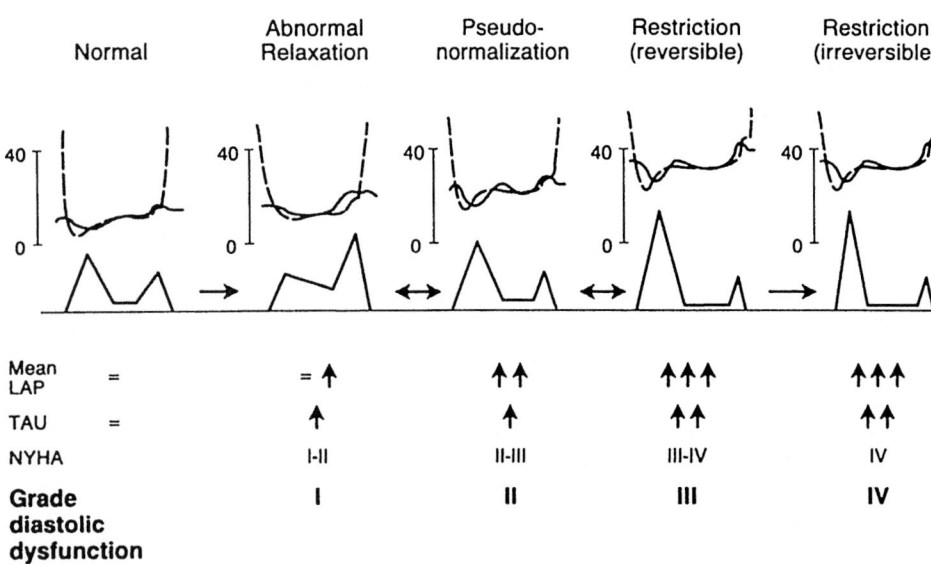

FIGURE 26.3 Proposed grading system for diastolic dysfunction based on progression of clinical disease patterns. Top row shows the high-fidelity left atrial and left ventricular pressure curves for the four grades of diastolic dysfunction, graded on a scale of I to IV, representing a progression from abnormal relaxation, pseudonormalization, restrictive (reversible), and restrictive (irreversible) disease. Below are the corresponding mitral flow velocity profiles; below these are the mean left atrial pressure (LAP), time constant of relaxation (TAU), and New York Heart Association (NYHA) class. Measurements are given in mm Hg. (From Nishimura RA, Tajik AJ. Evaluation of diastolic filling of the left ventricle in health and disease: Doppler echocardiography is the clinician's Rosetta stone. *J Am Coll Cardiol* 1997;30:8–18, with permission.)

Pulmonary Venous Velocity Patterns in Health and Diastolic Dysfunction

The pulmonary venous velocity pattern provides important adjunctive information to the transmitral pattern, particularly in distinguishing the normal transmitral pattern from the "pseudonormal" pattern (43) and evaluation of LV end diastolic pressures (96).

Pulmonary venous flow can be recorded by transthoracic echocardiography in 80% to 90% of cases (118,176) and by transesophageal echocardiography (119,177). The pulmonary venous velocity profile typically has three distinct waves (Fig. 26.2). ⚡ f71

Interpretation of Diastolic Filling Patterns

Using information from mitral inflow, pulmonary vein flow, color M-mode, and tissue Doppler imaging, four patterns of diastolic function can be determined (Fig. 26.2). These patterns are dependent on age and hemodynamic conditions and represent stages of relaxation and compliance abnormalities and filling pressures. A classification was proposed that diastolic dysfunction be graded in four stages that correlate with diastolic impairment and symptom class (212) (Fig. 26.3).

Normal Pattern
The normal filling pattern is seen in healthy subjects with normal relaxation, compliance, and filling pressures. Healthy individuals demonstrate a briskly accelerating E wave, relatively rapid deceleration, and an A wave significantly smaller in magnitude than the E wave. The E/A ratio is greater than 1, the mitral deceleration time is typically between 150 and 220 ms, and the IVRT less than 100 ms. The S/D ratio is generally greater than 1, and the AR wave should be less than 35 cm per second. The color M-mode propagation is relatively fast (greater than 45 cm per sec-

ond), and the tissue Doppler E_m is greater than 8 cm per second consistent with normal ventricular relaxation (16).

In young healthy subjects, there is a greater predominance of early diastolic filling due to the rapid "suction" effect of the ventricle (more enhanced relaxation with Vp greater than 55 cm per second and E_m greater than 10 cm per second) and little additional filling during atrial contraction. This results in an even greater E/A ratio with further shortening of the deceleration time. Because atrial contribution is minimal, the mitral inflow A wave and pulmonary vein AR are small. The S/D ratio may be less than 1, representing the large contribution of early filling.

Normal left-sided values with 95% confidence intervals with age are graphically shown in *e*Figures 26.3.1 and 26.3.2, and right- and left-sided normal values are listed in *e*Table 26.2.2 (4,84,92,120). *e*Figure 26.3.3 shows the left- and right-sided Doppler tracings in healthy subjects.

Delayed Relaxation Pattern (Stage I)
The delayed relaxation pattern is seen in patients with delayed LV relaxation but with relatively normal compliance and filling pressures (213). With normal aging and various pathologic states, the time constant of relaxation is lengthened, the E wave shows a slower acceleration and a lower peak velocity, a prolonged deceleration time (greater than 220 ms), and isovolumic relaxation time (greater than 100 ms). To the extent that emptying may not be complete by the end of diastasis, an increased left atrial volume is present at the time of atrial contraction, leading to a larger A wave, compensating in large part for the smaller E wave. Thus, the E/A ratio is less than 1 and concomitantly the S/D ratio is greater than 1, because if E is small, the corresponding D is small. Because relaxation is impaired, the color M-mode Vp is prolonged (less than 45 cm per second) and E_m is decreased (less than 8 cm per second).

Impaired relaxation may occur with normal or elevated filling pressures. If LV end diastolic pressure is normal, pulmonary vein AR is less than 35 cm per second; although if it is elevated, the AR is greater than 35 cm per second or the duration of AR is greater than the duration of the mitral inflow A duration (96).

This pattern is seen in normal aging (4,84), ischemia (214), hypertrophic cardiomyopathy (215,216), and secondary hypertrophy (217) and is usually seen in patients who typically have only mild symptoms or are asymptomatic (113) (*e*Fig. 26.3.4). It can also be seen with hypovolemia because of a decreased left atrial to LV pressure gradient with greater filling during atrial systole (15,218).

Pseudonormal Pattern (Stage II)

The pseudonormal pattern is difficult to recognize because it is similar to the normal pattern. As left atrial pressure increases further to compensate for deteriorating diastolic function, the peak E-wave velocity increases. Therefore, abnormalities of relaxation and compliance and elevated filling pressures are present. This is associated with a normal appearance of the transmitral inflow with an E/A ratio between 1 and 2, a deceleration time between 150 and 220 ms, and an isovolumic relaxation time between 60 and 100 ms (15,92,113) (*e*Fig. 26.3.4). One important feature to distinguish this pattern from normal is the pulmonary venous AR wave, which in pseudonormal filling displays a prolonged and increased AR greater than 35 cm per second (84), whereas the pulmonary vein S/D ratio could be normal or less than 1. The AR wave prominence may not be present if atrial systolic failure occurs, although the duration of AR greater than the mitral A wave may still occur. In addition, the Valsalva maneuver may be useful in differentiating normal from pseudonormal by reducing the preload, causing the normal-appearing E/A ratio to be greater than or equal to 0.5, and thus exposing a delayed relaxation pattern (4,92,170,219). Color M-mode propagation velocities and tissue Doppler imaging are particularly helpful to detect pseudonormal filling with a Vp less than 45 cm per second and E_m less than 8 cm per second (201).

Usually in patients with pseudonormal patterns, the left atrial size is increased, the LV function may be impaired or wall thickness increased, and the patient may have dyspnea (97,113). This pattern may represent an intermediate stage between impaired relaxation and restrictive filling as a result of disease progression, ischemia, or a change in loading conditions (15,100,113).

Restrictive Filling Pattern (Stage III)

The restrictive filling pattern is seen in the presence of severely reduced LV compliance and elevated filling pressures and ongoing delayed relaxation. It is characterized by a very elevated peak E-wave velocity with extremely rapid deceleration indicative of increased LV operating stiffness and diminutive (often absent) A wave (*e*Fig. 26.3.4). The E/A ratio is usually greater than 2, with a deceleration time less than 150

ms, and isovolumic relaxation time less than 60 ms (15). Pulmonary venous flow usually shows markedly blunted systolic flows with large and prolonged ARs (except in conditions of atrial systolic failure) (4). A pulmonary venous systolic fraction 0.40 to 0.55 of the of the sum of the systolic plus diastolic fraction is consistent with significant elevation of PCWP (96,220). Similar to pseudonormal patterns, the color M-mode propagation velocity and E_m are reduced.

Reduced filling due to increased ventricular stiffness may be counteracted by increases in heart rate, inotropic state, or most commonly left atrial pressure. This preload compensation dramatically changes the morphology of the E wave from a pattern consistent with delayed relaxation to one consistent with the restrictive pattern (221). Diastolic mitral and tricuspid regurgitation may occur as a result of ventricular pressure rising rapidly in a stiff ventricle and exceeding atrial pressure in mid- or late diastole (15).

The restrictive filling pattern is equivalent to the "square-root sign" or "dip and plateau" pattern seen in the ventricular pressure tracing at cardiac catheterization (92). The association between the restrictive filling pattern and the need for elevated filling pressures perhaps explains the poor prognosis connoted by the restrictive pattern (103). This pattern can be seen in patients with advanced stages of diastolic dysfunction due to restrictive, dilated, or ischemic cardiomyopathy, and usually the patients have dyspnea at rest and high New York Heart Association functional class (113). Severe enlargement and hypocontractility of the left atrium may be seen, and this pattern carries a poor prognosis in ischemic (222), dilated (223,224), and restrictive cardiomyopathies (103). In hypertrophic cardiomyopathy, there is a less clear prognostic potential of the filling patterns because of the complex interplay between systolic outflow tract obstruction, mitral regurgitation, and diastolic dysfunction (225).

Restrictive Filling Pattern (Stage IV)

As noted previously, restrictive filling patterns are associated with a poor prognosis for patients with various types of cardiac diseases. Additional prognostic information can be obtained in patients with restrictive filling patterns evaluated under different hemodynamic conditions. Failure to convert a restrictive mitral inflow filling pattern to a nonrestrictive pattern substantially increased the risk of death greater than twofold in a study of patients with chronic heart failure (226,227).

Estimating Left Atrial and Left Ventricular Filling Pressures

Transmitral inflow and pulmonary venous flow by Doppler echocardiography have been used to noninvasively estimate left heart filling pressures, including mean pulmonary capillary wedge and left atrial pressure and LV end diastolic pressure, primarily in patients with cardiac disease (96,97,220,228–230). A notable exception in the use of Doppler flow patterns to predict filling pressure is patients with hypertrophic cardiomyopathy in whom Doppler mitral flow patterns do not correlate well with LV filling pressures due mainly to the exaggerated relaxation abnormalities and other variables affecting diastolic function in this disease (225).

An increased E/A ratio, a shortened deceleration and isovolumic relaxation time, a decreased atrial filling fraction, a decreased pulmonary venous systolic fraction, an elevated and prolonged AR flow velocity, and increased left atrial volume may suggest an elevated mean left atrial pressure. Because these parameters are influenced by left atrial pressure and ventricular relaxation, these correlations work best for patients with abnormalities of LV relaxation in which left atrial pressure is the only variable. This includes mostly patients with structural heart disease. In the setting of isolated diastolic dysfunction with normal systolic function, mitral inflow and pulmonary venous inflow parameters are poorly related to LV filling pressures. By combining the mitral E wave, a variable that correlates modestly with left atrial pressure and one that is associated with ventricular relaxation (color M-mode propagation velocity or TDE early filling velocity), closer approximations of left atrial pressure can be obtained. ▼ f72

End diastolic LV pressure has been estimated by echocardiography independent of left atrial pressure. Several studies have shown that the difference between the duration of the pulmonary venous AR and transmitral inflow A-wave duration can be used as an estimate of elevated LV end diastolic pressure (96–98) (eFig. 26.3.5). When the duration of the pulmonary venous reversal wave is prolonged with respect to that of the forward mitral A-wave duration (greater than 20 to 30 ms), then the LV end diastolic pressure is usually elevated (greater than 15 mm Hg) (96). This variable has been shown to be relatively age independent (234) and not affected by mitral regurgitation (234a). Studies have demonstrated that the difference in duration between the pulmonary venous AR and mitral A wave of greater than or equal to 30 ms is a predictor of severity of disease in cardiac amyloidosis (235) and cardiac mortality in patients with coronary artery disease (236).

Clinical Presentation and Significance

Patients with impaired diastolic function present with the typical syndromes of congestive heart failure including dependent edema, limited exercise tolerance, ascites and effusions, orthopnea, and flash pulmonary edema. In general, the clinical examination is unreliable in differentiating systolic from diastolic dysfunction. The jugular veins are distended, and dependent pitting edema may be severe. Rales may be present on chest auscultation. Cardiac auscultation may demonstrate an S_3, S_4, or a pericardial knock (15,26). The typical clinical characteristic of patients with diastolic heart failure include the elderly, women, and those with hypertension, diabetes, and renal dysfunction (237). One study in Olmsted County, MN, of patients with dias-

tolic heart failure found that nearly 50% of patients were 80 years of age or older (238). The presentation of heart failure may be with flash pulmonary edema and hypertensive heart disease (239,240), advanced ischemic heart disease, or hypertensive hypertrophic cardiomyopathy (241). Those patients who do not respond to treatment for heart failure include patients with diseases such as aortic stenosis or hypertrophic cardiomyopathy, infiltrative cardiomyopathy, and constrictive pericarditis (242) (Table 26.1). Patients with diastolic heart failure may present with new onset of atrial fibrillation or flutter, especially with more advanced diastolic dysfunction (238,242a).

More specific signs of individual disease states are discussed in the following sections.

Management of Diastolic Heart Failure

The general goal of treatment is twofold: to reduce the variables responsible for the underlying diastolic dysfunction and to reduce the clinical manifestations of the process. Treatment consists of reducing elevated filling pressures, maintaining atrial contraction, decreasing heart rate, preventing ischemia, improving relaxation, and causing the regression of ventricular hypertrophy (28,62,243,244). Therapy must be targeted to the specific pathologic process as some medications may be inappropriate for certain conditions. For instance, a beta-blocker or calcium channel blocker would be preferable to an angiotensin-receptor blocker in patients with hypertrophic cardiomyopathy since the latter medication may contribute to LV outflow obstruction.

Diuretics produce symptomatic relief but should be used judiciously, as noncompliant ventricles, by definition, require higher pressures to achieve adequate filling. Nitrates may be beneficial secondary to their effects on reducing preload and ischemia (22). Beta-blocking agents slow heart rate, decrease myocardial oxygen demand, control blood pressure, and produce regression of LV hypertrophy. Calcium channel blockers have multiple benefits as negative chronotropic agents, controlling blood pressure, decreasing myocardial oxygen demand, dilating the coronary arteries, and regressing hypertrophy (26). Angiotensin-converting enzyme inhibitors and angiotensin-receptor blockers have direct and indirect effects. These include blood pressure control and substantial ventricular mass regression. The degree of myocardial mass regression of these agents appears more potent than any other antihypertensive agents for similar blood pressure reduction (245). Data have demonstrated improvement in diastolic function with lisinopril by reduction in myocardial fibrosis (including decreased collagen volume) independent of LV regression (246). Preliminary data support further investigation of nitric oxide donors, which produce improved myocardial relaxation (244,247).

Doppler flow patterns may be useful in guiding therapy (15) (eTable 26.2.3). Patients with abnormal relaxation with fusion of the E and A wave may need a calcium channel or beta-blocker to slow the heart rate, whereas patients with pseudonormal or restrictive filling may need diuretics or angiotensin-converting enzyme inhibitors to lower the elevated filling pressures. If there is a prolonged PR interval in the setting of dilated cardiomyopathy, dual-chamber pacing may be beneficial (248). There may be some additional benefit of the use in Doppler flow patterns in the evaluation of biventricular pacing (249).

Prognosis

Patients with congestive heart failure secondary to diastolic dysfunction generally have a better prognosis than patients with systolic dysfunction (250); however, they may have recurrent congestive heart failure and recurrent chest pain despite coronary revascularization (23,240). *e*Table 26.2.4 summarizes the mortality in a number of studies in patients with diastolic dysfunction. The prognosis of diastolic heart failure varies, depending on the population studied with an annual mortality varying from 1.3% to 17.5%, which is lower than patients with systolic dysfunction (19%) (22). The lower mortality with diastolic function has been shown in a large number of population-based studies including the Veterans Administration Cooperative Study and Coronary Artery Surgery Study (22,251). The addition of coronary artery disease in patients with congestive heart failure adds considerable risk to diastolic dysfunction; however, it does not approach the risk of patients with low ejection fractions (250). A study by Senni et al. showed similar mortality in older patients with diastolic and systolic dysfunction (238).

Large prospective epidemiologic studies have provided significant insight into the clinical outcomes of patients with diastolic heart failure. One study group of 2,498 patients with functional class II to IV symptoms and LV ejection fractions greater than or equal to 40% were analyzed from the Duke University Cardiovascular database. A 5-year mortality of 28% was observed with predictors of mortality in a multivariable model including advanced age, minority status, coronary artery disease, severe heart failure or lower ejection fraction, diabetes, and peripheral vascular disease (252). An ongoing study (Candesartan in Heart Failure, Assessment of Reduction in Mortality and Morbidity) will address the effect of an angiotensin II type I receptor blocker in patients with systolic and diastolic dysfunction (253).

SPECIFIC DISEASE STATES

Restrictive Cardiomyopathy

Classification

Restrictive cardiomyopathy is defined as a disease of the myocardium, which is characterized by "restrictive filling and reduced diastolic volume of either or both ventricles with normal or near-normal systolic function" (254). [⟁ f73] Systolic function may be normal in the early stage of disease, while wall thickness may be normal or increased depending on the etiology of the disease (254,261,262). The disease may be "idiopathic or associated with other disease" such as amyloidosis (254,261).

Despite this controversy of classification, in clinical practice, *cardiomyopathy* is a more loosely applied term. Dilated, hypertrophic, restrictive, and RV cardiomyopathies encompass the major categories of disease, although unclassified and specific cardiomyopathies (such as valvular, ischemic, hypertensive, and so forth) are also included (254). Restrictive cardiomyopathies are recognized as primary and secondary where the secondary forms include the specific heart muscle diseases in which the heart is affected as part of a multisystem disorder (e.g., infiltrative, storage, and noninfiltrative disease) (263).

A "working classification" of restrictive cardiomyopathy is shown in Figure 26.4 (261,263). Infiltrative cardiomyopathies can be further divided into interstitial and storage disorders. In interstitial diseases, the infiltrates localize to the interstitium (between myocardial cells), as with cardiac amyloidosis and sarcoidosis, whereas in storage disorders, the deposits are within cells, as with hemochromatosis and glycogen storage diseases (51). These secondary forms of restrictive cardiomyopathies are probably more common than the primary form (264) and display the classic restrictive hemodynamics only in their advanced form. The prototypical secondary restrictive cardiomyopathy is cardiac amyloidosis (51).

Anatomic Considerations

In idiopathic restrictive cardiomyopathy, pathologic studies have shown mild to moderate degrees of hypertrophy and fibrosis (259) with the hemodynamic findings unrelated to the histopathologic abnormalities detected (259). In cardiac amyloidosis (see the section Cardiac Amyloidosis), there is interstitial infiltration of amyloid fibrils in the ventricles and atria causing a firm, rubbery consistency of the heart (265,266), whereas in the endomyocardial diseases there is an endocardial fibrotic shell with extension into the myocardium (267).

Pathophysiology

The characteristic feature of restrictive cardiomyopathy is a marked increased stiffness of the myocardium or endocardium that causes the ventricular pressure to rise dramatically with only small changes in volume causing an upward shift of the LV pressure-volume relationship and a dip and plateau or square-root hemodynamic pattern (268,269). As mentioned, there is a controversy about whether this restrictive hemodynamic pattern is necessary (270,271) to be

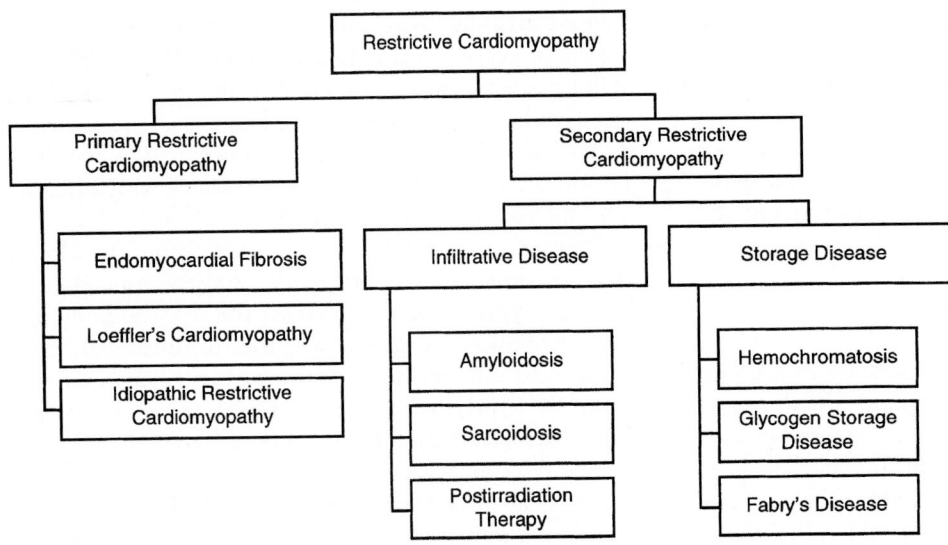

FIGURE 26.4 Working classification of restrictive cardiomyopathy. (From Leung DY, Klein AL. Restrictive cardiomyopathy; diagnosis and prognostic implications. In: Otto CM, ed. *Practice of clinical echocardiography.* Philadelphia: WB Saunders, 1997:474, with permission.)

included as a restrictive cardiomyopathy; however, the 1995 WHO/ISFC classification does include restrictive hemodynamics as an absolute criterion for the diagnosis. Both ventricles are affected with the restrictive process, but usually the pressures are higher on the left than the right (272), which may reflect the relatively decreased compliance of the left ventricle compared with the right ventricle. An exception may be tropical endomyocardial fibrosis in which the right ventricle may be predominantly involved (273).

Clinical Profile

The clinical signs and symptoms of restrictive cardiac diseases relate closely to the degree of left atrial hypertension required to compensate for poor ventricular filling (274). This gives rise to the typical clinical features of exercise intolerance in early cases and dyspnea at rest and symptoms of low cardiac output state such as fatigue in advanced cases (263). Left atrial dilatation, pulmonary congestion, distention of central veins, hepatic distention, ascites, peripheral edema, and anasarca are seen in advanced cases. Exertional chest pain is usually absent. Atrial fibrillation is common because of the atrial enlargement. Ventricular arrhythmias or heart block are not uncommonly present in advanced cases and are often the cause of death in these patients. Symptoms of the underlying multisystem disorder, if present, may also be evident (263). Examination may reveal jugular venous distention, S_4, or S_3 depending on the filling characteristics (275). Kussmaul's sign (272) can be detected, whereas apical retraction (as in constrictive pericarditis) is not seen (276).

In our experience, the main laboratory test to diagnose restrictive cardiomyopathy is echocardiography (4). Transthoracic or transesophageal echocardiography with respirometry has successfully been used to differentiate restriction from constriction (101,119). In patients with restriction, there is no significant respiratory variation as there is in

constriction (13,101). Newer imaging modalities, including TDE and color M-mode Doppler (15,16,121,123), appear promising to further distinguish these disorders. MRI and computed tomography (CT) scanning may also be useful to exclude pericardial thickness (124,277,278). Cine MRI may show abnormal patterns of filling in early and advanced stages of restrictive cardiomyopathy similar to echocardiography (279). MRI may also be capable of distinguishing tissue characteristics of infiltrative processes, such as amyloid, differentiating it from other forms of cardiomyopathy (163).

Management

The prognosis of restrictive cardiomyopathy depends on whether there is early or advanced stage of the disease as shown with cardiac amyloidosis (103). The prognosis is variable, but usually progressive (280). Diuresis may help with symptomatic relief, while angiotensin-converting enzyme inhibitors may be of benefit with LV dysfunction. Vasodilators should be used cautiously because they may cause hypotension. Reversible underlying conditions such as hemochromatosis should be addressed. Transplantation can be considered; however, often the restrictive cardiomyopathy is part of a systemic illness (281). Signs or symptoms of ischemia in children with restrictive cardiomyopathy predict sudden death and should be managed aggressively with beta-blockers, an implantable defibrillator, or consideration for transplantation (282).

Primary Restrictive Cardiomyopathy

Idiopathic Restrictive Cardiomyopathy

Idiopathic restrictive cardiomyopathy is a disease in patients with diastolic heart failure that is often characterized by familial transmission and the association with skeletal myopathies (259,283,284). It was first described by Benotti et al. (285), who described nine patients with heart failure, with elevated RV and LV filling pressures with normal systolic function and dip and plateau hemodynamic tracing.

Other investigators have described similar findings using strict hemodynamic criteria (270,286–289). Some series have excluded patients with hypertrophy, and others have not shown the dip and plateau pattern in all patients (271,284). Thus, there is a lack of consensus on the type of diastolic filling pattern and the degree of LV hypertrophy in this disease (259).

Anatomic Considerations

The diagnosis of this disease is confirmed by the lack of any specific pathology on endomyocardial biopsies or autopsy specimens. The atria are disproportionately large with normal or near-normal ventricular cavity size (eFig. 26.4.1A). The left ventricle shows normal systolic function and there may be hypertrophy of the left or right ventricles (259). Thrombi may be present in the atrial appendages (261). Histologic examination is unremarkable or shows nonspecific degenerative changes seen in other cardiomyopathies, including myocyte hypertrophy, interstitial fibrosis, and nuclear changes (259) (eFig. 26.4.1B). Some series have reported myofibrillar disarray, increased fibrosis, and some hypertrophy of myocytes (270,286–289). Fibrosis may occur in the sinoatrial and atrioventricular nodes (283).

Clinical Presentation

Idiopathic restrictive cardiomyopathy is usually a sporadic disease, but it can occur in families with autosomal dominant transmission. There may be a family history, the presence of a distal skeletal myopathy, and heart block in this condition, which has been reported in five generations of an Italian family (261,283,284). Another restrictive cardiomyopathy with autosomal dominance with variable penetrance is associated with Noonan's syndrome (291).

There may be differences in idiopathic restrictive cardiomyopathy in children compared with adults. In children, the disease may be more common in girls (292,293), and children may have a worse prognosis with the disease than adults (292,293).

Diagnosis

Cardiac catheterization, echocardiography, or both, and endomyocardial biopsy should be done to make the diagnosis. Atrial enlargement with nondilated ventricles with near-normal systolic function is uniformly present on echocardiography. In one series, the ejection fraction ranged from 40% to 55% in patients with advanced disease needing heart transplantation (294). Variable degrees of hypertrophy may be present (259,286,288,289). Cardiac catheterization and Doppler echocardiography may show restrictive hemodynamics; however, other patterns may be present as well

(259). Biopsy is important to exclude other diseases and to assess myocyte hypertrophy and interstitial fibrosis (259).

Differentiation between Restrictive Cardiomyopathy and Constrictive Pericarditis

It is important to differentiate idiopathic restrictive cardiomyopathy from secondary forms such as cardiac amyloidosis, as well as constrictive pericarditis, because of different treatment regimens and prognosis (259). As a result of the rapid early ventricular filling, a prominent 'y' descent is often seen in the jugular venous pulse and the RA pressure tracing. Left atrial pressure is usually greater than 15 mm Hg, right atrial pressure is greater than 7 mm Hg, and the pulmonary wedge pressure is greater than 12 mm Hg (295–297). LV end diastolic pressure is usually 5 mm Hg higher than the right-sided pressures (259), although the absence of this difference does not suggest constriction (298). Moderate pulmonary hypertension is usually present in advanced restrictive disease (274,299). In restrictive cardiomyopathy, the RV end diastolic pressure is often less than one-third of the peak RV systolic pressure (274,299). In early stage restrictive disease or with marked diuresis, these characteristic changes may only be unmasked by intravenous fluid challenge, exercise, or pharmacologic interventions (297,300). A comparison of hemodynamic abnormalities in restrictive and constrictive disease is shown in Table 26.3. The hemodynamic findings show much overlap in distinguishing these two similar conditions (13,301).

Management

Most small series show a protracted clinical course in adults, with a mean survival of 4 to 14 years (mean, 9 years) (285,288). Patients have symptoms of congestive heart failure, elevated jugular veins, and mitral and tricuspid regurgitation (288). Progressive heart failure that responds poorly to medical management and complete heart block requiring a pacemaker may occur (283,288). In one series, the mean follow-up time to transplantation or death was 117 months compared with 44 months for cardiac amyloidosis (284). In a large series of 94 patients with echocardiographically defined idiopathic restrictive cardiomyopathy, predictors of poor prognosis included advanced age, male gender, left atrial enlargement, and advanced functional class (302). The 5-year survival rate for this group was 64%. Heart transplantation can be considered in patients with idiopathic restrictive cardiomyopathy (284).

Löffler's Endocarditis

Löffler's endocarditis is considered to be part of the idiopathic hypereosinophilic syndrome that is characterized by a persistently elevated blood eosinophil count without recognizable cause, despite a careful workup with signs and symptoms of organ involvement, especially in the heart,

TABLE 26.3 DIFFERENTIAL DIAGNOSIS OF RESTRICTIVE CARDIOMYOPATHY AND CONSTRICTIVE PERICARDITIS

Type of evaluation	Restrictive cardiomyopathy	Constrictive pericarditis
Physical examination	Kussmaul's sign may be present	Kussmaul's sign usually present
	Apical impulse may be prominent	Apical impulse usually not palpable
	S$_3$ (advanced disease), S$_4$ (early disease)	Pericardial knock may be present
	Regurgitant murmurs common	Regurgitant murmurs uncommon
	Pulsus paradoxus absent	Pulsus paradoxus rare[a]
Electrocardiography	Low voltage (especially in amyloidosis), pseudoinfarction, left-axis deviation, atrial fibrillation, conduction disturbances common	Low voltage (<50%)
Chest radiography	Absent calcification	Calcification sometimes
Echocardiography	Small LV cavity with large atria	Normal wall thickness
	Increased wall thickness sometimes present (especially thickened interatrial septum in amyloidosis)	Pericardial thickening seen
	Thickened cardiac valves (amyloidosis)	Prominent early diastolic filling with abrupt displacement of interventricular septum
	Granular sparkling texture (amyloidosis)	
Doppler studies		
Mitral inflow	No respiration variation of mitral inflow E wave, IVRT	*With inspiration*
	E/A ratio ≥2	Decreased mitral inflow E wave, prolonged IVRT
	Short DT	*With expiration*, opposite changes
	Diastolic regurgitation	Short DT
		Diastolic regurgitation
Pulmonary vein	Blunted S/D ratio (0.5), prominent and prolonged AR	S/D ratio = 1
	No respiration variation D wave	*With inspiration*
		Decreased PV S and D waves
		With expiration, opposite changes
Tricuspid inflow	Mild respiration variation of tricuspid inflow E wave	*With inspiration*
	E/A ratio ≥2	Increased tricuspid inflow E wave, increased TR peak velocity
	TR peak velocity, no significant respiration change	*With expiration*, opposite changes
	Short DT with inspiration	Short DT
	Diastolic regurgitation	Diastolic regurgitation
Hepatic vein	Blunted S/D ratio, increased inspiratory reversals	*With inspiration*
		Minimally increased HV S and D
		With expiration, decreased diastolic flow and increased reversals
Inferior vena cava	Plethoric	Plethoric
Color M-mode	Slow flow propagation	Rapid flow propagation (≥100 cm/s)
Mitral annular motion	Low-velocity early filling (<8 cm/s)	High-velocity early filling (≥8 cm/s)
Cardiac catheterization	Dip and plateau	Dip and plateau
	LVEDP often >5 mm Hg greater than RVEDP, but may be identical	RVEDP and LVEDP usually equal
	RV systolic pressure >50 mm Hg	*With inspiration*
	RVEDP less than one-third of RV systolic pressure	Increase in RV systolic pressure
		Decrease in LV systolic pressure
		With expiration, opposite changes
Endomyocardial biopsy	May reveal specific cause of restrictive cardiomyopathy	May be normal or show nonspecific myocyte hypertrophy or myocardial fibrosis
Computed tomography/magnetic resonance imaging	Pericardium usually normal	Pericardium may be thickened

AR, atrial reversal flow velocity; DT, deceleration time; IVRT, isovolumic relaxation time; LV, left ventricular; LVEDP, left ventricular end diastolic pressure; RV, right ventricular; RVEDP, right ventricular end diastolic pressure; TR, tricuspid regurgitation.
[a]Unless effusive or subacute constrictive pericarditis is present.
Modified from Kushwaha SS, Fallon JT, Fuster V. Restrictive cardiomyopathy. *N Engl J Med* 1997;336:267–276, with permission.

nervous system, and bone marrow (274,311,312). Cardiac involvement occurs in more than 75% of the cases of the syndrome (303). ❥ f74

Clinical Manifestations

The typical presentation is a man less than 50 years of age who lives in a temperate climate and has the hypereosinophilic syndrome (274,305). Right- and left-sided congestive heart failure, mitral regurgitation, systemic embolism, cardiac enlargement on the chest radiography, and T-wave inversions on the electrocardiogram are the main clinical manifestations of this disorder, which depends on the stage of disease (264,317).

Echocardiography commonly demonstrates mural thrombosis (eFig. 26.4.3). There may be obliteration of the apex and immobility of the posterior leaflet of the mitral valve with entrapment against the thickened posterobasal endocardium, thus resulting in mitral regurgitation (264,318). These findings were described in a review of 29 patients with classic echocardiographic features of the hypereosinophilic syndrome (319). LV systolic function is often preserved, and restrictive physiology may be demonstrated by Doppler echocardiography, usually in the fibrotic phase (320).

Cardiac catheterization typically shows the dip and plateau physiology with reduced LV compliance because of the dense scarring of the ventricle, and mitral and tricuspid regurgitation may be present as well (303,312). Endomyocardial biopsy may be necessary to confirm the diagnosis; however, it may be difficult to obtain an adequate tissue sample (312).

Management

The treatment options depend on the stage of the disease; early Löffler's disease is treated medically with corticosteroids, whereas surgery is reserved for the fibrotic stages. Corticosteroids and hydroxyurea may be used to treat the myocarditis when associated with the hypereosinophilia (312,313,321). Also, interferon has been used in a limited number of patients with promising results (314,322). Standard supportive medical therapy should include digoxin, diuretics, afterload reducers, and anticoagulants (303,312). Surgical treatment involves debriding the fibrous plaque from the endocardial surface and replacement of the valves and pacemaker insertion (305,312,313).

Endomyocardial Fibrosis

Endomyocardial fibrosis is endemic to tropical and subtropical Africa and occurs less frequently in South America and Asia (300,323,324). It is a common cause of congestive heart failure and death in equatorial Africa, accounting for 15% to 25% of the deaths secondary to heart disease (274,305). Endomyocardial fibrosis involves both ventricles in 50% of the cases, followed by involvement of the left ventricle in 40% and right ventricle in 10% of the cases (274,307).

Endomyocardial fibrosis occurs in three distinct areas: the LV apex, subvalvular apparatus, and the RV apex (274,325). The fibrosis at the ventricular apex extends to the lower ventricular septum and to the posteromedial papillary muscle. The fibrosis also extends in the area behind the posterior mitral valve, causing tethering of the chordae tendineae and resulting in mitral regurgitation. The anterior leaflet of the mitral valve and the outflow tract is often spared. It also may involve the RV apex, causing impairment of filling of the tricuspid inflow and encasement of the papillary muscles of the tricuspid valve and resulting in tricuspid regurgitation (307,319).

A classification scheme according to the location of fibrosis was proposed by Shaper et al. (326). Usually, the right ventricle is obliterated more than the left ventricle (307).

Microscopically, there is a thick layer of collagen tissue over a layer of connective tissue in the endocardium, with granulation tissue extending into the myocardium (327).

Clinical Profile

The clinical presentation in the endomyocardial fibrosis depends on whether the left, right, or both ventricles are involved. The disease affects both male and female subjects, usually children and young adults (308). Left-sided disease results in pulmonary congestion, whereas right-sided disease results in right-sided heart failure simulating constrictive pericarditis. Often, mitral and tricuspid regurgitation is present because of the involvement of the valves. Atrial fibrillation is not uncommon, occurring in one-fourth of patients with endomyocardial fibrosis, especially when there is RV involvement. Embolism is a frequent finding with endomyocardial fibrosis. A pericardial and pleural effusion may also be present (274,305,324).

Two-dimensional echocardiography shows the obliteration of the apices of the ventricles and dilated atria, whereas Doppler echocardiography shows evidence of mitral and tricuspid regurgitation. The posterior leaflet shows decreased mobility in left-sided disease (274,305). The basal ventricle may be hypercontractile due to the obliterated apex (328). Cardiac catheterization and Doppler echocardiography may show the restrictive hemodynamics of the disease.

Management

The prognosis is poor in endomyocardial fibrosis, with progressive disease and death caused by heart failure, or sudden death (274,305,326). The 2-year mortality is between 35% and 50% in patients with advanced disease (308,329). Surgery may improve symptoms in the fibrotic stage with excision of the fibrous endocardium and repair or replacement of the mitral and tricuspid valves (314,330,331); operative mortality has been reported in the range of 15% to 25% (332,333). However, one study of 11 patients undergoing surgery with endocardial resection and valve replacement reported a 10-year survival of near 70% (334).

Secondary Restrictive Myocardial Diseases

Infiltrative Conditions

Interstitial Diseases

Cardiac Amyloidosis. Cardiac amyloidosis is the prototype of restrictive myocardial diseases and the most frequently encountered in clinical practice (51).

Clinical Presentation. Cardiac amyloidosis usually presents in men over 30 years of age (336,342) and occurs in older patients in the familial form (339). Patients with cardiac amyloidosis present with diastolic heart failure and the "stiff heart syndrome" resulting from amyloid infiltration. Patients may present with various degrees of progressive biventricular heart failure depending on the stage of disease as shown by two-dimensional and Doppler echocardiography (275). In early cardiac amyloidosis, patients may be asymptomatic, whereas patients with advanced disease have the typical evidence of restrictive cardiomyopathy with severe right-sided heart failure, ascites, and peripheral edema (305). During cardiac catheterization a square-root sign is present, and restrictive hemodynamics by Doppler echocardiography are detected only in the advanced stages of the disease (275). In addition, there may be an intermediate stage in which patients have more symptoms as left atrial pressure increases. Individual patients may actually evolve through the different stages of involvement (100). Often, it may be difficult to differentiate advanced cardiac amyloidosis from constrictive pericarditis (101,123). As the disease progresses, there are both systolic and diastolic heart failure (351). Chest pain resembling angina pectoris may also be present despite normal epicardial coronary arteries during cardiac catheterization (350), or there may be partial obliteration of the distal coronary arteries by amyloid infiltration (266,343,352). Involvement of the intramyocardial vessels may be an another explanation for this presentation (325,353). In 10% to 15% of cases, orthostatic hypotension is detected in patients with cardiac amyloidosis. This is secondary to amyloid infiltration of the autonomic nervous system with symptoms of syncope, diarrhea, lack of sweating, and impotence (337). Kidney, adrenal, and cardiac involvement with amyloid deposition may aggravate the postural hypotension. Refractory supraventricular and ventricular arrhythmias or conduction defects may also be another mode of presentation (354). Sudden death secondary to arrhythmias may also be the cause of death, especially in familial amyloidosis (339).

Physical examination may reveal an S_4 (early disease) or S_3 (advanced disease) on auscultation, depending on the stage of the illness (275). Mitral and tricuspid valvular regurgitation may also be present (51). There is evidence of biventricular heart failure with often predominant right-sided heart failure (305), an elevated jugular venous pulse with a prominent 'y' descent, hepatosplenomegaly, ascites, and peripheral edema, especially in advanced disease. The blood pressure may also be decreased.

The cardiac silhouette on chest radiography is usually enlarged in patients with advanced disease with evidence of pulmonary congestion (297). Electrocardiography typically is of low voltage and shows a pseudoinfarction pattern with Q waves simulating a myocardial infarction in the precordial leads (325,355). Arrhythmias especially atrial fibrillation are common (30% of patients) and a sick sinus syndrome may be present (325).

Atrioventricular conduction defects may be present, especially in familial amyloidosis associated with polyneuropathy (339). Also, ventricular arrhythmias consisting of

ventricular tachycardia may be present in advanced disease and may be a forewarning of death (343).

Investigations: Echocardiography. Two-dimensional and Doppler echocardiography is the procedure of choice in the noninvasive diagnosis, serial follow-up, and prognosis of patients with cardiac amyloidosis (51,100,103,180,275,351,356). Cardiac amyloidosis gives a distinctive appearance on two-dimensional echocardiography and is associated with abnormal LV and RV diastolic function. The findings of a normal or small LV cavity size with markedly thickened myocardium associated with a highly abnormal texture that is often described as "granular sparkling" in appearance is the classic presentation (51) (Fig. 26.5).

The sparkling granular appearance is thought to be caused by the acoustic mismatch between the highly reflective amyloid deposits in the endocardium, myocardium, and pericardium and the normal tissue (357). Moreover, autopsy and clinical biopsy series have demonstrated the presence of amyloid fibrils in the myocardium at the site of the granular sparkling echoes. Ultrasonic tissue characterization has been used to identify patients with cardiac amyloidosis (358).

Global LV systolic function is usually preserved in early disease, whereas systolic function is usually impaired in advanced disease. The interatrial septum and valve leaflets are also thickened. Both atria are enlarged, and small to moderate pericardial effusions are usually present (351,356).

Patients with cardiac amyloidosis have a low ratio of electrocardiographic voltage to LV wall thickness ratio, which is thought to be specific to cardiac amyloidosis and suggested to be predictive of clinical symptoms and prognosis (359,360). However, the usefulness of this ratio is limited by the presence of coexisting diseases that may result in decreased electrocardiographic voltage.

Management. The prognosis of cardiac amyloidosis is uniformly poor but does depend on the type of disease, with AL amyloidosis having the worse prognosis (335,336,338,339,342). In a series of over 800 patents with primary amyloidosis over a 10-year period, the median survival was 2.1 years (374). The treatment for cardiac amyloidosis (AL type) includes alkylating agents, such as melphalan and prednisone (374).

There have been two randomized trials of chemotherapy showing benefit in AL amyloid (341,375,376). A trial of 100 patients with primary amyloidosis using melphalan, prednisone, and colchicine showed improvement of systemic disease when the major features were not cardiac or renal (377). Colchicine has also been used to prevent amyloidosis associated with familial Mediterranean fever (374); however, there is no evidence that it halts the progression of amyloid deposition in primary amyloidosis. Dose-intensive melphalan with blood stem cell support is currently being evaluated (378).

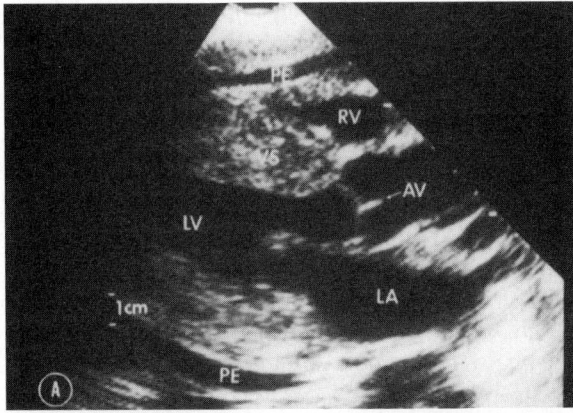
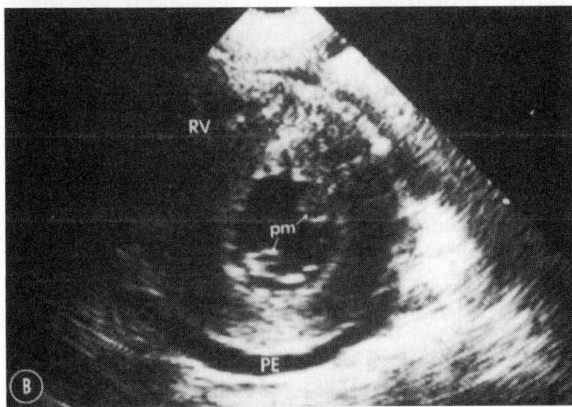
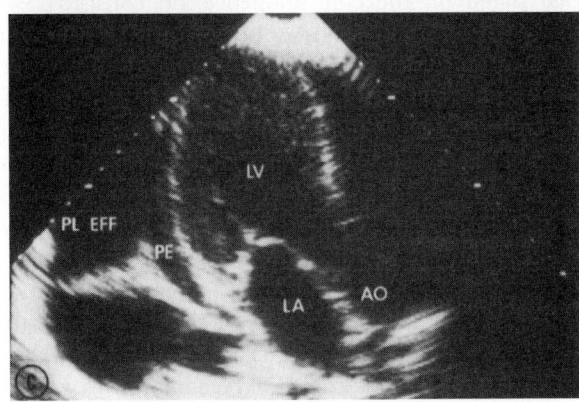

FIGURE 26.5 Parasternal long-axis **(A)**, short-axis **(B)**, and apical long-axis **(C)** views show typical echocardiographic features of advanced cardiac amyloidosis. Note left ventricle (LV) size is normal with markedly thickened ventricular walls [ventricular septum, 22 mm; posterior wall, 18 mm; and right ventricular (RV) free wall, 15 mm] and its characteristic granular sparkling appearance. Small pericardial effusion (PE) and left pleural effusion (PL EFF) are also present. AO, aorta; AV, aortic valve; LA, left atrium; pm, papillary muscle; VS, ventricular septum. (From Klein AL, Oh JK, Miller FA, et al. Two-dimensional and Doppler echocardiographic assessment of infiltrative cardiomyopathy. *J Am Soc Echocardiogr* 1988;1:48–59, with permission.)

Cardiac transplantation is generally not performed for patients with AL type amyloidosis, because this is a systemic illness with progressive amyloidosis in other organs (281). However, it has been considered in select patients without extracardiac disease (379,380). Liver transplanta-

tion has been suggested for the familial type (TTR variant) since the circulating TTR is produced in the liver. Thus, the new liver replaces the variant TTR with a normal TTR. There is no specific treatment for the senile type (381,382).

Avoidance of digoxin is recommended since digoxin-induced arrhythmias may occur because the digoxin may bind to the amyloid fibrils (305,383). However, it has been used to control heart rate in patients with atrial fibrillation with careful monitoring (336). Also, patients with cardiac amyloidosis may be sensitive to the negative inotropic effects of calcium channel blockers either because of their abnormal binding to amyloid fibrils or the vasodilator effects (305,384). Vasodilator agents and diuretics should be used judiciously because of the risk of postural hypotension. Pacemakers may be useful to treat symptomatic high atrioventricular block (385), and anticoagulation should be considered because of the risk of thrombus formation with atrial amyloid involvement and atrial standstill (171,386).

Cardiac Sarcoidosis. Sarcoidosis is a noncaseating granulomatous disorder of unknown etiology that may involve the lung, lymph nodes, skin, liver, spleen, parotid glands, and heart (387,388). Pulmonary manifestations are the predominant finding, with pulmonary hypertension and pulmonary fibrosis resulting in right-sided heart failure (389). Sarcoid granulomata are found in the myocardium at autopsy in up to 25% of the patients with sarcoidosis and are often clinically silent (390–393).

Clinical Manifestations. The clinical presentation of cardiac sarcoidosis is variable and may depend on the amount of myocardium replaced with granulomata and the amount and the location of scar tissue (264,394,396,398,399). Most patients are asymptomatic; however, rhythm abnormalities and conduction disorders may predominate (264,394). The most common arrhythmia is ventricular tachycardia (396,400,401), while complete heart block is the most common conduction disorder (393). Sudden death is the most feared complication (395,402) and occurs in 17% of patients when there is extensive myocardial involvement. Valvular dysfunction and pericardial effusions are less common manifestations in this disease (394,396,398,399).

Patients with congestive heart failure may show clinical features of restrictive cardiomyopathy, dilated cardiomyopathy, or both (393). Patients with marked disease may develop aneurysm formation and papillary dysfunction and mitral regurgitation (393,403). The electrocardiogram may show T-wave abnormalities, atrioventricular (AV) block, or Q waves mimicking myocardial infarction (393,404).

The echocardiographic findings consist of systolic and diastolic ventricular dysfunction, LV aneurysm formation, small to moderate pericardial effusions, and abnormal ventricular wall thickness (51,405–408). Regional wall motion abnormalities (suggestive of coronary artery disease) may be detected in the basal septum with sparing of the apex (409).

There may be RV dilatation and increased wall thickness consistent with cor pulmonale (389). LV diastolic function abnormalities may be present in 14% of patients with pulmonary sarcoidosis without evidence of cardiac disease, suggesting subclinical sarcoid cardiomyopathy (410).

Thallium-201 or gallium-67 scanning may show segmental defects suggestive of sarcoid infiltration (411–414). The gallium-67 uptake in the myocardium may be able to predict the efficacy of corticosteroids. MRI may also be useful to identify areas of high intensity in the LV septum and the free wall of the ventricle in the inflammatory phase, while detecting thinning and aneurysm formation in the chronic phase (415). The findings on MRI may be useful in guiding endomyocardial biopsy (416). Endomyocardial biopsy may be useful although the sensitivity is reported to be in the range of 20% to 30% and thus does not exclude the diagnosis if negative (393,404).

Management. The finding of pulmonary involvement with bilateral hilar adenopathy and evidence of myocardial disease may suggest sarcoidosis involving the heart in a young person (393). Echocardiography shows LV dilatation, regional wall motion abnormalities, or aneurysm formation (264,408). Treatment of sarcoidosis may include the use of corticosteroids, especially with myocardial involvement; conduction abnormalities and ventricular arrhythmias are present, however, this remains controversial (404,417–419). Permanent pacemakers may be needed to treat the conduction abnormalities (392,393). Implantable defibrillators may be needed to prevent sudden death (420,421), whereas heart transplantation is reserved for intractable heart failure (392,420).

Storage Diseases

Hemochromatosis. Hemochromatosis is an iron storage disease that affects the heart, pancreas, liver, gonads, and skin (433). Primary idiopathic hemochromatosis is an autosomal recessive disorder related to the human leukocyte antigen on chromosome 6, whereas secondary hemochromatosis results from hemoglobin synthesis abnormalities leading to ineffective erythropoiesis, chronic liver disease, excessive intake of iron, or multiple blood transfusions (433,434).

Clinical Presentation. Manifestations of cardiac involvement occur when there is a large amount of iron deposited over a long time period. One-third of patients manifest cardiac symptoms with evidence of congestive heart failure, supraventricular or ventricular arrhythmias, and conduction defects (433). One-third of patients die from cardiac involvement. A dilated or restrictive cardiomyopathy may be present with evidence of systolic and diastolic dysfunction. Cardiomegaly may be seen on chest radiography. Electrocardiographic findings have included arrhythmias, conduction disorders, and low voltages (51,433).

Echocardiography is a useful noninvasive technique in the assessment of cardiac involvement in primary hemochromatosis, detecting clinically occult heart involvement, following patients serially, and assessing LV function after phlebotomy (437–439) (*e*Fig. 26.5.6).

Olson et al. described 19 patients with primary hemochromatosis and demonstrated that 7 (37%) had chamber dilatation and systolic dysfunction secondary to the hemochromatosis, whereas 12 patients did not (440). Increased ventricular wall thickness and mass may also be observed, although Olson and coworkers suggested that increased ventricular wall thickness is not always present with cardiac hemochromatosis (440). Patterns consistent with dilated or restrictive cardiomyopathy have also been described in patients with primary hemochromatosis (441). Ventricular dysfunction and increased ventricular mass may normalize after successful venesection (441). The presence of systolic dysfunction usually signifies poor prognosis (439). Secondary hemochromatosis manifestations in the heart include increased LV wall thickness and mass, cavity dimension, and left atrial enlargement. Most patients have normal systolic function, and those with the depressed systolic function have the worst prognosis (442).

Other noninvasive tests, including CT scan or MRI, may be useful in demonstrating subclinical involvement of hemochromatosis (443). The MRI may show a low myocardial signal on the cine gradient-echo consistent with myocardial iron deposition. Endomyocardial biopsy may be useful to exclude the diagnosis, especially when the echocardiographic or clinical features are not evident (444,445). Laboratory tests show an elevated serum ferritin and increased ratio of plasma iron level to total iron-binding capacity, urinary iron, liver iron, and saturation of transferrin (445).

Management. Treatment by repeat phlebotomies in primary hemochromatosis or the use of chelating agents (desferrioxamine) in secondary hemochromatosis may result in improvement of the cardiac involvement, thus making early diagnosis important (433,446,447). Heart transplantation may be considered when the heart involvement is life-threatening (447) or combined heart and liver transplantation may be useful in patients with heart and liver failure (448).

Noninfiltrative Diseases

Carcinoid Heart Disease

Carcinoid heart disease is a rare cause of restrictive cardiomyopathy (462,463). Carcinoid syndrome results from metastatic carcinoid tumors that cause cutaneous flushing, diarrhea, bronchoconstriction, and fibrous endocardial plaques in the heart (464,465). Cardiac disease is detected by echocardiography in over 50% of patients with carcinoid syndrome, whereas clinically apparent heart disease with right-sided heart failure is detected in 25% of patients (464,466). ⬎ f75

Clinical Presentation. Carcinoid heart disease is difficult to diagnose until there is evidence of right-sided heart failure with an elevated jugular venous pulse with a prominent 'v' wave and tricuspid regurgitation (463). A systolic murmur along the left sternal border that shows inspiratory augmentation (tricuspid regurgitation) followed by an early diastolic sound and a diastolic rumble (tricuspid stenosis) may be detected. Also, there may be murmurs of pulmonic stenosis and regurgitation (464). Chest radiography may show cardiac enlargement, pleural effusions, and nodules. The pulmonary trunk is normal in size. The electrocardiogram is nonspecific with evidence of RA enlargement, nonspecific ST- and T-wave abnormalities, and sinus tachycardia (464). The hemodynamic findings are that of significant tricuspid regurgitation with a large RA 'v' wave and diastolic gradient (464).

Echocardiography is a sensitive technique to document the combined tricuspid and pulmonic abnormalities and RV overload, as well as to follow the progression and detect subclinical involvement (464,472).

Using echocardiography in one series, right-sided disease was detected in 66% of patients with carcinoid syndrome, and the patients with more severe valvular disease were more associated with higher levels of bradykinins and serotonin (466,473). In another series of 132 patients with carcinoid syndrome, Pellikka et al. found that 56% of patients had cardiac involvement, which was associated with higher levels of 5-hydroxy-indoleacetic acid. The 3-year survival of patients with echocardiographic evidence of carcinoid heart disease was reduced compared with those without cardiac involvement (464). Other studies have shown a correlation between posttreatment 5-hydroxy-indoleacetic acid levels and progression of disease assessed by an echocardiographic score of valvular involvement (474).

The echocardiographic features of cardiac involvement are remarkable (475). The tricuspid valve leaflets are thickened, shortened, and retracted and show incomplete coaptation and decreased excursion, resulting in stenosis and regurgitation. The pulmonic valve also shows thickening, retraction, and commissural fusion and stays open in a partly fixed position, resulting in both stenosis and regurgitation. The predominant lesions seen are tricuspid regurgitation and pulmonary stenosis (476) (*e*Fig. 26.5.9). Carcinoid plaques causing these lesions are usually seen on the ventricular surface of the tricuspid valve and the pulmonary artery surface of the pulmonary valve (476) (*e*Fig. 26.5.10). The Doppler findings show severe tricuspid regurgitation with a distinctive dagger-shaped Doppler spectral profile with an early peak pressure and rapid decline. In addition, the pressure half-time is prolonged, which is consistent with associated tricuspid stenosis (464). Also, there is evidence of RV volume overload from the associated tricuspid regurgitation (264). Transesophageal echocardiography may be useful in assessing the thickness of the valvular leaflets and the superficial wall layers on the cavity side of both atria (472,477).

Management. Carcinoid heart disease can be diagnosed in the presence of the right-sided heart findings with the classic systemic features. There may be urinary excretion of 5-hydroxy-indoleacetic acid, the principal metabolite of serotonin (463,476).

The long-term prognosis is poor, regardless of treatment modality (478). Chemotherapy may be partially effective in treating the hepatic metastasis, while removal of the primary tumor is rarely indicated. Occasionally, the liver metastasis is removed; more commonly, hepatic arterial embolization is performed (463,479). Medical therapy often includes digitalis and diuretics for mild congestive heart failure. The effects of the carcinoid syndrome can be treated with the use of somatostatin analogs, serotonin antagonists, and alpha-adrenergic blockers (463,480–482).

Interventional and surgical therapy has also been performed for patients with carcinoid valvular heart disease. Balloon valvuloplasty of the tricuspid stenosis and pulmonic stenosis can also be performed (483–486). Tricuspid valve replacement and pulmonary valvotomy is recommended with advanced disease (487,488). Implantation of a biologic valve or allograft is not recommended because of carcinoid developing on the new valve (463,476,489). Surgical mortality for symptomatic patients with severe valve disease is high (490); however, there can be marked improvement in symptoms in survivors (478).

Pericardial Disease

Clinical Presentations of Pericardial Disease

Acute Pericarditis

Inflammation of the layers of the pericardium, from any of myriad causes, yields a common clinical syndrome termed *acute pericarditis*. The causes of acute pericarditis are listed in Table 26.4. The classic symptom complex represents an important differential diagnosis in the assessment of chest pain presentations. However, the relatively common finding of pericardial inflammation at autopsy suggests that the majority of cases is subclinical.

Pathology. The histopathology of pericarditis is dependent on the underlying etiology. The majority of cases is manifested by hyperemia and increased microvascularity, polymorpholeukocyte accumulation, and fibrin deposition. Adhesions can form between the layers of the pericardium and between pericardium and adjacent structures such as pleura and mediastinum.

Clinical Presentation. Acute pericarditis classically presents with progressive, often severe, chest pain over hours.

TABLE 26.4 CAUSES OF ACUTE PERICARDITIS

Malignant tumor
Idiopathic pericarditis
Uremia
Bacteria infection
Anticoagulant therapy
Dissecting aortic aneurysm
Diagnostic procedures
Connective tissue disease
Postpericardiotomy syndrome
Trauma
Tuberculosis
Other
   Radiation
   Drugs inducing lupus-like syndrome
   Chylopericardium
   Postmyocardial infarction syndrome (Dressler's)
   Fungal infections
   Acquired immunodeficiency syndrome–related pericarditis

From Fowler NO. Pericardial disease. *Heart Dis Stroke* 1992;1:85–94, with permission.

This mechanical pain is typically postural, being worse on lying supine and relieved by sitting forward. It is often pleuritic and aggravated by coughing, motion, and swallowing. It is described as sharp, "stabbing," or "knife-like" in character. The pain my radiate to the neck and less frequently to the arms and back and even left shoulder, making differentiation from coronary ischemic pain more difficult. There is often a low-grade fever associated with viral and idiopathic pericarditis, while purulent pericarditis is associated with high fevers and systemic sepsis.

The presence of a pericardial rub is pathognomonic for pericarditis, although its absence does not exclude the syndrome. This "to and fro" rasping sound has a timing consistent with the cardiac cycle. It is best appreciated with the diaphragm of the stethoscope applied to the lower left sternal edge and is creaking in nature, like leather on leather. It is heard best with the patient leaning forward in end expiration. The sound classically has a triple cadence (520) with components related to (a) atrial systole, (b) ventricular systole, and (c) ventricular diastole. In 33% of the cases, the rub is biphasic, whereas in 10% it is monophasic. The intensity of the sound can be attenuated by subcutaneous tissue thickness and hyperinflated lung volume. Furthermore, the development of a pericardial effusion as part of the inflammatory syndrome can lead to waxing and waning of the rub over days, although a loud pericardial rub can be still be heard occasionally in the presence of a significant effusion. The sound should be differentiated from a pleural rub, which, although similar in character, is timed with the respiratory cycle; subcutaneous emphysema, which may be an associate in postsurgical or traumatic cases; and loud intracardiac murmurs such as ventricular septal defect.

Investigations. Electrocardiography represents the most useful diagnostic test in acute pericarditis (eFig. 26.5.14). Inflammation of the subepicardial myocardium is thought to be the mechanism producing ST- and T-wave changes, while inflammation of the atrium is thought to cause the PR-segment changes (521). The PR-segment deviations may precede the ST changes (522). In contrast to the regional ST changes of myocardial ischemia, pericarditis produces widespread electrocardiographic changes in limb and precordial leads. Four phases of electrocardiographic abnormalities have been recognized (Table 26.5) (521,523): Stage I, with ST elevation and upright T waves, is present in 90% cases. Over days, the ST changes resolve and the electrocardiogram may look normal (stage II). There may be further evolution to T-wave inversion (stage III) and finally to normal (stage IV).

The electrocardiographic abnormalities should be differentiated most importantly from acute myocardial ischemia. The ST changes are more widespread in pericarditis and have a typical saddle-shaped or upward concave appearance. Unlike myocardial infarction, there are no Q waves or loss of R-wave progression. The other important differential diagnosis of these electrocardiographic changes is the early repolarization pattern.

TABLE 26.5 FOUR-STAGE ("TYPICAL") ELECTROCARDIOGRAPHIC EVOLUTION OF ACUTE PERICARDITIS

Sequence stage	Leads of "epicardial" derivation: at least I, II, aV$_L$, aV$_F$, V$_3$–V$_6$			Leads reflecting "endocardial" potential: aV$_R$, often V$_1$, sometimes V$_2$		
	J-ST	T waves	PR segment	ST segment	T waves	PR segment
I	Elevated	Upright	Depressed or isoelectric	Depressed	Inverted	Elevated or isoelectric
II early	Isoelectric	Upright	Isoelectric or depressed	Isoelectric	Inverted	Isoelectric or elevated
II late	Isoelectric	Low to flat to inverted	Isoelectric or depressed	Isoelectric	Shallow to flat to upright	Isoelectric or elevated
III	Isoelectric	Inverted	Isoelectric	Isoelectric	Upright	Isoelectric
IV	Isoelectric	Upright	Isoelectric	Isoelectric	Inverted	Isoelectric

J-ST, junction of S (or T) wave with the end of the QRS complex.
Modified from Spodick DH. Electrocardiogram in acute pericarditis. Distributions of morphologic and axial changes by stages. *Am J Cardiol* 1974;33:470–474, with permission.

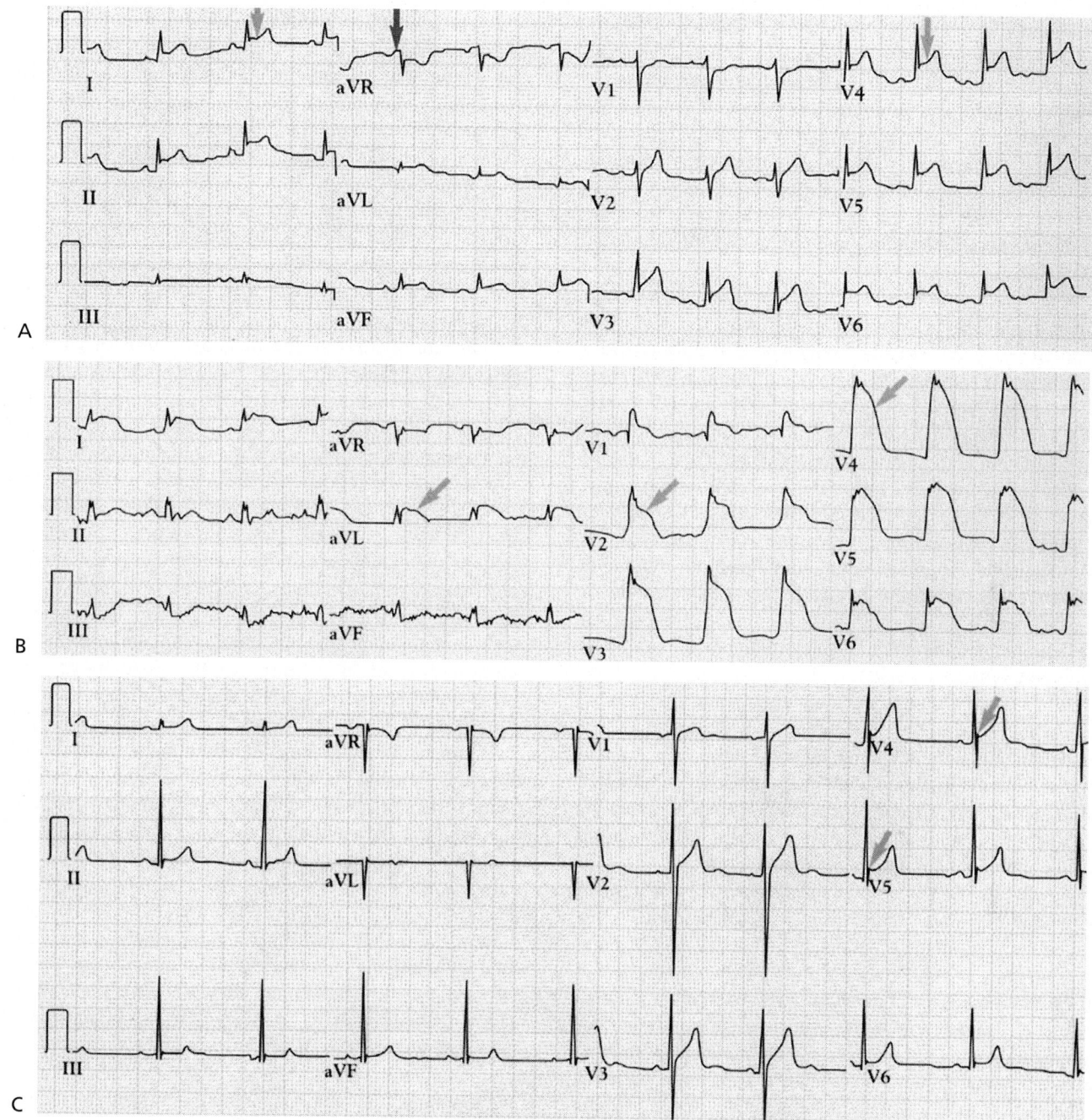

FIGURE 26.6 Differential diagnosis of acute pericarditis. **A:** Acute pericarditis. Note the upward concavity ST elevations in limb leads I, II, aVF, and aVL and in precordial leads V$_3$–V$_6$. (*left and right arrows*) and the PR segment elevation in aVR (*middle arrow*). **B:** Acute myocardial infarction. Note the convex ST elevation in leads I, aVL, V$_1$–V$_6$ (*left, right, middle arrows*), indicating a large anterior myocardial infarction. **C:** Early repolarization. Note the elevation of the J point (*right arrows*) with pseudonormalization of the ST segment in V$_4$–V$_6$. (From Aikat S, Ghaffari S. A review of pericardial diseases: clinical, ECG and hemodynamic features and management. *Cleve Clin J Med* 2000;67:903–914, with permission.)

Although it is difficult without clinical correlation, differentiation can be made by the presence of PR-segment elevation (especially aV$_R$) and ST elevation in V$_6$, which is uncommon in the early repolarization syndrome (524). Most patients with acute pericarditis remain in sinus rhythm (525) (Fig. 26.6).

Chest radiography contributes relatively little to the diagnosis of acute pericarditis. The presence of cardiomegaly may be seen in the minority of cases in which a significant pericardial effusion has accumulated. Laboratory analysis of blood often shows a modest leukocytosis and raised C-reactive protein and sedimentation rate.

Radionuclide scanning with In-111 (526) and Ga-67 (527,528) has been reported to be useful in identifying the pericardium as the source of an inflammatory syndrome of unknown diagnosis in some patients. Serum troponin I has been reported to be elevated in patients with ST elevation and acute pericarditis, reflecting a degree of myocardial injury (529). MRI, with gadolinium-diethylenetriamine-pentaacetic acid enhancement, has identified specific regions of the pericardium involved in the inflammatory process (530).

Diagnostic Algorithm. The following sequence has been proposed (531). All patients should have a complete history and physical examination, electrocardiography, and chest radiography. Diagnosis-specific testing may include tuberculin skin testing, rheumatoid factor and antinuclear antibody, and viral studies from pharyngeal and fecal swabs. In more complex cases (i.e., symptoms and signs lasting longer than 1 week, clinical evidence of tamponade, or purulent pericarditis), echocardiography, sputum and gastric aspirate for tubercle bacillus examination, and blood cultures *should be considered.* Pericardiocentesis (either percutaneous or surgical) is indicated for clinical tamponade, evidence for purulent pericarditis, high suspicion of tumor, or illness lasting longer than 1 week.

Pericardial Effusion

Pericardial effusion is diagnosed in routine echocardiographic practice in almost one in ten patients (532–534). Large pericardial effusions that develop slowly can be remarkably asymptomatic, while rapidly accumulating smaller effusions can present with tamponade.

Massive chronic pericardial effusion is a diagnosis ascribed to a syndrome consisting of a large pericardial effusion present for at least 3 months, not attributable to any systemic cause (535). This is an uncommon presentation of pericardial disease, accounting for 2.0% to 3.5% of all cases of large effusion (535). These effusions can be present for many years and were well tolerated in one series, with tamponade a rarity (536). However, in two series of patients, cardiac tamponade occurred in nearly 33% of the patients (535,537). In the larger study, 28 patients with large idiopathic chronic pericardial effusions were followed for a median of 7 years. Unexpected tamponade occurred in eight patients (29%) and pericardectomy was performed in 20 patients. Chronic nonspecific pericarditis was found in all patients evaluated by histology (537).

Clinical Presentation. Pericardial effusions that are not causing hemodynamic embarrassment to the heart are usually asymptomatic. Patients may describe dyspnea or dysphagia due to space-occupying effects in the chest. Physical compression may cause hoarseness (recurrent laryngeal nerve), hiccups (phrenic nerve), or nausea (diaphragm). Physical examination of patients with large effusions dem-

onstrates muffled heart sounds. Ewart's sign—dullness on auscultation under the left scapula—is a result of compression of the base of the left lung. This may be associated with coarse crepitations due to local atelectasis. Chest radiographic findings include cardiomegaly, which may be massive, often with a characteristic globular shape to the heart silhouette (*e*Fig. 26.6.1). The cardiac margins are unusually sharp, as the pericardium is free of the cardiac motion that usually blurs the silhouette radiographically. Electrocardiography demonstrates diminished QRS and T-wave voltages. Electrical alternans is a marker of massive pericardial effusion.

Echocardiography is the diagnostic tool of choice for pericardial effusion. Initially, M-mode was the standard, with a high sensitivity for posterior pericardial fluid (533). The advent of two-dimensional echocardiography has shown the various presentations of effusion, including circumferential, posterior, and loculated (Fig. 26.7). Loculated effusions are more common when scarring has supervened (e.g., postsurgical, posttrauma, postpurulent pericarditis). The size of effusions can be graded as small (less than 10 mm of echo-free space in systole and diastole), moderate (greater than or equal to 10 mm at least posteriorly), large (greater than or equal to 20 mm), or very large (compression of the heart) (538). Furthermore, two-dimensional echocardiography can give information about the nature of the fluid, suggesting the presence of fibrin, clot, tumor, air, and calcium. Care must be taken to differentiate pericardial fluid from pleural fluid and ascites. Left pleural effusions can be difficult to differentiate from pericardial fluid. By transthoracic echocardiography in the parasternal long-axis view, pericardial fluid can be seen to reflect at the posterior atrioventricular groove, while pleural fluid continues under the left atrium, posterior to the descending aorta. Spin-echo and cine MRI can also be used to assess the size and extent of simple and complex pericardial effusions similar to echocardiography (161). The effusions by MRI may tend to be larger than by echocardiography (539).

Management. The action taken after finding a significant pericardial fluid collection depends on the underlying etiology, the presence of hemodynamic compromise, and the volume of fluid. Pericardiocentesis may not be necessary in all cases, particularly when the diagnosis can be made based on other systemic features. Where doubt remains, particularly in cases in which malignancy or purulent pericarditis is suspected, pericardiocentesis is indicated. Hemodynamic compromise is an absolute indication for drainage (see following discussion).

Pericardial Tamponade

Fluid accumulation in the finite pericardial space causes an increase in pressure with subsequent cardiac compression. Tamponade is not a binary phenomenon, with a spectrum

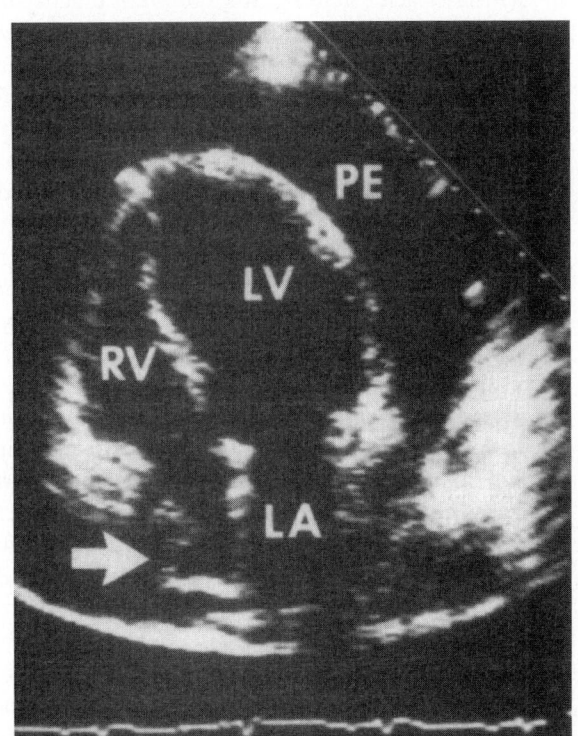
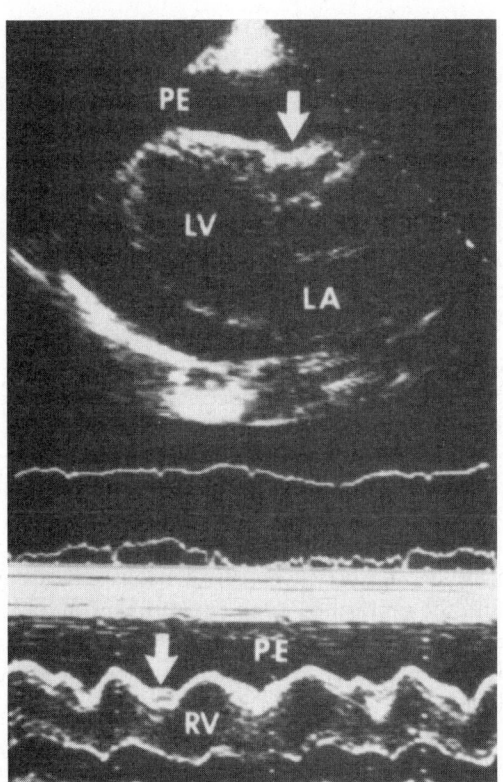

FIGURE 26.7   **A:** Apical four-chamber view of a large pericardial effusion (PE) with right atrial collapse (*arrow*). **B:** Parasternal long-axis view of a large PE with right ventricular (RV) collapse (*arrows*). LA, left atrium; LV, left ventricle. (From Schutzman JJ, Obarski TP, Pearce GL, et al. Comparison of Doppler and two-dimensional echocardiography for assessment of pericardial effusion. *Am J Cardiol* 1992;70:1353–1357, with permission.)

existing from mild cardiac compression and embarrassment to cardiovascular collapse.

Clinical Presentation. The spectrum of presentation of patients with cardiac tamponade ranges from dyspnea and edema to frank circulatory collapse. The classic triad of cardiac tamponade was described by Beck including hypotension, elevated jugular venous pressure, and distant heart sounds (547). Early tamponade is manifest by tachycardia, tachypnea and dyspnea, edema and elevated venous pressure, and quiet cardiomegaly. Examination of the central venous waveform shows a prominent 'x' descent and absence of the 'y' descent.

Pulsus paradoxus is examined using the stethoscope over the brachial pulse and measuring the pressure gap between the appearance of the Korotkoff's sounds during expiration only and their continuous presence. It is defined by a fall in systolic blood pressure of 10 mm Hg with inspiration, an exaggeration of the normal situation. False-positive pulsus paradoxus without cardiac tamponade may occur with obstructive lung disease, RV infarction, and pulmonary embolism, and a false-negative finding may occur with high LV pressures as with LV dysfunction or hypertrophy, severe hypotension, severe aortic regurgitation, or in the case of an atrial septal defect (548). ▼ f76

Investigations. Electrocardiography and chest radiography do not differentiate tamponade from noncompressive pericardial effusion. Large pericardial effusions allow "swinging" of the heart on its vascular pedicle, causing in some cases electrical alternans.

Echocardiography is a fast and noninvasive modality to accurately diagnose tamponade (519) (*e*Fig. 26.7.2, Table 26.6). The presence of pericardial fluid should be documented and its location defined. The classic signs of cardiac tamponade are RA and RV collapse (109,551,552). Postsurgical effusions may be loculated (e.g., behind the left atrium) and sometimes difficult to visualize from the transthoracic window. Indeed, if the diagnosis of tamponade is suspected in this scenario, transesophageal echocardiography is indicated (4). Two-dimensional echocardiography can also exclude pericardial masses and ventricular and valvular dysfunction as the cause of hemodynamic compromise. Doppler echocardiography allows direct quantitation of mitral and tricuspid inflows, pulmonary venous and systemic venous flows; and with the use of a nasal thermistor, variation with respiration can be assessed (553). ▼ f77

Pericardiocentesis. While preparing the equipment for pericardiocentesis, the patient in tamponade may be supported with cautious fluid loading and inotropes (such as

TABLE 26.6 ECHOCARDIOGRAPHIC FINDINGS IN PATIENTS WITH CARDIAC TAMPONADE

Abnormal inspiratory increase of right ventricular dimension with abnormal inspiratory decrease of left ventricular dimension
Inspiratory decrease of mitral valve DE excursion (M-mode) (anterior leaflet opening) and ejection fraction slope (initial anterior leaflet closing)
Right atrial collapse
Right ventricular early diastolic collapse
Left atrial collapse
"Flow paradoxus" with abnormal inspiratory increase of tricuspid valve flow and abnormal inspiratory decrease of mitral valve flow
Inferior vena cava plethora (failure to decrease proximal diameter by 50% or more on sniff or deep inspiration)

Modified from Fowler NO. Pericardial disease. *Heart Dis Stroke* 1992;1:85–94, with permission.

norepinephrine or isoproterenol). Percutaneous pericardiocentesis should be performed in an environment in which advanced cardiac life support equipment and personnel are immediately available. Historically, these procedures have been performed in the cardiac catheterization laboratory, with arterial and right-sided heart catheters in situ. More recently, the procedure has tended to be performed in the procedure room of the cardiac or intensive care unit, or even at the bedside, using echocardiographic guidance (555–557). Surgical drainage of the pericardium (either by a subxyphoid approach or using a complete pericardectomy) is indicated for loculated effusions, patients at risk of excessive bleeding, and in situations in which fluid has recurred after previous drainage procedures (558).

Echocardiography can demonstrate the most accessible window for passage of the needle (555,556,559). Historically, the subxyphoid approach has been used most commonly, with a long needle passed under the xiphoid and directed toward the left shoulder at a 30-degree angle to the skin. Echocardiography performed at the cardiac apex can often identify a window where the pericardium can be entered (usually in the sixth or seventh rib space in the anterior axillary line) without risk of cardiac puncture. A short needle is passed through the rib space under constant negative pressure until fluid is aspirated. It is important to confirm that the fluid aspirated is intrapericardial (i.e., the blood should not clot).

By either approach, once the pericardial space is reached a soft-tipped guidewire is passed and the needle removed. A multiholed catheter is then introduced and the pericardial fluid suctioned out. It is prudent to drain the fluid in steps of less than 1 L at a time to allow cardiovascular equilibrium to be restored at each stage and to avoid the rare complication of acute RV dilatation (560,561). Clinical improvement usually occurs after the aspiration of only 100 to 200 mL of fluid. The fluid should be drained completely, and specimens sent for chemistry, cytology, culture, and

acid-fast bacilli staining. It is common practice to leave the catheter in for some hours, connected to a free drainage bag, to allow further drainage as the patient assumes different postures. It is important to avoid allowing air into the pericardium because this is most uncomfortable for the patient.

Percutaneous pericardiocentesis is a rapid and safe procedure when performed by trained personnel (559). In a study of patients undergoing urgent pericardiocentesis following cardiac perforation, tamponade was relieved in 99% of patients. A major complication rate of 3% occurred and included pneumothorax and RV laceration. No deaths resulted directly from pericardiocentesis (562). A similar review of 245 pericardiocenteses performed in patients with postoperative effusions showed that anticoagulant therapy was the most common contributing factor to early pericardial effusions (less than 7 days), and postpericardiotomy syndrome contributed most often to late effusions (563). The rate of major complications from pericardiocentesis was 2% in this study.

Surgical Procedures. A median sternotomy or anterolateral thoracotomy approach provides good visualization for pericardial surgery including pericardiectomy for constrictive and effusive disease (564). However, less invasive procedures are available for drainage of pericardial effusions when pericardiocentesis is not feasible or recurrent fluid accumulates.

Subxyphoid pericardiectomy is a safe and efficacious method of draining large pericardial effusions. A small vertical incision is made in the upper epigastrium and the pericardium approached by posterior retraction of the diaphragm from the sternum. A pleuropericardial window is often created to allow ongoing drainage (565).

Alternative nonthoracotomy techniques for formation of a pericardial window include percutaneous pericardiotomy using an inflatable balloon from a subxyphoid approach (566–573) and a video-assisted thoracic surgical pericardiectomy. These procedures are effective for the management of malignant and other large pericardial effusions.

Constrictive Pericarditis

Dense fibrosis and adhesion of the parietal and visceral layers of the pericardium create a rigid "case" around the heart, limiting its filling and causing profound disturbances of cardiac function (eFig. 26.7.3). This final common pathway may be the end result of one (or more) of many etiologic agents including infections, postcardiac surgery, or radiation. The constrictive process can follow the etiology acutely, subacutely (months), or chronically (years) (538). The clinical presentation is well recognizable, with debilitating right-sided heart failure and a poor prognosis. Voluminous literature exists about the many methods of differentiating this constellation from that of restrictive cardiomyopathy, which presents with similar clinical signs and symptoms (Table 26.3).

Pathophysiology. The fundamental abnormality in constrictive pericarditis is limited filling and enhanced interventricular dependence of the heart because of the rigid encasement of the heart by thickened pericardium, effectively isolating it from the normal respiratory swings in pressure and allowing a finite filling volume for the ventricles (13). Within the pericardium, the myocardium is intrinsically normal (unless there is a combined abnormality such as in radiation myocarditis), with no specific abnormality of systolic or diastolic function. In constriction, the ventricle fills abruptly on valve opening (often more abruptly than normal due to elevated atrial filling pressures). However, in mid-diastole, the chambers reach the maximum volume that the constraining pericardium will allow, and filling abruptly ceases. This can be appreciated visually on two-dimensional echocardiography as wall motion ceases with a shudder in mid-diastole. In contrast, restrictive myocardial diseases involve abnormal ventricular filling from the onset of diastole, as the chamber relaxes slowly and stiffness increases with a compensatory increase in left atrial pressure (272).

However, it is the effect of respiration on cardiac flows that is the major hallmark for differentiating constrictive from restrictive cardiac diseases. As the heart is effectively isolated from the thorax by its rigid encasement, it does not experience marked respiratory swings in pressure. Thus, on inspiration, intrathoracic (and therefore pulmonary vein) pressure decreases, but left atrial pressure does not. Thus,

the pulmonary vein to left atrial pressure gradient that drives left atrial inflow diminishes, as does mitral inflow. The resultant decreased LV filling during diastole allows more room for RV filling because of a septal shift and enhanced ventricular interdependence and thus right-sided inflows increase. The exact opposite sequence occurs in expiration (4,13,101,102,166).

Filling pressures rise to compensate for the decrease in cardiac output via renal retention of salt and water. The finite space of the pericardium causes the filling pressure of the four chambers (and the pulmonary wedge pressure) to equalize. Intraventricular pressure recordings demonstrate the classical dip and plateau or square-root sign morphologies. The dip represents the abrupt early filling at atrioventricular valve opening related to high filling pressures and corresponds to a deep 'y' descent on the central venous tracing. The plateau phase represents a period of unchanging pressure and volume related to the finite volume of the pericardial encasement. The 'x' descent on the venous trace may also be prominent, as systolic emptying of the ventricles allows filling of the atria. The 'x' and 'y' descents are sometimes referred to as the *W pattern* (574) (Fig. 26.8).

Differentiating Restriction from Constrictive Pericarditis.

Hemodynamics. Cardiac catheterization has been traditionally the gold standard in distinguishing between these two similar diseases; however, there can be overlap of the hemodynamics (13). These hemodynamic findings have been shown in Table 26.3. Simultaneous recordings of the right and left heart pressures have revealed elevation and equal-

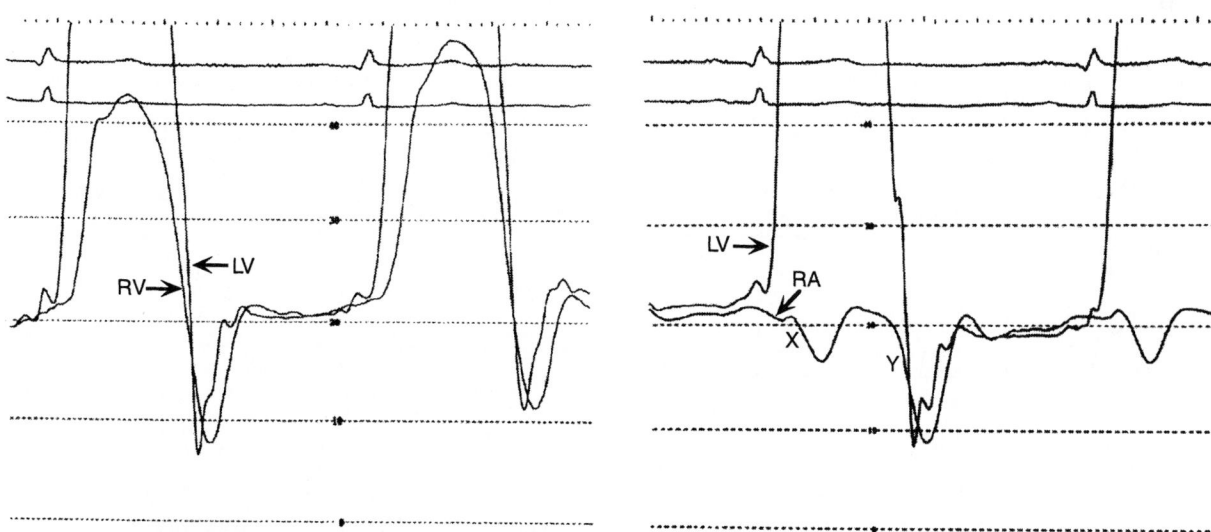

FIGURE 26.8 A,B: Simultaneous right ventricular (RV) and left ventricular (LV) pressure recordings demonstrating equalization of diastolic pressures and dip and plateau physiology. Simultaneous right atrial (RA) and LV pressure recordings demonstrating equalization during diastole and prominent 'x' and 'y' descents in the RA tracing. (From Vaitkus PT, Cooper KA, Shuman WP, et al. Images in cardiovascular medicine. Constrictive pericarditis. *Circulation* 1996;93:834–835, with permission.)

ization of pressures (within 5 mm Hg) of the RA, right ventricle diastolic, PCWP, and pre–'a' wave LV diastolic pressure. The RA pressure contour typically shows an M or W configuration with a preserved systolic 'x' descent and a prominent 'y' descent with small 'a' and 'v' waves. The RV and LV pressure tracings show a dip and plateau contour. The RV and pulmonary artery systolic pressures are mildly elevated, with a pressure of less than 50 mm Hg compared with a pressure greater than 50 mm Hg in restriction. Administration of saline over 6 to 8 minutes can enhance the classic findings of constriction in a patient with occult constriction (542). The respiratory changes in cardiac flows have been shown to be useful in the hemodynamic diagnosis of pericardial constriction. One study demonstrated that, although conventional hemodynamic variables failed to accurately diagnose constriction, differences between left and RV pressures on inspiration, a marker of ventricular interdependence, were highly specific and sensitive for the syndrome (301).

Echocardiography. There have been many M-mode and two-dimensional signs that have been used to differentiate these two conditions; however, these signs have proven to be nonspecific and insensitive (575–578). The important two-dimensional echocardiographic features of constriction that may provide clues to the diagnosis include pericardial thickening, myocardial tethering, a septal bounce with respiration, and inferior vena cava plethora (272,579).

Doppler Echocardiography. As described earlier, Doppler echocardiography with respirometry has emerged as a useful tool in these conditions (13,101,580). Limited ventricular filling and enhanced ventricular interaction account

for the Doppler findings in constrictive pericarditis, whereas decreased distensibility of the ventricles accounts for the Doppler findings in restriction (13).

The classic Doppler echocardiographic findings are shown in Figures 26.9 and 26.10. The similarities with restriction by Doppler echocardiography include a short deceleration time indicative of the dip and plateau hemodynamic pattern and limited filling. The main differences include enhanced respiratory variation in mitral inflow and pulmonary venous flow (greater than or equal to 25% at the onset of inspiration and expiration) in constriction, but not with restriction (unless a concomitant pericardial effusion accounting for respiratory variation is present). In restriction, there is a markedly blunted pulmonary venous systolic flow with greater diastolic forward flow indicative of a prominent 'y' descent and elevated left atrial pressures, whereas in constriction, there are usually both systolic and diastolic flows present (4) (Fig. 26.11). Because of enhanced ventricular interdependence, there is a decreased transtricuspid flow in expiration and enhanced expiratory flow reversals in the hepatic vein with constriction, while there are increased inspiratory flow reversals in restriction. Respiratory variation in the tricuspid regurgitation peak velocity and velocity duration has been noted in constriction but not in restriction (581). Superior vena cava Doppler can help distinguish respiratory variation of mitral inflow in patients with chronic obstructive lung disease and constrictive pericarditis (582). The systolic forward component of superior vena cava flow varies significantly with chronic obstructive lung disease, whereas there is little change with constrictive pericarditis. The newer modalities of color M-mode Doppler and TDE have provided comple-

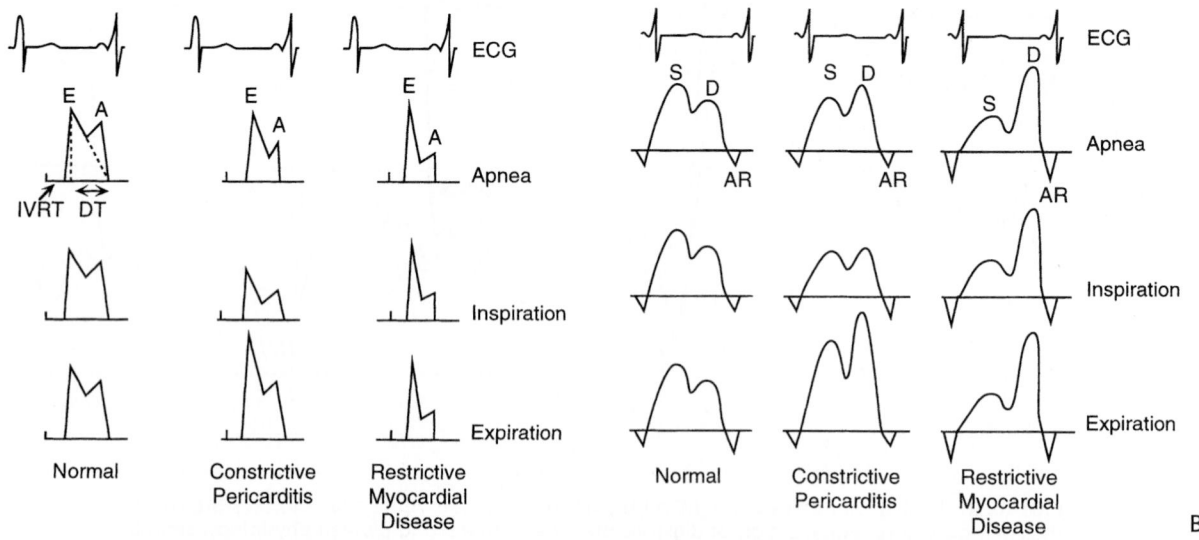

FIGURE 26.9 A,B: Left ventricular inflow velocities and pulmonary venous flow during different phases of respiration. (From Klein AL, Cohen GI. Doppler echocardiographic assessment of constrictive pericarditis, cardiac amyloidosis, and cardiac tamponade. *Cleve Clin J Med* 1992;59:278–290, with permission.)

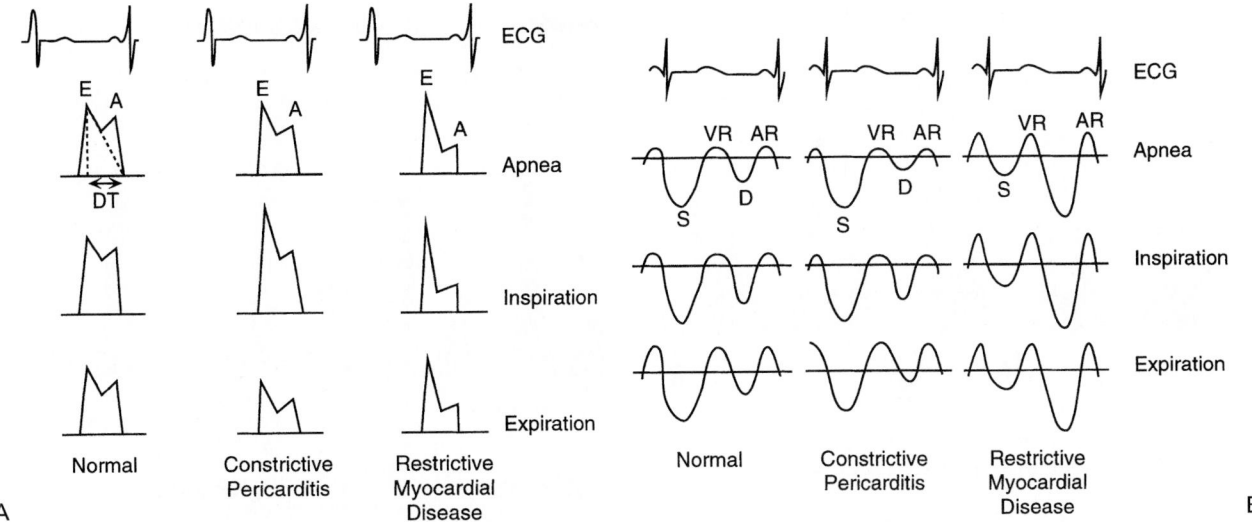

FIGURE 26.10 A,B: Right ventricular inflow velocities and hepatic venous flow during different phases of respiration. (From Klein AL, Cohen GI. Doppler echocardiographic assessment of constrictive pericarditis, cardiac amyloidosis, and cardiac tamponade. *Cleve Clin J Med* 1992;59:278–290, with permission.)

mentary information in the evaluation of patients with constrictive pericarditis (see the section Phases of Diastole) (121,123,206,583,583a) (*e*Fig. 26.11.1). Recently, in patients with constrictive pericarditis, the mitral inflow E/Em was shown to be inversely correlated with PCWP (annulus paradoxus).

There are several pitfalls in using Doppler echocardiography with respiratory monitoring in distinguishing constriction from restriction (*e*Table 26.6.1). Factors including depth of respiration, position of the sample volume, level of left atrial pressure, presence of concomitant myocardial disease, and atrial fibrillation may influence the accuracy of the diagnosis. Transesophageal echocardiography may be used to delineate the anatomy (pericardial thickening) as well as describe the physiology better than transthoracic echocardiography (101). In a large series of 192 patients undergoing transesophageal echocardiographic evaluation of complex diastolic function, 39% of patients had evidence of restrictive physiology, 30% had constriction, and 12% had mixed constriction and restriction, whereas the remainder had abnormal relaxation, pseudonormalization, or large pericardial effusion or tamponade (119). Preload reduction maneuvers may be useful in lowering the left atrial pressure to enhance the respiratory variation, whereas volume loading may be used if the filling pressures are decreased (584,585) (*e*Fig. 26.11.2). Mixed restriction and constriction may occur postirradiation and may have features of localized pericardial thickening with restrictive physiology (119). Also, atrial fibrillation may make it difficult to perform a Doppler evaluation of constriction and restriction; however, a series of 31 patients with constrictive pericarditis showed a similar respiratory variation of pulmonary venous flow and mitral inflow in patients with atrial fibrillation compared with normal sinus rhythm (586). Occasionally, ventricular pacing can be used to regularize the RR intervals in patients with atrial fibrillation. Constrictive pericarditis can also be evaluated in the operating room during mechanical ventilation. In a series of 15 patients, it was noted that positive pressure ventilation reverses the pattern of respiratory variation of the mitral inflow and pulmonary venous flow velocities (587).

Clinical Presentation. Patients with significant pericardial constriction present with congestive heart failure. Gross dependent edema, effusions and ascites (596), hepatic congestion with dysfunction, splenomegaly, poor exercise tolerance, and cachexia constitute anasarca, of which constriction is one of the few remaining causes in developed nations. Jugular venous distention is common with a prominent 'y' descent (Friedreich's sign) (597), and the classical Kussmaul's sign, a rise in central venous pressure with inspiration due to the inability of the right atrium to receive volume, is seen in some cases. The syndrome is relentless and progressive, responding poorly to conservative medical therapy.

Pulsus paradoxus is seen in one-third of cases. Auscultation of the chest reveals quiet heart sounds, often with a pericardial knock, which correlates with the abrupt cessation of early diastolic filling (E wave), when the ventricles reach their finite volume limit.

Electrocardiography demonstrates low voltages with nonspecific T-wave changes. Atrial fibrillation is seen in a minority of patients. Chest roentgenography may demonstrate "eggshell" calcification of the pericardium, particularly in tuberculous pericarditis, and pleural effusions (598).

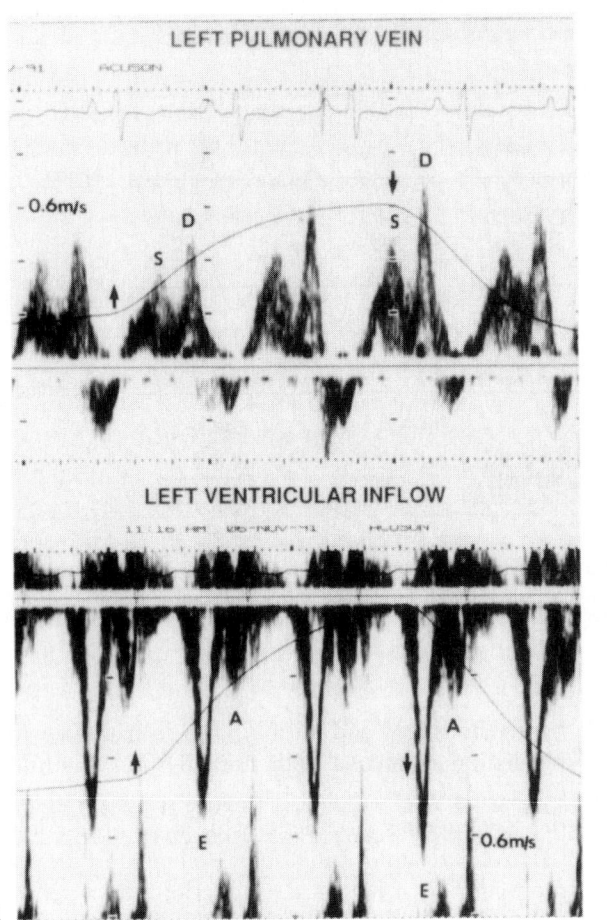

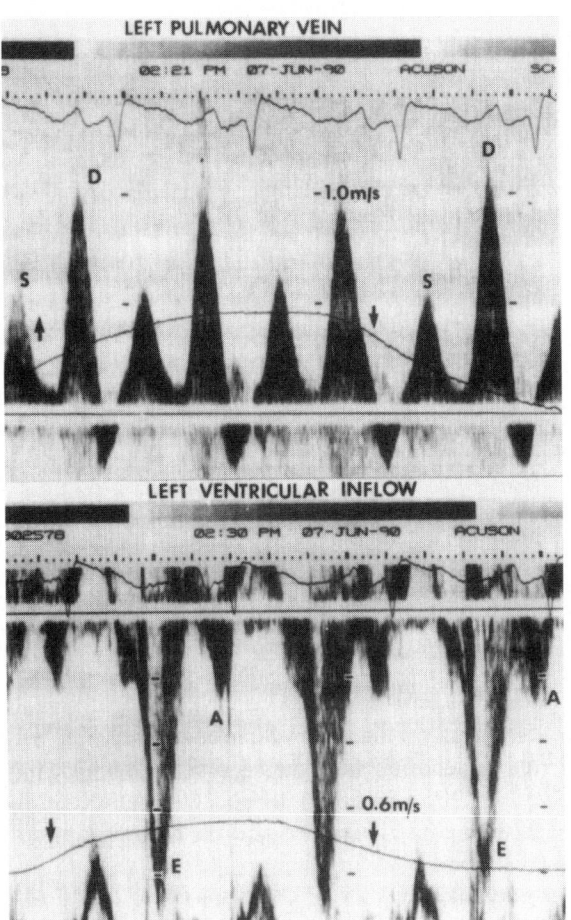

FIGURE 26.11 A: Constrictive pericarditis. Doppler transesophageal echocardiogram of the left upper pulmonary venous flow (*top*) and left ventricular inflow (*bottom*) in a 30-year-old man with constrictive pericarditis with respiratory monitoring with inspiration (*up arrow*) and expiration (*down arrow*). **B:** Restrictive cardiomyopathy. Doppler transesophageal echocardiogram of the left upper pulmonary venous flow (*top*) and left ventricular inflow (*bottom*) in a 64-year-old man with restrictive cardiomyopathy secondary to advanced cardiac amyloidosis during inspiration (*up arrow*) and expiration (*down arrow*). A, late filling velocity, D, peak diastolic; E, early filling; S, peak systolic. (From Klein AL, Cohen GI, Pietrolungo JF, et al. Differentiation of constrictive pericarditis from restrictive cardiomyopathy by Doppler transesophageal echocardiographic measurements of respiratory variations in pulmonary venous flow. *J Am Coll Cardiol* 1993;22:1935–1943, with permission.)

There may be variation in the presentation of constriction. These variants include localized constriction (localized scarring) (599), effusive constriction (after the pericardial fluid is drained), elastic constriction (thick pericardial fluid), latent or occult constriction (volume depleted), and transient constriction (600).

Treatment. Conservative medical management of constrictive pericarditis is at best palliative, with no substantial effect on the natural history of the disease. Diuretics decrease the intensity of fluid overload symptoms and atrioventricular blocking agents and antiarrhythmics are useful for the management of atrial fibrillation. Surgical pericardiectomy remains the only definitive management of this problem and should be

performed before calcification and myocardial involvement progress (102,601–603). ▼ f78

Specific Causes of Pericardial Disease

Idiopathic and Viral Pericarditis

The majority of cases of acute pericarditis has no specific cause detected and is designated idiopathic. Many of these cases represent acute viral pericarditis. Attacks of this syndrome follow the seasonal epidemics of enterovirus infection (coxsackie B and echovirus) (605). Proven viral cases are more likely to occur in immunocompromised hosts. Cytomegalovirus pericarditis has increased in frequency in association with immunocompromised hosts and early human immunodeficiency virus infection

(606–608). *e*Table 26.6.2 shows the most etiologies of infectious pericarditis.

Clinical Presentation. Idiopathic and viral pericarditis in the immunocompetent host is typically a self-limited illness, beginning with a nonspecific flu-like illness. There is often a history of a prodromal upper respiratory tract infection. There may be associated arthralgias and myalgias. Patients present with a syndrome of chest pain as described previously. The pain is often severe, distressing, and associated with sympathetic activation such as clamminess, pallor, and tremor. There is often an associated low-grade fever. Significant dyspnea is uncommon in simple cases, unless there is hemodynamic compromise by a large pericardial effusion or associated viral pneumonitis (609).

The specific diagnosis of viral pericarditis should be entertained in all cases, after other etiologic agents have been considered. However, the identification of the viral agent from serologic markers or from pericardial fluid occurs infrequently in clinical practice. A fourfold rise in serum antibody levels is highly suggestive of an underlying viral cause. Associated myocarditis is often associated with modest elevation of cardiac isoenzymes (529,605,610).

Pericardial collections in viral and idiopathic pericarditis are usually relatively small, being diagnosed and sized simply by transthoracic echocardiography. Having detected an effusion, it is important to exclude significant hemodynamic compromise or tamponade. Because of the relatively acute time frame of the fluid accumulation, tamponade may be present with only modest volumes of pericardial fluid. Pericardiocentesis is not usually indicated unless there is hemodynamic compromise, which occurs in up to 15% of cases of acute viral pericarditis (531). In a series of 57 patients, pericardial biopsy and fluid sampling identified cytomegalovirus in only four cases (607).

Uncomplicated acute pericarditis is a self-limited benign illness, with few sequelae and a course ranging from days to a few weeks. Complications are infrequent and include relapsing attacks of acute pericarditis (see following discussion), acute tamponade, acute myocarditis with ventricular dysfunction and late cardiomyopathy, and chronic constrictive pericarditis (609).

Management. Specific antiviral therapy is not indicated for viral idiopathic pericarditis in the immunocompetent host. Treatment is directed toward symptom relief. The mainstay of therapy has always centered on the oral antiinflammatory drugs, particularly aspirin (325 to 650 mg every 4 to 6 hours) or most often nonsteroidal antiinflammatory agents including ibuprofen (600 to 800 mg every 6 to 8 hours) (611). Indomethacin (25 to 50 mg four times per day) should be reserved in adults due to deleterious effects on coronary blood flow and myocardial infarcts. Thus, other nonsteroidal agents are commonly used. No specific studies have used the COX-2 inhibitor agents. Colchicine (0.6 mg

every 12 hours), with or without a load of 2 to 3 mg, may be used when added to the antiinflammatory agent or by itself in treating the initial attack or preventing recurrences (612–614). There is no role for antibiotics, unless purulent pericarditis has been documented. Systemic corticosteroid therapy with prednisone has been used in severe and intractable cases (609,615). Some patients may have recurrent or incessant pericarditis that may be related to an immunopathic etiology (616). Frequently, these patients may be corticosteroid dependent. Colchicine may be an effective drug to attempt to wean patients off corticosteroids (617).

Purulent Pericarditis

Management. A provisional diagnosis of purulent pericarditis is an indication for a drainage procedure, either percutaneous or preferably surgical. Complete clearance and lavage of the pericardial space should be attempted (636,639). Urgent bacterial, acid-fast, and fungal staining of the fluid, followed by complete culture is mandatory. Broad-spectrum antibiotic therapy should be narrowed on identification of the specific etiologic agent. Pericardectomy may be indicated in cases with significant pericardial adhesions to avoid late constriction.

Pericarditis Associated with Myocardial Infarction

Differentiation of pericardial chest pain from that of acute myocardial ischemia is important for the clinician. Pericarditis as an associate of acute myocardial infarction occurs in up to 30% of cases at autopsy (678,679), significantly complicating the situation. In life, pericarditis is observed clinically in 7% to 10% of acute infarcts (680,681). An incorrect diagnosis of primary pericarditis has important implications in this setting as it will most likely preclude the patient from receiving timely revascularization therapy. Conversely, an incorrect diagnosis of myocardial ischemia in the setting of simple acute pericarditis may lead to the patient suffering the consequences of thrombolytic or anticoagulant therapy. In 16 such cases reported in the decade ending in 1995, there has been one death (in a young man), one hemorrhagic tamponade, and two nonhemorrhagic effusions managed conservatively (682–687). Two forms of pericardial involvement have been observed in association with myocardial infarction.

Early Acute Pericarditis

Clinical Presentation. The clinical presentation of pericardial-type pain often occurs after the abatement of ischemic pain. This syndrome should be considered during each physical examination of the postinfarct patient. The presence of a pericardial rub is diagnostic, occurring more commonly than the pericardial pain. It is important to differentiate this sound from intracardiac murmurs, which may represent mechanical complications of infarction such as acute mitral regurgitation and ventricular rupture. The typical electrocardiographic changes of pericarditis are seen in a small minority of cases of postinfarct pericarditis (680). In a large retrospective series of autopsy-proven postinfarct regional pericarditis, a pattern of atypical T-wave evolution was observed: specifically at 48 hours, persistent upright T waves *or* normalization of transiently inverted T waves (690).

The clinical course of early postinfarct pericarditis is usually benign. However, pericarditis seems to be associated with larger transmural infarcts and therefore more complications. Despite this, poorer prognosis is not predicted by the presence of periinfarct pericarditis or effusions (688,689,691–693). In the Gruppo Italiano per lo Studio della Sopravvivenza nell'Infarto Miocardico (GISSI) trials of thrombolytic therapy for myocardial infarction, pericardial involvement was associated with a higher long-term mortality, but was not an independent risk factor when infarct size was considered (694). Further evidence that pericarditis is a by-product of more severe myocardial damage and not an independent prognostic factor is provided by the data from analysis of incidence of pericardial involvement in patients treated with thrombolytic therapy compared with those who did not receive this treatment. In the GISSI trials, the incidence of periinfarct pericarditis was halved by the use of thrombolytic therapy, and this effect was more pronounced with earlier institution of treatment (694,695).

Management. Management is symptomatic, with aspirin or nonsteroidal antiinflammatory drugs. Caution is recommended with the latter as there have been anecdotal reports of pronounced thinning and even rupture of infarct sites when these drugs have been used (696). For similar reasons, corticosteroid therapy (697) is not recommended.

Dressler's Syndrome. The second pericardial associate of myocardial infarction is the late-appearing Dressler's syndrome (698). Dressler suggested an incidence of 4% of infarct patients, but more recent studies have shown rates of 1% or less (699,700). Indeed, in patients treated with thrombolytics, this syndrome has been observed at rates of less than 0.5% (701).

Clinical Presentation. Dressler's syndrome of chest pain, pleurisy, pericarditis with friction rub, severe malaise, moderate fever, and leukocytosis occurs at 3 weeks to several months postinfarct (681). Pericardial collections of fluid are not uncommon and can be hemodynamically compromising.

Management. Consideration should be given to hospital admission, as these patients are often severely debilitated. Furthermore, recurrent ischemia, significant pericardial effusion, bacterial superinfection, and hemorrhagic complications need to be examined for and excluded. Anticoagulant therapy should be temporarily discontinued. Symptoms are relieved usually with aspirin or nonsteroidal antiinflamma-

tory drugs (see the section Acute Pericarditis for doses). Because of the recurrent nature of the syndrome and the possible immunologic nature of the insult, some authors recommend corticosteroid therapy (prednisone, 40 to 60 mg daily, tapering over a week) (702). Pericardiocentesis is indicated only for hemodynamic compromise or tamponade.

CONTROVERSIES AND PERSONAL PERSPECTIVES

Definition, Prevalence, and Utility of Diastolic Function

In 2001, the exact definition and prevalence of diastolic heart failure are controversial, as well as the appreciation of its importance in clinical practice. A good working definition of diastolic dysfunction has been proposed by the European Working Group (30), but modification of this definition has been proposed by other investigators and will likely continue to evolve (31,32,250).

The exact prevalence of diastolic function is still debatable (31,250,777). The prevalence of diastolic function has varied widely from 13% to 74% (250). The reasons for this heterogeneity include variability in the criteria, duration and chronicity of congestive heart failure, the effect of age, the presence of coronary artery disease, selection bias in obtaining the patients, the type of imaging modality, the variables for assessing systolic performance, and the timing of the study (250). Despite this variability, it is the authors' opinion that in a tertiary referral practice, elderly patients with hypertension and coronary disease commonly have diastolic heart failure, in keeping with the estimated 40% prevalence. A large population-based study (Cardiovascular Health Study) in older patients (66 to 103 years) found a prevalence of 55% of patients with heart failure and normal systolic function, and a total of 80% with normal or mildly reduced systolic function, especially in women (778).

Furthermore, the prognosis of patients with diastolic dysfunction is uncertain. The annual mortality was reported to vary from 1.3% to 17.5% (250). A worse prognosis is associated with older patients, men, coronary artery disease, and valvular heart disease (250). Relatively recent work in elderly patients (50% greater than 80 years age) with heart failure from Olmstead County showed similar poor prognosis in patients with normal (greater than or equal to 50%) or reduced systolic function. Despite the variability of these studies, the mortality of patients with diastolic dysfunction is generally lower than in patients with systolic dysfunction, with an annual mortality of 15% to 20% (24). It is the authors' opinion that it is important to recognize an episode of diastolic heart failure so that early detection of underlying causes and treatments can be initiated.

The newer noninvasive tools to diagnose diastolic function including TDE and color M-mode Doppler are less

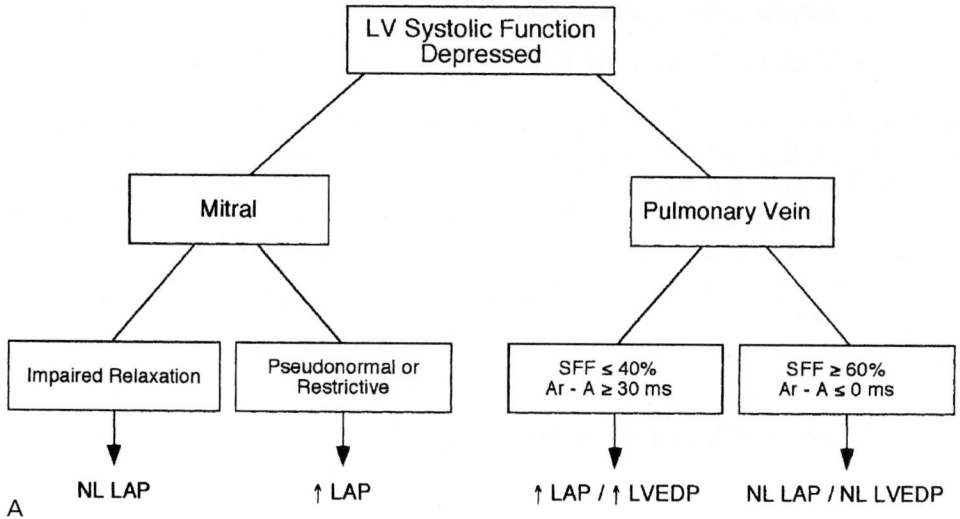

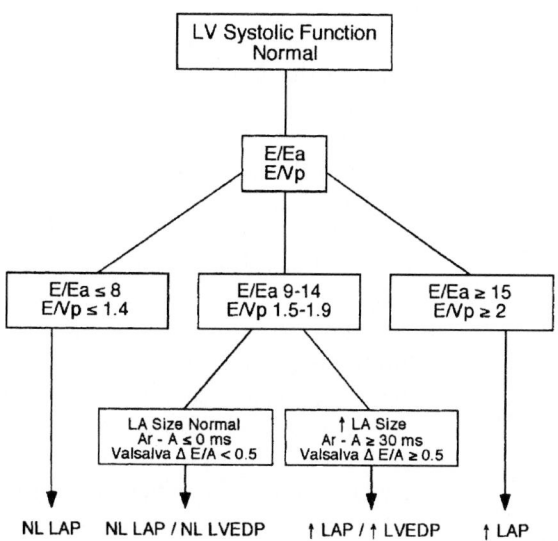

FIGURE 26.12 A: An algorithm for assessment of left atrial pressure and left ventricular end diastolic pressure (LVEDP) in patients with depressed LV systolic function. Ar-A, difference in duration of the atrial reversal wave (pulmonary vein) and of the atrial wave of mitral inflow; NL LAP, normal left atrial pressure; SFF, systolic filling fraction; ↑ LAP, increased left atrial pressure. **B:** Algorithm for estimation of LAP and LVEDP in individuals with normal LV systolic function using the new indices of diastolic function, mitral inflow E velocity (E), pulmonary vein velocity and left atrial size. Ea, early diastolic velocity at the mitral annulus; Vp, flow propagation velocity. (Adapted from Nagueh SF, Zoghbi WA. Clinical assessment of LV diastolic filling by Doppler echocardiography. *ACC Curr J Rev* 2001;10:45–49.)

load dependent than mitral inflow and pulmonary vein flow and have now been increasingly validated by hemodynamic standards. They may be useful especially in patients with isolated diastolic dysfunction, because they are more closely associated with myocardial relaxation. This will permit these techniques to be included into consensus and guideline papers in the measurement and reporting of diastolic dysfunction. The goal of determining diastolic function and estimating cardiac filling pressures in patients with depressed and normal systolic function by means of a comprehensive echocardiographic evaluation can be achieved for most patients (Fig. 26.12).

Treatment of Diastolic Function and the Need for Clinical Trials

The treatment of patients with diastolic heart failure is also controversial and limited to small studies (250). In fact, there have been no published clinical trials of patients with

diastolic heart failure; thus the treatment is highly empiric. It is not generally appreciated that Doppler echocardiography may be useful in guiding medical therapy depending on the filling pattern, LV dimensions, and etiology of diastolic function (15).

There are ongoing studies to evaluate the role of new therapies including angiotensin receptor blockers, beta-blockers, including carvedilol and nitric oxide donors in patients with diastolic heart failure (104). These studies will evaluate not just the hemodynamic, biochemical, and histologic effects on the myocardium, but also exercise capacity and prognosis (246,779). Recent studies have targeted the direct cellular mechanisms leading to diastolic dysfunction. Animal experiments have shown that diastolic function can be improved in senescent rat hearts through adenoviral gene transfer of sarcoplasmic reticulum Ca^{2+} ATPase protein (SERCA 2a) (780) and through the use of the advanced glycation end-product cross-link breaker (ALT-711) in older dogs (781).

THE FUTURE

There will be further recognition of the importance of diastolic function and the prevalence of diastolic heart failure, especially in the elderly. Future refinements in the noninvasive modalities will aid the consistent diagnosis of patients with diastolic dysfunction and elevated filling pressures, thus allowing for more uniform criteria for organization of large clinical trials. A diastolic stress test may be used as part of the assessment of patients with exertional dyspnea. There will be greater use of these newer modalities as part of the treatment algorithms for patients with diastolic dysfunction. There may be specific targeted therapies derived from the cellular, biochemical, neurohormonal, and physiologic mechanisms in these patients. There will be ongoing refinements in the differentiation of constrictive pericarditis and restriction. The genetic framework for all restrictive cardiomyopathies will aid in the assessment, prognosis, and treatment of these patients.

Controversies in Restrictive Cardiomyopathy and Constrictive Pericarditis

In 2001, the classification of restrictive cardiomyopathy still remains a controversial issue (see previous discussion) (269). The exact definition of restrictive cardiomyopathy has evolved over time and is not uniformly accepted by clinicians (255–259). Furthermore, there is still confusion about separating restrictive cardiomyopathy with diastolic heart failure from other cardiac diseases that manifest diastolic heart failure and restrictive hemodynamics (dip and plateau physiology) such as dilated cardiomyopathy with restrictive hemodynamics (263). The WHO/ISFC 1995 classification allays some of the confusion and preserves the old clinical entities of dilated, hypertrophic restrictive cardiomyopathies, and arrhythmogenic RV cardiomyopathy, but now considers the dominant pathophysiology or pathologic factors (254). Now, restrictive cardiomyopathy can be either idiopathic (which is rare) or more commonly be associated with an etiology (i.e., amyloidosis). Using this approach, restrictive cardiomyopathy is a disease within a large group of disorders which manifest diastolic heart failure.

There is also controversy about whether restrictive hemodynamics should be considered as a mandatory part of the disorder, as dictated by the 1995 WHO/ISFC classification (254). For example, as mentioned previously, cardiac amyloidosis may have an early (not restrictive) and advanced stage (restrictive) pattern (275). Similarly, hemochromatosis may present as a dilated cardiomyopathy in the majority of cases, and as a restrictive cardiomyopathy in others (439). It is the authors' opinion that a definite diagnosis of restrictive cardiomyopathy should show restrictive filling in a nondilated, nonhypertrophied ventricle with near-normal systolic function and dilated atria.

Differentiation of Restrictive Cardiomyopathy from Constrictive Pericarditis

Distinguishing restrictive cardiomyopathy from constriction is still an important clinical problem (119,166,269,272).

The importance of this distinction is that in restrictive cardiomyopathy, the disease is often treated medically and has a poor prognosis, whereas in constriction, the disease is treated with surgery and usually has a good prognosis (269). Furthermore, to highlight the importance of this differentiation, making the wrong diagnosis in sending a patient with restrictive cardiomyopathy for pericardial stripping is totally unacceptable and dangerous. Since the 1970s, there have been countless diagnostic tests that have been used to differentiate these two similar conditions (166,261). It is the authors' opinion that no single test is perfectly reliable in making the distinction, and good clinical judgment and a stepwise approach should be used (119). The history and physical examination often provide clues to the diagnosis but by no means are definitive. The history of a systemic disorder such as amyloidosis may favor restriction, whereas a history of idiopathic pericarditis or previous cardiac surgery may favor constriction. On the other hand, a history of radiation may show evidence of both constriction and restriction (119,269). It is also the authors' opinion that the noninvasive workup is most important in distinguishing restriction from constriction (15). In most patients, diastolic functional abnormalities can be adequately characterized using noninvasive modalities such as transthoracic echo, transesophageal echo with respirometry, and MRI (119). Furthermore, they have added new information regarding the actual structure and physiologic function of the myocardium and pericardium. MRI may be better suited to demonstrate the abnormal pericardial thickness, whereas echocardiography may show the physiologic abnormalities including interventricular dependence, limited filling, and dissociation between intrathoracic and intracardiac pressures. As with most tests, there may be some overlap (584); other noninvasive tools have also emerged such as color M-mode and tissue Doppler imaging to help distinguish these disorders (121). Finally, endomyocardial biopsy may be necessary for cases in which other modalities are inconclusive or ambiguous (295).

REFERENCES

1. Hirota Y. A clinical study of left ventricular relaxation. *Circulation* 1980;62:756–763.
2. Yellin EL, Nikolic S, Frater RW. Left ventricular filling dynamics and diastolic function. *Prog Cardiovasc Dis* 1990;32:247–271.
3. Thomas JD, Weyman AE. Echocardiographic Doppler evaluation of left ventricular diastolic function: physics and physiology *Circulation* 1991;84:977–990.
4. Klein AL, Cohen GI. Doppler echocardiographic assessment of constrictive pericarditis, cardiac amyloidosis, and cardiac tamponade. *Cleve Clin J Med* 1992;59:278–290.
5. Masui T, Finck S, Higgins CB. Constrictive pericarditis and restrictive cardiomyopathy: evaluation with MR imaging. *Radiology* 1992;182:369–373.
6. Wiggers CJ. *Physiology in health and disease*, 5th ed. Philadelphia: Lea & Febiger, 1949.
7. Gaasch WH, Quinones MA, Waisser E, et al. Diastolic compliance of the left ventricle in man. *Am J Cardiol* 1975;36:193–201.
8. Echeverria HH, Bilsker MS, Myerburg RJ, et al. Congestive heart failure: echocardiographic insights. *Am J Med* 1983;75:750–755.
9. Dougherty AH, Naccarelli GV, Gray EL, et al. Congestive heart failure with normal systolic function. *Am J Cardiol* 1984;54:778–782.
10. Soufer R, Wohlgelernter D, Vita NA, et al. Intact systolic left ventricular function in clinical congestive heart failure. *Am J Cardiol* 1985;55:1032–1036.
11. Nishimura RA, Housmans PR, Hatle LK, et al. Assessment of diastolic function of the heart: background and current applications of Doppler echocardiography. Part I. Physiologic and pathophysiologic features. *Mayo Clin Proc* 1989;64:71–81.
12. Nishimura RA, Abel MD, Hatle LK, et al. Assessment of diastolic function of the heart: background and current applications of Doppler echocardiography. Part II. Clinical studies. *Mayo Clin Proc* 1989;64:181–204.
13. Hatle LK, Appleton CP, Popp RL. Differentiation of constrictive pericarditis and restrictive cardiomyopathy by Doppler echocardiography. *Circulation* 1989;79:357–370.
14. Shah PM, Pai RG. Diastolic heart failure. *Curr Probl Cardiol* 1992;17:781–868.
15. Cohen GI, Pietrolungo JF, Thomas JD, et al. A practical guide to assessment of ventricular diastolic function using Doppler echocardiography. *J Am Coll Cardiol* 1996;27:1753–1760.
16. Garcia MJ, Thomas JD, Klein AL. New Doppler echocardiographic applications for the study of diastolic function. *J Am Coll Cardiol* 1998;32:865–875.
17. Garcia MJ, Ares MA, Asher C, et al. An index of early left ventricular filling that combined with pulsed Doppler peak E velocity may estimate capillary wedge pressure. *J Am Coll Cardiol* 1997;29:448–454.
18. Tei C, Nishimura RA, Seward JB, et al. Noninvasive Doppler-derived myocardial performance index: correlation with simultaneous measurements of cardiac catheterization measurements. *J Am Soc Echocardiogr* 1997;10:169–178.
19. Pai RG, Stoletniy LN. An integrated measure of left ventricular diastolic function based on relative rates of mitral E and A wave propagation. *J Am Soc Echocardiogr* 1999;12:811–816.
20. Palka P, Lange A, Fleming AD, et al. Differences in myocardial velocity gradient measured throughout the cardiac cycle in patients with hypertrophic cardiomyopathy, athletes and patients with left ventricular hypertrophy due to hypertension. *J Am Coll Cardiol* 1997;30:760–768.
21. Hatle LK, Sutherland GR. Regional myocardial function—a new approach. *Eur Heart J* 2000;21:1337–1357.
22. Cohn JN, Johnson G. Heart failure with normal ejection fraction: the V-HeFT study. Veterans Administration Cooperative Study Group. *Circulation* 1990;81[Suppl II]:III48–III53.
23. Brogan WC 3d, Hillis LD, Flores ED, et al. The natural history of isolated left ventricular diastolic dysfunction. *Am J Med* 1992;92:627–630.
24. Gaasch WH. Diagnosis and treatment of heart failure based on left ventricular systolic or diastolic dysfunction. *JAMA* 1994;271:1276–1280.
25. Little WC, Applegate RJ. Congestive heart failure: systolic and diastolic function. *J Cardiothorac Vasc Anesth* 1993;7[4 Suppl 2]:2–5.
26. Gaasch WH. Diastolic dysfunction of the left ventricle: importance to the clinician. *Adv Intern Med* 1990;35:311–340.
27. Little WC, Downes TR. Clinical evaluation of left ventricular diastolic performance. *Prog Cardiovasc Dis* 1990;32:273–290.
28. Brutsaert DL, Sys SU, Gillebert TC. Diastolic failure: pathophysiology and therapeutic implications. *J Am Coll Cardiol* 1993;22:318–325.
29. Thomas JD, Klein AL. Doppler-echocardiographic evaluation of diastolic function. In: Skorton DJ, Schelbert HR, Wolf GL, et al., eds. *Marcus cardiac imaging. A companion to Braunwald's Heart Disease.* Philadelphia: WB Saunders, 1996:336–365.
30. How to diagnose diastolic heart failure. European Study Group on Diastolic Heart Failure. *Eur Heart J* 1998;19:990–1003.
31. Vasan RS, Levy D. Defining diastolic heart failure: a call for standardized diagnostic criteria. *Circulation* 2000;101:2118–2121.
32. Grossman W. Defining diastolic dysfunction. *Circulation* 2000;101:2020–2021.
33. Wiggers CJ. Studies on the consecutive phases of the cardiac cycle. *Am J Physiol* 1921;56:415–459.
34. Brutsaert DL, Rademakers FE, Sys SU. Triple control of relaxation: implications in cardiac disease. *Circulation* 1984;69:190–196.
35. Brutsaert DL, Sys SU. Relaxation and diastole of the heart. *Physiol Rev* 1989;69:1228–1315.
36. Zile MR. Diastolic dysfunction: detection, consequences and treatment. Part 1: definition and determinants of diastolic function. *Mod Con Cardiovasc Dis* 1989;58:67–72.
37. Morgan JP, Erny RE, Allen PD, et al. Abnormal intracellular calcium handling, a major cause of systolic and diastolic dysfunction in ventricular myocardium from patients with heart failure. *Circulation* 1990;81[2 Suppl]:III21–III32.

38. Lorell BH, Apstein CS, Weinberg EO, et al. Diastolic function in left ventricular hypertrophy: clinical and experimental relationships. *Eur Heart J* 1990;11[Suppl G]:54–64.

39. Nikolic S, Yellin EL, Tamura K, et al. Passive properties of the canine left ventricle: diastolic stiffness and restoring forces. *Circ Res* 1988;62:1210–1222.

40. Flachskampf FA, Weyman AE, Guerrero JL, et al. Calculation of atrioventricular compliance from the mitral flow profile: analytic and in vitro study. *J Am Coll Cardiol* 1992;19:998–1004.

41. Keren G, Bier A, Sherez J, et al. Atrial contraction is an important determinant of pulmonary venous flow. *J Am Coll Cardiol* 1986;7:693–695.

42. Grimm RA, Leung DY, Black IW, et al. Left atrial appendage "stunning" after spontaneous conversion of atrial fibrillation demonstrated by transesophageal Doppler echocardiography. *Am Heart J* 1995;130:174–176.

43. Klein AL, Tajik AJ. Doppler assessment of pulmonary venous flow in healthy subjects and in patients with heart disease. *J Am Soc Echocardiogr* 1991;4:379–392.

44. Keren G, Meisner JS, Sherez J, et al. Interrelationship of mid-diastolic mitral valve motion, pulmonary venous flow, and transmitral flow. *Circulation* 1986;74:36–44.

45. Appleton CP, Carucci MJ, Henry CP, et al. Influence of incremental changes in heart rate on mitral flow velocity: assessment in lightly sedated, conscious dogs. *J Am Coll Cardiol* 1991;17:227–236.

46. Thomas JD, Flachskampf FA, Chen C, et al. Isovolumic relaxation time varies predictably with its time constant and aortic and left atrial pressures: implications for the noninvasive evaluation of ventricular relaxation. *Am Heart J* 1992;124:1305–1313.

47. Weiss JL, Frederikson JW, Weisfeldt ML. Hemodynamic determinants of the time-course of fall in canine left ventricular pressure. *J Clin Invest* 1976;58:751–760.

48. Raaf GL, Glantz S. Volume loading slows left ventricular isovolumic relaxation rate. Evidence of load-dependent relaxation in the intact dog heart. *Circ Res* 1981;48:813–824.

49. Lee CH, Vancheri F, Josen MS, et al. Discrepancies in the measurement of isovolumic relaxation time: a study comparing M-mode and Doppler echocardiography. *Br Heart J* 1990;64:214–218.

50. Lewis BS, Lewis N, Sapoznikov D, et al. Isovolumic relaxation period in man. *Am Heart J* 1980;100:490–499.

51. Klein AL, Oh JK, Miller FA, et al. Two-dimensional and Doppler echocardiographic assessment of infiltrative cardiomyopathy. *J Am Soc Echocardiogr* 1988;1:48–59.

52. Scalia GM, Greenberg NL, McCarthy PM, et al. Noninvasive assessment of the ventricular relaxation time constant (Tau) in humans by Doppler echocardiography. *Circulation* 1997;95:151–155.

53. Yamamoto K, Masuyama T, Doi Y, et al. Noninvasive assessment of left ventricular relaxation using continuous-wave Doppler aortic regurgitant velocity curve. Its comparative value to the mitral regurgitation method. *Circulation* 1995;91:192–200.

54. Brun P, Tribouilloy C, Duval AM, et al. Left ventricular flow propagation during early filling is related to wall relaxation: a color M-mode Doppler analysis. *J Am Coll Cardiol* 1992;20:420–432.

55. Ishida Y, Meisner JS, Tsujioka K, et al. Left ventricular filling dynamics: influence of left ventricular relaxation and left atrial pressure. *Circulation* 1986;74:187–196.

56. Choong CY, Abascal VM, Thomas JD, et al. Combined influence of ventricular loading and relaxation on the transmitral flow velocity profile in dogs measured by Doppler echocardiography. *Circulation* 1988;78:672–683.

57. Robinson TF, Factor SM, Sonnenblick EH. The heart as a suction pump. *Sci Am* 1986;254:84–91.

58. Suga H, Goto Y, Igarashi Y, et al. Ventricular suction under zero source pressure for filling. *Am J Physiol* 1986;251:H47–H55.

59. Yellin EL, Hori M, Yoran C, et al. Left ventricular relaxation in the filling and nonfilling intact canine heart. *Am J Physiol* 1986;250:H620–H629.

60. Thomas JD, Newell JB, Choong CYP, et al. Physical and physiological determinants of transmitral velocity: numerical analysis. *Am J Physiol* 1991;260(*Heart Circ Physiol* 29):H1718–H1730.

61. Pouleur H. Diastolic dysfunction and myocardial energetics. *Eur Heart J* 1990;11[Suppl C]:30–34.

62. Bonow RO, Udelson JE. Left ventricular diastolic dysfunction as a cause of congestive heart failure. Mechanisms and management. *Ann Intern Med* 1992;117:502–510.

63. Cunningham MJ, Apstein CS, Weinberg EO, et al. Deleterious effect of ouabain on myocardial function during hypoxia. *Am J Physiol* 1989;256:H681–H687.

64. Courtois M, Kovacs SJ Jr, Ludbrook PA. Transmitral pressure-flow velocity relation: importance of regional pressure gradients in the left ventricle during diastole. *Circulation* 1988;78:661–671.

65. Lorell BH, Grossman W. Cardiac hypertrophy: the consequences for diastole. *J Am Coll Cardiol* 1987;9:1189–1193.

66. Ling D, Rankin JS, Edwards CD, et al. Regional diastolic mechanics of the left ventricle in the conscious dog. *Am J Physiol* 1979;236:H323–H330.

67. Courtois M, Kovacs SJ Jr, Ludbrook PA. Physiological early diastolic intraventricular pressure gradient is lost during acute myocardial ischemia. *Circulation* 1990;81:1688–1696.

68. Janicki JS, Matsubara BB. Myocardial collagen and left ventricular diastolic dysfunction. In: Gaasch WH, LeWinter MM, eds. *Left ventricular diastolic dysfunction and heart failure*. Philadelphia: Lea & Febiger, 1994:125–140.

69. Matsubara B, Hennigar J, Janicki J. Structural and functional role of myocardial collagen. *Circulation* 1991;84:II-212.

70. Factor SM, Flomenbaum M, Zhao MJ, et al. The effects of acutely increased ventricular cavity pressure on intrinsic myocardial connective tissue. *J Am Coll Cardiol* 1988;12:1582–1589.

71. Lerman RH, Apstein CS, Kagan HM, et al. Myocardial healing and repair after experimental infarction in the rabbit. *Circ Res* 1983;53:378–388.

72. Gilbert JC, Glantz SA. Determinants of left ventricular filling and of the diastolic pressure-volume relation. *Circ Res* 1989;64:827–852.

73. Cheng CP, Igarashi Y, Little WC. Mechanism of augmented rate of left ventricular filling during exercise. *Circ Res* 1992;70:9–19.

74. Tyberg JV, Misbach GA, Glantz SA, et al. A mechanism for shifts in the diastolic, left ventricular, pressure-volume curve: the role of the pericardium. *Eur J Cardiol* 1978;7[Suppl]:163–175.

75. Thomas JD. Doppler echocardiography and left ventricular diastolic function. In: Gaasch WH, LeWinter MM, eds. *Left ventricular diastolic dysfunction and heart failure.* Philadelphia: Lea & Febiger, 1994:192–218.

76. Cheng CP, Freeman GL, Santamore WP, et al. Effect of loading conditions, contractile state, and heart rate on early diastolic left ventricular filling in conscious dogs. *Circ Res* 1990;66:814–823.

77. Toutouzas P, Stefanadis C, Boudoulas H. 1st international symposium on left atrial function: introduction. *Eur Heart J* 2000;2[Suppl]:K1–K3.

78. Ito T, Suwa M, Hirota Y, et al. Influence of left atrial function on Doppler transmitral and pulmonary venous flow patterns in dilated and hypertrophic cardiomyopathy: evaluation of left atrial appendage function by transesophageal echocardiography. *Am Heart J* 1996;131:122–130.

79. Pollick C, Taylor D. Assessment of left atrial appendage function by transesophageal echocardiography. Implications for the development of thrombus. *Circulation* 1991;84:223–231.

80. Lau VK, Sagawa K, Suga H. Instantaneous pressure volume relationship of right atrium during isovolumic contraction in the canine heart. *Am J Physiol* 1979;236:H672–H679.

81. Alexander J, Sunagawa K, Chang N, et al. Instantaneous pressure-volume relation of the ejecting canine left atrium. *Circ Res* 1987;61:209–219.

82. Nakatani S, Garcia MJ, Firstenberg MS, et al. Noninvasive assessment of left atrial maximum dP/dt by a combination of transmitral and pulmonary venous flow. *J Am Coll Cardiol* 1999;34:795–801.

83. Nishimura RA, Abel MD, Hatle LK, et al. Relation of pulmonary vein to mitral flow velocities by transesophageal Doppler echocardiography. Effect of different loading conditions. *Circulation* 1990;81:1488–1497.

84. Klein AL, Burstow DJ, Tajik AJ, et al. Effects of age on left ventricular dimensions and filling dynamics in 117 normal persons. *Mayo Clin Proc* 1994;69:212–224.

85. Plehn JF, Friedman BJ. Diastolic dysfunction in amyloid heart disease: restrictive cardiomyopathy or not? *J Am Coll Cardiol* 1989;13:54–56.

86. Harrison MR, Clifton GD, Pennell AT, et al. Effect of heart rate on left ventricular diastolic transmitral flow velocity patterns assessed by Doppler echocardiography in normal subjects. *Am J Cardiol* 1991;67:622–627.

87. Galderisi M, Benjamin EJ, Evans JC, et al. Impact of heart rate and PR interval on Doppler indexes of left ventricular diastolic filling in an elderly cohort (the Framingham Heart Study). *Am J Cardiol* 1993;72:1183–1187.

88. Walsh RA. Sympathetic control of diastolic function in congestive heart failure. *Circulation* 1990;82[2 Suppl]:I52–I58.

89. Panidis IP, Ross J, Munley B, et al. Diastolic mitral regurgitation in patients with atrioventricular conduction abnormalities: a common finding by Doppler echocardiography. *J Am Coll Cardiol* 1986;7:768–774.

90. Tanabe A, Mohri T, Ohga M, et al. The effects of pacing-induced left bundle branch block on left ventricular systolic and diastolic performances. *Jpn Heart J* 1990;31:309–317.

91. Xiao HB, Lee CH, Gibson DG. Effect of left bundle branch block on diastolic function in dilated cardiomyopathy. *Br Heart J* 1991;66:443–447.

92. Appleton CP, Hatle LK, Popp RL. Relation of transmitral flow velocity patterns to left ventricular diastolic function: new insights from a combined hemodynamic and Doppler echocardiographic study. *J Am Coll Cardiol* 1988;12:426–440.

93. Takahashi T, Iizuka M, Serizawa T, et al. Significance of left atrial pressure and left ventricular relaxation as determinants of left ventricular early diastolic filling flow in man. *Jpn Heart J* 1990;31:319–328.

94. DeMaria AN, Wisenbaugh TW, Smith MD, et al. Doppler echocardiographic evaluation of diastolic dysfunction. *Circulation* 1991;84[3 Suppl]:I288–I295.

95. Kuecherer HF, Kusumoto F, Muhiudeen IA, et al. Pulmonary venous flow patterns by transesophageal pulsed Doppler echocardiography: relation to parameters of left ventricular systolic and diastolic function. *Am Heart J* 1991;122:1683–1693.

96. Rossvoll O, Hatle LK. Pulmonary venous flow velocities recorded by transthoracic Doppler ultrasound: relation to left ventricular diastolic pressures. *J Am Coll Cardiol* 1993;21:1687–1696.

97. Appleton CP, Galloway JM, Gonzalez MS, et al. Estimation of left ventricular filling pressures using two-dimensional and Doppler echocardiography in adult patients with cardiac disease. Additional value of analyzing left atrial size, left atrial ejection fraction and the difference in duration of pulmonary venous and mitral flow velocity at atrial contraction. *J Am Coll Cardiol* 1993;22:1972–1982.

98. Brunazzi MC, Chirillo F, Pasqualini M, et al. Estimation of left ventricular diastolic pressures from precordial pulsed-Doppler analysis of pulmonary venous and mitral flow. *Am Heart J* 1994;128:293–300.

99. Hatle LK, Appleton CP, Popp RL. Differentiation of constructive pericarditis and restrictive cardiomyopathy by Doppler echocardiography. *Circulation* 1989;79:357–370.

100. Klein AL, Hatle LK, Taliercio CP, et al. Serial Doppler echocardiographic follow-up of left ventricular diastolic function in cardiac amyloidosis. *J Am Coll Cardiol* 1990;16:1135–1141.

101. Klein AL, Cohen GI, Pietrolungo JF, et al. Differentiation of constrictive pericarditis from restrictive cardiomyopathy by Doppler transesophageal echocardiographic measurements of respiratory variations in pulmonary venous flow. *J Am Coll Cardiol* 1993;22:1935–1943.

102. Oh JK, Hatle LK, Seward JB, et al. Diagnostic role of Doppler echocardiography in constrictive pericarditis. *J Am Coll Cardiol* 1994;23:154–162.

103. Klein AL, Hatle LK, Taliercio CP, et al. Prognostic significance of Doppler measures of diastolic function in cardiac amyloidosis. A Doppler echocardiography study. *Circulation* 1991;83:808–816.

104. Capomolla S, Febo O, Gnemmi M, et al. Beta-blockade

therapy in chronic heart failure: diastolic function and mitral regurgitation improvement by carvedilol. *Am Heart J* 2000;139:596–608.

105. Reinmuller R, Gurgan M, Erdmann E, et al. CT and MR evaluation of pericardial constriction: a new diagnostic and therapeutic concept. *J Thorac Imaging* 1993;8:108–121.

106. Fifer MA, Borow KM, Colan SD, et al. Early diastolic left ventricular function in children and adults with aortic stenosis. *J Am Coll Cardiol* 1985;5:1147–1154.

107. Spirito P, Maron BJ, Bellotti P, et al. Noninvasive assessment of left ventricular diastolic function: comparative analysis of pulsed Doppler ultrasound and digitized M-mode echocardiography. *Am J Cardiol* 1986;58:837–843.

108. Park JW, Warnecke H, Deng M, et al. Early diastolic left ventricular function as a marker of acute cardiac rejection: a prospective serial echocardiographic study. *Int J Cardiol* 1992;37:351–359.

109. Armstrong WF, Schilt BF, Helper DJ, et al. Diastolic collapse of the right ventricle with cardiac tamponade: an echocardiographic study. *Circulation* 1982;65:1491–1496.

110. Candell-Riera J, Garcia del Castillo H, Permanyer-Miralda G, et al. Echocardiographic features of the interventricular septum in chronic constrictive pericarditis. *Circulation* 1978;57:1154–1158.

111. Alam M, Wardell J, Andersson E, et al. Right ventricular function in patients with first inferior myocardial infarction: assessment by tricuspid annular motion and tricuspid annular velocity. *Am Heart J* 2000;139:710–715.

112. Sutherland GR, Kukulski T, Kvitting JE, et al. Quantitation of left-ventricular asynergy by cardiac ultrasound. *Am J Cardiol* 2000;86:4G–9G.

113. Appleton CP, Hatle LK. The natural history of left ventricular filling abnormalities: assessment by two-dimensional and Doppler echocardiography. *Echocardiography* 1992;9:437–457.

114. Himelman RB, Kircher B, Rockey DC, et al. Inferior vena cava plethora with blunted respiratory response: a sensitive echocardiographic sign of cardiac tamponade. *J Am Coll Cardiol* 1988;12:1470–1477.

115. Appleton CP, Jensen JL, Hatle LK, et al. Doppler evaluation of left and right ventricular diastolic function: a technical guide for obtaining optimal flow velocity recordings. *J Am Soc Echocardiogr* 1997;10:271–292.

116. Rakowski H, Appleton CP, Chan KL, et al. Canadian consensus recommendations for the measurement and reporting of diastolic dysfunction by echocardiography: from the Investigators of Consensus on Diastolic Dysfunction by Echocardiography. *J Am Soc Echocardiogr* 1996;9:736–760.

117. Jensen JL, Williams FE, Beilby BJ, et al. Feasibility of obtaining pulmonary venous flow velocity in cardiac patients using transthoracic pulsed wave Doppler technique. *J Am Soc Echocardiogr* 1997;10:60–66.

118. Williams MJ, McClements BM, Picard MH. Improvement of transthoracic pulmonary venous flow Doppler signal with intravenous injection of sonicated albumin. *J Am Coll Cardiol* 1995;26:1741–1746.

119. Klein AL, Canale MP, Rajagopalan N, et al. Role of transesophageal echocardiography in assessing diastolic dysfunction in a large clinical practice: a 9-year experience. *Am Heart J* 1999;138:880–889.

120. Klein AL, Leung DY, Murray RD, et al. Effects of age and physiologic variables on right ventricular filling dynamics in normal subjects. *Am J Cardiol* 1999;84:440–448.

121. Rajagopalan N, Garcia MJ, Rodriguez L, et al. Comparison of new Doppler echocardiographic methods to differentiate constrictive pericardial heart disease and restrictive cardiomyopathy. *Am J Cardiol* 2001;87:86–94.

122. Miyatake K, Yamagishi M, Tanaka N, et al. New method for evaluating left ventricular wall motion by color-coded tissue Doppler imaging: in vitro and in vivo studies. *J Am Coll Cardiol* 1995;25:717–724.

123. Garcia MJ, Rodriguez L, Ares M, et al. Differentiation of constrictive pericarditis from restrictive cardiomyopathy: assessment of left ventricular diastolic velocities in longitudinal axis by Doppler tissue imaging. *J Am Coll Cardiol* 1996;27:108–114.

124. Ling LH, Oh JK, Tei C, et al. Pericardial thickness measured with transesophageal echocardiography: feasibility and potential clinical usefulness. *J Am Coll Cardiol* 1997;29:1317–1323.

125. Vitarelli A, Gheorghiade M. Diastolic heart failure: standard Doppler approach and beyond. *Am J Cardiol* 1998;81:115G–121G.

126. Hausmann B, Muurling S, Stauch C, et al. Detection of diastolic dysfunction: acoustic quantification (AQ) in comparison to Doppler echocardiography. *Int J Card Imaging* 1997;13:301–310.

127. Chenzbraun A, Pinto FJ, Popylisen S, et al. Comparison of acoustic quantification and Doppler echocardiography in assessment of left ventricular diastolic variables. *Br Heart J* 1993;70:448–456.

128. Moidl R, Chevtchik O, Simon P, et al. Noninvasive monitoring of peak filling rate with acoustic quantification echocardiography accurately detects acute cardiac allograft rejection. *J Heart Lung Transplant* 1999;18:194–201.

129. Vignon P, Mor-Avi V, Weinert L, et al. Quantitative evaluation of global and regional left ventricular diastolic function with color kinesis. *Circulation* 1998;97:1053–1061.

130. Godoy IE, Mor-Avi V, Weinert L, et al. Use of color kinesis for evaluation of left ventricular filling in patients with dilated cardiomyopathy and mitral regurgitation. *J Am Coll Cardiol* 1998;31:1598–1606.

131. Tei C, Ling LH, Hodge DO, et al. New index of combined systolic and diastolic myocardial performance: a simple and reproducible measure of cardiac function—a study in normals and dilated cardiomyopathy. *J Cardiol* 1995;26:357–366.

132. Tei C, Dujardin KS, Hodge DO, et al. Doppler index combining systolic and diastolic myocardial performance: clinical value in cardiac amyloidosis. *J Am Coll Cardiol* 1996;28:658–664.

133. Dujardin KS, Tei C, Yeo TC, et al. Prognostic value of a Doppler index combining systolic and diastolic performance in idiopathic-dilated cardiomyopathy. *Am J Cardiol* 1998;82:1071–1076.

134. Kitzman DW, Higginbotham MB, Cobb FR, et al. Exercise intolerance in patients with heart failure and preserved left ventricular systolic function: failure of the Frank-Starling mechanism. *J Am Coll Cardiol* 1991;17:1065–1072.

135. Genovesi-Ebert A, Marabotti C, Palombo C, et al. Echo Doppler diastolic function and exercise tolerance. *Int J Cardiol* 1994;43:67–73.

136. Yuasa F, Sumimoto T, Takeuchi M, et al. Effects of left ventricular diastolic dysfunction on exercise capacity three to six weeks after acute myocardial infarction in men. *Am J Cardiol* 1995;75:14–17.

137. Sumimoto T, Jikuhara T, Hattori T, et al. Importance of left ventricular diastolic function on maintenance of exercise capacity in patients with systolic dysfunction after anterior myocardial infarction. *Am Heart J* 1997;133:87–93.

138. Belardinelli R, Georgiou D, Cianci G, et al. Exercise training improves left ventricular diastolic filling in patients with dilated cardiomyopathy. Clinical and prognostic implications. *Circulation* 1995;91:2775–2784.

139. Irace L, Iarussi D, Guadagno I, et al. Left ventricular function and exercise tolerance in patients with type II diabetes mellitus. *Clin Cardiol* 1998;21:567–571.

140. Warner JG Jr, Metzger DC, Kitzman DW, et al. Losartan improves exercise tolerance in patients with diastolic dysfunction and a hypertensive response to exercise. *J Am Coll Cardiol* 1999;33:1567–1572.

141. von Bibra H, Tuchnitz A, Klein A, et al. Regional diastolic function by pulsed Doppler myocardial mapping for the detection of left ventricular ischemia during pharmacologic stress testing: a comparison with stress echocardiography and perfusion scintigraphy. *J Am Coll Cardiol* 2000;36:444–452.

141a. Ha JW, Oh JK, Lulie F, et al. Changes of mitral inflow and annular velocities after exercise in middle aged healthy subjects [abstract]. *J Am Soc Echocardiogr* 2001;14:443.

142. Little WC, Downes TR, Applegate RJ. Invasive evaluation of left ventricular diastolic performance. *Herz* 1990;15:362–376.

143. Grossman W, McLaurin LP. Diastolic properties of the left ventricle. *Ann Intern Med* 1976;84:316–326.

144. Mirsky I. Assessment of diastolic function: suggested methods and future considerations. *Circulation* 1984;69:836–841.

145. Hammermeister KE, Warbasse JR. The rate of change of left ventricular volume in man. II. Diastolic events in health and disease. *Circulation* 1974;49:739–747.

146. Ohno M, Cheng CP, Little WC. Mechanism of altered patterns of left ventricular filling during the development of congestive heart failure. *Circulation* 1994;89:2241–2250.

147. Bonow RO. Radionuclide angiographic evaluation of left ventricular diastolic function. *Circulation* 1991;84[3 Suppl]:I208–I215.

148. Bonow RO, Vitale DF, Bacharach SL, et al. Asynchronous left ventricular regional function and impaired global diastolic filling in patients with coronary artery disease: reversal after coronary angioplasty. *Circulation* 1985;71:297–307.

149. Spirito P, Maron BJ, Bonow RO. Noninvasive assessment of left ventricular diastolic function: comparative analysis of Doppler echocardiographic and radionuclide angiographic techniques. *J Am Coll Cardiol* 1986;7:518–526.

150. Bonow RO, Bacharach SL, Green MV, et al. Impaired left ventricular diastolic filling in patients with coronary artery disease: assessment with radionuclide angiography. *Circulation* 1981;64:315–323.

151. Reduto LA, Wickemeyer WJ, Young JB, et al. Left ventricular diastolic performance at rest and during exercise in patients with coronary artery disease. Assessment with first-pass radionuclide angiography. *Circulation* 1981;63:1228–1237.

152. Bonow RO, Leon MB, Rosing DR, et al. Effects of verapamil and propranolol on left ventricular systolic function and diastolic filling in patients with coronary artery disease: radionuclide angiographic studies at rest and during exercise. *Circulation* 1982;65:1337–1350.

153. Betocchi S, Bonow RO, Bacharach SL, et al. Isovolumic relaxation period in hypertrophic cardiomyopathy: assessment by radionuclide angiography. *J Am Coll Cardiol* 1986;7:74–81.

154. Chen YT, Chang KC, Hu WS, et al. Left ventricular diastolic function in hypertrophic cardiomyopathy: assessment by radionuclide angiography. *Int J Cardiol* 1987;15:185–193.

155. Betocchi S, Losi MA, Piscione F, et al. Effects of dual-chamber pacing in hypertrophic cardiomyopathy on left ventricular outflow tract obstruction and on diastolic function. *Am J Cardiol* 1996;77:498–502.

156. Cuocolo A, Sax FL, Brush JE, et al. Left ventricular hypertrophy and impaired diastolic filling in essential hypertension. Diastolic mechanisms for systolic dysfunction during exercise. *Circulation* 1990;81:978–986.

157. Shepherd RF, Zachariah PK, Shub C. Hypertension and left ventricular diastolic function. *Mayo Clin Proc* 1989;64:1521–1532.

158. Quaife RA, Gilbert EM, Christian PE, et al. Effects of carvedilol on systolic and diastolic left ventricular performance in idiopathic dilated cardiomyopathy or ischemic cardiomyopathy. *Am J Cardiol* 1996;78:779–784.

159. Bonow RO. Effects of calcium-channel blocking agents on left ventricular diastolic function in hypertrophic cardiomyopathy and in coronary artery disease. *Am J Cardiol* 1985;55:172B–178B.

160. Nishimura RA, Schwartz RS, Holmes DR Jr, et al. Failure of calcium channel blockers to improve ventricular relaxation in humans. *J Am Coll Cardiol* 1993;21:182–188.

161. Sechtem U, Tscholakoff D, Higgins CB. MRI of the abnormal pericardium. *AJR Am J Roentgenol* 1986;147:245–252.

162. Furber A, Pezard P, Jeune JJ, et al. Radionuclide angiography and magnetic resonance imaging: complementary non-invasive methods in the diagnosis of constrictive pericarditis. *Eur J Nucl Med* 1995;22:1292–1298.

163. Celletti F, Fattori R, Napoli G, et al. Assessment of restrictive cardiomyopathy of amyloid or idiopathic etiology by magnetic resonance imaging. *Am J Cardiol* 1999;83:798–801.

164. Schulz-Menger J, Friedrich MG. Magnetic resonance imaging in patients with cardiomyopathies: when and why. *Herz* 2000;25:384–391.

165. Stark DD, Higgins CB, Lanzer P, et al. Magnetic resonance imaging of the pericardium: normal and pathologic findings. *Radiology* 1984;150:469–474.

166. Myers RB, Spodick DH. Constrictive pericarditis: clinical and pathophysiologic characteristics. *Am Heart J* 1999;138:219–232.

167. Hartiala JJ, Mostbeck GH, Foster E, et al. Velocity-encoded cine MRI in the evaluation of left ventricular diastolic function: measurement of mitral valve and pulmonary vein flow velocities and flow volume across the mitral valve. *Am Heart J* 1993;125:1054–1066.

168. Mantero A, Gentile F, Gualtierotti C, et al. Left ventricular diastolic parameters in 288 normal subjects from 20 to 80 years old. *Eur Heart J* 1995;16:94–105.

169. Appleton CP, Hatle LK, Popp RL. Relation of transmitral flow velocity patterns to left ventricular diastolic function: new insights from a combined hemodynamic and Doppler echocardiographic study. *J Am Coll Cardiol* 1988;12:426–440.

170. Dumesnil JG, Gaudreault G, Honos GN, et al. Use of Valsalva maneuver to unmask left ventricular diastolic function abnormalities by Doppler echocardiography in patients with coronary artery disease or systemic hypertension. *Am J Cardiol* 1991;68:515–519.

171. Plehn JF, Southworth J, Cornwell GGD. Brief report: atrial systolic failure in primary amyloidosis. *N Engl J Med* 1992;327:1570–1573.

172. Flachskampf FA, Weyman AE, Guerrero JL, et al. Influence of orifice geometry and flow rate on effective valve area: an in vitro study. *J Am Coll Cardiol* 1990;15:1173–1180.

173. Little WC, Ohno M, Kitzman DW, et al. Determination of left ventricular chamber stiffness from the time for deceleration of early left ventricular filling. *Circulation* 1995;92:1933–1939.

174. Hatle LK, Angelsen B. *Doppler ultrasound in cardiology: physical principles and clinical applications*, 2nd ed. Philadelphia: Lea & Febiger, 1985.

175. Flachskampf FA, Rodriguez LL, Chen C, et al. Analysis of mitral inertance: a factor critical for early transmitral filling. *J Am Soc Echocardiogr* 1993;6:422–432.

176. Jensen JL, Williams FE, Beilby BJ, et al. Feasibility of obtaining pulmonary venous flow velocity in cardiac patients using transthoracic pulsed wave Doppler technique. *J Am Soc Echocardiogr* 1997;10:60–66.

177. Vitarelli A, Gheorghiade M. Transthoracic and transesophageal echocardiography in the hemodynamic assessment of patients with congestive heart failure. *Am J Cardiol* 2000;86:36G–40G.

178. Appleton CP. Hemodynamic determinants of Doppler pulmonary venous flow velocity components: new insights from studies in lightly sedated normal dogs. *J Am Coll Cardiol* 1997;30:1562–1574.

178a. Smiseth OA, Thompson CR, Lohavanichbutr K, et al. The pulmonary venous systolic flow pulse—its origin and relationship to left atrial pressure. *J Am Coll Cardiol* 1999;34:802–809.

179. Scalia GM, Greenberg NL, McCarthy PM, et al. Inertial nature of pulmonary vein flow—invasive and Doppler correlations in humans [abstract]. *J Am Coll Cardiol* 1996;27[Suppl]:140A–141A.

180. Klein AL, Hatle LK, Burstow DJ, et al. Comprehensive Doppler assessment of right ventricular diastolic function in cardiac amyloidosis. *J Am Coll Cardiol* 1990;15:99–108.

181. Appleton CP, Hatle LK, Popp RL. Superior vena cava and hepatic vein Doppler echocardiography in healthy adults. *J Am Coll Cardiol* 1987;10:1032–1039.

182. Zoghbi WA, Habib GB, Quinones MA. Doppler assessment of right ventricular filling in a normal population. Comparison with left ventricular filling dynamics. *Circulation* 1990;82:1316–1324.

183. Stugaard M, Smiseth OA, Risoe C, et al. Intraventricular early diastolic filling during acute myocardial ischemia, assessment by multigated color M-mode Doppler echocardiography. *Circulation* 1993;88:2705–2713.

184. Stugaard M, Steen T, Lundervold A, et al. Visual assessment of intraventricular flow from colour M-mode Doppler images. *Int J Card Imaging* 1994;10:279–287.

185. Takatsuji H, Mikami T, Urasawa K, et al. A new approach for evaluation of left ventricular diastolic function: spatial and temporal analysis of left ventricular filling flow propagation by color M-mode Doppler echocardiography. *J Am Coll Cardiol* 1996;27:365–371.

186. Moller JE, Sondergaard E, Seward JB, et al. Ratio of left ventricular peak E-wave velocity to flow propagation velocity assessed by color M-mode Doppler echocardiography in first myocardial infarction: prognostic and clinical implications. *J Am Coll Cardiol* 2000;35:363–370.

187. Greenberg NL, Vandervoort PM, Thomas JD. Instantaneous diastolic transmitral pressure differences from color Doppler M-mode echocardiography. *Am J Physiol* 1996;271:H1267–H1276.

188. Thomas JD, Garcia MJ, Greenberg NL. Application of color Doppler M-mode echocardiography in the assessment of ventricular diastolic function: potential for quantitative analysis. *Heart Vessels* 1997;12[Suppl]:135–137.

189. Greenberg NL, Castro PL, Drinko J, et al. Effect of scanline orientation on ventricular flow propagation: assessment using high frame-rate color Doppler echocardiography. *Biomed Sci Instrum* 2000;36:203–208.

190. Beppu S, Izumi S, Miyatake K, et al. Abnormal blood pathways in left ventricular cavity in acute myocardial infarction. Experimental observations with special reference to regional wall motion abnormality and hemostasis. *Circulation* 1988;78:157–164.

191. Duval-Moulin AM, Dupouy P, Brun P, et al. Alteration of left ventricular diastolic function during coronary angioplasty-induced ischemia: a color M-mode Doppler study. *J Am Coll Cardiol* 1997;29:1246–1255.

192. Garcia MJ, Smedira NG, Greenberg NL, et al. Color M-mode Doppler flow propagation velocity is a preload insensitive index of left ventricular relaxation: animal and human validation. *J Am Coll Cardiol* 2000;35:201–208.

193. Trambaiolo P, Tonti G, Salustri A, et al. New insights into regional systolic and diastolic left ventricular function with tissue Doppler echocardiography: from qualitative analysis to a quantitative approach. *J Am Soc Echocardiogr* 2001;14:85–96.

194. Garcia MJ, Rodriguez L, Ares M, et al. Myocardial wall velocity assessment by pulsed Doppler tissue imaging: characteristic findings in normal subjects. *Am Heart J* 1996;132:648–656.

195. Garcia M, Thomas J. Tissue Doppler to assess diastolic left ventricular function. *Echocardiography* 1999;16:501–508.

196. Rodriguez L, Garcia M, Ares M, et al. Assessment of mitral annular dynamics during diastole by Doppler tissue imaging: comparison with mitral Doppler inflow in sub-

jects without heart disease and in patients with left ventricular hypertrophy. *Am Heart J* 1996;131:982–987.

197. Oki T, Tabata T, Yamada H, et al. Clinical application of pulsed Doppler tissue imaging for assessing abnormal left ventricular relaxation. *Am J Cardiol* 1997;79:921–928.

198. Sohn DW, Chai IH, Lee DJ, et al. Assessment of mitral annulus velocity by Doppler tissue imaging in the evaluation of left ventricular diastolic function. *J Am Coll Cardiol* 1997;30:474–480.

199. Nagueh SF, Sun H, Kopelen HA, et al. Hemodynamic determinants of the mitral annulus diastolic velocities by tissue Doppler. *J Am Coll Cardiol* 2001;37:278–285.

200. Firstenberg MS, Greenberg NL, Main ML, et al. Determinants of diastolic myocardial tissue Doppler velocities: influences of relaxation and preload. *J Appl Physiol* 2001;90:299–307.

201. Farias CA, Rodriguez L, Garcia MJ, et al. Assessment of diastolic function by tissue Doppler echocardiography: comparison with standard transmitral and pulmonary venous flow. *J Am Soc Echocardiogr* 1999;12:609–617.

202. Ommen SR, Nishimura RA, Appleton CP, et al. Clinical utility of Doppler echocardiography and tissue Doppler imaging in the estimation of left ventricular filling pressures: a comparative simultaneous Doppler-catheterization study. *Circulation* 2000;102:1788–1794.

202a. Arnold MF, Voigt JU, Kukulski T, et al. Does atrioventricular ring motion always distinguish constriction from restriction? A Doppler myocardial imaging study. *J Am Soc Echocardiogr* 2001;14:391–395.

203. Mankad S, Murali S, Kormos RL, et al. Evaluation of the potential role of color-coded tissue Doppler echocardiography in the detection of allograft rejection in heart transplant recipients. *Am Heart J* 1999;138:721–730.

204. Uematsu M, Miyatake K, Tanaka N, et al. Myocardial velocity gradient as a new indicator of regional left ventricular contraction: detection by a two-dimensional tissue Doppler imaging technique. *J Am Coll Cardiol* 1995;26:217–223.

205. Shimizu Y, Uematsu M, Shimizu H, et al. Peak negative myocardial velocity gradient in early diastole as a noninvasive indicator of left ventricular diastolic function: comparison with transmitral flow velocity indices. *J Am Coll Cardiol* 1998;32:1418–1425.

206. Palka P, Lange A, Donnelly JE, et al. Differentiation between restrictive cardiomyopathy and constrictive pericarditis by early diastolic Doppler myocardial velocity gradient at the posterior wall. *Circulation* 2000;102:655–662.

207. Derumeaux G, Loufoua J, Pontier G, et al. Tissue Doppler imaging differentiates transmural from nontransmural acute myocardial infarction after reperfusion therapy. *Circulation* 2001;103:589–596.

208. Urheim S, Edvardsen T, Torp H, et al. Myocardial strain by Doppler echocardiography. Validation of a new method to quantify regional myocardial function. *Circulation* 2000;102:1158–1164.

209. Greenberg NL, Lever H, Castro P, et al. Evaluation of segmental myocardial strain rate by tissue Doppler echocardiography in a feline model of hypertrophic cardiomyopathy. *J Am Coll Cardiol* 1999;33:458A.

210. Sutherland GR, Kukulski T, Voight JU, et al. Tissue Doppler echocardiography: future developments. *Echocardiography* 1999;16:509–520.

211. Stoylen A, Heimdal A, Bjornstad K, et al. Strain rate imaging by ultrasonography in the diagnosis of coronary artery disease. *J Am Soc Echocardiogr* 2000;13:1053–1064.

212. Nishimura RA, Tajik AJ. Evaluation of diastolic filling of left ventricle in health and disease: Doppler echocardiography is the clinician's Rosetta Stone. *J Am Coll Cardiol* 1997;30:8–18.

213. Yamamoto K, Redfield MM, Nishimura RA. Analysis of left ventricular diastolic function. *Heart* 1996;75:27–35.

214. Iliceto S, Amico A, Marangelli V, et al. Doppler echocardiographic evaluation of the effect of atrial pacing-induced ischemia on left ventricular filling in patients with coronary artery disease. *J Am Coll Cardiol* 1988;11:953–961.

215. Takenaka K, Dabestani A, Gardin JM, et al. Left ventricular filling in hypertrophic cardiomyopathy: a pulsed Doppler echocardiographic study. *J Am Coll Cardiol* 1986;7:1263–1271.

216. Bryg RJ, Pearson AC, Williams GA, et al. Left ventricular systolic and diastolic flow abnormalities determined by Doppler echocardiography in obstructive hypertrophic cardiomyopathy. *Am J Cardiol* 1987;59:925–931.

217. Otto CM, Pearlman AS, Amsler LC. Doppler echocardiographic evaluation of left ventricular diastolic filling in isolated valvular aortic stenosis. *Am J Cardiol* 1989;63:313–316.

218. Choong CY, Herrmann HC, Weyman AE, et al. Preload dependence of Doppler-derived indexes of left ventricular diastolic function in humans. *J Am Coll Cardiol* 1987;10:800–808.

219. Hurrell DG, Nishimura RA, Ilstrup DM, et al. Utility of preload alteration in assessment of left ventricular filling pressure by Doppler echocardiography: a simultaneous catheterization and Doppler echocardiographic study. *J Am Coll Cardiol* 1997;30:459–467.

220. Kuecherer HF, Muhiudeen IA, Kusumoto FM, et al. Estimation of mean left atrial pressure from transesophageal pulsed Doppler echocardiography of pulmonary venous flow. *Circulation* 1990;82:1127–1139.

221. Thomas JD, Choong CY, Flachskampf FA, et al. Analysis of the early transmitral Doppler velocity curve: effect of primary physiologic changes and compensatory preload adjustment. *J Am Coll Cardiol* 1990;16:644–655.

222. Oh JK, Ding ZP, Gersh BJ, et al. Restrictive left ventricular diastolic filling identifies patients with heart failure after acute myocardial infarction. *J Am Soc Echocardiogr* 1992;5:497–503.

223. Pinamonti B, Di Lenarda A, Sinagra G, et al. Restrictive left ventricular filling pattern in dilated cardiomyopathy assessed by Doppler echocardiography: clinical, echocardiographic and hemodynamic correlations and prognostic implications. Heart Muscle Disease Study Group. *J Am Coll Cardiol* 1993;22:808–815.

224. Rihal CS, Nishimura RA, Hatle LK, et al. Systolic and diastolic dysfunction in patients with clinical diagnosis of dilated cardiomyopathy. Relation to symptoms and prognosis. *Circulation* 1994;90:2772–2779.

225. Nishimura RA, Appleton CP, Redfield MM, et al. Noninva-

sive Doppler echocardiographic evaluation of left ventricular filling pressures in patients with cardiomyopathies: a simultaneous Doppler echocardiographic and cardiac catheterization study. *J Am Coll Cardiol* 1996;28:1226–1233.

226. Pozzoli M, Traversi E, Cioffi G, et al. Loading manipulations improve the prognostic value of Doppler evaluation of mitral flow in patients with chronic heart failure. *Circulation* 1997;95:1222–1230.

227. Pinamonti B, Zecchin M, Di Lenarda A, et al. Persistence of restrictive left ventricular filling pattern in dilated cardiomyopathy: an ominous prognostic sign. *J Am Coll Cardiol* 1997;29:604–612.

228. Stork TV, Muller RM, Piske GJ, et al. Noninvasive measurement of left ventricular filling pressures by means of transmitral pulsed Doppler ultrasound. *Am J Cardiol* 1989;64:655–660.

229. Vanoverschelde JL, Robert AR, Gerbaux A, et al. Noninvasive estimation of pulmonary arterial wedge pressure with Doppler transmitral flow velocity pattern in patients with known heart disease. *Am J Cardiol* 1995;75:383–389.

230. Nagueh SF, Middleton KJ, Kopelen HA, et al. Doppler tissue imaging: a noninvasive technique for evaluation of left ventricular relaxation and estimation of filling pressures. *J Am Coll Cardiol* 1997;30:1527–1533.

231. Nagueh SF, Kopelen HA, Quinones MA. Assessment of left ventricular filling pressures by Doppler in the presence of atrial fibrillation. *Circulation* 1996;94:2138–2145.

232. Gonzalez-Vilchez F, Ares M, Ayuela J, et al. Combined use of pulsed and color M-mode Doppler echocardiography for the estimation of pulmonary capillary wedge pressure: an empirical approach based on an analytical relation. *J Am Coll Cardiol* 1999;34:515–523.

233. Chirillo F, Brunazzi MC, Barbiero M, et al. Estimating mean pulmonary wedge pressure in patients with chronic atrial fibrillation from transthoracic Doppler indexes of mitral and pulmonary venous flow velocity. *J Am Coll Cardiol* 1997;30:19–26.

234. Klein AL, Abdalla I, Murray RD, et al. Age independence of the difference in duration of pulmonary venous atrial reversal flow and transmitral A-wave flow in normal subjects. *J Am Soc Echocardiogr* 1998;11:458–465.

234a. Rossi A, Cicoira M, Golia G, et al. Mitral regurgitation and left ventricular diastolic dysfunction similarly affect mitral and pulmonary vein flow Doppler parameters: the advantage of end-diastolic markers. *J Am Soc Echocardiogr* 2001;14:562–568.

235. Abdalla I, Murray RD, Lee JC, et al. Duration of pulmonary venous atrial reversal flow velocity and mitral inflow a wave: new measure of severity of cardiac amyloidosis. *J Am Soc Echocardiogr* 1998;11:1125–1133.

236. Dini FL, Dell'Anna R, Micheli A, et al. Impact of blunted pulmonary venous flow on the outcome of patients with left ventricular systolic dysfunction secondary to either ischemic or idiopathic dilated cardiomyopathy. *Am J Cardiol* 2000;85:1455–1460.

237. Devereux RB, Roman MJ, Liu JE, et al. Congestive heart failure despite normal left ventricular systolic function in a population-based sample: the Strong Heart Study. *Am J Cardiol* 2000;86:1090–1096.

238. Senni M, Tribouilloy CM, Rodeheffer RJ, et al. Congestive heart failure in the community: a study of all incident cases in Olmsted County, Minnesota, in 1991. *Circulation* 1998;98:2282–2289.

239. Gandhi SK, Powers JC, Nomeir AM, et al. The pathogenesis of acute pulmonary edema associated with hypertension. *N Engl J Med* 2001;344:17–22.

240. Kramer K, Kirkman P, Kitzman D, et al. Flash pulmonary edema: association with hypertension and reoccurrence despite coronary revascularization. *Am Heart J* 2000;140:451–455.

241. Grossman W. Diastolic dysfunction in congestive heart failure. *N Engl J Med* 1991;325:1557–1564.

242. Grossman W. Diastolic dysfunction and congestive heart failure. *Circulation* 1990;81[3 Suppl]:III1–III7.

242a. Ommen SR, Tsang TSM, Ammash NM, et al. Usefulness of serial echocardiographic parameters for predicting the subsequent occurrence of atrial fibrillation. *Am J Cardiol* 2001;87:1298–1301.

243. Litwin SE, Grossman W. Diastolic dysfunction as a cause of heart failure. *J Am Coll Cardiol* 1993;22[Suppl A]:49A–55A.

244. Mandinov L, Eberli FR, Seiler C, et al. Diastolic heart failure. *Cardiovasc Res* 2000;45:813–825.

245. Kahan T. The importance of left ventricular hypertrophy in human hypertension. *J Hypertens* 1998;16[Suppl]:S23–S29.

246. Brilla CG, Funck RC, Rupp H. Lisinopril-mediated regression of myocardial fibrosis in patients with hypertensive heart disease. *Circulation* 2000;102:1388–1393.

247. Matter CM, Mandinov L, Kaufmann PA, et al. Effect of NO donors on LV diastolic function in patients with severe pressure-overload hypertrophy. *Circulation* 1999;99:2396–2401.

248. Nishimura RA, Hayes DL, Holmes DR Jr, et al. Mechanism of hemodynamic improvement by dual-chamber pacing for severe left ventricular dysfunction: an acute Doppler and catheterization hemodynamic study. *J Am Coll Cardiol* 1995;25:281–288.

249. Breithardt OA, Stellbrink C, Franke A, et al. Echocardiographic evidence of hemodynamic and clinical improvement in patients paced for heart failure. *Am J Cardiol* 2000;86[9 Suppl 1]:K133–K137.

250. Vasan RS, Benjamin EJ, Levy D. Prevalence, clinical features and prognosis of diastolic heart failure: an epidemiologic perspective. *J Am Coll Cardiol* 1995;26:1565–1574.

251. Judge KW, Pawitan Y, Caldwell J, et al. Congestive heart failure symptoms in patients with preserved left ventricular systolic function: analysis of the CASS registry. *J Am Coll Cardiol* 1991;18:377–382.

252. O'Connor CM, Gattis WA, Shaw L, et al. Clinical characteristics and long-term outcomes of patients with heart failure and preserved systolic function. *Am J Cardiol* 2000;86:863–867.

253. Swedberg K, Pfeffer M, Granger C, et al. Candesartan in heart failure—assessment of reduction in mortality and morbidity (CHARM): rationale and design. Charm-Programme Investigators. *J Card Fail* 1999;5:276–282.

254. Richardson P, McKenna W, Bristow M, et al. Report of the 1995 World Health Organization/International Soci-

ety and Federation of Cardiology Task Force on the Definition and Classification of Cardiomyopathies. *Circulation* 1996;93:841–842.

255. Force WIT. Report of the WHO/ISFC Task Force on the definition and classification of cardiomyopathies. *Br Heart J* 1980;44:672–673.

256. Goodwin JF. Overview and classification of the cardiomyopathies. *Cardiovasc Clin* 1988;19:3–7.

257. Goodwin JF. The frontiers of cardiomyopathy. *Br Heart J* 1982;48:1–18.

258. Goodwin JF. Cardiomyopathies and specific heart muscle diseases. Definitions, terminology, classifications and new and old approaches. *Postgrad Med J* 1992;68[Suppl 1]:S3–S6.

259. Keren A, Popp RL. Assignment of patients into the classification of cardiomyopathies. *Circulation* 1992;86:1622–1633.

260. Johnson RA, Palacios I. Dilated cardiomyopathies of the adult (second of two parts). *N Engl J Med* 1982;307:1119–1126.

261. Kushwaha SS, Fallon JT, Fuster V. Restrictive cardiomyopathy. *N Engl J Med* 1997;336:267–276.

262. Angelini A, Calzolari V, Thiene G, et al. Morphologic spectrum of primary restrictive cardiomyopathy. *Am J Cardiol* 1997;80:1046–1050.

263. Leung DY, Klein AL. Restrictive cardiomyopathy: diagnosis and prognostic implications. In: Otto CM, ed. *The practice of clinical echocardiography*. Philadelphia: WB Saunders, 1997:473–493.

264. Click RL, Olson LJ, Edwards WD, et al. Echocardiography and systemic diseases. *J Am Soc Echocardiogr* 1994;7:201–216.

265. Roberts WC, Waller BF. Cardiac amyloidosis causing cardiac dysfunction: analysis of 54 necropsy patients. *Am J Cardiol* 1983;52:137–146.

266. Buja LM, Khoi NB, Roberts WC. Clinically significant cardiac amyloidosis. Clinicopathologic findings in 15 patients. *Am J Cardiol* 1970;26:394–405.

267. Spry CJ, Take M, Tai PC. Eosinophilic disorders affecting the myocardium and endocardium: a review. *Heart Vessels* 1985;1[Suppl]:240–242.

268. Abelmann WH, Lorell BH. The challenge of cardiomyopathy. *J Am Coll Cardiol* 1989;13:1219–1239.

269. Shabetai R. Controversial issues in restrictive cardiomyopathy. *Postgrad Med J* 1992;68[Suppl 1]:S47–S51.

270. Hirota Y, Kohriyama T, Hayashi T, et al. Idiopathic restrictive cardiomyopathy: differences of left ventricular relaxation and diastolic wave forms from constrictive pericarditis. *Am J Cardiol* 1983;52:421–423.

271. Hirota Y, Shimizu G, Kita Y, et al. Spectrum of restrictive cardiomyopathy: report of the national survey in Japan. *Am Heart J* 1990;120:188–194.

272. Appleton CP, Popp RL, Hatle LK. Differentiation of constrictive pericarditis and restrictive cardiomyopathy: general overview and new insights from two-dimensional and Doppler echocardiographic studies. In: Soler-Soler J, Permanyer-Miralda G, Sagrista-Sauleda J, eds. *Pericardial disease*. Dordrecht, The Netherlands: Kluwer, 1990:59–93.

273. Hirota Y. Restrictive cardiomyopathy, cardiac amyloidosis and hypereosinophilic heart disease. In: Abelman WH,

274. Braunwald E, eds. *Cardiomyopathies, myocarditis, and pericardial disease. Atlas of heart diseases.* Philadelphia: Current Medicine, 1995:5.1–5.15.

274. Child JS, Perloff JK. The restrictive cardiomyopathies. *Cardiol Clin* 1988;6:289–316.

275. Klein AL, Hatle LK, Burstow DJ, et al. Doppler characterization of left ventricular diastolic function in cardiac amyloidosis. *J Am Coll Cardiol* 1989;13:1017–1026.

276. Wynne J, Braunwald E. The cardiomyopathies and myocarditides. In: Braunwald E, ed. *Heart disease. A textbook of cardiovascular medicine*, 5th ed. Philadelphia: WB Saunders, 1997:1426–1434.

277. Oren RM, Grover-McKay M, Stanford W, et al. Accurate preoperative diagnosis of pericardial constriction using cine computed tomography. *J Am Coll Cardiol* 1993;22:832–838.

278. White CS. MR evaluation of the pericardium. *Top Magn Reson Imaging* 1995;7:258–266.

279. Soldo SJ, Norris SL, Gober JR, et al. MRI-derived ventricular volume curves for the assessment of left ventricular function. *Magn Reson Imaging* 1994;12:711–717.

280. Wilmshurst PT, Katritsis D. Restrictive cardiomyopathy. *Br Heart J* 1990;63:323–324.

281. Hosenpud JD, DeMarco T, Frazier OH, et al. Progression of systemic disease and reduced long-term survival in patients with cardiac amyloidosis undergoing heart transplantation. Follow-up results of a multicenter survey. *Circulation* 1991;84[5 Suppl]:III338–III343.

282. Rivenes SM, Kearney DL, Smith EO, et al. Sudden death and cardiovascular collapse in children with restrictive cardiomyopathy. *Circulation* 2000;102:876–882.

283. Fitzpatrick AP, Shapiro LM, Rickards AF, et al. Familial restrictive cardiomyopathy with atrioventricular block and skeletal myopathy. *Br Heart J* 1990;63:114–118.

284. Katritsis D, Wilmshurst PT, Wendon JA, et al. Primary restrictive cardiomyopathy: clinical and pathologic characteristics. *J Am Coll Cardiol* 1991;18:1230–1235.

285. Benotti JR, Grossman W, Cohn PF. Clinical profile of restrictive cardiomyopathy. *Circulation* 1980;61:1206–1212.

286. McManus BM, Bren GB, Robertson EA, et al. Hemodynamic cardiac constriction without anatomic myocardial restriction or pericardial constriction. *Am Heart J* 1981;102:134–136.

287. Arbustini E, Buonanno C, Trevi G, et al. Cardiac ultrastructure in primary restrictive cardiomyopathy. *Chest* 1983;84:236–238.

288. Siegel RJ, Shah PK, Fishbein MC. Idiopathic restrictive cardiomyopathy. *Circulation* 1984;70:165–169.

289. Keren A, Billingham ME, Weintraub D, et al. Mildly dilated congestive cardiomyopathy. *Circulation* 1985;72:302–309.

290. Gewillig M, Mertens L, Moerman P, et al. Idiopathic restrictive cardiomyopathy in childhood. A diastolic disorder characterized by delayed relaxation. *Eur Heart J* 1996;17:1413–1420.

291. Cooke RA, Chambers JB, Curry PV. Noonan's cardiomyopathy: a non-hypertrophic variant. *Br Heart J* 1994;71:561–565.

292. Lewis AB. Clinical profile and outcome of restrictive cardiomyopathy in children. *Am Heart J* 1992;123:1589–1593.

293. Cetta F, O'Leary PW, Seward JB, et al. Idiopathic restrictive cardiomyopathy in childhood: diagnostic features and clinical course. *Mayo Clin Proc* 1995;70:634–640.

294. Keren A, Billingham ME, Popp RL. Features of mildly dilated congestive cardiomyopathy compared with idiopathic restrictive cardiomyopathy and typical dilated cardiomyopathy. *J Am Soc Echocardiogr* 1988;1:78–87.

295. Schoenfeld MH. The differentiation of restrictive cardiomyopathy from constrictive pericarditis. *Cardiol Clin* 1990;8:663–671.

296. Appleton CP, Hatle LK, Popp RL. Demonstration of restrictive ventricular physiology by Doppler echocardiography. *J Am Coll Cardiol* 1988;11:757–768.

297. Shabetai R. Pathophysiology and differential diagnosis of restrictive cardiomyopathy. *Cardiovasc Clin* 1988;19:123–132.

298. Schoenfeld MH, Supple EW, Dec GW Jr, et al. Restrictive cardiomyopathy versus constrictive pericarditis: role of endomyocardial biopsy in avoiding unnecessary thoracotomy. *Circulation* 1987;75:1012–1017.

299. Vaitkus PT, Kussmaul WG. Constrictive pericarditis versus restrictive cardiomyopathy: a reappraisal and update of diagnostic criteria. *Am Heart J* 1991;122:1431–1441.

300. Seward JB. Restrictive cardiomyopathy: reassessment of definitions and diagnosis. *Curr Opin Cardiol* 1988;3:391–395.

301. Hurrell DG, Nishimura RA, Higano ST, et al. Value of dynamic respiratory changes in left and right ventricular pressures for the diagnosis of constrictive pericarditis. *Circulation* 1996;93:2007–2013.

302. Ammash NM, Seward JB, Bailey KR, et al. Clinical profile and outcome of idiopathic restrictive cardiomyopathy. *Circulation* 2000;101:2490–2496.

303. Parrillo JE. Heart disease and the eosinophil. *N Engl J Med* 1990;323:1560–1561.

304. Valiathan SM, Kartha CC. Endomyocardial fibrosis—the possible connection with myocardial levels of magnesium and cerium. *Int J Cardiol* 1990;28:1–5.

305. Spyrou N, Foale R. Restrictive cardiomyopathies. *Curr Opin Cardiol* 1994;9:344–348.

306. Davies J, Spry CJ, Sapsford R, et al. Cardiovascular features of 11 patients with eosinophilic endomyocardial disease. *QJM* 1983;52:23–39.

307. Ribeiro PA, Muthusamy R, Duran CM. Right-sided endomyocardial fibrosis with recurrent pulmonary emboli leading to irreversible pulmonary hypertension. *Br Heart J* 1992;68:326–329.

308. Gupta PN, Valiathan MS, Balakrishnan KG, et al. Clinical course of endomyocardial fibrosis. *Br Heart J* 1989;62:450–454.

309. Spry CJ, Tai PC. Studies on blood eosinophils. II. Patients with Löffler's cardiomyopathy. *Clin Exp Immunol* 1976;24:423–434.

310. deMello DE, Liapis H, Jureidini S, et al. Cardiac localization of eosinophil-granule major basic protein in acute necrotizing myocarditis. *N Engl J Med* 1990;323:1542–1545.

311. Fauci AS, Harley JB, Roberts WC, et al. NIH conference. The hypereosinophilic syndrome: clinical pathophysiologic, and therapeutic considerations. *Ann Intern Med* 1982;97:78–92.

312. Weller PF, Bubley GJ. The idiopathic hypereosinophilic syndrome. *Blood* 1994;83:2759–2779.

313. Arnold M, McGuire L, Lee JC. Loeffler's fibroplastic endocarditis. *Pathology* 1988;20:79–82.

314. Felice PV, Sawicki J, Anto J. Endomyocardial disease and eosinophilia. *Angiology* 1993;44:869–874.

315. Berger PB, Duffy J, Reeder GS, et al. Restrictive cardiomyopathy associated with the eosinophilia-myalgia syndrome. *Mayo Clin Proc* 1994;69:162–165.

316. Olsen EGJ, Spry CJF. Relation between eosinophilia and endomyocardial disease. *Prog Cardiovasc Dis* 1985;27:241–254.

317. Parrillo JE, Borer JS, Henry WL, et al. The cardiovascular manifestations of the hypereosinophilic syndrome; prospective study of 26 patients with review of the literature. *Am J Med* 1979;67:572–582.

318. Acquatella H, Schiller NB. Echocardiographic recognition of Chagas' disease and endomyocardial fibrosis. *J Am Soc Echocardiogr* 1988;1:60–68.

319. Ommen SR, Seward JB, Tajik AJ. Clinical and echocardiographic features of hypereosinophilic syndromes. *Am J Cardiol* 2000;86:110–113.

320. Acquatella H, Rodriguez-Salas LA, Gomez-Mancebo JR. Doppler echocardiography in dilated and restrictive cardiomyopathies. *Cardiol Clin* 1990;8:349–367.

321. Uetsuka Y, Kasahara S, Tanaka N, et al. Hemodynamic and scintigraphic improvement after steroid therapy in a case with eosinophilic heart disease. *Heart Vessels* 1990;5[Suppl]:8–12.

322. Butterfield JH, Gleich GJ. Interferon-alpha treatment of six patients with the idiopathic hypereosinophilic syndrome. *Ann Intern Med* 1994;121:648–653.

323. Connor DH, Somers K, Hutt MSR, et al. Endomyocardial fibrosis in Uganda (Davies' disease): part I: an epidemiologic, clinical, and pathologic study. *Am Heart J* 1967;74:687–709.

324. Valiathan MS. Endomyocardial fibrosis. *Natl Med J India* 1993;6:212–216.

325. Johnson RA, Palacios I. Nondilated cardiomyopathies. *Adv Intern Med* 1984;30:243–274.

326. Shaper AG, Hutt MS, Coles RM. Necropsy study of endomyocardial fibrosis and rheumatic heart disease in Uganda 1950–1965. *Br Heart J* 1968;30:391–401.

327. Chopra P, Narula J, Talwar KK, et al. Histomorphologic characteristics of endomyocardial fibrosis: an endomyocardial biopsy study. *Hum Pathol* 1990;21:613–616.

328. Berensztein CS, Pineiro D, Marcotegui M, et al. Usefulness of echocardiography and Doppler echocardiography in endomyocardial fibrosis. *J Am Soc Echocardiogr* 2000;13:385–392.

329. Barretto AC, da Luz PL, de Oliveira SA, et al. Determinants of survival in endomyocardial fibrosis. *Circulation* 1989;80:I177–I182.

330. Mady C, Pereira Barretto AC, de Oliveira SA, et al. Effectiveness of operative and nonoperative therapy in endomyocardial fibrosis. *Am J Cardiol* 1989;63:1281–1282.

331. de Oliveira SA, Pereira Barreto AC, Mady C, et al. Surgical treatment of endomyocardial fibrosis: a new approach. *J Am Coll Cardiol* 1990;16:1246–1251.

332. Uva MS, Jebara VA, Acar C, et al. Mitral valve repair in

patients with endomyocardial fibrosis. *Ann Thorac Surg* 1992;54:89–92.

333. Martinez EE, Venturi M, Buffolo E, et al. Operative results in endomyocardial fibrosis. *Am J Cardiol* 1989;63:627–629.

334. Schneider U, Jenni R, Turina J, et al. Long-term follow up of patients with endomyocardial fibrosis: effects of surgery. *Heart* 1998;79:362–367.

335. Kyle RA. Amyloidosis. *Circulation* 1995;91:1269–1271.

336. Gertz MA, Lacy MQ, Dispenzieri A. Amyloidosis. *Hematol Oncol Clin North Am* 1999;13:1211–1233.

336a. Liao R, Jain M, Teller P, et al. Infusion of light chains from patients with cardiac amyloidosis causes diastolic dysfunction in isolated mouse hearts. *Circulation* 2001;104:1594–1597.

337. Kyle RA, Greipp PR. Amyloidosis (AL): clinical and laboratory features in 229 cases. *Mayo Clin Proc* 1983;58:665–683.

338. Gertz MA, Kyle RA. Secondary systemic amyloidosis: response and survival in 64 patients. *Medicine* 1991;70:246–256.

339. Gertz MA, Kyle RA, Thibodeau SN. Familial amyloidosis: a study of 52 North American-born patients examined during a 30-year period. *Mayo Clin Proc* 1992;67:428–440.

340. Saraiva MJ. Transthyretin mutations in health and disease. *Hum Mutat* 1995;5:191–196.

341. Kronzon I, Fedor M, Schwartz D, et al. A 58-year-old man with shortness of breath, ascites and leg edema. *Circulation* 1996;94:1483–1488.

342. Gertz MA, Kyle RA. Primary systemic amyloidosis—a diagnostic primer. *Mayo Clin Proc* 1989;64:1505–1519.

343. Booth DR, Tan SY, Hawkins PN, et al. A novel variant of transthyretin, ^{59}Thr→Lys, associated with autosomal dominant cardiac amyloidosis in an Italian family. *Circulation* 1995;91:962–967.

344. Fredericksen T, Gotzsche H, Harboe N, et al. Familial primary amyloidosis with severe amyloid heart disease. *Am J Med* 1962;33:328–348.

345. Benson MD, Wallace MR, Tejada E, et al. Hereditary amyloidosis: description of a new American kindred with late onset cardiomyopathy. Appalachian amyloid. *Arthritis Rheum* 1987;30:195–200.

346. Jacobson DR, Pastore RD, Yaghoubian R, et al. Variant-sequence transthyretin (isoleucine 122) in late-onset cardiac amyloidosis in black Americans. *N Engl J Med* 1997;336:466–473.

347. Benson MD. Aging, amyloid, and cardiomyopathy. *N Engl J Med* 1997;336:502–504.

348. Olson LJ, Gertz MA, Edwards WD, et al. Senile cardiac amyloidosis with myocardial dysfunction. Diagnosis by endomyocardial biopsy and immunohistochemistry. *N Engl J Med* 1987;317:738–742.

349. Smith TJ, Kyle RA, Lie JT. Clinical significance of histopathologic patterns of cardiac amyloidosis. *Mayo Clin Proc* 1984;59:547–555.

350. Benson MD. Hereditary amyloidosis and cardiomyopathy. *Am J Med* 1992;93:1–2.

351. Cueto-Garcia L, Tajik AJ, Kyle RA, et al. Serial echocardiographic observations in patients with primary systemic amyloidosis: an introduction to the concept of early

(asymptomatic) amyloid infiltration of the heart. *Mayo Clin Proc* 1984;59:589–597.

352. Barth RF, Willerson JT, Buja LM, et al. Amyloid coronary artery disease, primary systemic amyloidosis and paraproteinemia. *Arch Intern Med* 1970;126:627–630.

353. Mueller PS, Edwards WD, Gertz MA. Symptomatic ischemic heart disease resulting from obstructive intramural coronary amyloidosis. *Am J Med* 2000;109:181–188.

354. Hesse A, Altland K, Linke RP, et al. Cardiac amyloidosis: a review and report of a new transthyretin (prealbumin) variant. *Br Heart J* 1993;70:111–115.

355. Dubrey SW, Cha K, Skinner M, et al. Familial and primary (AL) cardiac amyloidosis: echocardiographically similar diseases with distinctly different clinical outcomes. *Heart* 1997;78:74–82.

356. Siqueira-Filho AG, Cunha CL, Tajik AJ, et al. M-mode and two-dimensional echocardiographic features in cardiac amyloidosis. *Circulation* 1981;63:188–196.

357. Chiaramida SA, Goldman MA, Zema MJ, et al. Real-time cross-sectional echocardiographic diagnosis of infiltrative cardiomyopathy due to amyloid. *J Clin Ultrasound* 1980;8:58–62.

358. Chandrasekaran K, Aylward PE, Fleagle SR, et al. Feasibility of identifying amyloid and hypertrophic cardiomyopathy with the use of computerized quantitative texture analysis of clinical echocardiographic data. *J Am Coll Cardiol* 1989;13:832–840.

359. Carroll JD, Gaasch WH, McAdam KP. Amyloid cardiomyopathy: characterization by a distinctive voltage/mass relation. *Am J Cardiol* 1982;49:9–13.

360. Falk RH, Plehn JF, Deering T, et al. Sensitivity and specificity of the echocardiographic features of cardiac amyloidosis. *Am J Cardiol* 1987;59:418–422.

361. Chew C, Ziady GM, Raphael MJ, et al. The functional defect in amyloid heart disease. The "stiff heart" syndrome. *Am J Cardiol* 1975;36:438–444.

362. St. John Sutton MG, Reichek N, Kastor JA, et al. Computerized M-mode echocardiographic analysis of left ventricular dysfunction in cardiac amyloid. *Circulation* 1982;66:790–799.

363. Cueto-Garcia L, Reeder GS, Kyle RA, et al. Echocardiographic findings in systemic amyloidosis: spectrum of cardiac involvement and relation to survival. *J Am Coll Cardiol* 1985;6:737–743.

364. Tei C, Dujardin KS, Hodge DO, et al. Doppler index combining systolic and diastolic myocardial performance: clinical value in cardiac amyloidosis. *J Am Coll Cardiol* 1996;28:658–664.

365. Patel AR, Dubrey SW, Mendes LA, et al. Right ventricular dilation in primary amyloidosis: an independent predictor of survival. *Am J Cardiol* 1997;80:486–492.

366. Oh JK, Tajik AJ, Edwards WD, et al. Dynamic left ventricular outflow tract obstruction in cardiac amyloidosis detected by continuous-wave Doppler echocardiography. *Am J Cardiol* 1987;59:1008–1010.

367. Hongo M, Fujii T, Hirayama J, et al. Radionuclide angiographic assessment of left ventricular diastolic filling in amyloid heart disease: a study of patients with familial amyloid polyneuropathy. *J Am Coll Cardiol* 1989;13:48–53.

368. Hongo M, Hirayama J, Fujii T, et al. Early identification of amyloid heart disease by technetium-99m-pyrophosphate scintigraphy: a study with familial amyloid polyneuropathy. *Am Heart J* 1987;113:654–662.

369. Lekakis J, Nanas J, Moustafellou C, et al. Cardiac amyloidosis detected by indium-111 antimyosin imaging. *Am Heart J* 1992;124:1630–1631.

370. Gertz MA, Grogan M, Kyle RA, et al. Endomyocardial biopsy-proven light chain amyloidosis (AL) without echocardiographic features of infiltrative cardiomyopathy. *Am J Cardiol* 1997;80:93–95.

371. Gertz MA, Lacy MQ, Dispenzieri A. Amyloidosis: recognition, confirmation, prognosis, and therapy. *Mayo Clin Proc* 1999;74:490–494.

372. von Kemp K, Beckers R, Vandenweghe J, et al. Echocardiography and magnetic resonance imaging in cardiac amyloidosis. *Acta Cardiol* 1989;44:29–36.

373. Sechtem U, Higgins CB, Sommerhoff BA, et al. Magnetic resonance imaging of restrictive cardiomyopathy. *Am J Cardiol* 1987;59:480–482.

374. Gertz MA, Kyle RA. Amyloidosis: prognosis and treatment. *Semin Arthritis Rheum* 1994;24:124–138.

375. Skinner M, Anderson J, Wang M, et al. Treatment of patients with primary amyloidosis. In: Kisilevsky R, Benson MD, Frangione B, et al., eds. *Amyloid and amyloidosis 1993*. New York: Parthenon, 1994:232–234.

376. Kyle RA, Gertz MA, Garton JP, et al. Primary systemic amyloidosis (AL): randomized trial of colchicine vs melphalan and prednisone vs melphelan, prednisone, and colchicine. In: Kisilevsky R, Benson MD, Frangione B, et al., ed. *Amyloid and amyloidosis 1993*. New York: Parthenon, 1994:648–650.

377. Skinner M, Anderson J, Simms R, et al. Treatment of 100 patients with primary amyloidosis; a randomized trial of melphalan, prednisone, and colchicine versus colchicine alone. *Am J Med* 1996;100:290–298.

378. Comenzo RL, Vosburgh E, Falk RH, et al. Dose-intensive melphalan with blood stem-cell support for the treatment of AL (amyloid light-chain) amyloidosis: survival and responses in 25 patients. *Blood* 1998;91:3662–3670.

379. Dubrey S, Simms RW, Skinner M, et al. Recurrence of primary (AL) amyloidosis in a transplanted heart with four-year survival. *Am J Cardiol* 1995;76:739–741.

380. Pelosi F Jr, Capehart J, Roberts WC. Effectiveness of cardiac transplantation for primary (AL) cardiac amyloidosis. *Am J Cardiol* 1997;79:532–535.

381. Holmgren G, Ericzon BG, Groth CG, et al. Clinical improvement and amyloid regression after liver transplantation in hereditary transthyretin amyloidosis. *Lancet* 1993;341:1113–1116.

382. Skinner M, Lewis WD, Jones LA, et al. Liver transplantation as a treatment for familial amyloidotic polyneuropathy. *Ann Intern Med* 1994;120:133–134.

383. Rubinow A, Skinner M, Cohen AS. Digoxin sensitivity in amyloid cardiomyopathy. *Circulation* 1981;63:1285–1288.

384. Pollak A, Falk RH. Left ventricular systolic dysfunction precipitated by verapamil in cardiac amyloidosis. *Chest* 1993;104:618–620.

385. Wright JR, Calkins E. Clinical-pathologic differentiation of common amyloid syndromes. *Medicine* 1981;60:429–448.

386. Willens HJ, Levy R, Kessler KM. Thromboembolic complications in cardiac amyloidosis detected by transesophageal echocardiography. *Am Heart J* 1995;129:405–406.

387. Zelitch SR, Israel HL. Sarcoidosis. *Am Fam Physician* 1988;38:127–139.

388. Alton M, Juhlin-Dannfelt A, Pehrsson SK, et al. Sarcoid heart disease. *Sarcoidosis* 1992;9:147–149.

389. Rizzato G, Pezzano A, Sala G, et al. Right heart impairment in sarcoidosis: haemodynamic and echocardiographic study. *Eur J Respir Dis* 1983;64:121–128.

390. Silverman KJ, Hutchins GM, Bulkley BH. Cardiac sarcoid: a clinicopathologic study of 84 unselected patients with systemic sarcoidosis. *Circulation* 1978;58:1204–1211.

391. Gibbons WJ, Levy RD, Nava S, et al. Subclinical cardiac dysfunction in sarcoidosis. *Chest* 1991;100:44–50.

392. Sharma OP. Myocardial sarcoidosis. A wolf in sheep's clothing. *Chest* 1994;106:988–990.

393. Sharma OP, Maheshwari A, Thaker K. Myocardial sarcoidosis. *Chest* 1993;103:253–258.

394. Roberts WC, McAllister HA Jr, Ferrans VJ. Sarcoidosis of the heart. A clinicopathologic study of 35 necropsy patients (group 1) and review of 78 previously described necropsy patients (group 11). *Am J Med* 1977;63:86–108.

395. Bohle W, Schaefer HE. Predominant myocardial sarcoidosis. *Pathol Res Pract* 1994;190:212–217.

396. Jain A, Starek PJ, Delany DL. Ventricular tachycardia and ventricular aneurysm due to unrecognized sarcoidosis. *Clin Cardiol* 1990;13:738–740.

397. Angomachalelis N, Hourzamanis A, Vamvalis C, et al. Doppler echocardiographic evaluation of left ventricular diastolic function in patients with systemic sarcoidosis. *Postgrad Med J* 1992;68[Suppl 1]:S52–S56.

398. Ueda M, Fujimoto T, Shoji S, et al. Cardiac sarcoidosis. *Jpn Heart J* 1990;31:251–258.

399. Cepin D, McDonough M, James F. Cardiac sarcoidosis. A case with unusual manifestation. *Arch Intern Med* 1983;143:142–144.

400. Huang PL, Brooks R, Carpenter C, et al. Antiarrhythmic therapy guided by programmed electrical stimulation in cardiac sarcoidosis with ventricular tachycardia. *Am Heart J* 1991;121:599–601.

401. Winters SL, Cohen M, Greenberg S, et al. Sustained ventricular tachycardia associated with sarcoidosis: assessment of the underlying cardiac anatomy and the prospective utility of programmed ventricular stimulation, drug therapy and an implantable antitachycardia device. *J Am Coll Cardiol* 1991;18:937–943.

402. Kavanagh T, Huang S. Cardiac sarcoidosis: an unforeseen cause of sudden death. *Can J Cardiol* 1995;11:136–138.

403. Shammas RL, Movahed A. Sarcoidosis of the heart. *Clin Cardiol* 1993;16:462–472.

404. Sekiguchi M, Yazaki Y, Isobe M, et al. Cardiac sarcoidosis: diagnostic, prognostic, and therapeutic considerations. *Cardiovasc Drugs Ther* 1996;10:495–510.

405. Gregor P, Widimsky P, Sladkova T, et al. Echocardiography in sarcoidosis. *Jpn Heart J* 1984;25:499–508.

406. Kinney EL, Jackson GL, Reeves WC, et al. Thallium-scan myocardial defects and echocardiographic abnormalities in patients with sarcoidosis without clinical cardiac dysfunction. An analysis of 44 patients. *Am J Med* 1980;68:497–503.

407. Lewin RF, Mor R, Spitzer S, et al. Echocardiographic evaluation of patients with systemic sarcoidosis. *Am Heart J* 1985;110:116–122.

408. Burstow DJ, Tajik AJ, Bailey KR, et al. Two-dimensional echocardiographic findings in systemic sarcoidosis. *Am J Cardiol* 1989;63:478–482.

409. Valantine H, McKenna WJ, Nihoyannopoulos P, et al. Sarcoidosis: a pattern of clinical and morphological presentation. *Br Heart J* 1987;57:256–263.

410. Fahy GJ, Marwick T, McCreery CJ, et al. Doppler echocardiographic detection of left ventricular diastolic dysfunction in patients with pulmonary sarcoidosis. *Chest* 1996;109:62–66.

411. Tawarahara K, Kurata C, Okayama K, et al. Thallium-201 and gallium 67 single photon emission computed tomographic imaging in cardiac sarcoidosis. *Am Heart J* 1992;124:1383–1384.

412. Yamamoto N, Gotoh K, Yagi Y, et al. Thallium-201 myocardial SPECT findings at rest in sarcoidosis. *Ann Nucl Med* 1993;7:97–103.

413. Taki J, Nakajima K, Bunko H, et al. Cardiac sarcoidosis demonstrated by Tl-201 and Ga-67 SPECT imaging. *Clin Nucl Med* 1990;15:636–639.

414. Fields CL, Ossorio MA, Roy TM, et al. Thallium-201 scintigraphy in the diagnosis and management of myocardial sarcoidosis. *South Med J* 1990;83:339–342.

415. Riedy K, Fisher MR, Belic N, et al. MR imaging of myocardial sarcoidosis. *AJR Am J Roentgenol* 1988;151:915–916.

416. Matsuki M, Matsuo M. MR findings of myocardial sarcoidosis. *Clin Radiol* 2000;55:323–325.

417. Shiotani H, Miyazaki T, Matsunaga K, et al. Improvement of severe heart failure with corticosteroid therapy in a patient with myocardial sarcoidosis. *Jpn Circ J* 1991;55:393–396.

418. Schaedel H, Kirsten D, Schmidt A, et al. Sarcoid heart disease—results of follow-up investigations. *Eur Heart J* 1991;12[Suppl D]:26–27.

419. Shammas RL, Movahed A. Successful treatment of myocardial sarcoidosis with steroids. *Sarcoidosis* 1994;11:37–39.

420. Bajaj AK, Kopelman HA, Echt DS. Cardiac sarcoidosis with sudden death: treatment with the automatic implantable cardioverter defibrillator. *Am Heart J* 1988;116:557–560.

421. Paz HL, McCormick DJ, Kutalek SP, et al. The automated implantable cardiac defibrillator. Prophylaxis in cardiac sarcoidosis. *Chest* 1994;106:1603–1607.

422. Smith RL, Hutchins GM, Sack GH, et al. Unusual cardiac, renal and pulmonary involvement in Gaucher's disease. Intersitial glucocerebroside accumulation, pulmonary hypertension and fatal bone marrow embolization. *Am J Med* 1978;65:352–360.

423. Saraclar M, Atalay S, Kocak N, et al. Gaucher's disease with mitral and aortic involvement: echocardiographic findings. *Pediatr Cardiol* 1992;13:56–58.

424. Elstein D, Klutstein MW, Lahad A, et al. Echocardiographic assessment of pulmonary hypertension in Gaucher's disease. *Lancet* 1998;351:1544–1546.

425. Alizad A, Seward JB. Echocardiographic features of genetic diseases: part 2. Storage disease. *J Am Soc Echocardiogr* 2000;13:164–170.

426. Beutler E. Gaucher disease. *Curr Opin Hematol* 1997;4:19–23.

427. Dangel JH. Cardiovascular changes in children with mucopolysaccharide storage diseases and related disorders—clinical and echocardiographic findings in 64 patients. *Eur J Pediatr* 1998;157:534–538.

428. Fischer TA, Lehr HA, Nixdorff U, et al. Combined aortic and mitral stenosis in mucopolysaccharidosis type I-S (Ullrich-Scheie syndrome). *Heart* 1999;81:97–99.

429. Renteria VG, Ferrans VJ, Roberts WC. The heart in the Hurler syndrome: gross, histologic, and ultrastructural observations in five necropsy cases. *Am J Cardiol* 1976;38:487–501.

430. Gross DM, Williams JC, Caaprioli C, et al. Echocardiographic abnormalities in the mucopolysaccharide storage diseases. *Am J Cardiol* 1988;61:170–176.

431. Weinberg BA, Conces DJ Jr, Waller BF. Cardiac manifestations of noncardiac tumors. Part I: Direct effects. *Clin Cardiol* 1989;12:289–296.

432. Lestuzzi C, Biasi S, Nicolosi GL, et al. Secondary neoplastic infiltration of the myocardium diagnosed by two-dimensional echocardiography in seven cases with anatomic confirmation. *J Am Coll Cardiol* 1987;9:439–445.

433. Hauser SC. Hemochromatosis and the heart. *Heart Dis Stroke* 1993;2:487–491.

434. Buja LM, Roberts WC. Iron in the heart, etiology, and clinical significance. *Am J Med* 1971;51:209–221.

435. Olson LJ, Edwards WD, McCall JT, et al. Cardiac iron deposition in idiopathic hemochromatosis: histologic and analytic assessment of 14 hearts from autopsy. *J Am Coll Cardiol* 1987;10:1239–1243.

436. Cecchetti G, Binda A, Piperno A, et al. Cardiac alterations in 36 consecutive patients with idiopathic hemochromatosis: polygraphic and echocardiographic evaluation. *Eur Heart J* 1991;12:224–230.

437. Candell-Riera J, Lu L, Seres L, et al. Cardiac hemochromatosis: beneficial effects of iron removal therapy. An echocardiographic study. *Am J Cardiol* 1983;52:824–829.

438. Short EM, Winkle RA, Billingham ME. Myocardial involvement in idiopathic hemochromatosis. Morphologic and clinical improvement following venesection. *Am J Med* 1981;70:1275–1279.

439. Olson LJ, Baldus WP, Tajik AJ. Echocardiographic features in idiopathic hemochromatosis. *Am J Cardiol* 1987;60:885–889.

440. Olson LJ, Edwards WD, Holmes DR, et al. Endomyocardial biopsy in hemochromatosis: clinicopathologic correlates in six cases. *J Am Coll Cardiol* 1989;13:116–120.

441. Dabestani A, Child JS, Henze E, et al. Primary hemochromatosis: anatomic and physiologic characteristics of the cardiac ventricles and their response to phlebotomy. *Am J Cardiol* 1984;54:153–159.

442. Henry WL, Nienhuis AW, Wiener M, et al. Echocardiographic abnormalities in patients with transfusion-dependent anemia and secondary myocardial iron deposition. *Am J Med* 1978;64:547–555.

443. Blankenberg F, Eisenberg S, Scheinman MN, et al. Use of cine gradient echo (GRE) MR in the imaging of cardiac hemochromatosis. *J Comput Assist Tomogr* 1994;18:136–138.

444. Przybojewski JZ. Endomyocardial biopsy: a review of the literature. *Cathet Cardiovasc Diagn* 1985;11:287–330.

445. Porter J, Cary N, Schofield P. Haemochromatosis presenting as congestive cardiac failure. *Br Heart J* 1995;73:73–75.

446. Rivers J, Garrahy P, Robinson W, et al. Reversible cardiac dysfunction in hemochromatosis. *Am Heart J* 1987;113:216–217.

447. Westra WH, Hruban RH, Baughman KL, et al. Progressive hemochromatotic cardiomyopathy despite reversal of iron deposition after liver transplantation. *Am J Clin Pathol* 1993;99:39–44.

448. Case records of the Massachusetts General Hospital. Weekly clinicopathological exercises. Case 31-1994. A 25-year-old man with the recent onset of diabetes mellitus and congestive heart failure. *N Engl J Med* 1994;331:460–466.

449. Hwang B, Meng CC, Lin CY, et al. Clinical analysis of five infants with glycogen storage disease of the heart—Pompe's disease. *Jpn Heart J* 1986;27:25–34.

450. Olson LJ, Reeder GS, Noller KL, et al. Cardiac involvement in glycogen storage disease III: morphologic and biochemical characterization with endomyocardial biopsy. *Am J Cardiol* 1984;53:980–981.

451. Coleman RA, Winter HS, Wolf B, et al. Glycogen storage disease type III (glycogen debranching enzyme deficiency): correlation of biochemical defects with myopathy and cardiomyopathy. *Ann Intern Med* 1992;116:896–900.

452. Carvalho JS, Matthews EE, Leonard JV, et al. Cardiomyopathy of glycogen storage disease type III. *Heart Vessels* 1993;8:155–159.

453. Sakuraba H, Yanagawa Y, Igarashi T, et al. Cardiovascular manifestations in Fabry's disease. A high incidence of mitral valve prolapse in hemizygotes and heterozygotes. *Clin Genet* 1986;29:276–283.

454. Bass JL, Shrivastava S, Grabowski GA, et al. The M-mode echocardiogram in Fabry's disease. *Am Heart J* 1980;100:807–812.

455. Cohen IS, Fluri-Lundeen J, Wharton TP. Two dimensional echocardiographic similarity of Fabry's disease to cardiac amyloidosis: a function of ultrastructural analogy? *J Clin Ultrasound* 1983;11:437–441.

456. Tanaka H, Adachi K, Yamashita Y, et al. [Four cases of Fabry's disease mimicking hypertrophic cardiomyopathy]. *J Cardiol* 1988;18:705–718.

457. Pochis WT, Litzow JT, King BG, et al. Electrophysiologic findings in Fabry's disease with a short PR interval. *Am J Cardiol* 1994;74:203–204.

458. Linhart A, Palecek T, Bultas J, et al. New insights in cardiac structural changes in patients with Fabry's disease. *Am Heart J* 2000;139:1101–1108.

459. Matsui S, Murakami E, Takekoshi N, et al. Myocardial tissue characterization by magnetic resonance imaging in Fabry's disease. *Am Heart J* 1989;117:472–474.

460. von Scheidt W, Eng CM, Fitzmaurice TF, et al. An atypical variant of Fabry's disease with manifestations confined to the myocardium. *N Engl J Med* 1991;324:395–399.

461. Maben P, Evans R, Lin J, et al. Endomyocardial biopsy. Diagnosis of Fabry's disease in congestive cardiomyopathy. *J Kans Med Soc* 1983;84:556–557.

462. McGuire MR, Pugh DM, Dunn MI. Carcinoid heart disease. Restrictive cardiomyopathy as a late complication. *J Kans Med Soc* 1978;79:661–662, 665.

463. Strickman NE, Hall RJ. Carcinoid heart disease. In: Kapoor AS, Reynolds RD, ed. *Cancer and the heart.* New York: Springer Verlag, 1986:135–156.

464. Pellikka PA, Tajik AJ, Khandheria BK, et al. Carcinoid heart disease. Clinical and echocardiographic spectrum in 74 patients. *Circulation* 1993;87:1188–1196.

465. Robiolio PA, Rigolin VH, Wilson JS, et al. Carcinoid heart disease. Correlation of high serotonin levels with valvular abnormalities detected by cardiac catheterization and echocardiography. *Circulation* 1995;92:790–795.

466. Lundin L. Carcinoid heart disease. A cardiologist's viewpoint. *Acta Oncologica* 1991;30:499–502.

467. Millward MJ, Blake MP, Byrne MJ, et al. Left heart involvement with cardiac shunt complicating carcinoid heart disease. *Aust N Z J Med* 1989;19:716–717.

468. Blick DR, Zoghbi WA, Lawrie GM, et al. Carcinoid heart disease presenting as right-to-left shunt and congestive heart failure: successful surgical treatment. *Am Heart J* 1988;115:201–203.

468a. Connolly HM, Schaff HV, Mullany CJ, et al. Surgical management of left-sided carcinoid heart disease. *Circulation* 2001;104[Suppl 1]:I36–I40.

469. Lundin L, Funa K, Hansson HE, et al. Histochemical and immunohistochemical morphology of carcinoid heart disease. *Pathol Res Pract* 1991;187:73–77.

470. Waltenberger J, Lundin L, Oberg K, et al. Involvement of transforming growth factor-beta in the formation of fibrotic lesions in carcinoid heart disease. *Am J Pathol* 1993;142:71–78.

471. Ross EM, Roberts WC. The carcinoid syndrome: comparison of 21 necropsy subjects with carcinoid heart disease to 15 necropsy subjects without carcinoid heart disease. *Am J Med* 1985;79:339–354.

472. Lundin L, Landelius J, Andren B, et al. Transesophageal echocardiography improves the diagnostic value of cardiac ultrasound in patients with carcinoid heart disease. *Br Heart J* 1990;64:190–194.

473. Lundin L, Norheim I, Landelius J, et al. Carcinoid heart disease: relationship of circulating vasoactive substances to ultrasound-detectable cardiac abnormalities. *Circulation* 1988;77:264–269.

474. Denney WD, Kemp WE Jr, Anthony LB, et al. Echocardiographic and biochemical evaluation of the development and progression of carcinoid heart disease. *J Am Coll Cardiol* 1998;32:1017–1022.

475. Callahan JA, Wroblewski EM, Reeder GS, et al. Echocardiographic features of carcinoid heart disease. *Am J Cardiol* 1982;50:762–768.

476. Roberts WC. A unique heart disease associated with a unique cancer: carcinoid heart disease. *Am J Cardiol* 1997;80:251–256.

477. Le Metayer P, Constans J, Bernard N, et al. Carcinoid heart disease: two cases of left heart involvement diagnosed by transthoracic and transoesophageal echocardiography. *Eur Heart J* 1993;14:1721–1723.

478. Connolly HM, Nishimura RA, Smith HC, et al. Outcome of cardiac surgery for carcinoid heart disease. *J Am Coll Cardiol* 1995;25:410–416.

479. Ruszniewski P, Malka D. Hepatic arterial chemoembolization in the management of advanced digestive endocrine tumors. *Digestion* 2000;62[Suppl 1]:79–83.

480. Kvols LK. Metastatic carcinoid tumors and the malignant carcinoid syndrome. *Ann N Y Acad Sci* 1994;733:464–470.

481. Oates JA. The carcinoid syndrome. *N Engl J Med* 1986;315:702–704.

482. O'Toole D, Ducreux M, Bommelaer G, et al. Treatment of carcinoid syndrome: a prospective crossover evaluation of lanreotide versus octreotide in terms of efficacy, patient acceptability, and tolerance. *Cancer* 2000;88:770–776.

483. Mullins PA, Hall JA, Shapiro LM. Balloon dilatation of tricuspid stenosis caused by carcinoid heart disease. *Br Heart J* 1990;63:249–250.

484. Grant SC, Scarffe JH, Levy RD, et al. Failure of balloon dilatation of the pulmonary valve in carcinoid pulmonary stenosis. *Br Heart J* 1992;67:450–453.

485. Onate A, Alcibar J, Inguanzo R, et al. Balloon dilation of tricuspid and pulmonary valves in carcinoid heart disease. *Tex Heart Inst J* 1993;20:115–119.

486. Hargreaves AD, Pringle SD, Boon NA. Successful balloon dilatation of the pulmonary valve in carcinoid heart disease. *Int J Cardiol* 1994;45:150–151.

487. Lundin L, Hansson HE, Landelius J, et al. Surgical treatment of carcinoid heart disease. *J Thorac Cardiovasc Surg* 1990;100:552–561.

488. Knott-Craig CJ, Schaff HV, Mullany CJ, et al. Carcinoid disease of the heart. Surgical management of ten patients. *J Thorac Cardiovasc Surg* 1992;104:475–481.

489. Ohri SK, Schofield JB, Hodgson H, et al. Carcinoid heart disease: early failure of an allograft valve replacement. *Ann Thorac Surg* 1994;58:1161–1163.

490. Robiolio PA, Rigolin VH, Harrison JK, et al. Predictors of outcome of tricuspid valve replacement in carcinoid heart disease. *Am J Cardiol* 1995;75:485–488.

491. Glanzmann C, Huguenin P, Lutolf UM, et al. Cardiac lesions after mediastinal irradiation for Hodgkin's disease. *Radiother Oncol* 1994;30:43–54.

492. Vallebona A. Cardiac damage following therapeutic chest irradiation. Importance, evaluation and treatment. *Minerva Cardioangiol* 2000;48:79–87.

493. Brosius FC 3d, Waller BF, Roberts WC. Radiation heart disease. Analysis of 16 young (aged 15 to 33 years) necropsy patients who received over 3,500 rads to the heart. *Am J Med* 1981;70:519–530.

494. Botti RE, Driscol TE, Pearson OH, et al. Radiation myocardial fibrosis simulating constrictive pericarditis. A review of the literature and a case report. *Cancer* 1968;22:1254–1261.

495. Westerhof PW, van der Putte CJ. Radiation pericarditis and myocardial fibrosis. *Eur J Cardiol* 1976;4:213–218.

496. Bu'Lock FA, Mott MG, Oakhill A, et al. Left ventricular diastolic function after anthracycline chemotherapy in childhood: relation with systolic function, symptoms, and pathophysiology. *Br Heart J* 1995;73:340–350.

497. Mortensen SA, Olsen HS, Baandrup U. Chronic anthracycline cardiotoxicity: haemodynamic and histopathological manifestations suggesting a restrictive endomyocardial disease. *Br Heart J* 1986;55:274–282.

498. Schmitt K, Tulzer G, Merl M, et al. Early detection of doxorubicin and daunorubicin cardiotoxicity by echocardiography: diastolic versus systolic parameters. *Eur J Pediatr* 1995;154:201–204.

499. De Wolf D, Suys B, Verhaaren H, et al. Low-dose dobutamine stress echocardiography in children and young adults. *Am J Cardiol* 1998;81:895–901.

500. De Wolf D, Suys B, Maurus R, et al. Dobutamine stress echocardiography in the evaluation of late anthracycline cardiotoxicity in childhood cancer survivors. *Pediatr Res* 1996;39:504–512.

501. Suzuki J, Yanagisawa A, Shigeyama T, et al. Early detection of anthracycline-induced cardiotoxicity by radionuclide angiocardiography. *Angiology* 1999;50:37–45.

502. Tjeerdsma G, Meinardi MT, van Der Graaf WT, et al. Early detection of anthracycline induced cardiotoxicity in asymptomatic patients with normal left ventricular systolic function: autonomic versus echocardiographic variables. *Heart* 1999;81:419–423.

503. Siveski-Iliskovic N, Hill M, Chow DA, et al. Probucol protects against Adriamycin cardiomyopathy without interfering with its antitumor effect. *Circulation* 1995;91:10–15.

504. Singal PK, Siveski-Iliskovic N, Hill M, et al. Combination therapy with probucol prevents Adriamycin-induced cardiomyopathy. *J Mol Cell Cardiol* 1995;27:1055–1063.

505. Schurle DR, Evans RW, Cohlmia JB, et al. Restrictive cardiomyopathy in scleroderma. *J Kans Med Soc* 1984;85:49–50.

506. Moore K. *Clinically oriented anatomy*. Baltimore: Williams & Wilkins, 1982.

507. Holt JP. The normal pericardium. *Am J Cardiol* 1970;26:455–465.

508. Ishihara T, Ferrans VJ, Jones M, et al. Histologic and ultrastructural features of normal human parietal pericardium. *Am J Cardiol* 1980;46:744–753.

509. Wiegner AW, Bing OH, Borg TK, et al. Mechanical and structural correlates of canine pericardium. *Circ Res* 1981;49:807–814.

510. Nolan RD, Dusting GJ, Jakubowski J, et al. The pericardium as a source of prostacyclin in the dog, ox and rat. *Prostaglandins* 1982;24:887–902.

511. Miyazake T, Pride HP, Zipes DP. Prostaglandins in the pericardial fluid modulate neural regulation of cardiac electrophysiological properties. *Circ Res* 1990;66:163–175.

512. Lee MC, LeWinter MM, Freeman GL, et al. Biaxial mechanical properties of the pericardium in normal and volume overloaded dogs. *Am J Physiol* 1985;249:H222–H230.

513. Shabetai R. Pericardial and cardiac pressure. *Circulation* 1988;77:1–5.

514. Spodick DH. Macrophysiology, microphysiology, and anatomy of the pericardium: a synopsis. *Am Heart J* 1992;124:1046–1051.

515. Freeman GL, LeWinter MM. Pericardial adaptations during chronic cardiac dilation in dogs. *Circ Res* 1984;54:294–300.

516. Janicki JS. Influence of the pericardium and ventricular interdependence on left ventricular diastolic and systolic function in patients with heart failure. *Circulation* 1990;81[2 Suppl]:III15–III20.

517. Elzinga G, van Grondelle R, Westerhof N, et al. Ventricular interference. *Am J Physiol* 1974;226:941–947.

518. Appleton CP, Hatle LK, Popp RL. Cardiac tamponade and pericardial effusion: respiratory variation in transvalvular flow velocities studied by Doppler echocardiography. *J Am Coll Cardiol* 1988;11:1020–1030.

519. Burstow DJ, Oh JK, Bailey KR, et al. Cardiac tamponade: characteristic Doppler observations. *Mayo Clin Proc* 1989;64:312–324.

520. Spodick DH. Acoustic phenomena in pericardial disease. *Am Heart J* 1971;81:114–124.

521. Spodick DH. Electrocardiogram in acute pericarditis. Distributions of morphologic and axial changes by stages. *Am J Cardiol* 1974;33:470–474.

522. Baljepally R, Spodick DH. PR-segment deviation as the initial electrocardiographic response in acute pericarditis. *Am J Cardiol* 1998;81:1505–1506.

523. Spodick DH. Diagnostic electrocardiographic sequences in acute pericarditis. Significance of PR segment and PR vector changes. *Circulation* 1973;48:575–580.

524. Spodick DH. Differential characteristics of the electrocardiogram in early repolarization and acute pericarditis. *N Engl J Med* 1976;295:523–526.

525. Spodick DH. Arrhythmias during acute pericarditis: a prospective study of 100 consecutive cases. *JAMA* 1976;235:39–41.

526. Coupland DB, Terriff B, Fung AY, et al. The "hot halo" sign. Pyogenic pericarditis on In-111 leukocyte scintigraphy. *Clin Nucl Med* 1992;17:579–580.

527. Parry R, Akhtar N, Hartnell GG. Case report: unsuspected pericarditis diagnosed with gallium 67 scan. *Clin Radiol* 1993;48:332–333.

528. Kodama K, Igase M, Funada J, et al. Gallium-67 citrate scintigraphy in idiopathic pericarditis—report of a case. *Jpn Circ J* 1994;58:298–302.

529. Bonnefoy E, Godon P, Kirkorian G, et al. Serum cardiac troponin I and ST-segment elevation in patients with acute pericarditis. *Eur Heart J* 2000;21:832–836.

530. Matsuoka H, Hamada M, Honda T, et al. Precise assessment of myocardial damage associated with secondary cardiomyopathies by use of Gd-DTPA-enhanced magnetic resonance imaging. *Angiology* 1993;44:945–950.

531. Permanyer-Miralda G, Sagrista-Sauleda J, Soler-Soler J. Primary acute pericardial disease: a prospective series of 231 consecutive patients. *Am J Cardiol* 1985;56:623–630.

532. Berger M, Bobak L, Jelveh M, et al. Pericardial effusion diagnosed by echocardiography. Clinical and electrocardiographic findings in 171 patients. *Chest* 1978;74:174–179.

533. Horowitz MS, Schultz CS, Stinson EB, et al. Sensitivity and specificity of echocardiographic diagnosis of pericardial effusion. *Circulation* 1974;50:239–247.

534. Riba AL, Morganroth J. Unsuspected substantial pericardial effusions detected by echocardiography. *JAMA* 1976;236:2623–2625.

535. Soler-Soler J. Massive chronic pericardial effusion. In: Soler-Soler J, Permanyer-Miralda G, Sagrista-Sauleda J, ed. *Pericardial diseases—old dilemmas and new insights.* The Netherlands: Kluwer, 1990:153–165.

536. Fowler N. Chronic pericarditis. In: No F, ed. *The pericardium in health and disease.* Mount Kisco: Futura Publishing, 1985:217–334.

537. Sagrista-Sauleda J, Angel J, Permanyer-Miralda G, et al. Long-term follow-up of idiopathic chronic pericardial effusion. *N Engl J Med* 1999;341:2054–2059.

538. Spodick DH. Pericarditis, pericardial effusion, cardiac tamponade, and constriction. *Crit Care Clin* 1989;5:455–476.

539. Mulvagh SL, Rokey R, Vick GW, et al. Usefulness of nuclear magnetic resonance imaging for evaluation of pericardial effusions, and comparison with two-dimensional echocardiography. *Am J Cardiol* 1989;64:1002–1009.

540. Leimgruber PP, Klopfenstein HS, Wann LS, et al. The hemodynamic derangement associated with right ventricular diastolic collapse in cardiac tamponade: an experimental echocardiographic study. *Circulation* 1983;68:612–620.

541. Spodick DH. The normal and diseased pericardium: current concepts of pericardial physiology, diagnosis and treatment. *J Am Coll Cardiol* 1983;1:240–251.

542. Lorell BH, Grossman W. Profiles in constrictive pericarditis, restrictive cardiomyopathy and cardiac tamponade. In: Baim DS, Grossman W, eds. *Cardiac catheterization, angiography and intervention.* Baltimore: Williams & Wilkins, 1996:801–857.

543. Shabetai R. The pathophysiology of cardiac tamponade. *Cardiovasc Clin* 1976;7:67–89.

544. Gauchat HW, Katz LN. Observations of pulsus paradoxus (with special reference to pericardial effusions) I. Clinical. *Arch Intern Med* 1924;33:371–393.

545. Katz LN, Gauchat HW. Observations of pulsus paradoxus (with special reference to pericardial effusions) II. Experimental. *Arch Intern Med* 1924;33:371–393.

546. Fowler NO. Pulsus paradoxus. *Heart Dis Stroke* 1994;3:68–69.

547. Beck CS. Two cardiac compression triads. *JAMA* 1935;104:714–716.

548. Spodick DH. Cardiac tamponade: clinical characteristics, diagnosis and management. In: Spodick DH, ed. *The pericardium: a comprehensive textbook.* New York: Marcel Dekker, 1997.

549. Antman EM, Cargill V, Grossman W. Low-pressure cardiac tamponade. *Ann Intern Med* 1979;91:403–406.

550. Von Sohsten R, Kopistansky C, Cohen M, et al. Cardiac tamponade in the "new device" era: evaluation of 6999 consecutive percutaneous coronary interventions. *Am Heart J* 2000;140:279–283.

551. Kronzon I, Cohen ML, Winer HE. Diastolic atrial compression: a sensitive echocardiographic sign of cardiac tamponade. *J Am Coll Cardiol* 1983;2:770–775.

552. Singh S, Wann LS, Schuchard GH, et al. Right ventricular and right atrial collapse in patients with cardiac tamponade—a combined echocardiographic and hemodynamic study. *Circulation* 1984;70:966–971.

553. Schutzman JJ, Obarski TP, Pearce GL, et al. Comparison of Doppler and two-dimensional echocardiography for assessment of pericardial effusion. *Am J Cardiol* 1992;70:1353–1357.

554. Olson MC, Posniak HV, McDonald V, et al. Computed tomography and magnetic resonance imaging of the pericardium. *Radiographics* 1989;9:633–649.

555. Callahan JA, Seward JB, Nishimura RA, et al. Two-dimensional echocardiographically guided pericardiocentesis: experience in 117 consecutive patients. *Am J Cardiol* 1985;55:476–479.

556. Callahan JA, Seward JB, Tajik AJ. Cardiac tamponade: pericardiocentesis directed by two-dimensional echocardiography. *Mayo Clin Proc* 1985;60:344–347.

557. Salem K, Mulji A, Lonn E. Echocardiographically guided pericardiocentesis—the gold standard for the management of pericardial effusion and cardiac tamponade. *Can J Cardiol* 1999;15:1251–1255.

558. Schiavone WA, Rice TW. Pericardial disease: current diagnosis and management methods. *Cleve Clin J Med* 1989;56:639–645.

559. Tsang TS, Freeman WK, Sinak LJ, et al. Echocardiographically guided pericardiocentesis: evolution and state-of-the-art technique. *Mayo Clin Proc* 1998;73:647–652.

560. VanDyke WH, Cure J, Chakko CS, et al. Pulmonary edema after pericardiocentesis for cardiac tamponade. *N Engl J Med* 1983;309:595–596.

561. Armstrong WF, Feigenbaum H, Dillon JC. Acute right ventricular dilation and echocardiographic volume overload following pericardiocentesis for relief of cardiac tamponade. *Am Heart J* 1984;107:1266–1270.

562. Tsang TS, El-Najdawi EK, Seward JB, et al. Percutaneous echocardiographically guided pericardiocentesis in pediatric patients: evaluation of safety and efficacy. *J Am Soc Echocardiogr* 1998;11:1072–1077.

563. Tsang TS, Barnes ME, Hayes SN, et al. Clinical and echocardiographic characteristics of significant pericardial effusions following cardiothoracic surgery and outcomes of echo-guided pericardiocentesis for management: Mayo Clinic experience, 1979–1998. *Chest* 1999;116:322–331.

564. Flores RM, Jaklitsch MT, DeCamp MM Jr, et al. Video-assisted thoracic surgery pericardial resection for effusive disease. *Chest Surg Clin N Am* 1998;8:835–851.

565. Sugimoto JT, Little AG, Ferguson MK, et al. Pericardial window: mechanisms of efficacy. *Ann Thorac Surg* 1990;50:442–445.

566. Kouvaras G, Polydorou A, Hatziantoniou G. Percutaneous balloon pericardiotomy for management of cardiac tamponade in a patient with lung cancer and large pericardial effusion. *Acta Cardiol* 1994;49:549–553.

567. Fakiolas CN, Beldekos DI, Foussas SG, et al. Percutaneous balloon pericardiotomy as a therapeutic alternative for cardiac tamponade and recurrent pericardial effusion. *Acta Cardiol* 1995;50:65–70.

568. Vora AM, Lokhandwala YY, Kale PA. Echocardiography guided creation of balloon pericardial window. *Cathet Cardiovasc Diagn* 1992;25:164–165.

569. Galli M, Politi A, Pedretti F, et al. Percutaneous balloon pericardiotomy for malignant pericardial tamponade. *Chest* 1995;108:1499–1501.

570. Di Segni E, Lavee J, Kaplinsky E, et al. Percutaneous balloon pericardiostomy for treatment of cardiac tamponade. *Eur Heart J* 1995;16:184–187.

571. Bahl VK, Bhargava B, Chandra S. Percutaneous pericardiotomy using Inoue balloon catheter. *Cathet Cardiovasc Diagn* 1995;36:98–99.

572. Bahl VK, Juneja R, Wasir HS. Percutaneous balloon pericardiotomy for cardiac tamponade. *Indian Heart J* 1994;46:115–116.

573. Ziskind AA, Pearce AC, Lemmon CC, et al. Percutaneous balloon pericardiotomy for the treatment of cardiac tamponade and large pericardial effusions: description of technique and report of the first 50 cases. *J Am Coll Cardiol* 1993;21:1–5.

574. Grossman W, Baim D. *Cardiac catheterization, angiography and intervention.* Philadelphia: Lea & Febiger, 1991.

575. Candell-Riera J, Gutierrez-Palau L, Garcia-del-Castillo H, et al. "Atrial systolic notch" and "early diastolic notch" on the interventricular septal echogram in constrictive pericarditis. *J Am Coll Cardiol* 1985;5:1020–1021.

576. Chandraratna PA, Aronow WS, Imaizumi T. Role of echocardiography in detecting the anatomic and physiologic abnormalities of constrictive pericarditis. *Am J Med Sci* 1982;283:141–146.

577. D'Cruz IA, Dick A, Gross CM, et al. Abnormal left ventricular-left atrial posterior wall contour: a new two-dimensional echocardiographic sign in constrictive pericarditis. *Am Heart J* 1989;118:128–132.

578. Engel PJ, Fowler NO, Tei CW, et al. M-mode echocardiography in constrictive pericarditis. *J Am Coll Cardiol* 1985; 6:471–474.

579. Ling LH, Oh JK, Boonyaratavej S, et al. Diagnostic testing in 135 cases of constrictive pericarditis. *Circulation* 1996;94[Suppl I]:I-667.

580. Mertens LL, Denef B, De Geest H. The differentiation between restrictive cardiomyopathy and constrictive pericarditis: the impact of the imaging techniques. *Echocardiography* 1993;10:497–508.

581. Klodas E, Nishamura RA, Appleton CP, et al. Doppler evaluation of patients with constrictive pericarditis: use of tricuspid regurgitation velocity curves to determine enhanced ventricular interaction. *J Am Coll Cardiol* 1996;28:652–657.

582. Boonyaratavej S, Oh JK, Tajik AJ, et al. Comparison of mitral inflow and superior vena cava Doppler velocities in chronic obstructive pulmonary disease and constrictive pericarditis. *J Am Coll Cardiol* 1998;32:2043–2048.

583. Oki T, Tabata T, Yamada H, et al. Right and left ventricular wall motion velocities as diagnostic indicators of constrictive pericarditis. *Am J Cardiol* 1998;81:465–470.

583a. Ha JW, Oh JK, Ling LH, et al. Annulus paradoxus: transmitral flow velocity to mitral annular velocity ratio is inversely proportional to pulmonary capillary wedge pressure in patients with constrictive pericarditis. *Circulation* 2001;104:976–978.

584. Oh JK, Tajik AJ, Appleton CP, et al. Preload reduction to unmask the characteristic Doppler features of constrictive pericarditis: a new observation. *Circulation* 1997;95:796–799.

585. Klein AL, Al-Assaad AN, Pietrolungo JF, et al. Does rapid volume loading during transesophageal echocardiography differentiate constrictive pericarditis from restrictive cardiomyopathy? *J Am Soc Echocardiogr* 1994;S38:7C.

586. Tabata T, Kabbani SS, Murray RD, et al. Difference in the respiratory variation between mitral inflow and pulmonary venous flow Doppler velocities in patients with constrictive pericarditis. *J Am Soc Echocardiogr* 2000;13:435.

587. Abdalla IA, Murray RD, Awad HE, et al. Reversal of the pattern of respiratory variation of Doppler inflow velocities in constrictive pericarditis during mechanical ventilation. *J Am Soc Echocardiogr* 2000;13:827–831.

588. Pennell DJ, Underwood R. Magnetic resonance imaging of the heart. *Br J Hosp Med* 1993;49:90–95, 98–102.

589. Duvernoy O, Larsson SG, Thuren J, et al. Epicardial fat causing pitfalls in CT and MR imaging of the pericardium. *Acta Radiol* 1992;33:1–5.

590. Harasawa H, Li KS, Nakamoto T, et al. Ventricular coupling via the pericardium: normal versus tamponade. *Cardiovasc Res* 1993;27:1470–1476.

591. Frank H, Globits S. Magnetic resonance imaging evaluation of myocardial and pericardial disease. *J Magn Reson Imaging* 1999;10:617–626.

592. White RD, Zisch RJ. Magnetic resonance imaging of pericardial disease and paracardiac and intracardiac masses. In: Elliot LP, ed. *The fundamentals of cardiac imaging in children and adults*. Philadelphia: JB Lippincott, 1991:420–430.

593. White RD, Hardy PA, Van Dyke CW, et al. Diastolic dysfunction: dynamic MRI velocity-mapping of related flow patterns in the superior vena cava. *J Magn Reson Imaging* 1993;3[Suppl]:65.

594. O'Keeffe D, McCarthy P, O'Regan P. Computed tomography in constrictive pericarditis. *Ir Med J* 1984;77:172–174.

595. Hayashi H, Kawamata H, Machida M, et al. Tuberculous pericarditis: MRI features with contrast enhancement. *Br J Radiol* 1998;71:680–682.

596. Van der Merwe S, Dens J, Daenen W, et al. Pericardial disease is often not recognised as a cause of chronic severe ascites. *J Hepatol* 2000;32:164–169.

597. Abrams J. The jugular venous pulse. In: Abrams J, ed. *Essentials of cardiac physical diagnosis*. Philadelphia: Lea & Febiger, 1987:41–54.

598. Ling LH, Oh JK, Breen JF, et al. Calcific constrictive pericarditis: is it still with us? *Ann Intern Med* 2000;132:444–450.

599. Hasuda T, Satoh T, Yamada N, et al. A case of constrictive pericarditis with local thickening of the pericardium without manifest ventricular interdependence. *Cardiology* 1999;92:214–216.

600. Spodick DH. Constrictive pericarditis. In: Spodick DH, ed. *The pericardium: a comprehensive textbook*. New York: Marcel Dekker, 1997:214–259.

601. Aagaard MT, Haraldsted VY. Chronic constrictive pericarditis treated with total pericardiectomy. *Thorac Cardiovasc Surg* 1984;32:311–314.

602. Astudillo R, Ivert T. Late results after pericardectomy for constrictive pericarditis via left thoracotomy. *Scand J Thorac Cardiovasc Surg* 1989;23:115–119.

603. Tuna IC, Danielson GK. Surgical management of pericardial diseases. *Cardiol Clin* 1990;8:683–696.

604. Senni M, Redfield MM, Ling LH, et al. Left ventricular systolic and diastolic function after pericardiectomy in patients with constrictive pericarditis: Doppler echocardiographic findings and correlation with clinical status. *J Am Coll Cardiol* 1999;33:1182–1188.

605. Shabetai R. Acute pericarditis. *Cardiol Clin* 1990;8:639–644.

606. Saatci U, Ozen S, Ceyhan M, et al. Cytomegalovirus disease in a renal transplant recipient manifesting with pericarditis. *Int Urol Nephrol* 1993;25:617–619.

607. Campbell PT, Li JS, Wall TC, et al. Cytomegalovirus pericarditis: a case series and review of the literature. *Am J Med Sci* 1995;309:229–234.

608. Acierno LJ. Cardiac complications in acquired immunodeficiency syndrome (AIDS): a review. *J Am Coll Cardiol* 1989;13:1144–1154.

609. Spodick DH. Infectious pericarditis. In: Spodick DH, ed. *The pericardium: a comprehensive textbook*. New York: Marcel Dekker, 1997:260–290.

610. Newby LK, Ohman EM. Troponins in pericarditis: implications for diagnosis and management of chest pains patients. *Eur Heart J* 2000;21:798–800.

611. Sternbach GL. Pericarditis. *Ann Emerg Med* 1988;17:214–220.

612. Adler Y, Zandman-Goddard G, Ravid M, et al. Usefulness of colchicine in preventing recurrences of pericarditis. *Am J Cardiol* 1994;73:916–917.

613. Spodick DH. Diagnosis and management of acute non-effusive pericarditis. *Cardiol Board Rev* 1994;11:13–16.

614. Adler Y, Finkelstein Y, Guindo J, et al. Colchicine treatment for recurrent pericarditis. A decade of experience. *Circulation* 1998;97:2183–2185.

615. Melchior TM, Ringsdal V, Hildebrandt P, et al. Recurrent acute idiopathic pericarditis treated with intravenous methylprednisolone given as pulse therapy. *Am Heart J* 1992;123:1086–1088.

616. Fowler NO, Harbin ADD. Recurrent acute pericarditis: follow-up study of 31 patients. *J Am Coll Cardiol* 1986;7:300–305.

617. Brucato A, Cimaz R, Balla E. Prevention of recurrences of corticosteroid-dependent idiopathic pericarditis by colchicine in an adolescent patient. *Pediatr Cardiol* 2000;21:395–396.

618. Klacsmann PG, Bulkley BH, Hutchins GM. The changed spectrum of purulent pericarditis: an 86 year autopsy experience in 200 patients. *Am J Med* 1977;63:666–673.

619. Sagrista-Sauleda J, Barrabes JA, Permanyer-Miralda G, et al. Purulent pericarditis: review of a 20-year experience in a general hospital. *J Am Coll Cardiol* 1993;22:1661–1665.

620. Karim MA, Bach RG, Dressler F, et al. Purulent pericarditis caused by group B streptococcus with pericardial tamponade. *Am Heart J* 1993;126:727–730.

621. Luck PC, Helbig JH, Wunderlich E, et al. Isolation of *Legionella pneumophila* serogroup 3 from pericardial fluid in a case of pericarditis. *Infection* 1989;17:388–390.

622. Puleo JA, Matar FA, McKeown PP, et al. *Legionella* pericarditis diagnosed by direct fluorescent antibody staining. *Ann Thorac Surg* 1995;60:444–446.

623. Vietzke WM. Gonococcal arthritis with pericarditis. *Arch Intern Med* 1966;117:270–272.

624. Haggman DL, Rehm SJ, Moodie DS, et al. Nontyphoidal *Salmonella* pericarditis: a case report and review of the literature. *Pediatr Infect Dis* 1986;5:259–264.

625. Horowitz HW, Belkin RN. Acute myopericarditis resulting from Lyme disease. *Am Heart J* 1995;130:176–178.

626. Lam S, Greenberg R, Bank S. An unusual presentation of colon cancer: purulent pericarditis and cardiac tamponade

due to *Bacteroides fragilis. Am J Gastroenterol* 1995;90:1518–1520.

627. Rakita RM, Scerpella EG. A case of anaerobic pericarditis. *Clin Infect Dis* 1995;21:454.

628. Karp R, Meldahl R, McCabe R. *Candida albicans* purulent pericarditis treated successfully without surgical drainage. *Chest* 1992;102:953–954.

629. Schrank JH Jr, Dooley DP. Purulent pericarditis caused by *Candida* species: case report and review. *Clin Infect Dis* 1995;21:182–187.

630. Clenney TL, Hammond MD, McKeown PP, et al. Cardiac tamponade due to *Nocardia asteroides. Chest* 1993;103:641–642.

631. Kenney RT, Li JS, Clyde WA Jr, et al. Mycoplasmal pericarditis: evidence of invasive disease. *Clin Infect Dis* 1993;17[Suppl 1]:S58–S62.

632. van Ede AE, Meis JF, Koot RA, et al. Pneumopericardium complicating invasive pulmonary aspergillosis: case report and review. *Infection* 1994;22:102–105.

633. Moss W, Prince A. Pericarditis complicating meningococcal meningitis in a 7-month-old boy. *Clin Pediatr* 1994;33:169–171.

634. Hughes J, Goldsmith C, Shields MD, et al. Primary meningococcal pericarditis with cardiac tamponade in an infant. *J Infect* 1994;29:339–341.

635. Marik P. Pneumopyopericardium after penetrating chest injury. *AJR Am J Roentgenol* 1992;158:687–688.

636. Sato TT, Geary RL, Ashbaugh DG, et al. Diagnosis and management of pericardial abscess in trauma patients. *Am J Surg* 1993;165:637–641.

637. Smith DR. Pericarditis following blunt thoracic trauma. *Ala Med* 1995;64:6–8.

638. Maillier B, Chapoutot L, Metz D, et al. Late complication of blunt injuries of the thorax: acute pericarditis. Apropos of a case. *Ann Cardiol Angiol* 1993;42:253–255.

639. Sethi GK, Nelson RM, Jenson CB. Surgical management of acute septic pericarditis. *Chest* 1973;63:732–735.

640. Prager RL, Burney DP, Waterhouse G, et al. Pulmonary, mediastinal, and cardiac presentations of histoplasmosis. *Ann Thorac Surg* 1980;30:385–390.

641. Wheat LJ, Stein L, Corya BC, et al. Pericarditis as a manifestation of histoplasmosis during two large urban outbreaks. *Medicine* 1983;62:110–119.

642. Amundson DE. Perplexing pericarditis caused by coccidiomycosis. *South Med J* 1993;86:694–696.

643. Strang JI. Tuberculous pericarditis in Transkei. *Clin Cardiol* 1984;7:667–670.

644. Dalli E, Quesada A, Juan G, et al. Tuberculous pericarditis as the first manifestation of acquired immunodeficiency syndrome. *Am Heart J* 1987;114:905–906.

645. Kinney EL, Monsuez JJ, Kitzis M, et al. Treatment of AIDS-associated heart disease. *Angiology* 1989;40:970–976.

646. D'Cruz IA, Sengupta EE, Abrahams C, et al. Cardiac involvement, including tuberculous pericardial effusion, complicating acquired immune deficiency syndrome. *Am Heart J* 1986;112:1100–1102.

647. Sagrista-Sauleda J, Permanyer-Miralda G, Soler-Soler J. Tuberculous pericarditis: ten year experience with a prospective protocol for diagnosis and treatment. *J Am Coll Cardiol* 1988;11:724–728.

648. Fowler NO. Tuberculous pericarditis. *JAMA* 1991;266:99–103.

649. Desai HN. Tuberculous pericarditis. A review of 100 cases. *S Afr Med J* 1979;55:877–880.

650. Long R, Younes M, Patton N, et al. Tuberculous pericarditis: long-term outcome in patients who received medical therapy alone. *Am Heart J* 1989;117:1133–1139.

651. Peel A. Tuberculous pericarditis. *Br Heart J* 1948;10:195–222.

652. Maisch B, Maisch S, Kochsiek K. Immune reactions in tuberculosis and chronic constrictive pericarditis. Clinical data and diagnostic significance of antimyocardial antibodies. *Am J Cardiol* 1982;50:1007–1013.

653. Seino Y, Ikeda U, Kawaguchi K, et al. Tuberculous pericarditis presumably diagnosed by polymerase chain reaction analysis. *Am Heart J* 1993;126:249–251.

654. Rana BS, Jones RA, Simpson IA. Recurrent pericardial effusion: the value of polymerase chain reaction in the diagnosis of tuberculosis. *Heart* 1999;82:246–247.

655. Suwan PK, Potjalongsilp S. Predictors of constrictive pericarditis after tuberculous pericarditis. *Br Heart J* 1995;73:187–189.

656. Komsuoglu B, Gedik Y, Duman E. Tuberculous pericarditis in north-east Turkey. An echocardiographic study. *Materia Medica Polona* 1989;21:141–142.

657. Komsuoglu B, Goldeli O, Kulan K, et al. Tuberculous pericarditis in north-east Turkey. An echocardiographic study. *Acta Cardiol* 1994;49:157–163.

658. Dogan R, Demircin M, Sarigul A, et al. Diagnostic value of adenosine deaminase activity in pericardial fluids. *J Cardiovasc Surg* 1999;40:501–504.

659. Blake S, Bonar S, O'Neill H, et al. Aetiology of chronic constrictive pericarditis. *Br Heart J* 1983;50:273–276.

660. Hageman JH, D'Esopo ND, Glenn WW. Tuberculosis of the pericardium: a long-term analysis of forty-four proved cases. *N Engl J Med* 1964;270:327–332.

661. Ryoke T, Kakukawa H, Kunichika H, et al. Subacute tuberculous pericarditis with fibroelastic constriction diagnosed upon pericardiectomy. *Jpn Circ J* 2000;64:389–392.

662. Chen Y, Brennessel D, Johnson M, et al. Pericardial effusion in acquired immunodeficiency disease. *Arch Intern Med* 2000;160:2397–2398.

663. Wacker N, Merrill J. Uremic pericarditis in acute and chronic renal failure. *JAMA* 1954;156:764–765.

664. Rostand SG, Rutsky EA. Pericarditis in end-stage renal disease. *Cardiol Clin* 1990;8:701–707.

665. Marini PV, Hull AR. Uremic pericarditis: a review of incidence and management. *Kidney Int* 1975;7[Suppl 2]:163–166.

666. Rutsky EA, Rostand SG. Pericarditis in end-stage renal disease. Clinical characteristics and management. *Semin Dial* 1989;2:25–30.

667. Renfrew R, Buselmeier TJ, Kjellstrand CM. Pericarditis and renal failure. *Annu Rev Med* 1980;31:345–360.

668. Compty CM, Cohen SL, Shapiro FL. Pericarditis in chronic uremia and its sequels. *Ann Intern Med* 1971;75:173–183.

669. Osanloo E, Shaloub RJ, Cioffi RF, et al. Viral pericarditis in patients receiving hemodialysis. *Arch Intern Med* 1979;139:301–303.

670. Lindsay J Jr, Crawley IS, Callaway GM Jr. Chronic constrictive pericarditis following uremic hemopericardium. *Am Heart J* 1970;79:390–395.

671. Yoshida K, Shiina A, Asano Y, et al. Uremic pericardial effusion: detection and evaluation of uremic pericardial effusion by echocardiography. *Clin Nephrol* 1980;13:260–268.

672. Frommer JP, Young JB, Ayus JC. Asymptomatic pericardial effusion in uremic patients: effect of long-term dialysis. *Nephron* 1985;39:296–301.

673. Drueke T, Le Pailleur C, Zingraff J, et al. Uremic cardiomyopathy and pericarditis. *Adv Nephrol Necker Hosp* 1980;9:33–70.

674. Ribot S, Frankel HJ, Gielchinsky I, et al. Treatment of uremic pericarditis. *Clin Nephrol* 1974;2:127–130.

675. De Pace NL, Nestico PF, Schwartz AB, et al. Predicting success of intensive dialysis in the treatment of uremic pericarditis. *Am J Med* 1984;76:38–46.

676. Goldstein DH, Nagar C, Srivastava N, et al. Clinically silent pericardial effusions in patients on long-term hemodialysis. Pericardial effusions in hemodialysis. *Chest* 1977;72:744–747.

677. Luft FC, Gilman JK, Weyman AE. Pericarditis in the patient with uremia: clinical and echocardiographic evaluation. *Nephron* 1980;25:160–166.

678. Bean WB. Infarction of the heart. Clinical course and morphological findings. *Ann Intern Med* 1938;12:71–94.

679. Wartman WB, Hellerstein HK. The incidence of heart disease in 2000 consecutive autopsies. *Ann Intern Med* 1948;28:41–65.

680. Lichstein E, Liu HM, Gupta P. Pericarditis complicating acute myocardial infarction: incidence of complications and significance of electrocardiogram on admission. *Am Heart J* 1974;87:246–252.

681. Thadani U, Chopra MP, Aber CP, et al. Pericarditis after acute myocardial infarction. *BMJ* 1971;2:135–137.

682. Millaire A, de Groote P, Decoulx E, et al. Outcome after thrombolytic therapy of nine cases of myopericarditis misdiagnosed as myocardial infarction. *Eur Heart J* 1995;16:333–338.

683. Tilley WS, Harston WE. Inadvertent administration of streptokinase to patients with pericarditis. *Am J Med* 1986;81:541–544.

684. Ferguson DW, Dewey RC, Plante DA. Clinical pitfalls in the non-invasive thrombolytic approach to presumed acute myocardial infarction. *Can J Cardiol* 1986;2:146–151.

685. Blankenship JC, Almquist AK. Cardiovascular complications of thrombolytic therapy in patients with a mistaken diagnosis of acute myocardial infarction. *J Am Coll Cardiol* 1989;14:1579–1582.

686. Eriksen UH, Molgaard H, Ingerslev J, et al. Fatal haemostatic complications due to thrombolytic therapy in patients falsely diagnosed as acute myocardial infarction. *Eur Heart J* 1992;13:840–843.

687. Kahn JK. Inadvertent thrombolytic therapy for cardiovascular diseases masquerading as acute coronary thrombosis. *Clin Cardiol* 1993;16:67–71.

688. Galve E, Garcia-Del-Castillo H, Evangelista A, et al. Pericardial effusion in the course of myocardial infarction: incidence, natural history, and clinical relevance. *Circulation* 1986;73:294–299.

689. Widimsky P, Gregor P. Pericardial involvement during the course of myocardial infarction. A long-term clinical and echocardiographic study. *Chest* 1995;108:89–93.

690. Oliva PB, Hammill SC, Edwards WD. The electrocardiographic diagnosis of regional pericarditis in acute inferior myocardial infarction. *Eur Heart J* 1993;14:1683–1691.

691. Pierard LA, Albert A, Henrard L, et al. Incidence and significance of pericardial effusion in acute myocardial infarction as determined by two-dimensional echocardiography. *J Am Coll Cardiol* 1986;8:517–520.

692. Dubois C, Smeets JP, Demoulin JC, et al. Frequency and clinical significance of pericardial friction rubs in the acute phase of myocardial infarction. *Eur Heart J* 1985;6:766–768.

693. Tofler GH, Muller JE, Stone PH, et al. Pericarditis in acute myocardial infarction: characterization and clinical significance. *Am Heart J* 1989;117:86–92.

694. Correale E, Maggioni AP, Romano S, et al. Comparison of frequency, diagnostic and prognostic significance of pericardial involvement in acute myocardial infarction treated with and without thrombolytics. Gruppo Italiano per lo Studio della Sopravvivenza nell'Infarto Miocardico (GISSI). *Am J Cardiol* 1993;71:1377–1381.

695. Oliva PB, Hammill SC. The clinical distinction between regional postinfarction pericarditis and other causes of postinfarction chest pain: ancillary observations regarding the effect of lytic therapy upon the frequency of postinfarction pericarditis, postinfarction angina, and reinfarction. *Clin Cardiol* 1994;17:471–478.

696. Boden WE, Sadaniantz A. Ventricular septal rupture during ibuprofen therapy for pericarditis after acute myocardial infarction. *Am J Cardiol* 1985;55:1631–1632.

697. Toole JC, Silverman ME. Pericarditis of acute myocardial infarction. *Chest* 1975;67:647–653.

698. Dressler W. A post myocardial infarction syndrome: preliminary report of a complication resembling idiopathic recurrent benign pericarditis. *JAMA* 1956;160:1379–1383.

699. Broch OJ, Ofstad J. The post-myocardial infarction syndrome. *Acta Med Scand* 1960;166:281–290.

700. Lichstein E. The changing spectrum of post-myocardial infarction pericarditis. *Int J Cardiol* 1983;4:234–237.

701. Sharar A, Hod H, Barabash GM, et al. Disappearance of a syndrome: Dressler's syndrome in the era of thrombolysis. *Cardiology* 1994;85:255–258.

702. Gregoratos G. Pericardial involvement in acute myocardial infarction. *Cardiol Clin* 1990;8:601–608.

703. Dziadulewicz L, Shannon-Stone M. Postpericardiotomy syndrome: a complication of cardiac surgery. *AACN Clin Issues* 1995;6:464–470.

704. Engle MA, Klein AA, Hepner S, et al. The postpericardiotomy and similar syndromes. *Cardiovasc Clin* 1976;7:211–217.

705. Prince SE, Cunha BA. Postpericardiotomy syndrome. *Heart Lung* 1997;26:165–168.

706. Ofori-Krakye SK, Tyberg TI, Geha AS, et al. Late cardiac tamponade after open heart surgery: incidence, role of anticoagulants in its pathogenesis and its relationship to the

postpericardiotomy syndrome. *Circulation* 1981;63:1323–1328.

707. Veeragandham RS, Goldin MD. Surgical management of radiation-induced heart disease. *Ann Thorac Surg* 1998;65:1014–1019.

708. Stewart JR, Fajardo LF. Radiation-induced heart disease: an update. *Prog Cardiovasc Dis* 1984;27:173–194.

709. Stewart JR, Fajardo LF. Dose response in human experimental radiation induced heart disease. Application of the nominal standard dose (NSD) concept. *Radiology* 1971;99:403–408.

710. Tarbell NJ, Thompson L, Mauch P. Thoracic irradiation in Hodgkin's disease: disease control and long-term complications. *Int J Radiat Oncol Biol Phys* 1990;18:275–281.

711. Hancock EW. Heart disease after radiation. *N Engl J Med* 1983;308:588.

712. Arsenian MA. Cardiovascular sequelae of therapeutic thoracic radiation. *Prog Cardiovasc Dis* 1991;33:299–311.

713. Martin RG, Ruckdeschel JC, Chang P, et al. Radiation-related pericarditis. *Am J Cardiol* 1975;35:216–220.

714. Haas JM. Symptomatic constrictive pericarditis developing 45 years after radiation therapy to the mediastinum. A review of radiation pericarditis. *Am Heart J* 1969;77:89–95.

715. Ruckdeschel JC, Chang P, Martin RG, et al. Radiation-related pericardial effusions in patients with Hodgkin's disease. *Medicine* 1975;54:245–259.

716. Thar TL, Million RR. Complications of radiation treatment of Hodgkin's disease. *Semin Oncol* 1980;7:174–183.

717. Hancock EW. Subacute effusive-constrictive pericarditis. *Circulation* 1971;43:183–192.

718. Applefeld MM, Wiernik PH. Cardiac disease after radiation therapy for Hodgkin's disease: analysis of 48 patients. *Am J Cardiol* 1983;51:1679–1681.

719. Toyofuku M, Okimoto T, Tadehara F, et al. Cardiac disease late after chest radiotherapy for Hodgkin's disease: a case report. *Jpn Circ J* 1999;63:803–805.

720. Posner MR, Cohen GI, Skarin AT. Pericardial disease in patients with cancer. The differentiation of malignant from idiopathic and radiation-induced pericarditis. *Am J Med* 1981;71:407–413.

721. Piehler JM, Pluth JR, Schaff HV, et al. Surgical management of effusive pericardial disease. Influence of extent of pericardial resection on clinical course. *J Thorac Cardiovasc Surg* 1985;90:506–516.

722. Thadani U, Iveson JM, Wright V. Cardiac tamponade, constrictive pericarditis and pericardial resection in rheumatoid arthritis. *Medicine* 1975;54:261–270.

723. Goldenberg J, Ferraz MB, Pessoa AP, et al. Symptomatic cardiac involvement in juvenile rheumatoid arthritis. *Int J Cardiol* 1992;34:57–62.

724. Hara KS, Ballard DJ, Ilstrup DM, et al. Rheumatoid pericarditis: clinical features and survival. *Medicine* 1990;69:81–91.

725. Kelly CA, Bourke JP, Malcolm A, et al. Chronic pericardial disease in patients with rheumatoid arthritis: a longitudinal study. *QJM* 1990;75:461–470.

726. Langley RL, Treadwell EL. Cardiac tamponade and pericardial disorders in connective tissue diseases: case report and literature review. *J Natl Med Assoc* 1994;86:149–153.

727. Shikama N, Terano T, Hirai A. A case of rheumatoid pericarditis with high concentrations of interleukin-6 in pericardial fluid. *Heart* 2000;83:711–712.

728. Hakala M, Pettersson T, Tarkka M, et al. Rheumatoid arthritis as a cause of cardiac compression. Favourable long-term outcome of pericardiectomy. *Clin Rheumatol* 1993;12:199–203.

729. Di Franco M, Paradiso M, Mammarella A, et al. Diastolic function abnormalities in rheumatoid arthritis. Evaluation by echo Doppler transmitral flow and pulmonary venous flow: relation with duration of disease. *Ann Rheum Dis* 2000;59:227–229.

730. Oguz D, Ocal B, Ertan U, et al. Left ventricular diastolic functions in juvenile rheumatoid arthritis. *Pediatr Cardiol* 2000;21:374–377.

731. Leung WH, Wong KL, Lau CP, et al. Cardiac abnormalities in systemic lupus erythematosus: a prospective M-mode, cross-sectional and Doppler echocardiographic study. *Int J Cardiol* 1990;27:367–375.

732. Ehrenfeld M, Asman A, Shpilberg O, et al. Cardiac tamponade as the presenting manifestation of systemic lupus erythematosus. *Am J Med* 1989;86:626–627.

733. Ansari A, Larson PH, Bates HD. Cardiovascular manifestations of systemic lupus erythematosus: current perspective. *Prog Cardiovasc Dis* 1985;27:421–434.

734. Kahl LE. The spectrum of pericardial tamponade in systemic lupus erythematosus. Report of ten patients. *Arthritis Rheum* 1992;35:1343–1349.

735. Doherty NE, Siegel RJ. Cardiovascular manifestations of systemic lupus erythematosus. *Am Heart J* 1985;110:1257–1265.

736. Moder KG, Miller TD, Tazelaar HD. Cardiac involvement in systemic lupus erythematosus. *Mayo Clin Proc* 1999;74:275–284.

737. Badui E, Garcia-Rubi D, Robles E, et al. Cardiovascular manifestations in systemic lupus erythematosus. Prospective study of 100 patients. *Angiology* 1985;36:431–441.

738. Leung WH, Wong KL, Lau CP, et al. Association between antiphospholipid antibodies and cardiac abnormalities in patients with systemic lupus erythematosus. *Am J Med* 1990;89:411–419.

739. Zashin SJ, Lipsky PE. Pericardial tamponade complicating systemic lupus erythematosus. *J Rheumatol* 1989;16:374–377.

740. Coudray N, de Zuttere D, Bletry O, et al. M-mode and Doppler echocardiographic assessment of left ventricular diastolic function in primary antiphospholipid syndrome. *Br Heart J* 1995;74:531–535.

741. Kalke S, Balakrishanan C, Mangat G, et al. Echocardiography in systemic lupus erythematosus. *Lupus* 1998;7:540–544.

742. Janosik DL, Osborn TG, Moore TL, et al. Heart disease in systemic sclerosis. *Semin Arthritis Rheum* 1989;19:191–200.

743. Weiss S, Zyskind Z, Rosenthal T, et al. Cardiac involvement in progressive systemic sclerosis (P.S.S.)—an echocardiographic study. *Z Rheumatol* 1980;39:190–196.

744. Sattar MA, Guindi RT, Vajcik J. Pericardial tamponade and limited cutaneous systemic sclerosis (CREST syndrome). *Br J Rheumatol* 1990;29:306–307.

745. Abu-Shakra M, Koh ET, Treger T, et al. Pericardial effusion and vasculitis in a patient with systemic sclerosis. *J Rheumatol* 1995;22:1386–1388.

746. Gaffney FA, Anderson RJ, Nixon JV, et al. Cardiovascular function in patients with progressive systemic sclerosis (scleroderma). *Clin Cardiol* 1982;5:569–576.

747. Thompson AE, Pope JE. A study of the frequency of pericardial and pleural effusions in scleroderma. *Br J Rheumatol* 1998;37:1320–1323.

748. Purice S, Luca R, Vintila M, et al. Cardiac involvement in progressive systemic sclerosis and polymyositis: a comparative study in 116 patients. *Med Interne* 1989;27:209–213.

749. Armstrong GP, Whalley GA, Doughty RN, et al. Left ventricular function in scleroderma. *Br J Rheumatol* 1996;35:983–988.

750. Deswal A, Follansbee WP. Cardiac involvement in scleroderma. *Rheum Dis Clin North Am* 1996;22:841–860.

751. Lange K. Capillary permeability in myxedema. *Am J Med Sci* 1944;208:5–15.

752. Hardisty CA, Naik DR, Munro DS. Pericardial effusion in hypothyroidism. *Clin Endocrinol* 1980;13:349–354.

753. Davis PJ, Jacobson S. Myxedema with cardiac tamponade and pericardial effusion of "gold paint" appearance. *Arch Intern Med* 1967;120:615–619.

754. Kelly JK, Butt JC. Fatal myxedema pericarditis in a Christian scientist. *Am J Clin Pathol* 1986;86:113–116.

755. Steinberg AD. Myxedema and coronary artery disease—a comparative autopsy study. *Ann Intern Med* 1968;68:338–344.

756. Hamilton J. Myxedema heart disease. *Circulation* 1957;15:442–447.

757. Kerber RE, Sherman B. Echocardiographic evaluation of pericardial effusion in myxedema. Incidence and biochemical and clinical correlations. *Circulation* 1975;52:823–827.

758. Smolar E, Rubin J, Avramides A, et al. Cardiac tamponade in primary myxedema and review of literature. *Am J Med Sci* 1976;272:345–352.

759. Wilding G, Green HL, Longo DL, et al. Tumors of the heart and pericardium. *Cancer Treat Rev* 1988;15:165–181.

760. Thurber D, Edwards J, Achon R. Secondary malignant tumors of the pericardium. *Circulation* 1962;26:228–241.

761. Watanabe A, Sakata J, Kawamura H, et al. Primary pericardial mesothelioma presenting as constrictive pericarditis: a case report. *Jpn Circ J* 2000;64:385–388.

762. Buck M, Ingle JN, Giuliani ER, et al. Pericardial effusion in women with breast cancer. *Cancer* 1987;60:263–269.

763. Shepherd FA, Morgan C, Evans WK, et al. Medical management of malignant pericardial effusion by tetracycline sclerosis. *Am J Cardiol* 1987;60:1161–1166.

764. Osuch JR, Khandekar JD, Fry WA. Emergency subxiphoid pericardial decompression for malignant pericardial effusion. *Am Surg* 1985;51:298–300.

765. Cham WC, Freiman AH, Carstens PH, et al. Radiation therapy of cardiac and pericardial metastases. *Radiology* 1975;114:701–704.

766. Press OW, Livingston R. Management of malignant pericardial effusion and tamponade. *JAMA* 1987;257:1088–1092.

767. Davis S, Rambotti P, Grignani F. Intrapericardial tetracycline sclerosis in the treatment of malignant pericardial effusion: an analysis of thirty-three cases. *J Clin Oncol* 1984;2:631–636.

768. Shepherd FA, Ginsberg JS, Evans WK, et al. Tetracycline sclerosis in the management of malignant pericardial effusion. *J Clin Oncol* 1985;3:1678–1682.

769. Feigin DS, Fenoglio JJ, McAllister HA, et al. Pericardial cysts. A radiologic-pathologic correlation and review. *Radiology* 1977;125:15–20.

770. Bava GL, Magliani L, Bertoli D, et al. Complicated pericardial cyst: atypical anatomy and clinical course. *Clin Cardiol* 1998;21:862–864.

771. Gatzoulis MA, Munk MD, Merchant N, et al. Isolated congenital absence of the pericardium: clinical presentation, diagnosis, and management. *Ann Thorac Surg* 2000;69:1209–1215.

772. Saito R, Hotta F. Congenital pericardial defect associated with cardiac incarceration: case report. *Am Heart J* 1980;100:866–870.

773. Scalia GM, Stafford WJ, Burstow DJ, et al. Successful treatment of incessant atrial flutter with excision of congenital giant right atrial aneurysm diagnosed by transesophageal echocardiography. *Am Heart J* 1995;129:834–835.

774. Connolly HM, Click RL, Schattenberg TT, et al. Congenital absence of the pericardium: echocardiography as a diagnostic tool. *J Am Soc Echocardiogr* 1995;8:87–92.

775. Browning CA, Bishop RL, Heilpern RJ, et al. Accelerated constrictive pericarditis in procainamide-induced systemic lupus erythematosus. *Am J Cardiol* 1984;53:376–377.

776. Spodick DH. Drug and toxin-related pericardial disease. In: Spodick DH, ed. *The pericardium: a comprehensive textbook*. New York: Marcel Dekker, 1997:411–416.

777. Gardin JM, Arnold AM, Bild DE, et al. Left ventricular diastolic filling in the elderly: the cardiovascular health study. *Am J Cardiol* 1998;82:345–351.

778. Kitzman DW, Gardin JM, Gottdiener JS, et al. Importance of heart failure with preserved systolic function in patients > or = 65 years of age. CHS Research Group. Cardiovascular Health Study. *Am J Cardiol* 2001;87:413–419.

779. Roithinger FX, Punzengruber C, Wallner M, et al. The influence of ACE-inhibition on myocardial mass and diastolic function in chronic hemodialysis patients with adequate control of blood pressure. *Clin Nephrol* 1994;42:309–314.

780. Schmidt U, del Monte F, Miyamoto MI, et al. Restoration of diastolic function in senescent rat hearts through adenoviral gene transfer of sarcoplasmic reticulum Ca(2+)-ATPase. *Circulation* 2000;101:790–796.

781. Asif M, Egan J, Vasan S, et al. An advanced glycation end-product cross-link breaker can reverse age-related increases in myocardial stiffness. *Proc Natl Acad Sci U S A* 2000;97:2809–2813.

27

PULMONARY HYPERTENSION AND COR PULMONALE

CLARA I. RESTREPO
VICTOR F. TAPSON

OVERVIEW

Pulmonary arterial hypertension causes an increased pressure load on the right ventricle (RV) that subsequently results in the normal adaptive response of hypertrophy and dilation. Right ventricular failure occurs when the ventricle is unable to respond further to the hemodynamic burden (1). *Cor pulmonale* is defined as right ventricular hypertrophy, dilation, and dysfunction as a result of pulmonary hypertension secondary to a variety of chronic lung diseases (Table 27.1). Pulmonary hypertension may also develop in the absence of cardiac or pulmonary parenchymal disease.

INCIDENCE AND RISK FACTORS

Right ventricular failure is an important predictor of increased mortality in patients with chronic lung disease. It commonly occurs in individuals with COPD, which causes an estimated 70,000 deaths each year in the United States (20). A study of patients with COPD found that 40% had evidence of cor pulmonale at autopsy (1). Furthermore, in the National Institutes of Health (NIH) Primary Pulmo-

C. I. Restrepo: Department of Medicine, Division of Pulmonary and Critical Care Medicine, National Jewish Medical and Research Center, University of Colorado Health Sciences Center, Denver, Colorado
V. F. Tapson: Division of Pulmonary and Critical Care Medicine, Duke University Medical Center, Durham, North Carolina

TABLE 27.1 PULMONARY HYPERTENSION: NOMENCLATURE AND CLASSIFICATION

Pulmonary arterial hypertension
Primary pulmonary hypertension
  Sporadic
  Familial
Related to
  Collagen-vascular disease
  Congenital systemic to pulmonary shunts
  Portal hypertension
  Human immunodeficiency virus infection
  Drugs/toxins
    Anorexigens
    Other
  Persistent pulmonary hypertension of the newborn
  Other
Pulmonary venous hypertension
Left-sided atrial or ventricular heart disease
Left-sided valvular heart disease
Extrinsic compression of central pulmonary veins
  Fibrosing mediastinitis
  Adenopathy/tumors
Pulmonary venoocclusive disease
Other
Pulmonary hypertension associated with disorders of the respiratory system and/or hypoxemia
Chronic obstructive pulmonary disease
Interstitial lung disease
Sleep disordered breathing
Alveolar hypoventilation disorders
Chronic exposure to high altitude
Neonatal lung disease
Alveolar-capillary dysplasia
Other
Pulmonary hypertension due to chronic thromboembolic disease
Thromboembolic obstruction of proximal pulmonary arteries
Obstruction of distal pulmonary arteries
  Pulmonary embolism (thrombus, tumor, ova/parasites, foreign material)
  In situ thrombosis
  Sickle cell disease
Pulmonary hypertension due to disorders directly affecting the pulmonary vasculature
Inflammatory
  Schistosomiasis
  Sarcoidosis
  Other
Pulmonary capillary hemangiomatosis

nary Hypertension National Registry, mortality was found to correlate best with indices of right ventricular hemodynamic function (21). Cor pulmonale is also associated with increased morbidity in patients with chronic lung disease leading to reduced exercise tolerance, increased sensation of dyspnea, and reduced functional status (22). Other causes of cor pulmonale are less common. The incidence of PPH is estimated to be one to two cases per million in the general population (21). Pulmonary vascular disease that is clinically and pathologically indistinguishable from PPH can occur in association with human immunodeficiency virus infection, portal hypertension, cocaine inhalation,

monocrotaline (a compound from the plant *Crotalaria* that is found in bush tea), and drugs, including appetite suppressants and chemotherapeutic agents (23–27). In the 1960s, the anorexigenic agent aminorex was found to be associated with an increased risk of pulmonary hypertension (28). Use of the appetite suppressants fenfluramine and dexfenfluramine has been found to be associated with an increased risk of pulmonary hypertension (odds ratio 6.3) (27). This risk increased to an odds ratio of greater than 20 when the drugs were taken for more than 3 months, independent of body mass index. Other entities such as progressive systemic sclerosis and CREST (*c*alcification, *R*aynaud's, *e*sophageal dysmotility, *s*clerodactyly, and *t*elangiectasis) may present with progressive, severe pulmonary hypertension, often without associated parenchymal lung disease.

GENETICS OF PRIMARY PULMONARY HYPERTENSION

The genetics of PPH are becoming unraveled. Approximately 6% of patients with PPH have the familial variety. This disease is transmitted in the autosomal dominant manner with a risk of clinical expression of approximately 10% to 20% and demonstrates genetic anticipation. Studies of genetic linkage revealed that the locus for familial PPH is on chromosome 2q31–32. The known genes in this region have been surveyed for biologically plausible candidates. The results of a detailed genetic study of a large kindred of familial PPH patients has now provided additional information (28a). The gene that is associated with a unique member of the transforming growth factor-β (TGF-β) receptor family, known as *bone morphogenetic protein receptor II* (BMPR2), appears to be a likely candidate. Investigators have detected a missense mutation that involves a substitution of guanine for thymine at position 354 of *BMPR2*. This mutation was located in exon 3 of the gene and was present in all of the affected family members. More recently, it was discovered that the sporadic form of PPH is also associated with germline mutations of *BMPR2* (28b).

Bone morphogenetic proteins were previously identified as cellular products found in normal bone that promote ectopic bone formation and healing of fractures. Members of the TGF-β receptor superfamily of circulating proteins regulate growth and repair of tissue in all organs (28c,28d). Bone morphogenetic proteins exert their effects through the activation of receptors I and II, which are expressed adjacent to each other on cell surfaces and transduce intracellular signaling. The effect of activation of these receptors depends on the cell type and the circumstances and can result in either promotion or inhibition of growth. It appears that clinical PPH develops in only 10% to 20% of carriers of BMPR2 mutations; it has been speculated that gene modifiers, such as environmental factors, estrogens, or other mutations in unknown regulatory genes, may be required for clinical expression of the disease (28a). It may be that the normal function of bone morphogenetic receptor protein II in the pulmonary vasculature is antiproliferative. Based on these genetic discoveries, genetic testing and counseling will become increasingly important for PPH patients and their families.

PATHOPHYSIOLOGY

Mechanisms of Pulmonary Hypertension

Hypoxic Pulmonary Vasoconstriction

Alveolar hypoxia is a major contributor to the development of pulmonary hypertension. In 1947, Motley and associates (11) found in five human subjects that breathing 10% oxygen for 10 minutes caused increases in pulmonary artery pressure with a concomitant decrease in cardiac output as determined by the Fick method. This was subsequently confirmed, in 1952, by Fishman and colleagues (7) in the steady state, despite the finding that the application of the Fick principle by Motley and associates was found to be erroneous. Hypoxic pulmonary vasoconstriction involving small arteries and arterioles is thought to be a defense mechanism that determines local ventilation-perfusion ($\dot{V}/\dot{Q}$) relationships, as first suggested by von Euler and Liljestrand (12) in 1946. It is unclear, however, if the vasoconstriction is due specifically to the hypoxia or whether it is caused by vasoactive mediators, including prostaglandins, endothelin, bradykinin, acetylcholine, angiotensin, catecholamines, histamine, or serotonin, which lead to calcium influx (30).

In recent years, advances have been made in understanding the regulation of pulmonary vascular tone with the discovery of nitric oxide (NO). Endothelium-derived relaxation factor, discovered in 1980 (38), is produced by endothelial cells in a constitutive manner from arginine and is now identified as NO (39) or a nitroso compound that ultimately releases NO (40). NO synthase produces NO and citrulline from L-arginine, and the endothelial form of this enzyme depends on calcium and calmodulin to regulate NO production in a constitutive manner (41–43). Endothelium-dependent relaxation has been found in isolated pulmonary arteries from most mammalian species, including humans (44–48). Studies have demonstrated that inhibition of NO production by L-arginine analogs markedly enhances the pulmonary pressor response to acute hypoxic challenges, which demonstrates the role that NO has in regulating pulmonary vascular tone at rest and during acute hypoxia (49–53). In addition, impaired NO production or release by endothelial cells, or both, is seen in chronic hypoxic vasoconstriction (54–56). A number of mediators cause calcium influxes into vascular smooth mus-

cle cells, activating the endothelial constitutive NO synthase (43). Impairment of NO production allows for excessive vasoconstriction and reduces the ability of the pulmonary vasculature to relax.

Chronic vasoconstriction eventually leads to structural changes in the walls of the pulmonary vasculature. Changes in the vasculature begin to appear even 1 hour after the onset of hypoxia in experimental models (57). Although the mechanisms that lead to these changes are not fully understood, lack of NO production may allow mitogenesis and proliferation of cells within the vessel walls (55). The changes in the pulmonary vasculature include increases in the percentage of vessels with a muscular layer due to proliferation of vascular smooth muscle cells, medial hypertrophy, and eccentric intimal fibrosis (58). These changes may also allow for increased platelet aggregation and development of thrombi, causing further increases in PVR (58,59). As a result, the cross-sectional area of the pulmonary vasculature decreases, and pulmonary arterial hypertension is irreversible (30).

Myocardial Blood Flow

Inadequate blood supply to the RV may also contribute to the development of right ventricular failure. The RV responds to chronic increases in PVR with dilation and hypertrophy. With increases in muscle mass, oxygen demands increase (60,61). Oxygen also demands an increase in the LV with the development of systolic hypertension. Nonetheless, left ventricular coronary perfusion pressures are maintained or even increased because of increased diastolic pressures (60,62). Unlike the case with the LV, the perfusion (diastolic) pressure of the right coronary artery is unchanged or reduced when oxygen demands increase because right ventricular cardiac output remains unchanged or is diminished (62). In addition, the systolic component of right ventricular coronary blood flow is reduced due to the increase in chamber pressure that occurs with dilation of the RV (63).

The relationship between right coronary blood flow and right ventricular performance was studied in experimental animal models by Brooks et al. (37,64). Pigs were subjected to increases in pulmonary artery pressure by pulmonary artery occlusion. Right ventricular failure and shock developed at or above a pulmonary artery pressure of approximately 70 mm Hg. Hemodynamic collapse occurred at a lower pulmonary artery pressure when the right coronary was occluded. With reinstitution of coronary blood flow by a coronary artery perfusion pump, the RV could be resuscitated despite maintenance of high pulmonary artery pressures (37) (Fig. 27.1). This would also explain the findings that right ventricular failure and hemodynamic compromise are more likely to develop in patients with coronary artery disease in the setting of pulmonary embolism.

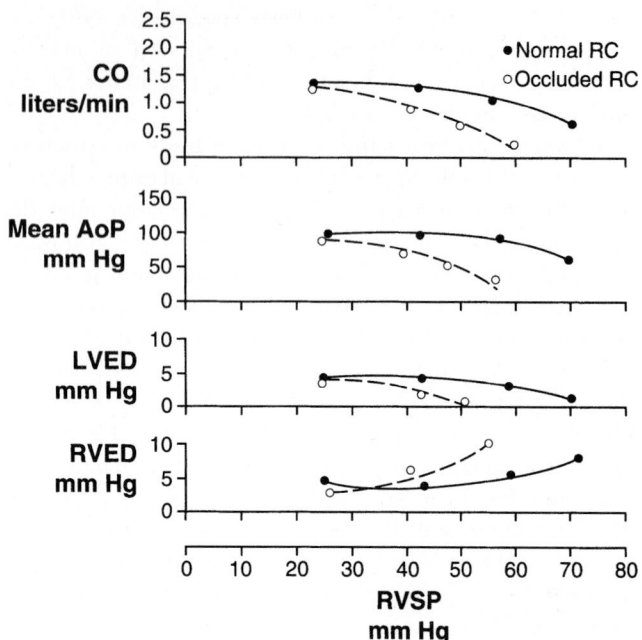

FIGURE 27.1 Effect of increasing right ventricular systolic pressure (RVSP) on cardiac output (CO), aortic pressure (AoP), left ventricular end diastolic pressure (LVED), and right ventricular end diastolic pressure (RVED). Solid lines join points with an intact right coronary artery (RC). Decompensation occurs at a much lower level of RVSP, with an occluded compared with intact RC. (From Brooks H, Kirk G, Vokonas P, et al. Performance of the right ventricle under stress: relation to right coronary flow. *J Clin Invest* 1971;50:2176–2182, with permission.)

Afterload and Preload

Increasing PVR increases afterload for the RV. By increasing preload and dilating, right ventricular function can improve via the Frank-Starling mechanism with increased cardiac output (29,65). Myocardial wall hypertrophy allows for reduction in wall stress and maintains adequate stroke volume. Spann and colleagues (66) showed that cardiac output and stroke volume were not different in cats who had pulmonary artery banding for 30 days compared with the normal control subjects. Nonetheless, right ventricular end diastolic volume and weight were significantly increased; in addition, contractile performance of the intact ventricles and isolated papillary muscles was reduced (66). Thus, normal hemodynamics were maintained by compensatory dilation and hypertrophy.

Chronic Obstructive Lung Disease and Interstitial Lung Disease

COPD and interstitial lung disease (ILD) are common causes of pulmonary parenchymal disease. In the United States, COPD is the most common pulmonary disease that results in right ventricular dysfunction, and it is a factor that adversely affects survival (1,30). In 1966, a Veterans Administration cooperative trial found that patients with

cor pulmonale had a 4-year mortality of 73% (67). These findings were reproduced by Lindsay and Read in 1972 (68), as well as by Traver and colleagues in 1979 (69).

Assessment of right ventricular systolic function is commonly done in patients with pulmonary disease by measuring the RVEF. Despite the variability of RVEF in patients with COPD, it has been shown that those with clinically evident cor pulmonale consistently have a reduced RVEF (70). In addition, patients without clinical cor pulmonale, but with a depressed RVEF, have severe obstructive ventilatory defects. In COPD patients with a history of cor pulmonale and elevated pulmonary artery pressure, the latter measure is inversely related to arterial oxygen tension, and increased PVR has been found to correlate with mortality (71). Therefore, it appears that increased right ventricular afterload leads to a depressed RVEF. Nonetheless, when right ventricular contractility was measured with load-independent methods, it did *not* appear to correlate with RVEF (72). Thus, RVEF may be a poor indicator of intrinsic contractility, although it is usually depressed in the setting of pulmonary artery hypertension.

The ILDs are disorders that cause thickening and fibrosis of the alveolar walls, resulting in disruption of the alveolar-capillary unit. The majority of these is of unknown etiology. The fibrosis can entrap segments of the pulmonary vasculature, compressing the vessels and subsequently leading to thrombosis and fibrous organization of the vessels with complete obliteration of some areas of the vasculature (73). This leads to hypoxemia from diffusion impairment and $\dot{V}/\dot{Q}$ mismatching. Patients with ILD die from respiratory failure or right ventricular failure. Initially, hyperventilation at rest allows for normal oxygenation, and desaturation occurs during exercise. As the disease progresses, oxygen consumption increases as the work of breathing increases, leading to hypoxemia at rest (1,30). Eventually, pulmonary artery hypertension develops that correlates with the degree of hypoxemia. The pulmonary artery pressure is moderately elevated in such patients until late in the disease. Again, as in their counterparts with COPD, pulmonary artery pressures are important predictors of survival (74). Sarcoidosis may result in significant parenchymal disease with hypoxemia and pulmonary hypertension. Alternatively, the predominant abnormality may appear to be intrinsic to the vasculature or due to compression/tethering of the vessels. Pulmonary hypertension may also result from left ventricular dysfunction in sarcoidosis.

Chronic Thromboembolic Pulmonary Hypertension

In normal patients without prior cardiopulmonary disease, acute pulmonary vascular obstruction results in an increase in PVR, pulmonary artery pressure, and right ventricular work (30). The degree of afterload increase is related to the degree of obstruction of the vascular bed, as well as the degree of vasoconstriction apparently due to vasoactive substances released from the thrombus. When previously healthy patients with pulmonary embolism were studied angiographically and hemodynamically, an increase in mean pulmonary artery pressure was found in 14 of 20 patients (95).

Patients with obstruction of greater than 25% of the vascular bed had increases in pulmonary artery pressures. Nonetheless, the mean pulmonary artery pressure did not exceed 40 mm Hg, even in patients with greater than 50% occlusion of the vascular bed. Therefore, a mean pulmonary artery pressure of greater than 40 mm Hg is rarely generated acutely by the previously normal, thin-walled RV. The RV dilates and increases its filling pressure, and there is a linear correlation between right atrial pressure (and pulmonary artery pressure) and the degree of obstruction by angiography (95). Patients with acute pulmonary embolism and mean pulmonary artery pressure greater than 40 mm Hg nearly always have prior cardiopulmonary disease (96). In such patients, less obstruction is required to increase the pulmonary artery pressure. In patients with right ventricular hypertrophy, however, no correlation is seen between the extent of obstruction and the elevation in pulmonary artery pressure (95). On the other hand, right atrial and pulmonary artery pressures correlate closely, indicating that the RV still makes use of its preload reserve in the setting of increased afterload (30).

Pulmonary Hypertension and Normal Lung Parenchyma

A number of entities can result in pulmonary hypertension in the absence of structural cardiac disease and with normal lung parenchyma. These include sleep apnea, chronic alveolar hypoventilation, high-altitude sickness, and neuromuscular disease. Chest wall and neuromuscular disease as well as sleep apnea are briefly discussed, offering some potential explanations for the resulting pulmonary hypertension.

Thoracic Cage Deformities and Neuromuscular Disease

Neuromuscular diseases, including muscular dystrophy, amyotrophic lateral sclerosis, postpolio syndrome, and numerous others, can result in respiratory failure, hypoxemia, and, occasionally, pulmonary hypertension (97), as may thoracic cage deformities including severe kyphoscoliosis. The management of hypoventilation in neuromuscular and chest wall disorders is based on the premise that preventing further reductions in alveolar ventilation during sleep will result in an improvement in nocturnal and subsequently daytime arterial blood gases, a reduction in pulmonary hypertension and cor pulmonale, and the prevention of premature death. Patients who have been previously disabled by profound dyspnea, sleep fragmentation, cor pul-

monale, and unstable respiratory failure have in many instances returned to full-time activities.

Hypoventilation and Sleep Apnea

Sleep apnea may lead to the development of pulmonary hypertension and right ventricular failure (98). In obstructive sleep apnea, airflow ceases as a result of complete occlusion of the upper airway despite continued activity of the inspiratory muscles. In central sleep apnea, airflow ceases because there is transient loss of central drive to the respiratory muscles. Most individuals with sleep apnea have a mixed obstructive and central picture. Obstructive apneas are often accompanied by intermittent elevations in pulmonary artery pressure above the baseline level that occur during wakefulness. The maximum increase in pulmonary artery pressure occurs at, or shortly after, the onset of arousal and ventilation, which usually coincides with the maximum extent of arterial oxyhemoglobin desaturation. Supplemental oxygen markedly attenuates but does not abolish these increases in pulmonary artery pressure. Hypoxia-induced pulmonary vasoconstriction certainly plays a role in the pathogenesis of these elevations in pulmonary artery pressure, but it is probably not the only contributing factor. Hypercapnia and acidosis can also induce pulmonary vasoconstriction, leading to elevations in pulmonary artery pressure (1). Thus, it is not surprising that elevations in pulmonary artery pressure are not completely abolished by supplemental oxygen. Although a number of factors contribute to the development of chronic hypercapnia and cor pulmonale in patients with obstructive sleep apnea, reversal of the obstruction alone is sufficient in most cases to alleviate symptoms and reverse right ventricular failure.

CLINICAL PROFILE: EVALUATION OF THE PATIENT WITH PULMONARY HYPERTENSION

History and Physical Examination

Because the development of right ventricular failure and pulmonary hypertension in the patient with chronic pulmonary disease has important prognostic implications, it is important to assess for symptoms that can herald such development. One of the main difficulties is that, in general, symptoms tend to develop gradually. In the NIH PPH Registry, a period of 2 to 5 symptomatic years before diagnosis was documented (99). This is also true of other chronic lung diseases including COPD.

Dyspnea is commonly reported early in the pulmonary patient. With the development of hypoxemia and right ventricular failure, this symptom increases in severity and is uniformly present in nearly all patients. Chest pain is also common and can be difficult to distinguish from angina. Orthopnea is relatively common in patients with severe

COPD, although it is not necessarily accompanied by worsening cardiac function. Orthopnea in these patients is believed to be related to hyperinflation of the lungs and the subsequent effects on ventricular function or reduction, or both, in venous return. Evidence of right ventricular dysfunction with increased venous and hepatic congestion can present with the development of early satiety, increasing lower extremity edema and fluid overload. Finally, in patients with PPH, Raynaud's phenomenon is common but also suggests the possibility of collagen-vascular disease. Presyncope and syncope are usually exertional in patients with severe pulmonary hypertension due to the inability to increase cardiac output in response to the increased demand.

Certain physical findings may suggest pulmonary hypertension or cor pulmonale, independent of their cause. The presence of a loud and occasionally palpable pulmonic valve closure sound is a common finding in patients with pulmonary hypertension. A parasternal or epigastric lift may be present due to the hypertrophied RV. With progression to cor pulmonale, tricuspid valvular regurgitation develops as a result of dilation of the RV, which causes a prominent jugular V wave. Progressive signs of chronic right ventricular dilation and failure include pulmonic valve insufficiency, a right ventricular third heart sound, jugular venous distention, hepatojugular reflux, hepatomegaly, lower extremity edema, ascites, and eventually anasarca.

Patients with cor pulmonale and pulmonary hypertension due to COPD invariably have findings that are associated with their obstructive lung disease, including decreased breath sounds and hyperinflation. Individuals with cor pulmonale secondary to ILD often have dry crackles at the lung bases. Auscultation of the lungs in PPH and chronic thromboembolic pulmonary hypertension are generally unremarkable, although bruits may be evident over the peripheral lung in the latter group. Clubbing is a common finding in chronic pulmonary disorders, particularly pulmonary fibrosis, cystic fibrosis, and other bronchiectatic disorders. It is also very common in individuals with pulmonary hypertension due to congenital heart disease. Cyanosis, either peripheral or central, may be present in individuals with hypoxemia due to advanced cardiopulmonary disease. Other pertinent physical findings include those associated with collagen-vascular disease, such as telangiectasias, sclerodactyly, or calcinosis, and findings that might suggest alveolar hypoventilation, such as muscle weakness, kyphoscoliosis, and extreme obesity. Algorithms for determining the presence and the cause of pulmonary hypertension are presented (Figs. 27.2 and 27.3).

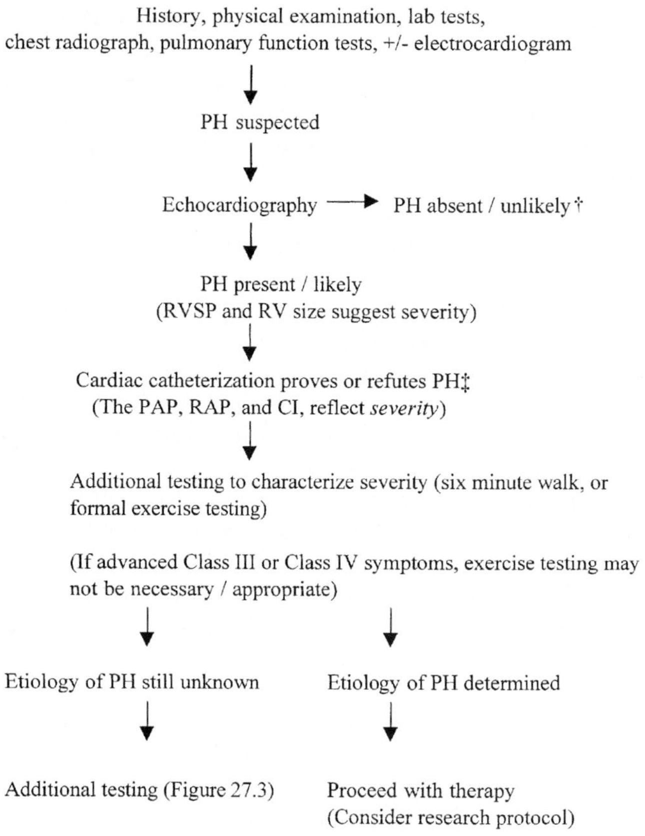

Electrocardiography

The electrocardiogram in the patient with pulmonary hypertension and cor pulmonale reveals evidence of right heart strain, including P-pulmonale, right-axis deviation, right ventricular hypertrophy, and a right ventricular strain pat-

FIGURE 27.2 An approach to the diagnosis of primary pulmonary hypertension (PH). CI, cardiac index; PAP, pulmonary artery pressure; RAP, right atrial pressure; RV, right ventricle; RVSP, right ventricular systolic pressure. [†]The absence of perceived tricuspid insufficiency by echocardiography may not absolutely exclude PH. [‡]Other tests may already have revealed potential etiology(ies) of PH. These tests may also strongly suggest the etiology. (From D'Alonzo GE, Dantzker DR. Diagnosing primary pulmonary hypertension. In: Rubin LJ, Rich S, eds. *Primary pulmonary hypertension.* New York: Marcel Dekker Inc, 1997:227–252, with permission.)

tern. In addition, atrial fibrillation, atrial flutter, and paroxysmal atrial tachycardia often occur in the setting of chronic pulmonary disorders. Although the electrocardiogram may not be sensitive in the presence of mild or early pulmonary hypertension, it is more often abnormal in those with advanced disease. In PPH patients, evidence of right heart strain appears to be present in approximately 80% of patients (99). However, particularly with the ready availability of echocardiography, electrocardiography does not offer much useful information regarding the cause or severity of pulmonary hypertension in the vast majority of settings.

Chest Radiography

The chest radiograph is an important tool in the evaluation of patients with suspected pulmonary hypertension or cor pulmonale (Fig. 27.4). It may be helpful in identifying parenchymal lung abnormalities such as pulmonary fibrosis

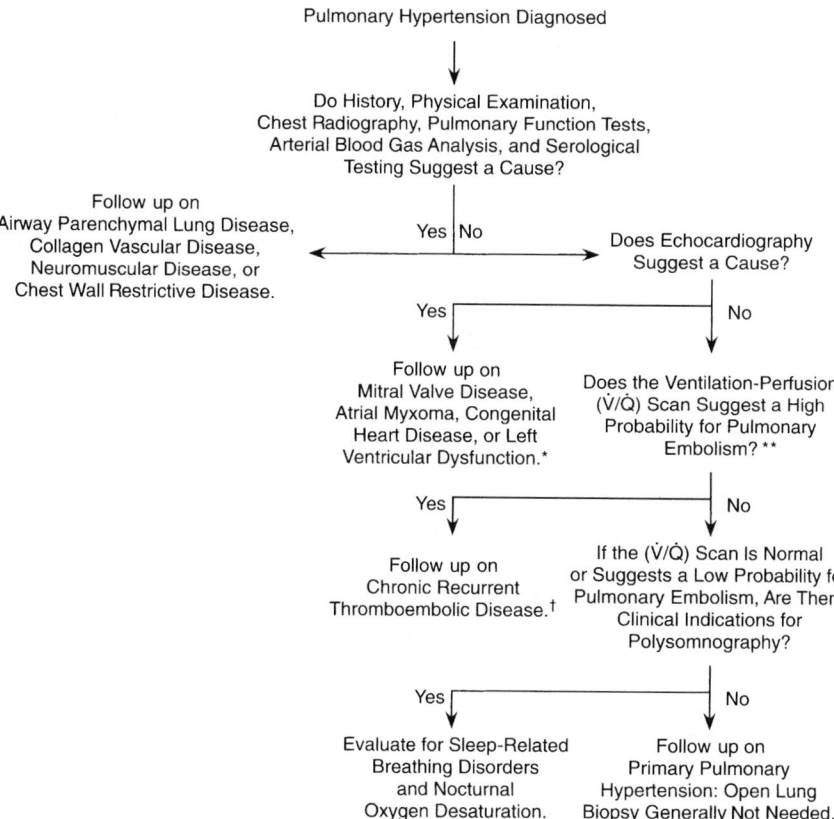

Pulmonary Hypertension Diagnosed

↓

Do History, Physical Examination, Chest Radiography, Pulmonary Function Tests, Arterial Blood Gas Analysis, and Serological Testing Suggest a Cause?

Yes | No

Follow up on Airway Parenchymal Lung Disease, Collagen Vascular Disease, Neuromuscular Disease, or Chest Wall Restrictive Disease.

Does Echocardiography Suggest a Cause?

Yes — Follow up on Mitral Valve Disease, Atrial Myxoma, Congenital Heart Disease, or Left Ventricular Dysfunction.*

No — Does the Ventilation-Perfusion (V̇/Q̇) Scan Suggest a High Probability for Pulmonary Embolism? **

Yes — Follow up on Chronic Recurrent Thromboembolic Disease.†

No — If the (V̇/Q̇) Scan Is Normal or Suggests a Low Probability for Pulmonary Embolism, Are There Clinical Indications for Polysomnography?

Yes — Evaluate for Sleep-Related Breathing Disorders and Nocturnal Oxygen Desaturation.

No — Follow up on Primary Pulmonary Hypertension: Open Lung Biopsy Generally Not Needed.

FIGURE 27.3 An approach to determining the cause of primary pulmonary hypertension. *Radionuclide ventriculography may be needed to confirm. **Spiral computed tomography may also suggest pulmonary embolism. In addition to emboli, a mosaic perfusion pattern may indicate chronic thromboembolic pulmonary hypertension. †Pulmonary angiography may be needed to confirm. (From D'Alonzo GE, Dantzker DR. Diagnosing primary pulmonary hypertension. In: Rubin LJ, Rich S, eds. *Primary pulmonary hypertension.* New York: Marcel Dekker Inc, 1997:227–252, with permission.)

or hyperinflation associated with emphysema. Skeletal abnormalities that may lead to right ventricular failure, such as kyphoscoliosis, can also be identified. In addition, the chest radiogram allows for assessment of cardiac size, especially of the RV. Abnormalities in distribution of pulmonary blood flow may offer clues to the presence of vascular obstruction due to thromboembolic disease. Prominence of the proximal pulmonary arteries is usually present in patients with pulmonary hypertension and may be accompanied by pruning of the distal vessels (100). Unlike classic

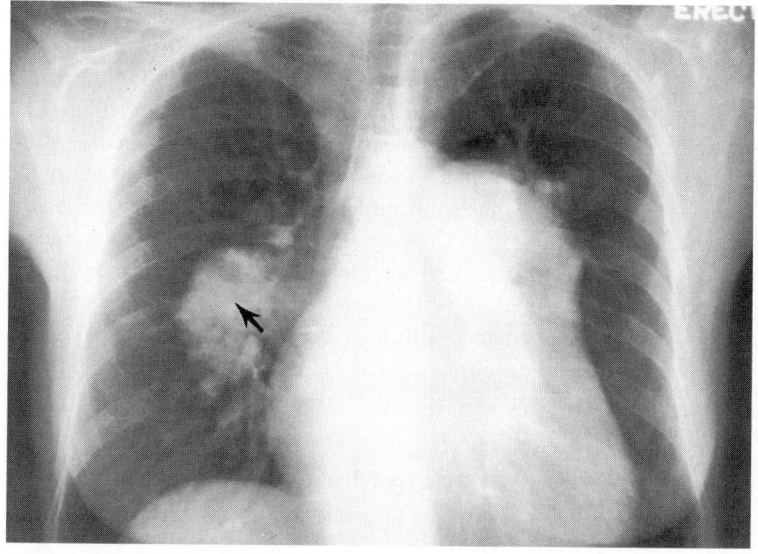

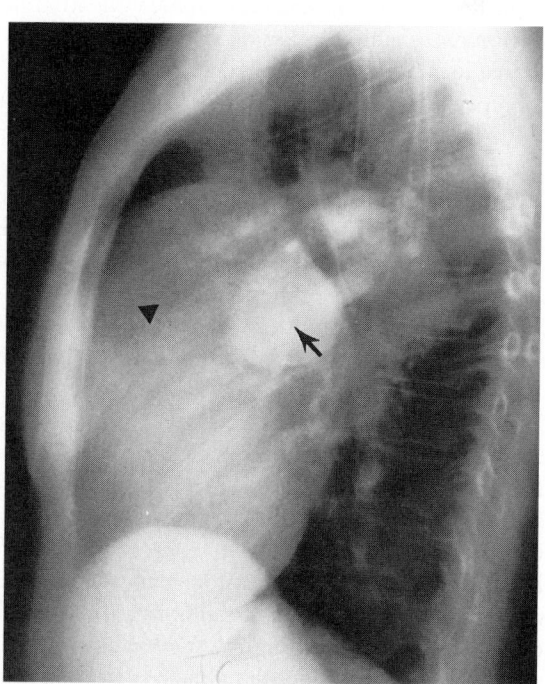

FIGURE 27.4 Chest radiograph in a patient with primary pulmonary hypertension. The proximal pulmonary arteries are dramatically enlarged. This is evident on the posteroanterior **(A)** and the lateral **(B)** views (*arrow*). The lateral film also reveals severe right ventricular enlargement (*arrowhead*).

PPH, even rarer entities such as pulmonary venoocclusive disease may be associated with interstitial infiltrates and Kerley B lines due to alveolar septal lymphatic edema.

Echocardiography: Anatomic Correlations and Clinical Use

Cor pulmonale is defined to some extent by structural changes of the RV including right ventricular hypertrophy and dilation. On gross inspection, right ventricular hypertrophy is usually defined as a posterior wall thickness of greater than or equal to 5 mm at the level of the inferior border of the posterior leaflet of the tricuspid valve, excluding the papillary muscles (102). However, the sensitivity of this measurement as an indicator of pulmonary hypertension has been shown on multiple occasions to be poor (103–106). The most accurate method to determine the presence of cor pulmonale pathologically includes measurement of the weight of the free wall of the RV and the ratio of the combined weight of the septum and the free left ventricular wall to the right ventricular weight (104). These measurements in normal adult hearts are right ventricular weight less than 65 g, combined ventricular weights less than 250 g, and the ratio (as defined above) of 2.3 to 3.3. Evidence of right ventricular failure, defined by the presence pathologically of chronic hepatic congestion, was seen in 27% of cases with a right ventricular weight of 75 to 99 g, in 64% of those with weights of 100 to 150 g, and in 93% of cases with weights greater than 150 g (107). Gross examination of the RV also reveals a change in its shape with the development of cor pulmonale. The volume of the RV appears to decrease relative to its mass; in addition, it becomes less C-shaped and more concentric, the so-called left ventricularization of the RV (107).

In the past, the echocardiographic evaluation of the RV was more difficult because of its crescentic shape and substernal location, which limited adequate visualization of its chambers and subjected it to near-field acoustic artifacts. With the advent of two-dimensional echocardiography—Doppler and color Doppler imaging—came a growing interest in right heart function and evaluation. The echocardiographic views that best depict right-sided anatomy include the apical four-chamber, the right ventricular inflow long-axis, the oblique short-axis, the subcostal, the long-axis pulmonary, the short-axis view of the great vessels, the angulated short-axis view of the pulmonary artery, and the short-axis ventricular view (108).

The ideal method to evaluate the RV in cor pulmonale adequately includes measurement of chamber sizes, volumes, flow, and pressures. The echocardiogram is helpful in establishing secondary causes for pulmonary hypertension, such as left ventricular dysfunction, mitral valve abnormalities, or congenital heart disease. Although echocardiography is not foolproof in detecting mild to moderate pulmonary hypertension, it is quite sensitive in detecting severe elevations in pulmonary artery pressure. Patients with pulmonary hypertension exhibit an early peak velocity on pulsed-wave Doppler patterns in the proximal pulmonary artery because of poor compliance of the pulmonary vascular bed (108). The majority of such patients has tricuspid regurgitation, thereby allowing a reasonably accurate estimate of pulmonary artery systolic pressure. In the absence of right ventricular outflow tract obstruction, the relationship of the squared peak velocity of the tricuspid jet multiplied by four (Bernoulli equation) equals the pressure gradient across the valve. In a study by Currie et al. (109), analyzable Doppler regurgitant velocities were accurate in 80% of patients with elevated right ventricular systolic pressures, compared with 57% of normal patients. Such predictions, however, are only accurate for outflow tract waveforms. Pulmonary artery flow patterns do not allow for accurate predictions of systolic pressures, but they do allow for accurate predictions of diastolic pressures (108). Pulmonary hypertension can also be estimated by studying the flow characteristics in the inferior vena cava, although this technique has not been studied prospectively. Other echocardiographic findings that are associated with pulmonary hypertension and cor pulmonale include the presence of a dilated pulmonary artery and dilation and hypertrophy of the RV, even though the posterior wall often is not adequately visualized. Diastolic flattening of the interventricular septum also occurs with progressive pulmonary hypertension, eventually leading to a concave septal configuration.

Because echocardiography is noninvasive, it is generally used early to determine the presence and severity of pulmonary hypertension and cor pulmonale. It is also extremely useful for following patients with established pulmonary hypertension after therapeutic interventions. Patients with markedly depressed RVEF measurements (10% or less) who have undergone lung transplantation appear to have considerable improvement of right ventricular function by echocardiography (110). Another study in patients who underwent pulmonary thromboendarterectomy for chronic thromboembolic pulmonary hypertension compared catheterization data with echocardiography. Strong correlations were seen between the maximal velocity of the regurgitant tricuspid jet by Doppler and the measurements of pulmonary artery pressures by cardiac catheterization postoperatively (111). Although transesophageal echocardiography can be used to evaluate the RV, there do not appear to be any major advantages with the latter technique for this particular indication. Three-dimensional echocardiography is being increasingly investigated, and although the technique has not yet been systematically investigated in patients with right ventricular dysfunction, this approach appears promising (112).

Nuclear Imaging Modalities

Ventriculography

The gold standard for the measurement of cardiac volumes and ejection fractions is usually considered to be contrast ventriculography. These measurements are normally calculated from geometric models that closely resemble the shape of the structure being studied (113). Nonetheless, unlike the left ventricle, the complex shape of the normal RV renders the methods that make use of such mathematical models prone to error. Additionally, in cor pulmonale, the changes in the shape of the RV can further invalidate measurements derived from models of the normal ventricle. Nuclear imaging techniques may overcome some of these difficulties because they are count based and relatively independent of the geometric constraints of the RV. Images in the septal left anterior oblique view are used in determining RVEF (114). Because inclusion of right atrial counts can falsely lower RVEF, the gated first-pass technique minimizes activity in adjacent structures. This technique performed with a multicrystal scintillation camera with high count rate capacities is the best way to measure RVEF.

Ventilation-Perfusion Scanning

When evaluating a patient with pulmonary hypertension, $\dot{V}/\dot{Q}$ scanning is only useful in differentiating whether the cause of the pulmonary hypertension is secondary to chronic thromboembolic disease (115). The latter patients typically have significant $\dot{V}/\dot{Q}$ abnormalities. The high-probability scans of such patients have at least one major perfusion defect. In contrast, patients with PPH generally have either normal or low-probability lung scans. Patients with cor pulmonale due to significant obstructive or restrictive lung diseases may have large perfusion defects, but these correlate with ventilation abnormalities. It is difficult to exclude thromboembolism using the $\dot{V}/\dot{Q}$ scan in the setting of severe COPD.

Computed Tomography

The use of computed tomographic (CT) scanning is increasingly being used to characterize the lung vasculature and parenchyma in patients with pulmonary hypertension. The pulmonary vasculature can be examined for thromboembolism, and the nature and extent of parenchymal disease can be evaluated. For example, patients with scleroderma and pulmonary hypertension may have variable degrees of interstitial disease; CT scanning may help determine whether the process is related primarily to pulmonary vascular involvement or to underlying fibrosis. The CT scan may reveal a mosaic perfusion pattern that suggests the presence of chronic thromboembolic pulmonary hypertension. In spite of the ability to visualize the pulmonary arteries with contrast-enhanced CT scanning, pulmonary arteriography should be performed if there is any question about proceeding with a potentially curable pulmonary thromboendarterectomy.

Pulmonary Arteriography

The role of the pulmonary arteriogram in the evaluation of the patient with pulmonary hypertension and cor pulmon-

ale is to diagnose thromboembolic disease, and it is especially useful if the $\dot{V}/\dot{Q}$ scan is nondiagnostic. In chronic thromboembolic disease, the arteriogram can reveal convex-bordered occlusions, stenoses, intravascular webs, and large central thrombi with filling defects and vessel cutoffs (116). The arteriogram in the PPH patient reveals dilation of the proximal vessels with pruning of the distal vessels. Performing pulmonary arteriography in patients with severe pulmonary hypertension carries a small risk, although it is generally safe in the absence of overt, severe right ventricular failure. In the NIH PPH Registry, 50 patients underwent the procedure without significant adverse events (99). One patient experienced transient hypotension. The risk is likely inversely proportional to the experience of the center performing the procedures (116). Pulmonary angioscopy may be necessary to determine the precise extent of thromboembolism (117).

Right Heart Catheterization

The gold standard for the diagnosis of pulmonary hypertension remains the right heart catheterization. This technique uses a thermodilution balloon catheter to measure right atrial, right ventricular, pulmonary artery, and pulmonary capillary wedge pressures (6). Patients with pulmonary arterial hypertension should have normal wedge pressures. The presence of an abnormal capillary wedge pressure usually requires left heart catheterization for further evaluation. In addition, right heart catheterization allows for comparisons between the oxygen saturations in the central veins, right atrium, RV, and pulmonary artery. This helps determine if a left-to-right shunt is present. The right heart catheterization may supplement the echocardiographic data in the diagnosis and evaluation of congenital heart disease.

PRINCIPLES OF MANAGEMENT

Oxygen

As was previously stated, a low arterial oxygen tension value is a predictor of reduced survival in patients with cor pulmonale. Supplemental oxygen not only relieves tissue hypoxia but can also reduce hypoxic pulmonary vasoconstriction, thereby reducing PVR, pulmonary artery pressures, and afterload. The reduction in such hemodynamic parameters might then allow right ventricular dysfunction to reverse. Two large trials have demonstrated the benefit of supplemental oxygen therapy in patients with hypoxemia and cor pulmonale: the Nocturnal Oxygen Therapy Trial Group (NOTT) (123) and the Medical Research Council Working Party (MRC) (124). The NOTT study enrolled 203 patients with hypoxemia and COPD at six treatment centers in the United States. The patients were randomized to continuous versus nocturnal oxygen therapy. Mortality

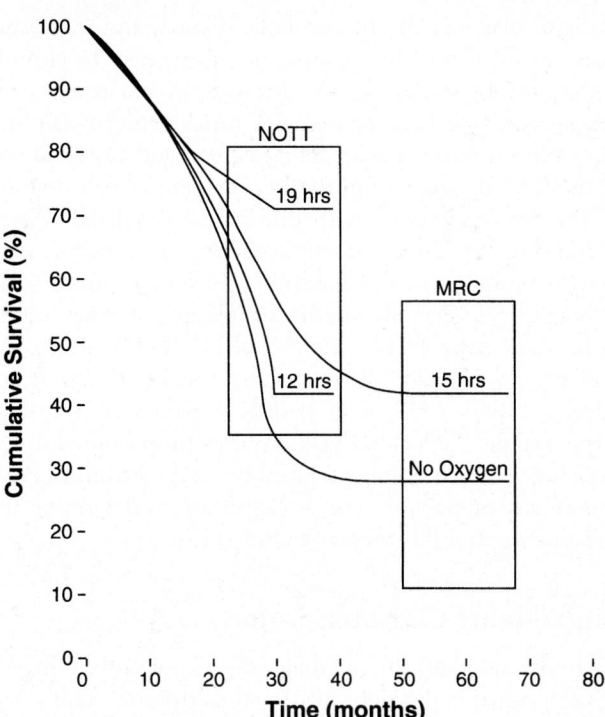

FIGURE 27.5 Composite graph of the British Medical Research Council Working Party (MRC) and the U.S. Nocturnal Oxygen Therapy Trial (NOTT) studies. Survival was poor with no oxygen, better with some oxygen, and best as they approached continuous oxygen (19 hours). (From Tiep BL. Long-term home oxygen therapy. *Clin Chest Med* 1990;11:505–521, with permission.)

was significantly reduced in patients who received continuous oxygen when compared with the other treatment group (Fig. 27.5). Nonetheless, statistically significant differences in mortality between each group were not evident when considering the specific subset of patients with altered pulmonary hemodynamics, despite an improvement in PVR with continuous oxygen therapy. ☜ f85

Treatment of Airflow Obstruction and Parenchymal Lung Disease

The therapy of patients with cor pulmonale due to COPD involves maximizing lung function. Several classes of drugs are used in patients with obstructive lung diseases for their bronchodilatory properties. Theophylline has been shown in animal models to have a bronchodilator effect and inotropic effects and to improve diaphragmatic contractility (126–128). The effects on ventricular function are attenuated by beta-receptor or calcium channel blockade (126). However, the use of this agent to improve diaphragmatic as well as cardiac function appears to be controversial in humans. Beta-adrenergic receptor agonists are primarily used for their bronchodilator properties. These are also vasodilators of the systemic and pulmonary vascular beds, although the latter effect does not appear to be clinically significant when used at standard doses via the inhaled

route. The development of tolerance with the use of these agents is common, and potential hemodynamic effects seem unlikely to be long term. These agents, including albuterol, salmeterol, terbutaline, and others, can be used for acute exacerbations of COPD or for chronic maintenance therapy. Ipratroprium bromide is also commonly used in the setting of acute and chronic airflow obstruction. A major advantage of this agent is the paucity of adverse effects, even at relatively high doses. Finally, steroid therapy plays a role in certain patients with obstructive as well as interstitial lung disease. Treatment of the underlying lung disease may improve airflow and potentially oxygenation, theoretically offering a chance for improvement in cor pulmonale.

Digoxin

The use of digoxin as an agent to improve cardiac contractility in patients with impaired right ventricular function is controversial. A randomized placebo-controlled trial studied the effect of digoxin on RVEF after 8 weeks of treatment in COPD patients (129). Improvement in RVEF was seen in those patients with concomitant left ventricular dysfunction, but not in individuals with isolated right ventricular dysfunction. In addition, digoxin does not improve cardiac function or oxygen consumption during exercise in patients with COPD (130). Finally, patients with chronic lung disease and gas exchange abnormalities tend to develop digoxin toxicity at lower serum levels than patients with right ventricular dysfunction without gas exchange abnormalities. Additional clinical trials would appear warranted.

Vasodilator Therapy

Because pulmonary arterial muscularization and vasoconstriction are believed to be major pathophysiologic mechanisms for the development of pulmonary hypertension and pressure overload of the RV, a number of vasodilator agents have been studied. Guidelines for their use are provided in *e*Tables 27.1.1 and 27.1.2 and in *e*Figure 27.5.1.

Calcium Channel Blockers

Calcium channel blockers have been the most widely tested and used group of drugs in patients with PPH. In such individuals, sustained improvement occurs in 25% to 30% (76,87). Nifedipine and diltiazem are the most commonly used, because verapamil has been shown to have negative inotropic effects. Typically, the patients who experience the most sustained improvement in hemodynamics during an acute vasodilator challenge are those who show improvement in symptoms and prolonged survival (76). However, these agents may also result in significant adverse effects such as hypotension, which can be life threatening in patients with severely compromised right ventricular function. Therefore, indiscriminate use of these agents should be avoided.

Data from the NIH PPH Registry suggested that patients with greatly depressed right ventricular function are at greatest risk of adverse outcomes with acute administration of vasodilators (131). If oral calcium channel blocker doses are changed in PPH patients who have already undergone right heart catheterization, the change should take place with careful monitoring of the blood pressure. In patients with other causes for pulmonary hypertension and cor pulmonale, the use of these agents is controversial. A study of 11 patients with COPD and cor pulmonale who were treated with nifedipine revealed no improvement in survival over age- and disease-matched control subjects despite improvements in PVR (132–134). Other studies have shown improvement in the hemodynamics of COPD patients, but these were accompanied by worsening of arterial oxygenation due to $\dot{V}/\dot{Q}$ mismatching. Therefore, treatment of COPD patients should be carefully considered on an individual basis. Other oral vasodilators have been evaluated. Despite a possible role of angiotensin-converting enzyme in the pathophysiology of pulmonary hypertension (135), the evaluation of inhibitors of this enzyme has not revealed significant benefit, and these drugs have not been studied in large prospective, randomized trials (136).

Prostacyclin

The use of prostacyclin (epoprostenol, PGI_2) as long-term therapy developed from observations of hemodynamic parameters during its acute administration (137). It has a very short half-life, and it is rapidly inactivated by the low gastric pH. Therefore, it must be given as a continuous intravenous infusion via a permanent indwelling catheter with a portable infusion pump. Substantial preliminary data (138,139) led to a large prospective, randomized multicenter trial that compared prostacyclin plus conventional therapy with conventional therapy alone in patients with class III and IV PPH (79). The patients who were treated with prostacyclin had significant improvements in exercise capacity, hemodynamics, and survival (Fig. 27.6). More recently, patients with severe pulmonary hypertension due to the scleroderma spectrum of diseases were randomized in a similar prospective trial (140). Improvement in exercise capacity and hemodynamics at 3 months was demonstrated in the prostacyclin cohort. Long-term benefits have also been reported, even in patients who have not demonstrated hemodynamic improvement during the acute infusion. The dose of the drug is increased, generally once or twice per week, and tolerance develops if it is not increased. The long-term effects have been suggested to be due not only to the vasodilator properties but also to antiplatelet or anti–smooth muscle proliferation properties. Adverse events are related to catheter-related infections and thrombosis and pump malfunction. Dose-related side effects include diar-

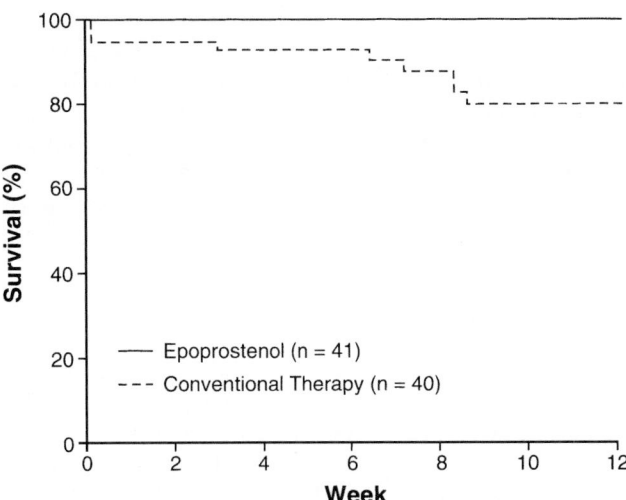

FIGURE 27.6 Survival among the 41 patients treated with epoprostenol and the 40 patients receiving conventional therapy. Data on patients who underwent transplantation during the 12-week study were censored at the time of transplantation. Estimates were made by the Kaplan-Meier product-limit method. The two-sided *p* value from the log-rank test was .003. Survival analysis with data on patients receiving transplants not censored at transplantation resulted in the same level of significance (two-sided *p* = .003 by the log-rank test). No deaths occurred in the epoprostenol group, and there were eight deaths in the conventional therapy group. [From Barst RJ, Rubin LJ, Long WA, et al. A comparison of continuous intravenous epoprostenol (prostacyclin) with conventional therapy for primary pulmonary hypertension. *N Engl J Med* 1996;334:296–301, with permission.]

rhea, jaw pain, flushing, and arthralgias. This drug should be administered by a team of individuals who are experienced with its use and aware of the time commitment that is required for proper teaching and maintenance. Alternatives to this form of prostacyclin are under investigation and include inhaled prostacyclin (141,142), nebulized iloprost (a prostacyclin analog) (142), and oral prostacyclin in the pill form (143). Subcutaneous prostacyclin delivered by a small pump (UT-15/Remodulin) is pending approval by the U.S. Food and Drug Administration.

Endothelin Antagonists

Because endothelin levels have been shown to be elevated in patients with PPH, and because the production and activity of this substance may be two of several important mechanisms in the development of pulmonary hypertension, endothelin antagonism has been studied as potential therapy in pulmonary arterial hypertension. Results in animal models with pulmonary hypertension have appeared to be favorable (144). Channick and colleagues (145) conducted a large randomized, double-blind, placebo-controlled multicenter trial that compared bosentan, an orally active antagonist receptor of both endothelin receptor subtypes (A and B). The Borg dyspnea index, 6-minute walk distance, WHO functional class, and PVR all improved to a statistically significant degree in patients who received the drug compared with placebo. Ultimately, it may prove most effective to combine this form of treatment with therapies that use other mechanisms of action for optimal therapy. Bosentan (Tracleer) was recently approved by the U.S. Food and Drug Administration for use in patients with New York Heart Association class III and IV PPH and those with pulmonary arterial hypertension due to the scleroderma spectrum of diseases.

Inhaled Nitric Oxide

Because abnormalities in NO production, regulation, and effect appear to be involved in the pathophysiology of pulmonary hypertension, its use as a therapeutic agent is being investigated. It is a selective pulmonary vasodilator (146,147), delivered via inhalation, with a short half-life. It appears to be useful as a "screening vasodilator" in the therapy of pulmonary hypertensive states (148). Two prospective randomized trials using inhaled NO in neonates with pulmonary hypertension revealed no reduction in mortality but a decrease in the need for more invasive therapy such as extracorporeal membrane oxygenation (149,150). The delivery of the inhaled gas has been a major obstacle in its use, because administration has been via ventilators or face masks. An ambulatory delivery system is being developed for the widespread use of inhaled NO, and it appears to be a promising alternative in the future (151,152). The effects of pulsed inhaled NO in eight patients with PPH revealed improvement in hemodynamic parameters over a short period of time (151). Long-term effects have not been studied, but a few patients have been maintained on this therapy.

Anticoagulation

Anticoagulation is recommended in the treatment of patients with pulmonary hypertension due to their increased risk of *in situ* thrombosis. In a subgroup of these patients, microscopic thrombi may play a role in the pathogenesis of the disease (152). In addition, these individuals appear to be at risk of thromboembolism due to right ventricular dilatation and dysfunction as well as relative immobility. A retrospective clinical trial and a nonrandomized prospective study have suggested improved survival with anticoagulation therapy (76,152). Despite the fact that heparin is beneficial in animal models of hypoxic pulmonary hypertension due to its inhibitory effects on smooth muscle proliferation (153), the drug of choice is warfarin; an international normalized ratio of 1.5 to 2.5 is considered therapeutic (76). The risk-benefit ratio has to be considered on an individual basis when using anticoagulant therapy.

Atrial Septostomy

Patients with PPH often begin to shunt blood from right to left as the pulmonary artery pressure rises. This is due to the opening of a patent foramen ovale. It is likely that, in some patients, this serves as a means by which to "unload" the RV to some degree. Creation of a shunt, atrial septostomy, has been performed as palliation in a few cases with severe PPH (154–156). In such patients, the RV is massively dilated, thereby encroaching on left ventricular filling. A right-to-left shunt is created in an attempt to improve forward output and allow for better filling of the left ventricle. The unfortunate tradeoff is the potential for causing profound systemic arterial hypoxemia or pulmonary edema by overloading the left ventricle. Therefore, this procedure is still considered investigational but may be used in extreme cases.

Surgical Treatment

Pulmonary Thromboendarterectomy

Thromboendarterectomy has been the treatment of choice for pulmonary hypertension that is associated with chronic thromboembolic disease. Anticoagulation should be instituted and inferior vena cava filters are recommended in patients with this entity, but the only means by which to alleviate symptoms and to have an impact on survival is surgery. Pulmonary thromboendarterectomy is performed via median sternotomy on cardiopulmonary bypass. The overall mortality continues to improve and is now less than 5%. The response to therapy is often impressive, with dramatic reversal of right ventricular dysfunction (157,158). Lung transplantation can be performed in patients in whom thrombi are too distal to extract.

Lung Transplantation

Lung transplantation and heart-lung transplantation are being used as surgical therapy for patients with a variety of pulmonary parenchymal and vascular disorders (159). Patients should be referred for evaluation for transplantation if class III or class IV symptoms are present. The length of the waiting list at a given center (generally 6 to 18 months) helps to determine the appropriate time for listing and transplantation. Patients with PPH or pulmonary arterial hypertension due to the scleroderma spectrum of diseases should undergo a trial of prostacyclin therapy by continuous infusion before proceeding to lung transplantation, because this drug has proved so efficacious in these settings. Single and bilateral lung transplantation, rather than heart-lung transplantation, are the procedures of choice due to the limited availability of organs. The RV has a tremendous capacity to recover in spite of severe dysfunction once the afterload posed by the abnormal pulmonary vasculature is removed. Single-lung transplants are done in all patients with pulmonary parenchymal disorders, except those with suppurative diseases such as cystic fibrosis, in which case bilateral lung transplantation is performed.

Most centers prefer bilateral lung transplantation for PPH as well. One advantage of the bilateral approach may be that the new lung is less likely to suffer from reperfusion pulmonary edema immediately after operation. Chronic rejection may also be more easily tolerated with a bilateral transplant than when the extremely abnormal native PPH lung remains (160). However, the waiting time on the list is shorter for a single-lung transplant, and a set of donor lungs can be offered to two patients when single-lung transplantation is used for PPH. Many transplant teams prefer the single-lung procedure. Heart-lung transplantation is reserved for patients with associated left heart disease or congenital heart disease with pulmonary hypertension when the atrial or ventricular septal defect cannot be repaired. Markedly depressed right ventricular function is not a contraindication to single or bilateral lung transplantation because right ventricular function improves considerably after transplantation (159). Right ventricular shape also appears to normalize after single and bilateral lung transplantation. One-year survival rates for lung transplantation are approximately 80%. Obliterative bronchiolitis (chronic rejection) is the major long-term complication of transplantation. Patients with PPH appear to have higher mortality as well as a higher frequency of obliterative bronchiolitis. Recurrence of the primary pulmonary disorder in the transplanted lung can occur in certain conditions but has not been reported in PPH.

SUMMARY

Pulmonary hypertension and cor pulmonale result in substantial morbidity and mortality. The etiologies are numerous because nearly any chronic lung disease can result in cor pulmonale. Other entities such as neuromuscular disease and thoracic cage abnormalities can result in hypoxemia and ultimately in pulmonary hypertension with right ventricular failure. Basic scientific efforts indicate the importance of growth factors and of smooth muscle proliferation in the pathogenesis of PPH. The diagnosis and an assessment of severity begin with the history and physical examination. Chest radiography and echocardiography may be useful in elucidating the etiology and severity of pulmonary hypertension, and pulmonary function testing may clarify the physiology and severity of underlying lung disease. Certain diseases such as chronic thromboembolic pulmonary hypertension require specific diagnostic testing, including $\dot{V}/\dot{Q}$ scanning and pulmonary arteriography. Helical CT scanning and MRI may be useful in diagnosing and characterizing the extent of this disease. Right heart catheterization remains the gold standard for quantifying the severity of pulmonary hypertension. Appropriate therapy involves treatment of underlying lung disease as well as direct measures to reduce pulmonary artery pressures without causing systemic hypotension. The prognosis depends

to some extent on the nature of the underlying disease. The underlying causes of pulmonary hypertension and cor pulmonale followed by the diagnostic and therapeutic approaches are described. Continuous intravenous prostacyclin has revolutionized the treatment of primary and some forms of secondary pulmonary hypertension. Finally, newer diagnostic and therapeutic modalities, some of which remain theoretical or unproven, are emphasized. The recently approved endothelin antagonist will likely be used in substantial numbers of patients with PPH and with pulmonary arterial hypertension due to scleroderma and related diseases.

CONTROVERSIES AND PERSONAL PERSPECTIVES

Despite tremendous progress in basic scientific and clinical research, pulmonary hypertension and cor pulmonale remain among the more difficult cardiopulmonary disorders to treat. Because (except in the case of PPH) they are the result of *other* disease processes, they may go clinically undetected for months or years, with the assumption that the COPD or ILD itself, for example, is responsible for the dyspnea, fatigue, and other clinical symptoms. The implications of missing the diagnosis of pulmonary hypertension and right ventricular failure are substantial. For PPH, prostacyclin and anticoagulation appear to improve mortality, and listing for transplantation is important because waiting lists are increasing in length. Patients with PPH are often young, do not have hypoxemia or abnormal pulmonary function testing early in the course of the disease process, and may not have glaring chest radiograph abnormalities. Thus, in the past, these individuals were often labeled as having psychogenic dyspnea until symptoms were quite advanced. Over the past decade, the level of awareness for PPH among cardiology and pulmonary specialists has increased, particularly with the advent of newer therapies. However, the diagnosis is more difficult for general practitioners, who may see only one case in a lifetime. It is appropriate for patients with PPH to be evaluated and followed at centers with expertise in this area, particularly as the disease advances.

Organizations such as the Pulmonary Hypertension Association have made tremendous progress in the education and support of patients with PPH. Their biannual conference is a very unique one, at which physicians as well as patients and their family members mutually attend lectures and conferences about pulmonary hypertension, ranging from drug therapy and lung transplantation to coping with a potentially fatal disease. Among the important controversies that clinicians continue to struggle with at present are the timing of the initiation of intravenous prostacyclin and the timing of lung transplantation. A massive effort is currently under way to evaluate all patients

THE FUTURE

The diagnostic and therapeutic approach to pulmonary hypertension and right ventricular failure will change substantially over the next 10 years. Noninvasive technology, including multidimensional echocardiography, ultrafast CT, and MRI techniques, will facilitate accurate characterization of right ventricular size and function, eliminating the need for invasive testing with cardiac catheterization. With the advent of this technology, evaluation of the RV and pulmonary circulation will, when necessary, be performed more frequently, permitting more effective assessment of therapeutic benefit. At the present time, the need for right heart catheterization for evaluation of pulmonary hypertension and cor pulmonale prevents rigorous accurate follow-up in these patients.

Clinical trials will be conducted, enabling better understanding of the utility of older treatment modalities, such as digoxin and other inotropes, on right ventricular function, as well as enhancing our knowledge base with regard to newer therapies, such as oral, subcutaneous, and inhaled prostacyclin; endothelin antagonism; and inhaled NO; and related therapies. Treatment of underlying lung disease that leads to cor pulmonale may become more feasible. Enhanced understanding of the role of various inflammatory mediators in primary pulmonary vascular disease as well as chronic fibrotic lung disorders will also have an impact on therapy. Surgical therapy will continue to become more sophisticated. Advances in lung transplantation (including xenotransplantation), pulmonary thromboendarterectomy, and lung volume reduction surgery for emphysema may lead to increases in survival in patients with end-stage lung disease. Perhaps direct right ventricular surgery with removal of hypokinetic myocardial tissue will enhance the function of the ventricle.

Our understanding of the basic biology of the vascular endothelium and its role in the development of pulmonary hypertension as well as the importance of its interaction with red blood cells is essential. The respective roles of platelet-derived growth factor B, TGFs, insulin-like growth factor-1, and basic fibroblast growth factor will be clarified, as will the regulation of endothelin and NO. The key elements of tissue repair and vascular remodeling will be elucidated. The relative role of the coagulation pathway in PPH will be essential to determine. The genetics of PPH are already becoming clearer. The *BMPR2*, a component of the TGF-β family, plays a key role in cell growth. This gene has been shown to be associated with familial PPH (28a). More recently, it has been discovered that the sporadic form of PPH is also associated with germline mutations of *BMPR2* in a significant minority of patients (28b). The importance of this gene and its relationship to pulmonary hypertension will be clarified. Regulation of gene expression may be a key method through which pulmonary hypertension can be controlled. The basic mechanisms that underlie hypoxic vasoconstriction are essential to understand; if this process can be unraveled, it may permit us to prevent right ventricular failure *completely*.

who have received intravenous prostacyclin in the past and to evaluate future patients prospectively to better characterize appropriate dosing of the drug and to examine the mortality and outcome. Although lung transplantation is the final therapeutic step for many patients with PPH and other patients with cor pulmonale, conquering the ultimate cause of death in many of these patients (chronic rejection) will be crucial. The genetics of PPH are being unraveled; this may contribute substantially to disease prevention and treatment in the future.

REFERENCES

1. Fishman AP. Chronic cor pulmonale. *Am Rev Respir Dis* 1976;114:775–794.
2. Cournand A. The historical development of the concepts of pulmonary circulation. In: Adams AR, Veith I, eds. *Pulmonary circulation.* New York: Grune & Stratton, 1959:1.
3. Cournand A, Ranges HA. Catheterization of the right auricle in man. *Proc Soc Exp Biol Med* 1941;46:462.
4. Bloomfield RA, Lauson HD, Cournand A, et al. Recording of right heart pressures in normal subjects and in patients with chronic pulmonary disease and various types of cardiocirculatory disorders. *J Clin Invest* 1946;25:639.
5. Fowler NO, Westcott RN, Scott RC. Normal pressure in the right heart and pulmonary artery. *Am Heart J* 1953;46:264.
6. Swan HJC, Ganz W, Forrester J, et al. Catheterization of the heart in man with the use of a flow-directed balloon-tipped catheter. *N Engl J Med* 1970;283:447–451.
7. Fishman AP, McClement J, Jimmelstein A, et al. Effects of acute anoxia on the circulation and respiration in patients with chronic pulmonary disease studied during the steady-state. *J Clin Invest* 1952;31:770–781.
8. Parker JO, Kelkar K, West RO. Hemodynamic effects of aminophylline in cor pulmonale. *Circulation* 1966;33:17–25.
9. Koziorowski A, Zielinski J, Maszczyk Z, et al. Effect of salbutamol on pulmonary circulation, ventilation and gas exchange in patients with chronic obstructive airways disease. Preliminary report. *Bull Physiopathol Respir* 1972;8:611–616.
10. Keller CA, Shepard JW, Chun DS, et al. Effects of hydralazine on hemodynamics, ventilation, and gas

exchange in patients with chronic obstructive pulmonary disease and pulmonary hypertension. *Am Rev Respir Dis* 1984;130:606–611.

11. Motley HL, Coumand A, Werko L, et al. The influence of short periods of induced anoxia upon pulmonary artery pressure in man. *Am J Physiol* 1947;150:315–320.

12. von Euler VS, Liljestrand G. Observations on the pulmonary arterial blood pressure in the cat. *Acta Physiol Scand* 1946;12:301–320.

13. Fishman AP. A century of primary pulmonary hypertension. In: Rubin LJ, Rich S, eds. *Primary pulmonary hypertension.* New York: Marcel Dekker Inc, 1997:1–17.

14. Dresdale DT, Schultz M, Michtom RJ. Primary pulmonary hypertension. I. Clinical and hemodynamic studies. *Am J Med* 1951;11:686–705.

15. Harris P. Influence of acetylcholine on the pulmonary artery pressure. *Br Heart J* 1957;19:272–286.

16. Wood P. Pulmonary hypertension with special reference to the vasoconstrictive factor. *Br Heart J* 1958;21:557–570.

17. Gurtner HP. Pulmonary hypertension, plexogenic pulmonary arteriopathy and the appetite depressant drug aminorex: post or propter? *Bull Eur Physiopathol Respir* 1979;15:897–923.

18. Hatano S, Strasser T. Primary pulmonary hypertension. *World Health Organ Tech Rep Ser* 1975:1–46.

19. Rich S. Executive summary of the World Symposium on PPH. 1999. Available at: http://www.who.int/ncd/cvd/pph.html.

20. McFadden E, Braunwald E. Cor pulmonale. In: Braunwald E, ed. *Heart disease: a textbook of cardiovascular medicine,* 3rd ed. Philadelphia: WB Saunders, 1988:1597–1616.

21. D'Alonzo GE, Barst RJ, Ayres SM, et al. Survival in patients with primary pulmonary hypertension. Results from a national prospective registry. *Ann Intern Med* 1991;115:343–349.

22. Weitzenblum E, Loiseau A, Hirth C, et al. Course of pulmonary hemodynamics in patients with chronic obstructive pulmonary disease. *Chest* 1979;75:656–662.

23. Petitpretz P, Brenot F, Azarian R, et al. Pulmonary hypertension in patients with human immunodeficiency virus infection: comparison with primary pulmonary hypertension. *Circulation* 1994;89:2722–2727.

24. Edwards BS, Weir EK, Edwards WD, et al. Coexistent pulmonary and portal hypertension: morphologic and clinical features. *J Am Coll Cardiol* 1987;10:1233–1238.

25. Schaiberger PH, Kennedy TC, Miller FC, et al. Pulmonary hypertension associated with long-term inhalation of "crank" methamphetamine. *Chest* 1993;104:614–616.

26. Tanaka Y, Bernstein ML, Mecham RP, et al. Site-specific responses to monocrotaline-induced vascular injury: evidence for two distinct mechanisms of remodeling. *Am J Respir Cell Mol Biol* 1996;15:390–397.

27. Abenhaim L, Moride Y, Brenot F, et al. Appetite-suppressant drugs and the risk of primary pulmonary hypertension. *N Engl J Med* 1996;335:609–616.

28. Kay JM, Smith P, Heath D. Aminorex and the pulmonary circulation. *Thorax* 1971;26:262–269.

28a. Newman JH, Wheeler L, Lane KB, et al. Mutations in the gene for bone morphogenetic protein receptor as a cause of primary pulmonary hypertension in a large kindred. *N Engl J Med* 2001;345:319–324.

28b. Thomson JR, Machado RD, Pauciulo MW, et al. Sporadic primary pulmonary hypertension is associated with germ-line mutations of the gene encoding BMPR-II, a receptor member of the TGF-β family. *J Med Genet* 2000;37:741–745.

28c. Zhou S, Kinzler KW, Vogelstein B. Going mad with *Smads. N Engl J Med* 1999;341:1144–1146.

28d. Massague J, Blain SW, Lo RS. TGF beta signaling in growth-control, cancer, and heritable disorders. *Cell* 2000;103:295–309.

29. Weber K, Janicki J, Shroff S, et al. The right ventricle: physiologic and pathophysiologic considerations. *Crit Care Med* 1983;11:323–328.

30. Schulman DS, Matthay RA. The right ventricle in pulmonary disease. *Cardiol Clin* 1992;10:111–138.

31. D'Amato AN, Galante JF, Smith WM. Hemodynamic response to treadmill exercise in normal subjects. *J Appl Physiol* 1966;23:631–640.

32. Epstein SE, Reiser GD, Stampfer M, et al. Characterization of the circulatory response to maximal upright exercise in normal subjects and patients with heart disease. *Circulation* 1967;35:1049–1062.

33. Glazier J, Hughes J, Maloney J, et al. Measurements of capillary dimensions and blood volume in rapidly frozen lungs. *J Appl Physiol* 1969;26:65–76.

34. Cromie JB. Correlation of anatomic pulmonary emphysema and right ventricular hypertrophy. *Am Rev Respir Dis* 1961;84:657–667.

35. Okada M, Ota T, Okada M, et al. Right ventricular dysfunction after major pulmonary resection. *J Thorac Cardiovasc Surg* 1994;108:503–511.

36. Fishman AP. Dynamics of the pulmonary circulation. In: Hamilton WF, Dow P, eds. *Handbook of physiology,* sec 2, vol 2. Washington, DC: American Physiological Society, 1963:1667.

37. Brooks H, Kirk E, Vokonas P, et al. Performance of the right ventricle under stress: relation to right coronary flow. *J Clin Invest* 1971;50:2176–2182.

38. Furchgott RF, Zawadzki JV. The obligatory role of endothelial cells in the relaxation of arterial smooth muscle by acetylcholine. *Nature* 1980;288:373–376.

39. Palmer RMJ, Ferrige AG, Moncada S. Nitric oxide release accounts for the biological activity of endothelium-derived relaxing factor. *Nature* 1987;327:524–526.

40. Myers PR, Minor RL Jr, Guerra R Jr, et al. Vasorelaxant properties of the endothelium-derived relaxing factor more closely resemble *S*-nitrosocysteine than nitric oxide. *Nature* 1990;345:161–163.

41. Palmer RMJ, Moncada S. A novel citrulline-forming enzyme implicated in the formation of nitric oxide by vascular endothelial cells. *Biochem Biophys Res Commun* 1989;158:348–352.

42. Moncada S, Palmer RMJ, Higgs EA. Nitric oxide: physiology, pathophysiology and pharmacology. *Pharmacol Rev* 1991;43:109–142.

43. Gaston B, Drazen JM, Loscalzo J, Stamler JS. The biology of nitrogen oxides in the airways. *Am J Respir Crit Care Med* 1994;149:538–551.

44. Chand N, Altura BM. Acetylcholine and bradykinin relax intrapulmonary arteries by acting on endothelial cells: role in lung vascular diseases. *Science* 1981;213:1376–1379.

45. Ignarro LJ, Burke TM, Wood KS, et al. Association between cyclic GMP accumulation and acetylcholine-elicited relaxation of bovine intrapulmonary artery. *J Pharmacol Exp Ther* 1984;228:682–690.

46. Satoh H, Inui J. Endothelial cell–dependent relaxation and contraction induced by histamine in the isolated guinea-pig pulmonary artery. *Eur J Pharmacol* 1984;97:321–324.

47. Tanaka DT, Grunstein MM. Vasoactive effects of substance P on isolated rabbit pulmonary artery. *J Appl Physiol* 1985;58:1291–1297.

48. Thom S, Hughes A, Martin G, Sever PS. Endothelium-dependent relaxation of isolated human arteries and veins. *Clin Sci* 1987;73:547–552.

49. Archer SL, Tolins JP, Raij L, Weir EK. Hypoxic pulmonary vasoconstriction is enhanced by inhibition of the synthesis of an endothelium-derived relaxing factor. *Biochem Biophys Res Commun* 1989;164:1198–1205.

50. Persson MG, Gustafsson LE, Wiklund NP, et al. Endogenous nitric oxide as a probable modulator of pulmonary circulation and hypoxic pressor response in vivo. *Acta Physiol Scand* 1990;140:449–457.

51. Robertson BE, Warren JB, Nye PC. Inhibition of nitric oxide synthesis potentiates hypoxic vasoconstriction in isolated rat lungs. *Exp Physiol* 1990;75:255–257.

52. Brashers VL, Peach MJ, Rose CE Jr. Augmentation of hypoxic pulmonary vasoconstriction in the isolated perfused rat lung by in vitro antagonists of endothelium-dependent relaxation. *J Clin Invest* 1988;82:1495–1502.

53. Adnot S, Raffestin B, Eddahibi S, et al. Loss of endothelium-dependent relaxant activity in the pulmonary circulation of rats exposed to chronic hypoxia. *J Clin Invest* 1991;87:155–162.

54. Liu SF, Crawley DE, Barnes PJ, Evans TW. Endothelium-derived relaxing factor inhibits hypoxic pulmonary vasoconstriction in rats. *Am Rev Respir Dis* 199;143:32–37.

55. Dinh-Xuan AT, Higgenbottam TW, Clelland CA, et al. Impairment of endothelium dependent pulmonary artery relaxation in chronic obstructive lung disease. *N Engl J Med* 1991;324:1539–1547.

56. Dinh-Xuan AT. Endothelial modulation of pulmonary vascular tone. *Eur Respir J* 1992;5:757–762.

57. Sobin S, Tremer H, Hardy J, et al. Changes in arteriole in acute and chronic hypoxic pulmonary hypertension and recovery in rat. *J Appl Physiol* 1983;55:1445–1455.

58. Voelkel NF, Tuder RM, Weir EK. Pathophysiology of primary pulmonary hypertension: from physiology to molecular mechanisms. In: Rubin LJ, Rich S, eds. *Primary pulmonary hypertension.* New York: Marcel Dekker Inc, 1997:83–133.

59. Moncada S, Glygewski R, Bunting S, Vane JR. An enzyme isolated from arteries transforms prostaglandin endoperoxides to an unstable substance that inhibits platelet aggregation. *Nature* 1976;263:663–665.

60. Aukland K, Kiil F, Kjekshus J. Relationship between ventricular pressures and right and left myocardial blood flow. *Acta Physiol Scand* 1967;70:116–126.

61. Gold F, Bache R. Transmural right ventricular blood flow during acute pulmonary artery hypertension in the sedated dog. *Circ Res* 1982;51:196–204.

62. Fixler D, Archie J, Ullyot D, et al. Effects of acute right ventricular systolic hypertension on regional myocardial blood flow in anesthetized dogs. *Am Heart J* 1973;85:491–500.

63. Lowensohn H, Khouri E, Gregg D, et al. Phasic right coronary artery blood flow in conscious dogs with normal and elevated right ventricular pressures. *Circ Res* 1976;39:760–765.

64. Brooks H, Holland R, Al-Sadir J. Right ventricular performance during ischemia: an anatomic and hemodynamic analysis. *Am J Physiol* 1977;233:H500–H513.

65. Sibbald W, Driedger A. Right ventricular function in acute disease states: pathophysiologic considerations. *Crit Care Med* 1983;11:339–345.

66. Spann J, Covell J, Eckbert D, et al. Contractile performance of the hypertrophied and chronically failing cat ventricle. *Am J Physiol* 1972;223:1150–1157.

67. Renzetti AD, McClement JH, Litt BD. The Veterans Administration cooperative study of pulmonary function. *Am J Med* 1966;41:115–129.

68. Lindsay D, Read J. Pulmonary vascular responsiveness in the prognosis of chronic obstructive lung disease. *Am Rev Respir Dis* 1972;105:242–249.

69. Traver GA, Cline MG, Burrows B. Predictors of mortality in chronic obstructive pulmonary disease. A 15 year follow-up study. *Am Rev Respir Dis* 1979;119:895–902.

70. Ellis J, Kirch D, Steele P. Right ventricular ejection fraction in severe chronic airway obstruction. *Chest* 1977;71:281–282.

71. Weitzenblum E, Hirth C, Ducolone A, et al. Prognostic value of pulmonary artery pressure in chronic obstructive pulmonary disease. *Thorax* 1981;36:752–758.

72. Brent B, Berger H, Matthay RA, et al. Physiologic correlates of right ventricular ejection fraction in chronic obstructive pulmonary disease. A combined radionuclide and hemodynamic study. *Am J Cardiol* 1982;50:255–262.

73. Crystal R, Gadek J, Ferrans V, et al. Interstitial lung disease: current concepts of pathogenesis, staging and therapy. *Am J Med* 1981;70:542–568.

74. Bishop J, Cross K. Physiologic variables and mortality in patients with various categories of chronic respiratory disease. *Bull Eur Physiopathol Respir* 1984;20;495–500.

75. Rubin LJ. Primary pulmonary hypertension. *N Engl J Med* 1997;336:111–117.

76. Rich S, Brundage BH. High-dose calcium channel–blocking therapy for primary pulmonary hypertension: evidence for long-term reduction in pulmonary arterial pressure and regression of right ventricular hypertrophy. *Circulation* 1987;76:135–141.

77. Weir EK, Rubin LJ, Ayres SM, et al. The acute administration of vasodilators in primary pulmonary hypertension: experience from the National Institutes of Health Registry on Primary Pulmonary Hypertension. *Am Rev Respir Dis* 1989;140:1623–1630.

78. Rich S, Kaufmann E, Levy PS. The effect of high doses of calcium-channel blockers on survival in primary pulmonary hypertension. *N Engl J Med* 1992;327:76–81.

79. Barst RJ, Rubin LJ, Long WA, et al. A comparison of continuous intravenous epoprostenol (prostacyclin) with con-

ventional therapy for primary pulmonary hypertension. *N Engl J Med* 1996;334:296–301.

80. Christman BW, McPherson CD, Newman JH, et al. An imbalance between the excretion of thromboxane and prostacyclin metabolites in pulmonary hypertension. *N Engl J Med* 1992;327:70–75.

81. Giaid A, Saleh D. Reduced expression of endothelial nitric oxide synthase in the lungs of patients with pulmonary hypertension. *N Engl J Med* 1995;333:214–221.

82. Franco-Obregon A, Urena J, Lopez-Barneo J. Oxygen-sensitive calcium channels in vascular smooth muscle and their possible role in hypoxic arterial relaxation. *Proc Natl Acad Sci U S A* 1995;92:4715–4719.

83. Eisenberg PR, Lucore C, Kaufmann L, et al. Fibrinopeptide levels indicative of pulmonary vascular thrombosis in patients with primary pulmonary hypertension. *Circulation* 1990;82:841–847.

84. Ingelsby TV, Singer JW, Gordon DS. Abnormal fibrinolysis in familial primary pulmonary hypertension. *Am J Med* 1973;55:5–14.

85. Tubbs PR, Levin RD, Shivey EK, et al. Fibrinolysis in familial primary pulmonary hypertension. *Am J Clin Pathol* 1979;71:384–387.

86. Geggel RV, Carvalho ACA, Hoyer LW, et al. von Willebrand factor: abnormalities in primary pulmonary hypertension. *ARRD* 1987;135:294–299.

87. Wagenvoort CA, Mulder PGH. Thrombotic lesions in primary plexogenic pulmonary arteriopathy. *Chest* 1993;103:844–849.

88. Badesch DB, Lee PDK, Parks WC, Stenmark KR. Insulin-like growth factor I stimulates elastin synthesis by bovine pulmonary arterial smooth muscle cells. *Biochem Biophys Res Commun* 1989;160:382–387.

89. Botney MD, Bahadori L, Gold LI. Vascular remodeling in primary pulmonary hypertension. Potential role for transforming growth factor B. *Am J Pathol* 1994;144:286–295.

90. Lindner V, Lappi DA, Baird A, et al. Role of basic fibroblast growth factor in vascular lesion formation. *Circ Res* 1991;63:106–113.

91. Pierce GF, Mustoe TA, Lingelbach J, et al. Platelet-derived growth factor B and transforming growth factors induce in vivo and in vitro tissue repair activities by unique mechanisms. *J Cell Biol* 1989;109:429–440.

92. Botney MD, Kaiser LR, Cooper JD, et al. Extracellular matrix protein gene expression in atherosclerotic hypertensive pulmonary arteries. *Am J Pathol* 1992;140:357–364.

93. Todorovich-Hunter L, Dodo J, Chongliang YE, et al. Increased pulmonary artery elastolytic activity in adult rats with monocrotaline-induced progressive hypertensive pulmonary vascular disease compared with infant rats with nonprogressive disease. *Am Rev Respir Dis* 1992;146:213–223.

94. Mandel J, Mark EJ, Hales CA. Pulmonary veno-occlusive disease. *Am J Respir Crit Care Med* 2000;162:1964–1973.

95. McIntyre K, Sasahara A. The hemodynamic response to pulmonary embolism in patients without prior cardiopulmonary disease. *Am J Cardiol* 1971;28:288–294.

96. McIntyre K, Sasahara A. Determinants of right ventricular function and hemodynamics after pulmonary embolism. *Chest* 1974;65:534–543.

97. Goldstein RS, Molotiu N, Skrastins R, et al. Reversal of sleep induced by hypoventilation and chronic respiratory failure by nocturnal negative pressure ventilation in patients with restrictive ventilatory impairment. *Am Rev Respir Dis* 1987;135:1049–1055.

98. Fletcher EC, Schaaf JW, Miller J, et al. Long-term cardiopulmonary sequelae in patients with sleep apnea and chronic lung disease. *Am Rev Respir Dis* 1987;135:525–533.

99. Rich S, Dantzker DR, Ayers SM. Primary pulmonary hypertension: a national prospective study. *Ann Intern Med* 1987;107:216–222.

100. Kanemoto N, Furuya H, Etoh T, et al. Chest roentgenograms in primary pulmonary hypertension. *Chest* 1979;96:45–49.

101. D'Alonzo GE, Dantzker DR. Diagnosing primary pulmonary hypertension. In: Rubin LJ, Rich S, eds. *Primary pulmonary hypertension.* New York: Marcel Dekker Inc, 1997:227–252.

102. Farb A, Burke AP, Virmani R. Anatomy and pathology of the right ventricle. *Cardiol Clin* 1992;10:1–21.

103. Astorri E, Chizzola A, Visioli A, et al. Right ventricular hypertrophy: a cytometric study on 55 human hearts. *J Mol Cell Cardiol* 1971;22:99.

104. Fulton RM, Hutchinson EC, Jones AM. Ventricular weight in cardiac hypertrophy. *Br Heart J* 1952;14:413.

105. Mitchell RS, Stanford RE, Silvers GW, et al. The right ventricle in chronic airway obstruction: a clinicopathologic study. *Am Rev Respir Dis* 1976;114:147.

106. Reiner L, Mazzoleni A, Rodriguez FL, et al. The weight of the human heart. *Arch Pathol* 1959;68:58.

107. Rahlf G. Chronic cor pulmonale: weight and intraventricular volume of the right ventricle in chronic pulmonary disease. *Virchows Arch* 1978;378:273.

108. Jaffe CC, Weltin G. Echocardiography of the right side of the heart. *Cardiol Clin* 1992;10:41–57.

109. Currie PJ, Seward JB, Chankl, et al. Continuous wave Doppler determination of right ventricular pressure: a simultaneous Doppler-catheterization study in 127 patients. *J Am Coll Cardiol* 1985;6:750–756.

110. Ritchie M, Waggoner AD, Davila-Roman VG, et al. Echocardiographic characterization of the improvement in right ventricular function in patients with severe pulmonary hypertension after lung transplantation. *J Am Coll Cardiol* 1993;22:1170–1174.

111. Chow LC, Dittrich HC, Hoit BD, et al. Doppler assessment of changes in right-sided cardiac hemodynamics after pulmonary thromboendarterectomy. *Am J Cardiol* 1988;61:1092–1097.

112. Bates JR, Tantengco MV, Ryan T, Feigenbaum H. A systematic approach to echocardiographic image acquisition and three-dimensional reconstruction with a subxiphoid rotational scan. *J Am Soc Echocardiogr* 1996:9:257–265.

113. Jain D, Zaret BL. Assessment of right ventricular function. Role of nuclear imaging techniques. *Cardiol Clin* 1992;10:23–29.

114. Jaffe CC, Ellis K. Angiographic determination of ventricular volume, shape and mass. *Curr Probl Radiol* 1974;4:1.

115. D'Alonzo GE, Bower JS, Dantzker DR. Differentiation of patients with primary and thromboembolic pulmonary hypertension. *Chest* 1984;85:457–461.

116. Auger WR, Fedullo PF, Moser KM, et al. Chronic major-vessel thromboembolic pulmonary artery obstruction: appearance at angiography. *Radiology* 1992;182:393–398.

117. Shure D, Gregoratos G, Moser KM. Fiberoptic angioscopy: role in the diagnosis of chronic pulmonary arterial obstruction. *Ann Intern Med* 1985;103:844–850.

118. Pattynama PMT, De Roos A, Van Der Wall EE, Van Voorthuisen AE. Evaluation of cardiac function with magnetic resonance imaging. *Am Heart J* 1994;128:595–607.

119. Mogelvang J, Stockholm KLT, Stubgaard M, et al. Assessment of right ventricular volumes by magnetic resonance imaging and by radionuclide angiography. *Am J Noninvasive Cardiol* 1991;5:321–327.

120. Helbing WA, Rebergen SA, Maliepaard C, et al. Quantification of right ventricular function with magnetic resonance imaging in children with normal hearts and with congenital heart disease. *Am Heart J* 1995;130:828–837.

121. Moulton MJ, Creswell LL, Ungacta FF, et al. Magnetic resonance imaging provides evidence for remodeling of the right ventricle after single-lung transplantation for pulmonary hypertension. *Circulation* 1996;94:II-312–II-319.

122. Sostman HD, Layish DT, Tapson VF, et al. Prospective comparison of helical CT and MR imaging in clinically suspected acute pulmonary embolism. *J Magn Reson Imaging* 1996;6:275–281.

123. Nocturnal Oxygen Therapy Trial Group. Continuous or nocturnal oxygen therapy in hypoxemic chronic obstructive lung disease. A clinical trial. *Ann Intern Med* 1980;93:391–398.

124. Medical Research Council Working Party. Long term domiciliary oxygen therapy in chronic hypoxic cor pulmonale complicating chronic bronchitis and emphysema: a clinical trial. *Lancet* 1981;1:681–685.

125. Weitzenblum E, Sautegeau A, Ehrhart M, et al. Long-term oxygen therapy can reverse the progression of pulmonary hypertension in patients with chronic obstructive pulmonary disease. *Am Rev Respir Dis* 1985;131:493–498.

126. Rutherford J, Vatner S, Braunwald E. Effects and mechanism of action of aminophylline on cardiac function and regional blood flow distribution in conscious dogs. *Circulation* 1981;63:378–387.

127. Aubier M, DeTroyer A, Sampton M, et al. Aminophylline improves diaphragmatic contractility. *N Engl J Med* 1981;305:249–252.

128. Matthay RA. Favorable cardiovascular effects of theophylline in COPD. *Chest* 1987;92:22S–26S.

129. Mathur P, Powles P, Pugsley S, et al. Effect of digoxin on right ventricular function in severe chronic airflow obstruction. *Ann Intern Med* 1981;95:283–287.

130. Brown S, Pakron F, Milne N, et al. Effects of digoxin on exercise capacity and right ventricular dysfunction during exercise in chronic airflow obstruction. *Chest* 1984;85:187–191.

131. Weir EK, Rubin LJ, Ayres SM, et al. The acute administration of vasodilators in primary pulmonary hypertension: experience from the National Institutes of Health Registry on Primary Pulmonary Hypertension. *Am Rev Respir Dis* 1989;140:1623–1630.

132. Morley TF, Zappasodi SJ, Belli A, Giudice JA. Pulmonary vasodilator therapy for chronic obstructive pulmonary disease and cor pulmonale. *Chest* 1987;92:71–76.

133. Saadjian A, Philip-Joet F, Arnaud A. Hemodynamic and oxygen delivery responses to nifedipine in pulmonary hypertension secondary to chronic obstructive lung disease. *Cardiology* 1987;74:196–204.

134. Agostoni P, Doria E, Galli C, et al. Nifedipine reduces pulmonary pressure and vascular tone during short- but not long-term treatment of pulmonary hypertension in patients with chronic obstructive pulmonary disease. *Am Rev Respir Dis* 1989;139:120–125.

135. Schuster DP, Crouch EC, Parks WC, et al. Angiotensin converting enzyme expression in primary pulmonary hypertension. *Am J Respir Crit Care Med* 1996;154:1087–1091.

136. Leier CV, Bambach D, Nelson S, et al. Captopril in primary pulmonary hypertension. *Circulation* 1983;67:155–161.

137. Rubin LJ, Groves BM, Reeves JT, et al. Prostacyclin-induced acute pulmonary vasodilation in primary pulmonary hypertension. *Circulation* 1982;66:334–338.

138. Barst RJ, Rubin LJ, McGoon MD, Caldwell EJ, et al. Survival in primary pulmonary hypertension with long-term continuous intravenous prostacyclin. *Ann Intern Med* 1994;121:409–415.

139. Rubin LJ, Mendoza J, Hood M, et al. Treatment of primary pulmonary hypertension with continuous intravenous prostacyclin (epoprostanol): results of a randomized trial. *Ann Intern Med* 1990;112:485–491.

140. Badesch DB, Tapson VF, McGoon MD, et al. Continuous intravenous epoprostenol for pulmonary hypertension due to the scleroderma spectrum of disease. *Ann Intern Med* 2000; 132:425–434.

141. Zobel G, Dacar D, Rodl S, Friehs I. Inhaled nitric oxide versus inhaled prostacyclin and intravenous versus inhaled prostacyclin in acute respiratory failure with pulmonary hypertension in piglets. *Pediatr Res* 1995;38:198–204.

142. Olschewski H, Walmrath D, Schermuly R, et al. Aerosolized prostacyclin and iloprost in severe pulmonary hypertension. *Ann Intern Med* 1996;124:820–824.

143. Saji T, Ozawa Y, Ishikita T, et al. Short-term hemodynamic effect of a new oral PGI_2 analogue, beraprost, in primary and secondary pulmonary hypertension. *Am J Cardiol* 1996;78:244–247.

144. Chen SJ, Chen YF, Meng QC, et al. Endothelin-receptor antagonist bosentan prevents and reverses hypoxic pulmonary vasoconstriction in rats. *J Appl Physiol* 1995;79:2122–2131.

145. Channick RN, Simonneau G, Sitbon O, et al. Effects of the dual endothelin-receptor antagonist bosentan in patients with pulmonary hypertension: a randomised placebo-controlled study. *Lancet* 2001;358:1119–1123.

146. Frostell C, Fratacci MD, Wain JC, et al. Inhaled nitric oxide, a selective pulmonary vasodilator reversing hypoxic pulmonary vasoconstriction. *Circulation* 1991;83:2038–2047.

147. Pepke-Zaba J, Higenbottam TW, Dinh-Xuan AT, et al. Inhaled nitric oxide as a cause of selective pulmonary vasodilatation in pulmonary hypertension. *Lancet* 1991;338:1173–1174.

148. Sitbon O, Brenot F, Denjean A, et al. Inhaled nitric oxide as a screening vasodilator agent in primary pulmonary hypertension: a dose-response study and comparison with prostacyclin. *Am J Respir Crit Care Med* 1995;151:384–389.

149. Neonatal Inhaled Nitric Oxide Study Group. Inhaled nitric oxide in full-term and nearly full-term infants with hypoxic respiratory failure. *N Engl J Med* 1997;336:597–604.

150. Roberts JD, Fineman JR, Morin FC III, et al. Inhaled nitric oxide and persistent pulmonary hypertension of the newborn. *N Engl J Med* 1997;336:605–610.

151. Channick RN, Newhart JW, Johnson FW, et al. Pulsed delivery of inhaled nitric oxide to patients with primary pulmonary hypertension: an ambulatory delivery system and initial clinical tests. *Chest* 1996;109:1545–1549.

152. Fuster V, Steele PM, Edwards WD, et al. Primary pulmonary hypertension: natural history and the importance of thrombosis. *Circulation* 1984;70:580–587.

153. Spence CR, Thompson BT, Janssens SP, et al. Effect of aerosol heparin on the development of hypoxic pulmonary hypertension in the guinea pig. *Am Rev Respir Dis* 1993;148:241–244.

154. Kerstein D, Levy PS, Hsu DT, et al. Blade balloon atrial septostomy in patients with severe primary pulmonary hypertension. *Circulation* 1995;91:2028–2035.

155. Nihill MR, D'Laughlin MP, Mullins CE. Effects of atrial septostomy in patients with terminal cor pulmonale due to pulmonary vascular disease. *Cath Cardiovasc Diag* 1991;24:166–172.

156. Austen WG, Morrow AG, Berry WB. Experimental studies of the surgical treatment of primary pulmonary hypertension. *J Thorac Cardiovasc Surg* 1964;48:448–455.

157. Shure D. Chronic thromboembolic pulmonary hypertension: diagnosis and treatment. *Semin Respir Crit Care Med* 1996;17:7.

158. Fedullo PF, Auger WR, Channick RN, et al. Chronic thromboembolic pulmonary hypertension. *Clin Chest Med* 1995;16:353–374.

159. Katayama Y, Cremona G, Wallwork J, et al. Transplantation for primary pulmonary hypertension. In: Rubin LJ, Rich S, eds. *Primary pulmonary hypertension.* New York: Marcel Dekker Inc, 1997:287–317.

160. Levine SM, Jenkinson SG, Bryan CL, et al. Ventilation-perfusion inequalities during graft rejection in patients undergoing single lung transplantation for primary pulmonary hypertension. *Chest* 1992;101:401–405.

28

VENOUS THROMBOEMBOLISM

VICTOR F. TAPSON

▼▼ **ADDITIONAL ELECTRONIC TOPICS**

Historical Perspective f86;   Molecular Defects f87;   Laboratory Testing f88;   Computed Tomography and Magnetic Resonance
Imaging f89;   Novel Anticoagulants and Experimental Models of Thrombosis f90;   Pulmonary Embolectomy and Catheter-Extraction Techniques f91

INCIDENCE

VTE constitutes a clinical spectrum encompassing DVT and
PE. This disorder occurs extraordinarily commonly in hospitalized patients particularly after major surgery, and the care
of these patients spans all specialties and subspecialties. PE
most commonly results from DVT occurring in the veins of
the proximal lower extremities—that is, including and proximal to the popliteal veins. Both DVT and PE are frequently
clinically unsuspected, leading to significant diagnostic and
therapeutic delays and accounting for substantial morbidity
and mortality. Although there are as many as 260,000
patients in the United States in whom VTE is diagnosed and
treated each year, more than half of the cases that actually
occur are never diagnosed, and as many as 600,000 cases
may therefore occur. Many patients dying from acute PE
have coexisting terminal illnesses; however, it would appear
that this disease entity is responsible for the deaths of 50,000
to 100,000 patients with an otherwise good prognosis, and
many of these deaths would appear preventable (20,21).
Autopsy studies have repeatedly documented the high frequency in which PE has gone unsuspected and undetected
(22). Despite advances in diagnostic technology and therapeutic approaches, VTE remains underdiagnosed, and prophylaxis continues to be dramatically underused (23).

RISK FACTORS AND PATHOPHYSIOLOGY

Risk Factors

The pathogenesis of DVT as proposed by Virchow is based
on several potential initiating events, including stasis,
venous injury, and hypercoagulability. Risk factors for
DVT are based on these processes (Table 28.1). Frequently
more than one risk factor is present, and knowledge of
these risk factors provides the rationale for both prophylaxis
and clinical suspicion.

   V. F. Tapson: Division of Pulmonary and Critical Care Medicine, Duke
University Medical Center, Durham, North Carolina

TABLE 28.1 RISK FACTORS FOR VENOUS THROMBOEMBOLISM

Clinical factors
   Age >40 yr
   History of venous thromboembolism
   Prior major surgical procedure/trauma
   Hip fracture
   Immobilization/paralysis
   Varicose veins
   Congestive heart failure
   Myocardial infarction
   Obesity
   Pregnancy/postpartum
   Oral contraceptive therapy
   Cerebrovascular accident
   Cancer
   Paroxysmal nocturnal hemoglobinemia
   Antiphospholipid antibody syndrome (including lupus
     anticoagulant)
Genetic/molecular factors
   Antithrombin III deficiency
   Factor V Leiden (activated protein C resistance)
   Protein C deficiency
   Protein S deficiency
   Prothrombin gene (G20210A) defect
   Dysfibrinogenemia
   Disorders of plasminogen
   Elevated factor VIII levels
   Elevated factor XI levels

Clinical Factors

Most venous thrombi arise in valve pockets, where blood flow tends to stagnate. The increased frequency of thrombosis with advanced age and immobilization further suggests the causal relationship between stasis and thrombogenesis. Immobility of any cause results in decreased venous return and stasis. Patients with acute cerebrovascular accidents commonly develop venous thrombi in the paralyzed lower extremity but only rarely in the unaffected limb. Acute paraplegia may be associated with a significantly increased risk of developing DVT, and the period of highest risk appears to be the first two weeks after the onset of the illness (24). Prolonged bedrest or long automobile or airplane trips may lead to the development of thromboemboli. The risk presented by air travel has been somewhat controversial (25–27). Although one recent trial suggests that the risk is not significant (25), more than 5 hours was the longest travel time evaluated, and this group of patients was not further subdivided. Thus, longer travel times were not independently analyzed. A more recent clinical trial does demonstrate a relationship between distance traveled and incidence of PE (27a). Obesity also appears to increase the risk of VTE. Information extrapolated from the Prospective Investigation of Pulmonary Embolism Diagnosis (PIOPED) suggests that the role of obesity as a risk factor requires further clarification; there were not enough patients with morbid obesity included to draw firm

conclusions (28). Immobility and resultant stasis are likely contributing factors. Age appears to increase mortality due to PE (29). This risk is particularly high in those with cardiac disease or cancer. It appears that PE is suspected premortem less commonly in the elderly patient (30).

Previous thromboembolic disease predicts a substantial risk of recurrence in the hospitalized patient. Surgical patients with a history of VTE who do not receive prophylaxis develop postoperative DVT in more than 50% of cases (31). Surgery itself places a patient at significantly increased risk. General surgery patients not receiving pharmacologic or mechanical prophylaxis have been shown to develop venography-proven DVT in as many as 19% of cases (32). Traditionally, heparin prophylaxis has been initiated perioperatively to prevent the development of intraoperative and early postoperative thrombosis. Patients undergoing spinal or pelvic surgery appear to be at particularly high risk (31). Total hip and total knee replacement patients not receiving prophylaxis develop DVT in more than 50% of cases (33). These orthopedic settings have been extensively investigated, prompted by clear evidence in clinical trials that low-molecular-weight heparin (LMWH) preparations are more effective than standard heparin in the setting of total joint replacement (33).

Lower extremity and pelvic trauma enhance the risk of DVT. Emboli are discovered at autopsy in as many as 60% of patients with fractures of the lower extremities (34), and mortality has been attributed to PE in 38% to 50% of patients dying after hip fracture (35). The duration of immobility after trauma influences the development of DVT. The frequency of autopsy-confirmed PE in patients surviving for less than 24 hours after trauma has been shown to be 3.3%, increasing to 5.5% in those surviving up to 7 days. Pulmonary emboli occurred in 18.6% of those surviving for a longer period (36). Other causes of venous trauma include placement of central venous catheters in the jugular, subclavian, or femoral veins. Clinically significant PE arising from upper extremity thrombosis can occur but is significantly less likely than from a lower extremity source.

Other disease processes are associated with a high risk of VTE. Autopsy studies as well as recent epidemiologic analyses suggest that patients with cardiac and malignant disease are particularly susceptible to VTE (29,37). Although myocardial infarction without anticoagulation resulted in a significant incidence of DVT, more recent therapeutic strategies have had a favorable impact (38). A reduction in the incidence of VTE resulting from the use of thrombolytic therapy was demonstrated in a number of large placebo-controlled trials for acute myocardial infarction, including the Gruppo Italiano per lo Studio della Streptochinasi nell'Infarto Miocardico and the second International Study of Infarct Survival (39,40). Patients with malignancies have an increased risk of developing VTE (41). Cancers of the pancreas, lung, stomach, genitourinary tract, and breast are associated with a particularly high risk of DVT and PE. In addition to thrombophilia, these disorders are frequently associated with significant weakness and decreased ambulation with venous stasis. Treatment with chemotherapy with resulting neutropenia and sepsis often necessitates hospitalization and bedrest, which contributes further to the high risk of VTE. A recent analysis based on data from the PIOPED trial revealed that of 399 patients with PE, 73 (18.3%) had cancer (29).

Pregnancy and the postpartum period are the most common settings in which women younger than age 40 develop DVT or PE. DVT develops in these settings five times more often than in women not on oral contraceptives (42). Thrombosis appears to be more common in the third trimester and postpartum than before delivery, but the risk is clearly significant throughout pregnancy (42). Delivery by cesarean section further increases the risk. Oral contraceptives are associated with the development of VTE (43). The risk increases with third-generation agents (agents containing desogestrel or gestodene as the progestin component) (44,45). In a clinical trial evaluating hormonal replacement therapy, it was determined that such therapy increased the incidence of VTE in women 45 to 64 years of age. It appears that an annual total of 16.5 cases of VTE out of 100,000 individuals may be attributed to hormonal replacement therapy (46). The risk of VTE also appears to be highest in the first year of exposure to hormonal replacement (47). Past use may not increase the risk (48). Although such therapy is associated with clear benefits, physicians should take risk factors for VTE into account before prescribing hormonal replacement therapy. A recent review of oral contraceptive use and VTE further emphasizes that, with the increased risk associated with third-generation progestins in combination preparations, these agents should not be the first choice for new users (49).

Disease states associated with the development of VTE include paroxysmal nocturnal hemoglobinuria, inflammatory bowel disease, homocystinuria, Behçet's syndrome, polycythemia, and thrombocythemia. Most intensive care unit patients can be considered at risk for VTE because of their multiple risk factors, including significant underlying disease, immobility, and the frequent presence of venous injury due to trauma. With few exceptions, these patients should receive some form of DVT prophylaxis, and a high index of suspicion for VTE should be maintained in appropriate clinical circumstances. Hospitalized general medical patients represent an increasingly ill population frequently requiring medical prophylaxis.

Gas Exchange and Hemodynamic Alterations in Acute Pulmonary Embolism

The hypoxemia occurring in the majority of patients with PE has been explained by various mechanisms. In patients without previous cardiopulmonary disease, regions with low ventilation-perfusion (V/Q) ratios and shunting secondary to perfusion of atelectatic areas are likely the dominant mechanisms of hypoxemia.

When emboli obstruct a significant portion of the pulmonary arterial bed, profound hemodynamic alterations occur. The impact of the embolic event depends on the extent of reduction of the cross-sectional area of the pulmonary vasculature as well as on the presence or absence of underlying cardiovascular disease. Submassive emboli in normal individuals may actually augment cardiac output (CO). Hypoxemia leads to an increase in sympathetic tone with systemic vasoconstriction and an increase in venous return with augmentation of stroke volume. With massive emboli, CO is diminished but may be sustained as the mean right atrial pressure increases. The ensuing increase in pulmonary vascular resistance impedes right ventricular outflow and reduces left ventricular preload. In a patient without previous cardiopulmonary disease, occlusion of 25% to 30% of the vascular bed by emboli is associated with a significant rise in pulmonary artery pressure (PAP). With increasing vascular obstruction, hypoxemia worsens, stimulating vasoconstriction and a further rise in PAP. More than 50% obstruction of the pulmonary arterial bed is usually present before substantial elevation of the mean PAP evolves. When the extent of obstruction of the pulmonary circulation approaches 75%, the right ventricle must generate a systolic pressure in excess of 50 mm Hg and a mean PAP of greater than 40 mm Hg to preserve pulmonary perfusion (52). The normal right ventricle is unable to achieve this and ultimately fails (52). Patients with underlying cardiopulmonary disease are more inclined to experience more substantial deterioration in CO than normal individuals in the setting of massive PE. A depressed CO *without* elevation of the right atrial pressure suggests cardiac dysfunction superimposed on PE. Right ventricular failure is more common in the setting of PE in patients with coronary artery disease (53). It is important to realize that although supportive measures may sustain a patient with massive embolism, any additional increment in embolic burden may be fatal.

CLINICAL PROFILE

The diagnostic technology for acute DVT has developed considerably with the evolution of convenient and inexpensive techniques such as compression ultrasound as well as highly accurate yet more expensive diagnostic modalities such as magnetic resonance imaging (MRI). For PE, V/Q scanning followed by pulmonary arteriography remains the gold standard approach to the diagnosis, although newer techniques such as MRI and helical computed tomography (CT) scanning are being used increasingly. The presence of risk factors together with the history and physical examination generally leads to further diagnostic testing in the setting of suspected VTE.

History and Physical Examination

The clinical diagnosis of both DVT and PE based on the history and physical examination are notoriously insensitive and nonspecific. Patients with lower extremity DVT often do not exhibit erythema, warmth, pain, swelling, or tenderness. These findings, however, although not specific for DVT, merit further evaluation. PE should always be considered whenever unexplained dyspnea is present. Dyspnea as well as pleuritic chest pain and hemoptysis are common in PE but are nonspecific. Anxiety, lightheadedness, and syncope are all symptoms that may be caused by PE but may also result from a number of other entities that result in hypoxemia or hypotension. Tachypnea and tachycardia are the most common signs of PE but are also nonspecific. PE should always be considered in the setting of syncope or sudden hypotension. The cardiac and pulmonary physical examinations are both nonspecific. The index of clinical suspicion does, however, become a more useful parameter when considered in conjunction with V/Q scanning (54). Diagnostic efforts directed at possible VTE may be appropriate despite alternative explanations if risk factors and the clinical setting are suggestive. Dyspnea, tachypnea, clear lung fields, and hypoxemia may often be attributed to a flare of chronic obstructive disease or asthma when underlying PE is present.

Chest Radiography, Ventilation-Perfusion Scanning, and Pulmonary Arteriography

Most patients with PE have abnormal but nonspecific findings on chest radiograph. Common radiographic findings include atelectasis, pleural effusion, pulmonary infiltrates, and mild elevation of a hemidiaphragm (56). Classic findings of pulmonary infarction such as Hampton's hump or decreased vascularity (Westermark's sign) are suggestive but infrequent. Normal chest radiograph findings in the setting of severe dyspnea and hypoxemia without evidence of bronchospasm or anatomic cardiac shunt are strongly suggestive of PE. The presence of a pleural effusion increases the likelihood of PE in young patients who present with acute pleuritic chest pain (62). Under most circumstances, however, the chest radiograph cannot be used to conclusively diagnose or exclude PE. Although exclusion of other processes such as pneumonia, pneumothorax, or rib fracture, which may cause symptoms similar to acute PE, is possible, PE may frequently coexist with other underlying lung diseases.

V/Q scanning should be performed when PE is suspected. Normal and high-probability scans are considered diagnostic. A normal perfusion scan rules out the diagnosis of PE with a high enough degree of certainty that further

diagnostic evaluation is unnecessary. Matching areas of decreased ventilation and perfusion in the presence of a normal chest radiograph generally represent a process other than PE. However, low- or intermediate-probability (nondiagnostic) scans are commonly found with PE, and in such situations further evaluation with pulmonary arteriography is often appropriate. Normal, high-, low-, and intermediate-probability lung scans are shown in Figures 28.1 through 28.4. In the PIOPED study, the use of V/Q scanning combined with clinical assessment of patients with suspected PE was prospectively evaluated (54). Patients with PE had scans that were high, intermediate, or low probability, but so did most patients without PE. Although the specificity of high-probability scans was 97%, the sensitivity was only 41%. Of interest, 33% of patients with intermediate-probability scans and 12% of patients with low-probability scans were diagnosed definitively with PE by pulmonary arteriography. When the clinical suspicion of PE was considered very high, PE was found to be present in 96% of patients with high-probability scans, 66% of patients with intermediate scans, and 40% of patients with low-probability scans. The diagnosis of PE should be rigorously pursued, even when the lung scan is low or intermediate probability, if the clinical scenario suggests PE. Therefore, although the V/Q scan may sometimes be diagnostic of PE or exclude the possibility with sufficient certainty, it is often nondiagnostic. Even in such circumstances, however, it may serve as a useful guide for limited pulmonary arteriography.

Pulmonary arteriography has remained the accepted gold standard technique for the diagnosis of PE. It is a very sensitive, specific, and safe test. Complications of pulmonary arteriography among 1,111 patients suspected of PE in the PIOPED study included death in 0.5% and major nonfatal complications in 1% (63). An alternative to pulmonary arteriography is to perform lower extremity studies when the lung scan is nondiagnostic, and if these are negative, the chances of significant PE or morbidity from a subsequent event appear unlikely (64). This practice is gaining acceptance and in patients with cardiopulmonary stability may be appropriate. Finally, pulmonary angiography has been performed at the bedside using a Swan-Ganz catheter (65). This may prevent the need to transport critically ill patients. A pulmonary arteriogram diagnostic of PE is shown in Figure 28.5.

Echocardiography in Acute Pulmonary Embolism

Other diagnostic techniques sometimes prove useful particularly in the setting of massive PE. Echocardiography, which can often be obtained more rapidly than either lung scanning or pulmonary arteriography, may reveal findings that strongly support hemodynamically significant PE (66). Studies of patients with documented PE have revealed that

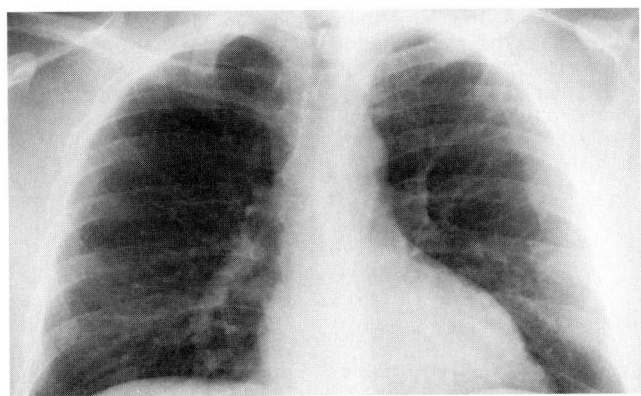

A

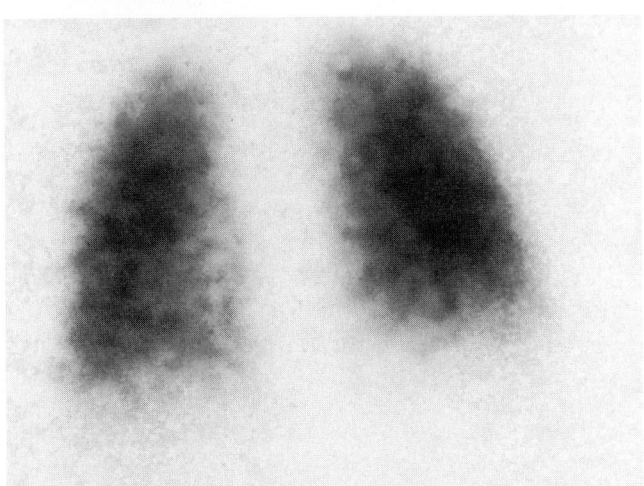

B

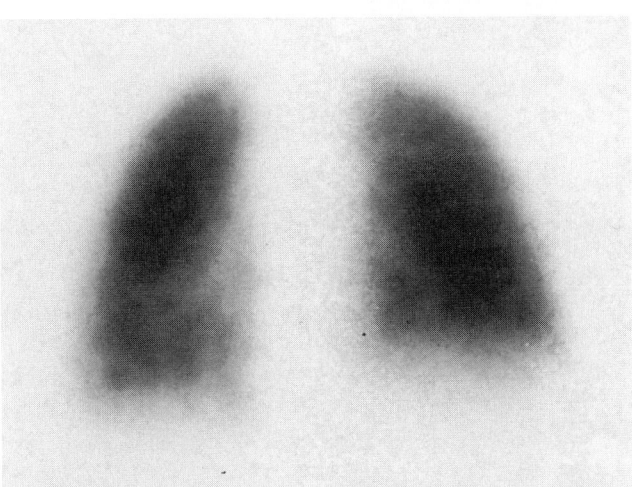

C

FIGURE 28.1 Normal ventilation-perfusion scan. Multiple views are always performed for the perfusion images; only the posterior view is shown in each of these cases. Ventilation scans are done as breath-hold, equilibrium, and washout phases; only one phase is shown in each of these cases. The chest radiograph **(A)**, ventilation scan **(B)**, and perfusion scan **(C)** are normal in this patient. Pulmonary embolism is excluded.

more than 80% of patients have imaging or Doppler abnormalities of right ventricular size or function that may suggest acute PE (66,67). Unfortunately, because patients with PE often have underlying cardiopulmonary disease such as chronic obstructive lung disease, neither right ventricular dilation nor hypokinesis can be reliably used even as indirect evidence of PE in such settings. Goldhaber and colleagues (68) demonstrated that echocardiography could be used to document improvement in right ventricular wall motion in patients with PE treated with recombinant tissue-type plasminogen activator (t-PA). Intravascular ultrasound imaging has been shown in both the experimental and clinical setting to adequately image large emboli (69–71). This procedure may be performed at the bedside. Although the technique may be less sensitive and specific and more time-consuming in the setting of smaller emboli, further investigation may be warranted.

Detection of Deep Venous Thrombosis

The available technology used to pursue the diagnosis of DVT has expanded over the past several decades. Each technique has advantages and limitations. Impedance plethysmography has been shown to be reliable for detection of DVT occurring above the knee. Early studies sug-

gested greater than 90% sensitivity and 97% specificity for DVT involving the proximal lower extremity, although less than 30% of isolated calf vein thromboses were detected (85,86). Other reports have emphasized the limitations of impedance plethysmography (41). In a more recent retrospective analysis at a university-based tertiary care center, impedance plethysmography was abnormal in only 37 of 56 patients, with proximal vein thrombosis confirmed by venography for a sensitivity of only 66% (87). The specificity was equally poor. Although this modality is sometimes portable, it does require access to the calf and thigh for electrode and cuff placement. The specificity is affected by disorders that obstruct venous outflow such as tumor or hematoma. External fixation or plaster immobilization of extremities reduces the usefulness of this technique. It is being used decreasingly.

Compression ultrasonography is a portable and accurate diagnostic technique for proximal lower extremity DVT. The sensitivity and specificity for symptomatic proximal DVT have been well above 90% in most recent clinical trials (88,89). Limitations include insensitivity for asymptomatic DVT, operator dependence, the inability to accurately distinguish acute from chronic DVT in symptomatic patients, and the insensitivity to calf vein thrombosis (90,91). A recent prospective evaluation of the utility

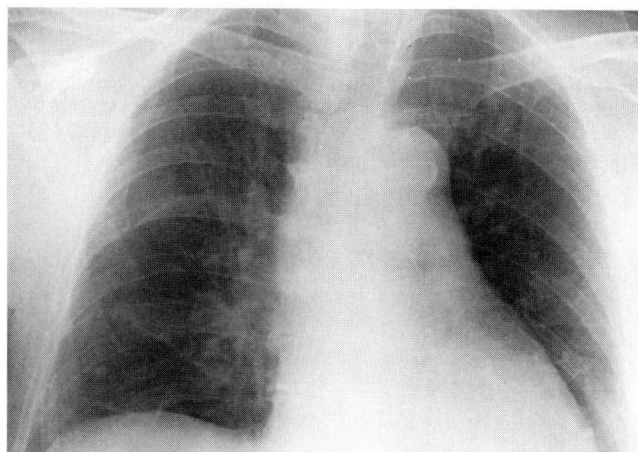

A

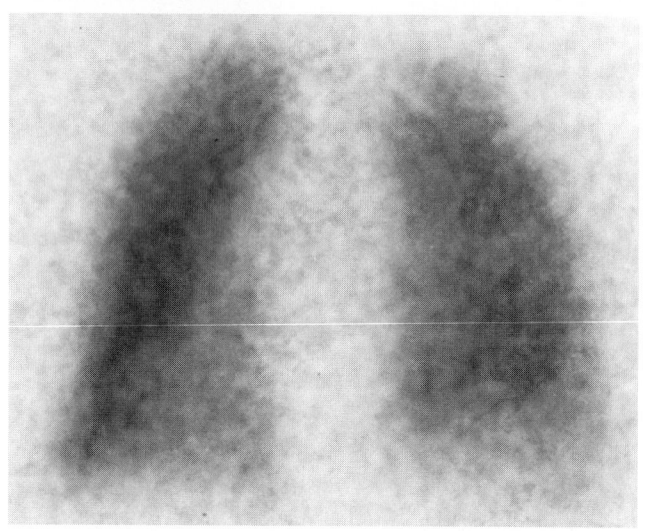

B

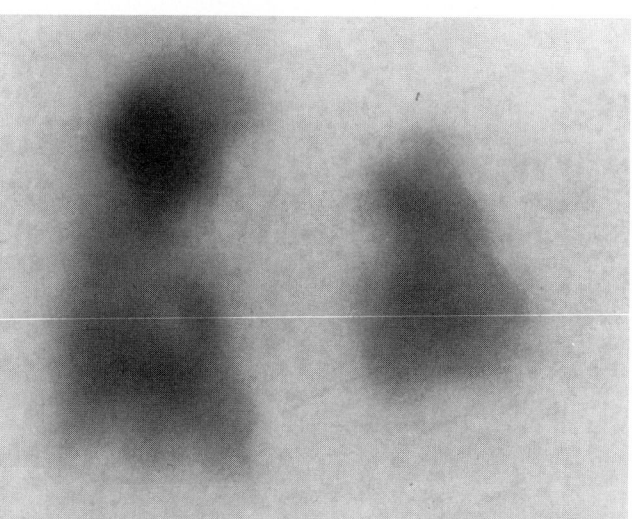

C

FIGURE 28.2 High-probability lung scan. This patient with metastatic cancer developed sudden dyspnea and unexplained hypoxemia after prolonged bedrest. The chest radiograph **(A)** reveals a right hilar mass. The ventilation scan **(B)** is normal, but the perfusion scan **(C)** demonstrates multiple bilateral perfusion defects, virtually diagnostic of pulmonary embolism.

of bilateral color Doppler ultrasound in asymptomatic high-risk (elective unilateral hip or knee replacement) patients revealed that ultrasound was only 38% sensitive for proximal DVT using contrast venography as the diagnostic standard (92). Compared with other technology, it is relatively inexpensive and is the preferred diagnostic modality for the straightforward case of symptomatic presumed proximal DVT.

Although contrast venography remains the gold standard technique for the diagnosis of DVT, it is less commonly performed since the advent of compression ultrasonography (93). Venography should be performed whenever noninvasive testing is nondiagnostic or impossible to perform. It is an invasive procedure that may result in superficial phlebitis or hypersensitivity reactions, but it is generally safe and accurate.

MRI is being increasingly used to diagnose DVT and appears to be an accurate noninvasive alternative to venography (94). A major advantage of this technique is excellent resolution of the inferior vena cava (IVC) and pelvic veins (95,96). Preliminary experience with this technique suggests that it is at least as accurate as contrast venography or ultrasound imaging and perhaps more sensitive than either for pelvic vein thrombosis. It offers the opportunity for simultaneous bilateral lower extremity imaging and appears to accurately distinguish acute from chronic DVT. It offers the additional advantage of lower extremity and lung imaging during the same session. DVT imaged by MRI is shown in Figure 28.4C.

At Duke University Medical Center, duplex ultrasound is commonly used as the first test to evaluate suspected acute DVT. MRI is frequently used subsequently when the ultrasound is nondiagnostic or to distinguish acute from chronic DVT. Another useful aspect of MRI lies in distinguishing other entities such as cellulitis or a Baker's cyst from acute DVT. The utility of this technique depends to a certain degree on the experience of the reader. Finally, helical CT scanning has been studied for suspected acute DVT. The contrast dye from the bolus injected for lung imaging is followed into the deep veins of the legs for viewing. Initial data are promising (97) and the utility of "CT venography" will be further studied in

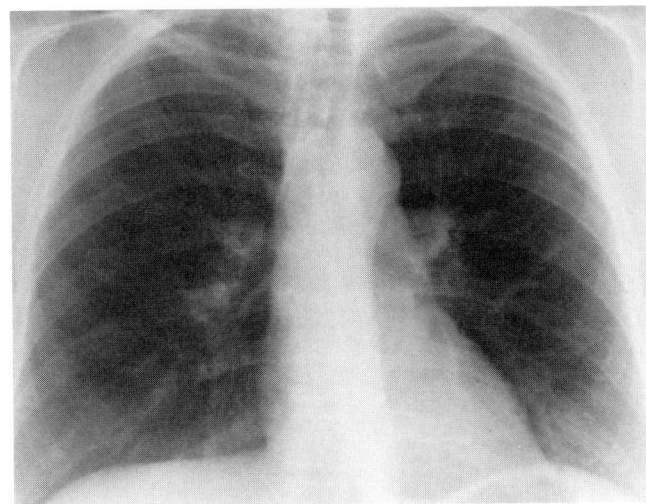

A

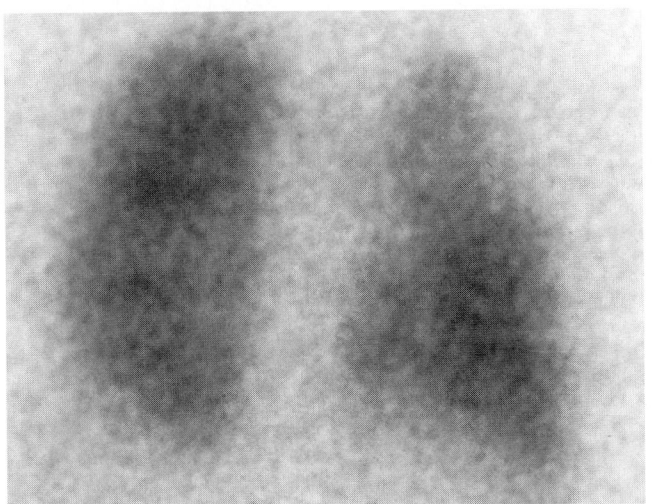

B

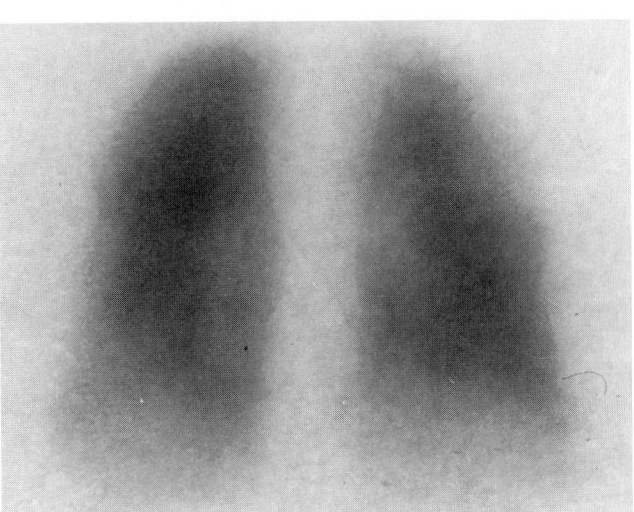

C

FIGURE 28.3 Low-probability lung scan. This patient had a significant smoking history and developed dyspnea with hemoptysis. The chest radiograph **(A)** reveals enlarged central pulmonary arteries consistent with pulmonary hypertension. The ventilation scan sequence revealed xenon retention consistent with chronic obstructive lung disease, and the image shown **(B)** demonstrates ventilation abnormalities, especially at the bases. Matched perfusion abnormalities were present on the perfusion scan **(C)**. Because of purulent sputum and a rapid response to bronchodilator therapy, pulmonary embolism was believed unlikely, and further evaluation was deemed unnecessary. Obstructive lung disease commonly results in nondiagnostic ventilation-perfusion scans. Further studies depend on level of clinical suspicion.

PIOPED II. These techniques may fit into diagnostic algorithms for DVT and PE, but these algorithms are institution-specific at present, depending on resources and expertise with certain techniques.

PRINCIPLES OF MANAGEMENT

Prophylaxis of Deep Venous Thrombosis

A significant reduction in the incidence of DVT can be achieved when patients at risk receive appropriate prophylaxis. Such preventive measures appear to be grossly underused. A review of the use of prophylaxis for DVT in 16 Massachusetts hospitals indicated that such therapy was administered to only 44% of high-risk patients in teaching hospitals and only 19% in nonteaching hospitals (98). The frequency of prophylaxis ranged from 9% to 56% among hospitals. Patients can be stratified according to DVT risk, and certain prophylactic measures are more appropriate for some patients than for others. In general, for medical patients at risk for DVT, subcutaneous heparin at 5,000 U every 8 to 12 hours is generally adequate. Intermittent pneumatic compression devices should be used in the unusual situation when such prophylactic doses of heparin are contraindicated. Both methods combined would be reasonable in patients deemed to be at exceptionally high risk, but an additional reduction in risk in such patients has not been well substantiated.

In the general surgery population, a number of prophylactic methods have been used. In a large metaanalysis, Colditz et al. (99) not only confirmed the value of prophylaxis to reduce the incidence of DVT but also suggested that intermittent pneumatic compression plus gradient compression stockings may result in the lowest incidence of postoperative DVT. Other combined treatments were associated with lower rates than heparin alone. Another overview of the results of randomized trials in surgical patients demonstrated the benefit of DVT prophylaxis (100). In this review of more than 70 randomized trials involving

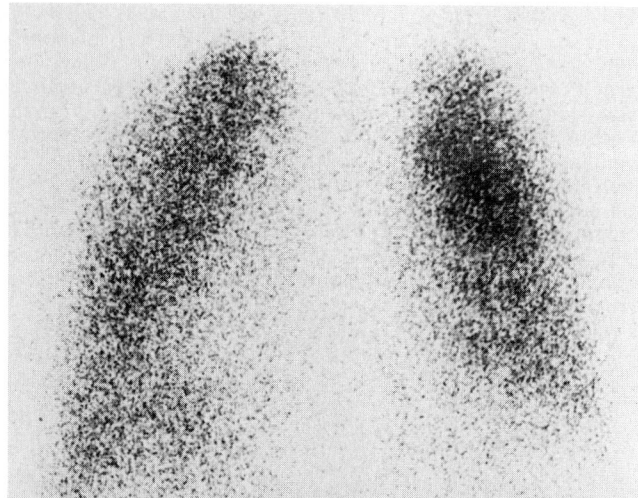

A

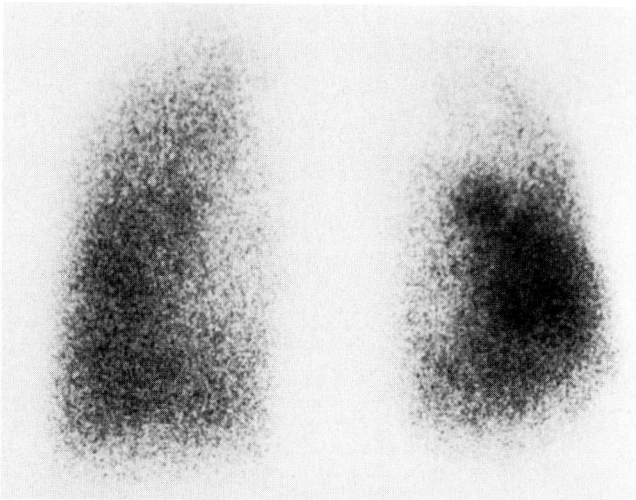

B

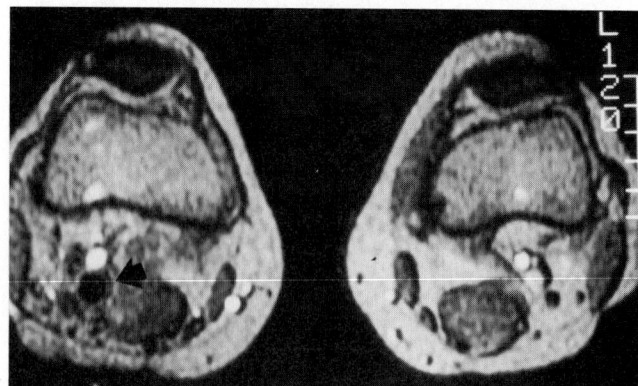

C

FIGURE 28.4 Intermediate probability. This patient developed sudden dyspnea and pleuritic chest pain after surgery. The chest radiograph (not shown) was clear. The ventilation scan **(A)** reveals a defect at the right base. The perfusion scan **(B)** reveals a solitary defect in the right upper lobe; this unmatched defect was not large enough to qualify as a high-probability reading. The clinical suspicion was high for pulmonary embolism, but pulmonary arteriography could not be performed because of significant renal insufficiency. Magnetic resonance imaging **(C)** was used to document proximal deep vein thrombosis of the right lower extremity. The completely occlusive thrombus (*arrow*) appears as a hypodense region adjacent to the high-intensity white signal representing normal arterial flow. The patient was heparinized for acute deep vein thrombosis (and presumed pulmonary embolism).

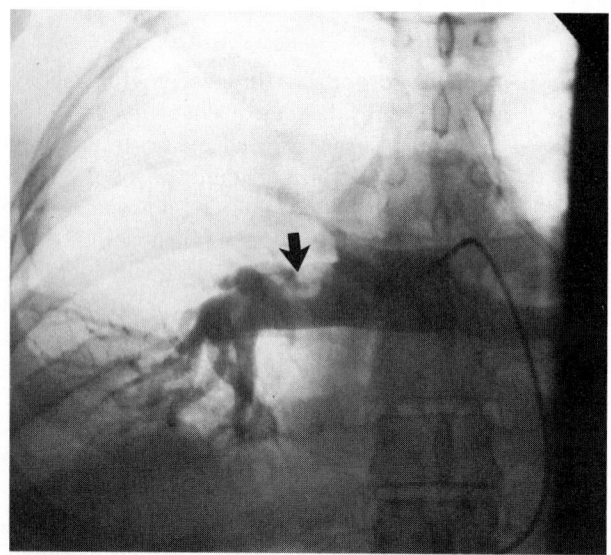

FIGURE 28.5 Pulmonary arteriography demonstrating acute pulmonary embolism. There is a large filling defect in the right pulmonary artery (*arrow*) and marked hypoperfusion to the right upper and middle lobes. A ventilation-perfusion scan had been performed and was nondiagnostic because of extensive air space disease in the right lung.

16,000 patients, it was demonstrated that perioperative use of subcutaneous heparin can prevent approximately half of all pulmonary emboli and approximately two-thirds of all DVT. ✔ f92

Anticoagulation Therapy

Anticoagulation has been proven to reduce mortality in acute PE. When VTE is diagnosed or strongly suspected, heparin therapy should be promptly instituted unless contraindications exist. Confirmatory testing should always be planned if anticoagulation is to be continued. Heparin exerts a prompt antithrombotic effect, preventing thrombus growth. Although it does not directly prevent the development of acute PE or dissolve thrombus, it allows the fibrinolytic system to act unopposed and more readily reduces the size of the thromboembolic burden (107). Although thrombus growth can be prevented, early recurrence can develop even in the setting of therapeutic anticoagulation.

With the institution of continuous intravenous heparin, the activated partial thromboplastin time (aPTT) should be aggressively followed at 6-hour intervals until it is consis-

TABLE 28.2 WEIGHT-BASED NOMOGRAM FOR HEPARIN THERAPY IN ACUTE VENOUS THROMBOEMBOLISM

Initial heparin dose = 80 U/kg bolus, then 18 U/kg per h

Subsequent modifications

aPTT		Heparin dose adjustment
(sec)	(times control)	
<35	<1.2	80 U/kg bolus, then increase by 4 U/kg per h
35 to 45	1.2 to 1.5	40 U/kg bolus, then increase by 2 U/kg per h
46 to 70	1.5 to 2.3	No change
71 to 90	2.3 to 3	Decrease infusion rate by 2 U/kg per h
>90	>3	Hold infusion 1 h, then decrease rate by 3 U/kg per h

aPTT, activated partial thromboplastin time.
From Dalen JE, Hirsh J, Guyatt GH. Sixth American College of Chest Physicians Consensus Conference on Antithrombotic Therapy. *Chest* 2001;119:1S–370S; and Raschke RA, Reilly BM, Guidry JR, et al. The weight-based heparin dosing nomogram compared with a "standard care" nomogram. *Ann Intern Med* 1993;119:874, with permission.

tently in the therapeutic range of 1.5 to 2.0 times control values (107). This range corresponds to a heparin level of 0.2 to 0.4 U per mL as measured by protamine sulfate titration. In general, heparin should be administered as an intravenous bolus of 5,000 U followed by a maintenance dose of at least 30,000 to 40,000 U per 24 hours by continuous infusion (108). The lower dose is administered if the patient is considered at high risk for bleeding. This aggressive approach decreases the risk of subtherapeutic anticoagulation, and although supratherapeutic levels are sometimes achieved initially, bleeding complications do not appear to be increased (109). More recent data continue to support aggressive heparin dosing. An alternative regimen consisting of a bolus of 80 U per kg followed by 18 U per kg per hour has been recommended (110). Further adjusting of the heparin dose should also be weight-based (Table 28.2). This weight-adjusted approach is recommended in the recent American College of Chest Physicians Consensus Conference on Antithrombotic Therapy (111). Warfarin therapy may be initiated as soon as the aPTT is therapeutic, and heparin should be maintained until a therapeutic international normalized ratio of 2.0 to 3.0 has been overlapped with a therapeutic aPTT for 2 consecutive days. Although proximal lower extremity thrombus is more likely to result in PE, calf thrombi should either be followed for proximal extension over 10 to 14 days with noninvasive testing, or anticoagulation should be instituted (112,113). Documented proximal DVT or PE should be treated for at least 3 months. Longer treatment is appropriate when significant risk factors persist. Both short- and long-term anticoagulation guidelines are outlined in the American College of Chest Physicians Consensus Conference guidelines (111).

A number of clinical trials have strongly suggested the efficacy and safety of LMWH for treatment of established acute proximal DVT using recurrent symptomatic VTE as the primary outcome measure (111,114–116). The inci-

dence of DVT and recurrent bleeding in these trials indicates that LMWH preparations are at least as effective and as safe as unfractionated heparin. These agents can be administered once or twice per day subcutaneously even at therapeutic doses and do not require monitoring of the aPTT. Antifactor X levels appear reasonable to monitor in certain settings such as in obese patients, in very small patients (less than 40 kg), and in those with renal insufficiency. There is no proven benefit in monitoring other patients. In two large randomized (Canadian and European) trials, therapy with LMWH was safely initiated at home or continued at home after a brief hospitalization (114,115). A number of outpatient studies have followed these two pivotal trials. Four metaanalyses examined the use of LMWH compared with unfractionated heparin in the initial treatment of acute proximal DVT (117–120). Although there was overlap between the analyses, they have helped to confirm the efficacy and safety of LMWH for the treatment of established DVT. The most recent of these studies has suggested a reduced mortality in patients treated with LMWH, although the precise reason for this is not absolutely clear (117). In the United States, at the present time, two LMWH preparations are FDA-approved for use in patients presenting with DVT with or without acute PE. Enoxaparin is approved for both inpatient and outpatient use at a dose of 1.0 mg per kg subcutaneously every 12 hours or at 1.5 mg per kg once daily for inpatient use. The latter regimens were both proven effective in a large study of inpatients in which both doses proved as effective and as safe as unfractionated heparin (121). The second preparation, tinzaparin, is administered as 175 U once daily, with FDA approval being based on therapy of inpatients. The latter treatment indication is the only approved use for this drug in this country at present. Neither enoxaparin nor tinzaparin is approved for use in patients presenting with acute PE, although tinzaparin has proven effective in a

TABLE 28.3 U.S. FOOD AND DRUG ADMINISTRATION–APPROVED INDICATIONS FOR SPECIFIC LOW-MOLECULAR-WEIGHT HEPARINS

	Low-molecular-weight heparin		
Indication[a]	Enoxaparin	Dalteparin	Tinzaparin
Patients presenting with acute DVT[b]	X		X
Prophylaxis for acute DVT in			
Total hip replacement	X	X	
Total knee replacement	X		
General abdominal surgery	X	X	
Hospitalized medical patients	X		
Acute coronary syndromes[c]	X	X	

DVT, deep venous thrombosis.
[a]It must be recognized that prophylactic doses differ from therapeutic doses.
[b]Enoxaparin is approved for use in both inpatients with DVT with or without pulmonary embolism at 1 mg/kg every 12 h or 1.5 mg/kg once daily and for outpatients (1 mg/kg every 12 h). The data supporting treatment with tinzaparin (175 units once daily) are based on studies of hospitalized patients. Neither drug is approved in patients presenting with acute pulmonary embolism.
[c]Unstable angina and non–ST-segment elevation myocardial infarction.

large, randomized European trial of patients with PE (122). The FDA-approved indications for the three LMWHs approved for use in the United States are shown in Table 28.3. It should be noted that the prophylactic doses of these agents differ from the doses used for treating active disease.

Complications of Anticoagulation

Complications of heparin include bleeding and heparin-induced thrombocytopenia (HIT). The rates of major bleeding in recent trials using heparin by continuous infusion or high-dose subcutaneous injection are less than 5% (33). HIT (defined as a platelet count of less than 150,000 per μL) typically develops 5 or more days after the initiation of heparin therapy, occurring in 5% to 10% of patients. The syndrome is caused by heparin-dependent immunoglobulin G antibodies that activate platelets via their crystallizable fragment receptors (130). It has been demonstrated that these antibodies recognize heparin complexed with platelet factor 4 (131). Visentin and associates (132) have shown that such antibodies also react with endothelial cells coated with platelet factor 4, and such potential antibody-mediated vascular injury may help to explain the predisposition of patients with HIT to thromboembolism when challenged with heparin. Positive platelet aggregation tests for antibodies to heparin may be present in the absence of significant thrombocytopenia, and such tests may be negative despite a progressive decrease in platelet count (130). If a patient is placed on heparin for VTE and the platelet count progressively decreases to 100,000 per μL or less, heparin therapy should be discontinued. The formation of heparin-dependent immunoglobulin G antibodies and the risk of HIT appears to be lower with this form of heparin. HIT occurred in 9 of 332 patients receiving standard unfractionated heparin

compared with none of 333 patients receiving enoxaparin (133). Eight of the nine patients receiving standard heparin developed one or more thrombotic events. However, it is important for clinicians to realize that HIT can occur with the use of either form of heparin. Newly developed solid-phase assays that use complexes of heparin and platelet factor 4 as targets for the detection of heparin-induced antibodies are much more sensitive than the serotonin-release test used in the above study (133). Both argatroban and lepirudin are approved by the FDA for the treatment of VTE in the setting of HIT.

Vena Cava Interruption

If heparin therapy cannot be continued, IVC filter placement can be undertaken to prevent lower extremity thrombus from embolizing to the lungs. These devices have been widely used for nearly two decades. The primary indications for filter placement include contraindications to anticoagulation, recurrent embolism while on adequate therapy, and significant bleeding complications during anticoagulation (134). Filters are sometimes placed in the setting of massive PE when it is believed that any further emboli might be lethal (135). A number of filter designs exist, but the Greenfield filter has been most widely used. Filters can be inserted via the jugular or femoral vein. These devices are effective and complications are unusual (135). Potential mechanisms of IVC filter failure include migration of the filter either distally or proximally to a point that no longer protects the vena cava, improper filter positioning allowing thrombi to bypass the filter, and formation of thrombosis proximal to the filter or on the proximal tip of the filter with subsequent embolization. Rare complications include clinically significant perforation of the IVC, cephalad migration, and displacement of the filter during insertion. IVC filters may rarely erode into the wall of the IVC.

Occasionally, IVC obstruction due to thrombosis at the filter site may occur. Deaths due to filter placement are exceedingly uncommon. In general, anticoagulation is continued when a filter is placed unless it is contraindicated.

Thrombolytic Therapy

The National Institutes of Health consensus guidelines for PE thrombolysis issued in 1980 recommended thrombolytic therapy for patients with obstruction of blood flow to a lobe or multiple pulmonary segments and for patients with hemodynamic compromise, regardless of the size of the PE (136). The recommendations for use of lytic therapy in PE have recently been carefully reviewed (137). Current guidelines are presented in Table 28.4. We favor the use of thrombolytic therapy in patients with hemodynamic instability (hypotension) or severely compromised oxygenation (138). Stable patients with a significant embolic load are individualized, often receiving treatment in the absence of absolute or relative contraindications. For example, strong arguments for thrombolytic therapy can be made when the perfusion defect by lung scan or pulmonary arteriogram is extensive (defect approaching the equivalent of one-half of the pulmonary vascular bed) even without clear hemodynamic instability. Another setting in which thrombolytic therapy may be considered is when extensive DVT accompanies a submassive PE. There are no clinical studies suggesting a reduction in mortality in the latter settings, and perhaps future clinical trials will clarify appropriate guidelines.

Acceleration of clot lysis in PE using thrombolytic therapy was first documented several decades ago (139–141). The multicenter, prospective, randomized Urokinase Pulmonary Embolism Trial evaluated 160 patients with arteriographically proven PE (55). Thrombolysis was accelerated in patients receiving urokinase compared with those on heparin when pulmonary arteriograms and lung perfusion scans were examined 24 hours after treatment. Thereafter, the difference between the two groups diminished, and by day 5 the improvement in each group was similar. There was no difference in the frequency of recurrent PE or mortality rate within 2 weeks of treatment. However, only 7% of the patients in the study were classified as having massive PE with shock. Although hemorrhagic complications in this trial were relatively high, further experience with thrombolytic therapy has suggested that adverse effects are reduced when venous cutdowns and unnecessary arterial phlebotomy are avoided. The second phase of this clinical trial also documented the efficacy of streptokinase administered over 24 hours. Finally, recombinant t-PA is approved for use in the treatment of PE and is administered as a 100-mg intravenous infusion delivered over 2 hours (142). Even shorter infusion durations have been evaluated, and future clinical trials may lead to wider acceptance of these regimens. At present, the above t-PA regimen is the most rapidly administered protocol that is currently approved for use.

Thrombolytic regimens approved by the FDA for the treatment of PE are presented in Table 28.5. Coagulation assays are unnecessary during thrombolysis because the approved regimens are administered as fixed doses. It is recommended that heparin be withheld until the thrombolytic infusion is completed. The aPTT is then determined, and heparin is initiated without a loading dose if this value is less than twice the upper limit of normal. If the aPTT exceeds this value, the test is repeated every 4 hours until it is safe to proceed with heparin. The method of delivery of thrombolytic agents has also been investigated. Although a number of investigators have used standard- or low-dose intrapulmonary arterial thrombolytic infusions to deliver a high concentration of drug in close proximity to the clot (143,144), intravenous therapy appears adequate in most cases (145). More direct techniques such as catheter-directed administration of intraembolic thrombolytic therapy are discussed below.

The use of thrombolytic therapy for DVT is more controversial. A comprehensive review of the literature suggests that use of streptokinase may be associated with a reduction in postphlebitic syndrome when used for acute DVT, although bleeding is increased with thrombolytic therapy (146). Future studies may clarify the role of thrombolytic therapy for DVT. It is reasonable to consider systemic thrombolytic therapy in patients with proximal occlusive DVT associated with significant swelling and symptoms when there are no absolute or relative contraindications. Although agents other than streptokinase have been stud-

TABLE 28.4 THROMBOLYTIC THERAPY IN VENOUS THROMBOEMBOLISM: POTENTIAL INDICATIONS

Hypotension related to pulmonary embolism[a]
Severe hypoxemia
Lobar or greater perfusion defect[b]
Right ventricular dysfunction associated with pulmonary embolism
Extensive deep venous thrombosis

[a]This indication is widely accepted. All indications require careful review of contraindications to thrombolytic therapy.
[b]National Institutes of Health Consensus 1980 (136). This indication is not widely accepted.

TABLE 28.5 THROMBOLYTIC THERAPY FOR ACUTE PULMONARY EMBOLISM: APPROVED REGIMENS

Streptokinase: 250,000 U i.v. (loading dose over 30 min), then 100,000 U/h for 24 h[a]
Urokinase: 2,000 U/lb i.v. (loading dose over 10 min), then 2,000 U/lb/h for 12 to 24 h[b]
Tissue-type plasminogen activator: 100 mg i.v. over 2 h

[a]Streptokinase administered over 24–72 h at this loading dose and rate has also been approved for use in patients with extensive deep venous thrombosis.
[b]Urokinase is not currently available in the United States.

TABLE 28.6 THROMBOLYTIC THERAPY FOR ACUTE PULMONARY EMBOLISM: CONTRAINDICATIONS

Absolute
  Intracranial tumor or hemorrhagic stroke
  Recent head trauma or cranial surgery
  Active or recent internal bleeding
Relative
  Thrombocytopenia or coagulopathy
  Uncontrolled severe hypertension
  Cardiopulmonary resuscitation
  Surgery or biopsy within the previous 10 days

TABLE 28.7 ACUTE MASSIVE PULMONARY EMBOLISM: THERAPEUTIC CONSIDERATIONS

Oxygen therapy
Intubation and mechanical ventilation
Intravenous heparin
Fluid administration
Norepinephrine or dopamine
Thrombolytic therapy
Catheter or suction cup embolectomy
Surgical embolectomy
Vena caval filter placement

ied, there are no firm dosing recommendations for them. Catheter-directed techniques have been used for the treatment of acute DVT (see Pulmonary Embolectomy and Catheter-Extraction Techniques).

Hemorrhage is the primary adverse effect associated with thrombolytic therapy and generally occurs at sites of invasive procedures such as pulmonary arteriography or arterial line placement (147). Thus, when thrombolytic therapy is administered, invasive procedures should be minimized. The most devastating complication associated with this form of treatment is the development of intracranial hemorrhage (148). Clinical trials have suggested that this occurs in significantly less than 1% of patients. Contraindications to systemic thrombolytic therapy in VTE are listed in Table 28.6. Bleeding related to thrombolytic therapy requires immediate diagnosis and management. Bleeding from vascular puncture sites should be addressed with manual compression followed by a pressure dressing. Intracranial bleeding requires immediate discontinuation of thrombolytics or heparin, and emergent neurologic and neurosurgical consultation should be obtained. A noncontrasted brain CT scan should be performed. Retroperitoneal hemorrhage may result from a vascular puncture above the inguinal ligament and may be life-threatening. Patients with severe or refractory bleeding should be transfused with 10 U of cryoprecipitate and 2 U of fresh frozen plasma, and heparin can be reversed with protamine.

Hemodynamic Management of Massive Pulmonary Embolism

Massive PE should always be suspected in the setting of the sudden onset of hypotension or extreme hypoxemia. The presence of electromechanical dissociation or sudden cardiac arrest should always make massive PE a consideration. If the patient is stable enough, V/Q scanning should be performed when possible. Although PE should be proven with either a high-probability V/Q scan (helical CT or MRI may also offer proof) and when necessary pulmonary arteriography, echocardiography may support the diagnosis of massive PE and may also suggest the need for aggressive intervention, including thrombolytic therapy (155). Once massive PE associated with hypotension and/or severe hypoxemia is sus-

pected, supportive treatment is immediately initiated. Intravenous saline should be infused rapidly but cautiously because right ventricular function is often markedly compromised. Dopamine or norepinephrine appear to be the favored choices of vasoactive therapy in massive PE and should be administered if the blood pressure is not rapidly restored (155). General guidelines for the approach to massive PE are offered in Table 28.7. Because death in this setting results from right ventricular failure, dobutamine has been recommended by some as a means by which to augment right ventricular output (156,157). A vasopressor such as norepinephrine combined with dobutamine might offer optimal results, and further exploration of such combined therapy would prove enlightening. Oxygen therapy is administered, and thrombolytic therapy is considered as described above. Intubation and institution of mechanical ventilation are instituted as needed to support respiratory failure.

CHRONIC THROMBOEMBOLISM

Although the vast majority of acute PE cases resolves with treatment, occasionally a substantial residual thromboembolic burden remains (158,159). In this setting, the clot becomes organized and adherent and is not amenable to thrombolysis. If the obstruction becomes extensive, pulmonary hypertension develops. This syndrome most commonly occurs in patients 40 to 70 years of age but can occur at any age. At least 50% of patients who develop chronic thromboembolic pulmonary hypertension have no documented history of DVT or PE. This feature greatly impedes the diagnosis. Most patients have no identifiable coagulopathy. Fatigue and dyspnea with exertion are the most common complaints. The nonspecific nature of these findings may substantially delay the correct diagnosis. The physical examination generally reveals a right ventricular heave, a loud pulmonary component of the second heart sound, and tricuspid regurgitation consistent with pulmonary hypertension. In more severe cases, a right ventricular third heart sound may be present. In 20% of patients, one or more murmurs may be auscultated over the lung fields.

Once the diagnosis is suspected, the diagnostic evaluation is generally revealing. The chest radiograph usually reveals right ventricular enlargement and enlarged main pulmonary arteries. Electrocardiographic changes are consistent with pulmonary hypertension. Arterial blood gases generally reveal hypoxemia with a widened A-a difference, although some patients may only demonstrate exercise-induced hypoxemia. Echocardiography documents pulmonary hypertension and enlargement of the right ventricle. It is prudent to perform chest CT scanning, which may reveal other rare causes of pulmonary hypertension such as mediastinal fibrosis; it may, in fact, demonstrate evidence of chronic thrombi. Helical CT scanning may be particularly useful in this regard. The V/Q scan is nearly always high probability for PE but occasionally is less impressive. Right heart catheterization and pulmonary arteriography are performed, both to establish the diagnosis with certainty and to determine operability. Pulmonary angioscopy frequently has proven complementary to arteriography in assessing these patients (160).

Although anticoagulation should be instituted and IVC filters are recommended in patients with chronic thromboembolic pulmonary hypertension, the only means by which to alleviate symptoms and impact on survival is with surgery. The group from the University of California at San Diego has had tremendous experience with evaluation and surgical therapy of these patients. Pulmonary thromboendarterectomy is performed via median sternotomy on cardiopulmonary bypass, and the overall mortality, which has continued to improve, is now less than 5%. Lung transplantation can be performed in patients in whom thrombi are too distal to extract.

CONTROVERSIES AND PERSONAL PERSPECTIVES

VTE is difficult to study in large randomized trials because of the varying presentations of acute PE and DVT, the difficulty with diagnosis, and the many different settings and specialties involved. A number of questions remain unanswered. Cost-effective approaches to the diagnosis and therapy of DVT and PE remain unclear. In view of the numerous controversies currently facing us, several groups such as the American College of Chest Physicians and the American Thoracic Society have taken steps to form consensus guidelines for areas in which substantial data exist and opinion and position statements to address issues and plan research strategies for areas that remain less clear (111,161,162).

Diagnostic Approach to Venous Thromboembolism

There are no firm consensus guidelines for the diagnostic approach to VTE. Critical pathways have been constructed by experts in the field for the diagnostic approach to DVT, for example, but these approaches suffer from institutional variability, availability of certain diagnostic studies, and lack of incorporation of newer technologies such as MRI. The American Thoracic Society has recently formulated consensus guidelines for the diagnostic approach to VTE (162). These include algorithms and the role of new technologies and account for institution-specific differences in approach.

The International Cooperative Pulmonary Embolism Registry represents the largest prospective PE registry ever undertaken (163). This effort has helped to answer a number of clinical questions and contribute to future strategies in clinical investigation. It has already enhanced international communication, which should increase the number and quality of international randomized clinical trials and help to unify the approach to VTE.

The roles of newer methods to diagnose DVT and PE such as MRI and helical CT scanning need to be clarified, and recommendations may change as the technology continues to improve. How often are venography and pulmonary arteriography still necessary? When should MRI be used in addition to, or instead of, ultrasonography? Can all patients with a negative helical CT be safely followed without therapy?

Screening and Prophylaxis

Determining a practical means by which to identify patients with recently characterized thrombophilias such as activated protein C resistance and determining their significance will facilitate the implementation of more meaningful prophylaxis and treatment protocols. Who should be screened for activated protein C resistance? Do patients with this disorder require lifelong prophylaxis? When should combined mechanical and pharmacologic prophylaxis be applied? What is the appropriate duration of prophylaxis in different clinical settings? What *are* the differences between the different LMWH compounds? Although the American College of Chest Physicians guidelines are useful, more data are needed to enhance their usefulness. *At present, recommendations in specific settings must be made for specific agents that have been studied in that setting.*

Therapeutic Approaches

A number of anticoagulation issues require clarification. The duration of therapy in different subsets of patients with VTE needs to be determined. Should patients with PE and without residual DVT be treated for a shorter period of time than patients with extensive DVT? Is it beneficial to use MRI to document the extent of DVT in every patient? Is it appropriate to repeat lower extremity studies in patients with DVT to help determine treatment duration? We are treating increasing numbers of outpatients, and this is simplified with the LMWH preparations. Which agents (and doses) are appropriate? Where do the direct thrombin inhibitors, selective factor X inhibitors, and TFPI fit in?

THE FUTURE

The future will be productive with regard to characterization of genetic risk factors, diagnosis, therapy, and prevention. The discovery of additional thrombophilic disorders appears inevitable, as does the development of standardized methods to screen patients for these. This, in turn, will undoubtedly affect current prophylaxis and treatment guidelines. Efforts currently under way include the PIOPED II, a prospective clinical trial evaluating the utility of helical CT scanning for suspected PE. Analysis of such data will assist in the delineation of appropriate algorithms for diagnosis. Nuclear imaging technology may improve, but the imaging of actual thromboses and emboli with MRI and CT appears to be much more promising. Our understanding of the utility of these techniques and the technology itself continue to evolve. The use of MRI, with its potential ability to distinguish acute from chronic thrombosis, may not only lead to more appropriate initiation of therapy but also may aid in the determination of the length and aggressiveness of therapy. CT scanning will become faster and undoubtedly more accurate. The latter techniques will likely replace arteriography and venography altogether. Hematologic studies such as the D-dimer may evolve into more useful techniques. The evolution of diagnostic technology will affect therapy. The ability to diagnose the presence and extent of acute DVT will permit refinement of treatment stratification. How issues such as extent of DVT, number of persisting risk factors, and specific therapeutic modality affect treatment duration should become more clearly defined. We are treating larger numbers of outpatients and using LMWHs. Newer agents such as direct thrombin inhibitors, selective factor X_a inhibitors, and TFPI, as well as more fibrin-specific thrombolytic agents, should have more clearly defined therapeutic roles. It is likely that we have an easier drug to use than warfarin. The means by which we monitor anticoagulation will improve. The roles of systemic and local thrombolytics, including indications, doses, duration of therapy, and delivery methods, need clarification. Guidelines for diagnostic and therapeutic approaches to VTE will become substantially more refined. It is very important to note that preventive efforts are of paramount importance. We are making strides in characterizing prolonged air travel as a risk factor for VTE. Paul Egermayer, a physician and VTE researcher, passed away in May 2001 in the midst of a very productive research career. This insightful and energetic individual wisely emphasized the importance of VTE prevention by stating that "the real problem is not the 10% of patients who survive long enough to receive treatment, but the 90% in the first hour after the event. For both groups, more systematic prophylaxis is clearly the way forward. Treatment is merely the ambulance waiting at the bottom of the cliff" (164).

What are appropriate guidelines for thrombolytic therapy in DVT and PE? Is one thrombolytic agent or regimen superior to others? When should acute pulmonary embolectomy be performed? Although some individuals believe that thrombolytic therapy should be reserved for patients with "hemodynamic compromise," the latter term is not clearly defined. I believe that patients with PE, extreme hypotension, and evidence of end-organ dysfunction, or those with extreme hypoxemia refractory to maximal oxygen therapy, should receive intravenous thrombolytic therapy even in the presence of certain "absolute contraindications" such as occult blood in the stool if other methods such as surgical embolectomy or catheter-based therapy are not immediately accessible. Even severe gastrointestinal bleeding can be controlled more easily than PE associated with shock. It is difficult to make blanket guidelines, and presence at the bedside may continue to be a prerequisite for rational decisions in such settings. Guidelines need to be investigated and clarified. The precise roles of systemic and local thrombolytic therapy and catheter-directed techniques, including indications, doses, duration of therapy, and delivery methods, all need clarification. The number of meaningful clinical trials planned and under way suggest that we may ultimately be able to resolve many of these controversies.

REFERENCES

1. Laennec RHT. *De l'auscultation mediate ou traite du diagnostic des maladies des poumons et du coeur*, vol. I. Paris: Brosson et Chaude, 1819.
2. Cruveilhier J. *Anatomic pathologique du corps humain*. Paris: JB Ballierre, 1828.
3. Virchow R von. Weitere Untersuchungen ueber die Verstopfung der Lungenarterien und ihre Folge. *Traube's Beitraege exp path u Physiol, Berlin* 1846;2:21.
4. Trousseau A. *Phlegmasia alba dolens. Clinique Medicale de l'Hotel Dieu de Paris*. London: The New Sydenham Society, 1865;3:94.
5. Luzzatto B. *Embolia dell' arteria polmonale*. Milan: Fratelli Richiedei ed., 1880.
6. Trendelenburg F. Uber die Operative Behandlurig der Embolie der Lungeroarterie. *Arch Klin Chirop* 1908;24:687.
7. Kirschner W. Ein durch die Trendelenburgsche Operation geheilter Fall von Embolie der Art Pulmonalis. *Arch Klin Chirop* 1924;48:312.

8. Ljungdahl M. Gibt es eine Chronische Embolistierung der Lungen Arterie? *Dtsch Arch Klin Med* 1928;102:1.

9. Moniz E, Carvallio L, Limer H. Angiopneumographic. *Presse Med* 1931;53:996.

10. Bauer G. A venographic study of thrombo-embolic problems. *Acta Chirop Scand* 1940;84[Suppl 65]:5.

11. Bauer G. Thrombosis: early diagnosis and abortive treatment with heparin. *Lancet* 1946;1:447.

12. Clason S. Three cases of pulmonary embolism following confinement, treated with heparin. *Acta Med Scand* 1941;107:131.

13. McLean J. The discovery of heparin. *Circulation* 1959;19:75.

14. Chrispin AR, Goodwin JF, Steiner RE. The radiology of obliterative pulmonary hypertension and thromboembolism. *Br J Radiol* 1963;36:705.

15. Williams JR, Wilcox C, Andrews GJ, Burns RR. Angiography in pulmonary embolism. *JAMA* 1963;184:473.

16. Sasahara AA, Stein M, Simon M, Littman D. Pulmonary angiography in the diagnosis of thromboembolic disease. *N Engl J Med* 1964;270:1075.

17. Stein PD, O'Connor JF, Dalen JE, et al. The angiographic diagnosis of acute pulmonary embolism. Evaluation of criteria. *Am Heart J* 1967;73:730.

18. Taplin GV, Johnson DE, Dore EK, Kaplan HS. Suspensions of radiolabeled albumin aggregates for photoscanning the liver, spleen and other organs. *J Nucl Med* 1964;5:259.

19. Wagner HN, Sabiston DC Jr, McAfee JG, et al. Diagnosis of massive pulmonary embolism in man by radioisotope scanning. *N Engl J Med* 1964;271:377.

20. Anderson FA, Wheeler HB. Venous thromboembolism: risk factors and prophylaxis. *Clin Chest Med* 1995;16:235.

21. Dalen JE, Alpert JS. Natural history of pulmonary embolism. *Prog Cardiovasc Dis* 1975;17:257.

22. Lindblad B, Eriksson A, Bergquist D. Autopsy-verified pulmonary embolism in a surgical department: analysis of the period from 1951 to 1988. *Br J Surg* 1991;78:849.

23. Bratzler DW, Raskob, GE, Murray CK, et al. Underuse of venous thromboembolism prophylaxis for general surgery patients. Physician practices in the community hospital setting. *Arch Intern Med* 1998;158:1909.

24. Lamb GC, Tomski MH, Kaufman J, et al. Is chronic spinal cord injury associated with increased risk of venous thromboembolism? *J Am Paraplegia Soc* 1993;16:153.

25. Kraaijenhagen RA, Haverkamp D, Koopman MMW, et al. Travel and risk of venous thrombosis. *Lancet* 2000;356:1492.

26. James, PB. Jet "leg," pulmonary embolism, and hypoxia. *Lancet* 1996;347:1697.

27. Bagshaw M. Jet "leg," pulmonary embolism, and hypoxia. *Lancet* 1996;348:415.

27a. Lapostolle F, Surget V, Borron SW, et al. Severe pulmonary embolism associated with air travel. *N Engl J Med* 2001;345:779–783.

28. Layish DT, DeLong DM, Tapson VF. Relationship between obesity and pulmonary embolism: a review of the PIOPED data. *Chest* 1996;110:53.

29. Carson JL, Kelley MA, Duffy A, et al. The clinical course of pulmonary embolism. *N Engl J Med* 1992;326:1240.

30. Goldhaber SZ, Hennekens CH, Evans DA, et al. Factors associated with correct antemortem diagnosis of major pulmonary embolism. *Am J Med* 1982;73:822.

31. Kakkar VV, Howe CT, Nicolaides AN, et al. Deep vein thrombosis of the legs: is there a "high risk" group? *Am J Surg* 1970;120:527.

32. Clagett GP, Reisch JS. Prevention of venous thromboembolism in general surgical patients: results of a meta-analysis. *Ann Surg* 1988;208:227.

33. Geerts WH, Heit JA, Clagett GP, et al. Prevention of venous thromboembolism. *Chest* 2001;119[Suppl]:132S.

34. Fisher M, Michele A, McCann W. Thrombophlebitis and pulmonary infarction associated with fractured hip. *Clin Res* 1963;11:407.

35. Fitts WT Jr, Lehr HB, Bitner RL, et al. An analysis of 950 fatal injuries. *Surgery* 1964;56:663.

36. Coon WW. Risk factors in pulmonary embolism. *Surg Gynecol Obstet* 1976;143:385.

37. Pineo GF, Brain MC, Gallus AS, et al. Tumors, mucus production and hypercoagulability. *Ann NY Acad Sci* 1974;230:262.

38. Handley AJ, Emerson PA, and Fleming PR. Heparin in the prevention of deep vein thrombosis after myocardial infarction. *BMJ* 1972;2:436.

39. Gruppo Italiano per lo Studio della Streptochinasi nell'Infarto Miocardico (GISSI). Effectiveness of intravenous thrombolytic treatment in acute myocardial infarction. *Lancet* 1986;1:397.

40. ISIS-2 Collaborative Group. Randomized trial of IV streptokinase, oral aspirin, both or neither among 17,187 cases of suspected acute myocardial infarction. *Lancet* 1988;2:349.

41. Rickles FR, Edwards RL. Activation of blood coagulation in cancer: Trousseau's syndrome revisited. *Blood* 1983;62:14.

42. Toglia MR, Weg JG. Current concepts: venous thromboembolism during pregnancy. *N Engl J Med* 1996;335:108.

43. Stadel BV. Oral contraceptives and cardiovascular disease. *N Engl J Med* 1981;305:672.

44. Weiss N. Third-generation oral contraceptives: how risky? *Lancet* 1995;346:1570.

45. World Health Organization Collaborative Study of Cardiovascular Disease and Steroid Hormone Contraception. Venous thromboembolic disease and combined oral contraceptives: results of international multicentre case-control study. *Lancet* 1995;346:1575.

46. Daly E, Vessey MP, Hawkins MM, et al. Risk of venous thromboembolism in users of hormone replacement therapy. *Lancet* 1996;348:977.

47. Jick H, Derby LE, Myers MW, et al. Risk of hospital admission for idiopathic venous thromboembolism among users of postmenopausal estrogens. *Lancet* 1996;348:981.

48. Grodstein F, Stampfer MJ, Goldhaber SZ, et al. Prospective study of exogenous hormones and risk of pulmonary embolism in women. *Lancet* 1996;348:983.

49. Vandenbroucke JP, Rosing J, Bloemenkamp KWM, et al. Oral contraceptives and the risk of venous thrombosis. *N Engl J Med* 2001;344:1527.

50. Seligsohn U, Lubetsky A. Genetic susceptibility to venous thrombosis. *N Engl J Med* 2001;344:1222.

51. Ridker PM, Hennekens CH, Lindpainter K, et al. Mutation in the gene coding for coagulation factor V and the risk of myocardial infarction, stroke, and venous thrombosis in apparently healthy men. *N Engl J Med* 1995;332:912.

52. Benotti JR, Dalen JE. The natural history of pulmonary embolism. *Clin Chest Med* 1984;5:403.

53. McIntyre KM, Sasahara AA. The ratio of pulmonary artery pressure to pulmonary vascular obstruction. *Chest* 1999;71:692.

54. The PIOPED investigators. Value of the ventilation/perfusion scan in acute pulmonary embolism. Results of the prospective investigation of pulmonary embolism diagnosis. *JAMA* 1990;263:2753.

55. The Urokinase Pulmonary Embolism Trial. A national cooperative study. *Circulation* 1973;47[Suppl II]:1.

56. Stein PD, Terrin ML, Hales CA, et al. Clinical, laboratory, roentgenographic, and electrocardiographic findings in patients with acute pulmonary embolism and no pre-existing cardiac or pulmonary disease. *Chest* 1991;100:598.

57. Green RM, Meyer TJ, Dunn M, Glassroth J. Pulmonary embolism in younger adults. *Chest* 1992;101:1507.

58. Bounameaux H, Cirafici P, DeMoerloose P, et al. Measurement of D-dimer in plasma as diagnostic aid in suspected pulmonary embolism. *Lancet* 1991;337:196.

59. Rowbotham BJ, Egerton-Vernon J, Whitaker AN, et al. Plasma cross-linked fibrin degradation products in pulmonary embolism. *Thorax* 1990;45:684.

60. Egermayer P, Town GI, Turner JG, et al. Usefulness of D-dimer, blood gas, and respiratory rate measurements for excluding pulmonary embolism. *Thorax* 1998;53:830.

60a. Wells PS, Anderson DR, Rodger M, et al. Excluding pulmonary embolism at the beside without diagnostic imaging: management of patients with suspected pulmonary embolism presenting to the emergency department by using a simple clinical model and D-dimer. *Ann Intern Med* 2001;135:98–107.

61. Ahearn GS, Bounameaux H. The role of the D-dimer in the diagnosis of venous thromboembolism. *Semin Respir Crit Care Med* 2000;21:521.

62. McNeil BJ, Hessel SJ, Branch WT, et al. Measures of clinical efficacy. III. The value of the lung scan in the evaluation of young patients with pleuritic chest pain. *J Nucl Med* 1976;17:163.

63. Stein PD, Athanasoulis C, Alavi A, et al. Complications and validity of pulmonary angiography in acute pulmonary embolism. *Circulation* 1992;85:462.

64. Hull RD, Raskob G, Ginsberg JS, et al. A noninvasive strategy for the treatment of patients with suspected pulmonary embolism. *Arch Intern Med* 1994;154:289.

65. Rosengarten PL, Tuxen DV, Weeks AM. Whole lung pulmonary angiography in the intensive care unit with two portable chest x-rays. *Crit Care Med* 1990;18:459.

66. Come PC. Echocardiographic evaluation of pulmonary embolism and its response to therapeutic interventions. *Chest* 1992;101:151S.

67. Kasper W, Meinertz T, Kersting F, et al. Echocardiography in assessing acute pulmonary hypertension due to pulmonary embolism. *Am J Cardiol* 1980;45:567.

68. Goldhaber SZ, Haire WD, Feldstein ML, et al. Alteplase versus heparin in acute pulmonary embolism: randomized trial assessing right ventricular function and pulmonary perfusion. *Lancet* 1993;341:507.

69. Tapson VF, Davidson CJ, Gurbel PA, et al. Rapid and accurate diagnosis of pulmonary emboli in a canine model using intravascular ultrasound imaging. *Chest* 1991;100:1410.

70. Tapson VF, Davidson CJ, Kisslo KB, et al. Rapid visualization of massive pulmonary emboli utilizing intravascular ultrasound. *Chest* 1994;105:888.

71. Ricou F, Nicod PH, Moser KM, Peterson KL. Catheter-based intravascular ultrasound imaging of chronic thromboembolic pulmonary disease. *Am J Cardiol* 1991;67:749.

72. Sostman HD, Layish DT, Tapson VF, et al. Prospective comparison of helical CT and MR imaging in clinically suspected acute pulmonary embolism. *J Magn Reson Imaging* 1996;6:275.

73. Touliopoulos P, Costello P. Helical (spiral) CT of the thorax. *Rad Clin North Am* 1995;33:843.

74. Remy-Jardin M, Remy J, Wattinne L, Giraud F. Central pulmonary thromboembolism: diagnosis with spiral volumetric CT with the single-breath-hold technique. Comparison with pulmonary angiography. *Radiology* 1992;185:381.

75. Goodman LR, Curtin JJ, Mewissen MW, et al. Detection of pulmonary embolism in patients with unresolved clinical and scintigraphic diagnosis: helical CT versus angiography. *AJR Am J Roentgenol* 1995;164:1369.

76. Remy-Jardin M, Remy J, Petyt L, et al. Diagnosis of acute pulmonary embolism with spiral CT: comparison with pulmonary angiography and scintigraphy (abstract). *Radiology* 1995;197(P):303.

77. Teigen CL, Maus TP, Sheedy PF, et al. Pulmonary embolism: diagnosis with contrast-enhanced electron-beam CT and comparison with pulmonary angiography. *Radiology* 1995;194:313.

78. van Rossum AB, Pattynama PM, Treurniat FE, et al. Spiral CT angiography for detection of pulmonary embolism: validation in 124 patients. *Radiology* 1995;197(P):303.

79. van Rossum AB, Treurniat FE, Kieft GJ, et al. Role of spiral volumetric computed tomographic scanning in the assessment of patients with clinical suspicion of pulmonary embolism and an abnormal ventilation perfusion scan. *Thorax* 1996;51:23.

80. Oser RF, Zuckerman DA, Gutirrez FR, Brink JA. Anatomic distribution of pulmonary embolism at pulmonary arteriography: implications for spiral and electron-beam CT. *Radiology* 1996;199:31.

81. Quinn MF, Lundell CJ, Klotz TA, et al. Reliability of selective pulmonary arteriography in the diagnosis of acute pulmonary embolism. *AJR Am J Roentgenol* 1987;149:469.

82. Goodman LR, Lipchik RJ. Diagnosis of acute pulmonary embolism: time for a new approach. *Radiology* 1996;199:25.

83. Teigen CL, Maus TP, Sheedy PF, et al. Pulmonary embolism: diagnosis with electron-beam CT. *Radiology* 1993;188:839.

84. Drucker EA, Rivitz SM, Shepard JO. Acute pulmonary embolism: assessment of helical CT. *Radiology* 1998;209:235.

85. Hull R, Hirsh J, Powers P. Impedance plethysmography: the relationship between venous filling and sensitivity and specificity for proximal vein thrombosis. *Circulation* 1978;58:898.

86. Hull R, van Aken WG, Hirsh J, et al. Impedance plethysmography using the occlusive cuff technique in the diagnosis of venous thrombosis. *Circulation* 1976;53:696.

87. Patterson RB. The limitations of impedance plethysmography in the diagnosis of acute DVT. *J Vasc Surg* 1989;9:725.

88. Anderson DR, Lensing AWA, Wells PS, et al. Limitations of impedance plethysmography in the diagnosis of clinically suspected deep-vein thrombosis. *Ann Intern Med* 1993;118:25.

89. Lensing AW, Levi MM, Buller HR, et al. Diagnosis of deep-vein thrombosis using an objective Doppler method. *Ann Intern Med* 1990;113:9.

90. White R, McGahan JP, Daschbach MM, Hartling MM. Diagnosis of deep-vein thrombosis using duplex ultrasound. *Ann Intern Med* 1989;111:297.

91. Cronan JJ, Leen V. Recurrent deep venous thrombosis: limitations of ultrasound. *Radiology* 1989;170:739.

92. Killewich LA, Bedford GR, Beach KW, Strandness DE. Diagnosis of deep venous thrombosis: a prospective study

comparing duplex scanning to contrast venography. *Circulation* 1989;79:810.

93. Davidson BL, Elliott CG, Lensing AWA. Low accuracy of color Doppler ultrasound in the detection of proximal leg vein thrombosis in asymptomatic high-risk patients. *Ann Intern Med* 1992;117:735.

94. Evans AJ, Tapson VF, Sostman HD, et al. The diagnosis of deep venous thrombosis: A prospective comparison of venography and magnetic resonance imaging. *Chest* 1992;102:120S.

95. Witty LA, Tapson VF, Evans AJ, et al. MRI versus ultrasound: a radiologic and clinical evaluation of DVT. *Am Rev Respir Dis* 1993;147:A998.

96. Burke B, Sostman HD, Carroll BA, Witty LA. The diagnostic approach to deep venous thrombosis: which technique? *Clin Chest Med* 1995;16:253.

97. Loud PA, Katz DS, Klippenstein DL, et al. Combined CT venography and pulmonary angiography in suspected thromboembolic disease: diagnostic accuracy for deep venous evaluation. *AJR Am J Roentgenol* 2000;174:61.

98. Anderson FA Jr, Brownell W, Goldberg RJ, et al. Physician practices in the prevention of venous thromboembolism. *Ann Intern Med* 1991;115:591.

99. Colditz GA, Tuden RL, Oster G. Rates of venous thrombosis after general surgery: combined results of randomised clinical trials. *Lancet* 1986;2:143.

100. Collins R, Scrimgeour A, Yusuf S, Peto R. Reduction in fatal pulmonary embolism and venous thrombosis by perioperative administration of subcutaneous heparin. *N Engl J Med* 1988;318:1162.

101. Tapson VF, Hull R. Management of venous thromboembolic disease: the impact of low-molecular-weight heparin. *Clin Chest Med* 1995;16:281.

102. Bergqvist D, Benoni G, Bjorgell O, et al. Low-molecular-weight heparin (enoxaparin) as prophylaxis against venous thromboembolism after total hip replacement. *N Engl J Med* 1996;335:696.

103. Comp PC, Spiro T, Friedman, RJ, et al. Prolonged enoxaparin therapy to prevent venous thromboembolism after primary hip or knee replacement. *J Bone Joint Surg* 2001;83A:336.

104. Samama MM, Cohen AT, Darmon J-Y, et al. A comparison of enoxaparin with placebo for the prevention of venous thromboembolism in acutely ill medical patients. *N Engl J Med* 1999;341:793.

105. Kleber FX, Witt C, Flosbach CW, et al. Study to compare the efficacy and safety of the low-molecular-weight heparin enoxaparin and standard heparin in the prevention of thromboembolic events in medical patients with cardiopulmonary diseases. *Ann Hematol* 1998;76[Suppl 1]:A93.

106. Lechler E, Schramm W, Flosbach CW, et al. The venous thrombotic risk in nonsurgical patients: epidemiological data and efficacy/safety profile of a low molecular weight heparin (enoxaparin). *Haemostasis* 1996;26[Suppl 2]:49.

107. Hirsh J, Dalen JE, Deykin D, Poller L. Heparin and low-molecular-weight heparin: mechanisms of action, pharmacokinetics, dosing, monitoring, efficacy and safety. *Chest* 2001;119[Suppl]:64S-94S.

108. Hull RD, Raskob GE, Hirsh J, et al. Continuous intravenous heparin compared with intermittent subcutaneous heparin in the initial treatment of proximal vein thrombosis. *N Engl J Med* 1986;315:1109.

109. Hull R, Raskob G, Rosenbloom D, et al. Optimal therapeutic level of heparin therapy in patients with venous thrombosis. *Arch Intern Med* 1992;152:1589.

110. Raschke RA, Reilly BM, Guidry JR, et al. The weight-based heparin dosing nomogram compared with a "standard care" nomogram. *Ann Intern Med* 1993;119:874.

111. Dalen JE, Hirsh J, Guyatt GH. Sixth American College of Chest Physicians Consensus Conference on Antithrombotic Therapy. *Chest* 2001;119:1S.

112. Lagerstedt CI, Olsson C-G, Fagher BO, Oqvist BW. Need for long-term anticoagulant treatment in symptomatic calf-vein thrombosis. *Lancet* 1985;2:515.

113. Moser KM, LeMoine JR. Is embolic risk conditioned by location of deep venous thrombosis? *Ann Intern Med* 1981;94:439.

114. Levine M, Gent M, Hirsh J, et al. A comparison of low molecular-weight-heparin administered primarily at home with unfractionated heparin administered in the hospital for proximal deep vein thrombosis. *N Engl J Med* 1996;334:677.

115. Koopman MM, Prandoni P, Piovella F, et al. Low molecular-weight-heparin versus heparin for proximal deep vein thrombosis. *N Engl J Med* 1996;334:682.

116. Tapson VF. Treatment of acute deep venous thrombosis and pulmonary embolism: use of low molecular weight heparin. *Semin Respir Crit Care Med* 2000;21:547.

117. Dolovich LR, Ginsberg JS, Douketis JD, et al. A meta-analysis comparing low molecular weight heparins with unfractionated heparin in the treatment of venous thromboembolism. *Arch Intern Med* 2000;160:181.

118. Siragusa S, Cosmi B, Piovella F, et al. Low-molecular-weight heparins and unfractionated heparin in the treatment of patients with acute venous thromboembolism: results of a meta-analysis. *Am J Med* 1996;100:269.

119. Lensing AWA, Prins MH, Davidson BL, Hirsh J. Treatment of deep venous thrombosis with low-molecular-weight heparins: a meta-analysis. *Arch Intern Med* 1995;155:601.

120. Leizorovicz A, Simonneau G, Decousus H, Boissel JP. Comparison of efficacy and safety of low molecular weight heparins and unfractionated heparin in initial treatment of deep venous thrombosis. *BMJ* 1994;309:299.

121. Merli G, Spiro T, Olsson C-G, Abildgaard U, et al. Subcutaneous enoxaparin once or twice daily compared with intravenous unfractionated heparin for treatment of venous thromboembolic disease. *Ann Intern Med* 2001;134:191.

122. Simmoneau G, Sors H, Charbonnier B, et al. A comparison of low-molecular-weight heparin with unfractionated heparin for acute pulmonary embolism. The THESEE Study Group. *N Engl J Med* 1997;337:663.

123. The Global Use of Strategies to Open Occluded Coronary Arteries (GUSTO) IIB Investigators. A comparison of recombinant hirudin with heparin for the treatment of acute coronary syndromes. *N Engl J Med* 1996;335:775.

124. Antman EM, for the TIMI 9B Investigators. Hirudin in acute myocardial infarction: thrombolysis and thrombin inhibition in MI (TIMI) 9B trial. *Circulation* 1996;94:911.

125. Gustafsson D, Elg M, Lenfors S, et al. Effects of inogatran, a new low molecular weight thrombin inhibitor, in rat models of venous and arterial thrombosis, thrombolysis and bleeding time. *Blood Coagul Fibrinolysis* 1996;7:69.

126. Roux S, Tschopp T, Baumgartner HR. Effects of napsagatran, a new synthetic thrombin inhibitor and of heparin in a

canine model of coronary artery thrombosis: comparison with an ex vivo annular perfusion chamber model. *J Pharmacol Exp Ther* 1996;277:71.

127. Valjii K, Arun K, Bookstein JJ. Use of a direct thrombin inhibitor (argatroban) during pulse-spray thrombolysis in experimental thrombosis. *J Vasc Interv Radiol* 1995;6:91.

128. Nicolini FA, Lee P, Malycky JL, et al. Selective inhibition of factor Xa during thrombolytic therapy markedly improves coronary artery patency in a canine model of coronary thrombosis. *Blood Coagul Fibrinolysis* 1996;7:39.

129. Abildgaard U. Relative roles of tissue factor pathway inhibitor and antithrombin in the control of thrombogenesis. *Blood Coagul Fibrinolysis* 1995;6[Suppl 1]:S45.

130. Kelton JG, Sheridan D, Santos A, et al. Heparin-associated thrombocytopenia: laboratory studies. *Blood* 1988;79:925.

131. Amiral J, Bridey F, Dreyfus M, et al. Platelet factor 4 complexed to heparin is the target for antibodies generated in heparin-induced thrombocytopenia. *Thromb Haemost* 1992;68:95.

132. Visentin GP, Ford SE, Scott JP, Aster RH. Antibodies from patients with heparin-induced thrombocytopenia/thrombosis are specific for platelet factor 4 complexed with heparin or bound to endothelial cells. *J Clin Invest* 1994;93:81.

133. Warkentin TE, Levine MN, Hirsh J, et al. Heparin-induced thrombocytopenia in patients treated with low-molecular-weight heparin or unfractionated heparin. *N Engl J Med* 1995;332:1330.

134. Greenfield LJ. Vena caval interruption and pulmonary embolectomy. *Clin Chest Med* 1984;5:495.

135. Becker DM, Philbrick JT, Selby JB. Inferior vena cava filters: indications, safety, effectiveness. *Arch Intern Med* 1992;152:1985.

136. Symposium: Thrombolytic therapy in thrombosis: a National Institutes of Health Consensus Development Conference. *Ann Intern Med* 1980;93:141.

137. Goldhaber SZ. Evolving concepts in thrombolytic therapy for pulmonary embolism. *Chest* 1992;101[Suppl]:183S.

138. Witty LA, Steinfeld AD, Tapson VF. Thrombolytic therapy in acute pulmonary embolism: physician attitudes. *Am Rev Respir Dis* 1993;147:A1000.

139. Johnson AJ, McCarthy WR. The lysis of artificially induced intravascular clots in man by intravenous infusion of streptokinase. *J Clin Invest* 1959;38:1627.

140. Miller GAH, Gibson RV, Sutton GC. Treatment of pulmonary embolism with streptokinase. *BMJ* 1969;1:812.

141. Sasahara AA, Cannilla JE, Belks JJ, et al. Urokinase therapy in clinical pulmonary embolism. *N Engl J Med* 1969;277:1168.

142. Goldhaber SZ, Kessler CM, Heit J, et al. A randomized controlled trial of recombinant tissue plasminogen activator versus urokinase in the treatment of acute pulmonary embolism. *Lancet* 1988;2:293.

143. Leeper KV Jr., Popovich J Jr., Lesser BA, et al. Treatment of massive acute pulmonary embolism. The use of low doses of intrapulmonary arterial streptokinase combined with full doses of systemic heparin. *Chest* 1988;93:234.

144. The UKEP study: multicentre clinical trial on two local regimens of urokinase in massive pulmonary embolism. The UKEP Study Research Group. *Eur Heart J* 1987;8:2.

145. Verstraete M, Miller GAH, Bounameaux H, et al. Intravenous and intrapulmonary recombinant tissue-type plasminogen activator in the treatment of acute massive pulmonary embolism. *Circulation* 1988;77:353.

146. Rogers LQ, Lutcher CL. Streptokinase therapy for deep vein thrombosis: a comprehensive review of the literature. *Am J Med* 1990;88:389.

147. Sane DC, Califf RM, Topol EJ, et al. Bleeding during thrombolytic therapy for acute myocardial infarction: mechanisms and management. *Ann Intern Med* 1989;111:1010.

148. Gore JM. Prevention of severe neurologic events in the thrombolytic era. *Chest* 1992;101:124S.

149. Gray HH, Morgan JM, Paneth M, Miller GAH. Pulmonary embolectomy: indications and results. *Br Heart J* 1987;57:572.

150. Greenfield LJ, Kimmell GO, McCurdy WC. Transvenous removal of pulmonary emboli by vacuum-cup catheter technique. *J Surg Res* 1969;9:347.

151. Timsit JF, Reynaud P, Meyer G, Sors H. Pulmonary embolectomy by catheter device in massive PE. *Chest* 1991;100:655.

152. Tapson VF, Gurbel PA, Royster R, et al. Pharmacomechanical thrombolysis of experimental pulmonary emboli: rapid low-dose intraembolic therapy. *Chest* 1994;106:1558.

153. Tapson VF, Davidson CJ, Bauman R, et al. Rapid thrombolysis of massive pulmonary emboli without systemic fibrinogenolysis: intra-embolic infusion of thrombolytic therapy. *Am Rev Respir Dis* 1992;145:A719.

154. Semba CP, Dake MD. Iliofemoral deep venous thrombosis: aggressive therapy with catheter-directed thrombolysis. *Radiology* 1994;191:487.

155. Tapson VF, Witty LA. Massive pulmonary embolism: diagnostic and therapeutic strategies. *Clin Chest Med* 1996;16:329.

156. Jardin F, Genevray B, Brunney D, Margairaz A. Dobutamine: a hemodynamic evaluation in pulmonary embolism shock. *Crit Care Med* 1985;13:1009.

157. Manier G, Castaing Y. Influence of cardiac output on oxygen exchange in acute pulmonary embolism. *Am Rev Respir Dis* 1992;145:130.

158. Shure D. Chronic thromboembolic pulmonary hypertension: diagnosis and treatment. *Semin Respir Crit Care Med* 1996;17:7.

159. Fedullo PF, Auger WR, Channick RN, et al. Chronic thromboembolic pulmonary hypertension. *Clin Chest Med* 1995;16:353.

160. Shure D, Gregoratos G, Moser KM. Fiberoptic angioscopy: role in the diagnosis of chronic pulmonary arterial obstruction. *Ann Intern Med* 1985;103:844.

161. American College of Chest Physicians Consensus Committee on Pulmonary Embolism. Opinions regarding the diagnosis and management of venous thromboembolism. *Chest* 1996;109:233.

162. Tapson VF, Carroll BA, Davidson BL, et al. The diagnostic approach to acute venous thromboembolism. Clinical Practice Guideline. American Thoracic Society. *Am J Respir Crit Care Med* 1999;160:1043.

163. Goldhaber SZ, Visani L. The International Cooperative Pulmonary Embolism Registry. *Chest* 1995;108:302.

164. Egermayer P. Silent pulmonary embolism. *Arch Intern Med* 2000;160:2218.

29

HYPERTROPHIC CARDIOMYOPATHY

WILLIAM J. MCKENNA
PERRY M. ELLIOTT

◥ ADDITIONAL ELECTRONIC TOPICS

OVERVIEW

Hypertrophic cardiomyopathy (HCM) is caused by mutations in genes that encode cardiac sarcomeric proteins. The disease is characterized by myocardial hypertrophy, most commonly affecting the interventricular septum, and disorganization (disarray) of cardiac myocytes and myofibrils. Myocardial fibrosis is common and may be associated with small-vessel disease. Twenty-five percent of patients have a dynamic left ventricular outflow tract gradient caused by the combined effects of rapid ventricular ejection, a narrowed outflow tract, and systolic anterior motion (SAM) of the mitral valve.

The characteristic pathology of HCM contributes to a spectrum of functional abnormalities that includes myocardial ischemia, diastolic dysfunction, ventricular and atrial arrhythmias, and congestive cardiac failure. Patients can present at any age with chest pain, dyspnea, palpitations, and syncope. The most important complication of the disease is sudden death, which occurs throughout life with an annual incidence (in referral populations) of 2% to 4% in children and adolescents and approximately 1% in adults. Other complications include thromboembolism, infective endocarditis, and conduction system disease. Clinical features associated with an increased risk of sudden death include nonsustained ventricular tachycardia (NSVT), syncope, a family history of sudden death, an abnormal exercise blood pressure response, and severe left ventricular hypertrophy.

The principal aims of management are the alleviation of symptoms and the prevention of sudden death. In patients with substantial left ventricular outflow tract obstruction, interventions that reduce the magnitude of the outflow tract gradient (e.g., disopyramide, beta-blockade, alcohol ablation of the interventricular septum, dual-chamber pacing, and surgery) often result in significant symptomatic improvement. Therapeutic options in patients without left ventricular outflow tract obstruction are more limited, but chest pain and, to a lesser extent, dyspnea may be alleviated by pharmacologic therapy. Clinical risk-stratification can identify the risk of sudden death

W. J. McKenna: Department of Cardiological Sciences, St. George's Hospital Medical School, London, United Kingdom
P. M. Elliott: Department of Cardiological Sciences, St. George's Hospital Medical School, London, United Kingdom

in most adults and many adolescents, allowing effective prophylactic treatment with an implantable cardioverter-defibrillator (ICD) or reassurance where appropriate.

ANATOMY

Macroscopic

HCM is defined by the presence of unexplained myocardial hypertrophy (1). In Teare's original series (13), myocardial hypertrophy was asymmetric, involving the interventricular septum more than the posterior or free wall of the left ventricle (Fig. 29.1). Subsequent studies have shown that, although asymmetric septal hypertrophy is present in approximately two-thirds of patients (70,71), virtually any pattern can occur. Hypertrophy confined to the left ventricular apex is uncommon, except possibly in Japanese patients (72). Isolated right ventricular hypertrophy is unreported. Macroscopically, the cut surface of involved myocardium has a characteristic appearance reminiscent of a uterine fibroid, with abnormally short and broad muscle fibers running in different directions. An additional feature occasionally seen during post mortem examination is a patch of subendocardial thickening on the septum caused by repeated contact with the anterior leaflet of the mitral valve.

Microscopic

The cardinal microscopic feature of HCM is myocyte disarray (70,71,73–76) (Fig. 29.2). This is recognized by a loss of the normal parallel arrangement of myocytes, with cells forming circles around foci of connective tissue. Individual myocytes may show marked variation in diameter and nuclear size and have abnormal intercellular connections.

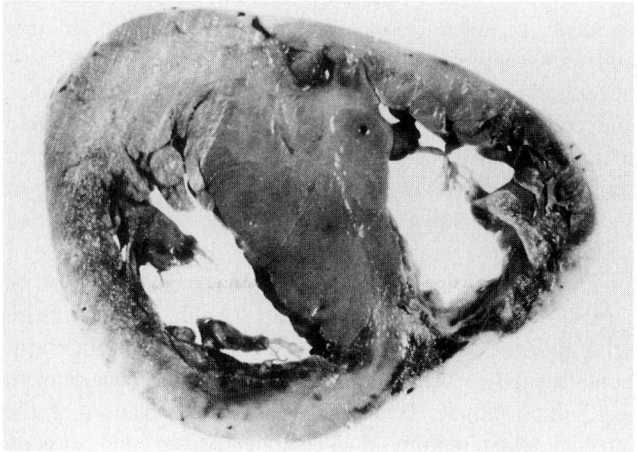

FIGURE 29.1 Myocardial section demonstrating the classical appearance of severe asymmetric septal hypertrophy in a patient with hypertrophic cardiomyopathy. (From Teare D. Asymmetrical hypertrophy of the heart in young adults. *Br Heart J* 1958;20:1–8, with permission.)

Myofibrillar architecture within cells is also disrupted—so-called myofibrillar disarray. Myocyte disarray is described in congenital heart disease, hypertension, and aortic stenosis, but in HCM it is typically more extensive, occupying 20% or more of at least one ventricular tissue block and more than 5% of total myocardium at post mortem examination. Disarray is often associated with myocardial fibrosis, ranging from extensive scarring in the interventricular septum, free wall of the left ventricle, and occasionally the left ventricular papillary muscles (77) to a more diffuse interstitial pattern (78). The demonstration of abnormal small intramural arteries (external diameter less than 1,500 mm) within fibrotic areas and in patients with ventricular dilatation and reduced systolic function (79,80) (Fig. 29.3) has suggested that contiguous myocardial scarring may be caused by myocardial ischemia. However, more recent data have shown that small-vessel disease may be just as widespread in patients without extensive fibrosis and may occur in the absence of myocardial hypertrophy (81).

PATHOPHYSIOLOGY

Molecular Genetics

HCM is usually familial, with autosomal dominant inheritance. Early reports of autosomal recessive patterns of transmission (31) have not been confirmed. A cardiac phenotype similar to that seen in HCM is described in association with a number of rare genetically determined disorders, including Friedreich's ataxia (chromosome 9) (82,83), neurofibromatosis (chromosome 17) (84), hereditary spherocytosis (chromosome 14) (85), aniridia with catalase deficiency (chromosome 11) (86), and Noonan's syndrome (chromosome 12) (87–89). Because the clinical phenotype of these disorders differs considerably from that seen in most patients with familial HCM, and none of the genes associated with these disorders encode known cardiac proteins, the identification of candidate genes in familial HCM has until quite recently relied on linkage analysis and a positional candidate gene approach. The first disease locus to be identified was situated in the chromosome 14q1 region in a large French Canadian family (36). The genes encoding the two cardiac myosin heavy chains (α and β) are arranged in tandem on chromosome 14 band q11.2-13, and further analysis involving this Canadian family revealed that each affected member had a missense mutation in exon 13 of the β-myosin heavy-chain gene (38). Since this discovery, numerous mutations in seven other genes that encode thick and thin filament sarcomeric proteins have been reported (Fig. 29.4): cardiac troponin T (chromosome 1), cardiac troponin I (chromosome 19), α-tropomyosin (chromosome 15), cardiac myosin-binding protein C (chromosome 11), the essential and regulatory myosin light chains (chromosomes 3 and 12, respectively), and cardiac actin (chromosome 15) (36–67). In addition, a

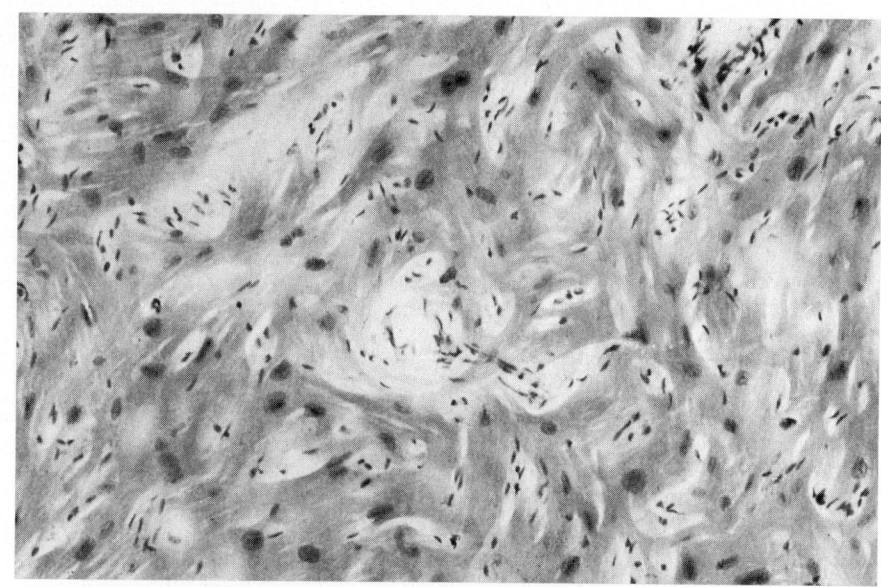

FIGURE 29.2 Myocyte disarray. Myocytes cross at right angles and display abnormal intercellular connections. Myocyte nuclei are large and of different sizes. Foci of fibrosis containing spindle-shaped connective-tissue cells are present. Evidence of marked disorganization of the intracellular myofibrillar structure is also seen (hematoxylin-eosin stain). (Courtesy of M. Davies, St. George's Hospital Medical School, London.)

locus on chromosome 7 has been identified in a large Irish family with HCM and Wolff-Parkinson-White syndrome (90,91), and a further unconfirmed mutation in the gene encoding another sarcomeric protein, Titin (chromosome 2) (68), has been reported. ❦ g02

Myocardial Ischemia

Several studies have shown that patients with HCM have reduced coronary flow reserve and metabolic evidence for myocardial ischemia during pacing and pharmacologic stress (119–125). It is likely that myocardial ischemia is the cause of chest pain and dyspnea in many individuals,

and limited data are available to suggest that myocardial ischemia may be a trigger for fatal ventricular arrhythmia (126,127). However, the clinical evaluation of patients with chest pain remains problematic. For example, whereas ST segment depression occurs in up to 40% of patients during exercise (118), lactate production during atrial pacing is seen in more than one-half of those with negative results of exercise tests. ST segment depression also occurs during ambulatory ECG monitoring in 25% of symptomatic young patients (128), but its metabolic significance in unknown. A number of pathophysiologic mechanisms have been suggested as causes of myocardial ischemia in patients with HCM (Table 29.1), but the predominant mechanism in individual patients is usually impossible to determine.

Diastolic Dysfunction

Several of the characteristic pathophysiologic features of HCM impair diastolic function, specifically, myocyte hypertrophy, myocyte and myofibrillar disarray, abnormal intracellular calcium metabolism, myocardial fibrosis, abnormal ventricular geometry, and myocardial ischemia (129–140). In a minority of patients, a restrictive hemodynamic picture may predominate, with marked elevation of filling pressures, biatrial dilatation, and predominantly right-sided signs, often in the absence of substantial myocardial hypertrophy (137,138). In the majority of cases, a mixed picture with slow relaxation and elevated end diastolic pressures is observed. Invasive hemodynamic studies have demonstrated a flat pressure-volume relationship with a response to off-loading similar to that seen in patients with constrictive pericarditis, suggesting the presence of increased pericardial or possibly myocardial constraint (140).

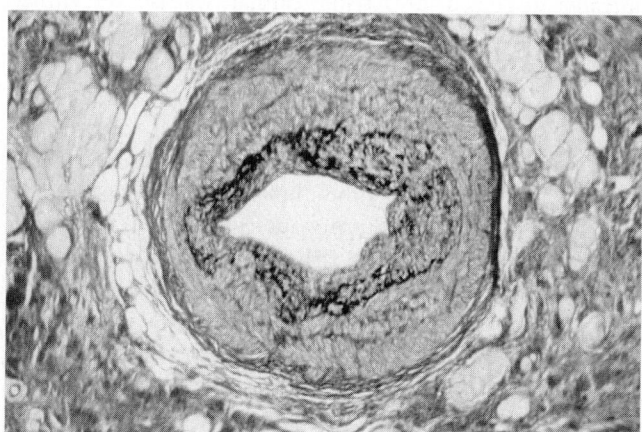

FIGURE 29.3 Section through a small artery demonstrating smooth-muscle disorganization in the intima and media, resulting in an abnormally high medial width–to-lumen ratio. In the adjacent myocardium, extensive replacement of myocytes by fibrous tissue can be seen (Elastica van Gieson stain). (Courtesy of M. Davies, St. George's Hospital Medical School, London.)

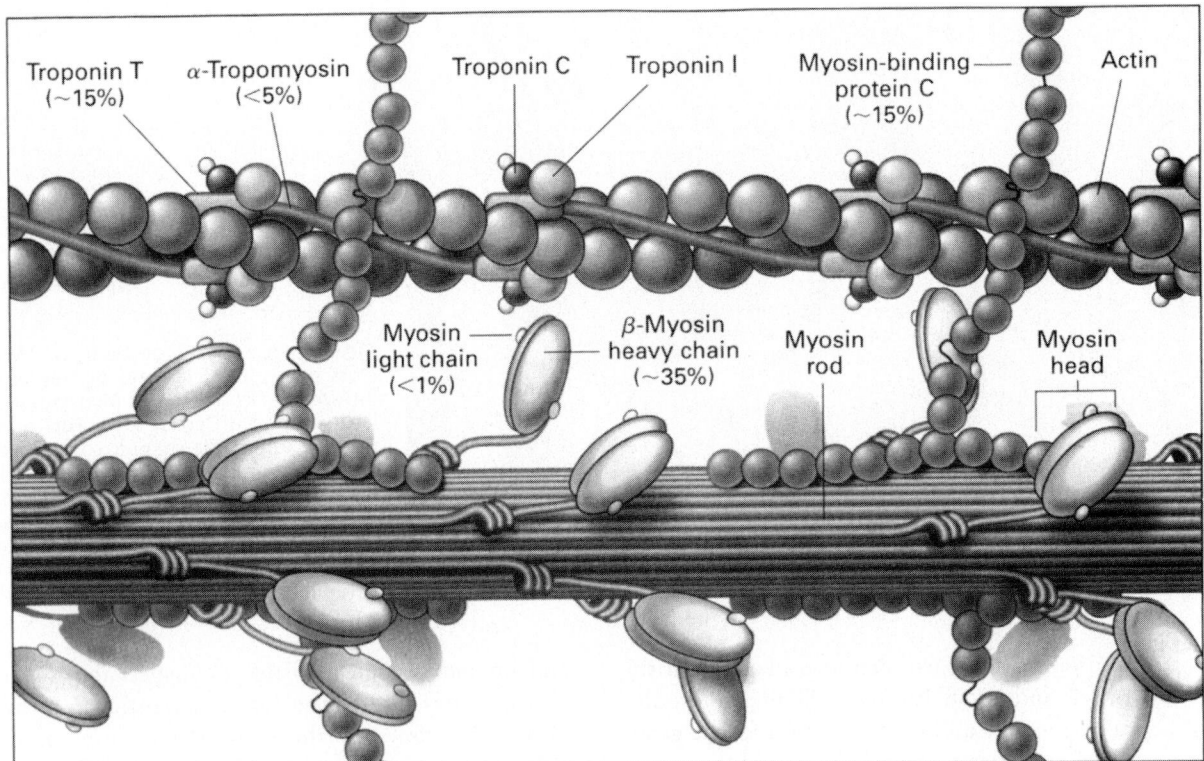

FIGURE 29.4 Structure of the human sarcomere. Cardiac contraction occurs as a consequence of actin-myosin interaction. This is initiated by the binding of calcium to the troponin complex (C, I, and T) and α-tropomyosin. Actin then stimulates adenosinetriphosphatase activity in the globular myosin head, resulting in the generation of contractile force. Cardiac myosin-binding protein C binds to myosin and modulates contraction. The estimated frequency of sarcomeric protein gene mutations that cause hypertrophic cardiomyopathy is shown. (From Spirito P, Seidman CE, McKenna WJ, et al. The management of hypertrophic cardiomyopathy. *N Engl J Med* 1997;336:775–785, with permission.)

CLINICAL PROFILE

Epidemiology

Whereas HCM occurs in all racial groups, most of the published literature comes from populations in North America, Europe, and Japan. Of five studies that have examined the prevalence of HCM (141–145), all but one suggest a preva-

TABLE 29.1 POTENTIAL MECHANISMS OF MYOCARDIAL ISCHEMIA IN HYPERTROPHIC CARDIOMYOPATHY

Increased myocardial oxygen demand
  Myocardial hypertrophy
  Diastolic dysfunction
  Myocyte disarray
  Left ventricular outflow obstruction
  Arrhythmia
Reduced myocardial perfusion
  Small-vessel disease
  Abnormal vascular responses
  Myocardial bridges
  Increased coronary vascular resistance

lence of 0.2% to 0.5% in the general population. The exception (144) was a disease surveillance study that examined the prevalence of HCM in a population of patients already suspected of having cardiac disease on clinical grounds.

Natural History

Ventricular hypertrophy usually develops during periods of rapid somatic growth, sometimes during the first year of life, but more typically during adolescence (101). De novo myocardial hypertrophy in early middle age is not reported, but the diagnosis of idiopathic or inappropriate left ventricular hypertrophy in patients older than 60 years is well described (146–150). The pattern of disease in this age group is said to differ from that observed in younger patients with HCM, in that symptoms occur late in life, the prognosis for most patients is relatively good, and many have mild hypertension. A number of morphologic differences are also described, including restricted anterior excursion of the mitral valve, mitral annular calcification, and a crescent-shaped left ventricular cavity. Whether the majority of patients with this so-called elderly phenotype has a separate disease entity reflecting a polygenic response to hypertrophic stimuli remains uncertain, but recently gathered data from families with mutations in the cardiac myosin-binding protein C gene have shown that a phenotype identical to that of young patients can be seen in older patients (63,102).

In most patients with HCM, progression of symptoms is slow and age related and associated with a gradual deterioration in left ventricular function. This course may end at any point in sudden death. Early data from referral institutions reported annual mortality rates of approximately 2% per annum in adults and 2% to 4% during childhood and adolescence (151–153). More recent data from regional and tertiary adult populations (154–159) suggest a lower figure of approximately 1% per annum. Sudden death in the first decade of life is thought to be relatively uncommon, although only limited data about this age group are available (160). In fewer than 10% of patients, rapid symptomatic deterioration may occur in association with progressive myocardial wall thinning, a reduction in systolic performance, and an increase in left ventricular end systolic dimensions (161). Survival in patients with late-onset disease has been thought to be relatively benign in comparison with younger patients, but in some families with myosin-binding protein C mutations, the rate of death or adverse cardiovascular events can be similar to that of the most severe troponin-T or β-myosin heavy-chain mutations once disease is expressed (*e*Figs. 29.4.1 and 29.4.2) (63,92–96,102).

Symptoms

Patients may present at any age with dyspnea, chest pain, unexplained syncope, or arrhythmia, or the disease may be identified after sudden death (13,14,20,28,151–162). Many patients have no or only minor symptoms, and in children and adolescents, the diagnosis is often made during family screening. Exertional chest pain occurs in up to 30% of adults, and many complain of atypical pain that is prolonged and occurs at rest and after meals (163). Dyspnea is common in adult patients, probably as a consequence of elevated pulmonary venous pressure resulting from impaired ventricular relaxation and filling. Patients less commonly present with paroxysmal nocturnal dyspnea and orthopnea, sometimes in the presence of apparently mild disease. The mechanism is uncertain, but myocardial ischemia or arrhythmia may be responsible.

Approximately 15% to 25% of patients experience syncope, and 20% complain of presyncope. In some, these symptoms are caused by paroxysmal arrhythmia, conduction system disease, or abnormal vascular responses during exercise, but in most cases, no underlying cause is identified even after extensive investigation. Recurrent unexplained syncope is associated with a higher incidence of sudden

death when it occurs during adolescence (151–153,162). Palpitations are a frequent complaint. Symptomatic cardiac contractions and ventricular ectopy are not uncommon, but most sustained palpitation is caused by supraventricular arrhythmia (151,152).

Examination

In the majority of patients with HCM, physical examination is unremarkable. Patients may have a rapid upstroke to the arterial pulse, occasionally followed by a secondary peak, reflecting hyperdynamic left ventricular contraction (13–15,20). The left ventricular impulse may be forceful, and a palpable left-atrial beat may be present. In approximately one-third of patients, a prominent 'a' wave is seen in the jugular venous pressure wave caused by reduced right ventricular compliance. On auscultation, the first and second heart sounds are usually normal, but a fourth heart sound, reflecting atrial systole into a poorly compliant left ventricle, may be heard in patients who are in sinus rhythm. Occasionally, reverse splitting of the second heart sound may be heard in patients who have severe left ventricular outflow tract obstruction. In one-fourth of patients, a systolic murmur caused by left ventricular outflow obstruction can be heard at the left sternal edge, radiating to the aortic and mitral areas, but not into the neck or axilla. A characteristic feature of the murmur is its dependence on ventricular volume. Physiologic and pharmacologic maneuvers that decrease afterload or venous return (e.g., standing, Valsalva's maneuver, administration of amyl nitrate) increase the intensity of the murmur, whereas interventions that increase afterload and venous return (e.g., squatting and administration of phenylephrine) reduce it. The majority of patients with significant left ventricular outflow gradients also has mitral regurgitation. This can be difficult to distinguish clinically from the outflow gradient (13,14), but its presence is suggested by the length of the murmur (starting 30 to 40 ms before the onset of the outflow gradient), radiation to the axilla, and, in patients with severe regurgitation, a mid-diastolic rumble. Rarely, a systolic murmur may be heard in the pulmonary area as a consequence of right ventricular outflow obstruction.

Electrocardiogram

Although ECG abnormalities occur in the majority of patients with HCM, no changes are specific to the disease (13–15,28,162,164–171). ECG evidence of right- and left-atrial enlargement is frequent. Voltage criteria for left ventricular hypertrophy in association with repolarization abnormalities are also common, but isolated increases in voltage without ST segment and T-wave changes are infrequent. Abnormal Q waves occur in 25% to 50% of patients (165–167), most commonly in the inferolateral leads and in young patients. ▼▼ g03

Echocardiograph

The first echocardiographic diagnostic criteria in HCM were established using M-mode imaging (23–30,179). They include ASH of the interventricular septum, SAM of the mitral valve, a small left ventricular cavity, septal immobility, and premature closure of the aortic valve. With the experience of two-dimensional echocardiography, diagnostic criteria have been broadened to include virtually any pattern of hypertrophy (Figs. 29.5 and 29.6). The proportion of patients with asymmetric and concentric hypertrophy depends on what definitions are used. When a septal to free-wall thickness ratio of 1.3:1.0 is used to define asymmetry (29), concentric hypertrophy accounts for only 1% to 2% of cases. However, this proportion rises to approximately 31% when a septal to free-wall thickness ratio of 1.5:1.0 is used (180). ⌔ g04

Criteria for abnormal wall thickness vary, but a wall thickness more than 2 standard deviations from the mean, corrected for age, sex, and height (typically = 1.5 cm in an adult) is generally accepted as diagnostic. Right ventricular hypertrophy is diagnosed when at least two right ventricular wall measurements exceed 2 standard deviations from the mean recorded in healthy subjects. Using this criterion, right ventricular hypertrophy occurs in more than one-third of patients with HCM (181).

Approximately 25% of patients with HCM have a resting pressure gradient between the body and outflow tract of the left ventricle (13–15,23–30). This is almost always accompanied by SAM of the anterior mitral valve leaflet and ASH (Fig. 29.7). Some patients who show no evidence of outflow obstruction at rest have gradients that can be provoked by physiologic and pharmacologic interventions that diminish left ventricular end diastolic volume or augment left ventricular contractility. The clinical relevance of provokable obstruction is uncertain, but some workers advocate the use of such maneuvers in patients with ASH but no resting SAM, or whenever dynamic outflow tract obstruction is clinically suspected. ⌔ g05

Mitral regurgitation occurs in almost all patients who have obstructive HCM, as a consequence of SAM and abnormal mitral leaflet coaptation (204). When no mitral valve abnormality other than SAM is present, a direct relationship exists between the pressure gradient and the severity of mitral regurgitation. In approximately 20% of patients with outflow gradients, mitral regurgitation is exacerbated by calcification of the mitral valve annulus, leaflet fibroelastosis caused by repeated traumatic septal contact, mitral valve prolapse, or rheumatic valve disease. Mitral regurgitation occurs in approximately 30% of patients with nonobstructive HCM but is usually mild and may be associated with leaflet abnormalities.

Conventional M-mode and two-dimensional indices of systolic function are typically normal or supranormal in both obstructive and nonobstructive HCM. However, regional systolic function may be reduced, particularly in

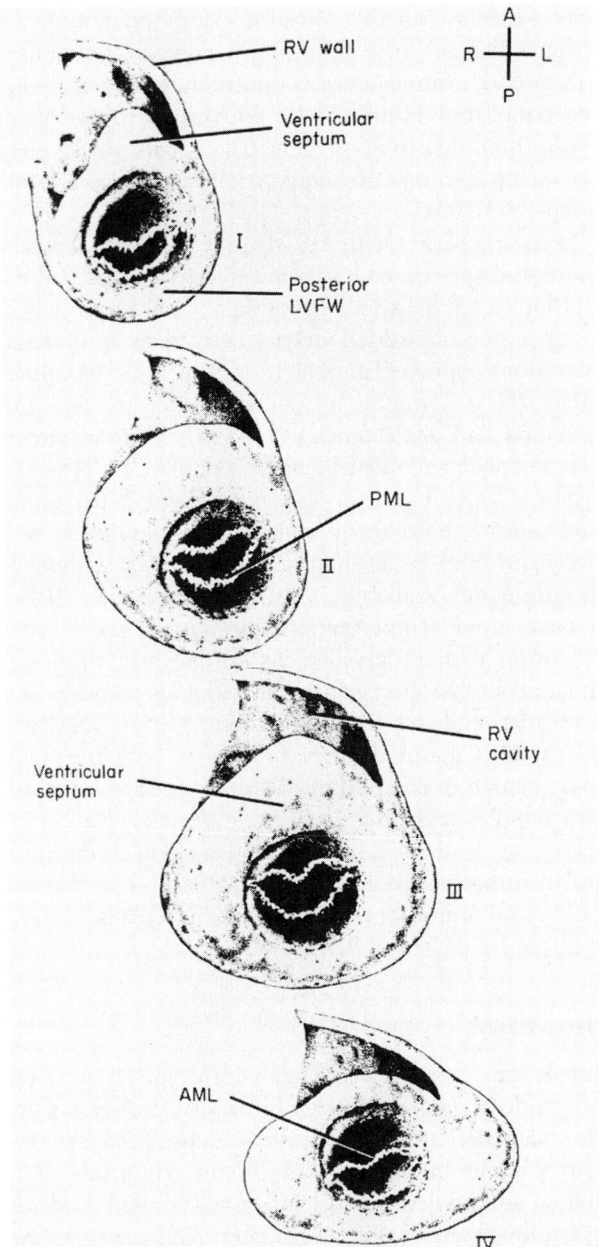

FIGURE 29.5 Maron classification. Artist's impression of four patterns of hypertrophy identified in 153 patients using two-dimensional echocardiography and shown on the short-axis plane at mitral valve level. I: Type I (10% of patients) hypertrophy confined to the anterior portion of the ventricular septum. II: Type II (20% of patients) hypertrophy involving the anterior and posterior septum. III: Type III (52% of patients) hypertrophy involving the anterior and posterior septum as well as the lateral free wall. IV: Type IV (18% of patients) hypertrophy involving left ventricular regions other than the anterior septum and the posterior free wall. A, anterior; AML, anterior mitral leaflet; L, patient's left; LVFW, left ventricular free wall; P, posterior; PML, posterior mitral leaflet; R, patient's right; RV, right ventricular. (From Maron BJ, Wolfson JK, Ciro E, et al. Relation of electrocardiographic abnormalities and patterns of left ventricular hypertrophy identified by 2-dimensional echocardiography in patients with hypertrophic cardiomyopathy. *Am J Cardiol* 1983;51:189–194, with permission.)

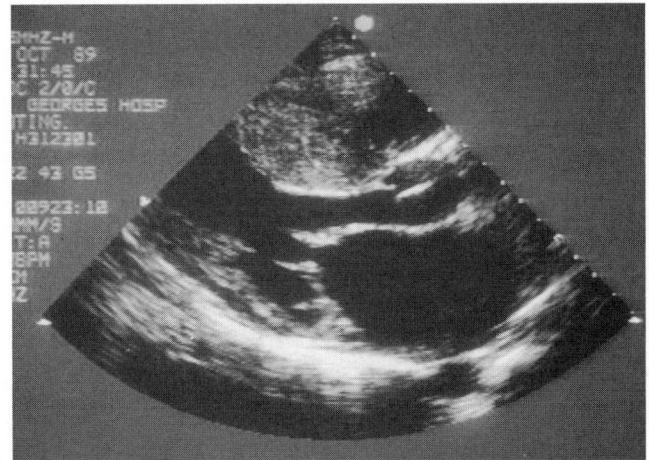

A

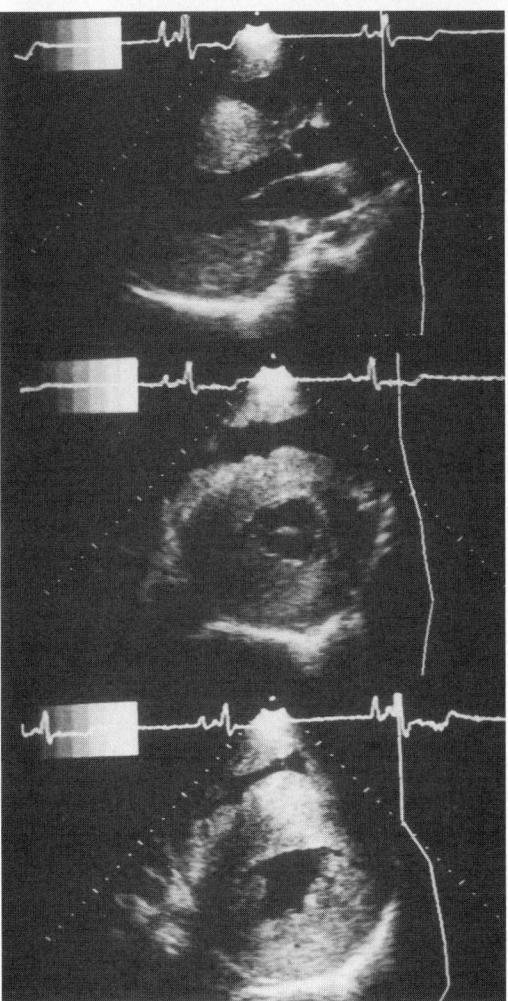

B

FIGURE 29.6 A: Two-dimensional echocardiogram in the parasternal long-axis view demonstrates asymmetric septal hypertrophy. **B:** Two-dimensional echocardiogram in the parasternal long- and short-axis view demonstrates severe concentric hypertrophy.

the interventricular septum, and indices of long-axis shortening are often abnormal (205–209). Thinning of hypertrophied myocardium and increases in end systolic dimensions occur in some adult patients as the disease progresses (161).

Early left ventricular filling velocities assessed using pulsed-wave Doppler imaging are, on average, very similar to control values, reflecting "pseudonormalization" of the transmitral Doppler filling pattern (210–212). E-wave deceleration time and isovolumic relaxation times are often increased. Pulmonary vein Doppler imaging often shows increased duration and peak velocity of the atrial reversal signal, reflecting increased left ventricular end diastolic pressure (210–212).

Cardiac Catheterization

Two-dimensional echocardiography has largely replaced cardiac catheterization in the diagnosis of HCM. Catheterization is indicated when the measurement of intracardiac pressures is likely to be useful in planning therapy (e.g., in patients who have severe mitral regurgitation), and for the exclusion of coronary atherosclerosis in older patients with chest pain. Left ventricular end diastolic pressure is often raised, secondary to increased stiffness and impaired relaxation. The characteristic left ventricular outflow gradient may be detected when careful pull-back across the aortic valve is performed (Fig. 29.8) or by measuring simultaneous aortic and left ventricular inflow pressures. An outflow gradient may be associated with an initial early spike in the aortic pressure wave, followed by a secondary dome-shaped tidal wave before the dichrotic notch (Fig. 29.8). In addition, the aortic pressure wave often fails to show postextrasystolic potentiation and may actually reduce in amplitude after an extrasystole. This phenomenon may reflect worsening of the outflow gradient during the potentiated post-extrasystolic beat. Right atrial and right ventricular pressures are usually normal, except in patients with significant right ventricular outflow gradients or severe restrictive physiology. Pulmonary capillary wedge pressure may be elevated, particularly when mitral regurgitation is severe. An increased 'v' wave can also be seen in the pulmonary capillary wedge tracing in the absence of significant mitral regurgitation, when reduced left atrial compliance is present. Resting cardiac output is usually normal or increased, except in patients with advanced disease and systolic impairment. Left ventricular angiography may show a septal bulge encroaching on the left ventricular outflow tract during systole, together with SAM of the anterior mitral valve leaflet and mitral regurgitation. In patients with hypertrophy that is confined to the left ventricular apex, the ventricular angiogram may show a characteristic spade-shaped appearance in the right anterior oblique projection. Coronary arteriography is usually normal, but obliteration of epicardial vessels and a "sawfish" appearance during systole are described (213,214).

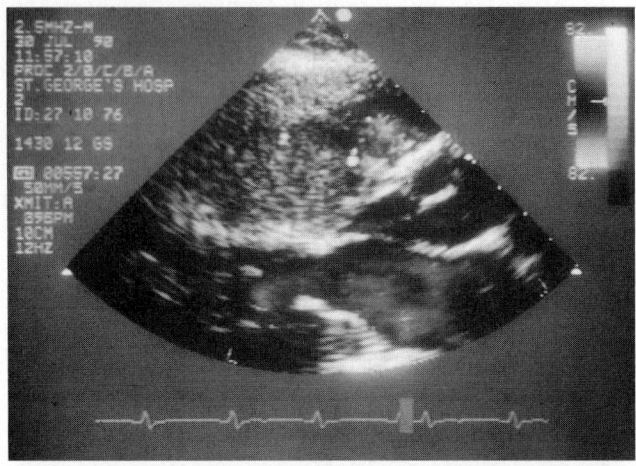

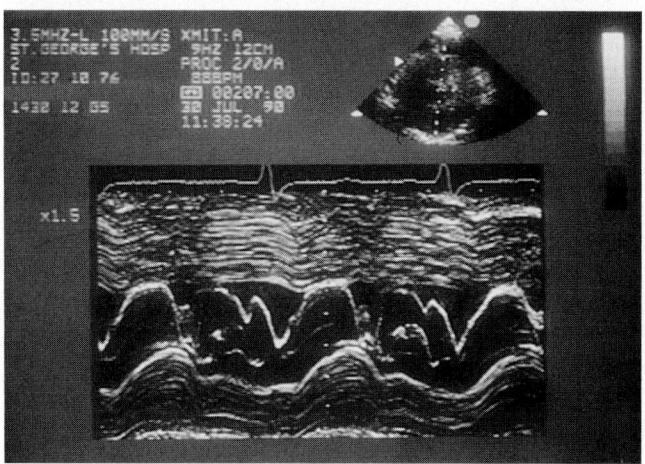

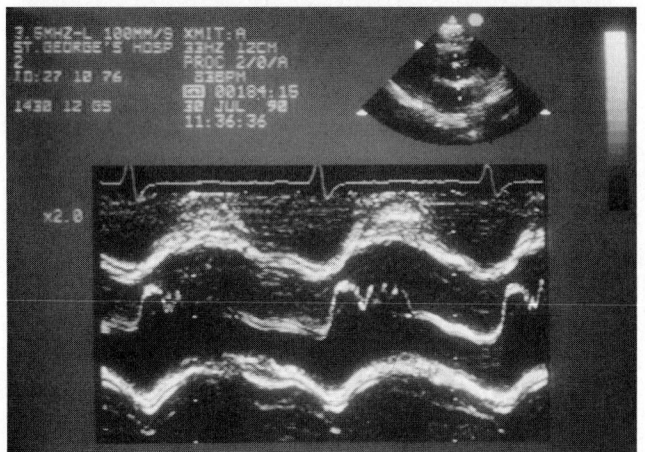

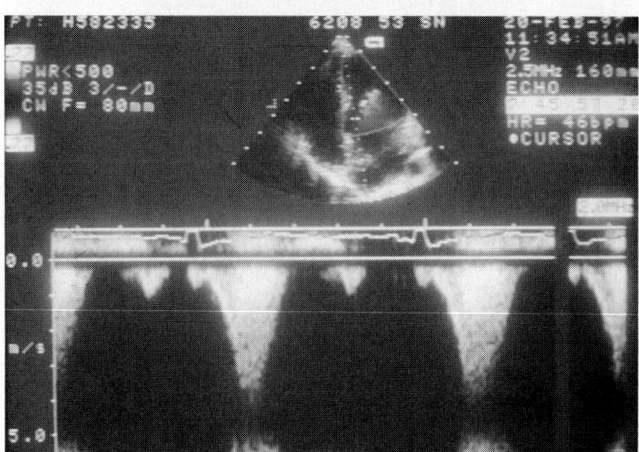

A   B   C   D

FIGURE 29.7 Sequence of four panels demonstrating **(A)** two-dimensional echocardiogram in the parasternal long-axis view that shows complete systolic anterior motion of the mitral valve and contact between the anterior mitral valve leaflet and the interventricular septum; **(B)** M-mode echocardiogram that shows asymmetric septal hypertrophy, systolic anterior motion of the mitral valve, and contact between the anterior mitral valve leaflet and the interventricular septum; **(C)** M-mode echocardiogram that shows mid-systolic closure of the aortic valve in a patient with left ventricular outflow obstruction; and **(D)** continuous-wave Doppler image that shows characteristic "dynamic" left ventricular outflow tract obstruction.

Although anecdotal reports have been made of improved symptoms in patients who undergo surgery for myocardial "bridges," the significance of systolic compression of epicardial or intramural vessels is uncertain, because data showing an association between sudden death and myocardial bridging in a highly selected cohort of young patients have not been confirmed by more recent studies (215,216).

Magnetic Resonance Imaging

In most patients with HCM, high-quality echocardiography suffices for diagnostic and therapeutic purposes, but magnetic resonance imaging may be useful in selected cases to assess right ventricular and apical involvement (eFig. 29.8.1). Technological advances have made it possible to use magnetic resonance imaging to assess structure,

regional function, myocardial perfusion, and myocardial energetics in a single study (228–232).

DIFFERENTIAL DIAGNOSIS

Existing diagnostic criteria for adults are based on the demonstration of unexplained left ventricular hypertrophy on echocardiography. That some individuals with HCM do not fulfill conventional echocardiographic criteria is, however, increasingly recognized. Because the probability of disease in a first-degree relative of a patient with HCM is 50%, minor ECG and echocardiographic abnormalities assume a far greater significance in the context of an affected family than in the general population. Based on this premise, new diagnostic criteria for HCM have been proposed (69) (Table 29.2). It is impor-

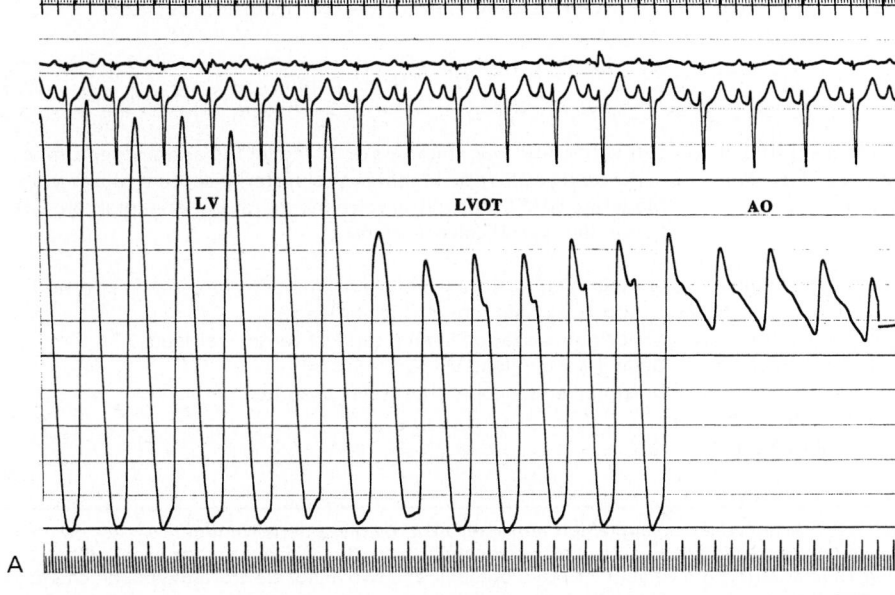

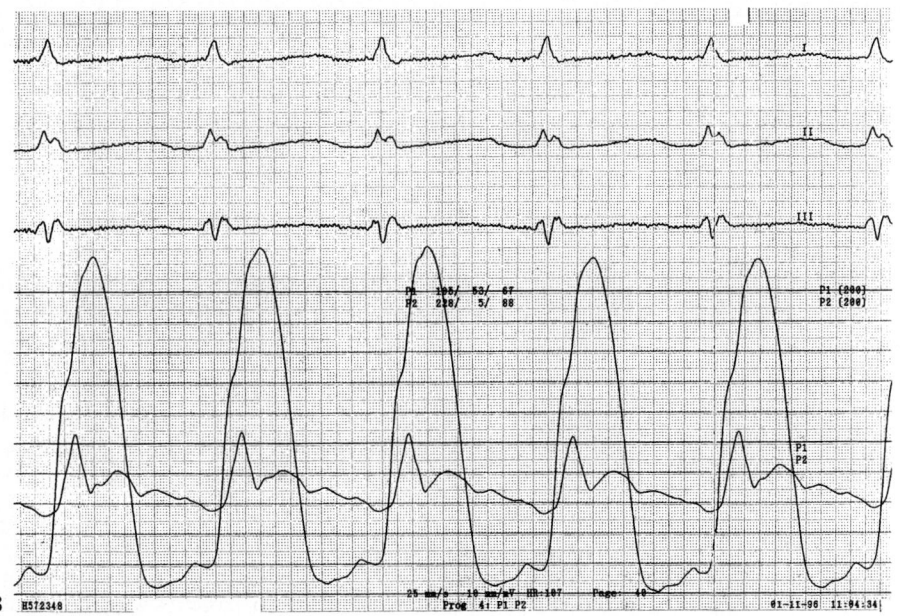

FIGURE 29.8 A: Pull-back pressure tracing shows sequential pressure pulses in the body of the left ventricle (LV), the left ventricular outflow tract (LVOT), and the aorta (AO). A pressure gradient exists between the body and outflow of the LV, and pulsus alternans is observed in the left ventricular pressure trace before the level of obstruction. **B:** Simultaneous LV (*upper trace*) and aortic (*lower trace*) pressure tracings in a patient with severe LV outflow obstruction. In the LV tracing, a prominent atrial contraction wave contributing to elevated LV end diastolic pressure can be seen. The aortic trace demonstrates a rapid upstroke with a second peak in late systole ("spike and dome") before the incisura. The notch on the upstroke of the LV pressure tracing corresponds approximately with the time of mitral leaflet–septal contact.

tant to realize that these criteria only apply to unexplained ECG and echocardiographic abnormalities in first-degree adult relatives. Diagnosis in children and adolescents, athletes, and adults with hypertension and obesity can present problems and requires specific consideration in each circumstance. A number of rare clinical syndromes overlap with idiopathic HCM (Table 29.3) and should also be considered in the differential diagnosis.

The Athletic Heart Syndrome

Although HCM is the commonest cause of death in young athletes (244,245), its diagnosis in individuals who regularly participate in competitive sports can be problematic

(246–250), because the physiologic changes brought on by athletic training can mimic HCM. Athletes who participate in events that combine both isometric and isotonic activities are most at risk of developing increased left ventricular wall thickness. Pure strength training is associated with an increase in left ventricular mass and wall thickness relative to the left ventricular cavity size, but strength training is rarely associated with an increase in absolute wall thickness (251). In a study of more than 900 elite athletes (246), fewer than 2% had a wall thickness greater than 13 mm, and none had a wall thickness greater than 16 mm. In female athletes, maximum wall thickness was less than or equal to 14 mm. A diagnosis of HCM in an elite athlete is more likely when an individual has left ventricular wall thickness exceeding these values and/or when the athlete is

TABLE 29.2 PROPOSED NEW DIAGNOSTIC CRITERIA FOR HYPERTROPHIC CARDIOMYOPATHY IN FIRST-DEGREE RELATIVES OF AFFECTED PATIENTS

Major criteria	Minor criteria
Echocardiography	
Left ventricular wall thickness ≥13 mm in the anterior septum or posterior wall or ≥15 mm in the posterior septum or free wall	Left ventricular wall thickness of 12 mm in the anterior septum or posterior wall or of 14 mm in the posterior septum or free wall
Severe SAM of the mitral valve (septal leaflet contact)	Moderate SAM of the mitral valve (no mitral leaflet–septal contact)
	Redundant mitral valve leaflets
Electrocardiography	
Left ventricular hypertrophy with repolarization changes (Romhilt-Estes)	Complete bundle branch block or (minor) interventricular conduction defects (in left ventricular leads)
T-wave inversion in leads I and aVL (≥3 mm) (with QRS-T wave axis difference ≥300), leads V_3–V_6 (≥ 3 mm), or leads II and III and aVF (≥5 mm)	Minor repolarization changes in left ventricular leads
Abnormal Q waves (>40 ms or >25% R wave) in at least two leads from II, III, aVF (in the absence of left anterior hemiblock), and V_1–V_4 or I, aVL, and V_5–V_6	Deep S wave in lead V_2 (>25 mm)
	Unexplained syncope, chest pain, dyspnea

aVF, augmented voltage unipolar left foot lead; aVL, augmented voltage unipolar left arm lead; SAM, systolic anterior motion.
Note: It is proposed that diagnosis of hypertrophic cardiomyopathy in first-degree relatives of patients with the disease be made based on the presence of one major criterion or two minor cardiographic criteria, or one minor echocardiographic and two minor electrocardiographic criteria.
From McKenna WJ, Spirito P, Desnos M, et al. Experience from clinical genetics in hypertrophic cardiomyopathy: proposal for new diagnostic criteria in adult members of affected families. *Heart* 1997;77:130–132.

symptomatic and has a family history of HCM and premature sudden death. The "athletic" ECG frequently displays voltage criteria for left ventricular hypertrophy, sinus bradycardia, and sinus arrhythmia. Although marked repolarization abnormalities are described in some elite athletes (252,253), they are uncommon and should always raise suspicion of myocardial disease. Echocardiographic features favoring HCM include small left ventricular cavity dimensions (athletes tend to have increased left ventricular end diastolic dimensions), left-atrial enlargement, left ventricular outflow gradients, and evidence on Doppler imaging of diastolic impairment. Recent data suggest that metabolic exercise testing may also be useful in differentiating athletic adaptation from HCM, with a peak oxygen consumption greater than 50 mL per minute per kg or more than 20%

TABLE 29.3 DIFFERENTIAL DIAGNOSIS OF UNEXPLAINED LEFT VENTRICULAR HYPERTROPHY (LVH)

Primary genetic disorders characterized by LVH
  Noonan's syndrome
  Friedreich's ataxia
  Lentiginosis
Exaggerated physiologic response
  Renal and Afro-Caribbean hypertension
  Athletic heart syndrome
  Obesity
Metabolic disorders
  Infants of diabetic mothers
  Amyloid
  Glycogen storage disease
  Mitochondrial myopathy
  Phaeochromocytoma
  Inborn errors of fatty-acid metabolism
  Fabry's disease

above the predicted maximum oxygen consumption that is highly suggestive of athletic adaptation (254).

PRINCIPLES OF CLINICAL MANAGEMENT

The main aims of clinical management in patients with HCM are to provide symptomatic relief and to prevent complications. In most cases, a relatively simple, noninvasive assessment that includes clinical history, echocardiography, ECG, 48-hour ambulatory ECG monitoring, and cardiopulmonary exercise testing is sufficient to identify patients who require specific treatments.

Symptomatic Therapy

Although pharmacologic therapy in patients with HCM is usually administered on an empirical basis, guided by subjective reporting of symptomatic improvement, the choice of therapy is influenced by left ventricular morphology and hemodynamics (eFig. 29.8.2). In patients with significant outflow obstruction, the principal aim of treatment is reduction of gradient using pharmacologic, surgical, or other means. Patients with outflow gradients or mitral regurgitation are also at increased risk of infective endocarditis, and standard antibiotic prophylaxis is recommended. Therapeutic options in patients without left ventricular outflow gradients are more limited, but pharmacologic therapy may improve chest pain and, to a lesser extent, dyspnea.

Obstructive Hypertrophic Cardiomyopathy

Patients who have moderate to severe left ventricular outflow tract obstruction may experience exertional chest pain, dyspnea, or syncope. Although some studies have suggested that up to 70% of patients improve with beta-blocker therapy, high doses are frequently required and side effects may be limiting (28,162). Furthermore, little convincing evidence exists that beta-blockers reduce the incidence of serious ventricular arrhythmias or sudden death (255). When beta-blockade alone is ineffective, the addition of disopyramide can be effective in reducing gradients and improving symptoms (256–258). Disopyramide should be titrated to patient's symptoms and the emergence of side effects, aiming for a maintenance dose of 400 to 600 mg daily. Data comparing beta-blockade and disopyramide are limited, but disopyramide may have a superior effect on exercise tolerance (258). In some patients, particularly elderly patients, anticholinergic side effects may preclude or limit the use of disopyramide. Recent data suggest that an alternative class I antiarrhythmic drug, cibenzoline, which has fewer anticholinergic side effects, may be equally effective (259). Verapamil is also used to treat symptoms in patients with outflow gradients, but its effect is unpredictable, and acute hemodynamic collapse is described in patients with substantial gradients or severe diastolic dysfunction.

Surgery should be considered in all patients with significant (i.e., greater than 50 mm Hg) outflow obstruction and symptoms refractory to medical therapy (260–267). The principal aim of surgical intervention is to eliminate SAM of the mitral valve and mitral leaflet–septal contact by widening the left ventricular outflow tract. The most commonly performed procedure is a ventricular septal myotomy-myectomy (Morrow procedure) performed using a transaortic approach. This procedure results in a significant reduction in outflow gradient in 95% of cases, reduced mitral regurgitation, and long-term symptomatic improvement in up to 70% of patients (260–267). Operative mortality rate figures in series reported elsewhere are of the order of 5% but are now probably less than 1% to 2% in centers with experienced surgeons. Complications such as atrioventricular block and ventricular septal defects do occur but have become less frequent with modification of surgical technique and the use of preoperative transesophageal echocardiography (268). Aortic regurgitation may occur in patients postoperatively but is not usually of hemodynamic significance (269).

Other techniques that have been advocated include myotomy alone (270) and mitral valve replacement (271). The latter option is controversial because of the subsequent risks of anticoagulation and prosthetic valve dysfunction, but mitral valve replacement may have a limited role in patients with other intrinsic mitral valve abnormalities. Mitral valve plication in conjunction with myotomy-myectomy has been advocated as an alternative to mitral valve replacement in patients who have elongation of the anterior mitral leaflet (272). More recently, elongation of the horizontal diameter of the mitral valve using a glutaraldehyde-preserved autologous pericardial patch has been advocated (273).

Although myotomy-myectomy remains the gold-standard interventional therapy for outflow tract obstruction, the procedure requires a level of expertise and support that are not universally available. Furthermore, additional comorbidities and patient reluctance may preclude this mode of therapy. Two novel approaches to gradient reduction have been recently evaluated. Several studies have suggested that dual-chamber pacing using a short programmed atrioventricular delay to ensure constant activation of the right ventricle from its apex improves symptoms in patients with left ventricular outflow tract gradients (eFig. 29.8.3) (274–283). Success depends on achieving an atrioventricular delay that gives maximum preexcitation while maintaining effective atrial transport. Although preliminary data indicated that pacing is capable of reducing gradients by approximately 50%, several multicenter trials have shown that pacemaker insertion is associated with a substantial placebo effect and little objective improvement in exercise capacity. Few comparative data are available for dual-chamber pacing and myectomy, but one small nonrandomized study has suggested that gradient reduction and exercise duration are greater after surgery (284). Nevertheless, a minority (10% to 20%) of patients do respond to pacing, and therefore pacemaker insertion remains an option in patients who have an unacceptable operative risk with myotomy-myectomy. Pacemaker insertion may also facilitate the use of higher doses of beta-blockers in some patients (280).

The second novel intervention involves selective injection of alcohol into one or more septal perforator branches of the left anterior descending coronary artery to create of localized septal scar (285–293). Published data suggest that the procedure-related mortality rate is lower than 1% in centers with experienced clinicians, but deaths due to conduction system damage and inadvertent injection of alcohol into other myocardial segments have occurred. The latter problem is minimized by the injection of intracoronary echo contrast agents before injection of alcohol to ensure that only the septal bulge at the point of mitral leaflet–septal contact is opacified. Alcohol injection is contraindicated if opacification is present in other regions of the myocardium, such as the distal septum, the right ventricle, or the papillary muscles. In contrast to the results of surgery, most patients develop right and not left bundle branch block after alcohol ablation. Higher degrees of AV block can occur transiently but persist in only 10% to 15% of patients. Prolonged or recurrent AV block after the procedure should prompt consideration of permanent dual-chamber pacing. Interim results suggest that left ventricular cavity dimensions increase slightly after alcohol ablation, but progressive ventricular dilatation and late arrhythmic complications have not yet been described. Results from the largest series show that gradients can be abolished or substantially reduced in 80% of patients. This reduction is paralleled by an improvement in symptom class and exercise tolerance.

Nonobstructive Hypertrophic Cardiomyopathy

Beta-blockade may improve chest pain and dyspnea, but patient response is usually suboptimal. Verapamil, often in high doses (240 to 480 mg per day), is a useful alternative, particularly in patients who experience exertional chest pain (294–297). The mechanism of action is uncertain, but verapamil can improve left ventricular relaxation and exercise tolerance. Data on its effect on myocardial perfusion are conflicting (297,298). Diltiazem (299) also has beneficial effects on symptoms and left ventricular function and provides a useful alternative to verapamil when side effects are problematic. Nifedipine (300) has been advocated, but the potential hazards of vasodilatation, particularly in patients with outflow gradients, preclude its general use. Although diuretics, sometimes in combination with beta-blockers or calcium antagonists, may alleviate symptoms caused by pulmonary congestion, their injudicious use can be dangerous, particularly in patients with severe diastolic impairment.

Supraventricular Arrhythmia

For the management of supraventricular arrhythmia, AF should be cardioverted; when this is not possible, control of the ventricular rate improves symptoms in most patients (177). AF in HCM is associated with a significant risk of thromboembolism, and anticoagulation therapy should be considered in all patients in whom AF is sustained or recurs frequently. Treatment is not usually indicated for other asymptomatic and self-limiting supraventricular arrhythmias, but if they are sustained or associated with symptoms, then specific medical therapy should be instituted. Treatment with low-dose amiodarone (1,000 to 1,400 mg weekly) is effective in maintaining sinus rhythm and in controlling the ventricular rate during breakthrough episodes. Beta-blockers with or without class III action may be useful, but class I agents are untested and potentially proarrhythmic.

Identification of High-Risk Patients

Patients who have HCM are prone to a number of potentially life-threatening complications, including sudden ventricular arrhythmia, thromboembolism, heart block, and congestive cardiac failure. Although the identification of patients who are at risk remains a clinical challenge, recent data show that high-risk patients can be identified and successfully treated.

Sudden death remains the greatest cause of premature death in patients with HCM (151–160). The underlying substrate for sudden death is complex and incompletely understood, but myocyte disarray and fibrosis—the microscopic hallmarks of the disease—provide the conditions for anisotropic conduction and reentry arrhythmia. Circumstantial evidence suggests that expression of this substrate is modified by factors such as myocardial ischemia, autonomic function, and abnormal vascular responses (119–127,301–307). Fortuitous ECG recordings made before sustained ventricular tachyarrhythmias in patients with HCM have shown that rapid AF may also act as a trigger to fatal arrhythmic events (178). In spite of this potent pathophysiologic substrate for sudden

death, survival data in both regional and tertiary center populations indicate that only a minority of patients are at sufficiently high risk to warrant consideration for prophylactic therapy (151–160). Therefore, identifying readily applicable clinical risk markers that allow patients to be stratified into high- and low-risk cohorts is the clinical goal.

Clinical Markers of Risk of Sudden Death

Patients with HCM and a history of sustained ventricular arrhythmia have a risk of a fatal event of approximately 10% per annum (157,308,309). Although this is much lower than the risk seen with some other cardiac diseases (310), patients with HCM who survive a cardiac arrest are often young and are, therefore, at risk for a longer period than most patients with coronary artery disease or congestive cardiac failure. Many sudden deaths occur in patients who have minor symptoms. Children and adolescents who have two or more first-degree relatives with HCM who died prematurely are at risk of dying suddenly themselves (127–129). Recurrent unexplained syncope in the young is also a highly specific marker of risk (28,151–153,311). Pooled data from two studies (174,175) indicate that in patients with HCM, NSVT is associated with an increased risk of sudden death, with a sensitivity of 69% and a specificity of 80%. However, its value as a risk marker is limited by a modest positive predictive accuracy of 22%, reflecting the fact that most patients with NSVT do not die suddenly and that the incidence of NSVT in children is low. More recently, some workers have suggested that NSVT is significant only when it is repetitive or when it occurs in symptomatic patients (312), but few data support this. The onset of AF has, in the past, been considered to be an adverse prognostic event. However, at least one prospective study has shown that the 5-year survival rate in patients with AF is similar to that in age- and sex-matched patients who remain in sinus rhythm (177).

Approximately 25% of patients with HCM have abnormal blood pressure responses during exercise (305). This phenomenon is associated with a family history of sudden death, small left ventricular cavity dimensions, and, in patients younger than 40 years, a higher mortality rate (306,313,314). The underlying mechanism for the abnormal response remains speculative, but some evidence suggests that inappropriate vasodilatation in nonexercising muscles is responsible (307). The presence of a pressure-dependent vasodepressor response in patients with HCM may explain the poor tolerance of paroxysmal arrhythmia or sinus tachycardia seen in some patients. In patients who have a particular susceptibility, systemic hypotension may also cause a fall in myocardial perfusion pressure, with consequent metabolic changes that trigger ventricular arrhythmia.

Data from cross-sectional studies and more recent large prospectively followed cohorts in regional and tertiary centers have shown that patients with severe hypertrophy (i.e., a wall thickness ≥30 mm) have an increased risk of sudden death (154,315–317). However, this marker is of limited value, because the majority of patients who die suddenly has wall thickness values less than 30 mm. To date, there is no conclusive evidence that left ventricular outflow obstruction is associated with sudden death, but a recent series has suggested that substantial gradients may be associated with the overall cardiovascular mortality rate (155).

Treatment of High-Risk Patients

There have been several obstacles to the construction of workable risk-stratification algorithms in patients who have HCM, most notably the low positive predictive accuracy of the majority of suggested risk markers for sudden death and the lack of data on the relative value of different risk markers. The latter problem has been difficult to study because of the relatively low incidence of HCM and the low annual event rates even within tertiary center populations. Some data suggest that a risk model based on a smaller number of easily assessed risk markers (specifically, NSVT, left ventricular wall thickness, abnormal blood pressure responses during exercise, family history of sudden death, and recurrent unexplained syncope) may allow identification of most high-risk patients with sufficient accuracy to permit rational decisions to be made about the necessity for prophylactic therapy (154) (Fig. 29.9). In this study, patients with two and three risk factors had an annual risk of sudden death of approximately 3% and 6%, respectively. Estimation of risk in patients with a single risk factor remains problematic, because the significance of a given risk factor may vary between individual patients, particularly in the context of a family history and syncope. Risk factors also have to be interpreted in the light of other features, such as patient age. Decision making in such patients inevitably has to be pragmatic and guided by physician experience and patient preference.

All patients who have spontaneous or exertional ventricular tachyarrhythmias should be considered for prophylactic ICD insertion (308–310,329,330). In patients who do not have a history of sustained ventricular tachycardia or cardiac arrest, the identification of two or more risk factors should also prompt consideration for prophylactic therapy. Low-dose amiodarone therapy has been shown to reduce sudden deaths in patients with NSVT (331) and in high-risk children (152), but evidence from multicenter ICD trials and reports of occasional deaths in patients with a history of ventricular tachycardia or ventricular fibrillation who were taking amiodarone has called into question its use as prophylactic therapy in patients considered to be at risk for sudden death. Because demographic and ethical considerations make a randomized study of ICD therapy in HCM extremely unlikely, patients should be offered the "best" therapy, which in most circumstances will be an ICD. Amiodarone continues to play a role in preventing potential triggers for sudden death or life-threatening arrhythmias, in particular paroxysmal AF and hemodynamically tolerated sustained monomorphic ventricular tachycardia. Other potential trigger factors, such as conduction system

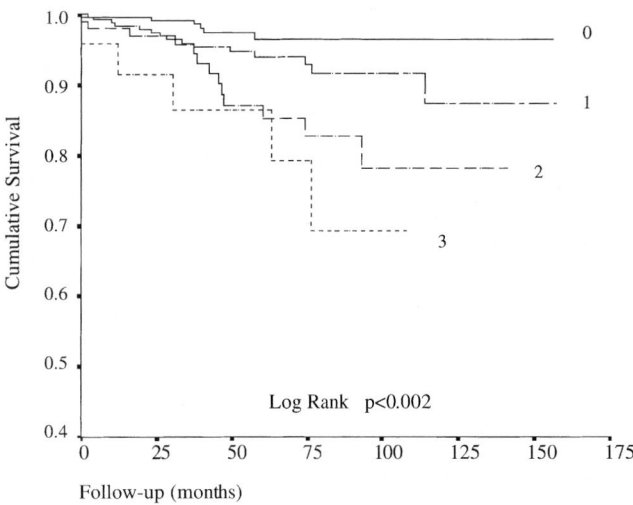

FIGURE 29.9 Kaplan-Meier survival curves in patients with zero, one, two, and three clinical risk factors. The risk factors used in this analysis were nonsustained ventricular tachycardia, family history of sudden death, recurrent unexplained syncope, and abnormal blood pressure during exercise (in patients younger than 40 years). (The original data set and the relationship between these risk factors and wall thickness are reported in Elliott PM, Gimeno Blanes JR, Mahon NG, et al. Relation between the severity of left ventricular hypertrophy and prognosis in patients with hypertrophic cardiomyopathy. *Lancet* 2001;357:420–424.)

disease, accessory pathways, and myocardial ischemia, should also be treated when possible.

Exercise and Hypertrophic Cardiomyopathy

Although 40% of HCM-associated sudden deaths occur after moderate to severe exertion (244,332), the increase in the relative risk of sudden death incurred by regular participation in vigorous exercise is unknown. No systematic data are available to prove that abstention from vigorous physical activity prevents death, but most clinicians agree that young patients with HCM should not participate in competitive sports. The 29th Bethesda Conference (333) has produced guidelines on the eligibility of patients with HCM for participation in sports. It is suggested that athletes with unequivocal HCM should be advised not to take part in most competitive events, regardless of symptoms or the presence of left ventricular outflow obstruction. Because of the risk of sudden death is higher in younger patients, participation of individuals older than 30 years should be assessed on the basis of recognized or potential clinical risk factors, bearing in mind that these guidelines are conservative and based on a consensus view of best practice rather than definitive proof.

CONTROVERSIES AND PERSONAL PERSPECTIVES

Over the past decade, considerable progress was made in unraveling the complex pathophysiology of HCM. We

THE FUTURE

Over the past decade, we learned that familial HCM is a genetically heterogeneous disease of the cardiac sarcomere, with variable penetrance and disease expression. One of the major challenges for the next decade is to unravel the complex mechanisms that determine disease expression and thereby develop new therapies that could modify the natural history of the condition. Other therapeutic challenges include the management of the disease in symptomatic patients who do not have left ventricular outflow tract obstruction and the refinement of risk-stratification algorithms, particularly in young patients and in patients who have a single risk factor.

know now that most cases are caused by mutations in genes that encode sarcomeric proteins, and that the spectrum of disease is even more diverse than was previously thought. Nevertheless, many questions relating to pathophysiology remain unanswered, in particular, questions involving the mechanisms that determine disease expression and penetrance. Clinical management of HCM has also progressed, specifically in relation to the treatment options for outflow tract obstruction and the identification and treatment of patients at high risk of sudden death. These advances clearly are good news for patients, but for clinicians they make the management of patients with HCM more, rather than less, challenging. Physicians must now offer specialist genetic counseling, detailed assessment of symptoms and pathophysiology, and a wide range of surgical and invasive cardiologic expertise. This means that the care of patients requires involvement of many specialists and will probably result in centralization of resources in centers with a special interest in "HCMology." The final result should be a major improvement in the outlook for patients with this capricious disease.

REFERENCES

1. Richardson P, McKenna W, Bristow M, et al. Report of the 1995 World Health Organization/International Society and Federation of Cardiology Task Force on the definition and classification of cardiomyopathies. *Circulation* 1996;93:841–842.
2. Liouville H. Retrecissement cardiaque sous aortique. *Gaz Med Paris* 1869;24:161.
3. Hallopeau L. Retrecissement ventriculo-aortique. *Gaz Med Paris* 1869;24:683.
4. Schmincke A. Ueber linkseitige musculöse conusstenosen. *Dtsch Med Wochenschr* 1907;33:2082.
5. Doane JC, Skversky NJ. Massive cardiac hypertrophy. *Am Heart J* 1944;28:816.
6. Whittle CH. "Idiopathic" hypertrophy of the heart in a young man. *Lancet* 1929;216:1354–1355.
7. Vulliamy DG. Idiopathic cardiac hypertrophy. *Br Heart J* 1947;9:161.
8. Mahon GS. Idiopathic hypertrophy of the heart with endocardial fibrosis. *Am Heart J* 1936;12:608–617.
9. Norris RF, Pote HH. Hypertrophy of the heart of unknown etiology in young adults: report of four cases with autopsies. *Am Heart J* 1946;32:599.
10. Evans W. Familial cardiomegaly. *Br Heart J* 1949;11:68–82.
11. Davies LG. A familial heart disease. *Br Heart J* 1952;14:206.
12. Brock R. Functional obstruction of the left ventricle. *Guys Hosp Rep* 1957;106:221.
13. Teare D. Asymmetrical hypertrophy of the heart in young adults. *Br Heart J* 1958;20:1–8.
14. Frank S, Braunwald E. Idiopathic hypertrophic subaortic stenosis: clinical analysis of 126 patients with emphasis on the natural history. *Circulation* 1968;37:759–788.
15. Goodwin JF, Hollman A, Cleland WP, et al. Obstructive cardiomyopathy simulating aortic stenosis. *Br Heart J* 1960;22:403–414.
16. Bercu BA, Diettert GA, Danforth WH, et al. Pseudoaortic stenosis produced by ventricular hypertrophy. *Am J Med* 1958;25:814.
17. Braunwald E, Brockenbrough EC, Frye RL. Studies on digitalis: a comparison of the effects of Ouabain on left ventricular dynamics in valvular aortic stenosis and hypertrophic subaortic stenosis. *Circulation* 1962;26:166.
18. Braunwald E, Morrow AG, Cornell WP, et al. Idiopathic hypertrophic subaortic stenosis: clinical, hemodynamic and angiographic manifestations. *Am J Med* 1960;29:924–945.
19. Brent LB, Aburano A, Fisher DL, et al. Familial muscular subaortic stenosis. *Circulation* 1960;21:167–180.
20. Wigle ED, Heimbecker RO, Gunton RW. Idiopathic ventricular septal hypertrophy causing muscular subaortic stenosis. *Circulation* 1962;26:325–340.
21. Neufield HN, Ongley PA, Edwards JE. Combined congenital subaortic and infundibular pulmonary stenosis. *Br Heart J* 1960;22:686–690.
22. Bevegard S, Jonsson B, Karloff I. Low subvalvular aortic and pulmonic stenosis caused by asymmetrical hypertrophic and derangement of muscle bundles of the ventricular wall. *Acta Med Scand* 1962;172:269–283.
23. Henry WL, Clarke CE, Epstein SE. Asymmetrical septal hypertrophy (ASH): echocardiographic identification of the pathognomonic anatomic abnormality of IHSS. *Circulation* 1973;43:225–233.
24. Henry WL, Clarke CE, Epstein SE. Asymmetrical septal hypertrophy the unifying link in the IHSS disease spectrum: observations regarding its pathogenesis, pathophysiology and course. *Circulation* 1972;46:897.
25. Shah PM, Gramiak R, Kramer DH. Ultrasound localization

of left ventricular outflow obstruction in hypertrophic obstructive cardiomyopathy. *Circulation* 1969;40:3–11.

26. Popp RL, Harrison DC. Ultrasound in the diagnosis and evaluation of therapy of idiopathic hypertrophic subaortic stenosis. *Circulation* 1969;40:905–914.

27. Abbassi AS, MacAlpin RN, Eber LM, et al. Echocardiographic diagnosis of idiopathic hypertrophic cardiomyopathy with outflow obstruction. *Circulation* 1972;46:897–904.

28. Maron BJ, Bonow RO, Cannon RO III, et al. Hypertrophic cardiomyopathy: interrelations of clinical manifestations, pathophysiology, and therapy. *N Engl J Med* 1987;316:780–789, 844–852.

29. Maron BJ, Gottdiener JS, Epstein SE. Patterns and significance of the distribution of left ventricular hypertrophy in hypertrophic cardiomyopathy: a wide angle, two-dimensional echocardiographic study of 125 patients. *Am J Cardiol* 1981;48:418–428.

30. Wigle ED, Sasson Z, Henderson MA, et al. Hypertrophic cardiomyopathy—the importance of the site and extent of hypertrophy: a review. *Prog Cardiovasc Dis* 1985;28:1–83.

31. Emanuel R, Withers R, O'Brien K. Dominant and recessive modes of inheritance in idiopathic cardiomyopathy. *Lancet* 1971;2:1065–1067.

32. Clark CE, Henry WL, Epstein SE. Familial prevalence and genetic transmission of idiopathic hypertrophic subaortic stenosis. *N Engl J Med* 1973;289:709–714.

33. Van Dorp WG, Ten Cate FJ, Vletter WB, et al. Familial prevalence of asymmetric septal hypertrophy. *Eur J Cardiol* 1976;4:349–357.

34. Greaves SC, Roche AHG, Neutze JM, et al. Inheritance of hypertrophic cardiomyopathy: a cross sectional and M-mode echocardiographic study of 50 families. *Br Heart J* 1987;58:259–266.

35. Maron BJ, Nichols PF, Pickle LW, et al. Patterns of inheritance in hypertrophic cardiomyopathy: assessment by M-mode and two-dimensional echocardiography. *Am J Cardiol* 1984;53:1087–1094.

36. Jarcho JA, McKenna WJ, Pare JA, et al. Mapping a gene for familial hypertrophic cardiomyopathy to chromosome 14q1. *N Engl J Med* 1989;321:1372–1378.

37. Tanigawa G, Jarcho JA, Kass S, et al. A molecular basis for familial hypertrophic cardiomyopathy: an α/β cardiac myosin heavy chain hybrid gene. *Cell* 1990;62:991–998.

38. Geisterfer-Lowrance AAT, Kass S, Tanigawa G, et al. A molecular basis for familial hypertrophic cardiomyopathy: a β-cardiac myosin heavy chain gene missense mutation. *Cell* 1990;62:999–1006.

39. Arai S, Matsuoka R, Hirayama K, et al. Missense mutation of the beta-cardiac myosin heavy chain gene in hypertrophic cardiomyopathy. *Am J Med Genetics* 1995;58:267–276.

40. Posen BM, Moolman JC, Corfield VA, et al. Clinical and prognostic evaluation of familial hypertrophic cardiomyopathy in two South African families with different cardiac beta-myosin heavy chain gene mutations. *Br Heart J* 1995;74:40–46.

41. Marian AJ, Roberts R. Molecular genetics of hypertrophic cardiomyopathy [review]. *Annu Rev Med* 1995;46:213–222.

42. Vosberg HP. Myosin mutations in hypertrophic cardiomyopathy and functional implications [review]. *Herz* 1994;19:75–83.

43. Epstein ND, Cohn GM, Cyran F, Fananapazir L. Differ-ences in clinical expression of hypertrophic cardiomyopathy associated with two distinct mutations in the β-myosin heavy chain gene. A $908_{Leu \to Val}$ mutation and a $403_{Arg \to Gln}$ mutation. *Circulation* 1992;86:345–352.

44. Hejtmancik JF, Brink PA, Towbin J, et al. Localisation of gene for familial hypertrophic cardiomyopathy to chromosome 14q1 in a diverse US population. *Circulation* 1991;83:1592–1597.

45. Nishi H, Kimura A, Harada H, et al. A myosin missense mutation, not a null allele, causes familial hypertrophic cardiomyopathy. *Circulation* 1995;91:2911–2915.

46. Marian AJ, Mares A Jr, Kelly DP, et al. Sudden cardiac death in hypertrophic cardiomyopathy: variability in phenotypic expression of beta-myosin heavy chain mutations. *Eur Heart J* 1995;16:368–376.

47. Rayment I, Holden HM, Sellers JR, et al. Structural interpretation of the mutations in the beta-cardiac myosin that have been implicated in familial hypertrophic cardiomyopathy. *Proc Natl Acad Sci U S A* 1995;92:3864–3868.

48. Dufour C, Dausse E, Fetler L, et al. Identification of a mutation near a functional site of the beta cardiac myosin heavy chain gene in a family with hypertrophic cardiomyopathy. *J Mol Cell Cardiol* 1994;26:1241–1247.

49. Hengstenberg C, Carrier L, Schwartz K, et al. Clinical and genetic heterogeneity of familial hypertrophic cardiomyopathy [review]. *Herz* 1994;19:84–90.

50. Hengstenberg C, Charron P, Isnard R, et al. Demonstration of a fifth locus in familial hypertrophic cardiomyopathies [in French]. *Arch Mal Coeur Vaiss* 1994;87:1655–1662.

51. Watkins H, Thierfelder L, Anan R, et al. Independent origin of identical beta cardiac myosin heavy chain mutations in hypertrophic cardiomyopathy. *Am J Hum Genet* 1993;53:1180–1185.

52. Thierfelder L, MacRae C, Watkins H, et al. A familial hypertrophic cardiomyopathy locus maps to chromosome 15q2. *Proc Natl Acad Sci U S A* 1993;90:6270–6274.

53. Yamauchi-Takihara K, Nakajima-Taniguchi C, Matsui H, et al. Clinical implications of hypertrophic cardiomyopathy associated with mutations in the alpha-tropomyosin gene. *Heart* 1996;76:63–65.

54. Nakajima-Taniguchi C, Matsui H, Nagata S, et al. Novel missense mutation in alpha-tropomyosin gene found in Japanese patients with hypertrophic cardiomyopathy. *J Mol Cell Cardiol* 1995;27:2053–2058.

55. Watkins H, Anan R, Coviello DA, et al. A de novo mutation in alpha-tropomyosin that causes hypertrophic cardiomyopathy. *Circulation* 1995;91:2302–2305.

56. Watkins H, McKenna WJ, Thierfelder L, et al. Mutations in the genes for cardiac troponin T and alpha-tropomyosin in hypertrophic cardiomyopathy. *N Engl J Med* 1995;332:1058–1064.

57. Thierfelder L, Watkins H, MacRae C, et al. Alpha-tropomyosin and cardiac troponin T mutations cause familial hypertrophic cardiomyopathy: a disease of the sarcomere. *Cell* 1994;77:701–712.

58. Coviello DA, Maron BJ, Spirito P, et al. Clinical features of hypertrophic cardiomyopathy caused by mutation of a "hot spot" in the alpha-tropomyosin gene. *J Am Coll Cardiol* 1997;29:635–640.

59. Watkins H, MacRae C, Thierfelder L, et al. A disease locus

for familial hypertrophic cardiomyopathy maps to chromosome 1q3. *Nat Genet* 1993;3:333–337.

60. Watkins H, Conner D, Thierfelder L, et al. Mutations in the cardiac myosin binding protein-C gene on chromosome 11 cause familial hypertrophic cardiomyopathy. *Nat Genet* 1995;11:434–437.

61. Bonne G, Carrier L, Bercovici J, et al. Cardiac myosin binding protein C gene splice acceptor site mutation is associated with familial hypertrophic cardiomyopathy. *Nat Genet* 1995;11:438–440.

62. Carrier L, Hengstenberg C, Beckmann JS, et al. Mapping of a novel gene for familial hypertrophic cardiomyopathy to chromosome 11. *Nat Genet* 1993;4:311–313.

63. Niimura H, Bachinski LL, Sangwatanaroj S, et al. Mutations in the gene for cardiac myosin-binding protein C and late-onset familial hypertrophic cardiomyopathy. *N Engl J Med* 1998;338:1248–1257.

64. Kimura A, Harada H, Park JE, et al. Mutations in the cardiac troponin I gene associated with hypertrophic cardiomyopathy. *Nat Genet* 1997;16:379–382.

65. Sanbe A, Nelson D, Gulick J, et al. In vivo analysis of an essential myosin light chain mutation linked to familial hypertrophic cardiomyopathy. *Circ Res* 2000;87:296–302.

66. Mogensen J, Klausen IC, Pedersen AK, et al. Alpha-cardiac actin is a novel disease gene in familial hypertrophic cardiomyopathy. *J Clin Invest* 1999;103:R39–R43.

67. Olson TM, Doan TP, Kishimoto NY, et al. Inherited and de novo mutations in the cardiac actin gene cause hypertrophic cardiomyopathy. *J Mol Cell Cardiol* 2000;32:1687–1694.

68. Satoh M, Takahashi M, Sakamoto T, et al. Structural analysis of the *titin* gene in hypertrophic cardiomyopathy: identification of a novel disease gene. *Biochem Biophys Res Commun* 1999;262:411–417.

69. McKenna WJ, Spirito P, Desnos M, et al. Experience from clinical genetics in hypertrophic cardiomyopathy: proposal for new diagnostic criteria in adult members of affected families. *Heart* 1997;77:130–132.

70. Davies MJ, McKenna WJ. Hypertrophic cardiomyopathy: pathology and pathogenesis. *Histopathology* 1995;26:493–500.

71. Maron BJ, Roberts WC. Quantitative analysis of cardiac muscle cell disorganisation in the ventricular septum of patients with hypertrophic cardiomyopathy. *Circulation* 1979;59:689–706.

72. Yamaguchi H, Ishimura T, Nishiyama S, et al. Hypertrophic nonobstructive cardiomyopathy with giant negative T-waves (apical hypertrophy): ventriculographic and echocardiographic features in 30 patients. *Am J Cardiol* 1979;44:401–412.

73. Van Noorden S, Olsen EG, Pearse AG. Hypertrophic obstructive cardiomyopathy: a histological, histochemical and ultrastructural study of biopsy material. *Cardiovasc Res* 1971;5:118–131.

74. Davies MJ. The current status of myocardial disarray in hypertrophic cardiomyopathy [editorial]. *Br Heart J* 1984;51:361.

75. Bulkley BH, Weisfeldt ML, Hutchins GM. Asymmetric septal hypertrophy and myocardial fibre disarray: features of normal developing, and malformed hearts. *Circulation* 1977;56:292–298.

76. Maron BJ, Sato N, Roberts WC, et al. Quantitative analysis of cardiac muscle cell disorganisation in the ventricular septum: comparison of fetuses and infants with and without congenital heart disease and patients with hypertrophic cardiomyopathy. *Circulation* 1979;60:685–696.

77. Maron BJ, Epstein SE, Roberts WC. Hypertrophic cardiomyopathy and transmural infarction without significant atherosclerosis of the extramural coronary arteries. *Am J Cardiol* 1979;43:1086–1102.

78. Factor SM, Butany J, Sole MJ, et al. Pathological fibrosis and matrix connective tissue in the subaortic myocardium of patients with hypertrophic cardiomyopathy. *J Am Coll Cardiol* 1991;17:1343–1351.

79. Maron BJ, Wolfson JK, Epstein SE, Roberts WC. Intramural ("small vessel") coronary artery disease in hypertrophic cardiomyopathy. *J Am Coll Cardiol* 1986;8:545.

80. Tanaka M, Fujiwara H, Onodera T, et al. Quantitative analysis of narrowings of intramyocardial small arteries in normal hearts, hypertensive hearts, and hearts with hypertrophic cardiomyopathy. *Circulation* 1987;75:1130–1139.

81. Varnava AM, Elliott PM, Sharma S, et al. Hypertrophic cardiomyopathy: the interrelation of disarray, fibrosis, and small vessel disease. *Heart* 2000;84:476–482.

82. Child JS, Perloff JK, Bach PM, et al. cardiac involvement in Friedreich's ataxia: a clinical study of 75 patients. *J Am Coll Cardiol* 1986;7:1370.

83. Campuzano V, Montermini L, Molto MD, et al. Friedreich's ataxia: autosomal recessive disease caused by an intronic GAA triplet repeat expansion. *Science* 1996;271:1423–1427.

84. Barker D, Wright E, Nguyen K, et al. Gene for von Recklinghausen neurofibromatosis is in the pericentric region of chromosome 17. *Science* 1987;236:1100.

85. Kimberling WJ, Taylor RA, Chapman RG, et al. Linkage and gene localisation of hereditary spherocytosis (HS). *Blood* 1978;52:859.

86. Gilgenkrantz S, Vigneron C, Gregoire MJ, et al. Association of del(11)(p15.1p12), aniridia, catalase deficiency and cardiomyopathy. *Am J Med Genet* 1982;13:39.

87. Burch M, Sharland M, Shinebourne E, et al. Cardiologic abnormalities in Noonan syndrome: phenotypic diagnosis and echocardiographic assessment of 118 patients. *J Am Coll Cardiol* 1993;22:1189–1192.

88. Burch M, Mann JM, Sharland M, et al. Myocardial disarray in Noonan syndrome. *Br Heart J* 1992;68:586–588.

89. Jamieson CR, van der Burgt I, Brady AF, et al. Mapping a gene for Noonan syndrome to the long arm of chromosome 12. *Nat Genet* 1994;8:357–360.

90. MacRae CA, Ghaisas N, Kass S, et al. Familial hypertrophic cardiomyopathy with Wolff-Parkinson-White syndrome maps to a locus on chromosome 7q3. *J Clin Invest* 1995;96:1216–1220.

91. Mehdirad AA, Fatkin D, DiMarco JP, et al. Electrophysiologic characteristics of accessory atrioventricular connections in an inherited form of Wolff-Parkinson-White syndrome. *J Cardiovasc Electrophysiol* 1999;10:629–635.

92. Watkins H, Rosenzweig A, Hwang DS, et al. Characteristics and prognostic implications of myosin missense mutations in familial hypertrophic cardiomyopathy. *N Engl J Med* 1992;326:1108–1114.

93. Anan R, Greve G, Thierfelder L, et al. Prognostic implications of novel beta cardiac myosin heavy chain gene mutations that cause familial hypertrophic cardiomyopathy. *J Clin Invest* 1994;93:280–285.

94. Marian AJ, Kelly D, Mares A Jr, et al. A missense mutation in the beta myosin heavy chain gene is a predictor of premature sudden death in patients with hypertrophic cardiomyopathy. *J Sports Med Phys Fitness* 1994;34:1–10.

95. Fananapazir L, Epstein ND. Genotype-phenotype correlations in hypertrophic cardiomyopathy: insights provided by comparisons of kindreds with distinct and identical beta-myosin heavy chain gene mutations. *Circulation* 1994;89:22–32.

96. Moolman JC, Corfield VA, Posen B, et al. Sudden death due to troponin T mutations. *J Am Coll Cardiol* 1997;29:549–555.

97. Redwood CS, Moolman-Smook JC, Watkins H. Properties of mutant contractile proteins that cause hypertrophic cardiomyopathy. *Cardiovasc Res* 1999;44:20–36.

98. Marian AJ, Wu Y, Lim DS, et al. A transgenic rabbit model for human hypertrophic cardiomyopathy. *J Clin Invest* 1999;104:1683–1692.

99. Geisterfer-Lowrance AA, Christe M, Conner DA, et al. A mouse model of familial hypertrophic cardiomyopathy. *Science* 1996;272:731–734.

100. Redwood C, Lohmann K, Bing W, et al. Investigation of a truncated cardiac troponin T that causes familial hypertrophic cardiomyopathy: Ca(2+) regulatory properties of reconstituted thin filaments depend on the ratio of mutant to wild–type protein. *Circ Res* 2000;86:1146–1152.

101. Maron BJ, Spirito P, Wesley Y, et al. Development or progression of left ventricular hypertrophy in children with hypertrophic cardiomyopathy: identification by two-dimensional echocardiography. *N Engl J Med* 1986;315:610–614.

102. Charron P, Dubourg O, Desnos M, et al. Clinical features and prognostic implications of familial hypertrophic cardiomyopathy related to the cardiac myosin-binding protein C gene. *Circulation* 1998;97:2230–2236.

103. Elliott PM, D'Cruz L, McKenna WJ. Late-onset hypertrophic cardiomyopathy caused by a mutation in the cardiac troponin T gene. *N Engl J Med* 1999;341:1855–1856.

104. Pfeufer A, Osterziel KJ, Urata H, et al. Angiotensin converting enzyme and heart chymase gene polymorphisms in hypertrophic cardiomyopathy. *Am J Cardiol* 1996;78:362–364.

105. Yoneya K, Okamoto H, Machida M, et al. Angiotensin converting enzyme gene polymorphism in Japanese patients with hypertrophic cardiomyopathy. *Am Heart J* 1995;130:1089–1093.

106. Lechin M, Quinones MA, Omran A, et al. Angiotensin converting enzyme genotypes and left ventricular hypertrophy in patients with hypertrophic cardiomyopathy. *Circulation* 1995;92:1808–1812.

107. Osterop AP, Kofflard MJ, Sandkuijl LA, et al. AT1 receptor A/C1166 polymorphism contributes to cardiac hypertrophy in subjects with hypertrophic cardiomyopathy. *Hypertension* 1998;32:825–830.

108. Ishanov A, Okamoto H, Watanabe M, et al. Angiotensin II type 1 receptor gene polymorphisms in patients with cardiac hypertrophy. *Jpn Heart J* 1998;39:87–96.

109. Brugada R, Kelsey W, Lechin M, et al. Role of candidate modifier genes on the phenotypic expression of hypertrophy in patients with hypertrophic cardiomyopathy. *J Investig Med* 1997;45:542–551.

110. Tesson F, Dufour C, Moolman JC, et al. The influence of the angiotensin I converting enzyme genotype in familial hypertrophic cardiomyopathy varies with the disease gene mutation. *J Mol Cell Cardiol* 1997;29:831–838.

111. Richard P, Charron P, Leclercq C, et al. Homozygotes for a R869G mutation in the beta-myosin heavy chain gene have a severe form of familial hypertrophic cardiomyopathy. *J Mol Cell Cardiol* 2000;32:1575–1583.

112. Richard P, Isnard R, Carrier L, et al. Double heterozygosity for mutations in the beta-myosin heavy chain and in the cardiac myosin binding protein C genes in a family with hypertrophic cardiomyopathy. *J Med Genet* 1999;36:542–545.

113. Ho CY, Lever HM, DeSanctis R, et al. Homozygous mutation in cardiac troponin T: implications for hypertrophic cardiomyopathy. *Circulation* 2000;102:1950–1955.

114. Pearse AGE. The histochemistry and electron microscopy of obstructive cardiomyopathy. In: Wolstenholme GEW, O'Connor M, eds. *Ciba Foundation symposium on cardiomyopathies*. London: J & A Churchill, 1964:132–164.

115. Kawai C, Yui Y, Hoshino T, et al. Myocardial catecholamines in hypertrophic and dilated (congestive) cardiomyopathy: a biopsy study. *J Am Coll Cardiol* 1983;2:834–840.

116. Brush JE, Eisenhofer G, Garty M, et al. Cardiac norepinephrine kinetics in hypertrophic cardiomyopathy. *Circulation* 1989;79:836–844.

117. Lefroy DC, de Silva R, Choudhury L, et al. Diffuse reduction of myocardial beta-adrenoceptors in hypertrophic cardiomyopathy: a study with positron emission tomography. *J Am Coll Cardiol* 1993;22:1653–1660.

118. Li S-T, Tack CJ, Fananapazir L, et al. Myocardial perfusion and sympathetic innervation in patients with hypertrophic cardiomyopathy. *J Am Coll Cardiol* 2000;35:1867–1873.

119. Cannon RO, Dilsizian V, O'Gara P, et al. Myocardial metabolic, hemodynamic, and electrocardiographic significance of reversible thallium-201 abnormalities in hypertrophic cardiomyopathy. *Circulation* 1991;83:1660–1667.

120. Pasternac A, Noble J, Streulens Y, et al. Pathophysiology of chest pain in patients with cardiomyopathies and normal coronary arteriograms. *Circulation* 1982;65:778.

121. Hanrath P, Montz R, Mathey D, et al. Correlation between myocardial thallium-201 kinetics, myocardial lactate metabolism and coronary angiographic findings in hypertrophic cardiomyopathy. *Z Kardiol* 1980;69:353–359.

122. Camici P, Chiriatti G, Lorenzoni R, et al. Coronary vasodilatation is impaired in both hypertrophied and non hypertrophied myocardium of patients with hypertrophic cardiomyopathy: a study with nitrogen-13 ammonia and positron emission tomography. *J Am Coll Cardiol* 1991;17:879–886.

123. Elliott PM, Rosano GMC, Gill JS, et al. Changes in coronary sinus pH during dipyridamole stress in patients with hypertrophic cardiomyopathy. *Heart* 1996;75:179–183.

124. Cannon RO, Rosing DR, Maron BJ, et al. Myocardial ischemia in patients with hypertrophic cardiomyopathy: contribution of inadequate vasodilator reserve and elevated left ventricular filling pressures. *Circulation* 1985;71:234–243.

125. Thompson DS, Naqvi N, Juul SM, et al. Effects of propranolol on myocardial oxygen consumption, substrate extraction, and haemodynamics in hypertrophic obstructive cardiomyopathy. *Br Heart J* 1980;44:488–498.

126. Nicod P, Polikar R, Peterson KL. Hypertrophic cardiomyopathy and sudden death. *N Engl J Med* 1988;318:1255–1257.

127. Dilsizian V, Bonow RO, Epstein SE, et al. Myocardial ischemia detected by thallium scintigraphy is frequently related to cardiac arrest and syncope in young patients with hypertrophic cardiomyopathy. *J Am Coll Cardiol* 1993;22:796–804.

128. Elliott PM, Kaski JC, Prasad K, et al. Chest pain during daily life in patients with hypertrophic cardiomyopathy: an ambulatory electrocardiographic study. *Eur Heart J* 1996;17:1056–1064.

129. Hanrath P, Mathey DG, Siegert R, et al. Left ventricular and filling patterns in different forms of left ventricular relaxation and filling patterns in different forms of left ventricular hypertrophy: an echocardiographic study. *Am J Cardiol* 1980;45:15–23.

130. Sanderson JE, Gibson DG, Brown DJ, et al. Left ventricular filling in hypertrophic cardiomyopathy. *Br Heart J* 1977;39:661–670.

131. Sanderson JE, Traill TA, St John Sutton MG, et al. Left ventricular relaxation and filling in hypertrophic cardiomyopathy. *Br Heart J* 1978;40:596–601.

132. Maron BJ, Spirito P, Green KJ, et al. Noninvasive assessment of left ventricular diastolic function by pulsed Doppler echocardiography in patients with hypertrophic cardiomyopathy. *J Am Coll Cardiol* 1987;10:733–742.

133. Betocchi S, Bonow RO, Bacharach SL, et al. Isovolumic relaxation period in hypertrophic cardiomyopathy: assessment by radionuclide angiography. *J Am Coll Cardiol* 1986;7:74–81.

134. Bonow RO, Frederick TM, Bacharach SL, et al. Atrial systole and left ventricular filling in hypertrophic cardiomyopathy: effect of verapamil. *Am J Cardiol* 1983;51:1386–1391.

135. Newman H, Sugrue DD, Oakley CM, et al. Relation of left ventricular function and prognosis in hypertrophic cardiomyopathy: an angiographic study. *J Am Coll Cardiol* 1985;5:1064–1074.

136. Chikamori T, Dickie S, Poloniecki JD, et al. Prognostic significance of radionuclide-assessed diastolic dysfunction in hypertrophic cardiomyopathy. *Am J Cardiol* 1990;65:478–482.

137. Waller BF, Maron BJ, Morrow AG, et al. Hypertrophic cardiomyopathy mimicking pericardial constriction or myocardial restriction. *Am Heart J* 1981;102:790–792.

138. McKenna WJ, Stewart JT, Nihoyannopoulos P, et al. Hypertrophic cardiomyopathy without hypertrophy: two families with myocardial disarray in the absence of increased myocardial mass. *Br Heart J* 1990;63:287–290.

139. Bonow RO, Dilsizian V, Rosing DR, et al. Verapamil induced improvement in left ventricular filling and increased exercise tolerance in patients with hypertrophic cardiomyopathy: short and long-term effects. *Circulation* 1985;72:853–864.

140. Pak PH, Maughan L, Baughman KL, et al. Marked discordance between dynamic and passive diastolic pressure: volume relations in idiopathic hypertrophic cardiomyopathy. *Circulation* 1996;94:52–60.

141. Hada Y, Sakamoto T, Amano K, et al. Prevalence of hypertrophic cardiomyopathy in a population of adult Japanese workers as detected by echocardiographic screening. *Am J Cardiol* 1987;59:183–184.

142. Savage DD, Castelli WP, Abbott RD, et al. Hypertrophic cardiomyopathy and its markers in the general population: the great masquerader revisited: the Framingham Study. *J Cardiovasc Ultrason* 1983;2:41–47.

143. Maron BJ, Gardin JM, Flack JM, et al. Prevalence of hypertrophic cardiomyopathy in a population of young adults: echocardiographic analysis of 4111 subjects in the CARDIA study. Coronary Artery Risk Development in (Young) Adults. *Circulation* 1995;92:785–789.

144. Codd MB, Sugrue DD, Gersh BJ, et al. Epidemiology of idiopathic dilated and hypertrophic cardiomyopathy: a population based study in Olmsted County, Minnesota, 1975–1984. *Circulation* 1989;80:564–572.

145. Maron BJ, Peterson EE, Maron MS, et al. Prevalence of hypertrophic cardiomyopathy in an outpatient population referred for echocardiographic study. *Am J Cardiol* 1994;73:577–580.

146. Topol EJ, Traill TA, Fortuin NJ. Hypertensive hypertrophic cardiomyopathy of the elderly. *N Engl J Med* 1985:312:277–283.

147. Faye WP, Taliercio CP, Ilstrup DM, et al. Natural history of hypertrophic cardiomyopathy in the elderly. *J Am Coll Cardiol* 1990;16:821–826.

148. Lewis JF, Maron BJ. Clinical and morphology expression of hypertrophic cardiomyopathy in patients > or = 65 years of age. *Am J Cardiol* 1994;73:1105–1111.

149. Chikamori T, Doi YL, Yonezawa Y, et al. Comparison of clinical features in patients greater than or equal to 60 years of age to those less than or equal 40 years of age with hypertrophic cardiomyopathy. *Am J Cardiol* 1990;66:875–878.

150. Whiting RB, Powell WJ, Dismore RE, et al. Idiopathic hypertrophic subaortic stenosis in the elderly. *N Engl J Med* 1971;285:196–200.

151. McKenna WJ, Deanfield J, Faruqui A, et al. Prognosis in hypertrophic cardiomyopathy: role of age and clinical, electrocardiographic and haemodynamic features. *Am J Cardiol* 1981;47:532–538.

152. McKenna WJ, Franklin RCG, Nihoyannopoulos P, et al. Arrhythmia and prognosis in infants, children and adolescents with hypertrophic cardiomyopathy. *J Am Coll Cardiol* 1988;11:147–153.

153. McKenna WJ, Deanfield JE. Hypertrophic cardiomyopathy: an important cause of sudden death. *Arch Dis Child* 1984;59:971–975.

154. Elliott PM, Poloniecki J, Dickie S, et al. Sudden death in hypertrophic cardiomyopathy: identification of high risk patients. *J Am Coll Cardiol* 2000;36:2212–2218.

155. Maron BJ, Casey SA, Poliac LC, et al. Clinical course of hypertrophic cardiomyopathy in a regional United States cohort. *JAMA* 1999;281:650–655.

156. Spirito P, Chiarella F, Carratino L, et al. Clinical course and prognosis of hypertrophic cardiomyopathy in an outpatients population. *N Engl J Med* 1989;320:749–755.

157. Cecchi F, Olivotto I, Montereggi A, et al. Hypertrophic cardiomyopathy in Tuscany: clinical course and outcome in an

unselected regional population. *J Am Coll Cardiol* 1995;26:1529–1536.

158. Cannan CR, Reeder GS, Bailey KR, et al. Natural history of hypertrophic cardiomyopathy: a population based study, 1976 through 1990. *Circulation* 1995;92:2488–2495.

159. Maron BJ, Olivotto I, Spirito P, et al. Epidemiology of hypertrophic cardiomyopathy-related death: revisited in a large non-referral-based patient population. *Circulation* 2000;102:858–864.

160. Maron BJ, Tajik AJ, Ruttenberg HD, et al. Hypertrophic cardiomyopathy in infants: clinical features and natural history. *Circulation* 1982;65:7–17.

161. Spirito P, Maron BJ, Bonow RO, et al. Occurrence and significance of progressive left ventricular wall thinning and relative cavity dilatation in hypertrophic cardiomyopathy. *Am J Cardiol* 1987;60:123–129.

162. Spirito P, Seidman CE, McKenna WJ, et al. The management of hypertrophic cardiomyopathy. *N Engl J Med* 1997;336:775–785.

163. Gilligan DM, Chan WL, Ang EL, et al. Effects of a meal on hemodynamic function at rest and during exercise in patients with hypertrophic cardiomyopathy. *J Am Coll Cardiol* 1991;18:429–436.

164. Savage DD, Seides SF, Clark CE, et al. Electrocardiographic findings in patients with obstructive and non-obstructive hypertrophic cardiomyopathy. *Circulation* 1978;58:402–409.

165. Maron BJ, Wolfson JK, Ciro E, et al. Relation of electrocardiographic abnormalities and patterns of left ventricular hypertrophy identified by 2-dimensional echocardiography in patients with hypertrophic cardiomyopathy. *Am J Cardiol* 1983;51:189–194.

166. Lemery R, Kleinebenne A, Nihoyannopoulos P, et al. Q-waves in hypertrophic cardiomyopathy in relation to the distribution and severity of right and left ventricular hypertrophy. *J Am Coll Cardiol* 1990;16:368–374.

167. Cosio FG, Moro C, Alonso M, et al. The Q-waves of hypertrophic cardiomyopathy. *N Engl J Med* 1980;302:96–99.

168. Panza JA, Maron BJ. Relation of electrocardiographic abnormalities to evolving left ventricular hypertrophy in hypertrophic cardiomyopathy during childhood. *Am J Cardiol* 1989;63:1258–1265.

169. Alfonso F, Nihoyannopoulos P, Stewart J, et al. Clinical significance of giant negative T waves in hypertrophic cardiomyopathy. *J Am Coll Cardiol* 1990;15:965–971.

170. Krikler DM, Davies MJ, Rowland E, et al. Sudden death in hypertrophic cardiomyopathy: associated accessory atrioventricular pathways. *Br Heart J* 1980;43:245–251.

171. Fananapazir L, Tracey CM, Leon MB, et al. Electrophysiological abnormalities in patients with hypertrophic cardiomyopathy: a consecutive analysis in 155 patients. *Circulation* 1989;80:1259.

172. Rosenweig A, Watkins H, Hwang D-S, et al. Preclinical diagnosis of familial hypertrophic cardiomyopathy by genetic analysis of blood lymphocytes. *N Engl J Med* 1991;325:1753–1760.

173. Al-Mahdawi S, Chamberlain S, Chojnowska L, et al. The electrocardiogram is a more sensitive indicator than echocardiography of hypertrophic cardiomyopathy in families with a mutation in the MYHA7 gene. *Br Heart J* 1994;72:105–111.

174. McKenna WJ, England D, Doi Y, et al. Arrhythmia in hypertrophic cardiomyopathy. 1: Influence on prognosis. *Br Heart J* 1981;46:168–172.

175. Maron BJ, Savage DD, Wolfson JK, et al. Prognostic significance of 24 hour ambulatory electrocardiographic monitoring in patients with hypertrophic cardiomyopathy: a prospective study. *Am J Cardiol* 1981;48:252–257.

176. Alfonso F, Frenneaux MP, McKenna WJ. Clinical sustained uniform ventricular tachycardia in hypertrophic cardiomyopathy: association with left ventricular apical aneurysm. *Br Heart J* 1989;61:178–181.

177. Robinson K, Frenneaux MP, Stockins B, et al. Atrial fibrillation in hypertrophic cardiomyopathy: a longitudinal study. *J Am Coll Cardiol* 1990;15:1279–1285.

178. Stafford WJ, Trohman RG, Bilsker M, et al. Cardiac arrest in an adolescent with atrial fibrillation and hypertrophic cardiomyopathy. *J Am Coll Cardiol* 1986;7:701–704.

179. Doi YL, McKenna WJ, Gehrke J, et al. M-mode echocardiography in hypertrophic cardiomyopathy: diagnostic criteria and prediction of obstruction. *Am J Cardiol* 1980;45:6–14.

180. Shapiro LM, McKenna WJ. Distribution of left ventricular hypertrophy in hypertrophic cardiomyopathy: a two-dimensional echocardiographic study. *J Am Coll Cardiol* 1983;2:437–444.

181. McKenna WJ, Kleinebenne A, Nihoyannopoulos O, et al. Echocardiographic measurement of right ventricular wall thickness in hypertrophic cardiomyopathy: relation to clinical and prognostic features. *J Am Coll Cardiol* 1988;11:351–358.

182. Doi YL, McKenna WJ, Oakley CM, et al. "Pseudo SAM" in patients with hypertensive heart disease. *Eur Heart J* 1983;4:838–845.

183. Maron BJ, Harding AM, Spirito P, et al. Systolic anterior motion of the posterior mitral valve leaflet: a previous unrecognized cause of dynamic subaortic obstruction in patients with hypertrophic cardiomyopathy. *Circulation* 1983;68:282–293.

184. Spirito P, Maron BJ. Patterns of systolic anterior motion of the mitral valve in hypertrophic cardiomyopathy: assessment by two-dimensional echocardiography. *Am J Cardiol* 1984;54:1039–1046.

185. Spirito P, Maron BJ. Significance of left ventricular outflow tract cross-sectional area in hypertrophic cardiomyopathy: a two-dimensional echocardiographic assessment. *Circulation* 1983;67:1100–1108.

186. Reis RL, Bolton MR, King JF, et al. Anterior-superior displacement of papillary muscles producing obstruction and mitral regurgitation in idiopathic hypertrophic subaortic stenosis. *Circulation* 1974;50[2 Suppl]:181–188.

187. Klues HG, Maron BJ, Dollar AL, et al. Diversity of structural mitral valve alterations in hypertrophic cardiomyopathy. *Circulation* 1992;85:1651–1660.

188. Klues HG, Roberts WC, Maron BJ. Morphological determinants of echocardiographic patterns of mitral valve systolic anterior motion in obstructive hypertrophic cardiomyopathy. *Circulation* 1993;87:1570–1579.

189. Klues HG, Proschan MA, Dollar AL, et al. Echocardiographic assessment of mitral valve size in obstructive hypertrophic cardiomyopathy: anatomic validation from mitral valve specimen. *Circulation* 1993;88:548–555.

190. Yock PG, Hatle L, Popp RL. Patterns and timing of Doppler-

detected intracavitary and aortic flow in hypertrophic cardiomyopathy. *J Am Coll Cardiol* 1986;8:1047–1058.

191. Wigle ED, Henderson M, Rakowski H, et al. Muscular (hypertrophic) subaortic stenosis (hypertrophic obstructive cardiomyopathy): the evidence for true obstruction to left ventricular outflow. *Postgrad Med J* 1986;62:531–536.

192. Levine RA, Vlahakes GJ, Lefebvre X, et al. Papillary muscle displacement causes systolic anterior motion of the mitral valve: experimental validation and insights into the mechanism of subaortic obstruction. *Circulation* 1995;91:1189–1195.

193. Pollick C, Rakowski H, Wigle ED. Muscular subaortic stenosis: the quantitative relationship between systolic anterior motion and the pressure gradient. *Circulation* 1984;69:43–49.

194. Sasson Z, Yock PG, Hatle LK, et al. Doppler echocardiographic determination of the pressure gradient in hypertrophic cardiomyopathy. *J Am Coll Cardiol* 1988;11:752–756.

195. Panza JA, Petrone RK, Fananapazir L, et al. Utility of continuous wave Doppler echocardiography in the noninvasive assessment of left ventricular outflow tract pressure gradient in patients with hypertrophic cardiomyopathy. *J Am Coll Cardiol* 1991;19:91–99.

196. Criley JM, Seigel RJ. Has "obstruction" hindered our understanding of hypertrophic cardiomyopathy? *Circulation* 1985;72:1148.

197. Murgo JP, Alter BR, Dorethy JF, et al. Dynamics of left ventricular ejection in obstructive and nonobstructive hypertrophic cardiomyopathy. *J Clin Invest* 1980;66:1369–1382.

198. Maron BJ, Epstein SE. Clinical significance and therapeutic implications of the left ventricular outflow tract pressure gradient in hypertrophic cardiomyopathy. *Am J Cardiol* 1986;58:1093–1096.

199. Criley JM, Siegel RJ. Obstruction is unimportant in the pathophysiology of hypertrophic cardiomyopathy. *Postgrad Med J* 1986;62:515–529.

200. Sugrue DD, McKenna WJ, Dickie S, et al. Relation between left ventricular gradient and relative stroke volume ejected in early and late systole in hypertrophic cardiomyopathy: assessment with radionuclide cineangiography. *Br Heart J* 1984;52:602–609.

201. Maron BJ, Nishimura RA, Danielson GK. Pitfalls in clinical recognition and a novel operative approach for hypertrophic cardiomyopathy with severe outflow obstruction due to anomalous papillary muscle. *Circulation* 1998;98:2505–2508.

202. Nakamura T, Matsubara K, Furukawa K, et al. Diastolic paradoxic jet flow in patients with hypertrophic cardiomyopathy: evidence of concealed apical asynergy with cavity obliteration. *J Am Coll Cardiol* 1992;19:516–524.

203. Sutsch G, Jenni R, Krayenbuhl HP. Left ventricular flow from apex to base during systole and isovolumic relaxation in a patient with hypertrophic cardiomyopathy and midventricular obstruction [review]. *Eur Heart J* 1991;12:1132–1139.

204. Wigle ED, Adleman AG, Auger P, et al. Mitral regurgitation in muscular subaortic stenosis. *Am J Cardiol* 1969;24:698.

205. Tabata T, Oki T, Yamada H, et al. Subendocardial motion in hypertrophic cardiomyopathy: assessment from long- and short-axis views by pulsed tissue Doppler imaging. *J Am Soc Echocardiogr* 2000;13:108–115.

206. Yamada H, Oki T, Tabata T, et al. Assessment of left ventricular systolic wall motion velocity with pulsed tissue Doppler imaging: comparison with peak dP/dt of the left ventricular pressure curve. *J Am Soc Echocardiogr* 1998;11:442–449.

207. Nakatani S, White RD, Powell KA, et al. Dynamic magnetic resonance imaging assessment of the effect of ventricular wall curvature on regional function in hypertrophic cardiomyopathy. *Am J Cardiol* 1996;77:618–622.

208. Dong SJ, MacGregor JH, Crawley AP, et al. Left ventricular wall thickness and regional systolic function in patients with hypertrophic cardiomyopathy: a three-dimensional tagged magnetic resonance imaging study. *Circulation* 1994;90:1200–1209.

209. Palka P, Lange A, Fleming AD, et al. Differences in myocardial velocity gradient measured throughout the cardiac cycle in patients with hypertrophic cardiomyopathy, athletes and patients with left ventricular hypertrophy due to hypertension. *J Am Coll Cardiol* 1997;30:760–768.

210. Nihoyannopoulos P, Karatasakis G, Frenneaux M, et al. Diastolic function in hypertrophic cardiomyopathy: relation to exercise capacity. *J Am Coll Cardiol* 1992;19:536–540.

211. Keren G, Maron BJ. Patterns of pulmonary venous and transmitral flow velocity in patients with hypertrophic cardiomyopathy. *J Am Soc Echocardiogr* 1995;8:494–502.

212. Nagueh SF, Lakkis NM, Middleton KJ, et al. Doppler estimation of left ventricular filling pressures in patients with hypertrophic cardiomyopathy. *Circulation* 1999;99:254–261.

213. Pichard AD, Mellor J, Teichholz LE, et al. Septal perforation compression (narrowing) in idiopathic hypertrophic subaortic stenosis. *Am J Cardiol* 1977;40:310–314.

214. Brugada P, Bar FW, de Zwaan C, et al. "Sawfish" systolic narrowing of the left anterior descending artery: an angiographic sign of hypertrophic cardiomyopathy. *Circulation* 1982;66:800–803.

215. Yetman AT, McCrindle BW, MacDonald C, et al. Myocardial bridging in children with hypertrophic cardiomyopathy: a risk factor for sudden death. *N Engl J Med* 1998;339:1201–1209.

216. Mohiddin SA, Begley D, Shih J, et al. Myocardial bridging does not predict sudden death in children with hypertrophic cardiomyopathy but is associated with more severe cardiac disease. *J Am Coll Cardiol* 2000;36:2270–2278.

217. O'Gara PT, Bonow RO, Maron BJ, et al. Myocardial perfusion abnormalities in patients with hypertrophic cardiomyopathy: assessment with thallium-201 emission computed tomography. *Circulation* 1987;76:1214–1223.

218. Yamada M, Elliott PM, Kaski JC, et al. Dipyridamole stress thallium-201 perfusion abnormalities in patients with hypertrophic cardiomyopathy: relationship to clinical presentation and outcome. *Eur Heart J* 1998;19:500–507.

219. Pitcher D, Wainwright R, Maisey M, et al. Assessment of chest pain in hypertrophic cardiomyopathy using exercise thallium-201 myocardial scintigraphy. *Br Heart J* 1980;44:650–656.

220. Rubin KA, Morrison J, Padnick MB, et al. Idiopathic hypertrophic subaortic stenosis: evaluation of anginal symp-

toms with thallium-201 myocardial imaging. *Am J Cardiol* 1979;44:1040–1045.

221. Von Dohlen TW, Prisant LM, Frank MJ. Significance of positive or negative thallium-201 scintigraphy in hypertrophic cardiomyopathy. *Am J Cardiol* 1989;64:498–503.

222. Choudhury L, Elliott P, Rimoldi O, et al. Transmural myocardial blood flow distribution in hypertrophic cardiomyopathy and effect of treatment. *Basic Res Cardiol* 1999;94:49–59.

223. Gould KL. Myocardial metabolism by positron emission tomography in hypertrophic cardiomyopathy [editorial]. *J Am Coll Cardiol* 1989;13:325–326.

224. Nienaber CA, Gambhir SS, Mody FV, et al. Regional myocardial blood flow and glucose utilisation in symptomatic patients with hypertrophic cardiomyopathy. *Circulation* 1993;87:1580–1590.

225. Grover-McKay M, Schwaiger M, Krivokapich J, et al. Regional myocardial blood flow and metabolism at rest in mildly symptomatic patients with hypertrophic cardiomyopathy. *J Am Coll Cardiol* 1989;13:317–324.

226. Perrone-Filardi P, Bacharach SL, Dilsizian V, et al. Regional systolic function, myocardial blood flow and glucose uptake at rest in hypertrophic cardiomyopathy. *Am J Cardiol* 1993;72:199–204.

227. Kagaya Y, Ishide N, Takeyama D, et al. Differences in myocardial fluro-18 2-deoxyglucose uptake in young versus old patients with hypertrophic cardiomyopathy. *Am J Cardiol* 1992;69:242–246.

228. Tadamura E, Yoshibayashi M, Yonemura T, et al. Significant regional heterogeneity of coronary flow reserve in paediatric hypertrophic cardiomyopathy. *Eur J Nucl Med* 2000;27:1340–1348.

229. Jung WI, Hoess T, Bunse M, et al. Differences in cardiac energetics between patients with familial and nonfamilial hypertrophic cardiomyopathy. *Circulation* 2000;101:E121.

230. Jung WI, Sieverding L, Breuer J, et al. 31P NMR spectroscopy detects metabolic abnormalities in asymptomatic patients with hypertrophic cardiomyopathy. *Circulation* 1998;97:2536–2542.

231. Mishiro Y, Oki T, Iuchi A, et al. Regional left ventricular myocardial contraction abnormalities and asynchrony in patients with hypertrophic cardiomyopathy evaluated by magnetic resonance spatial modulation of magnetization myocardial tagging. *Jpn Circ J* 1999;63:442–446.

232. White RD, Obuchowski NA, Gunawardena S, et al. Left ventricular outflow tract obstruction in hypertrophic cardiomyopathy: presurgical and postsurgical evaluation by computed tomography magnetic resonance imaging. *Am J Card Imaging* 1996;10:1–13.

233. Zeviani M, Gellera C, Antozzi C, et al. Maternally inherited myopathy and cardiomyopathy: association with mutation in mitochondrial DNA tRNALeu(UUR). *Lancet* 1991;338:143–147.

234. Sweeney MG, Brockington M, Weston MJ, et al. Mitochondrial DNA transfer RNA mutationLeu(UUR)A-G3260: a second family with myopathy and cardiomyopathy. *Q J Med* 1993;86:435–438.

235. Taniike M, Fukushima H, Yanagihara I, et al. Mitochondrial tRNAIle mutation in fatal cardiomyopathy. *Biochem Biophys Res Commun* 1992;186:47–53.

236. Channer KS, Channer JL, Campbell MJ, et al. Cardiomyopathy in the Kearns-Sayre syndrome. *Br Heart J* 1988;59:486–490.

237. Guenthard J, Wyker F, Fowler B, et al. Cardiomyopathy in respiratory chain disorders. *Arch Dis Child* 1995;72:223–226.

238. Sato W, Tanaka M, Sugiyama S, et al. Cardiomyopathy and angiopathy in patients with mitochondrial myopathy, encephalopathy, lactic acidosis, and stroke-like episodes. *Am Heart J* 1994;128:733–741.

239. Anan R, Nakagawa M, Miyata M, et al. Cardiac involvement in mitochondrial diseases: a study on 17 patients with documented mitochondrial DNA defects. *Circulation* 1995;91:955–961.

240. Gorlin RJ, Anderson RC, Blan M. Multiple lentigenes syndrome. *Am J Dis Child* 1969;117:652–662.

241. Somerville J, Bonham-Carter RE. The heart in lentiginosis. *Br Heart J* 1972;34:58–66.

242. Moynihan EJ, Polani PE. Progressive cardiomyopathic lentiginosis. *QJM* 1972;162:205.

243. Kolvekar S, Williams BT, Venn GE. Hypertrophic obstructive cardiomyopathy with LEOPARD (Moynihan's) syndrome: surgical treatment. *J R Soc Med* 1993;86:115–116.

244. Maron BJ, Roberts WC, McAllister HA, et al. Sudden death in young athletes. *Circulation* 1980;62:218–229.

245. Burke AP, Farb A, Virmani R, et al. Sports-related and non-sports related sudden cardiac death in young adults. *Am Heart J* 1991;121:568–575.

246. Pellicia A, Maron BJ, Spataro A, et al. The upper limit of physiologic cardiac hypertrophy in highly trained elite athletes. *N Engl J Med* 1991;324:295.

247. Shapiro LM, Kleinebenne A, McKenna WJ. The distribution of left ventricular hypertrophy in hypertrophic cardiomyopathy: comparison to athletes and hypertensives. *Eur Heart J* 1985;6:967–974.

248. Maron BJ, Pellicia A, Spirito P. Cardiac disease in young trained athletes: insights into methods for distinguishing athlete's heart from structural heart disease, with particular emphasis on hypertrophic cardiomyopathy. *Circulation* 1995;91:1569–1601.

249. Lewis JF, Spirito P, Pellicia A, et al. Usefulness of Doppler echocardiographic assessment of diastolic filling in distinguishing "athlete's heart" from hypertrophic cardiomyopathy. *Br Heart J* 1992;68:296–300.

250. Spirito P, Pellicia A, Proschan MA, et al. Morphology of the "athletes heart" assessed by echocardiography in 947 elite athletes representing 27 sports. *Am J Cardiol* 1994;74:802–806.

251. Pelliccia A, Spataro A, Caselli G, et al. Absence of left ventricular wall thickening in athletes engaged in intense power training. *Am J Cardiol* 1993;72:1048–1054.

252. Serra-Grima R, Estorch M, Carrio I, et al. Marked ventricular repolarization abnormalities in highly trained athletes' electrocardiograms: clinical and prognostic implications. *J Am Coll Cardiol* 2000;36:1310–1316.

253. Pelliccia A, Maron BJ, Culasso F, et al. Clinical significance of abnormal electrocardiographic patterns in trained athletes. *Circulation* 2000;102:278–284.

254. Sharma S, Elliott PM, Whyte G, et al. Utility of metabolic exercise testing in distinguishing hypertrophic cardiomyopathy from physiologic left ventricular hypertrophy in athletes. *J Am Coll Cardiol* 2000;36:864–870.

255. McKenna WJ, Chetty S, Oakley CM, et al. Arrhythmia in hypertrophic cardiomyopathy: exercise and 48 hour ambulatory electrocardiographic assessment with and without beta adrenergic blocking therapy. *Am J Cardiol* 1980;45:1–5.

256. Pollick C. Muscular subaortic stenosis: hemodynamic and clinical improvement after disopyramide. *N Engl J Med* 1982;307:997–999.

257. Pollick C, Kimball B, Henderson M, et al. Disopyramide in hypertrophic cardiomyopathy. I: Hemodynamic assessment after intravenous administration. *Am J Cardiol* 1988;62: 1248–1251.

258. Pollick C. Disopyramide in hypertrophic cardiomyopathy. II: Non-invasive assessment after oral administration. *Am J Cardiol* 1988;62:1252–1255.

259. Hamada M, Shigematsu Y, Ikeda S, et al. Class Ia antiarrhythmic drug cibenzoline: a new approach to the medical treatment of hypertrophic obstructive cardiomyopathy. *Circulation* 1997;96:1520–1524.

260. Morrow AG, Reitz BA, Epstein SE, et al. Operative treatment in hypertrophic subaortic stenosis: techniques and the results of pre and postoperative assessments in 83 patients. *Circulation* 1975;52:88–102.

261. Maron BJ, Epstein SE, Morrow AG. Symptomatic status and prognosis of patients after operation for hypertrophic cardiomyopathy: efficacy of ventricular septal myotomy/ myectomy. *Eur Heart J* 1983;4[Suppl F]:175–180.

262. Schulte HD, Bircks W, Loesse B. Surgical treatment of hypertrophic cardiomyopathy (HOCM): early and late results. In: Zipes DE, Rowlands DJ, eds. *Progress in cardiology*. Philadelphia: Lea and Febiger, 1989:183–194.

263. Williams WG, Wigle ED, Rakowski H, et al. Results of surgery for hypertrophic obstructive cardiomyopathy. *Circulation* 1987;76:V104–V108.

264. Rothlin ME, Gobet D, Habere T, et al. Surgical treatment versus medical treatment in hypertrophic obstructive cardiomyopathy. *Eur Heart J* 1983;4[Suppl F]:215–223.

265. McCully RB, Nishimura RA, Baily KR, et al. Hypertrophic obstructive cardiomyopathy: preoperative echocardiographic predictors of outcome after septal myectomy. *J Am Coll Cardiol* 1996;27:1491–1496.

266. Redwood DR, Goldstein RE, Hirshfeld J, et al. Exercise performance after septal myotomy and myectomy in patients with obstructive hypertrophic cardiomyopathy. *Am J Cardiol* 1979;44:215–220.

267. Schoendube FA, Klues HG, Reith S, et al. Long-term clinical and echocardiographic follow-up after surgical correction of hypertrophic obstructive cardiomyopathy with extended myectomy and reconstruction of the subvalvular mitral apparatus. *Circulation* 1995;92[9 Suppl]:II122–II127.

268. Grigg LE, Wigle ED, Williams WG, et al. Transesophageal Doppler echocardiography in obstructive hypertrophic cardiomyopathy: clarification of pathophysiology and importance in intraoperative decision making. *J Am Coll Cardiol* 1992;20:42–52.

269. Sasson Z, Prieur T, Skrobik Y, et al. Aortic regurgitation: a common complication after surgery for hypertrophic obstructive cardiomyopathy. *J Am Coll Cardiol* 1989;13:63–67.

270. Bigelow WG, Trimble AS, Wigle DE, et al. The treatment of muscular subaortic stenosis. *J Thorac Cardiov Surg* 1974;68:384–390.

271. McIntosh CL, Greenberg GJ, Maron BJ, et al. Clinical and hemodynamic results after mitral valve replacement in patients with hypertrophic cardiomyopathy. *Ann Thorac Surg* 1989;47:236–246.

272. McIntosh CL, Maron BJ, Cannon RO 3d, et al. Initial results of combined anterior mitral leaflet plication and ventricular septal myotomy-myectomy for relief of left ventricular outflow tract obstruction in patients with hypertrophic cardiomyopathy. *Circulation* 1992;86[5 Suppl]:II60–II67.

273. Kofflard MJ, van Herwerden LA, Waldstein DJ, et al. Initial results of combined anterior mitral leaflet extension and myectomy in patients with obstructive hypertrophic cardiomyopathy. *J Am Coll Cardiol* 1996;28:197–202.

274. Hassenstein P, Storch HH, Schmitz W. Results of electrical pacing in patients with hypertrophic obstructive cardiomyopathy [in German]. *Thoraxchir Vask Chir* 1975;23:496–498.

275. Duck HJ, Hutschenreiter W, Pankau H, et al. Atrial synchronous ventricular stimulation with reduced AV delay time as a therapeutic principle in hypertrophic obstructive cardiomyopathy [in German]. *Z Gesamte Inn Med* 1984;39:437–447.

276. McDonald K, McWilliams E, O'Keefe B, et al. Functional assessment of patients treated with permanent dual chamber pacing as a primary treatment for hypertrophic cardiomyopathy. *Eur Heart J* 1988;9:893–898.

277. Slade AKB, Sadoul N, Shapiro L, et al. DDD pacing in hypertrophic cardiomyopathy: a multicentre clinical experience. *Heart* 1996;75:44–49.

278. Jeanrenaud X, Goy JJ, Kappenberger L. Effects of dual-chamber pacing in hypertrophic obstructive cardiomyopathy. *Lancet* 1992;339:1318–1323.

279. Fananapazir L, Epstein ND, Curiel RV, et al. Long-term results of dual chamber (DDD) pacing in obstructive hypertrophic cardiomyopathy: evidence for progressive symptomatic and hemodynamic improvement and reduction of left ventricular hypertrophy. *Circulation* 1994;90:2731–2742.

280. Nishimura RA, Trusty JM, Hayes DL, et al. Dual chamber pacing for hypertrophic cardiomyopathy: a randomised double-blind crossover trial. *J Am Coll Cardiol* 1997;29:435–441.

281. Kappenberger L, Linde C, Daubert C, et al. Pacing in hypertrophic obstructive cardiomyopathy: a randomized crossover study. PIC Study Group. *Eur Heart J* 1997;18:1249–1256.

282. Gadler F, Linde C, Daubert C, et al. Significant improvement of quality of life following atrioventricular synchronous pacing in patients with hypertrophic obstructive cardiomyopathy: data from 1 year of follow-up. PIC Study Group. *Eur Heart J* 1999;20:1044–1050.

283. Maron BJ, Nishimura RA, McKenna WJ, et al. Assessment of permanent dual-chamber pacing as a treatment for drug-refractory symptomatic patients with obstructive hypertrophic cardiomyopathy: a randomized, double-blind, crossover study (M-PATHY). *Circulation* 1999;99:2927–2933.

284. Ommen SR, Nishimura RA, Squires RW, et al. Comparison of dual-chamber pacing versus septal myectomy for the treatment of patients with hypertrophic obstructive cardiomyopathy: a comparison of objective hemodynamic and exercise end points. *J Am Coll Cardiol* 1999;34:191–196.

285. Sigwart U. Non-surgical myocardial reduction for hypertrophic obstructive cardiomyopathy. *Lancet* 1995;346:211–214.

286. Lakkis NM, Nagueh SF, Dunn JK, et al. Nonsurgical septal reduction therapy for hypertrophic obstructive cardiomyopathy: one-year follow-up. *J Am Coll Cardiol* 2000;36:852–855.

287. Ruzyllo W, Chojnowska L, Demkow M, et al. Left ventricular outflow tract gradient decrease with non-surgical myocardial reduction improves exercise capacity in patients with hypertrophic obstructive cardiomyopathy. *Eur Heart J* 2000;21:770–777.

288. Faber L, Seggewiss H, Gleichmann U. Percutaneous transluminal septal myocardial ablation in hypertrophic obstructive cardiomyopathy: results with respect to intraprocedural myocardial contrast echocardiography. *Circulation* 1998;98:2415–2421.

289. Gietzen FH, Leuner CJ, Raute-Kreinsen U, et al. Acute and long-term results after transcoronary ablation of septal hypertrophy (TASH): catheter interventional treatment for hypertrophic obstructive cardiomyopathy. *Eur Heart J* 1999;20:1342–1354.

290. Nagueh SF, Lakkis NM, He ZX, et al. Role of myocardial contrast echocardiography during nonsurgical septal reduction therapy for hypertrophic obstructive cardiomyopathy. *J Am Coll Cardiol* 1998;32:225–229.

291. Knight C, Kurbaan AS, Seggewiss H, et al. Nonsurgical septal reduction for hypertrophic obstructive cardiomyopathy: outcome in the first series of patients. *Circulation* 1997;95:2075–2081.

292. Seggewiss H, Gleichmann U, Faber L, et al. Percutaneous transluminal septal myocardial ablation in hypertrophic obstructive cardiomyopathy: acute results and 3-month follow-up in 25 patients. *J Am Coll Cardiol* 1998;31:252–258.

293. Maron BJ. Role of alcohol septal ablation in treatment of obstructive hypertrophic cardiomyopathy. *Lancet* 2000;355:425–426.

294. Rosing DR, Kent KM, Maron BJ, et al. Verapamil therapy: a new approach to the pharmacological treatment of hypertrophic cardiomyopathy. II: Effects on exercise capacity and symptomatic status. *Circulation* 1979;60:1208–1213.

295. Hopf R, Kaltembach M. Verapamil treatment of hypertrophic cardiomyopathy. In: Kaltenbach M, Epstein SE, eds. *Hypertrophic cardiomyopathy: the therapeutic role of calcium antagonists.* New York: Springer-Verlag, 1982:163–166.

296. Bonow RO, Rosing DR, Bacharach SL, et al. Effects of verapamil on left ventricular systolic function and diastolic filling in patients with hypertrophic cardiomyopathy. *Circulation* 1981;64:787–796.

297. Udelson JE, Bonow RO, O'Gara PT, et al. Verapamil prevents silent myocardial perfusion abnormalities during exercise in asymptomatic patients with hypertrophic cardiomyopathy. *Circulation* 1989;79:1052–1060.

298. Gistri R, Cecchi F, Choudhury L, et al. Effect of verapamil on absolute myocardial blood flow in hypertrophic cardiomyopathy. *Am J Cardiol*ogy 1994;74:363–368.

299. Iwase M, Sobotata I, Takagi S, et al. Effects of diltiazem on left ventricular diastolic behaviour in patients with hypertrophic cardiomyopathy: evaluation with pulsed Doppler echocardiography. *J Am Coll Cardiol* 1987;9:1099.

300. Betocchi S, Cannon RO, Watson RM, et al. Effects of sublingual nifedipine on hemodynamics and systolic and diastolic function in patients with hypertrophic cardiomyopathy. *Circulation* 1985;72:1001–1007.

301. Counihan PJ, Fei L, Bashir Y, et al. Assessment of heart rate variability in hypertrophic cardiomyopathy: association with clinical and prognostic features. *Circulation* 1993;88:1682–1690.

302. Limbruno U, Strata G, Zucchi R, et al. Altered autonomic cardiac control in hypertrophic cardiomyopathy: role of outflow tract obstruction and myocardial hypertrophy. *Eur Heart J* 1998;19:146–153.

303. Fei L, Slade AK, Prasad K, et al. Is there increased sympathetic activity in patients with hypertrophic cardiomyopathy? *J Am Coll Cardiol* 1995;26:472–480.

304. Gilligan DM, Chan WL, Sbarouni E, et al. Autonomic function in hypertrophic cardiomyopathy. *Br Heart J* 1993;69:525–529.

305. Frenneaux MP, Counihan PJ, Caforio A, et al. Abnormal blood pressure response during exercise in hypertrophic cardiomyopathy. *Circulation* 1990;82:1995–2002.

306. Sadoul N, Prasad K, Elliott PM, et al. Prospective prognostic assessment of blood pressure response during exercise in patients with hypertrophic cardiomyopathy. *Circulation* 1997;96:2987–2991.

307. Counihan PJ, Frenneaux MP, Webb DJ, et al. Abnormal vascular responses to supine exercise in hypertrophic cardiomyopathy. *Circulation* 1991;84:686–696.

308. Elliott PM, Sharma S, Varnava A, et al. Survival after cardiac arrest or sustained ventricular tachycardia in patients with hypertrophic cardiomyopathy. *J Am Coll Cardiol* 1999;33:1596–1601.

309. Maron BJ, Shen WK, Link MS, et al. Efficacy of implantable cardioverter-defibrillators for the prevention of sudden death in patients with hypertrophic cardiomyopathy. *N Engl J Med* 2000;342:365–373.

310. Primo J, Geelen P, Brugada J, et al. Hypertrophic cardiomyopathy: role of the implantable cardioverter defibrillator. *J Am Coll Cardiol* 1998;31:1081–1085.

311. Nienaber CA, Hiller S, Spielmann RP, et al. Syncope in hypertrophic cardiomyopathy: multivariate analysis of prognostic determinates. *J Am Coll Cardiol* 1990;15:948–955.

312. Spirito P, Rapezzi C, Autore C, et al. Prognosis of asymptomatic patients with hypertrophic cardiomyopathy and nonsustained ventricular tachycardia. *Circulation* 1994;90:2743–2747.

313. Maki S, Ikeda H, Muro A, et al. Predictors of sudden cardiac death in hypertrophic cardiomyopathy. *Am J Cardiol* 1998;82:774–778.

314. Olivotto I, Maron BJ, Montereggi A, et al. Prognostic value of systemic blood pressure response during exercise in a community based population with hypertrophic cardiomyopathy. *J Am Coll Cardiol* 1999;33:2044–2051.

315. Spirito P, Maron BJ. Relation between extent of left ventricular hypertrophy and occurrence of sudden cardiac death in hypertrophic cardiomyopathy. *J Am Coll Cardiol* 1990;15:1521–1526.

316. Spirito P, Bellone P, Harris KM, et al. Magnitude of left ventricular hypertrophy and risk of sudden death in hypertrophic cardiomyopathy. *N Engl J Med* 2000;342:1778–1785.

317. Elliott PM, Gimeno Blanes JR, et al. Relation between the severity of left ventricular hypertrophy and prognosis in patients with hypertrophic cardiomyopathy. *Lancet* 2001;357:420–424.

318. Dritsas A, Sabarouni E, Gilligan D, et al. QT-interval abnormalities in hypertrophic cardiomyopathy. *Clin Cardiol* 1992;15:739–742.

319. Yanagisawa-Miwa A, Inoue I, Sugimoto T. Diurnal change in QT intervals in dilated and hypertrophic cardiomyopathy. *Am J Cardiol* 1991;67:1428–1430.

320. Fei L, Slade AK, Grace AA, et al. Ambulatory assessment of the QT interval in patients with hypertrophic cardiomyopathy: risk stratification and effect of low dose amiodarone. *Pacing Clin Electrophysiol* 1994;17:2222–2227.

321. Maron BJ, Leyhe MJ, Casey SA, et al. Assessment of QT dispersion as a prognostic marker for sudden death in a regional nonreferred hypertrophic cardiomyopathy cohort. *Am J Cardiol* 2001;87:114–115.

322. Yi G, Poloniecki J, Dickie S, et al. Can the assessment of dynamic QT dispersion on exercise electrocardiogram predict sudden cardiac death in hypertrophic cardiomyopathy? *Pacing Clin Electrophysiol* 2000;23:1953–1956.

323. Cripps TR, Counihan PJ, Frenneaux MP, et al. Signal averaged electrocardiography in hypertrophic cardiomyopathy. *J Am Coll Cardiol* 1990;15:956–961.

324. Kulakowski P, Counihan PJ, Camm AJ, et al. The value of time and frequency domain, and spectral temporal mapping analysis of the signal-averaged electrocardiogram in identification of patients with hypertrophic cardiomyopathy at increased risk of sudden death. *Eur Heart J* 1993;14:941–950.

325. Fananapazir L, Chang AC, Epstein SE, et al. Prognostic determinants in hypertrophic cardiomyopathy: prognostic evaluation of a therapeutic strategy based on clinical, Holter, hemodynamic and electrophysiological findings. *Circulation* 1992;86:730–740.

326. Wellens HJJ, Brugada P, Stevenson WG. Programmed electrical stimulation of the heart in patients with life threatening ventricular arrhythmias. What is the significance of induced arrhythmias and what is the correct stimulation protocol? *Circulation* 1985;72:1.

327. Saumarez RC, Camm AJ, Panagos A, et al. Ventricular fibrillation in hypertrophic cardiomyopathy is associated with increased fractionation of paced right ventricular electrocardiograms. *Circulation* 1992;86:467–474.

328. Saumarez RC, Slade AKB, Grace AA, et al. The significance of paced electrocardiogram fractionation in hypertrophic cardiomyopathy: a prospective study. *Circulation* 1995;91:2762–2768.

329. Silka MJ, Kron J, Dunnigan A, et al. Sudden cardiac death and the use of implantable cardioverter-defibrillators in pediatric patients. *Circulation* 1993;87:800–807.

330. Kron J, Oliver RP, Norsted S, et al. The automatic implantable cardioverter-defibrillator in young patients. *J Am Coll Cardiol* 1990;16:896–902.

331. McKenna WJ, Oakley CM, Krikler DM, et al. Improved survival with amiodarone in patients with hypertrophic cardiomyopathy and ventricular tachycardia. *Br Heart J* 1985;53:412–416.

332. Maron BJ, Robert WC, Epstein SE. Sudden death in hypertrophic cardiomyopathy: a profile of 78 patients. *Circulation* 1982;65:1388–1394.

333. Maron BJ, Isner JM, McKenna WJ. 26th Bethesda conference: recommendations for determining eligibility for competition in athletes with cardiovascular abnormalities. Task force 3: hypertrophic cardiomyopathy, myocarditis and other myopericardial diseases and mitral valve prolapse. *J Am Coll Cardiol* 1994;24:880–885.

ADULT CONGENITAL HEART DISEASE

ARIANE J. MARELLI
DOUGLAS S. MOODIE

▼▼ ADDITIONAL ELECTRONIC TOPICS

Intercirculatory Shunts g06;   Atrial Septal Defects: Prevalence and Anatomy g07;   Atrial Septal Defects: Outcome g08;   Ventricular Septal Defect: Prevalence and Anatomy g09;   Ventricular Septal Defect: Outcome g10;   Patent Ductus Arteriosus: Prevalence and Anatomy g11;   Patent Ductus Arteriosus: Outcome g12;   Pulmonary Stenosis: Prevalence and Anatomy g13;   Pulmonary Stenosis: Outcome g14;   Aortic Stenosis: Prevalence and Anatomy g15;   Aortic Stenosis: Outcome g16;   Aortic Coarctation: Prevalence and Anatomy g17;   Aortic Coarctation: Outcome g18;   Tetralogy of Fallot: Prevalence and Anatomy g19;   Tetralogy of Fallot: Outcome g20;   Pulmonary Atresia with Ventricular Septal Defect: Prevalence and Anatomy g21;   Pulmonary Atresia with Ventricular Septal Defect: Outcome g22;   Complete Transposition of the Great Arteries: Prevalence and Anatomy g23;   Complete Transposition of the Great Arteries: Outcome g24;   Right-Sided Ebstein's Anomaly: Prevalence and Anatomy g25;   Right-Sided Ebstein's Anomaly: Outcome g26;   Congenitally Corrected Transposition of the Great Arteries: Prevalence and Anatomy g27;   Congenitally Corrected Transposition of the Great Arteries: Outcome g28;   Univentricular Heart and Tricuspid Atresia: Prevalence and Anatomy g29;   Univentricular Heart and Tricuspid Atresia: Outcome g30

OVERVIEW

At the time of adulthood, native anatomy, physiology, and operative status converge to determine prognosis and surgical

   A. J. Marelli: Department of Medicine, McGill University Faculty of Medicine, Adult Congenital Heart Disease Unit, McGill University Health Center, Montreal, Canada
   D. S. Moodie: Department of Pediatrics, Ochsner Clinic Foundation, New Orleans, Louisiana

and medical management considerations. For common simple shunt lesions or single obstructive lesions of the right or left ventricular outflow tracts, early intervention for significant disease leads to optimal long-term results. When patients with complex lesions unoperated or palliated reach adulthood, physiologic repair may be feasible. The decision to proceed depends on the reversibility of deleterious physiology and the possibility of preventing further deterioration. The long-term complications of palliative shunts are pertinent, particularly for the first generation of patients who have undergone surgery. When physiologic repair has taken place, issues of concern in long-term follow-up include hemodynamic and arrhythmic complications and reoperation.

Adolescents and adults with congenital heart disease (CHD) are optimally cared for in specialized centers staffed by medical and pediatric cardiologists or cardiologists trained and committed to the care of adults with CHD as well as cardiac surgeons with skill in congenital heart surgery. These facilities should have easy access to specialists including those in cardiac anesthesia, obstetrics and gynecology, pulmonary disease, hematology, neurology, psychiatry, and genetic counseling.

The purpose of this chapter is to provide an overview of the issues that will be of major concern for physicians who are given the responsibility of following these patients as adults. We discuss a framework for clinical assessment and management at the time of presentation in adulthood. The role of invasive and noninvasive diagnostic modalities is reviewed. A problem-oriented discussion of the unoperated and operated lesions most likely to be encountered in this patient population is provided. Specialized issues pertinent to this population as a whole, such as Eisenmenger's syndrome, the medical management of cyanosis, endocarditis prophylaxis, exercise recommendations, pregnancy, and psychosocial issues, are summarized.

GLOSSARY

Complex lesions: A combination of lesions, the most common patterns of which, seen in adults, are described in this chapter.

Cyanosis: A blue discoloration of the mucous membranes resulting from an increase in the amount of reduced hemoglobin. Central cyanosis occurs when the circulation is mixed secondary to a right-to-left shunting. Cyanosis can be observed in unoperated and palliated patients with native cyanotic lesions.

Eisenmenger's complex: A term referring to flow reversal across a ventricular septal defect when pulmonary vascular resistance exceeds systemic levels.

Eisenmenger's physiology: A term used to designate the physiologic response in a broader category of lesions in which a right-to-left shunt occurs in response to an elevation in pulmonary vascular resistance.

Eisenmenger's syndrome: A term applied to common clinical features shared by patients with Eisenmenger's physiology. These findings in combination with the absence of left-to-right shunting make the patient inoperable.

Native lesions: The anatomic lesions at birth.

Palliative interventions: Increase or decrease pulmonary blood flow while a mixed circulation and cyanosis persist. Palliative surgical shunts aimed at increasing pulmonary blood flow are summarized in Table 31.1.

TABLE 31.1 SURGICAL PALLIATION OF CONGENITAL HEART LESIONS

Palliative surgical shunts	
Systemic venous-to-pulmonary artery shunts	
Classic Glenn	SVC to right PA
Bidirectional Glenn	SVC to right and left PA
Bilateral Glenn	Right and left SVC to right and left PA
Systemic arterial-to-pulmonary artery shunts	
Classic Blalock-Taussig	Subclavian artery to PA
Modified Blalock-Taussig	Subclavian artery to PA (prosthetic graft)
Pott's anastomosis	Descending aorta to left PA
Waterston's shunt	Ascending aorta to right PA

PA, pulmonary artery; SVC, superior vena cava.
Adapted from Marelli AJ, Mullen M. Congenital heart disease onward into adulthood. *Bailliere's Pediatr* 1996;4:192.

Physiologic repair: A term applied to procedures that result in total or near total anatomic and physiologic separation of the pulmonary and systemic circulations in complex cyanotic lesions. These patients are typically acyanotic.

Simple lesions: Shunt lesions or obstructive lesions of the right or left ventricular outflow tract that occur in isolation.

HISTORICAL PERSPECTIVE AND EPIDEMIOLOGY

Over the past four decades, the convergence of major advances in pediatric and medical cardiology as well as cardiovascular surgery has resulted in the survival of an increasingly large number of patients with complex structural heart lesions. Table 31.2 provides a historical perspective of primary operations for major disease categories. This chronologic listing of surgical interventions and their dates of introduction provides a basis for predicting the sequential rise in expected survival for patients with specific diseases.

TABLE 31.2 SURGICAL REPAIR OF COMPLEX CONGENITAL HEART LESIONS

1955	Tetralogy of Fallot
1959	Senning atrial baffle in TGA
1964	Mustard atrial baffle in TGA
1969	Rastelli right ventricle to pulmonary artery conduit
1971	Fontan anastomosis in tricuspid atresia
1975	Jatene arterial switch in TGA with ventricular septal defect
1983	Norwood reconstruction in hypoplastic left-sided heart syndrome
1984	Neonatal arterial switch in TGA with intact ventricular septum

TGA, transposition of the great arteries.
Adapted from Marelli AJ, Mullen M. Congenital heart disease onward into adulthood. *Bailliere's Pediatr* 1996;4:189.

Congenital cardiac malformations occur at a rate of 8 per 1,000 live births, corresponding to approximately 32,000 infants with newly diagnosed CHD each year in the United States. An estimated 20% die within the first year from life-threatening conditions, a substantial decrease from the reported 40% in the late 1960s (1). An approximate 80% of the first-year survivors live to reach adulthood in the current era (2–4). Coincident with improved survival in the neonatal and early childhood years, these numbers continue to grow with prevalence rates of adults with CHD in the United States estimated to be an approximate 800,000 (5).

PRESENTATION IN ADULTHOOD

The management of the young adult with CHD requires the clinician, at the end of his or her assessment, to determine the native anatomy, the surgical anatomy, the patient's physiology, and operative candidacy (Fig. 31.1) (6).

Understanding the details of the native and surgical anatomy is the cornerstone of appropriate management. Information obtained from objective diagnostic tests should complement that obtained from review of all previous available records. Reconsideration of the findings is imperative in delivering proper care, as the management of CHD has changed significantly over the last thirty years.

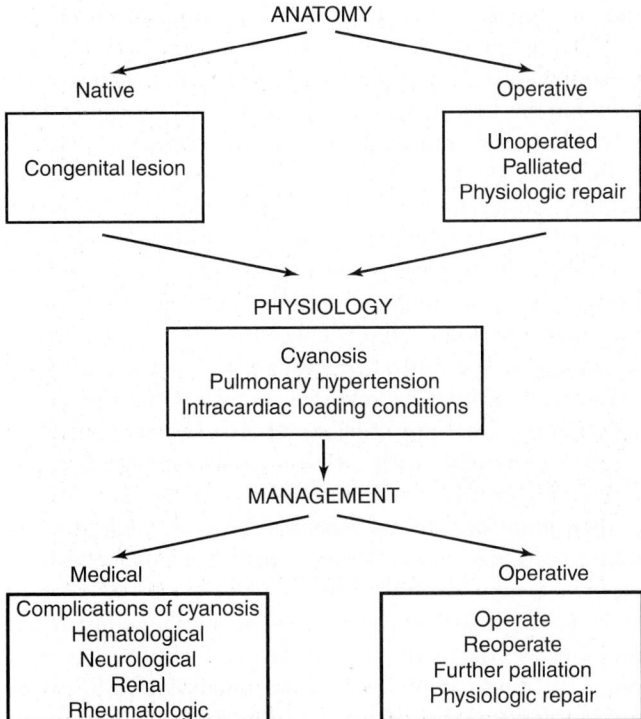

FIGURE 31.1 The goals of complete clinical assessment are to define anatomy and physiology to determine appropriate management. (From Marelli AJ. Congenital heart disease in adults. In: Goldman L, Bennett J. *Cecil's textbook of medicine.* Philadelphia: WB Saunders, 1999, with permission.)

Determination of the *physiology* includes two components. The first relates to the presence or absence of cyanosis, the medical complications that ensue, and the assessment of the pulmonary vascular bed. The second relates to the loading conditions of the cardiac chambers. Congenital heart lesions are classified as cyanotic or acyanotic (7). The presence or absence of pulmonary hypertension, with or without an increase in pulmonary vascular resistance, depends on the quantity and source of pulmonary blood flow. If forward flow from the right side of the heart is insufficient, native collaterals, surgical shunts, or both provide alternate sources of pulmonary blood flow. An increased volume load to the heart can result from intracardiac shunting or valvular regurgitation. An increase in pressure afterload can result from native or acquired stenosis of either outflow tracts or high pulmonary or systemic vascular resistance. It is the interaction between the pulmonary vascular bed and the heart that determines the patient's physiology.

Palliative interventions are defined as those operations that serve to either increase or decrease pulmonary blood flow while allowing a mixed circulation and cyanosis to persist. Palliative surgical shunts aimed at increasing pulmonary blood flow are summarized in Table 31.1. Systemic arterial-to-pulmonary artery shunts may result in a significant improvement in saturation levels but at the price of high levels of pulmonary blood flow and direct exposure of the pulmonary vascular bed to the high pressures of the systemic circulation (8). The possible long-term complications of these shunts include pulmonary hypertension, pulmonary artery stenosis, and volume overload of the ventricle receiving pulmonary venous return, making further surgical intervention more difficult or impossible. This is particularly true of large central shunts, the Pott's shunt, and Waterston's anastomosis. Well-sized Blalock-Taussig shunts can result in more controlled pulmonary flow, but may stenose over time and distort the pulmonary artery anatomy (9). These considerations provide the rationale for the current widespread use of systemic venous-to-pulmonary arterial shunts resulting in acceptable saturations with more balanced pulmonary blood flow and a lower transpulmonary pressure gradient (10). Surgical *pulmonary artery banding* is a palliative measure aimed at decreasing pulmonary blood flow and protecting the pulmonary vascular bed against direct exposure to systemic pressures. The pulmonary band is usually placed above the valve and below the pulmonary artery bifurcation. This procedure has been performed in patients with a ventricular septal defect (VSD) large enough to significantly increase pulmonary blood flow in the presence or absence of other complex lesions. In long-term follow-up, two issues are of concern. The first relates to distortion of the pulmonary artery trunk or at the bifurcation, with or without migration of the band. This can preclude or complicate adequate late repair, requiring reconstruction of the proximal pulmonary vascular bed. The second complication of the band has been observed in a subgroup of patients having a univentricular heart and transposition of the great arteries with a potentially or truly restrictive VSD. It has been suggested that banding the pulmonary trunk stimulates myocardial hypertrophy, promoting spontaneous reduction in the size of the bulboventricular foramen, leading to secondary subaortic stenosis. The surgical management of this is associated with a high mortality (11).

Physiologic repair is a term applied to procedures that result in total or near total anatomic, physiologic, or both anatomic and physiologic separation of the pulmonary and systemic circulations. Examples include repair of tetralogy of Fallot (TOF), the Senning's or Mustard's operation for transposition of the great arteries, and the Fontan operation for the single ventricle. Although an attempt is made to approximate normal physiology, long-term complications relating to prosthetic materials, valves, and conduits, as well as ventricular dysfunction, require careful and continued follow-up. These are discussed, where applicable, in the context of specific lesions.

DIAGNOSTIC TECHNIQUES: APPROACH, STRENGTHS, AND LIMITATIONS

Adequate use of the diagnostic tools assists in the determination of the anatomy, physiology, and operative status of the adult patient. A complete clinical assessment is essential and includes 12-lead electrocardiography, chest radiography, and baseline oxygen saturation. Serial use of these tests, Holter monitoring, and cardiorespiratory exercise testing are tailored to the individual patient. In this section, we describe the use of noninvasive imaging and cardiac catheterization as it pertains to adults with CHD.

Transthoracic Echocardiography

Two-dimensional and Doppler echocardiography is the cornerstone of imaging for diagnosis and follow-up of congenital lesions. The principle of segmental analysis of anatomy and hemodynamics underlies the echocardiographic examination of CHD in patients of all ages. The segmental approach to congenital cardiac disease (12) refers to sequential diagnosis of the major cardiac segments in a venous-to-arterial sequence, consistent with the development of the heart. Native and surgical anatomy is therefore described from inflow to outflow in keeping with the concept of a circulation in series. g31

Accurate assessment of complex congenital anatomy results from a careful interactive diagnostic search, which becomes progressively more specific and focused as the examination proceeds. This is particularly important during a patient's first examination, as echocardiography becomes the key to the future clinical and surgical management. In adults and older children in whom acoustic windows are more challenging, information can be maximized by adhering to three precautions: referring the patient to an echocardiographer who is familiar with congenital heart lesions and technically versatile with adults, providing as much information on the patient's history ahead of time, and referring the patient to the same laboratory for sequential examinations.

Complete spatial understanding of complex congenital lesions can be challenged by the limitations of two-dimensional echocardiography. Three-dimensional reconstruction of images acquired transthoracically offers unique imaging perspectives, more closely approximating surgical anatomy and optimizing surgical planning (14,15). Improved accuracy and spatial resolution of suboptimal data sets as well as the ability to quantitate cardiac function (16) are broadening the application of three-dimensional echocardiography (17).

Transesophageal Echocardiography

The transesophageal echocardiographic (TEE) examination is particularly useful in adults to maximize image acquisition when transthoracic acoustic windows are poor (18). TEE is routinely used to clarify and detail intracardiac anatomy when transthoracic echocardiography is problematic. By comparison with transthoracic imaging, TEE provides additional anatomic information for specific posterior and anterior congenital lesions. Anomalous pulmonary venous connections (19) and atrial septal defects (ASDs), in particular those of the sinus venosus type (20), and atrial septal aneurysms can be detected transthoracically but are best imaged using a combination of horizontal and vertical transesophageal planes. Integrity of atrial baffles and Fontan connections can sometimes only be inferred from abnormal flow patterns, using transthoracic imaging in adolescents and adults. Obstruction due to thrombus or progressive narrowing can clearly be seen using TEE. Assessment of complex atrioventricular anatomy and function can be enhanced using posterior acoustic windows. For central pulmonary vascular architecture, subaortic and supraaortic lesions, as well as ventriculoarterial conduit function, specific sites of obstruction can be clearly delineated with vertical transesophageal views. Proximal coronary artery anomalies and coronary fistulas at their point of exit and entry can be easily imaged using transesophageal views. Using transthoracic echocardiography, a patent ductus arteriosus (PDA) can be inferred from a turbulent flow pattern seen at the origin of the left pulmonary artery. In adolescents and adults, however, often the duct cannot be directly visualized. TEE can be used to confirm the diagnosis and exclude the presence of endarteritis (21). Palliative shunt anastomosis can be imaged and interrogated using a combination of transesophageal views. Difficulty in properly aligning the Doppler signal parallel to the shunt can hinder the ability to make a definitive diagnosis of an obstructed shunt. Aortic coarctation can be diagnosed using multiple transesophageal views, but accurate multilevel measurements of the arch and descending aorta often require the use of other complementary examinations.

Intraprocedural TEE has become increasingly important. Intraoperative TEE is used as an adjunct to complex intracardiac repair. In pediatric series, intraoperative TEE has been shown to affect surgical management of complex congenital lesions in up to 20% of cases (22,23). TEE is being routinely used during interventional catheter-guided atrial septal device closure (24) and coarctoplasty. Atrial baffle dilations can be guided using TEE. In addition, the electrophysiologist can be helped in guiding ablation catheters through the heart when abnormal native or surgical anatomy results in a distortion of the usual landmarks. This can be particularly useful for ablation therapy in patients with right-sided Ebstein's anomaly and congenitally corrected transposition of the great arteries, after Mustard's procedure for complete transposition of the great vessels and after the Fontan operation (18).

Magnetic Resonance Imaging and Computed Tomography

These imaging modalities are available in specialized centers and can be used as adjuncts to cardiac ultrasound and angiography. Magnetic resonance imaging (MRI) and ultrafast computed tomography (CT) can be particularly useful for detailed assessment of the aorta, branch pulmonary arteries, systemic-to-pulmonary artery shunts, and anomalous systemic venous connections (25,26). For patients with TOF repair, MRI is particularly useful to clarify anatomy and function of the pulmonary arteries and right ventricle (27). Judicious use of complementary noninvasive tools to elucidate anatomy allows a more focused application of cardiac catheterization.

Diagnostic Cardiac Catheterization

There are three principal indications for diagnostic studies most commonly performed before surgical or catheter-based intervention. These include assessment of pulmonary vascular bed, clarification of anatomy, and coronary angiography in patients over the age of 40 years. The study usually includes a saturation run for shunt calculations, right and left pressure measurements as needed, cardiac output measurements, and appropriate biplane cine angiographic views. Shunt quantification can usually be inferred from secondary chamber enlargement using noninvasive imaging. In instances in which an atrial or ventricular level shunt is of borderline significance or in which chamber enlargement is secondary to concomitant primary regurgitant lesions, pulmonary to systemic flow ratios should be directly measured. In assessing the pulmonary vascular bed, cardiac catheterization is indicated when there exists doubt

as to the etiology and potential reversibility of pulmonary vascular disease (28). Morphometric analysis of lung biopsy specimens and pulmonary wedge angiography can be used to quantify pulmonary vascular obstructive correlating obliterative vascular changes with hemodynamic abnormalities in the pulmonary circulation (29). ⚓ g32

INTERVENTIONAL CARDIAC CATHETERIZATION

Right and Left Ventricular Outflow Tract Obstruction

Pulmonary angioplasty is the procedure of choice for adults with congenital pulmonary valve stenosis (60). Long-term follow-up data of nearly 10 years demonstrates persistent resolution of the dynamic component of sub–pulmonary stenosis and no restenosis at the valvar level even for severe pulmonary stenosis (61,62). Pulmonary regurgitation is noted in an approximate 10% of patients and improves over time. Stents have been used in adults to relieve right ventricular pulmonary artery conduit obstruction (63) and peripheral pulmonary artery stenosis (64). The clinical usefulness of stents in the pulmonary arteries is particularly important in postoperative patients with TOF and truncus arteriosus with small pulmonary arteries. These patients may have peripheral pulmonary stenosis with severe pulmonary regurgitation after surgical repair. Stent placement with reduction in pulmonary artery pressure may reduce the amount of pulmonary regurgitation, decrease right ventricular dilatation and tricuspid regurgitation, and improve right ventricular function. ⚓ g33

Aortic coarctation can safely and effectively be treated with balloon dilation with or without stent implantation, particularly for adult patients with recoarctation after surgical repair (66,67). Incomplete relief is observed in 25% of patients with recoarctation versus 19% of patients with native coarctation (66). Restenosis remains a concern and appears to occur more frequently in children with native coarctation. The incidence of incomplete relief and restenosis is decreased in adolescents and adults with endovascular stent implantation (68). Aortic aneurysm formation is reported in 7% to 17% of adult patients (68,69), and aortic rupture occurs rarely. Percutaneous coarctoplasty is contraindicated in those with transverse arch hypoplasia.

LONG-TERM FOLLOW-UP AND MANAGEMENT OF THE MOST COMMON SPECIFIC LESIONS

A problem-oriented approach to the lesions most commonly encountered in this patient population, based on observations across the age groups (70), is provided. The patients presenting to adult cardiologists are a mixed population of operated and unoperated patients, the relative proportion of which will continue to vary, based on evolving therapeutic trends in pediatric cardiology. The discussion pertinent to each lesion is divided into three parts. Prevalence and Anatomy (see the CD-ROM and online versions of this text) provides epidemiologic information and reviews the anatomy necessary to understand diagnostic categories. Outcome (see the CD-ROM and online versions of this text) describes the clinical course and complications of the operated or unoperated patients, based on the pathophysiology of the lesion. Management provides a problem-oriented discussion of issues related to choice of medical or surgical therapy and surveillance of the patient presenting as an adult.

Isolated Shunt Lesions

Shunts at the atrial, ventricular, and great artery levels are some of the most commonly encountered lesions in children and adults. Hemodynamic complications of significant shunts relate to volume overload and chamber dilation of the primary chambers receiving the excess left-to-right shunt: the right side of the heart for patients with ASD and the left side of the heart for patients with VSD and PDA. Secondary complications result from valvular dysfunction and damage to the pulmonary vascular bed. The size and duration of the shunt determine the natural history and therefore the indications for closure. The degree of shunting is always a function not only of the size of the communication, but also a function of its location on biventricular compliance, the pulmonary and systemic vascular resistances, or both. Hemodynamic sequelae of shunts are typically clinically apparent or can be expected to occur when pulmonary-to-systemic flow ratios exceed 1.5 to 1.0; hence, the designation of a "significant shunt." It should be noted, however, that the diagnostic method used influences the clinical detectability of abnormal findings. For example, assessment of a mildly enlarged right ventricle may be variable between the physical examination, chest roentgenology, and cardiac ultrasound. Uncertainty about the physiologic significance of a borderline shunt can be minimized by integrating serial determinations from multiple clinically relevant diagnostic sources, rather than making management decisions based strictly on a calculated shunt value. Clinical decision making takes into consideration the patient's age, symptoms, and direct and indirect diagnostic information reflecting intracardiac and pulmonary hemodynamics.

Atrial Septal Defects

Management
The goal of management in patients with ASD is to prevent death, right-sided heart failure, atrial arrhythmia, and pulmonary hypertension (see the section Outcome for a description of complications). ASD closure may be achieved percutaneously (see previous discussion) or surgi-

cally. Uncomplicated secundum ASDs may be closed surgically in children and adults with minimal operative mortality, in the range of 1% to 3% (75) or less. The long-term prevention of death and complications is best achieved when ASD is closed before age 25 and when the systolic pressure in the main pulmonary artery measured at cardiac catheterization is less than 40 mm Hg. This results in a long-term mortality that is similar to age- and sex-matched control populations (75). Closure after age 40 in symptomatic patients with significant shunts improves survival, prevents deterioration in functional capacity (81), and improves exercise tolerance (82) when compared with patients treated medically. In contrast, surgical closure after age 40 does not reduce the risk of nonfatal cardiovascular complications, including supraventricular arrhythmias and cerebrovascular events (75,81). Age greater than 60 is not a contraindication to ASD closure in the presence of a significant shunt because up to 80% of patients show evidence of symptomatic improvement (83). ASD closure in asymptomatic patients with significant shunts between age 25 and 40 years is controversial (84), but is associated with a reduced incidence of atrial arrhythmia (85) and is undertaken in many centers with the expectation that long-term symptomatic deterioration is preventable (86).

Preoperative pulmonary artery pressure and the presence or absence of pulmonary vascular disease are important predictors of successful surgical outcome (75,80). Patients with a total pulmonary vascular resistance of less than 7 Wood units show improvement in New York Heart Association (NYHA) class, regression of symptoms, radiographic evidence of pulmonary artery enlargement, and electrocardiographic evidence of right ventricular hypertrophy, while a pulmonary vascular resistance greater than 15 Wood units is associated with a high surgical mortality (80). If pulmonary artery pressure, pulmonary vascular resistance, or both are greater than two-thirds systemic, there should be a net left-to-right shunt of at least 1.5:1.0 or evidence of reversibility during reactive pulmonary vascular reactivity studies before proceeding to surgical repair (87).

Patients who have had surgical closure of an uncomplicated ASD before age 25 have a favorable prognosis. Patients who are older at the time of repair require variable supervision depending on the presence and degree of preoperative and postoperative medical complications. Atrial fibrillation or flutter is more prevalent as the age of operation increases (85) and is present in up to 50% to 60% of patients over the age of 40, regardless of surgical status. In 60% to 70% of patients with preoperative arrhythmias, the rhythm persists postoperatively (75), particularly if surgery is undertaken after the age of 40 years (85). Ten percent to 25% of patients may develop new-onset atrial arrhythmias in spite of operation (75,81). Thromboembolic events including transient ischemic attacks or stroke are also observed in 5% to 10% of patients on long-term follow-up, regardless of surgical status (75,81). Atrial arrhythmias may be better tolerated postoperatively and should be managed with conventional therapy, including anticoagulants. Depending on the preoperative status, continued surveillance and conventional medical management of pulmonary hypertension and ventricular dysfunction in addition to acquired cardiac disease are necessary.

Ventricular Septal Defect

Management

For patients with VSD, management issues vary depending on the shunt size as manifested by volume overload of the left side of the heart and the presence or absence of pulmonary hypertension (see the section Outcome for a description of complications). The NHS-1 enrolled 1,280 patients with VSD from 1958 to 1969 (91). The overall 25-year survival rate for all patients managed with medical or surgical therapy is 87%, with mortality increasing with the severity of the VSD (90). Adult presentation is most frequently that of a small restrictive VSD, native or postsurgical, or that of a large unoperated VSD with Eisenmenger's complex (70).

Patients with Eisenmenger's complex can survive into the fourth decade (91). The focus of management for patients with Eisenmenger's complex centers around the medical complications of cyanosis. These include death due to intracardiac or pulmonary complications, prevention of infective endocarditis, and systemic complications related to the neurologic, hematologic, and renal systems. These issues are discussed in this chapter as part of a discussion of the medical complications of cyanosis applicable to all patients with Eisenmenger's syndrome.

Excluding those with Eisenmenger's physiology, the majority of unoperated patients have a small VSD and therefore have a favorable long-term prognosis (90). Late results after operative closure of isolated VSDs show residual patency in up to 20% of cases (96) but with only a 5% incidence of need for reoperation, indicating that most residual surgical defects are small (90). For patients with small residual defects, native or surgical management revolves around endocarditis prophylaxis and complications related to secondary valvular anomalies. Perimembranous defects may regress in size through aneurysm formation by engaging part of the septal tricuspid leaflet, resulting in secondary tricuspid insufficiency (97). Prolapse of the right or noncoronary cusp results in acquired aortic valve disease in approximately 2% of patients, regardless of surgical status (90). This occurs most frequently with subarterial outlet VSDs, but also with perimembranous and inlet defects (98). The surgical management of this group of patients is controversial and needs to take into account the location of the VSD, the degree of aortic regurgitation, and the patient's age (99,100). Hence, for a substrate of patients with small VSDs, the potential for progressive valvular insufficiency necessitates careful consideration and follow-up even after the defect is closed.

Patients with moderate pulmonary hypertension and operated or unoperated VSD require particular consideration. Fifteen percent of patients who had a large VSD in infancy or childhood, surgically closed when pulmonary vascular resistance was normal, are found to have indirect evidence of pulmonary hypertension on long-term follow-up, even in the absence of a residual shunt (90). These may represent a substrate of patients in whom factors responsible for triggering the development of pulmonary vascular disease are already engaged at time of VSD closure. When a VSD is present and appears small but the pulmonary pressure is moderately elevated, the left heart is enlarged, or both, there may have been partial closure of the VSD, either through a spontaneous reduction in size or through surgical intervention. One of two hemodynamic scenarios is possible: Either the pulmonary hypertension is "residual" from a previous large shunt and is not related to current shunt size or there is a significant moderate residual shunt, the closure of which may be beneficial (87,90). If surgical closure is contemplated and pulmonary artery pressure, pulmonary vascular resistance, or both are greater than two-thirds systemic, there should be a net left-to-right shunt of at least 1.5:1.0 or evidence of reversibility during pulmonary vascular reactivity studies before proceeding to surgical repair (87).

Sudden cardiac death after surgical repair of VSD occurs in 2% of patients (90,96). The etiology is unclear, and it remains surprising that even patients with small VSDs may be at risk for sudden cardiac death (90). It is reasonable, however, to consider age at operation and the presence of pulmonary hypertension as possible contributing factors. Abnormal myocardium long exposed to volume or pressure overload or both, with or without surgical scar, is likely to provide the substrate for arrhythmias and heart block. Rhythm disturbances after surgical closure of VSDs include tachyarrhythmias and conduction disturbances (90,96,101). Right bundle branch block is reported to occur in 30% to 60% of patients and appears independent of whether the VSD was repaired through an atrial or ventricular incision (90,96,101). Right bundle branch block with left-axis deviation is seen in 3% to 15% of patients (96,101). First-degree atrioventricular block occurs in approximately 10% of patients and the incidence of complete heart block on long-term follow-up is 1% to 3% (96,101). On 12-lead electrocardiography, couplets are observed in 18% of patients, while nonsustained ventricular tachycardia occurs in 5% of patients. Arrhythmia management should be symptom directed, with particular attention paid to reversible hemodynamic factors. Unexplained syncope is usually an indication for an electrophysiology study when Holter monitoring is unrevealing, and there are no exercise-induced arrhythmias.

Patent Ductus Arteriosus

Management

Most of the patients with moderate or large PDA have undergone ductal ligation in infancy (see the section Outcome for a description of complications). Typically, these patients have had the lesion repaired early enough that few sequelae can be expected to occur. If the clinical examination, electrocardiography, and chest radiography results are normal, surveillance requirements are minimal.

Adult patients with a PDA but without an audible murmur may come from one of two groups: those with Eisenmenger's physiology and irreversible pulmonary vascular obstructive disease, or those with a fortuitously discovered PDA on echocardiography. The management of patients with Eisenmenger's disease is as outlined for patients with VSD and Eisenmenger's physiology and is described later in this chapter (see Eisenmenger's Syndrome). Based on the observation that endocarditis has been documented in conjunction with an audible murmur, the current consensus is that the presence of a silent duct does not warrant closure unless endarteritis has occurred (87).

In all other patients, in the presence of a PDA with an audible murmur, the combined risk of endarteritis, left-sided heart failure, and late mortality provides the rationale for shunt closure (87). Between 1951 and 1984, 117 patients were seen at The Cleveland Clinic with a diagnosis of isolated PDA (107). Although the majority of patients was in NYHA class I or II on initial presentation, significantly higher mortality was found in the nonsurgical patient group. After a mean follow-up of 18 years, mortality occurred in 39% of the nonsurgical compared with 7% of the surgical group. Sixty percent of the patients who underwent ductal ligation reported symptomatic improvement compared with 19% of patients without ductal closure (107). These findings underscore the poor outcome of unoperated patients, even in the absence of significant symptoms at the time of presentation. If pulmonary artery pressure, pulmonary vascular resistance, or both are greater than two-thirds systemic, there should be a net left-to-right shunt of at least 1.5:1.0 or evidence of reversibility during pulmonary vascular reactivity studies before proceeding with PDA occlusion (87).

Options for ductal repair include surgical closure and transcatheter methods. Reported operative mortality varies from 0% to 8% (111–114). Calcification of the aortic end of the ductus and excessive bleeding if pulmonary hypertension is present may complicate the surgical approach and lead to incomplete ductal closure in adults (111,113). As described previously, transcatheter device closure or coil occlusion is considered the procedure of choice for PDA closure in adults (30,32–34,40,87).

Obstructive Lesions of the Right and Left Ventricular Outflow Tracts

The focus of the discussion that follows is on the most common single obstructive lesions of the pulmonary and aortic valves and aortic coarctation. Other anatomic variants are defined and referenced in the Prevalence and Anat-

omy section for each lesion. Obstructive lesions of the outflow tract are complicated by the secondary effects of pressure overload in the chamber proximal to the obstruction. In the presence of significant lesions, the inability to increase systemic or pulmonary blood flow in the face of a fixed obstruction, exercise intolerance, inadequate myocardial perfusion, ventricular arrhythmias, and sudden death requires monitoring, activity restriction, and timely intervention. Although recommendations for intervention are based on peak-to-peak gradients measured at cardiac catheterization, serial echocardiographic Doppler measurements can be used to assess initial disease and screen for significant changes in severity with the knowledge that cardiac catheterization–derived peak gradients correlate best with mean gradients obtained by echo-Doppler (115).

Pulmonary Stenosis

Management

For patients with pulmonary stenosis, indications for intervention should be tailored to symptoms, subjective and objective exercise tolerance, and the presence or absence of syncope and arrhythmias (see the section Outcome for a description of complications). Data from the NHS-1 and NHS-2 have been used to support recommendations for the management of valvar pulmonary stenosis (87,122). Intervention is usually indicated for severe lesions, defined as peak pulmonary gradients of greater than 80 mm Hg obtained on cardiac catheterization. Intervention is also indicated in patients with gradients greater than or equal to 50 mm Hg and symptoms. Conservative management is indicated for mild stenosis, defined as a gradient of less than 40 mm Hg. Unlimited athletic participation is allowed for asymptomatic patients with a peak echo-Doppler gradient of less than 50 mm Hg in patients with pulmonary stenosis (123).

The advent of balloon valvuloplasty for pulmonary valve obstruction has facilitated the decision to intervene in young patients, in whom the prospect of delaying or avoiding surgery with or without valve replacement is attractive (see previous discussion). Surgical valvulotomy remains a viable and safe alternative when valvuloplasty is not possible (124).

Aortic Stenosis

Management

For patients with aortic stenosis acquired as children, indications for intervention should be tailored to absolute gradients as well as symptoms (see the section Outcome for a description of complications). Data from the NHS-1 and NHS-2 can be used to support recommendations for the management of valvar aortic stenosis (87,132,133). Conservative management is generally indicated only for mild stenosis, defined as a peak cardiac catheterization gradient of less than 25 mm Hg, although close supervision is required because 20% of these patients are expected to require an intervention during long-term follow-up. The significant incidence of death during exercise in patients with severe aortic stenosis (134) underscores the need for close supervision and serial assessment for progression of disease. This is well reflected in the contrast between recommended exercise parameters for patients with pulmonic and aortic valve disease (123). Unlimited athletic participation is only allowed for asymptomatic patients with a peak echo-Doppler gradient of less than 20 mm Hg, and for patients with aortic stenosis, only if there are normal electrocardiogram and exercise test results. For patients in whom moderate or severe aortic stenosis is acquired during adulthood, indications for intervention are similar to those described for patients with other forms of acquired aortic valve disease described in Chapter 22.

In the absence of significant aortic insufficiency, transcatheter aortic valvotomy can be achieved successfully in children, although results are less uniform and less predictable than with pulmonary valvotomy (135). In young adults, aortic valvuloplasty can be considered as described previously. Calcification limits the procedural success, prompting consideration of well-established surgical alternatives described elsewhere in this text.

In patients with fixed fibromuscular subaortic stenosis, aortic regurgitation occurs in over 50% of cases (126) as the jet damages one or more of the leaflets of an otherwise normal valve. For these patients, surgical closure is indicated with resting gradients greater than 50 mm Hg, particularly in the presence of more than mild aortic insufficiency to prevent further deterioration of the valve (87,136).

Aortic Coarctation

Management

Intervention in patients with coarctation or recoarctation should be performed with gradients greater than 50 mm Hg documented by cardiac catheterization (145) (see the section Outcome for a description of complications). For patients with gradients above 20 mm Hg, the occurrence of symptoms, systemic hypertension, or both warrant consideration for intervention (87).

Surgical intervention is well established (141). Surgery is more hazardous in adults than in children. When patients of all ages are considered, perioperative death rates are 3% (141) or less. The incidence of paraplegia due to spinal cord injury is less than 1% and the preferred surgical approach is resection with end-to-end anastomosis of the descending aorta (119). This approach has the advantage of removing the site of cystic medial necrosis, which has been observed at the site of coarctation, thereby decreasing susceptibility to aneurysm formation and dissection (146). Recoarctation is least common when an end-to-end anastomosis is performed, but the prevalence varies from 11% requiring a reoperation (141) to as high as 30%, depending on the age of repair and the surgical approach used (147). Latent development of coronary artery disease (141) and systemic hypertension (147) require lifelong monitoring (142).

Percutaneous coarctoplasty is being increasingly used as an alternative to surgical intervention (see Interventional Cardiac Catheterization). It is the treatment of choice for focal recoarctation in adult patients who are previously operated. For adults with native coarctation, the choice of surgery or percutaneous coarctoplasty depends on the coarctation anatomy, the presence or absence of associated anomalies, as well as local expertise (87,148).

Complex Lesions

Tetralogy of Fallot

Management

Long-term management in the patient with TOF is focused on maximizing right ventricular function, the need for surgical or percutaneous intervention, and arrhythmia therapy (see the section Outcome for a description of complications). An unoperated or palliated adult with TOF should be considered for full repair. Candidacy for repair depends on the pulmonary vascular bed in a patient who has been palliated and on biventricular function in a patient who is unoperated. Indications for reoperation in a patient who has undergone physiologic repair most commonly include recurrent stenosis in the right ventricular outflow tract if the right ventricular pressure is greater than two-thirds systemic or if residual pulmonary stenosis occurs in combination with significant pulmonary regurgitation (87). Other indications include the presence of a significant residual VSD or significant aortic regurgitation. The indication for pulmonary valve replacement in a patient with asymptomatic significant pulmonary insufficiency remains controversial (159), but surgery is recommended when progressive right ventricular dilatation and dysfunction occur, particularly in the presence of significant arrhythmia.

Hemodynamic complications coexist with arrhythmias. The most contentious is the well-named *ectopic* ventricular beat, poorly understood and difficult to manage. Ventricular arrhythmias can be detected on a 12-lead electrocardiogram in 10% of patients, during an exercise test in 40% of patients, and during 24-hour Holter monitoring in 40% to 60% of patients (160,163). Although symptomatic patients with atrial or ventricular arrhythmia should be treated with antiarrhythmic therapy, it is not recommended to attempt suppression of ventricular ectopy in those who are without symptoms (164).

On 12-lead electrocardiography, a QRS duration of more than 180 ms correlates with right ventricular size, sustained monomorphic ventricular tachycardia, and sudden cardiac death (165,166). In addition to sustained ventricular tachycardia, severe right ventricular systolic hypertension (152,163) and significant pulmonary regurgitation (165) have both been implicated in sudden cardiac death, which is reported in up to 5% of patients after TOF repair (162). The presence of ventricular arrhythmia in combination with right ventricular pressure or volume overload conspires to increase the risk of sudden death more than either one alone, and therefore in the presence of either, the other should always be sought.

Monitoring of arrhythmias may be undertaken using 24-hour Holter monitoring and exercise testing every 1 to 2 years. Underlying hemodynamics, using two-dimensional and Doppler echocardiography, should be carefully and serially reassessed, particularly in the event of a change in frequency or complexity of ventricular ectopy. A reversible cause for a new-onset ventricular arrhythmia such as a rise in right ventricular pressure or a change in right ventricular function should not be missed. There is no role for routine electrophysiologic testing in the prevention of sudden death, but patients with unexplained syncope should be referred for detailed assessment in specialized centers. In addition to surgical or percutaneous intervention aimed at improving significant hemodynamic lesions, antiarrhythmic therapy, pacemakers, and implantable defibrillators may be indicated.

Pulmonary Atresia with Ventricular Septal Defect

Management

Staged reconstructive operations are now performed on a broad range of patients with PA-VSD, but long-term results of complex surgical management remain uncertain. Of adult survivors, two-thirds may be eligible for physiologic repair with low postoperative mortality and seemingly favorable outcome (167). Whether complex unifocalization techniques are destined to provide the best long-term follow-up remains to be seen, but consideration should be given to surgical management in specialized centers where expertise is available.

Complete Transposition of the Great Arteries

Management

In patients who have undergone Senning's or Mustard's operation arrhythmia management, systemic right ventricular dysfunction, and the need for reoperation constitute the key issues in long-term follow-up (see the section Outcome for a description of complications). Reoperation is performed in an approximate 20% of patients (181). The indications relate to baffle leak or obstruction, significant systemic tricuspid regurgitation, progressive left ventricular outflow tract obstruction, or rarely pulmonary venous obstruction (181).

Long-term follow-up reveals an increasing incidence of bradyarrhythmias and supraventricular tachyarrhythmias. Surveillance of arrhythmias should include Holter monitoring and exercise testing at regular intervals. Every attempt should be made to maintain the patient in sinus rhythm, using electrical cardioversion, medical therapy, or both. Pacemaker insertion should be considered in patients with symptomatic bradyarrhythmias. Transvenous pacing with fixation in the morphologic left ventricle (subpulmonary) may be required with or without antitachycardia pacing. Baffle integrity should always be verified to rule out obstruction or leak possibly giving rise to paradoxical emboli. Epicardial pacing is an alternative when ventricular access is hampered by small venous baffle channels. Referral for electrophysiologic studies should be considered in the event of unexplained syncope or arrhythmias unresponsive to medical therapy. Radiofrequency catheter ablation of supraventricular tachycardias can be performed in experienced specialized centers (182). The concurrent monitoring of hemodynamics is crucial. New arrhythmias should always prompt a search for a change in ventricular function or progressive atrioventricular valvar regurgitation requiring tricuspid valve replacement or repair. Trials are ongoing to examine if afterload reduction with angiotensin-converting enzyme inhibitors or receptor blockers may improve systemic right ventricular dysfunction.

For patients with unmanageable systemic right ventricular failure, atrial baffle takedown with a late arterial switch operation has been attempted as an alternative to heart transplantation (183–186). At the current time, mortality for this procedure is high, and much remains to be learned before this can be recommended. The problems delineated previously provide the rationale for the widespread application of the arterial switch operation whereby the left ventricle is reinstated to perform its destined systemic function, and the mismatch between morphology and function is restored. For the arterial switch operation, center-specific series are now emerging with encouraging results (187). Cumulative 15-year survival is over 85% and is expected to increase as improved early mortality makes an impact. The most common complication is neopulmonary stenosis, and thus far, arrhythmias and coronary complications are infrequent (187).

Right-Sided Ebstein's Anomaly

Management

In patients with Ebstein's anomaly, the indications for surgery are deterioration in functional class, progressive cardiomegaly or tricuspid regurgitation, and worsening cyanosis (87) (see the section Outcome for a description of complications). For surgical purposes, Carpentier has distinguished four types of Ebstein's anomalies emphasizing the mobility of the anterior leaflet of the tricuspid valve (type A and B) or its restricted motion (type B and C) as well as the variable degree of the septal leaflet displacement and the variable size and function of the atrialized right ventricle and the true right ventricle (194). Surgical options used in patients with Ebstein's anomaly include tricuspid valve replacement (195) or repair (194,196–198) of the tricuspid valve and closure of the atrial septal defect. Preservation of the native tricuspid valve and feasibility of tricuspid valvuloplasty depend on the size and mobility of the tricuspid leaflet used to construct a unicuspid right atrioventricular valve (194,196–198). Although early reports were associated with a mortality of 25% (193), more recent reports have shown early and late mortality of 3% to 14% with (195) or without (194,199) tricuspid valve replacement. In patients with high-risk preoperative anatomy the inclusion of a bidirectional cavopulmonary shunt decreases operative mortality (200). Addition of the Maze procedure in experienced centers is expected to reduce the incidence of atrial arrhythmias (201).

Congenitally Corrected Transposition of the Great Arteries

Management

In patients with congenitally corrected transposition of the great arteries, management issues relate to maintenance of systemic right ventricular function, treatment of heart block, and surgical correction of residual or associated lesions (see the section Outcome for a description of complications). Trials are ongoing to determine the effectiveness of afterload reduction in improving ventricular performance. Indications for surgery fall into one of three categories: pacemaker insertion, correction of associated VSD or pulmonary stenosis, and atrioventricular valve replacement or repair. Permanent pacing is usually required in the presence of complete heart block. DDD pacing is preferable to maximize ventricular filling in a systemic morphologic right ventricle. Surgical ablation of accessory pathways sometimes occurs fortuitously or with surgical intervention on the tricuspid valve. In the presence of a shunt, transvenous pacing is contraindicated because of the risk of paradoxical emboli. A VSD should be closed when the shunt is significant. Intervention or reintervention for pulmonary stenosis should be considered when the left ventricular outflow tract gradient exceeds 60 to 70 mm Hg. For uncomplicated congenitally corrected transposition of the great arteries, the timing of surgical intervention for atrioventricular valvular regurgitation remains controversial but should be considered in patients with moderate atrioventricular valve regurgitation in the face of worsening systemic right ventricular function. Early and late surgical mortality appears related to progressive ventricular failure. Postoperative survivorship correlates with a preoperative ventricular ejection fraction (208). A poor outcome occurs when preoperative ejection fraction is less than 40% to 45% (208).

Univentricular Heart and Tricuspid Atresia

Management

Patients with univentricular heart and tricuspid atresia require a detailed evaluation with noninvasive and invasive imaging techniques. Two-dimensional echocardiography and Doppler interrogation as well as MRI are used to determine ventricular and atrioventricular valve function, pulmonary artery pressure and resistance, and pulmonary anatomy. When biventricular repair is not feasible, patients may benefit from further palliation with a Glenn's shunt or may be eligible for the Fontan operation.

In both instances, a direct anastomosis is performed between the systemic venous and pulmonary circulations. The Glenn's anastomosis diverts part of the systemic venous return to the lungs, whereas the Fontan procedure and its variants divert the entire systemic venous circulation to the pulmonary vascular bed. Both are done with the goal of improving oxygenation and loading conditions of the systemic ventricle. Partial volume unloading of the single ventricle can be achieved with a bidirectional Glenn's anastomosis (215). Cavopulmonary shunts confer long-term benefit to ventricular function when compared with aortopulmonary shunts (216). Actuarial survival with Glenn's shunt is 84% and 66% at 10 and 20 years, respectively (10).

Fontan Operation

Since its first application in patients with tricuspid atresia in 1972, the Fontan procedure has undergone multiple modifications, resulting in improved surgical technique and expanded criteria for surgical candidacy. In its most recent anatomic variants, direct anastomosis between the systemic venous and the pulmonary circulations is achieved by bypassing the systemic venous ventricle (modified Fontan) or both the systemic venous atrium and ventricle (total cavopulmonary anastomosis) with or without a fenestration (217,218). In the absence of a pulsatile subpulmonary chamber, pulmonary pressures must necessarily be low. In the presence of a fenestration, the established communication between the Fontan conduit and the atrial cavity allows "decompression" of the pulmonary pressures maximizing flow through the pulmonary vascular bed. The goals of the Fontan operation are threefold: relief of cyanosis, maximal reduction of volume loading of the systemic ventricle, and maintenance of appropriate cardiac output. For optimal results, a successful Fontan operation requires preserved ventricular function, minimal atrioventricular valve regurgitation, unobstructed anastomosis between the systemic veins and the pulmonary arteries, as well as a low pulmonary vascular resistance. ❦ g34

EISENMENGER'S SYNDROME

Definition

The designation *Eisenmenger's syndrome* is not synonymous with pulmonary hypertension in a cyanotic patient with CHD. The term is reserved for patients in whom, in the presence of pulmonary vascular obstructive disease, pulmonary vascular resistance is fixed and irreversible. These findings in combination with the absence of left-to-right shunting make the patient inoperable in terms of physiologic repair or further palliation. It then becomes useful to designate the patient's physiology and its consequences as Eisenmenger's syndrome. The focus of management and therapy of chronic cyanotic heart disease is described.

Outcome and Cardiovascular Management

Survival into the seventh decade is rare but has been documented in Eisenmenger's patients (235,236) and is determined by the underlying cardiac condition and the medical complications of cyanosis. Mortality is high, and up to two-thirds of the deaths are sudden and unexpected. The etiology of sudden cardiac death remains poorly defined (235–237). Multiple factors including arrhythmias have been described. Symptomatic arrhythmia should be treated with individualized antiarrhythmic therapy depending on the presence or absence of ventricular dysfunction. An implantable defibrillator should be considered in patients with syncope and documented concurrent ventricular arrhythmia. The decision to use anticoagulants in patients with cyanosis is complicated by the presence of bleeding diathesis. Patients with atrial fibrillation should receive warfarin therapy with judicious monitoring of international normalized ratio levels.

MANAGEMENT OF CYANOTIC PATIENTS

Cyanosis is seen when persistent venous-to-arterial mixing results in hypoxemia. When cyanosis is not relieved, chronic hypoxemia and erythrocytosis result in systemic complications that require continued surveillance. Medical complications of cyanosis (238) are observed in unoperated or palliated adult patients with CHD. Hematologic, neurologic, renal, and rheumatic complications (236) and their management (239) are well described. Hematologic management is described here.

Hematologic complications (240) of chronic hypoxemia include erythrocytosis, iron deficiency, and bleeding diathesis. Erythrocytosis is different from polycythemia, which is the result of an increase in cellular mass not only of red cells, but also of white cells and platelets. Symptoms of hyperviscosity include headaches, faintness, dizziness, fatigue, altered mentation, visual disturbances, paresthesias, tinnitus, and myalgias. Patients with compensated erythrocytosis establish equilibrium hematocrit at higher levels in an iron-replete state with minimal symptoms. Patients with decompensated erythrocytosis manifest unstable rising hematocrit levels and experience severe hyperviscosity symptoms. In the iron-replete state, moderate to severe hyperviscosity symptoms may occur, typically when hematocrit levels are in excess of 65%.

Iron deficiency (241) is a common finding in cyanotic adult patients occurring because of inappropriate phlebotomy or excessive bleeding. Although normochromic erythrocytosis is not usually symptomatic at hematocrit levels of less than 65%, iron deficiency may manifest as symptoms similar to hyperviscosity at hematocrits well below 65%. If iron deficiency anemia is confirmed, careful iron replacement with 325 mg of ferrous sulfate or 65 mg of supplemental iron should be prescribed until an increase in hematocrit is detected, typically within 1 week. A significant and rapid increase in hematocrit is undesirable as it may exacerbate hyperviscosity symptoms, leading to phlebotomy, which can in turn worsen the iron deficiency (240).

Hemostatic abnormalities (240) have been documented in cyanotic patients with erythrocytosis and can occur in up to 20% of patients. In a minority of patients, hemoptysis or postoperative bleeding can be life-threatening. An elevated prothrombin and partial thromboplastin time, decreased levels of various coagulation factors, in addition to thrombocytopenia, and platelet disorders have been described (242,243). The management of bleeding diathesis is determined by the clinical circumstance, the severity, and the abnormal hemostatic parameters. Aspirin, heparin, and coumadin should be avoided unless indicated for chronic atrial fibrillation or in the presence of a mechanical prosthetic valve. Platelet transfusions, fresh frozen plasma, vitamin K, and cryoprecipitate and desmopressin can be used to treat severe bleeding.

Pulmonary thrombosis *in situ* and pulmonary hemorrhage have been described in up to 30% of patients with Eisenmenger's VSD who have CT scans of the chest (236,244). Typically, *in situ* thrombosis presents in a patient with a rapid clinical decline associated with progressive hypoxemia, marking the terminal stage of the disease. The tendency to form laminated thrombus in calcified, aneurysmal proximal pulmonary arteries is poorly understood. Currently, no benefit has been observed with the use of oral, intravenous, or intrapulmonary anticoagulants or from an attempt at pulmonary endarterectomy. The risk of bleeding and the potential for massive pulmonary hemorrhage continue to appear to outweigh the benefits of anticoagulation.

Neurologic complications (245), including cerebral hemorrhage, can occur secondary to hemostatic defects and can be seen after inappropriate use of anticoagulant therapy. Patients with right-to-left shunts may be at risk for paradoxical cerebral emboli. Focal brain injury may provide a nidus for brain abscess if bacteremia supervenes. Attention should be paid to the use of air filters in peripheral intravenous lines to avoid paradoxical emboli through a right-to-left shunt. Cyanotic adults are not at risk for cerebral arterial thrombosis (245). The occurrence of cerebrovascular accidents secondary to cerebral venous thrombosis in children (246,247) does not justify the presumed risk of cerebral arterial thrombosis in adults.

Phlebotomy is indicated under two sets of circumstances: for patients symptomatic of hyperviscosity in a nondehydrated state, most commonly when hematocrit levels exceed 65; and in asymptomatic patients with hematocrit levels greater than 65 before surgery to minimize postoperative bleeding. If symptoms occur with hematocrits of less than 65, evidence of iron deficiency should be sought. When indicated, removal of 500 mL of blood over 30 to 45 minutes followed by quantitative volume replacement with normal saline or dextran can be performed. Symptom control can be achieved with the removal of less than 2 L of blood and sometimes with as little as 250 mL. The procedure may be repeated every 24 hours until improvement occurs. An attempt should be made to achieve symptom control with the smallest quantity of blood removal to avoid iron deficiency. Prophylactic phlebotomy has no place in the prevention of cerebral arterial thrombosis (245,248). ❦ g35

SPECIALIZED ISSUES

Issues Pertinent to Patients Undergoing Noncardiac Surgery

Patients with acyanotic congenital lesions require routine intraoperative and postoperative care for noncardiac procedures. The intracardiac hemodynamics and arrhythmic complications are determined by the native and surgical anatomy. In patients with intracardiac shunts who are cyanotic or acyanotic, the risk of paradoxical embolization is increased (253). To avoid the introduction of air or particles into peripheral or central venous catheters, filters should be placed in intravenous lines, with care taken to avoid the introduction of air or bubbles (256). Other issues of concern include difficulties in venous and arterial access, appropriate volume and airway management, prevention of hemostatic anomalies as described previously, and precautionary measures in the administration of anesthesia (254,256–258). Because hemostatic defects correlate with the severity of hypoxemia and the degree of erythrocytosis, reduction in erythrocyte mass results in improved hemosta-

sis (255). Cyanotic patients undergoing surgery should have prophylactic phlebotomy if the hematocrit is greater than 65 to minimize bleeding. ❦ g36

Endocarditis

Prolonged survival of patients with complex CHD has resulted in a population at increased risk for developing infective endocarditis in unoperated and operated patients (260). Infection most commonly affects sites of turbulent blood flow (260) on the low-pressure side of gradients. Such sites include restrictive VSDs, PDA, the cleft mitral valve, aortic coarctation (most often at the site of an associated bicuspid aortic valve), and prosthetic shunts, valves, and conduits in the postoperative patient (261). These lesions may occur in combination in complex operated cyanotic heart disease. The risk of endocarditis associated with isolated low-pressure lesions in the right side of the heart is low in both simple and complex lesions (260).

Current recommendations for the prevention of bacterial endocarditis apply to most congenital heart lesions with the exception of the isolated secundum ASD, the surgically repaired atrial and ventricular or ductal shunt without residual shunt beyond 6 months after repair. These guidelines should be used for dental, oral, or respiratory procedures (262).

Pregnancy

The reported genetic transmission of maternal CHD to offspring varies from 4% (264) to as high as 16% (267). The conditions that result in the greatest risk to the mother and fetus include Eisenmenger's syndrome, severe pulmonary hypertension, severe left ventricular outflow tract obstruction, Marfan's syndrome with an enlarged aortic root, and heart failure resulting in NYHA class III or IV. Pregnancy in patients with Eisenmenger's syndrome is associated with mortality of up to 50% (268,269). Pregnancy in cyanotic CHD that excludes Eisenmenger's reaction results in a 3% incidence of maternal cardiovascular complications and a near 40% incidence of prematurity (264). These data support the recommendation that pregnancy should be avoided in patients with Eisenmenger's syndrome (87). When women with operated or unoperated CHD are studied as a group, live birth rates are 80% (270). In women after successful coarctation repair, in the presence of an arm-to-leg blood pressure gradient of less than 20 mm Hg, the incidence of preeclampsia is not increased (271). For patients with complex lesions, individual series have reported a total of nearly 250 pregnancies with no maternal mortality (272–275). Successful pregnancies have been reported in patients following surgically repaired transposition of the great arteries (265,272); congenitally corrected transposition of the great arteries (273); Ebstein's anomaly (266,274); and the Fontan operation (275).

TABLE 31.3 EXERCISE RECOMMENDATIONS IN ADULTS WITH CONGENITAL HEART DISEASE

Condition	Unrestricted	Low/moderate intensity[a]	Prohibited
Atrial septal defect[b]	No PHT, no arrhythmia; normal ventricular function	Pulmonary artery pressure >40 mm Hg *with* normal ETT; no arrhythmia	Eisenmenger's syndrome
Ventricular septal defect[b]	Small; no PHT; no arrhythmia; normal ventricular function	Moderate ventricular septal defect	Eisenmenger's syndrome
Patent ductus arteriosus[b]	Small; no PHT; no arrhythmia; normal ventricular function	Pulmonary artery pressure >40 mm Hg with normal ETT; no arrhythmia	Eisenmenger's syndrome
Coarctation[c]	Gradient ≤20 mm Hg arm to leg; normal blood pressure at rest and exercise	Gradient ≥20 mm Hg arm to leg with normal blood pressure and normal ETT	Gradient ≥50 mm Hg arm to leg or aortic aneurysm
Pulmonary stenosis	Gradient <50 mm Hg; no arrhythmia; normal ventricular function	Gradient ≥50 mm Hg	Gradient ≥70 mm Hg or ventricular arrhythmia
Aortic stenosis	Gradient ≤20 mm Hg; normal electrocardiogram; normal ETT; asymptomatic	Gradient >20 mm Hg with normal electrocardiogram; normal ETT; asymptomatic	Gradient ≥50 mm Hg or ventricular arrhythmia
Tetralogy of Fallot after repair	Normal RV pressure; no shunt; no arrhythmia	Increased RV pressure or moderate pulmonary regurgitation or supraventricular tachyarrhythmia	RV pressure ≥65% systemic or ventricular arrhythmia on ETT or severe pulmonary regurgitation
Mustard's or Senning's	—	No cardiomegaly, arrhythmia, or syncope; normal ETT	Cardiomegaly or arrhythmia at rest or exercise
Corrected transposition of the great arteries, unoperated	No cardiomegaly; mild TR; no arrhythmia; normal ETT	Moderate RV dysfunction, moderate TR; no arrhythmia	Severe TR or uncontrolled arrhythmia
Ebstein's	Mild Ebstein's; no arrhythmia; operated with mild TR	Moderate TR with no arrhythmia	Severe Ebstein's or uncontrolled arrhythmia
Fontan	—	Normal O$_2$ saturation with near normal ETT and ventricular function	Moderate/severe mitral regurgitation/TR or uncontrolled arrhythmia

ETT, exercise tolerance test; PHT, pulmonary hypertension; RV, right ventricle; TR, tricuspid regurgitation.
[a]Based on peak dynamic and static components of exercise during competition for individual sports (see credit line).
[b]Unoperated or 6 months after surgery.
[c]Unoperated or 1 year after surgery.
Based on guidelines recommended in Graham TP, Bricker TJ, James FW, et al: Task force 1: congenital heart disease, 26th Bethesda Conference. Eligibility for competition in athletes with cardiovascular abnormalities. *J Am Coll Cardiol* 1994;24:867.

Although small individual series are encouraging, complication rates remain significant even when close follow-up is undertaken in specialized centers. These patients should always be referred to experienced facilities when pregnancy is being considered. ▼ g37

Exercise

The goals of exercise evaluation are to assess functional results of therapeutic interventions and provide guidelines for athletic participation. Patients with residual hemodynamic lesions or unrepaired congenital cardiac anomalies should be evaluated on an annual basis with physical examination, electrocardiography, and cardiac ultrasound if indicated. Pertinent additional tests may include Holter monitoring and exercise testing. Attention should be directed to the detection of pulmonary hypertension, arrhythmias, myocardial dysfunction, and symptoms including exercise-induced syncope, chest pain, or dizziness. A series of guidelines have been proposed for major

groups of congenital heart defects, including shunt lesions, obstructive lesions, and unrepaired and repaired defects (123). These are summarized in Table 31.3.

Psychosocial Issues

In addition to physical defects, mental retardation syndromes and long-term neurologic consequences of cyanotic heart disease or cardiac surgery may be present in the young adult with CHD (263). In comparison with peers, young adults with CHD may choose a more dependent lifestyle with significant involvement of parents or other family members (280).

CONTROVERSIES AND PERSONAL PERSPECTIVES

This subspecialty of cardiology is in its infancy. There are more questions than answers. To date, for an individual

THE FUTURE

A new landscape in CHD care has been created in a way that would have been difficult to envisage a mere 50 years ago. The concepts of surgical palliation and repair evolved sequentially in progressively younger and younger patients. At the current time, our youngest patients are rapidly growing in numbers. They are most likely to have been operated and reoperated. The first intervention may have occurred as early as 24 hours of age. The efforts of pediatric cardiologists and congenital heart surgeons have resulted in one of the most rewarding achievements of twentieth-century medicine. The trends witnessed since the 1950s are shaping our direction as we engage the twenty-first century. We want these patients to stay alive as long and as *well* as possible, defying anatomy and phys-iology as we know it. They continuously bring us back to the reality of persistent, changing, and growing medical and surgical problems. Ultimately, these adults should be framing the pediatric perspective. What we need for this young specialty are data. We need to quantify where we are, rather than describe it. We need national and international databases. We need randomized trials. This should be given priority in parallel with the molecular biology that will enable prevention in the fetus and perhaps the embryo. We encourage our readers to understand the principles that govern current thinking so as to be equipped to follow the direction of a specialty in evolution. The big picture appears promising. We are watching. The color of the future is coming to light as it unfolds.

patient, the most controversial question has been to operate or not to operate? As surgical data accumulate, the consensus favors surgery. However, the same procedure in an infant and in an adult results in an operation with a different outcome, and can we use data generated in high-volume centers to make decisions about individual patients around the world? In the neonate and infant, current surgical strategy aims at intervening early enough to prevent exposure to deleterious physiology. In the adult, lifelong exposure to abnormal hemodynamics may offset the benefits of anatomic correction. On the other hand, a firm understanding of patient's anatomy may permit interventions that were previously not feasible. For both infants and adults, when physiologic repair has taken place, many issues of concern in long-term follow-up continue to exist, as described in this chapter. Right ventricular function and dysfunction take many forms in the numerous variants of CHD. Response to right ventricular remodeling and its prevention is undetermined. The right ventricle as a culprit for sudden cardiac death is atypical for adult cardiologists. The prevention of thromboembolic complications in a right-sided cardiopulmonary circulation without a subpulmonary ventricle is difficult. The organization of health care delivery for this group of patients remains our biggest challenge. Recommendations have been thoroughly laid out at the 32nd Bethesda conference (281,282). Their implementation remains variable. The importance of appropriate referral cannot be overemphasized. Even in patients with simple lesions, the decisions can be complex. Those with adequate training and experience are best suited to make management decisions that take into account the patient's needs and the reality of the medical environment where these needs can be met.

REFERENCES

1. Moller JH, Taubert KA, Allen HD, et al. Cardiovascular health and disease in children: current status. *Circulation* 1994;89:923–930.
2. Somerville J, Webb GD, Skorton DJ, et al. Medical center experiences, 22nd Bethesda Conference. Congenital heart disease after childhood: an expanding population. *J Am Coll Cardiol* 1991;69:18.
3. Deanfield JK. Adult congenital heart disease with special reference to the data on long-term follow-up of patients surviving to adulthood with or without surgical correction. *Eur Heart J* 1992;13:111–116.
4. Moller JH, Anderson RC. 1000 consecutive children with a cardiac malformation with 26 to 37 year follow-up. *Am J Cardiol* 1992;70:661–667.
5. Warnes CA, Liberthson R, Danielson GK, et al. Task force 1: the changing profile of congenital heart disease in adult life. *J Am Coll Cardiol* 2001;37:1170–1175.
6. Marelli AJ. Congenital heart disease in adults. In: Goldman L, Bennett J. *Cecil's textbook of medicine.* Philadelphia: WB Saunders, 1999.
7. Perloff JK. Formulation of the problem. *The clinical recognition of congenital heart disease.* Philadelphia: WB Saunders, 1994:1–8.
8. Cole RB, Muster AJ, Fixler DE, et al. Long-term results of aortopulmonary anastomosis for tetralogy of Fallot. *Circulation* 1971;18:263–271.
9. Stewart S, Alexson C, Manning J. Long-term palliation with the classic Blalock-Taussig shunt. *J Thorac Cardiovasc Surg* 1988;96:117–121.
10. Kopf GS, Laks H, Stansel HC, et al. Thirty-year follow-up of superior vena cava-pulmonary artery (Glenn) shunts. *J Thorac Cardiovasc Surg* 1990;100:662–671.
11. Rothman A, Lang P, Lock JE, et al. Surgical management of subaortic obstruction in single left ventricle and tricuspid atresia. *J Am Coll Cardiol* 1987;10:421–426.

12. Van Praagh R, Weinberg PM, Smith SD, et al. Malpositions of the heart. In: Adams FH, Emmanouilides GC, Riemenschneider TA, eds. *Moss' heart disease in infants, children, and adolescents.* Baltimore: Williams & Wilkins, 1989:530–580.

13. Levine RA, Jimoh MS, Cape EG, et al. Pressure recovery distal to a stenosis: potential cause of gradient "overestimation" by Doppler echocardiography. *J Am Coll Cardiol* 1989;13:706–715.

14. Salustri A, Spitaels S, McGhie J, et al. Transthoracic three-dimensional echocardiography in adult patients with congenital heart disease. *J Am Coll Cardiol* 1995;26:759–767.

15. Vogel M, Ho S, Lincoln C, et al. Three-dimensional echocardiography can simulate intraoperative visualization of congenitally malformed hearts. *Ann Thorac Surg* 1995;60:1282–1288.

16. Heusch A, Rubo J, Krogmann ON, et al. Volumetric analysis of the right ventricle in children with congenital heart defects: comparison of biplane angiography and transthoracic 3-dimensional echocardiography. *Cardiol Young* 1999;9:577–584.

17. Li J, Sanders SP. Three-dimensional echocardiography in congenital heart disease. *Curr Opin Cardiol* 1999;14:53–59.

18. Marelli AJ, Child JS, Perloff JK. Transesophageal echocardiography in congenital heart disease in the adult. *Cardiol Clin* 1993;3:505–520.

19. Ammash NM, Seward JB, Warnes CA, et al. Partial anomalous pulmonary venous connection: diagnosis by transesophageal echocardiography. *J Am Coll Cardiol* 1997;29:1351–1358.

20. Pascoe R, Oh J, Warnes C, et al. Diagnosis of sinus venosus atrial septal defect with transesophageal echocardiography. *Circulation* 1996;94:1049–1055.

21. Andrade A, Vargas-Barron J, Rijlaarsdam M, et al. Utility of transesophageal echocardiography in the examination of adult patients with patent ductus arteriosus. *Am Heart J* 1995;130:543–546.

22. O'Leary P, Hagler D, Seward J, et al. Biplane intraoperative transesophageal echocardiography in congenital heart disease. *Mayo Clin Proc* 1995;70:317–326.

23. Ungerleider R, Kisslo J, Greeley W, et al. Intraoperative echocardiography during congenital heart operations: experience from 1,000 cases. *Ann Thorac Surg* 1995;60:S539–S542.

24. Ewert P, Berger F, Daehnert I, et al. Transcatheter closure of atrial septal defects without fluoroscopy: feasibility of a new method. *Circulation* 2000;101:847–849.

25. Chung T. Assessment of cardiovascular anatomy in patients with congenital heart disease by magnetic resonance imaging. *Pediatr Cardiol* 2000;21:18–26.

26. Didier D, Ratib O, Beghetti M, et al. Morphologic and functional evaluation of congenital heart disease by magnetic resonance imaging. *J Magn Reson Imaging* 1999;10:639–655.

27. Helbing WA, de Roos A. Clinical applications of cardiac magnetic resonance imaging after repair of tetralogy of Fallot. *Pediatr Cardiol* 2000;21:70–79.

28. Berger RM. Possibilities and impossibilities in the evaluation of pulmonary vascular disease in congenital heart defects. *Eur Heart J* 2000;21:17–27.

29. Rabinovitch M. Pulmonary hypertension: pathophysiology as a basis for clinical decision making. *J Heart Lung Transplant* 1999;18:1041–1053.

30. Rashkind WJ, Mullins CE, Hellenbrand W, et al. Nonsurgical closure of patent ductus arteriosus: clinical application of the Rashkind PDA occluder system. *Circulation* 1987;75:583–592.

31. Bridges ND, Perry SB, Parness I, et al. Transcatheter closure of a large patent ductus arteriosus with the clamshell septal umbrella. *J Am Coll Cardiol* 1991;18:1297–1302.

32. Hosking MCK, Benson LN, Musewe N, et al. Transcatheter occlusion of the persistently patent ductus arteriosus. A forty-month follow-up and prevalence of residual shunting. *Circulation* 1991;84:2313–2317.

33. Lloyd TR, Fedderly R, Mendelsohn AM, et al. Transcatheter occlusion of patent ductus arteriosus with Gianturco coils. *Circulation* 1993;88:1412–1420.

34. Janorkar S, Goh T, Wilkinson J. Transcatheter closure of patent ductus arteriosus with the use of Rashkind occluders and/or Gianturco coils: long-term follow-up in 123 patients and special reference to comparison, residual shunts, complications, and technique. *Am Heart J* 1999;138:1176–1183.

35. Gray DT, Fyler DC, Walker AM, et al. Clinical outcomes and costs of transcatheter as compared with surgical closure of patent ductus arteriosus. The Patent Ductus Arteriosus Closure Comparative Study Group. *N Engl J Med* 1993;329:1517–1523.

36. Latson LA. Residual shunts after transcatheter closure of patent ductus arteriosus. A major concern or benign "techno-malady"? *Circulation* 1991;84:2591–2593.

37. Schenck MH, O'Laughlin MP, Rokey R, et al. Transcatheter occlusion of patent ductus arteriosus in adults. *Am J Cardiol* 1993;72:591–595.

38. Patel HT, Cao QL, Rhodes J, et al. Long-term outcome of transcatheter coil closure of small to large patent ductus arteriosus. *Catheter Cardiovasc Intervent* 1999;47:457–461.

39. Bilkis AA, Alwi M, Hasri S, et al. The Amplatzer duct occluder: experience in 209 patients. *J Am Coll Cardiol* 2001;37:258–261.

40. Thanopoulos BD, Hakim FA, Hiari A, et al. Further experience with transcatheter closure of the patent ductus arteriosus using the Amplatzer duct occluder. *J Am Coll Cardiol* 2000;35:1016–1021.

41. Hung J, Landzberg MJ, Jenkins KJ, et al. Closure of patent foramen ovale for paradoxical emboli: intermediate-term risk of recurrent neurological events following transcatheter device placement. *J Am Coll Cardiol* 2000;35:1311–1316.

42. Sievert H, Babic UU, Hausdorf G, et al. Transcatheter closure of atrial septal defect and patent foramen ovale with ASDOS device (a multi-institutional European trial). *Am J Cardiol* 1998;82:1405–1413.

43. Rao PS, Berger F, Rey C, et al. Results of transvenous occlusion of secundum atrial septal defects with the fourth generation buttoned device: comparison with first, second and third generation devices. International Buttoned Device Trial Group. *J Am Coll Cardiol* 2000;36:583–592.

44. Das GS, Harrison JK, O'Laughlin MP. The Angel Wings

Das devices for atrial septal defect closure. *Curr Interv Cardiol Rep* 2000;2:78–85.

45. Pedra CA, Pihkala J, Lee KJ, et al. Transcatheter closure of atrial septal defects using the Cardio-Seal implant. *Heart* 2000;84:320–326.

46. Chan KC, Godman MJ, Walsh K, et al. Transcatheter closure of atrial septal defect and interatrial communications with a new self expanding nitinol double disc device (Amplatzer septal occluder): multicentre UK experience. *Heart* 1999;82:300–306.

47. Berger F, Ewert P, Bjornstad PG, et al. Transcatheter closure as standard treatment for most interatrial defects: experience in 200 patients treated with the Amplatzer Septal Occluder. *Cardiol Young* 1999;9:468–473.

48. Hijazi ZM, Qi-Ling C, Patel HT, et al. Transesophageal echocardiographic results of catheter closure of atrial septal defect in children and adults using the Amplatzer device. *Am J Cardiol* 2000;85:1387–1390.

49. La Rosee K, Deutsch HJ, Schnabel P, et al. Thrombus formation after transcatheter closure of atrial septal defect. *Am J Cardiol* 1999;84:356–359.

50. Berger F, Vogel M, Alexi-Meskishvili V, et al. Comparison of results and complications of surgical and Amplatzer device closure of atrial septal defects. *J Thorac Cardiovasc Surg* 1999;118:674–678.

51. Qureshi SA. Selection of patients with secundum atrial septal defects for transcatheter device closure [editorial]. *Eur Heart J* 2000;21:510–511.

52. Lock JE, Block PC, McKay RC, et al. Transcatheter closure of ventricular septal defects. *Circulation* 1988;78:361–368.

53. Sideris EB, Walsh KP, Haddad JL, et al. Occlusion of congenital ventricular septal defects by the buttoned device. "Buttoned device" Clinical Trials International Register. *Heart* 1997;77:276–279.

54. Perry SB, Radtke W, Fellows KE, et al. Coil embolization to occlude aortopulmonary collateral vessels and shunts in patients with congenital heart disease. *J Am Coll Cardiol* 1989;13:100–108.

55. Florentine M, Wolfe RR, White RI Jr. Balloon embolization to occlude a Blalock-Taussig shunt. *J Am Coll Cardiol* 1984;3:200–202.

56. Gamillscheg A, Beitzke A, Stein JI, et al. Transcatheter coil occlusion of residual interatrial communications after Fontan procedure. *Heart* 1998;80:49–53.

57. Apostolopoulou SC, Papagiannis J, Hausdorf G, et al. Transcatheter occlusion of atrial baffle leak after mustard repair. *Catheter Cardiovasc Interv* 2000;51:305–307.

58. Perry SB, Rome J, Keane JF, et al. Transcatheter closure of coronary artery fistulas. *J Am Coll Cardiol* 1992;20:205–209.

59. Kambara AM, Pedra CA, Esteves CA, et al. Transcatheter embolization of congenital coronary arterial fistulas in adults. *Cardiol Young* 1999;9:371–376.

60. Chen CR, Cheng TO, Huang T, et al. Percutaneous balloon valvuloplasty for pulmonic stenosis in adolescents and adults. *N Engl J Med* 1996;335:21–25.

61. Teupe CH, Burger W, Schrader R, et al. Late (five to nine years) follow-up after balloon dilation of valvular pulmonary stenosis in adults. *Am J Cardiol* 1997;80:240–242.

62. Sadr-Ameli MA, Sheikholeslami F, Firoozi I, et al. Late results of balloon pulmonary valvuloplasty in adults. *Am J Cardiol* 1998;82:398–400.

63. Powell AJ, Lock JE, Keane JK, et al. Prolongation of RV-PA conduit life span by percutaneous stent implantation. Intermediate-term results. *Circulation* 1995;92:3282–3288.

64. Kreutzer J, Landzberg MJ, Preminger TJ, et al. Isolated peripheral pulmonary artery stenoses in the adult. *Circulation* 1996;93:1417–1423.

65. Rosenfeld HM, Landzberg MJ, Perry SB, et al. Balloon aortic valvuloplasty in the young adult with congenital aortic stenosis. *Am J Cardiol* 1994;73:1112–1117.

66. McCrindle BW, Jones TK, Morrow WR, et al. Acute results of balloon angioplasty of native coarctation versus recurrent aortic obstruction are equivalent. Valvuloplasty and Angioplasty of Congenital Anomalies (VACA) Registry Investigators. *J Am Coll Cardiol* 1996;28:1810–1817.

67. Magee AG, Brzezinska-Rajszys G, Qureshi SA, et al. Stent implantation for aortic coarctation and recoarctation. *Heart* 1999;82:600–606.

68. Harrison DA, McLaughlin PR, Lazzam C, et al. Endovascular stents in the management of coarctation of the aorta in the adolescent and adult: one year follow up. *Heart* 2001;85:561–566.

69. Fawzy ME, Sivanandam V, Galal O, et al. One- to ten-year follow-up results of balloon angioplasty of native coarctation of the aorta in adolescents and adults. *J Am Coll Cardiol* 1997;30:1542–1546.

70. Kaplan S. Natural and postoperative history across age groups. *Cardiol Clin* 1993;11:543–556.

71. Feldt R, Avasthey P, Yoshimasu F, et al. Incidence of congenital heart disease in children born to residents of Olmsted County, Minnesota, 1950–1969. *Mayo Clin Proc* 1971;46:794–784.

72. Feldt R, Porter C, Edwards W, et al. Defects of the atrial septum and the atrioventricular canal. In: Adams FH, Emmanouilides GC, Riemenschneider TA, eds. *Moss' heart disease in infants, children, and adolescents.* Baltimore: Williams & Wilkins, 1989:170–189.

73. Bizarro R, Callahan J, Feldt R, et al. Familial atrial septal defect with prolonged atrioventricular conduction. A syndrome showing the autosomal dominant pattern of inheritance. *Circulation* 1970;41:677–683.

74. Campbell M. Natural history of atrial septal defect. *Br Heart J* 1970;1970:820–826.

75. Murphy JG, Gersh BJ, McGoon MD, et al. Long-term outcome after surgical repair of isolated atrial septal defect. *N Engl J Med* 1990;323:1645–1650.

76. Liberthson RR. Severe mitral regurgitation: a common occurrence in the aging patient with secundum atrial septal defect. *Clin Cardiol* 1981;4:229–232.

77. Besterman E. Atrial septal defect with pulmonary hypertension. *Br Heart J* 1961;23:587–598.

78. Cherian F, Uthaman C, Durairaj M, et al. Pulmonary hypertension in isolated secundum atrial septal defect: high frequency in young patients. *Am Heart J* 1983;105:952–957.

79. Bedford D. The anatomical types of atrial septal defect. Their incidence and clinical diagnosis. *Am J Cardiol* 1960;6:568.

80. Steele PM, Fuster V, Cohen M, et al. Isolated atrial septal defect with pulmonary vascular obstructive disease: long term follow-up and prediction of outcome after surgical correction. *Circulation* 1987;76:1037–1042.

81. Konstantinides S, Geibel A, Olschewski M, et al. A comparison of medical and surgical therapy for atrial septal defect in adults. *N Engl J Med* 1995;333:469–473.

82. Marelli AJ, Alejos JC. Exercise response in atrial septal defect. *Prog Pediatr Cardiol* 1993;2:20–23.

83. St. John Sutton MG, Tajik AJ, McGoon DC. Atrial septal defect in patients ages 60 years or older: operative results and long-term postoperative follow-up. *Circulation* 1981;64:402–409.

84. Shah D, Azhar M, Oakley CM, et al. Natural history of secundum atrial septal defect in adults after medical or surgical treatment: a historical perspective study. *Br Heart J* 1994;71:224–228.

85. Gatzoulis MA, Freeman MA, Siu SC, et al. Atrial arrhythmia after surgical closure of atrial septal defects in adults. *N Engl J Med* 1999;340:839–846.

86. Gatzoulis M, Redington A, Somerville J, et al. Should atrial septal defects in adults be closed? *Ann Thorac Surg* 1996;61:657–659.

87. Therrien J, Dore A, Gersony W, et al. CCC Consensus Conference 2001 update: recommendations for the management of adults with congenital heart disease. Part I. *Can J Cardiol* 2001;17:940–959.

88. Hoffman JIE, Rudolph AM. The natural history of ventricular septal defects in infancy. *Am J Cardiol* 1965;16:634–653.

89. Graham TP, Bender HW, Spach MS. Ventricular septal defect. In: Adams FH, Emmanouilides GC, Riemenschneider TA, eds. *Moss' heart disease in infants, children, and adolescents.* Baltimore: Williams & Wilkins, 1989:189–209.

90. Kidd L, Driscoll DJ, Gersony WM, et al. Second natural history study of congenital heart defects: results of treatment of patients with ventricular septal defects. *Circulation* 1993;87:I-38–I-59.

91. Perloff J. Ventricular septal defect. In: *The clinical recognition of congenital heart disease.* Philadelphia: WB Saunders, 1994:396–440.

92. Moe D, Gentheroth W. Spontaneous closure of uncomplicated ventricular septal defect. *Am J Cardiol* 1987;60:674–680.

93. Sutherland G, Godman M, Smallhorn J, et al. Ventricular septal defects. Two dimensional echocardiographic and morphological correlations. *Br Heart J* 1982;47:316–328.

94. Abbott ME. *Congenital heart disease: Nelson's loose leaf medicine.* Vol. 5. New York: Nelson and Sons, 1932.

95. Rabinovitch M. Pulmonary hypertension. In: Adams FH, Emmanouilides GC, Riemenschneider TA, eds. *Moss' heart disease in infants, children, and adolescents.* Baltimore: Williams & Wilkins, 1989:856–886.

96. Moller JH, Patton C, Varco RL, et al. Late results (30 to 35 years) after operative closure of isolated ventricular septal defect from 1954 to 1960. *Am J Cardiol* 1991;68:1491–1497.

97. Hornberger LK, Sahn DJ, Krabill KA. Elucidation of the natural history of ventricular septal defects by serial Doppler color flow mapping studies. *J Am Coll Cardiol* 1989;13:1111–1118.

98. Rhodes LA, Keane JF, Keane JP, et al. Long follow-up (to 43 years) of ventricular septal defect with audible aortic regurgitation. *Am J Cardiol* 1990;66:340–345.

99. Moreno-Cabral R, Mamiya R, Nakamura F, et al. Ventricular septal defect and aortic insufficiency. Surgical treatment. *J Thorac Cardiovasc Surg* 1977;73:358–365.

100. Trusler G, Williams W, Smallhorn J, et al. Late results after repair of aortic insufficiency associated with ventricular septal defect. *J Thorac Cardiovasc Surg* 1992;103:276–281.

101. Blake W, Chung E, Wesley H, et al. Conduction defects, ventricular arrhythmias, and late death after surgical closure of ventricular septal defect. *Br Heart J* 1982;47:305–315.

102. Perloff JK. Patent ductus arteriosus. In: *The clinical recognition of congenital heart disease.* Philadelphia: WB Saunders, 1994:510–545.

103. Godtfredsen J, Wennerold A, Efsen F, et al. Natural history of vascular ring with clinical manifestations. A follow-up study of 11 unoperated cases. *Scand J Thorac Cardiovasc Surg* 1977;11:75.

104. Castaneda AR, Jonas R, Mayer JE, et al. *Vascular rings, slings and tracheal anomalies. Cardiac surgery of the neonate and infant.* Philadelphia: WB Saunders, 1994:397–409.

105. Krichenko A, Benson L, Burrows P, et al. Angiographic classification of the isolated, persistently patent ductus arteriosus and implications for percutaneous catheter occlusion. *Am J Cardiol* 1989;63:878–880.

106. Ohtsuka S, Kahihana M, Ishikawa T, et al. Aneurysm of patent ductus arteriosus in an adult case: findings of cardiac catheterization, angiography, and pathology. *Clin Cardiol* 1987;10:537.

107. Fisher R, Moodie D, Stera R, et al. Patent ductus arteriosus in adults—long-term follow up: nonsurgical versus surgical treatment. *J Am Coll Cardiol* 1986;8:280–284.

108. Campbell M. Natural history of persistent ductus arteriosus. *Br Heart J* 1968;30:4–13.

109. Houston A, Gnanapragasm J, Lim M, et al. Doppler ultrasound and the silent ductus. *Br Heart J* 1991;65:97–99.

110. Latson LA. Residual shunts after transcatheter closure of patent ductus arteriosus. A major concern or benign "techno-malady"? *Circulation* 1991;84:2591–2593.

111. Ng AS, Vlietstra RE, Danielson GK, et al. Patent ductus arteriosus in patients more than 50 years old. *Int J Cardiol* 1986;11:277–287.

112. Celermajer D, Sholler G, Hughes C, et al. Persistent ductus arteriosus in adults: a review of surgical experience with 25 patients. *Med J Aust* 1991;155:233–236.

113. Kron I, Harman P, Finkelmeier B, et al. The adult ductus: surgical results and long-term follow up. *Am J Surg* 1983;49:546–547.

114. John S, Muralidharan S, Jairaj P, et al. The adult ductus: review of surgical experience with 131 patients. *J Thorac Cardiovasc Surg* 1981;82:314–319.

115. Currie PJ, Hagler DJ, Seward JB. Instantaneous pressure gradient: a simultaneous Doppler and dual catheter correlative study. *J Am Coll Cardiol* 1986;7:800–806.

116. Perloff JK. Congenital pulmonary stenosis. In: *The clinical*

recognition of congenital heart disease. Philadelphia: WB Saunders, 1994:198–230.

117. Rocchini A, Emmanouilides G. Pulmonary stenosis. In: Adams FH, Emmanouilides GC, Riemenschneider TA, eds. *Moss' heart disease in infants, children, and adolescents.* Baltimore: Williams & Wilkins, 1989:308–338.

118. Marvin J, Mahoney L. Pulmonary atresia with intact ventricular septum. In: Adams FH, Emmanouilides GC, Riemenschneider TA, eds. *Moss' heart disease in infants, children, and adolescents.* Baltimore: Williams & Wilkins, 1989:338–348.

119. Drinkwater DC, Laks H, Perloff JK. *Surgical considerations: operation and reoperation: congenital heart disease in adults.* Philadelphia: WB Saunders, 1991:193–212.

120. Jones K, Smith D. The William elfin facies syndrome. *J Pediatr* 1975;86:718–723.

121. Li M, Coles J, McDonald A. Anomalous muscle bundle of the right ventricle: its recognition and surgical treatment. *Br Heart J* 1978;40:1040.

122. Hayes CJ, Gerson WM, Driscoll DJ. Second natural history of congenital heart defects: results of treatment of patients with pulmonary valvar stenosis. *Circulation* 1993;87:28–37.

123. Graham TP, Bricker JT, James FW, et al. Task force 1: congenital heart disease. *J Am Coll Cardiol* 1994;24:867–873.

124. Danielson GC, Exarhos ND, Weidman WH, et al. Pulmonic stenosis with intact ventricular septum. *J Thorac Cardiovasc Surg* 1971;61:228–237.

125. Friedman W. Aortic stenosis. In: Adams FH, Emmanouilides GC, Riemenschneider TA, eds. *Moss' heart disease in infants, children, and adolescents.* Baltimore: Williams & Wilkins, 1989:224–243.

126. Rohlicek CV, del Pino SF, Hosking M, et al. Natural history and surgical outcomes for isolated discrete subaortic stenosis in children. *Heart* 1999;82:708–713.

127. Choi JY, Sullivan ID. Fixed subaortic stenosis: anatomical spectrum and nature of progression. *Br Heart J* 1991;65:280–286.

128. Perloff JK. *Congenital aortic stenosis; congenital aortic regurgitation. The clinical recognition of congenital heart disease.* Philadelphia: WB Saunders, 1994:91–131.

129. de Sa M, Moshkovitz Y, Butany J, et al. Histologic abnormalities of the ascending aorta and pulmonary trunk in patients with bicuspid aortic valve disease: clinical relevance to the Ross procedure. *J Thorac Cardiovasc Surg* 1999;118:588–594.

130. Hahn RT, Roman MJ, Mogtader AH, et al. Association of aortic dilation with regurgitant, stenotic and functionally normal bicuspid aortic valves. *J Am Coll Cardiol* 1992;19:283–288.

131. Nistri S, Sorbo MD, Marin M, et al. Aortic root dilatation in young men with normally functioning bicuspid aortic valves. *Heart* 1999;82:19–22.

132. Keane J, Driscoll D, Gersony W, et al. Second natural history of congenital heart defects: results of treatment of patients with aortic valvar stenosis. *Circulation* 1993;87:16–27.

133. Wagner HR, Ellison RC, Keane JF. Clinical course in aortic stenosis. *Circulation* 1977;56:I-47–I-56.

134. Driscoll DJ, Edwards WD. Sudden unexpected death in children and adolescents. *J Am Coll Cardiol* 1985;5:118B–21B.

135. Rocchini AP, Beekman RH, Shachar BG, et al. Balloon aortic valvuloplasty: results of the valvuloplasty and angioplasty of congenital anomalies registry. *Am J Cardiol* 1990;65:784–789.

136. Brauner R, Laks H, Drinkwater DC Jr, et al. Benefits of early surgical repair in fixed subaortic stenosis. *J Am Coll Cardiol* 1997;30:1835–1842.

137. Fyler DC. Report of the New England regional infant cardiac program. *Pediatrics* 1980;65:375–461.

138. Perloff JK. *Coarctation of the aorta. The clinical recognition of congenital heart disease.* Philadelphia: WB Saunders, 1994:132–169.

139. Dungan WT, Char F, Gerald BE, et al. Pseudocoarctation of the aorta in childhood. *Am J Dis Child* 1970;119:401–406.

140. Campbell M. Natural history of coarctation of the aorta. *Br Heart J* 1970;32:633–640.

141. Cohen M, Fuster V, Steele PM, et al. Coarctation of the aorta: long-term follow-up and prediction of outcome after surgical correction. *Circulation* 1989;80:840–845.

142. Liberthson R, Pennington D, Jacobs M, et al. Coarctation of the aorta: review of 234 patients and clarification management problems. *Am J Cardiol* 1978;43:835–845.

143. Ong C, Canter C, Gutierrez F, et al. Increased stiffness and persistent narrowing of the aorta after successful repair of coarctation of the aorta: relationship to left ventricular mass and blood pressure at rest and with exercise. *Am Heart J* 1992;123:1594–1600.

144. Leandro J, Smallhorn J, Benson L, et al. Ambulatory blood pressure monitoring and left ventricular mass and function after successful surgical repair of coarctation of the aorta. *J Am Coll Cardiol* 1992;20:197–204.

145. Bashore TM, Lieberman EB. Aortic/mitral obstruction and coarctation of the aorta. *Cardiol Clin* 1993;11:617–641.

146. Isner JM, Donaldson RF, Fulton D, et al. Cystic medial necrosis in coarctation of the aorta: a potential factor contributing to adverse consequences observed after percutaneous balloon angioplasty of coarctation sites. *Circulation* 1987;75:689–695.

147. Presbitero P, Demarie D, Villani M, et al. Long term results (15–30 years) of surgical repair of aortic coarctation. *Br Heart J* 1987;57:462–467.

148. Gibbs JL. Treatment options for coarctation of the aorta. *Heart* 2000;84:11–13.

149. Lillehei CW, Cohen M, Warden HE. Direct vision intracardiac surgical correction of the tetralogy of Fallot, pentalogy of Fallot and pulmonary atresia defects: report of first ten cases. *Ann Surg* 1995;142:418–423.

150. Van Praagh R, Etienne L. Arthur Fallot and his tetralogy: a new translation of Fallot's summary and a modern reassessment of this anomaly. *Eur J Cardiothorac Surg* 1989;3:381–386.

151. Katz NM, Blackstone EH, Kirklin JW, et al. Late survival and symptoms after repair of tetralogy of Fallot. *Circulation* 1982;65:403–410.

152. Fuster V, McGoon DC, Kennedy MA, et al. Long-term evaluation (12 to 22 years) of open heart surgery for tetralogy of Fallot. *Am J Cardiol* 1980;46:635–642.

153. Nollert G, Fischlein T, Bouterwek S, et al. Long-term results of total repair of tetralogy of Fallot in adulthood: 35 years follow-up in 104 patients corrected at the age of 18 or older. *Thorac Cardiovasc Surg* 1997;45:178–181.

154. Murphy JG, Gersh BJ, Mair DD, et al. Long-term outcome in patients undergoing surgical repair of tetralogy of Fallot. *N Engl J Med* 1993;329:593–599.

155. Nollert G, Fischlein T, Bouterwek S, et al. Long-term survival in patients with repair of tetralogy of Fallot: 36-year follow-up of 490 survivors of the first year after surgical repair. *J Am Coll Cardiol* 1997;30:1374–1383.

156. Castaneda AR, Jonas R, Mayer JE, et al. *Tetralogy of Fallot: cardiac surgery of the neonate and infant.* Philadelphia: WB Saunders, 1994:215–235.

157. Presbitero P, Demarie D, Aruta E, et al. Results of total correction of tetralogy of Fallot performed in adults. *Ann Thorac Surg* 1988;46:297–301.

158. Joransen JA, Lucas RV, Moller JH. Postoperative haemodynamics in tetralogy of Fallot. A study of 132 children. *Br Heart J* 1979;41:33–39.

159. Therrien J, Siu SC, McLaughlin PR, et al. Pulmonary valve replacement in adults late after repair of tetralogy of Fallot: are we operating too late? *J Am Coll Cardiol* 2000;36:1670–1675.

160. Deanfield JE, McKenna WJ, Hallidie-Smith KA. Detection of late arrhythmia and conduction disturbance after correction of tetralogy of Fallot. *Br Heart J* 1980;44:248–253.

161. Roos-Hesselink J, Perlroth MG, McGhie J, et al. Atrial arrhythmias in adults after repair of tetralogy of Fallot. Correlations with clinical, exercise, and echocardiographic findings. *Circulation* 1995;91:2214–2219.

162. Garson AJ, Randall DC, Gillette PC, et al. Prevention of sudden death after repair of tetralogy of Fallot: treatment of ventricular arrhythmias. *J Am Coll Cardiol* 1985;6:221–227.

163. Garson A, Nihill MR, McNamara DG, et al. Status of the adult and adolescent after repair of tetralogy of Fallot. *Circulation* 1979;59:1232–1240.

164. Cullen S, Celermajer DS, Franklin RCG, et al. Prognostic significance of ventricular arrhythmia after repair of tetralogy of Fallot: a 12-year prospective study. *J Am Coll Cardiol* 1994;23:1151–1155.

165. Gatzoulis MA, Balaji S, Webber SA, et al. Risk factors for arrhythmia and sudden cardiac death late after repair of tetralogy of Fallot: a multicentre study. *Lancet* 2000;356:975–981.

166. Gatzoulis MA, Till JA, Somerville J, et al. Mechanoelectrical interaction in tetralogy of Fallot. QRS prolongation relates to right ventricular size and predicts malignant ventricular arrhythmias and sudden death. *Circulation* 1995;92:231–237.

167. Marelli AJ, Perloff JK, Child JS, et al. Pulmonary atresia with ventricular septal defect in adults. *Circulation* 1994;89:243–251.

168. Rastelli GC, Wallace RB, Ongley PA. Complete repair of transposition of the great arteries with pulmonary stenosis: a review and report of a case corrected by using a new surgical technique. *Circulation* 1969;39:83–95.

169. Castaneda AR, Norwood WI, Lang P. Transposition of the great arteries and intact ventricular septum: anatomical repair in the neonate. *Ann Thorac Surg* 1984;38:438–443.

170. Liebman J, Cullum L, Belloc N. Natural history of transposition of the great arteries: anatomy and birth and death characteristics. *Circulation* 1969;40:237–362.

171. Senning A. Surgical correction of transposition of the great vessels. *Surgery* 1959;45:966–975.

172. Mustard WT. Successful two-stage correction of transposition of the great vessels. *Surgery* 1964;55:469–473.

173. Flinn CJ, Wolff GS, Dick MI, et al. Cardiac rhythm after the Mustard operation for complete transposition of the great arteries. *N Engl J Med* 1984;310:1635–1638.

174. Gelatt M, Hamilton RM, McCrindle BW, et al. Arrhythmia and mortality after the Mustard procedure: a 30-year single-center experience. *J Am Coll Cardiol* 1997;29:194–201.

175. Gewillig M, Cullen S, Mertens B, et al. Risk factors for arrhythmia and death after mustard operation for simple transposition of the great arteries. *Circulation* 1991;84:III-187–III-192.

176. Hagler DJ, Ritter DG, Mair DD, et al. Right and left ventricular function after the mustard procedure in transposition of the great arteries. *Am J Cardiol* 1979;44:276–283.

177. Murphy JH, Barlai-Kovach MM, Mathews RA, et al. Rest and exercise right and left ventricular function late after the Mustard operation: assessment by radionuclide ventriculography. *Am J Cardiol* 1983;51:1520–1526.

178. Warnes CA, Somerville J. Transposition of the great arteries: late results in adolescents and adults after the Mustard procedure. *Br Heart J* 1987;58:148–155.

179. Gatzoulis MA, Walters J, McLaughlin PR, et al. Late arrhythmia in adults with the Mustard procedure for transposition of great arteries: a surrogate marker for right ventricular dysfunction? *Heart* 2000;84:409–415.

180. Garson AJ, Bink-Boelkens M, Hesslein PS. Atrial flutter in the young: a collaborative study of 380 cases. *J Am Coll Cardiol* 1985;6:871–878.

181. Cobanoglu A, Abbruzzese PA, Freimanis I, et al. Pericardial baffle complications following the Mustard operation. *J Thorac Cardiovasc Surg* 1984;87:371–378.

182. Kanter RJ, Papagiannis J, Carboni MP, et al. Radiofrequency catheter ablation of supraventricular tachycardia substrates after Mustard and Senning operations for d-transposition of the great arteries. *J Am Coll Cardiol* 2000;35:428–441.

183. Mee RBB. Severe right ventricular failure after Mustard or Senning operation. *J Thorac Cardiovasc Surg* 1986;92:385–390.

184. Chang AC, Wernovsky G, Wessel DL, et al. Surgical management of late right ventricular failure after Mustard or Senning repair. *Circulation* 1992;86:II-140–II-149.

185. Helvind MH, et al. Ventriculo-arterial discordance: switching the morphologically left ventricle into the systemic circulation after 3 months of age. *Eur J Cardiothorac Surg* 1998;14:173–178.

186. van Son JA, Reddy VM, Silverman NH, et al. Regression of tricuspid regurgitation after two stage arterial switch operation for failing systemic ventricle after atrial inversion operation. *J Thorac Cardiovasc Surg* 1996;111:342–347.

187. Haas F, Wottke M, Poppert H, et al. Long-term survival and functional follow-up in patients after the arterial switch operation. *Ann Thorac Surg* 1999;68:1692–1697.

188. Shiina A, Seward J, Edwards W, et al. Two-dimensional echocardiographic spectrum of Ebstein's anomaly: detailed anatomic assessment. *J Am Coll Cardiol* 1984;3:356–370.

189. Perloff JK. Ebstein's anomaly of the tricuspid valve. In: *The clinical recognition of congenital heart disease*. Philadelphia: WB Saunders, 1994:247–273.

190. Watson H. Natural history of Ebstein's anomaly of tricuspid valve in childhood and adolescence: an international co-operative study of 505 cases. *Br Heart J* 1974;36:417–427.

191. Celemajer D, Bull C, Till J, et al. Ebstein's anomaly: presentation and outcome from fetus to adult. *J Am Coll Cardiol* 1994;23:170–176.

192. Gentles T, Calder A, Clarkson P, et al. Predictors of long-term survival with Ebstein's anomaly of the tricuspid valve. *Am J Cardiol* 1992;69:377–381.

193. Giuliani E, Fuster V, Brandenburg R. The clinical features and natural history of Ebstein's anomaly of the tricuspid valve. *Mayo Clin Proc* 1979;54:163–173.

194. Carpentier A. A new reconstructive operation for Ebstein's anomaly of the tricuspid valve. *J Thorac Cardiovasc Surg* 1988;96:92–101.

195. Kiziltan HT, Theodoro DA, Warnes CA, et al. Late results of bioprosthetic tricuspid valve replacement in Ebstein's anomaly. *Ann Thorac Surg* 1998;66:1539–1545.

196. Mair D, Seward J, Driscoll D, et al. Surgical repair of Ebstein's anomaly: selection of patients and early and late operative results. *Circulation* 1985;72:72–76.

197. Hetzer R, Nagdyman N, Ewert P, et al. A modified repair technique for tricuspid incompetence in Ebstein's anomaly. *J Thorac Cardiovasc Surg* 1998;115:857–868.

198. van Son JA, Kinzel P, Mohr FW. Pericardial patch augmentation of anterior tricuspid leaflet in Ebstein's anomaly. *Ann Thorac Surg* 1998;66:1831–1832.

199. Augustin N, Schmidt-Habelmann P, Wottke M, et al. Results after surgical repair of Ebstein's anomaly. *Ann Thorac Surg* 1997;63:1650–1656.

200. Chauvaud S, Fuzellier JF, Berrebi AP, et al. Bi-directional cavopulmonary shunt associated with ventriculo- and valvuloplasty in Ebstein's anomaly: benefits in high risk patients. *Eur J Cardiothorac Surg* 1998;13:514–519.

201. Theodoro DA, Danielson GK, Porter CJ, et al. Right-sided maze procedure for right atrial arrhythmias in congenital heart disease. *Ann Thorac Surg* 1998;65:149–153.

202. Perloff JK. Congenitally corrected transposition of the great arteries. In: *The clinical recognition of congenital heart disease*. Philadelphia: WB Saunders, 1994:67–91.

203. Connely M, Liu P, Williams W, et al. Congenitally corrected transposition of the great arteries in the adult: functional status and complications. *J Am Coll Cardiol* 1996;27:1238–1243.

204. Dabizzi R, Barletta G, Caprioli G, et al. Coronary artery anatomy in corrected transposition of the great arteries. *J Am Coll Cardiol* 1988;12:486–491.

205. Presbitero P, Somerville J, Rabajoli F, et al. Corrected transposition of the great arteries without associated defects in adult patients: clinical profile and follow up. *Br Heart J* 1995;74:57–59.

206. Prieto LR, Hordof AJ, Secic M, et al. Progressive tricuspid valve disease in patients with congenitally corrected transposition of the great arteries. *Circulation* 1998;98:997–1005.

207. Esper W, Moodie D, Gill C, et al. Congenitally corrected transposition of the great vessels in adults. *J Am Coll Cardiol* 1983;1:663–670.

208. van Son J, Danielson G, Huhta J, et al. Late results of systemic atrioventricular valve replacement in corrected transposition. *J Thorac Cardiovasc Surg* 1995;109:642–653.

209. Perloff JK, Child JS. Survival patterns. In: Perloff JK, Child JS, eds. *Congenital heart disease in adults*. Philadelphia: WB Saunders, 1998.

210. Perloff JK. *The univentricular heart: the clinical recognition of congenital heart disease*. Philadelphia: WB Saunders, 1994:635–658.

211. Keith JD, Rowe RD, Ulad P. *Heart disease in infancy and childhood*. 2nd ed. New York: Macmillan, 1967.

212. Jordan JC, Sanders CA. Tricuspid atresia with prolonged survival. *Am J Cardiol* 1966;18:112.

213. Moodie DS, Ritter DG, Tajik AJ, et al. Long-term follow-up in the unoperated univentricular heart. *Am J Cardiol* 1984;53:1124–1128.

214. Moodie DS, Ritter DG, Tajik AH, et al. Long-term follow-up after palliative operation for univentricular heart. *Am J Cardiol* 1984;53:1648–1651.

215. Allgood NL, Alejos J, Drinkwater DC, et al. Effectiveness of the bidirectional Glenn shunt procedure for volume unloading in the single ventricle patient. *Am J Cardiol* 1994;74:834–836.

216. Gatzoulis MA, Munk MD, Williams WG, et al. Definitive palliation with cavopulmonary or aortopulmonary shunts for adults with single ventricle physiology. *Heart* 2000;83:51–57.

217. deLaval M, Kilner P, Gewillig M, et al. Total cavopulmonary connection: a logical alternative to atriopulmonary connection for complex Fontan operations. *J Thorac Cardiovasc Surg* 1988;96:682–695.

218. Lee C, Hartzell V, Danielson G, et al. Comparison of atriopulmonary versus atrioventricular connections for modified Fontan/Kreutzer repair of tricuspid valve atresia. *J Thorac Cardiovasc Surg* 1986;92:1038–1048.

219. Mair DD, Danielson GK, Schaff HU, et al. The Fontan procedure in adults: operative and late results with 121 patients. *J Am Coll Cardiol* 1994;28:119A.

220. Humes RA, Mair DD, Porter CJ, et al. Results of the modified Fontan operation in adults. *Am J Cardiol* 1988;612:602–604.

221. Grand GP, Mansell AL, Garofano RP, et al. Cardiorespiratory response to exercise after the Fontan procedure for tricuspid atresia. *Pediatr Res* 1988;24:1–5.

222. Driscoll DJ, Offord KP, Feldt RH, et al. Five to fifteen year Fallot after Fontan operation. *Circulation* 1992;85:469–496.

223. Carp H, Jayara MA, Vadhera R, et al. Epidural anaesthesia for cesarean delivery and vaginal birth after maternal Fontan repair reported two cases. *Anaesthes Analges* 1994;78:1190–1192.

224. Fredriksen PM, Therrien J, Veldtman G, et al. Lung function and aerobic capacity in adult patients following modified Fontan procedure. *Heart* 2001;85:295–299.

225. Harrison DA, Liu P, Walters JE, et al. Cardiopulmonary function in adult patients post-Fontan repair. *J Am Cardiol* 1995;26:1016–1021.

226. Porter CJ, Garson A. Incidence and management of dysrhythmia after Fontan procedure. *Herz* 1993;18:318–327.

227. Peters NN, Somerville J. Arrhythmias after the Fontan procedure. *Br Heart J* 1992;68:199–204.

228. Durongpisitkul K, Porter CJ, Cetta F, et al. Predictors of early- and late-onset supraventricular tachyarrhythmias after Fontan operation. *Circulation* 1998;98:1099–1107.

229. Deal BJ, Mavroudis C, Backer CL, et al. Impact of arrhythmia circuit cryoablation during Fontan conversion for refractory atrial tachycardia. *Am J Cardiol* 1999;83:563–568.

230. Mertens L, Hagler DJ, Sauer U, et al. Protein-losing enteropathy after the Fontan operation: an international multicenter study. PLE study group. *J Thorac Cardiovasc Surg* 1998;115:1063–1073.

231. Feldt RH, Driscoll DJ, Offord KP, et al. Protein-losing enteropathy after the Fontan operation. *J Thorac Cardiovasc Surg* 1996;112:672–680.

232. Monagle P, Cochrane A, McCrindle B, et al. Thromboembolic complications after Fontan procedures—the role of prophylactic anticoagulation. *J Thorac Cardiovasc Surg* 1998;115:493–498.

233. Balling G, Vogt M, Kaemmerer H, et al. Intracardiac thrombus formation after the Fontan operation. *J Thorac Cardiovasc Surg* 2000;119:745–752.

234. Rosenthal DN, Friedman AH, Kleinman CS, et al. Thromboembolic complications after Fontan operations. *Circulation* 1995;92[9 Suppl]:II-287–II-293.

235. Daliento L, Somerville J, Presbitero P, et al. Eisenmenger syndrome. Factors relating to deterioration and death. *Eur Heart J* 1998;19:1845–1855.

236. Niwa K, Perloff JK, Kaplan S, et al. Eisenmenger's syndrome in adults: ventricular septal defect, truncus arteriosus, univentricular heart. *J Am Coll Cardiol* 1999;34:223–232.

237. Cantor WJ, Harrison DA, Moussadji JS, et al. Determinants of survival and length of survival in adults with Eisenmenger syndrome. *Am J Cardiol* 1999;84:677–681.

238. Perloff JK. Systemic complications of cyanosis in adults with congenital heart disease. Hematologic derangements, renal function, and urate metabolism. *Cardiol Clin* 1993;11:689–699.

239. Therrien J, Marelli AJ. Medical management of cyanotic congenital heart disease in adults. *Contemp Treat Cardiovasc Dis* 1997;2:227–240.

240. Perloff JK, Rosove MH, Child JS, et al. Adults with cyanotic congenital heart disease: hematologic management. *Ann Intern Med* 1988;109:406–413.

241. Rosove MG, Perloff JK, Hocking WG, et al. Chronic hypoxaemia and decompensated erythrocytosis in cyanotic congenital heart disease. *Lancet* 1986;2:313–314.

242. Gill JC, Wilson AD, Brooks JE, et al. Loss of the largest von Willebrand factor multimers from the plasma of patients with congenital cardiac defects. *Blood* 1986;1967:758–761.

243. Rabinovitch M, Andrew M, Thom H, et al. Abnormal endothelial factor VIII associated with pulmonary hypertension and congenital heart defects. *Circulation* 1987;76:1043–1052.

244. Perloff JK, Rosove MH, Sietsema KE, et al. Cyanotic heart disease: a multisystem disorder. In: Perloff JK, Child JS, eds. *Congenital heart disease in adults*. Philadelphia: WB Saunders, 1998.

245. Perloff JK, Marelli AJ, Miner PD. Risk of stroke in adults with cyanotic congenital heart disease. *Circulation* 1994;87:1954–1959.

246. Phornphutkul C, Rosenthal A, Nadas AS, et al. Cerebrovascular accidents in infants and children with cyanotic congenital heart disease. *Am J Cardiol* 1973;32:329–334.

247. Cottrill CM, Kaplan S. Cerebral vascular accidents in cyanotic congenital heart disease. *Am J Dis Child* 1973;125:484–487.

248. Ammash N, Warnes CA. 1996. Cerebrovascular events in adults patients with cyanotic congenital heart disease. *J Am Coll Cardiol* 1996;28:768–772.

249. Ross EA, Perloff JK, Danovitch GM, et al. Renal function and urate metabolism in late survivors with cyanotic congenital heart disease. *Circulation* 1986;73:396–400.

250. Hopkins WE, Kelly DP. Angiotensin converting enzyme inhibitors in adults with cyanotic congenital heart disease. *Am J Cardiol* 1996;77:439–440.

251. Speziali G, Driscoll DJ, Danielson GK, et al. Cardiac transplantation for end-stage congenital heart defects: the Mayo Clinic experience. Mayo Cardiothoracic Transplant Team. *Mayo Clin Proc* 1998;73:923–928.

252. Ueno T, Smith JA, Snell GI, et al. Bilateral sequential single lung transplantation for pulmonary hypertension and Eisenmenger's syndrome. *Ann Thorac Surg* 2000;69:381–387.

253. Perloff JK, Marelli AJ, Miner PD. Neurological and psychosocial disorders in adults with congenital heart disease. *Heart Dis Stroke* 1992;1:218–224.

254. Perloff JK. Systemic complications of cyanosis in adults with congenital heart disease. Hematologic derangements, renal function, and urate metabolism. *Cardiol Clin* 1993;11:689–699.

255. Perloff JK, Rosove MH, Child JS, et al. Adults with cyanotic congenital heart disease: hematologic management. *Ann Intern Med* 1988;109:406–413.

256. Baum VC, Perloff JK. Anesthetic implications of adults with congenital heart disease. *Anesthes Analges* 1993;76:1342–1358.

257. Selsby DS, Sugden JC. Epidural anaesthesia for bilateral inguinal herniorrhaphy in Eisenmenger's syndrome. *Anaesthesia* 1989;44:130–132.

258. Stanger P, Lucas RB, Edwards JE. Anatomic factors causing respiratory distress and in cyanotic congenital heart disease. *Pediatrics* 1969;43:760–769.

259. Ammash NM, Connolly HM, Abel MD, et al. Noncardiac surgery in Eisenmenger syndrome. *J Am Coll Cardiol* 1999;33:222–227.

260. Li W, Somerville J. Infective endocarditis in the grown-up congenital heart (GUCH) population. *Eur Heart J* 1998;19:166–173.

261. Child JS. Infective endocarditis: risks and prophylaxis. *J Am Coll Cardiol* 1991;18:337–340.

262. Dajani AS, Taubert KA, Wilson W, et al. Prevention of bacterial endocarditis. Recommendations by the American Heart Association. *Circulation* 1997;96:358–366.

263. Perloff JK, Marelli AJ. Neurological and psychosocial disorders in adults with congenital heart disease. *Heart Dis Stroke* 1991;1:218–224.

264. Presbitero P, Somerville J, Stone S, et al. Pregnancy in cyanotic congenital heart disease. Outcome of mother and fetus. *Circulation* 1994;89:2673–2676.

265. Clarkson PM, Wilson NJ, Neutze JM, et al. Outcome of pregnancy after the Mustard operation for transposition of the great arteries with intact ventricular septum. *J Am Coll Cardiol* 1994;24:190–193.

266. Connolly HM, Warnes CA. Ebstein's anomaly: outcome of pregnancy. *J Am Coll Cardiol* 1994;23:1194–1198.

267. Whittemore R, Hobbins JC, Engle MA. Pregnancy and its outcome in women with and without surgical treatment of congenital heart disease. *Am J Cardiol* 1982;50:641.

268. Jones AM, Howitt G. Eisenmenger's syndrome in pregnancy. *BMJ* 1965;1:1627–1633.

269. Gleicher N, Midwall J, Hochberger D, et al. Eisenmenger's syndrome and pregnancy. *Obstet Gynecol Surv* 1979;34:721–741.

270. Whittemore R, Hobbins JC, Engle MA. Pregnancy and its outcome in women with and without surgical treatment of congenital heart disease. *Am J Cardiol* 1982;50:641–651.

271. Saidi AS, Bezold LI, Altman CA, et al. Outcome of pregnancy following intervention for coarctation of the aorta. *Am J Cardiol* 1998;82:786–788.

272. Genoni M, Jenni R, Hoerstrup SP, et al. Pregnancy after atrial repair for transposition of the great arteries. *Heart* 1999;81:276–277.

273. Therrien J, Barnes I, Somerville J. Outcome of pregnancy in patients with congenitally corrected transposition of the great arteries. *Am J Cardiol* 1999;84:820–824.

274. Donnelly JE, Brown JM, Radford DJ. Pregnancy outcome and Ebstein's anomaly. *Br Heart J* 1991;66:368–371.

275. Canobbio MM, Mair DD, van der Velde M, et al. Pregnancy outcomes after the Fontan repair. *J Am Coll Cardiol* 1996;28:763–767.

276. Sciscione AC, Callan NA. Pregnancy and contraception. *Cardiol Clin* 1993;4:701–709.

277. Bromley B, Estroff JA, Sanders SP, et al. Fetal echocardiography: accuracy and limitations in a population at high and low risk for heart defects. *Am J Obstet Gynecol* 1992;166:1473–1481.

278. Pitkin RM, Perloff JK, Koos BJ, et al. Pregnancy and congenital heart disease. *Ann Intern Med* 1990;112:445–454.

279. Sbarouni E, Oakley CM. Outcome of pregnancy in women with valve prostheses. *Br Heart J* 1994;71:196–201.

280. Kokkonen J, Paavilainen T. Social adaptation of young adults with congenital heart disease. *Int J Cardiol* 1992;36:23–29.

281. Webb GD, Williams RG. Care of the adult with congenital heart disease: introduction. *J Am Coll Cardiol* 2001;37:1166.

282. Strivastava D, Olson EN. Neurotrophin-3 knocks heart off Trk. *Nat Med* 1996;2:1069–1071.

THE HEART AND PREGNANCY

KENNETH L. BAUGHMAN

▼▼ *ADDITIONAL ELECTRONIC TOPICS*

OVERVIEW

Pregnancy normally induces significant physiologic adaptation in the cardiovascular system, including increases in heart rate, left ventricular size, stroke volume, and left ventricular mass. Systemic vascular resistance decreases during pregnancy. The maximal increase in hemodynamic burden for the pregnant patient is achieved at the end of the second trimester. Uterine contractions and the sympathetic discharge associated with delivery further increase cardiovascular demands on the pregnant patient, with the greatest increase in cardiac output achieved in the final stages of delivery. These alterations are resolved approximately 6 weeks after delivery. Moderate aerobic exercise during pregnancy is safe, increasing maximal aerobic power and the capacity for sustained submaximal exercise, as well as preserving aerobic capacity in late gestation.

Hypertension complicates 10% of pregnancies, is rarely due to secondary causes, and is classified as chronic hypertension, gestational hypertension, or preeclampsia. Preeclampsia, the most worrisome of these disorders, involves hypertension, proteinuria, edema, and possibly coagulopathy and liver dysfunction. If preeclampsia is severe, the condition may lead to eclampsia, a seizure disorder associated with high morbidity and mortality. The HELLP syndrome (*h*emolysis, *e*levated *l*iver function tests, and *l*ow *p*latelet levels) is a preeclampsia variant that has the same potential for malignant degeneration to eclampsia.

Peripartum cardiomyopathy is the presence of a new cardiomyopathy, without any other cause of congestive heart failure or preexisting heart muscle disorder, that appears in the final month of the pregnancy or in the first 5 months postpartum. Older patients, patients experiencing multibirth preg-

K. L. Baughman: Division of Cardiology, The Johns Hopkins University School of Medicine, Baltimore, Maryland

nancies, patients with toxemia, and patients carrying a first child are somewhat more likely to experience this condition. Most patients with this condition present within 1 to 2 months of delivery. Myocarditis is frequently found in patients who undergo endomyocardial biopsy early after presentation.

All forms of chronic anticoagulation may result in bleeding between the uterus and placenta and subsequent pregnancy loss. Heparin may cause osteoporosis if it is administered at a high dosage for long periods, and warfarin (Coumadin) may be associated with an embryopathy or central nervous system abnormality. Patients who require anticoagulants should receive heparin in the first trimester and in the terminal stages of pregnancy. Coumadin can usually be safely administered through the remainder of pregnancy until just before delivery.

Bioprosthetic heart valves frequently degenerate in and around the time of pregnancy and may require replacement. Pregnant patients who have mechanical prostheses have a lower live birth rate and higher incidence of thromboembolic complications.

Myocardial infarctions associated with pregnancy are unusual; however, pregnancy is associated with an increased incidence of vasospasm and coronary dissection. Pregnant patients are also predisposed to aortic dissection, particularly if they have aortic disease, including Marfan syndrome or Takayasu's syndrome.

Patients who have congenital heart disease, even if it is corrected, must be screened carefully before they become pregnant to ensure that their pulmonary vascular resistance, ventricular function, valvular insufficiency, prosthetic devices, and aortopathy will be able to tolerate the cardiovascular strains of pregnancy.

Tocolytic therapy consists of the use of β-sympathomimetic agents to decrease uterine contraction and allow fetal lung maturation. Approximately 5% of exposed fetuses develop pulmonary edema, which appears to be a capillary leak syndrome.

Because antiarrhythmic agents pose a significant risk to the patient and fetus, they must be chosen carefully.

GLOSSARY

Bioprosthesis: An artificial valve made of biologic material, including either homograft (human) or heterograft (pig) tissue.

Embryopathy: Damage to the embryo, usually as a result of maternal exposure, typically in the first trimester of pregnancy.

HELLP syndrome: Hemolysis, elevated liver function tests, and low platelet levels in pregnant patients. Considered to be a variant of preeclampsia.

Myocarditis: Inflammation of the myocardium, characterized by a significant inflammatory infiltrate associated with myocyte necrosis.

Peripartum cardiomyopathy: Cardiomyopathy appearing in the final month of pregnancy or the first 5 months postpartum, with no preexisting heart muscle disorder and absence of any other cause of congestive heart failure.

Preeclampsia: The appearance of hypertension, proteinuria, and edema in a patient of more than 20 weeks' gestation.

Teratogenic risk: Risk of an induced fetal abnormality, usually caused by maternal exposure in the first trimester of pregnancy.

Tocolytic therapy: Sympathomimetic therapy used to decrease uterine contractions; usually initiated to prolong gestation and increase fetal lung maturation.

INTRODUCTION

Cardiologists and internists are more and more often consulted in the management of cardiovascular complications associated with pregnancy. A greater number of women with known or potential cardiovascular disease are becoming pregnant, and cardiovascular complications in pregnant women are increasingly recognized.

This chapter discusses the normal morphologic and physiologic changes that occur during pregnancy, as well as the pathophysiology and management of hypertension associated with pregnancy and peripartum cardiomyopathy. Treatment of pregnant patients who have congenital heart disease or artificial heart valves and of those who require anticoagulation during pregnancy is outlined. Detection and management of coronary artery disease and coronary dissection, as well as the use of a cardiopulmonary bypass during pregnancy, is reviewed. Avoidance of fetal risk factors during pregnancy, including toxic drinking water, is addressed, as are the potential cardiac dangers of the use of tocolytic therapy to retard uterine contraction. Finally, management of both supraventricular and ventricular tachycardia in pregnancy is reviewed.

NORMAL PHYSIOLOGIC AND MORPHOLOGIC CHANGES IN PREGNANCY

Striking adaptations occur in the maternal cardiovascular system in response to pregnancy. An appreciation of these changes is mandatory to allow appropriate treatment of pregnant patients who have cardiovascular disease. Relatively accurate noninvasive techniques for measurement of maternal physiologic changes, including echocardiographic evaluation of the heart structure and function and respiratory gas exchange assessment of functional status, have improved our understanding of these alterations.

In 1992, Hunter and Robson (1) summarized hemodynamic and structural changes in maternal subjects based on many years of echocardiographic studies performed in their

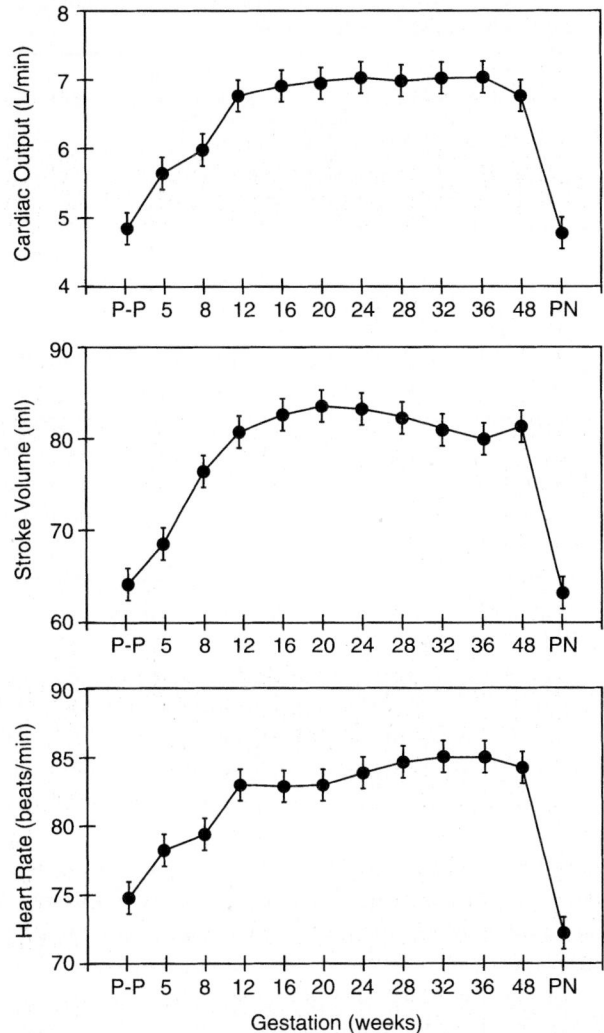

FIGURE 32.1 Serial echocardiographically determined changes in heart rate, stroke volume, and cardiac output during pregnancy and the early postpartum period. P-P, peripartum; PN, postnatal. (From Hunter S, Robson SC. Adaptation of the maternal heart in pregnancy. *Br Heart J* 1992;68:540–543, with permission.)

laboratory. Longitudinal studies of cardiac output began before conception and continued into the postnatal period. Cardiac output increases as early as 5 weeks after the last menstrual period and rises to 45% above baseline at 24 weeks' gestation. Increased cardiac output is achieved by an increase in heart rate, which rises progressively until 32 weeks' gestation, and in stroke volume, which begins to increase by 8 weeks and peaks as early as 20 weeks (Fig. 32.1). Twin pregnancies result in an additional 15% rise in cardiac output in mothers. The cardiovascular system is taxed further by stage 1 of labor, which is associated with an additional 12% increase in demand for cardiac output. This demand increases to a mean of 34% above the already increased baseline value as labor progresses to its final stages (Fig. 32.2). After-delivery stroke volume decreases by 2 weeks postpartum, but a small further reduction occurs up to 6 months after delivery. Notably, the stroke volume remains

at pregnancy levels for the first 2 days postpartum and then falls dramatically. Heart rate remains elevated for 2 days postpartum and returns to baseline by 10 days after delivery. Cardiac output similarly decreases from pregnancy levels to normal levels between 24 hours and 10 days postpartum.

The magnitude of these echocardiographic changes was documented by Mabie and associates (2), who repeated echocardiograms monthly for 18 pregnant patients from 8 to 11 weeks' gestation to 6 to 12 weeks postpartum. Cardiac output, as measured by pulsed Doppler studies, increased from 6.7 L per minute to 8.7 L per minute by 36 to 39 weeks and fell to 5.7 L per minute 2 weeks postpartum. Increases in heart rate and stroke volume of 29% and 18%, respectively, were documented. Additionally, left ventricular mass increased in association with an increased thickness of the left ventricular wall, which was maximal at 24 to 27 weeks. Vered and colleagues (3), in a similar echocardiographic analysis of 15 patients, noted that left ventricular mass increased from 172 to 186 g in association with increased body weight.

The structural changes noted by echocardiography are secondary to the alterations in intravascular volume and neurohumoral stimulation that are associated with pregnancy. Hess and Hess (4) summarized the physiologic fluid changes associated with pregnancy. Plasma volume increases approximately 40% and red blood cell volume 30% above baseline prepregnancy levels, resulting in mild relative anemia. Estrogen-mediated stimulation of the renin angiotensin axis results in increased renal tubular absorption of sodium and an increase in total body salt and water, contributing to the increased plasma volume. Systemic vascular resistance and diastolic blood pressure decrease as a result of changes in aortic compliance and arterial venous shunting in the uterus.

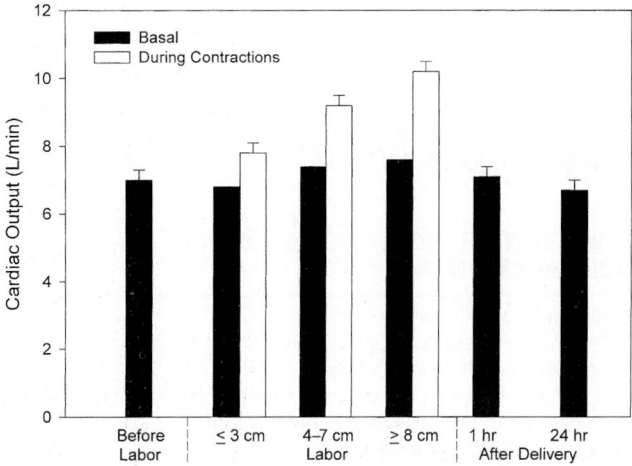

FIGURE 32.2 Normal labor-associated contractions increase cardiac output demands 12% to 34% above an already increased baseline cardiac output. (From Hunter S, Robson SC. Adaptation of the maternal heart in pregnancy. *Br Heart J* 1992;68:540–543, with permission.)

The normal physiologic changes associated with pregnancy result in alterations in the physical examination of the pregnant patient (Table 32.1). It is important to understand findings that are physiologic so that pathologic changes can be distinguished. Because of the increase in total body salt and water, as well as plasma volume, the jugular veins are often full, and the central venous pressure may be slightly increased. Similarly, the pregnant patient may have 1 to 2+ lower-extremity edema. As pregnancy progresses, increased uterus size forces both diaphragms upward, which may decrease pulmonary vital capacity and total lung volume. These mechanical changes may increase the work required for breathing. The previously documented changes in left ventricular size and mass, which are associated with increased volume, result in a mildly displaced and diffuse point of maximal impulse of the left ventricle and increased atrioventricular and aortic as well as pulmonic valve closure sounds. Because of the insulation of the atrioventricular sounds by the abdomen, only the aortic and pulmonic closure sounds are characteristically louder on examination. Increased flow through the pulmonic valve causes a characteristic "functional" early systolic murmur and slight widening of the physiologic variation of closure of the pulmonic component of the second heart sound. Ventricular gallop rhythms and diastolic murmurs are unexpected and serve as clues to anatomic or functional cardiac abnormalities. Occasionally, a normal physiologic diastolic murmur can be heard at the left sternal border in pregnant patients. This physiologic murmur is usually generated by increased diastolic flow through the internal mammary artery, located in the peristernal area and engorged with increased flow to the breasts of pregnant patients. This mammary souffle may persist in lactating mothers, even after delivery. The expected decrease in aortic diastolic pressure during pregnancy that is associated with the decreased systemic vascular resistance results in a widened pulse pressure (systolic pressure minus diastolic pressure) and pulsatile fingertips, warm hands, and occasional Quincke's sign in the extremity nail beds. These findings are also suggestive of aortic regurgitation that may be confused by the diastolic murmur of the mam-

TABLE 32.1 PHYSICAL FINDINGS DURING NORMAL PREGNANCY

Mild jugular venous distention
1–2+ Lower-extremity edema
Decreased breath sounds at bases
Upward and leftward deviation of point of maximal impulse
Volume-loaded ventricle (active precordium)
Increased valve closure sounds
"Flow" murmurs (pulmonic and aortic)
Mammary souffle (left sternal border)
Wide pulse pressure
Increased heart rate

TABLE 32.2 CHANGES IN NONINVASIVE TEST RESULTS THAT OCCUR DURING PREGNANCY

Test	Change
Electrocardiography	Leftward axis deviation
	Increased ventricular voltage
	Increased rate
	Repolarization changes
Chest x-ray film	Upward diaphragm displacement
	Horizontal heart placement
	Enlarged pulmonary silhouette
Echocardiography	Increased left ventricular diastolic dimension
	Increased left ventricular wall thickness
	Mild increase in contractility

mary souffle at the sternal border. Echocardiography may be required to distinguish the presence or absence of aortic valve disease.

The physiologic changes associated with pregnancy may also alter the results of noninvasive evaluations of the heart (Table 32.2). The increase in size and left ventricular mass seen by echocardiography has already been described in detail. The electrocardiogram may also be altered. Upward movement of the diaphragm is expected to result in a leftward shift of the electrical axis of ventricular depolarization, and increased ventricular mass may result in increased ventricular voltage. Although changes are altered relative to the subject's baseline values, most changes are not outside the normal limits of variability. Heart rate may be increased, particularly late in pregnancy, and atrial as well as ventricular arrhythmias may increase in frequency in patients predisposed to such events. Chest radiographic studies, which are rarely performed because of radiation risk to mother and fetus, reveal a mild increase in cardiac size, a horizontal shift of the heart that increases with the duration of pregnancy, and fullness of the left cardiac border and pulmonary vascular supply (5). ❦ g45

RADIATION AND PREGNANCY

X-rays produce direct and indirect damage to cells. Direct damage results from the effect of the high-energy radiation beam on cellular and molecular structure. Indirect damage is the result of ionized water and free radical generation. The strength and potential damage of x-rays are measured by the amount of ionic charge created per unit mass of air. One R (roentgen) creates more than 2 billion ion pairs per cm^3 of exposures to air. The absorbed dose of radiation is measured in rad, calculated by the energy imparted to tissue per unit mass of tissue. One rad is equivalent to the deposition of .01 J of energy per kg of tissue. One R of radiation usually produces 1 rad in tissue. Roentgen-equivalent-man (REM) is a measure of absorbed radiation modified by local tissue characteristics, which better delineate the risk of radiation damage to a given organ.

Radiation is harmful to all living tissue and particularly to the conceptus. Increasing radiation exposure is associated with a range of tissue defects, beginning with isolated cellular damage and progressing to growth impairment, structural deformity, neoplasia, and gonadal damage. Environmental radiation results in 50 to 100 mREM exposure during the 9 months of childbearing. The amount of radiation considered to be "safe" is unclear; however, virtually no data have demonstrated significant fetal damage after exposure to less than 1 rad (10).

Several features alter the amount of radiation exposure that occurs during radiologic procedures, including the nature of the radiation source, the equipment used, the size of the patient, the depth of the uterus and conceptus, and the distance from the area being investigated, as well as the extent of the radiologic study. The dose of radiation received by the uterus may vary by 50-fold, depending on these features and whether appropriate uterus shielding is performed.

The increased risk of development of a subsequent malignancy by children receiving radiation *in utero* was reported by the Childhood Cancer Research Group in 1956 and confirmed in 1975 (11). Bithell and Stewart (11) demonstrated a relative risk of 1.47 for the development of subsequent malignancy in children whose mothers underwent radiographs during pregnancy. Furthermore, the relative risk increased progressively from 1.26 for one film exposure to 2.32 for five or more x-rays, indicating a dose response. A first-trimester exposure resulted in a relative risk of malignancy of 8.95, falling to 1.25 and 1.41 in the second and third trimesters, respectively. The risk of childhood cancer from radiation exposure is displayed in *e*Table 32.2.1 (10).

The risk of radiation must be evaluated relative to the benefit to the mother. It is imperative that the clinician define (a) the dose of radiation to the conceptus, (b) the age and development of the conceptus, (c) the radiation risk from the radiation source, (d) the risk associated with delaying or not performing the test, and (e) the potential for alternative means of answering the question with nonradiation studies.

HYPERTENSION DURING PREGNANCY

High blood pressure may complicate as many as 10% of all pregnancies and remains a major cause of maternal and fetal morbidity and mortality (14,15). In normal pregnancy, diastolic blood pressure falls, often by as much as 10 mm Hg in the first and second trimesters as a result of decreased systemic vascular resistance and increased cardiac output. Blood pressure then increases gradually at or near term and may transiently rise higher than nonpregnant val-

ues in the immediate puerperium. Rarely is high blood pressure in pregnancy the result of secondary causes such as intrinsic renal disease, endocrinopathies, or renal vascular obstruction. The currently accepted categories for high blood pressure in pregnancy are (a) chronic hypertension, (b) gestational hypertension, and (c) preeclampsia, with or without preexisting high blood pressure.

Chronic high blood pressure is categorized as preexistent hypertension or a blood pressure of at least 140/90 mm Hg before 20 weeks' gestation. If the diastolic blood pressure is 110 mm Hg or greater, severe hypertension is diagnosed. Pregnant women with a diastolic blood pressure higher than 75 mm Hg in the second trimester and 95 mm Hg in the third trimester should be observed carefully (16). The maternal and fetal outcomes are good unless preeclampsia or abruptio placentae complicates the final stages of gestation. Clear evidence exists (17) that treatment of blood pressure of greater than 110 mm Hg (diastolic) during pregnancy lowers the risk of stroke and cardiovascular complications, although the benefit of lowering blood pressure in mild chronic hypertension during pregnancy is less clearly defined.

Gestational hypertension is defined as asymptomatic blood pressure elevation after 20 weeks' gestation. Unless this elevation of pressure reflects early preeclampsia or unrecognized chronic hypertension, the maternal and fetal outcomes are usually very good, even without treatment.

Preeclampsia is the most feared hypertensive disorder of pregnancy and may lead to life-threatening eclampsia, a convulsive disorder. Preeclampsia is characterized by hypertension, proteinuria (levels greater than 300 mg in 24 hours), and edema but may include coagulopathy and altered liver function in pregnant patients after 20 weeks' gestation (Table 32.3). Preeclampsia may be mild or severe, depending on the degree of blood pressure elevation and proteinuria. In preeclampsia, plasma volume and cardiac output fail to rise, and systemic resistance does not fall. This appears to be related to failure of the uterine spiral arteries to develop, preventing the anticipated arteriovenous shunting. Some researchers believe the primary abnormality causing preeclampsia is the result of prostaglandin deficiency; endothelial cell dysfunction; or immune,

TABLE 32.3 TYPICAL FINDINGS IN PATIENTS WITH PREECLAMPSIA

Definition
  Hypertension
  Proteinuria
  Edema
  Coagulopathy
  Liver dysfunction
After 20 wk gestation
Categories
  Mild
  Severe

genetic, or sodium/calcium membrane disorders. Schobel and colleagues (18) recently demonstrated that preeclampsia is associated with a dramatic increase in sympathetic nervous system activity. This conclusion was reached by evaluation of postganglionic sympathetic nerve activity in the blood vessels of skeletal muscles of preeclamptic patients, compared with those in pregnant and nonpregnant control subjects. Recently, investigators have demonstrated an increased level of platelet-activating factor (19) and plasma levels of prostaglandin isoforms (20) in preeclampsia subjects compared with levels in pregnant and nonpregnant control subjects. Dechend and coworkers (21) demonstrated angiotensin-1 receptor autoantibodies in preeclamptic patients and that these immunoglobulins may cause vascular smooth muscle cells to express tissue factor that may be responsible for placental infarction (often associated with preeclampsia). These observations may have ramifications for treatment. The maternal risks of preeclampsia include cerebral hemorrhage, pulmonary edema, disseminated intravascular coagulopathy, liver failure, renal failure, convulsions, and death. These risks are correlated with the severity of the complications and level of gestation at the onset of the condition. The fetus may suffer hypoxemia, acidosis, growth retardation, and death.

Mild preeclampsia may be managed at home; however, development of progressive symptoms such as headache, visual disturbances, and abdominal pain requires hospitalization (*e*Table 32.3.1). The use of antihypertensive or anticonvulsant therapy to treat mild preeclampsia remains questionable. Treatment of severe preeclampsia, on the other hand, may require termination of the pregnancy, regardless of fetal viability, if the mother's life is in jeopardy. Antihypertensive therapy should be initiated with hydralazine, labetalol, or nifedipine to lower mean blood pressure and diastolic blood pressure to 126 and 90 mm Hg, respectively. Because these patients are already volume-depleted, use of diuretics should be avoided. Intravenous magnesium should be given during labor and delivery and for 24 hours postpartum for patients who have severe preeclampsia to avoid convulsions.

There is no known mechanism for avoidance of preeclampsia, although sodium chloride restriction, diuretics, low-dose aspirin, and increased dietary calcium have been attempted.

A variant of preeclampsia, the HELLP syndrome, is characterized by minimal or no elevation of blood pressure, mild decreases in platelet levels, hemolysis, mild liver function abnormalities, and absence of renal impairment at the onset (*e*Table 32.3.2) (15,17). This syndrome may progress rapidly, resulting in hemolysis, thrombocytopenia, and liver failure. Recognition of this syndrome prepartum should prompt immediate delivery. O'Brien and coworkers (22) have suggested that corticosteroids may be of some benefit in this unusual disorder; however, recommendation of corticosteroid therapy is dependent on the outcome of pro-

spective randomized trials in affected patients. Both the HELLP syndrome and preeclampsia may occur up to 10 days postpartum.

Preeclampsia, the most devastating form of hypertension to affect the pregnant patient, has a unique pathophysiology and requires prompt and appropriate management for avoidance of serious complications to the mother and fetus. Use of antihypertension agents in pregnant women requires special consideration of the effect on the fetus and the uteroplacental unit, as well as on the mother. Cardiologists will likely increasingly be called on to assist in the management of this condition in a usually older, multigravida population.

TREATMENT OF HYPERTENSION DURING PREGNANCY

Medications commonly used to treat chronic, gestational, and preeclamptic hypertension are listed in Tables 32.4 and 32.5. Appropriate medical management of pregnancy-related hypertension depends on an understanding of the pathophysiology outlined in the previous sections. Some changes are unique to alterations in kidney handling of sodium and water.

TABLE 32.4 GUIDELINES FOR TREATING SEVERE HYPERTENSION NEAR TERM OR DURING LABOR

Regulation of blood pressure
   The degree to which blood pressure should be decreased is disputed; we recommend maintaining diastolic levels between 90 and 110 mm Hg.
Drug therapy
   Hydralazine administered intravenously is the drug of choice. Start with low doses (5 mg as an intravenous bolus), then administer 5 to 10 mg every 20 to 30 min to avoid precipitous decreases in pressure. Side effects include tachycardia and headache.
   Diazoxide is recommended for women whose hypertension is refractory to hydralazine. Use 30-mg miniboluses, because precipitous hypotension may result if higher doses are used. Side effects include arrest of labor and neonatal hypoglycemia.
   The experience with labetalol is growing, and some physicians use this agent, instead of diazoxide, as a second-line drug.
   Favorable results have been reported with calcium channel blockers. If magnesium sulfate is being infused, magnesium may potentiate the effects of calcium channel blockers, resulting in precipitous and severe hypotension.
   Refrain from using sodium nitroprusside, because fetal cyanide poisoning has been reported in animals. However, maternal well-being should dictate the choice of therapy.
Prevention of convulsions
   Parenteral magnesium sulfate is the drug of choice for preventing eclamptic convulsions. Therapy should be continued for 12 to 24 h postpartum, because one-third of women with eclampsia have convulsions during this period.

From Cunningham FG, Lindheimer MD. Hypertension in pregnancy. *N Engl J Med* 1992;326:927–932, with permission.

TABLE 32.5 ANTIHYPERTENSIVE DRUGS USED TO TREAT CHRONIC HYPERTENSION IN PREGNANT WOMEN

Alpha₂-adrenergic receptor agonists

Methyldopa is the most extensively used drug in this group. Its safety and efficacy are supported by evidence from randomized trials, and a 7.5-yr follow-up study has been made of children born to mothers treated with methyldopa.

Beta-adrenergic receptor antagonists

These drugs, especially atenolol and metoprolol, appear to be safe and efficacious when used in late pregnancy, but fetal growth retardation has been reported when treatment was started in early or mid-gestation. Fetal bradycardia can occur, and animal studies suggest that the fetus's ability to tolerate hypoxic stress may be compromised.

Alpha-adrenergic receptor and beta-adrenergic receptor antagonists

Labetalol appears to be as effective as methyldopa, but no follow-up studies have been conducted in children born to mothers given labetalol, and concern about maternal hepatotoxicity exists.

Arteriolar vasodilators

Hydralazine is frequently used as adjunctive therapy with methyldopa and beta-adrenergic receptor antagonists. Rarely, neonatal thrombocytopenia has been reported. Trials with calcium channel blockers look promising. The experience with minoxidil is limited, and this drug is not recommended.

Angiotensin-converting enzyme inhibitors

Captopril causes fetal death in diverse animal species, and several converting enzyme inhibitors have been associated with oligohydramnios and neonatal renal failure when administered to humans. *Do not use in pregnant women.*

Diuretics

Many authorities discourage the use of diuretics, but others continue these medications if they were prescribed before conception or if a woman with chronic hypertension appears quite sensitive to salt.

From Cunningham FG, Lindheimer MD. Hypertension in pregnancy. *N Engl J Med* 1992;326:927–932, with permission.

The mean increase in total body water and sodium during pregnancy is 6 to 8 L and 500 to 900 mEq, respectively, approximately one-half of which is extracellular (23). Many factors alter sodium excretion in pregnancy, of which a 50% increase in the glomerular filtration rate and elevated levels of progesterone and aldosterone are most important. The result is that more than 80% of all healthy pregnant women develop physiologic-dependent or generalized edema.

Edema may be a normal physiologic response; hypertension and preeclampsia are not. Hypertension in pregnancy is associated with increased rates of preterm delivery, perinatal mortality, and probably small-for-date babies and fetal neurologic impairment (16). Preeclampsia is a vascular abnormality, and the earliest manifestation, which occurs well before other manifestations of disease, can be demonstrated as an abnormal pressor response to infused angiotensin. Despite the increase in interstitial volume that occurs with preeclampsia, the intervascular volume is reduced, and oliguria and hemoconcentration are typically

present. There is no evidence that sodium restriction or diuretics prevent preeclampsia or other hypertensive complications of pregnancy, and use of such agents may cause additional volume contraction, alkalosis, electrolyte abnormalities, pancreatitis, and bleeding or hyponatremia in the neonate (16,23). Use of diuretics in women with preeclampsia should be avoided, and these agents are of limited benefit for treatment of pregnancy-related hypertension. Patients who have taken diuretics chronically before pregnancy or who are extremely sensitive to salt may derive some benefit from them (23).

Among agents used to treat chronic hypertension in pregnancy, Aldomet (methyldopa) is safe and preferable to other drugs. Randomized trials have demonstrated that Aldomet improves fetal survival significantly, and it is the only drug with long-term follow-up (7.5 years), in which no difference in health, physical, or intellectual outcomes was seen between patients who received treatment with this agent and those who did not (24,25). The use of beta-receptor–blocking agents, including oxprenolol, atenolol, and acebutolol, during pregnancy has been studied. Growth retardation, acute fetal distress, high perinatal mortality, and hypoglycemia, all early concerns, have been found to be nearly nonexistent in controlled trials, and use of these agents is now considered nearly as safe as administration of Aldomet (25,26). Type II calcium channel blockers, including nifedipine, nicardipine, and nitrindipine, are potent vasodilators and have been used to treat hypertension during pregnancy. Nifedipine may induce a rapid fall in blood pressure if given in high dose or sublingually, which may result in reflex tachycardia. Uterine blood flow is minimally affected by nitrindipine and nifedipine, and the drug may decrease uterine contractions as a result of its smooth muscle relaxant properties; therefore, it may serve as a successful tocolytic agent (27).

Angiotensin-converting enzyme (ACE) inhibitors are currently the agents of choice for use in nonpregnant patients who have cardiomyopathy or congestive heart failure and after myocardial infarction, but this class of antihypertensive drugs should *never* be used during pregnancy. Animal and human studies have demonstrated a high degree of morbidity and mortality in infants exposed to ACE inhibitors during pregnancy (28). Complications include growth retardation, renal failure, bone malformations, oligohydramnios, patent ductus arteriosis, pulmonary hypoplasia, respiratory distress syndrome, and neonatal death. The U.S. Food and Drug Administration has issued a warning against the use of ACE inhibitors during pregnancy after the first trimester (29). Most authorities favor avoiding these agents even in patients who are merely contemplating pregnancy.

Preeclampsia requires prompt control of accelerated hypertension. Because of its long history of use for preeclampsia, hydralazine remains the drug of choice for most physicians. The drug can be given intravenously, intramuscularly, or orally and titrated to achieve maximal effect (16). Labetalol combines alpha- and beta-blocking properties, can be given intravenously, and incurs a prompt response. Nifedipine has been used sublingually and, when compared with hydralazine in a small, controlled trial, resulted in improved blood pressure control (27). Type II calcium channel blockers are tocolytic, which may be advantageous for treatment of patients who have premature contractions but deleterious for patients in whom delivery should be hastened. Nitroprusside probably should be avoided because of the potential for thiocyanate accumulation. Magnesium sulfate has been demonstrated to be beneficial during preeclampsia and for up to 24 hours after delivery.

PERIPARTUM CARDIOMYOPATHY

Peripartum cardiomyopathy, a relatively infrequent dilated cardiomyopathy that occurs in women of reproductive age, is defined as "a disorder of heart muscle, which presents clinically with the onset of heart failure in the last month of pregnancy or the first 5 postpartum months" (30,31). Established diagnostic criteria include (a) absence of a determinable cause for cardiac failure, (b) absence of preexisting heart muscle disease, and (c) time limitations of onset of illness. Other causes of congestive heart failure in pregnancy should be ruled out, including congenital, valvular, infectious, metabolic, and toxic etiologies, as well as preeclampsia and pulmonary emboli, which may complicate late pregnancy and delivery. Some recent literature on this topic is tainted by the inclusion of patients who were in the last trimester of gestation rather than the final month. This expansion of the definition encompasses the response of patients with preexistent heart disease to the volume load imposed by pregnancy, which clouds the clinical observations about this unique disorder. Such patients should be excluded.

Peripartum cardiomyopathy complicates 1 in 1,300 to 1 in 4,000 deliveries in the United States (32,33). This condition may affect women of any race, age, or number of prior deliveries; however, pregnancies in older age, multigravida pregnancies, African-American race, and twin pregnancies are thought to represent predisposing features (Fig. 32.3).

The etiology of peripartum cardiomyopathy is unknown (*e*Table 32.5.1). Melvin and associates (34) in 1982 demonstrated myocarditis by endomyocardial biopsy in three of three patients presenting with peripartum cardiomyopathy. All three patients were treated with immunosuppressive therapy, and ventricular function improved in all three. Sanderson and associates (35) performed biopsies on 11 African women with peripartum cardiomyopathy in Nairobi and found healing myocarditis in five. Four patients with myocarditis during follow-up failed to improve, and no immunosuppressive treatment was given. O'Connell and coworkers (36) evaluated 14 consecutive patients with peripartum cardiomyopathy using endomyocardial biopsy, which revealed myocarditis in four (29%); all patients in whom the diagnosis of myocarditis was made underwent biopsy within 1 week of the onset of symptoms. Two of the four patients with myocarditis died, the condition of one stabilized, and the condition of one improved; none was treated with immunosuppressive therapy. Eight of these 14 patients presented before delivery, and these authors extended the window for diagnosis of peripartum cardiomyopathy to the last trimester of pregnancy, rather than to the last month, making their data difficult to interpret.

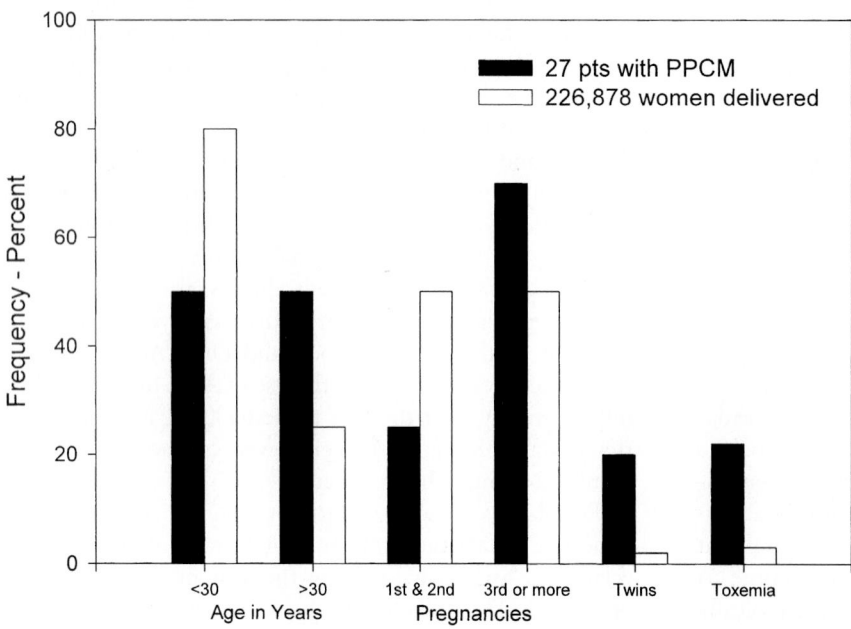

FIGURE 32.3 Risk factors for the development of peripartum cardiomyopathy (PPCM). pts, patients. (From Demakis JG, Rahimtoola SH. Peripartum cardiomyopathy. *Circulation* 1971;44:964–968, with permission.)

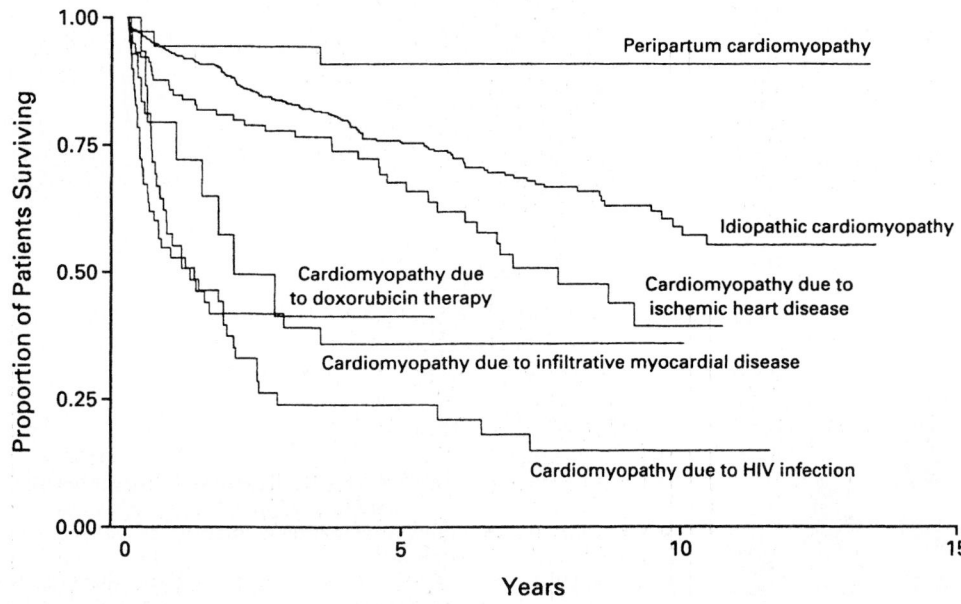

FIGURE 32.4 Adjusted Kaplan-Meier estimates of survival, according to the underlying cause of cardiomyopathy. Only idiopathic car-diomyopathy and cardiomyopathy resulting from causes for which survival was significantly different from that among patients with idiopathic cardiomyopathy are shown. HIV, human immunodeficiency virus. (From Felker GM, Thompson RE, Hare JM, et al. Underlying causes and long-term survival in patients with initially unexplained cardiomyopathy. *N Engl J Med* 2000; 342:1077–1084, with permission.)

Midei and coauthors (37) at The Johns Hopkins Hospital reported that 14 (78%) of 18 consecutive patients with peripartum cardiomyopathy had myocarditis found on endomyocardial biopsy. Felker and colleagues (38) expanded their study to include 42 women with peripartum cardiomyopathy who underwent biopsy. Despite a delay in biopsy of 1 to 2 weeks after presentation, the incidence of myocarditis remained high (62%). Additionally, the Johns Hopkins group demonstrated that the prognosis for mothers with peripartum cardiomyopathy is good relative to patients with idiopathic dilated cardiomyopathy (39) (Fig. 32.4). Of 42 patients included in that study, only three died (7%), and three underwent orthotopic heart transplantation (7%) (38). Ventricular function improved in most patients. In our experience, patients presenting early after delivery had more profound congestive heart failure and dramatic myocarditis found by endomyocardial biopsy, but they also had a greater chance of spontaneous resolution, even if they did not receive immunosuppressive therapy. These studies suggest that peripartum cardiomyopathy is immunologic in origin. Whether the inciting agent is an inapparent viral infection or an aberrant immunologic response to a placental or fetal antigen is unknown. As is true of the other cardiomyopathies that present with heart failure, patients with peripartum cardiomyopathy display elevated levels of tumor necrosis factor-α, interleukins, and apoptosis-signaling receptors (40).

Patients who have peripartum cardiomyopathy typically present with heart failure, which in our experience has been more profound near the time of delivery and more subtle in presentation when it occurs months later. Approximately 80% of patients present within the first 3 months postpartum (Fig. 32.5). Symptoms of heart failure may be particularly difficult to diagnose for patients in the last month of pregnancy and very early postpartum, when dyspnea,

edema, and fatigue may be the result of normal pregnancy and delivery. The physical findings of congestive heart failure are manifest, including jugular venous distention, rales, hepatic congestion, and edema. Patients presenting early may not have cardiomegaly, and the point of maximal impulse is frequently superiorly placed, in our experience.

The chest x-ray confirms the presence of pulmonary congestion and usually cardiomegaly. Echocardiography, which is mandatory in the evaluation of these patients, demonstrates markedly decreased contractility with variable degrees of cardiac enlargement (*e*Fig. 32.5.1). The results of electrocardiography are almost always abnormal and show nonspecific ST-T–wave changes. Right heart catheterization (if performed) reveals high filling pressures and decreased cardiac output that are compatible with cardiomyopathy. Only if the patient has multiple risk factors for coronary artery disease or is suspected of having a coronary dissection should coronary angiography be performed.

We do not perform endomyocardial biopsy or right heart catheterization on patients with peripartum cardiomyopathy unless they fail to show improvement in signs and symptoms of congestive heart failure and in echocardiographic ventricular function after 2 weeks of standard management therapy for congestive heart failure. Although endomyocardial biopsy can define the presence and severity of myocarditis in patients who have peripartum cardiomyopathy, it is unclear that this offers any therapeutic advantage, because immunosuppressive therapy is likely ineffective in influencing long-term left ventricular function (K. L. Baughman, *unpublished data*).

Standard management of heart failure should be applied to these patients postpartum, with careful attention to the potential influence of drugs on the uterus and, for patients in the last month of pregnancy, the fetus. Standard treatment includes afterload reduction therapy, diuresis, admin-

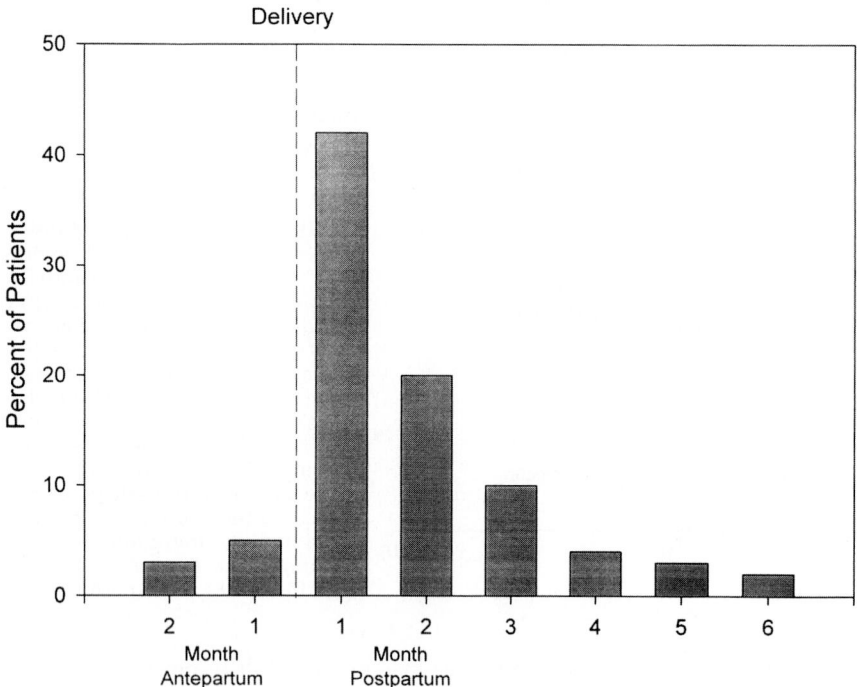

FIGURE 32.5 Peripartum cardiomyopathy. Most patients present with peripartum cardiomyopathy within 2 months of delivery. By definition, those presenting earlier than the last month of pregnancy do not have peripartum cardiomyopathy. (From Homans DC. Current concepts: peripartum cardiomyopathy. *N Engl J Med* 1985;312:1432–1437, with permission.)

istration of digoxin (if signs or symptoms of congestive heart failure persist despite preload and afterload reduction therapy), and anticoagulation therapy (if ventricular compromise persists).

In Demackus and coworkers' initial series (30,31), two groups of patient outcomes were categorized. Approximately one-half of the affected patients recovered normal heart size, and one-half still had cardiomegaly at 6 months' follow-up. Patients with persistent cardiomegaly had the same poor prognosis as patients with dilated cardiomyopathy; 80% died, with an average survival of 4.7 years after presentation. Of patients whose hearts returned to normal size, 14% died, none from cardiovascular disease. This pattern of survival has persisted in all subsequent studies, and, until recently, the prognosis for such patients was poor. Earlier recognition of peripartum cardiomyopathy due to the availability of echocardiography, more sophisticated standard therapy for congestive heart failure, and referral for full cardiac evaluation for patients who fail to respond to early heart failure management have likely improved the prognosis. Cole and associates (41) reported the echocardiographic evolution of peripartum cardiomyopathy compared with peripartum control subjects in 14 patients who presented with this entity. The left ventricular end diastolic volume index was 95 versus 67 mL per m², respectively; the end systolic volume index was 66 versus 27 mL per m², respectively; and left ventricular wall mass was 139 versus 96 g per m², with an ejection fraction of 29% versus 67%, respectively. Despite these findings, 13 of 14 patients improved early and rapidly with standard therapy, despite the fact that none of the five who underwent to endomyocardial biopsy had histologic myocarditis.

We routinely follow patients closely after presentation with peripartum cardiomyopathy. Most patients require hospitalization on presentation because of the severity of congestive heart failure symptoms. Appropriate therapy is administered until the patient's condition is stabilized. This can usually be accomplished with standard medical therapy, but occasionally extraordinary therapy is needed, including intraaortic balloon counterpulsation or use of a left ventricular assist device. Because the degree of reversibility of left ventricular dysfunction associated with peripartum cardiomyopathy is high, and because the patients are young, all means necessary should be applied to ensure the mother's survival. Once discharged from the hospital, patients are followed every 2 weeks with clinical evaluation and an echocardiogram until left ventricular function is stabilized and no longer improving. Echocardiograms are repeated at 3 months and 6 months postpartum. The ventricular function at 6 months will likely be the ventricular performance that the patient maintains. Vigorous activity and nursing are discouraged during this interval to avoid left ventricular stress, which might alter ventricular remodeling during recovery. No other noninvasive tests are helpful in follow-up, in our experience.

Recurrent pregnancies in patients who have experiences peripartum cardiomyopathy remain problematic. Demakis and Rahimtoola (31) reported that in 14 patients whose hearts returned to normal, eight patients attempted 21 subsequent pregnancies. Of these eight patients, three experienced transient cardiac decompensation responsive to heart failure management. Of the 13 patients whose hearts failed to recover, six attempted repeat pregnancy with three experiencing deterioration and death. Through a survey mechanism, Elkayam et al. (42) identified 44 patients who attempted 60 subsequent pregnancies after documented peripartum cardiomyopathy. Patients presenting in the last trimester—as opposed to the last month of pregnancy—were included. Of the 28 patients who normalized ventricular function at rest, there was a significant decrease in ejection fraction (from 56% to 49%), whereas 21% experienced congestive heart failure with subsequent pregnancies. Of the 16 patients with abnormal resting ventricular function, ejection fraction decreased (from 36% to 32%), and 44% developed symptomatic congestive heart failure with repeat pregnancy. Mortality was not noted in those with normalized ventricular function but was 19% in those with persistent dysfunction. Lampert (42a) studied ventricular reserve in patients with peripartum cardiomyopathy who normalized ventricular function. Ten patients were evaluated approximately 9 months after ventricular recovery from peripartum cardiomyopathy. These authors used an echocardiographic load and heart rate–independent mechanism to assess ventricular contractility and reserve in response to methoxamine and dobutamine infusion. Contractile reserve, even in patients with ventricular recovery, was impaired.

There are, therefore, three categories of patients after peripartum cardiomyopathy: those with persistent abnormal cardiac function, those with normal resting but abnormal cardiac reserve with stress, and those with normal resting and stress ventricular performance. For patients who do not recover left ventricular function, standard long-term management for congestive heart failure should be undertaken. For those whose congestive heart failure is unresponsive to treatment, cardiac transplantation can be done (42a,44) with a favorable long-term survival and morbidity comparable to that in age-matched control subjects. For patients with normal resting but abnormal stress ventricular response, pregnancy can be undertaken; however, cardiac decompensation may occur. Fortunately, this decompensation is usually responsive to medical management, and maternal mortality is not expected. In patients with normal resting and stress ventricular response after peripartum cardiomyopathy, repeat pregnancy can be undertaken with less risk of decompensation.

For patients who do not recover left ventricular function, standard long-term management for congestive heart failure should be undertaken. Cardiac transplantation can be done (43,44) for those whose congestive heart failure is unresponsive to treatment, with a favorable long-term survival and morbidity comparable to that in age-matched control subjects.

TRANSPLANTATION

The transplanted heart is denervated and may have limitations in ventricular dilatation, making the hemodynamic burden of pregnancy more difficult to manage (45). Cardiac transplant patients are usually hypertensive and hypercholesterolemic, and they face the potential that accelerated atherosclerosis will develop in the transplanted heart's coronary arteries, increasing the risk of cardiovascular compromise. Pregnancy may interrupt routine surveillance endomyocardial biopsy procedures because of the risk of fetal radiation exposure, thereby limiting the transplant cardiologist's ability to diagnose and treat rejection successfully before hemodynamic compromise develops. Immunosuppressive agents pose a potential risk to the fetus of genetic alterations and to the mother's renal function (cyclosporine) and bone, skin, and adrenal integrity (prednisone). Scott and colleagues (46) reviewed the literature and the University of Utah experience and polled other cardiac transplant centers to gather the experience of 30 posttransplant patients who became pregnant. Overall, 48% had chronic hypertension, 24% had preeclampsia, and 28% had preterm labor. Six episodes of rejection required increased immunosuppressive therapy, and nine required increased cyclosporine dosage to maintain therapeutic levels. Of 27 live births, ten infants were preterm (less than 36 weeks), five infants were small for gestational age, and four infants had neonatal complications. No congenital abnormalities were reported. Data from the National Transplantation Pregnancy Registry compiled by Branch and coworkers (47) confirmed a high incidence of premature and low-birth-weight infants born to 35 transplant recipients with 47 pregnancies. The risks appear to be similar in heart-lung transplant recipients (48). Pregnancy in cardiac transplant recipients must be considered high risk for mother and fetus and is discouraged.

ANTICOAGULATION AND PREGNANCY

Occasionally, pregnant patients require systemic anticoagulation for prophylaxis and treatment of venous or arterial thromboembolic disease or because of the presence of an artificial heart valve. Systemic anticoagulation exposes the mother and fetus to significant risks. Both heparin and warfarin may cause *in utero* placental bleeding, resulting in spontaneous abortion. Long-term systemic heparinization may cause osteoporosis. Heparin does not cross the placental barrier and has no effect on the fetus. Warfarin, on the other hand, does cross the placental membrane and causes fetal anticoagulation. More important, administration of warfarin during the first trimester may cause an embryopathy, and exposure at any time in gestation may cause central nervous system abnormalities in the fetus. Weeks 6 to 12 of gestation appear to be the critical time interval for embryopathy caused by warfarin exposure, resulting in nasal hypoplasia or stippled epiphysis. Central nervous system abnormalities caused by warfarin exposure include hemorrhage and dorsal or ventral midline dysplasia. Data concerning low-molecular-weight heparin are limited. Ellison and coauthors (50) reported a retrospective series of 57 pregnancies in 50 women and found a low incidence of complications with use of 40 mg of low-molecular-weight heparin once per day. Satisfactory antifactor X_a levels and prevention of thromboembolism were achieved (50).

Systemic heparinization during pregnancy traditionally has been thought to result in high risk to the fetus and mother. Ginsberg and Hirsh (51) reviewed the published literature in 1989 and reported a summary of 106 studies that evaluated 1,325 pregnancies in women who were receiving anticoagulation therapy. After excluding comorbid conditions, the risk of maternal death was 2.5% (7 of 278 patients) for women receiving heparin and 16.8% (95 of 567 patients) for patients treated with oral anticoagulants. These authors and colleagues (52) also carried out a prospective study of 77 women with 100 pregnancies, among whom heparin was given for prevention or treatment of venous thromboembolism in 98 pregnancies and because of a prosthetic valve replacement in two. The rates of prematurity, abortion, stillbirths, neonatal deaths, and congenital abnormalities are similar to those in normal populations. In addition, no symptomatic thromboembolisms and only two episodes of bleeding were seen after a mean of 18 weeks of treatment per pregnancy. As noted, few of these authors' patients received anticoagulation therapy for valvular disease or prosthesis. Osteoporosis is a potential complication of heparin therapy. Barbour and associates (53) performed a prospective study of heparin use in pregnant patients, using bone densitometry to evaluate osteoporosis. Of the 14 pregnant patients given heparin, 36% experienced a greater than 10% decrease in femur bone density measurements from baseline to immediately postpartum, compared with none of 14 pregnant control subjects who were not receiving heparin. The difference in bone density remained statistically significant at 6 months postpartum. These data confirm that one-third of pregnant patients treated with prolonged heparin are likely to develop osteoporosis, even at doses as low as 15,000 units per day. Additionally, patients rarely may develop heparin-associated antibodies during pregnancy, resulting in thrombosis and thrombocytopenia (54).

In their literature review, Ginsberg and Hirsh (51) reported warfarin embryopathy in 45 of 970 exposed fetuses and central nervous system abnormalities in 26 of 970 patients. Of 22 cases of heparin osteoporosis that have been reported, seven have occurred in pregnant patients. Development of osteoporosis may be related to total exposure and has been reported in patients receiving 15,000 to 20,000 units daily for more than 6 months.

Based on these data, most authors recommend systemic heparinization during the critical weeks 6 to 12 of gestation and in the last 2 weeks of pregnancy to allow rapid reversal for delivery. A dosage of 10,000 units twice per day subcutaneously is the recommended treatment. Activated partial thromboplastin time should be measured 6 hours after administration of heparin and should be 1.5 to 2.0 times control. Warfarin can be administered during the remainder of gestation with little risk of embryopathy.

PREGNANCY IN WOMEN WITH VALVE PROSTHESES

Cardiologists are often asked to evaluate and manage the condition of patients with prosthetic heart valves during pregnancy or to advise young women on the selection of an appropriate artificial valve, designed to maximize the potential for a future successful and uncomplicated pregnancy. However, limited data are available to assist in these tasks (*e*Table 32.5.3). g46

Recently, Vongpatanasin and colleagues (63) recommended that administration of warfarin be discontinued in patients attempting pregnancy and that administration of subcutaneous heparin be substituted, twice per day at a dose that prolongs the activated partial thromboplastin time by more than two times control 6 hours after administration. After week 12 of gestation, warfarin can be safely substituted until "the middle of the third trimester, after which warfarin should be discontinued and heparin resumed until delivery."

In summary, (a) pregnancy in a woman with an artificial valve prosthesis poses significant risks to the mother and fetus; (b) pregnancy is a hypercoagulable state, and valve thrombosis or thromboembolic complications are not rare, particularly in women with mechanical prostheses and especially in women with mitral valve replacement; (c) bioprostheses may degenerate in an accelerated fashion during or shortly after delivery; (d) maternal and fetal risks are increased by the presence of advanced congestive heart failure, and pregnancy is inadvisable for women with artificial heart valves and symptoms of significant heart failure; and (e) heparin cannot be recommended for use as the sole anticoagulating agent during pregnancy and should be combined with warfarin after week 12 of gestation for women with mechanical heart prostheses who require anticoagulation therapy.

CARDIOPULMONARY BYPASS DURING PREGNANCY

Severe native or prosthetic valvular heart disease and, rarely, symptomatic coronary atherosclerosis may require cardiac surgical intervention in pregnant women. A mortality rate as high as 20% may be seen among pregnant patients with native valvular heart disease and class III to IV congestive heart failure (64). Although balloon commissurotomy of mitral stenosis or percutaneous transluminal coronary angioplasty of coronary atherosclerosis may be beneficial for pregnant women who have appropriate mitral or coronary anatomy, most other valve and coronary disease patients require more than medical treatment and should undergo cardiopulmonary bypass.

Pomini and associates (65) examined 59 reports of cardiac surgery performed with the aid of cardiopulmonary bypass from 1958 through 1992. Cardiopulmonary bypass may compromise the placenta and fetus as a result of hypothermia, decreased arterial perfusion, and alterations in coagulation as well as acid-base balance. The reported fetal and maternal mortality rates were, respectively, 2.9% and 20.2% overall, but 0% and 12%, respectively, for the 40 most recently reported subjects (1975–1991). Hypothermia alters placental oxygen exchange and has been demonstrated to initiate uterine contractions. Embryo fetal mortality associated with hypothermic cardiopulmonary bypass was 24%, and mortality associated with normothermic perfusion was 0. Increased rates of pump flow diminished evidence of fetal cardiac distress, and higher-volume cardiopulmonary bypass flow is recommended, with the appropriate fetal monitoring to ensure adequacy. Therefore, normothermic bypass at high-flow volumes is recommended.

Additionally, it is recommended that patients whose pregnancies are past 20 weeks' gestation be positioned in the left lateral decubitus position during surgery to ensure that the uterus does not obstruct venous return as a result of direct inferior vena cava compression. Hyperkalemic arrest solutions may reach the fetal circulation and should be avoided, if possible. Finally, the duration of cardiopulmonary bypass should be minimized, and the operating room must be prepared for emergency cesarean section (65).

In summary, cardiopulmonary bypass may be necessary during pregnancy. To avoid maternal and particularly fetal complications, cardiopulmonary support should be high flow, normothermic, and initiated without hyperkalemic arrest. Surgery should be performed with the patient in the left lateral decubitus position if the pregnancy is past 20 weeks' gestation, and the operating room must be prepared for a potential emergency cesarean delivery.

MYOCARDIAL INFARCTION ASSOCIATED WITH PREGNANCY

Symptomatic coronary artery disease and myocardial infarction occur infrequently during pregnancy. Nevertheless, because pregnant patients may display spontaneous coronary artery dissection, and because the population of women attempting pregnancy is progressively older, cardiologists must be familiar with this potential problem. ▼ g47

PREGNANCY IN WOMEN WITH CONGENITAL OR ACQUIRED CARDIAC DISEASE

Women who have congenital or acquired cardiac disease with or without surgical correction should approach an obstetrician and a cardiologist for assistance in management of their condition during pregnancy. Siu and colleagues (76) examined prospectively the maternal and neonatal risks associated with pregnancy in women with known heart disease. Investigators at 13 Canadian cardiac and obstetric hospitals enrolled 562 consecutive patients and determined outcome in 599 pregnancies. Maternal cardiac complications (pulmonary edema, arrhythmia, stroke, or cardiac death) complicated 13% of pregnancies and were predicted by prior cardiac events or arrhythmia, poor functional class or cyanosis, left heart obstruction, and left ventricular systolic function. Patients experienced a 4%, 31%, or 68% risk of primary or secondary cardiac events with 0, 1, and more than 1 predictors. Neonatal complications occurred in 20% of pregnancies and were associated with poor functional class or cyanosis, left heart obstruction, anticoagulation, smoking, and multiple gestations. At the Royal Infirmary of Edenberg University, 50 years of experiences were reviewed; a decreasing incidence of rheumatic heart disease in pregnant women was seen (94% from 1928 through 1947 and 36% from 1968 through 1977). In the same time interval, the incidence of pregnant women presenting with congenital heart disease increased from 3.6% to 70.0% (77). Wooley and Sparks (78) summarized five clinical studies published between 1963 and 1977 that included a total of 490 patients who had congenital heart disease and were undergoing pregnancy, and reported a maternal mortality of 0.53% and a fetal mortality of 18.90%. Certain congenital defects were considered to place patients at a higher risk by these authors, including Eisenmenger's complex, pulmonary hypertension, and cyanotic cardiac defects. Aortopathy associated with Marfan syndrome and coarctation increased risks. Perloff (79) identified potential residual changes after congenital surgical correction that increased concern about maternal and fetal outcomes, including (a) residual elevation of pulmonary vascular resistance, (b) residual aortic stenosis or regurgitation, (c) persistent right or left ventricular dysfunction, (d) aortopathy after aorta or aortic valve repair or replacement, (e) uncertain capability of prosthetic material, and (f) cleft mitral valve residual defects after endocardial cushion repair (*e*Table 32.5.4). ▼ g48

CARDIOVASCULAR COMPLICATIONS OF TOCOLYTIC THERAPY

Tocolytic agents decrease uterine contractility and are used to prolong gestation, usually beyond week 34, to allow fetal lung maturation. These agents are used in up to 5% of all pregnancies. Drugs used include β-sympathetic agents such as terbutaline, isoxsuprine, ritodrine, salbutamol, and, recently, nifedipine (90). Physiologic effects from this class of agents include tachycardia and antidiuresis. In one study, as many as 4.4% of the female patients exposed to tocolytic drugs developed pulmonary edema (72). The peculiar nature of this life-threatening complication must be understood by the cardiologist for him or her to assist the obstetrician in intelligent management.

Pisani and Rosenow (91) reviewed 22 years of medical literature to report on 58 cases. Thirty-six percent of affected women were primigravida. The most commonly used agent was terbutaline (41%), followed by isoxsuprine (33%), ritodrine (17%), and salbutamol (10%). Corticosteroids were used in two-thirds of the patients to accelerate fetal lung maturation. The average duration of treatment was 54 hours, but the syndrome can appear after less than 24 hours' exposure, and in a few cases, symptoms began after drug discontinuation, although never more than 12 hours after administration of the drug was stopped. Patients complained of dyspnea (76%), chest pain (24%), and cough (17%). Affected women sometimes had fever (temperature higher than 38°C; 14%), were rarely hypotensive, and uniformly had pulmonary rales. Chest x-rays showed bilateral pulmonary infiltrates (81%) and rarely showed effusion. The mean PO_2 was only 50 mm Hg in patients in whom it was measured. Echocardiography revealed normal left ventricular function in only seven patients. Right heart catheterization demonstrated elevated filling pressures in only two of nine cases, and the cardiac index was greater than 61 minutes per m², on average.

Treatment includes discontinuation of tocolytic therapy and administration of supplemental oxygen and intravenous diuretics. Response is usually gratifying and rapid, within 12 hours. Maternal and fetal mortality is rare, unless the woman's condition is complicated by sepsis or full-blown acute respiratory distress syndrome. The etiology of tocolytic pulmonary edema remains unknown but does not appear to be related to myocardial failure and associated pulmonary congestion.

Other entities that may present similarly include peripartum cardiomyopathy, pulmonary embolism, aspiration with acute respiratory distress syndrome, pneumomediastinum, and amniotic fluid embolization. Amniotic fluid embolization, although rare (incidence of one in 8,000 to one in 80,000 deliveries), is associated with cardiovascular collapse, respiratory distress, disseminated intravascular coagulopathy, and coma and is rapidly fatal in more than 80% of patients (92).

The risks for development of tocolytic therapy pulmonary edema appear to be related in part to the dose, the number of agents used, and the form of delivery (intravenous vs. subcutaneous). Perry and colleagues (93) studied 8,709 women who were given continuous subcutaneous infusions of terbutaline to arrest preterm labor. Patients were followed daily in the hospital or at home. Pulmonary edema developed in only 0.32% (28 of 8,709 patients). Of the 28 patients affected, 17 were receiving one to three tocolytic agents and aggressive intravenous hydration. It appears that tocolytic therapy can be administered rela-

tively safely; however, patients receiving certain dosages, multiple drug infusions, and supplemental intravenous hydration must be watched carefully.

ARRHYTHMIAS IN PREGNANT WOMEN

Page (94), Cox and Gardner (26), and Rutherford (95) have recently reviewed the treatment of arrhythmias during pregnancy. The hemodynamic stress of pregnancy may exacerbate arrhythmias, and treatment of rhythm disorders poses a risk to the mother as well as to the fetus (96).

Pregnancy significantly alters drug absorption and metabolism as a result of (a) altered gastrointestinal motility, (b) expanded plasma volume, (c) decreased plasma protein, (d) progesterone-induced alterations of hepatic metabolism, and (e) increased renal blood flow. Therefore, frequent measurement of drug levels may be necessary. The teratogenic risk of drug exposure is greatest in the first trimester of pregnancy; use of drugs should be avoided during this time if possible. ⬩ g49

ANTIPHOSPHOLIPID SYNDROME

The antiphospholipid syndrome should be suspected in mothers with arterial or venous thrombosis, thrombocytopenia, neurologic disease, or recurrent abortion. Fetal loss is associated with thrombosis of the uteroplacental vasculature. Antiphospholipid antibodies recognize a plasma cofactor on the trophoblast and/or endothelial cell surface that produces a procoagulant state (102). Women with systemic lupus erythematosus who have the lupus anticoagulant or antiphospholipid antibodies have a greater than 60% chance of pregnancy loss, compared with a 15% loss among women with systemic lupus erythematosus who do not have these antibodies. It is believed that the antiphospholipid antibody results in placental infarction or thromboses, with subsequent pregnancy loss.

Silveria and coauthors (103) treated 11 consecutive patients who had positive anticardiolipin (antiphospholipid) assays and had experienced at least one pregnancy loss with prednisone and aspirin. This resulted in an improved live birth rate, from 15.6% before treatment to 100% after treatment, without significant adverse effects to the mother or fetus. Heparin, low-dose aspirin, and intravenous immunoglobulin have been proposed as treatment options for the antiphospholipid syndrome. In a prospective, double-blind, placebo-controlled trial involving only 50 patients who had antiphospholipid antibodies and three or more fetal losses, 75 mg per day of aspirin had no influence on the live birth rate compared with placebo (80% vs. 85%, respectively) (104). Similarly, Branch and colleagues (105) found no difference in maternal or fetal outcomes when intravenous immunoglobulin was added to a regimen including aspirin and heparin for patients who had antiphospholipid antibodies. Interruption of the anticardiolipin cycle of thrombosis may be important, because patients with this syndrome may develop ventricular diastolic dysfunction over the course of time (106).

CONTROVERSIES AND PERSONAL PERSPECTIVES

Peripartum cardiomyopathy remains a controversial area in the management of the pregnant or peripartum patient. Some authors have inappropriately reported patients in their series who showed evidence of congestive heart failure and cardiomyopathy earlier than the last month of pregnancy or later than 5 months after delivery. Inclusion of patients outside these parameters has tainted some of the data concerning the incidence of myocarditis, response to immunosuppressive agents, and outcome of individuals with this disorder. Not all authors agree that peripartum cardiomyopathy is associated with myocardial inflammation. Even those who believe that myocarditis is a component of peripartum cardiomyopathy have failed to recognize inflammation in all patients who underwent endomyocardial biopsy. Therefore, the etiology of the syndrome remains unknown. Assuming that the condition is associated with myocardial inflammation, the antigen to which the immune response is directed remains unknown. Even more controversial is the potential use of immunosuppressive agents. No prospective randomized trial involving patients with peripartum cardiomyopathy has been carried out on treatment with immunosuppressive therapy of patients with myocarditis proven by endomyocardial biopsy. It is also evident that in a high proportion of patients, peripartum cardiomyopathy, with or without myocarditis, resolves spontaneously. We have, therefore, taken the stance that once peripartum cardiomyopathy is recognized, patients should be treated with standard heart failure therapy for 2 weeks. If clear echocardiographic evidence of improvement in the myopathic state is seen, patients need not undergo endomyocardial biopsy. If the myopathic state does not improve or deteriorates, the patients undergo endomyocardial biopsy, and those with myocarditis are treated with immunosuppressive agents in hopes of improving left ventricular function. Patients with ejection fractions in the exceedingly low range (less than 15%) and those who are more than 4 months from delivery are unlikely to respond, even if myocarditis is demonstrated. Only patients in whom ventricular function does not return to normal after peripartum cardiomyopathy should be should be discouraged from additional pregnancies.

A second controversial area is the use of anticoagulants in pregnant patients. Some authors use heparin throughout the pregnancy to avoid any warfarin-related embryopathy or central nervous system abnormality. Other authors have observed such a low rate of embryopathy and central nervous system disorders with use of warfarin that the agent is used throughout the pregnancy, until delivery. Unless the patient declares her desire for a pregnancy and switches from warfarin to heparin before conceiving, most patients receiving chronic anticoagulants present to their physician already pregnant. These patients have already sustained most of the potential risk for embryopathy by the time the physician is aware of the pregnancy. On balance, the risk to the patient and fetus seems least if warfarin is discontinued before pregnancy is initiated and if heparin is used through at least the first 12 weeks of gestation. Thereafter, warfarin can be used until just before delivery, when heparin must be substituted to allow delivery without substantial bleeding.

The choice of artificial heart valves is a third controversial area of management in pregnant patients. Patients with bioprostheses have a much higher live birth rate and usually do not require chronic anticoagulation. However, the potential for degeneration of bioprostheses is associated with pregnancy and delivery. Mechanical prostheses do not degenerate but are associated with a higher rate of thromboembolic complications, including valve thrombosis and embolic phenomena in the central nervous system and periphery. Most of these thromboembolic complications have occurred in patients receiving inadequate heparin therapy. I favor the implantation of a mechanical prosthesis, even for the patient who desires a subsequent pregnancy. On the patient's declaration of the intention for pregnancy, conversion from warfarin to adequate heparin anticoagulation until after the first trimester, and then careful management of warfarin therapy, should diminish the potential for thromboembolic complications.

Not all clinicians are willing to follow patients who have undergone corrected congenital or acquired heart disease through pregnancy. These patients have often sustained life-threatening complications before surgery, and the surgery itself is usually high risk. Once patients have survived these risks, many clinicians are wary of the patient's decision to incur what some would consider an unnecessary additional risk. There is also the potential that the mother's genetic disorder may be passed on to any children. Other clinicians empathize with the patient's desire to bear and raise children despite the risk to the patient. We ensure that the patient is informed of the potential risk that her cardiac disorder could be transmitted to her offspring. If a patient is willing to accept this risk and we concur, a full cardiovascular evaluation is undertaken to evaluate the patient's cardiopulmonary capability to sustain the cardiovascular stress of normal pregnancy and delivery. Occasionally, the risk is determined to be too great, based on elevated pulmonary vascular resistance, high filling pressures, left or right ventricular dysfunction, or inadequate correction of congenital abnormalities. Most patients are willing to accept the decision to avoid pregnancy after a thorough evaluation.

THE FUTURE

An increased understanding of the pathophysiology of disorders such as preeclampsia and peripartum cardiomyopathy will lead to more effective therapies. With advances in vascular biology, more effective anticoagulation regimens can be used in patients who have thrombogenic abnormalities. More thorough prepregnancy cardiovascular evaluations, including stress or dobutamine echocardiography and magnetic resonance imaging, will better identify patients with acquired or corrected congenital heart disease who are able to proceed safely with pregnancy and delivery.

Little controversy exists about the risks of use of antiarrhythmic agents, regardless of the state of pregnancy. Drugs are infrequently used and when used are carefully chosen to avoid teratogenic and maternal problems.

FUTURE DIRECTIONS

It is likely that an increasing proportion of high-risk pregnancies will be undertaken by older women or women with preexisting heart disease. These factors will result in continued growth and development of the already strong relationships between physicians in cardiology and in high-risk obstetrics.

Because exercise in pregnancy has clear-cut advantages, it is appropriate for a larger proportion of pregnant patients to be involved in aerobic exercise.

It is likely that the etiology of preeclampsia will be discovered in the near future. An increased understanding of vascular biology and alterations of vascular biology that occur in pregnant women will allow an appropriate recognition of the underlying abnormality associated with this potentially fatal complication of pregnancy. Once the pathophysiology is understood, it is almost certain that an effective therapy can be introduced, significantly reducing maternal and fetal morbidity and mortality.

We are only beginning to understand the pathophysiology of peripartum cardiomyopathy. If the condition is associated with myocarditis, it seems logical that the etiology is immunologic. It is unlikely that the causative agent is viral and more likely that it is related to an altered placental antigen. Understanding the pathophysiology of the condition will allow better recognition and treatment of patients with this disorder. Once the pathophysiology is understood, it is anticipated that almost all patients who have peripartum cardiomyopathy will recover, as opposed to the approximately 50% recovery rate that is currently achieved.

Although new forms of anticoagulants are available, including low-molecular-weight heparin, antiplatelet agents, and platelet IIb/IIIa glycoprotein inhibitors, it is unlikely that any significant improvement will be made in the risk to patients who are pregnant and require anticoagulant therapy. Progress in this regard is again dependent on advances in vascular biology. Estrogen, progesterone, and other pregnancy-related hormone alterations that affect vascular and platelet reactivity may serve as a nidus for thrombus formation. Effective anticoagulant therapy depends on the physician understanding these alterations and providing appropriate interruption of pregnancy-related changes. Once these thrombogenic abnormalities are recognized and understood, it is expected that pregnancy can be more safely undertaken by women with mechanical valve prostheses. There is likely nothing that can alter the increased metabolic and calcium turnover in bioprostheses that are associated with pregnancy, and therefore the degeneration of these prostheses that is associated with pregnancy is likely to continue.

Although earlier correction of congenital and acquired heart disease is possible, it is unlikely that the early repair of these disorders will significantly alter the risk to the patient associated with pregnancy and delivery. More thorough prepregnancy cardiovascular evaluations, including stress or dobutamine echocardiography, and magnetic resonance imaging with or without exercise will likely better identify patients who are capable of proceeding safely with pregnancy and delivery.

Safer doses and durations of tocolytic therapy are already being used. The lack of understanding of pulmonary edema related to tocolytic therapy is the result primarily of inadequate investigation into the condition of these relatively rare patients. Despite the small number of patients who experience this disorder, the nature of the disorder can be ascertained, and appropriate treatment regimens can be designed.

The increased risk associated with use of antiarrhythmic agents has been recognized in nonpregnant patients. This risk is increased further with the pregnant state, because drug absorption and metabolism both alter in association with pregnancy. Therefore, drug therapy should be avoided if possible during pregnancy, and if it is used, agents without teratogenic risk or proarrhythmic potential are favored.

REFERENCES

1. Hunter S, Robson SC. Adaptation of the maternal heart in pregnancy. *Br Heart J* 1992;68:540–543.

2. Mabie WC, DiSessa TG, Crocker LG, et al. A longitudinal study of cardiac output in normal human pregnancy. *Am J Obstet Gynecol* 1994;170:849–856.

3. Vered Z, Poler SM, Gibson P, et al. Noninvasive detection of the morphologic and hemodynamic changes during normal pregnancy. *Clin Cardiol* 1991;14:327–334.

4. Hess DB, Hess LW. Management of cardiovascular disease in pregnancy. *Obstet Gynecol Clin North Am* 1992;19:679–695.

5. Elkayam U, Gleicher N. Changes in cardiac findings during normal pregnancy. In: Elkayam U, Gleiden N, eds. *Cardiac problems in pregnancy: diagnosis and management of maternal and fetal disease,* 2nd ed. New York: Alan R. Liss, 1990:31.

6. Sady MA, Haydon BB, Sady SP, et al. Cardiovascular response to maximal cycle exercise during pregnancy and at two and seven months post partum. *Am J Obstet Gynecol* 1990;162:1181–1185.

7. Lotgering FK, Struijk PC, Van Doorn MB, et al. Errors in predicting maximal oxygen consumption in pregnant women. *J Appl Physiol* 1992;72:562–567.

8. Lotgering FK, Struijk PC, Van Doorn MB, et al. Anaerobic threshold and respiratory compensation in pregnant women. *J Appl Physiol* 1995;78:1772–1777.

9. Wolfe LA, Walker RMC, Bonen A, et al. Effects of pregnancy and chronic exercise on respiratory responses to graded exercise. *J Appl Physiol* 1994;76:1928–1936.

10. Wegnerckileser RG, Saldana LR. *Exposure of the pregnant patient to diagnostic radiation: a guide to medical management.* Philadelphia: JB Lippincott, 1985.

11. Bithell JF, Stewart AM. Pre-natal irradiation and childhood malignancy: a review of British data from the Oxford survey. *Br J Cancer* 1975;31:271–287.

12. Rosenstein M. Organ doses in diagnostic radiology. *U.S. Department of Health, Education, and Welfare,* May 1976.

13. Elkayam U, Kawanishi D, Reid CL, et al. Contrast echocardiography to reduce ionizing radiation associated with cardiac catheterization during pregnancy. *Am J Cardiol* 1983;52:213–214.

14. Lindheimer MD. Hypertension in pregnancy. *Hypertension* 1993;22:127–137.

15. Sibai BM. Treatment of hypertension in pregnant women. *N Engl J Med* 1996;335:257–265.

16. Cunningham FG, Lindheimer MD. Hypertension in pregnancy. *N Engl J Med* 1992;326:927–932.

17. Collins R, Peto R, MacMahon S, et al. Blood pressure, stroke and coronary heart disease. 2. Short term reductions in blood pressure: overview of randomized drug trials in their epidemiologic context. *Lancet* 1990;335:827–838.

18. Schobel HP, Fischer T, Heuszer K, et al. Preeclampsia: a state of sympathetic overactivity. *N Engl J Med* 1996;335:1480–1485.

19. Rowland BL, Vermillion ST, Roudebush WE. Elevated circulating concentrations of platelet activating factor in preeclampsia. *Am J Obstet Gynecol* 2000;183:930–932.

20. McKinney ET, Shouri R, Hunt RS, et al. Plasma, urinary and salivary 8-epi-prostaglandin f2alpha levels in normotensive and preeclamptic pregnancies. *Am J Obstet Gynecol* 2000;183:874–877.

21. Dechend R, Homuth V, Wallukat G, et al. AT(1) receptor agonistic antibodies from preeclamptic patients cause vascular cells to express tissue factor. *Circulation* 2000;101:2382–2387.

22. O'Brien JM, Milligan DA, Barton JR. Impact of high-dose corticosteroid therapy for patients with HELLP (hemolysis, elevated liver enzymes, and low platelet count) syndrome. *Am J Obstet Gynecol* 2000;183:921–924.

23. Lindheimer MD, Katz AI. Sodium and diuretics in pregnancy. *N Engl J Med* 1976;288:891–894.

24. Cockburn J, Ounsted M, Moar VA, et al. Final report of study on hypertension during pregnancy: the effects of specific treatment on the growth and development of the children. *Lancet* 1982;647–649.

25. Sweit M. Antihypertensive drugs in pregnancy. *BMJ* 1985;291:3565–3566.

26. Cox JL, Gardner MJ. Treatment of cardiac arrhythmias during pregnancy. *Prog Cardiovasc Dis* 1993;36:137–178.

27. Childress CH, Katz VL. Nifedipine and its indications in obstetrics and gynecology. *Obstet Gynecol* 1994;83:616–624.

28. Shotan A, Widerhorn J, Hurst A, et al. Risks of angiotensin-converting enzyme inhibition during pregnancy: experimental and clinical evidence, potential mechanisms, and recommendations for use. *Am J Med* 1994;96:451–456.

29. Nightingale SL. From the Food and Drug Administration. *JAMA* 1992;267:2445.

30. Demakis JG, Rahimtoola SH. Peripartum cardiomyopathy. *Circulation* 1971;44:964–968.

31. Demakis JG, Rahimtoola SH, Sutton GC, et al. Natural course of peripartum cardiomyopathy. *Circulation* 1971;44:1053–1061.

32. Lampert MB, Lang RM. Peripartum cardiomyopathy. *Am Heart J* 1995;130:860–870.

33. Homans DC. Current concepts: peripartum cardiomyopathy. *N Engl J Med* 1985;312:1432–1437.

34. Melvin KR, Richardson PJ, Olsen EGJ, et al. Peripartum cardiomyopathy due to myocarditis. *N Engl J Med* 1982;307:731–734.

35. Sanderson JE, Olsen EGJ, Gate D. Peripartum heart disease: an endomyocardial biopsy study. *Br Heart J* 1986;56:285–291.

36. O'Connell JB, Costanzo-Nordin MR, Subramanian R, et al. Peripartum cardiomyopathy: clinical, hemodynamic, histologic and prognostic characteristics. *J Am Coll Cardiol* 1986;8:52–56.

37. Midei MG, DeMent SH, Feldman AM, et al. Peripartum myocarditis and cardiomyopathy. *Circulation* 1990;81:922–928.

38. Felker GM, Jaeger CJ, Klodas E, et al. Myocarditis and long-term survival in peripartum cardiomyopathy. *Am Heart J* 2000;140:785–791.

39. Felker GM, Thompson RE, Hare JM, et al. Underlying causes and long-term survival in patients with initially unexplained cardiomyopathy. *N Engl J Med* 2000;342:1077–1084.

40. Sliwa K, Skudicky D, Bergemann A, et al. Peripartum cardiomyopathy: analysis of clinical outcome, ventricular function, plasma levels of cytokines and Fas/APO-1. *J Am Coll Cardiol* 2000;35:701–705.

41. Cole P, Cook F, Plappert T, et al. Longitudinal changes in left ventricular architecture and function in peripartum cardiomyopathy. *Am J Cardiol* 1987;60:871–876.

42. Elkayam U, Tummala P, Rao K, et al. Maternal and fetal outcomes with subsequent pregnancies in women with peripartum cardiomyopathy. *N Engl J Med* 2001;344:1567–1571.

42a. Lampert MD, Winert L, Hibbard J, et al. Contractile reserve in patients with peripartum cardiomyopathy and recovered left ventricular function. *Am J Obstet Gynecol* 1997;176:189–195.

43. Rickenbacher PR, Rizeq MN, Hunt SA, et al. Long-term outcome after heart transplantation for peripartum cardiomyopathy. *Am Heart J* 1994;127:1318–1323.

44. Liljestrand J, Lindstrom B. Childbirth after post partum cardiac insufficiency treated with cardiac transplant. *Acta Obstet Gynecol Scand* 1993;72:406–408.

45. Laifer SA, Yeagley CJ, Armitage JM. Pregnancy after cardiac transplantation. *Am J Perinatol* 1994;11:217–219.

46. Scott JR, Wagoner LE, Olsen SL, et al. Pregnancy in heart transplant recipients: management and outcome. *Obstet Gynecol* 1993;82:324–327.

47. Branch KR, Wagoner LE, McGrory CH, et al. Risks of subsequent pregnancies on mother and newborn in female heart transplant recipients. *J Heart Lung Transplant* 1998;17:698–702.

48. Troche V, Ville Y, Fernandez H. Pregnancy after heart or heart-lung transplantation: a series of 10 pregnancies. *Br J Obstet Gynaecol* 1998;105:454–458.

49. Dajani AS, Bisno AL, Chung JK, et al. Prevention of bacterial endocarditis: recommendations by the American Heart Association. *JAMA* 1990;264:2919–2922.

50. Ellison J, Walker ID, Greer IA. Antenatal use of enoxaparin for prevention and treatment of thromboembolism in pregnancy. *BJOG* 2000;107:1116–1121.

51. Ginsberg JS, Hirsh J. Anticoagulants during pregnancy. *Annu Rev Med* 1989;40:79–86.

52. Ginsberg JS, Kowalchuk G, Hirsh J, et al. Heparin therapy during pregnancy: risks to the fetus and mother. *Arch Intern Med* 1989;149:2233–2236.

53. Barbour LA, Kick SD, Steiner JF, et al. A prospective study of heparin-induced osteoporosis in pregnancy using bone densitometry. *Am J Obstet Gynecol* 1994;170:862–869.

54. Calhoun BC, Hesser JW. Heparin-associated antibody with pregnancy: discussion of two cases. *Am J Obstet Gynecol* 1987;156:964–966.

55. Hanania G, Thomas D, Michel PL, et al. Pregnancy and prosthetic heart valves: a French cooperative retrospective study of 155 cases. *Eur Heart J* 1994;15:1651–1658.

56. Sbarouni E, Oakley CM. Outcome of pregnancy in women with valve prostheses. *Br Heart J* 1994;71:196–201.

57. Born D, Martinez EE, Almeida PAM, et al. Pregnancy in patients with prosthetic heart valves: the effects of anticoagulation on mother, fetus, and neonate. *Am Heart J* 1992;124:413–417.

58. Chan WS, Anand S, Ginsberg JS. Anticoagulation of pregnant women with mechanical heart valves: a systematic review of the literature. *Arch Intern Med* 2000;160(2):191–196.

59. Lev-Ran O, Kramer A, Gurevitch J, et al. Low-molecular-weight heparin for prosthetic heart valves: treatment failure. *Ann Thorac Surg* 2000;69(1):264–265.

60. Sadler L, McCowan L, White H, et al. Pregnancy outcomes and cardiac complications in women with mechanical, bioprosthetic and homograft valves. *BJOG* 2000;107(2):245–253.

61. Salazar E, Espinola N, Roman L, et al. Effect of pregnancy on the duration of bovine pericardial bioprostheses. *Am Heart J* 1999;137:714–720.

62. Mangione JA, Lourenco RM, dos Santos ES, et al. Long-term follow-up of pregnant women after percutaneous mitral valvuloplasty. *Catheter Cardiovasc Interv* 2000;50:413–417.

63. Vongpatanasin W, Hillis LD, Lange RA. Prosthetic heart valves. *N Engl J Med* 1996;335:407–416.

64. Sullivan HJ. Valvular heart surgery during pregnancy. *Surg Clin North Am* 1995;75:59–75.

65. Pomini F, Mercogliano D, Cavalletti C, et al. Cardiopulmonary bypass in pregnancy. *Ann Thorac Surg* 1996;61:259–268.

66. Sheikh AU, Harper MA. Myocardial infarction during pregnancy: management and outcome of two pregnancies. *Am J Obstet Gynecol* 1993;169:279–284.

67. Donnelly S, McKenna P, McGing P, et al. Myocardial infarction during pregnancy. *Br J Obstet Gynaecol* 1993;100:781–782.

68. Roth A, Elkayam U. Acute myocardial infarction associated with pregnancy. *Ann Intern Med* 1996;125:751–762.

69. Hennekens CH, Albert CM, Godfried SL, et al. Adjunctive drug therapy of acute myocardial infarction: evidence from clinical trials. *N Engl J Med* 1996;335:1660–1667.

70. Cowan NC, de Belder MA, Rothman MT. Coronary angioplasty in pregnancy. *Br Heart J* 1988;59:588–592.

71. Mather PJ, Hansen CL, Goldman B, et al. Postpartum multivessel coronary dissection. *J Heart Lung Transplant* 1994;13:533–537.

72. Coulson CC, Kuller JA, Bowes WA Jr. Myocardial infarction and coronary artery dissection in pregnancy. *Am J Perinatol* 1995;12:328–330.

73. Kearney P, Singh H, Huttr J, et al. Spontaneous coronary artery dissection: a report of three cases and review of the literature. *Postgrad Med J* 1993;69:940–945.

74. Rensing BJ, Kofflard M, van den Brand MJ, et al. Spontaneous dissections of all three coronary arteries in a 33-week-pregnant woman. *Catheter Cardiovasc Interv* 1999;48(2):207–210.

75. Pombar X, Strassner HT, Fenner PC. Pregnancy in a woman with class H diabetes mellitus and previous coronary artery bypass graft: a case report and review of the literature. *Obstet Gynecol* 1995;85:825–829.

76. Siu S, Sermer M, Colman JM, et al. Prospective multicenter study of pregnancy outcomes in women with heart disease. *Circulation* 2001;104:515–521.

77. Allan LD, Sharland GK, Milburn A, et al. Prospective diagnosis of 1,006 consecutive cases of congenital heart disease in the fetus. *J Am Coll Cardiol* 1994;23:1452–1458.

78. Wooley CF, Sparks EH. Congenital heart disease, heritable cardiovascular disease, and pregnancy. *Prog Cardiovasc Dis* 1992;35:41–60.

79. Perloff JK. Pediatric congenital cardiac becomes a postoperative adult: the changing population of congenital heart disease. *Circulation* 1973;47:606–619.

80. Pyeritz RE. Maternal and fetal complications of pregnancy in the Marfan syndrome. *Am J Med* 1981;71:784–790.

81. Pelliccia F, Cianfrocca C, Gaudio C, et al. Sudden death during pregnancy in hypertrophic cardiomyopathy. *Eur Heart J* 1992;13:421–423.

82. Oakley GDG, McGarry K, Limb DG, et al. Management of pregnancy in patients with hypertrophic cardiomyopathy. *BMJ* 1979;1:1749–1750.

83. Tang LCH, Chan SYW, Wong VCW, et al. Pregnancy in patients with mitral valve prolapse. *Int J Gynaecol Obstet* 1985;23:217–221.

84. Presbitero P, Somerville J, Stone S, et al. Pregnancy in cyanotic congenital heart disease: outcome of mother and fetus. *Circulation* 1994;89:2673–2676.

85. Connolly HM, Warnes CA. Ebstein's anomaly: outcome of pregnancy. *J Am Coll Cardiol* 1994;23:1194–1198.

86. Clarkson PM, Wilson NJ, Neutze JM, et al. Outcome of pregnancy after the Mustard operation for transposition of the great arteries with intact ventricular septum. *J Am Coll Cardiol* 1994;24:190–193.

87. Connolly HM, Grogan M, Warnes CA. Pregnancy among women with congenitally corrected transposition of great arteries. *J Am Coll Cardiol* 1999;33:1692–1695.

88. Lao TT, Sermer M, MaGee L, et al. *Am J Obstet Gynecol* 1993;169:540–545.

89. Al Kasab SM, Sabag T, Al Zaibag M, et al. Beta-adrenergic receptor blockade in the management of pregnant women with mitral stenosis. *Am J Obstet Gynecol* 1990;163:37–40.

90. Carr DB, Clark AL, Kernek K, et al. Maintenance oral nifedipine for preterm labor: a randomized clinical trial. *Am J Obstet Gynecol* 1999;181:822–827.

91. Pisani RJ, Rosenow EC 3d. Pulmonary edema associated with tocolytic therapy. *Ann Intern Med* 1989;110:714–718.

92. Morgan M. Amniotic fluid embolism. *Anaesthesia* 1979;34:20–32.

93. Perry KG, Morrison JC, Rust OA, et al. Incidence of adverse cardiopulmonary effects with low-dose continuous terbutaline infusion. *Am J Obstet Gynecol* 1995;173:1273–1277.

94. Page RL. Treatment of arrhythmias during pregnancy. *Am Heart J* 1995;130:871–876.

95. Rutherford JD. Management of cardiovascular disease during pregnancy. In: Smith TW, ed. *Cardiovascular therapeutics*. Philadelphia: WB Saunders, 1996:695–701.

96. American Academy of Pediatrics Committee on Drugs. The transfer of drugs and other chemicals into human milk. *Pediatrics* 1994;93:137–150.

97. Afridi I, Moise KJ Jr, Rokey R. Termination of supraventricular tachycardia with intravenous adenosine in a pregnant woman with Wolff-Parkinson-White syndrome. *Obstet Gynecol* 1992;80:481–483.

98. Brodsky M, Doria R, Allen B, et al. New-onset ventricular tachycardia during pregnancy. *Am Heart J* 1992;123:933–941.

99. Werler MM, Lammer EJ, Rosenberg L, et al. Maternal alcohol use in relation to selected birth defects. *Am J Epidemiol* 1991;134:691–698.

100. Werler MM, Mitchell AA, Shapiro S. The relation of aspirin use during the first trimester of pregnancy to congenital cardiac defects. *N Engl J Med* 1989;321:1639–1642.

101. Goldberg SJ, Lebowitz MD, Graver EJ, et al. An association of human congenital cardiac malformations and drinking water contaminants. *J Am Coll Cardiol* 1990;16:155–164.

102. Caruso A, De Carolis S, Di Simone N. Antiphospholipid antibodies in obstetrics: new complexities and sites of action. *Hum Reprod Update* 1999;5(3):267–276.

103. Silveria LH, Huggle CL, Jara LJ, et al. Prevention of anticardiolipin antibody–related pregnancy losses with prednisone and aspirin. *Am J Med* 1992;93:403–411.

104. Pattison NS, Chamley LW, Birdsall M, et al. Does aspirin have a role in improving pregnancy outcome for women with the antiphospholipid syndrome? A randomized controlled trial. *Am J Obstet Gynecol* 2000;183:1008–1012.

105. Branch DW, Peaceman AM, Druzin M, et al. A multicenter, placebo-controlled pilot study of intravenous immune globulin treatment of antiphospholipid syndrome during pregnancy. The Pregnancy Loss Study Group. *Am J Obstet Gynecol* 2000;182[1 Pt 1]:122–127.

106. Hasnie AMA, Stoddard MF, Gleason CB, et al. Diastolic dysfunction is a feature of the antiphospholipid syndrome. *Am Heart J* 1995;129:1009–1013.

34

END-OF-LIFE CARE

GARY S. FRANCIS

OVERVIEW

Life in the coronary care unit (CCU) is changing. Once a comfortable "laboratory" for conducting studies of physiology and pharmacology, as well as a bastion of medical education, the modern CCU has become a vastly different place over the course of the last 15 to 20 years. This is particularly true in large, tertiary teaching hospitals. The patients are older and sicker, and they have more multiorgan dysfunction than before. They frequently require multiple-team, interdisciplinary management. Patients who have routine, uncomplicated myocardial infarction continue to be admitted, but many such patients are now well cared for in large suburban hospitals by highly qualified cardiologists. Tertiary teaching hospitals more often receive elderly patients with highly complex conditions who are transferred on day 2 or 3 of acute myocardial infarction complicated by acute pulmonary edema, stroke, refractory ventricular tachycardia, cardiogenic shock, severe mitral regurgitation, ruptured interventricular septum, critical aortic stenosis, acute renal failure, sepsis, or some combination of the above. Such patients can usually be stabilized and their conditions managed, but they not uncommonly languish for days in the CCU, obtunded, unable to be easily weaned from the ventilator. Anxious families understandably become frus-

trated, and uncertainty about prognosis only serves to further fracture the bond between physicians and family members.

The dilemma is made worse by the inability of many patients to participate in the decision-making process. Families may be absent. Occasionally, competing interests and desires may emerge among family members. Decisions about the end of life are seemingly more complex in today's world. Resources are often constrained, and economic pressures exist to reduce the length of stay in the CCU. The overall daily charges for the CCU range from $2,000 to $10,000 per day. To put the economic burden into perspective, it is estimated that critical care costs in the United States are more than $80 billion per year, or approximately 1% of the gross domestic product (1). Of course, the high cost of care is a global problem, certainly not unique to the United States.

The aging CCU patient population, complexity of disease, high prevalence of multiorgan dysfunction, unrealistic expectations of patients and families, and persistence of taboos regarding discussions of the end of life in most cultures mean that physicians who work in the CCU must be familiar with certain guiding principles regarding the withholding and withdrawal of life-support systems. The decision to withhold or withdraw life-sustaining support from a critically ill patient is an increasingly difficult but necessary part of providing care in the CCU. The preciousness of human life is embedded in nearly every religion and culture. The natural tendency of every physician is to nurture the patient back to health, and therefore to preserve life without regard

G. S. Francis: Department of Cardiovascular Medicine, Coronary Intensive Care Unit, The Cleveland Clinic Foundation, Cleveland, Ohio

to age, cost, or other culturally imposed boundaries. It is clear that in a small number of cases, death is inescapable. In such cases, the wise physician turns attention to the family, while ensuring that the patient is made comfortable. But mostly there are gray zones, in which outcomes are uncertain and decisions about continued aggressive treatments are extremely difficult. Uncertainty becomes champion.

How are these decisions made? Who makes these decisions? What are the ethical principles that underlie these decisions? How does a physician actually withdraw life support? The goal of this chapter is to provide CCU physicians with practical advice that will help guide them through this difficult process.

HISTORICAL PERSPECTIVE

For many years, the ethical and legal consensus in the United States has been that patients and their surrogates have the right to refuse life-prolonging therapy. This stems from the common-law right of self-determination (the principles of autonomy), which was upheld by the U.S. Supreme Court in 1891 (2). Despite agreement on this general principle, dying patients in the United States frequently receive unwanted interventions (3,4). The patient's right to autonomy, though sacred and carefully guarded, sometimes competes with the staff member's skill in providing aggressive life-extending treatment. Physicians and nurses are often poorly trained in withholding or withdrawing intensive life support. It is sometimes easier for them to continue aggressive care than to struggle with the difficult decision to withdraw life support. This issue came to a head in the landmark case of Karen Ann Quinlan (1976), and the courts ultimately forged a legal consensus based on the principle of patient autonomy. This principle establishes the right of patients (or their surrogates) to determine which medical interventions to accept or refuse, even when the absence of treatment results in death. It was affirmed by the U.S. Supreme Court in the case of Nancy Cruzan in 1990. The court acknowledged that patients who die after life support is withheld or withdrawn die of the underlying disease process. Such deaths are not assisted suicides or euthanasia. The courts have also reasoned that the spouse and children are the most appropriate surrogates because they are best positioned to know the patient's feelings and desires about treatment.

In fact, next of kin are no better than physicians in estimating what the patient would want with regard to end-of-life care (5). Therefore, the physician, acting on behalf of the patient, must assess the validity of the surrogates' preferences and the commonality of belief structure. Friends or family members may hold power of attorney to make decisions for the patient, as directed by a living will or advanced directive. However, living wills have not had a major impact on decision-making or costs associated with end-of-life care, because they are so nonspecific. Patients frequently express different beliefs when they are healthy than when they face decisions about withdrawal of life-support measures (6). The U.S. Supreme Court has unanimously ruled that there is no constitutional right to physician-assisted suicide but has also effectively required all states to ensure that their laws do not obstruct the provision of palliative care—including the administration of drugs as needed to avoid pain at the end of life (7). The provision of morphine or other medications at the end of life to control pain and suffering has the full force of the judiciary behind it.

From a historical context, these rulings have come at a time when modern technology can sustain organ function for prolonged periods, and thus they are of great importance to physicians working in the CCU. Lay people, through the print media and television, have come to expect full recovery after illness. Families and patients often seem mystified when informed of the details of an illness and become alarmed when they realize that meaningful recovery may not be possible. The gap between family expectations and medical reality can only be closed by frequent empathetic and effective communication between the medical team, the family, and, when appropriate, the patient.

ETHICAL PRINCIPLES

Some fundamental principles of medical ethics have evolved over centuries and are generally accepted (Table 34.1).

Autonomy

The term *autonomy* is derived from the Greek words *auto* (self) and *nomos* (rule or law). The principle is the source of the common-law right of self-determination and lies behind the constitutional right of privacy. No right is held more sacred, and the U.S. Supreme Court has used this principle in asserting the right of patients to refuse life-saving treatment. If an adult patient is heavily sedated or unconscious, a surrogate decision-maker (usually a spouse or family member) should authorize decisions about care. Health care providers need to realize that

TABLE 34.1 FUNDAMENTAL PRINCIPLES OF MEDICAL ETHICS

Autonomy
Preservation of life
Alleviation of suffering
First do no harm
Justice: ensure that medical resources are allocated fairly
Telling the truth
The rule of double effect

decisions about care are in the hands of the patient, not the medical team. The attending physician and other members of the medical team determine treatment strategy on the basis of scientific principles and then decide on the best course of action based on discussion with the patient or the families. The patient (or the surrogate decision-maker) almost always accepts the team's advice, but the relationship is one of partnership, not paternalism. The ethical principle of autonomy states that the patient has a right to self-determination that supersedes the desires of the medical team—even if it means that death of the patient will result. In the United States, minors do not have autonomy under the law, and parents become the decision-makers.

The CCU environment doesn't always allow for the luxury of time, and lengthy discussions with multiple family members are sometimes not possible. Management of cardiogenic shock, recurrent ventricular fibrillation, acute pulmonary edema, or acute aortic dissection requires quick, reasoned actions. In such emergencies, the principle of preservation of life guides the physician, provided there are no antecedent instructions from the patient or family to withhold life support.

Although end-of-life issues are best discussed in the privacy of the outpatient clinic when the patient is medically stable, many patients misunderstand the process of advanced life support or are apprehensive about discussing death. This may be related to the nearly universal taboo against discussing death, which is particularly common among the older generation. A significant number of people prefer a less dominant autonomous role in end-of-life decisions and put their trust in their doctors and the health care system (8). To approach a critically ill patient in the CCU with heartless questions about cardiopulmonary resuscitation and intubation is a grotesque distortion of what should be a very private, reasoned dialogue. Trying to berate a sick patient into being autonomous near end of life is a tragic mistake. My practice is always to discuss end of life in the outpatient setting when possible. When this is not possible, which is often the case, it is helpful to talk to the patient alone at the bedside and attempt to have them understand and make distinctions between short-term aggressive care and prolonged life support.

In the end, the informed patient can usually make an autonomous decision. Physicians must guard against imposing their own values and should not slant the discussion in such a way as to mirror their own feelings about the end of life. It must be recognized that some cultures object to informing patients of a terminal diagnosis. It may be believed that the family, not the patient, should make life-support decisions. Violating a patient's cultural values should be avoided. This is a serious problem that defies a simple solution. It is often useful to have serious dialogue with the family and then the patient as

soon as possible—usually within 48 hours of admission to the CCU.

Preservation of Life

All physicians are aware of this ethical principle, and it requires no explanation. Problems may arise when preservation of life competes with beneficence or alleviation of suffering. For a dying patient, alleviation of suffering may be more important than prolonging the end of life. However, the sanctity of life is of great importance and has its roots in most religions of the world. Many believe that every second of life is sacred and must be preserved at all cost.

Alleviation of Suffering (Beneficence)

To restore health and relieve suffering is one of the most time-honored goals of physicians. It is the fundamental duty of all doctors. Beneficence supersedes the perceived beliefs of society or the personal values of the physician. Relief of suffering may supersede preservation of life (see the section Rule of Double Effect), particularly when death is inescapable.

First Do No Harm (Nonmaleficence)

Primum non nocere is an ancient principle of medicine and is embedded in the Hippocratic oath: "I will use treatment to help the sick according to my ability and judgment, but I will never use it to injure or wrong them." This principle underlies the physician's decision to recognize that death is inescapable and to proceed with comfort care. However, the Hippocratic oath's injunction to "do no harm" seldom applies in today's environment. It is unethical to continue aggressive care for patients who have no hope for recovery; the physician's goal is to provide comfort, not to prolong dying. Likewise, inappropriate drug use and the ordering of diagnostic tests that are potentially risky but not likely to help the patient are unethical under certain circumstances. On the other hand, there may be pressure from families to "keep going." Such a dilemma requires frequent and careful dialogue with the family. It may take days for some family members to realize that death is imminent. In the CCU, it isn't always possible to know when death is inescapable, and it is important for the physician to convey a sense of hope, when appropriate. Families and patients sometimes have unrealistic expectations and will request that "everything be done," even though the patient has little or no hope for meaningful recovery. Some families will put a highly spiritual spin on the problem and insist that the medical team should hold out for a "miracle." Often, the patient wants more aggressive care than the family (9). Physicians may be inaccurately overly pessimistic, whereas patients tend to be inaccurately overly optimistic (8). Frequent, careful assessment of the patient and the prognosis coupled with frequent communication with family becomes even more important.

An experienced CCU physician can often sense when multiorgan failure is beginning to emerge and is keenly aware of this when each day brings a new struggle to keep the patient alive. Such patients are often intubated, sedated, and unable to carry on meaningful dialogue. It is the physician who has specialized knowledge of the natural history of disease, not the family, and it is the physician who must use this powerful knowledge to help guide families when making decisions about withdrawal of life support. Families often want certainty, but there is no certainty in most instances, only judgments. Physicians should clearly describe what will likely happen if aggressive treatments are continued and contrast this information with what will likely happen if comfort care only is begun. A combination of objective quantitative information and the physician's judgment about outcome is better than either alone (8).

Justice: Ensure That Medical Resources Are Allocated Fairly

It is clear that some economically deprived populations are underserved and as a consequence may have higher morbidity and mortality rates. Decisions regarding care should be blind to economic circumstances, ethnicity, perceived societal views, political persuasion, gender, and age. As care becomes more rationed in our society, the principle of justice takes on more practical importance. Heart transplantation, for example, is a highly rationed form of treatment with generally accepted medical indications and contraindications. If a heart is transplanted into a patient who does not comply with treatment and who dies quickly of rejection, two people die: the noncompliant patient, and the anonymous patient on the transplant list who dies while waiting for a heart transplant. In our society, end-stage heart failure and the need for heart transplants occurs in cocaine dealers, prisoners, pedophiles, and wealthy elderly people who are beyond the usual age limit for heart transplantation. The principle of justice would assume that only medical need determines care. However, outcomes for heart transplantation are affected by social issues, medical compliance, age, family support, and underlying general health. If there were a surplus of donor hearts, decisions about who should receive a heart transplant would be less difficult. As all therapy becomes more rationed in an era of harsh cost-containment, the principle of justice becomes more applicable in the CCU. The principle of justice will become more difficult to apply as competition for scarce resources intensifies. Some evidence exists that justice has been ignored and that racial bias has entered the decision-making process (9).

Telling the Truth

Honest communication between physician and patient is very important and is a major principle of ethics in Western society (10). In some Asian societies, it is considered inappropriate to tell a patient that he or she has cancer; the stigma and fear associated with knowing one has cancer outweigh the active withholding of information about diagnosis and prognosis. In the United States, it is assumed that patients and families want to understand the diagnosis, prognosis, and risks and benefits of various diagnostic and therapeutic procedures, but the level of understanding desired by patients and families is highly variable (5). This principle is particularly important to uphold in the CCU, where the presence of many different teams and fellows can greatly fragment the care of the patient. It is important to try to personally explain to the patient the risks and benefits of cardiac catheterization, percutaneous coronary interventions, and cardiac surgery, fully understanding that someone else will obtain direct informed consent and will further expound on the risks and benefits of these procedures. Patients tend to view the CCU team and the attending physician as "their" doctors. This is who they see on rounds daily and know and trust most explicitly, and this is who should explain to the patient and family what diagnostic and therapeutic plans are evolving—what the strategy will be for the next 24 to 72 hours. Consultants may be asked to discuss the case with families on occasion. For example, when complex noncardiac complications occur, such as intracerebral hemorrhage or severe hypoxic encephalopathy, it is reasonable for the neurology team to have a discussion with the family. If an internist or family doctor has a long-standing relationship with the patient, that person should be consulted and engaged with the decision when possible.

Rule of Double Effect

The rule of double effect may be the ethical principle least understood by medical personnel and lay people. Many are not even aware of the principle. According to the rule of double effect, outcomes that would be morally wrong if intentionally provoked are permissible if foreseen but unintended (11–13). Specifically, administering opioids to treat a terminally ill patient's dyspnea or pain may be acceptable even if the medication contributes to or causes the patient's death. A harmful effect of treatment, even death, is permissible if death is not intended but occurs only as a side effect of a beneficial action. It is not uncommon for dying or terminally ill patients in the CCU to receive morphine as part of comfort care. It is usually given in small doses (an initial drip of 1 to 2 mg per hour or repeated boluses ranging from 10 to 30 mg per hour) to alleviate air hunger or dyspnea, supplemented by benzodiazepines to treat anxiety or agitation. Appropriate use of opioids for symptom control does not usually shorten life, and there is generally little or no need to invoke the rule of double effect (14).

The rule of double effect was developed by moral theologians of the Roman Catholic Church in the Middle Ages (15,16). The underlying logic is that it is impossible for a person to avoid all harmful actions. Failure to intervene to comfort a dying patient harms the patient by allowing treatable discomfort to continue. If the intent of treatment is to relieve suffering, the foreseen but unintended risk of earlier death is permissible. The U.S. Supreme Court has demonstrated support for this principle by requiring all states to ensure that their laws do not obstruct the provision of adequate palliative care, especially for alleviation of the physical discomfort of patients who are facing death (17,18). The physician's goal under these circumstances is to relieve the patient's discomfort (in this case, air hunger or dyspnea). Neither the physician nor the patient intends for the patient to die. If death occurs from the opioids (rare), it is foreseen but unintended. The rule of double effect and subsequent legal rulings supporting the principle have served to reassure physicians that prescribing morphine drips for terminally ill patients is morally and legally permissible and is the proper thing to do (19).

FAMILY CONFLICTS

The decision to withdraw advanced life-support measures is one of the most difficult decisions that clinicians and families must make. Often the prognosis is not absolutely certain. The patient's judgment should be involved when possible, although most patients who are on advanced life support are not mentally competent. Only a small minority are able to participate in the initial decision to limit treatment [4% in a surgical intensive care unit (ICU) vs. 27% in an oncology service] (20). It is important to provide hope to families, but hope is a double-edged sword. Hard questions need to be asked of families: What has been the family's experience with other dying patients? What do they consider "suffering"? What is their concept of "meaningful recovery"? The medical team should avoid offering guarantees and certainties regarding death or recovery. The worst thing a physician can do is give mixed messages or abdicate responsibility. Families need time to deal with the devastating thought of withdrawal of life-support systems and death. A useful tactic is to get the family together in a quiet, private room and discuss the issue at length. Give them room to vent. Allow the family to verbalize their grief. Make sure their spiritual needs are attended to by a hospital chaplain. Warring siblings with polarized desires for aggressive care versus comfort care are a particularly difficult problem, and an ethics consultation is usually in order. When our CCU team is first contemplating withdrawal of advanced life support, we take the following steps:

1. Determine the prognosis as carefully as possible. Unfortunately, Acute Physiologic Assessment and Chronic Health Evaluation (APACHE) scores do not apply to CCU patients. One must be able to deal with the uncertainty of dying.

2. Assess the patient's competence; engage them when possible. Patients receiving advanced life support are generally not mentally competent.

3. Discuss the case with the whole team and reach consensus about a decision. Nurses often have a more expansive knowledge of the family and the patient's needs and wants.

4. Do not rush the families! A useful strategy is to tell them that if things do not improve over the next 48 to 72 hours, withdrawal of life support may be appropriate. It should be stressed that repeated procedures and diagnostic tests can be uncomfortable and can be a form of suffering. Emphasize that comfort care may allow the patient to have a more peaceful and dignified death. The time-limited goal often allows the family time to contemplate a most difficult decision.

5. Families need assurances that comfort care will be maintained and that the CCU team will not abandon them. However, in some cases, transferring the patient out of the CCU after withdrawal of life support is appropriate, and this should be explained to the family in anticipation of such a move.

When family members or legal surrogates want "everything done," the medical team should comply with this request. A direct challenge by the medical team usually fails to convince the family of the futility of further treatment, but repeated, compassionate discussions can result in ethical decisions that will benefit the patient.

FUTILITY

The concept of medical futility has been controversial and remains vague. It attempts to establish the principle that physicians may use their judgment and skills to determine when treatment is futile. Once such a determination has been made, the physician can unilaterally withhold or withdraw treatment, even if the patient or family objects. The principle of autonomy is thus essentially expunged. Futility is not an objective entity but embraces many judgment-based values (21). There is no clear definition of medical futility (22). Such decisions, other than about physiologic futility (e.g., treating hypertension with an antibiotic) or an absolute inability to prevent death, always involve judging value. Whose value counts?

In reality, physicians can only frame choices for the patient; they cannot make unilateral decisions. Moreover, the courts have not recognized the right of physicians to act unilaterally in cases in which they believe further care would be futile (23). This is not to say that physicians do not recognize clinical situations in which care is futile. It simply means they cannot act unilaterally. Their obligation is to speak with the patient or the family, frame the issue, and have the patient or the family participate fully in the decision regarding further care. Judgments about anything other than physiologic futility are vague; imposed value judgments, imprecise definitions, a lack of concrete data, and great uncertainty about the definition of "futility" intervene. Communication of information to the family such as the success rate of resuscitation, long-term meaningful recovery, and likelihood of discharge from the hospital must be clear and consistent.

WITHHOLDING OR WITHDRAWAL OF LIFE-SUSTAINING THERAPY

Once the medical team and the patient or family has decided that the patient is dying and that further aggressive care is unwarranted, there is precious little guidance about how the process should be implemented. Physicians seem poorly trained in managing the transition from aggressive care to comfort care. The following steps should be considered:

- A final decision should be made after careful discussion with the patient (if appropriate), the family, and the nursing staff.
- Such patients are frequently intubated, and therefore a do-not-resuscitate order should also be written. If the patient is not intubated, a do-not-intubate order should be written.
- A morphine drip should be started. Patients in the CCU often suffer dyspnea as the primary discomfort, and morphine, 1 mg per hour, will usually alleviate this symptom. Presumed respiratory distress can be treated with a 5- to 10-mg bolus of morphine, followed by an increase in the infusion to 2 to 5 mg per hour.
- Conscious patients who manifest anxiety should be treated with intravenous lorazepam (1 to 4 mg every 30 minutes), and patients with delirium should be treated with intravenous haloperidol if necessary. If tolerance to these medications has developed, the hypnotic drug propofol may be used.
- Ventilation: in most cases, I prefer to leave the endotracheal tube in place while gradually decreasing the ventilator rate, positive end-expiratory pressure, oxygen therapy, and tidal volume until the patient is spontaneously breathing room air through the endotracheal tube. This way, secretions can be suctioned to prevent rattling, which may be perceived as suffering by the family. The gradual turning off of the ventilator (30 minutes to 3 hours) allows the family to spend time at the bedside if desired, but there is no merit in prolonging the dying process by very slow weaning over the course of many hours. Patients who are receiving neuromuscular blocking drugs should cease receiving such treatment before the ventilator is withdrawn. Such agents should not be introduced when the ventilator is being withdrawn, and neuromuscular function should be restored before life

support is withdrawn (24). It is believed that withdrawal of life support can ethically occur in the presence of pharmacologic neuromuscular blockade when death is expected to be rapid, but it is usually safest to stop neuromuscular blockade before withdrawing the ventilator, because assessment of comfort is impossible. When discontinuation of neuromuscular blockade is not possible because the burden on the family of waiting for neuromuscular blockade to wane exceeds the benefits of allowing better assessment of the patient's comfort level, sedatives and analgesics can be skillfully administered.

- Some patients or families will specifically request that the endotracheal tube be removed. This can be done after appropriate suctioning. Humidified air can be given to prevent drying of the airway.
- Pressors should be stopped.
- Intraaortic balloon pumps should be turned off.
- Antibiotic therapy should be stopped.
- Artificial nutrition should be stopped.
- Blood draws should be stopped.
- Intravenous fluids should be reduced and used to facilitate analgesics and sedation.
- Restraints should be removed, monitors discontinued, and alarms silenced.
- Excess secretions should be suctioned.

The median time between withdrawal of life support and death was 3.5 hours in one study but varied from 5 minutes to 5.5 days (25). Families should be told that death may not be instantaneous, and that patients are sometimes transferred to a palliative care ward where they will be kept comfortable. Rarely, patients may even spontaneously recover.

Withdrawal of artificial nutrition and hydration is often very difficult for health care workers and families to accept (26). However, both ethical guidelines and court decisions support the practice (27,28). Recent information supports the conclusion that tube feeding seldom achieves the intended medical aims and that it may cause, rather than prevent, suffering (29). Continued nutrition and hydration may lead to considerable volume overload and pulmonary edema in a patient who is not otherwise being monitored carefully (30). Emerging consensus now suggests that dying patients experience little or no discomfort on withdrawal of tube feedings, parenteral nutrition, and intravenous hydration (31).

There is a growing recognition that nephrologists should maintain a low threshold for initiating dialysis on a trial basis, and a similarly low threshold for discontinuing dialysis that fails to appreciably improve the quality of life. Death occurs, on average, 9.6 days after discontinuation of chronic dialysis treatment (32).

Lastly, it must be emphasized that forgoing life-sustaining treatment is usually not a single-point decision but one that evolves over the course of several days (20). In two large academic surgical ICUs (Moffitt-Long Hospital, San

TABLE 34.2 LIMITATIONS OF PROGNOSTIC MODELS FOR END-OF-LIFE DECISION-MAKING IN THE CORONARY CARE UNIT

Prognostic models give probabilities of survival or death rather than a "yes" or "no" answer; because of 95% confidence intervals, no model can statistically exclude survival even in the most severely ill patients.

Individual accuracy of these predictions depends on whether a specific patient's medical condition was reasonably well represented in the population from which the model was derived.

Most models derive their predictions from factors present at or shortly after admission to the intensive care unit and do not provide updated mortality estimates as the patient's condition changes.

Some patients have inherently unpredictable courses.

Conventional models of patients in the intensive care unit predict only hospital survival, not long-term survival, functional status, or quality of life after hospital discharge.

Modified from Faber-Lagendoer K, Lanken PN. Dying patients in the intensive care unit: foregoing treatment, maintaining care. *Ann Intern Med* 2000;133:886–893, with permission.

Francisco, and San Francisco General Hospital), the median time from ICU admission to death in patients undergoing withholding or withdrawal of life support varied from 4 to 8 days (median time period at Moffitt-Long Hospital and San Francisco General Hospital, respectively) (33). This suggests that it takes time for the decision to evolve and for the patient to die after the decision is made. However, surgical ICUs are quite different from CCUs. No such data are yet available from CCUs. At the Cleveland Clinic Foundation, the CCU mortality rate is 7.5%. Approximately one-half of the deaths result from withholding or withdrawing of life support, and one-half result from "natural" causes. Current prognostic models have limitations (Table 34.2) but should be used as an adjunct to the process of shared decision-making.

The withholding or withdrawal of life support is a difficult, often agonizing process. It requires careful scrutiny and rests on important ethical and legal principles that are continually evolving (34). There are no absolute guidelines for deciding when to withdraw advanced life support. Each patient and clinical situation must be considered in their own contexts. Frequent communication with patients, families, or legal surrogates; open sharing of data; and careful assessment of the changing prognosis are critical to the process.

EUTHANASIA

Euthanasia is the act of putting to death without pain a person suffering from an incurable and painful condition. It is a vague and emotionally provocative term and best describes an act such as giving a lethal injection. It is not to be confused with withholding or withdrawing life support in a dying patient. The U.S. Supreme Court has unanimously ruled that there is no constitutional right to physi-

cian-assisted suicide (euthanasia) (17,18). There is no constitutional right to suicide, and there is no legal or historical support for such a right. The right to abortion or the right to refuse treatment is different from the right to assisted suicide. Limiting physician-assisted suicide to terminally ill patients also has no basis in constitutional principles. Only 6% of medical students, house staff, or faculty physicians surveyed in one study were willing to terminate the life of a patient deliberately by administering medication to cause respiratory arrest, and only 1.1% of those surveyed were willing to do so if it causes a cardiac arrest (35). Of course, it is possible that these numbers might increase if legal restraints were removed. However, there is a long and impressive list, starting with Hippocrates and including leading physicians, philosophers, and biomedical ethicists, of professionals who are opposed to euthanasia. One humane alternative is to simulate a home environment for dying patients in the ICU (Table 34.3).

Strong popular support for euthanasia exists in Holland, which legalized euthanasia in 2000 (36). It is estimated that 5,000 to 10,000 Dutch citizens die each year after administration of a barbiturate followed by a lethal injection of a paralytic agent. In 1994, Oregon voters passed the Death with Dignity Act. This act does not permit euthanasia, but it allows state residents to receive prescriptions for self-administered lethal medications from their physicians. A 1-year follow-up indicated that only 23 patients received such prescriptions, 15 patients died after taking them, six died from underlying illness, and two patients who received such prescriptions were still alive (37). Some good has come out of the euthanasia movement—it has forced physicians to deal with death and dying.

TABLE 34.3 WAYS IN WHICH INTENSIVE CARE UNITS CAN SIMULATE A HOME ENVIRONMENT FOR DYING PATIENTS

Transportable aspects of a patient's home	Ways to provide these aspects in the intensive care unit
Privacy	Provide a private room / Close doors and curtains
Ready access to family	Suspend restrictive visiting hours / Provide comfortable chairs, recliners, and cots for family members in the patient's room
Access to patient's own possessions and amenities	Allow family to bring in favorite music, clothes, religious icons, food, and pets
Family serving as personal caregivers	When appropriate, allow family to assist with patient care
Access to religious rituals and spiritual support	Provide religious and spiritual resources / Encourage religious and other family rituals at the bedside before and after death

Modified from Faber-Lagendoer K, Lanken PN. Dying patients in the intensive care unit: foregoing treatment, maintaining care. *Ann Intern Med* 2000;133:886–893, with permission.

TABLE 34.4 PRINCIPLES OF A GOOD DEATH

To know when death is coming, and to understand what can be expected

To be able to retain control of what happens

To be afforded dignity and privacy

To have control over pain relief and other symptom control

To have a choice and control over where death occurs (at home or elsewhere)

To have access to information and expertise as necessary

To have access to any spiritual or emotional support required

To have access to hospice care in any location, not only in the hospital

To have control over who is present and who shares the end

To be able to issue advance directives that ensure wishes are respected

To have time to say goodbye and control over other aspects of timing

To be able to leave when it is time to go, and not to have life prolonged pointlessly

Modified from Brown M. A good death. Principles of palliative care are yet to be applied in acute hospitals. *BMJ* 2000;320:1206, with permission.

SUMMARY

People in the United States are uncomfortable discussing death. They do not know how to start the conversation and in some cases do not want to discuss it at all. People remain confused about what constitutes a "good death" (Table 34.4). A good death includes management of pain and symptoms, clear decision-making, preparation for death, and completion. The language is not always precise—a feeding tube is not the same as food and water.

Only frequent, clear, and open dialogue will overcome this hurdle. Eventually, society needs to understand end-of-life issues in a more realistic light and to realize that what they see on the television series *ER* does not mimic the real world. Patients will die despite our best efforts. Our job as physicians is to help patients and their families through the dying process, just as we help them achieve meaningful recovery.

CONTROVERSIES AND PERSONAL PERSPECTIVES

The concept of futility is controversial (21). It is supported by neither scientific principle nor the justice system. When continued aggressive life-support seems futile, it is best to discuss the likely outcome of continued support versus comfort care with the family. The final outcome—death—may be the same, but how the patient dies may be quite different. It is best that the family not perceive that the team is giving up, but rather that passive comfort care may be preferable to the potential suffering associated with continued life support. It must be stressed that such a decision is based on experience and judgment, not on the certainty of death. The family needs to understand and agree that the patient's best interests are served by such a strategy. Medical futility cannot be easily defined and is value-laden.

It has also been my personal experience that partial withdrawal of life support or "slow codes" confuse the issue and can prolong suffering. Decisions to withdraw or withhold life support should be complete. Only those measures that offer comfort should be continued.

THE FUTURE

We do a poor job of training our residents and fellows in end-of-life issues. Dying is part of living, and to ignore the management of dying is as grievous an error as ignoring methods of managing a major illness. We need to do a better job of educating our trainees and ourselves about these uncomfortable issues. At our institution, we have end-of-life small-group seminars as part of our didactic curriculum in the CCU. Bioethicists, pharmacists, and cardiologists assigned to the CCU participate in these lectures, which are often centered around a specific case history. We need to educate the public about death and dying. Expectations for individual patients must be framed carefully and repeatedly. Above all, families must be drawn into these important dialogues. Hope for meaningful recovery must in some cases be replaced with hope for comfort and caring.

REFERENCES

1. Snider G. Allocation of intensive care: the physician's role. *Am J Respir Crit Care Med* 1994;150:575–580.
2. Raffin TA. Ethics and withdrawal of support. In: Murray JF, Nadel JA, eds. *Textbook of Respiratory Medicine,* 2nd ed. Philadelphia: Saunders, 1994:2487–2503.
3. Solomon M, O'Donnell L, Jennings B, et al. Decisions near the end of life: professional views on life-sustaining treatments. *Am J Public Health* 1993;83:14–23.
4. A controlled trial to improve care for seriously ill hospitalized patients. The Study to Understand Prognoses and Preferences for Outcomes and Risks of Treatments (SUPPORT). The SUPPORT Principal Investigators [published erratum appears in *JAMA* 1996;275:1232]. *JAMA* 1995;274:1591–1598.
5. Puchalski CM, Zhong Z, Jacobs MM, et al. Patients who want their family and physician to make resuscitation decisions for them: observations from SUPPORT and HELP. Study to Understand Prognoses and Preferences for Outcomes and Risks of Treatments. Hospitalized Elderly Longitudinal Project. *J Am Geriatr Soc* 2000;48[Suppl]:S84–S90.
6. Rosenfeld KE, Wenger NS, Phillips RS, et al. Factors associated with change in resuscitation preference of seriously ill patients. The SUPPORT Investigators. Study to Understand Prognoses and Preferences for Outcomes and Risks of Treatments. *Arch Intern Med* 1996;156:1558–1564.
7. Burt RA. The Supreme Court speaks: not assisted suicide but a constitutional right to palliative care. *N Engl J Med* 1997;337:1234–1236.
8. Knaus WA, Harrell FE Jr, et al. The SUPPORT prognostic model: objective estimates of survival for seriously ill hospitalized adults. Study to Understand Prognoses and Preferences for Outcomes and Risks of Treatments. *Ann Intern Med* 1995;122:191–203.
9. Phillips RS, Hamel MB, Teno JM, et al. Race, resource use, and survival in seriously ill hospitalized adults. The SUPPORT Investigators. *J Gen Intern Med* 1996;11:387–396.
10. Bok S. *Lying: moral choice in public and private life.* New York: Pantheon Books, 1978:xxii, 326.
11. Decisions near the end of life. Council on Ethical and Judicial Affairs, American Medical Association. *JAMA* 1992; 276:2229–2233.
12. Good care of the dying patient. Council on Scientific Affairs, American Medical Association. *JAMA* 1996;275:474–478.
13. Quill TE, Dresser R, Brock DW. The rule of double effect: a critique of its role in end-of-life decision making. *N Engl J Med* 1997;337:1768–1771.
14. Thorns A, Sykes N. Opioid use in last week of life and implications for end-of-life decision-making [letter]. *Lancet* 2000;356:398–399.
15. Kenny AJP. *The anatomy of the soul: historical essays in the philosophy of mind.* Oxford: Basil Blackwell, 1973:ix, 146 [1].
16. Mangan J. A historical analysis of the principle of double effect. *Theol Studies* 1949;10:41–61.
17. Coleson RE. *Washington v. Glucksberg. Issues Law Med* 1997;13:315–321.
18. Coleson RE. *Vacco v. Quill. Issues Law Med* 1997;13:323–328.
19. Foley KM. Competent care for the dying instead of physician-assisted suicide [editorial]. *N Engl J Med* 1997;336:54–58.
20. Faber-Langendoen K, Bartels DM. Process of foregoing life-sustaining treatment in a university hospital: an empirical study. *Crit Care Med* 1992;20:570–577.
21. Helft PR, Siegler M, Lantos J. The rise and fall of the futility movement. *N Engl J Med* 2000;343:293–296.
22. Youngner SJ. Who defines futility? *JAMA* 1988;260:2094–2095.
23. Daar JF. Medical futility and implications for physician autonomy. *Am J Law Med* 1995;21:221–240.
24. Truog RD, Burns JP, Mitchell C, et al. Pharmacologic paralysis and withdrawal of mechanical ventilation at the end of life. *N Engl J Med* 2000;342:508–511.
25. Wilson WC, Smedira NG, Fink C, et al. Ordering and administration of sedatives and analgesics during the withholding and withdrawal of life support from critically ill patients. *JAMA* 1992;267:949–953.
26. Slomka J. What do apple pie and motherhood have to do with feeding tubes and caring for the patient? *Arch Intern Med* 1995;155:1258–1263.
27. Center H. *Guidelines on the termination of life-sustaining treatment and the care of the dying: a report.* Briarcliff Manor, NY: The Center, 1987:xii, 159.
28. Weir RF, Gostin L. Decisions to abate life-sustaining treatment for nonautonomous patients: ethical standards and legal liability for physicians after Cruzan. *JAMA* 1990;264:1846–1853.
29. Gillick MR. Rethinking the role of tube feeding in patients with advanced dementia. *N Engl J Med* 2000;342:206–210.
30. Rousseau P. Why give IV fluids to the dying? *Patient Care* 1992;26:71–74.
31. Brody H, Campbell ML, Faber-Langendoen K, Ogle KS. Withdrawing intensive life-sustaining treatment: recommendations for compassionate clinical management. *N Engl J Med* 1997;336:652–657.
32. Cohn LM, McCue JD, Germain M, et al. Dialysis discontinuation: a "good" death? *Arch Intern Med* 1995;155:42–47.
33. Smedira NG, Evans BH, Grais LS, et al. Withholding and withdrawal of life support from the critically ill. *N Engl J Med* 1990;322:309–315.
34. Ruark JE, Raffin TA. Initiating and withdrawing life support: principles and practice in adult medicine. *N Engl J Med* 1988;318:25–30.
35. Caralis PV, Hammond JS. Attitudes of medical students, housestaff, and faculty physicians toward euthanasia and termination of life-sustaining treatment. *Crit Care Med* 1992;20:683–690.
36. de Wachter MA. Active euthanasia in the Netherlands. *JAMA* 1989;262:3316–3319.
37. Chin AE, Hedberg K, Higginson GK, Fleming DW. Legalized physician-assisted suicide in Oregon: the first year's experience. *N Engl J Med* 1999;340:577–583.

THE HEART AND OTHER ORGAN SYSTEMS

ROBERT M. CALIFF

INTRODUCTION

Cardiovascular specialists are often consulted to evaluate patients with diseases that emanate from organ systems remote from the heart, but with substantial cardiac manifestations. At some point the cardiovascular system becomes a factor in most major systemic diseases. In this section, commonly encountered problems involving an interaction of the heart and other organ systems are reviewed. The goal is to focus on the cardiovascular manifestations of these problems without providing a comprehensive review of the illnesses per se.

Increasing attention is being focused on the interaction between the cardiovascular system and the central nervous system. Ranging from genetic diseases associated with neuromuscular degeneration to atherosclerotic disease of the cerebrovascular circulation, considerable knowledge about cardiovascular manifestations is required to understand the manifestations of neurologic disorders.

Myocarditis, endocarditis, and pericarditis are covered in detail in other portions of the book, but the enormous number of infectious causes of these problems, each with specific implications for treatment, requires discussion here. In addition, the rapidly growing knowledge base concerning the effects of the human immunodeficiency virus on the cardiovascular system will increasingly require the attention of cardiovascular specialists.

Although cardiovascular manifestations of rheumatic diseases are not common compared with atherosclerosis, some of the most striking cardiovascular problems arise from rheumatic diseases. The management of vasculitis, pericarditis, or aortic valve difficulties associated with rheumatic diseases requires a thorough understanding of both areas.

As with cerebrovascular disease, the basic approaches to atherosclerosis (medical management, percutaneous intervention, and surgical intervention) create a close tie between the most common type of renal disease and the cardiovascular system. In addition, the rapid growth of angiography with its associated problem of contrast nephropathy creates an iatrogenic condition requiring careful evaluation and treatment by the angiographer.

Finally, in many respects, cardiovascular disease is an endocrine disease in the sense that a major contributor to disease progression and outcome in cardiovascular diseases is the neuroendocrine status. In particular, diabetes has become the focus of activity in understanding factors associated with increased risk.

We hope that these sections in combination with specific disease-oriented chapters throughout the book will provide the reader with a comprehensive view of the interaction of the cardiovascular system with other organ systems in the development and progression of human disease.

R. M. Califf: Department of Medicine, Duke Clinical Research Institute, Durham, North Carolina

35A

THE HEART AND OTHER ORGAN SYSTEMS

Endocrine Systems and the Heart

MARCO ROFFI

INTRODUCTION

Cardiovascular involvement is frequent in endocrine disturbances. Clinical suspicion remains the most important step in diagnosing endocrine disorders—in particular, their cardiovascular manifestations, as they can be subtle and nonspecific. The purpose of this chapter is to summarize relevant interactions between endocrinologic diseases and the cardiovascular system to facilitate diagnostic recognition and to highlight management options.

THE THYROID

A relation between the thyroid and the heart has long been recognized (1). In the late 1700s, a patient with clinical fea-

tures of thyrotoxicosis including palpitations, irregular pulse, and dyspnea was described (2). In the early 1900s, a patient with "myxedema heart" was reported: The critical findings were enlarged cardiac silhouette, low electrocardiographic voltage, and bradycardia (3).

Thyroxine (T_4), a relatively inactive hormone, is the major secretory product of the thyroid gland. Triiodothyronine (T_3), the biologically active compound, is in large part derived from peripheral conversion of T_4 by the 5'-monodeiodinase enzyme. Therefore, alteration in T_3 plasma level may occur independently from thyroid function. Cardiovascular manifestations are frequent in thyroid dysfunction and may be the result of direct hormone effects at the cellular level, interactions with the sympathetic nervous system, or alterations of peripheral circulation and metabolism (4). At the cellular level, thyroid hormones act mainly through binding to specific nuclear receptors and activation of gene transcription (5). Additionally, they activate extranuclear sites as mitochondrial

M. Roffi: Department of Cardiovascular Medicine, The Cleveland Clinic Foundation, Cleveland, Ohio

and membrane-bound enzymes (6). Women are more likely to develop thyroid dysfunction, with an estimated 2.7% prevalence of hyperthyroidism and 1.9% prevalence of hypothyroidism in an unselected population (7).

Thyrotoxicosis

The terms *hyperthyroidism* and *thyrotoxicosis* can be differentiated but are frequently used interchangeably. Hyperthyroidism is defined as increased formation and release of thyroid hormones from the thyroid gland, whereas thyrotoxicosis describes the clinical syndrome that results from the thyroid hormone excess. The most frequent cause of thyrotoxicosis is Graves' disease, which accounts for 60% to 90% of cases and occurs among women ten times more frequently than men. This disorder is characterized by autoantibodies activating the thyroid-stimulating hormone (TSH) receptor. Other causes of thyrotoxicosis include toxic adenoma (Plummer's disease), toxic multinodular goiter, thyroiditis, and thyroid autonomy. Common symptoms of thyrotoxicosis are nervousness, emotional lability, sleep disturbances, tremor, diarrhea, heat intolerance, and weight loss. Clinical findings include goiter, exophthalmos, proximal muscle weakness, hyperreflexia, and occasionally pretibial myxedema. Thyrotoxicosis in the elderly might be particularly subtle and present with nonspecific symptoms such as weakness, weight loss, and apathy.

In subjects with preexisting thyroid autonomy, iodine administration (i.e., in the form of amiodarone or contrast agents) can result in iodine-induced thyrotoxicosis. Iodine deficiency, the presence of a goiter, and baseline low TSH levels have been considered risk factors for iodine-induced thyrotoxicosis. Accordingly, this disease is more frequently observed in areas with low iodine intake. An investigation in almost 800 patients from an iodine-deficient area undergoing coronary angiography showed that the risk of developing thyrotoxicosis was low (<0.3%) despite significant prevalence of low TSH levels (4%) and goiter (23%) (8). In contrast, amiodarone may induce thyrotoxicosis in up to 10% of iodine-deficient patients (9).

Cardiovascular Involvement

Thyrotoxic patients have increased mortality, primarily because of cardiovascular complications (10). Cardiovascular symptoms in this setting are frequently nonspecific. Palpitations are usually caused by sinus tachycardia and, occasionally, by atrial fibrillation. Exercise intolerance and dyspnea on exertion may be caused by a combination of inability to raise cardiac output and skeletal and respiratory muscle weakness. Cardiovascular involvement in the elderly may be limited to arrhythmias such as sinus tachycardia or atrial fibrillation, which occasionally trigger heart failure, angina, or both. The hemodynamic changes occurring in thyrotoxicosis are summarized in Table 35A.1 and include tachycardia, increased cardiac output and stroke volume, and

TABLE 35A.1 CARDIOVASCULAR HEMODYNAMICS IN THYROID DYSFUNCTION

	Thyrotoxicosis	Hypothyroidism
Systemic vascular resistance	↓	↑
Cardiac output	↑	↓
Systolic blood pressure	↑	↓ or →
Diastolic blood pressure	↓	↑ or →
Heart rate	↑	↓
Systolic function	↑	↓
Diastolic function	↑	↓
Blood volume	↑	↓

↑, increased; ↓, decreased; →, unchanged.

decreased systemic vascular resistance (11,12). In contrast to hypothyroidism, which is characterized by diastolic hypertension, hyperthyroidism is associated with systolic hypertension in the presence of normal or low diastolic blood pressure. It is speculated that isolated systolic hypertension is secondary to the inability of the vasculature to accommodate increased cardiac output and stroke volume (1).

Sympathetic Nervous System

Many of the cardiovascular signs and symptoms of thyrotoxicosis mimic those occurring in states of increased beta-adrenergic activity and respond to beta-blockade (13), suggesting an underlying dysfunction of the catecholamine metabolism or, alternatively, an increased sensitivity to catecholamines. However, patients with thyrotoxicosis have low or normal plasma catecholamine levels and normal urinary catecholamine excretion (14). Moreover, these patients have normal responses to catecholamine infusion (13). Finally, there is no conclusive evidence of increased beta-adrenergic receptor density in the myocardium, increased catecholamine turnover at neural synapses, or increased affinity of adrenergic receptor for catecholamines (15).

Ventricular Function

Short-term hyperthyroidism is associated with increased cardiac contractility and improved diastolic function (16,17) (Table 35A.1), which may be caused, at least in part, by augmented activity of the sarcoplasmic reticulum calcium ATPase pump (18). Both in humans (19) and animals (20), chronic thyrotoxicosis causes variable degrees of left ventricular hypertrophy (LVH). Thyroid hormones have been shown to induce cardiac protein synthesis, leading to the hypothesis that this is the trigger of LVH (21). However, beta-adrenergic blockade has been shown to block or reverse hypertrophy, suggesting that increased cardiac workload is the mediator of hypertrophy (22–24). In addition to the effects on the myocardium, thyroid hormones, specifically T_3, show vasodilator properties by acting directly on vascular smooth muscle cells, potentially explaining the decreased systemic vascular resistance observed in hyperthyroidism (25,26).

It remains a source of debate whether thyrotoxicosis per se may lead to heart failure. In the vast majority of cases, heart failure can be explained by the combination of underlying heart disease, arrhythmias, and/or chronically increased cardiac output. However, myocardial dysfunction has been described also in absence of underlying cardiac disease (27), even in children (28), and improvement in myocardial contractility after restoration of euthyroidism has been reported (29,30). Several factors may potentially contribute to heart failure in thyrotoxicosis. Diastolic function deteriorates in the course of the disease because of LVH and progressive LV stiffness, leading to filling impairment, particularly in the setting of tachycardia or atrial fibrillation (4). Additionally, thyrotoxicosis is associated with increased total blood volume and plasma volume (31). Occasionally, the decreased systemic resistance may overwhelm the cardiac capacity and cause high output failure. More frequently, however, the high-output state may unmask coronary artery disease, and heart failure is precipitated by ischemia. Myocardial ischemia in thyrotoxic patients has been described even in the absence of significant coronary artery disease, secondary to coronary vasospasms (32–34).

Arrhythmias

Sinus tachycardia at rest, during sleep, and during exercise is the most common arrhythmia in thyrotoxicosis (35,36). It is speculated that thyroid hormones have direct effects on the conduction system, possibly via cellular changes in cation transport, including a decrease of atrial excitation threshold, an increase of sinoatrial node firing, and a shortening of conduction tissue refractory time (11,37). Other common arrhythmias include atrial premature contractions and atrial fibrillation. Less frequently, patients present with paroxysmal atrial tachycardia and atrial flutter. Ventricular premature contractions and ventricular arrhythmias are rare.

Although thyrotoxicosis accounts for less than 5% of all cases of atrial fibrillation, this arrhythmia occurs in up to 15% of hyperthyroid patients (15). The ventricular rate response is frequently rapid because of increased atrioventricular node conduction. Atrial fibrillation related to thyrotoxicosis is more frequent in the elderly and in male subjects, probably reflecting their increased prevalence of intrinsic heart disease (38). Because this arrhythmia, particularly in the elderly, may be the only manifestation of thyrotoxicosis, thyroid hormone excess should always be excluded in patients with atrial fibrillation. Accordingly, one report showed subtle hyperthyroidism in 12.5% of elderly patients with atrial fibrillation previously considered idiopathic (39). One study, performed in patients 60 years of age or older, demonstrated that even patients with subclinical hyperthyroidism (i.e., asymptomatic but with low TSH) had a threefold higher risk of developing atrial fibrillation in the subsequent decade (40) (Fig. 35A.1). Major complications of thyrotoxic atrial fibrillation include heart failure and embolic events. In the absence of chronic atrial

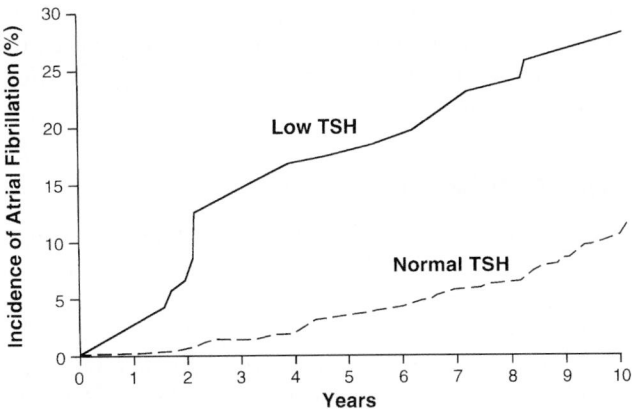

FIGURE 35A.1 Cumulative incidence of atrial fibrillation among subjects 60 years of age or older, according to serum thyroid-stimulating hormone (TSH) levels at baseline. Low TSH defined as ≤0.1 mU per L; normal TSH defined as >0.4 to 5.0 mU per L. (Adapted from Sawin CT, Geller A, Wolf PA, et al. Low serum thyrotropin concentrations as a risk factor for atrial fibrillation in older persons. *N Engl J Med* 1994;331:1249–1252.)

fibrillation or underlying heart disease, most patients convert spontaneously to sinus rhythm within 8 to 12 weeks of antithyroid treatment (41). Conversely, reversion into atrial fibrillation is likely in persistently thyrotoxic patients. Anticoagulation is indicated and cardioversion should be deferred until euthyroidism is restored.

Diagnosis and Therapy

Measurement of serum TSH is the most sensitive screening test for hyperthyroidism. An undetectable value is the hallmark of this thyroid dysfunction, whereas normal TSH levels virtually exclude the disease (42). Confirmation is usually sought measuring elevated serum free T_4 and free T_3. Beta-adrenergic blockers provide relief of symptoms such as tachycardia, tremor, anxiety, and heat intolerance. The nonselective agent propranolol has been traditionally used for this purpose but selective $beta_1$-adrenergic antagonists such as atenolol appear equally effective. If beta-blockers are contraindicated, calcium channel blockers such as verapamil or diltiazem can be administered as negative chronotropic agents (43). However, caution is warranted, as these agents may lead to hemodynamic instability by further reducing systemic vascular resistance and contractility. The thionamide derivatives propylthiouracil and methimazole are effective in decreasing thyroid hormone synthesis. Radioactive iodine is a valid alternative, particularly for older patients with moderate hyperthyroidism and goiter, for patients with prior allergic or toxic reaction to the antithyroid medication, and when frequent medication intake cannot be guaranteed. The disadvantages of radioactive iodine include a long latency of action and the fact that this therapy is ineffective in iodine-induced hyperthyroidism. Surgery is indicated in patients with large goiters causing airway obstruction or with malignant or equivocal nodules on fine-needle aspiration. Occasionally, surgery is necessary in severely hyperthyroid patients not responding to conservative treatment.

Hypothyroidism

Hypothyroidism is the clinical syndrome associated with decreased secretion of thyroid hormones. This condition reflects in over 90% of cases a disease of the gland itself (primary hypothyroidism). Rarely, hypothyroidism can be caused by pituitary disease (secondary hypothyroidism) or hypothalamic disease (tertiary hypothyroidism). The most frequent cause of hypothyroidism in adults is autoimmune thyroiditis, or Hashimoto's disease. Accordingly, women are more frequently affected. The slow and progressive nature of hypothyroidism often makes the diagnosis difficult. This is particularly true in elderly patients whose clinical manifestation may be limited to dry skin, weight gain, fatigue, and forgetfulness—all of which are easily explained by the aging process. Other complaints of hypothyroid patients include increased tiredness and sleep requirement, depressed mood, cold intolerance, constipation, and decreased exercise tolerance. Pleural effusions and pitting edema may occur in absence of heart failure.

Cardiovascular Involvement

Most hypothyroid patients present with nonspecific symptoms caused by psychological or skeletal muscle dysfunction. However, long-standing hypothyroidism may affect the cardiovascular system in several ways (Table 35A.1). Bradycardia is common, and pericardial effusion may occur in up to one-half of patients but rarely causes hemodynamic compromise (44). Both diastolic and systolic LV performance may be decreased (45), presumably because of alterations in calcium uptake and release by cardiac myocytes (18). Additionally, an increase in systemic vascular resistance is observed, possibly as the result of the lack of direct vasodilatory effect of thyroid hormones (25,26). Despite the fact that hypothyroid patients have symptoms suggesting a decreased sympathetic tone, plasma catecholamines are increased (46). The resulting hemodynamic changes are opposite but less marked than with thyrotoxicosis. Characteristic features include low cardiac output; decreased stroke volume, diastolic function, intravascular volume, and peripheral oxygen consumption; and increased systemic vascular resistance (47–49). Heart failure may occur when the metabolic demand cannot be matched by adequate cardiac output. As in patients with thyrotoxicosis, overt heart failure in hypothyroidism generally represents exacerbation of intrinsic cardiac disease. Rarely, however, hypothyroidism alone may cause cardiomyopathy (50). Therefore, unexplained heart failure should prompt determination of thyroid hormones. In the absence of underlying heart disease, the decreased myocardial contractility observed in hypothyroidism is generally reversible after hormone replacement (45,47), probably as a result of improved calcium handling in cardiac myocytes (18) and decreased systemic vascular resistance (47).

Risk Factors

Total cholesterol, low-density lipoprotein (LDL) cholesterol, very-low-density lipoprotein (VLDL) cholesterol, lipoprotein(a), and apolipoprotein B concentrations are often elevated in hypothyroidism; some patients have high serum triglyceride levels (1). It has been demonstrated that patients with hypothyroidism have an intrinsic LDL catabolism dysfunction, which is reversible after hormone replacement (51). Therefore, screening for this condition is mandatory when assessing patients with hyperlipidemia. The powerful interaction between thyroid hormones and lipid metabolism is highlighted by the fact that thyroid hormones have been used in the past as lipid-lowering agents. However, this strategy was associated with increased morbidity and mortality in patients after myocardial infarction (52).

Hypothyroidism is associated with increased prevalence of hypertension. In a review of 12 studies, the overall prevalence of hypertension was 21% (1). In large series of hypertensive patients, hypothyroidism accounted for 3% to 5% of the cases (53,54). Hypothyroid patients have a low-renin form of hypertension, and the mechanism remains unknown (54). The causal link between thyroid hormone deficiency and hypertension is confirmed by the fact that hormone replacement may lead to improvement of hypertension (54).

Coronary Artery Disease

Patients with hypothyroidism frequently have risk factors for coronary artery disease, but data to support the direct association between hypothyroidism and coronary artery disease are lacking (55). The suggestion that hypothyroidism may indeed represent an independent risk factor for coronary disease comes from a population-based cross-sectional study. In this analysis, women with subclinical hypothyroidism—defined as asymptomatic, with normal serum free T_4 and elevated TSH—had a higher prevalence of aortic atherosclerosis and myocardial infarction than euthyroid women (56). These observations are in agreement with previous case-control studies showing an association between subclinical hypothyroidism and coronary heart disease in elderly women (57,58). In contrast, a Finnish study addressing latent thyroid failure in both men and women found no association with coronary disease (59).

Diagnosis and Therapy

An elevated TSH combined with a low free T_4 is diagnostic of primary hypothyroidism. Antimicrosomal and antithyroglobulin antibodies are characteristic of Hashimoto's disease. Hypothyroidism is preferentially treated with thyroxine

TABLE 35A.2 EFFECTS OF AMIODARONE ON THYROID FUNCTION IN PATIENTS REMAINING EUTHYROID

Test	Treatment <3 mo	Treatment >3 mo
Thyroxine	Increased	Remains increased by up to 40% above baseline; may be in high reference range or modestly raised
Triiodothyronine	Decreased, usually to low reference range	Remains in low reference range or slightly low
Thyroid-stimulating hormone	Transient increase (up to 20 mU/L)	Normal, but may fluctuate with periods of high and low values

From Newman CM, Price A, Davies DW, et al. Amiodarone and the thyroid: a practical guide to the management of thyroid dysfunction induced by amiodarone therapy. *Heart* 1998;79:121–127, with permission.

because of its long half-life. In the elderly, as well as in patients with known or suspected coronary disease, it is prudent to start hormone substitution at a lower dosage. However, exacerbation of angina because of hormone replacement is rare (60) and responds well to beta-adrenergic blockade.

Amiodarone and Thyroid Dysfunction

Amiodarone is an iodine-rich benzofuran derivative with similar molecular structure to thyroid hormones. Organic iodine represents almost 40% of the molecular weight of amiodarone. A daily dose of 200 mg of amiodarone corresponds to an intake of 75 mg of organic iodide and generates approximately 7 mg of free iodine (61). Given the fact that the normal dietary requirement of iodine is 100 to 200 μg per day, amiodarone therapy is associated with an enormous iodide load, reflected in a 40-fold increase in plasma and urinary iodide levels (61). Because iodine is a necessary substrate for thyroid hormone synthesis but, at the same time, directly influences intrathyroidal processes, it is not surprising that over 50% of the patients on amiodarone have abnormal thyroid function test results, although most of them remain euthyroid (62). The predominant peripheral action of amiodarone on thyroid hormones is the inhibition of the deiodination of T_4 to T_3. As a result, the serum levels of T_4 increase and the levels of T_3 decrease (61,63) (Table 35A.2). In addition, high iodide availability initially inhibits thyroid hormone synthesis (the Wolff-Chaikoff effect) (64). During the first 3 months of therapy, TSH levels are commonly slightly elevated because of lack of feedback inhibition, due to the lowered T_3 levels, but they tend to normalize during long-term administration. Amiodarone-induced thyrotoxicosis (AIT) prevails in areas with low iodine intake, and hypothyroidism is more frequent in areas with high iodine intake. Whereas thyrotoxicosis can occur throughout the treatment period and even several months after treatment, hypothyroidism rarely develops beyond 18 months of initiation of therapy (65). Monitoring of thyroid function in this setting relies on TSH. If TSH is abnormal, free T_4 and free T_3 levels should be assessed to detect underlying gland dysfunction that may predispose to amiodarone-induced hyperthyroidism or hypothyroidism. Additional assessments are recommended at approximately 3 months and yearly thereafter.

A noniodinated analog of amiodarone, dronedarone, has been synthesized. Preliminary animal data show that this compound has similar electrophysiologic effects to amiodarone (66). The development of dronedarone or a similar compound will be followed with interest, because iodine deletion is expected to overcome endocrine side effects of amiodarone. However, extensive safety and efficacy data in animals are required before human testing.

Amiodarone-Induced Hypothyroidism

Hypothyroidism is a frequent sequela of amiodarone therapy, with a reported incidence ranging from 13% in iodine-replete countries to 6% in countries with low or intermediate iodine intake (63). Its occurrence is not related to the daily or cumulative dose of the drug. The risk of developing hypothyroidism is increased in the elderly and women, particularly in the setting of autoimmune thyroiditis. Accordingly, women on amiodarone with microsomal, thyroglobulin, or both autoantibodies have been shown to have more than a tenfold higher risk for subsequent hypothyroidism (65). Possible mechanisms leading to hypothyroidism in this setting include failure to escape the Wolff-Chaikoff effect and iodine-mediated exacerbation of preexisting autoimmune thyroid disease. TSH levels above 10 to 15 mU per L in patients on chronic amiodarone usually represent hypothyroidism. The diagnosis is confirmed by low T_4 or free T_4. The assessment of T_3 or free T_3 adds little information, because these parameters may be diminished in euthyroid patients on amiodarone. Once the diagnosis of hypothyroidism is established, the drug can be safely continued, if needed, and thyroxine replacement added in increasing doses at 4- to 6-week intervals until TSH returns within normal limits and symptoms resolve (63). If amiodarone is discontinued, recovery of thyroid function is influenced by the presence of thyroid antibodies. In fact, the absence of antibodies is associated with frequent recovery, mostly within a few months, whereas patients with thyroid antibodies usually do not recover normal thyroid function (63).

Amiodarone-Induced Thyrotoxicosis

In countries with high iodine intake, AIT is less frequent than hypothyroidism, with an estimated incidence of approximately 2%. In contrast, in the presence of iodine

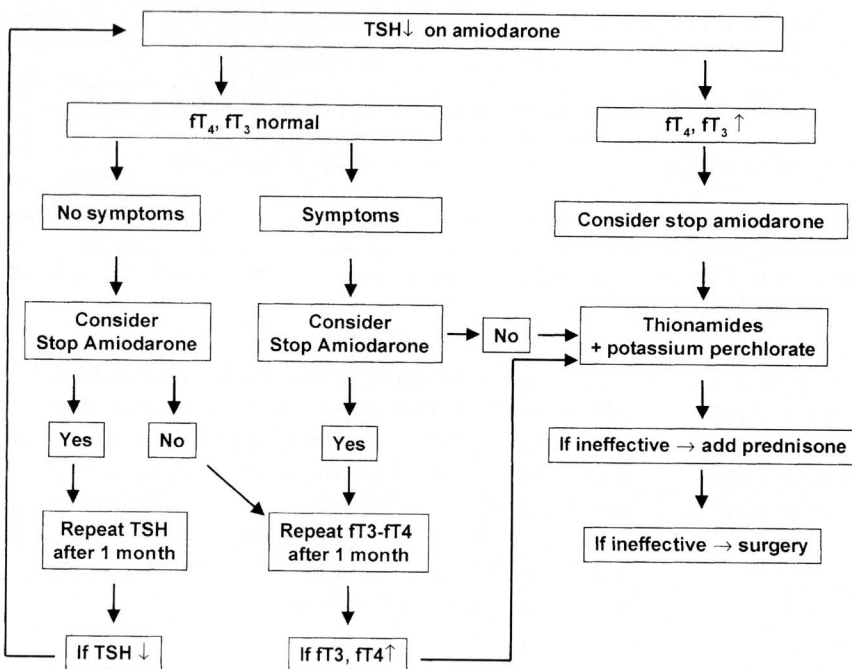

FIGURE 35A.2 Management algorithm for amiodarone-induced thyrotoxicosis. fT₃, free triiodothyronine; fT₄, free thyroxine; TSH, thyroid-stimulating hormone. (Courtesy of F. Cattaneo, MD, Lugano, Switzerland.)

deficiency, AIT may occur in up to 10% (9). Antiadrenergic effects of amiodarone may partially conceal thyrotoxic symptoms. AIT should be suspected in the presence of new or recurrent atrial arrhythmias or unexplained weight loss. Three pathophysiologic mechanisms have been associated with thyrotoxicosis in the setting of chronic amiodarone therapy (61). First, iodine may affect thyroid autoregulatory mechanisms and may lead, particularly in patients with underlying thyroid disease, to excessive hormone synthesis. Second, inflammatory destructive histologic changes and increased cytokines (e.g., interleukin-6) and thyroglobulin levels have been demonstrated in this setting, suggesting a direct cytotoxic effect of amiodarone (67). Third, it has been postulated that amiodarone may trigger an autoimmune response to the thyroid gland. Amiodarone should be discontinued whenever possible. The choice of treatment can be guided by distinction of two forms of AIT (68). In type I AIT patients have a goiter, positive thyroid antibodies, and abnormal (i.e., measurable or even high) 24-hour radioiodine uptake. Treatment consists of a combination of thionamides, propylthiouracil or methimazole, which inhibit hormone biosynthesis, and potassium perchlorate, which blocks thyroid iodide uptake (69,70). Patients with type II AIT have a normal thyroid and low radioiodine uptake. The efficacy of corticosteroids, alone or in combination with thionamides, has been convincingly demonstrated in this setting (68,71,72). However, because a mixed form of AIT is frequent, patients can be approached pragmatically with an initial combination of thionamides and potassium perchlorate, with corticosteroids being added after 2 weeks if no improvement occurs (Fig. 35A.2). In patients not responding to this therapy, lithium may be a valid alternative (73).

The cardiovascular risk associated with continuing amiodarone therapy is unknown, but the rate of remission following antithyroid drugs is decreased. However, discontinuation of the drug can be hazardous, particularly if the indications were ventricular arrhythmias, and thyrotoxicosis may take up to 8 months to subside (74). In addition, because of the extremely long terminal half-life of amiodarone, the use of beta-adrenergic antagonists is limited by the additive chronotropic and dromotropic effects, potentially leading to severe bradycardia, conduction abnormalities, or both. Because the high iodide plasma concentrations typically suppress iodine uptake in the thyroid, radioactive iodine treatment is not effective in this particular form of thyrotoxicosis. Subtotal thyroidectomy is the treatment of choice if pharmacologic regimens are ineffective (75,76). Surgery has been associated with low perioperative morbidity and mortality, even in the presence of thyroid storm, heart failure, and therapy-refractory arrhythmias (63,75,76).

THE ADRENAL GLAND

The cortex of the adrenal gland produces corticosteroid hormones, and the medulla—functionally a sympathetic ganglion—produces catecholamines. Clinical syndromes associated with adrenal hypersecretion and cardiovascular involvement include Cushing's syndrome and primary aldosteronism (Conn's syndrome) and result from excessive secretion of cortisol and mineralocorticoid, respectively. Cardiovascular involvement in adrenal insufficiency is mainly limited to its acute form (Addison's crisis) and is characterized by volume depletion, refractory hypotension, arrhythmias, and conduction abnormalities secondary to electrolyte disturbances.

Cushing's Syndrome

Cortisol, a central modulator of carbohydrate and protein metabolism, is synthesized in the adrenal cortex in response to pituitary adrenocorticotropic hormone (ACTH). The term *Cushing's syndrome* denotes glucocorticoid excess, which can be either endogenous or exogenous. ACTH-secreting pituitary tumor (Cushing's disease) accounts for approximately 80% of the cases of endogenous hypercorticism. In 10% of cases, an ectopic ACTH-producing tumor is identified (ectopic ACTH syndrome). Glucocorticoid excess is caused in another 10% of cases by adrenal pathologies such as adenoma, carcinoma, or bilateral hyperplasia.

Clinical Findings and Cardiovascular Risk

The characteristic findings in Cushing's syndrome include truncal obesity, abdominal striae, hypertension, osteoporosis, proximal muscle weakness, fatigue, and hyperglycemia. Concomitant androgen excess may lead to hirsutism and amenorrhea, and mineralocorticoid effect may cause hypokalemia. Early studies performed when no treatment was available showed that glucocorticoid excess is associated with premature atherosclerosis and increased cardiovascular morbidity and mortality (86). The risk profile of this population is characterized by a high prevalence of glucose intolerance or overt diabetes mellitus and hypertension (87). Additional cardiovascular risk factors include truncal obesity and hyperlipidemia. Hypertension has been related to volume expansion, increased production of vasoactive substances, and increased reactivity of vascular smooth muscle cells (88–90). LVH may be more frequent, more severe, or both in patients with Cushing's syndrome when compared with patients with essential hypertension (91). Despite surgical treatment, cardiovascular morbidity and mortality remain higher than in the general population (92), possibly because of residual obesity, insulin resistance, or both (93).

Diagnosis and Therapy

Diagnosis and treatment of Cushing's syndrome are complex and go beyond the scope of this textbook. In patients with clinical features suggestive of hypercorticism, screening can be performed with, among others, a 24-hour urine collection for free cortisol. Confirmatory tests include, among others, the dexamethasone suppression test or a second elevated free cortisol in a 24-hour urine sample (94). Specific treatment, which may include surgical removal or pharmacologic or radiation therapy, is chosen depending on the underlying process.

Primary Aldosteronism

Primary aldosteronism was first described in 1955 by Conn in a patient with an aldosterone-producing adrenal ade-

noma (95). This benign tumor is the most common cause of primary aldosteronism, accounting for approximately 65% of cases, whereas bilateral adrenal hyperplasia, also called *idiopathic hyperaldosteronism*, accounts for another 30% of cases. Primary aldosteronism has been considered the cause of hypertension in a minority of unselected hypertensive patients, with an incidence ranging between 0.05% and 2.20% (96). However, recent data suggest a higher prevalence of primary aldosteronism in the hypertensive population (97,98). Symptoms of primary aldosteronism are nonspecific and mainly result from potassium depletion. Neuromuscular involvement includes weakness, paralysis, cramps, tetany, and paresthesias.

Cardiovascular Manifestations

Primary aldosteronism is associated with moderate to severe hypertension (99). Acute mineralocorticoid administration induces renal sodium retention and potassium and hydrogen excretion, resulting in vascular volume expansion, hypokalemia, and metabolic alkalosis. Although hypertension is presumably related to sodium retention and volume expansion, chronic mineralocorticoid excess is associated with only mild hypervolemia due to escape mechanisms (99). Accordingly, peripheral edema is rare. Primary aldosteronism is associated with cardiac and vascular remodeling. Characteristic features include perivascular fibrosis, excessive LVH, and myocardial fibrosis (100,101).

Diagnosis and Therapy

Because mineralocorticoid excess does not produce specific symptoms, primary aldosteronism is a biochemical diagnosis. Diagnostic tests of choice include plasma renin activity, plasma aldosterone levels, aldosterone-to-renin ratio, and dexamethasone suppression test (102). The association of hypertension and hypokalemia, if not diuretic induced, is characteristic of primary aldosteronism and should prompt to appropriate analyses. However, mineralocorticoid excess may be present also in normokalemic subjects (97,98). Surgery is the treatment of choice in aldosterone-producing adenomas, but hypertension resolves only in approximately 35% to 50% of cases (96). As the rate of hypertension regression following bilateral adrenalectomy in idiopathic hyperplasia is even lower, therapy in this setting relies on the aldosterone antagonist spironolactone and a sodium-restricted diet.

Pheochromocytoma

The clinical presentation of pheochromocytoma is characterized by episodic catecholamine release. In approximately 90% of cases, pheochromocytomas are located in the adrenal glands (in less than 10% the process is bilateral), whereas extraadrenal tumors, originating from chromaffin tissue of any sympathetic paraganglion (paragangliomas), account for the remaining 10% of cases. Over 90% of pheochromocytomas are benign and cured by surgery with low operative mortality (103). After surgical resection, up to 25% of patients may remain hypertensive. Life-long follow-up is mandatory because the disease may show late recurrence (104). Familial forms are rare and associated with bilateral or extraadrenal involvement and occasionally with multiple endocrine neoplasia type II.

The classic presentation of pheochromocytoma consists of a paroxysm of the triad of palpitations, diaphoresis, and headache. These episodes begin abruptly, may last for minutes to hours, and subside gradually. Less common symptoms include orthostatic hypotension, anxiety, tremor, chest pain or abdominal pain, weakness, and weight loss. Because only a minority of patients presents with characteristic paroxysmal symptoms, the diagnosis is easily missed.

Cardiovascular Manifestations

Hypertension, one of the hallmarks of pheochromocytoma, is paroxysmal only in approximately one-half of the cases (105). Heart rate is frequently elevated during hypertensive episodes but may decrease because of reflex bradycardia, and usually no factors precipitating hypertensive episodes can be elicited. Prolonged exposure to high levels of catecholamines results in arterial and venous vasoconstriction and plasma volume contraction. Orthostatic hypotension may occur; possible mechanisms include plasma volume contraction and autonomous nervous system dysfunction (106). Electrocardiographic abnormalities are frequent but nonspecific and include T-wave abnormalities, signs of LVH, sinus tachycardia, and occasionally supraventricular ectopy and paroxysmal supraventricular tachycardia. In addition, particularly during hypertensive episodes, patients may show ischemic electrocardiographic changes. It has been postulated that pheochromocytoma affects the myocardium in the form of catecholamine-induced myocarditis, cardiomyopathy, or both (107,108). Tumor removal has been associated with regression of both LV dilatation and LVH (109–111).

Diagnosis

Because pheochromocytoma is the cause of hypertension in only approximately 0.1% of unselected patients (96), routine screening is not warranted. There is no gold standard to diagnose pheochromocytoma. Assessments of 24-hour urinary metanephrines and plasma metanephrines have shown comparable diagnostic sensitivity and specificity (112). Alternatively, plasma and urine metanephrines can be obtained during hypertensive paroxysm. Because only extreme elevations of plasma catecholamines affect blood pressure, normal levels in the setting of a hypertensive episode make pheochromocytoma highly unlikely. The great majority of pheochromocytomas are located in the abdo-

men and can be imaged by computed tomography or magnetic resonance imaging. Metaiodobenzylguanidine or octreotide scintigraphy may be useful for localization of metastatic, recurrent, or extraadrenal tumors.

Therapy

Surgery frequently represents the cure for pheochromocytoma. Adrenergic blockade for a few weeks is indicated before tumor resection, although on rare occasions urgent surgery may be necessary (Fig. 35A.3). The goal of preoperative treatment is adequate blood pressure control without inducing intolerable orthostatic hypotension. The alpha-blocker phenoxybenzamine, an irreversible noncompetitive antagonist predominantly of the alpha$_1$-receptors, has been the mainstay of preoperative and perioperative antihypertensive therapy (103,113). In patients intolerant to phenoxybenzamine, the alpha$_1$-selective antagonists prazosin, terazosin, or doxazosin have been used (103,113). To achieve optimal control of hypertension, tachyarrhythmias, and sinus tachycardia, beta-blockers can be added. However, beta-blockade should not be started if the patients are not pretreated with alpha-blockers. In fact, in the setting of high catecholamine levels, blockade of beta$_2$-mediated vasodilation can potentially lead to unopposed alpha$_1$-mediated vasoconstriction and exacerbation of hypertension. Frequently used drugs include the nonselective antagonist propranolol, beta$_1$-selective antagonists such as metoprolol or atenolol, and the mixed alpha/beta-blocker labetalol. However, because labetalol has a predominantly beta effect, additional alpha-blockade is usually required. In subjects with contraindications to beta-blockade, amiodarone can be used for tachyarrhythmia control. Severe hypertensive crisis may be acutely managed with intravenous nitroprusside or the alpha$_1$/alpha$_2$-blocker phentolamine. Several drugs can potentially trigger hypertension in pheochromocytoma and should, therefore, be avoided, including opiates, cocaine, tricyclic antidepressants, and metoclopramide (114).

ACROMEGALY AND GROWTH HORMONE DEFICIENCY

Growth hormone (GH) is produced and stored in large amounts in the pituitary gland. Direct GH effects include stimulation of lipolysis and gluconeogenesis. Indirect GH actions are mediated by insulin-like growth factor (IGF)-1. IGF-1, synthesized in hepatocytes and fibroblasts following GH stimulation, inhibits GH secretion in a classic feedback loop mechanism and acts as mediator of GH effects at the tissue level (i.e., it promotes chondrocytes proliferation and stimulates protein synthesis and glucose uptake in muscle cells). Stress, exercise, and a variety of neurogenic stimuli increase GH secretion. GH secretion persists throughout

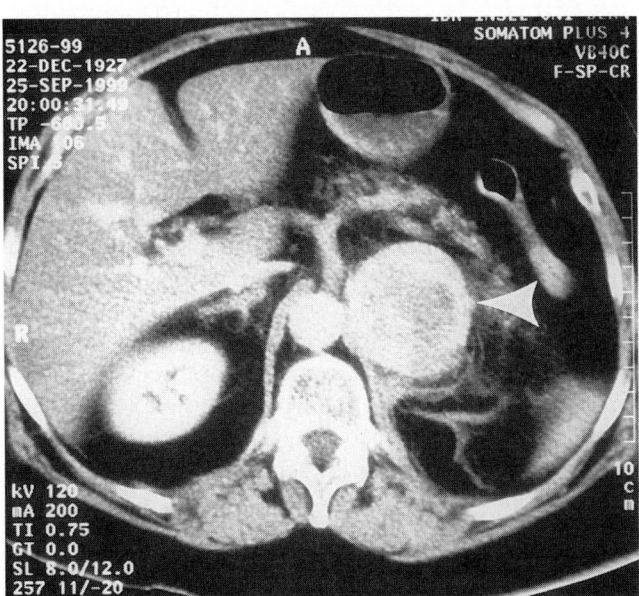

FIGURE 35A.3 Abdominal computed tomographic scan with contrast showing hemorrhagic transformation of a pheochromocytoma (*arrowhead*). The patient presented with lower back pain and extreme hemodynamic instability requiring emergency surgery. (Courtesy of E. Lipp, MD, Swiss Cardiovascular Center, Bern, Switzerland.)

life, reaching the maximum during puberty and then gradually declining in adulthood. In this book, the focus is exclusively on pituitary gland dysfunctions in the adult.

Acromegaly

Acromegaly is a rare disorder caused by a GH-secreting pituitary tumor, with an estimated incidence of approximately three per million (115). Excess GH secretion occurring during childhood leads to gigantismus. GH-producing tumors account for 10% to 15% of all pituitary neoplasms. Signs and symptoms are either caused by tumor mass effect (e.g., headaches, visual field defects, and hypopituitarism) or by GH excess (e.g., acral overgrowth, excessive sweating, and soft tissue swelling). Changes in facial appearance include enlargement of the lower jaw (prognathism), leading to malocclusion and increased spacing between the teeth and enlargement of the lips, tongue, nose, and sinuses. Progressive increase in shoe size and inability to wear rings are typical. Other features include sleep apnea, arthropathy, neuropathy, and cancer. Specifically, acromegalic patients have a three- to eightfold excess risk of colon cancer or premalignant polyps (116). Therefore, in these patients, screening with colonoscopy is recommended over the age of 50 years.

Cardiovascular Involvement

Despite the fact that cardiovascular symptoms are the leading feature at presentation in less than 5% of the patients,

overt cardiac disease may occurs in as many as 20% of acromegalic patients (117). GH excess is associated with a two- to threefold increase in mortality, mainly due to cardiovascular disease (118–120). Other causes include neoplastic and respiratory disorders. Hypertension is present in 25% to 35% of acromegalic patients, a three- to fourfold increase over the general population (117,121). The pathophysiology remains unknown, but its salt-sensitive nature suggests that, at least in part, it may be caused by a direct GH effect on the renal sodium pump leading to sodium retention (117,121). Glucose intolerance is present in up to 50% of the patients and overt diabetes mellitus in 10% to 25% (117). Diabetes resolves in two-thirds of patients after successful surgery (122). The lipid metabolism in acromegaly is characterized by hypertriglyceridemia (123), whereas no consistent findings on cholesterol abnormalities have been reported.

Electrocardiographic abnormalities are frequent and include ST-segment and T-wave depression, other signs of LVH, and, occasionally, conduction defects. Echocardiographic abnormalities, found in up to 80% of patients, include LVH and decreased systolic function (124,125). It has long been postulated that GH has trophic properties on the myocardium, but to date it remains a source of debate whether acromegalic cardiomyopathy exists. The assessment is complicated by frequent concomitant hypertension and/or coronary artery disease. However, echocardiographic studies in patients with acromegaly of recent onset and no associated cardiovascular abnormalities have demonstrated LVH, with or without associated diastolic dysfunction (126,127). These observations are in accordance with previous reports showing that less than 10% of patients with LVH and impaired LV function may have no evidence of hypertension or coronary artery disease (122,128). Additional arguments in favor of an acromegalic cardiomyopathy include the observation that LVH, LV dysfunction, or both may improve with treatment of GH excess (129,130). Moreover, both *in vitro* and *in vivo* animal models of GH excess have consistently demonstrated LV hypertrophic response and enhanced cardiac function (131,132). Finally, one autopsy series of acromegalic patients showed frequent myocardial interstitial fibrosis and inflammatory infiltrates (133). These observations suggest that, although most cardiac disease in acromegaly is explained by coexisting hypertension and/or coronary artery disease, a small proportion of patients may have a cardiomyopathy. It is speculated that elevated GH and/or IGF-1 levels may initially lead to LVH, followed by fibrosis, diastolic dysfunction, and later in the process, systolic dysfunction and overt heart failure (134).

Diagnosis and Therapy

Because GH is secreted in a pulsatile manner, random GH plasma levels are not useful in diagnosing acromegaly. IGF-

1 levels correlate with GH production and disease activity and represent the screening test of choice. Definitive diagnosis is made with the glucose tolerance test, showing no decrease of serum GH level following oral glucose load.

The goals of therapy are to reverse or prevent tumor mass effects and to reduce the long-term morbidity and mortality without incurring hypopituitarism. The current treatments for acromegaly include surgery, radiation therapy, and pharmacologic management. Among patients treated surgically, only 60% overall and less than one-half of those with large tumors can be cured (135,136). These low rates are explained by the fact that frequently, because of its extension and infiltrative nature, the tumor cannot be completely resected. Radiation therapy is characterized by delayed effect, poor efficacy, and a high incidence of panhypopituitarism (137). Preliminary data on stereotactic radiotherapy (gamma knife) appear promising, but its role in the treatment of acromegaly has yet to be demonstrated. Dopamine agonists, such as bromocriptine, cabergoline, or quinagolide (not available in the United States), adequately lower GH levels in only a minority of patients, and their adverse effects limit compliance (138). The somatostatin analogs octreotide and lanreotide inhibit the secretion of GH and are regarded by many authors as the first-line treatment of acromegaly. However, this drug class also leads to normalization of GH and IGF-1 levels only in approximately one-half of patients (139,140).

Pegvisomant is a recently developed, genetically engineered GH receptor antagonist. In the short run, this compound has been shown to be effective and well tolerated in over 100 patients with acromegaly (141). Should these promising results be confirmed in a large patient population with longer follow-up, GH receptor antagonism may become a useful tool for the medical management of acromegaly.

ANDROGENS AND THE CARDIOVASCULAR SYSTEM

Androgens in general, and testosterone in particular, are widely believed to be associated with a higher cardiovascular risk in men, probably because male gender itself is an established independent risk factor for cardiovascular disease. Additionally, the abuse of synthetic androgens in high doses by athletes and body builders has been associated with hypertension, cardiomyopathy, myocardial ischemia, and sudden death (188). However, a number of more recent reports challenge the assumption that androgen is detrimental for the cardiovascular system. Animal studies *in vitro* have shown that testosterone is a coronary vasodilator (189). This observation was reproduced in humans in a study showing that intracoronary administration of physiologic doses of testosterone increased coronary blood flow in men with ischemic heart disease (190). Accordingly, significant improvements in angina threshold have been demonstrated

in patients given supplemental intramuscular, oral, or intravenous testosterone (191,192). However, the doses used in these trials were supraphysiologic, raising concerns about potential side effects. The daily administration of small doses of testosterone to men with chronic stable angina was shown to prolong time to myocardial ischemia compared with placebo, and the magnitude of the benefit was comparable with the previous studies using higher testosterone doses (193). Additionally, castration resulted in a significant increase in aortic atherosclerosis in cholesterol-fed rabbits—a process that was markedly inhibited by testosterone replacement (194). In men without prior myocardial infarction referred for coronary angiography, a significant inverse correlation was found between plasma testosterone levels and extent of coronary disease, suggesting that low testosterone may represent a risk factor for coronary atherosclerosis (195). However, a number of prospective epidemiologic studies have failed to show a relationship between baseline testosterone levels and the subsequent development of coronary disease (196–198). The influence of androgens on serum lipids and glucose metabolism in men remains controversial (195,199,200). Currently no data exist on the effects of testosterone therapy on cardiovascular morbidity and mortality and on potential side effects such as growth in prostatic hyperplasia or prostatic cancer.

CONTROVERSIES AND PERSONAL PERSPECTIVES

Cardiovascular involvement is frequent in endocrine disease. However, it is often controversial whether hormonal imbalance has direct deleterious effects on the cardiovascular system or if cardiovascular involvement is caused by the increased prevalence of associated cardiovascular risk factors. Little is known about how hormones directly interact with the cardiovascular tissue and how they influence risk factors such as hypertension or hyperlipidemia.

In addition, it remains unproven whether therapy reduces cardiovascular morbidity and mortality in endocrine diseases other than diabetes mellitus. The fact that many endocrine disturbances are uncommon makes clinical research in this field difficult.

The potential for thyroid hormone and GH supplements in heart failure has been recognized. Data are limited; therefore, these therapies should be considered investigational. Equally controversial is the interaction between androgens, and specifically testosterone, and the cardiovascular system in men.

Notwithstanding the interest of these topics, we have to realize that frequently the most challenging step in endocrine disorders remains the diagnosis. Clinical suspicion is essential, as endocrine diseases and, in particular, their cardiovascular manifestations may present in a subtle and nonspecific way.

THE FUTURE

Amiodarone remains a cornerstone of antiarrhythmic therapy. However, its use is limited by side effects and, in particular, by frequent thyroid dysfunction. Preliminary animal data on a noniodinated analog of amiodarone have been encouraging. An iodine-free "amiodarone-like" compound without the disturbing endocrinologic side effects would be a major advance in cardiovascular medicine.

In the near future, newer innovative therapeutic modalities, including applications of pharmacogenomics, may modulate endocrinologic diseases before cardiovascular involvement. In addition, targeted therapy based on a patient's individual genetic profile may allow more selective and specific treatment of cardiovascular manifestations of endocrine diseases.

ACKNOWLEDGMENTS

The author wishes to acknowledge Dr. Fabio Cattaneo, Lugano, Switzerland, for his critical review of the manuscript. The author was supported by a research grant from the Swiss National Science Foundation.

REFERENCES

1. Gomberg-Maitland M, Frishman WH. Thyroid hormone and cardiovascular disease. *Am Heart J* 1998;135:187–196.
2. Parry CH. *Collection from the unpublished work of the late Caleb Hillier Parry.* London: Underwood, 1825:478.
3. Zondek H. Das Myxoedemherz. *Muench Med Wochenschr* 1918;65:1180–1183.
4. Polikar R, Burger AG, Scherrer U, et al. The thyroid and the heart. *Circulation* 1993;87:1435–1441.
5. Dillmann WH. Biochemical basis of thyroid hormone action in the heart. *Am J Med* 1990;88:626–630.
6. Segal J. Calcium is the first messenger for the action of thyroid hormone at the level of the plasma membrane: first evidence for an acute effect of thyroid hormone on calcium uptake in the heart. *Endocrinology* 1990;126:2693–2702.
7. Tunbridge WM, Evered DC, Hall R, et al. The spectrum of thyroid disease in a community: the Whickham survey. *Clin Endocrinol* 1977;7:481–493.
8. Hintze G, Blombach O, Fink H, et al. Risk of iodine–induced thyrotoxicosis after coronary angiography: an investigation in 788 unselected subjects. *Eur J Endocrinol* 1999;140:264–267.
9. Martino E, Safran M, Aghini–Lombardi F, et al. Environmental iodine intake and thyroid dysfunction during chronic amiodarone therapy. *Ann Intern Med* 1984;101:28–34.
10. Franklyn JA, Maisonneuve P, Sheppard MC, et al. Mortality after the treatment of hyperthyroidism with radioactive iodine. *N Engl J Med* 1998;338:712–718.
11. Woeber KA. Thyrotoxicosis and the heart. *N Engl J Med* 1992;327:94–98.
12. Klein I. Thyroid hormone and the cardiovascular system. *Am J Med* 1990;88:631–637.
13. Levey GS, Klein I. Catecholamine-thyroid hormone interactions and the cardiovascular manifestations of hyperthyroidism. *Am J Med* 1990;88:642–646.
14. Coulombe P, Dussault JH, Letarte J, et al. Catecholamines metabolism in thyroid diseases. I. Epinephrine secretion rate in hyperthyroidism and hypothyroidism. *J Clin Endocrinol Metab* 1976;42:125–131.
15. Klein I, Levey GS. The cardiovascular system in thyrotoxicosis. In: Braverman LE, Utiger RD, eds. *Werner & Ingbar's the thyroid: a fundamental and clinical text*, 8th ed. Philadelphia: Lippincott Williams & Wilkins, 2000:596–604.
16. Feldman T, Borow KM, Sarne DH, et al. Myocardial mechanics in hyperthyroidism: importance of left ventricular loading conditions, heart rate and contractile state. *J Am Coll Cardiol* 1986;7:967–974.
17. Mintz G, Pizzarello R, Klein I. Enhanced left ventricular diastolic function in hyperthyroidism: noninvasive assessment and response to treatment. *J Clin Endocrinol Metab* 1991;73:146–150.
18. Rohrer D, Dillmann WH. Thyroid hormone markedly increases the mRNA coding for sarcoplasmic reticulum Ca^{2+}-ATPase in the rat heart. *J Biol Chem* 1988;263:6941–6944.
19. Biondi B, Fazio S, Carella C, et al. Cardiac effects of long term thyrotropin-suppressive therapy with levothyroxine. *J Clin Endocrinol Metab* 1993;77:334–338.
20. Klein I, Ojamaa K. Thyroid hormone and the cardiovascular system: from theory to practice. *J Clin Endocrinol Metab* 1994;78:1026–1027.
21. Sanford CF, Griffin EE, Wildenthal K. Synthesis and degradation of myocardial protein during the development and regression of thyroxine-induced cardiac hypertrophy in rats. *Circ Res* 1978;43:688–694.
22. Klein I, Hong C. Effects of thyroid hormone on cardiac size and myosin content of the heterotopically transplanted rat heart. *J Clin Invest* 1986;77:1694–1698.
23. Klein I. Thyroxine–induced cardiac hypertrophy: time course of development and inhibition by propranolol. *Endocrinology* 1988;123:203–210.
24. Biondi B, Fazio S, Carella C, et al. Control of adrenergic overactivity by beta–blockade improves the quality of life in patients receiving long term suppressive therapy with levothyroxine. *J Clin Endocrinol Metab* 1994;78:1028–1033.
25. Ojamaa K, Klemperer JD, Klein I. Acute effects of thyroid hormone on vascular smooth muscle. *Thyroid* 1996;6:505–512.
26. Park KW, Dai HB, Ojamaa K, et al. The direct vasomotor effect of thyroid hormones on rat skeletal muscle resistance arteries. *Anesth Analg* 1997;85:734–738.

27. Ebisawa K, Ikeda U, Murata M, et al. Irreversible cardiomyopathy due to thyrotoxicosis. *Cardiology* 1994;84:274–277.

28. Cavallo A, Joseph CJ, Casta A. Cardiac complications in juvenile hyperthyroidism. *Am J Dis Child* 1984;138:479–482.

29. Bauerlein EJ, Chakko CS, Kessler KM. Reversible dilated cardiomyopathy due to thyrotoxicosis. *Am J Cardiol* 1992;70:132.

30. Sachs RN, Valensi P. Reversible cardiomyopathy due to thyrotoxicosis [letter; comment]. *Am J Cardiol* 1993;71:501.

31. Das KC, Mukherjee M, Sarkar TK, et al. Erythropoiesis and erythropoietin in hypo- and hyperthyroidism. *J Clin Endocrinol Metab* 1975;40:211–220.

32. Featherstone HJ, Stewart DK. Angina in thyrotoxicosis. Thyroid-related coronary artery spasm. *Arch Intern Med* 1983;143:554–555.

33. Bergeron GA, Goldsmith R, Schiller NB. Myocardial infarction, severe reversible ischemia, and shock following excess thyroid administration in a woman with normal coronary arteries. *Arch Intern Med* 1988;148:1450–1453.

34. Moliterno D, DeBold CR, Robertson RM. Case report: coronary vasospasm—relation to the hyperthyroid state. *Am J Med Sci* 1992;304:38–42.

35. Cacciatori V, Bellavere F, Pezzarossa A, et al. Power spectral analysis of heart rate in hyperthyroidism. *J Clin Endocrinol Metab* 1996;81:2828–2835.

36. Valcavi R, Menozzi C, Roti E, et al. Sinus node function in hyperthyroid patients. *J Clin Endocrinol Metab* 1992;75:239–242.

37. Freedberg AS, Papp JG, Williams EM. The effect of altered thyroid state on atrial intracellular potentials. *J Physiol* 1970;207:357–369.

38. Forfar JC, Caldwell GC. Hyperthyroid heart disease. *Clin Endocrinol Metab* 1985;14:491–508.

39. Forfar JC, Miller HC, Toft AD. Occult thyrotoxicosis: a correctable cause of "idiopathic" atrial fibrillation. *Am J Cardiol* 1979;44:9–12.

40. Sawin CT, Geller A, Wolf PA, et al. Low serum thyrotropin concentrations as a risk factor for atrial fibrillation in older persons. *N Engl J Med* 1994;331:1249–1252.

41. Nakazawa HK, Sakurai K, Hamada N, et al. Management of atrial fibrillation in the post-thyrotoxic state. *Am J Med* 1982;72:903–906.

42. Woeber KA. Update on the management of hyperthyroidism and hypothyroidism. *Arch Intern Med* 2000;160:1067–1071.

43. Roti E, Montermini M, Roti S, et al. The effect of diltiazem, a calcium channel-blocking drug, on cardiac rate and rhythm in hyperthyroid patients. *Arch Intern Med* 1988;148:1919–1921.

44. Kabadi UM, Kumar SP. Pericardial effusion in primary hypothyroidism. *Am Heart J* 1990;120:1393–1395.

45. Amidi M, Leon DF, DeGroot WJ, et al. Effect of the thyroid state on myocardial contractility and ventricular ejection rate in man. *Circulation* 1968;38:229–239.

46. Polikar R, Kennedy B, Ziegler M, et al. Plasma norepinephrine kinetics, dopamine-beta-hydroxylase, and chromogranin-A, in hypothyroid patients before and following replacement therapy. *J Clin Endocrinol Metab* 1990;70:277–281.

47. Graettinger JS, Muenster JJ, Checchia CS, et al. A correlation of clinical and hemodynamic studies in patients with hypothyroid. *J Clin Invest* 1958;19:502–510.

48. Crowley WF Jr, Ridgway EC, Bough EW, et al. Noninvasive evaluation of cardiac function in hypothyroidism. Response to gradual thyroxine replacement. *N Engl J Med* 1977;296:1–6.

49. Wieshammer S, Keck FS, Waitzinger J, et al. Left ventricular function at rest and during exercise in acute hypothyroidism. *Br Heart J* 1988;60:204–211.

50. MacKerrow SD, Osborn LA, Levy H, et al. Myxedema-associated cardiogenic shock treated with intravenous triiodothyronine. *Ann Intern Med* 1992;117:1014–1015.

51. Thompson GR, Soutar AK, Spengel FA, et al. Defects of receptor-mediated low density lipoprotein catabolism in homozygous familial hypercholesterolemia and hypothyroidism in vivo. *Proc Natl Acad Sci U S A* 1981;78:2591–2595.

52. The coronary drug project. Findings leading to further modifications of its protocol with respect to dextrothyroxine. The Coronary Drug Project Research Group. *JAMA* 1972;220:996–1008.

53. Anderson GH Jr, Blakeman N, Streeten DH. The effect of age on prevalence of secondary forms of hypertension in 4429 consecutively referred patients. *J Hypertens* 1994;12:609–615.

54. Streeten DH, Anderson GH Jr, Howland T, et al. Effects of thyroid function on blood pressure. Recognition of hypothyroid hypertension. *Hypertension* 1988;11:78–83.

55. Klein I, Ojamaa K. The cardiovascular system in hypothyroidism. In: Braverman LE, Utiger RD, eds. *Werner & Ingbar's the thyroid: a fundamental and clinical text*, 8th ed. Lippincott Williams & Wilkins, 2000:777–782.

56. Hak AE, Pols HA, Visser TJ, et al. Subclinical hypothyroidism is an independent risk factor for atherosclerosis and myocardial infarction in elderly women: the Rotterdam Study. *Ann Intern Med* 2000;132:270–278.

57. Tieche M, Lupi GA, Gutzwiller F, et al. Borderline low thyroid function and thyroid autoimmunity. Risk factors for coronary heart disease? *Br Heart J* 1981;46:202–206.

58. Dean JW, Fowler PB. Exaggerated responsiveness to thyrotrophin releasing hormone: a risk factor in women with coronary artery disease. *BMJ* 1985;290:1555–1561.

59. Heinonen OP, Gordin A, Aho K, et al. Symptomless autoimmune thyroiditis in coronary heart-disease. *Lancet* 1972;1:785–786.

60. Keating FR, Parkin TW, Selby JB. Treatment of heart disease associated with myxedema. *Prog Cardiovasc Dis* 1961;3:364.

61. Harjai KJ, Licata AA. Effects of amiodarone on thyroid function. *Ann Intern Med* 1997;126:63–73.

62. Albert SG, Alves LE, Rose EP. Thyroid dysfunction during chronic amiodarone therapy. *J Am Coll Cardiol* 1987;9:175–183.

63. Newman CM, Price A, Davies DW, et al. Amiodarone and the thyroid: a practical guide to the management of thyroid dysfunction induced by amiodarone therapy. *Heart* 1998;79:121–127.

64. Lambert MJ, Burger AG, Galeazzi RL, et al. Are selective increases in serum thyroxine (T_4) due to iodinated inhibitors of T_4 monodeiodination indicative of hyperthyroidism? *J Clin Endocrinol Metab* 1982;55:1058–1065.

65. Trip MD, Wiersinga W, Plomp TA. Incidence, predictability, and pathogenesis of amiodarone-induced thyrotoxicosis and hypothyroidism. *Am J Med* 1991;91:507–511.

66. Sun W, Sarma JS, Singh BN. Electrophysiological effects of dronedarone (SR33589), a noniodinated benzofuran derivative, in the rabbit heart: comparison with amiodarone. *Circulation* 1999;100:2276–2281.

67. Bartalena L, Grasso L, Brogioni S, et al. Serum interleukin–6 in amiodarone-induced thyrotoxicosis. *J Clin Endocrinol Metab* 1994;78:423–427.

68. Bartalena L, Brogioni S, Grasso L, et al. Treatment of amiodarone-induced thyrotoxicosis, a difficult challenge: results of a prospective study. *J Clin Endocrinol Metab* 1996;81:2930–2933.

69. Martino E, Aghini–Lombardi F, Mariotti S, et al. Treatment of amiodarone associated thyrotoxicosis by simultaneous administration of potassium perchlorate and methimazole. *J Endocrinol Invest* 1986;9:201–207.

70. Reichert LJ, de Rooy HA. Treatment of amiodarone induced hyperthyroidism with potassium perchlorate and methimazole during amiodarone treatment. *BMJ* 1989;298:1547–1548.

71. Wimpfheimer C, Staubli M, Schadelin J, et al. Prednisone in amiodarone-induced thyrotoxicosis. *BMJ* 1982;284:1835–1836.

72. Broussolle C, Ducottet X, Martin C, et al. Rapid effectiveness of prednisone and thionamides combined therapy in severe amiodarone iodine-induced thyrotoxicosis. Comparison of two groups of patients with apparently normal thyroid glands. *J Endocrinol Invest* 1989;12:37–42.

73. Dickstein G, Shechner C, Adawi F, et al. Lithium treatment in amiodarone-induced thyrotoxicosis. *Am J Med* 1997;102:454–458.

74. Leger AF, Massin JP, Laurent MF, et al. Iodine-induced thyrotoxicosis: analysis of eighty-five consecutive cases. *Eur J Clin Invest* 1984;14:449–455.

75. Brennan MD, van Heerden JA, Carney JA. Amiodarone-associated thyrotoxicosis (AAT): experience with surgical management. *Surgery* 1987;102:1062–1067.

76. Meurisse M, Hamoir E, D'Silva M, et al. Amiodarone-induced thyrotoxicosis: is there a place for surgery? *World J Surg* 1993;17:622–626; discussion 627.

77. Hamilton MA, Stevenson LW, Luu M, et al. Altered thyroid hormone metabolism in advanced heart failure. *J Am Coll Cardiol* 1990;16:91–95.

78. Hamilton MA, Stevenson LW, Fonarow GC, et al. Safety and hemodynamic effects of intravenous triiodothyronine in advanced congestive heart failure. *Am J Cardiol* 1998;81:443–447.

79. Moruzzi P, Doria E, Agostoni PG, et al. Usefulness of L-thyroxine to improve cardiac and exercise performance in idiopathic dilated cardiomyopathy. *Am J Cardiol.* 1994;73:374–378.

80. Moruzzi P, Doria E, Agostoni PG. Medium-term effectiveness of L-thyroxine treatment in idiopathic dilated cardiomyopathy. *Am J Med* 1996;101:461–467.

81. Holland FWD, Brown PS Jr, Weintraub BD, et al. Cardiopulmonary bypass and thyroid function: a "euthyroid sick syndrome." *Ann Thorac Surg* 1991;52:46–50.

82. Novitzky D, Cooper DK, Barton CI, et al. Triiodothyronine as an inotropic agent after open heart surgery. *J Thorac Cardiovasc Surg* 1989;98:972–977.

83. Klemperer JD, Klein I, Gomez M, et al. Thyroid hormone treatment after coronary-artery bypass surgery. *N Engl J Med* 1995;333:1522–1527.

84. Bennett–Guerrero E, Jimenez JL, White WD, et al. Cardiovascular effects of intravenous triiodothyronine in patients undergoing coronary artery bypass graft surgery. A randomized, double-blind, placebo-controlled trial. Duke T3 study group. *JAMA* 1996;275:687–692.

85. Jeevanandam V, Todd B, Regillo T, et al. Reversal of donor myocardial dysfunction by triiodothyronine replacement therapy. *J Heart Lung Transplant* 1994;13:681–687.

86. Plotz CM, Knowlton AI, Ragan C. The natural history of Cushing's syndrome. *Am J Med* 1952;13:597–614.

87. Ross EJ, Marshall–Jones P, Friedman M. Cushing's syndrome: diagnostic criteria. *QJM* 1966;35:149–192.

88. Soszynski P, Slowinska–Srzednicka J, Kasperlik–Zaluska A, et al. Endogenous natriuretic factors: atrial natriuretic hormone and digitalis-like substance in Cushing's syndrome. *J Endocrinol* 1991;129:453–458.

89. Mantero F, Boscaro M. Glucocorticoid-dependent hypertension. *J Steroid Biochem Mol Biol* 1992;43:409–413.

90. Yasuda G, Shionoiri H, Umemura S, et al. Exaggerated blood pressure response to angiotensin II in patients with Cushing's syndrome due to adrenocortical adenoma. *Eur J Endocrinol* 1994;131:582–588.

91. Sugihara N, Shimizu M, Kita Y, et al. Cardiac characteristics and postoperative courses in Cushing's syndrome. *Am J Cardiol* 1992;69:1475–1480.

92. Etxabe J, Vazquez JA. Morbidity and mortality in Cushing's disease: an epidemiological approach. *Clin Endocrinol* 1994;40:479–484.

93. Colao A, Pivonello R, Spiezia S, et al. Persistence of increased cardiovascular risk in patients with Cushing's disease after five years of successful cure. *J Clin Endocrinol Metab* 1999;84:2664–2672.

94. Meier CA, Biller BM. Clinical and biochemical evaluation of Cushing's syndrome. *Endocrinol Metab Clin North Am* 1997;26:741–762.

95. Conn JW. Primary aldosteronism, a new clinical syndrome. *J Lab Clin Med* 1955;45:3–17.

96. Dluhy RG, Williams GH. Endocrine hypertension. In: Wilson JD, Foster DW, Kronenberg HM, et al., eds. *Williams textbook of endocrinology*, 9th ed. Philadelphia: Saunders, 1998;729–749.

97. Fardella CE, Mosso L, Gomez–Sanchez C, et al. Primary hyperaldosteronism in essential hypertensives: prevalence, biochemical profile, and molecular biology. *J Clin Endocrinol Metab* 2000;85:1863–1867.

98. Gordon RD, Stowasser M, Tunny TJ, et al. High incidence of primary aldosteronism in 199 patients referred with hypertension. *Clin Exp Pharmacol Physiol* 1994;21:315–318.

99. Young WF Jr, Klee GG. Primary aldosteronism. Diagnostic evaluation. *Endocrinol Metab Clin North Am* 1988;17:367–395.

100. Rossi GP, Sacchetto A, Pavan E, et al. Remodeling of the left ventricle in primary aldosteronism due to Conn's adenoma. *Circulation* 1997;95:1471–1478.

101. Campbell SE, Diaz-Arias AA, Weber KT. Fibrosis of the human heart and systemic organs in adrenal adenoma. *Blood Press* 1992;1:149–156.

102. Vallotton MB. Primary aldosteronism. Part I. Diagnosis of primary hyperaldosteronism. *Clin Endocrinol* 1996;45:47–52.

103. Prys-Roberts C. Phaeochromocytoma—recent progress in its management. *Br J Anaesth* 2000;85:44–57.

104. van Heerden JA, Roland CF, Carney JA, et al. Long–term evaluation following resection of apparently benign pheochromocytoma(s)/paraganglioma(s). *World J Surg* 1990;14:325–329.

105. Bravo EL. Evolving concepts in the pathophysiology, diagnosis, and treatment of pheochromocytoma. *Endocrin Rev* 1994;15:356–368.

106. Levenson JA, Safar ME, London GM, et al. Haemodynamics in patients with phaeochromocytoma. *Clin Sci* 1980;58:349–356.

107. Scott I, Parkes R, Cameron DP. Phaeochromocytoma and cardiomyopathy. *Med J Aust* 1988;148:94–96.

108. McManus BM, Fleury TA, Roberts WC. Fatal catecholamine crisis in pheochromocytoma: curable cause of cardiac arrest. *Am Heart J* 1981;102:930–932.

109. Huddle KR, Kalliatakis B, Skoularigis J. Pheochromocytoma associated with clinical and echocardiographic features simulating hypertrophic obstructive cardiomyopathy. *Chest* 1996;109:1394–1397.

110. Gatzoulis KA, Tolis G, Theopistou A, et al. Cardiomyopathy due to a pheochromocytoma. A reversible entity. *Acta Cardiol* 1998;53:227–229.

111. Imperato-McGinley J, Gautier T, Ehlers K, et al. Reversibility of catecholamine-induced dilated cardiomyopathy in a child with a pheochromocytoma. *N Engl J Med* 1987;316:793–797.

112. Bravo EL. Plasma or urinary metanephrines for the diagnosis of pheochromocytoma? That is the question. *Ann Intern Med* 1996;125:331–332.

113. Hull CJ. Phaeochromocytoma. Diagnosis, preoperative preparation and anaesthetic management. *Br J Anaesth* 1986;58:1453–1468.

114. O'Connor DT. The adrenal medulla, catecholamines, and pheochromocytoma. In: Goldman L, Bennett JC, eds. *Cecil textbook of medicine*, 21st ed. Philadelphia: Saunders, 2000:1257–1262.

115. Molitch ME. Anterior pituitary. In: Goldman L, Bennett JC, eds. *Cecil textbook of medicine*, 21st ed. Philadelphia: Saunders, 2000:1208–1224.

116. Ron E, Gridley G, Hrubec Z, et al. Acromegaly and gastrointestinal cancer. *Cancer* 1991;68:1673–1677.

117. Molitch ME. Clinical manifestations of acromegaly. *Endocrinol Metab Clin North Am* 1992;21:597–614.

118. Wright AD, Hill DM, Lowy C, et al. Mortality in acromegaly. *QJM* 1970;39:1–16.

119. Alexander L, Appleton D, Hall R, et al. Epidemiology of acromegaly in the Newcastle region. *Clin Endocrinol* 1980;12:71–79.

120. Bengtsson BA, Eden S, Ernest I, et al. Epidemiology and long-term survival in acromegaly. A study of 166 cases diagnosed between 1955 and 1984. *Acta Med Scand* 1988;223:327–335.

121. Kraatz C, Benker G, Weber F, et al. Acromegaly and hypertension: prevalence and relationship to the renin-angiotensin-aldosterone system. *Klin Wochenschr* 1990;68:583–587.

122. Nabarro JD. Acromegaly. *Clin Endocrinol* 1987;26:481–512.

123. Nikkila EA, Pelkonen R. Serum lipids in acromegaly. *Metabolism* 1975;24:829–838.

124. Smallridge RC, Rajfer S, Davia J, et al. Acromegaly and the heart. An echocardiographic study. *Am J Med* 1979;66:22–27.

125. Martins JB, Kerber RE, Sherman BM, et al. Cardiac size and function in acromegaly. *Circulation* 1977;56:863–869.

126. Minniti G, Jaffrain–Rea ML, Moroni C, et al. Echocardiographic evidence for a direct effect of GH/IGF–I hypersecretion on cardiac mass and function in young acromegalics. *Clin Endocrinol* 1998;49:101–106.

127. Fazio S, Cittadini A, Biondi B, et al. Cardiovascular effects of short-term growth hormone hypersecretion. *J Clin Endocrinol Metab* 2000;85:179–182.

128. McGuffin WL Jr, Sherman BM, Roth F, et al. Acromegaly and cardiovascular disorders. A prospective study. *Ann Intern Med* 1974;81:11–18.

129. Thuesen L, Christensen SE, Weeke J, et al. The cardiovascular effects of octreotide treatment in acromegaly: an echocardiographic study. *Clin Endocrinol* 1989;30:619–625.

130. Chanson P, Timsit J, Masquet C, et al. Cardiovascular effects of the somatostatin analog octreotide in acromegaly. *Ann Intern Med* 1990;113:921–925.

131. Timsit J, Riou B, Bertherat J, et al. Effects of chronic growth hormone hypersecretion on intrinsic contractility, energetics, isomyosin pattern, and myosin adenosine triphosphatase activity of rat left ventricle. *J Clin Invest* 1990;86:507–515.

132. Cittadini A, Stromer H, Katz SE, et al. Differential cardiac effects of growth hormone and insulin-like growth factor-1 in the rat. A combined in vivo and in vitro evaluation. *Circulation* 1996;93:800–809.

133. Lie JT. Pathology of the heart in acromegaly: anatomic findings in 27 autopsied patients. *Am Heart J* 1980;100:41–52.

134. Lombardi G, Colao A, Marzullo P, et al. Is growth hormone bad for your heart? Cardiovascular impact of GH deficiency and of acromegaly. *J Endocrinol* 1997;155(Suppl 1):S33–37.

135. Swearingen B, Barker FG, Katznelson L, et al. Long-term mortality after transsphenoidal surgery and adjunctive therapy for acromegaly. *J Clin Endocrinol Metab* 1998;83:3419–3426.

136. Freda PU, Wardlaw SL, Post KD. Long-term endocrinological follow-up evaluation in 115 patients who underwent transsphenoidal surgery for acromegaly. *J Neurosurg* 1998;89:353–358.

137. Barkan AL, Halasz I, Dornfeld KJ, et al. Pituitary irradiation is ineffective in normalizing plasma insulin-like growth factor I in patients with acromegaly. *J Clin Endocrinol Metab* 1997;82:3187–3191.

138. Barkan AL. Acromegaly. Diagnosis and therapy. *Endocrinol Metab Clin North Am* 1989;18:277–310.

139. Ezzat S, Redelmeier DA, Gnehm M, et al. A prospective multicenter octreotide dose response study in the treatment of acromegaly. *J Endocrinol Invest* 1995;18:364–369.

140. Flogstad AK, Halse J, Bakke S, et al. Sandostatin LAR in acromegalic patients: long-term treatment. *J Clin Endocrinol Metab* 1997;82:23–28.

141. Trainer PJ, Drake WM, Katznelson L, et al. Treatment of acromegaly with the growth hormone-receptor antagonist pegvisomant. *N Engl J Med* 2000;342:1171–1177.

142. Salomon F, Cuneo RC, Hesp R, et al. The effects of treatment with recombinant human growth hormone on body composition and metabolism in adults with growth hormone deficiency. *N Engl J Med* 1989;321:1797–1803.

143. De Boer H, Blok GJ, Voerman HJ, et al. Body composition in adult growth hormone-deficient men, assessed by anthropometry and bioimpedance analysis. *J Clin Endocrinol Metab* 1992;75:833–837.

144. Stabler B, Turner JR, Girdler SS, et al. Reactivity to stress and psychological adjustment in adults with pituitary insufficiency. *Clin Endocrinol* 1992;36:467–473.

145. Rosen T, Bengtsson BA. Premature mortality due to cardiovascular disease in hypopituitarism. *Lancet* 1990;336:285–288.

146. Bates AS, Vant Hoff W, Jones PJ, et al. The effect of hypopituitarism on life expectancy. *J Clin Endocrinol Metab* 1996;81:1169–1172.

147. Cuneo RC, Salomon F, Watts GF, et al. Growth hormone treatment improves serum lipids and lipoproteins in adults with growth hormone deficiency. *Metabolism* 1993;42:1519–1523.

148. de Boer H, Blok GJ, Voerman HJ, et al. Serum lipid levels in growth hormone-deficient men. *Metabolism* 1994;43:199–203.

149. Rudling M, Norstedt G, Olivecrona H, et al. Importance of growth hormone for the induction of hepatic low density lipoprotein receptors. *Proc Natl Acad Sci U S A* 1992;89:6983–6987.

150. Beshyah SA, Johnston DG. Cardiovascular disease and risk factors in adults with hypopituitarism. *Clin Endocrinol* 1999;50:1–15.

151. Longobardi S, Cuocolo A, Merola B, et al. Left ventricular function in young adults with childhood and adulthood onset growth hormone deficiency. *Clin Endocrinol* 1998;48:137–143.

152. Colao A, Cuocolo A, Di Somma C, et al. Impaired cardiac performance in elderly patients with growth hormone deficiency. *J Clin Endocrinol Metab* 1999;84:3950–3955.

153. Cittadini A, Cuocolo A, Merola B, et al. Impaired cardiac performance in GH-deficient adults and its improvement after GH replacement. *Am J Physiol* 1994;267:E219–225.

154. Markussis V, Beshyah SA, Fisher C, et al. Detection of premature atherosclerosis by high-resolution ultrasonography in symptom-free hypopituitary adults. *Lancet* 1992;340:1188–1192.

155. Consensus guidelines for the diagnosis and treatment of adults with growth hormone deficiency: summary statement of the Growth Hormone Research Society Workshop on Adult Growth Hormone Deficiency. *J Clin Endocrinol Metab* 1998;83:379–381.

156. Chrisoulidou A, Beshyah SA, Rutherford O, et al. Effects of 7 years of growth hormone replacement therapy in hypopituitary adults. *J Clin Endocrinol Metab* 2000;85:3762–3769.

157. Jenkins PJ. Growth hormone and exercise. *Clin Endocrinol*, 1999;50:683–689.

158. Yarasheski KE, Zachwieja JJ, Campbell JA, et al. Effect of growth hormone and resistance exercise on muscle growth and strength in older men. *Am J Physiol* 1995;268:E268–276.

159. Deyssig R, Frisch H, Blum WF, et al. Effect of growth hormone treatment on hormonal parameters, body composition and strength in athletes. *Acta Endocrinol* 1993;128:313–318.

160. Deyssig R, Frisch H. Self–administration of cadaveric growth hormone in power athletes. *Lancet* 1993;341:768–769.

161. Cittadini A, Grossman JD, Napoli R, et al. Growth hormone attenuates early left ventricular remodeling and improves cardiac function in rats with large myocardial infarction. *J Am Coll Cardiol* 1997;29:1109–1116.

162. Grimm D, Cameron D, Griese DP, et al. Differential effects of growth hormone on cardiomyocyte and extracellular matrix protein remodeling following experimental myocardial infarction. *Cardiovasc Res* 1998;40:297–306.

163. Wollert KC, Drexler H. Growth hormone and insulin-like growth factor—friends of the infarcted heart? *Eur Heart J* 2000;21:1499–1501.

164. Friberg L, Werner S, Eggertsen G, et al. Growth hormone and insulin-like growth factor-1 in acute myocardial infarction. *Eur Heart J* 2000;21:1547–1554.

165. Fazio S, Sabatini D, Capaldo B, et al. A preliminary study of growth hormone in the treatment of dilated cardiomyopathy. *N Engl J Med* 1996;334:809–814.

166. Osterziel KJ, Strohm O, Schuler J, et al. Randomised, double-blind, placebo-controlled trial of human recombinant growth hormone in patients with chronic heart failure due to dilated cardiomyopathy. *Lancet* 1998;351:1233–1237.

167. Genth-Zotz S, Zotz R, Geil S, et al. Recombinant growth hormone therapy in patients with ischemic cardiomyopathy: effects on hemodynamics, left ventricular function, and cardiopulmonary exercise capacity. *Circulation* 1999;99:18–21.

168. Sivula A, Pelkonen R. Long-term health risk of primary hyperparathyroidism: the effect of surgery. *Ann Med* 1996;28:95–100.

169. Shane E. Parathyroid carcinoma. *Curr Ther Endocrinol Metab* 1994;5:522–525.

170. Palmer M, Adami HO, Bergstrom R, et al. Survival and renal function in untreated hypercalcaemia. Population-based cohort study with 14 years of follow-up. *Lancet* 1987;1:59–62.

171. Hedback G, Oden A. Increased risk of death from primary hyperparathyroidism—an update. *Eur J Clin Invest* 1998;28:271–276.

172. Wermers RA, Khosla S, Atkinson EJ, et al. Survival after the diagnosis of hyperparathyroidism: a population-based study. *Am J Med* 1998;104:115–122.

173. Soreide JA, van Heerden JA, Grant CS, et al. Survival after surgical treatment for primary hyperparathyroidism. *Surgery* 1997;122:1117–1123.

174. Stefenelli T, Mayr H, Bergler-Klein J, et al. Primary hyperparathyroidism: incidence of cardiac abnormalities and partial reversibility after successful parathyroidectomy. *Am J Med* 1993;95:197–202.

175. Barletta G, De Feo ML, Del Bene R, et al. Cardiovascular effects of parathyroid hormone: a study in healthy subjects and normotensive patients with mild primary hyperparathyroidism. *J Clin Endocrinol Metab* 2000;85:1815–1821.

176. Bernardi D, Bernini L, Cini G, et al. Asymmetric septal hypertrophy in uremic-normotensive patients on regular hemodialysis. An M-mode and two-dimensional echocardiographic study. *Nephron* 1985;39:30–35.

177. London GM, De Vernejoul MC, Fabiani F, et al. Secondary hyperparathyroidism and cardiac hypertrophy in hemodialysis patients. *Kidney Int* 1987;32:900–907.

178. Hara S, Ubara Y, Arizono K, et al. Relation between parathyroid hormone and cardiac function in long-term hemodialysis patients. *Miner Electrolyte Metab* 1995;21:72–76.

179. Sato S, Ohta M, Kawaguchi Y, et al. Effects of parathyroidectomy on left ventricular mass in patients with hyperparathyroidism. *Miner Electrolyte Metab* 1995;21:67–71.

180. Kosch M, Hausberg M, Vormbrock K, et al. Studies on flow-mediated vasodilation and intima-media thickness of the brachial artery in patients with primary hyperparathyroidism. *Am J Hypertens* 2000;13:759–764.

181. Kosch M, Hausberg M, Vormbrock K, et al. Impaired flow-mediated vasodilation of the brachial artery in patients with primary hyperparathyroidism improves after parathyroidectomy. *Cardiovasc Res* 2000;47:813–818.

182. Nilsson IL, Aberg J, Rastad J, et al. Endothelial vasodilatory dysfunction in primary hyperparathyroidism is reversed after parathyroidectomy. *Surgery* 1999;126:1049–1055.

183. Smith JC, Page MD, John R, et al. Augmentation of central arterial pressure in mild primary hyperparathyroidism. *J Clin Endocrinol Metab* 2000;85:3515–3519.

184. NIH conference. Diagnosis and management of asymptomatic primary hyperparathyroidism: consensus development conference statement. *Ann Intern Med* 1991;114:593–597.

185. Consensus conference. Diagnosis and management of asymptomatic primary hyperparathyroidism. National Institutes of Health. *Conn Med* 1991;55:349–354.

186. van Heerden JA, Grant CS. Surgical treatment of primary hyperparathyroidism: an institutional perspective. *World J Surg* 1991;15:688–692.

187. Chen H, Parkerson S, Udelsman R. Parathyroidectomy in the elderly: do the benefits outweigh the risks? *World J Surg* 1998;22:531–535.

188. Sullivan ML, Martinez CM, Gennis P, et al. The cardiac toxicity of anabolic steroids. *Prog Cardiovasc Dis* 1998;41:1–15.

189. Yue P, Chatterjee K, Beale C, et al. Testosterone relaxes rabbit coronary arteries and aorta. *Circulation* 1995;91:1154–1160.

190. Webb CM, McNeill JG, Hayward CS, et al. Effects of testosterone on coronary vasomotor regulation in men with coronary heart disease. *Circulation* 1999;100:1690–1696.

191. Rosano GM, Leonardo F, Pagnotta P, et al. Acute anti-ischemic effect of testosterone in men with coronary artery disease. *Circulation* 1999;99:1666–1670.

192. Webb CM, Adamson DL, de Zeigler D, et al. Effect of acute testosterone on myocardial ischemia in men with coronary artery disease. *Am J Cardiol* 1999;83:437–439.

193. English KM, Steeds RP, Jones TH, et al. Low-dose transdermal testosterone therapy improves angina threshold in men with chronic stable angina: a randomized, double-blind, placebo-controlled study. *Circulation* 2000;102:1906–1911.

194. Alexandersen P, Haarbo J, Byrjalsen I, et al. Natural androgens inhibit male atherosclerosis: a study in castrated, cholesterol–fed rabbits. *Circ Res* 1999;84:813–819.

195. Phillips GB, Pinkernell BH, Jing TY. The association of hypotestosteronemia with coronary artery disease in men. *Arterioscler Thromb* 1994;14:701–706.

196. Cauley JA, Gutai JP, Kuller LH, et al. Usefulness of sex steroid hormone levels in predicting coronary artery disease in men. *Am J Cardiol* 1987;60:771–777.

197. Barrett–Connor E, Khaw KT. Endogenous sex hormones and cardiovascular disease in men. A prospective population-based study. *Circulation* 1988;78:539–545.

198. Yarnell JW, Beswick AD, Sweetnam PM, et al. Endogenous sex hormones and ischemic heart disease in men. The Caerphilly prospective study. *Arterioscler Thromb* 1993;13:517–520.

199. Bagatell CJ, Heiman JR, Matsumoto AM, et al. Metabolic and behavioral effects of high-dose, exogenous testosterone in healthy men. *J Clin Endocrinol Metab* 1994;79:561–567.

200. Tripathy D, Shah P, Lakshmy R, et al. Effect of testosterone replacement on whole body glucose utilisation and other cardiovascular risk factors in males with idiopathic hypogonadotropic hypogonadism. *Horm Metab Res* 1998;30:642–645.

THE HEART AND OTHER ORGAN SYSTEMS

Hematologic and Oncologic Disorders and the Heart

PETER B. AMSTERDAM
DAVID M. YAMADA

▼ *ADDITIONAL ELECTRONIC TOPICS*
Heparin-Induced Thrombocytopenia: Pathophysiology g64

ANEMIA

Pathophysiology

Severe anemia (hemoglobin less than 7.0) results in profound hemodynamic and neurohormonal changes aimed at maintaining adequate oxygen delivery to vital organs (*e*Table 35B.0.1 and *e*Fig. 35B.0.1). Hemodynamic changes observed in patients with severe anemia include increased cardiac output, heart rate, and stroke volume and decreased systemic vascular resistance, mean arterial pressure, and cir-

culatory transit time (1). Neurohormonal changes include activation of the renin-angiotensin-aldosterone system and increases in vasopressin and norepinephrine release. Elevated levels of 2,3-diphosphoglycerate result in lower oxygen affinity for hemoglobin and hence greater tissue extraction of oxygen (2). All these adaptations correct with reversal of the anemia. Although healthy adults can sustain hemoglobin concentrations as low as 5 mg per dL without detrimental effects on tissue oxygenation (1), symptoms of fatigue may occur in anemia and resolve with transfusion (3). Although clinically significant myocardial ischemia is rare in otherwise healthy people, cardiac reserve is impaired (4). ▼ g65

In the most severe cases of anemia, congestive heart failure may develop and can resolve by simply correcting the

P. B. Amsterdam: Department of Cardiology, Grant Medical Center, Heart Care, Inc., Columbus, Ohio

D. M. Yamada: Department of Cardiovascular Medicine, Sarasota Memorial Hospital, Sarasota, Florida

anemia. *Congestive heart failure* is actually something of a misnomer in this case because most patients usually have normal or increased myocardial contractility. However, in some cases of protracted anemia, left ventricular systolic dysfunction can develop, and this, too, is reversed by correcting the anemia (7). When ventricular function remains preserved, the fluid retention in severe anemia appears to be caused by the neurohormonal activity (induction of the renin-angiotensin-aldosterone system and increased vasopressin release) that is caused by the decreased renal blood flow that occurs when low systemic arterial pressures result in a reflexive increase in renal vascular resistance.

Treatment

Guidelines have increasingly advised that routine transfusion using the *10/30 rule* (hemoglobin of 10 mg per dL or hematocrit of 30%) as a trigger should be avoided. [▼ g66] Both to reduce the risk to transfusion recipients and to conserve blood products, the overall status of the patient should be considered in addition to the specific measurements of hemoglobin or hematocrit. The primary reasons usually given for transfusion are to increase myocardial oxygen supply and to diminish the increased demand caused by the physiologic adaptations described previously. However, most evidence supports the concept that myocardial oxygen supply is maintained above a hemoglobin of 6 to 7 mg per dL (2) and that, at least in otherwise healthy individuals, administration of stored blood in mild anemia does not improve hemodynamics or tissue oxygenation. In a randomized clinical trial of critical care patients, those kept at a hemoglobin level of 7 to 9 mg per dL had a lower in-hospital mortality (p = .05) and a nonsignificantly (statistically) lower 30-day mortality compared with those kept at a hemoglobin of 10 to 12 mg per dL (8).

In anemia from acute blood loss, blood volume should be replaced first with crystalloid before determining if red cell transfusion is necessary, based on signs or symptoms. If blood loss can be anticipated, such as in elective surgery, arrangements should be made, if possible, for autologous blood donation. Finally, in chronic anemia, homologous blood transfusion should be the treatment of last resort: All other avenues, such as iron replacement or erythropoietin, should be tried before consideration of homologous transfusion, and then transfusion should only be performed for symptoms or signs attributable to the anemia. These symptoms include syncope, dyspnea, orthostatic hypotension, tachycardia, angina, or transient ischemic attacks (2).

The absence of definitive evidence concerning the point at which the increased myocardial oxygen demand creates a problem for patients with coronary artery disease makes practical criteria for cardiac patients difficult. No evidence exists that anemia in these patients predisposes to adverse cardiovascular events. Deleterious consequences of sending patients home after cardiopulmonary bypass or percutaneous intervention with hematocrit values between 21% and 30% have not been documented. One study suggests that, among patients with angina and anemia, low exercise capacity is caused more by anemia than by coronary disease when the hematocrit is below 25% (9). Therefore, the general guidelines of the American College of Physicians are recommended (*e*Figs. 35B.0.3 and 35B.0.4); only severe symptomatic anemia should be corrected with red cell transfusions, and only after nontransfusion therapy has been exhausted (2). In the setting of persistent refractory ischemia, packed red blood cells should be given to correct the anemia until the acute situation is stabilized. ▼ g67

A few specific causes of anemia merit special consideration from the cardiologist because of their relationship to cardiac disease. These include the hemoglobinopathies, including the thalassemias and sickle cell anemia, and hemolytic anemia related to heart disease.

Thalassemia

The thalassemias are diseases of the red blood cell resulting from decreased amounts of either the α (α-thalassemia) or β (β-thalassemia) chain components of hemoglobin, because of either absent or defective genes. The relative excess of the normal globin component leads to hemolysis and ineffective erythropoiesis. The thalassemic syndromes range from subclinical to life-threatening depending on the number and severity of the genetic defects. β-Thalassemia major, characterized by defects in both copies of the beta-globin gene, has been the best studied with regard to cardiac problems.

Cardiac disease, the most common cause of death in β-thalassemia major, develops because of multiple blood transfusions (which become necessary beginning at 4 to 6 months of age when beta-chain production supplants γ-chain production) rather than the disease itself. These blood transfusions, plus increased gastrointestinal absorption of iron, result in an iron-overload state, which leads to myocardial iron deposition, causing a restrictive cardiomyopathy, cardiac enlargement, ventricular dysfunction, and congestive heart failure. Both systolic and diastolic left ventricular dysfunction can occur (15). Arrhythmias (atrial and ventricular tachyarrhythmias and bradyarrhythmias, particularly involving atrioventricular block) may result from this cardiomyopathy or from hemosiderosis-related damage to the conduction system. Pericarditis is also commonly seen (16).

The advent of the iron-chelating agent deferoxamine in the mid-1970s resulted in an overall reduction in cardiac complications (17) and improvement in survival (18). Thus, deferoxamine, generally administered by continuous subcutaneous injection by a pump device, is a mainstay of medical treatment of β-thalassemia major. Allogeneic bone marrow transplant has been used as an alternative to long-term transfusion and iron chelation therapy (19).

Sickle Cell Disease

Sickle cell anemia is caused by a point mutation in the beta-globin gene, resulting in the substitution of valine for glutamate in the sixth amino acid of the protein. This change, in homozygous form, results in deoxygenated HbS polymerizing, distorting the shape of the red blood cell (sickling) and leading to occlusion of capillaries and end-organ damage. In addition, the abnormal hemoglobin results in a shortened life span of the erythrocyte, resulting in an anemia with reticulocytosis.

In contrast to β-thalassemia, cardiac complications of sickle cell anemia are not among the major causes of morbidity or mortality, although the heart is affected. Several studies using noninvasive imaging techniques have demonstrated abnormalities in sickle cell patients. Diastolic dysfunction, increased left ventricular mass and wall thickness, and enlargement of the cardiac chambers and aortic root are all common by echocardiography (20). Although resting EF is almost always normal (21,22), subtle abnormalities in load-independent parameters suggest underlying systolic dysfunction (21), and impaired EF response to exercise has been described (23). Right ventricular abnormalities and significant pulmonary hypertension are uncommon (21,24). Primary valvular disease is uncommon as well (24). Treatment involves addressing the underlying disease, including supportive therapy consisting of hydration, analgesics, oxygen, and transfusions when indicated. Newer therapies include hydroxyurea and allogeneic bone marrow transplant. ❦ g68

Hemolysis and Heart Disease

Hemolysis following valve replacement occurs mainly because of turbulence of blood flow and, in patients with mechanical valves, direct trauma to erythrocytes (29) (see Chapter 24). It is common, occurring in up to 50% of patients, although severe hemolysis is rare (30). Significant hemolysis is strongly indicative of valve dysfunction or a paravalvular leak (30) and may even be the presenting sign (31). The degree of hemolysis is directly related to severity of regurgitation. However, severe hemolysis necessitating repeat surgery in the absence of paravalvular leak or valve dysfunction has been reported (32). Risk factors for hemolysis include smaller prosthesis, mechanical valve versus bioprosthesis (29), double- versus single-valve replacement (30), suture type (33), and annular calcification (33). In addition to prosthetic valve disease, hemolysis has been reported following mitral valve repair, with native valve disease, and in patients following repair of ventricular septal defect (34). Diagnosis of hemolysis requires elevated lactate dehydrogenase, which is the most sensitive test and corre-

lates well with severity (35). Other laboratory evidence includes elevated reticulocytes, low haptoglobin, hemosiderinuria, anemia, and schistocytes seen on peripheral smear (30). Treatment is usually conservative, consisting of observation and iron and folate supplementation as needed. Beta-blockers may help by ameliorating shear stress (34). Transfusions may be required. Severe refractory anemia may necessitate repeat surgery.

DISORDERS WITH INCREASED BLOOD VISCOSITY

Polycythemia

Polycythemia is characterized by an increased concentration of circulating red blood cells. Absolute polycythemia represents an increase in red cell mass, whereas relative polycythemia denotes increased red cell concentration with normal red cell mass, due to reduced plasma volume. Absolute polycythemias may be characterized as primary (polycythemia vera) or secondary, caused by an increase in erythropoietin.

Polycythemia vera, caused by a neoplastic, clonal proliferation of hematopoietic stem cells, results in excess bleeding as well as thromboembolic complications in up to 60% of patients (36). These events include stroke, myocardial infarction, deep venous thrombosis, pulmonary embolism, and arterial embolism (36,37). Neurologic symptoms such as headache, dizziness, vision changes, and confusion may result from chronic decreased cerebral perfusion caused by elevated blood viscosity, rather than an acute event. Although thromboembolism tends to occur mainly in small vessels, aortic and cardiac intraventricular thrombi have been reported (38). Valvular lesions by echocardiography, usually thickening but occasionally distinct vegetations, occur commonly and are associated with thromboembolic events (39). Acute events are treated with phlebotomy and aspirin at a dose of approximately 300 mg per day (40). Chronic therapy includes phlebotomy (41), hydroxyurea (42), and interferon-α (43). Prophylaxis against thromboembolism with low-dose aspirin (75 mg per day) could be considered, although no randomized prospective trials of this have yet been conducted, and a higher risk for bleeding is incurred (40).

Secondary polycythemias may be caused by either an appropriate increase in erythropoietin secondary to hypoxia (such as in chronic obstructive pulmonary disease or congenital heart disease with right-to-left shunt; see Chapter 31) or an inappropriate increase in erythropoietin production due to an erythropoietin-producing tumor such as a renal cell carcinoma. Hematocrits tend to vary inversely with arterial oxygen saturation and in congenital heart disease have been reported to be as high as 85%. Clinical manifestations of secondary polycythemia are similar to those of polycythemia vera and can include thrombotic episodes and bleeding.

Polycythemia associated with smoking and chronic obstructive pulmonary disease is associated with a lower frequency of thromboembolic events compared with polycythemia vera, but events may occur in up to 40% of patients (36). The benefit of phlebotomy to reduce such events has not been conclusively proven (44). Exercise tolerance, however, has been shown to improve with phlebotomy to achieve a hematocrit in the range of 50%, but no further benefit seems to accrue by keeping hematocrit in the normal range (45). The mechanism may be caused by improved right ventricular performance due to decreased preload. Patients in clinical congestive heart failure receive more benefit than mildly symptomatic patients. To avoid significant hypovolemia, simultaneous volume expansion with normal saline may be required (41).

Relative, or spurious, polycythemia is defined by increased hematocrit with normal red cell mass, generally caused by either reduced plasma volume or the combination of high normal red cell volume and low normal plasma volume. Morbidity is not directly related to this condition; thus, phlebotomy is not warranted.

Essential Thrombocythemia

Essential thrombocythemia is a myeloproliferative disorder similar to polycythemia vera with clonal overexpression of a multipotent stem cell, but resulting predominantly in thrombocytosis rather than erythrocytosis (46). As in polycythemia, this condition results in both bleeding and thromboembolic complications, with 9% to 40% of patients experiencing one or more thrombotic events (47,48). Large vessel thrombosis is most common, but myocardial thrombosis has been reported (48). Because a history of a thrombotic event is a risk factor for future recurrence, patients suffering such events are usually started on cytoreductive therapy, which may include radiophosphorus, hydroxyurea, busulfan, or interferon-α (46,47). Platelet count does not correlate with thrombosis in most studies, and even young patients may have serious or even fatal thrombotic events (48). The benefit of prophylactic therapy, however, currently remains controversial (46,49).

HEMATOLOGIC EFFECTS OF CARDIAC DRUGS

Occasionally, drugs used to treat cardiovascular disorders may cause hematologic abnormalities such as anemia, neutropenia, and thrombocytopenia (*e*Table 35B.0.2). Antihypertensive drugs associated with rare untoward hematologic effects include captopril, which has been associated with leukopenia, neutropenia, and fatal pancytopenia (50). Thiazides have been associated with thrombocytopenia (51). Hemolytic anemia (51) and thrombocytopenia (52) have

been seen with use of alpha-methyldopa. Agranulocytosis has been reported after propranolol administration (53). Antiarrhythmic drugs have also been associated with hematologic abnormalities. Thrombocytopenia has been seen with digoxin use (52). Quinidine has been associated with hemolytic anemia and thrombocytopenia (52), and neutropenia and agranulocytosis have been reported with use of procainamide and tocainide (54). Use of the antiplatelet agent ticlopidine after coronary stent procedures has been associated with neutropenia, aplastic anemia, thrombocytopenia, and an incidence of thrombotic thrombocytopenic purpura of 1 in 1,600 to 5,000, resulting in over 250 deaths (55) and prompting recommendation of screening hematologic profiles while the patient remains on the drug (56). Clopidogrel is an alternative that has a safer hematologic profile, but nonetheless has been associated with thrombotic thrombocytopenic purpura (57). Hematologic abnormalities generally reverse with discontinuation of the offending agent.

Heparin-Induced Thrombocytopenia

Frequency

Perhaps one of the most commonly seen hematologic abnormalities caused by a cardiac drug in clinical practice is heparin-induced thrombocytopenia (HIT). Two types of HIT have been observed. Type I HIT is the more common, milder form, rarely resulting in platelet counts below 100,000. It occurs with a frequency of 10% to 25%, usually during the first 4 days of therapy, and resolves without serious sequelae despite continuation of heparin (58). A proaggregatory effect on platelets by heparin has been proposed as the mechanism for type I HIT. In contrast, type II HIT, a much more serious complication that is the subject of the remainder of this section, occurs with a frequency of approximately 1% to 5% of patients receiving heparin, usually 4 to 8 days after the start of heparin therapy (58). If there has been previous exposure to heparin, however, especially within the previous 3 months, onset may be much sooner, and therefore timing of thrombocytopenia alone cannot distinguish between HIT types I and II. The frequency with low-molecular-weight heparin is less than 1% (58).

Clinical Presentation

Thrombocytopenia occurs 4 to 8 days after the start of heparin and almost always drops to below 100,000, usually to a nadir of 30,000 to 50,000 (58,63). The platelet count decreases to less than 15,000 in only 5% of patients, in contrast to other drug-induced thrombocytopenias, in which nadirs are typically around 15,000 (64). Timing of thrombocytopenia has been documented to start as early as 2 days after initiation of therapy if recent previous exposure has occurred.

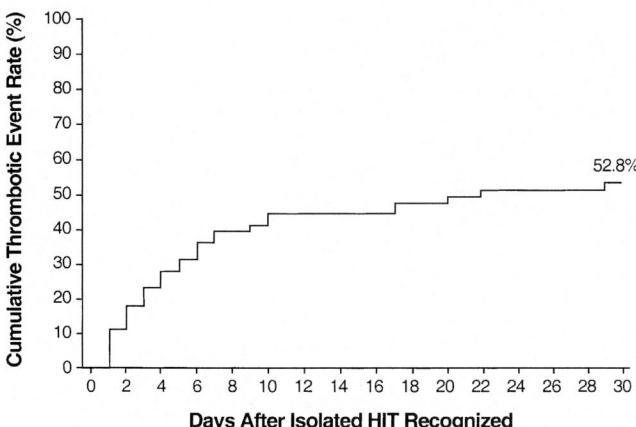

FIGURE 35B.1 Cumulative frequency of thrombotic events in patients with heparin-induced thrombocytopenia (HIT) presenting with isolated thrombocytopenia. (From Warkentin TE, Kelton JG. A 14-year study of heparin-induced thrombocytopenia. *Am J Med* 1996;101:502–507, with permission.)

Thrombosis occurs with a high frequency, anywhere from 25% to 80%, depending on the patient population and treatment initiated (58,65). Importantly, up to 50% of thrombotic events occur before HIT can be recognized by low platelet counts, and patients remain at increased risk for events up to 30 days after the syndrome has been identified, despite cessation of heparin (58,65) (Fig. 35B.1).

The types of thrombotic events that occur are almost always severe. Pulmonary embolism accounts for up to one-fourth of the events (65), followed by proximal deep venous thromboses, stroke, myocardial infarction, and otherwise rare events such as bilateral adrenal vein thrombosis, cavernous sinus thrombosis, and extremity or visceral arterial thrombosis (64,65). Death occurs in up to 10% to 20% of patients, despite cessation of heparin and initiation of appropriate treatment (63,66). Despite sometimes severe thrombocytopenia, hemorrhage is relatively rare in HIT, occurring in under 10% of patients (58,63). ⚡⚡ g69

Diagnosis

Because the HIT antibody may be found in the absence of any clinical sequelae (58), HIT remains a clinical diagnosis, requiring the following conditions: (1) occurrence of thrombocytopenia during heparin administration, (2) resolution of thrombocytopenia after heparin is discontinued, and (3) exclusion of other causes. Heparin resistance, a new thrombotic event, and laboratory evidence all help support the diagnosis.

Among the laboratory assays, the ^{14}C-serotonin release assay is the most sensitive and remains the current standard for laboratory diagnosis, although it is difficult to perform and time-consuming. It relies on detection of ^{14}C-serotonin when radiolabeled donor platelets are incubated with serum from a patient with HIT and heparin and has a sensitivity of approximately 94%, with a specificity of 90% to 100% (67). The platelet aggregation test uses platelet-rich plasma from both normal donors and patients incubated together. The test result is positive when platelet aggregation occurs when heparin but not buffer is added. This test is the easiest to perform, but usually has a sensitivity of only 50% (60). The sensitivity may approach that of the ^{14}C-serotonin release assay, however, when washed platelets from multiple donors are used, and different concentrations of heparin are used as well (60). The enzyme-linked immunosorbent assay test to detect IgG antibody is sensitive but not very specific because weak antibodies may be detected (60).

Functional laboratory assay results become negative an average of 3 months after resolution of the clinical syndrome, but may remain positive for as long as 14 months (63,68). Platelet counts return to normal after a mean of 4 to 6 days, but this may take as long as 2 weeks (63,64).

Treatment

Cessation of heparin is critical when the diagnosis of HIT is reasonably suspect. Because thrombotic complications may occur even after stopping heparin (58), additional anticoagulation should be strongly considered. Lepirudin, a recombinant derivative of hirudin, an anticoagulant originating from leeches, is currently the only drug approved by the U.S. Food and Drug Administration for treatment of HIT. It directly inhibits thrombin and is renally excreted. Two clinical trials have shown improvement compared with historical controls with respect to death (9% vs. 22%) and new thromboembolism (18% vs. 32%) (66,69). During the trials, new events were reduced from 5.1% per patient-day before treatment to 1.5% per patient-day during treatment. Bleeding was higher (44% vs. 27%), but there was no statistically significant increase in the requirement for transfusion (13% vs. 9%). Other agents that have been used include danaparoid, argatroban, and anacrod (59). Of note, argatroban is excreted normally in patients with renal failure. Low-molecular-weight heparin should not be used to treat HIT because of a high rate (up to 85%) of cross-reactivity with the antibody.

ONCOLOGIC DISORDERS AND THE HEART

Metastatic Disease Involving the Heart

Metastatic disease involving the heart is uncommon, but not rare. In contrast, primary tumors of the heart are exceedingly rare, with an incidence of less than 0.002% of all autopsies (70). Of 58,600 autopsies done between 1936 and 1960 as described in ten reports, the incidence of metastases to the heart was 1.1% of all cases (range, 0.2% to 6.0%) and 6.4% of all patients with malignancy (range,

2% to 21%) (71). In a study of 3,314 consecutive autopsies over a 14-year period at a single center, Abraham and colleagues reported a 2.9% incidence of metastatic malignancy involving the heart (70). Of the 3,314 cases, 24.3% revealed evidence of cancer, and of these cancer cases, 11.8% revealed evidence of metastatic cardiac involvement. The most common area of involvement was the myocardium (53.9%), followed by pericardium (28.4%), epicardium plus pericardium (13.7%), and endocardium (3.9%). However, other autopsy studies have indicated that the pericardium and epicardium are more common sites of metastasis than the myocardium (72).

The primary tumors resulting in cardiac metastases, in order of decreasing frequency, were lung (31.6%), lymphoma (15.8%), breast (13.7%), leukemia (13.7%), stomach (5.3%), melanoma (3.2%), liver (3.2%), colon (3.2%), and other tumors (10.5%) (70). These rates were dependent on the varying incidences of the primary tumors. To determine the propensity of a given tumor to metastasize to the heart, one large series examined the rate of cardiac metastases in autopsies showing evidence of each tumor. Malignancies with a high propensity for metastasis included leukemia (46% of all autopsies with leukemia showed cardiac involvement), melanoma (37%), thyroid (30%), lung (28%), sarcoma (26%), esophagus (23%), kidney (22%), lymphoma (22%), and breast (21%) (72).

Direct Effects of Tumors

Noncardiac tumors may either affect the heart directly, by actual infiltration of cardiac structures, or indirectly by thrombotic effects or secretion of mediators with cardiovascular effects (*e*Table 35B.0.3). Malignancy can involve the heart (including the pericardium) by a retrograde lymphatic route (carcinomas), hematogenously (carcinomas, sarcomas, lymphoma, leukemia, or melanoma), or by direct extension from contiguous structures (lung, breast, or esophageal carcinoma). Cardiac complications from direct effects of the tumor may occur by myocardial infiltration of tumor, pericardial infiltration causing effusion and tamponade, obstruction of the superior or inferior vena cava or right atrium, and pulmonary tumor emboli leading to elevated right-sided pressures and consequently right-sided heart failure (73). Cardiac complications are rarely the first signs of the malignancy; usually, the diagnosis of the primary tumor is well established before manifestation of cardiac involvement. It is also rare for cardiac metastases to occur without evidence of other metastases.

Myocardial Infiltration

Myocardial infiltration by metastases may be diagnosed by two-dimensional echocardiography or endomyocardial biopsy (74) (Fig. 35B.2), although most often it is discovered incidentally at autopsy. ECG findings are usually non-

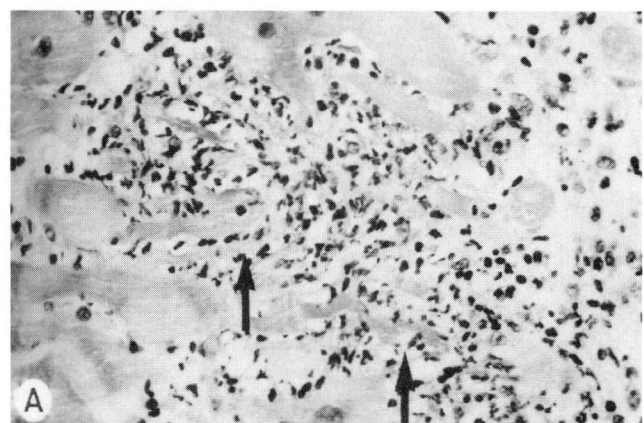
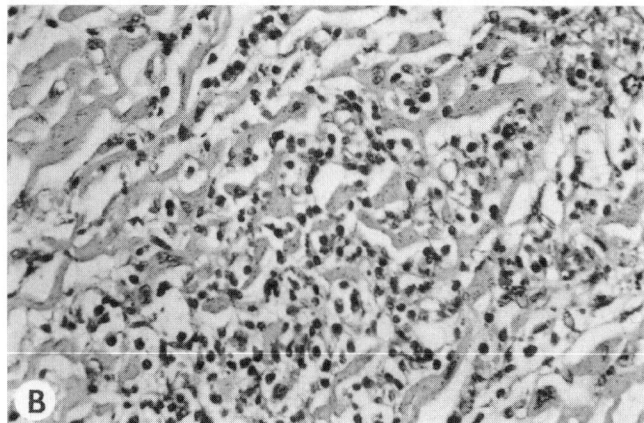

FIGURE 35B.2 A: Endomyocardial biopsy specimen in acute myelogenous leukemia showing myocardial infiltration by atypical hematopoietic cells and myocyte necrosis (*arrows*) (hematoxylin-eosin; ×400). **B:** Presence of immature myelogenous precursor cells is ascertained by chloroacetate esterase stain (×400). (From Flipse TR, Tazelaar HD, Holmes DR Jr. Diagnosis of malignant cardiac disease by endomyocardial biopsy. *Mayo Clin Proc* 1990;65:1415–1422, with permission.)

specific. Multiple reports exist, however, of persistent ST-segment elevation changes resembling those of myocardial infarction without other clinical evidence of myocardial infarction in patients with malignant myocardial infiltration, particularly if the epicardium is involved (75).

Myocardial infiltration by tumor is often clinically silent even when large amounts of myocardium are replaced by tumor, as in *charcoal heart* caused by metastatic malignant melanoma. However, clinical manifestations can include congestive heart failure (76), myocardial infarction (caused by tumor emboli, extrinsic compression, or ostial obstruction of coronary arteries) (77), and conduction disturbances (77,78). The pericardium is frequently also involved, and in these cases the clinical manifestations of pericardial disease predominate.

Treatment consists of addressing the underlying tumor; however, myocardial infiltration often represents an advanced state of the disease, in which treatment is ineffective. In cases of solitary cardiac metastases, surgical resection may be curative if the primary tumor has been controlled (79).

Pericardial Infiltration

Metastatic pericardial involvement, like myocardial involvement, is often asymptomatic and discovered as an incidental finding at autopsy. When clinically evident, pericardial disease is most often manifested by symptomatic pericardial effusion including tamponade. In rare cases pericardial tumor may encase the heart, leading to constriction. Initial diagnosis of pericardial disease is generally made by echocardiography, although occasionally computed tomographic scan may show disease when the echocardiography result was negative or may be necessary because of technically inadequate echocardiography (80).

When pericardial disease is discovered antemortem in cancer patients, malignant disease must be differentiated from idiopathic pericarditis and radiation-induced pericardial disease, both common in cancer patients. Clinical features helping to differentiate them include facial swelling in malignant pericardial disease; fever, pericardial friction rub, and improvement with nonsteroidal antiinflammatory drugs in idiopathic pericarditis; and constrictive pericarditis in radiation-induced disease. Cytologic examination of fluid is positive for malignant cells in 50% to 85% of cases (81). Bloody pericardial fluid with specific gravity greater than 1.016 and total protein greater than 3 mg per dL is also suggestive of malignant effusion.

Treatment of malignant pericardial effusions is only indicated in symptomatic patients. One retrospective, observational study of 93 consecutive patients revealed no difference in survival, duration of hospital stay, or hospital charges in less symptomatic patients managed conservatively initially compared with more symptomatic patients managed invasively. Furthermore, only 20% of the conservatively treated patients eventually required pericardiocentesis (82). Median survival after treatment is on the order of 3 to 4 months (81).

Treatment methods for malignant pericardial effusion include pericardiocentesis, pericardial sclerosis, systemic chemotherapy, radiotherapy, and surgery. Pericardiocentesis should be performed to relieve symptoms. Extended catheter drainage is associated with reduced recurrences compared with simple pericardiocentesis (81). Although pericardiocentesis alone can provide prolonged relief, symptomatic recurrence is frequent, up to 20% in one large series (81). Pericardial sclerosis may be performed using tetracycline. ▼ g70

Obstruction of Venous Inflow

Tumors may obstruct venous inflow into the heart, either by extrinsic compression or by direct invasion. Obstruction of the superior vena cava may result in the superior vena cava syndrome, which is caused in approximately 85% of cases by bronchogenic carcinoma, 10% by lymphomas, and the rest miscellaneous causes including benign etiologies (90). Extrinsic compression of the vein causes approximately 60% of cases and thrombosis the remainder.

In a retrospective review of 84 patients at a single center with superior vena cava syndrome, Perez and colleagues found that the most common presenting symptoms were shortness of breath (greater than 50%), facial swelling (43%), and swelling of the trunk or arms (40%). Chest pain, cough, and difficulty swallowing were also common and each occurred in approximately 20% of patients. Physical findings in decreasing order of frequency were trunk vein distention (67%), jugular vein distention (59%), facial edema (56%), tachypnea (40%), facial plethora (19%), cyanosis (15%), arm edema (9.5%), vocal cord paralysis (3.5%), and Horner's syndrome (2.3%) (90).

Treatment generally involves chemotherapy or radiation therapy or both. In this series, chemotherapy, radiation therapy, or both resulted in excellent or good symptomatic improvement in 70% of patients with bronchogenic carcinoma and 95% of patients with lymphoma. Percutaneous stenting has also been used to relieve symptoms of superior vena cava syndrome (91). ▼ g71

Indirect Effects of Tumors

Nonbacterial Thrombotic (Marantic) Endocarditis

Nonbacterial thrombotic endocarditis (NBTE) is a condition in which sterile vegetations, consisting of mostly fibrin and platelets but not inflammatory cells, develop on valve leaflets. In contrast to infectious endocarditis, there is no disruption of the underlying valve architecture. This condition is frequently, but not exclusively, associated with malignancy and may be seen in other debilitating conditions (73). One case report of NBTE of the mitral valve documents resolution of the vegetation 4 weeks after resection of a hepatic tumor (Fig. 35B.3). ▼ g72

NBTE is usually clinically silent and can be diagnosed by transthoracic echocardiography, although transesophageal echocardiography is more sensitive (96). However, embolism of vegetations can occur and have been shown to cause infarctions in the brain, myocardium, kidney, spleen, and thyroid gland (93,95).

Pheochromocytoma

Pheochromocytomas are neoplasms that arise from the adrenal medulla or preganglion cells and secrete norepinephrine and epinephrine. Clinical manifestations include hypertension (present in most, but not all, patients), which may be sustained (approximately 60% of cases) or episodic (approximately 40% of cases) (97).

Paroxysms or crises occur in more than 50% of patients and are characterized by headache, diaphoresis, palpitations,

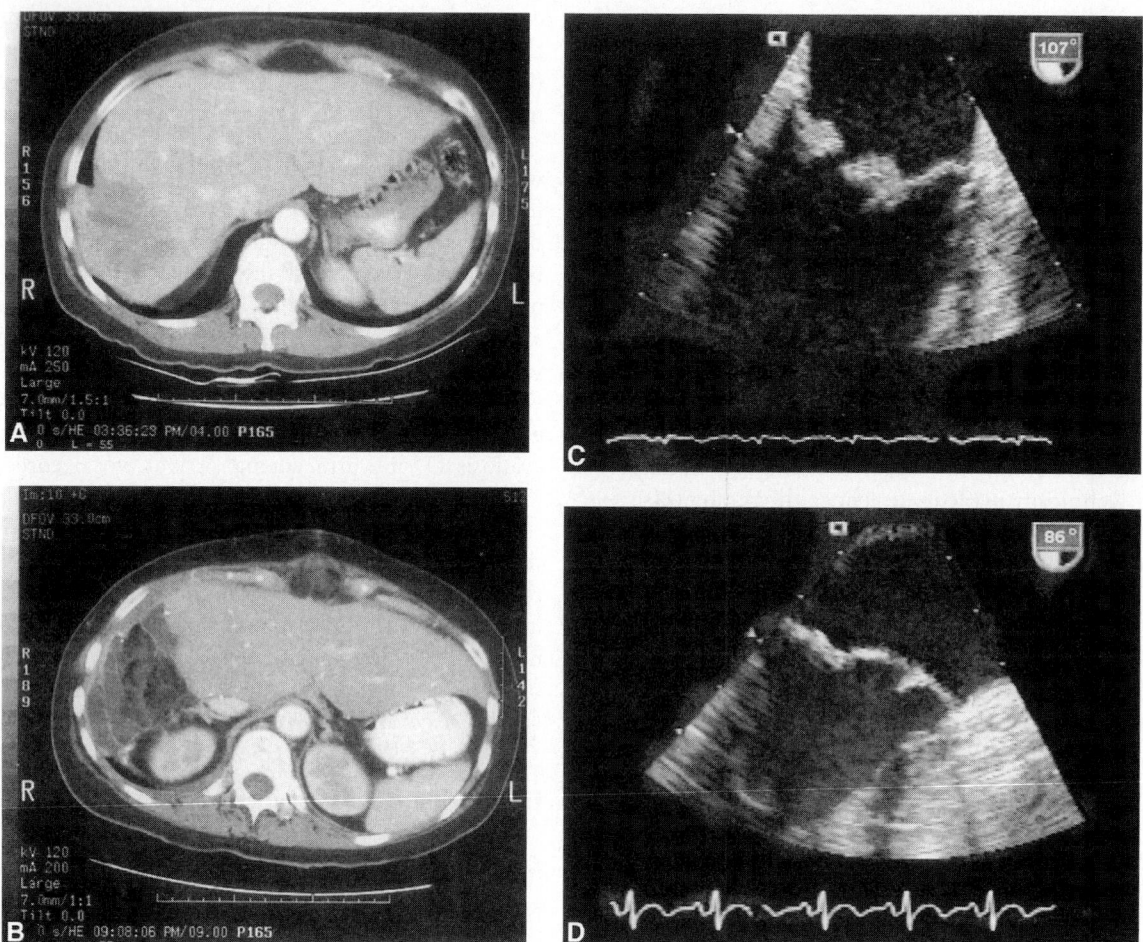

FIGURE 35B.3 Computed tomography scans of a hepatic tumor before **(A)** and after **(B)** resection. Transesophageal echocardiography demonstrating echodensities on the mitral valve consistent with vegetations **(C)**, and resolution of the abnormality 4 weeks after surgery **(D)**. (From Cockburn M, Swafford J, Mazur W, et al. Resolution of nonbacterial endocarditis after surgical resection of a malignant liver tumor. *Circulation* 2000;102:2671–2672, with permission.)

pallor or flushing, and elevated blood pressure, at times to severe levels. Effects on the heart can include arrhythmias, angina, and even myocardial infarction. In addition, focal areas of myocardial necrosis with contraction bands may occur, probably because of the toxic effects of catecholamines on myocytes, and may with time lead to cardiomyopathy and congestive heart failure (98). Reduced myo-cardial ^{123}I-metaiodobenzylguanidine uptake has been noted with pheochromocytoma, suggesting that the high circulating catecholamines may damage cardiac sympathetic nerve function (99).

The disorder may be suspected when hypertension is present in conjunction with symptoms or signs of a hyperadrenergic state, such as tachycardia, palpitations, sweating, paroxysmal anxiety attacks, or headache (100). However, because these signs are nonspecific and the disease is rare, many patients who are evaluated for the disease end up not having it. Diagnosis is by determination of urinary levels of vanillylmandelic acid, metanephrines, and unconjugated catecholamines. Treatment involves surgery if possible to remove the tumor. Before surgery, cardiovascular effects can be managed with alpha-adrenergic receptor blockers such as phenoxybenzamine or prazosin and beta-adrenergic blockers. Alpha-receptor blockade should be fully established before beta-blockade, because beta-blockade alone could lead to alpha-receptor–mediated vasoconstriction unopposed by beta$_2$-receptor–mediated vasodilation.

Carcinoid

Carcinoid tumors originate from amine precursor uptake and decarboxylase cells, and most commonly arise from the gastrointestinal tract. The tumors may secrete circulating chemical mediators such as serotonin and bradykinin, causing the carcinoid syndrome, which is characterized by flushing, diarrhea, wheezing, and episodic hypotension. Because these mediators are inactivated by the liver, carcinoid syndrome generally only develops if liver metastases are present or if the tumor is extraintestinal.

Cardiac abnormalities occur in approximately one-half of carcinoid syndrome cases. The cardiac lesion consists of a fibrous plaque made up of smooth muscle cells and collagen fibers in an acid mucopolysaccharide matrix (101). The lesions usually affect the right side of the heart only and may cause tricuspid valve and pulmonic valve dysfunction, typically tricuspid insufficiency and pulmonic stenosis. Although tricuspid valve surgery seems to result in symptomatic improvement in survivors of surgery, perioperative mortality is high (35% and 63% in two series) (102,103). ❦ g73

Cardiac Amyloidosis Secondary to Multiple Myeloma

Systemic amyloidosis occurs in approximately 10% of patients with multiple myeloma. When present, there is a high rate of cardiac involvement. One series reported amyloid-related cardiac failure in 40% of patients with systemic amyloidosis associated with myeloma (106). Clinical manifestations include congestive heart failure, arrhythmia, and restrictive cardiomyopathy. Definitive diagnosis must be made by endomyocardial biopsy, although the myeloma-involved heart has a characteristic, hyperrefractile appearance on echocardiography, which may assist in diagnosis. Other echocardiographic features include thickened ventricular walls, pericardial effusion, and thickening of multiple valves with regurgitation. Magnetic resonance imaging has also demonstrated promise in establishing the diagnosis noninvasively (107). Treatment is aimed at the underlying disease, in addition to using diuretics. There is anecdotal evidence that digoxin may be harmful because of heightened binding by amyloid fibrils in the heart, but systematic studies have failed to confirm this hypothesis (108). Coumadin may be beneficial, because intracardiac thrombi are frequently noted (108).

Cardiac Effects of Radiation Therapy for Cancer

Radiation therapy is used to treat many thoracic cancers and may cause injury to the heart and surrounding tissues (*e*Table 35B.0.4). The majority of patients with such radiation-induced heart disease (RIHD) have had Hodgkin's disease. Because they tend to be young at the time of treatment and are curable, they live long enough to develop the clinical sequelae of RIHD, many of which are delayed (109,110). However, patients irradiated for non-Hodgkin's lymphoma, esophageal carcinoma, thymoma, lung, and breast cancer have also developed RIHD. ❦ g74

Delayed onset pericardial disease is the most common form of RIHD. It may occur months to years after treatment, but often occurs within 12 months of therapy (114). One manifestation of disease may be a delayed acute pericarditis, with symptoms and findings typical of pericarditis including pleuritic chest pain, fever, pericardial rub, and ST-segment and T-wave abnormalities. Pericardial effusion is common and may result in tamponade (112). Case reports have suggested that corticosteroids may be helpful, although withdrawal of the corticosteroids may lead to recurrence (112). However, randomized controlled trials of corticosteroids in RIHD have not been performed to confirm this benefit.

The other form of delayed onset pericardial disease is chronic, consisting of either chronic effusion or constrictive pericarditis. Risk of constrictive pericarditis ranges from 4% to 20% in different series and depends on the amount of radiation given and the method of administration (112,113). The risk of constriction appears to be increased in patients in whom delayed acute pericarditis develops, especially if an effusion is present, with as many as 20% of such patients eventually developing constriction (112). Furthermore, a majority of patients with constriction previously had pericardial effusions. Treatment is pericardiectomy, although patients with constrictive disease caused by radiation therapy tend to do worse after pericardiectomy than those with constriction from other causes, with one series reporting a 12% 30-day mortality for patients undergoing pericardiectomy for any reason, but a 21% mortality in those who had the procedure for radiation-induced constriction (115).

Radiation therapy only rarely causes injury to the myocardium itself, which is of clinical importance. Pathologically, myocardial fibrosis may occur (116). Clinical sequelae are usually mild or absent (109). However, subtle impairment of left ventricular function at rest and especially with exercise may be seen with radionuclide techniques or echocardiography (117). The right ventricle may also be abnormally dilated or have wall motion abnormalities (118). Most patients do not have overt congestive heart failure; however, a restrictive cardiomyopathy may be present and in the worst cases lead to actual heart failure (112). Restrictive cardiomyopathy and constrictive pericarditis may both be present and may result in less than expected improvement after pericardiectomy, and may account for the poorer prognosis of radiation-treated patients after pericardiectomy (119). Chemotherapeutic agents, particularly anthracyclines, may potentiate the myocardial damage caused by radiation therapy (120).

Valvular heart disease may occur secondary to radiation therapy, probably secondary to endocardial fibrosis, causing valvular thickening and deformity (116,121). In a series of 129 patients treated with radiation for Hodgkin's disease, examined 5 to 13 years after treatment, Lund and colleagues found that 24% had valvular regurgitation, with the aortic valve involved most often, the mitral valve less often, and no cases of right-sided valvular abnormalities (122). Right-sided valvular disease, however, has been reported after radiation therapy (117,123). Although echocardiographic abnormalities are relatively common, clinically significant valvular heart disease is rare, with only three deaths occurring from valvular disease out of 635 patients in one series (113).

The risk of coronary artery disease is increased after radiation therapy to the chest, as shown by an autopsy study (116) and several case reports of coronary artery disease in irradiated patients who were young and without other risk factors (124,125). Angiographic assessment of the coronary arteries in such patients reveals frequent high-degree ostial stenosis of the right coronary artery and left main involvement (126). Boivin and colleagues reported a relative risk of death from myocardial infarction after mediastinal irradiation but not after chemotherapy, based on analysis of 4,665 patients treated for Hodgkin's disease with a mean of 7 years of follow-up (127). Coronary artery disease tends to appear late after radiation therapy and can be treated with coronary artery bypass surgery if necessary. However, because the left internal mammary artery is exposed to radiation, it may be difficult to dissect and may have a tendency to occlude prematurely (128). ❦ g75

Finally, radiation therapy to the chest may lead to conduction system abnormalities, including bundle branch block, and varying degrees of atrioventricular block, including complete heart block (111,129). Radiation may also affect pacemaker function, and therefore patients with pacemakers undergoing therapy should be closely monitored (130,131).

Effects of Chemotherapy on the Heart

Multiple chemotherapeutic agents cause cardiac toxicity (Table 35B.1), but the most widely recognized are the anthracyclines (e.g., doxorubicin and daunorubicin) used in treating leukemias, lymphomas, and solid tumors, because their main dose-limiting side effect is cardiac toxicity. Clinical manifestations of anthracycline-induced cardiac toxicity may be acute or chronic (132). Acute toxicity (occurring during or just after a single dose) is rare. Transient nonspecific ECG abnormalities are the most common manifestation, but arrhythmias such as supraventricular tachyarrhythmia or increased ventricular ectopy may be seen (133). These rarely are of clinical importance. Rare cases of acute left ventricular failure, pericarditis, fatal myocarditis, and sudden death have been reported (134,135). Chronic anthracycline-induced cardiac toxicity is more common and usually appears within 1 year of exposure (120). However, it may also become apparent after a prolonged, sometimes several-year, asymptomatic latent period. This has been particularly apparent in childhood survivors of cancer who are cured of their malignancy and live for long periods of time after treatment (136). ❦ g76

Clinically, cardiotoxicity can result in deterioration of systolic and diastolic left ventricular function as determined either by radionuclide techniques or echocardiography, which progresses to overt congestive heart failure in some patients (132,140). When overt congestive heart failure occurs, risk of mortality may be substantial, with reported mortality in patients with congestive heart failure ranging

TABLE 35B.1 CHEMOTHERAPEUTIC AGENTS AFFECTING THE HEART

Anthracyclines (doxorubicin, daunorubicin, etc.)
  Electrocardiographic abnormalities
  Arrhythmia
  Cardiomyopathy
  Congestive heart failure
Mitoxantrone
  Cardiomyopathy
5-Fluorouracil
  Angina
  Myocardial infarction
  Arrhythmia
  Left ventricular dysfunction
Cyclophosphamide, ifosfamide
  Hemorrhagic myopericarditis
  Severe reversible left ventricular dysfunction
Cisplatin
  Angina
  Myocardial infarction
Etoposide
  Angina
  Myocardial infarction
Amsacrine
  Nonspecific electrocardiographic changes
  Arrhythmia
  Congestive heart failure
Paclitaxel
  Sinus bradycardia
  Atrioventricular block
  Possible ischemia
  Cardiomyopathy (in combination with anthracyclines)
Cytosine arabinoside
  Arrhythmia
  Congestive heart failure
  Pericarditis
Interferon
  Arrhythmia
  Angina
  Myocardial infarction
  Cardiomyopathy
Interleukin-2
  Capillary leak syndrome
  Arrhythmia
  Angina
  Myocardial infarction
  Cardiomyopathy
  Myocarditis
Trastuzumab
  Cardiomyopathy

from 2.2% (141) to 43.0% (120). Clinical recovery with conventional heart failure therapy may occur in those who survive (141), including rare cases of complete reversal of left ventricular dysfunction (142). Prolonged infusions of drug (143), or more frequent dosing (144), may decrease toxicity for a given dose.

Prevention of anthracycline-induced cardiac toxicity is accomplished by monitoring for signs of myocardial damage using radionuclide angiocardiography, echocardiography, or both (*e*Table 35B.1.1). Schwartz and colleagues proposed guidelines for monitoring the EF of patients receiving doxorubicin, which were retrospectively validated by showing a lower incidence of clinical congestive heart failure in patients whose management was consistent with the guidelines (141). According to these guidelines, EF is determined by radionuclide angiocardiography at baseline. If the baseline EF is normal, then the second study should be at a cumulative dose level of 250 to 300 mg per m². If risk factors are present, the study is repeated at 400 mg per m², otherwise at 450 mg per m², and before all subsequent doses thereafter. If EF declines more than 10% during treatment to an absolute value less than 50%, then treatment is stopped. If baseline EF is greater than 30% but less than 50%, studies should be obtained before each dose, and treatment should be discontinued for a decrease in EF greater than 10% or an absolute EF less than 30%. If the baseline EF is less than 30%, anthracycline therapy should not be used (141). ▼ g77

Pharmacologic agents have been investigated for use as cardioprotectants during anthracycline therapy. Currently, only dexrazoxane (ICRF-187), an iron-chelating agent that reduces free radicals produced by anthracyclines, has been approved in the United States for use during doxorubicin therapy (132,149). It is approved for use in metastatic breast cancer in patients who have received more than 300 mg per m² of doxorubicin. Probucol, calcium antagonists, and beta-blockers have also been proposed as cardioprotective agents, but more work must be done in human prospective studies to determine if they are truly efficacious (132,150).

Several other anticancer drugs have been associated with cardiac toxicity. There appears to be an increased risk of cardiomyopathy with doxorubicin when given in combination with paclitaxel (for metastatic breast cancer). Such adverse synergy does not appear to occur with doxorubicin and docetaxel. One possible explanation is that paclitaxel may interfere with the elimination of doxorubicin (151). Rhythm disturbances such as sinus bradycardia and atrioventricular block have also been seen with paclitaxel administration; however, ischemic manifestations seen during treatment largely occurred in patients with preexisting cardiac disease (152). Trastuzumab, a monoclonal antibody against the HER2 receptor, also used to treat metastatic breast cancer, has led to a high incidence of congestive heart failure (up to 28%) when used in combination with anthracyclines (153). The mechanism of cardiac toxicity with trastuzumab is uncertain, but it has been demonstrated that the HER2 receptor is involved in myocyte survival pathways. Cardiac complications with 5-fluorouracil have been reported with an incidence of 1.6% to 3.0% (154). Adverse effects have included angina, myocardial infarction, arrhythmia, and reversible left ventricular dysfunction (154). Cyclophosphamide, when given in high doses such as those used for pre–bone marrow transplant regimens, may cause a hemorrhagic myopericarditis characterized by left ventricular dysfunction, congestive heart fail-

ure, and pericardial effusion that is often fatal (155). In those who survive, left ventricular function appears to recover (155). The closely related drug ifosfamide has also been shown, in high doses, to cause severe, reversible myocardial dysfunction (156). Myocardial ischemia and myocardial infarction have been attributed to cisplatinum and etoposide (157). Amsacrine has been associated with cardiac abnormalities such as nonspecific ECG changes, atrial and ventricular arrhythmias, and congestive heart failure in approximately 1.2% of patients administered the drug (158). Finally, pre–bone marrow transplant regimens involving high doses of combination chemotherapy, including cyclophosphamide and cytosine arabinoside, plus total body irradiation, have been associated with a high incidence of cardiac complications including arrhythmia, congestive heart failure, and pericarditis (159). ▼ g78

CONTROVERSIES AND PERSONAL PERSPECTIVES

Anemia

Whether patients with heart disease and mild anemia derive significant benefit from treating the anemia deserves further study. We believe that nontransfusion therapy, such as iron and folate, should be given to increase cardiac reserve, both for patients with obstructive coronary artery disease and particularly for patients with heart failure, because such a strategy in these patients is supported by prospective intervention data (161). The use of erythropoietin is likely to be cost effective only in patients with at least moderate anemia and severe heart failure requiring frequent hospitalization.

Heparin-Induced Thrombocytopenia

Laboratory testing for HIT remains controversial, because none of the tests is perfectly accurate. We recommend that the platelet aggregation test be performed first, because it is available in most laboratories and can be performed quickly and easily. When HIT is suspected, all heparin should be stopped even if the test result is pending or negative, given the potential devastating consequences of continuing heparin in the face of ongoing HIT. For patients with a negative platelet aggregation test result and a clinically high likelihood of the disease, the ¹⁴C-serotonin release assay or enzyme-linked immunosorbent assay test should be performed to confirm the diagnosis.

Whether alternative anticoagulation should be given to patients with HIT in the absence of thromboembolic complications is considered by some an issue of controversy. We believe that these patients should receive a direct thrombin inhibitor in addition to discontinuation of heparin, because of ongoing thrombin generation imparting risk of developing serious events. This therapy may be discontinued once platelet count returns to baseline. Further therapy with warfarin should be strongly considered, because some patients may develop thrombotic complications even after the platelet count returns to normal. In the presence of an established thrombotic event, warfarin should be given in the absence of contraindications. Warfarin therapy should always initially overlap with direct thrombin inhibition by several days to avoid paradoxical limb gangrene. Clinicians should be aware that lepirudin increases the prothrombin time. Direct factor X assays could be used to monitor warfarin therapy while the patient remains on lepirudin.

Malignant Pericardial Effusion

The optimal invasive treatment for malignant pericardial effusion is not well defined. We recommend initial treatment in symptomatic patients with a percutaneous approach, including use of extended catheter drainage. Sclerotherapy should be tried next if pericardiocentesis fails or becomes frequently required. Surgery should be offered after failure of the first two approaches, depending on the overall status of the patient, and if the patient is willing to accept the perioperative risk.

Chemotherapy and Cardiac Toxicity

Areas for continuing investigation include optimizing methods for early detection and prevention of cardiac toxicity, such as cardioprotective agents or particular dosing strategies. Although use of the cardioprotective agent dexrazoxane has been controversial because of concerns that it may reduce antitumor activity, this has not been a consistent finding in trials of this agent. Therefore, we think it is reasonable to use dexrazoxane in patients receiving high doses of doxorubicin or with borderline left ventricular function before therapy.

REFERENCES

1. Weiskopf RB, Viele MK, Feiner J, et al. Human cardiovascular and metabolic response to acute, severe isovolemic anemia [published erratum appears in *JAMA* 1998;280:1404]. *JAMA* 1998;279:217–221.
2. Welch HG, Meehan KR, Goodnough LT. Prudent strategies for elective red blood cell transfusion. *Ann Intern Med* 1992;116:393–402.
3. Toy P, Feiner J, Viele MK, et al. Fatigue during acute isovolemic anemia in healthy, resting humans. *Transfusion* 2000;40:457–460.
4. Kapoor RK, Kumar A, Chandra M, et al. Cardiovascular responses to treadmill exercise testing in anemia. *Indian Pediatr* 1997;34:607–612.
5. Lakhotia M, Shah PK, Gupta A, et al. Clinical assessment of autonomic functions in anemics. *J Assoc Physicians India* 1996;44:534–536.
6. Anand IS, Chandrashekhar Y, Wander GS, et al. Endothelium-derived relaxing factor is important in mediating the high output state in chronic severe anemia. *J Am Coll Cardiol* 1995;25:1402–1407.
7. Ho CH. The effect of transfusion on cardiac function in patients with chronic anemia. *Transfusion* 1997;37:1066–1069.
8. Hebert PC, Wells G, Blajchman MA, et al. A multicenter, randomized, controlled clinical trial of transfusion requirements in critical care. Transfusion Requirements in Critical Care Investigators, Canadian Critical Care Trials Group. *N Engl J Med* 1999;340:409–417.
9. Nagao K, Tsuchihashi K, Ura N, et al. Appropriate hematocrit levels of erythropoietin supplementary therapy in end-stage renal failure complicated by coronary artery disease. *Can J Cardiol* 1997;13:747–753.
10. Silverberg DS, Wexler D, Blum M, et al. The use of subcutaneous erythropoietin and intravenous iron for the treatment of the anemia of severe, resistant congestive heart failure improves cardiac and renal function and functional cardiac class, and markedly reduces hospitalizations. *J Am Coll Cardiol* 2000;35:1737–1744.
11. Linde T, Wikstrom B, Andersson LG, et al. Renal anaemia treatment with recombinant human erythropoietin increases cardiac output in patients with ischaemic heart disease. *Scand J Urol Nephrol* 1996;30:115–120.
12. Foley RN, Parfrey PS, Harnett JD, et al. The impact of anemia on cardiomyopathy, morbidity, and mortality in end-stage renal disease. *Am J Kidney Dis* 1996;28:53–61.
13. Wizemann V, Schafer R, Kramer W. Follow-up of cardiac changes induced by anemia compensation in normotensive hemodialysis patients with left-ventricular hypertrophy. *Nephron* 1993;64:202–206.

14. Conlon PJ, Kovalik E, Schumm D, et al. Normalization of hematocrit in hemodialysis patients does not affect silent ischemia. *Renal Fail* 2000;22:205–211.

15. Jessup M, Manno CS. Diagnosis and management of iron-induced heart disease in Cooley's anemia. *Ann N Y Acad Sci* 1998;850:242–250.

16. Vecchio C, Derchi G. Management of cardiac complications in patients with thalassemia major. *Semin Hematol* 1995;32:288–296.

17. Wacker P, Halperin DS, Balmer-Ruedin D, et al. Regression of cardiac insufficiency after ambulatory intravenous deferoxamine in thalassemia major. *Chest* 1993;103:1276–1278.

18. Olivieri NF, Nathan DG, MacMillan JH, et al. Survival in medically treated patients with homozygous beta-thalassemia. *N Engl J Med* 1994;331:574–578.

19. Lucarelli G, Galimberti M, Polchi P, et al. Marrow transplantation in patients with thalassemia responsive to iron chelation therapy. *N Engl J Med* 1993;329:840–844.

20. Lewis JF, Maron BJ, Castro O, et al. Left ventricular diastolic filling abnormalities identified by Doppler echocardiography in asymptomatic patients with sickle cell anemia. *J Am Coll Cardiol* 1991;17:1473–1478.

21. Martins W, Mesquita ET, Cunha DM, et al. Doppler echocardiographic study in adolescents and young adults with sickle cell anemia. *Arq Bras Cardiol* 1999;73:463–474.

22. Covitz W, Espeland M, Gallagher D, et al. The heart in sickle cell anemia. The Cooperative Study of Sickle Cell Disease (CSSCD). *Chest* 1995;108:1214–1219.

23. Covitz W, Eubig C, Balfour IC, et al. Exercise-induced cardiac dysfunction in sickle cell anemia. A radionuclide study. *Am J Cardiol* 1983;51:570–575.

24. Simmons BE, Santhanam V, Castaner A, et al. Sickle cell heart disease. Two-dimensional echo and Doppler ultrasonographic findings in the hearts of adult patients with sickle cell anemia. *Arch Intern Med* 1988;148:1526–1528.

25. Uzsoy N. Cardiovascular findings in patients with sickle cell anemia. *Am J Cardiol* 1964;13:320–328.

26. Val-Mejias J, Lee WK, Weisse AB, et al. Left ventricular performance during and after sickle cell crisis. *Am Heart J* 1979;97:585–591.

27. Martin CR, Johnson CS, Cobb C, et al. Myocardial infarction in sickle cell disease. *JAMA* 1996;88:428–432.

28. Vichinsky EP, Neumayr LD, Earles AN, et al. Causes and outcomes of the acute chest syndrome in sickle cell disease. National Acute Chest Syndrome Study Groups. *N Engl J Med* 2000;342:1855–1865.

29. Hammermeister KE, Sethi GK, Henderson WG, et al. A comparison of outcomes in men 11 years after heart-valve replacement with a mechanical valve or bioprosthesis. Veterans Affairs Cooperative Study on Valvular Heart Disease. *N Engl J Med* 1993;328:1289–1296.

30. Skoularigis J, Essop MR, Skudicky D, et al. Frequency and severity of intravascular hemolysis after left-sided cardiac valve replacement with Medtronic Hall and St. Jude Medical prostheses, and influence of prosthetic type, position, size and number. *Am J Cardiol* 1993;71:587–591.

31. Enzenauer RJ, Berenberg JL, Cassell PF Jr. Microangiopathic hemolytic anemia as the initial manifestation of porcine valve failure. *South Med J* 1990;83:912–917.

32. Brown MR, Hasaniya NW, Dang CR. Hemolytic anemia secondary to a porcine mitral prosthetic valve leaflet dissection. *Ann Thorac Surg* 1995;59:1573–1574.

33. Dhasmana JP, Blackstone EH, Kirklin JW, et al. Factors associated with periprosthetic leakage following primary mitral valve replacement: with special consideration of the suture technique. *Ann Thorac Surg* 1983;35:170–178.

34. Okita Y, Miki S, Kusuhara K, et al. Propranolol for intractable hemolysis after open heart operation. *Ann Thorac Surg* 1991;52:1158–1160.

35. Myhre E, Rasmussen K, Andersen A. Serum lactic dehydrogenase activity in patients with prosthetic heart valves: a parameter of intravascular hemolysis. *Am Heart J* 1970;80:463–468.

36. Schwarcz TH, Hogan LA, Endean ED, et al. Thromboembolic complications of polycythemia: polycythemia vera versus smokers' polycythemia. *J Vasc Surg* 1993;17:518–522.

37. Segura T, Serena J, Teruel J, et al. Cerebral embolism in a patient with polycythemia rubra vera. *Eur J Neurol* 2000;7:87–90.

38. Josephson GD, Tiefenbrun J, Harvey J. Thrombosis of the descending thoracic aorta: a case report. *Surgery* 1993;114:598–600.

39. Reisner SA, Rinkevich D, Markiewicz W, et al. Cardiac involvement in patients with myeloproliferative disorders. *Am J Med* 1992;93:498–504.

40. Willoughby S, Pearson TC. The use of aspirin in polycythaemia vera and primary thrombocythaemia. *Blood Rev* 1998;12:12–22.

41. Shah DM, Powers SR Jr, Bernard HR, et al. Increased oxygen uptake following phlebotomy and simultaneous fluid replacement in polycythemic patients. *Surgery* 1980;88:686–692.

42. Kaplan ME, Mack K, Goldberg JD, et al. Long-term management of polycythemia vera with hydroxyurea: a progress report. *Semin Hematol* 1986;23:167–171.

43. Sacchi S. The role of alpha-interferon in essential thrombocythaemia, polycythaemia vera and myelofibrosis with myeloid metaplasia (MMM): a concise update. *Leuk Lymphoma* 1995;19:13–20.

44. Ambrus JL, Ambrus CM, Dembinsky, W, et al. Thromboembolic disease susceptibility related to red cell membrane fluidity in patients with polycythemia vera and effect of phlebotomies. *J Med* 1999;30:299–304.

45. Weisse AB, Moschos CB, Frank MJ, et al. Hemodynamic effects of staged hematocrit reduction in patients with stable cor pulmonale and severely elevated hematocrit levels. *Am J Med* 1975;58:92–98.

46. Tefferi A, Hoagland HC. Issues in the diagnosis and management of essential thrombocythemia. *Mayo Clin Proc* 1994;69:651–655.

47. Fenaux P, Simon M, Caulier MT, et al. Clinical course of essential thrombocythemia in 147 cases. *Cancer* 1990;66:549–556.

48. McIntyre KJ, Hoagland HC, Silverstein MN, et al. Essential thrombocythemia in young adults. *Mayo Clin Proc* 1991;66:149–154.

49. Wehmeier A, Sudhoff T, Meierkord F. Relation of platelet abnormalities to thrombosis and hemorrhage in chronic

myeloproliferative disorders. *Semin Thromb Hemost* 1997;23:391–402.

50. Gavras I, Graff LG, Rose BD, et al. Fatal pancytopenia associated with the use of captopril. *Ann Intern Med* 1981;94:58–59.

51. Lundh B, Hasselgren KH. Hematological side effects from antihypertensive drugs. *Acta Med Scand Suppl* 1979;628:73–75.

52. Hackett T, Kelton JG, Powers P. Drug-induced platelet destruction. *Semin Thromb Hemost* 1982;8:116–137.

53. Nawabi IU, Ritz ND. Agranulocytosis due to propranolol. *JAMA* 1973;223:1376–1377.

54. Volosin K, Greenberg RM, Greenspon AJ. Tocainide associated agranulocytosis. *Am Heart J* 1985;109:1392–1393.

55. Bennett CL, Davidson CJ, Raisch DW, et al. Thrombotic thrombocytopenic purpura associated with ticlopidine in the setting of coronary artery stents and stroke prevention. *Arch Intern Med* 1999;159:2524–2528.

56. Love BB, Biller J, Gent M. Adverse haematological effects of ticlopidine. Prevention, recognition and management. *Drug Saf* 1998;19:89–98.

57. Bennett CL, Connors JM, Carwile JM, et al. Thrombotic thrombocytopenic purpura associated with clopidogrel. *N Engl J Med* 2000;342:1773–1777.

58. Warkentin TE, Levine MN, Hirsh J, et al. Heparin-induced thrombocytopenia in patients treated with low-molecular-weight heparin or unfractionated heparin. *N Engl J Med* 1995;332:1330–1335.

59. Brieger DB, Mak KH, Kottke-Marchant K, et al. Heparin-induced thrombocytopenia. *J Am Coll Cardiol* 1998;31:1449–1459.

60. Chong BH, Eisbacher M. Pathophysiology and laboratory testing of heparin-induced thrombocytopenia. *Semin Hematol* 1998;35[Suppl 5]:3–8.

61. Warkentin TE, Hayward CP, Boshkov LK, et al. Sera from patients with heparin-induced thrombocytopenia generate platelet-derived microparticles with procoagulant activity: an explanation for the thrombotic complications of heparin-induced thrombocytopenia. *Blood* 1994;84:3691–3699.

62. Denomme GA, Warkentin TE, Horsewood P, et al. Activation of platelets by sera containing IgG1 heparin-dependent antibodies: an explanation for the predominance of the Fc gamma RIIa "low responder" (his131) gene in patients with heparin-induced thrombocytopenia . *J Lab Clin Med* 1997;130:278–284.

63. Laster J, Cikrit D, Walker N, et al. The heparin-induced thrombocytopenia syndrome: an update. *Surgery* 1987;102:763–770.

64. Warkentin TE. Clinical presentation of heparin-induced thrombocytopenia. *Semin Hematol* 1998;35[Suppl 5]:9–16.

65. Warkentin TE, Kelton JG. A 14-year study of heparin-induced thrombocytopenia. *Am J Med* 1996;101:502–507.

66. Greinacher A, Janssens U, Berg G, et al. Lepirudin (recombinant hirudin) for parenteral anticoagulation in patients with heparin-induced thrombocytopenia. Heparin-Associated Thrombocytopenia Study (HAT) investigators. *Circulation* 1999;100:587–593.

67. Sheridan D, Carter C, Kelton JG. A diagnostic test for heparin-induced thrombocytopenia. *Blood* 1986;67:27–30.

68. Olinger GN, Hussey CV, Olive JA, et al. Cardiopulmonary bypass for patients with previously documented heparin-induced platelet aggregation. *J Thorac Cardiovasc Surg* 1984;87:673–677.

69. Greinacher A, Volpel H, Janssens U, et al. Recombinant hirudin (lepirudin) provides safe and effective anticoagulation in patients with heparin-induced thrombocytopenia: a prospective study. *Circulation* 1999;99:73–80.

70. Abraham KP, Reddy V, Gattuso P. Neoplasms metastatic to the heart: review of 3314 consecutive autopsies. *Am J Cardiovasc Pathol* 1990;3:195–198.

71. Fine G. *In:* Gould S, ed. *Neoplasms of the pericardium and heart.* 3rd ed. New York: Charles C. Thomas, 1968:875.

72. MacGee W. Metastatic and invasive tumours involving the heart in a geriatric population: a necropsy study. *Virchows Arch A Pathol Anat Histopathol* 1991;419:183–189.

73. Schoen FJ, Berger BM, Guerina NG. Cardiac effects of noncardiac neoplasms. *Cardiol Clin* 1984;2:657–670.

74. Flipse TR, Tazelaar HD, Holmes DR Jr. Diagnosis of malignant cardiac disease by endomyocardial biopsy. *Mayo Clin Proc* 1990;65:1415–1422.

75. Koiwaya Y, Nakamura M, Yamamoto K. Progressive ECG alterations in metastatic cardiac mural tumor. *Am Heart J* 1983;105:339–341.

76. Gouldesbrough DR, Carder PJ. Rapidly progressive cardiac failure due to lymphomatous infiltration of the myocardium. *Postgrad Med J* 1989;65:668–670.

77. Tamura A, Matsubara O, Yoshimura N, et al. Cardiac metastasis of lung cancer. A study of metastatic pathways and clinical manifestations. *Cancer* 1992;70:437–442.

78. Ciro A, Vincenti A, Bozzano A, et al. Cardiac involvement by non-Hodgkin's lymphoma: an unusual presentation of heart conduction disturbances. *Pacing Clin Electrophysiol* 1994;17:1561–1564.

79. Ravikumar TS, Topulos GP, Anderson RW, et al. Surgical resection for isolated cardiac metastases. *Arch Surg* 1983;118:117–120.

80. Isner JM, Carter BL, Bankoff MS, et al. Computed tomography in the diagnosis of pericardial heart disease. *Ann Intern Med* 1982;97:473–479.

81. Tsang TS, Seward JB, Barnes ME, et al. Outcomes of primary and secondary treatment of pericardial effusion in patients with malignancy. *Mayo Clin Proc* 2000;75:248–253.

82. Laham RJ, Cohen DJ, Kuntz RE, et al. Pericardial effusion in patients with cancer: outcome with contemporary management strategies. *Heart* 1996;75:67–71.

83. Shepherd FA, Morgan C, Evans WK, et al. Medical management of malignant pericardial effusion by tetracycline sclerosis. *Am J Cardiol* 1987;60:1161–1166.

84. Shepherd FA, Ginsberg JS, Evans WK, et al. Tetracycline sclerosis in the management of malignant pericardial effusion. *J Clin Oncol* 1985;3:1678–1682.

85. Buck M, Ingle JN, Giuliani ER, et al. Pericardial effusion in women with breast cancer. *Cancer* 1987;60:263–269.

86. Park JS, Rentschler R, Wilbur D. Surgical management of pericardial effusion in patients with malignancies. Com-

parison of subxiphoid window versus pericardiectomy. *Cancer* 1991;67:76–80.

87. Miller JI, Mansour KA, Hatcher CR Jr. Pericardiectomy: current indications, concepts, and results in a university center. *Ann Thorac Surg* 1982;34:40–45.

88. Mack MJ, Landreneau RJ, Hazelrigg SR, et al. Video thoracoscopic management of benign and malignant pericardial effusions. *Chest* 1993;103[Suppl]:390S–393S.

89. Ziskind AA, Pearce AC, Lemmon CC, et al. Percutaneous balloon pericardiotomy for the treatment of cardiac tamponade and large pericardial effusions: description of technique and report of the first 50 cases. *J Am Coll Cardiol* 1993;21:1–5.

90. Perez CA, Presant CA, Van Amburg ALD. Management of superior vena cava syndrome. *Semin Oncol* 1978;5:123–134.

91. Hochrein J, Bashore TM, O'Laughlin MP, et al. Percutaneous stenting of superior vena cava syndrome: a case report and review of the literature. *Am J Med* 1998;104:78–84.

92. Kane RD, Hawkins HK, Miller JA, et al. Microscopic pulmonary tumor emboli associated with dyspnea. *Cancer* 1975;36:1473–1482.

93. Chino F, Kodama A, Otake M, et al. Nonbacterial thrombotic endocarditis in a Japanese autopsy sample. A review of eighty cases. *Am Heart J* 1975;90:190–198.

94. Lange HW, Galliani CA, Edwards JE. Local complications associated with indwelling Swan-Ganz catheters: autopsy study of 36 cases. *Am J Cardiol* 1983;52:1108–1111.

95. Rosen P, Armstrong D. Nonbacterial thrombotic endocarditis in patients with malignant neoplastic diseases. *Am J Med* 1973;54:23–29.

96. Blanchard DG, Ross RS, Dittrich HC. Nonbacterial thrombotic endocarditis. Assessment by transesophageal echocardiography. *Chest* 1992;102:954–956.

97. Landsberg L, Young J. Pheochromocytoma. In: Wilson A, ed. *Harrison's principles of internal medicine.* 12th ed. New York: McGraw-Hill, 1991:1736.

98. Van Vliet PD, Burchell HB, Titus JL. Focal myocarditis associated with pheochromocytoma. *N Engl J Med* 1966;274:1102–1108.

99. Suga K, Tsukamoto K, Nishigauchi K, et al. Iodine-123-MIBG imaging in pheochromocytoma with cardiomyopathy and pulmonary edema. *J Nucl Med* 1996;37:1361–1364.

100. Ram CV. Pheochromocytoma. *Cardiol Clin* 1988;6:517–535.

101. Ferrans VJ, Roberts WC. The carcinoid endocardial plaque; an ultrastructural study. *Hum Pathol* 1976;7:387–409.

102. Connolly HM, Nishimura RA, Smith HC, et al. Outcome of cardiac surgery for carcinoid heart disease. *J Am Coll Cardiol* 1995;25:410–416.

103. Robiolio PA, Rigolin VH, Harrison JK, et al. Predictors of outcome of tricuspid valve replacement in carcinoid heart disease. *Am J Cardiol* 1995;75:485–488.

104. Robiolio PA, Rigolin VH, Wilson JS, et al. Carcinoid heart disease. Correlation of high serotonin levels with valvular abnormalities detected by cardiac catheterization and echocardiography. *Circulation* 1995;92:790–795.

105. Denney WD, Kemp WE Jr, Anthony LB, et al. Echocardiographic and biochemical evaluation of the development and progression of carcinoid heart disease. *J Am Coll Cardiol* 1998;32:1017–1022.

106. Kyle RA, Greipp PR. Amyloidosis (AL). Clinical and laboratory features in 229 cases. *Mayo Clin Proc* 1983;58:665–683.

107. Celletti F, Fattori R, Napoli G, et al. Assessment of restrictive cardiomyopathy of amyloid or idiopathic etiology by magnetic resonance imaging. *Am J Cardiol* 1999;83:798–801.

108. McCarthy RE 3rd, Kasper EK. A review of the amyloidoses that infiltrate the heart. *Clin Cardiol* 1998;21:547–552.

109. Arsenian MA. Cardiovascular sequelae of therapeutic thoracic radiation. *Prog Cardiovasc Dis* 1991;33:299–311.

110. Stewart JR, Fajardo LF, Gillette SM, et al. Radiation injury to the heart. *Int J Radiat Oncol Biol Phys* 1995;31:1205–1211.

111. Benoff LJ, Schweitzer P. Radiation therapy-induced cardiac injury. *Am Heart J* 1995;129:1193–1196.

112. Stewart JR, Fajardo LF. Radiation-induced heart disease: an update. *Prog Cardiovasc Dis* 1984;27:173–194.

113. Hancock SL, Donaldson SS, Hoppe RT. Cardiac disease following treatment of Hodgkin's disease in children and adolescents. *J Clin Oncol* 1993;11:1208–1215.

114. Martin RG, Ruckdeschel JC, Chang P, et al. Radiation-related pericarditis. *Am J Cardiol* 1975;35:216–220.

115. Cameron J, Oesterle SN, Baldwin JC, et al. The etiologic spectrum of constrictive pericarditis. *Am Heart J* 1987;113:354–360.

116. Brosius FCD, Waller BF, Roberts WC. Radiation heart disease. Analysis of 16 young (aged 15 to 33 years) necropsy patients who received over 3,500 rads to the heart. *Am J Med* 1981;70:519–530.

117. Pohjola-Sintonen S, Totterman KJ, Salmo M, et al. Late cardiac effects of mediastinal radiotherapy in patients with Hodgkin's disease. *Cancer* 1987;60:31–37.

118. Perrault DJ, Levy M, Herman JD, et al. Echocardiographic abnormalities following cardiac radiation. *J Clin Oncol* 1985;3:546–551.

119. Seifert FC, Miller DC, Oesterle SN, et al. Surgical treatment of constrictive pericarditis: analysis of outcome and diagnostic error. *Circulation* 1985;72:II264–II273.

120. Von Hoff DD, Layard MW, Basa P, et al. Risk factors for doxorubicin-induced congestive heart failure. *Ann Intern Med* 1979;91:710–717.

121. Warda M, Khan A, Massumi A, et al. Radiation-induced valvular dysfunction. *J Am Coll Cardiol* 1983;2:180–185.

122. Lund MB, Ihlen H, Voss BM, et al. Increased risk of heart valve regurgitation after mediastinal radiation for Hodgkin's disease: an echocardiographic study. *Heart* 1996;75:591–595.

123. Raviprasad GS, Salem BI, Gowda S, et al. Radiation-induced mitral and tricuspid regurgitation with severe ostial coronary artery disease: a case report with successful surgical treatment. *Cathet Cardiovasc Diagn* 1995;35:146–148.

124. Huff H, Sanders EM. Coronary-artery occlusion after radiation. *N Engl J Med* 1972;286:780.

125. Dunsmore LD, LoPonte MA, Dunsmore RA. Radiation-induced coronary artery disease. *J Am Coll Cardiol* 1986;8:239–244.

126. Orzan F, Brusca A, Conte MR, et al. Severe coronary artery disease after radiation therapy of the chest and mediastinum: clinical presentation and treatment. *Br Heart J* 1993;69:496–500.

127. Boivin JF, Hutchison GB, Lubin JH, et al. Coronary artery disease mortality in patients treated for Hodgkin's disease. *Cancer* 1992;69:1241–1247.

128. Schulman HE, Korr KS, Myers TJ. Left internal thoracic artery graft occlusion following mediastinal radiation therapy. *Chest* 1994;105:1881–1882.

129. Kereiakes DJ, Morady F, Ports TA. High-degree atrioventricular block after radiation therapy. *Am J Cardiol* 1983;51:1233–1234.

130. Katzenberg CA, Marcus FI, Heusinkveld RS, et al. Pacemaker failure due to radiation therapy. *Pacing Clin Electrophysiol* 1982;5:156–159.

131. Souliman SK, Christie, J. Pacemaker failure induced by radiotherapy. *Pacing Clin Electrophysiol* 1994;17:270–273.

132. Shan K, Lincoff AM, Young JB. Anthracycline-induced cardiotoxicity. *Ann Intern Med* 1996;125:47–58.

133. Steinberg JS, Cohen AJ, Wasserman AG, et al. Acute arrhythmogenicity of doxorubicin administration. *Cancer* 1987;60:1213–1218.

134. Bristow MR, Billingham ME, Mason JW, et al. Clinical spectrum of anthracycline antibiotic cardiotoxicity. *Cancer Treat Rep* 1978;62:873–879.

135. Wortman JE, Lucas VS Jr, Schuster E, et al. Sudden death during doxorubicin administration. *Cancer* 1979;44:1588–1591.

136. Lipshultz SE, Colan SD, Gelber RD, et al. Late cardiac effects of doxorubicin therapy for acute lymphoblastic leukemia in childhood. *N Engl J Med* 1991;324:808–815.

137. Kusuoka H, Futaki S, Koretsune Y, et al. Alterations of intracellular calcium homeostasis and myocardial energetics in acute Adriamycin-induced heart failure. *J Cardiovasc Pharmacol* 1991;18:437–444.

138. Rajagopalan S, Politi PM, Sinha BK, et al. Adriamycin-induced free radical formation in the perfused rat heart: implications for cardiotoxicity. *Cancer Res* 1988;48:4766–4769.

139. Singal PK, Iliskovic N. Doxorubicin-induced cardiomyopathy. *N Engl J Med* 1998;339:900–905.

140. Cottin Y, Touzery C, Coudert B, et al. Impairment of diastolic function during short-term anthracycline chemotherapy. *Br Heart J* 1995;73:61–64.

141. Schwartz RG, McKenzie WB, Alexander J, et al. Congestive heart failure and left ventricular dysfunction complicating doxorubicin therapy. Seven-year experience using serial radionuclide angiocardiography. *Am J Med* 1987;82:1109–1118.

142. Cohen M, Kronzon I, Lebowitz A. Reversible doxorubicin-induced congestive heart failure. *Arch Intern Med* 1982;142:1570–1571.

143. Shapira J, Gotfried M, Lishner M, et al. Reduced cardiotoxicity of doxorubicin by a 6-hour infusion regimen. A prospective randomized evaluation. *Cancer* 1990;65:870–873.

144. Anders RJ, Shanes JG, Zeller FP. Lower incidence of doxorubicin-induced cardiomyopathy by once-a-week low-dose administration. *Am Heart J* 1986;111:755–759.

145. Hashimoto I, Ichida F, Miura M, et al. Automatic border detection identifies subclinical anthracycline cardiotoxicity in children with malignancy. *Circulation* 1999;99:2367–2370.

146. Schmitt K, Tulzer G, Merl M, et al. Early detection of doxorubicin and daunorubicin cardiotoxicity by echocardiography: diastolic versus systolic parameters. *Eur J Pediatr* 1995;154:201–204.

147. Carrio I, Estorch M, Berna L, et al. Indium-111-antimyosin and iodine-123-MIBG studies in early assessment of doxorubicin cardiotoxicity. *J Nucl Med* 1995;36:2044–2049.

148. Cardinale D, Sandri MT, Martinoni A, et al. Left ventricular dysfunction predicted by early troponin I release after high-dose chemotherapy. *J Am Coll Cardiol* 2000;36:517–522.

149. Speyer JL, Green MD, Kramer E, et al. Protective effect of the bispiperazinedione ICRF-187 against doxorubicin-induced cardiac toxicity in women with advanced breast cancer. *N Engl J Med* 1988;319:745–752.

150. Siveski-Iliskovic N, Hill M, Chow DA, et al. Probucol protects against Adriamycin cardiomyopathy without interfering with its antitumor effect. *Circulation* 1995;91:10–15.

151. Sparano JA. Doxorubicin/taxane combinations: cardiac toxicity and pharmacokinetics. *Semin Oncol* 1999;26[Suppl 9]:14–19.

152. Rowinsky EK, Eisenhauer EA, Chaudhry V, et al. Clinical toxicities encountered with paclitaxel (Taxol). *Semin Oncol* 1993;20[Suppl 3]:1–15.

153. Feldman AM, Lorell BH, Reis SE. Trastuzumab in the treatment of metastatic breast cancer: anticancer therapy versus cardiotoxicity. *Circulation* 2000;102:272–274.

154. Schober C, Papageorgiou E, Harstrick A, et al. Cardiotoxicity of 5-fluorouracil in combination with folinic acid in patients with gastrointestinal cancer. *Cancer* 1993;72:2242–2247.

155. Gottdiener JS, Appelbaum FR, Ferrans VJ, et al. Cardiotoxicity associated with high-dose cyclophosphamide therapy. *Arch Intern Med* 1981;141:758–763.

156. Quezado ZM, Wilson WH, Cunnion RE, et al. High-dose ifosfamide is associated with severe, reversible cardiac dysfunction. *Ann Intern Med* 1993;118:31–36.

157. Airey CL, Dodwell DJ, Joffe JK, et al. Etoposide-related myocardial infarction. *Clin Oncol* 1995;7:135.

158. Weiss RB, Grillo-Lopez AJ, Marsoni S, et al. Amsacrine-associated cardiotoxicity: an analysis of 82 cases. *J Clin Oncol* 1986;4:918–928.

159. Trigg ME, Finlay JL, Bozdech M, et al. Fatal cardiac toxicity in bone marrow transplant patients receiving cytosine arabinoside, cyclophosphamide, and total body irradiation. *Cancer* 1987;59:38–42.

160. Sonnenblick M, Rosin A. Cardiotoxicity of interferon. A review of 44 cases. *Chest* 1991;99:557–561.

161. Schechter D, Nagler A. Recombinant interleukin-2 and recombinant interferon alpha immunotherapy cardiovascular toxicity. *Am Heart J* 1992;123:1736–1739.

THE HEART AND OTHER ORGAN SYSTEMS

The Heart and the Renal System

LYNDA ANNE SZCZECH
DEREK P. CHEW
JOSEPH A. COLADONATO
DONAL N. REDDAN

▼ ADDITIONAL ELECTRONIC TOPICS

Hyperparathyroidism g79;   Vitamin D g80;   Calcium and Phosphorus g81;   Uremic Pericarditis g82;   Exercise Electrocardiography g83;   Dobutamine Stress Electrocardiography g84;   Outcomes g85;   Renal Replacement Therapy in a Patient with Cardiac Disease g86;   Hemodialysis g87;   Hemodynamic Concerns g88;   Dysrhythmias g89;   Ischemia and High Output Cardiac Failure g90;   Peritoneal Dialysis g91;   Transplantation g92

OVERVIEW

Patients with renal impairment experience a disproportionate burden of cardiovascular morbidity and mortality, largely the result of accelerated atherogenesis, a hallmark characteristic of significant renal dysfunction (1–3). The

L. A. Szczech: Department of Medicine, Duke University Medical Center, Durham, North Carolina

D. P. Chew: Department of Cardiovascular Medicine, The Cleveland Clinic Foundation, Cleveland, Ohio

J. A. Coladonato: Department of Nephrology, Duke University Medical Center, Durham, North Carolina

D. N. Reddan: Department of Medicine/Nephrology, Duke University Medical Center, Durham, North Carolina

increased risk associated with renal impairment has a pervasive influence on outcomes across all aspects of cardiac disease including acute coronary syndromes, cardiac failure, coronary revascularization, and valvular heart disease. Furthermore, renal insufficiency is associated with adverse outcomes, with the magnitude of risk positively correlated with the degree of renal impairment (1,4). Consequently, among patients with end-stage renal disease (ESRD), cardiac mortality accounts for approximately one-half of all deaths, and of these, more than 50% occur as a result of acute myocardial infarction, with an incidence three to five times higher than the general population (5,6). Salient data from the 34,189 patient U.S. registry of long-term dialysis demonstrate that myocardial infarction was associated with a 59% 1-year, 73% 2-year, and 90% 5-year mortality (7). Further contributing to symptomatic myocardial ischemia is small vessel disease, reduced capillary density, volume overload, and altered myocyte bioenergetics. Hence, up to 27% of patients have myocardial ischemia without obstructive coronary artery disease. A greater prevalence and consequence of traditional coronary risk factors such as diabetes, lipid abnormalities, and hypertension underlie this increased risk (8–12). These risk factors are often coexistent and therefore synergistic in their potentiation of atherosclerosis in addition to their effect on renal dysfunction (2). Whether dialytic therapy directly contributes to the increased risk of coronary artery disease remains contentious (13).

Renal dysfunction contributes to perturbation in all components of vascular integrity, culminating in both an elevated bleeding risk and a thromboinflammatory state (14,15). Uremia is associated with chronic endothelial injury with increased tissue plasminogen activator and von Willebrand's factor release (16,17); elevated plasma levels of F1+2, thrombin–antithrombin complex, fibrinopeptide A, and D-dimer, implicating increased thrombin generation (18); and heightened factor VII coagulant activity that correlates with the increased cholesterol levels, triglyceride levels, and thrombin generation (17). Finally, chronic renal failure (CRF) is associated with a proinflammatory state, evidenced by elevated interleukin-1, tumor necrosis factor, and fibrinogen levels; monocyte activation; and increased tissue factor and metalloprotease expression (19,20). As a clinical marker of this inflammatory process, elevated C-reactive protein among end-stage renal patients is associated with up to a 5.5-fold risk of coronary artery disease and 4.5-fold risk of cardiovascular death (21).

Left ventricular (LV) hypertrophy and cardiac failure are also more prevalent among patients with significant renal impairment and are observed in approximately 35% to 40% of the renal dialysis population (9,22,23). Reports observe an increasing prevalence of cardiac failure among hemodialysis patients, corresponding to a similar increase in the prevalence of coronary artery disease (24). High-output states associated with arteriovenous fistulas, salt and water overload, and anemia further contribute to ventricular overload and LV hypertrophy, whereas chronic ischemia and increased myocardial oxygen demand, hyperparathyroidism, uremia, and malnutrition augment cardiomyocyte loss, fibrosis, and systolic dysfunction (25–29).

This chapter focuses on the effect of the numerous metabolic derangements associated with chronic renal insufficiency and ESRD including secondary hyperparathyroidism; vitamin D deficiency; and phosphorus, calcium, and lipid abnormalities. These disturbances may be causal in changes of cardiac structure and function responsible for the high cardiovascular morbidity and mortality within this population. Given the biochemical uniqueness of these patients, the diagnosis and treatment of cardiac disease among

patients with renal insufficiency present issues of interpretation and management. These issues, along with a description of the cardiovascular effects of renal replacement therapies, are also discussed.

METABOLIC CHANGES ASSOCIATED WITH CHRONIC RENAL FAILURE

Lipid Abnormalities

Abnormal lipid metabolism is common among patients with CRF (49) and contributes to the increase in cardiovascular events. These abnormalities are most prominent in the nephrotic syndrome in which marked elevations in the plasma levels of cholesterol, triglycerides, and lipoprotein(a) are common.

The two most common lipid abnormalities in the nephrotic syndrome are hypercholesterolemia and hypertriglyceridemia (50), possibly the result of increased hepatic synthesis of lipoproteins containing apolipoprotein B and cholesterol in response to the reduced plasma oncotic pressure (50,51). The severity of the hyperlipidemia is inversely related to the decrease in oncotic pressure (51), and albumin or dextran administration produces a rapid reduction in lipid levels (52). Alternate evidence suggests that reduced catabolism is primarily responsible for hypercholesterolemia among patients with the nephrotic syndrome (53) and is also a cause of the elevated triglyceride levels (49,50). The delipidation cascade in which very-low-density lipoproteins are converted to intermediate-density lipoproteins and then to low-density lipoproteins (LDL) by lipoprotein lipases is slowed in the nephrotic syndrome and with a trend toward reduced LDL receptor–mediated clearance of LDL and intermediate-density lipoproteins (54).

In concert with renal impairment, hyperlipidemia is a potent risk factor for cardiovascular disease (49,55). Compared with age-matched controls, a relative risk of 5.5 for death from coronary artery disease, 5.2 for myocardial infarction, and 2.8 for coronary death has been reported for nondiabetic nephrotic patients (56). The lipid abnormalities induced by the nephrotic syndrome reverse with resolution of the disease. The optimal treatment of patients with long-standing persistent nephrotic syndrome is uncertain because randomized trials have not been performed (49,50). The most successful lipid-lowering agents have been the 3-hydroxy-3-methylglutaryl coenzyme A reductase inhibitors and the bile acid sequestrants (49,50,57). Treatment with these agents should also extend to renal insufficiency patients with hyperlipidemia in the absence of nephrotic syndrome. Angiotensin-converting enzyme (ACE) inhibitors are another potential adjunctive therapy for hyperlipidemia since they lower 24-hour urine protein excretion (58,59) and are associated with a 10% to 20% decline in the plasma levels of total and LDL cholesterol and lipoprotein(a) (60). Similar findings have been shown with losartan, an angiotensin II receptor antagonist (61).

Hyperhomocystinemia

Homocysteine levels have been shown to be elevated two- to fourfold among patients with CRF (62–65). Moderate hyperhomocystinemia is a recognized independent risk factor for coronary artery disease and is a strong predictor of mortality among patients with established coronary artery disease (66–70). From prospective observational data, hyperhomocystinemia remains an independent risk factor for cardiovascular morbidity and mortality among the ESRD population, conferring a relative risk of 1% per μmol per L increase in total homocysteine concentration or a relative risk ratio of 1.5 for levels greater than 5 μmol per L (2,71).

Homocysteine metabolism is dependent on vitamin B_6, vitamin B_{12}, and folic acid. In renal failure, poor nutrition coupled with removal of water-soluble vitamins by dialysis may partially explain a tendency to deficiencies of these vitamins and the high prevalence of hyperhomocystinemia. In non-ESRD populations, treatment with folic acid alone or in combination with vitamins B_{12} and B_6 has been shown to lower homocysteine levels. Low doses of folic acid have been shown to lower homocysteine levels in non-ESRD patients; however, the effects have not been as pronounced in ESRD patients (72,73). To date, no prospective studies have reported the effect of lowering homocysteine levels on cardiovascular events, and this question requires further investigation.

Uremic Cardiomyopathy

Uremic syndrome is a multisystem deterioration including the cardiovascular, neurologic, hematologic, and immunologic systems. The pathophysiology of uremic syndrome is not completely understood but results from the retention of substances that are ordinarily removed by the kidneys, intake of dietary precursors, and derangements of hormonal and enzymatic homeostasis. The putative substance(s) or uremic toxins have not been clearly identified; however, several substances have been studied, including urea, PTH, beta$_2$-microglobulin, and middle molecules. Several factors may predispose or contribute to myocardial dysfunction in uremia, including hypertension, anemia, electrolyte disturbances, acidosis, hyperlipidemia, accelerated atherosclerosis, glucose intolerance, and malnutrition.

Abnormalities of LV structure and function are common among patients starting renal replacement therapy. Concentric LV hypertrophy is present in approximately 40% of ESRD patients starting dialysis (22,25,74). Twenty-seven percent of patients had LV dilatation and 18% had systolic dysfunction. These abnormalities occur early in CRF and progress rapidly as renal function deteriorates (75). Twenty-seven percent of patients with creatinine clearance greater than 50 mL per minute had LV hypertrophy and this increased to 31% and 45% for clearances between 25 and 50 mL per minute and less than 25 mL per minute, respectively.

Clinical cardiac failure is also common in ESRD patients with almost 50% having a history of cardiac failure before initiating dialysis (74). Congestive heart failure at the beginning of dialysis is an important predictor of cardiovascular and overall mortality in the ESRD population (median survival rate of 32 vs. 62 months) (74). Among ESRD patients, the incidence of valvular dysfunction is also elevated. Some studies note mitral or aortic valvular abnormalities in almost one-half of all patients with CRF. The most common reported abnormalities are mild to moderate mitral regurgitation secondary to LV dilatation and calcification. However, the prevalence of hemodynamically important valvular dysfunction is not well described in the literature thus far.

DIAGNOSIS AND MANAGEMENT OF ISCHEMIC HEART DISEASE AND CONGESTIVE HEART FAILURE AMONG PATIENTS WITH CHRONIC RENAL INSUFFICIENCY AND END-STAGE RENAL DISEASE

Diagnosis

Clinical history remains the cornerstone of diagnosis in stable and unstable coronary artery disease among patients with renal insufficiency. However, the prevalence of reduced physical capacity and significant comorbidities among these patients may somewhat obscure clinical manifestations of coronary artery disease. Similarly, specific interpretation of ECG changes is often limited by changes related to the presence of long-standing hypertension, LV hypertrophy, and electrolyte abnormalities. These factors may either falsely suggest or conceal the diagnosis of myocardial ischemia. These issues limit the diagnostic utility of the resting or exercise ECG in excluding significant myocardial ischemia among renal failure patients. The value of ambulatory ECG monitoring among patients on long-term dialysis also remains in question (87).

Cardiac Markers

Among patients with significant renal insufficiency, transient elevations in cardiac enzymes are commonly observed in the absence of clinical myocardial ischemia and are reported in up 72% of patients over long-term follow-up. The source of these enzyme elevations remains uncertain, but appears unrelated to the type of dialysis (peritoneal vs. hemodialysis) or the level of uremia. Elevations of these enzymes may be persistent, although often at low concen-

TABLE 35C.1 TROPONIN: IMPROVED SENSITIVITY FOR PREDICTING LONG-TERM ISCHEMIC EVENTS AMONG PATIENTS UNDERGOING RENAL DIALYSIS WITH HIGHER THRESHOLD TROPONIN LEVELS

		Troponin I >0.5 ng/mL	Troponin T >0.04 ng/mL	Troponin T >0.1 ng/mL	Troponin T >0.2 ng/mL
Roppolo	Sensitivity (%)	50	—	100	83
	Specificity (%)	100	—	56	91
	Positive predictive value (%)	100	—	24	56
	Negative predictive value (%)	94	—	100	98
Dierkes	Sensitivity (%)	—	45	83	—
	Specificity (%)	—	100	100	—

trations, with creatine kinase-MB (CKMB) fractions rarely exceeding 8%. Isolated elevation of the CKMB subfraction in the absence of demonstrable myocardial necrosis has also been observed. Nonspecific elevations of CK and CKMB contribute to a reduced diagnostic utility of these assays for confirming clinically significant ischemia (88). Similarly, serum myoglobin levels have limited diagnostic utility within this population because of the presence of these enzymes in skeletal muscle and its reduced renal clearance.

Cardiac troponin elevation is frequently observed among dialysis-dependent patients (30% to 50%), and less commonly, among patients with chronic renal impairment not requiring renal replacement (10% to 20%) (89). Troponin levels may also be directly influenced by hemodialysis. Consequently, reduced specificity and possibly sensitivity for myocardial ischemia has been reported within this population (90–93). Mild elevations in troponin T appear more common than in troponin I, suggesting that this assay may have greater specificity. Cross-reactivity with skeletal muscle enzymes may explain the high prevalence of troponin T elevation (89,93–95), although this is less of an issue with more recent assays (96). Nevertheless, troponin I or T among patients with symptomatic myocardial ischemia remains predictive of in-hospital mortality, whereas patients without troponin elevation appear to be at low risk (97,98). Increased troponin T on routine serial measurements of asymptomatic dialysis patients may also predict long-term adverse events, but this has not been consistently demonstrated (89,99–101). Among stable hemodialysis patients with and without known atherosclerosis, troponin T greater than 0.1 ng per mL has been associated with a sevenfold increase in long-term mortality (102). These studies demonstrate an acceptable sensitivity and improved specificity by adopting a higher threshold level. Conversely, among asymptomatic patients with renal insufficiency not requiring dialysis, the predictive utility of either troponin I or T remains low (89). Therefore, among patients with renal impairment, troponin elevation should be interpreted within the context of the clinical presentation, treatment with dialysis and the assay used, although adopting a

higher threshold level may improve diagnostic specificity (Table 35C.1).

Thallium Scintigraphy

The uses of diagnostic imaging studies overcome the issues of LV hypertrophy and repolarization abnormalities that confound the diagnosis of ischemia by ECG alone. However, the diagnostic utility of these noninvasive studies for coronary artery disease remains dependent on the cardiac work induced by either exercise or pharmacologic means. Consequently, among patients with renal failure, earlier studies have documented reduced utility of thallium scans for the diagnosis of coronary artery disease with a sensitivity and specificity as low as 37% and 75%, respectively (106). Furthermore, a low clinical value of thallium scans in predicting coronary artery disease and perioperative events in diabetic patients undergoing renal transplantation was initially observed. These results were attributable to a high prevalence of inadequate tests resulting from reduced exercise tolerance, inadequate heart rate response, concurrent beta-blockade, and the presence of LV hypertrophy (107–109).

More recent reports document substantially improved sensitivity and specificity of thallium-201 scans for the diagnosis of coronary artery disease and prediction of subsequent cardiac events. This improved diagnostic utility has been associated with the use of dipyridamole or combined dipyridamole and exercise testing in some studies, overcoming the issue of limited exercise capacity of these patients (110–112). Of note, Dahan et al. demonstrated a 92% sensitivity, 89% specificity, and 71% positive predictive value with dipyridamole and exercise thallium scanning in patients undergoing hemodialysis. Within this study, the negative predictive value of a normal scan was 91% during 2.8 years of follow-up (113).

Angiography and Contrast-Induced Nephropathy

The indications for coronary angiography within this population remain similar to the general population. However, in the patient with significant renal impairment not managed with renal replacement therapy, the additional risk of contrast-induced nephropathy bears careful consideration and preparation. Moreover, renal impairment is associated with a 3.3-fold increase in the overall complication rate during coronary angiography (120). Therefore, coronary angiography should be undertaken only when the anatomic information provided is essential to the planning of future management. Furthermore, technical considerations, such as the site of vascular access, bear careful consideration.

Contrast-induced nephropathy is a leading cause of in-hospital acute renal failure, occurring in less than 0.5% of patients undergoing coronary angiography. However, among patients with renal insufficiency, deterioration in renal function is reported to be between 10% and 40% of patients, depending on associated comorbidities (121–125). Of these patients, 75% experience complete recovery, whereas 10% require permanent dialysis. Factors clearly associated with worsening renal function are elevated baseline creatinine, volume depletion, diabetes, cardiac failure associated with a low output state, functioning renal allografts, the dose of contrast agent, and repeat contrast studies within 72 hours (126–128). Other potential contributing factors include hyperuricemia, anemia hypertension, and proteinuria (129). Age alone does not appear to increase the risk of contrast nephropathy (122).

Diabetes mellitus is a potent risk factor for the development of contrast-induced nephropathy, although most of this risk relates to the presence of associated diabetic nephropathy (130). In the diabetic patients with concurrent renal dysfunction, the risk is approximately fourfold that of diabetics without documented renal dysfunction, with an incidence of approximately 30%. In addition, the risk in diabetic patients appears greater for those with insulin-requiring diabetes than in those managed with oral therapy, although this may simply reflect the increased prevalence of diabetic nephropathy in the latter group. A strong correlation between dose and repeat administration of contrast and renal deterioration has been observed (123), although an independent relationship has not been universally demonstrated (122). Nevertheless, limiting the dose of contrast in these patients remains an important clinical practice. Low-osmolar agents are associated with less nephrotoxicity in animal models and fewer side effects clinically. However, a substantial difference between the low- and high-osmolality agents among relatively low-risk patients has not been consistently observed (131–133). Conversely, among high-risk patients, low-osmolar agents are associated with significantly lower rates of contrast-induced nephropathy (131). As with osmolarity, ionicity also appears to affect the development of contrast-induced nephropathy, again predominantly among patients with renal insufficiency (130). Therefore, the use of low-osmolar nonionic agents is advocated among those at substantial risk of contrast-induced nephropathy. ⚑ g93

Clinically, contrast nephropathy manifests as an increase in serum creatinine, occurring 24 to 48 hours after angiogra-

phy, peaking over 3 to 5 days, with slow resolution over 7 to 10 days. Oliguria is common among patients with reduced baseline renal function, with up to 50% of these patients requiring permanent dialysis. In addition, urinary sodium excretion is low, as is the fractional excretion of sodium (less than 1%). A persistent nephrogram on abdominal radiography and renal cortical attenuation on computed tomography are also frequently observed for more than 24 hours.

Maintenance of adequate intravascular volume status remains central in the prevention and management of contrast-induced nephropathy. Enhanced diuresis with either furosemide or mannitol has been shown to be of no greater efficacy compared with saline administration alone among patients with significant renal impairment (mean creatinine, 2.1 mg per dL) (141). Administration of 0.45% saline (1 mL per kg per hour) begun 12 hours before coronary angiography was associated with the lowest risk of renal insufficiency (11%) compared with either saline plus mannitol, 25 g (28%), or saline plus furosemide, 80 mg (40%) (141). Reports suggest that use of isotonic saline may be more efficacious (138). While improving urine output, the addition of diuretic agents may induce relative volume depletion and exacerbate nephrotoxicity (136,142). Forced diuresis with intravenous crystalloid infusion, furosemide, or mannitol, with or without dopamine, may also reduce the risk of contrast-induced nephropathy if a high level of urinary volume can be achieved (143). However, caution must be exercised in those with reduced cardiac function. Routine use of dopamine is not associated with a lower risk of contrast-induced nephropathy in high-risk populations (144). Vasodilation with endothelin-receptor antagonists appears to exacerbate contrast-induced nephropathy (139). By preventing renal vasoconstriction, calcium antagonists are a logical approach and have been shown to protect against reductions in glomerular filtration rate (GFR) and proteinuria. Similarly, the efficacy of alternate vasodilatory agents, such as atrial natriuretic peptide, adenosine, and theophylline, has been suggested in experimental models and some small human studies. A reduced rate of contrast-induced nephropathy has also been observed with ACE inhibition, but confirmation with larger studies is required for all of these agents (145). Interestingly, the preventive efficacy of acetylcysteine, an antioxidant administered together with intravenous saline, has been demonstrated. Among 83 patients with a mean creatine of 2.4 mg per dL, acetylcysteine, 600 mg twice daily administered for 1 day before and on the day of investigation, was associated with a small improvement in serum creatinine (0.4 mg per dL) compared with a small deterioration in renal function among controls (0.2 mg per dL; *p* <.001) (146).

Pharmacotherapy of Ischemic Heart Disease and Cardiac Failure

When considering the choice of pharmacotherapy for patients with renal insufficiency, several issues bear consideration. [⚐ g94] These include the relative efficacy of the specific agent within this population and the implications of reduced renal function on dosing regimens. Dose modifications for most therapies among patients with renal insufficiency have been described. Furthermore, among preuremic patients the effect of therapy on renal function in those not yet requiring renal replacement therapy and the prevention of deterioration in renal function should also be considered. However, most randomized trials assessing the long-term efficacy of therapies used in the management of cardiac conditions have excluded patients with moderate to severe renal insufficiency (creatinine greater than 2.5 mg per dL). Thus, in the absence of specific data, recommendations for the management of cardiac indications among patients with renal insufficiency follow the guidelines set forth for the general population. Nevertheless, the presence of renal impairment defines the high-risk nature of these patients, often warranting aggressive optimization of therapy.

Management of Hypertension

Control of hypertension is an important therapeutic goal for the prevention of LV failure and impeding the deterioration of function. Few data are available for guiding the choice of therapies among patients with renal insufficiency. Coexistent clinical indications may help guide therapy (e.g., beta-blockers among patients with ischemic heart disease). ACE inhibitors are of proven efficacy in the control of hypertension, may improve vascular distensibility (150), and also slow the progression of renal disease. Independent of their effects on blood pressure, these agents improve glomerular hemodynamics, reduce proteinuria, and antagonize the development of glomerular hypertrophy in patients with and without diabetes mellitus (151–157). Whether ACE inhibitors provide superior protection from renal deterioration in comparison with other agents is uncertain, but has also been suggested (158). Although calcium antagonists are also effective in the treatment of hypertension, the amlodipine arm of the African American Study of Kidney Disease and Hypertension Pilot Study (159) has been stopped. In this study, the use of this drug compared with ramipril and metoprolol was found to be relatively ineffective in preventing progression to dialysis and death among patients with severe proteinuria (L. Agodoa, *personal communication*, October 2000). Furthermore, renal-protective effects have also been documented among diabetic patients, mediated by improved renal blood flow, reduced glomerular hypertrophy, reduced proteinuria, and altered calcium metabolism with the kidney (160–163). Diuretic therapy is effective among patients with hypertension and fluid overload. Use of potassium-sparing diuretics in combination with ACE inhibitors should be avoided because of the risk of hyperkalemia. Thiazides may be ineffective among patients with a GFR less than 30 mL per minute.

Management of Acute Coronary Syndromes

In the absence of specific data within this high-risk patient subset, the management of acute coronary syndromes follows the guidelines developed for the general population. Mortality among patients presenting with acute coronary syndromes remains high, and underuse of therapies may account for some of this excess risk. Importantly, renal insufficiency is not a contraindication to the use of fibrinolytic therapy among patients presenting with ST-elevation myocardial infarction, but remains underused (164). No dose adjustment of any of the thrombolytic agents is required, and a marked increase in bleeding has not been observed in clinical trials. Nevertheless, attention to the established predictors of hemorrhagic risk should be maintained. Aspirin therapy is also indicated among patients presenting with acute coronary syndromes.

Because renal failure is considered a prothrombotic state, treatment with antithrombin therapy seems logical in the absence of specific data. With unfractionated heparin, titration of infusion doses to target activated partial thromboplastin time levels as defined within the general population is recommended. In contrast, despite the equivalent and possibly superior efficacy of low-molecular-weight heparins compared with unfractionated heparin within acute coronary syndrome patients, these trials have excluded those with significant renal impairment. Therefore, specific benefit among these patients has not been defined. The half-life of elimination for the low-molecular-weight heparins is significantly prolonged in the presence of renal impairment. Consequently, decreased frequency of dosing and monitoring of antifactor Xa levels are advocated, although specific dose-attenuation scales have not been defined. Although currently available direct thrombin inhibitors (bivalirudin) provide a useful alternative in those with heparin sensitivity, these agents also undergo renal elimination, and experience among patients with renal impairment is limited.

Trials evaluating glycoprotein IIb/IIIa inhibitors have excluded patients with significant renal impairment (creatinine greater than 2.0 to 2.5 mg per dL). Given the lack of randomized data in patients with significant renal impairment coupled with known underlying platelet dysfunction, use of these agents should be undertaken with caution and weighed carefully in the setting of acute coronary syndromes. Close attention to bleeding risk should be maintained. Both currently available small molecule antagonists (eptifibatide and tirofiban) undergo significant renal excretion and appear to be removed by dialysis. The adenosine diphosphate receptor antagonists are a useful alternative to aspirin, or in combination with aspirin among those receiving coronary stents. The degree of platelet inhibition provided by these agents among dialysis patients appears to be similar to that of the general population (165). Elimination of the adenosine diphosphate receptor antagonists clopidogrel and ticlopidine are by hepatic excretion, and dose attenuation is not required.

Management of Stable Coronary Artery Disease

Few randomized data are available to guide the choice of antianginal therapy among patients with renal insufficiency. Aspirin appears to increase skin bleeding time and reduce platelet aggregation by a greater degree in dialysis patients compared with healthy patients. Because of the known platelet defect associated with renal disease, the intermittent need for anticoagulation, and the high prevalence of clinical conditions known to be associated with adverse events following aspirin therapy, patients with renal disease receiving aspirin therapy as primary prevention should be monitored closely. In contrast, despite the lack of specific data, aspirin therapy is advocated as secondary prevention in all patients with coronary artery disease, based on compelling data within the general population. Among patients with renal impairment, beta-blockers are both safe and effective. As long-term therapy following myocardial infarction, treatment with beta-blockers is associated with mortality reductions among patients with renal insufficiency comparable with the general population. Chronic beta-blockade is associated with reduced renal blood flow and GFR, although these alterations in renal hemodynamics are usually minor and subclinical. Calcium antagonists are also effective in ischemic heart disease and can generally be administered without dose adjustment. Advantages with respect to the preservation of renal function have been suggested but require prospective validation. Nitrate preparations are also useful among patients with angina and renal insufficiency. However, given the prevalence of LV hypertrophy, these patients may be sensitive to preload reduction, which may be further exacerbated by dialysis. Ample evidence supports the aggressive treatment of hyperlipidemia, especially with 3-hydroxy-3-methylglutaryl coenzyme A reductase inhibitors, among patients with coronary artery disease within the general population. These recommendations have been extended to patients with renal insufficiency.

Management of Cardiac Failure

Within the general population, the benefit of ACE inhibition for the treatment of cardiac failure is well established. These agents are also advocated among patients with renal insufficiency. Specifically within the renal failure patient, ACE inhibitors have been shown to reduce LV hypertrophy and may improve vascular distensibility (150). Furthermore, among patients with a diverse array of cardiovascular

indications treated with ACE inhibition, mild to moderate renal impairment (creatinine 1.4 to 2.3 mg per dL) is associated with a greater mortality reduction compared with patients with normal renal function. Nevertheless, among patients at risk of acute renal insufficiency such as the elderly; patients who are substantially volume depleted; and those with bilateral renal artery stenosis, diabetes mellitus, hypertensive nephrosclerosis, and cardiac failure associated with renal impairment, ACE inhibitor therapy should be instituted with caution. In these conditions, GFR is often maintained in the face of reduced renal perfusion by afferent arteriolar vasodilation and efferent arteriolar vasoconstriction mediated by angiotensin II. By reducing systemic pressure and limiting this compensatory response, these agents may induce a marked decline in GFR. Deterioration in renal function is usually reversible, with dose reduction or cessation of therapy. Effects on renal hemodynamics and proteinuria are also similar to those observed with ACE inhibitors, suggesting the effect on the kidney is mediated by antagonizing the effect of angiotensin II rather than potentiation of bradykinin (166–170). However, specific evidence of renoprotective and cardioprotective effects remains to be demonstrated.

Beta-blockers are also indicated among patients with cardiac failure, although data specific to patients with renal insufficiency are limited. Extending beta-blockers to patients with end-stage cardiac failure awaiting cardiac transplantation does not appear to be associated with a significant deterioration in renal function (170). Caution should be exercised with the use of digoxin among patients undergoing hemodialysis because rapid reductions in plasma potassium, magnesium, and hydrogen ions lead to elevated ionized calcium concentrations potentially exposing patients to digoxin-induced arrhythmias. Although digoxin Fab fragments are useful in the treatment of digoxin-induced arrhythmias, renal elimination of the digoxin Fab fragment remains prolonged, requiring extended monitoring in these patients. Both digoxin and the Fab immune fragment are removed by continuous arteriovenous hemodialysis. Among the inotropic agents, specific benefits of dopamine with respect to renal function have been suggested but not substantiated by randomized studies.

Coronary Revascularization

The principles of revascularization among patients with renal impairment are similar to nonrenal patients, though the effect of renal disease on both short- and long-term outcomes bears careful consideration (Table 35C.2). Frequently, mechanical revascularization is essential for the management of acute coronary syndromes and to control angina resistant to medical therapy and should follow guidelines set forth within the general population in the absence of specific data. In particular, patients with cardiac failure or hemodynamic compromise as manifestations of

TABLE 35C.2 IN-HOSPITAL AND LATE MORTALITY AFTER CORONARY REVASCULARIZATION

Study	Year	Number	Mortality (%)					
			In-hospital	1 yr	2 yr	3 yr	4 yr	5 yr
Coronary artery bypass grafting								
Liu	2000	279	12.2					
Khaitan	2000	70	14.3					
Frenken	1999	45	4.4	10.0	27	33		33
Labrousse	1999	82	14.6	29.0		44		61
Simsir	1998	22	4.5		23			
Lazar	1997	117	13.6					
Jahangiri	1997	19	5.0	13.0	22	41		
Koyanagi	1997	23	0.0					17
Samuels	1996	44	23.0			34		
Reinhart	1995	60	—		66			
Owen	1994	21	9.0	16.0	55			
Ko	1993	16	19.0					
Batiuk	1991	25	20.0	5.0	23	30		
Blakeman	1990	26	0.0					
Deutch	1989	16	6.0					
Peper	1988	36	6.0					
Opsahl	1988	39	2.6	8.0	8			
Rostand	1988	20	20.0					
Marshall	1986	25	8.0	17.0		31		52
Laws	1986	10	10.0					
Monson	1980	22	9.0					
Francis	1980	10	10.0					
Percutaneous coronary intervention								
Rubenstein	2000	—	10.8	25.0				
Le Feuvre	1999	87	2.3	11.5				
Hang	1999	31	10.0	65.4				
Simsir	1998	19	5.3		21			
Marso	1996	23	4.0		63			
Koyangi	1994	20	0.0		10			
Reinhart	1995	64	4.0		49			
Ahmed	1994	21	14.0		33			
Khan	1989	17	12.0		41			

myocardial ischemia warrant more aggressive investigation and management.

Although the choice between revascularization strategies remains contentious within the general population, the poor long-term results associated with percutaneous coronary intervention has led many to recommend coronary artery bypass grafting as the preferred strategy for patients with significant renal impairment (171–173). However, with the continued evolution in mechanical revascularization strategies, of particular note coronary stenting, comparison of the relative benefits of each strategy among patients with ESRD requires prospective evaluation.

INVESTIGATION OF CARDIAC DISEASE BEFORE RENAL TRANSPLANTATION

Among patients undergoing renal transplantation, the incidence of coronary artery disease is increased and associated with a greater mortality, especially in high-risk groups (174,175). Risk stratification (176) and subsequent revas-

cularization appear to reduce long-term cardiac events (174). Therefore, a diagnostic strategy among these patients is warranted. Coronary angiography has commonly been advocated for the screening of coronary artery disease given its prevalence within this population. However, strategies among asymptomatic patients identifying intermediate- and low-risk groups may allow some patients to proceed to transplantation without invasive testing. Patients considered at intermediate risk include those older than 50 years or with diabetes in the absence of clinical cardiac disease and may warrant initial noninvasive investigations. Patients younger than 45 years, with no history of smoking, without diabetes for more than 25 years, and no ST-T–wave changes on ECG, again without clinical cardiac disease, appear to be at low risk of coronary artery disease, and transplantation without prior cardiac investigation may be safe (177). These recommendations have been set forth in the American Society of Transplant Physicians Guidelines for risk stratification before renal transplantation (Fig. 35C.1).

Similarly, parameters of LV function also correlate with long-term mortality after renal transplantation. In a study

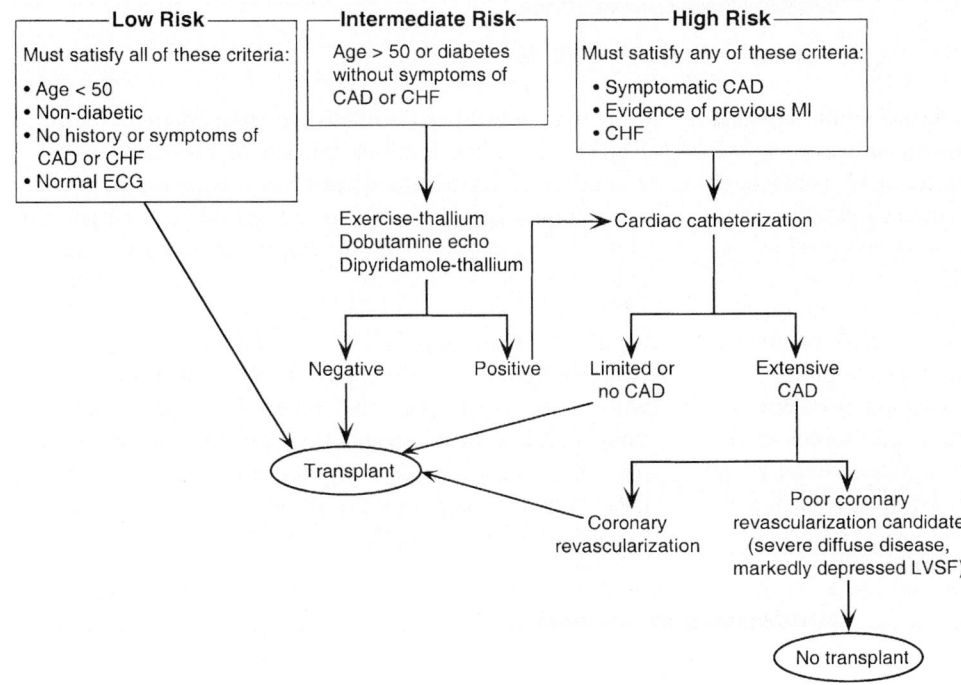

FIGURE 35C.1 American Society of Transplant Physicians Guidelines for risk stratification before renal transplant. CAD, coronary artery disease; CHF, congestive heart failure; ECG, electrocardiography; LVSF, left ventricular shortening fraction; MI, myocardial infarction.

of 141 patients undergoing echocardiography before transplantation, ejection fraction, end systolic and diastolic diameter, LV mass index, fractional shortening, and age were independent predictors of mortality. Not surprisingly, age and end systolic diameter were the strongest predictors of mortality (end systolic diameter risk ratio, 2.16; 95% confidence interval, 1.27 to 3.66, $p <.01$), whereas an association between LV mass index and mortality was also observed (178). However, whether targeting echocardiographic abnormalities provides improved survival in these cases requires validation.

Percutaneous Coronary Intervention

In comparison with the general population, earlier studies of coronary angioplasty among end-stage renal failure patients have reported reduced procedural and clinical success rates because of a substantial increase in vascular complications, long-term recurrent angina, myocardial infarction, restenosis, as well as in-hospital and long-term mortality (179–181). This excess in late adverse outcome extends to patients with chronic renal insufficiency, not requiring renal replacement therapy.

Developments in interventional practice, namely coronary stenting and novel adjunctive therapies, have led to some attenuation in the excess risk associated with renal impairment (182). Within a series of 362 patients, newer interventional techniques (coronary stenting in most patients) appear to be associated with an improved procedural success rate and reduced long-term death, myocardial infarction, or revascularization rates compared with balloon angioplasty, among patients with baseline creatinine greater than 1.5 mg per dL. However, coronary stenting has also been associated with an increased rate of in-hospital cardiac events compared with balloon angioplasty (stents 11% vs. percutaneous transluminal coronary angioplasty 5%) among dialysis patients. Within this study, target vessel revascularization at 1 year was required in 22% of dialysis-dependent patients receiving stents, a rate that was comparable with a contemporaneous non–renal failure population. Nevertheless, late mortality and disease progression resulted in a poor late event-free survival (183), whereas angiographic restenosis after coronary stenting remains elevated even among patients with mild to moderate renal impairment (184). Evidence supporting alternate interventional techniques such as rotational atherectomy is promising but limited to small observational studies.

Data supporting the use of glycoprotein IIb/IIIa inhibition specifically in the renal insufficiency patient are limited. Given the substantial benefit within the context of percutaneous coronary intervention, extrapolation of the results seen within the general population to those with significant renal impairment appears reasonable, although an increased risk of bleeding has been observed (185). Bedside tests of platelet aggregation may also prove useful in guiding therapy with these agents, although appropriate therapeutic targets for platelet inhibition within this population have yet to be defined.

With the continued evolution of interventional strategies, more recent evidence indicates an improvement in acute procedural results (186,187), although still inferior to the general population, and an increased rate of in-hospital major adverse events (10.8% rate of death, Q-wave myocardial infarction, and urgent coronary artery bypass graft-

THE FUTURE

Patients with both cardiac disease and renal insufficiency are increasing in prevalence, associated with an increase in the incidence of diabetes coupled with an aging population. Consequently, randomized trials of current and novel therapies addressing this high-risk population will provide specific clinical data to guide the management of these patients. Recognition of the heightened inflammatory, thrombotic, and metabolic processes contributing to cardiovascular disease within patients with renal insufficiency promises to provide important pathophysiologic information. Further, an understanding of the role of these mechanisms in the increased prevalence of cardiovascular disease among the population of patients with renal disease will provide insight into differential benefit from therapies such as revascularization procedures and pharmacologic management.

It has long been established that patients with ESRD have a tremendous burden of coronary artery and other cardiovascular disease. Increasing focus, however, is now being placed on the period in a patient's clinical course before the development of ESRD. The epidemiology of cardiovascular disease among patients with early renal insufficiency has not been fully explored. This population of patients has greater comorbidity and a unique pathobiology of disease that will require dedicated and focused study. A better understanding of the distribution and determinants of disease as well as the development of therapeutic strategies targeting the unique mechanisms is essential toward affecting the burden of cardiovascular disease in this population.

ing) persists. Long-term recurrent angina, myocardial infarction, and target vessel revascularization remain a problem with target vessel revascularization rates and mortality remaining in the range of 50% and 30%, respectively. Factors contributing to these adverse events include a higher degree of calcification, greater residual stenosis, and smaller vessel size, reflecting the diffuse atheromatous disease process (188,189). An increased intensity of prothrombotic and proinflammatory mechanisms as evidenced by increased fibrinogen levels has also been linked to the restenotic process and late events (189). Thus, whether contemporary catheter-based revascularization offers results comparable with coronary artery bypass grafting remains to be examined prospectively (190).

Coronary Artery Bypass Grafting

The adverse prognostic effect of renal insufficiency on the outcomes after coronary artery bypass grafting is well established and extends to include those with moderate renal dysfunction (creatinine greater than 2.5 mg per dL). In addition to an increased prevalence of risk factors such as extensive coronary artery disease, LV dysfunction, diabetes, and prior myocardial infarction, elevated blood urea nitrogen appears to impart increased risk of perioperative mortality and a low cardiac output postoperative state. The mortality risk associated with blood urea nitrogen may be partly attributable to the presence of associated comorbid conditions, such as uremia-induced platelet dysfunction and fluid, electrolyte, and acid–base disturbances contributing to perioperative cardiac failure and arrhythmias. Depressed immune function also increases the rate of infection. Therefore, patients with renal insufficiency experience

an increased incidence of prolonged ventilation, mediastinitis, and stroke, contributing to increased intensive care and in-hospital stays as well as an in-hospital mortality ranging from 4% to 14% or approximately three times the rate observed among the general population. Furthermore, combined coronary artery bypass grafting and valvular surgery appears to be associated with an even greater risk of in-hospital mortality (191).

Even within the general population, the incidence of renal failure after cardiac surgery ranges between 1% and 8% but is associated with a striking increase in operative mortality (63.7% vs. 4.3%, $p < .001$) (192). Similarly, myocardial infarction, mediastinitis, and reoperation for bleeding are also increased. Preexisting renal impairment, age, diabetes, and cardiac failure are important predictors of deterioration in renal function with approximately 25% of patients with preexisting mild or moderate renal insufficiency requiring permanent dialysis after cardiopulmonary bypass (192–194). Among renal transplant patients, a relatively small deterioration in renal function is also observed (195).

The use of peritoneal dialysis or hemodialysis on the day before surgery and after the operation is practiced in some centers. Minimizing fluid shifts and electrolyte disturbance during the procedure with intraoperative dialysis has also been suggested. Similarly, developments in operative technique and increased use of arterial conduits (196) may benefit these high-risk patients, while the minimally invasive surgery may prove a particular advance in renal failure patients, but this remains to be documented.

Although randomized comparisons are lacking, coronary artery bypass grafting appears to be associated with lower long-term mortality compared with patients receiving coronary stents or balloon angioplasty as observed in the United States Renal Data System database (61.2%, 70.6%, and 71.4%, respectively) (190). Nevertheless, the 22% mortality per year reported in more recent studies remains high (190,197–200). More recent reports of long-term survival do not differ substantially from earlier series. Furthermore, the presence of cardiac failure before coronary artery bypass grafting is associated with a three- to fourfold risk of increased late mortality (191,201). Thus, long-term survival after coronary artery bypass grafting is similar to the overall survival rates observed among dialysis patients regardless of revascularization (191,201–203). Whether revascularization provides a mortality benefit is uncertain and appears to depend not only on the extent of coronary artery disease, but also on the coexistent medical conditions within the individual patient.

REFERENCES

1. Foley RN, Parfrey PS, Sarnak MJ. Clinical epidemiology of cardiovascular disease in chronic renal disease. *Am J Kidney Dis* 1998;32:S112–S119.
2. Baigent C, Burbury K, Wheeler D. Premature cardiovascular disease in chronic renal failure. *Lancet* 2000;356:147–152.
3. Lindner A, Charra B, Sherrard DJ. Accelerated atherosclerosis in prolonged maintenance hemodialysis. *N Engl J Med* 1974;290:697–701.
4. McCullough PA, Soman SS, Shah SS, et al. Risks associated with renal dysfunction in patients in the coronary care unit. *J Am Coll Cardiol* 2000;36:679–684.
5. Held PJ, Port FK, Webb RL. Excerpts from United States Renal Data System 1995 Annual Data Report. *Am J Kidney Dis* 1995;26:S1–S186.
6. Lindholm A, Albrechtsen D, Frodin L. Ischemic heart disease—major cause of death and graft loss after renal transplantation in Scandinavia. *Transplantation* 1995;60:451–457.
7. Khaitan L, Sutter FP, Goldman SM. Coronary artery bypass grafting in patients who require long-term dialysis. *Ann Thorac Surg* 2000;69:1135–1139.
8. Parfrey PS, Foley RN, Rigatto C. Risk issues in renal transplantation: cardiac aspects. *Transplant Proc* 1999;31:291–293.
9. Parfrey PS, Foley RN. The clinical epidemiology of cardiac disease in chronic renal failure. *J Am Soc Nephrol* 1999;10:1606–1615.
10. Marso SP, Ellis SG, Gurm HS. Proteinuria is a key determinant of death in patients with diabetes after isolated coronary artery bypass grafting. *Am Heart J* 2000;139:939–944.
11. Ohashi H, Oda H, Ohno M. Lipoprotein(a) as a risk factor for coronary artery disease in hemodialysis patients. *Kidney Int Suppl* 1999;71:S242–S244.
12. Kronenberg F, Neyer U, Lhotta K. The low molecular weight apo(a) phenotype is an independent predictor for coronary artery disease in hemodialysis patients: a prospective follow-up. *J Am Soc Nephrol* 1999;10:1027–1036.
13. Foley RN, Parfrey PS, Harnett JD. Mode of dialysis therapy and mortality in end-stage renal disease. *J Am Soc Nephrol* 1998;9:267–276.
14. Remuzzi G. Bleeding in renal failure. *Lancet* 1988;1:1205–1208.
15. Sagripanti A, Barsotti G. Bleeding and thrombosis in chronic uremia. *Nephron* 1997;75:125–139.
16. Irish AB. Plasminogen activator inhibitor-1 activity in chronic renal disease and dialysis. *Metabolism* 1997;46:36–40.
17. Irish AB, Green FR. Factor VII coagulant activity (VIIc) and hypercoagulability in chronic renal disease and dialysis: relationship with dyslipidaemia, inflammation, and factor VII genotype. *Nephrol Dial Transplant* 1998;13:679–684.
18. Nakamura Y, Chida Y, Tomura S. Enhanced coagulation-fibrinolysis in patients on regular hemodialysis treatment. *Nephron* 1991;58:201–204.
19. Al-Saady NM, Leatham EW, Gupta S. Monocyte expression of tissue factor and adhesion molecules: the link with accelerated coronary artery disease in patients with chronic renal failure. *Heart* 1999;81:134–140.
20. Ebihara I, Nakamura T, Tomino Y. Metalloproteinase-9 mRNA expression in monocytes from patients with chronic renal failure. *Am J Nephrol* 1998;18:305–310.
21. Westhuyzen J, Healy H. Review: biology and relevance of C-reactive protein in cardiovascular and renal disease. *Ann Clin Lab Sci* 2000;30:133–143.
22. Foley RN, Parfrey PS, Harnett JD. Clinical and echocardiographic disease in patients starting end-stage renal disease therapy. *Kidney Int* 1995;47:186–192.
23. Parfrey PS, Foley RN, Harnett JD. Outcome and risk factors of ischemic heart disease in chronic uremia. *Kidney Int* 1996;49:1428–1434.
24. Churchill DN, Taylor DW, Cook RJ. Canadian Hemodialysis Morbidity Study. *Am J Kidney Dis* 1992;19:214–234.
25. Foley RN, Parfrey PS, Harnett JD. The prognostic importance of left ventricular geometry in uremic cardiomyopathy. *J Am Soc Nephrol* 1995;5:2024–2031.
26. Foley RN, Parfrey PS, Harnett JD. Hypocalcemia, morbidity, and mortality in end-stage renal disease. *Am J Nephrol* 1996;16:386–393.
27. Foley RN, Parfrey PS, Harnett JD. The impact of anemia on cardiomyopathy, morbidity, and mortality in end-stage renal disease. *Am J Kidney Dis* 1996;28:53–61.
28. Foley RN, Parfrey PS, Harnett JD. Hypoalbuminemia, cardiac morbidity, and mortality in end-stage renal disease. *J Am Soc Nephrol* 1996;7:728–736.
29. Rigatto C, Foley RN, Kent GM. Long-term changes in left ventricular hypertrophy after renal transplantation. *Transplantation* 2000;70:570–575.
30. Slatopolsky E, Delmez J. Pathogenesis of secondary hyperparathyroidism. *Miner Electrolyte Metab* 1995;21:91–96.
31. Brown EM, Wilkson RE, Eastman RC. Abnormal regulation of parathyroid hormone release by calcium in secondary hyperparathyroidism due to chronic renal failure. *J Clin Endocrinol Metab* 1982;54:172–179.
32. Llach F. Secondary hyperparathyroidism in renal failure: the trade-off hypothesis revisited. *Am J Kidney Dis* 1995;25:663–679.

33. Rostand SG, Drueke TB. Parathyroid hormone, vitamin D, and cardiovascular disease in chronic renal failure. *Kidney Int* 1999;56:383–392.

34. Wang R, Wu L, Karpinski E. The changes in contractile status of single vascular smooth muscle cells and ventricular cells induced by bPTH. *Life Sci* 1993;52:793–801.

35. Smogorezewski M. PTH, chronic renal failure and myocardium. *Miner Electrolyte Metab* 1995;21:55–62.

36. Ongino K, Burhkoff D, Bilezikian JP. The hemodynamic basis for the effects of parathyroid hormone and PTH-related protein. *Endocrinology* 1995;136:3024–3030.

37. Bro S, Olgaard K. Effects of excess PTH on nonclassical target organs. *Am J Kidney Dis* 1997;30:606–620.

38. Rostand SG, Drueke TB. Parathyroid hormone, vitamin D, and cardiovascular disease in chronic renal failure. *Kidney Int* 1999;56:383–392.

39. Rostand SG, Sanders C, Kirk KA. Myocardial calcification and cardiac dysfunction in chronic renal failure. *Am J Med* 1988;85:651–656.

40. Park CW, Oh YS, Shin YS. Intravenous calcitriol regresses myocardial hypertrophy in hemodialysis patients with secondary hyperparathyroidism. *Am J Kidney Dis* 1999;33:73–81.

41. Watson KE, Abrolat ML, Malone LL. Active serum vitamin D levels are inversely correlated with coronary calcification. *Circulation* 1997;96:1755–1760.

42. Shane E, Mancini D, Aaronson K. Bone mass vitamin D deficiency, and hyperparathyroidism in congestive heart failure. *Am J Med* 1997;103:197–207.

43. Coratelli P, Petrarulo F, Buongiorno E. Improvement in left ventricular function during treatment of hemodialysis patients with 25-OHD3. *Contrib Nephrol* 1984;41:433–437.

44. Lowrie EG, Lew NL. Death risk in hemodialysis patients: the predictive value of commonly measured variables and an evaluation of death rate differences between facilities. *Am J Kidney Dis* 1990;5:458–482.

45. Owen WF, Lowrie EG. C-reactive protein as an outcome predictor for maintenance hemodialysis patients. *Kidney Int* 1998;54:627–636.

46. Block GA, Hulbert-Shearon TE, Levin NW, et al. Association of serum phosphorus and calcium X phosphate product with mortality risk in chronic hemodialysis patients: a national study. *Am J Kidney Dis* 1998;31:607–617.

47. Goodman WG, Goldin J, Kuizon BD, et al. Coronary-artery calcification in young adults with end-stage renal disease who are undergoing dialysis. *N Engl J Med* 2000;342:1478–1483.

48. Mucsi I, Hercz G, Uldall R, et al. Control of serum phosphate without any phosphate binders in patients treated with nocturnal hemodialysis. *Kidney Int* 1998;53:1399.

49. Wheeler DC, Bernard DB. Lipid abnormalities in the nephrotic syndrome: causes, consequences, and treatment. *Am J Kidney Dis* 1994;23:331.

50. Appel G. Lipid abnormalities in renal disease. *Kidney Int* 1991;39:169.

51. Joven J, Villabona C, Vilella E. Abnormalities of lipoprotein metabolism in patients with the nephrotic syndrome. *N Engl J Med* 1990;323:579.

52. Baxter JH, Goodman HC, Allen JC. Effects of infusion of serum albumin on serum lipids and lipoproteins in nephrosis. *J Clin Invest* 1961;40:490.

53. Demant T, Mathes C, Gutlich K. A simultaneous study of the metabolism of apolipoprotein B and albumin in nephrotic patients. *Kidney Int* 1998;54:2064.

54. Vega GL, Toto RD, Grundy SM. Metabolism of low density lipoproteins in nephrotic dyslipidemia: comparison of hypercholesterolemia alone and combined hyperlipidemia. *Kidney Int* 1995;47:579.

55. Radhakrishnan J, Appel AS, Valeri A. The nephrotic syndrome, lipids, and risk factors for cardiovascular disease. *Am J Kidney Dis* 1993;22:135.

56. Ordonez JD, Hiatt RA, Killebrew EJ. The increased risk of coronary heart disease associated with nephrotic syndrome. *Kidney Int* 1993;44:638.

57. Rabelink AJ, Hene RJ, Erkelens DW. Effect of simvastatin and cholestyramine on lipoprotein profile in hyperlipidemia of nephrotic syndrome. *Lancet* 1988;2:1355.

58. Hollenberg NK, Raij L. Angiotensin-converting enzyme inhibition and renal protection. An assessment of implications for therapy. *Arch Intern Med* 1993;153:2426.

59. Brunner HR. ACE inhibitors in renal disease. *Kidney Int* 1992;42:462.

60. Keilani T, Schleuter WA, Levin ML. Improvement of lipid abnormalities associated with proteinuria using fosinopril, an angiotensin-converting enzyme inhibitor. *Ann Intern Med* 1993;118:246.

61. de Zeeuw D, Gansevoort RT, Dullaart RP. Angiotensin II antagonism improves the lipoprotein profile in patients with nephrotic syndrome. *Am J Kidney Dis* 1995;13[Suppl 1]:S53.

62. Bachman J, Tepel M, Raidt H. Hyperhomocystinemia and the risk for vascular disease in hemodialysis patients. *J Am Soc Nephrol* 1995;6:121–125.

63. Bostom AG, Shemin D, Lapane KL. Hyperhomocystinemia and traditional cardiovascular disease risk factors in end-stage renal disease patients on dialysis: a case-control study. *Atherosclerosis* 1995;114:93–103.

64. Chauveau P, Chadefaux B, Coude M. Hyperhomocystinemia as a risk factor for atherosclerosis in chronic uremic patients. *Kidney Int* 1993;43[Suppl 41]:S72–S77.

65. Massy AZ, Chadefaux-Vekemans B, Chevalier A. Hyperhomocystinemia: a significant risk factor for cardiovascular disease in renal transplant recipients. *Nephrol Dial Transplant* 1994;9:1103–1108.

66. Gotto AM. Hypertriglyceridemia: risks and perspectives. *Am J Cardiol* 1992;70:19H.

67. Clarke R, Daly L, Robinson K. Hyperhomocystinemia: an independent risk factor for vascular disease. *N Engl J Med* 1991;324:149–155.

68. Stampfer MJ, Malinow MR, Willett WC. A prospective study of plasma homocysteine and risk of myocardial infarction in US physicians. *JAMA* 1992;268:877–881.

69. Boushey CJ, Beresford SA, Omenn GS. A quantitative assessment of plasma homocysteine as a risk factor for vascular disease. *JAMA* 1995;274:1049–1057.

70. Nygard O, Nordrehaug JE, Refsum H. Plasma homocysteine levels and mortality in patients with coronary artery disease. *N Engl J Med* 1997;337:230–236.

71. Moustapha A, Naso A, Nahlawi M. Prospective study of

hyperhomocystinemia as an adverse cardiovascular risk factor in end-stage renal disease. *Circulation* 1998;97:138–141.

72. Bostom AG, Shemin D, Lapane KL. High dose B-vitamin treatment of hyperhomocystinemia in dialysis patients. *Kidney Int* 1996;49:147–152.

73. Wilcken DEL, Dudman NPB, Tyrrell PA. Folic acid lowers elevated plasma homocysteine in chronic renal insufficiency: possible implications for prevention of vascular disease. *Metabolism* 1988;37:697–701.

74. Harnett JD, Foley RN, Kent GM. Congestive heart failure in dialysis patients: prevalence, incidence, prognosis and risk factors. *Kidney Int* 1995;47:884–890.

75. Levin A, Singer J, Thomson CR. Prevalent left ventricular hypertrophy in the predialysis population: identifying opportunities for intervention. *Am J Kidney Dis* 1996;7:347–354.

76. Hampers CL, Schupak E. *Long-term hemodialysis. The management of the patient with chronic renal failure.* Orlando, FL: Grune & Stratton, 1967:81.

77. Comty CM, Cohen SL, Shapiro FL. Pericarditis in chronic uremia and its sequels. *Ann Intern Med* 1971;75:173–183.

78. Silverberg S, Oreopoulos DG, Wise DJ, et al. Pericarditis in patients undergoing long-term hemodialysis and peritoneal dialysis. *Am J Med* 1977;63:874–880.

79. Marini PV, Hull AR. Uremic pericarditis: a review of incidence and management. *Kidney Int Suppl* 1975;2:163–166.

80. Rostand SG, Rutsky EA. Pericarditis in end-stage renal disease. *Cardiol Clin* 1990;8:701–706.

81. Rutsky EA, Rostand SG. Treatment of uremic pericarditis and pericardial effusion. *Am J Kidney Dis* 1987;10:2–8.

82. Lundin AP. Recurrent uremic pericarditis: a marker of inadequate dialysis. *Semin Dial* 1990;3:5.

83. Rutsky EA, Rostand SG. Pericarditis in end-stage renal disease: clinical characteristics and management. *Semin Dial* 1989;2:25.

84. Emelife-Obi C, Chow MT, Qamar-Rohail H, et al. Use of a phosphorus-enriched hemodialysate to prevent hypophosphatemia in a patient with renal failure-related pericarditis. *Clin Nephrol* 1998;50:131.

85. Connors JP, Kleiger RE, Shaw RC, et al. The indications for pericardiectomy in the uremic pericardial effusion. *Surgery* 1976;80:689.

86. Ifudu O. Daily dialysis in hemodialysis patients with pericardial effusion: where are the data? *Int J Artif Organs* 1999;22:469.

87. Conlon PJ, Krucoff MW, Minda S. Incidence and long-term significance of transient ST segment deviation in hemodialysis patients. *Clin Nephrol* 1998;49:236–239.

88. Green TR, Golper TA, Swenson RD, et al. Diagnostic value of creatine kinase and creatine kinase MB isoenzyme in chronic hemodialysis patients: a longitudinal study. *Clin Nephrol* 1986;25:22–27.

89. Roppolo LP, Fitzgerald R, Dillow J. A comparison of troponin T and troponin I as predictors of cardiac events in patients undergoing chronic dialysis at a Veteran's Hospital: a pilot study. *J Am Coll Cardiol* 1999;34:448–454.

90. Frankel WL, Herold DA, Ziegler TW. Cardiac troponin T is elevated in asymptomatic patients with chronic renal failure. *Am J Clin Pathol* 1996;106:118–123.

91. Collinson PO, Hadcocks L, Foo Y. Cardiac troponins in patients with renal dysfunction. *Ann Clin Biochem* 1998;35:380–386.

92. George SK, Singh AK. Current markers of myocardial ischemia and their validity in end-stage renal disease. *Curr Opin Nephrol Hypertens* 1999;8:719–722.

93. Van Lente F, McErlean ES, DeLuca SA. Ability of troponins to predict adverse outcomes in patients with renal insufficiency and suspected acute coronary syndromes: a case-matched study. *J Am Coll Cardiol* 1999;33:471–478.

94. Musso P, Cox I, Vidano E. Cardiac troponin elevations in chronic renal failure: prevalence and clinical significance. *Clin Biochem* 1999;32:125–130.

95. Li D, Keffer J, Corry K, et al. Nonspecific elevation of troponin T levels in patients with chronic renal failure. *Clin Biochem* 1995;28:474–477.

96. Haller C, Zehelein J, Remppis A. Cardiac troponin T in patients with end-stage renal disease: absence of expression in truncal skeletal muscle. *Clin Chem* 1998;44:930–938.

97. Martin GS, Becker BN, Schulman G. Cardiac troponin-I accurately predicts myocardial injury in renal failure. *Nephrol Dial Transplant* 1998;13:1709–1712.

98. Ooi DS, Veinot JP, Wells GA. Increased mortality in hemodialyzed patients with elevated serum troponin T: a one-year outcome study. *Clin Biochem* 1999;32:647–652.

99. Stolear JC, Georges B, Shita A. The predictive value of cardiac troponin T measurements in subjects on regular haemodialysis. *Nephrol Dial Transplant* 1999;14:1961–1967.

100. Wayand D, Baum H, Schatzle GD. Cardiac troponin T and I in end-stage renal failure. *Clin Chem* 2000;46:1345–1350.

101. Mockel M, Schindler R, Knorr L. Prognostic value of cardiac troponin T and I elevations in renal disease patients without acute coronary syndromes: a 9-month outcome analysis. *Nephrol Dial Transplant* 1999;14:1489–1495.

102. Dierkes J, Domrose U, Westphal S, et al. Cardiac troponin T predicts mortality in patients with end-stage renal disease. *Circulation* 2000;102:1964–1969.

103. Murphy SW, Foley RN, Parfrey PS. Screening and treatment for cardiovascular disease in patients with chronic renal disease. *Am J Kidney Dis* 1998;32:S184–S199.

104. Morrow CE, Schwartz JS, Sutherland DE, et al. Predictive value of thallium stress testing for coronary and cardiovascular events in uremic diabetic patients before renal transplantation. *Am J Surg* 1983;146:331–335.

105. Philipson JD, Carpenter BJ, Itzkoff J, et al. Evaluation of cardiovascular risk for renal transplantation in diabetic patients. *Am J Med* 1986;81:630–634.

106. Marwick TH, Steinmuller DR, Underwood DA. Ineffectiveness of dipyridamole SPECT thallium imaging as a screening technique for coronary artery disease in patients with end-stage renal failure. *Transplantation* 1990;49:100–103.

107. Holley JL, Fenton RA, Arthur RS. Thallium stress testing does not predict cardiovascular risk in diabetic patients with end-stage renal disease undergoing cadaveric renal transplantation. *Am J Med* 1991;90:563–570.

108. Gelber CM, Diskin CJ, Claunch BC. Thallium-201 myo-

cardial imaging in patients on chronic hemodialysis. *Nephron* 1984;36:136–142.

109. DePuey EG, Guertler-Krawczynska E, Perkins JV. Alterations in myocardial thallium-201 distribution in patients with chronic systemic hypertension undergoing single-photon emission computed tomography. *Am J Cardiol* 1988;62:234–238.

110. Brown JH, Vites NP, Testa HJ. Value of thallium myocardial imaging in the prediction of future cardiovascular events in patients with end-stage renal failure. *Nephrol Dial Transplant* 1993;8:433–437.

111. Camp AD, Garvin PJ, Hoff J. Prognostic value of intravenous dipyridamole thallium imaging in patients with diabetes mellitus considered for renal transplantation. *Am J Cardiol* 1990;65:1459–1463.

112. de Lemos JA, Hillis LD. Diagnosis and management of coronary artery disease in patients with end-stage renal disease on hemodialysis. *J Am Soc Nephrol* 1996;7:2044–2054.

113. Dahan M, Viron BM, Faraggi M. Diagnostic accuracy and prognostic value of combined dipyridamole-exercise thallium imaging in hemodialysis patients. *Kidney Int* 1998;54:255–262.

114. Nally JV Jr. Cardiac disease in chronic uremia: investigation. *Adv Ren Replace Ther* 1997;4:225–233.

115. Murphy SW, Parfrey PS. Screening for cardiovascular disease in dialysis patients. *Curr Opin Nephrol Hypertens* 1996;5:532–540.

116. Reis G, Marcovitz PA, Leichtman AB. Usefulness of dobutamine stress echocardiography in detecting coronary artery disease in end-stage renal disease. *Am J Cardiol* 1995;75:707–710.

117. Herzog CA, Marwick TH, Pheley AM. Dobutamine stress echocardiography for the detection of significant coronary artery disease in renal transplant candidates. *Am J Kidney Dis* 1999;33:1080–1090.

118. Brennan DC, Vedala G, Miller SB. Pretransplant dobutamine stress echocardiography is useful and cost-effective in renal transplant candidates. *Transplant Proc* 1997;29:233–234.

119. Marwick TH, Lauer MS, Lobo A. Use of dobutamine echocardiography for cardiac risk stratification of patients with chronic renal failure. *J Intern Med* 1998;244:155–161.

120. Laskey W, Boyle J, Johnson LW. Multivariable model for prediction of risk of significant complication during diagnostic cardiac catheterization. The Registry Committee of the Society for Cardiac Angiography & Interventions. *Cathet Cardiovasc Diagn* 1993;30:185–190.

121. Scanlon PJ, Faxon DP, Audet AM, et al. ACC/AHA guidelines for coronary angiography. A report of the American College of Cardiology/American Heart Association Task Force on practice guidelines (Committee on Coronary Angiography). Developed in collaboration with the Society for Cardiac Angiography and Interventions. *J Am Coll Cardiol* 1999;33:1756–1824.

122. Rich MW, Crecelius CA. Incidence, risk factors, and clinical course of acute renal insufficiency after cardiac catheterization in patients 70 years of age or older. A prospective study. *Arch Intern Med* 1990;150:1237–1242.

123. Manske CL, Sprafka JM, Strony JT. Contrast nephropathy in azotemic diabetic patients undergoing coronary angiography. *Am J Med* 1990;89:615–620.

124. Porter GA. Contrast-associated nephropathy: presentation, pathophysiology and management. *Miner Electrolyte Metab* 1994;20:232–243.

125. Parfrey PS, Griffiths SM, Barrett BJ. Contrast material-induced renal failure in patients with diabetes mellitus, renal insufficiency, or both. A prospective controlled study. *N Engl J Med* 1989;320:143–149.

126. Davidson CJ, Hlatky M, Morris KG. Cardiovascular and renal toxicity of a nonionic radiographic contrast agent after cardiac catheterization. A prospective trial. *Ann Intern Med* 1989;110:119–124.

127. Ahuja TS, Niaz N, Agraharkar M. Contrast-induced nephrotoxicity in renal allograft recipients. *Clin Nephrol* 2000;54:11–14.

128. Taliercio CP, Vlietstra RE, Fisher LD, et al. Risks for renal dysfunction with cardiac angiography. *Ann Intern Med* 1986;104:501–504.

129. Deray G, Jacobs C. Radiocontrast nephrotoxicity. A review. *Invest Radiol* 1995;30:221–225.

130. Rudnick MR, Goldfarb S, Wexler L. Nephrotoxicity of ionic and nonionic contrast media in 1196 patients: a randomized trial. The Iohexol Cooperative Study. *Kidney Int* 1995;47:254–261.

131. Spinler SA, Goldfarb S. Nephrotoxicity of contrast media following cardiac angiography: pathogenesis, clinical course, and preventive measures, including the role of low-osmolality contrast media. *Ann Pharmacother* 1992;26:56–64.

132. Moore RD, Steinberg EP, Powe NR. Nephrotoxicity of high-osmolality versus low-osmolality contrast media: randomized clinical trial. *Radiology* 1992;182:649–655.

133. Lautin EM, Freeman NJ, Schoenfeld AH. Radiocontrast-associated renal dysfunction: a comparison of lower-osmolality and conventional high-osmolality contrast media. *Am J Roentgenol* 1991;157:59–65.

134. Shafi T, Chou SY, Porush JG. Infusion intravenous pyelography and renal function. Effects in patients with chronic renal insufficiency. *Arch Intern Med* 1978;138:1218–1221.

135. Larson TS, Hudson K, Mertz JI. Renal vasoconstrictive response to contrast medium. The role of sodium balance and the renin-angiotensin system. *J Lab Clin Med* 1983;101:385–391.

136. Weisberg LS, Kurnik PB, Kurnik BR. Risk of radiocontrast nephropathy in patients with and without diabetes mellitus. *Kidney Int* 1994;45:259–265.

137. Kamata K, Miyata N, Kasuya Y. Impairment of endothelium-dependent relaxation and changes in levels of cyclic GMP in aorta from streptozotocin-induced diabetic rats. *Br J Pharmacol* 1989;97:614–618.

138. Muller CH, Burkle G, Buttner HJ, et al. Prevention of contrast media-associated nephrotoxicity: comparison of 2 hydration regimens in 1,620 patients undergoing elective or urgent PTCA. *Eur Heart J* 2000;21[Suppl]:645.

139. Wang A, Holcslaw T, Bashore TM. Exacerbation of radiocontrast nephrotoxicity by endothelin receptor antagonism. *Kidney Int* 2000;57:1675–1680.

140. Quader MA, Sawmiller C, Sumpio BA. Contrast-induced nephropathy: review of incidence and pathophysiology. *Ann Vasc Surg* 1998;12:612–620.

141. Solomon R, Werner C, Mann D. Effects of saline, mannitol, and furosemide to prevent acute decreases in renal function induced by radiocontrast agents. *N Engl J Med* 1994;331:1416–1420.

142. Berns AS. Nephrotoxicity of contrast media. *Kidney Int* 1989;36:730–740.

143. Stevens MA, McCullough PA, Tobin KJ. A prospective randomized trial of prevention measures in patients at high risk for contrast nephropathy: results of the P.R.I.N.C.E. Study. Prevention of Radiocontrast Induced Nephropathy Clinical Evaluation. *J Am Coll Cardiol* 1999;33:403–411.

144. Gare M, Haviv YS, Ben-Yehuda A. The renal effect of low-dose dopamine in high-risk patients undergoing coronary angiography. *J Am Coll Cardiol* 1999;34:1682–1688.

145. Gupta RK, Kapoor A, Tewari S. Captopril for prevention of contrast-induced nephropathy in diabetic patients: a randomised study. *Indian Heart J* 1999;51:521–526.

146. Tepel M, van der Giet M, Schwarzfeld C, et al. Prevention of radiographic-contrast-agent-induced reductions in renal function by acetylcysteine. *N Engl J Med* 2000;343:180–184.

147. Fellner SK, Lang RM, Neumann A. Cardiovascular consequences of correction of the anemia of renal failure with erythropoietin. *Kidney Int* 1993;44:1309–1315.

148. Rostand SG. Coronary heart disease in chronic renal insufficiency: some management considerations. *J Am Soc Nephrol* 2000;11:1948–1956.

149. Massry SG, Smogorzewski M. Mechanisms through which parathyroid hormone mediates its deleterious effects on organ function in uremia. *Semin Nephrol* 1994;14:219–231.

150. London GM, Pannier B, Guerin AP. Cardiac hypertrophy, aortic compliance, peripheral resistance, and wave reflection in end-stage renal disease. Comparative effects of ACE inhibition and calcium channel blockade. *Circulation* 1994;90:2786–2796.

151. Becker GJ, Whitworth JA, Ihle BU. Prevention of progression in non-diabetic chronic renal failure. *Kidney Int Suppl* 1994;45:S167–170.

152. Hannedouche T, Landais P, Goldfarb B. Randomised controlled trial of enalapril and beta blockers in non-diabetic chronic renal failure. *BMJ* 1994;309:833–837.

153. Zucchelli P, Zuccala A, Gaggi R. Comparison of the effects of ACE inhibitors and calcium channel blockers on the progression of renal failure. *Nephrol Dial Transplant* 1995;10[Suppl 9]:46–51.

154. Kamper AL, Strandgaard S, Leyssac PP. Late outcome of a controlled trial of enalapril treatment in progressive chronic renal failure. Hard end-points and influence of proteinuria. *Nephrol Dial Transplant* 1995;10:1182–1188.

155. Maschio G. Low-protein diet and progression of renal disease: an endless story. *Nephrol Dial Transplant* 1995;10:1797–1800.

156. Ihle BU, Whitworth JA, Shahinfar S. Angiotensin-converting enzyme inhibition in nondiabetic progressive renal insufficiency: a controlled double-blind trial. *Am J Kidney Dis* 1996;27:489–495.

157. Lewis EJ, Hunsicker LG, Bain RP. The effect of angiotensin-converting-enzyme inhibition on diabetic nephropathy. The Collaborative Study Group. *N Engl J Med* 1993;329:1456–1462.

158. Giatras I, Lau J, Levey AS. Effect of angiotensin-converting enzyme inhibitors on the progression of nondiabetic renal disease: a meta-analysis of randomized trials. Angiotensin-Converting-Enzyme Inhibition and Progressive Renal Disease Study Group. *Ann Intern Med* 1997;127:337–345.

159. Wright JT, Kusek J, Toto RD, et al. Design and baseline characteristics of participants in the African American Study of Kidney Disease and Hypertension (AASK) Pilot Study. *Control Clin Trials* 1996;17:3S–16S.

160. Salvetti A, Mattei P, Sudano I. Renal protection and antihypertensive drugs: current status. *Drugs* 1999;57:665–693.

161. Epstein M. Calcium antagonists and the progression of chronic renal failure. *Curr Opin Nephrol Hypertens* 1998;7:171–176.

162. Parving HH, Tarnow L, Rossing P. Renal protection in diabetes—an emerging role for calcium antagonists. *Cardiology* 1997;88:56–62.

163. Neumayer HH, Gellert J, Luft FC. Calcium antagonists and renal protection. *Renal Failure* 1993;15:353–358.

164. Herzog CA. Acute myocardial infarction in patients with end-stage renal disease. *Kidney Int Suppl* 1999;71:S130–133.

165. Kaufman JS, Fiore L, Hasbargen JA, et al. A pharmacodynamic study of clopidogrel in chronic hemodialysis patients. *J Thromb Thrombolysis* 2000;10:127–131.

166. Gansevoort RT, de Zeeuw D. The antihypertensive and renal effects of angiotensin II receptor antagonists: remaining questions. *Curr Opin Nephrol Hypertens* 2000;9:57–61.

167. Uehara Y, Hirawa N, Kawabata Y. Angiotensin II subtype-1 receptor antagonists improve hemodynamic and renal changes without affecting glucose metabolisms in genetic rat model of non-insulin-dependent diabetes mellitus. *Am J Hypertens* 1999;12:21–27.

168. Taal MW, Brenner BM. ACE-I vs angiotensin II receptor antagonists: prevention of renal injury in chronic rat models. *J Hum Hypertens* 1999;13[Suppl 1]:S51–S56.

169. Mackenzie HS, Ots M, Ziai F. Angiotensin receptor antagonists in experimental models of chronic renal failure. *Kidney Int Suppl* 1997;63:S140–S143.

170. Pamboukian SV, Aminbakhsh A, Thompson CR. Carvedilol improves functional class in patients with severe left ventricular dysfunction referred for heart transplantation. *Clin Transplant* 1999;13:426–431.

171. Szczech LA, Reddan DN, Owen WF. Differential survival following coronary revascularization procedures among patients with renal insufficiency. *Kidney Int* 2001;60:292–299.

172. Rinehart AL, Herzog CA, Collins AJ. A comparison of coronary angioplasty and coronary artery bypass grafting outcomes in chronic dialysis patients. *Am J Kidney Dis* 1995;25:281–290.

173. Simsir SA, Kohlman-Trigoboff D, Flood R. A comparison of coronary artery bypass grafting and percutaneous transluminal coronary angioplasty in patients on hemodialysis. *Cardiovasc Surg* 1998;6:500–505.

174. Manske CL, Wang Y, Rector T. Coronary revascularisation in insulin-dependent diabetic patients with chronic renal failure. *Lancet* 1992;340:998–1002.

175. Lewis MS, Wilson RA, Walker K. Factors in cardiac risk stratification of candidates for renal transplant. *J Cardiovasc Risk* 1999;6:251–255.

176. Le A, Wilson R, Douek K. Prospective risk stratification in renal transplant candidates for cardiac death. *Am J Kidney Dis* 1994;24:65–71.

177. Manske CL, Thomas W, Wang Y. Screening diabetic transplant candidates for coronary artery disease: identification of a low risk subgroup. *Kidney Int* 1993;44:617–621.

178. McGregor E, Jardine AG, Murray LS, et al. Pre-operative echocardiographic abnormalities and adverse outcome following renal transplantation. *Nephrol Dial Transplant* 1998;13:1499–1505.

179. Ahmed WH, Shubrooks SJ, Gibson CM. Complications and long-term outcome after percutaneous coronary angioplasty in chronic hemodialysis patients. *Am Heart J* 1994;128:252–255.

180. Kahn JK, Rutherford BD, McConahay DR. Short- and long-term outcome of percutaneous transluminal coronary angioplasty in chronic dialysis patients. *Am Heart J* 1990;119:484–489.

181. Reusser LM, Osborn LA, White HJ. Increased morbidity after coronary angioplasty in patients on chronic hemodialysis. *Am J Cardiol* 1994;73:965–967.

182. Sharma SK, Cheema P, Andrews AS. Current status of PCI in patients with chronic renal failure on hemodialysis: acute and long-term results. *Eur Heart J* 2000;[Suppl]:646.

183. Le Feuvre C, Dambrin G, Helft G. Comparison of clinical outcome following coronary stenting or balloon angioplasty in dialysis versus non-dialysis patients. *Am J Cardiol* 2000;85:1365–1368.

184. Weinbrenner C, Tuischer J, Eldelmann F. Mild to moderate renal insufficiency promotes the risk of restenosis after stent implantation. *Eur Heart J* 2000;[Suppl]:391.

185. Frilling B, Zahn R, Fraiture B. Same efficacy but higher complication rates in patients with renal insufficiency treated with the IIb/IIIa-antagonists abciximab. *Circulation* 2000;102:II-615.

186. Hang CL, Chen MC, Wu BJ. Short- and long-term outcomes after percutaneous transluminal coronary angioplasty in chronic hemodialysis patients. *Catheter Cardiovasc Intervent* 1999;47:430–433.

187. Marso SP, Gimple LW, Philbrick JT. Effectiveness of percutaneous coronary interventions to prevent recurrent coronary events in patients on chronic hemodialysis. *Am J Cardiol* 1998;82:378–380.

188. Schwarz U, Buzello M, Ritz E, et al. Morphology of coronary atherosclerotic lesions in patients with end-stage renal failure. *Nephrol Dial Transplant* 2000;15:218–223.

189. Schoebel FC, Gradaus F, Ivens K. Restenosis after elective coronary balloon angioplasty in patients with end stage renal disease: a case-control study using quantitative coronary angiography. *Heart* 1997;78:337–342.

190. Herzog C, Ma J, Collins A. Long-term outcome of dialysis patients in the US after coronary artery bypass surgery, coronary angioplasty and coronary stenting. *Circulation* 2000;102:II-389.

191. Frenken M, Krian A. Cardiovascular operations in patients with dialysis-dependent renal failure. *Ann Thorac Surg* 1999;68:887–893.

192. Chertow GM, Lazarus JM, Christiansen CL, et al. Preoperative renal risk stratification. *Circulation* 1997;95:878–884.

193. Samuels LE, Sharma S, Morris RJ. Coronary artery bypass grafting in patients with chronic renal failure: a reappraisal. *J Cardiol Surg* 1996;11:128–133.

194. Mangano CM, Diamondstone LS, Ramsay JG, et al. Renal dysfunction after myocardial revascularization: risk factors, adverse outcomes, and hospital resource utilization. The Multicenter Study of Perioperative Ischemia Research Group. *Ann Intern Med* 1998;128:194–203.

195. Ferguson ER, Hudson SL, Diethelm AG. Outcome after myocardial revascularization and renal transplantation: a 25-year single-institution experience. *Ann Surg* 1999;230:232–241.

196. Koyanagi T, Nishida H, Endo M. Coronary artery bypass grafting in chronic renal dialysis patients: intensive perioperative dialysis and extensive usage of arterial grafts. *Eur J Cardiothorac Surg* 1994;8:505–507.

197. Marshall WG Jr, Rossi NP, Meng RL. Coronary artery bypass grafting in dialysis patients. *Ann Thorac Surg* 1986;42:S12–S15.

198. Opsahl JA, Husebye DG, Helseth HK, et al. Coronary artery bypass surgery in patients on maintenance dialysis: long-term survival. *Am J Kidney Dis* 1988;12:271–274.

199. Owen CH, Cummings RG, Sell TL. Coronary artery bypass grafting in patients with dialysis-dependent renal failure. *Ann Thorac Surg* 1994;58:1729–1733.

200. Jahangiri M, Wright J, Edmondson S. Coronary artery bypass graft surgery in dialysis patients. *Heart* 1997;78:343–345.

201. Khaitan L, Sutter RP, Goldman SM. Coronary artery bypass grafting in patients who require long-term dialysis. *Ann Thorac Surg* 2000;69:1135–1139.

202. Labrousse L, de Vincentiis C, Madonna F. Early and long term results of coronary artery bypass grafts in patients with dialysis dependent renal failure. *Eur J Cardiothorac Surg* 1999;15:691–696.

203. Anderson RJ, O'Brien M, McWhinney S. Renal failure predisposes patients to adverse outcome after coronary artery bypass surgery. VA Cooperative Study 5. *Kidney Int* 1999;55:1057–1062.

204. Koomans HA, Geers AB, Mees EJ. Plasma volume recovery after ultrafiltration in patients with chronic renal failure. *Kidney Int* 1984;26:848–854.

205. Mellander S, Oberg B. Transcapillary fluid absorption and other vascular reactions in the human forearm during reduction of the circulating blood volume. *Acta Physiol Scand* 1967;71:37–46.

206. Degoulet P, Reach I, Di Giulio S, et al. Epidemiology of dialysis induced hypotension. *Proc Eur Dial Transplant Assoc* 1981;18:133–138.

207. Jaraba M, Rodriguez-Benot A, Guerrero R, et al. Cardiovascular response to hemodialysis: the effects of uremia and dialysate buffer. *Kidney Int Suppl* 1998;68:S86–S91.

208. Aizawa Y, Ohmori T, Imai K. Depressant action of acetate upon the human cardiovascular system. *Clin Nephrol* 1977;8:477–480.

209. Iseki K, Onoyama K, Maeda T, et al. Comparison of hemodynamics induced by conventional acetate hemodialysis, bicarbonate hemodialysis and ultrafiltration. *Clin Nephrol* 1980;14:294–298.

210. Levine J, Falk B, Henriquez M. Effects of varying dialysate sodium using large surface area dialyzers. *Trans Am Soc Artif Intern Organs* 1978;24:139–141.

211. Stewart WK, Fleming LW, Manuel MA. Benefits obtained by the use of high sodium dialysate during maintenance haemodialysis. *Proc Eur Dial Transplant Assoc* 1972;9:111–118.

212. Henrich WL, Woodard TD, McPhaul JJ Jr. The chronic efficacy and safety of high sodium dialysate: double-blind, crossover study. *Am J Kidney Dis* 1982;2:349–353.

213. Churchill DN. Sodium and water profiling in chronic uraemia. *Nephrol Dial Transplant* 1996;11[Suppl 8]:38–41.

214. Henrich WL, Hunt JM, Nixon JV. Increased ionized calcium and left ventricular contractility during hemodialysis. *N Engl J Med* 1984;310:19–23.

215. Leunissen KM, van den Berg BW, van Hooff JP. Ionized calcium plays a pivotal role in controlling blood pressure during haemodialysis. *Blood Purif* 1989;7:233–239.

216. Rakash N, Danziger R. Dialysate magnesium concentration predicts the occurrence of intradialytic hypotension [abst]. *J Am Soc Nephrol* 1996;7:1496.

217. Sherman RA, Torres F, Cody RP. The effect of red cell transfusion on hemodialysis-related hypotension. *Am J Kidney Dis* 1988;11:33–35.

218. Ritz E, Bosch J, Henderson LW, et al. Hemofiltration and vascular stability. *Contrib Nephrol* 1982;32:200–217.

219. Chanard J, Brunois JP, Melin JP. Long-term results of dialysis therapy with a highly permeable membrane. *Artif Organs* 1982;6:261–266.

220. Locatelli F, Mastrangelo F, Redaelli B, et al. Effects of different membranes and dialysis technologies on patient treatment tolerance and nutritional parameters. The Italian Cooperative Dialysis Study Group. *Kidney Int* 1996;50:1293–1302.

221. Van Der Sande FM, Gladziwa U. Energy transfer is the single most important factor for the difference in vascular response between isolated ultrafiltration and hemodialysis. *J Am Soc Nephrol* 2000;11:1512–1517.

222. Hampl H, Paeprer H, Unger V. Hemodynamics during hemodialysis, sequential ultrafiltration and hemofiltration. *J Dialysis* 1979;3:51–71.

223. Renfrew R, Buselmeier TJ, Kjellstrand CM. Pericarditis and renal failure. *Annu Rev Med* 1980;31:345–360.

224. Wizemann V, Kramer W. Choice of ESRD treatment strategy according to cardiac status. *Kidney Int Suppl* 1988;24:S191–S195.

225. Shapira OM, Bar-Khayim Y. ECG changes and cardiac arrhythmias in chronic renal failure patients on hemodialysis. *J Electrocardiol* 1992;25:273–279.

226. D'Elia JA, Weinrauch LA, Gleason RE, et al. Application of the ambulatory 24-hour electrocardiogram in the prediction of cardiac death in dialysis patients. *Arch Intern Med* 1988;148:2381–2385.

227. Chazan J. Sudden death in patients with chronic renal failure on hemodialysis. *Dial Transplant* 1987;16:447–448.

228. Fantuzzi S, Caico S, Amatruda O, et al. Hemodialysis-associated cardiac arrhythmias: a lower risk with bicarbonate? *Nephron* 1991;58:196–200.

229. Morrison G, Michelson EL, Brown S. Mechanism and prevention of cardiac arrhythmias in chronic hemodialysis patients. *Kidney Int* 1980;17:811–819.

230. Burns CB, Scheinhorn DJ. Hypoxemia during hemodialysis. *Arch Intern Med* 1982;142:1350–1353.

231. Shinzato T, Miwa M, Nakai S, et al. Role of adenosine in dialysis-induced hypotension. *J Am Soc Nephrol* 1994;4:1987–1994.

232. Nakamura S, Uzu T, Inenaga T. Prediction of coronary artery disease and cardiac events using electrocardiographic changes during hemodialysis. *Am J Kidney Dis* 2000;36:592–599.

233. Steuer RR, Leypoldt JK, Cheung AK. Reducing symptoms during hemodialysis by continuously monitoring the hematocrit. *Am J Kidney Dis* 1996;27:525–532.

234. London GM, Parfrey PS. Cardiac disease in chronic uremia: pathogenesis. *Adv Ren Replace Ther* 1997;4:194–211.

235. Parfrey P, Foley R. Cardiac disease in dialysis patients. In: *Dialysis and transplantation.* Philadelphia: WB Saunders, 2000:221–236.

236. Bleyer AJ, Russell GB, Satko SG. Sudden and cardiac death rates in hemodialysis patients. *Kidney Int* 1999;55:1553–1559.

237. Deligiannis A, Paschalidou E, Sakellariou G, et al. Changes in left ventricular anatomy during haemodialysis, continuous ambulatory peritoneal dialysis and after renal transplantation. *Proceedings of the European Dialysis & Transplant Association—European Renal Association* 1985;21:185–189.

238. Mak RH, DeFronzo RA. Glucose and insulin metabolism in uremia. *Nephron* 1992;61:377–382.

239. Ramos JM, Heaton A, McGurk JG. Sequential changes in serum lipids and their subfractions in patients receiving continuous ambulatory peritoneal dialysis. *Nephron* 1983;35:20–23.

240. Prichard S. Major and minor risk factors for cardiovascular disease in peritoneal dialysis. *Periton Dial Int* 2000;20[Suppl 2]:S154–S159.

241. Dawnay A, Millar DJ. The pathogenesis and consequences of AGE formation in uraemia and its treatment. *Cell Mol Biol* 1998;44:1081–1094.

242. Burt RK, Gupta-Burt S, Suki WN. Reversal of left ventricular dysfunction after renal transplantation. *Ann Intern Med* 1989;111:635–640.

243. Rao KV, Andersen RC. Long-term results and complications in renal transplant recipients. Observations in the second decade. *Transplantation* 1988;45:45–52.

244. Braun WE. Long-term complications of renal transplantation. *Kidney Int* 1990;37:1363–1378.

245. Herzog CA, Ma JZ, Collins AJ. Long-term survival of renal transplant recipients in the United States after acute myocardial infarction. *Am J Kidney Dis* 2000;36:145–152.

246. Charnick SB, Nedelman JR, Chang CT, et al. Description of blood pressure changes in patients beginning cyclosporin A therapy. *Ther Drug Monit* 1997;19:17–24.

247. Amberger A, Hala M, Saurwein-Teissl M, et al. Suppressive effects of anti-inflammatory agents on human endo-

thelial cell activation and induction of heat shock proteins. *Mol Med* 1999;5:117–128.

248. Bouchard D, Despatis MA, Buluran J. Vascular effects of cyclosporin A and acute rejection in canine heart transplantation. *Ann Thorac Surg* 1997;64:1325–1330.

249. Jenkins JT, Boyle JJ, McKay IC. Vascular remodeling in intramyocardial resistance vessels in hypertensive human cardiac transplant recipients. *Heart* 1997;77:353–356.

250. Emeson EE, Shen ML. Accelerated atherosclerosis in hyperlipidemic C57BL/6 mice treated with cyclosporin A. *Am J Pathol* 1993;142:1906–1915.

251. Varghese Z, Fernando RL, Turakhia G, et al. Calcineurin inhibitors enhance low-density lipoprotein oxidation in transplant patients. *Kidney Int Suppl* 1999;71:S137–S140.

252. Murray BM, Paller MS, Ferris TF. Effect of cyclosporine administration on renal hemodynamics in conscious rats. *Kidney Int* 1985;28:767–774.

253. Scoble JE, Freestone A, Varghese Z. Cyclosporin-induced renal magnesium leak in renal transplant patients. *Nephrol Dial Transplant* 1990;5:812–815.

254. Zazgornik J, Shaheen FA, Kopsa H. Severe hyperkalaemia, hyperchloraemia, hyporeninaemia and hyperaldosteronism in a cyclosporin-treated renal-transplant patient. *Nephrol Dial Transplant* 1988;3:826–829.

255. Adu D, Turney J, Michael J, et al. Hyperkalaemia in cyclosporin-treated renal allograft recipients. *Lancet* 1983;2:370–372.

256. Katari SR, Magnone M, Shapiro R, et al. Clinical features of acute reversible tacrolimus (FK 506) nephrotoxicity in kidney transplant recipients. *Clin Transplant* 1997;11:237–242.

257. Jindal RM, Sidner RA, Milgrom ML. Post-transplant diabetes mellitus. The role of immunosuppression. *Drug Saf* 1997;16:242–257.

258. Tamura K, Fujimura T, Tsutsumi T, et al. Transcriptional inhibition of insulin by FK506 and possible involvement of FK506 binding protein-12 in pancreatic beta-cell. *Transplantation* 1995;59:1606–1613.

259. A comparison of tacrolimus (FK 506) and cyclosporine for immunosuppression in liver transplantation. The U.S. Multicenter FK506 Liver Study Group. *N Engl J Med* 1994;331:1110–1115.

THE HEART AND OTHER ORGAN SYSTEMS

Cardiac Manifestations of Selected Neurologic Disorders

KENNETH W. MAHAFFEY
DANIEL T. LASKOWITZ

OVERVIEW

Cardiac manifestations of neurologic disorders are common and diverse. Understanding the pathophysiology of cardiac and neurologic disorders is critical for physicians caring for patients with cardiovascular and neurologic disease states and investigators attempting to develop therapies and management strategies for disorders that have both central nervous system (CNS) and cardiovascular components. The importance of interactions between cardiology and neurology is exemplified by ongoing collaborative efforts between cardiologists and neurologists in several key clinical areas, including stroke prevention in atrial fibrillation, percutane-

ous intervention in cerebrovascular occlusive disease, and the use of thrombolytic and antiplatelet therapies in non-hemorrhagic stroke. Many of these specific issues are discussed in other chapters. In this chapter, the focus is on cardiac manifestations of specific CNS events and the cardiac anomalies associated with hereditary and acquired neuromuscular disorders.

CARDIAC MANIFESTATIONS OF CENTRAL NERVOUS SYSTEM EVENTS

It was more than 60 years ago that Beattie and colleagues recognized that the CNS had neurogenic input in cardiac arrhythmias (1). Soon after, Aschenbrenner and Bodechtel reported electrocardiographic (ECG) abnormalities in young patients with brain lesions and presumed normal cardiac structure (2). It is now commonly known that ECG

K. W. Mahaffey: Department of Cardiology, Duke Clinical Research Institute, Duke University Medical Center, Durham, North Carolina
D. T. Laskowitz: Department of Medicine, Duke University School of Medicine, Duke University Medical Center, Durham, North Carolina

abnormalities can occur in the setting of CNS abnormalities such as ischemic stroke, intracranial hemorrhage, seizure, headache, meningitis, encephalitis, and cranial trauma. Generally, these ECG features can be interpreted correctly in the setting of known or suspected neurologic disease. However, the erroneous diagnosis of primary cardiac disease can occur and, more importantly, result in inappropriate therapy or delay in proper treatment. Substantial work has been done to attempt to understand the pathophysiology of these cardiac manifestations.

Acute Ischemic Stroke

Cardiovascular complications are extremely common following stroke and represent a major form of morbidity. These complications may be caused by focal cerebral injury or may be a manifestation of preexisting cardiac disease, which is common in this patient population.

Several studies have documented a high prevalence of ECG changes and arrhythmias in patients presenting with acute ischemic stroke. Common ECG changes include QT prolongation, T-wave abnormalities, prominent U waves, and ST-segment abnormalities (*e*Table 35D.0.1) (3–7). Although ECG changes are common with ischemic stroke, interpretation of these studies is difficult, as the prevalence of asymptomatic coronary artery disease in patients with symptomatic cerebrovascular disease has been reported to be as high as 28% to 65% (8,9). Thus, cerebrovascular disease may be a marker for coronary artery disease that becomes clinically apparent during the physiologic stress of acute ischemic stroke. Few studies have systematically examined old tracings to establish if the ECG changes were new (10). There has been no definitive correlation between the presence of ECG changes and cerebral infarct location.

Arrhythmias are also common after acute ischemic stroke (*e*Table 35D.0.1). Atrial fibrillation has been most frequently described, although it is often unclear whether the atrial fibrillation was the cause of a cardioembolic event or secondary to cerebral infarction (3,10,11). Ventricular ectopy has also been frequently reported, although episodes of sustained ventricular tachycardia are distinctly uncommon. Atrioventricular (AV) block has been reported and has been attributed to excessive vagal stimulation (12). Intensive monitoring of patients presenting with acute stroke has increased the recognition of these arrhythmias, but this practice has not been shown to reduce morbidity or mortality. Because life-threatening arrhythmias in these patients are uncommon, it may be difficult to show a clear benefit. Prolonged cardiac monitoring, however, may be a useful diagnostic tool to help define the stroke etiology.

As many as 15% of patients with acute ischemic stroke may suffer a myocardial infarction (13,14). With the high coexistence between coronary artery and cerebrovascular disease, it is difficult to imply causality, although it is clear that there is a significantly increased morbidity in ischemic stroke patients who have a concurrent myocardial infarction.

Intracranial Hemorrhage

Byer et al. in 1947 first reported large T waves and QT prolongation in a patient with subarachnoid hemorrhage (15). The first systematic review of ECGs in patients with intracerebral or subarachnoid hemorrhage was done in 1954 and reported that QT prolongation, increased T-wave amplitude, and abnormal U waves were the most common abnormalities (16). Others have reported similar changes in small groups (*e*Table 35D.0.1) (17,18).   h04

The largest comparative series documenting specific ECG abnormalities in stroke patients included 150 stroke patients and 150 age- and sex-matched controls: 92% of stroke patients and 65% of controls had abnormal ECG results. Abnormal ECGs were found in 43 (98%) patients with intracranial hemorrhage. The most common ECG changes were QT prolongation, T-wave inversion, and prominent U waves. Few ECG findings characterized a particular stroke type. Atrial fibrillation was significantly more common in patients with cerebral embolus (47% vs. 9% for other stroke type), and QT prolongation was most common in patients with subarachnoid hemorrhage (71% vs. 39% for other stroke types). U waves were more common in patients with intracranial hemorrhage than in patients with other stroke types (25% vs. 8%). Prior ECG abnormalities were seen in 91% of stroke patients and 71% of controls. New ECG abnormalities at the time of stroke were identified in 74% of stroke patients and 14% of controls.

Supraventricular and ventricular arrhythmias as well as conduction abnormalities have been well documented in patients with intracranial hemorrhage (*e*Table 35D.0.1). Several observational series have reported arrhythmias in 47% to 90% of patients (10,11,21,22) and serious or life-threatening arrhythmias in 20% to 50% of patients with intracranial hemorrhage (21,23–25). However, because of diverse patient populations, the level of cardiac monitoring, and the severity of the disease state, the true incidence of specific arrhythmias is unknown.

The best data for the incidence of arrhythmias in stroke patients are from a large series reported by Di Pasquale and colleagues (21). Twenty-four-hour Holter monitor recordings were performed on 120 patients with subarachnoid hemorrhage: 96 of 107 patients (90%) with adequate recordings had arrhythmias. The most common arrhythmias were premature ventricular contractions (46%), sinus bradycardia (39%), sinus tachycardia (30%), sinus arrhythmia (30%), supraventricular premature complexes (27%), and sinoatrial block (21%) (*e*Table 35D.0.2).   h05

The implications of arrhythmias are important because they can cause hemodynamic compromise that may have adverse effects on cerebral perfusion or may increase the risk of further cerebral insult such as with atrial fibrillation. The presence of malignant ventricular arrhythmias or asystole has been reported as a univariable predictor of mortality after intracranial hemorrhage (10).

Management of Arrhythmias in Patients with Intracranial Hemorrhage or Ischemic Stroke

Management of patients with arrhythmias in the setting of intracranial hemorrhage has not been studied rigorously. Because of the high incidence of arrhythmias, continuous ECG monitoring is recommended, but there is no consensus about its required duration. Patients with QT prolongation should be monitored closely, and possible causative factors such as medications or electrolyte abnormalities should be identified and corrected. Patients with torsades de pointes have been treated with atrial or ventricular overdrive pacing or isoproterenol. Left stellate ganglion block has also been proposed in patients with recurrent arrhythmias (32).

Intracranial Hemorrhage and Electrocardiographic Changes Consistent with Acute Myocardial Infarction

Multiple cases of patients with intracranial hemorrhage and ECG changes consistent with acute myocardial infarction and normal coronary anatomy by cardiac catheterization or at autopsy have been reported (33–38). Although a rare clinical entity, physicians need to be aware that ECG changes and symptoms consistent with myocardial ischemia or acute infarction coexist with intracranial hemorrhage. ▼ h06

Mechanisms of Electrocardiographic Changes and Arrhythmias in Patients with Intracranial Hemorrhage or Ischemic Stroke

Substantial work in experimental models and humans has been done to try to understand the pathogenesis of the ECG changes seen in patients with cerebrovascular events. The first comprehensive report of CNS control of cardiovascular function was proposed more than a century ago by Jackson (39). The most widely accepted mechanism by which lesions in the CNS result in changes in the ECG is a direct result of alterations in the autonomic nervous system control on cardiac electrophysiology. Several other processes are considered contributory, including a direct effect on the myocardium, consequences of the associated hemodynamic derangements, electrolyte abnormalities, alterations in circulating catecholamine levels, or concurrent coronary artery disease. ▼ h07

The ECG changes seen in patients with CNS disorders are not completely explained by alterations in catechol-amine levels or changes in sympathetic or vagal tone. Patients with cerebrovascular disease are also at risk for cardiovascular disease. Hertzer and colleagues performed cardiac catheterization on 1,000 patients undergoing vascular surgery (64). In the subgroup of 295 patients with a primary diagnosis of cerebrovascular disease, 59% of the patients had significant coronary artery disease, and almost one-half (44%) of the patients without symptoms of coronary disease had significant stenosis, severe operable, or severe inoperable coronary atherosclerotic disease. Patients with coronary disease may manifest symptoms of cardiac ischemia and associated ECG changes during acute CNS processes. Transient coronary vasospasm may also contribute to the ECG changes. Abnormal electrolyte concentrations, particularly hypokalemia, may also contribute to some of the ECG findings seen in patients with intracranial hemorrhage. Vomiting is common in patients with increased intracranial pressure and elevated levels of circulating catecholamines, and cortisol may be responsible for the electrolyte abnormalities.

The pathogenic mechanism for arrhythmias has not been determined clearly. Experimental studies have demonstrated that injection of blood into the subarachnoid space is associated with the rapid onset of arrhythmias. Chronic elevations of intracranial pressure, however, typically cause bradyarrhythmias (65–67). Others have observed premature ventricular contractions and ventricular arrhythmias in anesthetized cats during stimulation of the hypothalamus, particularly the posterior hypothalamus (1). Based on these animal models and clinical observations, several mechanisms for the arrhythmias have been proposed. Sudden increases in intracranial pressure cause compression on the brainstem and diencephalic structures, which results in increased sympathetic or vagal stimulation of the heart. Alterations in cerebral vascular tone may cause changes in systemic hemodynamics. Underlying coronary artery disease and hypertensive heart disease, which are common in patients with cerebrovascular disease, may be contributing factors in some patients (11). Hypoxia caused by respiratory compromise, elevated catecholamines, and electrolyte imbalances, particularly hypokalemia, may also contribute to the arrhythmias (21).

Myocardial Damage in Patients with Intracranial Hemorrhage and Ischemic Stroke

Some controversy remains as to whether ECG abnormalities observed in patients with acute ischemic stroke or intracranial hemorrhage are caused solely by alterations in autonomic control or whether they represent primary myocardial changes. Experimental studies have shown pathologic myocardial changes after intracranial blood injection in mice (68,69). Focal myocardial lesions consisting of infiltrates of lymphocytes or histiocytes, which displaced or replaced short segments of myocardium, were seen in 45%

of rats with experimentally induced intracranial hemorrhage (70). Subendocardial hemorrhages have been reported after subarachnoid hemorrhage and stellate ganglion stimulation in animals (71,72). The incidence of these myocardial changes was dramatically reduced in rats treated with propranolol. Others have reported similar findings (73,74). Several investigators have shown focal necrosis, myofibrillar degeneration, and inflammatory cell infiltration in animals after catecholamine infusions or hypothalamic stimulation (73,75–81).

Despite numerous reports of patients with normal myocardium after stroke even in the presence of ECG changes (18,20,35,82), data from human autopsy series suggest that a subgroup of patients with acute ischemic stroke or intracranial hemorrhage may have abnormal myocardial pathology. In two autopsy series, 8% to 12% of patients with intracranial hemorrhage, tumor, infection, or head injury had foci of myocytolysis predominantly in the left ventricle, without evidence of infarction (63,83). Focal myocytolysis is often seen with myocardial infarction, but is a distinctive lesion. It was first reported by Schlesinger and Reiner (84). The characteristic features of myocytolysis are loss of sarcoplasm from focal areas of myocardium with retention of the cellular nuclei and sarcolemma. ❦ h08

Epilepsy

Cardiac arrhythmias are common during partial and generalized seizure activity and may be associated with significant morbidity and mortality. In several series, sinus tachycardia was the most common arrhythmia and was present during 97% of ictal episodes. By contrast, severe or life-threatening arrhythmias were present in only 5% of patients (90–93). There have been numerous reports of cardiac arrest and asystole associated with seizure activity, and undiagnosed seizure disorders have presented as unexplained syncope (94–98). ❦ h09

Migraine Headache

The precise etiology of migraine headaches is unknown. Migraine headaches are generally thought to be associated with arterial vasomotor and autonomic nervous system abnormalities. There are reports of typical angina-like chest pain and myocardial infarction in patients during the acute phase of a migraine headache. A generalized vasospastic disorder has been suggested to explain these findings (107,108). Ischemic ECG changes have been reported with normal coronary angiography, supporting coronary spasm as the cause of ischemia (107,108). Sympathetic function is impaired in some patients with migraine headaches (109). Several studies of ambulatory ECG monitoring have shown altered autonomic innervation of the heart in patients with migraine compared with controls (110–112).

Common medications used to treat migraine headaches can also have cardiac effects. Ergot compounds and sumatriptan are the two most common therapies used in aborting migraine headache. Dihydroergotamine has a high affinity for 5-HT_1, 5-HT_2, dopamine, and other catecholamine receptors (113). Ergotamine has been shown to precipitate coronary spasm and chest pain in patients with migraine (114). Sumatriptan has a more specific agonist of the presynaptic and postsynaptic $5\text{-HT}_{1B/D}$ receptor and works by constricting large intracranial vessels and blocking neurogenic inflammation (115). Sumatriptan has produced chest pain syndromes (116), and although it may affect blood pressure, the symptoms are generally not associated with ECG changes (117,118). Both agents have the potential for coronary vasoconstriction and are contraindicated in patients with ischemic heart disease or variant angina. Patients with multiple risk factors for ischemic heart disease should undergo evaluation for coronary artery disease, including ECG and stress testing before initiating therapy. Based on the success of sumatriptan, several oral second-generation triptans have also been developed, including zolmitriptan, rizatriptan, and naratriptan. Although experience with these newer agents is more limited and there are conflicting reports regarding their potential for coronary vasoconstriction, all of these drugs maintain the same precautions and contraindications as sumatriptan regarding administration to patients with coronary artery disease.

NEUROMUSCULAR DISORDERS WITH CARDIAC MANIFESTATIONS

Cardiac disease may be associated with the major types of diseases of the peripheral nerves, the neuromuscular junction, and the muscles with varying characteristics and severity. The cardiac manifestations and the clinical features of the neuromuscular disorders are heterogeneous. In some disorders, the most distinguishing feature is a cardiomyopathy, whereas in other disorders, conduction abnormalities are prominent (*e*Table 35D.0.3). The cardiac involvement can be minimal or life threatening. Several of the more common and clinically important diseases are reviewed here.

Disorders of Peripheral Nerves

Guillain-Barré Syndrome

Guillain-Barré syndrome is an acute autoimmune polyneuropathy that involves inflammation and demyelination of nerves and is classically characterized by ascending motor weakness and areflexia. The diagnosis is supported by a compatible clinical presentation, cerebral spinal fluid findings of albuminocytologic dissociation, and electrodiagnostic evidence of acute demyelination. Autonomic and cardiac complications in patients with Guillain-Barré syndrome are more common than generally recognized and may significantly complicate medical management.

Cardiac involvement in Guillain-Barré syndrome was initially described by Sir William Osler in 1892, who made the observation that some patients with "acute febrile neuritis" succumbed to "paralysis of the heart" (128). Cardiac arrhythmias are also common. Sinus tachycardia has been reported in 45% to 79% of patients (129). Bradyarrhythmias, sinus pauses, and asystole are also common and may portend cardiac arrest (130). Some authors recommend prophylactic pacemaker insertion for patients with clinically significant bradycardias or sinus pauses (131–133). Although bradyarrhythmias may occur spontaneously, patients often exhibit vagal hypersensitivity to suctioning, and care should be taken to preoxygenate adequately, suction gently, and administer atropine when appropriate.

Other arrhythmias and conduction abnormalities, although less common, have been described: atrial fibrillation, atrial flutter, paroxysmal atrial tachycardia, and ventricular tachycardia (130,131,134). Cardiac involvement usually parallels severity of disease, and patients at the highest risk for malignant arrhythmias are often ventilator dependent and have more fulminant disease progression. ECG abnormalities have also been described in Guillain-Barré syndrome, with nonspecific ST-T–wave changes observed most commonly (130).

Autonomic neuropathy is commonly associated with Guillain-Barré syndrome and may be associated with cardiac dysfunction. Early evidence of autonomic dysfunction may become clinically manifest as abnormalities of bladder function, gastroparesis, abnormal pseudomotor activity, or blood pressure lability. Formal autonomic testing has revealed subclinical evidence of neuropathy in two-thirds of patients with Guillain-Barré syndrome. It is difficult to get a true measure of the clinically relevant autonomic neuropathy in Guillain-Barré syndrome, as most of the published observations are case reports or small series. Hypertension is common, with a reported incidence of 5% to 79%. Clinically significant hypotension may also occur and is often exacerbated by impaired venous return to the heart caused by positive pressure ventilation and paralysis of the calf and abdominal musculature. The occurrence of dysautonomia in Guillain-Barré syndrome is most likely caused by a failure of baroreflex buffering mechanisms due to deafferentation of baroreceptor impulses.

Recognition of the features of early dysautonomia in the setting of Guillain-Barré syndrome is important. Patients with these symptoms are at increased risk for developing cardiac arrhythmias, especially AV block. Identification of this population with autonomic screening tests has met with limited success (135,136). It is probable that fulminant autonomic neuropathy with inflammation of the small intramyocardial nerves is responsible for the focal myocarditis described in Guillain-Barré syndrome (137). A dysautonomia-induced hypersympathetic state may also be responsible for acute reversible left ventricular dysfunction in these patients (138).

Friedreich's Ataxia

Friedreich's ataxia is an autosomal recessive neurodegenerative disease characterized by progressive ataxia, areflexia, proprioceptive loss, and upper motor neuron findings. When strict neurologic and genetic criteria for this disorder were met, cardiac involvement was reported in more than 90% of the patients (139,140). No correlation between severity of neurologic and cardiac disease has been confirmed.

The most common cardiac abnormality in patients with Friedreich's ataxia is concentric left ventricular hypertrophy (141,142). The cardiac pathology in this disorder is differentiated from genetic hypertrophic cardiomyopathy by the lack of cellular disorganization in the ventricular septum. Echocardiographic assessment of systolic and diastolic function is usually normal. The concentric hypertrophy associated with Friedreich's ataxia also tends to have a more benign course than hypertrophic cardiomyopathy, and malignant arrhythmias are distinctly uncommon (143).

A minority of patients with Friedreich's ataxia may develop a dilated cardiomyopathy associated with global hypokinesis. Although much less common than concentric left ventricular hypertrophy, this carries a worse prognosis, and patients usually experience progressive deterioration of cardiac function (144). Symptomatic atrial and ventricular arrhythmias are more common in this subgroup (139).

Peroneal Muscular Atrophy

Peroneal muscular atrophy includes two autosomal dominant genetic disorders collectively called *Charcot-Marie-Tooth neuropathy*. The clinical features include progressive distal lower extremity muscle weakness that begins in the second or third decade of life. Peroneal muscular atrophy does not normally involve the heart. Atrial flutter has been reported (145), but more common findings are conduction disturbances with complete heart block and right bundle branch block, which have been reported in several members of a family (146–148).

Disorders of the Neuromuscular Junction

Myasthenia Gravis

Myasthenia gravis is caused by an autoimmune process that results in a decrease in the number of acetylcholine receptors at the neuromuscular junction. It affects women more frequently than men and can appear at any age, with increased frequency in the third and fourth decades in women and the sixth and seventh decades in men. Weakness and fatigue are the classic symptoms, with weakness worsening after repeated use and improving after periods of rest.

Substantial data support the association with myocardial disease, particularly with malignant thymoma, although the nature and pathology of this process are unresolved. The cardiac abnormalities may represent a progressive autoimmune process or coincidental findings from other disease processes. Typical cardiac manifestations include nonspecific ECG changes, arrhythmias, and heart failure. The ECG changes have been reversed with neostigmine treatment. Drugs used to treat arrhythmias and cardiac disease, such as quinidine, procainamide, lidocaine, and calcium channel blockers, should be used with caution as they can exacerbate symptoms of myasthenia gravis (149,150).

Disorders of Muscle

Cardiac dysfunction is relatively common with primary disorders of muscle. In some circumstances, these cardiac abnormalities are potentially life-threatening, and cardiac evaluation is an important aspect of the clinical management of these patients. In Duchenne's muscular dystrophy, a dilated cardiomyopathy is present in virtually all patients by the age of 18 years, and management of associated heart failure is an important component of care. In other conditions, such as myotonic dystrophy and polymyositis, the conduction system is preferentially affected and may lead to clinically important arrhythmias or sudden cardiac death. Table 35D.1 summarizes the key neurologic features and cardiac manifestations of these primary muscle disorders.

Duchenne's and Becker's Muscular Dystrophy

Duchenne's muscular dystrophy is an X-linked recessive disorder with an incidence of 1:3,300 male births (151). This disorder, which is caused by a mutation in the dystrophin gene, usually presents in early childhood with severe and progressive muscle wasting. Death usually occurs by the third decade of life and is caused by respiratory and cardiac compromise.

Cardiac abnormalities are common in Duchenne's muscular dystrophy and include ECG changes, dilated cardiomyopathy, and arrhythmias. Up to 90% of patients with Duchenne's muscular dystrophy have characteristic electrographic abnormalities, which include the presence of tall precordial R waves, an increase in R/S ratio in V_1, and deep, narrow Q waves in the left precordial leads (152,153). Rhythm disturbances are also quite common. The majority of patients have sinus tachycardia, which may be either sustained or labile (14). AV block is less common but has been reported. Accelerated AV conduction may lead to a decrement in the PR interval (154). Dilated cardiomyopathy is also common in Duchenne's muscular dystrophy, and heart failure may be the terminal event in 10% of patients (155). Pathologically, patients with Duchenne's muscular dystrophy demonstrate extensive myocardial fibrosis, most prominently in the posterobasal left ventricular wall (154,156,157). There is usually selective sparing of the septum, right ventricle, and atrium. Degenerative changes of the conduction system have also been described (152). Given the absence of dystrophin in all cells, it is unclear why this pattern of selective myocardial involvement occurs.

Clinical management of cardiac complications in patients with Duchenne's muscular dystrophy is an important aspect of their care. In a large, longitudinal study of more than 300 patients, preclinical evidence of cardiac involvement was present in approximately one-fourth of patients younger than 6 years. Clinically apparent cardiomyopathy typically appeared by age 10 years and was present in virtually all patients by age 18 years (158). Surprisingly, given the prevalence and severity of these cardiac abnormalities, most patients usually remain relatively asymptomatic until late in the course of their disease. This may be because of the disproportionate involvement of the muscles of respiration and because these cardiac abnormalities develop slowly enough to allow some degree of compensation (159). In approximately 10% of patients, the proximal cause of death is directly referable to a cardiac cause (155). Female carriers are not usually symptomatic, although ECG abnormalities have been reported (160).

Becker's muscular dystrophy is a milder variant of Duchenne's muscular dystrophy, which is also caused by a mutation of the dystrophin gene. Becker's dystrophy is characterized by a much later onset of weakness and less fulminant progression. Only 10% of patients are wheelchair bound by the fifth decade of life (161). Cardiac abnormalities are similar to those seen in Duchenne's muscular dystrophy, although usually not as severe. Up to 75% of patients with Becker's muscular dystrophy develop cardiac abnormalities, although the majority of these are subclinical. A subset of patients may develop severe cardiomyopathy, often disproportionate to the degree of skeletal muscle weakness (162,163). It is usual for congestive heart failure to be a presenting symptom (164). Thus, longitudinal noninvasive assessment of cardiac function is warranted in patients with Becker's muscular dystrophy. When cardiac failure occurs, symptoms may develop precipitously. Initial management should include diuretics and afterload reduction. Because Becker's muscular dystrophy is associated with a near normal life expectancy, cardiac transplantation has been performed in these circumstances (165).

Myotonic Dystrophy

Myotonic dystrophy is characterized by myotonia, muscle weakness, frontal balding, cataracts, and gonadal dysfunction. It is an autosomal dominant disease, which is caused by an unstable triple repeat expansion in chromosome 19. A variety of cardiac disturbances have been associated with myotonic dystrophy, including conduction abnormalities, mitral valve prolapse, and cardiomyopathy. These usually

TABLE 35D.1 DISORDERS OF MUSCLE ASSOCIATED WITH CARDIAC MANIFESTATIONS

Disease	Genetic association	Neurologic and medical presentation	Cardiac manifestations
Duchenne's muscular dystrophy	X-linked recessive	Presents in early childhood with severe and disabling muscle wasting; pseudohypertrophy	ECG abnormalities: tall precordial R waves, deep narrow Q waves in left precordial leads. Rhythm abnormalities: sinus tachycardia, atrioventricular block, decreased PR interval. Anatomic abnormalities: myocardial fibrosis, dilated cardiomyopathy.
Becker's muscular dystrophy	X-linked recessive	Less fulminant course than Duchenne's muscular dystrophy; only 10% wheelchair bound by fifth decade of life	Similar to Duchenne's muscular dystrophy except less severe and often subclinical; dilated cardiomyopathy may be severe in a subset.
Myotonic dystrophy	Autosomal dominant caused by unstable triple repeat expansion in chromosome 19	Myotonia, muscle weakness, frontal balding, cataracts, and gonadal dysfunction	Conduction abnormalities: first-degree atrioventricular block, intraventricular conduction delay, left anterior hemiblock, right bundle branch block > left bundle branch block. Anatomic abnormalities: mitral valve prolapse, fibrosis and fatty infiltrate of sinoatrial and atrioventricular nodes, dilated cardiomyopathy.
Periodic paralysis	Autosomal dominant; usually present in the first decade of life; hyperkalemic form mapped to chromosome 17	Episodes of proximal > distal muscle weakness may be associated with hypokalemia or hyperkalemia; muscles of respiration rarely involved	ECG abnormalities and arrhythmias associated with alterations in serum potassium; ventricular tachycardia; prolonged QT interval.
Limb-girdle dystrophy	Variable: autosomal recessive and autosomal dominant variants have been reported	Muscle weakness begins in first to fourth decades, often first becoming symptomatic in the proximal lower extremities	Cardiac involvement uncommon, but ECG abnormalities, conduction disturbances, and cardiomyopathy with congestive heart failure have been reported.
Facioscapuloperoneal dystrophy	Autosomal dominant; mapped to long arm of chromosome 4	Facial weakness in first or second decade progressing to upper and lower extremities	Cardiac involvement uncommon; atrial standstill has been reported.
Scapuloperoneal	X-linked	Myopathy of shoulder girdle and distal lower extremities	Conduction abnormalities: complete heart block and sudden cardiac death reported in third and fourth decade.
Centronuclear myopathy	No definitive inheritance pattern	Ptosis, hyporeflexia, slowly progressive myopathy	Dilated cardiomyopathy, myocardial fibrosis, congestive heart failure, sudden cardiac death reported.
Polymyositis	No definitive inheritance pattern; triggered by viral infections, autoimmune	Proximal muscle weakness	Rhythm abnormalities common and include atrial fibrillation, atrial flutter, frequent atrial premature contractions, ventricular premature contractions; conduction abnormalities common; anatomic abnormalities include fibrosis, diffuse interstitial and perivascular mononuclear infiltrates, muscle fiber degeneration, mitral valve prolapse, and cardiomyopathy.
Kearns-Sayre syndrome	Mitochondrial cytopathy	Progressive external ophthalmoplegia, retinal pigmentary degeneration, myopathy	Conduction abnormalities include right bundle branch block, left anterior hemiblock, atrioventricular block. Sudden cardiac death reported; often selective infranodal involvement with normal PR interval.

ECG, electrocardiographic.

become clinically symptomatic several years after the onset of other symptoms associated with myotonic dystrophy.

Conduction disturbances account for the most common abnormality in this condition. Approximately 90% of patients with myotonic dystrophy eventually have ECG abnormalities (166). The most frequent abnormalities are first-degree AV block and intraventricular conduction delay (167,168). In one series, first-degree AV block was seen in

approximately two-thirds of patients, and one-third had right bundle branch block or left anterior hemiblock. Left bundle branch block was less common (169). These conduction disturbances are probably progressive, but only a few small longitudinal studies have evaluated the natural history.

Approximately one-fourth of patients have evidence of mitral valve prolapse, although the significance of this is unclear given the high prevalence of this condition in the general population (170,171). In one of the few series examining the cardiac pathology of patients with myotonic dystrophy, fibrosis and fatty infiltrate of the sinoatrial and AV nodes, conduction system, and ventricular walls were noted (172). Recognition of the high incidence of cardiac pathology plays an important role in the management of patients with myotonic dystrophy. In general, the cardiac abnormalities associated with myotonic dystrophy are relatively well tolerated, although 7% of patients have clinical evidence of heart failure, and sudden cardiac death has been reported (173,174).

Polymyositis

Polymyositis is a nonsuppurative inflammatory process of skeletal muscle and thought to be caused by genetic factors, viral infections, and autoimmune mechanisms. The heart is infrequently involved. The myocardium can have diffuse interstitial and perivascular mononuclear infiltrates, muscle fiber degeneration, and fibrosis (195,196). The conduction system, including the sinoatrial node, bundle of His, and left and right bundle branches, can be involved with similar histologic changes (197,198). Several series have found ECG changes and arrhythmias in more than one-half of the patients (199,200). ⟡ h10

Kearns-Sayre Syndrome

The mitochondrial myopathies are a heterogeneous collection of diseases characterized by abnormal muscle fibers. Cardiac involvement is rare. The Kearns-Sayre syndrome, however, is characterized by the triad of progressive external ophthalmoplegia, retinal pigmentary degeneration, and heart block (203). The syndrome is generally thought to be acquired, afflicting both sexes equally, with onset before the age of 20. Common features include ataxia, hearing loss, dementia, short stature, delayed secondary sexual characteristics, peripheral neuropathy, and endocrine abnormalities.

Cardiac abnormalities almost exclusively involve the conduction system. Characteristic conduction abnormalities are right bundle branch block, left anterior fascicular block, and atrioventricular block (204–206). A normal PR is common because of the selective infranodal involvement. Sudden death has been recognized, and pacemaker insertion is recommended (207).

CARDIOVASCULAR ABNORMALITIES IN NEURODEGENERATIVE DISEASES

Parkinson's Disease

Cardiovascular abnormalities are common in Parkinson's disease and may be challenging to manage. In particular, autonomic dysfunction is prevalent, and orthostatic hypotension often exacerbates postural instability, one of the hallmarks of this neurodegenerative disorder. Lewy bodies, the eosinophilic cytoplasmic inclusions characteristic of Parkinson's disease pathology, have been identified throughout the autonomic nervous system, including the hypothalamus, sympathetic system (thoracic intermediolateral nucleus and sympathetic ganglia), and parasympathetic system (dorsal vagal nucleus and parasympathetic nuclei). Of note, there is also evidence of cardiac sympathetic denervation, and Lewy bodies have been identified in the cardiac plexus (208). Myocardial imaging with ^{123}I-metaiodobenzylguanidine has demonstrated functional loss of cardiac sympathetic tone associated with these anatomic abnormalities (209). Interestingly, the marked decrease in myocardial ^{123}I-metaiodobenzylguanidine uptake appears to be specific for Parkinson's disease and may have some diagnostic value in differentiating atypical Parkinson's disease from other neurodegenerative disorders associated with extrapyramidal features (209). These abnormalities in cardiac autonomic tone seen in Parkinson's disease may also have contributed to several sporadic cases of sudden cardiac death associated with a prolonged QTc interval (210).

Alzheimer's Disease

Although less systematically studied, dysautonomia has also been described in Alzheimer's disease (211). Vascular disease is also associated with dementia and is often difficult to clinically distinguish from Alzheimer's disease. A large population-based study in Rotterdam explored the relationship between atherosclerosis and dementia. Evaluation of 284 demented patients and 1,698 healthy controls revealed that the odds ratio for Alzheimer's disease in those with severe disseminated atherosclerosis compared with those with normal vasculature was 3.0 (212). Although the biology for the association between atherosclerosis and Alzheimer's disease remains undefined, presence of the APOE4 allele appears to be a risk factor. Patients with atherosclerotic cerebrovascular disease and Alzheimer's disease have a higher prevalence of the apolipoprotein E_4 genotype.

CONTROVERSIES AND PERSONAL PERSPECTIVES

A large clinical interface between the practices of cardiology and neurology is becoming increasingly apparent. As cardiac and neurologic intensivists, we see this in a number of situations. The advent of specialized neurocritical care units in parallel with coronary care units is but one example. Another is the American Heart Association emphasis on diagnosis and treatment of "brain attack." We continue to focus on the breakdown of subspecialty barriers because with this approach we will optimize the clinical management of these patient populations.

THE FUTURE

Intensive collaboration between cardiologists and neurologists is ongoing and will result in incredible advances in our understanding of disease mechanisms and therapeutic interventions. Studies evaluating the ability of the brain to withstand ischemic insults, exploration of the use of glycoprotein IIb/IIIa inhibitors and other anticoagulants in patients with both cardiovascular and cerebrovascular disease, and investigation of diagnostic strategies with various biomarkers to diagnose stroke and myocardial infarction are being conducted. Furthermore, as the genetic basis of diseases continues to be unraveled, there will be tremendous opportunities to gain further understanding of the relationships between neuromuscular disorders and associated cardiac manifestations. Work in the basic sciences, clinical trials, and the important translation of scientific discoveries to the bedside will provide ample opportunity in the coming years for cardiologists and neurologists to work together on exciting projects.

REFERENCES

1. Beattie J, Brow GR, Long CNH. Physiological and anatomical evidence for the existence of nerve tracts connecting hypothalamus with spinal sympathetic centers. *Proc R Soc Lond Biol* 1930;106:253–275.
2. Aschenbrenner R, Bodechtel G. Uber EKG veranderungen bei hirntumorkranken. *Klin Wschr* 1938;17:298–302.
3. Dimant J, Grob D. Electrocardiographic changes and myocardial damage in patients with acute cerebrovascular accidents. *Stroke* 1977;8:448–455.
4. Ramani A, Shetty U, Kindaje GN. Electrocardiographic abnormalities in cerebrovascular accidents. *Angiology* 1990;41:681–686.
5. Yamour BJ, Sridharan MR, Rice JF, et al. Electrocardiographic changes in cerebrovascular hemorrhage. *Am Heart J* 1980;99:294–300.
6. Sainani GS, Andarkar SW. Electrocardiographic changes in cerebrovascular accidents. *Indian J Med Sci* 1976;30:331–333.
7. Miura T, Tsuchihashi K, Yoshida E, et al. Electrocardiographic abnormalities in cerebrovascular accidents. *Jpn J Med* 1984;23:22–26.
8. Rokey R, Rolak LA, Harati Y, et al. Coronary artery disease in patients with cerebrovascular disease: a prospective study. *Ann Neurol* 1984;16:50–53.
9. Hertzer NR, Young JR, Beven EG, et al. Coronary angiography in 506 patients with extracranial cerebrovascular disease. *Arch Intern Med* 1985;145:849–852.
10. Goldstein DS. The electrocardiogram in stroke: relationship to pathophysiological type and comparison with prior tracings. *Stroke* 1979;10:253–259.
11. Norris JW, Froggatt GM, Hachinski VC. Cardiac arrhythmias in acute stroke. *Stroke* 1978;9:392–396.
12. Chhetri MK, De B. Electrocardiographic changes in cerebrovascular accident. Role of vagal hyperactivity and intracranial hypertension. *Indian Heart J* 1965;17:347–355.
13. Chin PL, Kaminski J, Rout M. Myocardial infarction coincident with cerebrovascular accidents in the elderly. *Age Ageing* 1977;6:29–37.
14. Rogers FB. Unsuspected cardiac infarction with cerebrovascular accidents. *J Am Geriatr Soc* 1955;3:714–719.
15. Byer E, Ashman R, Toth LA. Electrocardiograms with large upright T-waves and long Q-T intervals. *Am Heart J* 1947;33:796–806.
16. Burch GE, Meyers R, Abildskov JA. A new electrocardiographic pattern observed in cerebrovascular accidents. *Circulation* 1954;9:719–723.
17. Fentz V, Gormsen J. Electrocardiographic patterns in patients with cerebrovascular accidents. *Circulation* 1962;25:22–28.
18. Wasserman F, Choquette G, Cassinelli R, et al. Electrocardiographic observations in patients with cerebrovascular accidents. *Am J Med Sci* 1956;231:502–510.
19. Stern S, Lavy S, Carmon A, et al. Electrocardiographic patterns in haemorrhagic stroke. *J Neurol Sci* 1969;8:61–67.
20. Cropp GJ, Manning GW. Electrocardiographic changes simulating myocardial ischemia and infarction associated with spontaneous intracranial hemorrhage. *Circulation* 1960;22:25–38.
21. Di Pasquale G, Pinelli G, Andreoli A, et al. Holter detection of cardiac arrhythmias in intracranial subarachnoid hemorrhage. *Am J Cardiol* 1987;59:596–600.
22. Lavy S, Yaar I, Melamed E, Stern S. The effect of acute stroke on cardiac functions as observed in an intensive stroke care unit. *Stroke* 1974;5:775–780.
23. Estanol Vidal B, Badui Dergal E, Cesarman E, et al. Cardiac arrhythmias associated with subarachnoid hemorrhage: prospective study. *Neurosurgery* 1979;5:675–680.
24. Sen S, Stober T, Burger L, et al. Long-term recording electrocardiogram in intracranial hemorrhage. *Jpn Heart J* 1982;23:659–661.
25. Mikolich JR, Jacobs WC, Fletcher GF. Cardiac arrhythmias in patients with acute cerebrovascular accidents. *JAMA* 1981;246:1314–1317.
26. Parizel G. Life-threatening arrhythmias in subarachnoid hemorrhage. *Angiology* 1973;24:17–21.
27. Estanol BV, Marin OS. Cardiac arrhythmias and sudden death in subarachnoid hemorrhage. *Stroke* 1975;6:382–386.
28. Carruth JE, Silverman ME. Torsades de pointes atypical ventricular tachycardia complicating subarachnoid hemorrhage. *Chest* 1980;78:886–888.

29. Sen S, Strober T, Burger L, et al. Recurrent torsades de pointes type ventricular tachycardia in intracranial hemorrhage. *Intensive Care Med* 1984;10:263–264.

30. Hust MH, Nitsche K, Hohnloser S, et al. Q-T prolongation and torsades de pointes in a patient with subarachnoid hemorrhage. *Clin Cardiol* 1984;7:44–48.

31. Chao CL, Chen WJ, Wu CC, et al. Torsades de pointes and T-wave alternans in a patient with brainstem hemorrhage. *Int J Cardiol* 1995;51:199–201.

32. Grossman MA. Cardiac arrhythmias in acute central nervous system disease. Successful management with stellate ganglion block. *Arch Intern Med* 1976;136:203–207.

33. Levine H. Non-specificity of the electrocardiogram associated with coronary artery disease. *Am J Med* 1953;15:344–354.

34. Katta SR, Berk WA. Hypertensive intracerebral hemorrhage simulating acute myocardial infarction. *Ann Emerg Med* 1992;21:1002–1005.

35. Menon S. Electrocardiographic changes simulating myocardial infarction in cerebrovascular accident. *Lancet* 1964;11:433–434.

36. Beard EF, Robertson JW, Robertson RCL. Spontaneous subarachnoid hemorrhage simulating acute myocardial infarction. *Am Heart J* 1959;58:755–759.

37. Kitching AD, Bernstein M, O'Kelly BF. Primary intracranial hemorrhage presenting as acute myocardial infarction: a contraindication to thrombolytic therapy. *CMAJ* 1994;150:519–522.

38. Ashby DW, Chadha JS. Electrocardiographic abnormalities simulating myocardial infarction in intracerebral hemorrhage and cerebral thrombosis. *Br Heart J* 1968;30:732–734.

39. Jackson HJ. On the anatomical and physiological localization of movements in the brain. In: Taylor J, ed. *Selected writings of John Hughlings Jackson*. London: Staples Press, 1958:37–76.

40. Fulton JF. *Functional localization in the frontal lobes and cerebellum*. London: Oxford University Press, 1949:66.

41. Kortiweg GCJ, Boeles JTF, TenCate J. Influence of stimulation of some subcortical areas on the electrocardiogram. *J Neurophysiol* 1957;20:100–107.

42. Manning JW, Cotten MD. Mechanism of cardiac arrhythmias induced by diencephalic stimulation. *Am J Physiol* 1962;203:1120–1124.

43. Fuster JM, Weinberg SJ. Bioelectrical changes of the heart cycle induced by stimulation of diencephalic regions. *Exp Neurol* 1960;2:26–39.

44. Weinberg SJ, Fuster JM. Electrocardiographic changes produced by localized hypothalamic stimulations. *Ann Intern Med* 1960;53:332–341.

45. Hoff EC, Kell JF, Carroll MN. Effects of cortical stimulation and lesions on cardiovascular function. *Physiol Rev* 1963;43:68–114.

46. Hockman CH, Mauck HP Jr, Hoff EC. ECG changes resulting from cerebral stimulation. II. A spectrum of ventricular arrhythmias of sympathetic origin. *Am Heart J* 1966;71:695–700.

47. Ruggiero DA, Mraovitch S, Granata AR, et al. A role of insular cortex in cardiovascular function. *J Comp Neurol* 1987;257:189–207.

48. Mesulam MM, Mufson EJ. Insula of the old world monkey. III: Efferent cortical output and comments on function. *J Comp Neurol* 1982;212:38–52.

49. Oppenheimer SM, Cechetto DF. Cardiac chronotropic organization of the rat insular cortex. *Brain Res* 1990;533:66–72.

50. Yanowitz F, Preston JB, Abildskov JA. Functional distribution of right and left stellate innervation to the ventricles. Production of neurogenic electrocardiographic changes by unilateral alteration of sympathetic tone. *Circ Res* 1966;18:416–428.

51. Ueda H, Yanai Y, Murao S, et al. Electrocardiographic and vectorcardiographic changes produced by electrical stimulation of the cardiac nerves. *Jpn Heart J* 1964;5:359–372.

52. Chapman WP, Livingston RB, Livingston KE. Frontal lobotomy and electrical stimulation of orbital surface of frontal lobes. *Arch Neurol Psych* 1949;62:701–716.

53. Chapman WP, Livingston KE, Poppen JL. Effect upon blood pressure of electrical stimulation of tips of temporal lobes in man. *J Neurophysiol* 1950;13:65–71.

54. Delgado JMR. Circulatory effects of cortical stimulation. *Physiol Rev* 1960;40:146–170.

55. Pool JL, Ransohoff J. Autonomic effects on stimulating rostral portion of cingulate gyri in man. *J Neurophysiol* 1949;12:385–392.

56. Oppenheimer SM, Gelb A, Girvin JP, et al. Cardiovascular effects of human insular cortex stimulation. *Neurology* 1992;42:1727–1732.

57. Svigelj V, Grad A, Tekavcic I, et al. Cardiac arrhythmia associated with reversible damage to insula in a patient with subarachnoid hemorrhage. *Stroke* 1994;25:1053–1055.

58. Hugenholz PG. Electrocardiographic changes typical for central nervous system disease after right radical neck dissection. *Am Heart J* 1967;74:438–441.

59. Porter RW, Kamikawa K, Greenhoot JH. Persistent electrocardiographic abnormalities experimentally induced by stimulation of the brain. *Am Heart J* 1962;64:815–820.

60. Melville KI, Blum B, Shister HE, et al. Cardiac ischemic changes and arrhythmias induced by hypothalamic stimulation. *Am J Cardiol* 1963;12:781–791.

61. Meyer JS, Stoica E, Pascu I, et al. Catecholamine concentrations in CSF and plasma of patients with cerebral infarction and haemorrhage. *Brain* 1973;96:277–288.

62. Grad A, Kiauta T, Osredkar J. Effect of elevated plasma norepinephrine on electrocardiographic changes in subarachnoid hemorrhage. *Stroke* 1991;22:746–749.

63. Connor RC. Heart damage associated with intracranial lesions. *BMJ* 1968;3:29–31.

64. Hertzer NR, Beven EG, Young JR, et al. Coronary artery disease in peripheral vascular patients. A classification of 1000 coronary angiograms and results of surgical management. *Ann Surg* 1984;199:223–233.

65. Smith M, Ray CT. Cardiac arrhythmias, increased intracranial pressure, and the autonomic nervous system. *Chest* 1972;61:125–133.

66. Estanol BV, Loyo MV, Mateos JH, et al. Cardiac arrhythmias in experimental subarachnoid hemorrhage. *Stroke* 1977;8:440–449.

67. Lacy PS, Earle AM. A small animal model for electrocardiographic abnormalities observed after an experimental subarachnoid hemorrhage. *Stroke* 1983;14:371–377.

68. Burch GE, Sun SC, Colcolough HL, et al. Acute myocardial lesions; following experimentally-induced intracranial hemorrhage in mice: a histological and histochemical study. *Arch Pathol* 1967;84:517–521.

69. Burch GE, Sohal RS, Sun SC, et al. Effects of experimental intracranial hemorrhage on the ultrastructure of the myocardium of mice. *Am Heart J* 1969;77:427–429.

70. Hunt D, Gore I. Myocardial lesions following experimental intracranial hemorrhage: prevention with propranolol. *Am Heart J* 1972;83:232–236.

71. Koskelo P, Punsar S, Sipila W. Subendocardial haemorrhage and ECG changes in intracranial bleeding. *BMJ* 1964;1:1479–1480.

72. Kay MP, McDonald RH, Randall WC. Systolic hypertension and subendocardial hemorrhages produced by electrical stimulation of the stellate ganglion. *Circ Res* 1961;9:1164–1170.

73. Mehes G, Papp G, Rajkovits K. Effect of adrenergic alpha- and beta-receptor blocking drugs on the myocardial lesions induced by sympathomimetic amines. *Acta Physiol Hung* 1967;32:175–184.

74. Lehr D, Krukowski M, Colon R. Electrolyte changes in isoproterenol-induced myocardial necrosis and the preventive effect of β-adrenergic blockade [abst]. *Fed Proc* 1965;24:561.

75. Raab W. Key position of catecholamines in functional and degenerative cardiovascular pathology. *Am J Cardiol* 1960;5:571–578.

76. Chappel CI, Rona G, Balazs T, et al. Comparison of cardiotoxic action of certain sympathetic amines. *Can J Biochem* 1969;37:35.

77. Szakacs JE, Mehlman B. Pathologic changes induced by l-norepinephrine. *Am J Cardiol* 1960;5:619–627.

78. Ferrans VJ, Hibbs RG, Black WC, et al. Isoproterenol-induced myocardial necrosis. A histochemical and electron microscopic study. *Am Heart J* 1964;68:71–90.

79. Bajusz E, Jasmin G. Influence of variations in electrolyte intake upon the development of cardiac necrosis produced by vasopressor amines. *Lab Invest* 1964;13:757–766.

80. Bloom S, Cancilla PA. Myocytolysis and mitochondrial calcification in rat myocardium after low doses of isoproterenol. *Am J Pathol* 1969;54:373–391.

81. Schenk EA, Moss AJ. Cardiovascular effects of sustained norepinephrine infusions. II. Morphology. *Circ Res* 1966;18:605–615.

82. Hersch C. Electrocardiographic changes in subarachnoid haemorrhage, meningitis, and intracranial space-occupying lesions. *Br Heart J* 1964;26:785–793.

83. Connor RC. Fuchsinophilic degeneration of myocardium in patients with intracranial lesions. *Br Heart J* 1970;32:81–84.

84. Schlesinger MJ, Reiner L. Focal myocytolysis of the heart. *Am J Pathol* 1955;31:443–459.

85. Greenhoot JH, Reichenbach DD. Cardiac injury and subarachnoid hemorrhage. A clinical, pathological, and physiological correlation. *J Neurosurg* 1969;30:521–531.

86. Hammermeister KE, Reichenbach DD. QRS changes, pulmonary edema, and myocardial necrosis associated with subarachnoid hemorrhage. *Am Heart J* 1969;78:94–100.

87. Castleman B. Case records of the Massachusetts General Hospital: Case 1-1970. *N Engl J Med* 1970;282:38–44.

88. Van Vliet PD, Burchell HB, Titus JL. Focal myocarditis associated with pheochromocytoma. *N Engl J Med* 1966;274:1102–1108.

89. Jenkins JS, Buckell M, Carter AB, et al. Hypothalamic-pituitary-adrenal function after subarachnoid hemorrhage. *BMJ* 1969;4:707–709.

90. Howell SJ, Blumhardt LD. ECG abnormalities in epileptics. *Neurology* 1988;38:1168.

91. Keilson MJ, Hauser WA, Magrill JP. Electrocardiographic changes during electrographic seizures. *Arch Neurol* 1989;46:1169–1170.

92. Keilson MJ, Hauser WA, Magrill JP, et al. ECG abnormalities in patients with epilepsy. *Neurology* 1987;37:1624–1626.

93. Keilson MJ, Magrill JP. Simultaneous ambulatory cassette EEG/ECG monitoring. In: Ebersole JS, ed. *Ambulatory EEG monitoring*. New York: Raven Press, 1989:171–193.

94. Wilder-Smith E. Complete atrio-ventricular conduction block during complex partial seizure. *J Neurol Neurosurg Psychiatry* 1992;55:734–736.

95. Liedholm LJ, Gudjonsson O. Cardiac arrest due to partial epileptic seizures. *Neurology* 1992;42:824–829.

96. Howell SJ, Blumhardt LD. Cardiac asystole associated with epileptic seizures: a case report with simultaneous EEG and ECG. *J Neurol Neurosurg Psychiatry* 1989;52:795–798.

97. Dasheiff RM, Dickinson LJ. Sudden unexpected death of epileptic patient due to cardiac arrhythmia after seizure. *Arch Neurol* 1986;43:194–196.

98. Reeves AL, Nollet KE, Klass DW, et al. The ictal bradycardia syndrome. *Epilepsia* 1996;37:983–987.

99. Earnest MP, Thomas GE, Eden RA, et al. The sudden unexplained death syndrome in epilepsy: demographic, clinical, and postmortem features. *Epilepsia* 1992;33:310–316.

100. Terrence CF Jr, Wisotzkey HM, Perper JA. Unexpected, unexplained death in epileptic patients. *Neurology* 1975;25:594–598.

101. Terrence CF, Rao GR, Perper JA. Neurogenic pulmonary edema in unexpected, unexplained death of epileptic patients. *Ann Neurol* 1981;9:458–464.

102. Falconer B, Rajs J. Post-mortem findings of cardiac lesions in epileptics: a preliminary report. *Forensic Sci Int* 1976;8:63–71.

103. Panidis IP, Morganroth J. Initiating events of sudden cardiac death. *Cardiovasc Clin* 1985;15:81–92.

104. Hirsch CS, Martin DL. Unexpected death in young epileptics. *Neurology* 1971;21:682–690.

105. Epstein MA, Sperling MR, O'Connor MJ. Cardiac rhythm during temporal lobe seizures. *Neurology* 1992;42:50–53.

106. Galimberti CA, Marchioni E, Barzizza F, et al. Partial epileptic seizures of different origin variably affect cardiac rhythm. *Epilepsia* 1996;37:742–747.

107. Wayne VS. A possible relationship between migraine and coronary artery spasm. *Aust N Z J Med* 1986;16:708–710.

108. Lafitte C, Even C, Henry-Lebras F, et al. Migraine and angina pectoris by coronary artery spasm. *Headache* 1996;36:332–334.

109. Pogacnik T, Sega S, Pecnik B, et al. Autonomic function

testing in patients with migraine. *Headache* 1993;33:545–550.

110. Appel S, Kuritzky A, Zahavi I, et al. Evidence for instability of the autonomic nervous system in patients with migraine headache. *Headache* 1992;32:10–17.

111. Rozentryt P, Durko A, Kozubski W, et al. Automatic regulation of sinus rhythm in patients with migraine. *Neurol Neurochir Pol* 1995;29:889–900.

112. Prusinski A, Trzos S, Rozentryt P, et al. Studies of heart rhythm variability in migraine. Preliminary communication. *Neurol Neurochir Pol* 1994;28[Suppl 1]:23–27.

113. Touchon J, Bertin L, Pilgrim AJ, et al. A comparison of subcutaneous sumatriptan and dihydroergotamine nasal spray in the acute treatment of migraine. *Neurology* 1996;47:361–365.

114. Snell NJ, Russell-Smith C, Coysh HL. Myocardial ischemia in migraine sufferers taking ergotamine. *Postgrad Med J* 1978;54:37–39.

115. Dechant KL, Clissold SP. Sumatriptan: a review of its pharmacodynamic and pharmacokinetic properties, and therapeutic efficacy in the treatment of migraine and cluster headache. *Drugs* 1992:43(S):776–798.

116. Walton-Shirley M, Flowers K, Whiteside JH. Unstable angina pectoris associated with Imitrex therapy. *Cathet Cardiovasc Diagn* 1995;34:188.

117. Paterna S, Parrinello G, Pinto A, et al. Effect of sumatriptan on facial temperature variations, blood pressure and electrocardiogram in healthy subjects and patients with migraine without aura. *Clin Ter* 1995;146:469–476.

118. Brown EG, Endersby CA, Smith RN, et al. The safety and tolerability of sumatriptan: an overview. *Eur Neurol* 1991;31:339–344.

119. Chandra R, Tandon RN, Singhal A. Reversible sick sinus syndrome with junctional and ventricular escape and fusion beats in a case of tuberculous meningitis. *Indian Heart J* 1981;33:37–39.

120. Brubakk O. Non-invasive assessment of cardiac function in meningitis. *Acta Med Scand* 1979;205:67–72.

121. Detsky AS, Salit IE. Complete heart block in meningococcemia. *Ann Emerg Med* 1983;12:391–393.

122. Bisht DB. Cardiac manifestations of encephalitis with special reference to ECG changes. *Indian Heart J* 1967;19:340–345.

123. De Keyser J, De Boel S, Ceulemans L, et al. Torsades de pointes as a complication of brainstem encephalitis. *Intensive Care Med* 1987;13:76–77.

124. Uemura A, Morimoto S, Hiramitsu S, et al. A case of brain stem encephalitis complicated with bifascicular block caused by rubella virus. *Kokyu To Junkan* 1992;40:499–503.

125. Hersch C. Electrocardiographic changes in head injuries. *Circulation* 1961;23:853–860.

126. Brunninkhuis LG. Electrocardiographic abnormalities suggesting myocardial infarction in a patient with severe cranial trauma. *Pacing Clin Electrophysiol* 1983;6:1336–1340.

127. Jacobson SA, Danufsky P. Marked EKG changes produced by experimental head trauma. *J Neuropath Exp Neurol* 1954;13:462–466.

128. Osler W. *The principles and practice of medicine.* New York: Appleton-Century-Crofts, 1892:777.

129. Krone A, Reuther P, Fuhrmeister U. Autonomic dysfunction in polyneuropathies: a report on 106 cases. *J Neurol* 1983;230:111–121.

130. Greenland P, Griggs RC. Arrhythmic complications in the Guillain-Barré syndrome. *Arch Intern Med* 1980;140:1053–1055.

131. Emmons PR, Blume WT, DuShane JW. Cardiac monitoring and demand pacemaker in Guillain-Barré syndrome. *Arch Neurol* 1975;32:59–61.

132. Narayan D, Huang MT, Mathew PK. Bradycardia and asystole requiring permanent pacemaker in Guillain-Barré syndrome. *Am Heart J* 1984;108:426–428.

133. Favre H, Foex P, Guggisberg M. Use of demand pacemaker in a case of Guillain-Barré syndrome. *Lancet* 1970;1:1062–1063.

134. Stewart IM. Arrhythmias in Guillain-Barré syndrome. *BMJ* 1973;2:665–666.

135. Winer JB, Hughes RA. Identification of patients at risk of arrhythmia in the Guillain-Barré syndrome. *QJM* 1988;68:735–739.

136. Flachenecker P, Mullges W, Wermuth P, et al. Eyeball pressure testing in the evaluation of serious bradyarrhythmias in Guillain-Barré syndrome. *Neurology* 1996;47:102–108.

137. Feiden W, Gerhard L, Borchard F. Neuritis cordis due to the acute polyneuritis of the Guillain-Barré syndrome. *Virchows Arch A Pathol Anat Histopathol* 1988;413:573–580.

138. Iga K, Himura Y, Izumi C, et al. Reversible left ventricular dysfunction associated with the Guillain-Barré syndrome: an expression of catecholamine cardiotoxicity? *Jpn Circ J* 1995;59:236–240.

139. Brumback RA, Panner BJ, Kingston WJ. The heart in Friedreich's ataxia. Report of a case. *Arch Neurol* 1986;43:189–192.

140. Child JS, Perloff JK, Bach PM, et al. Cardiac involvement in Friedreich's ataxia: a clinical study of 75 patients. *J Am Coll Cardiol* 1986;7:1370–1378.

141. Gottdiener JS, Hawley RJ, Maron BJ, et al. Characteristics of the cardiac hypertrophy in Friedreich's ataxia. *Am Heart J* 1982;103:525–531.

142. Smith ER, Sangalang VE, Heffernan LP, et al. Hypertrophic cardiomyopathy: the heart disease of Friedreich's ataxia. *Am Heart J* 1977;94:428–434.

143. Palagi B, Picozzi R, Casazza F, et al. Biventricular function in Friedreich's ataxia: a radionuclide angiographic study. *Br Heart J* 1988;59:692–695.

144. Alboliras ET, Shub C, Gomez MR, et al. Spectrum of cardiac involvement in Friedreich's ataxia: clinical, electrocardiographic and echocardiographic observations. *Am J Cardiol* 1986;58:518–524.

145. Leak D. Paroxysmal atrial flutter in peroneal muscular atrophy. *Br Heart J* 1961;23:326–328.

146. Littler WA. Heart block and peroneal muscular atrophy. *QJM* 1970;39:431–440.

147. Kay JM, Littler WA, Meade JB. Ultrastructure of the myocardium in familial heart block and peroneal muscular atrophy. *Br Heart J* 1972;34:1081–1084.

148. Lowry PJ, Littler WA. Peroneal muscular atrophy associated with cardiac conducting tissue disease: further observations. *Postgrad Med J* 1983;59:530–532.

149. Luomanmaki K, Hokkanen E, Heikkila J. Electrocardiogram in myasthenia gravis. Analysis of a series of 97 patients. *Ann Clin Res* 1969;1:236–245.

150. Gibson TC. The heart in myasthenia gravis. *Am Heart J* 1975;90:389–396.

151. Engel AG. Duchenne dystrophy. In: Engel AG, Banker BQ, eds. *Myology basic and clinical.* New York: McGraw Hill, 1986:1185–1240.

152. Sanyal SK, Johnson WW. Cardiac conduction abnormalities in children with Duchenne's progressive muscular dystrophy: electrocardiographic features and morphologic correlates. *Circulation* 1982;66:853–863.

153. Perloff JK. Cardiac rhythm and conduction in Duchenne's muscular dystrophy: a prospective study of 20 patients. *J Am Coll Cardiol* 1984;3:1263–1268.

154. Perloff JK, Roberts WC, de Leon AC Jr, et al. The distinctive electrocardiogram of Duchenne's progressive muscular dystrophy: an electrocardiographic-pathologic correlative study. *Am J Med* 1967;42:179–188.

155. Quinlivan RM, Dubowitz V. Cardiac transplantation in Becker muscular dystrophy. *Neuromuscul Disord* 1992;2:165–167.

156. Frankel KA, Rosser RJ. The pathology of the heart in progressive muscular dystrophy: epimyocardial fibrosis. *Hum Pathol* 1976;7:375–386.

157. Nomura H, Hizawa K. Histopathological study of the conduction system of the heart in Duchenne progressive muscular dystrophy. *Acta Pathol Jpn* 1982;32:1027–1033.

158. Nigro G, Comi LI, Politano L, et al. The incidence and evolution of cardiomyopathy in Duchenne muscular dystrophy. *Int J Cardiol* 1990;26:271–277.

159. Farah MG, Evans EB, Vignos PJ Jr. Echocardiographic evaluation of left ventricular function in Duchenne's muscular dystrophy. *Am J Med* 1980;69:248–254.

160. Perloff JK, Henze E, Schelbert HR. Alterations in regional myocardial metabolism, perfusion, and wall motion in Duchenne muscular dystrophy studied by radionuclide imaging. *Circulation* 1984;69:33–42.

161. Walton JN, Gardner-Medwin D. Progressive muscular dystrophy and the myotonic disorders. In: Walton J, ed. *Disorders of voluntary muscle.* 4th ed. Edinburgh: Churchill Livingstone, 1981:481–524.

162. Kinoshita H, Goto Y, Ishikawa M, et al. A carrier of Duchenne muscular dystrophy with dilated cardiomyopathy but no skeletal muscle symptoms. *Brain Dev* 1995;17:202–205.

163. Katiyar BC, Misra S, Somani PN, et al. Congestive cardiomyopathy in a family of Becker's X-linked muscular dystrophy. *Postgrad Med J* 1977;53:12–15.

164. Sakata C, Sunohara N, Nonaka I, et al. A case of Becker muscular dystrophy presenting cardiac failure as an initial symptom. *Rinsho Shinkeigaku* 1990;30:210–213.

165. Casazza F, Brambilla G, Salvato A, et al. Cardiac transplantation in Becker muscular dystrophy. *J Neurol* 1988;235:496–498.

166. Motta J, Guilleminault C, Billingham M, et al. Cardiac abnormalities in myotonic dystrophy. Electrophysiologic and histopathologic studies. *Am J Med* 1979;67:467–473.

167. Church SC. The heart in myotonia atrophica. *Arch Intern Med* 1967;119:176–181.

168. Fisch C. The heart in dystrophia myotonica. *Am Heart J* 1951;41:525–538.

169. Griggs RC, Davis RJ, Anderson DC, et al. Cardiac conduction in myotonic dystrophy. *Am J Med* 1975;59:37–42.

170. Gottdiener JS, Hawley RJ, Gay JA, et al. Left ventricular relaxation, mitral valve prolapse, and intracardiac conduction in myotonia atrophica: assessment by digitized echocardiography and noninvasive His bundle recording. *Am Heart J* 1982;104:77–85.

171. Hawley RJ, Gottdiener JS, Gay JA, et al. Families with myotonic dystrophy with and without cardiac involvement. *Arch Intern Med* 1983;143:2134–2136.

172. Nguyen HH, Wolfe JT III, Holmes DR Jr, et al. Pathology of the cardiac conduction system in myotonic dystrophy: a study of 12 cases. *J Am Coll Cardiol* 1988;11:662–671.

173. Harper PS. *Myotonic dystrophy.* Philadelphia: WB Saunders, 1979.

174. Orndahl G, Thulesius O, Enestrom S, et al. The heart in myotonic disease. *Acta Med Scand* 1964;176:479.

175. Egan TJ, Klein R. Hyperkalemic familial periodic paralysis. *Pediatrics* 1959;24:761–773.

176. Conn JW, Streeten DHP. Periodic paralysis. In: Stanbury JB, Fredrickson DS, Wyngaarden JB, eds. *The metabolic basis of inherited disease.* New York: McGraw-Hill, 1960:867–918.

177. Klein R, Ganelin R, Marks JF, et al. Periodic paralysis with cardiac arrhythmia. *J Pediatr* 1963;62:371–385.

178. Kastor JA, Goldreyer BN. Ventricular origin of bidirectional tachycardia. Case report of a patient not toxic from digitalis. *Circulation* 1973;48:897–903.

179. Lisak RP, Lebeau J, Tucker SH, et al. Hyperkalemic periodic paralysis and cardiac arrhythmias. *Neurology* 1972;22:810–815.

180. Fukuda K, Ogawa S, Yokozuka H, et al. Long-standing bidirectional tachycardia in a patient with hypokalemic periodic paralysis. *J Electrocardiol* 1988;21:71–75.

181. Jackson CE, Strehler DA. Limb-girdle muscular dystrophy: clinical manifestations and detection of preclinical disease. *Pediatrics* 1968;41:495–502.

182. Perloff JK, de Leon AC Jr, O'Doherty D. The cardiomyopathy of progressive muscular dystrophy. *Circulation* 1966;33:625–648.

183. Fairfax AJ, Lambert CD. Neurological aspects of sinoatrial heart blocks. *J Neurol Neurosurg Psychiatry* 1976;39:576–580.

184. James TN. Observations on the cardiovascular involvement, including the cardiac conduction system, in progressive muscular dystrophy. *Am Heart J* 1962;63:48–56.

185. Baldwin BJ, Talley RC, Johnson C, et al. Permanent paralysis of the atrium in a patient with facioscapulohumeral muscular dystrophy. *Am J Cardiol* 1973;31:649–653.

186. Caponnetto S, Pastorini C, Tirelli G. Persistent atrial standstill in a patient affected with facioscapulohumeral dystrophy. *Cardiologia* 1968;53:341–350.

187. Allensworth DC, Rice GJ, Lowe GW. Persistent atrial standstill in a family with myocardial disease. *Am J Med* 1969;47:775–784.

188. Waters D, Nutter DO, Hopkins LC, et al. Cardiac features of an unusual X-linked humeroperoneal neuromuscular disease. *N Engl J Med* 1975;293:1017–1022.

189. Thomas PK, Calne DB, Elliott CF. X-linked scapuloperoneal syndrome. *J Neurol Neurosurg Psychiatry* 1972;35:208–215.

190. Thomas PK, Schott GD, Morgan-Hughes JA. Adult onset scapuloperoneal myopathy. *J Neurol Neurosurg Psychiatry* 1975;38:1008–1015.

191. Sher JH, Rimalovski AB, Athanassiades TJ, et al. Familial centronuclear myopathy: a clinical and pathological study. *Neurology* 1967;17:727–742.

192. Verhiest W, Brucher JM, Goddeeris P, et al. Familial centronuclear myopathy associated with "cardiomyopathy." *Br Heart J* 1976;38:504–509.

193. Bethlem J, van Wijngaarden GK, Meijer AE, et al. Neuromuscular disease with type I fiber atrophy, central nuclei, and myotube-like structures. *Neurology* 1969;19:705–710.

194. Shafiq SA, Sande MA, Carruthers RR, et al. Skeletal muscle in idiopathic cardiomyopathy. *J Neurol Sci* 1972;15:303–320.

195. Kinney TD, Maher MM. Dermatomyositis: a study of five cases. *Am J Pathol* 1940;16:561–594.

196. Hill DL, Barrows HS. Identical skeletal and cardiac muscle involvement in a case of fatal polymyositis. *Arch Neurol* 1968;19:545–551.

197. Schaumburg HH, Nielsen SL, Yurchak PM. Heart block in polymyositis. *N Engl J Med* 1971;284:480–481.

198. Lynch PG. Cardiac involvement in chronic polymyositis. *Br Heart J* 1971;33:416–419.

199. Diessner GR, Howard FM Jr, Winkelmann RK, et al. Laboratory tests in polymyositis. *Arch Intern Med* 1966;117:757–763.

200. Gottdiener JS, Sherber HS, Hawley RJ, et al. Cardiac manifestations in polymyositis. *Am J Cardiol* 1978;41:1141–1149.

201. Babka JC, Pepine CJ. Hyperkinetic cardiovascular state in polymyositis. *Chest* 1973;64:243–246.

202. Winkelmann RK, Mulder DW, Lambert EH, et al. Course of dermatomyositis-polymyositis: comparison of untreated and cortisone-treated patients. *Mayo Clin Proc* 1968;43:545–556.

203. Kearns TP, Sayer GP. Retinitis pigmentosa, external ophthalmoplegia, and complete heart block. *Arch Ophthalmol* 1958;60:280–289.

204. Clark DS, Myerburg RJ, Morales RR, et al. Heart block in Kearns-Sayre syndrome, electrophysiologic-pathologic correlation. *Chest* 1975;68:727–730.

205. Roberts NK, Perloff JK, Kark RA. Cardiac conduction in the Kearns-Sayre syndrome (a neuromuscular disorder associated with progressive external ophthalmoplegia and pigmentary retinopathy). *Am J Cardiol* 1979;44:1396–1400.

206. Charles R, Holt S, Kay JM, et al. Myocardial ultrastructure and the development of atrioventricular block in Kearns-Sayre syndrome. *Circulation* 1981;63:214–219.

207. McComish M, Compston A, Jewitt D. Cardiac abnormalities in chronic progressive external ophthalmoplegia. *Br Heart J* 1976;38:526–529.

208. Wakabayashi K, Takahashi H. Neuropathology of autonomic nervous system in Parkinson's disease. *Eur Neurol* 1997;38[Suppl 2]:2–7.

209. Sato H, Serita T, Seto M, et al. Loss of ^{123}I-MIBG uptake in Parkinson's disease: assessment of cardiac sympathetic denervation and diagnostic value. *J Nucl Med* 1999;40:371–375.

210. Ishizaki F, Harada T, Yoshinaga H, et al. Prolonged QTc intervals in Parkinson's disease—relation to sudden death and autonomic dysfunction. *Shinkei Brain Nerve* 1996;48:443–448.

211. Francheschi M, Ferini-Strambi L, Minicucci F, et al. Signs of cardiac dysfunction during sleep in patients with Alzheimer's disease. *Gerontology* 1986;32:327–334.

212. Hofman A, Ott A, Breteler MM, et al. Atherosclerosis, apolipoprotein E, and prevalence of dementia and Alzheimer's disease in the Rotterdam Study. *Lancet* 1997;349:151–154.

35E

THE HEART AND OTHER ORGAN SYSTEMS

Cardiovascular Manifestations of Rheumatic Diseases

DAVID H. LEWIS

D. H. Lewis: Mid America Heart Institute, Kansas City, Missouri

OVERVIEW

The rheumatic diseases are a heterogeneous group of illnesses with protean manifestations and multisystem organ involvement. Although each individual disorder is relatively rare, together they represent important causes of morbidity and mortality worldwide. It is not at all unusual for specialists in cardiovascular medicine to encounter patients with these disorders in the office setting, hospital, or emergency department. Cardiac manifestations range from unusual to prominent (Table 35E.1) and from mild to dramatic. Occult cardiovascular involvement is common, is frequently detectable on noninvasive studies, and has important prognostic implications. Cardiovascular death is common, may be due to disease-specific cardiac involvement or secondary effects of disease on the heart, and underscores the importance of primary and secondary preventive strategies in this patient population (Table 35E.2).

TABLE 35E.1   INCIDENCE OF CLINICAL CARDIAC MANIFESTATIONS OF SELECT RHEUMATIC DISORDERS

Disorder	Pericardial	Valvular	Myocardial	Coronary	Arrhythmic
Systemic lupus erythematosus	25%	Rare	5%–10%	Rare	Rare
Rheumatoid arthritis	10%	Rare	Rare	Rare	Rare
Systemic sclerosis	7–16%	—	10%	—	10%
Kawasaki disease	Rare	1%	30%	23%,[a] 8%[b]	rare
Takayasu's disease	2%	7–20%	Rare	5–10%	5%
Ankylosing spondylitis	Rare	10–20%	Rare	Rare	10%
Churg-Strauss syndrome	20–32%	—	13–48%	Rare	Rare
Polyarteritis nodosa	2–5%	—	10%	5%	Rare
Giant cell arteritis/temporal arteritis	Rare	5–10%[c]	Rare	Rare	—
Wegener's granulomatosis	6–10%	Rare	2%	1%	1–2%
Polymyositis/dermatomyositis	7%	Rare	5%	—	6%

[a]Untreated.
[b]Treated.
[c]Valvular involvement secondary to aortic disease.

TABLE 35E.2   DISEASE INCIDENCE, FREQUENCY OF CARDIAC INVOLVEMENT, AND CAUSES OF DEATH IN PATIENTS WITH SELECT RHEUMATIC DISORDERS

Disorder	Annual incidence per million population	Clinical cardiac involvement	Cardiac involvement on autopsy	Most common causes of death
Systemic lupus erythematosus	40–80	50%	>60%	Renal, infection, **cardiac**
Rheumatoid arthritis	250–500	10–15%	>30%	**Cardiac**, infection, cancer
Systemic sclerosis	10	10%	>30%	Renal, **cardiac**, pulmonary
Kawasaki disease	105 (Japan); 5–15 (United States)	1–5%	>90%[a]	**Cardiac**
Takayasu's disease	2.6	20–30%	20–30%	**Cardiac**, stroke
Ankylosing spondylitis	73	10–20%	20%	**Cardiac**, stroke, pulmonary
Churg-Strauss syndrome	2.4	40–60%	>50%	**Cardiac**, renal, stroke
Polyarteritis nodosa	7	10–30%	>50%	Renal, stroke, **cardiac**
Giant cell arteritis	178[b]	5–10%[c]	5–10%[c]	**Cardiac**, stroke, renal
Wegener's granulomatosis	8.5	12–14%	>50%	Infection, **cardiac**, renal
Polymyositis/dermatomyositis	10	6–10%	>25%	Infection, cancer, **cardiac**

[a]Among those dying during the acute phase of the disease.
[b]Individuals older than 50 years.
[c]Valvular involvement secondary to aortic disease.

SYSTEMIC LUPUS ERYTHEMATOSUS

Systemic lupus erythematosus (SLE) is an autoimmune disorder characterized by antibodies against a variety of cellular antigens, resulting in multisystem organ dysfunction. Biett (1) first described the dermatologic manifestations of SLE in 1828. Nearly a half-century passed before it was recognized that SLE involved organs other than the skin, and not until a half-century after that was histopathologic proof of cardiac involvement systematically described by Libman and Sacks (2). Because of the protean manifestations of the disease, a diagnosis of SLE relies on the fulfillment, over time, of four criteria from a list of specific laboratory, histologic, and clinical findings (3). The most common presenting signs and symptoms are polyarthritis and dermatitis (4). ▼▼ h19

SLE is a pancarditis in which morbidity and mortality are the result of pericarditis, myocarditis, endocarditis, and coronary arteritis. More than 50% of patients with SLE experience clinical cardiovascular involvement during the course of the illness (8). Asymptomatic cardiac involvement is detected in a number of additional patients at autopsy. Cardiac involvement is rarely the initial presenting symptom of SLE (5).

Pericardial Involvement

Pericarditis is the most common cardiovascular manifestation of SLE. It has an estimated clinical frequency of 25% and autopsy frequency of 62% (9). Echocardiographically, pericardial abnormalities are present in 7% to 54% of asymptomatic individuals (10–13). Acute pericarditis is the only cardiovascular manifestation of SLE that is included in the diagnostic criteria for the disease (3), and it commonly occurs as part of a generalized serositis. It is also the only cardiovascular manifestation strongly related to disease activity, as assessed by clinical and laboratory variables (10). Histopathology of pericardial tissue reveals proliferation of the pericardial vessels, vasculitis, fibrosis, and fibrin stranding (14).

Pericarditis associated with SLE manifests clinically as chest discomfort that is frequently pleuritic and worse in the recumbent position. Examination may reveal fever, tachycardia, a pericardial friction rub, and diminished breath sounds as a result of concomitant pleuritis with effusion. Laboratory features include leukocytosis, elevated sedimentation rate, and elevated titers of anti–double-stranded DNA, which are indicative of active SLE. Chest radiography may reveal an enlarged cardiac silhouette and pleural effusion. Electrocardiography (ECG) typically reveals diffuse ST-segment elevation and PR-segment depression, except in lead aVR, where these findings are reversed. Pericardial fluid is exudative and characterized by high protein levels, normal glucose levels, a predominance of polymorphonuclear cells, low complement levels, and the ability to fix complement (15). The presence of LE cells and immune complexes in the pericardial fluid is not diagnostic, but it supports an immune-mediated cause of pericardial disease in patients with SLE (16).

Complications of pericarditis include pericardial tamponade, purulent pericarditis, and constrictive pericarditis. These entities are uncommon, but not rare, in SLE-induced pericarditis. Pericardial tamponade occurs in 0.25% to 2.50% of patients (6,9,14). It may be due to exuberant inflammation with translocation of fluid, hemorrhage, or, rarely, aortic dissection. Pericardiocentesis may be lifesaving in the critically ill patient, but a high rate of complications has been reported in this population. Pericardial window is the definitive procedure for treatment of patients with recurrence. SLE is an oft-quoted risk factor for purulent pericarditis, even though it occurs in only 0.250% to 0.375% of patients (6,9). Purulent pericarditis may be caused by hematologic seeding of an existing pericardial effusion or by direct extension from a penetrating endocardial abscess or empyema. *Staphylococcus aureus* is the most frequently encountered pathogen. Treatment includes surgical drainage and antibiotics. Constrictive pericarditis typically presents with signs and symptoms of right-sided heart failure, such as fatigue, dyspnea with exertion, jugular venous distention, hepatomegaly, ascites, and edema. Constrictive pericarditis, when severe, is best managed with pericardiectomy.

Valvular Involvement

Valvular pathology that is attributable to SLE is seen in nearly one-half of all patients in whom SLE is found at autopsy (9,17,18). Libman and Sacks (2) were the first to describe the pathognomonic valvular lesion of SLE. Gross (19) later described them as gray-pink and flat or raised clusters that may be found on either side of the valves, in the valve pockets, or adherent to the chordae or myocardium (Fig. 35E.1). Antiphospholipid antibodies have also been demonstrated within valvular lesions, leading some to suggest that endocardial damage and thrombosis may initiate lesion formation (20). ▼▼ h20

Clinically important valvular disease is much less common than asymptomatic disease detected by echocardiography or autopsy. Hemodynamically significant valvular disease may be caused by any combination of the following: valvulitis, fibrosis, infective or noninfective endocarditis, ischemic cardiomyopathy, papillary muscle dysfunction, and aortic dissection. Clinically important aortic regurgitation appears to be more frequent than mitral regurgitation, but the true incidence of each is unknown (9). Mitral stenosis, aortic stenosis, and right-sided valvular disease are all rare. Early reports of valve replacement in patients with SLE found an extremely high associated mortality, approaching 25% (25); however, recent reports have been more encouraging (26). Mechanical prostheses, biopros-

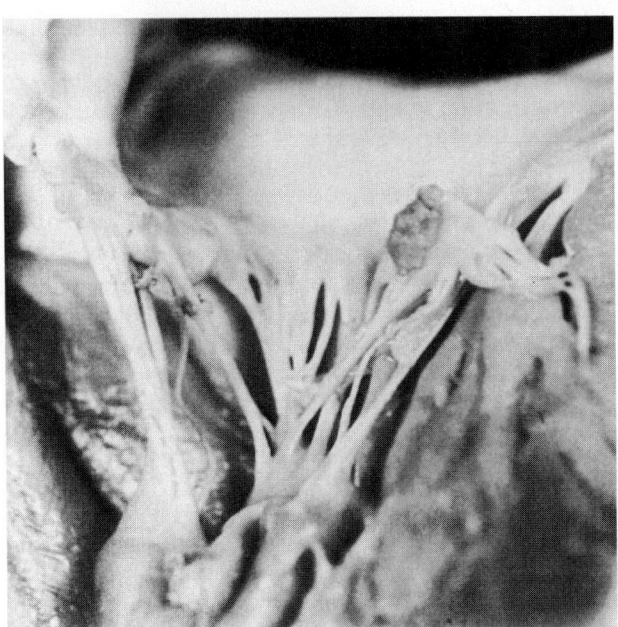

FIGURE 35E.1 Characteristic Libman-Sacks vegetation on the posterior cusp of the mitral valve. (From Cosh JA, Lever JV. *Rheumatic diseases and the heart.* Berlin: Springer-Verlag, 1988, with permission.)

thetic valves, and homografts have all been used to treat this condition. Patients with SLE are at high risk for hemorrhagic complications from anticoagulation therapy, because of the frequency of intracranial and pericardial disease in this population. However, they often have other indications for anticoagulation therapy, such as the antiphospholipid antibody syndrome with clinical thrombosis. Clearly, the choice of valvular prosthesis must be individualized.

The lesions of Libman-Sacks endocarditis act as a nidus for infective endocarditis. Clinical infective endocarditis occurs in 1% to 2% of SLE patients. At autopsy, it is found in nearly 5% (9). Patients with SLE and significant valvular dysfunction who are undergoing invasive medical or dental procedures are at moderate risk for infective endocarditis and should receive antibiotic prophylaxis, according to published guidelines (27).

Myocardial Involvement

Myocarditis is found commonly at autopsy of patients who had SLE. In the precorticosteroid era, myocarditis was found in nearly one-half of all SLE patients at autopsy (9). More recent autopsy series have shown a prevalence of less than 10% (18). When myocarditis is found, however, it typically involves only small patches of myocardium, and only 5% to 10% of SLE patients experience clinical myocarditis (9). Histopathology reveals perivascular and interstitial inflammation characterized by plasma cells, mononuclear cells, myocardial degeneration and regeneration, and, occasionally, necrosis. SLE is generally a cortico-

steroid-responsive disorder, but no randomized trials of the use of immunosuppressive therapy for myocarditis in patients with SLE have been performed. Trials of the use of immunosuppressive agents to treat other types of myocarditis have been disappointing. Endomyocardial biopsy should be considered when a patient with SLE develops severe myocarditis, to guide immunosuppressive therapy.

Congestive heart failure (CHF) is common and usually multifactorial in patients with SLE. It is the cause of death in 1% to 5% of patients with SLE (6,7). Ischemia, valvular heart disease, hypertension, and myocarditis may produce either systolic or diastolic dysfunction. Mild global left ventricular systolic dysfunction is present in 5% to 15% of patients with SLE (10,28). Echocardiography has detected abnormalities of myocardial relaxation in young, asymptomatic SLE patients (29,30). Other studies, however, have not reproduced this in normotensive SLE patients (31).

Coronary Involvement

Coronary artery disease (CAD) has become an increasingly important cause of morbidity and mortality among patients with SLE. Ischemic heart disease in patients with SLE presents, in order of decreasing frequency, as acute myocardial infarction (MI), CHF, sudden cardiac death, and angina pectoris. It is estimated that 3% to 15% of patients with SLE die from acute MI (7,32,33). Ischemic coronary events are attributed most frequently to coronary atherosclerosis, less frequently to coronary arteritis, and rarely to embolic phenomena involving the coronary circulation.

Coronary atherosclerosis is accelerated in patients with SLE. This likely is related to the effects of corticosteroids, the prevalence of traditional risk factors among patients with SLE, and coronary inflammation. The role of antiphospholipid antibodies in the pathogenesis of CAD and the occurrence of subsequent coronary events is controversial. Patients with SLE have a fivefold risk of acute MI, compared with age-matched control subjects (34). Women 35 to 44 years of age were found to have a relative risk of 52 (95% confidence interval, 21.6 to 98.5) for MI, compared with matched controls (32). Two groups have found a 40% prevalence of asymptomatic CAD in patients by nuclear stress testing (28,35). Autopsy studies have demonstrated a 50% prevalence of moderate to severe CAD both in general SLE populations (7) and in SLE patients less than 37 years of age (36). h21

RHEUMATOID ARTHRITIS

Rheumatoid arthritis (RA) is an autoimmune disorder of unknown etiology. It is characterized primarily by an erosive arthritis with progressive joint destruction, deformation, and immobility. RA has a prevalence of 1% worldwide and an annual incidence of 250 to 500 cases per

1 million individuals (43). The diagnosis relies on a variety of clinical, laboratory, and radiographic findings. Extraarticular manifestations are common but usually are overshadowed by joint involvement.

Four of the following criteria must be met for a diagnosis of RA to be indicated: morning stiffness that lasts at least 1 hour; arthritis affecting three or more joints; arthritis affecting the proximal interphalangeal, metacarpophalangeal, or wrist joints; symmetric arthritis; rheumatoid nodules; the presence of rheumatoid factor; and radiographic evidence of joint erosion or periarticular osteopenia (44). Symptoms should be present for 6 weeks before a diagnosis is made.

Caring for individuals with RA requires a multidisciplinary approach that includes the efforts of physicians, nurses, and physical and occupational therapists. Non–weight-bearing exercise, joint orthotics, and joint replacements may significantly improve patient function.

Steroids and nonsteroidal antiinflammatory drugs (NSAIDs), including cyclooxygenase-2 inhibitors, are the backbone of symptomatic therapy. Disease-modifying antirheumatic drugs include hydroxychloroquine, penicillamine, azathioprine, leflunomide, sulfasalazine, gold preparations, and methotrexate. Newer biologic response modulators, including etanercept and infliximab, which inhibit the activity of tumor necrosis factor-α, have been beneficial in patients who are resistant or intolerant to disease-modifying antirheumatic drugs. The use of etanercept in the treatment of heart failure is being investigated in the Randomized Etanercept North American Strategy to Study Antagonism of Cytokines trial. Conversely, concern has been raised regarding the safety of using cyclooxygenase-2 inhibitors in patients with cardiovascular disease. Anecdotal reports and initial clinical trial results suggest that these drugs have a potential prothrombotic effect, including an increased incidence of MI. Further study is required.

The profound morbidity associated with RA is undisputed. However, only recently has the substantial increase in mortality associated with the disease come to be appreciated. Standardized mortality ratios, which compare observed to expected event ratios in a population, reveal a greater than twofold increase in mortality among RA patients compared to that among epidemiologic controls (45). Cardiovascular disease is the most common cause of death in patients with RA (45–47).

Pericardial Involvement

Cardiac involvement in RA was first reported in 1881 by Charcot, who described a patient with clinical and autopsy evidence of pericarditis (48). Autopsy evidence of pericarditis is now recognized in nearly one-third of patients who have RA (49). Clinical pericarditis is much less common, occurring in fewer than 10% of patients who have RA in most series (49,50). Echocardiographic evidence of pericar-

dial disease occurs in 8% to 50% of asymptomatic RA patients (51–53) and may be more common among those with subcutaneous rheumatoid nodules (52). ☛ h22

Pericarditis may be asymptomatic and detected by physical examination, echocardiogram, or ECG. When symptoms are present, positional chest pain is most common, followed by dyspnea and swelling. NSAIDs or corticosteroids may be used for treatment, but trials comparing treatment strategies are lacking. Constrictive pericarditis has been reported in 0.64% of men and 0.06% of women (54). Tamponade is less common. Management of tamponade in patients with RA is complicated by a poor response to medical therapy and by frequent loculations. Pericardiocentesis may be attempted in patients with tamponade, but most patients with either tamponade or constrictive pericarditis eventually require pericardiectomy (55). Clinical predictors of poor outcome in patients with pericardial disease include advanced age, jugular venous distension, hypotension, and other extraarticular RA manifestations (50).

Valvular Involvement

Hemodynamically significant, histologically proven valvular involvement in RA is rare. Many of such patients reported in the literature showed evidence of superimposed rheumatic valvular heart disease. In 1941, Baggenstoss and Rosenberg (56) were the first to describe valvular disease in patients with RA. Roberts and coworkers (57) went on to describe in more detail the gross findings, noting firm, smooth, yellow deposits with a predilection for left-sided heart valves. Histologic changes may consist of bland fibrosis or may reveal inflammatory changes similar to rheumatoid nodules (57). Concurrent involvement of more than one valve is common among patients with valvular disease.

Myocardial Involvement

Rheumatoid nodules have been found within the myocardium of patients with RA. Sensitive echocardiographic techniques used to measure diastolic function have revealed abnormalities of myocardial relaxation in nearly 25% of patients with RA (53). However, clinical CHF and systolic dysfunction that can be attributed to RA are rare.

Coronary Involvement

Acute MI is common in patients with RA. This seems to reflect the high risk of MI in all adults, rather than a profound disease-specific increase in risk due to RA. A 51% excess in death due to ischemic heart disease was noted in one retrospective study (47), but another retrospective case-control series found an increase in MI only among RA patients who tested positive for rheumatoid factor (58), and other studies have found no increase in incidence of MI (46). In fact, autopsy series have actually suggested that patients with RA have a lower risk of MI than do control subjects, despite similar incidence of coronary atherosclerosis (59). The authors hypothesized that aspirin use may protect RA patients from coronary thrombosis. ▼ h23

SYSTEMIC SCLEROSIS

Background

Systemic sclerosis (SSc) is a rare connective-tissue disorder of unknown etiology, characterized by abnormal collagen deposition and fibrosis of the skin, viscera, and vasculature. Five- and 10-year survival rates are 70% and 50%, respectively (63,64), although wide ranges have been reported at different centers. Variables predicting a poor prognosis include male gender, advanced age at the time of diagnosis, and visceral involvement. Renal involvement portends the worst prognosis (5-year survival rate of 10%), followed by cardiac involvement (5-year survival rate of 40%) (64). ▼ h24

Cardiac dysfunction is common in patients with SSc. Symptomatic cardiac involvement occurs in approximately 10% of these patients, ECG and echocardiography detect abnormalities in 50%, and autopsy evidence of cardiac involvement is present in up to 80% (66–68). The presence of either occult or symptomatic evidence of cardiac involvement portends a poor prognosis. Clements and associates constructed a "cardiac score," based solely on the presence of left-axis deviation on ECG and the size of pericardial effusion, and found that this score was a strong independent predictor of survival in patients with SSc (69). Chest pain and shortness of breath are often ascribed to noncardiac causes, but their occurrence should prompt investigation into the possibility of cardiac involvement.

Pericardial Involvement

Pericardial disease is common in SSc; autopsy evidence of acute or chronic pericarditis is seen in 50% to 80% of patients (68,70,71), echocardiographic evidence in 10% to 40% of patients (72–74), and clinical evidence in 7% to 16% of patients (68,70). Pericardial effusion tends to be of little clinical importance, but it carries a poor prognosis if the effusion is large (greater than 200 mL). For reasons that are unclear, patients with large pericardial effusions frequently have progression to renal failure within 1 year (73,75). Pericardial fluid analysis typically reveals a bland exudate with high protein levels, high lactate dehydrogenase, normal immunoglobulin and complement levels, and a paucity of leukocytes (75,76). Patients may present with typical findings of acute pericarditis or may have nonspecific symptoms. Constrictive pericarditis is rare (67). Tamponade has been reported (77). Treatment of acute pericarditis consists of administration of NSAIDs and cor-

ticosteroids, but renal function should be closely monitored during therapy. Large effusions may require percutaneous or surgical drainage.

Valvular Involvement

Clinically important valvular heart disease is not a feature of SSc. Individual cases of severe valve dysfunction in patients with SSc have been reported, but without firm evidence of causation (78). Two echocardiographic studies involving unselected SSc patients have suggested that the prevalence of mild mitral regurgitation in this group is high, which may be related to papillary muscle fibrosis and dysfunction (74). Autopsy studies have demonstrated thickening of the mitral leaflets and chordae tendineae, but at levels no different than those in control subjects (68).

Myocardial Involvement

In 1943, Weiss (79) observed patchy myocardial fibrosis in patients with SSc, establishing sclerodermal heart disease as a clinical entity. Myocardial fibrosis has been found at autopsy in 37% to 81% of patients (67,68,80). Pathologic specimens reveal patchy areas of transmural fibrosis, which are not confined to epicardial coronary artery distributions. Areas of contraction-band necrosis, typical of myocardial ischemic injury followed by reperfusion, are well described. Myocardial injury may have a pathogenesis similar to that of the vasospasm-induced digital gangrene produced by Raynaud's phenomenon. This patchy fibrosis has, therefore, been termed the *myocardial Raynaud's phenomenon* (67). Support for this theory has been provided by investigators who have shown that cold-induced myocardial ischemia occurs in patients with SSc. This has been demonstrated by cold-induced echocardiographic wall motion abnormalities and abnormalities of thallium uptake (74,81). Interestingly, nondihydropyridine calcium channel antagonists and angiotensin-converting enzyme (ACE) inhibitors have been shown to blunt this response (82,83). Although such therapy is theoretically attractive, primary prevention of myocardial fibrosis and cardiac death with ACE inhibitors has not been studied in patients with SSc.

Diastolic dysfunction accompanied by echocardiographic evidence of impaired ventricular filling is common in patients with SSc (84,85). Myocardial fibrosis sufficient to produce systolic left ventricular dysfunction is uncommon but not rare and is mainly observed in autopsy studies. The prevalence of clinically apparent CHF has been reported to be 10% (86), but large series are lacking. Once thought to be contraindicated in patients with Raynaud's phenomenon, beta-blockers are now believed to be safe (87). Immunosuppressive treatment with corticosteroids is unlikely to be beneficial, because inflammation is rarely a major feature of this disease, and such treatment generally should be used only with the guidance of endomyocardial biopsy results. ❦ h25

KAWASAKI DISEASE

Dr. Tomisaku Kawasaki first examined a patient with what he called "mucocutaneous lymph node syndrome" in 1961, published a series of 50 cases in 1967, and reported it in English in 1974 (97). Kawasaki disease is an arteritis involving large, medium-sized, and small arteries and is associated with a mucocutaneous lymph-node syndrome (98). It is a disease of unknown etiology, with recognized perturbations of the cellular and humoral immune systems, and speculation of a viral or superantigen-driven pathologic inflammatory response (99). ❦ h26

Kawasaki disease is the number one cause of acquired heart disease in children in Japan and in North America. Although it is primarily a disease of children, arterial damage incurred during the acute phase of the illness may result in a high prevalence of early coronary events in affected adults. Advances in early treatment have allowed more patients with Kawasaki disease to survive into adulthood.

Pericardial Involvement

Autopsy series report pericarditis in 90% of patients who have died because of Kawasaki disease (103). Pericarditis is uncommonly reported in clinical series of patients with Kawasaki disease, suggesting that it is either commonly asymptomatic or underreported or that the autopsy series are not representative of the majority of patients. Echocardiographic studies report effusions in 30% of patients during the acute phase of the illness (104).

Valvular Involvement

Clinically evident valvular heart disease develops in the acute phase of Kawasaki disease in slightly more than 1% of patients (104–106). Valvulitis is detected at autopsy in 20% of patients (103). Ischemic papillary muscle dysfunction may also contribute to valvular dysfunction. Mitral regurgitation is most commonly seen, followed by aortic regurgitation. Severe valvular dysfunction requiring valve replacement has occurred, but most patients recover spontaneously. Valve dysfunction is more common among patients who have either prolonged fever or coronary aneurysm formation (106). The impact of intravenous immunoglobulin (IVIG) on valvular dysfunction in the acute phase of the illness has not been described.

Myocardial Involvement

Myocarditis, characterized by myocardial edema and polymorphonuclear leukocyte infiltration, is common in autopsy studies of patients with Kawasaki disease; it has an overall incidence of 45% and an incidence of 88% when death occurs between days 12 and 25 of the disease (103). Patients with myocarditis have tachycardia out of proportion to fever, a gallop rhythm, pulmonary congestion, and arrhythmia. The severity of myocarditis is not associated with the presence of coronary artery aneurysms (107). Left ventricle dimensions are increased and systolic function is abnormal in patients with Kawasaki disease in comparison with control subjects. Complete recovery is the rule, with normalization of ventricular function within 6 months in most patients (107,108). IVIG speeds recovery of myocardial function (108). CHF due to ischemia, infarction, or valvular heart disease may also occur. Heart transplantation has been required in some patients.

Coronary Involvement

Coronary artery aneurysm formation with subsequent myocardial ischemia and infarction is the most recognized and important cardiac complication of Kawasaki disease. MI is the leading cause of death in these patients. In untreated patients, 25% will develop coronary aneurysms in the acute phase of the illness (105). Within 2 years of detection, 50% of these patients will have complete angiographic resolution of the aneurysms. Giant aneurysms, those greater than 8 mm or more than four times the normal size of the vessel, occur in nearly 5% of patients and have special prognostic implications. As opposed to smaller aneurysms, giant aneurysms do not regress; frequently cause arterial remodeling, resulting in stenosis; and are prone to thrombosis, resulting in acute MI (Fig. 35E.2). More than one-third of infarctions may be silent, and more than two-thirds occur within the first year after the acute phase of the illness. Despite their young age, children with Kawasaki disease and acute MI have a 22% mortality rate (109).

IVIG has dramatically reduced the incidence of coronary aneurysms among patients with Kawasaki disease, from 23% to approximately 8% (110). High-dose aspirin administration is used until the febrile illness has passed, at which point the dose is reduced. In patients without coronary abnormalities, the aspirin may be discontinued 6 to 8 weeks after the acute phase of the illness. Patients with giant aneurysms or numerous smaller aneurysms should receive lifelong aspirin therapy, with or without coumadin. Frequency of clinical follow-up, ECG, echocardiography, and stress testing depends on the estimated risk of the patient. Patients with giant aneurysms, especially those with known coronary obstruction, require the most frequent follow-up (111).

Given the high cost and potential morbidity associated with coronary angiography, as well as the low incidence of coronary aneurysms since IVIG treatment came into use, routine angiography is not recommended in the acute illness, convalescent phase, or long-term follow-up of patients

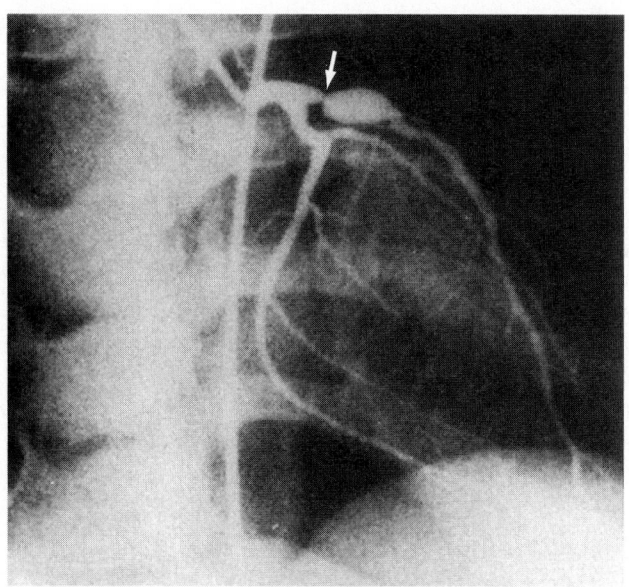

FIGURE 35E.2 Coronary angiogram revealing aneurysmal dilatation of the left anterior descending coronary artery with preceding focal stenosis (*arrow*). (Reprinted from Ino T, Akimoto K, Ohkubo M, et al. Application of percutaneous transluminal coronary angioplasty to coronary arterial stenosis in Kawasaki disease. *Circulation* 1996;93:1709–1715, with permission.)

with Kawasaki disease. In the acute and convalescent phases, echocardiography has been validated as the procedure of choice in detecting coronary aneurysms, with sensitivity of nearly 100% and specificity of 97% (112). Echocardiography performed by an experienced pediatric sonographer is recommended at the time of diagnosis, at 6 to 8 weeks, at 6 to 12 months, and when symptoms of ischemia are seen (111). Changes in patient size and artery characteristics limit the use of echocardiography beyond the first decade of life. Long-term follow-up with stress imaging procedures done at yearly intervals is recommended for patients with known stenoses and should be considered for patients with giant or multiple aneurysms. Dipyridamole-thallium testing is well validated and outperformed angiography in predicting future coronary events in one trial (113). Heart catheterization is indicated when noninvasive studies suggest the presence of flow-limiting coronary stenoses.

A number of therapeutic modalities have been used when patients with Kawasaki disease develop acute coronary syndromes or chronic ischemic heart disease. Thrombolysis has been used with good results to treat pediatric patients who have acute MI, unstable angina, and documented thrombosis in aneurysms (105). Coronary artery bypass graft surgery (CABG) is the procedure of choice for patients who require revascularization, but it is less effective in the very young patient. A recent series from Japan described surgical results in 100 patients who underwent CABG surgery, with 6.7 ± 4.5 years' follow-up. No intraoperative deaths occurred. Recurrent ischemia developed in 15% of patients, and 2% of patients died during the fol-

low-up period. One-year, 5-year, and 10-year graft patency rates were 94%, 82%, and 78% for arterial grafts and 82%, 63%, and 36% for venous grafts, respectively (114). The use of percutaneous coronary intervention (PCI) in this setting has been somewhat disappointing, characterized by high procedural mortality rates, frequent procedural failure, formation of new aneurysms, and high restenosis rates (115). There are no series that used state-of-the-art PCI with stents and glycoprotein IIb/IIIa antagonists.

Conduction System Involvement

Nonspecific ECG abnormalities are present in one-third of patients in the acute phase of the illness. Inflammation of the AV node, bundle of His, and bundle branches are present in 25% of patients at autopsy (103). Bradyarrhythmias and CHB may occur. Ventricular arrhythmias are more likely to be mediated by ischemia or infarction than by inflammation.

TAKAYASU'S DISEASE

Takayasu's disease is a chronic arteritis of the aorta, its major branches, pulmonary arteries, and coronary arteries. Takayasu, an ophthalmologist, first reported the ischemic retinal findings of the disorder in 1908. It is a rare disorder of unknown etiology with an annual incidence of 2.6 cases per 1 million individuals. It typically affects women of childbearing age, although cases affecting men are increasingly reported. Survival rates at 5 and 10 years are 91% and 84%, respectively. Clinical variables associated with poor outcome include hypertension, cardiac involvement, and poor functional capacity (116). Cardiac failure is the most common cause of death (116,117).

Diagnosis of Takayasu's disease relies on clinical, laboratory, and angiographic variables (118). Vascular bruits are the most common examination finding, followed by diminished or absent pulse. Claudication is the most common symptom, with upper extremity symptoms being more common than lower extremity symptoms (119). Arterial involvement includes, in order of decreasing frequency, the innominate and subclavian arteries, aorta, common carotid arteries, and renal arteries (120). Arterial lesions are occlusions or long, smooth stenoses more commonly than they are aneurysms or areas of ectasia.

Immunosuppression using corticosteroids and cytotoxic agents is the mainstay of medical therapy. A stepwise approach to medical therapy is advised, with initial corticosteroid therapy followed by the addition of cytotoxic agents, until clinical remission is achieved (119). No randomized, controlled trials of medical therapy have been performed, but observational data suggest that immunosuppression improves symptoms and may be associated with arterial lesion regression (119,121). Surgical and percutaneous revascularization of coronary and peripheral arteries has been described. In general, medical therapy may be pursued when symptoms are chronic and stable, but revascularization should be pursued when ischemia threatens life or limb.

Pericardial Involvement

During phases of clinical disease activity, patients may experience systemic findings such as fever, malaise, new arterial lesion formation, arterial tenderness, erythema nodosum, myalgias, arthralgias, weight loss, and night sweats. Pericarditis may occur as part of this symptom complex. Overall, however, pericarditis is uncommon in Takayasu's disease and has an estimated clinical frequency of only 2% (117). Cases of patients presenting with large effusions have been reported, and steroids have been used, with anecdotal success (122).

Valvular Involvement

Aortic regurgitation is common among patients with Takayasu's disease, is frequently severe, and is an independent predictor of mortality in these patients. Clinically detectable aortic regurgitation is present in 7% to 20% of patients (116,117,119,123). Aortic valve replacement is necessary in approximately 1% of patients. Regurgitation is usually the result of aortic root dilation and requires combined valve and root replacement. Leaflet thickening due to inflammation and subsequent fibrosis may contribute to valvular dysfunction (124).

Myocardial Involvement

CHF is the most common cause of death among patients with Takayasu's disease (116,117). CHF in these patients is usually multifactorial, with contributions from aortic regurgitation, hypertension, coronary involvement, and pulmonary artery involvement. Two-thirds of juvenile patients present in CHF, and one-third of adults experience heart failure (117). CHF with global left ventricular systolic dysfunction has been reported in the absence of hypertension or aortic regurgitation. When other markers of systemic inflammation are present, most of these patients exhibit myocarditis on endomyocardial biopsy, characterized by mononuclear cell infiltrate, necrosis, myocytolysis, and edema (125). Dramatic but anecdotal improvement has been noted after administration of corticosteroid therapy. Treatment with steroids must be done, with careful clinical follow-up, because of the capacity of steroids to increase sodium retention and raise blood pressure.

Coronary Involvement

Clinically important coronary artery involvement associated with Takayasu's disease occurs in 5% to 10% of patients (116,117). Three patterns of coronary involvement have been described: ostial stenosis; long, smooth stenoses; and aneurysm formation. The first two patterns predominate, and patients usually present with recent-onset exertional angina or non–ST-segment elevation MI (*e*Fig. 35E.2.1). Thrombosis of a coronary aneurysm resulting in abrupt vessel occlusion that presents as an ST-segment elevation MI is distinctly rare. Because of the frequency of occurrence of ostial stenosis, CABG has been the treatment of choice. However, graft survival is poor, which is likely a reflection of aortic disease at the proximal graft anastomosis. The high likelihood of subclavian artery disease precludes the use of internal thoracic artery grafts (126). When possible, surgery is delayed for these patients until medical therapy has induced remission of active aortic inflammation. PCI has been used with increasing frequency, but no large series are available that would allow the risk of procedural failure or restenosis to be estimated. Unprotected angioplasty of the left main coronary artery was undertaken in an 11-year-old girl in one case report. This is unconventional therapy, and the authors acknowledge that "acute obstruction is an inherent risk of PTCA [percutaneous transluminal coronary angioplasty] and can be deleterious in left coronary artery main stem lesions" (127).

Conduction System Involvement

ECG results are abnormal in 78% of patients with Takayasu's disease (117). The most common abnormality is left ventricular hypertrophy, followed by left atrial enlargement. These changes are frequently secondary to hypertension and aortic regurgitation, rather than to primary involvement of the conductive tissue. Holter monitoring of patients with Takayasu's disease reveals frequent ventricular ectopy in one-third and nonsustained ventricular tachycardia in 5%. The appearance of frequent ventricular ectopy during Holter monitoring is associated with echocardiographic evidence of aortic regurgitation and with the appearance of perfusion defects on thallium imaging. Patients who have Takayasu's disease and frequent ventricular ectopy have an increased risk of sudden cardiac death (128).

ANKYLOSING SPONDYLITIS

Ankylosing spondylitis is a seronegative spondyloarthropathy characterized by ankylosis and sacroiliitis, peripheral arthritis, iritis, and aortitis. It is a relatively common disorder, with a prevalence of 1% in white individuals (129). The pathogenesis is thought to have both heritable and environmental components. HLA-B27 is thought to be not only a marker of the disease, but pathologically involved. The diagnosis of ankylosing spondylitis is made on the basis of clinical and radiographic features. Cardiac involvement is associated with the presence of peripheral arthritis and with disease duration; it usually occurs after 10 to 20 years of disease (130). Heart disease is the most common cause of death among patients with ankylosing spondylitis (131). Reiter's syndrome, psoriatic arthritis, and inflammatory bowel disease have similar cardiac manifestations and are not discussed separately.

Pericardial Involvement

Pericarditis is rarely reported among patients with ankylosing spondylitis. Bulkley and coworkers, in a small autopsy series, found the pericardium to be normal in patients who had not had prior open heart surgery. Echocardiographic studies in unselected patients, however, have revealed a 5% to 10% incidence of pericardial thickening and effusion (132). Complicated pericardial disease would be reportable.

Valvular Involvement

Valvular heart disease occurs in approximately 10% of patients with ankylosing spondylitis (132–134). Pathology reveals fibrous thickening 1 to 2 cm superiorly and inferiorly from the aortic valve. Histopathology reveals adventitial scar, intimal proliferation, and inflammation of the vasa vasorum with lymphocytes and plasma cells (135). A "ridge" or "bump" of fibrous tissue may accumulate below the aortic valve on the membranous portion of the interventricular septum. Aortic regurgitation caused by fibrotic shortening of the aortic valve leaflets and aortic root dilatation occurs in approximately 8% of patients and may be severe. Mitral regurgitation due to extension of the fibrotic process to the anterior mitral leaflet has been reported (136). Mitral valve prolapse has been reported in as many as 10% of patients (132). Disease duration, advanced patient age, and the presence of peripheral arthritis predict valvular involvement. Echocardiography is a sensitive method for detection of preclinical valvular involvement, but whether early detection will affect late outcomes is unclear. Patients in whom careful clinical examination detects murmurs of aortic regurgitation should undergo echocardiography.

Myocardial Involvement

CHF is rarely reported among patients with ankylosing spondylitis, and systolic ventricular dysfunction is rare in the absence of ischemia, valvular heart disease, or hypertension. Diastolic dysfunction, however, has been found in up to 55% of patients (137). Diffuse myocardial connective tissue deposition in the absence of valvular heart disease, CAD, or hypertension has been observed histologically (137).

Coronary Involvement

Patients with ankylosing spondylitis do not appear to be at an increased risk for atheromatous CAD, and signifi-

cant inflammation of the epicardial coronary arteries has not been reported. Despite this, MI is an important cause of death in these patients, because of its high incidence in the general population (130). Extension of aortic pathology with ostial coronary artery narrowing presenting as stable angina has been reported in one patient with Reiter's syndrome (138).

Conduction System Involvement

Abnormalities of cardiac impulse formation or conduction are common among patients with ankylosing spondylitis and occur in 10% of patients (133). Sinus node dysfunction may be manifest as asymptomatic sinus pauses or sinus bradycardia (132,134). AV block is common, ranging from first-degree block to CHB. It is more common among patients with aortic regurgitation and occurs in as many as 44% of these patients (139). This is consistent with the known pathology of the disease, in which the fibrotic process extends into the interventricular septum, through which the conduction system traverses. Aortic regurgitation usually precedes heart block in the course of the disease (130). Bergfeldt and coauthors (140) studied a group of 223 consecutive men referred for pacemaker implantation and found 15 cases of ankylosing spondylitis, many of which were undiagnosed, suggesting that spondyloarthropathies may be an underappreciated cause of bradycardia.

CHURG-STRAUSS SYNDROME

Churg-Strauss syndrome (CSS) is characterized by eosinophil-rich and granulomatous inflammation that involves the respiratory tract and necrotizing vasculitis that affects small to medium-sized vessels, associated with asthma and eosinophilia (98). It is a rare disorder of unknown etiology, with an estimated annual incidence of less than one case per 100,000 individuals (141). Current therapy consists of administration of corticosteroids and cytotoxic agents, and the survival rate is 72% at 7 years (142). Cardiac involvement is a prominent feature of CSS; it occurs in 60% of patients in some studies and is the most common cause of death in most studies (142–145). Heart disease in patients with CSS is predictive of a poor outcome.

Pericardial Involvement

Clinically diagnosed pericarditis occurs in 20% to 32% of patients with CSS (142,145,146). Constrictive pericarditis and tamponade are rare but reported complications. Pericardial fluid may be bland or rich in eosinophils (147,148). Pericardial histopathology can be diagnostic and may reveal necrotizing granulomata, fibrosis, and prominent eosinophils. Acute management includes administration of corticosteroids and cytotoxic agents and drainage of the effusion when it causes hemodynamic compromise. Surgical creation of a pericardial window may be required for patients with recurrent disease and provides tissue for pathologic evaluation when the diagnosis is in doubt.

Valvular Involvement

Valvular heart disease is not a consequence of CSS.

Myocardial Involvement

Patients with CSS suffer considerable morbidity and mortality from CHF. Clinical evidence of CHF is present in 13% to 48% of patients (142,145). As noted earlier, cardiovascular disease is the most common cause of death among patients with CSS, and CHF is the most common cause of cardiovascular death. CHF that results from systolic dysfunction, diastolic dysfunction, and restrictive physiology may all be important. Ventricular thrombosis and thromboembolism resulting from underlying myocardial involvement have been reported (149).

Unlike many of the other connective tissue disorders and vasculitic syndromes, left ventricular dysfunction in association with CSS is frequently the result of primary myocardial involvement by the inflammatory process. Endomyocardial biopsy may show necrotizing granulomata and, frequently, eosinophils during the acute phase of the illness (*e*Fig. 35E.2.2) (150). Anecdotal reports are available of dramatic improvement in left ventricular function after immunosuppressive therapy is begun (150,151). Heart transplantation has been performed in a patient with CSS and fulminant myocarditis (152). Immunosuppression should be guided by endomyocardial biopsy, when possible, because fibrotic changes alone may be present if patients present late in the course of the illness (151).

Coronary Involvement

Autopsy evidence of coronary arteritis is present in more than one-half of patients with CSS (144). Acute MI is responsible for up to 20% of deaths in some series (143) (*e*Fig. 35E.2.3). Angiographic improvement of coronary arteritis after the start of medical therapy has been documented (153). Because of the difficulty in distinguishing between coronary arteritis and atherosclerotic CAD by angiography, corticosteroid therapy may be added to conventional therapy in select patients whose clinical course is stable and is strongly suggestive of arteritis.

Conduction System Involvement

Although ECG abnormalities are present in up to 50% of patients who have CSS, arrhythmias are uncommon. Those that have been reported are conduction abnormalities that appear in the setting of myocardial disease and respond to medical therapy (142).

POLYARTERITIS NODOSA

Polyarteritis nodosa (PAN) is a rare (154), nongranulomatous, necrotizing vasculitis of medium-sized and small arteries that is not accompanied by glomerulonephritis or microscopic angiitis (98). It is diagnosed by a combination of clinical and laboratory features, including weight loss, livedo reticularis, testicular pain, myalgias, neuropathy, diastolic hypertension, renal insufficiency, abnormal results of serologic testing for hepatitis B virus, and arteriographic or biopsy evidence of arteritis (155). Historically, survival rates have been only 13% 5 years after diagnosis (156). Advances in supportive care and medical treatment with corticosteroids and cyclophosphamide have improved the survival rate to 82% at 5 years (157). Death is usually the result of renal failure or infection. Cardiac involvement occurs in more than one-half of patients but is symptomatic in only 10% to 30% (154). The heart may be a direct target of the disease process, or it may be secondarily affected by hypertension, renal insufficiency, and corticosteroid use.

Pericardial Involvement

Clinically apparent pericarditis is uncommon in PAN and occurs in 2% to 5% of patients (154). At autopsy, however, pericarditis is observed in 27% of patients with PAN (158). It may be fibrous or fibrinous. Pericardial involvement complicated by purulent pericarditis, tamponade, or constrictive pericarditis would be worth reporting.

Valvular Involvement

PAN does not appear to be associated with valvular heart disease.

Myocardial Involvement

CHF is common among patients with PAN, occurring in 10% to 15%, but is usually secondary to associated hypertension, renal failure, or coronary involvement. Limited myocarditis has been reported in approximately 15% of patients with PAN at autopsy and is more common among patients with active arteritis (158). It is usually mild and of little clinical significance.

Coronary Involvement

Symptoms of coronary insufficiency occur in 4% to 15% of patients with PAN (154). Acute MI due to epicardial coronary artery necrotizing inflammation has been documented (*e*Fig. 35E.2.4) (159), but its exact incidence is unknown. Hypertension, corticosteroid use, and renal failure contribute to the high prevalence of atheromatous CAD among patients with PAN. Retrospective cohort series of patients with PAN report the occurrence of MI in 1% to 5% (154). MI in patients with PAN may be silent, or CHF may be the presenting symptom. PAN patients who present with chest pain and ST-segment elevation should be treated with either thrombolysis or primary coronary angioplasty, because occlusive lesions are typically caused by thrombus overlying areas of inflammation.

Pathologic evidence of coronary arteritis is more common than symptomatic disease and is found in one-half of all patients at autopsy (158). Arteritis begins with granulocytic infiltration of the vessel wall, followed by mononuclear cell predominance and then by fibrotic healing. Inflammation of epicardial coronary arteries may occur, but PAN more typically causes inflammatory lesions in intramyocardial coronary arteries (158). The clinical importance of this inflammation is unknown.

Conduction System Involvement

Autopsy evidence of involvement of the cardiac conduction system is commonly found in patients with PAN; however, clinically important arrhythmias are uncommon. Schrader and associates (158) reported sudden cardiac death to be the cause of death in 11% of their autopsy subjects, although detailed descriptions of the conductive tissue were not provided. Pathology of the AV nodal and SA nodal arteries, due to both ischemia and inflammation extending from the vessel into the conductive tissue, has also been implicated in clinical arrhythmias (*e*Fig. 35E.2.5) (160).

GIANT CELL (TEMPORAL) ARTERITIS

Giant cell arteritis (GCA) is a granulomatous arteritis of the aorta and its major branches that has a predilection for the extracranial branches of the carotid artery, often involves the temporal artery, and usually occurs in patients older than 50 years (98). The first case description is attributed to Hutchinson, in 1890 (161). The cause of GCA is not known, but it appears to be pathologic inflammation driven by a specific antigen and mediated by CD4+ lymphocytes, resulting in cytokine release and macrophage-induced oxidative damage (162). Diagnosis is based on clinical and pathologic criteria, including three of the following: age older than 50 years, new-onset headache, clinical abnormality of the temporal artery, elevated erythrocyte sedimentation rate, and diagnostic temporal artery biopsy (163). Its annual incidence in a predominantly white population is 17.8 in 100,000, but may reach 50.0 in 100,000 among elderly patients (164). Cardiac dysfunction occurs in 5% to 10% of patients with GCA (165). It is usually secondary to disease of the ascending aorta, rather than to primary cardiac involvement. Cardiac disease is the most common cause of death among patients with GCA (166).

Coronary Involvement

Coronary involvement in GCA appears to be rare, but it may be underreported. A number of case reports of histopathologically confirmed GCA of the coronary arteries have been published and summarized by Paulley (167), but the true incidence of coronary involvement is unknown. Acute MI has been reported (168). General angiographic predictors of arterial involvement by GCA include the presence of long, smooth stenoses; involvement of arch vessels; tapered occlusions; and the presence of skip lesions with diseased segments interspersed with normal segments (169). Traditional risk factors for the development of CAD are prevalent in patients with GCA. Hypertension has been noted in 43% of these patients, tobacco use in 14%, diabetes mellitus in 6%, and a positive family history of CAD in 31% (170). Risk factors should be aggressively treated, as should established CAD.

Aortic Involvement

Large arteries are involved in the cases of almost 15% of patients with GCA (171). The incidence of thoracic aortic aneurysms among these patients is 17.3-fold higher than that in the general population. On average, more than 5 years passes between diagnosis of GCA and diagnosis of aortic aneurysm. No clinical predictors of aneurysm development have been identified (165). Aortic dissection or rupture may occur. Despite this, life expectancy for patients with GCA is similar to that in the general population (165,166). Therefore, radiographic screening for aortic aneurysm in patients with GCA is not advocated. However, careful clinical examination may reveal evidence of aortic aneurysm or large-vessel involvement, and further evaluation in these patients is warranted.

Valvular Involvement

Aortic regurgitation has been described in 5% to 10% of patients with GCA. Histologic examination has shown that the valve itself is an innocent bystander. Aortic valve regurgitation is due to ascending aortic aneurysm formation with aortic root dilatation (Fig. 35E.3). Aortic valve replacement with aortic root reconstruction should be undertaken when patients develop large ascending aortic aneurysms or severe aortic regurgitation with either symptoms of CHF or signs of ventricular dysfunction.

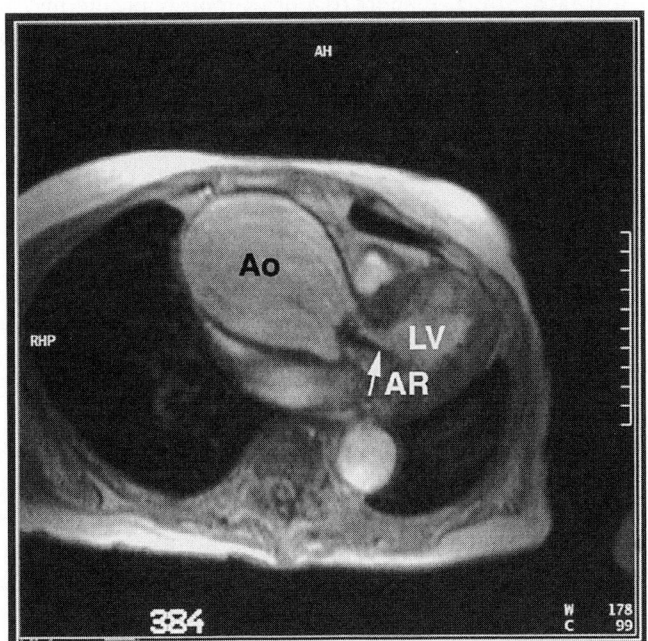
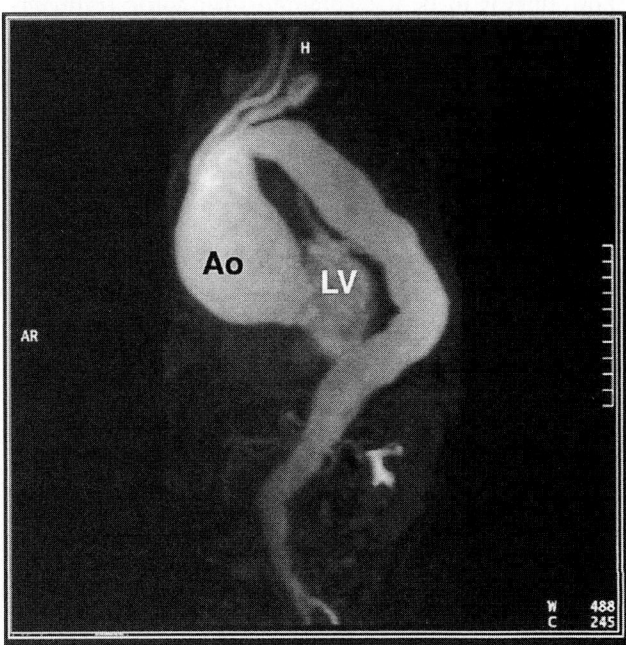

FIGURE 35E.3 Cross-sectional **(A)** and left anterior oblique **(B)** cardiac magnetic resonance images of a 72-year-old woman with giant cell arteritis/temporal arteritis, revealing an 8-cm ascending aortic aneurysm (Ao) and aortic regurgitant jet (AR, *arrow*). LV, left ventricle.

Pericardial involvement, myocardial involvement, or conduction system involvement in GCA with pathologic confirmation would be reportable.

WEGENER'S GRANULOMATOSIS

Wegener's granulomatosis (WG) is a rare systemic disorder of unknown etiology that is characterized by granulomatous inflammation involving the respiratory tract, necrotizing vasculitis of small and medium-sized vessels, and, commonly, necrotizing glomerulonephritis (98). Diagnosis relies on fulfillment of clinical criteria, including two or more of the following: nasal or oral inflammation, abnormal results of chest radiography, hematuria or red blood cell casts in urine, and granulomatous inflammation on examination of biopsy specimens. The presence of cytoplasmic patterned antineutrophil cytoplasmic antibody aids in diagnosis, but its pathologic role is uncertain. Once WG was almost uniformly fatal within months of diagnosis, but medical therapy with corticosteroids and cytotoxic agents has improved survival rates to 87% at 8 years (172). Despite this, patients with WG have standardized mortality ratios of more than 4, compared with the general population (173). Causes of death in these patients, in order of decreasing frequency, include infection, cardiovascular disease, renal failure, cancer, unknown causes, pulmonary disease, and stroke (173). Pulmonary and renal disease accounts for the majority of disease-related deaths. As the life expectancy for WG patients increases, cardiovascular disease is emerging as an important cause of morbidity and mortality. Cardiac involvement occurs in 12% to 14% of patients with WG (173,174).

Pericardial Involvement

Pericarditis is the most common cardiac manifestation of WG, occurring in one-half of patients with cardiac involvement (175) and in 6% to 10% of the overall patient population (172–174). It presents most commonly as acute pericarditis, but tamponade and constrictive pericarditis have been rarely reported (176,177). Histopathologic examination reveals fibrinous pericarditis with occasional pericardial granulomata (176,178). When pericarditis associated with WG is part of a systemic flare, it should be treated with initiation or intensification of steroid and cyclophosphamide therapy.

Valvular Involvement

Hemodynamically significant valvular dysfunction is uncommon, although not rare, in patients with WG. Clinical or autopsy evidence of valvulitis is found in 21% of patients with WG and cardiac involvement (175). Numerous case reports of severe aortic regurgitation with echocardiographic and histopathologic evidence of involvement by WG are available in the literature (176,179,180). Aortic valve leaflet perforation seems to have been reported with disproportionate frequency, relative to aortic regurgitation from other causes (181,182). Mitral valve regurgitation and stenosis appear to be less common than aortic regurgitation. When tissue is available from intraoperative or autopsy specimens, bland fibrosis with degeneration of collagen has been found more commonly than has active inflammation.

Myocardial Involvement

Myocarditis occurs in approximately 2% of patients with WG (174). Myocarditis may present as diffuse myocarditis, myocardial mass, or arrhythmia. Severe left ventricular systolic dysfunction due to myocarditis may respond to treatment with prednisone and cyclophosphamide, with resolution of symptoms and normalization of ventricular function (183). Kosovsky and associates (184) reported the case of a patient with a well-defined right ventricular mass, presenting as ventricular tachycardia, that was revealed on resection to be composed of granulomatous inflammatory tissue. Fauci and coauthors (174) also reported cases in which cardiomyopathy in patients with WG presented as ventricular tachycardia. On the basis of anecdotal improvements in left ventricular function that have been reported in patients with WG, it is reasonable to initiate or intensify immunosuppressive therapy in patients who present with new left ventricular systolic dysfunction, while standard heart failure therapy is started concurrently. This is particularly true if myocarditis occurs in conjunction with other signs or symptoms of active vasculitis.

Coronary Involvement

Coronary arteritis presenting as acute MI is rare but has been reported in patients with WG (185). Coronary arteritis at autopsy is present in one-half and evidence of MI in 11% of patients who have WG and known cardiac involvement (175). Histopathologic examination reveals epicardial arteritis with fibrinoid necrosis of the media and small-vessel fibrinoid occlusion (178). Patients with WG may, of course, have atheromatous CAD, and MI is a common cause of death in these patients (173).

Conduction System Involvement

A variety of arrhythmias have been described in patients with WG. CHB may be caused by granulomatous inflammation of the AV node, bundle of His, or bundle branches, or by inflammation of the artery to the AV node (175,178). Immunosuppressive therapy allowed pacemaker insertion to be avoided for one patient with CHB who had a stable ventricular response (177), and extraction of a pacemaker was possible for another patient (175). Sinus node dysfunction and atrial arrhythmias may be caused by inflammation of the sinus node artery or by extension of inflammation from overlying pericarditis. As noted, patients with WG and myocardial involvement may also present with ventric-

ular tachycardia. A short trial of temporary pacing may be considered for patients who have symptomatic bradycardia, while immunosuppressive therapy is initiated.

POLYMYOSITIS AND DERMATOMYOSITIS

Background

Polymyositis (PM) and dermatomyositis (DM) are inflammatory myopathies of unknown etiology. Diagnosis is based on fulfillment of clinical criteria put forth by Bohan and colleagues (186), which include proximal muscle weakness, serum enzyme abnormalities, abnormal results of electromyography, abnormal results on examination of muscle biopsy specimens, and, for diagnosis of DM, typical cutaneous manifestations. The survival rate is 73% at 8 years. The major causes of death are sepsis, malignancy, and cardiovascular disease (187). Cardiac involvement is the worst prognostic sign that may be found in patients with PM and DM (187). Symptoms suggesting cardiac involvement occur in 6% to 10% of patients.

Pericardial Involvement

Pericarditis is an uncommon but reported feature of PM and DM. Hochberg and colleagues (187) reported that 7% of the patients they followed for a mean time period of 8 years developed pericarditis. Echocardiography of unselected patients who have PM/DM reveals pericardial effusion in 8% (188). Complicated pericardial disease, such as purulent pericarditis, constrictive pericarditis, or tamponade, would be reportable.

Valvular Involvement

Clinically important valvular dysfunction is exceedingly rare in patients with PM/DM. ❦ h27

THERAPY

Primary prevention for patients with rheumatic diseases includes not only traditional risk-factor modification, but also minimization of cardiotoxic and atherogenic medications. Nonpharmacologic methods of prevention include smoking cessation, dietary changes, and exercise. Pharmacologic methods to prevent coronary events include 3-hydroxy-3-methylglutaryl coenzyme reductase inhibitors for hyperlipidemic patients, antihypertensive therapy for patients with hypertension, and aspirin and ramipril for high-risk patient groups. Newer immunomodulating therapies and cytotoxic agents may allow reduction of steroid doses, which may translate into a reduction in the incidence of manifest cardiac disease.

THE FUTURE

Progress in the treatment of the cardiac manifestations of the rheumatic diseases will require continued diligence, both at the bench and at the bedside. Basic research in immunology and the infectious diseases will, hopefully, provide insight into disease etiology and guide development of disease-specific therapies. Clinical research in rheumatology and cardiology may provide better treatment of established disease. Multicenter randomized controlled trials will be required to accrue adequate numbers of patients to draw firm conclusions with regard to detection and treatment of cardiovascular involvement in the rheumatic diseases.

Patients with established CAD and heart failure are candidates for secondary prevention strategies. These include nonpharmacologic methods such as sodium restriction, dietary changes, exercise, and smoking cessation. Secondary prevention for patients with CAD includes administration of aspirin and ACE inhibitors for all patients, beta-blockers for patients with a history of MI, and include 3-hydroxy-3-methylglutaryl coenzyme reductase inhibitors for patients with hyperlipidemia. Patients with chronic heart failure who have systolic left ventricular dysfunction benefit from ACE inhibitors, beta-blockers, digoxin, and diuretics. The optimal treatment of heart failure due to diastolic dysfunction is less well characterized; control of hypertension is paramount. Standard recommendations for use of revascularization, valvular surgery, pacemakers, and implantable cardioverter-defibrillators apply. No randomized controlled trials have evaluated any of these therapies specifically for use in patients with rheumatologic disease, and therefore therapy should be tailored to the individual patient.

The use of immunosuppressive therapy for patients with pericarditis, myocarditis, valvulitis, or coronary arteritis should be guided by adjunctive clinical, histologic, or laboratory evidence of inflammation, when possible. The treatment of myocarditis demands special attention, because trials addressing immunosuppressive therapy for "idiopathic" myocarditis have been disappointing. Endomyocardial biopsy may allow the clinician to distinguish between active inflammation and the subsequent fibrotic response that occurs in many of these illnesses. The rheumatic diseases, with few exceptions, are generally steroid-responsive. Immunosuppressive therapy should be considered when these patients present with biopsy-proven, symptomatic myocarditis.

CONTROVERSIES AND PERSONAL PERSPECTIVES

The rarity and clinical heterogeneity of both the cardiac and noncardiac manifestations of the rheumatic diseases have precluded prospective, randomized, controlled trials of therapeutic strategies. The clinician, therefore, is called on to draw from general principles of physiology and pharmacology, as well as the observational experience of the medical community, to guide individual patient care. This frequently involves a team approach, with internist, rheumatologist, cardiologist, and surgeon collaborating to benefit the patient.

The cardiac manifestations of the rheumatic diseases may be dramatic but more frequently are subtle, or patients may even be asymptomatic. The presence of these manifestations below the level of clinical detection belies their prognostic importance. The proper vigor with which to seek out cardiac involvement in these disorders remains to be defined. Careful attention should be paid to the cardiovascular system during physical examination and on any incidentally obtained studies.

REFERENCES

1. Biett T. Abrege pratique des maladies de la peau, d'apres les auteurs les plus estimes, et surtout d'apres des documens puises dans les lecanc cliniques de le docteur Biett. *Paris: Bechet* 1828:526.
2. Libman E, Sacks B. A hitherto undescribed form of valvular and mural endocarditis. *Arch Intern Med* 1924;33:294.
3. Tan EM, Cohen AS, Fries JF, et al. The 1982 revised criteria for the classification of systemic lupus erythematosus. *Arthritis Rheum* 1982;25:1271–1277.
4. Mills JA. Systemic lupus erythematosus. *N Engl J Med* 1994;330:1871–1879.
5. Fessel WJ. Systemic lupus erythematosus in the community: incidence, prevalence, outcome, and first symptoms; the high prevalence in black women. *Arch Intern Med* 1974;134:1027–1035.
6. Ward MM, Pyun E, Studenski S. Causes of death in systemic lupus erythematosus: long-term followup of an inception cohort. *Arthritis Rheum* 1995;38:1492–1499.
7. Abu-Shakra M, Urowitz MB, Gladman DD, et al. Mortality studies in systemic lupus erythematosus: results from a single center. I. Causes of death. *J Rheumatol* 1995;22:1259–1264.
8. Brigden W, Bywaters E, Lessof M, et al. The heart in systemic lupus erythematosus. *Br Heart J* 1960;22:1–16.
9. Doherty NE, Siegel RJ. Cardiovascular manifestations of systemic lupus erythematosus. *Am Heart J* 1985;110:1257–1265.

10. Leung WH, Wong KL, Lau CP, et al. Cardiac abnormalities in systemic lupus erythematosus: a prospective M-mode, cross-sectional and Doppler echocardiographic study. *Int J Cardiol* 1990;27:367–375.

11. Roldan CA, Shively BK, Crawford, MH. An echocardiographic study of valvular heart disease associated with systemic lupus erythematosus. *N Engl J Med* 1996;335:1424–1430.

12. Nihoyannopoulos P, Gomez PM, Joshi J, et al. Cardiac abnormalities in systemic lupus erythematosus: association with raised anticardiolipin antibodies. *Circulation* 1990;82:369–375.

13. Crozier IG, Li E, Milne MJ, et al. Cardiac involvement in systemic lupus erythematosus detected by echocardiography. *Am J Cardiol* 1990;65:1145–1148.

14. Kahl LE. The spectrum of pericardial tamponade in systemic lupus erythematosus: report of ten patients. *Arthritis Rheum* 1992;35:1343–1349.

15. Hunder GG, Mullen BJ, McDuffie FC. Complement in pericardial fluid of lupus erythematosus: studies in two patients. *Ann Intern Med* 1974;80:453–458.

16. Bidani AK, Roberts JL, Schwartz MM, et al. Immunopathology of cardiac lesions in fatal systemic lupus erythematosus. *Am J Med* 1980;69:849–858.

17. Klemperer P, Pollack A, Baehr D. Pathology of disseminated lupus erythematosus. *Arch Pathol* 1941;32:569–631.

18. Bulkley BH, Roberts WC. The heart in systemic lupus erythematosus and the changes induced in it by corticosteroid therapy: a study of 36 necropsy patients. *Am J Med* 1975;58:243–264.

19. Gross L. The cardiac lesions in Libman-Sacks disease with a consideration of its relationship to acute diffuse lupus erythematosus. *Am J Pathol* 1940;16:375–419.

20. Hojnik M, George J, Ziporen L, et al. Heart valve involvement (Libman-Sacks endocarditis) in the antiphospholipid syndrome. *Circulation* 1996;93:1579–1587.

21. Shapiro RF, Gamble CN, Wiesner KB, et al. Immunopathogenesis of Libman-Sacks endocarditis: assessment by light and immunofluorescent microscopy in two patients. *Ann Rheum Dis* 1977;36:508–516.

22. Roberts WC, High ST. The heart in systemic lupus erythematosus. *Curr Probl Cardiol* 1999;24(1):1–56.

23. Khamashta MA, Cervera R, Asherson RA, et al. Association of antibodies against phospholipids with heart valve disease in systemic lupus erythematosus. *Lancet* 1990;335:1541–1544.

24. Roldan CA, Shively BK, Lau CC, et al. Systemic lupus erythematosus valve disease by transesophageal echocardiography and the role of antiphospholipid antibodies. *J Am Coll Cardiol* 1992;20:1127–1134.

25. Dajee H, Hurley EJ, Szarnicki RJ. Cardiac valve replacement in systemic lupus erythematosus: a review. *J Thorac Cardiovasc Surg* 1983;85:718–726.

26. Galve E, Candell-Riera J, Pigrau C, et al. Prevalence, morphologic types, and evolution of cardiac valvular disease in systemic lupus erythematosus. *N Engl J Med* 1988;319:817–823.

27. Dajani AS, Taubert KA, Wilson W, et al. Prevention of bacterial endocarditis: recommendations by the American Heart Association. *Circulation* 1997;96(1):358–366.

28. Bruce I, Burns R, Gladman D, et al. A study of myocardial perfusion abnormalities in women with SLE. *J Rheumatol* 1998;25[Suppl 52]:72.

29. Leung WH, Wong KL, Lau CP, et al. Doppler echocardiographic evaluation of left ventricular diastolic function in patients with systemic lupus erythematosus. *Am Heart J* 1990;120(1):82–87.

30. Sasson Z, Rasooly Y, Chow CW, et al. Impairment of left ventricular diastolic function in systemic lupus erythematosus. *Am J Cardiol* 1992;69:1629–1634.

31. Winslow TM, Ossipov MA, Fazio GP, et al. The left ventricle in systemic lupus erythematosus: initial observations and a five-year follow-up in a university medical center population. *Am Heart J* 1993;125:1117–1122.

32. Manzi S, Meilahn EN, Rairie JE, et al. Age-specific incidence rates of myocardial infarction and angina in women with systemic lupus erythematosus: comparison with the Framingham Study. *Am J Epidemiol* 1997;145:408–415.

33. Rosner S, Ginzler EM, Diamond HS, et al. A multicenter study of outcome in systemic lupus erythematosus. II. Causes of death. *Arthritis Rheum* 1982;25:612–617.

34. Bruce IN, Gladman DD, Urowitz MB. Premature atherosclerosis in systemic lupus erythematosus. *Rheum Dis Clin North Am* 2000;26:257–278.

35. Hosenpud JD, Montanaro A, Hart MV, et al. Myocardial perfusion abnormalities in asymptomatic patients with systemic lupus erythematosus. *Am J Med* 1984;77:286–292.

36. Haider YS, Roberts WC. Coronary arterial disease in systemic lupus erythematosus: quantification of degrees of narrowing in 22 necropsy patients (21 women) aged 16 to 37 years. *Am J Med* 1981;70:775–781.

37. Petri M, Perez-Gutthann S, Spence D, et al. Risk factors for coronary artery disease in patients with systemic lupus erythematosus. *Am J Med* 1992;93:513–519.

38. Homcy CJ, Liberthson RR, Fallon JT, et al. Ischemic heart disease in systemic lupus erythematosus in the young patient: report of six cases. *Am J Cardiol* 1982;49:478–484.

39. James T, Rupe C, Monto R. Pathology of the cardiac conduction system in systemic lupus erythematosus. *Ann Intern Med* 1965;63:402–410.

40. Logar D, Kveder T, Rozman B, et al. Possible association between anti-Ro antibodies and myocarditis or cardiac conduction defects in adults with systemic lupus erythematosus. *Ann Rheum Dis* 1990;49:627–629.

41. Scott JS, Maddison PJ, Taylor PV, et al. Connective-tissue disease, antibodies to ribonucleoprotein, and congenital heart block. *N Engl J Med* 1983;309:209–212.

42. Deng JS, Bair LW Jr, Shen-Schwarz S, et al. Localization of Ro (SS-A) antigen in the cardiac conduction system. *Arthritis Rheum* 1987;30:1232–1238.

43. Wiles N, Symmons DP, Harrison B, et al. Estimating the incidence of rheumatoid arthritis: trying to hit a moving target? *Arthritis Rheum* 1999;42:1339–1346.

44. Arnett FC, Edworthy SM, Bloch DA, et al. The American Rheumatism Association 1987 revised criteria for the classification of rheumatoid arthritis. *Arthritis Rheum* 1988;31:315–324.

45. Wolfe F, Mitchell DM, Sibley JT, et al. The mortality of rheumatoid arthritis. *Arthritis Rheum* 1994;37:481–494.

46. Mutru O, Laakso M, Isomaki H, et al. Cardiovascular mortality in patients with rheumatoid arthritis. *Cardiology* 1989;76(1):71–77.

47. Myllykangas-Luosujarvi R, Aho K, Kautiainen H, et al. Cardiovascular mortality in women with rheumatoid arthritis. *J Rheumatol* 1995;22:1065–1067.

48. Charcot J. Clinical lectures on senile and chronic diseases. *New Sydenham Soc* 1881;95:172–175.

49. Kirk J, Cosh J. The pericarditis of rheumatoid arthritis. *QJM* 1969;38:397–423.

50. Hara KS, Ballard DJ, Ilstrup DM, et al. Rheumatoid pericarditis: clinical features and survival. *Medicine (Baltimore)* 1990;69(2):81–91.

51. Prakash R, Atassi A, Poske R, et al. Prevalence of pericardial effusion and mitral-valve involvement in patients with rheumatoid arthritis without cardiac symptoms: an echocardiographic evaluation. *N Engl J Med* 1973;289:597–600.

52. Bacon PA, Gibson DG. Cardiac involvement in rheumatoid arthritis: an echocardiographic study. *Ann Rheum Dis* 1974;33(1):20–24.

53. Maione S, Valentini G, Giunta A, et al. Cardiac involvement in rheumatoid arthritis: an echocardiographic study. *Cardiology* 1993;83:234–239.

54. Thould AK. Constrictive pericarditis in rheumatoid arthritis. *Ann Rheum Dis* 1986;45(2):89–94.

55. Thadani U, Iveson JM, Wright V. Cardiac tamponade, constrictive pericarditis and pericardial resection in rheumatoid arthritis. *Medicine (Baltimore)* 1975;54:261–270.

56. Baggenstoss A, Rosenberg E. Cardiac lesions associated with chronic infectious arthritis. *Arch Intern Med* 1941;67:241.

57. Roberts WC, Kehoe JA, Carpenter DF, et al. Cardiac valvular lesions in rheumatoid arthritis. *Arch Intern Med* 1968;122:141–146.

58. Gabriel S, Crowson C, O'Fallon W. Heart disease in rheumatoid arthritis (RA). *Arthritis Rheum* 1998;9[Suppl]:S132.

59. Davis RF, Engleman EG. Incidence of myocardial infarction in patients with rheumatoid arthritis. *Arthritis Rheum* 1974;17:527–533.

60. Karten I. Arteritis, myocardial infarction, and rheumatoid arthritis. *JAMA* 1969;210:1717–1720.

61. Swezey RL. Myocardial infarction due to rheumatoid arteritis: an antemortem diagnosis. *JAMA* 1967;199:855–857.

62. Ahern M, Lever JV, Cosh J. Complete heart block in rheumatoid arthritis. *Ann Rheum Dis* 1983;42:389–397.

63. Hesselstrand R, Scheja A, Akesson A. Mortality and causes of death in a Swedish series of systemic sclerosis patients. *Ann Rheum Dis* 1998;57:682–686.

64. Medsger T. Epidemiology of progressive systemic sclerosis. *Clin Rheum Dis* 1979;5(1):15–25.

65. Preliminary criteria for the classification of systemic sclerosis (scleroderma). Subcommittee for Scleroderma Criteria of the American Rheumatism Association Diagnostic and Therapeutic Criteria Committee. *Arthritis Rheum* 1980;23:581–590.

66. Deswal A, Follansbee WP. Cardiac involvement in scleroderma. *Rheum Dis Clin North Am* 1996;22:841–860.

67. Bulkley BH, Ridolfi RL, Salyer WR, et al. Myocardial lesions of progressive systemic sclerosis: a cause of cardiac dysfunction. *Circulation* 1976;53:483–490.

68. D'Angelo WA, Fries JF, Masi AT, et al. Pathologic observations in systemic sclerosis (scleroderma): a study of fifty-eight autopsy cases and fifty-eight matched controls. *Am J Med* 1969;46:428–440.

69. Clements PJ, Lachenbruch PA, Furst DE, et al. Cardiac score: a semiquantitative measure of cardiac involvement that improves prediction of prognosis in systemic sclerosis. *Arthritis Rheum* 1991;34:1371–1380.

70. McWhorter JE 4th, LeRoy EC. Pericardial disease in scleroderma (systemic sclerosis). *Am J Med* 1974;57:566–575.

71. Byers RJ, Marshall DA, Freemont AJ. Pericardial involvement in systemic sclerosis. *Ann Rheum Dis* 1997;56:393–394.

72. Ferri C, Bernini L, Bongiorni MG, et al. Noninvasive evaluation of cardiac dysrhythmias, and their relationship with multisystemic symptoms, in progressive systemic sclerosis patients. *Arthritis Rheum* 1985;28:1259–1266.

73. Smith JW, Clements PJ, Levisman J, et al. Echocardiographic features of progressive systemic sclerosis (PSS): correlation with hemodynamic and postmortem studies. *Am J Med* 1979;66(1):28–33.

74. Candell-Riera J, Armadans-Gil L, Simeon CP, et al. Comprehensive noninvasive assessment of cardiac involvement in limited systemic sclerosis. *Arthritis Rheum* 1996;39:1138–1145.

75. Satoh M, Tokuhira M, Hama N, et al. Massive pericardial effusion in scleroderma: a review of five cases. *Br J Rheumatol* 1995;34:564–567.

76. Gladman DD, Gordon DA, Urowitz MB, et al. Pericardial fluid analysis in scleroderma (systemic sclerosis). *Am J Med* 1976;60:1064–1068.

77. Choe W, Mehlman D. Mediastinal abnormalities in systemic sclerosis. *N Engl J Med* 2000;343:1771.

78. Yunus MB, Radford CM, Masi AT, et al. Aortic regurgitation in scleroderma. *J Rheumatol* 1984;11:384–386.

79. Weiss S, Stead EJ, Warren J, et al. Scleroderma heart disease with a consideration of certain other visceral manifestations of scleroderma. *Arch Intern Med* 1943;71:749.

80. Follansbee WP, Miller TR, Curtiss EI, et al. A controlled clinicopathologic study of myocardial fibrosis in systemic sclerosis (scleroderma). *J Rheumatol* 1990;17:656–662.

81. Alexander EL, Firestein GS, Weiss JL, et al. Reversible cold-induced abnormalities in myocardial perfusion and function in systemic sclerosis. *Ann Intern Med* 1986;105:661–668.

82. Kahan A, Devaux JY, Amor B, et al. Nifedipine and thallium-201 myocardial perfusion in progressive systemic sclerosis. *N Engl J Med* 1986;314:1397–1402.

83. Kahan A, Devaux JY, Amor B, et al. The effect of captopril on thallium 201 myocardial perfusion in systemic sclerosis. *Clin Pharmacol Ther* 1990;47:483–489.

84. Kazzam E, Caidahl K, Hallgren R, et al. Mitral regurgitation and diastolic flow profile in systemic sclerosis. *Int J Cardiol* 1990;29:357–363.

85. Giunta A, Tirri E, Maione S, et al. Right ventricular diastolic abnormalities in systemic sclerosis: relation to left ventricular involvement and pulmonary hypertension. *Ann Rheum Dis* 2000;59(2):94–98.

86. Janosik DL, Osborn TG, Moore TL, et al. Heart disease in systemic sclerosis. *Semin Arthritis Rheum* 1989;19:191–200.

87. Coffman JD, Rasmussen HM. Effects of beta-adrenoreceptor-blocking drugs in patients with Raynaud's phenomenon. *Circulation* 1985;72:466–470.

88. Follansbee WP, Curtiss EI, Medsger TA Jr, et al. Myocardial function and perfusion in the CREST syndrome variant of progressive systemic sclerosis: exercise radionuclide evaluation and comparison with diffuse scleroderma. *Am J Med* 1984;77:489–496.

89. Follansbee WP, Zerbe TR, Medsger TA Jr. Cardiac and skeletal muscle disease in systemic sclerosis (scleroderma): a high risk association. *Am Heart J* 1993;125(1):194–203.

90. James TN. De subitaneis mortibus. VIII. Coronary arteries and conduction system in scleroderma heart disease. *Circulation* 1974;50:844–856.

91. Follansbee WP, Curtiss EI, Rahko PS, et al. The electrocardiogram in systemic sclerosis (scleroderma): study of 102 consecutive cases with functional correlations and review of the literature. *Am J Med* 1985;79:183–192.

92. Ridolfi RL, Bulkley BH, Hutchins GM. The cardiac conduction system in progressive systemic sclerosis: clinical and pathologic features of 35 patients. *Am J Med* 1976;61:361–366.

93. Lev M, Landowne M, Matchar JC, et al. Systemic scleroderma with complete heart block: report of a case with comprehensive study of the conduction system. *Am Heart J* 1966;72(1):13–24.

94. Kostis JB, Seibold JR, Turkevich D, et al. Prognostic importance of cardiac arrhythmias in systemic sclerosis. *Am J Med* 1988;84:1007–1015.

95. Rankin AC, Osswald S, McGovern BA, et al. Mechanism of sustained monomorphic ventricular tachycardia in systemic sclerosis. *Am J Cardiol* 1999;83:633–636, A11.

96. Martinez-Taboada V, Olalla J, Blanco R, et al. Malignant ventricular arrhythmia in systemic sclerosis controlled with an implantable cardioverter defibrillator. *J Rheumatol* 1994;21:2166–2167.

97. Kawasaki T, Kosaki F, Okawa S, et al. A new infantile acute febrile mucocutaneous lymph node syndrome (MLNS) prevailing in Japan. *Pediatrics* 1974;54:271–276.

98. Jennette JC, Falk RJ, Andrassy K, et al. Nomenclature of systemic vasculitides: proposal of an international consensus conference. *Arthritis Rheum* 1994;37:187–192.

99. Barron KS, Shulman ST, Rowley A, et al. Report of the National Institutes of Health Workshop on Kawasaki Disease. *J Rheumatol* 1999;26(1):170–190.

100. Yanagawa H, Nakamura Y, Yashiro M, et al. Results of the nationwide epidemiologic survey of Kawasaki disease in 1995 and 1996 in Japan. *Pediatrics* 1998;102(6):E65.

101. Burns JC, Kushner HI, Bastian JF, et al. Kawasaki disease: a brief history. *Pediatrics* 2000;106(2):E27.

102. Dajani AS, Taubert KA, Gerber MA, et al. Diagnosis and therapy of Kawasaki disease in children. *Circulation* 1993;87:1776–1780.

103. Fujiwara H, Hamashima Y. Pathology of the heart in Kawasaki disease. *Pediatrics* 1978;61(1):100–107.

104. Takahashi M. Kawasaki syndrome (mucocutaneous lymph node syndrome). In: Emmanouilides G, ed. *Moss and Adams heart disease in infants, children, and adolescents: including the fetus and young adult.* Baltimore: Williams & Wilkins, 1995:1390–1399.

105. Kato H, Sugimura T, Akagi T, et al. Long-term consequences of Kawasaki disease: a 10- to 21-year follow-up study of 594 patients. *Circulation* 1996;94:1379–1385.

106. Akagi T, Kato H, Inoue O, et al. Valvular heart disease in Kawasaki syndrome: incidence and natural history. *Am Heart J* 1990;120:366–372.

107. Moran AM, Newburger JW, Sanders SP, et al. Abnormal myocardial mechanics in Kawasaki disease: rapid response to gamma-globulin. *Am Heart J* 2000;139:217–223.

108. Newburger JW, Sanders SP, Burns JC, et al. Left ventricular contractility and function in Kawasaki syndrome: effect of intravenous gamma-globulin. *Circulation* 1989;79:1237–1246.

109. Kato H, Ichinose E, Kawasaki T. Myocardial infarction in Kawasaki disease: clinical analyses in 195 cases. *J Pediatr* 1986;108:923–927.

110. Newburger JW, Takahashi M, Burns JC, et al. The treatment of Kawasaki syndrome with intravenous gamma globulin. *N Engl J Med* 1986;315:341–347.

111. Dajani AS, Taubert KA, Takahashi M, et al. Guidelines for long-term management of patients with Kawasaki disease. Report from the Committee on Rheumatic Fever, Endocarditis, and Kawasaki Disease, Council on Cardiovascular Disease in the Young, American Heart Association. *Circulation* 1994;89:916–922.

112. Capannari TE, Daniels SR, Meyer RA, et al. Sensitivity, specificity and predictive value of two-dimensional echocardiography in detecting coronary artery aneurysms in patients with Kawasaki disease. *J Am Coll Cardiol* 1986;7:355–360.

113. Miyagawa M, Mochizuki T, Murase K, et al. Prognostic value of dipyridamole-thallium myocardial scintigraphy in patients with Kawasaki disease. *Circulation* 1998;98:990–996.

114. Yoshikawa Y, Yagihara T, Kameda Y, et al. Result of surgical treatments in patients with coronary-arterial obstructive disease after Kawasaki disease. *Eur J Cardiothorac Surg* 2000;17:515–519.

115. Akagi T, Ogawa S, Ino T, et al. Catheter interventional treatment in Kawasaki disease: a report from the Japanese Pediatric Interventional Cardiology Investigation group. *J Pediatr* 2000;137:181–186.

116. Subramanyan R, Joy J, Balakrishnan KG. Natural history of aortoarteritis (Takayasu's disease). *Circulation* 1989;80:429–437.

117. Lupi-Herrera E, Sanchez-Torres G, Marcushamer J, et al. Takayasu's arteritis: clinical study of 107 cases. *Am Heart J* 1977;93(1):94–103.

118. Sharma BK, Jain S, Suri S, et al. Diagnostic criteria for Takayasu arteritis. *Int J Cardiol* 1996;54[Suppl]:S141–S147.

119. Kerr GS, Hallahan CW, Giordano J, et al. Takayasu arteritis. *Ann Intern Med* 1994;120:919–929.

120. Hoffman GS. Takayasu arteritis: lessons from the American National Institutes of Health experience. *Int J Cardiol* 1996;54[Suppl]:S99–S102.

121. Ishikawa K. Effects of prednisolone therapy on arterial angiographic features in Takayasu's disease. *Am J Cardiol* 1991;68:410–413.

122. Narita H, Ohte N, Yoneyama A, et al. Takayasu's arteritis accompanied with massive pericardial effusion: a case report. *Angiology* 1999;50:421–425.

123. Ishikawa K. Diagnostic approach and proposed criteria for the clinical diagnosis of Takayasu's arteriopathy. *J Am Coll Cardiol* 1988;12:964–972.

124. Kalangos A, Baldovinos A, Beghetti M, et al. Ascending aortic aneurysm associated with aortic insufficiency due to Takayasu's arteritis. *Ann Thorac Surg* 1999;68(1):248–250.

125. Talwar KK, Chopra P, Narula J, et al. Myocardial involvement and its response to immunosuppressive therapy in nonspecific aortoarteritis (Takayasu's disease): a study by endomyocardial biopsy. *Int J Cardiol* 1988;21:323–334.

126. Jolly M, Bartholomew JR, Flamm SD, et al. Angina and coronary ostial lesions in a young woman as a presentation of Takayasu's arteritis. *Cardiovasc Surg* 1999;7:443–446.

127. Lee HY, Rao PS. Percutaneous transluminal coronary angioplasty in Takayasu's arteritis. *Am Heart J* 1996;132:1084–1086.

128. Siburian G, Hashimoto Y, Numano F. Ventricular arrhythmias in Takayasu arteritis. *Int J Cardiol* 1993;40:243–249.

129. Carbone LD, Cooper C, Michet CJ, et al. Ankylosing spondylitis in Rochester, Minnesota, 1935–1989: is the epidemiology changing? *Arthritis Rheum* 1992;35:1476–1482.

130. Bergfeldt L, Edhag O, Vallin H. Cardiac conduction disturbances, an underestimated manifestation in ankylosing spondylitis: a 25-year follow-up study of 68 patients. *Acta Med Scand* 1982;212:217–223.

131. Khan MA, Khan MK, Kushner I. Survival among patients with ankylosing spondylitis: a life-table analysis. *J Rheumatol* 1981;8(1):86–90.

132. Alves MG, Espirito-Santo J, Queiroz MV, et al. Cardiac alterations in ankylosing spondylitis. *Angiology* 1988;39:567–571.

133. Lehtinen K. 76 Patients with ankylosing spondylitis seen after 30 years of disease. *Scand J Rheumatol* 1983;12(1):5–11.

134. O'Neill TW, King G, Graham IM, et al. Echocardiographic abnormalities in ankylosing spondylitis. *Ann Rheum Dis* 1992;51:652–654.

135. Bulkley BH, Roberts WC. Ankylosing spondylitis and aortic regurgitation: description of the characteristic cardiovascular lesion from study of eight necropsy patients. *Circulation* 1973;48:1014–1027.

136. Shah A. Echocardiographic features of mitral regurgitation due to ankylosing spondylitis. *Am J Med* 1987;82:353–356.

137. Brewerton DA, Gibson DG, Goddard DH, et al. The myocardium in ankylosing spondylitis: a clinical, echocardiographic, and histopathological study. *Lancet* 1987;1:995–998.

138. Hoogland YT, Alexander EP, Patterson RH, et al. Coronary artery stenosis in Reiter's syndrome: a complication of aortitis. *J Rheumatol* 1994;21:757–759.

139. Weed CL, Kulander BG, Massarella JA, et al. Heart block in ankylosing spondylitis. *Arch Intern Med* 1966;117:800–806.

140. Bergfeldt L, Edhag O, Vedin L, et al. Ankylosing spondylitis: an important cause of severe disturbances of the cardiac conduction system: prevalence among 223 pacemaker-treated men. *Am J Med* 1982;73:187–191.

141. Watts RA, Carruthers DM, Scott DG. Epidemiology of systemic vasculitis: changing incidence or definition? *Semin Arthritis Rheum* 1995;25(1):28–34.

142. Guillevin L, Cohen P, Gayraud M, et al. Churg-Strauss syndrome: clinical study and long-term follow-up of 96 patients. *Medicine (Baltimore)* 1999;78(1):26–37.

143. Chumbley LC, Harrison EG Jr, DeRemee RA. Allergic granulomatosis and angiitis (Churg-Strauss syndrome): report and analysis of 30 cases. *Mayo Clin Proc* 1977;52:477–484.

144. Churg J, Strauss L. Allergic granulomatosis, allergic angiitis, and periarteritis nodosa. *Am J Pathol* 1951;27:277–301.

145. Lanham JG, Elkon KB, Pusey CD, et al. Systemic vasculitis with asthma and eosinophilia: a clinical approach to the Churg-Strauss syndrome. *Medicine (Baltimore)* 1984;63(2):65–81.

146. Masi AT, Hunder GG, Lie JT, et al. The American College of Rheumatology 1990 criteria for the classification of Churg-Strauss syndrome (allergic granulomatosis and angiitis). *Arthritis Rheum* 1990;33:1094–1100.

147. Hasley PB, Follansbee WP, Coulehan JL. Cardiac manifestations of Churg-Strauss syndrome: report of a case and review of the literature. *Am Heart J* 1990;120:996–999.

148. Davison AG, Thompson PJ, Davies J, et al. Prominent pericardial and myocardial lesions in the Churg-Strauss syndrome (allergic granulomatosis and angiitis). *Thorax* 1983;38:793–795.

149. Lanham JG, Cooke S, Davies J, et al. Endomyocardial complications of the Churg-Strauss syndrome. *Postgrad Med J* 1985;61:341–344.

150. Frustaci A, Gentiloni N, Chimenti C, et al. Necrotizing myocardial vasculitis in Churg-Strauss syndrome: clinico-histologic evaluation of steroids and immunosuppressive therapy. *Chest* 1998;114:1484–1489.

151. Leung WH, Wong KK, Lau CP, et al. Myocardial involvement in Churg-Strauss syndrome: the role of endomyocardial biopsy. *J Rheumatol* 1989;16:828–831.

152. Thomson D, Chamsi-Pasha H, Hasleton P. Heart transplantation for Churg-Strauss syndrome. *Br Heart J* 1989;62:409–410.

153. Hellemans S, Dens J, Knockaert D. Coronary involvement in the Churg-Strauss syndrome. *Heart* 1997;77:576–578.

154. Lhote F, Guillevin L. Polyarteritis nodosa, microscopic polyangiitis, and Churg-Strauss syndrome: clinical aspects and treatment. *Rheum Dis Clin North Am* 1995;21:911–947.

155. Lightfoot RW Jr, Michel BA, Bloch DA, et al. The American College of Rheumatology 1990 criteria for the classification of polyarteritis nodosa. *Arthritis Rheum* 1990;33:1088–1093.

156. Frohnert PP, Sheps SG. Long-term follow-up study of periarteritis nodosa. *Am J Med* 1967;43(1):8–14.

157. Fauci AS, Katz P, Haynes BF, et al. Cyclophosphamide therapy of severe systemic necrotizing vasculitis. *N Engl J Med* 1979;301:235–238.

158. Schrader ML, Hochman JS, Bulkley BH. The heart in polyarteritis nodosa: a clinicopathologic study. *Am Heart J* 1985;109:1353–1359.

159. Odhav S, McKown K, Lohr KM. Polyarteritis nodosa pre-

senting as recurrent myocardial infarction [letter]. *Chest* 1994;105:1615.

160. Thiene G, Valente M, Rossi L. Involvement of the cardiac conducting system in panarteritis nodosa. *Am Heart J* 1978;95:716–724.

161. Hutchinson J. On a peculiar form of thrombotic arteritis of the aged which is sometimes productive of gangrene. *Arch Surg (London)* 1889–1890;1:323–329.

162. Weyand CM, Goronzy JJ. Pathogenic principles in giant cell arteritis. *Int J Cardiol* 2000;75[Suppl 1]:S9–S15, S17–S19.

163. Hunder GG, Bloch DA, Michel BA, et al. The American College of Rheumatology 1990 criteria for the classification of giant cell arteritis. *Arthritis Rheum* 1990;33:1122–1128.

164. Salvarani C, Gabriel SE, O'Fallon WM, et al. Epidemiology of polymyalgia rheumatica in Olmsted County, Minnesota, 1970–1991. *Arthritis Rheum* 1995;38:369–373.

165. Evans JM, O'Fallon WM, Hunder GG. Increased incidence of aortic aneurysm and dissection in giant cell (temporal) arteritis: a population-based study. *Ann Intern Med* 1995;122:502–507.

166. Matteson EL, Gold KN, Bloch DA, et al. Long-term survival of patients with giant cell arteritis in the American College of Rheumatology giant cell arteritis classification criteria cohort. *Am J Med* 1996;100:193–196.

167. Paulley JW. Coronary ischaemia and occlusion in giant cell (temporal) arteritis. *Acta Med Scand* 1980;208:257–263.

168. Lie JT, Failoni DD, Davis DC Jr. Temporal arteritis with giant cell aortitis, coronary arteritis, and myocardial infarction. *Arch Pathol Lab Med* 1986;110:857–860.

169. Stanson AW, Klein RG, Hunder GG. Extracranial angiographic findings in giant cell (temporal) arteritis. *AJR Am J Roentgenol* 1976;127:957–963.

170. Duhaut P, Pinede L, Demolombe-Rague S, et al. Giant cell arteritis and cardiovascular risk factors: a multicenter, prospective case-control study. Groupe de Recherche sur l'Arterite a Cellules Geantes. *Arthritis Rheum* 1998;41:1960–1965.

171. Klein RG, Hunder GG, Stanson AW, et al. Large artery involvement in giant cell (temporal) arteritis. *Ann Intern Med* 1975;83:806–812.

172. Hoffman GS, Kerr GS, Leavitt RY, et al. Wegener granulomatosis: an analysis of 158 patients. *Ann Intern Med* 1992;116:488–498.

173. Matteson EL, Gold KN, Bloch DA, et al. Long-term survival of patients with Wegener's granulomatosis from the American College of Rheumatology Wegener's Granulomatosis Classification Criteria Cohort. *Am J Med* 1996;101:129–134.

174. Fauci AS, Haynes BF, Katz P, et al. Wegener's granulomatosis: prospective clinical and therapeutic experience with 85 patients for 21 years. *Ann Intern Med* 1983;98(1):76–85.

175. Forstot JZ, Overlie PA, Neufeld GK, et al. Cardiac complications of Wegener granulomatosis: a case report of complete heart block and review of the literature. *Semin Arthritis Rheum* 1980;10:148–154.

176. Grant SC, Levy RD, Venning MC, et al. Wegener's granulomatosis and the heart. *Br Heart J* 1994;71(1):82–86.

177. Schiavone WA, Ahmad M, Ockner SA. Unusual cardiac complications of Wegener's granulomatosis. *Chest* 1985;88:745–748.

178. Allen DC, Doherty CC, O'Reilly DP. Pathology of the heart and the cardiac conduction system in Wegener's granulomatosis. *Br Heart J* 1984;52:674–678.

179. Yanda RJ, Guis MS, Rabkin JM. Aortic valvulitis in a patient with Wegener's granulomatosis. *West J Med* 1989;151:555–556.

180. Gerbracht DD, Savage RW, Scharff N. Reversible valvulitis in Wegener's granulomatosis. *Chest* 1987;92(1):182–183.

181. Fox AD, Robbins SE. Aortic valvulitis complicating Wegener's granulomatosis. *Thorax* 1994;49:1176–1177.

182. Leff RD, Hellman RN, Mullany CJ. Acute aortic insufficiency associated with Wegener granulomatosis. *Mayo Clin Proc* 1999;74:897–899.

183. Delevaux I, Hoen B, Selton-Suty C, et al. Relapsing congestive cardiomyopathy in Wegener's granulomatosis. *Mayo Clin Proc* 1997;72:848–850.

184. Kosovsky PA, Ehlers KH, Rafal RB, et al. MR imaging of cardiac mass in Wegener granulomatosis. *J Comput Assist Tomogr* 1991;15:1028–1030.

185. Gatenby PA, Lytton DG, Bulteau VG, et al. Myocardial infarction in Wegener's granulomatosis. *Aust N Z J Med* 1976;6:336–340.

186. Bohan A, Peter JB, Bowman RL, et al. Computer-assisted analysis of 153 patients with polymyositis and dermatomyositis. *Medicine (Baltimore)* 1977;56:255–286.

187. Hochberg MC, Feldman D, Stevens MB. Adult onset polymyositis/dermatomyositis: an analysis of clinical and laboratory features and survival in 76 patients with a review of the literature. *Semin Arthritis Rheum* 1986;15(3):168–178.

188. Gonzalez-Lopez L, Gamez-Nava JI, Sanchez L, et al. Cardiac manifestations in dermato-polymyositis. *Clin Exp Rheumatol* 1996;14:373–379.

189. Gottdiener JS, Sherber HS, Hawley RJ, et al. Cardiac manifestations in polymyositis. *Am J Cardiol* 1978;41:1141–1149.

190. Haupt HM, Hutchins GM. The heart and cardiac conduction system in polymyositis-dermatomyositis: a clinicopathologic study of 16 autopsied patients. *Am J Cardiol* 1982;50:998–1006.

191. Denbow CE, Lie JT, Tancredi RG, et al. Cardiac involvement in polymyositis: a clinicopathologic study of 20 autopsied patients. *Arthritis Rheum* 1979;22:1088–1092.

192. Larca LJ, Coppola JT, Honig S. Creatine kinase MB isoenzyme in dermatomyositis: a noncardiac source. *Ann Intern Med* 1981;94:341–343.

193. Schiff S, Moffatt R, Mandel WJ, et al. Acute myocardial infarction and recurrent ventricular arrhythmias in Behçet's syndrome. *Am Heart J* 1982;103:438–440.

194. Ozkan M, Emel O, Ozdemir M, et al. M-mode, 2-D and Doppler echocardiographic study in 65 patients with Behçet's syndrome. *Eur Heart J* 1992;13:638–641.

195. Bowness P, Hawley IC, Morris T, et al. Complete heart block and severe aortic incompetence in relapsing polychondritis: clinicopathologic findings. *Arthritis Rheum* 1991;34(1):97–100.

196. Ohta A, Yamaguchi M, Kaneoka H, et al. Adult Still's disease: review of 228 cases from the literature. *J Rheumatol* 1987;14:1139–1146.

197. Reginato AJ, Schumacher HR Jr, Baker DG, et al. Adult onset Still's disease: experience in 23 patients and literature review with emphasis on organ failure. *Semin Arthritis Rheum* 1987;17(1):39–57.

THE HEART AND OTHER
ORGAN SYSTEMS

The Heart and Infectious Diseases

ANDREW JAMES BOYLE

OVERVIEW

Infections of the heart are increasingly more prevalent and more serious causes of morbidity and mortality. Infective endocarditis is the most common clinically important entity and is occurring more frequently as greater numbers of prosthetic devices are being implanted into patients, predominantly in the form of valves, leads for pacemakers and defibrillators, and patches to repair various anatomic abnormalities (see Chapter 25). Although infectious myocarditis occurs less frequently than infectious endocarditis, it remains an important cause of both fulminant and chronic heart failure. Systemic infections, such as infection with the human immunodeficiency virus (HIV) and Chagas' disease, are common causes of profound heart failure, particularly in developing countries. A method for accurately diagnosing infectious myocarditis premortem remains elusive, and diagnosis currently relies largely on circumstantial evidence, such as increases in serum antibody titers. Newer techniques, such as gene amplification by reverse transcription polymerase chain reaction (rt-PCR) and nucleic acid hybridization of right ventricular endomyocardial biopsy (EMB) tissue, suffer from a lack of sensitivity. Furthermore, once the diagnosis of infectious myocarditis is made, treatment is mainly focused on providing hemodynamic support and symptom relief, as opposed to counteracting the pathogenic organism. Nevertheless, full recovery of cardiac function is common, although not uniform. Infectious pericarditis is also a common clinical cardiac infection (see Chapter 26).

Infectious pathogens have also been implicated as potential etiologic agents for the development of coronary atherosclerosis or restenosis after percutaneous coronary interventions. Although a causal relationship has yet to be established, this idea has given rise to several large prospective trials, which are currently ongoing.

CLINICAL PRESENTATION
IN INFECTIOUS MYOCARDITIS

There is a wide spectrum of clinical presentations associated with infectious myocarditis, ranging from a clinically silent

A. J. Boyle: Department of Heart Failure and Cardiac Transplantation, The Cleveland Clinic Foundation, Cleveland, Ohio

syndrome that ends in complete recovery to acutely or chronically decompensated irreversible heart failure that leads either to death or to heart transplantation. The symptoms of mild to moderate infectious myocarditis are relatively nonspecific, consisting of fever, sweats, or chills associated with mild dyspnea and palpitations. In severe cases of infectious myocarditis, symptoms relate to hypoperfusion and cardiac congestion, for example, mental status changes, limb or gut ischemia, and shortness of breath. Chest pain is relatively infrequent and usually results from accompanying pericarditis. The signs of infectious myocarditis are also nonspecific, and they include frequent atrial and ventricular extrasystoles, sinus tachycardia that is out of proportion to the degree of hyperthermia, and, in severe cases, more significant arrhythmias, a soft first heart sound, a third heart sound, and pulmonary edema. Varying degrees of atrioventricular heart block may develop transiently and usually resolve spontaneously and completely (1). In the majority of cases, the initial infection remains completely unrecognized, and full recovery of cardiac function ensues. However, for unclear reasons, the infectious insult leads in a minority of patients to progressive myocardial dysfunction either acutely or, more commonly, many years after the original insult. This is felt to be one of the more common etiologies for dilated cardiomyopathy (DCM), and it accounted for 12.8% of all cases in a recent study (2). Most commonly (in 51.2% of all cases), no etiology is discovered, and the cardiomyopathy is thus called *idiopathic*.

DIAGNOSIS OF INFECTIOUS MYOCARDITIS

In light of the lack of specific signs and symptoms for infectious myocarditis, accurate and early diagnosis of this condition relies on a high level of clinical suspicion in the practitioner. Often the earliest evidence of active myocarditis is nonspecific changes seen on the resting electrocardiogram. These changes usually involve the ST segment and the T wave, but, in severe cases, significant intraventricular conduction delays can develop, either transiently or permanently. A pseudoinfarction electrocardiographic pattern with Q waves and ST-segment elevation indicates a particularly poor prognosis and is often associated with a rapidly fatal course of the disease (3). Abnormal QRS morphology and left bundle branch block are also indicative of a worse prognosis, although clinical deterioration usually is the result of progressive congestive heart failure that occurs over a protracted time course (1). These electrocardiographic changes are more helpful when a baseline electrocardiogram is available for comparison.

Serum creatinine kinase levels, particularly the MB fraction (4), as well as both serum troponin I (5) and T levels (6), can be elevated as a reflection of ongoing myocardial necrosis resulting from the inflammatory process. The degree of elevation, and indeed whether these levels are elevated at all, is a function of the severity of the inflammatory insult and its acuity. Both the sensitivity and specificity of these markers of myonecrosis are particularly poor.

A documented fourfold rise in serum viral antibody titers from the acute to the convalescent stage of the infection is reasonable, but delayed, indirect evidence of viral infection does not assist in the management of the patient in the acute phase of the illness (7). A significant rise in virus-specific immunoglobulin M (IgM) antibody titers is an earlier serologic finding, although it is still not rapid enough to have therapeutic implications.

Various imaging modalities can also be used, with varying degrees of success, to assist in the diagnosis of acute infectious myocarditis. Echocardiography is of limited use and serves mainly to confirm left ventricular systolic dysfunction and to eliminate other potential etiologies, particularly valvular cardiomyopathies and anatomic abnormalities, such as atrial and ventricular septal defects. In antimyosin scintigraphy, a radiolabeled antimyosin antibody is infused and binds to cardiac myosin heavy chains that are exposed to the circulation. In highly selected patient populations, this diagnostic tool is reasonably specific, but it is less sensitive than EMB with immunohistologic analysis (8). However, the specificity of antimyosin scintigraphy is dramatically reduced in less selective populations, because a positive study is a reflection of active myonecrosis, regardless of its etiology, including myonecrosis that occurs after a myocardial infarction. For these reasons, this method has not been widely implemented. Similarly, gadolinium-enhanced magnetic resonance imaging has proven to be relatively sensitive in the detection of acute myocarditis (9). However, it lacks specificity, because abnormal myocardial enhancement reflects only active inflammation, regardless of the etiology, including inflammation that occurs after myocardial infarction and various other cardiomyopathic processes (10). Magnetic resonance imaging may play a more important role in the future, once effective and specific therapies have been discovered and serial assessments can be used to determine the adequacy of therapy.

The EMB remains the gold standard for diagnosis of acute viral myocarditis, despite its many imperfections. The Dallas criteria were created by a panel of cardiac pathologists in 1986 to standardize the pathologic requirements for a diagnosis of myocarditis (11). In brief, a diagnosis of myocarditis in this classification system requires the simultaneous finding of lymphocyte infiltration and myocyte necrosis (*e*Fig. 35F.0.1). Biopsy samples in which one criterion is met but not the other indicate borderline myocarditis. Despite this attempt to create worldwide uniformity in histologic diagnosis, there remains significant interobserver variability (12). Furthermore, lymphocytic myocarditis is a patchy disease that is unevenly distributed throughout the myocardium (13). In some patients, the pathologic myocardium is not easily accessible by the bioptome, which, by definition, is limited to sampling subendocardial tissue. Even when the inflammatory process involves the subendocardium, a tremendous sampling error may be present when only three to five biopsies are obtained (14). The rate of false-negative results of EMB is as high as 83% for individual biopsies and as high as 55% when five biopsy samples are obtained in a single patient with autopsy-proven myocarditis (13). In addition, there is a high rate of false-positive results of EMB because of the small numbers of lymphocytes that are normally present in the interstitium and because of the difficulty in distinguishing between lymphocytes and interstitial macrophages, fibroblasts, endothelial cells, and pericytes using light microscopy (15). Efforts to improve on this histologic classification system by adding a clinical perspective have not been widely accepted or implemented (16). Newer techniques developed to detect intramyocardial viral genome products in EMB samples using cloned DNA fragments that are complementary to the viral genome (*in situ* DNA hybridization) and rt-PCR have generally been successful (17,18). However, these techniques require adequate biopsy samples and thus suffer from significant sampling errors. Furthermore, they have yet to be implemented in the clinical setting, because few virus-specific therapies exist that could be initiated should a specific etiology be identified.

Because of the relatively low sensitivity and specificity of all of the aforementioned diagnostic studies, the diagnosis of myocarditis at this time and for the foreseeable future remains mainly a clinical one.

ETIOLOGIC AGENTS OF INFECTIONS IN THE HEART

Table 35F.1 lists pathogenic causes of acute infectious myocarditis.

Viruses

Enteroviruses

The enteroviruses, as their name implies, are a group of single-stranded RNA viruses pathogenic to the gastrointestinal and upper respiratory tracts. Individual species in this group, such as coxsackie A and B viruses, echovirus, and polioviruses, have been implicated as etiologic agents of viral myocarditis (19–21). Coxsackie B viruses (CBV) appear to be the most common pathogens. Serologic studies have revealed that 36% of all adults with acute myocarditis have demonstrable rises in either serum anti-CBV antibody titers or IgM (22,23). The full epidemiologic impact of CBV-induced myocarditis is difficult to assess because of the ubiquitous nature of this organism, as evidenced by the high rate of similar findings in control populations (22,23). Elements of the CBV genome have also

TABLE 35F.1 PATHOGENIC CAUSES OF ACUTE INFECTIOUS MYOCARDITIS

Viral
  Enteroviruses
    Coxsackie A virus (19)
    Coxsackie B virus
    Echovirus (20)
    Poliovirus (21)
  Herpesviruses
    Cytomegalovirus
    Epstein-Barr virus (54)
    Herpes simplex virus (56)
    Varicella-zoster virus (57)
  Human immunodeficiency virus
  Other viruses
    Hepatitis B virus (76)
    Hepatitis C virus (77)
    Adenovirus (56,219)
    Influenza A virus (78)
    Influenza B virus (79)
    Rabies virus (80)
    Parvovirus B19 (81)
    Mumps (82)
    Measles (83)
    Rubella (84)
Bacterial
  Chlamydia pneumoniae (109)
  Chlamydia psittaci (110)
  Corynebacterium diphtheriae (111)
  Whipple's disease (113)
  Neisseria meningitidis (120)
  Mycoplasma pneumoniae (121)
  Legionella pneumophila (122)
  Brucella melitensis (123)
  Salmonella typhi (124)
  Vibrio cholerae (125)
Spirochetal
  Lyme borreliosis
  Syphilis (125)
  Leptospira interrogans (139)
Rickettsial
  Rocky Mountain spotted fever (140)
  Q fever (142)
  Ehrlichiosis (143)
Fungal
  Aspergillus
  Candida albicans
  Histoplasma capsulatum
  Cryptococcus neoformans
  Coccidioides immitis
  Mucormycosis
Parasitic
  Chagas' disease
  Toxoplasma gondii (170–174)
  Trichinella spiralis (175)

been detected using rt-PCR in EMB of patients that met the Dallas criteria for diagnosis of acute myocarditis (17,24,25). The specificity of this finding is questionable, however, because of the unexpectedly high finding of enteroviral RNA on autopsy of patients who did not have cardiac disease (24). Furthermore, delineation of the exact viral species using this method is difficult, because significant nucleic acid sequence homology exists at the 5'-untranslated region of the RNA of all enteroviruses (26). However, probes do exist to species-specific regions of the RNA that are thus able to differentiate among various species using *in situ* hybridization.

In the majority of patients infected with CBV, cardiac manifestations are not found, although cardiac involvement has been estimated to be as high as 5.3% (27). Findings most frequently consist of asymptomatic and nonspecific electrocardiographic changes (28). In most cases, the signs and symptoms of infection are benign and resolve spontaneously. Some investigators have nevertheless proposed that some cases of nonischemic DCM may represent the end stage of either a previously detected (29) or undetected (30) enteroviral infection. Much of this speculation has arisen as a result of the frequent, although not uniform, detection of enteroviral RNA in EMB from patients who have nonischemic DCM without clinical evidence of myocarditis (18,24,30). In addition, recent studies have suggested that patients with DCM in whom persistent enteroviral RNA can be detected on EMB have a much poorer clinical prognosis (eFig. 35F.0.2) (25,31). However, because of the high prevalence of enteroviral infections in the community, these studies provide only circumstantial evidence of a link between enteroviral myocarditis and DCM without offering definitive proof. In fact, in one study, enteroviral RNA was detected more frequently in control patients undergoing either heart or lung transplantation for ischemic heart disease or primary lung disease than in patients with nonischemic DCM (30). This finding has been confirmed by another, similar study (32). The clinical association between enteroviral myocarditis and DCM, therefore, remains controversial and is yet to be proven.

Some investigators have suggested that enteroviruses have a potential role in the genesis of coronary atherosclerosis (33). However, the evidence is not very compelling, and the current focus of investigational attention has shifted toward more promising organisms.

Herpesviruses

Cytomegalovirus (CMV) is a double-stranded DNA herpesvirus readily identified in infected cells by its characteristic microscopic nuclear and paranuclear inclusion bodies. CMV is a ubiquitous organism that, in the immunocompetent host, commonly produces an asymptomatic primary infection, demonstrated by the presence of circulating anti-CMV antibodies in the majority of the population (34). Even in immunocompetent patients, CMV has been shown to cause myocarditis (35), albeit rarely. More commonly, however, as with all herpesviruses, CMV may remain latent intracellularly indefinitely in the host, until it is reactivated and leads to a systemic infection when the patient becomes immunocompromised, usually as a result of HIV infection,

neoplasia, immunosuppression for rheumatologic or pulmonary disease, or after transplantation (34,36). One component of this generalized infection may be acute CMV myocarditis, which can be adequately treated with ganciclovir (37,38). Systemic CMV infection has been associated with a higher rate of acute allograft rejection in the first 3 months after heart transplantation (39), although other studies have failed to confirm this finding (40,41). Furthermore, CMV has been associated with accelerated cardiac allograft vasculopathy, which is generally believed to be reflective of chronic allograft rejection (39,42). This hypothesis also remains controversial; other investigators have not been able to confirm the findings (43,44). Even more intriguingly, however, treatment of heart transplant recipients immediately postoperatively with ganciclovir appears to lower the incidence of allograft vasculopathy, regardless of whether the recipients developed a systemic CMV illness (45). ⚐ h34

Human Immunodeficiency Virus

Acquired immunodeficiency syndrome (AIDS) is the end stage of HIV infection. As the number of worldwide HIV infections has reached epidemic proportions, and because advances in medical therapies have prolonged survival of patients with AIDS and various opportunistic infections, the cardiac manifestations of this disease have become more apparent. These cardiac manifestations include the direct effects of HIV itself and effects resulting from opportunistic infections that arise as a consequence of a profoundly immunosuppressed state.

EMB-proven acute or chronic lymphocytic myocarditis is a frequent finding in patients with AIDS (58,59). Most frequently, this is a consequence of a superimposed opportunistic infection (36,58). HIV RNA and DNA have been detected in such biopsies but are usually very sparse, most often appearing in areas of myocardium where there is no inflammatory infiltrate or ongoing myonecrosis, and are frequently associated with other opportunistic pathogens (60,61). A causal relationship between HIV and myocarditis has therefore not been firmly established. It must be noted, however, that no pathogen is identified in a large percentage of cases of AIDS-associated cardiomyopathy (36), a finding not dissimilar to that among patients whose cardiomyopathy is not related to AIDS. Some investigators have proposed that AIDS-associated cardiomyopathy may result from antiretroviral therapy, specifically from administration of the nucleoside analogue azidothymidine (62,63). Multiple cytokines, vascular changes, nutritional deficiencies, and illicit drug use have also been implicated (64). However, regardless of the etiology of the cardiomyopathic process associated with AIDS, the diagnosis is a harbinger of an extremely poor clinical prognosis, irrespective of the adequacy of the anti-HIV therapy itself (eFig. 35F.0.3) (65).

Marantic endocarditis (66), infective endocarditis (usually found in intravenous drug users) (66), pericardial effusions (67), infective pericarditis (particularly that caused by *Mycobacterium tuberculosis* in Africa) (68), and pulmonary hypertension with cor pulmonale (69) are all infrequent findings in patients with HIV. Cardiac neoplasms also develop in these patients. Cardiac Kaposi's sarcomas are not usually isolated to the heart but rather are part of a widely metastatic process (70). They are usually asymptomatic and involve the subepicardium (*e*Fig. 35F.0.4) (70) or the pericardium, where they can lead to effusions (71). Most cases are discovered unexpectedly at autopsy. Cardiac non-Hodgkin's B-cell lymphoma is also usually associated with a widely disseminated malignant process in HIV patients, but it can be a primary lesion as well (72).

Accelerated coronary atherosclerosis has also been observed on autopsy of relatively young HIV patients, although a causal relationship has yet to be established (73). Recent studies have also implicated protease inhibitors, antiretroviral agents used to treat patients with HIV, in the development of coronary atherosclerosis (74,75); a profound deleterious effect on the serum lipid profile is the likely mechanism.

Bacteria

Rheumatic Fever

Acute rheumatic fever is characterized by a systemic inflammatory response that occurs approximately 3 weeks after an untreated group A streptococcal pharyngeal infection but never after a cutaneous infection. The incidence of acute rheumatic fever in the developed world is on the decline as a result of widespread use of antistreptococcal antibiotic therapy for upper respiratory tract infections and general improvements in living conditions. The same is not true in the developing world. Administration of appropriate antibiotic therapy during pharyngeal infection essentially eliminates the future risk of developing rheumatic fever (85).

The diagnosis of acute rheumatic fever is mainly a clinical one, using the revised Jones criteria of 1992 (86) (Table 35F.2). Evidence of two major criteria or one major criterion and at least two minor criteria is required for a presumptive diagnosis of acute rheumatic fever and is enhanced by either a history of a recent upper respiratory tract infection, a positive throat culture, or a positive antistreptococcal antibody test.

Rheumatic carditis can involve the endocardium, myocardium, or pericardium. Most commonly, there is variable involvement of the cardiac valves, particularly the mitral valve and its subvalvular apparatus, including papillary muscles and their attached chordae tendineae. Severe clinical decompensation is the exception rather than the rule. The most feared consequence of this pathologic process is

TABLE 35F.2 REVISED JONES CRITERIA FOR THE DIAGNOSIS OF ACUTE RHEUMATIC FEVER, 1992

Major criteria
Carditis
Polyarthritis
Chorea
Erythema marginatum
Subcutaneous nodules
Minor criteria
Arthralgia
Fever
Elevated erythrocyte sedimentation rate
Elevated C-reactive protein levels
First-degree atrioventricular block

Adapted from Guidelines for the diagnosis of rheumatic fever: Jones criteria, 1992 update. Special Writing Group of the Committee on Rheumatic Fever, Endocarditis, and Kawasaki Disease of the Council on Cardiovascular Disease in the Young of the American Heart Association. *JAMA* 1992;268:2069–2073, with permission.

chronic scarring that leads to mitral, and potentially aortic, valvular stenosis and/or regurgitation.

Treatment of mild cases is usually administration of high doses of aspirin (87). Corticosteroids can be added to this regimen for severe cases. To prevent recurrences of carditis and acute rheumatic fever, long-term, perhaps even lifelong, antibiotic prophylaxis involving administration of benzathine penicillin G intramuscularly every 3 weeks is recommended, although the duration of therapy should be individualized, depending on the patient's risk of recurrence (88).

Chlamydia pneumoniae

The chlamydiae are ubiquitous obligate intracellular gram-negative bacteria that have generated tremendous interest recently as a result of the purported association between *C. pneumoniae* and the development of coronary atherosclerosis. Seroepidemiologic studies initially demonstrated increased anti–*C. pneumoniae* antibody titers in patients who had acute myocardial infarctions (68%) or chronic angina (50%) as compared to control subjects (17%) (89). This concept, however, remains controversial—several studies have since confirmed this finding (90–92), but others have refuted it (93–95), mainly because of a prevalence of high seropositivity in the control groups of the latter studies. Nevertheless, the potential evidence supporting this association is strengthened by the vast majority of studies, which have readily demonstrated the presence of *C. pneumoniae* organisms in atherosclerotic plaques (96–98) but rarely in normal coronary arteries. This evidence is weakened, however, by the finding that although *C. pneumoniae* DNA could be detected in the presence of coronary atherosclerosis, it did not reflect either the extent or severity of the disease (99). In this study, *C. pneumoniae* DNA could be detected only at one site in one patient with severe diffuse atherosclerosis, whereas another patient with only mild coronary atherosclerosis had detectable DNA in every arterial segment examined. Furthermore, in contrast to CMV, no evidence exists to support an association between *C. pneumoniae* and the occurrence of restenosis after percutaneous coronary atherectomy (100).

The ability to detect *C. pneumoniae* in coronary atherosclerotic plaques does not prove that the organism plays a role in the genesis of the disease. The evidence would be more convincing if a reduction in cardiovascular events could be shown after eradication of the organism using antibiotic therapy. Thus far, one small study has demonstrated a fivefold reduction in cardiovascular events after short-term therapy with azithromycin in patients who had experienced a myocardial infarction (101). In the ROXIS study (Randomized Trial of Roxithromycin in Non–Q-Wave Coronary Syndromes), a small but statistically significant reduction in cardiovascular events at 30 days was found in patients who had unstable angina and were treated with roxithromycin, although this effect was not sustained to 90 days (102). The ACADEMIC study (Azithromycin in Coronary Artery Disease: Elimination of Myocardial Infection with *Chlamydia*) failed to show any benefit at 6 months in a lower-risk population of individuals with stable coronary disease who were treated with azithromycin, although the primary end point of cardiovascular events at 2 years has yet to be completed (103). Nevertheless, two large randomized, placebo-controlled trials using prolonged treatment courses of azithromycin are currently under way (WIZARD [Weekly Intervention with Zithromax (Azithromycin) for Atherosclerosis and Its Related Disorders] [104] and ACES [Azithromycin and Coronary Events Study] [105]). However, because antibiotics such as azithromycin produce key antiinflammatory effects by virtue of matrix metalloproteinase inhibition, it will not be possible to assert fully the role of *C. pneumoniae* in the atherosclerotic process on the basis of the aforementioned studies alone. At this juncture, therefore, insufficient data exist to justify the widespread use of antibiotic treatment in patients with coronary atherosclerosis. ⚡ h35

Spirochetes

Lyme Disease

Lyme disease is a systemic illness caused by the spirochete *Borrelia burgdorferi,* whose primary vector is the ixodid tick. Carditis is a common manifestation thought to occur in approximately 10% of all patients in the disseminated phase of the illness, often weeks to months after the initial infection (126,127). Because it can take as long as 8 weeks for serologic conversion to occur, signs and symptoms of Lyme borreliosis frequently precede positive serologic tests, and many false-negative results may be seen before seroconversion. The most common cardiac finding in patients with Lyme disease is varying degrees of atrioventricular heart

block, which can fluctuate from normal to first-degree atrioventricular block to complete heart block in the same patient within minutes (126,127). Although patients are often asymptomatic, some may become syncopal during periods of high-degree atrioventricular block and may benefit from temporary transvenous pacing (127,128). Permanent pacing is rarely indicated, and complete resolution of the conduction disturbance usually occurs within 1 to 2 weeks (126,127).

Less commonly, Lyme borreliosis can also cause acute myopericarditis (126,128,129), and *B. burgdorferi* has been isolated from EMB from patients with acute (128,130) and chronic (131) cardiomyopathies. Furthermore, patients with chronic DCM are more likely to have positive results of serologic testing for *B. burgdorferi* than are control subjects (132), although the association seems to be weak and has not been confirmed by other studies (133). This hypothesis is enhanced by the finding in one study that ceftriaxone reversed the cardiomyopathic process in 9 of 42 patients who were seropositive for *B. burgdorferi* (134), although other studies have been unable to demonstrate such a reversal (131,132). Suffice it to say, the evidence supporting an epidemiologic role for *B. burgdorferi* in DCM is very circumstantial, fails to prove causation, and is not currently the subject of major investigative efforts.

Current recommendations for treatment of Lyme disease carditis are listed in Table 35F.3 (135). Treatment during the early phase of the disease seems to eliminate the potential for development of future disseminated disease, including carditis (136). No evidence exists, however, demonstrating administration of appropriate antibiotic therapy after carditis has developed leads to more rapid resolution of the carditis, since Lyme disease carditis is usually self-limited, with complete recovery in most cases. Nevertheless, administration of antibiotic therapy is now common clinical practice, used mainly to prevent further dissemination of the disease, including avoidance of neurologic sequelae. Others have advocated the use of corticosteroids and salicylates for patients with severe cases (126,127), but

TABLE 35F.3 RECOMMENDATIONS FOR THE TREATMENT OF LYME CARDITIS

Early Lyme disease
  Doxycycline, 100 mg twice daily for 10–21 d; amoxicillin, 500 mg
    three times daily for 10–21 d
Lyme carditis
  Ceftriaxone, 2 g i.v. daily for 14 d
  Penicillin G, 20 million U i.v. daily for 14 d
Alternatives, for mild cases of Lyme carditis only
  Doxycycline, 100 mg orally twice daily for 14–21 d
  Amoxicillin, 500 mg three times daily for 14–21 d

Adapted from Rahn DW, Malawista SE. Lyme disease: recommendations for diagnosis and treatment. *Ann Intern Med* 1991;114:472–481, with permission.

this approach has not been proven by prospective studies to confer any therapeutic advantage.

Parasites

Chagas' Disease (Trypanosomiasis)

Chagas' disease is a protozoal infestation caused by *Trypanosoma cruzi* and is transmitted to humans in the feces of the reduviid bug as it bites. Chagas' disease is endemic to Central and South America, where more than 20 million people are currently estimated to be infected (154). More rarely, it may be transmitted by blood transfusions from a previously infected donor (155). The acute phase of the human disease is usually benign and clinically asymptomatic, with the exception of a mild fever, although acute myocarditis can be demonstrated by EMB in most patients and can be fatal (156). More commonly, a slowly progressive cardiomyopathic process ensues that may remain clinically unrecognized for more than 20 years (154). During this indeterminate phase, 30% to 40% of infected patients (and more than 80% of those who go on to develop a cardiomyopathy) develop cardiac conduction abnormalities due to extensive myocardial fibrosis. Right bundle branch block and left anterior hemiblock are the most frequently seen abnormalities and can progress to higher degrees of atrioventricular heart block (157).

Chronic Chagasic cardiomyopathy develops in approximately 10% to 30% of all infected patients. The pathogenesis of this disease remains highly controversial, but it is likely multifactorial, including a continued direct parasitic effect on the myocardium (158), autoimmune-mediated myocyte injury (159), and parasite-mediated microvascular endothelial injury resulting in compromised myocardial perfusion (159). Anatomically, Chagas' disease can be distinguished from other cardiomyopathies by the classical finding of apical thinning and aneurysm formation (*e*Fig. 35F.0.5) (154,157). Functionally, multiple segmental wall motion abnormalities are common, as is global systolic dysfunction (157), highlighting the need to rule out a coronary etiology for the cardiomyopathy. These apical aneurysms and their accompanying left ventricular systolic dysfunction place patients at risk for thromboembolism (160) and potentially lethal ventricular arrhythmias (161,162). Alternatively, the cardiomyopathic process may progress unrelentingly until the patient develops overt congestive heart failure, a harbinger of a very poor prognosis (*e*Fig. 35F.0.6) (163).

Antiparasitic therapy at this stage is generally thought to be ineffective, although recent studies have suggested that treatment may prevent disease progression in a minority of patients (164,165). Because the prognosis for these patients is relatively poor, it would seem appropriate to attempt one course of antiparasitic therapy in virtually all patients, although this is controversial. Despite the inflammatory nature of this disorder, immunosuppression is not advised because of the potential for reactivation of otherwise latent organisms (166). Because iatrogenic immunosuppression is routinely used to prevent rejection after heart transplantation, concerns have arisen with regard to the candidacy of patients with end-stage Chagasic cardiomyopathy for transplantation. However, successful heart transplantation can be performed if it is accompanied by careful follow-up with serologic testing to detect and treat any reactivation of the disease, which occurs at some point in nearly all patients (167,168). However, the higher incidence of malignant neoplasms that has been observed in these patients in comparison with control subjects is of great concern and may be related to parasite reactivation or to the specific antiparasitic therapy they received (169). Further follow-up studies are required to examine this issue.

MECHANISM OF INJURY IN VIRAL MYOCARDITIS

Current knowledge about the pathogenesis of viral myocarditis is derived almost exclusively from animal studies and remains controversial and incomplete (Fig. 35F.1). There are at least three phases of injury: (a) a direct effect of the viral pathogen on the myocyte, (b) an acute inflammatory response resulting in viral clearance and myocytolysis of infected cells, and (c) a chronic phase that occurs in animals that are unable to eradicate the virus. Although the time sequence in the murine viral myocarditis model is more rapid, it is generally thought to accurately reflect the sequence of events in humans.

The initial phase in this murine model is characterized by the direct cytotoxic effect of the virus on the myocyte during the first 4 days after inoculation. At this time, no inflammatory infiltrate is visualized histologically (179,180), yet myocyte necrosis is seen (*e*Fig. 35F.1.1) (179,181). This hypothesis is strongly supported by the finding that mice with severe combined immunodeficiency syndrome, which therefore have no B- or T-cell immunologic response, have widespread myonecrosis without accompanying inflammatory cells (182).

The second phase, which usually occurs from days 4 through 14, is characterized by a large increase in cytokine production that leads to severe inflammatory cell infiltration and myocyte necrosis (*e*Fig. 35F.1.1) (179). Similar cytokine elevations have also been observed in humans who have acute myocarditis (183). Natural killer cells appear in this inflammatory milieu on approximately day 4 and inhibit viral replication, which is also peaking at this time (184), resulting in cytolysis of infected cardiac myocytes (185). Viruses are also cleared via B lymphocyte–derived antiviral antibodies, which appear after day 4 with a rapidly rising titer (186,187). T lymphocytes are also crucial in this phase, and concentration of these cells peaks on days 7 through 14,

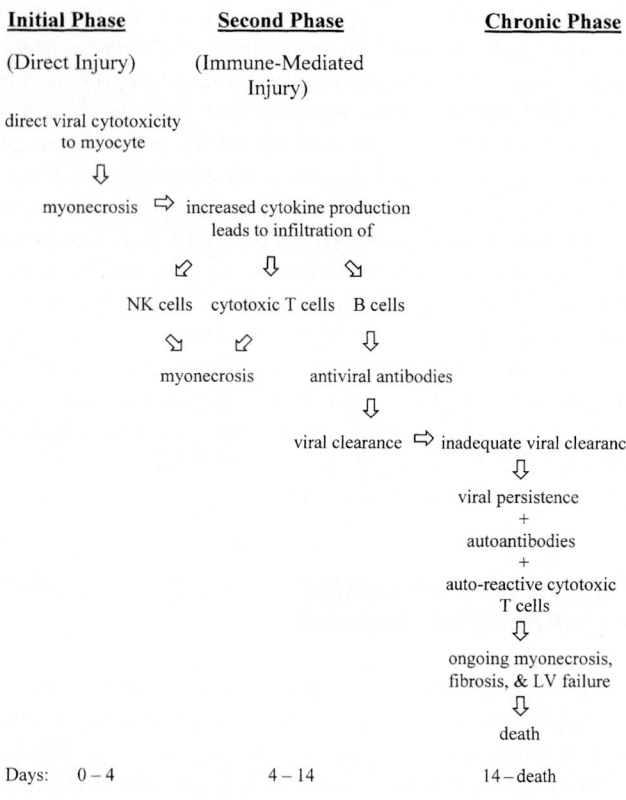

FIGURE 35F.1 Pathogenesis of acute infectious myocarditis. LV, left ventricular; NK, natural killer.

resulting in widespread myonecrosis of infected cells (188). The importance of lymphocytes to the process of virus load clearance has been confirmed in mice with severe combined immunodeficiency syndrome, in which viremia persisted throughout the duration of the study (182). T lymphocytes recognize viral proteins expressed on the surface of infected myocytes, resulting in further myocytolysis (189). However, T lymphocytes are not critical for virus load clearance and seem to play a role that is more harmful than helpful by increasing the severity of the resulting myonecrosis (180,190) and perhaps also by killing uninfected myocytes through autoimmune mechanisms (190,191). Therefore, in this model, humoral immunity is responsible for virus clearance, and cellular immunity inflicts much of the pathologic damage to the myocardium.

The chronic phase is characterized by progressive myocardial dysfunction and left ventricular dilation. Several different mechanisms have been proposed to explain this deterioration, but, in all likelihood, the process is multifactorial. With more sensitive diagnostic tools such as rt-PCR and *in situ* DNA hybridization, persistence of viral RNA has been demonstrated in the hearts of patients with chronic cardiomyopathy, raising the possibility that virus-specific immune-mediated damage is ongoing (18,24,192). Alternatively, ongoing myonecrosis may be caused either by autoantibodies, which cross-react between viral antigens and cardiac myocyte antigens (193–195), or by autoreactive cytotoxic T lymphocytes, which cross-react in a similar manner (191). In this scenario, uninfected cells are also irreversibly injured.

TREATMENT OF INFECTIOUS MYOCARDITIS

Treatment for both acute and chronic infectious myocarditis is generally aimed at reducing congestion, improving cardiac hemodynamics, and prolonging survival, irrespective of the etiology of the disease. Several guidelines exist and are updated regularly to assist in this endeavor (196,197). This topic is covered in greater detail in Chapters 91 and 92. However, it is important to note that, in murine models of acute myocarditis, high doses of digoxin increased mortality, presumably by increasing the production of various cytokines, in contrast to congestive heart failure from other etiologies (198).

Immunosuppression by means of corticosteroids, cyclosporine, azathioprine, or a combination was once advocated for the treatment of new-onset myocarditis. However, the Myocarditis Treatment Trial showed no survival benefit or improved myocardial recovery among patients who received immunosuppression (*e*Fig. 35F.1.2) (199). Nevertheless, no harmful effect from immunosuppression could be demonstrated, raising the possibility that patients with infectious myocarditis may have a poorer prognosis when they receive immunosuppression as a result of increased virus proliferation, whereas patients with a purely inflammatory or autoimmune etiology may in fact improve with such therapy. The ongoing European Study of Epidemiology and Treatment of Cardiac Inflammatory Diseases is addressing this issue by treating patients for whom viral etiologies have been identified with a specific antiviral agent, whereas patients in whom no viral etiology has been found are treated with corticosteroids (200). Immunosuppression has also been shown to be clinically ineffective when used to treat patients with DCM (201,202), although a more recent nonrandomized study has contradicted this finding (203).

Intravenous immunoglobulin therapy had also recently been advocated for patients with acute myocarditis, including pathogen-specific immunoglobulin (such as for CMV) (204) and nonspecific high-dose immunoglobulin (205–207). A recently completed randomized trial—Intervention in Myocarditis and Acute Cardiomyopathy—failed to demonstrate any therapeutic effect of intravenous immunoglobulin therapy (207a). Treatment of patients with acute myocarditis with immunomodulating agents such as interferon-α or thymomodulin, which reduces viral replication and myocardial inflammation, has been proposed (208,209). Although this suggestion is supported by results of a study using a murine model (210), larger randomized human studies are necessary before such treatment is widely implemented.

THE FUTURE

The greatest worldwide epidemiologic impact on infectious myocarditis could be achieved via improved living and health standards in the Third World, including methods for prevention of sexually transmitted diseases. Clearly, the incidence and prevalence of HIV and Chagasic cardiomyopathies could be significantly reduced with such measures.

Further investigations are currently under way to determine whether coronary atherosclerosis is truly an infectious disease. These results should be available within a few years and may alter the way in which this disease process is perceived. At the very least, it is likely that infectious diseases serve a facilitative role in promoting vascular inflammation and, in some patients, may represent the principal pathway to decompensation of vulnerable atherosclerotic plaque.

Specific antimicrobial therapy should always be tried when it is available. This is particularly true for patients infected with CMV, bacteria, spirochetes, rickettsiae, or parasites. However, the most common viral species have no specific antiviral therapy. Ribavirin, a nucleoside analog with potent nonspecific antiviral activity, has been shown to prevent the development of viral myocarditis in a murine model (211,212). Ribavirin was only effective, however, when it was administered before or at the same time that inoculation with the viral pathogen occurred. Any delay in the administration of the ribavirin rendered it useless, which may explain its apparent ineffectiveness in humans (212).

Infrequently, acute myocarditis may become fulminant and lead to circulatory collapse and cardiogenic shock. Such patients can be hemodynamically supported with extracorporeal membrane oxygenation (213) or ventricular-assist devices (214). Most patients can be successfully weaned from these devices within a few days, as ventricular function improves. If ventricular function does not improve, these devices can serve as a bridge to transplantation. Initial concerns about decreased survival after heart transplantation in the setting of active myocarditis (215) have been recently contradicted by a large retrospective analysis (216). However, a greater frequency of episodes of acute rejection, particularly in the first 4 months after transplantation, is observed in patients who have preoperative myocarditis (215,217), which may predispose them to an increased risk of transplant vasculopathy (218). At this juncture, it seems prudent to attempt to stabilize patients medically for as long as possible, to allow them a chance to recover ventricular function, or, at the very least, to perform transplantation in a less inflammatory or infectious milieu (214).

CONTROVERSIES AND PERSONAL PERSPECTIVES

A clinician's ability to accurately diagnose and specifically treat patients with acute infectious myocarditis has not progressed at the same rate as it has with other cardiac ailments. This stems from four fundamental difficulties associated with this disease process: (a) patients do not present to a physician before most of the damage is already done, (b) clinicians have a low index of suspicion for this disorder, (c) identifying the exact causative pathogen in a time-efficient manner is difficult, and (d) few specific therapies are available once a pathogen has been identified. Although the EMB remains the current gold standard for the diagnosis of acute infectious myocarditis, it will always suffer from a lack of sensitivity and specificity. The addition of rt-PCR and *in situ* DNA hybridization has enhanced this diagnostic modality, but they are targeted at identification of specific DNA sequences and thus require knowledge of which organisms should be sought. In light of the plethora of potential pathogens, such testing could become an expensive and time-consuming endeavor, like searching for the proverbial needle in a haystack. Furthermore, the lack of specific antimicrobial therapies renders the identification of the pathogen mainly an academic exercise. Therefore, it seems to me that any advancement in this field must begin with the development of either specific effective therapies against the offending pathogen or immunomodulatory therapies that would reduce the extent and severity of the immune-mediated injury. Only then will improvements in diagnostics become clinically meaningful.

REFERENCES

1. Morgera T, Di Lenarda A, Dreas L, et al. Electrocardiography of myocarditis revisited: clinical and prognostic significance of electrocardiographic changes. *Am Heart J* 1992;124:455–467.
2. Felker GM, Hu W, Hare JM, et al. The spectrum of dilated cardiomyopathy: the Johns Hopkins experience with 1,278 patients. *Medicine* 1999;78:270–283.
3. Take M, Sekiguchi M, Hiroe M, et al. Long-term follow-up of electrocardiographic findings in patients with acute myocarditis proven by endomyocardial biopsy. *Jpn Circ J* 1982;46:1227–1234.
4. Karjalainen J, Heikkila J. Acute pericarditis: myocardial

enzyme release as evidence for myocarditis. *Am Heart J* 1986;111:546–552.

5. Smith SC, Ladenson JH, Mason JW, et al. Elevations of cardiac troponin I associated with myocarditis: experimental and clinical correlates. *Circulation* 1997;95(1):163–168.

6. Lauer B, Niederau C, Kuhl U, et al. Cardiac troponin T in patients with clinically suspected myocarditis. *J Am Coll Cardiol* 1997;30:1354–1359.

7. See DM, Tilles JG. Viral myocarditis. *Rev Infect Dis* 1991;13:951–956.

8. Kuhl U, Lauer B, Souvatzoglu M, et al. Antimyosin scintigraphy and immunohistologic analysis of endomyocardial biopsy in patients with clinically suspected myocarditis: evidence of myocardial cell damage and inflammation in the absence of histologic signs of myocarditis. *J Am Coll Cardiol* 1998;32:1371–1376.

9. Friedrich MG, Strohm O, Schulz-Menger J, et al. Contrast media–enhanced magnetic resonance imaging visualizes myocardial changes in the course of viral myocarditis. *Circulation* 1998;97:1802–1809.

10. Frank H, Globits S. Magnetic resonance imaging evaluation of myocardial and pericardial disease. *J Magn Reson Imaging* 1999;10:617–626.

11. Aretz HT, Billingham ME, Edwards WD, et al. Myocarditis: a histopathologic definition and classification. *Am J Cardiovasc Pathol* 1987;1(1):3–14.

12. Shanes JG, Ghali J, Billingham ME, et al. Interobserver variability in the pathologic interpretation of endomyocardial biopsy results. *Circulation* 1987;75:401–405.

13. Hauck AJ, Kearney DL, Edwards WD. Evaluation of postmortem endomyocardial biopsy specimens from 38 patients with lymphocytic myocarditis: implications for role of sampling error. *Mayo Clin Proc* 1989;64:1235–1245.

14. Chow LH, Radio SJ, Sears TD, et al. Insensitivity of right ventricular endomyocardial biopsy in the diagnosis of myocarditis. *J Am Coll Cardiol* 1989;14:915–920.

15. Linder J, Cassling RS, Rogler WC, et al. Immunohistochemical characterization of lymphocytes in uninflamed ventricular myocardium: implications for myocarditis. *Arch Pathol Lab Med* 1985;109:917–920.

16. Lieberman EB, Hutchins GM, Herskowitz A, et al. Clinicopathologic description of myocarditis. *J Am Coll Cardiol* 1991;18:1617–1626.

17. Nicholson F, Ajetunmobi JF, Li M, et al. Molecular detection and serotypic analysis of enterovirus RNA in archival specimens from patients with acute myocarditis. *Br Heart J* 1995;74:522–527.

18. Jin O, Sole MJ, Butany JW, et al. Detection of enterovirus RNA in myocardial biopsies from patients with myocarditis and cardiomyopathy using gene amplification by polymerase chain reaction. *Circulation* 1990;82(1):8–16.

19. Grist NR, Bell EJ. Coxsackie viruses and the heart. *Am Heart J* 1969;77:295–300.

20. Shanmugam J, Raveendranath M, Balakrishnan KG. Isolation of ECHO virus type-22 from a child with acute myopericarditis: a case report. *Indian Heart J* 1986;38(1):79–80.

21. Jungeblut C, Edwards J. Isolation of poliomyelitis virus from the heart in fatal cases. *Am J Clin Pathol* 1951;21:601–623.

22. El-Hagrassy MM, Banatvala JE, Coltart DJ. Coxsackie-B-virus-specific IgM responses in patients with cardiac and other diseases. *Lancet* 1980;2(8205):1160–1162.

23. Bell EJ, McCartney RA. A study of Coxsackie B virus infections, 1972–1983. *J Hyg* 1984;93:197–203.

24. Ueno H, Yokota Y, Shiotani H, et al. Significance of detection of enterovirus RNA in myocardial tissues by reverse transcription–polymerase chain reaction. *Int J Cardiol* 1995;51:157–164.

25. Archard LC, Bowles NE, Cunningham L, et al. Molecular probes for detection of persisting enterovirus infection of human heart and their prognostic value. *Eur Heart J* 1991;12[Suppl D]:56–59.

26. Hyypia T. Etiological diagnosis of viral heart disease. *Scand J Infect Dis Suppl* 1993;88:25–31.

27. Coxsackie B5 virus infections during 1965: a report to the Director of the Public Health Laboratory Service from various laboratories in the United Kingdom. *BMJ* 1967;4:575–577.

28. Helin M, Savola J, Lapinleimu K. Cardiac manifestations during a Coxsackie B5 epidemic. *BMJ* 1968;3(610):97–99.

29. Levi G, Scalvini S, Volterrani M, et al. Coxsackie virus heart disease: 15 years after. *Eur Heart J* 1988;9:1303–1307.

30. Muir P, Nicholson F, Illavia SJ, et al. Serological and molecular evidence of enterovirus infection in patients with end-stage dilated cardiomyopathy. *Heart* 1996;76:243–249.

31. Why HJ, Meany BT, Richardson PJ, et al. Clinical and prognostic significance of detection of enteroviral RNA in the myocardium of patients with myocarditis or dilated cardiomyopathy. *Circulation* 1994;89:2582–2589.

32. Fujioka S, Koide H, Kitaura Y, et al. Molecular detection and differentiation of enteroviruses in endomyocardial biopsies and pericardial effusions from dilated cardiomyopathy and myocarditis. *Am Heart J* 1996;131:760–765.

33. Roivainen M, Alfthan G, Jousilahti P, et al. Enterovirus infections as a possible risk factor for myocardial infarction. *Circulation* 1998;98:2534–2537.

34. Lowry RW, Adam E, Hu C, et al. What are the implications of cardiac infection with cytomegalovirus before heart transplantation? *J Heart Lung Transplant* 1994;13:122–128.

35. Maisch B, Schonian U, Crombach M, et al. Cytomegalovirus associated inflammatory heart muscle disease. *Scand J Infect Dis Suppl* 1993;88:135–148.

36. Altieri PI, Climent C, Lazala G, et al. Opportunistic invasion of the heart in Hispanic patients with acquired immunodeficiency syndrome. *Am J Trop Med Hyg* 1994;51(1):56–59.

37. Gonwa TA, Capehart JE, Pilcher JW, et al. Cytomegalovirus myocarditis as a cause of cardiac dysfunction in a heart transplant recipient. *Transplantation* 1989;47(1):197–199.

38. Shabtai M, Luft B, Waltzer WC, et al. Massive cytomegalovirus pneumonia and myocarditis in a renal transplant recipient: successful treatment with DHPG. *Transplant Proc* 1988;20:562–563.

39. Grattan MT, Moreno-Cabral CE, Starnes VA, et al. Cytomegalovirus infection is associated with cardiac allograft rejection and atherosclerosis. *JAMA* 1989;261:3561–3566.

40. Boriskin YS, Booth JC, Corbishley CM, et al. Human cytomegalovirus and acute rejection after heart transplantation are not directly associated. *J Med Virol* 1996;50(1):59–70.

41. Ghisetti V, Barbui A, Rocci MP, et al. Detection of human cytomegalovirus myocardial involvement by polymerase chain reaction during systemic infection and correlation with pp65 antigenemia and DNAemia in infected heart recipients. *Transplantation* 1996;61:1072–1075.

42. McGiffin DC, Savunen T, Kirklin JK, et al. Cardiac transplant coronary artery disease: a multivariable analysis of pretransplantation risk factors for disease development and morbid events. *J Thorac Cardiovasc Surg* 1995;109:1081–1088.

43. Sharples LD, Caine N, Mullins P, et al. Risk factor analysis for the major hazards following heart transplantation: rejection, infection, and coronary occlusive disease. *Transplantation* 1991;52:244–252.

44. Gulizia JM, Kandolf R, Kendall TJ, et al. Infrequency of cytomegalovirus genome in coronary arteriopathy of human heart allografts. *Am J Pathol* 1995;147:461–475.

45. Valantine HA, Gao SZ, Menon SG, et al. Impact of prophylactic immediate posttransplant ganciclovir on development of transplant atherosclerosis: a post hoc analysis of a randomized, placebo-controlled study. *Circulation* 1999;100(1):61–66.

46. Sorlie PD, Nieto FJ, Adam E, et al. A prospective study of cytomegalovirus, herpes simplex virus 1, and coronary heart disease: the atherosclerosis risk in communities (ARIC) study. *Arch Intern Med* 2000;160:2027–2032.

47. Ridker PM, Hennekens CH, Stampfer MJ, et al. Prospective study of herpes simplex virus, cytomegalovirus, and the risk of future myocardial infarction and stroke. *Circulation* 1998;98:2796–2799.

48. Adler SP, Hur JK, Wang JB, et al. Prior infection with cytomegalovirus is not a major risk factor for angiographically demonstrated coronary artery atherosclerosis. *J Infect Dis* 1998;177(1):209–212.

49. Roivainen M, Viik-Kajander M, Palosuo T, et al. Infections, inflammation, and the risk of coronary heart disease. *Circulation* 2000;101:252–257.

50. Zhou YF, Leon MB, Waclawiw MA, et al. Association between prior cytomegalovirus infection and the risk of restenosis after coronary atherectomy. *N Engl J Med* 1996;335:624–630.

51. Speir E, Modali R, Huang ES, et al. Potential role of human cytomegalovirus and p53 interaction in coronary restenosis. *Science* 1994;265(5170):391–394.

52. Manegold C, Alwazzeh M, Jablonowski H, et al. Prior cytomegalovirus infection and the risk of restenosis after percutaneous transluminal coronary balloon angioplasty. *Circulation* 1999;99:1290–1294.

53. Carlsson J, Miketic S, Mueller KH, et al. Previous cytomegalovirus or *Chlamydia pneumoniae* infection and risk of restenosis after percutaneous transluminal coronary angioplasty. *Lancet* 1997;350(9086):1225.

54. Tyson AA Jr, Hackshaw BT, Kutcher MA. Acute Epstein-Barr virus myocarditis simulating myocardial infarction with cardiogenic shock. *South Med J* 1989;82:1184–1187.

55. Gray J, Wreghitt TG, Pavel P, et al. Epstein-Barr virus infection in heart and heart-lung transplant recipients: incidence and clinical impact. *J Heart Lung Transplant* 1995;14:640–646.

56. Martin AB, Webber S, Fricker FJ, et al. Acute myocarditis: rapid diagnosis by PCR in children. *Circulation* 1994;90(1):330–339.

57. Tsintsof A, Delprado WJ, Keogh AM. Varicella zoster myocarditis progressing to cardiomyopathy and cardiac transplantation. *Br Heart J* 1993;70(1):93–95.

58. Anderson DW, Virmani R, Reilly JM, et al. Prevalent myocarditis at necropsy in the acquired immunodeficiency syndrome. *J Am Coll Cardiol* 1988;11:792–799.

59. Beschorner WE, Baughman K, Turnicky RP, et al. HIV-associated myocarditis: pathology and immunopathology. *Am J Pathol* 1990;137:1365–1371.

60. Herskowitz A, Wu TC, Willoughby SB, et al. Myocarditis and cardiotropic viral infection associated with severe left ventricular dysfunction in late-stage infection with human immunodeficiency virus. *J Am Coll Cardiol* 1994;24:1025–1032.

61. Rodriguez ER, Nasim S, Hsia J, et al. Cardiac myocytes and dendritic cells harbor human immunodeficiency virus in infected patients with and without cardiac dysfunction: detection by multiplex, nested, polymerase chain reaction in individually microdissected cells from right ventricular endomyocardial biopsy tissue. *Am J Cardiol* 1991;68:1511–1520.

62. Domanski MJ, Sloas MM, Follmann DA, et al. Effect of zidovudine and didanosine treatment on heart function in children infected with human immunodeficiency virus. *J Pediatr* 1995;127(1):137–146.

63. Herskowitz A, Willoughby SB, Baughman KL, et al. Cardiomyopathy associated with antiretroviral therapy in patients with HIV infection: a report of six cases. *Ann Intern Med* 1992;116:311–313.

64. Lewis W. Cardiomyopathy in AIDS: a pathophysiological perspective. *Prog Cardiovasc Dis* 2000;43:151–170.

65. Currie PF, Jacob AJ, Foreman AR, et al. Heart muscle disease related to HIV infection: prognostic implications. *BMJ* 1994;309(6969):1605–1607.

66. Currie PF, Sutherland GR, Jacob AJ, et al. A review of endocarditis in acquired immunodeficiency syndrome and human immunodeficiency virus infection. *Eur Heart J* 1995;16[Suppl B]:15–18.

67. Hsia J, Ross AM. Pericardial effusion and pericardiocentesis in human immunodeficiency virus infection. *Am J Cardiol* 1994;74(1):94–96.

68. Cegielski JP, Ramiya K, Lallinger GJ, et al. Pericardial disease and human immunodeficiency virus in Dar es Salaam, Tanzania. *Lancet* 1990;335(8683):209–212.

69. Mesa RA, Edell ES, Dunn WF, et al. Human immunodeficiency virus infection and pulmonary hypertension: two new cases and a review of 86 reported cases. *Mayo Clin Proc* 1998;73(1):37–45.

70. Silver MA, Macher AM, Reichert CM, et al. Cardiac involvement by Kaposi's sarcoma in acquired immune deficiency syndrome (AIDS). *Am J Cardiol* 1984;53:983–985.

71. Vijay V, Aloor RK, Yalla SM, et al. Pericardial tamponade from Kaposi's sarcoma: role of early pericardial window. *Am Heart J* 1996;132:897–899.

72. Duong M, Dubois C, Buisson M, et al. Non-Hodgkin's lymphoma of the heart in patients infected with human immunodeficiency virus. *Clin Cardiol* 1997;20:497–502.

73. Joshi VV, Pawel B, Connor E, et al. Arteriopathy in children with acquired immune deficiency syndrome. *Pediatr Pathol* 1987;7:261–275.

74. Henry K, Melroe H, Huebsch J, et al. Severe premature coronary artery disease with protease inhibitors. *Lancet* 1998;351(9112):1328.

75. Vittecoq D, Escaut L, Monsuez JJ. Vascular complications associated with use of HIV protease inhibitors. *Lancet* 1998;351(9120):1959.

76. Mahapatra RK, Ellis GH. Myocarditis and hepatitis B virus. *Angiology* 1985;36:116–119.

77. Matsumori A, Yutani C, Ikeda Y, et al. Hepatitis C virus from the hearts of patients with myocarditis and cardiomyopathy. *Lab Invest* 2000;80:1137–1142.

78. Engblom E, Ekfors TO, Meurman OH, et al. Fatal influenza A myocarditis with isolation of virus from the myocardium. *Acta Med Scand* 1983;213(1):75–78.

79. Craver RD, Sorrells K, Gohd R. Myocarditis with influenza B infection. *Pediatr Infect Dis J* 1997;16:629–630.

80. Cheetham HD, Hart J, Coghill NF, et al. Rabies with myocarditis: two cases in England. *Lancet* 1970;1(7653):921–922.

81. Enders G, Dotsch J, Bauer J, et al. Life-threatening parvovirus B19–associated myocarditis and cardiac transplantation as possible therapy: two case reports. *Clin Infect Dis* 1998;26:355–358.

82. Ni J, Bowles NE, Kim YH, et al. Viral infection of the myocardium in endocardial fibroelastosis: molecular evidence for the role of mumps virus as an etiologic agent. *Circulation* 1997;95(1):133–139.

83. Frustaci A, Abdulla AK, Caldarulo M, et al. Fatal measles myocarditis. *Cardiologia* 1990;35:347–349.

84. Kriseman T. Rubella myocarditis in a 9-year-old patient. *Clin Pediatr* 1984;23:240–241.

85. Davis J, Schmidt W. Benzathine penicillin G: its effectiveness in prevention of streptococcal infections in a heavily exposed population. *N Engl J Med* 1957;256(8):339–342.

86. Guidelines for the diagnosis of rheumatic fever: Jones criteria, 1992 update. Special Writing Group of the Committee on Rheumatic Fever, Endocarditis, and Kawasaki Disease of the Council on Cardiovascular Disease in the Young of the American Heart Association. *JAMA* 1992;268:2069–2073.

87. Thatai D, Turi ZG. Current guidelines for the treatment of patients with rheumatic fever. *Drugs* 1999;57:545–555.

88. Lue HC, Wu MH, Wang JK, et al. Three- versus four-week administration of benzathine penicillin G: effects on incidence of streptococcal infections and recurrences of rheumatic fever. *Pediatrics* 1996;97:984–988.

89. Saikku P, Leinonen M, Mattila K, et al. Serological evidence of an association of a novel *Chlamydia*, TWAR, with chronic coronary heart disease and acute myocardial infarction. *Lancet* 1988;2(8618):983–986.

90. Saikku P, Leinonen M, Tenkanen L, et al. Chronic *Chlamydia pneumoniae* infection as a risk factor for coronary heart disease in the Helsinki Heart Study. *Ann Intern Med* 1992;116:273–278.

91. Thom DH, Grayston JT, Siscovick DS, et al. Association of prior infection with *Chlamydia pneumoniae* and angiographically demonstrated coronary artery disease. *JAMA* 1992;268(1):68–72.

92. Linnanmaki E, Leinonen M, Mattila K, et al. *Chlamydia pneumoniae*–specific circulating immune complexes in patients with chronic coronary heart disease. *Circulation* 1993;87:1130–1134.

93. Danesh J, Whincup P, Walker M, et al. *Chlamydia pneumoniae* IgG titres and coronary heart disease: prospective study and meta-analysis. *BMJ* 2000;321(7255):208–213.

94. Ridker PM, Kundsin RB, Stampfer MJ, et al. Prospective study of *Chlamydia pneumoniae* IgG seropositivity and risks of future myocardial infarction. *Circulation* 1999;99:1161–1164.

95. Nieto FJ, Folsom AR, Sorlie PD, et al. *Chlamydia pneumoniae* infection and incident coronary heart disease: the Atherosclerosis Risk in Communities Study. *Am J Epidemiol* 1999;150:149–156.

96. Kuo CC, Shor A, Campbell LA, et al. Demonstration of *Chlamydia pneumoniae* in atherosclerotic lesions of coronary arteries. *J Infect Dis* 1993;167:841–849.

97. Muhlestein JB, Hammond EH, Carlquist JF, et al. Increased incidence of *Chlamydia* species within the coronary arteries of patients with symptomatic atherosclerotic versus other forms of cardiovascular disease. *J Am Coll Cardiol* 1996;27:1555–1561.

98. Campbell LA, O'Brien ER, Cappuccio AL, et al. Detection of *Chlamydia pneumoniae* TWAR in human coronary atherectomy tissues. *J Infect Dis* 1995;172:585–588.

99. Thomas M, Wong Y, Thomas D, et al. Relation between direct detection of *Chlamydia pneumoniae* DNA in human coronary arteries at postmortem examination and histological severity (Stary grading) of associated atherosclerotic plaque. *Circulation* 1999;99:2733–2736.

100. Zhou YF, Csako G, Grayston JT, et al. Lack of association of restenosis following coronary angioplasty with elevated C-reactive protein levels or seropositivity to *Chlamydia pneumoniae*. *Am J Cardiol* 1999;84:595–598, A598.

101. Gupta S, Leatham EW, Carrington D, et al. Elevated *Chlamydia pneumoniae* antibodies, cardiovascular events, and azithromycin in male survivors of myocardial infarction. *Circulation* 1997;96:404–407.

102. Gurfinkel E, Bozovich G, Beck E, et al. Treatment with the antibiotic roxithromycin in patients with acute non-Q-wave coronary syndromes: the final report of the ROXIS Study. *Eur Heart J* 1999;20:121–127.

103. Anderson JL, Muhlestein JB, Carlquist J, et al. Randomized secondary prevention trial of azithromycin in patients with coronary artery disease and serological evidence for *Chlamydia pneumoniae* infection. The Azithromycin in Coronary Artery Disease: Elimination of Myocardial Infection with Chlamydia (ACADEMIC) study. *Circulation* 1999;99:1540–1547.

104. Dunne MW. Rationale and design of a secondary prevention trial of antibiotic use in patients after myocardial infarction: the WIZARD (Weekly Intervention with Zithromax [Azithromycin] for Atherosclerosis and Its Related Disorders) trial. *J Infect Dis* 2000;18[Suppl 3]:S572–S578.

105. Jackson LA. Description and status of the Azithromycin and Coronary Events Study (ACES). *J Infect Dis* 2000;18[Suppl 3]:S579–S581.

106. Otto CM, Kuusisto J, Reichenbach DD, et al. Characterization of the early lesion of "degenerative" valvular aortic stenosis: histological and immunohistochemical studies. *Circulation* 1994;90:844–853.

107. Juvonen J, Laurila A, Juvonen T, et al. Detection of *Chlamydia pneumoniae* in human nonrheumatic stenotic aortic valves. *J Am Coll Cardiol* 1997;29:1054–1059.

108. Nystrom-Rosander C, Thelin S, Hjelm E, et al. High incidence of *Chlamydia pneumoniae* in sclerotic heart valves of patients undergoing aortic valve replacement. *Scand J Infect Dis* 1997;29:361–365.

109. Bruu AL, Haukenes G, Aasen S, et al. *Chlamydia pneumoniae* infections in Norway 1981–87 earlier diagnosed as ornithosis. *Scand J Infect Dis* 1991;23:299–304.

110. Schinkel AF, Bax JJ, van der Wall EE, et al. Echocardiographic follow-up of *Chlamydia psittaci* myocarditis. *Chest* 2000;117:1203–1205.

111. Stockins BA, Lanas FT, Saavedra JG, et al. Prognosis in patients with diphtheric myocarditis and bradyarrhythmias: assessment of results of ventricular pacing. *Br Heart J* 1994;72:190–191.

112. Vlietstra RE, Lie JT, Kuhl WE, et al. Whipple's disease involving the pericardium: pathological confirmation during life. *Aust N Z J Med* 1978;8:649–651.

113. Silvestry FE, Kim B, Pollack BJ, et al. Cardiac Whipple disease: identification of Whipple bacillus by electron microscopy of a patient before death. *Ann Intern Med* 1997;126:214–216.

114. Elkins C, Shuman TA, Pirolo JS. Cardiac Whipple's disease without digestive symptoms. *Ann Thorac Surg* 1999;67(1):250–251.

115. James TN, Bulkley BH. Abnormalities of the coronary arteries in Whipple's disease. *Am Heart J* 1983;105:481–491.

116. Mendall MA, Goggin PM, Molineaux N, et al. Relation of *Helicobacter pylori* infection and coronary heart disease. *Br Heart J* 1994;71:437–439.

117. Patel P, Mendall MA, Carrington D, et al. Association of *Helicobacter pylori* and *Chlamydia pneumoniae* infections with coronary heart disease and cardiovascular risk factors. *BMJ* 1995;311(7007):711–714.

118. Folsom AR, Nieto FJ, Sorlie P, et al. *Helicobacter pylori* seropositivity and coronary heart disease incidence. Atherosclerosis Risk in Communities (ARIC) Study Investigators. *Circulation* 1998;98:845–850.

119. Whincup P, Danesh J, Walker M, et al. Prospective study of potentially virulent strains of *Helicobacter pylori* and coronary heart disease in middle-aged men. *Circulation* 2000;101:1647–1652.

120. Hardman JM, Earle KM. Myocarditis in 200 fatal meningococcal infections. *Arch Pathol* 1969;87:318–325.

121. Chen SC, Tsai CC, Nouri S. Carditis associated with *Mycoplasma pneumoniae* infection. *Am J Dis Child* 1986;140:471–472.

122. Armengol S, Domingo C, Mesalles E. Myocarditis: a rare complication during *Legionella* infection. *Int J Cardiol* 1992;37:418–420.

123. Lubani M, Sharda D, Helin I. Cardiac manifestations in brucellosis. *Arch Dis Child* 1986;61:569–572.

124. Akdeniz H, Tuncer I, Irmak H, et al. *Salmonella* myocarditis in a patient with Wolf-Parkinson-White syndrome that was confused with an inferior myocardial infarction. *Clin Infect Dis* 1997;25:736–737.

125. Leon F, Badui E, Campos A, et al. Cholera and myocarditis: a case report. *Angiology* 1997;48:545–549.

126. Steere AC, Batsford WP, Weinberg M, et al. Lyme carditis: cardiac abnormalities of Lyme disease. *Ann Intern Med* 1980;93(1):8–16.

127. McAlister HF, Klementowicz PT, Andrews C, et al. Lyme carditis: an important cause of reversible heart block. *Ann Intern Med* 1989;110:339–345.

128. Reznick JW, Braunstein DB, Walsh RL, et al. Lyme carditis: electrophysiologic and histopathologic study. *Am J Med* 1986;81:923–927.

129. Horowitz HW, Belkin RN. Acute myopericarditis resulting from Lyme disease. *Am Heart J* 1995;130(1):176–178.

130. de Koning J, Hoogkamp-Korstanje JA, van der Linde MR, et al. Demonstration of spirochetes in cardiac biopsies of patients with Lyme disease. *J Infect Dis* 1989;160(1):150–153.

131. Stanek G, Klein J, Bittner R, et al. Isolation of *Borrelia burgdorferi* from the myocardium of a patient with long-standing cardiomyopathy. *N Engl J Med* 1990;322:249–252.

132. Klein J, Stanek G, Bittner R, et al. Lyme borreliosis as a cause of myocarditis and heart muscle disease. *Eur Heart J* 1991;12[Suppl D]:73–75.

133. Rees DH, Keeling PJ, McKenna WJ, et al. No evidence to implicate *Borrelia burgdorferi* in the pathogenesis of dilated cardiomyopathy in the United Kingdom. *Br Heart J* 1994;71:459–461.

134. Gasser R, Dusleag J, Reisinger E, et al. Reversal by ceftriaxone of dilated cardiomyopathy *Borrelia burgdorferi* infection. *Lancet* 1992;339(8802):1174–1175.

135. Rahn DW, Malawista SE. Lyme disease: recommendations for diagnosis and treatment. *Ann Intern Med* 1991;114:472–481.

136. Steere AC, Hutchinson GJ, Rahn DW, et al. Treatment of the early manifestations of Lyme disease. *Ann Intern Med* 1983;99(1):22–26.

137. Jackman JD Jr, Radolf JD. Cardiovascular syphilis. *Am J Med* 1989;87:425–433.

138. Watt G, Padre LP, Tuazon M, et al. Skeletal and cardiac muscle involvement in severe, late leptospirosis. *J Infect Dis* 1990;162(1):266–269.

139. de Brito T, Morais CF, Yasuda PH, et al. Cardiovascular involvement in human and experimental leptospirosis: pathologic findings and immunohistochemical detection of leptospiral antigen. *Ann Trop Med Parasitol* 1987;81:207–214.

140. Bradford WD, Hackel DB. Myocardial involvement in Rocky Mountain spotted fever. *Arch Pathol Lab Med* 1978;102(7):357–359.

141. Walker DH, Paletta CE, Cain BG. Pathogenesis of myocarditis in Rocky Mountain spotted fever. *Arch Pathol Lab Med* 1980;104:171–174.

142. Raoult D, Tissot-Dupont H, Foucault C, et al. Q fever

1985–1998: clinical and epidemiologic features of 1,383 infections. *Medicine* 2000;79:109–123.

143. Jahangir A, Kolbert C, Edwards W, et al. Fatal pancarditis associated with human granulocytic ehrlichiosis in a 44-year-old man. *Clin Infect Dis* 1998;27:1424–1427.

144. Henochowicz S, Mustafa M, Lawrinson WE, et al. Cardiac aspergillosis in acquired immune deficiency syndrome. *Am J Cardiol* 1985;55:1239–1240.

145. Atkinson JB, Connor DH, Robinowitz M, et al. Cardiac fungal infections: review of autopsy findings in 60 patients. *Hum Pathol* 1984;15:935–942.

146. Walsh TJ, Hutchins GM, Bulkley BH, et al. Fungal infections of the heart: analysis of 51 autopsy cases. *Am J Cardiol* 1980;45:357–366.

147. Grossi P, Farina C, Fiocchi R, et al. Prevalence and outcome of invasive fungal infections in 1,963 thoracic organ transplant recipients: a multicenter retrospective study. Italian Study Group of Fungal Infections in Thoracic Organ Transplant Recipients. *Transplantation* 2000;70(1):112–116.

148. Williams AH. *Aspergillus* myocarditis. *Am J Clin Pathol* 1974;61:247–256.

149. Franklin WG, Simon AB, Sodeman TM. *Candida* myocarditis without valvulitis. *Am J Cardiol* 1976;38:924–928.

150. Lafont A, Wolff M, Marche C, et al. Overwhelming myocarditis due to *Cryptococcus neoformans* in an AIDS patient. *Lancet* 1987;2(8568):1145–1146.

151. Schwartz EL, Waldmann EB, Payne RM, et al. Coccidioidal pericarditis. *Chest* 1976;70:670–672.

152. Benbow EW, McMahon, RF. Myocardial infarction caused by cardiac disease in disseminated zygomycosis. *J Clin Pathol* 1987;40(1):70–74.

153. Berarducci L, Ford K, Olenick S, et al. Invasive intracardiac aspergillosis with widespread embolization. *J Am Soc Echocardiogr* 1993;6:539–542.

154. Hagar JM, Rahimtoola SH. Chagas' heart disease. *Curr Probl Cardiol* 1995;20:825–924.

155. Grant IH, Gold JW, Wittner M, et al. Transfusion-associated acute Chagas disease acquired in the United States. *Ann Intern Med* 1989;111:849–851.

156. Parada H, Carrasco HA, Anez N, et al. Cardiac involvement is a constant finding in acute Chagas' disease: a clinical, parasitological and histopathological study. *Int J Cardiol* 1997;60(1):49–54.

157. Hagar JM, Rahimtoola SH. Chagas' heart disease in the United States. *N Engl J Med* 1991;325:763–768.

158. Higuchi ML, de Brito T, Reis M, et al. Correlation between *Trypanosoma cruzi* parasitism and myocardial inflammatory infiltrate in human chronic Chagasic myocarditis: light microscopy and immunohistochemical findings. *Cardiovasc Pathol* 1993;2:101–106.

159. Rossi MA, Bestetti RB. The challenge of chagasic cardiomyopathy: the pathologic roles of autonomic abnormalities, autoimmune mechanisms and microvascular changes, and therapeutic implications. *Cardiology* 1995;86(1):1–7.

160. Samuel J, Oliveira M, Correa De Araujo RR, et al. Cardiac thrombosis and thromboembolism in chronic Chagas' heart disease. *Am J Cardiol* 1983;52(1):147–151.

161. Bestetti RB, Freitas OC, Muccillo G, et al. Clinical and morphological characteristics associated with sudden car-

diac death in patients with Chagas' disease. *Eur Heart J* 1993;14:1610–1614.

162. Milei J, Pesce R, Valero E, et al. Electrophysiologic-structural correlations in chagasic aneurysms causing malignant arrhythmias. *Int J Cardiol* 1991;32(1):65–73.

163. Carrasco HA, Parada H, Guerrero L, et al. Prognostic implications of clinical, electrocardiographic and hemodynamic findings in chronic Chagas' disease. *Int J Cardiol* 1994;43(1):27–38.

164. Viotti R, Vigliano C, Armenti H, et al. Treatment of chronic Chagas' disease with benznidazole: clinical and serologic evolution of patients with long-term follow-up. *Am Heart J* 1994;127(1):151–162.

165. de Andrade AL, Zicker F, de Oliveira RM, et al. Randomised trial of efficacy of benznidazole in treatment of early *Trypanosoma cruzi* infection. *Lancet* 1996;348(9039):1407–1413.

166. Sinagra A, Riarte A, Lauricella M, et al. Reactivation of experimental chronic *T. cruzi* infection after immunosuppressive treatment by cyclosporine A and betametasone. *Transplantation* 1993;55:1431–1434.

167. de Carvalho VB, Sousa EF, Vila JH, et al. Heart transplantation in Chagas' disease: 10 years after the initial experience. *Circulation* 1996;94:1815–1817.

168. Bocchi EA, Bellotti G, Mocelin AO, et al. Heart transplantation for chronic Chagas' heart disease. *Ann Thorac Surg* 1996;61:1727–1733.

169. Bocchi EA, Higuchi ML, Vieira ML, et al. Higher incidence of malignant neoplasms after heart transplantation for treatment of chronic Chagas' heart disease. *J Heart Lung Transplant* 1998;17:399–405.

170. Montoya JG, Jordan R, Lingamneni S, et al. Toxoplasmic myocarditis and polymyositis in patients with acute acquired toxoplasmosis diagnosed during life. *Clin Infect Dis* 1997;24:676–683.

171. Hofman P, Drici MD, Gibelin P, et al. Prevalence of *Toxoplasma* myocarditis in patients with the acquired immunodeficiency syndrome. *Br Heart J* 1993;70:376–381.

172. Jehn U, Fink M, Gundlach P, et al. Lethal cardiac and cerebral toxoplasmosis in a patient with acute myeloid leukemia after successful allogeneic bone marrow transplantation. *Transplantation* 1984;38:430–433.

173. Luft BJ, Billingham M, Remington JS. Endomyocardial biopsy in the diagnosis of toxoplasmic myocarditis. *Transplant Proc* 1986;18:1871–1873.

174. Ryning FW, McLeod R, Maddox JC, et al. Probable transmission of *Toxoplasma gondii* by organ transplantation. *Ann Intern Med* 1979;90(1):47–49.

175. Compton SJ, Celum CL, Lee C, et al. Trichinosis with ventilatory failure and persistent myocarditis. *Clin Infect Dis* 1993;16:500–504.

176. Merkel W. *Plasmodium falciparum* malaria: the coronary and myocardial lesions observed at autopsy in two cases of acute fulminating *P. falciparum* infection. *Arch Pathol* 1946;41:290–298.

177. Sadigursky M, Andrade ZA. Pulmonary changes in schistosomal cor pulmonale. *Am J Trop Med Hyg* 1982;31:779–784.

178. Miralles A, Bracamonte L, Pavie A, et al. Cardiac echinococcosis: surgical treatment and results. *J Thorac Cardiovasc Surg* 1994;107(1):184–190.

179. Shioi T, Matsumori A, Sasayama S. Persistent expression of cytokine in the chronic stage of viral myocarditis in mice. *Circulation* 1996;94:2930–2937.

180. Henke A, Huber S, Stelzner A, et al. The role of CD8+ T lymphocytes in coxsackievirus B3–induced myocarditis. *J Virol* 1995;69:6720–6728.

181. McManus BM, Chow LH, Wilson JE, et al. Direct myocardial injury by enterovirus: a central role in the evolution of murine myocarditis. *Clin Immunol Immunopathol* 1993;68:159–169.

182. Chow LH, Beisel KW, McManus BM. Enteroviral infection of mice with severe combined immunodeficiency: evidence for direct viral pathogenesis of myocardial injury. *Lab Invest* 1992;66(1):24–31.

183. Matsumori A, Yamada T, Suzuki H, et al. Increased circulating cytokines in patients with myocarditis and cardiomyopathy. *Br Heart J* 1994;72:561–566.

184. Godeny EK, Gauntt CJ. Involvement of natural killer cells in coxsackievirus B3–induced murine myocarditis. *J Immunol* 1986;137:1695–1702.

185. Seko Y, Shinkai Y, Kawasaki A, et al. Evidence of perforin-mediated cardiac myocyte injury in acute murine myocarditis caused by Coxsackie virus B3. *J Pathol* 1993;170(1):53–58.

186. Tomioka N, Kishimoto C, Matsumori A, et al. Effects of prednisolone on acute viral myocarditis in mice. *J Am Coll Cardiol* 1986;7:868–872.

187. Lodge PA, Herzum M, Olszewski J, et al. Coxsackievirus B-3 myocarditis: acute and chronic forms of the disease caused by different immunopathogenic mechanisms. *Am J Pathol* 1987;128:455–463.

188. Kishimoto C, Kuribayashi K, Fukuma K, et al. Immunologic identification of lymphocyte subsets in experimental murine myocarditis with encephalomyocarditis virus: different kinetics of lymphocyte subsets between the heart and the peripheral blood, and significance of Thy 1.2+ (pan T) and Lyt 1+, 23+ (immature T) subsets in the development of myocarditis. *Circ Res* 1987;61:715–725.

189. Seko Y, Tsuchimochi H, Nakamura T, et al. Expression of major histocompatibility complex class I antigen in murine ventricular myocytes infected with Coxsackievirus B3. *Circ Res* 1990;67:360–367.

190. Guthrie M, Lodge PA, Huber SA. Cardiac injury in myocarditis induced by coxsackievirus group B, type 3 in Balb/c mice is mediated by Lyt 2+ cytolytic lymphocytes. *Cell Immunol* 1984;88:558–567.

191. Huber SA, Lodge PA. Coxsackievirus B-3 myocarditis in Balb/c mice: evidence for autoimmunity to myocyte antigens. *Am J Pathol* 1984;116(1):21–29.

192. Klingel K, Hohenadl C, Canu A, et al. Ongoing enterovirus-induced myocarditis is associated with persistent heart muscle infection: quantitative analysis of virus replication, tissue damage, and inflammation. *Proc Natl Acad Sci U S A* 1992;89(1):314–318.

193. Neu N, Beisel KW, Traystman MD, et al. Autoantibodies specific for the cardiac myosin isoform are found in mice susceptible to coxsackievirus B3–induced myocarditis. *J Immunol* 1987;138:2488–2492.

194. Maisch B, Bauer E, Cirsi M, et al. Cytolytic cross-reactive antibodies directed against the cardiac membrane and viral proteins in coxsackievirus B3 and B4 myocarditis: characterization and pathogenetic relevance. *Circulation* 1993;87[Suppl 5]:IV49–IV65.

195. Lawson CM, O'Donoghue HL, Reed WD. Mouse cytomegalovirus infection induces antibodies which cross-react with virus and cardiac myosin: a model for the study of molecular mimicry in the pathogenesis of viral myocarditis. *Immunology* 1992;75:513–519.

196. HFSA guidelines for management of patients with heart failure caused by left ventricular systolic dysfunction: pharmacological approaches. Heart Failure Society of America. *Pharmacotherapy* 2000;20:495–522.

197. Consensus recommendations for the management of chronic heart failure: on behalf of the membership of the Advisory Council to Improve Outcomes Nationwide in Heart Failure. *Am J Cardiol* 1999;83[Suppl 2A]:1A–38A.

198. Matsumori A, Igata H, Ono K, et al. High doses of digitalis increase the myocardial production of proinflammatory cytokines and worsen myocardial injury in viral myocarditis: a possible mechanism of digitalis toxicity. *Jpn Circ J* 1999;63:934–940.

199. Mason JW, O'Connell JB, Herskowitz A, et al. A clinical trial of immunosuppressive therapy for myocarditis. The Myocarditis Treatment Trial Investigators. *N Engl J Med* 1995;333:269–275.

200. Hufnagel G, Pankuweit S, Richter A, et al. The European Study of Epidemiology and Treatment of Cardiac Inflammatory Diseases (ESETCID): first epidemiological results. *Herz* 2000;25:279–285.

201. Parrillo JE, Cunnion RE, Epstein SE, et al. A prospective, randomized, controlled trial of prednisone for dilated cardiomyopathy. *N Engl J Med* 1989;321:1061–1068.

202. Latham RD, Mulrow JP, Virmani R, et al. Recently diagnosed idiopathic dilated cardiomyopathy: incidence of myocarditis and efficacy of prednisone therapy. *Am Heart J* 1989;117:876–882.

203. Kuhl U, Schultheiss HP. Treatment of chronic myocarditis with corticosteroids. *Eur Heart J* 1995;16[Suppl O]:168–172.

204. Maisch B, Hufnagel G, Schonian U, et al. The European Study of Epidemiology and Treatment of Cardiac Inflammatory Disease (ESETCID). *Eur Heart J* 1995;16[Suppl O]:173–175.

205. Drucker NA, Colan SD, Lewis AB, et al. Gamma-globulin treatment of acute myocarditis in the pediatric population. *Circulation* 1994;89(1):252–257.

206. McNamara DM, Rosenblum WD, Janosko KM, et al. Intravenous immune globulin in the therapy of myocarditis and acute cardiomyopathy. *Circulation* 1997;95:2476–2478.

207. Takada H, Kishimoto C, Hiraoka Y. Therapy with immunoglobulin suppresses myocarditis in a murine coxsackievirus B3 model: antiviral and anti-inflammatory effects. *Circulation* 1995;92:1604–1611.

207a. McNamara D, Holubkov R, Starling RC, et al. Controlled trial of intravenous immune globulin in recent-onset dilated cardiomyopathy. *Circulation* 2001;103:2254–2259.

208. Miric M, Vasiljevic J, Bojic M, et al. Long-term follow up of patients with dilated heart muscle disease treated with

human leucocytic interferon alpha or thymic hormones: initial results. *Heart* 1996;75:596–601.

209. Stille-Siegener M, Heim A, Figulla HR. Subclassification of dilated cardiomyopathy and interferon treatment. *Eur Heart J* 1995;16[Suppl O]:147–149.

210. Matsumori A, Tomioka N, Kawai C. Protective effect of recombinant alpha interferon on coxsackievirus B3 myocarditis in mice. *Am Heart J* 1988;115:1229–1232.

211. Kishimoto C, Crumpacker CS, Abelmann WH. Ribavirin treatment of murine coxsackievirus B3 myocarditis with analyses of lymphocyte subsets. *J Am Coll Cardiol* 1988;12:1334–1341.

212. Ray CG, Icenogle TB, Minnich LL, et al. The use of intravenous ribavirin to treat influenza virus–associated acute myocarditis. *J Infect Dis* 1989;159:829–836.

213. Chen YS, Wang MJ, Chou NK, et al. Rescue for acute myocarditis with shock by extracorporeal membrane oxygenation. *Ann Thorac Surg* 1999;68:2220–2224.

214. Reiss N, el-Banayosy A, Posival H, et al. Management of acute fulminant myocarditis using circulatory support systems. *Artif Organs* 1996;20:964–970.

215. O'Connell JB, Dec GW, Goldenberg IF, et al. Results of heart transplantation for active lymphocytic myocarditis. *J Heart Transplant* 1990;9:351–355, discussion 355–356.

216. O'Connell JB, Breen TJ, Hosenpud JD. Heart transplantation in dilated heart muscle disease and myocarditis. *Eur Heart J* 1995;16[Suppl O]:137–139.

217. Hoyer S, Berglin E, Pettersson G, et al. Cardiac transplantation in patients with active myocarditis. *Transplant Proc* 1990;22:1450.

218. Kobashigawa JA, Miller L, Yeung A, et al. Does acute rejection correlate with the development of transplant coronary artery disease? A multicenter study using intravascular ultrasound. *J Heart Lung Transplant* 1995;14:S221–S226.

219. Lozinski GM, Davis GG, Krous HF, et al. Adenovirus myocarditis: retrospective diagnosis by gene amplification from formalin-fixed, paraffin-embedded tissues. *Hum Pathol* 1994;25:831–834.

SUBSTANCE ABUSE AND THE HEART

ROBERT A. KLONER
SHEREIF H. REZKALLA

OVERVIEW

Cocaine may be associated with myocardial ischemia and myocardial infarction (MI). A physician who sees a young person with an unexplained MI should consider cocaine use to be a possible cause. Cocaine may also cause hypertension, cardiomyopathy, arrhythmias, and sudden death. Whether coffee is associated with cardiovascular disease remains highly controversial. Anabolic steroids and

amphetamines have been associated with cases of MI. Excessive alcohol consumption causes dilated cardiomyopathy and hypertension, although small doses of alcohol may reduce coronary disease. Tobacco use is unquestionably a strong risk factor for coronary artery disease.

COCAINE CARDIOTOXICITY

Of the various substances of abuse that may affect the heart, cocaine has received the most attention over the last 10 years (1–9). This is largely a result of its widespread use, especially in large urban areas of the United States; the relative ease with which the substance can be obtained; and the

---

R. A. Kloner: Division of Cardiology, University of Southern California School of Medicine; and Heart Institute, Good Samaritan Hospital, Los Angeles, California
S. H. Rezkalla: University of Wisconsin Medical School, Madison, Wisconsin; and Department of Cardiology, Marshfield Clinic, Marshfield, Wisconsin

occurrence of sudden death among athletes who have used cocaine. In this section, we review the history of cocaine use, describe the basic science of the effect of cocaine use on the heart, detail the results of clinical and autopsy reports of cocaine use in humans, and describe the clinical approach to and therapy for patients who have cocaine cardiotoxicity.

History

It is estimated that approximately 5 to 6 million people in the United States use cocaine on a regular basis, that approximately 1 million are addicted, and that 25 to 30 million Americans have tried cocaine at least once (2,3). ▼▼ h52

Forms of Cocaine

Cocaine hydrochloride is a water-soluble form of cocaine in which the alkaloid extract of the *E. coca* plant is dissolved in hydrochloric acid to form a white crystalline powder (14,15). Because the white powder can be absorbed by the mucous membranes, intranasal insufflation (snorting) of this white powder is the most common route of administration. The powder also can be injected intravenously. Cocaine is not readily absorbed gastrointestinally, and the low pH of the gastric mucosa may inactivate the alkaloid (14,15).

Crack cocaine is produced by mixing cocaine powder with baking soda and water and then heating the results. The alkaloid base precipitates into a soft mass that hardens and is then smoked. The term "crack" derives from the cracking or popping sound heard when the cocaine crystals are prepared in this fashion.

Freebase cocaine is made by mixing the cocaine powder with a base (such as ammonia) and a solvent (such as ether). The alkaloid base or "free base" is extracted from the ether by evaporation. Like crack, freebase cocaine is smoked. The flammability of ether poses yet another danger in the preparation of this form of cocaine. Freebase use has declined as crack has become more available, and because crack does not pose the problem of flammability.

An estimated 90% of cocaine use in the United States is carried out through nasal snorting. In addition, approximately one-third of cocaine users have smoked crack. Less than 10% have injected the drug intravenously. Because cocaine is rapidly absorbed through the respiratory tract, smoking of either crack or freebase cocaine rapidly delivers cocaine to the circulation. Cocaine enters the brain within 6 to 8 seconds by the respiratory route (smoking) and within 10 to 15 seconds by an intravenous route. Snorting cocaine results in peak cocaine concentrations in 30 to 60 minutes (15). The amount of cocaine that can be absorbed through the nasal route may be self-limited to some extent because of vasoconstriction of the nasal mucosa induced by cocaine itself.

Cocaine is often combined with other substances, most commonly ethanol. An estimated 9 to 12 million individu-als use this combination on a recreational basis (16,17). Cocaethylene is the cocaine metabolite formed in the presence of ethyl alcohol and may be more potent than cocaine itself (see Cocaethylene).

Pharmacology

The pharmacology of cocaine is complex and has been the subject of a vast amount of basic science research during the last 10 years. First, cocaine is a local anesthetic. It blocks sodium and potassium channels (6) and thus blocks initiation and conduction of electrical impulses. This effect accounts for prolongation of electrocardiographic (ECG) intervals and decreases in cardiac contractility and may lead to a proarrhythmic effect (18). Second, cocaine blocks the reuptake of neurotransmitters at the presynaptic endings of nerves. As a result, neurotransmitters such as dopamine and norepinephrine accumulate in the synaptic cleft, which results in an intense sympathomimetic effect (6). This second major action of cocaine accounts for increases in heart rate, blood pressure, and contractility and, by stimulation of alpha receptors in the vasculature, contributes to vasoconstriction. A third pharmacologic action of cocaine that affects the cardiovascular system is a decrease in vagal tone, which also contributes to an increase in heart rate (19). Thus, on the one hand, cocaine may have a cardiodepressive effect resulting from its effect on sodium and potassium channels. On the other hand, it has a stimulatory effect because of its sympathomimetic properties. These opposing forces may result in very complex outcomes (20).

Controlled Studies of Administration of Cocaine in Humans

Cocaine is known to increase both heart rate and blood pressure in awake individuals. Fischman and coworkers (54) demonstrated a dose-related increase in these parameters when patients received intravenous cocaine. Although small doses did not have a significant effect, an intravenous injection of cocaine, 16 and 32 mg, resulted in a significant rise in both heart rate and blood pressure in human volunteers. The changes peaked at 10 minutes after administration and returned to baseline in approximately 1 hour.

To examine the acute effects of cocaine in humans, investigators administered low doses (2 mg per kg) of intranasal cocaine to patients in the cardiac catheterization laboratory (3,55–57). They observed increases in heart rate and blood pressure but only mild, diffuse reductions in coronary caliber (8% to 12% of normal), a 33% increase in coronary vascular resistance, and a 17% reduction in coronary sinus blood flow. Thus, even though myocardial oxygen demand increased—with an increase in double-product—these patients exhibited a decrease in coronary blood flow. It is likely that in cocaine abusers, who often use much higher doses than those administered in this controlled study, the imbalance in oxygen supply and demand is even worse. It was shown that the cocaine-induced coronary vasoconstriction could be reversed with the alpha adrenergic blocking agent phentolamine, suggesting that alpha-receptor stimulation by cocaine is a crucial aspect of the vasoconstriction. The vasoconstriction was worse at sites of atherosclerosis and could be relieved by nitroglycerin (58). The beta-blocker propranolol potentiated the cocaine-induced vasoconstriction, presumably because the beta receptors were blocked, leaving the alpha receptors unopposed. Investigators showed (59) that accumulation of cocaine metabolites may also contribute to coronary vasospasm. Addition of ethanol to intranasal cocaine did not worsen coronary vasospasm (16). Isolated human coronary arteries from patients undergoing cardiac transplantation have also been shown to undergo vasospasm when exposed to cocaine.

Administration of cocaine as a local anesthetic agent for use in laryngoscopy increased the frequency of ventricular premature beats (60). There have been occasional case reports of acute MI when intranasal cocaine was used as a topical anesthetic for nasal operative procedures. The effects of cocaine on human fetal left ventricles were studied (61). Cocaine reduced action potential amplitude, depressed the force of ventricular contraction, and then, at 90 minutes of exposure, resulted in electrical and mechanical arrest, which also suggests that cocaine has a direct cardiodepressant effect on cardiac muscle. And finally, we observed that when human blood is exposed to cocaine, in approximately one-half of the samples, platelet aggregation to adenosine diphosphate but not collagen or epinephrine is increased (Fig. 36.1) (47).

In summary, controlled studies in humans receiving low doses of intranasal cocaine showed that cocaine increases heart rate and blood pressure but causes coronary vasoconstriction at the same time. Thus, the potential for ischemia through an imbalance between oxygen supply and demand may occur, especially when even higher doses of cocaine are used.

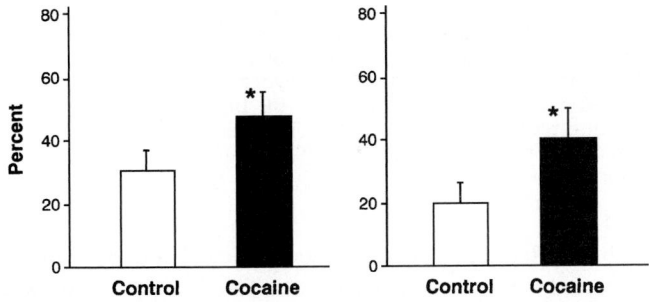

FIGURE 36.1 Platelet aggregation from humans (1 μg, adenosine diphosphate) after incubation with saline or cocaine. Peak aggregation (*left*) and aggregation at 15 minutes (*right*). Data are expressed as mean ± standard error of the mean; *p <.02. (From Rezkalla SH, Mazza JJ, Kloner RA, et al. Effects of cocaine on human platelets in healthy subjects. *Am J Cardiol* 1993;72:243–246.)

TABLE 36.1 CARDIOVASCULAR COMPLICATIONS OF COCAINE USE

Myocardial infarction and myocardial ischemia
Myocarditis
Cardiomyopathy: dilated and hypertrophic
Arrhythmias: tachy- and bradyarrhythmias
Hypertension
Aortic dissection
Endocarditis
Acceleration of atherosclerosis?

Cardiovascular Disease Associated with Cocaine Use

Most of our knowledge regarding the clinical complications of cocaine use in patients comes from clinical reports and autopsy studies. A number of cardiovascular diseases associated with cocaine use have been reported in the literature. These are summarized in Table 36.1, and mechanisms of cocaine action are illustrated in Fig. 36.2.

Acute Myocardial Infarction

Four possible causes of MI are related to cocaine use. (a) Coronary artery spasm is caused by the intense alpha-sympathetic stimulation associated with use of cocaine. (b) Thrombus formation was observed in 24% of patients in whom coronary artery disease was absent (62). Thrombus may have occurred on top of an area of vasospasm that was then relieved, and increased platelet aggregability may contribute (47). Thrombus formation may also occur on top of atherosclerotic narrowing (*e*Fig. 36.2.1). Plaque fracture or rupture, which is common in most Q-wave MIs, is usually not observed in cocaine-related infarcts (53,63). (c) Increased myocardial oxygen demand may occur in the presence of a fixed lesion. Chronic use of cocaine may cause an acceleration of atherosclerosis, resulting in atherosclerotic narrowing in young patients (53). The sympathomimetic responses of increased heart rate and blood pressure, in addition to the stenosis, may contribute to infarction. (d) Some combination of the above three may cause MI.

At least 114 cases of cocaine-related MI have been reported in the literature (64). Many more probably occur but are never reported. Clinical, angiographic, and autopsy features reveal some unique properties of cocaine-related infarction. MI after cocaine use typically occurs within 3 hours of use of cocaine, but this period ranges from minutes to a few days. The median time of onset of chest pain in the infarct patient depends on the route of administration (62). Onset of chest pain occurred at a median time of 30 minutes with intravenous use, 90 minutes with use of crack cocaine, and 135 minutes with nasal insufflation. In a study of 3,946 patients with acute MI (65), 38 patients reported cocaine use before the clinical presentation. The risk appears to be higher in the 60 minutes after cocaine

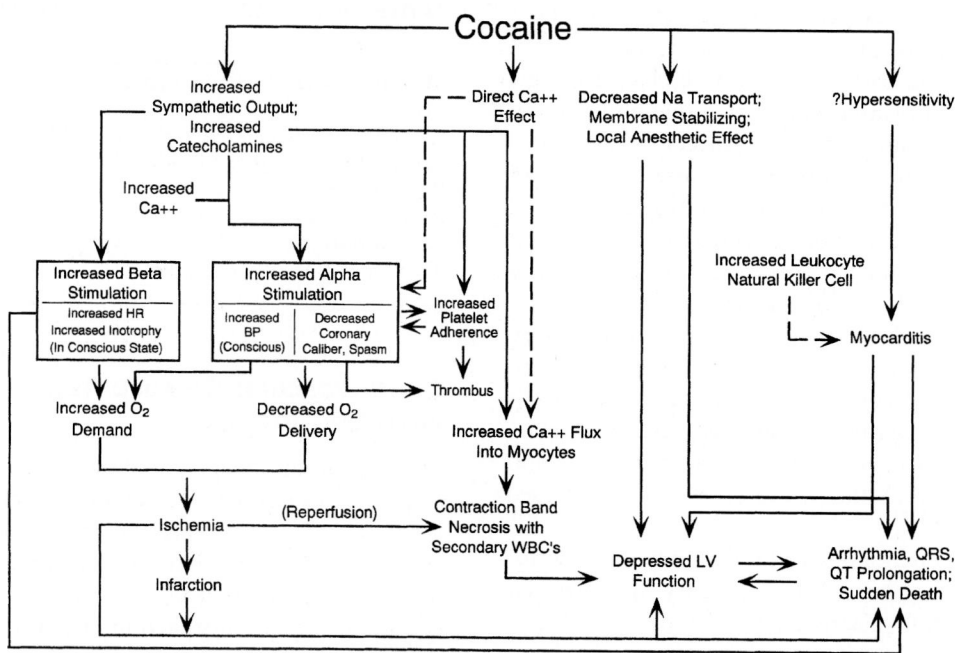

FIGURE 36.2 Schematic diagram describing potential mechanisms of the cardiotoxic effects of cocaine. Two primary mechanisms are suggested. First, cocaine inhibits presynaptic reuptake of catecholamines, resulting in a potentiation of the sympathetic nervous system and an increase in catecholamine levels. Second, cocaine inhibits sodium transport across the sarcolemmal membrane, leading to a membrane-stabilizing or local anesthetic effect that has been likened to a type I antiarrhythmic effect. In conscious preparations, increased sympathetic output and catecholamine levels result in an increase in heart rate and, in some studies, inotrophy, which can increase oxygen demand. α-Stimulation of blood vessels causes a vasoconstrictor response with increase in blood pressure in conscious preparations, also resulting in increased oxygen demand. α-Sympathetic stimulation decreases coronary artery caliber, increases coronary vascular resistance, and may lead to coronary spasm in both conscious and anesthetized preparations, thus reducing oxygen supply. Repetitive bouts of coronary spasm might alter or damage the endothelium, contributing to accelerated atherosclerosis, which has been reported with use of cocaine. Increased platelet aggregability has been reported with use of cocaine (and may be related to increased catecholamine levels), which can contribute to thrombus formation. All of these factors contribute to an imbalance between oxygen supply and demand and may thus lead to myocardial ischemia with subsequent infarction and associated left ventricular dysfunction and arrhythmias. Increased sympathetic output may also contribute to tachyarrhythmias. Catecholamine excess is known to lead to contraction-band formation, and this is thought to be related to calcium overload. Isner and Chokshi (1) postulated that cocaine may have a direct effect on calcium flux into blood vessels (and perhaps myocytes), leading to vasoconstriction that may be independent of the sympathetic nervous system (*dashed lines*). The local anesthetic effect of cocaine may cause direct depression of inotrophy (which in some studies surpasses any indirect positive inotropic response caused by sympathetic simulation) and can lead to a transient cardiomyopathic presentation. This local anesthetic effect can also lead to prolongation of electrocardiographic intervals, including QRS and QT duration, perhaps resulting in arrhythmias and sudden death, much like the proarrhythmic effects of agents such as quinidine. Hypersensitivity to cocaine has been postulated but not absolutely proved to be a cause of myocarditis. In addition, an increase in natural killer cell activity (which may be related to increased catecholamines) has been reported with cocaine and could lead to myocarditis. Scattered foci of myocarditis could lead to a cardiomyopathic presentation and form the nidus for arrhythmias. BP, blood pressure; HR, heart rate; LV, left ventricular; WBC's, white blood cells. (From Kloner RA, Hale S, Alker K, et al. The effects of acute and chronic cocaine use on the heart. *Circulation* 1992;85:407–419, with permission of the American Heart Association.)

administration, and it rapidly decreases after the first hour. In one study, the description of chest pain was typical: "pressure, crushing, squeezing, tightness, discomfort, heaviness, and in one case, sharp." Forty-four percent of patients had a history of chest pain (62). There may be a vasospastic component to some of these cases, as suggested by Holter monitoring studies of cocaine use (66). In 1988, at Montefiore Medical Center in Bronx, New York, 35 patients were admitted for chest pain associated with cocaine use. Of these, 11 developed infarction (67). Chest pain after the use of cocaine is not always caused by MI and may indicate the presence of angina or be noncardiac in nature.

In one report, the mean age of patients with acute MI associated with cocaine was 33 years, and 92% of patients were male (67). The most common associated risk factor was cigarette smoking. There does not appear to be any clear-cut dose relationship between the use of cocaine and development of MI. Chronic, occasional, and first-time users may develop infarction. The ECG was abnormal in 90% or more of patients in the emergency department. ECG abnormalities included ST segment elevation, T-wave inversion, and Q waves. Both Q- and non–Q-wave infarcts have been reported after cocaine use. High creatine kinase (CK) levels may be present as a result of trauma or rhabdomyolysis. Therefore, CK–MB elevation is needed to document damage to the myocardium (68). Cocaine users who develop coronary artery disease and MI tend to be older and to have multiple risk factors, such as smoking, compared with users who do not have evidence of coronary disease (69).

Coronary vasospasm has been well documented in only a few cocaine-related infarct patients. Coronary stenosis is present in 29%. Thrombosis is present in approximately one-fourth of the cases. In an analysis of 92 cases in which either coronary angiographic or coronary anatomic data were collected at autopsy (64), 38% of patients had normal coronary anatomy. Of these, 77% had infarcts of the anterior wall.

In a review of the literature (62), 22 of 91 cases of cocaine-induced infarction had some complication: six had congestive heart failure, three had cardiogenic shock, 11 had potentially life-threatening arrhythmias, three had ventricular fibrillation, six had ventricular tachycardia, and two had cardiac arrests. Three deaths occurred. In the series from Montefiore Hospital (67), among 22 patients with cocaine-related acute MI, no in-hospital deaths occurred, and only one episode of heart failure and ventricular tachycardia was seen. A case report of a patient who developed an intraventricular thrombus after cocaine-induced MI was recently described (70).

Management of Cocaine-Induced Myocardial Ischemia and Myocardial Infarction

No controlled, randomized, prospective trials clarify the best way to manage cocaine-induced ischemia or infarction. As stated earlier, not all episodes of chest pain associated with cocaine are necessarily MIs. The incidence of MIs associated with cocaine-induced chest pain was 0% to 31% in retrospective analysis and approximately 6% in prospective analyses (71). In addition, not all cocaine-related chest pain is necessarily ischemic; pleuritic pain has been reported. Chest radiographs should be obtained to rule out pneumothorax and pneumomediastinum, which have both been reported with cocaine use. Initiation of thrombolytic therapy should not be delayed while chest radiographs are awaited, however, unless physical examination strongly suggests conditions other than MI.

Patients who enter the emergency department with pain that suggests ischemia (but do not have evidence of infarc-

tion) after cocaine use should be observed (71–73). One report (71) favors a 12-hour observation period during which ECG and serial CK-MB measurements are obtained to rule out MI. Total creatine phosphokinase level elevation appears to occur in a significant number of cocaine users. This is an unreliable screening test for the detection of myocardial injury (74). Myoglobin level is not reliable in detecting MI secondary to cocaine use, but troponin-1 and CK-MB appear to have a good specificity (75). If possible, previous ECGs should be obtained, because cocaine users not infrequently also have early repolarization variants on their ECG or LV hypertrophy.

Medical therapies for cocaine-related chest pain that is ischemic (anginal) but is not infarction include nitroglycerin, oxygen, aspirin, and benzodiazepines (71–73). Verapamil or other calcium channel blockers and phentolamine may be considered if pain continues (71). If the ECG suggests MI, administration of thrombolytic agents (intravenous or intracoronary) (76) and aspirin should be considered. Some investigators (73) suggest the use of two-dimensional echocardiography to confirm regional wall motion abnormalities before thrombolysis is instituted in patients in whom ST segment elevation is not clearly present. Thrombolytic therapy has, in fact, been used successfully, but no contraindications, such as severe hypertension, intracerebral hemorrhage, or seizures, all of which may occur with cocaine, should be present. A few case reports have raised some safety issues regarding thrombolytic agents in the setting of cocaine. One death has occurred from intracerebral hemorrhage. Thus, primary angioplasty may be another approach. A recent case report described the efficacy of platelet glycoprotein IIb/IIIa inhibitor, given intravenously, with complete resolution of a thrombus in the coronary artery that was temporally related to use of crack cocaine (77). Primary coronary intervention has been tried in cocaine users with success (78). One 36-year-old cocaine user presented to the emergency department with acute MI and ventricular fibrillation. During emergency catheterization, a significant stenosis of the circumflex artery was found, and a coronary stent was successfully deployed. The authors noted that before the stent deployment, intense and frequent coronary spasms were seen.

Because beta-blockers may exacerbate coronary vasospasm in cocaine-induced coronary ischemia secondary to unopposed alpha-receptor stimulation, they should be used with extreme caution, if at all, in the acute setting. The available data are from scattered case reports, and no final conclusion has been drawn (79). At the time of the patient's discharge, however, beta-blockers should be considered part of routine postinfarction therapy. The benefits of beta-blockers may outweigh the potential risk of increasing the vasomotor tone, particularly because the cocaine effect should be gone by the time of discharge. If, however, the patient begins to use cocaine again after discharge, beta-blockers could worsen vasospasm. Labetalol might be a safer choice, but its primary effect is beta-blockade, not alpha-blockade, and therefore even this agent is controversial.

The best therapy for cocaine-induced ventricular arrhythmias remains to be determined. In experimental studies, sodium bicarbonate reverses QRS prolongation caused by cocaine (80). The use of lidocaine is debated, because lidocaine, a sodium channel blocker and local anesthetic, could theoretically worsen the proarrhythmic effect of cocaine. Some studies, however, suggest that lidocaine is safe when it is administered several hours after the use of cocaine.

Obviously, it is crucial that patients stop using cocaine and that they be educated about the dangers of this substance. Concern that cocaine may accelerate atherosclerosis is an additional reason to recommend drug rehabilitation programs.

Our own experience in an inner-city hospital was that acute MI occurring in an otherwise healthy young person may be related to cocaine, and a history of cocaine use and urine testing for cocaine should be considered. Urine testing may detect cocaine or its metabolites as long as 3 weeks after use. Various methods are used, including enzyme-multiplied immunoassay technique, gas chromatography, and mass spectrometry. A skin patch has recently been tested as an easy-to-use screening tool. When a young person has an MI, the physician should remember to ask whether the patient has been using cocaine (81).

Cocaine-Induced Cardiomyopathy and Myocarditis

Cases of transient congestive heart failure have occurred after use of cocaine (82). In some cases, this has involved global hypokinesis, typical of a cardiomyopathy, that may be accompanied by normal coronary angiograms (83,84). Clinically unrecognized reduction in LV function was reported in 7% of chronic cocaine users in one study (85). A case of recurrent dilated cardiomyopathy in a patient who quit and then began reusing cocaine was also reported (86).

In a controlled, randomized study, intracoronary cocaine or saline was administered to 20 patients during cardiac catheterization. Cocaine, but not saline infusion, led to an increase in LV end diastolic pressure and a decrease in LV ejection fraction (87). These findings suggest that cocaine can induce a global toxic effect on myocytes. Autopsy reports have described a mononuclear cell–type myocarditis in chronic cocaine users (88). Lymphocytes and macrophages were observed in the region of myocyte necrosis (eFig. 36.2.2). A second common morphologic finding among chronic cocaine users is the presence of contraction bands. Myocardial contraction-band necrosis occurs with catecholamine excess and calcium overload, as well as after reperfusion of ischemic tissue. In an experimental study involving rabbits, we observed that an acute infusion of cocaine caused foci of contraction-band necrosis in some of the animals (26).

As is true for MI, no controlled studies are available that clarify the best therapy for cocaine-induced cardiomyopathy. Limited data suggest that this condition may be reversible after cessation of cocaine use for 2 to 7 months. Administration of diuretics and angiotensin-converting enzyme inhibitors certainly should be considered.

In addition to dilated cardiomyopathy, LV hypertrophy has been reported with chronic cocaine use. It is presumably caused at least in part by the elevations in blood pressure that occur with cocaine (89).

Cocaine-Induced Hypertension

The hypertension induced by cocaine use is most likely secondary to the drug's sympathomimetic effect (90). Labetalol has been suggested as therapy because it blocks both alpha and beta receptors. This agent is primarily a beta-receptor blocker, however, and therefore unopposed alpha-receptor stimulation could increase both peripheral vascular and coronary vascular resistance. Calcium channel blockers and alpha-blocking agents such as prazosin and phentolamine might be a better choice.

Cocaine-Induced Arrhythmias

Case reports have described a variety of arrhythmias associated with cocaine use, including ventricular tachycardia, ventricular fibrillation and sudden death (2,91), and supraventricular arrhythmias (42). Ventricular arrhythmias may be associated with MI. One case report described a patient who developed ventricular tachycardia and fibrillation after using cocaine but who had no infarct and had normal coronary arteries at catheterization. After defibrillation, the ECG showed ST segment elevation in leads V_1 and V_2, suggesting that the arrhythmia may have been related to transmural ischemia (possibly caused by transient vasospasm). A case report of torsades de pointes in a patient with cocaine-related prolongation of the QT interval was described. On the basis of these and other case reports, six potential types of cocaine-induced arrhythmias in humans are thought to be likely: (a) those associated with structural damage (i.e., cocaine-induced MI or cardiomyopathy); (b) those caused by QT prolongation, the direct effect of cocaine on the myocardium; (c) those resulting from cocaine's sympathomimetic and vagolytic effects; (d) those resulting from cocaine-induced ischemia; (e) those caused by reperfusion after resolution of coronary artery vasospasm; and (f) those resulting from the systemic effects of cocaine, such as hyperthermia, seizures, and acidosis.

On rare occasions, bradyarrhythmias and sinus arrest have been described in cocaine users (92). This could be related to cocaine-induced myocardial ischemia. No controlled studies in humans have determined the best approach to cocaine-induced arrhythmia. In animal studies, sodium bicarbonate has been shown to reverse cocaine's prolongation of the QRS interval. Concerns about the use of beta-blockers have been described. Antiarrhythmic agents, such as lidocaine, procainamide, and quinidine, have the potential to compound cocaine's depressant effects on the conduction system and prolongation of the QT interval. Calcium channel blockers, such as nitrendipine and verapamil, have shown promise in experimental animal studies. If the arrhythmia is thought to be caused by ischemia or infarction, then the antiischemic and antiinfarction agents described earlier should be used to relieve ischemia.

Acceleration of Atherosclerosis Associated with Cocaine Use

Severe atherosclerosis of the coronary arteries has been described in young patients who died from cocaine (53). In one study (52), the average age of patients who developed cocaine-induced thrombus was only 29 years. It is important to remember, when interpreting these studies, that cocaine users tend also to be cigarette smokers, which might contribute to acceleration of atherosclerosis. An increase in adventitial mast cells within the atherosclerotic coronary arteries of cocaine users has been described (52). It was suggested that release of vasoactive substances by the mast cells could explain the acceleration of atherosclerosis in cocaine users (88). Elevation of catecholamine levels can increase low-density lipoprotein (LDL) uptake by the arterial wall. Hence, increases in catecholamine levels in cocaine users might also help explain this acceleration of atherosclerosis. Jones and colleagues (93) observed that cocaine had a direct toxic effect on coronary endothelium, resulting in endothelial denudation. Repetitive episodes of coronary vasospasm might also eventually lead to endothelial damage.

In addition to an acceleration of atherosclerosis, a few cases of intimal hyperplasia have been described as a cause for coronary narrowing (94,95). Another study (96) described thickening of intramural coronary arteries in young men who had ischemic chest pain related to cocaine use and had epicardial coronary arteries of normal appearance.

Miscellaneous Cardiac Conditions Reported with Cocaine Use

Cocaine use has been associated with aortic dissection, presumably because of the associated acute elevation of blood pressure (4), and intravenous cocaine use has been associated with bacterial endocarditis. It has been suggested that left-sided endocarditis is more common than right-sided endocarditis in this setting (4). Cocaine users are also prone to developing paravalvular abscesses.

The best way of avoiding cocaine-induced cardiovascular diseases is total abstinence. Various methods for treatment of cocaine addiction exist, including aversion therapy and narcotherapy. No long-term comparative studies on the usefulness of various programs are available, and the most optimistic success rate at 1 year is approximately 60%. It seems that greater efforts should be directed at preventing substance abuse before it starts, particularly in adolescents and in young adults.

Cocaine has also been shown to have a deleterious effect on other blood vessels, including peripheral (97,98), intestinal (99), and cerebral vessels (100,101). A summary of the effects of cocaine on the heart is shown in Fig. 36.2.

COCAETHYLENE

Cocaethylene is a pharmacologically active cocaine metabolite that has been detected in patients who simultaneously abuse cocaine and ethanol. It has been estimated that 9 to 12 million people in the United States use a combination of cocaine and ethanol (16,17), which accounts for more than 1,000 yearly deaths. The combination may be more toxic than either agent alone. Studies have suggested that their simultaneous use markedly increases the rate of sudden death (102), and that patients dying from the combination had cocaine blood concentrations lower (900 mg per mL) than those in patients dying of cocaine abuse alone (2,800 mg per mL), suggesting a synergistic effect (103). Other studies (104), however, have suggested that blood cocaine concentrations become elevated when oral ethanol is given to people snorting cocaine. Cocaethylene was more potent in killing mice than cocaine alone (105).

The mechanism whereby cocaethylene has such deleterious effects has been the subject of recent research. Combinations of cocaine and alcohol result in greater increases in heart rate, cardiac output, diastolic blood pressure, and myocardial depression than either agent alone (106–108). Although both cocaine and cocaethylene produced direct negative inotropic effects on isolated cardiac myocytes by decreasing the availability of calcium, the negative inotropic effect was more potent with cocaethylene, and this was related to an additional action, reduction of myofilament responsiveness to calcium (30).

Cocaethylene is more potent than cocaine in depressing contraction of myocardial cells in culture (17). In a study comparing cocaine, ethanol, and a combination of both, cocaine alone increased heart rate and blood pressure and, as previously observed, decreased coronary artery diameter (16). In patients receiving both substances, rate-pressure product increased, but coronary diameter increased as well. Therefore, ethanol did not potentiate the vasoconstrictor effect of cocaine; in fact, it appeared to counteract it. This study suggested that the combination of cocaine and alcohol probably does not exacerbate ischemia. However, the doses of cocaine used were low.

Although the exact mechanism whereby the combination of cocaine and ethanol causes increased rates of sudden death in humans remains to be elucidated, it is a deadly combination with which physicians should be familiar.

CAFFEINE AND COFFEE

Few areas in the medical literature are as confusing as the question of whether coffee and caffeine have deleterious effects on the cardiovascular system. Numerous studies describe data that conflict with others, and, in the end, it is difficult to draw conclusions. Recent reviews have described some of the difficulties in the papers published to date on this issue (109,110). Often, animal studies have used doses of caffeine that are "hundreds to thousands of times those achieved by normal human consumption." In addition, tolerance to caffeine is common in humans who regularly drink coffee, and most animal studies do not include conditioning protocols. Coffee and caffeine consumption is often associated with other variables and risk factors for coronary artery disease that are not always taken into account. For example, coffee consumption is more common among people with higher education levels and incomes, more common among white people, and more common among Catholics. It is less common among Mormons and Seventh Day Adventists, for religious reasons. Coffee is more commonly consumed among patients who are depressed and are experiencing anxiety and is commonly used by people who also smoke cigarettes. Most physiological studies in humans and animals test the effects of caffeine and relate this to coffee use. However, coffee may have compounds other than caffeine that can affect the cardiovascular system. Nevertheless, caffeine is an important compound in coffee that has been implicated in cardiovascular events.

Physiology of Caffeine Use

Caffeine is a methylxanthine found in a variety of products, including coffee, tea, chocolate, soft drinks, and many over-the-counter medications. Coffee is the predominant source of caffeine in the Western Hemisphere, and tea is the most common source in the rest of the world. Ninety-nine percent of caffeine from beverages is absorbed by the gastrointestinal tract and peaks in the serum within 30 to 60 minutes of ingestion. Caffeine is metabolized by the liver, and a very small percent is excreted unchanged by the kidneys.

Caffeine's major mechanism of action is to antagonize adenosine receptors. A second, less important action at the usual levels of consumption is phosphodiesterase inhibition. By antagonizing adenosine, caffeine blocks the vasodilatory effect of adenosine and adenosine's inhibitory effects on platelet aggregation, catecholamine levels, and renin release, as well as lipolysis. Thus, acute caffeine administration may increase blood pressure and increase levels of plasma catecholamine, renin (111), and free fatty acid. Tolerance devel-

ops within hours to days of caffeine use, and the effect of caffeine on any individual is highly dependent on the individual and the pattern of consumption.

In general, the effects of caffeine on heart rate and blood pressure in humans are quite variable, and contradicting statements about those effects can be found in the literature. In people who do not regularly drink caffeinated beverages, caffeine may initially increase blood pressure, but the effect is lessened or absent in those who regularly consume caffeine. In one study, a 10 mm Hg increase in blood pressure was seen after consumption of 3 to 5 mg per kg of caffeine. There was an initial *decrease* in heart rate during the first hour after consumption, followed by an *increase* from 2 to 3 hours after consumption (111). Prolonged exposure to caffeine results in tolerance, but chronic drinkers of caffeinated coffee may still exhibit small long-term increases in blood pressure, which seems to be worse among drinkers of boiled rather than filtered coffee (112,113). The increase in both systolic and diastolic blood pressure is more consistent in hypertensive patients, particularly in older men and women (114,115). In one study of 499 hypertensive men, the risk of thromboembolic stroke increased significantly in coffee drinkers (116). However, this finding requires confirmation in larger-scale epidemiologic studies.

Coffee and Coronary Heart Disease

Debate about whether coffee consumption and coronary heart disease are associated continues. Some epidemiologic studies suggest that they are, and that the prevalence of coronary disease increases among coffee drinkers, especially with intake of five or more cups of coffee per day. In a study of 1,130 male medical students older than 25 years, daily consumption of one to two cups of coffee resulted in a relative risk of coronary heart disease of 1.3; more than five cups of coffee daily increased the risk to 2.5 (117). The investigation did not fully control for all risk factors, but it did control for smoking. Other studies also suggested a relationship between increased coffee consumption and coronary events (118). Many studies (usually with a shorter period of follow-up), however, have been entirely negative. In a study of 45,589 men, daily consumption of four or more cups of coffee increased the risk of a cardiovascular event to only 1.04 (119). The study concluded that consumption of caffeinated coffee is in most cases unlikely to be a risk factor for cardiovascular disease.

A recent epidemiologic study suggested that tea drinking may reduce the risk of MI (120). In the Rotterdam study, tea drinking was associated with less atherosclerosis, as determined by radiographic examination of the abdominal aorta (121). This beneficial effect likely is secondary to the flavonoids present in tea and perhaps to other unknown products. Until the controversy regarding the effect of caffeinated coffee on coronary heart disease events is resolved, it might be prudent to limit patients with ischemic heart disease to fewer than four cups of coffee per day (122). Tea drinking, however, appears to be safe and may even be beneficial.

Coffee and Lipid Alterations

There is also ongoing debate about whether coffee increases serum cholesterol levels. Many of the studies that have shown a correlation between coffee consumption and increases in serum cholesterol levels have been performed outside the United States, whereas some of the studies that showed no association were performed in the United States.

It has been suggested that the method of brewing the coffee may be important. In some of the European studies, coffee was prepared by boiling, whereas in the United States, coffee is brewed mainly by filtering. Boiled coffee appears to have a greater adverse effect than filtered coffee on total serum cholesterol, LDL cholesterol, and apoprotein B levels. It has been postulated that the caffeine in coffee plays a minimal role in altering lipid levels, and that a surfactant in coffee (which is removed by filtration) is responsible for the elevation in lipid levels observed in some of the European studies (110,123). Other factors associated with boiled coffee that have been implicated in increasing serum lipids include cafestol and kahweal, two subfractions that can be found within the lipid fraction of coffee.

Studies in the United States did not report any increase in total or LDL cholesterol levels in patients who consumed filtered coffee (124,125). Thus, at least in the United States, the use of filtered coffee does not seem to cause an increase in cholesterol levels, and in European studies in which boiled coffee did seem to have this effect, a component other than caffeine appeared to be the culprit.

Coffee and Homocysteine Levels

Several studies have demonstrated a positive correlation between heavy coffee consumption and elevated homocysteine levels. These studies included drinking of filtered and unfiltered coffee (126–128). In a controlled crossover study, 64 healthy volunteers were randomly assigned to receive 1 L of unfiltered coffee daily for 2 weeks or to ingest a coffee-free diet (129). In the heavy coffee-drinking group, plasma fasting homocysteine levels were elevated by 10%. These studies were short-term studies and did not investigate whether a concomitant increase in cardiovascular events occurred. The results may, however, explain the reported increase in cardiovascular events among people who consume large amounts of coffee, particularly unfiltered coffee, in some studies.

Coffee and Arrhythmias

Although a common belief exists that caffeine can exacerbate arrhythmias, the evidence supporting this in humans is limited. Animal studies have examined this question, but studies demonstrating an association between caffeine and arrhythmia have usually involved doses that were several times higher than those ingested by humans.

One study demonstrated that caffeine had little or no effect on cardiac conduction in humans but might exacerbate underlying susceptibilities to arrhythmias (130). Although earlier studies found an increase in ventricular premature beats on the ECGs of patients who drank nine or more cups of coffee or the equivalent amount of tea (131), more recent studies have been negative.

In a study that examined the effect of caffeine on 50 patients with histories of symptomatic ventricular arrhythmias, continuous ECG recordings at rest and during exercise revealed no increase in ventricular arrhythmias after caffeine consumption, despite an increase in plasma norepinephrine and epinephrine levels (132). During programmed ventricular stimulation, the effect of caffeine varied among the patients. Some patients required an increase, others a decrease, and others no change in the extra stimuli needed to induce arrhythmias during exposure to caffeine (133). Although moderate caffeine ingestion produces a slight prolongation of QRS complexes seen on signal-averaged ECG (134), many studies suggest that moderate ingestion of caffeine does not exacerbate arrhythmias (135–137).

ANABOLIC STEROIDS AND CARDIOVASCULAR DISEASE

It is estimated that approximately 1 million Americans use anabolic steroids (138). Recent case reports suggest that anabolic steroids used primarily among bodybuilders may be associated with MI. Kennedy (139) described a 24-year-old bodybuilder who presented with 3 days of dull chest pain. He had been taking anabolic steroids, including oral stanozolol, intramuscular nandrolone, and intramuscular sustanon. He also had a history of smoking. The patient developed a lateral-wall MI, demonstrated by ECG and enzyme criteria. He was found to be hypertensive, his total serum cholesterol level was observed to be high, and his high-density lipoprotein (HDL) levels were observed to be low.

Acute MI was also reported in a young power lifter who was taking androgenic steroids (140). This patient had hypercholesterolemia, hyperaggregable platelets, and normal appearance of coronary arteries on angiography. Other cases have been documented in which MI, thrombotic occlusion of the coronary artery, and strokes were associated with use of anabolic steroids (140).

In a literature review on the link between anabolic steroids and atherogenic changes, anabolic steroids caused a 52% decrease in HDL levels, a 78% decrease in HDL b levels, and a 36% increase in LDL levels (141). Some studies reported depression of apolipoprotein A-1 and increases in apolipoprotein B. Commonly used anabolic steroids were stanozolol, oxandrolone, testosterone, methandrostenolone, nandrolone decanoate, and oxymetholone—usually in various combinations.

Changes in serum lipid levels after administration of anabolic steroids are rapid, occurring within days to a week. Lipid levels return to baseline approximately 3 to 5 weeks after cessation of anabolic steroid use, according to some reports, whereas other reports suggest that a prolonged residual effect may be seen, with lipid levels abnormal even at 6 months after steroid use has ended.

It has been estimated that the deleterious effects of anabolic steroid use on serum lipid levels might increase the risk of coronary heart disease to three to six times normal (141). The actual incidence of cardiovascular events among anabolic steroid users is probably underreported, however, and is limited to occasional case reports. Moreover, many young patients likely conceal their use of anabolic steroids when questioned. It is important to point out that physiologic doses of testosterone do not seem to adversely affect lipid levels. No effect on HDL levels was seen after administration of such doses in older men, and epidemiologic studies actually suggest a positive correlation between endogenous testosterone and HDL levels (142).

Exogenous steroids can also increase blood pressure (143) and hence cause LV hypertrophy and possibly increase thrombosis. A link between androgen use and thrombus formation is largely derived from experimental animal studies. In experimental thrombosis models, administration of exogenous androgens resulted in development of a larger experimental thrombus and reduced time to blood vessel occlusion (144–147). Use of exogenous androgens has also been reported to enhance platelet aggregation (148).

QT dispersion is increased in athletes who take anabolic steroids (149). QT dispersion reflects the heterogeneity of ventricular repolarization and is known to be associated with increased risk of ventricular arrhythmias. Atrial fibrillation was also reported in young athletes who abuse anabolic steroids (150).

AMPHETAMINES

Amphetamines are stimulants that are noncatecholamine sympathomimetic agents. Use of amphetamine and its derivatives may increase blood pressure and has been associated with lethal arrhythmias and MI (151–156). A 27-year-old man who developed an acute MI and ventricular fibrillation after intravenous amphetamine and was successfully cardioverted was shown to have normal coronary arteries during angiography (152). It was suggested that amphetamines might cause coronary artery vaso-

spasm followed by thrombus formation (157). Cases of cardiomyopathy have also been reported with use of amphetamines (158,159), including smoking of crystal amphetamine, or "ice" (159).

ECSTASY

Ecstasy is 3,4-methylendioxymethyamphetamine, a very popular designer drug that is gaining popularity among young adults. The drug has potent sympathomimetic properties and has been linked to a variety of vascular emergencies. Intracerebral hemorrhage, stroke, hypertension, ventricular arrhythmias, and even death have been described with use of the drug (160–162). The deaths reported after ecstasy use were related to massive cerebral hemorrhage and, less often, ventricular fibrillation.

PHENTERMINE-FENFLURAMINE (PHEN-FEN)

Phentermine is a nonsympathomimetic stimulant that inhibits the clearance of serotonin in the lungs. Fenfluramine is a sympathomimetic amine that promotes the release of serotonin (163). Both drugs in combination were widely used as anorexigenic agents for management of obesity. Shortly after their release, a variety of side effects were reported, including valvular regurgitation, primary pulmonary hypertension, endomyocardial fibrosis, and retroperitoneal hemorrhages.

In 1997, the cases of a group of 24 women who developed valvular heart disease after phentermine-fenfluramine therapy were reported (164). Twenty patients presented with various cardiovascular symptoms, and a new murmur was discovered in four patients during physical examination. The most common valvular abnormalities were mitral regurgitation and aortic regurgitation. The valves showed a glistening appearance on inspection (*e*Fig. 36.2.3). On histopathologic examination, proliferation of fibroblasts and an increase in extracellular matrix were found (*e*Fig. 36.2.4). These patients were young and had no previous histories of heart disease. Surgical intervention was performed in five patients.

Further epidemiologic studies confirmed a relationship between phentermine and fenfluramine and valvular regurgitant lesions, but to a much lesser extent (165–168). The incidence of valvular abnormalities ranges between 6% and 30% among patients who are taking phentermine-fenfluramine, with the most common lesion being aortic regurgitation. The incidence appears to be higher among patients who have undergone longer treatment with the drugs (169) and may regress after the cessation of therapy (170). The United States Department of Health and Human Services recommends that patients exposed to these medications undergo cardiovascular and echocardiographic examination, and that antibiotic prophylaxis be administered when appropriate (171).

A less common but more serious complication of phentermine-fenfluramine therapy is primary pulmonary hypertension (172). This occurs after exposure of at least a few months and has a 3-year survival rate of 50% (173). In one study, histologic examination at autopsy revealed intimal hyperplasia, medical hypertrophy, intimal fibroelastosis, and plexogenic arteriopathy of the pulmonary arteries (174).

Another rare complication of phentermine-fenfluramine therapy is restrictive cardiomyopathy secondary to endomyocardial fibrosis (175). A case report of ruptured retroperitoneal aneurysm had been described (176) and was felt to be secondary to enhanced sympathetic activity.

ALCOHOL

It is estimated that alcohol is consumed by two-thirds of the adult population in the United States, which makes alcohol one of the most widely used addictive drugs. It is also a unique substance in that a small amount may have some benefit on cardiovascular morbidity and mortality rates, but consumption of larger amounts can have devastating effects. The toxic effect of alcohol extends to the brain, liver, skeletal muscle, and many other organs. In this section, we focus on its cardiovascular effects.

Epidemiology

Approximately two-thirds of the adult population in the United States report alcohol consumption, and 10% of these are heavy drinkers. Men drink more than women, but women are more sensitive to the cardiac effects of alcohol. In one study, even though women drank only 60% of the lifetime alcohol dose consumed by men, they had a higher incidence of alcoholic cardiomyopathy (177). Alcohol consumption is also prevalent among adolescents, with rates ranging from 10% to 35% (178). It is more prevalent among young men than young women and among white students than black students; white male adolescents have the highest rate of consumption. Alcohol abuse is present in approximately 15% of the geriatric population. Depression, anxiety, and loneliness are some of the precipitating factors, and patients in that age group are more susceptible to the side effects of alcohol use (179).

Metabolism

Alcohol is absorbed from the stomach and small intestine. It is then distributed to tissues rich in water content and blood flow. Thus, the heart, liver, and brain are prime targets for alcohol's effects (180). In the liver, ethylalcohol is metabolized first to acetaldehyde and then to acetate. Acetate leaves the liver and is metabolized in extrahepatic tissues.

Cardiovascular Effects of Alcohol

Alcoholic Cardiomyopathy

Chronic ingestion of alcohol produces a decrease in both systolic and diastolic function of the myocardium. The condition is clinically indistinguishable from idiopathic dilated cardiomyopathy. Grossly, the myocardium is dilated and flabby, with diffuse areas of fatty degeneration and fibrosis (181). The condition is also histologically similar to idiopathic dilated cardiomyopathy, but the degree of myocyte hypertrophy and the extent of fibrosis are less pronounced (182). Ethanol and its metabolites, acetaldehyde and acetate, exert direct cardiac toxic effects. Although the nutritional deficiencies associated with alcoholism may play some role in alcoholic cardiomyopathy, they probably are not the only source; dietary supplementation fails to prevent the condition.

Initially, loss of the integrity of the sarcolemmal membrane occurs, resulting in loss of its function. This leads to an increase in the concentration of intracellular calcium. Animal studies showed that alcohol administration for 12 weeks led to a threefold increase in intracellular calcium (183). Furthermore, investigators found that administration of verapamil prevents alcohol-induced LV dysfunction (184). Ethanol also affects the sarcoplasmic reticulum, the mitochondria, and contractile protein synthesis and may produce oxygen free radicals (185,186). All of these adversely affect the structure and function of the myocardium.

The symptoms of alcoholic heart disease include dyspnea on exertion, orthopnea, fatigue, and peripheral edema. On examination, signs of right-sided and left-sided heart failure may be present. In addition, signs of chronic alcoholism, such as telangiectasia, spider angioma, and hepatic enlargement are a clue to the diagnosis. Chest radiography shows cardiomegaly and pulmonary congestion. A 12-lead ECG may show LV hypertrophy, nonspecific ST- and T-wave abnormality, and various cardiac arrhythmias.

One clue to the diagnosis of alcoholic myopathy is the presence of skeletal myopathy presenting as muscle weakness. Because the direct toxic effect of alcohol is usually exerted on the striated muscle, the effects are typically present in both heart and skeletal muscle. In a cross-sectional study (187), 24 patients with alcoholic cardiomyopathy were compared to chronic alcohol drinkers with normal heart function and to patients with idiopathic and ischemic cardiomyopathy. Only patients with alcoholic cardiomyopathy had significant skeletal myopathy as determined by muscle biopsy.

Individuals who drink alcohol may have various nutritional deficiencies, among them thiamine deficiency. Thiamine deficiency may lead to beriberi, which may also present with dilated cardiomyopathy. It is, however, distinct from pure alcoholic myopathy in that it is a form of high cardiac output failure (188). The two conditions may coexist.

The most sensitive and clinically useful tool in management and diagnosis of alcoholic cardiomyopathy is echocardiography. This technique usually reveals dilation of all chambers of the heart, and Doppler echocardiography shows valvular regurgitation, particularly of the mitral and tricuspid valves. Alcohol affects both systolic and diastolic function. Studies have shown a decrease in ejection fraction and stroke index (189). Doppler echocardiography is quite sensitive in evaluating diastolic dysfunction, even before the development of clinically evident dysfunction. Thirty-two alcohol users with no clinical evidence of cardiomyopathy were studied by Doppler echocardiography (190). Patients had a prolonged relaxation time, a decrease in peak early diastolic velocity, and a slower acceleration of early diastolic flow. Diastolic dysfunction, as detected by Doppler studies, may precede systolic dysfunction and may be the only manifestation seen in some patients with chronic alcoholism (191).

The hearts of alcoholic cardiomyopathy patients may have an increased uptake of antimyosin antibody, which may decrease after alcohol withdrawal (192). The natural history of alcoholic cardiomyopathy depends largely on the patient's drinking habits. If treatment is started early and the patient stops drinking, it may be partially reversible (193). Well-developed disease, however, is usually fatal if the patient continues to consume alcohol.

Treatment of alcoholic cardiomyopathy usually follows several paths. Treatment of the manifestation of congestive heart failure with angiotensin-converting enzyme inhibitors and diuretics is helpful. Nutritional deficiency, such as thiamine deficiency, and various electrolyte abnormalities, such as hypophosphatemia (194), hypomagnesemia, and hypokalemia, should be corrected. The mainstay of therapy is cessation of alcohol use. The earlier abstinence occurs in the course of the disease, the more pronounced is the benefit. In a group of patients with pure alcoholic cardiomyopathy (195), patients who abstained had a marked improvement in their ejection fraction, as measured by radionuclide angiography, and in their cardiothoracic ratio, as seen by chest radiography. Most of the improvement occurred in the first 6 months of abstinence, but improvement continued through up to 2 years of observation. Patients who did not abstain showed no improvement. In alcoholic cardiomyopathy, the benefit of abstinence from alcohol exceeds the benefits of medical therapy alone (196). The prognosis of alcoholic myopathy is similar to that of idiopathic dilated myopathy (197).

Hypertension

A link between alcohol use and high blood pressure has long been suspected (198). Social drinking is associated with a mild rise in systolic pressure, whereas those who drink heavily may have a substantial rise (199,200). Several mech-anisms have been proposed. However, the exact mechanism is not clear. This may, at least in part, explain the increase in LV mass. However, even alcoholic individuals who are normotensive may have an increase in LV mass (201). Blood pressure may normalize after a short period of abstinence.

Cardiac Arrhythmias

Alcohol use is associated with a variety of atrial and ventricular arrhythmias, regardless of whether the patient has overt alcoholic heart disease. Possible mechanisms include electrolyte imbalance, the hypercatecholamine states often seen during alcohol withdrawal, and a patchy delay in conduction that results in increased reentry (202). The QT-interval prolongation seen in alcoholic patients may be implicated in the genesis of ventricular arrhythmias (203). Atrial arrhythmias include premature atrial contractions, supraventricular tachycardia, and atrial flutter and fibrillation. Ventricular arrhythmias include premature ventricular depolarization and ventricular tachycardia or fibrillation. The most common arrhythmia, however, appears to be atrial fibrillation.

In a study of 32 episodes of cardiac arrhythmias in 24 patients who used alcohol, patients reported consuming alcohol every day for an extended period of time, yet had a marked increase in alcohol consumption on weekends or near holidays. No overt signs of alcoholic heart disease were seen. The most common arrhythmia noted was atrial fibrillation. The majority of episodes was seen in the hospital at the beginning of the week or after holidays; hence the term "holiday heart" (204).

In patients with new onset of atrial fibrillation, alcohol was responsible for 35% of the cases and up to two-thirds of the cases in patients younger than 65 years (205). It was also found to be an independent risk factor for recurrence of atrial fibrillation (206). Electrophysiologic testing in humans showed that alcohol enhances the vulnerability of normal hearts to induction of atrial flutter and fibrillation (207). The treatment is cessation of alcohol consumption; most rhythm disturbances disappear with little or no intervention.

Sudden Death

Heavy alcohol drinking is associated with an increase in sudden death. In one study, the increased incidence of sudden death was reported regardless of whether patients had coronary artery disease (208). The increase was also more pronounced in older age groups, regardless of social class. For nonsudden death, alcohol drinking had a biphasic effect, depending on the amount of alcohol consumed. Heavy drinkers were at a greater risk for death from noncardiovascular causes, particularly cirrhosis, accidents, and tobacco-related cancer. This increased risk was higher among women and among younger persons (209). Lighter drinkers, however, were at a lower risk for death from cardiovascular diseases, particularly coronary artery disease. In a prospective 13-year follow-up of 12,321 male British doctors, the consumption of one or two drinks each day was associated with a significantly lower mortality rate than that seen among heavy drinkers or nondrinkers (210). The mechanism of this benefit was not apparent in that study, yet it was postulated that a beneficial effect on coronary artery disease might be responsible.

Coronary Artery Disease

Heavy alcohol drinking is associated with an increased incidence of coronary artery disease and cardiovascular death. This is not surprising—such patients have an increased tendency for hypertension with increased cardiac muscle mass and hypertriglyceridemia, and they also tend to be smokers. Alcohol use is paradoxical; mild to moderate alcohol intake is associated with a decreased risk of MI and cardiovascular death. Various mechanisms contribute to that result, including the effect of alcohol consumption on HDL.

Investigators examined the relationship between alcohol ingestion and MI among 340 patients with MI, compared with an age- and sex-matched control group (211). Alcohol intake was inversely related to the risk of MI. Furthermore, a substantial component of that benefit resulted from an increase in HDL and its subfractions. It also appeared that this benefit derived from the alcohol itself and was not specific to any particular alcoholic drink (212). Most of this benefit is achieved by consumption of as little as half a drink per day (213,214). Other mechanisms that may play a role in this effect on coronary artery disease are the effects of alcohol on endogenous tissue–type plasminogen activator and on platelet function. In a study of 631 healthy male doctors, moderate drinking increased plasma levels of endogenous tissue plasminogen activator antigen (215). In addition, alcohol consumption resulted in the inhibition of platelet aggregation and prolongation of blocking time (216). These effects likely decrease the occurrence of coronary thrombosis in moderate alcohol drinkers.

What advice should physicians give their patients with regard to alcohol consumption? We must remember that alcohol is an addictive drug, and it may be difficult for some people to control their drinking. Heavy drinking increases overall mortality rates (217). Other risk factor modifications should be the priority in patients who have coronary artery disease. Mild alcohol drinking may, however, have a role in the subgroup of patients who have low HDL levels as the sole risk factor for coronary artery disease and in whom other measures to improve HDL levels have failed.

Alcohol Withdrawal

Alcohol withdrawal is usually managed in a quiet, supportive environment. The importance of close supervision cannot be understated. Benzodiazepines are the mainstay of therapy. Two cardiovascular effects commonly occur during alcohol withdrawal: significant hypertension and cardiac arrhythmias. They are likely related to the activation of the autonomic nervous system and usually subside spontaneously but may require a temporary pharmacologic intervention. In patients who have acute ischemic syndromes and are also experiencing alcohol withdrawal, control of blood pressure and heart rate is crucial. Liberal use of beta-blockers and intravenous nitroglycerin is recommended.

Prevention of Alcohol Addiction

Attempts to cure alcohol addiction are not always successful and often begin after many years of drinking, when significant health problems have already developed. Thus, efforts toward prevention of drinking should be the goal. Various programs are already in place that have had some success (218).

TOBACCO

A cigarette is a controlled device that delivers nicotine and many other substances to the human body. With each puff, approximately 100 μg of nicotine is absorbed through the lungs, with an average drug delivery of 1 to 2 mg of nicotine per cigarette. With the widespread use of smoking and its significant effects on the cardiovascular system, cigarette smoking has a major impact on public health.

Epidemiology

The number of tobacco smokers in the world exceeds 1.1 billion. Approximately 300 million smokers live in developed countries, and more than 800 million smokers live in developing countries. Globally, smoking is responsible for 3 million deaths per year, and this number is expected to reach 10 million per year in the year 2020, if current trends continue. It is estimated that 50 million Americans smoke on a regular basis. Although the overall number of adult smokers has decreased in the United States, smoking among teenage girls is on the rise. The prevalence of smoking among the African-American and Hispanic populations has surpassed that in the white population, but white smokers smoke more cigarettes per day, seem to be more addicted to smoking, and report more smoking-related illnesses than African-American and Hispanic smokers (219). Although some decline has been seen in the overall incidence of cigarette smoking in the United States, cigar smoking is on the rise, and smoking in general is not showing any significant decline in developing countries.

Tobacco Addiction

Drug addiction or dependency is described as "a behavioral pattern in which the use of a given psychoactive drug is given a sharply higher priority over other behaviors which once had a significantly higher value" (220). In other words, addiction is defined as loss of control over use of the drug and an inability to quit despite obvious risks associated with drug use. In the case of cigarette smoking, the drug is nicotine. Smokers report pleasure, relaxation, reduction of anxiety and stress, and improved attention after cigarette smoking (221). Within seconds of smoking a cigarette, nicotine is absorbed through the lung alveoli and taken up by the bloodstream to the brain and other tissues. In the brain, it acts at the nicotinic receptors, which are known to be increased in the brain tissues of smokers. As a result, dopamine, norepinephrine, acetylcholine, and endorphins are released. This results in the reported feelings of decreased anxiety and tension, pleasure and relaxation, and increased performance. Cigarette smoking may also be associated with a decrease in the enzyme monoamine oxidase, which is responsible for the breakdown of dopamine, in the brain (222). Thus, cigarette smoking not only increases the secretion of dopamine, but it also slows its metabolism.

With each cigarette smoked, tolerance to the effects of nicotine develops. But with abstinence at night, the effects are renewed, so that the first cigarette of the day produces the maximal psychological effect. When smoking ceases, symptoms of restlessness, irritability, impatience, and increased anxiety occur. Most symptoms gradually disappear in 1 to 2 weeks, but the desire to smoke may persist for a very long time.

Despite a recent controversy regarding whether cigarettes should be considered addictive, the balance of the arguments strongly suggests that they are (223). It has also been suggested that an individual's genetic composition may influence smoking behavior (224).

Cardiovascular Effects

The main components of cigarettes that exert cardiovascular effects are nicotine and carbon monoxide. The former may lead to the release of norepinephrine, which increases pulse rate, blood pressure, and platelet aggregability. It may also cause endothelial injury and adversely affect events that occur during atherosclerotic plaque rupture (225). Carbon monoxide displaces the oxygen from hemoglobin, interfering with oxygen delivery to cardiac tissue. Cigarette smoking has also been associated with hyperfibrinogenemia and low levels of HDL (226). These mechanisms lead to the devastating effects of smoking, regardless of the method used.

In a major epidemiologic study, 10,914 subjects were followed to assess the progression of atherosclerotic disease (227). Carotid ultrasounds were performed on the subjects, and the intimal medial thickness was measured at baseline and at 3 years of follow-up. Current smokers had a 50% increase in the rate of progression of atherosclerosis com-

pared to nonsmokers. Past smokers had a 25% increase in atherosclerosis. Even passive smokers who had never smoked had more progression than control subjects. The increase in the rate of atherosclerosis progression associated with smoking was more marked in diabetic and hypertensive patients.

Smoking results in an increase in heart rate and blood pressure. In a study of 135 healthy subjects, 24-hour ambulatory blood pressure monitoring revealed an increase in both heart rate and blood pressure (228). In addition to an increased cardiovascular risk profile, this increase in myocardial oxygen demand may increase, at least theoretically, anginal episodes in patients who already have coronary artery disease.

Active Smoking

Although cigarette smoking had long been suspected to increase the risk of cardiovascular diseases, the two were formally linked in 1958 (229). Subsequently, pathologic studies showed more-advanced coronary artery disease among heavy smokers than among light smokers (230). Smoking is associated with a two- to fourfold increase in coronary artery disease and an increased risk of MI and sudden death (231). Furthermore, if patients with MI continue to smoke, the rate of reinfarction and death also increases. The risk appears to be related to the duration of smoking and the number of cigarettes smoked per day. Smoking also has a synergistic effect with other coronary risk factors, particularly hypercholesterolemia.

Passive Smoking

Passive smoking is the involuntary inhalation of air contaminated by cigarette smoke. It affects both smokers and nonsmokers. Smokers have an increased risk of developing various cardiovascular effects, whereas nonsmokers may have an increased incidence of MI with chronic exposure and impaired cardiac performance with acute exposure. Investigators exposed patients who survived a first heart attack to passive smoking during an exercise stress test. During passive-smoking exposure, exercise tolerance decreased, time to recovery to baseline heart rate was prolonged, and the occurrence of cardiac arrhythmias increased (232).

Passive environmental smoking results in a 25% increase in the risk of coronary artery disease (233) and death (234) and is now estimated to be the third leading preventable cause of death after active smoking and alcohol abuse (235). Controlled studies showed that passive smoking impairs endothelial-dependent coronary vasodilation (236), and this is only partially reversible after exposure has ended (237). Passive smoking also leads to accelerated lipid peroxidation and accumulation of LDL cholesterol in human macrophages (238). These effects contribute to accelerated atherosclerosis (227) and subsequently to increased mortality rates (235). Educating smokers about the risk of passive smoking appears to be more important than ever in the face of these data.

Cigar and Pipe Smoking

Although cigarette smoking overall is on the decline in the United States, cigar smoking is rising. Regular cigar smokers who inhale smoke or are heavy smokers have an increased risk of coronary artery disease (239). One prospective study, however, suggested that the cardiovascular risk associated with cigars is less than that associated with cigarettes (240).

Smokeless Tobacco

Smokeless tobacco refers to tobacco snuff, chewing tobacco, and the recently introduced smokeless cigarette. Smokeless tobacco delivers an average amount of nicotine similar to smoking and may produce similar cardiovascular effects. In addition, chewing tobacco leads to a variety of cancerous and precancerous conditions, commonly oral leukoplakia (241). An epidemiologic study from Sweden, however, failed to show an increased risk of MI in people who use tobacco snuff (242).

Smoking Cessation

Smoking cessation includes three phases (243): preparation, intervention, and maintenance. The preparation phase primarily includes motivation of the patient. The intervention phase involves initiation of a specific method of smoking cessation, which ordinarily includes the daily use of nicotine gum or a patch and a gradual decrease in the dose of nicotine delivered. Other methods used alone or in combination are behavioral therapy, acupuncture, and hypnosis. The maintenance phase ensures that the patient continues to not smoke and includes stress reduction as an integral part of management, because the urge to return to smoking is accentuated by stressful conditions.

Nicotine patches are probably the most commonly used method of smoking cessation. Nicotine patches are safe, particularly because they deliver less nicotine in a slow, steady state, as opposed to the pulsatile nature of cigarette delivery. Investigators compared the effects of cigarette smoking, nicotine patches, and placebo patches on platelet aggregation in a crossover design (244). Smoking was associated with an increase in platelet activation, but nicotine patches were not. Use of nicotine patches should be limited to patients who have stable cardiovascular disease and avoided in patients who have unstable ischemic syndromes, because cases of MI during the use of such patches have been reported (245,246). The antidepressant drug bupropion is also effective in smoking

cessation and may even be more effective than nicotine-containing products (247).

Smoking Prevention

Despite the widespread availability of high-quality programs for smoking cessation, the rate of success is lower than desired. This low rate may result in part from the strongly addictive nature of tobacco use and the ease of obtaining cigarettes. Smoking prevention appears to be the best way to decrease the number of smokers and the incidence and prevalence of smoking-related illness (248). Every day, approximately 3,000 young people start smoking (249); individuals who do not smoke their first cigarettes as teenagers are less likely to start smoking as adults (250). School-based programs need to be initiated at an early phase in a child's education (251) to have an impact on the number of adult smokers.

CONTROVERSIES AND PERSONAL PERSPECTIVES

A few controversies still persist regarding substance abuse and the heart. Some of the controversy regarding how an acute dose of cocaine affects the heart depends on the model being studied. When cocaine is administered to awake, conscious animals and humans, the sympathomimetic effects predominate, with increases in heart rate and blood pressure. When the drug is administered to pentobarbital-anesthetized animals, the sympathomimetic effects appear to be masked and the cardiodepressive effects predominate. This has caused some confusion in the literature regarding the acute effects of cocaine on the heart. Some debate exists as to whether cocaine actually accelerates atherosclerosis, because many of the clinical reports suggesting such an effect involved patients who also have other risk factors, especially tobacco smoking. No general agreement exists regarding the best way to treat acute cocaine cardiotoxicity, and virtually no controlled studies have addressed this issue. The use of beta-blockers remains controversial. Although they decrease the heart rate and blood pressure, they block the beta receptors, leaving the alpha receptors unopposed, with the potential to worsen coronary artery vasospasm.

My personal observation (R.A.K.), in a large inner-city county hospital, is that cocaine cardiotoxicity is probably more common than we realize, especially in that type of environment. When a younger person presents with an acute MI, especially if other risk factors are not present, it is very important to remember to ask about a history of substance abuse, especially cocaine. Initially, patients may be reluctant to divulge this information. However, eventually, with compassionate persistence, the story often emerges. Patients then need to be educated about the hazards of sub-

THE FUTURE

The association between substance abuse and heart disease is one that has received increased attention, largely as a result of publicity surrounding the deaths of athletes and stars who have used drugs such as cocaine. Given the prevalence of drug abuse in this country, it is a topic that likely will remain important over the next decade. Its importance may vary, depending on which drugs are most used at a given point in time.

stance abuse. Most will not be aware that cocaine can affect the heart.

It is likely that the controversy regarding whether coffee and caffeine are deleterious to the cardiovascular system will continue for some time. Until the controversy is resolved, coffee should be consumed in moderation, especially by individuals with a history of coronary artery disease.

SUMMARY

Substance abuse remains an ongoing public health problem in the United States. Several common agents of abuse contribute to heart disease. The types and frequency of heart disease related to substance abuse probably vary depending on the prevalence and frequency of the type of drug being used. An acute dose of cocaine can have several adverse effects on the heart, including cardiodepressor effects, reductions in contractility and coronary artery blood flow, and conduction abnormalities, which are probably related to its local anesthetic properties. At the same time, cocaine has cardiostimulatory effects, increasing heart rate, blood pressure, contractility, ventricular excitability, and coronary vasoconstriction, related to its sympathomimetic and vagolytic effects. Cocaine has the potential for exacerbating ischemia in patients by increasing heart rate and blood pressure at the same time that it causes coronary vasoconstriction. The following common cardiovascular diseases have been associated with cocaine abuse in patients: acute MI and myocardial ischemia, dilated and hypertrophic cardiomyopathy, myocarditis, hypertension, arrhythmias, and possibly acceleration of atherosclerosis. Aortic dissection has been reported (286).

Controversy regarding the safety of caffeine and coffee use among coronary artery disease patients is ongoing. The consumption of filtered coffee does not cause an increase in cholesterol levels, whereas boiled coffee may negatively affect lipid levels. Moderate consumption of coffee probably is safe for most patients who have coronary artery disease. Anabolic steroid abuse has been associated with acute MI and lipid abnormalities. There are case reports of MI and cardiomyopathy after use of amphetamines. Small amounts of alcohol may have some benefit on cardiovascular morbidity and mortality rates, but excess use is associated with alcoholic cardiomyopathy, hypertension, arrhythmias, and sudden death.

Tobacco use is a risk factor for coronary artery disease. Both active smoking and exposure to passive smoke increase the risk of coronary artery disease events. Substance abuse associated with injection of intravenous material results in a risk of IE.

The best approach to long-term therapy for heart disease related to substance abuse is to avoid the deleterious substances. Rehabilitation programs play an important role in this regard. Specific therapies for cardiotoxicity in general are lacking. Anecdotal reports regarding therapy for acute ischemic cocaine cardiotoxicity favor nitrates, oxygen, aspirin, benzodiazepines, alpha-blockers, and possibly calcium channel blockers. If acute MI is present, use of thrombolytic agents and aspirin may be considered, unless contraindications such as severe hypertension, intracerebral hemorrhage, or seizures are present. Future studies are necessary to help clarify the best therapy for cocaine cardiotoxicity.

Primary prevention of substance abuse is clearly the most important goal for our society—although a formidable one, it is worth striving for. The cardiotoxicity of substance abuse is generally serious and potentially life-threatening, and treatment is far less optimal than preventing the behavior that causes disease in the first place.

ACKNOWLEDGMENT

We thank Alice Stargardt for a superb job and outstanding editorial assistance in preparing this chapter.

REFERENCES

1. Isner JM, Chokshi SK. Cardiac complications of cocaine abuse. *Annu Rev Med* 1991;42:33–38.
2. Kloner RA, Hale S, Alker K, et al. The effects of acute and chronic cocaine use on the heart. *Circulation* 1992;85:407–419.
3. Lange RA, Willard JE. The cardiovascular effects of cocaine. *Heart Dis Stroke* 1993;2:136–141.
4. Om A. Cardiovascular complications of cocaine. *Am J Med Sci* 1992;303:333–339.

5. Bunn WH, Giannini AJ. Cardiovascular complications of cocaine abuse. *Am Fam Physician* 1992;46:769–773.

6. Das G. Cardiovascular effects of cocaine abuse. *Int J Clin Pharmacol Ther Tox* 1993;31:521–528.

7. Perper JA, Van Thiel DH. Cardiovascular complications of cocaine abuse. *Recent Dev Alcohol* 1992;10:343–359.

8. Chakko S, Myerburg RJ. Cardiac complications of cocaine abuse. *Clin Cardiol* 1995;18:67–72.

9. Cregler LL. Cocaine: the newest risk factor for cardiovascular disease. *Clin Cardiol* 1991;14:449–456.

10. Billman GE. Cocaine: a review of its toxic actions on cardiac function. *Crit Rev Toxicol* 1995;25:113–132.

11. Rezkalla SH, Hale S, Kloner RA. Cocaine-induced heart disease. *Am Heart J* 1990;120:1403–1408.

12. Lewin L. *Phantastica, narcotics and stimulating drugs: their use and abuse.* New York: EP Dutton, 1931:79.

13. Isner JM, Estes NA 3d, Thompson PD, et al. Acute cardiac events temporary related to cocaine abuse. *N Engl J Med* 1986;315:1438–1443.

14. Warner EA. Cocaine abuse. *Ann Intern Med* 1993;119:226–235.

15. Warner EA. Is your patient using cocaine? Clinical signs that should raise suspicion. *Postgrad Med* 1995;98:173–180.

16. Pirwitz MJ, Willard JE, Landau C, et al. Influence of cocaine, ethanol, or their combination on epicardial coronary arterial dimensions in humans. *Arch Intern Med* 1995;155:1186–1191.

17. Welder AA, Grammas P, Melchert RB. Cellular mechanisms of cocaine cardiotoxicity. *Toxicol Lett* 1993;69:227–238.

18. Bauman JL, Grawe JJ, Winecoff AP, et al. Cocaine-related sudden cardiac death: a hypothesis correlating basic science and clinical observations. *J Clin Pharmacol* 1994;34:902–911.

19. Newlin DB. Effect of cocaine on vagal tone: a common factors approach. *Drug Alcohol Depend* 1995;37:211–216.

20. Kloner RA, Hale S. Unraveling the complex effects of cocaine on the heart. *Circulation* 1993;87:1046–1047.

21. Hale SL, Alker KJ, Rezkalla S, et al. Adverse effects of cocaine on cardiovascular dynamics, myocardial blood flow, and coronary artery diameter in an experimental model. *Am Heart J* 1989;118:927–933.

22. Stambler BS, Komamura K, Ihara T, et al. Acute intravenous cocaine causes transient depression followed by enhanced left ventricular function in conscious dogs. *Circulation* 1993;87:1687–1697.

23. Garfinkel A, Raetz SL, Harper RM. Heart rate dynamics after cocaine administration. *J Cardiovasc Pharmacol* 1992;19:453–459.

24. Hale SL, Alker KJ, Rezkalla SH, et al. Nifedipine protects the heart from the acute deleterious effects of cocaine if administered before but not after cocaine. *Circulation* 1991;83:1437–1443.

25. Abel FL, Wilson SP, Zhao RR, et al. Cocaine depresses the canine myocardium. *Circ Shock* 1989;28:309–319.

26. Gardin JM, Wong N, Alker K, et al. Acute cocaine administration induces ventricular regional wall motion and ultrastructural abnormalities in an anesthetized rabbit model. *Am Heart J* 1994;128:1117–1129.

27. Pagel PS, Power MW, Kenny D, et al. Cocaine depresses myocardial contractility and prolongs isovolumetric relaxation in conscious dogs with partial autonomic nervous system blockade. *J Cardiovasc Pharmacol* 1992;20:25–34.

28. Morcos NC, Fairhurst A, Henry WL. Direct myocardial effects of cocaine. *Cardiovasc Res* 1993;27:269–273.

29. Simkhovich BZ, Kloner RA, Alker KJ, et al. Time course of direct cardiotoxic effects of high cocaine concentration in isolated rabbit heart. *J Cardiovasc Pharmacol* 1994;23:509–516.

30. Qiu Z, Morgan JP. Differential effects of cocaine and cocaethylene on intracellular Ca^{2+} and myocardial contraction in cardiac myocytes. *Br J Pharmacol* 1993;109:293–298.

31. Fraker TD Jr, Temesy-Armos PN, Brewster PS, et al. Mechanism of cocaine-induced myocardial depression in dogs. *Circulation* 1990;81:1012–1016.

32. Vitullo JC, Karam R, Mekhail N, et al. Cocaine-induced small vessel spasm in isolated rat hearts. *Am J Pathol* 1989;135:85–91.

33. Perreault CL, Hague NL, Ransil BJ, et al. The effects of cocaine on intracellular CA^{2+} handling and myofilament Ca^{2+} responsiveness of ferret ventricular myocardium. *Br J Pharmacol* 1990;101:679–685.

34. Tomita F, Bassett AL, Myerburg RJ, et al. Effects of cocaine on sarcoplasmic reticulum in skinned rat heart muscle. *Am J Physiol* 1993;264:H845–H850.

35. Stambler BS, Morgan JP, Mietus J, et al. Cocaine alters heart rate dynamics in conscious ferrets. *Yale J Biol Med* 1991;64:143–153.

36. Hale SL, Lehmann MH, Kloner RA. Electrocardiographic abnormalities after acute administration of cocaine in the rat. *Am J Cardiol* 1989;63:1529–1530.

37. Przywara DA, Dambach GE. The direct actions of cocaine on cardiac cellular activity. *Circulation* 1988;78[Suppl II]:II-47(abst).

38. Billman GE, Lappi MD. The effects of cocaine on cardiac vagal tone before and during coronary artery occlusion: cocaine exacerbates the autonomic response to myocardial ischemia. *J Cardiovasc Pharmacol* 1993;22:869–876.

39. Kabas JS, Blanchard SM, Matsuyama Y, et al. Cocaine-mediated impairment of cardiac conduction in the dog: a potential mechanism for sudden death after cocaine. *J Pharmacol Exp Ther* 1990;252:185–191.

40. Schwartz AB, Janzen D, Jones RT, et al. Electrocardiographic and hemodynamic effects of intravenous cocaine in awake and anesthetized dogs. *J Electrocardiol* 1989;22:159–166.

41. Temesy-Armos PN, Fraker TD Jr, Brewster PS, et al. The effects of cocaine on cardiac electrophysiology in conscious, unsedated dogs. *J Cardiovasc Pharmacol* 1992;19:883–891.

42. Nanji AA, Filipenko JD. Asystole and ventricular fibrillation associated with cocaine intoxication. *Chest* 1984;85:132–133.

43. Watt TB, Pruitt RD. Cocaine-induced incomplete bundle branch block in dogs. *Circ Res* 1964;15:234–239.

44. Weidmann S. Effect of calcium ions and local anaesthetics on electrical properties of Purkinje fibres. *J Physiol (Lond)* 1955;129:568–582.

45. Grossie J. Ca-dependent action of cocaine on K current in freshly dissociated dorsal root ganglia from rats. *Am J Physiol* 1993;265[3 Pt 1]:C674–C679.

46. Togna G, Tempesta E, Togna AR, et al. Platelet responsiveness and biosynthesis of thromboxane and prostacyclin in

response to *in vitro* cocaine treatment. *Haemostasis* 1985;15:100–107.

47. Rezkalla SH, Mazza JJ, Kloner RA, et al. Effects of cocaine on human platelets in healthy subjects. A*m J Cardiol* 1993;72:243–246.

48. Heesch CM, Wilhelm CR, Ristich J, et al. Cocaine activates platelets and increases the formation of circulating platelet containing microaggregates in humans. *Heart* 2000;83:688–695.

49. Trulson ME, Epps LR, Joe JC. Cocaine: long-term administration depletes cardiac cellular enzymes in the rat. *Acta Anat* 1987;129:165–168.

50. Maillet M, Chiarasini D, Nahas G. Myocardial damage induced by cocaine administration of a week's duration in the rat. *Adv Biosci* 1991;80:187–197.

51. Kolodgie FD, Virmani R, Rice HE, et al. Intravenous cocaine accelerates atherosclerosis in cholesterol-fed New Zealand white rabbits. *J Am Coll Cardiol* 1990;15:217A(abst).

52. Kolodgie FD, Virmani R, Cornhill JF, et al. Increase in atherosclerosis and adventitial mast cells in cocaine abusers: an alternative mechanism of cocaine-associated coronary vasospasm and thrombosis. *J Am Coll Cardiol* 1991;17:1553–1560.

53. Dressler FA, Malekzadeh S, Roberts WC. Quantitative analysis of amounts of coronary arterial narrowing in cocaine addicts. *Am J Cardiol* 1990;65:303–308.

54. Fischman MW, Schuster CR, Resnekov L, et al. Cardiovascular and subjective effects of intravenous cocaine administration in humans. *Arch Gen Psychiatry* 1976;33:983–989.

55. Lange RA, Cigarroa RG, Yancy CW, et al. Cocaine-induced coronary-artery vasoconstriction. *N Engl J Med* 1989;321:1557–1562.

56. Lange RA, Cigarroa RG, Flores ED, et al. Potentiation of cocaine-induced coronary vasoconstriction by beta adrenergic blockade. *Ann Intern Med* 1990;112:897–903.

57. Flores ED, Lange RA, Cigarro RG, et al. Effect of cocaine on coronary artery dimensions in atherosclerotic coronary artery disease: enhanced vasoconstriction at sites of significant stenoses. *J Am Coll Cardiol* 1990;16:74–79.

58. Brogan WC 3d, Lange RA, Kim AS, et al. Alleviation of cocaine-induced coronary vasoconstriction by nitroglycerin. *J Am Coll Cardiol* 1991;18:581–586.

59. Brogan WC 3d, Lange RA, Glamann DB, et al. Recurrent coronary vasoconstriction caused by intranasal cocaine: possible role for metabolites. *Ann Intern Med* 1992;116:556–561.

60. Orr D, Jones I. Anaesthesia for laryngoscopy. *Anaesthesia* 1968;23:194–202.

61. Richards IS, Kulkarni AP, Bremner WF. Cocaine-induced arrhythmia in human foetal myocardium *in vitro*: possible mechanism for foetal death *in utero*. *Pharmacol Toxicol* 1990;66:150–154.

62. Hollander JE, Hoffman RS. Cocaine-induced myocardial infarction: an analysis and review of the literature. *J Emerg Med* 1992;10:169–177.

63. Virmani R, Robinowitz M, Smialek JE, et al. Cardiovascular effects of cocaine: an autopsy study of 40 patients. *Am Heart J* 1988;115:1068–1075.

64. Minor RL, Brook BD, Brown DD, et al. Cocaine-induced myocardial infarction in patients with normal coronary arteries. *Ann Intern Med* 1991;115:797–806.

65. Mittleman MA, Mintzer D, Maclure M, et al. Triggering of myocardial infarction by cocaine. *Circulation* 1999;99:2737–2741.

66. Nademanee K, Gorelick DA, Josephson MA, et al. Myocardial ischemia during cocaine withdrawal. *Ann Intern Med* 1989;111:876–880.

67. Amin M, Gabelman G, Buttrick P. Cocaine-induced myocardial infarction: a growing threat to men in their 30s. *Postgrad Med* 1991;90:50–55.

68. Rubin RB, Neugarten J. Cocaine-induced rhabdomyolysis masquerading as myocardial ischemia. *Am J Med* 1989;86:551–553.

69. Hollander JE, Shih RD, Hoffman RS, et al. Predictors of coronary artery disease in patients with cocaine-associated myocardial infarction. *Am J Med* 1997;102:158–163.

70. Lee H, Eisenberg M, Drew D, et al. Intraventricular thrombus after cocaine-induced myocardial infarction. *Am Heart J* 1995;129:403–405.

71. Hollander JE. The management of cocaine-associated myocardial ischemia. *N Engl J Med* 1995;333:1267–1272.

72. Om A, Ellahham S, DiSciascio G. Management of cocaine-induced cardiovascular complications. *Am Heart J* 1993;125:469–475.

73. Olshaker JS. Cocaine chest pain. *Emerg Clin North Am* 1994;12:391–396.

74. Counselman FL, McLaughlin EW, Kardon EM, et al. Creatine phosphokinase elevation in patients presenting to the emergency department with cocaine-related complaints. *Am J Emerg Med* 1997;15:221–223.

75. Hollander JE, Levitt MA, Young GP, et al. Effect of recent cocaine use on the specificity of cardiac markers for diagnosis of acute myocardial infarction. *Am Heart J* 1998;135:245–252.

76. Yao S-S, Spindola-Franco H, Menegus M, et al. Successful intracoronary thrombolysis in cocaine-associated acute myocardial infarction. *Cathet Cardiovasc Diagn* 1997;42:294–297.

77. Frangogiannis NG, Farmer JA, Lakkis NM. Tirofiban for cocaine-induced coronary artery thrombosis: a novel therapeutic approach. *Circulation* 1999;100:1939.

78. Shah DM, Dy TC, Szto GY, et al. Percutaneous transluminal coronary angioplasty and stenting for cocaine-induced acute myocardial infarction: a case report and review. *Cathet Cardiovasc Intervent* 2000;49:447–451.

79. Leikin JB. Cocaine and β-adrenergic blockers: a remarriage after a decade-long divorce? *Crit Care Med* 1999;27:688–689.

80. Wang RY. pH-dependent cocaine-induced cardiotoxicity. *Am J Emerg Med* 1999;17:364–369.

81. Hollander JE, Brooks DE, Valentine SM. Assessment of cocaine use in patients with chest pain syndromes. *Arch Intern Med* 1998;158:62–66.

82. Chokshi SK, Moore R, Pandian NG, et al. Reversible cardiomyopathy associated with cocaine intoxication. *Ann Intern Med* 1989;111:1039–1040.

83. Weiner RS, Lockhart JT, Schwartz RG. Dilated cardiomyopathy and cocaine abuse: report of two cases. *Am J Med* 1986;81:699–701.

84. Hogya PT, Wolfson AB. Chronic cocaine abuse associated with dilated cardiomyopathy. *Am J Emerg Med* 1990;8:203–204.

85. Bertolet BD, Freund G, Martin CA, et al. Unrecognized left ventricular dysfunction in an apparently healthy cocaine abuse population. *Clin Cardiol* 1990;13:323–328.

86. Willens HJ, Chakko SC, Kessler KM. Cardiovascular manifestations of cocaine abuse: a case of recurrent dilated cardiomyopathy. *Chest* 1994;106:594–600.

87. Pitts WR, Vongpatanasin W, Cigarroa JE, et al. Effects of the intracoronary infusion of cocaine on left ventricular systolic and diastolic function in humans. *Circulation* 1998;97:1270–1273.

88. Karch SB, Billingham ME. Coronary artery and peripheral vascular disease in cocaine users. *Coron Artery Dis* 1995;6:220–225.

89. Brickner ME, Willard JE, Eichhorn EJ, et al. Left ventricular hypertrophy associated with chronic cocaine abuse. *Circulation* 1991;84:1130–1135.

90. Clyburn EB, DiPette DJ. Hypertension induced by drugs and other substances. *Semin Nephrol* 1995;15:72–86.

91. Benchimol A, Bantell H, Dressen KB. Accelerated ventricular rhythm and cocaine abuse. *Ann Intern Med* 1978;88:519–520.

92. Castro VJ, Nacht R. Cocaine-induced bradyarrhythmia: an unsuspected cause of syncope. *Chest* 2000;117:275–277.

93. Jones LF, Tackett RL. Chronic cocaine treatment enhances the responsiveness of the left anterior descending coronary artery and the femoral artery to vasoactive substances. *J Pharmacol Exp Ther* 1990;255:1366–1370.

94. Simpson R, Edwards W. Pathogenesis of cocaine induced ischemic heart disease: autopsy findings in a 21-year-old man. *Arch Pathol Lab Med* 1986;110:479–484.

95. Roh LS, Hamele-Bena D. Cocaine-induced ischemic myocardial disease. *Am J Forensic Med Pathol* 1990;11:130–135.

96. Majid PA, Patel B, Kim HS, et al. An angiographic and histologic study of cocaine-induced chest pain. *Am J Cardiol* 1990;65:812–814.

97. Marder VJ, Mellinghoff IK. Cocaine and Buerger disease: is there a pathogenetic association? *Arch Intern Med* 2000;160:2057–2060.

98. Gutierrez A, England JD, Krupski WC. Cocaine-induced peripheral vascular occlusive disease: a case report. *Angiology* 1998;49:221–224.

99. Wattoo MA, Osundeko O. Cocaine-induced intestinal ischemia. *West J Med* 1999;170:47–49.

100. Kaufman MJ, Levin JM, Ross MH, et al. Cocaine-induced cerebral vasoconstriction detected in humans with magnetic resonance angiography. *JAMA* 1998;279:376–380.

101. Khellaf M, Fénelon G. Intracranial hemorrhage associated with cocaine abuse [letter]. *Neurology* 1998;50:1519–1520.

102. Rose S, Hearn WL, Hime GW, et al. Cocaine and cocaethylene concentrations in human postmortem cerebral cortex. *Neuroscience* 1990;16:14(abst).

103. Escobedo LG, Ruttenber AJ, Agocs MM, et al. Emerging patterns of cocaine use and the epidemic of cocaine overdose deaths in Dade County, Florida. *Arch Pathol Lab Med* 1991;115:900–905.

104. Perez-Reyes M, Jeffcoat R. Ethanol/cocaine interaction: cocaine and cocaethylene plasma concentrations and their relationship to subjective cardiovascular effects. *Life Sci* 1992;51:553–563.

105. Hearn WL, Rose S, Wagner J, et al. Cocaethylene is more potent than cocaine in mediating lethality. *Pharmacol Biochem Behav* 1991;39:531–533.

106. Uszenski RT, Gillis RA, Schaer GL, et al. Additive myocardial depressant effects of cocaine and ethanol. *Am Heart J* 1992;124:1276–1283.

107. Foltin RW, Fischman MW. Ethanol and cocaine interactions in humans: cardiovascular consequences. *Pharmacol Biochem Behav* 1988;31:877–883.

108. Farre M, de la Torre R, Llorente M, et al. Alcohol and cocaine interactions in humans. *J Pharmacol Exp Ther* 1993;266:1364–1373.

109. Chou T. Wake up and smell the coffee: caffeine, coffee, and the medical consequences. *West J Med* 1992;157:544–553.

110. Chou T, Benowitz NL. Caffeine and coffee: effects on health and cardiovascular disease. *Comp Biochem Physiol C Pharmacol Toxicol Endocrinol* 1994;109:173–189.

111. Robertson D, Frolich JC, Carr RK, et al. Effects of caffeine on plasma renin activity, catecholamines and blood pressure. *N Engl J Med* 1978;298:181–186.

112. van Dusseldorp M, Smits P, Thien T, et al. Effect of decaffeinated versus regular coffee on blood pressure: a 12-week, double-blind trial. *Hypertension* 1989;14:563–569.

113. van Dusseldorp M, Smits P, Lenders JW, et al. Boiled coffee and blood pressure: a 14-week controlled trial. *Hypertension* 1991;18:607–613.

114. Rachima-Maoz C, Peleg E, Rosenthal T. The effect of caffeine on ambulatory blood pressure in hypertensive patients. *Am J Hypertens* 1998;11:1426–1432.

115. Rakic V, Burke V, Beilin LJ. Effects of coffee on ambulatory blood pressure in older men and women: a randomized controlled trial. *Hypertension* 1999;33:869–873.

116. Hakim AA, Ross GW, Curb JD, et al. Coffee consumption in hypertensive men in older middle-age and the risk of stroke: the Honolulu Heart Program. *J Clin Epidemiol* 1998;51:487–494.

117. LaCroix AZ, Mead LA, Liang KY, et al. Coffee consumption and the incidence of coronary artery disease. *N Engl J Med* 1986;315:977–982.

118. Rosenberg L, Palmer JR, Kelly JP, et al. Coffee drinking and nonfatal myocardial infarction in men under 55 years of age. *Am J Epidemiol* 1988;128:570–578.

119. Grobbee DE, Rimm EB, Giovannucci E, et al. Coffee, caffeine, and cardiovascular disease in men. *N Engl J Med* 1990;323:1026–1032.

120. Sesso HD, Gaziano JM, Buring JE, et al. Coffee and tea intake and the risk of myocardial infarction. *Am J Epidemiol* 1999;149:162–167.

121. Geleijnse JM, Launer LJ, Hofman A, et al. Tea flavonoids may protect against atherosclerosis. The Rotterdam Study. *Arch Intern Med* 1999;159:2170–2174.

122. Lynn LA, Kissinger JF. Coronary precautions: should caffeine be restricted in patients after myocardial infarction? *Heart Lung* 1992;21:365–371.

123. Stavric B. An update on research with coffee/caffeine (1989–1990). *Food Chem Toxicol* 1992;30:533–555.

124. Rosmarin PC. Coffee and coronary heart disease: a review. *Prog Cardiovasc Dis* 1989;32:239–245.

125. Rosmarin PC, Applegate WB, Somes GW. Coffee consumption and serum lipids: a randomized, crossover clinical trial. *Am J Med* 1990;88:349–356.

126. Nygård O, Refsum H, Ueland PM, et al. Coffee consumption and plasma total homocysteine: the Hordaland Homocysteine Study. *Am J Clin Nutr* 1997;65:136–143.

127. El-Khairy L, Ueland PM, Nygård O, et al. Lifestyle and cardiovascular disease risk factors as determinants of total cysteine in plasma: the Hordaland Homocysteine Study. *Am J Clin Nutr* 1999;70:1016–1024.

128. Stolzenberg-Solomon RZ, Miller ER 3d, Maguire MG, et al. Association of dietary protein intake and coffee consumption with serum homocysteine concentrations in an older population. *Am J Clin Nutr* 1999;69:467–475.

129. Grubben MJ, Boers GH, Blom HJ, et al. Unfiltered coffee increases plasma homocysteine concentrations in healthy volunteers: a randomized trial. *Am J Clin Nutr* 2000;71:480–484.

130. Dobmeyer DJ, Stine RA, Leier CV, et al. The arrhythmogenic effects of caffeine in human beings. *N Engl J Med* 1983;308:814–816.

131. Prineas RJ, Jacobs DR Jr, Crow RS, et al. Coffee, tea and VPB. *J Chronic Dis* 1980;33:67–72.

132. Graboys TB, Blatt CM, Lown B. The effect of caffeine on ventricular ectopic activity in patients with malignant ventricular arrhythmia. *Arch Intern Med* 1989;149:637–639.

133. Chelsky LB, Cutler JE, Griffith K, et al. Caffeine and ventricular arrhythmias: an electrophysiological approach. *JAMA* 1990;264:2236–2240.

134. Donnerstein RL, Zhu D, Samson R, et al. Acute effects of caffeine ingestion on signal-averaged electrocardiograms. *Am Heart J* 1998;136:643–646.

135. Stamler JS, Goldman ME, Gomes J, et al. The effect of stress and fatigue on cardiac rhythm in medical interns. *J Electrocardiol* 1992;25:333–338.

136. Myers MG, Harris L. High dose caffeine and ventricular arrhythmias. *Can J Cardiol* 1990;6:95–98.

137. Myers MG. Caffeine and cardiac arrhythmias. *Ann Intern Med* 1991;114:147–150.

138. Welder AA, Melchert RB. Cardiotoxic effects of cocaine and anabolic-androgenic steroids in the athlete. *J Pharmacol Toxicol Methods* 1993;29:61–68.

139. Kennedy C. Myocardial infarction in association with misuse of anabolic steroids. *Ulster Med J* 1993;62:174–176.

140. Ferenchick GS. Anabolic/androgenic steroid abuse and thrombosis: is there a connection? *Med Hypotheses* 1991;35:27–31.

141. Glazer G. Atherogenic effects of anabolic steroids on serum lipid levels: a literature review. *Arch Intern Med* 1991;151:1925–1933.

142. Barrett-Connor EL. Testosterone and risk factors for cardiovascular disease in men. *Diabete Metab* 1995;21:156–161.

143. Rockhold RW. Cardiovascular toxicity of anabolic steroids. *Annu Rev Pharmacol Toxicol* 1993;33:497–520.

144. Uzunova AD, Ramey ER, Ramwell PW. Arachidonate-induced thrombosis in mice: effects of gender or testosterone and estradiol administration. *Prostaglandins* 1977;13:995–1002.

145. Penhos JC, Rabbani F, Myers A, et al. The role of gonadal steroids in arachidonate-induced mortality in mice. *Proc Soc Exp Biol Med* 1981;167:98–100.

146. Emms H, Lewis GP. Sex and hormonal influences on platelet sensitivity and coagulation in the rat. *Br J Pharmacol* 1985;86:557–563.

147. Myers A, Papadopoulos A, O'Day D, et al. Sexual differentiation of arachidonate toxicity in mice. *J Pharmacol Exp Ther* 1982;222:315–318.

148. Johnson M, Ramwell PW. Androgen mediated sex differences in platelet aggregation. *Physiologist* 1974;17:256(abst).

149. Stolt A, Karila T, Viitasalo M, et al. QT interval and QT dispersion in endurance athletes and in power athletes using large doses of anabolic steroids. *Am J Cardiol* 1999;84:364–366.

150. Sullivan ML, Martinez CM, Gallagher EJ. Atrial fibrillation and anabolic steroids. *J Emerg Med* 1999;17:851–857.

151. Carson P, Oldroyd K, Phadke K. Myocardial infarction due to amphetamine. *BMJ (Clin Res Ed)* 1987;294:1525–1526.

152. Dowling GP, McDonough ET 3d, Bost RO. "Eve" and "Ecstasy": a report of five deaths associated with the use of MDEA and MDMA. *JAMA* 1987;257:1615–1617.

153. Suarez RV, Riemersma R. "Ecstasy" and sudden cardiac death. *Am J Forensic Med Pathol* 1988;9:339–341.

154. Packe GE, Garton MJ, Jennings K. Acute myocardial infarction caused by intravenous amphetamine abuse. *Br Heart J* 1990;64:23–24.

155. Ragland AS, Ismail Y, Arsura EL. Myocardial infarction after amphetamine use. *Am Heart J* 1993;125:247–249.

156. Furst SR, Fallon SP, Reznik GN. Myocardial infarction after inhalation of methamphetamine [letter]. *N Engl J Med* 1990;323:1147–1148.

157. Bashour TT. Acute myocardial infarction resulting from amphetamine abuse: a spasm-thrombus interplay? *Am Heart J* 1994;128:1237–1239.

158. Jacobs LJ. Reversible dilated cardiomyopathy induced by methamphetamine. *Clin Cardiol* 1989;12:725–727.

159. Hong R, Matsuyama E, Nur K. Cardiomyopathy associated with the smoking of crystal methamphetamine. *JAMA* 1991;265:1152–1154.

160. McEvoy AW, Kitchen ND, Thomas DGT. Intracerebral haemorrhage in young adults: the emerging importance of drug misuse. *BMJ* 2000;320:1322–1324.

161. Perez JA Jr, Arsura EL, Strategos S. Methamphetamine-related stroke: four cases. *J Emerg Med* 1999;17:469–471.

162. Zahn KA, Li RL, Purssell RA. Cardiovascular toxicity after ingestion of "herbal ecstasy." *J Emerg Med* 1999;17:289–291.

163. Silvestry FE, St. John Sutton M. Anorectic therapy and valvular heart disease: a reappraisal. *Eur Heart J* 1999;20:917–920.

164. Connolly HM, Crary JL, McGoon MD, et al. Valvular heart disease associated with fenfluramine-phentermine. *N Engl J Med* 1997;337:581–588.

165. Jick H, Vasilakis C, Weinrauch LA, et al. A population-based study of appetite-suppressant drugs and the risk of cardiac-valve regurgitation. *N Engl J Med* 1998;339:719–724.

166. Khan MA, Herzog CA, St. Peter JV, et al. The prevalence of cardiac valvular insufficiency assessed by transthoracic echocardiography in obese patients treated with appetite-suppressant drugs. *N Engl J Med* 1998;339:713–718.

167. Burger AJ, Sherman HB, Charlamb MJ, et al. Low prevalence of valvular heart disease in 226 phentermine-fenfluramine protocol subjects prospectively followed for up to 30 months. *J Am Coll Cardiol* 1999;34:1153–1158.

168. Jick H. Heart valve disorders and appetite-suppressant drugs. *JAMA* 2000;283:1738–1740.

169. Jollis JG, Landolfo CK, Kisslo J, et al. Fenfluramine and phentermine and cardiovascular findings: effect of treatment duration on prevalence of valve abnormalities. *Circulation* 2000;101:2071–2077.

170. Cannistra LB, Cannistra AJ. Regression of multivalvular regurgitation after the cessation of fenfluramine and phentermine treatment. *N Engl J Med* 1998;339:771.

171. Centers for Disease Control and Prevention. Cardiac valvulopathy associated with exposure to fenfluramine or dexfenfluramine: US Department of Health and Human Services interim public health recommendations, November 1997. *JAMA* 1997;278:1729–1731.

172. Rich S, Rubin L, Walker AM, et al. Anorexigens and pulmonary hypertension in the United States: results from the Surveillance of North American Pulmonary Hypertension. *Chest* 2000;117:870–874.

173. Simonneau G, Fartoukh M, Sitbon O, et al. Primary pulmonary hypertension associated with the use of fenfluramine derivatives. *Chest* 1998;114:195S–199S.

174. Mark EJ, Patalas ED, Chang HT, et al. Fatal pulmonary hypertension associated with short-term use of fenfluramine and phentermine. *N Engl J Med* 1997;337:602–606.

175. Fowles RE, Cloward TV, Yowell RL. Endocardial fibrosis associated with fenfluramine-phentermine. *N Engl J Med* 1998;338:1316.

176. Sobel RM. Ruptured retroperitoneal aneurysm in a patient taking phentermine hydrochloride. *Am J Emerg Med* 1999;17:102–103.

177. Urbano-Marquez A, Estruch R, Fernandez-Sola J, et al. The greater risk of alcoholic cardiomyopathy and myopathy in women compared with men. *JAMA* 1995;274:149–154.

178. Johnson CC, Myers L, Webber LS, et al. Alcohol consumption among adolescents and young adults: the Bogalusa Heart Study, 1981 to 1991. *Am J Public Health* 1995;85:979–982.

179. Gambert SR. Alcohol abuse: medical effects of heavy drinking in late life. *Geriatrics* 1997;52:30–37.

180. Goldstein D. *The pharmacology of alcohol*. New York: Oxford University Press, 1983.

181. Piano MR, Schwertz DW. Alcoholic heart disease: a review. *Heart Lung* 1994;23:3–17.

182. Teragaki M, Takeuchi K, Takeda T. Clinical and histologic features of alcohol drinkers with congestive heart failure. *Am Heart J* 1993;125:808–817.

183. Polimeni PI, Otten MD, Hoeschen LE. *In vivo* effects of ethanol on the rat myocardium: evidence for a reversible, nonspecific increase of sarcolemmal permeability. *J Mol Cell Cardiol* 1983;15:113–122.

184. Wu S, White R, Wikman-Coffelt J, et al. The preventive effect of verapamil on ethanol-induced cardiac depression: phosphorus-31 nuclear magnetic resonance and high-pressure liquid chromatographic studies of hamsters. *Circulation* 1987;75:1058–1064.

185. Preedy VR, Atkinson LM, Richardson PJ, et al. Mechanisms of ethanol-induced cardiac damage. *Br Heart J* 1993;69:197–200.

186. Preedy VR, Siddiq T, Why H, et al. The deleterious effects of alcohol on the heart: involvement of protein turnover. *Alcohol* 1994;29:141–147.

187. Fernandez-Sola J, Estruch R, Grau JM, et al. The relation of alcoholic myopathy to cardiomyopathy. *Ann Intern Med* 1994;120:529–536.

188. Moushmoush B, Abi-Mansour P. Alcohol and the heart: the long-term effects of alcohol on the cardiovascular system. *Arch Intern Med* 1991;151:36–42.

189. Thomas AP, Rozanski DJ, Renard DC, et al. Effects of ethanol on the contractile function of the heart: a review. *Alcohol Clin Exp Res* 1994;18:121–131.

190. Kupari M, Koskinen P, Suokas A, et al. Left ventricular filling impairment in asymptomatic chronic alcoholics. *Am J Cardiol* 1990;66:1473–1477.

191. Lazarevic AM, Nakatani S, Neskovic AN, et al. Early changes in left ventricular function in chronic asymptomatic alcoholics: relation to the duration of heavy drinking. *J Am Coll Cardiol* 2000;35:1599–1606.

192. Ballester M, Martí V, Carrió I, et al. Spectrum of alcohol-induced myocardial damage detected by indium-111-labeled monoclonal antimyosin antibodies. *J Am Coll Cardiol* 1997;29:160–167.

193. Stöllberger C, Finsterer J. Reversal of dilated to hypertrophic cardiomyopathy after alcohol abstinence. *Clin Cardiol* 1998;21:365–367.

194. Machiels JP, Dive A, Donckier J, et al. Reversible myocardial dysfunction in a patient with alcoholic ketoacidosis: a role for hypophosphatemia. *Am J Emerg Med* 1998;16:371–373.

195. Jacob AJ, McLaren KM, Boon NA. Effects of abstinence on alcoholic heart muscle disease. *Am J Cardiol* 1991;68:805–807.

196. Gavazzi A, DeMaria R, Parolini M, et al. Alcohol abuse and dilated cardiomyopathy in men. The Italian Multicenter Cardiomyopathy Study Group. *Am J Cardiol* 2000;85:1114–1118.

197. Fauchier L, Babuty D, Poret P, et al. Comparison of long-term outcome of alcoholic and idiopathic dilated cardiomyopathy. *Eur Heart J* 2000;21:306–314.

198. Lian C. L'alcoolisme cause d'hypertension arterielle. *Bull Acad Natl Med* 1915;74:525–528.

199. Regan TJ. Alcohol and the cardiovascular system. *JAMA* 1990;264:377–381.

200. Moreira LB, Fuchs FD, Moraes RS, et al. Alcohol intake and blood pressure: the importance of time elapsed since last drink. *J Hypertens* 1998;16:175–180.

201. Manolio TA, Levy D, Garrison RJ, et al. Relation of alcohol intake to left ventricular mass: the Framingham Study. *J Am Coll Cardiol* 1991;17:717–721.

202. Koskinen P, Kupari M. Alcohol and cardiac arrhythmias. *BMJ* 1992;304:1394–1395.

203. Hendrickse MT. QT interval, autonomic neuropathy, and alcoholic liver disease. *Lancet* 1993;342:61.

204. Ettinger PO, Wu CF, De La Cruz C Jr, et al. Arrhythmias and the "holiday heart": alcohol-associated cardiac rhythm disorders. *Am Heart J* 1978;95:555–562.

205. Lowenstein SR, Gabow PA, Cramer J, et al. The role of alcohol in new-onset atrial fibrillation. *Arch Intern Med* 1983;143:1882–1885.

206. Koskinen P, Kupari M, Leinonen H. Role of alcohol in recurrences of atrial fibrillation in persons less than 65 years of age. *Am J Cardiol* 1990;66:954–958.

207. Engel TR, Luck JC. Effect of whiskey on atrial vulnerability and "holiday heart." *J Am Coll Cardiol* 1983;1:816–818.

208. Wannamethee G, Shaper AG. Alcohol and sudden cardiac death. *Br Heart J* 1992;68:443–448.

209. Klatsky AL, Armstrong MA, Friedman GD. Alcohol and mortality. *Ann Intern Med* 1992;117:646–654.

210. Doll R, Peto R, Hall E, et al. Mortality in relation to consumption of alcohol: 13 years' observations on male British doctors. *BMJ* 1994;309:911–918.

211. Gaziano JM, Buring JE, Breslow JL, et al. Moderate alcohol intake, increased levels of high-density lipoprotein and its subfractions, and decreased risk of myocardial infarction. *N Engl J Med* 1993;329:1829–1834.

212. Rimm EB, Klatsky A, Grobbee D, et al. Review of moderate alcohol consumption and reduced risk of coronary heart disease: is the effect due to beer, wine, or spirits. *BMJ* 1996;312:731–736.

213. Maclure M. Demonstration of deductive meta-analysis: ethanol intake and risk of myocardial infarction. *Epidemiol Rev* 1993;15:328–351.

214. Maclure M. Alcohol intake and risk of myocardial infarction. *N Engl J Med* 1994;330:1241–1242.

215. Ridker PM, Vaughan DE, Stampfer MJ, et al. Association of moderate alcohol consumption and plasma concentration of endogenous tissue-type plasminogen activator. *JAMA* 1994;272:929–933.

216. Rubin R, Rand ML. Alcohol and platelet function. *Alcohol Clin Exp Res* 1994;18:105–110.

217. Steinberg D, Pearson TA, Kuller LH. Alcohol and atherosclerosis. *Ann Intern Med* 1991;114:967–976.

218. Pentz MA, Dwyer JH, MacKinnon DP, et al. A multicommunity trial for primary prevention of adolescent drug abuse: effects on drug use prevalence. *JAMA* 1989;261:3259–3266.

219. Vander Martin R, Cummings SR, Coates TJ. Ethnicity and smoking: differences in white, black, Hispanic, and Asian medical patients who smoke. *Am J Prev Med* 1990;6:194–199.

220. Edwards G, Arif A, Hadgson R. Nomenclature and classification of drug- and alcohol-related problems: a WHO memorandum. *Bull World Health Organ* 1981;59:225–242.

221. Benowitz NL. Cigarette smoking and nicotine addiction. *Med Clin North Am* 1992;76:415–437.

222. Stephenson J. Clues found to tobacco addiction. *JAMA* 1996;275:1217–1218.

223. Schelling TC. Addictive drugs: the cigarette experience. *Science* 1992;255:430–433.

224. Carmelli D, Swan GE, Robinette D, et al. Genetic influence on smoking: a study of male twins. *N Engl J Med* 1992;327:829–833.

225. Falk E. Why do plaques rupture? *Circulation* 1992;86[Suppl 6]:III30–III42.

226. McCall MR, van den Berg JJ, Kuypers FA, et al. Modification of LCAT activity and HDL structure: new links between cigarette smoke and coronary heart disease risk. *Arterioscler Thromb* 1994;14:248–253.

227. Howard G, Wagenknecht LE, Burke GL, et al. Cigarette smoking and progression of atherosclerosis. The Atherosclerosis Risk in Communities (ARIC) Study. *JAMA* 1998;279:119–124.

228. Bolinder G, deFaire U. Ambulatory 24-h blood pressure monitoring in healthy, middle-aged smokeless tobacco users, smokers, and nontobacco users. *Am J Hypertens* 1998;11:1153–1163.

229. Hammond EC, Horn D. Smoking and death rates: report on forty-four months of follow-up of 187,783 men: II. Death rates by cause. *JAMA* 1958;166:1294–1308.

230. Auerbach O, Carter HW, Garfinkel L, et al. Cigarette smoking and coronary artery disease: a macroscopic and microscopic study. *Chest* 1976;70:697–705.

231. Lakier JB. Smoking and cardiovascular disease. *Am J Med* 1992;93[Suppl 1A]:8S–12S.

232. Leone A. Cardiovascular damage from smoking: a fact or belief? *Int J Cardiol* 1993;38:113–117.

233. He J, Whelton PK. Passive cigarette smoking increases risk of coronary heart disease. *Eur Heart J* 1999;20:1764–1765.

234. Steenland K. Risk assessment for heart disease and workplace ETS exposure among nonsmokers. *Environ Health Perspect* 1999;107[Suppl 6]:859–863.

235. Werner RM, Pearson TA. What's so passive about passive smoking? Secondhand smoke as a cause of atherosclerotic disease. *JAMA* 1998;279:157–158.

236. Sumida H, Watanabe H, Kugiyama K, et al. Does passive smoking impair endothelium-dependent coronary artery dilation in women? *J Am Coll Cardiol* 1998;31:811–815.

237. Raitakari OT, Adams MR, McCredie RJ, et al. Arterial endothelial dysfunction related to passive smoking is potentially reversible in healthy young adults. *Ann Intern Med* 1999;130:578–581.

238. Valkonen M, Kuusi T. Passive smoking induces atherogenic changes in low-density lipoprotein. *Circulation* 1998;97:2012–2016.

239. Satcher D. Cigars and public health. *N Engl J Med* 1999;340:1829–1831.

240. Wald NJ, Watt HC. Prospective study of effect of switching from cigarettes to pipes or cigars on mortality from three smoking related diseases. *BMJ* 1997;314:1860–1863.

241. Christen AG, McDaniel RK, McDonald JL Jr. The smokeless tobacco "time bomb." *Postgrad Med* 1990;87:69–74.

242. Huhtasaari F, Lundberg V, Eliasson M, et al. Smokeless tobacco as a possible risk factor for myocardial infarction: a population-based study in middle-aged men. *J Am Coll Cardiol* 1999;34:1784–1790.

243. Schwartz JL. Methods of smoking cessation. *Med Clin North Am* 1992;76:451–476.

244. Benowitz NL, Fitzgerald GA, Wilson M, et al. Nicotine effects on eicosanoid formation and hemostatic function: comparison of transdermal nicotine and cigarette smoking. *J Am Coll Cardiol* 1993;22:1159–1167.

245. Warner JG Jr, Little WC. Myocardial infarction in a patient who smoked while wearing a nicotine patch. *Ann Intern Med* 1994;120:695.

246. Arnaot MR. Treating heart disease: nicotine patches may not be safe. *BMJ* 1995;310:663–664.

247. Campbell IA. Smoking cessation. *Thorax* 2000;55[Suppl 1]:S28–S31.

248. Kessler DA. Nicotine addiction in young people. *N Engl J Med* 1995;333:186–189.

249. Lynch BS, Bonnie RJ, eds. *Growing up tobacco free: preventing nicotine addiction in children and youth.* Washington, DC: National Academy Press, 1994:8.

250. Department of Health and Human Services. *Preventing tobacco use among young people: a report of the Surgeon General.* Washington, DC: Government Printing Office, 1994:5–58.

251. Glynn TJ. Essential elements of school-based smoking prevention programs. *J Sch Health* 1989;59:181–188.

252. Thayer WS. Bacterial or infective endocarditis. *Edinb Med J* 1931;38:237–265.

253. Lerner PI, Weinstein L. Infective endocarditis in the antibiotic era. *N Engl J Med* 1966;274:199–206.

254. Griffin MR, Wilson WR, Edwards WD, et al. Infective endocarditis: Olmsted County, Minnesota, 1950 through 1981. *JAMA* 1985;254:1199–1202.

255. Hogevik H, Olaison L, Andersson R, et al. Epidemiologic aspects of infective endocarditis in an urban population: a 5-year prospective study. *Medicine* 1995;74:324–339.

256. Cherubin CE, Neu HC. Infective endocarditis at the Presbyterian Hospital in New York City from 1938–1967. *Am J Med* 1971;51:83–96.

257. El-Khatib MR, Wilson FM, Lerner AM. Characteristics of bacterial endocarditis in heroin addicts in Detroit. *Am J Med Sci* 1976;271:197–201.

258. Roberts R, Slovis CM. Endocarditis in intravenous drug abusers. *Emerg Med Clin North Am* 1990;8:665–681.

259. Sklaver AR, Hoffman TA, Greenman RL. Staphylococcal endocarditis in addicts. *South Med J* 1978;71:638–643.

260. Espersen F, Frimodt-Moller N. *Staphyloccus aureus* endocarditis. *Arch Intern Med* 1986;146:1118–1121.

261. Levine DP, Crane LR, Zervos MJ. Bacteremia in narcotic addicts at the Detroit Medical Center: II. Infectious endocarditis: a prospective comparative study. *Rev Infect Dis* 1986;8:374–396.

262. Graves MK, Soto L. Left-sided endocarditis in parenteral drug abusers: recent experience at a large community hospital. *South Med J* 1992;85:378–380.

263. Currie PF, Sutherland GR, Jacob AJ, et al. A review of endocarditis in acquired immunodeficiency syndrome and human immunodeficiency virus infection. *Eur Heart J* 1995;16(Suppl B):15–18.

264. Weisse AB, Heller DR, Schimenti RJ, et al. The febrile parenteral drug user: a prospective study in 121 patients. *Am J Med* 1993;94:274–280.

265. Ribera E, Miró JM, Cortés E, et al. Influence of human immunodeficiency virus 1 infection and degree of immunosuppression in the clinical characteristics and outcome of infective endocarditis in intravenous drug users. *Arch Intern Med* 1998;158:2043–2050.

266. Lukes AS, Bright DK, Durack DT. Diagnosis of infective endocarditis. *Infect Dis Clin North Am* 1993;7:1–8.

267. von Reyn CF, Levy BS, Arbeit RD, et al. Infective endocarditis: an analysis based on strict case definitions. *Ann Intern Med* 1981;94:505–518.

268. Durack DT, Lukes AS, Bright DK. New criteria for diagnosis of infective endocarditis: utilization of specific echocardiographic findings. Duke Endocarditis Service. *Am J Med* 1994;96:200–209.

269. Shively BK. Transesophageal echocardiography in endocarditis. *Cardiol Clin* 1993;11:437–446.

270. Rohmann S, Erbel R, Mohr-Kahaly S, et al. Use of transesophageal echocardiography in the diagnosis of abscess in infective endocarditis. *Eur Heart J* 1995;16[Suppl B]:54–62.

271. Alam M. Transesophageal echocardiography in critical care units: Henry Ford Hospital experience and review of the literature. *Prog Cardiovasc Dis* 1996;38:315–328.

272. Daniel WG, Mugge A, Martin RP, et al. Improvement in the diagnosis of abscesses associated with endocarditis by transesophageal echocardiography. *N Engl J Med* 1991;324:795–800.

273. Mills J, Abbott J, Utley JR, et al. Role of cardiac catheterization in infective endocarditis. *Chest* 1977;72:576–582.

274. Wiseman J, Rouleau J, Rigo P, et al. Gallium-67 myocardial imaging for the detection of bacterial endocarditis: concise communication. *Radiology* 1976;120:135–138.

275. Wong DW, Dhawan VK, Tanaka T, et al. Imaging endocarditis with TC-99m-labeled antibody: an experimental study. *J Nucl Med* 1982;23:229–234.

276. Besnier JM, Choutet P. Medical treatment of infective endocarditis: general principles. *Eur Heart J* 1995;16[Suppl B]:72–74.

277. DiNubile MJ. Short-course antibiotic therapy for right-sided endocarditis caused by *Staphylococcus aureus* in injection drug users. *Ann Intern Med* 1994;121:873–876.

278. Stamboulian D. Outpatient treatment of endocarditis in a clinic-based program in Argentina. *Eur J Clin Microbiol Infect Dis* 1995;14:648–654.

279. McAnulty JH, Rahimtoola SH. Surgery for infective endocarditis. *JAMA* 1979;242:77–79.

280. Katz NM. Current surgical treatment of valvular heart disease. *Am Fam Physician* 1995;52:559–568.

281. Acar J, Michel PL, Varenne O, et al. Surgical treatment of infective endocarditis. *Eur Heart J* 1995;16[Suppl B]:94–98.

282. Arbulu A, Thoms NW, Chiscano A, Wilson RF. Total tricuspid valvulectomy without replacement in the treatment of *Pseudomonas* endocarditis. *Surg Forum* 1971;22:162–164.

283. Arbulu A, Holmes RJ, Asfaw I. Surgical treatment of intractable right-sided infective endocarditis in drug addicts: 25 years experience. *J Heart Valve Dis* 1993;2:129–137.

284. Hughes CF, Noble N. Vegetectomy: an alternative surgical treatment for infective endocarditis of the atrioventricular valves in drug addicts. *J Thorac Cardiovasc Surg* 1988;95:857–861.

285. Delahaye F, Ecochard R, de Gevigney G, et al. The long term prognosis of infective endocarditis. *Eur Heart J* 1995;16[Suppl B]:48–53.

286. Rashid J, Eisenberg MJ, Topol EJ. Cocaine-induced aortic dissection. *Am Heart J* 1996;132:1301–1304.

ATHLETE'S HEART

PAUL D. THOMPSON
N. A. MARK ESTES III

▼ ADDITIONAL ELECTRONIC TOPICS

Effect of Exercise Training on Exercise Performance h53

OVERVIEW

Athlete's heart was first described by Henschen in 1899 and is now recognized as a constellation of clinical findings known as *the athletic heart syndrome*. These findings include sinus bradycardia, atrioventricular (AV) conduction delay, systolic flow murmurs, and cardiac chamber enlargement with normal or augmented function. All four cardiac chambers may be enlarged. Chamber enlargement may rarely exceed the upper limits of normal, but marked enlargement of the right ventricle or either atrium suggests a pathologic process. Clinical findings of the athletic heart syndrome are limited to athletes whose sports and training require a large aerobic or endurance exercise component. Left ventricular (LV) wall thickness can be slightly thickened, but this thickening is generally restricted to athletes with LV chamber enlargement and rarely reaches the thickness of pathological states such as hypertrophic cardiomyopathy (HCM). Physicians often are required to evaluate asymptomatic athletes before participation and to evaluate symptomatic athletes before permitting their return to vigorous exercise training. In these situations, the athletic heart syndrome must be differentiated from pathological conditions associated with cardiac complications during exercise, including HCM, coronary artery anomalies, aortic stenosis, right ventricular or LV cardiomyopathy in young athletes, and coronary artery disease in adults.

GLOSSARY

Athlete's heart or athletic heart syndrome: a constellation of clinical, electrocardiographic, and echocardiographic variants of normal found in well-trained athletes who participate in sports requiring prolonged aerobic exercise training.

Endurance or isotonic exercise: generally rhythmic, physical exertion (e.g., running, swimming, and bicycling) that requires significant, sustained increases in oxygen uptake.

External workrate: the amount of work an individual can perform on the environment. External workrate can be measured by oxygen uptake.

P. D. Thompson: Department of Cardiology, University of Connecticut School of Medicine, Farmington, Connecticut; and Department of Preventive Cardiology, Hartford Hospital, Hartford, Connecticut
N. A. M. Estes III: Department of Medicine, Tufts University School of Medicine, Boston, Massachusetts

Internal workrate: the myocardial oxygen consumption during exertion. Internal workrate can be estimated by the triple product (heart rate × systolic blood pressure × LV ejection time) or double product (heart rate × systolic blood pressure).

Maximal oxygen uptake ($\dot{V}O_2$max): the physiologic and highly reproducible upper limit of an individual's ability to extract and use oxygen during progressive isotonic exercise.

Onset of blood lactate accumulation (OBLA): the point during exercise at which the accumulation of lactate can be detected in blood samples. This point corresponds to an abrupt increase in the respiratory rate and often is referred to as the *anaerobic threshold.*

Relative workrate: the percentage of maximal oxygen uptake required to perform a certain physical task.

Strength exercise: physical exertion that requires lifting or moving objects against resistance. Strength exercises can result in motion against resistance (e.g., weightlifting) or require exertion against a fixed object, referred to as *isometric exercise.*

HISTORICAL PERSPECTIVE

The history of the athlete's heart is as clouded by myth and misinformation as the condition itself. Take, for example, the legend of Pheidippides, who reportedly ran 40 km (24 miles) from the battlefield at Marathon to Athens to announce the Athenians' victory over the Persians. After announcing the victory, he collapsed and died. This story provides a marvelous introduction to the risks of exercise, but it is probably not true. Pheidippides was more likely named Philippids or Phidippus. His run was not from Marathon to Athens to announce victory but from Athens to Sparta to solicit military aid, then back to Athens with the bad news that the Spartans were not coming. This distance was not 40 km but closer to 500 km (300 miles). Most distressing of all to those who cite this event, our runner, name uncertain, probably survived. Herodotus, the major historian of the event, never mentioned the runner's demise (1).

Similar confusion has plagued the concept of the athlete's heart—what we prefer to label *the athletic heart syndrome*—because this condition is often a constellation of findings. Indeed, as with the story of Pheidippides, the first telling was probably the most correct. Subsequent versions only distorted or embellished the truth.

The first description of the athletic heart syndrome was provided more than 100 years ago. Henschen used percussion of the chest to determine heart size in cross-country skiers before and after a ski race (2). His report in 1899 concluded that skiing produces a physiologic cardiac enlargement that enables the athlete's heart to perform more work than the heart of an untrained individual. He also noted that the right and left sides of the heart were enlarged. He concluded that this enlargement is due to athletic activity, and he called the

condition "the athlete's heart." Subsequent studies by a plethora of others using roentgenographic, echocardiographic, computerized tomographic, and magnetic resonance imaging techniques have confirmed Henschen's conclusion that exercise training produces a generalized cardiac enlargement.

Henschen also noted acute cardiac dilation after exhaustive exercise, and he attributed this dilation to cardiac failure. This conclusion has long been considered incorrect, although more recent echocardiographic studies have resurrected the possibility that prolonged, exhausting, competitive events such as triathlons may produce a cardiac fatigue typified by temporarily decreased LV contractility (3). Perhaps Henschen was not as wrong as previously thought.

How could Henschen, over 100 years ago and using a technique as crude as chest percussion, have reached such accurate conclusions? The answer is that he picked the right athletes, but this simple response obscures several principles critical to understanding the athletic heart syndrome. First, Henschen studied endurance-trained athletes. Strength-trained athletes such as weightlifters have increased cardiac dimensions, but their hearts' enlargement is related to body size and muscle mass (4). Only endurance-trained athletes or athletes training with endurance and strength modalities develop the athletic heart syndrome. Second, Henschen selected cross-country skiers—endurance athletes whose exercise uses arm and leg muscles. Cardiac dimensions and stroke volume are greatest in athletes whose training requires use of the most muscle mass.

NORMAL RESPONSE TO EXERCISE AND EXERCISE TRAINING

A basic understanding of the acute response to endurance exercise and of the exercise training response is useful in evaluating athletes with possible athletic heart syndrome.

Acute Response to Exercise

Compared to the general population, endurance athletes are characterized by a higher ability to perform maximal dynamic exercise. This ability can be measured as $\dot{V}O_2$max. $\dot{V}O_2$max is expressed as liters of oxygen per minute or is "normalized" for body weight as milliliters of oxygen per minute per kg of body weight. $\dot{V}O_2$max is physiologically limited by the ability of the cardiopulmonary system to deliver oxygen and the ability of the exercising muscles to use oxygen. Rearranging the Fick equation for cardiac output [cardiac output = volume of oxygen/arteriovenous oxygen difference ($\dot{V}O_2$/A-V O_2)] demonstrates that $\dot{V}O_2$max is the product of maximal cardiac output and the maximal A-V O_2 difference. Maximal cardiac output is the product of maximal heart rate and stroke volume. Because maximal heart rate among healthy individuals varies primarily by age, and because the ability to increase the A-V O_2 difference is limited, the major factor responsible for the higher $\dot{V}O_2$max among endurance athletes is an increased stroke volume. The clinical findings typical of the athletic heart syndrome are generally manifestations of this increased stroke volume.

Although higher $\dot{V}O_2$max values distinguish endurance athletes from sedentary individuals, $\dot{V}O_2$max is not a good discriminator of superior athletic performance among endurance athletes. This is because $\dot{V}O_2$max does not measure an individual's ability to maintain exertion over a long period of time. Other factors, including the athlete's mechanical efficiency and "anaerobic threshold," or OBLA, contribute to submaximal work capacity and are better discriminators of competitive exercise performance among athletes. Enhanced mechanical efficiency means that an athlete can perform a physical task while consuming less oxygen than a less efficient athlete. A higher OBLA means that the athlete can perform more mechanical work without producing lactate. OBLA indicates the onset of several factors that eventually reduce exercise capacity. OBLA is associated with a higher respiratory rate stimulated by the production of carbon dioxide from buffering lactic acid ($HLactate + HCO_3^- \rightarrow H_2CO_3 + lactate^- \rightarrow H_2O + CO_2$). In addition, the lactate production indicates a level of exertion requiring glycogen catabolism, and glycogen depletion is one potential limiting factor in endurance performance. Finally, lactic acid itself contributes to fatigue.

Acute cardiovascular adaptations to exercise in young, healthy subjects are mediated by several mechanisms. The increase in heart rate initially is due primarily to withdrawal of resting vagal tone. At approximately 50% of maximal heart rate, additional acceleration of heart rate is associated with increased sympathetic nerve activity and norepinephrine spillover into the circulation (5). Peak heart rate is estimated as 220 – age, but the standard deviation of this estimate is ± 11 to 22 beats/min (6). Therefore, the 95% confidence limits are ± 22 to 43 beats/min, and the range of normal can be 44 to 86 beats/min. These limits underscore the problem of estimating heart rate by age. Changes in stroke volume during exertion are influenced by body position. During supine exercise, the increase in stroke volume is due primarily to increases in end diastolic volume. During upright exercise, increases in stroke volume are produced by increases in end diastolic volume and decreases in end systolic volume (5). The increase in the A-V O_2 difference is produced by redistribution of blood from nonexercising tissue to the exercising musculature, increased extraction of oxygen over the exercising muscle bed, and hemoconcentration (5). Sweat loss is not required for this hemoconcentration, because plasma fluid moves into exercising muscle to produce the muscle swelling obvious in recently exercised muscle. These changes and the mediating mechanisms apply to young, healthy subjects such as those most likely to present with clinical findings of the athletic heart syndrome. Altered responses and different mechanisms are observed in elderly subjects and in patients with disease. ▼▼ h54

CLINICAL COMPONENTS OF THE ATHLETIC HEART SYNDROME

Variants Attributed to Enhanced Parasympathetic Tone

Several of the findings of the athletic heart syndrome (e.g., resting bradycardia, sinus arrhythmia, and AV conduction delay) are generally attributed to changes in the sympathetic nervous system with enhanced parasympathetic tone and reduced sympathetic tone. Of these two factors, enhanced parasympathetic tone is most important (13). These alterations in the sympathetic nervous system control are unlikely to be the entire explanation, however. The resting heart rates of endurance athletes remain lower than those of sedentary subjects, even after sympathetic nervous system control is theoretically eliminated in both groups with large doses of atropine and beta-adrenergic blockade; these circumstances suggest that other factors such as larger cardiac dimensions also contribute to the reduced heart rate (14,15). Similarly, athletes may demonstrate ST–T-wave

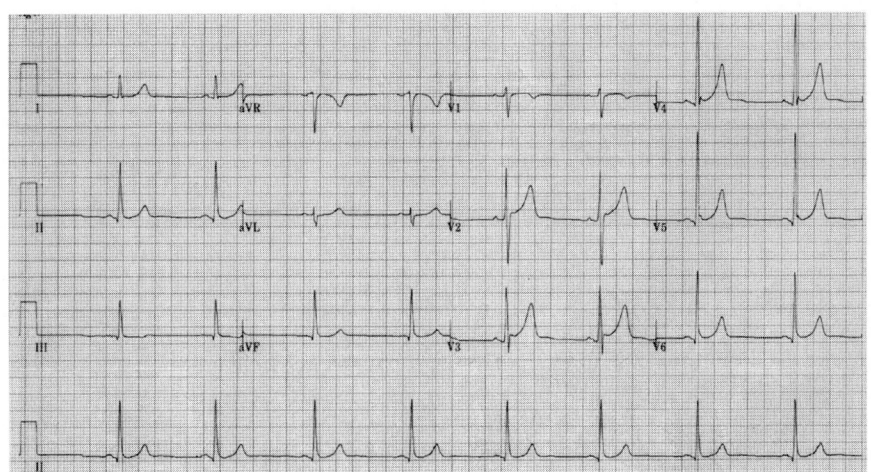

FIGURE 37.1 Electrocardiogram from a 53-year-old physician who has run a minimum of 60 km weekly for 40 years. The axis is 70 degrees—somewhat unusual in a healthy individual in this age group—and there is ST elevation of early repolarization in leads V_3–V_6.

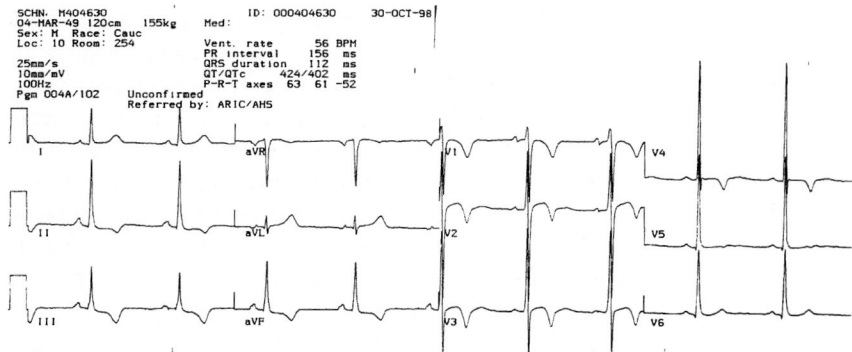

SCHN. M404630
04-MAR-49 120cm 155kg   Med:
Sex: M Race: Cauc
Loc: 10 Room: 254

ID: 000404630   30-OCT-98

Vent. rate   56 BPM
PR interval   156 ms
QRS duration   112 ms
QT/QTc   424/402 ms
P-R-T axes   63 61 -52

25mm/s
10mm/mV
100Hz
Pgm 004A/102   Unconfirmed
               Referred by: ARIC/AHS

FIGURE 37.2 Electrocardiogram (ECG) from a 49-year-old white physician showing diffuse T-wave inversions. He had run 58 to 108 km weekly and ridden a bicycle 32 km weekly for 20 years. The ECG was obtained when he volunteered for a study of healthy subjects. An echocardiogram showed left ventricular (LV) internal dimensions at end diastole and systole of 50 mm and 20 mm, respectively, and LV posterior and septal wall thickness of 12 mm each. He was not restricted from athletic competition.

changes of early repolarization and T inversions, which are also attributed to sympathetic nervous system alterations (Figs. 37.1 and 37.2). Some of the T-wave changes can be quite bizarre and may be similar to changes seen with conditions known to affect the parasympathetic nervous system, such as subarachnoid hemorrhage.

Nevertheless, not all extreme T-wave abnormalities in athletes are due to athletic heart syndrome. For example, among 26 Spanish athletes evaluated for negative T waves ≥2 mm, four were found to have HCM (16) (eFig. 37.2.1). Many of the changes typical of athletic heart syndrome (e.g., sinus arrhythmia and the ST changes of early repolarization) are also characteristic of young, healthy individuals, but they are more marked or more frequent in athletes and may persist into middle age among physically active subjects. All of these abnormalities in sinus rate, AV conduction, and the ST changes of early repolarization should resolve with exercise with its attendant withdrawal of vagal tone and increased sympathetic activity. This is not always true for marked T-wave inversions (16), however, so their failure to resolve does not necessarily imply a pathologic process.

Sinus Bradycardia

$\dot{V}O_2$max and maximal cardiac output are increased in endurance athletes, but there is little change in resting oxygen con-

sumption or cardiac output. Consequently, the larger resting stroke volume characteristic of endurance athletes permits a reduction in resting heart rate. Sinus bradycardia, generally defined as a heart rate <60 beats/min, is typical of athletic heart syndrome and reported in up to 91% of endurance athletes (17). Bradycardia in athletes can be profound, and a rate of 25 beats/min has been reported in one distance runner (18). In addition to sinus bradycardia, sinus pauses or "sinus arrest" of >2 seconds have been documented during sleep in endurance athletes (17) (Fig. 37.3).

Sinus Arrhythmia

Sinus arrhythmia refers to variation in sinus rate with respiration. Specifically, the sinus rate decreases slightly at the start of the expiratory phase of the respiratory cycle. Sinus arrhythmia is common in young, healthy subjects, but it is more marked in endurance athletes.

Atrioventricular Conduction Delay

First degree AV block, defined as a PR interval of >0.20 seconds, is reported in 10% to 33% of endurance athletes (19). Second degree AV block of the Mobitz I or Wenckebach pattern is characterized by progressive prolongation of the PR interval before a nonconducted P wave and is also

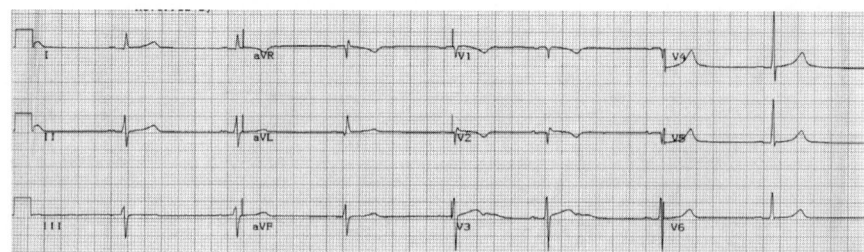

FIGURE 37.3 Electrocardiogram from a 36-year-old physician showing marked bradycardia of 46 beats/min, voltage criteria for left ventricular (LV) hypertrophy (note the ½ standard calibration), and a prolonged QT interval in lead V3. He was 180 cm (5'10") tall and weighed 67 kg (147 lb). He had played college lightweight American football and rowed in lightweight crew. Over the past 5 years, he had run 100 to 130 km weekly and competed in 42-km foot races. He was asymptomatic and had no family history of cardiac complications. His echocardiogram showed LV internal dimensions at end diastole and systole to be 54 and 37 mm, respectively. The LV posterior wall thickness was 10 mm, and the septal thickness was 11 mm. He was not restricted from athletic participation, despite the QT interval, because he was totally asymptomatic.

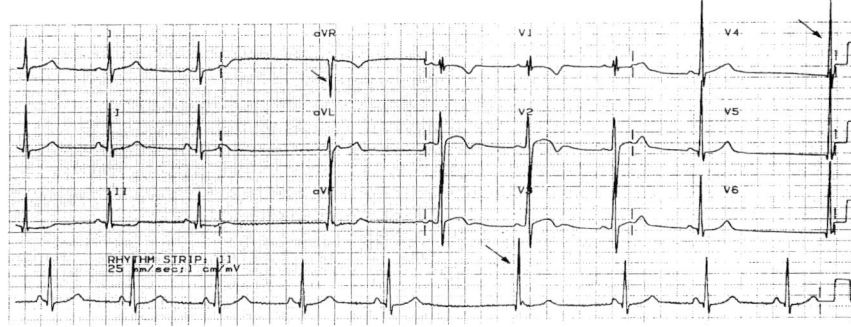

FIGURE 37.4 Electrocardiogram (ECG) from a 28-year-old man who had run 42 km in 2 hours and 17 minutes. He was evaluated for momentary chest discomfort felt in 1984, several days after the death of James Fixx, the author of *The Complete Book of Running*. The ECG shows an axis of 110 degrees, incomplete right bundle branch block, sinus pauses with junction "escape" beats (*arrows*), slight P-wave enlargement in lead II, increased precordial voltage, and biphasic T waves in V₂ and V₃. He was otherwise asymptomatic, had a normal echocardiogram, and was treated with reassurance. (Reproduced from Thompson PD. Cardiac evaluation of the young or old, competitive or recreational athlete. In: Strauss RH. *Sports medicine*, 2nd ed. Philadelphia: WB Saunders, 1991, with permission.)

seen more commonly in the athletic heart syndrome (19). Second degree AV block with Mobitz II appearance is characterized by a nonconducted P wave without preceding PR prolongation, but it is not typical of the athletic heart syndrome. Mobitz II block typically occurs at the level of the His-Purkinje system, whereas Mobitz I block is due to progressive slowing of conduction in the AV node. An AV block with Mobitz II appearance may occur in well-trained athletes due to enhanced vagal tone, but this is rare (17) (Fig. 37.4 and *e*Fig. 37.4.1). The presence of Mobitz II block should prompt a search for other causes and should be attributed to athletic training only if the athlete is asymptomatic and no other abnormalities are detected.

The prolongation of the AV interval and decrease in AV conduction velocity previously described may also unmask ventricular preexcitation—also known as Wolff-Parkinson-White (WPW) syndrome—when accompanied by symptomatic arrhythmia. Indeed, a WPW conduction pattern is more common in endurance athletes (19). Cardiologists should be cognizant of this fact when evaluating athletes for an asymptomatic WPW conduction pattern, because the risk of sudden death in asymptomatic subjects with this abnormality is low.

Vasovagal Syncope

Vasovagal syncope appears to occur more frequently in endurance-trained individuals because it is related, in part, to these athletes' enhanced vagal tone. Lower-body negative pressure is a research technique used to examine blood pressure control and an individual's response to orthostatic stress. Compared to nonathletes and strength-trained athletes, endurance-trained individuals have a reduced ability to maintain blood pressure during lower-body negative pressure (20). The clinical implications of this reduced ability are that endurance-trained individuals are more vulnera-

ble to vasovagal syncope or simple fainting and that positive tilt-table responses are almost the norm in well-trained endurance athletes. These athletes have a large venous capacity, enhanced vagal tone, and reduced sympathetic tone—all of which make them vulnerable to postural hypotension and a positive tilt-table response. Tilt-table results should not be interpreted as an adequate explanation for syncope in athletes, therefore, unless the clinical situation also strongly supports this explanation.

Electrocardiographic ST–T-Wave Changes

ST elevation of the early repolarization pattern is so common in endurance-trained athletes that it should be considered the norm rather than the exception. Persistent training into advanced age can preserve this pattern in older athletes. ST depression, in contrast, is rare and should prompt a search for other causes. Peaked, biphasic, and inverted T waves in the precordial leads are frequently seen in endurance athletes. The biphasic T waves typically occur in the precordial "transition" leads, where the QRS complex is changing from a primarily negative deflection in the right precordial leads to a primarily positive deflection in the left-sided leads. Deeply inverted T waves can also be normal in athletes, but they are rare and require the exclusion of significant disease (16). Of 952 healthy, Italian, national-caliber athletes, only 27 had marked T-wave inversions. Three-hundred seventy-five had abnormal or mildly abnormal electrocardiograms (ECGs), suggesting HCM in 11 and arrhythmogenic right ventricular cardiomyopathy in 16. Only one of these athletes actually had HCM, however (21).

Evidence of Cardiac Enlargement

Habitual endurance exercise produces a global cardiac enlargement that may affect the atria and ventricles. The

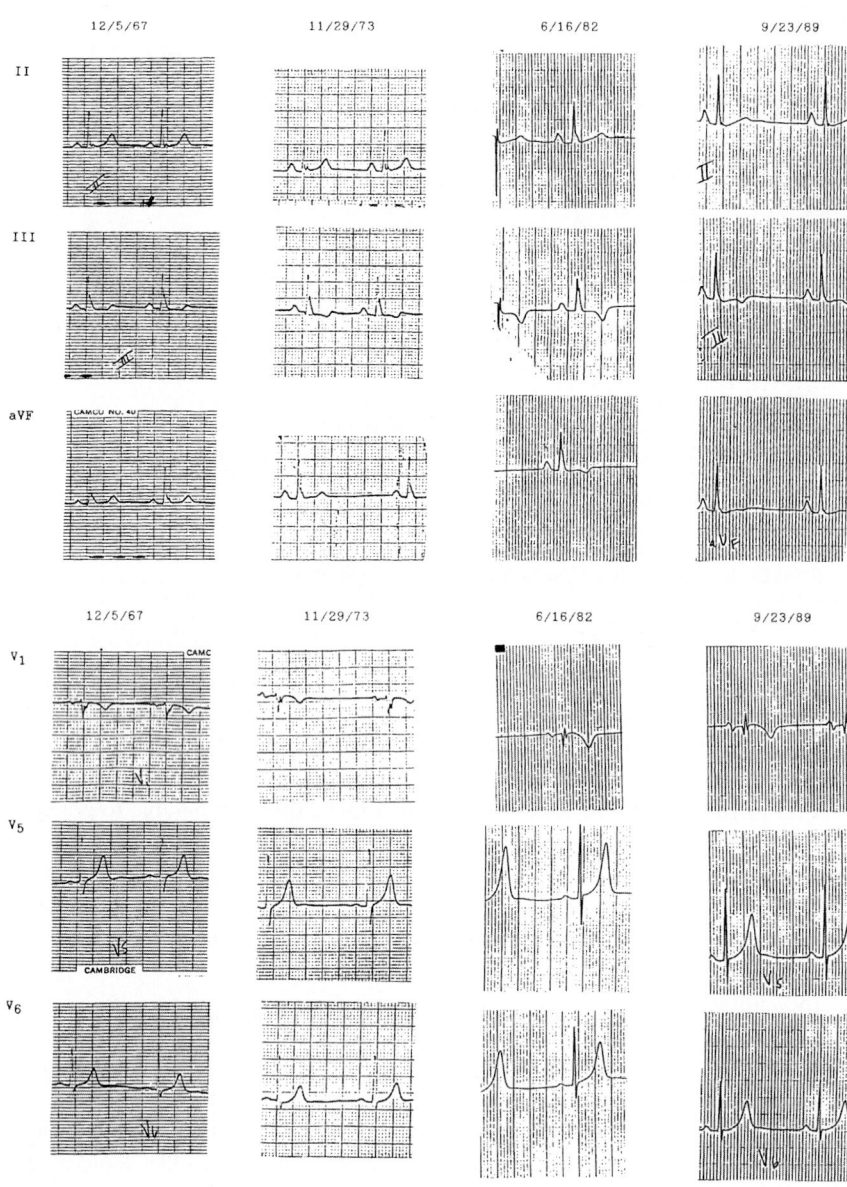

FIGURE 37.5 Selected leads from the serial electrocardiograms (ECGs) of a 42-year-old physician who began running in the late 1960s and progressed to running multiple 42-km foot races. The tracings show the development of the classic ECG of the athletic heart syndrome, including increased P-wave height (lead II), increased P-wave negativity (V$_1$), increased right-sided R wave (V$_1$), increased precordial voltage (V$_5$ and V$_6$). These developments suggest right and left atrial and ventricular enlargement, respectively. There are also progressive T-wave changes with increased precordial T waves (V$_5$ and V$_6$) and increasing negative T waves in the inferior leads (III and aVF). The presence of all of these findings in a single ECG is unusual, even among well-trained, elite athletes. This individual remains healthy in his mid-50s.

most consistent enlargement is seen in the LV chambers, where intracavity dimensions and, rarely, wall thickness, can be large enough to raise the suspicion of cardiac disease. Mild enlargement of both atria and the right ventricle can occur, but marked enlargement of these structures is suggestive of a disease process and is not observed in the athletic heart syndrome.

Electrocardiographic Evidence of Chamber Enlargement

The ECG in well-trained athletes may show mildly increased P-wave amplitude that suggests right atrial enlargement, P-wave notching that suggests left atrial enlargement, incomplete right bundle branch block

(IRBBB), and voltage criteria for right ventricular and LV hypertrophy (17) (Fig. 37.5).

Among endurance athletes, voltage criteria for right ventricular hypertrophy are noted in 18% to 69% of subjects (19). This ECG evidence for atrial and right ventricular enlargement does not usually suggest extreme enlargement, so marked evidence of atrial or right ventricular enlargement should prompt a search for pathologic causes. Similarly, although IRBBB is common, complete heart block generally is not accepted as part of the athletic heart syndrome (17).

In contrast to ECG evidence of atrial and right ventricular enlargement, the voltage criteria for LV hypertrophy can be extreme in endurance athletes (*e*Fig. 37.5.1). QRS voltage is greater in endurance athletes than in other subjects, even after adjusting for LV mass, suggesting that some of the extreme voltage seen in endurance-trained subjects is due to thinner chest walls (4).

Echocardiographic Evidence of Cardiac Enlargement

Echocardiography frequently is performed in evaluating symptoms in athletes, so it is important for clinicians to know the limits of cardiac enlargement produced by exercise training.

Thomas and Douglas have recently summarized the topic of echocardiographic dimensions in athletes (3). At least 59 studies have used echocardiography to examine cardiac dimensions in athletes (3). These studies consistently documented increased LV dimensions. Thirteen studies comparing right ventricular dimensions in athletes and controls demonstrated that the right ventricular transverse dimension was increased an average of 24% in the athletes (22 mm vs. 17 mm) (3). Fourteen studies comparing the left atria of athletes and controls demonstrated that the transverse dimension was 16% larger in the athletes. To our knowledge, only one study has documented a larger right atrial size in the athletes (3).

Pelliccia and colleagues have explored the upper limits of echocardiographic dimensions in athletes using data obtained in studies of Italian national athletes at the Institute of Sports Science in Rome. These authors examined LV wall thickness in 947 athletes, 209 of whom were women (22). Only 16 athletes (1.7%) had an LV wall thickness >12 mm, the upper limit of normal. Fifteen of these athletes participated in rowing or canoeing, sports that require isotonic and isometric effort and involve a large muscle mass. These 15 athletes represented 7% of the rowers and canoeists studied. The only other athlete with increased wall thickness was a cyclist. All athletes with increased wall dimensions had won medals in international competition. The largest wall thickness in any athlete was 16 mm. All of the female athletes had wall thicknesses less than 11 mm.

Six of the athletes with marked LV wall enlargement discontinued exercise training and were restudied after 40 to 240 (average = 90) days of reduced activity. Average wall thickness decreased from 12.8 ± 0.9 mm to 10.5 ± 0.4 mm, *p* <.05. Three of the athletes—none of whom had increased wall thickness—had localized apical hypertrophy suggestive of apical HCM, but none of these subjects had the marked apical T-wave abnormalities characteristic of this condition. All of the athletes with increased wall thickness also had increased cavity dimensions, which suggests that the increase in wall thickness in these subjects is an adaptation to maintain normal wall stress.

These results are extremely useful in differentiating the athletic heart syndrome from HCM. LV wall thickness >12 mm was unusual, even in elite athletes. Consequently, the presence of increased wall thickness in recreational or elite athletes should prompt a search for pathologic causes. No athlete had an LV wall thickness >16 mm, and values above this range should raise the possibility of HCM. Wall hypertrophy above the normal range was not observed in female athletes. All athletes with wall hypertrophy also demonstrated increased cavity dimensions, which are not seen in HCM or in other diseases with pathologic wall thickening. Finally, wall thickening in high-caliber athletes should regress with detraining.

In another study, Pelliccia et al. examined LV cavity dimensions in 1,300 elite athletes participating in 38 different sports (23). The LV end-diastolic diameter (LVEDD) was greater in male (55 mm) than in female (48 mm) athletes. The LVEDD was >55 mm (i.e., the upper limits of normal) in 45% of the athletes and exceeded 60 mm in 14% of the subjects. The largest cardiac dimensions by gender were 66 mm for a female athlete and 70 mm for a male athlete. Regression analysis demonstrated that body surface area (r = 0.76), heart rate (r = −0.37), and age (r = 0.29) correlated with the LVEDD, indicating that these three variables accounted for 60% of the variability in the LVEDD. Adding gender and the type of sport to these factors accounted for 72% of the variability. Age may function in this group as a surrogate for the duration of training, but this is not certain because age did not differ between athletes whose LVEDD was >60 mm or <60 mm. The sports that were most associated with an LVEDD ≥60 mm were cycling (49% of cycling athletes), ice hockey (42%), basketball (40%), rugby (39%), canoeing (39%), and rowing (34%). All are sports that require a large endurance component or a combination of moderate endurance training and increased body size. Systolic and diastolic function were normal in the athletes. Once again, few athletes had evidence of LV wall hypertrophy. Only 14 of the athletes (1.1%) had a septal thickness >12 mm, and only four athletes (0.3%) exceeded this posterior wall thickness. Wall thickness among all of the athletes correlated with cavity dimensions. Athletes with increased cavity dimensions also tended to have larger left atrial and aortic root dimensions. ❧ h55

Functional Cardiac Murmurs in Athletes

Both young and old endurance athletes often have functional cardiac murmurs created by cardiac adaptations to exercise training. Blood flow is laminar and without turbulence until a critical Reynolds number (Re) is exceeded. Re is determined by the following formula:

$$Re = \frac{\text{average velocity} \times \text{tube diameter} \times \text{fluid density}}{\text{fluid viscosity}}$$

Laminar flow is disrupted above an Re of 2,000, creating turbulence and murmurs. As previously discussed, endurance exercise training reduces resting heart rate, increases resting stroke volume, and enhances cardiac performance. Training does not change resting cardiac output, which is delivered via a slower heart rate and a larger stroke volume. Much of the larger stroke volume is delivered more vigorously in early systole by a more dynamic ventricle. This delivery increases blood velocity. The pulmonic and aortic valve orifices do not increase with exercise training, so the increased blood velocity produces early systolic "flow murmurs." Such flow murmurs in young athletes are due to flow across the pulmonic valve and often vary with respiration. Athletes aged 50 years and older may have mild sclerosis of the aortic valve leaflets, and their flow murmurs are often due to aortic valve sclerosis and the turbulence mentioned above. These murmurs are less "innocent" because they may progress to important aortic stenosis, especially in athletes with other risk factors for atherosclerosis such as hypercholesterolemia (26,27). Treatment of these risk factors may reduce the development of important aortic stenosis, but this has not been studied. Nevertheless, we often recommend 3-hydroxy-3-methylglutaryl coenzyme A (HMG CoA) reductase inhibitors in adult patients with noncritical aortic stenosis in the hope of preventing such progression.

EXERCISE-RELATED CARDIAC EVENTS

Clinicians are often required to differentiate the athletic heart syndrome from life-threatening cardiac disease and to make recommendations about the risks of exercise in individuals with diagnosed abnormalities. This section discusses the risks of exercise and the conditions associated with exercise-related cardiac events. There is little doubt that vigorous physical exertion increases the risk of cardiac events in children and adults with cardiovascular abnormalities. This increased risk of exertion has been quantified and documented conclusively only in adults in whom the risk of sudden death (28,29) and acute myocardial infarction (30–32) is increased by exercise. The data are less definitive in children, but the clinical association of exertion and sudden death in children with a variety of congenital and acquired cardiac diseases leaves little doubt that exercise has a provocative role in these events.

Pathology of Exertion-Related Cardiac Events

In contrast to the findings in adults, [▼ h56] atherosclerotic coronary artery disease is a rare cause of exercise-related deaths in younger subjects. The conditions associated with exercise-related sudden death in young athletes has been presented by Van Camp et al. with data from the National Center for Catastrophic Sports Injury Research (37). These authors examined 136 deaths in American athletes that occurred during or within 1 hour of sports participation.

TABLE 37.1 CARDIAC CAUSES OF DEATH IN HIGH SCHOOL AND COLLEGE ATHLETES[a] (n = 100)

	Men	Women
Hypertrophic cardiomyopathy[b]	50	1
Probable hypertrophic cardiomyopathy	5	0
Coronary artery anomalies[c]	11	2
Myocarditis	7	—
Aortic stenosis	6	—
Cardiomyopathy	6	—
Atherosclerotic coronary disease	2	1
Aortic rupture	2	—
Subaortic stenosis	2	—
Coronary aneurysm	—	1
Mitral prolapse	1	—
Right ventricular dysplasia	—	1
Cerebral arteriovenous malformation	—	1
Subarachnoid hemorrhage	—	1

[a]Adapted from Van Camp SP, Bloor CM, Mueller FO, et al. Nontraumatic sports death in high school and college athletes. *Med Sci Sports Exerc* 1995;27:641–647; and reproduced from Thompson PD. The cardiovascular risks of exercise. In: Thompson PD, ed. *Exercise and sports cardiology.* New York: McGraw-Hill, 2000, with permission.
[b]Three subjects also had coronary anomalies; one subject had Wolff-Parkinson-White syndrome.
[c]This category includes anomalous left coronary artery (LCA) from right sinus of Valsalva (n = 4); intramural left anterior descending (n = 4); anomalous LCA from pulmonary artery (n = 2); anomalous right coronary artery (RCA) from left sinus (n = 2); hypoplastic RCA (n = 2); and ostial ridge of the LCA (n = 2). Three subjects with coronary anomalies also had hypertrophic cardiomyopathy and are tabulated with that group.

Cardiac conditions were associated with 100 deaths, including HCM (50% of the cases), coronary artery anomalies (13%), myocarditis (7%), aortic stenosis (6%), and dilated cardiomyopathy (6%) (Table 37.1). The coronary artery anomalies included anomalous origin, intramyocardial course, and an ostial ridge at the coronary origin. Some coronary anomalies, such as an acute take-off of the artery from the aorta (41), may be overlooked or unappreciated during autopsy. Only one case was attributed to right ventricular dysplasia, contrasting with the findings in Italian subjects, as previously discussed. Other investigators have presented similar data for American athletes (42). ▼ h57

There are several clinically important lessons to learn from these pathologic studies of exercise-related events. Several of the conditions identified at autopsy could have been detected before death. These conditions include valvular and subvalvular aortic stenosis, Marfan syndrome as a cause of aortic rupture, and possibly HCM, although a murmur in the later condition is detected in only 25% of cases. Few of the victims were women, which is consistent with other observations that women are protected, to some extent, from sudden death (46).

Incidence of Exercise-Related Cardiac Event

Although vigorous exertion acutely increases the risk of sudden death during exercise for individuals with known or occult cardiac disease, it is important for clinicians to remember that the absolute risk of a cardiac event during exercise is extremely low. The estimated annual incidence of exercise-related deaths among high school and college athletes is only one death per 133,000 men and 769,000 women, respectively (37). These estimates include 36 noncardiac deaths and thereby overestimate the cardiac risks of athletic competition. The death rate is higher among college men than high school men (1.45 vs. 0.66 events per 100,000) for unclear reasons, but it may be related to cardiac size because cardiac size itself is a risk factor for cardiac death (47,48), and more mature athletes should have larger hearts. These reports do not provide any information on how many individuals with cardiac conditions were prohibited from participating in sports and thereby escaped an exercise-related complication.

The risk of exercise-related sudden death is considerably higher in adults because of the increased prevalence of coronary disease, but it has been estimated that there is only one death per year for every 15,000 to 18,000 asymptomatic middle-aged men (28,29). Published studies on adults have wide confidence limits, however, because they are based on few subjects. Using the 95% confidence limits from a study done in Rhode Island, the death rate may vary from one death per year for every 4,000 to 26,000 asymptomatic men (28).

PREPARTICIPATION SCREENING OF COMPETITIVE ATHLETES

There is ongoing debate about the value of screening competitive athletes and the extent to which such screening should go. It is critically important that cardiologists know the issues involved, because they are frequently asked to evaluate athletes with possible abnormalities detected during screening. Often, these abnormalities are bradycardia or functional murmurs and are of no significance, but on rare occasions, a completely asymptomatic athlete with a major cardiac abnormality is identified.

The American Heart Association has issued a medical and scientific statement on the cardiovascular preparticipation screening of competitive athletes (49). This document recommends a personal and family history and a physical examination before high school participation in sports, with the examination repeated at least every 4 years. This statement does not advocate routine echo- or electrocardiography. ❦ h58

Cardiac Examination of Competitive Athletes

The components of the cardiovascular examination are detailed elsewhere in this text, and a consensus statement on the components of the preparticipation cardiac exami-

nation has been published (49). The following section emphasizes clinical principles useful when examining athletes as part of a preparticipation examination or when evaluating athletes for suspected cardiac abnormalities.

Preparticipation Screening of Athletes

The preparticipation screening of athletes should include an inquiry about (a) exertional symptoms including chest discomfort, syncope, dyspnea, and fatigue; (b) a history of cardiac murmurs, hypertension or cardiac diagnoses; and (c) a family history of sudden death or of any of the conditions known to be associated with sudden death (49). The physical examination should include brachial artery blood pressure measurement, precordial auscultation with the athlete supine and standing, simultaneous palpation of the radial and femoral pulses to exclude coarctation, and an assessment for stigmata of Marfan syndrome.

Examining Athletes for Suspected Disease

The examination of athletes for suspected cardiac disease should be considerably more detailed than the preparticipation examination. Even with modern diagnostic techniques, the cardiac evaluation remains an important part of evaluating athletes. The severity of valvular lesions, for example, can be over- or underestimated by echocardiography, cardiac catheterization, and the physical examination. The best decisions are made when the results of several examination techniques are compared for agreement or discrepancies and the cardiologist does not rely on clinical, echocardiographic, or catheterization data alone. We have seen multiple athletes with clinical symptoms and physical examination findings of severe aortic stenosis that were not repaired because the catheterization data did not indicate a "critical" valve area. Mild, moderate, and severe aortic stenosis are classified as a calculated aortic valve area >1.5 cm^2, 1.0 to 1.5 cm^2, and <1.0 cm^2, respectively, but these values are not normalized for body surface area (53) and may severely underestimate the severity of the stenosis in large individuals. ❦ h59

CONTROVERSIES AND PERSONAL PERSPECTIVES

Our perspective on the athletic heart syndrome is indeed personal. One of us (P. D. T.) started training for competitive distance running events at age 12 and ultimately qualified for the 1972 U.S. Olympic Marathon Trials as a medical student. However, during the first year of medical school, he had a murmur detected during a demonstration of cardiac auscultation. His subsequent ECG showed marked LV hypertrophy and early repolarization changes, prompting an interest in cardiology and the medical prob-

THE FUTURE

The future of research and treatment of athletic heart syndrome, as with many aspects of medicine, will be greatly influenced by the revolution in genetic medicine. Molecular biologic approaches have already led to an understanding of the genetic basis for a number of cardiovascular conditions associated with cardiovascular complications during exercise. The genetic basis for HCM, arrhythmogenic right ventricular cardiomyopathy and the closely related Naxos disease, congenital long-QT syndromes, idiopathic ventricular fibrillation, familial atrial fibrillation, and familial dilated cardiomyopathy have all been partially elucidated. There will be an ongoing evolution of molecular biologic techniques and their application to the prediction, prevention, and treatment of cardiovascular disease. We foresee at least three ways in which this evolution may influence the cardiac care of athletes.

First, genetics will likely be used to predict which individuals with a disease phenotype are at risk for an exercise-related complication. HCM is the leading cause of exercise-related deaths among American athletes, and those with this condition are routinely restricted from athletic competition. There are reports, however, of athletes who have had successful athletic careers despite presence of the disease (58). Among the nonathletic population with HCM, those genetic mutations associated with a change in the electrical charge of their encoded amino acid in the myosin heavy chain appear to be associated with the greatest cardiac risk (59). Consequently, it may eventually be possible to predict by genetic analysis which athletes are or are not at risk of exercise-related events. Before such techniques can be used clinically, however, there will need to be widespread availability of the testing methods that are now available only for research, as well as careful clinical studies to determine the ability of genetic analysis to predict prognosis.

Second, genetics will be increasingly used to diagnose disease and may ultimately have a role in the preparticipation screening of athletes. This possibility is illustrated by the case report of a physically active 19-year-old woman who died after a near drowning. Molecular genetic screening of a sample of the deceased's myocardium demonstrated a novel genetic mutation of the long-QT 1 locus. The woman's 18-year-old sister had a similar mutation and was counseled about the risks of strenuous exercise, as well as the potential benefits of beta-adrenergic blockage (44).

Third, genetic analysis may help differentiate disease from normal physiologic adaptations to physical training. Some athletes appear to experience especially large changes in cardiac dimensions with endurance training. This response is influenced by genetic variants. The angiotensin-converting enzyme gene has two common variants. One variant, referred to as the *D*, or *deletion allele*, has a 287–base pair deletion and is associated with higher angiotensin-converting enzyme blood levels than the I or insertion allele. Among military recruits subjected to 10 weeks of intense physical training, echocardiographic changes in LV mass and ECG evidence of LV hypertrophy were greatest in individuals with the D allele (60). Additional genetic factors influencing the cardiac response to exercise training will undoubtedly be found. Knowledge of such variants may ultimately help in separating athletes with an excessive physiologic response to training from individuals with HCM.

---

lems of endurance athletes. The other author (N. A. M. E. III) developed his interest in athletic heart syndrome in part from his experiences as a secondary school and collegiate athlete. We have had the privilege of providing advice and medical care to hundreds of competitive athletes, including two medalists in the Olympic Marathon. The opportunity to combine our personal interest in athletics with our professions as cardiologists has enriched our academic careers.

In evaluating athletes for cardiac abnormalities, we make a strong distinction between abnormalities discovered during screening examinations and those discovered during the evaluation of symptoms. Most screening examinations do not detect real disease, but they do detect a high frequency of normal variants common in young, healthy subjects and part of the athletic heart syndrome. In our experience, physicians frequently overreact to mild abnormalities detected during screening because of legal concerns and the lack of appreciation for the magnitude of changes that can be produced by extreme endurance exercise.

On the other hand, symptomatic athletes require a thorough examination. We are repeatedly impressed with the number of well-known athletes who die during exercise after having presented with symptoms that were ignored or inadequately evaluated. Excluding important cardiac disease in symptomatic athletes may be the most efficient way to prevent exercise-related complications.

In evaluating symptoms, it is extremely important to evaluate any possible cardiovascular disease in the context of the athlete's total physical and psychological situation.

Many young, competitive athletes face enormous pressure from coaches, parents, and peers. Failure to achieve the desired level of success is extremely stressful on competitors at any age. Young athletes who present with fainting, for example, may be simply seeking a medical way out of a difficult, stressful situation. It is easier to claim a medical reason for failure than to simply not be good enough. We refer to this condition as *the athletic swoon syndrome*. Typically, this condition occurs in a young athlete in an individual sport who competes well when winning but collapses dramatically when losing, often within sight of the finish line. We do not mean to minimize the importance of this problem. The athlete often needs reassurance, both medically and personally, to place winning and losing in a more healthy perspective. Athletic swoon syndrome must be differentiated from true exercise-induced syncope and long-QT syndrome. True exercise-induced syncope is a threatening symptom associated with important cardiac disease, and patients with long-QT syndrome are occasionally misdiagnosed as having hysterical syncope (57).

We strongly recommend that individuals who serve as trainers and coaches or who officiate at sporting events should learn and update yearly their cardiopulmonary resuscitation skills. We also recommend that automatic defibrillators be available in areas where athletes train and compete. Coaches and officials are often present when athletes collapse. If properly trained in resuscitation and the use of automatic defibrillators, coaches and trainers may be able to resuscitate potential victims of exercise-related sudden death. We believe that competency in these skills should be a prerequisite for physical educators, coaches, and sports officials.

REFERENCES

1. Martin DE, Benario HW, Gynn RWH. Development of the marathon from Pheidippides to the present with statistics of significant races in the marathon: physiological, medical, epidemiological, and psychological studies. *Ann N Y Acad Sci* 1977;301:820–857.
2. Rost R. The athlete's heart. Historical perspectives—solved and unsolved problems. *Cardiol Clin* 1997;15:493–512.
3. Thomas LR, Douglas PS. Echocardiographic findings in athletes. In: Thompson PD, ed. *Exercise and sports cardiology*. New York: McGraw-Hill, 2000:43–70.
4. Longhurst JC, Kelly AR, Gonyea WJ, et al. Chronic training with static and dynamic exercise: cardiovascular adaptation, and response to exercise. *Circ Res* 1981;48:I171–I178.
5. Rowell LB. *Human circulation: regulation during physical stress*. New York: Oxford University Press, 1986.
6. Ferguson CM, Myers J, Froelicher VF. Overview of exercise testing. In: Thompson PD, ed. *Exercise and sports cardiology*. New York: McGraw-Hill, 2000:71–109.
7. Amsterdam EA, Hughes JL, DeMaria AN, et al. Indirect assessment of myocardial oxygen consumption in the evaluation of mechanisms and therapy of angina pectoris. *Am J Cardiol* 1974;33:737–743.
8. Wilmore JH, Costill DL. *Physiology of sport and exercise*. Champaign, IL: Human Kinetics, 1994.
9. Gobel FL, Norstrom LA, Nelson RR, et al. The rate-pressure product as an index of myocardial oxygen consumption during exercise in patients with angina pectoris. *Circulation* 1978;57:549–556.
10. Mitchell JH, Blomqvist G. Maximal oxygen uptake. *N Engl J Med* 1971;284:1018–1022.
11. Sadaniantz A, Yurgalevitch S, Zmuda JM, et al. One year of exercise training does not alter resting ventricular systolic or diastolic function. *Med Sci Sports Exerc* 1996;28:1345–1350.
12. Brooks G, Fahey TD, White TP. *Exercise physiology: human bioenergetics and its applications*. Mountain View, CA: Mayfield Publishing Co, 1996:281–299.
13. Kenney WL. Parasympathetic control of resting heart rate: relationship to aerobic power. *Med Sci Sports Exerc* 1985;17:451–455.
14. Lewis SF, Nylander E, Gad P, et al. Non-autonomic component in bradycardia of endurance trained men at rest and during exercise. *Acta Physiol Scand* 1980;109:297–305.
15. Smith ML, Hudson DL, Graitzer HM, et al. Exercise training bradycardia: the role of autonomic balance. *Med Sci Sports Exerc* 1989;21:40–44.
16. Serra-Grima R, Estorch M, Carrio I, et al. Marked ventricular repolarization abnormalities in highly trained athletes' electrocardiograms: clinical and prognostic implications. *J Am Coll Cardiol* 2000;36:1310–1316.
17. Estes NAM III, Link MS, Homoud M, et al. Electrocardiographic variants and cardiac rhythm and conduction disturbances in the athlete. In: Thompson PD, ed. *Exercise and sports cardiology*. New York: McGraw-Hill, 2000:211–232.
18. Chapman J. Profound sinus bradycardia in the athletic heart syndrome. *J Sports Med Phys Fit* 1981;22:294–298.
19. Huston TP, Puffer JC, Rodney WM. The athletic heart syndrome. *N Engl J Med* 1985;313:24–32.
20. Smith ML, Graitzer HM, Hudson DL, et al. Baroreflex function in endurance- and static exercise-trained men. *J Appl Physiol* 1988;64:585–591.
21. Pelliccia A, Maron BJ, Culasso F, et al. Clinical significance of abnormal electrocardiographic patterns in trained athletes. *Circulation* 2000;102:278–284.
22. Pelliccia A, Maron BJ, Spataro A, et al. The upper limit of physiologic cardiac hypertrophy in highly trained elite athletes. *N Engl J Med* 1991;324:295–301.
23. Pelliccia A, Culasso F, Di Paolo FM, et al. Physiologic left ventricular cavity dilatation in elite athletes. *Ann Intern Med* 1999;130:23–31.
24. Pelliccia A, Spataro A, Caselli G, et al. Absence of left ventricular wall thickening in athletes engaged in intense power training. *Am J Cardiol* 1993;72:1048–1054.
25. Pluim BM, Zwinderman AH, van der Laarse A, et al. The athlete's heart. A meta-analysis of cardiac structure and function. *Circulation* 2000;101:336–344.
26. Stewart BF, Siscovick D, Lind BK, et al. Clinical factors associated with calcific aortic valve disease. Cardiovascular Health Study. *J Am Coll Cardiol* 1997;29:630–634.
27. Wilmshurst PT, Stevenson RN, Griffiths H, et al. A case-control investigation of the relation between hyperlipidaemia and calcific aortic valve stenosis. *Heart* 1997;78:475–479.

28. Thompson PD, Funk EJ, Carleton RA, et al. Incidence of death during jogging in Rhode Island from 1975 through 1980. *JAMA* 1982;247:2535–2538.

29. Siscovick DS, Weiss NS, Fletcher RH, et al. The incidence of primary cardiac arrest during vigorous exercise. *N Engl J Med* 1984;311:874–877.

30. Mittleman MA, Maclure M, Tofler GH, et al. Triggering of acute myocardial infarction by heavy exertion: protection against triggering by regular exercise. *N Engl J Med* 1993;329:1677–1683.

31. Willich SN, Lewis M, Lowell H, et al. Physical exertion as a trigger of acute myocardial infarction. *N Engl J Med* 1993;329:1684–1690.

32. Giri S, Thompson PD, Kiernan FJ, et al. Clinical and angiographic characteristics of exertion-related acute myocardial infarction. *JAMA* 1999;282:1731–1736.

33. Ragosta M, Crabtree J, Sturner WQ, et al. Death during recreational exercise in the state of Rhode Island. *Med Sci Sports Exerc* 1984;16:339–342.

34. Siegel RJ, French WJ, Roberts WC. Spontaneous exercise testing: running as an early unmasker of underlying cardiac amyloidosis. *Arch Intern Med* 1982;342:345.

35. Thompson PD, Klocke FJ, Levine BD, et al. 26th Bethesda conference: recommendations for determining eligibility for competition in athletes with cardiovascular abnormalities. Task Force 5: coronary artery disease. *J Am Coll Cardiol* 1994;24:888–892.

36. Maron BJ, Roberts WC, McAllister HA, et al. Sudden death in young athletes. *Circulation* 1980;62:218–229.

37. Van Camp SP, Bloor CM, Mueller FO, et al. Nontraumatic sports death in high school and college athletes. *Med Sci Sports Exerc* 1995;27:641–647.

38. Thiene G, Nava A, Corrado D, et al. Right ventricular cardiomyopathy and sudden death in young people. *N Engl J Med* 1988;318:129–133.

39. Corrado D, Basso C, Schiavon M, et al. Screening for hypertrophic cardiomyopathy in young athletes. *N Engl J Med* 1998;339:364–369.

40. McKoy G, Protonotarios N, Crosby A, et al. Identification of a deletion in plakoglobin in arrhythmogenic right ventricular cardiomyopathy with palmoplantar keratoderma and woolly hair (Naxos disease). *Lancet* 2000;355:2119–2124.

41. Virmani R, Chun PK, Goldstein RE, et al. Acute takeoffs of the coronary arteries along the aortic wall and congenital coronary ostial valve-like ridges: association with sudden death. *J Am Coll Cardiol* 1984;3:766–771.

42. Maron BJ, Shirani J, Poliac LC, et al. Sudden death in young competitive athletes. Clinical, demographic, and pathological profiles. *JAMA* 1996;276:199–204.

43. Chiang CE, Roden DM. The long QT syndromes: genetic basis and clinical implications. *J Am Coll Cardiol* 2000;36:1–12.

44. Ackerman MJ, Tester DJ, Porter CJ, et al. Molecular diagnosis of the inherited long-QT syndrome in a woman who died after near-drowning. *N Engl J Med* 1999;341:1121–1125.

45. 26th Bethesda conference: recommendations for determining eligibility for competition in athletes with cardiovascular abnormalities. *J Am Coll Cardiol* 1994;24:845–899.

46. Kannel WB, Thomas E Jr. Sudden coronary death: the Framingham Study. *Ann N Y Acad Sci* 1982;382:3–21.

47. Cooper RS, Simmons BE, Castaner A, et al. Left ventricular hypertrophy is associated with worse survival independent of ventricular function and number of coronary arteries severely narrowed. *Am J Cardiol* 1990;65:441–445.

48. Kragel AH, Roberts WC. Sudden death and cardiomegaly unassociated with coronary, valvular, congenital or specific myocardial disease. *Am J Cardiol* 1988;61:659–660.

49. Maron BJ, Thompson PD, Puffer JC, et al. Cardiovascular preparticipation screening of competitive athletes. A statement for health professionals from the Sudden Death Committee (clinical cardiology) and Congenital Cardiac Defects Committee (cardiovascular disease in the young), American Heart Association. *Circulation* 1996;94:850–856.

50. Fuller CM, McNulty CM, Spring DA, et al. Prospective screening of 5,615 high school athletes for risk of sudden cardiac death. *Med Sci Sports Exerc* 1997;29:1131–1138.

51. Elliott VS. An exercise in prevention: echocardiograms for all. *Am Med News* 2000;Nov 27:29–32.

52. Maron BJ, Gardin JM, Flack JM, et al. Prevalence of hypertrophic cardiomyopathy in a general population of young adults: echocardiographic analysis of 4111 subjects in the CARDIA study. *Circulation* 1995;92:785–789.

53. Bonow RO, Carabello B, de Leon AC Jr, et al. Guidelines for the management of patients with valvular heart disease: executive summary. A report of the American College of Cardiology/American Heart Association Task Force on Practice Guidelines (Committee on Management of Patients with Valvular Heart Disease). *Circulation* 1998;98:1949–1984.

54. Perloff JK. *The clinical recognition of congenital heart disease.* Philadelphia: WB Saunders, 1970.

55. Chatterjee K. Physical examination. In: Topol E, ed. *Textbook of cardiovascular medicine.* Philadelphia: Lippincott-Raven, 1998:307–308.

56. Herbert PN, Bernier DN, Cullinane EM, et al. High-density lipoprotein metabolism in runners and sedentary men. *JAMA* 1984;252(8):1034–1037.

57. Viskin S, Fish R, Roth A, et al. Clinical problem-solving. QT or not QT? *N Engl J Med* 2000;343:352–356.

58. Maron BJ, Klues HG. Surviving competitive athletics with hypertrophic cardiomyopathy. *Am J Cardiol* 1994;73:1098–1104.

59. Watkins H, Rosenzweig A, Hwang DS, et al. Characteristics and prognostic implications of myosin missense mutations in familial hypertrophic cardiomyopathy. *N Engl J Med* 1992;326:1108–1114.

60. Montgomery HE, Clarkson P, Dollery CM, et al. Association of angiotensin-converting enzyme gene I/D polymorphism with change in left ventricular mass in response to physical training. *Circulation* 1997;96:741–747.

38

CARDIAC TRAUMA

SAMIR R. KAPADIA
ERIC J. TOPOL

OVERVIEW

Among young people, trauma is the most common cause of death, with cardiovascular mortality being the major contributor. Patients with injury to the thorax, blunt or penetrating, should be transferred rapidly to a trauma center for fast and expert surgical evaluation. In unstable patients, echocardiography helps to identify critical injury and facilitates early surgical exploration, which can be lifesaving. In more stable patients, the goal of evaluation is to rule out significant occult cardiac and thoracic great vessel injury. Echocardiography, computed tomographic (CT) scan, thoracoscopy, and magnetic resonance imaging (MRI) can make accurate diagnosis of these injuries. Although normal electrocardiography (ECG) helps to identify low-risk patients with blunt cardiac injuries, the significance of abnormal ECG and cardiac enzyme elevation in this setting remains unclear.

S. R. Kapadia: Department of Cardiology, University of Washington School of Medicine, Seattle, Washington
E. J. Topol: Department of Cardiovascular Medicine, The Cleveland Clinic Foundation, Cleveland, Ohio

INTRODUCTION

Trauma is a leading cause of death for young adults in the United States (1), with thoracic trauma accounting for 30% to 50% of 150,000 total deaths from trauma occurring annually (2–4). The heart and thoracic great vessels are commonly involved in blunt and penetrating trauma. Most serious injuries to these vital organs are rapidly fatal. Therefore, fast transport of the patients to trauma centers, rapid recognition of injury, and expeditious expert treatment are essential for better survival.

INJURY TO THE HEART

Classification of Cardiac Injury

Physical trauma to the heart can be penetrating or blunt. A penetrating injury results when a foreign object enters the body and pierces the heart. Blunt injury, on the other hand, results from physical forces acting externally on the body. Iatrogenic injuries to the heart and great vessels from invasive procedures are not uncommon. Electrical and radiation injury are other uncommon mechanisms of cardiovascular trauma.

Penetrating Cardiac Injury

Etiology

Penetrating wounds to the heart commonly result from puncture wounds, knife wounds, and gunshot wounds (16). Puncture wounds are caused by ice picks, needles, or pellets from an air gun or a distant shotgun, typically involving a single chamber. Knife injuries also frequently involve a single chamber, producing a slit-like defect. Small-caliber gunshot wounds can cause multiple-chamber perforations along with injuries to the great vessels. In contrast, large-caliber gunshot wounds result in fatal gaping cardiac defects.

Clinical Profile

Patients presenting to the emergency room (ER) with penetrating cardiac injury may be dead on arrival, alive but hemodynamically compromised, or hemodynamically stable. A few patients that are dead on arrival can be revived with resuscitative thoracotomy in the ER. Identifying this small subgroup of patients is important to conserve resources because the yield of indiscriminate resuscitative thoracotomy is very low (less than 5%). Patients who show some signs of life on transport have up to a 30% chance of successful resuscitation (20). Patients with stab wounds compared with gunshot wounds and patients presenting with cardiac tamponade have a better chance of survival.

In the second group of patients with hemodynamic compromise, it is important to recognize cardiac tamponade. Dyspnea, diaphoresis, agitation, confusion, apathy, or a feeling of strangling oppression should alert the physician to look for cardiac tamponade (21). Only 10% to 40% of trauma victims with tamponade present with the Beck's triad of hypotension, jugular distention, and muffled heart sounds (22). Neck vein distention may be absent due to accompanying hypovolemia. Pulsus paradoxus is neither sensitive nor specific for tamponade in this situation.

The third, more stable group should be examined in detail after primary assessment of airway, breathing, and circulation. The entry site is especially important with stab wounds. An entrance wound high on the right side is likely to involve the aorta and right atrium. Lower right and left parasternal wounds involve the right ventricle, whereas inferolateral left parasternal wounds typically signify left ventricle involvement (23). In a gunshot wound, the entry site may be deceptive. If the entry site involves the "danger zone" of Suer and Mordax, which includes the precordium, epigastrium, and superior mediastinum, cardiac injury is typically present (15). Trajectory of the gunshot should also be determined. If the trajectory suggests juxtacardiac passage, the physician should keep a high index of suspicion for cardiac injury.

Management

Rapid transport of the patient to the trauma center is essential for better outcome. The so-called scoop and run policy, without an attempt to stabilize the patient in the field, is the best approach (24). Even roadside thoracotomy done by medical teams flown to the scene is without benefit (25). Intubation is beneficial for patients with cardiac arrest or hemodynamic instability (26). Closed-chest cardiopulmonary resuscitation (CPR) is not only ineffective but also contraindicated if an impaling weapon is present. An intravenous line can be started en route to the hospital, although the role of intravenous fluids is controversial (27).

For patients who are dead on arrival, a diagnostic and therapeutic procedure is an ER thoracotomy with a goal to relieve tamponade, control hemorrhage, and restore cardiac function (28). After resuscitation, the patient should be rapidly transferred to the operating room for definitive surgery.

In patients with hemodynamic compromise, rapid operating room thoracotomy by a cardiothoracic trauma surgeon appears to be the most effective. The role of ER thoracotomy has been a constant source of debate but it should be restricted to patients who arrive in a moribund state or who rapidly deteriorate after arrival (29–32). ER thoracotomy with use of staples to control cardiac bleeding and to minimize risk of personal contamination from a needle stick remains controversial (33). Staples to the heart can enlarge the wound and at times are difficult to remove during definitive surgery. Definitive surgical treatment is detailed elsewhere, but the general principles are as follows (34). Myocardial rupture is repaired in all cases. With distal coronary artery injury, ligation is sufficient. Definitive valve or shunt surgery is usually deferred until later. Approach to a foreign body is variable, but most commonly only those projecting into cavities or involving the left ventricle are removed.

In hemodynamically stable patients or those stabilized with volume, transthoracic echocardiography (TTE) should be performed rapidly to diagnose pericardial effusion (PE). PE, however small, serves as a marker for cardiac penetration (35). When compared prospectively with a surgical gold standard (subxyphoid window), echocardiography has high specificity and sensitivity in diagnosing PE (36). It has rapidly become a modality of choice to assess patients with thoracic trauma (37). However, in the presence of hemothorax, its sensitivity is significantly decreased (38). Transesophageal echocardiography (TEE) can overcome this limitation of TTE, but in many patients it either is not feasible due to other injuries or is not expeditiously available and hence is of limited usefulness (39,40). Subxyphoid pericardial window was the traditional way to rule out PE in patients with suspected penetrating wound to the heart. It is best performed in the operating room under light general anesthesia. Although it is a safe procedure and provides a definitive diagnosis of hemopericardium (41–44), it is a surgical procedure that typically results in 75% to 80% negative explorations (43). The availability of TTE in the ER has significantly

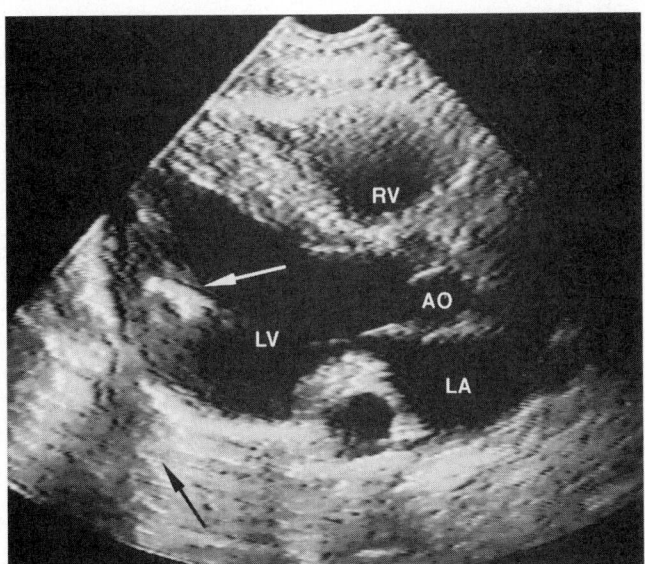

FIGURE 38.1 A transthoracic echocardiogram, a parasternal long-axis view, demonstrating a shotgun pellet (*white arrow*) in the distal posterior wall of the left ventricle. The pellet was identified years after the injury, and the patient was asymptomatic. Note how the pellet casts an acoustic shadow (*black arrow*). AO, aorta; LA, left atrium; LV, left ventricle; RV, right ventricle. (Courtesy of Dr. Carlos Antonio Da Mota Silveira and Dr. Roberto Pereira, Pernambuco University, Brazil.)

reduced the frequency of this operation, which is now used only in few difficult situations to complement echocardiography (45). Thoracoscopic pericardial window is another alternative that has been shown to be safe and effective in

diagnosing cardiac injury (46). However, echocardiography has other advantages in that it is a reliable tool to localize foreign bodies (Fig. 38.1) (47,48) and helps in diagnosing and monitoring structural abnormalities such as valvular regurgitations and shunts (Figs. 38.2 to 38.7) (49). Therefore, availability of TTE in the ER is shown to decrease time to definitive therapy, leading to a better outcome (50,51).

It is important to note that the ECG is not helpful in evaluating penetrating injury. It inconsistently shows injury pattern and if negative does not rule out significant injury (38,52). The chest x-ray may help by identifying patients with hemothorax who are difficult to image with ultrasound. But, other findings, such as an enlarged cardiac shadow or pneumopericardium, are infrequently present (53). Pericardiocentesis is not indicated for diagnosis in stable patients and can actually be harmful (54).

Blunt Cardiac Injury

In civilian life, the most common cause of blunt cardiac injury is a motor vehicular collision. Falls from heights, falling objects, direct trauma from assault, and blast injury are other less common causes. Injury patterns in motor vehicular collision are governed by the location of the individual in the vehicle and the direction of impact. In a front impact, abrupt deceleration against the steering wheel is the most common cause of cardiovascular trauma. Side impact generates a high shearing force, more commonly causing an aortic injury. Seat belts and air bags also play a major role in

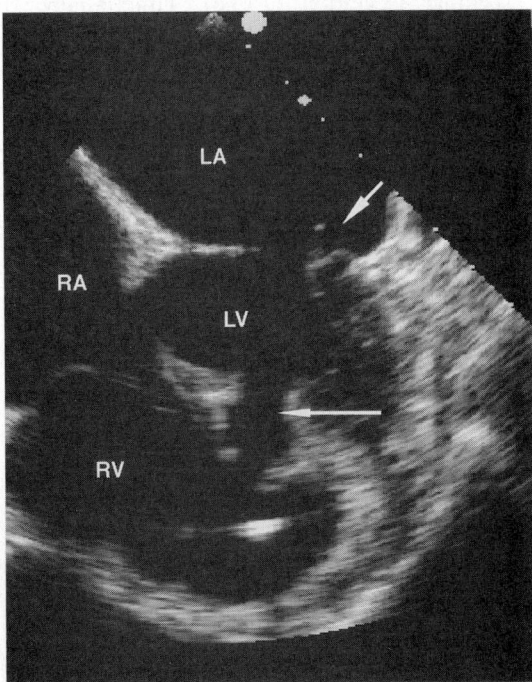
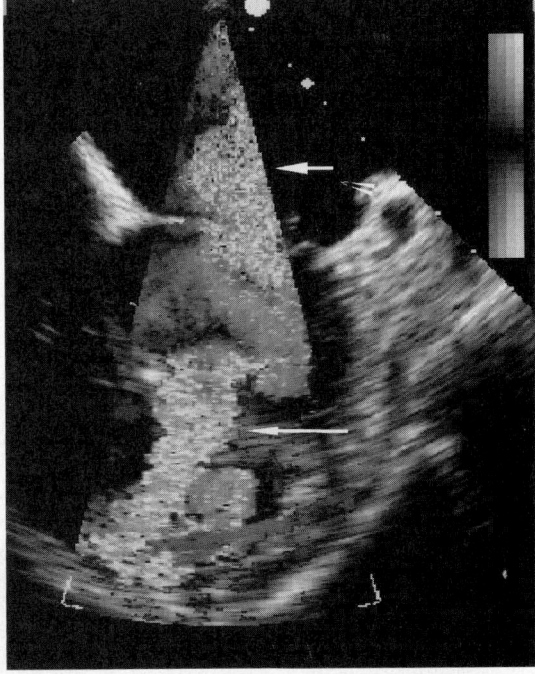

FIGURE 38.2 A transesophageal echocardiogram demonstrating a traumatic ventricular septal defect (*long arrow*) and mitral regurgitation (*short arrow*) from a gunshot wound. Swan-Ganz catheter is seen in the right ventricle (RV). LA, left atrium; LV, left ventricle; RA, right atrium. (From the DICOM demonstration DISC 96.)

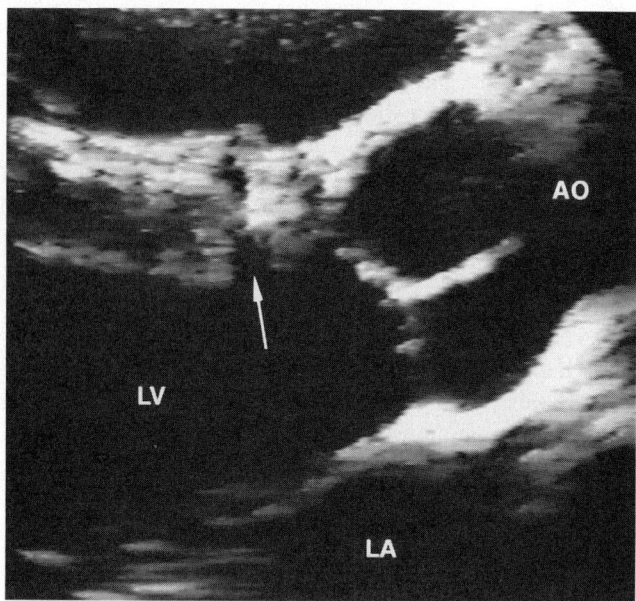

FIGURE 38.3 A transthoracic echocardiogram, a parasternal long-axis view, showing an interventricular septal defect (*arrow*) from a stab wound. This was successfully repaired. AO, aorta; LA, left atrium; LV, left ventricle. (Courtesy of Dr. Carlos Antonio Da Mota Silveira and Dr. Roberto Pereira, Pernambuco University, Brazil.)

determining the injury patterns. For unrestrained drivers, cardiac and aortic injury each occurs in approximately 20% of cases (65). Even in restrained drivers, significant thoracic injuries can still occur from contact with the steering wheel and from deceleration, but the number of deaths from thoracic injuries is significantly lower (66). The air bag has been associated with rupture of the right atrium (67).

Myocardial Contusion

Historical Perspective

Myocardial contusion was first noted by Burch in 1676 in an 8-year-old boy. In 1859, Schnabel noted hematoma

with right atrial tear in a 49-year-old man who died several hours after the blunt injury. In 1954 Burchell aptly observed "and always with heart contusion, arise both doubt and much confusion" (68). The confusion is still prevalent in literature, as myocardial contusion is a pathologic diagnosis without an accurate clinical counterpart (69). It implies a bruise to a segment of myocardium that reveals subepicardial and intramyocardial hemorrhage, disruption of myocardial fibers, cellular infiltration, and interstitial edema on histologic examination. The definition by some includes the presence of myocardial necrosis with or without bleeding into the myocardium (70). In strict pathologic terms, contusion should not include necrosis as its integral part. Therefore, *myocardial contusion* is considered a less favorable term to describe this injury pattern (71). *Commotio cordis* is a term used to describe fatal cardiac arrest without detectable structural damage to the heart as a result of blunt impact to chest (72). Various mechanisms, including ventricular fibrillation, have been proposed to explain this phenomenon (73).

Pathophysiology

Autopsy studies of patients who died of blunt cardiac injury show subendocardial and interstitial hemorrhage, large surrounding areas of focal myocardial edema, myofibrillar degeneration, myocytolysis, and infiltration with polymorphonuclear cells. In essence, it resembles myocardial infarction (MI). The few distinguishing features of blunt injury are the more abrupt demarcation between normal and abnormal, more hemorrhage, and more frequent cellular laceration (75,76). Functionally, these changes present with a decrease in myocardial contractility and cardiac output (77). Right ventricular ejection fraction is more commonly decreased, probably due to its anterior location and the acutely altered loading condition of the ventricle (78). At times, patients with mild injury present with regional wall motion abnormalities but negative chemical markers of myocardial necrosis. The term *cardiac concussion*

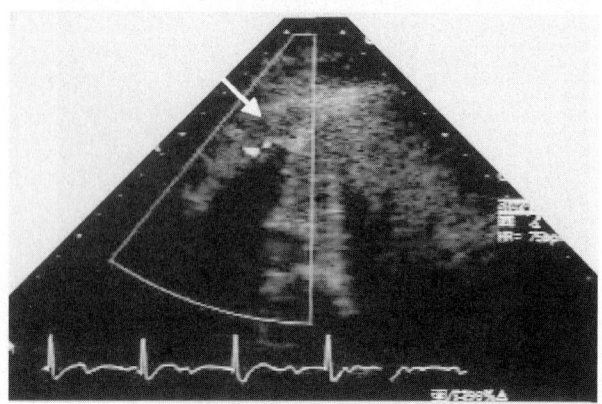
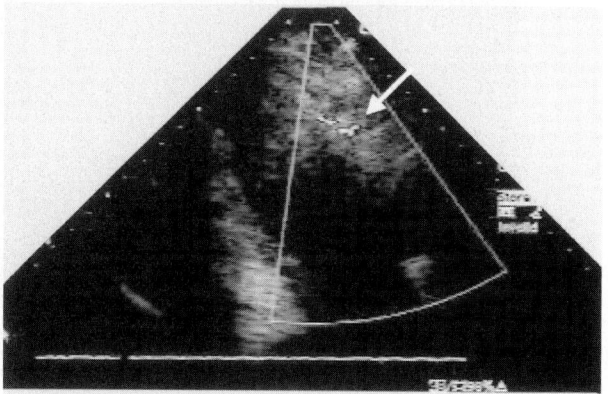

FIGURE 38.4 Patient with stab wound to the chest and right ventricle perforation. Perforation was repaired but on follow-up echocardiogram there was a very small pseudoaneurysm with some flow (*arrows*). Patient was conservatively managed without any complications.

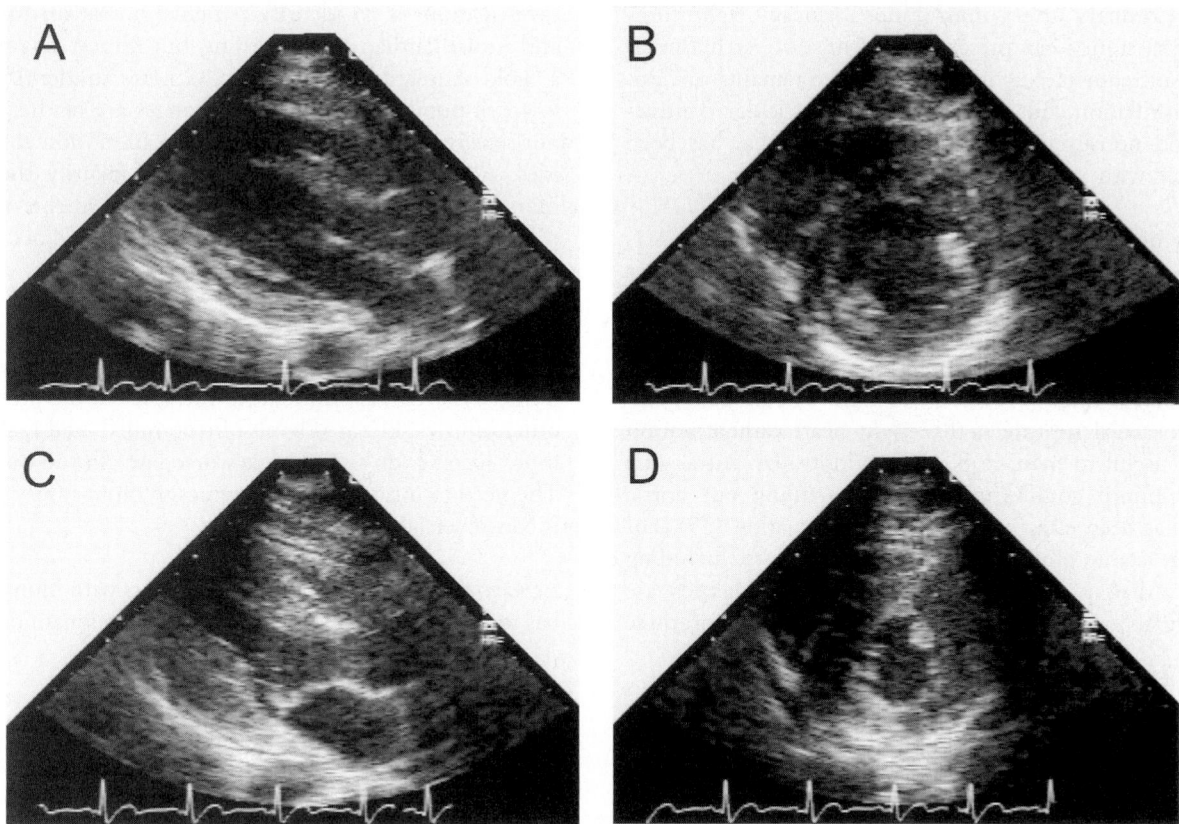

FIGURE 38.5 Patient with pneumatic staple gun injury to chest. Emergent echo in the emergency room initially did not demonstrate any pericardial effusion **(A,B)**, but while echocardiography was being performed (within 5 minutes), pericardial fluid accumulated **(C,D)**. (Courtesy of Dr. Riyad Karmy-Jones and Eric Sisk, University of Washington, Seattle.)

has been used to describe this. The mechanism is not known, but local factors that impair cardiac contractility, such as hematoma and focal inflammation, are considered to be responsible. These patients have excellent short- and long-term prognoses.

Clinical Profile

Cardiac contusion presents with a wide spectrum of severity. Patients with contusion can be hemodynamically unstable or stable. Pericardial tamponade and valvular regurgitation are important cardiac reasons for decompen-

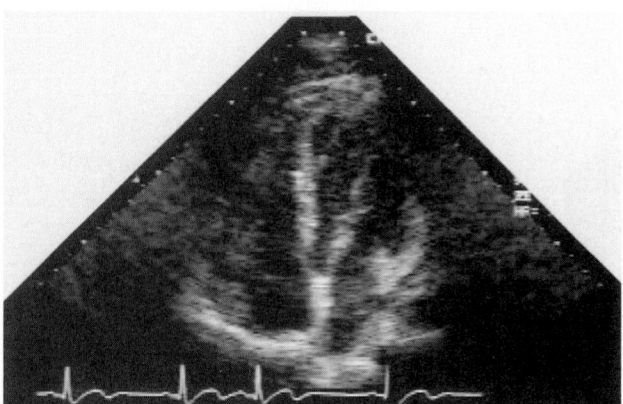
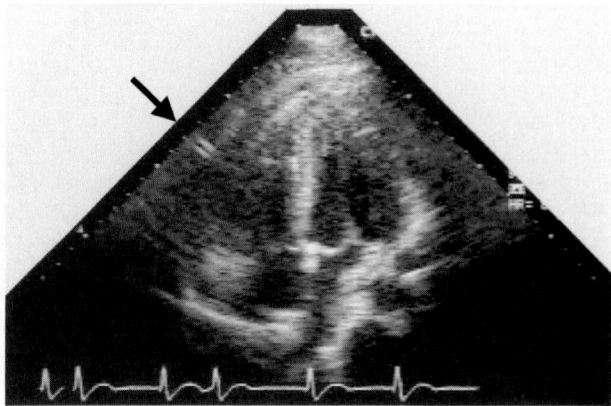

FIGURE 38.6 In the same patient, apical view showing increasing blood in the pericardium with a presence of staple in pericardium (*arrow*). Patient underwent emergent surgery. The needle was removed, and the right ventricle was successfully repaired.

sation. Coronary artery injury, most typically right coronary artery injury, can present with acute MI. Arrhythmias are not infrequent, but their significance remains unclear. Atrial fibrillation, but not premature ventricular contractions and nonsustained ventricular tachycardia, has been associated with a worse outcome (77). ❦ h76

Management

For hemodynamically unstable patients arriving after blunt chest trauma, echocardiography should be performed quickly. If echocardiography suggests a mechanical cause for hypotension, rapid appropriate surgical correction is mandatory. If there is severe ventricular dysfunction without myocardial rupture or PE, right heart catheterization may be useful to manage fluids and inotropes. Intraaortic balloon pump counterpulsation, after ruling out aortic injury, has been effectively used in this situation (79). For the more stable group, various diagnostic tests, including ECG, cardiac enzymes, and other imaging modalities, are available to quantify cardiac damage. The goal of these

investigations is to identify patients at risk of immediate and future cardiac complications, but no test is considered a "gold standard." A normal ECG helps to identify a very low-risk population, but ECG changes are neither specific nor sensitive to identify presence of wall motion abnormalities. Although echocardiography can identify these wall motion abnormalities, its role in management of stable patients after chest trauma has been questioned because the presence of wall motion abnormality does not signify a worse outcome in patients with normal ECG and enzymes (80). Cardiac enzymes, especially creatine kinase (CK) and isoenzyme of creatine kinase with muscle and brain subunits (CK-MB), are difficult to interpret in the presence of other injuries. Elevated levels of troponin T and I, although more specific, do not predict worse late clinical outcomes. The need to measure these enzymes in blunt injury patients is controversial (81,82).

Echocardiography. Approach to patients with blunt trauma has to be individualized according to hemodynamic stability

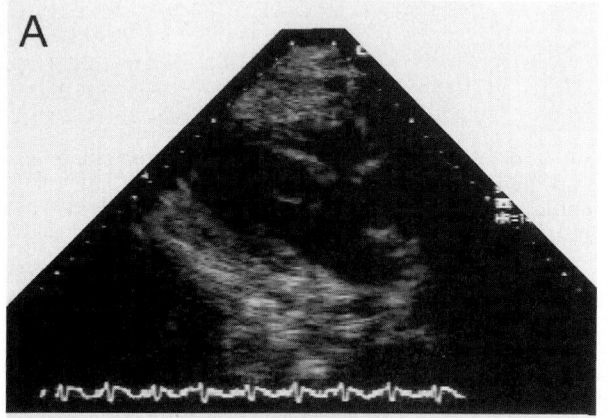

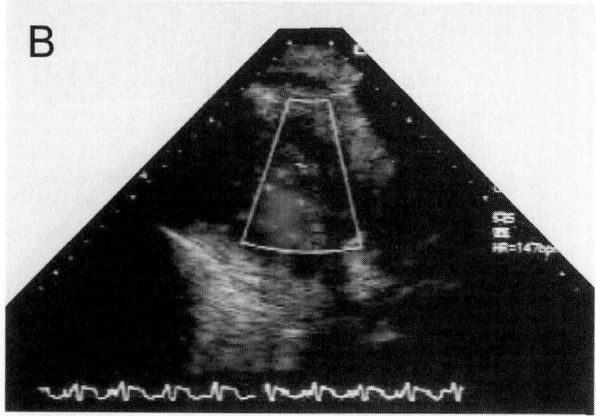

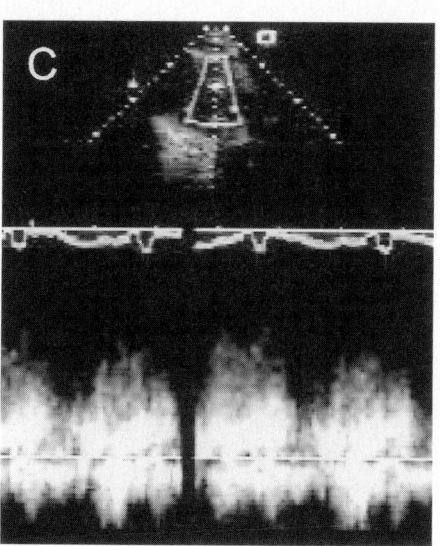

FIGURE 38.7 Patient with stab wound to chest with transsection of mid–left anterior descending artery (LAD) at the bifurcation and injury to the left ventricle. The patient had an emergency-room thoracotomy with ligation of LAD and diagonal branch. The left ventricle was successfully repaired in the operating room, and an intraaortic balloon pump was placed. There was mid and distal anteroseptal wall motion abnormality **(A)**. Abnormal flow was detected from the interventricular septum into the right ventricle **(B,C)**, which was diagnosed to be a coronary fistula (via a septal perforator) to right ventricular fistula by coronary angiography. (Courtesy of Dr. Riyad Karmy-Jones and Eric Sisk, University of Washington, Seattle.)

and other injuries. [✌ h77] In a hemodynamically stable patient, if no abnormalities are detected on initial detailed physical examination, ECG, and chest x-ray, the patient can be observed in the ER for 12 hours and then discharged. If the ECG shows nonspecific changes, 24 hours of observation with serial enzyme assay is advisable. If enzymes are negative after the period of observation the patient can be discharged without further investigations. If, on initial ECG, there are specific abnormalities or if the chest x-ray is abnormal, echocardiography should be performed to further assess cardiac injury. If the patient with suspected cardiac contusion has to be operated on for other injuries under general anesthesia, preoperative echocardiography and/or intraoperative invasive monitoring are recommended.

Prognosis

Late complications such as arrhythmia, aneurysm, pseudoaneurysm, heart failure, valvular regurgitation, and shunts have been reported but are rare. Although similarities are drawn between MI and cardiac contusion, there are significant differences that affect the outcome. Typically the trauma victims are younger and in good general health. Also, the underlying cause of myocardial damage (trauma) is episodic and not an ongoing process (atherosclerosis). So, the prognosis in these patients is much better than in those with MI (108).

Valve Injury

Valves are involved less commonly with blunt injury. Commonly involved valves are the aortic, mitral, and tricuspid, in that order. The pulmonary valve is rarely involved. Many patients have an underlying valvular pathology that predisposes them to rupture. The aortic valve is most vulnerable in the isovolumetric relaxation phase and the mitral valve in the isovolumetric contraction phase. Injury to the tricuspid valve occurs due to a sudden increase in hydrostatic pressure on the right side of the heart from venous compression (117). With blunt trauma, the aortic valve tears at the leading edge of the cusp, more commonly near the commissures (Fig. 38.8). Bioprosthetic valves are particularly at risk (118). Mitral valve injury includes rupture or avulsion of a papillary muscle (most common), rupture of chordae, or, rarely, a tear of the valve leaflets. Tricuspid injury leads to regurgitation from rupture of the anterior papillary muscle, tear in the anterior leaflet, or, rarely, tear of the septal leaflet (119–121).

Valvular injuries present with acute regurgitation. Acute aortic regurgitation can present with left ventricular failure without signs of wide pulse pressure. In mitral regurgitation, harsh pansystolic murmur radiating to the base rather than the axilla with an apical systolic thrill can be present (122). Tricuspid regurgitation presents with hypotension and signs of right heart failure. TEE helps to delineate the mechanism and severity of valvular regurgitation. Acute severe valvular regurgitation requires surgical reconstruction (119). For mild to moderate regurgitation, follow-up with rest or stress echocardiography is recommended (123). Endocarditis prophylaxis is recommended in all cases.

Coronary Artery Injury

Coronary artery injury is rare in patients who die of blunt injury (76,124). If a patient presents with clinical signs of acute MI, cardiac catheterization should be considered

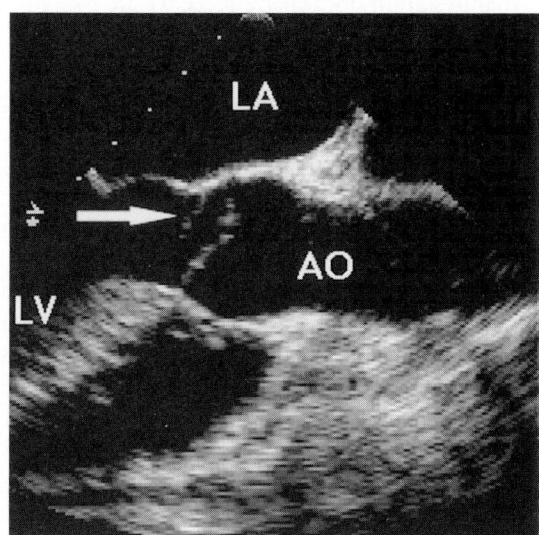
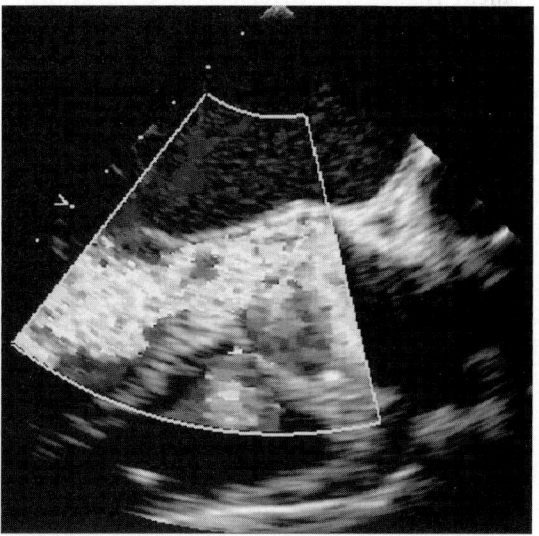

FIGURE 38.8 Aortic valve rupture from blunt injury due to a motor vehicle collision. The intraoperative transthoracic echocardiogram in long axis shows the flail left coronary cusp (*white arrow*) resulting in severe acute aortic regurgitation. AO, aorta; LA, left atrium; LV, left ventricle. (Courtesy of Dr. Ellen Mayer and Dr. Joseph Sabik, The Cleveland Clinic Foundation.)

(125,126). If coronary artery thrombosis is identified, percutaneous intervention or surgery should be considered depending on the clinical situation (127). Posttraumatic arteriovenous and arteriocameral fistulae have been reported.

Electrical Injury

Clinical Profile

Electrical injuries present with ventricular fibrillation, ventricular asystole, conduction system disturbances, transient myocardial ischemia, and myocardial damage. Cardiac arrest can be a primary ventricular fibrillation or secondary to prolonged respiratory center arrest or muscle paralysis. Electrical injury has a predilection for the conduction system for unclear reasons. It presents with sinoatrial or atrioventricular node dysfunction. MI can result from coronary artery spasm because angiography is frequently normal in these patients (130). It presents with increased enzyme levels and wall motion abnormalities. The ECG may show typical ST elevations, and Q waves can develop with evolution. QT prolongation has been noted in patients with electrical injury. This may be due to the direct effect of the current on myocardium or due to indirect effect from injury to the central nervous system.

Management

If the patient is in cardiopulmonary arrest, he or she should be resuscitated with standard advanced cardiac life support protocol. Due to low metabolic rate, survival after prolonged arrest is better in patients with electrical injury, especially from lightning, than from other causes (134). Lightning victims who do not suffer cardiac arrest have an excellent chance of recovery because subsequent arrest is uncommon. Therefore, when multiple victims are struck simultaneously with lightning, usual triage priorities should be reversed. Rescuers should give highest priority to patients in respiratory or cardiac arrest. Patients who regain their vitals after resuscitation have high survival rates (135).

After resuscitation, patients should be monitored for arrhythmia. They may develop significant tachycardia and hypertension due to catecholamine surge that may require beta-blocker therapy. Serial enzymes and echocardiography may help to estimate the extent of myocardial injury. Patients with significant myocardial damage should be monitored closely for complications. Treatment of post-MI complications is similar to that from other causes (136).

After AC shock, if the patients are stable and have a normal ECG, cardiac monitoring is not necessary (137). However, for patients struck by lightning, overnight monitoring is recommended, even if they are stable and have a normal ECG. If admission ECG is not normal (one-third of victims of electrical injury), irrespective of the cause of injury, echocardiographic assessment of left ventricular function and serial CK estimation are indicated (138).

Prognosis

The mortality with lightning injury is 20% to 30% (135). The mortality with domestic AC electrocution is difficult to estimate due to variability in severity of the shock. For every three significant injuries there is approximately one death (139). This amounts to 1,000 annual deaths in the United States (130). ECG abnormalities usually resolve in a few weeks (140). Ventricular dysfunction also improves in most patients (141). Patients tend to have a good long-term prognosis, but they should be monitored periodically for at least 1 year (137).

Radiation Injury

The heart was thought to be resistant to radiation injury in the first half of the twentieth century (142). High-dose radiation was delivered without proper cardiac shielding. Many reports of radiation-induced cardiac abnormalities changed the perception of safety of radiation to the heart. Radiation, when used in the treatment of mediastinal tumors, primarily Hodgkin's and non–Hodgkin's lymphoma, and spinal irradiation can cause cardiac abnormality in as many as 40% of patients (143). This awareness and the availability of better radiation techniques in the last decade have led to careful use of high-dose radiation to the chest with proper cardiac shielding. More than 30 Gy to the chest is usually not used. Therefore, the long-term effects of modern radiation may be less severe than before (144). However, due to better long-term survival of patients who received radiation in the past and delayed manifestation of cardiac effects, we are likely to continue to encounter these problems (145). The injuries due to radiation involve various cardiac structures and can cause acute or delayed manifestations.

Pericardium

Acute pericarditis due to radiation is rare (approximately 2% of total population undergoing chest radiation). Over the years, approximately one-half of the patients develop echocardiographically demonstrable abnormalities, and approximately 5% develop clinically significant pericardial disease (146,147). Clinical manifestations and management of radiation pericarditis are discussed in detail in Chapter 26.

Myocardium

Radiation causes progressive fibrin deposition and capillary destruction, leading to fibrosis in the myocardium (148). This leads to mild left ventricular dysfunction not requiring specific treatment (147,149). Coronary artery disease should be ruled out when significant systolic dysfunction of the left ventricle is identified. Restrictive cardiomyopathy has also been described from radiation treatment (150,151).

Valves

Valvular thickening is present in many patients after radiation treatment, but significant valvular disease is an infrequent sequela (147). The mean time from radiation to clinically recognizable valvular disease is approximately 10 years, and the symptoms develop approximately 5 years after that. Aortic and mitral replacement from radiation-induced sclerosis with significant aortic stenosis or mitral regurgitation has been reported (152). Pulmonary and tricuspid valve disease is even less common (153–155).

Conduction System

Nodal and infranodal conduction abnormalities occur with radiation injury. Although right bundle branch block is most common, complete heart block has been reported (150,154,156). Management of these abnormalities is similar to that from other causes.

Coronary Arteries

External radiation injury involves the proximal portion of coronary arteries (157–160). Left and right coronary ostia and proximal left anterior descending and left circumflex are involved in most cases. The lesions have an increased number of plasma cells with paucity of lipids (161). Large, bizarre fibroblasts are also present (162). Coronary disease commonly presents approximately 5 years after radiation but can present as late as 29 years (160). Predisposing factors other than the total dose of radiation are not clearly identified. Patients can present with any ischemic complication, such as angina, MI, arrhythmia, or heart failure. Children treated with chest radiation have a higher risk of MI (163). For significant left main stenosis, coronary artery bypass grafting with left internal mammary artery conduit is recommended, although surgery can be technically difficult due to excessive scarring. For other focal lesions, percutaneous transluminal coronary angioplasty can be useful. Intracoronary radiation is now used to treat recurring in-stent restenosis. The long-term effects of this type of therapy remain unknown (164,165).

INJURY TO THE GREAT VESSELS

Blunt Injury

Anatomic Considerations

Motor vehicular accidents are responsible for the majority of cases of aortic rupture (178). As the blood vessels are fixed by their branches to the chest wall, the direction of the pull determines the site of the tear. Aorta is fixed superiorly to the thoracic outlet and posteriorly to the chest wall. Vertical deceleration pulls the heart down and to the left, which causes shear on the right side, leading to a tear at the origin of the innominate artery. Horizontal deceleration causes shear at the aortic isthmus, the junction between the relatively mobile arch and the fixed descending aorta (183). Aortic injury can result in rupture, medial tear, and intramural hematoma or only intimal disruption. Rupture of the thoracic aorta causes immediate death in 75% to 90% of patients. Patients with contained ruptures have an unpredictable course, with up to 30% mortality in the first 24 hours (76,184). Patients with intimal flap or mural hematomas have a benign course.

Clinical Profile

Aortic rupture alone does not cause shock, as it quickly leads to exsanguination and death. Patients who arrive at the ER have sealed their defect with a clot. These patients may have reverse coarctation due to injury to the origin of subclavian artery, acute pseudocoarctation with upper-extremity hypertension, and increased pulse amplitude (182). Injury to the branches of the aortic arch can cause cerebral ischemia, but limb ischemia is rare due to a rich collateral supply (see Chapter 109) (185).

Management

In unstable patients with suspected aortic injury, the cause of bleeding should be ascertained and treated before aortic surgery (184,186). In stable patients with aortic rupture, chest x-ray can show mediastinal widening (8 cm or more), blurred aortic knob, shift of trachea or nasogastric tube when present, depressed left main bronchus of more than 40 degrees, presence of apical cap sign, obliteration of aortopulmonary window, and multiple rib or sternal fractures (187). These signs are present in 70% to 95% of cases (188). If the chest x-ray is abnormal, TEE is performed to confirm the diagnosis. TEE is sensitive and specific for the diagnosis of aortic intimal disruption, medial tear, and perivascular hematoma. The advantages over aortography are the bedside availability, the noninvasive nature of the study, and the ability to simultaneously evaluate the heart. However, its limitations are an occasional inability to pass the probe in patients with cervical injury, "blind spot" (this is the 3- to 5-cm portion of upper ascending aorta that is blinded by trachea) of ascending aorta, and operator variability (189). If TEE shows no abnormality, the patient should be observed, and chest x-ray should be repeated in 6 hours. If TEE shows rupture of the aorta, surgery is indicated. In patients with a small intramural hematoma or a small intimal flap, conservative medical management with close follow-up is justified. If TEE is nondiagnostic, other

THE FUTURE

Improvement in emergency services with a special effort for rapid patient transport to a well-equipped trauma center can save patients with serious cardiovascular trauma. TEE has significantly changed some of the protocols for evaluation of stable patients with thoracic injury, but more prospective studies are needed to better define its role. A consensus for the clinical definition of cardiac contusion is needed to avoid discrepancies in literature. Similarly, for better comparison of data from various institutions, a unified injury index should be used. Endovascular stent grafts may help in management of some injuries to thoracic great vessels.

imaging modalities are used. Magnetic resonance imaging is useful in this situation, as it gives an excellent definition of anatomy, including the arch vessels. Biplane aortogram is no longer considered to be the gold standard, as, depending on the plane of projection, tears and perivascular hematomas can be missed. It is an invasive procedure with occasional serious complications. CT scan has a high sensitivity for screening purposes and is a very useful imaging tool that is complementary to TEE (190–192). If the initial chest x-ray does not show any signs of aortic injury, further management should be guided by clinical judgment (193). TEE should be performed in patients older than 65 years with significant other injuries and comorbid factors.

In stable patients, nonoperative management of an intimal tear of the thoracic aorta or delayed operative management of full-thickness tear in patients with multiple injuries is favored. Use of beta-blockers to medically control shear stress by controlling heart rate and blood pressure appears to be effective in these patients.

Prognosis

Patients treated for thoracic aortic rupture with surgery have risk for paraplegia (4% to 10%) (194–196). Brain ischemia, MI, and other end-organ damage have been reported. Overall mortality is 10% to 25% when patients reach the hospital alive.

CONTROVERSIES AND PERSONAL PERSPECTIVES

The role of echocardiography is becoming clearer in the management of stable patients with penetrating cardiac injuries. TEE has proven to be useful in management of suspected great vessel injuries and is also useful in difficult situations to complement TTE. In the management of blunt trauma with stable hemodynamics, the role of echocardiography remains less clear, but it is extremely useful when structural problems need to be ruled out. Percutaneous interventions with stent grafts may find its role in management of a subgroup of patients with thoracic great vessel injuries. Coronary interventions have been success-

fully used in some cases of blunt trauma–related coronary thrombosis and closure. Thoracoscopy is also being more frequently used to assess the extent of injury in stable patients.

REFERENCES

1. National Center for Health Statistics, U.S. Department of Health and Human Services, Service PH. Advance report of final mortality statistics. *Monthly Vital Statistics Report,* 1992;43:1–76.
2. Mattox KL, Feliciano DV, Burch J, et al. Five thousand seven hundred sixty cardiovascular injuries in 4459 patients. Epidemiologic evolution 1958 to 1987. *Ann Surg* 1989;209:698–705.
3. Symbas PN. *Cardiothoracic trauma.* Philadelphia: WB Saunders, 1989.
4. Redelmeier DA, Tibshirani RJ. Association between cellular-telephone calls and motor vehicular collisions. *N Engl J Med* 1997;336:453–458.
5. Homer. *The Iliad.* New York: Macmillan, 1922.
6. Beck CS. Wounds of the heart. *Arch Surg* 1926;13:205–227.
7. Morgagni JB. De sedibus et causes morborum. Lipsiae sumptibus Leopoldi Vossii 1829. As quoted by Beck CS. Wounds of the heart. The technic of suture. *Arch Surg* 1926;13:205–227.
8. Larrey D. *Bull Sci Med* 1810;6:284.
9. Fischer G. Die Wunden des Herzens und des Hertzbeutels. *Arch Klin Chir* 1868;9:571.
10. Billroth T. Offenes Schreiben an Herr der Wittelshofer uver die erste mil gustingen susgange ausgefuhrte pylorectomie. *Weiner Med Wochensch* 1881;31:161.
11. Rehn L. Ueber Penetrerende Herzwunden und Herznaht. *Arch Klin Chir* 1897;55:315.
12. Hill LL. A report of a case of successful suturing of the heart, and table of other cases of suturing by different operators with various terminations and conclusions drawn. *Med Rec* 1902;62:846.
13. Dalton HC. Report of a case of stab wound of the pericardium, terminating in recovery after resection of a rib and suture of the pericardium. *Ann Surg* 1895;21:147–152.
14. Williams DH. Stab wound of heart and precordium: recovery-patient alive three years afterward. *Med Rec* 1897;51:437–439.

15. Karrel R, Shaffer MA, Franaszek JB. Emergency diagnosis, resuscitation, and treatment of acute penetrating cardiac trauma. *Ann Emerg Med* 1982;11:504–517.

16. Symbas PN, Symbas PJ. Missiles in the cardiovascular system. *Chest Surg Clin North Am* 1997;7:343–356.

17. Pate JW, Richardson RL Jr. Penetrating wounds of cardiac valves. *JAMA* 1969;207:309–311.

18. Cha EK, Mittal V, Allaben RD. Delayed sequelae of penetrating cardiac injury. *Arch Surg* 1993;128:836–839.

19. Espada R, Whisennand HH, Mattox KL, et al. Surgical management of penetrating injuries to the coronary arteries. *Surgery* 1975;78:755–760.

20. Ivatury RR, Shah PM, Ito K, et al. Emergency room thoracotomy for the resuscitation of patients with "fatal" penetrating injuries of the heart. *Ann Thorac Surg* 1981;32:377–385.

21. Porter JM, Page R, Wood AE, et al. Ventricular perforation associated with central venous introducer-dilator systems. *Can J Anaesth* 1997;44:317–320.

22. Rogers FB, Leavitt BJ. Upper torso cyanosis: a marker for blunt cardiac rupture. *Am J Emerg Med* 1997;15:275–276.

23. Wilson RF, Bassett JS. Penetrating wounds of the pericardium or its contents. *JAMA* 1966;195:513–518.

24. Ivatury RR, Nallathambi MN, Roberge RJ, et al. Penetrating thoracic injuries: in-field stabilization vs. prompt transport. *J Trauma* 1987;27:1066–1073.

25. Purkiss SF, Williams M, Cross FW, et al. Efficacy of urgent thoracotomy for trauma in patients attended by a helicopter emergency medical service. *J R Coll Surg Edinburgh* 1994;39:289–291.

26. Durham LA III, Richardson RJ, Wall MJ Jr, et al. Emergency center thoracotomy: impact of prehospital resuscitation. *J Trauma* 1992;32:775–779.

27. Bickell WH, Wall MJ Jr, Pepe PE, et al. Immediate versus delayed fluid resuscitation for hypotensive patients with penetrating torso injuries [see comments]. *N Engl J Med* 1994;331:1105–1109.

28. Henderson VJ, Smith RS, Fry WR, et al. Cardiac injuries: analysis of an unselected series of 251 cases. *J Trauma* 1994;36:341–348.

29. Mattox KL, Beall AC Jr, Jordan GL Jr, et al. Cardiorrhaphy in the emergency center. *J Thorac Cardiovasc Surg* 1974;68:886–895.

30. Blake DP, Gisbert VL, Ney AL, et al. Survival after emergency department versus operating room thoracotomy for penetrating cardiac injuries. *Am Surg* 1992;58:329–332.

31. Attar S, Suter CM, Hankins JR, et al. Penetrating cardiac injuries [see comments]. *Ann Thorac Surg* 1991;51:711–715; discussion 715–716.

32. Ivatury RR, Rohman M, Steichen FM, et al. Penetrating cardiac injuries: twenty-year experience. *Am Surg* 1987;53:310–317.

33. Macho JR, Markison RE, Schecter WP. Cardiac stapling in the management of penetrating injuries of the heart: rapid control of hemorrhage and decreased risk of personal contamination. *J Trauma* 1993;34:711–715.

34. Feliciano DV, Moore EE, Mattox KL. *Trauma*, 3rd ed. Stamford, CT: Appleton & Lange, 1996.

35. Bolton JW, Bynoe RP, Lazar HL, et al. Two-dimensional echocardiography in the evaluation of penetrating intrapericardial injuries. *Ann Thorac Surg* 1993;56:506–509.

36. Jimenez E, Martin M, Krukenkamp I, et al. Subxiphoid pericardiotomy versus echocardiography: a prospective evaluation of the diagnosis of occult penetrating cardiac injury. *Surgery* 1990;108:676–679.

37. Rozycki GS, Feliciano DV, Ochsner MG, et al. The role of ultrasound in patients with possible penetrating cardiac wounds: a prospective multicenter study. *J Trauma* 1999;46:543–551.

38. Meyer DM, Jessen ME, Grayburn PA. Use of echocardiography to detect occult cardiac injury after penetrating thoracic trauma: a prospective study. *J Trauma* 1995;39:902–907.

39. Chirillo F, Totis O, Cavarzerani A, et al. Usefulness of transthoracic and transoesophageal echocardiography in recognition and management of cardiovascular injuries after blunt chest trauma. *Heart* 1996;75:301–306.

40. Pearson GD, Karr SS, Trachiotis GD, et al. A retrospective review of the role of transesophageal echocardiography in aortic and cardiac trauma in a level I Pediatric Trauma Center. *J Am Soc Echocardiogr* 1997;10:946–955.

41. Andrade-Alegre R, Mon L. Subxiphoid pericardial window in the diagnosis of penetrating cardiac trauma. *Ann Thorac Surg* 1994;58:1139–1141.

42. Miller FB, Bond SJ, Shumate CR, et al. Diagnostic pericardial window. A safe alternative to exploratory thoracotomy for suspected heart injuries. *Arch Surg* 1987;122:605–609.

43. Brewster SA, Thirlby RC, Snyder WHD. Subxiphoid pericardial window and penetrating cardiac trauma. *Arch Surg* 1988;123:937–941.

44. Duncan AO, Scalea TM, Sclafani SJ, et al. Evaluation of occult cardiac injuries using subxiphoid pericardial window. *J Trauma* 1989;29:955–959.

45. Symbas NP, Bongiorno PF, Symbas PN. Blunt cardiac rupture: the utility of emergency department ultrasound. *Ann Thorac Surg* 1999;67:1274–1276.

46. Morales CH, Salinas CM, Henao CA, et al. Thoracoscopic pericardial window and penetrating cardiac trauma. *J Trauma* 1997;42:273–275.

47. Hassett A, Moran J, Sabiston DC, et al. Utility of echocardiography in the management of patients with penetrating missile wounds of the heart. *J Am Coll Cardiol* 1986;7:1151–1156.

48. Fry SJ, Picard MH, Tseng JF, et al. The echocardiographic diagnosis, characterization, and extraction guidance of cardiac foreign bodies. *J Am Soc Echocardiogr* 2000;13:232–239.

49. Porembka DT, Johnson DJ II, Hoit BD, et al. Penetrating cardiac trauma: a perioperative role for transesophageal echocardiography [see comments]. *Anesth Analg* 1993;77:1275–1277.

50. Plummer D, Brunette D, Asinger R, et al. Emergency department echocardiography improves outcome in penetrating cardiac injury. *Ann Emerg Med* 1992;21:709–712.

51. Rozycki GS, Feliciano DV, Schmidt JA, et al. The role of surgeon-performed ultrasound in patients with possible cardiac wounds. *Ann Surg* 1996;223:737–744.

52. Freshman SP, Wisner DH, Weber CJ. 2-D echocardiography: emergent use in the evaluation of penetrating precordial trauma. *J Trauma* 1991;31:902–905.

53. Demetriades D, van der Veen BW. Penetrating injuries of the heart: experience over two years in South Africa. *J Trauma* 1983;23:1034–1041.

54. Demetriades D, Rabinowitz B, Sofianos C. Emergency room thoracotomy for stab wounds to the chest and neck. *J Trauma* 1987;27:483–485.

55. Ivatury RR, Nallathambi MN, Rohman M, Stahl WM. Penetrating cardiac trauma. Quantifying the severity of anatomic and physiologic injury. *Ann Surg* 1987;205:61–66.

56. Coimbra R, Pinto MC, Razuk A, et al. Penetrating cardiac wounds: predictive value of trauma indices and the necessity of terminology standardization. *Am Surg* 1995;61:448–452.

57. Tyburski JG, Astra L, Wilson RF, et al. Factors affecting prognosis with penetrating wounds of the heart. *J Trauma* 2000;48:587–590.

58. Wall MJ Jr, Mattox KL, Chen CD, et al. Acute management of complex cardiac injuries. *J Trauma* 1997;42:905–912.

59. Harris DG, Papagiannopoulos KA, Pretorius J, et al. Current evaluation of cardiac stab wounds. *Ann Thorac Surg* 1999;68:2119–2122.

60. Asensio JA, Murray J, Demetriades D, et al. Penetrating cardiac injuries: a prospective study of variables predicting outcomes. *J Am Coll Surg* 1998;186:24–34.

61. Moreno C, Moore EE, Majure JA, et al. Pericardial tamponade: a critical determinant for survival following penetrating cardiac wounds. *J Trauma* 1986;26:821–825.

62. Schwengel RH, Bennett SK, Sequeira AJ, et al. Late presentation of left ventricular pseudoaneurysm and ventricular septal defect after surgery for penetrating cardiac injury. *Am Heart J* 1994;127:930–932.

63. Scott CH, Ferrari VA, Mittal S, et al. Diagnosis of a persistent coronary fistula after ventricular septal defect patch closure. *J Am Soc Echocardiogr* 1997;10:573–575.

64. Duque HA, Florez LE, Moreno A, et al. Penetrating cardiac trauma: follow-up study including electrocardiography, echocardiography, and functional test. *World J Surg* 1999;23:1254–1257.

65. Swierzewski MJ, Feliciano DV, Lillis RP, et al. Deaths from motor vehicle crashes: patterns of injury in restrained and unrestrained victims. *J Trauma* 1994;37:404–407.

66. Arajarvi E, Santavirta S, Tolonen J. Aortic ruptures in seat belt wearers. *J Thorac Cardiovasc Surg* 1989;98:355–361.

67. Lancaster GI, DeFrance JH, Borruso JJ. Air-bag-associated rupture of the right atrium [letter]. *N Engl J Med* 1993;328:358.

68. Symbas PN. Contusion of the heart. In: Symbas PN, ed. *Cardiothoracic trauma.* Philadelphia: WB Saunders, 1989:55–76.

69. RuDusky BM. More on myocardial contusion—with additional insight on myocardial concussion. *Chest* 1997;112:570–572.

70. Tenzer ML. The spectrum of myocardial contusion: a review. *J Trauma* 1985;25:620–627.

71. Mattox KL, Flint LM, Carrico CJ, et al. Blunt cardiac injury [editorial, see comments]. *J Trauma* 1992;33:649–650.

72. Maron BJ, Poliac LC, Kaplan JA, et al. Blunt impact to the chest leading to sudden death from cardiac arrest during sports activities. *N Engl J Med* 1995;333:337–342.

73. Bir CA, Viano DC. Biomechanical predictor of commotio cordis in high-speed chest impact. *J Trauma* 1999;47:468–473.

74. Pontillo D, Capezzuto A, Achilli A, et al. Bifascicular block complicating blunt cardiac injury. A case report and review of the literature [review]. *Angiology* 1994;45:883–890.

75. Saunders CR, Doty DB. Myocardial contusion. *Surg Gynecol Obstet* 1977;144:595–603.

76. Parmley LF, Marion WC, Mattingly TW, et al. Nonpenetrating traumatic injury to the heart. *Circulation* 1958;18:371–396.

77. McLean RF, Devitt JH, Dubbin J, et al. Incidence of abnormal RNA studies and dysrhythmias in patients with blunt chest trauma. *J Trauma* 1991;31:968–970.

78. Sutherland GR, Cheung HW, Holliday RL, et al. Hemodynamic adaptation to acute myocardial contusion complicating blunt chest injury. *Am J Cardiol* 1986;57:291–297.

79. Saunders CR, Doty DB. Myocardial contusion: effect of intra-aortic balloon counterpulsation on cardiac output. *J Trauma* 1978;18:706–708.

80. Dubrow TJ, Mihalka J, Eisenhauer DM, et al. Myocardial contusion in the stable patient: what level of care is appropriate? *Surgery* 1989;106:267–273; discussion 273–274.

81. RuDusky BM. Cardiac troponins in the diagnosis of myocardial contusion: an emerging controversy [letter, comment]. *Chest* 1997;112:858–860.

82. Kaups KL. Blunt cardiac injury [letter]. *Chest* 1996;110:1125–1126.

83. Potkin RT, Werner JA, Trobaugh GB, et al. Evaluation of noninvasive tests of cardiac damage in suspected cardiac contusion. *Circulation* 1982;66:627–631.

84. Karalis DG, Victor MF, Davis GA, et al. The role of echocardiography in blunt chest trauma: a transthoracic and transesophageal echocardiographic study. *J Trauma* 1994;36:53–58.

85. Hossack KF, Moreno CA, Vanway CW, et al. Frequency of cardiac contusion in nonpenetrating chest injury. *Am J Cardiol* 1988;61:391–394.

86. Mooney R, Niemann JT, Bessen HA, et al. Conventional and right precordial ECGs, creatine kinase, and radionuclide angiography in post-traumatic ventricular dysfunction. *Ann Emerg Med* 1988;17:890–894.

87. Healey MA, Brown R, Fleiszer D. Blunt cardiac injury: is this diagnosis necessary? [published erratum appears in *J Trauma* 1990;30:following 514]. *J Trauma* 1990;30:137–146.

88. Foil MB, Mackersie RC, Furst SR, et al. The asymptomatic patient with suspected myocardial contusion. *Am J Surg* 1990;160:638–642; discussion 642–643.

89. Sutherland GR, Driedger AA, Holliday RL, et al. Frequency of myocardial injury after blunt chest trauma as evaluated by radionuclide angiography. *Am J Cardiol* 1983;52:1099–1103.

90. Helling TS, Duke P, Beggs CW, Crouse LJ. A prospective evaluation of 68 patients suffering blunt chest trauma for evidence of cardiac injury. *J Trauma* 1989;29:961–965; discussion 965–966.

91. Tsung SH. Creatine kinase isoenzyme patterns in human tissue obtained at surgery. *Clin Chem* 1976;22:173–175.

92. Snow N, Richardson JD, Flint LM Jr. Myocardial contusion: implications for patients with multiple traumatic injuries. *Surgery* 1982;92:744–750.

93. Soliman MH, Waxman K. Value of a conventional approach to the diagnosis of traumatic cardiac contusion after chest injury. *Crit Care Med* 1987;15:218–220.

94. Biffl WL, Moore FA, Moore EE, et al. Cardiac enzymes are irrelevant in the patient with suspected myocardial contusion. *Am J Surg* 1994;168:523–527.

95. Bertinchant JP, Robert E, Polge A, et al. Release kinetics of cardiac troponin I and cardiac troponin T in effluents from isolated perfused rabbit hearts after graded experimental myocardial contusion. *J Trauma* 1999;47:474–480.

96. Bertinchant JP, Polge A, Mohty D, et al. Evaluation of incidence, clinical significance, and prognostic value of circulating cardiac troponin I and T elevation in hemodynamically stable patients with suspected myocardial contusion after blunt chest trauma. *J Trauma* 2000;48:924–931.

97. RuDusky BM. Cardiac troponins in the diagnosis of myocardial contusion [letter, comment]. *Chest* 1996;109:1413–1414.

98. Rodriguez A, Shatney C. The value of technetium99m pyrophosphate scanning in the diagnosis of myocardial contusion. *Am Surg* 1982;48:472–474.

99. Bodin L, Rouby JJ, Viars P. Myocardial contusion in patients with blunt chest trauma as evaluated by thallium 201 myocardial scintigraphy. *Chest* 1988;94:72–76.

100. Holness R, Waxman K. Diagnosis of traumatic cardiac contusion utilizing single photon-emission computed tomography. *Crit Care Med* 1990;18:1–3.

101. McCarthy MC, Pavlina PM, Evans DK, et al. The value of SPECT-thallium scanning in screening for myocardial contusion. *Cardiovasc Intervent Radiol* 1991;14:238–240.

102. Pandian NG, Skorton DJ, Doty DB, et al. Immediate diagnosis of acute myocardial contusion by two-dimensional echocardiography: studies in a canine model of blunt chest trauma. *J Am Coll Cardiol* 1983;2:488–496.

103. King RM, Mucha P Jr, Seward JB, et al. Cardiac contusion: a new diagnostic approach utilizing two-dimensional echocardiography. *J Trauma* 1983;23:610–614.

104. Shapiro MJ, Yanofsky SD, Trapp J, et al. Cardiovascular evaluation in blunt thoracic trauma using transesophageal echocardiography (TEE). *J Trauma* 1991;31:835–839.

105. Garcia-Fernandez MA, Lopez-Perez JM, Perez-Castellano N, et al. Role of transesophageal echocardiography in the assessment of patients with blunt chest trauma: correlation of echocardiographic findings with the electrocardiogram and creatine kinase monoclonal antibody measurements. *Am Heart J* 1998;135:476–481.

106. Gendreau MA, Triner WR, Bartfield J. Complications of transesophageal echocardiography in the ED. *Am J Emerg Med* 1999;17:248–251.

107. Thanigaraj S, Perez JE. Diagnosis of cardiac rupture with the use of contrast-enhanced echocardiography. *J Am Soc Echocardiogr* 2000;13:862–865.

108. Sturaitis M, McCallum D, Sutherland G, et al. Lack of significant long-term sequelae following traumatic myocardial contusion. *Arch Intern Med* 1986;146:1765–1769.

109. Kato K, Kushimoto S, Mashiko K, et al. Blunt traumatic rupture of the heart: an experience in Tokyo. *J Trauma* 1994;36:859–863.

110. Moront M, Lefrak EA, Akl BF. Traumatic rupture of the interventricular septum and tricuspid valve: case report. *J Trauma* 1991;31:134–136.

111. Rao G, Garvey J, Gupta M, et al. Atrial septal defect due to blunt thoracic trauma. *J Trauma* 1977;17:405–406.

112. Fulda G, Brathwaite CE, Rodriguez A, et al. Blunt traumatic rupture of the heart and pericardium: a ten-year experience (1979–1989). *J Trauma* 1991;31:167–172.

113. Shalaby RI, Rajendran U, Regunathan R. Blunt traumatic rupture of the heart: case report and selected review. *Ann Thorac Cardiovasc Surg* 1999;5:123–129.

114. Calhoon JH, Hoffmann TH, Trinkle JK, et al. Management of blunt rupture of the heart. *J Trauma* 1986;26:495–502.

115. Carrillo EH, Heniford BT, Dykes JR, et al. Cardiac herniation producing tamponade: the critical role of early diagnosis. *J Trauma* 1997;43:19–23.

116. Meng RL, Straus A, Milloy F, et al. Intrapericardial diaphragmatic hernia in adults. *Ann Surg* 1979;189:359–366.

117. Bailey PL, Peragallo R, Karwande SV, et al. Mitral and tricuspid valve rupture after moderate blunt chest trauma. *Ann Thorac Surg* 2000;69:616–618.

118. Rumisek JD, Robinowitz M, Virmani R, et al. Bioprosthetic heart valve rupture associated with trauma. *J Trauma* 1986;26:276–279.

119. van Son JA, Danielson GK, Schaff HV, et al. Traumatic tricuspid valve insufficiency. Experience in thirteen patients. *J Thorac Cardiovasc Surg* 1994;108:893–898.

120. Chiu WC, Shindler DM, Scholz PM, et al. Traumatic tricuspid regurgitation with cyanosis: diagnosis by transesophageal echocardiography. *Ann Thorac Surg* 1996;61:992–993.

121. Holper K, Hahnel C, Augustin N, et al. Operative correction of traumatic tricuspid insufficiency. *Herz* 1996;21:172–178.

122. Ronan JA Jr, Steelman RB, DeLeon AC Jr, et al. The clinical diagnosis of acute severe mitral insufficiency. *Am J Cardiol* 1971;27:284–290.

123. Leung DY, Griffin BP, Stewart WJ, et al. Left ventricular function after valve repair for chronic mitral regurgitation: predictive value of preoperative assessment of contractile reserve by exercise echocardiography. *J Am Coll Cardiol* 1996;28:1198–1205.

124. Banzo I, Montero A, Uriarte I, et al. Coronary artery occlusion and myocardial infarction: a seldom encountered complication of blunt chest trauma. *Clin Nucl Med* 1999;24:94–96.

125. Patel R, Samaha FF. Right coronary artery occlusion caused by blunt trauma. *J Invasive Cardiol* 2000;12:376–378.

126. Liedtke AJ, Allen RP, Nellis SH. Effects of blunt cardiac trauma on coronary vasomotion, perfusion, myocardial mechanics, and metabolism. *J Trauma* 1980;20:777–785.

127. Ginzburg E, Dygert J, Parra-Davila E, et al. Coronary artery stenting for occlusive dissection after blunt chest trauma [review, 16 refs]. *J Trauma* 1998;45:157–161.

128. Andrews CJ, Darveniza M. Telephone-mediated lightning injury: an Australian survey. *J Trauma* 1989;29:665–671.

129. Eriksson A, Ornehult L. Death by lightning. *Am J Forensic Med Pathol* 1988;9:295–300.

130. James TN, Riddick L, Embry JH. Cardiac abnormalities demonstrated postmortem in four cases of accidental electrocution and their potential significance relative to nonfatal electrical injuries of the heart. *Am Heart J* 1990;120:143–157.

131. Thompson JC, Ashwal S. Electrical injuries in children [review]. *Am J Dis Child* 1983;137:231–235.

132. Chandra NC, Siu CO, Munster AM. Clinical predictors of myocardial damage after high voltage electrical injury. *Crit Care Med* 1990;18:293–297.

133. Xenopoulos N, Movahed A, Hudson P, et al. Myocardial injury in electrocution. *Am Heart J* 1991;122:1481–1484.

134. Taussig HB. "Death" from lightning and the possibility of living again. *Am Sci* 1969;57:306–316.

135. Cooper MA. Lightning injuries: prognostic signs for death. *Ann Emerg Med* 1980;9:134–138.

136. Kirchmer JT Jr, Larson DL, Tyson KR. Cardiac rupture following electrical injury. *J Trauma* 1977;17:389–391.

137. Carleton SC. Cardiac problems associated with electrical injury. *Cardiol Clin* 1995;13:263–266.

138. Solem L, Fischer RP, Strate RG. The natural history of electrical injury. *J Trauma* 1977;17:487–492.

139. Bernstein T. Electrical injury: electrical engineer's perspective and an historical review. *Ann N Y Acad Sci* 1994;720:1–10.

140. Kleiner JP, Wilkin JH. Cardiac effects of lightning stroke. *JAMA* 1978;240:2757–2759.

141. McGill MP, Kamp TJ, Rahko PS. High-voltage injury resulting in permanent right heart dysfunction. *Chest* 1999;115:586–587.

142. Warren S. Effects of radiation on the cardiovascular system. *Arch Pathol* 1942;34:1070–1079.

143. Vallebona A. Cardiac damage following therapeutic chest irradiation. Importance, evaluation and treatment [review, 69 refs]. *Minerva Cardioangiol* 2000;48:79–87.

144. Glanzmann C, Huguenin P, Lutolf UM, et al. Cardiac lesions after mediastinal irradiation for Hodgkin's disease. *Radiother Oncol* 1994;30:43–54.

145. Zinzani PL, Gherlinzoni F, Piovaccari G, et al. Cardiac injury as late toxicity of mediastinal radiation therapy for Hodgkin's disease patients. *Haematologica* 1996;81:132–137.

146. Hancock SL, Donaldson SS, Hoppe RT. Cardiac disease following treatment of Hodgkin's disease in children and adolescents. *J Clin Oncol* 1993;11:1208–1215.

147. Kreuser ED, Voller H, Behles C, et al. Evaluation of late cardiotoxicity with pulsed Doppler echocardiography in patients treated for Hodgkin's disease. *Br J Haematol* 1993;84:615–622.

148. Corn BW, Trock BJ, Goodman RL. Irradiation-related ischemic heart disease. *J Clin Oncol* 1990;8:741–750.

149. Applefeld MM, Wiernik PH. Cardiac disease after radiation therapy for Hodgkin's disease: analysis of 48 patients. *Am J Cardiol* 1983;51:1679–1681.

150. Arsenian MA. Cardiovascular sequelae of therapeutic thoracic radiation. *Prog Cardiovasc Dis* 1991;33:299–311.

151. Gottdiener JS, Katin MJ, Borer JS, et al. Late cardiac effects of therapeutic mediastinal irradiation. Assessment by echocardiography and radionuclide angiography. *N Engl J Med* 1983;308:569–572.

152. Mittal S, Berko B, Bavaria J, et al. Radiation-induced cardiovascular dysfunction. *Am J Cardiol* 1996;78:114–115.

153. Gustavsson A, Eskilsson J, Landberg T, et al. Late cardiac effects after mantle radiotherapy in patients with Hodgkin's disease. *Ann Oncol* 1990;1:355–363.

154. Pohjola-Sintonen S, Totterman KJ, Salmo M, et al. Late cardiac effects of mediastinal radiotherapy in patients with Hodgkin's disease. *Cancer* 1987;60:31–37.

155. Knight CJ, Sutton GC. Complete heart block and severe tricuspid regurgitation after radiotherapy. Case report and review of the literature [see comments, review]. *Chest* 1995;108:1748–1751.

156. Cohen SI, Bharati S, Glass J, et al. Radiotherapy as a cause of complete atrioventricular block in Hodgkin's disease. An electrophysiological-pathological correlation. *Arch Intern Med* 1981;141:676–679.

157. Om A, Ellahham S, Vetrovec GW. Radiation-induced coronary artery disease [review]. *Am Heart J* 1992;124:1598–1602.

158. Brosius FCD, Waller BF, Roberts WC. Radiation heart disease. Analysis of 16 young (aged 15 to 33 years) necropsy patients who received over 3,500 rads to the heart. *Am J Med* 1981;70:519–530.

159. Boivin JF, Hutchison GB, Lubin JH, et al. Coronary artery disease mortality in patients treated for Hodgkin's disease. *Cancer* 1992;69:1241–1247.

160. McEniery PT, Dorosti K, Schiavone WA, et al. Clinical and angiographic features of coronary artery disease after chest irradiation. *Am J Cardiol* 1987;60:1020–1024.

161. McReynolds RA, Gold GL, Roberts WC. Coronary heart disease after mediastinal irradiation for Hodgkin's disease. *Am J Med* 1976;60:39–45.

162. Fajardo LF, Stewart JR, Cohn KE. Morphology of radiation-induced heart disease. *Arch Pathol* 1968;86:512–519.

163. Hancock SL, Tucker MA, Hoppe RT. Factors affecting late mortality from heart disease after treatment of Hodgkin's disease. *JAMA* 1993;270:1949–1955.

164. Williams DO, Sharaf BL. Intracoronary radiation: it keeps on glowing. *Circulation* 2000;101:350–351.

165. Taylor AJ, Gorman PD, Farb A, et al. Long-term coronary vascular response to (32)P beta-particle-emitting stents in a canine model. *Circulation* 1999;100:2366–2372.

166. Davis GK, Au J, Roberts D. Myocardial perforation associated with the use of the Gensini ventriculography catheter. *Int J Cardiol* 1996;53:103–106.

167. Katta S, Akosah K, Stambler B, et al. Atrioventricular fistula: an unusual complication of endomyocardial biopsy in a heart transplant recipient. *J Am Soc Echocardiogr* 1994;7:405–409.

168. Flynn MS, Aguirre FV, Donohue TJ, et al. Conservative management of guidewire coronary artery perforation with pericardial effusion during angioplasty for acute inferior myocardial infarction. *Cathet Cardiovasc Diagn* 1993;29:285–288.

169. Von Sohsten R, Kopistansky C, Cohen M, et al. Cardiac tamponade in the 'new device' era: evaluation of 6999 consecutive percutaneous coronary interventions. *Am Heart J* 2000;140:279–283.

170. Manga P, Singh S, Brandis S. Left ventricular perforation during percutaneous balloon mitral valvuloplasty. *Cathet Cardiovasc Diagn* 1992;25:317–319.

171. Collier PE, Goodman GB. Cardiac tamponade caused by central venous catheter perforation of the heart: a preventable complication. *J Am Coll Surg* 1995;181:459–463.

172. Ingle RJ. Rare complications of vascular access devices [review]. *Semin Oncol Nurs* 1995;11:184–193.

173. Reese JC. Cardiac tamponade caused by central venous catheter perforation of the heart: a preventable complication [letter, comment]. *J Am Coll Surg* 1996;182:558.

174. Morgan CD, Marshall SA, Ross JR. Catheter drainage of the pericardium: its safety and efficacy. *Can J Surg* 1989;32:331–334.

175. Thakur RK, Klein GJ, Yee R, et al. Complications of radiofrequency catheter ablation: a review [review]. *Can J Cardiol* 1994;10:835–839.

176. Krischer JP, Fine EG, Davis JH, et al. Complications of cardiac resuscitation. *Chest* 1987;92:287–291.

177. Mattana J, Singhal PC. Determinants of elevated creatine kinase activity and creatine kinase MB-fraction following cardiopulmonary resuscitation. *Chest* 1992;101:1386–1392.

178. Baker PB, Keyhani-Rofagha S, Graham RL, et al. Dissecting hematoma (aneurysm) of coronary arteries. *Am J Med* 1986;80:317–319.

179. Machii M, Inaba H, Nakae H, et al. Cardiac rupture by penetration of fractured sternum: a rare complication of cardiopulmonary resuscitation. *Resuscitation* 2000;43:151–153.

180. Gavant ML, Flick P, Menke P, et al. CT aortography of thoracic aortic rupture. *AJR Am J Roentgenol* 1996;166:955–961.

181. Childs D, Wilkes RG. Puncture of the ascending aorta—a complication of subclavian venous cannulation [letter]. *Anaesthesia* 1986;41:331–332.

182. Calhoon JH, Grover FL, Trinkle JK. Chest trauma. Approach and management [review]. *Clin Chest Med* 1992;13:55–67.

183. Hunt JP, Baker CC, Lentz CW, et al. Thoracic aorta injuries: management and outcome of 144 patients. *J Trauma* 1996;40:547–555.

184. Pate JW, Fabian TC, Walker W. Traumatic rupture of the aortic isthmus: an emergency? [review]. *World J Surg* 1995;19:119–125.

185. George SJ. Transoesophageal echocardiography in chest trauma [letter]. *Br J Anaesth* 1996;76:336–337.

186. Kipfer B, Leupi F, Schuepbach P, et al. Acute traumatic rupture of the thoracic aorta: immediate or delayed surgical repair? *Eur J Cardiothoracic Surg* 1994;8:30–33.

187. Burney RE, Gundry SR, Mackenzie JR, et al. Chest roentgenograms in diagnosis of traumatic rupture of the aorta. Observer variation in interpretation. *Chest* 1984;85:605–609.

188. Smith MD, Cassidy JM, Souther S, et al. Transesophageal echocardiography in the diagnosis of traumatic rupture of the aorta [see comments]. *N Engl J Med* 1995;332:356–362.

189. Vlahakes GJ, Warren RL. Traumatic rupture of the aorta [editorial; comment]. *N Engl J Med* 1995;332:389–390.

190. Feliciano DV, Rozycki GS. Advances in the diagnosis and treatment of thoracic trauma. *Surg Clin North Am* 1999;79:1417–1429.

191. Tomiak MM, Rosenblum JD, Messersmith RN, et al. Use of CT for diagnosis of traumatic rupture of the thoracic aorta. *Ann Vasc Surg* 1993;7:130–139.

192. LeBlang SD, Dolich MO. Imaging of penetrating thoracic trauma [review, 64 refs]. *J Thorac Imaging* 2000;15:128–135.

193. Pretre R, Chilcott M. Blunt trauma to the heart and great vessels. *N Engl J Med* 1997;336:626–632.

194. Mauney MC, Tribble CG, Cope JT, et al. Is clamp and sew still viable for thoracic aortic resection? *Ann Surg* 1996;223:534–540.

195. von Oppell UO, Dunne TT, De Groot KM, et al. Spinal cord protection in the absence of collateral circulation: meta-analysis of mortality and paraplegia. *J Card Surg* 1994;9:685–691.

196. Von Oppell UO, Brink J, Hewitson J, et al. Acute traumatic rupture of the thoracic aorta. A comparison of techniques. *S Afr J Surg* 1996;34:19–24.

39

CARDIAC NEOPLASMS

WILLIAM C. ROBERTS

OVERVIEW

Primary cardiac tumors involving the heart may be either benign or malignant. Most of the benign tumors are myxomas, which are most commonly located in the left atrium. Primary malignant neoplasms usually involve the myocardium and the interior of the cardiac cavities, whereas metastatic neoplasms to the heart most commonly involve the pericardium, and pericardial effusion and constriction are the most common consequences. Computed tomography

(CT) and magnetic resonance imaging (MRI) are becoming the most useful instruments of precision to diagnose cardiac tumors. A number of nonneoplastic conditions in the heart or pericardium are frequently mistaken for cardiac neoplasms, including pericardial cysts, teratoma, lipomatous hypertrophy of the atrial septum, papillary fibroelastoma, thrombi, and sarcoid. There are a number of cardiac consequences of malignancy, including radiation heart disease, cardiac hemorrhages, cardiac infection, and cardiac adiposity of the corticosteroid-treated heart, cardiac hemosiderosis, and anthracycline chemotherapy. Carcinoid heart disease is a unique type of heart disease associated with a unique type of cancer.

W. C. Roberts: Baylor Heart and Vascular Center, Baylor University Medical Center, Dallas, Texas

TABLE 39.1   PRIMARY BENIGN NEOPLASMS OF THE HEART (1976–1993)

Tumor[a]	Total	Surgical	Autopsy	Age ≤15 yr at diagnosis
Myxoma	114	102	12	4
Rhabdomyoma	20	6	14	20
Fibroma	20	18	2	13
Hemangioma	17	10	7	2
Atrioventricular nodal	10	0	10	2
Granular cell	4	0	4	0
Lipoma	2	2	0	0
Paraganglioma	2	2	0	0
Myocytic hamartoma	2	2	0	0
Histiocytoid cardiomyopathy	2	0	2	2
Inflammatory pseudotumor	2	2	0	1
Fibrous histiocytoma	1	0	1	0
Epithelioid hemangioendothelioma	1	1	0	0
Bronchogenic cyst	1	1	0	0
Teratoma	1	0	1	1
Totals	199	146 (73%)	53 (27%)	45 (23%)

[a]Excludes papillary fibroelastoma and lipomatous hypertrophy of the atrial septum.
Modified from Burke A, Virmani R. *Atlas of tumor pathology. Tumors of the heart and great vessels.* Washington, DC: Armed Forces Institute of Pathology, 1996:231.

HISTORICAL PERSPECTIVE

In the last 40 years, cardiac neoplasms have progressed from clinical curiosities described primarily in numerous case reports, with diagnosis mainly at autopsy, to fairly rapid antemortem diagnosis and frequent curative operative therapy. Diagnosis has been greatly facilitated by two-dimensional echocardiography and, in select cases, the use of MRI or CT.

CLASSIFICATION

There is no perfect classification for cardiac neoplasms. Like any organ or tissue, neoplasms involving the heart may be primary or secondary. The primary ones may be benign or malignant, and the secondary or metastatic ones are, by definition, malignant. The metastatic neoplasms are far more frequent than are the primary neoplasms by at least a 30:1 ratio (1,2). The various frequencies of the primary benign and primary malignant tumors vary from report to report, approximately 0.1% to 0.3% in most autopsy series. A list of primary benign neoplasms gathered by investigators at the Armed Forces Institute of Pathology is presented in Table 39.1; primary malignant tumors encountered are listed in Table 39.2 (3). The frequencies of the metastatic neoplasms also vary from report to report, but nearly all studies have listed carcinoma of the lung as the most commonly encountered metastatic tumor at autopsy, with cancer of the breast, followed by lymphoma

TABLE 39.2   PRIMARY MALIGNANT TUMORS OF THE HEART (1976–1993)

Tumor	Total	Surgical	Autopsy	Age ≤15 yr at diagnosis
Sarcoma	137 (95%)	116	21	11 (8%)
Angiosarcoma	33	22	11	1
Unclassified	33	30	3	3
Fibrous histiocytoma	16	16	0	1
Osteosarcoma	13	13	0	0
Leiomyosarcoma	12	11	1	1
Fibrosarcoma	9	9	0	1
Myxosarcoma	8	8	0	1
Rhabdomyosarcoma	6	2	4	3
Synovial	4	4	0	0
Liposarcoma	2	0	2	0
Schwannoma	1	1	0	0
Lymphoma	7 (5%)	1	6	0
Totals	144 (100%)	117 (81%)	27 (19%)	11 (8%)

Modified from Burke A, Virmani R. *Atlas of tumor pathology. Tumors of the heart and great vessels.* Washington, DC: Armed Forces Institute of Pathology, 1996:231.

TABLE 39.3 METASTATIC NEOPLASMS IN THE HEART AT NECROPSY IN THE ORDER OF FREQUENCY OF CANCERS ENCOUNTERED

Primary tumor	Total autopsies	Metastases to heart[a]
1. Lung	1,037	180 (17)
2. Breast	685	70 (10)
3. Lymphoma	392	67 (17)
4. Leukemia	202	66 (33)
5. Esophagus	294	37 (13)
6. Uterus	451	36 (8)
7. Melanoma	69	32 (46)
8. Stomach	603	28 (5)
9. Sarcoma	159	24 (15)
10. Oral cavity and tongue	235	22 (9)
11. Colon and rectum	440	22 (5)
12. Kidney	114	12 (11)
13. Thyroid gland	97	9 (9)
14. Larynx	100	9 (9)
15. Germ cell	21	8 (38)
16. Urinary bladder	128	8 (6)
17. Liver and biliary tract	325	7 (2)
18. Prostate gland	171	6 (4)
19. Pancreas	185	6 (3)
20. Ovary	188	2 (1)
21. Nose (interior)	32	1 (3)
22. Pharynx	67	1 (1)
23. Miscellaneous	245	0
Totals	6,240	653 (10)

[a]Numbers in parentheses are percentages.
Modified from Burke and Virmani, who combined studies of McAllister HA and Fenoglio JJ Jr. *Tumors of the cardiovascular system. Atlas of tumor pathology.* Washington, DC: Armed Forces Institute of Pathology, 1978:111–119; and Mukai J, Shinkai T, Tominaga K, et al. The incidence of secondary tumors of the heart and pericardium: a 10-year study. *Jpn J Clin Oncol* 1988;18:195–201.

TABLE 39.4 METASTATIC NEOPLASMS IN THE HEART AT NECROPSY: ORDER OF FREQUENCY OF METASTASES OF EACH DIFFERENT PRIMARY TUMOR

Primary tumor	Number of autopsies	Percent with metastases to heart
1. Melanoma	100	46
2. Germ cell	100	38
3. Leukemia	100	33
4. Lymphoma	100	17
5. Lung	100	17
6. Sarcoma	100	15
7. Esophagus	100	13
8. Kidney	100	11
9. Breast	100	10
10. Mouth and tongue	100	9
11. Thyroid gland	100	9
12. Uterus	100	8
13. Urinary bladder	100	6
14. Stomach	100	5
15. Colon and rectum	100	5
16. Prostate gland	100	4
17. Pancreas	100	3
18. Nose (interior)	100	3
19. Ovary	100	1
20. Pharynx	100	1
21. Miscellaneous	100	0

These percentages were obtained by combining studies by McAllister HA and Fenoglio JJ Jr. *Tumors of the cardiovascular system. Atlas of tumor pathology.* Washington, DC: Armed Forces Institute of Pathology, 1978;111–119; and Mukai K, Shinkai T, Tominaga K, et al. The incidence of secondary tumors of the heart and pericardium: a 10-year study. *Jpn J Clin Oncol* 1988;18:195–201.

and leukemia, as the next leading causes (Table 39.3). The order of frequency of metastases is different, however, if the frequency of each different type of tumor with metastasis to the heart is determined. For example, Table 39.4 lists the frequencies of metastases to the heart in each of 100 cases of 20 separate tumors: Melanoma has the highest frequency of metastases to the heart followed by malignant germ cell tumor, leukemia, lymphoma, cancer of the lung, and then the various sarcomas (3).

LOCATION OF CARDIAC NEOPLASMS

Cardiac neoplasms may involve only the endocardium, only the myocardium, only the epicardium, or various combinations (Fig. 39.1). By far, the most common location of metastatic cardiac neoplasm is the epicardium. Neoplasms limited to parietal pericardium without extension into the epicardium are not considered cardiac neoplasms. The epicardial tumor deposits may be multifocal or single, or they may be extensive and essentially diffuse or nearly so. Likewise, the intramyocardial masses may be focal or multifocal. The most common locations for intramyocardial masses are the left ventricular free wall and the ventricular septum, the portions of the heart, of course, with the greatest myocardial mass. The endocardial neoplasms are the intracavitary ones. They may involve a single cardiac cavity or more than one. They may be limited to either the right or left side of the heart, or they may involve both. Intracavitary tumors produce obstruction to inflow into the heart or into a ventricular cavity or outflow from a ventricular cavity. The intracavitary neoplasms are the ones that may partially dislodge and produce either pulmonary or systemic emboli or both. The intracavitary deposits have the potential of producing the triad of obstruction, embolization, and constitutional symptoms.

TECHNIQUES FOR DIAGNOSING CARDIAC NEOPLASMS

Symptoms and Physical Signs

The signs and symptoms produced by the various cardiac neoplasms are determined primarily by the tumor's location in the heart. Physical examination is rarely diagnostic (4–7). ▼ h78

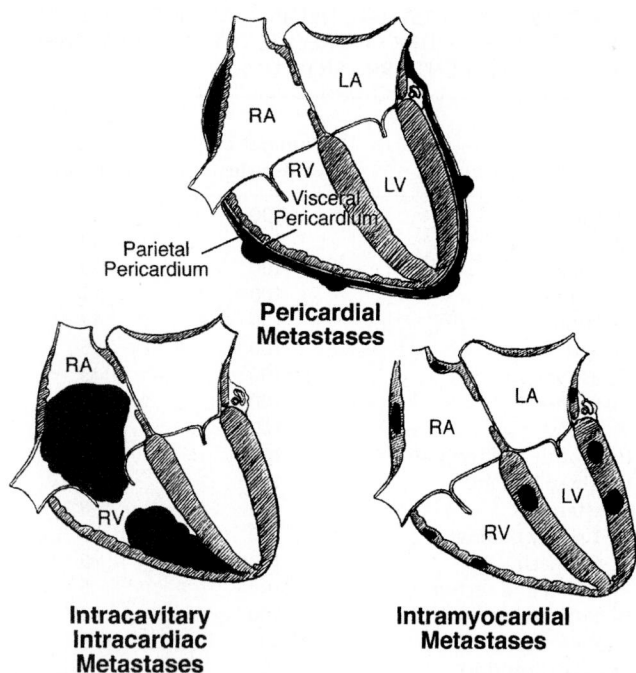

FIGURE 39.1 Diagram showing various locations of cardiac neoplasms involving the heart. LA, left atrium; LV, left ventricle; RA, right atrium; RV, right ventricle.

Electrocardiography

The electrocardiogram (ECG) result is usually nonspecific (8,9), but it could be far more useful than has been appreciated in the past. The problem has been that the ECG may be recorded when diagnosis is first considered, but subsequent ECGs are not taken frequently toward the end of the patient's life. One study (8) compared findings on ECG in patients with malignant lymphoma who had cardiac lymphoma to another group of patients with lymphoma who did not have cardiac involvement. The percentage with abnormal tracings (62%) was similar in each of the two groups. Fewer than one-half of the patients had more than one ECG during the entire illness. Findings included sinus tachycardia, low-voltage, ectopic tachycardia (including atrial fibrillation), atrial flutter, atrial tachycardia, atrial ventricular block (including prolonged PR interval), second- and third-degree block, premature ventricular complexes, right- or left-axis deviation, right bundle branch block, T-wave abnormalities, and ST-T–wave changes of usually nonspecific nature. The sudden development of some of these ECG findings in a patient who previously lacked these changes suggests cardiac involvement.

Radiography

The chest radiograph may be helpful, particularly when an epicardial neoplasm is present (10). Enlargement of the cardiac silhouette, mediastinal widening, a hilar mass, or an irregular contour of the cardiac silhouette may suggest peri-

cardial involvement. Calcium within an intracardiac neoplasm can be seen, on occasion, by chest radiography or fluoroscopy. The lung fields may have a paucity of pulmonary markings in patients with large right atrial or right ventricular neoplasms. Patients with neoplasms in the left atrium may have pulmonary changes similar to those in mitral stenosis. Likewise, left ventricular neoplasms causing obstruction to left ventricular inflow or outflow may produce similar pulmonary arterial vascular changes.

Echocardiography

More cardiac tumors today are diagnosed by echocardiography (Table 39.5), at least initially, than by any other instrument of precision. Diagnosis of left atrial myxoma has been one of the principal uses of echocardiography since the introduction of the technique (11–15). The classic left atrial myxoma is a mobile echogenic mass that is in the body of the left atrium in ventricular systole and passes into the mitral orifice in ventricular diastole. Occasionally, echocardiography detects a left atrial myxoma that is small or not close to the mitral orifice; therefore, it is clinically silent. Although it is usually possible to detect intracardiac tumors with transthoracic echocardiography, the transesophageal examination produces, as a rule, spectacular images and makes diagnosis, particularly of atrial masses, relatively easy (16,17). The transesophageal examination not only offers a higher sensitivity for detecting left atrial tumors, for example, but also permits a clearer picture of the attachment or stalk of the tumor and more precise characterization of the size, shape, and location of the mass. A major advantage of echocardiography is its ability to provide serial studies. Thus, by this technique, one may see progressive increase in size of a neoplasm or detect recurrence once the initial tumor is excised. The echocardiogram also has been useful in detecting intracardiac tumors other than myxomas, including rhabdomyomas and rhabdomyosarcomas, neoplasms that occur primarily in infants and are located usually in the ventricles. The echocardiogram is also helpful in detecting metastases to the heart. This is particularly true in neoplasms that migrate up the inferior vena cava into the right side of the heart, such as renal cell carcinoma or adrenal cell carcinoma. Echocardiography, particularly transesophageal, has been extremely helpful in detecting mediastinal or extracardiac masses, which may compress the cardiac structure.

Computed Tomography

CT is useful in diagnosing cardiac tumors (18,19); it may be especially useful in defining the degree of intramyocardial extension or the lack thereof and whether the tumor is present in adjacent extracardiac structures. Ultrafast CT appears to be particularly well suited for assessing intracardiac masses.

TABLE 39.5 IMAGING TECHNIQUES FOR THE DIAGNOSIS OF CARDIAC TUMORS

	Radiography	Computed tomography	Angiography	Magnetic resonance imaging	Echocardiography
Primary benign tumors					
Myxoma	+	++	+++	++++	+++++
Pericardial cyst	++	+++	0	+++++	+
Lipoma	+	+++	+	+++++	+++
Fibroelastoma	0	0	0	+++	+++++
Rhabdomyoma	0	+	+	++++	+++++
Fibroma	0	+		++++	++++
Primary malignant tumors					
Sarcoma	+	++	++	+++++	+++
Mesothelioma	+	+++	+	+++++	++
Lymphoma	++	+++	+	+++++	++
Secondary tumors					
Direct extension	+	+++	++	+++++	+++
Venous extension	0	+	+++	++++	++++
Metastatic spread	+	++	+	++++	++

0, of no use; +, of limited use; ++, may be of use; +++, useful; ++++, very useful; +++++, preferred diagnostic tool.
From Salcedo EE, Cohen GI, White RD, et al. Cardiac tumors: diagnosis and management. *Curr Prob Cardiol* 1992;17:75–137, with permission.

Magnetic Resonance Imaging

Compared with CT, MRI appears to be of greater value in delineating cardiac tumors (20). It may be able to depict the size, shape, and surface characteristics of the tumor more clearly than CT. This technique also can provide information regarding tissue composition that can help to differentiate neoplasms from thrombi.

Angiography

A cardiac catheterization and selective angiography are no longer necessary in all patients with cardiac neoplasms because adequate preoperative information can usually be obtained by echocardiography, CT, or MRI. For cases in which the latter three techniques have not fully defined the location and attachment of the neoplasm, in which all four chambers of the heart have not been well delineated, or in which another type of cardiac condition is suspected (such as coronary arterial narrowing), then cardiac catheterization with angiography might be necessary. Angiography in patients with cardiac neoplasms is particularly useful in detecting compression or displacement of cardiac cavities or large masses and the magnitude of the intracavitary filling defects. The most frequent angiographic findings are intracavitary filling defects, which may be either fixed or mobile, lobulated or smooth, and attached over a broad base or by a narrow stalk. Coronary angiography is sometimes helpful in visualizing the vascular supply of the neoplasm and the relation of the neoplasm to the coronary arteries. The vascular pattern is not helpful, however, in differentiating benign from malignant tumors. In contrast to the other diagnostic techniques, cardiac catheterization can be a bit risky in patients with intracardiac neoplasms, because the catheter may dislodge a fragment of the tumor

with resulting embolus. Thus, the noninvasive techniques are preferred before cardiac catheterization in a patient suspected of having an intracardiac mass. The transseptal approach to the left atrium is not advised if a left atrial tumor is suspected, because the stalk of the left atrial myxoma is usually attached to the fossa ovale membrane, where the transseptal catheter courses.

SPECIFIC BENIGN PRIMARY CARDIAC NEOPLASMS

Myxoma

Myxomas are by far the most common type of primary cardiac tumor; 75% of them are located in the left atrial cavity (*e*Fig. 39.1.1), approximately 23% in the right atrial cavity (Fig. 39.2), and approximately 2% in a ventricular cavity (21–33). On rare occasion, the tumor is present in more than one cavity. Generally, when located in the left atrium, the neoplasm produces symptoms when it reaches approximately 7 cm in size. Those in the right atrium that produce symptoms are usually approximately twice as large and sometimes several-fold larger. The cell of origin of the myxoma is still unclear (22,34–36). How fast atrial myxomas grow has never been clarified. An attempt to answer this question was provided by a study that examined the size of recurrent myxomas and divided that size in grams by the interval between the first and second operations (37). It was estimated that recurrent left atrial myxomas grow an average of 0.15 cm per month or 1.80 cm per year, or an average of 1.2 g per month or 14.0 g per year. Whatever the exact growth rate may be, both recurrent and initial left atrial myxomas appear to grow rather rapidly (38,39). Morphologic diagnosis of myxoma is readily

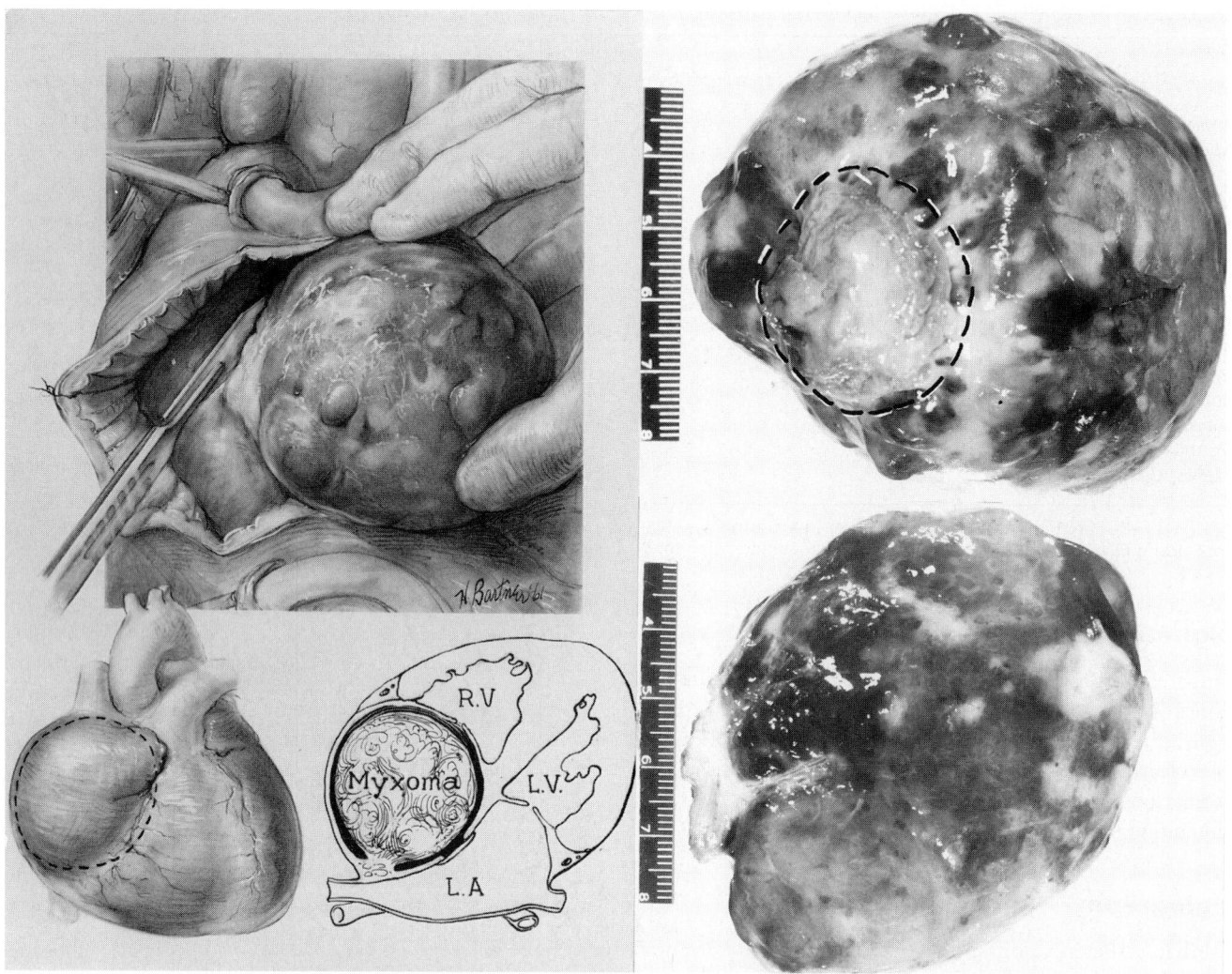

FIGURE 39.2 Myxoma excised from the right atrium of a 46-year-old man (S61-980) who had had evidence of cardiac dysfunction for 12 years. The tumor was attached to the atrial septum by a relatively small stalk (surrounded by dashed circle, *upper right*). The myxoma weighed 142 g, and its largest diameter was 8 cm. A view of the cut section of the tumor is shown in the lower right. LA, left atrium; LV, left ventricle; RV, right ventricle.

made by gross inspection, and their appearance is clearly different from thrombi. The surface is smooth but irregular, shiny, and usually multicolored. Although there are exceptions (29–32,40–43), attachment is nearly always to the atrial septum if the tumor is in the left atrium, and the stalk is most commonly much smaller than the maximal diameter of the mass. On occasion, the site of attachment to the atrial septum is broad. The mean age of patients with sporadic myxoma is 56 years, and at least 75% are women. During the last 10 years at Baylor University Medical Center in Dallas, 15 left atrial myxomas have been excised—14 were in women.

Familial cardiac myxomas constitute approximately 10% of all myxomas, and they appear to have an autosomal dominant transmission (44). These occur in younger patients (mean age, 25) and have less female gender predominance. The myxomas in the familial syndrome are much more liable (50% of the time) to be multiple and to have a ventricular cavity location (13% as compared with <1% in the nonfamilial or sporadic patients with myxomas). These patients typically have exterior facial freckling; they have noncardiac myxomas (breast or skin) and also endocrine neoplasms. Both the NAME (nevi, atrial myxoma, neurofibromata, ephelides) and the LAMB (lentigines, atrial myxoma, and balloon nevi) syndromes are associated with the familial variety of cardiac myxoma. Chromosomal abnormalities for atrial myxoma on chromosome 2 (Carney's) and chromosome 12 (*Ki-ras* genes) have been described.

Myxomas probably present the most varied clinical picture of all primary cardiac neoplasms (4–6,23,25,26,45). Several major syndromes have been observed, including presentation with signs of emboli, obstruction to blood flow, and various constitutional syndromes. Fragments of tumor located in the right side of the heart may embolize to the lungs, and of those in the left side of the heart, of course, to various systemic organs. Diagnosis may be made, on occasion, by finding typical myxomatous endothelial-like cells, which are elongated and spindle shaped with round or oval nuclei and prominent nucleoli, in surgically removed emboli.

Obstruction to blood flow may occur at the orifice of any valve, most commonly of course, the mitral valve. Interference with flow through the mitral orifice may mimic signs of mitral stenosis, including signs of pulmonary congestion, diastolic apical rumble, opening snap, and accentuated first heart sounds. A murmur of mitral regurgitation may also be present as a result of chronic damage to the valve leaflets or to interference with proper closure of the valve by tumor. Differentiation between left atrial tumor and primary mitral stenosis is suggested by the influence of position on symptoms and on the intensity of the precordial murmurs and the opening snap.

The constitutional symptoms associated with atrial myxomas include fever, weight loss, Raynaud's phenomenon, digital clubbing, anemia, elevated erythrocyte sedimentation rate, elevated leukocyte count, decreased platelet count, positive seroreactive protein, and abnormal serum proteins (usually increased gamma globulins). These constitutional symptoms may mimic infective endocarditis, collagen vascular disease, or occult malignancy. A myxoma also may become infected (46).

The proper treatment of myxoma in any cavity of the heart is operative resection, because no medicine is known to shrink myxomas or to prevent their continued growth (21,27,33). Some surgeons advise a biatrial approach for full visualization of both sides of the heart and then complete removal of a left or right atrial myxoma, excising the full thickness of the atrial septum if the neoplasm is attached to the region of the fossa ovalis. If a large portion of the atrial septum is removed, a patch must be used to close the defect. Because fragmentation and embolization of the tumor are ever-present threats, vigorous palpation and other manipulations of the heart should be avoided until cardiopulmonary bypass is initiated. Most surgeons induce ventricular standstill with cardioplegia solution before manipulating the heart to reduce the possibility of fragmentation of portions of the tumor. Left atrial myxomas have been removed successfully during pregnancy. On occasion, an atrioventricular valve has been so traumatized by the tumor prolapsing through it during ventricular diastole that valve excision and replacement are necessary. Fortunately, recurrences of atrial myxomas are rare, and if they do recur, it is usually within a 4-year period (38,39).

Rhabdomyoma

The most common cardiac neoplasm in infants and children is rhabdomyoma (47). There is some question about whether this particular tumor is a true neoplasm or a hamartoma. These neoplasms are usually multiple, most often involve the ventricular myocardium, and project into the cavity or move freely as a pedunculated mass (48–50). Associated tuberous sclerosis is present in approximately one-third of the patients. The diagnosis is suggested by the presence of yellow-brown angiofibromas (adenoma sebaceum) on the face, sublingual fibromas around the fingernails, café au lait spots, and subcutaneous nodules. Presenting symptoms may be caused by obstruction to inflow to or outflow from the ventricles, arrhythmias, atrioventricular block, pericardial effusion, and even sudden death (51). These neoplasms may mimic pulmonic valve stenosis and produce hypoxic spells, resembling those seen in tetralogy of Fallot. These neoplasms are usually readily diagnosed by echocardiography, angiography, or MRI. Prenatal detection of intracardiac rhabdomyoma by intrauterine echocardiography has been reported. The occurrence of more than one tumor does not prevent operative intervention. On rare occasions, these tumors have produced ventricular tachycardia in infants, and this arrhythmia has disappeared following successful operative removal.

Fibroma

Fibromas are usually within a ventricular wall (intramural) (3,52) (*e*Fig. 39.2.1). Most also occur in infants and children. Calcific deposits may be present within the neoplasm. Sudden death has occurred in approximately one-third of the patients, presumably the result of a conduction defect, arrhythmia, or obstruction to outflow from a ventricle. Left axis deviation has been seen on ECG. Total or partial resection of the neoplasm may relieve obstruction with an excellent probability of long-term survival.

Lipoma

Lipomas involving the heart may be extremely small and represent incidental necropsy findings or they may be massive (53–56). The largest cardiac neoplasm ever reported apparently was an intrapericardial lipoma. They may be mistaken for pericardial cysts, cause pericardial effusion, or they may be asymptomatic and suggested by a widened mediastinum on chest radiography. Intramyocardial lipomas are encapsulated and usually small. Lipomas also have been located on cardiac valves, where they may simulate vegetations or myxomas (55). MRI permits preoperative identification of these fatty tumors.

Hemangioma

Hemangiomas are best diagnosed by coronary angiography, which yields a characteristic "tumor blush." Spontaneous resolution without treatment has been reported. Total excision usually is not possible.

SPECIFIC MALIGNANT PRIMARY CARDIAC NEOPLASMS

Angiosarcoma

Nearly all primary malignant cardiac neoplasms are sarcomas; the most frequent is angiosarcoma (57–62), which characteristically originates from the right atrium or from the epicardium of the right atrium. The large quantity of vascular channels within these tumors and the subsequent large quantity of blood flowing through them may produce a continuous precordial murmur. Approximately 25% of all angiosarcomas are, at least in part, intracavitary with valvular obstruction and cause right-sided heart failure and pericardial tamponade with a hemorrhagic-type fluid. The course is rapid, with widespread metastases, and operative intervention is usually unsuccessful.

Rhabdomyosarcoma

Rhabdomyosarcoma is the second most frequent primary sarcoma of the heart, and, like angiosarcoma, it is most

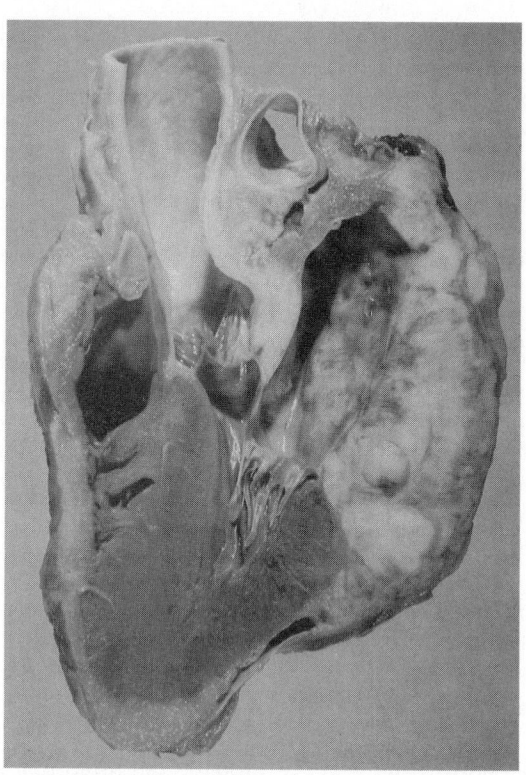

FIGURE 39.4 Cardiac histiocytic lymphoma in a 64-year-old woman (A77-172) who had had evidence of congestive heart failure for 7 months. The cause of the heart failure was not apparent until necropsy. The wall of the left atrium is massively thickened by the neoplasm. (From Roberts CS, Gottdiener JS, Roberts WC. Clinically undetected cardiac lymphoma causing congestive heart failure. *Am Heart J* 1990;120:1239–1242, with permission.)

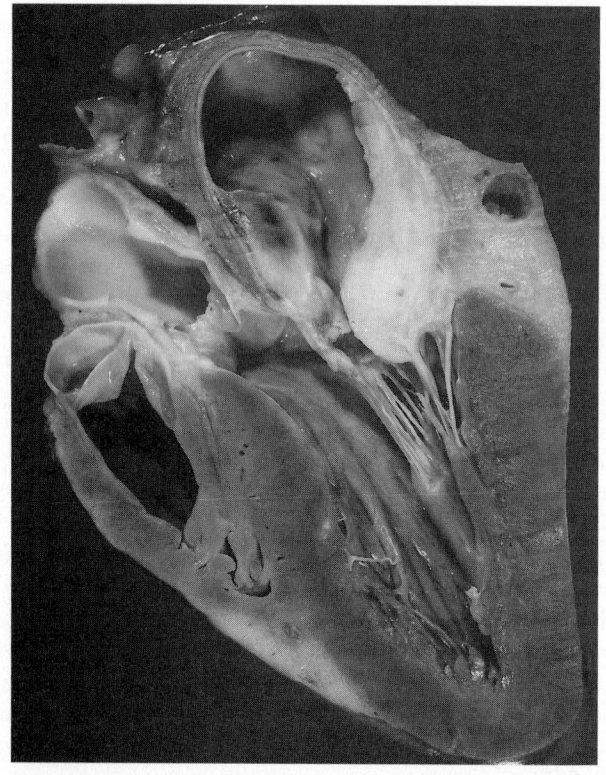

FIGURE 39.3 Primary cardiac sarcoma, undifferentiated type, causing mitral stenosis in a 46-year-old woman (A90-2) who had been well until 8 months before death. Cardiac catheterization disclosed a 20 mm Hg mean diastolic gradient between the pulmonary artery wedge position and the left ventricle. The right ventricular pressure was 105/18 mm Hg. The neoplasm was located in the walls of the left atrium and in both arteries and posterior mitral leaflets. (From Domanski MJ, Delaney TF, Kleiner DE Jr, et al. Primary sarcoma of the heart causing mitral stenosis. *Am J Cardiol* 1990;66:893–895, with permission.)

common in male subjects (63–65). In contrast to angiosarcoma, however, no single cardiac chamber has a predilection for this neoplasm. Indeed, the neoplasm may be in all four cardiac chambers, or at least in more than one, and obstruction may occur in one or more valve orifices. Again, prognosis is poor, survival is short, and operative intervention is usually futile.

Miscellaneous Neoplasms

Fibrosarcoma, liposarcoma, primary malignant lymphoma, and occasional sarcomas of other cell types constitute the remaining but infrequent primary malignant coronary neoplasms (66–69) (Fig. 39.3, *e*Fig. 39.3.1, and Fig. 39.4). All of these neoplasms may obstruct valvular orifices or obliterate chambers, produce peripheral emboli, or both (70). Hypertrophic cardiomyopathy has been suggested by heavy tumorous infiltrations of the ventricular septum (71).

METASTATIC NEOPLASMS TO THE HEART

Metastatic or secondary tumors of the heart with a primary in another body organ or tissue are far more frequent than are primary tumors of the heart (72). The secondary tumors are far more commonly carcinomas than sarcomas, simply because carcinomas are far more common. Diagnosis can be suspected whenever cardiac manifestations occur in a patient diagnosed with a primary tumor in an organ or tissue other than the heart. The development of cardiac enlargement, tachycardia, arrhythmias, or heart failure in the presence of neoplasm elsewhere in the body is highly suggestive of cardiac metastases. Only rarely is metastatic tumor limited to the heart. Thus, the presence of metastatic tumor in the heart usually indicates widespread metastases in a number of body organs. On rare occasion, cardiac involvement may be the first or only expression of a noncardiac primary neoplasm. The most common sign is tamponade (73). Direct invasion of the heart via the vena cava or pulmonary veins may lead to obstruction of an atrioventricular valve, as well as to pulmonary or systemic emboli or both (74–76).

Carcinoma of the lung and carcinoma of the breast tend to invade the parietal pericardium and then the visceral pericardium, leading to myocardial constriction, pericardial effusion, or both (*e*Fig. 39.4.1). Another common presentation of cancer of the lung is invasion of the pulmonary veins within the lung, with spread of the cancer within the lumen of the pulmonary veins into the left atrium. From there, the cancer in turn can continue into the mitral orifice, sometimes causing obstruction of that orifice (77,78) (Fig. 39.5). Metastatic cancer from the lung to the adrenal

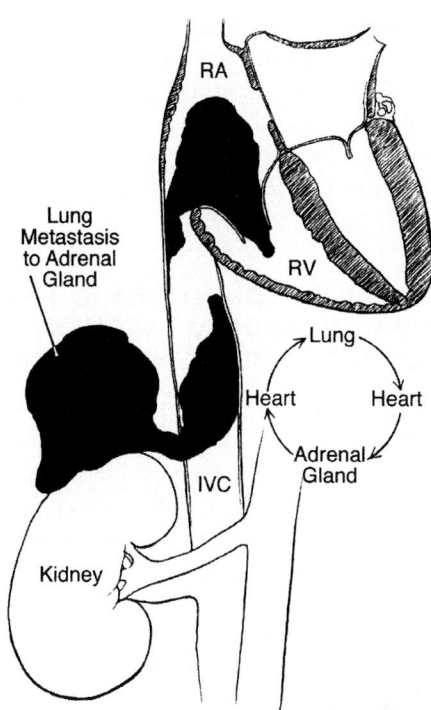

FIGURE 39.6 Diagram of metastatic cancer of the lung to the right adrenal gland with extension into the inferior vena cava (IVC) and then into the right side of the heart in a 57-year-old man (DCVAH 84A-121). Echocardiography showed the right atrial mass, which prolapsed through the tricuspid valve in atrial systole. RA, right atrium; RV, right ventricle.

gland also may extend into the inferior vena cava and then into the right side of the heart (Fig. 39.6), just as primary adrenal gland or renal cancer can (79). Cancer of the lung or breast surrounding the main right or left pulmonary artery can lead to pulmonary arterial obstruction (80).

Melanoma has the highest frequency of metastases to the heart per 100 cases of any neoplasm (81,82). The metastases may be anywhere in the heart; usually, melanotic metastases invade the walls of all four cardiac chambers, the epicardium, and the endocardium (*e*Fig. 39.6.1). The cancers in these patients are in so many organs that the presence of the neoplasm in the heart is almost incidental. Resection of an intracardiac melanoma has been accomplished (83).

Leukemia commonly invades the heart (84). In the days before platelet transfusions, extensive hemorrhages into the myocardial walls and into the endocardium and epicardium were commonly found in patients with fatal leukemia of various types. Histologically, leukemic infiltration between myocardial cells is quite common, and sometimes gross deposits of leukemic cells are visible within the heart. A few patients with leukemia present with pericardial effusion, which is usually hemorrhagic. Large calcific deposits in the right side of the heart have been reported (85).

Lymphoma also has a high frequency of metastases to the heart (86–89). Nearly 25% of patients with lymphomas

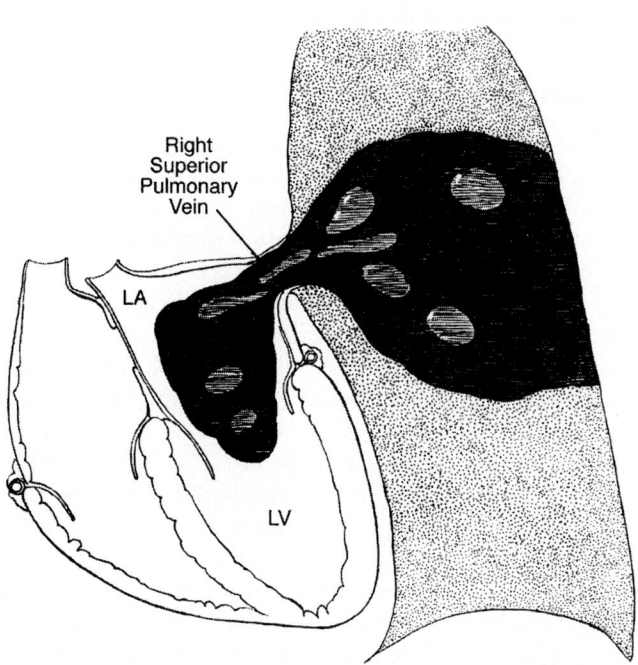

FIGURE 39.5 Sarcoma, undifferentiated type, in lung (primary uncertain, possibly in pulmonary vein) in a 29-year-old woman (A21-83) in whom echocardiography disclosed the tumor in the left atrium moving about "like a yo-yo." The left lung and its left atrial extension were operatively excised. LA, left atrium; LV, left ventricle.

of various types have lymphoma involving the epicardium, myocardium, or endocardium, or combinations. In contrast to leukemic involvement, the lymphomatous deposits are usually grossly discernible.

Some cancers, like osteogenic sarcoma, may have calcium within them (90–92) (*e*Fig. 39.6.2).

NONNEOPLASTIC CONDITIONS IN THE HEART OR PERICARDIUM FREQUENTLY MISTAKEN FOR CARDIAC NEOPLASM

Pericardial Cyst

Pericardial or mesothelial cysts are the most frequent benign "tumors" of the pericardium. These cysts are generally asymptomatic and found on routine chest radiography (93). Approximately one-fourth of the patients, however, develop various symptoms including chest pain, dyspnea, cough, and tachycardia, as a consequence of a pericardial cyst. The cysts are usually outside the pericardial cavity and, therefore, they really should not be considered cardiac tumors.

Teratoma

Teratomas are actually extracardiac in at least 99% of the cases but still within the pericardial cavity (94–96) (*e*Fig. 39.6.3). They arise and receive their blood supply from the ascending aorta or pulmonary trunk, presumably through the vasa vasorum. Most are found in infants and children and primarily in female subjects. Recurrent serous pericardial effusion in children should suggest intrapericardial teratoma. Because these tumors may become quite large, they may cause compression of various cardiac chambers and resulting symptoms.

Lipomatous Hypertrophy of the Atrial Septum

Massive fatty infiltration of the atrial septum is an extremely common condition occurring almost exclusively in persons over 50 years of age and usually over 65 years of age (97) (Fig. 39.7). These lesions are essentially limited to obese people, and they are always associated with enormous quantities of subepicardial adipose tissue, particularly enormous amounts of adipose tissue in the atrioventricular sulci. These hearts are almost always so fat that they float in water (98). Normally, the atrial septum is less than 1 cm in thickness. In patients with lipomatous hypertrophy of the atrial septum, the atrial septum cephalad to the fossa ovale may be as thick as 7 cm, and the portion of atrial septum caudal to the fossa ovale may be as thick as 4 cm. Enormous infiltration of fat into the atrial septum may be associated with atrial arrhythmias. The importance of lipomatous hypertrophy of the atrial septum in the context

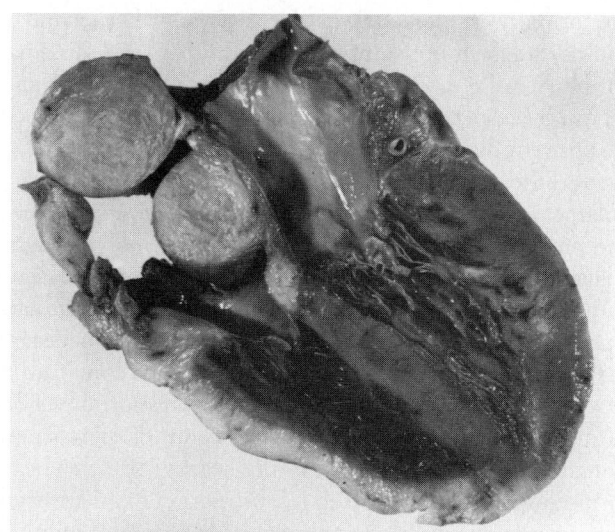

FIGURE 39.7 Lipomatous hypertrophy of the atrial septum in a 74-year-old woman (GT 77A-42) with huge fatty deposits in the atrial septum (except for the fossa ovale area). [From Shirani J, Roberts WC. Clinical, electrocardiographic and morphologic features of massive fatty deposits ("lipomatous hypertrophy") in the atrial septum. *J Am Coll Cardiol* 1993;22:226–238, with permission.]

of cardiac tumors is that these patients should not be operated on to remove fat from the atrial septum. The treatment is simply weight loss. These fatty deposits may be diagnosed by echocardiography, CT, or MRI (99,100). Fat in the subepicardial adipose tissue has been confused by echocardiography with pericardial effusion (101).

Papillary Fibroelastomas

Papillary fibroelastomas are small avascular growths with multiple papillary fronds usually limited to cardiac valves (mainly the aortic and mitral valves), and they are common in older persons (102). They consist of fibrous tissue covered by an elastic membrane, which in turn is covered by endocardium. Occasionally (approximately 15% of cases), they also occur on left ventricular or ventricular septal mural endocardium (103–112), particularly in patients with small or relatively small ventricular cavities, such as in patients with hypertrophic cardiomyopathy (103,109) or mitral stenosis with or without aortic valve stenosis (107,110,111). When located on the aortic valve, papillary fibroelastomas are usually found on the ventricular aspects of the cusps in the more central portions. They also occur on the aortic aspects of these cusps, usually near the margins (113–116). On the mitral valve leaflets, they are usually on the atrial aspects near the margins (117–124). In patients with hypertrophic cardiomyopathy or mitral stenosis, they may be on the ventricular aspects of the anterior mitral leaflet and sometimes on mural endocardium, particularly over the papillary muscles. These lesions may be the result of contact of one valve leaflet with another or one mural endocardial surface with another.

A number of patients have been reported with papillary fibroelastomas and stroke (115–118,122,123,125–129). Whether the stroke was truly connected with the cardiac fibroelastomas is debatable. Some patients have been in their 20s or 30s without other predisposing features or findings commonly associated with cerebral infarction, and the occurrence of stroke in the younger age group is suggestive of a connection. In contrast to myxoma, in which myxomatous material has been seen in systemic emboli, however, histologic findings of papillary fibroelastomas have not been observed in a cerebral artery in a patient with stroke and cardiac papillary fibroelastomas. Furthermore, the papillary fibroelastomas are firmly attached to valvular or mural endocardium, and dislodgement of a fibroelastoma therefore would appear unlikely. Thrombus, however, is occasionally superimposed on papillary fibroelastomas, and it may be that the thrombus is the material that is dislodged and responsible for the stroke.

Additionally, angina pectoris (129), acute myocardial infarction (130–134), and sudden death (130,135) have been observed in patients with cardiac papillary fibroelastomas, mainly on the aortic valve. These papillary growths may obstruct an aortic ostium of a coronary artery (136,137). On rare occasion, papillary fibroelastomas have been observed on the right side of the heart, mainly the tricuspid valve (138–141).

Papillary fibroelastomas have been operatively excised from the cardiac valve, mural endocardium, or both in patients with evidence of stroke or other peripheral events, and a few patients have had cardiac valve replacement (107,109,111,112,115,116,118–120,125,126,133,137,139, 141). When papillary fibroelastomas are detected by echocardiography in asymptomatic patients, operative excision rarely appears warranted.

Thrombi

Thrombi within an intracardiac cavity may be indistinguishable from neoplasm by echocardiography or radiography. Grossly, however, they are very different.

Sarcoid

When located in myocardium, sarcoid granuloma may grossly resemble neoplasm (142–144).

CONSEQUENCES OF THERAPY FOR NEOPLASMS IN THE HEART OR MEDIASTINUM

Radiation Heart Disease

Radiation heart disease was first recognized after radiation therapy for Hodgkin's disease (145–148). Some of the earlier patients with Hodgkin's disease received 8,000 rad,

which adversely affected the pericardium, myocardium, and endocardium. The most common manifestation of radiation heart disease is pericardial effusion. Fibrin deposits occur on both the visceral and parietal aspects of the pericardia. Because coronary arteries are located in subepicardial adipose tissue, they often receive the effects of radiation. Many patients have been reported to have coronary arterial narrowing at a very young age after radiation therapy, particularly patients with Hodgkin's disease. The intimal plaques resulting from radiation heart disease cannot be distinguished from plaques occurring from typical atherosclerosis. The distinguishing feature of radiation heart disease involving the coronary arteries is extensive fibrous thickening of the adventitia, and also loss, focally or diffusely, of internal and external elastic membranes, particularly the latter. Narrowing of coronary ostia also is common in radiation heart disease. In addition, radiation can cause considerable scarring within the subepicardial adipose tissue. The second most common manifestation of radiation heart disease is mural endocardial thickening, most commonly of the right atrium and ventricle, but focally also in the left ventricle. The third most common manifestation of radiation heart disease is interstitial fibrosis; depending on the portal of entry, it usually involves the anterior wall of the right ventricle more than any other portion of the heart.

Cardiac Hemorrhages

Thrombocytopenia, particularly if persistent, often results in focal epicardial, myocardial, and mural endocardial hemorrhages. If the hemorrhages are located in conduction tissue, various degrees of heart block or arrhythmias may be the consequence.

Cardiac Infection

The most common cardiac infections today in cancer patients are myocardial abscesses and mural endocardial and epicardial abscesses. These are particularly prevalent in patients with prolonged leukopenia (149,150). Patients having unsuccessful bone marrow transplantation are particularly prone to these infections, which usually are produced by fungi, not bacteria. Gas gangrene may involve the heart as well as most other body organs and tissues (151).

Cardiac Adiposity or the Corticosteroid-Treated Heart

Patients with various types of cancers, particularly those with leukemia and lymphoma, and those developing cancer after transplantation of one or more body organs, usually receive corticosteroid therapy for prolonged periods. The consequence is excessive deposition of fat in the heart, mainly in the subepicardial areas (152). These hearts may become so fatty that they float in water (buffalo hump of the heart), and this excessive subepicardial adipose tissue may simulate pericardial effusion.

Cardiac Hemosiderosis

Normally, the human body contains approximately 4 g of iron. If the deposits increase to approximately 25 g, iron deposits are then usually found within myocardial cells. Patients who receive 100 units of blood without associated bleeding diatheses can acquire approximately 25 g of iron within the body organs and tissues. This situation may exist in some patients with cancer, particularly leukemia, and the result is cardiac hemosiderosis (153). These patients may be asymptomatic, or they may develop features of dilated cardiomyopathy with heart failure. At times, ventricular arrhythmias may be a consequence. Myocardial restriction as a result of myocardial ironic deposits has occurred, but dilatation is far more common (154).

Anthracycline Chemotherapy (Doxorubicin and Daunorubicin)

Cardiac toxicity is a well-recognized complication of doxorubicin and daunorubicin therapy and is frequently the dose-limiting factor in their administration (155–157). Clinical toxicity is usually manifested by evidence of impaired left ventricular systolic function. Morphologic signs of toxicity may be present when clinical signs of toxicity are absent.

A UNIQUE HEART DISEASE ASSOCIATED WITH A UNIQUE CANCER: CARCINOID HEART DISEASE

Carcinoid tumors are never primary in the heart, and they rarely metastasize to the heart (158). Nevertheless, patients with ileal, bronchial, or ovarian carcinoid, when hepatic metastases are present, often develop distinctive lesions in the heart, particularly in the right side (159–163) (Fig. 39.8). The distinctive lesions consist of deposits of fibrous tissue devoid of elastic fibers on the ventricular aspect of the tricuspid valve leaflets and on the arterial aspect of the pulmonic valve leaflets. Occasionally, deposits also are seen on the ventricular aspects of the mitral leaflets and, rarely and usually to a small extent, on the aortic aspects of the aortic valve cusps. These lesions may result in tricuspid regurgitation and stenosis and pulmonic valve stenosis and regurgitation. Surprisingly, patients with carcinoid heart disease, compared with patients with metastatic carcinoid disease without carcinoid heart disease, have similar life spans after diagnosis of the carcinoid syndrome. The syndrome is diagnosed primarily by the presence of facial flushing and diarrhea.

Ross and Roberts (162) studied at necropsy 36 patients with metastatic carcinoid: 21 (57%) with and 15 (43%)

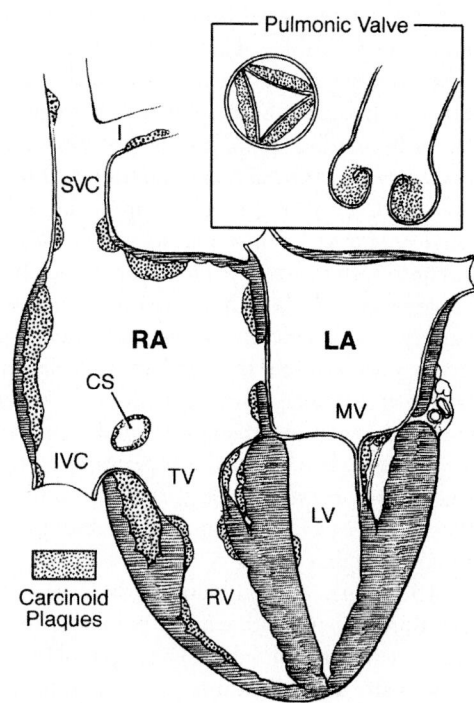

FIGURE 39.8 Diagram showing location of carcinoid fibrous plaques in carcinoid heart disease. CS, coronary sinus ostium; I, innominate vein; IVC, inferior vena cava; LA, left atrium; LV, left ventricle; MV, mitral valve; RA, right atrium; RV, right ventricle; SVC, superior vena cava; TV, tricuspid valve. (From Ross EM, Roberts WC. The carcinoid syndrome: comparison of 21 necropsy subjects with carcinoid heart disease to 15 necropsy subjects without carcinoid heart disease. *Am J Med* 1986;79:339–354, with permission.)

without carcinoid heart disease. The two groups were similar in mean age (54 vs. 55 years), duration of clinical illness (4.7 vs. 6.3 years), body weight (50 vs. 52 kg), systemic blood pressure (117/77 vs. 128/77 mm Hg), blood hematocrit levels (37% vs. 36%), total serum protein levels (6.0 g per dL), and serum albumin levels (2.2 vs. 2.6 g per dL). The two groups differed in the frequency of the presence of precordial murmurs consistent with tricuspid regurgitation, pulmonic stenosis, or both (95% vs. 13%); cardiomegaly by chest radiography (38% vs. 0%); low voltage on ECG (47% vs. 0%); and location of the primary site of the carcinoid tumor. Total ECG 12-lead QRS voltage was similar in each group (105 vs. 132 mm; 10 mm = 1 mV). Of the patients with carcinoid heart disease, 43% died of cardiac causes; none of those without carcinoid heart disease died of cardiac causes. Of the 21 subjects with carcinoid heart disease, seven had left-sided cardiac involvement, but in none was it of functional significance. Thus, although carcinoid heart disease frequently is the cause of death in patients with the carcinoid syndrome, the development of carcinoid heart disease is not related to the duration of symptoms of the carcinoid syndrome.

All of the 21 patients with carcinoid heart disease studied by Ross and Roberts (162) had involvement of both tri-

THE FUTURE

Improvement of chemotherapy will almost certainly improve outcome of primary and metastatic cancer involving the heart.

cuspid and pulmonic valves by carcinoid plaques, and 19 also had carcinoid plaques on the mural endocardium of the right atrium and usually also on the mural endocardium of the right ventricle. The number of subjects with right-sided valvular dysfunction as a consequence of the carcinoid plaques on the valvular leaflets is less certain because of the relative difficulty in diagnosing by auscultation mild degrees of tricuspid and pulmonic valve dysfunction. In 2 of the 21 subjects with right-sided carcinoid heart disease, the degree of morphologic involvement of both valves was minimal, and valvular function clearly was not affected. Of the remaining 19 subjects, 18 had precordial systolic, diastolic, or both kinds of murmurs of grade 2/6 or greater intensity. ❦ h79

CONTROVERSIES AND PERSONAL PERSPECTIVES

Benign cardiac tumors should constantly be kept in mind because so many of them are entirely curable by operative therapy. It is not bad to overlook metastatic cancer to the heart, because virtually no cancers metastasize to the heart without metastasizing to other body organs and usually multiple other body organs. Cardiac tumors, whether primary or secondary, can simulate more common types of cardiac disease, and this fact should always be kept in mind.

REFERENCES

1. Lam KY, Dickens P, Chan ACL. Tumors of the heart. A 20-year experience with review of 12485 consecutive autopsies. *Arch Pathol Med* 1993;117:1027–1031.
2. Reynan K. Frequency of primary tumors of the heart. *Am J Cardiol* 1996;77:107.
3. Burke A, Virmani R. *Atlas of tumor pathology.* Third Series, Fascicle 16. *Tumors of the heart and great vessels.* Washington, DC: Armed Forces Institute of Pathology, 1996:231.
4. Goodwin JF. The spectrum of cardiac tumors. *Am J Cardiol* 1968;21:307–314.
5. Harvey WP. Clinical aspects of cardiac tumors. *Am J Cardiol* 1968;21:328.
6. Salcedo EE, Cohen GI, White RD, et al. Cardiac tumors: diagnosis and management. *Curr Prob Cardiol* 1992;17:75–137.
7. Roberts WC, Spray TL. Pericardial heart disease. *Curr Prob Cardiol* 1977;2:1–71.
8. Roberts WC, Glancy DL, DeVita VT Jr. Heart in malignant lymphoma (Hodgkin's disease, lymphosarcoma, reticulum cell sarcoma and mycosis fungoides). A study of 196 autopsy cases. *Am J Cardiol* 1968;22:85–107.
9. Lindsay J Jr, Goldberg SD, Roberts WC. Electrocardiogram in neoplastic and hematologic disorders. In: Rios JD, ed. *Clinical electrocardiographic correlations.* Philadelphia: FA Davis, 1977:225–242.
10. Steiner RE. Radiologic aspects of cardiac tumors. *Am J Cardiol* 1968;21:344–356.
11. Bass NM, Sharratt GJP. Left atrial myxoma diagnosed by echocardiography with observation on tumor movement. *Br Heart J* 1973;35:1332.
12. Giuliani ER, Lemur F, Schattenberg T. Unusual echocardiographic findings in a patient with left atrial myxoma. *Mayo Clin Proc* 1978;53:469.
13. Obeid AI, Marvasti M, Parker F, et al. Comparison of transthoracic and transesophageal echocardiography in diagnosis of left atrial myxoma. *Am J Cardiol* 1989;63:1006–1008.
14. Pernod J, Piwnica A, Duret JC. Right atrial myxoma: an echocardiographic study. *Br Heart J* 1978;40:201.
15. Meller J, Teichholz LE, Pichard AD, et al. Left ventricular myxoma: echocardiographic diagnosis and review of the literature. *Am J Med* 1977;63:816–823.
16. Reeder GS, Khandheria BK, Seward JB, et al. Transesophageal echocardiography and cardiac masses. *Mayo Clin Proc* 1991;66:1101–1109.
17. Mugge A, Daniel WG, Haverich A, et al. Diagnosis of noninfective cardiac mass lesions by two-dimensional echocardiography: comparison of the transthoracic and transesophageal approaches. *Circulation* 1991;83:70–78.
18. Monocada R, Baker M, Salinas M, et al. Diagnostic role of computed tomography in pericardial heart disease: congenital defects, thickening, neoplasms, and effusions. *Am Heart J* 1982;103:263–282.
19. Bateman TM, Sethna DH, Whiting JS, et al. Comprehensive noninvasive evaluation of left atrial myxomas using cardiac cine computed tomography. *J Am Coll Cardiol* 1987;9:1180–1183.
20. Boxer RA, LaCorte MA, Singh S, et al. Diagnosis of cardiac tumors in infants by magnetic resonance imaging. *Am J Cardiol* 1985;56:831–832.
21. Bahnson HT, Spencer FC, Andrus EC. Diagnosis and treatment of intracavitary myxomas of the heart. *Ann Surg* 1957;145:915–926.
22. Ferrans VJ, Roberts WC. Structural features of cardiac myxomas. Histology, histochemistry, and electron microscopy. *Hum Pathol* 1973;4:111–146.
23. Peters MN, Hall RJ, Cooley DA, et al. The clinical syndrome of atrial myxoma. *JAMA* 1974;230:695–701.

24. Morgan DL, Palazola J, Reed W, et al. Left heart myxomas. *Am J Cardiol* 1977;40:611–614.

25. St. John Sutton MG, Mercier L-A, Giuliani ER, et al. Atrial myxomas: a review of clinical experience in 40 patients. *Mayo Clin Proc* 1980;55:371–376.

26. Markel ML, Waller BF, Armstrong WF. Cardiac myxoma: a review. *Medicine* 1987;66:114–125.

27. Murphy MC, Sweeney MS, Putnam JB Jr, et al. Surgical treatment of cardiac tumors: a 25-year experience. *Ann Thorac Surg* 1990;49:612–618.

28. Tazelaar HD, Locke TJ, McGregor CGA. Pathology of surgically excised primary cardiac tumors. *Mayo Clin Proc* 1992;67:957–965.

29. Burke AP, Virmani R. Cardiac myxomas: a clinicopathologic study. *Am J Clin Pathol* 1994;100:671–680.

30. Morrow AG, Kahler RL, Reis RL. Primary myxoma of the right ventricle. Clinical, hemodynamic and angiographic findings before and following operative treatment. *Am J Med* 1966;40:954–960.

31. Hickie JB, Gibson H, Windsor HM. "The wrecking ball": right atrial myxoma. *Med J Aust* 1970;2:82–86.

32. Hada Y, Wolfe C, Murray GF, et al. Right ventricular myxoma. Case report and review of phonocardiographic and auscultatory manifestations. *Am Heart J* 1980;100:871–877.

33. Schaff HV, Mullany CJ. Surgery for cardiac myxomas. *Semin Thorac Cardiovas Surg* 2000;12:77–88.

34. Chopra P, Ray R, Airan B, et al. Appraisal of histogenesis of cardiac myxoma: our experience of 78 cases and review of literature. *Indian Heart J* 1999;51:69–74.

35. Pucci A, Gagliardotto P, Zanini C, et al. Histopathologic and clinical characterization of cardiac myxoma: review of 53 cases from a single institution. *Am Heart J* 2000;140:134–138.

36. Lindner V, Edah-Tally S, Chakfe N, et al. Cardiac myxoma with glandular component: case report and review of the literature. *Pathol Res Pract* 1999;195:267–272.

37. Malekzadeh S, Roberts WC. Growth rate of left atrial myxoma. *Am J Cardiol* 1989;64:1075–1076.

38. Shinfeld A, Katsumata T, Westaby S. Recurrent cardiac myxoma: seeding or multifocal disease? *Ann Thorac Surg* 1998;66:285–288.

39. Bortolotti U, Scioti G, Guglielmi C, et al. Recurrent myxoma of the left ventricle. Case report and review of the literature. *J Cardiovasc Surg* 1999;40:233–235.

40. Das AK, Reddy KS, Suwanjindar P, et al. Primary tumors of the aorta. *Ann Thorac Surg* 1996;62:1526–1528.

41. Chakfe N, Kretz JG, Valentin P, et al. Clinical presentation and treatment options for mitral valve myxoma. *Ann Thorac Surg* 1997;64:872–877.

42. Murphy DP, Glazier DB, Krause TJ. Mitral valve myxoma. *Ann Thorac Surg* 1997;64:1169–1170.

43. Thongcharoen P, Laksanabunsong P, Thongtang V. Left ventricular outflow tract obstruction due to a left ventricular myxoma: a case report and review of the literature. *J Med Assoc Thailand* 1997;80:799–806.

44. Singh SD, Lansing AM. Familial cardiac myxoma—a comprehensive review of reported cases. *J Kentucky Med Assoc* 1996;94:96–104.

45. Panos A, Kalangos A, Sztajzel J. Left atrial myxoma presenting with myocardial infarction. Case report and review of the literature. *Int J Cardiol* 1997;62:73–75.

46. Revankar SG, Clark RA. Infected cardiac myxoma. Case report and literature review. *Medicine* 1998;77:337–344.

47. Chan HSL, Sonley MJ, Moes CAF, et al. Primary and secondary tumors of childhood involving the heart, pericardium, and great vessels: a report of 75 cases and review of the literature. *Cancer* 1985;56:825–836.

48. Fenoglio JJ Jr, McAllister HA, Ferrans VJ. Cardiac rhabdomyoma: a clinico-pathologic and electron microscopic study. *Am J Cardiol* 1976;38:241–251.

49. Smythe JF, Dyck JD, Smallhorn JF, et al. Natural history of cardiac rhabdomyoma in infancy and childhood. *Am J Cardiol* 1990;66:1247–1249.

50. Burke AP, Virmani R. Cardiac rhabdomyoma: a clinico-pathologic study. *Mod Pathol* 1991;4:70–74.

51. Biancaniello TM, Meyer RA, Gaum WE, et al. Primary benign intramural ventricular tumors in children: pre- and post-operative electrocardiographic, echocardiographic, and angiocardiographic evaluation. *Am Heart J* 1982;103:852–857.

52. Williams DB, Danielson GK, McGoon DC, et al. Cardiac fibroma: long-term survival after excision. *J Thorac Cardiovasc Surg* 1982;84:230–236.

53. Estevez JM, Thompson DS, Levinson JP. Lipoma of the heart. Review of the literature and report of 2 autopsied cases. *Arch Pathol* 1964;77:638–642.

54. Moulton AL, Jaretzki A III, Bowman FO Jr, et al. Massive lipoma of the heart. *N Y State J Med* 1976;76:1820–1825.

55. Dollar AL, Wallace RB, Kent KM, et al. Mitral valve replacement for mitral lipoma associated with severe obesity. *Am J Cardiol* 1989;64:1405–1407.

56. Shirani J, Roberts WC. Epicardial lipoma. *Am Heart J* 1993;126:1030.

57. Bear PA, Moodie DS. Malignant primary cardiac tumors. The Cleveland Clinic Experience, 1956–1986. *Chest* 1987;92:860–862.

58. Putman JB Jr, Sweeney MS, Colon R, et al. Primary cardiac sarcomas. *Ann Thorac Surg* 1991;51:906–910.

59. Burke AP, Cowan D, Virmani R. Primary sarcomas of the heart. *Cancer* 1992;69:387–395.

60. Glancy DL, Morales JB, Roberts WC. Angiosarcoma of the heart. *Am J Cardiol* 1968;21:413–419.

61. Herrmann MA, Shankerman RA, Edwards WD, et al. Primary cardiac angiosarcoma: a clinicopathologic study of six cases. *J Thorac Cardiovasc Surg* 1992;103:655–664.

62. Butany J, Yu W. Cardiac angiosarcoma: two cases and a review of the literature. *Can J Cardiol* 2000;16:197–205.

63. Shrivastava S, Jacks JJ, White RS, et al. Diffuse rhabdomyomatosis of the heart. *Arch Pathol Lab Med* 1977;101:78–90.

64. Hajar R, Roberts WC, Folger GM Jr. Embryonal botryoid rhabdomyosarcoma of the mitral valve. *Am J Cardiol* 1986;57:376.

65. Hui KS, Green LK, Schmidt WA. Primary cardiac rhabdomyosarcoma: definition of a rare entity. *Am J Cardiovasc Pathol* 1988;2:19–29.

66. Pessotto R, Silvestre G, Luciani GB, et al. Primary cardiac leiomyosarcoma: seven-year survival with combined surgical and adjuvant therapy. *Int J Cardiol* 1997;60:91–94.

67. Babatasi G, Massetti M, Galateau F, et al. Leiomyosarcoma of the pulmonary veins extending into the left atrium or left atrial leiomyosarcoma: multimodality therapy. *J Thorac Cardiovasc Surg* 1998;116:665–667.

68. Minardi G, Pulignano G, Sentinelli S, et al. Left atrial leiomyosarcoma: double occurrence and double recurrence—report of one case. *J Am Soc Echocardiogr* 1998;11:1171–1176.

69. Department of Pathology, Northwestern Memorial Hospital, Chicago, IL 60611, USA. Epithelioid and spindle-celled leiomyosarcoma of the heart. Report of 2 cases and review of the literature. *Arch Pathol Lab Med* 1999;123:782–788.

70. Domanski MJ, Delaney TF, Kleiner DE Jr, et al. Primary sarcoma of the heart causing mitral stenosis. *Am J Cardiol* 1990;66:893–895.

71. Isner JM, Falcone MW, Virmani R, et al. Cardiac sarcoma causing "ASH" and simulating coronary heart disease. *Am J Med* 1979;66:1025–1030.

72. Abraham DP, Reddy V, Gattusa P. Neoplasms metastatic to the heart: review of 3314 consecutive autopsies. *Am J Cardiovasc Pathol* 1990;3:195–198.

73. Adenle AD, Edwards JE. Clinical and pathologic features of metastatic neoplasms of the pericardium. *Chest* 1982;81:166–169.

74. MacLowry JD, Roberts WC. Metastatic choriocarcinoma of the lung: invasion of pulmonary veins with extension into the left atrium and mitral orifice. *Am J Cardiol* 1966;18:938–941.

75. Labib SB, Schick EC Jr, Isner JM. Obstruction of right ventricular outflow tract caused by intracavitary metastatic disease: analysis of 14 cases. *J Am Coll Cardiol* 1992;19:1664–1668.

76. Domanski MJ, Cunnion RE, Fernicola DJ, et al. Fatal cor pulmonale caused by extensive tumor emboli in the small pulmonary arteries without emboli in the major pulmonary arteries or metastases in the pulmonary parenchyma. *Am J Cardiol* 1993;72:233–234.

77. Onuigbo WI. Direct extension of cancer between pulmonary veins and the left atrium. *Chest* 1972;62:444–446.

78. Weg IL, Mehra S, Azueta V, et al. Cardiac metastasis from adenocarcinoma of the lung. Echocardiographic-pathologic correlation. *Am J Med* 1986;80:108–112.

79. Kadir S, Coulam CM. Intracaval extension of renal cell carcinoma. *Cardiovasc Intervent Radiol* 1980;3:180–183.

80. Waller BF, Fletcher RD, Roberts WC. Carcinoma of the lung causing pulmonary arterial stenosis. *Chest* 1981;79:589–591.

81. Glancy DL, Roberts WC. The heart in malignant melanoma: a study of 70 autopsy cases. *Am J Cardiol* 1968;21:555–571.

82. Waller BV, Gottdiener JS, Virmani R, et al. The "charcoal heart": melanoma to the cor. *Chest* 1980;77:671–676.

83. Chen RH, Gaos CM, Frazier OH. Complete resection of a right atrial intracavitary metastatic melanoma. *Ann Thorac Surg* 1996;61:1255–1257.

84. Roberts WC, Bodey GP, Wertlake PT. The heart in acute leukemia: a study of 420 autopsy cases. *Am J Cardiol* 1968;21:388–412.

85. Waller BF, Roberts WC. Systolic clicks caused by rocks in the right heart chambers. *Am Heart J* 1981;102:459–460.

86. Roberts WC, Glancy DL, DeVita VT Jr. Heart in malignant lymphoma (Hodgkin's disease, lymphosarcoma, reticulum cell sarcoma and mycosis fungoides): a study of 196 autopsy cases. *Am J Cardiol* 1968;22:85–107.

87. McDonnell PJ, Mann RB, Bulkley BH. Involvement of the heart by malignant lymphoma: a clinicopathologic study. *Cancer* 1982;49:944–951.

88. Roberts CS, Gottdiener JS, Roberts WC. Clinically undetected cardiac lymphoma causing congestive heart failure. *Am Heart J* 1990;120:1239–1242.

89. Moore JA, DeRan BP, Minor R, et al. Transesophageal echocardiographic evaluation of intracardiac lymphoma. *Am Heart J* 1992;124:514–516.

90. Seibert KA, Rettenmier CW, Waller BF, et al. Osteogenic sarcoma metastatic to the heart. *Am J Med* 1982;73:136–141.

91. Burke AP, Virmani R. Osteosarcomas of the heart. *Am J Surg Pathol* 1991;15:289–295.

92. Zanella M, Falconieri G, Bussani R, et al. Polypoid osteosarcoma of the left atrium: report of a new case with autopsy confirmation and review of the literature. *Ann Diag Pathol* 1998;2:167–172.

93. Feigin DS, Fenoglio JJ, McAllister HA, et al. Pericardial cysts: a radiologic-pathologic correlation and review. *Radiology* 1977;125:15–20.

94. Reynolds JL, Donahue JK, Pearce CW. Intrapericardial teratoma: a cause of acute pericardial effusion in infancy. *Pediatrics* 1969;4:71–78.

95. DeGeeter B, Kretz JG, Nisand I, et al. Intrapericardial teratoma in a newborn infant: use of fetal echocardiography. *Ann Thorac Surg* 1983;35:664–666.

96. Brabham KR, Roberts WC. Cardiac-compressing intrapericardial teratoma at birth. *Am J Cardiol* 1989;63:386–387.

97. Shirani J, Roberts WC. Clinical, electrocardiographic and morphologic features of massive fatty deposits ("lipomatous hypertrophy") in the atrial septum. *J Am Coll Cardiol* 1993;22:226–238.

98. Roberts WC, Roberts JD. The floating heart of the heart too fat to sink: analysis of 55 necropsy patients. *Am J Cardiol* 1983;52:1286–1289.

99. Applegate PM, Taijk AJ, Ehman RL, et al. Two-dimensional echocardiographic and magnetic resonance imaging observations in massive lipomatous hypertrophy of atrial septum. *Am J Cardiol* 1987;59:489–491.

100. Kindman LA, Wright A, Tye T, et al. Lipomatous hypertrophy of the interatrial septum: characterization of transesophageal and transthoracic echocardiography, magnetic resonance imaging, and computed tomography. *J Am Soc Echocardiogr* 1988;1:450–454.

101. Isner JM, Carter BL, Roberts WC, et al. Subepicardial adipose tissue producing echocardiographic appearance of pericardial effusion. Documentation by computed tomography and necropsy. *Am J Cardiol* 1983;51:565–569.

102. Fisbein MC, Ferrans VJ, Roberts WC. Endocardial papillary elastofibromas. Histologic, histochemical, and electron microscopical findings. *Arch Pathol* 1975;99:335–341.

103. Roberts WC. Valvular, subvalvular, and supravalvular aortic stenosis: morphologic features. *Cardiovasc Clin* 1973;5:97–126.

104. Heath D, Thompson IM. Papillary "tumors" of the left ventricle. *Br Heart J* 1965;29:950–954.

105. Burn CG, Bishop MB, Davies JNP. A stalked papillary tumor of the mural endocardium. *Am J Clin Pathol* 1969;51:344–346.

106. Flotte T, Pinar H, Feiner H. Papillary elastofibroma of the left ventricular septum. *Am J Surg Pathol* 1980;4:585–588.

107. Almagro UA, Perry LS, Choi H, et al. Papillary fibroelastoma of the heart. Report of six cases. *Arch Pathol Lab Med* 1982;106:318–321.

108. Ong LS, Nanda NC, Barold SS. Two-dimensional echocardiographic detection and diagnostic features of left ventricular papillary fibroelastoma. *Am Heart J* 1982;103:917–918.

109. Topol EJ, Biern RO, Reitz BA. Cardiac papillary fibroelastoma and stroke. Echocardiographic diagnosis and guide to excision. *Am J Med* 1986;80:129–132.

110. Kalman JM, Lubicz S, Brennan JB, et al. Multiple cardiac papillary fibroelastoma and rheumatic heart disease. *Aust N Z J Med* 1991;21:744–746.

111. Bedi HS, Sharma VK, Mishra M, et al. Papillary fibroelastoma of the mitral valve associated with rheumatic mitral stenosis. *Eur J Cardiothorac Surg* 1995;9:54–55.

112. Allen KB, Goldin M, Mitra R. Transaortic video-assisted excision of a left ventricular papillary fibroelastoma. *J Thorac Cardiovasc Surg* 1996;112:199–201.

113. Campbell M, Carling W. Sudden death due to a fibrinous polyp of the aortic valve. *Guy's Hosp Rep* 1934;84:41–42.

114. Gopal A, Li Mandri G, King DL, et al. Aortic valve papillary fibroelastoma: a diagnosis by transthoracic echocardiography. *Chest* 1994;105:1885–1887.

115. Ragni T, Grande AM, Cappuccio G, et al. Embolizing fibroelastoma of the aortic valve. *Cardiovasc Surg* 1994;2:639–641.

116. Shahian DM, Labib SB, Chang G. Cardiac papillary fibroelastoma. *Ann Thorac Surg* 1995;59:538–541.

117. Fowles RE, Miller DC, Ebgert BM, et al. Systemic embolization from a mitral valve papillary endocardial fibroma detected by two-dimensional echocardiography. *Am Heart J* 1981;102:128–130.

118. Groton ME, Soltanzadeh H. Mitral valve fibroelastoma. *Ann Thorac Surg* 1989;47:605–607.

119. Gallo R, Kumar N, Prabhakar G, et al. Papillary fibroelastoma of mitral valve chorda. *Ann Thorac Surg* 1993;55:1576–1577.

120. Shapira OM, Williamson WA, Dugan JM. Papillary fibroelastoma of the mitral valve. *Cardiovasc Surg* 1993;1:599–601.

121. Mann J, Parker DJ. Papillary fibroelastoma of the mitral valve: a rare cause of transient neurological deficits. *Br Heart J* 1994;71:6.

122. Pinelli G, Carteaux JP, Mertes PM, et al. Mitral valve tumor revealed by stroke. *J Heart Valve Dis* 1995;4:199–201.

123. Zamora RL, Adelberg DA, Berger AS, et al. Branch retinal artery occlusion caused by a mitral valve papillary fibroelastoma. *Am J Ophthalmol* 1995;119:325–329.

124. Colucci V, Alberti A, Bonacina E, et al. Papillary fibroelastoma of the mitral valve: a rare cause of embolic events. *Tex Heart Inst J* 1995;22:327–331.

125. McFadden PM, Lacy JR. Intracardiac papillary fibroelastoma: an occult cause of embolic neurologic deficit. *Ann Thorac Surg* 1987;43:667–669.

126. Brown RD Jr, Khandheria BK, Edwards WD. Cardiac papillary fibroelastoma: a treatable cause of transient ischemic attack and ischemic stroke detected by transesophageal echocardiography. *Mayo Clinic Proc* 1995;70:863–868.

127. Nighoghossian N, Trouillas P, Perinetti M, et al. Lambl's excrescence: an uncommon cause of cerebral embolism. *Rev Neurol* 1995;151:583–585.

128. Kasarskis EJ, O'Connor W, Earle G. Embolic stroke from cardiac papillary fibroelastomas. *Stroke* 1988;19:1171–1173.

129. Zull DN, Diamond M, Beringer D. Angina and sudden death resulting from papillary fibroelastoma of the aortic valve. *Ann Emerg Med* 1985;14:470–473.

130. Marvasti MA, Obeid AT, Cohen PS, et al. Successful removal of papillary endocardial fibroma. *Thorac Cardiovasc Surg* 1983;31:254–255.

131. Richard J, Castello R, Dressler FA, et al. Diagnosis of papillary fibroelastoma of the mitral valve complicated by non-Q wave infarction with apical thrombus: transesophageal and transthoracic echocardiography study. *Am Heart J* 1993;126:710–712.

132. Etienne Y, Jobic Y, Houel JF, et al. Papillary fibroelastoma of the aortic valve with myocardial infarction: echocardiographic diagnosis and surgical excision. *Am Heart J* 1994;127:443–445.

133. Eckstein FS, Chafers HJ, Grote J, et al. Papillary fibroelastoma of the aortic valve presenting with myocardial infarction. *Ann Thorac Surg* 1995;60:206–208.

134. Grote J, Mugge A, Schfers JH, et al. Multiplane transesophageal echocardiography detection of a papillary fibroelastoma of the aortic valve causing myocardial infarction. *Eur Heart J* 1995;16:426–429.

135. Harris LS, Adelson L. Fatal coronary embolism from a myxomatous polyp of the aortic valve: an unusual cause of sudden death. *Am J Clin Pathol* 1965;43:61–64.

136. Boone S, Higginson LA, Walley VM. Endothelial papillary fibroelastoma arising in and around the aortic sinus, filling the ostium of the right coronary artery. *Arch Pathol Lab Med* 1992;116:135–137.

137. Mazzucco A, Bortolotti U, Thiene G, et al. Left ventricular fibroelastoma with coronary embolization. *Eur J Cardiothorac Surg* 1989;3:471–473.

138. Anderson KR, Fiddler FI, Lie JR. Congenital papillary tumor of the tricuspid valve: an unusual cause of right ventricular outflow obstruction in a neonate with trisomy E. *Mayo Clin Proc* 1977;52:665–669.

139. Wolfe JT III, Finck SJ, Safford RE, et al. Tricuspid valve papillary fibroelastoma: echocardiographic characterization. *Ann Thorac Surg* 1991;51:116–118.

140. Neerukonda SK, Jantz RD, Vijay NK, et al. Pulmonary embolization of papillary fibroelastoma arising from the tricuspid valve. *Tex Heart Inst J* 1991;18:132–135.

141. Ganjoo AK, Johnson WD, Gordon RT, et al. Tricuspid papillary fibroelastoma causing syncopal episodes. *J Thorac Cardiovasc Surg* 1996;112:551–553.

142. Roberts WC, McAllister HA Jr, Ferrans VJ. Sarcoidosis of the heart: a clinicopathologic study of 35 necropsy

patients (group I) and review of 78 previously described necropsy patients (group II). *Am J Med* 1977;63:86–108.

143. Virmani R, Bures JC, Roberts WC. Cardiac sarcoidosis: a major cause of sudden death in young individuals. *Chest* 1980;77:423–428.

144. Shirani J, Roberts WC. Subepicardial myocardial lesions. *Am Heart J* 1993;125:1346–1352.

145. Morton DL, Kagar AR, Roberts WC, et al. Pericardiectomy for radiation-induced pericarditis with effusion. *Ann Thorac Surg* 1969;8:195–208.

146. McReynolds RA, Gold GL, Roberts WC. Coronary heart disease after mediastinal irradiation for Hodgkin's disease. *Ann J Med* 1976;60:39–45.

147. Brosius FC III, Waller BF, Roberts WC. Radiation heart disease: analysis of 16 young (aged 15 to 33 years) necropsy patients who received over 3,500 rad to the heart. *Am J Med* 1981;70:519–530.

148. Harvey LAC, DeMaio SJ, Roberts WC. Radiation-induced cardiovascular disease including stenosis of coronary ostium, coronary and carotid arteries, and aortic valve. *Baylor Univ Med Center Proc* 1994;7:33–36.

149. Ihde DC, Roberts WC, Marr KC, et al. Cardiac candidiasis in cancer patients. *Cancer* 1978;41:2364–2371.

150. Ross EM, Macher AM, Roberts WC. *Aspergillus fumigatus* thrombi causing total occlusion of both coronary arterial ostia, all four major epicardial coronary arteries and coronary sinus and associated with purulent pericarditis. *Am J Cardiol* 1985;56:499–500.

151. Roberts WC, Berard CW. Gas gangrene of the heart in clostridial septicemia. *Am Heart J* 1967;74:482–488.

152. Bulkley BH, Roberts WC. The heart in systemic lupus erythematosus and the changes induced in it by corticosteroid therapy: a study of 36 necropsy patients. *Am J Med* 1975;58:243–264.

153. Buja LM, Roberts WC. Iron in the heart: etiology and clinical significance. *Am J Med* 1971;51:209–221.

154. Cutler DJ, Isner JM, Bracey AW, et al. Hemochromatosis heart disease: an unemphasized cause of potentially reversible restrictive cardiomyopathy. *Am J Med* 1980;69:923–928.

155. Buja LM, Ferrans VJ, Mayer RJ, et al. Cardiac ultrastructural changes induced by daunorubicin therapy. *Cancer* 1973;32:771–788.

156. Buja LM, Ferrans VJ, Roberts WC. Drug-induced cardiomyopathies. *Adv Cardiol* 1974;13:330–348.

157. Isner JM, Ferrans VJ, Cohen SR, et al. Clinical and morphologic cardiac findings after anthracycline chemotherapy: analysis of 64 patients studied at necropsy. *Am J Cardiol* 1983;51:1167–1174.

158. Schlegel PJ, Kralios AC, Terreros DA, et al. Malignant carcinoid tumor with myocardial metastases. *Am J Med* 1990;89:690–692.

159. Roberts WC, Sjoerdsma A. The cardiac disease associated with carcinoid syndrome (carcinoid heart disease). *Am J Med* 1964;36:5–34.

160. Roberts WC, Mason DT, Wright LD Jr. The non-distensible right atrium of carcinoid disease of the heart. *Am J Clin Pathol* 1965;44:627–631.

161. Ferrans VJ, Roberts WC. The carcinoid endocardial plaque: an ultrastructural study. *Hum Pathol* 1976;7:387–409.

162. Ross EM, Roberts WC. The carcinoid syndrome: comparison of 21 necropsy subjects with carcinoid heart disease to 15 necropsy subjects without carcinoid heart disease. *Am J Med* 1986;79:339–354.

163. Oates JA. The carcinoid syndrome. *N Engl J Med* 1986;315:702–704.

164. Callahan JA, Wroblewski EM, Reeder GS, et al. Echocardiographic features of carcinoid heart disease. *Am J Cardiol* 1982;50:762–768.

165. Howard RJ, Drobac M, Rider WD, et al. Carcinoid heart disease: diagnosis by two-dimensional echocardiography. *Circulation* 1982;66:1059–1065.

ROLE OF THE CARDIOLOGY CONSULTANT

SAEED R. SHAIKH
MYLAN C. COHEN
KIM A. EAGLE

▼▼ *ADDITIONAL ELECTRONIC TOPICS*

OVERVIEW

The relationship between generalists and specialists and the role that each has in the overall care of patients has become an increasingly important issue in health care delivery and is undergoing dramatic changes. *Consultation* is the act of seeking advice regarding diagnosis and management, and *referral* is transferal of the patient to another physician for a specific therapy or management of a particular medical problem while the primary (or referring physician) provides general care. Consultation may be a major component of a cardiologist's practice, but a consultant's good clinical judgment only has an impact on a patient's care if recommendations are communicated effectively.

S. R. Shaikh: Department of Cardiology, Maine Medical Center, Portland, Maine

M. C. Cohen: Division of Cardiology, University of Vermont College of Medicine, Burlington, Vermont; and Maine Medical Center, Portland, Maine

K. A. Eagle: Department of Internal Medicine/Cardiology, University of Michigan Medical School, Ann Arbor, Michigan

During consultation, ideally, there should be an exchange of information between the primary physician and the cardiology consultant, as well as coordination of care that ensures that patients receive care from the physician who is most likely to be able to provide a favorable outcome at the lowest cost. The consultant should determine whether the clinical situation is an emergency or whether it is urgent or elective. Emergency or urgent consultations should be discussed with the primary physician. It is important for the consultant to verify all information communicated by the physician. The most important component of successful cardiology consultation is effective communication with patients and primary physicians. The consultant should provide contingency plans and remember that follow-up increases compliance with recommendations.

Preoperative risk assessment is a frequent reason for cardiac consultation. As morbidity and mortality related to noncardiac surgery steadily decrease, cardiovascular management strategies that are known to improve long-term outcomes should guide decision making in the perioperative setting. Several factors may limit the predictive value of the clinical indices. There is extensive published data on the role of radionuclide perfusion imaging for preoperative risk stratification. Stress echocardiography is also evolving as a valuable tool for identifying high-risk patients. Risk reduction is the cornerstone of preoperative evaluation and management. Medical treatment and coronary revascularization procedures, when used appropriately, may significantly reduce perioperative cardiac events.

The preoperative cardiac consultation also represents an opportunity to initiate or modify cardiac care, including primary and secondary preventive measures. A stepwise approach to perioperative cardiac risk assessment, as set forth by recent joint American College of Cardiology (ACC) and American Heart Association (AHA) guidelines, should be used.

HISTORICAL PERSPECTIVE

Physicians have collaborated in the care of patients since antiquity. Hippocratic writings dating back to 400 BC refer to the importance of consultation in challenging medical cases (1). In 1927 (for the first edition of his textbook), Cecil explained why the work required more than one author:

> The rapid growth of medical science during the last few years has made it almost impossible for a single individual to master the entire field. In Internal Medicine, as in other branches of human knowledge, the age of specialism has of necessity arrived, and some of our ablest practitioners even devote themselves in great measure to one disease . . . (2)

In 1940, approximately 1,000 American physicians considered themselves to be heart specialists, but few of them had received formal training in cardiology (3). Earlier in the twentieth century, possession of an electrocardiograph (ECG) defined a physician as a cardiovascular specialist. With the trend toward specialization, the number of cardiovascular specialists has increased substantially. Today, cardiologists still fill the traditional roles of teachers, researchers, and care providers, but the field has diversified to include endeavors from molecular biology to disease prevention to cardiac imaging to coronary intervention (3). In 1965, the number of self-designated cardiologists was 1,901. The ACC on its fiftieth anniversary reported 25,214 members, including 34 masters and 20,525 fellows (4). In 1999 and 2000, there were 190 cardiology training programs and 2,164 trainees (5). Burgeoning numbers of cardiovascular specialists have contributed to substantial advances in cardiovascular knowledge and patient care.

Foot and associates (6) studied the effects of the changing demographics of the U.S. population on the cardiology workforce. They estimated that the U.S. population would reach 275 million in 2000, 297 million in 2010, and 397 million in 2030. As a result of the World War II baby boom, the population is aging, and the number of senior citizens (age >65 years) will increase from 12.6% to 20.0% of the population between 2000 and 2030. Due to the increasing prevalence of heart disease, deaths from heart disease are projected to increase by 128% between 2000 and 2050 (6). This suggests that demand for cardiovascular specialists in the future will increase. Unless a revolutionary breakthrough in the management of cardiovascular diseases occurs, this demand will be evident in the next 5 to 10 years and will continue until at least 2030. ▼⟋ h82

RELATIONSHIP TO REFERRING PHYSICIANS

Generalists and surgeons usually have some knowledge and experience in treating patients with cardiovascular diseases, and therefore thresholds for referral to a cardiologist will vary. Referral may be influenced by a practitioner's level of diagnostic certainty (9), the availability of consultants (10), and the accessibility of diagnostic tests (11). Ongoing changes in the American health care system are likely to influence the route by which patients reach the care of a cardiovascular specialist, and self-referral by patients likely will be dramatically reduced if development of managed care continues to its logical conclusion. The Physician Workforce Advisory Committee of the ACC performed a membership survey to quantify the amount of cardiovascular care provided by noncardiologist primary care physicians. Figure 41.1 summarizes the type of cardiovascular procedures performed by the primary care physicians. The most commonly performed procedure was ECG; 44% of internists performed exercise stress tests, compared with less than 18% of family practitioners. Primary care physicians indicated that 29% to 52% of their patients with cardiovascular disease or cardiovascular risk factors also saw a cardiologist (*e*Fig. 41.1.1). On the other hand, cardiologists perform a significant amount of the primary care. Cardiologists indicated that they were the primary care source for 30% of their patients and primary care providers for 13% of patients not seen for cardiac diagnoses (12). ▼⟋ h83

Whether the additional training and experience of cardiologists translate to improved cardiovascular outcomes has not been firmly established. We know that for a controlled population, specialists use more resources than do primary care providers (19). An important question is whether the increased cost of care incurred by specialists translates into improved outcomes. Schreiber and colleagues (20) reviewed a prospective cohort of 890 consecutive patients discharged with a diagnosis-related group diagnosis of unstable angina from William Beaumont Hospital (Royal Oak, Michigan). They compared 225 patients treated by internists with 665 patients treated by cardiologists with regard to patterns of use of established pharmacotherapies for unstable angina, diagnostic testing, and clinical out-

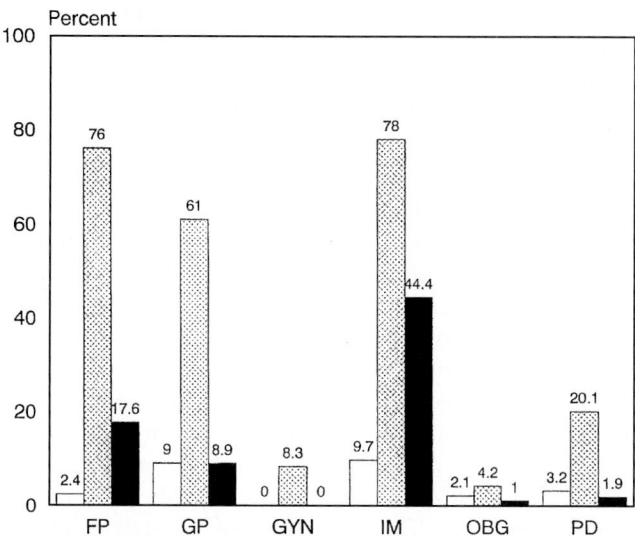

FIGURE 41.1 Frequency with which noninvasive cardiovascular procedures are performed by primary care specialists. Crosshatched bars, electrocardiography; solid bars, exercise stress tests; open bars, echocardiography. FP, family practitioner; GP, general practitioner; GYN, gynecologist; IM, internal medicine; OBG, obstetrician-gynecologist; PD, pediatrician. (From Vetrovec GW, Gardin JM, Gregory JJ, et al. Adult cardiovascular physician resources and needs assessment. *J Am Coll Cardiol* 1995;26:1125–1132, with permission.)

come. Patients treated by internists had a prior cardiac history less frequently (53% vs. 80%, *p* <.001). Cardiologists were more likely to use aspirin (78% vs. 68%, *p* = .032), heparin (84% vs. 67%, *p* <.001), and beta-adrenergic blocking agents (30% vs. 18%, *p* <.004) in initial management. Exercise tests were undergone less frequently by cardiologist-treated patients (22% vs. 37%, *p* <.001), but catheterization (61% vs. 27%, *p* <.0001) and angioplasty (40% vs. 7%, *p* <.0001) were undergone more frequently. Patients with unstable angina whose care was directed by internists experienced a trend toward increased hospital mortality (4.0% vs. 1.8%, *p* = .06), although the incidence of myocardial infarction (MI), length of stay, and hospital charges were similar (20).

These observations support a previous study by Greenfield and coworkers (19) that indicated that cardiologists tend to use more expensive diagnostic techniques. Interestingly, patients of cardiologists were older, had worse functional status and well-being scores, and had more chronic diagnoses than patients of general internists (21). In another investigation, Greenfield and colleagues (22) found no evidence that specialists achieved better long-term outcomes than generalists for patients with non–insulin-dependent diabetes mellitus or hypertension. It is possible that this may be the result of the very common nature of these illnesses and of good dissemination of information related to optimal care of these conditions.

Improved dissemination of information from clinical trials was advocated by Ayanian and coauthors (23), based on the finding that internists and family practitioners are less aware of or less certain about important advances in the treatment of MI. They surveyed 1,211 cardiologists, internists, and family practitioners in two states about four treatments demonstrated by randomized clinical trials to improve survival after MI (thrombolytic therapy, immediate and long-term use of aspirin, and long-term use of beta-blockers) and two treatments for which such evidence is lacking (diltiazem for patients with pulmonary congestion and prophylactic lidocaine). They asked physicians about the effect of each treatment on survival and the likelihood that they would prescribe each class of drugs. Cardiologists believed more strongly than internists and family physicians that survival was improved by the four beneficial treatments and were more likely to prescribe these drugs (*p* <.001). With regard to thrombolytic agents, for example, 94% of cardiologists said they were very likely to use these medications to treat an acute MI, compared with 82% of internists and 77% of family practitioners. On the other hand, cardiologists were less likely than internists and family practitioners to believe there was benefit associated with the two treatments for which the trials showed no survival benefit. Cardiologists were significantly less likely to prescribe these drugs (*p* <.001); only approximately 5% of cardiologists reported that they were very likely to use prophylactic lidocaine, compared with 13% of internists and more than 16% of family practitioners. ☛ h84

In a retrospective study of 327 patients with MI, management of hyperlipidemia for secondary prevention of coronary disease was shown to vary by physician specialty. Only 30% of patients with LDL levels greater than 130 mg per dL who were followed in a general internal medicine clinic received a cholesterol-lowering agent, compared with 55% of patients who were followed in a cardiology clinic (*p* <.008). This Veterans Affairs Health Care System–based study, in which access to drug treatment was equal among all patients, implies that patients observed by cardiologists are likely to have better outcomes, in part as a result of better secondary prevention (25). More recently, Stafford and Blumenthal (26) examined specialty differences in cardiovascular disease prevention practices. Using a national survey of office visits, they analyzed 30,929 adult visits to 1,521 physicians selected at random. When analysis was controlled for patient and visit characteristics, the likelihood that preventive services would be provided was higher for cardiologists than for general internists [adjusted odds ratio (OR), 1.65; 95% confidence interval (CI), 1.44 to 1.89].

Currently, there is a paucity of empirical evidence to support guidelines with regard to indications for and timing of cardiovascular consultations. This suggests that more research is needed that documents outcomes for patients with many types of medical problems who are treated by generalists and specialists in various systems of care. Cardiologists should take an active role in fostering research that evaluates patient outcomes for a variety of cardiovascular conditions. Cardiologists can also educate referring physicians and should make themselves available to discuss clinical situations with referring physicians. Such a process may facilitate patient care and allow primary care physicians to appreciate nuances of patient presentations that justify referral, even in the presence of guidelines that suggest that the role of the cardiologist in patient care is limited.

Conversely, the cardiologist is a subspecialist with training in internal medicine. The cardiologist might seek the assistance of a generalist or other specialist for care beyond the cardiologist's usual practice. This interchange may be an important educational opportunity for both physicians: The generalist or other medical specialist may gain insight into cardiologic problems and management, and the cardiologist has an opportunity to learn about new approaches in other specialties (8).

REASONS FOR REFERRAL AND CONSULTATION

Although the terms "consultation" and "referral" are often used interchangeably, their definitions are distinct. *Consultation* is the act of seeking advice regarding diagnosis and/or management (14). Such an exchange between the primary physician and the consultant may be formal (an appointment for an outpatient visit is made or an order for an inpatient consultation is written in the medical record) or informal (the "curbside consult," consisting of conversation regarding a patient between two physicians either in the hallway or by phone). A patient, a patient's family, or an insurance company may also seek a "second opinion." These are usually alluded to as "confirmatory consults." *Referral* represents transferal of the patient to another physician for a specific therapy or management of a particular medical problem while the primary (or referring physician) provides general care (14).

In cardiology practice, it is quite common for primary physicians to cede the care of the patient to the cardiologist when cardiovascular problems predominate. This represents *transferal of care*, which makes the cardiologist responsible for a patient's overall care during that hospitalization. In this situation, it is prudent for the primary care physician to continue observing the patient to remain abreast of clinical developments during the hospitalization. This maintains continuity of care and helps provide guidance regarding noncardiac problems and complex medicosocial decisions such as end-of-life issues. Finally, on discharge, the cardiologist should ideally send a letter to the primary care provider describing the patient's hospital course and a cardiac management plan as well as outstanding medical issues.

Referral and consultation rates vary widely, even for family physicians and nurse practitioners within the same practice. The rate at which a practitioner orders consulta-

tion in a specialty area increases in relation to the diagnostic certainty at the time of the consultation (9). Diagnostic certainty may be related to a referring practitioner's knowledge in a specialty field (implying that greater knowledge in a specialty leads to more consultations in that field). Studies have shown that referral rates range from 1.5% to 11% of patient visits in the family practice setting (27–30). In the managed care era, we can expect an increase in research evaluating the costs and effectiveness of calling on different types of physicians, with special focus on comparisons between generalists and specialists (31). Kaiser Permanente, a large health maintenance organization that provides health care services to 25% of the total population in northern California, has reported declines in consultation request rates with the introduction of the hospitalist system (32). Little information is available regarding referral to specific specialties. However, 10% of referrals from the University of Missouri–Columbia Department of Family and Community Medicine (14) and 6.8% of referrals from general internal medicine at University Hospital in Boston (33) were for cardiology services, and 11.9% of patients at Family Medical Center at the University Hospital in Seattle were referred to cardiology (34).

Consultation with a cardiologist may be sought to establish or confirm a diagnosis, to review or suggest specific management options for a known medical problem, to perform or interpret diagnostic tests, to perform a therapeutic procedure, or to clarify prognosis or cardiovascular risk associated with noncardiac tests and procedures. Depending on the severity of the patient's of illness and the urgency of the questions being asked of the consultant, patients may be evaluated in the outpatient setting (e.g., office, preadmission testing clinic, emergency department, or free-standing diagnostic imaging center) or inpatient setting (e.g., ward or specialized care or intensive care unit). The expectation is that the patient-physician relationship will terminate when the service requested by the primary care physician is complete. However, consultation may require multiple patient visits over an extended period of time, depending on the nature of the medical problem (35). Alternatively, a primary care physician may not feel that formal consultation is required and may desire only to confirm impressions or plans that have already been formulated. This type of informal consultation occurs frequently and involves a brief telephone call, e-mail, or hallway conversation.

ROLE OF THE CARDIOLOGY CONSULTANT

The opinions and reports of the Judicial Council of the American Medical Association, published in 1960 (36), contain one of the most comprehensive lists of the responsibilities of a consultant. This document lists nine ethical principles of consultation, six pertaining to the role of the consultant:

- The attending physician has the overall responsibility for the patient's treatment.
- The consultant should not assume the primary care of the patient without consent of the referring physician.
- The consultation should be done punctually.
- Discussions during consultation should be with the referring physician and only with the patient by prior consent of the referring physician.
- Conflicts of opinion should be resolved by second consultation or withdrawal of the consultant; however, the consultant has the right to render an opinion to the patient in the presence of the referring physician.

More than 40 years later, these tenets remain the guiding principles for the conduct of a successful consultant.

Evaluation

The first tasks for the cardiology consultant are to establish what question the primary physician would like to have answered and to establish the urgency of the consultation (37). Frequently, the question has not been clearly communicated by the primary care physician, and at other times, the consultant may overlook the question. If the issue prompting consultation is not clear, direct contact with the primary care physician can help to avoid consultations that do not meet the primary care physician's needs. Whether a scheduled patient is to be seen in the office or in the hospital, the consultant should determine whether the clinical situation is an emergency or whether it is urgent or elective.

The consultant's evaluation of a patient begins with a detailed medical history, physical examination, and review of data that may have already been obtained by the referring physician. It is important to "look for yourself" (37). Consultations are rarely requested to obtain assistance in interpreting already available data (38), but a careful review of the patient's chart is imperative for a complete consultation. This review should include obtaining outside records, pursuing unreturned laboratory workups, and personally reviewing ECGs, echocardiograms, and radiographs. Previous angiographic and hemodynamic data should also be reviewed personally. The New York Heart Association has classified the components of a complete cardiovascular evaluation and diagnosis of disease into the following categories: etiology, anatomy, physiology, cardiac status and prognosis, and specific recommendations (39). A complete cardiac diagnosis will likely include one or more of these categories. Based on this evaluation, tests may occasionally be repeated or new tests recommended. ▼ह h85

Communication

After the initial patient evaluation and the formulation of a management plan, [▼ह h86] the cardiology consultant must record his or her findings in the medical chart and communicate an assessment and recommendations to the primary physician who requested the consultation or referred the patient to the cardiologist. Opinions should be expressed in as brief a manner as appropriate. When writing in the hospital chart, it may be sufficient to merely note the history already provided and add components not already documented (38). This preliminary note may serve to communicate the initial assessment and recommendations to the medical team and to supplement a conversation between the consultant and primary physician. However, this brief note may be inadequate from the standpoint of medicolegal documentation and for documentation reimbursement purposes (see Documentation Compliance with Federal Health Programs). Although a long list of possible diagnoses with references to the medical literature may be of academic interest, lengthy intellectual discussions are unlikely to be read. Nevertheless, a copy of one or two key references, preferably from top-tier subspecialty journals, left at the front of the chart may be greatly appreciated. The cardiology consultant should share expertise with brevity, clarity, and lack of condescension (*e*Fig. 41.1.3). Also, whether the consultant or the primary physician will execute the recommendations or arrange the pertinent tests should be either clearly stated in the note or verbally communicated. Specific recommendations should be made, with contingency plans (37). The primary physician should be able to copy recommendations directly to the order sheet if he or she is in agreement. By anticipating potential problems, contingencies allow for brief management strategies to be in place if a patient's status changes (8). ▼ह h87

Documentation Compliance with Federal Health Programs

In its February 1999 Comprehensive Plan for Program Integrity, the federal agency that administers Medicare and Medicaid, the Health Care Financing Administration (HCFA), stated that "Our program integrity goal is straightforward . . . to pay the right amount, to a legitimate provider, for covered, reasonable and necessary services, provided to an eligible beneficiary . . ." (43). Accurate and complete medical records are absolutely essential to ensure high-quality patient care and an efficient and smooth process for the submission and reimbursement of claims. One of the most important principles is to verify that the current procedure terminology codes indicating the services provided match the services rendered and that *ICD-9* (*International Classification of Diseases, Ninth Revision*) codes indicating diagnosis support the services provided. The consultant must also be able to prove the scope of medical history covered, the extent of the physical examination, and the complexity of the decision making. HCFA's evaluation and management documentation guidelines define exactly how much documentation must be provided for each type of encounter. Detailed description of these guidelines is beyond the scope of this text and is available through the American College of Physicians or can be found as part of Medicare billing rules (44).

Extensive documentation is also supposed to improve patient care. However, HCFA's complex evaluation and management requirements may also result in omission of critical information from the patient's chart while the physician attempts to document trivial details (45). However, the reality is that a consultant must comply with HCFA's burdensome evaluation and management rules or risk the consequences.

Effective Consultation

Certain aspects of a consultant's role may influence whether recommendations are carried out by the requesting physician. Literature on this subject is limited and is available primarily from academic institutions. One measure of consultative quality is compliance with the consultant's recommendations. In one study, compliance with the consultant's advice ranged from 54% to 77% in academic centers (36). A study in a military teaching center reported that 90% of the recommendations were followed, implying higher compliance in nonacademic institutions (46).

Most research on the consultative process confirms the importance of good communication. In one study, disagreement occurred between the primary physician and the consultant on the issues of a consultation in 14% of cases (37). No specific question may be asked in 24% of preoperative consultations, and consultants may ignore explicit questions in 12% of cases (47). Direct contact between the consultant and the physician ordering the consultation can clarify misperceptions and has been associated with increased compliance with recommendations (46).

Compliance with recommendations decreases as the number of suggestions increases. Sears and Charlson (48) found that compliance was highest in their series of 202 general medicine consultations when five or fewer recommendations were made, regardless of the severity of the illness. The inverse relationship between number of recommendations and compliance has been observed in other studies (46,49). Identifying essential recommendations leads to greater compliance. Pupa and colleagues (46) found that labeling recommendations as "crucial" led to more than 90% compliance, even when the recommendations were contained in a long list of other suggestions. Verbal communication of high-priority recommendations is extremely effective. Recommendations should be as specific as possible so that physicians less familiar with cardiovascular tests and medications can copy suggestions directly to the order sheet in the chart (37). Horwitz and associates (50) found 100% compliance with recommendations for pharmacologic therapy when dose and duration were included in the consultant's note; compliance fell to 85%

when only dose or duration was specified and to 65% when neither was stated (*p* <.001).

Thus, when composing a consultative note in the chart, one might consider listing the impression and plan at the top to gain greater attention. Brief bullets are often more effective than long sentences. Recommendations may be divided into those aimed at making a diagnosis and those used for further management or therapy.

An effective consultant may also benefit from an organized referral evaluation team. The structure of this team greatly varies according to the size of the referral base and the consultant's practice. For example, a single cardiologist in a multispecialty group may have nurse practitioners and physician assistants as a part of his referral team compared to multiple cardiologists in a single specialty group. Another variation in the practice of cardiology pertains to physicians being on staff at an academic medical center where medical housestaff and cardiology fellows may play an important role in accepting, evaluating, and treating a patient. One of the most important elements of providing consultative services, regardless of the structure of the team, is appropriate acceptance followed by expedited evaluation and cohesive management. This can be achieved by providing easy access to the referring physician and delegating responsibility among the members of the referral evaluation team.

Follow-Up and Prevention

Many cardiovascular conditions require follow-up, which allows the cardiologist to adjust medications and assess response to therapy. Examples include management of severe hypertension and hyperlipidemia, cardiomyopathy, and inoperable CAD. Several studies have shown the importance of follow-up in gaining greater compliance with recommendations (47,51). Horwitz and colleagues (50) found that when more than one follow-up note was written, consultation had an effect on diagnosis in 92% of cases and an effect on management in 84% of cases. When one or no follow-up note was written, effects on diagnosis were noted in only 74% of cases (*p* <.001), and effects on management were observed in only 56% of cases (*p* <.001). A final job for the consultant is to ensure continuity of the patient's care for cardiac problems after discharge. A letter to the primary physician is often indicated to better coordinate the long-term management plan (36). ◥ h88

PREOPERATIVE EVALUATION

Advances in surgical and anesthetic techniques and an aging patient population have resulted in more complex procedures being performed in greater numbers of patients with higher likelihood of significant cardiovascular disease. Consultation may be sought for a history of cardiovascular disease, hypertension, or chest pain, or in the presence of a murmur, arrhythmia, or abnormal ECG results (51–53). Preoperative cardiac consultations are also frequently obtained for patients who have high pretest likelihood of CAD or in patients undergoing a high-risk noncardiac surgery.

Although consultation may occur in the office, on the ward, or in the postanesthesia care unit, recent greater emphasis on outpatient surgery or admission of patients on the morning of the planned surgical procedure has led to more frequent evaluations in a preadmission testing clinic (53). After noncardiac surgery, patients with cardiovascular disease require surveillance for cardiac complications, particularly for the first 48 hours after surgery, although the risk of MI may persist for at least 5 to 6 days after surgery (54). Particular attention to good consultative techniques is warranted, because it has been suggested that compliance with consultant recommendations is lower for preoperative consultation than for consultations performed in other settings (55). ❦ h89

Epidemiology of Postoperative Myocardial Infarction

Of the 27 million men and women who have surgery each year in the United States, 1 million have perioperative cardiac complications, which result in approximately $20 billion in costs of in-hospital and long-term care (75). Over the course of the next 25 years, it is estimated that 37 million patients will undergo an operation, and 12 million of those will be older than 65 years. As a result, perioperative mortality will increase substantially, resulting in an approximate cost of $40 billion by the year 2018 (76).

The overall risk of postoperative MI is low overall (<1%) (77,78). A history of MI increases the chance of sustaining a recurrent perioperative MI to approximately 6% (79). The risk of MI peaks within the first 3 postoperative days. Von Knorring (80) prospectively analyzed a cohort of surgical patients and found that 87% of perioperative MIs occur within the first 3 postoperative days, with peak incidence on postoperative day 2. Most postoperative MIs are non–Q-wave MIs and are usually detected in the first 24 hours after the operation, probably as a result of increased surveillance using frequent ECG and measurement of cardiac enzymes (81–83).

Because atherosclerosis is a diffuse process, patients with peripheral vascular disease often have CAD. In a study seeking to define the relationship between CAD and peripheral vascular disease, 1,000 patients undergoing peripheral vascular reconstruction at The Cleveland Clinic underwent preoperative coronary angiography; only 14% had normal coronary arteries (68). Several other studies have correlated coronary angiographic findings with different types of vascular diseases. The incidence of severe CAD among patients with abdominal aortic aneurysms is 52% to 82%, and the incidence among patients with peripheral

occlusive disease is 47% to 60% (84). In a random sample of 6,895 Medicare patients undergoing major vascular surgery, perioperative mortality was 7.3% for aortic surgery and 5.8% for infrainguinal vascular surgery (85). Eagle and coworkers (86) identified 3,368 patients from the Coronary Artery Survival Study (CASS) registry who underwent noncardiac surgery, after a mean follow-up of 4.1 years. In patients with CAD who have not undergone revascularization, abdominal, vascular, thoracic, and head and neck surgery each had a combined rate of death and MI of more than 4%, with the highest event rate in vascular surgery patients (rate of perioperative MI, 8.5%; mortality rate, 2.8%). Therefore, the substantially higher cardiac morbidity and mortality among patients with nonrevascularized CAD who are undergoing vascular surgery mandates the need for an aggressive risk stratification strategy. ❦ h90

Pathophysiology

Alterations in the balance of clotting and fibrinolytic systems, varying as a function of the magnitude of the surgery, create a "prothrombotic milieu" (*e*Fig. 41.1.4) in the postoperative period that predisposes the patient to thrombotic complications such as deep vein thrombosis, stroke, and MI (91). The stress response is a physiologic measure of the magnitude of the surgery and surgical factors such as urgency, blood loss, and perioperative fluid shifts, which have been shown to influence perioperative cardiac events (90).

To date, very few studies have attempted to elucidate the pathophysiologic mechanism of postoperative MI. Traditionally, oxygen supply–demand mismatch has been invoked as the pathophysiologic mechanism of postoperative MI. However, plaque rupture followed by intracoronary thrombosis may also be a causative mechanism in patients who experience fatal MI. Cohen and Aretz (91) identified 26 patients who had sustained a fatal postoperative MI out of a total of 1,841 autopsies. They found that plaque rupture was present in almost one-half (46%) of the patients. In another study, Dawood and associates (92) found evidence of plaque rupture in 23 (55%) of 42 patients who died after noncardiac surgery. Therefore, in addition to oxygen supply-demand mismatch, plaque rupture followed by coronary thrombosis may also be an important pathophysiologic mechanism, and multiple strategies likely are required to lower the risk of postoperative MI.

Clinical Prediction

Several groups have stratified surgical risk based on patient characteristics. First, Dripps and colleagues (93) assigned a physical status class to patients, before administration of anesthesia, over a 10-year period (1947–1957). This physical status index is still used by the American Society of Anesthesiologists (ASA; *e*Table 41.0.3) (94) and has been validated in a large cohort of patients (95). However, the index is subjective and may be less predictive in some subsets of patients, such as elderly patients, obese patients, and patients with prior MI or mild systemic disease (96). Goldman and coworkers (57) developed a multifactorial index to assess the cardiac risk of noncardiac surgery in 1,001 consecutive general surgery patients (57) (*e*Table 41.0.4). To adjust risk estimates for a specific planned surgical procedure, Detsky and colleagues (97) developed a modified index of perioperative cardiac risk. They altered several features of Goldman's original index, based on the authors' clinical experiences (*e*Table 41.0.5). ▼ h91

Several factors may limit the predictive value of these clinical indices. When estimating surgical risk, relevant factors (patient-specific, institution-specific, and procedure-specific) must be considered. These considerations, as well as the desire to increase predictive accuracy, have led to investigation of noninvasive tests to help assess preoperative risk to the patients in an incremental fashion.

Stress Testing and Assessment of Left Ventricular Function

One of the first noninvasive technologies used in preoperative cardiac risk stratification was exercise treadmill testing, because poor functional capacity in patients with CAD is associated with an increased incidence of subsequent cardiac events. The positive predictive value for postoperative death and MI of abnormal results of an exercise stress test ranges from 5% to 25%. The negative predictive value of normal results of a maximal study exceeds 90% (102). An important limitation of exercise testing in preoperative evaluation of noncardiac surgery is patients' inability to perform optimal level of exercise in 30% to 50% of cases (102). This does not preclude obtaining important functional information, and estimates of perioperative risk can be determined in patients who can exercise. Numerous studies have examined the usefulness of exercise stress testing as a preoperative diagnostic tool in men, and the results may not be reliable when applied to women (75). Exercise stress testing has a lower overall accuracy among women compared with that among men because of the higher prevalence of ECG changes with hyperventilation or position change among women. Table 41.1, from the ACC/AHA guidelines, illustrates selected studies of preoperative exercise testing before major noncardiac surgery (103).

Several studies suggest that inability to perform even modest levels of exercise identifies a high-risk subset of patients (61,101,102). McPhail and associates (61) demonstrated that patients who achieved greater than 85% predicted maximal heart rate during exercise testing had a postoperative cardiac complication rate (cardiac death, MI, CHF, malignant ventricular ectopic activity) of 6%, whereas patients who achieved less than 85% of their predicted maximal heart rate had a complication rate of 24%.

In addition, Gerson and colleagues (104) showed that inability to perform 2 minutes of supine bicycle exercise to raise the heart rate above 99 beats/min was a good predictor of perioperative pulmonary, cardiac, and combined cardiopulmonary complications (104).

Investigators have also assessed resting and exercise left ventricular function using RVG and echocardiography. Initial studies showed a relationship between decreased left ventricular systolic function and adverse cardiac events (105–111). However, subsequent studies (112–116) failed to show a statistically significant relationship between resting left ventricular ejection fraction (LVEF) and the development of perioperative adverse cardiac events. Thus, taken together, the data indicate that resting LVEF is a relatively insensitive and nonspecific marker for postoperative MI and cardiac death, however poorly left ventricular systolic function or diastolic dysfunction may predict postoperative CHF. Similar findings have been reported with echocardiography, although results have not been uniform across studies (117). More recently, Rhode and coauthors (118) studied the incremental value of transthoracic echocardiography after consideration of clinical data for prediction of cardiac complications after a major noncardiac surgery in 570 patients. In univariate analyses, preoperative systolic function was associated with postoperative MIs (OR, 2.8; 95% CI, 1.1 to 7.0). In logistic regression analysis, models with echocardiographic variables predicted major cardiac complications much better than those that included only clinical variables. Studies of exercise LVEF (104,119) also have indicated that resting LVEF and exercise-induced wall motion abnormalities are insensitive predictors of postoperative MI and cardiac death.

Long-Term Prognostic Value of Perfusion Imaging

Because the prevalence of CAD is high among patients with peripheral vascular disease, patients undergoing peripheral vascular surgery remain at increased risk of cardiac events in subsequent years, even if they remain event-free during the immediate postoperative period (127). Hendel and colleagues (141) evaluated 360 patients, of whom 327 patients underwent vascular surgery. Operative death and nonfatal MI occurred in 4.9% and 6.7%, respectively. A cardiac event (nonfatal MI or cardiac death) occurred in 14.4% of patients with a transient thallium defect, compared to 1% among patients with normal results of scanning (*p* <.001). Multivariate analysis revealed that the best predictor of perioperative events was the presence of a reversible thallium defect. Late cardiac events occurred in 53 (15.2%) surgical survivors or nonsurgically treated patients who were followed for a mean of 31 months. Patients with a fixed perfusion abnormality had a 24% late-event rate, compared with 4.9% among patients

TABLE 41.1 SUMMARY OF STUDIES EXAMINING THE VALUE OF PREOPERATIVE EXERCISE TESTING BEFORE MAJOR NONCARDIAC SURGERY

Study, year	N	Patients with abnormal test results (%)	Criteria for abnormal test results	Events	Predictive value		Event	Comments
					Positive	Negative		
Peripheral vascular surgery or abdominal aortic aneurysm repair								
McCabe et al., 1981 (201)	314	36	STD, CP, or A	38% (15/39)	81% (13/16)	91% (21/23)	D, M, I, H, A	
Cutler et al., 1981 (59)	130	39	STD	7% (9/130)	16% (8/50)	99% (79/80)	D, M	<75% MPHR increased risk
Arous et al., 1984 (202)	808	17	STD	NR	21% (19/89)	NR	D, M	
Gardine et al., 1985 (203)	86	48	STD	11% (2/19)	11% (1/9)	90% (9/10)	D, M	
Von Knorring, 1986 (204)	105	25	STD, A, or CP	3% (3/105)	8% (2/26)	99% (78/79)	D, M	
Leppo et al.,[a] 1987 (63)	60	28	STD	12% (7/60)	25% (3/12)	92% (44/48)	D, M	Exercise test results used to refer patients for revascularization
Hanson et al., 1988 (205)	74	57	STD	3% (1/37)	5% (1/19)	100% (18/18)	D, M	
McPhail et al.,[a] 1988 (61)	100	70	<85% MPHR	19% (19/100)	24% (17/70)	93% (28/30)	D, M, A, F	<85% MPHR, p = .04; STD, p is NS
Urbinati et al., 1994 (206)	121	23	STD	0	0/28	100% (93/93)	D, M	Carotid endarterectomy patients. STD predicted late death
Peripheral vascular surgery or major noncardiac surgery								
Carliner et al., 1985 (60)	200	16	STD	16% (32/200)	16% (5/32)	93% (157/168)	D, M	5 METs (NS)

A, cardiac arrhythmia; CP, chest pain; D, death; F, failure; H, hypotension; I, myocardial ischemia; M, myocardial infarction; MET, metabolic equivalent; MPHR, maximum predicted heart rate; NR, not reported; NS, not significant; STD, exercise-induced electrocardiographic ischemia.
Note: In references 201, 202, 203, and 205, the total no. of patients undergoing peripheral vascular surgery was less than the total no. tested.
[a]Studies with prospective collection of postoperative electrocardiogram and cardiac enzymes.
Modified from Eagle KA, Brundage BH, Chaitman BR, et al. Guidelines for perioperative cardiovascular evaluation for noncardiac surgery: report of the American College of Cardiology/American Heart Association Task Force on Practice Guidelines (Committee on Perioperative Cardiovascular Evaluation for Noncardiac Surgery). *J Am Coll Cardiol* 1996;27:910–948, with permission.

with normal results of the dipyridamole-thallium study (p <.01). Cox regression analysis showed that a fixed thallium defect was the most powerful predictor of late events and increased the relative risk by almost fivefold. A history of CHF was the only significant clinical variable that contributed additional value to knowledge of the presence of a fixed defect. Life-table analysis confirmed the strong relationship between fixed defects and cardiac event–free survival (p <.0001).

Younis and coworkers (142) also evaluated late outcomes among 131 patients scheduled for peripheral vascular surgery. Two years after surgery, the actuarial event-free survival rate for patients with thallium redistribution was approximately 50%. Urbinati and colleagues (207) evaluated early and late cardiac events among 106 patients with neither history nor symptoms of CAD who underwent exercise thallium myocardial perfusion imaging before carotid endarterectomy. No cardiac deaths or MIs occurred within 30 days of surgery. However, actuarial survival without coronary events was 51% among patients with positive

results of stress test and thallium redistribution, compared with 98% among patients without such results (p <.01) by 7 years (Fig. 41.2).

Among 172 patients who were followed for a mean of 21 ± 14 months after elective vascular surgery, event-free survival was significantly less for patients with abnormal MIBI scans than for those with normal scan results (74% vs. 96%; p <.0001). After controlling for other clinical factors using Cox proportional hazards models, abnormal results of an MIBI study (relative risk, 3.7; 95% CI, 1.2 to 11.4) and MIBI-detected ischemia (relative risk, 2.7; 95% CI, 1.2 to 6.1) remained significant predictors of increased risk of late cardiac events (143). More recently, Cohen and associates (144) reported long-term prognostic significance of preoperative dipyridamole technetium-99m MIBI scanning in vascular surgery patients. They followed 153 patients for as long as 4 years after the dipyridamole MIBI scan to determine nuclear imaging predictors of death and MI. The only statistically significant predictor of death and MI visible on dipyridamole MIBI scanning was abnormal-

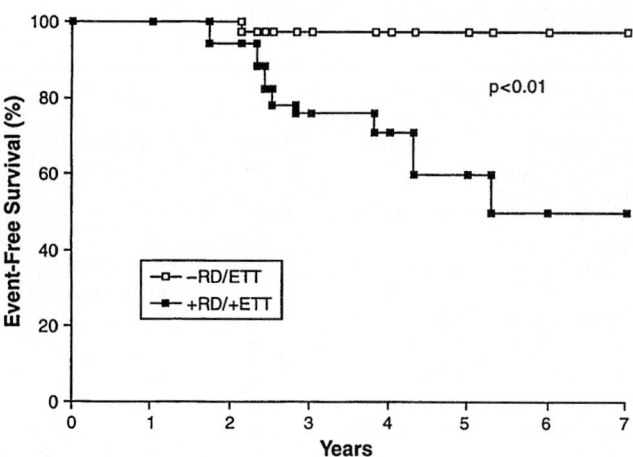

FIGURE 41.2 Long-term follow-up in patients undergoing exercise thallium-201 imaging before carotid endarterectomy. *p* <.01. ETT, positive stress electrocardiogram; RD, reversible defects.

ity in the left anterior descending artery territory (adjusted relative risk, 2.9; 95% CI, 1.2 to 7.3).

Stress Echocardiography

Several reports have evaluated the accuracy of pharmacologic stress echocardiography in identifying patients who are at risk for postoperative cardiac events (65,66,145–150) (Table 41.2). Most studies have used dobutamine, although dipyridamole has also been used. The populations examined predominantly have been patients undergoing vascular surgery. Only one study has blinded clinicians to the echocardiographic results (147). In the other studies, results

affected management, including decisions about whether to perform preoperative coronary angiography and coronary revascularization. Among the studies of preoperative dobutamine echocardiography, the positive predictive value for MI and death ranged from 7% to 23%; the negative predictive value was 100% in all but one study. The severity of wall motion changes at low-dose dobutamine infusion may be especially important. Furthermore, Poldermans and coworkers (151) have shown that stress-induced ischemia on dobutamine echocardiography is predictive of late cardiac events after vascular surgery. Recently, Ballal and coauthors (152) reported long-term cardiac outcome in 233 vascular surgery patients who underwent preoperative dobutamine stress echocardiography. Late events occurred in 36 patients after a mean follow-up of 28 months. New or worsening regional wall motion abnormality was predictive of these events, even after the analysis was adjusted for clinical variables and left ventricular dysfunction (relative risk, 3.3; *p* = .001).

A metaanalysis of published reports on preoperative pharmacologic stress risk stratification identified ten reports on dipyridamole–thallium-201 scintigraphy and five on dobutamine stress echocardiography (153). Random effect models were used to calculate the summary OR and 95% CIs. The summary OR for death or MI and secondary cardiac end points were greater for dobutamine-induced echocardiographic dyssynergy (14- to 24-fold) than for dipyridamole-thallium defect redistribution (fourfold). However, wide CIs were noted with dobutamine echocardiography (Fig. 41.3). Therefore, the published experience with stress echocardiography is not as extensive as that with radionuclide perfusion imaging, but the literature to date

TABLE 41.2 SUMMARY OF STUDIES EXAMINING THE VALUE OF DOBUTAMINE STRESS ECHOCARDIOGRAPHY (ECG) FOR PREOPERATIVE RISK ASSESSMENT

Study, year	Patients with ischemia who underwent surgery, no. (%)	Events,[a] no. (%)	Criteria for abnormal test results	Predictive value[b]		Comments
				Positive[a]	Negative	
Lane et al., 1991 (66)	38 (50)	3 (8%)	New WMA	16% (3/19)	100% (19/19)	Vascular and general surgery
Lalka et al., 1992 (145)	60 (50)	9 (15%)	New or worsening WMA	23% (7/30)	93% (28/30)	Multivariate analysis
Eichelberger et al., 1993 (146)	75 (36)	2 (3%)	New or worsening WMA	7% (2/27)	100% (48/48)	Managing physicians blinded to DSE results
Langan et al., 1993 (147)	74 (24)	3 (4%)	New WMA or ECG changes	17% (3/18)	100% (56/56)	
Poldermans et al., 1993 (148)	131 (27)	5 (4%)	New or worsening WMA	14% (5/35)	100% (96/96)	Multivariate analysis; managing physicians blinded to DSE results
Davila-Roman et al., 1993 (149)	88 (23)	2 (2%)	New or worsening WMA	10% (2/20)	100% (68/68)	Included long-term follow-up

DSE, dobutamine stress echocardiogram; WMA, wall motion abnormality.
[a]Myocardial infarction or death.
[b]Numbers in parentheses are no. of patients/total no. in each group.
Reprinted from Eagle KA, Brundage BH, Chaitman BR, et al. Guidelines for perioperative cardiovascular evaluation for noncardiac surgery: report of the American College of Cardiology/American Heart Association Task Force on Practice Guidelines (Committee on Perioperative Cardiovascular Evaluation for Noncardiac Surgery). *J Am Coll Cardiol* 1996;27:910–948, with permission.

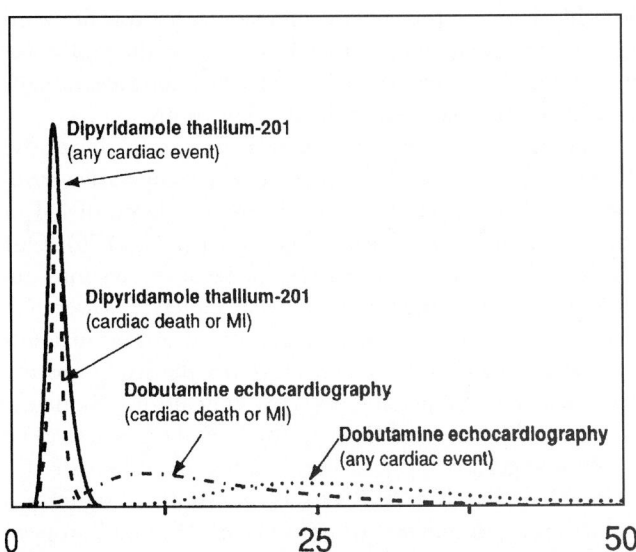

FIGURE 41.3 Summary odds ratio and 95% confidence intervals for risk stratification of patients undergoing pharmacologic stress perfusion and echocardiographic imaging, as determined by metaanalytic confidence profile method. Because of larger sample sizes, narrower confidence profiles are seen for dipyridamole–thallium-201 perfusion imaging than for dobutamine stress echocardiography, although point estimates for the summary odds ratio are greater using echocardiography. MI, myocardial infarction. [From Shaw LJ, Eagle KA, Gersh BJ, et al. Meta-analysis of intravenous dipyridamole–thallium-201 (1985–1994) for risk stratification before vascular surgical candidates. *J Am Coll Cardiol* 1996;27:787–798, with permission.]

suggests that dobutamine stress echocardiography is a valuable risk stratification modality.

Perioperative Evaluation of Other Cardiac Conditions

To this point, we have considered the evaluation of the patient only in terms of the presence or absence of significant CAD and the implications for prognosis. However, preoperative cardiac consultation is sought for a variety of indications, including CHF, murmurs, and arrhythmias (51–53).

CHF is an important harbinger of poor postoperative outcome (64,65,161). Therefore, great effort should be made to identify and treat unsuspected heart failure by performing a careful history and physical examination. It is important to identify the mechanism of CHF, because systolic dysfunction, diastolic dysfunction, and valvular abnormalities all can cause this syndrome, and management of each of these disease entities is significantly different. Determination of etiology may have prognostic implications (103).

Cardiac murmurs are common. The cardiology consultant must determine etiology and distinguish significant murmurs from those that are not clinically important. Severe aortic stenosis conveys high risk (57) and may justify postponement or cancellation of surgery. Rarely, percutaneous balloon aortic valvuloplasty may be justified in a patient who is not a candidate for aortic valve replacement, which is the preferred treatment before noncardiac surgery (103). Mild or moderate mitral stenosis requires monitoring to maintain reasonable control of heart rate to reduce the risk of pulmonary congestion associated with a decreased diastolic filling period. Patients with severe mitral stenosis may benefit from balloon mitral valvuloplasty or open surgical repair before high-risk noncardiac surgery (103). Patients with regurgitant lesions may benefit from heart-rate control, antibiotic prophylaxis, or afterload reduction, depending on the etiology and severity of the lesions. Patients with prosthetic valves should receive appropriate antibiotic prophylaxis for endocarditis (162). In addition, patients with mechanical prosthetic valves require careful management of coagulation and may need a short course of intravenous heparin therapy.

Cardiac arrhythmias and conduction disturbances are common in the perioperative period (56,86,163). Although both supraventricular and ventricular arrhythmias have been associated with increased risk of adverse postoperative cardiac events, they are probably markers for underlying cardiopulmonary disease that places a patient at higher risk. Perioperative atrial fibrillation is a common arrhythmia, especially after intrathoracic surgical procedures; direct atrial irritation may be the operative mechanism. Because of the increased catecholamine state that occurs in the immediate postoperative period, it may not be possible to maintain sinus rhythm, and therapy should be directed at heart-rate control and anticoagulation, if indicated (164). Cardioversion is usually reserved for hemodynamically compromising atrial fibrillation. Most arrhythmias are not malignant, but their presence can expose underlying disease that may compromise the patient (e.g., new atrial fibrillation with rapid ventricular response that precipitates ischemia and subsequent CHF). Patients with conduction disease and no history of high-grade atrioventricular block generally do well. However, high-grade atrioventricular block may require insertion of a temporary pacing wire. Transcutaneous pacing allows rapid response to sudden and hemodynamically significant heart block (106). ▼ h92

Risk Reduction

Risk reduction is the cornerstone of preoperative evaluation and management. Generally, interventions aimed at reducing perioperative cardiac risk can be classified as perioperative monitoring, medical therapy, or preoperative revascularization. In preoperative monitoring, the role of pulmonary artery catheters has been studied, although not extensively. The effect of various medical therapies, including beta-blockers, alpha-adrenergic agents, and calcium channel blockers has been reported. Preoperative coronary revascularization to decrease cardiac risk has also been studied, but most of the data have been observational.

There is some evidence that optimization of preoperative hemodynamics may be beneficial (165), and careful perioperative hemodynamic monitoring may decrease cardiac morbidity (166). However, Bender and associates (167) randomly assigned 104 patients to one of two groups: a group in which all patients received a pulmonary artery catheter and a group in which only patients with accepted indications for pulmonary artery catheterization received such a catheter. The authors demonstrated no significant difference in rates of intraoperative and postoperative complications or mortality between the two groups. Valentine and colleagues (168) reported a randomized trial studying the routine use of pulmonary artery catheters in 120 patients undergoing aortic surgery. They found no significant reduction in morbidity and a higher rate of intraoperative cardiac events among patients who had a pulmonary artery catheter. Overall, the routine use of pulmonary arterial catheters in the initial care of surgical patients has been discouraged (167–170). Consultants should be aware that insertion of a pulmonary artery catheter, by itself, does not constitute a cure. It is only by obtaining vital information that is used to guide therapy and interpreting that information correctly that the pulmonary artery catheter may prove useful (170). Furthermore, a retrospective analysis of data for patients who underwent abdominal aortic surgery revealed that risk of cardiac arrest was higher when no daily rounds were made by an intensive care unit physician (OR, 2.9; 95% CI, 1.2 to 7.0) (171). Therefore, careful postoperative management of critical patients by an intensivist and sound decision making based on clinical and procedural data are the only monitoring strategies that may be recommended.

Several studies suggest that beta-blockade may be beneficial in the perioperative period and long term in patients who have undergone noncardiac surgery (172–174). The first well-designed trial randomly assigned 200 patients undergoing noncardiac surgery to receive atenolol or placebo. Atenolol was used intravenously before and immediately after surgery and orally thereafter for the duration of the hospitalization. No difference was noted in the perioperative MI or death, but the overall mortality after discharge from the hospital was significantly reduced among patients who received atenolol (0% vs. 8% at 6 months; $p <.001$; 3% vs. 14% at 1 year; $p = .005$; 10% vs. 21% at 2 years) (172). However, the placebo group had a higher risk profile as a result of unequally distributed risk factors. More recently, Poldermans and coworkers (174) performed a randomized trial involving 173 high-risk patients in whom inducible regional wall motion abnormalities were seen on dobutamine stress echocardiography to assess the effect of perioperative bisoprolol on the incidence of cardiac events within 30 days after a major vascular surgery. The primary end point of cardiac death and MI occurred in two patients (3.4%) in the bisoprolol group versus 18 patients (34%) in the group of patients who received standard care without

beta-blockers ($p <.001$). This dramatic reduction in events may be partly attributed to selection bias; the study was performed in a high-risk cohort in which an exceptionally high event rate was seen in the placebo group.

Administration of nitroglycerin in the perioperative period may decrease the incidence of intraoperative myocardial ischemia, but reduction in the incidence of MI or cardiac death has not been demonstrated (175,176). One small study evaluated the efficacy of use of intravenous diltiazem in patients undergoing vascular surgery. A lower incidence of myocardial ischemia was noted among patients who were receiving diltiazem. However, the study was too small for it to be possible to draw conclusions about the effect of diltiazem on MI or death (177). Perioperative use of alpha$_2$-agonists has also been studied in few small randomized trials that failed to demonstrate a significant reduction in postoperative events (178,179). In a European multicenter trial, 2,801 patients with known CAD who were undergoing noncardiac surgery were assigned to receive intravenous mivazerol (an alpha$_2$-agonist that reduces postganglionic noradrenaline availability and sympathetic efferent output) or placebo. Mivazerol failed to reduce the overall rate of death and MI. However, among a preselected cohort of patients with known CAD who were undergoing vascular surgery, a reduced risk of death and MI was seen in the mivazerol group (relative risk, 0.67; 95% CI, 0.45 to 0.98) (180). Further study of the alpha-adrenergic agents may, therefore, be warranted. Presumably, these medical interventions could prevent postoperative adverse cardiac events that are preceded by tachycardia and ECG evidence of ischemia (181,182).

Interventions aimed at increasing oxygen supply through increased oxygen delivery (183) or improved blood flow via intraaortic balloon counterpulsation (IABP) may reduce postoperative cardiac morbidity and mortality (183–185). Arafa and associates (186) analyzed 344 patients undergoing cardiac operations who required perioperative use of IABP, with a mean follow-up of 7.45 years. On regression analysis, timing of IABP insertion was identified as an independent predictor of early (30-day) mortality ($p <.05$) and late death ($p <.05$). Survival analysis demonstrated significantly improved survival among patients who received an IABP preoperatively ($p <.02$). These studies may justify allowing preoperative IABP a more liberal role in treatment of high-risk patients undergoing cardiac surgery.

There are no randomized trials to evaluate the protective role of percutaneous coronary revascularization before noncardiac surgery. Studies by Golden and colleagues (187) and Younis and coworkers (136) suggest that coronary intervention in patients identified as high risk by myocardial perfusion scintigraphy may improve cardiac outcomes. Retrospective analysis of data regarding the role of use of percutaneous transluminal coronary angioplasty (PTCA) for preoperative revascularization has been reported (188–

190). All three studies reported a low incidence of perioperative cardiac events after noncardiac surgery. However, these studies did not define a clear indication for PTCA, and they also lacked a control arm, making interpretation of the results difficult. A recent study that used an administrative database of patients who underwent noncardiac surgery revealed that PTCA was associated with significant reduction in perioperative cardiac events (191). Interestingly, the percutaneous revascularization procedure reduced risk only if it was performed more than 90 days before surgery. This finding suggests that PTCA immediately before surgery may not confer protection against perioperative cardiac events, and that the immediate postprocedure period is probably not the optimal time for noncardiac surgery. Coronary stenting before noncardiac surgery presents a unique clinical dilemma because of the risk of acute stent thrombosis and bleeding complications associated with postprocedure anticoagulation. Kaluza and colleagues (192) studied 40 patients who underwent noncardiac surgery less than 6 weeks after coronary stent placement. Seven MIs and eight deaths occurred, all in patients who underwent surgery fewer than 14 days after coronary stenting. Judging by ECG and by enzymatic and angiographic evidence, stent thrombosis accounted for most of the fatal events. Therefore, postponing elective noncardiac surgery for at least 4 weeks after coronary stenting should allow completion of a mandatory antiplatelet regimen, thereby reducing the risk of postoperative cardiac events.

Studies have shown that patients who have undergone recent CABG before noncardiac surgery have postoperative cardiac morbidity and mortality rates that are similar to those among patients who have no clinical evidence of CAD (193–195). Manske and colleagues (196) performed a randomized trial in which patients with coronary disease who were scheduled to undergo renal transplantation were assigned to receive medical therapy or CABG. Although a 57% reduction in cumulative probability of unstable angina, MI, or death at 12 months was observed among patients who underwent revascularization compared with that among medically treated patients and the study was terminated early, loss to follow-up and small size limit the study's usefulness. A similar randomized trial involving patients who had peripheral vascular disease has not been performed. However, the CASS registry provided a unique opportunity to evaluate the outcome of patients with CAD who were either medically managed or had undergone CABG and subsequently underwent noncardiac surgery. Eagle and colleagues (86) evaluated 3,368 patients, of whom 1,546 were undergoing abdominal, vascular, or head and neck surgeries. Among the patients who underwent these high-risk procedures, a dramatic reduction in event rates and fewer deaths (1.7% vs. 3.3%; *p* = .03) and MI (0.8% vs. 2.7%; *p* = .002) were seen in the CABG group than in the medically treated group. Rihal and associates (197) analyzed data from the CASS registry to examine the long-term outcomes of 1,834 patients undergoing noncardiac surgery. For patients treated with CABG, the Kaplan-Meier 8-year and 16-year survival rates were 72% and 41%, respectively; for the medically treated group, the corresponding survival rates were 57% and 34%, respectively (*p* <.0001). However, the benefits were limited to patients with three-vessel CAD and inversely related to LVEF. These data may suggest that the relatively high short-term risks of CABG may be outweighed by the long-term benefits, even though the overall long-term survival rates among patients with peripheral vascular disease remain poor. Finally, in a recently published analysis of the Bypass Angioplasty Revascularization Investigation trial, patients randomly assigned to undergo CABG or PTCA who underwent noncardiac surgery during the follow-up period were evaluated for perioperative cardiac events (198). After an average of 29 months of follow-up, low perioperative event rates were associated with both of the revascularization procedures (1.6% in each group), suggesting that coronary revascularization of either type may reduce the event rate of cardiac complications after noncardiac surgery (199).

Certain issues regarding risk reduction remain unresolved: (a) the lack of randomized trials that evaluate preoperative coronary revascularization and the optimal timing for the revascularization procedure, (b) the optimal timing and duration of perioperative beta-blocker therapy and the usefulness of beta-blockers to treat patients undergoing nonvascular surgery and low-risk patients, and (c) the role of alpha-adrenergic agents and the usefulness of their addition to perioperative beta-blocker therapy.

Stepwise Approach to Preoperative Cardiac Risk Assessment

The ACC and the AHA have jointly produced guidelines, based on current knowledge, for cardiac evaluation [✌ h93] before noncardiac surgery. A general strategy for preoperative cardiac risk assessment is summarized in Figure 41.4. Ideally, this strategy should be applied in the outpatient setting for elective surgery. A stepwise approach to risk stratification includes the following (103):

1. Determine whether the patient has undergone coronary revascularization in the past 5 years. Prior coronary revascularization probably reduces the cardiac risk associated with noncardiac surgery (70,71).
2. Determine whether the patient has had an adequate, favorable prior cardiac evaluation in the past 2 years. If there have been no new intercurrent symptoms, it may not be necessary to repeat costly testing.
3. Determine whether the patient has an unstable coronary syndrome or a major clinical predictor of risk (e.g., decompensated heart failure, significant arrhythmias, severe valvular disease), which usually leads to cancellation or

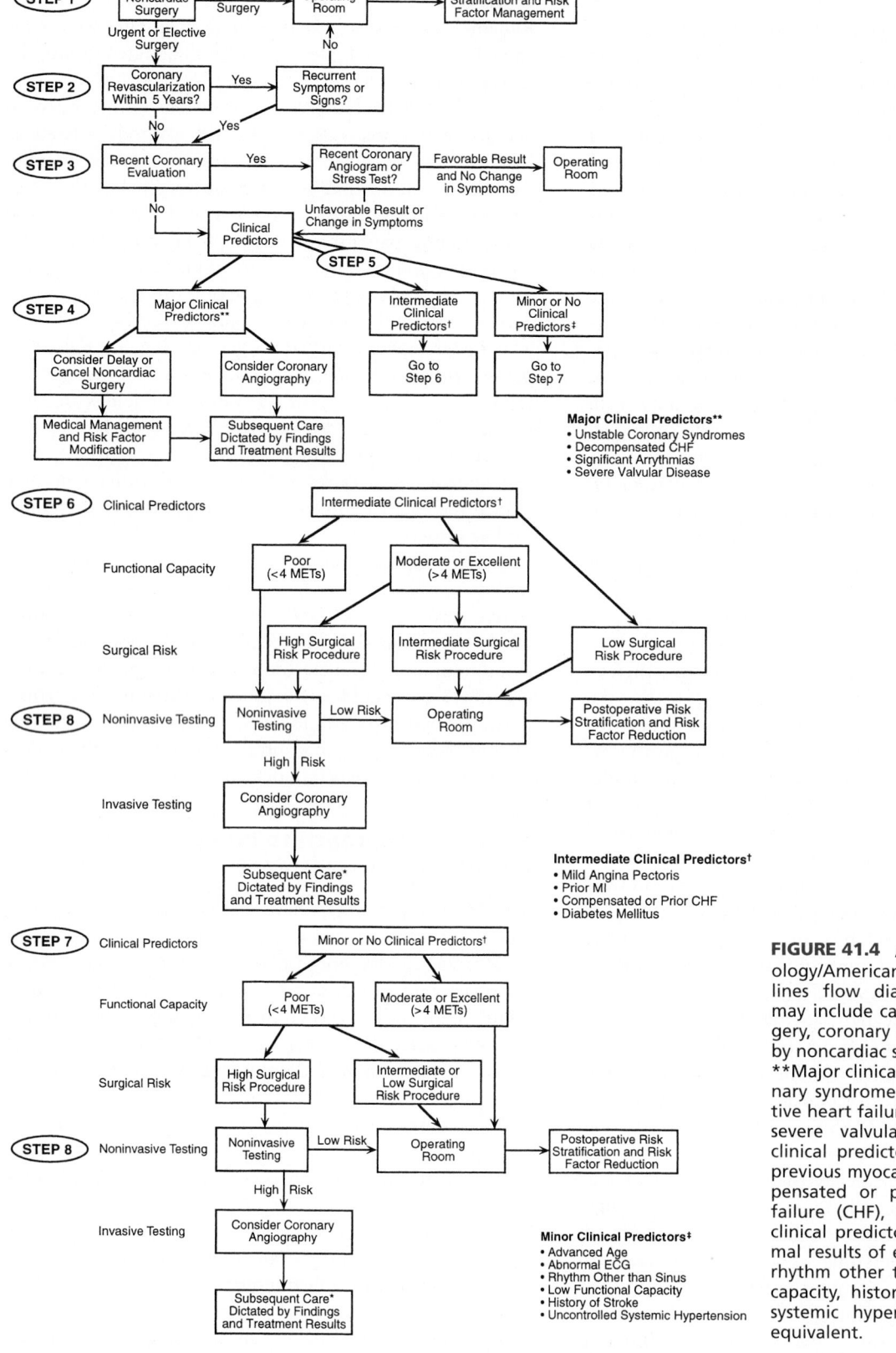

FIGURE 41.4 American College of Cardiology/American Heart Association Guidelines flow diagram. *Subsequent care may include cancellation or delay of surgery, coronary revascularization followed by noncardiac surgery, or intensified care. **Major clinical predictors: unstable coronary syndromes, decompensated congestive heart failure, significant arrhythmias, severe valvular disease. †Intermediate clinical predictors: mild angina pectoris, previous myocardial infarction (MI), compensated or previous congestive heart failure (CHF), diabetes mellitus. ‡Minor clinical predictors: advanced age, abnormal results of electrocardiography (ECG), rhythm other than sinus, low functional capacity, history of stroke, uncontrolled systemic hypertension. MET, metabolic equivalent.

delay of surgery until the problem has been diagnosed and treated.

4. Determine whether the patient has intermediate clinical predictors of risk (e.g., prior MI recognized by history or by ECG, angina pectoris, compensated or prior heart failure, and diabetes mellitus). Consider the patient's functional capacity and surgery-specific risk.

5. Patients who have no major predictors but who have intermediate predictors of clinical risk and at least moderate functional capacity generally may undergo intermediate risk surgery with low probability of perioperative MI or death. Conversely, patients with poor functional capacity (inability to exercise at 4 metabolic equivalents) or who have multiple markers of risk and who are undergoing higher-risk surgery should undergo noninvasive evaluation to further stratify risk. If the anticipated risk of surgery is high and results of noninvasive testing show abnormalities that suggest significant CAD, coronary angiography, followed by coronary revascularization if appropriate, should be considered.

6. Noncardiac surgery is generally safe for patients with neither major nor intermediate predictors of clinical risk and at least moderate functional capacity.

7. Use results of the preoperative evaluation, including noninvasive testing in selected patients, to determine further preoperative management. Use information gained during preoperative evaluation and careful postoperative surveillance to tailor long-term therapy and follow-up.

To date there have been no large prospective studies of preoperative cardiac risk reduction, in part because of the difficulties associated with designing and carrying out such investigations (74). Because of the lack of sufficient sound evidence, the decision to perform coronary angiography based on preoperative noninvasive cardiac testing remains difficult, controversial, and costly. The ACC/AHA guidelines for perioperative cardiovascular evaluation before noncardiac surgery do not address whether coronary angiography should be performed in response to specific test results (103). Therefore, using a modification of the *Delphi method* (a term sometimes used to describe a reiterative process by which consensus panels make recommendations), Cohen and Eagle (200) offered an expert opinion regarding the indications for preoperative coronary angiography when results of noninvasive tests are known. There was agreement that catheterization should be performed for

(a) ischemia seen on exercise ECG in a patient with a blood pressure drop greater than 10 mm Hg; (b) stress perfusion scan reversibility in greater than or equal to one-half of SPECT slices; and (c) ischemia seen on stress echocardiography in more than five segments, more than two coronary artery zones, or four left anterior descending coronary artery segments. Therefore, in general, coronary angiography should be performed in the appropriate clinical context, based on results of noninvasive tests that indicate large zones of myocardial ischemia, and should not be performed for patients who have limited ischemia without other significant clinical findings.

CONTROVERSIES AND PERSONAL PERSPECTIVES

Cardiology consultants frequently provide perioperative cardiac care. Evidence supports selective screening and efforts at cardiac risk reduction. "Universal precautions," including intensified antiischemic medical regimens and close hemodynamic monitoring, combined with constantly improving surgical and anesthetic techniques, may make preoperative cardiac risk assessment less cost-effective. In this context, surgery may be considered just one of many potential triggers of cardiac morbidity and mortality with which a person may come in contact during daily life. The preoperative cardiac consultation may, therefore, represent an opportunity to initiate or modify cardiac care, including primary and secondary preventive measures. The consultant should assess and suggest management for risk factors for CAD (e.g., hypertension and hyperlipidemia) and heart failure. Further evaluation may be appropriate after the patient has recovered from surgery. The physician responsible for the long-term care of the patient should receive pertinent information obtained during the perioperative consultation (103). One of the most important aspects of a consultation is referral back to the primary care provider. This ensures that the physician responsible for the overall medical needs of the patient remains involved in the individual's care. Also, the primary care provider may have the benefit of long-term follow-up, providing more insight into the social and psychological aspects of patient care. Lastly, referral back to the primary care provider helps strengthen the relationship between the consultant and the referring physician, which may result in continued referrals to the consultant's practice.

THE FUTURE

Regardless of the political and economic environment in which medicine is practiced, successful cardiology consultation requires more than proficiency in taking histories, examination, and test interpretation. The ideal consultant "informs without patronizing, educates without lecturing, and directs without ordering. . . ." (36). Cardiology consultants might gain from the adage: "Successful consultation depends on the '3 A's': affability, availability, and ability—in that order!"

REFERENCES

1. Hippocrates. *Precepts*. Jones WHS, trans. Cambridge: Harvard University Press, 1962.
2. When does a generalist need a specialist? *J Gen Intern Med* 1996;11(4):247–248.
3. Ullyot DJ. President's page: cardiology manpower. *J Am Coll Cardiol* 1994;23:1516–1517.
4. Lewis RP. The ACC at 50. *J Am Coll Cardiol* 2000;35:1061–1066.
5. Education update: training programs in United States in adult cardiology. *J Am Coll Cardiol* 1997;34:1231–1261.
6. Foot FK, Lewis RP, Pearson TP, et al. Demographics and cardiology. *J Am Coll Cardiol* 2000;35:1067–1081.
7. Rudd P. Contrasts in academic consultation. *Ann Intern Med* 1981;94:537–538.
8. Lee TH, Goldman L. Role of the consultant. In: Breslow MJ, Miller CF, Rogers M, eds. *Perioperative management*. St. Louis: Mosby, 1990:46–51.
9. Calman NS, Hyman RB, Litch W. Variability in consultation rates and practitioner level of diagnostic accuracy. *J Fam Pract* 1976;3:163–169.
10. Roland M, Morris R. Are referrals by general practitioners influenced by the availability of consultants? *BMJ* 1988;297:599–600.
11. Sulke AN, Paul VE, Taylor CJ, et al. Open access exercise electrocardiography: a service to improve management of ischaemic heart disease by general practitioners. *J R Soc Med* 1991;84:590–594.
12. Vetrovec GW, Gardin JM, Gregory JJ, et al. adult cardiovascular physician resources and needs assessment. *J Am Coll Cardiol* 1995;26:1125–1132.
13. Schappert SM, Nelson C. National ambulatory medical survey: 1995–96 summary. *Vital Health Stat 13* 1999;142:1–14.
14. Goldstein S, Pearson TA, Colwill JM, et al. The relationship between cardiovascular specialists and generalists. Task Force 4. *J Am Coll Cardiol* 1994;24:304–312.
15. St. Clair EW, Oddone EZ, Waugh RA, et al. Assessing housestaff diagnostic skills using a cardiology patient simulator. *Ann Intern Med* 1992;117:751–756.
16. Mangione S, Nieman LZ, Gracely E, et al. The teaching and practice of cardiac auscultation during internal medicine and cardiology training: a nationwide survey. *Ann Intern Med* 1993;119:47–54.
17. Norcin JJ, Lipner RS, Benson JA Jr, et al. An analysis of the knowledge base of practicing internists as measured by the 1980 recertification examination. *Ann Intern Med* 1985;102:385–389.
18. Ely JW, Levinson W, Elder NC, et al. Perceived causes of family physicians' errors. *J Fam Pract* 1995;40:337–344.
19. Greenfield S, Nelson EC, Zubkoff M, et al. Variations in resource utilization among medical specialties and systems of care: results from the medical outcomes study. *JAMA* 1992;267:1624–1630.
20. Schreiber TL, Elkhatib A, Grines CL, et al. Cardiologist versus internist management of patients with unstable angina: treatment patterns and outcomes. *J Am Coll Cardiol* 1995;26:577–582.
21. Kravitz RL, Greenfield S, Rogers W, et al. Differences in the mix of patients among medical specialties and systems of care: results from the medical outcomes study. *JAMA* 1992;267:1617–1623.
22. Greenfield S, Rogers W, Mangotich M, et al. Outcomes of patients with hypertension and non–insulin dependent diabetes mellitus treated by different systems and specialties: results from the medical outcomes study. *JAMA* 1995;274:1436–1444.
23. Ayanian JZ, Hauptman PJ, Guadagnoli E, et al. Knowledge and practices of generalist and specialist physicians regarding drug therapy for acute myocardial infarction. *N Engl J Med* 1994;331:1136–1142.
24. Jollis JG, DeLong ER, Peterson ED, et al. Outcome of acute myocardial infarction according to the specialty of the admitting physician. *N Engl J Med* 1996;335:1880–1887.
25. Whyte JJ, Filly AL, Jollis JG. Treatment of hyperlipidemia by specialists versus generalists as secondary prevention of coronary artery disease. *Am J Cardiol* 1997;80:1345–1347.
26. Stafford RS, Blumenthal D. Specialty differences in cardiovascular disease prevention practices. *J Am Coll Cardiol* 1998;32:1238–1243.
27. Geyman JP, Brown TC, Rivers K. Referrals in family practice: a comparative setting by geographic region and practice setting. *J Fam Pract* 1976;3:163–167.
28. Mayer TR. Family practice referral patterns in a health maintenance organization. *J Fam Pract* 1982;14:315–319.
29. Schmidt DD. Referral patterns in an individual family practice. *J Fam Pract* 1977;5:401–403.
30. Lawler FH, Purvis JR, Glenn JK, et al. Physician referrals from a rural family practice residency clinic: a pilot study. *Fam Pract Res J* 1990;10:19–26.
31. Greenfield S. Dividing up the turf: generalists versus specialists. *J Gen Intern Med* 1996;11:245–246.

32. Craig DE, Harkta L, Likosky WH, et al. Implementation of the hospitalist system in a large health maintenance organization: the Kaiser Permanente experience. *Ann Intern Med* 1999;130:355–359.

33. Byrd JC, Moskowitz MA. Outpatient consultation: interaction between the general internist and the specialist. *J Gen Intern Med* 1987;2:93–98.

34. Schneeweiss R, Ellsbury K, Hart LG, et al. The economic impact and multiplier effect of a family practice clinic on an academic medical center. *JAMA* 1989;262:370–375.

35. Mendenhall RC, Lewis CE, DeFlorio GP, et al. A national study of medical and surgical specialties: an empirical approach to the classification of patient care. *JAMA* 1979;241:2180–2185.

36. Gross RJ, Caputo GM. General medical consultation service. In: Gross RJ, Caputo GM, eds. *Medical consultation,* 3rd ed. Baltimore: William & Wilkins, 1998:1–8.

37. Goldman L, Lee TH, Rudd P. Ten commandments for effective consultations. *Arch Intern Med* 1983;143:1753–1755.

38. Lee TH, Pappius EM, Goldman L. Impact of inter-physician communication on the effectiveness of medical consultations. *Am J Med* 1983;74:106–112.

39. The Criteria Committee of the New York Heart Association. *Nomenclature and criteria for diagnosis of diseases of the heart and great vessels,* 8th ed. New York: New York Heart Association/Little, Brown and Company, 1979.

40. Patterson RE, Horowitz SF. Importance of epidemiology and biostatistics in deciding clinical strategies for using diagnostic tests: a simplified approach using examples from coronary artery disease. *J Am Coll Cardiol* 1989;13:1653–1665.

41. Fletcher GF, Balady G, Froelicher VF, et al. Exercise standards: a statement for healthcare professionals from the American Heart Association. *Circulation* 1995;91:580–615.

42. Ryan TJ, Anderson JL, Antman EM, et al. ACC/AHA guidelines for the management of patients with acute myocardial infarction: a report of the American College of Cardiology/American Heart Association Task Force on Practice Guidelines (Committee on Management of Acute Myocardial Infarction). *J Am Coll Cardiol* 1996;28:1328–1428.

43. What the internist needs to know about the compliance requirements of the federal health programs. ACP-ASIM Publication, April 1999.

44. Maguire NJ, ed. *Medicare billing rules from A to Z.* Rockville, MD: Part B News Group Publishers, 2000.

45. Silk AD. Why we need help finding a solution to the E/M crisis. *ACP-ASIM Observer* Sep 2000:6–7.

46. Pupa LE Jr, Coventry JA, Hanley JF, et al. Factors affecting compliance for general medicine consultations to non-internists. *Am J Med* 1986;81:508–514.

47. Rudd P, Siegler M, Byyny RL. Perioperative diabetic consultation: a plea for improved training. *J Med Educ* 1978;53:590–596.

48. Sears CL, Charlson ME. The effectiveness of a consultation: compliance with initial recommendations. *Am J Med* 1983;74:870–876.

49. Mackenzie TB, Popkin MK, Callies AL, et al. The effectiveness of cardiology consultation: concordance with diagnostic and drug recommendations. *Chest* 1981;79:16–22.

50. Horwitz RI, Henes CG, Horwitz SM. Developing strategies for improving the diagnostic and management efficacy of medical consultations. *J Chronic Dis* 1983;36:213–218.

51. Ferguson RP, Rubinstien E. Preoperative medical consultations in a community hospital. *J Gen Intern Med* 1987;2:89–92.

52. Greenfield S, Linn LS, Putrill N, et al. Reverse consultations: the profiles of patients referred from subspecialists to generalists. *J Chron Dis* 1983;36:883–889.

53. Dudley JC, Brandenburg JA, Hartley LH, et al. Last-minute preoperative cardiology consultations: epidemiology and impact. *Am Heart J* 1996;131:245–249.

54. Goldman L. Cardiac risks and complications of noncardiac surgery. *Ann Intern Med* 1983;98:504–513.

55. Klein LE, Levine DM, Moore RD, et al. The preoperative consultation: response to internists' recommendations. *Arch Intern Med* 1983;143:743–744.

56. Detsky AS, Abrams HB, McLaughlin JR, et al. Predicting cardiac complications in patients undergoing noncardiac surgery. *J Gen Intern Med* 1986;1:211–219.

57. Goldman L, Caldera DL, Nussbaum SR, et al. Multifactorial index of cardiac risk in noncardiac surgical procedures. *N Engl J Med* 1977;297:845–850.

58. Velanovich V. Preoperative screening electrocardiography. *South Med J* 1994;87(4):431–434.

59. Cutler BS, Wheeler HB, Paraskos JA, et al. Applicability and interpretation of electrocardiographic stress testing in patients with peripheral vascular disease. *Am J Surg* 1981;141:501–506.

60. Carliner NH, Fisher ML, Plotnick GD, et al. Routine preoperative exercise testing in patients undergoing major noncardiac surgery. *Am J Cardiol* 1985;56:51–58.

61. McPhail NV, Calvin JE, Shariatmadar A, et al. The use of preoperative exercise testing to predict cardiac complications after arterial reconstruction. *J Vasc Surg* 1988;7:60–68.

62. Boucher CA, Brewster DC, Darling RC, et al. Determination of cardiac risk by dipyridamole-thallium imaging before peripheral vascular surgery. *N Engl J Med* 1985;312:389–394.

63. Leppo J, Plaja J, Gionet M, et al. Noninvasive evaluation of cardiac risk before elective vascular surgery. *J Am Coll Cardiol* 1987;9:269–276.

64. Lane SE, Lewis SM, Pippin JJ, et al. Predictive value of quantitative dipyridamole-thallium scintigraphy in assessing cardiovascular risk after vascular surgery in diabetes mellitus. *Am J Cardiol* 1989;64:1275–1279.

65. Tischler MD, Lee TH, Hirsch AT, et al. Prediction of major cardiac events after peripheral vascular surgery using dipyridamole echocardiography. *Am J Cardiol* 1991;68:593–597.

66. Lane RT, Sawada SG, Segar DS, et al. Dobutamine stress echocardiography for assessment of cardiac risk before noncardiac surgery. *Am J Cardiol* 1991;68:976–977.

67. Tomatis LA, Fierens EE, Verbrugge GP. Evaluation of surgical risk in peripheral vascular disease by coronary arteriography: a series of 100 cases. *Surgery* 1972;71:429–435.

68. Hertzer NR, Beven EG, Young JR, et al. Coronary artery disease in peripheral vascular patients: a classification of

1000 coronary angiograms and results of surgical management. *Ann Surg* 1984;199:223–233.

69. Eagle KA, Coley CM, Newell JB, et al. Combining clinical and thallium data optimizes preoperative assessment of cardiac risk before major vascular surgery. *Ann Intern Med* 1989;110:859–866.

70. Foster ED, Davis KB, Carpenter JA, et al. Risk of noncardiac operation in patients with defined coronary disease: the Coronary Artery Surgery Study (CASS) registry experience. *Ann Thorac Surg* 1986;41:42–50.

71. Huber KC, Evans MA, Bresnahan JF, et al. Outcome of noncardiac operations in patients with severe coronary artery disease successfully treated preoperatively with coronary angioplasty. *Mayo Clin Proc* 1992;67:15–21.

72. Cohen MC, McKenna C, Lewis SM, et al. Requirements for controlled clinical trials of preoperative cardiovascular risk reduction. *Control Clin Trials* 1995;16:89–95.

73. Brener S, Cohen MC, Talley JD, et al. Striking hospital to hospital variation in pre-operative cardiac work-up for patients referred for major non-cardiac surgery. *Circulation* 1995;92:I-679.

74. Baron JF, Mundler O, Bertrand M, et al. Dipyridamole-thallium scintigraphy and gated radionuclide angiography to assess cardiac risk before abdominal aortic surgery. *N Engl J Med* 1994;330:663–669.

75. Liu LL, Wiener-Kronish JP. Preoperative cardiac evaluation of women for noncardiac surgery. *Cardiol Clin* 1998;16:59–66.

76. Mangano DT. Perioperative cardiac morbidity, epidemiology, costs, problems and solutions. *West J Med* 1994;161:87–89.

77. Steen PA, Tinker JH, Tarhan S. Myocardial reinfarction after anesthesia and surgery. *JAMA* 1978;239:2566–2570.

78. Tarhan S, Moffitt EA, Taylor WF, et al. Myocardial infarction after general anesthesia. *JAMA* 1972;220:1451–1454.

79. Abraham SA, Coles NA, Coley CM, et al. Coronary risk of noncardiac surgery. *Prog Cardiovasc Dis* 1991;34:205–234.

80. von Knorring J. Postoperative myocardial infarction: a prospective study in a risk group of surgical patients. *Surgery* 1981;90:55–60.

81. Raby KE, Goldman L, Creager MA, et al. Correlation between preoperative ischemia and major cardiac events after peripheral vascular surgery. *N Engl J Med* 1989;321:1296–1300.

82. Charlson ME, MacKenzie CR, Ales KL, et al. The postoperative electrocardiogram and creatine kinase: implications for diagnosis of myocardial infarction after non-cardiac surgery. *J Clin Epidemiol* 1989;42:25–34.

83. Charlson ME, MacKenzie CR, Ales KL, et al. Surveillance for postoperative myocardial infarction after noncardiac operations. *Surg Gynecol Obstet* 1988;167:407–414.

84. Potyk DK. Cardiac evaluation and risk reduction in patients undergoing major vascular operations. *West J Med* 1994;161:50–56.

85. Fleisher LA, Eagle KA, Shaffer T, et al. Perioperative- and long-term mortality rates after major vascular surgery: the relationship to preoperative testing in the Medicare population. *Anesth Analg* 1999;89:849–855.

86. Eagle KA, Charanjit SR, Mickel MC, et al. Cardiac risk of noncardiac surgery: influence of coronary disease and type of surgery in 3368 operations. *Circulation* 1997;96:1882–1887.

87. Becker RC, Underwood DA. Myocardial infarction in patients undergoing noncardiac surgery. *Cleve Clin J Med* 1987;321:1296–1300.

88. Backer CL, Tinker JH, Robertson DM, et al. Myocardial reinfarction following local anesthesia for ophthalmic surgery. *Anesth Analg* 1980;59:257–262.

89. McAuley CE, Watson CG. Elective inguinal herniorrhaphy after myocardial infarction. *Surg Gynecol Obstet* 1984;159:36–38.

90. Wirthlin DJ, Cambria RP. Surgery specific considerations in a cardiac patient undergoing noncardiac surgery. *Prog Cardiovasc Dis* 1998;40:453–468.

91. Cohen MC, Aretz TH. Histological analysis of coronary artery lesions in fatal postoperative myocardial infarction. *Cardiovasc Pathol* 1999;8:133–139.

92. Dawood MM, Gupta DK, Southern J, et al. Pathology of fatal myocardial infarction: implications regarding pathophysiology and prevention. *Int J Cardiol* 1996;321:1296–1300.

93. Dripps RD, Lamont A, Eckenhoff JE. The role of anesthesia in surgical mortality. *JAMA* 1961;178:261–266.

94. American Society of Anesthesiologists. I. New classification of physical status. *Anesthesiology* 1963;24:111.

95. Vacanti CJ, VanHouten RJ, Hill RC. A statistical analysis of the relationship of physical status to postoperative mortality in 68,388 cases. *Anesth Analg* 1970;49:564–566.

96. Owens WD, Felts JA, Spitznagel EL Jr. ASA physical status classifications: a study of consistency of ratings. *Anesthesiology* 1978;49:239–243.

97. Detsky AS, Abrams HB, Forbath N, et al. Cardiac assessment for patients undergoing noncardiac surgery: a multifactorial clinical risk index. *Arch Intern Med* 1986;146:2131–2134.

98. Zeldin RA. Assessing cardiac risk in patients who undergo noncardiac surgical procedures. *Can J Surg* 1984;27:402–404.

99. Gerson MC, Hurst JM, Hertzberg VS, et al. Cardiac prognosis in noncardiac geriatric surgery. *Ann Intern Med* 1985;103:832–837.

100. Jeffrey CC, Kunsman J, Cullen DJ, et al. A prospective evaluation of cardiac risk index. *Anesthesiology* 1983;58:462–464.

101. Gilbert K, Larocque BJ, Patrick LT. Prospective evaluation of cardiac risk indices for patients undergoing noncardiac surgery. *Ann Intern Med* 2000;133:356–359.

102. Chaitman BR, Miller DD. Perioperative cardiac evaluation for noncardiac surgery noninvasive cardiac testing. *Prog Cardiovasc Dis* 1998;40:405–418.

103. Eagle KA, Brundage BH, Chaitman BR, et al. Guidelines for perioperative cardiovascular evaluation for noncardiac surgery: report of the American College of Cardiology/American Heart Association Task Force on Practice Guidelines (Committee on Perioperative Cardiovascular Evaluation for Noncardiac Surgery). *J Am Coll Cardiol* 1996;27:910–948.

104. Gerson MC, Hurst JM, Hertzberg VS, et al. Prediction of cardiac and pulmonary complications related to elective abdominal and noncardiac thoracic surgery in geriatric patients. *Am J Med* 1990;88:101–107.

105. Pasternack PF, Imparato AM, Bear G, et al. The value of radionuclide angiography as a predictor of perioperative myocardial infarction in patients undergoing abdominal aortic aneurysm resection. *J Vasc Surg* 1984;1:320–325.

106. Pasternack PF, Grossi EA, Baumann FG, et al. The value of silent myocardial ischemia monitoring in the prediction of perioperative myocardial infarction in patients undergoing peripheral vascular surgery. *J Vasc Surg* 1989;10:617–625.

107. Kazmers A, Cerqueira MD, Zierler RE. The role of preoperative radionuclide left ventricular ejection fraction for risk assessment in carotid surgery. *Arch Surg* 1988;123:416–419.

108. Mosley JG, Clarke JM, Ell PJ, et al. Assessment of myocardial function before aortic surgery by radionuclide angiocardiography. *Br J Surg* 1985;72:886–887.

109. Fletcher JP, Antico VF, Gruenewald S, et al. Risk of aortic aneurysm surgery as assessed by preoperative gated heart pool scan. *Br J Surg* 1989;76:26–28.

110. Fiser WP, Thompson BW, Thompson AR, et al. Nuclear cardiac ejection fraction and cardiac index in abdominal aortic surgery. *Surgery* 1983;94:736–739.

111. Lazor L, Russell JC, DaSilva J, et al. Use of the multiple uptake gated acquisition scan for the preoperative assessment of cardiac risk. *Surg Gynecol Obstet* 1988;167:234–238.

112. Kazmers A, Cerqueira MD, Zierler RE. The role of preoperative radionuclide ejection fraction in direct abdominal aortic aneurysm repair. *J Vasc Surg* 1988;8:128–136.

113. Kazmers A, Cerqueira MD, Zierler RE. Perioperative and late outcome in patients with left ventricular ejection fraction of 35% or less who require major vascular surgery. *J Vasc Surg* 1988;8:307–315.

114. McEnroe CS, O'Donnell TF Jr, Yeager A, et al. Comparison of ejection fraction and Goldman risk factor analysis to dipyridamole-thallium 201 studies in the evaluation of cardiac morbidity after aortic aneurysm surgery. *J Vasc Surg* 1990;11:497–504.

115. Franco CD, Goldsmith J, Veith FJ, et al. Resting gated pool ejection fraction: a poor predictor of perioperative myocardial infarction in patients undergoing vascular surgery for infrainguinal bypass grafting. *J Vasc Surg* 1989;10:656–661.

116. McCann RL, Wolfe WG. Resection of abdominal aortic aneurysm in patients with low ejection fractions. *J Vasc Surg* 1989;10:240–244.

117. Halm EA, Browner WS, Tubau JF, et al. Echocardiography for assessing cardiac risk in patients having noncardiac surgery. Study of Perioperative Ischemia Research Group. *Ann Intern Med* 1996;125:433–441.

118. Rhode LE, Polanczyk CA, Goldman L, et al. Usefulness of transthoracic echocardiography as a tool for risk stratification of patients undergoing major noncardiac surgery. *Am J Cardiol* 2001;87:505–509.

119. Freeman WK, Gibbons RJ, Shub C. Preoperative assessment of cardiac patients undergoing noncardiac surgical procedures. *Mayo Clin Proc* 1989;64:1105–1117.

120. Gage AA, Bhayana JN, Balu V, Hook N. Assessment of cardiac risk in surgical patients. *Arch Surg* 1977;112:1488–1492.

121. McPhail NV, Ruddy TD, Calvin JE, et al. A comparison of dipyridamole-thallium imaging and exercise testing in the prediction of postoperative cardiac complications in patients requiring arterial reconstruction. *J Vasc Surg* 1989;10:51–55.

122. Iskandrian AS, Heo J, Kong B, et al. Effect of exercise level on the ability of thallium-201 tomographic imaging in detecting coronary artery disease: analysis of 461 patients. *J Am Coll Cardiol* 1989;14:1477–1486.

123. Waters TA, Botwinick EH, Dae MW. Comparison of findings on preoperative dipyridamole scintigraphy and intraoperative transesophageal echocardiography. *J Am Coll Cardiol* 1991;18:93–100.

124. Brown KA. Prognostic value of nuclear cardiology technique. In: Gerson MC, ed. *Cardiac nuclear medicine,* 3rd ed. New York: McGraw-Hill, 1987:619–654.

125. Lette J, Waters D, Lapointe J, et al. Usefulness of the severity and extent of reversible perfusion defects during thallium-dipyridamole imaging for cardiac risk assessment before noncardiac surgery. *J Am Coll Cardiol* 1989;64:276–281.

126. Levinson JR, Boucher CA, Coley CM, et al. Usefulness of semiquantitative analysis of dipyridamole-thallium-201 redistribution for improving risk stratification before vascular surgery. *Am J Cardiol* 1990;66:406–410.

127. Eagle KA, Singer DE, Brewster DC, et al. Dipyridamole-thallium scanning in patients undergoing vascular surgery: optimizing preoperative evaluation of cardiac risk. *JAMA* 1987;257:2185–2189.

128. Zarich SW, Cohen MC, Lane SE, et al. Routine preoperative dipyridamole 201 thallium imaging in diabetic patients undergoing vascular surgery. *Diabetes Care* 1996;19:355–360.

129. L'Italien GJ, Paul SD, Hendel RC, et al. Development and validation of a Bayesian model for perioperative cardiac risk assessment in a cohort of 1,081 vascular surgical candidates. *J Am Coll Cardiol* 1996;27:779–786.

130. Brown KA, Rimmer J, Haisch C. Noninvasive cardiac risk stratification of diabetic and nondiabetic uremic renal allograft candidates using dipyridamole-thallium-201 imaging and radionuclide ventriculography. *Am J Cardiol* 1989;64:1017–1021.

131. Camp AD, Garvin PJ, Hoff J, et al. Prognostic value of intravenous dipyridamole thallium imaging in patients with diabetes mellitus considered for renal transplantation. *Am J Cardiol* 1990;65:1459–1463.

132. Iqbal A, Gibbons RJ, McGoon MD, et al. Noninvasive assessment of cardiac risk in insulin-dependent diabetic patients being evaluated for pancreatic transplantation using thallium-201 myocardial perfusion scintigraphy. *Transplant Proc* 1991;23:1690–1691.

133. Coley CM, Field TS, Abraham SA, et al. Usefulness of dipyridamole-thallium scanning for preoperative evaluation of cardiac risk for nonvascular surgery. *Am J Cardiol* 1992;69:1280–1285.

134. Shaw L, Miller DD, Kong BA, et al. Determination of perioperative cardiac risk by adenosine thallium-201 myocardial imaging. *Am Heart J* 1992;124:861–869.

135. Takase B, Younis LT, Byers SL, et al. Comparative prognostic value of clinical risk indexes, resting two-dimensional echocardiography, and dipyridamole stress thallium-201

myocardial imaging for perioperative cardiac events in major nonvascular surgery patients. *Am Heart J* 1993; 126:1099–1106.

136. Younis L, Stratmann H, Takase B, et al. Preoperative clinical assessment and dipyridamole thallium-201 scintigraphy for prediction and prevention of cardiac events in patients having major noncardiovascular surgery and known or suspected coronary artery disease. *Am J Cardiol* 1994;74:311–317.

137. Van Damme H, Pierard L, Gillian D, et al. Cardiac risk assessment before vascular surgery: a prospective study comparing clinical evaluation, dobutamine stress echocardiography and dobutamine Tc-99m tomoscintigraphy. *Cardiovasc Surg* 1997;5:54–64.

138. Bry JD, Belkin M, O'Donnell TF Jr, et al. An assessment of the positive predictive value and cost-effectiveness of dipyridamole myocardial scintigraphy in patients undergoing vascular surgery. *J Vasc Surg* 1994;19:112–121.

139. Elliott BM, Robinson JG, Zellner JL, et al. Dobutamine-201Tl imaging: assessing cardiac risk associated with vascular surgery. *Circulation* 1991;84:54–60.

140. Geleijnse ML, Elhendy A, Fioretti PM, et al. Dobutamine stress myocardial perfusion imaging. *J Am Coll Cardiol* 2000;36:2017–2027.

141. Hendel RC, Whitfield SS, Villegas BJ, et al. Prediction of late cardiac events by dipyridamole thallium imaging in patients undergoing elective vascular surgery. *Am J Cardiol* 1992;70:1243–1249.

142. Younis LT, Aguirre F, Byers S, et al. Perioperative and long-term prognostic value of intravenous dipyridamole thallium scintigraphy in patients with peripheral vascular disease. *Am Heart J* 1990;119:1287–1292.

143. Stratmann HG, Younis LT, Wittry MD, et al. Dipyridamole technetium-99m sestamibi myocardial tomography in patients evaluated for elective vascular surgery: prognostic value for perioperative and late cardiac events. *Am Heart J* 1996;131:923–929.

144. Cohen MC, Siewers S, Dickens J, et al. Long-term prognostic significance of MIBI-SPECT in vascular surgery patients. *J Nucl Cardiol* 2000;7:59(abst).

145. Lalka SG, Sawada SG, Dalsing MC, et al. Dobutamine stress echocardiography as a predictor of cardiac events associated with aortic surgery. *J Vasc Surg* 1992;15:831–840.

146. Eichelberger JP, Schwarz KQ, Black ER, et al. Predictive value of dobutamine echocardiography just before noncardiac vascular surgery. *Am J Cardiol* 1993;72:602–607.

147. Langan EM 3d, Youkey JR, Franklin DP, et al. Dobutamine stress echocardiography for cardiac risk assessment before aortic surgery. *J Vasc Surg* 1993;18:905–911.

148. Poldermans D, Fioretti PM, Forster T, et al. Dobutamine stress echocardiography for assessment of perioperative cardiac risk in patients undergoing major vascular surgery. *Circulation* 1993;87:1506–1512.

149. Davila-Roman VG, Waggoner AD, Sicard GA, et al. Dobutamine stress echocardiography predicts surgical outcome in patients with an aortic aneurysm and peripheral vascular disease. *J Am Coll Cardiol* 1993;21:957–963.

150. Poldermans D, Arnese M, Fioretti PM, et al. Improved cardiac risk stratification in major vascular surgery with dobutamine-atropine stress echocardiography. *J Am Coll Cardiol* 1995;26:648–653.

151. Poldermans D, Arnese M, Fioretti PM, et al. Sustained prognostic value of dobutamine stress echocardiography for late cardiac events after major noncardiac vascular surgery. *Circulation* 1997;95:53–58.

152. Ballal RS, Kapadia S, Secknus M, et al. Prognosis of patients with vascular disease after clinical evaluation and dobutamine stress echocardiography. *Am Heart J* 1999;137:468–474.

153. Shaw LJ, Eagle KA, Gersh BJ, et al. Meta-analysis of intravenous dipyridamole thallium-201 (1985–1994) for risk stratification before vascular surgical candidates. *J Am Coll Cardiol* 1996;27:787–798.

154. Mangano DT, Browner WS, Hollenberg M, et al. Association of perioperative myocardial ischemia with cardiac morbidity and mortality in men undergoing noncardiac surgery. The Study of Perioperative Ischemia Research Group. *N Engl J Med* 1990;323:1781–1788.

155. Fleisher LA, Rosenbaum SH, Nelson AH, et al. Preoperative dipyridamole thallium imaging and ambulatory electrocardiographic monitoring as a predictor of perioperative cardiac events and long-term outcome. *Anesthesiology* 1995;83:906–917.

156. Fleisher LA, Rosenbaum SH, Nelson AH, et al. The predictive value of preoperative silent ischemia for postoperative ischemic cardiac events in vascular and nonvascular surgery patients. *Am Heart J* 1991;122:980–986.

157. McPhail NV, Ruddy TD, Barber GG, et al. Cardiac risk stratification using dipyridamole myocardial perfusion imaging and ambulatory ECG monitoring prior to vascular surgery. *Eur J Vasc Surg* 1993;7:151–155.

158. Kirwin JD, Ascer E, Gennaro M, et al. Silent myocardial ischemia is not predictive of myocardial infarction in peripheral vascular surgery patients. *Ann Vasc Surg* 1993;7:27–32.

159. Knight AA, Hollenberg M, London MJ, et al. Perioperative myocardial ischemia: importance of the preoperative ischemic pattern. *Anesthesiology* 1988;68:681–688.

160. Moore EH, Greenberg RW, Merrick SH, et al. Coronary artery calcifications: significance of incidental detection on CT scans. *Radiology* 1989;172:711–716.

161. Cooperman M, Pflug B, Martin EW Jr, et al. Cardiovascular risk factors in patients with peripheral vascular disease. *Surgery* 1978;84:505–509.

162. Dajani AS, Taubert KA, Wilson W, et al. Prevention of bacterial endocarditis: recommendations by the American Heart Association. *JAMA* 1997;96:358–366.

163. Hollenberg M, Mangano DT, Browner WS, et al. Predictors of postoperative myocardial ischemia in patients undergoing noncardiac surgery. The Study of Perioperative Ischemia Research Group. *JAMA* 1992;268:205–209.

164. Bach DS. Management of specific medical conditions in the perioperative period. *Prog Cardiovasc Dis* 1998;40:469–476.

165. Berlauk JF, Abrams JH, Gilmour IJ, et al. Preoperative optimization of cardiovascular hemodynamics improves outcome in peripheral vascular surgery: a prospective, randomized clinical trial. *Ann Surg* 1991;214:289–297.

166. Rao TL, Jacobs KH, El-Etr AA. Reinfarction following

anesthesia in patients with myocardial infarction. *Anesthesiology* 1983;59:499–505.

167. Bender JS, Smith MA, Jones CE. Routine use of pulmonary artery catheterization does not reduce morbidity or mortality of elective vascular surgery: results of prospective randomized trial. *Ann Surg* 1997;226:229–236.

168. Valentine RJ, Duke ML, Inman MH, et al. Effectiveness of pulmonary artery catheters in aortic surgery. *J Vasc Surg* 1998;27:203–211.

169. Connors AF Jr, Speroff T, Dawson NV, et al. The effectiveness of right heart catheterization in the initial care of critically ill patients. SUPPORT Investigators. *JAMA* 1996;276:889–897.

170. Bender JS. When is a pulmonary artery catheter needed in a care of surgical patient? *Adv Surg* 1999;32:365–384.

171. Provost PJ, Jenckes MW, Dorman T, et al. Organizational characteristics of intensive care units related to outcomes of abdominal aortic surgery. *JAMA* 1999;281:1310–1317.

172. Pasternack PF, Grossi EA, Baumann FG, et al. Beta blockade to decrease silent myocardial ischemia during peripheral vascular surgery. *Am J Surg* 1989;158:113–116.

173. Mangano DT, Layug EL, Wallace A, et al. Effect of atenolol on mortality and cardiovascular morbidity after noncardiac surgery. The Multicenter Study of Perioperative Ischemia Research Group. *N Engl J Med* 1996;335:1713–1720.

174. Poldermans D, Boersma E, Bax JJ, et al. The effect of bisoprolol on perioperative mortality and myocardial infarction in high risk patients undergoing vascular surgery. *N Engl J Med* 1999;341:1789–1794.

175. Coriat P, Daloz M, Bousseau D, et al. Prevention of intraoperative myocardial ischemia during noncardiac surgery with intravenous nitroglycerin. *Anesthesiology* 1984;61:193–196.

176. Dodds TM, Stone JG, Coromilas J, et al. Prophylactic nitroglycerin infusion during noncardiac surgery does not reduce perioperative ischemia. *Anesth Analg* 1993;76:705–713.

177. Godet G, Coriat P, Baron JF, et al. Prevention of intraoperative myocardial ischemia during noncardiac surgery with intravenous diltiazem: a randomized trial versus placebo. *Anesthesiology* 1987;66:241–245.

178. Ellis JE, Drijers, Pedlow S, et al. Premedication with oral and transdermal clonidine provides safe and effective sympatholysis. *Anesth Analg* 1994;79:1133–1140.

179. Stuhmeier KD, Mainzer B, Cierpka J, et al. Small, oral dose of clonidine reduces the risk of intraoperative myocardial ischemia in patients having vascular surgery. *Anesthesiology* 1996;85:706–712.

180. Oliver MF, Goldman L, Julian DJ, et al. Effect of mivazerol on perioperative cardiac complications during noncardiac surgery in patients with coronary heart disease: The European Mivazerol Trial (EMIT). *Anesthesiology* 1999;91:951–961.

181. Mangano DT, Wong MG, London MJ, et al. Perioperative myocardial ischemia in patients undergoing noncardiac surgery. II. Incidence and severity during the 1st week after surgery. The Study of Perioperative Ischemia (SPI) Research Group. *J Am Coll Cardiol* 1991;17:851–857.

182. Landesberg G, Luria MH, Cotev S, et al. Importance of long-duration postoperative ST-segment depression in cardiac morbidity after vascular surgery. *Lancet* 1993;341:715–719.

183. Boyd O, Grounds RM, Bennett ED. A randomized clinical trial of the effect of deliberate perioperative increase of oxygen delivery on mortality in high-risk surgical patients. *JAMA* 1993;270:2699–2707.

184. Georgeson S, Coombs AT, Eckman MH. Prophylactic use of the intra-aortic balloon pump in high-risk cardiac patients undergoing noncardiac surgery: a decision analytic view. *Am J Med* 1992;92:665–678.

185. Siu SC, Kowalchuk GJ, Welty FK, et al. Intra-aortic balloon counterpulsation support in the high-risk cardiac patient undergoing urgent noncardiac surgery. *Chest* 1991;99:1342–1345.

186. Arafa OE, Pederson TH, Sevnnevig JL, et al. Intraaortic balloon pump in open heart operations: 10 year follow up and risk analysis. *Ann Thorac Surg* 1998;65:741–747.

187. Golden MA, Whittemore AD, Donaldson MC, et al. Selective evaluation and management of coronary artery disease in patients undergoing repair of abdominal aortic aneurysms: a 16-year experience. *Ann Surg* 1990;212:415–420.

188. Allen JR, Helling TS, Hartzler GO. Operative procedures not involving the heart after percutaneous transluminal coronary angioplasty. *Surg Gynecol Obstet* 1991;173:285–288.

189. Elmore JR, Hallett JW Jr, Gibbons RJ, et al. Myocardial revascularization before abdominal aortic aneurysmorrhaphy: effect of coronary angioplasty. *Mayo Clin Proc* 1993;68:637–641.

190. Gottlieb A, Banoub M, Sprung J, et al. Perioperative cardiovascular morbidity in patients with coronary artery disease undergoing vascular surgery after percutaneous transluminal coronary angioplasty. *J Cardiothorac Vasc Anethesiol* 1998;12:501–506.

191. Posner KL, Van Norman GA, Chan V. Adverse cardiac outcomes after noncardiac surgery in patients with prior percutaneous transluminal coronary angioplasty. *Anesth Analg* 1999;89:553–560.

192. Kaluza GL, Joseph J, Lee JR, et al. Catastrophic outcomes of noncardiac surgery soon after coronary stenting. *J Am Coll Cardiol* 2000;35:1288–1294.

193. Cruchley PM, Kaplan JA, Hug CC Jr, et al. Noncardiac surgery in patients with prior myocardial revascularization. *Can Anaesth Soc J* 1983;30:629–634.

194. Mahar LJ, Steen PA, Tinker JH, et al. Perioperative myocardial infarction in patients with coronary artery disease with and without aorta–coronary artery bypass grafts. *J Thorac Cardiovasc Surg* 1978;76:533–537.

195. Reul GJ Jr, Cooley DA, Duncan JM, et al. The effect of coronary bypass on the outcome of peripheral vascular operations in 1093 patients. *J Vasc Surg* 1986;3:788–798.

196. Manske CL, Wang Y, Rector T, et al. Coronary revascularisation in insulin-dependent diabetic patients with chronic renal failure. *Lancet* 1992;340:998–1002.

197. Rihal CS, Eagle KA, Mickel MC, et al. Surgical therapy for coronary artery disease among patients with combined coronary artery and peripheral vascular disease. *Circulation* 1995;91:46–53.

198. Hassan SA, Haltky MA, Boothroyd D, et al. Outcomes of noncardiac surgery after coronary artery bypass surgery or

coronary angioplasty in the Bypass Angioplasty Revascularization Investigation (BARI). *Am J Med* 2001;110:260–266.

199. Rihal CS. The role of myocardial revascularization preceding surgery. *Prog Cardiovasc Dis* 1998;40:383–404.

200. Cohen MC, Eagle KA. Expert opinion regarding cardiac catheterization prior to noncardiac surgery. *Am Heart J* 1997;134:321–329.

201. McCabe CJ, Reidy NC, Abbott WM, et al. The value of electrocardiogram monitoring during treadmill testing for peripheral vascular disease. *Surgery* 1981;89:183–186.

202. Arous EJ, Baum PL, Cutler BS. The ischemic exercise test in patients with peripheral vascular disease: implications for management. *Arch Surg* 1984;119:780–783.

203. Gardine RL, McBride K, Greenberg H, et al. The value of cardiac monitoring during peripheral arterial stress testing in the surgical management of peripheral vascular disease. *J Cardiovasc Surg* 1985;26:258–261.

204. von Knorring J, Lepantalo M. Prediction of perioperative cardiac complications by electrocardiographic monitoring during treadmill exercise testing before peripheral vascular surgery. *Surgery* 1986;99:610–613.

205. Hanson P, Pease M, Berkoff H, et al. Arm exercise testing for coronary artery disease in patients with peripheral vascular disease. *Clin Cardiol* 1988;11:70–74.

206. Urbinati S, Di Pasquale G, Andreoli A, et al. Preoperative noninvasive coronary risk stratification in candidates for carotid endarterectomy. *Stroke* 1994;25:2022–2027.

207. Cutler BS, Leppo JA. Dipyridamole thallium 201 scintigraphy to detect coronary artery disease before abdominal aortic surgery. *J Vasc Surg* 1987;5:91–100.

208. Fletcher JP, Antico VF, Gruenewald S, et al. Dipyridamole-thallium scan for screening of coronary artery disease prior to vascular surgery. *J Cardiovasc Surg* 1988;29:666–669.

209. Sachs RN, Tellier P, Larmignat P, et al. Assessment by dipyridamole-thallium-201 myocardial scintigraphy of coronary risk before peripheral vascular surgery. *Surgery* 1988;103:584–587.

210. Mangano DT, London MJ, Tubau JF, et al. Dipyridamole thallium-201 scintigraphy as a preoperative screening test: a reexamination of its predictive potential. Study of Perioperative Ischemia Research Group. *Circulation* 1991;84:493–502.

211. Strawn DJ, Guernsey JM. Dipyridamole thallium scanning in the evaluation of coronary artery disease in elective abdominal aortic surgery. *Arch Surg* 1991;126:880–884.

212. Watters TA, Botvinick EH, Dae MW, et al. Comparison of the findings on preoperative dipyridamole perfusion scintigraphy and intraoperative transesophageal echocardiography: implications regarding the identification of myocardium at ischemic risk. *J Am Coll Cardiol* 1991;18:93–100.

213. Lette J, Waters D, Cerino M, et al. Preoperative coronary artery disease risk stratification based on dipyridamole imaging and a simple three-step, three-segment model for patients undergoing noncardiac vascular surgery or major general surgery. *Am J Cardiol* 1992;69:1553–1558.

214. Madsen PV, Vissing M, Munck O, et al. A comparison of dipyridamole thallium 201 scintigraphy and clinical examination in the determination of cardiac risk before arterial reconstruction. *Angiology* 1992;43:306–311.

215. Brown KA, Rowen M. Extent of jeopardized viable myocardium determined by myocardial perfusion imaging best predicts perioperative cardiac events in patients undergoing noncardiac surgery. *J Am Coll Cardiol* 1993;21:325–330.

216. Kresowik TF, Bower TR, Garner SA, et al. Dipyridamole thallium imaging in patients being considered for vascular procedures. *Arch Surg* 1993;128:299–302.

MEDICAL ECONOMICS IN CARDIOVASCULAR MEDICINE

DANIEL B. MARK

▼ ADDITIONAL ELECTRONIC TOPICS

Major Medical Cost Concepts h94;   Medical Cost: General Considerations h95;   Medical Cost: Terminology h96;   Medical Cost: Measurement h97;   Medical Cost: Methodology of Cost Studies h98;   Structural Framework h99;   Perspectives of Cost Analysis i01;   Resource Use and Cost Measurement i02;   Time Effects on Cost i03;   Generalizability i04;   Medical Cost: Cost Drivers i05;   Cost-Effectiveness Analysis i06;   Types of Analyses i07;   Standards for Economic Analysis i08;   Other Pharmacologic Agents i09;   Disease Management Approaches i10;   Cigarette Smoking i11;   Hypertension i12;   Physical Inactivity and Cardiac Rehabilitation i13;   Multiple Risk Factor Interventions i14

OVERVIEW

During the late 1960s and 1970s (an era that has been euphemistically termed the *open checkbook era* in health care), hospitals and doctors in the United States were paid essentially what they charged. Competition on price was nonexistent, but competition among hospitals to have the most modern, technologically up-to-date facilities was fierce. The resulting double-digit annual escalation in health care costs alarmed policy makers and private businesses and led to the first concerted efforts to control the growth of medical spending (1).

The failure of modest efforts at medical cost control during the 1970s and 1980s convinced many payers that the medical establishment would not voluntarily become fiscally accountable. In the late 1980s, the business and insurance communities began an aggressive bid for control of health care costs and increased accountability in medicine, catching the profession largely by surprise (2). Many physicians had assumed that the value of the U.S. health care system was self-evident and hence that their dominant role in it was assured. Others believed that pathophysiologic reasoning or personal experience and judg-

ment were sufficient to justify a course of action, regardless of the cost. Still others regarded any discussion of costs as demeaning to the profession. These attitudes largely became untenable when multiple outcome studies in the 1980s demonstrated that physicians practicing in different areas of the country made remarkably different management decisions for similar patients (3,4). Other studies from this period reported that doctors across the country performed significant numbers of unnecessary surgical procedures, particularly coronary bypass surgery. Together, variability of practice and appropriateness of care studies suggested the presence of substantial waste in the medical care system and demonstrated that physicians and hospitals by themselves had no incentives to develop a more standardized and efficient mode of practice.

Managed care can trace its origins back to the 1930s, but it first gained serious national attention during the 1970s as a method of controlling escalating health care costs. It was not until the late 1980s, with costs continuing to rise unabated and the medical establishment's prestige and credibility in tatters, that managed care began its exponential growth phase. Two major factors have driven this expansion: (a) the failure of health care reform efforts during the first term of the Clinton administration and (b) the demand by large employers for their employee health care costs to start

D. B. Mark: Department of Cardiology, Duke University Medical Center, Durham, North Carolina

shrinking rather than growing. For a brief period in the 1990s, managed care became the *de facto* national health care reform policy in the United States. However, because it is driven by market interests rather than carefully crafted policy, it does not address many key issues (such as access to care and funding of medical research and education). Furthermore, managed care will not be successful in the long-term control of medical spending. Between 1999 and 2006, medical costs in the United States are expected to double. The pressure from payers to resist these increases is therefore likely to intensify in the next 5 years. For clinicians to be partners in shaping the future of medicine during the critical period to come, they must understand the outcomes of medical care and its costs. The purpose of this chapter is to provide a general introduction to the key concepts of medical cost analysis and to review current knowledge about the economic consequences of cardiovascular diagnostic and therapeutic technologies.

ECONOMIC STUDIES OF CARDIOVASCULAR DISEASE

Acute Coronary Syndromes

General Considerations

Acute coronary syndromes (acute MI, unstable angina) share a common pathophysiology, similar clinical manifestations, a need for hospital-based management in the vast majority of cases, and a self-limited course that typically extends 30 to 60 days from presentation (47,48). After this period, most (surviving) patients cycle back to a stabler phase of coronary disease. The economic analysis of acute coronary syndromes and their treatments therefore is primarily focused on the events during the critical initial phase of presentation and care, particularly those that occur during the initial hospitalization.

Conceptually, the cost of hospitalization for an acute coronary syndrome can be divided into four major resource/cost components (Fig. 42.1). In patients who are eligible for reperfusion therapy, the reperfusion strategy selected (i.e., either thrombolytic therapy or direct coronary angioplasty) is a major cost component. Although streptokinase is relatively inexpensive (at approximately $300 per dose), t-PA, recombinant tissue plasminogen activator (rt-PA), and TNK all cost more than $2,000 per dose, and the procedural costs of direct PTCA are even higher. A second component is the routine hospital stay that is required for the patient with an uncomplicated course. For acute MI patients in the United States, this typically includes 1 or 2 days in the intensive care unit and 3 or 4 days more in a step-down or regular hospital floor setting. For unstable angina, the course is typically shorter. The primary cost components for this type of care are the hospital room costs and the associated ancillary care costs (such as laboratory testing, medications administered, consultations obtained, radiology testing performed, and so on). A third major component is the risk stratification strategy selected. For many patients in the United States with acute coronary syndromes, diagnostic coronary angiography is the principal mode of risk stratification. Use of coronary revascularization techniques has been shown to track the use of coronary angiography with a fair degree of predictability (49). The need for revascularization is a major predictor of higher hospital costs (50). For some patients, one of several noninvasive testing strategies can be used. These may eventually lead to coronary angiography and revascularization or may permit the patient to be discharged without such testing being performed.

The last category of cost components for patients with acute coronary syndrome is complications. These are of several different types and have varying cost implications. The reperfusion strategy selected, for example, can induce a variety of complications, including minor bleeding (which may have no discernible cost effects) and major bleeding (which may induce a significant extra cost). Coronary angiography in the anticoagulated patient may lead to a major groin hematoma or other vascular complications, which in turn require additional days of care, testing, and consultation. Thrombolytic and anticoagulant drugs may

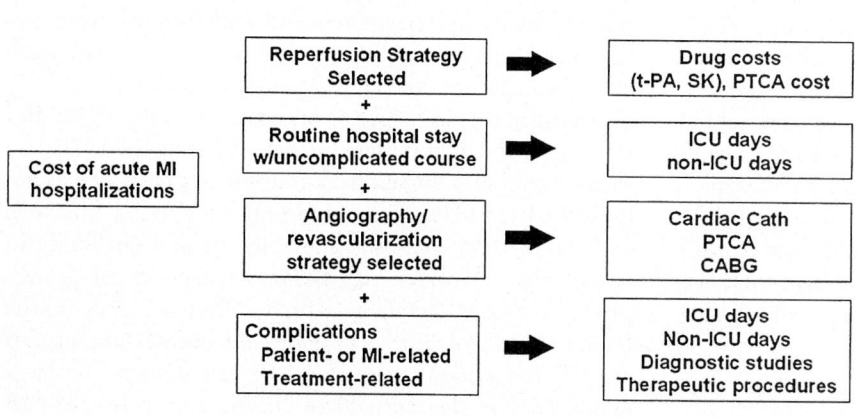

FIGURE 42.1 Cost components for an acute coronary syndrome hospitalization. CABG, coronary artery bypass graft surgery; ICU, intensive care unit; MI, myocardial infarction; PTCA, percutaneous transluminal coronary angioplasty; SK, streptokinase; t-PA, tissue plasminogen activator.

induce gastrointestinal bleeding, sometimes because of previously undiagnosed gastrointestinal comorbidity. The acute coronary syndrome itself may produce complications (e.g., heart failure, arrhythmias, and recurrent ischemia). Costs related to complications can be substantial and are difficult to predict.

Thrombolytic Therapy

The benefits of thrombolytic therapy in acute MI are firmly established (51). Of the approximately 16 studies that have been published on the cost effectiveness of thrombolytic therapy, most are now of historical interest because of their age or because of changes in the standard of practice, or both (52). Four thrombolytic strategy comparisons are of current relevance: streptokinase versus no reperfusion therapy, t-PA versus streptokinase, t-PA versus rt-PA or TNK, and rt-PA versus rt-PA with abciximab. As of 2001, the U.S. market share for streptokinase was only approximately 4%, that for t-PA was approximately 44%, and rt-PA and TNK were equivalent at approximately 25% each. Outside of the United States, streptokinase remains the most widely used thrombolytic agent (53). ▼ i15

GUSTO I clearly established that t-PA was superior to intravenous streptokinase in establishing Thrombolysis in Myocardial Infarction flow grade 3 (TIMI-3) coronary flow and in saving lives (56). Because the cost of t-PA is substantially higher than that of streptokinase, the question that directly emerged from the clinical results of GUSTO I was whether the added benefits of accelerated t-PA were sufficient to justify the added costs of this regimen. It is important to note that from a patient perspective (assuming that the patient does not bear the added cost of t-PA), the choice of thrombolytic regimen virtually always favors t-PA on medical grounds alone (i.e., additional survivors minus additional disabling strokes). On the other hand, from the fee-for-service hospital perspective, t-PA is usually a losing financial proposition, because the added costs of the therapy are often not reflected in the reimbursement received. The one added survivor per 100 generated by t-PA is a statistical survivor, and the individual patient who is actually "lost" when streptokinase is used in lieu of t-PA cannot be identified clinically and is therefore invisible to the hospital. Furthermore, most of the added life-years generated by t-PA, as is discussed below, occur after patients are discharged from the hospital.

In a detailed prospective economic analysis, the GUSTO I trial estimated that cumulative medical costs (hospital costs plus physician fees) at 1 year averaged $24,575 for streptokinase patients and $24,990 for t-PA patients exclusive of the costs of the thrombolytic agent (22). When the average wholesale drug costs for the two agents were added in, the incremental lifetime (undiscounted) costs for each patient who received t-PA was $2,845. Using the empiric 1-year GUSTO survival data,

additional data from the Duke Cardiovascular Database, and statistical modeling, we projected a life expectancy for t-PA patients of 15.41 years versus 15.27 for the streptokinase patients, an undiscounted increase in life expectancy for t-PA of 0.14 years per patient. This result can be more intuitively restated as follows: The one extra patient per 100 saved with accelerated t-PA lives an average of 14 additional years.

With an increased life expectancy of 0.14 years of life per patient for t-PA patients and an increased cost of $2,845 per patient, the incremental cost-effectiveness ratio for t-PA (discounted at 5%) was $32,678 per year of life saved (22). Because the average thrombolytic drug cost to hospitals is lower than the average wholesale prices for the two drugs, we substituted a cost of $270 for the streptokinase and $2,216 for the 100 mg t-PA and repeated the calculations. These lower drug costs yielded a cost-effectiveness ratio of $27,115 per year of life saved (22).

The GUSTO III trial compared rt-PA with t-PA and found no difference in major cardiovascular events (including death, stroke, and bleeding) out to 1 year (57). The costs of these two agents are the same, and although the nursing time and ancillary costs associated with a double-bolus regimen are likely smaller than with a bolus and 90-minute infusion, inefficiencies in the care process would likely eliminate these small theoretical savings.

TNK-tPA was compared with rt-PA in 16,999 patients in the Assessment of the Safety and Efficacy of a New Thrombolytic Regimen (ASSENT) 2 Study (58). Mortality was identical in the two arms as was intracranial hemorrhage. Bleeding complications and need for blood transfusion were modestly reduced by TNK. The cost of TNK is the same as that of t-PA, and the single-bolus administration regimen is attractive to a busy emergency department, if not cost saving. A formal economic analysis of ASSENT 2 has not been performed.

The GUSTO V trial compared rt-PA with half-dose rt-PA plus full-dose abciximab in 16,588 patients (59). The combination regimen reduced nonfatal reinfarction but did not alter 30-day mortality. The rt-PA plus abciximab regimen also reduced urgent revascularization but increased bleeding, although strokes and intracranial hemorrhage rates were equivalent. A cost analysis of this trial is currently under way.

Primary Percutaneous Coronary Reperfusion

A quantitative overview of all the randomized trials conducted through 1996 showed that there was a strong possibility that direct angioplasty was superior to thrombolytic therapy in saving lives (60). Furthermore, comparison of hospital charges in the Primary Angioplasty in Myocardial Infarction I (PAMI I) study and estimated hospital costs in the Mayo Clinic Randomized Trial both suggested that direct angioplasty might also be a less expensive reperfusion strategy (61–63). However, of the ten trials included in the overview, nine were quite small. The largest, by far, was GUSTO II.

Although the small randomized trials had established that dedicated experienced operators could achieve excellent results with primary angioplasty, the GUSTO II study was meant to evaluate whether the technique was practically suited for larger-scale implementation in the cardiovascular community. GUSTO II compared accelerated t-PA and primary angioplasty. A total of 1,138 patients were enrolled (1994–1995) in the trial from 57 hospitals in nine countries (64). The 30-day results of this trial showed a statistically significant 33% reduction in the primary outcome event (the combination of death, nonfatal MI, and disabling stroke) for primary angioplasty. However, at the end of 6 months of follow-up, the 30-day benefit had attenuated by approximately 50%, and the intention-to-treat comparison was no longer statistically significant. The small differences observed in mortality and nonfatal MI, both favoring direct angioplasty, were not statistically significant. However, the study was not powered to detect such differences.

The principal resource use data from the U.S. portion of the trial showed the expected extra procedures in the direct angioplasty group (65). Importantly, the rate of diagnostic angiography was approximately 70% in the accelerated t-PA group. This is consistent with the rates observed in GUSTO I and reflects the predominant choice among U.S. GUSTO investigators in the use of angiography as a primary risk stratification tool after MI. At the end of the initial hospitalization, direct angioplasty showed a $900 cost advantage in the use of hospital resources, whereas accelerated t-PA had a $600 cost advantage in the use of physician resources, leaving a net cost advantage for direct angioplasty of approximately $300 (*p* >.05) (65). At the end of the 6-month follow-up period, the net cost advantage of direct angioplasty had fallen to approximately $100.

One of the main limitations of the direct angioplasty reperfusion strategy is that only approximately 20% of U.S. hospitals have catheterization facilities, and many of these are not staffed 24 hours a day (66). Building new interventional catheterization laboratories, training new personnel to staff them, and providing 24-hour coverage would substantially increase the long-term per-case cost of the procedure over that calculated in the GUSTO II analysis (67).

The Myocardial Infarction Triage Intervention registry performed an observational comparison of 1,050 patients who received direct angioplasty with 2,095 patients who received thrombolytic therapy (65% t-PA, 32% streptokinase, 3% other) (68). This community-based study found no mortality benefit for angioplasty, but, in contrast to the GUSTO II economic analysis, it found that the thrombolytic group had 13% lower costs at 3 years.

More recently, the percutaneous approach to acute MI patients has been modified to include stenting and the use

of glycoprotein (GP) IIb/IIIa inhibitors. Stenting versus PTCA has been compared in six randomized trials, five of which were quite small (see Chapter 18). The largest, STENT PAMI, randomized 900 patients to stent over balloon PTCA (69). Only approximately 5% of patients received a GP IIb/IIIa inhibitor. At 1 month, the stent group had a nonsignificant increase in mortality and a nonsignificant decrease in reinfarction. The major difference in outcome was a lower rate of target vessel repeat revascularization seen in the stent arm (10 per 100 fewer at 6 months). Cohen and colleagues (70) performed an economic analysis of STENT PAMI. The index hospital costs in the stent arm were approximately $2,000 higher, due primarily to the extra costs of the stents used. The decreased need for follow-up procedures saved approximately half that amount over the first year of follow-up. In addition, the avoidance of recurrent angina and repeat procedures was associated with a small utility benefit for the stent patients. Thus, with a net cost of approximately $1,000 per patient and a utility advantage of 0.02, the cost per QALY added with stenting was $65,000 using the technology available during the trial. With the current repertoire of longer stents that allow a reduction in the total number of stents placed, the equipment cost of the stent arm in STENT PAMI would have been lower and the cost per QALY would have been less than $30,000, using the assumptions of the investigators.

The benefits of adding abciximab to primary PTCA were evaluated in 483 MI patients enrolled in the ReoPro and Primary PTCA Organization and Randomized Trial (71). No significant benefit was seen for the addition of abciximab to PTCA on death or reinfarction out to 6 months. Urgent target vessel repeat revascularization was significantly reduced, but any target vessel revascularization was not. In addition, major bleeding and the need for transfusion were increased by abciximab.

The benefits of adding abciximab to primary stenting in acute MI were tested in the Controlled Abciximab and Device Investigation to Lower Late Angioplasty Complications (CADILLAC) trial. This trial enrolled 2,665 acute MI patients who were within 12 hours of symptom onset and who were deemed eligible for stenting. Randomization used a factorial design: balloon PTCA versus stent and abciximab versus no abciximab. In contrast to STENT PAMI, this trial showed a nonsignificant mortality benefit for stenting over PTCA. The addition of abciximab reduced ischemia and ischemia-driven target revascularization for stent and for PTCA patients. The Abciximab before Direct Angioplasty and Stenting in Myocardial Infarction Regarding Acute and Long-term Follow-up (ADMIRAL) trial randomized 300 acute MI patients who were undergoing acute coronary intervention with stenting to abciximab or placebo (72). At 30 days, the abciximab arm had a 49% lower mortality, a 49% lower incidence of reinfarction, and a 58% reduction in target vessel revascularization. Major bleeding was not increased by abciximab, although minor bleeding was. At 6 months, the abciximab arm had a 5.4% absolute decrease in the need for revascularization.

Neither CADILLAC nor ADMIRAL has yet reported economic data (73). Given that bolus plus 12-hour infusion therapy with abciximab adds approximately $1,400 to the cost of care, examination of resource use patterns and associated costs will be an important aspect of final interpretation of these data. At present, it appears that percutaneous revascularization is a clinically acceptable but less available and more expensive alternative to thrombolytic therapy.

Coronary Angiography and Predischarge Risk Stratification

Several randomized trials have now compared different forms of invasive and conservative management strategies for patients with acute coronary syndromes. The TIMI IIIB trial compared these two strategies in 1,473 patients (74). Early invasive management involved routine angiography at 18 to 48 hours after presentation. Early conservative management used angiography only if certain high-risk indicators were present. At 6 weeks, the two strategies had identical rates of death and MI. Hospital stay was shortened for the invasive arm, and rehospitalization for recurrent unstable angina was also reduced in this arm. Veterans Affairs Non–Q-Wave Infarction Strategies in Hospital (VANQWISH), in contrast, found that early conservative management in 920 patients with non–Q-wave MI was associated with lower mortality at hospital discharge and at 12 months (75). In the conservative arm of TIMI IIIB and of VANQWISH, catheterization was used in approximately half of the assigned patients. In contrast, in Fragmin and Fast Revascularization during Instability in Coronary Artery Disease (FRISC) II, only 10% of patients from the conservative arm received catheterization (76). If such an extreme conservative strategy is the comparator, invasive therapy has clearly demonstrable benefits in patients with acute coronary syndrome. What is less clear is whether a policy that uses angiography approximately half the time is inferior to one that uses it almost all the time. The most recent clinical trial to address this issue is the TACTICS-TIMI 18 study (77). At 6 months, death was equivalent in the two arms and there was an approximately 2 per 100 reduction in the rate of MI in the invasive arm. A cost analysis of this trial found that the invasive arm was modestly more expensive during the index hospitalization ($14,660 vs. $12,667) but less expensive during the first 6 months of follow-up ($6,063 vs. $7,203) (78). Thus, cumulative costs at 6 months were equivalent. ▼ i16

Antithrombin Therapy

Small randomized trials of heparin versus no heparin in patients with unstable angina or non–Q-wave MI have shown a reduction in short-term death and nonfatal MI. Consequently, heparin has been adopted as a standard of care for these patients in the early phase of their presentation (47).

Recent work has centered on identifying more potent antithrombin agents that would improve on the results obtained with heparin. The most promising new antithrombin at present is bivalirudin. Kong and colleagues (81) performed a metaanalysis of six trials that compared this agent with standard heparin therapy in elective percutaneous revascularization (4,603 patients) and in acute coronary syndrome (1,071 patients). Overall, at 30 days, bivalirudin reduced the risk of death or MI by 27% (p = .02). In addition, bivalirudin was associated with a 59% decrease in major bleeding. These data suggest at least equivalent effectiveness with heparin and better safety. Two ongoing large phase III trials are testing bivalirudin in percutaneous coronary revascularization and acute coronary syndromes, respectively. Both trials are including prospective economic analyses.

Several studies have been conducted using low-molecular-weight heparins in patients with acute coronary syndromes. The first such study, FRISC, reported a benefit for dalteparin but had some important design limitations that made it difficult to interpret the study for current cardiovascular practice. In the FRISC II trial, patients with acute coronary syndrome were randomized to dalteparin plus aspirin versus aspirin alone for approximately 1 month (82). At 6 days, the dalteparin arm had a significant reduction in death or MI, but these differences did not persist at the 6-month follow-up.

A second agent, enoxaparin, has been compared with unfractionated heparin in more than 7,000 patients in the Efficacy and Safety of Subcutaneous Enoxaparin in Non-Q-Wave Coronary Events (ESSENCE) (3,171 patients) and TIMI IIB (3,910 patients) trials. Metaanalysis of these two trials showed a 23% reduction in death or MI at 8 days that persisted at 6 weeks (83). In the ESSENCE trial, these benefits lasted out to 1 year. The economic analysis of ESSENCE showed that the low-molecular-weight heparin strategy was associated with a drug cost of $155 per patient (2.5 days of therapy) in the United States. After taking this cost into account, the enoxaparin strategy was associated with a cost savings of $760 to $1,170 per patient shifted from standard unfractionated heparin therapy because of a reduction in use of invasive procedures and length of stay (84).

Antiplatelet Therapy

As reviewed elsewhere in this text, a number of new compounds have been developed that block the platelet GP IIb/IIIa receptor, thereby providing potent inhibition of platelet aggregation. Three compounds have been approved for clinical use in the United States: abciximab (in patients undergoing or planned for percutaneous revascularization), eptifibatide, and tirofiban. The GUSTO IV trial surprisingly failed to show a benefit of abciximab therapy in patients with non–ST-elevation acute coronary syndrome (85). Tirofiban has been tested in two trials, Platelet Receptor Inhibition in Ischemic Syndrome Management (PRISM) and Platelet Receptor Inhibition in Ischemic Syndrome Management in Patients Limited by Unstable Signs and Symptoms (PRISM-PLUS).

The PRISM trial tested tirofiban without heparin and found a significant mortality reduction but no effect on MI or refractory ischemia at 30 days (86). However, the same tirofiban plus aspirin with no heparin regimen had the highest mortality in PRISM-PLUS, and this arm was stopped prematurely (87). Thus, many believe that the mortality benefit in PRISM was not a real finding. With no mortality benefit and also no effect on MI, there is little effectiveness in PRISM to use as the basis for a cost-effectiveness analysis.

In PRISM-PLUS, investigators were "encouraged" to refer patients to coronary angiography between 48 and 96 hours after enrollment, and 90% of patients underwent catheterization. This protocol-guided care represented a substantial shift from usual practice for most of the participating sites and creates difficulties in assessing the economic impact of the tirofiban plus heparin regimen. To date, no formal cost-effectiveness analysis of the entire PRISM-PLUS trial has been performed. Based on the 1.8% absolute reduction in mortality and 2.9% absolute reduction in MI at 6 months for the tirofiban plus heparin arm and a mean infusion duration of 71 hours (total cost of tirofiban infusion is approximately $1,000 to $1,100), it is likely that a formal cost-effectiveness analysis would find this therapy to be economically attractive.

The Platelet Glycoprotein IIb/IIIa in Unstable Angina: Receptor Suppression Using Integrilin Therapy (PURSUIT), with 10,948 patients, is the largest trial of an intravenous GP IIb/IIIa inhibitor in patients with non–ST-segment elevation acute coronary syndrome. At 30 days, the eptifibatide arm had a 1.5% absolute reduction in death or MI compared with placebo ($p = .04$) (88). A detailed prospective economic substudy in the 3,522 U.S. patients enrolled in PURSUIT showed two major findings (89). First, with a diagnostic catheterization rate of 85% as background, the addition of eptifibatide did not alter the use of invasive cardiac procedures or hospital length of stay. Second, with a cost for the eptifibatide regimen ranging from $1,217 (average wholesale price) to $1,014 (hospital discounted price) and an incremental increase in life expectancy of 0.11 years attributable to eptifibatide therapy in U.S. patients, the cost per year of life added was between $13,700 and $16,500. This fulfills criteria cited earlier for an economically attractive therapy.

Coronary Revascularization

In the United States, it is estimated that approximately 1.3 million diagnostic cardiac catheterizations, approximately 553,000 coronary artery bypass surgeries, and 926,000 percutaneous interventional procedures (on 528,000 patients) are performed annually (based on 1998 figures) (90). ⚡ i17

Percutaneous Coronary Revascularization

In the Evaluation of PTCA to Improve Long-Term Outcome by c7E3 GPIIb/IIIa Receptor Blockade (EPILOG) multicenter randomized trial, which involved 2,792 patients undergoing nonemergent balloon PTCA in 1995 and 1996, mean length of stay was 3.3 days; mean hospital costs were $7,600 with physician fees (from the Medicare Fee Schedule) of $1,400, yielding a total initial medical cost of $9,000 (97). Costs for follow-up hospitalizations and procedures to 6 months were $3,400, so that cumulative 6-month medical costs totaled $12,400. As noted earlier, PTCA costs can be systematically examined by separating them into four categories (Table 42.1). Patient characteristics can alter the costs of coronary angioplasty through their effects on the complexity of the procedure, the likelihood of success, and the rate of complications, early (e.g., abrupt closure) and late (e.g., restenosis). Patients with American College of Cardiology/American Heart Association type B2 or C lesions, for example, tend to have higher procedure-related costs because the procedure is less often successful, and, even when it is initially successful, the results are less often durable (98). In the Duke database, costs for angioplasty were lowest for one-vessel disease, intermediate for two-vessel disease, and highest for three-vessel disease (99). The Bypass Angioplasty Revascularization Investigation (BARI) study confirmed these findings and also reported that costs associated with an angioplasty strategy in diabetic patients were substantially higher than those for nondiabetics ($9,500 more for diabetics with 2-vessel disease vs. nondiabetics, more than $40,000 more for 3-vessel disease after 5 years of follow-up) (100). In a consecutive series of 1,258 patients who underwent percutaneous revascularization at The Cleveland Clinic between November 1992 and June 1993, the strongest clinical predictors of increased cost were admission for acute MI (91% increase), recent MI (17% increase), more complex lesion morphology based on the American College of Cardiology/American Heart Association classification (≥12% increase), diabetes (12% increase), and the number of diseased vessels (9% increase per vessel) (101).

In a private insurance claims database, Topol and coworkers (102) found that hospital charges for PTCA were higher in older patients, in women, and in individuals with a history of prior MI. In summary, the most consistent patient-related predictors of higher initial hospital costs for percutaneous coronary intervention (PCI) are acuity of presentation, complexity of treated lesions, presence of diabetes, more extensive coronary disease, and older age. Some of these predictors, in turn (e.g., age, diabetes), may

TABLE 42.1 MAJOR CATEGORIES OF MEDICAL COST DRIVERS

Patient-related factors
  Age
  Sex
  Cardiac disease severity (e.g., ejection fraction, extent of coronary artery disease)
  Cardiac comorbidity (cardiac disease other than the principal condition under study)
  Noncardiac comorbidity
Treatment-related factors
  Aggressive versus conservative management
  Complications
Provider-related factors
  Quality of care
  Efficiency of care
  Preferred management styles
Geographic/economic factors
  Labor costs
  Supply costs

be surrogates for unmeasured aspects of disease severity or lesion complexity.

Treatment-related factors can also have a large effect on PCI costs. Ellis and colleagues (101) found that decision delay (delay between admission and diagnostic angiography or between diagnostic angiography and revascularization) was associated with an 86% increase in hospital costs and that weekend delay (postponed procedure due to a weekend) was related to a 61% increase. In a separate analysis, combined angiography and PTCA increased hospital costs by $850 versus separate procedures (98). Reeder and coworkers at the Mayo Clinic found that failed PTCA more than doubled hospital charges (due primarily to referral for CABG) relative to initially successful procedures (103,104). Use of adjunctive procedures and pharmacologic agents has a substantial influence on the cost picture of PTCA. In The Cleveland Clinic study, urgent CABG increased costs 83% and intraaortic balloon pump use increased costs by 42% (101). Costs were also increased with the use of transluminal extraction catheter atherectomy (40% increase), Rotablator (25% increase), stents (25% increase), perfusion balloons (12% increase), directional coronary angioplasty (10% increase), and laser (7% increase). In the EPILOG randomized trial, use of abciximab (with low-dose heparin) increased index hospital costs by a net of approximately $600 (97). Average cost for the drug itself was approximately $1,450 per patient, and reduced complications offset some, but not all, of that initial cost. In the Evaluation of Platelet IIb/IIIa Inhibitor for Stenting Trial (EPISTENT), the cost of stenting added approximately $2,200 to the hospital costs (not counting professional fees), and stenting with abciximab added $3,600 (105). Thus, the main procedural determinants of PCI costs are related primarily to extra therapies that are used to prevent or treat complications.

With regard to provider-related factors, care at a teaching hospital was associated with lower charges for PCI in one study (102). The physician who performed the procedure was a major cost driver in 250 consecutive patients treated at the University of California at San Francisco, with a $4,400 cost increase from lowest-cost to highest-cost physician (98). This difference appeared to reflect a behavioral pattern by the more expensive operators of using more catheterization laboratory resources. No differences were found with lower-cost operators in patient characteristics, lesion characteristics, success rate, or complications. Shook and colleagues (106) found that high-volume operators (≥50 cases/year) averaged slightly lower hospital costs compared with low-volume operators ($7,977 vs. $8,278, $p = .07$) despite greater complexity and risk of procedures done by the high-volume operators. Geographic factors have also been identified as an important source of cost variability, with the western region of the United States having the highest charges and the Midwest having the lowest for balloon PTCA (102).

Coronary Artery Bypass Graft Surgery

The costs of CABG surgery have been studied for approximately two decades. During this time, the technical aspects of the procedure as well the postprocedure care and the long-term outcomes have changed substantially. Therefore, only the more recent literature is of relevance to current practice. The most recent national cost figures for bypass surgery come from an analysis by Cowper and coworkers (107) at Duke Medical Center of the 1990 Medicare database. At that time, the average hospital costs for an admission for bypass surgery were $23,000. With an additional $10,000 in physician fees (i.e., charges), the total cost of an isolated bypass surgery was approximately $30,000. In 2001 figures, this equates to a cost of approximately $41,000. The distribution of costs for the initial hospitalization included 37% for intensive care unit and regular care rooms, 21% for operating room, and 42% for laboratory/supply/pharmacy and other departments.

A number of studies have evaluated the determinants of the cost of CABG. Patient characteristics typically account for no more than 25% of the total variance in hospital costs for this procedure. In an analysis of 604 patients treated at Duke, factors identified as predictive of higher costs included older age ($p < .0001$), female gender ($p < .005$), black race ($p < .19$), lower ejection fraction ($p < .0001$), prior bypass surgery ($p < .0001$), more extensive coronary disease ($p < .01$), prior CABG ($p < .0001$), and diabetes ($p < .03$) (108). In 807 patients treated at Emory University, patient predictors of higher cost included higher angina class ($p = .02$), previous MI ($p = .03$), older age ($p = .0001$), heart failure ($p = .001$), and a higher number of diseased vessels ($p = .0001$) (109). Diabetes was a marginally significant predictor of higher costs ($p = .07$). However, in the BARI study, diabetic patients who underwent CABG had 5-year costs that were $15,000 higher than those of their nondiabetic counterparts (100). In contrast, there was no difference in cost between patients with two- and three-vessel disease who were undergoing CABG in BARI.

Two procedural factors have been associated with higher CABG costs: need for additional invasive procedures, such as valvular surgery or coronary angiography, and use of internal mammary artery grafts (107). Perioperative complications are a major source of increased hospital costs for CABG. Complications identified as important cost drivers in the Emory study included adult respiratory distress syndrome, pneumonia, septicemia, major arrhythmias, neurologic events, and bleeding that required reexploration (109). Patients with no complications had a mean hospital cost of $16,776 (1990 dollars). Patients with one of the above complications had hospital costs of $17,794, patients with three complications had costs of $23,624, and patients with five complications had costs of $50,609.

Analysis of the national Medicare data has indicated that hospital-level provider-related factors account for approximately 17% of the total variation in bypass surgery costs, independent of patient-level factors (107). Analysis of determinants of CABG costs at Duke Medical Center showed that the attending surgeon was the single most important determinant of cost (108). Median hospital cost for the most expensive surgeon was $15,000, whereas the corresponding figure for the least expensive surgeon was $10,800.

As with coronary angioplasty, the costs for coronary bypass surgery are a moving target. Nationally, length of stay for this procedure has decreased substantially over the last decade, in part because of the pressures of managed care. Progress with minimally invasive coronary artery bypass surgery (MICAB) has raised the possibility of further reductions in cost (110). Investigators from Johns Hopkins University reported length-of-stay and cost figures for MICAB that are comparable to those of percutaneous interventional procedures ($7,803 for PTCA, $13,415 for stent, $11,623 for MICAB) (111). However, the technology is still in its developmental phase, and its true role in the panoply of revascularization options will likely not be defined for at least several more years.

Two trials have compared medical therapy with percutaneous revascularization. The Angioplasty Compared to Medical Therapy (ACME) trial found a very modest improvement among 212 patients with single-vessel disease in exercise treadmill time and physical functioning in the PTCA arm (112). A preliminary economic analysis of ACME was conducted but has not yet been published. The second Randomized Intervention Treatment of Angina (RITA-2) trial found that PTCA improved angina and exercise test performance but had a slight excess of procedure-related MIs. Quality of life was significantly better for the PTCA arm at 1 year, but these benefits attenuated by 3

years (113). At least part of this attenuation appears due to late revascularization procedures in the medical arm. An economic analysis of RITA-2 has not yet been published.

The Asymptomatic Ischemia Pilot randomized 558 patients with clinically stable coronary disease and documented ischemia to one of three treatment strategies: angina-guided medical care, ischemia-guided medical care, and revascularization. The ischemia-guided therapy was adjusted on the basis of repeated ambulatory monitoring studies. The principal medical regimens used in this pilot study were either atenolol-nifedipine or diltiazem-isosorbide. Patients who were randomized to revascularization received either PTCA or CABG at the discretion of the principal investigator. Although an economic analysis was not initially planned for this study, we performed a *post hoc* analysis using the available resource use data along with cost estimates taken from the GUSTO I analysis (114). At the end of 3 months, the average costs for the revascularization patients were $13,400, compared with $1,500 for the angina-guided patients and $900 for the ischemia-guided patients. However, between 3 months and 2 years, the costs for the medical arms significantly exceeded those for the revascularization arm, primarily because of an increased need for revascularization procedures and rehospitalizations. At the end of 2 years, the cumulative costs for the angina-guided strategy were $7,735, those for the ischemia-guided strategy were $8,575, and those for the revascularization strategy were $16,782. No empiric data were collected past 2 years in the Asymptomatic Ischemia Pilot. However, taking the second-year costs as the best estimate of annual costs for each treatment arm, a simple linear extrapolation (discounting future costs at a 3% rate) suggested that at 10 years the medical arms would have cumulative costs of approximately $23,500 and the revascularization arm would average $25,300. However, good empiric data on resource use patterns after 5 years in a modern cohort of CAD patients does not exist.

Two randomized trials have compared the costs of coronary angioplasty and coronary bypass surgery in patients with multivessel coronary disease in the United States. The clinical outcomes from these trials are reviewed in Chapter 16. The Emory Angioplasty Surgery Trial (EAST) enrolled 392 patients between 1987 and 1990 (115). Patients were followed every 6 months for 3 years. Hospital costs were estimated from hospital bills, with charges converted to costs using department-level cost-charge ratios (116). Physician fees for care at Emory were obtained from physician bills (i.e., charges). Hospital cost data were not collected for outside (i.e., non-Emory) hospitalization. Instead, Emory costs were applied to the follow-up hospitalizations reported on follow-up contacts. Costs were all deflated to 1987 dollars. For the initial hospitalization, hospital costs were $11,684 (median, $10,290) for PTCA and $14,579 (median, $13,991) for CABG ($p <.0001$) (116). With physician fees added in, total initial costs were $16,223 for

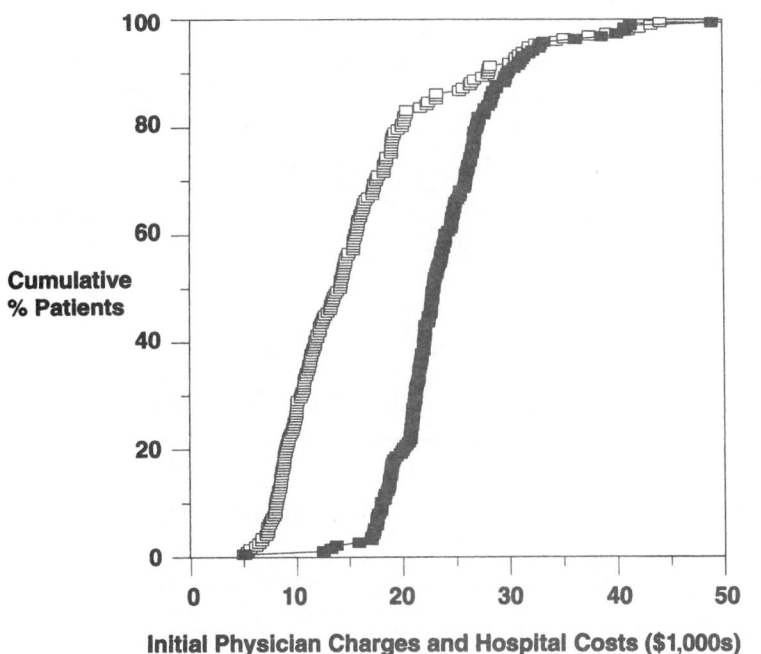

FIGURE 42.2 Cumulative distribution plot of total initial costs (hospital and physician) by treatment group in the Emory Angioplasty versus Surgery Trial. CABG, coronary artery bypass graft surgery; PTCA, percutaneous transluminal coronary angioplasty. [From Weintraub WS, Mauldin PD, Becker E, et al. A comparison of the costs of and quality of life after coronary angioplasty or coronary surgery for multivessel coronary disease: results from the Emory Angioplasty versus Surgery Trial (EAST). *Circulation* 1995;92:2831–2840, with permission.]

PTCA and $24,005 for CABG (*p* <.0001) (Fig. 42.2). At the end of 3 years, cumulative costs for the PTCA arm were $23,734 versus $25,310 for CABG (*p* <.0001) (Fig. 42.3). Thus, PTCA costs initially constituted 68% of CABG costs but after 3 years had risen to 94% of these costs (116). In multiple regression analysis, the major correlates of initial medical costs were randomization to CABG, heart failure, and male gender (Table 42.2). Regression analysis of 3-year costs identified ejection fraction, hypertension, and male gender as the major cost correlates. Assignment to CABG

was no longer an independent predictor. Between 3 and 8 years, the CABG patients had $2,700 of extra medical costs versus $4,700 for the PTCA arm. With 8 years of follow-up, total costs were $46,348 for the CABG arm and $44,491 for the PTCA arm (*p* = .37) (117).

BARI enrolled 1,829 patients with multivessel CAD between 1988 and 1991 in 18 centers (118). The BARI Substudy of Economics and Quality of Life was conducted in 7 of the 18 enrolling sites and collected cost data on 934 of the 1,829 total patients randomized in the trial (100).

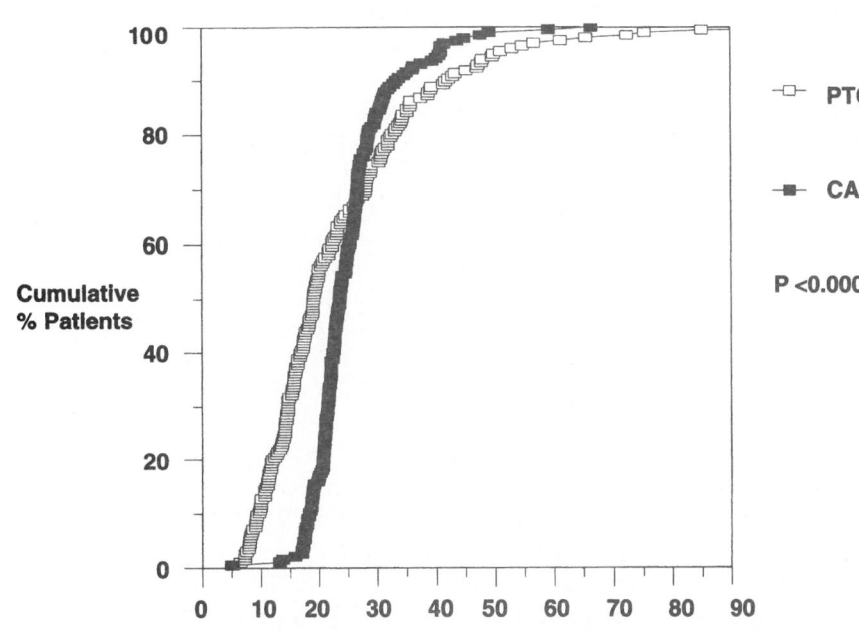

FIGURE 42.3 Cumulative distribution plot of 3 years of costs by treatment group in the Emory Angioplasty versus Surgery Trial. CABG, coronary artery bypass graft surgery; PTCA, percutaneous transluminal coronary angioplasty. [From Weintraub WS, Mauldin PD, Becker E, et al. A comparison of the costs of and quality of life after coronary angioplasty or coronary surgery for multivessel coronary disease: results from the Emory Angioplasty versus Surgery Trial (EAST). *Circulation* 1995;92:2831–2840, with permission.]

TABLE 42.2 MAJOR COST CORRELATES IN EMORY ANGIOPLASTY SURGERY TRIAL

Variable	Cost	*p*
Correlates of initial hospital and physician costs		
Surgical group	$7,725	<.01
Heart failure	$6,766	.01
Older age (per yr)	$122	.01
Male	$2,777	.01
Hypertension	$1,934	.04
Angina class	$622	.08
Correlates of 3-yr cumulative costs[a]		
Ejection fraction (per %)	–$115	.01
Hypertension	$3,289	.01
Male	$3,465	.02
Angina class	$834	.08

[a]Surgical group no longer significant independent correlate.
From Weintraub WS, Mauldin PD, Becker E, et al. A comparison of the costs of and quality of life after coronary angioplasty or coronary surgery for multivessel coronary disease: results from the Emory Angioplasty versus Surgery Trial (EAST). *Circulation* 1995;92:2831–2840, with permission.

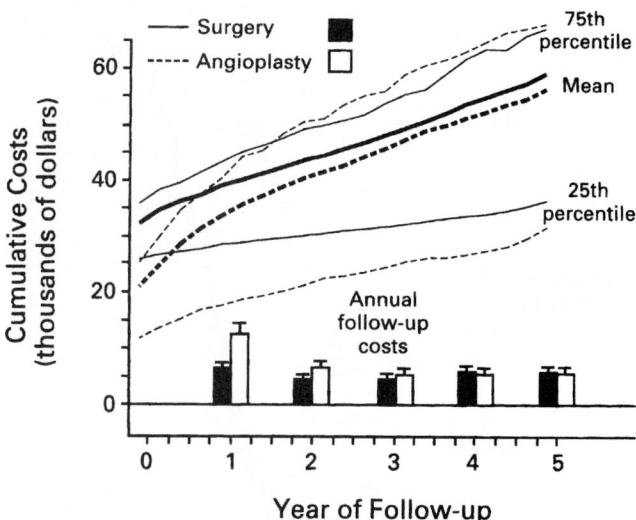

FIGURE 42.4 Cumulative cost at quarterly intervals for patients in Bypass Angioplasty Revascularization Investigation Substudy of Economics and Quality of Life. The thick lines indicate mean cumulative costs. The lighter lines represent twenty-fifth and seventy-fifth percentiles of the cumulative costs. The bars at the bottom show the mean (±2 standard error) follow-up costs accrued over the prior year. (From Hlatky MA, Rogers WJ, Johnstone I, et al. Medical care costs and quality of life after randomization to coronary angioplasty or coronary bypass surgery. *N Engl J Med* 1997;336:92–99, with permission.)

Detailed cost data were collected on all hospitalizations (regardless of diagnosis) as well as outpatient visits to ten different types of health care providers and outpatient cardiac tests and procedures. Medication use was also collected in this trial. Initial length of stay was 9 days for the PTCA arm and 13.3 days for the CABG arm. Hospital costs were $14,415 versus $21,534, and physician fees were $6,698 versus $10,813 (100) (Fig. 42.4). In follow-up, PTCA patients averaged 3.1 readmissions versus 2.7 for CABG patients. Total inpatient follow-up costs (hospital plus physician) were $27,439 for PTCA and $19,529 for CABG. Number of outpatient visits was equivalent for the two therapies, as were outpatient costs ($1,656 vs. $1,617). The PTCA patients took an average of 4.1 cardiac medicines at a cumulative 5-year cost of $4,948. The CABG patients averaged 4.0 cardiac medicines at a cost of $3,670. Outpatient diagnostic testing was equivalent in the two treatments, but CABG patients had a slightly higher rate of nursing home admission (3.2% vs. 2.6%) with higher associated costs ($1,027 vs. $265). After 5 years of follow-up, total discounted costs in the CABG arm were 5% greater than those for PTCA ($58,889 vs. $56,225) (Fig. 42.4). In subgroup analyses, patients with two-vessel disease had significantly lower costs with angioplasty ($52,390 vs. $58,498 for CABG), whereas angioplasty costs were actually higher than those of bypass surgery in patients with three-vessel disease ($60,918 vs. $59,430).

Cost analysis of the British Randomized Intervention Treatment of Angina trial of 1,011 patients confirmed the findings of EAST and BARI (119). The initial costs (estimated in British pounds) of treating with PTCA were approximately 52% those of CABG, but at the end of 2 years PTCA costs were 80% those of CABG. Follow-up in this trial out to 10 years is planned.

Coronary Stents

Coronary artery stents have undergone an exponential increase in usage since 1994. Data from 18 high-volume interventional programs participating in the National Cardiovascular Network showed that 6% of interventional cases at these institutions involved stents in 1994; by 1996, that proportion had risen to 39%, and current usage averages more than 70% (120).

To date, five randomized trials have compared a strategy of primary stenting versus conventional balloon PTCA (with stent backup if necessary) in stable patients with lesions of 20 mm or less in large target vessels (≥3.0 mm): the Stent Restenosis Study I (STRESS I), Belgian Netherlands Stent Study (BENESTENT) I, BENESTENT II, the Optimum Percutaneous Transluminal Coronary Angioplasty Compared with Routine Stent Strategy (OPUS) trial, and the Doppler Endpoint Stenting International Investigation (121–125). The clinical data from these trials are reviewed in Chapter 80. Most important, these trials did not show any significant differences between initial stent and initial PTCA strategies in mortality, nonfatal MI, stroke, or anginal symptoms. The principal benefit of stenting that emerged from these trials was a reduction in repeat revascularization rates. In BENESTENT II, which used a heparin-coated Palmaz-Schatz stent and a ticlopidine-aspirin antithrombotic regimen in lieu of the earlier aspirin-warfarin regimen, 14% of PTCA patients and 9% of stent patients required a repeat revascularization procedure out

TABLE 42.3 COMPARISON OF STENT AND PERCUTANEOUS TRANSLUMINAL CORONARY ANGIOPLASTY (PTCA) COSTS AT DUKE HOSPITAL

Cost category	Stent, 9/95–6/96 (n = 384)	PTCA, 9/95–6/96 (n = 159)	*p* Value
Catheter laboratory			
Balloons	$1,759	$1,479	<.001
Stents	$3,629	$169	<.001
Abciximab	$661	$817	.15
Guide catheter/wire	$481	$490	.64
Dye	$556	$504	.04
Other costs	$2,694	$2,765	.82
Total	$9,780	$6,224	<.001
Rooms			
Routine	$1,309	$1,419	.88
Step-down/intensive care unit	$1,368	$1,402	.79
Pharmacy	$302	$289	.89
Laboratory	$385	$345	.01
Emergency room	$787	$756	.35
Catheter laboratory	$9,780	$6,224	<.001
Other	$871	$1,100	.90
In-hospital costs	$14,802	$11,534	<.001
Professional fee	$1,863	$1,816	<.001
Total in-hospital costs	$16,665	$13,350	<.001

From Peterson ED, Cowper PA, Delong ER, et al. Acute and long-term cost implications of coronary stenting. *J Am Coll Cardiol* 1999;33:1610–1613, with permission.

to 6 months (125). These results are important not only because of the substantial reduction in clinical restenoses achieved in the stent arm but also because of the very substantial improvement in outcomes reflected in the PTCA arm statistics relative to earlier trial results.

Sukin and coworkers (126) compared 1995 practice in 78 patients who underwent coronary stenting at the Beth Israel Hospital with earlier data from the STRESS I trial (1991–1993). The major temporal trends observed in the use of coronary stenting included use of more stents and more adjunctive balloons per patient to achieve "optimal stent deployment." The associated catheterization laboratory costs rose from $3,012 in STRESS I to $5,209, a $2,197 increase. Stenting of large lesions or multiple lesions increased catheterization laboratory costs by an additional $2,000 relative to single-lesion stenting.

Peterson and colleagues (127) compared hospital costs of stenting with those of balloon PTCA at Duke Hospital from 1995 to 1996 (Table 42.3). Compared with PTCA, stenting costs were $3,600 more per case in catheterization laboratory resources and $3,300 higher in total hospital costs (127). Over the next 6 months, however, stent patients were rehospitalized less often (22% vs. 34%) and had less frequent need for repeat revascularization (9% vs. 26%). Thus, at 6 months, the costs for the two strategies were equal ($19,600 vs. $19,800), and this economic parity was maintained out to 1 year.

The OPUS-1 trial tested whether routine coronary stenting was superior to optimum PTCA with provisional stenting in 479 patients with one-vessel disease (123). In the routine stenting arm, patients averaged 1.2 stents, whereas in the optimum PTCA arm they averaged 0.5 stents, and 37% of patients in this arm required stent implantation. Use of abciximab was low in both arms (13% to 14%). Index hospital length of stay was similar in the two arms (2.5 to 2.6 days). The procedural costs were higher for routine stenting ($5,455 vs. $4,219, *p* <.001), and total initial hospital costs were correspondingly higher for the stent arm: $9,234 versus $8,434 (*p* <.001). Follow-up cardiac events out to 6 months were higher in the PTCA arm (123). In particular, target vessel repeat revascularization occurred in 10% for the PTCA arm versus 3% for stenting and any repeat revascularization procedure in 15% of the PTCA arm versus 5% of the stent arm. Hospital readmissions were twice as frequent for PTCA-arm patients. These follow-up costs offset the extra initial costs of routine stenting so that at 6 months, the stent group had slightly lower cumulative costs ($10,206 vs. $10,490 for PTCA). A bootstrap simulation yielded a net 6-month cost savings for routine stenting in 69% of 1,000 replications, with a mean savings of $268.

Comparisons of PTCA with stenting must also be interpreted in the larger context of a comparison of percutaneous revascularization (including stenting and PTCA) versus CABG and medicine. Several trials have compared a percutaneous revascularization strategy with routine stenting to CABG. The Arterial Revascularization Therapies Study randomized 1,205 patients with multivessel CAD to stent versus CABG (128). At 1 year, there was no significant difference in mortality, stroke, or MI. Repeat revascularization occurred in 16.8% of stent patients versus 3.5% of CABG patients. Initial procedural costs (based on European practices and prices and converted to U.S. dollars) were lower in the stent arm ($6,400 vs. $10,700). At 1 year, these differences had narrowed somewhat because of the extra repeat procedures in the stent arm: $10,700 for the stent arm versus $13,600 for the CABG arm ($p < .001$). The relevance of these cost data for U.S. practice is uncertain given the unexpectedly low cost estimates for CABG. The Canadian/European Surgery or Stent study has been reported in abstract form, and an economic analysis of this trial is anticipated. The ongoing Clinical Outcomes Utilizing Revascularization and Aggressive Drug Evaluation (COURAGE) trial is comparing optimal medical therapy with a strategy of PCI, and an economic analysis of this trial is planned.

Heart Failure

Approximately 4.7 million Americans carry a diagnosis of heart failure, and more than 550,000 new cases are identified each year (90). Approximately 70% of cases are due to coronary disease, with hypertension the next most common underlying disorder (129). The annual hospitalization volume for heart failure now approaches 1 million (1998 figure), with an associated annual cost in excess of $3.7 billion. The prevalence of heart failure rises with increasing age, and it is the single most frequent cause of hospitalization in the Medicare population (age ≥65) (90). After a first admission for heart failure, Medicare patients have a 44% chance of being readmitted at least once within 6 months (130).

Costs of Medical Care of Heart Failure

To analyze the costs of heart failure and their determinants, it is useful to look at three cost components (Fig. 42.5): maintenance care, care for episodes of decompensation, and procedures to reverse the heart failure state. Maintenance care includes the use of medications and routine medical follow-up for the patient with a stable, well-compensated course. The goals of maintenance therapy are to reduce symptoms and improve functional status to the extent possible, to improve survival, and to decrease the need for repeat hospitalizations. Periodically, patients with heart failure enter a state of decompensation; this may occur gradually as a result of progressive myocardial dysfunction or more abruptly (e.g., because of complicating arrhythmias, excess intake of dietary sodium, infection, or inappropriate cessation or reduction of medical therapy). The three most common causes of need for hospitalization in patients with congestive heart failure (CHF) are uncontrolled ischemia, uncontrolled atrial fibrillation, and increasing pulmonary or peripheral edema. Although not all hospitalizations for CHF can be eliminated without reversing the underlying heart failure state, some interventions have been proven to reduce the need for such admissions. Whether the efficiency of admissions for heart failure can also be improved (with a consequent reduction in costs) remains largely undefined. Finally, there are a growing number of nonpharmacologic interventions whose goal is to stabilize or even reverse the heart failure state. These include cardiac transplantation, use of various mechanical assistive devices, and CABG (with or without left ventricular reconstruction).

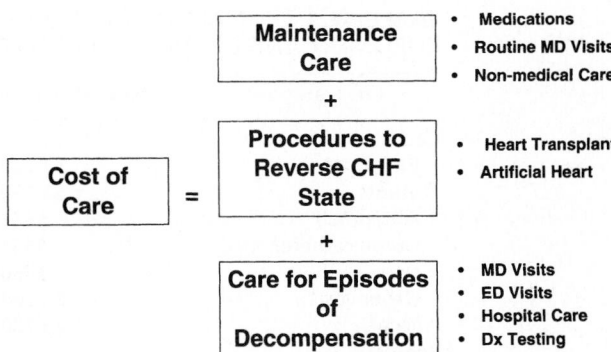

FIGURE 42.5 Cost components for heart failure care. CHF, congestive heart failure; Dx, diagnosis; ED, emergency department; MD, doctor of medicine.

The costs of care for a typical group of patients with heart failure consist of a mix of costs due to maintenance care and costs for treatment of decompensation. Only very small numbers of patients (2,360 in 2000) undergo cardiac transplantation (90). No "natural history" cost studies of heart failure have been done, and therefore it is difficult to define the cost of the disorder independently of the interventions used to treat it. Overall annual costs for patients with advanced heart failure, including inpatient and outpatient care and outpatient medications (including ACE inhibitor therapy), averaged $22,500 in the Fosinopril Efficacy/Safety Trial (FIRST) study and $21,100 in the Washington University trial (131,132). Patients with New York Heart Association (NYHA) class IV had higher costs than those with class III; costs were also increased for patients with renal insufficiency and with diabetes (131).

Digoxin

Digoxin is one of the oldest pharmacologic interventions in cardiovascular medicine, but its clinical effectiveness remains controversial. The National Institutes of Health DIG trial found no survival benefit for digoxin but a significant 6% reduction in the need for hospitalization (133). Using DRG-based Medicare reimbursement rates, Eisenstein and colleagues (133) performed a cost analysis of the DIG trial. Digoxin patients averaged fewer all-cause (1.9 vs. 2.0, $p = .01$) and heart-failure (0.6 vs. 0.8, $p = .001$) hospitalizations. Digoxin patients had higher total medical costs ($12,648 vs. $12,362, $p = .001$). Heart-failure costs were lower ($3,122 vs. $4,130, *p* = .001), but non–heart-failure costs were higher. PTCAs were more frequent in the digoxin arm, suggesting that these patients improved enough clinically to be treated more aggressively for their CAD. The average cost of the digoxin therapy over a mean of 37 months was $163. A cost-effectiveness analysis of this trial is planned.

Angiotensin-Converting Enzyme Inhibitors

ACE inhibitor therapy is recognized as one of the foundations of modern medical therapy for heart failure (134). A number of large-scale clinical trials have clearly demonstrated that ACE inhibitors prolong survival in patients with heart failure due to systolic dysfunction. However, none of these trials included prospective measurement of costs. Two U.S. studies have used decision analysis models to estimate the cost effectiveness of this form of therapy (135,136).

Glick and colleagues (135) used primary data to form the Studies of Left Ventricular Dysfunction (SOLVD) treatment trial (mild to moderate heart failure and ejection fraction <35%) to model the cost effectiveness of enalapril therapy. The model evaluated 48-month outcomes (from the available empiric data) and projected lifetime outcomes. Analysis was done from a societal perspective, and costs were expressed in 1992 U.S. dollars. On the health-benefit side, this study estimated that patients who were randomized to enalapril gained 0.14 discounted years of life and 0.11 discounted quality-adjusted years of life during the 4-year follow-up of the trial. The life expectancy of these patients was estimated at 6.5 to 7.0 years, and over this period enalapril was projected to add 0.30 discounted years and 0.21 discounted QALYs.

On the cost side, enalapril patients averaged $11,840 in discounted costs of hospitalization, enalapril therapy, and outpatient visits during the 4 years of the study. The corresponding cost for the placebo patients was $12,560. Thus, during the trial period, enalapril saved $720 per patient (135). Importantly, these savings occurred during the first 18 months of the trial, and costs after this point were similar. Over the projected life expectancy of the study cohort, enalapril patients had discounted costs of $22,000 and placebo patients had costs of $21,975. The lifetime incremental cost of enalapril therapy was therefore projected to be $25 per patient.

During the 4 years of the trial, enalapril improved survival and reduced medical costs. Projecting these data out to a lifetime cost-effectiveness perspective, enalapril saved an added life-year for $80 and an added QALY for $115 (135). These data demonstrate that, at a minimum, ACE inhibitor therapy with enalapril in mild to moderate CHF is in the "best buy" category of cost effectiveness. For several reasons, it is likely that in this population ACE inhibitor therapy is actually cost saving over the patient's lifetime. First, sensitivity analysis on the long-term effects of enala-

pril shows that if the drug continued to reduce hospitalizations after 18 months it would be cost saving (135). Second, the average wholesale price for a year's supply of enalapril, 20 mg per day, is $475. The advent of generic captopril makes an ACE inhibitor available for a substantially lower cost and would, therefore, make the therapy cost saving over a lifetime. Finally, the cost assigned to follow-up hospitalizations was based on HCFA DRG reimbursement rates and may have, therefore, underestimated the fair cost of such an event (and, hence, the value of preventing it). ▼ i18

Beta-Blocking Agents

Two important randomized trials reported that beta-blocker therapy in heart failure produces a clinically important and statistically significant reduction in mortality and hospitalization. The Metoprolol CR/XL Randomized Intervention Trial in Congestive Heart Failure (MERIT-HF) randomized 3,991 patients with class II or greater heart failure and an ejection fraction of 0.40 or less to metoprolol CR/XL or placebo (141). With an average follow-up of 1 year, metoprolol reduced death or heart transplantation by 32%. All-cause hospitalization was reduced from 33% to 29% (*p* = .004), and days in hospital were reduced from 6.1 to 5.1 per patient (*p* = .004). The discounted retail cost of metoprolol XL/CR therapy ranges from $20 per month for the 50-mg dosage ($240 per year) to $54 per month for the 200-mg dosage ($650 per year). Although a formal cost analysis of MERIT-HF has not yet been reported, the cost of metoprolol therapy should be largely offset by the approximate 1-day average reduction in hospital stay.

The Cardiac Insufficiency Bisoprolol Study II (CIBIS II) enrolled 2,647 patients with heart failure in class III or IV with an ejection fraction of 35% or less (142). All-cause mortality was reduced 34% by bisoprolol (*p* <.001). All-cause hospitalization was reduced 20% from 34% to 33% (*p* <.001). An economic analysis of CIBIS II is planned. In contrast, the Beta-Blocker Evaluation of Survival Trial randomized 2,708 class III or IV heart failure patients to bucindolol or placebo (143). At an average of 2 years, there was no significant effect on mortality overall, although nonblack patients had a survival advantage. Hospitalization was reduced by 8% in the bucindolol group (*p* = .08).

Economic analysis of the smaller U.S. Carvedilol Heart Failure Trials Program was performed using a Markov decision model, clinical data from the trials, and published cost data (144). Trial data were projected out to a lifetime perspective. Projected lifetime costs of conventional CHF care in this model were $28,750. Costs for the carvedilol strategy were $36,420, or $7,600 more than conventional therapy. Carvedilol was projected to extend life expectancy by 0.31 to 0.95 years per patient over the life expectancy without such therapy (6.7 years). This range reflects different assumptions about the persistence of therapeutic benefit. The corresponding cost effectiveness of carvedilol therapy ranged from $30,000 per life-year added to $13,000 per life-year added. Current (2001) discounted retail price for carvedilol is approximately $90 per month, or $1,080 per year.

Surgical Approaches to Heart Failure

Invasive approaches that have been used to reduce or reverse the heart failure state include CABG (with or without ventricular reconstruction), heart transplantation, and left ventricular assist devices (LVADs).

For patients with ischemic cardiomyopathy, CABG has offered a theoretically attractive but controversial approach. Although registry data suggest a more favorable survival with CABG than with medical therapy, no randomized trial has validated these observations (145). Randomized trial and registry data from the 1970s comparing CABG and medicine demonstrated a magnification in absolute terms of the survival benefits of surgery in patients with impaired left ventricular function (146). Whether these observations extend to patients with advanced heart failure (NYHA class III) and a severely impaired left ventricle (ejection fraction <35%) remains uncertain. In recent years, clinicians at some centers have begun using "viability" radiologic studies such as positron emission tomography or perfusion imaging to identify the subset with substantial ischemic viable myocardium who are presumed most likely to benefit from a high-risk CABG. The Surgical Treatment for Ischemic Heart Failure (STICH) trial will be the first large-scale randomized trial of modern surgical versus optimal modern medical therapy in these difficult patients and will include an economic evaluation as well as substudies to define whether preoperative viability screening is of benefit (145).

Heart transplantation offers a radical but effective therapy for a small subset of patients with advanced heart failure. Although it has been estimated that there are more than 40,000 patients a year with advanced heart failure who could benefit from cardiac replacement therapy, only approximately 2,300 donor hearts are available each year for transplantation. This shortage of available organs relative to organs needed creates some major inefficiencies in the care of patients on the heart transplant list. The availability of a suitable heart for a given patient is, of course, unpredictable, and because available organs are allocated on an illness severity-based priority scale, doctors face an incentive to keep their candidate patients hospitalized in the intensive care unit with intravenous inotropes and a balloon pump to preserve their position at the top of the list. As a consequence, patients may wait for months in the hospital.

No high-quality modern cost data on transplantation have been published, but claims (charge) data are available (147). In 1999, charges per transplant patient averaged $303,000 through the end of the first year (corresponding costs are likely to be approximately half that amount). Hos-

pital charges were $181,000, physician charges $23,000, and organ procurement $24,000. Follow-up care averaged $40,000, and immunosuppressive therapy charges were $11,400. The average medical charges for care after the first year (including angiography, biopsies, and drug therapy) are approximately $24,000. Thus, cumulative 5-year charges for heart transplantation are currently approximately $400,000 (representing probably approximately $200,000 in medical costs). Although no modern cost-effectiveness analysis of heart transplantation has been done, heart transplantation currently has a 1-year survival rate of more than 90% and a posttransplant life expectancy of approximately 9 to 11 years. This represents a huge increment in life-years over medical treatment of advanced heart failure, and the cost per added life-year is therefore likely to fall securely in the economically attractive zone.

Several LVADs have been approved by the U.S. Food and Drug Administration as a bridge to transplant. The acquisition cost of these devices is high, currently $50,000 to $75,000 (not counting costs of implantation or follow-up care). One small observational study suggests that, when used as a bridge to transplant, these devices pay for themselves (148). Of 90 consecutive patients on the heart transplant list who received LVAD, 44 were discharged to home to await their transplant. The cost for pretransplant care at home was $13,200, versus $165,200 for inpatient care. In addition, 30% of the outpatients resumed working, and all were independent in activities of daily living.

The more controversial aspects of LVAD use is as "destination therapy." As noted earlier, more than 40,000 patients a year could be candidates for this form of therapy if it is approved by the U.S. Food and Drug Administration. The Randomized Evaluation of Mechanical Assistance Therapy for Congestive Heart Failure (REMATCH) trial randomized class IV patients who were ineligible for transplantation to the HeartMate vented electric LVAD or optimal medical therapy (149). If this study shows a survival advantage for the LVAD, a wider indication for these devices could add more than $5 billion to the annual health care budget in the United States. For reference, the total annual cost for heart transplantation in the United States is approximately $700 million, but this figure is constrained by the lack of more donor hearts. An economic analysis of REMATCH is planned.

Prevention of Coronary Heart Disease and Its Complications

Clinically overt CHD has a prevalence of approximately 7 million persons in the United States and is the most common cause of death in this and other industrialized countries (90). It is also a major cause of morbidity and resulting disability. Approximately 2.0 to 2.3 million individuals with CHD in the United States have limitations in their daily activities as a result of the disease. CHD accounts for more than 2.2 million hospital admissions per year and over 10 million outpatient medical visits. The direct medical costs of caring for coronary disease patients in the United States have been estimated at $47.5 billion, and the cost to society of the loss in productivity due to morbidity and premature mortality has been assessed at $43 billion (90). For many years, it has been hypothesized that prevention might be a more cost-effective way of reducing the clinical and economic sequelae of CHD than treatment of symptomatic or decompensated disease. As discussed elsewhere in this text, epidemiologic studies have identified a set of major modifiable risk factors for CHD, and clinical trials have been conducted to define the relationship between modification of these risk factors and subsequent outcome. *Primary prevention* is usually defined as prevention in individuals at risk for the disease but without any clinical evidence that the disease has actually developed. *Secondary prevention* is prevention in patients with clinically manifest disease. In primary prevention, the risk factors that have been most often targeted are hypercholesterolemia, smoking, hypertension, diabetes, and physical inactivity. In secondary prevention programs, in addition to these risk factors, major emphasis is given to the use of aspirin, beta-blockers, and ACE inhibitors in appropriate patients. The medical effectiveness of these interventions is discussed in detail elsewhere. In this section, we review the available work on their economic implications.

In general, effective prevention programs for CHD improve outcomes at a net increased cost (154). Secondary prevention programs usually have more favorable cost-effectiveness ratios than do primary programs. Some clinicians find this counterintuitive because, they argue, prevention programs are usually less expensive on a per-patient basis than is treatment with expensive high-technology therapies. Although this may be true, the total economic picture is very substantially influenced by the number of individuals who must be treated to prevent a single death or major complication. Because risk factors for CHD only define a propensity for future disease, many individuals who are enrolled in primary prevention programs never develop the disease and consequently cannot benefit from the interventions being applied. In contrast, secondary prevention programs target individuals with an established propensity to development of disease-related complications. Consequently, the number needed to treat to prevent one adverse event is small. For example, using data from the West of Scotland trial (largely a primary prevention population), prevention of one additional death by cholesterol reduction with a statin agent would require treating 166 patients for 5 years (155). Using data from the Cholesterol and Recurrent Events (CARE) study of patients with established CHD and modestly elevated cholesterol, prevention of one death would require treating 91 patients for 5 years (156). Using the Scandinavian Simvastatin Survival Study (4S) results in patients with CHD and very elevated cholesterol levels, only 29 patients would have required 5

years of statin therapy to prevent one death (157). Because the direct costs of statin therapy would be similar in the preceding three examples, it is clear that the largest "bang for the buck" (and the most favorable cost-effectiveness ratio) would be obtained in treating the highest-risk patients.

Hypercholesterolemia

Numerous observational studies have established a strong dose-response relationship between total cholesterol levels and CHD risk. The National Cholesterol Education Program has established a target desirable level of less than 220 mg per dL for adults without evidence of clinical CHD. The corresponding low-density lipoprotein (LDL) cholesterol level is less than 130 mg per dL. Earlier primary prevention trials tested diet and pharmacologic regimens that were able to achieve reductions in total cholesterol of approximately 10%. Associated reductions in all-cause mortality were small and largely nonsignificant. Consequently, early cost-effectiveness analysis based on these clinical data generally concluded that cholesterol reduction as a primary prevention strategy was not economically attractive (158).

The West of Scotland Coronary Prevention Study (WOSCOPS) found that primary prevention with pravastatin at 40 mg per day reduced total cholesterol by 20% relative to placebo in 4,159 men older than age 45 years with LDL cholesterol levels of 155 mg per dL or greater. Pravastatin patients experienced a 22% reduction in all-cause mortality ($p = .051$) (155). Over 4.9 years of follow-up, for every 1,000 patients shifted to the pravastatin arm, there were five fewer deaths, 19 fewer MIs, 14 fewer diagnostic catheterizations, and eight fewer revascularization procedures. An economic analysis using British costs and the WOSCOPS data has been published (159). This analysis estimated that treating 10,000 men such as those in the trial would prevent the development of CHD in approximately 300. The pravastatin therapy cost $3,700 per patient for 5 years and saved approximately $100 per patient as a result of reduced procedures and complications. Life expectancy was increased by pravastatin by 0.10 years, and the cost per year of life added was $32,600.

A cost-effectiveness model of cholesterol-lowering strategies in the United States reported that primary prevention with a statin compared with diet therapy has a cost-effectiveness ratio ranging from $54,000 per QALY to $1.4 million per QALY depending on patient risk level (160). Importantly, the WOSCOPS economic model did not assume a preexisting secondary prevention program (i.e., wait to treat patients once they manifest clinical CAD), which may explain part of the difference with this U.S. model.

The Air Force/Texas Coronary Atherosclerosis Prevention Study randomized 6,605 subjects without clinical CAD and with average cholesterol levels to lovastatin or placebo (161). Over 5 years of therapy, lovastatin reduced acute coronary events by 37% ($p < .001$). In absolute terms, for every 1,000 patients shifted to lovastatin therapy there were four fewer cardiovascular deaths, 26 fewer MIs, 16 fewer unstable angina admissions, and 31 fewer revascularization procedures. The cumulative 5-year cost of lovastatin therapy was $4,654 per patient, and there was a $524 cost offset due to reduced cardiac events and procedures (net cost of drug therapy $4,130). A cost-effectiveness analysis of this trial has not yet been reported.

The National Cholesterol Education Program has identified an LDL cholesterol of less than 100 mg per dL as optimal in patients with evidence of CHD. Although a number of important secondary prevention trials have been published, two of the most useful for assessing economic impact are the 4S and the CARE trial. The 4S randomized 4,444 patients of both sexes aged 35 to 60 years with a history of angina or prior MI and total cholesterol of 210 to 310 mg per dL to adjusted-dose simvastatin or placebo (157). The majority of patients received 20 mg simvastatin, and 37% required 40 mg per day. Over a median of 5.4 years, simvastatin decreased total cholesterol by 25% and LDL cholesterol by 35% and decreased total mortality by 30% (*p* = .0003) (157). The study also observed a 37% reduction in the need for revascularization in the simvastatin arm (*p* <.0001). In a subsequent analysis, the 4S investigators reported that simvastatin therapy reduced hospitalizations for acute cardiovascular disease, including revascularization (81% of which were CABG), by 26% (*p* <.0001). Over the course of the study, total hospital days due to cardiovascular disease were reduced by 5,138 days in the simvastatin arm (*p* <.0001). The beneficial effect of simvastatin on hospitalization first became evident after 10 months of therapy and became statistically significant after 22 months. No effect was seen on the use of antianginal or other cardiovascular drugs.

Using U.S.-derived reimbursement rates as cost weights, the 4S investigators estimated that the observed reduction in hospitalizations would equal a $3,872 reduction in average cost per patient treated with simvastatin (162). With a wholesale price for simvastatin over the trial averaging $4,400 per patient ($4,879 undiscounted), the net cost of simvastatin therapy was estimated to be $528 per patient over the trial or $0.28 per day (an offset of 88% of the drug's cost). The cost of repeat laboratory measurement of lipids and transaminases (three to four in the first year, annually after year 1) added a discounted cost of $250 per patient or an additional $0.13 per day. Thus, the total net cost of the simvastatin strategy was estimated at $778 per patient over a mean of 1,915 days of follow-up (approximately $148 per year). As noted earlier, the benefits of simvastatin on follow-up medical care take 10 months to become clinically detectable and appear to increase progressively as treatment is continued.

Three separate cost-effectiveness analyses have been conducted using the data from the 4S trial. One was done from a Swedish perspective (163); two others were conducted

from a U.S. perspective. Schwartz (164) estimated a cost per year of life saved of $18,100 with a cost per QALY saved of $15,100, assuming that costs and benefits only occurred for the duration of the trial. Extrapolating to a lifetime perspective yielded a cost per year of life saved of $5,800, with a cost per QALY saved of $6,100. The most recently published analysis used the empiric data from 4S in a Markov model to evaluate cost effectiveness of therapy for different subgroups (165). In this analysis, costs were derived from four hospitals in Sweden that had patient-based cost-accounting systems. Swedish costs were converted to U.S. dollars. The patient's work status, measured every 6 months, was used to estimate productivity costs saved by simvastatin. This analysis estimated that for 59-year-old men, the cost effectiveness of 5 years of simvastatin therapy was $5,400 per year of life saved; the corresponding figure for 59-year-old women was $10,500. Adding in the productivity costs related to time lost from work saved by simvastatin improved the cost-effectiveness ratios to $1,600 for men and $5,100 for women (165). Extensive sensitivity analyses showed that statin therapy was very economically attractive under a wide range of assumptions.

The CARE study evaluated pravastatin versus placebo in 4,159 patients who were 3 to 20 months post-MI and who had a total cholesterol of less than 240 mg per dL and an LDL cholesterol of 115 to 174 mg per dL (156). Like in other statin trials, pravastatin reduced total cholesterol by 20% and LDL cholesterol by 28%. Death and nonfatal MI were reduced by 24%. The mean cost for 6 years of pravastatin therapy in CARE was $5,500, which was partially offset by a $1,660 savings from reduced cardiac events and procedures (166). A cost-effectiveness model using the CARE data estimated that to add a life-year with pravastatin therapy would cost between $16,000 and $31,000.

Other Pharmacologic Secondary Preventions

Long-term aspirin therapy is the mainstay of secondary prevention efforts in patients with manifest coronary disease (193). The clinical effectiveness is substantial, and the cost is minimal. Therefore, although aspirin use has not been the subject of a formal economic analysis, this therapy clearly belongs in the "best buy" category of medical intervention. Despite these attractive characteristics, much evidence exists that aspirin is underused in patients with coronary disease (194). Long-term use of beta-blockers after MI was modeled by Goldman and colleagues (195). Based on the earlier (prethrombolytic) beta-blocker trials, they estimated cost-effectiveness ratios of less than $15,000 per life-year added, with ratios less than $5,000 for moderate- or high-risk patients. Their model projected a 6-year course of therapy, with 25% mortality reductions by beta-blockers in years 1 to 3, 7% reduction in years 4 to 6, and gradual attenuation of treatment benefit over a subsequent 9-year period. Based on the data from the Survival and

THE FUTURE

New approaches are needed in this area to meet the demands for information and for relevant measures of medical value. Three major areas need intensive work over the next few years. The first is to improve methods for costing out medical care accurately but efficiently (i.e., with a relatively low cost of data collection). The second is to develop new measures of value that do not require extrapolation out to a lifetime perspective. These measures would not preclude traditional cost-effectiveness analysis but could be used to supplement it. The third area is education of medical practitioners about medical economics. It is only by getting practi-tioners to use cost data on a daily basis, asking questions about it and challenging it, that we will get better data and ultimately better value-based medical decision making.

In the final analysis, no economic model can dictate how many resources society should expend on health care and what types of health care should be given priority. These are political and ethical questions that transcend medicine. However, the medical profession must constantly strive to achieve better outcomes at an acceptable cost and to continue the dramatic pace of technological advances set over the last century.

Ventricular Enlargement trial, Tsevat and colleagues (196) developed a decision model to assess the cost effectiveness of captopril therapy in 50- to 80-year-old survivors of acute MI with an ejection fraction of 40% or less. Under the assumption that survival benefits of captopril persisted for more than 4 years, these investigators estimated cost-effectiveness ratios of $10,400 per QALY or less (1991 dollars), depending on age. Analysis of the cost effectiveness of early lisinopril use in acute MI based on GISSI-3 data yielded a cost-effectiveness ratio of $2,300 (U.S.) per 6-week death avoided (197). Assuming that the clinical benefits observed in GISSI-3 were sustained over a 10- to 15-year life expectancy, these data suggest that 6 weeks of ACE inhibitor therapy for all post-MI patients may fall into a "best buy" category of economic attractiveness.

CONTROVERSIES AND PERSONAL PERSPECTIVES

As recently as the early 1990s, medical economics was viewed as a scholarly academic discipline that was largely irrelevant to the practice of medicine. Cost is now one of the dominant issues in almost all medical decisions, although it is the controlling issue in only a minority. Demands by payers that medicine demonstrate its value (benefits produced for dollars spent) have thrust economists into the mainstream of the revolution that is currently reshaping medical practice. However, just as clinicians found themselves woefully unprepared to prove the medical benefits of their decisions, economists were unprepared to provide the pragmatic sorts of data that are now required of them. As was discussed earlier, medical economics is principally concerned with matters related to the efficient societal allocation of scarce resources. Economists have paid little attention to measuring the cost of health care, preferring to discuss the abstract notion of "opportunity cost" while leaving the more pragmatic measurement issues to the accountants. Payers and policy makers, however, are not interested in theories or abstract problems of resource allocation. Instead, they wish to understand the costs of care and how they can be reduced or at least controlled. Clinicians are also not interested in theoretical economic exercises. They want to be able to prove that the care they provide their patients is worth the money it costs. Cost-effectiveness ratios are the economists' measure of value and have some important strengths. However, the need to frame all cost-effectiveness ratios in terms of dollars required to add an extra QALY (9) often stretches the available clinical and cost data beyond credibility.

REFERENCES

1. Mark DB. Medical economics for interventional cardiology. In: Topol EJ, ed. *Textbook of interventional cardiology*. Philadelphia: WB Saunders, 1999:889–909.
2. Anders G. *Health against wealth: HMOs and the breakdown of medical trust*. New York: Houghton Mifflin, 1996.
3. Wennberg JE, Freeman JL, Culp WJ. Are hospital services rationed in New Haven or over-utilised in Boston? *Lancet* 1987;1:1185–1189.
4. Wennberg JE. Outcomes research, cost containment, and the fear of health care rationing. *N Engl J Med* 1990;323:1202–1204.
5. Finkler SA. *Essentials of cost accounting for health care organizations*. Gaithersburg, MD: Aspen Publishers, 1994.
6. Stewart RD. *Cost estimating*, 2nd ed. New York: John Wiley and Sons, 1991.
7. Feldstein PJ. *Health care economics*, 4th ed. Albany, NY: Delmar Publishers, 1993.
8. Fuchs VR. *The health economy*. Cambridge, MA: Harvard University Press, 1986.

9. Gold MR, Siegel JE, Russell LB, et al. *Cost-effectiveness in health and medicine.* New York: Oxford University Press, 1996.

10. Drummond MF, O'Brian B, Stoddart GL, et al. *Methods for the economic evaluation of health care programmes,* 2nd ed. Oxford, UK: Oxford University Press, 1997.

11. Detsky AS, Naglie IG. A clinician's guide to cost-effectiveness analysis. *Ann Intern Med* 1990;113:147–154.

12. Eisenberg JM. Clinical economics. A guide to the economic analysis of clinical practices. *JAMA* 1989;262:2879–2886.

13. Finkler SA. The distinction between costs and charges. *Ann Intern Med* 1982;96:102–109.

14. Shwartz M, Young DW, Siegrist RB. The ratio of costs to charges: how good a basis for estimating costs? *Inquiry* 1995;32:476–481.

15. Ashby JL. The accuracy of cost measures derived from Medicare cost report data. *Hospital* 1992;3:1–8.

16. Hsiao WC, Braun P, Yntema D, et al. Estimating physicians' work for a resource-based relative-value scale. *N Engl J Med* 1988;319:835–841.

17. Adams ME, McCall NT, Gray DT, et al. Economic analysis in randomized control trials. *Med Care* 1992;30:231–243.

18. Drummond MF, Davies L. Economic analysis alongside clinical trials: revisiting the methodological issues. *Int J Tech Assess Health Care* 1991;7:561–573.

19. Rigby K, Silagy C, Crockett A. Can resource use be extracted from randomized controlled trials to calculate costs? *Int J Tech Assess Health Care* 1996;12:714–720.

20. Freemantle N, Drummond M. Should clinical trials with concurrent economic analyses be blinded? *JAMA* 1997;277:63–64.

21. Ellwein LB, Drummond MF. Economic analysis alongside clinical trials. *Int J Tech Assess Health Care* 1996;12:691–697.

22. Mark DB, Hlatky MA, Califf RM, et al. Cost effectiveness of thrombolytic therapy with tissue plasminogen activator as compared with streptokinase for acute myocardial infarction. *N Engl J Med* 1995;332:1418–1424.

23. Feit F, Mueller HS, Braunwald E, et al. Thrombolysis in Myocardial Infarction (TIMI) phase II trial: outcome comparison of a "conservative strategy" in community versus tertiary hospitals. *J Am Coll Cardiol* 1990;16:1529–1534.

24. Every NR, Larson EB, Litwin PE, et al. The association between on-site cardiac catheterization facilities and the use of coronary angiography after acute myocardial infarction. *N Engl J Med* 1993;329:546–551.

25. Blustein J. High-technology cardiac procedures. The impact of service availability on service use in New York State. *JAMA* 1993;270(3):344–349.

26. Pilote L, Miller DP, Califf RM, et al. Determinants of the use of coronary angiography and revascularization after thrombolysis for acute myocardial infarction. *N Engl J Med* 1996;335:1198–1205.

27. Jollis JG, Delong ER, Peterson ED, et al. Outcome of acute myocardial infarction according to the specialty of the admitting physician. *N Engl J Med* 1996;335:1880–1887.

28. Mark DB, Naylor CD, Hlatky MA, et al. Use of medical resources and quality of life after acute myocardial infarc-

tion in Canada versus the United States. *N Engl J Med* 1994;331:1130–1135.

29. Laupacis A, Feeny D, Detsky AS, et al. How attractive does a new technology have to be to warrant adoption and utilization?: tentative guidelines for using clinical and economic evaluations. *Can Med Assoc J* 1992;146:473–481.

30. Mason J, Drummond M, Torrance G. Some guidelines on the use of cost effectiveness league tables. *BMJ* 1993;306:570–572.

31. Sox HC Jr, Blatt MA, Higgins MC, et al. *Medical decision making.* Boston: Butterworth, 1988.

32. Cohen BJ. Is expected utility theory normative for medical decision making? *Med Decis Making* 1996;16:1–6.

33. Nease RF. Do violations of the axioms of expected utility theory threaten decision analysis? *Med Decis Making* 1996;16:399–403.

34. Torrance GW. Measurement of health state utilities for economic appraisal. A review. *J Health Econ* 1986;5:1–30.

35. Torrance GW. Utility approach to measuring health-related quality of life. *J Chronic Dis* 1987;40:595–600.

36. Patrick DL, Erickson P. *Health status and health policy: quality of life in health care evaluation and resource allocation.* New York: Oxford University Press, 1993.

37. Tengs TO, Meyer G, Siegel JE, et al. Oregon's Medicaid ranking and cost-effectiveness. *Med Decis Making* 1996;16:99–107.

38. Ubel PA, Loewenstein G, Scanlon D, et al. Individual utilities are inconsistent with rationing choices: a partial explanation of why Oregon's cost-effectiveness list failed. *Med Decis Making* 1996;16:108–116.

39. Hadorn DC. Setting health care priorities in Oregon: cost-effectiveness meets the rule of rescue. *JAMA* 1991;265:2218–2225.

40. Ubel PA, DeKay ML, Baron J, et al. Cost-effectiveness analysis in a setting of budget constraints: is it equitable? *N Engl J Med* 1996;334:1174–1177.

41. Task force on principles for economic analysis of health care technology. Economic analysis of health care technology: a report on principles. *Ann Intern Med* 1995;123:61–70.

42. Torrance GW, Blaker D, Detsky AS, et al. Canadian guidelines for economic evaluation of pharmaceuticals. *PharmacoEconomics* 1996;9:535–559.

43. Langley PC. The November 1995 revised Australian guidelines for the economic evaluation of pharmaceuticals. *PharmacoEconomics* 1996;9:341–352.

44. Weinstein MC, Siegel JE, Gold MR, et al., for the Panel on Cost-Effectiveness in Health and Medicine. Recommendations of the Panel on Cost-Effectiveness in Health and Medicine. *JAMA* 1996;276:1253–1258.

45. Russell LB, Gold MR, Siegel JE, et al., for the Panel on Cost-Effectiveness in Health and Medicine. The role of cost-effectiveness analysis in health and medicine. *JAMA* 1996;276:1172–1177.

46. Siegel JE, Weinstein MC, Russell LB, et al., for the Panel on Cost-Effectiveness in Health and Medicine. Recommendations for reporting cost-effectiveness analyses. *JAMA* 1996;276:1339–1341.

47. Braunwald E, Antman EM, Beasley JW, et al. ACC/AHA guidelines for the management of patients with unstable

angina and non–ST-segment elevation myocardial infarction: executive summary and recommendations. A report of the American College of Cardiology/American Heart Association task force on practice guidelines (Committee on the Management of Patients with Unstable Angina). *Circulation* 2000;102:1193–1209.

48. Mark DB. Assessment of prognosis in patients with coronary artery disease. In: Roubin GS, Califf RM, O'Neill WW, et al., eds. *Interventional cardiovascular medicine: principles and practice*, 2nd ed. New York: Churchill Livingstone, 2001 (in press).

49. Pilote L, Califf RM, Sapp S, et al. Regional variation across the United States in the management of acute myocardial infarction. *N Engl J Med* 1995;333:565–578.

50. Weintraub WS, Mauldin PD, Talley JD, et al. Determinants of hospital charges and costs in acute myocardial infarction: a report from the Myocardial Infarction Cost Study (MICS) group. *Am J Managed Care* 1996;2:977–986.

51. Collins R, Peto R, Baigent C, et al. Aspirin, heparin, and fibrinolytic therapy in suspected acute myocardial infarction. *N Engl J Med* 1997;336:847–860.

52. Mark DB. Economic analysis methods and endpoints. In: Califf RM, Mark DB, Wagner GS, eds. *Acute coronary care in the thrombolytic era*. St. Louis: Mosby–Year Book, 1995:167–182.

53. Armstrong PW, Collen D. Fibrinolysis for acute myocardial infarction: current status and new horizons for pharmacological reperfusion, Pt 1. *Circulation* 2001;103:2862–2866.

54. Naylor CD, Bronskill S, Goel V. Cost-effectiveness of intravenous thrombolytic drugs for acute myocardial infarction. *Can J Cardiol* 1993;9(6):553–558.

55. Krumholz HM, Pasternak RC, Weinstein MC, et al. Cost effectiveness of thrombolytic therapy with streptokinase in elderly patients with suspected acute myocardial infarction. *N Engl J Med* 1992;327:7–13.

56. The GUSTO Investigators. An international randomized trial comparing four thrombolytic strategies for acute myocardial infarction. *N Engl J Med* 1993;329:673–682.

57. Topol EJ, Ohman EM, Armstrong PW, et al. Survival outcomes 1 year after reperfusion therapy with either alteplase or reteplase for acute myocardial infarction: results from the Global Utilization of Streptokinase and t-PA for Occluded Coronary Arteries (GUSTO) III trial. *Circulation* 2000;102:1761–1765.

58. Single-bolus tenecteplase compared with front-loaded alteplase in acute myocardial infarction: the ASSENT-2 double-blind randomised trial. *Lancet* 1999;354:716–722.

59. Topol EJ. Reperfusion therapy for acute myocardial infarction with fibrinolytic therapy or combination reduced fibrinolytic therapy and platelet glycoprotein IIb/IIIa inhibition: the GUSTO V randomised trial. *Lancet* 2001;357:1905–1914.

60. Weaver WD, Simes RJ, Betriu A, et al. Comparison of primary coronary angioplasty and intravenous thrombolytic therapy for acute myocardial infarction: a quantitative review. *JAMA* 1997;278:2093–2098.

61. Grines CL, Browne KF, Marco J, et al. A comparison of immediate angioplasty with thrombolytic therapy for acute myocardial infarction. *N Engl J Med* 1993;328:673–679.

62. Gibbons RJ, Holmes DR, Reeder GS, et al. Immediate angioplasty compared with the administration of a thrombolytic agent followed by conservative treatment for myocardial infarction. *N Engl J Med* 1993;328:685–691.

63. Reeder GS, Bailey KR, Gersh BJ, et al. Cost comparison of immediate angioplasty versus thrombolysis followed by conservative therapy for acute myocardial infarction: a randomized prospective trial. *Mayo Clin Proc* 1994;69:5–12.

64. The GUSTO IIb Angioplasty Substudy Investigators. An international randomized trial of 1138 patients comparing primary coronary angioplasty versus tissue plasminogen activator for acute myocardial infarction. *N Engl J Med* 1997;336:1621–1628.

65. Mark DB, Granger CB, Ellis SG, et al. Costs of direct angioplasty versus thrombolysis for acute myocardial infarction: results from the GUSTO II randomized trial. *Circulation* 1996;94:168A.

66. Faxon DP, Heger JW. Primary angioplasty—enduring the test of time. *N Engl J Med* 1999;341:1464–1465.

67. Lieu TA, Lundstrom RJ, Ray GT, et al. Initial cost of primary angioplasty for acute myocardial infarction. *J Am Coll Cardiol* 1996;28:882–889.

68. Every NR, Parsons LS, Hlatky MA, et al., for the Myocardial Infarction Triage and Intervention Investigators. A comparison of thrombolytic therapy with primary coronary angioplasty for acute myocardial infarction. *N Engl J Med* 1996;335:1253–1260.

69. Mayou R, Blackwood R, Bryant B, et al. Cardiac failure: symptoms and functional status. *J Psychosom Res* 1991;35(4/5):399–407.

70. Cohen DJ, Taira DA, Berezin RH, et al. Cost-effectiveness of coronary stenting in acute myocardial infarction: results from the STENT PAMI trial. *Circulation* 2001 (*in press*).

71. Brener SJ, Barr LA, Burchenal JE, et al. Randomized, placebo-controlled trial of platelet glycoprotein IIb/IIIa blockade with primary angioplasty for acute myocardial infarction. ReoPro and Primary PTCA Organization and Randomized Trial (RAPPORT) Investigators. *Circulation* 1998;98:734–741.

72. Montalescot G, Barragan P, Wittenberg O, et al. Platelet glycoprotein IIb/IIIa inhibition with coronary stenting for acute myocardial infarction. *N Engl J Med* 2001;344(25):1895–1903.

73. Degeare VS, Dangas G, Stone GW, et al. Interventional procedures in acute myocardial infarction. *Am Heart J* 2001;141:15–24.

74. Effects of tissue plasminogen activator and a comparison of early invasive and conservative strategies in unstable angina and non–Q-wave myocardial infarction. Results of the TIMI IIIB trial. Thrombolysis in myocardial ischemia. *Circulation* 1994;89:1545–1556.

75. Boden WE, O'Rourke RA, Crawford MH, et al. Outcomes in patients with acute non–Q-wave myocardial infarction randomly assigned to an invasive as compared with a conservative management strategy. Veterans Affairs Non–Q-Wave Infarction Strategies in Hospital (VANQWISH). *N Engl J Med* 1998;338:1785–1792.

76. Invasive compared with non-invasive treatment in unstable coronary-artery disease: FRISC II prospective randomised multicentre study. *Lancet* 1999;354:708–715.

77. Cannon CP, Weintraub WS, Demopoulos LA, et al. Comparison of early invasive and conservative strategies in patients with unstable coronary syndromes treated with the glycoprotein IIb/IIIa inhibitor tirofiban. *N Engl J Med* 2001;344:1879–1887.

78. Weintraub WS. *Economics of the TACTICS-TIMI 18 trial.* Orlando, FL: American College of Cardiology 50th Annual Scientific Session, 2001.

79. Selby JV, Fireman BH, Lundstrom RJ, et al. Variation among hospitals in coronary angiography practices and outcomes after myocardial infarction in a large health maintenance organization. *N Engl J Med* 1996;335:1888–1896.

80. Kuntz KM, Tsevat J, Goldman L, et al. Cost-effectiveness of routine coronary angiography after acute myocardial infarction. *Circulation* 1996;94:957–965.

81. Kong DF, Topol EJ, Bittl JA, et al. Clinical outcomes of bivalirudin for ischemic heart disease. *Circulation* 1999;100:2049–2053.

82. Long-term low-molecular-mass heparin in unstable coronary-artery disease: FRISC II prospective randomised multicentre study. *Lancet* 1999;354:701–707.

83. Antman EM, Cohen M, Radley D, et al. Assessment of the treatment effect of enoxaparin for unstable angina/non–Q-wave myocardial infarction. TIMI 11B-ESSENCE meta-analysis. *Circulation* 1999;100:1602–1608.

84. Mark DB, Cowper PA, Berkowitz S, et al. Economic assessment of low molecular weight heparin (enoxaparin) versus unfractionated heparin in acute coronary syndrome patients: results from the ESSENCE randomized trial. *Circulation* 1998;97:1702–1707.

85. The GUSTO IV-ACS Investigators. Effect of glycoprotein IIb/IIIa receptor blocker abciximab on outcome in patients with acute coronary syndromes without early coronary revascularisation: the GUSTO IV-ACS randomised trial. *Lancet* 2001;357(9272):1915–1924.

86. Platelet Receptor Inhibition in Ischemic Syndrome Management (PRISM) Study Investigators. A comparison of aspirin plus tirofiban with aspirin plus heparin for unstable angina. *N Engl J Med* 1998;338:1498–1505.

87. Platelet Receptor Inhibition in Ischemic Syndrome Management in Patients Limited by Unstable Signs and Symptoms (PRISM-PLUS) Study Investigators. Inhibition of the platelet glycoprotein IIb/IIIa receptor with tirofiban in unstable angina and non–Q-wave myocardial infarction. *N Engl J Med* 1998;338:1488–1497.

88. PURSUIT Trial Investigators. Platelet glycoprotein IIb/IIIa in unstable angina: receptor suppression using Integrilin therapy. Inhibition of platelet glycoprotein IIb/IIIa with eptifibatide in patients with acute coronary syndromes. *N Engl J Med* 1998;339:436–443.

89. Mark DB, Harrington RA, Lincoff AM, et al. Cost effectiveness of platelet glycoprotein IIb/IIIa inhibition with eptifibatide in patients with non-ST elevation acute coronary syndromes. *Circulation* 2000;101:366–371.

90. American Heart Association. *Heart and stroke statistical update. 2000.* Dallas: American Heart Association, 2001.

91. Wennberg JE, Freeman JL, Shelton RM, et al. Hospital use and mortality among Medicare beneficiaries in Boston and New Haven. *N Engl J Med* 1989;321:1168–1173.

92. Verrilli DK, Welch G. The impact of diagnostic testing on therapeutic interventions. *JAMA* 1996;275:1189–1191.

93. Chassin MR, Kosecoff J, Park RE, et al. Does inappropriate use explain geographic variations in the use of health care services? A study of three procedures. *JAMA* 1987;258:2533–2537.

94. McGlynn EA, Naylor CD, Anderson GM, et al. Comparison of the appropriateness of coronary angiography and coronary artery bypass graft surgery between Canada and New York State. *JAMA* 1994;272(12):934–940.

95. Hux JE, Naylor CD, the Steering Committee of the Provincial Adult Cardiac Care Network of Ontario. Are the marginal returns of coronary artery surgery smaller in high-rate areas? *Lancet* 1996;348:1202–1207.

96. Wong JB, Sonnenberg FA, Salem DN, et al. Myocardial revascularization for chronic stable angina: an analysis of the role of percutaneous transluminal coronary angioplasty based on data available in 1989. *Ann Intern Med* 1990;113:852–871.

97. Lincoff AM, Mark DB, Tcheng JE, et al. Economic assessment of platelet glycoprotein IIb/IIIa receptor blockade with abciximab and low-dose heparin during percutaneous coronary revascularization: results from the EPILOG randomized trial. Evaluation in PTCA to improve long-term outcome with abciximab GP IIb/IIIa blockade. *Circulation* 2000;102:2923–2929.

98. Heidenreich PA, Chou TM, Amidon TM, et al. Impact of the operating physician on costs of percutaneous transluminal coronary angioplasty. *Am J Cardiol* 1996;77:1169–1173.

99. Mark DB, Gardner LH, Nelson CL, et al. Long-term costs of therapy for CAD: a prospective comparison of coronary angioplasty, coronary bypass surgery and medical therapy in 2258 patients. *Circulation* 1993;88[Pt 2]:I-480.

100. Hlatky MA, Rogers WJ, Johnstone I, et al. Medical care costs and quality of life after randomization to coronary angioplasty or coronary bypass surgery. *N Engl J Med* 1997;336:92–99.

101. Ellis SG, Miller DP, Brown KJ, et al. In-hospital costs of percutaneous coronary revascularization: critical determinants and implications. *Circulation* 1995;92:741–747.

102. Topol EJ, Ellis SG, Cosgrove DM, et al. Analysis of coronary angioplasty practice in the United States with an insurance-claims data base. *Circulation* 1993;87(5):1489–1497.

103. Reeder GS, Krishan I, Nobrega FT, et al. Is percutaneous coronary angioplasty less expensive than bypass surgery? *N Engl J Med* 1984;311:1157–1162.

104. Reeder GS. Angioplasty and the cost of myocardial revascularization: has its promise been fulfilled? *Int J Cardiol* 1987;15:287–292.

105. Topol EJ, Mark DB, Lincoff AM, et al. Outcomes at 1 year and economic implications of platelet glycoprotein IIb/IIIa blockade in patients undergoing coronary stenting: results from a multicentre randomised trial. *Lancet* 1999;354:2019–2024.

106. Shook TL, Sun GW, Burstein S, et al. Comparison of percutaneous transluminal coronary angioplasty outcome and hospital costs for low-volume and high-volume operators. *Am J Cardiol* 1996;77:331–336.

107. Cowper PA, Delong ER, Peterson ED, et al. Geographic variation in resource use for coronary artery bypass surgery. *Med Care* 1997;35:320–333.

108. Smith LR, Milano CA, Molter BS, et al. Preoperative determinants of postoperative costs associated with coronary artery bypass graft surgery. *Circulation* 1994;90:II-124–II-128.

109. Mauldin PD, Weintraub WS, Becker ER. Predicting hospital costs for first-time coronary artery bypass grafting from preoperative and postoperative variables. *Am J Cardiol* 1994;74:772–775.

110. Westaby S, Benetti FJ. Less invasive coronary surgery: consensus from the Oxford meeting. *Ann Thorac Surg* 1996;62:924–931.

111. Fonger JD, Nicholson CF, Sussman MS, et al. Cost analysis of current therapies for limited coronary artery revascularization. *Circulation* 1996;94:324A.

112. Parisi AF, Folland ED, Hartigan P. A comparison of angioplasty with medical therapy in the treatment of single-vessel coronary artery disease. *N Engl J Med* 1992;326:10–16.

113. Pocock SJ, Henderson RA, Clayton T, et al. Quality of life after coronary angioplasty or continued medical treatment for angina: three-year follow-up in the RITA-2 trial. Randomized intervention treatment of angina. *J Am Coll Cardiol* 2000;35:907–914.

114. Pepine CJ, Mark DB, Bourassa MG, et al. Cost estimates for treatment of cardiac ischemia [from the Asymptomatic Cardiac Ischemia Pilot (ACIP) study]. *Am J Cardiol* 1999;84:1311–1316.

115. King SB III, Lembo NJ, Weintraub WS, et al. A randomized trial comparing coronary angioplasty with coronary bypass surgery. *N Engl J Med* 1994;331:1044–1050.

116. Weintraub WS, Mauldin PD, Becker E, et al. A comparison of the costs of and quality of life after coronary angioplasty or coronary surgery for multivessel coronary disease: results from the Emory Angioplasty versus Surgery Trial (EAST). *Circulation* 1995;92:2831–2840.

117. Weintraub WS, Becker ER, Mauldin PD, et al. Costs of revascularization over eight years in the randomized and eligible patients in the Emory Angioplasty versus Surgery Trial (EAST). *Am J Cardiol* 2000;86:747–752.

118. The BARI Investigators. Comparison of coronary bypass surgery with angioplasty in patients with multivessel disease. *N Engl J Med* 1996;335:217–225.

119. Sculpher MJ, Seed P, Henderson RA, et al. Health service costs of coronary angioplasty and coronary artery bypass surgery: the Randomised Intervention Treatment of Angina (RITA) trial. *Lancet* 1994;344:927–930.

120. Peterson ED, Lansky AJ, Anstrom KJ, et al. Evolving trends in interventional device use and outcomes: results from the National Cardiovascular Network database. *Am Heart J* 2000;139:198–207.

121. Serruys PW, de Jaegere P, Kiemeneij F, et al. A comparison of balloon-expandable-stent implantation with balloon angioplasty in patients with coronary artery disease. *N Engl J Med* 1994;331(8):489–495.

122. Pepine CJ, Holmes DR, Block PC, et al. ACC expert consensus document: coronary artery stents. *J Am Coll Cardiol* 1996;28:782–794.

123. Weaver WD, Reisman MA, Griffin JJ, et al. Optimum percutaneous transluminal coronary angioplasty compared with routine stent strategy trial (OPUS-1): a randomised trial. *Lancet* 2000;355:2199–2203.

124. Di Mario C, Moses JW, Anderson TJ, et al. Randomized comparison of elective stent implantation and coronary balloon angioplasty guided by online quantitative angiography and intracoronary Doppler. DESTINI Study Group (Doppler Endpoint Stenting International Investigation). *Circulation* 2000;102:2938–2944.

125. Serruys PW, van Hout B, Bonnier H, et al. Randomised comparison of implantation of heparin-coated stents with balloon angioplasty in selected patients with coronary artery disease (Benestent II). *Lancet* 1998;352:673–681.

126. Sukin CA, Baim DS, Caputo RP, et al. The impact of optimal stenting techniques on cardiac catheterization laboratory resource utilization and costs. *Am J Cardiol* 1997;79:275–280.

127. Peterson ED, Cowper PA, Delong ER, et al. Acute and long-term cost implications of coronary stenting. *J Am Coll Cardiol* 1999;33:1610–1618.

128. Serruys PW, Unger F, Sousa JE, et al. Comparison of coronary-artery bypass surgery and stenting for the treatment of multivessel disease. *N Engl J Med* 2001;344(15):1117–1124.

129. Smith WM. Epidemiology of congestive heart failure. *Am J Cardiol* 1985;55:3A–8A.

130. Krumholz HM, Parent EM, Tu N, et al. Readmission after hospitalization for congestive heart failure among Medicare beneficiaries. *Arch Intern Med* 1997;157:99–104.

131. Schulman KA, Buxton MJ, Glick H, et al. Results of the economic evaluation of the FIRST study: a multinational prospective economic evaluation. *Int J Tech Assess Health Care* 1996;12:698–713.

132. Rich MW, Beckham V, Wittenberg C, et al. A multidisciplinary intervention to prevent the readmission of elderly patients with congestive heart failure. *N Engl J Med* 1995;333:1190–1195.

133. Eisenstein EL, Yusuf S, Bourassa M, et al. What is the economic value of digoxin therapy in congestive heart failure patients? Results from the DIG trial. *Circulation* 2001 (in press).

134. Konstam MA, Dracup K, Baker DW, et al. Clinical practice guideline XI: heart failure: evaluation and care of patients with left-ventricular systolic dysfunction. AHCPR 1994;No. 94-0612.

135. Glick H, Cook J, Kinosian B, et al. Costs and effects of enalapril therapy in patients with symptomatic heart failure: an economic analysis of the Studies of Left Ventricular Dysfunction (SOLVD) treatment trial. *J Cardiac Failure* 1995;1:371–380.

136. Paul SD, Kuntz KM, Eagle KA, et al. Costs and effectiveness of angiotensin converting enzyme inhibition in patients with congestive heart failure. *Arch Intern Med* 1994;154:1143–1149.

137. McMurray J, Davie A. The pharmacoeconomics of ACE inhibitors in chronic heart failure. *PharmacoEconomics* 1996;9:188–197.

138. Kleber FX. Socioeconomic aspects of ACE inhibition in the secondary prevention in cardiovascular diseases. *Am J Hypertens* 1994;7:112S–116S.

139. van Hout BA, Wielink G, Bonsel GJ, et al. Effects of ACE inhibitors on heart failure in the Netherlands: a pharmacoeconomic model. *PharmacoEconomics* 1993;3:387–397.

140. Hart W, Rhodes G, McMurray J. The cost effectiveness of enalapril in the treatment of chronic heart failure. *Br J Med Econ* 1993;6:91–98.

141. Hjalmarson A, Goldstein S, Fagerberg B, et al. Effects of controlled-release metoprolol on total mortality, hospitalizations, and well-being in patients with heart failure: the Metoprolol CR/XL Randomized Intervention Trial in congestive heart failure (MERIT-HF). MERIT-HF Study Group. *JAMA* 2000;283:1295–1302.

142. CIBIS II Investigators. The Cardiac Insufficiency Bisoprolol Study II (CIBIS-II): a randomised trial. *Lancet* 1999;353:9–13.

143. A trial of the beta-blocker bucindolol in patients with advanced chronic heart failure. *N Engl J Med* 2001;344:1659–1667.

144. Delea TE, Vera-Llonch M, Richner RE, et al. Cost effectiveness of carvedilol for heart failure. *Am J Cardiol* 1999;83:890–896.

145. Jones RH. Is it time for a randomized trial of surgical treatment of ischemic heart failure? *J Am Coll Cardiol* 2001;37:1210–1213.

146. Bounous EP Jr, Mark DB, Pollock BG, et al. Surgical survival benefits for coronary disease patients with left ventricular dysfunction. *Circulation* 1988;78[Suppl I]:I151–I157.

147. Evans RW. Economic impact of mechanical cardiac assistance. *Prog Cardiovasc Dis* 2000;43:81–94.

148. Morales DL, Catanese KA, Helman DN, et al. Six-year experience of caring for forty-four patients with a left ventricular assist device at home: safe, economical, necessary. *J Thorac Cardiovasc Surg* 2000;119:251–259.

149. Rose EA, Moskowitz AJ, Packer M, et al. The REMATCH trial: rationale, design, and end points. Randomized evaluation of mechanical assistance for the treatment of congestive heart failure. *Ann Thorac Surg* 1999;67:723–730.

150. Rich MW, Gray DB, Beckham V, et al. Effect of a multidisciplinary intervention of medication compliance in elderly patients with congestive heart failure. *Am J Med* 1996;101:270–276.

151. Weinberger M, Oddone EZ, Henderson WG, for the Veterans Affairs Cooperative Study Group on Primary Care and Hospital Readmission. Does increased access to primary care reduce hospital readmissions? *N Engl J Med* 1996;334:1441–1447.

152. Philbin EF, Rocco TA, Lindenmuth NW, et al. The results of a randomized trial of a quality improvement intervention in the care of patients with heart failure. The MIS-CHF Study Investigators. *Am J Med* 2000;109:443–449.

153. West JA, Miller NH, Parker KM, et al. A comprehensive management system for heart failure improves clinical outcomes and reduces medical resource utilization. *Am J Cardiol* 1997;79:58–63.

154. Weinstein MC. Economics of prevention. The costs of prevention. *J Gen Intern Med* 1990;5[Suppl]:S89–S92.

155. Shepherd J, Cobbe SM, Ford I, et al. Prevention of coronary heart disease with pravastatin in men with hypercholesterolemia. *N Engl J Med* 1995;333:1301–1307.

156. Sacks FM, Pfeffer MA, Moye LA, et al. Cholesterol and Recurrent Events (CARE). *N Engl J Med* 1996;335:1001–1009.

157. Scandinavian Simvastatin Survival Study Group. Randomised trial of cholesterol lowering in 4444 patients with coronary heart disease: the Scandinavian Simvastatin Survival Study (4S). *Lancet* 1994;344:1383–1389.

158. Morris S, McGuire A, Caro J, et al. Strategies for the management of hypercholesterolaemia: a systematic review of the cost-effectiveness literature. *J Health Serv Res Policy* 1997;2:231–250.

159. Caro J, Klittich W, McGuire A, et al. International economic analysis of primary prevention of cardiovascular disease with pravastatin in WOSCOPS. West of Scotland Coronary Prevention Study. *Eur Heart J* 1999;20:263–268.

160. Prosser LA, Stinnett AA, Goldman PA, et al. Cost-effectiveness of cholesterol-lowering therapies according to selected patient characteristics. *Ann Intern Med* 2000;132:769–779.

161. Downs JR, Clearfield M, Weis S, et al. Primary prevention of acute coronary events with lovastatin in men and women with average cholesterol levels: results of AFCAPS/TexCAPS. Air Force/Texas Coronary Atherosclerosis Prevention Study. *JAMA* 1998;279:1615–1622.

162. Pedersen TR, Kjekshus J, Berg K, et al. Cholesterol lowering and the use of healthcare resources: results of the Scandinavian Simvastatin Survival Group. *Circulation* 1996;93:1796–1802.

163. Jonsson B, Johannesson M, Kjekshus J, et al. Cost-effectiveness of cholesterol lowering: results from the Scandinavian Simvastatin Survival Study (4S). *Eur Heart J* 1996;17:1001–1007.

164. Schwartz JS. Economics and cost-effectiveness in evaluating the value of cardiovascular therapies. Comparative economic data regarding lipid-lowering drugs. *Am Heart J* 1999;137:S97–S104.

165. Johannesson M, Jonsson B, Kjekshus J, et al. Cost effectiveness of simvastatin treatment to lower cholesterol levels in patients with coronary heart disease. *N Engl J Med* 1997;336:332–336.

166. Tsevat J, Kuntz KM, Orav EJ, et al. Cost-effectiveness of pravastatin therapy for survivors of myocardial infarction with average cholesterol levels. *Am Heart J* 2001;141:727–734.

167. Tsevat J. Impact and cost-effectiveness of smoking interventions. *Am J Med* 1992;93:43S–47S.

168. Cummings SR, Rubin SM, Oster G. The cost-effectiveness of counseling smokers to quit. *JAMA* 1989;261:75–79.

169. Oster G, Huse DM, Delea TE, et al. Cost-effectiveness of nicotine gum as an adjunct to physician's advice against cigarette smoking. *JAMA* 1986;256:1315–1318.

170. Krumholz HM, Cohen BJ, Tsevat J, et al. Cost-effectiveness of a smoking cessation program after myocardial infarction. *J Am Coll Cardiol* 1993;22:1697–1702.

171. Rigotti NA, McKool KM, Shiffman S. Predictors of smoking cessation after coronary artery bypass graft surgery: results of a randomized trial with 5-year follow-up. *Ann Intern Med* 1994;120:287–293.

172. Taylor CB, Houston-Miller N, Killen JD, et al. Smoking cessation after acute myocardial infarction: effects of a

nurse-managed intervention. *Ann Intern Med* 1990; 113:118–123.

173. Psaty BM, Smith NL, Siscovick DS, et al. Health outcomes associated with antihypertensive therapies used as first-line agents: a systematic review and meta-analysis. *JAMA* 1997;277:739–745.

174. Insua JT, Sacks HS, Lau TS, et al. Drug treatment of hypertension in the elderly: a meta-analysis. *Ann Intern Med* 1994;121:355–362.

175. Mulrow CD, Cornell JA, Herrera CR, et al. Hypertension in the elderly: implications and generalizability of randomized trials. *JAMA* 1994;272:1932–1938.

176. Neal B, MacMahon S, Chapman N. Effects of ACE inhibitors, calcium antagonists, and other blood-pressure–lowering drugs: results of prospectively designed overviews of randomised trials. Blood Pressure Lowering Treatment Trialists' Collaboration. *Lancet* 2000;356:1955–1964.

177. Pahor M, Psaty BM, Alderman MH, et al. Health outcomes associated with calcium antagonists compared with other first-line antihypertensive therapies: a meta-analysis of randomised controlled trials. *Lancet* 2000;356:1949–1954.

178. Weinstein MC, Stason WB. *Hypertension: a policy perspective*. Cambridge, MA: Harvard University Press, 1976.

179. Littenberg B, Garber AM, Sox HC Jr. Screening for hypertension. *Ann Intern Med* 1990;112:192–202.

180. Edelson JT, Weinstein MC, Tosteson AN, et al. Long-term cost-effectiveness of various initial monotherapies for mild to moderate hypertension. *JAMA* 1990;263:407–413.

181. Littenberg B. A practice guideline revisited: screening for hypertension. *Ann Intern Med* 1995;122:937–939.

182. Massie BM. Analyses of cost effectiveness in the management of essential hypertension: what they can and what they do not teach us. *Clin Cardiol* 1996;19:810–816.

183. Hatziandreu EI, Koplan JP, Weinstein MC, et al. A cost-effectiveness analysis of exercise as a health promotion activity. *Am J Public Health* 1988;78:1417–1421.

184. O'Connor GT, Buring JE, Yusuf S, et al. An overview of randomized trials of rehabilitation with exercise after myocardial infarction. *Circulation* 1989;80:234–244.

185. Oldridge NB, Guyatt GH, Fischer ME, et al. Cardiac rehabilitation after myocardial infarction: combined experience of randomized clinical trials. *JAMA* 1988;260:945–950.

186. Dennis C, Houston-Miller N, Schwartz RG, et al. Early return to work after uncomplicated myocardial infarction. Results of a randomized trial. *JAMA* 1988;260:214–220.

187. Picard MH, Dennis C, Schwartz RG, et al. Cost-benefit analysis of early return to work after uncomplicated acute myocardial infarction. *Am J Cardiol* 1989;63:1308–1314.

188. Oldridge N, Furlong W, Feeny D, et al. Economic evaluation of cardiac rehabilitation soon after acute myocardial infarction. *Am J Cardiol* 1993;72:154–161.

189. Haskell WL, Alderman EL, Fair JM, et al. Effects of intensive multiple risk factor reduction on coronary atherosclerosis and clinical cardiac events in men and women with coronary artery disease: the Stanford Coronary Risk Intervention Project (SCRIP). *Circulation* 1994;89:975–990.

190. Superko HR. Sophisticated primary and secondary atherosclerosis prevention is cost effective. *Can J Cardiol* 1995;11:35–1140.

191. DeBusk RF, Miller NH, Superko R, et al. A case-management system for coronary risk factor modification after acute myocardial infarction. *Ann Intern Med* 1994;120:721–729.

192. Miller NH, Warren D, Myers D. Home-based cardiac rehabilitation and lifestyle modification: the MULTIFIT model. *J Cardiovasc Nurs* 1996;11:76–87.

193. Antiplatelet Trialist's Collaboration. Collaborative overview of randomized trials of antiplatelet therapy. I. Prevention of death, myocardial infarction, and stroke by prolonged antiplatelet therapy in various categories of patients. *BMJ* 1994;308:81–106.

194. Krumholz HM, Radford MJ, Ellerbeck EF, et al. Aspirin for secondary prevention after acute myocardial infarction in the elderly: prescribed use and outcomes. *Ann Intern Med* 1996;124:292–298.

195. Goldman L, Sia STB, Cook EF, et al. Costs and effectiveness of routine therapy with long-term beta-adrenergic antagonists after acute myocardial infarction. *N Engl J Med* 1988;319:152–157.

196. Tsevat J, Duke D, Goldman L, et al. Cost-effectiveness of captopril therapy after myocardial infarction. *J Am Coll Cardiol* 1995;26:914–919.

197. Franzosi MG, Maggioni AP, Santoro E, et al. for the GISSI-3 trial. Cost-effectiveness analysis of an early lisinopril use in patients with acute myocardial infarction: results from GISSI-3 trial. *J Am Coll Cardiol* 1997;29:49A.

198. Goldman L. Cost-effective strategies in cardiology. In: Braunwald E, ed. *Heart disease: a textbook of cardiovascular medicine*. Philadelphia: WB Saunders, 1992:1694–707.

44

DATABASES IN CARDIOLOGY

MICHAEL S. LAUER
EUGENE H. BLACKSTONE

▼▼ ADDITIONAL ELECTRONIC TOPICS

Types of Database Elements i19;   Data Dictionaries and Metadata i20;   Database Standards i21;   Coding Systems i22;   Data Exchange i23;   Database Management Systems i24;   Data Quality i25;   Missing Data i26;   Methods of Dealing with Missing Data i27;   Data Credibility i28;   Risk Adjustment and Measurement of Case Mix i29;   Overcoming Bias i30;   Incorporating Guidelines into Clinical Databases i31;   Survival Analyses i32;   Modern Multivariable Techniques i33;   Duke Databank for Cardiovascular Disease i34;

OVERVIEW

A clinical database is a systematic collection of observations related to patients and/or clinical processes. With the advent of relatively inexpensive and sophisticated computer technology, databases can be used for information retrieval, case finding, description of cohorts, and predictive modeling of outcomes and risks. Databases are increasingly being used for a process known as *outcomes management*, or technology of experience. According to outcomes management, predefined standards and coding systems are used to describe systematically all patients and outcomes encountered. Large databases are then used to identify variances in outcome that may be related to processes in patient care. Although this process is potentially very powerful for identifying and improving deficiencies in patient care, it suffers from a number of inherent methodologic difficulties.

Databases in cardiology have been developed and described in five major settings: (a) population-based studies, such as the Framingham Heart Study, which are used to describe risk factors for and the natural history of cardiovascular disease in the community; (b) disease-oriented registries, which describe care processes for and outcomes of patients with specific problems, such as acute myocardial infarction; (c) procedure- or technology-oriented registries; (d) government-mandated and administrational databases; and (e) registries derived from randomized clinical trials.

M. S. Lauer: Department of Cardiovascular Medicine, The Cleveland Clinic Foundation, Cleveland, Ohio
E. H. Blackstone: Department of Thoracic and Cardiovascular Surgery, The Cleveland Clinic Foundation, Cleveland, Ohio

Newer database technologies, including the development of object-oriented databases, along with the computerized medical record, represent means by which clinical database methods can be incorporated into routine clinical care.

GLOSSARY

American Standard Code for Information Interchange (ASCII): A code representing English characters and numbers with each letter assigned a number from 0 to 127 (7-bit ASCII) or 0 to 255 (8-bit ASCII) that is independent of machine (computer) and operating systems. A more universal standard is ISO Latin-1, used on the World Wide Web.

Attributional validity: Whether an apparent association between a variable and an outcome reflects reality as opposed to confounding by an unknown or unconsidered covariate.

Case-control study: A study design in which patients with and without a certain outcome are identified and then compared with respect to an exposure variable of interest.

Case-mix adjustment: Identifying and controlling for patient-specific factors over which physicians and health care institutions have no control and that may explain variances in outcome.

Categorical variable: A variable that can have only a finite set of values.

Clinical model concept: A model whereby outcomes are related to patients factors, physician plan factors, and hospital execution factors.

Coding system: A system for describing outcomes, clinical findings, and therapies according to a standardized format (e.g., Current Procedural Terminology; International Classification of Diseases, Ninth Revision, Clinical Modification; Systemized Nomenclature of Medicine).

Cohort study: A study design in which a population cohort is prospectively defined and divided according to the presence or absence of an exposure variable of interest and then followed over time for the occurrence of prespecified outcomes.

Colinearity: Spurious associations or lack of associations in a multivariable model due to excessive correlation of covariates with one another.

Computerized patient record: A type of clinical database in which an electronic medium is used to capture, process, analyze, and retrieve values for variables representing the entire clinical process.

Content validity: Appropriate and complete selection of covariates in a predictive model.

Continuous variable: A variable that can have an infinite set of values.

Cox proportional hazards model: A multivariable model that relates the log of the unspecified hazard function ratio between groups of patients to a linear equation.

Data dictionary: A set of uniform definitions for data elements.

Data element: A specific piece of organized information about a person or event.

Database design: A model according to which data elements are linked logically to one another.

Database management system: A set of computer programs that manage access to, modification of, and analyses of a database.

Database standards: Agreed-on methods for defining terms and interfaces, thus allowing cross-communication between databases.

Extensible Markup Language (XML): A formal, concise, human-legible machine (computer)- and operating system–independent language that describes both data entities (objects) and the behavior of computer programs (XML Processor) to understand and present them. This is achieved through markup, which encodes (tags) a description of the entity's storage layout and logical structure.

External Data Representation (XDR): A standard for describing and encoding data in a fashion that is machine (computer)- and operating system–independent. It uses a language to describe data formats (structure) and has been particularly useful in exchange of so-called binary data (data, such as real numbers, that are not human-readable).

Face validity: The clinical sense of a prediction model—that is, the model makes sense given current understanding.

Field: A placeholder for a specific value regarding a person or event; synonymous with *variable*.

Flatfile: A single data table that contains columns representing variables and rows representing bases of observations, for example, individuals. The table has no structural information about the data values themselves.

Hazard function: The instantaneous risk of a time-related event.

Hierarchical database: A database model based on a nested root-subordinate segment structure.

Interaction: Also known as *effect modification* or *modulation*; a situation in which the strength of association between one variable and an outcome is affected by another variable; to be distinguished from confounding, in which an association between a variable and an outcome is only a reflection of the association between another variable with the index variable and with outcome.

Internet: A complex system of worldwide interacting computer networks.

Logistic regression model: A multivariable prediction model in which the log of the odds of a time-fixed outcome event is related to a linear equation.

Metadata: Data about data—that is, information describing other data. Metadata in one context may be data in another, in effect metadata describing metadata. In a database context, metadata is usually considered the structural information associated with both data and the database organization.

Object-oriented database: A database model in which complex data structures (objects) are used that consist of both values for variables and instructions for operations to be performed on the data.

Outcomes management: A process by which clinical processes and outcomes are recorded systematically in large databases and then analyzed to detect variances in outcome that can be improved by altering those processes.

Overfitting: Using too many covariates for the number of outcome events in a multivariable predictive model; can lead to spurious or incorrect associations.

Predictive modeling: A process by which a clinical database is used to describe mathematically the likelihood of outcome events, given a set of values for variables of a new patient.

Predictive validity: How well a multivariable predictive model predicts outcome in a database separate from the one from which the model was derived.

Relational database: A database model that consists of multiple cross-referenced tables that can be linked together by set(s) of user-defined "linking variables" and queried using Structured Query Language.

Reliability: Reproducibility or stability of data measures.

Semistructured data: Complex data elements whose contextual structures are embedded along with the values for variables, rather than being dependent on an external data structure. As such, the data elements are simultaneously independent self-defining entities and self-organizing given a specific query.

Spreadsheet: A table of values arranged in rows and columns in which values at row-column intersections (called *cells*) can have predefined relationships with other cells. Data structure accompanies the spreadsheet.

Time-oriented database: A database model in which time is the organizing theme to facilitate temporal reasoning based on temporal attributes (duration) and temporal relations to other data (temporal order).

Validity: How well a data element or predictive model reflects what is really supposed to be measured or predicted.

World Wide Web: A technology by which access to the Internet is made easy by use of graphical hypertext-linked interfaces.

INTRODUCTION

In the late 1940s and early 1950s, epidemiologists from the U.S. Public Health Service and academic cardiologists and internists in the Boston area collaborated to develop a population-based database of cardiovascular disease in Framingham, Mass. (1,2). The early development of the Framingham Heart Study database was fraught with difficulties (3): Methods of population sampling were not well developed, the natural history of coronary artery disease (CAD) was poorly understood, the clinical manifestations of CAD were known to only partially reflect pathologic events, the modern "computer era" had not yet begun, and modern biostatistical science was in its infancy. Nonethe-

less, the investigators successfully assembled a cohort of more than 5,000 adults who have now been systematically followed for nearly 50 years (1); later in the 1970s, a new cohort based on the offspring and spouses of offspring of the original cohort was assembled and continues to be followed (4). Numerous analyses of the characteristics and outcomes of the participants in the Framingham Heart and Offspring studies have yielded invaluable insights into the risk factors, pathogenesis, and natural history of cardiovascular disease (5); the Framingham and other population-based databases continue to be fruitful sources for cardiovascular investigators today (6–14).

The Framingham Heart Study is illustrative of many of the attributes of a successful database (15). The database was assembled and continues to be maintained by a large, multidisciplinary team with involvement of clinicians, classic epidemiologists, computer engineers, and biostatisticians; they have been able to depend on adequate and stable funding. The goals of the database were well-defined, leading to high-quality, focused data collection. Efforts have been consistently made to keep the database relevant, with appropriate addition, alteration, and deletion of data fields as new technologies and understanding of disease processes change the questions that investigators wish to answer. Finally, and perhaps most important, dynamic and strong leaders have championed the development, implementation, use, and analyses of the database as well as publicly advocated its benefits.

With the advent of the computer, large databases became possible in clinical environments as well. Early examples of clinical databases included the Duke Databank for Cardiovascular Disease (16), which was established in 1969, and the Coronary Artery Surgery Study database (17). Today, clinical databases have expanded into multiple areas of practice and investigation, presenting tremendous opportunities for improving knowledge about and care of patients with cardiovascular disease but also frustrating developers and users with numerous technical and inherent design problems.

This chapter reviews population-based and clinical databases, with particular attention to their applications in cardiology. The use of these databases for clinical investigation, quality assessment, and outcomes analyses are explored.

WHAT IS A DATABASE? DATABASE TECHNOLOGY, TERMS, AND DEFINITIONS

A clinical database is a systematic collection of facts about individual patients or clinical events (Table 44.1). Facts about a person or event might include, for example, last name, patient identifier, birth date, heart rate at the time of admission, or medications used.

Computer-based databases divide these facts into (a) what the fact is, which can be termed a *variable* or in specific

TABLE 44.1 BASIC CONCEPTS OF DATABASE CONSTRUCTION

Concept	Description	Types

Fields (variables)	Factor information about a particular subject or patient; requires data definitions (metadata)	Discrete (categorical)
		  Dichotomous (yes/no)
		  Ordinal (e.g., New York Heart Association functional class)
		  Polytomous (lists)
		Continuous

Management system	Computer programs that manage access to and use of databases	Multiple services required:
		  Data sharing
		  Consistency, error checks
		  Security
		  Protection and backup
		  Timeliness
		  Standards for entry
		  Query engine
		  Temporal attributes
		  Extensibility

Design	Model by which variables are logically linked to one another	Flatfile Spreadsheet Relational Object-oriented Time-oriented Semistructured
Focus	Orientation of developers and questions of interest	Disease Population Procedure/therapy/device Computerized patient record Values for variables of all health care–related data

contexts a *field* or *column name*; (b) the specific *value* for the variable for an individual patient; and (c) *structural* information, including the name of the data element, unique identifier for the data element, version, authorization information, language, definition, obligation (whether the data element is required or not), data type (e.g., numerical or character), limits (e.g., age cannot be less than 0 or more than 120), author (who or what obtained and recorded the information), time stamp, temporal attributes, and many other attributes of the variable and value. All these properties of a clinical fact constitute a data element either implicitly in most traditional databases or explicitly in semistructured data.

A collection of data elements that relate to one specific person or clinical event constitutes a *patient record*. Thus, a clinical database can be thought of as a potentially limitless collection of patient records consisting of data elements. In the simplest database designs, the patient record may constitute a single row in a table, with one or more columns of variables containing data for that patient.

Focuses of Clinical Databases

Clinical databases can have one of two primary focus types: (a) disease- or population-oriented or (b) procedure-, ther-

apy-, or device-specific (15). Both of these types of databases are used in cardiology. The Framingham Heart Study, the Nurses' Health Study (18), the Cardiovascular Health Study (19), and a hospital-based computerized patient record are examples of population-oriented databases. The Duke Databank for Cardiovascular Disease (16) is a disease-oriented database that is focused primarily on CAD. The National Heart, Lung, and Blood Institute angioplasty registry (20) and the Cardiac Transplant Research Database (21) are examples of procedure-oriented databases.

Structure and Content of Clinical Databases

Determination of the size, structure, and content of clinical databases has been a major source of frustration, in part because no standards for these existed before the modern computer age. Dolin points out that any database that is to be used for assessment of outcomes must contain information in three key areas: input, intervention, and outcome (25). Input data include demographics, family history, reproductive history, social history, types of episodes and encounters (e.g., ambulatory, emergency, critical care), signs and symptoms, diagnoses, and test results. Intervention data include information on medications, immunizations, operations, procedures, functional assessment, and socioeconomic assessment. Outcomes data include death, disability, discomfort, drug toxicity, and dollar costs; the last includes service costs, hospital days, and days of missed work. Some validated data already exist for assessing outcomes in specific situations; an example would be the Acute Physiology, Age, Chronic Health Evaluation III for analyses of outcomes in noncoronary critical care units (26). ▼ i35

Database Designs

A *database design* refers to the model that describes which data fields are logically linked to one another (41); the most commonly cited database designs are flatfile, spreadsheet, hierarchical, relational, and object-oriented. The simplest design is a single table of values called a *flatfile*. A flatfile is non–self-documenting, requiring a separate data dictionary to accompany the data file. The next simplest design is the spreadsheet. It is superior to the flatfile in containing not only self-documentation, such as column headings, but also in allowing in-place associations to be established among the data cells themselves. A major limitation of flatfiles and spreadsheets is that they have primarily been proprietary products requiring either export in a more universal form or the definition of a software driver that permits direct communication.

One of the earliest database designs was the *hierarchical* model. This consisted of linkage of multiple collections of similar information into a tree structure, with a root and child nodes like branches and ending with leaf nodes. In effect this model acts as a collection of index cards in which each card has a small number of variables (e.g., demographics) about one patient. A major disadvantage of this database design is that hierarchies are rather arbitrary. For example, one might think of the heart as the root of a hierarchy of the cardiovascular system. However, one could imagine it also in the domains of infectious disease (bacterial endocarditis), developmental disorders, neuroendocrine function, a hierarchy of surgical procedures, and many others. Thus, use of a single hierarchy rapidly becomes limiting. Today, hierarchical database models have been extended to polyhierarchical models, which are of interest in medical nomenclature.

A database model that ties together multiple tables of information provides more flexibility and is called a *relational model*. Relational databases allow for very efficient and powerful storage of large quantities of information (38,42). The multiple tables in a relational database are linked together by user-defined cross-references, or "linking variables" (Fig. 44.1). As an example, a database might be designed to contain a patient's name and the name of the primary physician. In a hierarchical or flatfile design, the name of the primary physician would have to be individually entered for each patient; thus, the names of physicians who care for more than one patient might have to be entered multiple times. A relational database would have a separate table with the names and characteristics of all primary physicians; thus, when it comes time for the user to enter the name of the primary physician, he or she can simply refer to the primary physician table and, using a "pick list," click the appropriate name. Data entry is therefore easier and of better quality. The relational database also allows one to modify a data element in one table with assurance that the same data element in other tables will be automatically updated without a need to alter programs that use the data.

Relational databases are, however, static repositories of data. Imagine a database that could note that an entered value for a glucose tolerance test was well above the normal range and therefore set into motion a predetermined sequence of activities, such as paging the physician, printing a diabetic diet based on patient characteristics, discovering a clinical trial of pancreatic islet transplantation, or a host of other functions. This is possible in *object-oriented* databases. Objects contain not only data, but also *instructions* as to what might be done with them given that certain data values are present. A major modern challenge in clinical database technology has been to define an object model of medicine and all its accompanying behaviors. ⚐ i36

WHAT ARE THE USES OF CLINICAL DATABASES?

Fundamental Uses of Clinical Databases

As described by Safran (63), there are four fundamental uses of clinical databases: (a) results reporting, (b) case finding, (c) cohort description, and (d) predictive modeling. *Results reporting* refers to the ability to retrieve information about a specific patient or procedure; this is the type of activity by which practicing clinicians would most often interact with, or at least "seek rewards" from, a clinical data repository. Case finding involves looking for patients with similar problems or outcomes as a patient of interest, often to direct management based on prior individual experiences. Cohort description seeks to simply describe a group of patients or procedures based on a common set of attributes. Finally, prediction modeling involves applying sophisticated analytical methods to describe changes or associations that can lend insight into the natural history of disease processes, the effects of different clinical interventions, and/or quality of care within given institutions or by specific providers. It is this use of databases that presents the most powerful, and perhaps also the most controversial, benefit of computerized clinical information technology.

Case for Outcomes Management

In the 1988 Shattuck Lecture to the Annual Meeting of the Massachusetts Medical Society, Paul Ellwood advocated the nationwide adoption of outcomes management, which he described as a new "technology of patient experience" (27). Work by Wennberg and others (64–66), which showed tremendous variation of practice patterns without clear differences in patient outcome, has caused the public and third-party payers to demand better-quality information by which the clinical effectiveness of various interventions and providers can be systematically studied. Practice variation is a ubiquitous problem in medicine; within cardiology, recent evaluations of the Global Utilization of Streptokinase and Tissue Plasminogen Activator for Occluded Coronary Arteries database, for example, have revealed marked

ID#	Lastname	Age	Gender	Physician
22005	Jones	45	M	Lauer
22006	Smith	52	F	Fortin

ID#	PCW	PAS	PAD
22005	23	62	27
22006	12	25	13

Physician	Gender	Institution
Lauer	M	Cleveland Clinic
Fortin	M	Duke University

FIGURE 44.1 Schematic of a relational database. Tables are linked to one another by linking variables (in this case, ID# and Physician). Data entry of "Physician" into the first table is made easy by linking to data available in the third table.

geographic variation of management of postinfarct patients within the United States and among countries (67–69), with varying differences in clinical outcomes. In addition to patients and payers, physicians too are frustrated by their inability to accurately and quantitatively predict the impact of their care on patient outcomes, as good-quality data from randomized controlled trials simply do not exist for many common clinical scenarios (70). To help solve these problems, the process of outcomes management would seek to use high-quality data based on real patient experiences to help physicians, payers, and patients make the most rational choices.

Ellwood described four processes by which outcomes management occurs (*e*Table 44.1.2): (a) adoption of database standards and clinical guidelines; (b) routine systematic measurements of patient outcomes at appropriate times (or follow-up); (c) pooling of clinical, outcome, and financial data into enormous databases; and (d) careful analyses and dissemination of results of these analyses to appropriate parties.

The enormous databases to be used in the outcomes management process may be organized according to the *clinical model concept* (Fig. 44.2), as described by Steen (71). This model divides clinical encounters into four sets of data elements: (a) patient factors, (b) physician plan, (c) hospital execution, and (d) outcome measures. Patient factors are extremely important to recognize and codify properly, as they represent variables that are related to outcome but over which providers have little or no control. These include specific disease entities, comorbidities, socioeconomic background, compliance, and satisfaction. The physician plan has two major components, namely, an assessment of diagnostic probabilities and an assessment of the urgency of action needed to address them. Between the physician plan and outcomes are hospital execution factors; no matter how excellent a physician's assessment and plan are, if hospital systems fail to respond to them in an efficient and timely way, adverse outcomes may result. For example, an emergency room physician may quickly and accurately diagnose acute myocardial infarction and appropriately prescribe thrombolysis, but if pharmacy, transport, and clerical staff are not properly organized, there may still be significant delays in implementing therapy. Outcome measures include not only standard mortality and morbidity measures, but also "softer" end points such as quality of life and costs of care.

Analyses of enormous databases can be used to achieve a number of objectives (72). These include assessment of patient risk based on clinical characteristics and medical test results, risk-adjustment assessment of quality of care, postmarketing drug surveillance, assessment of resource consumption, analyzing and improving clinical decision making, identifying and correcting variations in physician practice, and aiding in collaborative clinical research projects.

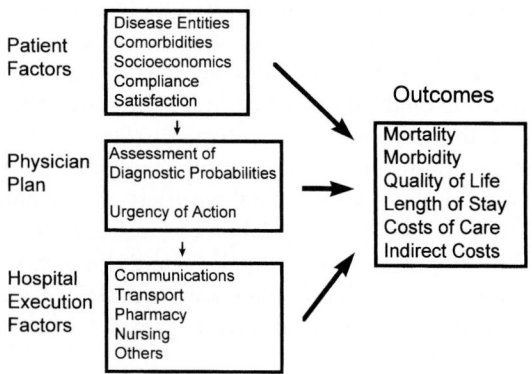

FIGURE 44.2 The clinical concept model. Patient factors, physician plan, and hospital execution factors all play a role in determining patient outcomes.

Why Not Just Use Randomized Controlled Trials to Determine Clinical Effectiveness? Bias and Unexplained Confounders

A major component of outcomes management is determination, based on analyses of large observational clinical databases, of how outcomes are associated with physician plan and hospital execution factors after "adjusting for" patient factors. Some have argued, though, that using observational databases to assess the impacts of therapies or behaviors under physician or patient control is inherently flawed and that randomized trials can appropriately answer these questions (73). This belief is held so strongly that one major textbook on clinical epidemiology (74) recently stated, "If you find that a study was not randomized, we'd suggest that you stop reading it and go on to the next article." Indeed, today the randomized controlled trial is considered by many to be the gold standard method of assessing the relative impact of different therapies.

The main strengths of randomized controlled trials are reviewed by Moses (75): (a) assembly of a single, well-defined inception cohort; (b) elimination of potential biases and confounding, particularly those caused by unknown or unmeasurable factors; and (c) adherence to well-defined clinical care and data collection protocols with vigorous quality assurance and safety mechanisms in place. However, as reviewed by Califf (76), clinical trials suffer from several inherent limitations: (a) they are expensive and sometimes very time-consuming; (b) therapies change such that by the time trial results are reported, new technologies become available that may replace the methods used; (c) many patients, particularly those with comorbidities or the elderly, are excluded; (d) trials are performed more often in patients at tertiary referral centers, raising generalizability questions; and (e) the benefits of a therapy as noted in the ideal conditions of a clinical trial may not necessarily apply to the "real world" of clinical care. Furthermore, some clinical treatment questions simply cannot be answered with randomized trials. For example, a study found that a prolonged door-to-balloon time was associated with a higher mortality among patients undergoing primary angioplasty for acute myocardial infarction (77). It is difficult to imagine that the validity of this finding could be tested by a controlled trial in which patients would be randomized to an immediate versus a delayed angioplasty (70).

Causes of Bias

Although some have found that analyses of clinical databases can lead to conclusions that are consistent with those from presumably unbiased randomized clinical trials (78–80), the presence of bias remains a major impediment to the widespread acceptance of clinical databases as a valid source of insights on clinical effectiveness (73,75,81). There are many potential reasons for bias. Data that are systematically missing because of patient or condition-specific reasons can lead to serious misinterpretations, as described above. Patients who visit a given health facility less frequently because they are less ill or because they "shop around" for care may have fewer data available (27). Patients may be selected for treatment or interventions for reasons that, no matter how ostensibly comprehensive a database is, are simply not adequately captured. For example, some patients may not receive therapies because they are "too sick," making it appear that healthier patients do worse than they really do after undergoing those therapies. Definitions of disease and the nature of therapies are often unstable over time, making comparisons between time eras difficult (82). For example, both medical and surgical therapies for CAD have changed dramatically over the past 15 to 20 years, making comparisons between them problematic if assessed over long periods. Because of more intensive screening and treatment of coronary risk factors, some patients with milder forms of disease may be identified now, whereas they may have been missed in years past. Measurement bias may occur because patients in different groups have certain variables measured in different ways (83). ▼ i37

Randomized Trials and Observational Studies: Empirical Evidence

Even setting aside all the arguments that biases and confounding can be overcome, critics of treatment assessments based on observational analyses point to studies in which observational data inflated positive treatment effects when compared with randomized trials (79,104–108). These comparisons were based on studies done in the 1970s and 1980s, when database technology and analytical methods were less developed than they are today. Benson and Hartz performed a systematic comparison of results of randomized trials and observational studies that were published between 1985 and 1998 (79). Figure 44.3 shows their analyses of cardiac treatments based on eight articles; in nearly all cases, randomized trials and observational studies

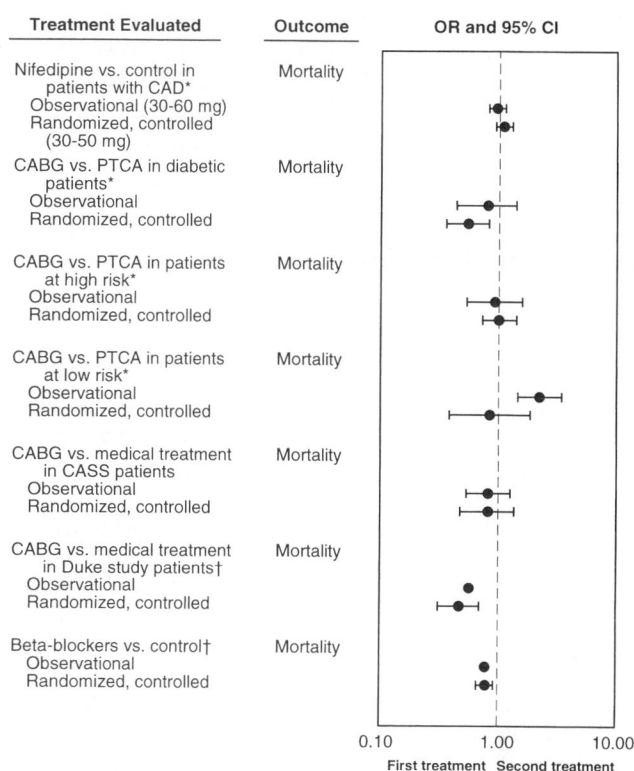

FIGURE 44.3 Results of observational studies and randomized, controlled trials of cardiologic treatments. The figure is based on data from eight articles. *, studies that reported relative risks rather than odds ratios; †, studies that reported neither a confidence interval nor a *p* value for the odds ratio; CABG, coronary artery bypass graft surgery; CAD, coronary artery disease; CASS, Coronary Artery Surgery Study; CI, confidence interval; Duke, Duke Databank for Cardiovascular Disease; OR, odds ratio; PTCA, percutaneous transluminal coronary angioplasty. [From Benson K, Hartz AJ. A comparison of observational studies and randomized, controlled trials (see comments). *N Engl J Med* 2000;342:1878–1886, with permission.]

yielded remarkably similar results. The one discrepant comparison involved low-risk patients undergoing bypass surgery or angioplasty; the authors suggested that the unusually low bypass surgery mortality rate in the randomized trial might have explained the difference.

A similar comparison of randomized trials and observational studies was also reported by Concato and colleagues (80). Based on published metaanalyses, they compared the results of 14 randomized trials and nine cohort observational studies that assessed the impact of treatment of hypertension on occurrence of coronary heart disease events. The randomized trials, which enrolled a total of 36,894 patients, found a positive treatment effect (risk ratio, 0.86; 95% confidence interval, 0.78 to 0.96). The cohort studies, which described a much larger patient sample of 418,343 patients, found a remarkably similar positive treatment effect (risk ratio, 0.77; 95% confidence interval, 0.75 to 0.80). Another comparison of 14 randomized trials and seven cohort studies that evaluated the impact of antihypertensives treatment on stroke again found remarkably similar positive treatment effects; for the randomized trials the risk ratio was 0.58 (95% confidence interval, 0.50 to 0.67), whereas for the cohort studies the risk ratio was 0.62 (95% confidence interval, 0.60 to 0.65).

ANALYTICAL METHODS

Univariable Methods

The fundamental goal of any data analysis is to describe an association between an exposure and an outcome. An exposure could be a treatment or a characteristic, such as cholesterol level, whereas an outcome could be mortality or morbidity or the result of a blood test.

Three analytical approaches are commonly used to establish associations between exposures and outcomes. In a *cohort study,* a group of patients is prospectively assembled and then classified according to the presence or absence of an exposure variable of interest, after which time the patients are followed for the occurrence of an outcome event. In a *case-control* study, patients are selected according to whether or not the outcome occurred and are then compared for the presence or absence of an exposure variable. In a *clinical trial,* a group of patients is assembled and then treatments assigned, typically by random allocation, after which patients are followed for the occurrence of outcome events. In reality, a clinical trial is a kind of cohort study.

When comparing continuous variables between two groups (e.g., blood pressure with and without treatment), commonly used statistical tests include the Student's *t* test when the variables are normally distributed (i.e., follow a gaussian bell-shape curve) and the Wilcoxon rank sum test when an assumption of normal distribution cannot be made. When three or more groups are being compared, the analogous tests are analysis of variance and the Kruskal-Wallis test. The purpose of these statistical tests is to determine whether any apparent association between the exposure and outcome are merely due to chance; the probability that the association is merely due to chance is expressed as the *p* value.

When comparing categoric variables, the commonly used statistical test is the chi-square test, which again determines whether an apparent association between an exposure and an outcome are due to chance. Often it is more helpful to describe the magnitude of difference between groups. This is done by calculating relative risk differences, absolute risk differences, number needed to treat to prevent one outcome event, and their confidence intervals (see Chapter 43).

Multivariable Methods

Analyses of large clinical databases usually involve multivariable regression techniques. Multivariable regressions are used to develop models by which outcomes can be pre-dicted or to evaluate the impact of particular variables of interest on outcome after considering potential confounding or interaction from other variables. The development of regression models includes four key steps (71): (a) population selection, (b) outcome selection, (c) type of regression, and (d) variable selection. Other critical aspects of model development include formal testing for goodness of fit and validity as well as assessment for possible interactions (132).

The type of regression model chosen depends in large part on the outcome variable of interest. Many analyses are interested in binary outcomes such as death, occurrence of a major nonfatal cardiac event, or readmission to the hospital within a given time. If the outcome is time-independent (e.g., in-hospital mortality, readmission any time within 30 days), then logistic regression is the most common type of model chosen (133). The logistic model seeks to predict outcomes according to a linear equation:

$$\log \text{Odds}_{event} = \alpha + \beta_1 x_1 + \beta_2 x_2 + \beta_3 x_3 + \ldots + \beta_i x_i$$

where

$\text{Odds} = (\text{probability}_{event})/(1 - \text{probability}_{event})$,
α = y-intercept,
$x_1, x_2, x_3, \ldots, x_i$ are variables chosen for the model (e.g., age, gender, number of diseased coronary arteries), and
$\beta_1, \beta_2, \beta_3, \ldots, \beta_i$ are "parameter coefficients," which are estimates based on examination of the data relating each variable to the $\log \text{Odds}_{event}$ after adjusting for all other covariates.

Logistic regression modeling consists of estimating values and standard errors of parameter coefficients based on observed outcomes in a selected data set. Although much of the work of modeling is performed by computers using powerful statistics packages (e.g., PROC LOGISTIC of the SAS System, Cary, NC), the validity of the models developed depend largely on appropriate model specification and variable selection by the investigators. Models can be built in a number of ways, including simple inclusion of all variables, forward or backward selection, and cluster analyses; the method of model building used can have a significant impact on results (134).

When the outcome is time-dependent, such as time free of death or major nonfatal cardiac events, survival analyses are used. The most popularly used multivariable model for survival outcomes is the Cox proportional hazards regression (135). The hazard function of an event describes the instantaneous risk of its occurrence. Cox proposed that if the ratio of the hazard functions between different groups (known as the *hazard ratio* or *relative risk*) can be assumed to remain constant over time, then the hazard ratio can be modeled:

$$\log [\text{Hazard}_{event}(x,t)/\text{Hazard}_{event}(0)] = \alpha + \beta_1 x_1 + \beta_i x_i + \beta_3 x_3 + \ldots + \beta_i x_i$$

where $\text{Hazard}_{event}(x,t)$ refers to the hazard function at time t given circumstances $(x_1, x_2, x_3, \ldots, x_i)$ and $\text{Hazard}_{event}(0)$ is the hazard function for a hypothetical patient where all x_1, x_2, x_3, . . . , x_i are equal to 0. Analogous to the logistic regression model, each parameter coefficient estimates the association between its associated variable and the log of the hazard ratio after adjusting for all other covariates considered. Also, models can be built according to forward and backward selection techniques. ⌖ i38

When the outcome of interest is a continuous variable, such as length of stay or cost of care, linear regression techniques are often used for predictive modeling:

$$\text{Outcome} = \alpha + \beta_1 x_1 + \beta_2 x_2 + \beta_3 x_3 + \ldots + \beta_i x_i$$

Linear regression models are derived using the "least squares technique," by which parameter estimates are derived that minimize the squares of the differences between actual and predicted outcome values.

Problems with Multivariable Models

Multivariable regression, when properly performed, allows for powerful analyses of large datasets. However, failure to consider inherent limitations and assumptions on which the models are built can lead to serious misinterpretation or invalid results (Table 44.2). Serious error can result from a number of problems: (a) model overfitting, (b) inappropriate use of a linear model, (c) violation of proportional hazards, (d) failure to test for interaction, (e) inappropriate variable selection techniques, (f) colinearity of variables, and (g) excessively influential observations (139). ⌖ i39

Interaction is an exceedingly important phenomenon that is often ignored. When the strength of association between an outcome and one particular variable is affected, the level of another variable, "effect modification," or interaction is present. For example, heparin dose is associated with risk of bleeding in most patients, but this association is much stronger in lower-weight patients than in obese patients. In this case, there is an interaction of body weight with heparin dose regarding the outcome of bleeding risk. Unlike confounding or bias, which potentially can invalidate an apparent association, interaction is of great clinical interest and should be actively sought by investigators when developing multivariate models. ⌖ i40

Model Validation Techniques

Even when the above problems are appropriately avoided or dealt with, multivariable models may still not be valid predictors of outcome. Several different types of validity need to be considered (60). *Face validity* refers to the clinical sense that a model has. For example, many models of risk of valve surgery do not include endocarditis as a covariate because in many series this is a relatively uncommon occurrence. Nonetheless, most surgeons would argue that endocarditis is an important predictor of outcome. *Content validity* depends on the appropriate and complete selection

TABLE 44.2 LIMITATIONS OF MULTIVARIABLE ANALYSES

Type of limitation	Description and possible solutions
Model overfitting	Too few outcome events for number of covariates
	Use no more than one covariate per ten events
Inappropriate linear assumption	Linear model incorrect
	Test with goodness-of-fit or examination of residuals
	Use nonlinear techniques or transformations
Violation of proportional hazards assumption	Ratio of hazard function between groups fails to remain constant over time
	Use hazards analyses
	Time interaction terms
	Divide into arbitrary time periods
Failure to account for interaction	One or more variables may modify the strength of association between outcome and another variable
	Incorporate interaction terms in analyses
Inappropriate variable selection	Forward and backward analyses may not reflect clinical reality
	Important covariates missing
	Consider sequential models, principal components/cluster analyses
Colinearity	Covariates closely associated with one another
	Test with variance inflation factors or cross-correlation matrices
Excessively influential observations	Formally test

of covariates that are related to outcome. Closely related to this is *attributional validity*, which relates to whether an apparent independent association between a variable and an outcome is really true or whether it is confounded by a covariate that was not considered in the model. Thus, different "risk-adjusted" outcomes among different operators may be real or may exist because not enough variables were considered for adequate risk adjustment.

Predictive validity refers to how well a model actually predicts outcome. Within the database studied, there are formal methods for testing the ability of a multivariate model to accurately discriminate high-risk subjects from low-risk subjects. For example, for a binary, time-independent outcome in a logistic regression model, the c-index, or area under the receiver operating characteristic curve, is often reported: A value of 1.0 implies perfect discrimination, whereas one of 0.5 is consistent with nothing better than random chance. Hosmer and Lemeshow (133) have derived a "goodness-of-fit" statistic that tests the validity of logistic models. The predictive validity of linear regression models can be measured using the model R^2 statistic: This reflects what proportion of the variance of the outcome variable can be explained by the variables included in the model. For example, many models of left ventricular mass in populations report R^2 values of well under 0.5, suggesting that many of the important determinants of this variable are either not known or not yet accurately measured.

Another dimension of predictive validity is how well a regression model predicts outcomes in datasets different from that upon which it was derived. For example, one can study a series of coronary interventions and come up with a prediction model of adverse events. To test the validity of the model, it can be used to predict the likelihood of events in a different set of patients. Some investigators will formally report results from "test sets" and "validation sets," which are two entirely different groups of patients from which multivariate predictive models are derived and then tested. There are also methods, such as the "jackknife" and "bootstrap," by which model derivation and validation can be performed on the same dataset (145).

DATABASES IN CARDIOLOGY

Many cardiology-oriented clinical databases have been developed and are actively used today. This section is not meant to be exhaustive; it provides a brief summary of how some of these databases have been developed and are being applied. Cardiology databases can be roughly divided into five major types: (a) population-based epidemiologic studies; (b) disease-oriented registries; (c) technology- and procedure-focused registries; (d) administrative, financial, and government-sanctioned databases that relate to cardiac issues; and (e) databases derived from randomized clinical trials (Table 44.3).

Population-Based Studies

Framingham Heart Study

The Framingham Heart and Offspring studies are prototypic population-based cardiovascular epidemiologic databases (1 to 5,156). The original cohort consisted of 5,209 adults between ages 18 and 62 years. Since the late 1940s this group has been invited back every 2 years for serial examinations that have consisted of a detailed medical history, physical examination, electrocardiogram, laboratory studies, and imaging studies. In the 1970s, offspring and spouses of the offspring of the original cohort formed a second group of approximately 7,000 adults for the Framingham Offspring Study. This group has been invited for follow-up examinations every 4 years. One of the major strengths of the study has been the nearly complete follow-up with high-quality descriptions of outcome events. Over the past few decades new technologies have been incorporated into the study, including echocardiography, exercise testing, Holter monitoring, heart rate variability analyses, carotid Doppler studies, and sophisticated genetic tests.

The concepts of risk factors, or characteristics that define high-risk subsets of populations initially free of disease, and multivariate risk formulation, according to which risk could be attributed to multiple risk factors, were first coined by Dawber and Kannel (156) and have been exten-

TABLE 44.3 EXAMPLES OF DATABASES IN CARDIOLOGY

Type of database	Examples
Population-based studies	Framingham Heart Study
	Physicians' Health Study
	Nurses' Health Study
	Cardiovascular Health Study
Disease-oriented registries	National Registries of Myocardial Infarction
	Minnesota Heart Survey
	Duke Databank for Cardiovascular Disease
Technology- and procedure-oriented registries	Cardiac Transplant Research Database
	United Network for Organ Sharing database
	National Heart, Lung, and Blood Institute registries on percutaneous transluminal angioplasty and new technologies
	Northern New England Cardiovascular Disease Study Group
	Surgeons' National Database
	Veterans' Affairs Cardiac Surgery Database
	The Cleveland Clinic Foundation Exercise Stress Laboratory Database
Administrative and abstracted based on administrative databases	New York State Cardiac Surgery Database
	Health Care Financing Administration Cardiovascular Care Project
	American College of Cardiology
Randomized clinical trial registries	Global Utilization of Streptokinase and Tissue Plasminogen Activator for Occluded Coronary Arteries trials
	Thrombolysis in Myocardial Ischemia trials
	Coronary Artery Surgery Study
	Scandinavian Simvastatin Survival Study

sively developed over several decades. Despite criticism of the epidemiologic method (157,158), work derived from the Framingham Heart Study database has formed the foundation for much of our understanding of the nature of atherosclerotic cardiovascular disease. The epidemiologic method continues to be a valid source of valuable insights in the 1990s, as evidenced, for example, by recent Framingham Heart Study work in the areas of lipid abnormalities (159), homocysteine metabolism (160), risk factor clustering (161), echocardiographic left ventricular mass (162), coronary heart disease risk prediction instruments (163), and mortality risks associated with atrial fibrillation (9,164). As an example of the ongoing power and relevance of the Framingham Heart Study, independent investigators recently found that the Framingham risk prediction instrument accurately identified absolute coronary heart disease risk in a cohort of British hypertensive men (165).

Physicians' and Nurses' Health Studies

The Physicians' Health Study was originally conceived as a randomized trial of aspirin and β-carotene for prevention of coronary heart disease events and cancer among 22,071 male physicians aged 40 to 84 years (164). The aspirin part of the trial was stopped prematurely due to a marked reduction in coronary events among those participants randomized to aspirin (166). However, the database derived from the Physicians' Health Study has been quite comprehensive and has been used to examine a number of issues, including the prognostic importance of endogenous tissue-type plasminogen activator (167), homocysteine (167), C-reactive protein (168), fibrinogen (169), ACE gene polymorphisms (170), adhesion molecules (171,172), and lipoprotein(a) (173).

The Nurses' Health Study was started in 1976 as a prospective study of 121,700 female registered nurses aged 30 to 55 years (174). A questionnaire was sent to the nurses covering information about age, weight, height, smoking, cardiac history, reproductive history, drug use, dietary and other lifestyle habits, and other factors. Every 2 years, subjects were sent a repeat questionnaire to update their data. The Nurses' Health Study database represents a very large population sample of women; very good quality follow-up, careful verification of outcome events, and large numbers of outcome events have allowed for a number of powerful analyses. The database has been used to examine the importance of obesity (175), smoking (176), and lack of postmenopausal hormone replacement (18) as cardiovascular risk factors in women (19,177). Recent work from the Nurses' Health Study has included reports on the prognostic significance of whole grain, saturated fat, nut, dietary fiber, and egg consumption (178–183); weight cycling (184); abdominal adiposity (185); use of calcium channel blockers for hypertension (186); intake of folate and vitamin B_6 from dietary sources and supplements (187); and physical activity (188,189).

Cardiovascular Health Study

The Cardiovascular Health Study is a population-based study of coronary heart disease and stroke among adults aged 65 years or older. This database has been developed because of the well-documented aging of the U.S. population and the fact that much of the morbidity and mortality associated with cardiovascular disease occur among older adults. By routinely performing diagnostic studies among asymptomatic elder adults, the database is designed to learn more about "subclinical" cardiovascular disease and its association with overt clinical events, as well as to learn more about conventional and hypothesized risk factors for cardiovascular disease. The cohort includes 5,201 ambulatory subjects who were recruited in 1989 and 1990 from four field centers: Forsyth County, North Carolina; Sacramento County, California; Allegheny County, Pennsylvania; and Washington County, Maryland, with the coordinating center located at the University of Washington, Seattle. Cohorts were assembled by random sampling from Medicare eligibility lists. Examinations included detailed home health, dietary, and psychosocial interviews as well as mea-

surement of blood pressure, height, weight, physical activity, functional status, and neurologic function; spirometry; electrocardiography; echocardiography (190); carotid ultrasonography; and blood laboratory studies. Early reports from this study yielded valuable insights on cardiovascular in the elderly, with, for example, reports on the population prevalence of atrial fibrillation (191) and on determinants of left ventricular mass (192). Recent reports have addressed the prognostic importance of aspirin use (193), silent myocardial infarction (194), ankle-arm index (195), daytime sleepiness (196), and carotid artery intima and media thickening as detected by ultrasound (197).

Disease-Oriented Registries

Myocardial Infarction Registries

The National Registry of Myocardial Infarction was organized in 1990 as a postmarketing survey of the treatment of myocardial infarction in 1,073 U.S. hospitals (198). Participation in the study is voluntary, although hospitals are encouraged to enter data on consecutive patients irrespective of presentation or treatment. For each patient, a simple one-page form is filled out and sent to a central data coordinating center; the form covers demographics, presentation of illness, electrocardiographic findings, treatment, clinical course, including complications, and status at time of hospital discharge. To ensure data quality, all data abstractors undergo training, and internal computer audits are present to check for inconsistencies, missing data, and out-of-range values. In the first 3 years of activity, the registry recorded data on 240,989 patients with acute myocardial infarction. The database was first used to examine treatment patterns in clinical practice outside the settings of clinical trials (175), use of thrombolytic drugs in elderly patients (199), and the association between thrombolytic therapy and myocardial rupture (200). Recent work from this registry and from its successor, National Registry of Myocardial Infarction 2, which now includes close to 1 million patients, has included reports on prevalence of primary angioplasty (201,202), door-to-needle time (203,204), door-to-balloon time (77), bundle branch block (205,206), myocardial infarction without chest pain (207), procedural volume and outcome (208), economics of myocardial care (209,210), risks for intracranial hemorrhage (211), early use of ACE inhibitors (212), seasonal distribution of myocardial infarction (213), and outcomes in blacks (214) and women (215).

Technology- and Procedure-Oriented Registries

Cardiac Transplantation Databases

The Cardiac Transplant Research Database was initiated in 1990 when 25 major cardiac transplant centers agreed to share data on the clinical characteristics and outcomes of patients undergoing cardiac transplantation. Each center was responsible for completing coded forms and sending them to a central data processing center at the University of Alabama at Birmingham. During computer entry, all data were checked for validity with range and inconsistency checks, and all missing or "suspicious" data elements were forwarded back to the original centers for correction and completion. During the first 18 months of operation, data on 911 patients were collected and used to identify risk factors for death after heart transplantation (21). This database has subsequently been used to rigorously study a number of issues related to outcome after heart transplantation, including donor-specific characteristics associated with outcome (221), pretransplantation risk factors (138), influence of human leukocyte antigen mismatching (222), risks for late recurrent rejection (223), and impact of trends in practice on outcome after transplantation (224). The Cardiac Transplant Research Database has been used to develop predictive software by which clinicians can very quickly compare potential transplant recipients to previous recipients to predict long-term outcome and thereby use the database to make more efficacious point-of-care decisions (225). Recent reports have addressed cardiac allograft vasculopathy (226) and the prognostic importance of pretransplantation body mass (227).

Angioplasty and Percutaneous Revascularization Registries

The first percutaneous transluminal coronary angioplasty was performed by Gruntzig et al. (228) in Zurich, Switzerland, September 16, 1977, with data on four patients presented at the American Heart Association meeting in November of that year. Less than 2 years later, in March 1979, the National Heart, Lung, and Blood Institute established a percutaneous transluminal coronary angioplasty registry through which a centralized accumulation of data obtained from multiple centers would allow for a rapid and systematic assessment of procedure-related outcomes (20). The registry collected data on 3,248 patients who underwent angioplasty at 105 different centers between 1977 and 1981; after September 1981, consecutive cases were no longer recorded. In 1985, 15 centers that contributed to the original registry cooperated to form a second registry that recorded data on all patients undergoing angioplasty between August 1985 and May 1986.

The structure of the original registry has been described by Mullin et al. (20) and is illustrative of the multidisciplinary team approach required for a database to be successful. The overall administration and policy making for the registry came from the Cardiac Diseases Branch of the National Heart, Lung, and Blood Institute Program Office. A steering committee, made up of both elected and appointed investigators, met several times a year to review

policy and scientific direction. Collection, verification, storage, and analysis of all data were performed at a central data-coordinating center at the University of Pittsburgh.

Because of the increasing use of new devices, particularly coronary stents, a new registry known as *New Approaches to Coronary Intervention* was established with the aid of the National Heart, Lung, and Blood Institute in the early 1990s (229,230). This database has been used to study a number of important issues, including the association of use of new technologies with outcome (229), coronary artery size (231), and the impact of race (232).

Cardiac Surgery Databases

In 1986, the Health Care Financing Administration encouraged public release of crude mortality statistics for coronary bypass grafting (233). Because of concern that administrative and financial databases that were being used to assess mortality after coronary artery bypass grafting did not have the richness of clinical detail to provide fair, risk-adjusted measures of outcome, a number of groups assembled clinically oriented databases. The Northern New England Cardiovascular Disease Study Group collected data since 1987 on more than 60,000 patients undergoing coronary bypass surgery in the five northern New England hospitals performing the procedure (234–236). Data were collected on demographic data, cardiac and angiographic variables, priority of surgery, and comorbidities using the Charlson comorbidity index (88). Results of interim data reports are given to participating centers and surgeons in the hope that feedback will result in changes of processes that can lead to better outcome. The study group has noted improvements in risk-adjusted mortality and in reducing costs, improving patient satisfaction, and matching patient expectations with outcomes (237–239). Recent publications from this database have included reports on operator volumes and outcomes (240), obesity (241), preoperative aspirin use (242), and mediastinitis (243).

In 1989, the Society of Thoracic Surgeons established a national database for cardiac surgery (244). It may well be the largest cooperative database of its kind in medicine, with more than 500 participating sites and more than 1.5 million patients. The national data warehouse and analysis center are located in the Duke Clinical Research Institute. The database is voluntary, and in the first 10 years of its existence, data have largely been acquired from community-based cardiac surgery practices and only a few university-based academic practices. Because of its political clout and the adoption of its data elements for statewide and payor quality initiatives, its generalizability has become greater as academic institutions have joined its ranks.

The major strength of the Society of Thoracic Surgery database is in very high numbers. However, to attract continuing participation, the number of data elements collected from participants has been reduced to a core number that appear to influence outcome, and for the most common operations. Recent major publications have focused on risk adjustment, logistic regression models of early risk after coronary artery bypass grafting (245), and cardiac valve replacement (246).

The Cleveland Clinic Foundation Stress Laboratory Database

Beginning in September 1990, all patients undergoing stress testing at The Cleveland Clinic Foundation had their medical histories, medication lists, and exercise test results entered prospectively and immediately on-line into a computerized database (247,248). An early application of the database was to assess whether an association exists between exercise hypertension and angiographic severity of coronary disease (249). By linking stress test results with the Social Security Death Index (250,251), the database has been used to describe the prognostic importance of a number of exercise test findings, including exercise capacity (248), chronotropic incompetence (252), and an attenuated heart rate recovery (253,254).

Administrative, Financial, and Government Databases

New York State Cardiac Surgery Database

Beginning in 1989, all centers performing coronary artery bypass grafting in the state of New York were required by the New York State Department of Health to provide data on a quarterly basis on all patients undergoing the procedure; with these data, risk factors for death and the calculation of hospital-based adjusted mortality rates were reported (255). Each hospital was provided feedback regarding its own actual and expected mortality rates. After 4 years, a significant reduction in risk-adjusted mortality was noted (256), with subset analyses suggesting that the improvement in outcome may have been related to centers responding to data reports by making positive changes in personnel and processes (257). At one cardiac surgery program with a very high reported risk-adjusted mortality, initial frustration with the database gave way to a careful, systematic evaluation of outcome at that center (258). The program directors were able to identify the primary source of their high mortality rates, namely, emergency cases, especially those with recent acute myocardial infarction. They deliberately worked to change the processes by which these patients were managed, with many more patients receiving intraaortic balloon pumps before going to the operating room. Since making these changes, this program has noted a marked decline in its risk-adjusted mortality. Other investigators have suggested, however, that the apparent improvements in outcome since the establishment of the database reporting system may be more due to rejection of

high-risk patients, with some of them being referred out-of-state to other centers (257,259).

The story of the New York State Cardiac Surgery Database took an interesting twist in 1991, when *Newsday*, invoking the Freedom of Information Act, successfully sued the New York State Department of Health for surgeon-specific mortality data (260). Since then, operator-specific mortality data have been publicly released yearly, with each surgeon assigned a risk-adjusted mortality rate and a notation as to whether that mortality rate is statistically better, the same, or worse than average. Interestingly, the public release of surgeon-specific mortality data has had little impact on cardiologists' referral patterns (261). Topol and Califf (262) point out that the extension of traditional risk-adjustment data modeling methods to individual operators, or "scorecard medicine," raises a number of concerns, including (a) failure to account for outcomes other than mortality; (b) difficulty establishing an appropriate reference group; (c) limited sample sizes with small numbers of outcome events for each surgeon; (d) difficulty with risk adjustment and appropriate weighting of variables, as well as "rewarding" operators for taking on very high-risk patients; and (e) logistical problems with proper collection and maintenance of costly data. The American College of Cardiology has already taken steps to address these problems not only through the publication of guidelines but also through the establishment and maintenance of a national database of cardiac procedures (263).

Medicare, the Health Care Financing Administration, and the Cardiovascular Care Project

The process by which Medicare monitors and attempts to improve quality of care among its beneficiaries has undergone a marked change during the past 5 to 15 years, with less emphasis on identifying and removing "bad apples" and more on affecting mainstream care processes (61,264). The Cardiovascular Care Project represents an effort by many different physicians, health service researchers, and professional societies to identify and measure a variety of "quality of care indicators" for patients presenting with acute myocardial infarction and for those undergoing myocardial revascularization. Examples of quality indicators for acute myocardial infarction include percentage of eligible patients receiving therapies such as aspirin, thrombolysis, ACE inhibitors, and beta-blockers; percentage of smoking patients who receive smoking cessation counseling; and percentage of patients who undergo or are scheduled to undergo some form of stress testing or cardiovascular imaging at the time of discharge. A four-state pilot study from this project reported multiple opportunities for improvement among Medicare myocardial infarction patients (265). A number of important reports about quality of myocardial infarction care (266,267) have more recently appeared based on this database, including publications about why "America's best hospitals" have lower myocardial infarction mortality rates (268), the importance of physician specialty (269), the use of beta-blockers (270,271), and the impact of mental illness on the use of cardiovascular procedures (272).

Databases Derived from Randomized Clinical Trials

Although randomized clinical trials are designed to answer specific therapeutic questions, investigators often use them to assemble large observational databases that can be used to study natural history, prognosis, diagnostic questions, and outcomes related to interventions other than those tested. A prototypical example of this is the Coronary Artery Surgery Study, from which a large database was created of 24,959 patients with suspected or known coronary disease who were admitted to one of 15 clinical centers between 1974 and 1979 (273). Although the study results regarding the impact of coronary bypass surgery were published nearly 15 years ago (274), the database emanating from that study continues to provide insight regarding the prognosis of patients with coronary heart disease (275). Some clinical trial registries, such as that of the Studies of Left Ventricular Dysfunction, include patients who were not included in the trial itself (276). Other examples of clinical trial registries being used as observational databases for answering questions unrelated to the trial itself include an analysis of gender and management of acute myocardial infarction from the Myocardial Infarction Triage and Intervention Registry (277); an analysis of the impact of race, age, and sex on management of unstable angina from the Thrombolysis in Myocardial Ischemia III Registry (278); and an analysis on the impact of elevated blood pressure on presentation mortality and stroke outcomes after acute myocardial infarction from the Global Utilization of Streptokinase and Tissue Plasminogen Activator for Occluded Coronary Arteries Registry (279). More recent observational studies based on clinical trial databases include reports on the combination of aspirin and ACE inhibitors in patients with coronary disease (101) and on the impact of diabetes and lesion characteristics among patients undergoing myocardial revascularization (280).

CONTROVERSIES AND PERSONAL PERSPECTIVES

Formally organized databases have existed in cardiology for more than 50 years, even predating the modern computer age. The last 5 to 10 years have witnessed an explosion in database numbers and sizes, such that very large databases now exist in virtually all areas of clinical cardiology. The use of these databases to analyze the importance of patient characteristics and clinical test results for predicting long- and short-term risks is well-established. In the realm of therapeutics, however, there remains considerable controversy, with some strongly believing that the real-world effects of drugs and procedures can be validly assessed by careful analyses of observational databases, whereas others argue that therapeutic effectiveness and safety can only be measured with randomized, controlled trials. There will always be skepticism of database models that describe risk-adjusted outcome, especially for those individuals and institutions where the outcomes appear to be poor. Clinical science is very complex, and clinical knowledge continues to explode; thus, one can always argue that case mix can never be wholly adequately adjusted for. Improvement of analytical methods and ways to identify and adjust for bias and confounding must remain a high priority within the clinical database and research communities.

Once it is widely accepted that, when properly analyzed, observational databases can be used to assess the impacts of treatments on outcomes, it will then become, we believe, incumbent on the cardiology community to implement Ellwood's technology of experience into routine clinical care. This means careful design and universal use of computerized patient records as well as computerized recording of the nature and outcomes of all cardiac procedures. Considerable investment will be required to purchase hardware and software; employ support personnel; and train and support clinical researchers who will have the skills, enthusiasm, time, and resources needed to appropriately analyze observational databases and disseminate their results. The existence of large databases, along with the rapidly improving technologies to develop, store, manipulate, and analyze them, means that we owe our future patients nothing less.

THE FUTURE

The future of clinical databases in clinical cardiology is uncertain. Academic cardiologists will likely continue to nurture and develop population-based, disease-oriented, and procedure-oriented registries, and these will continue to provide new and valuable insights into the nature and optimal management of cardiovascular disease. Some of these databases are growing to truly humongous sizes, allowing for previously unimagined statistical power. Professional societies, such as the American College of Cardiology, are also actively developing databases for outcomes assessment. However, it is very unclear how computerized databases will be used at the level of routine clinical care. It is hoped that academic and clinical leaders will successfully champion the enormous benefits of the "power of information." One cardiac surgeon who has successfully used a clinical database to improve his outcomes may have seen the future: "'Playing by the numbers' has radically changed the way people involved think about their jobs. We have moved from feeling out of control to feeling in control, from being reactive to being proactive, and from not knowing to beginning to know" (237).

REFERENCES

1. Dawber TR, Meadors GR, Moore FE. Epidemiologic approaches to heart disease: the Framingham Heart Study. *Am J Publ Health* 1951;41:279–286.
2. Dawber TR, Kannel WB, Lyell LP. An approach to longitudinal studies in a community: the Framingham Heart Study. *Ann N Y Acad Sci* 1963;107:539–556.
3. Dawber TR. *The Framingham study: the epidemiology of atherosclerotic disease.* Cambridge, MA: Harvard University Press, 1980.
4. Kannel WB. An investigation of coronary heart disease in families: the Framingham Offspring Study. *Am J Epidemiol* 1979;110:281–290.
5. Kannel WB. Clinical misconceptions dispelled by epidemiological research. *Circulation* 1995;92:3350–3360.
6. Lauer MS, Okin PM, Larson MG, et al. Impaired heart rate response to graded exercise. Prognostic implications of chronotropic incompetence in the Framingham Heart Study [see comments]. *Circulation* 1996;93:1520–1526.
7. Culleton BF, Larson MG, Wilson PW, et al. Cardiovascular disease and mortality in a community-based cohort with mild renal insufficiency. *Kidney Int* 1999;56:2214–2219.
8. Chen L, Chen MH, Larson MG, et al. Risk factors for syncope in a community-based sample (the Framingham Heart Study). *Am J Cardiol* 2000;85:1189–1193.
9. Benjamin EJ, Wolf PA, D'Agostino RB, et al. Impact of atrial fibrillation on the risk of death: the Framingham Heart Study [see comments]. *Circulation* 1998;98:946–952.
10. Lloyd-Jones DM, Martin DO, Larson MG, et al. Accuracy of death certificates for coding coronary heart disease as the cause of death [see comments]. *Ann Intern Med* 1998;129:1020–1026.
11. Lauer MS, Larson MG, Evans JC, et al. Association of left ventricular dilatation and hypertrophy with chronotropic incompetence in the Framingham Heart Study. *Am Heart J* 1999;137:903–909.
12. Singh JP, Larson MG, O'Donnell CJ, et al. Association of hyperglycemia with reduced heart rate variability (the Framingham Heart Study). *Am J Cardiol* 2000;86:309–312.
13. O'Donnell CJ, Lindpaintner K, Larson MG, et al. Evidence for association and genetic linkage of the angiotensin-converting enzyme locus with hypertension and blood pressure in men but not women in the Framingham Heart Study [see comments]. *Circulation* 1998;97:1766–1772.
14. Vasan RS, Larson MG, Benjamin EJ, et al. Congestive heart failure in subjects with normal versus reduced left ventricular ejection fraction: prevalence and mortality in a population-based cohort. *J Am Coll Cardiol* 1999;33:1948–1955.
15. Pryor DB, Califf RM, Harrell FE Jr, et al. Clinical data bases. Accomplishments and unrealized potential. *Med Care* 1985;23:623–647.
16. Pryor DB, Harrell FE Jr, Lee KL, et al. Estimating the likelihood of significant coronary artery disease. *Am J Med* 1983;75:771–780.
17. Lundberg ED, McBride R, Rawson TE, et al. C2: a data base management system developed for the Coronary Artery Surgery Study (CASS) and other clinical studies. *J Med Syst* 1982;6:501–518.
18. Stampfer MJ, Willett WC, Colditz GA, et al. A prospective study of postmenopausal estrogen therapy and coronary heart disease. *N Engl J Med* 1985;313:1044–1049.
19. Fried LP, Borhani NO, Enright P, et al. The Cardiovascular Health Study: design and rationale. *Ann Epidemiol* 1991;1:263–276.
20. Mullin SM, Passamani ER, Mock MB. Historical background of the National Heart, Lung, and Blood Institute Registry for Percutaneous Transluminal Coronary Angioplasty. *Am J Cardiol* 1984;53:3C–6C.
21. Bourge RC, Naftel DC, Costanzo-Nordin MR, et al. Pretransplantation risk factors for death after heart transplantation: a multiinstitutional study. The Transplant Cardiologists Research Database Group. *J Heart Lung Transplant* 1993;12:549–562.
22. Feinstein AR. Clinical biostatistics. XII. On exorcising the ghost of Gauss and the curse of Kelvin. *Clin Pharmacol Ther* 1971;12:1003–1016.
23. Wiederhold G. *Database design.* New York: McGraw-Hill, 1983.
24. Kahn MG. Clinical databases and critical care research. *Crit Care Clin* 1994;10:37–51.

25. Dolin RH. Outcome analysis: considerations for an electronic health record. *MD Comput* 1997;14:50–56.

26. Knaus WA, Wagner DP, Draper EA, et al. The APACHE III prognostic system. Risk prediction of hospital mortality for critically ill hospitalized adults [see comments]. *Chest* 1991;100:1619–1636.

27. Ellwood PM. Shattuck lecture—outcomes management. A technology of patient experience. *N Engl J Med* 1988;318:1549–1556.

28. McDonald CJ, Hammond WE. Standard formats for electronic transfer of clinical data. *Ann Intern Med* 1989;110:333–335.

29. Chute CG, Cohn SP, Campbell KE, et al. The content coverage of clinical classifications. For The Computer-Based Patient Record Institute's Work Group on Codes & Structures. *J Am Med Inform Assoc* 1996;3:224–233.

30. Cote RA. Ending classification versus nomenclature controversy. *Med Inf (Lond)* 1983;8:1–4.

31. Activities CoPaH. *International classification of diseases, ninth revision, clinical modification (ICD-9-CM).* Ann Arbor, MI, 1993.

32. *International classification of diseases, tenth revision (ICD-10).* Geneva: World Health Organization, 1992.

33. Cote RA, Rothwell DJ, Palotay JL, Beckett RS, eds. *SNOMED international.* Northfield, IL: College of American Pathologists, 1994.

34. *Unified medical language system, 4th experimental edition, version 1.3.* Bethesda, MD: National Library of Medicine, 1992.

35. Kirschner CG, Burkett RD, Coy JJA, et al. *Physician's current procedural terminology.* Chicago: American Medical Association, 1993.

36. *NANDA nursing diagnoses: definitions and classification.* Philadelphia: North American Nursing Diagnosis Association, 1992–1993.

37. Shortliffe EH, Perreault LE, Wiederhold G, et al. *Medical informatics: computer applications in health care.* Reading, Mass.: Addison Wesley, 1990.

38. Murphy GF. *Computer-based patient records—a unifying principle.* Philadelphia: WB Saunders, 1996.

39. Shahar Y. Dimensions of time in illness: an objective view. *Ann Intern Med* 2000;132:45–53.

40. McHugh J, Abiteboul S, Goldman R, et al. Lore: a database management system for semistructured data. *SIGMOD Record* 1997;26:54–66.

41. Date CJ. *An introduction to database systems.* Reading, MA: Addison Wesley, 1990.

42. Lee N, Millman A, Osborne M, et al. ABC of medical computing. Storing and managing data on a computer. *BMJ* 1995;311:562–565.

43. Blum RL. Displaying clinical data from a time-oriented database. *Comput Biol Med* 1981;11:197–210.

44. Pinciroli F, Combi C, Pozzi G, et al. Dissemination, standardization and user-flexibility in implementing TOMRs for cardiology. *Proc Annu Symp Comput Appl Med Care* 1991:391–395.

45. Combi C, Shahar Y. Temporal reasoning and temporal data maintenance in medicine: issues and challenges. *Comput Biol Med* 1997;27:353–368.

46. Kirklin JW, Vicinanza SS. Metadata and computer-based patient records. *Ann Thorac Surg* 1999;68:S23–S24.

47. Goldman R, McHugh J, Widom J. From semistructured data to XML: migrating the Lore data model and query language. *Proceedings of the 2nd International Workshop on the Web and Databases (WebDB '99), Philadelphia* 1999:1–7.

48. McDonald CJ, Hui SL. The analysis of humongous databases: problems and promises. *Stat Med* 1991;10:511–518.

49. Wagner MM, Hogan WR. The accuracy of medication data in an outpatient electronic medical record. *J Am Med Inform Assoc* 1996;3:234–244.

50. Choi BC. Sensitivity and specificity of a single diagnostic test in the presence of work-up bias [see comments]. *J Clin Epidemiol* 1992;45:581–586.

51. Iezzoni LI, Foley SM, Daley J, et al. Comorbidities, complications, and coding bias. Does the number of diagnosis codes matter in predicting in-hospital mortality? [see comments]. *JAMA* 1992;267:2197–2203.

52. Jencks SF, Williams DK, Kay TL. Assessing hospital-associated deaths from discharge data. The role of length of stay and comorbidities [see comments]. *JAMA* 1988;260:2240–2246.

53. Iezzoni LI. Using administrative diagnostic data to assess the quality of hospital care. Pitfalls and potential of ICD-9-CM. *Int J Technol Assess Health Care* 1990;6:272–281.

54. Little RJA, Rubin DA. *Statistical analysis with missing data.* New York: John Wiley & Sons, 1987.

55. Roth PL, Switzer FSI, Switzer D. Missing data in multi-item scares: a Monte Carlo analysis of missing data techniques. *Org Res Methods* 1999;2:211–232.

56. Rubin DB, Schenker N. Multiple imputation in health-care databases: an overview and some applications. *Stat Med* 1991;10:585–598.

57. Rubin DB. Multiple imputation after 18+ years. *J Am Stat Assoc* 1996;91:473–489.

58. Efron B. Missing data, imputation, and the bootstrap. *J Am Stat Assoc* 1994;89:463–479.

59. Demlo LK. Measuring health care effectiveness. Research and policy implications. *Int J Technol Assess Health Care* 1990;6:288–294.

60. Daley J. Criteria by which to evaluate risk-adjusted outcomes programs in cardiac surgery. *Ann Thorac Surg* 1994;58:1827–1835.

61. Jencks SF. Accuracy in recorded diagnoses [editorial; comment]. *JAMA* 1992;267:2238–2239.

62. Feinstein AR. Clinical biostatistics. VII. The rancid sample, the tilted target, and the medical poll-bearer. *Clin Pharmacol Ther* 1971;12:134–150.

63. Safran C. Electronic patient records and clinical research. In: Bemmel J, McCray AT (eds), *Yearbook of Medical Informatics.* Stuttgart, Germany: Schattauer, 1995:98–102.

64. Wennberg JE. The paradox of appropriate care. *JAMA* 1987;258:2568–2569.

65. Wennberg J, Gittelsohn. Small area variations in health care delivery. *Science* 1973;182:1102–1108.

66. Park RE, Brook RH, Kosecoff J, et al. Explaining variations in hospital death rates. Randomness, severity of illness, quality of care [see comments]. *JAMA* 1990;264:484–490.

67. Pilote L, Califf RM, Sapp S, et al. Regional variation across the United States in the management of acute myocardial infarction. GUSTO-1 Investigators. Global Utilization of Streptokinase and Tissue Plasminogen Activator for

Occluded Coronary Arteries [see comments]. *N Engl J Med* 1995;333:565–572.

68. Mark DB, Naylor CD, Hlatky MA, et al. Use of medical resources and quality of life after acute myocardial infarction in Canada and the United States [see comments]. *N Engl J Med* 1994;331:1130–1135.

69. Van de Werf F, Topol EJ, Lee KL, et al. Variations in patient management and outcomes for acute myocardial infarction in the United States and other countries. Results from the GUSTO trial. Global Utilization of Streptokinase and Tissue Plasminogen Activator for Occluded Coronary Arteries. *JAMA* 1995;273:1586–1591.

70. Lauer MS. Primary angioplasty—time is of the essence [editorial; comment]. *JAMA* 2000;283:2988–2989.

71. Steen PM. Approaches to predictive modeling. *Ann Thorac Surg* 1994;58:1836–1840.

72. Tierney WM, McDonald CJ. Practice databases and their uses in clinical research. *Stat Med* 1991;10:541–557.

73. Pocock SJ, Elbourne DR. Randomized trials or observational tribulations? [editorial; comment]. *N Engl J Med* 2000;342:1907–1909.

74. Sackett DL, Richardson WS, Rosenberg W, et al. *Evidence based medicine: how to practice and teach EBM.* New York: Churchill Livingstone, 1997.

75. Moses LE. Measuring effects without randomized trials? Options, problems, challenges. *Med Care* 1995;33:AS8–A14.

76. Califf RM, Pryor DB, Greenfield JC Jr. Beyond randomized clinical trials: applying clinical experience in the treatment of patients with coronary artery disease. *Circulation* 1986;74:1191–1194.

77. Cannon CP, Gibson CM, Lambrew CT, et al. Relationship of symptom-onset-to-balloon time and door-to-balloon time with mortality in patients undergoing angioplasty for acute myocardial infarction [see comments]. *JAMA* 2000;283:2941–2947.

78. Hlatky MA. Using databases to evaluate therapy. *Stat Med* 1991;10:647–652.

79. Benson K, Hartz AJ. A comparison of observational studies and randomized, controlled trials [see comments]. *N Engl J Med* 2000;342:1878–1886.

80. Concato J, Shah N, Horwitz RI. Randomized, controlled trials, observational studies, and the hierarchy of research designs [see comments]. *N Engl J Med* 2000;342:1887–1892.

81. Kunz R, Oxman AD. The unpredictability paradox: review of empirical comparisons of randomised and non-randomised clinical trials. *BMJ* 1998;317:1185–1190.

82. Byar DP. Why data bases should not replace randomized clinical trials. *Biometrics* 1980;36:337–342.

83. Rosati RA, Lee KL, Califf RM, et al. Problems and advantages of an observational data base approach to evaluating the effect of therapy on outcome. *Circulation* 1982;65:27–32.

84. *American Hospital Association Division of Quality Control Management: coding clinic for ICD-9-CM.* Chicago: American Hospital Association, 1990.

85. Edwards FH, Clark RE, Schwartz M. Practical considerations in the management of large multiinstitutional databases. *Ann Thorac Surg* 1994;58:1841–1844.

86. Knaus WA, Draper EA, Wagner DP, et al. An evaluation of outcome from intensive care in major medical centers. *Ann Intern Med* 1986;104:410–418.

87. Horn SD, Horn RA. Reliability and validity of the severity of illness index. *Med Care* 1986;24:159–178.

88. Charlson ME, Pompei P, Ales KI, MacKenzie CR. A new method of classifying prognostic comorbidity in longitudinal studies: development and validation. *J Chron Dis* 1987;373–383.

89. Lee KL, Woodlief LH, Topol EJ, et al. Predictors of 30-day mortality in the era of reperfusion for acute myocardial infarction. Results from an international trial of 41,021 patients. GUSTO-I Investigators [see comments]. *Circulation* 1995;91:1659–1668.

90. Califf RM, Harrell FE Jr, Lee KL, et al. Changing efficacy of coronary revascularization. Implications for patient selection. *Circulation* 1988;78:1185–1191.

91. Hltaky MA, Califf RM, Harrell FE, et al. Comparison of predictions based on observational data with the results of randomized controlled trials of coronary artery bypass surgery. *J Am Coll Cardiol* 1988;1:237–245.

92. Jencks SF, Dobson A. Refining case-mix adjustment. The research evidence. *N Engl J Med* 1987;317:679–686.

93. Iezzoni LI. Using risk-adjusted outcomes to assess clinical practice: an overview of issues pertaining to risk adjustment. *Ann Thorac Surg* 1994;58:1822–1826.

94. Mark DH. Race and the limits of administrative data. *JAMA* 2001;285:337–338.

95. Jencks SF, Daley J, Draper D, et al. Interpreting hospital mortality data. The role of clinical risk adjustment. *JAMA* 1988;260:3611–3616.

96. D'Agostino RB Jr. Propensity score methods for bias reduction in the comparison of a treatment to a non-randomized control group. *Stat Med* 1998;17:2265–2281.

97. Rubin DB. Estimating causal effects from large data sets using propensity scores. *Ann Intern Med* 1997;127:757–763.

98. Joffe MM, Rosenbaum PR. Invited commentary: propensity scores. *Am J Epidemiol* 1999;150:327–333.

99. Psaty BM, Heckbert SR, Koepsell TD, et al. The risk of myocardial infarction associated with antihypertensive drug therapies [see comments]. *JAMA* 1995;274:620–625.

100. Connors AF Jr, Speroff T, Dawson NV, et al. The effectiveness of right heart catheterization in the initial care of critically ill patients. SUPPORT Investigators [see comments]. *JAMA* 1996;276:889–897.

101. Peterson JG, Topol EJ, Sapp SK, et al. Evaluation of the effects of aspirin combined with angiotensin-converting enzyme inhibitors in patients with coronary artery disease. *Am J Med* 2000;109:371–377.

102. Poses RM, McClish DK, Smith WR, et al. Results of report cards for patients with congestive heart failure depend on the method used to adjust for severity. *Ann Intern Med* 2000;133:10–20.

103. Peterson ED, DeLong ER, Muhlbaier LH, et al. Challenges in comparing risk-adjusted bypass surgery mortality results: results from the Cooperative Cardiovascular Project. *J Am Coll Cardiol* 2000;36:2174–2184.

104. Chalmers TC, Matta RJ, Smith H Jr, et al. Evidence favoring the use of anticoagulants in the hospital phase of acute myocardial infarction. *N Engl J Med* 1977;297:1091–1096.

105. Chalmers TC, Celano P, Sacks HS, et al. Bias in treatment assignment in controlled clinical trials. *N Engl J Med* 1983;309:1358–1361.

106. Sacks H, Chalmers TC, Smith H Jr. Randomized versus historical controls for clinical trials. *Am J Med* 1982;72:233–240.

107. Miller JN, Colditz GA, Mosteller F. How study design affects outcomes in comparisons of therapy. II: Surgical. *Stat Med* 1989;8:455–466.

108. Colditz GA, Miller JN, Mosteller F. How study design affects outcomes in comparisons of therapy. I: Medical. *Stat Med* 1989;8:441–454.

109. Braunwald E, Antman EM, Beasley JW, et al. ACC/AHA guidelines for the management of patients with unstable angina and non-ST-segment elevation myocardial infarction. A report of the American College of Cardiology/American Heart Association Task Force on Practice Guidelines (Committee on the Management of Patients with Unstable Angina). *J Am Coll Cardiol* 2000;36:970–1062.

110. O'Rourke RA, Brundage BH, Froelicher VF, et al. American College of Cardiology/American Heart Association Expert Consensus document on electron-beam computed tomography for the diagnosis and prognosis of coronary artery disease. *J Am Coll Cardiol* 2000;36:326–340.

111. Eagle KA, Guyton RA, Davidoff R, et al. ACC/AHA guidelines for coronary artery bypass graft surgery: a report of the American College of Cardiology/American Heart Association Task Force on Practice Guidelines (Committee to Revise the 1991 Guidelines for Coronary Artery Bypass Graft Surgery). American College of Cardiology/American Heart Association. *J Am Coll Cardiol* 1999;34:1262–1347.

112. Crawford MH, Bernstein SJ, Deedwania PC, et al. ACC/AHA guidelines for ambulatory electrocardiography. A report of the American College of Cardiology/American Heart Association Task Force on Practice Guidelines (Committee to Revise the Guidelines for Ambulatory Electrocardiography). Developed in collaboration with the North American Society for Pacing and Electrophysiology. *J Am Coll Cardiol* 1999;34:912–948.

113. Gibbons RJ, Chatterjee K, Daley J, et al. ACC/AHA/ACP-ASIM guidelines for the management of patients with chronic stable angina: a report of the American College of Cardiology/American Heart Association Task Force on Practice Guidelines (Committee on Management of Patients with Chronic Stable Angina) [published erratum appears in *J Am Coll Cardiol* 1999;34:314]. *J Am Coll Cardiol* 1999;33:2092–2197.

114. Scanlon PJ, Faxon DP, Audet AM, et al. ACC/AHA guidelines for coronary angiography. A report of the American College of Cardiology/American Heart Association Task Force on Practice Guidelines (Committee on Coronary Angiography). Developed in collaboration with the Society for Cardiac Angiography and Interventions. *J Am Coll Cardiol* 1999;33:1756–1824.

115. Leape LL. Institute of Medicine medical error figures are not exaggerated [comment]. *JAMA* 2000;284:95–97.

116. Leape LL, Woods DD, Hatlie MJ, et al. Promoting patient safety by preventing medical error [editorial; see comments]. *JAMA* 1998;280:1444–1447.

117. Bates DW, Leape LL, Cullen DJ, et al. Effect of computerized physician order entry and a team intervention on prevention of serious medication errors [see comments]. *JAMA* 1998;280:1311–1316.

118. Berwick DM, Leape LL. Reducing errors in medicine [editorial; see comments]. *BMJ* 1999;319:136–137.

119. Leape L. Lucian Leape on the causes and prevention of errors and adverse events in health care [interview by Peter I. Buerhaus]. *Image J Nurs Sch* 1999;31:281–286.

120. Leape LL. Reporting of medical errors: time for a reality check. *Qual Health Care* 2000;9:144–145.

121. McDonald CJ. Protocol-based computer reminders, the quality of care and the non-perfectibility of man. *N Engl J Med* 1976;295:1351–1355.

122. McDonald CJ, Wilson GA, McCabe GP Jr. Physician response to computer reminders. *JAMA* 1980;244:1579–1581.

123. McDonald CJ, Hui SL, Smith DM, et al. Reminders to physicians from an introspective computer medical record. A two-year randomized trial. *Ann Intern Med* 1984;100:130–138.

124. Safran C, Rind DM, Davis RB, et al. Guidelines for management of HIV infection with computer-based patient's record. *Lancet* 1995;346:341–346.

125. Tierney WM, Miller ME, McDonald CJ. The effect on test ordering of informing physicians of the charges for outpatient diagnostic tests [see comments]. *N Engl J Med* 1990;322:1499–1504.

126. Rosati RA, McNeer JF, Starmer CF, et al. A new information system for medical practice. *Arch Intern Med* 1975;135:1017–1024.

127. Payne TH, Savarino J, Marshall R, et al. Use of a clinical event monitor to prevent and detect medication errors. *Proc AMIA Annu Symposium* 2000;6:40–44.

128. Bates DW, Kuperman GJ, Rittenberg E, et al. A randomized trial of a computer-based intervention to reduce utilization of redundant laboratory tests [see comments]. *Am J Med* 1999;106:144–150.

129. Allison PD. *Survival analysis using the SAS System.* Cary, NC: SAS Institute, 1995.

130. Hosmer DW, Lemeshow S. *Applied survival analysis: regression modeling of time to event data.* New York: John Wiley & Sons, 1999.

131. Kalbfleisch JD, Prentice RL. *The statistical analysis of failure time data.* New York: John Wiley & Sons, 1980.

132. Harrell FE Jr, Lee KL, Mark DB. Multivariable prognostic models: issues in developing models, evaluating assumptions and adequacy, and measuring and reducing errors. *Stat Med* 1996;15:361–387.

133. Hosmer DW, Lemeshow S. *Applied logistic regression.* New York: Wiley, 1989.

134. Marshall G, Grover FL, Henderson WG, et al. Assessment of predictive models for binary outcomes: an empirical approach using operative death from cardiac surgery. *Stat Med* 1994;13:1501–1511.

135. Cox DR. Regression methods and life tables [with discussion]. *J R Stat Soc B* 1972;34:187–220.

136. Gilpin EA, Koziol JA, Madsen EB, et al. Periods of differing mortality distribution during the first year after acute myocardial infarction. *Am J Cardiol* 1983;52:240–244.

137. Blackstone EH, Naftel DC, Turner ME Jr, et al. The decomposition of time-varying hazard into phases, each incorporating a separate stream on concomitant information. *J Am Stat Soc* 1986;81:615–624.

138. Kobashigawa JA, Kirklin JK, Naftel DC, et al. Pretransplantation risk factors for acute rejection after heart transplantation: a multiinstitutional study. The Transplant Cardiologists Research Database Group. *J Heart Lung Transplant* 1993;12:355–366.

139. Concato J, Feinstein AR, Holford TR. The risk of determining risk with multivariable models. *Ann Intern Med* 1993;118:201–210.

140. Harrell FE Jr, Lee KL, Califf RM, et al. Regression modelling strategies for improved prognostic prediction. *Stat Med* 1984;3:143–152.

141. Christensen E. Multivariate survival analysis using Cox's regression model. *Hepatology* 1980;7:1346–1358.

142. Andersen PK. Testing goodness of fix of Cox's regression and life model. *Biometrics* 1982;38:67–77.

143. Harrell FE Jr, Lee KL, Matchar DB, Reicher TA. Regression models for prognostic prediction: advantages, problems, and selected solution. *Cancer Treat Res* 1985;69:1071–1077.

144. Krumholz HM. Mathematical models and the assessment of performance in cardiology [editorial; see comments]. *Circulation* 1999;99:2067–2069.

145. Efron B, Gong G. A leisurely look at the bootstrap, the jackknife, and cross-validation. *Am Statistician* 1983;37:36–48.

146. Burnham KP, Anderson DR. *Model selection and inference: a practical information-theoretic approach.* New York: Springer, 1998.

147. Akaike H. A Bayesian analysis of the minimum AIC procedure. *Ann Inst Stat Math* 1978;30:9–14.

148. Chipman HA, George EI, McCulloch RE. Bayesian CART model search. *J Am Stat Assoc* 1998;93:935–960.

149. Loh WY, Vanichsetakul N. Tree-structured classification via generalized discriminant analysis. *J Am Stat Assoc* 1988;83:715–725.

150. Binder DA. Bayesian cluster analysis. *Biometrika* 1978;65:31–38.

151. Yarnold PR, Soltysik RC, Lefevre F, et al. Predicting in-hospital mortality of patients receiving cardiopulmonary resuscitation: unit-weighted MultiODA for binary data. *Stat Med* 1998;17:2405–2414.

152. Ripley BD. Neural networks and related methods for classification. *J R Stat Soc* 1994;56:409–456.

153. Ennis M, Hinton G, Naylor D, et al. A comparison of statistical learning methods on the GUSTO database. *Stat Med* 1998;17:2501–2508.

154. Lippmann RP, Shahian DM. Coronary artery bypass risk prediction using neural networks [see comments]. *Ann Thorac Surg* 1997;63:1635–1643.

155. Tu JV, Weinstein MC, McNeil BJ, et al. Predicting mortality after coronary artery bypass surgery: what do artificial neural networks learn? The Steering Committee of the Cardiac Care Network of Ontario. *Med Decis Making* 1998;18:229–235.

156. Dawber TR, Kannel WB, Revotskie N, et al. Some factors associated with the development of coronary heart disease: six years' follow-up experience in the Framingham Study. *Am J Publ Health* 1959;49:1349–1356.

157. Stehbens WE. The quality of epidemiological data in coronary heart disease and atherosclerosis [see comments]. *J Clin Epidemiol* 1993;46:1337–1346.

158. Stehbens WE. Limitations of the epidemiological method in coronary heart disease [letter]. *Int J Epidemiol* 1991;20:818–820.

159. Kannel WB, Wilson PW. Efficacy of lipid profiles in prediction of coronary disease. *Am Heart J* 1992;124:768–774.

160. Selhub J, Jacques PF, Bostom AG, et al. Association between plasma homocysteine concentrations and extracranial carotid-artery stenosis [see comments]. *N Engl J Med* 1995;332:286–291.

161. Wilson PW, Kannel WB, Silbershatz H, et al. Clustering of metabolic factors and coronary heart disease. *Arch Intern Med* 1999;159:1104–1109.

162. Levy D, Garrison RJ, Savage DD, et al. Prognostic implications of echocardiographically determined left ventricular mass in the Framingham Heart Study [see comments]. *N Engl J Med* 1990;322:1561–1566.

163. Wilson PW, D'Agostino RB, Levy D, et al. Prediction of coronary heart disease using risk factor categories [see comments]. *Circulation* 1998;97:1837–1847.

164. Benjamin EJ, Levy D, Vaziri SM, et al. Independent risk factors for atrial fibrillation in a population-based cohort. The Framingham Heart Study. *JAMA* 1994;271:840–844.

165. Haq IU, Ramsay LE, Yeo WW, et al. Is the Framingham risk function valid for northern European populations? A comparison of methods for estimating absolute coronary risk in high risk men [see comments]. *Heart* 1999;81:40–46.

166. Group SCotPHSR. Final report on the aspirin component of the ongoing Physicians' Health Study. Steering Committee of the Physicians' Health Study Research Group [see comments]. *N Engl J Med* 1989;321:129–135.

167. Ridker PM, Vaughan DE, Stampfer MJ, et al. Endogenous tissue-type plasminogen activator and risk of myocardial infarction [see comments]. *Lancet* 1993;341:1165–1168.

168. Ridker PM, Glynn RJ, Hennekens CH. C-reactive protein adds to the predictive value of total and HDL cholesterol in determining risk of first myocardial infarction [see comments]. *Circulation* 1998;97:2007–2011.

169. Ma J, Hennekens CH, Ridker PM, et al. A prospective study of fibrinogen and risk of myocardial infarction in the Physicians' Health Study. *J Am Coll Cardiol* 1999;33:1347–1352.

170. Zee RY, Ridker PM, Stampfer MJ, et al. Prospective evaluation of the angiotensin-converting enzyme insertion/deletion polymorphism and the risk of stroke [see comments]. *Circulation* 1999;99:340–343.

171. Ridker PM, Hennekens CH, Roitman-Johnson B, et al. Plasma concentration of soluble intercellular adhesion molecule 1 and risks of future myocardial infarction in apparently healthy men [see comments]. *Lancet* 1998;351:88–92.

172. de Lemos JA, Hennekens CH, Ridker PM. Plasma concentration of soluble vascular cell adhesion molecule-1 and subsequent cardiovascular risk. *J Am Coll Cardiol* 2000;36:423–426.

173. Ariyo A, Hennekens CH, Stampfer MJ, et al. Lipoprotein (a), lipids, aspirin, and risk of myocardial infarction in the Physician's Health Study. *J Cardiovasc Risk* 1998;5:273–278.

174. Manson JE, Colditz GA, Stampfer MJ, et al. A prospective study of obesity and risk of coronary heart disease in women [see comments]. *N Engl J Med* 1990;322:882–889.

175. Willett WC, Manson JE, Stampfer MJ, et al. Weight, weight change, and coronary heart disease in women. Risk within the 'normal' weight range [see comments]. *JAMA* 1995;273:461–465.

176. Willett WC, Green A, Stampfer MJ, et al. Relative and absolute excess risks of coronary heart disease among women who smoke cigarettes. *N Engl J Med* 1987;317:1303–1309.

177. Tell GS, Fried LP, Hermanson B, et al. Recruitment of adults 65 years and older as participants in the Cardiovascular Health Study [see comments]. *Ann Epidemiol* 1993;3:358–366.

178. Liu S, Stampfer MJ, Hu FB, et al. Whole-grain consumption and risk of coronary heart disease: results from the Nurses' Health Study [see comments]. *Am J Clin Nutr* 1999;70:412–419.

179. Liu S, Manson JE, Stampfer MJ, et al. Whole grain consumption and risk of ischemic stroke in women: a prospective study. *JAMA* 2000;284:1534–1540.

180. Hu FB, Stampfer MJ, Manson JE, et al. Dietary saturated fats and their food sources in relation to the risk of coronary heart disease in women [see comments]. *Am J Clin Nutr* 1999;70:1001–1008.

181. Hu FB, Stampfer MJ, Manson JE, et al. Frequent nut consumption and risk of coronary heart disease in women: prospective cohort study [see comments]. *BMJ* 1998;317:1341–1345.

182. Wolk A, Manson JE, Stampfer MJ, et al. Long-term intake of dietary fiber and decreased risk of coronary heart disease among women. *JAMA* 1999;281:1998–2004.

183. Hu FB, Stampfer MJ, Rimm EB, et al. A prospective study of egg consumption and risk of cardiovascular disease in men and women. *JAMA* 1999;281:1387–1394.

184. Field AE, Byers T, Hunter DJ, et al. Weight cycling, weight gain, and risk of hypertension in women. *Am J Epidemiol* 1999;150:573–579.

185. Rexrode KM, Carey VJ, Hennekens CH, et al. Abdominal adiposity and coronary heart disease in women [see comments]. *JAMA* 1998;280:1843–1848.

186. Michels KB, Rosner BA, Manson JE, et al. Prospective study of calcium channel blocker use, cardiovascular disease, and total mortality among hypertensive women: the Nurses' Health Study [see comments]. *Circulation* 1998;97:1540–1548.

187. Rimm EB, Willett WC, Hu FB, et al. Folate and vitamin B6 from diet and supplements in relation to risk of coronary heart disease among women [see comments]. *JAMA* 1998;279:359–364.

188. Hu FB, Sigal RJ, Rich-Edwards JW, et al. Walking compared with vigorous physical activity and risk of type 2 diabetes in women: a prospective study. *JAMA* 1999;282:1433–1439.

189. Hu FB, Stampfer MJ, Colditz GA, et al. Physical activity and risk of stroke in women. *JAMA* 2000;283:2961–2967.

190. Gardin JM, Wond ND, Bommer W, et al. Echocardiographic design of a multicenter investigation of free-living elderly subjects: the Cardiovascular Health Study. *J Am Soc Echocardiogr* 1992;5:63–72.

191. Furberg CD, Psaty BM, Manolio TA, et al. Prevalence of atrial fibrillation in elderly subjects (the Cardiovascular Health Study). *Am J Cardiol* 1994;74:236–241.

192. Gardin JM, Siscovick D, Anton-Culver H, et al. Sex, age, and disease affect echocardiographic left ventricular mass and systolic function in the free-living elderly. The Cardiovascular Health Study. *Circulation* 1995;91:1739–1748.

193. Kronmal RA, Hart RG, Manolio TA, et al. Aspirin use and incident stroke in the Cardiovascular Health Study. CHS Collaborative Research Group [see comments]. *Stroke* 1998;29:887–894.

194. Sheifer SE, Gersh BJ, Yanez ND III, et al. Prevalence, predisposing factors, and prognosis of clinically unrecognized myocardial infarction in the elderly. *J Am Coll Cardiol* 2000;35:119–126.

195. Newman AB, Shemanski L, Manolio TA, et al. Ankle-arm index as a predictor of cardiovascular disease and mortality in the Cardiovascular Health Study. The Cardiovascular Health Study Group. *Arterioscler Thromb Vasc Biol* 1999;19:538–545.

196. Newman AB, Spiekerman CF, Enright P, et al. Daytime sleepiness predicts mortality and cardiovascular disease in older adults. The Cardiovascular Health Study Research Group [see comments]. *J Am Geriatr Soc* 2000;48:115–123.

197. O'Leary DH, Polak JF, Kronmal RA, et al. Carotid-artery intima and media thickness as a risk factor for myocardial infarction and stroke in older adults. Cardiovascular Health Study Collaborative Research Group [see comments]. *N Engl J Med* 1999;340:14–22.

198. Rogers WJ, Bowlby LJ, Chandra NC, et al. Treatment of myocardial infarction in the United States (1990 to 1993). Observations from the National Registry of Myocardial Infarction. *Circulation* 1994;90:2103–2114.

199. Gurwitz JH, Gore JM, Goldberg RJ, et al. Recent age-related trends in the use of thrombolytic therapy in patients who have had acute myocardial infarction. National Registry of Myocardial Infarction [see comments]. *Ann Intern Med* 1996;124:283–291.

200. Becker RC, Gore JM, Lambrew C, et al. A composite view of cardiac rupture in the United States National Registry of Myocardial Infarction [see comments]. *J Am Coll Cardiol* 1996;27:1321–1326.

201. Barron HV, Rundle A, Gurwitz J, et al. Reperfusion therapy for acute myocardial infarction: observations from the National Registry of Myocardial Infarction 2. *Cardiol Rev* 1999;7:156–160.

202. Canto JG, Rogers WJ, Zhang Y, et al. The association between the on-site availability of cardiac procedures and the utilization of those services for acute myocardial infarction by payer group. The National Registry of Myocardial Infarction 2 Investigators. *Clin Cardiol* 1999;22:519–524.

203. Goldberg RJ, Mooradd M, Gurwitz JH, et al. Impact of time to treatment with tissue plasminogen activator on morbidity and mortality following acute myocardial infarction (the second National Registry of Myocardial Infarction). *Am J Cardiol* 1998;82:259–264.

204. Lambrew CT, Bowlby LJ, Rogers WJ, et al. Factors influencing the time to thrombolysis in acute myocardial infarction. Time to Thrombolysis Substudy of the National Registry of Myocardial Infarction-1. *Arch Intern Med* 1997;157:2577–2582.

205. Go AS, Barron HV, Rundle AC, et al. Bundle-branch block and in-hospital mortality in acute myocardial infarction. National Registry of Myocardial Infarction 2 Investigators. *Ann Intern Med* 1998;129:690–697.

206. Shlipak MG, Go AS, Frederick PD, et al. Treatment and outcomes of left bundle-branch block patients with myocardial infarction who present without chest pain. National Registry of Myocardial Infarction 2 Investigators [see comments]. *J Am Coll Cardiol* 2000;36:706–712.

207. Canto JG, Shlipak MG, Rogers WJ, et al. Prevalence, clinical characteristics, and mortality among patients with myocardial infarction presenting without chest pain. *JAMA* 2000;283:3223–3229.

208. Canto JG, Every NR, Magid DJ, et al. The volume of primary angioplasty procedures and survival after acute myocardial infarction. National Registry of Myocardial Infarction 2 Investigators. *N Engl J Med* 2000;342:1573–1580.

209. Sada MJ, French WJ, Carlisle DM, et al. Influence of payor on use of invasive cardiac procedures and patient outcome after myocardial infarction in the United States. Participants in the National Registry of Myocardial Infarction. *J Am Coll Cardiol* 1998;31:1474–1480.

210. Canto JG, Rogers WJ, French WJ, et al. Payer status and the utilization of hospital resources in acute myocardial infarction: a report from the National Registry of Myocardial Infarction 2. *Arch Intern Med* 2000;160:817–823.

211. Gurwitz JH, Gore JM, Goldberg RJ, et al. Risk for intracranial hemorrhage after tissue plasminogen activator treatment for acute myocardial infarction. Participants in the National Registry of Myocardial Infarction 2 [see comments]. *Ann Intern Med* 1998;129:597–604.

212. Michaels AD, Maynard C, Every NR, et al. Early use of ACE inhibitors in the treatment of acute myocardial infarction in the United States: experience from the National Registry of Myocardial Infarction 2. National Registry of Myocardial Infarction 2 participants. *Am J Cardiol* 1999;84:1176–1181.

213. Spencer FA, Goldberg RJ, Becker RC, et al. Seasonal distribution of acute myocardial infarction in the second National Registry of Myocardial Infarction [see comments]. *J Am Coll Cardiol* 1998;31:1226–1233.

214. Taylor HA Jr, Canto JG, Sanderson B, et al. Management and outcomes for black patients with acute myocardial infarction in the reperfusion era. National Registry of Myocardial Infarction 2 Investigators. *Am J Cardiol* 1998;82:1019–1023.

215. Vaccarino V, Parsons L, Every NR, et al. Sex-based differences in early mortality after myocardial infarction. National Registry of Myocardial Infarction 2 Participants [see comments]. *N Engl J Med* 1999;341:217–225.

216. Hlatky MA, Pryor DB, Harrell FE Jr, et al. Factors affecting sensitivity and specificity of exercise electrocardiography. Multivariable analysis. *Am J Med* 1984;77:64–71.

217. Harris PJ, Harrell FE Jr, Lee KL, et al. Survival in medically treated coronary artery disease. *Circulation* 1979;60:1259–1269.

218. Mark DB, Nelson CL, Califf RM, et al. Continuing evolution of therapy for coronary artery disease. Initial results from the era of coronary angioplasty. *Circulation* 1994;89:2015–2025.

219. Califf RM, Harrell FE Jr, Lee KL, et al. The evolution of medical and surgical therapy for coronary artery disease. A 15-year perspective [see comments]. *JAMA* 1989;261:2077–2086.

220. Jones RH, Kesler K, Phillips HRD, et al. Long-term survival benefits of coronary artery bypass grafting and percutaneous transluminal angioplasty in patients with coronary artery disease. *J Thorac Cardiovasc Surg* 1996;111:1013–1025.

221. Young JB, Naftel DC, Bourge RC, et al. Matching the heart donor and heart transplant recipient. Clues for successful expansion of the donor pool: a multivariable, multiinstitutional report. The Cardiac Transplant Research Database Group. *J Heart Lung Transplant* 1994;13:353–364; discussion 364–365.

222. Jarcho J, Naftel DC, Shroyer TW, et al. Influence of HLA mismatch on rejection after heart transplantation: a multi-institutional study. The Cardiac Transplant Research Database Group. *J Heart Lung Transplant* 1994;13:583–595; discussion 595–596.

223. Kubo SH, Naftel DC, Mills RM Jr, et al. Risk factors for late recurrent rejection after heart transplantation: a multi-institutional, multivariable analysis. Cardiac Transplant Research Database Group. *J Heart Lung Transplant* 1995;14:409–418.

224. Rodeheffer RJ, Naftel DC, Stevenson LW, et al. Secular trends in cardiac transplant recipient and donor management in the United States, 1990 to 1994. A multi-institutional study. Cardiac Transplant Research Database Group. *Circulation* 1996;94:2883–2889.

225. Bourge RC. Predicting outcome after cardiac transplantation: lessons from the Cardiac Transplant Research Database. *J Heart Lung Transplant* 1997;12:136–145.

226. Costanzo MR, Naftel DC, Pritzker MR, et al. Heart transplant coronary artery disease detected by coronary angiography: a multiinstitutional study of preoperative donor and recipient risk factors. Cardiac Transplant Research Database. *J Heart Lung Transplant* 1998;17:744–753.

227. Grady KL, White-Williams C, Naftel D, et al. Are preoperative obesity and cachexia risk factors for post heart transplant morbidity and mortality: a multi-institutional study of preoperative weight-height indices. Cardiac Transplant Research Database (CTRD) Group. *J Heart Lung Transplant* 1999;18:750–763.

228. Gruntzig AR, Senning A, Siegenthaler WE. Nonoperative dilatation of coronary-artery stenosis: percutaneous transluminal coronary angioplasty. *N Engl J Med* 1979;301:61–68.

229. King SB III, Yeh W, Holubkov R, et al. Balloon angioplasty versus new device intervention: clinical outcomes. A comparison of the NHLBI PTCA and NACI registries [see comments]. *J Am Coll Cardiol* 1998;31:558–566.

230. Steenkiste AR, Baim DS, Sipperly ME, et al. The NACI Registry: an instrument for the evaluation of New Approaches to Coronary Intervention. The NACI Investigators. *Cathet Cardiovasc Diagn* 1991;23:270–281.

231. Saucedo JF, Popma JJ, Kennard ED, et al. Relation of coronary artery size to one-year clinical events after new device angioplasty of native coronary arteries (a New Approach to Coronary Intervention [NACI] Registry Report). *Am J Cardiol* 2000;85:166–171.

232. Marks DS, Mensah GA, Kennard ED, et al. Race, baseline characteristics, and clinical outcomes after coronary intervention: the New Approaches in Coronary Interventions (NACI) registry. *Am Heart J* 2000;140:162–169.

233. Edwards FH, Clark RE, Schwartz M. Coronary artery bypass grafting: the Society of Thoracic Surgeons National Database experience [see comments]. *Ann Thorac Surg* 1994;57:12–19.

234. O'Connor GT, Plume SK, Olmstead EM, et al. A regional prospective study of in-hospital mortality associated with coronary artery bypass grafting. The Northern New England Cardiovascular Disease Study Group [see comments]. *JAMA* 1991;266:803–809.

235. Malenka DJ, O'Connor GT. The Northern New England Cardiovascular Disease Study Group: a regional collaborative effort for continuous quality improvement in cardiovascular disease. *Jt Comm J Qual Improv* 1998;24:594–600.

236. Nugent WC. Innovative uses of a cardiothoracic database. *Ann Thorac Surg* 1999;68:359–361; discussion 374–376.

237. Nugent WC, Schults WC. Playing by the numbers: how collecting outcomes data changed by life. *Ann Thorac Surg* 1994;58:1866–1870.

238. Davidow SL. Physicians taking the lead to improve patient care. *Jt Comm J Qual Improv* 1999;25:145–152.

239. McGrath PD, Malenka DJ, Wennberg DE, et al. Changing outcomes in percutaneous coronary interventions: a study of 34,752 procedures in northern New England, 1990 to 1997. Northern New England Cardiovascular Disease Study Group. *J Am Coll Cardiol* 1999;34:674–680.

240. McGrath PD, Wennberg DE, Malenka DJ, et al. Operator volume and outcomes in 12,998 percutaneous coronary interventions. Northern New England Cardiovascular Disease Study Group. *J Am Coll Cardiol* 1998;31:570–576.

241. Birkmeyer NJ, Charlesworth DC, Hernandez F, et al. Obesity and risk of adverse outcomes associated with coronary artery bypass surgery. Northern New England Cardiovascular Disease Study Group. *Circulation* 1998;97:1689–1694.

242. Dacey LJ, Munoz JJ, Johnson ER, et al. Effect of preoperative aspirin use on mortality in coronary artery bypass grafting patients. Northern New England Cardiovascular Disease Study Group. *Ann Thorac Surg* 2000;70:1986–1990.

243. Braxton JH, Marrin CA, McGrath PD, et al. Mediastinitis and long-term survival after coronary artery bypass graft surgery. Northern New England Cardiovascular Disease Study Group. *Ann Thorac Surg* 2000;70:2004–2007.

244. Ferguson TB Jr, Dziuban SW Jr, Edwards FH, et al. The STS National Database: current changes and challenges for the new millennium. Committee to Establish a National Database in Cardiothoracic Surgery, The Society of Thoracic Surgeons. *Ann Thorac Surg* 2000;69:680–691.

245. Shroyer AL, Plomondon ME, Grover FL, et al. The 1996 coronary artery bypass risk model: the Society of Thoracic Surgeons Adult Cardiac National Database. *Ann Thorac Surg* 1999;67:1205–1208.

246. Jamieson WR, Edwards FH, Schwartz M, et al. Risk stratification for cardiac valve replacement. National Cardiac Surgery Database. Database Committee of The Society of Thoracic Surgeons. *Ann Thorac Surg* 1999;67:943–951.

247. Lauer MS, Pashkow FJ, Snader CE, et al. Gender and referral for coronary angiography after treadmill thallium testing. *Am J Cardiol* 1996;78:278–283.

248. Snader CE, Marwick TH, Pashkow FJ, et al. Importance of estimated functional capacity as a predictor of all-cause

mortality among patients referred for exercise thallium single-photon emission computed tomography: report of 3,400 patients from a single center. *J Am Coll Cardiol* 1997;30:641–648.

249. Lauer MS, Pashkow FJ, Harvey SA, et al. Angiographic and prognostic implications of an exaggerated exercise systolic blood pressure response and rest systolic blood pressure in adults undergoing evaluation for suspected coronary artery disease. *J Am Coll Cardiol* 1995;26:1630–1636.

250. Boyle CA, Decoufle P. National sources of vital status information: extent of coverage and possible selectivity in reporting [see comments]. *Am J Epidemiol* 1990;131:160–168.

251. Curb JD, Ford CE, Pressel S, et al. Ascertainment of vital status through the National Death Index and the Social Security Administration. *Am J Epidemiol* 1985;121:754–766.

252. Lauer MS, Francis GS, Okin PM, et al. Impaired chronotropic response to exercise stress testing as a predictor of mortality. *JAMA* 1999;281:524–529.

253. Cole CR, Blackstone EH, Pashkow FJ, et al. Heart-rate recovery immediately after exercise as a predictor of mortality. *N Engl J Med* 1999;341:1351–1357.

254. Nishime EO, Cole CR, Blackstone EH, et al. Heart rate recovery and treadmill exercise score as predictors of mortality in patients referred for exercise ECG. *JAMA* 2000;284:1392–1398.

255. Hannan EL, Kilburn H Jr, O'Donnell JF, et al. Adult open heart surgery in New York State. An analysis of risk factors and hospital mortality rates [see comments]. *JAMA* 1990;264:2768–2774.

256. Hannan EL, Kilburn H Jr, Racz M, et al. Improving the outcomes of coronary artery bypass surgery in New York State. *JAMA* 1994;271:761–766.

257. Omoigui NA, Miller DP, Brown KJ, et al. Outmigration for coronary bypass surgery in an era of public dissemination of clinical outcomes [see comments]. *Circulation* 1996;93:27–33.

258. Dziuban SW Jr, McIlduff JB, Miller SJ, et al. How a New York cardiac surgery program uses outcomes data. *Ann Thorac Surg* 1994;58:1871–1876.

259. Byer MJ. Saints hearts. *New York Times* 1992;Sect. 23.

260. Zinman D. Heart surgeons rated: State reveals patient-mortality records. *Newsday* 1991:34.

261. Hannan EL, Stone CC, Biddle TL, et al. Public release of cardiac surgery outcomes data in New York: what do New York state cardiologists think of it? [corrected and republished article originally printed in *Am Heart J* 1997;134:55–61]. *Am Heart J* 1997;134:1120–1128.

262. Topol EJ, Califf RM. Scorecard cardiovascular medicine. Its impact and future directions [see comments]. *Ann Intern Med* 1994;120:65–70.

263. Weintraub WS, McKay CR, Riner RN, et al. The American College of Cardiology National Database: progress and challenges. American College of Cardiology Database Committee. *J Am Coll Cardiol* 1997;29:459–465.

264. Jencks SF, Wilensky GR. The health care quality improvement initiative. A new approach to quality assurance in Medicare [see comments]. *JAMA* 1992;268:900–903.

265. Ellerbeck EF, Jencks SF, Radford MJ, et al. Quality of care for Medicare patients with acute myocardial infarction. A

four-state pilot study from the Cooperative Cardiovascular Project [see comments]. *JAMA* 1995;273:1509–1514.

266. Marciniak TA, Ellerbeck EF, Radford MJ, et al. Improving the quality of care for Medicare patients with acute myocardial infarction: results from the Cooperative Cardiovascular Project [see comments]. *JAMA* 1998;279:1351–1357.

267. Holmboe ES, Meehan TP, Radford MJ, et al. What's happening in quality improvement at the local hospital: a statewide study from the Cooperative Cardiovascular Project. *Am J Med Qual* 2000;15:106–113.

268. Chen J, Radford MJ, Wang Y, et al. Do "America's best hospitals" perform better for acute myocardial infarction? [see comments]. *N Engl J Med* 1999;340:286–292.

269. Chen J, Radford MJ, Wang Y, et al. Care and outcomes of elderly patients with acute myocardial infarction by physician specialty: the effects of comorbidity and functional limitations. *Am J Med* 2000;108:460–469.

270. Krumholz HM, Radford MJ, Wang Y, et al. National use and effectiveness of beta-blockers for the treatment of elderly patients after acute myocardial infarction: National Cooperative Cardiovascular Project [published erratum appears in *JAMA* 1999;281:37]. *JAMA* 1998;280:623–629.

271. Chen J, Marciniak TA, Radford MJ, et al. Beta-blocker therapy for secondary prevention of myocardial infarction in elderly diabetic patients. Results from the National Cooperative Cardiovascular Project. *J Am Coll Cardiol* 1999;34:1388–1394.

272. Druss BG, Bradford DW, Rosenheck RA, et al. Mental disorders and use of cardiovascular procedures after myocardial infarction [see comments]. *JAMA* 2000;283:506–511.

273. National Heart, Lung, and Blood Institute Coronary Artery Surgery Study. A multicenter comparison of the effects of randomized medical and surgical treatment of mildly symptomatic patients with coronary artery disease, and a registry of consecutive patients undergoing coronary angiography. *Circulation* 1981;63:I1–81.

274. Coronary Artery Surgery Study (CASS): a randomized trial of coronary artery bypass surgery. Survival data. *Circulation* 1983;68:939–950.

275. Emond M, Mock MB, Davis KB, et al. Long-term survival of medically treated patients in the Coronary Artery Surgery Study (CASS) Registry. *Circulation* 1994;90:2645–2657.

276. Bangdiwala SI, Weiner DH, Bourassa MG, et al. Studies of Left Ventricular Dysfunction (SOLVD) Registry: rationale, design, methods and description of baseline characteristics. *Am J Cardiol* 1992;70:347–353.

277. Kudenchuk PJ, Maynard C, Martin JS, et al. Comparison of presentation, treatment, and outcome of acute myocardial infarction in men versus women (the Myocardial Infarction Triage and Intervention Registry) [see comments]. *Am J Cardiol* 1996;78:9–14.

278. Stone PH, Thompson B, Anderson HV, et al. Influence of race, sex, and age on management of unstable angina and non-Q-wave myocardial infarction: the TIMI III Registry. *JAMA* 1996;275:1104–1112.

279. Aylward PE, Wilcox RG, Horgan JH, et al. Relation of increased arterial blood pressure to mortality and stroke in the context of contemporary thrombolytic therapy for acute myocardial infarction. A randomized trial. GUSTO-I Investigators. *Ann Intern Med* 1996;125:891–900.

280. Brooks MM, Jones RH, Bach RG, et al. Predictors of mortality and mortality from cardiac causes in the bypass angioplasty revascularization investigation (BARI) randomized trial and registry. For the BARI Investigators. *Circulation* 2000;101:2682–2689.

MEDICAL ERRORS AND QUALITY OF CARE IN CARDIOVASCULAR MEDICINE

ERIC J. TOPOL
ROBERT M. CALIFF

OVERVIEW

Quality of care is linked with achieving the best outcomes for patients, but the term is a complex one that can mean access to care, the appropriateness of procedures or tests, absence of errors, or patient satisfaction level. It is difficult to measure, particularly when one deviates from using mortality as the principal outcome, because of the intrinsic difficulties of risk-adjustment modeling. Despite some of these limitations, the

E. J. Topol: Department of Cardiovascular Medicine, The Cleveland Clinic Foundation, Cleveland, Ohio
R. M. Califf: Department of Medicine, Duke Clinical Research Institute, Durham, North Carolina

use of "report cards" or "scorecards" is more commonplace than ever for evaluating managed care organizations, individual hospitals, and, in some cases, even the physicians themselves.

Much is being done to improve the methodology of assessing quality, and this will help make the process more acceptable and meaningful. One of the major issues that has emerged is the remarkable expense required to collect data at community and academic centers for such analytical work to be performed. For several cardiovascular procedures and diagnoses—including coronary artery bypass grafting (CABG), percutaneous transluminal coronary intervention (PCI), and acute myocardial infarction (MI)—the relationship of volume to operator or hospital has turned out to be a pivotal index for outcomes. Consistently, across the procedures and diagnoses, low volume reflects suboptimal quality. Although one solution is to regionalize centers ("centers of excellence"), an alternative is to have risk-adjusted modeling data available to secure the level of care provided by low-volume operators. Mortality is only one outcome that needs to be considered and, although easier to measure, should not override key morbidity outcomes such as stroke, MI, or functional status. On the other hand, the best measurement of overall quality related to outcomes may be considered the total mortality of the population seen in a health system rather than the mortality for a particular segment such as bypass surgery or acute MI. The focus on medical errors by the Institute of Medicine (IOM) report in 1999 brought these issues to the forefront (1–5). For the field to further evolve, report cards of the report cards will need to be assessed on a frequent basis. A major objective in the field is to drive quality to an unprecedented high level.

HISTORICAL PERSPECTIVE

Although the quality of medical care has been considered since the beginning of the medical profession, Florence Nightingale is generally credited with the fundamental insights in her book *Notes on Hospitals*, published in 1863 (6). In this review of hospitals in London and the United Kingdom, she noted a 91% death rate in the 24 hospitals in London as compared with 40% in 55 county and regional facilities. She recommended sweeping changes in operation and location of the London hospitals and was a veritable pioneer to advance the quality of medical care (6,7). Her vision of the field is well exemplified by her writing:

> Accurate hospital statistics are much more rare than is generally imagined, and at best they only give the mortality which has taken place in the hospitals, and take no cognizance of those cases which are discharged in a hopeless condition, to die immediately afterwards, a practice which is followed to a much greater extent by some hospitals than others.
>
> We have known incurable cases discharged from one hospital, to which the deaths ought to have been accounted and received into another hospital, to die there in a day or two after admission, thereby lowering the mortality rate of the first at the expense of the second (6).

Ironically, nearly 135 years later, we are still coping with many of the same issues—suboptimal data collection, lack of adequate follow-up, interhospital transfer of high-risk patients who do not "show" on report card instruments, and less-than-expected accountability.

In 1914, Ernest Amory Codman, a surgeon in Boston, formed his own hospital known as End-Result Hospital, based on the philosophy that hospitals should study their mortality rates and that hospitals with the lowest adjusted mortality should be able to charge the highest rates (8,9). He told the Philadelphia Medical Society the following:

> We must formulate some method of hospital report showing as nearly as possible what are the results of the treatment obtained at different institutions. This report must be made out and published by each hospital in a uniform manner, so that comparison will be possible. With such a report as a starting point, those interested can begin to ask questions as to the management and efficiency (8).

Despite these pioneering concepts, Codman's hospital went bankrupt, and the idea was not adopted. This may be telling, as the cost of collecting data for report cards is a significant burden.

Intuitively, the need for risk adjustment of relevant patient demographic features is essential for comparison of outcomes. However, it was Roemer and colleagues (10) in 1968, and later Iezzoni and others (9,11), who demonstrated the critical need of adjustment for severity of illness.

Substantial national attention was drawn to quality assessment when the U.S. Health Care Financing Administration (HCFA) began publishing hospital mortality rates in 1986 (12,13). There was substantial concern over the risk adjustment used in this project, given the limited data in the Medicare administrative billing database (9,14); ultimately, HCFA stopped the release of hospital mortality reports (12). This, too, is a telling historical anecdote. The difficulties in risk adjustment are significant, and this indeed represents a formidable challenge for the future of quality assessment. In the early 1990s, Chelimsky (15) noted that there was much more interest in the cost of health care than in quality. Clearly, the lay press, as represented by *The New York Times*, focused on cost and access rather than quality indicators. But in recent years, although cost continues to be a central factor, there has been considerable research dedicated to the quality of medical care (16–20). In some instances, there has been application of relatively crude assessment tools in clinical practice; as a result, the field has been quite controversial. Some cardiologists and internists have the sense that quality assessment is simply a means of camouflage to reduce costs; others feel they are being harassed by such efforts. Nevertheless, if quality assessment is properly done in cardiovascular medicine, there is significant potential improvement in patient care (21).

DEFINITION OF QUALITY OF CARE

General

Despite the fact that quality of care became a standard phrase in the late 1990s, the operational definition of *quality* has been a source of confusion and difference of opinion. The IOM (22–25) defined *quality* as the "degree to which health services for individuals and populations increase the likelihood of desired health outcomes and are consistent with current professional knowledge." The technical excellence of the care that is provided, with special emphasis on the physician-patient relationship, is a common theme for most definitions of *quality of care*. Two factors drive the technical quality—the appropriateness of the services provided and the skill with which the appropriate care is performed.

One reason why cardiovascular medicine has been a major focus of quality efforts is that the most obvious health outcome—death—is common in patients with identified cardiac disease. This ease of measurement coupled with the high cost of cardiovascular care has made cardiology a focal point for quality measurement activities.

The determination of quality depends to some extent on the perspective of the person for whom the assessment is done. Patients, health care providers, and policy makers tend to have somewhat different, though considerably overlapping, concepts regarding quality. Patients tend to focus on the nature of the interactions with providers, including personal attention, courteous behavior, and prompt service, elements of what has been termed *patient satisfaction*. A major issue is the view that patients, as consumers, should have all of the information necessary to make judgments about the value of medical services, the concept of "patient-centered care" (22).

In contrast, providers tend to emphasize the technical aspects of quality, including whether correct decisions regarding diagnostic or therapeutic strategies have been made and whether those strategies have been executed with proper skill and knowledge. Policy makers and managers of health plans or health benefits organizations are most interested in measures of health and satisfaction of the overall population rather than a single measure of health. Integrating these different perspectives can be a daunting task, and most quality assessments tend to emphasize one of the three perspectives. Ultimately, quality of care is evaluated at three different levels—structure, process, and outcome (26).

Clinical practice guidelines are a pivotal part of defining quality on an evidence basis, with a list of class IA, IB, II, and III recommendations. By simply counting the number of times such recommendations are followed as a proportion of the number of opportunities, one can derive a quality measure which should relate quite nicely to outcomes.

Structure

The *structure* of a health care system refers to the characteristics of physicians, other health care providers, and the facilities in which they deliver health care. For cardiology practice, the critical structural characteristics comprise the specialty status, practice organization, availability of facilities for noninvasive and invasive testing and therapeutic intervention, and the types of disease management programs. Recent information has demonstrated that both spe-

cialty status (27) and environment, such as teaching or financial status of hospitals (28,29), have an influence on mortality. These studies reinforce the component of structure for determining quality of care.

Process

The "time-honored" method of peer review has been the morbidity and mortality conference. In this approach, when a poor outcome occurred, the patient's care was reviewed in front of a peer group. This approach suffered from lack of consistency and frequently did not provide the type of information that could lead to systematic improvement in the delivery of care. In a sense, quality assessment has followed the same course as clinical investigation: from anecdote to systematic quantitative assessment.

An appealing approach to measurement of quality is to determine when it is known that one diagnostic or therapeutic strategy is superior to an alternative and to measure how often the preferred strategy is used rather than the inferior strategy (26). "Doing the right thing at the right time" in concept can be measured relatively easily, and because multiple patient encounters occur, this sort of process measurement has a frequency of events high enough to allow for meaningful quantitative measures. Thus, measurement of the proportion of post-MI patients treated with aspirin and beta-blocker drugs has become a standard method of assessing quality.

The use of statins in patients with atherosclerosis and low-density lipoprotein of more than 100 mg per dL is a useful index. A recent report by Bradley and colleagues (30) on beta-blockers after acute MI highlights the process issues. Eight representative hospitals across the United States were selected to prospectively study the use of beta-blockers (Table 45.1). The range of improvement varied between 30% and −21%. The key factors characterizing improvement were administrative support, support and leadership among clinicians, use of data, explicit goals, and the proper design and execution of initiatives to affect change (30).

Another increasingly used measure is the time from admission to the emergency department to the administration of thrombolytic therapy. In patients with congestive heart failure, the proportion of patients with left ventricular function measurements and the proportion of patients receiving angiotensin-converting enzyme inhibitors among those with reduced systolic function comprise data-derived explicit process measures.

This approach of using explicit process-based criteria derived from results of randomized trials has increasingly supplanted traditional peer review, which consisted of a review of the chart by an independent expert to assess the degree to which care of the patient seemed to reflect community standards with nonquantitative feedback to individual practitioners. The weaknesses of this nonquantitative,

TABLE 45.1   LISTING OF STUDY HOSPITALS

| Site | Staffed beds | Beta-blocker use rate, patients, %[a] | | Absolute change in beta-blocker use (% points) | Beta-blocker use rating | |
		Baseline	Follow-up		Improvement	Follow-up
California	271	43	73	+30	High	High
Ohio	428	47	69	+22	High	High
Florida	629	56	68	+12	High	High
California	263	39	46	+7	Average	Medium
New York	231	61	67	+6	Average	High
Arkansas	275	29	35	+6	Average	Low
Missouri	708	63	47	−16	Low	Medium
Minnesota	110	66	45	−21	Low	Medium

[a]Beta-blocker use rates were calculated as the number of patients who received beta-blockers at discharge divided by the total number of patients discharged from each hospital during the relevant (baseline or follow-up) period.

implicit assessment are obvious. The lack of consistency increases the chance of arbitrary use of the information for negative feedback rather than providing standards by which self-improvement can be made.

Brook and colleagues (26) described the rationale for the subjective approach. An expert or a "peer" reviews the documentation in the medical record. The first question asked in the examination is whether the basic approach to patient care was adequate by community standards. The second question is whether a different approach to care would have improved the outcome. Finally, these two elements are put together to determine whether the overall quality of care was "acceptable." Multiple problems have been encountered with this approach, including difficulty identifying peers or experts to perform the review (excellent practitioners spend their time caring for patients and not reviewing others' charts) and inadequacies in the typical medical record in terms of providing the best information for quality assessment.

An appealing method that combines process and intermediate measures of outcomes is to identify a physiologic outcome that would fall within an excellent, acceptable, or unacceptable range based on what is known about the disease pathophysiology and its management (26). An example of this type of measure is the assessment of hemoglobin A_{1C} in patients with diabetes. It is assumed that excellent care for diabetes will result in low hemoglobin A_{1C} levels, although multiple methods of achieving these levels might be acceptable practice (diet, exercise, insulin, oral hypoglycemic agents). Therefore, a quality assessment might simply consist of measuring the proportion of patients seen by a practitioner for longitudinal care with acceptable hemoglobin A_{1C} measures.

This approach can be extrapolated to populations of patients by evaluating the proportion of patients meeting the physiologic target. Variation in compliance would be expected in a population, and therefore an acceptable range of uncontrolled diabetic patients could be defined based on community data. The proportion of patients with adequately controlled blood pressure or stable weight could

also be quantified and compared using benchmarking methods. Of course, these measures are subject to gaming in the same way as complex outcome measures, by steering high-risk patients for poor outcomes or poor compliance away from the practice (21).

Appropriateness

A more formal means of assessing whether the "right thing was done at the right time" is to evaluate its appropriateness. Whether a diagnostic or interventional procedure was properly indicated and needed is an alternative assessment of process. To determine the "appropriateness" of a medical procedure, it is necessary to have the circumstances judged by an independent group of health care professionals, with access to the medical records and relevant laboratory information. Ratings of appropriateness have been used for CABG, PCI, coronary angiography, and other cardiovascular procedures (31–34). However, it is cumbersome to review the patients on a case-by-case basis. The qualitative and subjective aspects, in trying to assess whether the accepted criteria or indications have been met, can be difficult to resolve. Accordingly, a considerable proportion of the procedures performed for patients wind up being scored as "uncertain." Still, the level of appropriateness of a given procedure may be used as an index of quality of a given hospital, health care system, or even operator.

Medical Errors

One of the most controversial areas to have been highlighted in recent years is that of medical errors. The IOM report issued in 2000 (initially issued in 1999) (1) set off considerable debate in the medical community and peer-reviewed medical literature (2–5). The report claims that at least 44,000 to 98,000 deaths occur in American hospitals each year that are attributable to medical errors. The IOM notes a "cycle of inaction" and calls for prevention of errors and resultant injuries, along with better accountability and dedicated research. In review of the literature surrounding the report, it is clear that medical errors constitute a problem. But what remains unclear is whether the magnitude of the problem has been exaggerated. On one hand, noted authorities such as Brennan (2) and McDonald et al. (3) have questioned the report's accuracy and potential for harm itself. Others such as Leape (4) and Meyer et al. (5) stand firm behind the report. Of note, Meyer et al. represent the Agency for Healthcare Research and Quality, which stands to gain considerable federal funding for research in this area. Much of the debate is related to the data from which the potential error death toll is extrapolated, such as a 1984 study of New York hospitals, and a 1991 to 1992 study in Colorado and Utah hospitals (2). For example, postoperative hemorrhages are classified as "errors" when most physicians would not consider this as an appropriate categorization. Another example of potential miscalculation was that of medication errors that were attributable to drug abuse rather than an iatrogenic cause (3). The IOM report calls for a future 50% reduction in the incidence of errors, but there is no accurate incidence available in a general medical population. Some data suggest that safety has already improved from the 4% to 5% rate of injury reported in California in 1976 to the 2.9% in Colorado and Utah in 1992 (2).

Recently, Hayward and Hofer (34a) estimated the number of deaths from medical errors in the United States to be 5,000 to 15,000 per year. The gross discrepancy (one-tenth of the IOM estimate) was attributed to inaccurate definitions of what constitutes a medical error. Hayward and Hofer looked at 111 in-hospital deaths at seven Veterans Administration hospitals between 1995 and 1996 and concluded that a very small proportion (0.5%) of patients would have lived at least 3 months in good health if optimal care was delivered.

Despite the media attention and headline-grabbing nature of the IOM report and the flurry of additional edi-

torials, the positive side is more focus and attention to the issue of quality of care. Many examples have been developed in cardiovascular medicine. MI, which has the greatest profile of conditions in the field, has been the subject of several recent papers on errors in medication (35–41a) and of media coverage. The alarming newspaper coverage of one of the first reports of errors in fibrinolytic dosing in acute MI read "up to 25% of heart attack patients who are given the two most widely used clotbusting drugs during heart attacks get the wrong doses, doubling their death rates."

It is particularly confounding to analyze medication errors in the treatment of acute MI, because patients die before they can receive the complete dose, and this could be wrongly classified as an "error." In Figure 45.1, a report from the Global Utilization of Streptokinase and Tissue Plasminogen Activator for Occluded Coronary Arteries (GUSTO) III trial by Goodman et al. highlights the association between deviation in planned dosing and mortality, both for alteplase and reteplase (35). The difficult issue, however, is to establish cause and effect, and none of the studies to date was prospectively defined to address this pivotal question. It seems logical that bolus fibrinolytic agents such as reteplase or tenecteplase may reduce errors in dosing, as compared with the complex regimen of accelerated alteplase, which required a 90-minute infusion and different doses of the drug in three discrete phases (bolus, initial 30 minutes, next 60 minutes). Similarly, excessive dosing could result in intracranial hemorrhage or other life-threatening bleeding complications. As with the overall problem of medical errors, we can be assured that there is indeed a problem, but the precise quantification is quite difficult with fibrinolytics in acute MI.

It should be noted that the IOM report and related studies have focused only on in-patient medical errors. Although these are relatively easier to measure (despite controversy over definitions), important errors also occur in the

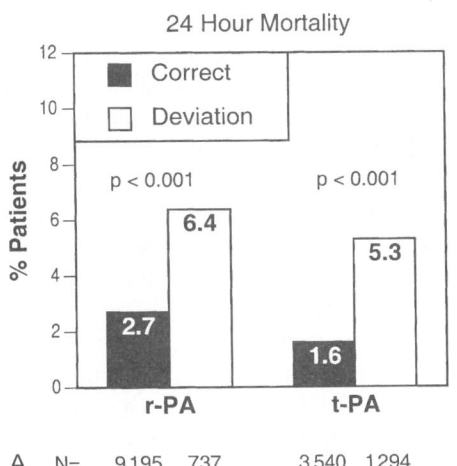

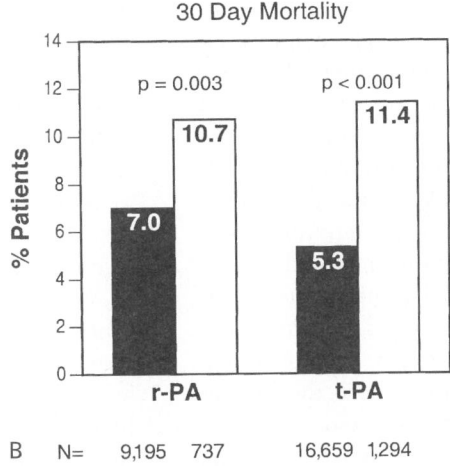

FIGURE 45.1 Mortality at 24 hours **(A)** and 30 days **(B)** in the GUSTO III trial by correct or incorrect fibrinolytic dosing. r-PA, reteplase; t-PA, alteplase. (From Goodman S, et al. Presented at the American College of Cardiology, March 2001, with permission.)

outpatient arena, and those represent a major challenge for our health care system.

Outcomes

The concept that medical outcomes should be the gold standard of quality assessment is not difficult. However, a number of problems with collection and assessment of the relevant data severely limit the degree to which outcomes can be used in the current environment. Several studies found that when both process and outcomes are measured with adequate power, the two indicators point in the same direction (26). The list of potential key outcomes include mortality, morbidity, cost, and patient satisfaction.

Mortality

Mortality is the most appealing outcome to use in the assessment of quality in cardiovascular disease. It is easy to measure and difficult to manipulate. Additionally, as compared with many other medical problems, mortality is the critical outcome in the treatment of most cardiovascular problems.

Only certain cardiovascular diagnoses or procedures have an appreciable risk of mortality to make them suitable for a parameter of quality assessment. In patients who present with either acute MI or congestive heart failure or who undergo cardiac transplantation or coronary artery bypass surgery, the proportion of expected deaths may be adequate to use this as a benchmark of the quality of care. But for the common diagnoses such as unstable angina, evaluation of chest discomfort, or procedures such as percutaneous coronary revascularization, the fatality rates are too low for meaningful assessment. Thus, despite its importance, death is rare enough that in most circumstances adequate numbers of deaths cannot be accumulated to develop statistically robust estimates.

Furthermore, although statistical models to predict mortality have been developed more extensively for cardiovascular procedures and problems than for other medical conditions, the majority of the variance in mortality cannot be explained by known factors. Accordingly, considerable debate remains about whether differences observed in mortality outcomes between systems, practices, or practitioners represent differences in quality, differences in risk status of the population before treatment, or random variation.

Beyond the problem of low incidence and potential of random variance, mortality may not be the most important outcome to assess for a given diagnosis or procedure. For example, with percutaneous revascularization, the occurrence of periprocedural MI and the need for emergency bypass surgery or repeat PCI are much more common adverse outcomes than mortality. Furthermore, the durability of the procedure is reflected by the avoidance of the need for repeat procedures during extended follow-up,

along with the patient being symptom-free. In such patients, an assessment of mortality does not indicate the important outcomes that one needs to know to adjudicate the quality of a particular center or even operator.

There are certain instances in which mortality and morbidity may not track. For example, in a center where patients undergo CABG with a low mortality but with a heightened risk of perioperative stroke or mediastinitis, one could be misled by the low occurrence of fatal outcomes. Indeed, Silber and colleagues (42) identified a poor correlation between nonfatal and fatal complications of CABG in 57 hospitals and nearly 17,000 patients. Of note, this study also suggested that sites that record details of medical care may be the ones with the lowest operative mortality.

Major Morbidity

Major morbidity has advantages as a measure of quality in that it is more common and it is usually detectable in the medical record. However, the imperfections of major morbidity result from variability in definition, degree of documentation, and adjustment models. Although the general concept of MI or stroke is intuitively obvious, the actual classification of individual cases is highly variable. The diagnosis of MI is dependent on timely measurement of enzymes and electrocardiograms, the type of enzyme assay used (creatinine kinase-MB, troponin), and appropriate interpretation of the data with recording in the medical record. Particularly with cardiovascular procedures, there is a well-described bias of the person performing the procedure to minimize procedure-related difficulties; in clinical trials of percutaneous interventional procedures, detection of nonfatal MI by the practitioner occurs at much lower rates than does detection by a clinical events committee (43). Additionally, uncertainty concerning the accuracy of statistical models to adjust for differences in baseline risk for death is multiply compounded in the prediction of nonfatal events.

Cost

The use of cost as a measure of quality is controversial. In the in-patient setting, costs are increasingly measured for administrative reasons to ensure the financial viability of hospitals. Because patients are also concerned about cost, it is reasonable to consider that high-quality physicians or practices might be defined as providing excellent outcomes or evidence of excellent process at a reasonable cost. Outpatient costs are more difficult to obtain and have not become a commonly used measure for comparative data.

With the availability of extensive financial data in some centers, it is often easier to measure hospital and professional costs rather than clinical outcomes. Such indices as length of stay or cost per case have been increasingly used in recent years but may not accurately reflect quality of care. Ideally, the best outcomes can be achieved at the lowest cumulative cost. Interestingly, the state of Pennsylvania technology assessment program showed an inverse correlation between hospital costs and outcomes for coronary artery bypass surgery (44) that was not expected. The centers with the lowest cost tended to also achieve the best outcomes. Whether this will occur with other diagnoses, procedures, and even for this particular operation in other health care systems remains to be seen. The economy of scale with high volume may be a principal driving factor when there is a direct relationship between quality and cost. At times, use of "big ticket" items such as stents or abciximab may be linked to much higher costs but would be expected to provide reduced risk of ischemic complications.

Patient Satisfaction

Patient satisfaction, like cost, has become a standard administrative measure to ensure that practices remain economically viable. It can be measured quickly and efficiently, just as satisfaction with other services can be measured in our society. Large numbers can be aggregated to allow accurate statistical comparisons to be made.

However, little relationship exists between the satisfaction of the patient with the encounter and the technical quality of care delivered. A patient undergoing an uncomplicated percutaneous intervention that was not indicated in the first place may have felt that the care was excellent, but the judgment about whether the procedure was indicated requires substantial medical knowledge. Patient satisfaction is typically rated via questionnaires and may be difficult to interpret. The parameter that seems to drive this in a favorable direction is time with the physician and the sense that the physician is giving the patient undivided attention and utmost priority. However, factors such as parking at the hospital, the cafeteria, accommodations, reading materials in the waiting room, the service orientation of ancillary personnel, and many others play a role in the composite experience. Therefore, patient satisfaction is an important parameter to survey, but its relationship with clinical outcomes is not established. It is possible that the three different indices of clinical outcomes, cost, and patient satisfaction may go in different directions. For the low-volume center that is characterized by exquisite customer service and long physician and physician extender visits, for example, there may be excellent patient satisfaction but excessive costs and suboptimal outcomes. Nevertheless, with health care plans that rely on patient subscription, this may be one of the most important indices to evaluate a program's success.

METHODS OF MEASUREMENT

The validity of proposed measures of quality cannot be understood without a thorough knowledge of the source of data. A major problem with interpretation of much of the data made available to the public has been the reliance on inaccurate sources of data and extrapolation beyond the limits of the data. Because most of the medical record consists of handwritten notes, there is no available method of aggregating information that captures the interaction between the health care provider and the patient in most systems. Consequently, administrative databases or medical record reviews have formed the basis for most quality assessments.

Administrative Databases

Administrative databases designed to allow patient billing and tracking for financial reasons provide excellent information concerning demographics, procedures, and survival. However, this information does not reflect the modifying medical information concerning severity of illness, complications, or medical outcomes other than death. Multiple studies have demonstrated that the clinical information contained in administrative databases is incomplete and often erroneous and misleading. Comparisons of insurance claims information with clinical databases have demonstrated poor concordance rates in classifying patient diagnosis, ranging from 0.09 for unstable angina to 0.83 for diabetes (45).

Administrative databases such as Medicare or those at state departments of health are especially attractive to use because they contain large data sets with the sufficient outcomes needed to analyze the relationship of a hospital or clinician to outcomes. However, these databases were frequently not designed to perform such an analysis and may be quite insufficient with respect to missing data. Often, only mortality data are available with limited demographic information. These typically represent retrospective ad hoc assessments. Many of the data, if not all that have been entered, have not, ironically, been quality-assured except for the financial component. More recently, using an administrative database to prospectively capture relevant data, such as is ongoing in New York for PCI procedures, is a powerful means of combining large numbers of patients, outcomes, and establishing the relationship.

Medical Record Review

Although administrative or claims databases certainly have problems, the medical record itself has many deficiencies that make chart audit a suboptimal exercise. The nomenclature used to describe similar phenomena varies from practitioner to practitioner. Pertinent negatives are frequently not mentioned so that the reviewer must assume that if a finding or procedure is not mentioned in the medical record, it was not evaluated or done. In an adverse event reporting study, a chart audit missed more than half of adverse events related to medications (46). On the other hand, physician reporting of adverse events in the same study was equally remiss for identifying the outcomes but twice as likely to detect the important, preventable events. The physician-reporting mechanism was considered less costly: $15,000 compared with $54,000 (46). This study emphasizes some of the pivotal shortcomings of chart review—its lack of accuracy and high cost.

Clinical Databases

Very few clinical databases are used in concurrent patient care. Such databases tend to have considerably more information that is relevant, with data having more likely been verified by source medical record or other documentation, and are easier to work with. A clinical database can take the form of a single center's results, a clinical trial, or a consortium of sites. Prospective randomized clinical trials are emerging as a powerful tool to provide information on outcomes between different health care systems or regions (47,48).

Risk Adjustment

Although it seems that determining the severity of illness for patient groups and performing risk adjustment might be straightforward, this has not proved to be the case (49–51). There is considerable debate about what constitutes the clinical vital facts; whether to use administrative data alone or incorporate relevant laboratory data; and the value of further clinical data that can be obtained only via the time-consuming, labor-intensive, and expensive abstraction of medical records. Several proprietary commercial severity measures have been used (eTable 45.1.1). Of these, the MedisGroups has been adopted by Pennsylvania for the "consumer guide" for CABG; the Acute Physiology and Chronic Health Evaluation III "physiology score" has been widely used to assess quality of care for intensive care units. Of note, direct comparisons of these four severity measures showed considerable variance, with only about 80% of patients receiving similar rankings between severity tools (49).

The discriminatory power of a particular model for risk adjustment can be assessed by comparing c-statistics, which are equivalent to area under receiver-operating characteristic curves (50). Pine and colleagues (51) showed that a model that relies solely on administrative data compares favorably (good concordance) to one that incorporates administrative, laboratory, and clinically extracted data, with an area under receiver-operating characteristic curves of approximately 0.85. This remains controversial, as many studies have demonstrated the added value of the laboratory and additional clinical data. Nevertheless, review of these data is instructive to highlight some of the difficulties encountered in performing risk adjustment of patients, even for mortality outcomes.

WHO IS MEASURING QUALITY?

Because participants in health care ranging from the patient to the practitioner to the health care administrator are interested in quality, considerable overlap exists in the assignment of responsibility of its assessment. An understanding of the roles currently assumed by various organizations could allow the practitioner to develop an approach to responding to the demands and needs of the various constituents.

Centers for Medicare and Medicaid Services

As the largest single payer for health care delivery in the United States, the government has been concerned with the quality of medical care since its beginning. The evolution of thinking about how to assess quality has been propelled by the initiative that the Centers for Medicare and Medicaid Services (formerly HCFA) has taken in making risk-adjusted data for such procedures as CABG or cardiac transplantation available to the public. The public availability of this information has also allowed for ascertainment of outcome data for various constituents to use for benchmarking and advertising. Given that the clinical information contained in the Centers for Medicare and Medicaid Services database reflects diagnoses recorded for billing purposes, this approach has been highly controversial (14,52) and, ultimately, for in-hospital mortality data the practice was abandoned in 1993.

National Committee on Quality Assurance

The National Committee on Quality Assurance (NCQA) was founded in 1979 as an effort to establish a system of quality assessment by national managed care organizations (35). In addition to a primary interest in the importance of quality assessment, this organization was provided as an alternative to government intervention. With grant funding, the NCQA became independent of the national managed care organizations and its board was altered to provide a societal perspective on quality. One perspective on the NCQA is that it represents the most powerful single organization through which employers can participate in the assessment and the improvement of large health plans.

The method by which the NCQA accredits health plans includes a review of operations and an assessment using the Health Plan Employer Data and Information Set (HEDIS). HEDIS is a continually evolving set of measures designed to assess quality, access, and satisfaction in addition to critical issues in finances and administration. The measures are simple, and the HEDIS measures in use in 1996 included only whether cholesterol screening was used as a cardiovascular outcome measure. In *e*Table 45.1.2, a version of HEDIS is provided. More disease-specific measures are currently being added to the system. In a review of the NCQA, Iglehart (53) reported that the organization is growing and making a difference despite the rudimentary nature of the instruments being used and concern about the cost by managed care organization administrators.

State agencies (peer review organizations) have focused on quality assurance in the practice of medicine but have generally not collected large data sets on particular diagnoses or procedures. Some exceptions are highlighted in the subsequent section on outcome assessment by procedure.

Agency for Healthcare Research and Quality

In the United States, the new federal agency responsible for quality health care is the Agency for Healthcare Research and Quality, formerly the Agency for Health Care Policy and Research. The agency has solid government funding and an ambitious agenda to improve the country's health care delivery.

State Agencies

In the late 1980s, New York State instituted mandatory reporting of baseline characteristics and outcomes in patients undergoing CABG. Since then, percutaneous interventional procedures have been added to the mandatory reporting scheme. This approach has caused substantial controversy both because of the public disclosure of this information and because of uncertainty about whether this system has actually improved care. Pennsylvania and California have instituted similar programs for producing outcome report cards for acute myocardial infarction and revascularization procedures.

Regional Efforts

The Northern New England Group has organized major hospitals performing coronary revascularization in the New England region, with a goal of improving quality through the collection and dissemination of process and outcome data. A common database has been developed and used to provide scorecards for outcomes, and serial measures of process have been used to document improvement in the quality of care.

Cities

A number of metropolitan areas have now developed business coalitions interested in assessing the quality of medical care. This approach was quite visible in Cleveland with the organization known as the Cleveland Health Quality Choice. Formed in the early 1990s by the Cleveland Met-

ropolitan Business Coalition to facilitate selection of hospitals, the 30 centers were ranked on a quarterly basis for risk-adjusted mortality for five different diagnoses (50), including acute MI and congestive heart failure. The data were published in the newspaper along with other indices such as patient satisfaction and length of stay. Ultimately, the rating system was terminated when the costs of accruing the data specific to the project became unacceptable to some of the large hospital providers.

Managed Care Organizations

Individual managed care organizations typically provide individual assessments of quality and satisfaction, but the major method of ensuring accountability is external accreditation. The HEDIS measures (*e*Table 45.1.2) administered by the NCQA have become the standard, although these measures have almost no relevance to the care of patients with cardiovascular disease.

Professional Societies

Although professional societies can provide standards for quality assessment, the responsibility of professional societies to guard the welfare of their members makes actual assessment of the quality of individual practitioners difficult. An approach adopted by the American College of Cardiology focuses on the development of standards for data collection that will allow the assessment of structure, process, and outcome measures (54). The Society of Thoracic and Cardiovascular Surgeons is far ahead of the American College of Cardiology, and output from their database has been linked to driving better quality at institutions throughout the United States.

Individual Hospitals

The interest of individual hospitals in quality measures has been primarily to promote excellence in the quest for managed care contracts or public attention. However, in this process substantial progress has been made at the local level in the ascertainment and aggregation of major procedural outcomes. The major mechanism of quality assessment in this manner has been the use of clinical databases. The American College of Cardiology is playing a major role in focusing commercial database sponsors on common nomenclature and collection of baseline clinical data that will allow for adjustment according to baseline risk.

The National Hospital Network provides one example of a large group of hospitals that have organized for contracting purposes and to that end have developed common standards for data capture. This database provides reports to individual institutions, benchmarking them against other institutions in the network with regard to patient characteristics, choices of procedures, and outcomes. The database has provided substantial documentation of a wide variation in practice patterns related to choice of devices, even in high-volume institutions.

QUALITY OUTCOMES FOR PARTICULAR CARDIOVASCULAR PROCEDURES AND DIAGNOSES

Coronary Artery Bypass Surgery

The most extensively studied medical procedure for relationship of volume to outcome is bypass surgery. The procedure is ideal for scorecard analysis because it is frequently performed, it carries an appreciable risk of mortality, and there has been extensive refinement of the features that are important for risk adjustment. Luft and coworkers (55–57) pioneered much of this effort and were among the first to document the inverse relationship between hospitals with low volume and high mortality in the late 1970s. In the mid-1980s, the HCFA and Veterans Affairs hospitals began reporting hospital CABG activity and risk-adjusted mortality on an annual basis to the public (9,12,13,21,58). As early as 1989, Hannan and colleagues (59) from New York State noted that the surgeon's annual volume was even more critical a determinant than the hospital volume of CABG for risk-adjusted mortality. In 1991, two influential studies from the Northeast demonstrated the extensive interhospital, interoperator, and geographic variability for CABG risk-adjusted mortality outcomes (60,61). There has been considerable effort and clinical investigation in the Northeast on this topic, especially in New York, Pennsylvania, and northern New England (59–61).

In New York, a pivotal study in 1990 described the statewide Cardiac Surgery Reporting System and tracking of the 28 hospitals performing CABG, with four hospitals demonstrating mortality rates that were significantly higher than expected—one with a death rate of 14.3% and only 63 cases during a 6-month period in 1989 (62). These data attracted considerable attention in December 1991, when a newspaper sued the State Department of Public Health for access to the operator- and hospital-specific data. A supreme court in New York ruled that the citizens of the state have a right to know these data and granted the newspaper access, setting a national precedent for public disclosure of not only hospital-specific but also physician-specific crude and risk-adjusted mortality data (21,63).

The findings in New York of certain hospital outliers were replicated in other parts of the country (62,64). Pooling seven studies that examined the relationship between hospital volume and mortality outcome for CABG, Sowden and coworkers (65) showed that the adjusted relative risk of dying was between 0.44 and 0.83 for surgery in a high-volume hospital (cutoff of high volume ranging from 150 to 223 cases per year). Of interest, in Ontario,

Canada, where there are no low-volume hospitals (all performed more than 300 cases per year in 1992 and 1993), there were no outliers and the in-hospital mortality was consistently low in all nine hospitals (66). These findings certainly provide a foundation for the call for "regionalization" that many of the studies have beckoned (57,64,66,67). Of note, in contrast to California there is considerable lack of a regionalized approach. In California, 91% of patients are within 25 miles of a center that offers bypass surgery, as compared with 82% in New York and 60% in Canada (67). Along with this, in 1987 to 1989, 31% of California hospitals performed fewer than 100 CABGs per year, as compared with 10% in New York and 0% in Canada (67).

The tracking of hospital- and operator-specific risk-adjusted mortality has been associated with a reduction in mortality not only in New York and northern New England but also in Massachusetts, where there is no centralized tracking (68–71). Hannan and colleagues (68) reported a New York statewide 41% decrease in risk-adjusted CABG mortality (from 4.2% to 2.5%) from 1989 to 1992. This mortality decline could not be explained by shifts of patients from low-volume to high-volume surgeons, changes in patient mix, or improvement of performance of surgeons with low volumes (69). Rather, it was suggested the improvement was related to the influx of new cardiac surgeons with better results and the exodus of some low-volume surgeons with high risk-adjusted mortality (69). As with New York, O'Connor and colleagues (70) reported a 24% reduction in mortality from 1987 to 1993 for patients undergoing surgery in Maine, New Hampshire, and Vermont. Quite comparable to the improved cardiac mortality observed in New York, in Massachusetts the observed mortality rates decreased from 4.7% to 3.3% from 1990 to 1994 (71), despite the absence of statewide reporting of outcomes.

The relationship of surveillance reporting systems and improvement of outcomes has fueled considerable controversy and has important implications on regional and national health care policy (72–74). It remains unclear that a statewide report card directly influences outcomes because the CABG mortality rate has decreased on a national level (72). Green and Wintfeld (74) harshly criticized the claims of the New York State Department of Health's first physician-specific mortality report by objecting to the validity of the risk-adjusted mortality model, changing of definitions from any in-hospital death to in-hospital death within 30 days, and changing in coding of key risk factors (renal failure, congestive heart failure, chronic obstructive pulmonary disease, and low ejection fraction). Examples that they cited were a 350% to 600% increase in coding of renal failure (with a change in definition to creatinine of more than 2.5 mg per dL instead of dialysis) and increase in coding of chronic lung disease from 2% to 53% (74).

Chassin and members of the New York State Department of Health (75,76) strongly objected to these critique points and quantitatively assert that the reduction of CABG is real and attributable to the reporting system. Omoigui and coworkers (77) from The Cleveland Clinic Foundation showed that patients from New York State outmigrated to The Cleveland Clinic with increased frequency during the period of the statewide reporting system, and these patients were distinctly higher risk. However, the number of patients who were shown to outmigrate from New York could not have accounted for the marked reduction in CABG-related mortality during the period under study (75–77); perhaps it accounted for a small contribution (75–78).

The statewide reporting mechanism of CABG results has also been available in Pennsylvania since 1990 with

hospital and professional charge data, in addition to hospital- and physician-specific outcome data (Fig. 45.2) (44). Recently, Schneider and Epstein (79) surveyed Pennsylvanian cardiologists and cardiac surgeons and claimed that the state's *Consumer Guide to Coronary Artery Bypass Surgery* has limited credibility and raised concern that such a guide could have an unfavorable effect on access to CABG for the most severely ill patients who need surgery the most.

The New York CABG database has offered a window to the effect of managed care insurance (80). Recently, Peterson et al. used the New York CABG database to analyze access to care and elderly patient outcome (81). This group of investigators also examined the difficulties of risk adjustment for comparing CABG mortality results (82). The refinement of risk-adjusted indices for CABG has continued with work by Ivanov et al. (83).

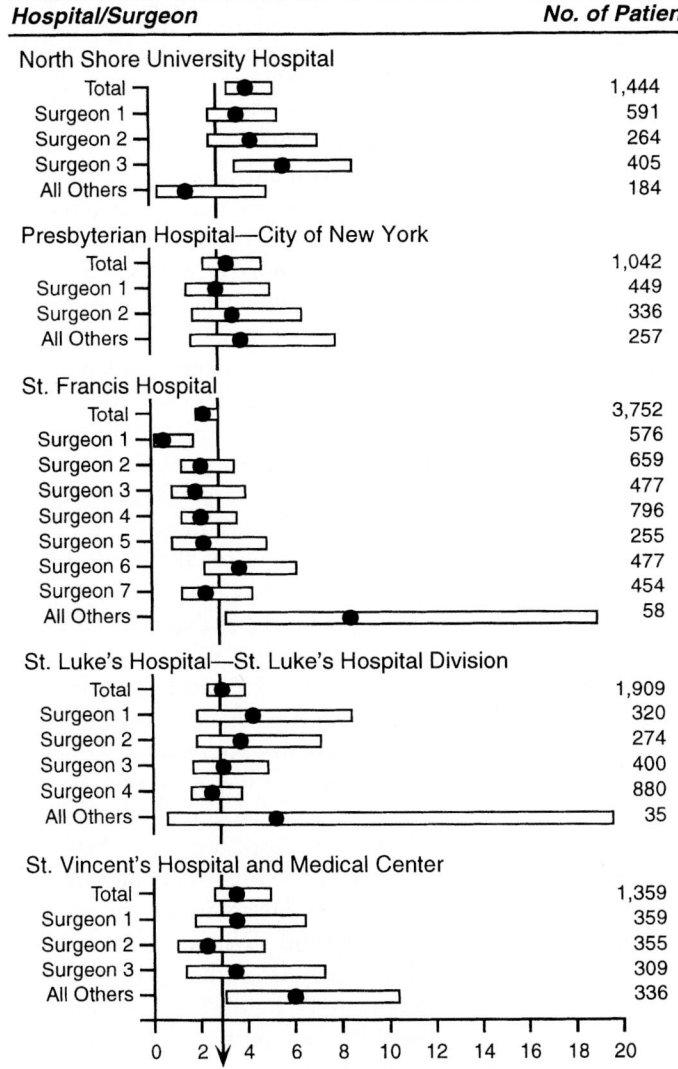

FIGURE 45.2 Risk-adjusted coronary artery bypass surgery mortality data (black dots are point estimates) with 95% confidence intervals (*horizontal bars*) for representative hospitals in Downstate New York. (From Topol EJ, Block PC, Holmes DR, et al. Readiness for the scorecard era in cardiovascular medicine. *Am J Cardiol* 1995;75:1170–1173, with permission.)

In summary, report cards on CABG have been extensively used in many parts of the country, but their true effects on favorably modulating mortality are not completely accepted. This particular operation has been the "front-runner" in the field for hospital- and physician-specific outcomes and the testing grounds for public disclosure. Surely the lessons learned from the experience and controversies will be instructive in other procedures and diagnoses in cardiovascular medicine.

Percutaneous Coronary Intervention

PCI has been more difficult to study and produce scorecards for because, although the procedure is very frequently performed, the mortality is quite low (approximately 1% or less) and the morbidities of emergency bypass surgery or MI are difficult to define, especially in a post hoc analysis of a large administrative database (84). Nevertheless, the studies that have been reported parallel the findings of CABG, with a clear-cut inverse relationship of hospital and operator volume and adverse outcomes. Hannan and associates (85) studied more than 5,800 patients in New York State to delineate a multivariate risk-adjusted model. One of the first activity-to-volume relationship studies was performed by Ritchie and colleagues (86), who showed, using nearly 25,000 procedures in the state of California during 1989, that urgent CABG was progressively more likely as hospital percutaneous transluminal coronary angioplasty (PTCA) volumes fell below 200 per year. Further, in patients having PTCA related to a principal diagnosis of acute MI, the relationship of hospital volume to adverse outcomes was exaggerated in hospitals with an annual volume of fewer than 200; the death or urgent CABG rate was 12.4%.

The Society for Cardiac Angiography and Interventions reported on more than 19,500 consecutive patients in 48 hospitals in North America. Most of the hospitals performed more than 200 PTCAs per year, and the major finding was fewer major complications in centers performing more than 400 procedures per year (a 44% risk reduction, risk-adjusted) (87). Of note, if the threshold of 400 cases is used, these data suggest a 2-fold reduction in mortality, a 10-fold reduction in emergency CABG, and an 18-fold reduction in periprocedural MI (87).

The relationship of hospital volume to major complications was studied by Jollis and colleagues (88) using the Medicare database of more than 217,000 patients. As shown in Figure 45.3, there was a definite relationship of hospital volume and mortality as well as the rate of CABG during the index hospitalization. Of note, the patients undergoing PTCA in hospitals without surgical backup had the highest mortality (9.9%), which may be attributed in part to a higher proportion of primary PTCA for acute MI.

Operator-specific results in PCI have been studied by many groups, and parallel trends of a volume to outcome relationship have been shown (87–93). Ellis and associates

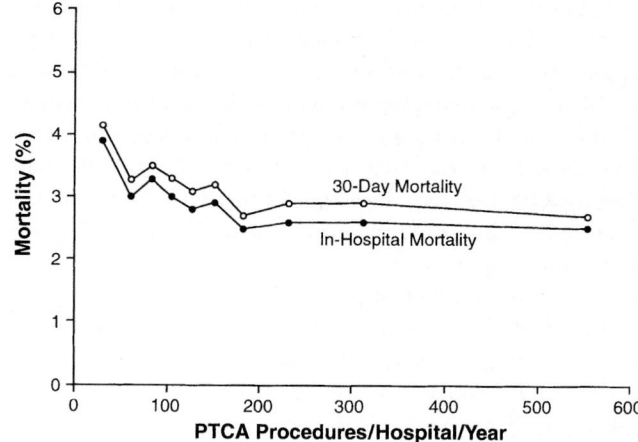

FIGURE 45.3 Mortality among Medicare beneficiaries who underwent percutaneous transluminal coronary angioplasty (PTCA) from 1987 through 1990, according to the volume of PTCA procedures at the hospitals where they were treated. The points on the curves correspond to the mortality rates among patients treated at hospitals with volumes of 1 to 46, 47 to 70, 71 to 93, 94 to 114, 115 to 137, 138 to 166, 167 to 206, 207 to 261, 262 to 371, and 372 to 987 procedures per year. (From Jollis JG, Peterson ED, DeLong ER, et al. The relation between the volume of coronary angioplasty procedures at hospitals treating Medicare beneficiaries and short-term mortality. *N Engl J Med* 1994;331:1625–1629, with permission.)

(90) pointed out some of the difficulties in categorizing a "poor" operator or outliers with a database of nearly 5,000 procedures. By using a 50 cases per year dichotomization for low- and high-volume operators, Shook and colleagues (92) demonstrated a near doubling of emergency bypass surgery (2.1% vs. 3.9% for low-volume operators) and significant differences in length of stay as well as hospital costs. The 2001 guidelines for the American College of Cardiology/American Heart Association call for a minimum of 75 cases per year (94). Still, it is estimated that in the United States, 55% of physicians perform fewer than 75 procedures per year and 46% of hospitals perform fewer than the recommended 400 per year (95).

The data set from New York State for all 62,670 patients undergoing PCI between 1991 and 1994 is illuminating and further corroborates the volume relationship (96). As shown in Figure 45.4, patients undergoing PCI by cardiologists with annual volumes of fewer than 75 cases had a substantial rise in same-day bypass surgery need. Risk-adjusted mortality was unfavorably affected in hospitals with annual PTCA volumes of fewer than 600. Although not as striking, the relationship of activity and mortality outcomes by hospital and operator was similar. The New York State data have been made available to the public (97). These data provide independent verification of the critical relationship of major complications and PTCA hospital and physician volume.

Much recent work has reinforced the operator-volume and outcome correlation in PCI (98–119). A prototypic example of the relationship was reported by McGrath et al. (119) involving 167,208 Medicare patients in 1,003 hospi-

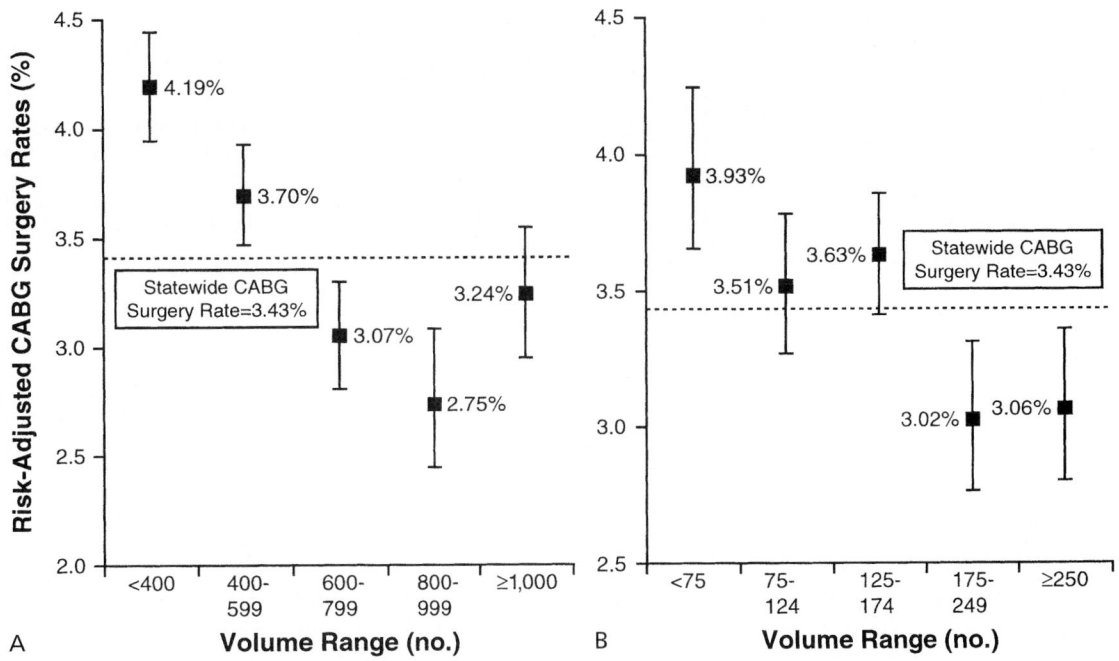

FIGURE 45.4 A: Risk-adjusted coronary artery bypass grafting (CABG) surgery rates for different hospital percutaneous transluminal coronary angioplasty volume ranges. Data presented as mean, with 95% confidence intervals indicated by the vertical bars. **B:** Risk-adjusted CABG surgery rates for different cardiologists' percutaneous transluminal coronary angioplasty volume ranges. Data presented as mean, with 95% confidence intervals indicated by the vertical bars. (From Hannan EL, Racz M, Ryan TJ, et al. Coronary angioplasty volume-outcome relationships for hospitals and cardiologists. *JAMA* 1997;277:892–898, with permission.)

tals and 6,534 operator-physicians. The need for CABG by operator volume and the hospital volume–mortality relationships are presented in Figure 45.5. Although the operator volume did not affect mortality and the hospital volume was not associated with urgent CABG use, the relationships that were found appear to be quite convincing and reinforced by the bulk of the other parallel studies.

Acute Myocardial Infarction

The risk-adjusted modeling for acute MI in the reperfusion era was addressed by Lee and colleagues (120) and in a large Medicare cohort by Normand and associates (121). Many states and regions have begun to analyze outcomes for acute MI by hospital. In December 1993, the state of California published the California Hospital Outcome Project, which provided extensive data for the diagnosis and outcome for patients presenting with acute MI for every hospital in the state. Representative data are summarized in *e*Table 45.1.3 (122,123). Beyond the outcome of mortality, important parameters such as the time to treatment, the use of thrombolytic therapy or catheter-based reperfusion, and the use of aspirin and other adjunctive medications are reflective of the quality of care for MI

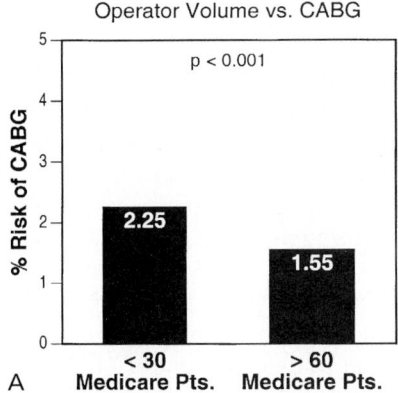

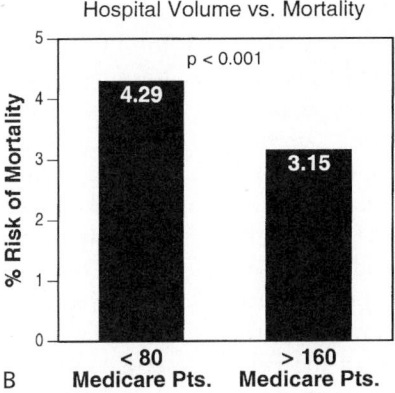

FIGURE 45.5 Rates of coronary artery bypass grafting (CABG) **(A)** or 30-day mortality **(B)** after percutaneous transluminal coronary intervention according to annual physician percutaneous coronary intervention volume among Medicare beneficiaries. (Data from McGrath PD, Wennberg DE, Dickens JD Jr, et al. Relation between operator and hospital volume and outcomes following percutaneous coronary interventions in the era of the coronary stent. *JAMA* 2000;284:3139–3144.)

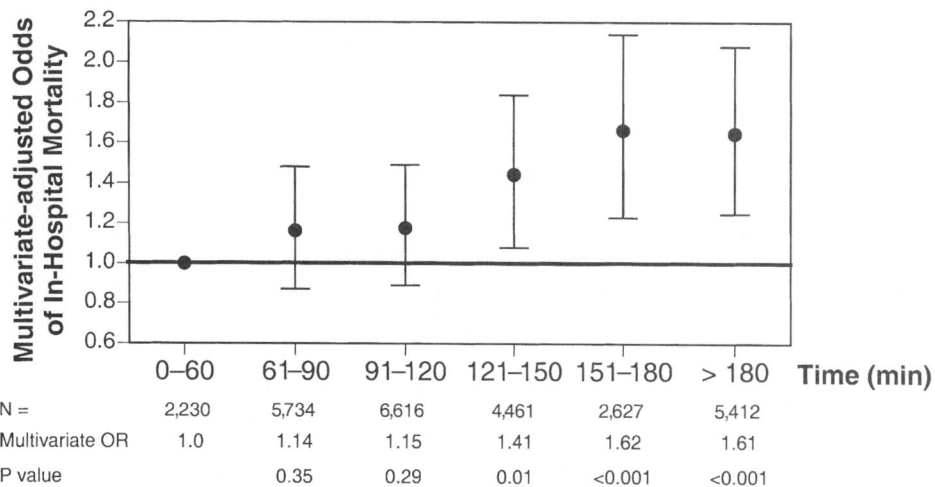

FIGURE 45.6 Multivariate-adjusted relationship between door-to-balloon time and mortality (χ^2 trend = 99.5; p <.01). Error bars indicate 95% confidence intervals. *Door time* refers to arrival at the hospital; *balloon time* refers to the time of first balloon inflation of the primary angioplasty procedure. OR, odds ratio. (From Cannon CP, Gibson CM, Lambrew CT, et al. Relationship of symptom-onset-to-balloon time and door-to-balloon time with mortality in patients undergoing angioplasty for acute myocardial infarction. *JAMA* 2000;283:2941–2947, with permission.)

patients (121). Significant regional and global variability exists in the use of angiography, PTCA, adjunct medications, and outcomes (46,47). Interestingly, the availability or age of the patient appears to be driving most of the coronary angiography performed after MI in the United States, rather than the expected medical indication of recurrent ischemia (124). The care pattern is affected by not only whether a primary care physician is involved but also improved when a noninvasive or invasive cardiologist is involved (27,125–127) and is affected by the type of hospital (128,129). The tremendous variability in practice patterns, even in the United States, with limited long-term data for large populations, underscores the uncertainty as to the appropriate level of aggressiveness.

Two studies suggested that involvement of a cardiologist in the care of a patient with acute MI may have a particularly beneficial impact on survival (27,130–134). In the Medicare study performed by Jollis and coworkers, involving 8,241 patients in four states in 1992, a significant relationship of risk-adjusted mortality reduction was demonstrated according to the specialty of the admitting physician. The odds reduction of mortality of approximately 12% to 15% for a cardiologist versus a primary care physician (Fig. 45.6) is noteworthy, as this represents at least as much of a benefit that has been targeted in several large-scale MI intervention trials (135–138). Willison et al. and others provide data and insight to reinforce Jollis' report (139–141). Consistent with the mortality effects was the use of evidence-based medications such as beta-blockade, aspirin, and angiotensin-converting enzyme inhibitors. A similar pattern of physician specialty and outcome was found for patients with unstable angina (142). An analysis of superior outcomes for MI in the 40 "top" heart hospitals reinforced the use of evidence-based treatment (lytics, aspirin, beta-blockade) as a marker for improved quality of care (143). Like the critique of scorecards, a point of vulnerability is the validity of the risk-adjusted modeling for making key comparisons in these

large administrative data sets. Of interest, if the gradient of mortality reduction of 10% to 15% (or more) can be achieved through improvement of process, such as the reduction of time to thrombolytic treatment by 1 hour on average associated with a 15% reduction of 30-day mortality, then meaningful improvement in outcomes can be derived and anticipated in the most common killer of patients in Western society today.

Outcomes research in acute MI reperfusion has been very helpful in demonstrating the importance of door-to-balloon time, hospital volume, and mortality. Using the National Registry of Myocardial Infarction data in 27,080 patients and multivariate adjustment, Cannon et al. showed the striking direct relationship of door-to-balloon and the odds ratio of mortality (Fig. 45.6) (144). Furthermore, these investigators went on to show the hospital volume–mortality relationship with primary angioplasty (Fig. 45.7) (144). Using the National Registry database from 1994 to 1999 in 62,299 patients, Magid et al. provided a comprehensive analysis of both thrombolytic therapy and primary angioplasty (145). As summarized in Figure 45.8, low-volume hospitals (fewer than 16 patients per year) had the longest door-to-balloon time and achieved similar in-hospital mortality for lytics or catheter-based reperfusion. On the other hand, the high-volume MI centers had better door-to-balloon times and better results for PCI compared with lytics (p <.001 for a strategy-hospital volume interaction) (145). Tu and colleagues have taken the field a step further by analyzing MI outcomes in 98,194 patients treated by 5,374 physicians in Canada (146). A strong inverse relationship between average annual volume of MI cases treated by the admitting physician and mortality rate was demonstrated (Fig. 45.9) (146).

The health care system and type of hospital have also been the subject of study for MI outcome research. The advantages of teaching and academic centers (147,148), those that have on-site revascularization (149) and Medi-

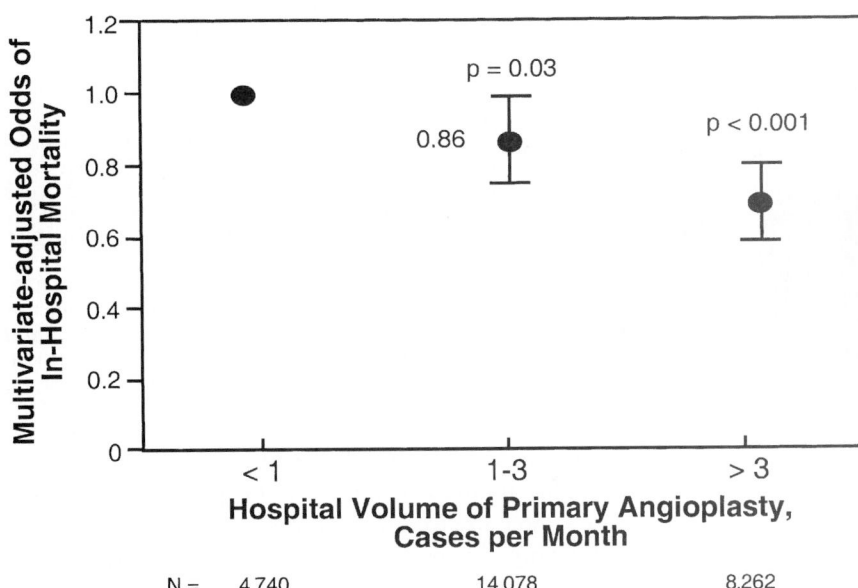

FIGURE 45.7 Multivariate-adjusted relationship between institutional volume of primary angioplasty cases and mortality. (From Cannon CP, Gibson CM, Lambrew CT, et al. Relationship of symptom-onset-to-balloon time and door-to-balloon time with mortality in patients undergoing angioplasty for acute myocardial infarction. *JAMA* 2000;283:2941–2947, with permission.)

care compared with the Veterans Health Administration (150,151), have all been explored.

COMMON THEMES AND PROBLEMS

Process versus Outcome

The debate about whether quality of care measurements should focus on the process of care or outcomes remains highly controversial. Advocates of measuring process point to the near impossibility of being certain that outcomes can be risk-adjusted and to the huge costs of measuring outcomes other than death. Furthermore, difficulty with com-

mon definitions and the ease of gaming the system with regard to nonfatal outcomes continue to produce substantial difficulty in the assessment of outcomes. Finally, the large number of outcomes that must be identified to discern differences in quality produces a fundamental limitation for the system.

Some have advocated that clinical trials should be used to establish efficacy and that outcome research should be used to determine the most effective way of delivering a diagnostic therapy or strategy. When these components have been evaluated in adequately sized studies, measurement of how often appropriate practices are used provides a method of measuring quality that is firmly based in empirical methodology and does not require adjustment for dif-

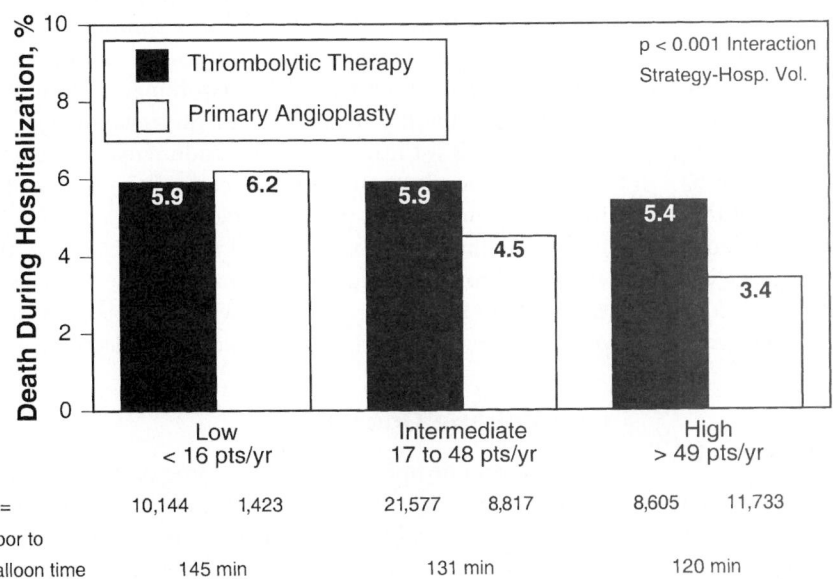

FIGURE 45.8 Rates of death during hospitalization for patients with acute myocardial infarction treated with thrombolytic therapy versus primary angioplasty, stratified by hospital primary angioplasty volume. *Door time* refers to arrival at the hospital; *balloon time* refers to the time of first balloon inflation of the primary angioplasty procedure. (From Magid DJ, Calonge BN, Rumsfeld JS, et al., for the National Registry of Myocardial Infarction 2 and 3 Investigators. Relation between hospital primary angioplasty volume and mortality for patients with acute MI treated with primary angioplasty vs thrombolytic therapy. *JAMA* 2000;284:3131–3138, with permission.)

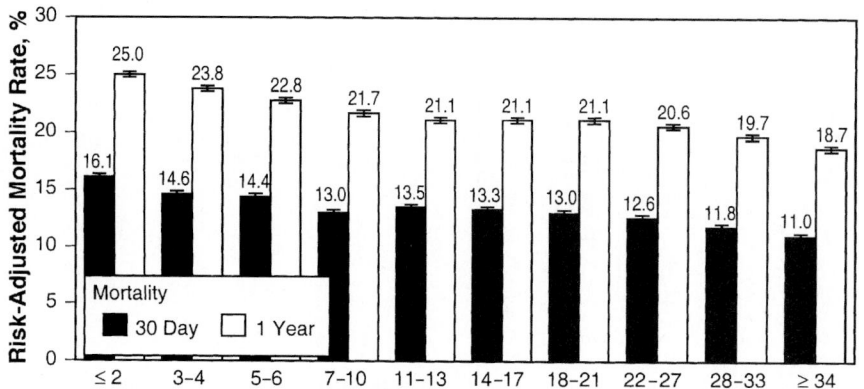

FIGURE 45.9 Risk-adjusted acute myocardial infarction mortality rates at 30 days and 1 year by deciles of annual volume of acute myocardial infarction patients treated by admitting physician. Error bars indicate 95% confidence intervals for mortality rates. (Adapted from Tu JV, Austin PC, Chan BTB. Relationship between annual volume of patients treated by admitting physician and mortality after acute myocardial infarction. *JAMA* 2001;285:3116–3122, with permission.)

ferences in baseline characteristics of patients seen by one practice compared with another.

Volume versus Outcome

The relationship between volume and outcome has been at the center of discussion because it is an easy structural measure to record and to assess in an aggregate manner. The fundamental observation that "practice makes perfect" seems to be a verifiable observation across multiple medical practices and procedures. This relationship seems to hold not only for individual practitioners, but also for institutions.

However, volume is not the only determinant of quality, and empirically, differences in volume account for only a modest amount of differences in outcomes observed. Nevertheless, almost all adequately sized studies indicate that focus on a particular medical problem or procedure as evidenced by high volume tends to be associated with better outcome; therefore, when all other factors are equal with regard to medical outcomes, one would prefer to be cared for by a high-volume clinician in a high-volume facility.

A particularly interesting issue in the volume-outcome relationship is the extent to which the proper environment can allow the low-volume clinician to achieve adequate or excellent outcomes. For example, interventional laboratories in which a high-volume operator is physically present may allow many low-volume operators to thrive with oversight and help from a more experienced person. Similarly, although cardiologists provide care for acute MI, which has a more consistent evidence base for appropriate use of therapies and better outcomes than what internists or family practitioners provide, it is also likely that a coronary care unit supervised by a cardiology intensivist can allow equal or better quality of care with multiple lower-volume generalists admitting patients.

Individual versus Institutional Assessment

Arguments can be made that oversight agencies should concern themselves with aggregate measures of performance of practice groups or institutions, allowing internal assessments to govern the behavior of individual practitioners. This approach has the advantage of providing adequate sample size to discern differences and of allowing for high-quality, low-volume operators to perform within groups that can monitor quality in groups of patients. It also seems apparent that holding groups responsible for outcomes will allow the natural selection process to occur, as groups will not want poor performers to drag down the overall group effort, and it is likely that gravitation toward development of shared expertise would occur. This approach is already being used in the assessment of managed care organizations by the NCQA and in the assessment of institutions by managed care organizations in the determination of which practices are awarded contracts.

Multifactorial Understanding of Outcomes

The science of determining the reasons for the variability in underlying risk that can affect outcome is in an early stage of development. In the past, this science was mostly limited by the inability to aggregate large amounts of data, but this restriction is no longer a problem. The most fundamental limitation remains difficulty accessing true clinical information, because little of it is recorded in a computerized format. Statistical methodology, including multivariable regression analysis and neural networking, continues to develop, but for the most part, an understanding of the empirical basis for reaching a conclusion remains elusive to most practitioners, and statistical concepts are even more foreign to most administrators and patients. Finally, an understanding of the biologic and clinical constructs that are critical to the prediction of outcomes generally falls far short of desired accuracy, even with the best statistical methodology and careful prospective data collection.

Low-Volume Operator

The low-volume operator or low-volume provider presents a special problem with regard to statistical assessment. In the absence of a sufficient number of cases, a few bad outcomes will give unreliably high point estimates of event rates. Additionally, practitioners with low volume may have the appearance of excellent outcomes due to chance. A useful rule of thumb is that when no complications have been observed, an approximation for the upper ninety-fifth percentile of the confidence interval is $3/N$, where N is the number of patients treated.

Fundamentally, the numbers demonstrate that determining complication rates or outcomes with confidence is nearly impossible in the low-volume situation. This conclusion limits the number of options. Because it is known that low-volume operators have worse outcomes, they could simply be banned; this approach is not likely to succeed in the current environment. A second option would be to allow low-volume operators to avoid statistical assessment until an adequate number of cases had been recorded. An alternate option would set up a "buddy," or pairing, configuration of operators as long as the group volume was adequate for statistical assessment. This approach would promote peer review as the main method of controlling quality in the low-volume operator, with substantial motivation through peer pressure.

New Operator

In an environment focused on assessment of quality, the training of new operators requires special consideration. The lack of experience and volume would be expected to lead to less sufficient process and outcome measures. Teachers and teaching institutions put themselves at risk in this situation. An evaluation of this problem leads to the inevitable conclusion that special allowances need to be made for teaching institutions, but the measurement of process and outcomes provides a motivation for providing top-notch teaching rather than "laissez-faire" training programs.

Difficulty of Data Collection

Substantial information exists to validate the concept that a hierarchy of accuracy of clinical data exists. Prospective clinical databases provide the highest level of data reliability, followed by chart review, administrative reports, and self-audit. Several studies provide substantial insight into the difficulties with self-audit. A review of the literature on reported complications of carotid endarterectomy revealed that studies with only individual surgeon assessment of the patient found only a 2.3% rate of death or major complications, whereas multiauthored reports showed a 5.5% rate and reports with specific assessments by internists or neurologists revealed a 7.7% rate of death or major complications (152). Similarly, when cardiologists report rates of nonfatal MI after percutaneous intervention, much lower rates are observed with self-report than with individual assessment (43). Extensive data are available comparing self-report with core laboratory assessment of procedural anatomic results indicating a similar phenomenon: Practitioners have diffi-

culty of bias when reporting on their own care (153). Administrative databases provide low-quality, but comprehensive data. In one report (45), agreement rates between clinical and claims databases varied from 0.83 for diabetes diagnosis to 0.09 for unstable angina, with a wide variety of values in between. All of these findings point to the fact that the ideal data system does not currently exist. The limitations of these systems should be acknowledged in quality reports, but too often this issue is forgotten.

Cost

The cost of collecting data specific for quality assessment is much higher than anticipated. For hospitals that are responsible to provide their data to multiple payers, this burden can be overwhelming. In Pennsylvania, where extensive data are required to submit for patients, the cost per case for specific data collection was estimated to be $17.43, or representing approximately $100,000 per year (51). In comparison, to participate in the Cleveland Health Quality Choice program of rating risk-adjusted mortality for five diagnoses, it costs The Cleveland Clinic Foundation more than $450,000 per year for chart abstractors, data management, and quality assurance. Thus, the cost of the collection of the data can be quite imposing and represents a major obstacle to the widespread use and acceptance of serial quality assessments. Efforts to reduce the costs by using electronic means of capturing the data, from both the administrative database and the laboratory, with avoidance of chart review, are under way (51).

Auditing

The difficulties with statistical modeling to adjust for differences in baseline characteristics have been reviewed elsewhere. Regardless of the method used, when the results in one practice differ from the results in another practice, whether the different outcomes resulted from differences in medical care, the play of chance, or a greater severity of underlying illness from one practice to another cannot be determined with certainty. Fortunately, it has been the experience of most outcome assessors that when major differences in outcomes occur, the differences in quality are measurable on multiple levels. Even when high-quality statistical models are available, the ability to game the system can be substantial. As reviewed for bypass surgery in New York State, concern exists about practices ensuring that maximum severity of illness is coded so that the observed versus expected numbers will be as favorable as possible (74).

Rewarding High Risk

Another special problem is the frequent inability of statistical models to account adequately for those who care for specially high-risk populations. Inner-city or extremely rural populations may have worse outcomes due to difficulty with compliance or resources. These sorts of variables are frequently not collected or accounted for. It has been proposed that special consideration should be given to practices voluntarily caring for identifiable high-risk populations. In the context of gaming the system, this approach would reduce the current incentive to steer high-risk patients away from practices undergoing substantial outcome scrutiny or financial pressures. Outcome models frequently neglect recording critical information about patients transferred from one institution to another.

CONTROVERSIES AND PERSONAL PERSPECTIVES

The public entitlement for complete information on hospitals and physicians has been validated by the supreme court in New York, but the most important concern is that the public accesses quality information about the quality of care. Many clinical, statistical, and logistic problems, summarized in *e*Table 45.1.4, largely remain unresolved. Although public release of meaningful data can be supported, the most critical obstacle is whether and how such data can be generated. The public expectations of assessing the quality of care have been raised in the last few years. In a State of the Union address, former President Bill Clinton stated the following:

> We have evidence that more efficient delivery of health care doesn't decrease quality. . . . Pennsylvania discovered that patients who were charged $21,000 for coronary artery bypass surgery received as good or better care as patients who were charged $84,000 for the same procedure in the same state. High prices simply don't always equal good quality (49).

Clearly, the amalgamation of cost and quality into the "value" of health care has become a principal competitive concept, for one health care system to prevail against another. However, the data for the quality component are too often "soft," with such components as patient satisfaction indices heavily relied on. Even for comparing cardiac services between hospitals or health care systems, it is very difficult to get an authentic quantitative evaluation of interventional cardiology, bypass surgery, electrophysiology and pacing, management of acute MI and heart failure, and all the other facets of a heart center. Paradoxically, in this world of a high density of information that is immediately electronically available for business, sports, and news, we are still lacking the critical data that would be necessary for decisions on health care.

Assuming that one can strive to generate worthwhile data, there is also the controversy about whether the data have an impact on improving the quality of care. With CABG the best-case scenario for measuring outcomes and assessing and adjusting risk, the debate continues as to whether the 40% reduction in mortality in CABG throughout New York State was a direct result of detailed quality assessment. Transfer of high-risk patients outside a particular medical system continues to be studied (154).

Operator- or physician-specific outcome data are perhaps most controversial of all because the inadequacies of sample size magnify the problems of interpreting these data. Nonetheless, such data have been used for cardiac surgeons in New York State and in Pennsylvania. Ultimately, for low-volume operators to assert their capabilities to deliver excellent care, it will be essential to demonstrate lack of complications on a risk-adjusted basis.

FUTURE DIRECTIONS

As was expressed by Nightingale more than a century ago, there is a need for better accountability in medicine. Via the study of quality parameters, it is hoped that health care systems, hospitals, and physicians will accept more responsibility for maintaining data and disclosing the data in suitable circumstances. Surely checks on process, such as monitoring the proportion of patients with proven coronary disease and hypercholesterolemia who are not getting secondary prevention therapy or the number of patients with heart failure not on an angiotensin-converting enzyme inhibitor, will be worthwhile. Internally, medical centers should consider developing risk-adjusted models for such procedures as CABG and percutaneous revascularization to monitor groups of physicians over an extended period, such that the number of operations or procedures is suitable for analysis.

Many factors suggest that the future of quality assessment will continue to be mired with controversy (155–161). The cost of information about quality care (162,163) and the cost of not delivering quality care (164) will remain contentious. The risks of risk adjustment (165–167) and release to the public of such data (168–172) remain unsettled issues. Fundamental issues such as defining the optimal way to measure quality (173–178), appropriateness of procedures (179,180), and physician competence (181,182) lie at the heart of debate and will continue to evolve over time. Without question, the effect of simply studying quality can have a salutary outcome (183), and as clinical trials continue to address major, unanswered dilemmas it becomes easier to judge whether evidence-based medicine is being practiced (184). A major, penetrating issue is individual physician and institution accountability. Kassirer, a former editor of the *New England Journal of Medicine*, claims we remain in a state of "pseudoaccountability" (185) and that hospitals need to heal themselves (186). Much of Iglehart's review of the American health care system (187) and the insight of Shine, who directs the IOM (188) and the International Practitioners Data Bank (189), reinforce this perspective. The recent British Royal Infirmary Inquiry and Report underscored the nature of pseudoaccountability

THE FUTURE

Electronic data retrieval, ultimately via Internet entry, will greatly facilitate collection and analysis of data. There will be steady refinement of risk adjustment for each of the major diagnoses and procedures in cardiovascular medicine (e.g., acute MI, heart failure, atrial fibrillation, CABG, PCI). Ultimately, the goal of measuring quality and stepwise reduction of medical errors will be increasingly achieved over time.

recounting the deaths of brain-damaged children (in 167 of 1,827 children undergoing cardiac surgery in a 12-year period) and the media characterized the "club" atmosphere with reluctance to accept criticism that allowed poor surgical standards to continue undetected for years (190–192). Certainly, in our quest to improve the quality of care and to avoid medical errors in cardiovascular medicine, there will need to be deep commitment for not only improving the data accountability and measurement instruments, but also the "teeth," or active steps towards privileging, credentializing, and close surveillance of hospital and physicians.

REFERENCES

1. Kohn LT, Corrigan JM, Donaldson MS, eds. *To err is human: building a safer health system.* Washington, DC: National Academy Press, 2000.
2. Brennan TA. The Institute of Medicine report on medical errors—could it do harm? *N Engl J Med* 2000;342:1123–1125.
3. McDonald CJ, Weiner M, Hui SL. Deaths due to medical errors are exaggerated in Institute of Medicine report. *JAMA* 2000;284:93–94.
4. Leape LL. Institute of Medicine medical error figures are not exaggerated. *JAMA* 2000;284:95–96.
5. Meyer G, Lewin DI, Eisenberg J. To err is preventable: medical errors and academic medicine. *Am J Med* 2001;110:597–603.
6. Nightingale F. *Notes on hospitals,* 3rd ed. London: Longman, Green, Longman, Roberts and Green, 1863.
7. Iezzoni LI. 100 Apples divided by 15 red herrings: a cautionary tale from the mid-19th century on comparing hospital mortality rates. *Ann Intern Med* 1996;124:1079–1085.
8. Codman EA. The product of a hospital. *Surg Gynecol Obstet* 1914;18:491–496.
9. Hammermeister KE. Risk, predicting outcomes, and improving care. *Circulation* 1995;91:899–900.
10. Roemer MI, Moustafa AT, Hopkins CE. A proposed hospital quality index: hospital death rates adjusted for case severity. *Health Serv Res* 1968;3:96–118.
11. Iezzoni LI. Measuring the severity of illness and case mix. In: Goldfield N, Nash DB, eds. *Providing quality care: the challenge to clinicians.* Philadelphia: American College of Physicians, 1989:70–105.
12. Brinkley J. US releasing lists of hospitals with abnormal mortality rates. *The New York Times* March 12, 1986:1.
13. Health Care Financing Administration. *Medicare hospital mortality information,* vol. I, 1986. Washington, DC: US Government Printing Office, 1987. HCFA Publication No. 01-002.
14. Blumberg MS. Comments on HCFA hospital death rate statistical outliers. *Health Serv Res* 1987;21:715–740.
15. Chelimsky E. The political debate about health care: are we losing sight of quality? *Science* 1993;262:525–528.
16. Brook RH, Kamberg CJ, McGlynn EA. Health systems reform and quality. *JAMA* 1996;276:476–480.
17. Flitcraft A. A report card for report cards. *Ann Intern Med* 1995;123:800–802.
18. Nash DB. Quality of measurement or quality of medicine. *JAMA* 1995;273:1537–1538.
19. Kerr EA, Mittman BS, Hays RD, et al. Quality assurance in capitated physician groups: where is the emphasis? *JAMA* 1996;276:1236–1239.
20. Dauphinee WD. Assessing clinical performance: where do we stand and what might we expect? *JAMA* 1995;274:741–743.
21. Topol EJ, Califf RM. Scorecard cardiovascular medicine. *Ann Intern Med* 1994;120:65–70.
22. Blumenthal D. Part I: quality of care—what is it? *N Engl J Med* 1996;335:891–894.
23. Lohr KN, Donaldson MS, Harris-Wehling J. Medicare: a strategy for quality assurance. V. Quality of care in a changing health care environment. *Qual Rev Bull* 1992;18:120–126.
24. Lohr KN, ed. *Medicare: a strategy for quality assurance.* Washington, DC: National Academy Press, 1990.
25. Donabedian A. The quality of care: how can it be assessed? *JAMA* 1988;260:1743–1748.
26. Brook RH, McGlynn EA, Cleary PD. Part 2: measuring quality of care. *N Engl J Med* 1996;335:966–970.
27. Jollis JG, DeLong ER, Peterson ED, et al. Outcome of acute myocardial infarction according to the specialty of the admitting physician. *N Engl J Med* 1996;335:1880–1887.
28. Kahn KL, Rogers WH, Rubenstein LV, et al. Measuring quality of care with explicit process criteria before and after implementation of the DRG-based prospective payment system. *JAMA* 1990;264:1969–1973.
29. Burstin HR, Lipsitz SR, Udvarhelyi IS, Brennnan TA. The effect of hospital financial characteristics on quality of care. *JAMA* 1993;270:845–849.
30. Bradley, EH, Holmboe ES, Mattera JA, et al. A qualitative study of increasing beta-blocker use after myocardial infarction. *JAMA* 2001;285:2604–2611.

31. Tu JV, Naylor CD, Kumar D, et al., the Steering Committee of the Cardiac Care Network of Ontario. Coronary artery bypass graft surgery in Ontario and New York State: which is right? *Ann Intern Med* 1997;126:13–19.

32. Phelps CE. The methodologic foundations of studies of the appropriateness of medical care. *N Engl J Med* 1993;329:1241–1245.

33. McGlynn EA, Naylor CD, Anderson GM, et al. Comparison of the appropriateness of coronary angiography and coronary artery bypass graft surgery between Canada and New York State. *JAMA* 1994;272:934–940.

34. Leape LL, Hilborne LH, Schwartz JS, et al., the Working Group of the Appropriateness Project of the Academic Medical Center Consortium. The appropriateness of coronary artery bypass graft surgery in academic medical centers. *Ann Intern Med* 1996;125:8–18.

34a. Hayward RA, Hofer TP. Estimating hospital deaths due to medical errors. Preventability is in the eye of the reviewer. *JAMA* 2001;286:415–420.

35. Goodman SG, Barr A, Granger C, et al. Medication errors and outcomes with fixed double-bolus r-PA versus bolus plus weight-adjusted infusion t-PA fibrinolysis: the GUSTO-III experience. *J Am Coll Cardiol* 2001;37[suppl]:351A.

36. Gurwitz JH, Gore JM, Goldberg RJ, et al. Risk for intracranial hemorrhage after tissue plasminogen activator treatment for acute myocardial infarction. Participants in the National Registry of Myocardial Infarction 2. *Ann Intern Med* 1998;129:597–604.

37. Vorchheimer DA, Baruch L, Thompson TD, Kukin M. North American vs non-North American use in GUSTO-I: impact of protocol deviation on mortality benefit of tPA. *Circulation* 1997;96[Suppl]:I-535.

38. Coulter SA, McCabe CH, Giugliano RP, et al. Dosing errors and outcomes in patients receiving single bolus compared to bolus + infusion thrombolytic regimens: an InTIME-II Study. *Circulation* 1999;100[Suppl]:I-791.

39. Granger CB, Alexander JH, Armstrong PW. Caution needed in interpreting the impact of dosing errors: a case study from ASSENT-2. *Circulation* 2000;102[Suppl]:II-590.

40. Cannon CP. Multimodality reperfusion therapy for acute myocardial infarction. *Am Heart J* 2000;140:707–716.

41. Seyedroudbari A, Kessler ER, Mooss AN, et al. Time to treatment and cost of thrombolysis: a multicenter comparison of tPA and rPA. *J Thromb Thrombolysis* 2000;9:303–308.

41a. Sternberg S. Study finds heart-drug errors. *USA Today* March 9, 2000:1A.

42. Silber JH, Rosenbaum PR, Schwartz S, et al. Evaluation of the complication rate as a measure of quality of care in coronary artery bypass graft surgery. *JAMA* 1995;274:317–323.

43. Topol EJ. Caveats about elective coronary stenting. *N Engl J Med* 1994;331:539–541.

44. The Pennsylvania Health Care Cost Containment Council. *Coronary artery bypass graft surgery*. Technical Report. Vol. II, 1991. Harrisburg, PA: 1994.

45. Jollis JG, Ancukiewicz M, DeLong ER, et al. Discordance of databases designed for claims payment versus clinical information systems. *Ann Intern Med* 1993;119:844–850.

46. O'Neil AC, Petersen LA, Cook EF, et al. Physician report-

ing compared with medical-record review to identify adverse medical events. *Ann Intern Med* 1993;119:370–376.

47. Pilote L, Califf RM, Sapp S, et al. Regional variability in the United States for the management of acute myocardial infarction: insights from the GUSTO trial. *N Engl J Med* 1995;333:565–572.

48. Van de Werf F, Topol EJ, Lee KL, et al., for the GUSTO Investigators. Variations in patient management and outcome for acute myocardial infarction in the United States and other countries. *JAMA* 1995;273:1586–1591.

49. Iezzoni LI, Ash AS, Shwartz M, et al. Predicting who dies depends on how severity is measured: implications for evaluating patient outcomes. *Ann Intern Med* 1995;123:763–770.

50. Pine M, Norusis M, Jones B, Rosenthal GE. Predictions of hospital mortality rates: a comparison of data sources. *Ann Intern Med* 1997;126:347–354.

51. Iezzoni LI. How much are we willing to pay for information about quality of care? *Ann Intern Med* 1997;126:391–393.

52. US General Accounting Office, Health, Education, and Human Services Division. *Employers and individual consumers want additional information on quality.* Washington, DC: U.S. General Accounting Office, 1995. GAO/HFHS-95-201.

53. Iglehart JK. The national committee for quality assurance. *N Engl J Med* 1996;335:995–999.

54. Ritchie JL, Forrester JS, Fye WB. 28th Bethesda Conference: practice guidelines and the quality of care. *J Am Coll Cardiol* 1997;29:1125–1179.

55. Luft HS, Bunker JP, Enthovea AC. Should operations be regionalized? The empirical relationship between surgical volume and mortality. *N Engl J Med* 1979;301:1364–1369.

56. Luft H. The relation between surgical volume and mortality: an exploration of causal factors and alternative models. *Med Care* 1980;15:941–959.

57. Macrid SC, Luft HS, Huar SS. Selecting categories of patients for regionalization: implications of the relationship between volume and outcome. *Med Care* 1980;24:148–158.

58. Medicare hospital mortality information, 1986. Washington, DC: U.S. Department of Health and Human Services, Health Care Financing Administration, 1987. HFCA publication No. 01-002.

59. Hannan EL, O'Donnell JF, Kilburn H Jr, et al. Investigation of the relationship between volume and mortality for surgical procedures performed in New York State hospitals. *JAMA* 1989;262:503–510.

60. O'Connor GT, Plume SK, Olmstead EM, et al., for the New England Cardiovascular Disease Study Group. A regional prospective study of in-house mortality associated with coronary artery bypass grafting. *JAMA* 1991;266:803–809.

61. Williams SV, Nash DB, Goldfarb N. Differences in mortality from coronary artery bypass graft surgery at five teaching hospitals. *JAMA* 1991;266:811–815.

62. Hannan EL, Kilburn H Jr, O'Donnell JF, et al. Adult open heart surgery in New York State. *JAMA* 1990;264:2768–2774.

63. Topol EJ, Block PC, Holmes DR, et al. Readiness for the

scorecard era in cardiovascular medicine. *Am J Cardiol* 1995;75:1170–1173.

64. Luft HS, Romano PS. Chance, continuity, and change in hospital mortality rates. *JAMA* 1993;270:331–337.

65. Sowden AJ, Deeks JJ, Sheldon TA. Volume and outcome in coronary artery bypass graft surgery: true association or artefact. *BMJ* 1995;311:151–155.

66. Tu JV, Naylor CD, the Steering Committee of the Provincial Adult Cardiac Care Network of Ontario. Coronary artery bypass mortality rates in Ontario: a Canadian approach to quality assurance in cardiac surgery. *Circulation* 1996;94:2429–2433.

67. Grumbach K, Anderson GM, Luft HS, et al. Regionalization of cardiac surgery in the United States and Canada: geographic access, choice, and outcomes. *JAMA* 1995;274:1282–1288.

68. Hannan EL, Kilburn H Jr, Racz M, et al. Improving the outcomes of coronary artery bypass surgery in New York State. *JAMA* 1994;271:761–766.

69. Hannan EL, Siu AL, Kumar D, et al. The decline in coronary artery bypass graft surgery mortality in New York State. *JAMA* 1995;273:209–213.

70. O'Connor GT, Plume SK, Olmstead EM, et al. A regional intervention to improve the hospital mortality associated with coronary artery bypass graft surgery. *JAMA* 1996;275:841–846.

71. Ghali WA, Ash AS, Hall RE, Moskowitz MA. Statewide quality improvement initiatives and mortality after cardiac surgery. *JAMA* 1997;277:379–382.

72. Jencks SF. Can large-scale interventions improve care? *JAMA* 1997;277:419–420.

73. O'Connor GT, Plume SK, Olmstead EM, et al., for the Northern New England Cardiovascular Disease Study Group. A regional intervention to improve the hospital mortality associated with coronary artery bypass graft surgery. *JAMA* 1996;275:841–846.

74. Green J, Wintfeld N. Report cards on cardiac surgeons: assessing New York State's approach. *N Engl J Med* 1995;332:1229–1232.

75. Chassin MR, Hannan EL, DeBuono BA. Benefits and hazards of reporting medical outcomes publicly. *N Engl J Med* 1996;334:394–398.

76. Chassin MR. Part 3: Improving the quality of care. *N Engl J Med* 1996;335:1060–1063.

77. Omoigui NA, Miller DP, Brown KJ, et al. Outmigration for coronary bypass surgery in an era of public dissemination of clinical outcomes. *Circulation* 1996;93:27–33.

78. Cooley DA. Building shelters: Safeguards in public disclosure of outcomes data. *Circulation* 1996;93:1–3.

79. Schneider EC, Epstein AM. Influence of cardiac surgery performance reports on referral practices and access to care. *N Engl J Med* 1996;335:251–256.

80. Erickson LC, Torchiana DF, Schneider EC, et al. The relationship between managed care insurance and use of lower-mortality hospitals for CABG surgery. *JAMA* 2000;283:1976–1982.

81. Peterson ED, DeLong ER, Jollis JG, et al. The effects of New York's bypass surgery provider profiling on access to care and patient outcomes in the elderly. *J Am Coll Cardiol* 1998;32:993–999.

82. Peterson ED, DeLong ER, Muhlbaier LH, et al. Challenges in comparing risk-adjusted bypass surgery mortality results. Results from the Cooperative Cardiovascular Project. *J Am Coll Cardiol* 2000;36:2174–2184.

83. Ivanov J, Tu JV, Naylor CD. Ready-made, recalibrated, or remodeled? Issues in the use of risk indexes for assessing mortality after coronary artery bypass graft surgery. *Circulation* 1999;99:2098–2104.

84. Lindsay J, Pinnow EE, Popma JJ, et al. Obstacles to outcomes analysis in percutaneous transluminal coronary revascularization. *Am J Cardiol* 1995;76:168–172.

85. Hannan EL, Arani DT, Johnson LW, et al. Percutaneous transluminal coronary angioplasty in New York State. *JAMA* 1992;268:3092–3097.

86. Ritchie JL, Phillips KA, Luft HS. Coronary angioplasty. Statewide experience in California. *Circulation* 1993;88:2735–2743.

87. Kimmel SE, Berlin JA, Laskey WK. The relationship between coronary angioplasty procedure volume and major complications. *JAMA* 1995;274:1137–1142.

88. Jollis JG, Peterson ED, DeLong ER, et al. The relation between the volume of coronary angioplasty procedures at hospitals treating Medicare beneficiaries and short-term mortality. *N Engl J Med* 1994;331:1625–1629.

89. Ryan TJ. The critical question of procedure volume minimums for coronary angioplasty. *JAMA* 1995;274:1169–1170.

90. Ellis SG, Omoigui N, Bittl JA, et al. Analysis and comparison of operator-specific outcomes in interventional cardiology: from a multicenter database of 4860 quality-controlled procedures. *Circulation* 1996;93:431–439.

91. Califf RM, Jollis JG, Peterson ED. Operator-specific outcomes: a call to professional responsibility. *Circulation* 1996;93:403–406.

92. Shook TL, Sun GW, Burstein S, et al. Comparison of percutaneous transluminal coronary angioplasty outcome and hospital costs for low-volume and high-volume operators. *Am J Cardiol* 1996;77:331–336.

93. Heidenreich PA, Chou TM, Amidon TM, et al. Impact of operating physician on costs of percutaneous transluminal coronary angioplasty. *Am J Cardiol* 1996;77:1169–1173.

94. Smith SC, Dove JT, Jacobs AK, et al. ACC/AHA Guidelines for percutaneous coronary intervention (revision of the 1993 PTCA guidelines). A report of the American College of Cardiology/American Heart Association Task Force on Practice Guidelines (Committee to Revise the 1993 Guidelines for Percutaneous Transluminal Coronary Angioplasty). *Circulation* 2001;103:3019–3041.

95. Dickens JD Jr, McGrath PD, Siewers AE, et al. AHA/ACC guidelines for percutaneous coronary interventions (PCIs): are recommendations for procedure volume being followed? *Circulation* 1999;100:I-393.

96. Hannan EL, Racz M, Ryan TJ, et al. Coronary angioplasty volume-outcome relationships for hospitals and cardiologists. *JAMA* 1997;277:892–898.

97. Shine KI, Spencer FC. *Angioplasty in New York State 1994.* Albany, NY: New York State Department of Health, 1996:1–10.

98. Ryan TJ. Stents: expanding the case for volume minimums in interventional cardiology [editorial; comment]. *J Am Coll Cardiol* 1998;32:977–999.

99. Kastrati A, Neumann F-J, Schömig A. Operator volume and outcome of patients undergoing coronary stent placement. *J Am Coll Cardiol* 1998;32:970–976.

100. Ritchie JL, Maynard C, Chapko MK, et al. Association between percutaneous transluminal coronary angioplasty volumes and outcomes in the Healthcare Cost and Utilization Project 1993–1994. *Am J Cardiol* 1999;83:493–497.

101. Ellis SG, Miller D, Keys TF, et al. Comparing physician-specific two-year patient outcomes after coronary angiography: methodologic issues and results. *J Am Coll Cardiol* 1999;33:1278–1285.

102. Nash IS. Improving outcomes of percutaneous coronary intervention [editorial]. *Am Heart J* 1999;137:979–982.

103. McGrath PD, Malenka DJ, Wennberg DE, et al., for the Northern New England Cardiovascular Disease Study Group. Changing outcomes in percutaneous coronary interventions. *J Am Coll Cardiol* 1999;34:674–680.

104. O'Connor GT, Malenka DJ, Quinton H, et al., for the Northern New England Cardiovascular Disease Study Group. Multivariate prediction of in-hospital mortality after percutaneous coronary interventions in 1994–1996. *J Am Coll Cardiol* 1999;34:681–691.

105. Moscucci M, O'Connor GT, Ellis SG, et al. Validation of risk adjustment models for in-hospital percutaneous transluminal coronary angioplasty mortality on an independent data set. *J Am Coll Cardiol* 1999;34:692–697.

106. Ritchie JL, Maynard C, Every NR, Chapko MK. Coronary artery stent outcomes in a Medicare population: less emergency bypass surgery and lower mortality rates in patients with stents. *Am Heart J* 1999;138:437–440.

107. Jollis JG. Practice still makes perfect [editorial]. *Am Heart J* 1999;138:394–395.

108. Becker ER, Cohen D, Culler SD, et al. Benchmarking cardiac catheterization laboratories: the impact of patient age, gender and risk factors on variable costs, device costs, total time and procedural time in 53 catheterization laboratories. *J Invasive Cardiol* 1999;11:533–542.

109. Perrins J. Quality assurance in interventional cardiology. *Heart* 1999;82[Suppl II]:II23–II26.

110. Hannan EL. Percutaneous coronary interventions: heed the American College of Cardiology volume recommendations, but strive to improve quality [editorial; comment]. *J Am Coll Cardiol* 1999;34:1481–1483.

111. Malenka DJ, McGrath PD, Wennberg DE, et al., for the Northern New England Cardiovascular Disease Study Group. The relationship between operator volume and outcomes after percutaneous coronary interventions in high volume hospitals in 1994–1996. The Northern New England experience. *J Am Coll Cardiol* 1999;34:1471–1480.

112. Gilchrist IC, Gardner LH, Muhlestein JB, et al. Effect of institutional volume and academic status on outcomes of coronary interventions: the IMPACT-II experience. *Am Heart J* 1999;138:976–982.

113. Peterson ED, Lansky AJ, Anstrom KJ, et al., for the National Cardiovascular Network. Evolving trends in interventional device use and outcomes: results from the National Cardiovascular Network database. *Am Heart J* 2000;139:198–207.

114. Ho V. Evolution of the volume-outcome relation for hospitals performing coronary angioplasty. *Circulation* 2000; 101:1806–1811.

115. Holmes Jr DR, Berger PB, Garratt KN, et al. Application of the New York State PTCA mortality model in patients undergoing stent implantation. *Circulation* 2000;102:517–522.

116. Cohen DJ, Becker ER, Culler SD, et al. Impact of patient characteristics, complications, and facility volume on the costs and time of cardiac catheterization and coronary angioplasty in 70 catheterization laboratories. *Am J Cardiol* 2000;86:595–601.

117. Maynard C, Every NR, Chapko MK, Ritchie JL. Outcomes of coronary angioplasty procedures performed in rural hospitals. *Am J Med* 2000;108:710–713.

118. Mathew V, Gersh BJ. Coronary interventions: keeping score. *Am J Med* 2000;108:748–750.

119. McGrath PD, Wennberg DE, Dickens JD Jr, et al. Relation between operator and hospital volume and outcomes following percutaneous coronary interventions in the era of the coronary stent. *JAMA* 2000;284:3139–3144.

120. Lee KL, Woodlief L, Topol EJ, et al. Predictors of 30-day mortality in the era of reperfusion for acute myocardial infarction: results from an international trial of 41,021 patients. *Circulation* 1995;91:1659–1668.

121. Normand SL, Glickman ME, Sharma RG, McNeil BJ. Using admission characteristics to predict short-term mortality from myocardial infarction in elderly patients. *JAMA* 1996;275:1322–1328.

122. Office of Statewide Hospital Planning and Development. *Annual report. California hospital outcomes project.* Vols. 1–3. San Francisco: Office of Statewide Hospital Planning and Development, December, 1993.

123. Wagner EH. The cost-quality relationship. Do we always get what we pay for? *JAMA* 1994;272:1951–1952.

124. Pilote L, Miller DP, Califf RM, et al. Determinants of the use of coronary angiography and revascularization after thrombolysis for acute myocardial infarction in the United States. *N Engl J Med* 1996;335:1198–1205.

125. Di Salvo TG, Paul SD, Lloyd-Jones D, et al. Care of acute myocardial infarction by noninvasive and invasive cardiologists: procedure use, cost and outcome. *J Am Coll Cardiol* 1996;27:262–269.

126. Goldman L. The value of cardiology. *N Engl J Med* 1996;335:1918–1919.

127. Nash IS, Nash DB, Fuster V. Do cardiologists do it better? *J Am Coll Cardiol* 1997;29:475–478.

128. Selby JV, Fireman BH, Lundstrom RJ, et al. Variation among hospitals in coronary angiography practices and outcomes after myocardial infarction in a large health maintenance organization. *N Engl J Med* 1996;335:1888–1896.

129. Bernard AM, Hayward RA, Rosevear J, et al. Comparing the hospitalizations of transfer and non-transfer patients in an academic medical center. *Acad Med* 1996;71:262–266.

130. *Focus on heart attack in southeastern Pennsylvania. A 1993 summary report for health benefits purchasers, health care providers, policy-makers, and consumers.* Harrisburg, PA: Pennsylvania Health Care Cost Containment Council, 1996.

131. *Focus on heart attack in central and northeastern Pennsylvania. A 1993 summary report for health benefits purchasers, health care providers, policy-makers, and consumers.* Harrisburg, PA: Pennsylvania Health Care Cost Containment Council, 1996.

132. *Focus on heart attack in western Pennsylvania. A 1993 summary report for health benefits purchasers, health care providers, policy-makers, and consumers.* Harrisburg, PA: Pennsylvania Health Care Cost Containment Council, 1996.

133. *Focus on heart attack in Pennsylvania: research methods and results.* Harrisburg, PA: Pennsylvania Health Care Cost Containment Council, 1996.

134. *Focus on heart attack in Pennsylvania: the technical report—1993.* Parts A and B. Harrisburg, PA: Pennsylvania Health Care Cost Containment Council, 1996.

135. ISIS-3 (Third International Study of Infarct Survival) Collaborative Group. ISIS-3: a randomized comparison of streptokinase vs tissue plasminogen activator vs anistreplase and of aspirin plus heparin vs aspirin alone among 41,299 cases of suspected acute myocardial infarction. *Lancet* 1992;339:753–770.

136. Gruppo Italiano per lo Studio della Sopravvivenza nell'Infarto Miocardico. GISSI-2: a factorial randomised trial of alteplase versus streptokinase and heparin versus no heparin among 12,490 patients with acute myocardial infarction. *Lancet* 1990;336:65–71.

137. The GUSTO Investigators. An international randomized trial comparing four thrombolytic strategies for acute myocardial infarction. *N Engl J Med* 1993;329:673–682.

138. The GUSTO IIa Investigators. Randomized trial of intravenous heparin versus recombinant hirudin for acute coronary syndromes. *Circulation* 1994;90:1631–1637.

139. Willison DJ, Soumerai SB, McLaughlin TJ, et al. Consultation between cardiologists and generalists in the management of acute myocardial infarction. *Arch Internal Med* 1998;158:1778–1783.

140. Casale PN, Jones JL, Wolf FE, et al. Patients treated by cardiologists have a lower in-hospital mortality for acute myocardial infarction. *J Am Coll Cardiol* 1998;32:885–889.

141. Nash IS, Corrato RR, Dlutowski MJ, et al. Generalist versus specialist care for acute myocardial infarction. *Am J Cardiol* 1999;83:650–654.

142. Schreiber TL, Elkhatib A, Grines CL, et al. Cardiologist versus internist management of patients with unstable angina: treatment patterns and outcomes. *J Am Coll Cardiol* 1995;26:577–582.

143. Chen J, Radford MJ, Wang Y, et al. Do "America's best hospitals" perform better for acute myocardial infarction? *N Engl J Med* 1999;340:286–292.

144. Cannon CP, Gibson CM, Lambrew CT, et al. Relationship of symptom-onset-to-balloon time and door-to-balloon time with mortality in patients undergoing angioplasty for acute myocardial infarction. *JAMA* 2000;283:2941–2947.

145. Magid DJ, Calonge BN, Rumsfeld JS, et al., for the National Registry of Myocardial Infarction 2 and 3 Investigators. Relation between hospital primary angioplasty volume and mortality for patients with acute MI treated with primary angioplasty vs thrombolytic therapy. *JAMA* 2000;284:3131–3138.

146. Tu JV, Austin PC, Chan BTB. Relationship between annual volume of patients treated by admitting physician and mortality after acute myocardial infarction. *JAMA* 2001;285:3116–3122.

147. Matsui K, Polanczyk CA, Gaspoz J-M, et al. Management of patients with acute myocardial infarction at five academic medical centers: clinical characteristics, resource utilization, and outcome. *J Invest Med* 1999;47:134–140.

148. Allison JJ, Kiefe CI, Weissman NW, et al. Relationship of hospital teaching status with quality of care and mortality for Medicare patients with acute MI. *JAMA* 2000;284:1256–1262.

149. Alter DA, Naylor CD, Austin PC, Tu JV. Long-term MI outcomes at hospitals with or without on-site revascularization. *JAMA* 2001;285:2101–2108.

150. Petersen LA, Normand S-LT, Daley J, McNeil BJ. Outcome of myocardial infarction in Veterans Health Administration patients as compared with Medicare patients. *N Engl J Med* 2000;343:1934–1941.

151. Fihn SD. Does VA health care measure up [editorial]? *N Engl J Med* 2000;343:1963–1965.

152. Rothwell P, Warlow C. Is self-audit reliable? *Lancet* 1995;346:1623.

153. Topol EJ, Nissen S. Our preoccupation with coronary luminology: the dissociation between clinical and angiographic findings in ischemic heart disease. *Circulation* 1995;92:2333–2342.

154. Dudley RA, Johansen KL, Brand R, et al. Selective referral to high-volume hospitals. Estimating potentially avoidable deaths. *JAMA* 2000;283:1159–1166.

155. Blumenthal D, Epstein AM. Part 6: the role of physicians in the future of quality management. *N Engl J Med* 1996;335:1328–1331.

156. Teistein PS. Credentialing for coronary interventions—practice makes perfect. *Circulation* 1997;95:2467–2470.

157. Ellis SG, Weintraub W, Holmes D, et al. Relation of operator volume and experience to procedural outcome of percutaneous coronary revascularization at hospitals with high interventional volumes. *Circulation* 1997;96:2479–2484.

158. Jollis JG, Peterson ED, Nelson CL, et al. Relationship between physician and hospital coronary angioplasty volume and outcome in elderly patients. *Circulation* 1997;95:2485–2491.

159. Firshein J. US employers ignore hospital mortality data. *Lancet* 1997;349:1459.

160. Green J, Wintfeld N, Krasner M, et al. In search of America's best hospitals—the promise and reality of quality assessment. *J Am Coll Cardiol* 1997;277:1152–1155.

161. Carlsen W. Physicians' files could be unsealed—assembly considers opening records. *San Francisco Chronicle*, News Section, A1, Monday, May 5, 1997.

162. Nash IS, Nash DB, Fuster V. Do cardiologists do it better? *J Am Coll Cardiol* 1997;29:475–478.

163. Iezzoni LI. How much are we willing to pay for information about quality of care? *Ann Intern Med* 1997;126:391–393.

164. Taylor Jr DH, Whellan DJ, Sloan FA. Effects of admission

to a teaching hospital on the cost and quality of care for Medicare beneficiaries. *N Engl J Med* 1999;340:293–299.

165. Iezzoni LI. The risks of risk adjustment. *JAMA* 1997;278:1600–1607.

166. Hofer TP, Hayward RA, Greenfield S, et al. The unreliability of individual physician "report cards" for assessing the costs and quality of care of a chronic disease. *JAMA* 1999;281:2098–2105.

167. Bindman AB. Can physician profiles be trusted [editorial]? *JAMA* 1999;281:2142–2143.

168. Davies HTO, Marshall MN. Public disclosure of performance data: does the public get what the public wants [comment]? *Lancet* 1999;353:1639–1640.

169. Baldwin L-M, Hart LG, Oshel RE, et al. Hospital peer review and the National Practitioner Data Bank. Clinical privileges action reports. *JAMA* 1999;282:349–355.

170. Epstein AM. Public release of performance data. A progress report from the front [editorial]. *JAMA* 2000;283:1884–1886.

171. Schneider EC, Epstein AM. Use of public performance reports. A survey of patients undergoing cardiac surgery. *JAMA* 1998;279:1638–1642.

172. Marshall MN, Shekelle PG, Leatherman S, Brook RH. The public release of performance data. What do we expect to gain? A review of the evidence [review]. *JAMA* 2000;283:1866–1874.

173. Peabody JW, Luck J, Glassman P, et al. Comparison of vignettes, standardized patients, and chart abstraction. A prospective validation study of 3 methods for measuring quality. *JAMA* 2000;283:1715–1722.

174. Shine KI. Closing the gap in quality health care for Americans. *Circulation* 2000;101:2325–2327.

175. Bodenheimer T. The American health care system. The movement for improved quality in health care. *N Engl J Med* 1999;340:488–492.

176. Rawlins M. In pursuit of quality: the National Institute for Clinical Excellence. *Lancet* 1999;353:1079–1082.

177. O'Connor GT, Eagle KA. How do we know how well we are doing [editorial; comment]? *J Am Coll Cardiol* 1998;32:1000–1001.

178. Bodenheimer T. The American health care system. Physicians and the changing medical marketplace. *N Engl J Med* 1999;340:584–588.

179. Bernstein SJ, Brorsson B, Åberg T, et al., on behalf of the SECOR/SBU Project Group. Appropriateness of referral of coronary angiography patients in Sweden. *Heart* 1999;81:470–477.

180. Shekelle PG. Are appropriateness criteria ready for use in clinical practice? [editorial]. *N Engl J Med* 2001;344:677–678.

181. Bindman AB. Can physician profiles be trusted? [editorial]. *JAMA* 1999;281:2142–2143.

182. Wass V, Van der Vleuten C, Shatzer J, Jones R. Assessment of clinical competence. *Lancet* 2001;357:945–949.

183. Casalino LP. The unintended consequences of measuring quality on the quality of medical care. *N Engl J Med* 1999;341:1147–1150.

184. Sackett DL, Straus SE, for Firm A of the Nuffield Department of Medicine. Finding and applying evidence during clinical rounds. The "evidence cart." *JAMA* 1998;280:1336–1338.

185. Kassirer JP. Pseudoaccountability. *Ann Intern Med* 2001;134:587–590.

186. Kassirer JP. Hospitals, heal yourselves [editorial]. *N Engl J Med* 1999;340:309–310.

187. Iglehart JK. The American health care system. Medicare. *N Engl J Med* 1999;340:327–332.

188. Shine KI. Closing the gap in quality health care for Americans. *Circulation* 2000;101:2325–2327.

189. Baldwin L-M, Hart LG, Oshel RE, et al. Hospital peer review and the National Practitioner Data Bank. Clinical privileges action reports. *JAMA* 1999;282:349–355.

190. The British Royal Infirmary Inquiry. Final report, July, 2001. http://www.bristol-inquiry.org.uk/final_report/report/sec1_conclusions_.htm.

191. Rumbelow H. Q & A on Bristol babies report. *The London Times*, July 18, 2001.

192. Beller GA. Presidential address: quality of cardiovascular care in the U.S. *J Am Coll Cardiol* 2001;38:587–594.

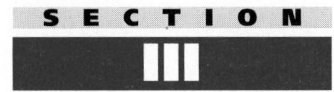
CARDIOVASCULAR IMAGING

JAMES D. THOMAS

PRINCIPLES OF IMAGING

JAMES D. THOMAS

OVERVIEW

Accurate imaging is essential to assess cardiac anatomy, function, perfusion, and metabolism, and revolutionary advances have been seen in the past 20 years, primarily because of improvements in computer technology and digital signal processing. The heart may be imaged using x-rays [radiography, angiography, computed tomography (CT)], gamma rays (radionuclide imaging, positron emission technology), sound waves (Doppler echocardiography), and the magnetic properties of the hydrogen nucleus [magnetic resonance imaging (MRI)]. Tests may be compared by their ability to detect and exclude disease (sensitivity and specificity, respectively), but the predictive value of the test depends largely on the prevalence of the disorder in the

J. D. Thomas: Department of Cardiovascular Imaging, The Cleveland Clinic Foundation, Cleveland, Ohio

population being tested (Bayesian analysis). Computer processing is important both in generating images and in enhancing the images for display (smoothing and edge enhancement); Fourier transformation is commonly used to analyze the frequency content of images and data in Doppler echocardiography, MRI, and radionuclide ventriculography. Digital image storage is becoming feasible with reductions in computer costs and agreement on the Digital Imaging and Communications in Medicine (DICOM) Standard for medical image exchange. The massive storage requirements may be reduced by careful clinical editing of studies and with digital compression algorithms. All-digital storage and transmission will greatly enhance the value of cardiac studies and facilitate telemedicine.

GLOSSARY

Convolution: Altering a pixel based on the values of surrounding pixels.

DICOM: Digital Imaging and Communications in Medicine, a formatting standard to allow the exchange of medical images.

Digital compression: Recording an image to require less storage. *Lossless* compression does not change the appearance at all (but yields little compression), whereas *lossy* compression yields greater savings (but with some alteration of the image).

Doppler principle: Ultrasound signals have their frequency shifted in proportion to the blood velocity.

Fourier analysis: Analysis of the frequency content of an image or signal.

Gamma ray: High-energy photon produced by nuclear decay.

Nuclear magnetic resonance: Spinning or precessing of certain nuclei (typically the hydrogen proton) in the presence of a magnetic field.

Photons: "Particles" of electromagnetic radiation.

Piezoelectric: A property of matter that converts electricity into vibration and vice versa.

Point processing: Altering an image gray scale, pixel by pixel.

Positron: Positive electron (antimatter); when it encounters an electron, both are annihilated and two 511-keV photons are emitted in opposite directions, forming the physical basis for positron emission tomography.

X-ray: High-energy photon produced by rearrangement of an atom's electron cloud.

INTRODUCTION

High-fidelity imaging is required to understand cardiovascular anatomy, function, metabolism, and blood flow more than any other organ system in the body. The fine structure

and complex motion of the heart demand imaging modalities with high temporal and spatial resolution. Fortunately, intensive research in physics, pharmacology, and computer processing over the past 50 years has led to dramatic improvements in our ability to characterize and quantify disorders of the cardiovascular system. The next 11 chapters describe in greater detail the clinical aspects of the major cardiovascular imaging modalities: radiography, echocardiography, angiography, nuclear cardiology, and MRI. As a prelude, this chapter describes many of the concepts common to each of these techniques, including image generation, computer processing, assessment of diagnostic accuracy, and the emerging area of digital storage and transmission. An understanding of the physical background of these methods will help the reader to understand better the clinical applications described in later chapters.

Here we consider four broad ways to acquire images of the heart: x-ray transmission, radionuclide emission, ultrasonic reflection, and nuclear magnetic resonance. Although these techniques share many features, together they span virtually all of classical and quantum physics. This chapter can only touch on these topics, and the reader is referred to a number of excellent texts for greater detail (1–9).

What Is Imaging?

In a broad sense, imaging displays the differential interaction of energy with matter to discern structure or function. For instance, the printed page reflects fewer photons from dark letters, allowing them to be seen against the photon-rich white page. Similarly, radiography exploits the fact that more x-rays are absorbed by bone than by soft tissue, and echocardiography displays the reflection of ultrasonic energy from the border of two tissues with different acoustic impedances. Radionuclide techniques are slightly different in that they deliver an energy source (the radioactive compound) to the body, where it is concentrated in structures of interest and then localized by external detectors. MRI defines the differential distribution of weak magnetic characteristics within the body.

Basic Concepts

A number of terms and concepts are common to all imaging modalities.

Resolution

Resolution can have several meanings in imaging. *Spatial resolution* reflects the smallest separation that two objects can be distinguished. For example, in radiography, spatial resolution is measured with a grid of finely spaced lines. The densest packing of lines that can be distinguished is reported as the number of line pairs per centimeter. For radiography, resolution is relatively constant across the field of view. This is not true for echocardiography, which typically has greater resolution in the near field than in the far field, because of the divergence of the ultrasound beam. Furthermore, in echocardiography, resolution is *anisotropic*, that is, better in the axial direction (along a scan line) than in the lateral direction (across scan lines). One must also take care to distinguish the physical resolution of the imaging modality from the resolution of a video or computer display (commonly used in nuclear imaging, echocardiography, MRI, and digital angiography). The spacing of the picture elements (*pixels*) on the screen may be greater or lesser than the physical resolution. This screen resolution typically is stated in the number of pixels across the screen in the horizontal and vertical direction (640×480 is typical for low-end computer monitors; $1,024 \times 1,024$ for high-resolution digital angiography; and $2,048 \times 2,048$ or even higher for digital radiographic and mammographic images). The functional spatial resolution is always the lesser of the physical and screen resolutions.

Temporal resolution reflects the frequency with which an image is generated, usually stated in frames per second. Plain film radiographs are typically taken as single images, but temporal resolution may still be relevant because the *shutter speed* (the time the film is actually exposed to x-rays) determines whether rapid movements (such as prosthetic valve motion) can be "frozen" in the image. There often is a trade-off between temporal and spatial resolution. Echocardiograms can be generated more frequently, but this usually requires that the density of scan lines per image be reduced. The data for a multigated nuclear scan can be divided into shorter temporal "bins," but this reduces the amount of data available for each image, reducing the signal-to-noise ratio and spatial resolution.

Resolution issues are also important in the calculation of cardiac blood velocity (by Doppler echocardiography or MRI). Velocity resolution reflects the smallest difference in velocity that can be discerned, whereas temporal resolution is the frequency with which the velocity data are updated. Just as with images, there usually is a trade-off between velocity and temporal resolution. Increasing the frequency of display reduces the velocity resolution and vice versa.

Dimensionality

The heart is a four-dimensional structure, possessing three spatial dimensions of shape and one temporal dimension of motion. Most imaging modalities have two spatial dimensions (i.e., a picture, such as a radiograph or an echocardiographic image). M-mode echocardiography displays structures along a single line in the heart (like an ice pick), and so is a one-dimensional display. Magnetic resonance, CT, and some nuclear and echocardiographic studies are intrinsically three-dimensional (3-D), although the display may be on a two-dimensional (2-D) screen. Because motion is critical to many cardiac diagnoses, most modalities include the temporal dimension, typically with a series

of 2-D or 3-D images. Plain film radiographs and some nuclear studies do not show motion.

Transmission versus Tomographic Imaging

Two-dimensional images of the heart can be generated by either *transmission* or *tomographic* techniques. In transmission imaging, the full thickness of the heart is projected onto a screen, whereas a tomogram displays structures lying within a single plane of the heart. For most applications, tomographic imaging (used in MRI, CT, echocardiography, and many nuclear tests) is preferable, because there is no interference from overlying structures. For angiography, however, transmission imaging is actually an advantage, because the full course of the vessel can be visualized, something no single tomographic plane could do. Indeed, in magnetic resonance angiography, the 3-D data set is projected onto a plane to generate a transmission image for easier diagnosis.

IMAGING WITH ELECTROMAGNETIC RADIATION: X-RAYS AND GAMMA RAYS

Radiography uses x-rays delivered externally to image the body, whereas nuclear imaging uses gamma rays produced inside the body. There is in fact no physical difference between x-rays and gamma rays, both being forms of high-energy electromagnetic radiation. The only distinctions are historic and etiologic: Gamma rays by definition are produced by radioactive decay within the atomic nucleus, whereas x-rays are produced by processes in the electron cloud surrounding the nucleus. As detailed in the CD-ROM and online versions of this chapter, electromagnetic radiation is characterized by frequency and wavelength, the product of which is equal to the speed of light (299,792 km per second) and an energy, which is proportional to the frequency. Table 46.1 shows typical values for a range of electromagnetic radiation.

TABLE 46.1 ELECTROMAGNETIC RADIATION

Radiation	Frequency (Hz)	Wavelength (m)	Energy (eV)
AM radio	1.00×10^6	300	4.14×10^{-9}
^{1}H in 1T field	4.26×10^7	7.04	1.76×10^{-7}
FM radio	1.00×10^8	3.00	4.14×10^{-7}
Microwave oven	2.45×10^9	1.22×10^{-1}	1.01×10^{-5}
Infrared	4.29×10^{14}	7.00×10^{-7}	1.78
Green light	6.00×10^{14}	5.00×10^{-7}	2.48
Ultraviolet	1.00×10^{15}	3.00×10^{-7}	4.13
Diagnostic x-ray	1.45×10^{19}	2.07×10^{-11}	6.00×10^4
Technetium-99m gamma ray	3.38×10^{19}	8.87×10^{-12}	1.40×10^5
β+ β− gamma ray	1.23×10^{20}	2.43×10^{-12}	5.11×10^5
Therapeutic gamma ray	4.80×10^{21}	6.25×10^{-14}	2.00×10^7
Cosmic rays	6.00×10^{21}	5.00×10^{-14}	2.49×10^7

Nature of Electromagnetic Radiation

Quantum mechanics has taught us that electromagnetic radiation can be thought of as being made up of either waves or particles (10). ❦ i94

Photon Attenuation

The net effect of Compton scattering and the photoelectric effect is to remove a certain percentage of the incident photons for each centimeter of tissue they pass through. This percentage is determined by the linear attenuation coefficient μ (cm^{-1}), which causes the intensity of an x-ray beam to decrease exponentially with distance traveled through the body. The critical factor for x-ray imaging is that the attenuation coefficient μ varies for different tissues in the body, being low for lung, intermediate for soft tissue, and high for bone and radiographic contrast media such as barium and iodine. The coefficient μ further varies inversely with photon energy (generally), yielding deeper penetration for higher energy photons.

As a beam of photons passes through the body, the rate of attenuation changes as they pass through tissue with variable attenuation coefficient μ. Figure 46.1 shows the photon intensity as a function of depth of travel into the tissue, which decays most rapidly when $\mu = 5$ (arbitrary units). The 2-D image that results from the passage of x-rays thus has lost all information about the distribution of matter along the x-ray path. CT techniques (see Computed Tomography) must be used to reconstruct the 3-D distribution of μ.

Note that attenuation has different implications for x-ray and nuclear imaging. In radiography, all diagnostic information results from differential attenuation of the x-ray beams

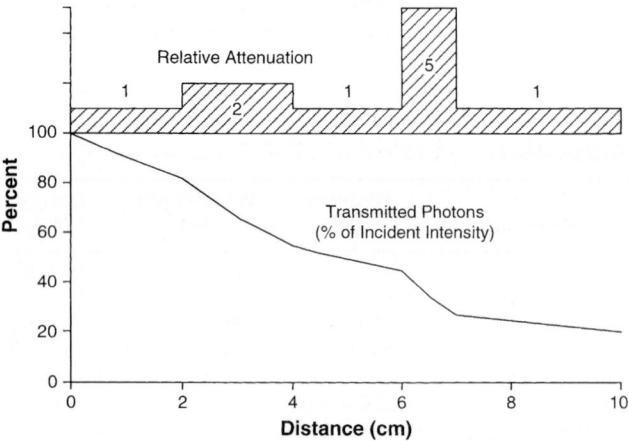

FIGURE 46.1 Impact of linear attenuation coefficient (μ) on the rate of photon intensity decay. A beam of photons (with 100% intensity) enters the tissue at 0 cm, losing intensity in proportion to μ (upper bar graph, units arbitrary). Only 21% of the incident photons traverse the entire tissue without absorption or scattering. Each of the segments is an exponential curve with a decay constant proportional to μ. (Adapted from Fozzard HA, et al. *The heart and cardiovascular system*, 2nd ed. New York: Raven, 1992:628, with permission.)

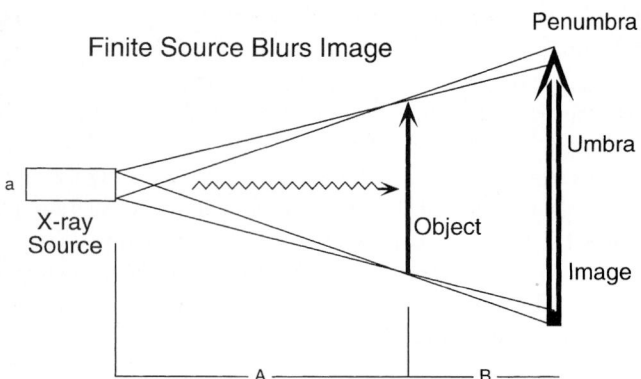

FIGURE 46.2 Geometric limits to x-ray resolution. The finite size of the x-ray source (a) leads to a penumbra around solid objects of *aB/A*. (Adapted from Fozzard HA, et al. *The heart and cardiovascular system*, 2nd ed. New York: Raven, 1992:630, with permission.)

passing through the body. In nuclear medicine, by contrast, the photons themselves are similar to x-rays, but it is their distribution *within* the body that is of interest. Ideally, there should be no attenuation at all to maximize the diagnostic information available at the surface, but short of this, attenuation should be as uniform as possible.

The distinctive features of radiography and nuclear medicine are discussed.

Imaging with X-Rays

Geometric Limits to X-Ray Image Resolution

The second major determinant of x-ray image quality relates to the finite size of the x-ray source. Within the x-ray tube, the anode is beveled at a small angle (7 to 13 degrees), so that the x-rays, emitted at right angles to the electron beam, appear to arise from a small focal spot, perhaps 1 mm^2 in area. As shown in Figure 46.2, even this small spot may blur the image. For a focal spot *a* cm in diameter, positioned *A* cm from the patient with the film *B* cm from the patient, the width of blurring will be *aB/A*. To minimize this, one seeks as small a focal spot as possible, limited principally by anode heat. Similarly, *B* should be as small as possible, but this is usually dictated by patient size. Finally, resolution can be improved by positioning the focal spot as far from the patient as possible (large *A*), but since x-ray density declines as $1/A^2$, a trade-off exists between signal-to-noise ratio and blurring.

Nuclear Imaging

Nuclear imaging uses trace quantities of radioactive isotopes to produce high-energy photons inside the body. The internal distribution of the radioactive compound is based on its *chemical* properties, giving it affinity for specific anatomic or pathologic structures (bone, blood, myocardium, for example). Localization and quantification of photon production gives diagnostic information about these structures.

TABLE 46.2 CHARACTERISTICS OF
DIAGNOSTIC RADIOISOTOPES

Isotope	Decay mode	Half-life	Photon energy (keV)[a]
^{99m}Tc	Isomeric transition	6.0 h	140
^{201}Tl	Electron capture	73.0 h	69–83
^{133}Xe	β–	5.3 d	81
^{82}Rb	β+	1.25 min	511 (2)
^{11}C	β+	20.5 min	511 (2)
^{15}O	β+	2.0 min	511 (2)
^{18}F	β+	1.8 h	511 (2)

β–, beta-emission; β+, positron emission; (2), 2 photons of 511 keV
are emitted.
[a]Photon energies are for the principal decay mode. There usually are other emissions of lesser frequency.

In general, the isotopes of nuclear medicine can be
divided into two broad types, those that produce single
photons when they disintegrate and those that produce
pairs of oppositely directed photons. Table 46.2 lists the
decay mechanism and photon energy of several important
isotopes, the details of which are provided on the CD-
ROM and online versions of this chapter.

Radioactive Decay Rates

The number of disintegrations per second in an isotope is
proportional to the amount of the isotope and to a decay
constant λ, which expresses the likelihood of a given atom
decaying per second. Another common way to characterize
the decay rate is the half-time $t_{1/2}$, the time required for half
of the isotope to decay. It is related to λ by

$$t_{1/2} = 0.693/\lambda$$

The half-time of an isotope has important practical and
safety impacts. If $t_{1/2}$ is too long, then a large dose of the
isotope will have to be given to the patient to get adequate
images, leading to excessive long-term exposure unless the
compound is cleared from the body chemically (e.g., via the
kidneys). If $t_{1/2}$ is too short, however, the isotope may be
impossible to transport: Many positron emitters have a $t_{1/2}$
measured in minutes and must be generated by an on-site
cyclotron.

Imaging the Emitted Gamma Rays

The Anger gamma camera uses a large sodium iodide (NaI)
crystal that emits light by the photoelectric effect in proportion to the energy of an impinging high-energy photon.
This provides a means of not only counting the photons,
but also of identifying the isotopes from which they arise.
When a scintillation event occurs, it is "seen" by several
photomultiplier tubes behind the NaI crystal, triangulating
the position of the discharge before computer storage (Fig.
46.3). ▼ i95

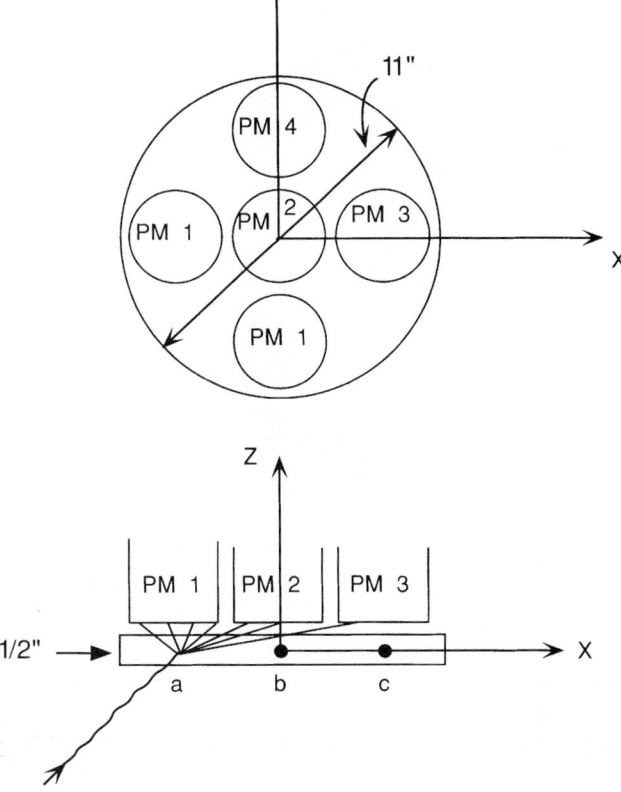

FIGURE 46.3 Schematic diagram of the Anger camera. The different output magnitudes from the photomultiplier (PM) tubes
allow localization of the impinging gamma ray.

Positron Emission Tomography

Imaging with positron emitters offers both advantages and
disadvantages over single-photon imaging. The major disadvantage is that most positron sources have very short
half-lives and thus must be made at the imaging site by a
nearby cyclotron. An exception to this is rubidium-82,
which can be eluted from a generator similar to techne-
tium-99m and thus stored for some time.

The major advantage of positron imaging is that each
decay event generates two high-energy photons (511 keV)
directed 180 degrees from each other (Fig. 46.4). Using a
ring of gamma cameras surrounding the patient, these photons will be detected simultaneously by two cameras, and
the disintegration must have occurred on a line between
them, allowing truly tomographic images to be obtained
(13). Further refinement is possible by measuring the tiny
difference in reception time for the two "simultaneous"
photons, localizing the disintegration event along the line
connecting the detectors. Unfortunately, the incredible
speed of light (30 cm per nanosecond) and the finite temporal resolution of the simultaneity circuits (approximately
300 picosecond) limits localization to approximately 5 cm.
Although this alone is not sufficiently accurate, it does aid
in the statistical reconstruction from multiple events (14).

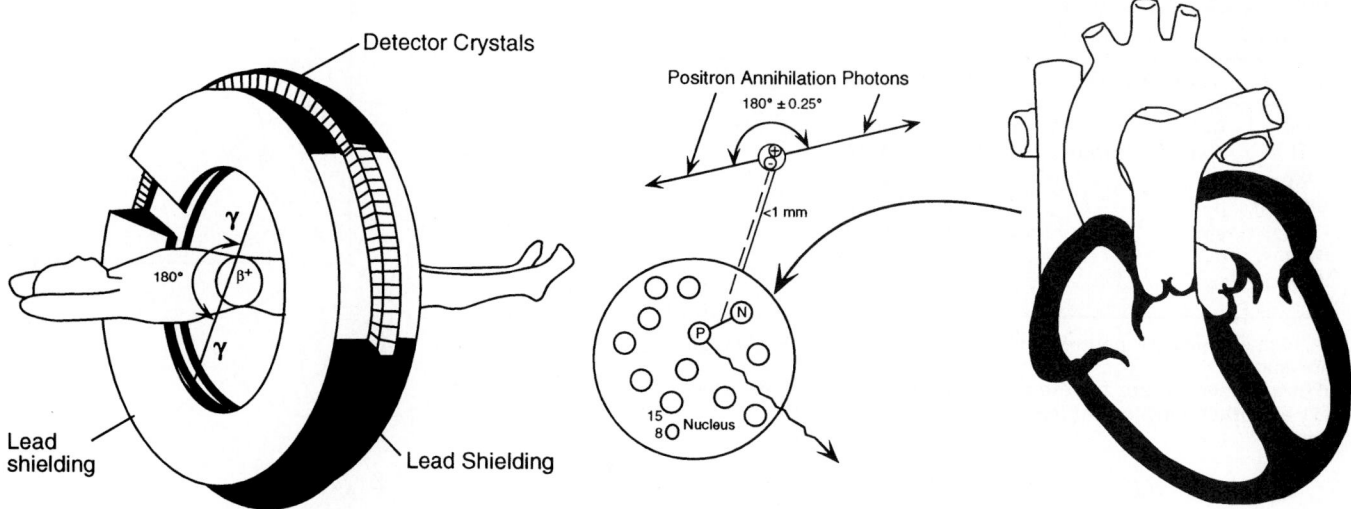

FIGURE 46.4 Positron emission tomography. The simultaneous detection of two photons localizes the disintegration to a line connecting the two detectors.

Further refinement in electronic hardware may improve this performance in the future.

IMAGING WITH ULTRASOUND

We now turn from imaging modalities that use high-energy photons to the use of high-frequency sound waves, which have a much longer wavelength and slower propagation than the photons considered previously. In addition, the speed of sound c is not constant like the speed of light, but rather varies with the medium through which it is passing. For typical soft tissue, this speed is approximately 1,540 m per second or 1.54 mm per μs (Table 46.3), and, as with electromagnetic radiation, there is an inverse relationship between wavelength λ and frequency f: $\lambda = c/f$.

Interaction of Ultrasound with Matter

The important interactions to consider are attenuation, reflection, refraction, and scattering. Like electromagnetic radiation, ultrasound suffers an exponential decrease in amplitude as it passes through homogeneous tissue. Atten-

TABLE 46.3 ULTRASONIC PARAMETERS

Tissue	Velocity (m/sec)	Attenuation (cm^{-1})	Impedance (10^4 kg/m^2 sec)
Blood	1,580	0.0198	1.6
Bone	2,240	3.01	3.8–7.4
Fat	1,450	0.100	1.4
Muscle	1,580	0.193	1.7
Lung	—	—	0.26
Plasma	—	0.0069	1.5
Water	1,480	—	—

uation varies with tissue type (Table 46.3) and is faster at higher frequencies, limiting the frequency that can be used clinically in echocardiography (15).

Whenever a sound wave encounters a boundary between two types of tissue, the energy partially reflected with the remainder transmitted into the second tissue, the proportion being determined by the difference in acoustic impedance Z of the two tissues, defined as the product of sound velocity and tissue density, $Z = \rho c$. For relatively large, flat boundaries, the amount of reflected energy I_R is given by

$$I_R = I_i \, [(Z_2 - Z_1)/(Z_2 + Z_1)]^2$$

where I_i is the incident intensity and Z_1 and Z_2 are the impedances for the two tissues (16) (Table 46.3). Boundaries with a large difference in impedance reflect much more energy than those between tissues with similar acoustic properties. For instance, the heart–lung interface reflects 54% of the incident ultrasound, whereas the blood–myocardium boundary reflects less than 0.1%. ▼ i96

Echocardiographic Imaging

In echocardiography, short pulses of ultrasound are attenuated, scattered, and refracted as they pass through tissue, with a small amount of energy reflected from deep structures to the transducer. Assuming the velocity of sound c to be constant in soft tissue (1,540 m per second), the depth d of a reflector is given by the time delay Δt between transmission of the ultrasound pulse and receipt of the echo: $d = c\Delta t/2$, the factor of 2 entering because Δt includes time *to* and *from* the object, approximately 13 μs per cm of depth (Fig. 46.5).

Echo Basics: *Time = Depth*

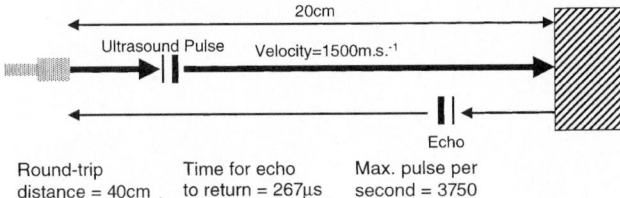

Round-trip distance = 40cm   Time for echo to return = 267µs   Max. pulse per second = 3750

- For depth d, time t, and speed of sound c (1500 – 1540 m/sec):
- $d = ct/2 \approx 77t$ (d in cm, t in ms)
- Maximal pulse repetition frequency: $PRF = c/2d \approx 77/d$

FIGURE 46.5 Basics of echocardiographic imaging. Because of the relatively fixed speed of sound in tissue, the delay in echo return can be translated into the distance to the reflection.

Display Modes

As discussed in Chapter 49, echo signals can be displayed in various formats. In M-mode echocardiography, repeated echo pulses are made along a single scan line, and the processed envelope is drawn vertically on the output video with subsequent envelopes displaced rightward, so that the horizontal axis of the display corresponds to time while the vertical axis relates to distance from the chest wall (Fig. 46.6).

In 2-D or sector scanning, echo interrogations are made sequentially throughout a 60- to 90-degree sector, fanning out from the transducer, typically approximately 100 scan lines per frame. For a 20-cm imaging depth, pulses can be emitted every 260 µs, allowing a 100–scan-line frame to be formed in 26 ms, and a display rate of over 38 frames per second. With parallel processing, up to four scan lines can

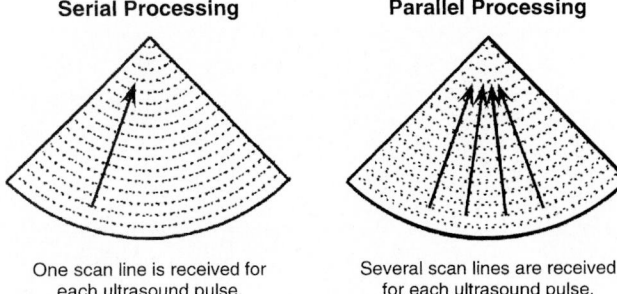

FIGURE 46.7 Serial versus parallel processing. By analyzing several scan lines simultaneously through parallel processing, frame rate can be significantly improved.

be displayed simultaneously, allowing frame rates over 150 per second (Fig. 46.7).

Tissue Harmonic Imaging

One of the greatest advances in echocardiographic image quality in the past years has been the development of tissue harmonic imaging. When ultrasound waves propagate through tissue, their frequency content does not remain constant, but rather shifts to increasing amounts of higher frequencies [17]. ▾ i97

Figure 46.8 shows the impact of harmonic imaging in a patient with mitral stenosis, demonstrating improved endocardial definition and imaging of the subvalvular apparatus. Clinical tests on this modality have shown improved contrast between the wall and cavity [18] without adverse effect on valve thickness [19].

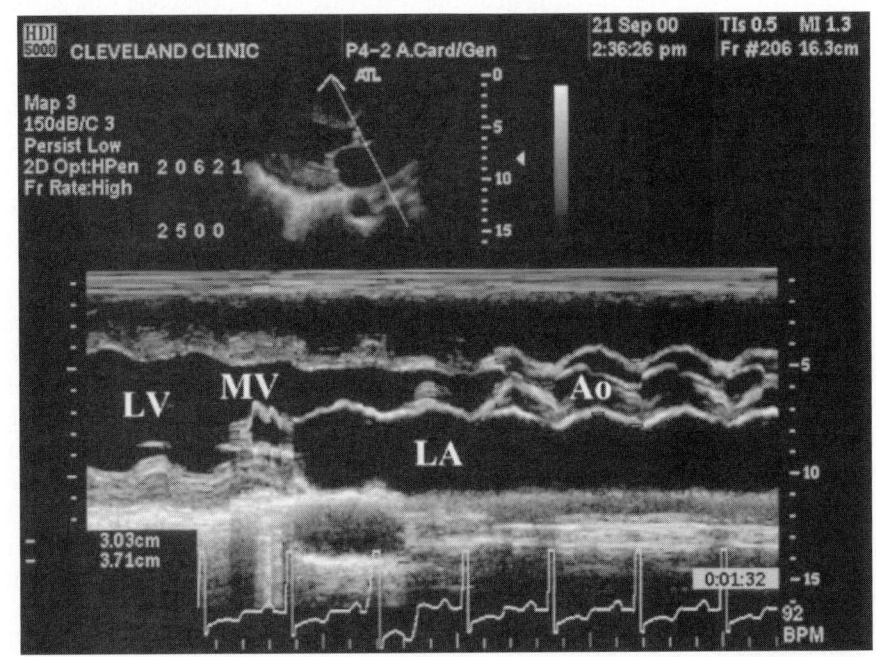

FIGURE 46.6 M-mode echocardiographic imaging. The M-mode display shows depth vertically and time horizontally. Ao, aorta; LA, left atrium; LV, left ventricle; MV, mitral valve.

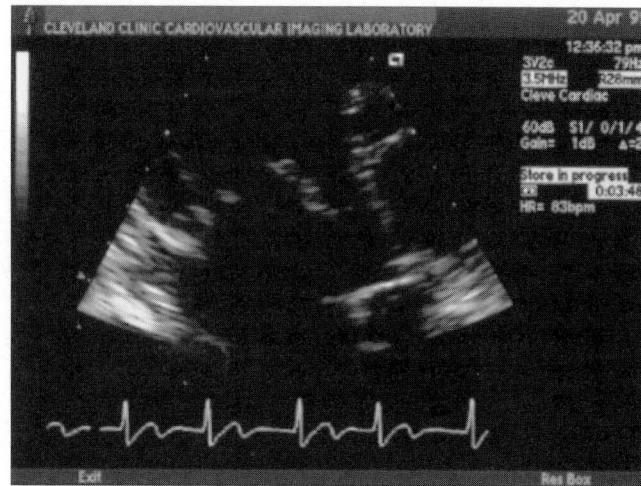
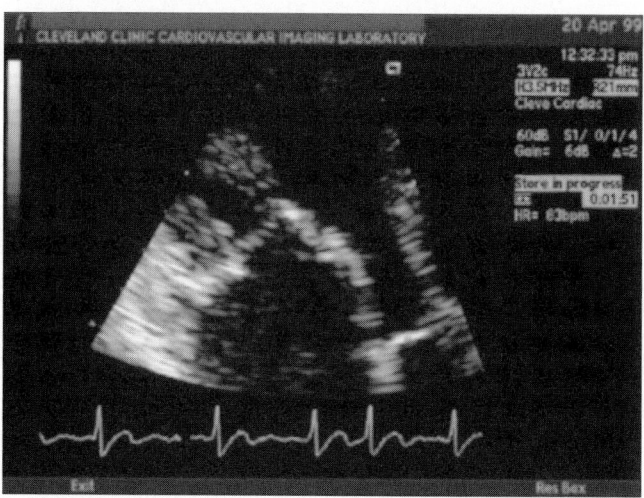

FIGURE 46.8   Impact of harmonic imaging in a patient with mitral stenosis. **A:** Fundamental. **B:** Harmonic.

Doppler Echocardiography

Exploitation of the Doppler principle to define intracardiac blood velocity adds enormous value to echocardiographic imaging (20,21). It is based on the observation that sound reflected from moving objects is frequency shifted in proportion to the ratio of object velocity v and sound velocity c: $f_d = 2vf_0/c$, where f_0 is the transducer frequency and f_d is the amount of the Doppler shift. The factor 2 occurs because the frequency is shifted when the sound hits the moving particle and again when it is reradiated by scattering. Only the component of particle velocity parallel to the ultrasound beam affects the Doppler shift (Fig. 46.9). For a particle moving at an angle θ to the scan line, the Doppler shift is proportional to the cosine of θ: 30-degree misalignment leads to a 13% velocity underestimation.

- *Sound transmitted from a moving object:*

$$\frac{\Delta f}{f} = \frac{v}{c}$$

- *Sound reflected from a moving object*

$$\frac{\Delta f}{f} = \frac{2v}{c}$$

- *....from an object moving at angle θ*

$$\frac{\Delta f}{f} = \frac{2v \cos \theta}{c}$$

- *Rearranging..........*

$$v = \frac{c \, \Delta f}{2f \cos \theta}$$

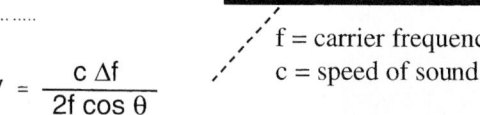

f = carrier frequency
c = speed of sound

FIGURE 46.9   Determinants of the Doppler shift. When sound is emitted from a moving object, the frequency is shifted in proportion to the velocity. For reflected sound, the factor 2 occurs because this shift occurs on absorption and reflection. Only the component of velocity parallel to the sound wave contributes to the Doppler shift.

In general, three different types of Doppler processing are available on contemporary echocardiographic equipment: continuous wave Doppler, pulsed Doppler, and Doppler flow mapping ("color Doppler"). Each is processed differently and discussed in detail on the CD-ROM and online versions of this chapter.

MAGNETIC RESONANCE IMAGING

The third physical principle used in cardiac imaging, nuclear magnetic resonance, is less familiar than electromagnetic and sonic radiation, but its physical basis has been well defined in the last half-century, an understanding of which helps in the appreciation of clinical MRI. Pauli first suggested the existence of microscopic magnetic moments within atomic nuclei in 1924. Studies of this phenomenon in the presence of external magnetic and electromagnetic fields by Purcell and Bloch in 1946 were landmarks and led to the two sharing the Nobel Prize for physics in 1952.

Physical Principles

Although many nuclei are magnetic, by far the most important to medical imaging is the single hydrogen proton (^{1}H), both because of its abundance and its high sensitivity to external influences. An individual proton in an external magnetic field of strength B_0 spins or *precesses* about the magnetic field at the *Larmor frequency*, f, proportional to the strength of the external field B_0 and the magnetogyric ratio γ, a constant specific to each nuclear species: $f = \gamma B_0 / 2\pi$. For the hydrogen proton, $\gamma/2\pi$ is 42.58 MHz per Tesla (Fig. 46.10), where Tesla is a standard unit of magnetic field strength, equivalent to 10,000 Gauss, an older unit. Typical MRI magnets have field strengths from 0.5 to 4.0 T. By way of comparison, the earth's magnetic field strength

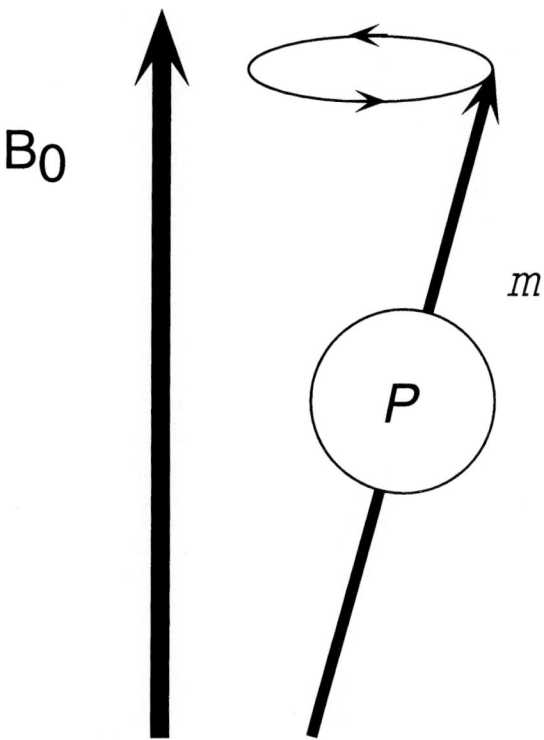

FIGURE 46.10 Precession. Nuclei with odd numbers of protons and neutrons are weakly magnetic with magnetic moment μ, ^{1}H being most important. In a strong magnetic field (strength B_0), a few protons line up; in a 1T field (3,000 × earth), <0.001% are aligned. If these "aligned" protons are tipped out of alignment, they will precess like a wobbling top at 42.6 MHz per Tesla. This Larmor frequency is proportional to the magnetic field, critical to magnetic resonance imaging. (Adapted from Fozzard HA, et al. *The heart and cardiovascular system*, 2nd ed. New York: Raven, 1992:639, with permission.)

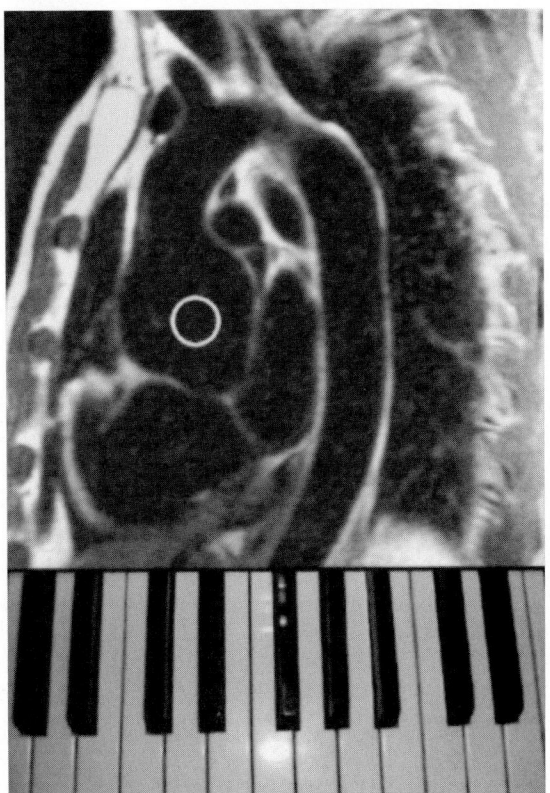

FIGURE 46.11 Localizing the magnetic resonance imaging signal. By varying the strength of the magnetic field across the image, the proton precessional frequency varies, allowing them to be localized by Fourier analysis, much like a piano note can be localized.

is approximately 0.3 Gauss or 3×10^{-5} T, and thus a proton in the Earth's magnetic field will precess at approximately 1,280 Hz.

Localizing the Signal

The final issue to contend with is localizing a particular magnetic signal within the body. Because all protons in a magnetic field B_0 will precess with the same frequency $f = \gamma B_0/2\pi$ (except for minuscule variations related to the local chemical environment and exploited in magnetic resonance spectroscopy), there is no way for an external receiver to distinguish where the signals are arising. It is possible, however, to make the precessional frequency a function of position by varying the magnetic field across the patient during the readout period. If a magnetic gradient G_x is applied across the region of interest in the x-direction, the precessional frequency will be $f = \gamma(B_0 + xG_x)/2\pi$, and protons at high x values will ring at a higher frequency than those at low x values. By analyzing the frequency content of the received signal, it is possible to distinguish regions with different x-coordinates (in much the same way that it is possi-

ble to tell whether the right or left end of the piano keyboard has been struck simply by listening to the pitch of the emitted note; Fig. 46.11). This process is intimately involved with Fourier transform theory (see Application of Fourier Analysis in Cardiac Imaging, later in this chapter).

COMPARISON OF TECHNIQUES

The preceding physical descriptions and the subsequent chapters show there are a host of diagnostic tests available for most cardiovascular disorders. To choose among them in the workup of a given patient, one may apply any of several criteria, such as cost, safety, accuracy, and availability of the test. Also of critical importance is the likelihood that a particular disease is actually present in the patient.

Sensitivity and Specificity

Two key parameters for the accuracy of a test are its sensitivity and specificity. In general, *sensitivity* refers to the likelihood that a patient with a given disease will have a positive test result, whereas *specificity* is the likelihood that a patient without that disease will have a negative test result. We can divide patients into four general classes: true-positive results (TP, patient with disease has a positive test result), true-negative results (TN, patient without disease has a negative test result), false-positive results (FP, patient without disease has a positive test result), and false-negative results (FN, patient with disease has a negative test result). Sensitivity then is defined as TP/(TP + FN), whereas specificity is TN/(TN + FP). Closely related to these concepts are the positive and negative predictive values for a test. The positive predictive value is the proportion of patients with positive test results who, in fact, have the disease: TP/(TP + FP), whereas the negative predictive value reflects patients with a negative test result who are free of the disease: TN/(TN + FN). Overall accuracy of the test is given by the percentage of patients who have the proper test result: (TP + TN)/(TP + TN + FP + FN).

Critical to rational use of sensitivity and specificity figures is knowing the prevalence of disease in the test population. For example, a test with a specificity of 95% sounds very accurate, but in a population whose prevalence is only 1:1,000, there will be 50 false-positive test results for every patient who actually has the disease.

Bayesian Analysis

To determine the true value of a test in a given patient population, one uses Bayesian analysis. If the prevalence of a finding in a given population is p, then the likelihood of being free of that disease is $1 - p$. Sensitivity and specificity data can then be used to derive the positive and negative predictive value for a given p:

$$\text{Positive predictive value} = Se \cdot p/[Se \cdot p + (1 - Sp)(1 - p)]$$

$$\text{Negative predictive value} = Sp \cdot p/[Sp \cdot p + (1 - Se)(1 - p)].$$

Thus, when the prevalence of a disease is low, a test must have extraordinarily good specificity for most of the positive test results not to represent false-positive results. Alternatively, one may solve for the prevalence of disease at which the predictive value positive for a test is 0.5 (equal odds of disease vs. false-positive result), given by $p = (1 - Sp)/(1 + Se - Sp)$. Thus, for a test with equal sensitivity and specificity, this break-even point for predictive value positive is given by a prevalence of $1 - Sp$. It is often unwise to perform tests in populations with either a very low prevalence of disease (high proportion of false-positive test results) or a very high prevalence (most negative test results are false negative).

Receiver-Operator Curve Analysis

Often a test may produce a continuum of parameter values, and it is unclear what threshold should be used to

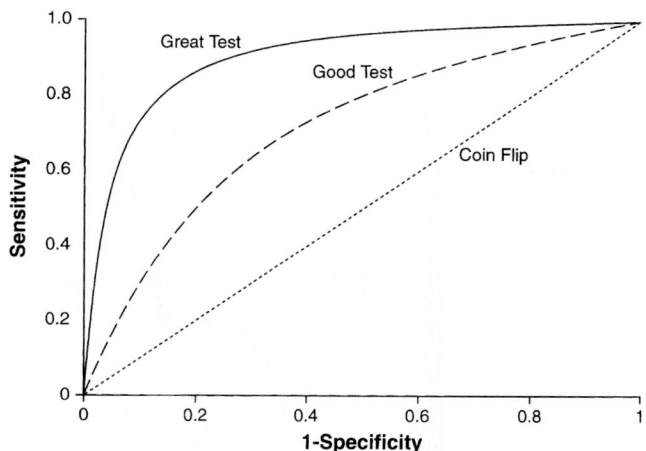

FIGURE 46.12 Receiver-operator curve analysis. For tests with continuous output parameters, there is a trade-off between sensitivity and specificity based on the choice of the cutoff to declare a test result positive. The closer a test result approaches the ideal of 100% sensitivity and specificity (*upper left corner*), the better the test.

determine whether a disease is present. If the threshold is set too low, this results in an unacceptable number of false-positive readings, whereas a threshold set too high will miss many patients with disease. A receiver-operator curve is useful for determining the optimal test threshold as well as judging the overall value of the test. In receiver-operator curve analysis (Fig. 46.12), one specificity is plotted along the *x*-axis, while sensitivity is plotted along the *y*-axis with various points plotted corresponding to alternative test thresholds. A test that is entirely without value (such as flipping a coin) produces a diagonal line between (0,0) and (1,1). There is always a trade-off between sensitivity and specificity of a test as the threshold is altered, but generally the optimal point is the one that is closest to the upper left-hand corner of the receiver-operator box (0,1). The area under the receiver-operator curve (or between the receiver-operator curve and the line of identity) is a measure of the overall worth of the test, and tests that approach the ideal are those that are skewed strongly to the upper left-hand corner.

Economic Analysis

With the current restraints on health care expenditures, the cost of a diagnostic test must be considered in judging its overall worth. Unfortunately, determining the cost-effectiveness of a diagnostic test (in terms such as the cost per additional quality year of life) is more difficult than a therapeutic maneuver (25). With a therapeutic intervention, there is a discrete encounter with a well-defined cost and an outcome that can be tracked from that point forward. With a diagnostic test, however, a physician must act on the test, putting a cloud of therapeutic uncertainty between the diagnostic test and the outcome. Furthermore, this evaluation does not in any way account for the significant reassurance that a patient may feel by having a negative test outcome.

PRACTICAL ASPECTS OF DIGITAL IMAGING

The foregoing indicates that much of contemporary cardiac imaging relies on digital acquisition and processing, but until relatively recently, the final image was usually stored in analog format: 35-mm film for angiography, videotape for echocardiography, and cut film for radiography and nuclear cardiology. Increasingly, however, images are being stored in digital format for review, analysis, and archiving. Among the advantages of digital storage are the following (66,67): (a) individual components of an examination (e.g., cine runs in angiography, echocardiographic views) can be quickly reviewed without needing to search through the entire study; (b) prior examinations are available for side-by-side comparison with the current study; (c) studies can be reviewed by clinicians throughout the hospital; (d) images can be transferred instantaneously to other institutions for consultation or referral (68,69); (e) spatial, temporal, and other calibration data can be stored with the study, facilitating quantitative off-line analysis; (f) sophisticated image-processing algorithms can be readily applied to the original data; (g) images can be duplicated without degradation; (h) long-term archiving can be accomplished without loss of quality; and (i) costs may be lower than with analog techniques. To accomplish this goal has required agreement on formatting standards, dramatic improvement in the cost-effectiveness of computers and networks, and agreement within the clinical community as to the degree of data compression that will be allowable.

Digital Imaging at The Cleveland Clinic Foundation

The year 2000 marked the time that digital storage became a reality in the echocardiography and catheterization laboratories. Figure 46.13 shows the current architecture in use for digital echocardiography in our laboratory. All echo machines in the inpatient and outpatient laboratories, operating rooms, and regional satellite facilities are capable of digital output of still images and loops in the DICOM format using a standard TCP/IP network (100 MB per second for the local machines, 1.54-MB per second T1 lines for the regional facilities). For portable studies performed outside the high-speed network, studies can be stored temporarily on the machine's hard disk for later network export or stored on a magneto-optical disk for "sneaker netting" onto the archive. Within the echo laboratory, all image traffic is handled over a network that is isolated by switches so as not to degrade performance of

the remainder of the cardiology network. A typical study in our laboratory contains 30 to 80 single-cycle cine loops with an additional 10 to 20 still frames of spectral Doppler and M-mode tracings, yielding an average study size of approximately 60 MB. With 160 studies performed daily, this requires 10 GB of storage daily or approximately 2.5 TB of storage annually. To handle this enormous storage need while providing rapid review of recent studies (access times less than 30 seconds), data sets are initially stored on a local hard drive with almost 1 TB of storage, where they remain for 30 to 60 days. Simultaneously, data are also copied to a long-term digital tape archive providing 160-TB storage with 2- to 3-minute access time. All of this is controlled by a dedicated software program running on several viewing stations in the laboratory. A similar architecture is used in the catheterization laboratory with a dedicated network providing access to up to 60 angiographic studies performed daily and stored using the DICOM standard and lossless JPEG encoding.

SUMMARY

The theory underlying cardiac imaging techniques spans a wide range of physical principles, from low-energy photons (magnetic resonance) to high-energy photons (radiography and nuclear medicine) to acoustic energy (ultrasound). With each of these methods, there are fundamental trade-offs to be made in terms of spatial resolution, temporal resolution, acquisition time, and radiation exposure, trade-offs that often become clearer when studied in terms of the spectral content of signals using Fourier analysis. Finally, combining data from any of these imaging modalities with techniques of digital image processing may provide new ways for automated image analysis and understanding.

CONTROVERSIES AND PERSONAL PERSPECTIVES

Each year brings dramatic new developments in cardiac imaging. Since the physical interaction of photons, ultrasound, and magnetism with matter has changed little, most of these improvements result from enhancement in the computer processing of these data. Extrapolating to the future, we can only expect this to continue. Moore's law states that, over the past 50 years, computer processing power (per unit cost) doubled every 18 months. Had the auto industry shown similar productivity gains, the cost of a new car would be less than 1 cent. Since the mid-1990s, the trend toward all-digital acquisition and storage for radiography, angiography, and echocardiography has become reality, with practical solutions available from several vendors. For the most part, however, these solutions

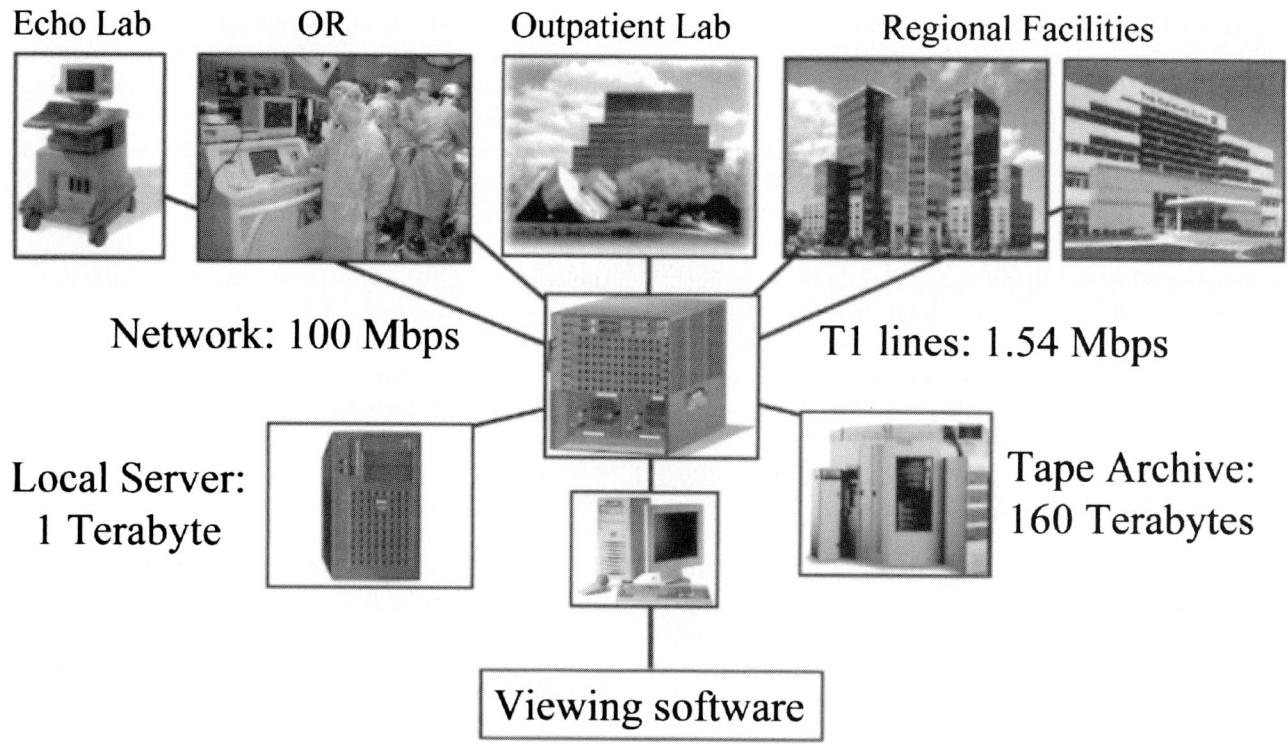

Echo Lab   OR   Outpatient Lab   Regional Facilities

Network: 100 Mbps   T1 lines: 1.54 Mbps

Local Server: Tape Archive:
1 Terabyte   160 Terabytes

Viewing software

FIGURE 46.13 Implementation of digital echocardiography at The Cleveland Clinic Foundation in 2001. High-speed networks connect more than 30 echocardiographs to a central server and archive. See text for details. OR, operating room.

are isolated from each other and are not generally available throughout the hospital. If we are to achieve true intervendor, intermodality utility, the medical community must insist on adherence to both the letter and spirit of DICOM: DICOM should be output (by disk, network, or both) by each imaging machine and read by all information management systems. In this way, the end-user can choose components based solely on quality and price performance without concern for interoperability. In the next 5 years, we can expect solutions to emerge that can read multiple modalities and deliver these quickly to the practitioner's screen, allowing the easy integration of echo, nuclear, catheterization, and MRI data to guide management of the patient.

Digital storage and transmission should also make health care more economical by reducing the need for duplicate studies. Patients will carry their medical records and images with them, initially on compact disk but perhaps soon on a small holographic card. Images will be transmittable via telephone, satellite, or the Internet, allowing remote consultation and timely referral. Equally important is extracting as much data as we can from any given study. In this regard, several modalities (ultrasound, MRI, and nuclear imaging) are touting themselves as "one-stop shopping" for cardiac structure, function, and perfusion. Of the three, ultrasound permits the least expensive assessment of chamber size, global and regional ventricular func-

tion, and valvular stenosis and regurgitation. With the development of stress echocardiography and novel contrast agents, myocardial perfusion may similarly be measurable. Unfortunately, echocardiography has been used traditionally in a largely qualitative fashion; it is hoped that the trend toward quantitative processing of color Doppler velocities and regional wall motion will continue. Nuclear imaging has seen great improvement in the last two decades and represents the current gold standard for myocardial perfusion and metabolism. Positron emission tomographic scanning is uniquely informative, but so expensive as to be confined to a few large medical centers. In this era of cost containment, it is hard to imagine widespread dissemination of this technology. MRI provides high-resolution isotropic 3-D data throughout the body without the restriction of echocardiographic windows. With improvements, the large epicardial coronary arteries may be routinely imaged, contrast may assess myocardial perfusion, and spectrographic techniques may detect ischemia. Like positron emission tomography, though, the large capital investment and operating expense of MRI will likely limit it to specialized applications in major medical centers. More recently, computed tomography with spiral scanning techniques has allowed rapid acquisition of gated cardiac images, allowing excellent visualization of the aorta and proximal coronaries at considerably lower cost and complexity than MRI.

THE FUTURE

The next decade will see continued technical progress in all cardiac imaging modalities, but economic forces will increasingly force clinicians to choose between examinations. Those tests that provide the most comprehensive assessment of the heart at the least cost will prosper, whereas others may see diminished use. A great challenge is the routine exchange of digital studies both within and between institutions. Vendors and professional societies have agreed on the DICOM standard for this exchange, but implementation remains incomplete. The medical community must insist on adherence to standards if global interoperability is ever to be achieved.

REFERENCES

1. Collins SM, Skorton DJ, eds. *Cardiac imaging and image processing.* New York: McGraw-Hill, 1985.
2. Chandra R. *Introductory physics of nuclear medicine.* Philadelphia: Lea & Febiger, 1982.
3. Coulam CM, Erickson JJ, Rollo FD, et al., eds. *The physical basis of medical imaging.* New York: Appleton-Century-Crofts, 1981.
4. Gifford D. *A handbook of physics for radiologists and radiographers.* New York: Wiley, 1984.
5. Weyman AE. *Cross-sectional echocardiography,* 2nd ed. Philadelphia: Lea & Febiger, 1994.
6. Stark DD, Bradley WG Jr. *Magnetic resonance imaging.* St. Louis: Mosby, 1988.
7. Meredith WJ. *Fundamental physics of radiology.* Bristol: J. Wright, 1977.
8. James AE Jr, Anderson JH, Higgins CB, eds. *Digital image processing in radiology.* Baltimore: Williams & Wilkins, 1985.
9. Skorton DJ, et al., eds. *Marcus' cardiac imaging,* 2nd ed. Philadelphia: WB Saunders, 1996.
10. Saxon D. *Elementary quantum mechanics.* San Francisco: Holden-Day, 1968:1–16.
11. Curry TS III, Dowdey JE, Murry RC Jr. *Christensen's introduction to the physics of diagnostic radiology.* Philadelphia: Lea & Febiger, 1984.
12. Wachsmann F, Drexler G. *Graphs and tables for use in radiology.* New York: Springer-Verlag, 1976.
13. Ell PJ, Holman BL, eds. *Computed emission tomography.* New York: Oxford University Press, 1982.
14. Budinger TF. Time-of-flight positron emission tomography: status relative to conventional PET. *J Nucl Med* 1983;24:73–78.
15. Miller JG, Yuhus DE, Mimbs JW, et al. Ultrasonic tissue characterization: correlation between biochemical and ultrasonic indices of myocardial injury. *Proc IEEE Ultrasonics Symp* 1976;76:33–43.
16. Wells PNT. *Biomedical ultrasonics.* New York: Academic Press, 1977.
17. Thomas JD, Rubin DN. Tissue harmonic imaging: why does it work? *J Am Soc Echocardiogr* 1998;11:803–808.
18. Rubin DN, Yazbek N, Garcia MJ, et al. The qualitative and quantitative effects of harmonic echocardiographic imaging on endocardial edge definition and side-lobe artifacts. *J Am Soc Echocardiogr* 2001 (*in press*).
19. Prior DL, Jaber WA, Homa DA, et al. Impact of tissue harmonic imaging on the assessment of rheumatic mitral stenosis. *Am J Cardiol* 2000;86:573–576.
20. Hatle L, Angelsen B. *Doppler ultrasound in cardiology: physical principles and clinical applications.* Philadelphia: Lea & Febiger, 1982.
21. Goldberg SJ. *Doppler echocardiography.* Philadelphia: Lea & Febiger, 1988.
22. Kasai C, Namekawa K, Koyano A, et al. Real-time two-dimensional blood flow imaging using an autocorrelation technique. *IEEE Trans Sonics and Ultrasonics* 1985;32:458–464.
23. Fukushima E, Roeder SBW. *Experimental pulse NMR.* Reading, MA: Addison-Wesley, 1981.
24. Bushong SC. *Magnetic resonance imaging.* St. Louis: C. V. Mosby, 1988.
25. Doubilet P, Weinstein MC, McNeil BJ. Use and misuse of the term "cost-effective" in medicine. *N Engl J Med* 1986;314:253–256.
26. Pratt WK. *Digital image processing.* New York: Wiley, 1978:593–598.
27. Ophir J, Maklad NF. Digital scan converters in diagnostic ultrasound imaging. *Proceedings of the IEEE* 1979;67:79.
28. Leavitt SC, Hunt BF, Larsen HG. A scan conversion algorithm for displaying ultrasound images. *Hewlett-Packard J* 1983;34:30–34.
29. Rosenfield A, Kak AC. *Digital picture processing,* 2nd ed. New York: Academic Press, 1982.
30. Skorton DJ, McNary CA, Child JS, et al. Digital image processing of two-dimensional echocardiograms: identification of the endocardium. *Am J Cardiol* 1981;48:479.
31. Zwehl W, Levy R, Garcia E, et al. Validation of a computerized edge detection algorithm for quantitative two-dimensional echocardiography. *Circulation* 1983;68:1127.
32. Collins SM, Skorton DJ, Geiser EA, et al. Computer assisted edge detection in two-dimensional echocardiography: comparison with anatomic data. *Am J Cardiol* 1984;53:1980.
33. Delp EJ, Buda AJ, Swastek MR, et al. The analysis of two-dimensional echocardiograms using a time varying image approach. In: *Computers in cardiology.* Long Beach, CA: IEEE Computer Society, 1982:391–394.
34. Parker DL, Pryor TA, Ridges JD. Enhancement of two-dimensional echocardiographic images by lateral filtering. *Comput Biomed Res* 1979;12:265.
35. Garcia E, Gueret P, Bennett M, et al. Real-time computer-

ization of two-dimensional echocardiography. *Am Heart J* 1981;101:783–792.

36. Jenkins JM, Qian G, Besozzi M, et al. Computer processing of echocardiographic images for automated edge detection of left ventricular boundaries. In: *Computers in cardiology*. Long Beach, CA: IEEE Computer Society, 1981:391–394.

37. Brennecke R, Hahne H-J, Wessel A, et al. Computerized enhancement techniques for echocardiographic sector scans. In: *Computers in cardiology*. Long Beach, CA: IEEE Computer Society, 1981:7–11.

38. Horn BKP, Schunck BG. Determining optical flow. *Artificial Intelligence* 1981;17:185–203.

39. Mailloux GE, Bleau A, Bertrand M, et al. Measurement of heart motion from two-dimensional echocardiograms. In: *Computers in cardiology*. Long Beach, CA: IEEE Computer Society, 1986:397–400.

40. Mailloux GE, Langlois F, Bertrand M, et al. Analysis of heart motions from two-dimensional echocardiograms by velocity field decomposition. In: *Computers in cardiology*. Long Beach, CA: IEEE Computer Society, 1987:441–444.

41. Thomas JD, Higginbotham RD, Waxman AM, et al. Real-time echocardiographic noise reduction, border extraction, and velocity derivation. In: *Computers in cardiology*. Long Beach, CA: IEEE Computer Society, 1988:129–132.

42. Fujita M, Sasayama S, Kawai C, et al. Automatic processing of cine ventriculograms for analysis of regional myocardial function. *Circulation* 1981;63:1065.

43. Mancini GBJ, Norris SL, Peterson KL, et al. Quantitative assessment of segmental wall motion abnormalities at rest and after atrial pacing using digital intravenous ventriculography. *J Am Coll Cardiol* 1983;2:70.

44. Spear JR, Sandor T, Als AV, et al. Computerized image analysis for quantitative measurement of vessel diameter from cineangiograms. *Circulation* 1983;68:453.

45. Kirkeeide RL, Fung P, Smalling RW, et al. Automated evaluation of vessel diameter from arteriograms. In: *Computers in cardiology*. Long Beach, CA: IEEE Computer Society, 1982:215–218.

46. Okada RD, Kirshenbaum HD, Kushner FG. Observer variance in the qualitative evaluation of left ventricular wall motion and the quantitation of left ventricular ejection fraction using rest and exercise multigated blood pool imaging. *Circulation* 1980;61:128.

47. Reiber JHC, Lie SP, Simoons ML, et al. Clinical validation of fully automated computation of ejection fraction from gated equilibrium blood-pool scintigrams. *J Nucl Med* 1983;24:1099.

48. Bacharach SL, Green MV, Vitale D, et al. Optimum Fourier filtering of cardiac data: a minimum error method. *J Nucl Med* 1983;24:1176.

49. Frais MA, Botvinick EH, Shosa DW, et al. Phase image characterization of ventricular contraction in right and left bundle branch block. *Am J Cardiol* 1982;50:95–105.

50. Ratib O, Henze E, Schon H, et al. Phase analysis of radionuclide ventriculograms for the detection of coronary artery disease. *Am Heart J* 1982;104:1.

51. Eiho S, Matsumoto N, Kuwahara M, et al. 3-D reconstruction and display of moving heart shapes from MRI data. In: *Computers in cardiology*. Long Beach, CA: IEEE Computer Society, 1987:349–352.

52. Zhang L, Geiser EL. An approach to optimal threshold selection on a sequence of two-dimensional echocardiographic images. *IEEE Trans Biomed Eng* 1982;BME-29:577–585.

53. Buda AJ, Delp EJ, Meyer CR, et al. Automatic computer processing of 2-dimensional echocardiograms. *Am J Cardiol* 1983;52:384–349.

54. Adam D, Hareuveni O, Sideman S. Semiautomated border tracking of cine echocardiographic ventricular images. *IEEE Trans Med Imaging* 1987;MI-6:266–271.

55. Angermann CE, Hart RJ, Spes CH, et al. Computerized quantitative evaluation of the endocardium in serial two-dimensional echocardiograms of the left ventricular short axis. In: *Computers in cardiology*. Long Beach, CA: IEEE Computer Society, 1987:437–440.

56. Brinkley JF. Knowledge driven ultrasonic three-dimensional organ modelling. *IEEE Trans Pattern Analysis Machine Intelligence* 1985;PAMI-7:431–441.

57. Bracewell RN. *The Fourier transform and its applications*. New York: McGraw-Hill, 1978.

58. Brigham EO. *The fast Fourier transform*. Englewood Cliffs, NJ: Prentice-Hall, 1974.

59. Arfken G. *Mathematical methods for physicists*. New York: Academic Press, 1985.

60. Thomas JD, Hagege AA, Choong CY, et al. Improved accuracy of echocardiographic endocardial borders by spatiotemporal filtered Fourier reconstruction: description of the method and optimization of the cutoffs. *Circulation* 1988;77:415–428.

61. Mansfield P, Morris PG. *NMR imaging in biomedicine*. New York: Academic Press, 1982.

62. Kumar A, Welti D, Ernst RR. NMR Fourier zeugmatography. *J Magnet Res* 1975;16:69.

63. Lee JKT, Sagel SS, Stanley RJ, eds. *Computed body tomography*. New York: Raven, 1983.

64. Brooks RA, DiCharo G. Theory of image reconstruction in computed tomography. *Radiology* 1975;117:561–572.

65. Gordon R, Herman GT. Three-dimensional reconstruction from projections: a review of algorithms. *Int Rev Cytol* 1974;38:111–151.

66. Thomas JD, Khandheria BK. Digital formatting standards in medical imaging: a primer for echocardiographers. *J Am Soc Echocardiogr* 1994;7:100–104.

67. Thomas JD, Nissen SE. Digital storage and transmission of cardiovascular images: what are the costs, benefits and timetable for conversion? *Heart* 1996;76:13–17.

68. Alboliris ET, Berdusis K, Fisher J, et al. Transmission of full-length echocardiographic images over ISDN for diagnosing congenital heart disease. *Telemedicine J* 1996;2:251–258.

69. Sobczyk WL, Solinger RE, Rees AH, et al. Transtelephonic echocardiography: successful use in a tertiary pediatric referral center. *J Pediatr* 1993;122:S84–S88.

70. Nissen SE, Pepine CJ, Bashore TM, et al. Cardiac angiography without cine film: erecting a "tower of Babel" in the cardiac catheterization laboratory (American College of Cardiology position statement). *J Am Coll Cardiol* 1994;24:834–837.

71. Kerensky RA, Cusma JT, et al. American College of Car-

diology/European Society of Cardiology International Study of Angiographic Data Compression Phase I: the effect of lossy data compression on recognition of diagnostic features in digital coronary angiography. *J Am Coll Cardiol* 2000;35:1370–1379.

72. Thomas JD. The DICOM image formatting standard: what it means for echocardiographers. *J Am Soc Echocardiogr* 1995;8:319–327.

73. Karson TH, Chandra S, Morehead AJ, et al. JPEG compression of digital echocardiographic images: impact on image quality. *J Am Soc Echocardiogr* 1995;8:306–318.

74. Thomas JD, Chandra S, Karson TH, et al. Digital compression of echocardiograms: impact on quantitative interpretation of color Doppler velocity. *J Am Soc Echocardiogr* 1996;9:606–615.

75. Karson TH, Zepp RC, Chandra S, et al. Digital storage of echocardiograms offers superior image quality to analog storage even with 20:1 digital compression: results of the Digital ERA (Echo Record Access) study. *J Am Soc Echocardiogr* 1996;9:769–778.

76. Cosman PC, Davidson HC, Bergin CJ, et al. Thoracic CT images: effect of lossy image compression on diagnostic accuracy. *Radiology* 1994;190:517–524.

77. Rebolo MS, Furuie SS, Munhoz AC, et al. Lossy compression in nuclear medicine images. *Proc Annu Symp Computer Appl Med Care* 1993;12:824–828.

78. Soble JS, Yurow G, Brar R, et al. Comparison of MPEG digital video with super VHS tape for diagnostic echocardiographic readings. *J Am Soc Echocardiogr* 1998;11:819–825.

79. Main ML, Foltz D, Firstenberg MS, et al. Real-time transmission of full-motion echocardiography over a high-speed data network: impact of data rate and network quality of service. *J Am Soc Echocardiogr* 2000;13:764–770.

80. Goldberg MA, Pivovarov M, Mayo-Smith WW, et al. Application of wavelet compression to digitized radiographs. *AJR Am J Roentgenol* 1994;163:463–468.

PLAIN FILM EXAMINATION OF THE CHEST

LAWRENCE M. BOXT

▼▼ **ADDITIONAL ELECTRONIC TOPICS**
The Chest Film Itself: Image Quality i98;   Pulmonary Venous Hypertension i99

OVERVIEW

The value of plain film examination of the heart and lungs lies in its availability, long history of clinical utility, and ability to display acute and chronic changes in a safe and convenient manner. Diagnosis is based on identification and characterization of variance in the appearance of structures on chest film from their expected normal appearance. Interpretation of the chest radiograph involves systematic evaluation of the quality of the examination, the position of the patient undergoing examination, as well as the radiographic changes encountered in the examination. The validity and significance of observed abnormalities depend on a belief in the physiologic or technical basis for their presence. Attention to these factors allows extraction of pertinent, reliable evidence of pathophysiologic mechanisms that allows the observer to make cardiovascular diagnoses, as well as to assess the instant physiologic status of the patient at the time of examination.

L. M. Boxt: Department of Clinical Radiology, Albert Einstein College of Medicine of Yeshiva University, Bronx, New York; and Department of Radiology, Beth Israel Medical Center, New York, New York

GLOSSARY

Cardiac contour: The borders of the cardiac silhouette are formed by portions of the cardiac chambers and aorta and pulmonary artery; in oblique view, different border-forming chambers are accentuated or brought into view. Analysis of chamber and great artery abnormality is based on systematic estimation of the appearance of these contours. Evaluation begins by dividing the cardiac silhouette into the left and right heart borders. The left heart border is composed of the aortic arch, main pulmonary artery, left atrial appendage, and left ventricular portion. The right heart border is composed of the superior vena cava, ascending aorta, and right atrial portion.

Cardiac position: This describes the position of the heart within the chest. In general, it is determined by estimating where the bulk of the cardiac silhouette resides. We expect the cardiac apex and bulk of the ventricular myocardium to lie just slightly off the midline, toward the left (levocardia). Thus, *mesocardia* and *dextrocardia* describe the heart as straddling over toward the right with respect to an imaginary line drawn in the chest midline. *Dextrocardia* refers to the presence of a heart in the right chest resulting from an abnormality of embryologic cardiac rotation. It is frequently associated with congenital heart disease. *Dextroposition* describes a heart in the right chest, caused by noncardiac abnormalities that affect the normally formed heart.

Cardiac rotation: The heart and proximal great arteries are contained by the pericardium and fixed in the superior mediastinum and at the diaphragm. Right atrial, ventricular, or both atrial and ventricular dilatation produces (looking from below) clockwise rotation of the heart and great vessels, so that the appearance of the left heart border in postero-anterior view is altered. The superior mediastinal silhouette is narrow as the superior vena cava rotates toward the midline, and the mid-left heart border becomes more convex as the dilated right ventricular outflow forms the left heart border.

Left ventricular configuration: Hearts that appear unusual may be morphologically normal. However, many abnormal hearts share a common appearance: The contour of the left ventricular portion of the left heart border appears greater in curvature than expected. This appearance of the left-sided heart contour is found in a variety of congenital and acquired forms of heart disease. It is a sensitive "case finder" or indicator of cardiac abnormality. However, it is nonspecific and requires appreciation of other radiographic or clinical findings for more precise cardiac diagnosis.

Pulmonary edema: This term refers to the characteristic inhomogeneous appearing infiltrates found with alveolar edema. It represents the severe end of the spectrum of the radiographic changes of pulmonary venous hypertension. The earliest radiographic finding in elevated left atrial pressure is indistinct lower lobe pulmonary vessels.

Pulmonary vascularity: The radiographic appearance of the pulmonary arteries and veins closely correlates with left atrial pressure and the regional distribution of water in the lungs. This general term refers to the caliber of the larger pulmonary arteries and veins in a chest radiograph. Comparison of left-sided vessels with those on the right, upper with lower vessels, and central with peripheral vessels is commonly used to differentiate failure from pneumonia and shunt from pulmonary hypertension.

Shunt vascularity: This subcategory of pulmonary vascularity refers to the status of the pulmonary arteries in individuals with left-to-right shunts. In particular, it refers to increase in the caliber of the entire pulmonary arterial tree, from main pulmonary artery segment, to peripheral subsegmental pulmonary arterial branches. Vessels are sharp, demonstrate normal peripheral branching, and extend further toward the pleura.

INTRODUCTION

Plain film examination of the chest is nearly always employed to determine the presence of heart disease and to help establish its etiology and severity. The development and use of angiographic, nuclear, and tomographic cardiac imaging technologies (echocardiography, computed tomography, and magnetic resonance imaging) have changed but not excluded the role of plain film radiography in the management of these patients. Characteristic changes in the atrial and ventricular portions of the cardiac contour reflect change in their chamber volume and myocardial mass. Similarly, changes in the contours formed by the great arteries and veins of the chest reflect altered pressure and blood flow. Evaluation of these changes provides the substrate for constructing a differential diagnosis or to assess the severity and often etiology of the cardiac dysfunction.

This chapter is designed to assist clinicians in the use of plain film examination of adult patients with acquired and congenital heart disease. Conventionally, chapters describe radiographic abnormalities in an organized list of cardiovascular conditions. This format can be excellent if the reader knows the answer before asking the question (i.e., if you know the patient has mitral stenosis, then reference to such a chapter provides a source for review of the literature concerning radiographic diagnosis and so on). However, as is more often the case, one does not know the plain film diagnosis; rather, one has acquired a list of positive (and negative) radiographic findings and is in need of an outline of differential diagnoses. In other words, the role of the chest film examination has changed in the management of patients with cardiovascular disease. The examination is performed more to evaluate the instant physiologic status of the patient. This change in use is not surprising, considering the rapid advance in noninvasive cardiovascular imaging. On the other hand, there remains a great deal of diagnostic information contained in plain film examination that can and does benefit the clinician.

This chapter is organized based on radiographic abnormality [i.e., the cardiac silhouette in the postero-anterior (PA) chest film is divided into left and right heart borders and the pulmonary vascularity]. The left heart border contains the aortic arch, pulmonary artery, left atrial appendage, and left ventricular contours. The right heart border contains the superior vena cava, ascending aorta, and right atrial contours. The parenchymal pulmonary vascularity is described in terms of the appearance of the pulmonary vessels. Thus, entrée into cardiovascular diagnosis and differential diagnosis is based on identification of an abnormality or constellation of abnormalities. This approach is useful, especially if one does not know the diagnosis before interpretation of the examination.

After describing the normal appearance of the cardiopulmonary structures, the range of abnormalities of that portion of the chest film is characterized and the differential diagnosis of congenital and acquired cardiovascular disease based on those specific changes is presented. That is, many different diseases may produce individual specific changes in the chest film, but more specific diagnosis may be made or a differential diagnosis ordered by evaluation of the particular constellation of findings present. In other words, rather than review the radiographic findings of a series of cardiovascular lesions, I describe particular radiographic abnormalities, explain how these changes may represent the effect of a congenital abnormality or acquired pathophysiologic mechanism, and then use these findings to construct a differential diagnosis. This is a clinically relevant approach, and it more effectively demonstrates the utility and limitations of chest film examination.

As the reader will appreciate, the utility of plain film examination in the evaluation of adult patients with congenital heart disease is emphasized. This is an important area of rapid growth. This chapter should aid clinicians who encounter such a patient or have an established practice containing many such individuals. Few non–plain film images are included in this chapter; only a few relevant images are included to reinforce mechanisms of radiographic changes in the plain film. One final note on the interpretation of plain chest films. In many cases, one may observe major "obvious" findings that form the basis for an anatomic diagnosis. Further careful analysis of the image, however, often reveals other subtler observations that correlate with the major findings. The constellation of all findings allows the observer to assess not only the disease and its severity, but also to assess the confidence the individual has in that diagnosis.

HISTORY OF CHEST RADIOGRAPHY IN CARDIAC DISEASE

Wilhelm Conrad Roentgen discovered x-rays on November 8, 1895 (1). Immediately after his discovery, physicians around the world began using this new tool in the evaluation of bone fractures and abnormalities of the gastrointestinal tract. Within months of the discovery, application of the "new photography" to chest examination was reported. Williams (2) reported fluoroscopic examination of a patient with cardiomegaly and described the findings for pericardial effusion. Early examinations were crude and dangerous by today's standards. For example, Walsh (3) published a text that included a chest film demonstrating the position and dimensions of the heart. The exposure required 20 minutes and was obtained using a 30-in. focus-film (x-ray tube–to-film) distance.

A report of heart size in healthy individuals (4) was published in 1902; by 1909 (5), a review of the normal appearance of the heart, the size and appearance of the heart in patients with aortic and mitral valvular disease, and a thoracic aortic aneurysm was published. The measurement of the cardiothoracic ratio (the quotient of the transverse diameter of the heart divided by the greatest transverse chest diameter) was introduced by Danzer (6) in 1919. In his paper, he also noted that the normal ratio is probably greater in children. Radiographic demonstration of pericardial calcification (7) and rheumatic valvular calcification (8) were reported in the early 1920s. Evaluation of changes in cardiac size, as determined by computation of the area of the cardiac silhouette in PA chest film examinations of patients with valvular heart disease, myocarditis, systemic hypertension, and hyperthyroidism (9,10) became routine during the latter half of the decade.

Seeking to gain improved insight into the sensitivity of chest film examination for detecting cardiac disease, Ungerleider and Gubner (11) reviewed the PA chest films of 1,460 healthy individuals and published nomograms for normal transverse diameter and radiographic area of the heart, an indicator of cardiac volume.

The clinical value of plain film examination of the heart was pointed out by Paul Dudley White in an address to the American Roentgen Ray Society in 1929 (12). He emphasized that radiographic examination of the heart provided the most accurate available means of estimating cardiac size and detecting unsuspected pericardial calcification and aortic aneurysms. Furthermore, he praised the technique for its ability to estimate atrial and ventricular chamber enlargement and to provide clinical information in patients too obese or emphysematous for accurate physical examination of the heart. Although there are other imaging modalities, the value of plain chest film examination remains high, and in terms of clinically relevant information obtained, the cost to perform, and patient risk, it remains an integral means of cardiac diagnosis.

THE HEART AND GREAT ARTERIES

Cardiac Position

The heart lies just to the left of midline, and the bulk of the ventricular myocardium is in the left chest (Fig. 47.1). The position of the heart within the chest depends on cardiac looping and intrathoracic rotation, as well as the presence of skeletal, pulmonary, and diaphragmatic lesions. In situs solitus, a right-sided heart secondary to a noncardiac abnormality is called *dextroposition* (*e*Fig. 47.1.1). This term implies an abnormal position of the heart in the absence of an intrinsic cardiac abnormality. Dextroposition may be caused by abnormalities of the bony thorax (scoliosis, deformities of the sternum or ribs), the lungs (pulmonary agenesis, pneumonectomy, right pneumothorax, chronic volume loss, scimitar syndrome), eventration, or diaphragmatic hernia.

The diagnosis of pneumothorax is made by identification of the visceral pleural line. Only large pneumothoraces produce complete lung collapse and significant mediastinal shift. The roentgenographic density of the ipsilateral collapsing lung changes little until lung volume is greatly reduced (20). In a pneumothorax of any size, shift away

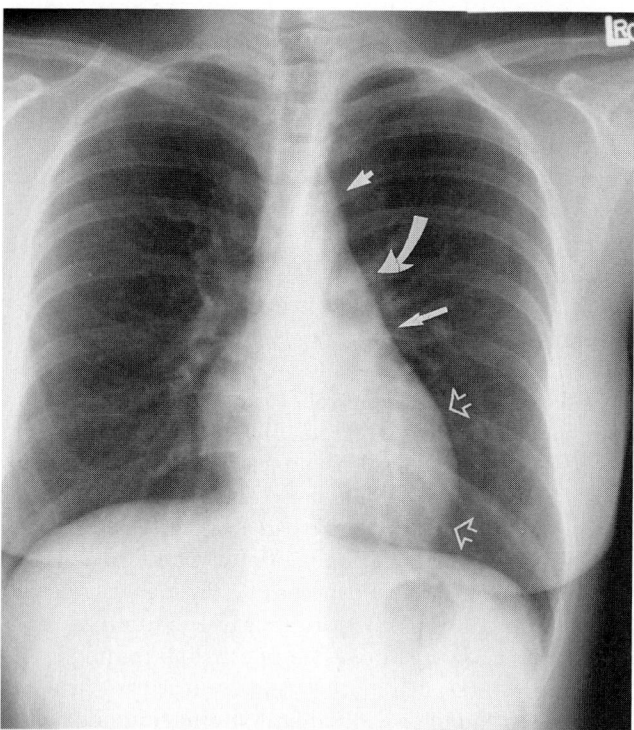

FIGURE 47.1 Normal postero-anterior chest film from a 35-year-old woman. The contours of the left heart border include the aortic arch (*short arrow*), the pulmonary artery segment (*curved arrow*), the concave left atrial appendage segment (*long arrow*), and the gentle curvature of the left ventricular segment (*open arrows*). The lower right heart border is derived from the lateral border of the right atrium.

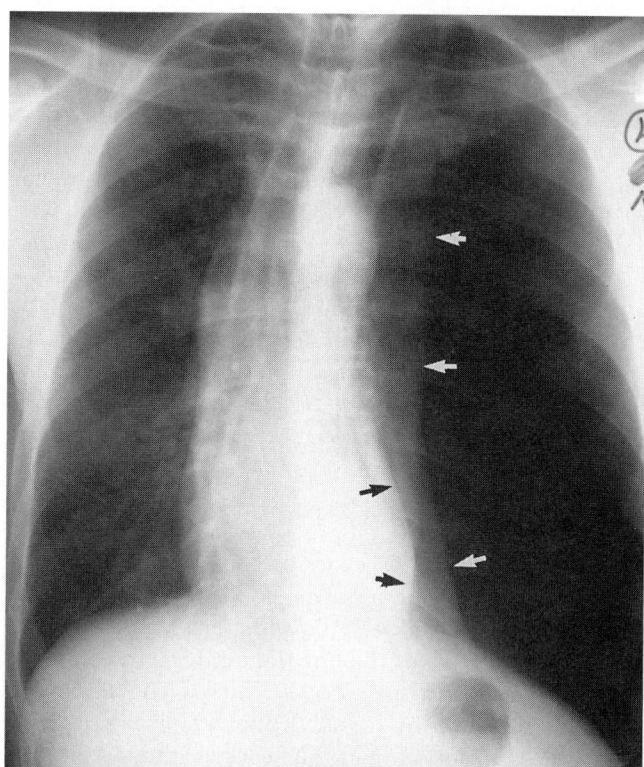

FIGURE 47.2 Tension pneumothorax in a 30-year-old man. The left ventricular contour is medial (*black arrows*) to the line of the pleura (*white arrows*) against the air-filled left chest. The heart and mediastinal structures are shifted toward the right. Notice the flattened left diaphragm.

from that side is inevitable because pressure in the normal hemithorax remains relatively more negative. Such a circumstance must be differentiated from a tension pneumothorax, in which there is a check valve mechanism, which allows air into the pleural space during inspiration, but prevents its egress during expiration. In tension pneumothorax, one finds inspiratory shift of the heart and mediastinum away from the side of the pneumothorax associated with ipsilateral diaphragmatic depression (Fig. 47.2). Eventration of the diaphragm is a congenital failure of the muscular development of one or both diaphragms (21). Unless occurring in neonates (21,22), this condition does not cause symptoms.

The scimitar syndrome (23–25) is an unusual malformation consisting of partial or total anomalous pulmonary venous return of the right lung veins to the inferior vena cava just above or below the diaphragm. It is frequently associated with hypoplasia of the right lung and right pulmonary artery. Frequently, bronchial anomalies and anomalous arterial blood supply to the right lung from the aorta are found (26). PA chest films demonstrate a slight decrease in the size of the right bony thorax and a shift of the heart and mediastinal structures to the right. The characteristic anomalous vein, or scimitar (after the Turkish curved sword), shows a vertical course toward the right cardio-

phrenic angle, closely paralleling the right atrial border (*e*Fig. 47.2.1). Depending on the degree of right lung hypoplasia, the scimitar may project through the heart or in the right pericardial area.

Cardiac Situs

Cardiac atrial situs is assumed to be solitus in the presence of thoracoabdominal situs concordance and abdominal situs solitus. Thus, identification of a right-sided liver and left-sided gastric air bubble establishes normal abdominal situs (Fig. 47.1). Thoracic situs is reliably determined by analysis of the trachea and lungs (27). That is, the morphologic left lung has two lobes (and therefore no minor fissure) and a longer left main bronchus over which the morphologic left pulmonary artery passes proximal to the origin of the left upper lobe bronchus. The morphologic right lung has three lobes (and thus a minor fissure). The right bronchus travels a short course before the origin of the right upper lobe bronchus. The morphologic right pulmonary artery lies anterior and slightly inferior to the right bronchus. Under these circumstances, atrial situs solitus (i.e., morphologic right atrium on the right and morphologic left atrium on the left) can be assumed. The position of the aortic arch or cardiac apex cannot be used to ascer-

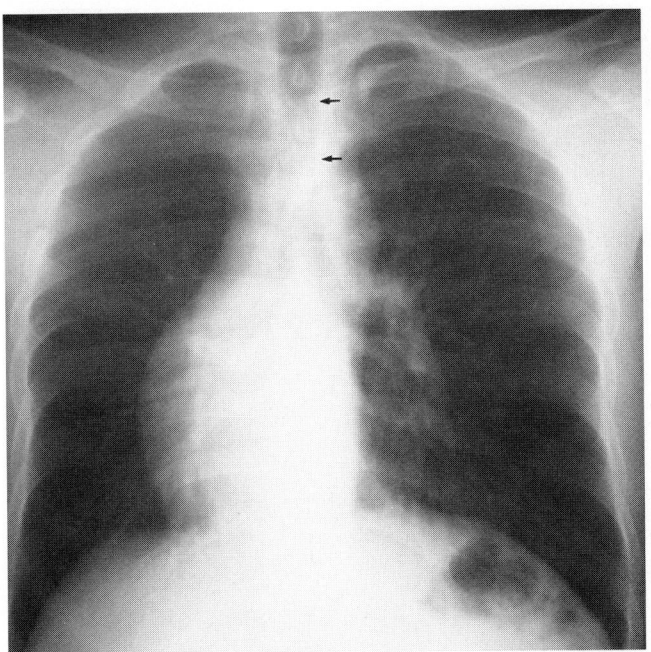

FIGURE 47.3 A 21-year-old man with isolated dextrocardia. The heart and lungs are normal. The cardiac apex is in the right chest. The trachea (*arrows*) is midline.

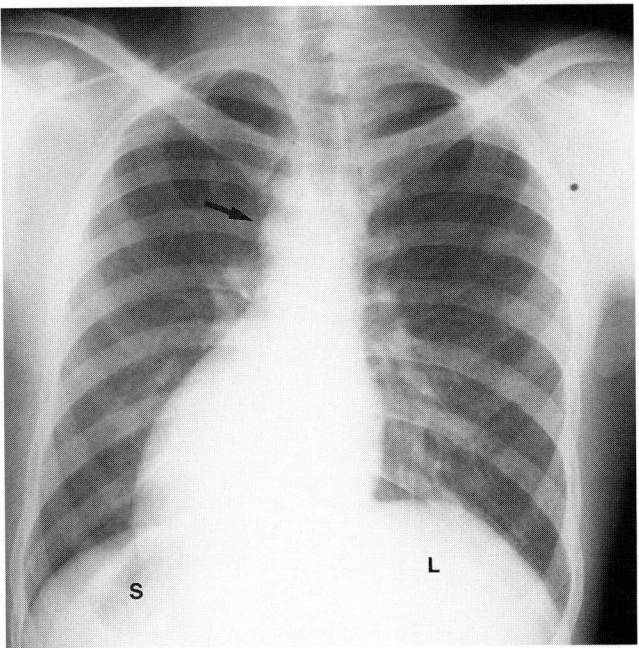

FIGURE 47.4 A 30-year-old man with complete situs inversus. The liver (L) is on the left, and the stomach bubble (S) is on the right. The aortic arch (*arrow*) and cardiac apex are on the right.

tain thoracic situs. Patients with atrial situs solitus may have an isolated right aortic arch or the bulk of their myocardial mass in the right chest (situs solitus with dextrocardia, isolated dextrocardia) in the absence of any other abnormality (Fig. 47.3). Atrial situs inversus is deduced by concordance between inverted abdominal viscera and lung morphology (Fig. 47.4).

Aortic Arch and Ascending Aorta

The normal aortic arch passes to the left, displacing the trachea toward the right (Fig. 47.1). Measurement of the true caliber of the aorta is difficult on plain chest examination because both contours are not visualized in frontal projection. The left border of the descending thoracic aorta is visualized in the PA radiograph, but the right border is not. The contour of the ascending aorta should not extend to the right beyond the vascular pedicle of the right hilum or shadow of the superior vena cava. Enlargement of the ascending aorta is characterized by increased curvature of the middle third of the mid-right heart border or by a forward bulge of the anterior border of the aorta, as viewed on lateral examination (Fig. 47.5). The aortic arch diameter (28) is the sum of the distances measured between the midline and the right-most ascending aortic contour and left-most aortic shadow, measured above the base of the heart. The diameter of the aortic arch may vary in healthy individuals between 1.8 and 3.8 cm but must not exceed 4.0 cm. However, the ascending aorta, for which there are no "normal" values, is most frequently enlarged in disease.

The proximal descending thoracic aorta may be identified as a straight line seen through the cardiac silhouette running parallel to the spine in continuity with the inferior, medial aspect of the aortic arch. Usually this line is to the left of the spine, but the proximal portion may be right-sided in cases of right aortic arch. Unless situs inversus is present, the aorta in cases of left and right aortic arch enters the abdomen through the left-sided aortic hiatus.

Discrete, rim-like calcification of the aorta and aortic arch is usually a sign of degenerative intimal change, most often resulting from atherosclerosis (eFig. 47.5.1). The distance between visualized calcification and the outer aortic contour is an estimation of aortic wall thickness; its measurement may be helpful in evaluating acute and chronic changes. If care is taken to consider the effects of supine versus upright examination, and the effects of tangential visualization of the heart and aorta in oblique or anteroposterior versus PA examination, then the distance between intimal calcification and the outer wall of the aorta should be no greater than 10 mm (29). This sign is valuable in the descending aorta but may be of limited value in analysis of the more proximal aortic arch as a result of technical problems described previously.

When there is a right aortic arch, the convex shadow of the aortic arch lies on the right side of the superior mediastinum, displacing the tracheal air column to the left (Fig. 47.6). Right aortic arches may be classified (30–32) by whether the arch is anterior or posterior to the esophagus. This distinction is important, because the heart is characteristically normal when a posterior arch is present. The

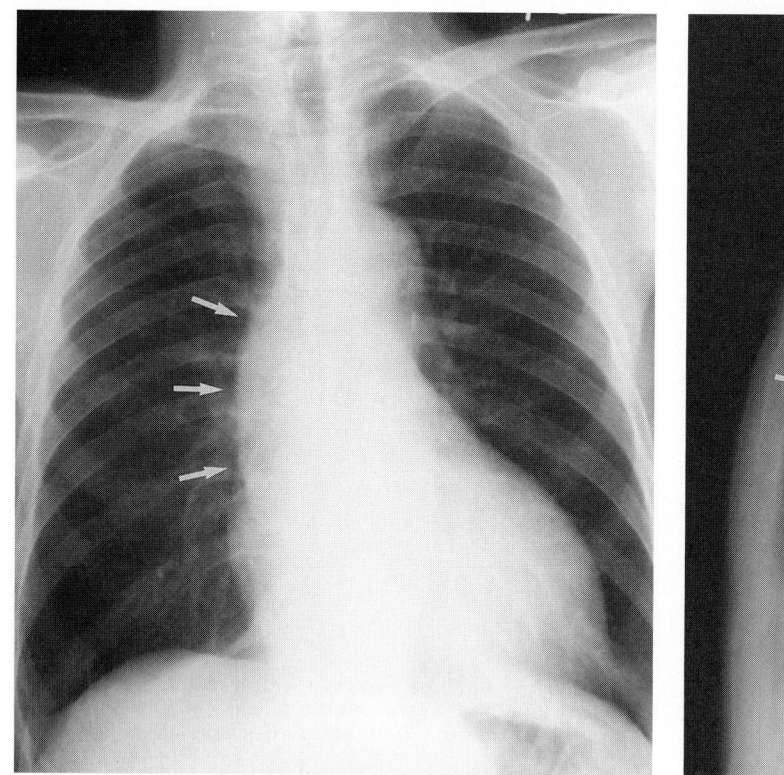
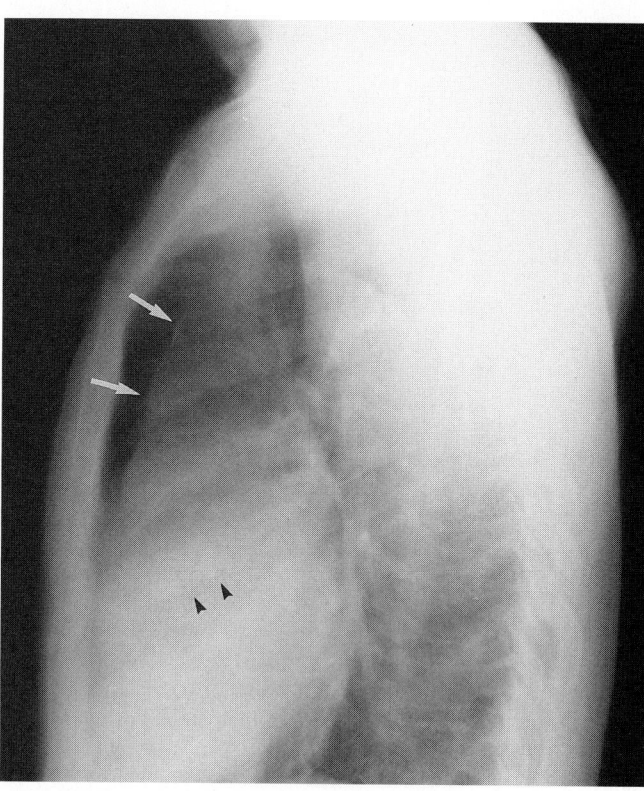

FIGURE 47.5 A 60-year-old man with degenerative calcific aortic stenosis. **A:** Postero-anterior examination shows increased rounding of the left ventricular portion of the left heart border and dilatation of the ascending aorta (*arrows*). **B:** Lateral examination shows aortic valvular calcification (*arrowheads*) in the center of the cardiac silhouette and filling of the retrosternal air space by the dilated, calcified (*arrows*) ascending aorta. The left ventricle is not dilated.

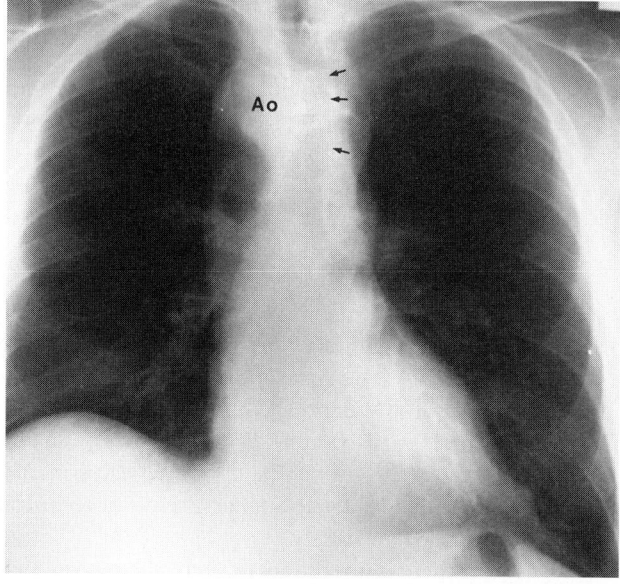
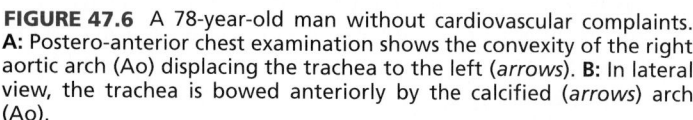
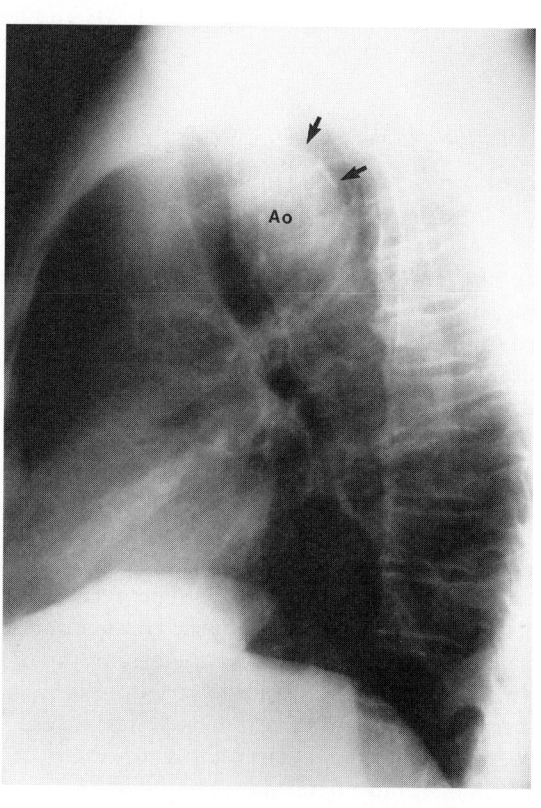

FIGURE 47.6 A 78-year-old man without cardiovascular complaints. **A:** Postero-anterior chest examination shows the convexity of the right aortic arch (Ao) displacing the trachea to the left (*arrows*). **B:** In lateral view, the trachea is bowed anteriorly by the calcified (*arrows*) arch (Ao).

presence of an anterior arch is almost universally associated with congenital heart disease. This distinction is made by evaluation of the lateral chest radiograph. In the posterior right aortic arch, found in approximately 0.1% of the population (33,34), there is a large retroesophageal defect produced by the junction of the posterior right aortic arch with the descending aorta, causing anterior bowing of the tracheal air shadow. This form of right aortic arch is usually asymptomatic and frequently associated with an aberrant left subclavian artery.

The anterior aortic arch is frequently associated with mirror-image branching. That is, the first branch from the aortic arch is a left-sided innominate trunk, followed by the right common carotid and right subclavian arteries. In this case, there is no retroesophageal component, and thus, no anterior bowing of the tracheal air column (*e*Fig. 47.6.1). There is a significant association between this form of right aortic arch and congenital heart disease. Between 18% (35) and 34% (33) of patients with tetralogy of Fallot (TOF), 33% (36) and 60% (33) of patients with truncus arteriosus, and 4.9% (24) and 6.7% (33,37) of patients with D-transposition of the great arteries have this form of right aortic arch. Unoperated survival of individuals with these lesions into adulthood is uncommon. However, differentiation among these lesions can be made based on the appearance of the superior mediastinum, the pulmonary artery segment, and the pulmonary vasculature. In patients with TOF one finds a small pulmonary artery segment and decreased pulmonary vascularity; in D-transposition and persistent truncus arteriosus, the pulmonary artery segment is not found on the left heart border, and there is increased pulmonary vascularity.

Increase in the caliber of the aortic arch segment may be caused by changes in the aortic wall, often associated with more generalized changes in the aorta or by localized increase in vessel caliber. The former class of diseases includes atherosclerosis and systemic hypertension. They often result in a "prominent" appearing aortic arch, but one not necessarily dilated to pathologic size. Focal atherosclerotic aneurysms of the distal aortic arch or proximal descending aorta may present in association with other localized areas of increase in aortic caliber. Diseases resulting in focal dilatation of the aortic arch include aortic dissection and posttraumatic aortic pseudoaneurysm formation (*e*Fig. 47.6.2).

Atherosclerosis is the most common cause of descending aortic aneurysm (38–40). These aneurysms are typically located just distal to the origin of the left subclavian artery and appear as fusiform enlargement of the aortic contour (*e*Fig. 47.6.3). Focal aneurysmal enlargement of the aorta may be difficult to differentiate from diffuse aortic ectasia or from focal mediastinal or pulmonary masses. Most often, however, these aneurysms project into the left chest. Displacement of the distal trachea is most often caused by increased caliber of the proximal portion of the aortic arch as well as by masses within the superior mediastinum, medially located with respect to the aortic arch (*e*Fig. 47.6.4).

A high index of suspicion is the most important factor in diagnosing aortic dissection (29). In the appropriate clinical setting, an abnormal chest radiograph lends support to this diagnosis. However, the aortic arch, and in fact the entire chest film examination itself, may appear normal in the presence of an aortic dissection (41). When the aortic arch is involved, one frequently finds widening of the distal portion of the arch, beyond the origin of the left subclavian artery; the aortic arch is abnormal in 80% to 90% of patients with dissection involving the arch (42). Intimal aortic calcification separated by more than 6 (29,43) to 10 (44–46) mm from the outer contour of the arch shadow is an excellent indicator of intramural hemorrhage and dissection. One must keep in mind, however, that calcification in a more proximal portion of the aortic arch may be projected medial to the outer contour of the distal arch, and that calcification of mural thrombus or inflammatory thickening of the aortic wall may produce a false-positive diagnosis. Any subtle or questionable finding becomes significant when a change in appearance from a previous examination is demonstrated (Fig. 47.7).

Diminution of the aortic arch segment may be real, as seen in patients with coarctation of the aorta, or apparent, as in the case of individuals with increased pulmonary blood flow in left-to-right shunts. In the former circumstance, there is tubular hypoplasia of the distal aortic arch proximal to the actual area of focal coarctation. The resulting narrow aorta presents as a small, inapparent aortic arch segment (*e*Fig. 47.7.1). The focal coarctation presents as a concave (to the right) notch in the proximal descending aorta, immediately below the aortic arch. The descending aortic shadow can usually be followed from below in a cephalad direction just to the left of the spine, continuous with the aortic arch shadow. In patients with coarctation, the shadow of the descending aorta is interrupted caudad to its continuity with the aortic arch. Rib notching (*e*Figs. 47.7.1 and 47.7.2) is a reliable sign of retrograde collateral flow to the postcoarctation aorta by dilated intercostal arteries.

The hearts of patients with corrected transposition of the great arteries have discordant atrioventricular and ventriculoarterial relations. The systemic venous return is as expected, to the right-sided morphologic right atrium. Blood drains across a right-sided mitral valve to the right-sided morphologic left ventricle, which supports a right-sided main pulmonary artery. Pulmonary venous blood returns to the left-sided left atrium, across a left-sided tricuspid valve, and into the left-sided morphologic right ventricle, which supports a left-sided aortic valve and ascending aorta. The left-sided ascending aorta in these patients produces an aortic arch segment that is typically longer and more convex than that found in the normal segment (47–49). Furthermore, although the hilar pulmonary

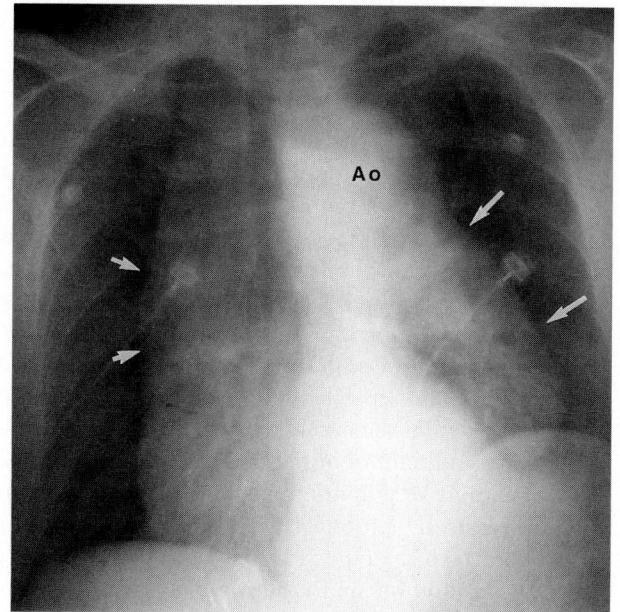
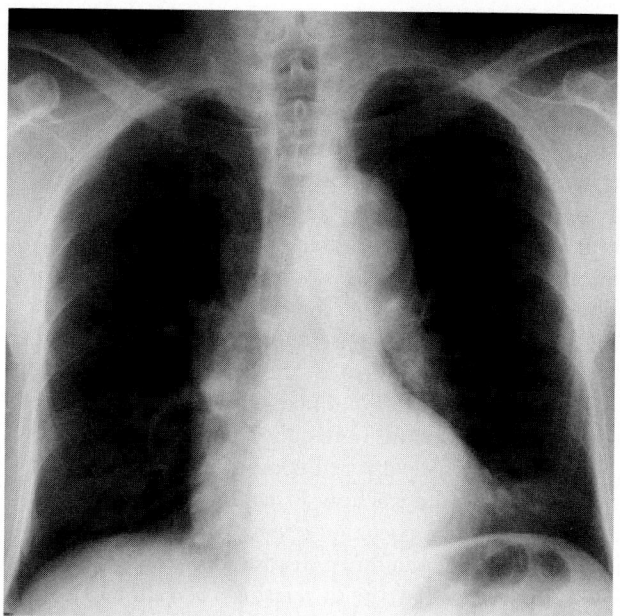

FIGURE 47.7 A 71-year-old hypertensive man awakened from sleep with midscapular back pain. **A:** Postero-anterior chest examination shows marked widening of the mediastinum, particularly involving the ascending aorta (*short arrows*), the aortic arch (Ao), and descending aorta (*long arrows*). **B:** Postero-anterior examination from 18 months earlier.

arteries may appear normal, the main pulmonary artery segment of the left heart border is not seen (*e*Fig. 47.7.3). Mesocardia and dextrocardia are relatively common in corrected transposition of the great arteries. Mirror-image patterns of this anomaly occur in situs inversus (in which the convex upper right cardiac contour is produced by the ascending aorta).

Increase in the prominence of the ascending aortic segment on frontal examination may be a sign of increase in aortic caliber or tortuosity of the aorta itself. Poststenotic dilatation of the aorta may be found in aortic stenosis (50) (*e*Fig. 47.7.4). More generalized dilatation of the ascending aorta may be found in aortic insufficiency or in dissection of the aorta. In systemic hypertension, or in long-standing atherosclerosis, the aorta may become mildly dilated and "meander" through the mediastinum, causing increase in the curvature of the ascending aorta on frontal examination. Whether the aorta is dilated or tortuous, these changes may not always be readily apparent on the frontal examination. If the predominant direction of the aortic curve is anteriorly into the anterior mediastinum, then the retrosternal space on the lateral examination will become filled and reveal this abnormality (*e*Fig. 47.7.5).

Superior Vena Cava

The superior vena cava is formed by the junction of the left and right brachiocephalic veins dorsal to the right first sternochondral articulation, behind the right border of the sternum. As it descends in the anterior mediastinum, it makes a slight curve convex to the right and dorsalward before emp-

tying into the right atrium at the level of the third costal cartilage ventrally and the seventh thoracic vertebra dorsally. The superior vena cava forms the upper half of the right heart border on the frontal radiograph. The caval shadow is fairly straight and lies parallel to and to the right of the tracheal air column. It extends from the inferior edge of the clavicle to its insertion into the right atrium. At its inferior extension, its insertion into the right atrium, there is a break in the contour of the right heart border, representing the superior aspect of the curve of the right atrium.

The superior vena cava may be displaced to the right by a dilated or tortuous ascending aorta, giving the observer the impression of a widened superior mediastinum. Masses in the superior mediastinum cause extrinsic compression of the cava, resulting in the superior vena cava syndrome. In this circumstance, the cava may actually be displaced medially (to the left) by the mass. More distal caval obstruction (secondary to lymphadenopathy or mediastinal fibrosis) may result in dilatation of the cava and innominate veins, resulting in widening of the mediastinum with prominent curvature of the superior right heart border. Similarly, the functional obstruction and resulting elevation of caval pressure caused by pericardial constriction may present with a dilated superior vena cava. Because there is no obstructing valve in the superior vena cava, elevation of right atrial pressure—such as that found in severe tricuspid regurgitation or right ventricular failure of any etiology—is transmitted back, resulting in dilatation of the azygos vein, and if severe enough, the cava itself.

Dilatation of the azygos vein is found in patients with interruption of the inferior vena cava with azygos continuation. PA chest examination reveals a prominent rounded contour adjacent to the right hilum, at the junction of the distal trachea and origin of the right mainstem bronchus (*e*Fig. 47.7.6). In individuals with isolated lesions, the chest film is otherwise unremarkable. This condition (27,51,52) is frequently associated with polysplenia and left isomerism (bilateral left-sidedness), but may be found as an isolated lesion in adults. Failure of development of the intrahepatic portion of the inferior vena cava results in passage of lower extremity and abdominal venous return to the heart via the dilated azygos vein. Persistence of the superior vena cava (*e*Fig. 47.7.7) results from failure of the obliteration of the left anterior cardinal vein. It most frequently drains to the coronary sinus and right atrium, resulting in no hemodynamic insult. In approximately 15% of cases, the right superior vena cava may be absent.

Increased blood flow through the superior vena cava results in its dilatation and increase in the curvature of the superior right cardiomediastinal silhouette. This may be found in children with intracerebral arteriovenous malformations, or in individuals with total anomalous pulmonary venous connection above the heart. In the latter entity, both the left and right superior mediastinal contours are convex; the left contour is dilated by the draining vertical vein and the right by the dilated superior vena cava (*e*Fig. 47.7.8). These individuals have a characteristic "snowman" configuration of the heart and mediastinum and increased caliber of their pulmonary artery segment and parenchymal pulmonary arteries, evidence of left-to-right shunt.

In individuals with right-sided heart dilatation, the heart rotates (looking from below) in a clockwise manner, bringing the bulk of the cardiac mass into the left chest and causing the superior vena cava to come to lie over the spine, resulting in a narrow-appearing superior mediastinum. This is common in patients with atrial septal defect (ASD) or in patients with pulmonary hypertension and secondary tricuspid regurgitation.

Main and Central Pulmonary Arteries

The main pulmonary artery and pulmonary valve are supported by the right ventricular infundibulum and thus lie cephalad and to the left of the aortic valve. The pulmonary artery segment of the left heart border is composed of the main pulmonary and proximal portion of the left pulmonary artery (Fig. 47.1). The right pulmonary artery originates from the main pulmonary artery, passing over the roof of the left atrium to enter the right lung. The right hilum is slightly caudad with respect to the left hilum. The main pulmonary artery then passes over the left mainstem bronchus to become the left pulmonary artery. Because, in PA projection, a portion of the main pulmonary artery segment is derived from the proximal left pulmonary artery, accurate measurement of the caliber of the main pulmonary artery in this view is inaccurate. The main pulmonary

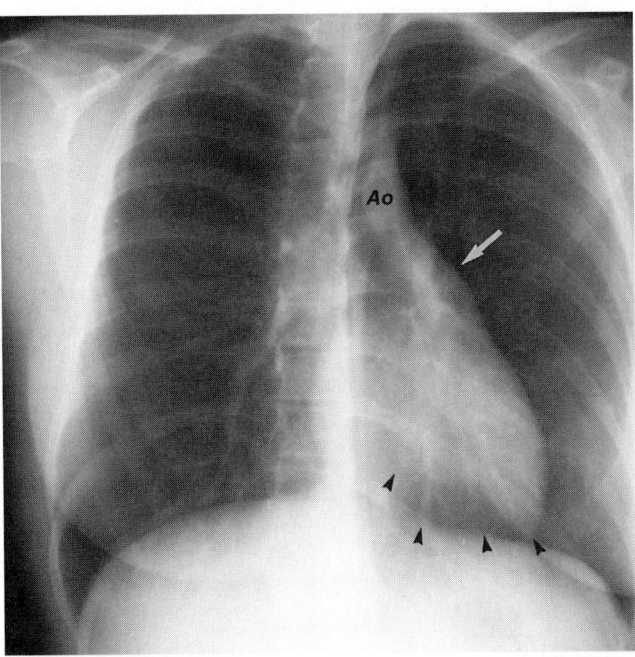

FIGURE 47.8 Normal right anterior oblique chest film of the same woman in Figure 47.1. The pulmonary artery (*arrow*) lies beneath the aortic arch (Ao). Left pulmonary artery branches (*arrowheads*) are seen projected through the heart.

artery is best viewed in shallow right anterior oblique projection (Fig. 47.8), which has the effect of rotating the proximal left pulmonary artery posteriorly, away from the cardiac contour. The pulmonary artery appears as a smooth convexity above the upper portion of the right ventricular contour, paralleling the distal trachea and left main bronchus. In individuals with normal pulmonary artery pressure and no left-to-right or right-to-left shunt [i.e., left ventricular output equals right ventricular output (Qp:Qs = 1.0)], the size of the pulmonary artery segment should be nearly the same side as the aortic arch segment on the PA radiograph. As the main pulmonary artery ascends and curves to become the left pulmonary artery, it runs away from the sternum to leave a retrosternal clear space behind (Fig. 47.9).

Often, both lateral and medial borders of the left pulmonary artery may be visualized through the heart, descending in the left chest. The right pulmonary artery shadow on lateral examination is identified as a round density anterior to the tracheal air column at the level of the carina. The left pulmonary artery is visualized in cross-section just as it passes over the left bronchus, behind and slightly superior to the right pulmonary artery.

On PA view, the right descending pulmonary artery is found running from the right hilum parallel to the right heart border. Its widest point is distal to the origin of the right middle lobe artery. At this level, the contour of the artery is sharply outlined against the air-filled lung on its right and by the air-filled right mainstem bronchus along

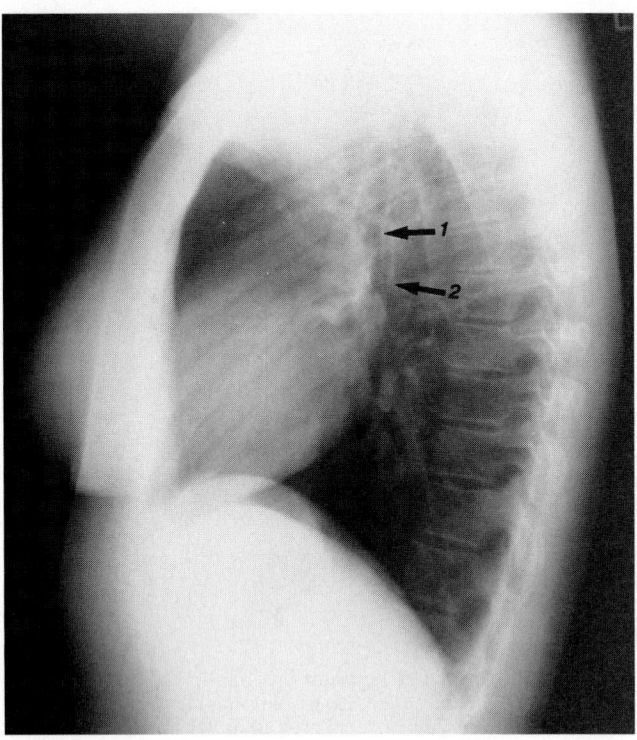

FIGURE 47.9 Normal lateral chest film of the same woman shown in Figure 47.1 and Figure 47.8. The retrosternal space is air filled. The right pulmonary artery lies anterior to the trachea. The right upper lobe bronchus (*arrow 1*) and left upper lobe bronchus (*arrow 2*) are labeled.

its left border. In patients with pulmonary hypertension, the caliber of the artery is greater than 16 mm in men and 15 mm in women (53).

Pulmonary Vasculature

The majority of right and left hilar opacities is formed by the right and left pulmonary arteries, respectively. In the infant and adolescent, the left hilum may be obscured by the superimposed thymus and pulmonary trunk. Beyond each hilum, the intrapulmonary arteries extend in a tree-like branching pattern, gradually tapering with each division. It is abnormal for a pulmonary vessel to change caliber abruptly. The branching pulmonary arteries and veins should be identified nearly two-thirds the distance from the hilum to the pleural surface. Beyond this region, the spatial resolution of the chest film technique is inadequate to resolve individual vessels.

The distribution of the pulmonary vessels is uniform in both the left and right lungs, as well as between upper and lower lung zones. In general, the pulmonary arteries appear to converge at the hila, and the pulmonary veins course toward the left atrium to enter the cardiac silhouette at a level lower than the arteries. In healthy individuals, there is a normal, gravity-dependent perfusion gradient from pulmonary apex to base. Furthermore, alveolar air pressure in the upper lung segments narrows and collapses upper lobe capillaries and pulmonary veins, increasing upper lobe pulmonary resistance. In the upright position, therefore, lower lobe perfusion is four times that of the upper lobes. Thus, the intrapulmonary vessels of the lower lobes carry greater pulmonary blood flow and appear larger radiographically. When in the supine position, the normal apex-to-base gravitational gradient is lost; in its place, a similar gravitational anterior-to-posterior lung segment gradient develops. Therefore, when supine, the radiographic appearance of the pulmonary vessels is altered; one observes an increase in the caliber of the upper lobe pulmonary arteries (which lie relatively posterior) with respect to the lower lobe vessels (which are now relatively anterior).

The intrapulmonary arteries are sharply outlined by the air-filled lung and appear to branch in a relatively regular pattern as they extend toward the chest wall. The interstitial connective tissues of the lung invest the pulmonary arteries and veins, lymphatics, bronchi and bronchioles, and nerves. Connective tissue supports the alveolar spaces and forms the interlobar septa that delineate the pulmonary lobules. The pulmonary interstitium does not produce identifiable shadows on plain chest film examination but may be identified by an overall, faint homogeneous density to the space between parenchymal pulmonary arteries and veins. The normal pulmonary interstitium should not appear "busy" or filled with radiographic density not conforming to any vascular structure.

Increased Pulmonary Blood Flow

Because left ventricular output should equal right ventricular output, the main pulmonary artery and aortic arch segments of the left heart border should be approximately the same size. Patients experiencing hypermetabolic states, including fever, pregnancy (54,55), and hyperthyroidism (56,57) or those experiencing hyperkinetic, nonhypermetabolic conditions such as anemia (58,59), arteriovenous fistula (60,61), and beriberi (62,63) all exhibit increased preload with a reduction in afterload, resulting in cardiac chamber dilatation with increased caliber of the pulmonary vascular markings (*e*Fig. 47.9.1). If the increase in ventricular filling pressure is great enough, symptoms of congestive failure occur even though myocardial contractility is normal. Maintenance of increased cardiac output in the face of congestive heart failure is referred to as *high output cardiac failure.*

In circumstances of increased pulmonary artery blood flow, pressure, or both, the main pulmonary artery segment appears increased in size with respect to the aortic arch. In patients with left-to-right shunts, the difference in size is a function of the difference in blood flow carried by the two vessels. Therefore, small left-to-right shunts may not be identified by plain film examination. In patients with increased pulmonary artery pressure, the greater pulmonary

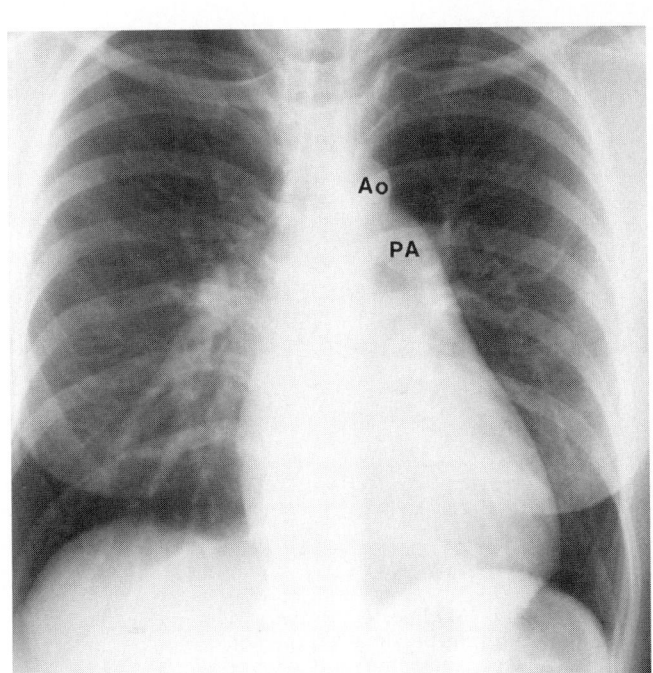

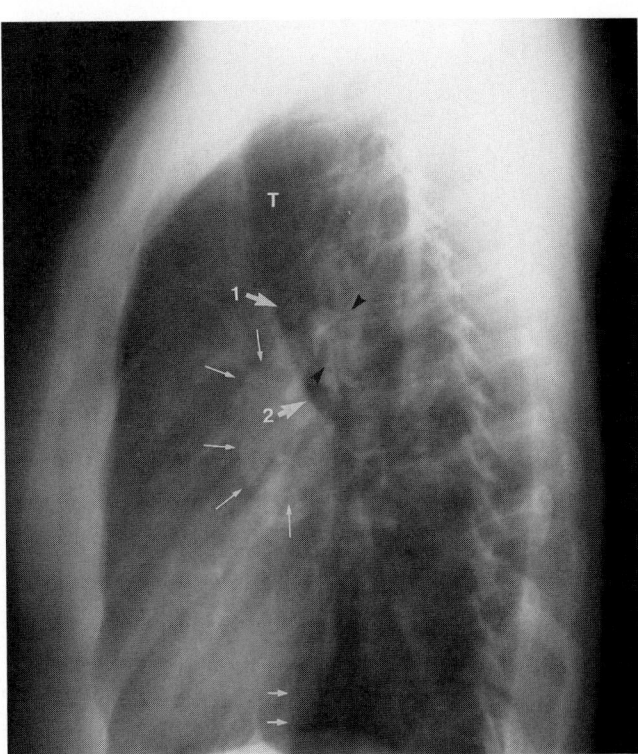

A

B

FIGURE 47.10 A 46-year-old woman with secundum atrial septal defect. Mean pulmonary artery pressure is 20 mm Hg. **A:** The heart lies in the left chest. The pulmonary artery segment (PA) is greater in caliber than the aortic arch (Ao). The pulmonary artery branches of both lungs are all dilated, sharp edged, and extend nearly to the pleura. The narrow superior mediastinum and decreased concavity in the middle of the left heart contour are caused by cardiac rotation secondary to right heart dilatation. Furthermore, as the heart rotates, the left bronchus no longer crosses the left heart border. **B:** In lateral view, the retrosternal space is filled by the dilated right ventricle and proximal pulmonary artery. The orifices of the right upper lobe bronchus (*arrow 1*) and left upper lobe bronchus (*arrow 2*) are in line with the tracheal air column (T), a sign of normal left atrial volume. The right (*long arrows*) and left (*arrowheads*) pulmonary arteries are dilated. Analysis of the relation between the inferior vena cava (*short arrows*) and the posterior left ventricular border reveals no left ventricular enlargement.

artery caliber may be the result of increased distension. Differentiation between increased pressure and increased flow may be difficult, but in general, the two may be identified by further analysis of the pulmonary vascular tree (53).

Shunt vascularity may be characterized by increase in the size of the entire roentgenographically visualized pulmonary tree (Fig. 47.10). That is, not only are the central main and proximal hilar left and right pulmonary arteries dilated, but the branch parenchymal vessels are increased in size. Furthermore, the pulmonary artery branches appear sharp and are visualized far beyond the usual two-thirds of the way between hilum and chest wall. The vessels in both the upper and lower lobes appear to be dilated to the same degree as well. Depending on the adequacy of roentgenologic technique, and the depth of the individual's inspiratory effort, dilated, sharp, branching vessels may be seen far into the posterior pulmonary sulci and out to the lateral chest wall pleura on PA and lateral views. The increased arterial flow in shunt lesions is matched by an increase in the size of the draining pulmonary veins.

The differential diagnosis of increase in the caliber of the main pulmonary artery segment depends on associated cardiac and pulmonary vascular changes. Adolescents and young adults (especially women) under 30 years of age commonly have an isolated *prominence* or increase in caliber of the main pulmonary artery segment (*e*Fig. 47.10.1) without any abnormality of the central or parenchymal pulmonary arteries, and without any cardiac chamber abnormality. These individuals, in fact, have no cardiac or pulmonary abnormality and thus represent a normal anatomic variant.

Idiopathic dilatation of the pulmonary artery (64,65) (*e*Fig. 47.10.2) is a benign condition that does not affect cardiac function. It is characterized by prominence of the pulmonary artery segment and proximal pulmonary arteries with normal or slightly increased heart size. In this lesion, pulmonary insufficiency is frequently associated, resulting in a typical murmur and dilatation of the right ventricle.

If enlargement of the pulmonary artery segment is associated with shunt vascularity, then a left-to-right shunt

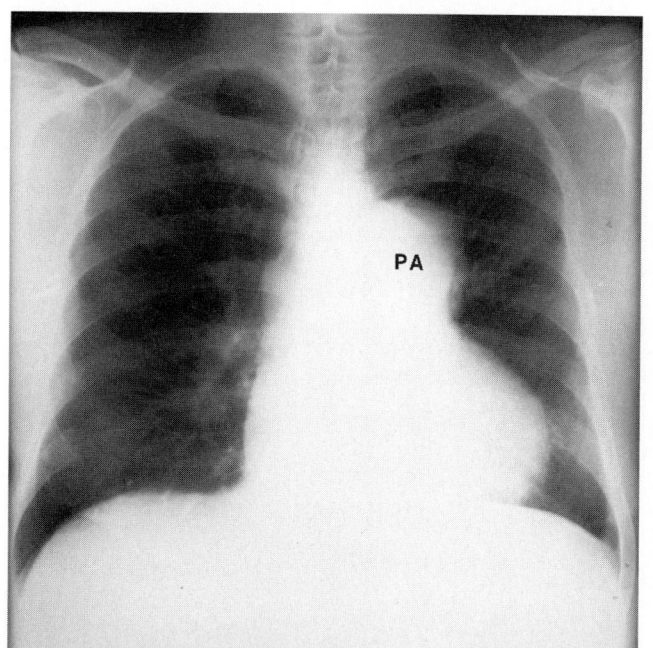
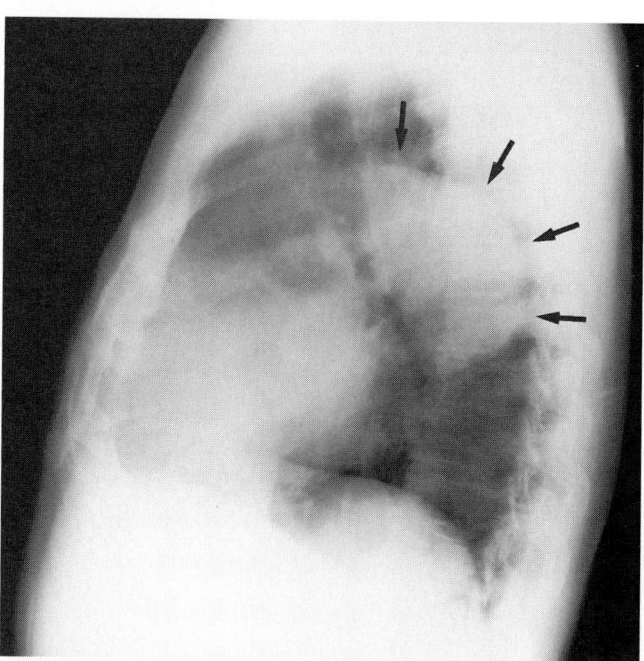

FIGURE 47.11 A 61-year-old man with valvular pulmonic stenosis. **A:** In postero-anterior view, the dilated pulmonary artery segment (PA) is apparent and obscures the proximal left pulmonary artery. The contour of the right atrium is normal. **B:** In lateral view, the aneurysmal dilation of the main and left pulmonary artery (*arrows*) is better viewed.

should be considered. Disparity between the caliber of the central pulmonary arteries and the peripheral branches indicates pulmonary hypertension. Dilatation of the pulmonary artery in the face of normal pulmonary vascular markings should raise the possibility of valvular pulmonic stenosis. Valvar pulmonic stenosis is usually congenital in origin and frequently bicuspid in nature (66). It is a common congenital cardiac malformation in adult patients. In these patients, there is dilatation of the pulmonary artery segment and classically that of the proximal left pulmonary artery as well (*e*Fig. 47.10.3). The caliber of the pulmonary artery segment does not correlate with the gradient across the valve. If right ventricular hypertension results in tricuspid regurgitation, then right atrial and ventricular dilatation occurs, and the heart rotates into the left chest. Otherwise, the heart usually appears normal in size. Longstanding turbulence in the main and left pulmonary artery may result in aneurysmal pulmonary arterial dilatation (Fig. 47.11). Identifying normal appearing parenchymal pulmonary arterial branches (the consequence of the normal pulmonary blood flow) helps differentiate the appearance of valvular pulmonic stenosis from pulmonary hypertension.

Shunt Lesions in Adults

Adult survival with secundum ASD is the rule. Secundum ASD is the most common congenital cardiac lesion diagnosed in adult patients. In a review of 412 patients with

ASD, 45% were more than 20 years old at the time of diagnosis (67). Sixty-five percent of these patients were female; 35% were male. The radiographic appearance of uncomplicated secundum ASD is characterized by normal or near normal overall cardiac size, changes in the heart contours secondary to cardiac rotation, and pulmonary arterial changes caused by the increased pulmonary blood flow. In these patients, right atrial and ventricular dilatation rotates the heart and shifts it into the left chest. The superior mediastinum is relatively narrow, and the lucency of the left bronchus runs parallel to the convex curve of the mid-left heart border. The pulmonary artery segment and both central left and right pulmonary arteries are dilated. Furthermore, the parenchymal branch pulmonary arteries are sharply defined, dilated, and visualized further toward the pleura than in normal individuals. Both the left ventricle and left atrium are typically normal in size.

Changes in myocardial compliance and pulmonary vascular resistance play an important role in the radiographic appearance of adults with ASD. The decreased compliance of older ventricular myocardium, especially if further reduced by superimposed myocardial ischemia, results in decreased myocardial compliance, resulting in elevation of left atrial pressure, further increasing the left-to-right shunt across the atrial septum. This causes progressive elevation of pulmonary arteriolar tone, resulting in increased pulmonary vascular resistance and the radiographic appearance of pulmonary hypertension. In a review of 311 patients with ASD who underwent cardiac catheterization (67), 31% had pulmonary hypertension (mean PA pressure greater than 20 mm Hg). Pulmonary hypertension was found to increase in incidence with increasing age; from 14% of patients under 20 years of age to 53% of patients greater than 30 years of age had pulmonary hypertension.

The chest radiograph of patients with ASD and pulmonary hypertension displays relative paucity of peripheral pulmonary artery branches and abrupt change in caliber of the central pulmonary arteries, typical of the generalized changes of pulmonary hypertension. However, careful inspection reveals that although sparse, upper lobe as well as lower lobe vessels are enlarged, and that branching vessels often may be identified farther out toward the pleura than in other patients with non–shunt-related causes of pulmonary hypertension. The size of these vessels reflects the sequelae of the increased blood flow of the shunt. Their number is an indication of the reduced cross-sectional area of the pulmonary bed (*e*Fig. 47.11.1).

Progressive, severe mitral regurgitation is found in 15% of patients with ASD (68–70). In these patients, left atrial (and left ventricular) dilatation (71) confuses the picture, making it difficult to radiographically differentiate ASD from other shunts. An unusual cause of left atrial enlargement in adult patients with ASD is Lutembacher's syndrome (ASD with coexisting rheumatic mitral stenosis). The picture may be complicated further in cases in which left atrial pressure is elevated, resulting in radiographic changes of pulmonary venous hypertension and left atrial enlargement superimposed on shunt vascularity (*e*Fig. 47.11.2).

Most patients with patent ductus arteriosus (PDA) present early in childhood. Those who survive their first year of life are generally asymptomatic. Among 804 patients with PDA seen in one series (72), 37 (4.6%) reached 50 years of age. Of these, 35 had exclusively left-to-right shunts, and 28 of the 35 (80%) were women. The mean age at diagnosis in this group was 49 years (range, 19 to 73 years). PDA may rarely be diagnosed in patients more than 50 years old (73,74). If the shunt is small, the heart may appear normal. The right ventricle dilates if there is pulmonary hypertension or heart failure. The central pulmonary arteries are dilated, and occasionally, one may see aneurysmal dilatation of one pulmonary artery or another (75). In adult patients with shunt vascularity, the radiographs of individuals with PDA often exhibit dilatation of the ascending aorta (*e*Fig. 47.11.3), an indication of the extracardiac shunt. Calcification of the ductus arteriosus itself is of limited value; it does not necessarily indicate whether the duct is patent or occluded (75). Calcification of the ligamentum arteriosus, however, implies closure of the duct.

If pulmonary hypertension persists, the chest film reflects changes in the appearance of the heart. Signs of right ventricular hypertrophy and pulmonary hypertension (dilatation of the central pulmonary arteries with diminished caliber of the peripheral vessels) dominate the film. Reversal of the shunt results in a decrease in cardiomegaly.

Spontaneous closure or surgical repair in childhood both decrease the prevalence of ventricular septal defect (VSD) in the adult population. VSD is found in 0.5% of adults (76,77) and 10.0% of adult patients with congenital heart disease (78). Adult patients with VSD may be classified (79) based on the size of their defects. Patients with small defects (with mean pulmonary arterial pressure less than 20 mm Hg) are usually treated medically and appear not to develop progressive pulmonary vascular changes. Patients with larger defects (mean PA pressure greater than or equal to 20 mm Hg) are more likely to undergo surgical repair, as well as develop Eisenmenger's syndrome (79). Patients with Eisenmenger's syndrome have four times the risk of death compared with patients with normal pulmonary artery pressure (80).

There is marked variation in the chest film appearance of individuals with VSD, depending on the size of the defect and the pulmonary resistance. An adult with a small VSD may have a nearly normal examination, with only a suggestion of dilatation of the pulmonary artery segment (*e*Fig. 47.11.4). Individuals with larger defects have the typical appearance of shunt vascularity, with dilatation of the left atrium and both right and left ventricles. In the face of cardiac rotation secondary to right ventricular enlargement, left ventricular dilatation may be difficult to assess. The right atrial contour should appear normal as it is not dilated. The aorta should appear normal or slightly decreased in size (*e*Fig. 47.11.5). If pulmonary resistance exceeds systemic resistance and the shunt reverses, then the heart may appear normal or small or demonstrate rotation resulting from right atrial and ventricular dilatation. The typical appearance of pulmonary hypertension—dilated central pulmonary arteries and constricted peripheral vessels—is expected.

Pulmonary Hypertension

In patients with pulmonary arterial hypertension, the more distal pulmonary artery branches are vasoconstricted. Therefore, not only are the visualized parenchymal pulmonary artery branches smaller in caliber than normal, but fewer (of the more peripheral pulmonary artery branches) are visualized. There is an apparent disparity between the appearance of the dilated central and hilar pulmonary arteries and the more peripheral vessels (Fig. 47.12). Not only is the appearance of gradual taper in caliber between the central and peripheral vessels lost, but the space between peripheral vessels appears to be increased. Thus, the "ratio" of central pulmonary artery to peripheral branch pulmonary artery caliber is greatly increased, and the lungs appear "blacker."

The chest films of patients with pulmonary hypertension secondary to left-to-right shunts present an interesting

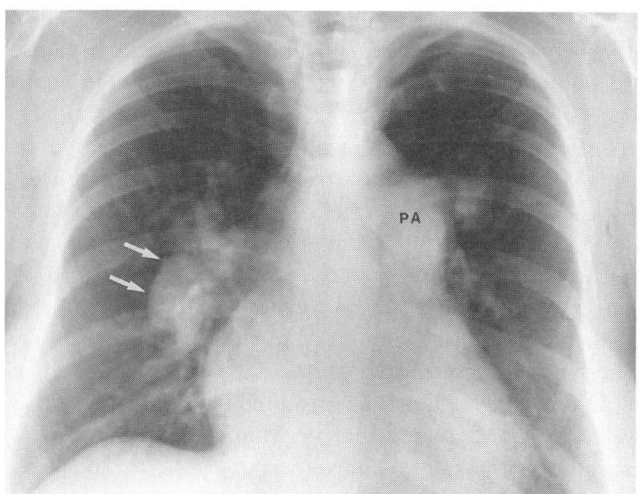

FIGURE 47.12 A 45-year-old woman with unexplained pulmonary hypertension. The pulmonary artery segment (PA) and descending right pulmonary artery (*arrows*) are markedly enlarged. Note the abrupt change in caliber of the peripheral pulmonary arterial branches beyond the right hilum. Right atrial and ventricular dilatation are indicated by the pronounced contour of the lower right heart border and rotation of the heart into the left chest.

hybrid picture. Their predominant vascular appearance is that of central pulmonary arterial enlargement with constricted peripheral vessels (i.e., that of pulmonary hypertension). However, close inspection of the vasoconstricted peripheral parenchymal pulmonary artery branches reveals that sharply defined branches are identified going far out into the periphery of the lung (i.e., findings of both shunt and hypertensive constricted vessels are evident).

Decreased Pulmonary Blood Flow

Diagnosing decreased pulmonary blood flow may be difficult. When right ventricular cardiac output is decreased, the size of the main pulmonary artery and the pulmonary arterial segment of the left heart border appear decreased in caliber. The caliber of the central and hilar pulmonary arterial branches, as well as the parenchymal pulmonary arterial segments, is decreased. The parenchymal pulmonary arterial segments appear normal, but the overall appearance of the lung is that of greater spacing among the arterial segments, and increased "blackness" of the pulmonary parenchyma. Regions of the lung distal to a focal branch pulmonary artery stenosis may appear focally darker, resulting from the focal perfusion defect. Without good data describing the normal caliber of pulmonary arterial branches, objective plain film changes may be hard to detect and differentiation between normal caliber and mild to moderately decreased blood may not be reliable.

The limited differential diagnosis of adult patients with decreased pulmonary blood flow includes TOF, pulmonary atresia with VSD (PAVSD), Ebstein's anomaly, and tricuspid atresia.

Most patients with TOF die before the end of their second decade. Only 11% are alive at 20 years, 6% at 30 years, and 3% at 40 years (81,82). Survival to adulthood in patients without prior surgical palliation or repair appears to be associated with early development of collateral circulation to the lungs and progressive narrowing of an initially mild infundibular stenosis with age (83). Decreased pulmonary blood flow results in a small main pulmonary artery segment with commensurate decrease to normal caliber of all visualized pulmonary arterial branches (*e*Fig. 47.12.1). Systemic-to-pulmonary arterial collaterals appear as unusually shaped radiographic densities among the normally distributed arterial branches. Not uncommonly, collateralization is asymmetric, so that the pulmonary arterial branches in one lung are greater in caliber than in the other. Generalized cardiomegaly is frequently found in adult patients with TOF. Cardiomegaly was found in 25% (83) of adult patients without previous surgical intervention. Among patients followed after surgical repair, postoperative cardiomegaly was reported in 85% (84) and 42% (85). Aneurysm of the right ventricular outflow after patch repair is uncommon, but may be associated with residual distal obstruction (86) or pulmonary insufficiency leading to right ventricular enlargement (*e*Fig. 47.12.2). Right aortic arch was the most frequently reported anomaly (83,84). PAVSD may be regarded as a severe variant of TOF. However, in PAVSD, pulmonary blood flow is maintained via systemic-to-pulmonary artery collaterals. Thus, radiographically, these patients may differ from those with TOF (Fig. 47.13). In the former, the main pulmonary artery segment of the left heart border is smaller and often concave, as opposed to only diminished in caliber in patients with TOF. Furthermore, collateralization to the lungs in patients with TOF is usually only from the bronchial arteries, and that in PAVSD is via larger systemic-to-pulmonary artery collaterals (87–89). Hence, asymmetry in pulmonary blood flow as well as the radiographic appearance of larger collateral vessels is usually found in patients with PAVSD. The incidence of right aortic arch is approximately 40% in these patients (90), greater than the expected 33% in patients with TOF.

In patients with Ebstein's malformation, the tricuspid valve is displaced into the right ventricle, resulting in "atrialization" of a portion of the right ventricle (91–93). Tricuspid regurgitation dilates the "true" right atrium as well as the "atrialized" right ventricle, causing right-sided enlargement and cardiac rotation (*e*Fig. 47.13.1). The right atrium may become markedly enlarged, filling the retrosternal space on lateral examination. The main pulmonary artery segment is normal to small, and the parenchymal pulmonary artery segments are normal to decreased in caliber (94). Left atrial size is generally normal, but, depending on the amount of right-to-left shunting across the atrial septum, there may be evidence of mild pulmonary vascular congestion.

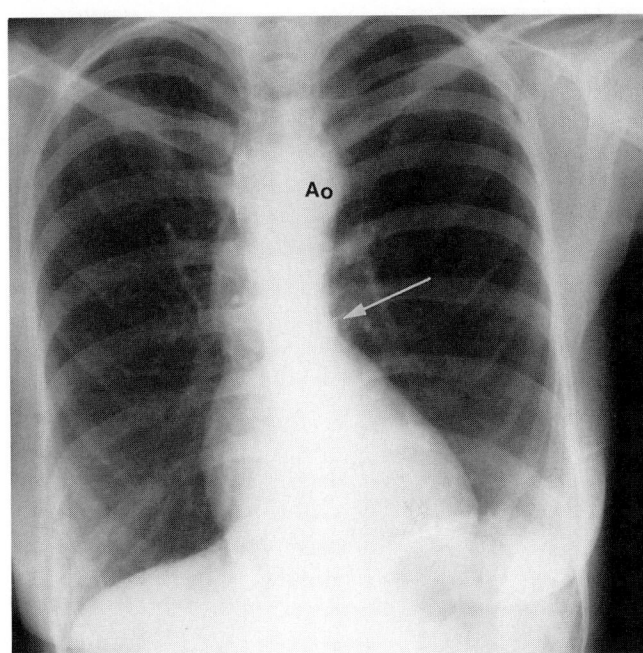

FIGURE 47.13 A 28-year-old woman with pulmonary atresia with ventricular septal defect. There is a left aortic arch (Ao). The pulmonary artery segment is concave (*arrow*), and the parenchymal pulmonary artery segments are decreased in caliber.

The chest film appearance of the heart in patients with tricuspid atresia depends on the relationship of the great arteries, the presence or absence of a VSD, and the state of the pulmonary valve (95,96). In patients with normally related great arteries with associated pulmonic stenosis, the main pulmonary artery segment appears small, and parenchymal pulmonary artery branches are decreased in caliber (*e*Fig. 47.13.2). In the presence of transposition of the great arteries or in patients with normally related great arteries and a large VSD without pulmonic stenosis, pulmonary blood flow may appear increased. Right-to-left shunting across the interatrial septum causes left atrial dilatation with or without evidence of left atrial hypertension. Left ventricular enlargement is characteristic in these patients.

Left Atrium and Left Atrial Appendage

The left atrial appendage is a long, finger-like extension of the left atrium. It wraps around the left side of the base of the heart to form the left heart border between the main pulmonary artery segment and the superior portion of the left ventricular contour. When left atrial pressure and volume are normal, this segment of the left heart border is concave.

The body of the left atrium lies in the midline, superior and posterior to the left ventricle, and beneath the tracheal bifurcation. In lateral view, the superior posterior border of the heart is formed by the left atrium. Early or mild

enlargement of the left atrium may be detected as enlargement of the left atrial appendage (i.e., straightening of this segment of the left heart border). Subsequent enlargement of the atrium results in convexity of the left atrial appendage portion of the left heart border and development of a double density in the midportion of the cardiac silhouette (representing the dilated, blood-filled left atrium). The double density is characterized by identification of its right lateral border medial to the right atrial portion of the right cardiac border. Displacement of the left bronchus can be recognized by analysis of the lateral examination. The right upper lobe bronchus originates just after the tracheal bifurcation. The left main bronchus travels for several centimeters before the origin of the left upper lobe bronchus. The plane of the tracheal bifurcation is nearly parallel to the coronal, so that when viewed in lateral, the ostia of the right and left upper lobe bronchi have a directly superior-inferior relationship. Thus, if one can draw a straight line passing through the distal tracheal air column and the centers of the right and left upper lobe bronchi, then the left atrium is not enlarged.

Left Atrial Enlargement

Analogous to the left ventricle, the left atrium is a muscular cardiac chamber, albeit thinner. Therefore, smaller increases in volume and pressure manifest as changes in the shape of the left atrium and, therefore, its radiographic appearance. Increased left atrial pressure or volume increases the size of the left atrium. Radiographically, this is manifested by change in the contour of the left atrium, extrinsic compression of adjacent structures, and change in the radiographic appearance of the chamber. Furthermore, depending on the severity and chronicity of the disease processes resulting in the elevation of left atrial pressure and volume, characteristic pulmonary vascular findings may exist.

Straightening of the left atrial appendage segment between the level of the main pulmonary artery and left ventricular segments on the left border of the heart is the earliest and most sensitive radiographic sign of elevated left atrial pressure or volume (Fig. 47.14). Continued left atrial enlargement results in convexity of this segment beyond the lower, left ventricular contour, and then identification of a double density to the right of the spine on the PA examination (*e*Fig. 47.14.1). This represents displacement of the right inferior border of the left atrium caused by enlargement of the left atrial body. This is associated with a discrete convex bulge to the superior posterior cardiac contour below the carina on the lateral examination. The distance between the midpoint of the double density and the midpoint of the left mainstem bronchus (the left atrial dimension) is less than 7.5 cm in the adult man and less than 7.0 cm in the adult woman. Enlargement is a good sign of previous rheumatic disease. Enlargement of the left atrium results in posterior dis-

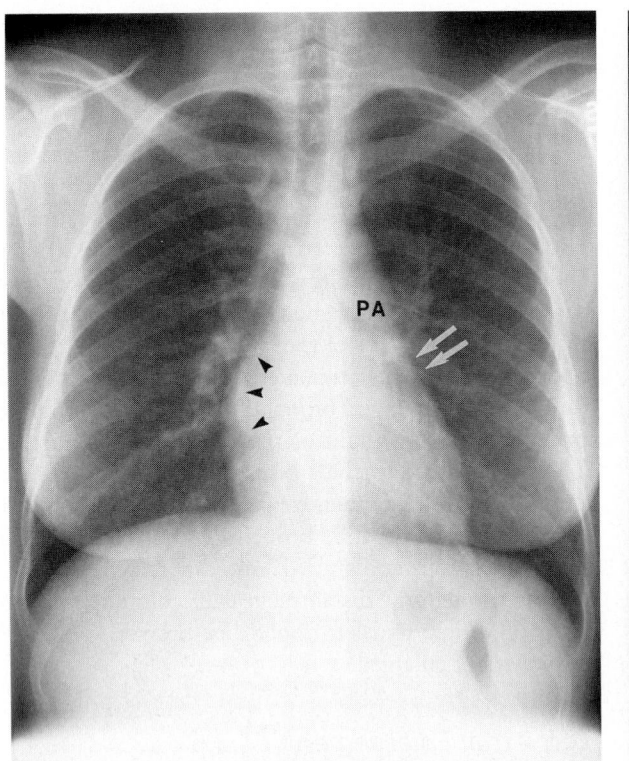
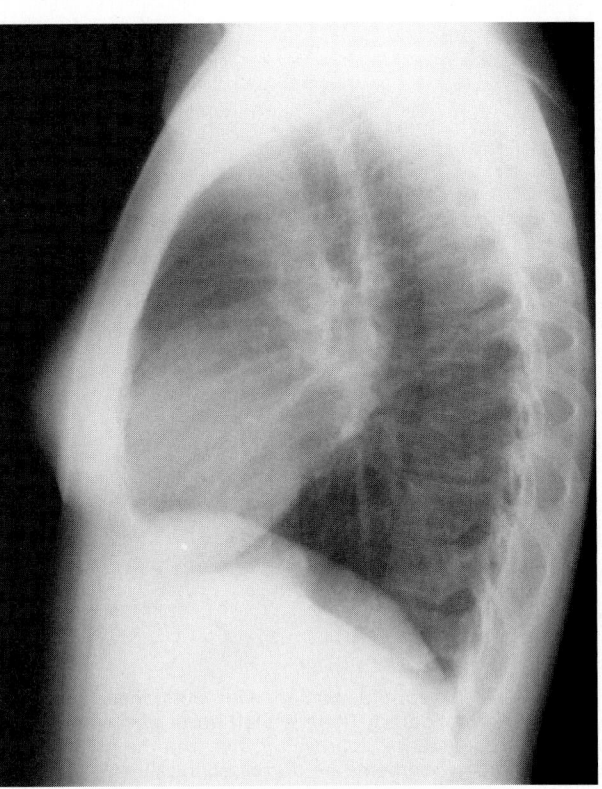

FIGURE 47.14 A 37-year-old woman with rheumatic mitral stenosis. **A:** Postero-anterior examination demonstrates straightening of the left atrial appendage portion of the left heart border (*arrows*). The right border of the left atrium (*arrowheads*) appears to approach the right cardiac contour. There is indistinctness of the pulmonary vessels, including the descending right pulmonary artery. The caliber of the upper lobe vessels is greater than that in the lower lung zones. The pulmonary artery segment (PA) is larger than the aortic arch segment. The left ventricle is normal. **B:** There is fullness in the superior posterior cardiac space, but no displacement of the left bronchus.

placement of the left bronchial tree (97), and in chronic cases of left atrial enlargement, elevation of the left main bronchus (98). On the frontal radiograph, the normally observed carinal angle of approximately 75 degrees may be increased to 90 degrees or more. However, care must be taken in considering this observation. Without a previous PA chest examination for comparison, it is difficult to judge small differences from normal. In the lateral view, a sensitive marker of left atrial enlargement is posterior displacement of the left bronchus. Normally, a straight line constructed by connecting the centers of the right and left upper lobe bronchi, when extended superiorly, should pass within the main tracheal air column. In cases of left atrial enlargement, this line extends outside of the trachea. Care must be taken to make this observation only in true lateral radiographs. When the left atrium is enlarged, it produces a superior, posterior mass behind the heart and under the tracheal carina. Often the mass extends inferiorly, producing a second contour along the posterior aspect of the heart. Although no longer in common practice, barium esophagography is a sensitive technique for demonstrating the extrinsic compression of the esophagus by the dilated left atrium. Severe left atrial enlargement results in merging of the left atrial contour

with the right atrial contour on the right border of the heart on PA examination.

Differential Diagnosis of Left Atrial Enlargement

Left atrial enlargement is most frequently caused by left atrial obstruction in chronic rheumatic mitral stenosis. Early roentgenologic changes in these patients may be limited to left atrial enlargement. With time and progressive increase in the mitral valvular gradient, signs of pulmonary venous hypertension and eventually pulmonary hypertension are seen. Untreated, mitral stenosis may cause chronic parenchymal pulmonary hemorrhage, resulting in hemosiderosis, nodular calcific (predominately lower lung zone) densities. The pulmonary hypertension associated with mitral stenosis may eventually result in right ventricular failure. Left atrial and left atrial appendage calcification is frequently associated with chronic mitral stenosis. Calcium deposits are most often found within the endocardial or subendocardial layers of the myocardium, but may also be found in organized thrombus adherent to the atrial wall (111), appearing as a curvilinear circumferential calcific shell (112,113). Left atrial enlargement may also be found in other forms of left atrial obstruction, including left atrial myxoma and congenital mitral stenosis.

Increased left atrial volume results in left atrial enlargement. Chronic mitral valvular regurgitation often results in massive left atrial enlargement. Increased pulmonary blood flow, as seen in VSD and PDA, results in left atrial dilatation. It is important to remember that increased pulmonary blood flow does not necessarily result in left atrial enlargement. The left atrium is of normal size in patients with ASD. In these individuals, the increased pulmonary blood flow reaching the left atrium divides between flow across both the mitral valve and atrial defect, resulting in increased blood flow through the left atrium, but normal atrial volume.

The etiology of left atrial enlargement can be distinguished by analysis of associated findings in the chest examination. Left atrial enlargement associated with left atrial outflow obstruction is associated with a normal-appearing left ventricle and findings associated with chronic pulmonary venous hypertension (i.e., interstitial edema, redistribution, and evidence of pulmonary hypertension). Atrial tumors often calcify. Left atrial enlargement resulting from mitral regurgitation is associated with left ventricular enlargement and a conspicuous absence of significant pulmonary venous changes. Most notably absent is any sign of pulmonary hypertension, nearly always found in patients with chronic mitral stenosis. Shunt lesions resulting in left atrial enlargement present most notably with shunt vascularity and enlargement of the central and peripheral pulmonary arterial segments.

Left Ventricular Free Wall and Left Ventricle

In a normal heart (situs solitus, D-loop, normally related great arteries), the left ventricle lies posterior to and slightly to the left of the right ventricle. The plane of the tricuspid valve (and thus, the right ventricular inflow) lies to the right of the plane of the mitral valve (the left ventricular inflow). The shape of the left ventricle is best approximated by a prolate ellipsoid (114,115) or football. The ventricular long axis is rotated approximately 25 to 30 degrees clockwise from the coronal plane, and 10 to 20 degrees caudal to the axial. The apex of the normal left ventricle points down, anteriorly, and to the left. Thus, in PA, the inferior portion of the left heart border is formed by the anterolateral wall of the left ventricle, the portion of the left ventricular myocardium lateral to the interventricular sulcus. In lateral view (Fig. 47.9), the lower one-half of the posterior border of the heart is formed by the free wall of the left ventricle. When the right ventricle is not enlarged, the shadows of the inferior vena cava and the posterior border of the heart intersect approximately 2 cm above the level of the diaphragm (Figs. 47.9 and 47.14B) (116).

Left Ventricular Enlargement and the Left Ventricular Configuration

In adults, the appearance of the left heart border may change in the absence of left ventricular dilatation. In this circumstance, the heart assumes in the PA view a so-called

left ventricular configuration (117); i.e., there is an increase in the curvature of the left ventricular contour and aortic arch segment of the left heart border, between which are sandwiched normal (and thus relatively concave appearing) left atrial appendage and pulmonary artery segments (eFig. 47.14.5). Although this configuration may be found in individuals with healthy hearts, its recognition may be helpful in identifying patients with subtle and significant heart disease.

The left ventricular configuration is associated with increased left ventricular wall stress, including volume-loaded, pressure-loaded, ischemic, and cardiomyopathic left ventricular myocardium. In the absence of a lateral chest examination, identification of the left ventricular contour is useful as a case finder or entry point into a differential diagnosis. Left ventricular obstruction, whether caused by asymmetric subaortic septal hypertrophy, congenital or acquired aortic stenosis, coarctation of the aorta, or essential hypertension (Fig. 47.15), may present with this configuration. Associated other observations will help to differentiate among these lesions. For example, the ventricular appearance associated with a small aortic arch segment, with or without the presence of rib notching, may be diagnostic of coarctation of the aorta. If the aortic arch segment appears prominent or enlarged, one might consider the diagnosis of systemic hypertension. When the ascending aorta is volume loaded, its lateral contour is directed toward the right. When this is associated with a left ventricular configuration, then aortic regurgitation (eFig. 47.15.1) is a likely diagnosis. Calcification of the aortic valve (118) is almost always found on plain chest film examination in patients with clinically significant degenerative calcific aortic stenosis. In patients with congenitally bicuspid aortic valve, calcification is almost universally present but may not be apparent on plain chest films. Patients with rheumatic aortic stenosis may not have the calcification found in cases of nonrheumatic disease.

In some patients with ischemic heart disease, the only morphologic abnormality identifiable on PA chest examination may be the left ventricular configuration. However, in most of these individuals, elevated left ventricular filling pressure manifests radiographically as elevation of pulmonary venous pressure. Depending on the severity and chronicity of the ischemia, one may find only subtle signs of indistinctness of lower lobe vessels or mild redistribution. The left atrium may be normal in size, allowing the chest film to retain a typical convex-concave-convex appearance. Similarly, patients with other abnormalities that result in abnormal left ventricular diastolic compliance, including cardiomyopathy, may present with the left ventricular configuration, with or without evidence of pulmonary venous hypertension.

The addition of the lateral view aids in differentiation between a dilated and nondilated (and potentially hypertrophied) left ventricle and adds information about the

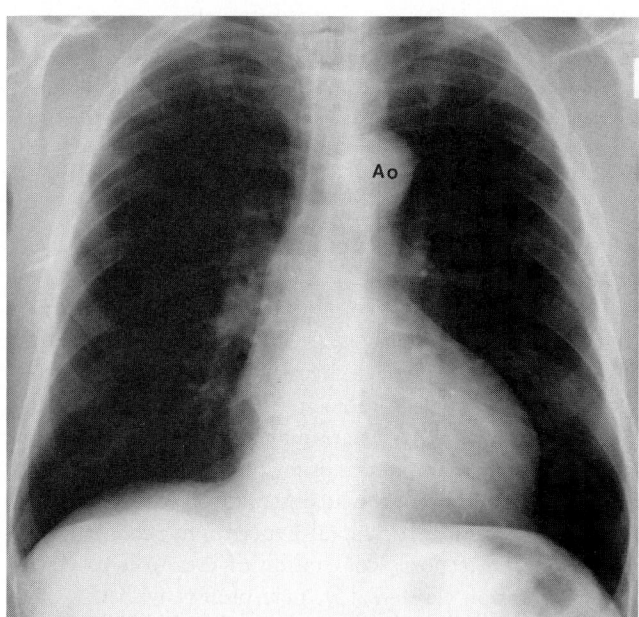

FIGURE 47.15 A 69-year-old man with essential hypertension. In postero-anterior view, the left ventricular contour is rounder and extends farther toward the left chest wall than is normal. Visualization of more than half the circumference of the aortic arch segment (Ao) increases its apparent size, accentuating the concavity of the pulmonary artery and left atrial appendage segments. The lateral view (not shown) demonstrates normal left ventricular volume.

presence or absence of intracardiac (aortic) valvular calcification. The left ventricular configuration with a normal-sized heart may be found in patients with aortic stenosis. If calcification of the aortic valve is found in the presence of a left ventricular configuration and a normal-sized heart, then the diagnosis of valvular aortic stenosis is assured. The left ventricular configuration with left ventricular dilatation, as determined from the lateral view, is often associated with aortic regurgitation. The ascending aorta usually dilates toward the right in PA view. However, if the aorta dilates in an anterior direction, then the ascending aortic segment of the right heart border on PA view may appear normal, but on lateral view, the retrosternal air space fills, confirming the presence of a dilated aorta.

Left ventricular dilatation increases the roundness of the lower left cardiac border (*e*Fig. 47.15.2). The apex of the heart may appear to be displaced in a downward direction. In films obtained during deep inspiration, the left ventricular apex may not be separated from the left diaphragm. In both oblique and lateral examination, the inferior posterior cardiac border extends posterior to the inferior vena caval shadow filling the retrocardiac space, and the heart appears to increase in size inferiorly, causing extrinsic compression of the superior aspect of the gastric air bubble. Hoffman and Rigler (116) found that the relationship between inferior vena cava and left ventricle on

lateral chest film may provide important information concerning left ventricular size. If the posterior border of the left ventricle extends more than 1.8 cm posteriorly to the border of the inferior vena cava when measured at 2 cm cephalad to the crossing of the right hemidiaphragm and inferior vena cava, then one may presume with certainty that the left ventricle is enlarged. Care must be taken, however, to perform this measurement in true lateral views; measurement in oblique chest examinations results in erroneous interpretation (119).

Global left ventricular enlargement is commonly found in patients with left ventricular ischemia, aortic or mitral regurgitation, or cardiomyopathy. This appearance may be mimicked by a pericardial effusion. In patients with ventricular ischemia, the left ventricle dilates to maintain wall stress, and left atrial pressure increases to maintain ventricular filling at increased end diastolic pressure. Depending on the duration and severity of the ventricular ischemia and the compliance of the left atrial myocardium, one might expect to find patients with myocardial ischemia in whom there is left ventricular dilatation with left atrial hypertension in the absence of left atrial dilatation. Chronic left ventricular ischemia results in dilatation of the left atrium as well as the left ventricle.

In patients with chronic aortic regurgitation, left ventricular dilatation becomes pronounced and progressive (120). In these individuals, the volume-loaded left ventricle unloads into the ascending aorta, resulting in the typical picture of left ventricular and ascending aortic dilatation (*e*Fig. 47.15.1). The dilatation of the ascending aorta may appear as an increase in the curvature of the ascending aortic segment of the mid-right heart border, or in the lateral view, present as filling of the retrosternal air space by the dilated ascending aorta (Fig. 47.5B). Generally, these individuals have normal left ventricular filling pressures and, therefore, present with a normal-sized left atrium and no evidence of left atrial hypertension.

In acute mitral regurgitation, the left ventricle and left atrium do not dilate in the face of the rapid increase in volume. Rather, these individuals present radiographically with normal-sized hearts and marked left atrial hypertension, caused by the systolic emptying of the left ventricle through the left atrium and into the pulmonary veins, with the resultant dramatic increase in pulmonary venous pressure (Fig. 47.16). However, in chronic mitral regurgitation, both the left atrium and left ventricle adapt to the increased volume load and dilate. Increased left atrial volume results in near normal left atrial and thus pulmonary venous pressure. The chest radiographs of patients with chronic mitral regurgitation demonstrate dilatation of both the left atrium and left ventricle in the absence of significant pulmonary venous hypertension (Fig. 47.17). In fact, although the left atrium in chronic mitral regurgitation is generally the largest encountered radiographically [greater in size than that found in mitral stenosis (120)], the disparity between the

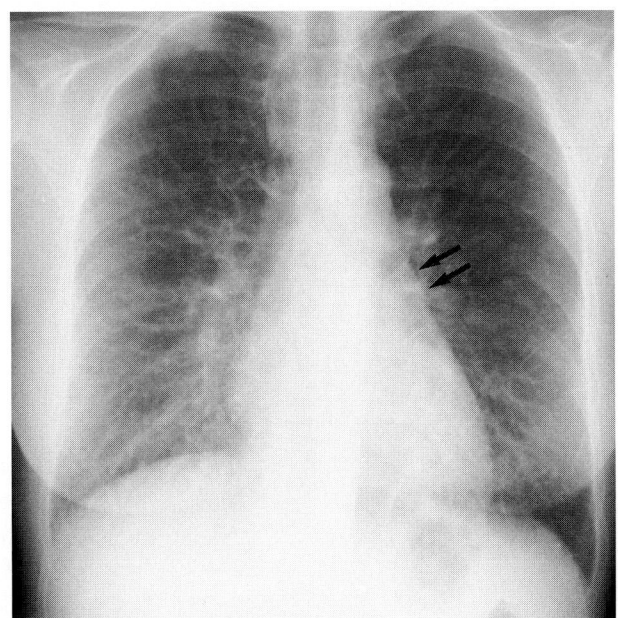 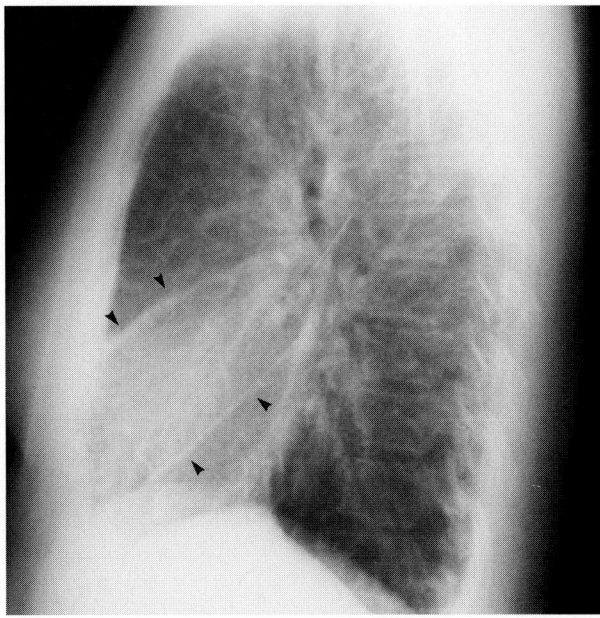

A

B

FIGURE 47.16 A 52-year-old woman experiencing an acute myocardial infarction. **A:** The heart is not enlarged. The left atrial appendage segment of the left heart contour (*arrows*) is straightened. Notice the moderate to severe bilateral interstitial edema obscuring the pulmonary vascular markings and the increase in caliber of upper lobe vessels. **B:** In lateral view, all vascular markings are indistinct, and the interlobar fissures are thickened (*arrowheads*), containing edema fluid. The left ventricle is not dilated. Although the left atrial appendage segment is straightened on the postero-anterior view, the left bronchus is not posteriorly displaced in lateral, indicating the mildness of left atrial enlargement.

size of the left atrium and the paucity of pulmonary venous change is most pronounced.

Left Ventricular Aneurysm

Focal aneurysmal dilatation of a portion of the ventricular wall is found in between 8% and 12% of patients who sustain an acute myocardial infarction (121). The overwhelming majority of left ventricular aneurysms is caused by ischemic heart disease (*e*Fig. 47.17.1). Ventricular aneurysms are localized, permanent, blood-filled dilatations of the left ventricle (122). Gradual bulging (expansion) of the involved (thinned) portion of the LV wall (123–125) results in a true aneurysm with a wide mouth. Nearly all anterolateral and apical aneurysms are true aneurysms (126) (*e*Fig. 47.17.2). False aneurysms (pseudoaneurysms) are the result of contained cardiac rupture. The wall of a false aneurysm is fibrous, containing blood clot, but without myocardium present. Nearly 50% of false aneurysms are posterior in location.

Occasionally, the inferior border of the heart appears abnormal (*e*Fig. 47.17.3). When the aneurysm is large, it can be identified in more than one projection. Whether they appear as focal or global contour abnormalities, left ventricular aneurysms frequently have curvilinear, rim-like calcifications (*e*Figs. 47.17.2, 47.17.3, and Fig. 47.18) immediately subjacent to their abnormal curvature, result-

ing from dystrophic calcification of the underlying infarcted ventricular myocardium (111). On occasion, a ventricular aneurysm may be detected on the lateral radiograph (127) as a retrosternal or superior soft tissue border (*e*Fig. 47.17.2B) produced by the wall of the aneurysm silhouetting against the midline cardiac shadow. False ventricular aneurysms may not be directly differentiated from true aneurysms on plain film examination. Location is not an absolute means of differentiating between true and false aneurysms.

A close relationship between the presence and extent of coronary arterial calcification and the presence and severity of coronary atherosclerosis (128,129,132,133) has been known for years. However, the only reasonably sensitive means of detection of coronary calcification had been cardiac fluoroscopy (130,131,134), a decidedly operator-dependent technique. Thus, investigation of coronary calcification as a detector of coronary atherosclerosis and quantitation of the degree and distribution of calcification as a function of clinical status and prognosis were severely limited. Although limited in its sensitivity, coronary calcification may be detected on plain chest film examination by evaluation of a triangular area located on the left mid-heart border, bordered medially by the vertebral column, inferiorly by a horizontal line drawn from the vertebral column to the top of the left ventricular portion of the left heart border, and diagonally by connecting the former two bor-

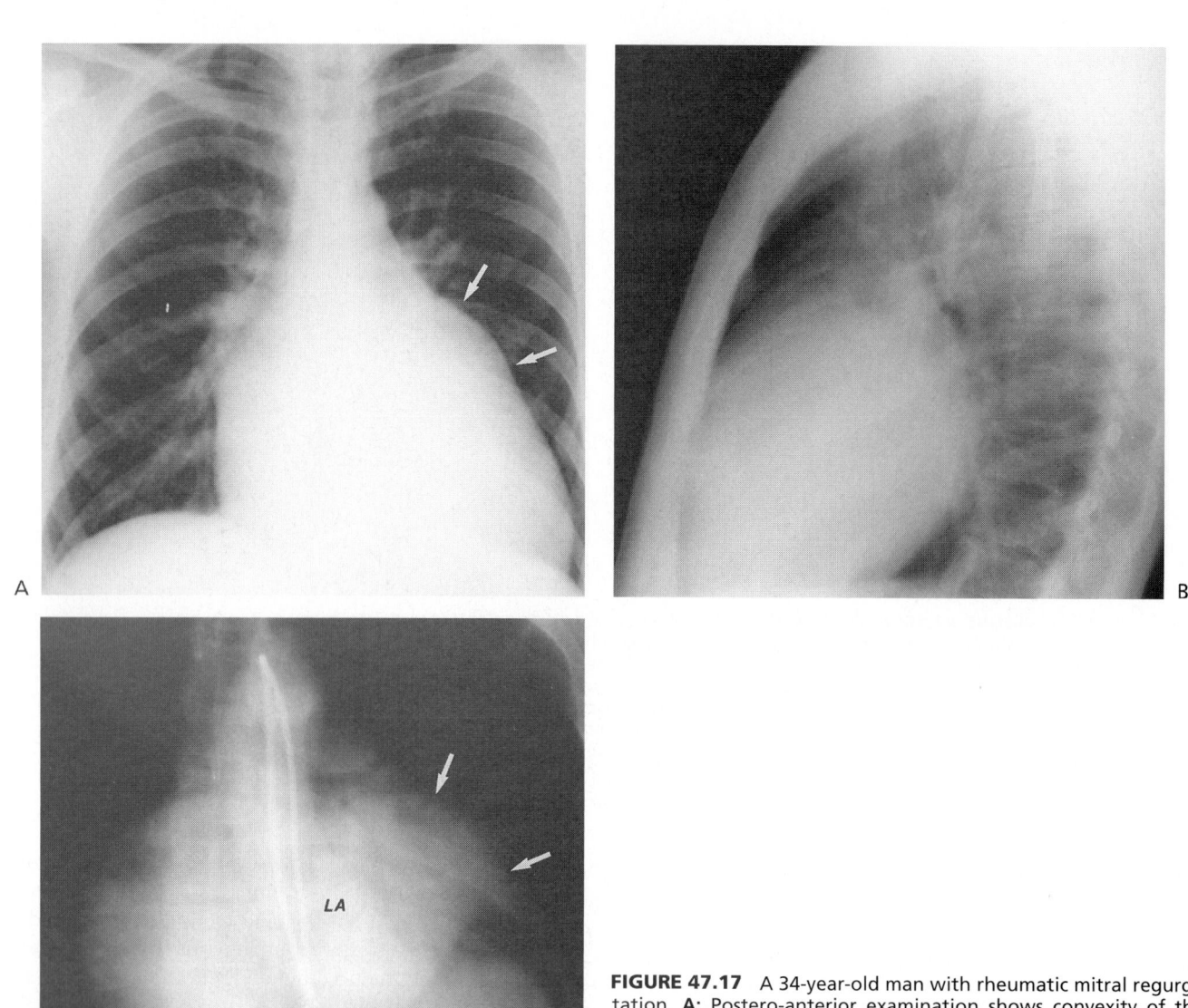

FIGURE 47.17 A 34-year-old man with rheumatic mitral regurgitation. **A:** Postero-anterior examination shows convexity of the dilated left atrial appendage segment (*arrows*) and displacement of the left ventricular contour toward the left chest wall. The pulmonary vascular markings are only mildly indistinct. **B:** Lateral view shows filling of the retrocardiac space by the dilated left atrium and ventricle. **C:** Postero-anterior image from a retrograde left ventriculogram demonstrates the dilated opacified left atrium (LA) and left atrial appendage (*arrows*).

ders (135). These authors found coronary calcification or a strong suspicion of coronary calcification within this triangle in 42% of patients with fluoroscopically detected coronary calcification (*e*Fig. 47.18.1).

Pericardial Effusion

Nonspecific change in the appearance of the lower left heart contour may be an indication of pericardial disease, most commonly pericardial effusion. Small pericardial effusions may not be detected by plain film examination. The greater the accumulation of fluid, the more apparent the change in cardiac contour, and the greater the confidence one has in making the diagnosis. The pericardium is an

Erlenmeyer flask–shaped fibrous bag consisting of the visceral pericardium, the parietal pericardium, and the normally occurring 20 to 60 mL of fluid collection between them. The normal visceral pericardium (or epicardium) covers the external surface of the heart. Beneath the visceral pericardium is either myocardium or epicardial fat. This layer extends for short distances along the pulmonary veins, the superior vena cava below the azygos vein, the inferior vena cava, the ascending aorta to a point 20 to 30 mm above the root, and the main pulmonary artery as far as its bifurcation. It then reflects on itself to become the parietal pericardium, which is a 1-mm-thick outer fibrous layer composed of dense collagen lined on the inside by a monolayer of mesothelial cells.

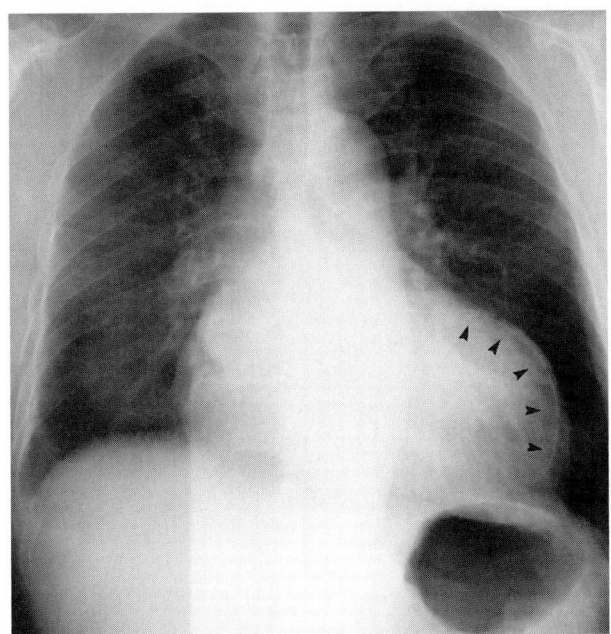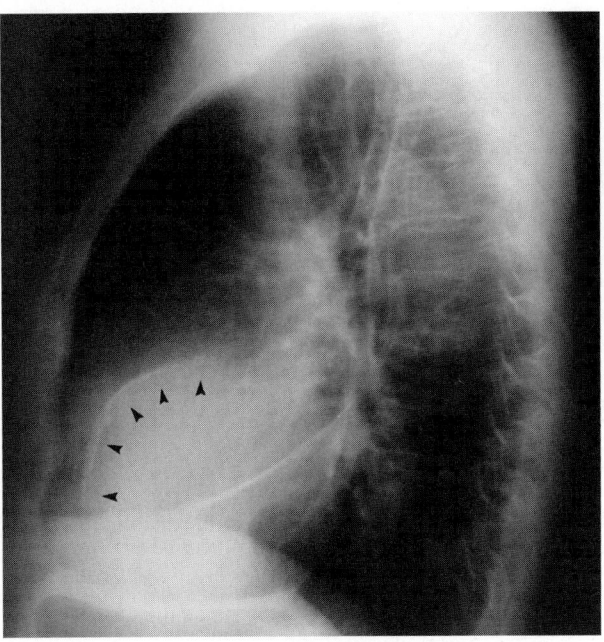

FIGURE 47.18 A 53-year-old man with chronic stable angina. **A:** Postero-anterior view of the chest shows mild pulmonary venous hypertension and enlargement of the left ventricular contour. Curvilinear calcification of the distal interventricular septum (*arrowheads*) defines the extent of a previous myocardial infarction. **B:** In lateral view, the calcification (*arrowheads*) is superimposed on the cardiac mass.

On the lateral chest radiograph, the normal pericardium may occasionally be seen as a 1- to 2-mm-thick curved stripe anterior to the heart set between more radiolucent mediastinal fat anteriorly and epicardial fat posteriorly. The visceral pericardium is normally thin and is therefore not visualized separately by any imaging modality.

An abrupt asymmetric increase in the dimension of the cardiac silhouette without specific chamber enlargement suggests the diagnosis of pericardial effusion. Frequently, the asymmetric change in configuration occurs along the right atrial contour of the right heart border (*e*Fig. 47.18.2), suggesting loculation of fluid about the right atrium. Filling of the retrosternal space, effacement of the normal cardiac borders, development of a "flask" or "water-bottle" cardiac configuration, and bilateral hilar overlay are characteristic of a larger pericardial collection (Fig. 47.19). The epicardial fat pad "sign" is positive when, visualized in the lateral projection, an anterior pericardial stripe (bordered by epicardial fat posteriorly and mediastinal fat anteriorly) is thicker than 2 mm. This sign is diagnostic of pericardial disease (136) (Fig. 47.20). Because there is abundant fat between the pericardium and the pleura at the cardiac apex, a positive epicardial fat pad may also be seen in the frontal projection. This is usually seen as an elliptical stripe internal to and paralleling the lower left heart border. This radiolucent line may migrate toward or away from the cardiac border with changes in the amount of pericardial fluid (137,138). Although diagnostically valuable in many patients, reliance on the plain film diagnosis of pericardial

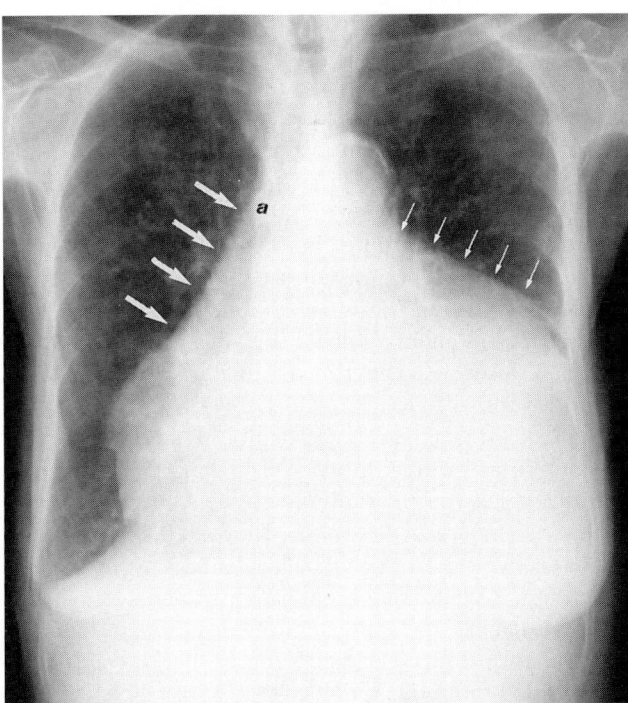

FIGURE 47.19 An 87-year-old woman with chronic renal failure. The silhouette of the heart is globular in shape. The density of the fluid collection is defined by the attachments of the pericardium to the ascending aorta (*thick arrows*) above the azygos vein (a) and to the top of the pulmonary artery (*thin arrows*). The pulmonary hila are hidden.

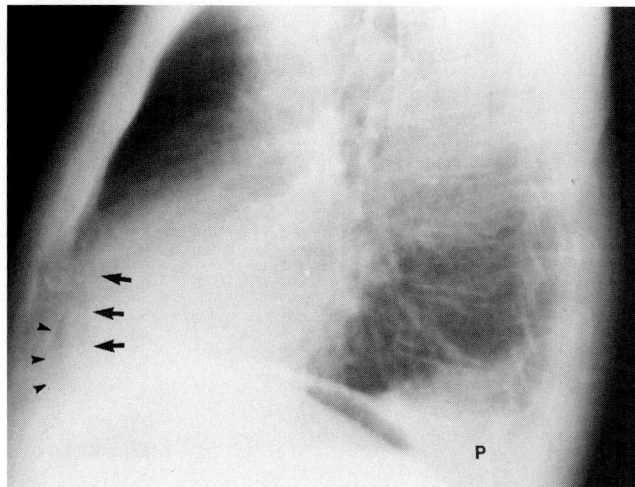

FIGURE 47.20 A 52-year-old man with pericardial and pleural effusion, lateral view. The lucency of the epicardial fat (*arrows*) is separated from the lucency of the pericardial fat (*arrowheads*) by the density of fluid in the pericardial space. A small left pleural effusion (P) silhouettes the posterior left hemidiaphragm.

effusion has been largely supplanted by echocardiography and other cross-sectional imaging techniques.

Pericardial Calcification

Constrictive pericarditis is usually the result of a chronic pericardial insult. The greatest number of cases are of unknown etiology, presumably secondary to an inapparent viral pericarditis (139). Outside the United States, the most common cause is probably tuberculosis or fungal etiology (140). Other causes of nontuberculous disease include connective tissue disorders such as rheumatoid arthritis (141) and systemic lupus erythematosus (142), hemodialysis-treated chronic renal failure (143,144), and neoplastic infiltration of the pericardium, most commonly secondary to carcinoma of the lung or breast, lymphoproliferative malignancies, and melanoma (145). Pericardial constriction may occur months to years after mediastinal irradiation, usually performed to treat Hodgkin's disease (127) or breast carcinoma. Constrictive pericarditis had been considered a rare complication of cardiac surgery (146), especially in those cases in which the pericardium was left open. However, more recent experience (147) has shown a 0.2% incidence of constrictive pericarditis following cardiac surgery (148).

Pericardial calcification is not pathognomonic for pericardial constriction. However, extensive calcification is found in nearly one-half of patients and strongly suggests pericardial constriction of infectious etiology (149,150) (*e*Fig. 47.20.1). Pericardial calcification appears as irregular, large loci, distributed on both the left and right of the midline, reflecting the distribution of the pericardial space (151). Although the heart in most patients with constrictive pericarditis is usually enlarged, it is not unusual for the heart size to be normal

(152). Coexisting pericardial effusion may increase the apparent heart size, but indirect findings associated with increased right-sided pressure (i.e., dilatation of the superior vena cava and azygos vein) help suggest the diagnosis. These radiographic findings are common to both constrictive pericarditis and restrictive cardiomyopathy.

Pericardial Cyst

Most pericardial cysts appear as sharply demarcated masses near the right cardiophrenic angle (*e*Fig. 47.20.2). They may be found in other mediastinal locations, including at the left cardiophrenic angle. The borders of the cysts are usually round, but a pointed upper border may also be seen. This is thought to be due to drooping of the cysts originating higher in the mediastinum into the cardiophrenic region (153). Pericardial diverticula can be suggested on plain films and fluoroscopy by their change in contour and size during deep inspiration (154,155).

Congenital Partial Absence of the Pericardium

As described previously, the heart is fixed within the middle mediastinum by the pericardial attachments. Any interruption of this fixation results in distortion of the normal cardiac silhouette. The characteristic plain film findings (156) are usually present in complete absence of the left pericardium and include displacement of the left ventricle and pulmonary arteries toward the left side (*e*Fig. 47.20.3). The individual cardiac segments that make up the left heart border may be more clearly defined and separated than usual. Both the medial and lateral borders of the main pulmonary artery may be visualized more clearly because of an absence of the anterior pericardial reflection between the aorta and the pulmonary artery. In partial pericardial defects, varying degrees of prominence of the pulmonary artery or left atrial appendage or both may be seen, whereas the heart retains its normal position in the thorax (156).

In an asymptomatic patient the characteristic plain film findings may be sufficient to make the diagnosis. However, because plain film findings are frequently subtle and nonspecific, the condition often goes unrecognized (157). In a series of six patients only two had the diagnosis suggested on plain chest radiography (157). None of the 15 patients diagnosed with congenital absence of the pericardium during unrelated cardiac or thoracic surgery reported in the Mayo Clinic series had the diagnosis suggested on preoperative chest radiography (158).

Right Ventricle

The right ventricle is an anterior, midline structure. The right medial border is limited by the anterior atrioventricular ring containing the tricuspid valve. To the left, the ventricle is limited by the anterior interventricular sulcus containing the left anterior descending coronary artery. Thus, in PA projection, the right ventricle does not form a cardiac border. In lateral projection, the right ventricle fills the inferior retrosternal air space; the free wall of the right ventricle lies directly subjacent to the inferior half of the sternum (Fig. 47.9).

Right ventricular hypertrophy may alter the appearance of the lower left cardiac contour and cardiac apex on PA view. The cardiac apex may be lifted from the diaphragm, and the curvature of the left ventricular contour may become more rounded. In the absence of another associated lesion (such as induced tricuspid regurgitation), right ventricular hypertrophy does not cause right ventricular dilatation. In PA projection, right ventricular dilatation causes (as viewed from below) clockwise rotation of the heart (*e*Fig. 47.20.4). This has the effect of altering the superior portion of the lower third of the left heart contour. As the heart rotates, the relative concavity of the left atrial appendage segment is rotated posteriorly and medially, and the right ventricular outflow tract and anterior interventricular sulcus are displaced laterally and come to form that portion of the left heart border. This portion of the left heart border appears fuller than in the healthy heart. This change can be differentiated from left ventricular and left atrial enlargement by recognition of the increased distance between the left main bronchus (which itself does not appear elevated on frontal examination or displaced on lateral examination) and the left heart border itself. In addition, in cases of right ventricular dilatation, other signs of heart and mediastinal rotation usually occur. The most important of these is medial displacement of the superior vena caval shadow; this results in disappearance of the vertical line of the superior vena cava over the spine. In lateral view, changes in the size of the right ventricular chamber manifest as filling of the retrosternal clear space and posterior displacement of the left ventricle, as manifested by posterior displacement of the inferior posterior heart border toward the spine.

Right ventricular dilatation may be observed in patients with left-to-right shunts or malformations of the tricuspid valve or primary abnormalities of the right ventricular myocardium (159,160) (*e*Fig. 47.20.5). More commonly, however, they result from right ventricular dysfunction caused by left-sided heart problems, pulmonary disease, and primary or secondary right ventricular myocardial disease. The most common cause of right-sided heart failure is chronic left-sided heart failure (161). The common denominator of this and other left-sided heart problems causing right ventricular dysfunction is chronic left atrial hypertension transmitted back to the pulmonary veins, capillaries, and arteries. Similar cardiac changes may be found in cor pulmonale, the syndrome of right ventricular hypertrophy, dilatation, and failure resulting from pulmonary hypertension secondary to lung disease (162). Although the condition may be acute, as seen in sudden massive pulmonary thromboembolism (163,164), it most often develops

chronically, resulting from hypoxia-induced pulmonary arteriolar vasoconstriction or fibrosis of the pulmonary vascular bed (165,166).

Right Atrium

The convexity of the lower right heart border on PA examination is formed by the lateral wall of the right atrium. Estimation of right atrial enlargement is difficult on plain films of the chest. Few linear measurements of the radiographic size of the right atrium have clinical significance. There is no good way to reliably differentiate patients with right atrial enlargement from those without (167). The chamber overlaps the right ventricle, and when the right ventricle is enlarged (which is the case in most conditions causing right atrial enlargement), determination of right atrial size can be difficult. On lateral examination, posterior displacement of the inferior vena caval shadow is a very specific finding.

Isolated enlargement of the right atrium is uncommon. Enlargement secondary to volume loading is most often the case, usually caused by tricuspid regurgitation (*e*Fig. 47.20.4 and Fig. 47.21). The most common cause of tricuspid regurgitation is pulmonary hypertension of any etiology. In these cases, the diagnosis is made by observation

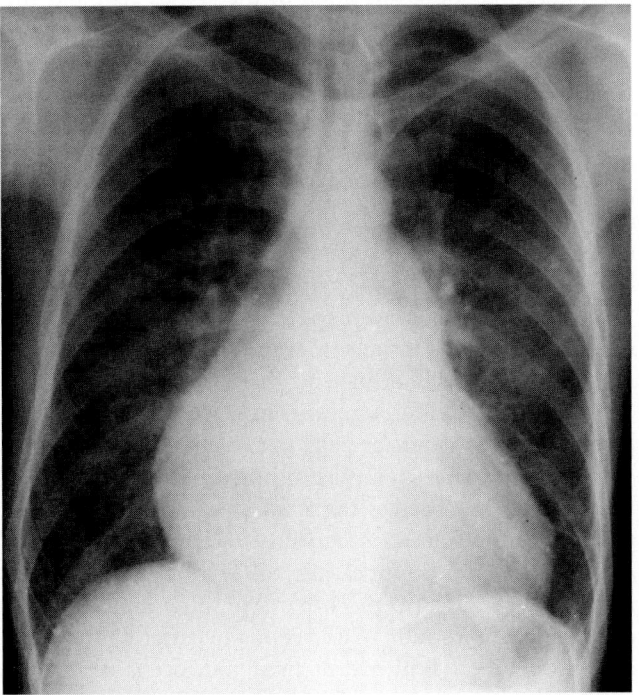

FIGURE 47.21 A 56-year-old woman with rheumatic mitral stenosis and secondary tricuspid regurgitation. The pulmonary artery segment is enlarged. The right atrial contour of the right heart border is increased in convexity. Convexity of the left atrial appendage section of the left heart border and pulmonary vascular redistribution are evident. Visualized lower lobe vessels are acutely smaller in caliber than the hilar pulmonary arteries. The left ventricle is normal.

THE FUTURE

This is the future. Over the past 25 years, a revolution in the practice of cardiac imaging has occurred. It is becoming mainstream practice for chest radiography to be acquired and archived in digital format and displayed electronically on a video monitor. In a post-future era, we can expect to see better interconnectivity among imaging devices and their networks, as well as among cardiac imagers themselves. This will increase the availability of previous examinations and allow easier comparison of current examinations with other imaging modalities. Along with a more sophisticated approach to the issues of privacy and broad public access, access to diagnostic imagery will be broadened, increasing net-work volume and maintaining pressure for network growth and evolution. Credit card–based access to all medical imagery and the means of transferring image studies, supporting the availability of rapid second opinions, will change the manner in which we manage patients with cardiovascular disease. As society becomes wired for broadband cable as well as ground-based and satellite-based Internet services, expect to see rapid growth in the use of distant reviewing stations for interpretation of centrally obtained diagnostic imagery. The film library will continue its evolution from storage facility to networking hub for distribution of electronic imagery.

of associated evidence of changes in the central and peripheral pulmonary arteries. Until right ventricular failure supervenes, right atrial dilatation in the absence of right ventricular dilatation is found. By the time the right ventricle has failed, clockwise rotation of the heart has occurred, and other findings associated with right atrial hypertension are found, including dilatation of the azygos vein and the presence of pleural or pericardial effusion or ascites.

Marked dilatation of the right atrium may be found in congenital tricuspid regurgitation or Ebstein's anomaly. More severe tricuspid regurgitation is found in individuals with more severe tricuspid valvular malformations. Depending on how much of systemic cardiac output is derived from right-to-left shunting across the interatrial septum, varying degrees of left ventricular enlargement may be found.

In patients with tricuspid atresia, there is no antegrade filling of the right ventricle from the right atrium. Furthermore, in nearly 75% of patients there is pulmonic stenosis or a restrictive VSD, resulting in decreased pulmonary blood flow and an overall normal-sized heart (*e*Fig. 47.21.1). The tricuspid valve obstruction and obligatory right-to-left shunt across the atrial septum results in right atrial dilatation (increased curvature of the right atrial border) and a normal-appearing to slightly enlarged left atrium. Depending on the size of the shunt and left atrial compliance, mild pulmonary venous hypertension may be evident. The left ventricle in these patients is dilated (it receives both systemic and pulmonary blood flow). The dilated ascending aorta increases the curvature of the right upper cardiac border directly and by lateral displacement of the superior vena cava. In approximately 25% of patients with tricuspid atresia, there is associated transposition of the great arteries, resulting in a less specific radiographic picture of increased pulmonary circulation and left atrial and ventricular enlargement without the characteristic increase in right atrial convexity.

CONTROVERSIES AND PERSONAL PERSPECTIVES

There is little that is controversial about chest film examination of the heart. The role of the chest film has shifted in the past half century from a central role in cardiac diagnosis and patient management to more of a barometer of patient physiologic status. This reflects the increase of more sensitive and accurate imaging modalities, rather than the limited accuracy of plain film examination. In an era of advancing invasive means of monitoring physiologic status, the role of the chest film for assessment of cardiac chamber pressure will wane. However, there is still no better means than the plain chest film for displaying the presence and location of the myriad devices used for the monitoring of an intensive care unit or recovery room patient.

The form of image obtained from chest examination has begun to change. The evolution in electronic imaging that began in the 1970s and 1980s has produced reliable means of acquiring high-resolution imagery, high-volume means of archiving these images, and tools for distributing the data to sites around the hospital and community. As institutions have felt the pinch for space, the cumbersome radiology film library has evolved into an electronic library for examinations obtained with filmless systems. These studies arrive at the library via network and are archived for the short- or long-term on magnetic or optical disc. The file room now serves as the distribution center for direction of collected imagery to reading terminals, where algorithms may be applied to manipulate image data, and for the purpose of enhancing the appearance of the heart and pulmonary vascularity. The era of the 14-in. × 17-in. plain film is nearly over. Although the electronic revolution in radiologic imaging and archiving always raises the issue of automated image evaluation, we still have not reached that level of sophistication. The wide variation in physiologic statuses of individuals, as well as the potential artifacts and overlying hardware in and around an acutely ill individual in an intensive care unit, has confounded attempts to automate image evaluation. For the foreseeable future, humans will probably continue to interpret and report the results of these examinations.

REFERENCES

1. Roentgen WR. Uber eine neue art von strehlen. *Sitzber Physik Med Ges Wurtzberg* 1885;December:132–141.
2. Williams FH. Notes on x rays in medicine. *Trans Assoc Am Physicians* 1896;11:375–382.
3. Walsh D. *The roentgen rays in medical work*. New York: William Wood, 1898:102–109.
4. Abrams A. Roentgen rays in pulmonary disease. *JAMA* 1902;38:1142–1147.
5. Clayton TA, Merrill WH. Orthodiagraphy in the study of the heart and great vessels. *Am J Med Sci* 1909;138:549–562.
6. Danzer CS. The cardiothoracic ratio: an index of cardiac enlargement. *Am J Med Sci* 1919;157:513–521.
7. Case JT. Pericarditis calculosa. *JAMA* 1923;80:236–240.
8. Cutler EC, Sosman MC. Calcification in the heart and pericardium. *AJR Am J Roentgenol* 1924;12:312–320.
9. Eyster JAE. The size of the heart in the normal and in organic heart disease. *Radiology* 1927;8:300–306.
10. Eyster JAE. Determination of cardiac hypertrophy by roentgen ray methods. *Arch Intern Med* 1928;41:667–682.
11. Ungerleider HE, Gubner R. Evaluation of heart size measurements. *Am Heart J* 1942;24:494–510.
12. White P. Observations on the clinical value of the roentgen ray in the diagnosis of cardiovascular disease. *AJR Am J Roentgenol* 1930;4:353–357.
13. Wilkinson GA, Fraser RG. Roentgenography of the chest. *Appl Radiol* 1975;4:41–49.
14. Lynch PA. A different approach to chest roentgenography: triad technique (high kilovoltage, grid, wedge filter). *AJR Am J Roentgenol* 1965;93:965–971.
15. Naeye RL. Kyphoscoliosis and cor pulmonale. A study of the pulmonary vascular bed. *Am J Pathol* 1961;38:561–573.
16. Reid L. Pathological changes in the lungs in scoliosis. In: Zorab PA, ed. *Symposium on scoliosis*, 2nd ed. New York: Longman, 1969.
17. Bjure J, Grimby G, Kasalicky J, et al. Respiratory impairment and airway closure in patients with untreated idiopathic scoliosis. *Thorax* 1970;25:451–456.
18. Wooler GH, Mashhour YAS, Garcia JB, et al. Pectus excavatum. *Thorax* 1969;24:557–562.
19. Backer OG, Brunner S, Larsen V. Radiologic evaluation of funnel chest. *Acta Radiol* 1961;55:249–256.
20. Dornhorst AC, Pierce JW. Pulmonary collapse and consolidation: the role of collapse in the production of lung field shadows and the significance of segments in inflammatory lung disease. *J Fac Radiol* 1954;5:276–281.
21. Chin EF, Lynn RB. Surgery of eventration of the diaphragm. *J Thorac Surg* 1956;32:6–14.
22. Paris F, Blasco E, Canto A, et al. Diaphragmatic eventration in infants. *Thorax* 1973;28:66–72.
23. Kiely B, Filler J, Stone S, et al. Syndrome of anomalous venous drainage of the right lung to the inferior vena cava. *Am J Cardiol* 1967;20:102–116.
24. Jue KL, Amplatz K, Adams P Jr, et al. Anomalies of great vessels associated with lung hypoplasia. *Am J Dis Child* 1966;111:35–44.
25. Dupuis C, Charaf LAC, Breviere G-M, et al. The "adult" form of scimitar syndrome. *Am J Cardiol* 1992;70:502–507.
26. Neill CA, Ferencs S, Sabiston DC, et al. The familial occurrence of hypoplastic right lung with systemic arterial supply and venous drainage. Scimitar syndrome. *Bull Johns Hopkins Hosp* 1960;107:1–20.
27. Van Mierop LHS, Eisen S, Schiebler GL. The radiographic appearance of the tracheobronchial tree as an indicator of visceral situs. *Am J Cardiol* 1970;26:432–435.
28. Baron MG. Radiologic notes in cardiology: dissecting aneurysm of the aorta. *Circulation* 1971;43:933–943.
29. Crawford ES. The diagnosis and management of aortic dissection. *JAMA* 1990;264:2537–2541.
30. Stewart JR, Kincaid OW, Titus JL. Right aortic arch: plain film diagnosis and significance. *AJR Am J Roentgenol* 1966;97:377–389.
31. Shuford WH, Sybers RG, Edwards FK. The three types of right aortic arch. *AJR Am J Roentgenol* 1970;109:67–74.
32. Felson B, Palayew MJ. Two types of right aortic arch. *Radiology* 1963;81:745–759.
33. Hastreiter AR, D'Cruz IA, Cantez T. Right-sided aorta. *Br Heart J* 1966;28:722–737.
34. Liechty JD, Shields TW, Anson BJ. Variations pertaining to the aortic arches and their branches. *Q Bull Northwest Univ Med Sch* 1957;31:136–143.
35. Keith JD, Rowe RD, Vlad P. *Heart disease in infancy and childhood*. New York: Macmillan, 1958.
36. Tandon R, Hauck AJ, Nadas AS. Persistent truncus arteriosus. A clinical, hemodynamic and autopsy study of nineteen cases. *Circulation* 1963;28:1050–1060.
37. Elliott LP, Neufeld HN, Anderson RC, et al. Complete transposition of the great vessels. I. Anatomic study of sixty cases. *Circulation* 1963;27:1105–1117.
38. DeBakey ME, Noon GP. Aneurysms of the thoracic aorta. *Mod Concept Cardiovasc Dis* 1975;44:53–82.
39. Joyce JW, Fairbairn JF II, Kinkaid OW, et al. Aneurysms of the thoracic aorta. *Circulation* 1964;29:176–181.
40. Dillon ML, Young WG, Sealy WC. Aneurysms of the descending thoracic aorta. *Ann Thorac Surg* 1967;3:430–438.
41. Stein HL, Steinberg I. Selective aortography, the definitive technique for diagnosis of dissecting aneurysm of the aorta. *AJR Am J Roentgenol* 1968;102:333–348.
42. Slater EE, DeSanctis RW. Clinical recognition of dissecting aortic aneurysm. *Am J Med* 1976;60:625–633.

43. Dow J, Roebuck EJ, Cole F. Dissecting aneurysms of the aorta. *Br J Radiol* 1966;39:915–927.

44. Earnest F IV, Muhm JR, Sheedy PF II. Roentgenographic findings in thoracic aortic dissection. *Mayo Clin Proc* 1979;54:43–50.

45. Eyler WR, Clark MD. Dissecting aneurysms of the aorta: roentgen manifestations including a comparison with other types of aneurysms. *Radiology* 1965;85:1047–1057.

46. Beachley MC, Ranniger K, Roth FJ. Roentgenographic evaluation of dissecting aneurysms of the aorta. *AJR Am J Roentgenol* 1974;121:617–625.

47. Ellis K, Morgan BC, Blumenthal S, et al. Congenitally corrected transposition of the great vessels. *Radiology* 1962;79:35–50.

48. Carey LS, Ruttenberg HD. Roentgenographic features of congenital corrected transposition of the great vessels. *AJR Am J Roentgenol* 1964;92:623–651.

49. Tonkin IL, Kelley MJ, Bream PR, et al. The frontal chest film as a method of suspecting transposition complexes. *Circulation* 1976;53:1016–1025.

50. Jarchow BH, Kinkaid OW. Poststenotic dilatation of the ascending aorta: its occurrence and significance as a roentgenologic sign of aortic stenosis. *Proc Mayo Clin* 1961;36:23–33.

51. Moller JH, Nakib A, Anderson RC, et al. Congenital cardiac disease associated with polysplenia. *Circulation* 1967;36:789–799.

52. Rose V, Izukawa I, Moes CAF. Syndromes of asplenia and polysplenia. A review of cardiac and non-cardiac malformations in 60 cases with special reference to diagnosis and prognosis. *Br Heart J* 1975;37:840–852.

53. Abrams HL. Radiologic aspects of increased pulmonary artery pressure and flow: preliminary observations. *Stanford Med Bull* 1956;14:97–111.

54. Atkins AFJ, Watt JM, Milan P, et al. A longitudinal study of cardiovascular dynamics throughout pregnancy. *Eur J Obstet Gynecol Reprod Biol* 1981;12:215–224.

55. Katz R, Karliner JS, Resnik R. Effects of a natural volume overload state (pregnancy) on left ventricular performance in normal human subjects. *Circulation* 1978;58:434–441.

56. Merillion JP, Passa P, Chastre J, et al. Left ventricular function and hyperthyroidism. *Br Heart J* 1982;46:137–143.

57. Grossman W, Robin NI, Johnson LW, et al. The enhanced myocardial contractility of thyrotoxicosis. *Ann Intern Med* 1971;74:869–874.

58. Duke M, Abelmann WH. The hemodynamic response to chronic anemia. *Circulation* 1969;39:503–515.

59. Graettinger JS, Parsons RL, Campbell JA. A correlation of clinical and hemodynamic studies in patients with mild and severe anemia with and without congestive heart failure. *Ann Intern Med* 1963;58:617–626.

60. Burckhardt D, Stalder GA, Ludin H, et al. Hyperdynamic circulatory state due to Osler-Weber-Rendu disease with intrahepatic arteriovenous fistulas. *Am Heart J* 1973;85:797–800.

61. Anderson CB, Codd JR, Graff RA, et al. Cardiac failure and upper extremity arteriovenous dialysis fistulas. *Arch Intern Med* 1976;136:292–297.

62. Weiss S, Wilkinson RW. The nature of the cardiovascular disturbances in nutritional deficiency states (beriberi). *Ann Intern Med* 1937;11:104–148.

63. Akram H, Maslowski AH, Smith BL, et al. The haemodynamic, histopathological and hormonal features of alcoholic beriberi. *Q J Med* 1981;50:359–375.

64. Deshmukh M, Guvenc S, Bentivoglio L, et al. Idiopathic dilatation of the pulmonary artery. *Circulation* 1960;21:710–716.

65. Gould L, Reddy CVR, Gomprecht RF. Idiopathic dilatation of the pulmonary artery with pulmonic insufficiency. *Am J Med* 1974;57:139–142.

66. Jeffery RF, Moller JH, Amplatz K. The dysplastic pulmonary valve: a new roentgenographic entity. *AJR Am J Roentgenol* 1972;114:322–339.

67. Hamilton WT, Haffajee CI, Dalen JE, et al. Atrial septal defect secundum: clinical profile with physiologic correlates in children and adults. In: Roberts WC, ed. *Congenital heart disease in adults*. Philadelphia: FA Davis, 1979:267–277.

68. Boucher CA, Liberthson RR, Buckley MJ. Secundum atrial septal defect and significant mitral regurgitation. Incidence, management, and morphologic basis. *Chest* 1979;75:697–702.

69. Davies MJ. Mitral valve in secundum atrial septal defect. *Br Heart J* 1981;46:126–128.

70. Liberthson RR, Boucher CA, Fallon JT, et al. Severe mitral regurgitation: a common occurrence in the aging patient with secundum atrial septal defect. *Clin Cardiol* 1981;4:229–232.

71. Sanders C, Bittner V, Nath PH, et al. Atrial septal defect in older adults: atypical radiographic appearances. *Radiology* 1988;167:123–127.

72. Marquis RM, Miller HC, McCormack RJM, et al. Persistence of ductus arteriosus with left to right shunt in the older patient. *Br Heart J* 1982;48:469–484.

73. Woodruff WW III, Gabliani G, Grant AO. Patent ductus arteriosus in the elderly. *South Med J* 1983;76:1436–1437.

74. Ng AS, Vliestra RC, Smith HC, et al. Patent ductus arteriosus in patients over age 50 years [abstr]. *J Am Coll Cardiol* 1984;3:599.

75. Margulis AR, Figley MF, Stern AM. Unusual roentgen manifestations of patent ductus arteriosus. *Radiology* 1954;63:334–345.

76. Keith JD, Rose V, Collins G, et al. Ventricular septal defect. Incidence, morbidity, and mortality in various age groups. *Br Heart J* 1971;33:81–87.

77. Hoffman JIE. Natural history of congenital heart disease: problems in its assessment with special reference to ventricular septal defects. *Circulation* 1968;37:97–125.

78. Engle MA. Ventricular septal defect: status report of the seventies. *Cardiovasc Clin* 1972;4:281–304.

79. Corone P, Doyon F, Gaudeau JS, et al. Natural history of ventricular septal defect: a study involving 790 cases. *Circulation* 1977;55:908–915.

80. Kidd L, Driscoll DJ, Gersony WM, et al. The second natural history study of congenital heart disease: results of treatment of patients with ventricular septal defect. *Circulation* 1993;87[Suppl 2]:138–151.

81. Child JS, Perloff JK. Natural survival patterns. In: Perloff JK, Childs JS, eds. *Congenital heart disease in adults*. Philadelphia: WB Saunders, 1991:21.

82. Perloff JK. *The clinical recognition of congenital heart disease*, 3rd ed. Philadelphia: WB Saunders, 1987:404.

83. Higgins CB, Mulder DG. Tetralogy of Fallot in the adult. *Am J Cardiol* 1972;29:837–846.

84. Hu DCK, Seward JB, Puga FJ, et al. Total correction of tetralogy of Fallot at age 40 years and older: long-term follow-up. *J Am Coll Cardiol* 1985;5:40–44.

85. Garson A Jr, Nihill MR, McNamara DG, et al. Status of the adult and adolescent after repair of tetralogy of Fallot. *Circulation* 1979;59:1232–1240.

86. Ascuitto RJ, Ross-Ascuitto NT, Markowitz RI, et al. Aneurysms of the right ventricular outflow tract after tetralogy of Fallot repair: role of radiology. *Radiology* 1988;167:115–119.

87. Rabinovitch M, Herrera-DeLeon V, Casteneda AR. Growth and development of the pulmonary vascular bed in patients with tetralogy of Fallot with or without pulmonary atresia. *Circulation* 1981;64:1234–1248.

88. Diethelm E, Soto B, Nath PH, et al. The pulmonary vascularity in patients with pulmonary atresia and ventricular septal defect. *RadioGraphics* 1985;5:243–254.

89. Tadavarthy SM, Klugman J, Casteneda-Zuniga WR, et al. Systemic-to-pulmonary collaterals in pathologic states. *Radiology* 1982;144:55–59.

90. Warnes CA. Tetralogy of Fallot and pulmonary atresia/ ventricular septal defect. *Cardiol Clin North Am* 1993;11:643–650.

91. Anderson KR, Lie JT. Pathologic anatomy of Ebstein's anomaly of the heart revisited. *Am J Cardiol* 1978;41:739–745.

92. Lev M, Liberthson RR, Joseph RH, et al. The pathologic anatomy of Ebstein's disease. *Arch Pathol* 1970;90:334–343.

93. Zuberbuhler JR, Allwork SP, Anderson RH. The spectrum of Ebstein's anomaly of the tricuspid valve. *J Thorac Cardiovasc Surg* 1979;77:202–211.

94. Amplatz K, Lester RG, Schiebler GL, et al. The roentgenologic features of Ebstein's anomaly of the tricuspid valve. *AJR Am J Roentgenol* 1959;81:788–794.

95. Wittenborg MH, Neuhauser EBD, Sprunt WH. Roentgenographic findings in congenital tricuspid atresia with hypoplasia of the right ventricle. *AJR Am J Roentgenol* 1951;66:712–727.

96. Marder SN, Seaman WB, Scott WG. Roentgenologic considerations in the diagnosis of congenital tricuspid atresia. *Radiology* 1953;61:174–182.

97. Chen JTT, Behar VS, Morris JJ Jr, et al. Correlation of roentgen findings with hemodynamic data in pure mitral stenosis. *AJR Am J Roentgenol* 1968;102:280–292.

98. Lane EJ Jr, Whalen JP. A new sign of left atrial enlargement: posterior displacement of the left bronchial tree. *Radiology* 1969;93:279–284.

99. West JB. Regional differences in gas exchange in the lung of erect man. *J Appl Physiol* 1962;17:893–898.

100. West JB, Dollery CT, Naimark A. Distribution of blood flow in isolated lung; relation to vascular and alveolar pressures. *J Appl Physiol* 1964;19:713–724.

101. Editorial. Pulmonary edema. *Lancet* 1976;2:350–351.

102. Harrison MO, Conte PJ, Heitzman ER. Radiological detection of clinically occult cardiac failure following myocardial infarction. *Br J Radiol* 1971;44:265–272.

103. Don C, Johnson R. The nature and significance of peri-

104. Grainger RG. Interstitial pulmonary edema and its radiological diagnosis. A sign of pulmonary venous and capillary hypertension. *Br J Radiol* 1958;31:201–217.

105. Trapnell DH. The peripheral lymphatics of the lung. *Br J Radiol* 1963;36:660–672.

106. West JB, Dollery CT, Heard BE. Increased pulmonary vascular resistance in the dependent zone of the isolated dog lung caused by perivascular edema. *Circ Res* 1965;17:191–206.

107. Chait A. Interstitial pulmonary edema. *Circulation* 1972;45:1323–1330.

108. Fleischner FG. The butterfly pattern of acute pulmonary edema. *Am J Cardiol* 1967;20:39–46.

109. Richman SM, Godar TJ. Unilateral pulmonary edema. *N Engl J Med* 1961;264:1148–1149.

110. Gurney JW, Goodman LR. Pulmonary edema localized in the right upper lobe accompanying mitral regurgitation. *Radiology* 1989;171:397–399.

111. Freundlich LM, Lind TA. Calcification of the heart and great vessels. *CRC Crit Rev Clin Radiol Nucl Med* 1975;6:171–216.

112. Leonard JJ, Katz S, Nelson D. Calcification of the left atrium: its anatomic location, diagnostic significance, and roentgenologic demonstration. *N Engl J Med* 1957;256:629–633.

113. Matsuyama S, Watabe T, Kuribayashi S, et al. Plain film diagnosis of thrombosis of the left atrial appendage in mitral valve disease. *Radiology* 1983;146:15–20.

114. Arvidsson A. Angiocardiographic determination of left ventricular volume. *Acta Radiol* 1961;56:321–338.

115. Dodge HT, Sandler H, Ballew DW, et al. The use of biplane angiocardiography for the measurement of left ventricular volume in man. *Am Heart J* 1960;60:762–776.

116. Hoffman RB, Rigler LG. Evaluation of left ventricular enlargement in the lateral projection of the chest. *Radiology* 1965;85:93–100.

117. Elliott LP, Schiebler GL. The normal cardiovascular silhouette. In: *The x-ray diagnosis of congenital heart disease in infants, children, and adults*. Springfield, IL: Charles C. Thomas, 1979.

118. Lehman JS, Florence H, Schimert AP, et al. Acquired aortic valvular stenosis. *Radiology* 1963;81:24–37.

119. Bachman DM, Ellis K, Austin JHM. The effects of minor degrees of obliquity on the lateral chest radiograph. *Radiol Clin North Am* 1978;16:465–485.

120. Carlsson E, Gross R, Hold RG. The radiological diagnosis of cardiac valvular insufficiencies. *Circulation* 1977;55:921–933.

121. Abrams DL, Edelist A, Luria MH, et al. Ventricular aneurysm. *Circulation* 1963;27:164–169.

122. Kittridge RD, Cameron A. Abnormalities of left ventricular wall motion and aneurysm formation. *AJR Am J Roentgenol* 1972;116:110–124.

123. Vladover Z, Coe JI, Edwards JE. True and false left ventricular aneurysms. Propensity for the latter to rupture. *Circulation* 1975;51:567–572.

124. Higgins CB, Lipton MJ, Johnson AD, et al. False aneurysms of the left ventricle. *Radiology* 1978;127:21–27.

125. Spindola-Franco H, Kronacher N. Pseudoaneurysm of the

left ventricle. Radiographic and angiocardiographic diagnosis. *Radiology* 1978;127:29–34.

126. Buehler DL, Stinson EB, Oyer PE, et al. Surgical treatment of aneurysms of the inferior left ventricle. *J Thorac Cardiovasc Surg* 1979;78:74–78.

127. Kittredge RD, Gamboa B, Kemp HG. Radiographic visualization of left ventricular aneurysms on lateral chest film. *AJR Am J Roentgenol* 1976;126:1140–1146.

128. Tampas JP, Soule AB. Coronary artery calcification. Its incidence and significance in patients over forty years of age. *AJR Am J Roentgenol* 1966;97:369–376.

129. Eggen DA, Strong JP, McGill HC. Coronary calcification: relationship to clinically significant coronary lesions and race, sex, and tomographic distribution. *Circulation* 1965;32:948–955.

130. Bartel AG, Chen JT, Peter RH, et al. The significance of coronary calcification detected by fluoroscopy. *Circulation* 1974;49:1247–1253.

131. Kelley MJ, Huang EK, Langou RA. Correlation of fluoroscopically detected coronary artery calcification with exercise stress testing in asymptomatic men. *Radiology* 1978;129:1–6.

132. Warburton RK, Tampas JP, Soule AB, et al. Coronary artery calcification: its relationship to coronary artery stenosis and myocardial infarction. *Radiology* 1968;91:109–115.

133. Hamby RI, Tabrah F, Wisoff HC. Coronary artery calcification: clinical implications and angiographic correlates. *Am Heart J* 1974;87:565–570.

134. Margolis JR, Chen JTT, Kong Y, et al. The diagnostic and prognostic significance of coronary artery calcification. *Radiology* 1980;137:609–616.

135. Souza AS Jr, Bream PR, Elliott LP. Chest film detection of coronary artery calcification. The value of the CAC triangle. *Radiology* 1978;129:7–10.

136. Lane EJ Jr, Carsky EW. Epicardial fat: lateral plain film analysis in normals and in pericardial effusion. *Radiology* 1968;91:1–5.

137. Kremens V. Demonstration of the pericardial shadow on routine chest roentgenograms: new roentgen finding. *Radiology* 1955;64:72–80.

138. Carsky EW, Maucori RA, Azimi F. The epicardial fat pad sign. *Radiology* 1980;137:303–308.

139. Blake S, Bonar S, O'Neill H, et al. Aetiology of chronic constrictive pericarditis. *Br Heart J* 1983;50:273–276.

140. Stewart JR, Fajardo LF. Radiation-induced heart disease: an update. *Prog Cardiovasc Dis* 1984;27:173–194.

141. Arthur A, Oskvig R, Basta LL. Calcific rheumatoid constrictive pericarditis with cardiac failure treated by pericardiectomy. *Chest* 1973;64:769–771.

142. Bulkley BH, Roberts WC. The heart in systemic lupus erythematosus and the changes induced in it by corticosteroid therapy. A study of 36 necropsy patients. *Am J Med* 1975;58:243–264.

143. Wacker W, Merrill JP. Uremic pericarditis in acute and chronic renal failure. *JAMA* 1954;156:764–765.

144. Schupak E, Merrill JP. Experience with long-term intermittent hemodialysis. *Ann Intern Med* 1965;62:509–518.

145. Deloran L, Thurber MD, Jesse E, et al. Secondary malignant tumors of the pericardium. *Circulation* 1962;26:228–241.

146. Clements SD, Hurst JW. Medical care before, during and after coronary bypass surgery. In: Hurst JW, ed. *The heart, update II*. New York: McGraw-Hill, 1980:261–269.

147. Masui T, Finck S, Higgins CB. Constrictive pericarditis and restrictive cardiomyopathy: evaluation with MR imaging. *Radiology* 1992;182:369–373.

148. Fowler NO. Constrictive pericarditis: new aspects. *Am J Cardiol* 1982;50:1014–1017.

149. Cooper DKC, Sturridge MF. Constrictive pericarditis following coxsackie virus infection. *Thorax* 1976;31:472–474.

150. Auerbach O. Pleural, peritoneal, and pericardial tuberculosis. *Am Rev Tuberc* 1950;61:845–861.

151. MacGregor JH, Chen JTT, Chiles C, et al. The radiographic distinction between pericardial and myocardial calcification. *AJR Am J Roentgenol* 1987;148:675–677.

152. Pulvaneswary M, Singham KT, Singh J. Constrictive pericarditis. Clinical, hemodynamic, and radiologic correlation. *Aust Radiol* 1982;26:53–59.

153. Feigin DS, Fenoglio JJ, McAllister HA, et al. Pericardial cysts: a radiologic-pathologic correlation and review. *Radiology* 1977;125:15–20.

154. Lam CR. Pericardial celomic cysts. *Radiology* 1947;48:239–243.

155. Loehr WM. Pericardial cysts. *AJR Am J Roentgenol* 1952;68:584–609.

156. Ellis K, Leeds NE, Himmelstein A. Congenital deficiencies in partial pericardium: review with two new cases including successful diagnosis by plain roentgenography. *AJR Am J Roentgenol* 1959;82:125–137.

157. Nasser WK, Helmen C, Tavel ME, et al. Congenital absence of the left pericardium: clinical, electrocardiographic, radiographic, hemodynamic, and angiographic findings in six cases. *Circulation* 1970;41:469–478.

158. van Son JAM, Danielson GK, Hartzell V. Congenital partial and complete absence of the pericardium. *Mayo Clin Proc* 1993;68:743–747.

159. Uhl HSM. A previously undescribed congenital myocardial malformation of the right ventricle. *Bull Johns Hopkins Hosp* 1952;91:197–205.

160. Ostermeyer J. Uhl's disease: partial parchment right ventricle. *Virchows Arch Pathol Anat Histol* 1974;362:185–194.

161. Thompson WP, White PD. The commonest cause of hypertrophy of the right ventricle: left ventricular strain and failure. *Am Heart J* 1936;12:641–649.

162. Chronic cor pulmonale. Report of an expert committee. *WHO Tech Rep Ser* 1961;213:1.

163. Dalen JE, Banas JS Jr, Brooks HL, et al. Resolution rate of acute pulmonary embolism in man. *N Engl J Med* 1969;280:1194–1199.

164. McIntyre KM, Sasahara AA. The hemodynamic response to pulmonary embolism in patients without prior cardiopulmonary disease. *Am J Cardiol* 1971;28:288–294.

165. Fishman A. Chronic cor pulmonale. *Am Rev Respir Dis* 1976;114:775–794.

166. Fishman A. Pulmonary hypertension and cor pulmonale. In: Fishman A, ed. *Pulmonary diseases and disorders*, 2nd ed. New York: McGraw-Hill, 1988:999–1048.

167. Klatte EC, Tampas JP, Campbell JA. Evaluation of right atrial size. *Radiology* 1963;81:48–53.

EXERCISE ELECTROCARDIOGRAPHY

PETER M. OKIN

▼⟋ **ADDITIONAL ELECTRONIC TOPICS**

OVERVIEW

Exercise electrocardiography (ECG) is the most widely used method for assessment of the presence and severity of coronary artery disease. Clinical confidence in the exercise ECG has been eroded by the limited sensitivity and predictive value of standard ST-segment depression criteria and by the overapplication of Bayesian principles to interpretation of the exercise ECG in comparison with other noninvasive modalities. However, the development of new approaches to analysis of the ST-segment response to exercise, including the heart rate (HR)–adjusted indices of ST-segment depression (the ST/HR slope and ST/HR index) and treadmill exercise scores, has led to a resurgence of clinical and research interest in the exercise ECG. These methods improve the accuracy of the exercise ECG for the identification and quantification of coronary artery disease and improve risk stratification in both asymptomatic low-risk subjects and symptomatic patients with coronary artery disease. Application of HR-adjusted techniques has been supported by theoretical and experimental evidence that relates the magnitude of ischemic ST depression at peak exercise to both the area of ischemic territory and the degree of myocardial oxygen supply-demand mismatch as reflected by changing HR. Novel approaches to analysis of the ECG during exercise, including changes in QRS complex duration and high-frequency content and assessment of HR responses during both exercise and recovery, hold promise for future improvements in test performance.

GLOSSARY

Bayesian analysis: Relation of test performance to the prevalence of disease in a population.

Chronotropic response index: Fraction of HR reserve achieved with exercise, adjusted by the fraction of metabolic reserve achieved.

P. M. Okin: Division of Cardiology, Weill Medical College of Cornell University, New York, New York

ETT: Exercise tolerance test or exercise electrocardiogram.

J-point: Junction of the end of the QRS complex and the beginning of the ST segment.

Rate-recovery loop: Plots of ST-segment depression as a function of HR during both exercise and recovery.

ST/HR index: Maximal change in ST-segment depression with exercise, divided by the total change in HR.

ST/HR slope: Linear regression–based calculation of maximal rate of change in ST-segment depression as a function of change in HR during exercise.

INTRODUCTION

Exercise ECG, or the exercise tolerance test (ETT), is the most widely used and widely available technique for the investigation of known or suspected coronary artery disease. It has been estimated that 6 to 8 million treadmill tests are performed annually in the United States. Nonetheless, clinical confidence in the simple ETT has been eroded by the limited sensitivity and predictive value of standard ECG criteria. However, new approaches to analysis of the ETT have been developed over the past 15 years that improve the accuracy of the exercise ECG to levels found with use of more expensive and less widely available imaging methods. This chapter reviews the development of exercise ECG; gives a brief review of the pathophysiologic basis for exercise-induced ST-segment depression; provides detailed information on the performance, interpretation, and applications of the ETT; and addresses the controversies and future directions in exercise ECG.

PERFORMING AN EXERCISE ELECTROCARDIOGRAM

Indications and Contraindications

The most widely accepted indications for ETT are in patients with known or suspected coronary artery disease, in whom ETT is used to determine the likelihood of coronary artery disease, to assess the likelihood of anatomic or functionally severe disease that may be of prognostic importance, to determine functional capacity, and to assess the effects of therapy (39,40). Although indications for the exercise ECG continue to evolve, a joint committee of the American College of Cardiology and American Heart Association has published categories of indications for the ETT based on published literature (39). Their classification includes conditions that are generally accepted as indications for exercise testing, conditions for which the test may be indicated, and conditions for which the ETT is generally considered to have marginal value (Table 48.1). Clini-

---

TABLE 48.1 INDICATIONS FOR EXERCISE ELECTROCARDIOGRAPHY

Clearly indicated
  Diagnosis of CAD in men with atypical symptoms
  Patient has known CAD; assess prognosis and functional capacity
  Symptomatic, recurrent, exercise-induced arrhythmias
  Patient has experienced an uncomplicated myocardial infarction; evaluate prognosis and functional capacity
  Patient has undergone coronary artery revascularization; evaluation recommended
Possibly indicated
  Diagnosis of CAD in woman with typical or atypical angina
  Diagnosis of CAD in patient taking digitalis
  Diagnosis of CAD in patient with complete right bundle branch block
  Patient has CAD or heart failure; evaluate functional capacity and response to therapy
  Patient has variant angina; evaluation recommended
  Patient has known CAD; serial evaluation recommended
  Asymptomatic man who is older than 40 yr and in a high-risk occupation, who has two or more risk factors for CAD, or who is sedentary and plans to begin a vigorous exercise program; evaluation recommended
  Asymptomatic patient after coronary revascularization; annual evaluation recommended
  Selected patients with valvular heart disease; evaluate functional capacity
Probably not indicated
  Asymptomatic patient with isolated ventricular ectopy; evaluation recommended
  Patient is enrolled in a cardiac rehabilitation program; serial evaluation recommended
  Diagnosis of CAD in patient with left bundle branch block or ventricular preexcitation (Wolff-Parkinson-White) syndrome on resting electrocardiography
  Asymptomatic man or woman; evaluation recommended
  Man or woman with chest pain of noncardiac etiology; evaluation recommended

---

CAD, coronary artery disease.
Adapted from Schlant RC, Blomqvist CG, Brandenburg RO, et al. Guidelines for exercise testing: a report of the American College of Cardiology/American Heart Association Task Force on Assessment of Cardiovascular Procedures (Subcommittee on Exercise Testing). *J Am Coll Cardiol* 1986;8:725, with the permission of Elsevier Science, Inc.

cal contraindications to performing diagnostic exercise ECG include acute myocardial infarction, unstable angina before a period of stabilization, uncompensated severe congestive heart failure, advanced atrioventricular (AV) block or life-threatening arrhythmias, acute myocarditis or pericarditis, severe aortic stenosis, severe resting hypertension, and any medical condition that precludes the patient's walking safely on the treadmill. The presence of left bundle branch block, left ventricular hypertrophy with strain, ventricular preexcitation (Wolf-Parkinson-White syndrome), or permanent ventricular pacing on the ECG is a contraindication to use of the exercise ECG for diagnostic purposes, because of the uncertain diagnostic value of additional ST-segment changes in these settings, but these factors do not preclude use of the ETT to assess exercise performance or to evaluate the risk of arrhythmia, when indicated.

Equipment and Personnel

Exercise tests [▼❯ j06] should be performed under the supervision of a physician who has been trained to conduct exercise tests. The degree of supervision required is primarily dependent on the type of patient being tested and can range from direct performance of the test for patients who are at higher risk of complications (e.g., those who have unstable angina after stabilization, who have congestive heart failure, or who have a high risk of arrhythmias) to assigning the performance of the test to an appropriately trained exercise physiologist or a specialist in patients at lower risk. In all cases, a physician should be immediately available during the exercise test.

Treadmill Protocol

Most exercise ECG laboratories in the United States use a treadmill rather than a bicycle ergometer for stress testing. The advantages of the treadmill lie in the greater familiarity of most people in this country with walking and the ability to increase both speed and grade of the treadmill to increase workload. Although a number of excellent treadmill protocols are available for use, by far the most commonly used protocols are the original protocol of Bruce (43) and modifications of this protocol. The Cornell protocol, originally developed in our laboratory to produce the smaller HR increments between stages that are necessary for calculation of the ST/HR slope (44), is a more graded modification of the Bruce protocol that divides each standard stage into 2-minute half-stages. To allow adequate warm-up time and to allow more patients to be able to exercise for a period of time adequate for calculating the ST/HR slope, the protocol begins with a 2-minute stage 0 at 1.7 miles per hour and 0% grade, with a 2-minute stage 0.5 at 1.7 miles per hour at a 5% grade, before reaching the usual starting point of the Bruce protocol (1.7 miles per hour and a 10% grade) (*e*Table 48.1.1).

Lead Systems

The number and types of leads used in exercise ECG vary widely, but with the advent of modern recording devices, most stress laboratories monitor and record at least three leads during the test. Although the use of all 12 conventional leads is becoming more common, almost all of the useful diagnostic ST-segment information from these leads is present in limb leads II, III, and aVF and precordial leads V_3 to V_6. Bipolar lead systems that include one electrode in the V_5 position provide additional diagnostic information; bipolar lead CM_5 is the most sensitive for ST-segment changes (11) and is particularly important in optimal recording of the ST/HR slope (45). ▼❯ j07

Indications for Test Termination

The general indications for terminating an exercise test are outlined in Table 48.2. In the absence of symptoms or signs that warrant termination of the exercise ECG, patients should exercise with 100% of age-predicted target HR as the goal. Although use of 100% of the age-predicted target HR as an indication for terminating an exercise test may prevent the accurate assessment of functional exercise capacity in patients able to exercise beyond this point, in general, achievement of greater than 85% of target HR provides an adequate level of stress for diagnostic exercise ECG (10). Various equations have been used to relate target HR to age, but the simplest and most commonly used are 220 − age and 200 − (age/2). Although angina alone is not an absolute indication for test termination, progressively worsening typical anginal symptoms are a reason to stop the test, as are any other symptoms that limit further walking on the treadmill.

ST-segment elevation in the absence of Q waves is consistent with possible transmural injury and a reason for immediate termination of the ETT. In contrast, ST-

TABLE 48.2 GENERAL INDICATIONS FOR TERMINATING AN EXERCISE TEST

Achievement of target heart rate (see text for definitions)
Progressive angina
Other limiting symptoms (dyspnea, fatigue, lightheadedness, claudication)
ST-segment elevation >2 mm (in leads without a resting Q wave)
Severe ST-segment depression (see text)
Nonsustained ventricular tachycardia (three or more sequential ventricular premature contractions)
New onset of atrial fibrillation, atrial flutter, or of a supraventricular tachycardia
Development of second- or third-degree atrioventricular block
Development of a new left bundle branch block
A 10–mm Hg drop in systolic blood pressure
Extreme elevation of systolic or diastolic blood pressure
A progressive drop in heart rate with continued exercise
Equipment problems, such as loss of electrocardiographic signal

---

segment depression alone is rarely an indication for cessation of the exercise test. Indeed, only marked ST depression (>3 mm of additional ST depression compared with baseline) would warrant test termination in the absence of other findings. New sustained tachyarrhythmias are clearly an indication for stopping the test, as is the development of second- or third-degree heart block. Routine diagnostic stress tests should also be halted if nonsustained ventricular tachycardia is seen, unless the patient is undergoing the test expressly for evaluation of the possibility of exercise-induced ventricular tachycardia with the extra precautions taken of having a second physician in attendance, intravenous access, and additional leads to a synchronous cardiodefibrillator. Other relative indications for terminating the ETT include development of a new left bundle branch block that precludes further evaluation of ST-segment changes, a 10–mm Hg or greater drop in systolic blood pressure, an extreme elevation of systolic or diastolic blood pressure, a progressive decrease in HR with exercise, or significant equipment problems, such as loss of the ECG signal.

Other Applications of Stress Testing

Performance of an exercise test for indications other than routine assessment of the presence or severity of coronary artery disease or evaluation of functional capacity deserves comment. After uncomplicated myocardial infarction, exercise testing is frequently performed to assess functional capacity and to help stratify risk (46). When exercise testing is performed early after myocardial infarction (i.e., before discharge or within 2 to 3 weeks of the infarction), submaximal symptom-limited testing is recommended (40), to a target HR of 140 beats/min or a metabolic equivalent of 7 in patients younger than 40 years and to a maximum HR of 130 beats/min or a metabolic equivalent of 5 in patients 40 years and older. A full symptom-limited maximal test is appropriate more than 3 weeks after myocardial infarction. Exercise ECGs are also commonly performed to evaluate the risk of exercise-induced tachyarrhythmias in patients who have exercise-related presyncope or syncope. Because of the risk of inducing a hemodynamically significant arrhythmia in these settings, the ETT should be performed with at least one (and preferably two) physicians present, with intravenous access, and with leads connected to a defibrillator.

Exercise ECG is also frequently used after percutaneous transluminal angioplasty to stratify risk and aid in the assessment of restenosis and appears to be well tolerated (47,48). However, reports of acute stent thrombosis associated with exercise testing soon after stent placement (49) raise the question of whether exercise testing should be performed in the immediate post-stent period. Until further data become available, caution should be used in the performance of exercise testing soon after the placement of

intracoronary stents, with strong consideration given to the use of pharmacologic stress if early noninvasive assessment is indicated (49).

INTERPRETATION OF THE EXERCISE ELECTROCARDIOGRAM

ST-Segment Depression Criteria

To fully appreciate the ST-segment excursions that occur during the transient ischemia associated with exercise in patients with coronary artery disease requires some understanding of the ST-segment changes that occur during exercise in healthy subjects (Fig. 48.1). At baseline, most healthy subjects will have ST segments that are either at the isoelectric level or slightly elevated as a result of physiologic early repolarization of the J-point. As HR increases, progressive J-point or junctional depression occurs, with resultant rapidly upsloping ST segment (50,51). After exercise is terminated, the J-point depression tends to resolve quickly (usually within the first 2 minutes), as does the rapidly upsloping ST-segment depression. In contrast, the ST-segment depression associated with subendocardial ischemia is more likely to be horizontal or downsloping but may also be slowly upsloping (Fig. 48.2) (10,51). With progressive exercise, increasing HR, and the resulting increasing myocardial oxygen demand, the magnitude of ischemic ST-segment depression will increase, and the ST depression is more likely to be horizontal or downsloping. Placing the patient in the supine position immediately after exercise may accentuate ischemic ST-segment depression. However, ischemic ST depression may occur during exercise only, emphasizing the importance of adequate skin preparation before electrode placement. In a small percentage of cases, ischemic ST-segment depression will be seen during recovery only (52), especially when the patient is placed in the supine

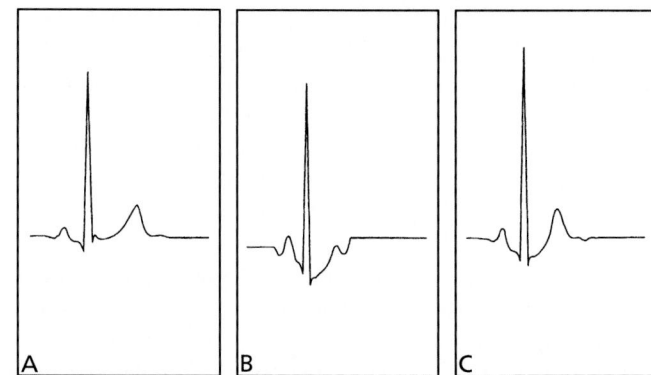

FIGURE 48.1 Progression of ST-segment changes that occur in healthy subjects from isoelectric at baseline **(A)** to J-point depression with rapidly upsloping ST-segment depression at peak exercise **(B)** and rapid resolution of the ST changes in recovery **(C)**.

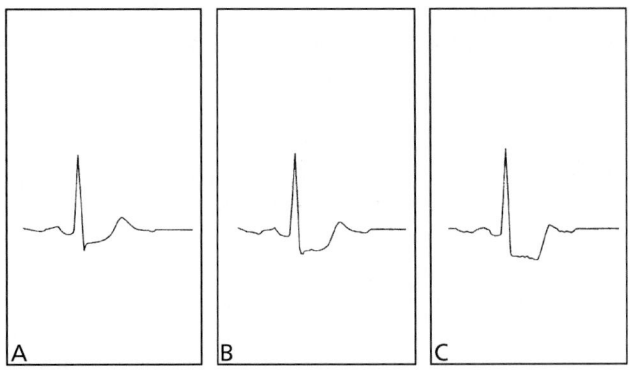

FIGURE 48.2 Comparison of the different patterns of ST depression. **A:** Slowly upsloping ST-segment depression. **B:** Horizontal ST-segment depression. **C:** Downsloping ST-segment depression.

position, but isolated recovery-phase ischemic ST-segment depression is less common when patients remain in the upright position after exercise. In rare instances of exercise-induced transmural ischemia or injury, ST-segment elevation similar to that seen during the acute injury of myocardial infarction may also occur. ▾☞ j08

The actual measurement of ST-segment deviation on the exercise ECG is most accurately performed by the computerized systems that are widely in use today, but accurate ST-segment measurements can be performed by hand if careful attention is paid to proper selection of the correct measurement points. In measurement of ST deviation, the PQ segment is usually chosen as the isoelectric point, which some computerized systems choose by scanning before the QRS complex for the 10-ms interval with the lowest slope, and ST-segment depression should be measured at 60 ms after the J-point. Computer systems are capable of accurately measuring ST deviation to the nearest 10 μV, and careful hand measurements using calipers or a magnifying graticule can readily achieve a precision of 25 μV for ST measurements (54). However, when computer measurements are used, it is important to recognize that motion artifact, electrical interference, and changes in QRS or atrioventricular conduction can interfere with PQ segment and J-point determinations and introduce error into the computerized ST measurements. Therefore, physicians should routinely compare the raw ECG signal with the computer-averaged or median beats used to perform ST measurements before accepting the computer measurements as accurate.

Standard Test Criteria

Assessment of the magnitude and configuration of ST-segment depression on the exercise ECG provides the basis for the standard ST depression criteria that are commonly in use. A positive test result based on standard ST depression criteria has been routinely defined as the achievement of 0.1 mV (100 μV) or more of horizontal or downsloping

ST-segment depression at peak exercise or in early recovery compared with the baseline pre-exercise ECG (10,39,40). However, as is discussed later, these criteria have only limited test sensitivity for the presence of coronary artery disease and variable performance for identification of anatomically severe disease and for risk stratification (10–16,20–23,45,55). Additional factors that can affect the likelihood that coronary artery disease or multivessel disease will be detected in the presence of traditional criteria include the magnitude, time of onset, duration, and number of leads with ST depression. Although inclusion of upsloping ST depression of greater than or equal to 0.1 mV or 0.15 mV has been suggested as an additional component of standard criteria, to increase sensitivity for the detection of coronary artery disease (56,57), the incorporation of upsloping ST depression also lowers test specificity (10,20,55,56). As a consequence, we consider the presence of upsloping ST-segment depression of 1 mm (0.1 mV) or more to be an "equivocal" test response by standard criteria.

Heart Rate–Adjusted Criteria

HR adjustment of the magnitude of ST-segment depression is a rational, physiologic approach to interpretation of the ETT. Two related but distinct methods of HR adjustment of ST-segment depression seen during exercise have evolved: the linear regression–based ST/HR slope and the simpler ST/HR index. The ST/HR slope method was originally developed in England (58) and Hungary (59) and has subsequently been applied to treadmill exercise, using computerized ST-segment measurements, and further refined in our laboratory at Cornell (20–23,25,44,45,51,54). The ST/HR slope is calculated from the maximal rate of change of ST depression relative to HR during the period of active ischemia that accompanies end-exercise (Fig. 48.3). The ST/HR index, originally described by Detrano and coworkers (60), represents the average change of ST depression relative to HR change over the entire course of exercise, which underestimates the maximal ST/HR slope because it includes a large change in HR before any ischemia occurs (Fig. 48.3). Both of these methods specifically do not consider any ST depression that occurs during the postexercise recovery period.

Calculations of the ST/HR slope and ST/HR index are illustrated in Figure 48.3. Measurement of the ST/HR slope is determined by linear regression analysis to relate the measured amount of ST-segment depression in each lead to the HR at the end of each stage of exercise and at peak exercise. Because the maximal rather than the average rate of change is sought, linear regression analysis is performed from the end of exercise to progressively earlier intermediate stage data points, using HR as the independent variable and ST depression as the dependent variable. The highest ST/HR slope with a statistically significant

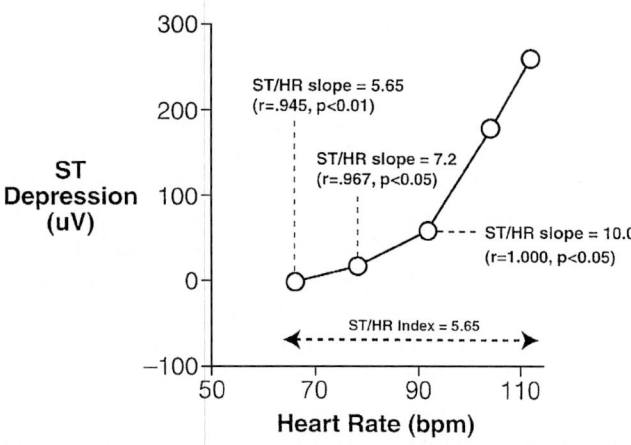

FIGURE 48.3 Calculation of the ST/heart rate (HR) slope. Progressive ST-segment depression in lead CM5 (shown as a positive magnitude on the vertical axis) is plotted against exercise HR in a patient with three-vessel coronary artery disease. This case illustrates the linear relation of ST-segment depression to HR as peak exercise is approached. As a result, the slope of the line relating the final three data points by linear regression is higher than the slope of lines incorporating earlier data points. When more than one linear correlation is statistically significant, the greatest value (in this case, 10.0) is taken as the test result for that patient. Note that the value obtained by simply dividing the total change in ST-segment depression by the total change in HR (the ST/HR index) markedly underestimates the true ST/HR slope. (Reprinted from Okin PM, Kligfield P. Heart rate adjustment of ST depression and performance of the exercise electrocardiogram: a critical evaluation. *J Am Coll Cardiol* 1995;25:1726, with the permission of Elsevier Science, Inc.)

correlation coefficient is taken as the test finding for that lead (in µV per beat per minute). After calculation of the maximal ST/HR slope for each lead, the highest ST/HR slope among all the leads (including bipolar lead CM$_5$, but excluding aVR, aVL, and V$_1$) is taken as the final test result (45,54). The ST/HR index is derived by dividing the maximal change in ST-segment depression during exercise by the total change in HR from rest to peak effort (45,60). Initial studies from our laboratory (20) established parti-

tion values, with specificities of 95% in healthy subjects, of more than 2.40 µV per beat per minute for the ST/HR slope and more than 1.60 µV per beat per minute for the ST/HR index for the identification of coronary artery disease. Partition values of more than 6.0 µV per beat per minute (ST/HR slope) and more than 3.3 µV per beat per minute (ST/HR index) have been established for the identification of three-vessel, left main, and functionally severe coronary artery disease (45).

Analysis of the behavior of ST-segment depression as a function of HR during both exercise and recovery using the rate-recovery loop (21,22,45) can elicit additional diagnostic and prognostic information from the ETT. Physiologic correlates of rate-recovery loop patterns can be found in the initial observations of Detry and Bruce and associates (61,62), which compare myocardial ischemia during exercise and recovery. They found a close linear relation of ST-segment depression during exercise to myocardial oxygen demand, as reflected by the tension-time index, among patients with coronary artery disease. During recovery, however, this relation was nonlinear, with similar ST-segment depressions observed at lower tension-time indexes than those seen during exercise. Additional support for this approach is found in reports of cases of subendocardial ischemia that continue into the recovery period with persistent ST-segment depression that remains greater relative to HR during early recovery than during the development of ischemia (63,64). Rate-recovery loops are constructed by plotting ST-segment deviation, with reference to changing HR, throughout treadmill exercise and recovery (Fig. 48.4). Healthy subjects typically exhibit a clockwise loop of ST-segment depression as a function of HR during exercise and recovery, whereas patients with coronary artery disease commonly exhibit a counterclockwise loop. Quantification of the degree of abnormal rate-recovery loop behavior by integrating the difference in ST depression between exercise and recovery phases from peak-exercise to the end of 3 minutes of the recovery phase

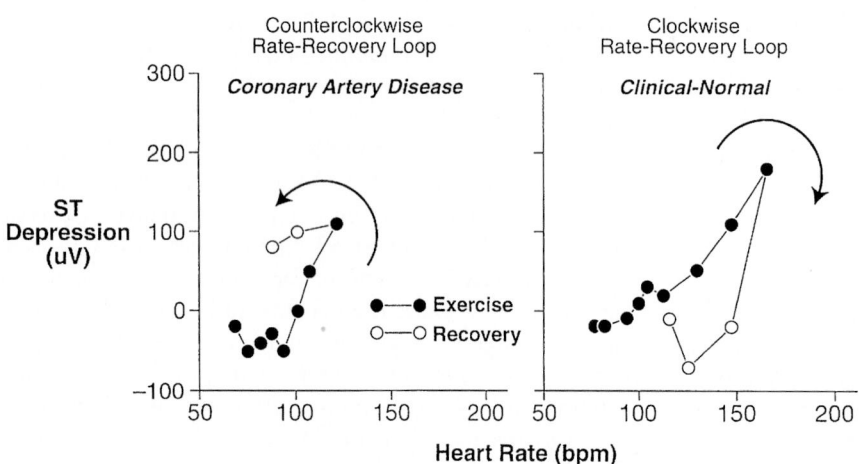

FIGURE 48.4 ST-segment deviation as a function of heart rate during exercise and recovery, with ST-segment depression shown in the upward direction and ST-segment elevation shown in the downward direction. Typical rate-recovery loops are shown for a clinically normal subject (*right*) and a patient with coronary artery disease (*left*). Despite a greater magnitude of ST-segment depression at peak exercise in the clinically normal subject, there is a clockwise pattern of ST-segment depression relative to heart rate during recovery; the patient with coronary artery disease has the opposite, counterclockwise pattern. (Reprinted from Okin PM, Kligfield P. Heart rate adjustment of ST depression and performance of the exercise electrocardiogram: a critical evaluation. *J Am Coll Cardiol* 1995;25:1726, with permission of Elsevier Science, Inc.)

TABLE 48.3 TREADMILL EXERCISE SCORES

Hollenberg exercise score (16)

$$\text{Exercise score} = \frac{\text{area (J-point + ST slope) V}_5 \times 12/RV_5 + \text{area (J-point + ST slope)aVF}}{\text{exercise duration} \times \text{fraction of maximal predicted heart rate}}$$

(where exercise duration is in min and R-wave amplitudes are in mm)

Duke treadmill score (26)

$$\text{Treadmill score} = \text{exercise duration} - (5 \times \text{ST deviation}) - (4 \times \text{TM angina index})$$

[where exercise duration is in min; ST deviation is in mm; and TM (treadmill) angina index = 0 for no angina, 1 for nonlimiting angina, or 2 for exercise-limiting angina]

can further stratify the presence and severity of coronary artery disease (23a).

Treadmill Exercise Scores

Numerous investigators have used either multivariate analyses or Bayesian theory to produce clinical scores in an attempt to improve the accuracy of the ETT (16,26,65–68). However, many of these methods incorporated clinical and catheterization data that make the contribution of the exercise test unclear. Two methods that have used data only from the ETT are the Hollenberg exercise score (16) and the Duke treadmill score (Table 48.3) (26,65). The Hollenberg exercise score quantifies the ECG response to exercise by measuring the cumulative area of ST depression and ST slope in leads V_5 and aVF during exercise and recovery, which is then normalized for R-wave height and workload (exercise duration and HR). The Duke treadmill score is a simple quantitative score, derived using a Cox regression model in a training sample of more than 1,400 patients, that includes exercise duration and weighted measures of ST-segment deviation and an angina score. The prognostic value of this score has been validated for ambulatory patients (26) and for patients undergoing angiography (65).

Chronotropic Response to Exercise

Independent of evidence of myocardial ischemia, an attenuated HR response to exercise, a measure of chronotropic incompetence, has been associated with the presence and severity of coronary artery disease (25,75) and has been shown to be a predictor of both coronary heart disease events and of total mortality (24,76,76a). Different measures of chronotropic response to exercise have been used to assess the adequacy of HR response, including simple measures such as peak exercise HR, percentage of target HR achieved, and change in HR during exercise. In addition, simple and HR-adjusted ST-segment depression criteria can be corrected for an attenuated HR response to exercise by adjustment of these measurements for the fraction of HR reserve achieved during exercise, which is the change in

HR during exercise divided by the difference between 100% of age-predicted target HR and the HR at standing rest (25). A more complex measure is the chronotropic response index (24,25), which adjusts the fraction of HR reserve achieved for workload as measured by the fraction of metabolic reserve. HR changes during the recovery phase of the exercise test have also been demonstrated to provide prognostic information. A delayed decrease in HR after exercise, or abnormal HR recovery, predicts all-cause mortality among healthy adults and in patients referred for exercise testing, independent of evidence of inducible ischemia and beyond the predictive value of exercise-phase changes in HR (25a,76b,76c).

Blood Pressure Changes

Among patients with coronary artery disease, failure to increase systolic blood pressure to 120 mm Hg or higher and a sustained decrease in systolic blood pressure of 10 mm Hg or more both have been associated with an increased likelihood of anatomically extensive disease. However, other conditions can produce a blunted blood pressure response to exercise, such as obstruction of left ventricular outflow, hypovolemia, left or right ventricular dysfunction, cardioactive medications, and vigorous exercise. In contrast, although an exaggerated blood pressure response to exercise has been clearly associated with an increased risk of developing hypertension at rest and with a greater prevalence of left ventricular hypertrophy (77), the prevalence of coronary artery disease appears to be similar among patients who do and those who do not have exercise hypertension (210 mm Hg or higher in men and 190 mm Hg or higher in women) (78). Moreover, an exaggerated systolic blood pressure response to exercise appears to be associated with a lower likelihood of anatomically severe disease and with a lower 2-year overall mortality rate (78).

In the postexercise recovery phase, a progressive decline in systolic blood pressure is usually seen. Failure of systolic blood pressure to decline normally during early recovery, as measured by an increased ratio (greater than 0.90) of systolic blood pressure during the first 3 minutes of recovery to peak exercise systolic blood pressure, has been reported to be useful in the diagnosis of coronary artery disease (79). However, an increased ratio is also seen in patients who have hypertension and no significant coronary obstructions (79), and additional studies have not substantiated a high sensitivity of this ratio for coronary artery disease (80). Further study of the utility of blood pressure changes in improving the accuracy of the diagnosis of coronary artery disease by ETT is necessary before the routine application of these criteria can be recommended.

Rhythm and Conduction Changes

The ETT can be used to evaluate the risk for significant abnormalities of cardiac rhythm and conduction under appropriate conditions. Exercise-induced ventricular premature contractions (VPCs) are common, increase in prevalence with age, are more frequent, and may be associated with a somewhat worse prognosis in patients with coronary artery disease (81). In contrast, neither the abolition of VPCs with increasing exercise nor development of VPCs only during the postexercise recovery period appear to be of clinical significance, and the appearance of nonsustained ventricular tachycardia during exercise testing does not appear to convey an increased short-term risk (82). The development of sustained ventricular tachycardia during exercise testing in patients who have coronary artery disease is most commonly the result of myocardial ischemia and can be prevented by treatment of the underlying ischemia. Exercise testing can play an important adjunctive role to electrophysiologic studies in the evaluation of patients with exercise-induced ventricular tachycardia in whom the presumptive mechanisms are after-depolarizations or enhanced automaticity and who have no obvious structural heart disease. A left bundle branch block morphology and termination of ventricular tachycardia with vagal maneuvers or adenosine strongly suggest that delayed after-depolarizations are the cause of the tachycardia. Exercise-induced supraventricular arrhythmias occur in 4% to 8% of patients, increase in frequency with age, and do not reflect the presence of coronary artery disease.

Changes in AV and intraventricular conduction may occur during exercise. Rarely, exercise testing can elicit second-degree AV block in patients with exertional fatigue or dyspnea, but more commonly, AV conduction is enhanced with exercise as a result of increased sympathetic tone and increased circulating catecholamines. Exercise-induced, rate-related development of right or left bundle branch block is relatively rare; it is not associated with an increased incidence of underlying coronary artery disease in younger subjects (younger than 40 years), but it appears to be associated with coronary artery disease in older subjects. When right bundle branch block is seen on resting ECG, exercise-induced ST-segment depression in leads V_1 to V_4 commonly occurs and is not diagnostic for coronary artery disease; ST-segment depression in the inferior leads and leads V_5 and V_6 is consistent with ischemia. ST-segment changes in the presence of a left bundle branch block are best considered nondiagnostic for coronary artery disease. ⚘ j09

Drugs and Hormonal Effects

Cardioactive drugs and sex hormones can significantly affect interpretation of the ETT. Drugs that blunt the HR and blood pressure response to exercise, such as beta-blockers, diltiazem, and verapamil, may delay or diminish ST-segment depression during exercise and reduce the sensitivity of standard test criteria. Although the sensitivity of HR-adjusted criteria appears to be less affected by these medications (45), failure to produce ischemia during exercise that is the result of medication limits the diagnostic accuracy of any noninvasive modality. Conversely, digitalis preparations can produce ST-segment changes in the absence of heart disease, significantly decreasing the specificity of ETT criteria that are based on ST-segment changes. Similarly, both endogenous and exogenous estrogens and progesterones have been implicated in abnormal ST-segment responses that are seen in healthy women (83,84). Moreover, the administration of estrogens can increase the magnitude of ST-segment depression in men and women with ischemic disease (23,83,84), and consideration of estrogen status significantly improves the overall accuracy of the ETT in women (85). Although numerous investigators have reported lower accuracy when standard ST-segment depression criteria are used for women than when these criteria are used for men, whether these differences are better explained by lower test sensitivity or lower specificity in women remains controversial (23). Although the mechanisms of ST-segment changes in response to cyclic hormonal variations remain to be determined (23,83,84), notably, both the ST/HR index and ST/HR slope provide diagnostic accuracy that is similar in men and women, despite these potential limitations (23).

APPLICATIONS AND TEST PERFORMANCE OF THE EXERCISE ELECTROCARDIOGRAM

Identification of Coronary Artery Disease

The diagnosis of coronary artery disease remains the most frequent indication for exercise testing with standard ST depression criteria; achievement of at least 0.1 mV of additional horizontal or downsloping ST-segment depression is the most common diagnostic criterion. However, utility of the standard ETT for this purpose has been limited by the relatively low sensitivity and poor predictive accuracy of standard criteria (10,11,20,45,55). Although the exact performance of any test is difficult to determine because of the influence of study design, population selection, and referral bias (45,55,86–88), a metaanalysis assessing the sensitivity and specificity of the ETT in 24,074 patients evaluated in 147 consecutively published reports provides some important insights into the performance of standard ST depression criteria (55). Using 50% luminal obstruction at angiography as the diagnostic standard for coronary artery disease, the weighted mean sensitivity was 68% (range, 23% to 100%), and mean specificity was 77% (range, 17% to 100%); when upsloping ST depression was considered to be abnormal, test specificity was significantly reduced (from 80% to 73%), but sensitivity increased by a similar amount (8%). Predictably, use of these criteria for the identification of multivessel disease or left-main or triple-vessel disease was associated with higher sensitivity (mean, 81% and 86%, respectively) but also was associated with lower test specificity (mean, 66% and 53%) (89). ✌ j10

Although some controversy persists over the value of HR-adjusted criteria (see the section Controversies and Personal Perspectives), the great majority of published studies that have adhered to proscribed requirements for ST-segment depression measurements have demonstrated that the ST/HR slope and the simple ST/HR index improve performance of the ETT as a tool for recognizing coronary artery disease. Early studies of the ST/HR slope by Elamin and colleagues (58), using an individually tailored bicycle ergometry protocol, demonstrated 100% specificity and 100% sensitivity for the detection of coronary artery disease; however, subsequent investigators have failed to reproduce this perfect test performance. Initial studies from our laboratory, using computerized ST measurements at 60 ms after the J-point and the Cornell modification of the Bruce protocol, derived criteria for the ST/HR slope and the ST/HR index that yielded a 95% specificity when used for clinically normal subjects, similar to the specificity of standard test criteria used for the same subjects (20). Test sensitivity of these criteria in separate groups of patients with clinical angina and with angiographically proven coronary artery disease were 94% and 95%, respectively, for the ST/HR slope and 88% and 93%, respectively, for the ST/HR index, all of which are significantly greater than the 68% sensitivity of use of standard ST-segment depression criteria for these populations (20). Moreover, these new criteria maintained similar specificity to standard criteria among patients in whom no significant obstruction was demonstrated by angiography (ST/HR slope, 72%; ST/HR index, 61%; standard criteria, 56%). Compared with standard test criteria, rate-recovery loops have demonstrated similarly high specificity in healthy subjects (95% vs. 93%), similar specificity in patients in whom no significant coronary obstruction was demonstrated by angiography (71% vs. 71%), and better sensitivity for the detection of coronary artery disease (93% vs. 74%) (21). Additional studies of the ST/HR slope from our laboratory and from investigators in Japan, Europe, and the United States have confirmed that the performance of this method in detecting coronary

artery disease is superior (45). Improved accuracy for the detection of coronary artery disease has also been found in association with the simple ST/HR index in most but not all studies from other centers (45,53,60,68).

Detection of Anatomically and Functionally Severe Coronary Artery Disease

The poorer prognosis of patients with multivessel, and in particular three-vessel or left-main, coronary artery disease has made recognition of these patients a clinical priority. A metaanalysis of the cases of 12,030 patients that involved 60 consecutively published reports, comparing the ETT with findings at coronary angiography, found a weighted mean sensitivity of 81% (range, 40% to 100%) and mean specificity of 66% (range, 17% to 100%) for multivessel disease and mean sensitivity of 86% and specificity of 53% for three-vessel or left-main disease (89). In this metaanalysis, use of HR adjustment of ST depression was independently associated with improved specificity of the ETT for identification of three-vessel or left-main coronary artery disease (89). Factors that have been found to improve the performance of standard test criteria for these purposes include use of 2 mm or greater horizontal or downsloping ST-segment depression, early test positivity (Bruce stage 2 or earlier), and persistence of test positivity 8 minutes or more into recovery, all of which improve test specificity. In addition, both the Duke treadmill score and a consensus score that includes clinical variables have been shown to provide useful information for the recognition of anatomically severe coronary artery disease (89a,89b).

Studies from multiple investigators have demonstrated that both the ST/HR slope and the ST/HR index improve performance of the ETT for the identification of multivessel coronary artery disease. In early studies from our laboratory, standard test criteria identified multivessel coronary artery disease with a sensitivity of 76%, which is significantly lower than the 97% sensitivity associated with an ST/HR slope greater than 2.4 and than the 94% sensitivity associated with an ST/HR index greater than 1.6, with similar differences in test sensitivity for three-vessel disease (20). Similarly, when criteria that are specifically designed for the identification of three-vessel disease are used, the ST/HR slope significantly improves performance of the ETT for diagnosis of anatomically or functionally severe coronary artery disease, compared with standard test criteria. An ST/HR slope of more than 6.0 μV per beat per minute significantly improves ETT identification of three-vessel or left-main coronary artery disease and has been shown to be more accurate than standard criteria for assessment of the anatomic extent of coronary obstruction, as alternatively defined by high Duke jeopardy scores or Gensini scores (45,90–92). Further, as a functional consequence of extensive coronary obstruction, high ST/HR slopes have been found to correlate with large decreases in left ventricular ejection fraction during exercise and with abnormal results of thallium imaging (91,92). However, the simple ST/HR index does not appear to consistently improve performance of the exercise ECG for identification of extensive coronary artery disease, compared with standard test criteria (45).

Risk Stratification and Assessment of Prognosis

Although the value of screening asymptomatic subjects for coronary artery disease remains controversial because of the poor predictive value of positive test findings in populations in which the prevalences of disease is low (18,19,22,93,94), numerous studies have documented the ability of the ETT to stratify risk in low-risk populations (12,13,22,69,70,95). An ischemic ST-segment response to exercise as judged by standard criteria was a significant predictor of cardiac morbidity and mortality in the overall population of the Seattle Heart Watch (13) and in a referred group of clinically normal male Air Force personnel (12). However, standard test criteria did not significantly concentrate risk among the large subset of asymptomatic healthy subjects in Seattle (13), did not concentrate risk in a nonreferred subset of healthy pilots and astronauts undergoing exercise testing as part of routine preflight assessment (12), was not predictive of coronary events in more than 3,000 asymptomatic men and women in the Framingham Offspring Study (Fig. 48.5) (22), and was not predictive of coronary heart disease mortality in 5,940 asymptomatic men from the usual-care arm of the Multiple Risk Factor Intervention Trial (MRFIT) (Fig. 48.6) (95).

In contrast, an ST/HR index greater than 1.60 µV per beat per minute significantly concentrated the risk of primarily nonfatal coronary events in asymptomatic men and women in the Framingham Offspring Study (Fig. 48.5) and stratified the risk of coronary heart disease death in MRFIT (Fig. 48.6) (22,95). In both studies, risk concentration by the ST/HR index was independent of age and additional cardiac risk factors and, in the Framingham Offspring Study, was similar in men and in women. An ST/HR index of more than 3.3 µV per beat per minute, previously demonstrated to be associated with anatomically extensive coronary artery disease (90,92), was associated with a nearly tenfold increase in risk of coronary death in MRFIT (95). In addition, an abnormal rate-recovery loop, both alone and in combination with the ST/HR index, and a blunted HR response to exercise, independent of ST depression findings, improved risk stratification by the ETT in the Framingham Offspring Trial (22,24). Perhaps most important, the decreased 7-year coronary mortality associated with an abnormal ST/HR index that was seen in the special-intervention group of MRFIT, compared with that in the usual-care group, suggests that this methodology can be used to identify men who are at increased risk of coronary death and will benefit from an aggressive risk factor–reduction program (95a).

The ETT can also be used to stratify risk among symptomatic patients who have known or presumed coronary artery disease (26,65,76,76c,96). In 4,083 medically treated patients from the Coronary Artery Survival Study registry, a high-risk subset with an annual mortality rate greater than 5% was identified when patients had positive results of standard testing and an exercise workload less than Bruce stage 1; a low-risk subset with an annual mortality rate less than 1% was identified by the ability to exercise to at least stage 3 of the Bruce protocol with a negative ST-segment response (96). The Duke treadmill exercise score (26,65,76c,96a) provides additional risk stratification to supplement that provided by ST-segment depression criteria among inpatients who have undergone angiography, outpatients who have suspected coronary artery disease, and patients who have resting ST-T–wave abnormalities. Further, among 1,300 symptomatic patients in whom coronary artery disease was demonstrated by angiography, the ST/HR index improved risk stratification by the Duke treadmill score and clinical variables and was an independent predictor of cardiac death in both men and women (97).

The prognostic value of standard ST-segment depression criteria after myocardial infarction has been well studied. In a metaanalysis of post–myocardial infarction exercise testing, Froelicher and coauthors (46) found exercise-induced ST-segment depression, poor effort tolerance, and an abnormal systolic blood pressure response to exercise to be associated with an increased risk of adverse outcome. The prognostic value of ST-segment changes after myocardial infarction in an era in which thrombolytic medications are available remains uncertain, because outcomes are similar in patients with and those without ischemic ST-segment changes (98). However, an inability to perform a predischarge low-level exercise test appears to be associated with a poor prognosis after myocardial infarction, independent of the use of thrombolytic agents (46,98). Independent of ECG, thallium imaging, or echocardiographic evidence of myocardial ischemia, attenuated HR changes, both during exercise and in the postexercise recovery phase, have been demonstrated to stratify the risk of all-cause mortality in asymptomatic subjects and in patients undergoing diagnostic exercise testing (24,24a,25a,76a–76c). An impaired chronotropic response to exercise, defined as failure to achieve 85% of target HR or a low chronotropic index, is associated with a 1.8- to 2.2-fold increased risk of all-cause mortality, after the analysis has been adjusted for confounding variables (24a). A delayed decrease in HR during the first minute of recovery provides similar risk concentration for overall mortality, even when exercise-phase HR responses were taken into account (25a).

Test Performance in Women

Among the problems associated with use of the standard ETT is the lower overall test accuracy for the identification

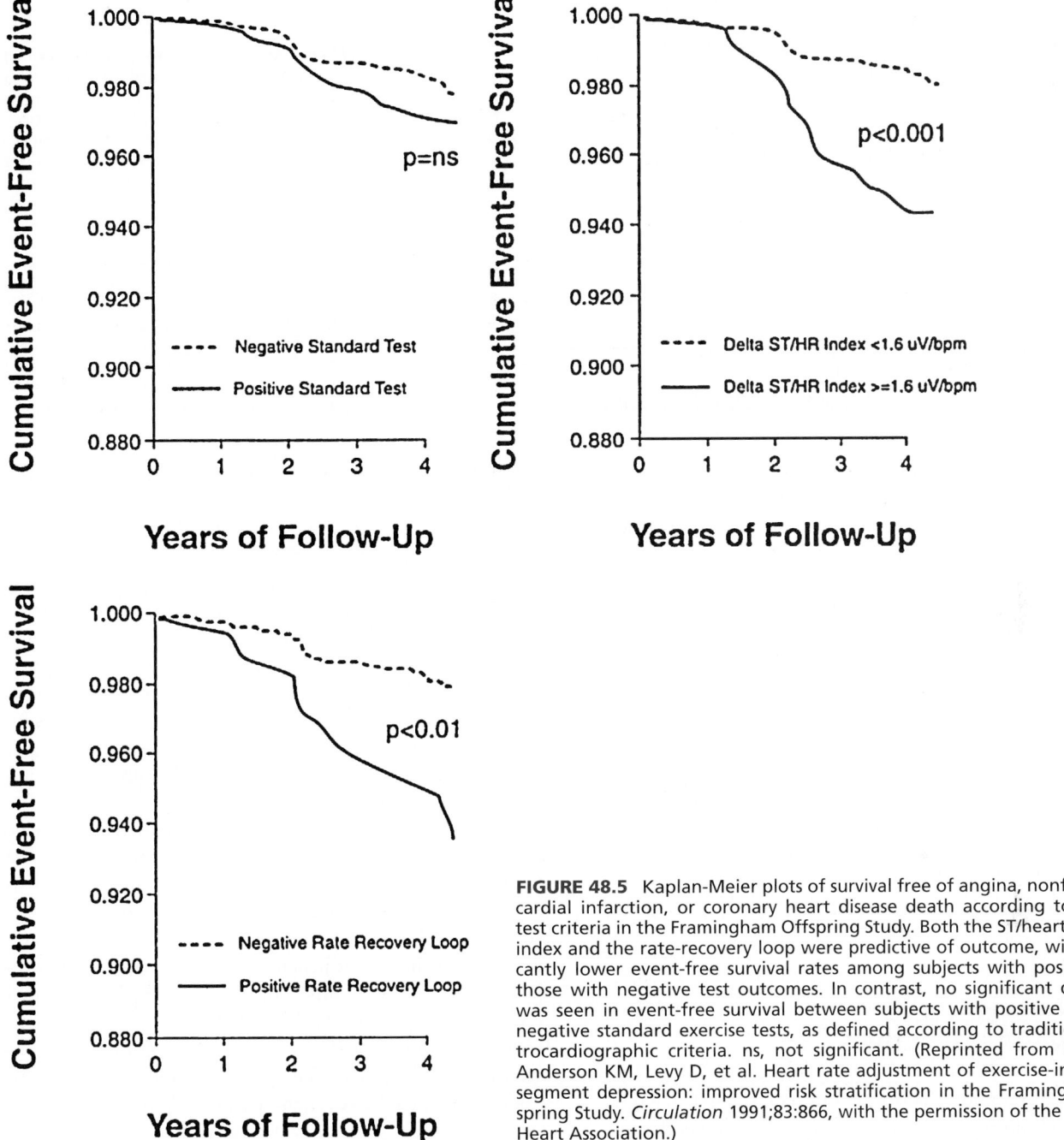

FIGURE 48.5 Kaplan-Meier plots of survival free of angina, nonfatal myocardial infarction, or coronary heart disease death according to exercise test criteria in the Framingham Offspring Study. Both the ST/heart rate (HR) index and the rate-recovery loop were predictive of outcome, with significantly lower event-free survival rates among subjects with positive than those with negative test outcomes. In contrast, no significant difference was seen in event-free survival between subjects with positive and with negative standard exercise tests, as defined according to traditional electrocardiographic criteria. ns, not significant. (Reprinted from Okin PM, Anderson KM, Levy D, et al. Heart rate adjustment of exercise-induced ST segment depression: improved risk stratification in the Framingham Offspring Study. *Circulation* 1991;83:866, with the permission of the American Heart Association.)

of coronary artery disease in women compared with that in men. However, it remains unclear whether the decreased test performance among women is a result of lower test sensitivity or of lower specificity. In a large subgroup of men and women from the Coronary Artery Survival Study who were matched for age, prevalence, and severity of coronary artery disease (99), no significant difference was seen in test sensitivity between women and men (76% vs. 78%), but specificity was significantly lower among women (64% vs. 73%). Barolsky and associates (100) reported similarly lower specificities when the test was used for women com-

pared with its use for men (68% vs. 89%), with no significant gender differences in sensitivity (60% vs. 65%). However, when patients taking digitalis preparations were excluded from these analyses, standard ST-segment depression criteria had identical 95% specificity but lower sensitivity with use for women than with use for men (50% vs. 64%). We have found similar differences in sensitivity of standard test criteria between women and men (51% vs. 67%), with matched specificities of 96% (23). Morise and colleagues (85) found lower overall test accuracy among women, which was the result of a combination of lower

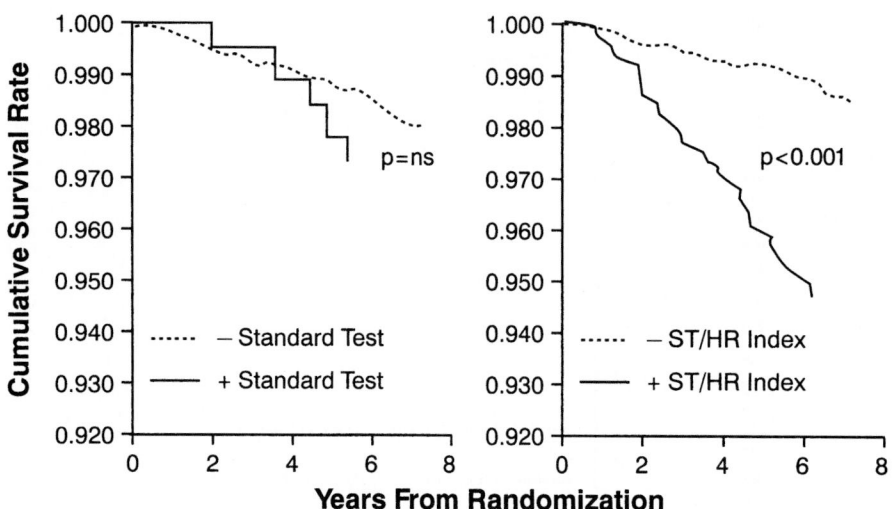

FIGURE 48.6 Kaplan-Meier plots of cumulative survival according to exercise test criteria in 5,940 asymptomatic men from the usual-care arm of the Multiple Risk Factor Intervention Trial. An abnormal ST/heart rate (HR) index identified a group of men with a significantly lower 7-year survival rate. In contrast, no significant difference was seen in survival rates between men with positive and with negative standard exercise test responses. ns, not significant. (Reprinted from Okin PM, Grandits G, Rautaharju P, et al. Prognostic value of heart rate adjustment of exercise-induced ST segment depression in the Multiple Risk Factor Intervention Trial. *J Am Coll Cardiol* 1996;27:1437, with the permission of Elsevier Science, Inc.)

sensitivity and specificity associated with use for women than that associated with use for men. ⚡ j11

Independent of these findings, adjustment or correction of ST depression by HR clearly improves test performance in women (23,68,101). In a study of 620 patients (23), we found that, compared with use of non-gender-specific test criteria in both sexes, use of gender-specific test criteria with high specificity improved sensitivity of the ST/HR slope for the identification of coronary artery disease in women from 84% to 91%, with no decrease in sensitivity in men. Compared with standard criteria, the increase in sensitivity provided by HR adjustment was significantly greater among women than among men, both for the detection of any coronary obstruction (40% vs. 21%) and for the identification of three-vessel coronary artery disease (50% vs. 9%) (*e*Fig. 48.6.1). Thus, at the present time, we recommend use of HR-adjusted criteria for improved test accuracy in women.

CONTROVERSIES AND PERSONAL PERSPECTIVES

Although most studies performed to date suggest that HR adjustment improves performance of ST-segment depression criteria in diagnosis of coronary artery disease, some controversy remains (45,53). Initial reports from England reporting perfect test accuracy for the ST/HR slope (58) were met with well-deserved skepticism. These studies and other early reports documenting the expected imperfect performance of this technique severely hindered acceptance of HR adjustment of ST-segment depression, as did more recent studies that reported no improvement in sensitivity with use of the simple ST/HR index (53). However, these studies did not reproduce the methods previously used, and it has subsequently been shown that improved accuracy of HR-adjusted methods is strongly dependent on exercise protocol, number of ECG leads, the time of ST-segment

measurement relative to the , and the precision and accuracy of ST-segment measurement (44,45,51,54,71). Recent reports have demonstrated that HR adjustment improves risk stratification compared with standard test criteria in many different studies from various other centers (22,95,97), further highlighting the utility of these methods. Although final acceptance of these methods will require even further study in clinically more diverse populations, it should be emphasized that no study has demonstrated *lower* sensitivity of HR-adjusted ST depression criteria compared with standard test criteria, and numerous manufacturers have incorporated ST/HR slope calculation into their clinical ETT systems (54).

The diagnostic utility of the ETT in patients who have some resting ECG abnormalities and in patients who are receiving digoxin is variable, so caution must be used in applying ST-segment depression criteria under these circumstances. We have found that the high sensitivity and specificity of the HR-adjusted ST-segment depression criteria appear to be maintained in patients who have isolated ST-segment depression and in whom minor intraventricular conduction delays are seen on the resting ECG. In contrast, we have observed that administration of digoxin can produce marked ST-segment depression during exercise, even in healthy subjects with normal results of resting ECGs who have normal results of ETTs during exercise while they are not receiving digoxin. However, we do not have enough data to assess the performance of these criteria in patients with left ventricular hypertrophy (demonstrated by ECG or echocardiography); ongoing studies will help to address this gap in our knowledge. As a consequence, at the present time I would advocate the use of imaging modalities in conjunction with ECG criteria in diagnosis for patients who have left ventricular hypertrophy and patients who are receiving digitalis preparations.

My own perspective is that exercise ECG is not optimally used in current practice. In large part because of limited confidence in the accuracy of the simple ETT, the

THE FUTURE

The development of new ECG criteria that have increased sensitivity at high specificity based on precise computer-based measurements is essential to improving the performance of the ETT. The increased accuracy seen with incorporation of measures of chronotropic incompetence in analysis of the ETT (24,25) suggests that further improvements in test performance may be achievable with better adjustment of ST-segment depression for HR changes that occur with exercise. Additional refinements in the ETT may be achieved by the combination of HR-adjusted ST-segment depression criteria with less-expensive imaging modalities, such as stress echocardiography, to increase accuracy and localize ischemia. Novel and interesting approaches to ETT analysis, based on examination of ECG findings that are distinct from the ST segment itself, also hold promise. These include measures of amplitude, duration, and frequency content of the QRS complex and measures of duration and dispersion of repolarization during exercise. Development and further refinement of computerized methods are needed before many of these new approaches can be adequately evaluated and used in clinical practice.

number of nuclear and echocardiographic imaging stress tests performed in the United States has increased dramatically. Although these methods provide important localizing information and are clearly indicated in situations in which performance of the exercise ECG is known to be poor, I believe that imaging stress tests are overused for the routine assessment of patients who have known or suspected coronary artery disease. It is also clear that exercise testing in general is inappropriately applied in large numbers of low-risk patients who undergo screening stress tests as part of annual physical examinations. The appropriate application of Bayesian analysis to these populations demonstrates that the large number of false-positive test responses (regardless of the test used) is a consequence of the extremely low pretest likelihood of disease and leads to further noninvasive and invasive testing at substantial cost and some risk to these patients. A better understanding of the limitations and indications of exercise testing and application of the more accurate HR-adjusted ST-segment depression criteria hold promise for improvement of the use and accuracy of the exercise ECG in clinical practice.

REFERENCES

1. Feil H, Seigel M. Electrocardiographic changes during attacks of angina pectoris. *Am J Med Sci* 1928;175:225.
2. Hellerstein HK, Katz L. The electrical effects of injury at various myocardial locations. *Am Heart J* 1948;36:184.
3. Master AM, Oppenheimer EJ. A simple exercise tolerance test for circulatory efficiency with standard tables for normal individuals. *Am J Med Sci* 1929;177:223.
4. Master AM, Jaffe HL. The electrocardiographic changes after exercise in angina pectoris. *J Mt Sinai Hosp* 1941;7:629.
5. Wood FC, Wolferth CC. Angina pectoris: the clinical and electrocardiographic phenomena of the attack and their comparison with the effects of experimental temporary coronary occlusion. *Arch Intern Med* 1931;47:339.
6. Katz I, Landt H. Effect of standardized exercise on the four-lead electrocardiogram: its value in the study of coronary disease. *Am J Med Sci* 1935;189:346.
7. Riseman JEF, Waller J, Brown M. The electrocardiogram during attacks of angina pectoris: its characteristics and diagnostic significance. *Am Heart J* 1940;19:683.
8. Yu PNG, Soffer A. Studies of electrocardiographic changes during exercise (modified double two-step test). *Circulation* 1952;6:183.
9. Bruce RA. Evaluation of functional capacity and exercise tolerance of cardiac patients. *Mod Concepts Cardiovasc Dis* 1956;25:321.
10. Goldschlager N, Selzer A, Cohn K. Treadmill stress tests as indicators of the presence and severity of coronary artery disease. *Ann Intern Med* 1976;85:277.
11. Chaitman BR, Bourassa MG, Wagniart P, et al. Improved efficiency of treadmill exercise testing using a multiple lead ECG system and basic hemodynamic response. *Circulation* 1978;57:71.
12. Froelicher VF, Thomas MM, Pillow C, et al. Epidemiologic study of asymptomatic men screened by maximal treadmill testing for latent coronary artery disease. *Am J Cardiol* 1974;34:770.
13. Bruce RA, Hossack KF, DeRouen TA, et al. Enhanced risk assessment for primary coronary heart disease events by maximal exercise testing: 10 years experience of the Seattle Heart Watch Study. *J Am Coll Cardiol* 1983;2:565.
14. Sheffield LT, Holt JH, Lester FM, et al. On-line analysis of the exercise electrocardiogram. *Circulation* 1969;40:935.
15. Simoons ML. Optimal measurements for detection of coronary artery disease by exercise electrocardiography. *Comput Biomed Res* 1977;10:483.
16. Hollenberg M, Zoltick JM, Go M, et al. Comparison of a quantitative treadmill score with standard electrocardiographic criteria in screening asymptomatic young men for coronary artery disease. *N Engl J Med* 1985;313:600.
17. Kligfield P, Okin PM. Evolution of the exercise electrocardiogram. *Am J Cardiol* 1994;73:1209.
18. Rifkin RD, Hood WB Jr. Bayesian analysis of electrocardiographic exercise stress testing. *N Engl J Med* 1977;297:681–686.

19. Diamond GA, Forrester JS. Analysis of probability as an aid in the clinical diagnosis of coronary artery disease. *N Engl J Med* 1979;300:1350.

20. Kligfield P, Ameisen O, Okin PM. Heart rate adjustment of ST segment depression for improved detection of coronary artery disease. *Circulation* 1989;79:245.

21. Okin PM, Ameisen O, Kligfield P. Recovery phase patterns of ST segment depression in the heart rate domain: identification of coronary artery disease by the rate recovery loop. *Circulation* 1989;80:533.

22. Okin PM, Anderson KM, Levy D, et al. Heart rate adjustment of exercise-induced ST segment depression: improved risk stratification in the Framingham Offspring Study. *Circulation* 1991;83:866.

23. Okin PM, Kligfield P. Gender-specific criteria and performance of the exercise electrocardiogram. *Circulation* 1995;92:1209.

23a. Lehtinen R, Sievänen H, Viik J, et al. Accurate detection of coronary artery disease by integrated analysis of the ST segment/heart rate patterns during the exercise and recovery phase of the exercise electrocardiography test. *Am J Cardiol* 1996;78:1002.

24. Lauer MS, Okin PM, Larson MG, et al. Impaired heart rate response to graded exercise: prognostic implications of chronotropic incompetence in the Framingham Heart Study. *Circulation* 1996;93:1520.

24a. Lauer MS, Francis GS, Okin PM, et al. Impaired chronotropic response to exercise as a predictor of mortality. *JAMA* 1999;281:524.

25. Okin PM, Lauer MS, Kligfield P. Chronotropic response to exercise: improved performance of ST segment depression criteria after adjustment for heart rate reserve. *Circulation* 1996;94:3226.

25a. Cole CR, Blackstone EH, Pashkow FJ, et al. Heart rate recovery immediately after exercise as a predictor of mortality. *N Engl J Med* 1999;341:1351.

26. Mark DB, Shaw L, Harrell FE, et al. Prognostic value of a treadmill exercise score in outpatients with suspected coronary artery disease. *N Engl J Med* 1991;325:849.

27. Michaelides A, Ryan J, Van Fossen D, et al. Exercise-induced QRS prolongation in patients with coronary artery disease: a marker of myocardial ischemia. *Am Heart J* 1993;126:1320.

27a. Stoletniy LN, Pai RG. Value of QT dispersion in interpretation of the exercise stress test in women. *Circulation* 1997;96:904.

28. Guyton RA, McClenathan JH, Newman GE, et al. Significance of subendocardial ST segment elevation caused by coronary stenosis in the dog. *Am J Cardiol* 1977;40:373.

29. Holland RP, Brooks H. Precordial and epicardial surface potentials during myocardial ischemia in the pig: a theoretical and experimental analysis of the TQ and ST segments. *Circ Res* 1975;37:471.

30. Holland RP, Brooks H. TQ-ST segment mapping: critical review and analysis of current concepts. *Am J Cardiol* 1977;40:110.

31. Mirvis DM, Ramanathan KB, Wilson JL. Regional blood flow correlates of ST segment depression in tachycardia-induced myocardial ischemia. *Circulation* 1986;73:365.

32. Wilson RF, Marcus ML, Christensen BV, et al. Accuracy of exercise electrocardiography in detecting physiologically significant coronary arterial lesions. *Circulation* 1991;83:412.

33. Okin PM, Kligfield P. Solid angle theory and heart rate adjustment of ST segment depression for the identification and quantification of coronary artery disease. *Am Heart J* 1994;127:658.

34. Kitamura K, Jorgensen CR, Gobel FL, et al. Hemodynamic correlates of myocardial oxygen consumption during upright exercise. *J Appl Physiol* 1972;32:516.

35. Hoffman JIE. Maximal coronary flow and the concept of coronary vascular reserve. *Circulation* 1984;70:153.

36. Lipscomb K, Hooten S. Effect of stenotic dimensions and blood flow on the hemodynamic significance of model coronary arterial stenoses. *Am J Cardiol* 1978;42:781.

37. Gordon JB, Ganz P, Nabel EG, et al. Atherosclerosis influences the vasomotor response of epicardial coronary arteries to exercise. *J Clin Invest* 1989;83:1946.

38. Nabel EG, Selwyn AP, Ganz P. Paradoxical narrowing of atherosclerotic coronary arteries induced by increases in heart rate. *Circulation* 1990;81:850.

39. Gibbons RJ, Balady GJ, Beasley JW, et al. ACC/AHA guidelines for exercise testing: executive summary. A report of the American College of Cardiology/American Heart Association Task Force on Practice Guidelines (Committee on Exercise Testing). *Circulation* 1997;96:345.

40. Fletcher GF, Balady G, Froelicher VF, et al. Exercise standards: a statement for healthcare professionals from the American Heart Association. *Circulation* 1995;91:580.

41. Pina IL, Balady GJ, Hanson P, et al. Guidelines for clinical exercise testing laboratories: a statement for healthcare professionals from the committee on exercise and rehabilitation, American Heart Association. *Circulation* 1995;91:912.

42. Mason RE, Likar I. A new system of multiple lead exercise electrocardiography. *Am Heart J* 1966;71:196.

43. Bruce RA, Blackmon JR, Jones JW, Strait G. Exercise testing in adult normal subjects and cardiac patients. *Pediatrics* 1963;32[Suppl]:742.

44. Okin PM, Ameisen O, Kligfield P. A modified treadmill protocol for computer-assisted analysis of the ST segment/heart rate slope: methods and reproducibility. *J Electrocardiol* 1986;19:311.

45. Okin PM, Kligfield P. Heart rate adjustment of ST depression and performance of the exercise electrocardiogram: a critical evaluation. *J Am Coll Cardiol* 1995;25:1726.

45a. Michaelides AP, Psomadaki ZD, Dilaveris PE, et al. Improved detection of coronary artery disease by exercise electrocardiography with the use of right precordial leads. *N Engl J Med* 1999;340:340.

46. Froelicher VF, Perdue S, Pewen W, et al. Application of meta-analysis using an electronic spread sheet to exercise testing in patients after myocardial infarction. *Am J Med* 1987;83:1045.

47. Balady GJ, Leitschuh ML, Jacobs AK, et al. Safety and clinical use of exercise testing one to three days after percutaneous transluminal angioplasty. *Am J Cardiol* 1992;69:1259.

48. Laarman G, Luitjen HE, van Zeyl LG, et al. Assessment of silent restenosis and long-term follow-up after successful angioplasty in single vessel coronary artery disease: the value of quantitative exercise electrocardiography and

quantitative coronary angiography. *J Am Coll Cardiol* 1990;16:578.

49. Samuels B, Schumann J, Kiat H, et al. Acute stent thrombosis associated with exercise testing after successful percutaneous transluminal coronary angioplasty. *Am Heart J* 1995;130:1120.

50. Simoons ML, Hugenholtz PG. Gradual changes of ECG waveform during and after exercise in normal subjects. *Circulation* 1975;52:570.

51. Okin PM, Bergman G, Kligfield P. Effect of ST segment measurement point on performance of standard and heart rate–adjusted ST segment criteria for the identification of coronary artery disease. *Circulation* 1991;84:57.

52. Lachterman B, Lehmann KG, Abrahamson D, et al. Recovery only ST-segment depression and the predictive accuracy of the exercise test. *Ann Intern Med* 1990;112:11.

53. Lachterman B, Lehmann KG, Detrano R, et al. Comparison of ST segment/heart rate index to standard ST criteria for analysis of exercise electrocardiogram. *Circulation* 1990;82:44.

54. Okin PM, Kligfield P. Computer-based implementation of the ST segment/heart rate slope. *Am J Cardiol* 1989;64:926.

55. Gianrossi R, Detrano R, Mulvihill D, et al. Exercise-induced ST depression in the diagnosis of coronary artery disease: a meta analysis. *Circulation* 1989;80:87.

56. Rijneke RD, Ascoop CA, Talmon JL. Clinical significance of upsloping ST segments in exercise electrocardiography. *Circulation* 1980;61:671.

57. Ascoop CA, Distelbrink CA, DeLong P. Clinical value of quantitative analysis of ST slope during exercise. *Br Heart J* 1977;39:212.

58. Elamin MS, Mary DA, Smith DR, et al. Prediction of severity of coronary artery disease using slope of submaximal ST segment/heart rate relationship. *Cardiovasc Res* 1980;14:681.

59. Berenyi I, Hajduczki S, Baszoremenyi E. Quantitative evaluation of exercise-induced ST segment depression for estimation of degree of coronary artery disease. *Eur Heart J* 1984;5:289.

60. Detrano R, Salcedo E, Passalaqua M, et al. Exercise electrocardiographic variables: a critical appraisal. *J Am Coll Cardiol* 1986;8:836.

61. Detry JMR, Bruce RA. Effects of nitroglycerin on maximal oxygen intake and exercise electrocardiogram in coronary heart disease. *Circulation* 1971;43:155.

62. Detry JMR, Piette F, Brasseur LA. Hemodynamic determinants of exercise ST segment depression in coronary patients. *Circulation* 1970;42:593.

63. Parker JO, Chiong MA, West RO, et al. Sequential alterations in myocardial lactate metabolism, ST segments, and left ventricular function during angina induced by atrial pacing. *Circulation* 1969;40:113.

64. Tomoike H, Franklin D, McKown D, et al. Regional myocardial dysfunction and hemodynamic abnormalities during strenuous exercise in dogs. *Circ Res* 1978;42:487.

65. Mark DB, Hlatky MA, Harrell FE, et al. Exercise treadmill score for predicting prognosis in coronary artery disease. *Ann Intern Med* 1987;106:793.

66. Froelicher VF, Lehmann KG, Thomas R, et al. The electrocardiographic stress test in a population with reduced workup bias: diagnostic performance, computerized interpretation, and multivariable prediction. *Ann Intern Med* 1998;1:965.

67. Do D, West JA, Morise A, et al. A consensus approach to diagnosing coronary artery disease based on clinical and exercise test data. *Chest* 1997;111:1742.

68. Robert AR, Melin JA, Detry JMR. Logistic discriminant analysis improves diagnostic accuracy of exercise testing for coronary artery disease in women. *Circulation* 1991;83:1202.

69. Gordon DJ, Ekelund LG, Karon JM, et al. Predictive value of the exercise tolerance test for mortality in North American men: the Lipid Research Clinics Mortality Follow-up Study. *Circulation* 1986;74:252.

70. Rautaharju PM, Prineas RJ, Eifler WJ, et al. Prognostic value of exercise electrocardiogram in men at high risk of future coronary heart disease: Multiple Risk Factor Intervention Trial experience. *J Am Coll Cardiol* 1986;8:1.

71. Okin PM, Bergman G, Kligfield P. Measurement variables for optimal performance of the ST integral. *J Am Coll Cardiol* 1993;22:168.

72. Bonoris PE, Greenberg PS, Christison GW, Castellanet MJ, et al. Evaluation of R wave changes vs. ST segment depression in stress testing. *Circulation* 1978;57:904.

73. de Caprio L, Cuomo S, Vigorito C, et al. Influence of heart rate on exercise-induced R-wave amplitude changes in coronary patients and normal subjects. *Am Heart J* 1984;107:61.

74. Pettersson J, Pahlm O, Edenbrandt L, et al. Changes in high-frequency QRS components are more sensitive than ST-segment deviation for detecting acute coronary occlusion. *J Am Coll Cardiol* 2000;36:1827.

75. Brenner SJ, Pashkow FJ, Harvey SA, et al. Chronotropic response to exercise predicts angiographic severity in patients with suspected or stable coronary artery disease. *Am J Cardiol* 1995;76:1228.

76. Ellestad MH, Wan MKC. Predictive implications of stress testing: follow-up of 2700 subjects after maximal treadmill stress testing. *Circulation* 1975;51:363.

76a. Lauer MS, Mehta R, Pashkow FJ, et al. Association of chronotropic incompetence with echocardiographic ischemia and prognosis. *J Am Coll Cardiol* 1998;32:1280.

76b. Cole CR, Foody JM, Blackstone EH, et al. Heart rate recovery after submaximal exercise testing as a predictor of mortality in a cardiovascularly healthy cohort. *Ann Intern Med* 2000;132:552.

76c. Nishime EO, Cole CR, Blackstone EH, et al. Heart rate recovery and treadmill exercise score as predictors of mortality in patients referred for exercise ECG. *JAMA* 2000;284:1392.

77. Lauer MS, Levy D, Anderson KM, et al. Is there a relationship between exercise systolic blood pressure response and left ventricular mass? The Framingham Heart Study. *Ann Intern Med* 1992;116:203.

78. Lauer MS, Pashkow FJ, Harvey SA, et al. Angiographic and prognostic implications of an exaggerated exercise systolic blood pressure response and rest systolic blood pressure in adults undergoing evaluation for suspected coronary artery disease. *J Am Coll Cardiol* 1995;26:1630.

79. Wray Amon K, Richards KL, Crawford MH. Usefulness of

the postexercise response to systolic blood pressure in the diagnosis of coronary artery disease. *Circulation* 1984;70:951.

80. Acanfora D, De Caprio L, Cuomo S, et al. Diagnostic value of the ratio of recovery systolic blood pressure to peak exercise systolic blood pressure for the detection of coronary artery disease. *Circulation* 1988;77:1306.

81. Udall JA, Ellestad MH. Predictive implications of ventricular premature contractions associated with treadmill stress testing: a follow-up of 6,500 patients after maximal treadmill stress testing. *Circulation* 1977;56:985.

82. Yang JC, Wesley RC, Froelicher VF. Ventricular tachycardia during routine treadmill testing. *Arch Intern Med* 1991;151:349.

83. Jaffe MD. Effect of oestrogens on postexercise electrocardiograms. *Br Heart J* 1977;38:1299.

84. Clark PI, Glasser SP, Lyman GH, et al. Relation of results of exercise stress tests in young women to phases of the menstrual cycle. *Am J Cardiol* 1988;61:197.

85. Morise AP, Dalal JN, Duval RD. Value of a simple measure of estrogen status for improving the diagnosis of coronary artery disease in women. *Am J Med* 1993;94:491.

86. Ransohoff DF, Feinstein AR. Problems of spectrum and bias in evaluating the efficacy of diagnostic test. *N Engl J Med* 1978;299:926.

87. Hlatky MA, Pryor DB, Harrell FE, et al. Factors affecting sensitivity and specificity of exercise electrocardiography. *Am J Med* 1984;77:64.

88. Okin PM, Kligfield P. Population selection and performance of the exercise ECG for the identification of coronary artery disease. *Am Heart J* 1994;127:296.

89. Detrano R, Gianrossi R, Mulvihill D, et al. Exercise-induced ST segment depression in the diagnosis of multivessel coronary artery disease: a meta analysis. *J Am Coll Cardiol* 1989;14:1501.

89a. Shaw LJ, Peterson ED, Kesler KL, et al. Use of a prognostic treadmill score in identifying coronary disease subgroups. *Circulation* 1998;98:1622.

89b. Do D, Morise A, Atwood AE, et al. An agreement approach to predict severe angiographic coronary artery disease with clinical and exercise test data. *Am Heart J* 1997;134:672.

90. Okin PM, Kligfield P, Ameisen O, et al. Identification of anatomically extensive coronary artery disease by the exercise electrocardiographic ST segment/heart rate slope. *Am Heart J* 1988;115:1002.

91. Finkelhor RS, Newhouse KE, Vrobel TR, et al. The ST segment/heart rate slope as a predictor of coronary artery disease: comparison with quantitative thallium imaging and conventional ST segment criteria. *Am Heart J* 1986;112:296.

92. Kligfield P, Okin PM, Ameisen O, et al. Correlation of the exercise ST/HR slope in stable angina pectoris with anatomic and radionuclide cineangiographic findings. *Am J Cardiol* 1985;56:418.

93. Epstein SE, Quyyumi AA, Bonow RO. Sudden cardiac death without warning: possible mechanisms and implications for screening asymptomatic populations. *N Engl J Med* 1989;321:320.

94. Detrano R, Froelicher VF. A logical approach to screening for coronary artery disease. *Ann Intern Med* 1987;106:846.

95. Okin PM, Grandits G, Rautaharju P, et al. Prognostic value of heart rate adjustment of exercise-induced ST segment depression in the Multiple Risk Factor Intervention Trial. *J Am Coll Cardiol* 1996;27:1437.

95a. Okin PM, Prineas RJ, Grandits G, et al. Heart rate adjustment of exercise-induced ST segment depression identifies men who benefit from a risk factor reduction program. *Circulation* 1997;96:2899.

96. Weiner DA, Ryan TJ, McCabe CH, et al. Prognostic importance of a clinical profile and exercise test in medically treated patients with coronary artery disease. *J Am Coll Cardiol* 1984;3:772.

96a. Kwok JM, Miller TD, Christian TF, et al. Prognostic value of a treadmill exercise score in symptomatic patients with nonspecific ST-T abnormalities on resting ECG. *JAMA* 1999;282:1047.

97. Shaw LJ, Kesler KL, DeLong ER, et al. Is the prognostic value of ST depression improved with heart rate adjustment? *Circulation* 1996;94(1):567.

98. Chaitman BR, McMahon RP, Terrin M, et al. Impact of treatment strategy on predischarge exercise test in the Thrombolysis in Myocardial Infarction (TIMI) II Trial. *Am J Cardiol* 1993;71:131.

99. Weiner DA, Ryan TJ, McCabe CH, et al. Exercise stress testing: correlations among history of angina, ST segment response and prevalence of coronary artery disease in the Coronary Artery Surgery Study (CASS). *N Engl J Med* 1979;301:230.

100. Barolsky SM, Gilbert CA, Faruqui A, et al. Differences in electrocardiographic response to exercise of women and men: a non-Bayesian factor. *Circulation* 1979;60:1021.

101. Deckers JW, Rensing BJ, Tijssen JG, et al. A comparison of methods of analysing exercise tests for diagnosis of coronary artery disease. *Br Heart J* 1989;62:438.

TRANSTHORACIC ECHOCARDIOGRAPHY

REBECCA L. SMITH
JAMES D. THOMAS

▼ **ADDITIONAL ELECTRONIC TOPICS**

INTRODUCTION AND HISTORY

Echocardiography (cardiac ultrasound) is the most powerful diagnostic tool in cardiology. Although technically demanding, its diagnostic accuracy, cost effectiveness, availability, and noninvasive nature have made it the largest cardiovascular expense item in the Medicare budget. ▼ j23

MODALITIES OF ECHOCARDIOGRAPHY

M-mode echocardiography was the first form of cardiac ultrasound (Fig. 49.1), in which a single beam is directed toward the heart and reflected signals are displayed on a strip chart or oscillograph at high data rates (>1,000 Hz in early machines, 200 Hz in most contemporary machines). Two-dimensional echocardiography (Fig. 49.2) is created by sweeping an ultrasound beam back and forth through an arc either mechanically or by phased-array transducer. Minimizing the depth of interrogation or the width of the sector scan can enhance the frame rate. Structural resolution is dependent on imaging depth and transducer frequency. Transducer focus improves resolution in the focal zone, at the expense of greater divergence for deeper structures.

ECHOCARDIOGRAPHIC EVALUATION OF THE CARDIAC CHAMBERS

Left Ventricle

Left ventricular (LV) evaluation is probably the single most important clinical application of echocardiography. A com-

---

R. L. Smith: Department of Cardiovascular Medicine, The Cleveland Clinic Foundation, Cleveland Ohio

J. D. Thomas: Department of Cardiovascular Imaging, The Cleveland Clinic Foundation, Cleveland, Ohio

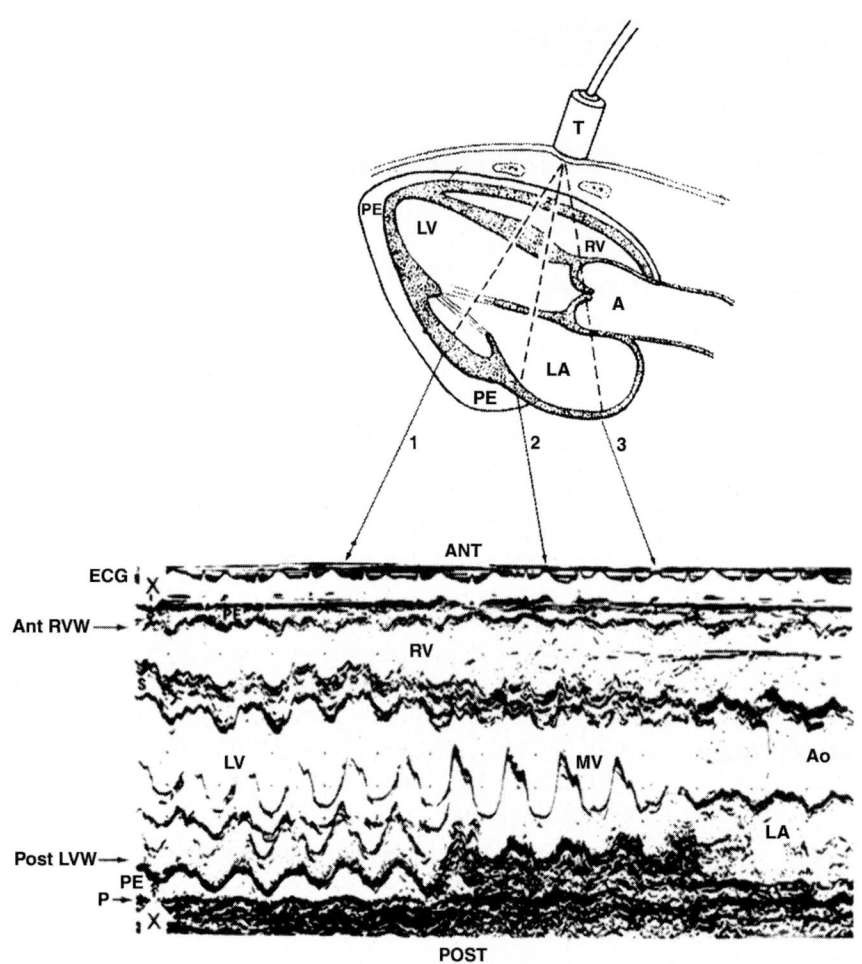

FIGURE 49.1 M-mode echocardiogram displaying motion along a single scan line within the heart. Here, the transducer (T) is swept from the left ventricular level (*left side of scan*) to the mitral valve level (*middle*) and up to the left atrial level (*right*). A, aorta; Ao, aorta; ANT, anterior; ECG, electrocardiogram; LA, left atrium; LV, left ventricle; MV, mitral valve; P, pericardium; PE, pericardial effusion; POST, posterior; RV, right ventricle; RVW, right ventricular wall. (From Cheitlin MD, Sokolow M, McIlroy MB. *Clinical cardiology*, 6th ed. Norwalk, CT: Appleton & Lange, 1993, with permission.)

bined M-mode, two-dimensional, and Doppler evaluation of the LV can provide reliable information about overall systolic function, regional wall motion, and ventricular mass and geometry.

Evaluation of Global Systolic Function of the Left Ventricle

Reliable determinations of LV function require the qualitative and quantitative evaluation of images taken from several standard windows. Typically, the LV is first viewed in the parasternal long-axis and short-axis planes (Fig. 49.2). From these, M-mode tracings are generated. If quantitation of M-mode tracings is used clinically, the American Society of Echocardiography recommends obtaining these from the parasternal short axis in the two-dimensional M mode (12,13) (Fig. 49.3).

M-Mode Evaluation

Standard M-mode measurements are shown in Figure 49.4. Fractional shortening by M mode is given by left ventricular diameter at end diastole ($LVED_d$) – left ventricular diameter at end systole ($LVES_d$)/$LVED_d$ where ED_d is the LV minor

axis in diastole and ES_d in systole. Normally, fractional shortening is approximately 50% and is considered clearly abnormal when it falls below 30% (8,14). Another M-mode measurement is the E-point septal separation (15,16) (a marker of LV dysfunction when it exceeds 7 mm).

A further M-mode guide to overall LV function is aortic root motion, largely reflecting the atrial filling curve (17,18). With normal cardiac output, change in atrial volume moves the aorta anteriorly approximately 14 mm, but with low stroke volume, the aorta barely moves (19). This also yields information about diastolic function. In youth, most atrial emptying occurs early in diastole, with atrial contraction accounting for less than 30% of the total. Hypertrophy and aging slow early passive relaxation, and therefore the majority (up to 70%) of emptying occurs late in diastole at the time of atrial contraction. Finally, aortic valve (AV) opening yields useful information about LV function, opening fully when stroke volume is normal but incompletely when stroke volume falls.

Apical Window Imaging

After the parasternal images, the left ventricle is displayed along its long axis from the apical impulse location, with axial rotation of the transducer producing any number of long-axis

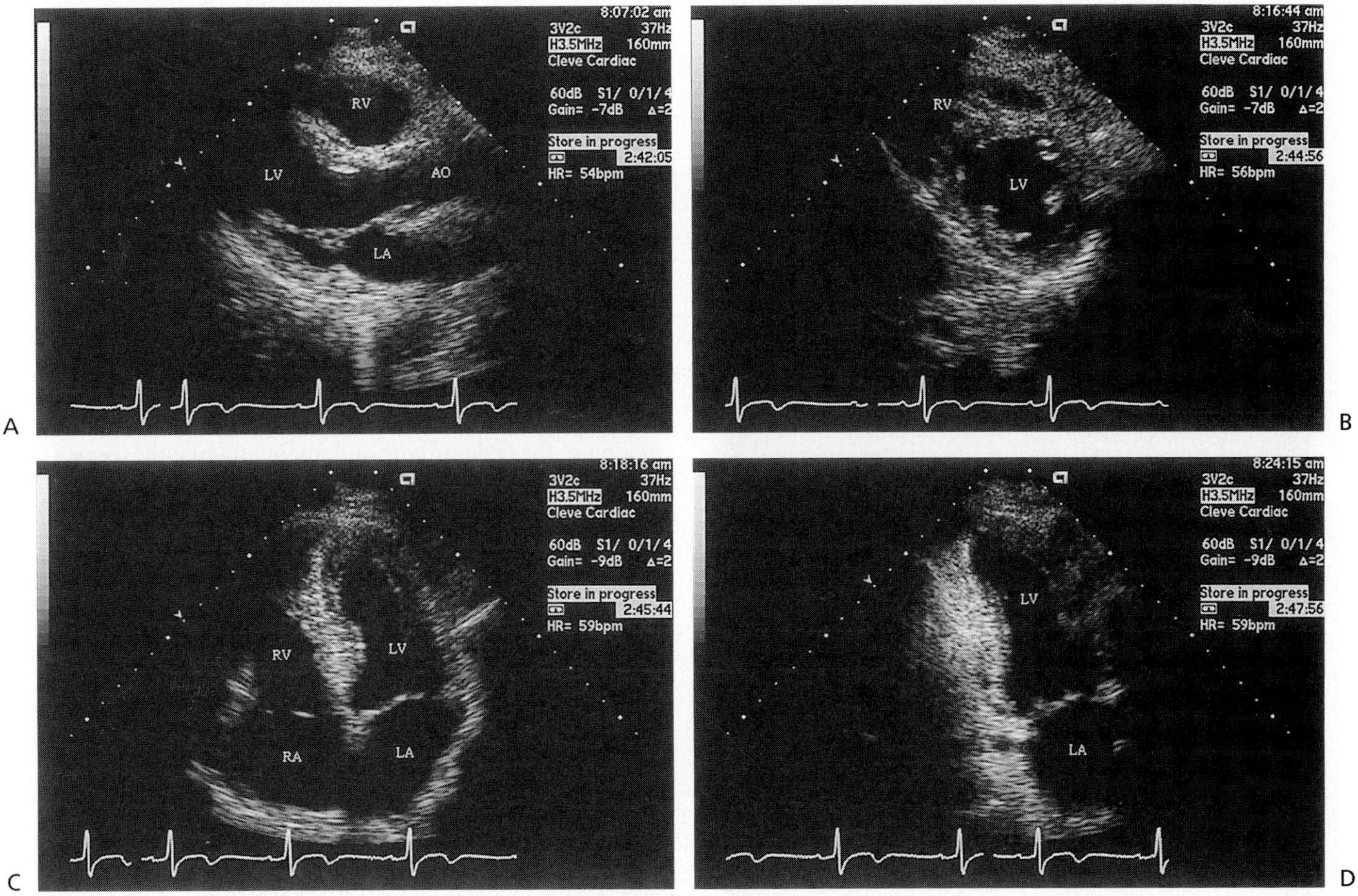

FIGURE 49.2 Two-dimensional echocardiography. Four standard views. **A:** Parasternal long axis. **B:** Parasternal short axis. **C:** Apical four chamber. **D:** Apical two chamber. AO, aorta; LA, left atrium; LV, left ventricle; RA, right atrium; RV, right ventricle.

views. However, the standard examination typically includes the apical four- and two-chamber views (orthogonal to each other, Fig. 49.2) and the apical long-axis view (20,21).

The four-chamber view (20) displays the midseptum and inferolateral LV wall and shows the right ventricle (RV) at its widest point, including the moderator band. At the cardiac base, the mitral and tricuspid valves (TVs) are shown, with the TV being displaced approximately 1 cm more apically than the MV by the membranous septum. The atria are shown partitioned by the interatrial septum. Posterior transducer angulation reveals the coronary sinus and papillary muscles. Anterior angulation shows the LV outflow tract. To enhance endocardial definition, ultrasonic contrast agents that cross the lungs intact (unlike agitated saline contrast) can be used. Because ultrasound energy can destroy these bubbles, intermittent insonification (e.g., once per cardiac cycle) permits the development of greater contrast effects in the myocardium and the cavity. Further contrast augmenta-

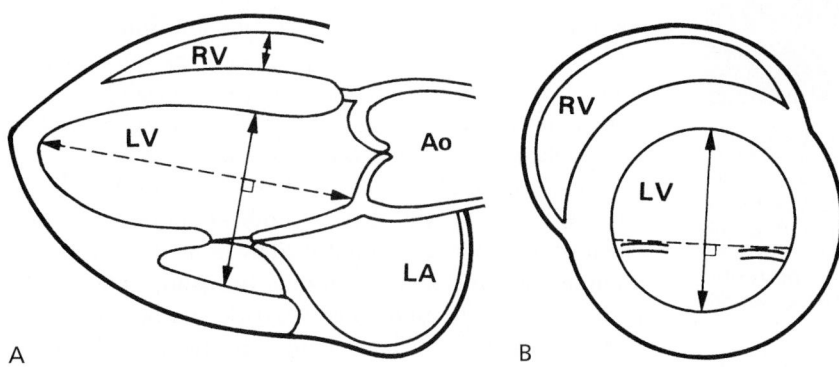

FIGURE 49.3 Quantitation of left ventricular size. Measurement sites recommended by the American Society of Echocardiography (12). **A:** Parasternal long-axis view. **B:** Parasternal short-axis view. Ao, aorta; LA, left atrium; LV, left ventricle; RV, right ventricle. (Reproduced with permission of the American Society of Echocardiography.)

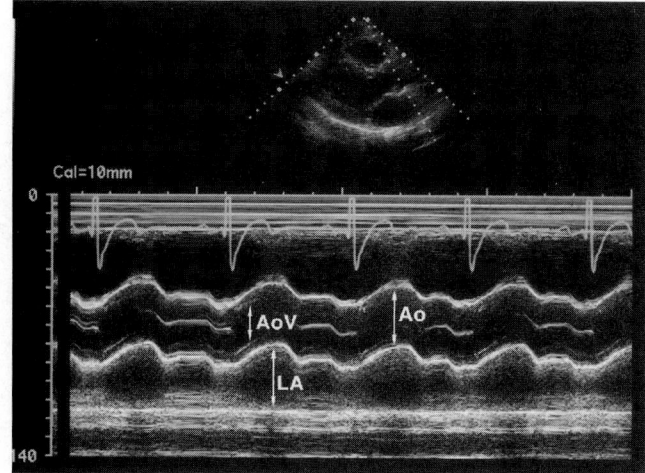

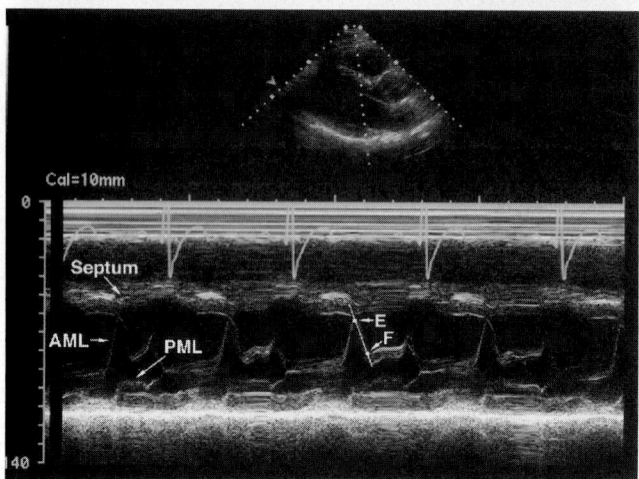

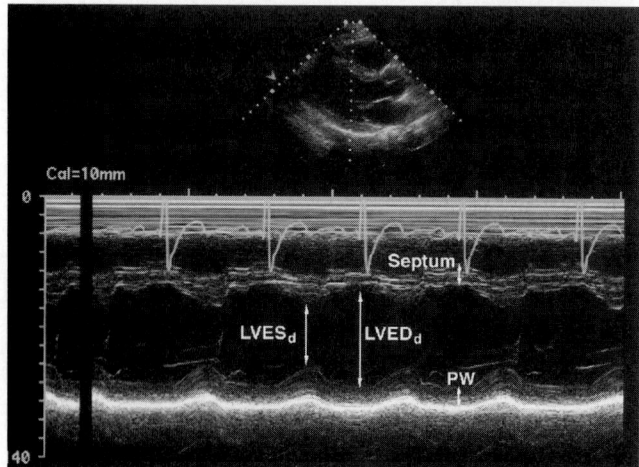

FIGURE 49.4 Standard measurements from M mode. Shown are sweeps at the aortic level **(A)**, mitral valve level **(B)**, and left ventricular level **(C)**. AML, anterior mitral leaflet; Ao, aortic root diameter; AoV, opening of aortic valve; EF, E to F slope (rate of closure of mitral valve); LA, end systolic left atrial diameter; LVED$_d$, left ventricular diameter at end diastole; LVES$_d$, left ventricular diameter at end systole; PML, posterior mitral leaflet; PW, posterior wall thickness; SEPTUM, septal thickness.

tion is gained by displaying the second harmonic of the transmitted ultrasound carrier frequency.

The shape of a healthy left ventricle is a truncated ellipsoid with the long axis roughly twice the length of the short axis. As the heart decompensates, it assumes a more globular shape (22) (*e*Fig. 49.4.1). Diastolic wall thickness is viewed in absolute terms (approximately 1 cm is normal, >1.2 cm is considered hypertrophied) and relative to LV cavity size, with a radius-thickness ratio that is typically about 2:1. The distribution of hypertrophy is important. In secondary hypertrophy (e.g., from hypertension or outflow obstruction), the increase in wall thickness is uniform or concentric, whereas it is typically confined to the septum in asymmetric hypertrophy. Regional LV function is assessed by looking for inward motion of the endocardium and, more importantly, segmental thickening. Myocardial texture is also informative. Scar formation results in a thin bright segment, and infiltrative disease yields increased reflectance in approximately half of such cases. Geometric uniformity is another useful feature and becomes important after infarction. LV remodeling in its extreme form involves an entire region in an aneurysm (*e*Fig. 49.4.2), which is distinguished from simple dysfunction by deformity throughout the cardiac cycle. Generally, all endocardial segments should move inward synchronously, with incoordinate contraction suggesting at least moderate LV dysfunction. However, it can also be seen with left bundle branch block (23) or RV pacing. Finally, the longitudinal motion of the heart can be observed by the descent of the cardiac base (annular plane) toward the nearly fixed cardiac apex (24). A decrease in this parameter is often the first sign of nascent cardiomyopathy.

Quantitation of Left Ventricular Function

Although automated methods of measurement have been developed for assessing LV function (25), the standard method remains manual border tracing (26–28). Although ejection fraction (EF) is commonly estimated by visual inspection, this is prone to error and interobserver variability.

M-mode measurements of LV function (29–32) are limited because they use a single LV short-axis dimension, generally assuming a long-axis–short-axis ratio of 2:1 to extrapolate information to three dimensions. Unfortunately, many pathologic states introduce regional asymmetry or alter the ratio toward unity. Because volume is a cube function of dimension, errors are compounded (26,33,34). In contrast, two-dimensional volumes and mass compare favorably to those that are obtained from angiography and autopsy, but only if care is taken to optimize data acquisition and analysis (12).

The best apical images are usually obtained with the patient lying in the left recumbent position. Image enhancement can be accomplished by using a mattress with a removable panel and positioning the sonographer to the patient's left. A foreshortened ventricle can be avoided by maximizing the visualized long axis. Because the heart

BY METHOD OF DISKS (MODIFIED SIMPSON'S RULE)

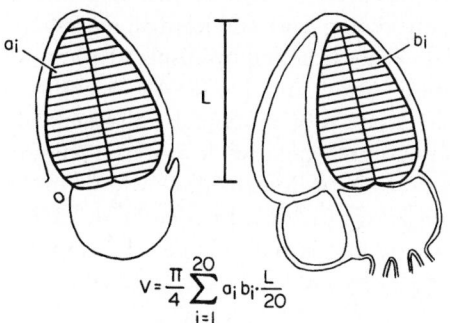

$$V = \frac{\pi}{4} \sum_{i=1}^{20} a_i\, b_i \cdot \frac{L}{20}$$

BY SINGLE PLANE AREA LENGTH

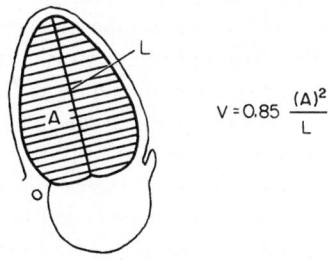

$$V = 0.85\, \frac{(A)^2}{L}$$

FIGURE 49.5 Left ventricular (LV) volume determination. The biplane method of disks (*upper panels*) requires orthogonal two- and four-chamber apical views and is more accurate in asymmetric hearts than the single-plane method shown below. In symmetric ventricles, the single-plane method is almost as accurate as the biplane one. [Reproduced with permission from the American Society of Echocardiography (26).]

moves with respiration, images should be obtained during unforced suspended expiration. ⚐ j24

The biplane method of disks (referred to less precisely as *modified Simpson's rule*) most closely predicts angiographic volumes (21,26–28). The single-plane area length is also suitable, provided that the ventricle is symmetric (35) (Fig. 49.5). These algorithms are applied to orthogonal apical two- and four-chamber views. The apical four-chamber view (21) should display the true LV apex, showing neither the aorta nor the coronary sinus while maximizing RV size. The two-chamber view should not include any portion of the RV, aorta, or right atrium (RA) (Fig. 49.2).

LV mass computed from two-dimensional images is more reproducible and anatomically rational than M-mode values but is still limited by relatively wide standard deviations (±35 g for 95% confidence intervals) (36,37). The truncated ellipsoid and area-length methods are both recommended by the American Society of Echocardiology for mass determination (12,38).

Wall Thickness and Left Ventricular Mass

Hypertrophy is defined anatomically as an increase in the mass of the ventricular myocardium, but wall thickness often serves as its surrogate. Initially obtained from M mode (45), wall thickness is usually determined from two-dimensional images

with normal values from 0.6 to 1.1 cm. Wall thickness should be measured at the onset of the QRS (rather than in diastasis), because atrial contraction may thin the wall considerably. Analogously, if filling volume is greatly reduced (e.g., in cardiac tamponade), the wall becomes thickened despite normal mass and a dilated ventricle may have increased mass with normal thickness. To overcome the shortcomings of simple wall thickness, actual mass can be estimated. However, M-mode formulas (29,46–48) suffer the same theoretical limitation as the cube method of estimating LV volume, especially in hearts with asymmetric thickening (49). Despite this, the Framingham Study has used M-mode methods to yield valuable insight into the electrocardiographic (ECG) criteria for hypertrophy (47,50,51) and the adverse prognosis of ventricular hypertrophy (52).

Most two-dimensional methods for determining LV mass (12,36–38) are similar because they combine a short-axis estimation of wall thickness with an estimation of ventricular length. The difference between the endocardial and epicardial volumes multiplied by the specific gravity of myocardium (1.05 g per mL) yields myocardial mass. Even two-dimensional methods have relatively wide 95% confidence bounds (±25 g) (34,36,37). ⚐ j25

Two-Dimensional Echocardiography in Ischemic Heart Disease

Myocardial infarction produces regional akinesis within seconds of coronary occlusion. The presence of scarring (thinning and increased brightness) indicates an old infarction. The interface between contracting and akinetic tissue forms a visually distinctive "hinge point." The diffuse hypokinesis of ischemic cardiomyopathy can be difficult to distinguish from primary myocardial disease.

To localize segmental wall motion abnormalities in a standardized format, the American Society of Echocardiography has recommended dividing the ventricle into 16 segments (12). Grading of these segments generates a wall motion score index that has been shown to have prognostic value (71). A diastolic deformity, sharply demarcated, indicates aneurysm formation. Hypokinesis without wall thinning suggests ischemia rather than completed infarction, but the specificity of this is not high. Echocardiography is valuable in the assessment of chest pain (72–76), because a normal echocardiogram makes cardiac ischemia unlikely. The reliability and speed in detecting ischemic hypokinesis have led to the use of echocardiography in conjunction with exercise and pharmacologic stress testing (see Chapter 50).

Complications of Myocardial Infarction: Recognition by Echocardiography

Many of the complications of myocardial infarction can be diagnosed by a bedside echocardiogram. LV thrombi occur frequently in the setting of extensive anteroapical infarction and rarely in inferior infarction. They can appear within days of the infarction and typically are highly mobile. Older thrombi tend to have smooth surfaces and a texture like liver and may have a layered appearance (eFig. 49.5.1). The more mobile and irregular the surface of the thrombus, the higher the risk of embolization (77–80). Thrombi can be difficult to differentiate from apical trabeculations, which may be pronounced in cardiomyopathy (81).

Postinfarction aneurysms are characterized by a wall motion abnormality with a diastolic deformity. The ability of echocardiography to delineate aneurysm is emphasized (82–84) (eFig. 49.4.2).

Pseudoaneurysms, which result from frank wall rupture or cardiorrhexis, are actually composed of pericardium, which confines the rupture. Because only small ruptures in the wall are compatible with survival, pseudoaneurysms tend to have narrow necks, in contrast to the more open neck of true aneurysms (see Chapter 19). Pseudoaneurysms typically form at the infero-posterior base of the heart, are usually accompanied by pericardial effusion (85), and carry a poor prognosis if unrepaired.

Abrupt myocardial rupture into the pericardial sac is rapidly fatal, although slower accumulations can allow time for surgery. Most postinfarction pericardial effusions are either due to local inflammation (early) or Dressler's syndrome (late). The incidence of pericardial effusions has ranged from 6% (86) to 37% (87) after infarction, and there is poor correlation with physical signs of pericarditis. Ventricular septal defect is a contained cardiorrhexis (88–92), typically at the anteroapex for left coronary infarction and the inferior base for right coronary infarction.

Mitral regurgitation (MR) is regularly encountered as a periinfarction complication (22,88). Papillary muscle rupture is always disabling and may be rapidly fatal (93,94) (eFig. 49.5.2). Because of cross support of the chordae, free motion of the liberated papillary muscle can sometimes be inapparent. Therefore, any patient with severe heart failure and unexpectedly good ventricular function after infarction should have papillary muscle rupture considered. Less severe MR is also commonly seen after myocardial infarction, typically due to the abnormal wall motion displacing or undermining the papillary muscle (see Chapter 51).

RV infarction can be seen in approximately 40% of inferior infarctions (95,96), with injury ranging from subclinical depression to severe RV dysfunction causing a low-output state with high mortality. RV infarction is characterized by ventricular enlargement, decreased descent of the base, and inferior vena cava (IVC) plethora (95,96). Elevation of right-sided filling pressures can cause right-to-left shunting through a patent foramen ovale and can be easily documented by the passage of saline microbubbles across the interatrial septum.

Cardiomyopathies: Their Recognition by Echocardiography

Dilated, hypertrophic, and restrictive cardiomyopathies can be characterized by two-dimensional echocardiography.

Congestive cardiomyopathy shows spherical cavitary dilatation (LV volume often >250 mL), normal wall thickness, and poor wall thickening and endocardial motion (eFig. 49.4.1). M-mode echocardiography displays mitral-septal E-point separation, poor mitral and AV opening, and decreased systolic aortic root motion. Involvement of the right heart is important because it implies pulmonary hypertension and RV cardiomyopathy, which independently worsen prognosis (97,98). In spite of an EF of less than 30%, cardiac output (stroke volume × heart rate) may be normal due to tachycardia and the large end diastolic volume.

Early signs of cardiomyopathy are a decrease in the descent of the cardiac base (24), an increase in sphericity (24), and a rise in end systolic volume index (40,42). This latter value is highly useful in detecting early cardiomyopathy because the end systolic volume tends to be more sensitive to contractility than the preload volume (35). An end systolic volume index that exceeds 30 mL per m^2 indicates significant global dysfunction. In valve disease, patients whose end systolic volume index exceeded 60 mL per m^2 (40) had a much poorer outcome than did other patients. Similarly, in ischemic cardiomyopathy the value of 45 mL per m^2 segregates patients with poor outcome.

In South America, a congestive or a segmental cardiomyopathy raises the possibility of Chagas' disease (99), in which insect-borne *Trypanosoma cruzi* eventually leads to damage of the myocardium. It may appear as global dysfunction or as an apical aneurysm that, unlike coronary disease, spares the interventricular septum. Less commonly, the inferior base can be the site of segmentally isolated thinning and scar formation.

Hypertrophic Cardiomyopathies

Primary hypertrophic cardiomyopathies are characterized by increased LV mass without apparent etiology, such as hypertension or aortic stenosis, and can be asymmetric or symmetric (100–103). In asymmetric septal hypertrophy (ASH), the increased wall thickness is typically localized in the basal septum (101) (eFig. 49.5.3A,B), and, although it is clearly heritable, there is variable expressivity among affected family members. An unusual variation of ASH is apical hypertrophy (so-called Yamaguchi's disease) (104,105) (eFig. 49.5.3C). When dynamic outflow tract obstruction accompanies ASH, hypertrophic obstructive cardiomyopathy is present (106–108). Findings that are consistent with obstruction may be noted echocardiographically at rest or with provocation by amyl nitrite, exercise, or inotropic stimulation (100). Fully developed hypertrophic obstructive cardiomyopathy consists of ASH, systolic anterior motion of the MV, crowding of the LV outflow tract by the mitral apparatus and septum, partial mid-systolic closure or notching of the AV, and mitral annular calcification.

Secondary LV hypertrophy (LVH) is most commonly due to hypertension and conveys a poor prognosis (52). The sensitivity of M-mode echocardiography for detecting LVH is clearly superior to ECG (50), but two-dimensional echocardiography has superior reproducibility.

Restrictive Cardiomyopathy

Restrictive cardiomyopathies are more difficult to diagnose than hypertrophic or congestive states, but echocardiography remains the most effective diagnostic test. The most common restrictive state is the small stiff heart of diabetes (109). It is clinically inapparent in the majority of diabetics but may lead to pulmonary congestion in association with regional ischemia.

Amyloid heart disease is rare (110–112) and carries a poor prognosis (113). Amyloid infiltration is characterized echocardiographically by increased LV wall thickness and a peculiar glittering or scintillating appearance of the myocardium (*e*Fig. 49.5.4). Superficially, amyloid heart disease can resemble typical LVH (110). Contractile function is nearly normal or mildly depressed, and the left atrium (LA) is usually enlarged. The presence of these findings along with typical clinical signs or symptoms (e.g., low ECG voltage, neuropathy) should prompt a gingival or rectal biopsy.

Unclassified Cardiomyopathy

Ventricular noncompaction is a rare form of ventricular dysplasia that results from intrauterine arrest in endomyocardial morphogenesis (114,115). It involves the LV or the LV and RV, most commonly in association with other congenital malformations, but occasionally in isolation (116). The myocardium is characterized by numerous prominent, excessive trabeculations with deep intertrabecular recesses. Noncompaction most commonly affects the apical, mid-inferior, and mid-lateral segments (117).

Left Ventricular Masses

Nonthrombotic masses of the left ventricle are quite rare, but approximately 25% are malignant (33% angiosarcomas, 20% rhabdomyosarcomas, 10% mesotheliomas, and 11% fibrosarcomas with melanomas reported) (118). In the pediatric population, the most common tumors are rhabdomyomas associated with tuberous sclerosis. *e*Figure 49.5.5 shows a three-dimensional image of an apical mass, found to be a benign lipoma at surgery. Nonmalignant lesions include myxomas and fibroelastomas, and both have considerable embolic potential. Myxomas can occur anywhere in the left ventricular cavity, whereas fibroelastomas usually occur on the MV or valvular apparatus.

Endomyocardial fibrosis is a disease of the impoverished living in North Africa and South America. It is associated with restriction of LV and RV filling by obliteration of one or both cardiac apices by a thrombotic fibrocalcific process (119). The disease can also occur in relation to eosinophilia (Loeffler's or Davies' disease) and eosinophilic leukemia. In addition to the unique appearance of the apices, the atria are strikingly enlarged, with mitral and tricuspid regurgitation (TR) complicating the picture. Its recognition depends on a high degree of clinical suspicion and a characteristic echocardiographic appearance. In South America, a surgical approach has been developed that debulks fibrotic material from the apex and restores LV compliance.

Right Ventricle

Imaging the RV is an essential portion of a comprehensive echocardiographic evaluation, as occult right heart disease may occur as a result of left-sided pathology.

Right Ventricular Wall Thickness, Contractile Function, and Size

RV wall thickness, assessed from the parasternal or subcostal windows, should be only 3 to 4 mm thick, with 5 mm considered hypertrophied (13,45,120). In contrast to the elliptical LV, the shape of the RV frustrates volumetric measurement. It has been described as a pyramid with a triangular base or as a teapot. The tomographic nature of echocardiography makes imaging this irregular-shaped organ in a single plane impractical (56,120–124). One simple analog is the parasternal M-mode diameter of the RV, although a more accurate dimension can be obtained from a two-dimensional image. The size of the normal RV is considerably less than the left ventricle, whether imaged from the parasternal long axis, the parasternal short axis, or the apical four-chamber view (Fig. 49.2). In the latter view, the LV should form the cardiac apex. If the RV even shares the apex, RV dilatation should be suspected.

To assess RV contractility visually, careful adjustments of instrument settings may be needed to detect RV inward systolic motion or wall thickening accurately. Most M-mode images are of the RV outflow tract region, which may not be representative of the whole chamber.

RV volume and EF can be estimated by the area-length algorithm applied from the apical four-chamber or subcostal views (122–124). This correlates reasonably well ($r = 0.83$) with radionuclide scanning for EF (121), although absolute volumes are significantly underestimated. The four-chamber area-length RV-LV volume ratio should be approximately 0.6, but it increases to greater than 1.1 in cor pulmonale (125).

Descent of the RV base toward the fixed apex is easily seen in the subcostal and four-chamber views and, if depressed, is a sensitive indicator of RV systolic dysfunction (124). Descent of the RV base was 0.7 ± 0.2 cm in patients with hemodynamically significant RV infarction, 1.3 ± 0.4 cm in those with ECG evidence but without hemodynamic compromise, and 2.0 ± 0.2 cm in a group of 20 normal control patients (*p* <.001). Doppler tissue imaging has yielded similar results in normal subjects (126).

Segmental Abnormalities of the Right Ventricle

The most common segmental RV abnormality results from RV infarction, usually in the setting of inferior wall myocardial infarction (95), and may lead to a lethal low-output syndrome even when LV damage is not extensive. In RV infarction, there is cavity enlargement (96) with mid-anterior and inferior wall akinesis or even aneurysm by two-dimensional imaging. A hinge point may differentiate infarcted from normal segments, and the descent of the RV base is impaired (95). The degree of RV dilatation and IVC plethora provides clues to the hemodynamic severity of RV infarction (95).

Endocardial fibrosis (with or without eosinophilia) can also segmentally affect the RV. The apex fills with fibrothrombotic matter, resulting in RV restriction, TR, and atrial enlargement (99,119).

Right Ventricular Tumors and Masses

RV masses can be primary, metastatic, or embolic in nature (127,128). Generally, the same masses that affect the LV can also involve the RV. Myxomas are the most common benign RV tumors and tend to be larger because they are detected later. Primary malignant tumors are very rare and are usually angiosarcomas. Metastatic melanoma can occur, but usually very late in the course of the disease. More commonly, tumors reach the right heart by propagating through the venae cavae. Hepatic, renal, and adrenal tumors can present in this manner, and a malignant thymoma that obstructs RV inflow has been observed. Such masses can be surgically palliated.

The most important propagating masses are embolic thrombi from the lower extremities (129). These thrombi, which may present as a localized mobile RV mass, are generally less reflective than malignant masses. RV enlargement and pulmonary hypertension suggest multiple pulmonary emboli. These masses may remain in the right heart, embolize to the lungs, or rarely cross a patent foramen ovale (130). These thrombi generally have an ominous prognosis and require aggressive medical or surgical intervention.

Conditions Associated with Right Ventricular Dilatation

RV volume overload without pulmonary hypertension is seen in atrial septal defect (ASD), tricuspid insufficiency, and pulmonary insufficiency, in which cases the RV enlarges to form the cardiac apex. RV contractile function is usually preserved, and wall thickness remains normal. In ASD, the pulmonary artery is also enlarged. *e*Figure 49.5.6 shows a suprasternal view of the aortic arch and pulmonary artery bifurcation. If the right pulmonary artery is of normal caliber, pulmonary hypertension and left-to-right shunts of any magnitude are unlikely. Similarly, the short-axis basal precordial view is the best window for evaluating the size of the main pulmonary artery.

An ASD can be further confirmed by saline contrast injection, showing a negative contrast jet in the RA or right-to-left shunt flow in the LA. Sometimes the defect itself can be seen, especially with color Doppler, which may also show discrepant flow through the RV and LV outflow tracts (121). Congenital absence of the pericardium may cause RV enlargement (131) due to rotation of the heart, but with a small pulmonary artery, low pulmonary pressure, and a normal contrast study. RV enlargement may also be caused by severe TR, most commonly due to LV dysfunction, rheumatic disease, endocarditis, and primary pulmonary hypertension. Two-dimensional signs of TR include leaflet flail or malcoaptation, although color Doppler is the most reliable modality.

Chronically elevated pulmonary vascular resistance leads to cor pulmonale with a dilated apex-forming RV (125), mild to moderate RV hypertrophy, and a dilated IVC that is unresponsive to respiration. A patent foramen ovale (20–30% of patients) may show right-to-left shunting with contrast injection. The etiology usually is chronic obstructive lung disease but may be chronic pulmonary embolism, cystic fibrosis, bronchiectasis, connective tissue disease, adult respiratory distress syndrome, asthma, sarcoid, obesity with sleep apnea, or chronic pulmonary infection.

Echocardiographic features of primary pulmonary hypertension are similar to those of cor pulmonale but with greater RV hypertrophy and septal flattening (*e*Fig. 49.5.7), often preceding IVC plethora. Pulmonary hypertension from congenital heart disease (atrial or ventricular septal defect) may cause severe RVH, but right heart failure may be minimal early on. In the end stage, it may be difficult to distinguish ASD/Eisenmenger complex from primary pulmonary hypertension with a patent foramen ovale.

Isolated RV dilatation may be seen in arrhythmogenic RV dysplasia (parchment ventricle or Uhl's disease) (132). Features of RV dysplasia include a thin RV wall, increased epicardial fat, aneurysms of the RV free wall, and a prominent moderator band with complex attachment to the septum and RV free wall. Spontaneous fatal ventricular arrhythmias may be seen with this condition.

In Ebstein's anomaly, the septal leaflet of the TV is displaced toward the RV apex, leaving an "atrialized ventricle" behind the valve (*e*Fig. 49.5.8). Contraction during systole may cause right-to-left shunting across a patent foramen and cyanosis (133,134).

ECHOCARDIOGRAPHY OF THE ATRIA

Left Atrium

The LA serves reservoir, conduit, and booster pump functions for blood that enters the LV. It is commonly involved in pathologic processes, including dilation, thromboembolic and neoplastic disease, extrinsic compression, and fibrillation, each of which is well assessed by echocardiography.

Echocardiographic Assessment of Left Atrial Volume and Function

The standard parasternal M-mode image yields the anterior-to-posterior dimension of the LA (Fig. 49.4), typically the smallest, perhaps because of confinement between the sternum and the spine (135). This dimension is the least sensitive to enlargement but, when increased, is highly specific.

Because this single anterior-to-posterior dimension may underestimate overall LA size, volume estimates are preferred, requiring two sector scans, preferably orthogonal apical planes. The area-length formula has shown good correlation ($r = 0.82$–0.98) with angiography and contrast computed tomographic scanning (66,135), with some underestimation (up to 23%) but good reproducibility (95% confidence interval = 10 mL). Normal values throughout the cardiac cycle are shown in *e*Table 49.0.1 (65,68). Maximal volume occurs at end systole and averages 40 mL, falling to 25 mL after passive and active emptying. For a normal LV stroke volume of 65 mL, approximately 25 mL is reservoir emptying and 40 mL is conduit flow from the pulmonary veins. In the healthy young heart, only 10 mL atrial transport occurs with atrial contraction, the rest entering by passive flow early in diastole. With aging, the amount of active atrial transport more than doubles.

Atrial fibrillation causes progressive LA enlargement (136), which may be prevented by cardioversion (137). In rheumatic disease, LA diameter is predictive of atrial fibrillation (138) and the restoration of atrial function after cardioversion (139). However, the recurrence of lone atrial fibrillation appears to be independent of atrial diameter (140). Atrial volume has not been used in these studies.

Left Atrial Thrombi, Masses, and Tumors

Left atrial thrombi are common but must be large to be identified by transthoracic echocardiography (TTE). This is especially true of the left atrial appendage, which usually requires transesophageal interrogation (141).

The most common LA tumor is myxoma (*e*Fig. 49.5.9), a benign mass that most commonly arises from the inferior limb of the fossa ovalis. It can present with embolism or obstruction to mitral inflow. Myxomas may be encapsulated or highly mobile and amorphous, with the latter at highest risk for peripheral emboli. Encapsulated myxomas may have clear spaces (cysts) and highly reflective patches (bone). Attachment is typically by a stalk to the interatrial septum and may be biatrial. The attachment of amorphous myxomas is broader based, with a highly mobile, less reflective tip. Malignant LA tumors include fibrosarcoma, liposarcoma, and osteogenic sarcoma that may metastasize through the pulmonary vein.

ECHOCARDIOGRAPHY OF THE CARDIAC VALVES

Echocardiography images the cardiac valves as does no other modality, providing high temporal and spatial resolution while relating valve structure to surrounding structures. Doppler is also critical to valve interrogation. It is discussed in detail in Chapter 51.

Evaluation of the Mitral Valve

Historically, the mitral valve was the first structure to be identified by echocardiography (3–5,145). An integrated investigation of the MV includes an M-mode tracing, several two-dimensional views, a Doppler evaluation, and, if needed, transesophageal imaging (141).

The anterior mitral leaflet is highly mobile and quite echogenic, whereas the posterior leaflet is somewhat less apparent (Fig. 49.2). Images are acquired from the parasternal, apical, and subcostal regions. By M mode, an M-shaped pattern of MV motion is seen, reflecting first passive rapid filling and second atrial contraction, with near closure during diastasis, although blood may still pass from pulmonary veins to LV using the atrium as a conduit (65). Final closure results from atrial inflow deceleration and isovolumic LV contraction (Fig. 49.4).

By two-dimensional imaging in the short-axis plane (Fig. 49.2), the MV is an ovoid orifice. In the long-axis plane, it resembles clapping hands moving freely in diastole, but forming a stable coaptation plane in systole. The MV and annulus descend with the cardiac base to assist left atrial filling.

Normal mitral leaflets are thin (<2 mm), although somewhat thicker at points of chordal attachment to the free margin (primary chordae) and leaflet body (secondary chordae). Transducer frequencies of greater than 2.5 MHz are required for adequate resolution. The papillary muscles can be seen in the short-axis view at four and eight o'clock with highly variable anatomy. From the apical four-chamber view, posterior angulation (typically showing the coronary sinus) is necessary to show the papillary muscles and chordae. Normal chordae appear fragmented unless they are thickened and fused by fibrosis or calcification. The mitral annulus has been shown to be nonplanar (saddle-shaped) and highly dynamic by three-dimensional imaging. On two-dimensional imaging annular diameter and calcification can be noted.

Mitral Pathology

Mitral Stenosis

From the earliest days of echocardiography (4), MS has been recognized by altered motion of the valve due to commissural fusion and chordal shortening. MS severity can be assessed on M mode by measuring the delay in diastolic closure (E-F slope). A normal value is greater than 60 mm per second; a slope of less than 10 mm per second indicates severe MS (146). By two-dimensional echocardiography, the leaflets dome into the ventricle throughout diastole (*e*Fig. 49.5.11). In short axis, the mitral orifice can be reliably measured by direct planimetry (146,147), with an area of less than 1 cm² defining severe MS. Doppler quantitation methods are discussed in Chapter 51.

Indirect signs of MS severity include chordal shortening, leaflet calcification, LA enlargement, LV underloading, and right heart involvement (pulmonary hypertension). Progression cannot be accurately predicted, although those with mild MS and aortic insufficiency progress slightly faster (148).

Mitral Regurgitation

Regurgitant lesions may be structurally more subtle than stenotic ones, with Doppler (see Chapter 51) playing an even more dominant role. Nevertheless, careful structural interrogation is critical to evaluating MR.

Rheumatic Mitral Regurgitation

In rheumatic disease, the posterior leaflet is fixed and shortened, allowing the anterior leaflet to override it on closure and resulting in posteriorly directed MR. The degree of malcoaptation is predictive of MR severity (160).

Mitral Valve Prolapse

The original clinical, auscultatory, and angiographic descriptions of mitral valve prolapse (MVP) (161,162) were rapidly supplemented by echocardiographic studies (163–165), which contributed to an "epidemic" of MVP by overly liberal diagnostic criteria.

Although MVP has a classic appearance by M mode (mid- or pansystolic posterior motion), up to 23% of healthy asymptomatic women may be diagnosed by these criteria (165). Two-dimensional echocardiography yielded a similar diagnostic prevalence until Levine et al. (166) demonstrated that the mitral annulus was saddle-shaped (nonplanar). Thus, leaflets may appear to close above the annulus in the apical four-chamber view (cutting through the low points of the annulus), while being normally oriented in a long-axis view (through the high points of the annulus). Current diagnosis of MVP rests on this long-axis displacement, although anatomic variability dictates that the full anterior leaflet and each of the three posterior scallops be thoroughly interrogated (*e*Fig. 49.5.13).

MVP is also associated with myxomatous leaflet thickening and redundancy, with the tips sometimes being club-like, with a ground-glass appearance extending onto the chordae. The degree of MV deformity has been related to chest pain, arrhythmias, endocarditis, systemic emboli, and chordal rupture (167). Extreme prolapse may be difficult to differentiate from frank chordal rupture or endocarditis.

ECHOCARDIOGRAPHY OF THE AORTIC VALVE

Aortic Valve

Normal Aortic Valve

M-mode echocardiography of the AV and root demonstrates leaflet closure at the midpoint of the aortic root and opening throughout systole to the walls of the aortic root, producing a "box-like" M-mode waveform. Fine systolic vibrations can be seen and correspond to a normal flow murmur. Failure to achieve or sustain full opening implies decreased stroke volume. Abrupt early closure may be caused by fixed subvalvular stenosis (*e*Fig. 49.5.14), and subsequent reopening in later systole may imply dynamic subvalvular obstruction. The coapted leaflets move parallel to the aortic root in diastole, with vibrations suggesting valve disruption or endocarditis. Eccentricity on closure typically indicates a congenital bicuspid valve (*e*Fig. 49.5.15).

Normally, the aortic root moves more than 7 mm anteriorly in systole, with fair concordance to stroke volume independent of LV EF (e.g., an underfilled LV with normal EF causes decreased root motion). Augmented motion of the root despite reduced aortic leaflet separation is typical of mitral insufficiency. Slowed posterior motion of the root in early diastole with augmented presystolic movement is analogous to the delayed relaxation pattern of mitral inflow. In restrictive states, root motion is flat, reflecting reduced stroke volume.

Two-dimensional imaging of the normal AV demonstrates three thin leaflets, opening as a circular orifice and closing as a three-pointed star with slight central thickening. The left coronary cusp is adjacent to the left atrial appendage, the left main coronary artery, and the pulmonary valve and artery. The right lies just posterior to the RV outflow tract, close to the septal attachment of the TV. The noncoronary cusp sits above the RA and the interatrial septum. Aortic diameter is largest at the sinuses of Valsalva and should not exceed 3.5 cm.

Aortic Stenosis

In severe AS, the M mode shows dense persistent echoes with little systolic separation (168) (*e*Fig. 49.5.16). Aortic sclerosis without stenosis shows dense echoes, but at least one leaflet will move rapidly or will vibrate, indicating a peak systolic gradient below 50 mm Hg. M mode also shows secondary features of AS such as LVH and LA enlargement.

Cusp separation by two-dimensional imaging is helpful if it is less than 8 mm or more than 12 mm but poorly predictive between 8 and 12 mm (169). Leaflet doming, post-stenotic aortic dilatation, and LVH are predictive of significant AS, although none approaches the utility of Doppler-derived pressure gradient and valve area (169–172).

The severe calcification of senile AS is nonspecific as to underlying pathology. In younger patients, bicuspid valves show eccentric opening and only two moving leaflets. On closure of the valve, three commissures may be seen due to raphe formation between two leaflets, usually the left and right. Rheumatic AS shows commissural fusion and leaflet retraction and is generally associated with rheumatic mitral disease. Senile calcification typically begins in the aortic annulus, spreading centrally into the leaflets.

Subvalvular and Supravalvular Stenosis

Fixed subvalvular stenosis is occasionally encountered in the adult population (173–175), often with prior ventricular septal defect. The subvalvular membrane is a narrow ridge in the distal septum (*e*Fig. 49.5.14). Because the narrowing may be difficult to appreciate by inspection, Doppler remains the definitive quantitative modality. Dynamic subvalvular stenosis is discussed above under Normal Aortic Valve. Supravalvular AS is rarely seen in adults. Features include narrowing above and affixed to the valve leaflets, aortic insufficiency, enlarged coronary arteries (sometimes obstructed), and severe hypertrophy (176).

Aortic Regurgitation

Aortic regurgitation (AR) can be seen with diastolic fluttering of the anterior mitral leaflet by M mode (177), a sign largely supplanted by Doppler. With severe acute AR, M mode may show early closure of the MV (178), indicating precarious hemodynamics and a need for urgent pharmacologic or surgical intervention (178). Henry et al. (179) have suggested that an LV end systolic dimension of greater than 55 mm predicts poor operative results—a concept challenged by Fioretti et al. (180), perhaps due to improvements in myocardial preservation at surgery. Assessment of AR severity by two-dimensional echocardiography has not been adequately studied (181). Posteriorly directed AR may reverse the diastolic curvature of the anterior mitral leaflet (182), but no two-dimensional sign replaces a quantitative Doppler examination (177,183) (see Chapter 51).

Senile calcification typically results in mild AR. Rheumatic disease causes leaflet retraction and a central AR jet. Bicuspid aortic valves may have significant AR due to leaflet prolapse, usually of a conjoined anterior leaflet. Endocarditis may cause acute severe AR, recognized as mobile echoes prolapsing into the LV outflow tract. Transesophageal echocardiography (TEE) has greatly improved detection of aortic vegetations (184). AR can arise from subaortic membrane jets that undermine valve integrity. Myxomatous disease can cause AV prolapse. In Marfan dis-

ease (*e*Fig. 49.5.17), isolated dilation of the sinuses of Valsalva causes traction on the aortic commissures and a central jet of AR (185). Other aortic diseases that are associated with AR include dissection, sinus of Valsalva aneurysms, aortoannular ectasia, and aneurysms due to atherosclerosis, syphilis, and ankylosing spondylitis. As discussed in Chapter 52, TEE is preferred for emergent diagnosis (186). Small perimembranous ventricular septal defects may close in childhood but leave behind AR. Doubly committed subarterial ventricular septal defect is also associated with aortic regurgitation.

Tricuspid Valve

The TV has anterior, septal, and posterior leaflets; the latter two are somewhat variable in size and position. M mode from the parasternal window with rightward and inferior angulation is useful for timing. Two-dimensional imaging can be recorded from the parasternal long- and short-axis and apical four-chamber views for anatomic and Doppler evaluation. The TV is apically displaced by the membranous septum, which is useful in identifying the TV in congenital heart disease. Transesophageal imaging offers relatively little advantage, especially for measuring TR velocity (187).

Tricuspid Insufficiency

Contemporary echocardiography confirms Sir James Mackenzie's claim, made in 1908, that TR is ubiquitous. Present in 80% of normal subjects and nearly all cardiac patients, this "abnormality" usually is just a convenient means to estimate pulmonary artery pressure (188). Pathologic TR causes RV and RA enlargement, paradoxical septal motion, and systolic IVC pulsation from retrograde flow. M mode shows paradoxical septal motion, with anterior systolic motion of the septum related to the exaggerated RV stroke volume. M mode can also record systolic IVC expansion, which should not be confused with respiratory fluctuations. By two-dimensional imaging, RV dilatation can be seen, although quantitation is imprecise (125) and hyperdynamic function can be seen due to the augmented stroke volume (24,236). RA enlargement is common and is related to TR duration and severity and the presence of atrial fibrillation. With severe TR, the normal leftward bulging of the interatrial septum is reversed (189).

The most common cause of significant TR is RV failure from high LV filling pressures, with annular dilatation and failure of leaflet coaptation (190). Rheumatic TR rarely exists without MV involvement. It is characterized by leaflet thickening, commissural fusion and calcification, and chordal shortening. Myxomatous MV disease may be accompanied by tricuspid prolapse (191), but severe TR is uncommon unless there is chordal rupture (192). RV biopsy may rarely cause iatrogenic chordal rupture (193). Endocarditis (usually due to intravenous drug use) causes bulky prolapsing vegetations and flail leaflets (194) (*e*Fig. 49.5.18). Metastatic liver carcinoid causes TV leaflet shortening with more regurgitation than stenosis (159). Ebstein's anomaly commonly causes severe TR (133) (*e*Fig. 49.5.8).

Tricuspid Stenosis

Tricuspid stenosis may be due to rheumatic disease, carcinoid syndrome, or prolapsing RA tumors. Two-dimensional planimetry is not reliable, making Doppler the mainstay of quantitation.

Pulmonary Valve and Artery

Pulmonary valve pathology is common in congenital disease but is rarely acquired. M-mode and two-dimensional imaging are limited to leaflet inspection (often difficult) and pulmonary artery dilatation. The M mode in pulmonary stenosis (PS) shows an exaggerated diastolic "'a' wave" caused by powerful RA contraction opening or doming the pulmonary valve. By two-dimensional imaging, PS shows systolic leaflet doming, variable leaflet thickening, poststenotic dilation of the main PA with decreased pulsations, and variable RV hypertrophy. PS must be distinguished from subpulmonic stenosis and double-chamber RV that results from prior ventricular septal defect.

Trivial pulmonary regurgitation (PR) is present in most healthy persons. Severe PR rarely occurs from prior tetralogy of Fallot repair, endocarditis (195), or carcinoid (159). Moderate PR can result from pulmonary hypertension (Graham Steell's murmur).

Infective Endocarditis

Echocardiography is essential to the diagnosis and management of patients with infective endocarditis (IE). Early studies of echocardiography and IE used the criteria of Von Reyn et al. (196) for diagnosis. New echocardiographic criteria for diagnosing IE have been prospectively tested by the Duke Endocarditis Service (197,198). In these studies, echocardiography increased the sensitivity for detecting IE from 51% to 80%, although TEE was required to visualize the vegetations in 41% of cases.

Two-Dimensional Imaging

In a metaanalysis of 16 early studies (641 patients), O'Brien and Geiser (201) reported a mean sensitivity of 79% for two-dimensional detection of vegetations and 52% for M mode, with vegetations as small as 3 mm reported by two-dimensional imaging (200). More recently, however, the reported sensitivity of TTE has dropped to 62% despite equipment improvement (184,202–207), reflecting less biased case selection and the fact that these studies used TEE (sensitivity of 92%).

Sanfilippo et al. (208) retrospectively studied 204 patients with IE, showing that larger (>10 mm) mobile noncalcified vegetations were predictive of antibiotic failure, congestive heart failure, embolization, surgery, and death. Size was highly predictive of complications: 10% for 6-mm vegetations, 50% at 11 mm, and almost 100% at 16 mm.

Right-Sided Infective Endocarditis

Tricuspid IE (usually *Staphylococcus aureus*) typically occurs in intravenous drug users (221) and causes large vegetations that are equally well detected by TTE and TEE (187). Multiplane TEE may be of value for the very rare pulmonic vegetations (195).

PERICARDIAL DISORDERS

Echocardiography detects virtually all pericardial effusions (222,223) and is the diagnostic test of choice (224), providing important hemodynamic data as well. Normally, there is less than 20 mL pericardial fluid (225), barely detected during systole by M mode. The high temporal resolution of M mode is valuable in assessing pericardial motion and RA and RV dynamics. The parietal pericardium is highly echogenic.

Two-Dimensional Echocardiography

Two-dimensional echocardiography and Doppler are key in assessing pericardial disease, with small effusions first seen above the RA. The normal systolic torsion of the heart is lost when inflammation causes adhesions between the pericardial layers. Pericardial fat may mimic effusion (226), typically seen anterior to the heart. D'Cruz and Hoffman (227) have described an ellipsoidal formula for estimating effusion size, although effusions typically are graded as small (separation seen throughout the cardiac cycle), medium, and large (typically >2 cm circumferentially). Although transudates, exudates, and blood appear similar, septations suggest chronicity.

Tamponade

Tamponade is a continuum of hemodynamic embarrassment, often associated with large effusions (228–235), although small rapid accumulation can be life threatening. Characteristic echocardiographic features are listed in Table 49.1. The heart is usually small, unless previously enlarged (229), and respirophasic ventricular interdependence is seen. The RV enlarges with inspiration and the LV with expiration, the echocardiographic equivalent of pulsus paradoxus (229,236). RV diastolic collapse and RA invagination (>one-third of cardiac cycle) are seen (229,230,232,233) (*e*Fig. 49.5.20). Central venous pressure (CVP) can be estimated

TABLE 49.1 TWO-DIMENSIONAL ECHOCARDIOGRAPHIC FINDINGS IN TAMPONADE

Large effusion
Right atrial (RA) expiratory collapse
Right ventricular (RV) expiratory compression or collapse
IVC plethora with diminished respiratory response
Left atrial compression
Small chamber volumes
Reciprocal size changes between RV and LV and excursion between MV and TV

Sensitivity, specificity, and positive and negative predictive values

	Sen	Spec	PPV	NPV
Size (large vs. moderate)	—	97	45	99
RV compression	48	95	38	99
RA compression	55	88	10	99
IVC plethora	97	66	7	99

IVC, inferior vena cava; LV, left ventricular; MV, mitral valve; NPV, negative predictive value; PPV, positive predictive value; TV, tricuspid valve.

from IVC dynamics (231). If CVP is normal, the IVC is greater than 17 mm and decreases by more than 5 mm during inspiration. With elevated CVP, typical of tamponade, the IVC exceeds 20 mm and respiratory change is blunted (231,237) (*e*Fig. 49.5.21), a sign that is less useful with mechanical ventilation (238).

Loculated Effusion

Following pericardiotomy, effusions may be loculated, making the diagnosis of tamponade and differentiation from pleural effusions difficult. Many two-dimensional signs of tamponade (such as RA invagination) may be absent if the hematoma is not localized to that area. Postcardiotomy (Dressler's) syndrome may develop days to weeks after surgery and requires a high degree of clinical suspicion to diagnose.

Pleural versus Pericardial Effusion

Left pleural effusions can be distinguished by their posterior location, passing behind the descending aorta. Large bilateral pleural effusions may occasionally cause tamponade that is responsive to drainage (239).

Pericardial Thickening and Constriction

Pericardial thickening is common, although constriction is rare. Thickening and adhesion are distinguished from simple effusion by the parallel (rather than damped) motion of the epicardium and visceral pericardium with the parietal pericardium. Pericardial constriction is a continuum of hemodynamic impairment, which may overlap with tamponade and (when the visceral layer is primarily involved) may have a component of restriction. By M mode, a septal notch may be seen in early diastole around the time of the pericardial knock (between S_2 and S_3) (240,241). Two-

dimensional echocardiography may show extensive adhesion and a diastolic septal bounce (237), which may resemble left bundle branch block or RV pacing. IVC plethora is usually seen (231,237) unless the patient is severely dehydrated. In the four-chamber view, the ventricles appear elongated, and the atria are globally enlarged. Brief constrictive phases may be seen with resolution of simple effusions. Table 49.2 lists two-dimensional signs of constriction, distinct from restrictive cardiomyopathy. Malignancy often causes pericardial effusions and pericardial studding, and frank-mass effect may be seen.

Congenital Abnormalities

Complete absence of the pericardium causes RV enlargement and paradoxical septal motion (144). Partial absence may cause LV herniation through the defect with coronary compression and myocardial infarction. Pericardial cysts are difficult to localize by echocardiography due to their lateral position (242).

Aorta and Great Vessels

Despite the primacy of TEE, TTE is useful in assessing the great vessels. The aortic root and ascending aorta are well seen in the parasternal long- and short-axis views. Coronary

TABLE 49.2 PERICARDIAL CONSTRICTION FINDINGS ON TWO-DIMENSIONAL ECHOCARDIOGRAPHY

Pericardial thickening and adhesion: lack of "sliding"; heart motion transmitted to other organs ("tugging")
Septal bounce: abrupt transient rightward movement
Inferior vena cava plethoric and unresponsive; hepatic veins dilated
Left and right ventricle size decreased; heart tubular in shape
Mild biatrial enlargement

artery ostia can be visualized (*e*Fig. 49.5.22), sometimes allowing for diagnosis of coronary anomalies and Kawasaki's disease.

Aortic Aneurysm

Symmetric sinus of Valsalva aneurysms (243,244) may be seen in Marfan syndrome. Echocardiographic enlargement of the root beyond 55 mm should generally prompt surgery. Ascending aortic dilatation may be poststenotic or atherosclerotic in origin, requiring high parasternal and right parasternal imaging to observe. The descending thoracic aorta can be seen in the long- and short-axis parasternal views posterior to the AV groove. The left and right pulmonary arteries may be seen in the short-axis view. The suprasternal notch allows visualization of the transverse and descending aorta as well as the origins of the innominate, left common carotid, and left subclavian vessels. In the apical views, posterior angulation often produces long- (two-chamber) and short- (four-chamber) axis views of the thoracic aorta. Atheroma and aneurysms of the abdominal aorta may be seen subcostally to the left of and deep to the IVC (245). Thoracic aortic dissection with effusion can also be imaged from the left paraspinal window, although TEE is the preferred method to assess the aorta (246).

Great Veins

The IVC is seen subcostally, crossing the diaphragm just after receiving the confluence of the hepatic veins. Its size and response to respiration predict RA pressure (247,248). If the vessel loses 50% of its initial expiratory diameter during deep inspiration (while lying supine with the knees bent), RA pressure is considered normal. The superior vena cava can be seen from a suprasternal notch plane orthogonal to the aortic arch view, allowing Doppler interrogation of its flow.

CONTROVERSIES AND PERSONAL PERSPECTIVES

TTE is the single most useful imaging test in cardiology. Its use has grown tremendously over the last 10 years. However, this examination is not performed and interpreted uniformly—a fact that has attracted unfavorable attention to the potential overuse of echocardiography in the United States. Particularly appalling is the lack of quantitation in many echocardiographic reports. Echocardiography is quantitative in nature—calibration marks are included on every screen, and the Digital Imaging and Communications in Medicine (DICOM) standard allows them to be stored digitally; yet, echocardiograms too often are interpreted in general categoric terms.

Of the emerging echocardiographic (distinct from Doppler) technologies, three are most noteworthy: three-dimensional imaging, contrast echocardiography, and harmonic imaging. Three-dimensional reconstruction has been available commercially for several years and is a valuable tool in quantifying chamber size and visualizing cardiac structures. Nevertheless, it has failed to penetrate the clinical arena completely, primarily because of the prolonged acquisition and display times. With the development of real-time three-dimensional acquisition, however, examination time could become shorter, as all structural data could be captured in a data set from a single cardiac cycle. True three-dimensional display remains problematic, but even scanning the data with properly oriented two-dimensional planes would be of great value.

Recent advances in echocardiography have resulted in improvements in image quality, especially for patients whose echocardiographic examination was previously suboptimal. Intravenous contrast agents are now available for LV opacification and endocardial border detection. Guidelines for the use of ultrasonic contrast in echocardiography have been published (269). Intravenous contrast agents should be used to provide additional diagnostic information for the detection of cardiac disease in difficult-to-image patients. They have been shown to be especially beneficial in obese patients, those with lung disease, and individuals who are receiving mechanical ventilation.

Use of harmonic frequencies to image tissue and contrast agents can further enhance image quality. In contrast harmonics, the harmonic frequency energy is generated on reflection of the ultrasound wave from the microbubble contrast agent. In tissue harmonics, the energy is gradually generated as the ultrasound wave propagates through the tissue. Essential to the utility of tissue-generated harmonic frequencies is their origin beyond the chest wall and their nonlinear relation to the fundamental frequency energy strength. These characteristics ensure that the echocardiograms that are most likely to produce artifact are least likely to produce harmonic waves (270). It is anticipated that harmonic imaging will become the standard for assessment of regional and global LV function in difficult-to-image patients.

Contrast agents that cross the lungs to opacify the LV cavity and myocardium combined with novel imaging techniques (e.g., transmitting at 2 MHz but receiving at 4 MHz) allow myocardial perfusion to at least be assessed in a binary sense (presence of coronary occlusion, occurrence of reperfusion). This may greatly assist in the detection and management of acute coronary syndromes. Even more exciting is the possibility of quantifying regional perfusion and flow reserve, an achievement that would bring echocardiography close to the holy grail of "one-stop shopping" that is claimed by other modalities.

THE FUTURE

Over the next 10 years, the field of echocardiography will be under intense pressure as cost containment leads to decreased reimbursement. This is ironic, because the value of the test should grow enormously as contrast, three-dimensional, and digital technologies mature. Although videotape will still be used, digital storage would allow retrieval throughout the hospital and transmission anywhere in the world, eliminating repetition of tests. Adherence to international formatting standards is critical. Attesting to the value of echocardiography are plans for a permanent ultrasound machine aboard the International Space Station for scientific research and for medical diagnosis.

REFERENCES

1. Feigenbaum H. Evolution of echocardiography. *Circulation* 1996;93:1321–1327.
2. Hertz CH. Ultrasonic engineering in heart diagnosis. *Am J Cardiol* 1967;19:6–17.
3. Edler I. Ultrasound cardiogram in mitral valve disease. *Acta Chir Scand* 1956;111:230.
4. Edler I. Ultrasonic cardiogram in mitral stenosis. *Acta Med Scand* 1957;159:85.
5. Edler I. Ultrasound cardiography in mitral valve stenosis. *Am J Cardiol* 1967;19:18–31.
6. Joyner CR Jr, Hey EB Jr, Johnson J, Reid JM. Reflected ultrasound in the diagnosis of tricuspid stenosis. *Am J Cardiol* 1967;19:66–73.
7. Feigenbaum H. *Echocardiography.* Philadelphia: Lea & Febiger, 1972.
8. Feigenbaum H. *Echocardiography,* 5th ed. Philadelphia: Lea & Febiger, 1994.
9. Ziskin MC. Fundamental physics of ultrasound and its propagation in tissue. *Radiographics* 1993;13:705–709.
10. Goldstein A. Overview of the physics of US. *Radiographics* 1993;13:701–704.
11. Geiser E. Physics and instrumentation. In: Skorton DJ, ed. *Marcus cardiac imaging: a companion to Braunwald's heart disease.* Philadelphia: WB Saunders, 1996:273–291.
12. Schiller NB, Shah PM, Crawford M, et al. Recommendations for quantitation of the left ventricle by two-dimensional echocardiography. American Society of Echocardiography Committee on Standards, Subcommittee on Quantitation of Two-Dimensional Echocardiograms. *J Am Soc Echocardiogr* 1989;2:358–367.
13. Schnittger I, Gordon EP, Fitzgerald PJ, Popp RL. Standardized intracardiac measurements of two-dimensional echocardiography. *J Am Coll Cardiol* 1983;2:934–938.
14. Weyman A. *Principles and practice of echocardiography,* 2nd ed. Philadelphia: Lea & Febiger, 1994.
15. Massie BM, Schiller NB, Ratshin RA, Parmley WW. Mitral-septal separation: new echocardiographic index of left ventricular function. *Am J Cardiol* 1977;39:1008–1016.
16. Child JS, Krivokapich J, Perloff JK. Effect of left ventricular size on mitral E point to ventricular septal separation in assessment of cardiac performance. *Am Heart J* 1981;101:797–805.
17. Djalaly A, Schiller NB, Poehlmann HW, et al. Diastolic aortic root motion in left ventricular hypertrophy. *Chest* 1981;79:442–445.
18. Strunk BL, Fitzgerald JW, Lipton M, et al. The posterior aortic wall echocardiogram. Its relationship to left atrial volume change. *Circulation* 1976;54:744–750.
19. Pratt RC, Parisi AF, Harrington JJ, Sasahara AA. The influence of left ventricular stroke volume on aortic root motion: an echocardiographic study. *Circulation* 1976;53:947–953.
20. Silverman NH, Schiller NB. Apex echocardiography. A two-dimensional technique for evaluating congenital heart disease. *Circulation* 1978;57:503–511.
21. Silverman NH, Ports TA, Snider AR, et al. Determination of left ventricular volume in children: echocardiographic and angiographic comparisons. *Circulation* 1980;62:548–557.
22. Van Dantzig JM, Delemarre BJ, Koster RW, et al. Pathogenesis of mitral regurgitation in acute myocardial infarction: importance of changes in left ventricular shape and regional function. *Am Heart J* 1996;131:865–871.
23. Dillon JC, Chang S, Feigenbaum H. Echocardiographic manifestations of left bundle branch block. *Circulation* 1974;49:876–880.
24. Simonson JS, Schiller NB. Descent of the base of the left ventricle: an echocardiographic index of left ventricular function [see comments]. *J Am Soc Echocardiogr* 1989;2:25–35.
25. Lang RM, Vignon P, Weinert L, et al. Echocardiographic quantification of regional left ventricular wall motion with color kinesis [see comments]. *Circulation* 1996;93:1877–1885.
26. Schiller NB, Acquatella H, Ports TA, et al. Left ventricular volume from paired biplane two-dimensional echocardiography. *Circulation* 1979;60:547–555.
27. Folland ED, Parisi AF, Moynihan PF, et al. Assessment of left ventricular ejection fraction and volumes by real-time, two-dimensional echocardiography. A comparison of cineangiographic and radionuclide techniques. *Circulation* 1979;60:760–766.
28. Starling MR, Crawford MH, Sorensen SG, et al. Comparative accuracy of apical biplane cross-sectional echocardiography and gated equilibrium radionuclide angiography for estimating left ventricular size and performance. *Circulation* 1981;63:1075–1084.
29. Corya BC, Rasmussen S, Knoebel SB, Feigenbaum H. M-mode echocardiography in evaluating left ventricular function and surgical risk in patients with coronary artery disease. *Chest* 1977;72:181–185.
30. Fortuin NJ, Hood WP Jr, Craige E. Evaluation of left ven-

tricular function by echocardiography. *Circulation* 1972; 46:26–35.

31. Kisslo J, Wolfson S, Ross A, et al. Ultrasound assessment of left ventricular function following aortocoronary saphenous vein bypass grafting. *Circulation* 1973;48:III-156–III-161.

32. McDonald IG, Feigenbaum H, Chang S. Analysis of left ventricular wall motion by reflected ultrasound. Application to assessment of myocardial function. *Circulation* 1972;46:14–25.

33. Germain P, Roul G, Kastler B, et al. Inter-study variability in left ventricular mass measurement. Comparison between M-mode echography and MRI. *Eur Heart J* 1992;13:1011–1019.

34. Collins HW, Kronenberg MW, Byrd BF III. Reproducibility of left ventricular mass measurements by two-dimensional and M-mode echocardiography. *J Am Coll Cardiol* 1989;14:672–676.

35. Sagawa K, Suga H, Shoukas AA, Bakalar KM. End-systolic pressure/volume ratio: a new index of ventricular contractility. *Am J Cardiol* 1977;40:748–753.

36. Byrd BF III, Finkbeiner W, Bouchard A, et al. Accuracy and reproducibility of clinically acquired two-dimensional echocardiographic mass measurements. *Am Heart J* 1989;118:133–137.

37. Kuecherer HF, Kee LL, Modin G, et al. Echocardiography in serial evaluation of left ventricular systolic and diastolic function: importance of image acquisition, quantitation, and physiologic variability in clinical and investigational applications. *J Am Soc Echocardiogr* 1991;4:203–214.

38. Schiller NB. Considerations in the standardization of measurement of left ventricular myocardial mass by two-dimensional echocardiography. *Hypertension* 1987;9:II33–35.

39. Kuecherer H. Importance of image acquisition, quantitation, and physiological variability in clinical and investigational applications. *J Am Soc Echocardiogr* 1991;4:203–214.

40. Borow KM, Green LH, Mann T, et al. End-systolic volume as a predictor of postoperative left ventricular performance in volume overload from valvular regurgitation. *Am J Med* 1980;68:655–663.

41. Hammermeister KE, DeRouen TA, Dodge HT. Variables predictive of survival in patients with coronary disease. Selection by univariate and multivariate analyses from the clinical, electrocardiographic, exercise, arteriographic, and quantitative angiographic evaluations. *Circulation* 1979;59:421–430.

42. White HD, Norris RM, Brown MA, et al. Left ventricular end-systolic volume as the major determinant of survival after recovery from myocardial infarction. *Circulation* 1987;76:44–51.

43. Moye LA, Pfeffer MA, Braunwald E. Rationale, design and baseline characteristics of the survival and ventricular enlargement trial. SAVE investigators. *Am J Cardiol* 1991;68:70D–79D.

44. Volpi A, De Vita C, Franzosi MG, et al. Determinants of 6-month mortality in survivors of myocardial infarction after thrombolysis. Results of the GISSI-2 data base. The Ad Hoc Working Group of the Gruppo Italiano Per lo Studio Della Sopravvivenza Nell'Infarto Miocardico (GISSI)-2 Data Base. *Circulation* 1993;88:416–429.

45. Sahn DJ, DeMaria A, Kisslo J, Weyman A. Recommendations regarding quantitation in M-mode echocardiography: results of a survey of echocardiographic measurements. *Circulation* 1978;58:1072–1083.

46. Troy BL, Pombo J, Rackley CE. Measurement of left ventricular wall thickness and mass by echocardiography. *Circulation* 1972;45:602–611.

47. Devereux RB, Alonso DR, Lutas EM, et al. Echocardiographic assessment of left ventricular hypertrophy: comparison to necropsy findings. *Am J Cardiol* 1986;57:450–458.

48. Devereux RB, Lutas EM, Casale PN, et al. Standardization of M-mode echocardiographic left ventricular anatomic measurements. *J Am Coll Cardiol* 1984;4:1222–1230.

49. Teichholz LE, Kreulen T, Herman MV, Gorlin R. Problems in echocardiographic volume determinations: echocardiographic-angiographic correlations in the presence or absence of asynergy. *Am J Cardiol* 1976;37:7–11.

50. Devereux RB, Casale PN, Eisenberg RR, et al. Electrocardiographic detection of left ventricular hypertrophy using echocardiographic determination of left ventricular mass as the reference standard. Comparison of standard criteria, computer diagnosis and physician interpretation. *J Am Coll Cardiol* 1984;3:82–87.

51. Casale PN, Devereux RB, Kligfield P, et al. Electrocardiographic detection of left ventricular hypertrophy: development and prospective validation of improved criteria. *J Am Coll Cardiol* 1985;6:572–580.

52. Levy D, Garrison RJ, Savage DD, et al. Prognostic implications of echocardiographically determined left ventricular mass in the Framingham Heart Study [see comments]. *N Engl J Med* 1990;322:1561–1566.

53. Schroder KM, Sapin PM, King DL, et al. Three-dimensional echocardiographic volume computation: in vitro comparison to standard two-dimensional echocardiography. *J Am Soc Echocardiogr* 1993;6:467–475.

54. Sapin PM, Schroeder KD, Smith MD, et al. Three-dimensional echocardiographic measurement of left ventricular volume in vitro: comparison with two-dimensional echocardiography and cineventriculography [see comments]. *J Am Coll Cardiol* 1993;22:1530–1537.

55. Sapin PM, Schroder KM, Gopal AS, et al. Comparison of two- and three-dimensional echocardiography with cineventriculography for measurement of left ventricular volume in patients. *J Am Coll Cardiol* 1994;24:1054–1063.

56. Jiang L, Siu SC, Handschumacher MD, et al. Three-dimensional echocardiography. In vivo validation for right ventricular volume and function. *Circulation* 1994;89:2342–2350.

57. Gopal AS, King DL, Katz J, et al. Three-dimensional echocardiographic volume computation by polyhedral surface reconstruction: in vitro validation and comparison to magnetic resonance imaging. *J Am Soc Echocardiogr* 1992;5:115–124.

58. Gopal AS, Keller AM, Rigling R, King DL. Left ventricular volume and endocardial surface area by three-dimensional echocardiography: comparison with two-dimensional echocardiography and nuclear magnetic resonance imaging in normal subjects. *J Am Coll Cardiol* 1993;22:258–270.

59. Gopal AS, Keller AM, Shen Z, et al. Three-dimensional

echocardiography: in vitro and in vivo validation of left ventricular mass and comparison with conventional echocardiographic methods [see comments]. *J Am Coll Cardiol* 1994;24:504–513.

60. Gopal AS, Shen Z, Sapin PM, et al. Assessment of cardiac function by three-dimensional echocardiography compared with conventional noninvasive methods. *Circulation* 1995;92:842–853.

61. King DL, Gopal AS, Keller AM, et al. Three-dimensional echocardiography. Advances for measurement of ventricular volume and mass. *Hypertension* 1994;23:I172–179.

62. Byrd BF III, Wahr D, Wang YS, et al. Left ventricular mass and volume/mass ratio determined by two-dimensional echocardiography in normal adults. *J Am Coll Cardiol* 1985;6:1021–1025.

63. Byrd BF III. Left ventricular mass and volume/mass ratio in a normal population determined by two-dimensional echocardiography. *J Am Coll Cardiol* 1985;5:1021.

64. Diethelm L, Simonson JS, Dery R, et al. Determination of left ventricular mass with ultrafast CT and two-dimensional echocardiography. *Radiology* 1989;171:213–217.

65. Gutman J, Wang YS, Wahr D, Schiller NB. Normal left atrial function determined by 2-dimensional echocardiography. *Am J Cardiol* 1983;51:336–340.

66. Kircher B, Abbott JA, Pau S, et al. Left atrial volume determination by biplane two-dimensional echocardiography: validation by cine computed tomography. *Am Heart J* 1991;121:864–871.

67. Wahr DW, Wang YS, Schiller NB. Left ventricular volumes determined by two-dimensional echocardiography in a normal adult population. *J Am Coll Cardiol* 1983;1:863–868.

68. Wang Y, Gutman JM, Heilbron D, et al. Atrial volume in a normal adult population by two-dimensional echocardiography. *Chest* 1984;86:595–601.

69. Mickelson JK, Byrd BF III, Bouchard A, et al. Left ventricular dimensions and mechanics in distance runners. *Am Heart J* 1986;112:1251–1256.

70. Himelman RB, Chung WS, Chernoff DN, et al. Cardiac manifestations of human immunodeficiency virus infection: a two-dimensional echocardiographic study. *J Am Coll Cardiol* 1989;13:1030–1036.

71. Nishimura RA, Reeder GS, Miller FA Jr, et al. Prognostic value of predischarge 2-dimensional echocardiogram after acute myocardial infarction. *Am J Cardiol* 1984;53:429–432.

72. Gibson RS, Bishop HL, Stamm RB, et al. Value of early two dimensional echocardiography in patients with acute myocardial infarction. *Am J Cardiol* 1982;49:1110–1119.

73. Kan G, Visser CA, Lie KI, Durrer D. Early two-dimensional echocardiographic measurement of left ventricular ejection fraction in acute myocardial infarction. *Eur Heart J* 1984;5:210–217.

74. Kumar A, Minagoe S, Chandraratna PA. Two-dimensional echocardiographic demonstration of restoration of normal wall motion after acute myocardial infarction. *Am J Cardiol* 1986;57:1232–1235.

75. Roberts CS, Maclean D, Maroko P, Kloner RA. Early and late remodeling of the left ventricle after acute myocardial infarction. *Am J Cardiol* 1984;54:407–410.

76. Stamm RB, Gibson RS, Bishop HL, et al. Echocardiographic detection of infarct-localized asynergy and remote asynergy during acute myocardial infarction: correlation with the extent of angiographic coronary disease. *Circulation* 1983;67:233–244.

77. Haugland JM, Asinger RW, Mikell FL, et al. Embolic potential of left ventricular thrombi detected by two-dimensional echocardiography. *Circulation* 1984;70:588–598.

78. Reeder GS, Tajik AJ, Seward JB. Left ventricular mural thrombus: two-dimensional echocardiographic diagnosis. *Mayo Clin Proc* 1981;56:82–86.

79. Visser CA, Kan G, David GK, et al. Two dimensional echocardiography in the diagnosis of left ventricular thrombus. A prospective study of 67 patients with anatomic validation. *Chest* 1983;83:228–232.

80. Visser CA, Kan G, Meltzer RS, et al. Long-term follow-up of left ventricular thrombus after acute myocardial infarction. A two-dimensional echocardiographic study in 96 patients. *Chest* 1984;86:532–536.

81. Keren A, Billingham ME, Popp RL. Echocardiographic recognition and implications of ventricular hypertrophic trabeculations and aberrant bands. *Circulation* 1984;70:836–842.

82. Arvan S, Varat MA. Persistent ST-segment elevation and left ventricular wall abnormalities: a 2-dimensional echocardiographic study. *Am J Cardiol* 1984;53:1542–1546.

83. Matsumoto M, Watanabe F, Goto A, et al. Left ventricular aneurysm and the prediction of left ventricular enlargement studied by two-dimensional echocardiography: quantitative assessment of aneurysm size in relation to clinical course. *Circulation* 1985;72:280–286.

84. Wong M, Shah PM. Accuracy of two-dimensional echocardiography in detecting left ventricular aneurysm. *Clin Cardiol* 1983;6:250–254.

85. Kaul S, Josephson MA, Tei C, et al. Atypical echocardiographic and angiographic presentation of a postoperative pseudoaneurysm of the left ventricle after repair of a true aneurysm. *J Am Coll Cardiol* 1983;2:780–784.

86. Wunderink RG. Incidence of pericardial effusions in acute myocardial infarctions. *Chest* 1984;85:494–496.

87. Kaplan K, Davison R, Parker M, et al. Frequency of pericardial effusion as determined by M-mode echocardiography in acute myocardial infarction. *Am J Cardiol* 1985;55:335–337.

88. Lindower P, Embrey R, Vandenberg B. Echocardiographic diagnosis of mechanical complications in acute myocardial infarction. *Clin Intensive Care* 1993;4:276–283.

89. Drobac M, Gilbert B, Howard R, et al. Ventricular septal defect after myocardial infarction: diagnosis by two-dimensional contrast echocardiography. *Circulation* 1983;67:335–341.

90. Recusani F, Raisaro A, Sgalambro A, et al. Ventricular septal rupture after myocardial infarction: diagnosis by two-dimensional and pulsed Doppler echocardiography. *Am J Cardiol* 1984;54:277–281.

91. Keren G, Sherez J, Roth A, et al. Diagnosis of ventricular septal rupture from acute myocardial infarction by combined 2-dimensional and pulsed Doppler echocardiography. *Am J Cardiol* 1984;53:1202–1203.

92. Eisenberg PR, Barzilai B, Perez JE. Noninvasive detection by Doppler echocardiography of combined ventricular septal rupture and mitral regurgitation in acute myocardial infarction. *J Am Coll Cardiol* 1984;4:617–620.

93. Nishimura RA, Schaff HV, Shub C, et al. Papillary muscle rupture complicating acute myocardial infarction: analysis of 17 patients. *Am J Cardiol* 1983;51:373–377.

94. Nishimura RA, Shub C, Tajik AJ. Two dimensional echocardiographic diagnosis of partial papillary muscle rupture. *Br Heart J* 1982;48:598–600.

95. Goldberger JJ, Himelman RB, Wolfe CL, Schiller NB. Right ventricular infarction: recognition and assessment of its hemodynamic significance by two-dimensional echocardiography. *J Am Soc Echocardiogr* 1991;4:140–146.

96. Sharpe DN, Botvinick EH, Shames DM, et al. The noninvasive diagnosis of right ventricular infarction. *Circulation* 1978;57:483–490.

97. Unverferth DV, Magorien RD, Moeschberger ML, et al. Factors influencing the one-year mortality of dilated cardiomyopathy. *Am J Cardiol* 1984;54:147–152.

98. Lewis JF, Webber JD, Sutton LL, et al. Discordance in degree of right and left ventricular dilation in patients with dilated cardiomyopathy: recognition and clinical implications. *J Am Coll Cardiol* 1993;21:649–654.

99. Acquatella H, Schiller NB, Puigbo JJ, et al. M-mode and two-dimensional echocardiography in chronic Chagas' heart disease. A clinical and pathologic study. *Circulation* 1980;62:787–799.

100. Abbasi AS, MacAlpin RN, Eber LM, Pearce ML. Echocardiographic diagnosis of idiopathic hypertrophic cardiomyopathy without outflow obstruction. *Circulation* 1972;46:897–904.

101. Maron BJ, Nichols PFd, Pickle LW, et al. Patterns of inheritance in hypertrophic cardiomyopathy: assessment by M-mode and two-dimensional echocardiography. *Am J Cardiol* 1984;53:1087–1094.

102. Maron BJ. Asymmetry in hypertrophic cardiomyopathy: the septal to free wall thickness ratio revisited. *Am J Cardiol* 1985;55:835–838.

103. Nair CK, Kudesia V, Hansen D, et al. Echocardiographic and electrocardiographic characteristics of patients with hypertrophic cardiomyopathy with and without mitral anular calcium. *Am J Cardiol* 1987;59:1428–1430.

104. Maron BJ, Bonow RO, Seshagiri TN, et al. Hypertrophic cardiomyopathy with ventricular septal hypertrophy localized to the apical region of the left ventricle (apical hypertrophic cardiomyopathy). *Am J Cardiol* 1982;49:1838–1848.

105. Kereiakes DJ, Anderson DJ, Crouse L, Chatterjee K. Apical hypertrophic cardiomyopathy. *Am Heart J* 1983;105:855–856.

106. Maron BJ, Harding AM, Spirito P, et al. Systolic anterior motion of the posterior mitral leaflet: a previously unrecognized cause of dynamic subaortic obstruction in patients with hypertrophic cardiomyopathy. *Circulation* 1983;68:282–293.

107. Spirito P, Maron BJ. Patterns of systolic anterior motion of the mitral valve in hypertrophic cardiomyopathy: assessment by two-dimensional echocardiography. *Am J Cardiol* 1984;54:1039–1046.

108. Yock PG, Hatle L, Popp RL. Patterns and timing of Doppler-detected intracavitary and aortic flow in hypertrophic cardiomyopathy. *J Am Coll Cardiol* 1986;8:1047–1058.

109. Bouchard A, Sanz N, Botvinick EH, et al. Noninvasive assessment of cardiomyopathy in normotensive diabetic patients between 20 and 50 years old. *Am J Med* 1989;87:160–166.

110. Sedlis SP, Saffitz JE, Schwob VS, Jaffe AS. Cardiac amyloidosis simulating hypertrophic cardiomyopathy. *Am J Cardiol* 1984;53:969–970.

111. Siqueira-Filho AG, Cunha CL, Tajik AJ, et al. M-mode and two-dimensional echocardiographic features in cardiac amyloidosis. *Circulation* 1981;63:188–196.

112. Nicolosi GL, Pavan D, Lestuzzi C, et al. Prospective identification of patients with amyloid heart disease by two-dimensional echocardiography. *Circulation* 1984;70:432–437.

113. Klein AL, Hatle LK, Taliercio CP, et al. Prognostic significance of Doppler measures of diastolic function in cardiac amyloidosis. A Doppler echocardiography study. *Circulation* 1991;83:808–816.

114. Allenby PA, Gould NS, Schwartz MF, Chiemmongkoltip P. Dysplastic cardiac development presenting as cardiomyopathy. *Arch Pathol Lab Med* 1988;112:1255–1258.

115. Jenni R, Goebel N, Tartini R, et al. Persisting myocardial sinusoids of both ventricles as an isolated anomaly: echocardiographic, angiographic, and pathologic anatomical findings. *Cardiovasc Intervent Radiol* 1986;9:127–131.

116. Agmon Y, Connolly HM, Olson LJ, et al. Noncompaction of the ventricular myocardium. *J Am Soc Echocardiogr* 1999;12:859–863.

117. Oechslin EN, Jost CH, Rojas JR, et al. Long-term follow-up of 34 adults with isolated left ventricular noncompaction: a distinct cardiomyopathy with poor prognosis. *J Am Coll Cardiol* 2000;36:493–500.

118. Ports TA, Cogan J, Schiller NB, Rapaport E. Echocardiography of left ventricular masses. *Circulation* 1978;58:528–536.

119. Acquatella H, Schiller NB, Puigbo JJ, et al. Value of two-dimensional echocardiography in endomyocardial disease with and without eosinophilia. A clinical and pathologic study. *Circulation* 1983;67:1219–1226.

120. Cooper MJ, Teitel DF, Silverman NH, Enderlein M. Comparison of M-mode echocardiographic measurement of right ventricular wall thickness obtained by the subcostal and parasternal approach in children. *Am J Cardiol* 1984;54:835–838.

121. Silverman NH, Hudson S. Evaluation of right ventricular volume and ejection fraction in children by two-dimensional echocardiography. *Pediatr Cardiol* 1983;4:197–203.

122. Levine RA, Gibson TC, Aretz T, et al. Echocardiographic measurement of right ventricular volume. *Circulation* 1984;69:497–505.

123. Starling MR, Crawford MH, Sorensen SG, O'Rourke RA. A new two-dimensional echocardiographic technique for evaluating right ventricular size and performance in patients with obstructive lung disease. *Circulation* 1982;66:612–620.

124. Kaul S, Tei C, Hopkins JM, Shah PM. Assessment of right ventricular function using two-dimensional echocardiography. *Am Heart J* 1984;107:526–531.

125. Himelman RB, Struve SN, Brown JK, et al. Improved recognition of cor pulmonale in patients with severe chronic obstructive pulmonary disease. *Am J Med* 1988;84:891–898.

126. Isaaz K, Munoz del Romeral L, Lee E, Schiller NB. Quantitation of the motion of the cardiac base in normal subjects by Doppler echocardiography. *J Am Soc Echocardiogr* 1993;6:166–176.

127. Ports TA, Schiller NB, Strunk BL. Echocardiography of right ventricular tumors. *Circulation* 1977;56:439–447.

128. Lee CC, Celik C, Lajos TZ. Excision of papillary fibroelastoma arising from the septal leaflet of the tricuspid valve. *J Cardiol Surg* 1995;10:589–591.

129. Nellessen U, Daniel WG, Matheis G, et al. Impending paradoxical embolism from atrial thrombus: correct diagnosis by transesophageal echocardiography and prevention by surgery. *J Am Coll Cardiol* 1985;5:1002–1004.

130. Higgins JR, Strunk BL, Schiller NB. Diagnosis of paradoxical embolism with contrast echocardiography. *Am Heart J* 1984;107:375–377.

131. Payvandi MN, Kerber RE. Echocardiography in congenital and acquired absence of the pericardium. An echocardiographic mimic of right ventricular volume overload. *Circulation* 1976;53:86–92.

132. Marcus FI, Fontaine G. Arrhythmogenic right ventricular dysplasia/cardiomyopathy: a review. *Pacing Clin Electrophysiol* 1995;18:1298–1314.

133. Ports TA, Silverman NH, Schiller NB. Two-dimensional echocardiographic assessment of Ebstein's anomaly. *Circulation* 1978;58:336–343.

134. Silverman NH, Gerlis LM, Horowitz ES, et al. Pathologic elucidation of the echocardiographic features of Ebstein's malformation of the morphologically tricuspid valve in discordant atrioventricular connections. *Am J Cardiol* 1995;76:1277–1283.

135. Schabelman S, Schiller NB, Silverman NH, Ports TA. Left atrial volume estimation by two-dimensional echocardiography. *Cathet Cardiovasc Diagn* 1981;7:165–178.

136. Sanfilippo AJ, Abascal VM, Sheehan M, et al. Atrial enlargement as a consequence of atrial fibrillation. A prospective echocardiographic study [see comments]. *Circulation* 1990;82:792–797.

137. Welikovitch L, Lafreniere G, Burggraf GW, Sanfilippo AJ. Change in atrial volume following restoration of sinus rhythm in patients with atrial fibrillation: a prospective echocardiographic study. *Can J Cardiol* 1994;10:993–996.

138. Diker E, Aydogdu S, Ozdemir M, et al. Prevalence and predictors of atrial fibrillation in rheumatic valvular heart disease. *Am J Cardiol* 1996;77:96–98.

139. Mattioli AV, Tarabini Castellani E, Vivoli D, et al. Restoration of atrial function after atrial fibrillation of different etiological origins. *Cardiology* 1996;87:205–211.

140. Rostagno C, Olivo G, Comeglio M, et al. Left atrial size changes in patients with paroxysmal lone atrial fibrillation. An echocardiographic follow-up. *Angiology* 1996;47:797–801.

141. Schiller NB, Foster E, Redberg RF. Transesophageal echocardiography in the evaluation of mitral regurgitation. The twenty-four signs of severe mitral regurgitation. *Cardiol Clin* 1993;11:399–408.

142. Kaplan JD, Evans GT Jr, Foster E, et al. Evaluation of electrocardiographic criteria for right atrial enlargement by quantitative two-dimensional echocardiography. *J Am Coll Cardiol* 1994;23:747–752.

143. Armstrong WF, Feigenbaum H, Dillon JC. Echocardiographic detection of right atrial thromboembolism. *Chest* 1985;87:801–806.

144. Felner JM, Churchwell AL, Murphy DA. Right atrial thromboemboli: clinical, echocardiographic and pathophysiologic manifestations. *J Am Coll Cardiol* 1984;4:1041–1051.

145. Fagard R, Aubert A, Lysens R, et al. Noninvasive assessment of seasonal variations in cardiac structure and function in cyclists. *Circulation* 1983;67:896–901.

146. Nichol PM, Gilbert BW, Kisslo JA. Two-dimensional echocardiographic assessment of mitral stenosis. *Circulation* 1977;55:120–128.

147. Wann LS, Weyman AE, Feigenbaum H, et al. Determination of mitral valve area by cross-sectional echocardiography. *Ann Intern Med* 1978;88:337–341.

148. Sagie A, Freitas N, Padial LR, et al. Doppler echocardiographic assessment of long-term progression of mitral stenosis in 103 patients: valve area and right heart disease. *J Am Coll Cardiol* 1996;28:472–479.

149. Abascal VM, Wilkins GT, O'Shea JP, et al. Prediction of successful outcome in 130 patients undergoing percutaneous balloon mitral valvotomy [see comments]. *Circulation* 1990;82:448–456.

150. Wilkins GT, Weyman AE, Abascal VM, et al. Percutaneous balloon dilatation of the mitral valve: an analysis of echocardiographic variables related to outcome and the mechanism of dilatation. *Br Heart J* 1988;60:299–308.

151. Fatkin D, Roy P, Morgan JJ, Feneley MP. Percutaneous balloon mitral valvotomy with the Inoue single-balloon catheter: commissural morphology as a determinant of outcome. *J Am Coll Cardiol* 1993;21:390–397.

152. Carpentier AF, Pellerin M, Fuzellier JF, Relland JY. Extensive calcification of the mitral valve anulus: pathology and surgical management. *J Thorac Cardiovasc Surg* 1996;111:718–729; discussion 729–730.

153. D'Cruz I, Panetta F, Cohen H, Glick G. Submitral calcification or sclerosis in elderly patients: M mode and two dimensional echocardiography in "mitral anulus calcification." *Am J Cardiol* 1979;44:31–38.

154. Gabor GE, Mohr BD, Goel PC, Cohen B. Echocardiographic and clinical spectrum of mitral anular calcification. *Am J Cardiol* 1976;38:836–842.

155. Labovitz AJ, Nelson JG, Windhorst DM, et al. Frequency of mitral valve dysfunction from mitral anular calcium as detected by Doppler echocardiography. *Am J Cardiol* 1985;55:133–137.

156. Nair CK, Thomson W, Ryschon K, et al. Long-term follow-up of patients with echocardiographically detected mitral anular calcium and comparison with age- and sex-matched control subjects. *Am J Cardiol* 1989;63:465–470.

157. Himelman RB, Helms CA, Schiller NB. Is parathormone a cardiac toxin in uremia? *Int J Card Imaging* 1988;3:209–215.

158. D'Cruz IA, Madu EC. Progression to calcific mitral stenosis in end-stage renal disease. *Am J Kidney Dis* 1995;26:956–959.

159. Himelman RB, Schiller NB. Clinical and echocardiographic comparison of patients with the carcinoid syndrome with and without carcinoid heart disease. *Am J Cardiol* 1989;63:347–352.

160. Wann LS, Feigenbaum H, Weyman AE, Dillon JC. Cross-sectional echocardiographic detection of rheumatic mitral regurgitation. *Am J Cardiol* 1978;41:1258–1263.

161. Allen H, Harris A, Leatham A. Significance and prognosis of an isolated late systolic murmur: a 9- to 22-year follow-up. *Br Heart J* 1974;36:525–532.

162. Barlow JB, Pocock WA. Mitral valve prolapse, the specific billowing mitral leaflet syndrome, or an insignificant non-ejection systolic click [editorial]. *Am Heart J* 1979;97:277–285.

163. Kerber RE, Isaeff DM, Hancock EW. Echocardiographic patterns in patients with the syndrome of systolic click and late systolic murmur. *N Engl J Med* 1971;284:691–693.

164. Dillon JC, Haine CL, Chang S, Feigenbaum H. Use of echocardiography in patients with prolapsed mitral valve. *Circulation* 1971;43:503–507.

165. Markiewicz W, Stoner J, London E, et al. Mitral valve prolapse in one hundred presumably healthy young females. *Circulation* 1976;53:464–473.

166. Levine RA, Triulzi MO, Harrigan P, Weyman AE. The relationship of mitral annular shape to the diagnosis of mitral valve prolapse. *Circulation* 1987;75:756–767.

167. Nishimura RA, McGoon MD, Shub C, et al. Echocardiographically documented mitral-valve prolapse. Long-term follow-up of 237 patients. *N Engl J Med* 1985;313:1305–1309.

168. Chin ML, Bernstein RF, Child JS, Krivokapich J. Aortic valve systolic flutter as a screening test for severe aortic stenosis. *Am J Cardiol* 1983;51:981–985.

169. Godley RW, Green D, Dillon JC, et al. Reliability of two-dimensional echocardiography in assessing the severity of valvular aortic stenosis. *Chest* 1981;79:657–662.

170. Stoddard MF, Hammons RT, Longaker RA. Doppler transesophageal echocardiographic determination of aortic valve area in adults with aortic stenosis. *Am Heart J* 1996;132:337–342.

171. Teirstein P, Yeager M, Yock PG, Popp RL. Doppler echocardiographic measurement of aortic valve area in aortic stenosis: a noninvasive application of the Gorlin formula. *J Am Coll Cardiol* 1986;8:1059–1065.

172. Yeager M, Yock PG, Popp RL. Comparison of Doppler-derived pressure gradient to that determined at cardiac catheterization in adults with aortic valve stenosis: implications for management. *Am J Cardiol* 1986;57:644–648.

173. Choi JY, Sullivan ID. Fixed subaortic stenosis: anatomical spectrum and nature of progression. *Br Heart J* 1991;65:280–286.

174. Kitchiner D, Jackson M, Malaiya N, et al. Morphology of left ventricular outflow tract structures in patients with subaortic stenosis and a ventricular septal defect. *Br Heart J* 1994;72:251–260.

175. Kleinert S, Geva T. Echocardiographic morphometry and geometry of the left ventricular outflow tract in fixed subaortic stenosis. *J Am Coll Cardiol* 1993;22:1501–1508.

176. Braunstein PW Jr, Sade RM, Crawford FA Jr, Oslizlok PC. Repair of supravalvar aortic stenosis: cardiovascular morphometric and hemodynamic results. *Ann Thorac Surg* 1990;50:700–707.

177. Landzberg JS, Pflugfelder PW, Cassidy MM, et al. Etiology of the Austin Flint murmur. *J Am Coll Cardiol* 1992;20:408–413.

178. Botvinick EH, Schiller NB, Wickramasekaran R, et al. Echocardiographic demonstration of early mitral valve closure in severe aortic insufficiency. Its clinical implications. *Circulation* 1975;51:836–847.

179. Henry WL, Bonow RO, Borer JS, et al. Observations on the optimum time for operative intervention for aortic regurgitation. I. Evaluation of the results of aortic valve replacement in symptomatic patients. *Circulation* 1980;61:471–483.

180. Fioretti P, Roelandt J, Bos RJ, et al. Echocardiography in chronic aortic insufficiency. Is valve replacement too late when left ventricular end-systolic dimension reaches 55 mm? *Circulation* 1983;67:216–221.

181. Vandenbossche JL, Massie BM, Schiller NB, Karliner JS. Relation of left ventricular shape to volume and mass in patients with minimally symptomatic chronic aortic regurgitation. *Am Heart J* 1988;116:1022–1027.

182. Robertson WS, Stewart J, Armstrong WF, et al. Reverse doming of the anterior mitral leaflet with severe aortic regurgitation. *J Am Coll Cardiol* 1984;3:431–436.

183. Pflugfelder PW, Landzberg JS, Cassidy MM, et al. Comparison of cine MR imaging with Doppler echocardiography for the evaluation of aortic regurgitation. *AJR Am J Roentgenol* 1989;152:729–735.

184. Shively BK, Gurule FT, Roldan CA, et al. Diagnostic value of transesophageal compared with transthoracic echocardiography in infective endocarditis. *J Am Coll Cardiol* 1991;18:391–397.

185. Freed C, Schiller NB. Echocardiographic findings in Marfan's syndrome. *West J Med* 1977;126:87–90.

186. Schiller N. Transesophageal echocardiography. In: Skorton DJ, ed. *Marcus cardiac imaging: a companion to Braunwald's heart disease*. Philadelphia: WB Saunders, 1996:533–566.

187. San Roman JA, Vilacosta I, Zamorano JL, et al. Transesophageal echocardiography in right-sided endocarditis [see comments]. *J Am Coll Cardiol* 1993;21:1226–1230.

188. Schiller NB. Pulmonary artery pressure estimation by Doppler and two-dimensional echocardiography. *Cardiol Clin* 1990;8:277–287.

189. Kusumoto FM, Muhiudeen IA, Kuecherer HF, et al. Response of the interatrial septum to transatrial pressure gradients and its potential for predicting pulmonary capillary wedge pressure: an intraoperative study using transesophageal echocardiography in patients during mechanical ventilation. *J Am Coll Cardiol* 1993;21:721–728.

190. Sagie A, Schwammenthal E, Padial LR, et al. Determinants of functional tricuspid regurgitation in incomplete tricuspid valve closure: Doppler color flow study of 109 patients. *J Am Coll Cardiol* 1994;24:446–453.

191. Werner JA, Schiller NB, Prasquier R. Occurrence and significance of echocardiographically demonstrated tricuspid valve prolapse. *Am Heart J* 1978;96:180–186.

192. Bonmassari R, Nicolosi GL, Disertori M. [Tricuspid insufficiency with rupture of the chordae tendineae caused by closed thoracic trauma: evaluation by transesophageal

echocardiography. Description of a case.] *G Ital Cardiol* 1994;24:763–768.

193. Lewen MK, Bryg RJ, Miller LW, et al. Tricuspid regurgitation by Doppler echocardiography after orthotopic cardiac transplantation. *Am J Cardiol* 1987;59:1371–1374.

194. Hausen B, Albes JM, Rohde R, et al. Tricuspid valve regurgitation attributable to endomyocardial biopsies and rejection in heart transplantation. *Ann Thorac Surg* 1995;59:1134–1140.

195. Winslow T, Foster E, Adams JR, Schiller NB. Pulmonary valve endocarditis: improved diagnosis with biplane transesophageal echocardiography. *J Am Soc Echocardiogr* 1992;5:206–210.

196. Von Reyn CF, Levy BS, Arbeit RD, et al. Infective endocarditis: an analysis based on strict case definitions. *Ann Intern Med* 1981;94:505–518.

197. Bayer AS, Ward JI, Ginzton LE, Shapiro SM. Evaluation of new clinical criteria for the diagnosis of infective endocarditis [see comments]. *Am J Med* 1994;96:211–219.

198. Durack DT, Lukes AS, Bright DK. New criteria for diagnosis of infective endocarditis: utilization of specific echocardiographic findings. Duke Endocarditis Service [see comments]. *Am J Med* 1994;96:200–209.

199. Hirschfeld DS, Schiller N. Localization of aortic valve vegetations by echocardiography. *Circulation* 1976;53:280–285.

200. Gilbert BW, Haney RS, Crawford F, et al. Two-dimensional echocardiographic assessment of vegetative endocarditis. *Circulation* 1977;55:346–353.

201. O'Brien JT, Geiser EA. Infective endocarditis and echocardiography. *Am Heart J* 1984;108:386–394.

202. Mugge A, Daniel WG, Frank G, Lichtlen PR. Echocardiography in infective endocarditis: reassessment of prognostic implications of vegetation size determined by the transthoracic and the transesophageal approach. *J Am Coll Cardiol* 1989;14:631–638.

203. Jaffe WM, Morgan DE, Pearlman AS, Otto CM. Infective endocarditis, 1983–1988: echocardiographic findings and factors influencing morbidity and mortality [see comments]. *J Am Coll Cardiol* 1990;15:1227–1233.

204. Burger AJ, Peart B, Jabi H, Touchon RC. The role of two-dimensional echocardiology in the diagnosis of infective endocarditis [corrected] [published erratum appears in *Angiology* 1991 Sep;42(9):765]. *Angiology* 1991;42:552–560.

205. Daniel WG, Mugge A, Martin RP, et al. Improvement in the diagnosis of abscesses associated with endocarditis by transesophageal echocardiography [see comments]. *N Engl J Med* 1991;324:795–800.

206. Sochowski RA, Chan KL. Implication of negative results on a monoplane transesophageal echocardiographic study in patients with suspected infective endocarditis [see comments]. *J Am Coll Cardiol* 1993;21:216–221.

207. Shapiro SM, Young E, De Guzman S, et al. Transesophageal echocardiography in diagnosis of infective endocarditis [see comments]. *Chest* 1994;105:377–382.

208. Sanfilippo AJ, Picard MH, Newell JB, et al. Echocardiographic assessment of patients with infectious endocarditis: prediction of risk for complications. *J Am Coll Cardiol* 1991;18:1191–1199.

209. Peterson SP, Schiller N, Stricker RB. Failure of two-dimensional echocardiography to detect *Aspergillus* endocarditis. *Chest* 1984;85:291–294.

210. Lichtlen PR, Gahl K, Daniel WG. [Infectious endocarditis: clinical aspects and diagnosis.] *Schweiz Med Wochenschr* 1984;114:1566–1575.

211. Birmingham GD, Rahko PS, Ballantyne FD. Improved detection of infective endocarditis with transesophageal echocardiography. *Am Heart J* 1992;123:774–781.

212. Daniel WG, Mugge A, Grote J, et al. Comparison of transthoracic and transesophageal echocardiography for detection of abnormalities of prosthetic and bioprosthetic valves in the mitral and aortic positions. *Am J Cardiol* 1993;71:210–215.

213. Alton ME, Pasierski TJ, Orsinelli DA, et al. Comparison of transthoracic and transesophageal echocardiography in evaluation of 47 Starr-Edwards prosthetic valves. *J Am Coll Cardiol* 1992;20:1503–1511.

214. Zabalgoitia M, Garcia M. Pitfalls in the echo-Doppler diagnosis of prosthetic valve disorders. *Echocardiography* 1993;10:203–212.

215. Rohmann S, Erbel R, Darius H, et al. Prediction of rapid versus prolonged healing of infective endocarditis by monitoring vegetation size. *J Am Soc Echocardiogr* 1991;4:465–474.

216. Mugge A. Echocardiographic detection of cardiac valve vegetations and prognostic implications. *Infect Dis Clin North Am* 1993;7:877–898.

217. Heinle S, Wilderman N, Harrison JK, et al. Value of transthoracic echocardiography in predicting embolic events in active infective endocarditis. Duke Endocarditis Service. *Am J Cardiol* 1994;74:799–801.

218. Akins EW, Slone RM, Wiechmann BN, et al. Perivalvular pseudoaneurysm complicating bacterial endocarditis: MR detection in five cases. *AJR Am J Roentgenol* 1991;156:1155–1158.

219. Karalis DG, Bansal RC, Hauck AJ, et al. Transesophageal echocardiographic recognition of subaortic complications in aortic valve endocarditis. Clinical and surgical implications. *Circulation* 1992;86:353–362.

220. Leung DY, Cranney GB, Hopkins AP, Walsh WF. Role of transesophageal echocardiography in the diagnosis and management of aortic root abscess. *Br Heart J* 1994;72:175–181.

221. Hecht SR, Berger M. Right-sided endocarditis in intravenous drug users. Prognostic features in 102 episodes. *Ann Intern Med* 1992;117:560–566.

222. Feigenbaum H, Zaky A, Grabhorn LL. Cardiac motion in patients with pericardial effusion. A study using reflected ultrasound. *Circulation* 1966;34:611–619.

223. Feigenbaum H, Zaky A, Waldhausen JA. Use of ultrasound in the diagnosis of pericardial effusion. *Ann Intern Med* 1966;65:443–452.

224. Eisenberg MJ, Dunn MM, Kanth N, et al. Diagnostic value of chest radiography for pericardial effusion [see comments]. *J Am Coll Cardiol* 1993;22:588–593.

225. Horowitz MS, Schultz CS, Stinson EB, et al. Sensitivity and specificity of echocardiographic diagnosis of pericardial effusion. *Circulation* 1974;50:239–247.

226. Rifkin RD, Isner JM, Carter BL, Bankoff MS. Combined posteroanterior subepicardial fat simulating the echocar-

diographic diagnosis of pericardial effusion. *J Am Coll Cardiol* 1984;3:1333–1339.

227. D'Cruz IA, Hoffman PK. A new cross sectional echocardiographic method for estimating the volume of large pericardial effusions. *Br Heart J* 1991;66:448–451.

228. Eisenberg MJ, Oken K, Guerrero S, et al. Prognostic value of echocardiography in hospitalized patients with pericardial effusion. *Am J Cardiol* 1992;70:934–939.

229. Schiller NB, Botvinick EH. Right ventricular compression as a sign of cardiac tamponade: an analysis of echocardiographic ventricular dimensions and their clinical implications. *Circulation* 1977;56:774–779.

230. Schiller NB. Echocardiography in pericardial disease. *Med Clin North Am* 1980;64:253–282.

231. Himelman RB, Kircher B, Rockey DC, Schiller NB. Inferior vena cava plethora with blunted respiratory response: a sensitive echocardiographic sign of cardiac tamponade. *J Am Coll Cardiol* 1988;12:1470–1477.

232. Armstrong WF, Schilt BF, Helper DJ, et al. Diastolic collapse of the right ventricle with cardiac tamponade: an echocardiographic study. *Circulation* 1982;65:1491–1496.

233. Singh S, Wann LS, Schuchard GH, et al. Right ventricular and right atrial collapse in patients with cardiac tamponade—a combined echocardiographic and hemodynamic study. *Circulation* 1984;70:966–971.

234. Kronzon I, Cohen ML, Winer HE. Diastolic atrial compression: a sensitive echocardiographic sign of cardiac tamponade. *J Am Coll Cardiol* 1983;2:770–775.

235. D'Cruz IA, Constantine A. Problems and pitfalls in the echocardiographic assessment of pericardial effusion. *Echocardiography* 1993;10:151–166.

236. Ho GM, Eisenberg MJ, Schiller NB. Variation of blood flow in the thoracic aorta during cardiac tamponade. *Am Heart J* 1994;128:190–193.

237. Himelman RB, Lee E, Schiller NB. Septal bounce, vena cava plethora, and pericardial adhesion: informative two-dimensional echocardiographic signs in the diagnosis of pericardial constriction. *J Am Soc Echocardiogr* 1988;1:333–340.

238. Jue J, Chung W, Schiller NB. Does inferior vena cava size predict right atrial pressures in patients receiving mechanical ventilation? *J Am Soc Echocardiogr* 1992;5:613–619.

239. Klopfenstein HS, Wann LS. Can pleural effusions cause tamponade-like effects? *Echocardiography* 1994;11:489–492.

240. Tei C, Child JS, Tanaka H, Shah PM. Atrial systolic notch on the interventricular septal echogram: an echocardiographic sign of constrictive pericarditis. *J Am Coll Cardiol* 1983;1:907–912.

241. Gibson TC, Grossman W, McLaurin LP, et al. An echocardiographic study of the interventricular septum in constrictive pericarditis. *Br Heart J* 1976;38:738–743.

242. Hynes JK, Tajik AJ, Osborn MJ, et al. Two-dimensional echocardiographic diagnosis of pericardial cyst. *Mayo Clin Proc* 1983;58:60–63.

243. Eisenberg MJ, Rice SA, Paraschos A, et al. The clinical spectrum of patients with aneurysms of the ascending aorta. *Am Heart J* 1993;125:1380–1385.

244. Dev V, Goswami KC, Shrivastava S, et al. Echocardiographic diagnosis of aneurysm of the sinus of Valsalva. *Am Heart J* 1993;126:930–936.

245. Eisenberg MJ, Geraci SJ, Schiller NB. Screening for abdominal aortic aneurysms during transthoracic echocardiography. *Am Heart J* 1995;130:109–115.

246. Banning AP, Masani ND, Ikram S, et al. Transoesophageal echocardiography as the sole diagnostic investigation in patients with suspected thoracic aortic dissection. *Br Heart J* 1994;72:461–465.

247. Popp RL, Yock PG. Noninvasive intracardiac pressure measurement using Doppler ultrasound [editorial]. *J Am Coll Cardiol* 1985;6:757–758.

248. Simonson JS, Schiller NB. Sonospirometry: a new method for noninvasive estimation of mean right atrial pressure based on two-dimensional echographic measurements of the inferior vena cava during measured inspiration. *J Am Coll Cardiol* 1988;11:557–564.

249. Cahalan MK, Ionescu P, Melton HE Jr, et al. Automated real-time analysis of intraoperative transesophageal echocardiograms. *Anesthesiology* 1993;78:477–485.

250. Gorcsan J 3rd, Denault A, Gasior TA, et al. Rapid estimation of left ventricular contractility from end-systolic relations by echocardiographic automated border detection and femoral arterial pressure. *Anesthesiology* 1994;81:553–562; discussion 27A.

251. Perez JE, Waggoner AD, Barzilai B, et al. On-line assessment of ventricular function by automatic boundary detection and ultrasonic backscatter imaging [see comments]. *J Am Coll Cardiol* 1992;19:313–320.

252. Stewart WJ, Rodkey SM, Gunawardena S, et al. Left ventricular volume calculation with integrated backscatter from echocardiography. *J Am Soc Echocardiogr* 1993;6:553–563.

253. Sutherland GR, Stewart MJ, Groundstroem KW, et al. Color Doppler myocardial imaging: a new technique for the assessment of myocardial function. *J Am Soc Echocardiogr* 1994;7:441–458.

254. Miyatake K, Yamagishi M, Tanaka N, et al. New method for evaluating left ventricular wall motion by color-coded tissue Doppler imaging: in vitro and in vivo studies. *J Am Coll Cardiol* 1995;25:717–724.

255. Marini C, Picano E, Varga A, et al. Cyclic variation in myocardial gray level as a marker of viability in man. A videodensitometric study. *Eur Heart J* 1996;17:472–479.

256. Vitale DF, Bonow RO, Gerundo G, et al. Alterations in ultrasonic backscatter during exercise-induced myocardial ischemia in humans. *Circulation* 1995;92:1452–1457.

257. Davison G, Hall CS, Miller JG, et al. Ultrasonic tissue characterization of end-stage dilated cardiomyopathy. *Ultrasound Med Biol* 1995;21:853–860.

258. Meltzer RS, Ohad DG, Reisner S, et al. Quantitative myocardial ultrasonic integrated backscatter measurements during contrast injections. *J Am Soc Echocardiogr* 1994;7:1–8.

259. Perez JE, Miller JG, Wickline SA, et al. Quantitative ultrasonic imaging: tissue characterization and instantaneous quantification of cardiac function. *Am J Cardiol* 1992;69:104H–111H.

260. Popp RL. Recent experience with ultrasonic tissue characterization. *Am J Cardiol* 1992;69:112H–116H.

261. Lythall DA, Gibson DG, Kushwaha SS, et al. Changes in myocardial echo amplitude during reversible ischaemia in humans. *Br Heart J* 1992;67:368–376.

262. Ismail S, Jayaweera AR, Skyba DM, et al. Integrated backscatter and digital acquisition during myocardial contrast echocardiography: is there an advantage over conventional echocardiography for intracoronary injections? *J Am Soc Echocardiogr* 1995;8:453–464.

263. Salustri A, Roelandt J. Three dimensional reconstruction of the heart with rotational acquisition: methods and clinical applications. *Br Heart J* 1995;73[5 Suppl 2]:10-5.

264. Delabays A, Pandian NG, Cao QL, et al. Transthoracic real-time three-dimensional echocardiography using a fan-like scanning approach for data acquisition: methods, strengths, problems, and initial clinical experience. *Echocardiography* 1995;12:49–59.

265. Flachskampf FA, Franke A, Job FP, et al. Three-dimensional reconstruction of cardiac structures from transesophageal echocardiography. *Am J Card Imaging* 1995;9:141–147.

266. Salustri A, Becker AE, van Herwerden L, et al. Three-dimensional echocardiography of normal and pathologic mitral valve: a comparison with two-dimensional transesophageal echocardiography. *J Am Coll Cardiol* 1996;27:1502–1510.

267. Levine RA, Weyman AE, Handschumacher MD. Three-dimensional echocardiography: techniques and applications. *Am J Cardiol* 1992;69:121H–130H; discussion 131H–134H.

268. Roelandt JR, ten Cate FJ, Vletter WB, Taams MA. Ultrasonic dynamic three-dimensional visualization of the heart with a multiplane transesophageal imaging transducer. *J Am Soc Echocardiogr* 1994;7:217–229.

269. Mulvagh SL, DeMaria AN, Feinstein SB, et al. Contrast echocardiography: current and future applications. *J Am Soc Echocardiogr* 2000;13:331–342.

270. Thomas JD, Rubin DN. Tissue harmonic imaging: why does it work? *J Am Soc Echocardiogr* 1998;11:803–808.

50

STRESS ECHOCARDIOGRAPHY

THOMAS H. MARWICK

▼▼ ADDITIONAL ELECTRONIC TOPICS

OVERVIEW

Stress echocardiography provides a means of identifying myocardial ischemia by detection of stress-induced wall motion abnormalities on comparison of pre-stress and post-stress images. The technological revolution of ultrasound and digital technology has driven the development of this modality from a research to a clinical tool. However, interpretation of these studies remains subjective, and the

learning curve of skills required to use this modality must be considered.

Echocardiography may be combined with various stressors and used in a variety of environments. The test is patient friendly because it is rapidly performed and inexpensive. The accuracy of stress echocardiography in detecting significant coronary stenoses ranges from 80% to 90%, depending on the population studied, and the specificity is high. The accuracy exceeds that of exercise electrocardiography (ECG), especially in subgroups among whom the latter is unreliable (e.g., women and patients with left ventricular hypertrophy), and the accuracy is comparable with that of stress myocardial perfusion scintigraphy. The need

T. H. Marwick: Department of Medicine, University of Queensland, Princess Alexandra Hospital, Brisbane, Queensland, Australia

to induce ischemia limits the accuracy of stress echocardiography in detecting coronary artery disease (CAD) in patients who exercise submaximally or who are on antianginal therapy. However, the detection of ischemia may prove to be of value in using this test for prognostic evaluation or for monitoring the efficacy of therapy. Use of dobutamine echocardiography for identification of viable myocardium following myocardial infarction is another application that has moved this modality into the arena of assisting decision making in the management of CAD. Similarly, this test may provide useful data for the management of valvular and primary myocardial disease.

Stress echocardiography has been refined significantly over the last 3 years, and progress is likely to continue at a rapid pace. Endocardial border detection has been facilitated by harmonic imaging and contrast echocardiography. Tissue Doppler imaging and acoustic quantification techniques have been used to develop a quantitative approach to interpretation that is likely to become more sophisticated. The next major step is likely to be routine or selective use of echocontrast agents to permit acquisition of both left ventricular (LV) function and perfusion data at rest and after stress.

GLOSSARY

Coronary steal: A situation in which a vasodilator increases runoff to a normal branch, thus reducing the driving pressure in an artery proximal to a stenosis and causing ischemia because of reduced blood flow across the stenosis.

Echocardiographic contrast agents: Injectable compounds comprising gas-filled microbubbles approximately the size of or smaller than erythrocytes that increase the reflected signal of the cardiac structures in which they are located.

Myocardial tissue Doppler imaging: Use of Doppler principle to examine myocardial rather than blood flow velocity.

Sensitivity: Proportion of patients with CAD correctly identified as abnormal.

Single-photon emission computed tomography (SPECT): A means of acquiring and portraying scintigraphic data in a tomographic fashion.

Specificity: Proportion of patients without CAD correctly identified as normal.

Viable myocardium: Myocardial segments characterized by reduced function at rest but potentially recoverable either spontaneously (*stunned*) or with revascularization [usually associated with reduced myocardial perfusion (i.e., *hibernating myocardium*)].

INTRODUCTION

The use of exercise testing to provoke ischemic symptoms, ECG changes, and assess exercise capacity for the purpose of evaluating CAD dates back to the 1950s (1). However, while the exercise ECG is the most commonly accepted functional test for the diagnosis of CAD, there are situations in which it is inappropriate. First, patients who either cannot exercise or exercise submaximally account for 30% to 40% of patients presenting for functional testing (2). These patients are best studied using the combination of pharmacologic stress with various imaging techniques for the diagnosis of coronary disease. Second, even if the patient is able to exercise, the ECG may be uninterpretable because of repolarization abnormalities. In these circumstances, the ability of the patient to exercise is exploited by the combination of exercise testing with an imaging modality.

The use of stress imaging tests is not restricted to the diagnosis of coronary disease. As the ability to perform revascularization has improved, there has been a need to evaluate coronary disease on a functional basis, both to understand the site of ischemic tissue (and hence the likely culprit lesion) and to distinguish between ischemic, infarcted, and viable myocardium. Exercise ECG testing is unable to provide these data, which mandate the use of imaging. Similarly, the management of non–coronary heart disease, including valvular heart disease, primary myocardial disease, and some obstructive lesions may be facilitated by an appreciation of functional responses to stress. ☙ j38

PATHOPHYSIOLOGY

Detection of Ischemia by Echocardiography

The normal response of the left ventricle to increasing workload is a uniform increase of regional wall motion, thickening, and a reduction of end-systolic LV cavity size, with minimal changes of diastolic size during exercise or vasodilation (20). These changes return to baseline usually within minutes of the conclusion of the stress (21).

The distinction between resting and stress-induced wall motion abnormalities (Table 50.1) fundamentally differentiates prior myocardial infarction, identified by resting akinesis or dyskinesis, from induced ischemia, characterized by either new or worsening wall motion abnormalities. This effect of ischemia on regional ventricular function has been well defined with microcrystals (22), as well as with echocardiography (23,24). A more subtle index of myocardial ischemia is delayed contraction (25). The presence of LV enlargement following stress identifies severe ischemia or other serious heart muscle diseases. The time course of offset of regional myocardial dysfunction is variable and probably reflects the severity and duration of ischemia. Wall motion abnormalities may rapidly recover following the cessation of stress (26,27) but may also persist for 30 minutes or longer (9), especially if stunning is induced.

The presence of regional systolic dysfunction is usually caused by CAD, although cardiomyopathic processes may

TABLE 50.1 INTERPRETATION OF EXERCISE AND PHARMACOLOGIC STRESS ECHOCARDIOGRAPHY

Characterization of tissue	Resting function	Low-dose	Peak/poststress function
Normal	Normal	Normal	Hyperkinetic
Ischemic	Normal	Normal (ischemic with severe coronary artery disease)	Reduction vs. rest Reduction vs. adjacent segments Delayed contraction
Viable, nonischemic	Rest WMA	Improvement	Sustained improvement
Viable, ischemic	Rest WMA	Improvement	Reduction (compared with low-dose)
Infarction	Rest WMA	No change	No change

WMA, wall motion abnormalities (severe hypokinesis, akinesis, dyskinesis).

be regional rather than global. Resting wall motion abnormalities may not necessarily indicate the presence of transmural infarction; hypokinetic segments may be partially infarcted (especially the subendocardium) or viable (28). Viable segments may recover spontaneously (if the tissue is stunned) or following revascularization (if the myocardium is hibernating) (29,30). The presence of residual viable tissue is more common in hypokinetic than akinetic segments and least common in dyskinetic segments (31). Viable myocardium augments function in response to inotropic stimulation, and this response may be detected using echocardiography, as discussed in the section Identification of Myocardial Viability. Probably, both stunned and hibernating tissue contribute to chronic LV dysfunction due to CAD, and the conventional stress echo interpretation algorithm has been modified by the application of these findings to the clinical arena (Table 50.1).

METHODOLOGY OF STRESS ECHOCARDIOGRAPHY

Stress Testing Modalities

Exercise Stress

The use of stress echocardiography in patients with known or suspected CAD *who are able to exercise* usually incorporates exercise stress. The choice of modalities in this respect is between the treadmill and cycle ergometry, which may be upright or supine. During exercise, heart rate, blood pressure, and inotropic state all increase, in proportion to the increase of cardiac work. During upright exercise, venous return is relatively reduced, and LV end diastolic volume and pressure are similarly less than they would be during supine exercise (36). ◥⋎ j39

The merits and limitations of treadmill and bicycle stress are summarized in Table 50.2. In general, treadmill exercise is more widely accepted among patients and physicians in the United States. On the basis of peak and poststress imaging on the bicycle, it has been identified that a small reduction of sensitivity is possible if postexercise imaging is used. Lower workloads are attainable with bicycle than treadmill exercise, which

needs to be traded off against the benefits of peak exercise imaging on the bicycle. It is currently not possible to identify an optimal approach for exercise echocardiography, and the decision between bicycle and treadmill exercise is dependent on local expertise and, to some extent, on the nature of the clinical question in each individual patient. The acquisition of multiple images at peak stress is attractive for making assessments of the functional severity of coronary stenoses, and peak exercise imaging is attractive for assessment of valvular lesions. Moreover, the performance of imaging during stress may facilitate definition of the ischemic threshold.

Sympathomimetic Stressors

Hemodynamic Response

The response to dobutamine is summarized in Figure 50.1. Generally, peak heart rates of 120 to 140 beats/min are attainable (42), this corresponding to at least 85% of age-predicted heart rate in most patients. The systolic blood pressure usually increases by 30 to 40 mm Hg, with peak pressures of 170 to 180 mm Hg, and peak rate-pressure products of approximately 20,000. However, considerable variability occurs between different patients with respect to both the extent and speed of these hemodynamic responses.

Side Effects

Many patients requiring dobutamine stress are elderly and have serious noncardiac diseases or even severe CAD and LV dysfunction. Despite the use of high doses of these agents, serious complications occur in approximately 3 in 1,000 (43).

TABLE 50.2 ADVANTAGES AND DISADVANTAGES OF TREADMILL VERSUS BICYCLE STRESS FOR EXERCISE ECHOCARDIOGRAPHY

	Treadmill	Bicycle
Acceptance	Familiar to patient and physicians	Unfamiliarity
Adequacy of stress	Patients stress maximally	Premature termination due to leg fatigue Dependent on patient compliance
Imaging	Postexercise	Peak and postexercise

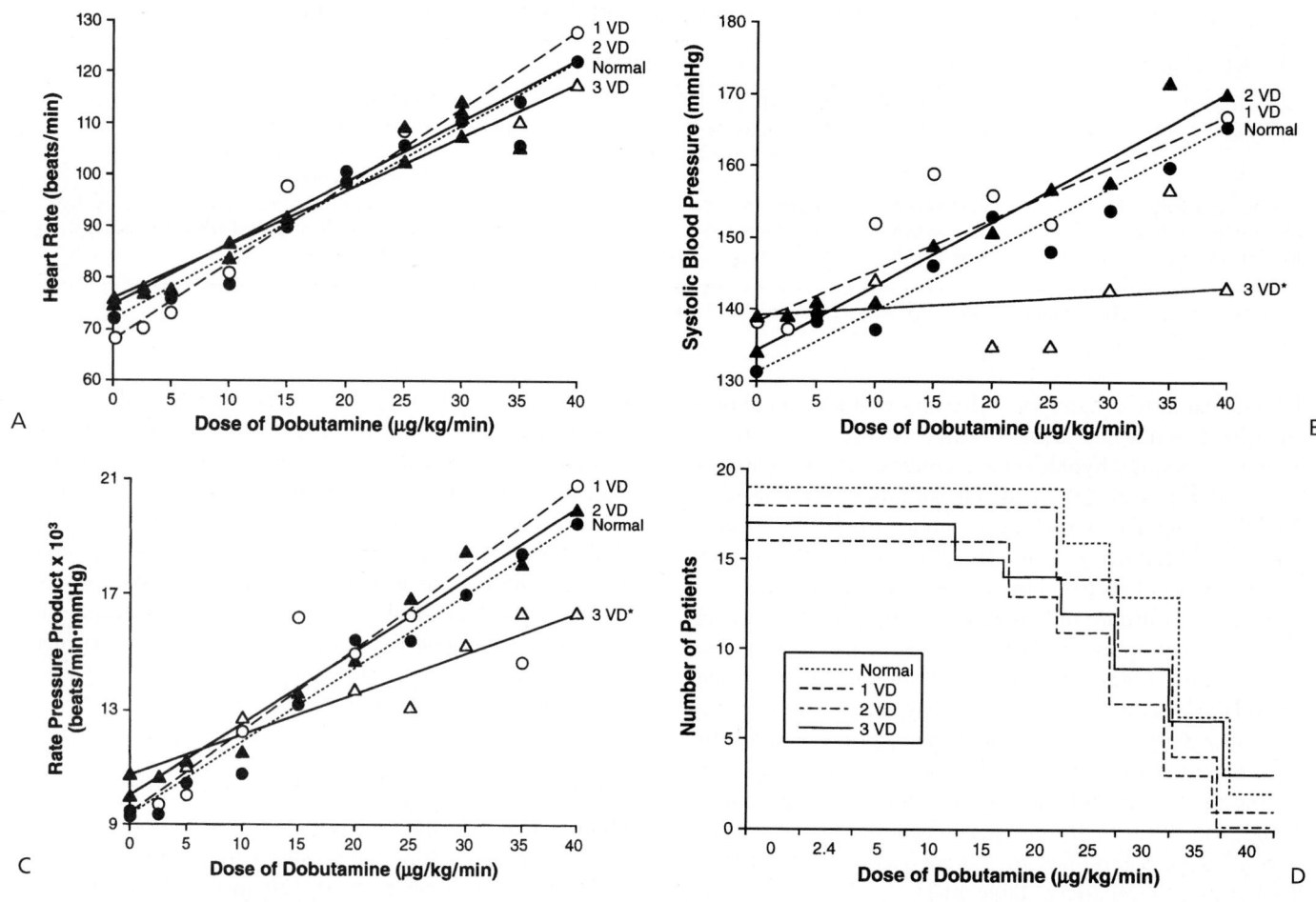

FIGURE 50.1 Hemodynamic responses to dobutamine, including heart rate **(A)**, systolic blood pressure **(B)**, and rate-pressure product **(C)**, according to the extent of coronary artery disease. **D:** The number of patients undergoing testing at each dose level of dobutamine, according to disease extent. 1 VD, one-vessel disease; 2 VD, two-vessel disease; 3 VD, three-vessel disease. (From Cohen JL, Greene TO, Ottenweller J, et al. Dobutamine digital echocardiography for detecting coronary artery disease. *Am J Cardiol* 1991;67:1311–1318, with permission.)

Administration Protocol

The protocol for dobutamine administration is empiric. Initially, a peak dose of 20 μg per kg per minute was used with myocardial perfusion imaging (44) and later echocardiography (45). The currently employed high-dose protocols (to 40 μg per kg per minute) were initially described by Sawada and Cohen (42,46) and seem to be more sensitive than lower dose protocols (47), although low-dose protocols provide adequate stress if the duration of each stage is longer (e.g., 5 rather than 3 minutes) (48). Atropine has been combined with dobutamine at peak dose if the heart-rate target is not attained (49) and more recently has been administered earlier in an attempt to shorten test duration (50). When evidence of myocardial viability is being sought, it is important to recognize that augmentation of function may occur at lower doses of dobutamine, and some authors have suggested specific low-dose protocols (e.g., to 12.5 μg per kg per minute in 2.5-μg increments) for this purpose. However, the practice of our laboratory has been to use a single standard protocol (including high

dose), which offers the versatility of identifying both viability and ischemia, while at the same time providing a study of acceptable length (Fig. 50.2). A rare exception is the situation in which peak dose is considered unsafe (e.g., history of hemodynamic instability); while caution should be exercised, the test appears safe for studying patients with severe LV dysfunction (51–53). Moreover, as discussed later in the chapter (see Extent and Severity of Disease), the biphasic response is the most reliable marker of recovery of LV function, and the detection of this usually requires a high-dose protocol. At present, none of the dobutamine protocols is clearly superior to the others, and the main consideration should be to ensure the adequacy of stress. ▼ j40

Vasodilator Stress

Hemodynamic Response

The hemodynamic effects of these stressors are minor. Blood pressure is little influenced by vasodilator stressors, although hypotension may occur. There may be a small

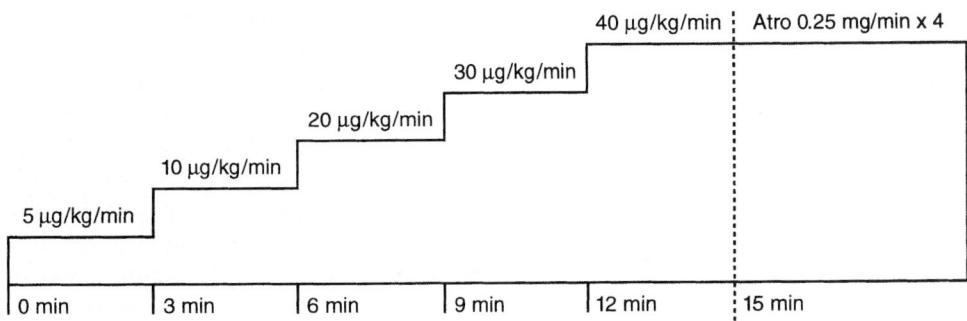

FIGURE 50.2 Dobutamine-atropine infusion protocol. Atro, atropine. (From Otto K. *Practice of clinical echocardiography*. Philadelphia: WB Saunders, 1996, with permission.)

increment of heart rate, which may occur in response to various side effects.

Side Effects

Serious side effects occur in approximately 1 in 1,000 patients. The most common side effects of dipyridamole and adenosine are headache and dyspnea, respectively (58,59). The speed of onset and potency of adenosine render its side effects less well tolerated, but these effects resolve rapidly with cessation of the drug. Both techniques are contraindicated in patients with untreated atrioventricular block and bronchospastic disorders, and abstinence from xanthene-containing foods and drugs is required before either stress.

Administration Protocol

The standard dipyridamole dose for myocardial perfusion imaging is 0.56 mg per kg administered over 4 minutes. For stress echocardiography, this dose induces ischemia only in patients with severe coronary disease. Thus, 0.56 mg per kg is administered first, but if ischemia is not induced, an additional 0.28 mg per kg is administered over 2 minutes. Atropine may be added if the response to dipyridamole is negative (60), and imaging is continued over 16 minutes. In some laboratories, dipyridamole is reversed with aminophylline. Although this is not usually necessary, aminophylline is useful for reversing the effect of dipyridamole in the presence of significant side effects. However, if aminophylline is needed for the treatment of severe ischemia, the supervising physician should be aware that the effect of dipyridamole may last longer than that of aminophylline, leading patients to become ischemic after they have left the stress laboratory.

The standard dose of adenosine for myocardial perfusion imaging is 0.14 mg per kg per minute intravenously over 4 minutes. This is also the most widely used dose for stress echocardiography, although both higher and lower doses have been studied. Although analogous to the dose of dipyridamole, higher dose protocols are constrained by dose-limiting side effects.

Selection of the Optimal Stress Agent

Pharmacologic stressors enhance the feasibility of imaging, but they have a number of important disadvantages

(Table 50.3). Generally, comparable levels of sensitivity are obtainable, although the performance of submaximal stress due to side effects is an important limitation. If a patient can exercise, we believe that he or she should undergo exercise echocardiography, unless the test has been performed for other reasons than the detection of myocardial ischemia (e.g., in specialized situations in which viability or coronary spasm are being evaluated). The development of new technologies such as tissue Doppler imaging, automated border detection, and contrast echocardiography have made pharmacologic stressors more attractive than exercise, but whether the incremental data offered by the addition of these features justifies the disadvantages of using a pharmacologic stressor in all patients remains to be established.

The type of pharmacologic stress may also be the source of debate. The frequency of side effects with dipyridamole and dobutamine stress is comparable, but the contraindications of each test are different. Thus, patients with asthma or untreated conduction system disease might be better tested using dobutamine echocardiography, whereas dipyridamole stress would be preferable in those with serious arrhythmias or severe hypertension. Most patients do not fall into these categories, so that either stressor might be used. In this situation, the choice might be based on physician preference, cost (dobutamine costs considerably less than dipyridamole in the United States, but the situation is reversed in Europe), and the clinical question to be addressed. If this relates to the diagnosis of coronary disease, the sensitivity of dobutamine echocardiography is somewhat greater than that of dipyridamole echocardiography, especially in patients with single-vessel disease. On the other hand, if the main interest is in prognostic evalua-

TABLE 50.3 BENEFITS OF EXERCISE OVER PHARMACOLOGIC STRESS

Evaluates exercise capacity
Correlates symptoms with physical workload
ST-segment evaluation
Cardiac workload is greater with exercise
Prognostic information
Probably greater sensitivity for ischemia

tion, the agents are both attractive, and certainly a wealth of information is available regarding dipyridamole echocardiography as a prognostic test (see Prognostic Considerations in Coronary Artery Disease).

Imaging Techniques

Stress echocardiography is almost universally performed using transthoracic echocardiography, although transesophageal imaging is sometimes used in the setting of poor image quality. The procedure brings together facilities for stress testing, echocardiography, and at least two and sometimes three personnel including physician, sonographer, and nurse. To use all of these resources efficiently, there is a need to limit the duration of activities that precede and follow the stress, during which time all resources are required. Consequently, it is not possible to perform an exhaustive echocardiographic examination in the context of stress echocardiography. Nonetheless, a screening M-mode and color Doppler examination should be performed at the beginning of every study. If more complex (e.g., valvular) problems are identified, these issues should be analyzed by echocardiography at another time. Using this approach, it should be possible to perform a treadmill echocardiogram in approximately 35 minutes, a bicycle stress echocardiogram in 45 minutes, and a dobutamine stress echocardiogram in approximately 1 hour.

Analysis of digital loops is beneficial for the interpretation of all forms of stress echo. Side-by-side comparison of cine loops in a split-screen display permits easy comparison of regional wall motion at rest and stress, and frame-by-frame review facilitates definition of the endocardium as well as evaluation of the temporal sequence of contraction. The disadvantage of this approach, however, is the finite number of views that can be compared using the quad-screen display and the presentation of single cardiac cycles. Consequently, review of the videotape is an important part of stress echocardiographic interpretation (76). j41

Interpretation of Stress Echocardiography

Qualitative Approaches

A qualitative approach is currently used for the interpretation of stress echocardiography. Using a segmental model of the left ventricle, each segment is compared before, during, and after stress. It is important in this evaluation that myocardial thickening is examined wherever possible, in preference to myocardial motion, which may occur due to translational movement, or tethering. Table 50.1 illustrates the criteria used to identify ischemia, myocardial viability, and myocardial scar. In general, ischemia is identified by the development of a new or worsening wall motion abnormality. Subtle indices of ischemia include delayed contrac-

tion; a temporal evaluation of myocardial contraction can be appreciated by stepping through individual freeze-frame images in the digital cine loop. Stress-induced LV enlargement is often a marker of multivessel coronary disease, and changes of ventricular shape as well as size are useful diagnostic clues to ischemia. As summarized by Table 50.1, myocardial viability is characterized by improvement of a dyssynergic zone in response to *low-dose* dobutamine. It is especially important that myocardial thickening is sought in patients with extensive infarction, as tethering can induce wall motion in nonviable segments. The most specific indicator of myocardial viability in the setting of hibernation is deterioration of this zone showing initial augmentation in response to increasing dobutamine dose, the "biphasic" response (81). In contrast, stunned myocardium augments functioning in response to low-dose dobutamine, but does not subsequently deteriorate. The presence of augmentation at *peak doses* of dobutamine is a nonspecific response, which is poorly predictive of myocardial viability.

The subjectivity of current approaches to the interpretation of stress echocardiography is the greatest shortcoming of this technique. This has two major manifestations: first, the need for training, and, second, the problems posed for reproducibility of the test. The importance of training in stress echocardiography was studied by a comparison of experts in stress echocardiography and skilled echocardiographers without stress echocardiography experience (82). The experts demonstrated a significantly greater accuracy than the other echocardiographers, but after a training period, during which the trainees were instructed using 100 studies, this difference in accuracy became insignificant (Fig. 50.3). This training period may not need to be as long as 6 months, and we and others (83) have documented enhancement in reviewer accuracy over a 3-day course, during which fewer than 70 studies were reviewed. However, once this level of skill is attained, we believe that a regular workload is required to prevent it from attenuating. Finally, even among expert readers, while the concordance of interpretations within the same center is high (84), concordance between different centers may be less than or equal to 80% (85). Uniform interpretive criteria have reduced but still not avoided this problem of discordance (86). As this is particularly a problem in studies of poor technical quality, and in patients with milder forms of coronary disease, it is not surprising that technical advances including harmonic imaging and digital display have further improved observer agreement (87), although this remains imperfect.

To control issues related to subjectivity and concordance between observers, we review stress echocardiograms systematically. Quad-screen displays are first examined to assess their quality and the presence of technical limitations (e.g., gating problems); in technically limited studies, more reliance will need to be based on analysis of the videotape.

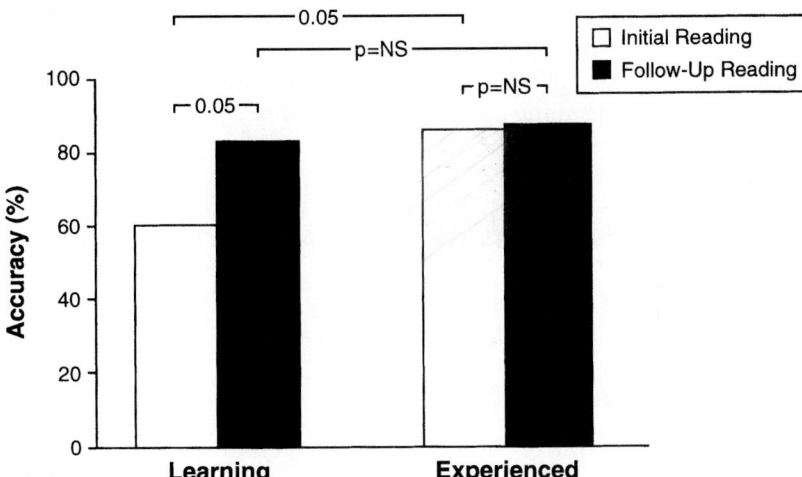

FIGURE 50.3 The learning curve of stress echocardiography. Over 6 months and 100 supervised echos, the trainees increased their accuracy from approximately 60% to 80%. NS, not significant.

Resting images are then examined in each view, using the American Society of Echocardiography 16-segment model to score regional wall motion (Fig. 50.4). Global function may be assessed subjectively by calculation of a wall motion scoring index or by measurement of the ejection fraction. The rest and stress images are then compared. The first step is to check for the presence of LV enlargement and shape changes, which are global indicators of ischemia, and in the case of the former, of multivessel disease. Each segment is then scored and compared with the equivalent segment at rest to identify the site, extent, and severity of abnormal function. If a bicycle or dobutamine stress study is used, the ischemic threshold is an important clue to the severity of ischemia. The report should therefore describe the site,

extent, and severity of scar and ischemia, the global LV function before and after stress, and the presence of other abnormalities.

Quantitative Approaches

Given the limitations of the qualitative approach, a quantitative approach would seem desirable. Global systolic indices (e.g., ejection fraction or volumes) have limited value, as they are usually abnormal only in the setting of severe ischemia. Wall motion scoring is semiquantitative, but is similar to the standard qualitative approach. Quantitative techniques may be used for the measurement of radial or longitudinal function (Table 50.4).

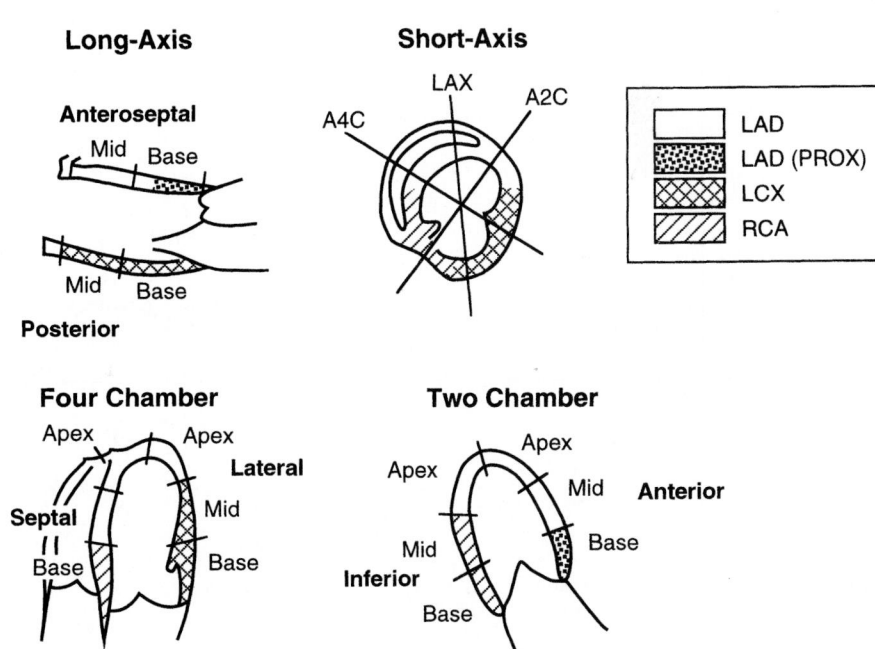

FIGURE 50.4 Systematic evaluation of the left ventricle using the 16-segment model of the American Society of Echocardiography. Each segment must be scored individually at rest and during, after, or both during and after stress. LAD, left anterior descending coronary artery; LAX, long axis; LCX, left circumflex coronary artery; PROX, proximal; RCA, right coronary artery.

TABLE 50.4 QUANTITATIVE TECHNIQUES FOR THE EVALUATION OF STRESS ECHOCARDIOGRAPHY

	Radial	Longitudinal
Displacement	Centerline Acoustic quantification	M-mode
Thickening	Anatomic M-mode	Backscatter
Velocity (including velocity gradient)	Tissue Doppler	Tissue Doppler, strain
Timing	Tissue Doppler	Tissue Doppler

Myocardial displacement may be measured in the short- or long-axis dimension. Although long-axis shortening is easily measured using M-mode echocardiography and the timing of long-axis contraction may be altered by ischemia (88), this is not specific for the location of ischemia. The centerline approach is well established as a means of measuring regional function (Fig. 50.5) and has been applied to the interpretation of stress echocardiograms (89). Using this technique, radial excursion is measured by tracing of the endocardial surface (thickening is sometimes possible to measure by tracing of endocardial and epicardial surfaces) at peak diastole and peak systole, and compared with a normal range. There are three major limitations with this technique. First, many stress echocardiograms are not of satisfactory quality to provide excellent border definition, although this has improved in the era of harmonic imaging. Second, the approach requires compensation for trans-

lational or rotational cardiac movement, and methodologies for compensating for these technical issues are not well defined. Third, the process of tracing the wall is time consuming and not applicable in a busy clinical laboratory. ▼ j42

DIAGNOSIS OF CORONARY ARTERY DISEASE

Influences on Accuracy of Stress Echocardiography

Adequacy of Stress

The use of stress testing is inherent to all functional tests for the diagnosis of coronary disease. Failure to stress the heart maximally will not engender either maximal coronary hyperemia (used for myocardial perfusion imaging) or ischemia (used for stress echocardiography and ECG analysis). Thus, failure to stress the patient maximally will be associated with reduced sensitivity, especially for milder coronary disease. Indeed, in our experience of exercise echocardiography, apart from the number and severity of coronary stenoses, the only predictor of false-negative results was failure to obtain 85% of age-predicted maximum heart rate (101). As discussed previously, patients who are unable to exercise, or likely to exercise submaximally, should undergo pharmacologic stress testing.

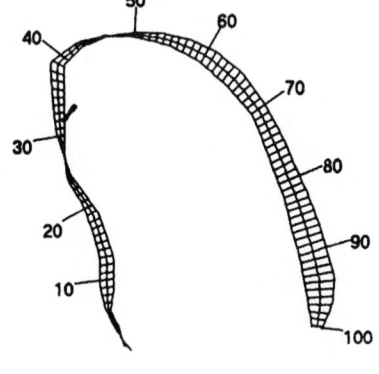

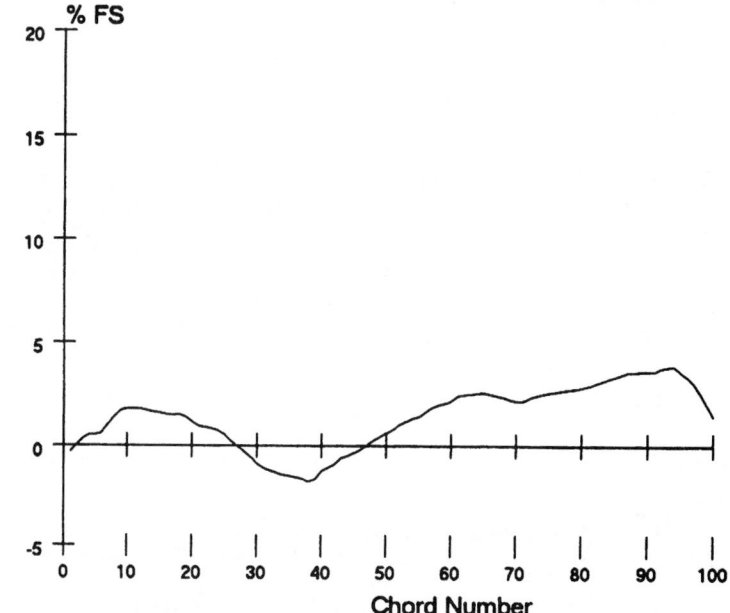

FIGURE 50.5 Quantitative stress echocardiography. A centerline is drawn between diastolic and systolic images and the excursion compared with a normal population. Endo., endocardial; FS, fractional shortening. (From Marwick T, ed. *Stress echocardiography*. New York: Kluwer, 1994, with permission.)

The use of pharmacologic stress testing may be particularly useful in patients with previous myocardial infarction and resting wall motion abnormalities. In these situations, the identification of ischemia may be facilitated by the availability of low-dose augmentation in viable tissue (102), which may not be appreciated during exercise testing. This topic is discussed further in a later section (see Identification of Myocardial Viability).

Echocardiographic Considerations

Image quality is probably more important during stress echocardiography than during alternative stress imaging techniques. Poor image quality reduces concordance between expert observers (85), and likely reduces the accuracy of the test, if not for the identification of coronary disease (101) then at least the ability to recognize multivessel disease. Not all segments of the myocardium are equally well visualized; the lateral wall is usually parallel with the ultrasound beam in the apical four-chamber view, and the endocardium may be poorly defined, with consequent effects on the sensitivity for left circumflex disease. Fortunately, this problem has been improved by the development of lateral gain correction techniques as well as harmonic imaging. The basal inferoposterior walls are particularly difficult to interpret due to tethering to the plane of the mitral valve and poor endocardial definition. Wall motion abnormalities involving the latter segments should be identified only if adjacent segments are abnormal (103).

As discussed in a previous section, stress echocardiography is interpreted qualitatively and subjectively, and several interpretive factors may influence the accuracy of the data. First, a low threshold for identifying wall motion abnormalities (e.g., identification of minor stress-induced wall motion abnormalities as ischemic, or identification of failure to enhance function as being indicative of ischemia) is attended by a high sensitivity, but a correspondingly low specificity. Interpreter bias may also be an important source of inaccuracy. It is important that the echocardiographic data are interpreted independent of the clinical and stress testing data; failure to do so may compromise accuracy (particularly the specificity). The experience of the reader is obviously an important determinant of accuracy during stress echocardiography. Factors responsible for false-negative and false-positive results are summarized in Table 50.5.

Exercise Echocardiography

The feasibility of exercise echocardiography in the more recent studies has been approximately 100%. In significant studies of exercise echocardiography (greater than 100 patients), the sensitivity and specificity range from 74% to 97% and 64% to 86%, respectively (Table 50.5.1) (27,101,104–109). Some variability is apparent, for the reasons discussed previously. The effect of differing criteria of

TABLE 50.5 CAUSES OF FALSE-NEGATIVE AND FALSE-POSITIVE STRESS ECHOCARDIOGRAM RESULTS

False-negative results	False-positive results
Inadequate stress	Overinterpretation, interpreter bias
Antianginal therapy	Localized basal inferior wall abnormalities
Mild coronary artery disease	Abnormal septal motion (left bundle branch block, post–coronary artery bypass grafting)
Left circumflex disease	
Poor image quality	Cardiomyopathies
Delayed images post-stress	Hypertensive responses to stress

stenosis significance is well illustrated in the study by Robertson (9), which showed a sensitivity of 100% but a specificity of 75%, using a cutoff including more severe lesions (e.g., greater than 75% diameter) in the sensitivity group. This cutoff makes it highly likely that any patient with anatomically defined disease would have ischemia, whereas patients with less than 75% stenoses may indeed have ischemia, particularly if the stenosis is in the 50% to 75% range.

Using a 50% stenosis diameter cutoff at quantitative angiography, Shiekh reported a sensitivity of 81% and a specificity of 92% (110), and patients with single-vessel coronary disease and inducible wall motion abnormalities had a stenosis diameter of 1.0 mm, compared with patients without inducible ischemia in spite of detectable stenoses, among whom the diameter was 1.7 mm. A similar study by Agati et al. (111) used quantitative wall motion analysis to define abnormal function and identified an absolute lumen diameter of 0.7 mm, corresponding to an 85% diameter stenosis, as best predictive of inducible wall motion abnormalities, although the sensitivity of exercise echocardiography in that study may have been compromised by the quantitative criteria used for defining a positive test result. ⌖ j43

Pharmacologic Stress Echocardiography

Dobutamine Stress Echocardiography

Significant studies (greater than 100 patients) of dobutamine stress echocardiography show a range of sensitivity of between 61% and 95%, whereas that for specificity ranged from 51% to 95% (Table 50.5.2) (3,46,61,106,113–123). Again, some variability in the reported accuracy of the test is apparent. The addition of atropine increases sensitivity (49), as does the use of transesophageal echocardiography (77), although the feasibility of the latter is limited, as discussed previously.

At quantitative coronary angiography (124–126), the optimal correlates of a positive dobutamine test result are a lumen diameter of 1.07 mm, percent diameter stenosis of 52%, and percent area stenosis of 75%, and minimal lumen diameter has the best predictive value for a positive dobutamine stress test result (sensitivity 94%, specificity 75%, odds ratio 51) (124). Stenoses less than 1 mm in diameter can be identified with a sensitivity of 86% (125,126). However, although quantitative angiography deals with the problem of reproducibility of angiographic interpretation, it still has the limitation of being an anatomic measure of disease severity, which may not necessarily correlate with functional indices. One such parameter that takes into account collateral flow is myocardial fractional flow reserve, which is calculated as the ratio of mean hyperemic distal coronary to aortic pressure. The magnitude of wall motion abnormalities correlated more closely with functional than anatomic markers of lesion severity, and dobutamine echocardiography was found to be a more sensitive marker of ischemia in lesions involving larger (greater than 2.6 mm in diameter) vessels than smaller vessels (125).

Some of the earlier studies of dobutamine echocardiography (46,117) show a sensitivity above the usual level (Table 50.5.2), suggesting a decrement in the accuracy of dobutamine stress since its inception, reflecting clinical application of the test. As the technique is applied for clinical decision making, referral bias to angiography may inflate sensitivity but produce more adverse findings for specificity (127). Moreover, dobutamine is not a very robust stress, and sensitivity is likely to be compromised if the cardiac workload is reduced by medical therapy or dose-limiting side effects. Comparison of the quoted ranges (Tables 50.5.1 and 50.5.2) suggests that the sensitivity of dobutamine echocardiography is somewhat less than exercise echocardiography, but its specificity is slightly greater. In studies in which exercise and pharmacologic stress echocardiography were performed in the same patients, the accuracy of stress echocardiography has been comparable with either stressor (106,128–132). In situations in which stress is submaximal because of side effects with pharmacologic agents, exercise is superior. Clearly, the converse is true when patients are unable to exercise maximally and a pharmacologic agent is more desirable. Nonetheless, the hemodynamic effects of the agents are different, so that the markers of severe (including left main) disease including LV cavity dilation and marked ST-segment depression occur more often with exercise than with dobutamine echocardiography (133). Because exercise is a more potent stress on the heart, a greater extent of abnormal wall motion may be induced, and this may compensate for the more difficult imaging with exercise (130,132). As discussed previously, a number of features favor the use of exercise testing over pharmacologic techniques, provided that the patient can exercise maximally.

Vasodilator Stress Echocardiography

The ranges for the sensitivity and specificity of dipyridamole and adenosine stress echocardiography for the detection of CAD are 61% to 81% and 90% to 94%, respectively (Table 50.5.3) (60,61,106,119–121,123,134,135). The low-dose dipyridamole protocol (0.56 mg per kg) is associated with low sensitivity. For the high-dose and adenosine protocols, more variability is present than for any of the other stressors, reflecting variations in the populations studied. The inclusion in some studies of patients with prior myocardial infarction has inflated the sensitivity of adenosine echocardiography, but the sensitivity of patients without prior infarction is only approximately 60% (136,137). Likewise, populations with a high prevalence of extensive coronary disease are associated with a high sensitivity, but single-vessel disease is more difficult to detect using this technique (137).

The type of pharmacologic agent to select in a patient who is unable to exercise maximally remains a source of debate. Studies comparing dobutamine and vasodilator agents in the same patients have shown that the sensitivity of dobutamine is somewhat higher than that of dipyridamole echocardiography, this difference being mainly attributable to patients with single-vessel disease (Table 50.5.4) (61,106,119,121,138). In an environment in which most of the studies are being performed for diagnostic purposes, dobutamine is probably more attractive as some patients may have single-vessel disease. In situations in which the main interest is prognostic evaluation, the agents are both attractive, and certainly a wealth of information is available regarding dipyridamole echocardiography as a prognostic test (see Prognostic Considerations in Coronary Artery Disease). Other factors influencing this decision, such as side effects and cost, have been discussed earlier (see Selection of the Optimal Stress Agent).

Important Limitations in the Diagnostic Use of Stress Echocardiography

Extent and Severity of Disease

Stress echocardiography is effective for the detection of severe coronary stenoses, as these are usually associated with more extensive wall motion abnormalities (125). Extensive coronary disease is also marked by an early onset of ischemia, at a low heart rate and rate-pressure product, or at a low dose of pharmacologic stressor. However, the sensitivity of stress echocardiography for single-vessel CAD has been quite limited in several studies and is probably less than that of myocardial perfusion scintigraphy. This reflects the need for ischemia to involve a significant extent of myocardium for the stress echocardiogram to be positive, which may not be fulfilled if the involved vessel is small or distal or if the stenosis is only mildly flow limiting.

The presence of extensive areas of ischemia, the development of global ventricular dysfunction (reduction of ejection fraction or LV enlargement), or both indicate the presence of multivessel disease (144). However, while the predictive value of these findings is high, the predictive value of their absence is dependent on the resting LV function. In patients with a history of previous myocardial infarction, the sensitivity of stress echocardiography for recognition of multivessel disease (effectively, "ischemia at a distance") is approximately 80% to 85%. In contrast, the sensitivity for multivessel disease in patients without previous infarction is approximately 50% (145). These data contrast with a sensitivity greater than 70% in this situation using myocardial perfusion scintigraphy (146). However, when the extent of ischemia defined by dobutamine echocardiography and perfusion scintigraphy was compared with the angiographic extent of disease (a modified Gensini score), the extent was comparable, and both underestimated the disease extent (137).

The identification of ischemia within areas of resting wall motion abnormalities is difficult, because of the problems posed by identification of minor gradations of wall motion in the setting of abnormal function. Comparison of the regional findings of exercise echocardiography and SPECT have shown this to be an important cause of discordant diagnoses (109). The problem is probably less during dobutamine stress because ischemic segments with abnormal resting function often show a biphasic response (102).

These aspects represent a fundamental limitation of an ischemia-based technique. Their solution will require either a more sensitive tool for assessment of wall motion or combination with a perfusion marker such as contrast echocardiography.

Site of Disease

Although the extent of coronary disease has an important influence on the accuracy of functional testing in general, the location of coronary disease may have important implications for the sensitivity of stress echocardiography in particular. The allocation of segments to particular vascular territories is ambiguous, especially in the apex (usually assumed to be within the territory of the left anterior descending coronary artery) and the posterior wall (usually assumed to be supplied by the left circumflex). Using exercise echocardiography, Marwick (145) reported regional sensitivities of 77% for the anterior descending, 67% for the left circumflex, and 70% for the right coronary, and Hecht (147) reported respective sensitivities of 95%, 78%, and 81%. However, Armstrong (148) reported a 22% sensitivity for the recognition of left circumflex disease, and Pozzoli (149) reported a sensitivity of 45% at this site. The sensitivity for circumflex disease may be limited by difficulties in the evaluation of the lateral wall due to unfavorable imaging characteristics.

COMPARISON WITH OTHER TECHNIQUES

Comparison with Stress Electrocardiography

The presence of ST-segment depression in response to exercise remains the simplest and most widely used test for the documentation of myocardial ischemia. However, the proportion of patients in whom adequate exercise is achieved

and the ST segment is interpretable is less than 50% in many tertiary referral centers. In patients with left bundle branch block, ECG changes with stress are nondiagnostic (150). In patients with LV hypertrophy or resting ST- and T-wave changes, additional ST-segment changes are not specific markers for coronary disease, although the sensitivity of ECG (and hence the predictive value of a negative test result) is debated (151,152).

In patients who are unable to exercise maximally, the use of exercise testing is attended by inadequate sensitivity (153). Even if pharmacologic stress testing is performed, the combination of these stresses with ECG alone has limitations with respect to sensitivity (154–156).

In those who can exercise and have an interpretable ECG, exercise echocardiography has benefits in both sensitivity and specificity (17,101,109,157). This greater sensitivity of exercise echocardiography over the exercise ECG is not surprising in view of the earlier occurrence of wall motion abnormalities than ST-segment changes during stress; these data are analogous to those reported for thallium imaging. However, as it would be financially and logistically impossible to replace diagnostic exercise testing with imaging, we have sought subgroups in whom the standard stress test is unreliable, despite an interpretable ECG. These groups might include women and patients with LV hypertrophy.

The accuracy of exercise ECG in women has been extensively debated. Depending on the population studied, either the sensitivity or the specificity may be compromised (158–161). Although some of the differences from stress testing in men may be caused by lower disease prevalence, these results are influenced by non-Bayesian factors, including the presence of milder coronary disease in women than men, the likelihood of submaximal stress, and intrinsic gender-based differences in the ST-segment response. A number of large studies have now shown that the accuracy of stress echocardiography is not compromised in women (114,135,162,163), and these results are superior to those of the exercise ECG, even after correction for referral bias. A cost analysis suggested that the use of exercise echo as an initial test caused more initial expense but was cheaper in the long run because of the avoidance of unnecessary angiograms in patients with false-positive ECG responses (162).

Comparison with Nuclear Imaging

Despite competition from echocardiography, perfusion scintigraphy [▼ j44] remains the most widely performed stress imaging test in the United States, and its use continues to increase.

Comparison of Stress Perfusion Imaging and Stress Echocardiography

Studies of the accuracy of SPECT myocardial perfusion scintigraphy have shown that this technique has a sensitivity greater than 90% for the detection of CAD (166). However, they also show that the specificity is approximately 70%, partly reflecting the phenomenon of posttest referral bias (127) as well as the problems of false-positive results related to image artifacts. In a metaanalysis, the superior sensitivity of SPECT was balanced by a greater specificity with echocardiography, so that the accuracy of the techniques was comparable (167). However, although the analytic technique permitted correction of a number of population-based factors that influence the accuracy of diagnostic testing, including the prevalence of prior infarction and multivessel coronary disease, comparisons between separate studies of myocardial perfusion imaging and stress echocardiography are difficult, not the least because of the different level of maturity of the investigations, which affects the posttest referral bias effect. An alternate design involves head-to-head comparison in the same patients, in the presence of an additional test (e.g., coronary angiography) to act as the arbiter of which result is correct, even though this design has the disadvantage of studying a selected population who are undergoing angiography (168).

A number of large studies have compared the results of stress echocardiography and perfusion scintigraphy in the same patients using various stressors (109,115,118, 137,149,169–171) (Table 50.5.5). Comparisons of vasodilator stress echocardiography and perfusion scintigraphy have confirmed the insensitivity of adenosine stress, particularly for single-vessel disease. When exercise and dobutamine stress are used, however, the sensitivities of the two techniques have also been shown to be comparable, with most studies showing a minor benefit for perfusion scintigraphy. The slightly lower sensitivity of stress echocardiography than perfusion scintigraphy may reflect superiority of perfusion imaging (which does not require the development of ischemia in a metabolic or functional sense) for the identification of patients with single-vessel disease. For similar reasons, patients on therapy with antianginal agents may be better studied using perfusion scintigraphy (as ischemia does not need to be induced for the test result to be positive) than stress echocardiography. As discussed in the section on limitations, perfusion scintigraphy appears to be significantly more sensitive for the recognition of multivessel disease as such (146) and may be superior in the detection of ischemia in the setting of resting wall motion abnormalities, in which circumstance the recognition of worsening wall motion may be difficult (109). These issues cannot be measured by consideration of sensitivity and specificity. Finally, scintigraphy can be expected to be superior in patients with poor echocardiographic windows (e.g., due to pulmonary disease).

On the other hand, there appears to be a particular benefit of echocardiography over perfusion scintigraphy with respect to specificity. This difference is most marked in patients with LV hypertrophy and left bundle branch block. Breast attenuation artifacts and other issues have led to lower reported levels of accuracy of perfusion imaging in women, and the results of a metaanalysis suggest this may be a group better studied with stress echocardiography (172). Finally, stress echocardiography is versatile, rapidly performed, and less expensive than perfusion imaging. In situations in which other cardiac problems are present as well as ischemia (e.g., valvular, pericardial diseases), the selection of stress echocardiography avoids duplicate testing.

Practical Considerations

The selection between SPECT and stress echocardiography is influenced by numerous factors, some of which are summarized in Table 50.6. Of these, the most important is local expertise. Thus, at a center with an excellent nuclear laboratory and an echocardiographer inexperienced in stress echocardiography, the selection of the latter test would likely engender unfavorable results. The converse is true of facilities without the requisite nuclear experience.

TABLE 50.6 ADVANTAGES AND DISADVANTAGES OF STRESS ECHOCARDIOGRAPHY AND MYOCARDIAL PERFUSION SCINTIGRAPHY

Consideration		Stress echocardiography	Myocardial perfusion imaging
Application	Versatility	++	−
	Cost	++	−
	Credentialing	−	++ (Nuclear Regulatory Commission)
Interpretation	Training/quality control	±	±
	Artifacts	+ (better with contrast?)	+ (better with sestamibi?)
	Quantitation	−	++
Clinical value	Sensitivity	80–85%	90%
	Specificity	85%	70%
	Prognostic value	+	++ (established role)
	Familiarity	±	++
	Ancillary data	++	−

Comparison with Magnetic Resonance Imaging

Modern MRI protocols promise to deliver information of gross cardiac anatomy, details of structure, function, and perfusion, all of which are of value in the diagnosis and evaluation of ischemic heart disease and are discussed in another chapter (see Chapter 54). There is no question that MRI can provide information of similar accuracy to echocardiography during stress, both for identification of ischemia (3) and assessment of viable myocardium (173). The problems with the widespread application of this technology relate to issues of feasibility, access, and cost. It seems most likely that in the future, technically difficult studies will be performed using MRI, and that this modality will be especially useful for evaluation of complex problems such as detection of viable myocardium in severe LV dysfunction.

USE OF STRESS ECHOCARDIOGRAPHY IN MANAGEMENT DECISIONS

Evaluation of Patients undergoing Myocardial Revascularization

Patients undergoing myocardial revascularization procedures should have some documentation of the presence and site of ischemia (174). Although stress echocardiography can accurately localize disease, the assumptions inherent in allocating territories of the heart to individual coronary vessels may compromise its ability to designate a "culprit" lesion. This is particularly problematic if multivessel disease is present, in which case the most ischemic territory is most commonly detected.

Following both surgical (175,176) and percutaneous revascularization (177), stress echocardiography appears to have similar accuracy to its use in patients with native disease. However, its use in asymptomatic patients may be limited by Bayesian considerations.

Identification of Myocardial Viability

Background

In a number of acute animal models of myocardial stunning, the use of sympathomimetic amines such as isoproterenol and dobutamine have been shown to reverse regional LV dysfunction in stunned myocardium (178). The same response appears to be applicable to chronic ischemic LV dysfunction, which is often considered to be truly hibernating tissue. In the presence of dysfunctional but viable myocardium, regional function is enhanced by the inotropic effect of low-dose dobutamine (usually 5 to 10 µg per kg per minute), which enhances calcium cycling before dobutamine-induced tachycardia increases oxygen consumption and leads to ischemia. Dipyridamole also exerts similar effects at low dose, the mechanism of which is ill defined; increasing myocardial turgor has been suggested to produce a mini-Starling effect, and augmentation of coronary flow has also been suggested. Viable myocardium supplied by a patent infarct-related vessel (generally corresponding to stunned myocardium) demonstrates a sustained improvement during the infusion. Viable tissue supplied by a stenosed infarct-related artery (which may involve stunned or hibernating tissue) is characterized by an initial improvement followed by deterioration of regional function as the chronotropic effect becomes more prominent and myocardial work increases (Table 50.1).

Accuracy for Detection of Improvement after Revascularization

In regions predicted to be viable by low-dose dobutamine echocardiography early (less than 2 weeks) after "incomplete" infarction (non–Q-wave infarcts, and infarction treated with lytic therapy), improvement may be observed spontaneously (179,180). Several studies have addressed the accuracy of dobutamine echocardiography to predict regional functional recovery at follow-up (179–185), although most studies involve small patient numbers (Table 50.6.1). Later after myocardial infarction, myocardial hibernation might be expected to constitute an important source of reversible dysfunction in preference to myocardial stunning. Comparisons with positron emission tomography (PET) have suggested that a dobutamine response is more likely in the presence of preserved myocardial perfusion (stunning) than in the situation of a perfusion metabolism mismatch (hibernation) (181). Dobutamine echocardiography has been effective for the prediction of myocardial viability in this group of patients (186–188), possibly because recurrent episodes of myocardial stunning are an important source of viable tissue late following infarction (189). The evidence base for the accuracy of dobutamine echocardiography for the prediction of regional functional recovery after revascularization is larger (Table 50.6.1). In these studies, the sensitivity of dobutamine stress to identify an improvement of systolic function in response to revascularization ranged from 69% to 86%, with a range of specificity from 57% to 100%.

Comparison of Stress Echocardiography with Other Techniques for Identification of Viable Myocardium

The ability of dobutamine echocardiography and other techniques to predict recovery of regional function (Fig. 50.6) has been compared in metaanalyses (190,191) and direct comparison in individual patients. Both analyses suggest that the accuracy of dobutamine echocardiography for identification of viable myocardium is equivalent to that of

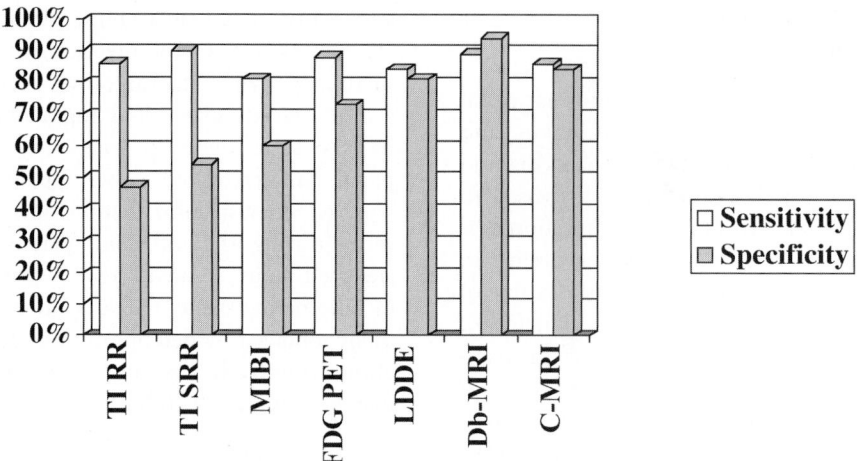

FIGURE 50.6 Prediction of viability (defined as recovery of regional function after revascular-ization) using thallium rest redistribution (Tl RR), thallium stress rest reinjection (Tl SRR), Tc-99m sestamibi (MIBI), positron emission tomography (FDG PET), low-dose dobutamine echocardiog-raphy (LDDE), dobutamine magnetic resonance imaging (Db-MRI), and contrast-enhanced MRI (C-MRI) for the detection of viable myocardium. (Modified from Bax JJ, Wijns W, Cornel JH, et al. Accuracy of currently available techniques for prediction of functional recovery after revascular-ization in patients with left ventricular dysfunction due to chronic coronary artery disease: com-parison of pooled data. *J Am Coll Cardiol* 1997;30:1451–1460; Kim RJ, Wu E, Rafael A, et al. The use of contrast-enhanced magnetic resonance imaging to identify reversible myocardial dysfunc-tion. *N Engl J Med* 2000;343:1445–1453; and Baer FM, Theissen P, Schneider CA, et al. Dobu-tamine magnetic resonance imaging predicts contractile recovery of chronically dysfunctional myocardium after successful revascularization. *J Am Coll Cardiol* 1998;31:1040–1048.)

thallium-201 reinjection imaging (188,192–202). In com-parison with thallium imaging, dobutamine echocardiog-raphy was similarly somewhat less sensitive but substantially more specific. Pierard demonstrated that the prediction of myocardial viability using low-dose dobu-tamine echocardiography correlated with PET in 79% of segments (181). Similar levels of correlation have been reported from other centers (203); in our experience, although dobutamine echocardiography is less sensitive than PET, it is more specific (204). Finally, as mentioned previously, the accuracy of dobutamine echo and MRI are similar, especially if good echo images are obtained (173).

Prediction of Recovery of Functional Capacity

The evidence base regarding the accuracy of tests for pre-diction of myocardial viability is based on comparison with recovery of regional LV function. However, decision mak-ing regarding revascularization in patients with LV dysfunc-tion is more influenced by the likelihood of improving ejection fraction, functional capacity, and quality of life.

Although ejection fraction is the most widely used index of global LV function and an important predictor of out-come, it is not a good marker for recovery of viable tissue, as it is load dependent and influenced by changes elsewhere in the heart. Hypercontractility in uninvolved regions of the myocardium may compensate for regional dysfunction; when these dysfunctional segments improve after revascu-larization, the compensating segments may resume normal

function and the ejection fraction may remain unchanged. Nonetheless, improvement of ejection fraction can be expected if sufficient viable tissue is identified before revas-cularization; if greater than 25% of segments are viable (205) or if there is an improvement of ejection fraction with low-dose dobutamine (206), a significant (5%) improvement in ejection fraction can be predicted with an accuracy greater than 80%. Clearly, the response to revas-cularization is also dependent on a number of other vari-ables, including the adequacy of revascularization target vessels, the overall status of the ventricle (very large ventri-cles are unlikely to recover dramatically), and the extent of scar tissue (thinned tissue is unlikely to recover). The extent of data regarding the ability to predict global functional recovery with dobutamine echocardiography is still limited. In patients with severe LV dysfunction, improvement in exercise capacity was predicted by the extent of viable myo-cardium, but PET appeared superior to dobutamine echocardiography (207). Extensive (greater than 25%) via-bility has also been associated with increased functional class after revascularization (208).

Prediction of Prognosis after Revascularization

Several observational studies have shown viable myocar-dium to be prognostically important. Medical treatment of patients with viable myocardium is associated with adverse outcome, whereas myocardial revascularization has been shown to improve survival in patients with viable tissue

2nd Edition

Textbook of Cardiovascular Medicine

Eric J. Topol
Editor

Robert M. Califf
Jeffrey Isner
Eric N. Prystowsky
Judith Swain
James Thomas
Paul Thompson
James B. Young
Associate Editors

Steven Nissen
Consulting Editor
CD-ROM

Donna Bressan
Managing Editor

Dear Readers,

Thank you for purchasing the second edition of the Textbook of Cardiovascular Medicine. We are very pleased to provide you with the first truly interactive learning resource in this field.

The product you have just purchased includes a textbook with a CD-ROM bound in the back. The book and the CD-ROM are an integrated unit, each providing invaluable support for the other. Content for the print textbook focuses on clinical material providing all of the essential information needed for daily practice. Content on the CD-ROM presents expanded versions of the print chapters plus additional chapters that incorporate more detailed mechanistic and basic science information. The CD-ROM also contains more than 1000 digital images – most in color – plus more than 250 angio and echo loops and 25 heart sounds. All of this has been designed to provide you with the most comprehensive interactive reference source available in the field of cardiovascular medicine.

We have provided you with a wide-array of cross-referencing between the print product and the supplemental material that appears in electronic form. This has been done by way of an icon (see below). Content icons are followed by a locator number. To access supplemental electronic information, simply open the CD-ROM and type in the locator number; this will take you directly to the appropriate information. Figures and tables that appear on the CD-ROM are cross-referenced in the print product with an e-number. To access these, simply type in the e-number and you will be taken directly to that information.

Our pioneering effort in developing a medical textbook with true digital interface will hopefully meet the challenge of comprehensively covering an ever-burgeoning field, while at the same time providing a handy traditional tool for clinical issues. We hope that the extraordinary array of supportive digital multimedia material will prove to be a truly enriching and exciting educational resource.

Sincerely,

Eric J. Topol, MD
Editor in Chief

Icon as it appears in the text:

9500 Euclid Avenue, Desk F25, Cleveland, Ohio 44195 • *Phone:* 216-445-9490 • *Fax:* 216-445-9595 • *E mail:* topole@ccf.org

Published by Lippincott-Williams and Wilkins Publishers • *A Wolters Kluwer Company*

(209). Relatively recent data suggest that this effect is related to the extent of viable tissue (210).

PROGNOSTIC CONSIDERATIONS IN CORONARY ARTERY DISEASE

Stable Chronic Coronary Artery Disease

In addition to information regarding the presence of ischemia and scar, exercise and pharmacologic stress testing offer adjunctive information that may be of prognostic significance. [⚑ j45] With exercise, these include exercise capacity, hemodynamic responses to exercise, and the ST-segment response. However, although ECG evidence of ischemia carries incremental prognostic value, most prognostic information derives from echocardiographic evidence of ischemia. Similarly, although prognostic analysis of stress testing data has shown reduced exercise capacity to be a strong predictor of adverse outcome, the presence of ischemia at stress echocardiography adds significant prognostic information. With dobutamine, the rate pressure product at the onset of ischemia is important, and the equivalent measure using dipyridamole stress testing (dipyridamole time) is also of prognostic value. However, as discussed previously, the ECG component of both dipyridamole and dobutamine stress testing is rather insensitive (154,155), and the development of hypotension during these tests is not meaningful prognostically.

Many patients who present for exercise testing are either unable to exercise or exercise submaximally, and these individuals have a high cardiac event rate (221). From the prognostic standpoint, the detection of ischemia during either dobutamine or dipyridamole stress is analogous to its development during exercise stress. Likewise, the detection of ischemia during dobutamine stress (relative risk 5.6) was a stronger predictor of outcome than most clinical variables and superior to the prognostic significance of significant coronary stenoses (215). Although ejection fraction is recognized as an important predictor of cardiac events, the change of ejection fraction in response to dobutamine does not appear to be predictive of outcome (222). Similar findings have been reported using dipyridamole echocardiography; in the largest reported study, death and hard events were predicted by the presence of a positive dipyridamole echo test result, together with ECG positivity and angina (135,220). In particular, the degree of stress required to induce ischemia (evidenced by the dipyridamole time) was most predictive of hard events, whereas total events were predicted by the wall motion score at peak stress, reflecting the extent of both ischemia and infarction. Moreover, a number of studies have reported that the stress data are not only independent of other variables, but also incremental to the information obtained clinically (135,211,212).

Stress echocardiography offers important prognostic material in patients with chronic stable coronary disease (*e*Table 50.6.2). The presence and time of onset of ischemia is clearly associated with increased events, and these data are adjunctive to exercise capacity and ST-segment changes. Unfortunately, only limited comparisons are available between stress echocardiography and perfusion scintigraphy in terms of their ability to predict events; these data suggest that the techniques are comparable (223).

Postinfarct Risk Stratification

The factors predicting outcome following myocardial infarction include ejection fraction and the presence and extent of ischemic and viable myocardium. All of these may be identified using stress echocardiography, and a number of large studies have gathered prognostic data using stress echocardiography in postinfarction patients (224–230) (Table 50.6.3). Most of these data have been obtained with pharmacologic stress, with only two small studies with exercise echocardiography (231,232). This may reflect reluctance to perform exercise stress in the early postinfarct period. In contrast to patients with chronic stable coronary disease, cardiac events more commonly occur than in patients without evidence of ischemia (reflecting the risk associated with LV dysfunction), but hard events occur in greater than 50% of those with positive stress echocardiographic results.

The timing of postinfarct risk stratification is a critical consideration as recurrent cardiac events may occur early after infarction. Because dipyridamole leads to a negligible increment of cardiac workload, this stress is attractive for early stress testing. In a report of a group of 250 patients who were studied with dipyridamole echocardiography 3 days following myocardial infarction (226), ischemia at dipyridamole stress testing was predictive of both total and hard events. In a multivariate model, the combination of both echocardiographic evidence of ischemia and angina was the strongest predictor of subsequent events, followed by ischemia alone, and anterior infarction.

As discussed in the previous section, hibernating myocardium may be identified by dobutamine echocardiography, with an accuracy of approximately 80% for the prediction of functional recovery (Table 50.6.1). However, while the presence of this tissue is a positive feature if it is revascularized, it is associated with cardiac events if left unrevascularized; this finding appears to be the case whether this finding is identified by either PET (233–235) or dobutamine echocardiography (52).

In the evaluation of patients following myocardial infarction, the influence of resting wall motion abnormalities on the identification of ischemia is an important limitation of the interpretation of stress echocardiography. As discussed previously, this reflects the difficulty of judging minor deteriorations in the severity of wall motion abnormalities, which may denote the presence of myocardial ischemia. However, it should be emphasized that this problem concerns homozonal ischemia, and the presence of previous infarction does not compromise the ability to recognize ischemia in another zone. The ability of stress echocardiography to recognize heterozonal ischemia may explain the ability of stress echocardiography to predict events in postinfarction patients. In a small study from the Thoraxcenter (265), the presence of ischemia at thallium scintigraphy was not predictive of total cardiac events over 2 years of follow-up, whereas ischemia at stress echocardiography was associated with a significantly worse prognosis than the absence of ischemia. Although this study involved few hard events, these findings imply that the interpretive challenge of resting wall motion abnormalities may not constitute a major limitation. Additional comparative data are needed between stress echocardiography and scintigraphy in this group.

Peripheral Vascular Disease

Anatomic evidence of CAD is present in over 80% of patients with aortic, lower limb, and cerebral vascular disease (236). However, the challenge of preoperative risk stratification is that although *anatomic* coronary disease is highly prevalent, serious perioperative cardiac complications are infrequent. For example, cardiac death and myocardial infarction occurs in 5% of unselected patients who have not undergone myocardial revascularization before undergoing vascular surgery (237). The identification of this small subgroup is a major challenge on Bayesian grounds, as the low pretest probability of an event influences the posttest probability, irrespective of the results of testing. This problem may at least in part be addressed by clinical evaluation (e.g., using Eagle's criteria for assigning the risk of a cardiac event). Patients with none of these factors (diabetes, age greater than 70 years, angina, myocar-

dial infarction, or heart failure) have a negligible risk of cardiac complications, irrespective of the results of stress testing (238).

The inability of most of these patients to exercise maximally necessitates the use of pharmacologic stress testing. Just as perfusion scintigraphy has shown to be effective in predicting outcome in patients with vascular disease (239–243), a number of studies have shown dipyridamole and dobutamine echocardiography to be predictive of perioperative cardiac events (Table 50.6.4) (244–251), and echocardiographic test results appear to be at least as predictive as those performed with nuclear imaging (252). The largest experience of the use of stress echocardiography for risk stratification of patients undergoing vascular surgery has been reported from the Thoraxcenter in Rotterdam. In the initial report of 136 patients, physicians looking after these vascular patients were blinded to the results of dobutamine echocardiography. During perioperative follow-up, five patients died, and ten suffered cardiac events; dobutamine echocardiography was positive in all patients with cardiac events and was the strongest predictor of events. In a multivariate model, only dobutamine echocardiography (odds ratio, 95; 95% confidence interval, 11 to 822) and age were predictive of cardiac complications.

In many studies of risk stratification, although a negative test result renders a cardiac complication unlikely, a positive result generally confers 20% to 30% risk of a cardiac complication. Risk stratification may be enhanced by considering the ischemic threshold (i.e., the cardiac workload necessary to induce myocardial ischemia). Using dobutamine stress (250), a low ischemic threshold rather than extensive ischemia was seen in patients suffering events, including death and infarction. The extent and time of onset of ischemia during dipyridamole echocardiography are also associated with cardiac events (245). The combination of clinical evaluation and the presence and threshold of ischemia may be integrated into a patient care algorithm as illustrated in Figure 50.7. First, the

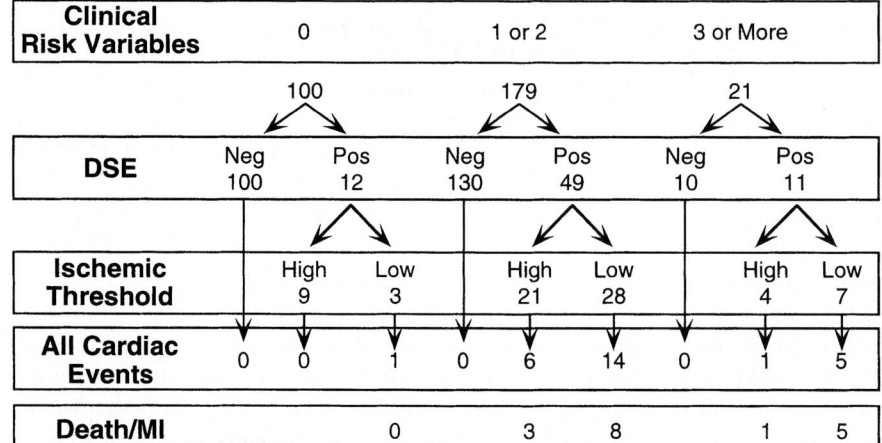

FIGURE 50.7 Integration of clinical data with ischemic threshold to dobutamine to predict events in patients undergoing vascular surgery. DSE, dobutamine stress echocardiography; MI, myocardial infarction; Neg, negative; Pos, positive. (From Poldermans D, Arnese M, Fioretti PM, et al. Improved cardiac risk stratification in major vascular surgery with dobutamine-atropine stress echocardiography. *J Am Coll Cardiol* 1995;26:648–653, with permission.)

patient is stratified on clinical grounds. If the patient has clinical risk variables, he or she should undergo a dobutamine stress echocardiogram, and if this result is negative for ischemia, even if scar is present, the patient should proceed to surgery. If ischemia develops, a decision should be made as to its severity, based more on the ischemic threshold than the extent of ischemia. Patients with limited areas of ischemia, only appearing at peak dose, can probably safely proceed to surgery. Those with more extensive ischemia or that occurring at a low dose should either have an alteration of surgical planning or be considered for cardiac catheterization.

In summary, stress echocardiography offers useful prognostic data. More material needs to be obtained for the comparison between stress echocardiography and perfusion scintigraphy for prognostic purposes, both with respect to accuracy and cost effectiveness.

CONTROVERSIES AND PERSONAL PERSPECTIVES

The use of stress echocardiography as a diagnostic tool is supported by a large evidence base. Although studies of the learning curve have been presented, there are limited data reflecting the accuracy of this technique outside of the hands of experts. However, the future of this technique is likely to be influenced by the balance between the training requirements of this methodology and technical developments. The growth of this methodology has

been so dramatic that many studies are likely being performed by individuals with limited training in this discipline. The need for training and quality control in this, as in other diagnostic techniques, warrants attention. However, the development of new quantitative approaches may improve the reproducibility and robustness of this technique. Of the new technologies, myocardial Doppler and contrast echocardiography are most likely to offer lasting contributions.

Apart from the impetus of technological development, the driving forces behind the growth of stress echocardiography have been practical. In comparison with nuclear imaging, stress echocardiography is relatively inexpensive to perform; there are no disposables, equipment is cheaper, and less processing is required. A less costly test was attractive to the patient and insurer in the conventional fee-for-service model of care, but is even more so for the physician and hospital in the current era of managed care and capitation. Finally, although the new dual-isotope techniques are shorter to perform than the older thallium techniques, stress echocardiography is versatile and patient friendly. The results are available immediately after testing, and the equipment is relatively inexpensive and portable, enabling the service to be offered in the physician's office or at a satellite clinic.

As in other fields of medicine, the challenge of the future will be to balance the technological and financial forces supporting the growth of stress echocardiography with the need to maintain quality.

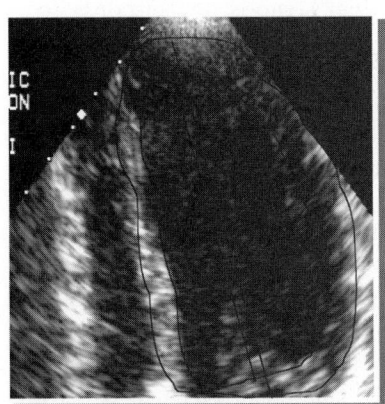 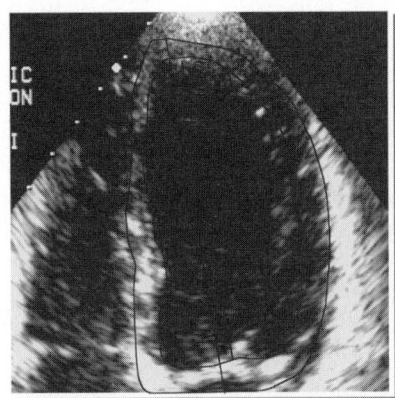

REST   EF = 62%   POST EXERCISE   EF = 50%

Contractile Reserve (CR) = -12%

FIGURE 50.8 Determination of left ventricular contractile reserve in a patient with severe mitral regurgitation and preserved resting function (*left*). After exercise (*right*), the left ventricular cavity increases and ejection fraction (EF) falls. Despite normal left ventricular size and function at rest, this response implies that the ventricle is becoming compromised.

THE FUTURE

Quantitative Techniques for Interpretation of Stress Echocardiography

The development of harmonic imaging and contrast echocardiography has improved border detection to the extent that this is no longer the greatest limitation of the technique. Instead, the issue of training and expertise has become the most pressing problem, and a feasible quantitative approach to interpretation is needed. There is no doubt that, although Doppler myocardial imaging of longitudinal motion and integrated backscatter-based approaches are currently feasible, further developments will be needed before quantitation becomes a routine component of the interpretation of stress echocardiography.

Ancillary Techniques for Detecting Ischemia

The detection of myocardial ischemia is currently dependent on the detection of stress-induced wall motion abnormalities. As discussed in the limitations section, this may cause problems with the recognition of multivessel disease as such, the detection of single-vessel coronary disease, and the distinction of ischemia and scar. Techniques that detect more subtle evidence of ischemia, such as myocardial contrast echocardiography and analysis of cyclic backscatter variation, may supplement these findings and may indeed exceed the sensitivity of two-dimensional echocardiography alone for the detection of coronary disease.

Non–air-filled echocardiographic contrast agents traverse the lungs to reach high concentration in the left-sided heart chambers and thereby may enhance the reflectivity of the myocardium. Although these agents do not currently conform to the characteristics of diffusible tracers, analysis of the degree of myocardial opacification corresponds to the concentration of tracer and therefore gives a semiquantitative measure of regional myocardial perfusion. This field has developed a large evidence base, but for the purposes of this topic, it is important to recognize that myocardial contrast echocardiography has already been successfully applied during stress by several authors (253). Importantly, it has been shown to improve the sensitivity of the technique for recognizing all involved vascular territories in patients with multivessel disease. Although the application of the technique is currently constrained by technical complexity, it seems likely that the use of myocardial contrast will facilitate detection of coronary disease by examination of both wall motion and perfusion at stress echocardiography.

When myocardium becomes ischemic, its reflectivity changes. Using video densitometry, Picano et al. have shown that the backscatter profile of ischemic myocardium during angioplasty is altered before the development of wall motion abnormalities (254). Other authors have demonstrated that cyclic variation of backscatter is preserved in akinetic but viable myocardium (94,255). These findings remain to be applied to the routine clinical arena and at present are limited by considerations pertaining to image quality.

Use in Noncoronary Heart Diseases

The stress echocardiography literature mostly pertains to the detection of myocardial ischemia. However, the functional response to stress is important in the evaluation of myocardial and valvular heart diseases, and the importance of stress echocardiography for this purpose is likely to grow. Patients at risk for anthracycline toxicity may be detected using stress echocardiography (256,257). Similarly, loss of contractile reserve in response to stress also appears to be a marker of impending contractile dysfunction in patients with LV volume loading related to mitral regurgitation (Fig. 50.8) (258).

In patients with valvular stenosis, the response to stress may differentiate the interrelated influences of ventricular function and valvular disease on the production of gradients. The finding of a low gradient in a patient with aortic stenosis may reflect the influence of reduced ventricular function. Dobutamine echocardiography is able to distinguish a low-output state due to myocardial disease from tight aortic stenosis (Fig. 50.9) (259). Similarly, patients with latent LV outflow tract obstruction may demonstrate exercise-induced outflow tract obstruction in response to exercise or amyl nitrite (260).

Finally, measurement of tricuspid regurgitant velocity may be used to calculate pulmonary artery pressure after exercise. Exercise-induced pulmonary hypertension is a common pathway of cardiac decompensation following stress and may be a particularly useful measurement in patients with apparently moderate mitral stenosis at rest but marked decompensation with stress. The development of this response may correlate with a marked increment of diastolic gradient with exercise.

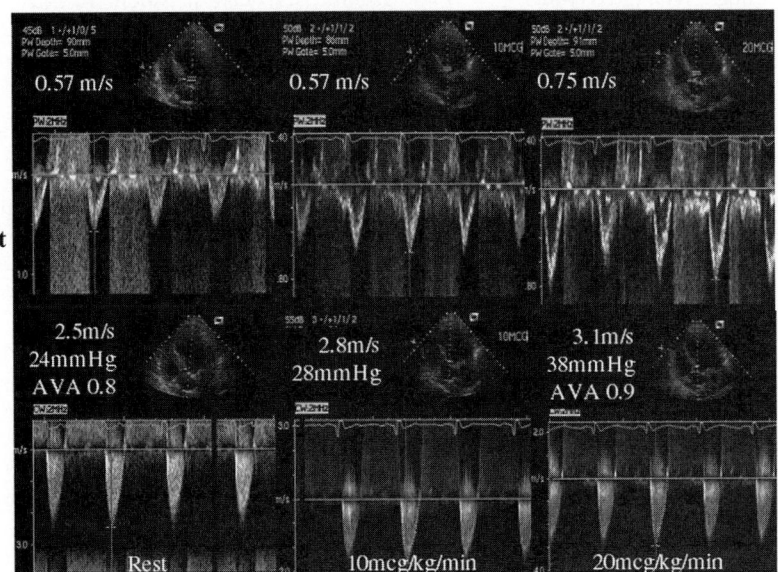

LV outflow tract

0.57 m/s   0.57 m/s   0.75 m/s

Aortic valve

2.5m/s   2.8m/s   3.1m/s
24mmHg   28mmHg   38mmHg
AVA 0.8   AVA 0.9

Rest   10mcg/kg/min   20mcg/kg/min

FIGURE 50.9 Application of dobutamine echocardiography to low output aortic stenosis. Resting Doppler measurements show a low gradient in the setting of left ventricular (LV) dysfunction. The increment of the valvular gradient (which exceeds that of the LV outflow tract velocity) signifies a primary valvular problem. AVA, aortic valve area.

REFERENCES

1. Masters AM. The two-step test of myocardial function. *Am Heart J* 1935;495–510.
2. Marwick TH. Current status of non-invasive techniques for the diagnosis of myocardial ischemia. *Acta Clin Belg* 1992;47:1–5.
3. Nagel E, Lehmkuhl HB, Bocksch W, et al. Noninvasive diagnosis of ischemia-induced wall motion abnormalities with the use of high-dose dobutamine stress MRI: comparison with dobutamine stress echocardiography. *Circulation* 1999;99:763–770.
4. van Rugge FP, van der Wall EE, Spanjersberg SJ, et al. Magnetic resonance imaging during dobutamine stress for detection and localization of coronary artery disease. Quantitative wall motion analysis using a modification of the centerline method. *Circulation* 1994;90:127–138.
5. Baer FM, Voth E, LaRosee K, et al. Comparison of dobutamine transesophageal echocardiography and dobutamine magnetic resonance imaging for detection of residual myocardial viability. *Am J Cardiol* 1996;78:415–419.
6. Vuille C, Weyman AE. Left ventricle I: general considerations, assessment of chamber size and function. In: Weyman AE, ed. *Principles and practice of echocardiography.* Philadelphia: Lea & Febinger, 1994:575–624.
7. Mason SJ, Weiss JL, Weisfeldt ML, et al. Exercise echocardiography: detection of wall motion abnormalities during ischemia. *Circulation* 1979;59:50–59.
8. Wann LS, Faris JV, Childress RH, et al. Exercise cross-sectional echocardiography in ischemic heart disease. *Circulation* 1979;60:1300–1308.
9. Robertson WS, Feigenbaum H, Armstrong WF, et al. Exercise echocardiography: a clinically practical addition in the evaluation of coronary artery disease. *J Am Coll Cardiol* 1983;2:1085–1091.
10. Berberich SN, Zager JR, Plotnick GD, et al. A practical approach to exercise echocardiography: immediate postexercise echocardiography. *J Am Coll Cardiol* 1984;3:284–290.
11. Heng MK, Simard M, Lake R, et al. Exercise two-dimensional echocardiography for diagnosis of coronary artery disease. *Am J Cardiol* 1984;54:502–507.
12. Ginzton LE, Conant R, Brizendine M, et al. Exercise subcostal two-dimensional echocardiography: a new method of segmental wall motion analysis. *Am J Cardiol* 1984;53:805–811.
13. Limacher MC, Quinones MA, Poliner LR, et al. Detection of coronary artery disease with exercise two-dimensional echocardiography. Description of a clinically applicable method and comparison with radionuclide ventriculography. *Circulation* 1983;67:1211–1218.
14. Crawford MH, Petru MA, Amon KW, et al. Comparative value of 2-dimensional echocardiography and radionuclide angiography for quantitating changes in left ventricular performance during exercise limited by angina pectoris. *Am J Cardiol* 1984;53:42–46.
15. Visser CA, van der Wieken RL, Kan G, et al. Comparison of two-dimensional echocardiography with radionuclide angiography during dynamic exercise for the detection of coronary artery disease. *Am Heart J* 1983;106:528–534.
16. Maurer G, Nanda NC. Two dimensional echocardiographic evaluation of exercise-induced left and right ventricular asynergy: correlation with thallium scanning. *Am J Cardiol* 1981;48:720–727.
17. Armstrong WF, O'Donnell J, Dillon JC, et al. Complementary value of two-dimensional exercise echocardiography to routine treadmill exercise testing. *Ann Intern Med* 1986;105:829–835.
18. Gould KL, Schelbert HR, Phelps ME, et al. Noninvasive assessment of coronary stenoses with myocardial perfusion imaging during pharmacologic coronary vasodilatation. V. Detection of 47 percent diameter coronary stenosis with intravenous nitrogen-13 ammonia and emission-com-

puted tomography in intact dogs. *Am J Cardiol* 1979;43:200–208.

19. White CW, Wright CB, Doty DB, et al. Does visual interpretation of the coronary arteriogram predict the physiologic importance of a coronary stenosis? *N Engl J Med* 1984;310:819–824.

20. Kraunz RF, Kennedy JW. Ultrasonic determination of left ventricular wall motion in normal man. Studies at rest and after exercise. *Am Heart J* 1970;79:36–43.

21. Koike A, Itoh H, Doi M, et al. Beat-to-beat evaluation of cardiac function during recovery from upright bicycle exercise in patients with coronary artery disease. *Am Heart J* 1990;120:316–323.

22. Tennant R, Wiggers CJ. The effect of coronary occlusion on myocardial contraction. *Am J Physiol* 1935;112:351–361.

23. Kerber RE, Martins JB, Marcus ML. Effect of acute ischemia, nitroglycerin and nitroprusside on regional myocardial thickening, stress and perfusion. Experimental echocardiographic studies. *Circulation* 1979;60:121–129.

24. Kerber RE, Marcus ML, Wilson R, et al. Effects of acute coronary occlusion on the motion and perfusion of the normal and ischemic interventricular septum. *Circulation* 1976;54:928–935.

25. Takayama M, Norris RM, Brown MA, et al. Postsystolic shortening of acutely ischemic canine myocardium predicts early and late recovery of function after coronary artery reperfusion. *Circulation* 1988;78:994–1007.

26. Presti CF, Armstrong WF, Feigenbaum H. Comparison of echocardiography at peak exercise and after bicycle exercise in evaluation of patients with known or suspected coronary artery disease. *J Am Soc Echo* 1988;1:119–126.

27. Ryan T, Segar DS, Sawada SG, et al. Detection of coronary artery disease with upright bicycle exercise echocardiography. *J Am Soc Echo* 1993;6:186–197.

28. Armstrong WF. "Hibernating" myocardium: asleep or part dead? *J Am Coll Cardiol* 1996;28:530–535.

29. Kloner RA, Przyklenk K, Patel B. Altered myocardial states: the stunned and hibernating myocardium. *Am J Med* 1986;86[Suppl 1A]:14–17.

30. Rahimtoola SH. The hibernating myocardium. *Am Heart J* 1989;117:2113–2115.

31. Fudo T, Kambara H, Hashimoto T, et al. F-18 deoxyglucose and stress N-13 ammonia positron emission tomography in anterior wall healed myocardial infarction. *Am J Cardiol* 1988;61:1191–1197.

32. Nesto RW, Kowalchuk GJ. The ischemic cascade: temporal sequence of hemodynamic, electrocardiographic and symptomatic expressions of ischemia. *Am J Cardiol* 1987;59:23C–30C.

33. Aroesty JM, McKay RG, Heller GV, et al. Simultaneous assessment of left ventricular systolic and diastolic dysfunction during pacing-induced ischemia. *Circulation* 1985;71:889–900.

34. Wijns W, Serruys PW, Slager CJ, et al. Effect of coronary occlusion during percutaneous transluminal angioplasty in humans on left ventricular chamber stiffness and regional diastolic pressure-radius relations. *J Am Coll Cardiol* 1986;7:455–463.

35. Armstrong WF. Echocardiography in coronary artery disease. *Prog Cardiovasc Dis* 1988;30:267–288.

36. Flamm SD, Taki J, Moore R, et al. Redistribution of regional and organ blood volume and effect on cardiac function in relation to upright exercise intensity in healthy human subjects. *Circulation* 1990;81:1550–1559.

37. Marwick TH. How to perform stress echocardiography. Practical aspects. In: Marwick TH, ed. *Stress echocardiography*. Dordrecht: Kluwer, 1994.

38. Fujita T, Ajisaka R, Matsumoto R. Isoproterenol infusion stress two-dimensional echocardiography in diagnosis of coronary artery disease in elderly patients: comparison with the other stress testing methods. *Jpn Heart J* 1986;27:287–297.

39. Vasu MA, O'Keefe DD, Kapellakis GZ, et al. Myocardial oxygen consumption: effects of epinephrine, isoproterenol, dopamine, norepinephrine, and dobutamine. *Am J Physiol* 1978;235:H237–H241.

40. Ruffolo RR, Spradlin TA, Pollock GD, et al. Alpha and beta effects of the stereoisomers of dobutamine. *J Pharm Exp Ther* 1981;219:447–452.

41. Young M, Pan W, Weisner J. Characterization of arbutamine: a novel catecholamine stress agent for diagnosis of coronary artery disease. *Drug Dev Res* 1994;32:19–28.

42. Cohen JL, Greene TO, Ottenweller J, et al. Dobutamine digital echocardiography for detecting coronary artery disease. *Am J Cardiol* 1991;67:1311–1318.

43. Secknus MA, Marwick TH. Evolution of dobutamine echocardiography protocols and indications: safety and side effects in 3,011 studies over 5 years. *J Am Coll Cardiol* 1997;29:1234–1240.

44. Mason JR, Palac RT, Freeman ML, et al. Thallium scintigraphy during dobutamine infusion: nonexercise-dependent screening test for coronary disease. *Am Heart J* 1984;107:481–485.

45. Berthe C, Pierard LA, Hiernaux M, et al. Predicting the extent and location of coronary artery disease in acute myocardial infarction by echocardiography during dobutamine infusion. *Am J Cardiol* 1986;58:1167–1172.

46. Sawada SG, Segar DS, Ryan T, et al. Echocardiographic detection of coronary artery disease during dobutamine infusion. *Circulation* 1991;83:1605–1614.

47. Mazeika PK, Nadazdin A, Oakley CM. Dobutamine stress echocardiography for detection and assessment of coronary artery disease. *J Am Coll Cardiol* 1992;19:1203–1211.

48. Weissman NJ, Nidorf SM, Guerrero JL, et al. Optimal stage duration in dobutamine stress echocardiography. *J Am Coll Cardiol* 1995;25:605–609.

49. McNeill AJ, Fioretti PM, el-Said SM, et al. Enhanced sensitivity for detection of coronary artery disease by addition of atropine to dobutamine stress echocardiography. *Am J Cardiol* 1992;70:41–46.

50. Lewandowski TJ, Armstrong WF, Bach DS. Reduced test time by early identification of patients requiring atropine during dobutamine stress echocardiography. *J Am Soc Echocardiogr* 1998;11:236–242.

51. Cornel JH, Balk AH, Boersma E, et al. Safety and feasibility of dobutamine-atropine stress echocardiography in patients with ischemic left ventricular dysfunction. *J Am Soc Echocardiogr* 1996;9:27–32.

52. Williams MJ, Odabashian J, Lauer MS, et al. Prognostic value of dobutamine echocardiography in patients with

left ventricular dysfunction. *J Am Coll Cardiol* 1996;27:132–139.

53. Poldermans D, Rambaldi R, Bax JJ, et al. Safety and utility of atropine addition during dobutamine stress echocardiography for the assessment of viable myocardium in patients with severe left ventricular dysfunction. *Eur Heart J* 1998;19:1712–1728.

54. Picano E, Lattanzi F. Dipyridamole echocardiography. A new diagnostic window on coronary artery disease. *Circulation* 1991;83:III19–III26.

55. Rossen JD, Quillen JE, Lopez AG, et al. Comparison of coronary vasodilation with intravenous dipyridamole and adenosine. *Am J Cardiol* 1991;18:485–491.

56. Wilson RF, Wyche K, Christensen BV, et al. Effects of adenosine on human coronary arterial circulation. *Circulation* 1990;82:1595–1606.

57. Picano E. Dipyridamole-echocardiography test: historical background and physiologic basis. *Eur Heart J* 1989;10:365–376.

58. Picano E, Marini C, Pirelli S, et al. Safety of intravenous high-dose dipyridamole echocardiography. The Echo-Persantine International Cooperative Study Group. *Am J Cardiol* 1992;70:252–258.

59. Cerqueira MD, Verani MS, Schwaiger M, et al. Safety profile of adenosine stress perfusion imaging: results from the Adenoscan Multicenter Trial Registry. *J Am Coll Cardiol* 1994;23:384–389.

60. Picano E, Pingitore A, Conti U, et al. Enhanced sensitivity for detection of coronary artery disease by addition of atropine to dipyridamole echocardiography. *Eur Heart J* 1993;14:1216–1222.

61. Ostojic M, Picano E, Beleslin B, et al. Dipyridamole-dobutamine echocardiography: a novel test for the detection of milder forms of coronary artery disease. *J Am Coll Cardiol* 1994;23:1115–1122.

62. Kamp O, De Cock CC, Kupper AJ, et al. Simultaneous transesophageal two-dimensional echocardiography and atrial pacing for detecting coronary artery disease. *Am J Cardiol* 1992;69:1412–1416.

63. Lambertz H, Kreis A, Trumper H, et al. Simultaneous transesophageal atrial pacing and transesophageal two-dimensional echocardiography: a new method of stress echocardiography. *J Am Coll Cardiol* 1990;16:1143–1153.

64. Stempfle HU, Kruger TM, Brandl BC, et al. Simultaneous transesophageal echocardiography and atrial pacing: assessment of the functional significance of coronary artery disease before surgical treatment of an abdominal aneurysm. *Clin Invest* 1994;72:206–208.

65. Norris LP, Stewart RE, Jain A, et al. Biplane transesophageal pacing echocardiography compared with dipyridamole thallium-201 single-photon emission computed tomography in detecting coronary artery disease. *Am Heart J* 1993;126:676–685.

66. Iliceto S, Sorino M, D'Ambrosio G, et al. Detection of coronary artery disease by two-dimensional echocardiography and transesophageal atrial pacing. *J Am Coll Cardiol* 1985;5:1188–1197.

67. Pasternac A, Gorlin R, Sonnenblick EH, et al. Abnormalities of ventricular motion induced by atrial pacing in coronary artery disease. *Circulation* 1972;45:1195–1205.

68. Kotler MN, Jacobs LE. Transesophageal atrial pacing or pharmacologic stress testing in detection of coronary artery disease in patients who are unable to undergo exercise stress testing. *J Am Coll Cardiol* 1990;16:1154–1157.

69. Marangelli V, Iliceto S, Piccinni G, et al. Detection of coronary artery disease by digital stress echocardiography: comparison of exercise, transesophageal atrial pacing and dipyridamole echocardiography. *J Am Coll Cardiol* 1994;24:117–124.

70. Iliceto S, Amico A, Marangelli V, et al. Doppler echocardiographic evaluation of the effect of atrial pacing-induced ischemia on left ventricular filling in patients with coronary artery disease. *J Am Coll Cardiol* 1988;11:953–961.

71. Song JK, Park SW, Kang DH, et al. Diagnosis of coronary vasospasm in patients with clinical presentation of unstable angina pectoris using ergonovine echocardiography. *Am J Cardiol* 1998;82:1475–1478.

72. Song JK, Park SW, Kim JJ, et al. Values of intravenous ergonovine test with two-dimensional echocardiography for diagnosis of coronary artery spasm. *J Am Soc Echocardiogr* 1994;7:607–615.

73. Previtali M, Ardissino D, Barberis P, et al. Hyperventilation and ergonovine tests in Prinzmetal's variant angina pectoris in man. *Am J Cardiol* 1989;63:17–20.

74. Song JK, Lee SJ, Kang DH, et al. Ergonovine echocardiography as a screening test for diagnosis of vasospastic angina before coronary angiography. *J Am Coll Cardiol* 1996;27:1156–1161.

75. Morales MA, Lombardi M, Distante A, et al. Ergonovine-echo test to assess the significance of chest pain at rest without ECG changes. *Eur Heart J* 1995;16:1361–1366.

76. Attenhofer CH, Pellikka PA, Oh JK, et al. Is review of videotape necessary after review of digitized cine-loop images in stress echocardiography? A prospective study in 306 patients. *J Am Soc Echocardiogr* 1997;10:179–184.

77. Prince CR, Stoddard MF, Morris GT, et al. Dobutamine two-dimensional transesophageal echocardiographic stress testing for detection of coronary artery disease. *Am Heart J* 1994;128:36–41.

78. Agati L, Renzi M, Sciomer S, et al. Transesophageal dipyridamole echocardiography for diagnosis of coronary artery disease. *J Am Coll Cardiol* 1992;19:765–770.

79. Caidahl K, Kazzam E, Lidberg J, et al. New concept in echocardiography: harmonic imaging of tissue without use of contrast agent. *Lancet* 1998;352:1264–1270.

80. Franke A, Hoffmann R, Kuhl HP, et al. Non-contrast second harmonic imaging improves interobserver agreement and accuracy of dobutamine stress echocardiography in patients with impaired image quality. *Heart* 2000;83:133–140.

81. Afridi I, Kleiman NS, Raizner AE, et al. Dobutamine echocardiography in myocardial hibernation. Optimal dose and accuracy in predicting recovery of ventricular function after coronary angioplasty. *Circulation* 1995;91:663–670.

82. Picano E, Lattanzi F, Orlandini A, et al. Stress echocardiography and the human factor: the importance of being expert. *J Am Coll Cardiol* 1991;17:666–669.

83. Varga A, Picano E, Dodi C, et al. Madness and method in stress echo reading. *Eur Heart J* 1999;20:1271–1275.

84. Oberman A, Fan PH, Nanda NC, et al. Reproducibility of two-dimensional exercise echocardiography. *J Am Coll Cardiol* 1989;14:923–928.

85. Hoffmann R, Lethen H, Marwick T, et al. Analysis of interinstitutional observer agreement in interpretation of dobutamine stress echocardiograms. *J Am Coll Cardiol* 1996;27:330–336.

86. Hoffmann R, Lethen H, Marwick T, et al. Standardized guidelines for the interpretation of dobutamine echocardiography reduce interinstitutional variance in interpretation. *Am J Cardiol* 1998;82:1520–1524.

87. Hoffmann R, Poldermans D, van der Meer P, et al. The maturing of stress echocardiography: improved intercenter agreement in interpretation of dobutamine stress echocardiograms using new techniques. *Eur Heart J* 2001 (in press).

88. Henein MY, Gibson DG. Long axis function in disease. *Heart* 1999;81:229–231.

89. Ginzton LE, Conant R, Brizendine M, et al. Quantitative analysis of segmental wall motion during maximal upright dynamic exercise: variability in normal adults. *Circulation* 1986;73:268–275.

90. Lang RM, Vignon P, Weinert L, et al. Echocardiographic quantitation of regional left ventricular wall motion with color kinesis. *Circulation* 1996;93:1877–1885.

91. Koch R, Lang RM, Garcia MJ, et al. Objective evaluation of regional left ventricular wall motion during dobutamine stress echocardiographic studies using segmental analysis of color kinesis images. *J Am Coll Cardiol* 1999;34:409–419.

92. Chan J, Wahi SCP, Marwick TH. Anatomical M-mode: a novel technique for the quantitative evaluation of regional wall motion analysis during stress echocardiography. *Int J Cardiol Imaging* 2000;16:247–255.

93. Feinberg MS, Gussak HM, Davila-Roman VG, et al. Dissociation between wall thickening of normal myocardium and cyclic variation of backscatter during inotropic stimulation. *Am J Cardiol* 1996;77:515–520.

94. Milunski MR, Mohr GA, Perez JE, et al. Ultrasonic tissue characterization with integrated backscatter: acute myocardial ischemia, reperfusion, and stunned myocardium in patients. *Circulation* 1989;80:491–503.

95. Bach DS, Armstrong WF, Donovan CL, et al. Quantitative Doppler tissue imaging for assessment of regional myocardial velocities during transient ischemia and reperfusion. *Am Heart J* 1996;132:721–725.

96. Wilkenshoff UM, Sovany A, Wigstrom L, et al. Regional mean systolic myocardial velocity estimation by real-time color Doppler myocardial imaging: a new technique for quantifying regional systolic function. *J Am Soc Echocardiogr* 1998;11:682–692.

97. Pasquet A, Armstrong G, Beachler L, et al. Analysis of segmental myocardial Doppler velocity as a quantitative adjunct to exercise echocardiography. *J Am Soc Echocardiogr* 1999;12:901–912.

98. Pasquet A, Armstrong G, Rimmerman CM, et al. Correlation of myocardial Doppler velocity response to exercise with independent evidence of myocardial ischemia by dual isotope single photon emission computed tomography. *Am J Cardiol* 2000;85:536–542.

99. Cain P, Baglin T, Case C, et al. Application of tissue Doppler to interpretation of dobutamine echocardiography: comparison with quantitative coronary angiography. *Am J Cardiol* 2001;87:525–531.

100. Topol EJ, Nissen SE. Our preoccupation with coronary luminology. The dissociation between clinical and angiographic findings in ischemic heart disease. *Circulation* 1995;92:2333–2342.

101. Marwick TH, Nemec JJ, Pashkow FJ, et al. Accuracy and limitations of exercise echocardiography in a routine clinical setting. *J Am Coll Cardiol* 1992;19:74–81.

102. Senior R, Lahiri A. Enhanced detection of myocardial ischemia by stress dobutamine echocardiography utilizing the "biphasic" response of wall thickening during low and high dose dobutamine infusion. *J Am Coll Cardiol* 1995;26:26–32.

103. Bach DS, Muller DW, Gros BJ, et al. False positive dobutamine stress echocardiograms: characterization of clinical, echocardiographic and angiographic findings. *J Am Coll Cardiol* 1994;24:928–933.

104. Crouse LJ, Harbrecht JJ, Vacek JL, et al. Exercise echocardiography as a screening test for coronary artery disease and correlation with coronary arteriography. *Am J Cardiol* 1991;67:1213–1218.

105. Hecht HS, DeBord L, Sotomayor N, et al. Supine bicycle stress echocardiography: peak exercise imaging is superior to postexercise imaging. *J Am Soc Echocardiogr* 1993;6:265–271.

106. Beleslin BD, Ostojic M, Stepanovic J, et al. Stress echocardiography in the detection of myocardial ischemia. Head-to-head comparison of exercise, dobutamine, and dipyridamole tests. *Circulation* 1994;90:1168–1176.

107. Roger VL, Pellikka PA, Oh JK, et al. Stress echocardiography. Part I. Exercise echocardiography: techniques, implementation, clinical applications, and correlations. *Mayo Clin Proc* 1995;70:5–15.

108. Armstrong WF, O'Donnell J, Ryan T, et al. Effect of prior myocardial infarction and extent and location of coronary disease on accuracy of exercise echocardiography. *J Am Coll Cardiol* 1987;10:531–538.

109. Quinones MA, Verani MS, Haichin RM, et al. Exercise echocardiography versus 201Tl single-photon emission computed tomography in evaluation of coronary artery disease. Analysis of 292 patients. *Circulation* 1992;85:1026–1031.

110. Sheikh KH, Bengtson JR, Helmy S, et al. Relation of quantitative coronary lesion measurements to the development of exercise-induced ischemia assessed by exercise echocardiography. *J Am Coll Cardiol* 1990;15:1043–1051.

111. Agati L, Arata L, Luongo R, et al. Assessment of severity of coronary narrowings by quantitative exercise echocardiography and comparison with quantitative arteriography. *Am J Cardiol* 1991;67:1201–1207.

112. Badruddin SM, Ahmad A, Mickelson J, et al. Supine bicycle versus post-treadmill exercise echocardiography in the detection of myocardial ischemia: a randomized single-blind crossover trial. *J Am Coll Cardiol* 1999;33:1485–1490.

113. Elhendy A, Geleijnse ML, van Domburg RT, et al. Gender differences in the accuracy of dobutamine stress echocar-

diography for the diagnosis of coronary artery disease. *Am J Cardiol* 1997;80:1414–1418.

114. Dionisopoulos PN, Collins JD, Smart SC, et al. The value of dobutamine stress echocardiography for the detection of coronary artery disease in women. *J Am Soc Echocardiogr* 1997;10:811–817.

115. Marwick T, D'Hondt AM, Baudhuin T, et al. Optimal use of dobutamine stress for the detection and evaluation of coronary artery disease: combination with echocardiography or scintigraphy, or both? *J Am Coll Cardiol* 1993;22:159–167.

116. Ling LH, Pellikka PA, Mahoney DW, et al. Atropine augmentation in dobutamine stress echocardiography: role and incremental value in a clinical practice setting. *J Am Coll Cardiol* 1996;28:551–557.

117. Marcovitz PA, Armstrong WF. Accuracy of dobutamine stress echocardiography in detecting coronary artery disease. *Am J Cardiol* 1992;69:1269–1273.

118. Takeuchi M, Araki M, Nakashima Y, et al. Comparison of dobutamine stress echocardiography and stress thallium-201 single-photon emission computed tomography for detecting coronary artery disease. *J Am Soc Echocardiogr* 1993;6:593–602.

119. Anthopoulos LP, Bonou MS, Kardaras FG, et al. Stress echocardiography in elderly patients with coronary artery disease: applicability, safety and prognostic value of dobutamine and adenosine echocardiography in elderly patients. *J Am Coll Cardiol* 1996;28:52–59.

120. Pingitore A, Picano E, Colosso MQ, et al. The atropine factor in pharmacologic stress echocardiography. Echo Persantine (EPIC) and Echo Dobutamine International Cooperative (EDIC) Study Groups. *J Am Coll Cardiol* 1996;27:1164–1170.

121. San Roman JA, Vilacosta I, Castillo JA, et al. Dipyridamole and dobutamine-atropine stress echocardiography in the diagnosis of coronary artery disease. Comparison with exercise stress test, analysis of agreement, and impact of antianginal treatment. *Chest* 1996;110:1248–1254.

122. Hennessy T, Diamond P, Holligan B, et al. Correlation of myocardial histologic changes in hibernating myocardium with dobutamine stress echocardiographic findings. *Am Heart J* 1998;135:952–959.

123. Beleslin BD, Ostojic M, Djordjevic-Dikic A, et al. Integrated evaluation of relation between coronary lesion features and stress echocardiography results: the importance of coronary lesion morphology. *J Am Coll Cardiol* 1999;33:717–726.

124. Baptista J, Arnese M, Roelandt JR, et al. Quantitative coronary angiography in the estimation of the functional significance of coronary stenosis: correlations with dobutamine-atropine stress test. *J Am Coll Cardiol* 1994;23:1434–1439.

125. Bartunek J, Marwick TH, Rodrigues AC, et al. Dobutamine-induced wall motion abnormalities: correlations with myocardial fractional flow reserve and quantitative coronary angiography. *J Am Coll Cardiol* 1996;27:1429–1436.

126. Segar DS, Brown SE, Sawada SG, et al. Dobutamine stress echocardiography: correlation with coronary lesion severity as determined by quantitative angiography. *J Am Coll Cardiol* 1992;19:1197–1202.

127. Roger VL, Pellikka PA, Bell MR, et al. Sex and test verification bias. Impact on the diagnostic value of exercise echocardiography. *Circulation* 1997;95:405–410.

128. Previtali M, Lanzarini L, Fetiveau R, et al. Comparison of dobutamine stress echocardiography, dipyridamole stress echocardiography and exercise stress testing for diagnosis of coronary artery disease. *Am J Cardiol* 1993;72:865–870.

129. Cohen JL, Ottenweller JE, George AK, et al. Comparison of dobutamine and exercise echocardiography for detecting coronary artery disease. *Am J Cardiol* 1993;72:1226–1231.

130. Marwick TH, D'Hondt AM, Mairesse GH, et al. Comparative ability of dobutamine and exercise stress in inducing myocardial ischaemia in active patients. *Br Heart J* 1994;72:31–38.

131. Dagianti A, Penco M, Agati L, et al. Stress echocardiography: comparison of exercise, dipyridamole and dobutamine in detecting and predicting the extent of coronary artery disease. *J Am Coll Cardiol* 1995;26:18–25.

132. Rallidis L, Cokkinos P, Tousoulis D, et al. Comparison of dobutamine and treadmill exercise echocardiography in inducing ischemia in patients with coronary artery disease. *J Am Coll Cardiol* 1997;30:1660–1668.

133. Attenhoffer CH, Pellikka PA, Oh JK, et al. Comparison of ischemic response during exercise and dobutamine echocardiography in patients with left main coronary artery disease. *J Am Coll Cardiol* 1996;27:1171–1177.

134. Picano E, Severi S, Lattanzi F. The diagnostic and prognostic value of echo-dipyridamole in patients with suspected coronary disease. *Giornale Italiano di Cardiologia* 1991;21:621–632.

135. Severi S, Picano E, Michelassi C, et al. Diagnostic and prognostic value of dipyridamole echocardiography in patients with suspected coronary artery disease. Comparison with exercise electrocardiography. *Circulation* 1994;89:1160–1173.

136. Zoghbi WA, Cheirif J, Kleiman NS, et al. Diagnosis of ischemic heart disease with adenosine echocardiography. *J Am Coll Cardiol* 1991;18:1271–1279.

137. Marwick T, Willemart B, D'Hondt AM, et al. Selection of the optimal nonexercise stress for the evaluation of ischemic regional myocardial dysfunction and malperfusion. Comparison of dobutamine and adenosine using echocardiography and 99mTc-MIBI single photon emission computed tomography. *Circulation* 1993;87:345–354.

138. Fragasso G, Lu C, Dabrowski P, et al. Comparison of stress/rest myocardial perfusion tomography, dipyridamole and dobutamine stress echocardiography for the detection of coronary disease in hypertensive patients with chest pain and positive exercise test. *J Am Coll Cardiol* 1999;34:441–447.

139. Zabalgoitia M, Gandhi DK, Abi-Mansour P, et al. Transesophageal stress echocardiography: detection of coronary disease in patients with normal left ventricular contractility. *Am Heart J* 1991;122:1456–1463.

140. Anselmi M, Golia G, Marino P, et al. Usefulness of transesophageal atrial pacing combined with two-dimensional echocardiography (echo-pacing) in predicting the presence and site of residual jeopardized myocardium after uncom-

plicated acute myocardial infarction. *Am J Cardiol* 1994;73:534–538.

141. Michael TA, Antonescu A, Bhambi B, et al. Accuracy and usefulness of atrial pacing in conjunction with transthoracic echocardiography in the detection of cardiac ischemia. *Am J Cardiol* 1996;77:187–190.

142. Matthews RV, Haskell RJ, Ginzton LE, et al. Usefulness of esophageal pill electrode atrial pacing with quantitative two-dimensional echocardiography for diagnosing coronary artery disease. *Am J Cardiol* 1989;64:730–735.

143. Lee CY, Pellikka PA, McCully RB, et al. Nonexercise stress transthoracic echocardiography: transesophageal atrial pacing versus dobutamine stress. *J Am Coll Cardiol* 1999;33:506–511.

144. Olson CE, Porter TR, Deligonul U, et al. Left ventricular volume changes during dobutamine stress echocardiography identify patients with more extensive coronary artery disease. *J Am Coll Cardiol* 1994;24:1268–1273.

145. Marwick TH, Nemec JJ, Stewart WJ, et al. Diagnosis of coronary artery disease using exercise echocardiography and positron emission tomography: comparison and analysis of discrepant results. *J Am Soc Echocardiogr* 1992;5:231–238.

146. O'Keefe JH Jr, Barnhart CS, Bateman TM. Comparison of stress echocardiography and stress myocardial perfusion scintigraphy for diagnosing coronary artery disease and assessing its severity. *Am J Cardiol* 1995;75:25D–34D.

147. Hecht HS, DeBord L, Shaw R, et al. Digital supine bicycle stress echocardiography: a new technique for evaluating coronary artery disease. *J Am Coll Cardiol* 1993;21:950–956.

148. Armstrong W, O'Donnell W, Ryan T, et al. Effect of prior myocardial infarction and extent and location of coronary disease on accuracy of exercise echocardiography. *J Am Coll Cardiol* 1987;10:531–538.

149. Pozzoli MM, Fioretti PM, Salustri A, et al. Exercise echocardiography and technetium 99m MIBI single photon emission computed tomography in the detection of coronary artery disease. *Am J Cardiol* 1991;67:350–355.

150. Whinnery JE, Froelicher VF, Stuart AJ. The electrocardiographic response to maximal treadmill exercise in asymptomatic men with left bundle branch block. *Am Heart J* 1977;94:316–320.

151. Miranda CP, Lehmann KG, Froelicher VF. Correlation between resting ST segment depression, exercise testing, coronary angiography and long-term prognosis. *Am Heart J* 1991;122:1617–1626.

152. Kansal S, Roitman D, Sheffield LT. Stress testing with ST depression at rest. *Circulation* 1976;54:636–639.

153. Cumming GR. Yield of ischemic exercise electrocardiograms in relation to exercise intensity in a normal population. *Br Heart J* 1972;34:919–923.

154. Mairesse GH, Marwick TH, Vanoverschelde JL, et al. How accurate is dobutamine stress electrocardiography for detection of coronary artery disease? Comparison with two-dimensional echocardiography and technetium-99m methoxyl isobutyl isonitrile (MIBI) perfusion scintigraphy. *J Am Coll Cardiol* 1994;24:920–927.

155. Chambers CE, Brown KA. Dipyridamole-induced ST segment depression during thallium-201 imaging in patients with coronary artery disease: angiographic and hemodynamic determinants. *J Am Coll Cardiol* 1988;12:37–41.

156. Villanueva FS, Smith WH, Watson DD, et al. ST-segment depression during dipyridamole infusion, and its clinical, scintigraphic and hemodynamic correlates. *Am J Cardiol* 1992;69:445–448.

157. Ryan T, Vasey CG, Presti CF, et al. Exercise echocardiography: detection of coronary artery disease in patients with normal left ventricular wall motion at rest. *J Am Coll Cardiol* 1988;11:993–999.

158. Hung J, Chaitman BR, Lam J, et al. Noninvasive diagnostic test choices for the evaluation of coronary artery disease in women: a multivariate comparison of cardiac fluoroscopy, exercise electrocardiography and exercise thallium myocardial perfusion scintigraphy. *J Am Coll Cardiol* 1984;4:8–16.

159. Okin PM, Kligfield P. Gender-specific criteria and performance of the exercise electrocardiogram. *Circulation* 1995;92:1209–1216.

160. Cumming GR, Dufresne C, Kich L, et al. Exercise electrocardiogram patterns in normal women. *Br Heart J* 1973;35:1055–1061.

161. Sketch MH, Mohiuddin SM, Lynch JD, et al. Significant sex differences in the correlation of electrocardiographic exercise testing and coronary arteriograms. *Am J Cardiol* 1975;36:169–173.

162. Marwick TH, Anderson T, Williams MJ, et al. Exercise echocardiography is an accurate and cost-efficient technique for the detection of coronary artery disease in women. *J Am Coll Cardiol* 1995;26:335–341.

163. Secknus MA, Marwick TH. Influence of gender on physiologic response and accuracy of dobutamine echocardiography. *Am J Cardiol* 1997;80:721–724.

164. Gibbons RJ, Miller TD. Equilibrium radionuclide angiography. In: Skorton DJ, Schelbert HR, Wolf GL, et al., eds. *Marcus' cardiac imaging: a companion to Braunwald's heart disease.* Philadelphia: WB Saunders, 1996:941–962.

165. Gould KL. Noninvasive assessment of coronary stenoses by myocardial perfusion imaging during pharmacologic coronary vasodilation. 1. Physiologic basis and experimental validation. *Am J Cardiol* 1978;41:267–278.

166. Mahmarian J, Boyce T, Goldberg R, et al. Quantitative exercise thallium-201 single photon emission computed tomography for the enhanced diagnosis of ischemic heart disease. *J Am Coll Cardiol* 1990;15:318–325.

167. Fleischmann KE, Hunink MG, Kuntz KM, et al. Exercise echocardiography or exercise SPECT imaging? A meta-analysis of diagnostic test performance. *JAMA* 1998;280:913–920.

168. Simek CL, Watson DD, Smith WH, et al. Dipyridamole thallium-201 imaging versus dobutamine echocardiography for the evaluation of coronary artery disease in patients unable to exercise. *Am J Cardiol* 1993;72:1257–1262.

169. Oosterhuis WP, Breeman A, Niemeyer MG, et al. Patients with a normal exercise thallium-201 myocardial scintigram: always a good prognosis? *Eur J Nucl Med* 1993;20:151–158.

170. San Roman JA, Rollan MJ, Vilacosta I, et al. [Echocardiography and MIBI-SPECT scintigraphy during dobutamine infusion in the diagnosis of coronary disease]. *Rev Esp Cardiol* 1995;48:606–614.

171. Huang PJ, Ho YL, Wu CC, et al. Simultaneous dobutamine stress echocardiography and thallium-201 perfusion imaging for the detection of coronary artery disease. *Cardiology* 1997;88:556–562.

172. Kwok Y, Kim C, Grady D, et al. Meta-analysis of exercise testing to detect coronary artery disease in women. *Am J Cardiol* 1999;83:660–666.

173. Baer FM, Theissen P, Crnac J, et al. Head to head comparison of dobutamine-transesophageal echocardiography and dobutamine-magnetic resonance imaging for the prediction of left ventricular functional recovery in patients with chronic coronary artery disease. *Eur Heart J* 2000;21:981–991.

174. Topol EJ, Ellis SG, Cosgrove DM, et al. Analysis of coronary angioplasty practice in the United States with an insurance-claims data base. *Circulation* 1993;87:1489–1497.

175. Sawada SG, Judson WE, Ryan T, et al. Upright bicycle exercise echocardiography after coronary artery bypass grafting. *Am J Cardiol* 1989;64:1123–1129.

176. Elhendly A, Geleijnse ML, Roelandt JR, et al. Assessment of patients after coronary artery bypass grafting by dobutamine stress echocardiography. *Am J Cardiol* 1996;77:1234–1236.

177. Hecht HS, DeBord L, Shaw R, et al. Usefulness of supine bicycle stress echocardiography for detection of restenosis after percutaneous transluminal coronary angioplasty. *Am J Cardiol* 1993;71:293–296.

178. Ellis SG, Wynne J, Braunwald E, et al. Response of reperfusion-salvaged, stunned myocardium to inotropic stimulation. *Am Heart J* 1984;107:13–19.

179. Smart SC, Sawada S, Ryan T, et al. Low-dose dobutamine echocardiography detects reversible dysfunction after thrombolytic therapy of acute myocardial infarction. *Circulation* 1993;88:405–415.

180. Watada H, Ito H, Oh H, et al. Dobutamine stress echocardiography predicts reversible dysfunction and quantitates the extent of irreversibly damaged myocardium after reperfusion of anterior myocardial infarction. *J Am Coll Cardiol* 1994;24:624–630.

181. Pierard LA, De Landsheere CM, Berthe C, et al. Identification of viable myocardium by echocardiography during dobutamine infusion in patients with myocardial infarction after thrombolytic therapy: comparison with positron emission tomography. *J Am Coll Cardiol* 1990;15:1021–1031.

182. Previtali M, Poli A, Lanzarini L, et al. Dobutamine stress echocardiography for assessment of myocardial viability and ischemia in acute myocardial infarction treated with thrombolysis. *Am J Cardiol* 1993;72:124G–130G.

183. Bolognese L, Antoniucci D, Rovai D, et al. Myocardial contrast echocardiography versus dobutamine echocardiography for predicting functional recovery after acute myocardial infarction treated with primary coronary angioplasty. *J Am Coll Cardiol* 1996;28:1677–1683.

184. Poli A, Previtali M, Lanzarini L, et al. Comparison of dobutamine stress echocardiography with dipyridamole stress echocardiography for detection of viable myocardium after myocardial infarction treated with thrombolysis. *Heart* 1996;75:240–246.

185. Varga A, Ostojic M, Djordjevic-Dikic A, et al. Infra-low dose dipyridamole test. A novel dose regimen for selective assessment of myocardial viability by vasodilator stress echocardiography. *Eur Heart J* 1996;17:629–634.

186. Cigarroa CG, deFilippi CR, Brickner ME, et al. Dobutamine stress echocardiography identifies hibernating myocardium and predicts recovery of left ventricular function after coronary revascularization. *Circulation* 1993;88:430–436.

187. La Canna G, Alfieri O, Giubbini R, et al. Echocardiography during infusion of dobutamine for identification of reversibly dysfunction in patients with chronic coronary artery disease. *J Am Coll Cardiol* 1994;23:617–626.

188. Arnese M, Cornel JH, Salustri A, et al. Prediction of improvement of regional left ventricular function after surgical revascularization. A comparison of low-dose dobutamine echocardiography with 201Tl single-photon emission computed tomography. *Circulation* 1995;91:2748–2752.

189. Vanoverschelde JL, Wijns W, Depre C, et al. Mechanisms of chronic regional postischemic dysfunction in humans. New insights from the study of noninfarcted collateral-dependent myocardium. *Circulation* 1993;87:1513–1523.

190. Stewart S. Current theories and therapies relating to acute myocardial infarction and reperfusion injury. *Intens Crit Care Nursing* 1992;8:104–112.

191. Bonow RO. Identification of viable myocardium. *Circulation* 1996;94:2674–2680.

192. Marzullo P, Parodi O, Reisenhofer B, et al. Value of rest thallium-201/technetium-99m sestamibi scans and dobutamine echocardiography for detecting myocardial viability. *Am J Cardiol* 1993;71:166–172.

193. Charney R, Schwinger ME, Chun J, et al. Dobutamine echocardiography and resting-redistribution thallium-201 scintigraphy predicts recovery of hibernating myocardium after coronary revascularization. *Am Heart J* 1994;128:864–869.

194. Kostopoulos KG, Kranidis AI, Bouki KP, et al. Detection of myocardial viability in the prediction of improvement in left ventricular function after successful coronary revascularization by using the dobutamine stress echocardiography and quantitative SPECT rest-redistribution-reinjection 201Tl imaging after dipyridamole infusion. *Angiology* 1996;47:1039–1046.

195. Qureshi U, Nagueh SF, Afridi I, et al. Dobutamine echocardiography and quantitative rest-redistribution 201Tl tomography in myocardial hibernation. Relation of contractile reserve to 201Tl uptake and comparative prediction of recovery of function. *Circulation* 1997;95:626–635.

196. Nagueh SF, Vaduganathan P, Ali N, et al. Identification of hibernating myocardium: comparative accuracy of myocardial contrast echocardiography, rest-redistribution thallium-201 tomography and dobutamine echocardiography. *J Am Coll Cardiol* 1997;29:985–993.

197. Senior R, Glenville B, Basu S, et al. Dobutamine echocardiography and thallium-201 imaging predict functional improvement after revascularisation in severe ischaemic left ventricular dysfunction. *Br Heart J* 1995;74:358–364.

198. Perrone-Filardi P, Pace L, Prastaro M, et al. Assessment of myocardial viability in patients with chronic coronary artery

disease. Rest-4-hour-24-hour 201Tl tomography versus dobutamine echocardiography. *Circulation* 1996;94:2712–2719.

199. Bax JJ, Cornel JH, Visser FC, et al. Prediction of recovery of myocardial dysfunction after revascularization. Comparison of fluorine-18 fluorodeoxyglucose/thallium-201 SPECT, thallium-201 stress-reinjection SPECT and dobutamine echocardiography. *J Am Coll Cardiol* 1996;28:558–564.

200. Haque T, Furukawa T, Takahashi M, et al. Identification of hibernating myocardium by dobutamine stress echocardiography: comparison with thallium-201 reinjection imaging. *Am Heart J* 1995;130:553–563.

201. Vanoverschelde JL, D'Hondt AM, Marwick T, et al. Head-to-head comparison of exercise-redistribution-reinjection thallium single-photon emission computed tomography and low-dose dobutamine echocardiography for prediction of reversibility of chronic left ventricular ischemic dysfunction. *J Am Coll Cardiol* 1996;28:432–442.

202. Elsasser A, Muller KD, Vogt A, et al. Assessment of myocardial viability: dobutamine echocardiography and thallium-201 single-photon emission computed tomographic imaging predict the postoperative improvement of left ventricular function after bypass surgery. *Am Heart J* 1998;135:463–475.

203. Chan RKM, Lee KJ, Calafiore P, et al. Comparison of dobutamine echocardiography and positron emission tomography in patients with chronic ischemic left ventricular dysfunction. *J Am Coll Cardiol* 1996;27:1601–1607.

204. Pasquet A, Williams MJ, Secknus MA, et al. Correlation of preoperative myocardial function, perfusion, and metabolism with postoperative function at rest and stress after bypass surgery in severe left ventricular dysfunction. *Am J Cardiol* 1999;84:58–64.

205. Cornel JH, Bax JJ, Elhendy A, et al. Biphasic response to dobutamine predicts improvement of global left ventricular function after surgical revascularization in patients with stable coronary artery disease: implications of time course of recovery on diagnostic accuracy. *J Am Coll Cardiol* 1998;31:1002–1010.

206. Pasquet A, Lauer MS, Williams MJ, et al. Prediction of global left ventricular function after bypass surgery in patients with severe left ventricular dysfunction. Impact of pre-operative myocardial function, perfusion, and metabolism. *Eur Heart J* 2000;21:125–136.

207. Marwick TH, Zuchowski C, Lauer MS, et al. Functional status and quality of life in patients with heart failure undergoing coronary bypass surgery after assessment of myocardial viability. *J Am Coll Cardiol* 1999;33:750–758.

208. Bax JJ, Poldermans D, Elhendy A, et al. Improvement of left ventricular ejection fraction, heart failure symptoms and prognosis after revascularization in patients with chronic coronary artery disease and viable myocardium detected by dobutamine stress echocardiography. *J Am Coll Cardiol* 1999;34:163–169.

209. Afridi I, Grayburn PA, Panza JA, et al. Myocardial viability during dobutamine echocardiography predicts survival in patients with coronary artery disease and severe left ventricular systolic dysfunction. *J Am Coll Cardiol* 1998;32:921–926.

210. Meluzin J, Cerny J, Frelich MS, et al. Prognostic value of the amount of dysfunctional but viable myocardium in revascularized patients with coronary artery disease and left ventricular dysfunction. *J Am Coll Cardiol* 1998;32:912–920.

211. Krivokapich J, Child JS, Gerber RS, et al. Prognostic usefulness of positive or negative exercise stress echocardiography for predicting coronary events in ensuing twelve months. *Am J Cardiol* 1993;71:646–651.

212. Marwick TH, Mehta R, Arheart K, et al. Use of exercise echocardiography for prognostic evaluation of patients with known or suspected coronary artery disease. *J Am Coll Cardiol* 1997;30:83–90.

213. McCully RB, Roger VL, Mahoney DW, et al. Outcome after normal exercise echocardiography and predictors of subsequent cardiac events: follow-up of 1,325 patients. *J Am Coll Cardiol* 1998;31:144–149.

214. Syed MA, Al Malki Q, Kazmouz G, et al. Usefulness of exercise echocardiography in predicting cardiac events in an outpatient population. *Am J Cardiol* 1998;82:569–573.

215. Poldermans D, Fioretti PM, Boersma E, et al. Dobutamine-atropine stress echocardiography and clinical data for predicting late cardiac events in patients with suspected coronary artery disease. *Am J Med* 1994;97:119–125.

216. Kamaran M, Teague SM, Finkelhor RS, et al. Prognostic value of dobutamine stress echocardiography in patients referred because of suspected coronary artery disease. *Am J Cardiol* 1995;76:887–891.

217. Marcovitz PA, Shayna V, Horn RA, et al. Value of dobutamine stress echocardiography in determining the prognosis of patients with known or suspected coronary artery disease. *Am J Cardiol* 1996;78:404–408.

218. Chuah SC, Pellikka PA, Roger VL, et al. Role of dobutamine stress echocardiography in predicting outcome in 860 patients with known or suspected coronary artery disease. *Circulation* 1998;97:1474–1480.

219. Poldermans D, Fioretti PM, Boersma E, et al. Long-term prognostic value of dobutamine-atropine stress echocardiography in 1737 patients with known or suspected coronary artery disease: a single-center experience. *Circulation* 1999;99:757–762.

220. Picano E, Severi S, Michelassi C, et al. Prognostic importance of dipyridamole-echocardiography test in coronary artery disease. *Circulation* 1989;80:450–457.

221. Krone RJ, Gillespie JA, Weld FM, et al. Low-level exercise testing after myocardial infarction: usefulness in enhancing clinical risk stratification. *Circulation* 1985;71:80–89.

222. Mazeika PK, Nadazdin A, Oakley CM. Prognostic value of dobutamine echocardiography in patients with high pretest likelihood of coronary artery disease. *Am J Cardiol* 1993;71:33–39.

223. Olmos LI, Dakik H, Gordon R, et al. Long-term prognostic value of exercise echocardiography compared with exercise 201Tl, ECG, and clinical variables in patients evaluated for coronary artery disease. *Circulation* 1998;98:2679–2686.

224. Bolognese L, Rossi L, Sarasso G, et al. Silent versus symptomatic dipyridamole-induced ischemia after myocardial

infarction: clinical and prognostic significance. *J Am Coll Cardiol* 1992;19:953–959.

225. Picano E, Landi P, Bolognese L, et al. Prognostic value of dipyridamole echocardiography early after uncomplicated myocardial infarction: a large-scale, multicenter trial. The EPIC Study Group. *Am J Med* 1993;95:608–618.

226. Chiarella F, Domenicucci S, Bellotti P, et al. Dipyridamole echocardiographic test performed 3 days after an acute myocardial infarction: feasibility, tolerability, safety and in-hospital prognostic value. *Eur Heart J* 1994;15:842–850.

227. Picano E, Pingitore A, Sicari R, et al. Stress echocardiographic results predict risk of reinfarction early after uncomplicated acute myocardial infarction: large-scale multicenter study. Echo Persantine International Cooperative (EPIC) Study Group. *J Am Coll Cardiol* 1995;26:908–913.

228. Carlos ME, Smart SC, Wynsen JC, et al. Dobutamine stress echocardiography for risk stratification after myocardial infarction. *Circulation* 1997;95:1402–1410.

229. Sicari R, Picano E, Landi P, et al. Prognostic value of dobutamine-atropine stress echocardiography early after acute myocardial infarction. Echo Dobutamine International Cooperative (EDIC) Study. *J Am Coll Cardiol* 1997;29:254–260.

230. Picano E, Sicari R, Landi P, et al. Prognostic value of myocardial viability in medically-treated patients with global left ventricular dysfunction early after acute uncomplicated myocardial infarction: a dobutamine stress echocardiographic study. *Circulation* 1998;98:1078–1084.

231. Applegate RJ, Dell'Italia LJ, Crawford MH. Usefulness of two-dimensional echocardiography during low-level exercise testing early after uncomplicated acute myocardial infarction. *Am J Cardiol* 1987;60:10–14.

232. Ryan T, Armstrong WF, O'Donnell JA, et al. Risk stratification after acute myocardial infarction by means of exercise two-dimensional echocardiography. *Am Heart J* 1987;114:1305–1316.

233. Lee KS, Marwick TH, Cook SA, et al. Prognosis of patients with left ventricular dysfunction, with and without viable myocardium after myocardial infarction: relative efficacy of medical therapy and revascularization. *Circulation* 1994;90:2687–2694.

234. Yoshida K, Gould KL. Quantitative relation of myocardial infarct size and myocardial viability by positron emission tomography to left ventricular ejection fraction and 3-year mortality with and without revascularization. *J Am Coll Cardiol* 1993;22:984–997.

235. Di Carli MF, Davidson M, Little R, et al. Value of metabolic imaging with positron emission tomography for evaluating prognosis in patients with coronary artery disease and left ventricular dysfunction. *Am J Cardiol* 1994;73:527–533.

236. Hertzer NR, Beven EG, Young JR, et al. Coronary artery disease in peripheral vascular patients. A classification of 1000 coronary angiograms and results of surgical management. *Ann Surg* 1984;199:223–233.

237. Mangano DT, London MJ, Tubau JF, et al. Dipyridamole thallium-201 scintigraphy as a preoperative screening test: a reexamination of its predictive capacity. *Circulation* 1991;84:493–502.

238. Eagle KA, Brundage BH, Chaitman BR, et al. Guidelines for perioperative cardiovascular evaluation for noncardiac surgery: report of the ACC/AHA Task Force on Practice Guidelines. *J Am Coll Cardiol* 1996;27:910–948.

239. Eagle KA, Singer DE, Brewster DC, et al. Dipyridamole thallium scanning in patients undergoing vascular surgery. Optimizing preoperative evaluation of cardiac risk. *JAMA* 1987;257:2185–2189.

240. Boucher CA, Brewster DC, Darling RC, et al. Determination of cardiac risk by dipyridamole thallium imaging before peripheral vascular surgery. *N Engl J Med* 1985;312:389–394.

241. Eagle KA, Coley CM, Newell JB, et al. Combining clinical and thallium data optimizes preoperative assessment of cardiac risk before major vascular surgery. *Ann Intern Med* 1989;110:859–866.

242. Younis LT, Aguirre F, Byers S, et al. Perioperative and long-term prognostic value of intravenous dipyridamole thallium scintigraphy in patients with peripheral vascular disease. *Am Heart J* 1990;119:1287–1292.

243. McFalls EO, Doliszny KM, Grund F, et al. Angina and persistent exercise thallium defects: independent risk factors in elective vascular surgery. *J Am Coll Cardiol* 1993;21:1347–1352.

244. Tischler MD, Lee TH, Hirsch AT. Prediction of major cardiac events after peripheral vascular surgery using dipyridamole echocardiography. *Am J Cardiol* 1991;68:593–599.

245. Sicari R, Picano E, Lusa AM, et al. The value of dipyridamole echocardiography in risk stratification before vascular surgery: a multicenter study. *Eur Heart J* 1995;16:842–847.

246. Miyazono Y, Kisanuki A, Toyonaga K, et al. Usefulness of adenosine triphosphate-atropine stress echocardiography for detecting coronary artery stenosis. *Am J Cardiol* 1998;82:290–294.

247. Pasquet A, D'Hondt AM, Verhelst R, et al. Comparison of dipyridamole stress echocardiography and perfusion scintigraphy for cardiac risk stratification in vascular surgery patients. *Am J Cardiol* 1998;82:1468–1474.

248. Poldermans D, Fioretti PM, Forster T, et al. Dobutamine stress echocardiography for assessment of perioperative cardiac risk in patients undergoing major vascular surgery. *Circulation* 1993;87:1506–1512.

249. Poldermans D, Fioretti PM, Forster T, et al. Dobutamine-atropine stress echocardiography for assessment of perioperative and late cardiac risk in patients undergoing major vascular surgery. *Eur J Vasc Surg* 1994;8:286–293.

250. Poldermans D, Arnese M, Fioretti PM, et al. Improved cardiac risk stratification in major vascular surgery with dobutamine-atropine stress echocardiography. *J Am Coll Cardiol* 1995;26:648–653.

251. Ballal RS, Kapadia S, Secknus MA, et al. Prognosis of patients with vascular disease after clinical evaluation and dobutamine stress echocardiography. *Am Heart J* 1999;137:469–475.

252. Shaw LJ, Eagle KA, Gersh BJ, et al. Meta-analysis of intravenous dipyridamole-thallium-201 imaging (1985 to 1994) and dobutamine echocardiography (1991 to 1994)

for risk stratification before vascular surgery. *J Am Coll Cardiol* 1996;27:787–798.

253. Porter TR, Xie F, Kilzer K, et al. Detection of myocardial perfusion abnormalities during dobutamine and adenosine stress echocardiography with transient myocardial contrast imaging after minute quantities of intravenous perfluorocarbon-exposed sonicated dextrose albumin. *J Am Soc Echocardiogr* 1996;9:779–786.

254. Picano E, Faletra F, Marini C, et al. Increased echodensity of transiently asynergic myocardium in humans: a novel echocardiographic sign of myocardial ischemia. *J Am Coll Cardiol* 1993;21:199–207.

255. Milunski MR, Mohr GA, Wear KA, et al. Early identification with ultrasonic integrated backscatter of viable but stunned myocardium in dogs. *J Am Coll Cardiol* 1989;14:462–471.

256. Weesner KM, Bledsoe M, Chauvenet A, et al. Exercise echocardiography in the detection of anthracycline cardiotoxicity. *Cancer* 1991;68:435–438.

257. Fukazawa R, Ogawa S, Hirayama T. Early detection of anthracycline cardiotoxicity in children with acute leukemia using exercise-based echocardiography and Doppler echocardiography. *Jpn Circ J* 1994;58:625–634.

258. Leung DY, Griffin BP, Stewart WJ, et al. Left ventricular function after valve repair for chronic mitral regurgitation: predictive value of preoperative assessment of contractile reserve by exercise echocardiography. *J Am Coll Cardiol* 1996;28:1198–1205.

259. deFilippi CR, Willett DL, Brickner ME, et al. Usefulness of dobutamine echocardiography in distinguishing severe from non-severe valvular aortic stenosis in patients with depressed left ventricular function and low transvalvular gradients. *Am J Cardiol* 1995;75:191–194.

260. Marwick TH, Nakatani S, Haluska B, et al. Provocation of left ventricular outflow tract gradients with amyl nitrite and exercise in hypertrophic cardiomyopathy. *Am J Cardiol* 1995;75:805–809.

261. Smart SC, Bhatia A, Hellman R, et al. Dobutamine-atropine stress echocardiography and dipyridamole sestamibi scintigraphy for the detection of coronary artery disease: limitations and concordance. *J Am Coll Cardiol* 2000;36:1265–1273.

262. Furukawa T, Haque T, Takahashi M, et al. An assessment of dobutamine echocardiography and end-diastolic wall thickness for predicting post-revascularization functional recovery in patients with chronic coronary artery disease. *Eur Heart J* 1997;18:798–806.

263. Monin JL, Garot J, Scherrer-Crosbie M, et al. Prediction of functional recovery of viable myocardium after delayed revascularization in postinfarction patients: accuracy of dobutamine stress echocardiography and influence of long-term vessel patency. *J Am Coll Cardiol* 1999;34:1012–1019.

264. Rossi E, Citterio F, Vescio MF, et al. Risk stratification of patients undergoing peripheral vascular revascularization by combined resting and dipyridamole echocardiography. *Am J Cardiol* 1998;82:306–310.

265. van Daele ME, McNeil AJ, Fioretti PM, et al. Prognostic value of dipyridamole sestamibi single-photon emission computed tomography and dipyridamole stress echocardiography for new cardiac events after an uncomplicated myocardial infarction. *J Am Soc Echocardiogr* 1994;7:379–380.

51

DOPPLER ASSESSMENT

FRANK A. FLACHSKAMPF

▼▼ ADDITIONAL ELECTRONIC TOPICS

OVERVIEW

Doppler echocardiography measures blood flow velocities. From flow velocities, pressure gradients can be calculated by the simplified Bernoulli equation in valvular and other stenoses. Doppler echocardiography has the highest sensitivity in the detection of valvular regurgitation of all diagnostic techniques, and regurgitant lesions can be graded at least semiquantitatively by several Doppler techniques. Using additional echocardiographic data, it is possible to obtain reliable estimates of cardiac output, systolic pulmonary artery pressure, and the magnitude of cardiac shunts. Doppler data can identify pathologic changes in diastolic left ventricular function, and the restrictive mitral flow pattern is associated with a reduced prognosis in various cardiac diseases. Doppler has an important role in diagnosing structural complications of myocardial infarction, aortic dissection, pulmonary embolism, cardiac tamponade, and other life-threatening cardiac diseases. Finally, tissue Dop-

F. A. Flachskampf: Department of Medicine, Medizinische Klinik II, University Erlangen–Nürnberg, Erlangen, Germany

pler allows analysis of regional myocardial velocities and contraction and elongation (strain).

GLOSSARY

Aliasing: The maximal velocity unambiguously identifiable by pulsed (and color) Doppler is the aliasing velocity, which depends on the pulse repetition frequency, the frame rate, the sampling depth, and the carrier frequency (see Chapter 46 for more details).

Color Doppler flow mapping: A Doppler display that codes blood flow velocities by colors (red toward the transducer and blue away from the transducer) and superimposes this color map on the two-dimensional image. Thus, a cross-sectional display of blood flow velocities is created. Color Doppler is a way of simultaneously displaying Doppler data from multiple sites in an easily interpretable way. This modality serves for quick orientation about pathologic blood flow (turbulence, regurgitation, shunt flows) and for analysis of valvular regurgitation.

Continuous wave Doppler: A Doppler modality that measures velocities along one scan line. Any velocities are measured unequivocally, but along the scan line there is no spatial resolution. This modality serves to measure the high velocities encountered in valvular stenosis or regurgitation.

Flow profile: The plot of flow velocities measured by pulsed or continuous wave Doppler over time (e.g., diastole for the mitral valve). Essentially synonymous with spectral Doppler display.

Gradient: Pressure drop (or difference) across a restrictive orifice (e.g., a valve).

Jet: A flow stream created by discharge from a narrow orifice (e.g., valvular regurgitation occurs as a jet).

Orifice: See Restrictive orifice.

Pressure half-time: The time that it takes for a pressure gradient to decay to half of its peak value. The pressure half-time is used to evaluate mitral stenosis and aortic regurgitation.

Pulsed wave Doppler: A Doppler modality that measures blood flow velocity in a specific region, the *sample volume*. Thus, unlike continuous wave Doppler, pulsed wave Doppler allows the choice of the site of measurement. The tradeoff is that the maximal unequivocally identifiable velocity is limited (see Aliasing).

Restrictive orifice: Narrowing in the path of flow stream. Stenotic and regurgitant lesions are restrictions to forward and backward flow, respectively. Restrictive orifices have a geometric or anatomic orifice area, which is the smallest cross-sectional area between the solid boundaries of the lesion, and an effective area, which is the smallest cross section of the jet created by such a lesion.

Sample volume: The volume of blood or tissue from which an average velocity is measured by pulsed Doppler. Technically, the length of the sample volume depends on the pulse length (the number of ultrasound wavelengths in one pulse),

and the axial position of the sample volume along the cursor depends on the range gate, which defines which time interval is allowed to elapse between transmit and receive. Spatial position and sample volume length can be chosen by the operator, and angle correction is also possible.

Spectral Doppler: Display of continuous or pulsed wave Doppler plotting blood flow velocity against time.

Strain: The deformation (lengthening or shortening) of myocardium during the cardiac cycle. It is dimensionless (e.g., a strain of 0.2 means a 20% elongation). Strain rate (strain divided by corresponding time, in 1/s units) is measurable by tissue Doppler between two chosen points in the myocardium by subtracting the tissue velocities at these points and dividing by the distance between the points. From strain rate, strain is obtained by temporal integration.

Stroke length, stroke distance: Synonymous with velocity-time integral.

Tissue Doppler: Pulsed or color Doppler modality measuring the velocity of solid cardiac structures (e.g., the movement of the myocardium with respect to the transducer over the heart cycle). Typically, these are low-velocity (rarely exceeding 20 cm per second), relatively high-amplitude signals, in contrast to transvalvular blood velocity measured by classic pulsed and color Doppler, which even in healthy subjects reaches 1 m per second and more and has relatively low amplitudes.

Turbulence: Characteristic of flow under certain conditions (especially at high velocities) in which fluid particle velocity and direction change rapidly and chaotically.

Velocity-time integral: The area enclosed by the envelope (the boundary) of the spectral pulsed or continuous wave Doppler display (unit, centimeters). This term is synonymous with stroke length.

FROM DOPPLER SIGNALS TO HEMODYNAMICS: BASIC CONCEPTS

The Doppler Signal

The Doppler signal contains the following data: the Doppler frequency shift, the intensity of the signal, and the audio signal.

The Doppler frequency shift (between emitted and received ultrasound) quantifies the instantaneous velocity component of the moving reflectors (usually blood cells) toward or away from the transducer (in centimeters per second) at a site determined by the sample volume of the pulsed Doppler or along the scan line in continuous wave Doppler. The display of this instantaneous velocity over time is called the *spectral Doppler display* (Fig. 51.1). Usually, an electrocardiographic (ECG) signal is also displayed for the purpose of timing. The occurrence of flow faster than normal (in stenotic lesions), of flow in the opposite direction than normal (in regurgitant lesions), or of flow where

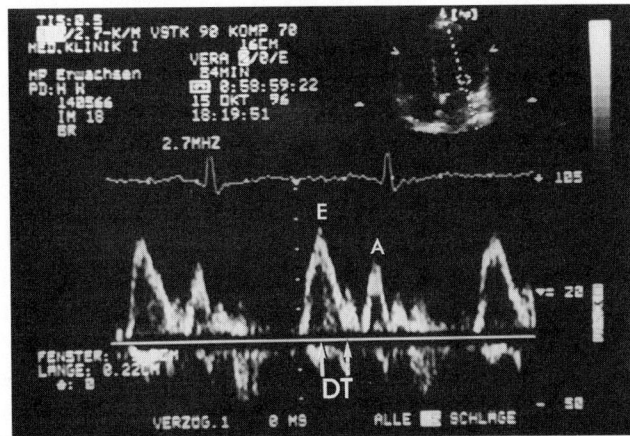

A

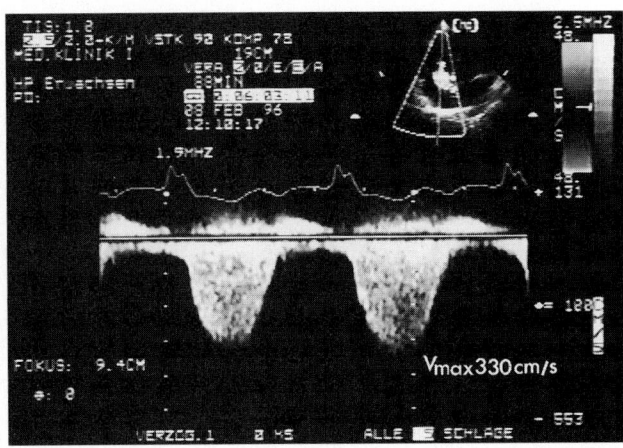

B

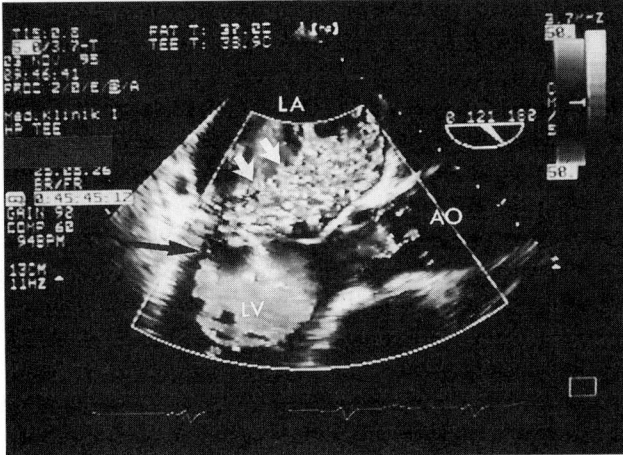

C

FIGURE 51.1 Pulsed, continuous, and color flow Doppler. **A:** Normal transmitral flow pattern. The sample volume is positioned at the tip of the mitral leaflets. Diastolic transmitral flow in sinus rhythm consists of an early, usually larger and higher E wave (E), and a late, usually smaller, A wave (A). Deceleration time (DT, *arrows*) of the E wave is the time between peak E-wave velocity and cessation of E wave. **B:** Continuous wave Doppler of tricuspid regurgitation in pulmonary hypertension. The maximal regurgitant velocity (v_{max}) of 330 cm per second implies a maximal systolic pressure gradient between the right ventricle and right atrium of 44 mm Hg, and, hence, a systolic pulmonary pressure of 44 mm Hg plus central venous pressure. **C:** Transesophageal color Doppler flow mapping of severe mitral regurgitation due to a posterior flail leaflet. The left atrium (LA) is on top. A proximal convergence zone (*black arrow*) is seen, as well as the eccentric, anteriorly directed turbulent jet in the left atrium (*white arrows*). AO, ascending aorta; LV, left ventricle.

usually no flow exists (in shunt lesions) can be detected. If velocities are integrated over time, the time velocity integral is obtained (in centimeters). With color Doppler, multiple measurements at different sites in the heart cavities are made simultaneously and represented qualitatively in colors (Fig. 51.1). Velocities toward the transducer are represented in shades of red and away from the transducer in shades of blue. Rapid variations in velocity, as in turbulent flow, are characterized by an admixture of green, which changes red hues to yellow and blue hues to cyan (17).

The intensity (amplitude) of the signal is represented in shades of gray in the spectral display. It is related to the number of scatterers (red blood cells) found within the sample volume moving with the measured velocity. Characteristically, if a pulsed Doppler sample volume is positioned in a region where all scatterers move with approximately the same velocity, the result is a bright, narrow bandwidth display of this velocity over time. The width of the signal reflects the variation in velocity within the sample volume. The brightest line is the *modal* velocity, which is the velocity most frequently measured by the Doppler device in the sample volume (Fig. 51.1). This is important when calculating flow rates from cross-sectional areas and pulsed Doppler data. In contrast, continuous wave spectral displays are filled with white signals up to the maximal velocity, the

envelope. The reason for this is that the continuous wave Doppler device measures velocities along a whole scan line, so that all flow velocities that the scan line encounters are represented.

Experienced echocardiographers use the audible signal to optimize the angulation of the transducer. The magnitude of the Doppler shift for usual carrier frequencies lies within the audible range (under 20 kHz). Therefore, high pitch corresponds to high blood flow velocity, and purity of tone to a narrow range of flow velocities.

Use of Doppler Signals to Evaluate Obstruction to Flow

Valvular stenoses and other obstructions to blood flow (e.g., left ventricular outflow tract obstruction) can be quantified by Doppler. The mainstay of this evaluation is the calculation of maximal and mean pressure gradients across an obstruction from transstenotic blood flow velocities by the *simplified Bernoulli equation*:

$$\Delta p = 4v^2$$

(Δp, pressure drop in millimeters of mercury; v, velocity in meters per second)

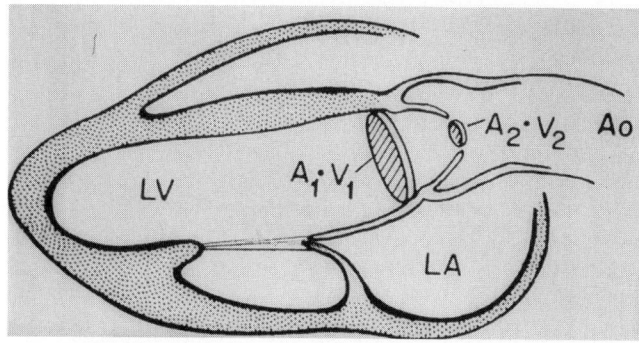

FIGURE 51.2 Schematic drawing of the continuity principle. By virtue of the conservation of mass between the left ventricular outflow tract and the aortic valve, the flow rate in the outflow tract ($A_1 \times v_1$, where A_1 is outflow tract area and v_1 is average blood flow velocity in the outflow tract) and the flow rate across the aortic valve ($A_2 \times v_2$, where A_2 is aortic valve area and v_2 is average velocity across the aortic valve) are equal. Hence, $A_2 = A_1 \times v_1/v_2$. For this calculation, the outflow tract is taken to be circular and calculated from outflow tract diameter D as $A_1 = \pi \times D^2/4$. AO, ascending aorta; LA, left atrium; LV, left ventricle. (From Weyman AE. *Principles and practice of echocardiography*, 2nd ed. Philadelphia: Lea & Febiger, 1994, with permission.)

Another way to quantify stenoses is the calculation of effective stenotic orifice area, which is usually accomplished by the continuity equation (Fig. 51.2): $A_{EFF} = A_1 \times TVI_1/TVI_{MAX}$, where A_{EFF} is the effective stenotic orifice area, A_1 is the area of the flow cross section, usually calculated as $\pi \times d^2/4$, where d is the left ventricular outflow tract diameter, TVI_1 is time velocity integral at another flow cross section (by pulsed wave Doppler), usually the left ventricular outflow tract, and TVI_{MAX} is the transstenotic time velocity integral (by continuous wave Doppler). Instead of time velocity integrals, the maximal transstenotic velocity and the maximal velocity in the outflow tract can be used.

Quantification of Regurgitant Lesions

Regurgitation is easily identified by spectral or color Doppler, but difficult to quantify. The *area of the regurgitant jet* by color Doppler is the easiest way to grade severity but does not reliably differentiate moderate and severe regurgitation. Useful other approaches are measurement of the proximal jet diameter immediately at the origin of the jet and the proximal flow convergence zone concept.

Quantification of Cardiac Output

Stroke volume across any flow cross section and thus across any valve can in theory be calculated by multiplying the time velocity integral across that valve by valve orifice area. Unfortunately, neither is easily and reliably measured. Usually, stroke volume (and, hence, by multiplication with heart rate, cardiac output) is measured by multiplying the time velocity integral of the pulsed Doppler signal of sys-

tolic transaortic flow by the aortic orifice area (calculated by $\pi \times d^2/4$, where d is aortic annulus diameter).

CLINICAL DOPPLER EXAMINATION

General Considerations

Modern echo machines have imaging transducers with incorporated Doppler capabilities and show the Doppler cursor or sample volume in the current 2-D image. Additionally, guidance is provided by the audio output. However, in difficult continuous wave Doppler examinations (e.g., in aortic stenosis), a dedicated, stand-alone transducer without imaging frequently is superior to the combined 2-D and Doppler transducer for technical reasons and because of the smaller transducer face size (e.g., for use with the suprasternal window). Furthermore, although carrier frequency for imaging ideally should be as high as possible to optimize spatial resolution, for pulsed Doppler there is a trade-off between spatial resolution and the maximal unambiguously identifiable flow velocity at a given range. Therefore, transducers often operate at a lower carrier frequency in Doppler mode than in imaging mode.

The following practical points should be observed:

1. The interrogating beam should be aligned with the direction of flow. This is difficult even using 2-D–guided Doppler, because the third dimension is missing. It is better to change the transducer position to enable optimal alignment than to use the angle correction option. Although angle correction is possible in available Doppler devices, it is likely to introduce more error than it corrects, unless the true direction of flow is evident, as in a vessel imaged in a long axis. Fortuitously, in truly turbulent flow, which is present in severe valvular stenosis and in left-sided regurgitation, high flow velocities occur in all spatial directions; therefore, optimal alignment is less critical in these instances. A few heart cycles should be recorded, especially in the presence of atrial fibrillation.

2. The visual and the audio output should be used to optimize the signal (see Instrument Settings, later in this chapter).

3. Timing of the Doppler signal should be compared with the corresponding ECG. For example, the mitral regurgitation signal, which may be mistaken for an aortic stenosis signal, begins earlier (immediately after mitral valve closure) than the aortic ejection signal. If the origin of the continuous Doppler signal is unclear, the timing of a 2-D–guided pulsed Doppler signal in relation to the ECG should be obtained for orientation.

4. The pitfalls include that clear flow velocity recordings by Doppler cannot be created *ex nihilo* (but they can represent a flow that was not intended to be recorded). An exception is mirror artifacts, which are created by high

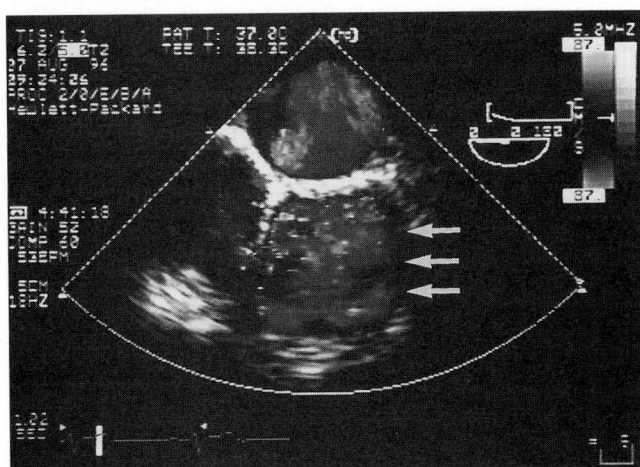

FIGURE 51.3 Phantom flow in the descending aorta. On top, the true descending aorta is seen by transesophageal echo with color Doppler imaging. At the twofold distance, a second lumen with phantom flow is seen (*arrows*). This "double-barrel" appearance of the descending aorta is frequently found and represents a mirror artifact, which can be misdiagnosed as dissection.

amplitude signals (or too high gain) and which duplicate an existing signal with inverse sign or reverberations of color Doppler signals, which also duplicate real existing flow at a manifold of the real depth (Fig. 51.3). An important example of the latter is *phantom flow* in transesophageal color Doppler images of the descending aorta, resulting in a *double-barrel* descending aorta. Conversely, there is never proof that the recorded velocities are truly the highest ones that exist, because there is always the possibility of false placement or malalignment of the echo beam. Thus, to minimize the first type of error, ECG timing, 2-D orientation, and characteristics of the flow profile should always be checked. Practically, the most important error is misreading mitral regurgitation for aortic stenosis. The second type of error is minimized by carefully using all echo windows, patience, and clinical judgment. If doubts remain, it is preferable to state that the echo examination is suboptimal than to report possibly false values without this caveat.

5. Normal values for forward flow velocities are, of course, dependent on cardiac output and heart rate, and in some instances also on other factors. For instance, the ratio of early to late velocity of transmitral flow decreases with age, as does the ratio of diastolic to systolic peak velocity of pulmonary venous flow. Minimal or trace regurgitation by color and pulsed Doppler is frequently seen in all valves without clinical evidence of heart disease. The incidence increases with age.

The Routine Examination

The Doppler examination is an integral part of the routine echocardiographic examination. However, specific pathologies (as in aortic stenosis or congenital heart disease) frequently require use of additional echo windows and additional examination time.

In the parasternal views, because the left heart flows are approximately orthogonal to the echo beam, velocity measurements are not practical. However, color Doppler reveals the occurrence and direction of mitral and aortic regurgitation. The width of these jets is well assessed in parasternal long-axis views, and the minimal cross section in appropriate basal short-axis views. Subaortic obstruction and ventricular septal defects can also be detected by color Doppler. Short-axis views at the aortic root level allow both pulsed or continuous wave Doppler and color Doppler assessment of the right ventricular inflow and outflow tract, including tricuspid and pulmonary forward and, if present, regurgitant flow. Congenital anomalies such as atrial septal defects, membranous ventricular septal defects, or a patent ductus arteriosus may also be detected.

In the routine examination, mitral and aortic valves and the left ventricular outflow tract should be examined by color Doppler in parasternal long-axis views. Also, color Doppler recordings of the tricuspid and pulmonary valves should be obtained in basal short-axis views.

The apical views are ideally suited to record left ventricular inflow and outflow velocities. Transmitral flow is well assessed in four-chamber and two-chamber views. Flow velocities in the left ventricular outflow tract, at the aortic valve level, and in the first centimeters of the ascending aorta are recorded in the apical long-axis view. The four-chamber view also allows measurement of tricuspid flow. Furthermore, atrial and ventricular septal defects (especially of the muscular type) may be detected by color Doppler in the apical four-chamber view. Pulmonary venous flow may be interrogated in a slightly cranially angulated four-chamber view in the right upper pulmonary vein. In the routine examination, a transmitral flow profile should be obtained by pulsed Doppler at the leaflet tips (where transmitral velocities are highest); if cardiac output calculations are to be made, a recording at the mitral annulus level should also be obtained. Mitral regurgitation is sought by color Doppler in all apical views. A transaortic flow profile and an outflow tract profile are recorded by pulsed Doppler. An additional continuous wave Doppler recording of outflow tract and aortic valve is valuable to exclude an obstruction that may have been overlooked by 2-D imaging. Color Doppler of the outflow tract should also be recorded to exclude aortic regurgitation. The tricuspid valve is examined by color Doppler for the presence of regurgitation; if present, the maximal regurgitant velocity is recorded by continuous wave Doppler. By the simplified Bernoulli equation, the maximal systolic pressure difference between right ventricle and right atrium can be calculated from the maximal tricuspid regurgitant velocity. This is an estimate of maximal right ventricular, and, thus, pulmonary, pressure. The pressure difference either can be reported as such, or 10 mm Hg can be added as an estimate of right atrial pressure, or right atrial pressure can be assessed clinically by the collapse level of the neck veins. Further, a color Doppler map of flows in the proximity of the interatrial septum should be obtained to rule out atrial septal defect.

The subcostal views are rarely optimal windows for Doppler examination except for atrial septal defects, in which the echo beam orientation is more appropriate than in the apical four-chamber view. Routinely, the interatrial septum should be examined by color Doppler to rule out atrial septal defect. The subcostal views, however, provide a valuable alternative if more cranial windows are insufficient (e.g., in aortic stenosis). Aortic coarctation and aortic stenosis should be evaluated from the suprasternal position, which in adults often is difficult to use except with a dedicated continuous wave probe.

Transesophageal Doppler

Transesophageal echo offers a full set of echo windows for the 2-D and Doppler examination that are almost never obstructed (36). Evidently, transmitral flow can be studied under ideal conditions and even eccentric regurgitant jets are well depicted by color Doppler. Aortic regurgitation is well seen by color Doppler from transesophageal windows, especially long-axis views (at 130 to 160 degrees) of the left ventricular outflow tract. It is difficult, however, to obtain a good alignment of transvalvular aortic flow with the echo beam; this is best done from a transgastric position by rotating from the left ventricular short axis to a long-axis view or using maximal anteflexion of the instrument in the stomach. Tricuspid flow is also sometimes difficult to align with the echo beam. Continuous wave Doppler of the tricuspid valve may be contaminated with a mitral regurgitation signal, since the echo beam always first traverses the left atrium before reaching the tricuspid valve. The pulmonary valve is mostly not well visualized transesophageally. Transesophageal echo offers a unique access to measuring emptying and filling velocities in the left atrial appendage, which are related to thromboembolic risk. Furthermore, pulmonary venous flow is easily interrogated either in the left upper or right upper pulmonary vein. Being the diagnostic procedure of choice in the setting of aortic dissection, entry and reentry jets and flow in the true and false lumen can be examined by transesophageal echocardiography. Given the excellent visibility of the interatrial septum, a color Doppler examination for an atrial septal defect should be performed. The sensitivity of transesophageal color Doppler for a patent foramen ovale, however, is inferior to that of contrast echo. If cardiac embolism is suspected, especially in atrial fibrillation, a pulsed Doppler recording of left atrial appendage flows should be obtained. Flow

velocities in the ascending and descending aorta can be visualized by color Doppler, while absolute velocity values are unreliable because of the large angle between flow direction and echo beam.

Normal Transvalvular and Pulmonary Venous Flow Velocity Signals

The normal transmitral flow velocity signal consists of an early (E) wave, which is produced by the rapid decrease in left ventricular pressure caused by relaxation below the level of left atrial pressure (Fig. 51.4). E-wave upslope reflects the rapid growth of the early diastolic atrioventricular pressure gradient. When this pressure gradient ceases to exist, deceleration ensues, which reflects largely the passive compliance of the left ventricle and the left atrium, with a steep deceleration if compliance is low and a slow deceleration if compliance is high. The E wave in sinus rhythm is followed by the late diastolic atrial (A) wave, which is the result of atrial contraction and occurs after the ECG P wave. It reflects atrial contraction force and elastic properties of the left ventricle and atrium at end diastole.

Aortic flow velocities have an approximately triangular shape, with a slightly more rapid upslope than downslope (Fig. 51.4). The slopes reflect left ventricular contraction and relaxation and aortic resistance. Aortic flow ends before mitral flow begins, and the time between aortic valve closure and mitral flow onset is the isovolumic relaxation time (normally, approximately 60 ms). Conversely, mitral valve closure occurs before the onset of aortic flow (isovolumic contraction time).

Tricuspid forward velocities form an early diastolic wave and a late wave after atrial contraction, analogous to the transmitral flow pattern (Fig. 51.4). Transtricuspid flow velocities are the lowest of all valves, because the tricuspid valve has the largest orifice area. Pulmonary forward flow is represented by an approximately triangular-shaped systolic velocity signal with a symmetric upslope and deceleration. A steep upslope or a mid-systolic notch are typical of pulmonary hypertension.

Pulmonary venous flow velocities in sinus rhythm have a systolic and a diastolic portion directed toward the left atrium and a short low-velocity retrograde wave after atrial contraction (Fig. 51.4). Systolic and diastolic inflow velocities in young individuals are approximately equal. Diastolic inflow velocities decrease with age and in general behave as the transmitral E wave, because in diastole the atrium acts largely as a passive conduit. Note that peak diastolic pulmonary venous velocity follows peak transmitral E-wave velocity by approximately 50 ms (40), again because early diastolic left ventricular relaxation initiates transmitral left ventricular inflow, which in turn gives rise to pulmonary venous diastolic inflow.

Normal values for the flow velocities obtained during routine examination are given in Table 51.1.

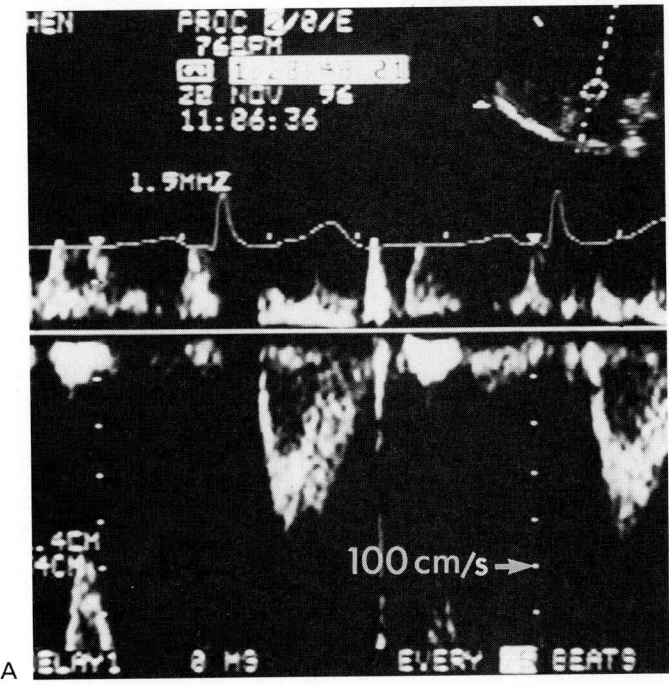

A

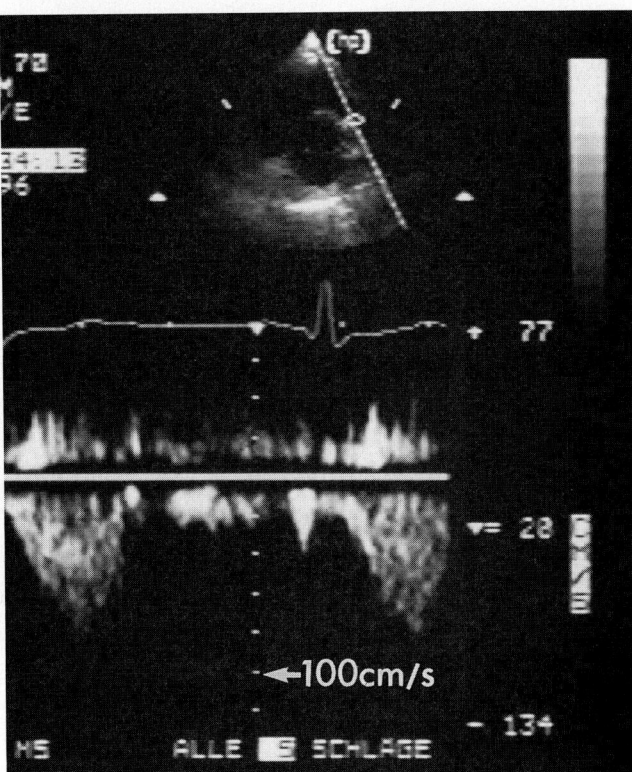

B

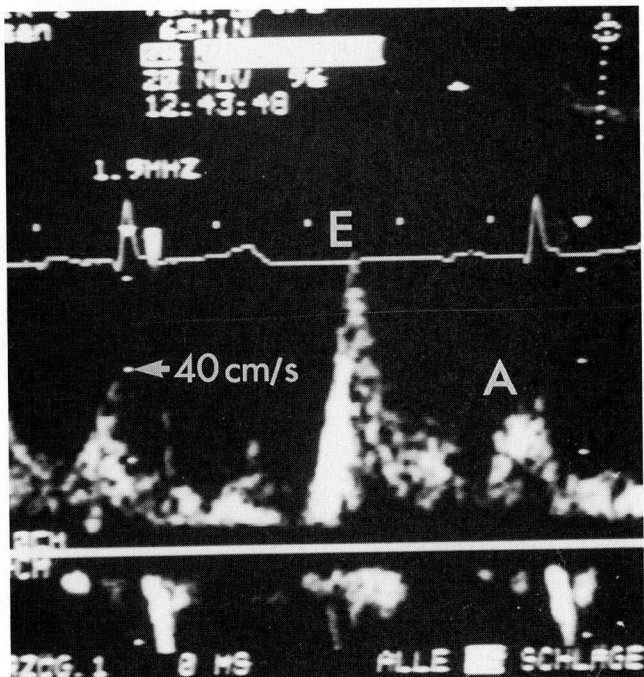

C

FIGURE 51.4 Normal flow velocity profiles by pulsed Doppler. (See Figure 51.1 for normal transmitral profile.) **A:** Normal transaortic flow pattern. The sample volume is positioned at the aortic valve annulus in an apical long-axis view. **B:** Normal transpulmonary flow. The sample volume is positioned in the pulmonary valve in a basal parasternal short-axis view. **C:** Normal transtricuspid flow pattern. The sample volume is positioned at the tricuspid leaflet tips in an apical four-chamber view. A, late atrial wave; E, early inflow wave. (*continued*)

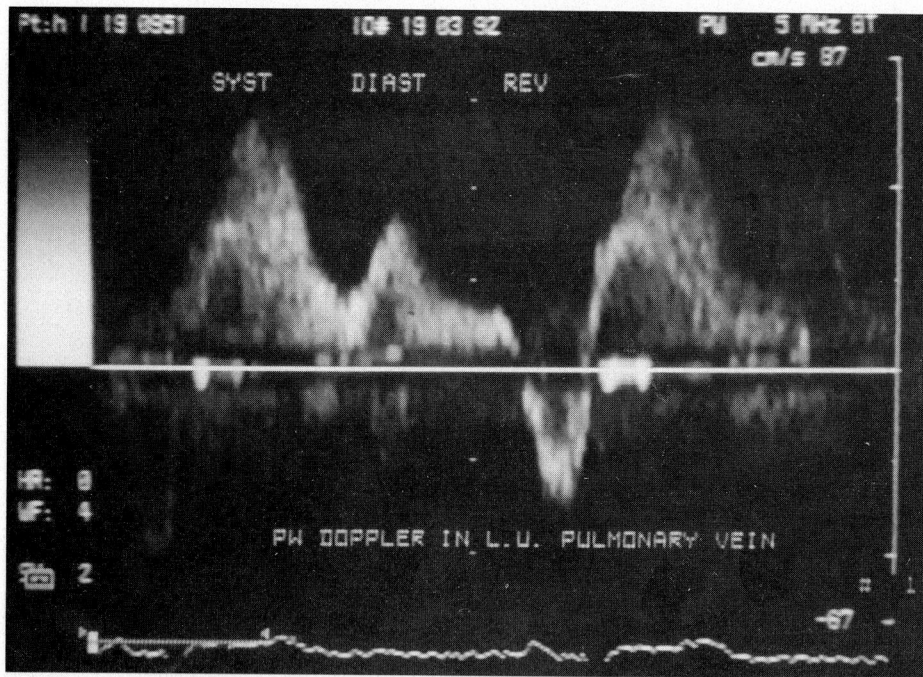

FIGURE 51.4 *Continued* **D:** Normal pulmonary venous inflow pattern from the left upper pulmonary vein by transesophageal Doppler. Systolic (SYST) and diastolic (DIAST) inflow into the left atrium is seen, as well as a short reverse (REV) wave representing atrial contraction.

TABLE 51.1 NORMAL VALUES FOR FLOW VELOCITIES IN ADULTS COMPILED FROM SEVERAL REFERENCES (17,18,66,116,117)[a]

Intracardiac flow velocities		
	Maximal velocity (m/sec)	**Range**
Mitral valve	0.9 (E wave)	0.6–1.3
	0.5 ± 0.1 (A wave)	
Aortic valve	1.35	1.0–1.7
Tricuspid valve	0.5 (E wave)	0.3–0.7
Pulmonary valve	0.75	0.6–0.9
Left ventricular outflow tract	0.9	0.7–1.1
Left upper pulmonary venous inflow	0.6 ± 0.2 (systolic wave)	
	0.4 ± 0.1 (diastolic wave)	

Flow velocities and mean gradients across valve prostheses		
	v_{max} (m/sec)	**Mean gradient (mm Hg)**
Aortic position		
Starr-Edwards	3.1 ± 0.5	24.0 ± 4.0
St. Jude Medical	2.1 ± 0.6 (No. 31)	10 ± 6 (No. 31)
	3.0 ± 0.6 (No. 19)	17 ± 7 (No. 19)
Björk-Shiley	2.8 ± 0.9 (No. 21)	21.0 ± 7.0 (No. 19)
	1.9 ± 0.2 (No. 29)	1.3 ± 0.6 (No. 29)
Carpentier-Edwards bioprostheses	2.8 ± 0.7 (No. 19)	16.5 ± 1.4 (No. 21)
	2.4 ± 0.4 (No. 31)	9.9 ± 1.0 (No. 29)
Hancock bioprostheses	2.4 ± 0.4	11.0 ± 2.3
Mitral position		
Starr-Edwards	1.9 ± 0.4	4.6 ± 2.4
St. Jude Medical	1.6 ± 0.3	3.5 ± 1.3
Björk-Shiley	1.6 ± 0.3	2.9 ± 1.6
Carpentier-Edwards bioprostheses	1.8 ± 0.2	6.5 ± 2.1
Hancock bioprostheses	1.5 ± 0.3	4.3 ± 2.1
Tricuspid position		
Starr-Edwards	1.3 ± 0.2	3.1 ± 0.8
Björk-Shiley (case reports)	1.3	3.2
St. Jude Medical	1.2 ± 0.3	2.7 ± 1.1
Bioprostheses	1.3 ± 0.2	3.2 ± 1.1

[a]Values are dependent on cardiac output, heart rate, age, and other factors, and therefore must be judged in the clinical context.

ACQUIRED VALVULAR HEART DISEASE

Mitral Valve

Mitral stenosis is best assessed in one of the apical views. Continuous wave Doppler recordings of transmitral flow should be obtained; in atrial fibrillation, at least a short and long diastolic period should be recorded to document the range of occurring gradients. The mean gradient and the pressure half-time should be calculated (Fig. 51.5). The latter is calculated from the downslope of the E wave or the single diastolic wave in atrial fibrillation. It is the time of decay from maximal velocity of flow (immediately after mitral valve opening) to $1/\sqrt{2}$ of the maximal velocity (the $1/\sqrt{2}$ factor is due to the quadratic relation between pressure drop and velocity in Bernoulli equation). The pressure half-time (PHT, in milliseconds) is relatively robust against changes in cardiac output and heart rate; a useful empiric

relationship exists with mitral valve area (MVA, in centimeters squared), given by MVA = 220/PHT (41). However, pressure half-time also depends on left atrial and left ventricular compliance and the maximal pressure gradient. j64

Severity of mitral stenosis is graded as from invasively obtained pressure gradients or Gorlin areas. It has been reported that some amount of stretch of the orifice with increasing stroke volume may occur in patients with mild or moderate, not heavily calcified, mitral stenosis (45).

Mitral regurgitation should be evaluated by color Doppler using all available windows, especially the apical views. If doubtful by color Doppler, it should be confirmed by pulsed Doppler, with the sample positioned on the atrial side of the mitral valve. Mitral regurgitant jets often are eccentric, hugging the atrial walls (Fig. 51.1). Mitral valve prolapse creates jets directed toward the back side of the prolapsing leaflet, while flail mitral leaflets direct the jet to

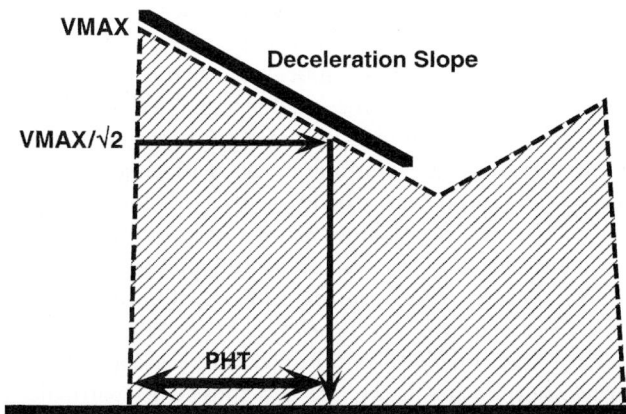

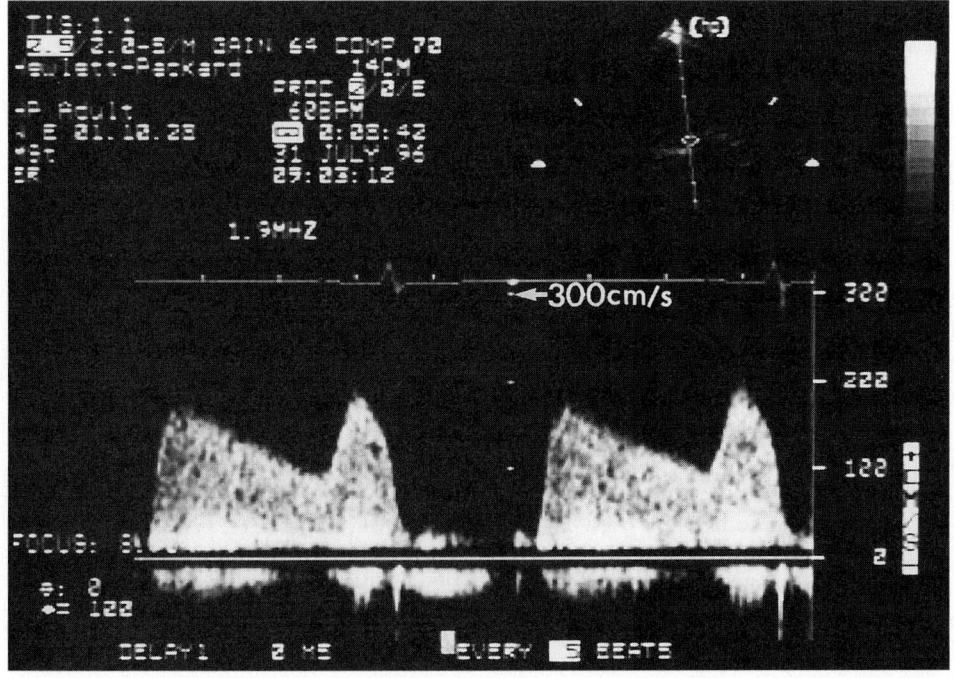

FIGURE 51.5 A: Schematic drawing of measurement of time-velocity integral and pressure half-time (PHT) in mitral stenosis. VMAX, maximal early diastolic velocity. The area surrounded by the dotted line is the time-velocity integral. See text for details. **B:** Transmitral flow by apical continuous wave Doppler in mitral stenosis with preserved sinus rhythm. Peak gradient is 15 mm Hg, mean gradient is 9 mm Hg, and pressure half-time is 228 ms, corresponding to an orifice area of 1 cm².

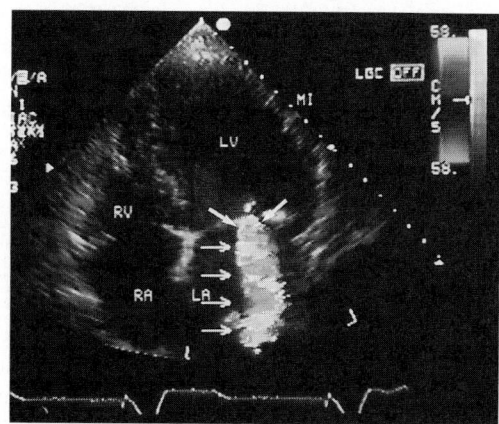

FIGURE 51.6 Measurement of proximal diameter of a severe mitral regurgitant jet (*horizontal arrows*). The proximal diameter is marked by the oblique arrows. Apical four-chamber view. LA, left atrium; LV, left ventricle; RA, right atrium; RV, right ventricle.

the opposite side (Fig. 51.1). Mitral regurgitation caused by left ventricular dilatation usually results in central jets (46). Planimetry or eyeballing of maximal color Doppler jet size yields a rough estimate of severity. Division by left atrial area in the same view to *normalize* jet size has been proposed and is particularly convenient for eyeballing [with cutoff values of 20% and 40% of left atrial size (47)], but lacks theoretical justification. By transesophageal echo, where the atrium is not visualized fully in single views, the cutoff values for planimetry are 3 and 6 cm² (48). Eccentric, wall-hugging jets are underestimated by an average of 40% by the jet area method (27). Whereas very small and very large jets are usually well identified, the intermediate severities are impossible to reliably grade by color jet area. Two color Doppler–based approaches have been well validated and are clinically practical, if image quality is good (in particular, using transesophageal echocardiography):

1. Measurement of the proximal jet diameter. The smallest diameter of the jet should be measured, which is within millimeters of its origin (Fig. 51.6). The plane should be sought where the minimal diameter is largest. Jet diameter greater than 7 mm indicates severe regurgitation (49,50).

2. The proximal convergence zone method. Although cutoff values have not been extensively validated, maximal regurgitant flow rates greater than 150 mL per second and effective regurgitant orifice areas greater than 0.3 cm² indicate grade III or IV mitral regurgitation (21,51). Because of enhanced image quality, this approach works particularly well with transesophageal echocardiography (*e*Fig. 51.2.5).

A number of additional signs are helpful in grading mitral regurgitation. Severe mitral regurgitation creates a continuous wave signal that has a *shoulder* in late systole instead of the symmetric, parabolic appearance of less severe mitral regurgitation. This is due to rapidly increasing

end systolic pressure in the left atrium in this circumstance. Pulmonary venous flow recordings show a reduction in the systolic portion of pulmonary venous inflow into the left atrium. In severe mitral regurgitation, the systolic portion of pulmonary venous flow may even be reversed and merge with the end diastolic retrograde flow wave, showing blood being pushed back into the pulmonary vein by the inflow of blood from the left ventricle into the atrium (Fig. 51.7). In eccentric jets, it may be useful to sample both upper pulmonary veins to detect flow reversal (52). Although this sign is quite sensitive, it is not very specific, because impaired systolic pulmonary venous inflow also occurs in atrial fibrillation or impaired systolic function.

Aortic Valve

For the assessment of a stenotic aortic valve, three parameters should be obtained in the best possible quality: the transvalvular continuous wave Doppler, the subaortic pulsed Doppler, and the left ventricular outflow tract diameter (Fig. 51.8). Continuous wave Doppler signals should be recorded at least from two, preferably from three or more, windows (apical, subcostal, suprasternal, right parasternal), to ensure that the maximal velocities have been detected. Mean and maximal pressure gradients are calculated from the continuous wave tracing. In atrial fibrillation, several beats should be analyzed. A slowed early systolic rise in flow velocities across the aortic valve, resulting in an approximately symmetric upslope and downslope, indicates severe stenosis, analogous to the clinical finding of pulsus tardus in this condition (Fig. 51.9). Effective orifice area has traditionally been assumed to be independent of cardiac output and heart rate and thus to be particularly valuable in impaired left ventricular function, when a low-pressure gradient can reflect mild obstruction, low stroke

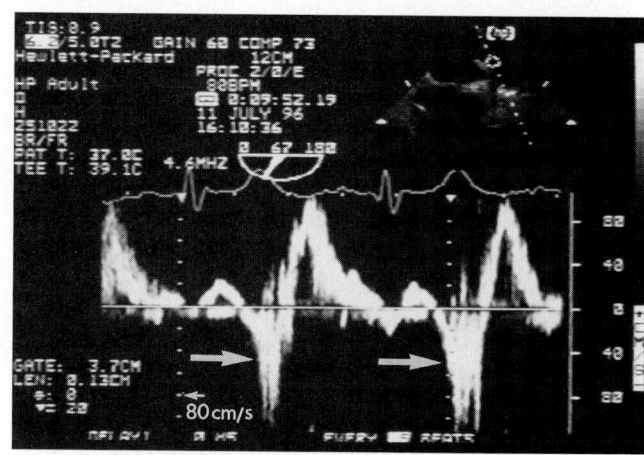

FIGURE 51.7 Pulmonary venous flow in the presence of severe mitral regurgitation. Registration by transesophageal pulsed Doppler from the left upper pulmonary vein. There is only a small positive systolic wave, followed by reversed systolic flow (*arrows*). Diastolic atrial inflow velocities are increased.

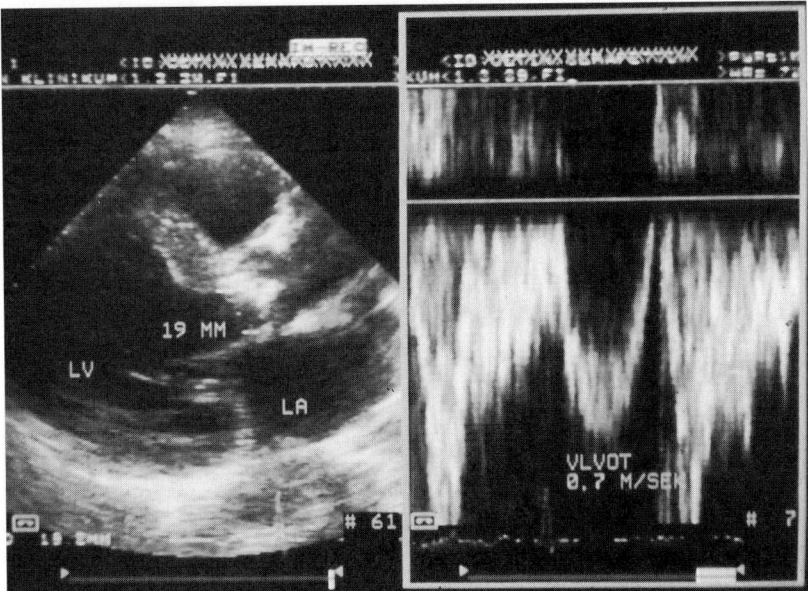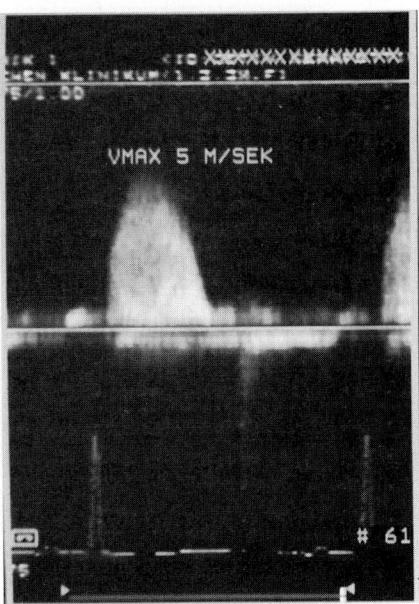

FIGURE 51.8 Aortic valve area calculation by the continuity principle (*top left*). Measurement of left ventricular outflow tract diameter in a parasternal long-axis view (19 mm, corresponding to an area of 2.8 cm²). **Middle:** Pulsed wave Doppler recording in the left ventricular outflow tract. **Right:** Continuous wave Doppler recording of transstenotic flow velocities. By the continuity equation, an aortic valve area of 0.4 cm² was calculated.

volume, or both. Subaortic pulsed wave tracings and the left ventricular outflow tract diameter (D) are necessary to calculate the effective orifice area (A_{EFF}) by the continuity equation. It is valid to use the maximal velocities from continuous wave Doppler (v_{MAX}) and subaortic pulsed wave Doppler (v_{LVOT}) instead of the time velocity integrals: $A_{EFF} = \frac{1}{4}\pi \times D^2 \times v_{LVOT}/v_{MAX}$. However, it has been reported that in some patients with aortic stenosis, orifice area is flow dependent and stretches with increasing cardiac output between 10% and 20% (23,24).

If Doppler-derived parameters of aortic stenosis are in conflict with other clinical data, the following sources of error should be checked:

(a) Doppler gradient too high: misreading the mitral regurgitation signal for aortic stenosis (check timing of velocities); neglect of high proximal velocities, as in aortic regurgitation or high cardiac output; pressure recovery; atrial fibrillation with high beat-to-beat variation in gradient. ⌦ j65

(b) Doppler gradient too low: missing the maximal signal (use all available windows). ⌦ j66

Aortic regurgitation is the most difficult valvular lesion to evaluate. The best parameter to assess severity is the size of the regurgitant jet by color Doppler in the left ventricular outflow tract (Fig. 51.10). Both the height in parasternal long-axis views or the area in short-axis views are used and normalized to the diameter or area of the left ventricular outflow tract, respectively. Twenty percent and 60% of

the left ventricular outflow tract area (25% and 65% of the left ventricular outflow tract diameter) are the cutoff values for mild, moderate, and severe regurgitation (56). Another useful parameter is the pressure half-time of the continuous wave Doppler of regurgitant flow (57) (*e*Fig. 51.10.1). This is sometimes difficult to record and may necessitate an orientation of the transducer different from the optimal orientation for recording forward transaortic flow velocity. The shorter the pressure half-time and the more rapidly pressure equalizes between the ascending aorta and the left ventricle, the more severe the aortic regurgitation. Values less than 300 ms indicate severe aortic regurgitation. ⌦ j67

Additionally, the presence of a holodiastolic flow signal on pulsed Doppler recordings from the ascending, descending, or (from the subcostal window) abdominal aorta (or a large systemic artery) can be taken as a sign of at least moderate aortic regurgitation (Fig. 51.11).

Tricuspid Valve

The tricuspid valve is examined in the apical four-chamber view, in a basal parasternal short-axis view, or in the (parasternal) right ventricular inflow view. The mean pressure gradient is calculated from continuous wave or pulsed wave Doppler recordings in analogy to transmitral gradients. The pressure half-time may be used for serial measurements, but its use to calculate orifice areas has not been validated in the tricuspid valve. Tricuspid regurgitation is best detected by color Doppler in the apical (or subcostal) four-chamber view (Fig. 51.12). By continuous wave Dop-

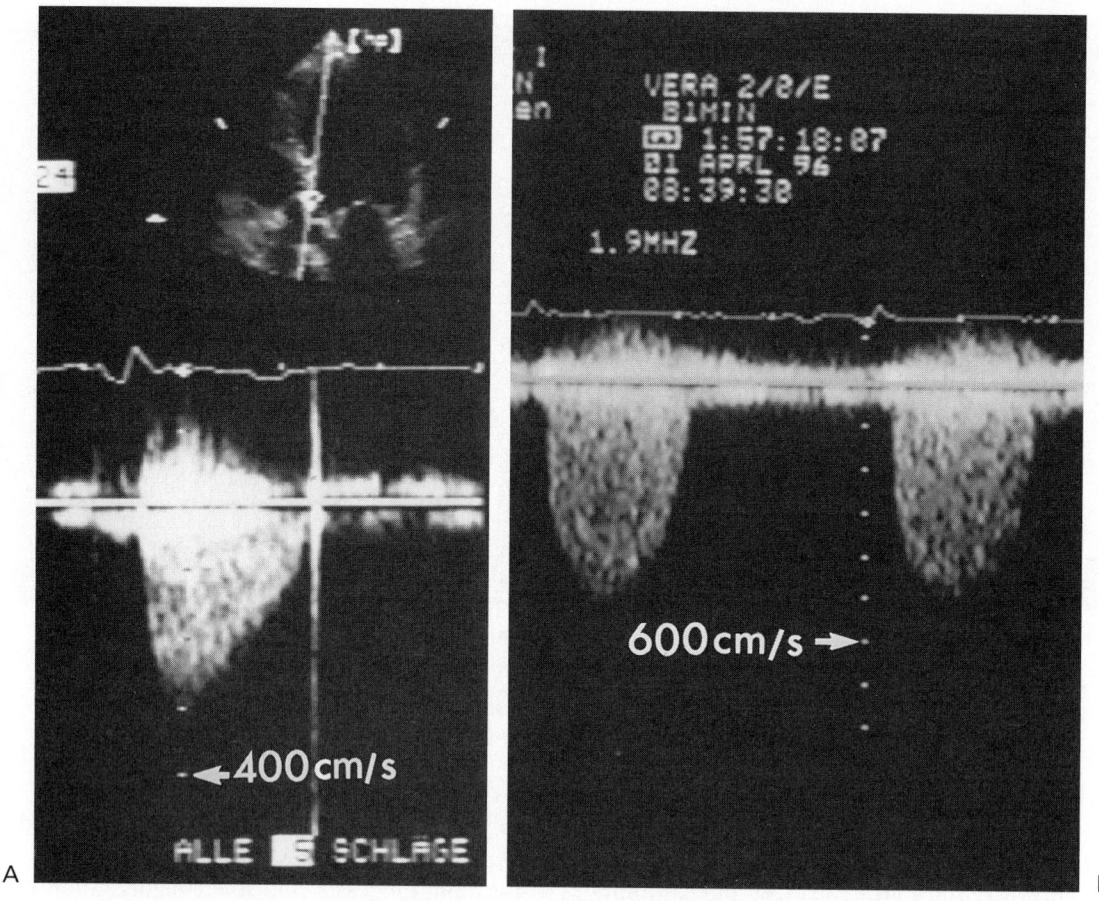

FIGURE 51.9 A: Moderate aortic stenosis with a triangular shape and steep upslope, and **(B)** severe aortic stenosis, with a parabolic shape and a slow upslope.

pler, it produces a systolic regurgitant velocity spectrum of parabolic shape, similar to mitral regurgitation. As in mitral regurgitation, in severe tricuspid insufficiency there is a rapid late systolic decay of regurgitant velocities because of high end systolic right atrial pressure. The maximal regurgitant velocity is important to diagnose the presence of pulmonary hypertension.

Pulmonary Valve

The pulmonary valve is best examined in the parasternal basal short-axis view or alternatively in a subcostal short-axis view. Minimal pulmonary regurgitation is frequent in individuals without clinical evidence of cardiac disease. The color Doppler representation of an eccentric pulmonary regurgitant jet may be misread as a membranous ventricular septal defect signal. Pulmonary stenosis is evaluated reliably by the mean transvalvular gradient from continuous wave Doppler.

Aortic Pathology

From the suprasternal window, flow velocity in the ascending and descending aorta can be sampled. Aortic coarctation can be visualized by turbulence, and the gradient measured directly (*e*Fig. 51.12.1). However, although the simplified Bernoulli equation in general is well applicable, it may underestimate the true pressure drop in long, tunnel-like obstructions, or overestimate the pressure drop in the presence of high proximal velocities or downstream pressure recovery. In aortic dissection, transesophageal evaluation is the procedure of choice. Color Doppler flow in the true lumen is usually brighter than in the false lumen, where it may be absent if stasis and thrombosis have ensued. Thus, color flow mapping should be used to confirm the existence of a true and a false lumen. Entry and reentry tears of the intima may also be detected (Fig. 51.13).

PROSTHETIC HEART VALVES

Obstruction

Pulsed and continuous wave measurement of forward flow velocities across valvular prostheses is usually well obtainable even if 2-D image quality is impaired by prosthetic artifacts. Opening and closing clicks are seen on the spectral Doppler display as narrow, bright vertical lines (Fig. 51.14). Mean gra-

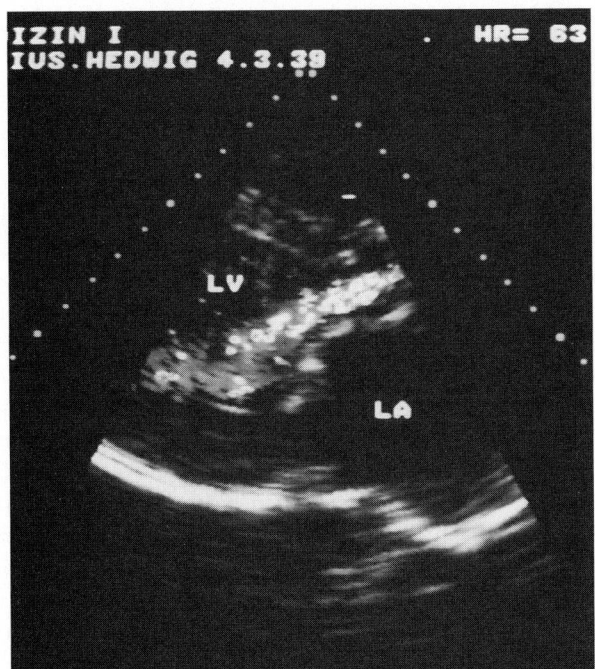

FIGURE 51.10 Aortic regurgitation. Color Doppler flow mapping in a parasternal long-axis view. The regurgitant jet is depicted in the left ventricular outflow tract and left ventricle, hugging the anterior mitral leaflet. LA, left atrium; LV, left ventricle.

dients should be calculated in the same way as described for native stenotic valves (60). Contrary to these, however, there is some degree of obstruction inherent in all prosthetic valves. The limits of normalcy are difficult to define mainly for two reasons: the influence of prosthesis design, and the match or mismatch of the implanted valve and the implantation site. The different prosthesis types and sizes involve different degrees of obstruction (e.g., the caged-ball Starr-Edwards prosthesis is much more obstructive than the St. Jude Medical valve). Normal values for transprosthetic flow velocities or

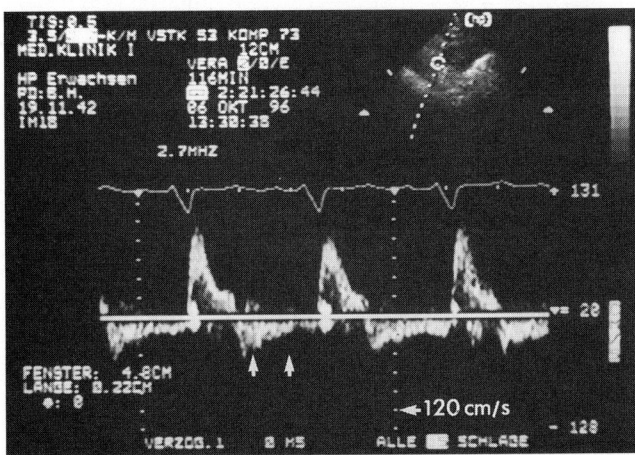

FIGURE 51.11 Holodiastolic flow reversal (*arrows*) in the descending aorta in severe aortic regurgitation. Pulsed Doppler recording from the suprasternal notch.

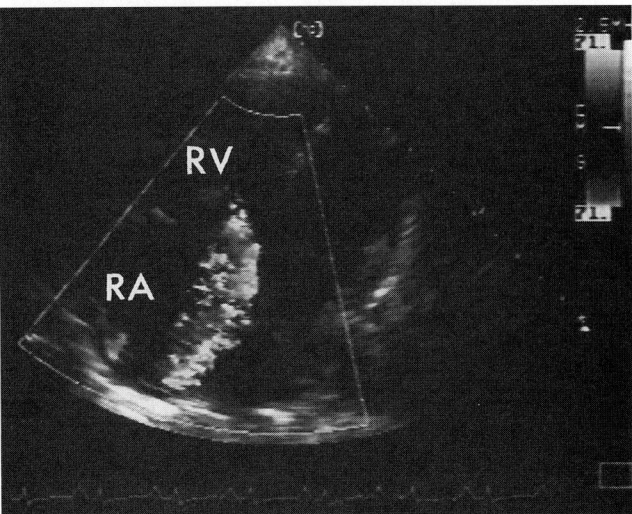

FIGURE 51.12 Moderate tricuspid regurgitation by color Doppler (apical four-chamber view). RA, right atrium; RV, right ventricle.

gradients have been published, but because of the additional dependency on cardiac output and heart rate, these values offer only an orientation (61). Furthermore, especially the bileaflet valves by their design create high local gradients and pressure recovery downstream (62–64). ▼ j68

Mismatch obstruction results from the implantation of a prosthesis that is too small for the site and patient. This is mainly a problem in aortic valve replacement. For example, the effective orifice areas of ring size number 21 and smaller prostheses would be considered mild to moderate aortic stenosis in a native valve (see following discussion). This type of obstruction must be differentiated from new prosthetic obstruction due to thrombosis or pannus by comparison with earlier studies, by transesophageal echocardiography, or by fluoroscopy.

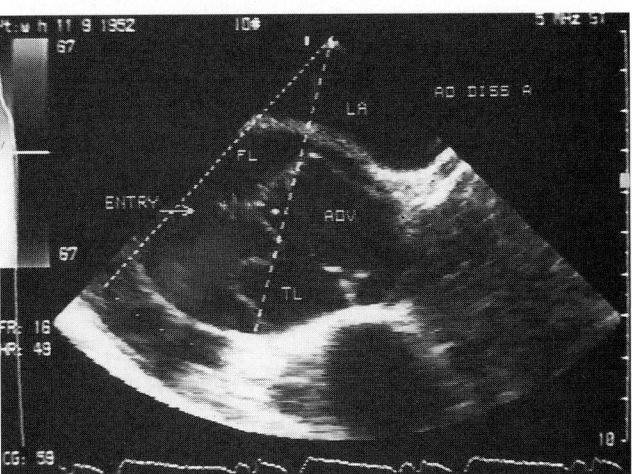

FIGURE 51.13 Aortic dissection (DeBakey type I/Stanford type A). Transesophageal image of the dilated ascending aorta (5 cm). An intimal flap is seen separating a false lumen (FL) from the true lumen (TL). A small entry jet is seen by color Doppler (ENTRY). LA, left atrium.

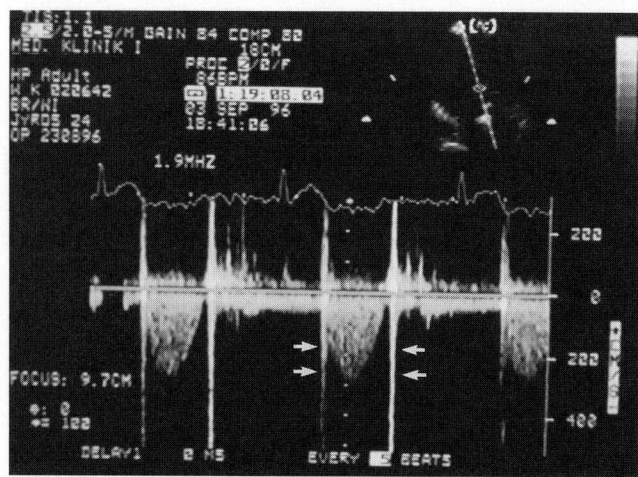

FIGURE 51.14 Aortic prosthetic forward flow in a normal mechanical bileaflet prosthesis (JYROS), with clicks (*arrows*).

Note that pressure recovery and mismatch mainly create problems in the interpretation of velocities across *aortic prostheses.* ▼ j69

For the reasons cited, it is important to document the baseline velocities or gradients of valvular prostheses postoperatively for later comparison. In bioprostheses, because of the well-described degenerative changes, an increase in obstruction with time may be expected.

Regurgitation

All mechanical prostheses, except for the caged-ball Starr-Edwards valve, exhibit some amount of in-built transvalvular leakage, which is intended to prevent the formation of microthrombi at the hinge points and to preclude sticking of the occluder in the closed position. Depending on the prosthesis type, typical spatial orientation patterns of the regurgitant jets are present (70) (Fig. 51.15). Bioprostheses, too, almost invariably present some transvalvular regurgitation. Wear-and-tear lesions in bioprostheses may lead to unpredictable, sudden increases in the severity of regurgitation. In addition to transvalvular regurgitation, paravalvular leakage is frequent in prosthetic valves (Fig. 51.16). ▼ j70

Although aortic regurgitation is more easily identifiable, aortic prostheses are less well examined even by transesophageal echo than mitral prostheses. The principles outlined for the assessment of native aortic regurgitation apply.

EVALUATION OF CARDIAC FUNCTION

Systolic Left Ventricular Function

The most straightforward Doppler parameter of systolic left ventricular function is cardiac output. In the presence of mitral regurgitation, the rate of increase of regurgitant velocities can be used to calculate the rise of the pressure

gradient between the left ventricle and the left atrium throughout systole. This allows one to obtain an estimate of the rise of pressure in the left ventricle (dP/dT). ▼ j71

Diastolic Left Ventricular Function

Diastolic left ventricular function is in itself heterogeneous, comprising active (relaxation) and passive (chamber stiffness) characteristics of the left ventricle. It is characterized in classic hemodynamics by the diastolic time course of pressure and volume. Several parameters obtainable by Doppler have been proposed to evaluate left ventricular diastolic function (74,75). The most time honored is isovolumic relaxation time (the time from aortic valve closure to mitral valve opening; *e*Fig. 51.16.5), which depends on the velocity of myocardial relaxation (classically characterized by the time constant τ), the end systolic pressure level of the aorta, and the early diastolic pressure level of the left atrium. Positioning the continuous wave Doppler beam in an apical long-axis view between left ventricular inflow and outflow, the end of outflow and the onset of inflow can be read from the spectral display.

Intensive interest has focused on the characteristics of the mitral flow profile. Left ventricular filling in sinus rhythm occurs in two phases: an early E wave, which is caused by the pressure difference between the left atrium and the left ventricle, and a late A wave, which is caused by atrial contraction. In young healthy persons, maximal E velocity is slightly higher than A wave velocity. The following factors decrease the E wave: age, heart rate (in heart rates over 100 beats/min, there is generally E and A wave fusion), slowed left ventricular relaxation, and decreased left atrial pressure. Moreover, the site of measurement is important (E/A ratio is lower at the mitral annulus than at the leaflet tips). Increased left atrial pressure, conversely, increases maximal E wave velocity. Maximal A wave velocity depends on left atrial contraction and late diastolic left ventricular compliance. Because the E/A ratio is multifactorial, caution is necessary to interpret it, since *filling is not function.* ▼ j72

Presence of the restrictive mitral inflow pattern (E/A greater than 1.5), in particular presence of a short E wave deceleration time (less than 150 ms), has been convincingly shown to imply high pulmonary capillary pressure, impaired functional class, and bad prognosis in postinfarction patients (83,84), in dilated cardiomyopathy (85,86), in cardiac amyloidosis (87), and others (88). It can be shown theoretically that the slope of deceleration directly reflects the net compliance of the left atrium and left ventricle lumped together (36,37). Hence, a stiff diastolic ventricle leads to rapid E wave deceleration. ▼ j73

Right-Sided Heart Function and Pulmonary Hypertension

Right-sided heart output can be calculated at the pulmonary valve level by multiplying the pulmonary time velocity

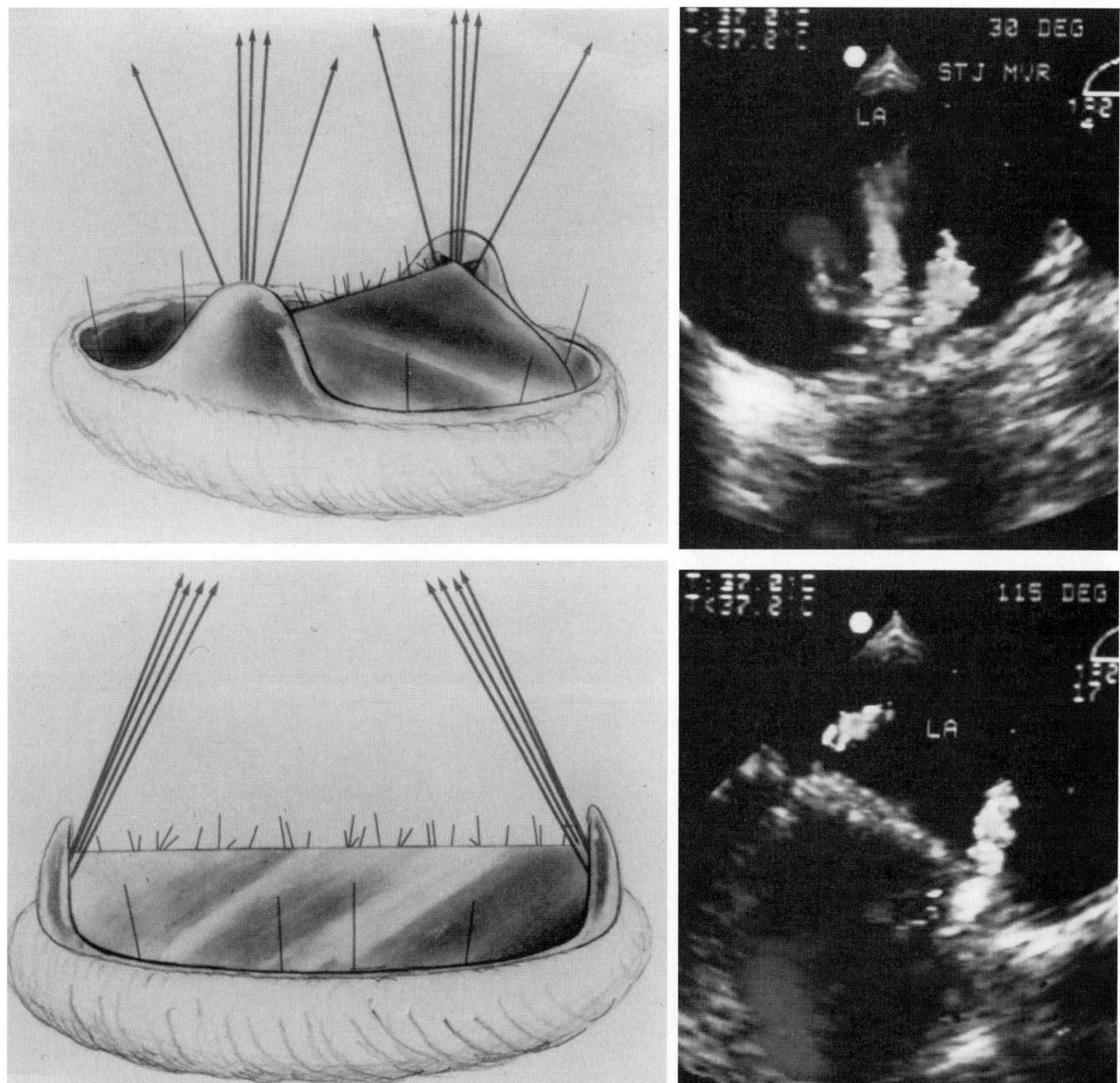

FIGURE 51.15 Normal regurgitant flow patterns of mechanical valves. **A:** St. Jude Medical bileaflet prosthesis. Normal regurgitation mainly occurs at the hinge points of the leaflets. Depending on the view of the valve, typical diverging and converging jet patterns occur. **Left:** Schematic drawing. **Right:** Flow imaging by transesophageal color Doppler. **B:** Medtronic-Hall tilting-disc prosthesis. Normal regurgitation mainly occurs across the central orifice. **Left:** Schematic drawing. **Right:** In the closed position, a normal central transvalvular regurgitation (NTVR) and a medial small paravalvular leak (PVL) are seen. SR, sewing ring. **C:** Björk-Shiley tilting-disc prosthesis in the mitral position with small peripheral normal regurgitant jets occurring between occluder and valve ring. LA, left atrium; LV, left ventricle; RA, right atrium; RV, right ventricle. (From Flachskampf FA, Guerrero JL, O'Shea JP, et al. Patterns of normal transvalvular regurgitation in mechanical valve prostheses. *J Am Coll Cardiol* 1991;18:1493–1498, with permission.) (*continued*)

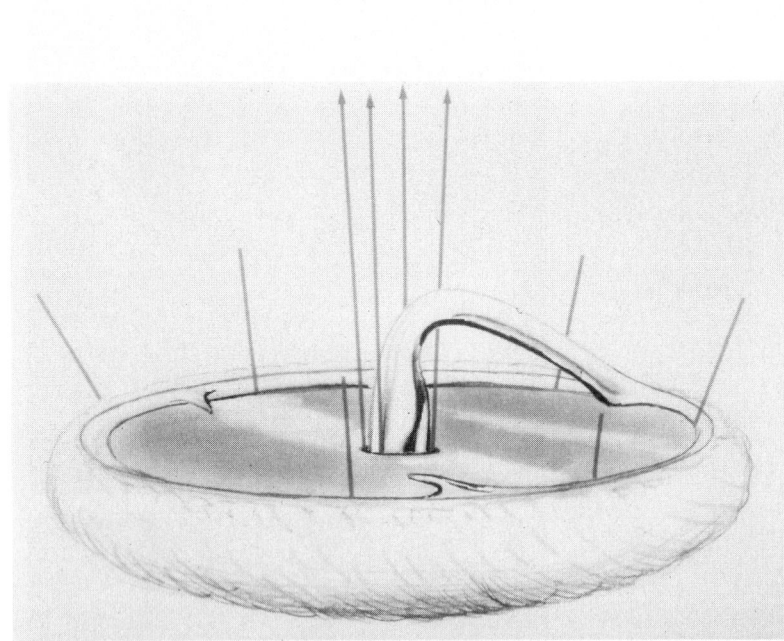

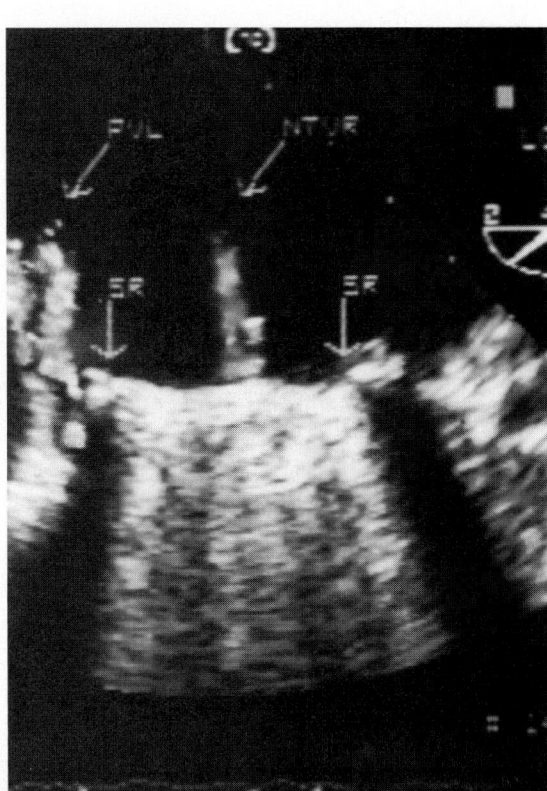

B

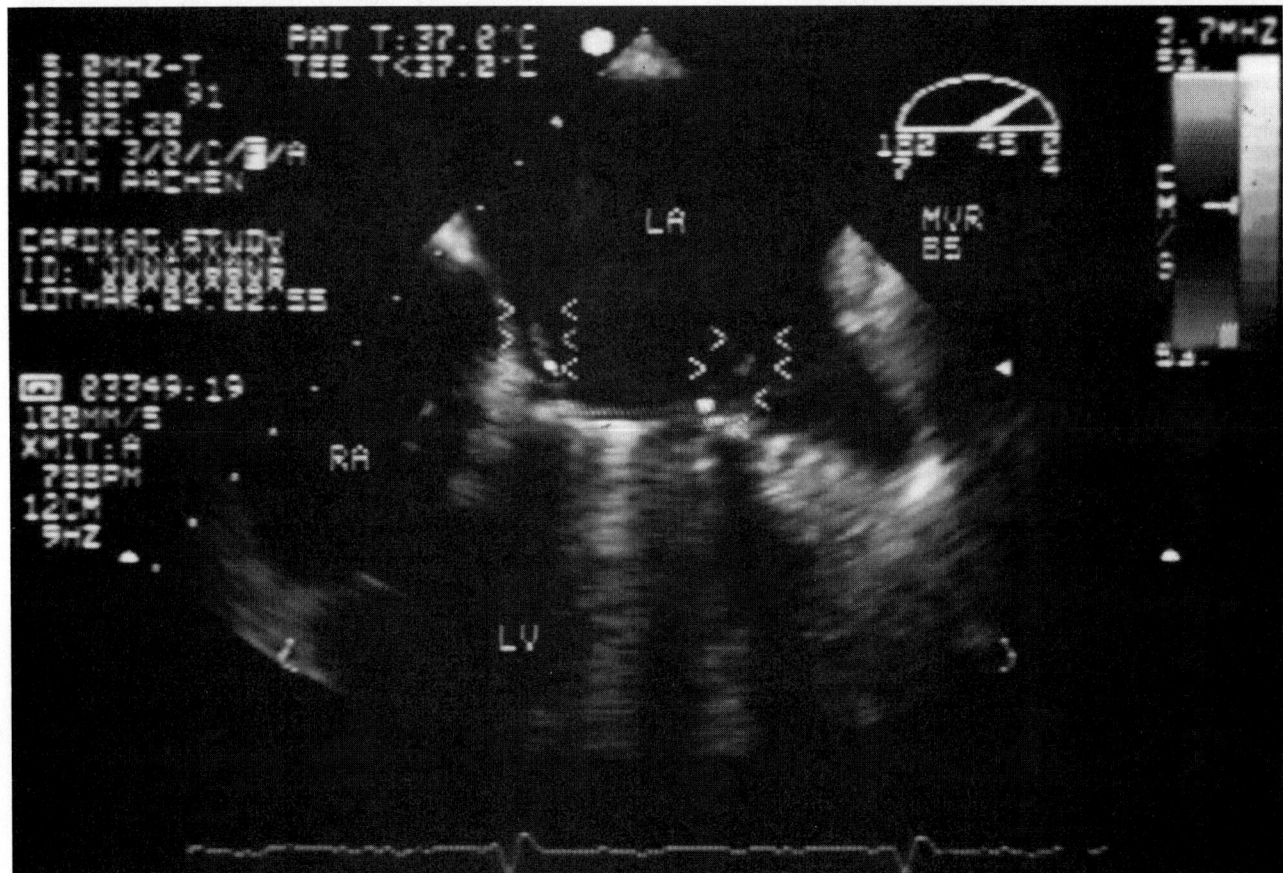

C

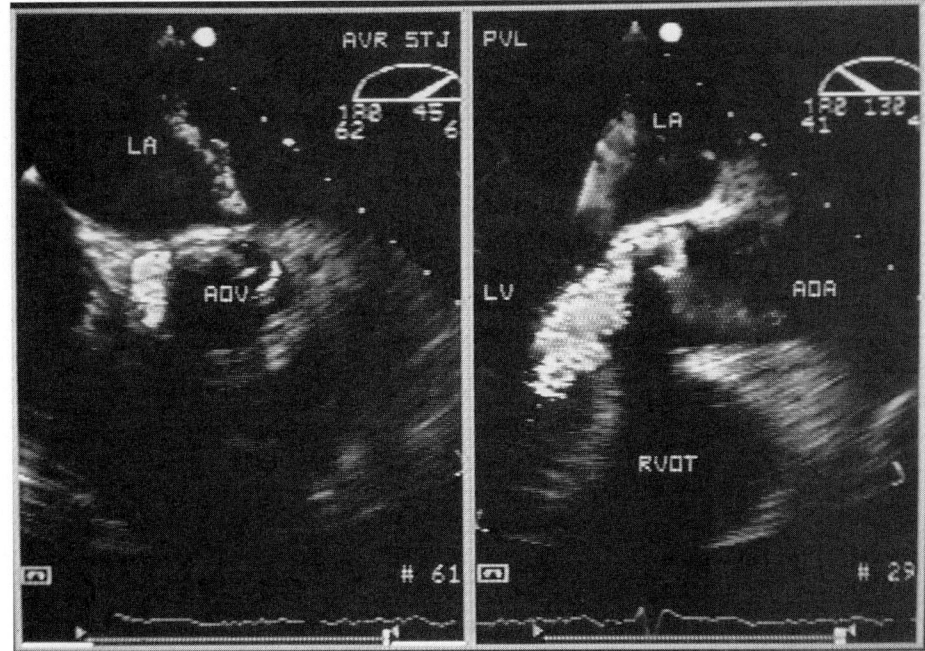

FIGURE 51.16 Paravalvular leakage by color Doppler. Paravalvular leakage of aortic St. Jude Medical prosthesis (AOV) in a short-axis (*left*) and long-axis (*right*) transesophageal view. The leakage cross section and the paravalvular path of the leakage are well seen. AOA, ascending aorta; LA, left atrium; LV, left ventricle; RVOT, right ventricular outflow tract. (From Flachskampf FA, Hoffmann R, Verlande M, et al. Initial experience with a multiplane transesophageal echotransducer: assessment of diagnostic potential. *Eur Heart J* 1992;13:1201–1206, with permission.)

integral by the orifice area of the pulmonary valve ($\pi d^2/4$, where d is the diameter of the pulmonary annulus). The presence of pulmonary hypertension is easiest to assess from tricuspid regurgitation, which is present in almost all patients with pulmonary hypertension and particularly common in acute pulmonary hypertension due to pulmonary embolism. Peak tricuspid regurgitant velocity by continuous wave Doppler is converted to the maximal pressure drop during systole between the right ventricle and the right atrium by the simplified Bernoulli equation. Either this pressure drop can be taken as an estimate of pulmonary systolic pressure or an estimate of right atrial v wave pressure can be added by observing the collapse level of the jugular veins. Some echocardiographers simply add 10 mm Hg to the maximal ventriculoatrial pressure drop. ❦ j74

Left Atrial Appendage Flow

In sinus rhythm, the left atrial appendage shows four brief flow waves: a small emptying wave in early diastole and a larger one during atrial contraction after the P wave of the ECG. Both emptying waves are followed by a filling wave of similar velocity (*e*Fig. 51.16.12). Peak emptying and filling velocities occur immediately before and after the QRS complex and average 64 and 46 cm per second, respectively, in healthy individuals (93). These velocities can be recorded by transesophageal pulsed Doppler, with the sample volume well in the appendage cavity. In nonvalvular atrial fibrillation, although the transmitral A wave is absent and therefore there is no net effect of atrial contraction detectable at the mitral valvular level, emptying and filling velocities of the appendage still are well detectable in most

patients. This is because the appendage encloses a small blood volume, on which the decreased wall motion during fibrillation still imparts enough acceleration to create inward and outward flow. In patients with large atria, especially in long-standing mitral stenosis, and apparently in rare cases of *left atrial appendage standstill* in sinus rhythm (94), these velocities are absent: The appendage is a static pouch, and these conditions are associated with frequent thrombus formation and thromboembolic events. Appendage flow velocities have been used with success retrospectively to stratify the thromboembolic risk of patients with nonvalvular atrial fibrillation, with peak velocities less than 25 cm per second indicating a higher risk and therefore a strong argument for anticoagulation (95).

DOPPLER EVALUATION OF CORONARY ARTERY DISEASE

Impairment of left ventricular relaxation precedes systolic wall motion abnormalities in acute myocardial ischemia. Acute transmitral E/A ratio decrease has been documented during percutaneous transluminal coronary angioplasty balloon inflation (63). Similarly, during dobutamine stress echo, a decrease in peak E wave velocity and in E wave acceleration ratio was shown to be an excellent predictor of coronary artery disease superior to the detection of wall motion abnormalities (96). However, this has not been seen in exercise stress echo, presumably because after treadmill exercise the change to a supine position for the echo examination led to an increase in preload, blunting the response of filling parameters (97).

If depressed systolic left ventricular function is present after myocardial infarction, a decreased cardiac output can be measured. Doppler signs of impaired diastolic function are discussed in the section on Diastolic Left Ventricular Function, earlier in this chapter. The presence of a restrictive pattern (E/A greater than 1.5, E wave deceleration time less than 150 ms; eFigs. 51.16.8 and 51.16.9) after myocardial infarction is associated with a poor life expectancy, even if controlled for systolic variables such as ejection fraction (74). Two large randomized placebo-controlled pharmacologic intervention trials in postinfarction patients with reduced systolic function have attempted to analyze diastolic function by echo. In the Studies of Left Ventricular Dysfunction (SOLVD) trial, a decrease in E/A ratio under enalapril was ascribed to a reduction in atrial pressure due to a favorable influence of enalapril on ventricular remodeling and hypertrophy (98). In the Doppler Flow and Echocardiography in Functional Cardiac Insufficiency: Assessment of Nisoldipine Therapy (DEFIANT) trial, a small increment in E wave velocity and a small reduction in isovolumic relaxation time were seen under the calcium antagonist nisoldipine, and this was ascribed to improvement in left ventricular relaxation (99). It is ironic that these trials interpret opposite echo findings as indicative of a favorable pharmacologic influence on diastolic function.

Doppler has an important role in the identification of some structural complications of myocardial infarction, especially in septal rupture leading to a ventricular septal defect located mostly in the apical half of the septum and in acute mitral regurgitation after papillary muscle rupture. In left ventricular pseudoaneurysm, Doppler recordings at the rupture site reveal biphasic flow, with flow into the pseudoaneurysm during both systole and after atrial contraction, and flow from the pseudoaneurysm into the ventricle during early to mid-diastole (100) (eFig. 51.16.12). ☞ j75

DOPPLER EVALUATION OF THE CARDIOMYOPATHIES, CARDIAC TAMPONADE, AND THE TRANSPLANTED HEART

Dilated Cardiomyopathy

Apart from measuring a reduced cardiac output, Doppler examination is useful to estimate systolic pulmonary pressure by the peak tricuspid regurgitation velocity (see Right-Sided Heart Function and Pulmonary Hypertension, earlier in this chapter), to assess mitral regurgitation, and to evaluate the transmitral filling pattern. A restrictive pattern (E/A greater than 1.5, E wave deceleration time less than 150 ms) indicates high filling pressures and a reduced left ventricular compliance and is associated with a poor prognosis (103,104). Because mitral annular motion is reduced,

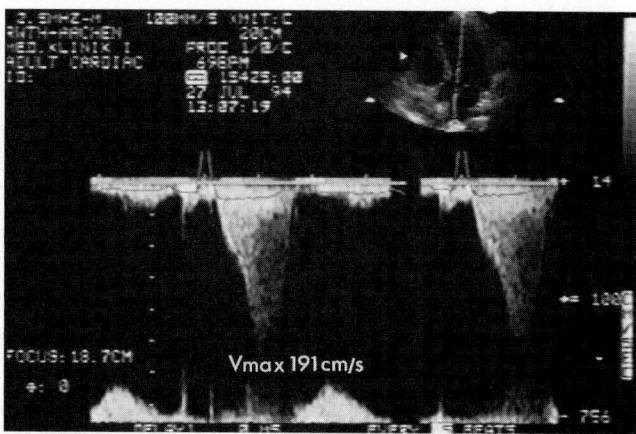

FIGURE 51.17 Left ventricular outflow tract obstruction in hypertrophic obstructive cardiomyopathy recorded by continuous wave Doppler from the apical window. A typical profile with a late systolic peak is recorded, which is well distinguished from the frequently concomitant mitral regurgitation.

systolic pulmonary venous inflow is also reduced in comparison with diastolic inflow.

Hypertrophic Cardiomyopathy

The main task of the Doppler examination is to detect and assess left ventricular outflow obstruction. For this purpose, a continuous wave Doppler recording with the echo beam passing through the left ventricular outflow tract in the apical long-axis view should be obtained. Hypertrophic obstructive cardiomyopathy characteristically produces a sabre-shaped, late-peaking systolic velocity profile different from the (mostly also present) mitral regurgitation in the continuous wave Doppler examination, which begins earlier and exhibits an earlier steep velocity increase (Fig. 51.17). Because continuous wave Doppler has no range resolution, the diagnosis should be confirmed by moving the sample volume of the pulsed Doppler systematically along the interventricular septum from the midventricle to the aortic valve to map the velocities toward the aortic valve. If intraventricular obstruction is present, this is seen in the pulsed Doppler recording, as the systolic velocities at the location of the obstruction abruptly exceed the range limit of the pulsed Doppler. Color Doppler typically shows turbulence in the left ventricular outflow tract. ☞ j76

Constrictive and Restrictive Cardiomyopathy

The transmitral flow profile in constrictive and restrictive cardiomyopathies is frequently characterized by tall and short E waves and small A waves (the restrictive pattern) and a short isovolumic relaxation time. In constrictive pericarditis, but not in restrictive cardiomyopathy, accentuated influence of respiration on cardiac flow velocities is present during inspira-

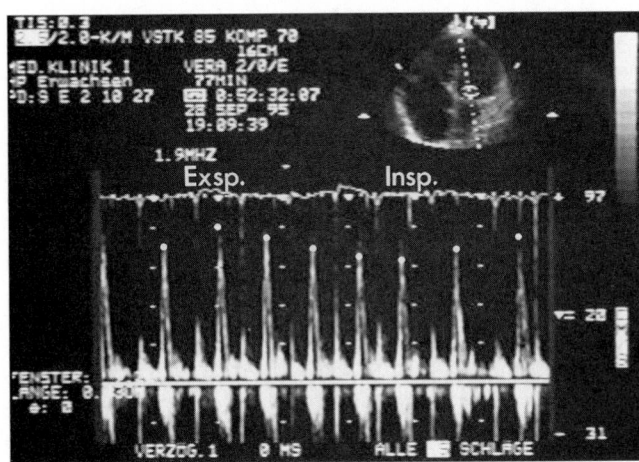

FIGURE 51.18 Transmitral flow profiles in constrictive pericarditis. A "restrictive" transmitral flow pattern with high and short E waves is seen. Peak E-wave velocities show pathologic respiratory variation (greater than 10%) with a decrease during inspiration (Insp.). Exsp., expiration.

tion (a 10% inspiratory decrease in peak transmitral E wave velocity is seen in healthy subjects), transmitral flow velocities decrease, transtricuspid flow velocities increase, and left ventricular relaxation time also increases (Fig. 51.18). Recording is best done at a slow sweep speed to obtain several respiration cycles on one sweep. However, because inspiration image quality often is impaired, reliable documentation of this pattern frequently is difficult. The pulmonary venous flow in constrictive pericarditis decreases in inspiration, and this effect is more marked for diastolic than for systolic pulmonary venous inflow.

Restrictive cardiomyopathy exhibits no marked respiratory variation in mitral flow velocities and is characterized by particularly short mitral and tricuspid pressure half-times. Often, systolic mitral and tricuspid regurgitation are present following the E wave (105). There is usually at least moderate pulmonary hypertension, and ventricular walls are frequently thickened (e.g., in cardiac amyloidosis), which represents the most frequent and classical form of restrictive cardiomyopathy.

Cardiac Tamponade

The Doppler characteristics of cardiac tamponade resemble those of constrictive pericarditis. There is a marked (30% to 40%) inspiratory decrease of transmitral, transaortic, and diastolic pulmonary venous inflow velocities (corresponding to the clinical finding of pulsus paradoxus), and an even more pronounced (greater than 80%) increase in transtricuspid (and transpulmonic) flow velocities. Left ventricular isovolumic relaxation time increases in inspiration.

CONTROVERSIES AND PERSONAL PERSPECTIVES

Although a tremendous success story, some problems in the echo-Doppler assessment of valvular stenosis and regurgitation remain. One fundamental limitation in the present quantitative Doppler approaches to regurgitation is the characterization of spatially complex three-dimensional flow velocity fields in the heart by severely limited data. For instance, a single pulsed Doppler sample volume is used in transvalvular flow rate calculations, or a 2-D color Doppler map in the proximal convergence method. These problems may ultimately be overcome by real-time, three-dimensional, multigated, pulsed Doppler. In the assessment of stenotic lesions, future three-dimensional echo capabilities could help solve the pressure recovery dilemma and reconcile the discrepancies between effective and geometric orifice areas by combining spatial morphologic and functional data. However, it is mostly the effect on myocardial function rather than the valvular lesion per se that clinically matters most, in particular in chronic regurgitant lesions. Thus, the quest for the single magic number representing the severity of a valvular lesion is misleading. A set of parameters measuring both valvular and myocardial function will be needed to fully characterize such lesions.

Much interest has focused on Doppler parameters of diastolic left ventricular function. A set of Doppler parameters (isovolumic relaxation time, E/A ratio, E deceleration, A wave duration, pulmonary venous reverse flow, and so

THE FUTURE

Several developments in particular will permit better calculation of flow rates. *Unwrapping* of high velocities will enable full mapping of the velocity field of regurgitant jets. Thus, jet momentum could be calculated, and because momentum is conserved in the cross sections of a jet, flow rate at the regurgitant orifice can be derived. Moreover, the length of the jet's laminar core has a fairly constant relationship with the diameter of the regur-

gitant orifice; measurement of the length of the laminar core would therefore allow estimation of regurgitant orifice size and, hence, severity of regurgitation (21). Automated integration of color Doppler velocities in two or three dimensions and three-dimensional Doppler of the proximal convergence zone are two other developments (*e*Fig. 51.18.3), and use of Doppler power (amplitude squared) for flow calculations is a third (115).

forth) used cautiously together with other echo data generally allows prediction of elevated diastolic left ventricular pressures. However, because systolic and diastolic myocardial function are interrelated and both pervasively load dependent, the search for the one parameter exclusively reflecting *diastolic function* (itself an ill-defined term) is inadequate, and data should always be viewed in clinical and hemodynamic perspective.

REFERENCES

1. Doppler C. Über das farbige Licht der Doppelsterne und einiger anderer Gestirne des Himmels. *Abhandlungen der Königlich-Böhmischen Gesellschaft der Wissenschaften* 1842;2:465–483.
2. Satomura S. Ultrasonic Doppler method for the inspection of cardiac functions. *J Acoust Soc Am* 1957;29:1181–1185.
3. Franklin DL, Schlegal WA, Rushmer RF. Blood flow measured by Doppler frequency shift of backscattered ultrasound. *Science* 1961;134:564–565.
4. Peronneau P, Deloche A, Bui-Mong-Hung, et al. Debitmetrie ultrasonore: Développements et applications expérimentales. *Eur Surg Res* 1969;1:147–156.
5. Baker DW. Pulsed ultrasonic Doppler blood-flow sensing. *IEEE Trans Sonics Ultrasonics* 1970;SU-17:170–185.
6. Holen J, Aaslid R, Landmark K, et al. Determination of pressure gradient in mitral stenosis with a non-invasive ultrasound Doppler technique. *Acta Med Scand* 1976;19:455–460.
7. Hatle L, Angelsen BA, Tromsdal A. Non-invasive assessment of aortic stenosis by Doppler ultrasound. *Br Heart J* 1980;43:284–292.
8. Brandestini MA, Howard EA, Weiler EB, et al. The synthesis of echo and Doppler in M-mode and sectorscan. *Proc Annu Meet AIUM* 1979;125:704.
9. Namekawa K, Kasai C, Koyano A. Imaging of blood flow using autocorrelation. *Ultrasound Med Biol* 1982;8:138.
10. Bommer W, Miller L. Real-time two-dimensional color flow Doppler-enhanced imaging in the diagnosis of cardiovascular disease. *Am J Cardiol* 1982;49:944.
11. Kasai C, Namekawa K, Koyano A, et al. Real-time two dimensional blood flow imaging using an autocorrelation technique. *IEEE Trans Sonic Ultrasonic* 1985;32:458.
12. Side CD, Gosling RG. Non-surgical assessment of cardiac function. *Nature* 1971;232:335–336.
13. Stegall HF, Stone HL, Bishop VS, et al. A catheter-tip pressure and velocity sensor. *Proc 20th Am Conf Eng Med Biol* 1967;27:4.
14. Benchimol A, Stegall HF, Gartlan JL. A new method to measure phasic coronary blood velocity in man. *Am Heart J* 1971;81:93–101.
15. Reid JM, Davis DL, Ricketts HJ, et al. A new Doppler flowmeter system and its operation with catheter mounted transducers. In: Reneman RS, ed. *Cardiovascular applications of ultrasound*. New York: Elsevier, 1974:108–124.
16. McDicken WN, Sutherland GR, Moran CM, et al. Colour Doppler velocity imaging of the myocardium. *Ultrasound Med Biol* 1992;18:651–654.
17. Weyman AE. *Principles and practice of echocardiography*, 2nd ed. Philadelphia: Lea & Febiger, 1994.
18. Hatle L, Angelsen B. *Doppler ultrasound in cardiology*, 2nd ed. Philadelphia: Lea & Febiger, 1985.
19. Yoganathan AP, Cape EG, Sung HW, et al. Review of hydrodynamic principles for the cardiologist: applications to the study of blood flow and jets by imaging techniques. *J Am Coll Cardiol* 1988;12:1344–1353.
20. Teirstein PS, Yock PG, Popp RL. The accuracy of Doppler ultrasound measurement of pressure gradients across irregular, dual, and tunnel-like obstructions to blood flow. *Circulation* 1985;72:577–584.
21. Diebold B, Delouche A, Delouche P, et al. In vitro flow mapping of regurgitant jets. Systematic description of free jet with laser Doppler velocimetry. *Circulation* 1996;94:158–169.
22. Recusani F, Bargiggia GS, Yoganathan AP, et al. A new method for quantification of regurgitant flow rate using color flow imaging of the flow convergence region proximal to a discrete orifice: an in vitro study. *Circulation* 1991;83:594–604.
23. Vandervoort P, Rivera JM, Mele D, et al. Application of color Doppler flow mapping to calculate effective regurgitant orifice area. An in vitro study and initial clinical observations. *Circulation* 1993;88:1150–1156.
24. Barclay SA, Eidenvall L, Karlsson M, et al. The shape of the proximal isovelocity surface area varies with regurgitant orifice size and distance from orifice: computer simulation and model experiments with color M-mode technique. *J Am Soc Echocardiogr* 1993;6:433–445.
25. Burwash IG, Pearlman AS, Kraft CD, et al. Flow dependence of measures of aortic stenosis severity during exercise. *J Am Coll Cardiol* 1994;24:1342–1350.
26. Voelker W, Reul H, Nienhaus G, et al. Comparison of valvular resistance, stroke work loss, and Gorlin valve area for quantification of aortic stenosis. An in vitro study in a pulsatile aortic flow model. *Circulation* 1995;91:1196–1204.
27. Akamatsu S, Ueda N, Terzawa E, et al. Mitral prosthetic dehiscence with laminar regurgitant flow signals assessed by transesophageal echocardiography. *Chest* 1993;104:1911–1913.
28. Thomas JD, Liu CM, Flachskampf FA, et al. Quantification of jet flow by momentum analysis: an in vitro Doppler color flow study. *Circulation* 1990;81:247–259.
29. Chen C, Thomas JD, Anconina J, et al. Impact of impinging wall jet on color Doppler quantification of mitral regurgitation. *Circulation* 1991;84:712–720.
30. Schwammenthal E, Chen C, Benning F, et al. Dynamics of mitral regurgitant flow and orifice area. Physiologic application of the proximal flow convergence method: clinical data and experimental testing. *Circulation* 1994;90:307–322.
31. Reimold SC, Maier SE, Fleischmann KE, et al. Dynamic nature of the aortic regurgitant orifice area during diastole in patients with chronic aortic regurgitation. *Circulation* 1994;89:2085–2092.
32. Rodriguez L, Thomas JD, Monterroso V, et al. Validation of the proximal flow convergence method: calculation of orifice area in patients with mitral stenosis. *Circulation* 1993;88:1157–1165.
33. Fisher DC, Sahn DJ, Friedman MJ, et al. The mitral valve

orifice method for noninvasive two-dimensional echo Doppler determinations of cardiac output. *Circulation* 1983;67:872–877.

34. Dittmann H, Jacksch R, Voelker W, et al. Accuracy of Doppler echocardiography in quantification of left to right shunts in adult patients with atrial septal defect. *J Am Coll Cardiol* 1988;11:338–342.

35. Sun JP, Stewart WJ, Pu M, et al. Automated cardiac output measurement by spatiotemporal integration of color Doppler data. *Circulation* 1997;75:932–939.

36. Flachskampf FA, Decoodt P, Fraser AG, et al. Recommendations for performing transesophageal echocardiography. *Eur J Echocardiogr* 2001 (*in press*).

37. von Bibra H, Sutherland G, Becher H, et al. Clinical evaluation of left heart Doppler contrast enhancement by a saccharide-based transpulmonary contrast agent. The Levovist Cardiac Working Group. *J Am Coll Cardiol* 1995;25:500–508.

38. Iliceto S, Caiati C, Aragona P, et al. Improved Doppler signal intensity in coronary arteries after intravenous peripheral injection of a lung-crossing contrast agent (SHU 508A). *J Am Coll Cardiol* 1994;23:184–190.

39. Masugata H, Cotter B, Peters B, et al. Assessment of coronary stenosis severity and transmural perfusion gradient by myocardial contrast echocardiography. Comparison of gray-scale B-mode with power Doppler imaging. *Circulation* 2000;102:1427–1433.

40. Keren G, Sonnenblick EH, LeJemtel TH. Mitral annulus motion: relation to pulmonary venous and transmitral flows in normal subjects and in patients with dilated cardiomyopathy. *Circulation* 1988;78:621–629.

41. Hatle L, Angelsen B, Tromsdal A. Noninvasive assessment of atrioventricular pressure half-time by Doppler ultrasound. *Circulation* 1989;6:1096–1104.

42. Flachskampf FA, Weyman AE, Gillam L, et al. Aortic regurgitation shortens Doppler pressure half-time in mitral stenosis: theoretical analysis, in vitro modelling, and clinical evidence. *J Am Coll Cardiol* 1990;16:396–404.

43. Flachskampf FA, Weyman AE, Guerrero JL, et al. Calculation of atrioventricular compliance from the mitral flow profile: analytical and in vitro study. *J Am Coll Cardiol* 1992;19:998–1004.

44. Thomas JD, Weyman AE. Doppler mitral pressure half-time: a clinical tool in search of theoretical justification. *J Am Coll Cardiol* 1987;10:923–929.

45. Voelker W, Berner A, Regele B, et al. Effect of exercise on valvular resistance in patients with mitral stenosis. *J Am Coll Cardiol* 1993;22:777–782.

46. Stewart WJ, Currie PJ, Salcedo EE, et al. Evaluation of mitral leaflet motion by echocardiography and jet direction by Doppler color flow mapping to determine the mechanism of mitral regurgitation. *J Am Coll Cardiol* 1992;20:1353–1361.

47. Helmcke F, Nanda NC, Hsiung MC, et al. Color Doppler assessment of mitral regurgitation with orthogonal planes. *Circulation* 1987;75:175–183.

48. Castello R, Lenzen P, Aguirre F, et al. Quantitation of mitral regurgitation by transesophageal echocardiography with Doppler color flow mapping: correlation with cardiac catheterization. *J Am Coll Cardiol* 1992;19:1516–1521.

49. Tribouilloy C, Shen WF, Quéré JP, et al. Assessment of severity of mitral regurgitation by measuring regurgitant jet width at its origin with transesophageal Doppler color flow imaging. *Circulation* 1992;85:1248–1253.

50. Mele D, Vandervoort P, Palacios I, et al. Proximal jet size by Doppler color flow mapping predicts severity of mitral regurgitation. Clinical studies. *Circulation* 1995;91:746–754.

51. Rivera JM, Vandervoort PM, Thoreau DH, et al. Quantification of mitral regurgitation with the proximal flow convergence method: a clinical study. *Am Heart J* 1992;124:1289–1296.

52. Klein L, Bailey AS, Cohen GI, et al. Importance of sampling both pulmonary veins in grading mitral regurgitation by transesophageal echocardiography. *J Am Soc Echocardiogr* 1993;6:115–123.

53. Baumgartner H, Stefenelli T, Niederberger J, et al. "Overestimation" of catheter gradients by Doppler ultrasound in patients with aortic stenosis: a predictable manifestation of pressure recovery. *J Am Coll Cardiol* 1999;33:1655–1661.

54. Garcia D, Pibarot P, Dumesnil JG, et al. Assessment of aortic valve stenosis severity. A new index based on the energy loss concept. *Circulation* 2000;101:765–771.

55. Grayburn PA, deFilippi CR, Willett DL, et al. Usefulness of dobutamine echocardiography in distinguishing severe from nonsevere valvular aortic stenosis in patients with depressed left ventricular function and low transvalvular gradients. *Am J Cardiol* 1995;75:191–194.

56. Perry GJ, Helmcke F, Nanda NC, et al. Evaluation of aortic insufficiency by Doppler color flow mapping. *J Am Coll Cardiol* 1987;9:952–959.

57. Teague SM, Heinsimer JA, Anderson JL, et al. Quantification of aortic regurgitation utilizing continuous wave Doppler ultrasound. *J Am Coll Cardiol* 1986;8:592–599.

58. Griffin BA, Flachskampf FA, Reimold SC, et al. Relationship of aortic regurgitation velocity slope and pressure half-time to severity of aortic regurgitation under changing haemodynamic conditions. *Eur Heart J* 1994;15:681–685.

59. Griffin BG, Flachskampf FA, Siu S, et al. The effects of regurgitant orifice size, chamber compliance, and systemic vascular resistance on aortic regurgitant velocity slope and pressure half-time. *Am Heart J* 1991;122:1049–1056.

60. Burstow DJ, Nishimura RA, Bailey KR, et al. Continuous wave Doppler echocardiographic measurement of prosthetic valve gradients. A simultaneous Doppler-catheter correlative study. *Circulation* 1989;80:504–514.

61. Bech-Hanssen O, Wallentin I, Larsson S, et al. Reference Doppler echocardiographic values for St. Jude Medical, Omnicarbon, and Biocor prosthetic valves in the aortic position. *J Am Soc Echocardiogr* 1998;11:466–477.

62. Baumgartner H, Khan S, DeRobertis M, et al. Discrepancies between Doppler and catheter gradients in aortic prosthetic valves in vitro. A manifestation of localized gradients and pressure recovery. *Circulation* 1990;82:1467–1475.

63. Vandervoort PM, Greenberg NL, Powell KA, et al. Pressure recovery in bileaflet heart valve prostheses. Localized high velocities and gradients in central and side orifices with implications for Doppler-catheter gradient relation

in aortic and mitral position. *Circulation* 1995;92:3464–3472.

64. Bech-Hanssen O, Caidahl K, Wallentin I, et al. Aortic prosthetic valve design and size: relation to Doppler echocardiographic findings and pressure recovery—an in vitro study. *J Am Soc Echocardiogr* 2000;13:39–50.

65. Baumgartner H, Schima H, Kühn P. Effect of prosthetic valve malfunction on the Doppler-catheter gradient relation for bileaflet aortic valve prostheses. *Circulation* 1993;87:1320–1327.

66. Wiseth R, Levang OW, Sande E, et al. Hemodynamic evaluation by Doppler echocardiography of small (<21 mm) prostheses and bioprostheses in the aortic valve position. *Am J Cardiol* 1992;70:240–246.

67. Geibel A, Kasper W, Fraedrich G, et al. Limitation der Doppler-Echokardiographie in der Beurteilung von Aortenklappenprothesen. *Z Kardiol* 1993;82:175–180.

68. Chafizadeh ER, Zoghbi WA. Doppler echocardiographic assessment of the St. Jude Medical prosthetic valve in the aortic position using the continuity equation. *Circulation* 1991;83:213–223.

69. Rosenzweig BP, Kronzon I, Feit F, et al. Systolic antegrade tricuspid blood flow—a sign of severe prosthetic valve stenosis. *Am Heart J* 1988;115:693–696.

70. Flachskampf FA, Guerrero JL, O'Shea JP, et al. Patterns of normal transvalvular regurgitation in mechanical valve prostheses. *J Am Coll Cardiol* 1991;18:1493–1498.

71. Flachskampf FA, Hoffmann R, Franke A, et al. Does multiplane transesophageal echocardiography improve the assessment of prosthetic valve regurgitation? *J Am Soc Echocardiogr* 1995;8:70–78.

72. Yoshida K, Yoshikawa J, Akasaka T, et al. Value of acceleration flow signals proximal to the leaking orifice in assessing the severity of prosthetic mitral valve regurgitation. *J Am Coll Cardiol* 1992;19:333–338.

73. Bargiggia GS, Bertucci C, Recusani F, et al. A new method for estimating left ventricular dP/dT by continuous wave Doppler echocardiography: validation studies at catheterization. *Circulation* 1989;80:1287–1292.

74. Appleton CP, Jensen JL, Hatle LK, et al. Doppler evaluation of left and right ventricular diastolic function: a technical guide for obtaining optimal flow velocity recordings. *J Am Soc Echocardiogr* 1997;10:271–291.

75. Oh JK, Appleton CP, Hatle LK, et al. The noninvasive assessment of left ventricular diastolic function with two-dimensional and Doppler echocardiography. *J Am Soc Echocardiogr* 1997;10:246–270.

76. Appleton CP, Hatle LK, Popp RL. Relation of transmitral flow velocity patterns to left ventricular diastolic function: new insights from a combined hemodynamic and Doppler echocardiographic study. *J Am Coll Cardiol* 1988;12:426–440.

77. Labovitz AJ, Lewen MK, Morton K, et al. Evaluation of left ventricular systolic and diastolic dysfunction during transient myocardial ischemia produced by angioplasty. *J Am Coll Cardiol* 1987;10:748–755.

78. Choong CY, Herrmann HC, Weyman AE, et al. Preload dependence of Doppler-derived indexes of left ventricular diastolic function in humans. *J Am Coll Cardiol* 1987;10:800–808.

79. Kuecherer HF, Kusumoto F, Muhiudeen IA, et al. Pulmonary venous flow patterns by transesophageal pulsed Doppler echocardiography: relation to parameters of left ventricular systolic and diastolic function. *Am Heart J* 1991;122:1683–1693.

80. Hoit BD, Shao Y, Gabel M, et al. Influence of loading conditions and contractile state on pulmonary venous flow. Validation of Doppler velocimetry. *Circulation* 1992;86:651–659.

81. Rossvoll O, Hatle L. Pulmonary venous flow velocities recorded by transthoracic Doppler ultrasound: relation to left ventricular diastolic pressures. *J Am Coll Cardiol* 1993;21:1687–1696.

82. Hoffmann R, Lambertz H, Thoenissen G, et al. Altered left ventricular diastolic function post atrial pacing in coronary artery disease and left ventricular hypertrophy: further insights by pulmonary venous flow analysis. *Eur Heart J* 1994;15:1096–1105.

83. Oh JK, Ding ZP, Gersh BJ, et al. Restrictive left ventricular diastolic filling identifies patients with heart failure after acute myocardial infarction. *J Am Soc Echocardiogr* 1992;5:497–503.

84. Pozzoli M, Capomolla S, Sanarico M, et al. Doppler evaluations of left ventricular diastolic filling and pulmonary wedge pressure provide similar prognostic information in patients with systolic dysfunction after myocardial infarction. *Am Heart J* 1995;129:716–725.

85. Pinamonti B, Di Lenarda A, Sinagra G, Camerini F, and The Heart Muscle Disease Study Group. Restrictive left ventricular filling pattern in dilated cardiomyopathy assessed by Doppler echocardiography: clinical, echocardiographic and hemodynamic correlations and prognostic implications. *J Am Coll Cardiol* 1993;22:808–815.

86. Vanoverschelde JLJ, Raphael DA, Robert AR, et al. Left ventricular filling in dilated cardiomyopathy: relation to functional class and hemodynamics. *J Am Coll Cardiol* 1990;15:1288–1295.

87. Klein AL, Hatle LK, Taliercio CP, et al. Prognostic significance of Doppler measures of diastolic function in cardiac amyloidosis. A Doppler echocardiographic study. *Circulation* 1991;83:808–816.

88. Xie GY, Berk MR, Smith MD, et al. Prognostic value of Doppler transmitral flow patterns in patients with congestive heart failure. *J Am Coll Cardiol* 1994;24:132–139.

89. Brun P, Tribouilloy C, Duval AM, et al. Left ventricular flow propagation during early filling is related to wall relaxation: a color M-mode Doppler analysis. *J Am Coll Cardiol* 1992;20:420–432.

90. Stugaard M, Smiseth OA, Risöe C, et al. Intraventricular early diastolic filling during acute myocardial ischemia. Assessment by multigated color M-mode Doppler echocardiography. *Circulation* 1993;88:2705–2713.

91. Steine K, Stugaard M, Smiseth O. Mechanisms of retarded apical filling in acute ischemic left ventricular failure. *Circulation* 1999;99:2048–2054.

92. Jiang L, Stewart WJ, King ME, et al. An improved method for estimation of pulmonary artery pressure using Doppler velocity time intervals. *J Am Coll Cardiol* 1984;3:613.

93. Kortz RAM, Delemarre BJ, van Dantzig JM, et al. Left atrial appendage blood flow determined by transesoph-

ageal echocardiography in healthy subjects. *Am J Cardiol* 1993;71:976–981.

94. Pozzoli M, Febo O, Torbicki A, et al. Left atrial appendage dysfunction: a cause of thrombosis? Evidence by transesophageal echocardiography-Doppler studies. *J Am Soc Echoardiogr* 1991;4:435–441.

95. Mügge A, Kühn H, Nikutta P, et al. Assessment of left atrial appendage function by biplane transesophageal echocardiography in patients with nonrheumatic atrial fibrillation: identification of a subgroup of patients at increased embolic risk. *J Am Coll Cardiol* 1994;23:599–607.

96. El-Said EM, Roelandt JRTC, Fioretti PM, et al. Abnormal left ventricular early diastolic filling during dobutamine stress Doppler echocardiography is a sensitive indicator of significant coronary artery disease. *J Am Coll Cardiol* 1994;24:1618–1624.

97. Presti CM, Walling AD, Montemayor I, et al. Influence of exercise-induced myocardial ischemia on the pattern of left ventricular diastolic filling: a Doppler echocardiographic study. *J Am Coll Cardiol* 1991;18:75–82.

98. Greenberg B, Quinones MA, Koilpillai C, et al., for the SOLVD Investigators. Effects of long-term enalapril therapy on cardiac structure and function in patients with left ventricular dysfunction. Results of the SOLVD echocardiography substudy. *Circulation* 1995;91:2573–2581.

99. DEFIANT Research Group. Improved diastolic function with the calcium antagonist nisoldipine (coat-core) in patients post myocardial infarction: results of the DEFIANT study. *Eur Heart J* 1992;13:1496–1505.

100. Roelandt JRTC, Sutherland GR, Yoshida K, et al. Improved diagnosis and characterization of left ventricular pseudoaneurysm by Doppler color flow imaging. *J Am Coll Cardiol* 1988;13:807–811.

101. Iliceto S, Marangelli V, Memmola C, et al. Transesophageal Doppler echocardiography evaluation of coronary blood flow velocity in baseline condition and during dipyridamole-induced coronary vasodilation. *Circulation* 1991;83:61–69.

102. Isaaz K, Bruntz JF, Ethevenot G, et al. Noninvasive assessment of coronary flow dynamics before and after coronary angioplasty using transesophageal Doppler. *Am J Cardiol* 1993;72:1238–1242.

103. Vanoverschelde JLJ, Raphael DA, Robert AR, et al. Left ventricular filling in dilated cardiomyopathy: relation to functional class and hemodynamics. *J Am Coll Cardiol* 1990;15:1288–1295.

104. Pinamonti B, Di Lenarda A, Sinagra G, et al., and The Heart Muscle Disease Study Group. Restrictive left ventricular filling pattern in dilated cardiomyopathy assessed by Doppler echocardiography: clinical, echocardiographic and hemodynamic correlations and prognostic implications. *J Am Coll Cardiol* 1993;22:808–815.

105. Hatle LK, Appleton CP, Popp RL. Differentiation of constrictive pericarditis and restrictive cardiomyopathy by Doppler echocardiography. *Circulation* 1989;79:357–370.

106. Lambertz H, Sigmund M, Hoffmann R, et al. Transesophageal Doppler analysis of pulmonary venous flow in cardiac transplant recipients. *Am Heart J* 1991;121:623–626.

107. Valantine HA, Appleton CP, Hatle LK. A hemodynamic and Doppler echocardiographic study of ventricular function in longterm cardiac allograft recipients: etiology and prognosis of restrictive/constrictive physiology. *Circulation* 1989;79:66–75.

108. Desruennes M, Corcos T, Cabrol A, et al. Doppler echocardiography for the diagnosis of acute cardiac allograft rejection. *J Am Coll Cardiol* 1988;12:63–70.

109. Miyatake K, Yamagishi M, Tanaka N, et al. New method for evaluating left ventricular wall motion by color-coded tissue Doppler imaging: in vitro and in vivo studies. *J Am Coll Cardiol* 1995;25:717–724.

110. Sutherland GR, Stewart MJ, Groundstroem KWE, et al. Color Doppler myocardial imaging: a new technique for the assessment of myocardial function. *J Am Soc Echocardiogr* 1994;7:441–458.

111. Hatle L, Sutherland G. Regional myocardial function—a new approach. *Eur Heart J* 2000;21:1337–1357.

112. Derumeaux G, Ovize M, Loufoua J, et al. Assessment of nonuniformity of transmural myocardial velocities by color-coded tissue Doppler imaging: characterization of normal, ischemic, and stunned myocardium. *Circulation* 2000;101:1390–1395.

113. Armstrong G, Pasquet A, Fukamachi K, et al. Use of peak systolic strain as an index of regional left ventricular systolic function: comparison with tissue Doppler velocity during dobutamine stress and myocardial ischemia. *J Am Soc Echocardiogr* 2000;13:731–737.

114. Sohn DW, Chai IH, Lee DJ, et al. Assessment of mitral annulus velocity by Doppler tissue imaging in the evaluation of left ventricular diastolic function. *J Am Coll Cardiol* 1997;30:474–480.

115. Buck T, Mucci RA, Guerrero JL, et al. The power-velocity integral at the vena contracta. A new method for direct quantification of regurgitant volume flow. *Circulation* 2000;102:1053–1061.

116. Castello R, Pearson AC, Lenzen P, et al. Evaluation of pulmonary venous flow by transesophageal echocardiography in subjects with a normal heart: comparison with transthoracic echocardiography. *J Am Coll Cardiol* 1991;18:65–71.

117. Connolly HM, Miller FA, Taylor CL, et al. Doppler hemodynamic profiles of 82 clinically and echocardiographic normal tricuspid valve prostheses. *Circulation* 1993:88:2722–2727.

TRANSESOPHAGEAL ECHOCARDIOGRAPHY

BRIAN P. GRIFFIN

▼ ADDITIONAL ELECTRONIC TOPICS

OVERVIEW

Transesophageal echocardiography (TEE) is an important tool in the evaluation of cardiac structure and function and for assessing the thoracic aorta. With TEE, images are acquired from an esophageal or gastric imaging window rather than from the chest wall (*e*Table 52.0.1). This is advantageous as the heart and aorta lie very close to the esophagus throughout much of its course. Esophageal imaging is therefore possible with a higher frequency transducer than is usually possible with transthoracic imaging. This and the absence of air-filled lung tissue in the imaging window allow improved image resolution. TEE images the heart from behind, which allows excellent resolution of posterior structures such as the atria, interatrial septum, and aorta as compared with transthoracic imaging. The posterior imaging approach is also advantageous in circumventing acoustic shadowing from strong reflectors of ultrasound such as prosthetic valves.

B. P. Griffin: Cardiovascular Training Program, Department of Cardiovascular Medicine, The Cleveland Clinic Foundation, Cleveland, Ohio

TEE is invasive, as the transducer must be inserted into the esophagus and stomach. This usually requires local anesthesia and intravenous sedation. It is more consumptive of physician time, more expensive, and has less patient acceptance than transthoracic imaging. Transthoracic echocardiography (TTE) can provide adequate clinical information in many instances and is therefore usually acquired first. TEE is performed if additional information is required or if transthoracic image quality is suboptimal. In most adult echocardiography laboratories, less than 10% of all studies are performed by the transesophageal approach (*e*Fig. 52.0.1) (1,2). Major current indications for TEE are shown in *e*Table 52.0.2.

ANATOMIC CONSIDERATIONS

The esophagus is approximately 25 cm in length and extends from the pharynx to the stomach (Fig. 52.1). The esophagus is narrowest at the junction with the pharynx. This is the most difficult area to cross when passing a transesophageal transducer. The esophagus descends vertically and slightly to the left, passing behind the trachea, left mainstem bronchus, left atrium, and left ventricle before passing through the diaphragm. The ascending aorta and

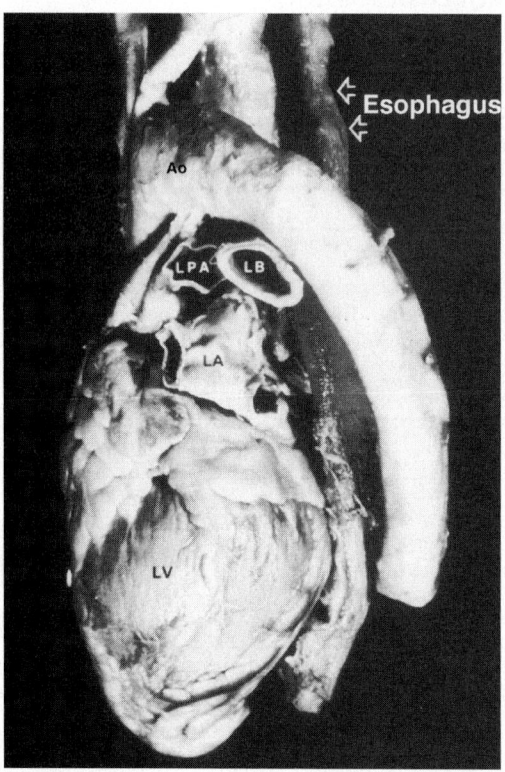

FIGURE 52.1 Anatomic specimen showing relationship of esophagus to heart and aorta. Ao, aorta; LA, left atrium; LB, left main bronchus; LPA, left pulmonary artery; LV, left ventricle. (From Weyman AE. *Principles and practice of echocardiography*, 2nd ed. Philadelphia: Lea & Febiger, 1994, with permission.)

arch lie anterior to the esophagus (*e*Fig. 52.1.1). The air-filled trachea and left mainstem bronchus interpose between the esophagus and portion of the ascending aorta and ascending arch and cause a "blind spot" in imaging the aorta from the transesophageal window. The esophagus twines around the descending aorta. It lies medial to the aorta in the midthorax, whereas the aorta lies behind it at the level of diaphragm. Therefore, the esophageal transducer must be rotated while imaging the descending aorta to keep it in view.

TECHNOLOGY: TRANSDUCERS AND PROBES

TEE requires the use of a special esophageal probe that interfaces with a conventional cardiac ultrasound system. The esophageal probes currently in use consist of an ultrasound transducer(s) mounted at the end of a flexible gastroscope from which the fiberoptic cables and suction capability have been removed (*e*Fig. 52.1.2). The transducers typically used are phased-array and multielement and operate at multiple frequencies from 3.5 to 7.0 MHz. These probes are capable of performing all Doppler modalities, and M-mode, and two-dimensional imaging. The length of the gastroscope is typically 100 cm. The transducer represents the fixed portion of the probe. Adult transducers vary in length from 27 to 45 mm, are 14 to 17 mm wide, and are approximately 11 mm thick. The gastroscope cable is approximately 10 mm wide in adult probes. TEE probes 7 mm in diameter are now available and allow imaging even in infants as small as 3 kg (12). Esophageal probes have the standard gastroscope controls that allow remote movement of the transducer at the tip anteriorly, posteriorly, and to both sides. Specific positioning of the probe requires (a) advancing or withdrawing the probe within the esophagus, (b) rotation of the esophageal probe, and (c) manipulation of the tip of the probe using the controls described above (*e*Fig. 52.1.3).

Initially, esophageal probes consisted of a single transducer (*e*Fig. 52.1.2) mounted perpendicular to the long axis of the gastroscope. With this monoplane probe, cross-sectional or horizontal images of the heart are obtained, although additional imaging planes are possible by manipulation of the transducer tip. Biplane probes consist of two transducers mounted orthogonally on the probe (13). Multiplane probes are now standard with the major ultrasound systems (14,15). With this probe, the transducer is rotated either mechanically or electronically around a central axis through 180 degrees (Fig. 52.2). The horizontal transducer position is, by convention, at 0 degrees, whereas the longitudinal position is at 90 degrees. Planes not easily available with either the monoplane or biplane probe are available at intermediate degrees of rotation. The precise degree of rotation of the transducer is displayed graphically on the image.

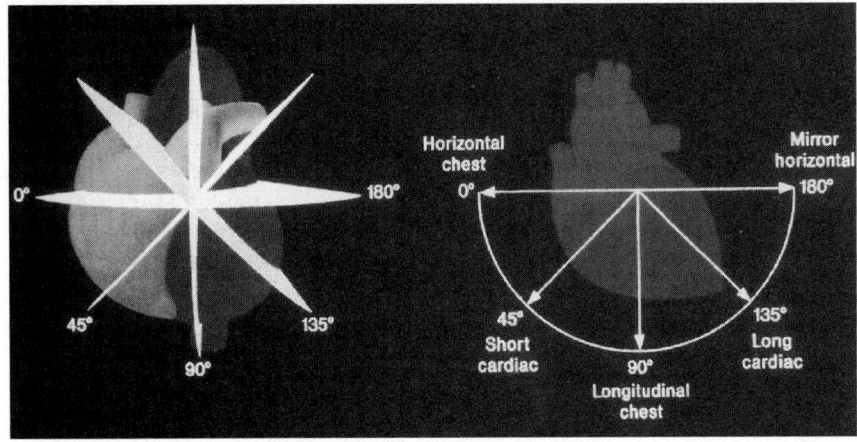

FIGURE 52.2 Scan planes of biplane and multiplane transducers. With the monoplane probe, the transducer is usually fixed and can image only in the transverse plane at zero degrees. Biplane probes have an additional transducer mounted to image in the longitudinal orientation at 90 degrees. In multiplane imaging, the transducer may rotate so that many additional imaging planes in between the transverse and longitudinal and mirror image of the transverse planes may be obtained. (From Khandheria BK. Transesophageal echocardiography in the evaluation of prosthetic valves. *Cardiol Clin* 1993;11:427–436, with permission.)

TECHNIQUE OF TRANSESOPHAGEAL ECHOCARDIOGRAPHY

TEE is performed in a manner similar to upper gastrointestinal endoscopy and requires experience in the safe intubation of the esophagus and stomach. Only operators who have adequate training in esophageal intubation and in echocardiography should perform this procedure.

Patient Selection

Patients should fast for at least 4 hours before the procedure (*e*Table 52.0.4). A detailed history should be obtained first, paying attention to a history of dysphagia, esophageal problems, and drug allergies. As the esophageal probe is passed blindly in TEE, any disorder of the esophagus that might interfere with the passage of the probe or that may lead to injury by the probe is considered a contraindication (Table 52.1). All oral prostheses and dentures are removed, and intravenous access is acquired. Blood pressure and electrocardiographic monitoring and oximetry are undertaken throughout the study. Resuscitation equipment, suction, and oxygen should be readily available. Although TEE may be performed without either pharyngeal anesthesia or seda-

TABLE 52.1 CONTRAINDICATIONS TO TRANSESOPHAGEAL ECHOCARDIOGRAPHY

1. Significant dysphagia of unknown origin
2. Significant esophageal pathology
   Esophageal diverticulum (Zenker's)
   Invasive esophageal tumor
   Esophageal stricture—undilated
   Esophageal tear, fistula, or rupture
   Severe esophagitis or ulceration
   Esophageal varices especially if recent bleed
3. Instability of the cervical vertebrae
4. Fasting <4 h
5. Uncooperative patient

tion, both of these increase patient comfort and facilitate a thorough examination (16).

Anesthesia and Sedation

Pharyngeal anesthesia helps reduce retching and gagging on probe insertion. The pharynx is sprayed with lidocaine or benzocaine. The patient may also gargle viscous lidocaine 2% for additional anesthetic effect. The effects of anesthesia are apparent within a few minutes and persist for 30 to 45 minutes after the procedure. Patients should not eat or drink during this period because of the risk of aspiration. At The Cleveland Clinic, we use both a narcotic and a benzodiazepine agent for sedation. Meperidine at a dose of 12.5 to 50.0 mg is given intravenously for its anxiolytic action. We usually start by giving 12.5 or 25.0 mg, increasing the dose as necessary while monitoring the effects on heart rate, blood pressure, and oximetry. For additional sedation and amnestic action, we give midazolam in an initial dose of 0.5 to 1.0 mg. Incremental doses are given every 3 minutes until the required effect has occurred or the vital signs suggest that further medication is contraindicated. Midazolam is a short-acting drug that has a half-life of 1 to 4 hours and that is active within 5 minutes. It can cause respiratory depression. Specific antagonists are now available: Reversed for midazolam and Naloxone for meperidine. These should be available for use in the event of significant respiratory depression or other adverse event. Additional sedative medication may be required throughout the procedure to maintain patient comfort. Ambulatory patients should be accompanied so that they do not have to drive home under the influence of sedative and narcotic drugs.

Need for Antibiotic Prophylaxis

Upper gastrointestinal endoscopy is associated with bacteremia in 4% to 8% of reported series and in 45% of patients after esophageal dilatation (17). Many patients undergoing TEE have valvular or other lesions that pose a risk for endocarditis. Individual case reports have suggested that TEE was a causative factor in the development of endocarditis (18). Several studies involving a total of 522 patients have failed to detect significant bacteremia of oral flora associated with the TEE procedure or of clinical infection at follow-up (19–21). Therefore, the risk of endocarditis with TEE in experienced hands seems low. Routine prophylaxis for the procedure is not indicated. We do not routinely give antibiotic prophylaxis for patients with valve prostheses. Antibiotic coverage may be considered if the intubation is unexpectedly difficult or traumatic.

Probe Insertion

The probe is usually inserted by having the patient assume a lateral decubitus position while maintaining flexion of the neck. The probe is guided into the upper esophagus, and then the patient is asked to swallow. As the patient swallows, the probe is gently but firmly advanced into the distal esophagus. A bite block is inserted between the teeth to protect the probe, except in edentulous patients. Probe insertion in the ventilated patient is performed with the patient in the supine position. Probe passage is facilitated by removing nonessential tubes in the oropharynx, flexion of the neck, and manual advancement of the tongue and anterior pharyngeal wall in an anterior direction. The probe should never be forcibly advanced because this risks causing an esophageal tear. If the probe does not pass smoothly, assistance from an endoscopist should be sought. At the end of the procedure, the patient should be monitored until vital signs have returned to basal or at least normal values and the sedation has begun to wear off. The probe is washed and then sterilized by immersion in an antimicrobial solution (Cidex, Surgikos Inc.) for 20 minutes. The probe is rinsed and allowed to air dry.

SAFETY AND COMPLICATIONS OF TRANSESOPHAGEAL ECHOCARDIOGRAPHY

Although TEE is invasive and is often performed on critically ill patients, successful intubation is possible in more than 98% of appropriately selected patients, and complications are uncommon (*e*Fig. 52.2.1) (1,2). Inability to pass the probe is most often due to operator inexperience, patient noncompliance, and, rarely, pathologic lesions in the esophagus. Once successful probe passage has occurred, early cessation of the procedure occurs in less than 1% of cases. This is most often due to patient intolerance of the probe rather than the onset of a complication (1). The complication rate of TEE varies with the setting in which it is performed and the experience of the opera-

tor. TEE in the emergency room is reported to have a higher complication rate, likely due to the acuity of illness in this setting (22).

Major Complications

Major complications such as death, esophageal perforation, serious arrhythmia, congestive heart failure, and laryngospasm are uncommon and occur in less than 0.3% of patients (1). One death was reported out of 3,827 consecutive patients examined in one series. This was due to arrhythmia after the procedure in a patient with autopsy-proven myocarditis (2). Another death was reported in a series of 10,419 patients. This was due to esophageal perforation in a patient with unsuspected neoplasm that had invaded the esophagus (1). A third death after TEE has been reported in a patient with acute aortic dissection in whom aortic rupture occurred during a bout of severe retching and nausea after probe insertion (23). Serious esophageal injury may occur, and both esophageal perforation and tear have been reported (24). Absence of significant damage to the mucosal lining of the esophagus after prolonged TEE examination has been demonstrated in animals (25). Laryngospasm and severe bronchospasm occasionally occur because of aspiration of anesthetic agents or lubricants used for probe insertion and rarely from inadvertent passage of the probe into the airway (26).

Minor Complications

Minor complications such as transient hypoxia, hypotension, hypertension, angina, bronchospasm, atrioventricular block, supraventricular tachycardia, and nonsustained ventricular arrhythmia occur in less than 3% of cases (2). Transient vocal cord paralysis has been noted in patients undergoing neurosurgical procedures who were studied in the upright position (27). Compression of anomalous vascular structures by the esophageal probe has also been reported (28). Sore throat and mild dysphagia is common after the procedure and rarely is prolonged for more than 24 hours. Toxic and allergic reactions to the drugs used in patient preparation occur but are uncommon. The most common reaction encountered is methemoglobinemia in susceptible subjects receiving topical anesthesia (29).

Technical Problems

A number of technical factors may affect the quality of the TEE examination. These include air in the esophagus and stomach and poor contact between the probe and the esophagus. Distorted anatomy from prior surgery, a tortuous aorta, or a large hiatal hernia may also interfere with imaging. Problems with the probe during the procedure such as mechanical or electronic failure occur but are uncommon (1,30).

IMAGING PLANES

The esophageal window imposes a number of challenges in imaging the heart and related structures in a standard format. The esophagus is not usually precisely aligned with the true long and short axis of the heart (Fig. 52.3). Furthermore, the relationship between the esophagus and cardiac structures is variable. Standard imaging planes have been described for TEE. However, the maneuvers required to acquire them are not always predictable but are facilitated by multiplane technology. Interpretation of esophageal images is often challenging initially despite their high quality. The orientation of the images is different to TTE, as the images are acquired from behind rather than from the front of the heart. The multiple imaging planes available and the ability to resolve structures rarely visible with other imaging modalities add to the initial difficulty. TEE requires a familiarity with the three-dimensional anatomy of the heart and aorta as imaged from the esophagus. This can best be obtained by performance of multiple procedures while supervised by an experienced operator. The transesophageal examination is usually goal-oriented. Specific questions unanswered by the prior transthoracic study are first addressed, followed by a comprehensive evaluation of other structures. It is important to follow a standard examination format encompassing all major cardiac structures and the aorta so that a complete examination is always performed.

Base of the Heart

At approximately 30 cm from the incisors, the probe lies behind the left atrium and the base of the heart. In the transverse plane at this level, the aortic valve is seen in cross-section, with portions of the left and right atrium and interatrial septum (Fig. 52.4). Withdrawing the probe slightly from this view allows imaging of the left atrial appendage, the superior vena cava, the right ventricular outflow tract, ostia of the coronary vessels and the main pulmonary artery to its bifurcation, and a portion of the right pulmonary artery. The proximal portion of the ascending aorta is imaged in this view but it and the distal portions of the left pulmonary artery are difficult to image because of the interposition of air-filled large airways. The longitudinal imaging plane at this level provides important images of the great vessels, interatrial septum, left atrial appendage, and pulmonary veins. When the transducer is rotated to the left, a two-chamber view of the left atrium and left ventricle is seen. The left atrial appendage and the left pulmonary veins are often most easily imaged in this view. The mitral valve is also well seen in this view, and mitral regurgitation may be sought here. With clockwise rotation of the probe around its long axis, the right ventricular outflow tract, pulmonary valve, and main pulmonary artery may be imaged. With additional clockwise rotation,

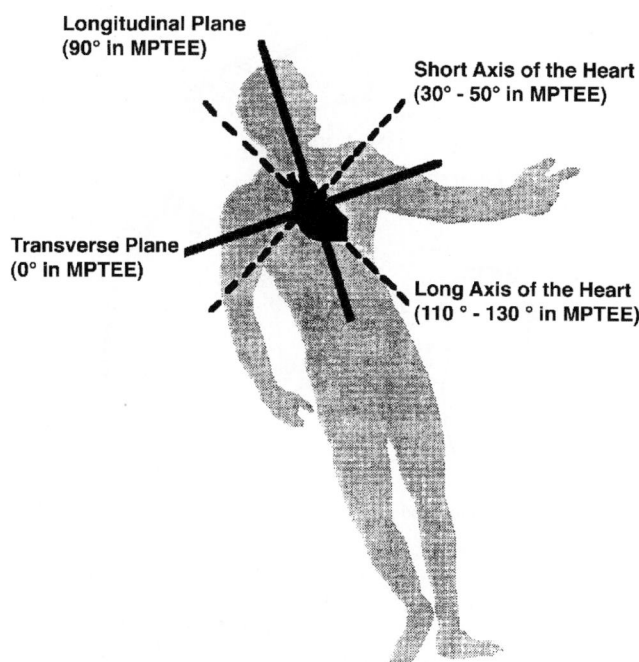

FIGURE 52.3 Relationship of horizontal and vertical vectors of the heart to those of the body and esophagus. The transverse (0-degree) and longitudinal (90-degree) esophageal imaging planes do not parallel the true short and long axis of the heart, which are imaged at 30 to 50 degrees and 110 to 130 degrees, respectively. The true short and long axis varies with individual habitus. MPTEE, multiplane transesophageal echocardiography. (From Schneider AT, Hsu TL, Schwartz S, Pandian NG. Single, biplane, multiplane, and three-dimensional transesophageal echocardiography. Echocardiographic-anatomic correlations. *Cardiol Clin* 1993;11:361–387, with permission.)

the aortic valve and ascending aorta are seen. This view is important in the evaluation of the ascending aorta particularly with regard to dissection and in assessing aortic regurgitation. Finally, with further clockwise rotation, the right atrium, interatrial septum, and superior vena cava may be imaged. This plane is important in the detection of a communication at the atrial level and in assessing pathology of the superior vena cava. Multiplane imaging is especially useful at this level in allowing the true long and short axis of the aortic valve and ascending aorta to be obtained. Typically, the true short axis is seen at approximately 30 to 60 degrees and the true long axis at 120 to 150 degrees (*e*Fig. 52.4.1).

Midesophageal Views

By advancing the probe into the midesophagus beyond the base of the heart, portions of both atria and ventricles, the interventricular septum, and the mitral and tricuspid valves are seen in the transverse imaging plane (Fig. 52.4). A four-chamber view is acquired at this level by flexing the probe posteriorly. This view is similar to the apical four-chamber view acquired transthoracically, except that the imaging plane does not cut through the true apex. This

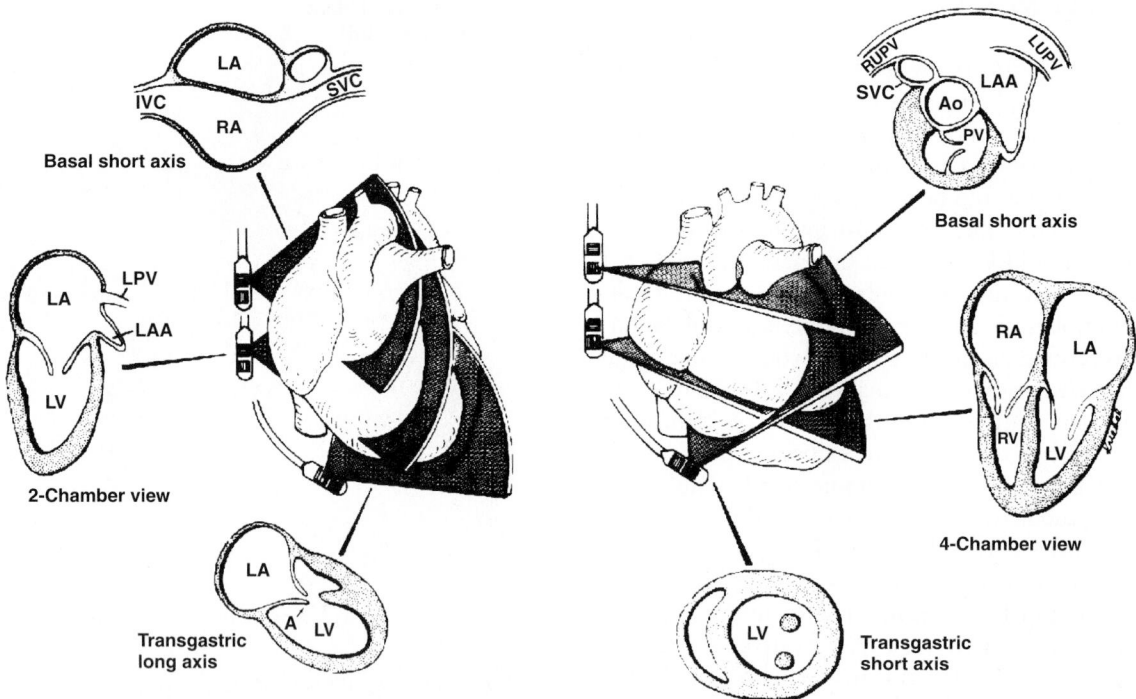

FIGURE 52.4 Transverse **(A)** and longitudinal **(B)** imaging planes at base of the heart, midesophagus, and transgastric windows. A, anterior leaflet of the mitral valve; Ao, aorta; IVC, inferior vena cava; LA, left atrium; LAA, left atrial appendage; LPV, left pulmonary vein; LUPV, left upper pulmonary vein; LV, left ventricle; PV, pulmonary valve; RA, right atrium; RUPV, right upper pulmonary vein; RV, right ventricle; SVC, superior vena cava. (From Fisher EA, Stahl JA, Budd JH, Goldman ME. Transesophageal echocardiography: procedures and clinical application. *J Am Coll Cardiol* 1991;18:1333–1348, with permission.)

represents an inherent limitation of transesophageal imaging in the acquisition of ventricular volumes and in the detection of apical thrombus. This imaging plane is helpful in detecting regurgitation at the mitral and tricuspid valves and in global assessment of ventricular function. With slight counterclockwise rotation of the transducer, the left ventricular outflow tract and the proximal ascending aorta are seen. Longitudinal imaging at this level produces a two-chamber image of the heart already described. Multiplane images at this level are useful in distinguishing the individual leaflets of the mitral valve and the scallops of the posterior leaflet and in detecting eccentric jets of mitral regurgitation. Optimal differentiation between anterior and posterior mitral leaflet pathology is at approximately 140 degrees, whereas the full extent of the mitral closure line, from medial to lateral commissure, is at approximately 50 degrees.

Transgastric Views

To obtain the transgastric series of views, the probe is advanced into the stomach. Generally, the tip of the probe must be flexed to bring the transducer in contact with the mucosa of the gastric fundus. In the transverse plane, a short-axis view of the left and right ventricle is acquired

(Fig. 52.4). With increased anteflexion of the probe, the base of the heart and the mitral and tricuspid valves are imaged, whereas lesser degrees of anteflexion bring the image more toward the apex. This view allows an assessment of regional and global left ventricular function. The mitral valve apparatus and leaflets are also well seen in this view. This view is most often used when ventricular function is being monitored. A longitudinal view at this level allows the mitral valve and the left ventricle to be imaged in long axis. The anterior and inferior walls are well seen, as are the papillary muscles and chordae. The true apex of the heart is most likely to be displayed in this view. Rotation of the probe in the long axis frequently allows the left ventricular outflow tract to be aligned with the Doppler cursor so that a Doppler evaluation of the aortic valve and left ventricular outflow tract may be performed. Further rotation allows examination of the right ventricle and outflow tract. Multiplane imaging at this level facilitates the evaluation of the left ventricular outflow tract and examination of the tricuspid valve and its component leaflets. Another series of images is frequently possible by passing the probe further into the stomach and anteflexing (the deep transgastric view). In this view, the transducer is close to the apex, and the images obtained simulate those acquired in a transthoracic five-chamber or subcostal view.

This view often optimizes Doppler interrogation of the aortic valve and outflow tract.

Aorta

The aorta may be examined from the ascending aorta to below the diaphragm (Fig. 52.5). The examination of the ascending aorta has already been described. The distal portion of the ascending aorta cannot be examined using the transverse plane because of the interposition of the trachea. The longitudinal and multiplane imaging planes may allow an additional area of imaging, but not all of the ascending aorta can be identified. The descending aorta is evaluated by rotating the probe to the left and posteriorly at midesophageal level. The aorta is seen in cross-section using the transverse transducer at this level and in long axis using the longitudinal transducer. More distal portions of the aorta are examined by advancing the probe, whereas the proximal portions of the descending aorta are imaged by withdrawing the probe and rotating anteriorly and to the left to keep the aorta in view. As the probe is withdrawn to approximately 20 to 25 cm, the transverse arch and distal portions of the ascending aorta are seen. The transverse plane cuts the arch in long axis at this level, and the longitudinal plane provides a short-axis view. The proximal portions of the left subclavian and other head and neck vessels may be imaged with a longitudinal or multiplane transducer. Examination of the aortic arch is usually performed last, as the probe often elicits a gag reflex at this level, even in well-prepared patients.

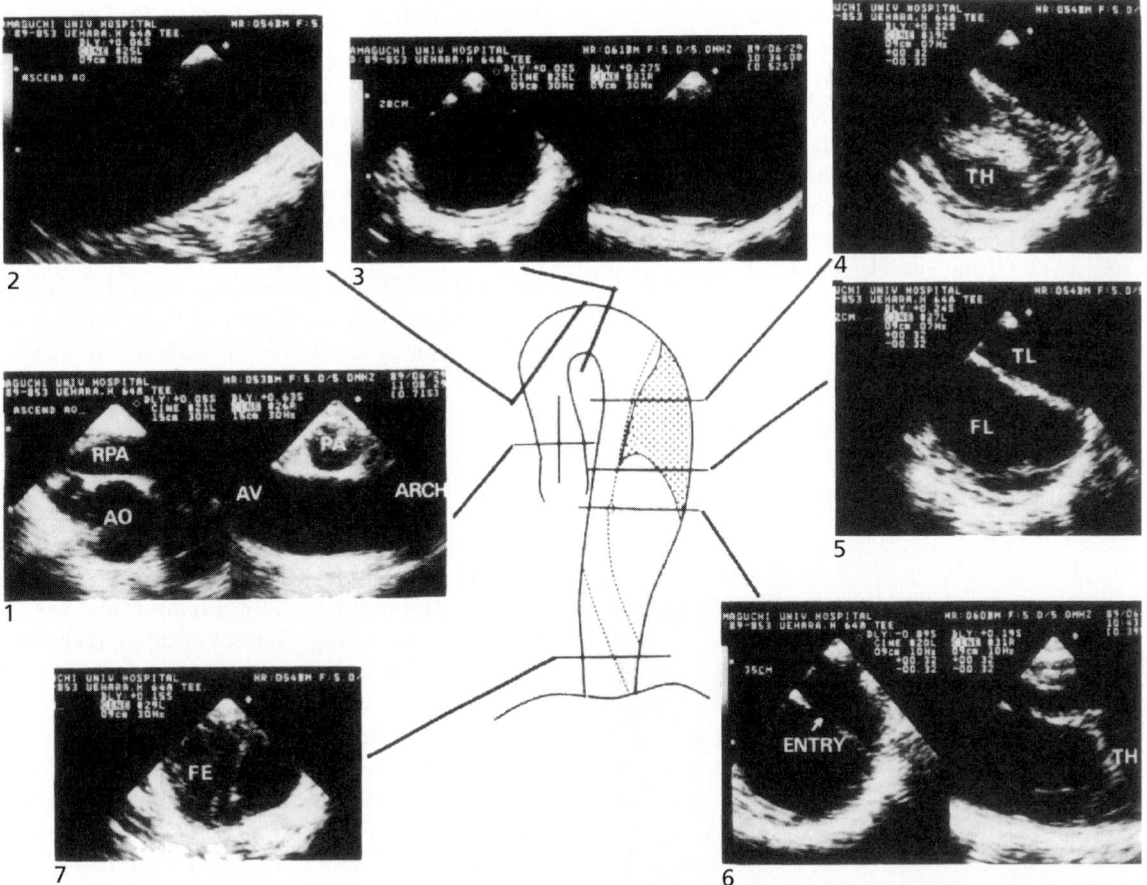

FIGURE 52.5 Imaging planes of aorta. Biplane imaging planes of the aorta illustrated in a patient with dissection flap confined to the distal aorta. **Panel 1:** Transverse (*left*) and longitudinal plane (*right*) images of the ascending aorta. **Panel 2:** Transverse plane image of the aortic arch. **Panel 3:** Transverse (*left*) and longitudinal (*right*) plane images of the proximal descending aorta at the junction with the arch. **Panels 4–7:** Transverse (**panels 4–7**) and longitudinal (**panel 6,** *right*) plane images of the aortic dissection flap and its variable orientation in various portions of the descending aorta. AO, aorta; AV, aortic valve; Entry, communication between true and false lumen; FL, false lumen; PA, pulmonary artery; RPA, right pulmonary artery; TH, thrombus; TL, true lumen. (From Matsuzaki M, Toma Y, Kusukawa R. Clinical applications of transesophageal echocardiography. *Circulation* 1990;82:709–722, with permission.)

INDICATIONS FOR TRANSESOPHAGEAL ECHOCARDIOGRAPHY

Left and Right Atria

Atrial Thrombus

TEE is now the technique of choice in the evaluation of atrial thrombus (*e*Fig. 52.5.1 and Fig. 52.6) and is superior to TTE in detecting atrial appendage thrombus (31,32). Left atrial thrombus is associated with mitral stenosis, atrial dilatation, atrial fibrillation, left ventricular dysfunction, or a combination of these factors (33) and is an independent risk factor for thromboembolism (34). The sensitivity and specificity of TEE in the detection of thrombus in both the body and appendage (32) of the left atrium are excellent and have exceeded 90% in a number of large series with surgical validation (35), as compared with less than 50% for TTE. TEE has shown that patients with atrial flutter are also at risk for development of atrial thrombus and are thus at risk of embolization especially with cardioversion (36). Patients with atrial fibrillation and mitral valve disease frequently undergo ligation of the atrial appendage. TEE has shown that flow may persist into the atrial appendage despite surgical ligation in more than one of three patients and who therefore remain at risk of thrombus formation and embolization from the atrial appendage. (37). TEE is also superior to TTE in the detection of right atrial thrombus (38).

Spontaneous Contrast

TEE often identifies swirling echoes of spontaneous contrast in the left atrium or appendage, especially in those with atrial fibrillation or atrial thrombus (*e*Fig. 52.6.1)

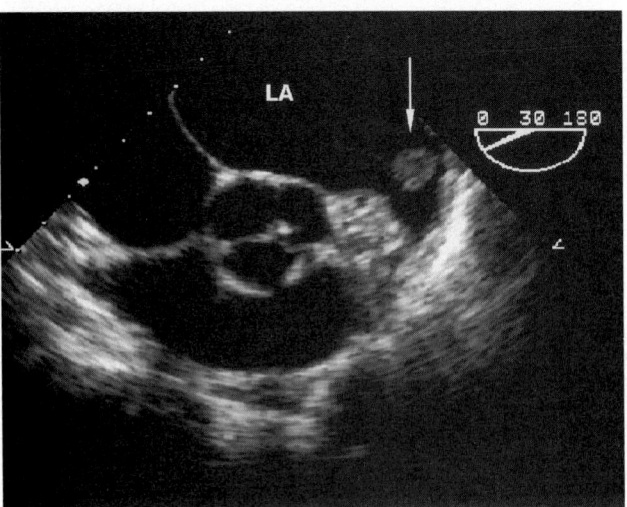

FIGURE 52.6 Left atrial appendage thrombus (*arrow*). LA, left atrium.

(39). This is reported in as many as 20% of all patients undergoing TEE but is rarely seen in TTE (39,40). The level of intensity of the contrast varies within the atrium and appendage and is most dense in areas of lowest flow such as the atrial appendage. The precise mechanism of its generation is uncertain but is thought to relate to rouleaux formation of red blood cells in areas of low flow (40,41). This theory is supported by the reduced incidence of this phenomenon after successful dilatation of stenotic mitral valves (42). Anticoagulation has not been shown to affect the prevalence or intensity of spontaneous contrast (40,41). Spontaneous contrast in the left atrium is an independent risk factor for systemic embolization in both mitral stenosis and nonvalvular atrial fibrillation (41,43). Spontaneous contrast occurs in 2% of patients with sinus rhythm and is an independent risk factor for stroke (44).

Transesophageal Echocardiography Screening before Mitral Valvuloplasty and Cardioversion

Atrial thrombus poses a risk for embolization during percutaneous mitral valvuloplasty and electrical cardioversion of atrial fibrillation (52). TEE has been used to screen for atrial thrombus before these procedures. TEE detected atrial thrombus in 26% of 19 patients being considered for balloon valvuloplasty of the mitral valve, only one of which was detected by TTE (53). Patients with atrial thrombus detected by TEE were excluded from the procedure. TEE has also been used to allow early cardioversion of patients with chronic atrial fibrillation without the standard 3 to 4 weeks of systemic anticoagulation. In one prospective study of TEE cardioversion, left atrial thrombus was found in 15% of 233 patients with atrial fibrillation of unknown or prolonged duration (39). Cardioversion was performed without a prolonged interval of anticoagulation in those without evidence of atrial thrombus and no embolic complications were recorded (39). A prospective randomized trial of prolonged anticoagulation versus TEE cardioversion (Assessment of Cardioversion Using Transesophageal Echocardiography study) (54) has been completed. The embolic event rate in both the TEE and conventional group were lower than expected and similar. Although inadequately powered to show a difference between the two strategies, this study convincingly demonstrates a low embolic event rate associated with TEE-guided cardioversion. TEE cardioversion was associated with a shorter duration of anticoagulation but not with a greater likelihood of remaining in sinus rhythm (55). TEE cardioversion appears to be particularly cost-effective in patients with increased risk of hemorrhage with anticoagulation (56). Thromboembolic complications have been reported in patients who were cardioverted despite TEE results that were negative for atrial thrombus but who were inadequately anticoagulated (57). Temporary deterioration of atrial function after return of normal sinus rhythm with subsequent thrombus formation and embolization is postulated to account for these embolic events rather than embolization of thrombus undetected by TEE (46,48,58). The deterioration in atrial function occurs even with chemical cardioversion (59) and does not occur after delivery of a shock to the atrium in patients with normal sinus rhythm (60). The deterioration in atrial function is less after atrial flutter conversion as compared with atrial fibrillation (61). Anticoagulation for a number of weeks is indicated after cardioversion even when TEE does not show atrial thrombus to minimize the risk of embolism after the procedure.

Interatrial Septum

Atrial Septal Defect

TEE is the technique of choice in the diagnosis of abnormalities of the interatrial septum. The atrial septum is visualized in the long-axis view of the base of the heart. TEE is especially useful in the detection of small atrial septal defects (less than 5 mm) (62) and of sinus venosus defects. In one study, TEE detected all sinus venosus defects, whereas only 25% were detected by TTE (63). Anomalous drainage of pulmonary veins, which often accompanies sinus venosus–type defects, is also reliably detected by TEE (63). TEE measurements of anatomic size and shunt flow compare well with those measured at the time of surgery (64).

Patent Foramen Ovale

Patent foramen ovale occurs in 25% to 30% of the normal population and is more commonly found in those with unexplained stroke (*e*Fig. 52.6.3) (65,66). The latter finding and the TEE demonstration of passage of a paradoxical embolus through a patent foramen ovale support its causative role in cerebral embolism (Fig. 52.7) (67). TEE is highly sensitive and specific in the detection of patent foramen ovale and is superior to TTE (68). In one study, TEE detected all of the defects subsequently found at autopsy (69). In another study, patent foramen ovale was detected by TEE in 22% of patients and only in 8% by TTE (70). Contrast venous injection is useful in the detection of right-to-left shunting, whereas color-flow imaging is the method of choice in detecting left-to-right shunting (71). Both color-flow and contrast techniques are performed in practice. Characteristics of patent foramen ovale by TEE that predict an increased likelihood of embolic event include larger size and increased shunt flow across the defect (72).

Atrial Septal Aneurysm

Atrial septal aneurysm (ASA) is also a risk factor for cerebral embolism and is detected more frequently by TEE than by conventional echocardiography (73). ASA occurs in 2.2% of the population and is associated with a single patent foramen ovale or rarely with multiple fenestrations

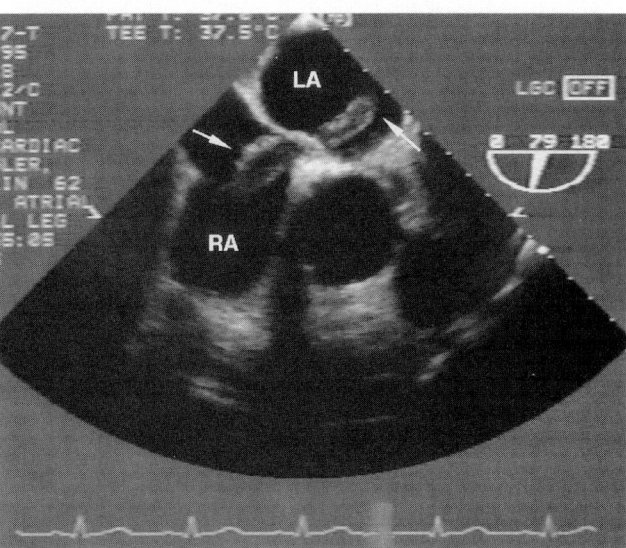

FIGURE 52.7 Embolus in transit across a patent foramen ovale (*arrows*). LA, left atrium; RA, right atrium.

(74,75). It is three times more common in those with a history of cerebral ischemia (74). The embolic risk of this condition is due to the associated shunt or rarely to thrombus formation within the aneurysm, which occurs in 1% of patients with ASA (76). An ASA is recognized by the finding of a redundant highly mobile outpouching of the atrial septum that is at least 10 mm wide and 15 mm long. (Fig. 52.8). In a multicenter study, TEE detected 195 patients with this entity, whereas only half of these were detected by TTE (76). Half of the patients had evidence of an atrial shunt, whereas embolic events had occurred in 44%.

Other Atrial Abnormalities

The membrane of cor triatriatum is particularly well-delineated by TEE. Atrial tumors such as myxomas are usually well-characterized by TTE. TEE is useful when there is diagnostic uncertainty and is superior in detecting the site of attachment to the wall and the composition of the tumor (*e*Fig. 52.8.1) (77). It is also useful in elucidating the nature of other masses suspected by TTE and in distinguishing them from normal variants.

Endocarditis

Diagnosis

Echocardiography is now an integral part of the evaluation of suspected endocarditis (78). TEE is more sensitive in diagnosing endocarditis, as it provides better resolution of vegetations than TTE. In one study, TTE detected 63% of vegetations, whereas TEE detected all of them (Fig. 52.9) (79). In that study, TTE had equivalent diagnostic accuracy to TEE in detection of vegetations greater than 11 mm but

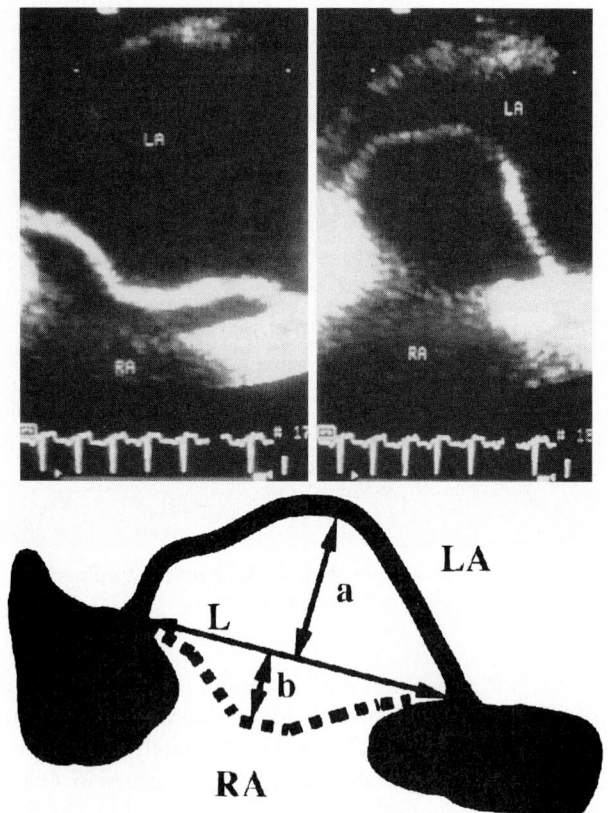

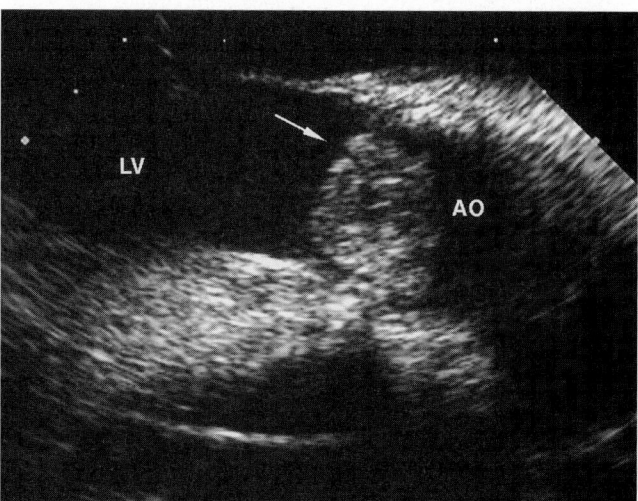

FIGURE 52.9 Long-axis view of fungal vegetation of aortic valve (*arrow*). AO, aorta; LV, left ventricle.

FIGURE 52.8 Mobile atrial septal aneurysm by transesophageal echocardiography. Bottom panel illustrates measurements. a and b, maximal extent of oscillation into left and right atrium, respectively; L, length; LA, left atrium; RA, right atrium. (From Mugge A, Daniel WG, Angermann C, et al. Atrial septal aneurysm in adult patients. A multicenter study using transthoracic and transesophageal echocardiography. *Circulation* 1995;91:2785–2792, with permission.)

only detected 25% of vegetations less than 5 mm in size and 69% of vegetations of a size between 6 and 10 mm. In other studies in which the ability of TEE and TTE to detect vegetations has been compared, the sensitivity of TTE has varied from 25% to 60%, whereas that of TEE has varied from 87% to 100% (79–81). Both TEE and TTE have a reported specificity in the diagnosis of vegetations of more than 90% (81,82). The superiority of TEE in the detection of prosthetic endocarditis is even greater than for native-valve disease (*e*Fig. 52.9.1). The sensitivity of TEE and TTE in detecting prosthetic endocarditis is more than 80% and less than 45%, respectively (83,84). Vegetations on the tricuspid valve are detected with equal frequency by TEE and TTE (85). However, endocarditis of the pulmonary valve is more often recognized by TEE than by TTE (86), as is endocarditis at unusual sites such as on pacemaker wires (87).

Complications

TEE is more reliable than TTE in detecting perforation of a valve leaflet in endocarditis (88). TEE can detect pyogenic

complications of endocarditis such as abscess and fistula formation (Fig. 52.10 and *e*Fig. 52.10.1) more readily than TTE (89,90). These complications are associated with increased mortality, usually require operative intervention for successful treatment, and occur in approximately one-third of endocarditis cases. They occur most often with staphylococcal infections of the aortic valve and in prosthetic endocarditis (89,91,92). The sensitivity of TEE in the detection of abscess or infected pseudoaneurysm has been reported at 87% to 100%, whereas that of TTE has varied from 28% to 43% (89,92) (Fig. 52.10). TEE is more reliable (100% sensitive) than TTE (32% sensitive) in the detection of endocarditis in patients with *Staphylococcus aureus* sepsis. Endocarditis may exist in 25% of such patients and when present carries a fivefold increase in mortality as compared with sepsis without endocarditis (93). TEE has also been shown to be both useful and cost-effective in following patients with catheter-associated sepsis to determine the duration of antibiotic treatment (94).

Predictive Value and Usefulness of Transesophageal Echocardiography in Endocarditis

Failure of TEE to detect vegetations in suspected endocarditis has a high negative predictive value. In one study, no evidence of endocarditis was noted on TEE in 65 of 105 patients with suspected endocarditis (95). Of these 65, definite endocarditis developed in only five (7%) on subsequent follow-up. However, TEE may fail to detect endocarditis early in the course of the illness or after embolization of a vegetation. Serial studies are indicated if the clinical suspicion is high despite an initially negative TEE. Many findings on native and prosthetic valves may simulate vegetations. These include degenerative changes such as

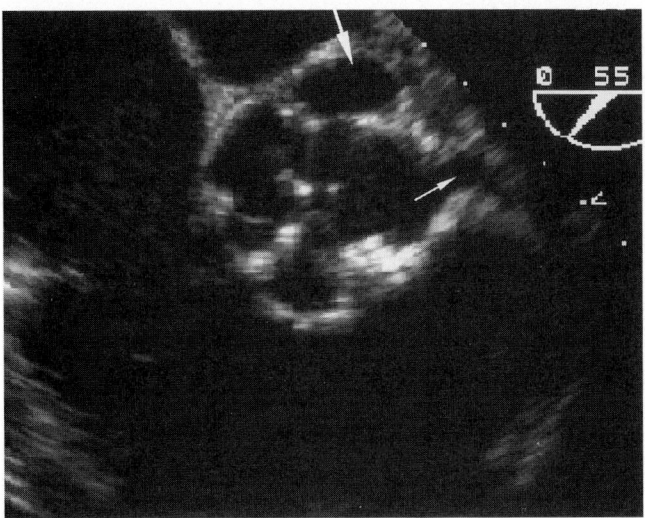

FIGURE 52.10 Short-axis view of abscess (*wide arrow*) of native aortic valve detected by multiplane transesophageal echocardiography. Left main coronary is shown by the narrow arrow.

Lambl's excrescences on the aortic valve or suture material in the case of prostheses. Comparison with prior studies is very useful in these instances. Because of the high sensitivity, specificity, and negative predictive value of TEE in the detection of endocarditis, it has been advocated as the technique of choice in the evaluation of this condition. In one study, the addition of TEE to clinical criteria increased the case detection rate from 50% using clinical criteria to 100% with TEE (96). In a study addressing the incremental usefulness of transthoracic and TEE over clinical criteria in the diagnosis of endocarditis (97), TEE was incrementally useful in patients with intermediate or high probability of disease based on clinical criteria and TTE and in those with suspected prosthetic endocarditis. TEE and TTE were equivalent in excluding endocarditis in patients with a low likelihood of endocarditis on clinical grounds. Another study has indicated that in native-valve endocarditis, an adequate TTE without evidence of endocarditis was highly accurate in excluding this diagnosis (98). TEE has been shown to improve the diagnosis of native-valve endocarditis based on the Duke criteria and TTE in 11% of the study patients, most of whom had an intermediate likelihood of disease (99).

Disease of the Aorta

TEE has become the technique of choice in many institutions in the diagnosis of acute dissection because of its high sensitivity, portability, and speed with which the diagnosis may be made (101). It is also used in diagnosis of aortic trauma and aortic atheroma. TEE is less often used as the primary diagnostic technique in evaluating other aortic pathologies, such as saccular aneurysm, which are effectively imaged by competing technologies such as

computed tomography scanning and magnetic resonance imaging (MRI).

Aortic Dissection

TEE has been used as the sole diagnostic tool in the evaluation of suspected dissection, with excellent results (102). In one study of 45 patients who underwent TEE for evaluation of suspected dissection, only one required a further study for additional information (103). None of the 24 patients without evidence of dissection on their initial examination required additional investigation of their aorta over 2 years of follow-up. Other imaging modalities used in the assessment of aortic dissection include MRI, angiography, and computed tomography scanning (104). *e*Table 52.1.1 provides a summary of the relative strengths and weaknesses of these imaging tests in the diagnosis of dissection and its complications.

Diagnosis of Dissection

TEE has been reported to be more than 95% sensitive in the detection of aortic dissection in multiple studies (Fig. 52.11) (105–107). The detection rate reported is somewhat less for dissection involving the ascending aorta mainly because of the blind spot in the distal ascending aorta and proximal arch already described (105,108). The detection rate is also lower in patients who have had prior surgery of the aorta (109), when the dissection flap is very localized, or when the false lumen is thrombosed (110,111). The reported specificity of TEE in the detection of aortic dissection has varied from 68% to 100% (105–107,112). Studies that have shown perfect specificity have generally included only patients in whom the diagnosis was already established, whereas those with low specificity have used monoplane probes or less stringent criteria for diagnosis (106). False positives are most common in the ascending aorta and are often due to reverberation simulating a dissection flap (106,113). These may be minimized by the use of a biplane or multiplane probe (114). M-mode echocardiography is useful in timing and localizing reverberation (115). The presence of a flow disturbance on color-flow mapping at the site of the supposed dissection flap increases the likelihood of a true diagnosis. Recourse to other confirmatory techniques such as MRI or angiography should be made if the diagnosis is indeterminate by TEE (104). Operator experience is an important determinant of overall specificity.

Assessment of Prognostic Features and Complications of Dissection

TEE provides important information concerning prognosis, complications, and surgical intervention in aortic dissection. Aortic dissection is most conveniently classified based on the presence (type A) or absence (type B) of a

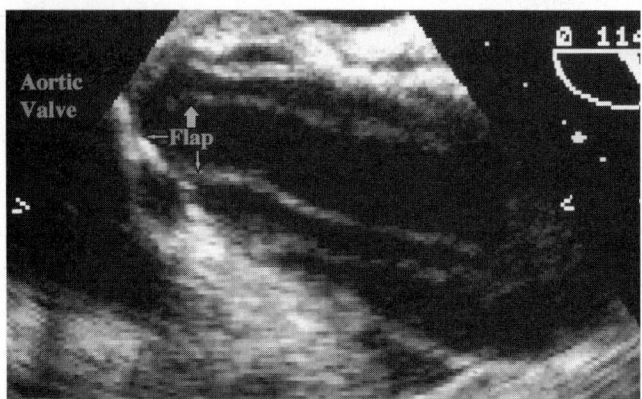

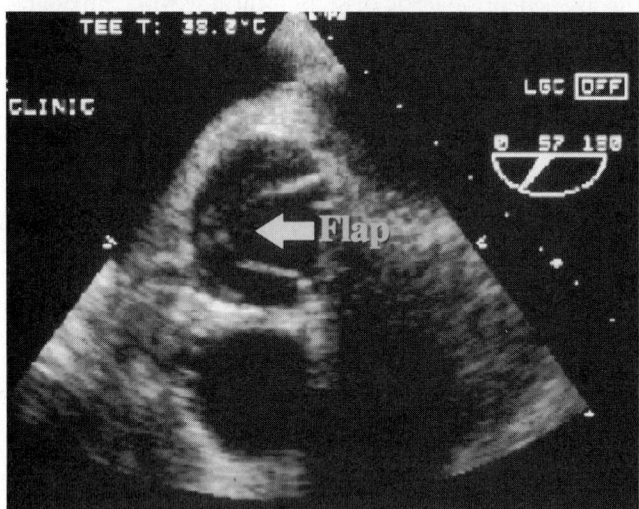

FIGURE 52.11 Aortic dissection with flap in ascending aorta. **A:** Long axis. **B:** Short axis.

dissection flap in the ascending aorta. This classification is important prognostically. Type A aneurysms are considered for urgent surgery, whereas type B aneurysms are initially treated medically. The accuracy of classification of dissection by TEE has varied from 89% to 100% (102,112). Detection of the primary tear between the true and false lumen is important, as surgical plication of this communication may reduce and even obliterate flow in the false lumen and thus reduce the risk of late rupture. The primary entry site is most often in the ascending aorta and is detected in 73% to 89% of type A dissections (102,107). Other sites of communication between true and false lumen are frequently detected by TEE (*e*Fig. 52.11.1).

Thrombus in the false lumen, a favorable prognostic feature, is also accurately detected by TEE. Important complications of dissection such as pericardial effusion, cardiac tamponade, the mechanism and severity of aortic regurgitation, and involvement of the coronary ostia are also accurately diagnosed by TEE. In one study, TEE correctly identified six of seven dissections involving the coronary ostia that were confirmed surgically (112). TEE can also

detect other causes of chest pain when dissection is excluded. These include other aortic abnormalities and myocardial ischemia or infarction (116).

Limitations of Transesophageal Echocardiography in Dissection

Side branches, the head and neck vessels, and involvement of the abdominal aorta and branches and the distal coronaries are often not visualized by TEE. These are rarely crucial to surgical intervention for acute type A dissection. Supplemental imaging of the abdominal and head and neck vessels is possible with subcostal and suprasternal TTE. In chronic dissection, angiography and other imaging studies such as MRI may be performed to define the coronary anatomy and involvement of other branch vessels if surgery is planned.

Aortic Trauma

TEE has become an important tool in the rapid evaluation of aortic injury after major trauma. Aortic trauma most often involves the aortic isthmus just distal to the ligamentum arteriosum. Subadventitial disruption requires immediate surgical intervention and is recognized echocardiographically as a dense, thick, mobile flap that represents the disrupted intima and media. Asymmetric aortic enlargement is seen in this area due to the formation of a pseudoaneurysm. TEE can be performed rapidly and safely in trauma patients and is accurate in the detection of significant aortic disruption (122). Sensitivity and specificity of more than 90% have been reported in a number of studies of TEE in aortic trauma patients (122,123).

Aortic Atherosclerosis

Aortic atheroma is seen as echodense thickening of the intimal surface with superimposed thrombus or calcification in many instances. Involvement of the aorta varies from discrete plaques to diffuse thickening. TEE detection and classification of aortic atheromatous plaque shows good agreement with the pathologic findings (124). Aortic atheroma is most commonly seen in the descending thoracic aorta, less often in the aortic arch, and least often in the ascending aorta (125). Aortic atheroma on TEE is a sensitive marker of significant coronary disease (126) and of extensive peripheral vascular and carotid disease (127). Plaque in the aortic arch of more than 4 mm in thickness by TEE was an independent risk factor for ischemic stroke in one study (128). This risk appears to be lowered to a greater degree by oral anticoagulation rather than by antiplatelet drugs (129,130). Other studies have indicated that aortic atheroma on TEE increases the risk of perioperative stroke in patients undergoing bypass surgery and of atherogenic embolism after other procedures (131,132). The morphology of the plaque has independent predictive value. The likelihood of an embolic event is greatest with complex mobile plaque and least with sessile plaque (*e*Fig. 52.11.2). In one study, complex atherosclerotic plaque was seen in 7% of 556 consecutive patients being evaluated by TEE. Systemic thromboembolism subsequently occurred in 73% of these patients but only in 12% of those with sessile plaque (133). Protruding atheroma was an independent risk factor for stroke in another study (134). Complex atheroma has been shown to be associated with a high prevalence of high-intensity transient signals in cerebral arteries, which further supports its role in cerebral embolism (135). The presence of spontaneous contrast in the aorta is an independent embolic risk factor (136) as well as a risk factor for cardiac mortality (137). Recently, mobile thrombus has been detected by TEE in younger patients with systemic embolism in the absence of diffuse aortic atheroma. Underlying atherosclerosis at the insertion site of the thrombus has been demonstrated histologically in patients who have undergone surgical removal of the thrombus (138).

Other Aortic Conditions

TEE can characterize thoracic aneurysms involving the sinuses of Valsalva and the ascending and descending aorta. It is useful in improving the resolution of sinus of Valsalva aneurysm and in detecting communication with individual cardiac chambers.

Native-Valve Disease

Transthoracic imaging can usually provide a complete anatomic and hemodynamic profile of abnormal valves. TEE is used in addition when improved resolution of valve structure is needed or when the hemodynamic severity of a regurgitant lesion is in question. Assessment of valve lesions to determine their suitability for repair or reconstruction is an increasing indication for TEE during cardiac surgery.

Mitral Valve

TEE is highly sensitive and specific in the detection of flail mitral valve leaflets and chordae and is superior to TTE in differentiating flail leaflets from vegetations (139,140). TEE is also superior in defining the mechanism of regurgitation, the site of regurgitation, the likelihood of repair, and a subset of patients at greatest risk for the development of complications such as systolic motion of the mitral valve after repair for myxomatous disease (141–143). It is more sensitive than either TTE or angiography in the detection of mitral regurgitation (Fig. 52.12). In one study, mitral regurgitation was present on TEE in 25% of patients in whom it could not be detected by TTE, and in 14% of these patients the regurgitation was at least of moderate

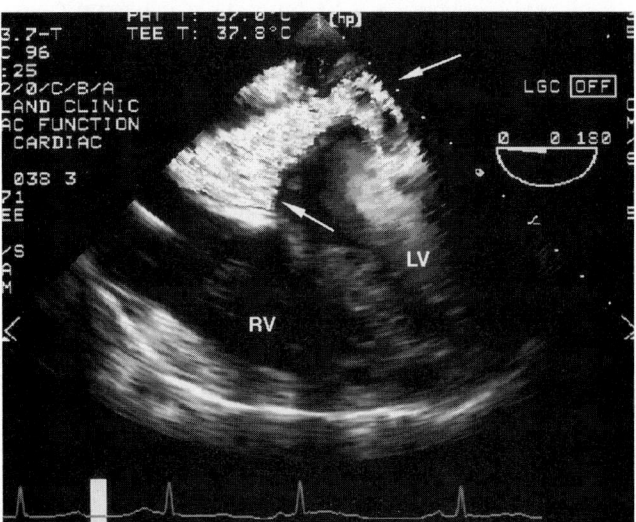

FIGURE 52.12 Severe anteriorly directed mitral regurgitation due to a flail posterior leaflet (*arrows*) imaged in the transverse four-chamber view. LV, left ventricle; RV, right ventricle.

severity (144). The superior ability of TEE to detect mitral regurgitation is most marked in critically ill ventilated patients with acute ischemia or infarction (145). TEE is superior to transthoracic echo in the detection of papillary muscle rupture in this population (146). Multiplane TEE is superior to TTE in the detection of eccentric regurgitant jets (114). The size of the regurgitant jet on color-flow mapping often appears larger by TEE than by TTE (147). This discrepancy is attributable to the proximity of the jet to the transducer and the higher carrier frequency of the Doppler used by TEE. When the area of high-velocity turbulent, or "mosaic," flow alone is used in the assessment of regurgitant severity, a good correlation with angiographic grading is noted (148).

Parameters other than regurgitant jet size are available with TEE in assessing severity of mitral regurgitation. These include the size of the regurgitant jet at its origin and the size of the area of flow acceleration just proximal to the regurgitant orifice (proximal flow convergence area). Both of these relate well to the size of the regurgitant orifice area and are less dependent on loading conditions than regurgitant jet area or length (149,150). Analysis of pulmonary vein flow is a useful parameter in confirming the severity of mitral regurgitation. High-quality Doppler recordings of both left and right pulmonary veins are readily obtained by TEE (151,152). Systolic flow reversal in a pulmonary vein is an accurate marker of severe mitral regurgitation. Blunting of the systolic flow is suggestive of significant mitral regurgitation in the setting of normal ventricular function and normal sinus rhythm but is unreliable otherwise (153). Quantification of mitral regurgitation is usually possible by TEE with methods based on both pulsed Doppler and the proximal flow convergence area with TEE (154,155). Planimetry of the mitral orifice in cross-section in mitral stenosis is more difficult with TEE than with TTE but is sometimes possible with multiplane imaging.

Aortic and Other Valves

Multiplane TEE has facilitated imaging of the aortic valve and allows the true long and short axis to be acquired. High-resolution images obtained by this technique are useful in diagnosing a bicuspid valve or other structural abnormality when TTE is uncertain (*e*Fig. 52.12.1). In a recent study with operative corroboration, multiplane TEE was significantly better than TTE at detection of bicuspid aortic valves, with a sensitivity of 87% and specificity of 97% in their detection (156). Subaortic stenosis, especially subaortic membrane, is often better imaged by TEE than by TTE (*e*Fig. 52.12.2) (157). Interrogation of the aortic valve with continuous-wave Doppler in the standard TEE imaging planes is more difficult than with transthoracic imaging. Planimetry of the aortic valve orifice is also feasible in many instances with multiplane transducers, and excellent agreement has been reported between the valve area planimetered by TEE and that measured at cardiac catheterization or by TTE (158). TEE provides excellent images of the tricuspid and pulmonary valve. However, the anterior situation of these structures in the chest allows adequate imaging in most circumstances by TTE, with little incremental benefit from TEE.

Prosthetic Valves

TEE allows improved resolution of prosthetic leaflets and regurgitation both at mechanical and bioprostheses as compared with TTE (83,159). In one study of 148 prosthetic valves (113 bioprostheses and 35 mechanical prostheses) in which abnormality was confirmed pathologically, TEE and TTE were 86% and 57% sensitive, respectively, in the detection of abnormalities (83). TEE was superior to TTE in the detection of abnormalities at mechanical prostheses (83% vs. 22%), bioprostheses (87% vs. 65%), aortic prostheses (77% vs. 50%), and mitral prostheses (97% vs. 65%) (83). TEE may detect thrombus in patients with mechanical mitral valves that is clinically unsuspected but that is a risk factor for thromboembolic events (160).

Prosthetic Regurgitation

A small amount of regurgitation occurs normally at mechanical prostheses by design. This is readily detected by TEE and less often by TTE. The pattern of regurgitation is specific to individual prosthetic types and is usually easily differentiated from abnormal regurgitation by the relative low velocity, short duration, and small size of the normal jets (161). Abnormal regurgitation at mitral prostheses is more reliably detected by TEE than TTE, but TEE's superiority in this regard is less for aortic prostheses (159,162).

TEE is also more accurate than TTE in defining the origin of the prosthetic regurgitation (162,163). Prosthetic regurgitation, especially when paravalvular, is associated with intravascular hemolysis (Fig. 52.13). Regurgitant jets that produce a high shear stress on red blood cells and consequent hemolysis may be characterized using TEE (164). Structural abnormalities leading to regurgitation such as flail bioprosthetic leaflets are more also more reliably detected by TEE than by TTE (84).

Prosthetic Stenosis

TEE is an important diagnostic tool in the assessment of prosthetic stenosis, especially at mechanical valves. Although TTE is used to characterize the valve gradients, TEE provides incremental information on structural abnormalities of the valve leaflets or sewing ring once stenosis is suspected. TEE is especially useful in the detection of thrombus on the prosthetic leaflets (165). Thrombus may not be apparent on TTE and may occur despite normal prosthetic gradients. In one study, TEE detected thrombus on a mechanical valve in 13% of 114 patients in whom it was unsuspected by TTE (165). In another study, TEE detected all eight prosthetic thrombi (100%), whereas TTE detected only one (13%) of them (83). TEE is useful in prediction of the response of thrombus to thrombolytic treatment, which is more likely to be successful with nonobstructive thrombus rather than when the thrombus is completely occluding the prosthesis (166). It is also useful in detecting resolution of thrombus after thrombolytic infusion and the need for further thrombolytic infusion (167). TEE also helps in identifying thrombus from pannus at mechanical valve prostheses (168,169). The high resolution of TEE may detect features on prosthetic valves of uncertain significance, which are not seen with other imaging modalities. Microbubbles are frequently seen emanating from mechanical prostheses, especially at mitral tilting-disc prostheses. These are thought to be due to cavitation of erythrocytes and are often a normal finding (170). Filamentous strands have also been detected on mechanical and even biologic prostheses (171,172). The precise nature and significance of these strands are uncertain.

CONTROVERSIES AND PERSONAL PERSPECTIVES

A major controversy with regard to TEE is when should it be used as a primary diagnostic modality. TEE provides incremental information to that obtained by clinical examination and TTE in many selected instances of endocarditis, source of embolism, prosthetic dysfunction, disease of the aorta, native-valve disease, and atrial fibrillation. As outlined already, in specific situations such as suspected prosthetic endocarditis, the value of a TEE is such that it should

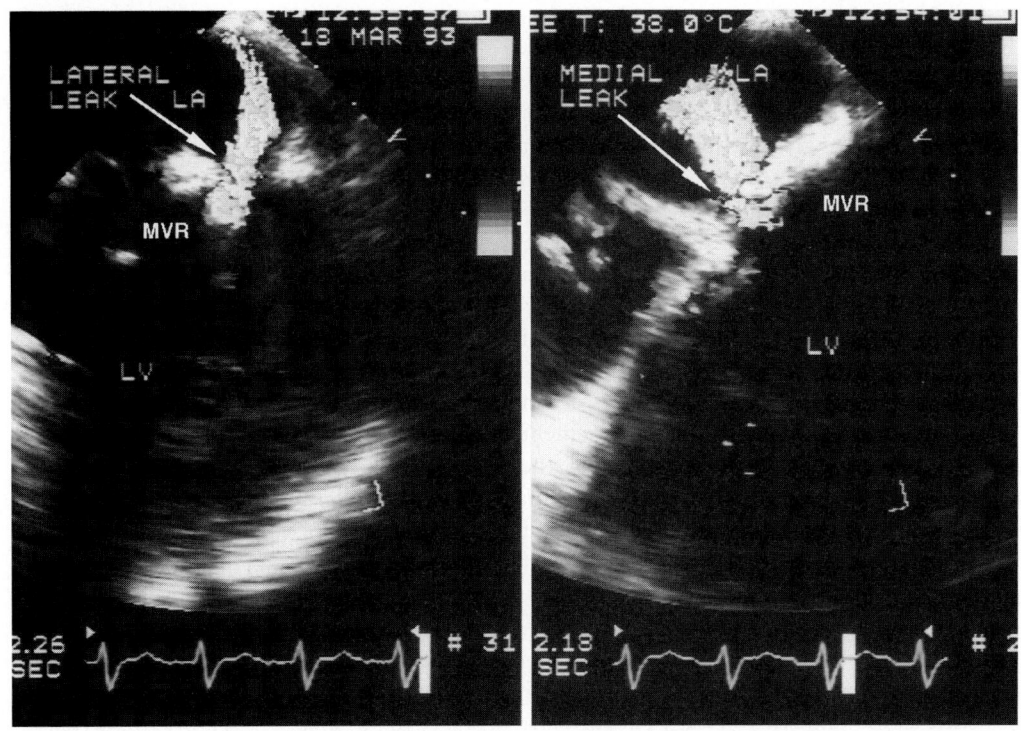

FIGURE 52.13 Two periprosthetic regurgitant leaks [lateral, **(A)**; medial, **(B)**] at a mitral mechanical prosthesis (MVR) demonstrated by multiplane transesophageal echocardiography. LA, left atrium; LV, left ventricle.

THE FUTURE

Three-Dimensional Reconstruction

Multiple high-quality tomograms of the heart and aorta may be sequentially acquired with multiplane transesophageal transducers. Technological advances have led to the more rapid acquisition and reconstruction of images (239). These may be reconstructed by computer to derive a three-dimensional dataset. Three-dimensional reconstruction is of most value in the assessment of complex structures such as the mitral valve and in congenital heart disease (240) and in accurate estimation of chamber volume. Three-dimensional TEE may be especially useful in percutaneous interventional procedures such as closure of complex congenital shunts (241) and in assessing the mitral orifice in balloon valvuloplasty (242). The complex anatomy of the regurgitant orifice in myxomatous mitral valve disease may be reliably demonstrated and measured with three-dimensional TEE (239,243). Real-time acquisition of three-dimensional images is currently under investigation. This has the potential to greatly facilitate volumetric evaluation of the patient and to accelerate image acquisition. Once the three-dimensional dataset has been obtained, multiple tomograms through the heart may be generated later. Three-dimensional color Doppler is currently under investigation and appears to have potential in improving the detection and quantification of eccentric regurgitant jets (244). Although three-dimensional TEE is of great potential use, its diagnostic usefulness in a clinical setting is not sufficiently well-established for it to be used in routine clinical practice.

Miniaturization

The progress of TEE has been marked by increased miniaturization of the transducer and probe. Pediatric probes capable of imaging even neonates are currently available. Recently, transducers capable of passage through the nasopharynx have become available. Because of size constraints these have limited capabilities and are under investigation as an adjunct to monitoring left ventricle function in the ICU setting (245). Smaller transducers have the advantage of easier passage and have the potential to increase the patient acceptability of transesophageal imaging and reduce the need for conscious sedation in its use.

be considered part of the normal workup. In other situations, such as in patients with stroke and atrial fibrillation, although TEE may detect a potential embolic source, it is unlikely to alter management, as the patient will most likely require chronic anticoagulation anyway. The usefulness and need for TEE in such situations are highly controversial. For instance, in the setting of embolic stroke, cost-effectiveness models have supported the use of TEE as a primary diagnostic modality (180). However, clinical variables have proven more predictive of outcome than TEE information in other studies of stroke in atrial fibrillation (179). TEE is an extremely accurate diagnostic tool. However, because of its invasiveness and cost, both economically and in physician time, it should be reserved for those situations in which information from it will likely alter patient management substantially. This will vary with the competency of the operator both in TTE and TEE in an individual institution and with variation in management algorithms in different institutions. Currently, TEE represents less than 10% of all studies performed in echocardiography laboratories. Although the indications for TEE have grown, improvement in TTE technology such as in contrast agents and harmonic imaging have reduced the need for TEE in many other situations such as the difficult-to-image patient. The proportion of echocardiograms being performed as TEE has not changed substantially over the last number of years, and this trend seems likely to continue.

REFERENCES

1. Daniel WG, Erbel R, Kasper W, et al. Safety of transesophageal echocardiography. A multicenter survey of 10,419 examinations. *Circulation* 1991;83:817–821.
2. Seward JB, Khanderia BK, Oh JK, et al. Critical appraisal of transesophageal echocardiography: limitations, pitfalls and complications. *J Am Soc Echocardiographr* 1992;5:288–305.
3. Side CD, Gosling RG. Non-surgical assessment of cardiac function. *Nature* 1971;232:335.
4. Frazin L, Talano JV, Stephanides L, et al. Esophageal echocardiography. *Circulation* 1976;54:102–108.
5. Hisanaga K, Hisanaga A, Jehie Y, et al. Transesophageal pulsed Doppler echocardiography. *Lancet* 1979;1:53–54.
6. Hanrath P, Kremer P, Langenstein BA, et al. Transosophageeale Echokardiographie: Ein neues Verfahren zur dynamischen Ventrikelfunktionsanalyse. *Dtsch Med Wochenschr* 1981;106:523–525.
7. Souquet J, Hanrath P, Zitelli L, et al. Transesophageal phased array for imaging the heart. *IEEE Trans Biomed Eng* 1982;29:707–712.
8. Schluter M, Langenstein BA, Hanrath P, et al. Assessment of transesophageal pulsed Doppler echocardiography in the detection of mitral regurgitation. *Circulation* 1982;66:784–789.
9. de Bruijn NP, Clements FM, Kisslo JA. Intraoperative transesophageal color flow mapping: initial experience. *Anesth Analg* 1987;66:386–390.
10. Omoto R, Kyo S, Matsumura M, et al. Bi-plane color transesophageal Doppler echocardiography (color TEE): its advantages and limitations. *Int J Cardiac Imaging* 1989;4:58.
11. Flachskampf FA, Hoffman R, Verlande M, et al. Initial experience with a multiplane transesophageal transducer: assessment of diagnostic potential. *Eur Heart J* 1992;13:1201–1206.
12. Gentles TL, Rosenfeld HM, Sanders SP, et al. Pediatric biplane transesophageal echocardiography: preliminary experience. *Am Heart J* 1994;128:1225–1233.
13. Seward JB, Khandheria BK, Edwards WD, et al. Biplanar transesophageal echocardiography: anatomic correlations, image orientation, and clinical applications. *Mayo Clin Proc* 1990;65:1193–1213.
14. Seward JB, Khanheria BJ, Freeman WK, et al. Multiplane transesophageal echocardiography: image orientation, examination technique, anatomic correlations, and clinical applications. *Mayo Clin Proc* 1993;68:523–551.
15. Schneider AT, Hsu TL, Schwartz S, et al. Single, biplane, multiplane, and three-dimensional transesophageal echocardiography. Echocardiographic-anatomic correlations. *Cardiol Clin* 1993;11:361–387.
16. Aeschbacher BC, Portner M, Fluri M, et al. Midazolam premedication improves tolerance of transesophageal echocardiography. *Am J Cardiol* 1998;81:1022–1026.
17. Shorvon PJ, Eykyn SJ, Cotton PB. Gastrointestinal instrumentation, bacteraemia, and endocarditis. *Gut* 1983;24:1078–1093.
18. Foster E, Kusumoto FM, Sobois M, et al. Streptococcal endocarditis temporarily related to transesophageal echocardiography. *J Am Soc Echocardiographr* 1990;3:424–427.
19. Nikutta P, Mantey-Steirs F, Becht I, et al. Risk of bacteremia induced by transesophageal echocardiography. Analysis of 100 consecutive procedures. *J Am Soc Echocardiographr* 1992;5:168–172.
20. Pongratz G, Henneke KH, von der Grun M, et al. Risk of endocarditis in transesophageal echocardiography. *Am Heart J* 1993;125:190–193.
21. Shyu KG, Hwang JJ, Tzou SS, et al. Prospective study of blood cultures during transesophageal echocardiography. *Am Heart J* 1992;124:1541–1544.
22. Gendreau MA, Triner WR, Bartfield J. Complications of transesophageal echocardiography in the ED. *Am J Emerg Med* 1999;17:248–251.
23. Silvey SV, Stoughton TL, Pearl W, et al. Rupture of the outer partition of aortic dissection during transesophageal echocardiography. *Am J Cardiol* 1991;68:286–287.
24. Dewhirst WE, Stragand JJ, Fleming BM. Mallory-Weiss tear complicating intraoperative transesophageal echocardiography in a patient undergoing aortic valve replacement. *Anesthesiology* 1990;73:777–778.
25. O'Shea JP, Southern JF, D'Ambra MN, et al. Effect of prolonged transesophageal echocardiographic imaging and probe manipulation on the esophagus—an echocardiographic-pathologic study. *J Am Coll Cardiol* 1991;17:1426–1429.
26. Chan KL, Cohen GI, Sochowski RA, et al. Complications of transesophageal echocardiography in ambulatory adult patients. *J Am Soc Echocardiographr* 1991;4:577–582.

27. Cucchiara RF, Nugent M, Seward JB, et al. Air embolism in upright neurosurgical patients: detection and localization by two-dimensional transesophageal echocardiography. *Anesthesiology* 1984;60:353–355.

28. Frommelt PC, Stuth EA. Transesophageal echocardiography in total anomalous pulmonary venous drainage: hypotension caused by compression of the pulmonary venous confluence during probe passage. *J Am Soc Echocardiogr* 1994;76:652–654.

29. Marcovitz PA, Williamson BD, Armstrong WF. Toxic methemoglobinemia caused by topical anesthetic given before transesophageal echocardiography. *J Am Soc Echocardiogr* 1991;4:615–618.

30. Kronzon I, Cziner DG, Katz ES, et al. Buckling of the tip of the transesophageal echocardiography probe: a potentially dangerous technical malfunction. *J Am Soc Echocardiogr* 1992;5:176–177.

31. Shrestha NK, Moreno FL, Narciso FV, et al. Two-dimensional echocardiographic diagnosis of left atrial thrombus in rheumatic heart disease: a clinicopathologic study. *Circulation* 1983;67:341–347.

32. Aschenberg W, Schluter M, Kremer P, et al. Transesophageal two-dimensional echocardiography for the detection of left atrial appendage thrombus. *J Am Coll Cardiol* 1986;7:163–166.

33. Brickner ME, Friedman DB, Cigarroa CG, et al. Relation of thrombus in the left atrial appendage by transesophageal echocardiography to clinical risk factors for thrombus formation. *Am J Cardiol* 1994;7:391–393.

34. Leung DY, Davidson PM, Cranney GB, et al. Thromboembolic risks of left atrial thrombus detected by transesophageal echocardiogram. *Am J Cardiol* 1997;79:626–629.

35. Manning WJ, Weintraub RM, Wakomonski CA, et al. Accuracy of transesophageal echocardiography for identifying left atrial thrombi. A prospective intraoperative study. *Ann Intern Med* 1995;123:817–822.

36. Irani WN, Grayburn PA, Afridi I. Prevalence of thrombus, spontaneous echo contrast, and atrial stunning in patients undergoing cardioversion of atrial flutter. A prospective study using transesophageal echocardiography. *Circulation* 1997;95:962–966.

37. Katz ES, Tsiamtsiouris T, Applebaum RM, et al. Surgical left atrial appendage ligation is frequently incomplete: a transesophageal echocardiographic study. *J Am Coll Cardiol* 2000;36:468–471.

38. Schwartzbard AZ, Tunick PA, Rosenzweig BP, et al. The role of transesophageal echocardiography in the diagnosis and treatment of right atrial thrombi. *J Am Soc Echocardiogr* 1999;12:64–69.

39. Manning WJ, Silverman DI, Keighley CS, et al. Transesophageal echocardiographically facilitated early cardioversion from atrial fibrillation using short-term anticoagulation: final results of a prospective 4.5 year study. *J Am Coll Cardiol* 1995;25:1354–1361.

40. Daniel WG, Nellessen V, Schroder E, et al. Left atrial spontaneous contrast in mitral valve disease: an indicator for an increased thromboembolic risk. *J Am Coll Cardiol* 1988;11:1204–1211.

41. Black IW, Hopkins AP, Lee LCL, et al. Left atrial spontaneous echo contrast: a clinical and echocardiographic analysis. *J Am Coll Cardiol* 1991;18:398–404.

42. Leung DY, Black IW, Cranney GB, et al. Resolution of left atrial spontaneous echocardiographic contrast after percutaneous mitral valvuloplasty: implications for thromboembolic risk. *Am Heart J* 1995;129:65–70.

43. Leung DY, Black IW, Cranney GB, et al. Prognostic implications of left atrial spontaneous echo contrast in nonvalvular atrial fibrillation. *J Am Coll Cardiol* 1994;24:755–762.

44. Sadanandan S, Sherrid MV. Clinical and echocardiographic characteristics of left atrial spontaneous echo contrast in sinus rhythm. *J Am Coll Cardiol* 2000;35:1932–1938.

45. Pollick C, Taylor D. Assessment of left atrial appendage function by transesophageal echocardiography. Implications for the development of thrombus. *Circulation* 1991;84:223–231.

46. Fatkin D, Kelly RP, Feneley MP. Relations between left atrial appendage blood flow velocity, spontaneous echocardiographic contrast and thromboembolic risk in vivo. *J Am Coll Cardiol* 1994;23:961–969.

47. Verhorst PM, Kamp O, Visser CA, et al. Left atrial appendage flow velocity assessment using transesophageal echocardiography in nonrheumatic atrial fibrillation and systemic embolism. *Am J Cardiol* 1993;71:192–196.

48. Grimm RA, Stewart WJ, Maloney JD, et al. Impact of electrical cardioversion for atrial fibrillation on left atrial appendage function and spontaneous echo contrast characterization by simultaneous transesophageal echocardiography. *J Am Coll Cardiol* 1993;22:1359–1366.

49. Kamp O, Verhorst PM, Welling RC, et al. Importance of left atrial appendage flow as a predictor of thromboembolic events in patients with atrial fibrillation. *Eur Heart J* 1999;20:979–985.

50. Verhorst PM, Kamp O, Welling RC, et al. Transesophageal echocardiographic predictors for maintenance of sinus rhythm after electrical cardioversion of atrial fibrillation. *Am J Cardiol* 1997;79:1355–1359.

51. Goldman ME, Pearce LA, Hart RG, et al. Pathophysiologic correlates of thromboembolism in nonvalvular atrial fibrillation: I. Reduced flow velocity in the left atrial appendage (The Stroke Prevention in Atrial Fibrillation [SPAF-III] study). *J Am Soc Echocardiogr* 1999;12:1080–1087.

52. Arnold AZ, Mick MJ, Mazurek RP, et al. Role of prophylactic anticoagulation for direct current cardioversion in patients with atrial fibrillation or atrial flutter. *J Am Coll Cardiol* 1992;19:851–855.

53. Kronzon I, Tunick PA, Glassman E, et al. Transesophageal echocardiography to detect atrial clots in candidates for percutaneous transseptal mitral balloon valvuloplasty. *J Am Coll Cardiol* 1990;16:1320–1322.

54. Klein AL, Grimm RA, Black IW, et al. Assessment of cardioversion using transesophageal echocardiography compared to conventional therapy: the ACUTE Randomized Pilot Study [abstract]. *Circulation* 1994;90:I–24.

55. Klein AL, Grimm RA, Black IW, et al. Cardioversion guided by transesophageal echocardiography: the ACUTE Pilot Study. A randomized, controlled trial. Assessment of cardioversion using transesophageal echocardiography [see comments]. *Ann Intern Med* 1997;126:200–209.

56. Seto TB, Taira DA, Tsevat J, et al. Cost-effectiveness of transesophageal echocardiographic-guided cardioversion: a decision analytic model for patients admitted to the hospital with atrial fibrillation. *J Am Coll Cardiol* 1997;29:122–130.

57. Black IW, Fatkin D, Sagar KB, et al. Exclusion of atrial thrombus by transesophageal echocardiography does not preclude embolism after cardioversion of atrial fibrillation. A multicenter study. *Circulation* 1994;89:2509–2513.

58. Grimm RA, Stewart WJ, Black IW, et al. Should all patients undergo transesophageal echocardiography before electrical cardioversion of atrial fibrillation? *J Am Coll Cardiol* 1994;23:533–541.

59. Antonielli E, Pizzuti A, Bassignana A, et al. Transesophageal echocardiographic evidence of more pronounced left atrial stunning after chemical (propafenone) rather than electrical attempts at cardioversion from atrial fibrillation. *Am J Cardiol* 1999;84:1092–1096, A9–A10.

60. Sparks PB, Kulkarni R, Vohra JK, et al. Effect of direct current shocks on left atrial mechanical function in patients with structural heart disease. *J Am Coll Cardiol* 1998;31:1395–1399.

61. Grimm RA, Stewart WJ, Arheart K, et al. Left atrial appendage "stunning" after electrical cardioversion of atrial flutter: an attenuated response compared with atrial fibrillation as the mechanism for lower susceptibility to thromboembolic events. *J Am Coll Cardiol* 1997;29:582–589.

62. Hausmann D, Daniel WG, Mugge A, et al. Value of transesophageal color Doppler echocardiography for detection of different types of atrial septal defect in adults. *J Am Soc Echocardiogr* 1992;5:481–488.

63. Kronzon I, Tunick PA, Freedberg RS, et al. Transesophageal echocardiography is superior to transthoracic echocardiography in the diagnosis of sinus venosus atrial septal defect. *J Am Coll Cardiol* 1991;17:537–542.

64. Rittoo D, Sutherland GR, Shaw TR. Quantification of left-to-right shunting and defect size after balloon mitral commissurotomy using biplane transesophageal echocardiography, color flow Doppler mapping, and the principle of proximal flow convergence. *Circulation* 1993;87:1591–1603.

65. Hagen PT, Scholz DG, Edwards WD. Incidence and size of patent foramen ovale during the first 10 decades of life. An autopsy study of 965 normal hearts. *Mayo Clin Proc* 1984;59:17–20.

66. Lechat P, Mas JL, Lascault G, et al. Prevalence of patent foramen ovale in patients with stroke. *N Engl J Med* 1988;318:1148–1152.

67. Meacham RR III, Headley AS, Bronze MS, et al. Impending paradoxical embolism. *Arch Intern Med* 1998;158:438–448.

68. Pearson AC, Labovitz AJ, Tatineni S, et al. Superiority of transesophageal echocardiography in detecting cardiac source of embolism in patients with cerebral ischemia of uncertain etiology. *J Am Coll Cardiol* 1991;17:66–72.

69. Schneider B, Zienkiewicz T, Jansen V, et al. Diagnosis of patent foramen ovale by transesophageal echocardiography and correlation with autopsy findings. *Am J Cardiol* 1996;77:1202–1209.

70. Hausmann D, Mugge A, Becht I, et al. Diagnosis of patent foramen ovale by transesophageal echocardiography and association with cerebral and peripheral embolic events. *Am J Cardiol* 1992;70:668–672.

71. de Belder MA, Tourikis L, Griffith M, et al. Transesophageal contrast echocardiography and color flow mapping: methods of choice for the detection of shunts at the atrial level? *Am Heart J* 1992;124:1545–1550.

72. Steiner MM, Di Tullio MR, Rundek T, et al. Patent foramen ovale size and embolic brain imaging findings among patients with ischemic stroke. *Stroke* 1998;29:944–948.

73. Pearson AC, Nagelhout D, Castello R, et al. Atrial septal aneurysm and stroke: a transesophageal echocardiographic study. *J Am Coll Cardiol* 1991;18:1223–1229.

74. Agmon Y, Khandheria BK, Meissner I, et al. Frequency of atrial septal aneurysms in patients with cerebral ischemic events. *Circulation* 1999;99:1942–1944.

75. Burstow DJ, McEniery PT, Stafford EG. Fenestrated atrial septal aneurysm: diagnosis by transesophageal echocardiography. *J Am Soc Echocardiogr* 1990;3:499–501.

76. Mugge A, Daniel WG, Angermann C, et al. Atrial septal aneurysm in adult patients. A multicenter study using transthoracic and transesophageal echocardiography. *Circulation* 1995;91:2785–2792.

77. Mugge A, Daniel WG, Haverick A, et al. Diagnosis of non-infective cardiac mass lesions by two-dimensional echocardiography: comparison of transthoracic and transesophageal approaches. *Circulation* 1991;83:70–78.

78. Durack DT, Lukes AS, Bright DK. New criteria for diagnosis of infective endocarditis: utilization of specific echocardiographic findings. Duke Endocarditis Service. *Am J Med* 1994;96:200–209.

79. Erbel R, Rohmann S, Drexler M, et al. Improved diagnostic value of echocardiography in patients with infective endocarditis by transesophageal approach. A prospective study. *Eur Heart J* 1988;9:43–53.

80. Birmingham GD, Rahko PS, Ballantyne F III. Improved detection of infective endocarditis with transesophageal echocardiography. *Am Heart J* 1992;123:774–781.

81. Shapiro SM, Young E, De Guzman S, et al. Transesophageal echocardiography in diagnosis of infective endocarditis. *Chest* 1994;105:377–382.

82. Shively BK, Gurule FT, Roldan CA, et al. Diagnostic value of transesophageal compared with transthoracic echocardiography in infective endocarditis. *J Am Coll Cardiol* 1991;18:391–397.

83. Daniel WG, Mugge A, Grote J, et al. Comparison of transthoracic and transesophageal echocardiography for detection of abnormalities of prosthetic and bioprosthetic valves in the mitral and aortic positions. *Am J Cardiol* 1993;71:210–215.

84. Zabalgoitia M, Herrera CJ, Chaudhry FA, et al. Improvement in the diagnosis of bioprosthetic valve dysfunction by transesophageal echocardiography. *J Heart Valve Dis* 1993;2:595–603.

85. San Roman JA, Vilacosta I, Zamorano JL, et al. Transesophageal echocardiography in right-sided endocarditis. *J Am Coll Cardiol* 1993;21:1226–1230.

86. Shapiro SM, Young E, Ginzton LE, et al. Pulmonic valve endocarditis as an underdiagnosed disease: role of transesophageal echocardiography. *J Am Soc Echocardiogr* 1992;5:48–51.

87. Vilacosta I, Sarria C, San Roman JA, et al. Usefulness of transesophageal echocardiography for diagnosis of infected transvenous permanent pacemakers. *Circulation* 1994;89:2684–2687.

88. De Castro S, Cartoni D, d'Amati G, et al. Diagnostic accuracy of transthoracic and multiplane transesophageal

echocardiography for valvular perforation in acute infective endocarditis: correlation with anatomic findings. *Clin Infect Dis* 2000;30:825–826.

89. Daniel WG, Mugge A, Martin R, et al. Improvement in the diagnosis of abscesses associated with endocarditis by transesophageal echocardiography. *N Engl J Med* 1991;324:795–800.

90. Karalis DG, Bansal RC, Hauck AJ, et al. Transesophageal echocardiographic recognition of subaortic complication in aortic valve endocarditis: clinical and surgical implications. *Circulation* 1992;86:353–362.

91. Rohmann S, Erbel R, Mohr-Kahaly S, et al. Use of transesophageal echocardiography in the diagnosis of abscess in infective endocarditis. *Eur Heart J* 1995;16:54–62.

92. Leung DY, Cranney GB, Hopkins AP, et al. Role of transesophageal echocardiography in the diagnosis and management of aortic root abscess. *Br Heart J* 1994;72:175–181.

93. Fowler VG Jr, Li J, Corey GR, et al. Role of echocardiography in evaluation of patients with Staphylococcus aureus bacteremia: experience in 103 patients. *J Am Coll Cardiol* 1997;30:1072–1078.

94. Rosen AB, Fowler VG Jr, Corey GR, et al. Cost-effectiveness of transesophageal echocardiography to determine the duration of therapy for intravascular catheter-associated Staphylococcus aureus bacteremia. *Ann Intern Med* 1999;130:810–820.

95. Sochowski RA, Chan KL. Implication of negative results on a monoplane transesophageal echocardiographic study in patients with suspected infective endocarditis. *J Am Coll Cardiol* 1993;21:216–221.

96. Bayer AS, Ward JI, Gintzon LE, et al. Evaluation of new clinical criteria for the diagnosis of infective endocarditis. *Am J Med* 1994;96:211–219.

97. Lindner JR, Case RA, Dent JM, et al. Diagnostic value of echocardiography in suspected endocarditis. An evaluation based on the pretest probability of disease. *Circulation* 1996;93:730–736.

98. Irani WN, Grayburn PA, Afridi I. A negative transthoracic echocardiogram obviates the need for transesophageal echocardiography in patients with suspected native valve active infective endocarditis. *Am J Cardiol* 1996;78:101–103.

99. Roe MT, Abramson MA, Li J, et al. Clinical information determines the impact of transesophageal echocardiography on the diagnosis of infective endocarditis by the duke criteria. *Am Heart J* 2000;139:945–951.

100. Rohmann S, Erbel R, Darius H, et al. Prediction of rapid versus prolonged healing of infective endocarditis by monitoring vegetation size. *J Am Soc Echocardiogr* 1991;4:465–474.

101. Adachi H, Omoto R, Kyo S, et al. Emergency surgical intervention of acute aortic dissection with the rapid diagnosis by transesophageal echocardiography. *Circulation* 1991;84:III14–19.

102. Simon P, Owen AN, Havel M, et al. Transesophageal echocardiography in the emergency surgical management of patients with aortic dissection. *J Thorac Cardiovasc Surg* 1992;103:1113–1117.

103. Banning AP, Masani ND, Ikram S, et al. Transesophageal echocardiography as the sole diagnostic investigation in patients with suspected thoracic aortic dissection. *Br Heart J* 1994;72:461–465.

104. Cigarrao JE, Isselbacher EM, DeSanctis RW, et al. Diagnostic imaging in the evaluation of suspected aortic dissection. Old standards and new directions. *N Engl J Med* 1993;328:35–43.

105. Erbel R, Engberding R, Daniel W, et al. Echocardiography in diagnosis of aortic dissection. *Lancet* 1989;1:457–481.

106. Nienaber CA, Spielman RP, Kodolitsch YV, et al. Diagnosis of thoracic aortic dissection. Magnetic resonance imaging versus transesophageal echocardiography. *Circulation* 1992;85:434–447.

107. Nienaber CA, von Kodolitsch Y, Nicolas V, et al. The diagnosis of thoracic aortic dissection by noninvasive imaging procedures. *N Engl J Med* 1993;328:1–9.

108. Bansal RC, Chandrasekaran K, Ayala K, et al. Frequency and explanation of false negative diagnosis of aortic dissection by aortography and transesophageal echocardiography. *J Am Coll Cardiol* 1995;25:1393–1401.

109. Deutsch HJ, Sechtem U, Meyer H, et al. Chronic aortic dissection: comparison of MR imaging and transesophageal echocardiography. *Radiology* 1994;192:845–850.

110. Adachi H, Kyo S, Takamoto S, et al. Early diagnosis and surgical intervention of acute aortic dissection by transesophageal color flow mapping. *Circulation* 1990;82[Suppl IV]:19–23.

111. Svensson LG, Labib SB, Eisenhauer AC, et al. Intimal tear without hematoma: an important variant of aortic dissection that can elude current imaging techniques. *Circulation* 1999;99:1331–1336.

112. Ballal RS, Nanda NC, Gatewood R, et al. Usefulness of transesophageal echocardiography in assessment of aortic dissection. *Circulation* 1991;84:1903–1914.

113. Applebe AF, Walker PG, Yeoh JK, et al. Clinical significance and origin of artifacts in transesophageal echocardiography of the thoracic aorta. *J Am Coll Cardiol* 1993;21:754–760.

114. Omoto R, Kyo S, Matsumura M, et al. Evaluation of biplane color Doppler transesophageal echocardiography in 200 consecutive patients. *Circulation* 1992;85:1237–1247.

115. Evangelista A, Garcia-del-Castillo H, Gonzalez-Alujas T, et al. Diagnosis of ascending aortic dissection by transesophageal echocardiography: utility of M-mode in recognizing artifacts. *J Am Coll Cardiol* 1996;27:102–107.

116. Chan KL. Usefulness of transesophageal echocardiography in the diagnosis of conditions mimicking aortic dissection. *Am Heart J* 1991;122:495–504.

117. Harris KM, Braverman AC, Gutierrez FR, et al. Transesophageal echocardiographic and clinical features of aortic intramural hematoma. *J Thorac Cardiovasc Surg* 1997;114:619–626.

118. Vilacosta I, San Roman JA, Ferreiros J, et al. Natural history and serial morphology of aortic intramural hematoma: a novel variant of aortic dissection. *Am Heart J* 1997;134:495–507.

119. Mohr-Kahaly S, Erbel R, Kearney P, et al. Aortic intramural hemorrhage visualized by transesophageal echocardiography: findings and prognostic implications. *J Am Coll Cardiol* 1994;23:658–664.

120. Atar S, Nagai T, Birnbaum Y, et al. Transesophageal echocardiographic Doppler findings in patients with penetrating aortic ulcers. *Am J Cardiol* 1999;83:133–135.

121. Vilacosta I, San Roman JA, Aragoncillo P, et al. Penetrating atherosclerotic aortic ulcer: documentation by transesophageal echocardiography. *J Am Coll Cardiol* 1998;32:83–89.

122. Smith MD, Cassidy JM, Souther S, et al. Transesophageal echocardiography in the diagnosis of traumatic rupture of the aorta. *N Engl J Med* 1995;332:356–362.

123. Vignon P, Gueret P, Vedrinne JM, et al. Role of transesophageal echocardiography in the diagnosis and management of traumatic aortic disruption. *Circulation* 1995;92:2959–2968.

124. Vaduganathan P, Ewton A, Nagueh SF, et al. Pathologic correlates of aortic plaques, thrombi and mobile "aortic debris" imaged in vivo with transesophageal echocardiography. *J Am Coll Cardiol* 1997;30:357–363.

125. Tunick PA, Kronzon I. Atheromas of the thoracic aorta: clinical and therapeutic update. *J Am Coll Cardiol* 2000;35:545–554.

126. Tribouilloy C, Shen WF, Peltier M, et al. Noninvasive prediction of coronary artery disease by transesophageal echocardiographic detection of thoracic aortic plaque in valvular heart disease. *Am J Cardiol* 1994;74:258–260.

127. Nihoyannopoulos P, Joshi J, Athanasopoulos G, et al. Detection of atherosclerotic lesions in the aorta by transesophageal echocardiography. *Am J Cardiol* 1993;71:208–212.

128. Amarenco P, Cohen A, Tzourio C, et al. Atherosclerotic disease of the aortic arch and the risk of ischemic stroke. *N Engl J Med* 1994;331:1474–1479.

129. Ferrari E, Vidal R, Chevallier T, et al. Atherosclerosis of the thoracic aorta and aortic debris as a marker of poor prognosis: benefit of oral anticoagulants. *J Am Coll Cardiol* 1999;33:1317–1322.

130. Dressler FA, Craig WR, Castello R, et al. Mobile aortic atheroma and systemic emboli: efficacy of anticoagulation and influence of plaque morphology on recurrent stroke. *J Am Coll Cardiol* 1998;31:134–138.

131. Katz ES, Tunick PA, Rusinek H, et al. Protruding aortic atheromas predict stroke in elderly patients undergoing cardiopulmonary bypass: experience with intraoperative transesophageal echocardiography. *J Am Coll Cardiol* 1992;20:70–77.

132. Bansal RC, Pauls GL, Shankel SW. Blue digit syndrome: transesophageal echocardiographic identification of thoracic aortic plaque-related thrombi and successful outcome with warfarin. *J Am Soc Echocardiogr* 1993;6:319–323.

133. Karalis DG, Chandrasekaran K, Victor MF, et al. The recognition and embolic potential of intraaortic atherosclerotic debris. *J Am Coll Cardiol* 1991;17:73–78.

134. Tunick PA, Perez JL, Kronzon I. Protruding atheromas in the thoracic aorta and systemic embolization. *Ann Intern Med* 1991;115:423–427.

135. Rundek T, Di Tullio MR, Sciacca RR, et al. Association between large aortic arch atheromas and high-intensity transient signals in elderly stroke patients. *Stroke* 1999;30:2683–2686.

136. Finkelhor RS, Youssefi ME, Lamont WE, et al. Embolic risk based on aortic atherosclerotic morphologic features and aortic spontaneous echocardiographic contrast. *Am Heart J* 1999;137:1088–1093.

137. Steinberg EH, Madmon L, Wesolowsky H, et al. Prognostic significance of spontaneous echo contrast in the thoracic aorta: relation with accelerated clinical progression of coronary artery disease. *J Am Coll Cardiol* 1997;30:71–75.

138. Laperche T, Laurian C, Roudaut R, et al. Mobile thromboses of the aortic arch without aortic debris. A transesophageal echocardiographic finding associated with unexplained arterial embolism. The Filiale Echocardiographie de la Societe Francaise de Cardiologie. *Circulation* 1997;96:288–294.

139. Hozumi T, Yoshikawa J, Yoshida K, et al. Direct visualization of ruptured chordae tendineae by transesophageal two-dimensional echocardiography. *J Am Coll Cardiol* 1990;16:1315–1319.

140. Sochowski RA, Chan KL, Ascah KJ, et al. Comparison of accuracy of transesophageal versus transthoracic echocardiography for the detection of mitral valve prolapse with ruptured chordae tendineae (flail mitral leaflet). *Am J Cardiol* 1991;67:1251–1255.

141. Foster GP, Isselbacher EM, Rose GA, et al. Accurate localization of mitral regurgitant defects using multiplane transesophageal echocardiography. *Ann Thorac Surg* 1998;65:1025–1031.

142. Maslow AD, Regan MM, Haering JM, et al. Echocardiographic predictors of left ventricular outflow tract obstruction and systolic anterior motion of the mitral valve after mitral valve reconstruction for myxomatous valve disease. *J Am Coll Cardiol* 1999;34:2096–2104.

143. Enriquez-Sarano M, Freeman WK, Tribouilloy CM, et al. Functional anatomy of mitral regurgitation: accuracy and outcome implications of transesophageal echocardiography. *J Am Coll Cardiol* 1999;34:1129–1136.

144. Castello R, Fagan L Jr, Lenzen P, et al. Comparison of transthoracic and transesophageal echocardiography for assessment of left-sided valvular regurgitation. *Am J Cardiol* 1991;68:1677–1680.

145. Smith MD, Cassidy JM, Gurley JC, et al. Echo Doppler evaluation of patients with acute mitral regurgitation: superiority of transesophageal echocardiography with color flow imaging. *Am Heart J* 1995;129:967–974.

146. Stoddard MF, Keedy DL, Kupersmith J. Transesophageal echocardiographic diagnosis of papillary muscle rupture complicating acute myocardial infarction. *Am Heart J* 1990;120:690–692.

147. Smith MD, Harrison MR, Pinton R, et al. Regurgitation jet size by transesophageal compared with transthoracic Doppler color flow imaging. *Circulation* 1991;83:79–86.

148. Castello R, Lenzen P, Aquirre F, et al. Variability in the quantitation of mitral regurgitation by Doppler color flow mapping: comparison of transthoracic and transesophageal studies. *J Am Coll Cardiol* 1992;20:433–438.

149. Recusani F, Bargiggia GS, Yoganathan AP, et al. A new method for quantification of regurgitant flow rate using color Doppler flow imaging of the flow convergence region proximal to a discrete orifice: an in vitro study. *Circulation* 1991;83:594–604.

150. Tribouilloy C, Shen WF, Auere JP, et al. Assessment of severity of mitral regurgitation by measuring regurgitant jet width at its origin with transesophageal Doppler color flow mapping. *Circulation* 1992;85:1248–1253.

151. Castello R, Pearson AC, Lenzen P, et al. Effect of mitral regurgitation on pulmonary venous velocities derived from transesophageal echocardiography color-guided pulsed Doppler imaging. *J Am Coll Cardiol* 1991;17:1499–1506.

152. Klein AL, Obarski TP, Stewart WJ, et al. Transesophageal Doppler echocardiography of pulmonary venous flow: a new marker of mitral regurgitation severity. *J Am Coll Cardiol* 1991;18:518–526.

153. Pu M, Griffin BP, Vandervoort PM, et al. The value of assessing pulmonary venous flow velocity for predicting severity of mitral regurgitation: a quantitative assessment integrating left ventricular function. *J Am Soc Echocardiogr* 1999;12:736–743.

154. Pu M, Griffin BP, Vandervoort PM, et al. Intraoperative validation of mitral inflow determination by transesophageal echocardiography: comparison of single-plane, biplane and thermodilution techniques. *J Am Coll Cardiol* 1995;26:1047–1053.

155. Pu M, Vandervoort PM, Griffin BP, et al. Quantification of mitral regurgitation by the proximal convergence method using transesophageal echocardiography. Clinical validation of a geometric correction for proximal flow constraint. *Circulation* 1995;92:2169–2177.

156. Espinal M, Fuisz AR, Nanda NC, et al. Sensitivity and specificity of transesophageal echocardiography for determination of aortic valve morphology. *Am Heart J* 2000;139:1071–1076.

157. Widimsky P, Ten Cate FJ, Vletter W, et al. Potential applications for transesophageal echocardiography in hypertrophic cardiomyopathies. *J Am Soc Echocardiogr* 1992;5:163–167.

158. Stoddard MF, Acre J, Liddell NE, et al. Two-dimensional transesophageal echocardiographic determination of aortic valve area in adults with aortic stenosis. *Am Heart J* 1991;122:1415–1422.

159. Nellessen U, Schnittger I, Appleton CP, et al. Transesophageal two-dimensional echocardiography and color Doppler flow velocity mapping in the evaluation of cardiac valve prosthesis. *Circulation* 1988;78:848–855.

160. Laffort P, Roudaut R, Roques X, et al. Early and long-term (one-year) effects of the association of aspirin and oral anticoagulant on thrombi and morbidity after replacement of the mitral valve with the St. Jude medical prosthesis: a clinical and transesophageal echocardiographic study. *J Am Coll Cardiol* 2000;35:739–746.

161. Flachskampf FA, O'Shea JP, Griffin BP, et al. Patterns of transvalvular regurgitation in normal mechanical prosthetic valves. *J Am Coll Cardiol* 1991;18:1493–1498.

162. Chaudhry FA, Herrera C, DeFrino PF, et al. Pathologic and angiographic correlations of transesophageal echocardiography in prosthetic heart valve dysfunction. *Am Heart J* 1991;122:1057–1064.

163. Karalis DG, Chandrasekaran K, Ross JJ Jr, et al. Single-plane transesophageal echocardiography for assessing function of mechanical or bioprosthetic valves in the aortic valve position. *Am J Cardiol* 1992;69:1310–1315.

164. Garcia MJ, Vandervoort PM, Stewart WJ, et al. Mechanism of hemolysis with mitral prosthetic regurgitation: a study using transesophageal echo and fluid dynamic simulation. *J Am Coll Cardiol* 1996;27:399–406.

165. Gueret P, Vignon P, Fournier P, et al. Transesophageal echocardiography for the diagnosis and management of nonobstructive thrombosis of mechanical mitral valve prosthesis. *Circulation* 1995;91:103–110.

166. Ozkan M, Kaymaz C, Kirma C, et al. Intravenous thrombolytic treatment of mechanical prosthetic valve thrombo-

sis: a study using serial transesophageal echocardiography. *J Am Coll Cardiol* 2000;35:1881–1889.

167. Young E, Shapiro SM, French WJ, et al. Use of transesophageal echocardiography during thrombolysis with tissue plasminogen activator of a thrombosed prosthetic mitral valve. *J Am Soc Echocardiogr* 1992;5:153–158.

168. Barbetseas J, Nagueh SF, Pitsavos C, et al. Differentiating thrombus from pannus formation in obstructed mechanical prosthetic valves: an evaluation of clinical, transthoracic and transesophageal echocardiographic parameters. *J Am Coll Cardiol* 1998;32:1410–1417.

169. Lin SS, Tiong IYH, Asher CR, et al. Prediction of thrombus-related mechanical prosthetic valve dysfunction using transesophageal echocardiography. *Am J Cardiol* 2000;86:1097–1101.

170. Orsinelli DA, Pasierski TJ, Pearson AC. Spontaneously appearing microbubbles associated with prosthetic cardiac valves detected by transesophageal echocardiography. *Am Heart J* 1994;128:990–996.

171. Isada LR, Torelli JN, Stewart WJ, et al. Detection of fibrous strands on prosthetic mitral valves with transesophageal echocardiography: another potential embolic source. *J Am Soc Echocardiogr* 1994;7:641–645.

172. Orsinelli DA, Pearson AC. Detection of prosthetic valve strands by transesophageal echocardiography: clinical significance in patients with suspected cardiac source of embolism. *J Am Coll Cardiol* 1995;26:1713–1718.

173. Come PC, Riley MF, Bivas NK. Roles of echocardiography and arrhythmia monitoring in the evaluation of patients with suspected systemic embolism. *Ann Neurol* 1983;13:527–531.

174. Sansoy V, Abbott RD, Jayaweera AR, et al. Low yield of transthoracic echocardiography for cardiac source of embolism. *Am J Cardiol* 1995;75:166–169.

175. DeRook FA, Comess KA, Albers GW, et al. Transesophageal echocardiography in the evaluation of stroke. *Ann Intern Med* 1992;117:922–932.

176. Lee RJ, Bartzokis, Yeoh TK, et al. Enhanced detection of intracardiac sources of cerebral emboli by transesophageal echocardiography. *Stroke* 1991;22:734–739.

177. Comess KA, DeRook FA, Beach KW, et al. Transesophageal echocardiography and carotid ultrasound in patients with cerebral ischemia: prevalence of findings and recurrent stroke risk. *J Am Coll Cardiol* 1994;23:1598–1603.

178. O'Brien PJ, Thiemann DR, McNamara RL, et al. Usefulness of transesophageal echocardiography in predicting mortality and morbidity in stroke patients without clinically known cardiac sources of embolus. *Am J Cardiol* 1998;81:1144–1151.

179. Stollberger C, Chnupa P, Kronik G, et al. Transesophageal echocardiography to assess embolic risk in patients with atrial fibrillation. ELAT Study Group. Embolism in left atrial thrombi [see comments]. *Ann Intern Med* 1998;128:630–638.

180. McNamara RL, Lima JA, Whelton PK, et al. Echocardiographic identification of cardiovascular sources of emboli to guide clinical management of stroke: a cost-effectiveness analysis. *Ann Intern Med* 1997;127:775–787.

181. Rauh G, Fischereder M, Spengel FA. Transesophageal echocardiography in patients with focal cerebral ischemia of unknown cause. *Stroke* 1996;27:691–694.

182. Hata JS, Ayres RW, Biller J, et al. Impact of transesophageal echocardiography on the anticoagulation management of

patients admitted with focal cerebral ischemia. *Am J Cardiol* 1993;72:707–710.

183. Goldman M, Kronzon I, Goldstein SA, et al. Value of transesophageal echocardiography: results in 3,001 patients. *Circulation* 1994;90:I–20.

184. Tardif JC, Vannon MA, Taylor K, et al. Delineation of extended lengths of coronary arteries by multiplane transesophageal echocardiography. *J Am Coll Cardiol* 1994;24:909–919.

185. Samdarshi TE, Nanda NC, Gatewood RP Jr, et al. Usefulness and limitations of transesophageal echocardiography in the assessment of proximal coronary artery stenosis. *J Am Coll Cardiol* 1992;19:572–580.

186. Yamagishi M, Yasu T, Ohara K, et al. Detection of coronary blood flow associated with left main coronary artery stenosis by transesophageal Doppler color flow echocardiography. *J Am Coll Cardiol* 1991;17:87–93.

187. Yoshida K, Yoshikawa J, Hozumi T, et al. Detection of left main coronary artery stenosis by transesophageal color Doppler and two-dimensional echocardiography. *Circulation* 1990;81:1271–1276.

188. Firstenberg MS, Greenberg NL, Lin SS, et al. Transesophageal echocardiography assessment of severe ostial left main coronary stenosis. *J Am Soc Echocardiogr* 2000;13:696–698.

189. Calafiore PA, Raymond R, Schiavone W, et al. Precise evaluation of a complex coronary arteriovenous fistula: the utility of transesophageal color Doppler. *J Am Soc Echocardiogr* 1989;2:337–341.

190. Kosar E, Chandraratna PA. Assessment of coronary artery aneurysms with multiplane transesophageal echocardiography. *Am Heart J* 1997;133:526–533.

191. Skiles JA, Griffin BP. Transesophageal echocardiographic (TEE) evaluation of ventricular function. *Cardiol Clin* 2000;18:681–697.

192. Agati L, Renzi M, Sciomer S, et al. Transesophageal dipyridamole echocardiography for diagnosis of coronary artery disease. *J Am Coll Cardiol* 1992;19:765–770.

193. Frohwein S, Klein JL, Lane A, et al. Transesophageal dobutamine stress echocardiography in the evaluation of coronary artery disease. *J Am Coll Cardiol* 1995;25:823–829.

194. Hoffmann R, Kleinhans E, Lambertz H, et al. Transesophageal pacing echocardiography for detection of restenosis after percutaneous transluminal coronary angioplasty. *Eur Heart J* 1994;15:823–831.

195. Panza JA, Laurienzo JM, Curiel RV, et al. Transesophageal dobutamine stress echocardiography for evaluation of patients with coronary artery disease. *J Am Coll Cardiol* 1994;24:1260–1267.

196. Panza JA, Curiel RV, Laurienzo JM, et al. Relation between ischemic threshold measured during dobutamine stress echocardiography and known indices of poor prognosis in patients with coronary artery disease. *Circulation* 1995;92:2095–2101.

197. Madu EC. Transesophageal dobutamine stress echocardiography in the evaluation of myocardial ischemia in morbidly obese subjects. *Chest* 2000;117:657–661.

198. Redberg RF, Sobol Y, Chou TM, et al. Adenosine-induced coronary vasodilation during transesophageal Doppler echocardiography. Rapid and safe measurement of coronary flow reserve ratio can predict significant left anterior descending coronary stenosis. *Circulation* 1995;92:190–196.

199. Iliceto S, Caiati C, Aragona P, et al. Improved Doppler signal intensity in coronary arteries after intravenous peripheral injection of a lung-crossing contrast agent (SHU 508A). *J Am Coll Cardiol* 1994;23:184–190.

200. Caiati C, Aragona P, Iliceto S, et al. Improved Doppler detection of proximal left anterior descending coronary artery stenosis after intravenous injection of a lung-crossing contrast agent: a transesophageal Doppler echocardiographic study. *Am J Cardiol* 1996;77:1164–1168.

201. Isaaz K, Bruntz JF, Paris D, et al. Abnormal coronary flow velocity pattern in patients with left ventricular hypertrophy, angina pectoris, and normal coronary arteries: a transesophageal Doppler echocardiographic study. *Am Heart J* 1994;128:500–510.

202. Tomochika Y, Tanaka N, Wasaki Y, et al. Assessment of flow profile of left anterior descending coronary artery in hypertrophic cardiomyopathy by transesophageal pulsed Doppler echocardiography. *Am J Cardiol* 1993;72:1425–1430.

203. Stumper OF, Elzenga NJ, Hess J, et al. Transesophageal echocardiography in children with congenital heart disease: an initial experience. *J Am Coll Cardiol* 1990;16:433–441.

204. Weintraub R, Shiota T, Elkadi T, et al. Transesophageal echocardiography in infants and children with congenital heart disease. *Circulation* 1992;86:711–722.

205. Marelli AJ, Child JS, Perloff JK. Transesophageal echocardiography in congenital heart disease in the adult. *Cardiol Clin* 1993;11:505–520.

206. Vargas-Barron J, Rijlaardsam M, Romero-Cardenas A, et al. Transesophageal echocardiography in adults with congenital cardiopathies. *Am Heart J* 1993;126:426–432.

207. Sreeram N, Sutherland GR, Geuskens R, et al. The role of transoesophageal echocardiography in adolescents and adults with congenital heart defects. *Eur Heart J* 1991;12:231–240.

208. Stumper O, Vargas-Barron J, Rijlaarsdam M, et al. Assessment of anomalous systemic and pulmonary venous connections by transesophageal echocardiography in infants and children. *Br Heart J* 1991;66:411–418.

209. Sreeram N, Stumper OF, Kaulitz R, et al. Comparative value of transthoracic and transesophageal echocardiography in the assessment of congenital abnormalities of the atrioventricular junction. *J Am Coll Cardiol* 1990;16:1205–1214.

210. Gnanapragasam JP, Houston AB, Doig WB, et al. Transesophageal echocardiographic assessment of fixed subaortic obstruction in children. *Br Heart J* 1991;66:281–284.

211. Kaulitz R, Oliver F, Stumper W, et al. Comparative values of the precordial and transesophageal approaches in the echocardiographic evaluation of atrial baffle function after an atrial correction procedure. *J Am Coll Cardiol* 1990;16:686–694.

212. Stumper O, Sutherland GR, Geuskens R, et al. Transesophageal echocardiography in evaluation and management after a Fontan procedure. *J Am Coll Cardiol* 1991;17:1152–1160.

213. Fyfe DA, Kline CH, Sade RM, et al. Transesophageal echocardiography detects thrombus formation not identified by transthoracic echocardiography after the Fontan operation. *J Am Coll Cardiol* 1991;18:1733–1737.

214. Heidenreich PA, Stainback RF, Redberg RF, et al. Transesophageal echocardiography predicts mortality in critically ill patients with unexplained hypotension. *J Am Coll Cardiol* 1995;26:152–158.

215. Foster E, Schiller NB. The role of transesophageal echocardiography in critical care: UCSF experience. *J Am Soc Echocardiogr* 1992;5:368–374.

216. Khoury AF, Afridi I, Quinones MA, et al. Transesophageal echocardiography in critically ill patients: feasibility, safety, and impact on management. *Am Heart J* 1994;127:1363–1371.

217. Oh JK Seward JB, Khandheria BK, et al. Transesophageal echocardiography in critically ill patients. *Am J Cardiol* 1990;66:1492–1495.

218. Font VE, Obarski TP, Klein AL, et al. Transesophageal echocardiography in the critical care unit. *Cleve Clin J Med* 1991;43:315–322.

219. Vandenberg BF, Rath LS, Stuhlmuller P, et al. Estimation of left ventricular cavity area with an on-line, semiautomated echocardiographic edge detection system. *Circulation* 1992;86:159–166.

220. Smith MD, Mac Phail B, Harrison MR, et al. Value and limitations of transesophageal echocardiography in determination of left ventricular volumes and ejection fraction. *J Am Coll Cardiol* 1992;19:1213–1222.

221. Kochar GS, Jacobs LE, Kotler MN. Right atrial compression in postoperative cardiac patients: detection by transesophageal echocardiography. *J Am Coll Cardiol* 1990;16:511–516.

222. Stoddard MF, Longaker RA. The role of transesophageal echocardiography in cardiac donor screening. *Am Heart J* 1993;125:1676–1681.

223. Garcia-Fernandez MA, Lopez-Perez JM, Perez-Castellano N, et al. Role of transesophageal echocardiography in the assessment of patients with blunt chest trauma: correlation of echocardiographic findings with the electrocardiogram and creatine kinase monoclonal antibody measurements. *Am Heart J* 1998;135:476–481.

224. Redberg RF, Tucker KJ, Cohen TJ, et al. Physiology of blood flow during cardiopulmonary resuscitation. A transesophageal echocardiographic study. *Circulation* 1993;88:534–542.

225. Tucker KJ, Redberg RF, Schiller NB, et al. Active compression-decompression resuscitation: analysis of transmitral flow and left ventricular volume by transesophageal echocardiography in humans. Cardiopulmonary Resuscitation Working Group. *J Am Coll Cardiol* 1993;22:1485–1493.

226. van der Wouw PA, Koster RW, Delemarre BJ, et al. Diagnostic accuracy of transesophageal echocardiography during cardiopulmonary resuscitation. *J Am Coll Cardiol* 1997;30:780–783.

227. Wittlich N, Erbel R, Eichler A, et al. Detection of central pulmonary artery thromboemboli by transesophageal echocardiography in patients with severe pulmonary embolism. *J Am Soc Echocardiogr* 1992;5:515–524.

228. Chan RK, Johns JA, Calafiore P. Clinical implications of the morphological features of central pulmonary artery thromboemboli shown by transesophageal echocardiography. *Br Heart J* 1994;72:58–62.

229. Russo A, De Luca M, Vigna C, et al. Central pulmonary artery lesions in chronic obstructive pulmonary disease: a transesophageal echocardiography study. *Circulation* 1999;100:1808–1815.

230. Goldstein SA, Campbell AN. Mitral stenosis: evaluation and guidance of valvuloplasty by transesophageal echocardiography. *Cardiol Clin* 1993;11:409–425.

231. Lee KS, Tuzcu EM, Elliott JM, et al. Rapid development of left atrial thrombus associated with percutaneous mitral valvuloplasty. *Cathet Cardiovasc Diagn* 1994;33:345–348.

232. Tumbarello R, Sanna A, Cardu G, et al. Usefulness of transesophageal echocardiography in the pediatric catheterization laboratory. *Am J Cardiol* 1993;71:1321–1325.

233. Dhillon R, Thanopoulos B, Tsaousis G, et al. Transcatheter closure of atrial septal defects in adults with the Amplatzer septal occluder. *Heart* 1999;82:559–562.

234. Rubin DC, Ziskind AA, Hawke MW, et al. Transesophageal echocardiographically guided percutaneous biopsy of a right atrial cardiac mass. *Am Heart J* 1994;127:935–936.

235. Pytlewski G, Georgeson S, Burke J, et al. Endomyocardial biopsy under transesophageal echocardiographic guidance can be safely performed in the critically ill cardiac transplant recipient. *Am J Cardiol* 1994;73:1019–1020.

236. Stumper O, Witsenburg M, Sutherland GR, et al. Transesophageal echocardiographic monitoring of interventional cardiac catheterization in children. *J Am Coll Cardiol* 1991;18:1506–1514.

237. Erbel R, Bednarczyk I, Pop T, et al. Detection of dissection of the aortic intima and media after angioplasty of coarctation of the aorta. An angiographic, computer tomographic, and echocardiographic comparative study. *Circulation* 1990;81:805–814.

238. Jordaens LJ, Vandenbogaerde JF, Van de Bruaene P, et al. Transesophageal echocardiography for insertion of a physiological pacemaker in early pregnancy. *Pacing Clin Electrophysiol* 1990;13:955–957.

239. Abraham TP, Warner JG Jr, Kon ND, et al. Feasibility, accuracy, and incremental value of intraoperative three-dimensional transesophageal echocardiography in valve surgery. *Am J Cardiol* 1997;80:1577–1582.

240. Marx GR, Fulton DR, Pandian NG, et al. Delineation of site, relative size and dynamic geometry of atrial septal defects by real-time three-dimensional echocardiography. *J Am Coll Cardiol* 1995;25:482–490.

241. Acar P, Saliba Z, Bonhoeffer P, et al. Influence of atrial septal defect anatomy in patient selection and assessment of closure with the Cardioseal device: a three-dimensional transoesophageal echocardiographic reconstruction. *Eur Heart J* 2000;21:573–581.

242. Applebaum RM, Kasliwal RR, Kanojia A, et al. Utility of three-dimensional echocardiography during balloon mitral valvuloplasty. *J Am Coll Cardiol* 1998;32:1405–1409.

243. Breburda CS, Griffin BP, Pu M, et al. Three-dimensional echocardiographic planimetry of maximal regurgitant orifice area in myxomatous mitral regurgitation: intraoperative comparison with proximal flow convergence. *J Am Coll Cardiol* 1998;32:432–437.

244. De Simone R, Glombitza G, Vahl CF, et al. Three-dimensional color Doppler: a clinical study in patients with mitral regurgitation. *J Am Coll Cardiol* 1999;33:1646–1654.

245. Greim CA, Brederlau J, Kraus I, et al. Transnasal transesophageal echocardiography: a modified application mode for cardiac examination in ventilated patients. *Anesth Analg* 1999;88:306–311.

246. Cremer M. Ueber die direkte Ableitung der Aktiensstrome des menschlichen herzens vom Oesophagus und uber das Elektokariogramm des fotus. *Munchen Med Wschmsr* 1906;53:811–813.

53

NUCLEAR IMAGING TECHNIQUES

AMI E. ISKANDRIAN
MARIO S. VERANI

▽ ADDITIONAL ELECTRONIC TOPICS

GLOSSARY

Attenuation: The reduction in the intensity of radiation that occurs when it passes through matter.

Background subtraction: Subtraction of nontarget counts from the target area; for example, left ventricular counts

A. E. Iskandrian: Department of Medicine and Radiology, Section of Nuclear Cardiology, Division of Cardiovascular Disease, University of Alabama School of Medicine, Birmingham, Alabama

M. S. Verani: Department of Medicine (Cardiology), The Methodist Hospital, Houston, Texas

– background counts = background subtracted left ventricular counts.

Becquerel (Bq): The SI unit of radioactivity, equal to 1 disintegration per second. 1 mCi = 37 mBq.

Biologic half-life: The time interval over which the body eliminates one-half of a given amount of substance through biologic processes.

Compton scattering: The loss in photon energy that results from scattering by collision with electrons.

Effective half-life: The combined half-life of physical decay and biologic elimination.

mCi: The unit of activity that gives 3.7×10^{10} disintegrations per second.

Physical half-life: The time interval over which radioactivity decreases to exactly one-half.

Rad: Radiation absorbed dose.

Radioactive disintegration or decay: A process whereby an unstable nucleus becomes more stable by emitting charged particles.

Radionuclide generator: A system for producing short-lived isotopes by eluting a daughter radionuclide with short half-life from a parent radionuclide with a long half-life.

Rem: Roentgen equivalent, man. Dose in rem equals dose in rad for x-rays and for gamma rays.

Shielding: Any heavy materials used to block radiation.

Spatial resolution: Ability of a gamma camera to distinguish activities very close to each other; for example, separating lines.

Temporal resolution: Ability of a system to separate activities sequentially; for example, framing rate in first-pass study.

IMAGING TECHNIQUES AND PROTOCOLS

The cardiac nuclear imaging techniques that have been applied to clinical imaging are summarized in *e*Table 53.0.2. At present, the most commonly used nuclear cardiac imaging procedure is myocardial perfusion imaging with the gated SPECT technique.

Imaging Protocols

Nuclear cardiac images can be acquired either at rest or during stress (exercise or pharmacologic). When the perfusion tracer is injected at peak stress, a separate rest injection is often required if a Tc-99m labeled tracer (such as tetrofosmin or sestamibi) is used. Tl-201 images are obtained shortly after stress and repeated 4 hours later. Defects that are present during stress and improve 4 hours later (measured with Tl-201) or at rest (measured with Tc-99m tracers) denote myocardial ischemia, whereas lack of improvement denotes either scar or resting hypoperfusion. Reinjection of a small dose of Tl-201 (1 mCi) after the 4-hour redistribution images are taken aids in distinguishing between ischemia and scar: Ischemic but viable areas improve after reinjection, whereas myocardial scar does not (27,28). A hybrid protocol (the dual isotope technique) uses a rest injection of Tl-201, followed by imaging, which is then followed by an injection within 1 hour of injection of a Tc-99m tracer during stress (29). In patients who are unable to exercise, pharmacologic stress with dipyridamole, adenosine, or dobutamine has been used successfully. With proper administration and monitoring, all three of these

drugs are quite safe, although side effects are very common during the test (30,31).

DETECTION AND EVALUATION OF CORONARY ARTERY DISEASE

In the past decade, myocardial perfusion imaging with SPECT has evolved into the preeminent noninvasive technique for assessment of coronary artery disease (CAD). Although RNA during stress remains a useful technique in selected patients, it is most often used in the risk-stratification of patients who have experienced myocardial infarction (MI) or heart failure.

Myocardial Perfusion Imaging

The basic principle underlying the detection of CAD by perfusion imaging is a differential blood flow distribution through the left ventricular myocardium, with a normal flow (and normal tracer uptake) in the myocardium perfused by normal coronary arteries and *relatively* diminished flow (and diminished tracer uptake) in regions perfused by stenotic vessels. A perfusion abnormality may be present at rest in patients with previous MI or fibrosis, or in patients with high-grade (>85% of the luminal diameter) coronary stenoses. However, most functionally significant coronary stenoses, including severe ones, are associated with normal resting myocardial blood flow and, hence, normal resting perfusion images. Consequently, to demonstrate these stenoses, it is necessary to perform imaging of these patients during stress.

During maximal exercise or pharmacologic stress, blood flow increases through the normal coronary arteries but increases less or even fails to increase (occasionally, it decreases) in vessels with significant (>50% of the luminal diameter) stenoses. This diminished coronary flow reserve in stenotic vessels is not an all-or-none phenomenon; rather, the flow reserve decreases gradually as the severity of the coronary stenosis progresses. The most severe stenoses (>85%) typically have no flow reserve left. ⮞ j99

Exercise Myocardial Perfusion Imaging

The most common indications for exercise perfusion imaging are listed in Table 53.1. ⮞ k01

Recent reports have confirmed the diagnostic utility of perfusion imaging in patients with normal and with abnormal resting ECG results (35). The information provided by myocardial perfusion scintigraphy during stress transcends the mere categorization of the test results as normal or abnormal. On the basis of the location of the perfusion abnormality, one can infer which arteries are involved. It has been shown that stenoses involving the left anterior descending artery generally lead to a larger perfusion defect

TABLE 53.1 INDICATIONS FOR EXERCISE PERFUSION SCINTIGRAPHY

Diagnosis of coronary artery disease
   Stable angina or chest pain of uncertain origin
   Unstable angina, after initial stabilization
   Positive exercise electrocardiogram without symptoms
   Screening of high-risk, asymptomatic patients
   Patients who are referred for exercise electrocardiographic testing but have an abnormal resting echocardiogram that hampers evaluation of ischemia
   Prior nondiagnostic exercise electrocardiogram test
Assessment of functional importance of known coronary stenoses
   Borderline stenoses (40% to 70%) by coronary angiography
   Assessment of culprit lesion before coronary angioplasty
   Stenoses of small branches or of distal location
Assessment of therapeutic benefits
   After percutaneous coronary intervention
   After coronary artery bypass surgery
   After medical therapy
Risk-stratification
   Stable angina
   Unstable angina
   Post–myocardial infarction
   Preoperative risk
Demonstration of myocardial ischemia in patients with angiographically normal coronary arteries.

Modified from Iskandrian AS, Verani MS. *Nuclear cardiac imaging: principles and applications.* Philadelphia: FA Davis, 1996, with permission.

than stenoses in the right coronary or circumflex arteries (36,37) (*e*Fig. 53.0.4). Patients with multivessel CAD have larger perfusion defects than patients with single-vessel disease (38). In addition to the extent of hypoperfusion, the

reversibility of the defects needs to be assessed during the redistribution (in the case of Tl-201) or the rest images (in the case of the Tc-99m tracers). It is important to assess also the severity of tracer uptake reduction in the stress and rest or redistribution images. Transient cavity dilation during exercise or pharmacologic stress and increased Tl-201 lung uptake during stress are powerful predictors of poor prognosis (25,33).

The use of exercise perfusion scintigraphy to screen asymptomatic patients is controversial. It certainly cannot be recommended across the board, but it may be very useful in selected populations who are at increased risk for CAD despite being asymptomatic (Fig. 53.1). For example, the test is useful in patients with a conglomerate of risk factors and in adolescents or young adults who have familial hypercholesterolemia (39). Middle-aged siblings of patients who have had an MI also are at increased risk for cardiac events and are good candidates for a stress perfusion study (40).

An extensive review of published studies that used exercise Tl-201 qualitative planar scintigraphy, which included 52 publications and 5,160 patients (41), shows an overall sensitivity and specificity of 83% and 88%, respectively. Several studies assessed the value of quantitative Tl-201 planar scintigraphy during exercise for the diagnosis of CAD (24). The mean sensitivity and specificity are 90% and 80%, respectively. With exercise Tl-201 SPECT, the average sensitivity and specificity are 89% and 76%, respectively, by qualitative analysis (24).

A comparison between qualitative and quantitative analyses of Tl-201 SPECT images has not shown a major difference in sensitivity or specificity between these two

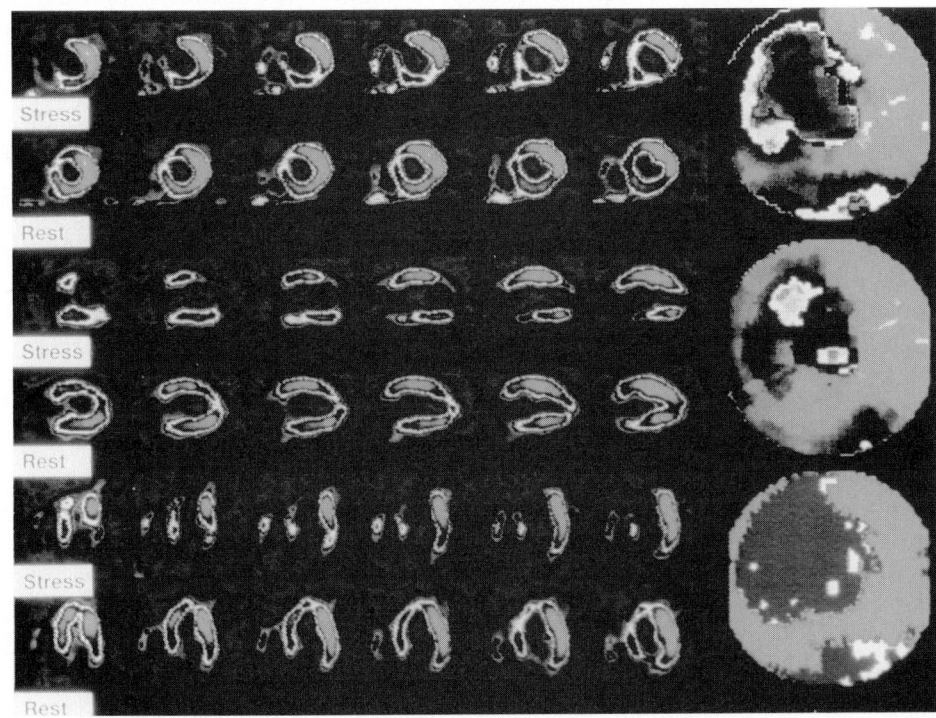

FIGURE 53.1 Technetium-99m single-photon emission computed tomographic images during exercise and at rest in a 52-year-old diabetic male who was asymptomatic. The images during stress depict large defects involving the anterior wall, septum, apex, and inferior and posterolateral walls, with substantial improvement at rest. Subsequent coronary angiography showed severe proximal left anterior descending (90%) and left circumflex (75%) stenoses.

techniques (38,42–45). However, detection of the individual coronary arteries involved may be moderately improved by quantitative analysis. This is particularly true for detection of circumflex artery stenoses and coronary stenoses of moderate severity (between 50% and 75% of the luminal diameter) (45).

Use of Technetium-99m Perfusion Tracers in the Diagnosis of Coronary Angiography Disease

The newer Tc-99m flow tracers represent a substantial improvement in nuclear cardiac imaging. The more favorable physical characteristics of Tc-99m, such as an optimal emission energy for imaging with gamma cameras, and less physical scatter and shorter half-life (which allows administration of a much higher tracer dose) than Tl-201, are definite advantages of these agents. Interestingly, the few studies that have direct compared Tl-201 with Tc-99m sestamibi, teboroxime, or tetrofosmin have not shown an overall superiority for detection of CAD with any of these newer agents. The overall sensitivity of Tc-99m sestamibi using planar imaging is 87%, with a specificity of 62% and a normalcy rate of 92%. When SPECT imaging is used, the overall sensitivity and specificity are 90% and 74%, respectively (24). As mentioned, Tc-99m sestamibi imaging during stress has also been used in combination with Tl-201 resting imaging (dual isotope imaging). With this strategy, a sensitivity of 91% and specificity of 75% have been found by Berman and coworkers (29).

Because the Tc-99m–labeled agents undergo less attenuation than agents labeled with Tl-201, they may be particularly useful for patients who are prone to attenuation artifacts, such as women with large breasts or breast implants and obese individuals (46). Tc-99m teboroxime has been used with planar imaging and with SPECT imaging. Despite its high myocardial extraction rate and its good correlation with determination of myocardial flow using microspheres, it has a very short residence time in the myocardium, rendering SPECT imaging a challenging proposition. The initial favorable reports (which indicated an average sensitivity of 87% and specificity of 62% with either planar or SPECT imaging) (47,48) notwithstanding, this tracer is not currently used for clinical imaging. New research has focused on the idea of measuring absolute myocardial blood flow using dynamic imaging with teboroxime (49).

Tetrofosmin is another attractive Tc-99m–labeled perfusion agent. A high concordance rate has been found between this agent and Tl-201, both with planar and SPECT imaging (50,51). As is the case for sestamibi, the sensitivity and specificity of tetrofosmin imaging appear to be comparable, but not superior, to those of Tl-201 imaging. In the largest reported series, from a phase III multicenter trial, that used planar imaging and included 252

patients from ten centers in the United States and Europe, tetrofosmin and Tl-201 had similar sensitivity and specificity for CAD detection. Other studies have confirmed the diagnostic accuracy of tetrofosmin (52–55) and confirmed that it is comparable to sestamibi (56).

Furofosmin is another Tc-99m–labeled compound that has been tested in the United States but has not received FDA approval. In a large multicenter trial comparing Tc-99m furofosmin SPECT with Tl-201 SPECT during exercise, an overall agreement in the results of 86% was found (57).

The principal advantage of the Tc-99m tracers is that they can be administered in higher doses, and, hence, high-quality images are feasible even for large or obese individuals and women with large breasts. Another very attractive feature is the ability to gate the SPECT images, which allows an evaluation of the global and regional ventricular function by observation of the motion of the perfused ventricular walls. These agents also enable assessment of left and right ventricular function during the injection of the Tc-99m tracers by first-pass RNA.

Pharmacologic Perfusion Imaging

Approximately 20% to 30% of patients with suspected or documented CAD are unable to perform an exercise stress test and, thus, are good candidates for pharmacologic stress imaging. Other clinical conditions for which pharmacologic stress imaging is appropriate are listed in Table 53.2. Adenosine produces maximal or near-maximal coronary vasodilation through its agonistic effect on the adenosine A2 receptors located in the coronary arterial wall. Dipyridamole has an indirect vasodilator effect, through the inhibition of the cellular reuptake and metabolism of adenosine (24,30), leading to an increase in the interstitial and perimembrane levels of adenosine. The principal difference between these two agents, which have similar hemodynamic effects (24), is the much shorter half-life of adenosine. Both produce frequent side effects, but the reported experience in large numbers of patients has indicated that both are quite safe when properly used (58–60). Investigators in Japan have used intravenous adenosine triphosphate as yet another option for pharmacologic stressor (61,62).

TABLE 53.2 INDICATIONS FOR PHARMACOLOGIC PERFUSION IMAGING

Patient unable to exercise
Preoperative risk-stratification
Early postinfarct risk-stratification
Left bundle branch block
Presence of fixed-rate ventricular pacemaker

Modified from Verani MS. Pharmacologic stress myocardial perfusion imaging. *Curr Probl Cardiol* 1993;18(8):481–525.

Studies comparing dipyridamole or adenosine Tl-201 scintigraphy with exercise Tl-201 scintigraphy have indicated excellent agreement between these stressors. The overall reported sensitivity with dipyridamole Tl-201 planar imaging is 82%, with a specificity of 75%. These values are slightly higher with SPECT imaging (89% and 78%, respectively). The average sensitivity of adenosine Tl-201 SPECT is 88%, with a specificity of 85% (24,30). Clinical studies have shown similar values when adenosine or dipyridamole is combined with Tc-99m sestamibi or tetrofosmin (63–65). Both adenosine and dipyridamole can be combined with a submaximal exercise test. The main advantage of such a combination is the decrease in splancnic uptake, which improves the quality of the images, especially with Tc-99m agents (66,67).

Adenosine and dipyridamole are contraindicated in patients who have active asthma or severe chronic obstructive pulmonary disease with wheezing. In these patients, dobutamine is a proven adequate stressor, with reported sensitivity ranging from 80% to 97% and specificity ranging from 74% to 89%, in combination with SPECT (24). Although a curious antagonism has been described between dobutamine and sestamibi in animal experiments (68), the reported sensitivity of this combination of agents in clinical patients is high thus far (69,70).

Causes of False-Negative Results of Myocardial Perfusion Scintigraphy

Table 53.3 lists several of the possible causes of false-negative myocardial perfusion images. Among these, the most frequent are an inadequate exercise stress test and concomitant administration of antiischemic medications. It must be emphasized that the gold standard for determination of diagnostic accuracy of perfusion imaging has traditionally been coronary angiography. The potential weaknesses of this gold standard have long been emphasized (71). It is not unusual for lesions that are considered "significant" by angiography to have a normal flow reserve. It is thus not surprising that some of them are also associated with normal myocardial perfusion images.

TABLE 53.3 CAUSES OF FALSE-NEGATIVE RESULTS OF SCANS

Inadequate exercise stress
Administration of antiischemic medications
Non–flow-limiting coronary stenoses
Overlap circulation
Collateral circulation
Hypoperfusion in segments with attenuation
Incorrect interpretation of angiograms
Incorrect interpretation of scans
Poor-quality images
"Balanced" hypoperfusion
Delay in obtaining thallium-201 stress images

Modified from Iskandrian AS, Verani MS. *Nuclear cardiac imaging: principles and applications.* Philadelphia: FA Davis, 1996, with permission.

TABLE 53.4 CAUSES OF FALSE-POSITIVE RESULTS OF SCANS

Regional photon attenuation
Poor technique
Conduction abnormalities[a]
Cardiomyopathies[a]
Coronary vasospasm[a]
Coronary anomalies[a]
Microvascular disease[a]
Recanalized coronary occlusion[a]
Posttest referral bias
Gold-standard pitfalls

[a]Causes "real" defects. The term *false-positive* is used in comparison with absence of stenoses as seen on coronary angiography.
Modified from Iskandrian AS, Verani MS. *Nuclear cardiac imaging: principles and applications.* Philadelphia: FA Davis, 1996.

Causes of False-Positive Myocardial Perfusion Images

Table 53.4 lists some of the causes that may be associated with false-positive results of imaging. Among them, the most important is photon attenuation, which may have a different impact on different myocardial walls. ⌖ k02

RISK ASSESSMENT

Risk Assessment in Patients with Stable Symptoms

Cardiac events are defined either as "hard" (death or MI) or "soft" (e.g., increasing angina, the need for coronary revascularization, or the need for hospitalization). [⌖ k03] The predictors of hard and soft events may be different—in fact, the predictors of death may also differ from those of MI. For example, ischemic manifestation may predict an ischemic event such as acute MI or unstable angina, and left ventricular function or the overall extent of perfusion defect may predict death (81). Clinical, angiographic, and exercise variables have been identified that separate high- and low-risk groups for cardiac events. Califf and associates developed a risk-factor prediction chart that used age, gender, lipid profile, smoking history, systolic blood pressure, presence of diabetes or left ventricular hypertrophy, and fibrinogen level to separate patients into those with <1% risk of events and those with a 25% probability of having events during the 5 years after assessment (82).

Early planar imaging and subsequent SPECT (using Tl-201– and Tc-99m–based tracers) in thousands of patients in multiple trials has yielded a strong message regarding the prognostic value of such tests. The message is consistent whether the imaging is done with exercise or with pharmacologic stress testing. Simply stated, perfusion imaging can separate patients at low risk from those at high risk. The relevance of such a conclusion on patient management is equally strong, because the condition of patients at low risk

TABLE 53.5 STRESS PERFUSION PREDICTORS OF RISK IN MEDICALLY TREATED PATIENTS WITH STABLE ANGINA

Large zone of ischemia
Large zone of fixed defects
Perfusion abnormality in more than one vascular territory
Increased lung uptake
Left ventricular dilation (transient or fixed)
Left ventricular ejection fraction (by gated single-photon emission computed tomography)

may be managed conservatively, without the need of coronary angiography or coronary interventions, whereas at least subgroups of high-risk patients may benefit from coronary revascularization (34,83–119).

The major prognostic variables are listed in Table 53.5. The available data strongly suggest the following ten points:

1. Normal stress images have a very high negative predictive value; hard event rate (death or nonfatal MI) is less than 1% per year (87,88,96,101,104,105).
2. Accordingly, the rate of coronary angiography is often very low in patients who have normal results of imaging (86,89,95,96,99,105).
3. The event rate is significantly higher (mean, 12-fold) in patients with abnormal results of imaging, based on review of data from more than 12,000 patients (*e*Fig. 53.1.2) (96,105).
4. The event rate among patients who have abnormal results of imaging increases as a function of the severity of the perfusion abnormality. Patients with severe abnormality are at higher risk than patients with mild abnormality (85,96,105,109). The results are true in men and in women (90,102,115).
5. The results of exercise and pharmacologic stress testing using Tl-201, sestamibi, or tetrofosmin are comparable (96,105). The risk may be slightly higher among patients with normal results of dobutamine sestamibi imaging, possibly because ischemia is underestimated or because of a higher risk among the patient population in whom the use of dobutamine was studied (68).
6. Stress perfusion imaging provides statistically significant incremental information to support that provided by clinical evaluation, treadmill exercise testing, and coronary angiography (34,85,96).
7. The use of gated SPECT perfusion imaging enhances the prognostic power of imaging by incorporating left ventricular functional data, such as LVEF and left ventricular volumes, with perfusion data.
8. Diagnostic strategies based on the use of stress perfusion imaging as the initial test followed by selective referral of high-risk patients to coronary angiography are more cost-effective than routine use of coronary angiography on all patients. This advantage is accompanied by at least similar outcome (113–115).
9. The perfusion pattern may predict the type of subsequent events. Large fixed defects often predict cardiac death, and large reversible defects predict MI and total hard events (death plus MI) and, as expected, the need for coronary revascularization (34,104,105).
10. The "warranty" period associated with normal or mildly abnormal results of imaging depends on pretest likelihood of CAD; in high-risk patients and patients with established CAD, the test needs to be repeated at 18 to 24 months after revascularization, or earlier if symptoms change. In low-risk and intermediate-risk groups, the test needs to be repeated at 5 and at 3 years, respectively (85,96,105). ▼ k04

Risk Assessment: Noncardiac Surgery

The American College of Cardiology (ACC)/American Heart Association (AHA) Task Force report on guidelines for perioperative cardiovascular evaluation for noncardiac surgery reaffirmed the importance of clinical evaluation in risk assessment (81). [▼ k05] Major predictors of increased perioperative risk include recent acute MI, unstable angina pectoris, decompensated congestive heart failure, significant arrhythmias, high degree of atrioventricular block and severe valvular disease. Intermediate predictors include mild angina pectoris, prior MI, compensated or prior congestive heart failure, and diabetes mellitus. Minor predictors include advanced age, abnormal resting ECG, normal rhythm on ECG, low functional capacity, history of stroke, and uncontrolled systemic hypertension.

High-risk surgical procedures include a major emergency operation, such as aortic and other major vascular surgery, and peripheral vascular surgery, especially in elderly patients. Intermediate-risk procedures include carotid endarterectomy, head and neck surgery, and intraperitoneal, intrathoracic, orthopedic, and prostate surgery. Low-risk procedures include endoscopic procedures, superficial procedures, cataract removal, and breast surgery.

Patients who are at low risk, especially if they are undergoing a low-risk surgical procedure, may not need preoperative stress testing. Surgery should be avoided, whenever possible, in patients who have experienced recent MI or unstable angina pectoris, until the clinical condition has been stabilized; if surgery must be performed, then coronary angiography is recommended. In many other patients, stress testing is indicated. The greatest amount of experience by far is in the use of pharmacologic perfusion imaging with dipyridamole or adenosine (126–136). Mangano and Goldman (124) summarized the results of large studies published in the literature (*e*Table 53.5.1). The results show that among patients in whom no evidence of ischemia is found, the event rate is extremely low (2%); on the other hand, among patients who have reversible defects, the event rate is 18% (relative risk, 9.0). These general conclusions are concordant with those of multiple other studies that involved smaller number of patients. Most of these studies did not include quantitative analysis to assess the size of jeopardized ischemic myocardium, although Brown and Rowen (134) demonstrated that the risk of perioperative events increased in proportion to the degree of abnormality (assessed as the number of abnormal segments on dipyridamole planar Tl-201 imaging).

The ACC/AHA guidelines recommend coronary angiography should be performed in patients for whom the results of noninvasive testing indicate a high risk of cardiac events (presence of a large area of ischemia, perfusion defects in multiple vascular territories, left ventricular dilatation, or increased lung Tl-201 uptake) or who have angina pectoris that is unresponsive to medical therapy (class I indication) (81). Among other patients, either coronary angiography is not indicated or there is a divergence of opinion about whether such testing is indicated. Patients in whom left ventricular dysfunction is demonstrated by clinical evaluation or by the results of measurement of EF and patients who have extensive fixed perfusion defects are at risk of developing congestive heart failure or serious ventricular arrhythmias during the perioperative period. The risk of ischemic events in these patients is low, but the long-term outcome is poor because of the underlying left ventricular dysfunction. Thus, extensive fixed perfusion defects do not have the same implication as reversible defects in the short run, but they do have an impact on long-term prognosis (24,81).

A randomized study showed that bisoprolol (a selective beta$_1$-blocker) reduced the perioperative (137) death/MI rate from 34% in the control group to 3.4% in the treatment group for high-risk patients with ischemia who are undergoing high-risk vascular surgery. ✌ k06

EVALUATION OF PATIENTS AFTER PERCUTANEOUS TRANSLUMINAL CORONARY ANGIOPLASTY AND CORONARY ARTERY BYPASS GRAFT SURGERY

Nuclear techniques are very useful in the selection of patients for whom coronary revascularization is appropriate, in the evaluation of the results of revascularization interventions, and to ascertain the presence of recurrent myocardial ischemia early or late after revascularization. Ideally, coronary revascularization should be reserved for patients in whom myocardial ischemia has been documented, especially those patients who have large ischemic areas involving multiple vascular territories and patients who have transient cavity dilation or increased lung uptake of Tl-201 during stress testing; these are the characteristics that identify patients who are at high risk for future events if they do not undergo revascularization. Conversely, patients who have normal myocardial perfusion during stress testing or who have only small perfusion defects

TABLE 53.6 MECHANISMS OF PERFUSION DEFECTS AFTER REVASCULARIZATION

After PCI
  Residual stenosis of dilated artery
  Restenosis
  Side-branch occlusion
After CABG
  Graft disease (occlusion or stenosis)
After either PCI or CABG
  Remote or periprocedure infarct
  Incomplete revascularization
  Disease progression

CABG, coronary artery bypass graft; PCI, percutaneous coronary intervention.

involving one vascular territory (especially if the defect is fixed) are not in a high-risk category; in general, the condition of these patients should be managed medically. However, patients who present with heart failure or angina in whom the perfusion scans show only fixed defects should undergo reinjection of Tl-201 (or a separate rest redistribution protocol), because some of these defects may further improve after reinjection, which is characteristic of myocardial ischemia and viable myocardium (138). Fixed defects accompanied by mild to moderate reduction in tracer activity are consistent with viable myocardium and often improve after revascularization (139).

Substantial resolution of myocardial ischemia with amelioration of perfusion defects is the rule after successful percutaneous transluminal coronary angioplasty (PTCA) or coronary artery bypass graft (CABG) surgery (140–148). However, residual perfusion defects are common after coronary revascularization. The possible mechanisms of these defects are summarized in Table 53.6. The indications for perfusion imaging after PTCA or CABG are summarized in Table 53.7.

TABLE 53.7 INDICATIONS FOR POSTREVASCULARIZATION PERFUSION IMAGING

PCI
  Early (<2 wk)
    Uncertain or suboptimal results
    Symptoms
  Late (>2 wk)
    Recurrence of symptoms
    Silent ischemia before PCI
    Multivessel disease with incomplete revascularization
    High risk of coronary lesions
CABG
  Recurrence of symptoms
  Incomplete revascularization
  Poor distal run-off
  Silent ischemia before CABG surgery
  Patient asymptomatic 3 to 5 yr after revascularization

CABG, coronary artery bypass graft; PCI, percutaneous coronary intervention.

Myocardial Perfusion Imaging after Percutaneous Transluminal Coronary Angioplasty

The ideal time to perform stress perfusion imaging after PTCA is controversial. Some authors have suggested that defects that occur very early after successful PTCA may later resolve (145). Others, however, have suggested that perfusion defects that appear early after PTCA are in fact highly predictive of late restenosis (143,146). It may be appropriate to delay myocardial perfusion imaging for 2 to 4 weeks after angioplasty. Alternatively, only patients with recurrent symptoms could be targeted for repeat myocardial perfusion imaging, although Hecht and colleagues (147) showed a similar rate of restenosis (61% vs. 59%) in asymptomatic and symptomatic patients, respectively, after PTCA (*e*Fig. 53.1.6). In both groups of patients, exercise perfusion imaging was highly accurate for detection of restenosis.

Myocardial Perfusion Imaging after Coronary Artery Bypass Graft Surgery

Contrary to PTCA, in which restenosis usually occurs within the first 3 to 6 months after the intervention, patients with CABG have a high early patency rate (90% at 1 year), with an attrition rate of 2% per year from years 1 to 7 and then 5% per year for years 7 to 12. At the end of 10 years, only approximately 40% of saphenous vein grafts are open and have a normal appearance. In contrast, internal mammary grafts have a patency rate of 85% to 95% after 7 to 10 years. Improved myocardial perfusion with normalization of ischemic perfusion defects is the rule after CABG (148), although residual defects after CABG resulting from the mechanisms listed in Table 53.6 are not infrequent. Myocardial perfusion imaging is also an effective way to assess graft patency after CABG. A new perfusion defect early (within the first 1 or 2 years) after CABG suggests a graft problem or incomplete revascularization, whereas defects appearing late (>5 years after CABG) suggest either graft disease or CAD progression (148). Tl-201 SPECT is very useful in the prognostic evaluation of patients who are examined late after CABG (149–152). The indications for perfusion imaging after CABG are listed in Table 53.7.

ACUTE CORONARY SYNDROMES

The main indications for nuclear imaging in acute coronary syndromes are listed in Table 53.8. ▼▼ k07

Because of the associated long myocardial retention and slow washout, Tc-99m–labeled tracers have been used to measure the size of MI and myocardial salvage. Injection of the tracer before thrombolytic therapy or primary angioplasty is initiated defines the area of myocardium at risk, even when the images are obtained several hours later. These images can be compared to a second set of images

TABLE 53.8   USES OF NUCLEAR IMAGING IN ACUTE CORONARY SYNDROMES

Detection of acute MI
Measurement of the size of MI
Assessment of myocardial salvage in response to thrombolytic therapy or primary angioplasty
Measurement of left ventricular ejection fraction
Identification of the culprit artery in patients with unstable angina pectoris
Triage of patients who present with chest pain in the emergency department
Risk assessment in patients with unstable angina pectoris
Risk assessment after acute MI
Detection of complications of acute MI
Viability assessment

MI, myocardial infarction.

obtained several days later. The defect size reduction reflects the degree of myocardial salvage, and the final defect size reflects the area of residual necrosis. Further reduction in the size of a perfusion defect has been reported in approximately 70% of patients after 6 months, even without coronary intervention (154). Several studies have shown substantial variability in both the area at risk and the degree of salvage in patients with acute infarction. In general, both the area at risk and the absolute amount of salvaged myocardium are larger in patients with anterior than inferior or posterior MI (although, in relative terms, the percentage of salvage may be similar). The size of the defect seen on predischarge scan correlates well with indices of left ventricular function such as EF and end systolic volume and is also an important predictor of survival (155,156). ▼▼ k08

In many institutions, chest pain units have been established within the emergency department to screen for patients who need admission and monitoring and to identify those who may be discharged or need early stress testing. The precise algorithm varies from center to center, but generally patients with nondiagnostic ECG ST/T changes undergo clinical evaluation and serial cardiac enzymes measurements (including creatine kinase/MB and troponin I or T). When the results of these tests are negative, the patients undergo rest or exercise perfusion imaging (or both), depending on the probability of CAD. Injection of a tracer during chest pain or shortly after has shown perfusion defects in many patients with acute MI or unstable angina pectoris and nondiagnostic ECG changes. Varetto and colleagues (162) observed perfusion defects in 27 of 30 patients who subsequently were demonstrated to have acute coronary syndromes, but in 0 of 34 patients who subsequently showed no evidence of CAD. Hilton et al. (160) reported events in only 1 of 70 patients who had normal scans but in 71% of 32 patients with abnormal scans. The group of investigators (164) at the Medical College of Virginia have reported their extensive experience with emergency department imaging. Their pioneering work suggests that acute perfusion imaging may be an important addition to current screening modalities in the acute setting.

Risk Assessment

The risk among patients with acute MI for future cardiac events depends on the size of the infarction, clinical findings (e.g., third heart sound gallop, age, gender, presence of diabetes mellitus, rales, hypotension, serious ventricular arrhythmias, recurrent ischemia, infarction extension), LVEF and the results of coronary angiography (extent of CAD), exercise results, and imaging variables. Several studies made in the 1980s concluded that stress perfusion imaging (exercise or pharmacologic) (166,167) and the LVEF determined by RNA (168) performed in patients who had uncomplicated acute MI could stratify patients into low- and high-risk groups. These studies were carried out in the prethrombolytic era. For example, Gibson et al. (166) reported that 50% of patients who had multiple perfusion defects in more than one vascular territory or abnormal lung Tl-201 uptake on predischarge exercise testing subsequently experienced cardiac events. On the other hand, the event rate was only 6% in patients who had either a normal scan or fixed defects in the territory of the infarction. Other studies have also shown that stress perfusion imaging is clearly superior to ST segment changes in detecting multivessel disease in such patients. One of the most important markers of prognosis, judging by the results of the Multicenter Postinfarction Research group (168), has been the radionuclide-measured resting LVEF. In this study, patients with an EF >40% had a low event rate, whereas patients with an EF <40% had a significantly higher event rate, especially those with an EF <30%. In more recent studies involving patients who received thrombolytic therapy, the LVEF was still a strong predictor of outcome, but fewer patients had left ventricular dysfunction (Fig. 53.2) (169–171).

In the thrombolytic era, early studies have suggested that SPECT perfusion imaging is less accurate in risk assessment (172,173). However, more recent studies using exercise testing combined with quantitative Tl-201 imaging have shown that the size of the perfusion defect as well as the extent of ischemia and the LVEF are independent predictors of cardiac events. The perfusion data had incremental value to the LVEF (174). In nonselected patients who had acute infarcts, one-half of whom had thrombolytic therapy, Mahmarian et al. (175,176) showed that traditional variables of perfusion imaging, such as the size of the perfusion abnormality and the extent of reversibility during adenosine SPECT Tl-201 imaging, were still important predictors of prognosis. Another important observation from the latter study is that the LVEF provided incremental value to the size of the perfusion defect (*e*Fig. 53.2.1). This observation is pertinent because the Tc-99m–labeled tracers allow simultaneous assessment of both the perfusion defect and the LVEF. Several studies have shown that pharmacologic vasodilatation with adenosine or dipyridamole is safe as early as 48 hours after an acute MI. A recent comparison between dipyridamole and submaximal exercise testing, both associated with SPECT imaging, showed the pharma-

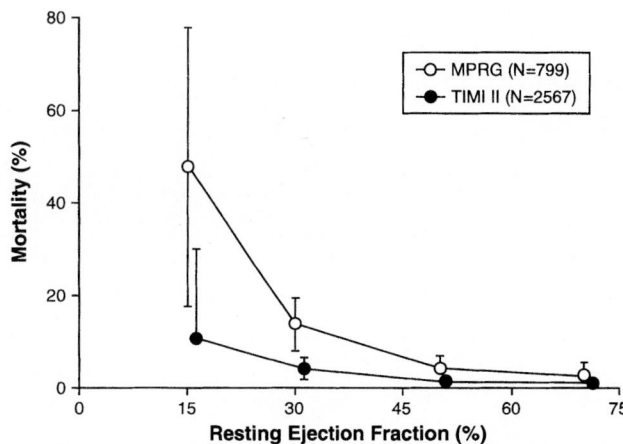

FIGURE 53.2 The relationship between resting left ventricular ejection fraction and survival in patients who have experienced acute myocardial infarction. The results from patients who received thrombolytic therapy [Thrombolysis in Myocardial Infarction phase II study (TIMI II)] are contrasted with those from the Multicenter Postinfarction Research Group (MPRG). [From Zaret BL, Wackers FJ, Terrin ML, et al. Value of radionuclide rest and exercise left ventricular ejection fraction in assessing survival of patients after thrombolytic therapy for acute myocardial infarction: results of Thrombolysis in Myocardial Infarction (TIMI) phase II study. *J Am Coll Cardiol* 1995;26:73–79, with permission.]

cologic approach to be at least as good as exercise imaging, if not better (177). Another recent report has suggested that aggressive antiischemic therapy involving either revascularization or medical therapy substantially reduces perfusion defect size and may improve outcomes in these patients (178). Early testing may expedite the decision-making process and decrease hospitalization time. The relative value of vasodilator perfusion imaging compared with early exercise perfusion testing, however, remains unclear. There are no data on the safety of high-dose dobutamine perfusion imaging in risk assessment. The importance of perfusion imaging in risk assessment is emphasized in the new ACC/AHA guidelines on management of the condition of patients who have acute MI (179). The VANQWISH trial, which involved patients with non–Q-wave MI, used Tl-201 imaging as a risk-stratifying modality to identify patients randomly assigned to a conservative strategy who might have a high risk for cardiac events. These patients could cross-over to revascularization. The results of the Veterans Affairs Non-Q-Wave Infarction Strategies in Hospital trial suggested that a noninvasive strategy, in which assessment was performed by perfusion imaging, led to better outcomes than an invasive strategy (180). Recently published guidelines for management of non–Q-wave MI and unstable angina suggest that a noninvasive risk assessment strategy is appropriate for stable patients (181).

Unstable Angina Pectoris

The indications for nuclear testing include differentiation between cardiac and noncardiac chest pains in patients

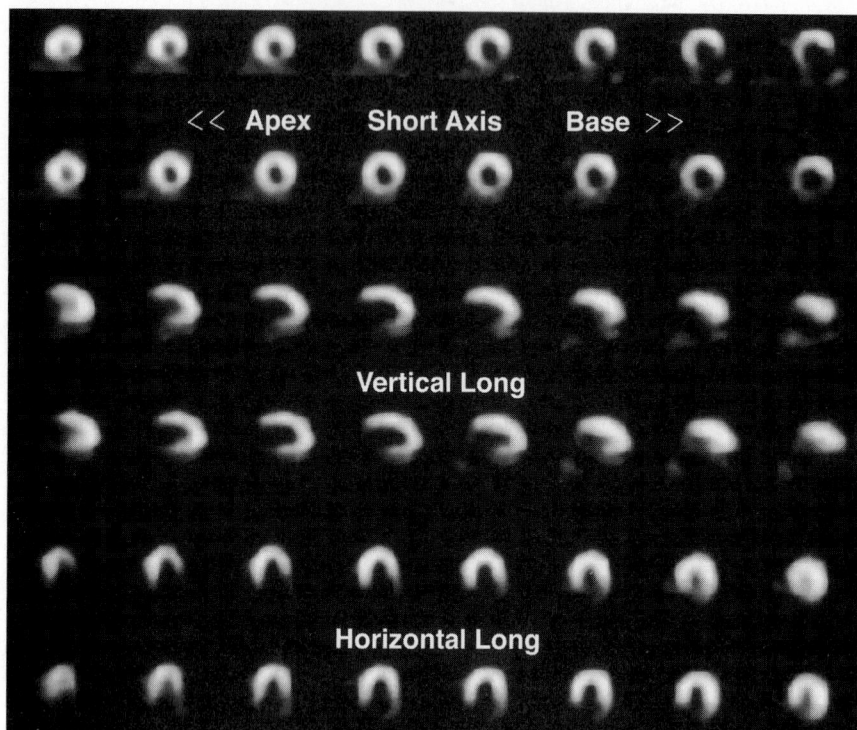

<< **Apex**   **Short Axis**   **Base** >>

Vertical Long

Horizontal Long

FIGURE 53.3 Resting single-photon emission computed tomographic technetium-99m sestamibi images obtained during spontaneous chest pain in a patient with unstable angina pectoris. The images show a large perfusion defect in the inferolateral regions (*first*, *third*, and *fifth rows*). The second set of images, obtained 24 hours later during an angina-free period, show partial redistribution (*second, fourth,* and *sixth rows*). Each set shows short-axis, vertical long-axis, and horizontal long-axis slices.

with equivocal presentations, and risk assessment. Injection of Tc-99m–labeled tracers while the patient is at rest during or shortly after chest pain can be very helpful in determining the cardiac etiology of pain and, more specifically, the culprit vessel (Fig. 53.3). According to Bilodeau et al. (157), this method had a sensitivity of 62% and a specificity of 88% (ST segment shifts had a sensitivity of 38% only).

The guidelines on unstable angina pectoris suggest that in the following patients coronary angiography may be indicated: patients with previous MI or revascularization, those who fail to stabilize on medical therapy, those with high-risk clinical findings seen on noninvasive testing, and those with significant heart failure or left ventricular dysfunction (182). For patients who can be stabilized with medical therapy, a more conservative approach, using noninvasive testing, is generally preferable (181–186). Routine use of coronary angiography for all patients is not only expensive but also exposes many patients to unnecessary risk and interventions. Noninvasive risk-stratification can identify the patients most likely to benefit from additional invasive procedures.

Several studies have shown that myocardial perfusion imaging appears to be superior to ST segment response. For example, Brown et al. (183) found that the cardiac event rate was 26% in patients with reversible defects and 3% in those with no reversible defects; Stratmann et al. (184) found that the cardiac event rate was 25% in patients with reversible defects and 2% in those with normal scans; Madsen et al. (186) found a cardiac event rate

of 21% in patients with reversible defects and 3% in patients with no reversible defects. Therefore, stress perfusion imaging may be used to risk-stratify patients with unstable angina who had no occurrence of ischemia for 48 to 72 hours while receiving medical therapy. Patients who are classified as high risk on the basis of scan results need coronary angiography, and patients classified as low risk can be treated medically.

MYOCARDIAL VIABILITY

Clinical Use of Nuclear Imaging in the Assessment of Myocardial Viability

Several different tracers and protocols can be used for the assessment of myocardial viability (*e*Table 53.8.3). [✈ k09] The presence of redistribution on Tl-201 images taken 4 hours after stress is indicative of myocardial ischemia and hence viability. However, regions with absent or incomplete redistribution may still be viable and may improve after revascularization (139,140). Early attempts to overcome this problem used 12- to 36-hour delayed imaging after the stress Tl-201 injection (203). Although filling in of defects in this late redistribution image identifies additional areas of viable myocardium, a considerable number of viable regions are still missed. Moreover, because of the typically poor count statistics associated with the 24-hour delayed Tl-201 images, interpretation of these studies may be difficult.

Tl-201 reinjection after the redistribution images may circumvent some of the deficiencies of the latter. As initially described by Dilsizian et al. (27), approximately 50% of defects that may appear fixed at 4 hours improve after reinjection, and most of these regions also show improved function after revascularization.

Although the identification of stress-induced ischemia is a superior indication of viable myocardium (204), incompletely resolved ischemia may also present as a persistent defect (scar) (139,140,203)—hence the current use of resting 4-hour redistribution Tl-201 imaging. It is recognized that asynergic myocardial regions perfused by coronaries with high-grade stenosis may display resting hypoperfusion (hibernating myocardium) during resting Tl-201 imaging (27,28,205,206). These defects may fill in over the course of the next several hours, thereby demonstrating viable myocardium (*e*Fig. 53.3.4). It has also been shown that the higher the regional uptake of Tl-201, the more likely it is that the region is viable. Conversely, regions with very low uptake during rest redistribution or stress reinjection are likely to contain predominant scarring. An arbitrary 50% or 60% Tl-201 uptake, relative to that in normal regions, is a clinically useful threshold to differentiate between viable and nonviable myocardium (28,206–208). However, the identification of viable regions by rest redistribution Tl-201 imaging is still less than ideal, and positive and negative predictive accuracies range from 45% to 79% and 62% to 80%, respectively (205,209,210).

Clinical Use of Technetium-99m Sestamibi in the Assessment of Myocardial Viability

Because Tc-99m sestamibi undergoes only minimal redistribution at 4 hours after the injection, sestamibi has been considered by some to be less useful for detecting viable myocardium than Tl-201 (211,212). More recently, Udelson and associates (207) and Kauffman and coauthors (213) compared sestamibi uptake, after a resting injection, with Tl-201 uptake in the rest redistribution images. Under those conditions, these authors found very similar sestamibi and Tl-201 activities. A sestamibi activity >60% of maximal uptake had a positive predictive value of 80% and a negative predictive value of 96% for improvement in regional dyssynergy after revascularization. Dilsizian and colleagues (28) have also compared sestamibi uptake at 1 hour and 4 hours after a resting injection and observed that 40% of the segments had improved uptake over the course of time. These authors also compared sestamibi and Tl-201 uptakes by quantitative analysis, which markedly improved the concordance between these two tracers for viability detection. Recent investigations comparing the levels of Tc-99m sestamibi in perfusion defects with the extent of historically viable myocardium have indicated a high degree of correlation

between the uptake of this tracer and the amount of viable myocardium (214,215).

Nitrate-Augmented Perfusion Imaging

Nitroglycerin administration may improve myocardial perfusion either by increasing coronary collateral flow or by dilating the stenosis slightly. Thus, it is not surprising that administration of nitroglycerin may improve perfusion defects. Galli et al. (216) reported that administration of nitroglycerin before sestamibi injection while the patient was at rest improved detection of myocardial viability. It has also been shown that nitrate administration before Tl-201 reinjection improved detection of viable myocardium (217). Therefore, nitroglycerin administration before either sestamibi or Tl-201 injection may further improve detection of myocardial viability (217,218).

Clinical Use of Fatty Acids for Detection of Myocardial Viability

Recent reports have suggested that iodine-123 iodophenyl-pentadecanoic acid (I-123 IPPA) may be a good marker for use in detection of myocardial viability (219,220). Iskandrian et al. (220) have reported a 91% agreement between IPPA and rest redistribution Tl-201 SPECT (Fig. 53.4). A recent multicenter trial (221) evaluated the utility of I-123 IPPA for predicting substantial increases in LVEF (=10%) after CABG in patients with a depressed preoperative LVEF (<40%). On multivariate analysis, the number of segments that were viable by IPPA was the most important predictor of recovery of function after revascularization.

Another fatty acid that has been used, especially in Japan, for evaluation of myocardial viability is I-123-beta-methyl-*p*-iodophenylpentadecanoic acid (I-123-BMIPP). This agent has a structure that is remarkably similar to IPPA, with the addition of a methyl radical. However, it possesses a longer residence time intracellularly and therefore allows more convenient imaging. Although I-123-BMIPP has not yet been well studied as a viability marker, it has been suggested that areas with discordant BMIPP/Tl-201 uptake (greater decrease in BMIPP than Tl-201) are likely to show increased F-18-FDG uptake, a marker of myocardial viability (222).

Clinical Use of Positron Emission Tomography for Assessment of Myocardial Viability

At the present time, PET is probably the best technique for the assessment of myocardial viability. The best predictor of viable myocardium is a mismatch between flow (measured by oxygen-15 H$_2$O, nitrogen-15 NH3, or rubidium-82) and glucose metabolism (assessed by F-18-FDG) (208,223). Recently, F-18-FDG has been successfully imaged using

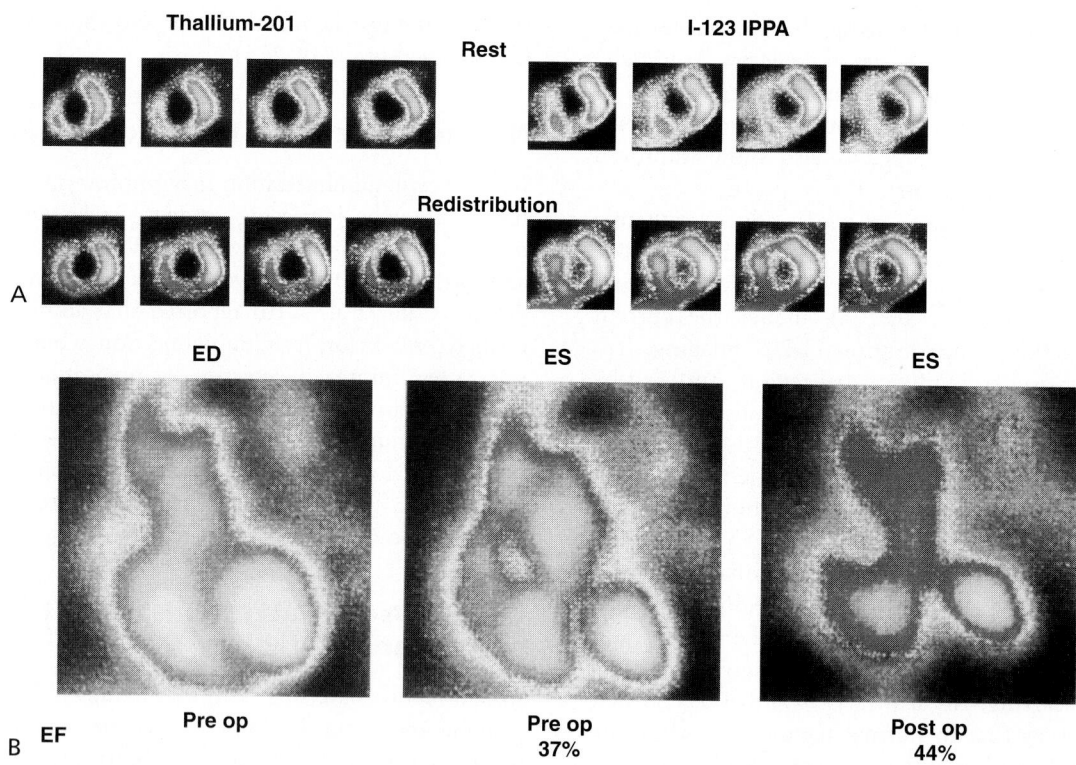

FIGURE 53.4 A: Rest-redistribution thallium-201 tomographic images and 5- and 30-minute iodine-123 iodophenylpentadecanoic acid (I-123 IPPA) tomographic images from a patient with severe three-vessel disease and left ventricular dysfunction. The thallium-201 and I-123 IPPA images reveal reversible defects. The reversibility is better seen with I-123 IPPA. **B:** This patient had improvement in left ventricular function after coronary artery bypass grafting. ED, end diastole; EF, ejection fraction; ES, end systole. (From Iskandrian AS, Powers J, Cave V, et al. Assessment of myocardial viability by dynamic tomographic iodine 123 iodophenylpentadecanoic acid imaging: comparison with rest-redistribution thallium-201 imaging. *J Nucl Cardiol* 1995;2:101–109, with permission.)

standard SPECT cameras mounted with a special high-energy (511-KeV) collimator (224). Although the feasibility of this technique has been demonstrated, the quality of the F-18-FDG SPECT images is not as good as that of images obtained with PET. Moreover, the radiopharmaceutical cost remains a serious impediment to widespread clinical use of F-18-FDG.

Other investigators have used PET imaging with carbon-11 acetate as an indicator of myocardial oxidative metabolism, which potentially could be a good marker of viability (225). The clearance of rubidium-82 has also been proposed as a marker of viability, but there is limited experience with this approach (226). A new protocol has been proposed to assess myocardial viability with low-dose dobutamine sestamibi SPECT (227,228). At this time, only preliminary data have been reported with this technique (229).

RECENT DEVELOPMENTS IN NUCLEAR CARDIOLOGY

A number of guidelines on training, competency, certification, and accreditation of radionuclide users and laboratories are now available. A variety of educational programs are also sponsored by the American Society of Nuclear Cardiology, including an annual scientific meeting. The new developments are summarized in Table 53.9. Newer generations of solid-state gamma cameras, nonimaging detectors, and micro-PET and micro-SPECT will enhance clinical and research applications of nuclear cardiology, including the ability to study myocardial metabolism and gene expression in small animals. Improvements in software to correct for attenuation, scatter, and depth resolution have been made, and such methods may be used at the present time (Table 53.9). ❦ k10

TABLE 53.9 RECENT DEVELOPMENTS IN NUCLEAR CARDIOLOGY

Hardware and software
New tracers
New stress agents
Molecular and vascular imaging
New applications

Adapted from Iskandrian AE, Verani MS, eds. Bar Harbor Invitation Meeting 2000. *J Nucl Cardiol* 2001;8(2):224–316, with permission.

THE FUTURE

We believe the future will bring about important changes in the way that nuclear cardiology is practiced. First, newer tracers will be available that will allow imaging to be target-specific for studying myocardial perfusion, myocardial hypoxemia, myocardial necrosis, myocarditis, myocardial metabolism, sympathetic innervation, ventricular function, and coronary atherosclerosis. Targeting gene expression with specific nuclear markers will allow imaging of genetically engineered animal models and, later, of human beings. It may become possible to image vulnerable plaques in diverse arteries. Second, SPECT imaging will be used routinely with attenuation/scatter and depth resolution compensation, as well as with gating, three-dimensional imaging, and absolute quantification. These advances will increase the precision of the technique and improve quantification.

Third, there will be increased applications of nuclear imaging in other groups of patients, such as patients with life-threatening ventricular arrhythmias, patients with congestive heart failure, asymptomatic patients who are at high risk, and in the evaluation of effects of therapeutic interventions such as gene therapy, lipid-lowering therapy, antianginal medications, and hormone-replacement therapy. Fourth, the quality of the nuclear images will improve through standardization of procedures, quality assurance measures, and certification and credentialing programs. Last, managed-care organizations will recognize that nuclear procedures are cost-effective for selecting patients who will benefit most from coronary angiography and percutaneous procedures and patients in whom routine coronary angiography is not justified.

CONTROVERSIES AND PERSONAL PERSPECTIVES

Three perfusion tracers are currently approved for routine clinical use: Tl-201, Tc-99m sestamibi, and Tc-99m tetrofosmin. All three tracers are useful in the assessment of diagnosis, risk-stratification, and myocardial viability.

The Tc-99m–labeled tracers provide significantly better image quality than Tl-201 and allow attenuation/scatter correction and first-pass RNA studies. The results with attenuation/scatter correction with Tl-201 are not yet convincing. The importance of EF measurement suggests that gated SPECT should be used in all patients. Today, >70% of perfusion studies are performed using Tc-99m–labeled tracers, and >90% are performed using gating; this is a remarkable change in a relatively short period of time.

For viability assessment, rest redistribution Tl-201 imaging provides a measure of hibernation (rest hypoperfusion) that, arguably, is not obtainable by Tc-99m–labeled tracers. The role played by ischemia in recovery of function, however, suggests that a stress rather than a resting study is needed for these patients. A hybrid protocol using rest redistribution Tl-201 and stress Tc-99m–labeled tracers may provide a complete assessment (*e*Fig. 53.4.1) (235).

The strongest asset of nuclear imaging is the ability to provide quantitative measurements (e.g., EF, area of myocardium at risk, and infarct size). This is best achieved by tomographic imaging enhanced by gated perfusion imaging and by performing attenuation/scatter depth resolution compensation. Emerging techniques are likely to expand the applications beyond perfusion and function to include metabolic, receptor, and atherosclerosis imaging,

and ultimately the ability to identify unstable plaques and gene expression.

Some argue that nuclear testing is prohibitively expensive, which it is in comparison to exercise ECG. However, cost is a market-driven value, and cost-effectiveness is a better index than cost.

Regarding the choice of stress modality, exercise continues to be preferred because of the known prognostic variables associated with stress ECG and exercise tolerance. From the standpoint of diagnostic accuracy, however, pharmacologic stress imaging appears to be at least equivalent to exercise imaging. Moreover, the image variables that indicate increased risk by exercise stress (e.g., large defects, multivessel defects, transient ischemia dilation, and LVEF and left ventricular size) are also powerful risk predictors when observed with pharmacologic imaging.

REFERENCES

1. Beller GA, Glover DK, Edwards NC, et al. Tc-99m sestamibi uptake and retention during myocardial ischemia and reperfusion. *Circulation* 1993;87:2033–2042.
2. Beller Watson DD, Ackell P, et al. Time course of thallium-201 redistribution after transient myocardial ischemia. *Circulation* 1980;61:791–797.
3. Gerson MC, Millard RW, Roszell NJ, et al. Kinetic properties of Tc-99m-Q12 in canine myocardium. *Circulation* 1994;89:1291–1300.
4. Glover DK, Ruiz M, Edwards NC, et al. Comparison between thallium-201 and Tc-99m sestamibi uptake during adenosine-induced vasodilation as a function of coronary stenosis severity. *Circulation* 1995;91:813–820.

5. Grunwald AM, Watson DD, Holzgrefe HH Jr, et al. Myocardial thallium-201 kinetics in normal and ischemic myocardium. *Circulation* 1981;64:610–618.

6. Jain D, Wackers FJ, Mattera J, et al. Biokinetics of 99m Tc tetrofosmin, a new myocardial perfusion imaging agent: implications for a one day imaging protocol. *J Nucl Med* 1993;34:1254–1259.

7. Lee J, Chae SC, Lee K, et al. Biokinetics of thallium-201 in normal subjects: comparison between adenosine, dipyridamole, dobutamine, and exercise. *J Nucl Med* 1994;35:535–541.

8. Leppo JA, Okada RD, Strauss HW, et al. Effect of hyperemia on thallium-201 redistribution in normal canine myocardium. *Cardiovasc Res* 1985;19:679–685.

9. Leppo JA, Meerdink DJ. Comparison of the myocardial uptake of a technetium-labeled isonitrile analogue and thallium. *Circ Res* 1989;65:632–639.

10. Melon PG, Beanlands RS, DeGrado TR, et al. Comparison of technetium-99m sestamibi and thallium-201 retention characteristics in canine myocardium. *J Am Coll Cardiol* 1992;20:1277–1283.

11. Moore CA, Cannon J, Watson DD, et al. Thallium-201 kinetics in stunned myocardium characterized by severe postischemic systolic dysfunction. *Circulation* 1990;81:1622–1632.

12. Nielsen AP, Morris KG, Murdock R, et al. Linear relationship between the distribution of thallium-201 and blood flow in ischemic and nonischemic myocardium during exercise. *Circulation* 1980;61:797–801.

13. Okada RD, Glover D, Gaffney T, et al. Myocardial kinetics of Tc-99m-hexakis-2-methoxy-2-methylpropyl-isonitrile. *Circulation* 1988;77:491–498.

14. Piwnica-Worms D, Chiu ML, Kronauge JF. Divergent kinetics of 201Tl and 99mTc-SESTAMIBI in cultured chick ventricular myocytes during ATP depletion. *Circulation* 1992;85:1531–1541.

15. Pohost GM, Okada RD, O'Keefe DD, et al. Thallium redistribution in dogs with severe coronary artery stenosis of fixed caliber. *Circ Res* 1981;48:439–446.

16. Garcia EV. Imaging guidelines for nuclear cardiology procedures. *J Nucl Cardiol* 1996;3:G1–G46.

17. Germano G, Kiat H, Kavanagh PB, et al. Automatic quantification of ejection fraction from gated myocardial perfusion SPECT. *J Nucl Cardiol* 1995;36:2138–2147.

18. DePuey EG, Parmett S, Ghesani M, et al. Comparison of Tc-99m sestamibi and Tl-201 gated perfusion SPECT. *J Nucl Cardiol* 1999;6:278–285.

19. Nichols K, Lefkowitz D, Faber T. Echocardiographic validation of gated SPECT ventricular function measurements. *J Nucl Med* 2000;41:1308–1314.

20. He ZX, Cwajg E, Preslar JS, et al. Accuracy of left ventricular ejection fraction determined by gated myocardial perfusion SPECT with Tl-201 and Tc-99m sestamibi: comparison with first pass radionuclide angiography. *J Nucl Cardiol* 1999;6:412–417.

21. Cwajg E, Cwajg J, He ZX, et al. Gated myocardial perfusion tomography for the assessment of left ventricular function and volumes: comparison with echocardiography. *J Nucl Med* 1999;40:1857–1865.

22. Vaduganathan P, He ZX, Vick G, et al. Evaluation of left ventricular wall motion, volumes, and ejection fraction by gated myocardial tomography with technetium 99m-labeled tetrofosmin: a comparison with cine magnetic resonance imaging. *J Nucl Cardiol* 1999;6:3–10.

23. Port SC, Wackers FJ. Clinical application of radionuclide angiography. *J Nucl Cardiol* 1995;2:551–558.

24. Iskandrian AS, Verani MS. *Nuclear cardiac imaging: principles and applications.* Philadelphia: FA Davis, 1996.

25. Beller G. *Clinical nuclear cardiology.* Philadelphia: Saunders, 1995.

26. Gerson M. *Cardiac nuclear medicine,* 2nd ed. New York: McGraw-Hill, 1991.

27. Dilsizian V, Rocco TP, Freedman NM, et al. Enhanced detection of ischemic but viable myocardium by the reinjection of thallium after stress-redistribution imaging. *N Engl J Med* 1990;323:141–146.

28. Dilsizian V, Arrighi JA, Diodati JG, et al. Myocardial viability in patients with chronic coronary artery disease: comparison of Tc-99m sestamibi with thallium reinjection and F-18-fluorodeoxyglucose. *Circulation* 1994;89:578–587.

29. Berman DS, Kiat H, Friedman JD, et al. Separate acquisition rest thallium-201/stress technetium-99m sestamibi dual-isotope myocardial perfusion single-photon emission computed tomography: a clinical validation study. *J Am Coll Cardiol* 1993;22:1455–1464.

30. Verani MS. Pharmacologic stress myocardial perfusion imaging. *Curr Prob Cardiol* 1993;18:481–525.

31. Iskandrian AS, Verani MS, Heo J. Pharmacologic stress testing: mechanisms of action, hemodynamic responses, and results in detection of coronary artery disease. *J Nucl Cardiol* 1994;1:94–111.

32. DiRocco RJ, Rumsey WL, Kuczynski BL, et al. Measurement of myocardial blood flow using a co-injection technique for technetium-99m teboroxime, technetium-96-sestamibi and thallium-201. *J Nucl Med* 1992;33:1152–1159.

33. Brown KA. Prognostic value of thallium-201 myocardial perfusion imaging: a diagnostic tool comes of age. *Circulation* 1991;83:363–381.

34. Hachamovitch R, Berman DS, Kiat H, et al. Exercise myocardial perfusion SPECT in patients without known coronary artery disease: incremental prognostic value and use in risk stratification. *Circulation* 1996;93:905–914.

35. Nallamothu N, Ghods M, Heo J, et al. Comparison of thallium-201 single photon emission computed tomography and electrocardiographic response during exercise in patients with normal rest electrocardiographic results. *J Am Coll Cardiol* 1995;25:830–836.

36. Mahmarian JJ, Pratt CM, Boyce TM, et al. The variable extent of jeopardized myocardium in patients with single vessel disease: quantification by thallium-201 single photon emission computed tomography. *J Am Coll Cardiol* 1991;17:355–362.

37. Gallik DM, Obermueller SD, Swarna US, et al. Simultaneous assessment of myocardial perfusion and left ventricular function during transient coronary occlusion. *J Am Coll Cardiol* 1995;25:1529–1538.

38. Mahmarian JJ, Boyce TM, Goldberg RK, et al. Quantitative exercise thallium-201 single-photon emission computed tomography for the enhanced diagnosis of ischemic heart disease. *J Am Coll Cardiol* 1990;15:318–329.

39. Mouratidis B, Vaughan-Neil EF, Gilday DL, et al. Detection of silent coronary artery disease in adolescents and young adults with familial hypercholesterolemia by single-photon emission computed tomography thallium-201 scanning. *Am J Cardiol* 1992;70:1109–1112.

40. Blumenthal RS, Becker DM, Moy TF, et al. Exercise thallium tomography predicts future clinically manifest coronary heart disease in a high-risk asymptomatic population. *Circulation* 1996;93:915–923.

41. Detrano R, Janosi A, Lyons KP, et al. Factors affecting sensitivity and specificity of a diagnostic test: the exercise thallium scintigram. *Am J Med* 1988;84:699–710.

42. DePasquale EE, Nody AC, DePuey EG, et al. Quantitative rotational thallium-201 tomography for identifying and localizing coronary artery disease. *Circulation* 1988;77:316–327.

43. Kasabali B, Woodard ML, Bekerman C, et al. Enhanced sensitivity and specificity of thallium-201 imaging for the detection of regional ischemic coronary disease by combining SPECT with "bull's-eye" analysis. *Clin Nucl Med* 1989;14:484–491.

44. Tamaki N, Yonekura Y, Mukai T, et al. Stress thallium-201 trans-axial emission computed tomography: quantitative versus qualitative analysis for evaluation of coronary artery disease. *J Am Coll Cardiol* 1984;4:1213–1221.

45. Mahmarian JJ, Verani MS. Exercise thallium-201 perfusion scintigraphy in the assessment of ischemic heart disease. *Am J Cardiol* 1991;67:2D–11D.

46. Taillefer R, Depuey EG, Udelson JE, et al. Comparative diagnostic accuracy of Tl-201 and Tc-99m sestamibi SPECT imaging (perfusion and ECG-gated SPECT) in detecting coronary artery disease in women. *J Am Coll Cardiol* 1997;29:69–77.

47. Burns RJ, Iles IS, Fung AY, et al. The Canadian exercise technetium-99m-labeled teboroxime single photon emission computed tomographic study. *J Nucl Cardiol* 1995;2:117–125.

48. Seldin DW, Johnson LL, Blood DK, et al. Myocardial perfusion imaging with technetium-99m SQ 30217: comparison with thallium-201 and coronary anatomy. *J Nucl Med* 1989;30:312–319.

49. Smith AM, Gullberg GT, Christian PE, et al. Kinetic modeling of teboroxime using dynamic SPECT imaging of a canine model. *J Nucl Med* 1994;35:484–495.

50. Rigo P, Leclercq B, Itti R, et al. Tc-99m-tetrofosmin myocardial imaging: a comparison with thallium-201 and angiography. *J Nucl Med* 1994;35:587–593.

51. Zaret BL, Rigo P, Wackers FJ, et al. Myocardial perfusion imaging with Tc-99m tetrofosmin: comparison to Tl-201 and coronary angiography in a phase III multicenter trial. Tetrofosmin International Trial Study Group. *Circulation* 1995;91:313–319.

52. Sridhara BS, Braat S, Rigo P, et al. Comparison of myocardial perfusion imaging with technetium-99m tetrofosmin versus thallium-201 in coronary artery disease. *Am J Cardiol* 1993;72:1015–1019.

53. Takahashi N, Tamaki N, Tadamura E, et al. Combined assessment of regional perfusion and wall motion in patients with coronary artery disease with technetium 99m tetrofosmin. *J Nucl Cardiol* 1994;1:29–38.

54. Cuocolo A, Nicolai E, Soricelli A, et al. Technetium 99m-labeled tetrofosmin myocardial tomography in patients with coronary artery disease: comparison between adenosine and dynamic exercise stress testing. *J Nucl Cardiol* 1996;3:194–203.

55. Sullo P, Cuocolo A, Nicolai E, et al. Quantitative exercise technetium-99m tetrofosmin myocardial tomography or the identification and localization of coronary artery disease. *Eur J Nucl Med* 1996;23:648–655.

56. Flamen P, Bossuyt A, Franken PR. Technetium-99m tetrofosmin in dipyridamole-stress myocardial SPECT imaging: intra-individual comparison with technetium-99m-sestamibi. *J Nucl Med* 1995;36:2009–2015.

57. Hendel RC, Verani MS, Miller DD, et al. Diagnostic utility of tomographic myocardial perfusion imaging with technetium-99m furifosmin (Q12) compared with thallium-201: results of a phase III multicenter trial. *J Nucl Cardiol* 1996;3:291–300.

58. Ranhosky A, Kempthorne-Rawson J. The safety of intravenous dipyridamole thallium myocardial perfusion imaging. Intravenous Dipyridamole Thallium Imaging Study Group. *Circulation* 1990;81:1205–1209.

59. Abreu A, Mahmarian JJ, Nishimura S, et al. Tolerance and safety of pharmacologic coronary vasodilation with adenosine in association with thallium-201 scintigraphy in patients with suspected coronary artery disease. *J Am Coll Cardiol* 1991;18:730–735.

60. Cerqueira MD, Verani MS, Schwaiger M, et al. Safety profile of adenosine stress perfusion imaging: results from the Adenoscan Multicenter Trial Registry. *J Am Coll Cardiol* 1994;23:384–389.

61. Miyagawa M, Kumano S, Sekiya M, et al. Thallium-201 myocardial tomography with intravenous infusion of adenosine triphosphage in diagnosis of coronary artery disease. *J Am Coll Cardiol* 1995;26:1196–1201.

62. Takeishi Y, Takahashi N, Fujiwara S, et al. Myocardial tomography with technetium-99m-tetrofosmin during intravenous infusion of adenosine triphosphate. *J Nucl Med* 1998;39:582–586.

63. Cuocolo A, Sullo P, Pace L, et al. Adenosine coronary vasodilation in coronary artery disease: technetium-99m tetrofosmin myocardial tomography versus echocardiography. *J Nucl Med* 1997;38:1089–1094.

64. Nicolai E, Cuocolo A, Pace L, et al. Adenosine coronary vasodilation quantitative technetium 99m methoxy isobutyl isonitrile myocardial tomography in the identification and localization of coronary artery disease. *J Nucl Cardiol* 1996;3:9–17.

65. He ZX, Iskandrian AS, Gupta NC, et al. Assessing coronary artery disease with dipyridamole technetium-99-m tetrofosmin SPECT: a multicenter trial. *J Nucl Med* 1997;38:44–48.

66. Pennell DJ, Mavrogeni SI, Forbat SM, et al. Adenosine combined with dynamic exercise for myocardial perfusion imaging. *J Am Coll Cardiol* 1995;25:1300–1309.

67. Jamil G, Ahlberg A, Elliott MD, et al. Impact of limited treadmill exercise on adenosine Tc-99m sestamibi single-photon emission computed tomographic myocardial perfusion imaging in coronary artery disease. *Am J Cardiol* 1999;84:400–403.

68. Calnon DA, Glover DK, Beller GA, et al. Effects of dobutamine stress on myocardial blood flow, 99mTc sestamibi uptake and systolic wall thickening in the presence of coronary artery stenoses: implications for dobutamine stress testing. *Circulation* 1997;96:2353–2360.

69. Marwick T, D'Hondt AM, Baudhuin T, et al. Optimal use of dobutamine stress for the detection and evaluation of coronary artery disease: combination with echocardiography or scintigraphy, or both? *J Am Coll Cardiol* 1993;22:159–167.

70. Iftikhar I, Koutelou M, Mahmarian JJ, et al. Simultaneous perfusion tomography and radionuclide angiography during dobutamine stress. *J Nucl Med* 1996;37:1306–1310.

71. White CW, Wright CB, Doty DB, et al. Does visual interpretation of the coronary arteriogram predict the physiologic importance of a coronary stenosis? *N Engl J Med* 1984;310:819–824.

72. Ficaro EP, Fessler JA, Shreve PD, et al. Simultaneous transmission/emission myocardial perfusion tomography: diagnostic accuracy of attenuation-corrected 99mTc-sestamibi single-photon emission computed tomography. *Circulation* 1996;93:463–473.

73. Ficaro EP, Fessler JA, Ackerman RJ, et al. Simultaneous transmission-emission thallium-201 cardiac SPECT: effect of attenuation correction in myocardial tracer distribution. *J Nucl Med* 1995;36:921–931.

74. Hendel RC, Berman DS, Cullom SJ, et al. Multicenter clinical trial to evaluate the efficacy of correction for photon attenuation and scatter in SPECT myocardial perfusion imaging. *Circulation* 1999;99:2742–2749.

75. Prvulovich EM, Lonn AH, Bomanji JB, et al. Effect of attenuation correction on myocardial thallium-201 distribution in patients with a low likelihood of coronary artery disease. *Eur J Nucl Med* 1997;24:266–275.

76. Chuoraqui P, Livschitz S, Sharir T, et al. Evaluation of an attenuation correction method for thallium-201 myocardial perfusion tomographic imaging of patients with low likelihood of coronary artery disease. *J Nucl Cardiol* 1998;5:369–377.

77. Vaduganathan P, He ZX, Raghavan C, et al. Detection of left anterior descending coronary artery stenosis in patients with left bundle branch block: exercise, adenosine or dobutamine imaging? *J Am Coll Cardiol* 1996;28:543–550.

78. Fuster V, Badimon L, Badimon JJ, et al. The pathogenesis of coronary artery disease and the acute coronary syndromes (1). *N Engl J Med* 1992;326(4):242–250.

79. Fuster V, Badimon L, Badimon JJ, et al. The pathogenesis of coronary artery disease and the acute coronary syndromes (2). *N Engl J Med* 1992;326(5):310–318.

80. Leor J, Poole WK, Kloner RA. Sudden cardiac death triggered by an earthquake. *N Engl J Med* 1996;334:413–419.

81. ACC/AHA guidelines for preoperative cardiovascular evaluation of noncardiac surgery. *Circulation* 1996;93:1280–1317.

82. Califf RM, Armstrong PW, Carver JR, et al. Stratification of patients into high, medium and low risk subgroups for purposes of risk factor management. Task Force 5. *J Am Coll Cardiol* 1996;27:964–1047.

83. Abdel Fattah A, Kamal AM, Pancholy S, et al. Prognostic implications of normal exercise tomographic thallium images in patients with angiographic evidence of significant coronary artery disease. *Am J Cardiol* 1994;74:769–771.

84. Schalet BD, Kegel JG, Heo J, et al. Prognostic implications of normal exercise SPECT thallium images in patients with strongly positive exercise electrocardiograms. *Am J Cardiol* 1993;72:1201–1203.

85. Iskandrian AS, Chae SC, Heo J, et al. Independent and incremental prognostic value of exercise single-photon emission computed tomographic (SPECT) thallium imaging in coronary artery disease. *J Am Coll Cardiol* 1993;22:665–670.

86. Bateman JM, O'Keefe JH Jr, Dong VM, et al. Coronary angiographic rates after stress single photon emission computed tomographic scintigraphy. *J Nucl Cardiol* 1995;2:217–223.

87. Machecourt J, Longere P, Fagret D, et al. Prognostic value of thallium-201 single photon emission computed tomographic myocardial perfusion imaging according to extent of myocardial defect: study in 1,926 patients with follow-up at 33 months. *J Am Coll Cardiol* 1994;23:1096–1106.

88. Marie PY, Danchin N, Durand JF, et al. Long-term prediction of major ischemic events by exercise thallium-201 single photon emission computed tomography: incremental prognostic value compared with clinical, exercise testing, catheterization and radionuclide angiographic data. *J Am Coll Cardiol* 1995;26:879–886.

89. Nallamothu N, Pancholy SB, Lee KR, et al. Impact on exercise single-photon emission computed tomographic thallium imaging on patient management and outcome. *J Nucl Cardiol* 1995;2:334–338.

90. Pancholy SB, Fattah AA, Kamal AA, et al. Independent and incremental prognostic value of exercise single-photon emission computed tomographic imaging in women. *J Nucl Cardiol* 1995;2:110–116.

91. Patterson RE, Eisner RL, Horowitz SF. Comparison of cost-effectiveness and utility of exercise ECG, single photon emission computed tomography, positron emission tomography, and coronary angiography for diagnosis of coronary artery disease. *Circulation* 1995;91:54–65.

92. Patillo RW, Fuchs S, Johnson J, et al. Predictors of prognosis by quantitative assessment of coronary angiography, single photon emission computed tomographic thallium imaging, and treadmill exercise testing. *Am Heart J* 1996;131:582–590.

93. Pollock SG, Abbott RD, Boucher CA, et al. Independent and incremental prognostic value of tests performed in hierarchical order to evaluate patients with suspected coronary artery disease: validation of models based on these tests. *Circulation* 1992;85:237–248.

94. Nallamothu N, Araujo L, Russel J, et al. Prognostic value of simultaneous perfusion and function assessment using Tc-99m sestamibi. *Am J Cardiol* 1996;78:562–563.

95. Berman DS, Hachamovitch R, Kiat H, et al. Incremental value of prognostic testing in patients with known or suspected ischemic heart disease: a basis for optimal utilization of exercise Tc-99m sestamibi myocardial perfusion single-photon emission computed tomography. *J Am Coll Cardiol* 1995;26:639–647.

96. Beller GA, Zaret BL. Contributions of nuclear cardiology to diagnosis and prognosis of patients with coronary artery disease. *Circulation* 2000;101:1465–1478.

97. Boyne TS, Koplan BA, Parsons WJ, et al. Predicting adverse outcome with exercise SPECT technetium-99m sestamibi imaging in patients with suspected or known coronary artery disease. *Am J Cardiol* 1997;79:270–274.

98. Brown KA. Prognosis in stable coronary artery disease. In: Zaret BL, Beller GA, eds. *Nuclear cardiology: state of the art and future directions*, 2nd ed. St. Louis: Mosby, 1999:331–345.

99. Brown KA. Prognostic value of myocardial perfusion imaging: state of the art and new developments. *J Nucl Cardiol* 1996;35:516–537.

100. Chatziioannou SN, Moore WH, Ford PV, et al. Prognostic value of myocardial perfusion imaging in patients with high exercise tolerance. *Circulation* 1999;99:867–872.

101. Gibbons RJ, Hodge DO, Berman DS, et al. Long-term outcome of patients with intermediate-risk exercise electrocardiograms who do not have myocardial perfusion defects on radionuclide imaging. *Circulation* 1999;100:2140–2145.

102. Hachamovitch R, Berman DS, Kiat H, et al. Exercise myocardial perfusion SPECT in patients without known coronary artery disease: incremental prognostic value and use in risk stratification. *Circulation* 1996;93:905–914.

103. Hachamovitch R, Berman DS, Kiat H, et al. Incremental prognostic value of adenosine stress myocardial perfusion single-photon emission computed tomography and impact on subsequent management in patients with or suspected of having myocardial ischemia. *Am J Cardiol* 1997;80:426–433.

104. Hachamovitch R, Berman DS, Shaw LJ, et al. Incremental prognostic value of myocardial perfusion single photon emission computed tomography for the prediction of cardiac death. *Circulation* 1998;97:535–543.

105. Iskander S, Iskandrian AE. Risk assessment using single-photon emission computed tomographic technetium-99m sestamibi imaging. *J Am Coll Cardiol* 1998;32:57–62.

106. Kang X, Berman DS, Lewin HC, et al. Incremental prognostic value of myocardial perfusion single photon emission computed tomography in patients with diabetes mellitus. *Am Heart J* 1999;138:1025–1032.

107. Amanullah AM, Berman DS, Erel J, et al. Incremental prognostic value of adenosine myocardial perfusion single-photon emission computed tomography in women with suspected coronary artery disease. *Am J Cardiol* 1998;82:725–730.

108. Marie PY, Danchin N, Branly F, et al. Effects of medical therapy on outcome assessment using exercise thallium-201 single photon emission computed tomography imaging. *J Am Coll Cardiol* 1999;34:113–121.

109. Marwick TH, Shaw LJ, Lauer MS, et al. The noninvasive prediction of cardiac mortality in men and women with known or suspected coronary artery disease. Economics of Noninvasive Diagnosis (END) Study Group. *Am J Med* 1999;106:172–178.

110. O'Keefe JH Jr, Bateman TM, Ligon RW, et al. Outcome of medical versus invasive treatment strategies for non-high-risk ischemic heart disease. *J Nucl Cardiol* 1998;5:28–33.

111. Olmos LI, Dakik H, Gordon R, et al. Long-term prognostic value of exercise echocardiography compared with exercise 201TI, ECG, and clinical variables in patients evaluated for coronary artery disease. *Circulation* 1998;98:2679–2686.

112. Sharir T, Germano G, Kavanagh PB, et al. Incremental prognostic value of post-stress left ventricular ejection fraction and volume by gated myocardial perfusion single photon emission computed tomography. *Circulation* 1999;100:1035–1042.

113. Shaw LJ, Hachamovitch R, Berman DS, et al. The economic consequences of available diagnostic and prognostic strategies for the evaluation of stable angina patients: an observational assessment of the value of pre-catheterization ischemia. Economics of Noninvasive Diagnosis (END) Multicenter Study Group. *J Am Coll Cardiol* 1999;33:661–669.

114. Shaw LJ, Hachamovitch R, Peterson ED, et al. Using an outcomes-based approach to identify candidates for risk stratification after exercise treadmill testing. *J Gen Intern Med* 1999;14:1–9.

115. Shaw LJ, Heller GV, Travin MI, et al. Cost analysis of diagnostic testing for coronary artery disease in women with stable chest pain. *J Nucl Cardiol* 1999;6:559–569.

116. Shaw LJ, Peterson ED, Shaw LK, et al. Use of a prognostic treadmill score in identifying diagnostic coronary disease subgroups. *Circulation* 1998;98:1622–1630.

117. Vanzetto G, Halimi S, Hammoud T, et al. Prediction of cardiovascular events in clinically selected high-risk NIDDM patients: prognostic value of exercise stress test and thallium 201 single-photon emission computed tomography. *Diabetes Care* 1999;22(1):19–26.

118. Vanzetto G, Ormezzano O, Fagret D, et al. Long-term additive prognostic value of thallium-201 myocardial perfusion imaging over clinical and exercise stress test in low to intermediate risk patients. *Circulation* 1999;100:1521–1527.

119. Iskandrian AE, Verani MS, eds. *New developments in nuclear cardiac imaging.* New York: Futura, 1998.

120. Pitt B, Waters D, Brown WV, et al. Aggressive lipid-lowering therapy compared with angioplasty in stable coronary artery disease. *N Engl J Med* 1999;341:70–76.

121. Hasdai D, Gibbons RJ, Holmes DR, et al. Coronary endothelial dysfunction in humans is associated with myocardial perfusion defects. *Circulation* 1997;96:3390–3395.

122. Schachinger V, Britten MB, Zeiher AM. Prognostic impact of coronary vasodilator dysfunction on adverse long-term outcome of coronary heart disease. *Circulation* 2000;101:1899–1906.

123. Suwaidi JA, Hamasaki S, Higano ST, et al. Long-term follow-up of patients with mild coronary artery disease and endothelial dysfunction. *Circulation* 2000;101:948–954.

124. Mangano DT, Goldman L. Preoperative assessment of patients with known or suspected coronary disease. *N Engl J Med* 1995;333:1750–1756.

125. Lee TH, Marcantonio ER, Mangione CM, et al. Derivation and prospective validation of a simple index for prediction of cardiac risk of major non cardiac surgery. *Circulation* 1999;100:1043–1049.

126. Hendel RC, Whitfield SS, Villegas BJ, et al. Prediction of late cardiac events by dipyridamole thallium imaging in patients undergoing elective vascular surgery. *Am J Cardiol* 1992;70:1243–1249.

127. Emlein G, Villegas B, Dahlberg S, et al. Left ventricular cavity size determined by preoperative dipyridamole thallium scintigraphy as a predictor of late cardiac events in vascular surgery patients. *Am Heart J* 1996;131:907–914.

128. Eagle KA, Coley CM, Newell JB, et al. Combining clinical and thallium data optimizes preoperative assessment of cardiac risk before major vascular surgery. *Ann Intern Med* 1989;110:859–866.

129. Hendel RC, Chen MH, L'Italien GJ, et al. Sex differences in perioperative and long-term cardiac event-free survival in vascular surgery patients: an analysis of clinical and scintigraphic variables. *Circulation* 1995;91:1044–1051.

130. Lette J, Waters D, Cerino M, et al. Preoperative coronary artery disease risk stratification based on dipyridamole imaging and a simple three-step, three-segment model for patients undergoing noncardiac vascular surgery or major general surgery. *Am J Cardiol* 1992;69:1553–1558.

131. Mangano DT, London MJ, Tubau JF, et al. Dipyridamole thallium-201 scintigraphy as a preoperative screening test: a reexamination of its predictive potential. Study of Perioperative Ischemia Research Group. *Circulation* 1991;84:493–502.

132. Stratmann HG, Younis LT, Wittry MD, et al. Dipyridamole technetium-99m sestamibi myocardial tomography in patients evaluated for elective vascular surgery: prognostic value for perioperative and late cardiac event. *Am Heart J* 1996;131:923–929.

133. Boucher CA, Brewster DC, Darling RC, et al. Determination of cardiac risk by dipyridamole-thallium imaging before peripheral vascular surgery. *N Engl J Med* 1985;312:389–394.

134. Brown KA, Rowen M. Extent of jeopardized viable myocardium determined by myocardial perfusion imaging best predicts perioperative cardiac events in patients undergoing noncardiac surgery. *J Am Coll Cardiol* 1993;21:325–330.

135. Bry JD, Belkin M, O'Donnell TF Jr, et al. An assessment of the positive predictive value and cost-effectiveness of dipyridamole myocardial scintigraphy in patients undergoing vascular surgery. *J Vasc Surg* 1994;19:112–121.

136. Baron JF, Mundler O, Bertrand M, et al. Dipyridamole-thallium scintigraphy and gated radionuclide angiography to assess cardiac risk before abdominal aortic surgery. *N Engl J Med* 1994;330:663–669.

137. Poldermans D, Boersma E, Bax JJ, et al. The effect of bisoprolol on perioperative mortality and myocardial infarction in high-risk patients undergoing vascular surgery. *N Engl J Med* 1999;341:1789–1794.

138. Bax JJ, Wijns W, Cornel JH, et al. Accuracy of currently available techniques for prediction of functional recovery after revascularization in patients with left ventricular dysfunction due to chronic coronary artery disease: comparison of pooled data. *J Am Coll Cardiol* 1997;30:1451–1460.

139. Cloninger KG, DePuey EG, Garcia EV, et al. Incomplete redistribution in delayed thallium-201 single photon emission computed tomographic (SPECT) images: an overestimation of myocardial scarring. *J Am Coll Cardiol* 1988;12:955–963.

140. Verani MS, Tadros S, Raizner AE, et al. Quantitative analysis of thallium-201 uptake and washout before and after transluminal coronary angioplasty. *Int J Cardiol* 1986;13:109–124.

141. Hirzel HO, Nuesch K, Gruentzig AR, et al. Short and long-term changes in myocardial perfusion after percutaneous transluminal coronary angioplasty assessed by thallium-201 exercise scintigraphy. *Circulation* 1981;63:1001–1007.

142. Scholl JM, Chaitman BR, David PR, et al. Exercise electrocardiography and myocardial scintigraphy in the serial evaluation of the results of percutaneous transluminal coronary angioplasty. *Circulation* 1982;66:380–390.

143. Jain A, Mahmarian JJ, Borges-Neto S, et al. Clinical significance of perfusion defects by thallium-201 single photon emission tomography following oral dipyridamole early after coronary angioplasty. *J Am Coll Cardiol* 1988;11:970–976.

144. Iskandrian AS, Lemlek J, Ogilby JD, et al. Early thallium imaging after percutaneous transluminal coronary angioplasty: tomographic evaluation during adenosine-induced coronary hyperemia. *J Nucl Med* 1992;33:2086–2089.

145. Manyari DE, Knudston M, Kloiber R, et al. Sequential thallium-201 myocardial perfusion studies after successful percutaneous transluminal coronary artery angioplasty: delayed resolution of exercise-induced scintigraphic abnormalities. *Circulation* 1988;77:86–95.

146. Hardoff R, Shefer A, Gips S, et al. Predicting late restenosis after coronary angioplasty by very early (12 to 24 h) thallium-201 scintigraphy: implications with regard to mechanism of late coronary restenosis. *J Am Coll Cardiol* 1990;15:1486–1492.

147. Hecht HS, Shaw RE, Chin HL, et al. Silent ischemia after coronary angioplasty: evaluation of restenosis and extent of ischemia in asymptomatic patients by tomographic thallium-201 exercise imaging and comparison with symptomatic patients. *J Am Coll Cardiol* 1991;17:670–677.

148. Lakkis NM, Mahmarian JJ, Verani MS. Exercise thallium-201 single photon emission computed tomography for evaluation of coronary artery bypass graft patency. *Am J Cardiol* 1995;76:107–111.

149. Palmas W, Bingham S, Diamond GA, et al. Incremental prognostic value of exercise thallium-201 myocardial single-photon emission computed tomography late after coronary artery bypass surgery. *J Am Coll Cardiol* 1995;25:403–409.

150. Lauer MS, Lytle B, Pashkow F, et al. Prediction of death and myocardial infarction by screening with exercise-thallium testing after coronary-artery-bypass grafting. *Lancet* 1998;351:615–622.

151. Nallamothu N, Johnson JH, Bagheri B, et al. Utility of stress single-photon emission computed tomography (SPECT) perfusion imaging in predicting outcomes after coronary artery bypass grafting. *Am J Cardiol* 1997;80:1517–1521.

152. Miller TD, Christian TF, Hodge DO, et al. Prognostic value of exercise thallium-201 imaging performed within 2 years of coronary artery bypass graft surgery. *J Am Coll Cardiol* 1998;31:848–854.

153. Johnson LL, Schofield L, Mastrofrancesco P, et al. Tc-99m glucarate uptake in swine model of limited flow plus increased demand. *J Nucl Cardiol* 2000;7:590–598.

154. Galli M, Marcassa C, Bolli R, et al. Spontaneous delayed recovery of perfusion and contraction after the first 5 weeks after anterior infarction: evidence for the presence of hibernating myocardium in the infarcted area. *Circulation* 1994;90:1386–1397.

155. Christian TF, Schwartz RS, Gibbons RJ. Determinants of infarct size in reperfusion therapy for acute myocardial infarction. *Circulation* 1992;86:81–90.

156. Gibbons RJ, Verani MS, Behrenbeck T, et al. Feasibility of tomographic Tc-99m-hexakis-2-methoxy-2-methylpropyl-

isonitrile imaging for the assessment of myocardial area at risk and the effect of treatment in acute myocardial infarction. *Circulation* 1989;80:1277–1286.

157. Bilodeau L, Theroux P, Gregoire J, et al. Technetium-99m sestamibi tomography in patients with spontaneous chest pain: correlation with clinical, electrocardiographic and angiographic findings. *J Am Coll Cardiol* 1991;18:1684–1691.

158. Hakki AH, Iskandrian AS, Kane SA, et al. Thallium-201 myocardial scintigraphy and left ventricular function at rest in patients with rest angina pectoris. *Am Heart J* 1984;108;326–332.

159. Hakki AH, Nestico PF, Heo J, et al. Relative prognostic value of rest thallium-201 imaging, radionuclide ventriculography and 24 hour ambulatory electrocardiographic monitoring after acute myocardial infarction. *J Am Coll Cardiol* 1987;10:25–32.

160. Hilton TC, Thompson RC, Williams HJ, et al. Technetium-99m sestamibi myocardial perfusion imaging in the emergency room evaluation of chest pain. *J Am Coll Cardiol* 1994;23:1016–1022.

161. Gregoire J, Theroux P. Detection and assessment of unstable angina using myocardial perfusion imaging: comparison between technetium-99m sestamibi SPECT and 12-lead electrocardiogram. *Am J Cardiol* 1990;66:42E–46E.

162 Varetto T, Cantalupi D, Altieri A, et al. Emergency room technetium-99m sestamibi imaging to rule out myocardial ischemic events in patients with nondiagnostic electrocardiograms. *J Am Coll Cardiol* 1993;22:1804–1808.

163. Heller GV, Stowers SA, Hendel RC, et al. Clinical value of acute rest technetium-99m tetrofosmin tomographic myocardial perfusion imaging in patients with acute chest pain and nondiagnostic electrocardiograms. *J Am Coll Cardiol* 1998;31:1011–1017.

164. Kontos MC, Jesse RL, Anderson FP, et al. Comparison of myocardial perfusion imaging and cardiac troponin I in patients admitted to the emergency department with chest pain. *Circulation* 1999:99:2073–2078.

165. Goldman L, Cook EF, Johnson PA, et al. Prediction of the need for intensive care in patients who come to emerging departments with acute chest pain. *N Engl J Med* 1996;334:1498–1504.

166. Gibson RS, Watson DD, Craddock GB, et al. Prediction of cardiac events after uncomplicated myocardial infarction: a prospective study comparing predischarge exercise thallium-201 scintigraphy and coronary angiography. *Circulation* 1983;68:321–336.

167. Leppo JA, O'Brien J, Rothendler JA, et al. Dipyridamole-thallium-201 scintigraphy in the prediction of future cardiac events after acute myocardial infarction. *N Engl J Med* 1984;310:1014–1018.

168. Multicenter Postinfarction Research Group. Risk stratification and survival after myocardial infarction. *N Engl J Med* 1983;309:331–336.

169. Cerqueira MD, Maynard C, Ritchie JL, et al. Long-term survival in 618 patients from the Western Washington Streptokinase in Myocardial Infarction trials. *J Am Coll Cardiol* 1992;20:1452–1459.

170. Zaret BL, Wackers FJ, Terrin ML, et al. Assessment of global and regional left ventricular performance at rest and during exercise after thrombolytic therapy for acute myocardial infarction: results of the Thrombolysis in Myocardial Infarction (TIMI) II Study. *Am J Cardiol* 1992;69:1–9.

171. Zaret BL, Wackers FJ, Terrin ML, et al. Value of radionuclide rest and exercise left ventricular ejection fraction in assessing survival of patients after thrombolytic therapy for acute myocardial infarction: results of Thrombolysis in Myocardial Infarction (TIMI) phase II study. The TIMI Study Group. *J Am Coll Cardiol* 1995;26:73–79.

172. Krone RJ, Gregory JJ, Freedland KE, et al. Limited usefulness of exercise testing and thallium scintigraphy in evaluation of ambulatory patients several months after recovery from an acute coronary event: implications for management of stable coronary heart disease. Multicenter Myocardial Ischemia Research Group. *J Am Coll Cardiol* 1994;24:1274–1281.

173. Moss AJ, Goldstein RE, Hall WJ, et al. Detection and significance of myocardial ischemia in stable patients after recovery from an acute coronary event. Multicenter Myocardial Ischemia Research Group. *JAMA* 1993;269:2379–2385.

174. Dakik HA, Mahmarian JJ, Kimball KT, et al. Prognostic value of exercise 201Tl tomography in patients treated with thrombolytic therapy during acute myocardial infarction. *Circulation* 1996;94:2735–2742.

175. Mahmarian JJ, Pratt CM, Nishimura S, et al. Quantitative 201Tl single-photon emission computed tomography for the early assessment of patients surviving acute myocardial infarction. *Circulation* 1993;87:1197–1210.

176. Mahmarian JJ, Mahmarian AC, Marks GF, et al. Role of adenosine thallium-201 tomography for defining long-term risk in patients after acute myocardial infarction. *J Am Coll Cardiol* 1995;25:1333–1340.

177. Brown KA, Heller GV, Landin RS, et al. Early dipyridamole (99m) Tc-sestamibi single photon emission computed tomographic imaging 2 to 4 days after acute myocardial infarction predicts in-hospital and post discharge cardiac events: comparison with submaximal exercise imaging. *Circulation* 1999;100:2060–2066.

178. Dakik HA, Kleiman NS, Farmer JA, et al. Intensive medical therapy versus coronary angioplasty for suppression of myocardial ischemia in survivors of acute myocardial infarction: a prospective, randomized pilot study. *Circulation* 1998;98:2017–2023.

179. Ryan TJ, Anderson JL, Antman EM, et al. ACC/AHA guidelines for the management of patients with acute myocardial infarction: a report of the American College of Cardiology/American Heart Association Task Force on Practice Guidelines (Committee on Management of Acute Myocardial Infarction). *J Am Coll Cardiol* 1996;28:1328–1428.

180. Boden WE, O'Rourke RA, Crawford MH, et al. Outcomes in patients with acute non-Q wave myocardial infarction randomly assigned to an invasive as compared with a conservative management strategy. Veterans Affairs Non-Q-Wave Infarction Strategies in Hospital (VANQWISH) Trial Investigators. *N Engl J Med* 1998;338:1785–1792.

181. Braunwald E, Antman EM, Beasley JW, et al. ACC/AHA guidelines for the management of patients with unstable angina and non-ST-segment elevation myocardial infarction: executive summary and recommendations. *Circulation* 2000;102:1193–1209.

182. Braunwald E, Mark DB, Jones RH, et al. Clinical practice guideline. Unstable angina: diagnosis and management. AHCPR publication no. 94-0602. Rockville, MD: Agency for Health Care Policy and Research, U.S. Department of Health and Human Services, 1994.

183. Brown KA. Prognostic value of thallium-201 myocardial perfusion imaging in patients with unstable angina who respond to medical treatment. *J Am Coll Cardiol* 1991;17:1053–1057.

184. Stratmann HG, Younis LT, Wittry MD, et al. Exercise technetium-99m myocardial tomography for the risk stratification of men with medically treated unstable angina pectoris. *Am J Cardiol* 1995;76:236–240.

185. Butman SM, Olson HG, Gardin JM, et al. Submaximal exercise testing after stabilization of unstable angina pectoris. *J Am Coll Cardiol* 1984;4:667–673.

186. Madsen JK, Stubgaard M, Utne HE, et al. Prognosis with thallium-201 scintigraphy in patients admitted with chest pain without confirmed acute myocardial infarction. *Br Heart J* 1988;59:184–189.

187. Cerqueira MD, Harp GD, Ritchie JL. Quantitative gated blood pool tomographic assessment of regional ejection fraction: definition of normal limits. *J Am Coll Cardiol* 1992;20:934–941.

188. Corbett JR. Gated blood pool SPECT. In: Depuey EG, Berman DS, Garcia EV, eds. *Cardiac SPECT imaging.* New York: Raven Press, 1995:257.

189. Jones RH, Johnson SH, Bigelow C, et al. Exercise radionuclide angiocardiography predicts cardiac death in patients with coronary artery disease. *Circulation* 1991;84:I52–I58.

190. Pryor DB, Harrell FE, Lee KL, et al. Prognostic indicators from radionuclide angiography in medically treated patients with coronary artery disease. *Am J Cardiol* 1984;53:18–22.

191. Lee KL, Pryor DB, Pieper KS, et al. Prognostic value of radionuclide angiography in medically treated patients with coronary artery disease: a comparison with clinical and catheterization variables. *Circulation* 1990;82:1705–1717.

192. Upton MT, Rerych SK, Newman GE, et al. Detecting abnormalities in left ventricular function during exercise before angina and ST-segment depression. *Circulation* 1980;62:341–349.

193. Shaw LJ, Heinle SK, Borges-Neto S, et al. Prognosis by measurements of left ventricular function during exercise. *J Nucl Med* 1998;39:140–146.

194. Bonow RO, Kent KM, Rosing DR, et al. Exercise-induced ischemia in mildly symptomatic patients with coronary artery disease and preserved left ventricular function: identification of subgroups at risk of death during medical therapy. *N Engl J Med* 1984;311:1339–1345.

195. Borer JS, Bacharach SL, Green MV, et al. Real-time radionuclide cineangiography in the noninvasive evaluation of global and regional left ventricular function at rest and during exercise in patients with coronary artery disease. *N Engl J Med* 1977;296:839–844.

196. DePace NL, Iskandrian AS, Hakki AH, et al. Value of left ventricular ejection fraction during exercise in predicting the extent of coronary artery disease. *J Am Coll Cardiol* 1983;1:1002–1010.

197. Gibbons RJ, Zinsmeister AR, Miller TD, et al. Supine exercise electrocardiography compared with exercise radionuclide angiography in noninvasive identification of severe coronary artery disease. *Ann Intern Med* 1990;112:743–749.

198. Iskandrian AS, Hakki AH, Goel IP, et al. The use of rest and exercise radionuclide ventriculography in risk stratification in patients with suspected coronary artery disease. *Am Heart J* 1985;110:864–872.

199. Supino PG, Borer JS, Herrold EM, et al. Prognostication in 3-vessel coronary artery disease based on left ventricular ejection fraction during exercise. *Circulation* 1999;100:924–932.

200. Borer JS, Hochreiter C, Herrold E, et al. Prediction of indications for valve replacement among asymptomatic or minimally symptomatic patients with chronic aortic regurgitation and normal left ventricular performance. *Circulation* 1998;97:525–534.

201. Verani MS, Lacy JL, Guidry GW, et al. Quantification of left ventricular performance during transient coronary occlusion at various anatomic sites in humans: a study using tantalum-178 and Multiwire gamma camera. *J Am Coll Cardiol* 1992;19:297–306.

202. Zaret BL, Jain D. Continuous monitoring of left ventricular function with miniaturized non-imaging detectors. In: Zaret BL, Beller GA, eds. *Nuclear cardiology: state of the art and future directions,* 2d ed. St. Louis: Mosby, 1999.

203. Kiat H, Berman DS, Maddahi J, et al. Late reversibility of tomographic myocardial thallium-201 defects: an accurate marker of myocardial viability. *J Am Coll Cardiol* 1988;12:1456–1463.

204. Kitsiou AN, Srinivasan G, Quyyumi AA, et al. Stress-induced reversible and mild-to-moderate irreversible thallium defects: are they equally accurate for predicting recovery of regional left ventricular function after revascularization? *Circulation* 1998;98:501–508.

205. Iskandrian AS, Hakki AH, Kane SA, et al. Rest and redistribution thallium-201 myocardial scintigraphy to predict improvement in left ventricular function after coronary arterial bypass grafting. *Am J Cardiol* 1983;51:1312–1316.

206. Bonow RO, Dilsizian V, Cuocolo A, et al. Identification of viable myocardium in patients with chronic coronary artery disease and left ventricular dysfunction: comparison of thallium scintigraphy with reinjection and PET imaging with 18F-fluorodeoxyglucose. *Circulation* 1991;83:26–37.

207. Udelson JE, Coleman PS, Metherall J, et al. Predicting recovery of severe regional ventricular dysfunction: comparison of resting scintigraphy with thallium-201 and Tc-99m sestamibi. *Circulation* 1994;89:2552–2561.

208. Di Carli M, Asgarzadie F, Schelbert HR, et al. Quantitative relation between myocardial viability and improvement in heart failure symptoms after revascularization in patients with ischemic cardiomyopathy. *Circulation* 1995;92:3436–3444.

209. Ragosta M, Beller GA, Watson DD, et al. Quantitative planar rest-redistribution thallium-201 imaging in detection of myocardial viability and prediction of improvement in left ventricular function after coronary bypass surgery in patients with severely depressed left ventricular function. *Circulation* 1993;87:1630–1641.

210. Mori T, Minamiji K, Kurogane H, et al. Rest-injected thallium-201 imaging for assessing viability of severe asynergic regions. *J Nucl Med* 1991;32:1718–1724.

211. Cuocolo A, Pace L, Ricciardelli B, et al. Identification of viable myocardium in patients with chronic coronary artery

disease: comparison of thallium-201 scintigraphy with reinjection and technetium-99m-methoxyisobutyl isonitrile. *J Nucl Med* 1992;33:505–511.

212. Marzullo P, Sambuceti G, Parodi O. The role of sestamibi scintigraphy in the radioisotopic assessment of myocardial viability. *J Nucl Med* 1992;33:1925–1930.

213. Kauffman GJ, Boyne TS, Watson DD, et al. Comparison of rest thallium-201 imaging and rest technetium-99m sestamibi imaging for assessment of myocardial viability in patients with coronary artery disease and severe left ventricular dysfunction. *J Am Coll Cardiol* 1996;27:1592–1597.

214. Medrano R, Lowry RW, Young JB, et al. Assessment of myocardial viability with 99mTc sestamibi in patients undergoing cardiac transplantation: a scintigraphic/pathological study. *Circulation* 1996;94:1010–1017.

215. Dakik HA, Howell JF, Lawrie GM, et al. Assessment of myocardial viability with 99mTc-sestamibi tomography before coronary artery bypass graft surgery: correlation with histopathology and postoperative improvement in cardiac function. *Circulation* 1997;96:2017–2023.

216. Galli M, Marcassa C, Imperta A, et al. Effects of nitroglycerin by technetium-99m sestamibi tomoscintigraphy on resting regional myocardial hypoperfusion in stable patients with healed myocardial infarction. *Am J Cardiol* 1994;74:843–848.

217. He ZX, Medrano R, Hays JT, et al. Nitroglycerine-augmented 201Tl reinjection enhances detection of reversible myocardial hypoperfusion: a randomized, double-blind, parallel, placebo-controlled trial. *Circulation* 1997;95:1799–1805.

218. He ZX, Verani MS. Evaluation of myocardial viability by myocardial perfusion imaging: should nitrates be used? *J Nucl Cardiol* 1998;5:527–532.

219. Murray G, Schad N, Ladd W, et al. Metabolic cardiac imaging in severe coronary disease: assessment of viability with iodine 123-I-iodophenylpentadecanoic acid and multicrystal gamma camera, and correlation with biopsy. *J Nucl Med* 1992;33:1269–1277.

220. Iskandrian AS, Powers J, Cave V, et al. Assessment of myocardial viability by dynamic tomographic iodine 123 iodophenylpentadecanoic acid imaging: comparison with rest-redistribution thallium-201 imaging. *J Nucl Cardiol* 1995;2:101–109.

221. Verani MS, Taillefer R, Iskandrian AE, et al. 123I-IPPA SPECT for the prediction of enhanced left ventricular function after coronary bypass graft surgery. Multicenter IPPA Viability Trial Investigators. 123I-iodophenylpentadecanoic acid. *J Nucl Med* 2000;41:1299–1307.

222. Tamaki N, Kawamoto M. The use of iodinated free fatty acids for assessing fatty acid metabolism. *J Nucl Cardiol* 1994;1:S72–S78.

223. Schelbert HR. Merits and limitations of radionuclide approaches to viability and future developments. *J Nucl Cardiol* 1994;1:S86–S96.

224. Sandler MP, Videlefsky S, Delbeke D, et al. Evaluation of myocardial ischemia using a rest metabolism/stress perfusion protocol with fluorine-18 deoxyglucose/technetium-99m MIBI and dual-isotope simultaneous-acquisition single-photon emission computed tomography. *J Am Coll Cardiol* 1995;26:870–878.

225. Henes CG, Bergmann SR, Walsh MN, et al. Assessment of myocardial oxidative metabolic reserve with positron emission tomography and carbon-11 acetate. *J Nucl Med* 1989;30:1489–1499.

226. Gould KL, Yoshida K, Hess MJ, et al. Myocardial metabolism of fluorodeoxyglucose compared to cell membrane integrity for the potassium analogue rubidium-82 for assessing infarct size in man by PET. *J Nucl Med* 1991;32:1–9.

227. Iskandrian AE, Acio E. Methodology of a novel myocardial viability protocol. *J Nucl Cardiol* 1998;5:206–209.

228. Leoncini M, Marcucci G, Sciagrà R, et al. Nitrate-enhanced gated Tc-99m sestamibi SPECT for evaluating regional wall motion at baseline and during low dose dobutamine infusion inpatients with chronic coronary artery disease and left ventricular dysfunction: comparison with two-dimensional echocardiography. *J Nucl Cardiol* 2000;7:426–431.

229. Duncan BH, Ahlberg AW, Marini D, et al. Regional left ventricular response to low dose dobutamine infusion during ECG-gated Tc-99m sestamibi SPECT image acquisition accurately predicts global left ventricular function after revascularization in patients with coronary artery disease and left ventricular dysfunction. *J Am Coll Cardiol* 2000;35:446A(abst).

230. Okada RD, Johnson G III, Nguyen KN, et al. 99mTc-HL91 "hot spot" detection of ischemic myocardium *in vivo* by gamma camera imaging. *Circulation* 1998;97:2557–2566.

231. Riou L, Ghezzi C, Mouton O, et al. Cellular uptake mechanisms of 99mTcN-NOET in cardiomyocytes from newborn rats: calcium channel interaction. *Circulation* 1998;98:2591–2597.

232. Shryock JC, Snowdy S, Baraldi G, et al. A2A-adenosine receptor reserve for coronary vasodilation. *Circulation* 1998;98:711–718.

233. Vanzetto G, Glover DK, Ruiz M, et al. 99mTc-N-NOET myocardial uptake reflects myocardial blood flow and not viability in dogs with reperfused acute myocardial infarction. *Circulation* 2000;101:2424–2429.

234. Iskandrian AE, Verani MS, eds. Bar Harbor Invitation Meeting 2000. *J Nucl Cardiol* 2001;8(2):224–316.

235. Narula J, Dawson MS, Singh BK, et al. Noninvasive characterization of stunned, hibernating, remodeled and nonviable myocardium in ischemic cardiomyopathy. *J Am Coll Cardiol* 2000;36:1913–1919.

MAGNETIC RESONANCE IMAGING

PAULO R. SCHVARTZMAN
RICHARD D. WHITE

OVERVIEW

Cardiovascular (CV) magnetic resonance imaging (MRI) is uniquely well suited for the morphologic and physiologic evaluation of a wide range of acquired and congenital disease processes affecting the heart, pericardium, and great arteries and veins of the thorax. Its technological diversity permits MRI to provide four-dimensional (three spatial dimensions over the dimension of time) imaging of the CV system based on definition of high-detail anatomy, histologic characterization, intracardiac or intravascular blood flow, cardiac chamber contraction and filling, regional myocardial mechanics, and tissue perfusion. Already, CV MRI has established itself as a valuable noninvasive diagnostic imaging tool within the clinical arena, with its application largely limited by actual or perceived expense, lack of availability of dedicated CV MRI services compared with other imaging services (e.g., echocardiography), unportability of equipment to ill patients, diffi-

culty in monitoring patients on life support or during induced stress, and contraindication to imaging certain implanted devices (e.g., pacemaker). Nevertheless, CV MRI has evolving roles being established in the following groups of CV diseases: (a) thoracic aortic disease (e.g., aortic dissection); (b) ischemic heart disease [e.g., determination of viability and post–myocardial infarction (MI) complications]; (c) myocardial disease [e.g., right ventricular cardiomyopathy (CM)]; (d) pericardial disease (e.g., constrictive pericarditis); (e) thrombi and masses (e.g., cardiac tumor); (f) adult congenital heart disease (CHD) (e.g., great vessel abnormality); (g) valvular heart disease (e.g., aortic regurgitation); and (h) pulmonary artery disease (e.g., pulmonary hypertension). The future of CV MRI will depend on (a) establishment of an important role in the evaluation of ischemic heart disease or related conditions (e.g., possibly by providing comprehensive profiles of the pertinent parameters); (b) unique definitions of aspects of CV diseases (e.g., myocardial characterization, load-independent measure of myocardial function, noninvasive arterial wall imaging), leading to high morbidity and mortality in this country; (c) cooperative efforts between services dealing with diagnostic imaging of CV diseases; or (d) all of these.

P. R. Schvartzman: Departments of Cardiovascular Imaging and Radiology, The Cleveland Clinic Foundation, Cleveland, Ohio
R. D. White: Department of Medicine, Division of Radiology, The Cleveland Clinic Foundation, Cleveland, Ohio

SPECIFIC CLINICAL APPLICATIONS

For the purpose of this discussion, application of MRI to CV diseases presenting in the adult are addressed.

Ischemic Heart Disease

Assessment of Global Ventricular Function

Multiphasic MRI techniques have been used to estimate impaired EF as a result of ischemic heart disease. End diastolic and end systolic images of the LV have been obtained to evaluate EF and the resulting values derived, using the area-length method to correlate with those obtained by single-plane and biplane LV ventriculography (e.g., R = 0.79 and R = 0.95 for parallel and perpendicular to the interventricular septum, respectively) (73,74). Nevertheless, in the presence of LV asymmetry caused by MI with remodeling, formulas for calculating LV volumes by geometric models have serious limitations (107).

After MI, LVEF values (determined from transaxial MRI, obtained using a multiphasic multilevel S-E technique) have been shown to correlate well with those from radionuclide or contrast LV ventriculography (108). However, the correlation varied with the damaged region, described by primary coronary artery distribution (e.g., R = 0.87 for right coronary artery and R = 0.48 for left anterior descending distributions). A semiquantitative measure of global post-MI LV function, based on segmental wall motion scoring from transaxial multiphasic multilevel images, also correlated regionally with ventriculographic EF values (e.g., R = 0.96 for left anterior descending and R = 0.62 for right coronary artery distributions) (38). Such regional variations have been attributed to the limitations of orthogonal imaging, including poor visualization of the undersurface of the LV adjacent to the diaphragm. This limitation is overcome when short-axis imaging is used.

Multilevel-multiphasic MRI for EF determination in patients with ischemic heart disease can be performed more efficiently and with better temporal resolution using cine (68,71,76). In patients imaged within 7 days of acute MI using cine, LVEF by MRI has been shown to correlate better with EF by contrast ventriculography (e.g., R = 0.94) than with EF by radionuclide ventriculography (e.g., R = 0.82) (109).

Despite its advantages, MRI continues to have difficulties in gaining acceptance in the assessment of ventricular volumes and function in patients with ischemic heart disease because of a lack of general availability of dedicated CV MRI services with full capabilities for performing the functional aspects of cardiac imaging, and the wider availability and general familiarity with echo (107). Although the precision and the reproducibility of echo measurements are less than those achieved with MRI, echo information generally can be relied on for clinical management.

Assessment of Regional Ventricular Function

Abnormal wall motion, and more specifically abnormal systolic thickening, in the LV indicates diminished regional myocardial function (110). Regional myocardial wall thickening abnormalities are frequently observed on MRI in association with ischemic heart disease, starting as early as 5 minutes after coronary artery occlusion (111).

Compared with other criteria, such as increased myocardial intensity and adjacent intracavitary blood signal, regional wall motion abnormality appears to be the most predictive and specific MRI finding associated with either a recent or remote MI (112). By analyzing the outline of the endocardial and epicardial borders on images acquired at various segments of the cardiac cycle using the different multiphasic MRI techniques, regions of hypokinesia, akinesia, or dyskinesia, accompanied by increasing degrees of impaired wall thickening, can be defined clinically (69,80,108). For the detection of a recent MI, using a multiphasic multilevel S-E MRI technique, sensitivity, specificity, and accuracy are improved when wall motion abnormalities are used along with myocardial intensity increase (e.g., 93%, 80%, and 87%, respectively) rather than intensity increase alone (e.g., 80%, 80%, and 80%, respectively) (113).

Regions of decreased LV systolic wall thickening caused by ischemic heart disease can be identified and quantitated using the various multiphasic S-E MRI techniques. Employing transaxial imaging and a multiphasic multilevel S-E MRI technique, absolute and percent wall thickening has been assessed in various cardiac diseases, including ischemic heart disease; MRI consistently demonstrated decreased systolic wall thickening measurements in regions damaged by MI when compared with normal myocardial regions in the same patients, and with the LV wall in normal individuals (38,79). When concurrent multilevel multiphasic S-E MRI and 2-D echo examinations of patients with a single MI were evaluated using a segment-by-segment point scoring of residual wall thickening, most of the LV segments, representing the left anterior descending distribution, showed significant agreement (38). In experimentally evaluating regional LV contractility in comparison with histochemical evidence of MI, determinations of mean maximal percent systolic thickening have been found to be significantly decreased in induced MI regions; with high sensitivity and moderate specificity, the same MRI approach identified reduced systolic wall thickening in segments recognized as akinetic or dyskinetic by LV ventriculography in patients with a history of MI (114).

More so than multiphasic S-E techniques, cine is suited to the evaluation of regional ventricular function in patients with ischemic heart disease (69,80,109,110). Assessments of LV wall motion by cine in patients with coronary artery disease (CAD) have correlated well with results of echo or LV ventriculography (80); impaired systolic wall thickening has proved to be a very specific marker of

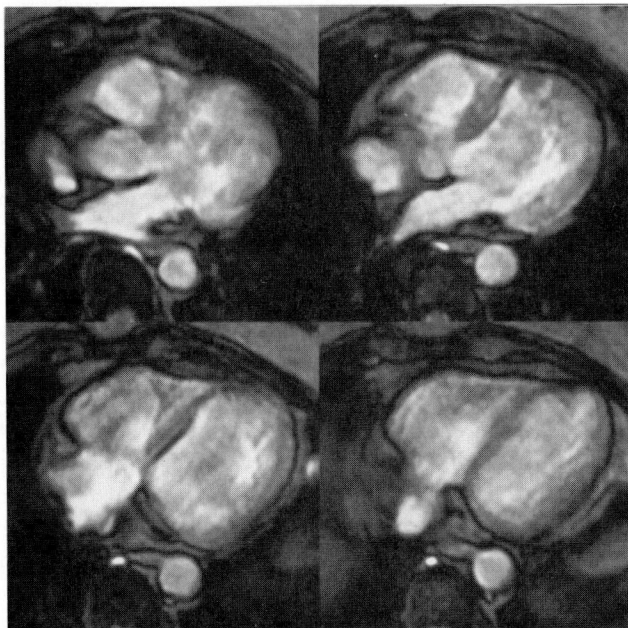

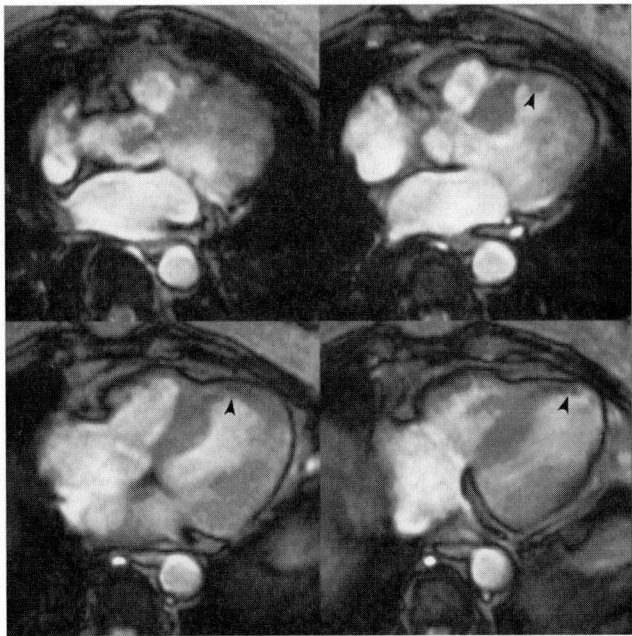

FIGURE 54.1 Regional myocardial dysfunction from coronary artery disease (cine; transaxial). From end diastole **(A)** to end systole **(B)**, four adjacent levels of the left ventricle reveal decreased anteroseptal and anteroapical wall thickening (*arrowheads*) from disease of the left anterior descending coronary artery.

regional myocardial dysfunction (Fig. 54.1). Compared with contrast ventriculography, the concordance in regional wall motion has been similar for both cine (e.g., 69%) and radionuclide ventriculography (e.g., 65%) (109). Although a multilevel cine series gives the advantage of full representation of the ventricles, when patients with suspected CAD have been studied using only biplane cine and biplane LV ventriculography, 96% agreement in the right anterior oblique view and 92% agreement in the left anterior oblique view have been demonstrated (115).

Absence of systolic wall thickening in the presence of passive inward wall motion, which is potentially mistaken for hypokinetic viable myocardium on ventriculography, is detectable in MI regions on MRI because of direct LV wall visualization. Wall thickening of greater than 2 mm has been measured in all regions of the normal LV on cine; less thickening has been demonstrated at sites of prior MI (80,116–118). Cine has proved to be more accurate than echo in the measurement of LV systolic wall thickening (119).

More recently, myocardial tagging has been used to provide unique functional information about regions of MI and compensatory changes of noninfarcted portions of the LV (*e*Fig. 54.1.1) (120). In patients with one-vessel disease leading to an acute MI, reduced intramyocardial circumferential shortening has been noted throughout the LV, including remote noninfarcted regions (121). Using SPAMM, LV dilatation and eccentric hypertrophy from remodeling have been shown to be associated with persistent differences in segmental function and wall stress between adjacent and remote noninfarcted myocardium (121).

Although the determination of wall motion, thickening, and mechanics by these forms of multiphasic MRI may eventually play an important role in the accurate detection and functional characterization of myocardial ischemia in patients with suspected or known CAD (122), their routine clinical use has been limited because of the aforementioned reasons.

Complications and Natural History of Myocardial Infarction

Tissue characterization by MRI has shown an inverse relationship between relaxation times and flow during experimental coronary artery occlusion (123). Acute MI is characterized by prolonged T1 and T2 (111–113,124). The alteration in relaxation times, and the associated signal increase, in acutely infarcted myocardium seems to primarily represent edema resulting from acute, irreversible ischemia (125). In addition, following an acute MI, maximum T1 values are observed at 2 weeks after the event, suggesting that cellular infiltration also contributes significantly to the appearance (126). However, other factors (e.g., hemorrhage, loss of myocyte membrane integrity, increased triglyceride content, free radicals, changes in magnetic susceptibility) also presumably contribute to the prolonged relaxation times (127).

Although an *in vivo* determination of these relaxation times is calculated from signal intensities detected on MRI, intensity does not depend only on T1 and T2 but, rather, is related to other physiologic characteristics (e.g., movement). Therefore, image-derived quantitation of the relaxation times for clinical purposes is influenced by hemodynamics and by cardiac and respiratory motions; hence, the obtained values for relaxation times differ from *ex vivo* measurements and are less reliable (111–113).

Nevertheless, increase in relative myocardial intensity is routinely seen as early as 30 minutes, but almost certainly 3 to 6 hours, after coronary occlusion when MI has occurred (113,124). The intensity reaches a maximum after 3 days, but then tends to decline after 20 days (113,128). Because T2 is prolonged, helping to enhance intensity in the region of an acute MI, the contrast between the MI region and normal regions is optimized on T2-weighted images (113,124).

Regional increase in S-E myocardial intensity, indicating acute MI (Fig. 54.2), has corresponded with the ECG location of the MI (113), enzymatic indicators (129), the presence of hypokinetic segments on ventriculography (113,129), and nuclear perfusion defects at rest (130). Although this characteristic pattern of myocardial S-E intensity is often noted in clinical cases during the first 2 weeks after MI, there are pitfalls in the clinical application of alterations in signal intensity (112). Increased myocardial intensity on T2-weighted images may be difficult to distinguish from slowly moving intraventricular blood (131), and it has been noted that T2 prolongation might not be a specific marker for acute MI and can also be observed in abnormally perfused myocardial segments of patients with unstable angina (132). In addition, increased intensity may often be seen in normal individuals, thereby reducing its value as a marker of MI. Thus, although the increased intensity of MI regions on S-E MRI can be considered a sensitive finding, it is of low specificity (112).

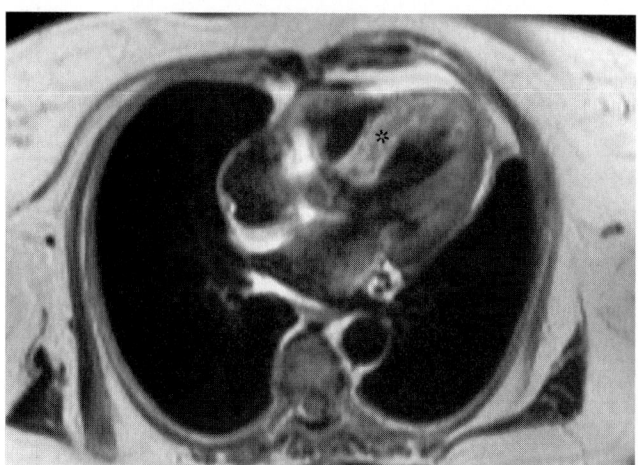

FIGURE 54.2 Regional increase in myocardial intensity from acute myocardial infarction (T2-weighted spin-echo; transaxial). Increased myocardial signal intensity in interventricular septum and anterior wall (*asterisk*) is caused by edema from an acute myocardial infarction.

Findings consistent with hemorrhagic MI have also been detected *ex vivo* on S-E imaging (133). Regions of decreased signal intensity, histologically proven to be hemorrhage, have been noted adjacent to or within the central zone of increased intensity that represents acute MI; good correlation has been found between the volume of hemorrhage measured at postmortem examination and the volume of such decreased signal intensity. The decreased myocardial intensity results from T2 enhancement produced by deoxyhemoglobin (134).

The use of Gd chelates enhances the ability to visualize a region of MI on T1-weighted S-E images (66,135,136), and it may also result in a higher specificity in detecting MI (137). Gd chelates at lower doses mainly shorten T1 of the myocardium and, because of the different washout rates, increase the contrast between MI and normal regions on T1-weighted images. *Ex vivo* MRI of perfused hearts using Gd chelates has shown increased contrast between normal and reperfused ischemic myocardium, when compared with both nonreperfused ischemic hearts after Gd chelate administration and reperfused ischemic hearts not given Gd chelate (138). However, this distinction has been less evident on S-E MRI performed *in vivo*.

The appearance of an acute MI after the injection of contrast media is regulated by whether images are acquired during the initial or early passage of the contrast media through the heart or during the equilibrium phase (66). The appearance also depends on the age of the MI, the dose of the medium, and the sequences applied (107). During the first pass, there is delayed entrance of the contrast medium into the ischemic region. Consequently, the region supplied by an occluded artery shows lower signal intensity than normal myocardium during the first few minutes after injection of a Gd chelate (107) (*e*Fig. 54.2.1). On the other hand, there is greater enhancement of intensity of the MI region using T1-weighted images acquired during the equilibrium phase of distribution, because of a delayed washout of the medium in the occluded area or the enlarged extracellular space of the MI region (135,136); the differentiation persists 30 minutes after injection (137).

Although in patients, significantly greater myocardial intensity enhancement results from Gd chelate (i.e., 66% to 70% increase) in regions of MI when compared with normal regions (i.e., 20% to 35% increase) on T1-weighted images (136,137), it is not true on T2-weighted images (139). Because contrast between acute MI and normal regions is increased (e.g., 6% and 39% before and after Gd chelate, respectively), improved clinical discrimination has been possible, allowing for a more accurate diagnosis of MI (135,137,138). A new delayed-enhancement MRI technique (Turbo FLASH with inversion recovery) has been applied to study both acute and chronic MI after the administration of Gd chelate and has shown an excellent correlation with TTC staining histology in animal models (139). The sequence is employed 15 to 30 minutes after

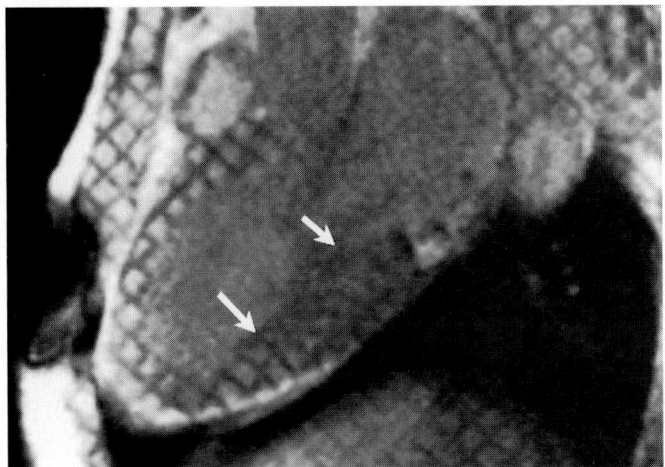 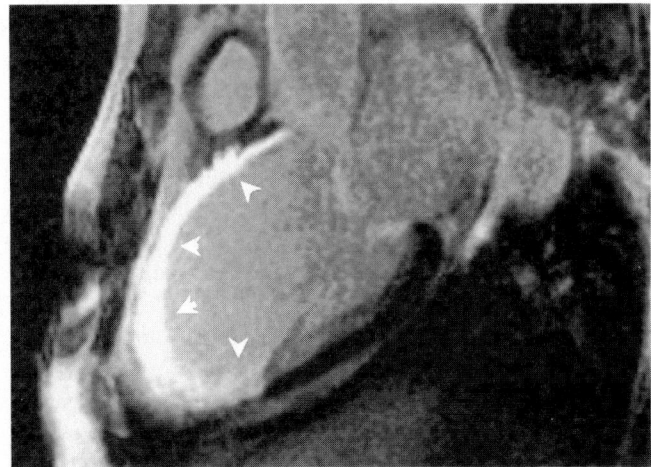

FIGURE 54.3 Delayed-enhancement magnetic resonance image of chronic myocardial infarction [spatial modulation of magnetization (SPAMM); Turbo FLASH with inversion recovery; long axis]. At end systole a SPAMM image **(A)** demonstrates contraction (*arrows*) (deformation of grid pattern with change from square to diamond shape) of the left ventricle inferior wall. Delayed-enhancement image **(B)** demonstrates transmural hyperenhancement of the anterior wall, apex, and apical inferior wall (*arrowheads*) caused by myocardial necrosis, corresponding to the area of absent contraction on the SPAMM image.

the injection of a double dose (0.2 mmol per kg) of gadolinium-diethylenetriaminepentaacetic acid (Gd-DTPA), and the area of necrosis is delineated as an area of hyperenhancement and viable myocardium as an area of nulled signal (Fig. 54.3 and *e*Fig. 54.3.1).

Although a number of experimental and clinical studies have shown that MRI contrast agents improve the demarcation between acute or subacute MI and normal myocardium, it has been accomplished for a chronic MI (140). In addition, despite encouraging initial results, it has been shown that signal intensities measured 25 minutes after Gd chelate administration differentiate reperfused from non-reperfused MI when the delayed-enhancement technique is employed (140). In patients status-post thrombolytic therapy for acute MI, measured intensity ratios 6 to 8 minutes after injection of Gd chelate have been shown to be significantly different from those of MI regions subtended by occluded coronary arteries, indicating that assessment of the early dynamics of contrast enhancement using Gd chelates may identify successful reperfusion (138). It has also been shown that the morphologic appearance of contrast enhancement by Gd chelates may identify the presence or absence of reperfusion; reperfusion leads to no enhancement, whereas lack of reperfusion may be visualized as a hyperenhancement (140,141).

Chronic MI produces regions characterized by shortened T2 and decreased intensity on routine S-E and G-E imaging consistent with the replacement of myocardium with fibrous tissue (142). On ultrafast for first-pass assessment, 50% enhancement of chronic MI regions, compared with 134% in normal regions, has been observed after Gd chelate administration; the MI site on MRI corresponded with the location of wall motion abnormality on echo (143).

In addition to increased relaxation times, other morphologic MRI features of MI are valuable diagnostic parameters. Areas of thinning of the LV wall caused by remote MI are sharply demarcated from myocardium that is of normal thickness (130,142,144). Regional abnormalities are delineated better on systolic images than on diastolic images, because there is an accentuated disparity in the wall thickness. Compared with increased myocardial intensity and abnormal cavitary signal, relative regional wall thinning has been found to be the most predictive and specific marker for the presence of an acute MI during clinical evaluation by MRI (112).

Damage to the LV wall segments is often indicated by intracavitary stagnant blood and thrombotic material (*e*Fig. 54.3.2). These intracavitary areas appear as abnormal signal on S-E and cine MRI (49,77,145). With S-E MRI, the differentiation between these two causes of such signal may be made, as described earlier, from multiple S-E magnitude-data images or the corresponding phase-display images. The presence of even-echo rephasing or significant motion-dependent phase changes indicates slow blood flow; the absence of these changes accompanies thrombus (146). On cine, their differentiation is achieved by finding fluctuating areas of intermediate signal loss (i.e., indicating slow blood flow) or fixed lower intensity areas (i.e., indicating thrombus) on the image loop (63) (*e*Fig. 54.3.3).

Because of its therapeutic and prognostic importance, MI sizing by MRI has been pursued. *Ex vivo* and *in vivo* measurements of relative MI size (i.e., percent LV), based on changes in myocardial signal parameters such as intensity on T2-weighted images after experimental coronary artery occlusion, have correlated closely with postmortem estimates (147). However, S-E imaging without the administration of contrast has tended to overestimate MI size and to demonstrate abnormal intensity extending well beyond the margins of the MI found on pathologic evaluation, suggesting that T2-weighted S-E MRI depicts not only MI damage but also some reversibly injured myocardium (148). In addition, MRI-determined MI size has correlated well with microsphere-determined reduction of blood flow of 25% or more (122). But with the new delayed-enhancement technique, an excellent correlation has been shown between MRI images and histology, either in acute or chronic MI (139).

Clinical MI size determinations, based on intensity at a mean of 9 days after the acute onset of symptoms, have been shown to correlate well with the region of severe hypokinesia visualized by ventriculography (113). Good agreement has been found between MI sizing based on T1 MRI maps and assessment by infarct-avid scintigraphy and ventriculography 5 to 7 days after MI (149). In addition, mean MI volume, based on signal changes, correlated well with segmentally quantitated dysfunction by ventriculography. In the setting of a recent MI, studied 5 to 20 days after the acute event, T2-weighted S-E MRI allows for the direct assessment of MI location and size (150).

A good correlation between MI size measured with contrast-enhanced MRI and enzymatically determined MI size, 3 to 7 days after the acute event, has been demonstrated (151). Also, Gd chelates produce markedly increased myocardial intensity that correlates well with extent of acute or chronic MI on the delayed-enhancement MRI (139,140).

Another approach to evaluate MI may well be a correlation with the extent of regional wall thinning. Clinically, MI size has been measured based on regional LV wall thinning and dysfunction noted on multiphasic multilevel S-E MRI, and the resulting values correlated inversely with EF determinations by ventriculography (e.g., R = 0.88) (108). Nevertheless, significant reduction in MI size, based on myocardial signal on S-E MRI with (152) or without (153) contrast enhancement, has been shown in patients who did, compared with those who did not, receive intravenous streptokinase within hours of the onset of chest pain related to an acute MI.

MRI is also capable of detecting long-term sequelae of MI. Complications of acute MI including ventricular aneurysm (eFig. 54.3.4), ventricular septal perforation (154), mitral regurgitation, and LV thrombus also can be readily demonstrated by MRI (107,122). Post-MI LV aneurysms are identified as outwardly protruding myocardial wall segments associated with marked transmural thinning and occasionally mural thrombus (142,144). A true aneurysm (i.e., relatively wide neck,) can usually be differentiated from a pseudoaneurysm (i.e., relatively narrow neck), based on the relative size of the communication between the aneurysmal cavity and the main LV cavity (155,156) (eFigs. 54.3.5 and 54.3.6).

Although therapy is focused on minimizing the deleterious remodeling process in the LV after MI, imaging modalities have not been routinely used to guide or to assess the effect of this therapy (107). MRI used to show remodeling of the LV after acute MI (157), and attenuation of the remodeling process in response to drug therapy has been documented experimentally (158). In patients, cine has provided accurate quantification of myocardial mass of the abnormally shaped LV caused by a transmural MI (159).

In spite of the recognition that MRI can be used to evaluate many aspects of MI, there has been limited clinical use of it for these purposes (107). Perhaps the reason for this is that LV shape changes and complications after acute MI are well shown by echo, although MRI is able to produce a 3-D view of the LV and define with extreme accuracy the extension and size of MI.

Assessment of Ischemia

Myocardial ischemia, like MI, is associated with increased myocardial signal as a result of prolonged relaxation times (160), and correlations have been observed between increases in T1 and T2 and the increase in tissue water content (161). However, in the clinical setting, the detection of myocardial intensity changes from induced reversible ischemia, moreover ischemia at rest, has not been reliable without the administration of Gd chelate. In contrast to irreversibly injured myocardium, reversibly ischemic myocardium does not necessarily alter myocardial relaxation times or intensity in the early phase. In unstable angina, S-E MRI has occasionally shown significantly increased T2 in reversibly ischemic myocardium. It also failed to distinguish reversibly from irreversibly ischemic regions, as determined by nuclear perfusion imaging (132). The detection of acute ischemia with unenhanced MRI does not occur until several hours after coronary occlusion.

The detection of myocardial ischemia by any imaging modality frequently requires some form of stress to induce disparity in blood flow between normal and potentially ischemic regions. In more recent years, pharmacologic stress has been applied in MRI for detection of functional abnormalities in patients with CAD, because physical exercise during MRI is difficult because of space restriction and it results in motion artifact. The agents used for this purpose increase flow by causing either direct coronary vasodilation or secondary vasodilatation caused by augmented myocardial oxygen requirements, or both; regional myocardial dysfunction is then caused by either an absolute decrease in regional perfusion (i.e., coronary steal phenomenon) or inadequate increase in flow relative to augmented oxygen requirements (i.e., increased myocardial work) (107).

Using ultrafast, the assessment of myocardial blood flow in normal, reversibly ischemic and irreversibly ischemic myocardium, at rest and during dipyridamole-induced hyperemia, has been validated experimentally (102). With dipyridamole as the vasodilator, a direct relation has been found between myocardial blood flow and signal intensity

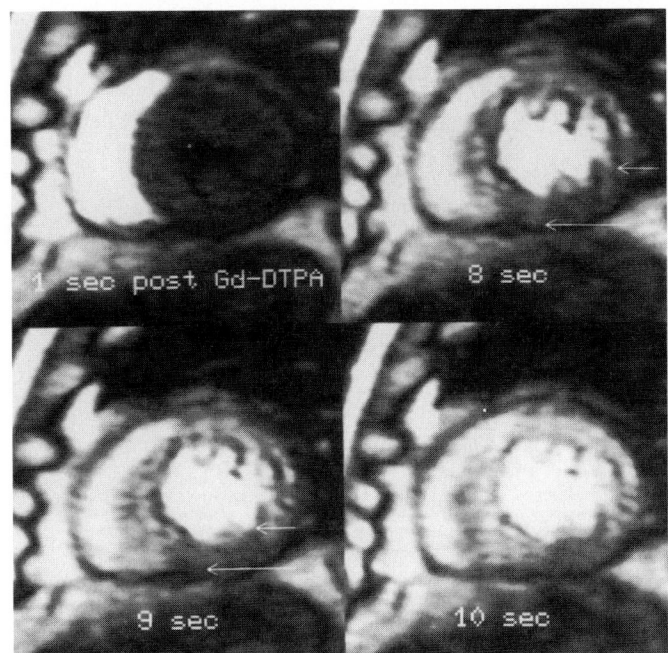

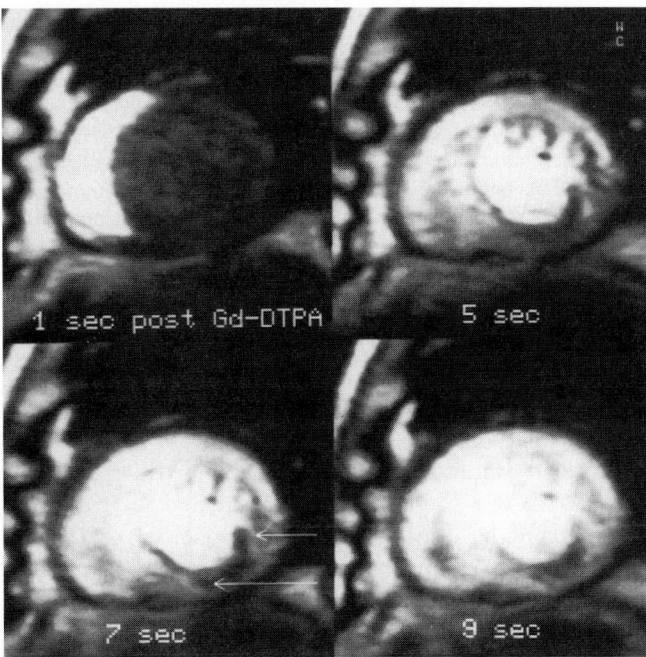

A

B

FIGURE 54.4 Dipyridamole-induced hypoperfusion in myocardial ischemia (ultrafast, short axis). On sequential diastolic images at rest **(A)**, only a moderate lack of signal enhancement is detected in the posterior wall of the left ventricle (*arrows*); this is caused by asymptomatic retrograde-filled occlusion of the right coronary artery. Following administration of dipyridamole **(B)**, resulting in angina, decreased signal intensity around the subendocardial layers (*arrows*) of the posterior wall is clearly differentiated from the higher signal intensity of the normal myocardium. Gd-DTPA, gadolinium-diethylenetriaminepentaacetic acid. (From Wilke N, Jerosch-Herold M, Stillman AE, et al. Concepts of myocardial perfusion imaging in magnetic resonance imaging. *Magn Reson Q* 1994;10:249, with permission.)

after administration of Gd chelates (162). These experimental studies have stimulated the application of ultrafast in patients with CAD.

Applying ultrafast to patients with or without the use of pharmacologic stress, myocardial regions perfused by a severely stenosed coronary artery can be detected by an abnormal pattern of change in myocardial intensity. Several differences in intensity versus time curves between the normally perfused segments and the segments supplied by stenotic arteries have been observed after the bolus administration of Gd chelates (163). Some investigators have qualitatively observed an abnormal delay in signal increase of the hypoperfused myocardium; these areas have been shown to correlate well with abnormal areas shown on nuclear perfusion imaging (*e*Fig. 54.3.7) (106). Others have shown that regions with reduced perfusion can be quantitatively characterized on ultrafast, as areas of reduced peak intensity and diminished upslope of the intensity versus time curve compared with normal myocardium (163).

Ultrafast for the resting assessment of patients with CAD before and after revascularization has demonstrated improvement in peak intensity and rate of signal increase in myocardium perfused by the treated vessel (163). However, ultrafast has more often been used during the peak effects of dipyridamole (Fig. 54.4) (164). When patients with CAD have been studied using Gd chelate-enhanced

ultrafast and dipyridamole stress, sensitivity, specificity, and accuracy of 65%, 76%, and 74%, respectively, have been noted (104).

The limitation of all studies using ultrafast imaging is that the LV can be only partially sampled (usually 3 to 5 anatomic levels) while maintaining adequate temporal resolution (image at each level at 2- to 3-second intervals), whereas higher speed methods would allow multislice tomography to generate a 3-D perspective. Experimentally, EPI has been used to monitor the first pass of Gd chelates in hearts of normal animals and those with coronary occlusion (103) but has not yet been applied clinically. The results in animals and in humans suggest that perfusion imaging by MRI could become an important tool in the diagnosis of ischemic heart disease. A conclusion about the importance of perfusion MRI in relation to nuclear perfusion studies must await further publications (107).

An alternative to the assessment of perfusion abnormalities for the assessment of myocardial ischemia is the detection of reversible LV contractile dysfunction by multiphasic MRI. Multiphasic MRI may show regional LV dysfunction associated with induced reversible ischemia. In patients with known CAD and induced defects on nuclear perfusion examinations, corresponding regional LV functional abnormalities have been noted on MRI after administration of dipyridamole; these wall motion abnormalities occurred at the site of more extensive thallium defects and were associated with chest pain and more severe CAD (164). The 84% sensitivity and 89% specificity of dipyridamole-stress cine resembles that of stress nuclear perfusion imaging for detecting hemodynamically significant stenoses at coronary arteriography (165).

Compared with dipyridamole, dobutamine appears to be a more appropriate agent for eliciting wall motion abnormalities; dobutamine infusion is well tolerated during MRI (166). Cine has been used to visualize wall motion or wall-thickening abnormalities in the potentially ischemic myocardium provoked by dobutamine (Fig. 54.5) (117,166). In patients with CAD studied by both dobutamine-stress cine and nuclear perfusion imaging, comparison of perfusion defects and wall motion abnormalities showed 90% agreement (117,167). Studies of patients referred for coronary arteriography have shown that dobutamine-stress cine can identify wall motion abnormalities by such quantitative analysis with sensitivity, specificity, and accuracy of 91%, 80%, and 90%, respectively; the sensitivity for detection of one-vessel disease was 88%, two-vessel disease 91%, and three-vessel disease 100% (168). Dobutamine-stress MRI has been compared with dobutamine-stress echo and showed similar accuracy, but when echo images were suboptimal, the MRI accuracy was significantly higher than echo (169). Furthermore, dobutamine-stress MRI has been used in patients with poor acoustic window and not well suited for second harmonic stress echo, generating an accuracy of 83% when compared with coronary angiography (170).

Myocardial tagging may improve the accuracy of MRI with dobutamine stress to detect regional dysfunction, including that limited to the subendocardium. However, to date, this application has been largely investigational in animal models.

Stress MRI is becoming an important tool for diagnosis of myocardial ischemia due to its capability of excellent spatial resolution and been able to define the endocardial border with high accuracy (166–170).

Assessment of Myocardial Viability

The distinction between viable and nonviable myocardium after MI is an important determinant of therapeutic options. The effectiveness of MRI in assessing the complete area at risk following acute coronary occlusion may depend on the use of MRI contrast agents to delineate the volume of jeopardized myocardium. Work in animal models has shown that the region of increased myocardial intensity correlates with the bed of myocardium at risk in reperfused myocardium, when Gd chelate is injected after 5 minutes of reperfusion (171). Also, with late injection (e.g., 15 to 30 minutes), an excellent correlation is noted if the delayed-enhancement technique is employed (139,140).

Ultrafast, during administration of Gd chelates, has been shown to provide clear differentiation between an occlusive

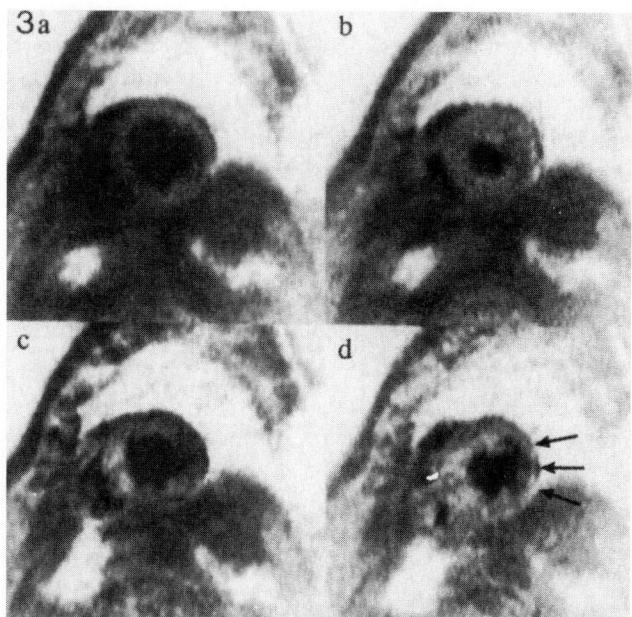

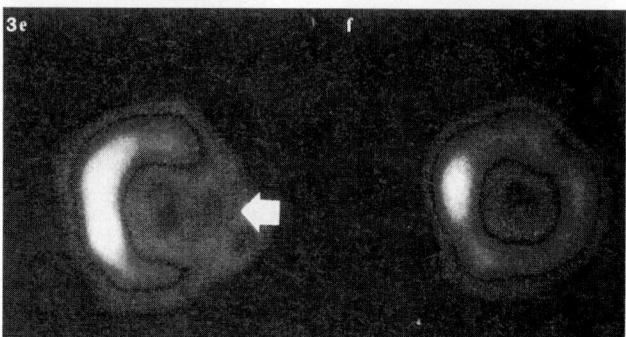

FIGURE 54.5 Dobutamine-induced contractile dysfunction in myocardial ischemia (cine and thallium single photon emission computed tomography, short axis). On end diastolic **(left, 3a, 3c)** and end systolic **(right, 3b, 3d)** cine images (displayed in negative format) at rest **(above)**, baseline contraction is normal in all regions of the left ventricle. During dobutamine administration **(below, 3c, 3d)**, decreased systolic motion and wall thickening are noted in the lateral free wall of the left ventricle (*arrows*); these are caused by left circumflex coronary artery disease. Corresponding thallium single photon emission computed tomography images during stress **(3e)** and after redistribution **(3f)** demonstrate a reversible lateral free-wall perfusion defect (*large arrow*) corresponding to the wall motion abnormality on cine. (From Pennell DJ, Underwood SR, Manzara CC, et al. Magnetic resonance imaging during dobutamine stress in coronary artery disease. *Am J Cardiol* 1992;70:34, with permission.)

(i.e., nonenhancing) and a reperfused (i.e., enhancing) MI (172) and between reversible and irreversible injuries in reperfused myocardium in experimental models (173). Although reperfused reversibly injured myocardium shows no significant difference in intensity compared with normal myocardium, irreversibly injured reperfused myocardium shows a substantial increase in intensity during equilibrium, probably as a result of greater distribution space for the contrast media in the jeopardized region because of expansion of the extracellular space (173). An occlusive MI shows a significantly greater enhancement of the peripheral zone than of the central zone, whereas reperfused MI shows homogeneous enhancement of the injured zone (173). EPI has also been used to compare the first pass of a Gd chelate in occluded and reperfused MI (174).

These studies performed in various animal models have been promising in characterizing different types of myocardial injuries, and studies in patients with an occlusive MI or a reperfused MI have shown that contrast-enhanced MRI with a delayed-enhancement technique is effective in differentiating between these two types of myocardial injury (175). When clinical results of delayed enhancement have been compared with positron emission tomography and dobutamine-stress echo, concordant results have been observed, and a correlation has been observed between the amount of enhancement transmurally and the percentage of nonviable segments determined by both techniques (176).

The capability of basic forms of MRI such as cine to provide functional information about myocardium in combination with assessment of diastolic wall thickness and systolic wall thickening makes it suitable for identification of myocardial viability (177). Regional end diastolic wall thickness of less than 6 mm and end systolic wall thickening of less than 1 mm on cine have been identified as features of nonviable myocardium, as defined by nuclear perfusion or metabolism imaging (178,179). A comparison of cine with low-dose dobutamine stress with positron emission tomography in patients with chronic MI showed that use of these parameters was accurate in assessing myocardial viability; wall thickening was found to be a better predictor (e.g., 96% positive predictive value) of residual metabolic activity than was end diastolic wall thickness

(Fig. 54.6) (179). Cine and transesophageal echo with dobutamine stress have been assessed for their relative ability to detect induced contraction reserve; when results of each were compared against segmental assessments of viability by positron emission tomography, the sensitivities were 81% and 77% and the specificities were 100% and 94%, respectively (180).

Direct Assessment of Coronary Arteries

Noninvasive visualization of the coronary arteries is one of the ultimate challenges for MRI (122). Imaging of the coronary arteries by MRI has received a great deal of attention since the beginning of clinical CV MRI (181). Visualization of the coronary arteries with standard MRI approaches has been erratic and limited to the proximal segments of the vessels (181,182); only occasionally have readily recognizable vascular abnormalities been identified. Nevertheless, in the cardiac cycle between rapid filling in early diastole and atrial systole, there is a period of relative diastasis with high coronary flow; this has become a target for the many more recently introduced approaches to MRI of the coronary arteries employing static versus dynamic, structural versus flow-based, 2-D versus 3-D, and other variations (183).

Although angiographic forms of MRI are routinely used clinically for evaluation of the carotid and intracerebral vasculature, the great vessels of the chest and abdomen, and the arteries and veins of the extremities (40), angiography of the coronary arteries by MRI remains investigational. This is because of the greater technical difficulties related to the relatively small size of these arteries, their complex 3-D

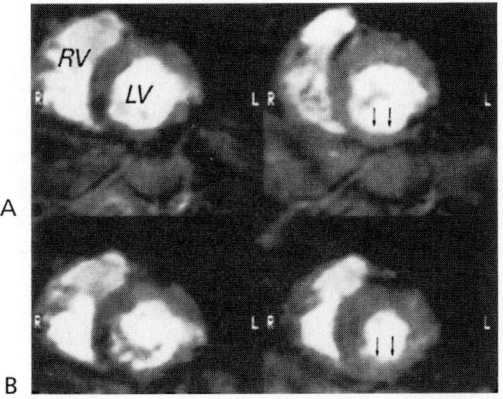
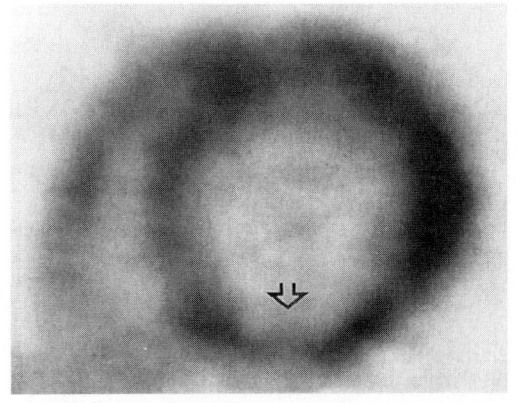

FIGURE 54.6 Post–myocardial infarction myocardial viability (cine and fluorine-18-fluorodeoxy-glucose positron emission tomography; short axis). Despite an inferior myocardial infarction (*closed arrows*), viability in the injured region is represented on end diastolic (**left**) and end systolic (**right**) cine images by dobutamine-induced systolic wall thickening (**B**) of the akinetic-appearing inferior wall at rest (**A**). The positron emission tomographic image (**C**) demonstrates preserved metabolism in the same region (*open arrow*). [From Baer FM, Voth E, Schneider CA, et al. Comparison of low-dose dobutamine-gradient-echo magnetic resonance imaging and positron emission tomography with (18F) fluorodeoxyglucose in patients with chronic coronary artery disease: a functional and morphological approach to the detection of residual myocardial viability. *Circulation* 1995;91:1006, with permission.]

anatomy, normal cyclic variations in coronary flow, competing signal from neighboring blood pools, and their constantly changing position within the chest caused by cardiac and respiratory motion (107,122). To overcome these obstacles, several approaches have been proposed and have already achieved some success (183). To date, the greatest experience has been with 2-D G-E MRI with fat saturation to eliminate signal from adjacent adipose tissue and segmented k-space acquisition, allowing imaging at one level during a breath-hold to avoid excessive blurring from respiratory motion (184).

With the 2-D G-E approach, good visualization of all major vessels in healthy subjects has been reported (185), and good correlation between measurements made by MRA and coronary arteriography has been established (186). In patients with CAD, occluded coronary arteries have appeared on such MRA images as absent flow signal distal to the occlusion, while high-grade stenoses showed signal loss in the area of stenosis with visualization of the vessel distally (Fig. 54.7). Initial clinical work with the approach resulted in optimism about identifying hemodynamically significant stenoses (i.e., ≥50% narrowing) of major coronary arteries. Using selective coronary arteriography as the gold standard, MRI-based angiography had 90% sensitivity and 92% specificity for identifying a diseased epicardial coronary artery on blinded analysis, although correspondence between lesion location within an individual coronary artery was not assessed; the corre-

sponding positive and negative predictive values were 85% and 95%, respectively (187). The sensitivity and specificity of the technique were, respectively, 100% and 100% for the left main coronary artery, 87% and 92% for the left anterior descending artery, 71% and 90% for the left circumflex coronary artery, and 100% and 78% for the right coronary artery (187). Subsequent work, using the same approach (188) or a 3-D approach with respiratory compensation (189), however, showed much poorer results, which were attributable to patient selection biasing, independent evaluation, technique differences, and experience of the interpreter. More recently, contrast-enhanced 3-D approaches with breath holding have shown great promise (183).

The present spatial resolution and loss of signal caused by turbulence preclude accurate prediction of coronary artery stenosis severity by MRA. It has been shown that it is not possible to identify stenotic vessels based on quantification of signal intensity; no significant difference in signal was found between vessel segments of a normal coronary artery and vessel segments proximal to a significant stenosis (190). Nevertheless, MRA can be used to noninvasively identify patency of infarcted artery (191).

High-resolution MRI of the human coronary atheroma has developed significantly in the last years. The feasibility of imaging the coronary artery and determining the plaque content has been demonstrated (192). Although the plaque lipid material and the fibrous cap were identified in this

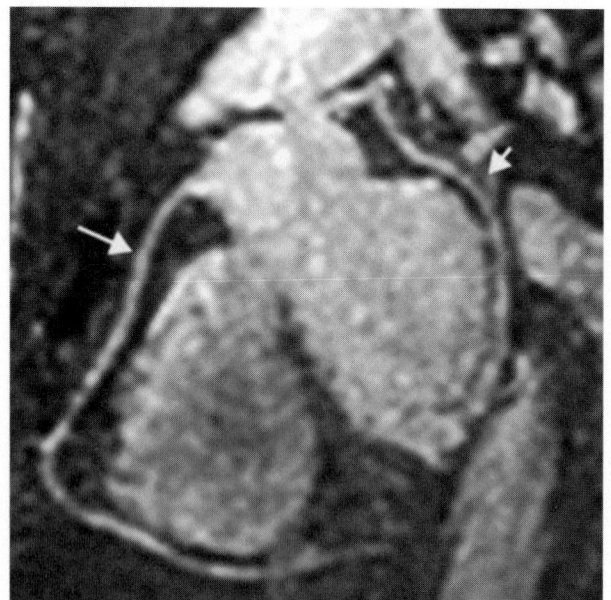
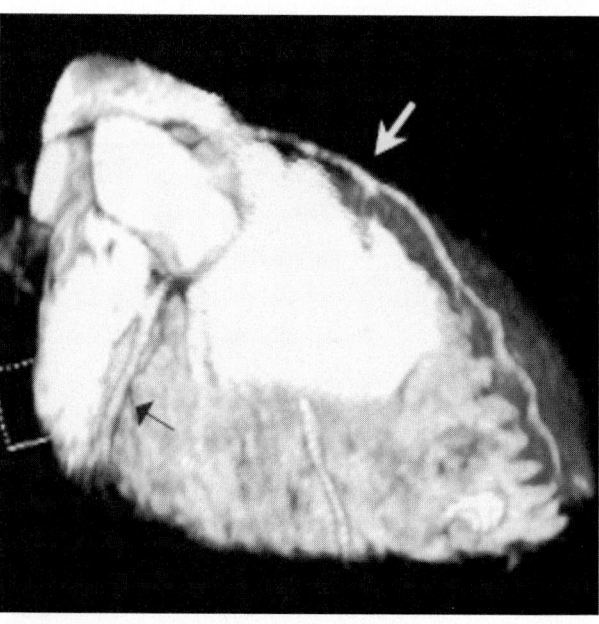

FIGURE 54.7 Magnetic resonance angiography of normal coronary artery (breath-hold, three-dimensional, segmented echo-planar imaging magnetic resonance angiography; maximal intensity projection). A maximal intensity projection image **(A)** demonstrates widely patent normal right coronary artery (*long arrow*) and left circumflex artery (*short arrow*). A volume-rendered reconstruction **(B)** of the same data set delineates the normal left anterior descending coronary artery (*white arrow*) and right coronary artery (*black arrow*). (Courtesy of Debiao Li, Ph.D., Northwestern University, Chicago, IL.)

preliminary work, further studies are needed to prove the applicability in a large population of this new and interesting technique to determine the morphology of the coronary plaques. In addition, its role relative to advancements in CT (subsecond multidetector scanning), which has also shown promise for plaque characterization, is unclear.

In addition to the morphologic approaches, an MRI method for evaluating flow in coronary vessels has been described (183,193). Results have indicated the feasibility of MRI for measuring flow in the native or simulated coronary arteries (194). Segmented velocity mapping has since been used to measure flow in the coronary arteries in healthy subjects; adenosine was used to increase coronary flow by severalfold, and an increase in velocity was shown (195). Others showed the feasibility of assessing increased coronary flow velocity using breath-hold velocity mapping or TOF EPI, during hand-grip exercise or after dipyridamole (196). Finally, coronary flow reserve in the left anterior descending coronary artery has been measured in an animal model (197) and in patients with CAD undergoing cardiac catheterization with validation by intracoronary Doppler velocity and flow measurements (198). Thus, MRI may become a noninvasive technique to demonstrate reduced coronary flow reserve caused by hemodynamically significant coronary arterial stenoses.

Encouraging initial results with MRI evaluation of coronary artery bypass graft (CABG) patency has been noted. S-E MRI has been used to assess patency of CABGs; an accuracy of 84% to 95% for detection of graft patency and 72% to 85% for graft occlusion was demonstrated (199,200). After studies with the S-E technique, cine was used to assess CABG patency, with the expectation that the associated signal enhancement of flowing blood would improve evaluation. Cine achieved adequate sensitivities (88% to 93%), specificities (86% to 100%), and overall predictive accuracies (89% to 91%) for patency (201,202). Subsequently, velocity mapping was applied to the measurement of flow in internal mammary artery grafts (203) or aortocoronary vein grafts (204); the normal flow patterns for coronary artery grafts is biphasic with peaks in both diastole and systole. The potential of MRA to evaluate CABG patency has been recognized (Fig. 54.8).

MRA provides a new approach to the evaluation of the patency of coronary vessels. While preliminary work with small numbers of patients has been described, large population studies are needed to see how this new technique will ultimately perform. High-resolution coronary MRI is a new and exciting technique that might be able to discriminate the plaque content, but further studies in this area are also needed, including correlation with histologic specimens.

Valvular Heart Disease

Until the advent of the multiphasic techniques, MRI could provide little valuable information about valvular heart dis-

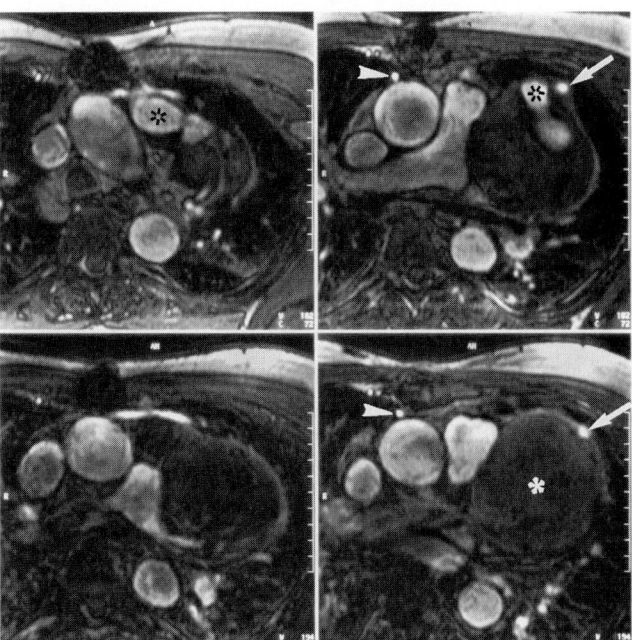

FIGURE 54.8 Coronary artery bypass graft patency and occlusion (contrast-enhanced, three-dimensional magnetic resonance angiography; oblique-transaxial). While patency of an internal mammary artery graft to the left coronary system (*arrows*) and a saphenous vein graft to the right coronary system (*arrowheads*) is confirmed, mid-graft occlusion of an aneurysmal, thrombus-filled saphenous vein graft to the left coronary system (*asterisks*) is detected.

ease (64); for the most part, only indirect signs were offered by S-E MRI. Because of signal enhancement of the intracardiac and intravascular blood pools, morphologic changes of the leaflets may be demonstrated better on cine (63).

MRI generally produces less information about valvular disease than is offered by Doppler echo. However, MRI has the following advantages: Its 3-D nature makes it operator independent; it may be less susceptible to missing or underestimating eccentrically directed flow through a diseased valve; and it is free from geometric assumptions if cardiac chamber volumes are to be calculated (205). Echo has the advantage of providing true real-time imaging, whereas dynamic MRI techniques provide image loops composed of multiple averaged cardiac cycles. Nevertheless, in the setting of stenosis, thickening and calcification, decreased excursion or doming, and fusion of leaflets have been observed on MRI; predisposition to regurgitation, vegetation, prolapse, and flail can be detected on MRI (205).

Abnormalities of the adjacent chambers are easily detected with MRI. In the presence of stenosis (205), focal dilatation of the distal recipient chamber, concentric hypertrophy of a proximal ventricle, and generalized dilatation of a proximal atrium have been described; with regurgitation present (205,206), generalized dilatation of the proximal and distal chambers and eccentric hypertrophy of an associated ventricle have been noted.

The flow disturbances associated with valvular heart disease are also detectable by MRI. S-E MRI identifies abnormally increased signal caused by stagnant flow within a chamber proximal or distal to a diseased valve, especially an atrioventricular valve; on cine, the same flow disturbance creates an ill-defined cloud of low signal (49,63). On the other hand, in the setting of turbulence, a discrete jet of signal void extending from the diseased valve into the otherwise signal-enhanced recipient chamber characterizes poststenotic or regurgitant flow on cine (62,205,206). Such signal-void jets must be differentiated from physiologic signal loss from normal antegrade flow and from normal inflow, respectively (205–207). Jets from these valvular problems are easily detected and are distinguishable based on their direction of propagation and time of appearance (63).

The semiquantitative or quantitative dynamic MRI assessment of the severity of flow disturbance caused by valve disease has been approached by several methods (205–207). The methods are based on the following measurements: (a) valve leaflet separation (208); (b) proximal convergent flow signal-void dimensions (209); (c) distal flow signal-void jet dimensions [e.g., length, area, or volume (absolute or relative to receiving chamber)] (207,210–213); (d) ventricular volumetrics (205,214); (e) transvalvular flow velocity (215); and (f) net volume flow (62,216).

Mitral Valve

Mitral Stenosis

The following anatomic abnormalities of mitral stenosis (MS) have been described by MRI: thickened leaflets with reduced diastolic opening, enlarged left atrium, abnormal left atrial signal, and abnormal diastolic transmitral signal (208,217).

A signal-void jet begins at the site of the mitral valve level and extends into the cavity of the LV during diastole on cine (205–207). More so than for the evaluation of regurgitation, evaluation of MS by cine is limited by the need for differentiation between the physiologic signal loss resulting from normal antegrade transvalvular flow and the abnormal flow through the stenotic mitral valve (*e*Fig. 54.8.1). However, some studies indicate that significant MS can be easily detected and semiquantitatively evaluated using cine (208,217).

Dynamic MRI has demonstrated its ability to quantitatively evaluate physiologic abnormalities associated with MS. The following have been assessed: valve leaflet separation (R = 0.81 vs. area by Doppler by pressure half-time method) (208), relative distal signal-void jet area (R = 0.77 vs. peak trans-valve gradient by catheterization) (207), and peak trans-valve gradient (R = 0.89 vs. gradient by Doppler) (218).

Mitral Regurgitation

The anatomic abnormalities of mitral regurgitation on MRI resemble those of MS; however, dilatation of the LV is present (205–207).

Mitral regurgitation is readily identified on cine because of the signal-void jet of turbulent flow extending from the mitral valve level into the left atrial cavity during systole (Fig. 54.9). Based on the detection of a jet, mitral regurgitation is identified with a high degree of accuracy (94% to 100% sensitivity and 95% to 100% specificity vs. color Doppler) (210,219,220).

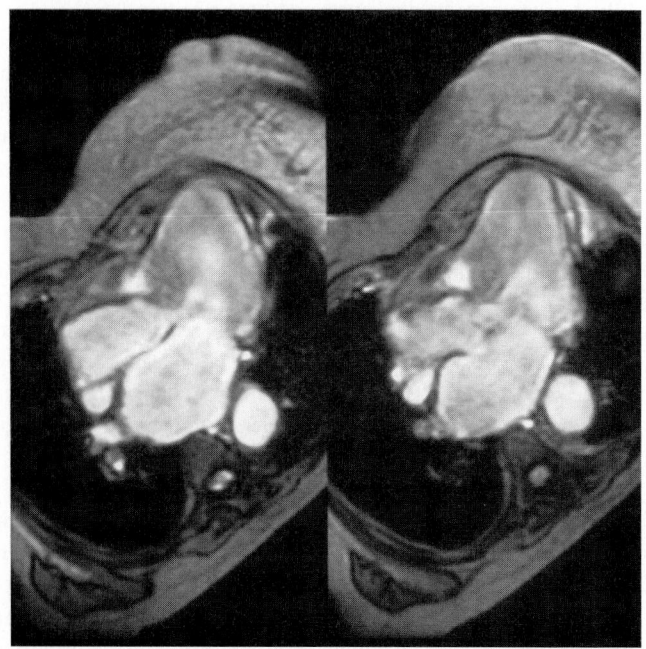
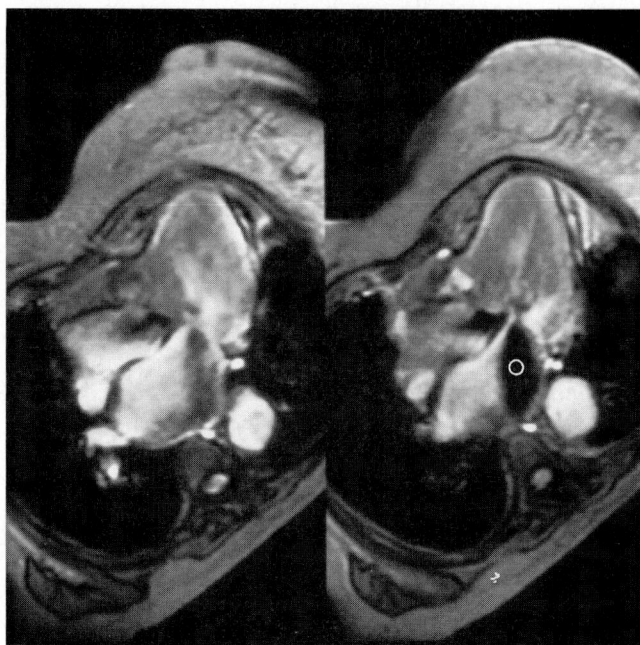

A   B

FIGURE 54.9 Mitral regurgitation (cine; left ventricle outflow tract). From end diastole **(A)** to mid-systole **(B)**, mitral regurgitation becomes identified by a signal-void jet of turbulent flow (*open circle*) extending from the mitral valve level into the left atrial cavity.

Quantitative physiologic assessment by dynamic MRI has included the following: distal signal-void jet grade [70% concordance vs. grade by color Doppler (221) and R = 0.77 vs. ventriculography (220)]; distal signal-void jet size [length, R = 0.74 vs. color Doppler (220); absolute area, R = 0.71 vs. color Doppler (220); relative area, R = 0.74 to 0.87 vs. color Doppler (219,220); volume, R = 0.84 vs. regurgitant volume by cine volumetric analysis (210,213)]; volumetric regurgitant fraction [R = 0.84 vs. ventriculography (221)]; volume-flow regurgitant fraction [R = 0.87 to 0.96 vs. grading by color Doppler (222,223)]; and combined volumetric and volume-flow regurgitant fraction [R = 0.96 vs. ventriculography (223)].

Aortic Valve

Aortic Stenosis

Anatomic abnormalities of aortic stenosis (AS) evaluated by MRI have included concentric LV hypertrophy, dilatation of the ascending aorta, reduced aortic valve area [R = 0.75 by S-E vs. catheterization or Doppler (224)], and mean difference by velocity mapping of 0.2 cm^2 versus catheterization by Gorlin formula and of 0.1 cm^2 versus Doppler by continuity equation (225). A double-oblique cine image taken through the aortic valve plane best demonstrates the cusps and their coaptation and serves to differentiate acquired AS from congenital AS with a bicuspid aortic valve. Because of its proven accuracy for quantifying LV mass (67,68), MRI may also be used to monitor the effects of AS on the LV before and after surgical repair or balloon valvuloplasty.

On cine, a signal-void jet of AS extends from the level of the aortic valve outward until its hemodynamic effects are dissipated within the blood pool of the ascending aorta (Fig. 54.10 and *e*Fig. 54.10.1). AS jets are usually observed on cine throughout most of systole; however, some physiologic signal-void jets normally appear transiently just beyond the aortic valve after the initial opening of its leaflets. Nevertheless, significant AS can be detected using cine, and when there is a pressure gradient across the aortic valve, the severity of pressure drop and the length of the area of signal loss on cine show significant correlation (205–207). Mild, moderate, and severe AS can be differentiated based on jet size, but at pressure gradients above approximately 60 mm Hg, no further size increase is noted (207).

Dynamic MRI has proved its ability to quantitatively evaluate physiologic abnormalities associated with AS. The following have been assessed: absolute distal signal-void jet length [R = 0.86 vs. peak trans-valve gradient by catheterization (207)] and peak trans-valve gradient [R = 0.96 vs. gradient by Doppler (225) and R = 0.67 to 0.97 vs. catheterization (225,226)].

Aortic Regurgitation

On MRI, the anatomic abnormalities of aortic regurgitation (AR) resemble those of AS, but instead of concentric hypertrophy, there is dilatation of the LV (205–207).

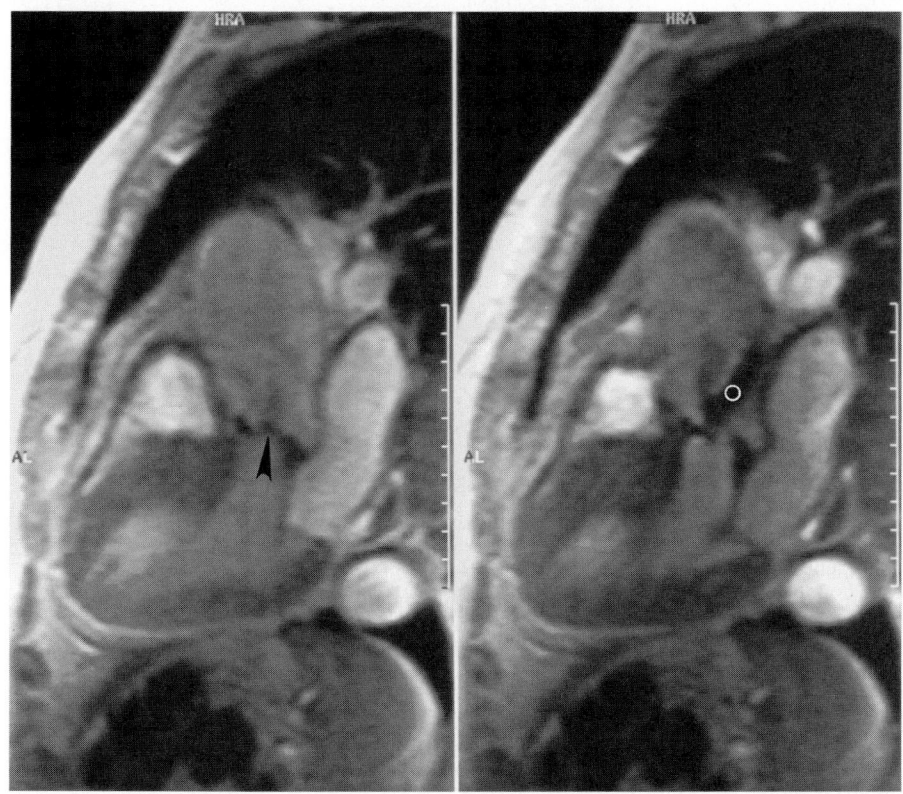

FIGURE 54.10 Aortic stenosis (cine; left ventricle outflow tract). From end diastole **(left)** to mid-systole **(right)**, a signal-void jet of turbulent flow (*open circle*), representing aortic stenosis, develops beyond the thickened aortic valve leaflets (*arrowhead*). HRA, high right atrium.

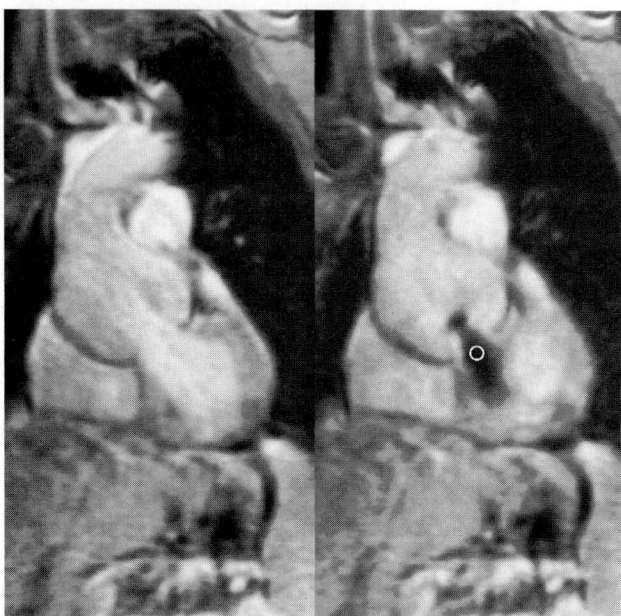

FIGURE 54.11 Aortic regurgitation (cine; oblique-coronal). A signal-void jet of aortic regurgitation (*open circle*) is seen extending from the dilated aortic root into the left ventricle cavity during diastole.

The signal-void jet of AR on cine has been fully described and evaluated for its potential to stage the severity of disease (Fig. 54.11 and *e*Figs. 54.10.1 and 54.11.1) (205–207). Qualitative assessment by cine has also involved proximal flow convergence detection (227) (87% sensitivity and 100% specificity vs. aortography) (209) and distal signal-void jet detection (89% to 92% sensitivity and 93% to 98% specificity vs. Doppler) (210). Velocity mapping has also received a great deal of attention for physiologic evaluation of AR, largely by assessing total reverse flow (62,205–207).

For quantitative physiologic assessment, dynamic MRI has been used for proximal convergent flow signal-void area (significantly greater than for all grades by echo) (209); distal signal-void jet grade (93% concordance vs. grade by aortography) (228); distal signal-void jet size [area significantly greater than for moderate to severe vs. normal to mild 2-D echo grades (229)]; volume R = 0.84 versus regurgitant volume by cine volumetrics (210,212), significantly greater than for moderate versus mild and for severe versus moderate 2-D echo grades (210); volumetric regurgitant fraction (significantly greater than for moderate to severe versus normal to mild 2-D echo grades) (212); volume-flow regurgitant fraction [R = 0.97 to 98 vs. cine volumetrics (216,229); R = 0.80 vs. grading by aortography (230)] (Fig. 54.12).

Tricuspid and Pulmonic Valves

Little work has specifically dealt with the issues of acquired right-sided valvular heart disease, although the value of

MRI in assessing congenital tricuspid, including Ebstein's anomaly or pulmonic valve disease, has been described (231). The principles correspond to the aforementioned for assessment of acquired left-sided valvular heart disease by MRI.

Volume-flow regurgitant fraction of pulmonic regurgitation has been validated (R = 0.93 vs. cine volumetrics) (232).

Prosthetic Valves

Normally Functioning Prosthesis
Studies *in vitro* and *in vivo* have shown that patients with artificial heart valves can be safely examined in high-field magnets (43,45). On MRI, little image distortion outside the immediate area of the prosthetic valve and no patient discomfort have been observed in related studies (233).

Abnormally Functioning Prosthesis
When the diagnostic value of cine for detecting regurgitation in prosthetic valves has been compared with that of transesophageal color Doppler echo, excellent (e.g., 96%) agreement between the methods in distinguishing physiologic from pathologic regurgitation was observed (234). In addition, quantitative physiologic evaluation of the severity of regurgitation has been promising [75% concordance of grade vs. grade by Doppler (234); R = 0.85 distal signal-

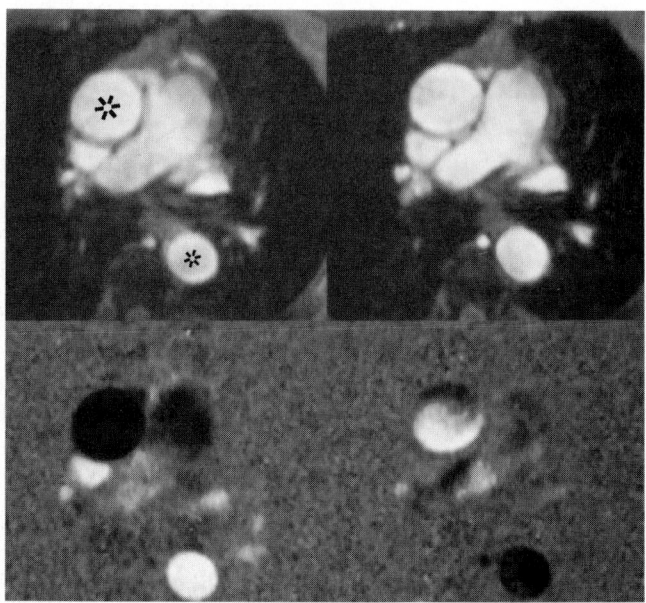

FIGURE 54.12 Aortic regurgitation (velocity mapping; oblique-transaxial). Corresponding to the magnitude data cine images (*above*) are the mid-systolic image (*left*) and mid-diastolic image (*right*) from velocity mapping (*below*). In systole, rapid antegrade-cranial flow in the ascending aorta (*large asterisk*) and antegrade-caudal systolic flow in the descending aorta (*small asterisk*) are represented by intense black and white shades, respectively. Because of significant aortic regurgitation, retrograde flow patterns are demonstrated in the thoracic aorta in diastole.

void jet length, and R = 0.91 distal signal-void jet vs. Doppler (234)].

Myocardial Disease

Nonischemic myocardial disease (CM) is represented by the group of diseases in which the dominant feature is pathology of the myocardium unrelated to ischemic, hypertensive, congenital, valvular, or pericardial diseases. Of the variety of schemes that have been proposed for classifying the CMs, the following categorization is helpful: (a) dilated CM causing ventricular dilatation, contractile dysfunction; (b) hypertrophic CM associated with inappropriate hypertrophy of the LV, often with asymmetric septal involvement and usually with preserved contractile function, despite frequent regional impairment; (c) restrictive CM characterized by impaired diastolic filling; and (d) RV CM causing dilatation and regionally or globally impaired contractility of the RV related to dysplasia, with partial to total replacement of the myocardium by variable amounts of adipose and fibrosis tissue.

Dilated Cardiomyopathy

MRI can readily define the abnormally enlarged cavity size and globally depressed function (*e*Fig. 54.12.1) of the LV and RV in cases of dilated CM (70,235). In contrast to healthy subjects, patients with dilated CM fail to demonstrate a gradient of progressively increasing systolic wall thickening from base to apex and have significantly decreased EF on cine (83,236), although improvement in LVEF from afterload reduction by angiotensin-converting enzyme inhibitor therapy has been demonstrated (237). The effects of such therapy on diastolic dysfunction have also been assessed using cine in patients suffering from dilated CM with and without MR; analysis of LV time-volume curves revealed improvements in both peak filling rate to end diastolic volume ratios and EF in the group without, but not in the group with, mitral regurgitation (238).

End systolic LV wall stress determined from cine has been determined to be abnormally elevated in patients with dilated CM, and inversely proportional to regional EF (239). In patients with dilated CM, significant increase in peak systolic wall stress, compared with normal values, has also been demonstrated (83). However, decreased end systolic wall stress following afterload reduction by angiotensin-converting enzyme inhibitor therapy has been shown using cine (237).

Myocardial tagging has been used in the assessment of the mechanical effects of surgical ventricular remodeling (*e*Fig. 54.12.2) for treatment of LV failure; reshaping of the LV wall and improvement in contraction with surgery has been demonstrated.

Hypertrophic Cardiomyopathy

Various patterns of LV hypertrophy in hypertrophic CM (Fig. 54.13) have been defined using MRI (240). Unfortu-

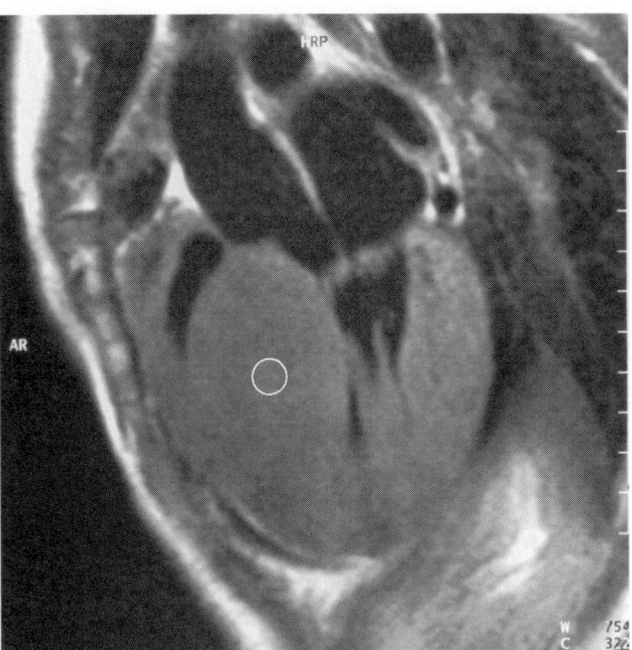

FIGURE 54.13 Left ventricular hypertrophy in hypertrophic cardiomyopathy (T1-weighted spin-echo; left ventricle outflow tract). Severe hypertrophy of the left ventricle wall, especially in the interventricular septum (*open circle*), is demonstrated.

nately, S-E signal characteristics of the myocardium in hypertrophic CM have not been shown to differ from those found in healthy subjects or in patients with physiologic LV hypertrophy (241). Pathophysiologic characteristics associated with hypertrophic CM have also been demonstrated with MRI; in the setting of this condition, cine has been used to evaluate asymmetric LV systolic wall thickening, subaortic poststenotic flow related to systolic anterior motion of the anterior mitral leaflet, and related mitral regurgitation (Fig. 54.14 and *e*Fig. 54.14.1) (242,243).

Pronounced heterogeneous reductions in circumferential, longitudinal, and 3-D shortening, with the septal impairment exceeding the free-wall impairment, have been described in hypertrophic CM using MRI (Fig. 54.15) (244,245). Accentuated heterogeneity in strain rate, increasing in diastole, has also been demonstrated in hypertrophic CM (246). The degree of contractile dysfunction has been correlated with both its abnormal geometry (e.g., flattened to negative septal curvature) (247) and the severity of internal histopathology (i.e., myocardial fibrosis and myofiber disarray) (248). Using cine to evaluate RV time-volume curves in hypertrophic CM, abnormally depressed peak-filling rates and filling fractions have been demonstrated; these changes suggested diastolic dysfunction from associated restrictive physiology (249). Contrast-enhanced ultrafast has been used to study cases of hypertrophic CM; decreased diastolic first-pass enhancement of the septal myocardium correlated with increased amounts of characteristic histopathology (e.g., intramyocardial small vessel narrowing) (250).

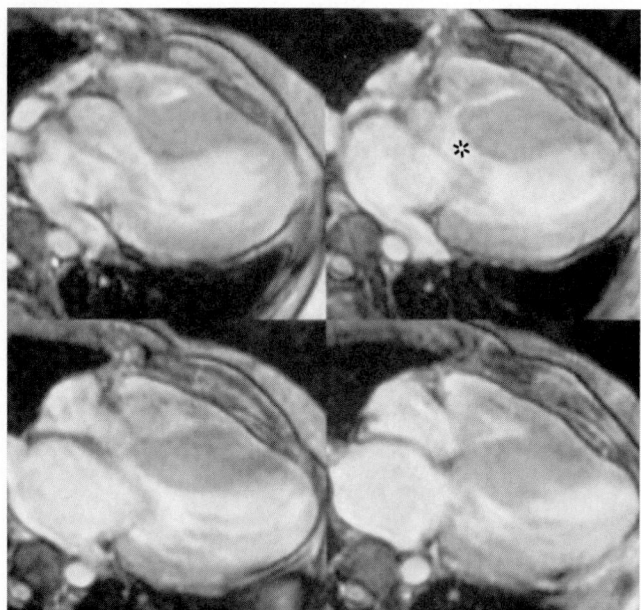

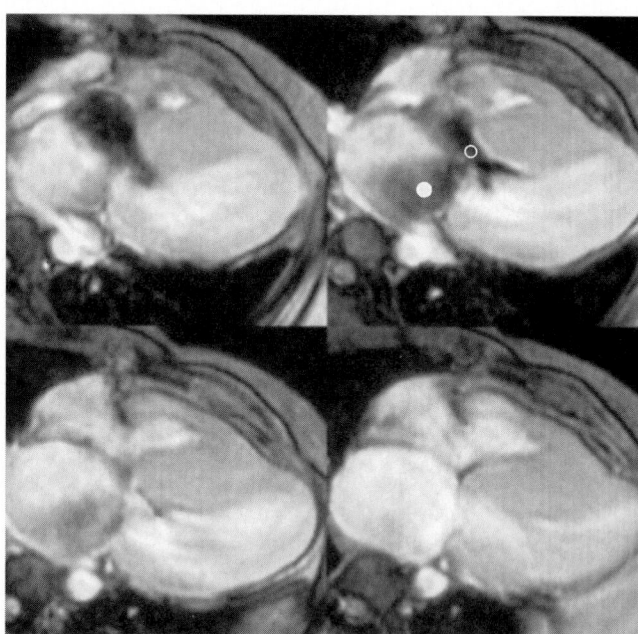

A

B

FIGURE 54.14 Subaortic poststenotic flow in hypertrophic cardiomyopathy (cine; horizontal long axis). On adjacent end diastolic images **(A)**, asymmetric left ventricle hypertrophy is noted; it results in fixed narrowing of the left ventricle outflow tract (*asterisk*). Because of systolic anterior motion of the anterior mitral leaflet in mid-systole **(B)**, abnormal subaortic signal void (*open circle*), representing stenosis, and left atrial signal void (*closed circle*), representing mitral regurgitation, develop.

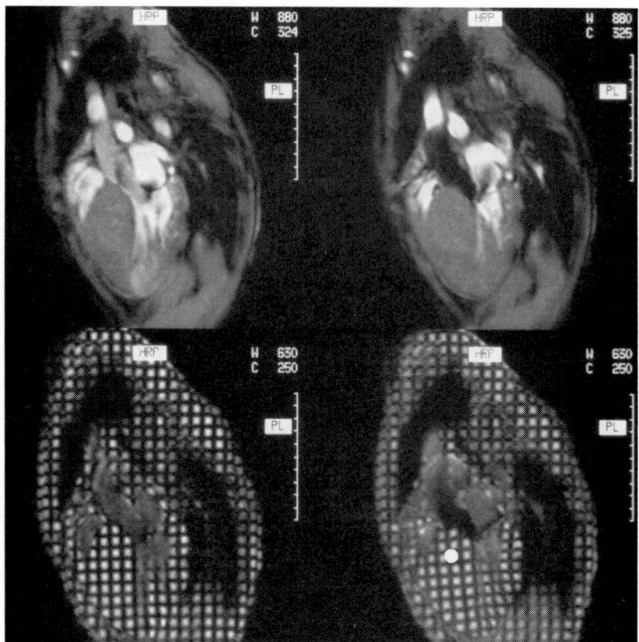

FIGURE 54.15 Regional variation in myocardial function in hypertrophic cardiomyopathy (cine and spatial modulation of magnetization; left ventricle outflow tract). With morphologic and hemodynamic abnormalities demonstrated on end diastolic cine (*above, left*) and end systolic cine (*above, right*) images, corresponding myocardial spin-tagging images (*below*) provide information about regional left ventricle function. Minimal deformation of the grid in the interventricular septum (*closed circle*), compared with the free wall, indicates its markedly impaired systolic mechanics.

Restrictive Cardiomyopathy

In cases of diastolic dysfunction caused by restrictive CM, rather than constrictive pericarditis, MRI is valuable in demonstrating the absence of abnormal pericardial thickening in the presence of indirect findings of impaired ventricular filling (e.g., dilatation of the inferior vena cava and right atrium) (251). MRI of cardiac amyloidosis (Fig. 54.16), a classic cause of restrictive physiology, has revealed increased thickness of the LV wall without cavity dilatation (252). Similar anatomic findings, in combination with slightly increased myocardial signal intensity, have been observed in some deposition diseases (e.g., Fabry's disease) resulting in diastolic dysfunction (253). However, for the most part, the myocardium of restrictive CM has normal MRI properties (e.g., T2) (254). There are notable exceptions in the setting of hemochromatosis: Prominent susceptibility-related loss of signal within the myocardium caused by iron deposition, especially on G-E images, has been demonstrated (255). Sarcoid heart disease, another potential cause of restrictive CM, is manifested on MRI in its acute inflammatory phase as discrete areas of high intensity that are associated with increased wall thickness within the LV septal and free wall myocardium (256) and chronically as focal areas of pronounced wall thinning, possibly with aneurysm formation, in the same LV wall regions (*e*Fig. 54.16.1).

An abnormally delayed pattern of ventricular filling caused by diastolic dysfunction associated with restrictive

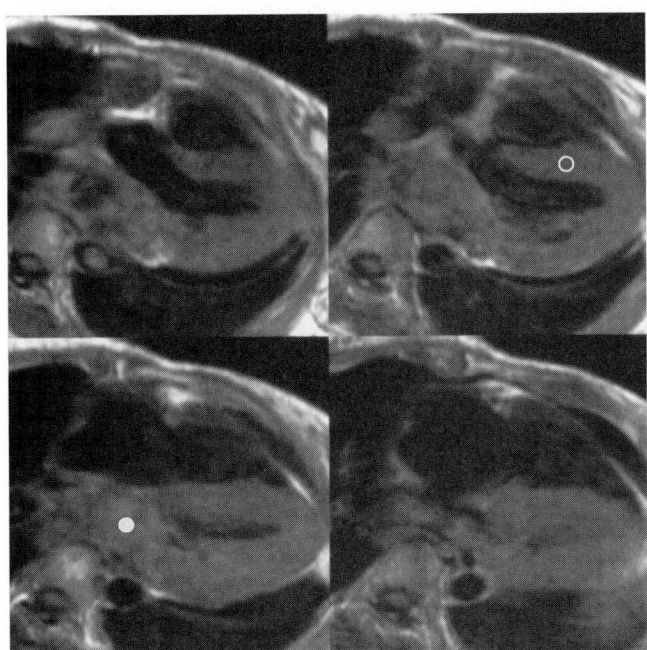

FIGURE 54.16 Cardiac amyloidosis (T1-weighted spin-echo; horizontal long axis). Generalized increase in left ventricle wall thickness (*open circle*), caused by protein deposition, is noted. Restrictive physiology is suggested by the presence of abnormal flow signal in the dilated left atrial cavity (*closed circle*).

CM can be evaluated qualitatively or quantitatively using cine (257). In the initial stages of restrictive CM, sluggish early ventricular filling is noted with or without mild impairment of systolic function; late restrictive CM, on the other hand, is characterized by rapid early, but abruptly terminated late filling of the ventricles (as in constrictive pericarditis) and with significantly impaired systolic emptying of the ventricles (unlike constrictive pericarditis). Velocity mapping of ventricular myocardium has been used to demonstrate reduction in mean peak early diastolic velocity related to LV stiffening with aging (258).

By measuring the rate of flow across the tricuspid and mitral annuli in diastole, velocity mapping has been proposed as a method for assessing diastolic dysfunction, as found in restrictive CM (259). Using velocity mapping, abnormal flow patterns in the superior vena cava have been demonstrated in restrictive CM; a progressively decreasing ratio of peak flow in systole relative to that in diastole is found with worsening restrictive physiology, but such ratios do not differentiate restrictive CM from constrictive pericarditis (260).

Right Ventricular Cardiomyopathy

Along with dilatation of the cavity of the RV, thinning of its wall in regions of fibrosis (Fig. 54.17) and increased signal intensity in regions of replacement of its myocardium with fat (*e*Fig. 54.17.1) have been well demonstrated in advanced cases of RV CM (arrhythmogenic RV dysplasia) using MRI (261,262). Greater reduction in RVEF and

more pronounced structural and histologic changes in the RV, including evidence of fatty replacement of the myocardium, have been more often demonstrated in the setting of RV CM than with inducible ventricular tachycardia (263). Regional wall motion abnormalities, compatible with milder focal dysplasia, have been observed using cine in patients with the diagnosis of idiopathic RV outflow tract tachycardia (*e*Fig. 54.17.2) (264).

Pericardial Disease

To an acute injury, the pericardial sac responds with one of the following reactions: (a) congestion; (b) increased exudation of fluid into the sac; (c) exudation of both fibrin and acute inflammatory cells into the sac; or (d) a combination of these reactions (the composition of the pericardial fluid that results depends on the cause of pericardial insult). Pericarditis, an inflammation of the pericardial surfaces, has many infectious and noninfectious causes.

Effusion and Tamponade

The normal pericardium and the contained physiologic fluid appear on MRI as only a thin (usually 2 mm or less) curvilinear line situated between the epicardial and pericardial fat. MRI has an advantage over CT in differentiating a small pericardial effusion from pericardial thickening because different acquisition schemes may be employed in MRI to appreciate and characterize fluid (265).

Simple pericardial effusions are visualized on S-E MRI as low-intensity regions between the cardiac surface with its epicardial fat and the outwardly displaced pericardial fat (265,266). Because of cardiac motion, the signal intensity from simple pericardial effusions is less than that from simple pleural effusions (265–267). Although characterized by low signal intensity on T1-weighted images, its signal intensity may increase on T2-weighted images; this is particularly true of the most dependent portions of the pericardial effusion. Whereas simple pericardial effusions produce high signal intensity on G-E MRI and when imaged with cine, they demonstrate mobility and changing distribution during the cardiac cycle (267) (Fig. 54.18).

Assessment of the distribution and general size of a simple pericardial effusion using MRI has shown good overall correlation with that by 2-D echo (266). However, when fluid volume has been quantitated by both techniques, the pericardial effusion has tended to measure larger by MRI (268). In fact, MRI has been shown to detect small pericardial effusions not visualized by echo, and to be better for detecting fluid located superiorly in the aortic pericardial reflection or superior pericardial recess, medially at the border of the right atrium, and posteriorly at the LV apex (266,268).

Because of T1 shortening from their high protein or cell content, complex pericardial effusions typically exhibit greater signal intensity than simple pericardial effusions on

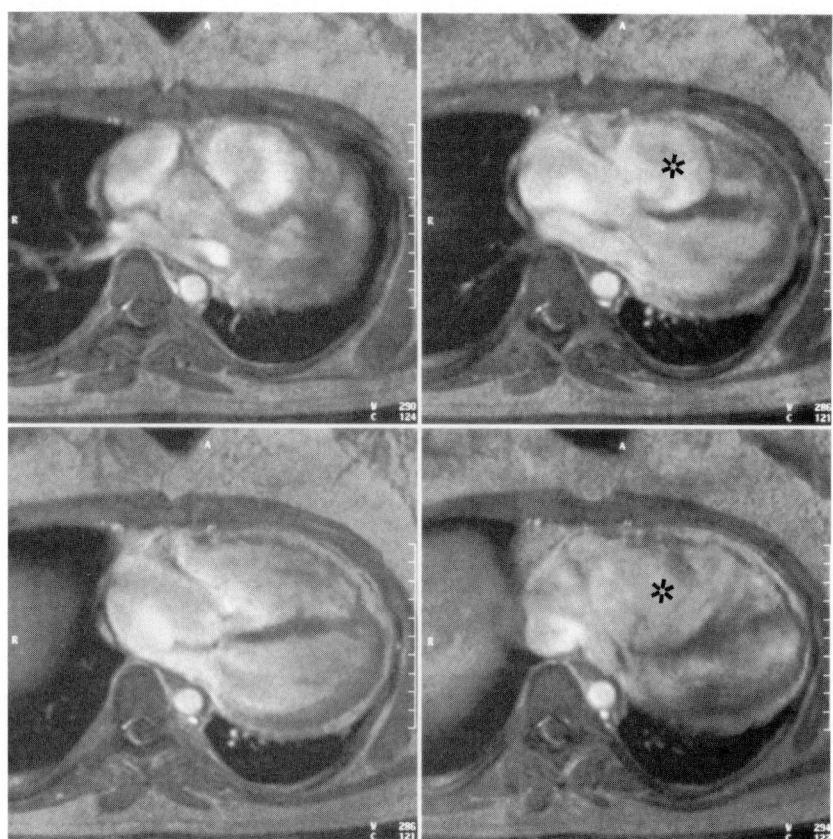

FIGURE 54.17 Arrhythmogenic right ventricle dysplasia (cine; transaxial). Marked dilatation of the cavity of the right ventricle (*asterisks*) and thinning of its wall in regions of fibrosis is shown on adjacent images.

T1-weighted S-E MRI (266,267). Thus, on S-E MRI, regions of moderately increased signal within complex effusions probably represent exudate made relatively immobile by fibrinous material that has adhered to the pericardium.

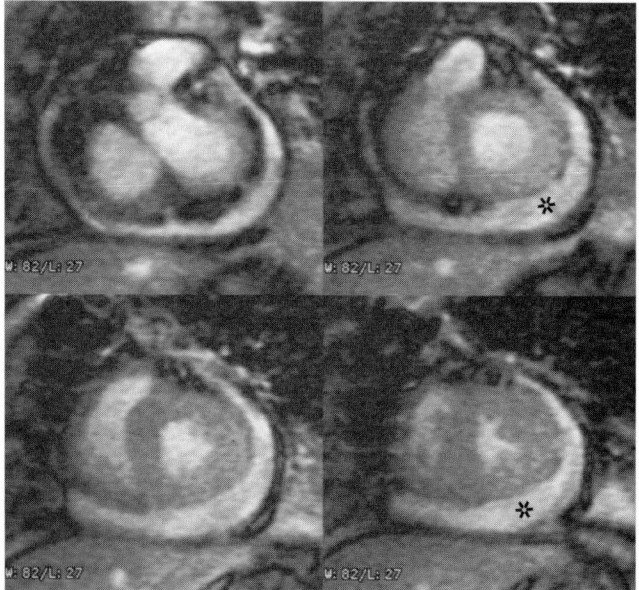

FIGURE 54.18 Simple pericardial effusion (cine, short axis). The bright appearance of the fluid (*asterisks*) separating the epicardial surfaces of the cardiac chambers from the dark-appearing pericardium indicates its simple nature.

With exudative pericardial effusions, both the pericardium and pericardial adhesions may have greater signal intensities than a normal pericardium (266,269).

Hemopericardium and pericardial hematoma can generally be distinguished from other types of effusions because of the high, at times extremely intense, signal of the paramagnetic blood products on S-E MRI (266). However, these hemorrhagic pericardial effusions often contain areas of both medium and high signal intensity, reflecting the variable age of the bloody material (*e*Fig. 54.18.1) (266,269). Although hemorrhagic effusions have been shown to have significantly greater effusion-to-myocardial signal intensity ratios than nonhemorrhagic effusions on T1-weighted S-E MRI, differences in hematocrit are not reliably appreciated (270).

MRI appears to be superior to echo in defining the nature and extent of processes causing clinical signs of cardiac chamber compromise from hemopericardium (265,269); compression of the cardiac chambers by hematoma indicates pericardial tamponade (267).

Pericarditis and Constriction

The low intensity of the pericardium on S-E MRI is explained partly by the presence of a phase discontinuity artifact. The shearing action between the visceral and parietal pericardium presumably results in a large local velocity variation, causing a reduction in signal intensity in the voxels

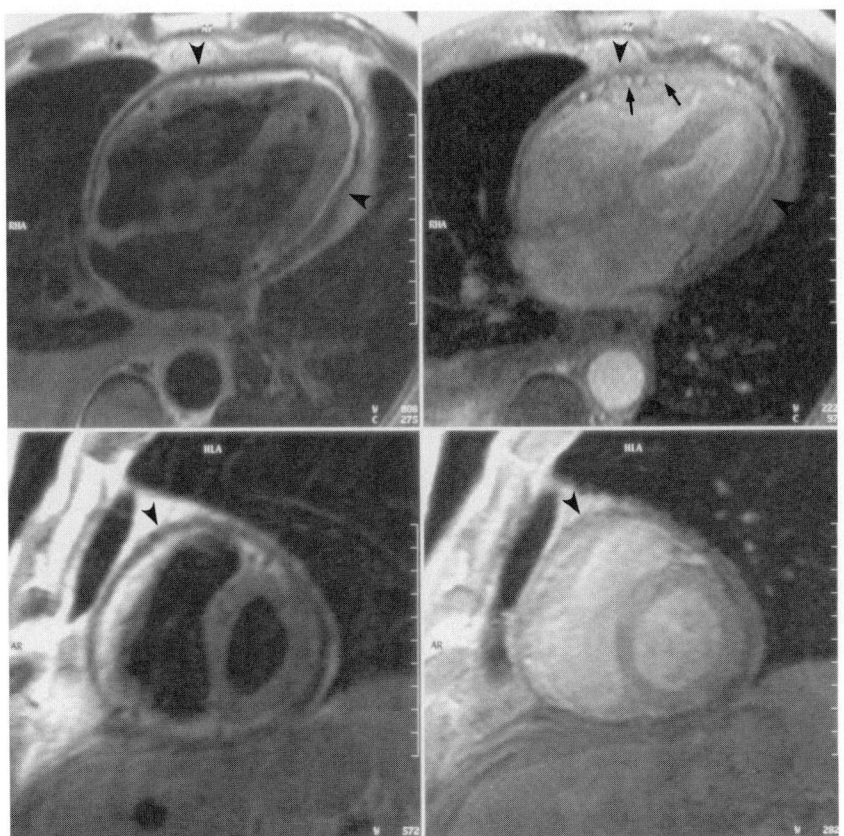

FIGURE 54.19 Pericarditis (subacute tuberculosis) (T1-weighted, spin-echo, and cine; horizontal long axis and short axis). Well shown on both the dark-blood **(left)** and bright-blood **(right)** images is the abnormally thickened pericardium (*arrowheads*) encasing the cardiac chambers, especially the ventricles, which appear compressed. The high concentration of small epicardial vessels along the right ventricular wall (*arrows*) is consistent with its inflammatory stage.

spanning the pericardium (271). Absence of the low-intensity pericardial line on S-E MRI implies that the normal transpericardial shearing motion is also absent in that region (269). This change is caused by primary or secondary abnormalities of the pericardium (e.g., inflammatory disease).

Because MRI provides excellent direct visualization of the pericardium, it can readily define the presence and extent of pericardial thickening. Measuring pericardial thickness is of great value in the diagnosis of constrictive pericarditis; however, the presence of pericardial thickening does not indicate constriction. Pericardial thickening has been noted on MRI in several other clinical settings (e.g., after cardiac surgery) (266). Both pericardial thickening and effusion have been demonstrated in the setting of uremic or infectious pericarditis; because of inflammatory changes associated with both of these conditions, the pericardial signal is generally increased on S-E MRI, and adhesions between the irregularly thickened visceral and parietal pericardium may be detected (Fig. 54.19). Nevertheless, MRI can be used effectively in the differentiation between constrictive pericarditis and restrictive CM (266,269,272), both of which may result in similar clinical presentations; although restrictive CM could demonstrate pericardial effusion, it would not generally reveal significant pericardial thickening.

Although in constrictive pericarditis, increased thickness of the pericardium is evident on MRI (251,266,269,272), the associated conical or tubular narrowing of the generally

nonhypertrophied ventricles, resulting from compression and confinement by the thick pericardium, is more specific for the diagnosis (Fig. 54.20). Secondary changes, such as atrial enlargement, systemic vein dilatation, hepatomegaly, ascites, and occasionally pleural effusion, may also be noted on MRI. When found in association with the appropriate clinical syndrome, these abnormal anatomic findings are strongly supportive of the diagnosis of constrictive pericarditis, with 93% accuracy documented (251). Unfortunately, MRI has not been able to differentiate reliably between fibrous tissue and calcification and, consequently, is of limited value compared with CT in the evaluation of calcification of the pericardium in the setting of calcific pericarditis (265).

Cases of constrictive pericarditis may be evaluated functionally with MRI. Absolute and relative systolic wall thickening of the LV, measured with multiphasic S-E MRI, have not been found to be significantly different from that in normal volunteers (79). Cine is more useful than S-E techniques in functionally evaluating cases of diastolic dysfunction and in defining qualitatively or quantitatively the specific pathophysiologic abnormalities associated with constrictive pericarditis (63,267). Because of the higher temporal resolution provided with this technique, the abrupt limitation of late diastolic filling of the ventricles because of the abnormally thickened and confining pericardium in constrictive pericarditis is distinguishable from the delayed diastolic filling patterns of the ventricles caused by

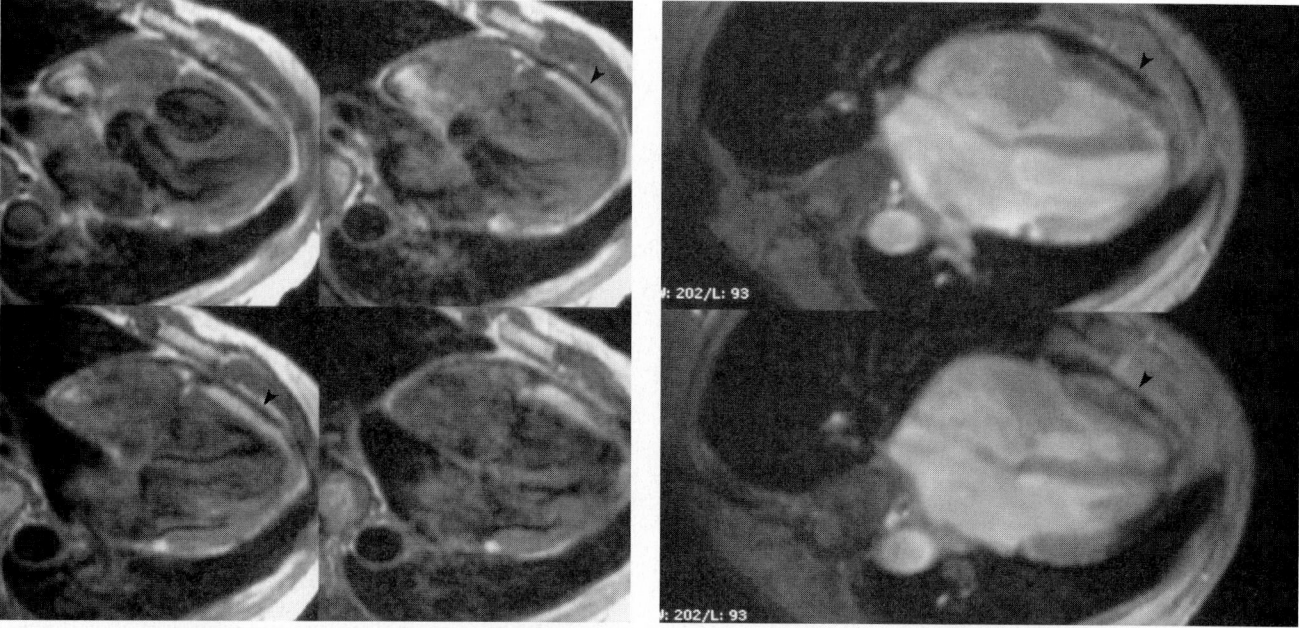

FIGURE 54.20 Constrictive pericarditis (T1-weighted, spin-echo, and cine; horizontal long axis). Constrictive pericarditis is manifested at adjacent levels on spin-echo **(A)** and cine **(B)** images by a thickened fibrotic and calcified pericardium (*arrowheads*), conical compression of the ventricles, biatrial dilatation, and abnormal intracardiac flow signal caused by diastolic dysfunction.

restrictive CM in the absence of significant pericardial thickening.

Using velocity mapping, abnormal flow patterns in the superior vena cava have been demonstrated in cases of constrictive pericarditis (260); improvement in diastolic return with pericardial stripping can be documented. In both healthy subjects and patients with right-sided disease, systemic venous flow measured without respiratory gating closely resembles its flow at end expiration (96).

Aortic Disease

Complete and timely imaging of the thoracic aorta is essential in that some disease entities are potentially life threatening and require prompt surgical intervention. The best surgical approach will be based on a complete depiction and understanding of the anatomy, which necessarily includes the thoracic aortic configuration and caliber, aortic wall characteristics, arch vessel origins, and descriptions of the aortic valve and the paraaortic structures.

MRI is now assuming an increasing and distinct role in furthering the evaluation and diagnosis of diseases of the thoracic aorta (273). In fact, the majority of CV MRI studies are currently performed for the evaluation of thoracic aortic disease (17). The ability of MRI to noninvasively depict abnormalities in anatomy or physiology in the thoracic aorta in multiple oblique planes or 3-D makes it ideally suited for initial diagnosis, monitoring during medical therapy, and postoperative assessment (273–275). Other parameters that are important to address in the evaluation of patients with thoracic aortic disease (e.g., origin

of the coronary arteries) can also be evaluated effectively with MRI.

In addition, MRI provides a highly specific and sensitive method for detecting postoperative complications from thoracic aortic surgery (57,276,277). These complications include periprosthetic valve leak, graft infection, extension or development of dissection, rupture, or aneurysmal expansion.

Aneurysm

Accurate identification of the size, location, and extent of a thoracic aortic aneurysm is essential for management, preoperative planning, and follow-up; large aneurysms of the thoracic aorta should be surgically corrected because of the increased risk of spontaneous rupture when the diameter exceeds 5 cm. Thoracic aortic aneurysms are categorized as being either true aneurysms, meaning that all three mural layers of the aortic wall are involved, or as pseudoaneurysms, in which there has been a break in the intima, and possibly media, leaving only the remaining wall to contain the intraaortic blood pool. These forms of aneurysm are characteristically represented by fusiform (i.e., circumferential enlargement of the involved segment) or saccular (i.e., asymmetric or focal outpouching of the involved segment) dilatations, respectively. The saccular configuration connotes a less stable condition than the other configuration. These characteristics of a thoracic aortic aneurysm can be easily delineated with MRI for planning of therapy or for clinical monitoring (273,276). In addition, because of the abilities of MRI to depict the configuration and associated mural changes, it is critical in differentiating the various etiologies of thoracic aortic aneurysms (278).

On MRI, atherosclerotic aneurysms may be found in any portion of the thoracic aorta and are characterized by fusiform enlargement, usually over long segments (Fig. 54.21). The aortic wall is thickened and irregular, secondary to atherosclerotic plaque (279). Mural calcification is common and is manifested by areas of focal signal absence on both S-E and cine, although it is better seen on CT. Intraluminal thrombus also is common and may be difficult to distinguish from atherosclerotic plaque, although thrombus usually has a smooth internal border as opposed to atherosclerosis, which typically is irregular (273,276). In atherosclerotic aneurysms involving the ascending portion, the sinotubular junction and aortic valve function usually are preserved—important characteristics appreciated on MRI.

Aortic aneurysms that may occur secondary to aortic valvular disease are also characterized by relative preservation of the aortic root and sinotubular junction on MRI (273,276). In cases of AS, the aneurysmal dilation usually is limited to the midascending aorta where the poststenotic flow effects are most prominent (226). In AR, aneurysmal dilation of the thoracic aorta typically involves the ascending aorta but extends into the transverse arch because of the "water hammer" effect and, in long-standing cases, also

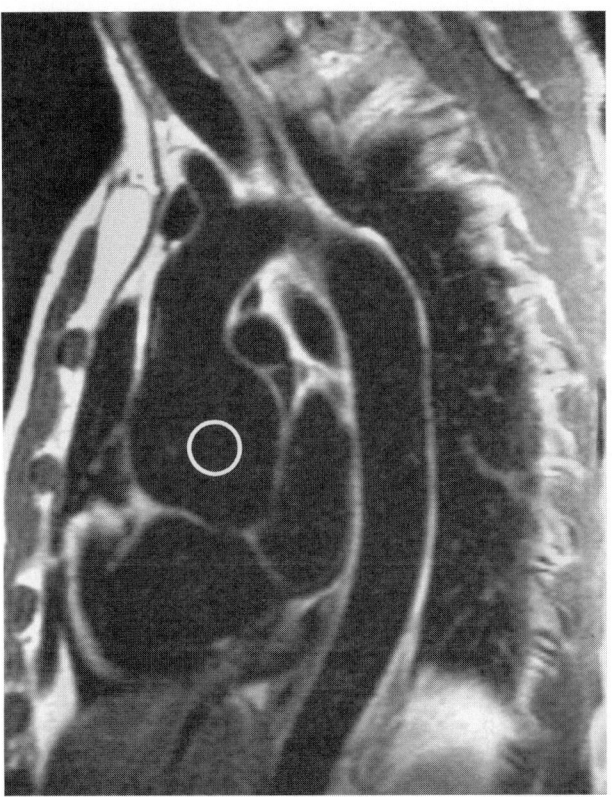

FIGURE 54.22 Annuloaortic ectasia of the aortic root (T1-weighted, spin-echo; left anterior oblique). An "onion-bulb" dilatation of the proximal ascending aorta and sinuses of Valsalva (*open circle*), associated with pronounced effacement of the sinotubular junction, is noted.

may involve the descending thoracic aorta; often there is slight effacement of the sinotubular junction and dilatation of the aortic root in primary AR because of their relationship (228).

Equally important in the case of aneurysms involving the ascending aorta is the appreciation of annuloaortic ectasia that leads to characteristic "onion bulb" dilatation of the proximal ascending aorta and sinuses of Valsalva from pronounced effacement of the sinotubular junction (*e*Fig. 54.11.1 and Fig. 54.22) (273,276). Indicating cystic medial necrosis, detection of annuloaortic ectasia on MRI connotes a worsened prognosis; Marfan syndrome and other connective tissue disorders characteristically result in weakening of the aortic wall, as a result of cystic medial necrosis. Typically, the associated dilation of the aortic root leads to suboptimal coaptation of the aortic valve cusps as the aortic annulus dilates and ultimately to significant AR. More serious and potentially ominous complications include ascending aortic dissection, rupture, or both (280).

Another configuration of thoracic aortic aneurysms that is important to identify on MRI is saccular dilatation from a mycotic or pseudoaneurysm. Mycotic aneurysms result from weakening of the aortic wall by infection (278), although pseudoaneurysms typically are caused by trauma (e.g., automobile accidents) and occur most commonly at

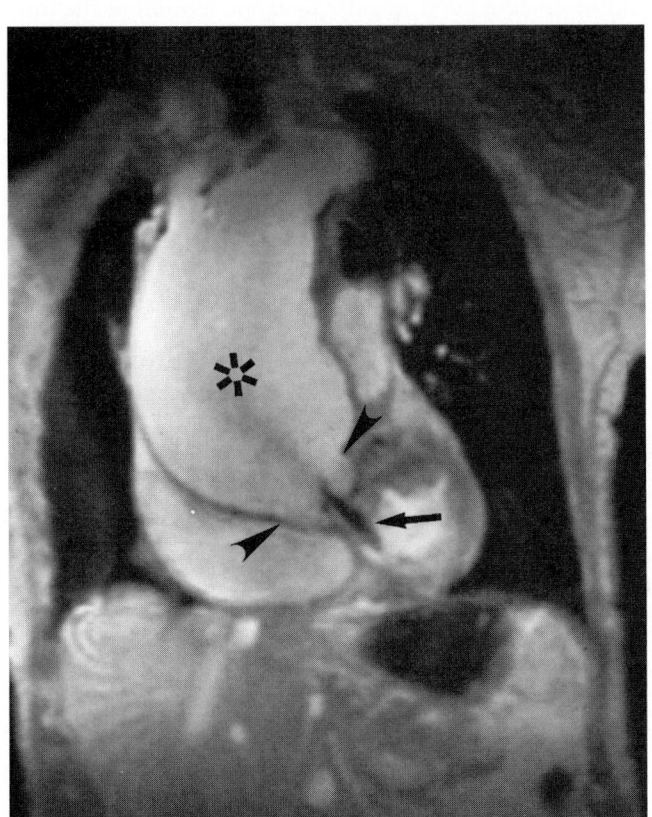

FIGURE 54.21 Atherosclerotic aneurysm (cine; oblique-coronal). Despite marked dilatation of the ascending aorta (*asterisk*), there is preservation of the sinotubular junction (*arrowheads*). Aortic regurgitation is also seen (*arrow*).

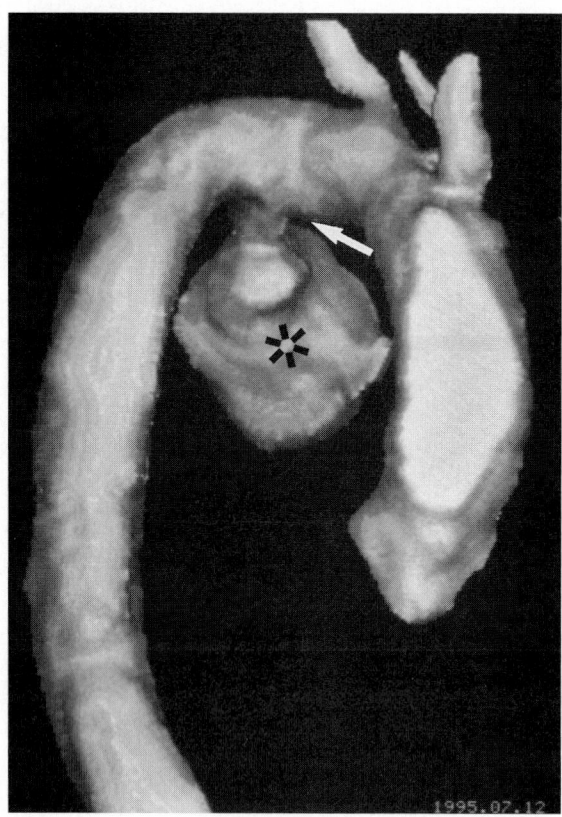

FIGURE 54.23 Aortic pseudoaneurysm (magnetic resonance angiography surface reconstruction). A saccular outpouching (*asterisk*) from the undersurface of the aortic arch communicates with the aortic lumen through a narrow neck (*arrow*), indicating disruption of the layers of the aortic wall.

the level of the ligamentum arteriosum or after surgery at anastomotic or cannulation sites (Fig. 54.23) (281).

Dissection

Dissections are classified according to either the Stanford or DeBakey systems. The important distinction to be made clinically is whether the dissection flap involves the ascending aorta with or without transverse arch involvement (Stanford A; DeBakey I and II) (*e*Fig. 54.23.1) or both the distal arch beyond the left subclavian artery origin and the descending aorta (Stanford B; DeBakey III) (*e*Fig. 54.23.2). This distinction is important because the involvement of the ascending aortic is associated with a higher mortality and generally requires urgent surgical repair.

MRI is a highly sensitive and specific technique for the detection of aortic dissection that has proven to be superior to conventional angiography, CT, and transthoracic echo (282). It also has been compared with transesophageal echo; both techniques have demonstrated a similar high sensitivity (e.g., 98% to 100%), but MRI has a significantly higher specificity (e.g., 98% to 100%) than transesophageal echo (e.g., 68% to 77%) in high-risk populations (282). The advantages of MRI include an ability to evaluate not

just the intravascular space and walls of the aorta, but also the extravascular space, which may yield further information, particularly in regard to more serious complications of aortic dissection (273). Nonetheless, most agree that transesophageal echo—because of its portability, speed, and ability to image in real time—is the preferred method of evaluation in the subset of unstable patients, such as those in the emergency room and intensive care settings.

The goals of MRI in aortic dissections, both acute and chronic, are to identify the intimal flap, its extent, orientation, and involvement with aortic arch branch vessels and coronary arteries, the location of entry and reentry tears of the intima, and to assess for areas of flow and thrombus within the false channel (273). In addition, potential complications such as pleural effusion, pericardial tamponade, and AR must be assessed.

Whether by S-E or cine imaging, aortic dissection is characterized by the inwardly displaced intraluminal intimal flap, surrounded by rapid flow within the true channel and usually slower flow, with or without thrombus formation in the false channel (Fig. 54.24) (273,282,283). Both primary and secondary tears of the intimal flap may be difficult to identify on the static images unless they are relatively large. Dynamic flow-based images (i.e., cine, SPAMM, or velocity mapping) are useful adjuncts to identify these sites of flow between the true and false channels and to observe the frequently dynamic motion of the intimal flap (*e*Fig. 54.24.1) (273,284).

The patterns of flow within each channel can be further qualitatively or quantitatively assessed with these MRI techniques for the purposes of planning surgical repairs or interventional procedures (e.g., fenestration) in which the adequacy of blood supply to vital organs is often an issue (284). Velocity mapping, in particular, may identify retrograde patterns of flow within the false channel that may potentiate retrograde extension of a simple type B dissection into the arch and ascending aorta.

A common hurdle is the distinction between a thrombosed false channel within a chronic dissection from an intraluminal thrombus adherent to the wall of an aneurysm. These are not always possible to differentiate, as a chronic intraluminal thrombus may neoepithelialize, giving the appearance of an intimal flap overlying the chronic thrombus (273,284). Signs that have been reported to be more consistent with a diagnosis of thrombosed false channel associated with dissection are a compressed or eccentric patent channel and extensive thrombus with associated wall thickening over a length greater than 7 cm; these signs are easily appreciated on MRI (284).

The entity of noncommunicating dissecting intramural hematoma is being detected with increasing frequency with the development of tomographic imaging, including MRI. Technically, this may be described as dissection of the aortic wall without intimal rupture or tear; the etiology is unknown, but presumably is related to a weakening of the

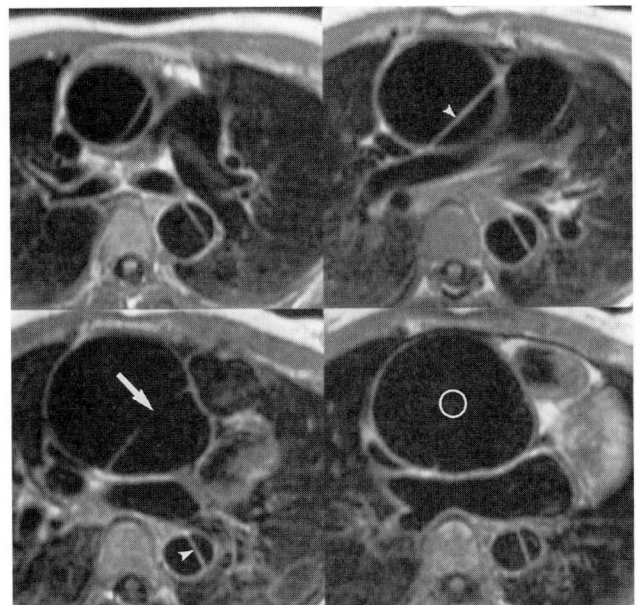 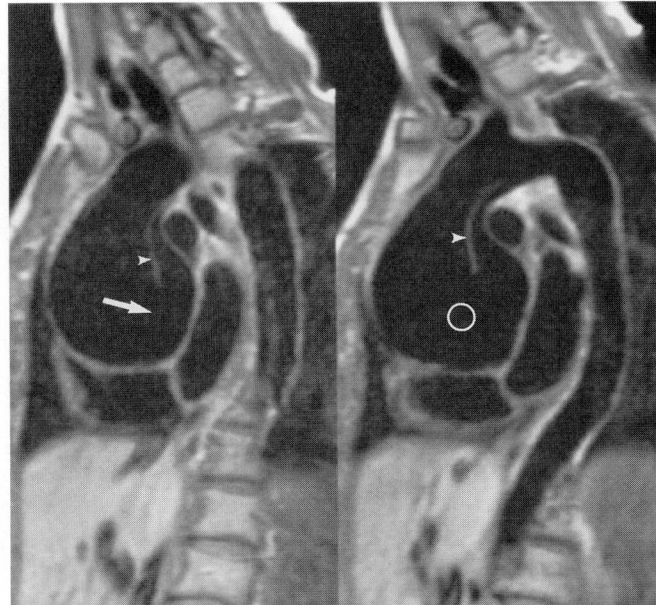

FIGURE 54.24 Aortic dissection (T1-weighted spin-echo; transaxial and left anterior oblique). Type A dissection of the aorta is manifested on representative transaxial **(A)** and oblique **(B)** images by the inwardly displaced intimal flap (*arrowheads*), extending from the dilated aortic root (*open circle*) to the descending thoracic aorta, and a large proximal intimal tear (*arrows*).

media. Clinically, the presentation is almost always similar to that of aortic dissection; the diagnosis of an intramural hematoma is entertained, once communicating aortic dissection has been excluded. On MRI designed to exclude communicating aortic dissection, an intramural hematoma is identified as a smooth crescentic to circumferential area of thickened aortic wall without evidence of blood flow in the false channel (e.g., velocity-dependent phase changes on velocity mapping or displacement of saturation bands on SPAMM) (284–286). Depending on the age of the hematoma, the area of thickening may be isointense or hyperintense relative to skeletal muscle on S-E MRI; the signal intensity is relatively isointense in the acute phase, and then becomes greatest in the subacute stages (Fig. 54.25) (286). If intramural bleeding stops, the intramural hematoma resolves with decreasing thickness and returns to S-E isointensity in the more chronic stages.

At present, there is only limited knowledge regarding the natural course of an intramural hematoma. However, complete resolution or evolution to dissection have been demonstrated on MRI (285,286). Involvement of the ascending aorta by intramural hematoma has been shown to predispose the development of communicating aortic dissection in most cases; rebleeding before development of communicating dissection has been detected based on S-E intensity changes (285,286).

Atherosclerosis

The first attempt at MRI of atherosclerotic plaque involved the use of postmortem specimens of excised peripheral artery (287); good correlation between the morphology of the plaques on MRI and on histology was demonstrated. Atherosclerotic lesions were seen as vessel wall thickening with overall intermediate signal intensity, except in areas of calcium and lipids, where there were focally decreased and increased signal, respectively (287). Since these early studies, images obtained with more advanced MRI protocols in experimental models have proved to be useful in identifying various wall components in atheromatous artery samples on the basis of chemical composition, molecular motion, diffusion, physical state, or water content (288). These differences may be particularly important in determining the contributing factors related to plaque rupture, which depend strongly on the presence of soft lipid and collagenous fibers (289). Some studies using image processing have also shown that it may be possible to identify and quantify the types of materials present in atherosclerotic plaque (290,291).

High-resolution MRI has shown excellent contrast between fatty plaque components (i.e., foam cells, loose necrosis, and cholesterol) and solid components; signal loss in images was seen at locations where calcium existed (288,289). Experimental work has shown the potential of MRI to demonstrate (a) the variable nature of the collagen cap with underlying lipid-rich regions in more vulnerable plaques; (b) anatomic response of the atherosclerotic plaque to *in vitro* angioplasty; (c) the relationship between the nature of the lipids inside atheromatous plaques and the severity of vessel obstruction; and (d) "aging" changes of thrombi.

In the clinical setting, MRI currently has the capability of routinely providing valuable information regarding the

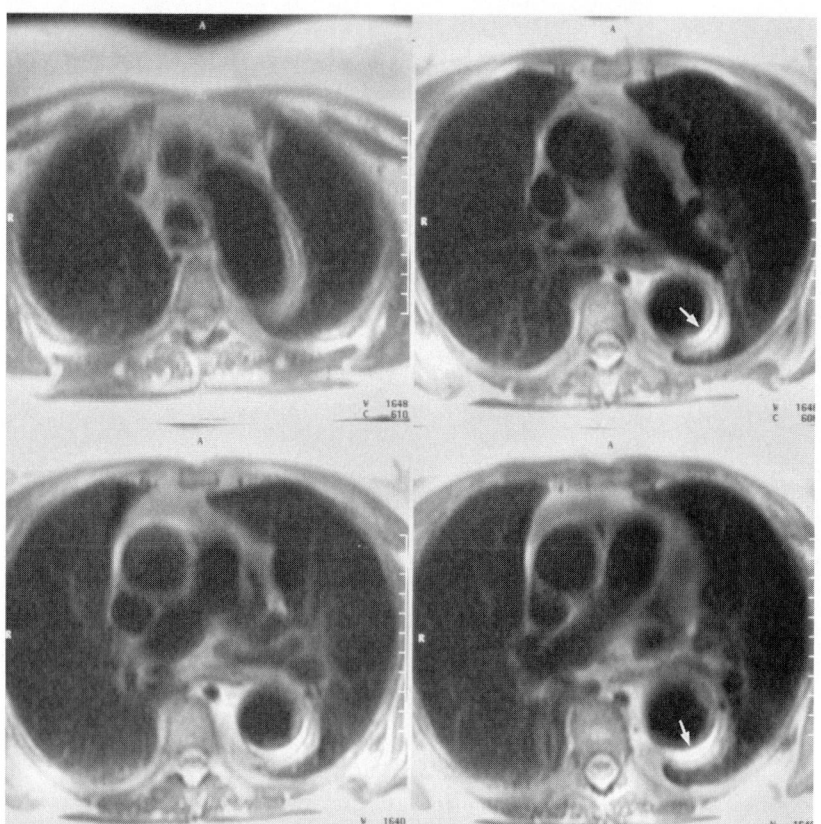

FIGURE 54.25 Intramural hematoma of the thoracic aorta (T1-weighted spin-echo; transaxial). A smooth crescentic collection within the wall of the descending thoracic aorta (*arrows*) indicates an intramural hematoma; its extremely bright signal intensity indicates its subacute nature.

patency of the arterial lumen, as well as the status of the arterial wall in patients with atherosclerotic vascular disease (40). Atherosclerotic lesions in humans consist of eccentric or concentric mural thickening with luminal narrowing and discrete plaques protruding into the vessel lumen. Although early studies using standard S-E techniques yielded promising results, limitations in detecting calcified plaques by MRI were revealed (292).

Good accuracy of MRA for depicting peripheral stenoses and occlusions has been demonstrated clinically (60,293). However, because minor luminal irregularities, ulcers, or aneurysms may all lead to significant local turbulence and resultant intraluminal signal loss in the absence of an angiographically significant narrowing, an imperfect concordance between MRI and conventional forms of angiography may result. Nevertheless, measurements of the degree of stenosis on projectional MRA images have been shown to correlate reasonably well with conventional angiographic techniques (294). However, there are limitations that potentially interfere with clinical characterization of adjacent atherosclerotic plaques.

A penetrating atherosclerotic ulcer is an MRI-detectable entity, occupying an as yet uncertain place in the spectrum of aortic atherosclerotic disease (279). It usually appears as a shallow, wide-necked ulceration of an atheroma that extends through the intima to disrupt the underlying media; the mid- and distal descending aorta are the most common sites.

Pulmonary Artery Disease

Few options have been available for diagnosing disease of the pulmonary artery. The gold standard for diagnosis has been pulmonary artery catheterization with or without angiography. MRI has many unique capabilities that make it preferable to other noninvasive imaging methods and to angiography for the evaluation of some abnormalities of the pulmonary artery system. Aside from depicting intrinsic pulmonary artery disease, MRI is an ideal imaging method for evaluating the secondary effects of adjacent extravascular disease.

Pulmonary Emboli

Because all therapies for pulmonary emboli (PE) pose significant risks, an accurate diagnosis of such disease is mandatory before the initiation of treatment. For the diagnosis of PE, there has been no single noninvasive and accurate imaging procedure. Imaging by ventilation-perfusion scintigraphy is safe, but accurate interpretation in the presence of lung disease or cardiac conditions is reduced. Consequently, many individuals with suspected PE ultimately come to angiography because of diagnostic evaluations.

Because of the signal void of normally flowing blood, thrombus within a pulmonary artery can usually be readily discerned on systolic S-E images; the intensity of thrombus is variable, depending on its age. Because cases of pulmonary artery hypertension (PAH) are often present with symptoms requiring evaluation for suspected PE, and because abnormal systolic intravascular signal may also be caused by slow blood flow in PAH, the need for differentiation of thrombus from slow blood flow in MRI is common. This can be accomplished by noting that, unlike slow blood flow, a thrombus from PE demonstrates no even-echo rephasing on multiple S-E images, and no change in distribution on multiphasic images (295,296). Although it can be used to demonstrate a thrombus in a larger pulmonary artery, it is unlikely that S-E MRI can at the current time be considered reliable for the evaluation of PE beyond the level of a segmental pulmonary artery (296). Phase-display imaging may also be useful in detecting the phase changes related to slowly flowing blood and the absence of such phase changes related to a fixed thrombus.

Cine and SPAMM are adjuncts to S-E imaging, which potentially increase the diagnostic yield and capabilities for characterization of PE (296–298). In general, an intravascular thrombus from PE is manifested by a fixed area of signal void or preservation of saturation band patterns, respectively, which can be differentiated from the appearance of the surrounding flowing blood (Fig. 54.26). A complicating factor in thrombus detection would be slow blood flow caused by pulmonary artery obstruction by the thrombus or from superimposed PAH because of slow blood flow (296,297). PE diagnosed by cine has been shown to correspond to the locations of angiographic abnormalities and mismatched ventilation-perfusion defects on scintigraphy and has been able to assess the age of the embolic mass (299).

Although some potential to identify the age of the thrombotic material within a pulmonary artery by MRI has been realized, it is more practically used for monitoring resolution of clotting during anticoagulation therapy. MRA techniques have created pleasing images of the branching pulmonary artery system, and the capability of reliably demonstrating PE is now being done (300).

Pulmonary Hypertension

The ability of S-E MRI to distinguish normally flowing from slowly flowing blood and slowly flowing blood from fixed intravascular lesions (e.g., thrombus caused by PE) indicates its value as an alternative to catheterization in assessing PAH. The increased risk of catheterization plus angiography for the diagnosis or exclusion of PE in cases of PAH has also emphasized the potential of MRI for this purpose.

Initially, the primary use of S-E MRI in evaluation of PAH was the description of secondary changes (301). Anatomic findings include RV hypertrophy in proportion to the pulmonary artery pressures; reversal of septal curvature

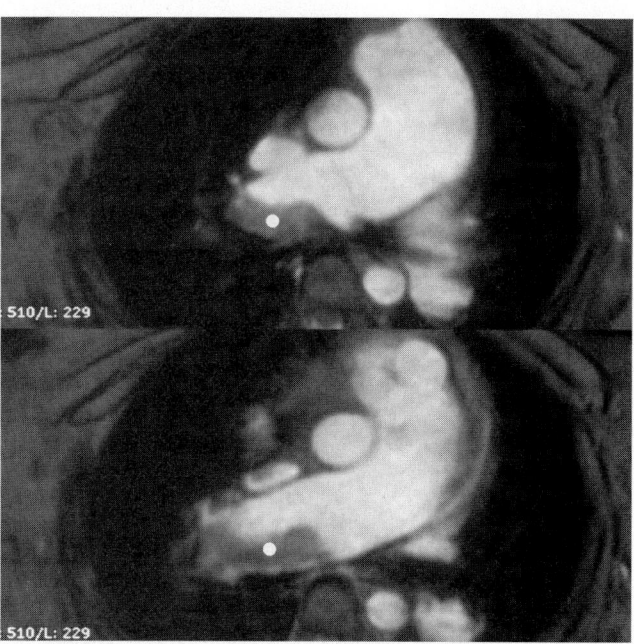

FIGURE 54.26 Intravascular thrombus from pulmonary emboli (cine; transaxial). Adjacent levels both demonstrate a fixed lobular area of relative signal void (*closed circles*), surrounded by flow enhancement, in the right central pulmonary artery; it represents pulmonary emboli.

when pulmonary artery pressures approximate systemic pressures; and pulmonary artery dilatation (Fig. 54.27).

In PAH, substantial elevation in pulmonary vascular resistance and dilatation of the pulmonary artery system result in diminished velocity of blood flow; the intensity of such abnormal intravascular signal has a direct linear relationship with the amount of pulmonary vascular resistance, showing the ability of S-E MRI to provide information about the severity of PAH (302). Combined use of multiple S-E and multiphasic techniques permits further description of the characteristic pulmonary artery signal patterns typically found in the setting of PAH (*e*Fig. 54.27.1) (295). Because of the presence of even-echo rephasing, as well as its fluctuating distribution during the cardiac cycle, abnormal intravascular signal from slow blood flow can be distinguished from that of intraluminal thrombus or tumor (295,303). Phase-display and cine images can also be used to properly identify abnormal intravascular signal from slowly flowing blood in PAH, through demonstration of velocity-dependent phase changes and saturation-related diffuse intermediate signal loss, respectively (296,297).

Pulmonary artery distensibility has been studied with S-E MRI in healthy subjects and in patients with PAH; distensibility was found to be significantly reduced in cases with PAH (304). When velocity mapping of the pulmonary artery flow was performed, all cases of PAH had totally irregular antegrade flow in systole with large velocity variations across the vessel lumen. PAH was also associated with abnormally slow net forward flow, but with

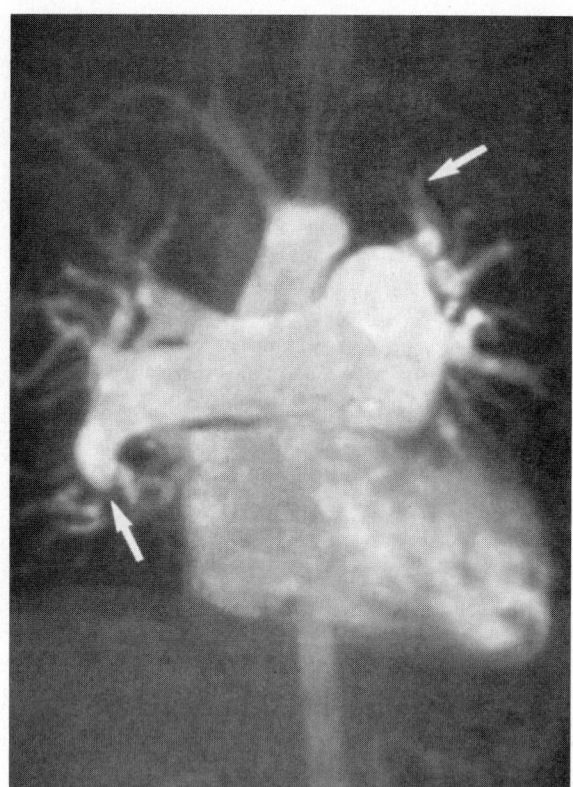

FIGURE 54.27 Pulmonary artery (PA) dilatation of pulmonary artery hypertension (contrast-enhanced three-dimensional magnetic resonance angiography; coronal). Marked dilatation of the main PA and each central PA is noted. Beyond the hilar regions, rapid tapering of PA branch caliber (*arrows*) is indicative of pulmonary artery hypertension.

earlier velocity peaking than in healthy subjects; abnormally large retrograde flow was noted in systole and diastole in PAH.

The multipotentiality of MRI is clearly evident in the assessment of patients undergoing evaluation for possible lung transplantation or for monitoring following this surgery. Improved RV function and enhanced pulmonary artery flow in transplanted lungs have been shown (305,306).

Thrombi and Masses

MRI has proved to be extremely valuable in assessing mass lesions located in the cardiac chambers or myocardium or adjacent to the heart in the pericardium, mediastinum, or lung (307). S-E MRI images provide excellent anatomic detail, sufficient for assessment of the extent of such lesions, indicating their site of origin, as well as the secondary effects on adjacent structures. Cine may provide additional information concerning their movement relative to the cardiac chambers; this insight may provide a better appreciation of sites of attachment and influence on myocardial and valve function (267). This anatomic and functional information has an important role in planning therapy for thrombi and cardiac masses (308).

MRI has been shown to outperform echo in demonstrating the presence, location (i.e., paracardiac vs. intramural vs. intracavitary), and extent of mass lesions (308,309). In a significant proportion of cases referred from echo to MRI for evaluation of a suspected cardiac mass lesion, the presence of a lesion is excluded by MRI (309). Thus, MRI can be used effectively in combination with echo to increase the certainty of diagnosis and plan therapy (267).

In addition to providing important morphologic data, MRI has the potential to assess the tissue composition of mass lesions. As is true elsewhere in the body, the use of both T1- and T2-weighted S-E images allows for some general degree of tissue characterization (308,311). Because lipomatous tissues have a uniquely short T1 and their signal intensity resembles that of subcutaneous fat on S-E imaging, cardiac lipomas have a relatively high signal intensity on T1-weighted images and a moderate signal intensity on T2-weighed images (267,310). Cystic cardiac lesions typically have long T1 and T2 relaxation times, resulting in a low signal intensity on T1-weighted images and a high signal intensity on T2-weighted images (266,307,310). Most soft-tissue cardiac tumors have T1 and T2 relaxation times that are much shorter than those of cystic fluid, yet T1 and T2 are long enough to produce a relatively low signal intensity on T1-weighted images and high signal intensity on T2-weighted images (267,307).

Like tumors elsewhere in the body, cardiac tumors have increased water content, resulting in prolongation of T1 and T2 relaxation times (267). The effects of edema in the surrounding tissue may make the distinction between the tumor and the surrounding tissues difficult. In addition, the presence of hemorrhage or necrosis within a tumor may alter its appearance. To complicate matters further, dense fibrous tissue and areas of calcification, possibly resulting from therapy, produce a low signal intensity on T1- or T2-weighted images because of a relative paucity of mobile protons.

Gd-DTPA accumulates in tumors more than in myocardium, improving detection and anatomic delineation of cardiac tumors (267,311). Enhancement helps to distinguish neoplasms from nonvascular masses, because the tumor must have a capillary blood supply to accumulate the extracellular contrast agent. However, similar to other organ systems, cardiac neoplasms show variable degrees of enhancement, and the kinetics are not specific for benignancy or malignancy. Thus, the early hope that MRI would permit the differentiation of benign from malignant masses has not been fulfilled.

Intracardiac Thrombi

The accuracy of MRI in the diagnosis of an LV thrombus is comparable with angiography, CT, and echo (145,146,267). Interpretation of S-E MRI is complicated by the presence of intraventricular flow signal, resulting from stagnant blood within areas of LV dysfunction. The demonstration of even-echo rephasing or phase shifts in regions of slowly flowing blood is helpful in excluding the diagnosis of a thrombus (267). Similarly, cine can exploit flow-related enhancement to distinguish slow flow from a thrombus (146) (*e*Fig. 54.3.3).

Nevertheless, the signal intensities of intracardiac thrombi on S-E MRI have been variable and not reliably distinguishable from those of nonthrombotic masses (307,309).

Primary Cardiac Tumors

The exclusion or verification of the presence of an intracardiac mass suggested by a prior echo has been a frequent indication for MRI (267); this complementary role of MRI in the evaluation of intracardiac masses is now well established in clinical practice. Frequently, MRI excludes the presence of an intracardiac mass initially suggested by echo. In some cases, MRI identifies an anatomic variant (e.g., distortion of cardiac anatomy by a pectus deformity) as the source of the false-positive echo result (309).

The ability of MRI to identify a variety of benign or malignant tumors primarily involving the cardiac chambers is well known (307,308,312). Studies comparing MRI with echo have indicated that MRI more clearly demonstrates the relationship of masses to normal intracardiac structures and extension into adjacent vasculature or the mediastinum (312,313). When MRI confirms the presence of a mass, definition of anatomy is the most useful parameter for establishing a specific diagnosis (267,307,312). For example, the location of the mass within the left atrium is the main criterion for differentiation between myxoma (i.e., almost always arises from the interatrial septum) and

thrombus (i.e., usually occurs near the posterolateral wall or atrial appendage).

MRI tissue characteristics of intracardiac masses add some specificity to their diagnoses (267). Myxomas typically appear brighter than myocardium on T2-weighted S-E MRI because of their increased T2 relaxation times (307) (*e*Fig. 54.27.2). Variability in the appearance of myxomas may reflect their variable composition of water-rich myxomatous tissue (long T2; high signal intensity) versus fibrous tissue and calcification (short T2, low proton density; low intensity). Similarly, fibromas show decreased signal intensity relative to myocardium (*e*Fig. 54.27.3). Lipomatous hypertrophy or lipomas of the interatrial septum have the distinctive short T1 and high signal intensity of adipose tissue (Fig. 54.28). Various other benign intracardiac masses have been described.

The pattern of invasion by intracardiac malignancies is also well defined using MRI, which permits more accurate diagnosis and description than angiography, CT, or echo (267). MRI findings in cases of intracardiac malignancies have correlated extremely well with findings from surgical exploration or postmortem examination (313).

Various primary intracardiac malignancies have been detected by MRI (267,307). Angiosarcomas are typically found in the region of the right atrioventricular groove and are associated with significant pericardial disease, including complex effusion (Fig. 54.29).

Anatomic relationships between primary paracardial tumors and the heart are well demonstrated on MRI (267). Signal intensity differences between tumor (long T1 and long T2), myocardium (long T1 and short T2), and peri-

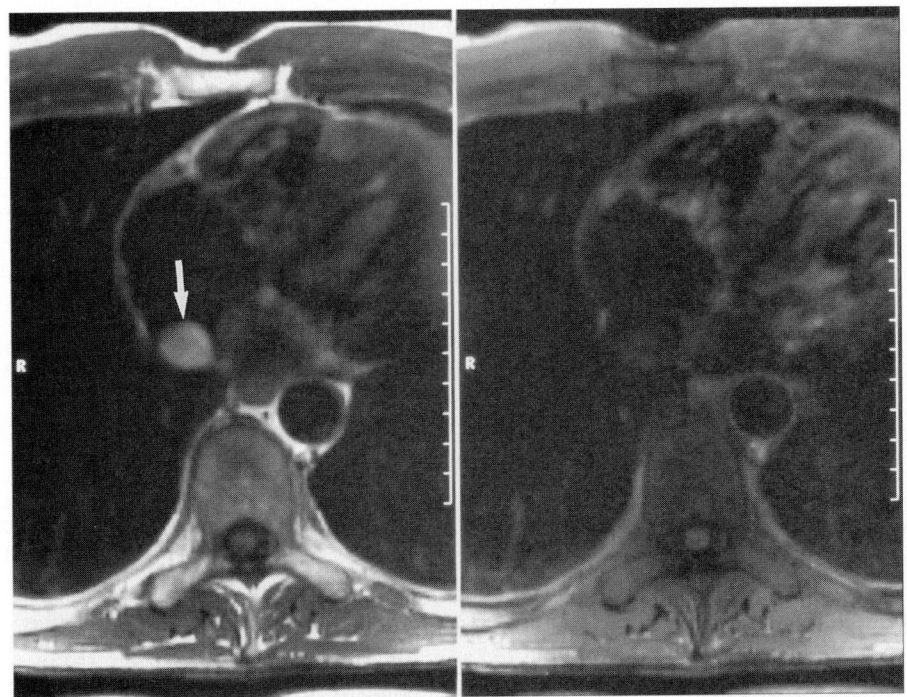

FIGURE 54.28 Atrial lipoma (T2-weighted spin-echo; transaxial). Because of its fatty composition, the signal intensity of the relatively bright, rounded intracardiac lipomatous mass (*arrow*) within the right atrium **(left)** is suppressed with application of fat-saturation techniques **(right)**.

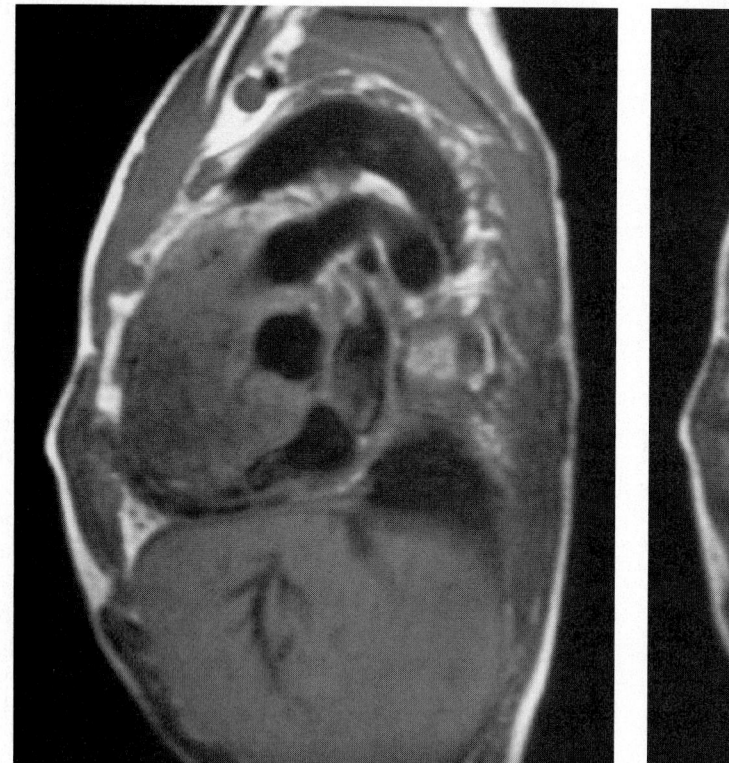
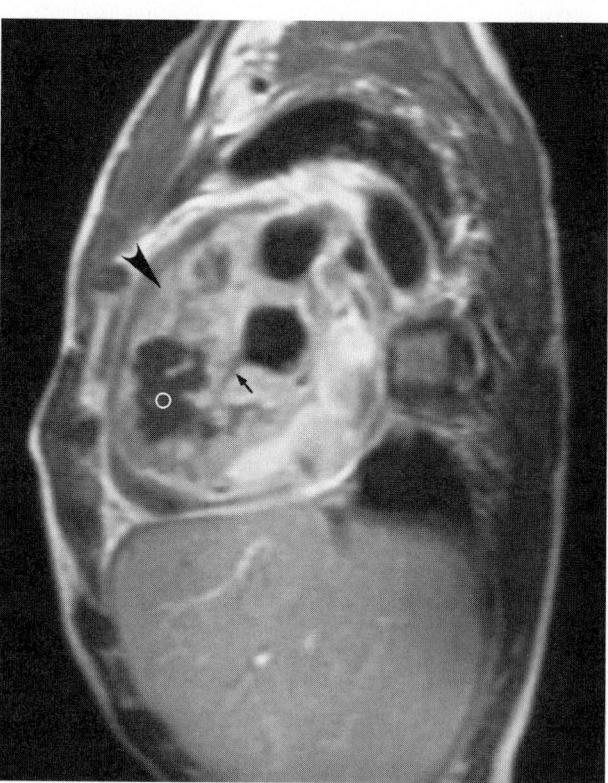

FIGURE 54.29 Angiosarcoma (T1-weighted spin-echo; short axis). Although the mass created by this primary cardiac tumor is easily seen in the right atrioventricular groove before administration of gadolinium chelate **(A)**, the use of contrast enhancement demonstrates peripheral hyperperfusion (*arrowhead*) and its central zone of necrosis (*open circle*) **(B)**; encasement of the right coronary artery (*arrow*) is better seen after injection of the magnetic resonance imaging contrast agent.

cardial and epicardial fat (short T1 and intermediate T2) provide excellent image contrast. Furthermore, MRI is useful in differentiating a variety of benign intrapericardial lesions from extrapericardial masses (314). Paracardiac masses external to the pericardial sac are often benign and their characteristics are easily appreciated on MRI (267).

Secondary Tumors

Secondary intracardiac malignancies may involve the cardiac chambers via intravascular or transmural extension. Few have been described by MRI (267).

Secondary paracardiac malignancies, including tumors directly extending or metastasizing to the pericardium or pericardial space, are well seen on MRI (315). Unfortunately, their MRI tissue characteristics are nonspecific (long T1 and long T2) (*e*Fig. 54.29.1). Masses abutting the pericardium with penetration can be easily differentiated from those in which there is direct extension of the tumor to involve the pericardium or myocardium. Compression of the cardiac chambers, interposition of the masses between the spine and the left atrium, and extension of the invasive tumors through the wall of a cardiac chamber are readily demonstrated by S-E MRI. Cine can

aid in assessing the extension of such tumors into the pericardium or cardiac chambers because of the appreciation of the relative motion of these structures. Various secondary paracardiac tumors have been evaluated using MRI (315,316).

Congenital Heart Disease

Despite the plethora of reports demonstrating MRI to be an accurate modality for diagnosing many forms of CHD (231,317), its role in this area remains largely supportive to echo. In particular, in adults with CHD, the diagnostic information provided by transthoracic echo is often incomplete because of the larger body, associated chest deformities, and paucity of adequate imaging windows (318,319). This provides the incentive for using MRI and transesophageal echo, but MRI has the advantage over transesophageal echo of imaging in any desired plane chosen by the operator to include the structures of interests and related anatomy, thereby becoming useful for clarification of complex structural relations in space.

The unique role of MRI in the assessment of adult CHD is primarily in (a) noninvasive shunt quantitation; (b) pursuit of hard to find lesions; (c) evaluation of complex anomalies; (d) assessment of congenital great vessel disease; and (e) postoperative assessment.

Noninvasive Shunt Quantitation

Direct quantitation of the amount of shunting as an indicator of the anatomic size of a defect is a useful parameter for planning corrective surgery. For this purpose, ventricular volumes can be accurately determined directly from a series of cine image loops encompassing the full extent of the RV and LV (69). For an atrial septal defect with left-to-right shunting, shunt quantitation can be accomplished with cine in the absence of associated valvular insufficiency or additional shunts by evaluating the difference between the larger RV and smaller LV stroke volumes. Shunt volume for a ventricular septal defect could theoretically be derived by subtraction of the smaller RV stroke volume from the larger LV stroke volume. However, it has been found that RV stroke volume may also be increased in such left-to-right shunts, depending on the location of the ventricular septal defect (154). Therefore, the ventricular volume method may not be as accurate in the setting of a ventricular septal defect.

Some of the previously mentioned limitations of ventricular volume analysis for shunt quantitation may be overcome using volume-flow analysis of great artery flow with velocity mapping. With this approach, quantitation of shunt size can be accomplished by measurement of net blood flow volumes within the main pulmonary artery and ascending aorta over a cardiac cycle. Shunts produce discrepant pulmonary and systemic arterial flows, with the former exceeding the latter in left-to-right shunts, and the converse in right-to-left shunts (Fig. 54.30) (320). This difference can be expressed either in absolute terms (e.g., shunt volume) or in relative terms (e.g., Qp/Qs). Values for shunting derived by volume-flow analysis have correlated well with the results from cardiac catheterization or nuclear first-pass ventriculography (320).

Pursuit of Hard-to-Find Lesions

Echo provides a rapid, repeatable method for assessing the anatomy and functional significance of a simple congenital defect. Therefore, it remains the mainstay of noninvasive assessment of congenital heart disease. Nevertheless, some lesions remain elusive to echo in an adult. Examples of simple lesions often hard to find in the adult on echo, even when a transesophageal approach is used, are sinus venous atrial septal defect and partial anomalous pulmonary venous return (Fig. 54.31) (318,319).

Evaluation of Complex Anomalies

To capitalize on the anatomy that MRI demonstrates, application of the segmental approach has proven to be useful to characterize complex CHD in the adult (317–

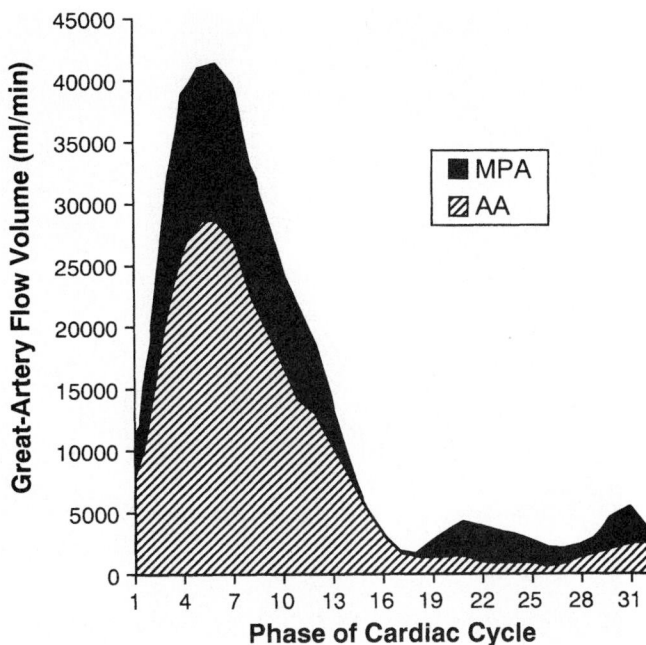

FIGURE 54.30 Flow-volume analysis of atrial septal defect with left-to-right shunting. Volume-flow analysis using velocity mapping permits direct measurement of great artery volume flows over the cardiac cycle after integration of the areas under the curves resulting from plotting of mean instantaneous volume flows passing through a cross section of each artery. The relative difference in volume flow between the main pulmonary artery (MPA), representing systemic stroke volume plus shunt volume, and the ascending aorta (AA), representing only stroke volume, may be used to derive a quantitative measure of left-to-right shunting, such as Qp/Qs. (From White RD. Magnetic resonance imaging of congenital heart disease. In: Pohost GM, ed. *Cardiovascular applications of magnetic resonance.* New York: Futura Publishing, 1993:59, with permission.)

319,321). Although the morphology of the appendages may be helpful, the received veins generally offer the best clues as to the nature of the atria visualized on MRI; the normal state (atrial situs solitus) is easily distinguishable from the inverted condition (atrial situs inversus), and both conditions can be easily differentiated from classic isomerism (situs ambiguus with either bilateral right-sidedness or left-sidedness). The ventricular positions define the bulboventricular loop; in the dextro (D)-loop, the normal state, the morphologic RV is situated to the right of the morphologic LV, and the reverse occurs with a levo (L)-loop. The morphologic RV, generally the more trabeculated, is characterized by the infundibulum separating the semilunar and atrioventricular valves, whereas the LV, generally the smoother walled, has its atrioventricular valve in fibrous continuity with the associated semilunar valve. Definition of the relationship of the great arteries is also part of the segmental approach, and it is clearly demonstrated with MRI; normally, the ascending aorta is located posteriorly and to the right of the main pulmonary artery, but the relationship is more difficult to define in the setting of atresia of either great artery. This relationship is disrupted with

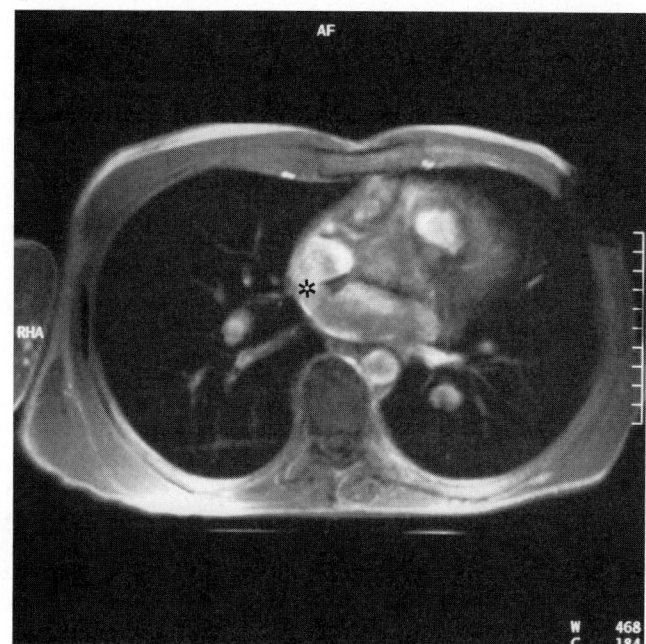
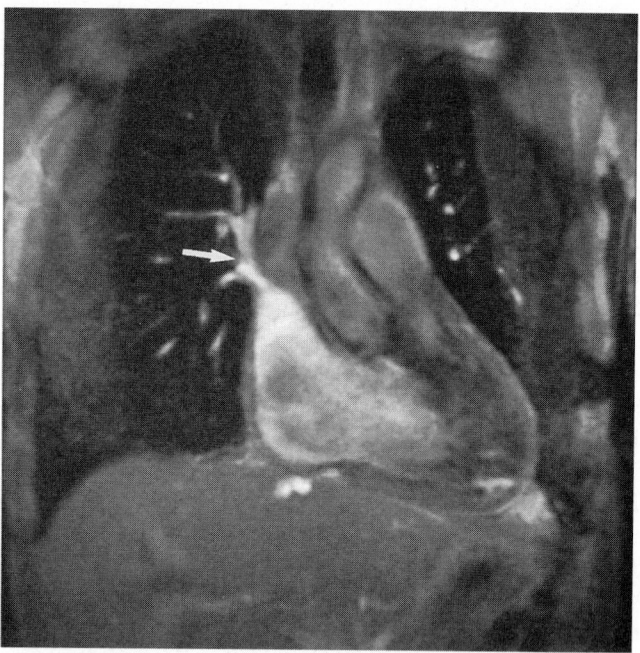

FIGURE 54.31 A hard-to-find sinus venosus atrial septal defect (cine; transaxial and oblique-coronal). High in the sinus venosus portion of the interatrial septum, immediately below the confluence of the superior vena cava with the right atrium, an atrial septal defect (*asterisk*) is noted **(A)**. The frequently associated anomalous return of the right upper pulmonary vein (*arrow*), in this case to the lower superior vena cava, is also demonstrated **(B)**.

transposition variants, whereby the ascending aorta may become positioned anterior-rightward (D-transposition), anterior-leftward (L-transposition), or alongside the main pulmonary artery. With generally high sensitivity at high specificity levels, MRI may be used to detect abnormalities of visceroatrial situs, venoatrial connection, atrioventricular connection, bulboventricular loop, ventriculoarterial connection, and great artery relationship (Fig. 54.32) (319,321).

Assessment of Congenital Great Vessel Disease

Imaging of the great arteries and veins by conventional echo can be problematic in adults, because imaging windows are limited by the surrounding lungs (318,319). Because MRI does not require an imaging window, the great vessels and their connections are visualized with the same clarity as cardiac structures.

Congenital Abnormalities of the Aorta

Coarctation

Defining the anatomy of coarctation is important, and for this reason MRI is of particular value (318). With MRI, the whole of the thoracic and abdominal aorta can be visualized with precise anatomic detail. Thus, MRI is a sensitive tool in the investigation of coarctation; the type of coarctation and the severity of stenosis can be seen easily on these images (Fig. 54.33 and *e*Fig. 54.33.1) (317,322). Other details, including the length of the stenotic segment, the

presence of arch or isthmic hypoplasia, the relationship of the coarctation to the aortic arch branches, and the presence of a ductus, are also accurately demonstrated.

Although the anatomy and degree of luminal stenosis are clearly visible on S-E images, a pressure gradient cannot be determined. However, the use of cine can both detect basic hemodynamic alterations resulting from stenosis and the resulting pressure gradient and provide further valuable insight into the collateralization from the nature of the turbulent downstream jet (231,318,323). Specifically, a low-signal jet can be visualized passing through and distal to the area of a significant stenosis, although this signal loss must be differentiated from normal signal decrease caused by antegrade flow (323). However, in the setting of complete or high-grade narrowing, flow may be primarily through collaterals and a transcoarctation jet may not be present. Velocity mapping allows quantitative assessment of the coarctation severity based on measurement of transstenosis velocity (99,324). In addition to the site and severity of aortic narrowing, other abnormalities associated with coarctation (e.g., collateral vessels and poststenotic dilatation) may be seen with MRI.

MRI is particularly valuable when applied on a serial basis during regular follow-up of patients who have undergone coarctation repair; it can provide high-resolution images of the repair site and determine the extent of recoarctation (317,318). In patients who have undergone balloon dilatation of either a native coarctation or recoarctation, MRI provides an ideal serial investigation to

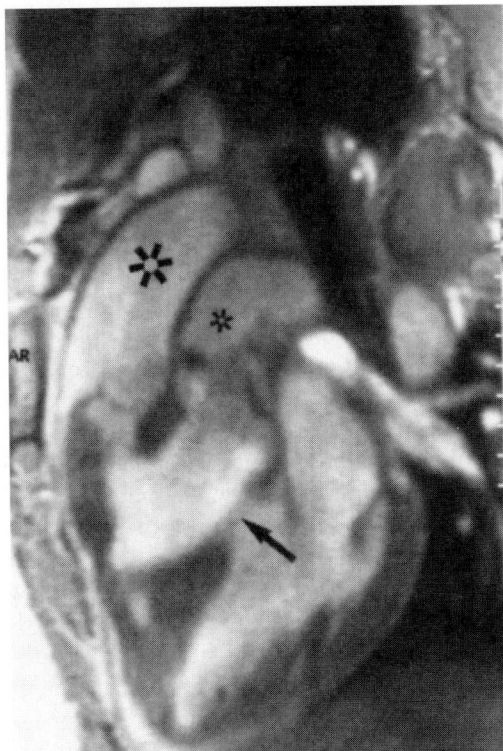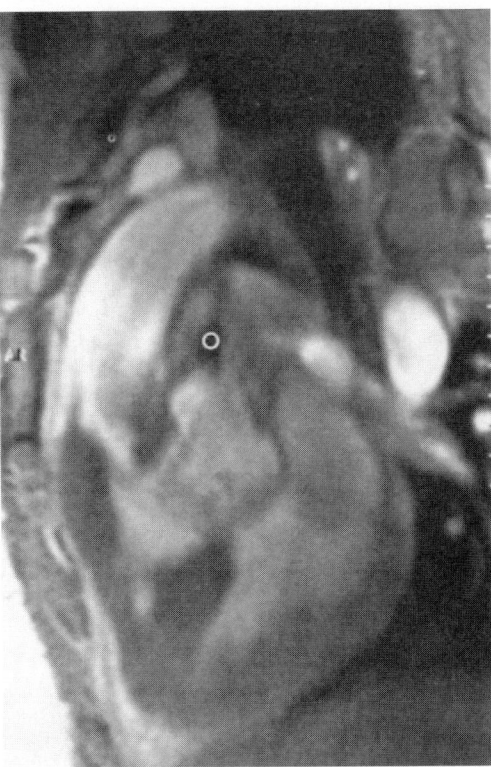

FIGURE 54.32 Complex congenital heart disease with abnormal ventriculoarterial connection and great artery relationship (cine; oblique-sagittal). In communication with an anatomic left ventricle through a muscular ventricular septal defect (*arrow*) is a small hypertrophic anatomic right ventricle, giving rise to both the aorta (*large asterisk*) and the main pulmonary artery (*small asterisk*) in a transposed arrangement. Valvular pulmonic stenosis is manifested by a signal-void jet (*open circle*).

watch for the development of aneurysm formation at the dilatation site.

Aortic Arch Branching Abnormalities

The value of MRI in the detection of congenital anomalies of the aorta has been well established (322,325). The morphology of the arch, its branching pattern, and its effect on adjacent structures can be recorded with a high degree of detail.

All types of vascular rings and the various anomalous branching patterns of the aortic arch (e.g., double aortic arch) are reliably seen on MRI (324,325). In older patients, or in those who have undergone surgery, MRI shows arch anomalies with greater clarity than transthoracic echo (322). Three-dimensional displays are often valuable for visually relating or connecting in a single image the often tortuous and obliquely oriented arterial components of a vascular ring (326).

Congenital Pulmonary Artery Abnormalities

Because MRI is not limited by the acoustic penetration of ultrasound or by the vascular access required for angiography, visualization of central pulmonary vessels (whether a true pulmonary artery or one arising from systemic-to-pulmonary collaterals) can be readily imaged with a high

degree of spatial resolution (318,327). The origin, size, and morphology of these vessels can be determined with relative ease using MRI. Stenoses of the main pulmonary artery and central arteries are detected better using cine than S-E imaging; pulmonary artery stenoses result in flow disturbances manifested by jets of signal void on cine (328).

Although MRI accurately delineates the anatomy of the central pulmonary artery system and can identify the aortic origin of major collateral vessels, it often fails to demonstrate the intrapulmonary segments of the arteries and collaterals, thus making the diagnosis of peripheral pulmonic stenoses difficult (319). Although evaluation of the pulmonary artery system within the lungs may be problematic for MRI, evaluation of the main pulmonary artery and central arteries appears to be as accurate as angiography and more accurate than transthoracic echo.

Congenital Abnormalities of the Pulmonary and Systemic Veins

Although the proximal portions of the pulmonary veins near their insertions into the left atrium are usually easily demonstrated with S-E MRI, G-E imaging has the advantage of displaying flow-related signal enhancement within the veins, thereby readily identifying them within the lungs

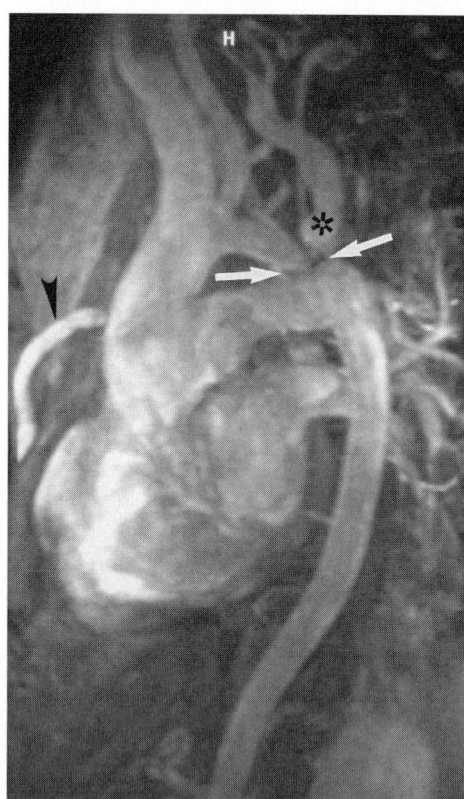

FIGURE 54.33 Complete interruption of the aorta (contrast-enhanced, three-dimensional magnetic resonance angiography; maximal intensity projection). Immediately beyond the stenotic origin of the dilated left subclavian artery (*asterisk*), there is complete interruption of the juxtaductal region of the aortic isthmus (*arrows*). A large internal mammary artery (*arrowhead*) serves as a systemic collateral vessel.

(329). Consequently, cine or MRA is preferable to S-E MRI for the identification of anomalous pulmonary venous drainage, and it may aid in the diagnosis of congenital abnormalities of the systemic veins (330).

MRI has been shown to be effective for demonstration of all types of anomalous pulmonary venous connections, comparable with or more accurate than echo and angiography (321,329,330). In addition to showing anomalous connections (*e*Fig. 54.33.2), venous stenosis or stenosis at an anastomotic site is accurately demonstrated. Reduced sensitivity for detecting the return connections of the pulmonary veins by S-E imaging, compared with G-E MRI or MRA, is probably related to the aforementioned inherent limitations in this technique.

Postoperative Assessment

As more patients with CHD undergo corrective surgery and survive longer, postoperative clinical evaluation becomes increasingly important. MRI is an important adjunct to echo and an alternative to angiography for morphologic examination of CHD after surgery (318,319). The combination of capabilities described earlier for the

evaluation of anatomic aspects makes MRI uniquely suited for this pursuit. In contrast to echo, MRI is not severely restricted by postoperative scarring.

The course and patency of extracardiac shunts (e.g., Blalock-Taussig shunt) may be well visualized using S-E or G-E MRI (331), with G-E images more sensitive to identification of blood flow through vascular structures and differentiation between vessels and airway. MRI is somewhat less important for the evaluation of intracardiac postsurgical changes because its morphology is demonstrated as well or better with echo. However, in those instances in which an echo does not provide sufficient intracardiac detail, such as in older patients, MRI remains an important alternative diagnostic modality (330,332).

Important postoperative anatomic features of various surgical procedures for CHD (e.g., Fontan procedure for tricuspid atresia) have been successfully detected and delineated using S-E MRI (331,332). Cine has also been used successfully for postoperative evaluation of CHD patients (330); it has the advantage over S-E MRI of improved differentiation between blood vessels and air-filled structures. Finally, using cine, postoperative complications (e.g., peripatch leak after defect repair) have also been detected based on the presence of signal-void jets. However, the artifacts from metallic surgical materials are more prominent on G-E imaging than on S-E imaging because of greater sensitivity of the former to local magnetic field inhomogeneities, and this may increasingly hinder adequate visualization of structures using cine.

With an increasing number of interventional therapeutic devices, such as umbrellas, coils, and stents, as well as surgical materials being placed for therapy in patients with CHD, there may be increasing limitations of the postoperative diagnostic capabilities of MRI because of increasing problems related to artifacts (319).

CONTROVERSIES AND PERSONAL PERSPECTIVES

In several large institutions, such as ours, MRI has been actively applied to the routine clinical evaluation of a variety of CV diseases over a number of years. In some clinical settings, MRI has gained great acceptance and is now regarded as the diagnostic imaging procedure of choice, whereas in other settings, the yield has been disappointing and MRI is regarded as, at most, an infrequently used adjunct to other modalities, such as echo. Based on our experience, which includes over 1,700 clinical CV MRI examinations per year, a practical weighting of the relative value of MRI, compared with state-of-the-art echo and ECG-referenced multidetector CT, is presented in Table 54.1; in this weighting, relative study cost, portability, and clinical stability of the patient are considered.

Probably more than any other modality currently available, MRI has the potential to contribute to the improved

TABLE 54.1 PRACTICAL VALUE OF CARDIOVASCULAR MAGNETIC RESONANCE IMAGING RELATIVE TO OTHER AVAILABLE NONINVASIVE DIAGNOSTIC IMAGING MODALITIES BY DISEASE GROUP

	Magnetic resonance imaging	Echocardiography	Computed tomography
Ischemic heart disease			
Reversible			
Induced	++++	++++	0
Stunned/hibernating	++++	++++	0
Irreversible			
Acute (e.g., acute myocardial infarction	++++	+++	+
Chronic (e.g., post–myocardial infarction aneurysm)	++++	+++	++
Valvular heart disease			
Stenosis	+++	++++	+
Regurgitation	+++	++++	0
Myocardial disease			
Dilated cardiomyopathy	++++	++++	+
Hypertrophic cardiomyopathy	+++	++++	++
Restrictive cardiomyopathy	+++	++++	+
Right ventricular cardiomyopathy	++++	+	++
Pericardial disease			
Effusion and tamponade	++++	++++	++
Pericarditis and constriction	++++	+++	++
Aortic disease			
Aneurysm	++++	++	+++
Dissection			
Acute: rule out ascending dissection	++++	++++	++++
Acute: rule out descending dissection	++++	+++	++++
Acute: equivocal initial study or presurgical planning	++++	++	++++
Nonacute: uncomplicated	++++	++	+++
Nonacute: complicated	++++	++	+++
Intramural hematoma	++++	++	++++
Pulmonary artery disease			
Pulmonary emboli	++	0	++++
Pulmonary hypertension	+++	++	+++
Thrombi and masses			
Intracardiac	++++	++++	+++
Extracardiac	++++	++	++++
Adult congenital heart disease			
Simple cardiac abnormality	++++	++++	++
Complex cardiac abnormality	++++	++	+++
Great vessel abnormality	++++	++	+++

0, no significant useful information; ++++, maximal amount of useful information.

understanding of CV diseases based on diagnostic imaging; this potential is now rapidly gaining increased attention by the medical community and manufacturers of medical imaging equipment. For this potential to be realized, however, several types of obstacles must be overcome.

Not the least of these obstacles is the current medical environment with its increasing emphasis on cost containment and capitated reimbursement; in this environment, expensive technology, in particular MRI, has already been targeted. Included in this environment are (a) pressures on ordering physicians to avoid use of CV MRI, even when it is thought to be the best first-line diagnostic imaging study and possibly the only one needed, because the charge per examination is relatively greater (e.g., approximately $200 more than transesophageal echo and $600 more than CT at

our institution); (b) increasing demands on physicians involved in CV MRI to pursue clinical productivity in more basic diagnostic imaging areas, where reimbursement may be better established; (c) greater and greater limitations on research time and institutional support for needed clinical investigation in CV MRI; and (d) decreasing availability of MRI equipment for CV imaging because of reduced numbers of scanners or increasing limitations on scheduled scan time for greater patient throughput.

Another obstacle has been largely created by the MRI community itself. It is the problem related to lack of a history of meaningful large clinical studies dealing with outcome and efficacy. Since the advent of clinical MRI, research has rewarded the development of cutting-edge technology in which only alterations in acquisition and

THE FUTURE

With diseases of the CV system cumulatively representing the number one killer in the United States, there is a need for better understanding of the fundamental histologic, anatomic, and physiologic manifestations of disease processes affecting the heart and vasculature. Technical advances, applicable to the assessment of the CV system, may facilitate MRI's gaining a more significant role in evaluating these areas. Because MRI permits direct high-resolution, 3-D visualization of the myocardium, it can potentially characterize the myocardium based on assessments of tissue composition, geometry, perfusion, contraction, and relaxation and filling.

It is difficult to determine which, if any, of the expensive technologic advancements currently under investigation in MRI might have a future role in CV imaging. Current research and development with high-field spectroscopic MRI (333), interventional MRI (334), metabolic MRI contrast agents (335), and high-resolution vessel-wall characterization (289) may eventually find clinical applications to future work in CV MRI.

postprocessing schemes along with the speculation, but no proof, of improved clinical care have been sufficient to gain recognition in the form of grant funding, support from manufacturers, and relatively unchallenged acceptance of written reports for publication in peer-reviewed journals. In an area with such seemingly endless technologic potential as MRI, this tendency has created a rewarding path of least resistance in clinical investigation with a heavy emphasis on uniqueness and individualism. An unfortunate outcome that now hinders the future of CV MRI has been the passive discouragement of large multicenter patient studies addressing the clinical value of information about CV diseases provided by the more widely available, nonproprietary, and validated MRI techniques; the common argument against past efforts to develop such outcomes and efficacy studies is the anticipation of technologic obsolescence by the time of their completion. Consequently, there is currently little ammunition to fight off cost-containment efforts directed against CV MRI.

Finally, another obstacle that must be overcome is the issue of "ownership," whether it be that dealing with control of patients or of equipment. MRI is an expensive technology, with scanner costs alone exceeding those of echo and CT by approximately tenfold and twofold, respectively. Siting costs in MRI, which in some circumstances match equipment costs, greatly add to the relatively greater expense of MRI compared with other imaging modalities, especially echo with its negligible siting needs. Although the manufacturers of medical imaging equipment are now demonstrating the ability to reduce the costs of purchasing and installing MRI systems, there appears to be a limit to which the costs can be reduced before the research and development of MRI is no longer regarded as being economically viable. In addition, as long as MRI continues to evolve, the regular allocation of significant funds for hardware and software upgrades, along with the significant routine maintenance costs, will have to be factored annually into institutional budgets. Therefore, a state-of-the-art MRI will probably need to be viewed increasingly, from an economic standpoint, as a technology that is most appropriate for larger medical facilities.

In the case of CV MRI, its potential will be best realized at major CV centers, if it is regarded as an institutional effort, and the leadership responsibility is shared among the following groups: (a) radiology, (b) adult and pediatric cardiology, and (c) cardiothoracic and vascular surgery. To this common effort, radiology departments can contribute expertise in the application of general imaging and MRI principles and in the interpretation and use of the resulting data; experience with quality assurance of an MRI facility; oversight of the performance of routine CV imaging and non-CV issues that arise; and direction in the implementation of new acquisition and postprocessing schemes originating from the general imaging and MRI communities. Adult and pediatric cardiology departments can contribute to the identification of new medical applications of MRI to the evaluation of acquired and congenital CV diseases; leadership in overseeing the monitoring and the manipulations (e.g., stress testing) of patients during physiologic CV MRI examinations; expertise in the interpretation and use of physiologic data from MRI and its correlation with other findings, such as from echo; and experience in conducting meaningful large clinical research studies of CV diseases using MRI. Finally, cardiothoracic and vascular surgery, the clinical groups probably profiting the most to date from CV MRI, can contribute to the identification of new applications of MRI to the presurgical and postsurgical evaluation of CV diseases; expertise in the interpretation and use of morphologic data from MRI; and leadership in exploring the possibility of less invasive surgical therapies, incorporating indirect anatomic visualization by MRI rather than direct surgical visualization. This type of cooperative effort should allow MRI to develop further as a valuable clinical tool for the evaluation of CV diseases.

REFERENCES

1. Bloch F, Hanson WW, Packsard ME. Nuclear induction. *Phys Rev* 1946;69:127.

2. Purcell EM, Torry HC, Pound RV. Resonance absorption by nuclear magnetic movements in a solid. *Phys Rev* 1946;69:37.

3. Mansfield P, Grannell PK. NMR "diffraction" in solids? *J Phys C: Solid State Phys* 1973;6:L422.

4. Lauterbur PC. Image formation by induced local interactions: examples employing nuclear magnetic resonance. *Nature* 1973;242:190.

5. Damadian AR, Goldsmith M, Minkoff L. NMR in cancer. XVI. FONAR image of the live human body. *Physiol Chem Phys* 1977;9:97.

6. Alfidi RJ, Haaga JR, El Yousel SJ, et al. Preliminary experimental results in humans and animals with a superconducting, whole-body nuclear magnetic resonance scanner. *Radiology* 1982;143:175.

7. Herfkens RJ, Higgins CB, Hricak H, et al. Nuclear magnetic resonance imaging of the cardiovascular system: normal and pathologic findings. *Radiology* 1983;147:749.

8. Dinsmore RE, Wismer GL, Levine RA. Magnetic resonance imaging of the heart: positioning and gradient angle selection for optimal imaging planes. *AJR Am J Roentgenol* 1984;143:1135.

9. Sechtem U, Pflugfelder PW, White RD, et al. Cine MR imaging: potential for the evaluation of cardiovascular function. *AJR Am J Roentgenol* 1987;148:239.

10. Firmin DN, Naylor GL, Klipstein RH, et al. *In vivo* validation of MR velocity imaging. *J Comput Assist Tomogr* 1987;11:751.

11. Haase A, Matthaei D, Hanicke W, et al. FLASH imaging: rapid NMR imaging using low flip-angle pulses. *J Magn Reson* 1986;67:258.

12. Atkinson DJ, Edelman RR. Cineangiography of the heart in a single breath hold with a segmented turboFLASH sequence. *Radiology* 1991;178:357.

13. Rzedzian RR, Pykett IL. Instant images of the human heart using a new, whole-body MR imaging system. *AJR Am J Roentgenol* 1987;149:245.

14. Zerhouni EA, Parish DM, Rogers WJ, et al. Human heart: tagging with MR imaging—a method for noninvasive assessment of myocardial motion. *Radiology* 1988;169:59.

15. Pelc NJ, Herfkens RJ, Pelc LR. Three-dimensional analysis of myocardial motion and deformation with phase contrast cine MRI. *Magn Reson Med* 1992;11:18.

16. Edelman RR, Mattle HP, Atkinson DJ, et al. MR angiography. *AJR Am J Roentgenol* 1990;154:937.

17. White RD, Ehman RL, Weinreb JC. Cardiovascular MR imaging: current level of clinical activity. *J Magn Reson Imaging* 1992;2:365.

18. Koutcher JA, Burt CT. Principles of imaging by nuclear magnetic resonance. *J Nucl Med* 1984;25:371.

19. Mezrich R. A perspective on k-space. *Radiology* 1995;195:297.

20. Chien D, Edelman RR. Ultrafast imaging using gradient echoes. *Magn Reson Q* 1991;7:31.

21. Crooks LE, Barker B, Chang H, et al. Magnetic resonance imaging strategies for heart studies. *Radiology* 1984;153:459.

22. Simonetti O, Finn JP, White RD, et al. Black-blood T2-weighted inversion-recovery MR imaging of the heart. *Radiology* 1996;199:49.

23. Stemerman DH, Krinsky GA, Lee VS, et al. Thoracic aorta: rapid black-blood MR imaging with half-Fourier rapid acquisition with relaxation enhancement with or without electrocardiographic triggering. *Radiology* 1999;213:185.

24. Schulen V, Schick F, Loichat J, et al. Evaluation of k-space segmented cine sequences for fast functional cardiac imaging. *Invest Radiol* 1996;31:512.

25. von Schulthess GK, Higgins CB. Blood flow imaging with MR: spin-phase phenomenon. *Radiology* 1985;157:687.

26. Lenz GW, Haacke EM, Masaryk TJ. In plane vascular imaging: pulse sequence design and strategy. *Radiology* 1988;166:875.

27. Nayler GL, Firmin DN, Longmore DB. Blood flow imaging by cine magnetic resonance. *J Comput Assist Tomogr* 1986;10:715.

28. Underwood SR, Firman DN, Klipstein RH, et al. Magnetic resonance velocity mapping: clinical application of a new technique. *Br Heart J* 1987;57:404.

29. Axel L, Dougherty L. Heart wall motion: improved method of spatial modulation of magnetization of MR imaging. *Radiology* 1989;172:349.

30. Frahm J, Merboldt KD, Bruhn H, et al. 0.3-Second FLASH MRI of the human heart. *Magn Reson Med* 1990;13:150.

31. Atkinson DJ, Burstein D, Edelman RR. First-pass cardiac perfusion: evaluation with ultrafast MR imaging. *Radiology* 1990;174:757.

32. Edelman RR, Wielopolski P, Schmitt F. Echo-planar MR imaging. *Radiology* 1994;192:600.

33. Lanzer P, Barta C, Botvinick EH, et al. ECG-synchronized cardiac MR imaging: method and evaluation. *Radiology* 1985;155:681.

34. Foo TK, Bernstein MA, Aisen AM, et al. Improved ejection fraction and flow velocity estimates with use of view sharing and uniform repetition time excitation with fast cardiac techniques. *Radiology* 1995;195:471.

35. Wood ML, Henkelman RM. MR imaging artifacts from periodic motion. *Med Phys* 1985;12:143.

36. Runge VM, Clanton JN, Partain CL, et al. Respiratory gating in magnetic resonance imaging at 0.5 Tesla. *Radiology* 1984;151:521.

37. Bailes DR, Gilderdale DJ, Bydder GM, et al. Respiratory ordered phase encoding (ROPE): a method for reducing respiratory motion artifacts in MR imaging. *J Comput Assist Tomogr* 1985;9:835.

38. White RD, Cassidy MM, Cheitlin MD, et al. Segmental evaluation of left ventricular wall motion after myocardial infarction: magnetic resonance imaging versus echocardiography. *Am Heart J* 1988;115:166.

39. Listerud J. First principles of magnetic resonance angiography. *Magn Reson Q* 1991;7:136.

40. Finn PF, Goldmann A, Edelman RR. Magnetic resonance angiography in the body. *Magn Reson Q* 1992;8:1.

41. Prince MR. Gadolinium-enhanced MR aortography. *Radiology* 1994;191:155.

42. Roy OZ. Technical note: summary of cardiac fibrillation thresholds for 60 Hz currents and voltages applied directly to the heart. *Med Biol Eng Comput* 1980;18:657.

43. Shellock FG, Kanal E. Guidelines and recommendations for MR imaging safety and patient management. III. Questionnaire for screening patients before MR procedures. *J Magn Reson Imaging* 1994;4:749.

44. Hug J, Nagel E, Bornstedt A, et al. Coronary arterial stents: safety and artifacts during MR imaging. *Radiology* 2000;216:781.

45. Edwards MB, Taylor KM, Shellock FG. Prosthetic heart valves: evaluation of magnetic field interactions, heating, and artifacts at 1.5 T. *J Magn Reson Imaging* 2000;12:363.

46. Axel L. Blood flow effects in magnetic resonance imaging. *AJR Am J Roentgenol* 1984;143:1157.

47. Bradley WG, Waluch V. Blood flow: magnetic resonance imaging. *Radiology* 1985;154:443.

48. Valk PE, Hale JD, Crooks LE, et al. MRI of blood flow: correlation of image appearance with spin-echo phase shift and signal intensity. *AJR Am J Roentgenol* 1986;146:931.

49. Von Schulthess GK, Fisher MR, Crooks LE, et al. Gated MR imaging of the heart: intracardiac signal in patients and healthy subjects. *Radiology* 1985;157:125.

50. Schultz CL, Alfidi RJ, Nelson AD, et al. The effect of motion on two-dimensional Fourier transformation magnetic resonance images. *Radiology* 1984;152:117.

51. Ehman RL, Felmlee JP. Flow artifact reduction in MRI: a review of the roles of gradient moment nulling and spatial presaturation. *Magn Reson Med* 1990;14:293.

52. Bradley WG, Waluch V. NMR even echo rephasing in slow laminar flow. *J Comput Assist Tomogr* 1984;8:594.

53. von Schulthess GK, Augustiny N. Calculation of T2 values versus phase imaging for the distinction between flow and thrombus in MR imaging. *Radiology* 1987;164:549.

54. Rapoport S, Sostman HD, Pope C, et al. Venous clots: evaluation with MR imaging. *Radiology* 1987;162:527.

55. White EM, Edelman RR, Wedeen VJ, et al. Intravascular signal in MR imaging: use of phase display for differentiation of blood-flow signal from intraluminal disease. *Radiology* 1986;161:245.

56. Dinsmore RE, Wedeen VJ, Miller SW, et al. MRI of dissection of the aorta: recognition of the intimal tear and differential flow velocities. *AJR Am J Roentgenol* 1986;146:1286.

57. White RD, Ullyot DJ, Higgins CB. MR imaging of the aorta after surgery for aortic dissection. *AJR Am J Roentgenol* 1988;150:87.

58. Mirowitz SA, Lee JKT, Gutierrez FR, et al. Normal signal-void patterns in cardiac cine MR images. *Radiology* 1990;176:49.

59. Evans AJ, Blinder RA, Herfkens RJ, et al. Effects of turbulence on signal intensity in gradient echo images. *Invest Radiol* 1988;23:512.

60. Yucel EK, Anderson CM, Edelman RR, et al. Magnetic resonance angiography. *Circulation* 1999;100:2284.

61. Suzuki J, Caputo GR, Kondo, et al. Cine MR imaging of valvular heart disease: display and imaging parameters affect the size of the signal void by valvular regurgitation. *AJR Am J Roentgenol* 1990;155:723.

62. Ohnishi S, Fukui S, Kusuoka H, et al. Assessment of valvular regurgitation using cine magnetic resonance imaging coupled with phase compensation technique: comparison with Doppler color flow mapping. *Angiology* 1992;43:913.

63. White RD, Paschal CB, Tkach JA, et al. Functional cardiovascular evaluation by magnetic resonance imaging. *Top Magn Reson Imaging* 1990;2:31.

64. Higgins CB, Byrd BF, McNamara MT, et al. Magnetic resonance imaging of the heart: a review of the experience in 172 subjects. *Radiology* 1985;155:671.

65. Saloner D, Selby K, Anderson CM. MRA studies of arterial stenosis: improvements by diastolic acquisition. *Magn Reson Med* 1994;31:196.

66. Higgins CB, Saeed M, Wendland MF, et al. Contrast media for cardiothoracic MR imaging. *J Magn Reson Imaging* 1993;3:265.

67. Keller AM, Peshock RM, Malloy CR, et al. In vivo measurement of myocardial mass using nuclear magnetic resonance imaging. *J Am Coll Cardiol* 1986;8:113.

68. Sakuma H, Fujita N, Foo TK, et al. Evaluation of LV volumes and mass with breathhold cine MR imaging. *Radiology* 1993;188:377.

69. Higgins CB, Holt W, Pflugfelder P, et al. Functional evaluation of the heart with magnetic resonance imaging. *Magn Reson Med* 1988;6:121.

70. Sechtem U, Pflugfelder PW, Gould RG, et al. Measurement of right and left ventricular volumes in healthy individuals with cine MRI imaging. *Radiology* 1987;163:697.

71. Pattynama PMT, Lamb HJ, van der Velde EO, et al. Left ventricular measurements with cine and spin-echo MR imaging: a study of reproducibility with variance component analysis. *Radiology* 1993;187:261.

72. Longmore DB, Klipstein RH, Underwood SR, et al. Dimensional accuracy of magnetic resonance in studies of the heart. *Lancet* 1985;1:1360.

73. Stratemeier EJ, Thompson R, Brady TJ, et al. Ejection fraction determination by MR imaging: comparison with left ventricular angiography. *Radiology* 1986;158:775.

74. von Rossum AC, Visser FC, van Eenige MJ, et al. Magnetic resonance imaging of the heart for determination of ejection fraction. *Int J Cardiol* 1988;18:53.

75. Dulce MC, Mostbeck GH, Friese KK, et al. Quantitation of the left ventricular volumes and function with cine MR imaging: comparison of geometric models with three-dimensional data. *Radiology* 1993;188:371.

76. Semelka RC, Tomei E, Wagner S, et al. Interstudy reproducibility of dimensional and functional measurements between cine magnetic resonance studies in the morphologically abnormal left ventricle. *Am Heart J* 1990;119:1367.

77. Buser PT, Auffermann W, Holt WW, et al. Noninvasive evaluation of global left ventricular function with use of cine nuclear magnetic resonance. *J Am Coll Cardiol* 1989;13:1294.

78. van Rossum AC, Visser FC, Sprenger M, et al. Evaluation of magnetic resonance imaging for determination of left ventricular ejection fraction and comparison with angiography. *Am J Cardiol* 1988;62:628.

79. Sechtem U, Sommerhoff BA, Markiewicz W, et al. Regional left ventricular wall thickening by magnetic resonance imaging: evaluation in normal persons and patients with global and regional dysfunction. *Am J Cardiol* 1987;59:145.

80. Pflugfelder PW, Sechtem UP, White RD, et al. Quantification of regional myocardial function by rapid cine MR imaging. *AJR Am J Roentgenol* 1988;150:523.

81. Reichek N. Magnetic resonance imaging for assessment of myocardial function. *Magn Reson Q* 1991;7:255.

82. Dulce MC, Higgins CB. Evaluation of ventricular dimensions and function with magnetic resonance imaging. *Am J Card Imaging* 1994;8:168.

83. Wagner S, Auffermann W, Buser P, et al. Functional description of the left ventricle in patients with volume overload, pressure overload, and myocardial disease using cine magnetic resonance imaging. *Am J Card Imaging* 1991;5:87.

84. Clark NR, Reichek N, Bergey P, et al. Circumferential myocardial shortening in the normal human left ventricle: assessment by magnetic resonance imaging using spatial modulation of magnetization. *Circulation* 1991;84:67.

85. Moore CC, O'Dell WG, McVeigh ER, et al. Calculation of three-dimensional left ventricular planes from bipolar tagged MR images. *J Magn Reson Imaging* 1992;2:165.

86. Buchalter MB, Weiss JL, Rogers WJ, et al. Noninvasive quantification of left ventricular rotational deformation in normal humans using magnetic resonance imaging myocardial tagging. *Circulation* 1990;81:1236.

87. Lima JAC, Jeremy R, Guier W, et al. Accurate systolic wall thickening by nuclear magnetic resonance imaging with tissue tagging: correlation with sonomicrometers in normal and ischemic myocardium. *J Am Coll Cardiol* 1993;21:1741.

88. Beyar R, Weiss JL, Shapiro EP, et al. Small apex-to-base heterogeneity in radius-to-thickness ratio by three-dimensional magnetic resonance imaging. *Am J Physiol* 1993;264:H133.

89. Rademakers FE, Rogers WJ, Guier WH, et al. Relation of regional cross-fiber shortening to wall thickening in the intact heart: three-dimensional strain analysis by NMR tagging. *Circulation* 1994;89:1174.

90. Pelc LR, Sayre J, Yun K, et al. Evaluation of myocardial motion tracking with cine-phase contrast magnetic resonance imaging. *Invest Radiol* 1994;29:1038.

91. Karwatowski SP, Mohiaddin RH, Yang GZ, et al. Regional myocardial velocity imaging by magnetic resonance in patients with ischemic heart disease. *Br Heart J* 1994;72:332.

92. Bazille A, Guttman MA, McVeigh ER, et al. Impact of semiautomated versus manual image segmentation errors on myocardial strain calculation by magnetic resonance tagging. *Invest Radiol* 1994;29:427.

93. Edelman RR, Mattle HP, Kleefield J, et al. Quantification of blood flow with dynamic MR imaging and presaturation bolus tracking. *Radiology* 1989;171:551.

94. Sondergaard L, Stahlberg F, Thomsen C, et al. Accuracy and precision of MR velocity mapping in measurement of stenotic cross-sectional area, flow rate, and pressure gradient. *J Magn Reson Imaging* 1993;3:433.

95. Kilner PJ, Firmin DN, Rees RS, et al. Valve and great vessel stenosis: assessment with MR jet velocity mapping. *Radiology* 1991;178:229.

96. Mohiaddin RH, Wann SL, Underwood R, et al. Vena caval flow: assessment with cine MR velocity mapping. *Radiology* 1990;177:537.

97. Mohiaddin RH, Amanuma M, Kilner PJ, et al. MR phase-shift velocity mapping of mitral and pulmonary venous flow. *J Comp Assist Tomogr* 1991;15:237.

98. Mostbeck GH, Caputo GR, Higgins CB. MR measurement of blood flow in the cardiovascular system. *AJR Am J Roentgenol* 1992;159:453.

99. Mohiaddin RH, Longmore DB. Functional aspects of cardiovascular nuclear imaging: techniques and application. *Circulation* 1993;88:264.

100. Sloth E, Houlind KC, Oyre S, et al. Three-dimensional visualization of velocity profiles in the human main pulmonary artery with magnetic resonance phase-velocity mapping. *Am Heart J* 1994;128:1130.

101. Rebergen SA, van der Wall EE, Doornbos J, et al. Magnetic resonance measurement of velocity and flow: technique, validation, and cardiovascular applications. *Am Heart J* 1993;126:1439.

102. Wilke N, Simm C, Zhang J, et al. Contrast enhanced first pass myocardial perfusion imaging: correlation between myocardial blood flow in dogs at rest and during hyperemia. *Magn Reson Med* 1993;29:485.

103. Wendland MF, Saeed M, Masui T, et al. Echo-planar MR imaging of normal and ischemic myocardium with gadodiamide injection. *Radiology* 1993;186:535.

104. Eichenberger AC, Schuiki E, Kochli VD, et al. Ischemic heart disease: assessment with gadolinium-enhanced ultrafast MR imaging and dipyridamole stress. *J Magn Reson Imaging* 1994;4:425.

105. van Rugge FP, Boreel JJ, van der Waal EE, et al. Cardiac first pass and myocardial perfusion in normal subjects assessed by subsecond Gd-DTPA enhanced MR imaging. *J Comput Assist Tomogr* 1991;15:965.

106. Wilke N, Jerosch-Herold M, Stillman AE, et al. Concepts of myocardial perfusion imaging in magnetic resonance imaging. *Magn Reson Q* 1994;10:249.

107. Steffens JC, Sakuma H, Bourne MW, et al. Magnetic resonance imaging in ischemic heart disease. *Am Heart J* 1996;132:156.

108. White RD, Holt WW, Cheitlin MD, et al. Estimation of the functional and anatomical extent of myocardial infarction using magnetic resonance imaging. *Am Heart J* 1988;115:740.

109. Meese RB, Spritzer CE, Negro-Villar R, et al. Detection, characterization and functional assessment of reperfused Q-wave myocardial infarction by cine magnetic resonance imaging. *Am J Cardiol* 1990;66:1.

110. Matheijssen NAA, De Roos A, Doornbos J, et al. Left ventricular wall motion analysis in patients with acute myocardial infarction using magnetic resonance imaging. *Magn Reson Imaging* 1993;11:485.

111. Tscholakoff D, Higgins CB, McNamara MT, et al. Early-phase myocardial infarction: evaluation of MR imaging. *Radiology* 1986;159:667.

112. Filipchuk NG, Peschock RM, Malloy CR, et al. Detection and localization of recent myocardial infarction by magnetic resonance imaging. *Am J Cardiol* 1986;58:214.

113. Johnston DL, Thompson RC, Liu P, et al. Magnetic resonance imaging during acute myocardial infarction. *Am J Cardiol* 1986;57:1059.

114. Peshock RM, Rokey R, Malloy CM, et al. Assessment of myocardial systolic wall thickening using nuclear magnetic resonance imaging. *J Am Coll Cardiol* 1989;4:653.

115. Lotan CS, Cranney GB, Bouchard A, et al. The value of

cine nuclear magnetic resonance imaging for assessing regional ventricular function. *J Am Coll Cardiol* 1989;14:1721.

116. Peshock RM, Rokey R, Malloy CM, et al. Assessment of myocardial systolic wall thickening using nuclear magnetic resonance imaging. *J Am Coll Cardiol* 1989;14:653.

117. Baer FM, Voth E, Theissen P, et al. Gradient-echo magnetic resonance imaging during incremental dobutamine infusion for the localization of coronary artery stenoses. *Eur Heart J* 1994;15:218.

118. Underwood SR, Rees RSO, Savage PE, et al. Assessment of regional left ventricular function by magnetic resonance. *Br Heart J* 1986;56:334.

119. Fedele F, Scopinaro F, Montesano DI, et al. Characterization of reversible myocardial dysfunction by magnetic resonance imaging. *Herz* 1994;19:210.

120. Kramer CM, Lima JA, Reichek N, et al. Regional differences in function within noninfarcted myocardium during left ventricular remodeling. *Circulation* 1993;88:1279.

121. Kramer CM, Rogers WJ, Theobald TM, et al. Remote noninfarcted region dysfunction soon after anterior myocardial infarction: a magnetic resonance tagging study. *Circulation* 1996;94:660.

122. van der Wall EE, de Roos A, van Voorthuisen AE, et al. Magnetic resonance imaging: a new approach for evaluating coronary artery disease. *Am Heart J* 1991;121:1203.

123. Ratner AV, Okada RD, Newell JB, et al. The relationship between proton nuclear magnetic resonance relaxation parameters and myocardial perfusion with acute arterial occlusion and reperfusion. *Circulation* 1985;72:823.

124. McNamara MT, Higgins CB, Schechtmann N, et al. Detection and characterization of acute myocardial infarction in man with use of gated magnetic resonance. *Circulation* 1985;71:717.

125. Wesbey G, Higgins CB, Lanzer P, et al. Imaging and characterization of acute myocardial infarction in vivo by gated nuclear magnetic resonance. *Circulation* 1984;69:125.

126. Been M, Smith MA, Ridgway JP, et al. Serial changes in the T1 magnetic relaxation parameter after myocardial infarction in man. *Br Heart J* 1988;59:1.

127. Canby RC, Reeves RC, Evanochko WT, et al. Proton nuclear magnetic resonance relaxation times in severe myocardial ischemia. *J Am Coll Cardiol* 1987;10:412.

128. Wisenberg G, Prato FS, Carroll SE, et al. Serial nuclear magnetic resonance imaging of acute myocardial infarction with and without reperfusion. *Am Heart J* 1988;115:510.

129. Krauss XH, Van der Wall EE, Van der Laarse A, et al. Magnetic resonance imaging of myocardial infarction: correlation with enzymatic, angiographic, and radionuclide findings. *Am Heart J* 1991;122:1274.

130. Krauss XH, Van der Wall EE, Doornbos J, et al. The value of nuclear magnetic resonance imaging in patients with a recent myocardial infarction: comparison with planar thallium-201 scintigraphy. *Cardiovasc Intervent Radiol* 1989;12:119.

131. Fisher MR, McNamara MT, Higgins CB. Acute myocardial infarction: MR evaluation in 29 patients. *AJR Am J Roentgenol* 1987;148:247.

132. Ahmad J, Johnson RF, Fawcett HD, et al. Magnetic resonance imaging in patients with unstable angina: comparison with acute myocardial infarction and normals. *Magn Reson Imaging* 1988;6:527.

133. Lotan C, Miller SK, Bouchard A, et al. Detection of myocardial hemorrhage using 1H NMR imaging at 1.5 T. *J Am Coll Cardiol* 1989;13:48A.

134. Brooks RA, Battocletti JH, Sances A, et al. Nuclear magnetic relaxation in blood. *IEEE Trans Biomed Eng* 1975;1:12.

135. de Roos A, Doornbos J, van der Wall EE, et al. MR imaging of acute myocardial infarction: value of Gd-DTPA. *AJR Am J Roentgenol* 1988;150:531.

136. Eichstaedt HW, Felix R, Dougherty FC, et al. Magnetic resonance imaging (MRI) in different stages of myocardial infarction using the contrast agent gadolinium-DTPA. *Clin Cardiol* 1986;9:527.

137. Dulce MC, Duerinckx AJ, Hartiala J, et al. MR imaging of the myocardium using nonionic contrast medium: signal intensity changes in patients with subacute myocardial infarction. *AJR Am J Roentgenol* 1993;160:963.

138. van Rossum AC, Visser FC, van Eenige MJ, et al. Value of gadolinium-diethylene-triamine pentaacetic acid dynamics in magnetic resonance imaging of acute myocardial infarction with occluded and reperfused coronary arteries after thrombolysis. *Am J Cardiol* 1990;65:845.

139. Kim RJ, Fieno DS, Parrish TB, et al. Relationship of MRI contrast delayed-enhancement to irreversible injury, infarct age and contractile function. *Circulation* 1999;100:1992.

140. Fieno DS, Kin RJ, Chen EL, et al. Contrast-enhanced magnetic resonance imaging of myocardium at risk: distinction between reversible and irreversible injury throughout infarct healing. *J Am Coll Cardiol* 2000;36:1985.

141. Van der Wall EE, Van Dijkman PRM, De Roos A, et al. Diagnostic significance of gadolinium-DTPA (diethylene-triamine penta-acetic acid) enhanced magnetic resonance imaging in thrombolytic therapy for acute myocardial infarction: its potential in assessing reperfusion. *Br Heart J* 1990;63:12.

142. McNamara MT, Higgins CB. Magnetic resonance imaging of chronic myocardial infarcts in man. *AJR Am J Roentgenol* 1986;146:316.

143. Van Rugge FP, Van der Wall EE, Van Dijkman PRM, et al. Usefulness of ultrafast magnetic resonance imaging in healed myocardial infarction. *Am J Cardiol* 1992;70:1233.

144. Higgins CB, Lanzer P, Stark D, et al. Imaging by nuclear magnetic resonance in patients with chronic ischemic heart disease. *Circulation* 1984;69:523.

145. Dooms GC, Higgins CB. MR imaging of cardiac thrombi. *J Comput Assist Tomogr* 1986;10:415.

146. Sechtem U, Theissen P, Heindel W, et al. Diagnosis of left ventricular thrombi by magnetic resonance imaging and comparison with angiocardiography, computed tomography and echocardiography. *Am J Cardiol* 1989;64:1195.

147. Rokey R, Verani MS, Bolli R, et al. Myocardial infarct size quantification by MR imaging early after coronary artery occlusion in dogs. *Radiology* 1986;158:771.

148. Bouchard A, Reeves RC, Cranney G, et al. Assessment of myocardial infarct size by means of T2-weighted 1H nuclear magnetic imaging. *Am Heart J* 1989;117:281.

149. Turnbull LW, Ridgway JP, Nicoll JJ, et al. Estimating the size of myocardial infarction by magnetic resonance imaging. *Br Heart J* 1991;66:359.

150. Johns JA, Leavitt MB, Newell JB, et al. Quantitation of acute myocardial infarct size by nuclear magnetic resonance imaging. *J Am Coll Cardiol* 1990;15:143.

151. Holman ER, Van Jonbergen HPW, Van Dijkman PRM, et al. Comparison of magnetic resonance imaging studies with enzymatic indexes of myocardial necrosis for quantification of myocardial infarct size. *Am J Cardiol* 1993;71:1036.

152. De Roos A, Matheijssen NA, Doornbos J, et al. Assessment of myocardial infarct size after reperfusion therapy using gadolinium-DTPA-enhanced magnetic resonance imaging. *Radiology* 1990;176:517.

153. Wisenberg G, Finnie KJ, Jablonsky G, et al. Nuclear magnetic resonance and radionuclide angiographic assessment of acute myocardial infarction in a randomized trial of intravenous streptokinase. *Am J Cardiol* 1988;62:1011.

154. Sechtem U, Pflugfelder P, Cassidy MC, et al. Ventricular septal defect: visualization of shunt flow and determination of shunt size by cine MR imaging. *AJR Am J Roentgenol* 1987;149:689.

155. Ahmad M, Johnson RF, Fawcett HD, et al. Left ventricular aneurysm in short axis: a comparison of magnetic resonance, ultrasound and thallium-201 SPECT images. *Magn Reson Imaging* 1987;5:293.

156. Gomberg J, Feinsmith N, Askenase A, et al. Visualization of a left ventricular pseudoaneurysm with magnetic resonance imaging. *Am J Card Imaging* 1989;3:146.

157. Shapiro EP, Rogers WJ, Beyar R, et al. Determination of left ventricular mass by magnetic resonance imaging in hearts deformed by acute infarction. *Circulation* 1989;79:706.

158. Saeed M, Wendland MF, Seelos K, et al. Effect of cilazapril on regional left ventricular wall thickness and chamber dimensions following acute myocardial infarction: *in vivo* assessment using MRI. *Am Heart J* 1992;123:1472.

159. Blackwell GG, Pohost GM. The evolving role of MRI in the assessment of coronary artery disease. *Am J Cardiol* 1995;75:750.

160. Williams ES, Kaplan JI, Thatcher F, et al. Prolongation of proton spin lattice relaxation times in regionally ischemic tissue from dog hearts. *J Nucl Med* 1980;21:449.

161. Scholz TD, Martins JB, Skorton DJ. NMR relaxation times in acute myocardial infarction: relative influence of tissue water and fat content. *Magn Reson Med* 1992;23:89.

162. Miller DD, Holmvang G, Gill JB, et al. MRI detection of myocardial perfusion changes by gadolinium-DTPA infusion during dipyridamole hyperemia. *Magn Reson Med* 1989;10:246.

163. Manning WJ, Atkinson DJ, Grossman W, et al. First-pass nuclear magnetic resonance imaging studies using gadolinium DTPA in patients with coronary artery disease. *J Am Coll Cardiol* 1991;18:959.

164. Pennell DJ, Underwood SR, Longmore DB. Detection of coronary artery disease using MR imaging with dipyridamole. *J Comput Assist Tomogr* 1990;14:167.

165. Baer FM, Smolarz K, Theissen P, et al. Identification of hemodynamically significant coronary artery stenoses by dipyridamole-magnetic resonance imaging and 99mTc-methoxy-isobutyl-isonitrile-SPECT. *Int J Card Imaging* 1993;9:133.

166. Pennell DJ, Underwood SR, Manzara CC, et al. Magnetic resonance imaging during dobutamine stress in coronary artery disease. *Am J Cardiol* 1992;70:34.

167. Baer FM, Voth E, Theissen P, et al. Gradient-echo magnetic resonance imaging during incremental dobutamine infusion for the localization of coronary artery stenoses. *Eur Heart J* 1994;15:218.

168. Van Rugge FP, Van der Wall EE, Spanjersberg SJ, et al. Magnetic resonance imaging during dobutamine stress for detection and localization of coronary artery disease: quantitative wall motion analysis using a modification of the centerline method. *Circulation* 1994;90:127.

169. Baer FM, Theissen P, Crnac J, et al. Head to head comparison of dobutamine-trans-esophageal echocardiography and dobutamine-magnetic resonance imaging for the prediction of left ventricular functional recovery in patients with chronic coronary artery disease. *Eur Heart J* 2000;21:981

170. Hundley WG, Hamilton CA, Thomas MS. Utility of fast cine magnetic resonance imaging and display for the detection of myocardial ischemia in patients not well suited for second harmonic stress echocardiography. *Circulation* 1999;100:1697.

171. Schaefer S, Malloy CR, Katz J. Gadolinium-DTPA-enhanced nuclear magnetic resonance imaging of reperfused myocardium: identification of the myocardial bed at risk. *J Am Coll Cardiol* 1988;12:1064.

172. Masui T, Saeed M, Wendland MF, et al. Occlusive and reperfused myocardial infarcts: MR imaging differentiation with nonionic Gd-DTPA-BMA. *Radiology* 1991;181:77.

173. Saeed M, Wendland MF, Takehara Y, et al. Reversible and irreversible injury in the reperfused myocardium: differentiation with contrast material enhanced MR imaging. *Radiology* 1990;175:633.

174. Yu KK, Saeed M, Wendland MF, et al. Real-time dynamics of an extravascular magnetic resonance contrast medium in acutely infarcted myocardium using inversion recovery and gradient-recalled echo-planar imaging. *Invest Radiol* 1992;27:927.

175. Hillenbrand HB, Kim RJ, Parker MA, et al. Early assessment of myocardial salvage by contrast-enhanced magnetic resonance imaging. *Circulation* 2000;102:1678.

176. Schvartzman PR, Rodriguez L, Brunken RD, et al. Non-viable myocardium grade on delayed-enhancement MRI correlates inversely with amount of viable myocardium on dobutamine stress echocardiography and positron emission tomography. *Circulation* 2000;102:II-808.

177. Peshock RM. Assessing myocardial viability with magnetic resonance imaging. *Am J Card Imaging* 1992;6:237.

178. Baer FM, Smolarz K, Jungehulsing M, et al. Chronic myocardial infarction: assessment of morphology, function and perfusion by gradient-echo magnetic resonance imaging and technetium-99m methoxyisobutyl-isonitrile-SPECT. *Am Heart J* 1992;123:636.

179. Baer RM, Voth E, Schneider CA, et al. Comparison of low dose dobutamine-gradient-echo magnetic resonance imaging and positron emission tomography with [18F] fluorodeoxyglucose in patients with chronic coronary artery disease: a functional and morphological approach to the detection of residual myocardial viability. *Circulation* 1995;91:1006.

180. Baer FM, Voth E, LaRosee K, et al. Comparison of dobutamine transesophageal echocardiography and dobutamine magnetic resonance imaging for detection of residual myocardial viability. *Am J Cardiol* 1996;78:415.

181. Paulin S, von Schulthess GK, Fossel E, et al. MR imaging of the aortic root and proximal coronary arteries. *AJR Am J Roentgenol* 1987;148:665.

182. Alfidi RJ, Masaryk TJ, Haacke EM, et al. MR angiography of peripheral, carotid, and coronary arteries. *AJR Am J Roentgenol* 1987;149:1097.

183. Duerinckx AJ. Coronary MR angiography. *Radiol Clin North Am* 1999;37:273.

184. Edelman RR, Manning WJ, Burstein D, et al. Coronary arteries: breath-hold MR angiography. *Radiology* 1991;181:641.

185. Manning WJ, Li W, Boyle NG, et al. Fat suppressed breath-hold magnetic resonance coronary angiography. *Circulation* 1993;87:94.

186. Pennell DJ, Keegan J, Firmin DN, et al. Magnetic resonance imaging of the coronary arteries: techniques and preliminary results. *Br Heart J* 1993;70:315.

187. Manning WJ, Li W, Edelman RR. A preliminary report comparing magnetic resonance coronary angiography with conventional angiography. *N Engl J Med* 1993;328:828.

188. Duerinckx AJ, Urman MK. Two-dimensional coronary MR angiography: analysis of initial clinical results. *Radiology* 1994;193:731.

189. Post JC, van Rossum AC, Hofman MBM, et al. Three-dimensional respiratory-gated MR angiography of coronary arteries: comparison with conventional coronary angiography. *AJR Am J Roentgenol* 1996;166:1399.

190. Rogers WJ, Kramer CM, Simonetti OP, et al. Quantification of human coronary stenoses by magnetic resonance angiography. *Proc Soc Magn Reson* 1994;1:370.

191. Hundley WG, Clarke GD, Landau C, et al. Noninvasive determination of infarct artery patency by cine magnetic resonance angiography. *Circulation* 1995;91:1347.

192. Fayad ZA, Fuster V, Fallon JT, et al. Noninvasive in vivo human coronary artery lumen and wall imaging using black-blood magnetic resonance imaging. *Circulation* 2000;102:506.

193. Underwood SR, Firmin DN, Klipstein RH, et al. The assessment of coronary artery bypass grafts using magnetic resonance imaging with velocity mapping. *Br Heart J* 1987;57:193.

194. Keegan J, Firmin D, Gatehouse P, et al. The application of breathhold phase velocity mapping techniques to the measurement of coronary artery blood flow velocity: phantom data and initial in vivo results. *Magn Reson Med* 1994;31:526.

195. Edelman RR, Manning WL, Gervino E, et al. Flow velocity quantification in human coronary arteries with fast breathhold MR angiography. *J Magn Reson Imaging* 1993;3:699.

196. Poncelet B, Weisskopf RM, Wedeen VJ, et al. Time of flight quantification of coronary flow with echo-planar MRI. *Magn Reson Med* 1993;30:447.

197. Clarke GD, Eckels R, Chaney C, et al. Measurement of absolute epicardial coronary artery flow and flow reserve with breath-hold phase-contrast magnetic resonance imaging. *Circulation* 1995;91:2627.

198. Hundley WG, Lange RA, Clarke GD, et al. Assessment of coronary arterial flow and flow reserve in humans with magnetic resonance imaging. *Circulation* 1996;93:1502.

199. White RD, Caputo GR, Mark AS, et al. Coronary artery bypass graft patency: noninvasive evaluation with MR imaging. *Radiology* 1987;164:681.

200. Rubinstein RI, Askenase AD, Thickman D, et al. Magnetic resonance imaging to evaluate patency of aortocoronary bypass grafts. *Circulation* 1987;76:786.

201. White RD, Pflugfelder PW, Lipton MJ, et al. Coronary artery bypass grafts: evaluation of patency with cine MR imaging. *AJR Am J Roentgenol* 1988;150:1271.

202. Aurigemann GP, Reichek N, Axel L, et al. Noninvasive determination of coronary artery bypass graft patency by cine magnetic resonance imaging. *Circulation* 1989;80:1595.

203. Debatin JF, Strong JA, Sostman HD, et al. MR characterization of blood flow in native and grafted internal mammary arteries. *J Magn Reson Imaging* 1993;3:443.

204. Galjee MA, van Rossum AC, Doesburg T, et al. Value of magnetic resonance imaging in assessing patency and function of coronary artery bypass grafts: an angiographically controlled study. *Circulation* 1996;93:660.

205. Globits S, Higgins CB. Assessment of valvular heart disease by magnetic resonance imaging. *Am Heart J* 1995;129:369.

206. Underwood SR, Klipstein RH, Firmin DN, et al. Magnetic resonance assessment of aortic and mitral regurgitation. *Br Heart J* 1986;56:453.

207. Mitchell L, Jenkins JPR, Watson Y, et al. Diagnosis and assessment of mitral and aortic valve disease by cine-flow magnetic resonance imaging. *Magn Reson Imaging* 1989;12:181.

208. Casolo GC, Zampa V, Rega L, et al. Evaluation of mitral stenosis by cine magnetic resonance imaging. *Am Heart J* 1992;123:1252.

209. Yoshida K, Yoshikawa J, Hozumi T, et al. Assessment of aortic regurgitation by acceleration flow signal void proximal to the leaking orifice in cine magnetic resonance imaging. *Circulation* 1991;83:1951.

210. Wagner S, Auffermann W, Buser P, et al. Diagnostic accuracy and estimation of the severity of valvular regurgitation from the signal void on cine magnetic resonance imaging. *Am Heart J* 1989;118:760.

211. DeRoos A, Reichek N, Axel L, et al. Cine MR imaging in aortic stenosis. *J Comput Assist Tomogr* 1989;13:421.

212. Pflugfelder PW, Landzberg JS, Cassidy MM, et al. Comparison of cine MR imaging with Doppler echocardiography for evaluation of aortic regurgitation. *AJR Am J Roentgenol* 1989;152:729.

213. Pflugfelder PW, Sechtem U, White RD, et al. Noninvasive evaluation of mitral regurgitation by analysis of left atrial signal loss in cine magnetic resonance. *Am Heart J* 1989;117:1113.

214. Sechtem U, Pflugfelder PW, Cassidy MM, et al. Mitral and aortic regurgitation: quantification of regurgitant volumes with cine MR imaging. *Radiology* 1988;167:425.

215. Kilner PJ, Manzara CC, Mohiaddin RH, et al. Magnetic resonance velocity mapping in mitral and aortic valve stenosis. *Circulation* 1993;87:1239.

216. Dulce MC, Mostbeck GH, O'Sullivan M, et al. Severity of aortic regurgitation: interstudy reproducibility of measurements with velocity-encoded cine MR imaging. *Radiology* 1992;185:235.

217. Hill JA, Akins EW, Fitzsimmons JR, et al. Mitral stenosis: imaging by nuclear magnetic resonance. *Am J Cardiol* 1986;57:352.

218. Heidenreich PA, Steffens J, Fujita N, et al. Evaluation of mitral stenosis with velocity-encoded cine-magnetic resonance imaging. *Am J Cardiol* 1995;75:365.

219. Aurigemma G, Reichek N, Schiebler M, et al. Evaluation of mitral regurgitation by cine magnetic resonance imaging. *Am J Cardiol* 1990;66:621.

220. Glogar D, Globits S, Neuhold A, et al. Assessment of mitral regurgitation by magnetic resonance imaging. *Magn Reson Imaging* 1989;7:611.

221. Nishimura T, Yamada N, Itoh A, et al. Cine MR imaging in mitral regurgitation: comparison with color Doppler flow imaging. *AJR Am J Roentgenol* 1989;153:721.

222. Fujita N, Chazouilleres AF, Hartiala JJ, et al. Quantification of mitral regurgitation by velocity-encoded cine nuclear magnetic resonance imaging. *J Am Coll Cardiol* 1994;2:951.

223. Hundley WG, Li HF, Willard JE, et al. Magnetic resonance imaging assessment of the severity of mitral regurgitation: comparison with invasive techniques. *Circulation* 1995;92:1151.

224. Kupari M, Hekali P, Keto P, et al. Assessment of aortic valve area in aortic stenosis by magnetic resonance imaging. *Am J Cardiol* 1992;70:952.

225. Sondergaard L, Hildebrandt P, Lindvig K, et al. Valve area and cardiac output in aortic stenosis: quantitation by magnetic resonance velocity mapping. *Am Heart J* 1993;127:1156.

226. Eichenberger AC, Jenni R, von Schulthess GK. Aortic valve pressure gradients in patients with aortic valve stenosis: quantitation with velocity-encoded cine MR imaging. *AJR Am J Roentgenol* 1993;160:971.

227. Cranney GB, Benjelloun H, Perry GJ, et al. Rapid assessment of aortic regurgitation and left ventricular function using cine nuclear magnetic resonance imaging and the proximal convergence zone. *Am J Cardiol* 1993;71:1074.

228. Nishimura F. Oblique cine MRI for the valuation of aortic regurgitation: comparison with cine angiography. *Clin Cardiol* 1992;15:73.

229. Honda N, Machida K, Hashimoto M, et al. Aortic regurgitation: quantitation with MR imaging velocity mapping. *Radiology* 1993;186:189.

230. Sondergaard L, Lindvig K, Hildebrandt P, et al. Quantitation of aortic regurgitation by magnetic resonance velocity mapping. *Am Heart J* 1993;125:1081.

231. Wexler L, Higgins CB. The use of magnetic resonance imaging in adult congenital heart disease. *Am J Cardiol Imaging* 1995;9:15.

232. Rebergen SA, Chin JGJ, Ottenkamp J, et al. Pulmonary regurgitation in the late postoperative follow-up of tetralogy of Fallot. *Circulation* 1993;88:2257.

233. Randall PA, Kohman LJ, Scalzetti EM, et al. Magnetic resonance imaging of prosthetic cardiac valves *in vitro* and *in vivo*. *Am J Cardiol* 1988;62:973.

234. Deutsch HJ, Bachmann R, Sechtem U, et al. Regurgitant flow in cardiac valve prostheses: diagnostic value of gradient echo nuclear magnetic resonance imaging in reference to transesophageal two-dimensional color Doppler echocardiography. *J Am Coll Cardiol* 1992;19:1500.

235. Doherty NE, Fujita N, Caputo GR, et al. Measurement of right ventricular mass in normal and dilated cardiomyopathic ventricles using cine magnetic resonance imaging. *Am J Cardiol* 1992;69:1223.

236. Buser PT, Aufferman W, Holt WW, et al. Noninvasive evaluation of global left ventricular function with use of cine nuclear magnetic resonance. *J Am Coll Cardiol* 1989;13:1294.

237. Doherty NE, Seelos KC, Suzuki J-I, et al. Application of cine nuclear magnetic resonance imaging for sequential evaluation of response to angiotensin-converting enzyme inhibitor therapy in dilated cardiomyopathy. *J Am Coll Cardiol* 1992;19:1294.

238. Fujita N, Hartiala J, O'Sullivan M, et al. Assessment of left ventricular diastolic function in dilated cardiomyopathy with cine magnetic resonance imaging: effect of an angiotensin converting enzyme inhibitor, benazepril. *Am Heart J* 1993;125:171.

239. Fujita N, Duerinckx AJ, Higgins CB. Variation in left ventricular regional wall stress with cine magnetic resonance imaging: normal subjects versus dilated cardiomyopathy. *Am Heart J* 1993;125:1337.

240. Park JH, Kim YM, Chung JW, et al. MR imaging of hypertrophic cardiomyopathy. *Radiology* 1992;185:441.

241. Been M, Kean D, Smith MA, et al. Nuclear magnetic resonance in hypertrophic cardiomyopathy. *Br Heart J* 1985;54:48.

242. White RD, Obuchowski NA, Gunawardena S, et al. Left ventricular outflow tract obstruction in hypertrophic cardiomyopathy: pre- and post-operative evaluation by computed tomography magnetic resonance imaging. *Am J Cardiol Imaging* 1996;1:1.

243. Sardanelli F, Molinari G, Petillo A, et al. MRI in hypertrophic cardiomyopathy: a morphofunctional study. *J Comput Assist Tomogr* 1993;17:862.

244. Kramer CM, Reichek N, Ferrari V, et al. Regional heterogeneity of function in hypertrophic cardiomyopathy. *Circulation* 1994;90:186.

245. Dong SJ, MacGregor JH, Crawley AP, et al. Left ventricular wall thickness and regional systolic function in patients with hypertrophic cardiomyopathy: a three-dimensional tagged magnetic resonance imaging study. *Circulation* 1994;90:1200.

246. Beach GM, Wedeen VJ, Weisskoff RM, et al. Intramural mechanics in hypertrophic cardiomyopathy: functional mapping with strain-rate MR imaging. *Radiology* 1995;197:117.

247. Nakatani S, White RD, Powell KA, et al. Dynamic magnetic resonance imaging assessment of the effect of ventricular wall curvature on regional function in hypertrophic cardiomyopathy. *Am J Cardiol* 1996;77:618.

248. White RD, Lever HM, Murphy DJ, et al. MRI-tagging measurements of impaired regional LV-midwall contractility correlate with histopathology in hypertrophic obstructive cardiomyopathy. *J Am Coll Cardiol* 1993;21(Suppl A):266A.

249. Suzuki JI, Chang JM, Caputo GR, et al. Evaluation of right ventricular early diastolic filling by cine nuclear magnetic resonance imaging in patients with hypertrophic cardiomyopathy. *J Am Coll Cardiol* 1991;18:120.

250. White RD, Chow KC, Hardy PA, et al. Improved characterization of myocardial histopathology in hypertrophic obstructive cardiomyopathy with bolus-first-pass ultrafast MRI. *Circulation* 1993;88(Suppl I):I.

251. Masui T, Finck S, Higgins CB. Constrictive pericarditis and restrictive cardiomyopathy: evaluation with MR imaging. *Radiology* 1992;182:369.

252. von Kemp K, Beckers R, Vandenweghe J, et al. Echocardiography and magnetic resonance imaging in cardiac amyloidosis. *Acta Cardiol* 1989;1:29.

253. Matsui S, Murakami E, Takekoshi N, et al. Myocardial tissue characterization by magnetic resonance imaging in Fabry's disease. *Am Heart J* 1989;117:472.

254. Sechtem U, Higgins CB, Sommerhoff BA, et al. Magnetic resonance imaging of restrictive cardiomyopathy. *Am J Cardiol* 1987;59:480.

255. Blankenberg F, Eisenberg S, Scheinman MN, et al. Use of cine gradient echo (GRE) MR in the imaging of cardiac hemochromatosis. *J Comput Assist Tomogr* 1994;18:136.

256. Riedy K, Fisher MR, Belic N, et al. MR imaging of myocardial sarcoidosis. *AJR Am J Roentgenol* 1988;151:915.

257. Soldo SJ, Norris SL, Gober JR, et al. MRI-derived ventricular volume curves for the assessment of left ventricular function. *Magn Reson Imaging* 1994;12:711.

258. Karwatowski SP, Mohiaddin R, Yang GZ, et al. Assessment of regional left ventricular long-axis motion with MR velocity mapping in healthy subjects. *J Magn Reson Imaging* 1994;4:151.

259. Hartiala JJ, Mostbeck GH, Foster E, et al. Velocity-encoded cine MRI in the evaluation of left ventricular diastolic function: measurement of mitral valve and pulmonary vein flow velocities and flow volume across the mitral valve. *Am Heart J* 1993;125:1054.

260. White RD, Hardy PA, VanDyke CW, et al. Diastolic dysfunction: dynamic MRI velocity-mapping of related flow patterns in the superior vena cava. *J Magn Reson Imaging* 1993;3:65.

261. Blake LM, Scheinman MM, Higgins CB. MR features of arrhythmogenic right ventricular dysplasia. *AJR Am J Roentgenol* 1994;162:809.

262. Ricci C, Longo R, Pagnan L, et al. Magnetic resonance imaging in right ventricular dysplasia. *Am J Cardiol* 1992;70:1589.

263. Auffermann W, Wichter T, Breithardt G, et al. Arrhythmogenic right ventricular disease: MR imaging vs angiography. *AJR Am J Roentgenol* 1993;161:549.

264. Carlson MD, White RD, Trohman RG, et al. Right ventricular outflow tract ventricular tachycardia: detection of previously unrecognized anatomical abnormalities using cine magnetic resonance imaging. *J Am Coll Cardiol* 1994;24:720.

265. Olson MC, Posniak HV, McDonald V, et al. Computed tomography and magnetic resonance imaging of the pericardium. *Radiographics* 1989;9:633.

266. Sechtem U, Tscholakoff D, Higgins CB. MRI of the abnormal pericardium. *AJR Am J Roentgenol* 1986;147:245.

267. White RD, Zisch RJ. Magnetic resonance imaging of pericardial disease and paracardiac and intracardiac masses. In: Elliott LP, ed. *The fundamentals of cardiac imaging in children and adults.* Philadelphia: Lippincott, 1991:420.

268. Mulvagh SL, Rokey R, Vick GW, et al. Usefulness of nuclear magnetic resonance imaging for evaluation of pericardial effusions, and comparison with two-dimensional echocardiography. *Am J Cardiol* 1989;64:1002.

269. Stark DD, Higgins CB, Lanzer P, et al. Magnetic resonance imaging of the pericardium: normal and pathologic findings. *Radiology* 1984;150:469.

270. Rokey R, Vick GW III, Bolli R, et al. Assessment of experimental pericardial effusion using nuclear magnetic resonance imaging techniques. *Am Heart J* 1991;121:1161.

271. Henkelman RM, Bronskill MJ. Artifacts in magnetic resonance imaging. *Rev Magn Reson Med* 1987;2:77.

272. Soulen RL, Stark DD, Higgins CB. Magnetic resonance imaging of constrictive pericardial disease. *Am J Cardiol* 1985;55:480.

273. Link KM, Loehr SP, Baker DM, et al. Magnetic resonance imaging of the thoracic aorta. *Semin Ultrasound CT MRI* 1993;14:91.

274. White RD, Obuchowski NA, VanDyke CW, et al. Thoracic aortic disease: evaluation using a single MRA volume series. *J Comput Assist Tomogr* 1994;18:843.

275. Bogren HG, Buonocore MH. Blood flow measurements in the aorta and major arteries with MR velocity mapping. *J Magn Reson Imaging* 1994;4:119.

276. White RD, Higgins CB. Magnetic resonance imaging of thoracic vascular disease. *J Thorac Imaging* 1989;4:34.

277. Auffermann W, Olofsson P, Stoney R, et al. MR imaging of complications of aortic surgery. *J Comput Assist Tomogr* 1987;11:982.

278. Tennant WG, Hartnell GG, Baird RN, et al. Inflammatory aortic aneurysms: characteristic appearance on magnetic resonance imaging. *Eur J Vasc Surg* 1992;6:399.

279. Yucel EK, Steinberg FL, Egglin TK, et al. Penetrating aortic ulcers: diagnosis with MR imaging. *Radiology* 1990;177:779.

280. Banki JHZ, Meiners LC, Barentsz JO, et al. Detection of aortic dissection by magnetic resonance imaging in adults with Marfan's syndrome. *Int J Cardiol Imaging* 1992;8:249.

281. Woodard PK, Patz EF, Sostman HD. Pseudoaneurysms at aortic cannulation site after coronary artery bypass graft: MR findings. *J Comput Assist Tomogr* 1992;16:883.

282. Nienaber CA, von Kodolitsch Y, Nicolas V, et al. The diagnosis of thoracic aortic dissection by noninvasive imaging procedures. *N Engl J Med* 1993;328:1.

283. Nienaber CA, Spielmann RP, von Kodolitsch Y, et al. Diagnosis of thoracic aortic dissection: magnetic resonance imaging versus transesophageal echocardiography. *Circulation* 1992;85:434.

284. Flamm SD, VanDyke CW, White RD. MR Imaging of the thoracic aorta. *Magn Reson Imaging Clin N Am* 1996;4:217.

285. Nienaber CA, von Kodolitsch Y, Petersen B, et al. Intramural hemorrhage of the thoracic aorta: diagnostic and therapeutic implications. *Circulation* 1995;92:1465.

286. Murray JG, Manisali M, Flamm SD, et al. Intramural

hematoma of the thoracic aorta: MRI findings and their prognostic implications. *Radiology* 1997;204:349.

287. Crooks L, Sheldon P, Kaufman L, et al. Quantification of obstructions in vessels by nuclear magnetic resonance (NMR). *IEEE Trans Nucl Sci* 1982;NS-29:1181.

288. Vinitski S, Consigny PM, Shapiro MJ, et al. Magnetic resonance chemical shift imaging and spectroscopy of atherosclerotic plaque. *Invest Radiol* 1991;26:703.

289. Toussaint JF, LaMuraglia GM, Southern JF, et al. Magnetic resonance images lipid, fibrous, calcified, hemorrhagic, and thrombotic components of human atherosclerosis in vivo. *Circulation* 1996;94:932.

290. Merickel MB, Carman CS, Brookeman JR, et al. Image analysis and quantifications of atherosclerosis using MRI. *Comput Med Imaging Graph* 1991;15:207.

291. Martin AJ, Gotlieb AI, Henkelman RM. High-resolution MR imaging of human arteries. *J Magn Reson Imaging* 1995;5:93.

292. Wesbey GE, Higgins CB, Amparo EG, et al. Peripheral vascular disease: correlation of MR imaging and angiography. *Radiology* 1985;156:733.

293. Mulligan SA, Matsuda TM, Lanzer P, et al. Peripheral arterial occlusive disease: prospective comparison of MR angiography and color duplex US with conventional angiography. *Radiology* 1991;178:695.

294. Yucel EK, Kaufman JA, Geller SC, et al. Atherosclerotic occlusive disease of the lower extremity: prospective evaluation with two-dimensional time-of-flight MR angiography. *Radiology* 1993;187:637.

295. White RD, Winkler ML, Higgins CB. MR imaging of pulmonary arterial hypertension and pulmonary emboli. *AJR Am J Roentgenol* 1987;149:15.

296. Hatabu H, Gefter WB, Konishi J, et al. Magnetic resonance approaches to the evaluation of pulmonary vascular anatomy and physiology. *Magn Reson Q* 1991;7:208.

297. Posteraro RH, Sostman HD, Spritzer CE, et al. Cine-gradient-refocused MR imaging of central pulmonary emboli. *AJR Am J Roentgenol* 1989;152:465.

298. Schiebler ML, Holland GA, Hatabu H, et al. Suspected pulmonary embolism: prospective evaluation with pulmonary MR angiography. *Radiology* 1993;189:125.

299. Sostman HD, Layish DT, Tapson VF, et al. Prospective comparison of helical CT and MR imaging in clinically suspected acute pulmonary embolism. *J Magn Reson Imaging* 1996;6:275.

300. Grist TM, Sostman HD, MacFall JR, et al. Pulmonary angiography with MR imaging: preliminary clinical experience. *Radiology* 1993;189:523.

301. Bouchard A, Higgins CB, Byrd BF, et al. Magnetic resonance imaging in pulmonary arterial hypertension. *Am J Cardiol* 1985;56:938.

302. von Schulthess GK, Fisher MR, Higgins CB. Pathologic blood flow in pulmonary vascular disease as shown by gated magnetic resonance imaging. *Ann Intern Med* 1985;103:317.

303. Frank H, Globits S, Glogar D, et al. Detection and quantification of pulmonary artery hypertension with MR imaging: results in 23 patients. *AJR Am J Roentgenol* 1993;161:27.

304. Bogren HG, Klipstein RH, Mohiaddin RH, et al. Pulmonary artery distensibility and blood flow patterns: a magnetic resonance study of normal subjects and of patients with pulmonary arterial hypertension. *Am Heart J* 1989;118:990.

305. Mohiaddin RH, Paz R, Theodoropoulos S, et al. Magnetic resonance characterization of pulmonary arterial blood flow after single lung transplantation. *J Thorac Cardiovasc Surg* 1991;101:1016.

306. Patel SR, Kirby TJ, McCarthy PM, et al. Lung transplantation: the Cleveland Clinic experience. *Cleve Clin J Med* 1993;60:303.

307. Schvartzman PR, White RD. Imaging of cardiac and paracardiac masses. *J Thorac Imaging* 2000;15:265.

308. Lund JT, Ehman RL, Julsrud PR, et al. Cardiac masses: assessment by MR imaging. *AJR Am J Roentgenol* 1989;152:469.

309. Winkler M, Higgins CB. Suspected intracardiac masses: evaluation with MR imaging. *Radiology* 1987;165:117.

310. Brown JJ, Barakos JA, Higgins CB. Magnetic resonance imaging of cardiac and paracardiac masses. *J Thorac Imaging* 1989;4:58.

311. Niwa K, Tashima K, Terai M, et al. Contrast-enhanced magnetic resonance imaging of cardiac tumors in children. *Am Heart J* 1989;118:424.

312. Go RT, O'Donnell JK, Underwood DA, et al. Comparison of gated cardiac MRI and 2D echocardiography of intracardiac neoplasms. *AJR Am J Roentgenol* 1985;145:21.

313. Freedberg RS, Kronzon I, Rumancik WM, et al. The contribution of magnetic resonance imaging to the evaluation of intracardiac tumors diagnosed by echocardiography. *Circulation* 1988;77:96.

314. Gamsu G, Stark D, Webb WR, et al. Magnetic resonance imaging of benign mediastinal masses. *Radiology* 1984;151:709.

315. Barakos JA, Brown JJ, Higgins CB. MR imaging of secondary cardiac and paracardiac lesions. *AJR Am J Roentgenol* 1989;153:47.

316. Gomes AS, Lois JF, Child JS, et al. Cardiac tumors and thrombus: evaluation with MR imaging. *AJR Am J Roentgenol* 1987;149:895.

317. Link KM, Lesko NM. Magnetic resonance imaging in the evaluation of congenital heart disease. *Magn Reson Q* 1991;7:173.

318. Simpson IA, Sahn DJ. Adult congenital heart disease: use of transthoracic echocardiography versus magnetic resonance imaging scanning. *Am J Card Imaging* 1995;9:29.

319. Hirsch R, Kilner PJ, Connelly MS, et al. Diagnosis in adolescents and adults with congenital heart disease: prospective assessment of individual and combined roles of magnetic resonance imaging and transesophageal echocardiography. *Circulation* 1994;90:2937.

320. Rees S, Firmin D, Mohiaddin R, et al. Application of flow measurements by magnetic resonance velocity mapping to congenital heart disease. *Am J Cardiol* 1989;64:953.

321. Kersting-Sommerhoff BA, Diethelm L, Stanger P, et al. Evaluation of complex congenital ventricular anomalies with magnetic resonance imaging. *Am Heart J* 1990;120:133.

322. Gomes AS, Lois JF, George B, et al. Congenital abnormalities of the aortic arch: MR imaging. *Radiology* 1987;165:691.

323. Simpson IA, Chung KJ, Glass RF, et al. Cine magnetic resonance imaging for evaluation of anatomy and flow relations in infants and children with coarctation of the aorta. *Circulation* 1988;78:142.

324. Kilner PJ, Firmin DN, Rees RS, et al. Valve and great vessel stenosis: assessment with MR jet velocity mapping. *Radiology* 1991;178:229.

325. Kersting-Sommerhoff BA, Sechtem UP, Fisher MR, et al. MR imaging of congenital anomalies of the aortic arch. *AJR Am J Roentgenol* 1987;149:9.

326. VanDyke CW, White RD. Congenital abnormalities of the thoracic aorta presenting in the adult. *J Thorac Imaging* 1994;9:230.

327. Vick GW, Rokey R, Huhta JC, et al. Nuclear magnetic resonance imaging of the pulmonary arteries, subpulmonary region, and aorticopulmonary shunts: a comparative study with two-dimensional echocardiography and angiography. *Am Heart J* 1990;119:1103.

328. Rees RSO, Somerville J, Underwood SR, et al. Magnetic resonance imaging of the pulmonary arteries and their systemic connections in pulmonary atresia: comparison with angiographic and surgical findings. *Br Heart J* 1987;58:621.

329. Takayuki M, Seelos KC, Kersting-Sommerhoff K, et al. Abnormalities of the pulmonary veins: evaluation with MRI imaging and comparison with cardiac angiography and echocardiography. *Radiology* 1991;181:645.

330. Chung KJ, Simpson IA, Newman R, et al. Cine magnetic resonance imaging for evaluation of congenital heart disease: role in pediatric cardiology compared with echocardiography and angiography. *J Pediatr* 1988;113:1028.

331. Kersting-Sommerhoff BA, Seelos KC, Hardy C, et al. Evaluation of surgical procedures for cyanotic congenital heart disease by using MR imaging. *AJR Am J Roentgenol* 1990;155:259.

332. Rees S, Somerville J, Warnes C, et al. Comparison of magnetic resonance imaging with echocardiography and radionuclide angiography in assessing cardiac function and anatomy following Mustard's operation for transposition of the great arteries. *Am J Cardiol* 1988;61:1316.

333. Hetherington HP, Luney DJE, Vaughan JT, et al. 3D 31P spectroscopic imaging of the human heart at 4.1 T. *Magn Reson Med* 1995;33:427.

334. Jolesz FA, Blumenfeld SM. Interventional use of magnetic resonance imaging. *Magn Reson Q* 1994;10:85.

335. Weissleder R, Bogdanov A, Papisov M. Drug targeting in magnetic resonance imaging. *Magn Reson Q* 1992;8:55.

POSITRON EMISSION TOMOGRAPHY

MARKUS SCHWAIGER
SIBYLLE I. ZIEGLER

OVERVIEW

Positron emission tomography (PET) represents the most advanced scintigraphic imaging technique developed for *in vivo* quantification of cardiac physiology and biochemistry. The state-of-the-art PET instrumentation allows delineation of regional tracer activity with high spatial (4 to 8 mm) and temporal resolution (few seconds per image). A large number of radiopharmaceuticals have been developed to study myocardial perfusion, energy metabolism, and autonomic innervation of the heart. Initial research applications included assessment of fatty acid and glucose metabolism, followed by the quantification of regional myocardial perfusion in patients with coronary artery disease (CAD). More recently, newer tracers such as radiolabeled beta-receptor antagonists allow the presynaptic and postsynaptic evaluation of sympathetic cardiac innervation. Metabolic imaging with fluorine-18-fluorodeoxyglucose (F-18-FDG) has emerged as an important clinical application for assessment of tissue viability in patients with impaired left ventricular function with well-validated diagnostic and prognostic information. F-18-FDG has also been used in combination with single-photon emission computed tomography (SPECT)

imaging to exploit the physiologic information, without the need for expensive imaging technology such as PET. PET, in combination with perfusion tracers, provides accurate diagnosis and localization of CAD. The development of less costly PET imaging devices and new radiopharmaceuticals for specific tissue characterization is needed to ensure that PET remains a competitive research and clinical tool in cardiology.

GLOSSARY

Polar map: Planar representation of tracer accumulation in the left ventricular myocardium, determined by volumetric sampling of the scintigraphic data.

Tracer: Very small amount of substance, labeled with a radioactive isotope, and the decay can be detected externally.

Transmission scan: Measurement of photon attenuation using external sources. Data are used for correction of emission data.

HISTORICAL PERSPECTIVE

PET was developed as a noninvasive method for quantitative imaging of tissue tracer distribution *in vivo* (autoradiography). Three important technical requirements contribute

M. Schwaiger: Department of Nuclear Medicine, Klinikum Rechts der Isar, Technische Universität München, München, Germany

S. I. Ziegler: Department of Nuclear Medicine, Technische Universität München, München, Germany

to this method: the labeling of a biologic substance with short-lived positron emitters, the detection of the annihilation radiation, and the reconstruction of the two-dimensional tracer distribution in transversal slices through the body. Radiopharmacy, instrumentation, and data processing have evolved since the discovery of artificial radioactivity by I. Curie and F. Joliot in 1934. Radioactive isotopes such as carbon-11 (C-11), nitrogen-13 (N-13), or F-18 became available in the late 1930s and early 1940s after the development of the cyclotron by E. O. Lawrence and were used in biologic (1) and the first human studies (2). The advantage of using coincidence measurements for collimation became apparent and was implemented for the first time in a positron probe by Brownell (3) and in a positron scanner for brain studies by Aronow (4). Short-lived radionuclides proved useful for metabolic studies and the first cyclotron that was dedicated to medical application was installed at the Hammersmith Hospital in 1955. With the tomographic imaging of single photon emitters, Kuhl introduced transverse section scanning using a backprojection algorithm (1963) (5). These advances in reconstruction also promoted the development of tomographs for positron imaging in the early 1970s, when the research group of Hoffmann, Phelps, and Ter Pogossian at Washington University built the first positron emission tomograph for brain imaging (6).

PET was introduced in the 1970s as a new imaging modality in cardiology by investigators at Washington University in St. Louis (7). Initial studies used metabolic tracers such as F-18-FDG and C-11 palmitate for the noninvasive characterization of myocardial substrate metabolism. These investigations took advantage of the availability of biologically active tracers labeled with short-lived isotopes such as C-11 and F-18 and demonstrated the ability of PET to describe the interaction of various substrates for cardiac energy metabolism. With the introduction of flow markers such as N-13 ammonia and oxygen-15 (O-15) water, the application of PET shifted toward the evaluation of myocardial perfusion primarily in patients with CAD. Since then, the technical advances of PET have allowed sophisticated biochemical and physiologic investigations of the heart, using a large number of radiopharmaceuticals to examine not only flow and metabolism, but also the autonomic innervation of the heart. The method provides quantitative measurements of spatial as well as temporal distribution of radioactivity within the blood and myocardium. Although other imaging modalities provide similar information, PET should be considered the most validated and accurate tool to measure myocardial perfusion and to allow quantitative tissue characterization assessing various aspects of cardiac function.

This chapter reviews the current role of PET in the functional evaluation of CAD and other cardiovascular disorders. Established clinical applications, as well as experimental concepts, are discussed. Finally, the results obtained with PET are compared with those derived from SPECT

and other imaging modalities to define the clinical role of PET in cardiology.

IMAGING PRINCIPLES

Imaging of regional tracer concentration is accomplished by the unique properties of positron decay and annihilation. Positron-emitting radionuclides have a nuclear imbalance characterized by an excess of protons. To restore stability to the nuclear structure, a proton is converted to a neutron, and a positron is emitted. This energetic positron traverses a few millimeters through the tissue until it becomes thermalized by electrostatic interaction between the electrons and the atomic nuclei of the media and combines with a free electron to form a two-particle atom-like entity called a *positronium*. The positronium quickly decays by annihilation, which converts the positron and electron mass into energy and generates a pair of gamma rays. Conservation of energy and momentum of the positronium before annihilation require the photons to travel in nearly opposite directions (180 degrees apart) with an energy of 511 keV each (Fig. 55.1). The opposed photons from positron decay can be detected by using pairs of colinearly aligned detectors. Gamma rays interact with these aligned detectors within a predefined time window and are registered as radioactive events (coincidence counting). The detector pairs of a PET system are installed in a ring-like pattern, which allows measurement of radioactivity along lines through the organ of interest at a series of angles and radial distances. This angular information is used to reconstruct tomographic images of regional radioactivity distribution. State-of-the-art PETs consist of multiple, closely

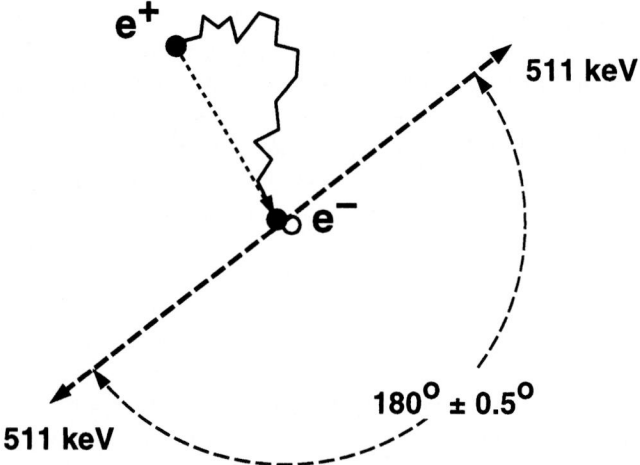

FIGURE 55.1 Positron emission and decay. The energetic positron (e+) travels several millimeters in the tissue before it combines with an electron (e−). The positron and electron annihilate, resulting in two opposing gamma rays with 511 keV each. See text for details.

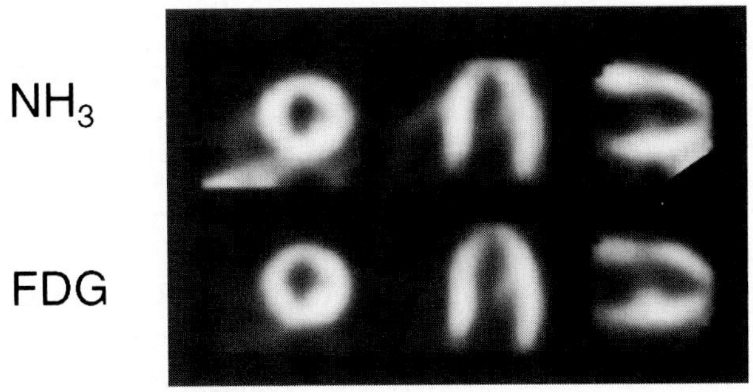

FIGURE 55.2 Positron emission tomographic images of normal volunteer with nitrogen-13 ammonia (NH₃) and fluorine-18-fluorodeoxyglucose (FDG).

packed rings of detectors that enable simultaneous imaging of several image planes.

Because the left ventricular wall is approximately 10 mm thick, high spatial resolution is necessary for the quantitative analysis of tissue tracer concentration (Fig. 55.2). The spatial resolution of PET approaches 5 to 7 mm in all axes and is expected to improve to approximately 2 to 3 mm in the future. Myocardial movement and change in wall thickness during the cardiac cycle affect the image resolution. PET data quality can be improved by ECG gated acquisitions (8).

Correction of photon attenuation is a prerequisite for tracer distribution measurements in the heart to avoid artifacts caused by tissue surrounding the heart. External sources are used to perform a transmission scan, which allows estimates of regional attenuation factors. Ring or rotating pin sources made of positron emitters are used for this purpose (9,10).

The PET detector system has to perform linearly over a wide range of count rates and allow for short scan time intervals to monitor the rapid uptake and release of tracers. Most of the current commercial tomographs use block detectors made of scintillation crystals (bismuth germanate) and photomultipliers (11). New detector materials such as lutetium oxyorthosilicate and lutetium aluminum perov-skite may improve imaging performance at a reasonable cost. Lutetium oxyorthosilicate has a shorter scintillation light-decay time, higher light output, and approximately the same attenuation length compared with bismuth germanate (12).

Collimators have been designed for imaging 511-keV gamma rays from positron emitters with SPECT systems. Although spatial resolution (15 to 20 mm) and detection efficiency (eight times less) are lower in these systems compared with PET, good imaging quality can be achieved for cardiac studies. The concept of dual-head SPECT cameras without collimators in coincidence mode was introduced. By exploiting the electronic collimation inherent in coincidence detection, sensitivity is increased. Using conventional nuclear medicine instrumentation could facilitate the widespread use of imaging positron emitters (13,14).

PRINCIPLES OF RADIONUCLIDE PRODUCTION AND RADIOCHEMISTRY

C-11, N-13, O-15, and F-18 are the most common positron-emitting radionuclides, all of which have a short physical half-life ranging from 122 seconds for O-15 to 110 minutes for F-18 (Table 55.1).

These radionuclides do not occur naturally; they must be produced using a nuclear reaction. The predominant and most efficient production method is to modify the nuclear structure of specific stable radionuclides by accelerated particle bombardment with either protons or deuterons. A cyclotron is a particle accelerator used most often for radioisotope production in PET imaging (15,16).

Few positron-emitting radionuclides are generator produced. A generator consists of a parent–daughter radionuclide pair in an apparatus that permits a separation and extraction of the daughter compound from the parent. The daughter radionuclide is replenished continuously by decay of the parent. The most common generator system in cardiology is strontium-82/rubidium-82 (17). The preparation of radiopharmaceuticals for PET requires a dedicated

TABLE 55.1 TRACERS COMMONLY AVAILABLE FOR CARDIAC POSITRON EMISSION TOMOGRAPHIC APPLICATIONS

Radionuclide	Physical half-life	Radiopharmaceutical	Application
Rubidium-82	76 sec	Rubidium	Flow
Oxygen-15	120 sec	Water	Flow
Nitrogen-13	10 min	Ammonia	Flow
Carbon-11	20 min	Palmitate	Fatty acid metabolism
		Acetate	Oxygen consumption
		Hydroxyephedrine	Catecholamine uptake
		CGP-12177	Beta-receptor density
Fluorine-18	110 min	Deoxyglucose	Glucose metabolism
		Misonidazole	Hypoxia
		FTHA	Fatty acid metabolism

FTHA, 14(R,S)-[18F]-fluoro-6-thiaheptadecanoic acid.

radiopharmaceutical facility. Because of the short half-lives of the isotopes, novel adaptations of sometimes complex synthetic procedures are needed to prepare useful amounts of molecules. Because there are positron-emitting radionuclides of oxygen, carbon, and nitrogen, it is theoretically possible to label any organic compound of interest, whether it is a natural substance or a synthetic drug. Fluorine, although not often found in naturally occurring molecules, can be readily substituted for a hydrogen or hydroxyl group and is a favorite of radiochemists designing new pharmaceuticals. With these four radionuclides a large number of positron-emitting tracers can be synthesized and used in clinical studies.

TRACER KINETIC MODELING

Current PET instrumentation allows for the acquisition of scintigraphic data, with high temporal resolution necessary for the description of tracer kinetics in myocardial and vascular structures. In contrast to other organs, the large blood chambers of the right and left ventricle allow simultaneous measurements of radioactivity in blood and tissue. Several studies have validated the accuracy of this approach for the noninvasive determination of the arterial input function without the need for arterial blood sampling (18).

Combining temporal sequencing of activity changes in blood and myocardium, tracer tissue uptake rates as well as clearance of activity from tissue can be quantitated (19). Depending on the radiopharmaceutical used, tracer kinetic models can be used to derive estimates of myocardial blood flow, metabolic rate, and tissue tracer retention. The most commonly used kinetic models are two- or three-compartment models. Although physiologic processes are more complicated than can be described by such simple models, limitations in counting statistics and duration of data acquisition require a simplification of the physiologic process with such models. Please refer to references 19 and 20, both excellent reviews that discuss details of tracer kinetic modeling.

ASSESSMENT OF MYOCARDIAL BLOOD FLOW

Flow Tracer

Blood flow tracers can be classified based on their physiologic behavior. O-15 water, for example, represents a freely diffusable tracer that washes in and out of myocardial tissue as a function of blood flow. The first-pass extraction of O-15 water in the heart is not diffusion limited, nor is O-15 water tissue extraction affected by any metabolic pathways (21–23) (Fig. 55.3).

The second group of flow markers are radiotracers, which are retained in myocardial tissue proportional to myocardial

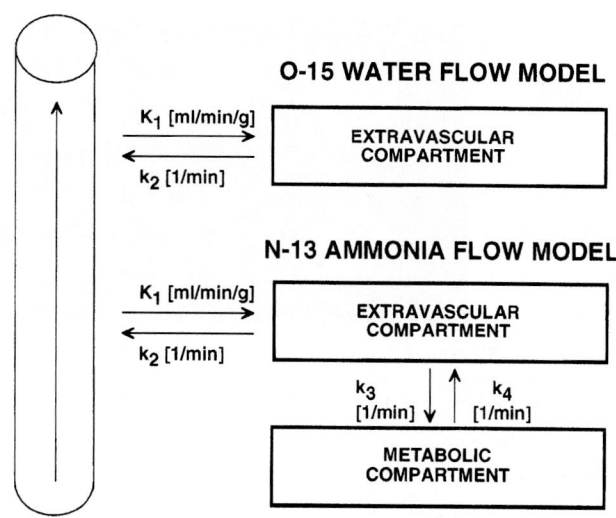

FIGURE 55.3 Schematic diagram illustrating the compartment models for oxygen-15 water (*top*) and nitrogen-13 ammonia (*bottom*).

blood flow. For these radiopharmaceuticals, the initial tracer extraction (first-pass extraction) and their tissue retention are important factors defining their suitability as blood flow tracers. N-13 ammonia is highly extracted by myocardial tissue in the form of N-13 ammonia (24–26). Within the tissue, the tracer can either back diffuse into the vascular space or be trapped in the form of N-13 glutamine.

Ionic tracers such as rubidium-82, rubidium-81, or potassium-38 display similar tracer kinetics to thallium-201 (27). Initial extraction of these compounds ranges between 50% and 70%. For both N-13 ammonia retention and ionic tracer extraction, a nonlinear relationship exists between blood flow and tissue tracer extraction (27,28).

Clinical Application

Qualitative Assessment of Regional Myocardial Blood Flow

Initial applications of PET for the detection of CAD consisted of the visual assessment of regional myocardial tracer distribution under rest and stress conditions (29–33). In most studies, pharmacologic stress testing has been used to assess coronary reserve (29). The advantage of this approach is the standardized stress procedure, which can be performed in the PET gantry without moving the patient between rest and stress imaging (34).

The most commonly used tracers are rubidium-82 and N-13 ammonia (24,32). With rubidium-82, the rest/stress protocol can be completed in approximately 1 hour, whereas N-13 ammonia blood flow studies require approximately 2 hours. Extensive clinical data exist with both radiopharmaceuticals to document the high diagnostic

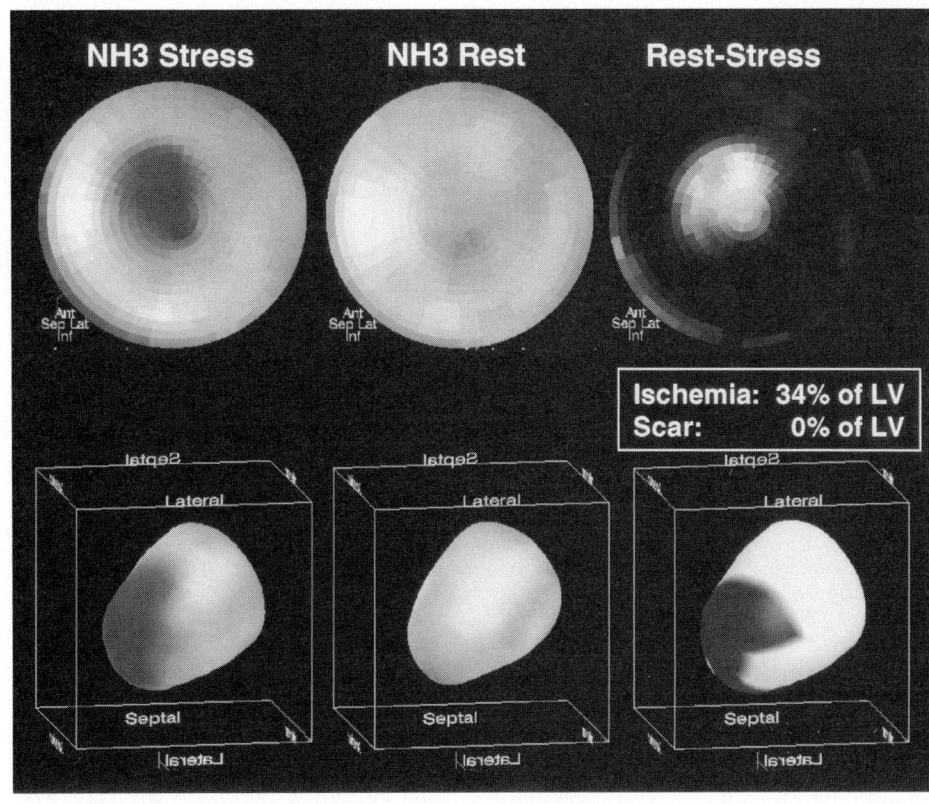

FIGURE 55.4 Polar maps (*top*) and three-dimensional visualization (*bottom*) of nitrogen-13 ammonia (NH₃) uptake in a patient with a stress-induced defect. Results provide semi-quantitative assessment of ischemic and scar tissue. LV, left ventricle.

accuracy with sensitivity and specificity values ranging from 85% to 95%. Demer et al. demonstrated that there is little difference between the use of either tracer for the detection of CAD (33). Most studies used visual data analysis similar to the methods used routinely for thallium-201 or technetium-99m sestamibi SPECT imaging (25,30,35,36). Automated techniques for semiquantitative data analysis, similar to those used for SPECT imaging, have also been developed for PET flow studies (37,38) (Fig. 55.4).

Although PET investigations are more expensive than conventional SPECT imaging or stress echocardiography, data by Patterson et al. (39) indicate that the use of PET in the diagnostic workup of patients with suspected CAD may be cost-effective, especially when patients with low and intermediate pretest likelihood for CAD are evaluated.

Demer et al. demonstrated that the severity of perfusion abnormalities determined by PET imaging correlated with the angiographically predicted coronary reserve measurements for a given vascular territory (33). More recently, Gould et al. reported a significant gradient in regional perfusion from base to apex in patients with mild but diffuse arteriographic disease, suggesting greater downstream flow abnormalities in the absence of regional limiting stenoses (40).

In addition to the diagnosis of CAD, the follow-up of patients with CAD by noninvasive means is of clinical interest (41). Longitudinal studies evaluating the effect of therapeutic or lifestyle interventions provide objective outcome criteria and are especially important in patients con-

sidered at high risk for progression of disease severity. Gould et al. have used PET and angiography to follow 20 patients undergoing cholesterol-lowering diets over 5 years. The semiquantitative PET parameters describing severity and extent of stress-induced perfusion abnormalities indicated much more profound changes following therapy as compared with angiographic criteria (Fig. 55.5). The relative magnitude of changes in size and severity of PET perfusion abnormalities was comparable with or greater than the magnitude of changes in percent diameter stenosis, absolute stenosis lumen area, or stenosis flow reserve documented by quantitative coronary arteriography (42).

Quantitative Assessment of Myocardial Blood Flow

The potential of PET for the quantitative assessment of myocardial blood flow represents a major advantage over SPECT imaging. Such measurements provide flow estimates in milliliters per minute per 100 g of tissue, which can be used to assess myocardial microcirculation under resting and stress conditions as well as before and after pharmacologic interventions. For such flow measurements, dynamic data acquisition is necessary to describe arterial input function as well as tissue response.

Oxygen-15 Water

O-15 water can be administered either as bolus injection or O-15–labeled CO_2 inhalation (22,23,43,44). Radiolabeled

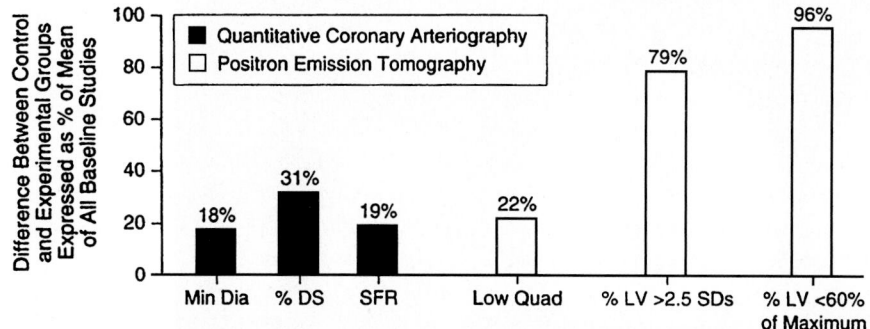

FIGURE 55.5 Comparison of changes by positron emission tomography and quantitative coronary arteriography. The positron emission tomography measures were myocardial quadrant with the lowest average activity (Low Quad), percentage of left ventricle (LV) outside 2.5 standard deviations of normals, and percentage of LV activity less than 60% of maximal activity. Measurements by quantitative coronary arteriography were minimum absolute lumen diameter (Min Dia), percent diameter stenosis (% DS), and stenosis flow reserve (SFR) derived from the integrated effects of absolute lumen diameter, % DS, and cumulative length effects based on fluid dynamic equations. The absolute difference in changes between the control and experimental groups was expressed as a percentage of the mean of each measurement at baseline for all patients. (From Gould KL, Ornish D, Scherwitz L, et al. Changes in myocardial perfusion abnormalities by positron emission tomography after long-term, intense risk factor modification. *JAMA* 1995;274:894–901, with permission.)

CO_2 is rapidly converted to water in lung tissue and transported to the heart as O-15 water. Both approaches use the uptake as well as washout of radioactivity from the myocardium, assuming a constant partition coefficient (0.80 to 0.90) of water between vascular and tissue space (Fig. 55.3). The water method also assumes homogeneous tissue within the region of interest used for quantitation of myocardial blood flow. To delineate myocardial tissue boundaries, the blood pool contribution has to be removed from O-15 water studies. For this purpose, a separate inhalation of O-15–labeled CO is commonly used (23). More recently, spectral analysis of dynamic O-15 water has been shown to allow for delineation of myocardial structures. The tracer kinetic model approach for O-15 water flow measurement includes a term correcting for the geometric distortion caused by limited image resolution provided by PET (partial volume effect, activity cross-contamination) (21,23,45). The use of O-15 water (as a blood flow marker) has been validated in various animal models and has demonstrated close agreement with microsphere flow measurements (45–47). Correction of flow values with the perfused tissue fraction leads to a determination of an index describing the relative amount of perfused tissue within a myocardial segment (48). In addition, methods have been developed to quantify not only flow, but also oxygen metabolism using O-15 water (49).

Nitrogen-13 Ammonia
Several approaches have been introduced to describe the myocardial kinetics of N-13 ammonia using a compartmental model that relates the N-13 activity in the vascular, free intracellular, and metabolic space (50–52) (Fig. 55.3). Assuming the first transit extraction (EF) of N-13 ammonia is approximately 100%, the model estimate (K_1) serves

as a quantitative index of perfusion (F) ($F = K_1 \times EF$) (24). These methods have been validated in the animal laboratory comparing N-13 ammonia perfusion measurements with microsphere measurements as a gold standard, or with O-15 reference PET measurements (46,52,53).

Other Tracers (Rubidium-82, Copper-62 PTSM, Potassium-38)
Rubidium-82 has been proposed for quantitative flow measurements (54,55). Data in the animal model and preliminary clinical results demonstrate the feasibility of using this radiopharmaceutical for quantitative flow measurements. Copper-62 PTSM [pyruvaldehyde bis(N4-methyl)thiosemicarbazone] has also been used for the assessment of myocardial blood flow (56). Quantitative flow estimates are limited because of the rapid sequestration of activity in red blood cells, which alters the arterial input function and the availability of tracer to tissue.

Clinical Application

The quantitation of regional coronary flow reserve has been advocated by Gould et al. for the functional assessment of the severity of coronary artery stenosis in patients with CAD (57). The parameter flow reserve describes not only the functional significance of a given coronary lesion but also vascular reactivity and collateral blood flow in the poststenotic vascular territories. Such functional measurements complement the anatomic description of CAD and link the morphologic alterations of epicardial arteries with perfusion patterns assessed at the level of microcirculation. Limitations of angiographic characterization of CAD are widely appreciated because of the complex three-dimensional nature of atherosclerotic plaques as well as considerable interobserver variability in angiographic data interpretation (41,57–59).

PET approaches have been extensively validated in animals and in healthy volunteers. There is good reproducibility of blood flow measurements under resting as well as stress conditions in volunteers and patients with CAD, as shown by the consistent measurements of coronary reserve values (60,61). Coronary flow reserve over 2.5 times resting flow must be considered *normal* based on the standard deviation of measurements in individuals at low likelihood of CAD (62,63).

A relationship between coronary reserve measurements and age in subjects without CAD has been demonstrated (64,65). However, there are other factors, such as left ventricular hypertrophy, hypertension, and syndrome X, which may affect coronary reserve measurements in the absence of vascular abnormalities defined by angiography (66). Animal and clinical data have indicated that arterial hyperten-

sion leads to reduced coronary flow reserve. It also has been shown, using PET, that therapy of patients with arterial hypertension may improve regional coronary reserve measurements (67).

Relationship Between Positron Emission Tomography Flow Measurements and Angiographic Assessment of Coronary Artery Disease

In patients with CAD, coronary flow reserve measurements are reduced (62,68–71). A correlation between the severity of coronary artery disease and severity of flow reserve impairment has been documented (62,70–72) (Fig. 55.6).

Detection of Preclinical Coronary Artery Disease by Flow Measurements

Comparing the incidence of abnormal coronary flow reserve with the severity of stenosis, as defined by quantitative angiography, reveals a high sensitivity of coronary flow

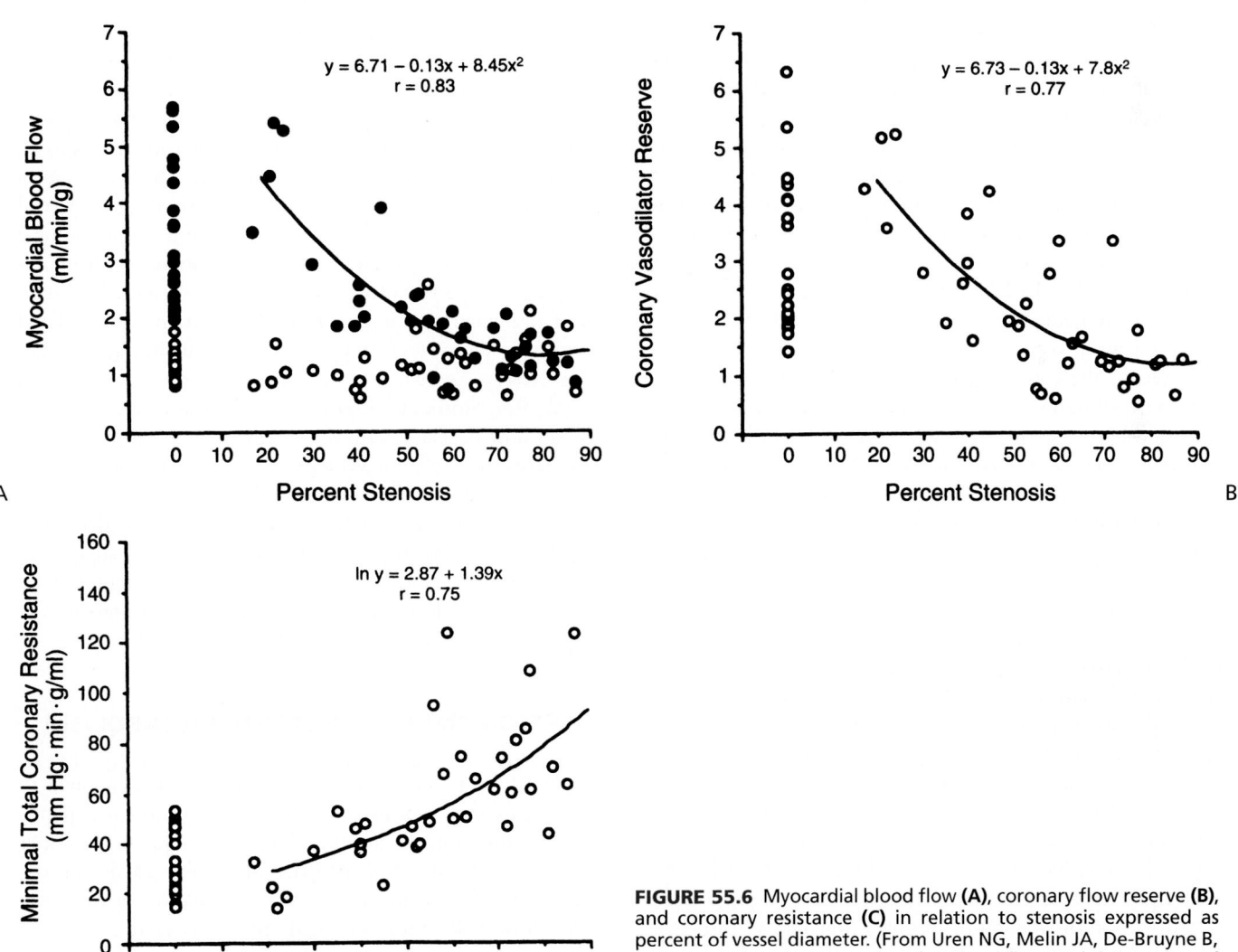

FIGURE 55.6 Myocardial blood flow **(A)**, coronary flow reserve **(B)**, and coronary resistance **(C)** in relation to stenosis expressed as percent of vessel diameter. (From Uren NG, Melin JA, De-Bruyne B, et al. Relation between myocardial blood flow and the severity of coronary-artery stenosis. *N Engl J Med* 1994;330:1782–1788, with permission.)

reserve measurements for the detection of severe coronary artery stenosis (greater than 95%). The high incidence (approximately 30%) of abnormal coronary flow reserve in territories with only mild CAD is surprising as defined by angiography (63). These data have been confirmed by several laboratories, indicating that coronary flow reserve with pharmacologic stress agents may provide more sensitive means to detect early CAD than angiographic criteria alone (62,73). This hypothesis has been addressed by several investigators (74–77), who have demonstrated that coronary flow reserve was abnormal in asymptomatic male patients without clinical evidence of myocardial ischemia, but at high risk for the development of CAD based on risk factor profile. A significant relationship between the impairment of coronary flow reserve and plasma cholesterol, low-density lipoprotein, high-density lipoprotein, and oxidized low-density lipoprotein has been reported. Coronary flow reserve has been shown to be reduced in young men with familial hyperlipidemia, especially with combined abnormalities in cholesterol and triglyceride serum levels (phenotype IIB) (78). Furthermore, reduction of flow reserve has been observed in asymptomatic patients with insulin-dependent and non–insulin-dependent diabetes mellitus (74). The pathophysiologic mechanism of the reduced coronary flow reserve in territories with no or only mild angiographic evidence of stenoses is not yet known but may represent a complex interplay of vascular alterations, as well as endothelial dysfunction (79). The hemodynamic response to dipyridamole or adenosine can be modified by alpha- or beta-receptor blockade enhancing the range of coronary flow measurements (80,81). First results using cold pressor stress testing in combination with PET confirm the results obtained in the catheterization laboratory using intracoronary acetylcholine infusion (82,83). In addition, mental stress has been used to investigate coronary vascular reactivity in normal and CAD patients, which demonstrated reduced flow response in this patient group (84).

PET measurements have been used to assess the acute and chronic effect of smoking on dipyridamole-induced flow changes. Smoking during the PET study decreased the dipyridamole-induced hyperemia and coronary reserve (77). The effects of smoking on coronary vascular reactivity can be reversed by intravenous L-arginine (82) or administration of the antioxidant vitamin C (77).

Cardiovascular conditioning is thought to favorably alter the natural history of CAD. Czernin et al. (85) investigated patients undergoing a short-term exercise and diet program. The beneficial effect of this program on heart rate, blood pressure, and cholesterol was associated with a significant increase in flow reserve. Pharmacologic therapy with lipid-lowering drugs (simvastatin, fluvastatin) is associated with improvement of coronary flow reserve (86–88). Guethlin et al. reported a delayed response when flow measurements at 2 months were compared with those obtained at 6 months after initiation of lipid-lowering therapy. These

data suggest that other factors than only lipid serum levels may be responsible for the beneficial effects of statins on vascular reactivity.

Quantitative regional flow measurements may be useful in preclinical CAD, identifying abnormal vascular reactivity as an early marker of the atherosclerotic process with diagnostic and prognostic value (76,89). In advanced disease PET provides a means to monitor pharmacologic interventions as well as to assess the effect of regional revascularization by percutaneous coronary intervention and surgery (90–98).

Other Cardiovascular Diseases

Quantitative flow measurements with PET have been used in patients with cardiac transplantation to study coronary physiology in this patient population. Several studies have indicated that coronary reserve is maintained in the cardiac transplant patient (69,99). Wolpers et al. (100) also demonstrated a relationship between angiographic evidence of vasculopathy and PET flow reserve. In contrast to angiography, flow reserve values were homogeneously reduced, suggesting a diffuse obstruction of the microvascular bed in patients with posttransplant vasculopathy. Quantitative PET flow measurements were also performed in patients with cardiomyopathy (101). Patients with hypertrophic cardiomyopathy display a reduced coronary reserve, which not only affects the hypertrophied interventricular septum but also the free lateral wall (68). These findings indicate that the pathophysiologic process involving the myocardium of patients with hypertrophic cardiomyopathy may not be limited to the hypertrophied interventricular septum (68). In patients with dilated cardiomyopathy, there appears to be a reduction in coronary flow reserve, which may provide prognostic information (102,103). Studies by Merlet et al. (104) indicate that PET blood flow measurements are in close agreement with invasive assessment of flow velocity by Doppler methods in this patient population. Furthermore, data by Parodi et al. (105) show that the flow response to pacing and dipyridamole is altered in patients with dilated cardiomyopathy, suggesting endothelial dysfunction. This hypothesis is supported by data reporting decreased flow response to cold pressor testing in this patient population (106).

ASSESSMENT OF SUBSTRATE METABOLISM

Several PET radiopharmaceuticals have been developed to investigate the myocardial energy metabolism that depends on the oxidation of various substrates (Table 55.1). Under fasting conditions, the majority of cardiac adenosine triphosphate production relies on the oxidation of free fatty acids (107,108). Free fatty acids are avidly extracted by the myocardium where long-chain acyl-coenzyme A (CoA) is rapidly formed. Activated fatty acids are used in the synthesis of triglycerides or phospholipids. The majority of acyl-

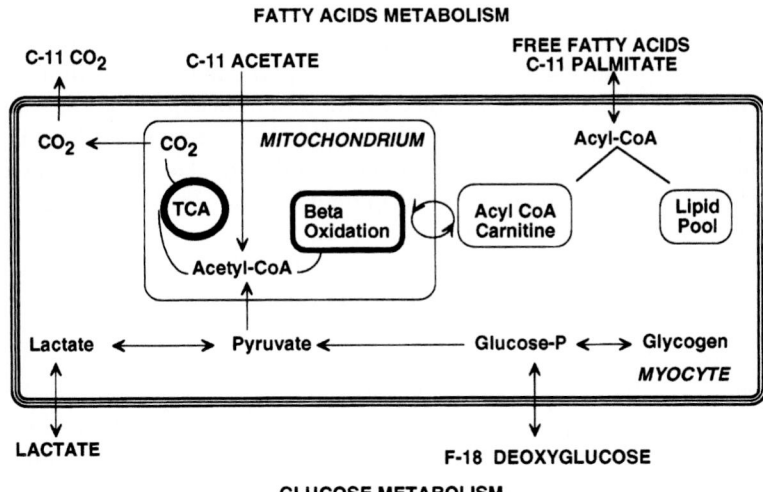

FIGURE 55.7 Conceptual model illustrating metabolic fate of various substrates in the myocardium. Acyl-CoA, acyl-coenzyme A; TCA, tricarboxylic acid cycle.

CoA, however, is transported via the carnitine shuttle into the mitochondria where beta-oxidation takes place (Fig. 55.7). The end product of beta-oxidation is acetyl-CoA, which enters the tricarboxylic acid cycle, the final pathway of oxidative metabolism of all substrates. In the presence of high free fatty acid and low insulin plasma levels, only a small amount of glucose is extracted by the myocardium. However, in the postprandial state, glucose transport into the cell is enhanced and the glycolytic rate is increased. But even after carbohydrate loading, only approximately 30% to 50% of overall cardiac substrate metabolism depends on oxidative metabolism of glucose (109). During physical exercise, plasma lactate levels increase and contribute to myocardial energy metabolism (110).

Aside from the physiologic increase of glycolysis in the postprandial state, glycolysis plays an important role during and after myocardial ischemia. Experimental studies have shown that myocardial glucose transport and metabolism are upregulated during myocardial ischemia with production and release of lactate (111,112). However, after ischemic episodes, glycolysis remains enhanced, with evidence of oxidative and nonoxidative use of exogenous glucose. There is preliminary evidence that enhanced myocardial oxidative glucose metabolism persists after an ischemic episode, most likely because of an upregulation of glucose transport (113–115). Biopsy studies in patients with severe CAD and chronic dysfunction of left ventricular segments have shown increased glycogen storage, as evidence of chronic alterations of glucose metabolism in hibernating myocardium (116). Such a metabolic pattern may reflect cell dedifferentiation in repetitively ischemic myocardium with predominant glycolytic metabolism (117) as a protective mechanism to avoid cell death in the form of apoptosis or acute necrosis (118).

Fatty Acid Metabolism

The first radiopharmaceutical used in combination with PET for the assessment of regional cardiac metabolism was C-11 palmitate. Experimental studies changing cardiac workload or cardiac substrate availability demonstrated changes in C-11 palmitate kinetics (119). To avoid the complexity of substrate interaction defining the relative contribution of long-chain fatty acids and carbohydrates to overall oxidative metabolism, C-11 acetate has been proposed as an alternative probe to describe oxidative metabolism. C-11 acetate is converted to C-11 acetyl-CoA in the mitochondria and enters the TCA cycle. C-11 activity equilibrates within TCA cycle intermediates and C-11 activity clears from the myocardium in the form of $C-11–CO_2$ (Fig. 55.7). Several studies have indicated that C-11 acetate kinetics, as assessed by dynamic PET imaging, correlate closely with myocardial oxygen consumption. Kinetics of C-11 acetate are only sparsely affected by substrate interactions and thus allow quantification of myocardial oxygen consumption, yielding parameters of oxidative metabolism as well as blood flow (120–124).

Glucose Metabolism

F-18-FDG traces transmembranous transport, as well as phosphorylation of exogenous glucose (125,126). F-18-FDG-6-phosphate does not enter any further metabolic pathways but accumulates in myocardium proportional to glucose transport and phosphorylation (127,128). Experimental studies in isolated rabbit septum as well as canine models demonstrated a close relationship of FDG uptake and exogenous glucose metabolism measured by Fick's principle (128). However, FDG molecules display different affinities for glucose transport and phosphorylation than the glucose molecule. To correct this discrepancy, a correction term is necessary for the quantification of exogenous glucose use of the myocardium by FDG. This correction term (lumped constant) is assumed to be constant under physiologic and most pathophysiologic conditions. More recent data, however, indicate that under rapidly changing conditions the lumped constant may actually change as a function of altered affinities for glucose transport, as well as for the hexokinase reaction (129). Exogenous glucose use can be quantified using a simple fitting procedure of FDG myocardial kinetics and parametric display of regional metabolic data (130). The comparison of C-11 acetate uptake and clearance with regional FDG kinetics in normal volunteers demonstrated an inhomogeneity of regional glucose use in the heart (131). Regional FDG uptake is increased in the lateral wall of the left ventricle and slightly decreased in the area of intraventricular septum (132). FDG measurements have been performed to evaluate cardiac glucose metabolism in patients with insulin-dependent and non–insulin-dependent diabetes mellitus. In patients with insulin-dependent diabetes, there was no significant difference in overall glucose use as compared with a control population, if insulin was substituted by an euglycemic-insulin clamp (133–135). The quantitative nature of the PET measurements allows for *in vivo* studies under varying conditions to study the relationship of insulin and glucose metabolism in heart and skeletal muscle (136).

Clinical Application of Metabolic Imaging

Ischemic Heart Disease

Specific changes in regional substrate use can occur during acute myocardial ischemia and in patients with chronic ischemic heart disease as demonstrated by PET imaging (137–140). Myocardial ischemia results in impaired oxidative metabolism of fatty acids and increased myocardial glucose use (112). Comparing regional myocardial FDG uptake and myocardial blood flow, as assessed by microspheres during acute myocardial ischemia, showed a dissociation of myocardial blood flow and glucose use (112). In severe ischemia, however, both blood flow and glucose use are reduced, whereas there is evidence for increased FDG uptake during moderate ischemia. Marshall et al. were the first to investigate the relationship of increased FDG uptake in patients with acute myocardial infarction and clinical signs of ongoing ischemia, as well as electrocardiographic changes (141). This study indicated that in a considerable number of patients with acute myocardial infarction, residual metabolic activity could be demonstrated in the infarct territory, which was associated with a higher incidence of postinfarct angina and electrocardiographic signs of recurrent ischemia.

Metabolic Evaluation of Dysfunctioning Myocardium

Animal and clinical studies using FDG as metabolic tracer have shown that reversible left ventricular dysfunction (stunned, hibernating myocardium) is associated with maintained or even increased tissue FDG uptake (137,140,142). Experimental data support the notion that reversible chronic left ventricular dysfunction in patients with advanced CAD does not represent ongoing ischemia but downregulation of function (118,143). There are two experimental conditions that may serve as a model for the clinical presentation of reversible dysfunction in ischemic heart disease. First, transient ischemia with restoration of blood flow leads to slow functional recovery on the basis of *stunning* (144). Second, chronic reduction of blood flow in the animal model is associated with metabolic adaptive changes that minimize the imbalance of oxygen supply and demand, limiting the development of irreversible cell injury (hibernation) (145,146). There is increasing evidence that similar mechanisms are involved in the pathophysiology of reversible chronic dysfunction in patients with advanced CAD (147,148). Rahimtoola (147) first described this condition as *hibernating myocardium*. His definition included chronic reduction of blood flow as a culprit for the observed dysfunction, implying chronic ischemia. However, subsequent studies with PET have shown that blood flow either can be normal or only slightly decreased in dysfunctioning viable myocardium. Vanoverschelde et al. demonstrated near normal perfusion in collateral-dependent viable, but dysfunctioning, myocardium distal to an occluded coronary artery. Sophisticated measurements of blood flow corrected for tissue loss (perfused tissue fraction) also indicate that dysfunctioning myocardium may not be limited by oxygen supply under resting conditions (48,149). Based on these results, there is ongoing discussion as to whether reversible left ventricular dysfunction in severe ischemic heart disease reflects repetitive stunning or hibernation (143). The clinical situation in most patients is characterized by a heterogeneous ischemic injury, consisting of necrosis or scar in the subendocardium surrounded by viable but compromised tissue. The dynamic nature of ischemic heart disease renders these segments ischemic during daily life activities, which may lead to repetitive stunning. On the other hand, severe flow restriction may result in chronic hypoperfusion fulfilling the original criteria of hibernation. One can speculate that both conditions coexist in patients with advanced CAD and impairment of left ventricular function (150). From a clinical point of view, the pathophysiologic discussion is less important because many studies have shown that revascularization results in functional improvement of both stunned and hibernating myocardium (150). Therefore, differentiation between reversible and irreversible dysfunction in patients with severe impairment of left ventricular function has become a major clinical question for the decision-making process concerning revascularization. Qualitative evaluation of PET flow studies demonstrated decreased N-13 ammonia and increased FDG uptake (mismatch) in viable myocar-

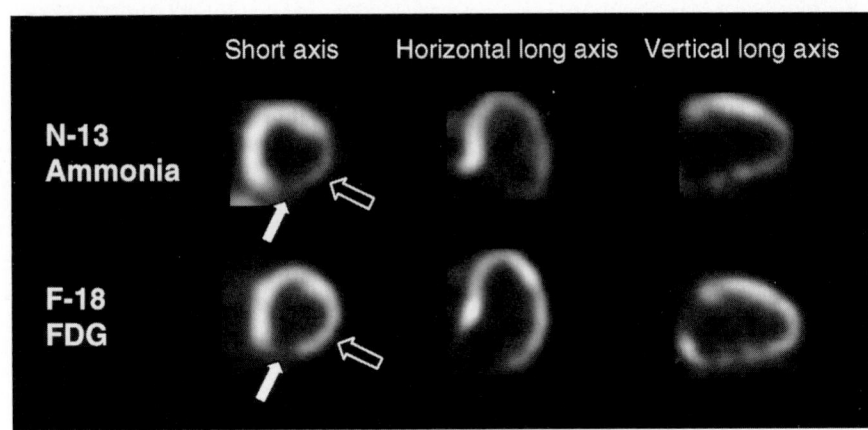

FIGURE 55.8 Positron emission tomographic images using nitrogen-13 ammonia and fluorine-18-fluorodeoxyglucose (F-18-FDG) of a patient with a perfusion to metabolism mismatch pattern (hibernating myocardium, *open arrows*) and scar (*filled arrows*).

dium, which has been considered the scintigraphic hallmark of hibernation (140) (Fig. 55.8). Although such a pattern suggests reduced blood flow, the intensity of tracer uptake depends not only on flow, but also on left ventricular wall thickness (partial volume effect). Therefore, reduction of N-13 ammonia uptake may reflect wall thinning or an admixture of viable and scarred myocardium (151). Flow measurements with O-15 water are less sensitive to partial volume effects, but may overestimate transmural flow (152). In contrast, the FDG signal indicates a relatively higher FDG extraction compared with N-13 ammonia. Using information on both blood flow and glucose metabolism, sensitive specific identification of viable myocardium can be performed. This was first shown by Tillisch et al. (140), who compared relative FDG uptake in patients with advanced CAD and impaired regional and global function before and after revascularization. This study demonstrated that maintained FDG uptake in dysfunctioning segments with reduced flow is associated with functional recovery after revascularization, whereas segments with concordantly decreased flow and metabolism did not recover after restoration of blood flow. Subsequently, a large number of similar studies confirmed the predictive value of FDG imaging. Table 55.2 summarizes clinical PET results,

which were collected from several laboratories documenting the high predictive value of PET metabolic imaging for tissue recovery after revascularization. In all studies, recovery of regional function after revascularization served as the gold standard for tissue viability. It has been shown that functional recovery of hibernating myocardium may require several months (150,153).

Comparison with Other Imaging Modalities

Numerous investigations exist comparing regional FDG uptake with electrocardiographic criteria, standard thallium-201 and Tc-99m flow agents, imaging stress echocardiography, and MRI imaging (154,155). Early observations of discrepant results between FDG distribution and thallium-201 redistribution patterns emphasized the limitations of thallium-201 redistribution imaging for assessment of tissue viability, which are partly overcome by reinjection techniques (156). Tc-99m sestamibi also provides clinically useful information on tissue viability. In combination with nitrate application, the predictive value of Tc-99m sestamibi imaging can be enhanced. Comparing scintigraphic data with those obtained after positive inotropic interventions, it appears that tracer retention provides more sensitive markers of viable myocardium, whereas assessment of

TABLE 55.2 PREDICTIVE VALUE OF VIABILITY ASSESSMENT

Reference	Patients	Dysfunctional segments	Predictive accuracy (%)	Positive predictive accuracy (%)	Negative predictive accuracy (%)
Tillisch (140)	17	67	88	85	92
Tamaki (212)	22	46	78	78	78
Tamaki (213)	11	56	82	80	100
Marwick (211)	16	85	74	68	79
Lucignani (210)	14	54	91	95	80
Carrel (209)	21	23	83	84	75
Gropler (169)	16	53	81	79	83
vom Dahl (151)	37	45	80	69	84
Total	154	429	82	82	83

TABLE 55.3 PROGNOSIS OF POSITRON EMISSION TOMOGRAPHY

		References	Number	Left ventricular ejection fraction (%)	Complication
Hibernating	Drug therapy	Tamaki (160)	31	—	12 (39%)
		Eitzman (158)	18	33	9 (50%)
		Maddahi (159)	17	24	7 (41%)
Scarred	Drug therapy	Tamaki (160)	17	—	1 (6%)
		Eitzman (158)	24	32	3 (13%)
		Maddahi (159)	33	24	3 (9%)
Hibernating	Percutaneous transluminal coronary angioplasty or coronary artery bypass grafting	Eitzman (158)	26	36	3 (12%)
		Maddahi (159)	26	25	3 (12%)
Scarred	Percutaneous transluminal coronary angioplasty or coronary artery bypass grafting	Eitzman (158)	14	37	1 (7%)
		Maddahi (159)	17	25	1 (6%)

contactile reserve is associated with higher specificity for reversible myocardial dysfunction (156,157).

Prognostic Significance of Metabolic Imaging

Aside from the predictive value of FDG for tissue recovery, the prognostic information provided by FDG uptake in segments with reduced perfusion as assessed by N-13 ammonia PET has been emphasized by several groups (Table 55.3). Retrospective data analysis revealed a high incidence of cardiovascular complications in patients with decreased blood flow, but maintained FDG uptake in patients who did not undergo revascularization (158–160). In contrast, the incidence of cardiovascular complications was similar in groups with scintigraphic evidence of scar or normal myocardium, regardless of whether they were revascularized. These data indicate that the mismatch pattern identifies a subgroup of patients at increased risk for cardiovascular complications. The prognostic information appears independent of the traditional markers such as left ventricular ejection fraction or New York Heart Association classification, which were not different among the investigated subgroups. Survival was significantly higher in revascularized patients with mismatch, as demonstrated by DiCarli et al. (161,162).

The degree of functional recovery of patients after revascularization can be predicted based on the scintigraphic pattern, as well as extent of mismatch (151,162). DiCarli et al. reported an 80% likelihood of functional improvement in the presence of mismatch exceeding 18% of the left ventricle. Pagano et al. indicated that the extent of viability correlates not only with functional recovery, but also survival (163). Furthermore, delay of revascularization in these patients is associated with increased mortality, confirming the prognostic significance of the identification of viable, but jeopardized, myocardium (164). Patients with severe left ventricular dysfunction are at higher risk for complications associated with revascularization. Dreyfus et al. (165) reported that assessment of tissue viability in such patients before surgery improves the selection process for revascularization with low perioperative mortality. Haas et al. (166) confirmed this prognostic role of PET by comparing short-

and midterm survival after surgical revascularization in two groups of patients with three-vessel disease and impaired left ventricular function. Attempts to exploit the clinical significance of the FDG signal by less costly means included the use of high-energy collimators for SPECT systems and coincidence circuitry in gamma cameras. Initial results indicate the feasibility of such approaches with comparable diagnostic and prognostic performance (157,167).

Carbon-11 Acetate in the Assessment of Tissue Viability

Regional FDG uptake is modulated by plasma substrate levels and hormonal milieu. Many patients with CAD have diabetes mellitus or prediabetic conditions affecting glucose tolerance. Therefore, the image quality following oral glucose loading and intravenous injection of FDG is limited in some patients undergoing tissue viability studies (133). As an alternative, C-11 acetate has been proposed for the assessment of residual oxidative metabolism in patients with severe CAD. Studies by Gropler et al. demonstrated that C-11 acetate may also be useful in the assessment of tissue viability in patients with chronic stable CAD (168,169). More recently, Gerber et al. applied C-11 acetate kinetics to investigate the relationship between flow and oxygen consumption in patients with unstable angina. Reversible dysfunctioning myocardium displayed normal flow and oxygen consumption, suggesting the presence of stunning in these patients (170). C-11 acetate serves as an alternative to FDG imaging. However, the assessment of C-11 acetate kinetics requires dynamic data acquisition and sophisticated image processing, limiting widespread clinical use (168,169).

Metabolic Imaging in Patients with Other Cardiovascular Diseases

Dilated Cardiomyopathy

C-11 palmitate has been used to study fatty acid metabolism in patients with dilated cardiomyopathy. Observations by Geltman revealed a heterogeneous fatty acid metabolism in patients with dilated cardiomyopathy in the presence of relatively homogeneous perfusion, as measured with thallium-201 scintigraphy (171). Kelly et al. (172) addressed the role of C-11 palmitate in probing mitochondrial enzyme defects resulting in an impairment of beta-oxidation. These investigators were able to demonstrate that oxidation of C-11 acetate was dissociated from that of C-11 palmitate in patients affected with this enzyme disorder. As discussed previously, C-11 acetate allows the noninvasive assessment of myocardial oxygen consumption (173). This tracer approach can be used to probe myocardial oxygen consumption in healthy as well as diseased cardiac muscle. In addition, this technique can be used to assess right ventricular oxygen consumption, as demonstrated by Hicks et al., who described a close relationship between right ventricular acetate kinetics in patients and pulmonary artery pressure (174). Wolpers et al. first introduced the concept of noninvasively assessing myocardial efficiency by PET as defined by external work of the left ventricle divided by oxygen consumption (175). Such a parameter allows the assessment of the link between mechanical performance and metabolic demand under various pathophysiologic conditions as well as after therapeutic interventions (122,176).

Beanlands et al. applied this method in patients with cardiomyopathy before and after therapy with dobutamine and nitroprusside (177). Myocardial efficiency increased after both pharmacologic interventions. In both instances, the improvement in cardiac efficiency was most related to changes in left ventricular afterload. More recently, Beanlands et al. demonstrated the beneficial effect of beta-blockade (metoprolol) on metabolic left ventricular performance in heart failure patients using C-11 acetate (122).

ASSESSMENT OF AUTONOMIC INNERVATION

Tracer approaches are uniquely suited to the assessment of specific tissue function. Although tracers have been developed for the parasympathetic nervous system, the sparse cholinergic innervation of the left ventricle limits the presynaptic evaluation of this system *in vivo*. Therefore, most imaging approaches focus on the scintigraphic delineation of the presynaptic and postsynaptic sympathetic nervous systems because the left and right ventricles are densely innervated by sympathetic fibers. Figure 55.9 displays the nerve terminal, which is an important functional unit of the sympathetic nervous system.

Postganglionic sympathetic fibers travel along vascular structures on the surface of the heart. On entering the myocardial wall, the fibers branch into multiple sympathetic varicosities. These nerve terminals include vesicles, which represent the storage pool for neurotransmitters, enzymes, and other proteins (178). Norepinephrine, the predominant cardiac neurotransmitter, is synthesized from the amino acid tyrosine by several enzymatic steps (Fig. 55.9) and is released on nerve stimulation by exocytosis. Several receptor systems have been postulated to exist on the membrane of the presynaptic nerve terminal, modulating norepinephrine release. As much as 80% of the norepinephrine that is released from the nerve terminal is taken up via a mechanism known as *uptake 1*. Reuptake is an important mechanism to regulate the norepinephrine concentration in the extraneuronal space. A fraction of the released norepinephrine diffuses back into the vascular space where it can be measured as norepinephrine spillover in the coronary sinus venous blood (179). Only a small amount of

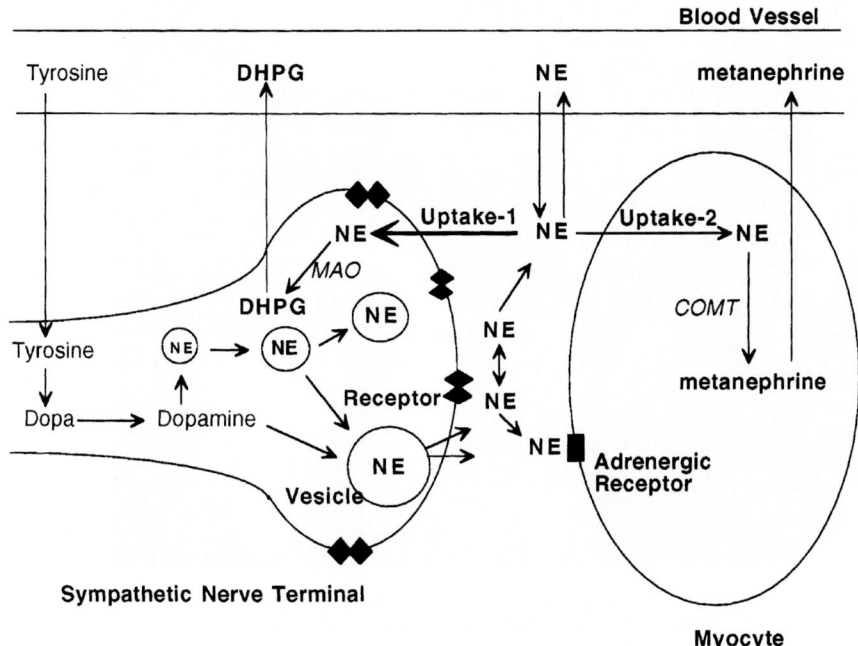

FIGURE 55.9 Conceptual model of sympathetic nerve terminal. COMT, catechol-*O*-methyl transferase; DHPG, 3,4-dihydroxyphenylglycol; MAO, monoamine oxidase; NE, norepinephrine.

norepinephrine in the synaptic cleft activates receptors on the surface of the myocytes or enters cardiac cells directly (uptake 2 mechanism). Norepinephrine undergoes rapid metabolism in neuronal and extraneuronal tissue. Metabolism of the neurotransmitter in the neuronal tissue is mediated by the enzyme monoamine oxidase, while extraneuronal norepinephrine is metabolized by the catechol-*O*-methyltransferase enzyme system.

Imaging of Presynaptic Nerve Terminals

The use of radiolabeled norepinephrine or analogs appears to be most promising for the visualization of the sympathetic nerve terminals. C-11 hydroxyephedrine (HED) has been synthesized at the University of Michigan (Fig. 55.10) (180). This norepinephrine analog is taken up by the nerve terminal but is not metabolized by the intraneuronal enzyme systems. The myocardial retention of this tracer reflects the activity of uptake 1 mechanism and, to a lesser degree, the storage of norepinephrine in nerve terminals (181). In contrast, the more recently introduced compound C-11 epinephrine is not only taken up by the nerve terminal, but also stored in the vesicles of nerve terminals (182). A further analog of epinephrine is phenylephrine, which enters the nerve terminal via uptake 1, but is primarily metabolized by the monoamine oxidase enzyme system (183). Phenylephrine, therefore, allows the evaluation of the enzymatic integrity of the nerve terminal. Other radiopharmaceuticals for the characterization of the presynaptic nerve terminal include F-18 dopamine and F-18 norepinephrine, as well as MBBG (metabromobenzylguanidine) (184–186).

Clinical Application

Initial clinical applications of C-11 HED show excellent image quality with high contrast between myocardial tracer activity and blood pool, as well as lung tissue surrounding the heart (Fig. 55.10). The specificity of the tracer approach for neuronal tissue has been well documented by studies in cardiac transplant patients, which showed a marked reduction of tracer uptake, suggesting only little nonspecific binding of this tracer (181), which allows for quantitative image analysis (187). Studies in transplant patients at various time points following surgery indicate partial reinnervation of transplanted myocardium by retention of C-11 HED in the anterior septal segments of the left ventricle in transplant recipients several

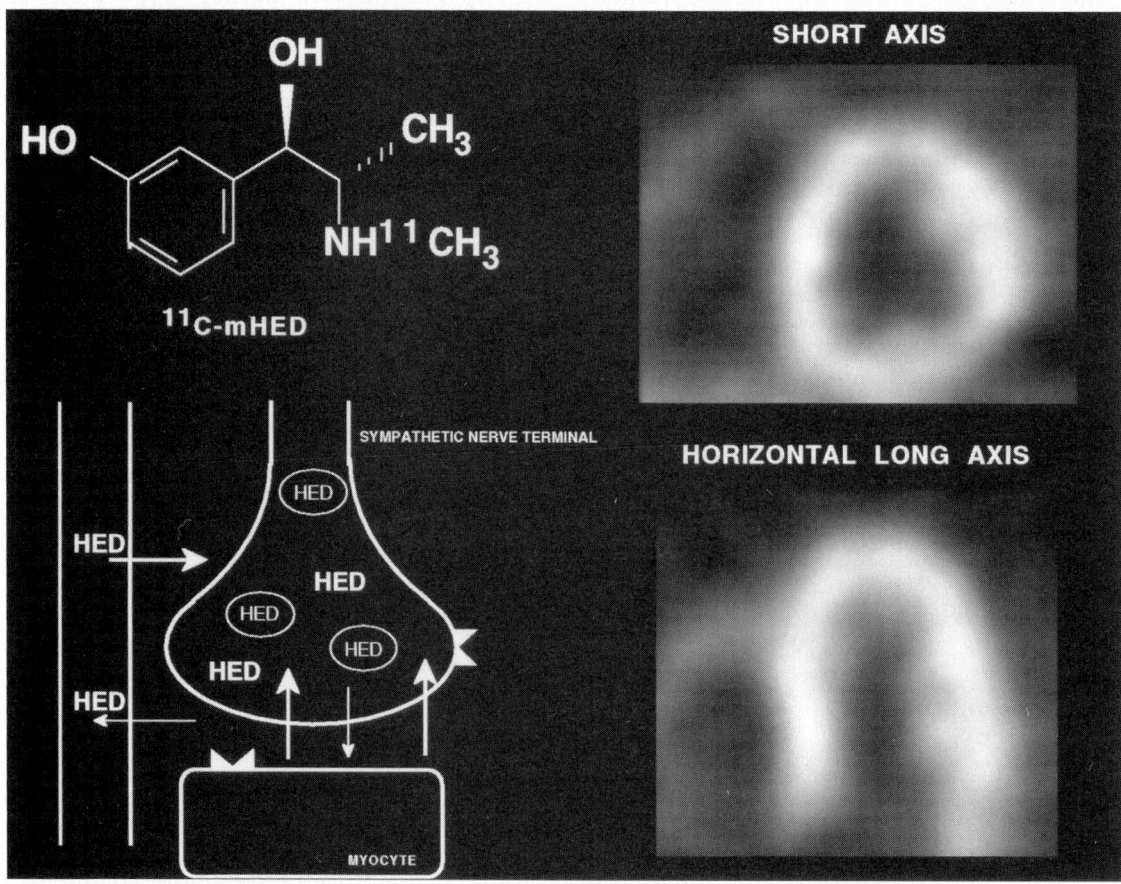

FIGURE 55.10 Illustration of molecular structure of carbon-11 hydroxyephedrine (HED), a model of the uptake mechanism, and positron emission tomographic images of the tracer in a healthy volunteer, showing homogeneous distribution of the tracer.

years after operation (188). These data suggested for the first time that regional reinnervation occurs in the human transplant. First results comparing this scintigraphic pattern with heart rate variability suggest that the partial reinnervation of the left ventricle is associated with electrophysiologic evidence of functional reinnervation (189–191). Allman et al. used C-11 HED in the assessment of patients with acute myocardial infarction undergoing thrombolytic therapy (192). Experimental data indicated that the extent of neuronal damage following transient ischemia is larger than the area of tissue necrosis. Wolpers et al. demonstrated a decreased retention fraction of C-11 HED in reperfused canine myocardium, suggesting a high sensitivity of neurons to ischemic injury. Similar data have been observed in the clinical setting (193). The area of neuronal dysfunction, as evidenced by C-11 HED defects, was significantly larger than the area of perfusion abnormalities in patients with acute myocardial infarction and correlated closely with the area of risk as assessed by Tc-99m sestamibi imaging in the same patients, confirming the experimental data (194). C-11 HED PET studies were also performed in patients with diabetic neuropathy. These studies revealed a correlation between the results of autonomic nervous system testing and the abnormalities of HED distribution. The finding that regional cardiac denervation represents a heterogeneous process in patients with diabetic neuropathy was surprising. C-11 hydroxyephedrine defects were most severe in the apical segments of the left ventricle and least severe in the proximal segments of the left ventricle (195–197). Comparison of neuronal dysfunction and blood flow measurements by PET revealed impaired vasodilator response in diabetic patients (198).

Preliminary studies suggest the possible role of HED imaging in patients with congestive heart failure. Several investigators demonstrated decreased HED uptake in patients with severely impaired left ventricular function, suggesting neuronal damage in this patient population (199,200). Again this process appears to be heterogeneous with pronounced abnormalities in the apical segments of the left ventricle.

Postsynaptic Receptor Sites

The development of radiotracers and the initial clinical validation of tracer methods for the visualization of the adrenergic receptor system have been initiated by Syrota et al. The specific visualization of cardiac beta-receptors became possible by the successful radiosynthesis of a more hydrophilic beta-receptor antagonist (CGP-12177). This nonselective C-11–labeled beta-receptor antagonist provided excellent image quality of the postsynaptic binding sites in the heart (201). A tracer kinetic model approach has yielded estimates of receptor densities in agreement with *in vitro* beta-receptor density assessments (202). Clinical validation of this approach confirmed the *in vitro* demonstrated reduction of beta-receptor density in patients with congestive heart fail-

ure. This approach has also been adapted by Camici et al. and used in patients with hypertrophic cardiomyopathy, arrhythmogenic right ventricular cardiomyopathy, and syndrome X (203–206). These PET studies demonstrated a reduction in beta-receptor density as well as presynaptic function in patients with hypertrophic cardiomyopathy. The reduced beta-receptor density was not limited to the intraventricular septum, but included the entire left ventricular myocardium, suggesting a global change in beta-receptor density. These initial studies using beta-receptor antagonists for visualization of the adrenergic receptor system indicate the potential of PET imaging in monitoring pathophysiologic alterations in beta-receptor density and in probing the effect of various pharmacologic interventions on the sympathetic neurotransmission (207).

SUMMARY OF CURRENT STATUS

The improved imaging technology of PET, including attenuation correction and high spatial resolution, allows for the highly accurate detection of CAD. Coronary reserve measurements may be useful in the early detection of vascular abnormalities and follow-up of therapeutic interventions designed to halt or reverse CAD. Finally, such measurements can serve as end points in the evaluation of new drugs altering endothelial function.

Assessment of tissue viability has become an important application for PET in cardiology. Metabolic imaging documented the high incidence of reversible dysfunction in patients with severe CAD. These PET findings resulted in increasing diagnostic efforts to identify viable myocardium by various methods. At the current time, PET must be considered the reference method for identification of tissue viability with established diagnostic and prognostic value. In patients with high-risk interventions and in transplant candidates, PET best supports the selection process for revascularization. Finally, new tracer approaches designed to map cardiac innervation may not only prove useful in clinical research assessing neurophysiology of various cardiovascular disorders, but also provide important prognostic information in patients with congestive heart failure.

CONTROVERSIES AND PERSONAL PERSPECTIVES

PET imaging of the heart provides important clinical information and promising new avenues for clinical research. The quantitative nature, as well as the in-depth validation, of this technology, makes it an attractive research tool. For example, PET represents the most validated noninvasive method to quantitate regional myocardial perfusion. Although there are defined clinical indications for the use of regional quantification of myocardial perfusion, there are many scientific

THE FUTURE

The future clinical role of PET depends primarily on the development of simplified PET methods, centralized distribution of radiopharmaceuticals, and the clinical acceptance and integration of complex physiologic information.

It is expected that PET and SPECT technology will overlap in the future, and the uniqueness and usefulness of clinical information provided by each of these modalities will define their place in clinical cardiology.

questions regarding coronary physiology and cardiac microcirculation, which can be addressed noninvasively by PET. However, this technology is not widely available and requires a well-developed academic infrastructure to exploit its research potential. It is expected that physiologic parameters beyond flow will gain importance in the future. It is, however, difficult to predict whether the resolution of scintigraphic methods will ever permit the study of the vascular wall of the coronary arteries. Specific tracers, which provide high contrast for a given physiologic process (e.g., thrombocytes activation inflammation), may enable imaging of vulnerable coronary plaques. In addition, tracer approaches may be useful in the monitoring of gene expression (208). Emphasis on further development of molecular imaging by PET clearly depends on basic cardiovascular research, providing new insights into the cell signaling and receptor systems. Tracer approaches are uniquely suited to study physiologic and biochemical consequences of altered cell interaction, providing *functional genomics*. This potential to characterize the phenotype may not only apply to human studies but may also be especially attractive for research in transgenic animals.

Metabolic imaging with PET provided the first insights into the adaptive processes in response to repetitive cellular stress (e.g., ischemia). Based on clinical observations in hibernating myocardium, new experimental models are being developed to study the consequences of ischemia on myocardial substrate metabolism using molecular biology approaches. Similar interaction between imaging of human pathology and experimental work can be envisioned for other systems modifying cardiac performance—for instance, autonomic innervation of the failing heart.

There seems to be a gap between the technical potential of modern imaging modalities and the integration of functional information in the clinical decision-making process. Despite advances in functional imaging, physiologic and biochemical signals are often too complex to be readily accepted and exploited in daily patient care.

ACKNOWLEDGMENTS

The authors appreciate the excellent secretarial help of Gabriele Sonoda and thank Dr. S. Nekolla and Ngoc Nguyen for the careful preparation of illustrations.

REFERENCES

1. Buchanan J, Hastings A. The use of isotopically marked carbon in the study of intermediary metabolism. *Physiol Rev* 1946;26:120–155.
2. Tobias C, Lawrence J, Roughton F. The elimination of carbon monoxide from human body with reference to the possible conversion of carbon monoxide to carbon dioxide. *Am J Physiol* 1945;145:253–263.
3. Brownell G, Sweet W. Localization of brain tumors with positron-emitters. *Nucleonics* 1953;11:40–45.
4. Aronow S. Positron scanning. In: Hine G, ed. *Instrumentation in nuclear medicine.* New York: Academic, 1967:461–483.
5. Kuhl D, Edwards R. Image separation radioisotope scanning. *Radiology* 1963;80:653–661.
6. Phelps M, Hoffman E, Mullani N, et al. Application of annihilation coincidence detection to transaxial reconstruction tomography. *J Nucl Med* 1975;16:210–224.
7. Hoffman EJ, Phelps ME, Weiss ES, et al. Transaxial tomographic imaging of canine myocardium with 11C-palmitic acid. *J Nucl Med* 1977;18:57–61.
8. Porenta G, Kuhle W, Sinha S, et al. Parameter estimation of cardiac geometry by ECG-gated PET imaging: validation using magnetic resonance imaging and echocardiography. *J Nucl Med* 1995;36:1123–1129.
9. Meikle S, Dahlbom M, Cherry S. Attenuation correction using count-limited transmission data in positron emission tomography. *J Nucl Med* 1993;34:143–150.
10. Thompson CJ, Ranger N, Evans AC, et al. Validation of simultaneous PET emission and transmission scans. *J Nucl Med* 1991;32:154–160.
11. Spinks TJ, Araujo LI, Rhodes CG, et al. Physical aspects of cardiac scanning with a block detector positron tomograph. *J Comput Assist Tomogr* 1991;15:893–904.
12. Cherry SR. Recent advances in instrumentation for positron emission tomography. *Nucl Instr Meth* 1994;A348:577–582.
13. Sandler MP, Bax JJ, Patton JA, et al. Fluorine-18-fluorodeoxyglucose cardiac imaging using a modified scintillation camera. *J Nucl Med* 1998;39:2035–2043.
14. Hasegawa S, Uehara T, Yamaguchi H, et al. Validity of 18F-fluorodeoxyglucose imaging with a dual-head coincidence gamma camera for detection of myocardial viability. *J Nucl Med* 1999;40:1884–1892.
15. Hoop B, Laughlin JS, Tilbury RS. Cyclotrons in nuclear medicine. In: Hine GJ, Sorensen JA, eds. *Instrumentation in nuclear medicine.* New York: Academic Press, 1974:407.
16. Fowler JS, Wolf AP. Positron emitter-labeled compounds: priorities and problems. In: Phelps ME, Mazziotta JC,

Schelbert HR, eds. *Positron emission tomography and autoradiography: principles and applications for the brain and heart.* New York: Raven Press, 1986:391.

17. Gennaro GP, Bergner B, Muller WR, et al. A radionuclide generator and infusion system for pharmaceutical quality Rb-82. In: *American Chemical Society Symposium Series No. 241, Radionuclide generators: new systems for nuclear medicine applications.* American Chemical Society, 1984.

18. Weinberg I, Huang S, Hoffman E, et al. Validation of PET-acquired input functions for cardiac studies. *J Nucl Med* 1988;29:241–247.

19. Godfrey K. *Compartmental models and their application.* New York: Academic Press, 1983.

20. Huang SC, Phelps ME. Principles of tracer kinetic modeling in positron emission tomography and autoradiography. In: Phelps ME, Mazziotta JC, Schelbert HR, eds. *Positron emission tomography and autoradiography: principles and applications for the brain and heart.* New York: Raven Press, 1986:287–346.

21. Iida H, Kanno I, Takahashi A, et al. Measurement of absolute myocardial blood flow with $H_2^{15}O$ and dynamic positron emission tomography. Strategy for quantification in relation to the partial-volume effect. *Circulation* 1988;78:104–115.

22. Araujo LI, Lammertsma AA, Rhodes CG, et al. Noninvasive quantification of regional myocardial blood flow in coronary artery disease with oxygen-15-labeled carbon dioxide inhalation and positron emission tomography. *Circulation* 1991;83:875–885.

23. Bergmann S, Herrero P, Markham J, et al. Non-invasive quantitation of myocardial blood flow in human subjects with oxygen-15 labeled water and positron emission tomography. *J Am Coll Cardiol* 1989;14:639–652.

24. Schelbert HR, Phelps ME, Huang S-C, et al. N-13 ammonia as an indicator of myocardial blood flow. *Circulation* 1981;63:1259–1272.

25. Schelbert H, Phelps M, Hoffman E, et al. Regional myocardial perfusion assessed with N-13 labeled ammonia and positron emission computerized axial tomography. *Am J Cardiol* 1979;43:209–218.

26. Bergmann SR, Hack S, Tewson T, et al. The dependence of accumulation of 13NH3 by myocardium on metabolic factors and its implications for quantitative assessment of perfusion. *Circulation* 1980;61:34–43.

27. Mullani NA, Goldstein RA, Gould KL, et al. Myocardial perfusion with rubidium-82. I. Measurement of extraction fraction and flow with external detectors. *J Nucl Med* 1983;24:898–906.

28. Krivokapich J, Huang S, Phelps M, et al. Dependence of $^{13}NH_3$ myocardial extraction and clearance on flow and metabolism. *Am J Physiol* 1982;242:H536–542.

29. Gould K. Assessment of coronary stenoses with myocardial perfusion imaging during pharmacologic coronary vasodilation. *Am J Cardiol* 1978;42:761–768.

30. Stewart RE, Schwaiger M, Molina E, et al. Comparison of rubidium-82 positron emission tomography and thallium-201 SPECT imaging for detection of coronary artery disease. *Am J Cardiol* 1991;67:1303–1310.

31. Tamaki N, Yonekura Y, Senda M, et al. Myocardial positron computed tomography with 13N-ammonia at rest and during exercise. *Eur J Nucl Med* 1985;11:246–251.

32. Gould KL, Goldstein RA, Mullani NA, et al. Noninvasive assessment of coronary stenoses by myocardial perfusion imaging during pharmacologic coronary vasodilation. VIII. clinical feasibility of positron cardiac imaging without a cyclotron using generator-produced rubidium-82. *J Am Coll Cardiol* 1986;7:775–789.

33. Demer LL, Gould KL, Goldstein RA, et al. Assessment of coronary artery disease severity by positron emission tomography. Comparison with quantitative arteriography in 193 patients. *Circulation* 1989;79:825–835.

34. Chan SY, Brunken RC, Czernin J, et al. Comparison of maximal myocardial blood flow during adenosine infusion with that of intravenous dipyridamole in normal men. *J Am Coll Cardiol* 1992;20:979–985.

35. Go RT, Marwick TH, MacIntyre WJ, et al. A prospective comparison of rubidium-82 PET and thallium-201 SPECT myocardial perfusion imaging utilizing a single dipyridamole stress in the diagnosis of coronary artery disease [see comments]. *J Nucl Med* 1990;31:1899–1905.

36. Tamaki N, Yonehura Y, Senda M, et al. Value and limitation of stress thallium-201 single photon positron computed tomography: comparison with nitrogen-13 ammonia positron tomography. *J Nucl Med* 1988;29:1181–1188.

37. Porenta G, Kuhle W, Czernin J, et al. Semiquantitative assessment of myocardial blood flow and viability using polar map displays of cardiac PET images. *J Nucl Med* 1992;33:1628–1636.

38. Laubenbacher C, Rothley J, Sitomer J, et al. An automated analysis program for the evaluation of cardiac PET studies: initial results in the detection and localization of coronary artery disease using nitrogen-13-ammonia. *J Nucl Med* 1993;34:968–978.

39. Patterson RE, Eisner RL, Horowitz SF. Comparison of cost-effectiveness and utility of exercise ECG, single photon emission computed tomography, positron emission tomography, and coronary angiography for diagnosis of coronary artery disease. *Circulation* 1995;91:54–65.

40. Gould KL, Nakagawa Y, Nakagawa K, et al. Frequency and clinical implications of fluid dynamically significant diffuse CAD manifest as graded, longitudinal, base-to-apex myocardial perfusion abnormalities by noninvasive PET. *Circulation* 2000;101:1931–1939.

41. Gould KL, Martucci JP, Goldberg DI, et al. Short-term cholesterol lowering decreases size and severity of perfusion abnormalities by positron emission tomography after dipyridamole in patients with coronary artery disease: a potential noninvasive marker of healing coronary endothelium. *Circulation* 1994;89:1530–1538.

42. Gould KL, Ornish D, Scherwitz L, et al. Changes in myocardial perfusion abnormalities by positron emission tomography after long-term, intense risk factor modification. *JAMA* 1995;274:894–901.

43. Iida H, Takahashi A, Ono Y, et al. Quantitative and noninvasive measurement of myocardial blood flow using H2-15O and dynamic positron emission tomography. *J Nucl Med* 1986;27:976.

44. Hermansen F, Rosen S, Fath-Ordoubadi F, et al. Measurement of myocardial blood flow with oxygen-15 labeled water: comparison of different administration protocols. *Eur J Nucl Med* 1998;25:751–759.

45. Bergmann SR, Fox K, Rand A, et al. Quantification of

regional myocardial blood flow with H215-0. *Circulation* 1984;70:724–733.

46. Muzik O, Beanlands RS, Hutchins GD, et al. Validation of nitrogen-13-ammonia tracer kinetic model for quantification of myocardial blood flow using PET. *J Nucl Med* 1993;34:83–91.

47. Bol A, Melin JA, Vanoverschelde JL, et al. Direct comparison of [13N]ammonia and [15O]water estimates of perfusion with quantification of regional myocardial blood flow by microspheres. *Circulation* 1993;87:512–525.

48. Iida H, Tamura Y, Kitamura K, et al. Histochemical correlates of 15O-water-perfusable tissue fraction in experimental canine studies of old myocardial infarction. *J Nucl Med* 2000;41:1737–1745.

49. Katoh C, Ruotsalainen U, Laine H, et al. Iterative reconstruction based on median root prior in quantification of myocardial blood flow and oxygen metabolism. *J Nucl Med* 1999;40:862–867.

50. Krivokapich J, Smith GT, Huang S-C, et al. 13N ammonia myocardial imaging at rest and with exercise in normal volunteers: quantification of absolute myocardial perfusion with dynamic positron emission tomography. *Circulation* 1989;80:1328–1337.

51. Hutchins G, Schwaiger M, Rosenspire K, et al. Noninvasive quantification of regional myocardial blood flow in the human heart using N-13 ammonia and dynamic positron emission tomographic imaging. *J Am Coll Cardiol* 1990;15:1032.

52. Choi Y, Huang SC, Hawkins RA, et al. A simplified method for quantification of myocardial blood flow using nitrogen-13-ammonia and dynamic PET. *J Nucl Med* 1993;34:488–497.

53. Choi Y, Huang SC, Hawkins RA, et al. Quantification of myocardial blood flow using 13N-ammonia and PET: comparison of tracer models. *J Nucl Med* 1999;40:1045–1055.

54. Herrero P, Markham J, Shelton ME, et al. Noninvasive quantification of regional myocardial perfusion with rubidium-82 and positron emission tomography. *Circulation* 1990;82:1377–1386.

55. deKemp RA, Ruddy TD, Hewitt T, et al. Detection of serial changes in absolute myocardial perfusion with 82Rb PET. *J Nucl Med* 2000;41:1426–1435.

56. Herrero P, Markham J, Weinheimer CJ, et al. Quantification of regional myocardial perfusion with generator-produced 62Cu-PTSM and positron emission tomography. *Circulation* 1993;87:173–183.

57. Gould K, Kirkeeide R, Buchi M. Coronary flow reserve as a physiologic measure of stenosis severity. *J Am Coll Cardiol* 1990;15:459–474.

58. Mancini JGB, Williamson PR, DeBoe SF. Effect of coronary stenosis severity on variability of quantitative arteriography and implications for interventional trials. *Am J Cardiol* 1992;69:806–807.

59. Wilson RF, Marcus ML, White CW. Prediction of the physiologic significance of coronary arterial lesions by quantitative lesion geometry in patients with limited coronary artery disease. *Circulation* 1987;75:723–732.

60. Sawada S, Muzik O, Beanlands RSB, et al. Interobserver and interstudy variability of myocardial blood flow and flow-reserve measurements with nitrogen 13 ammonia-labeled positron emission tomography. *J Nucl Cardiol* 1995;2:413–422.

61. Kaufmann PA, Gnecchi-Ruscone T, Yap JT, et al. Assessment of the reproducibility of baseline and hyperemic myo-cardial blood flow measurements with 150-labeled water PET. *J Nucl Med* 1999;40:1848–1856.

62. Beanlands RS, Muzik O, Melon P, et al. Noninvasive quantification of regional myocardial flow reserve in patients with coronary atherosclerosis using nitrogen-13 ammonia positron emission tomography. Determination of extent of altered vascular reactivity. *J Am Coll Cardiol* 1995;26:1465–1475.

63. Muzik O, Duvernoy C, Beanlands R, et al. Assessment of diagnostic performance of quantitative flow measurements in normal subjects and patients with angiographically documented CAD by means of nitrogen-13 ammonia and using PET. *J Am Coll Cardiol* 1998;31:534–540.

64. Czernin J, Muller P, Chan S, et al. Influence of age and hemodynamics on myocardial blood flow and flow reserve. *Circulation* 1993;88:62–69.

65. Uren NG, Camici PG, Melin JA, et al. Effect of aging on myocardial perfusion reserve. *J Nucl Med* 1995;36:2032–2036.

66. Rosen SD, Uren NG, Kaski JC, et al. Coronary vasodilator reserve, pain perception, and sex in patients with syndrome X. *Circulation* 1994;90:50–60.

67. Parodi O, Neglia D, Sambuceti G, et al. Regional myocardial blood flow and coronary reserve in hypertensive patients. The effect of therapy. *Drugs* 1992;1:48–55.

68. Camici P, Chiriatti G, Lorenzoni R, et al. Coronary vasodilation is impaired in both hypertrophied and nonhypertrophied myocardium of patients with hypertrophic cardiomyopathy: a study with nitrogen-13 ammonia and positron emission tomography. *J Am Coll Cardiol* 1991;17:879–886.

69. Krivokapich J, Stevenson LW, Kobashigawa J, Huang, et al. Quantification of absolute myocardial perfusion at rest and during exercise with positron emission tomography after human cardiac transplantation. *J Am Coll Cardiol* 1991;18:512–517.

70. Uren NG, Melin JA, De-Bruyne B, et al. Relation between myocardial blood flow and the severity of coronary-artery stenosis. *N Engl J Med* 1994;330:1782–1788.

71. DiCarli M, Czernin J, Hoh CK, et al. Relation among stenosis severity, myocardial blood flow, and flow reserve in patients with coronary artery disease. *Circulation* 1995;91:1944–1951.

72. Araujo LI. Myocardial perfusion and metabolic changes associated with transient episodes of ischemia in patients with coronary artery disease as assessed by positron emission tomography. *Coron Artery Dis* 1990;1:54–106.

73. Uren NG, Marraccini P, Gistri R, et al. Altered coronary vasodilator reserve and metabolism in myocardium subtended by normal arteries in patients with coronary artery disease. *J Am Coll Cardiol* 1993;22:650–658.

74. Pitkanen OP, Nuutila P, Raitakari OT, et al. Coronary flow reserve is reduced in young men with IDDM. *Diabetes* 1998;47:248–254.

75. Raitakari O, Pitkänen O-P, Lehtimäki T, et al. In vivo low density lipoprotein oxidation relates to coronary reactivity in young men. *J Am Coll Cardiol* 1997;30:97–102.

76. Duvernoy C, Meyer C, Seifert-Klauss V, et al. Gender differences in myocardial blood flow dynamics: lipid profile and hemodynamic effects. *J Am Coll Cardiol* 1999;33:463–470.

77. Kaufmann PA, Gnecchi-Ruscone T, di Terlizzi M, et al. Coronary heart disease in smokers: vitamin C restores coronary microcirculatory function. *Circulation* 2000;102:1233–1238.

78. Pitkanen OP, Nuutila P, Raitakari OT, et al. Coronary flow

reserve in young men with familial combined hyperlipidemia. *Circulation* 1999;99:1678–1684.

79. Maseri A, Crea F, Cianflone D. Myocardial ischemia caused by distal coronary vasoconstriction [editorial]. *Am J Cardiol* 1992;70:1602–1605.

80. Bottcher M, Czernin J, Sun K, et al. Effect of beta 1 adrenergic receptor blockade on myocardial blood flow and vasodilatory capacity. *J Nucl Med* 1997;38:442–446.

81. Rosen SD, Lorenzoni R, Kaski JC, et al. Effect of alpha1-adrenoceptor blockade on coronary vasodilator reserve in cardiac syndrome X. *J Cardiovasc Pharmacol* 1999;34:554–560.

82. Campisi R, Czernin J, Schoder H, et al. L-Arginine normalizes coronary vasomotion in long-term smokers. *Circulation* 1999;99:491–497.

83. Bottcher M, Botker HE, Sonne H, et al. Endothelium-dependent and -independent perfusion reserve and the effect of L-arginine on myocardial perfusion in patients with syndrome X. *Circulation* 1999;99:1795–1801.

84. Schoder H, Silverman DH, Campisi R, et al. Effect of mental stress on myocardial blood flow and vasomotion in patients with coronary artery disease. *J Nucl Med* 2000;41:11–16.

85. Czernin J, Barnard RJ, Sun KT, et al. Effect of short-term cardiovascular conditioning and low-fat diet on myocardial blood flow and flow reserve. *Circulation* 1995;92:197–204.

86. Huggins G, Pasternack R, Alpert N, et al. Effects of short-term treatment of hyperlipidemia on coronary vasodilator function and myocardial perfusion in regions having substantial impairment of baseline dilator reverse. *Circulation* 1998;98:1291–1296.

87. Guethlin M, Kasel AM, Coppenrath K, et al. Delayed response of myocardial flow reserve to lipid-lowering therapy with fluvastatin. *Circulation* 1999;99:475–481.

88. Baller D, Notohamiprodjo G, Gleichmann U, et al. Improvement in coronary flow reserve determined by positron emission tomography after 6 months of cholesterol-lowering therapy in patients with early stages of coronary atherosclerosis. *Circulation* 1999;99:2871–2875.

89. Schachinger V, Britten MB. Prognostic impact of coronary vasodilatory dysfunction on adverse long-term outcome of coronary heart disease. *Circulation* 2000;101:1899–1906.

90. Kitsiou AN, Bacharach SL, Bartlett ML, et al. 13N-ammonia myocardial blood flow and uptake: relation to functional outcome of asynergic regions after revascularization. *J Am Coll Cardiol* 1999;33:678–686.

91. Bogaert J, Maes A, Bosmans H, et al. Functional recovery of subepicardial myocardial tissue in transmural myocardial infarction after successful reperfusion: an important contribution to the improvement of regional and global left ventricular function. *Circulation* 1999;99:36–43.

92. Rimoldi O, Burns SM, Rosen SD, et al. Measurement of myocardial blood flow with positron emission tomography before and after transmyocardial laser revascularization. *Circulation* 1999;100[Suppl II]:134–138.

93. Hughes GC, Kypson AP, St. Louis JD, et al. Improved perfusion and contractile reserve after transmural laser revascularization in a model of hibernating myocardium. *Ann Thorac Surg* 1999;67:1714–1720.

94. Schneider CA, Voth E, Moka D, et al. Improvement of myocardial blood flow to ischemic regions by angiotensin-converting enzyme inhibition with quinaprilat IV: a study using [¹⁵O] water dobutamine stress positron emission tomography. *J Am Coll Cardiol* 1999;34:1005–1011.

95. Kosa I, Blasini R, Schneider-Eicke J, et al. Early recovery of coronary flow reserve after stent implantation as assessed by PET. *J Am Coll Cardiol* 1999;34:1036–1041.

96. Spyrou N, Khan MA, Rosen SD, et al. Persistent but reversible coronary microvascular dysfunction after bypass grafting. *Am J Physiol* 2000;261:H2634–H2640.

97. Campisi R, Czernin J, Schoder H, et al. Effects of long-term smoking on myocardial blood flow, coronary vasomotion, and vasodilator capacity. *Circulation* 1998;98:119–125.

98. Gnecchi-Ruscone T, Bernard X, Pierre P, et al. Effect of naratriptan on myocardial blood flow and coronary vasodilator reserve in migraineurs. *Neurology* 2000;55:95–99.

99. Senneff MJ, Hartman J, Sobel BE, et al. Persistence of coronary vasodilator responsivity after cardiac transplantation. *Am J Cardiol* 1993;71:333–338.

100. Wolpers HG, Koster C, Burchert W, et al. Coronary reserve after orthotopic heart transplantation: quantification with N-13 ammonia and positron emission tomography. *Z Kardiol* 1995;84:112–120.

101. Tadamura E, Yoshibayashi M, Yonemura T, et al. Significant regional heterogeneity of coronary flow reserve in paediatric hypertrophic cardiomyopathy. *Eur J Nucl Med* 2000;27:1340–1348.

102. van den Heuvel AF, van Veldhuisen DJ, van der Wall EE, et al. Regional myocardial blood flow reserve impairment and metabolic changes suggesting myocardial ischemia in patients with idiopathic dilated myopathy. *J Am Coll Cardiol* 2000;35:19–28.

103. Shikama N, Himi T, Yoshida K, et al. Prognostic utility of myocardial blood flow assessed by N-13 ammonia positron emission tomography in patients with idiopathic cardiomyopathy. *Am J Cardiol* 1999;84:434–439.

104. Merlet P, Mazoyer B, Hittinger L, et al. Assessment of coronary reserve in man: comparison between positron emission tomography with oxygen-15-labeled water and intracoronary Doppler technique. *J Nucl Med* 1993;34:1899–1904.

105. Parodi O, De-Maria R, Oltrona L, et al. Myocardial blood flow distribution in patients with ischemic heart disease or dilated cardiomyopathy undergoing heart transplantation. *Circulation* 1993;88:509–522.

106. Drzezga A, Blasini R, Ziegler S, et al. Coronary microvascular reactivity to sympathetic stimulation in patients with idiopathic dilated cardiomyopathy. *J Nucl Med* 2000;41:837–844.

107. Liedtke AJ. Alterations of carbohydrate and lipid metabolism in the acutely ischemic heart. *Prog Cardiovasc Dis* 1981;23:321–336.

108. Taegtmeyer H. Myocardial metabolism. In: Phelps ME, Mazziotta JC, Schelbert HR, eds. *Positron emission tomography and autoradiography: principles and applications for the brain and heart.* New York: Raven Press, 1986:149–195.

109. Depre C, Vanoverschelde JL, et al. Glucose for the heart. *Circulation* 1999;99:578–588.

110. Gertz EW, Wisneski JA, Stanley WC, et al. Myocardial substrate utilization during exercise in humans. Dual carbon-labeled carbohydrate isotope experiments. *J Clin Invest* 1988;82:2017–2025.

111. Opie LH. Effects of regional ischemia on metabolism of glucose and fatty acids. Relative rates of aerobic and anaero-

bic energy production during myocardial infarction and comparison with effects of anoxia. *Circ Res* 1976;38[Suppl 1]:I52–74.

112. Kalff V, Schwaiger M, Nguyen N, et al. The relationship between myocardial blood flow and glucose uptake in ischemic canine myocardium determined with fluorine-18-deoxyglucose. *J Nucl Med* 1992;33:1346–1353.

113. Sun DQ, Nguyen N, DeGrado TR, et al. Ischemia induces translocation of the insulin-responsive glucose transporter GLUT4 to the plasma membrane of cardiac myocytes. *Circulation* 1994;89:793–798.

114. Young LH, Russell RR 3rd, Yin R, et al. Regulation of myocardial glucose uptake and transport during ischemia and energetic stress. *Am J Cardiol* 1999;83:24H–30H.

115. Egert S, Nguyen N. The contribution of alpha-adrenergic and beta-adrenergic stimulation on ischemia-induced GLUT4 and GLUT1 translocation in the isolated perfused rat heart. *Circ Res* 1998;84:1407–1415.

116. Borgers M, Thoné F, Wouters L, et al. Structural correlates of regional myocardial dysfunction in patients with critical coronary artery stenosis: chronic hibernation? *Cardiovasc Pathol* 1993;2:237–245.

117. Ausma J, Schaart G, Thone F, et al. Chronic ischemic viable myocardium in man: aspects of dedifferentiation. *Cardiovasc Pathol* 1995;4:29–37.

118. Depre C. Metabolic aspects of programmed cell survival and cell death in the heart. *Cardiovasc Res* 2000;45:538–548.

119. Schelbert H, Henze E, Schon H, et al. C-11 palmitic acid for the noninvasive evaluation of regional myocardial fatty acid metabolism with positron computed tomography. IV. In vivo demonstration of impaired fatty acid oxidation in acute myocardial ischemia. *Am Heart J* 1983;106:736–750.

120. Buxton DB, Schwaiger M, Nguyen A, et al. Radiolabeled acetate as a tracer of myocardial tricarboxylic acid cycle flux. *Circ Res* 1988;63:628–634.

121. Brown MA, Marshall DR, Sobel BE, et al. Delineation of myocardial oxygen utilization with carbon-11 labeled acetate. *Circulation* 1987;76:687–696.

122. Beanlands RS, Nahmias C, Gordon E, et al. The effects of beta(1)-blockade on oxidative metabolism and the metabolic cost of ventricular work in patients with left ventricular dysfunction: a double-blind, placebo controlled, positron emission tomography study. *Circulation* 2000;102:2070–2075.

123. Buck A, Wolpers HG, Hutchins GD, et al. Effect of carbon-11-acetate recirculation on estimates of myocardial oxygen consumption by PET [see comments]. *J Nucl Med* 1991;32:1950–1957.

124. Gropler RJ, Siegel BA, Geltman EM. Myocardial uptake of carbon-11-acetate as an indirect estimate of regional myocardial blood flow. *J Nucl Med* 1991;32:245–251.

125. Sokoloff L, Reivich M, Kennedy C, et al. The (14C) deoxyglucose method for the measurement of local cerebral glucose utilization: theory, procedure and normal values in the conscious and anesthetized albino rat. *J Neurochem* 1977;28:897–916.

126. Phelps ME, Huang SC, Hoffman EJ, et al. Tomographic measurement of local cerebral glucose metabolic rate in humans with (F-18)2-fluoro-2-deoxy-D-glucose: validation of method. *Ann Neurol* 1979;6:371–388.

127. Krivokapich J, Huang SC, Phelps ME, et al. Estimation of rabbit myocardial metabolic rate for glucose using fluorodeoxyglucose. *Am J Physiol* 1982;243:H884–H894.

128. Krivokapich J, Huang SC, Selin CE, et al. Fluorodeoxyglucose rate constants, lumped constant, and glucose metabolic rate in rabbit heart. *Am J Physiol* 1987;252:H777–787.

129. Hariharan R, Bray M, Ganim R, et al. Fundamental limitations of [18F]2-deoxy-2-fluoro-D-glucose for assessing myocardial glucose uptake. *Circulation* 1995;91:2435–2444.

130. Patlak CS, Blasberg RG. Graphical evaluation of blood-to-brain transfer constants from multiple-time uptake data. Generalizations. *J Cereb Blood Flow Metab* 1985;5:584–590.

131. Hicks RJ, Herman WH, Wolfe E, et al. Regional variation in oxidative and glucose metabolism in the normal heart: comparison of PET-derived C-11 acetate and FDG kinetics. *J Nucl Med* 1990;31:774.

132. Gropler RJ, Lee KJ, Moerlein SM, et al. Regional variation in myocardial accumulation of 18F-fluorodeoxyglucose in fasted normal subjects. *J Am Coll Cardiol* 1990;15:81A.

133. vom Dahl J, Herman WH, Hicks RJ, et al. Myocardial glucose uptake in patients with insulin-dependent diabetes mellitus assessed quantitatively by dynamic positron emission tomography. *Circulation* 1993;88:395–404.

134. Ohtake T, Yokoyama I, Watanabe T, et al. Myocardial glucose metabolism in noninsulin-dependent diabetes mellitus patients evaluated by FDG-PET. *J Nucl Med* 1995;36:456–463.

135. Knuuti MJ, Nuutila P, Ruotsalainen U, et al. Euglycemic hyperinsulinemic clamp and oral glucose load in stimulating myocardial glucose utilization during positron emission tomography. *J Nucl Med* 1992;33:1255–1262.

136. Takala TO, Nuutila P, Knuuti J, et al. Insulin action on heart and skeletal muscle glucose uptake in weight lifters and endurance athletes. *Am J Physiol* 1999;27:E706–711.

137. Schwaiger M, Fishbein MC, Block M, et al. Metabolic and ultrastructural abnormalities during ischemia in canine myocardium: non-invasive assessment by positron emission tomography. *J Mol Cell Cardiol* 1987;19:259–269.

138. Marshall RC, Huang SC, Nash WW, et al. Assessment of the (18F)fluorodeoxyglucose kinetic model in calculations of myocardial glucose metabolism during ischemia. *J Nucl Med* 1983;24:1060–1064.

139. Schelbert HR, Henze E, Phelps ME, et al. Assessment of regional myocardial ischemia by positron-emission computed tomography. *Am Heart J* 1982;103:588–597.

140. Tillisch J, Brunken R, Marshall R, et al. Reversibility of cardiac wall motion abnormalities predicted by positron tomography. *N Engl J Med* 1986;314:884–888.

141. Marshall RC, Tillisch JH, Phelps ME, et al. Identification and differentiation of resting myocardial ischemia and infarction in man with positron computed tomography 18F-labeled fluorodeoxyglucose and N-13 ammonia. *Circulation* 1981;64:766–778.

142. Vanoverschelde JL, Wijns W, Depre C, et al. Mechanisms of chronic regional postischemic dysfunction in humans. New insights from the study of noninfarcted collateral-dependent myocardium. *Circulation* 1993;87:1513–1523.

143. Wijns W, Vatner SF. Hibernating myocardium. *N Engl J Med* 1998;339:173–181.

144. Camici PG, Wijns W, Borgers M, et al. Pathophysiological mechanisms of chronic reversible left ventricular dysfunction due to coronary artery disease (hibernating myocardium). *Circulation* 1997;96:3205–3214.

145. Pantely GA, Malone SA, Rhen WS, et al. Regeneration of

myocardial phosphocreatine in pigs despite continued moderate ischemia. *Circ Res* 1990;67:1481–1493.

146. Schulz R. Hibernating myocardium. *Heart* 2000;84:587–594.

147. Rahimtoola SH. The hibernating myocardium. *Am Heart J* 1989;117:211–221.

148. Braunwald E, Kloner R. The stunned myocardium: prolonged, postischemic ventricular dysfunction. *Circulation* 1982;66:1146–1149.

149. Yamamoto Y, de Silva R, Rhodes C, et al. A new strategy for the assessment of viable myocardium and regional myocardial blood flow using 15O-water and dynamic positron emission tomography. *Circulation* 1992;86:167–178.

150. Haas F, Augustin N, Holper K, et al. Time course and extent of improvement of dysfunctioning myocardium in patients with coronary artery disease and severely depressed left ventricular function after revascularization: correlation with positron emission tomographic findings. *J Am Coll Cardiol* 2000;36:1927–1934.

151. vom Dahl J, Eitzman DT, al-Aouar ZR, et al. Relation of regional function, perfusion, and metabolism in patients with advanced coronary artery disease undergoing surgical revascularization. *Circulation* 1994;90:2356–2366.

152. Gerber BL, Melin JA, Bol A, et al. Nitrogen-13-ammonia and oxygen-15-water estimates of absolute myocardial perfusion in left ventricular ischemic dysfunction. *J Nucl Med* 1998;39:1655–1662.

153. Vanoverschelde JL, Depre C, Gerber BL, et al. Time course of functional recovery after coronary artery bypass graft surgery in patients with chronic left ventricular ischemic dysfunction. *Am J Cardiol* 2000;85:1432–1439.

154. Baer FM, Voth E, Schneider CA, et al. Comparison of low-dose dobutamine-gradient-echo magnetic resonance imaging and positron emission tomography with [18F]fluorodeoxyglucose in patients with chronic coronary artery disease. A functional and morphological approach to the detection of residual myocardial viability. *Circulation* 1995;91:1006–1015.

155. Bax JJ, Wijns W, Cornel JH, et al. Accuracy of currently available techniques for prediction of functional recovery after revascularization in patients with left ventricular dysfunction due to chronic coronary artery disease: comparison of pooled data. *J Am Coll Cardiol* 1997;30:1451–1460.

156. Dilsizian V, Rocco TP, Freedman NM, et al. Enhanced detection of ischemic but viable myocardium by the reinjection of thallium after stress-redistribution imaging [see comments]. *N Engl J Med* 1990;323:141–146.

157. Bax JJ, Poldermans D, Elhendy A. 18-Fluorodeoxyglucose imaging with positron emission tomography and single photon emission computed tomography: cardiac applications. *Semin Nucl Med* 2000;30:281–298.

158. Eitzman D, Al-Aouar Z, Kanter H, et al. Clinical outcome of patients with advanced coronary artery disease following positron emission tomography viability studies. *J Am Coll Cardiol* 1992;20:559–565.

159. Maddahi J, DiCarli M, Davidson M, et al. Prognostic significance of PET assessment of myocardial viability in patients with left ventricular dysfunction. *J Am Coll Cardiol* 1992;19:142A.

160. Tamaki N, Yonekura Y, Yamashita K, et al. Prognostic value of an increase in fluorine-18 deoxyglucose uptake in patients with myocardial infarction: comparison with stress thallium imaging. *J Am Coll Cardiol* 1993;22:1621–1627.

161. DiCarli MF, Davidson M, Little R, et al. Value of metabolic imaging with positron emission tomography for evaluating prognosis in patients with coronary artery disease and left ventricular dysfunction. *Am J Cardiol* 1994;73:527–533.

162. DiCarli MF, Asgarzadie F, Schelbert HR, et al. Quantitative relation between myocardial viability and improvement in heart failure symptoms after revascularization in patients with ischemic cardiomyopathy. *Circulation* 1995;92:3436–3444.

163. Pagano D, Lewis ME, Townend JN, et al. Coronary revascularization for postischaemic heart failure: how myocardial viability affects survival. *Heart* 1999;82:684–688.

164. Beanlands R, Hendry P, Masters R, et al. Delay in revascularization is associated with increased mortality rate in patients with severe left ventricular dysfunction and viable myocardium on fluorine 18-fluorodeoxyglucose positron emission tomography imaging. *Circulation* 1998;98[Suppl 19]:II51–II56.

165. Dreyfus GD, Duboc D, Blasco A, et al. Myocardial viability assessment in ischemic cardiomyopathy: benefits of coronary revascularization. *Ann Thorac Surg* 1994;57:1402–1407.

166. Haas F, Hähnel C, Sebening F, et al. Effect of preoperative PET viability on peri- and postoperative risk. *J Am Coll Cardiol* 1996;27:300A.

167. Fukuchi K, Sago M, Nitta K, et al. Attenuation correction for cardiac dual-head gamma camera coincidence imaging using segmented myocardial perfusion SPECT. *J Nucl Med* 2000;41:919–925.

168. Gropler RJ, Geltman EM, Sampathkumaran K, et al. Functional recovery after coronary revascularization for chronic coronary artery disease is dependent on maintenance of oxidative metabolism. *J Am Coll Cardiol* 1992;20:569–577.

169. Gropler RJ, Geltman EM, Sampathkumaran K, et al. Comparison of carbon-11-acetate with fluorine-18-fluorodeoxyglucose for delineating viable myocardium by positron emission tomography. *J Am Coll Cardiol* 1993;22:1587–1597.

170. Gerber BL, Wijns W, Vanoverschelde JL, et al. Myocardial perfusion and oxygen consumption in reperfused noninfarcted dysfunctional myocardium after unstable angina: direct evidence for myocardial stunning in humans. *J Am Coll Cardiol* 1999;34:1939–1946.

171. Geltman E. Metabolic findings in cardiomyopathies. In: *Cardiac imaging: a companion to Braunwald's heart disease.* Philadelphia: WB Saunders, 1991:1244–1255.

172. Kelly D, Mendelsohn N, Sobel B, et al. Detection and assessment by positron emission tomography of a genetically determined defect in myocardial fatty acid utilization (long-chain acyl-CoA dehydrogenase deficiency). *Am J Cardiol* 1993;71:738–744.

173. Buxton DB, Nienaber CA, Luxen A, et al. Noninvasive quantitation of regional myocardial oxygen consumption in vivo with [1-11C]acetate and dynamic positron emission tomography. *Circulation* 1989;79:134–142.

174. Hicks RJ, Kalff V, Savas V, et al. Assessment of right ventricular oxidative metabolism by positron emission tomography with C-11 acetate in aortic valve disease. *Am J Cardiol* 1991;67:753–757.

175. Wolpers GH, Buck A, Nguyen N, et al. An approach to ventricular efficiency by use of carbon-11 labeled acetate and positron emission tomography. *J Nucl Cardiol* 1994;1:262–269.

176. Bengel FM, Permanetter B, Ungerer M, et al. Non-invasive estimation of myocardial efficiency using positron emission tomography and carbon-11 acetate—comparison between

the normal and failing human heart. *J Nucl Med* 2000;41:837–844.

177. Beanlands RS, Bach DS, Raylman R, et al. Acute effects of dobutamine on myocardial oxygen consumption and cardiac efficiency measured using carbon-11 acetate kinetics in patients with dilated cardiomyopathy. *J Am Coll Cardiol* 1993;22:1389–1398.

178. Francis GS. Modulation of peripheral sympathetic nerve transmission. *J Am Coll Cardiol* 1988;12:250–254.

179. Goldstein D, Brush Jr J, Eisenhofer G, et al. In vivo measurement of neuronal uptake of norepinephrine in the human heart. *Circulation* 1988;78:41–48.

180. Rosenspire K, Haka M, Jewett D, et al. Synthesis and preliminary evaluation of 11C-meta-hydroxyephedrine: a false transmitter agent for heart neuronal imaging. *J Nucl Med* 1990;31:1328–1334.

181. Schwaiger M, Kalff V, Rosenspire K, et al. The noninvasive evaluation of the sympathetic nervous system in the human heart by PET. *Circulation* 1990;82:457–464.

182. Munch G, Nguyen N, Nekolla S, et al. Evaluation of sympathetic nerve terminals using C-11 epinephrine and C-11 hydroxyephedrine and PET. *Circulation* 2000;101:516–523.

183. Corbett J, Chiao P-C, del Rosario R, et al. Mapping neuronal enzyme function of the human heart with C-11 phenylephrine. *J Nucl Med* 1994;35:109P.

184. Goldstein D, Eisenhofer G, Dunn B, et al. Positron emission tomographic imaging of cardiac sympathetic innervation using 6-18F-fluorodopamine: initial findings in humans. *J Am Coll Cardiol* 1993;22:1961–1971.

185. Ding Y, Fowler J, Dewey S, et al. Comparison of high specific activity (–) and (+)-6-18F-fluoronorepinephrine and 6-18F-fluorodopamine in baboons: heart uptake, metabolism and the effect of desipramine. *J Nucl Med* 1993;34:619–629.

186. Valette H, Loc'h C, Mardon K, et al. Bromine-76-metabromobenzylguanidine: a PET radiotracer for mapping sympathetic nerves of the heart. *J Nucl Med* 1993;34:1739–1744.

187. Caldwell JH, Kroll K, Li Z, et al. Quantitation of presynaptic cardiac sympathetic function with carbon-11-meta-hydroxyephedrine. *J Nucl Med* 1998;39:1327–1334.

188. Schwaiger M, Hutchins GD, Kalff V, et al. Evidence for regional catecholamine uptake and storage sites in the transplanted human heart by positron emission tomography. *J Clin Invest* 1991;87:1681–1690.

189. Ziegler S, Frey A, Uberfuhr P, et al. Assessment of myocardial reinnervation in cardiac transplants by positron emission tomography: functional significance tested by heart rate variability. *Clin Sci* 1996;91[Suppl]:126–128.

190. Uberfuhr P, Frey AW, Ziegler S, et al. Sympathetic reinnervation of sinus node and left ventricle after heart transplantation in humans: regional differences assessed by heart rate variability and positron emission tomography. *J Heart Lung Transplant* 2000;19:317–323.

191. Bengel FM, Ueberfuhr P, Ziegler SI, et al. Serial assessment of sympathetic reinnervation after orthotopic heart transplantation. A longitudinal study using PET and C-11 hydroxyephedrine. *Circulation* 1999;99:1866–1871.

192. Allman KC, Wieland DM, Muzik O, et al. Carbon-11 hydroxyephedrine with positron emission tomography for serial assessment of cardiac adrenergic neuronal function after acute myocardial infarction in humans. *J Am Coll Cardiol* 1993;22:368–375.

193. Wolpers H, Nguyen N, Rosenspire K, et al. C-11 hydroxyephedrine as marker for neuronal dysfunction in reperfused canine myocardium. *Coronary Artery Disease* 1991;2:923–929.

194. Matsunari I, Schricke U, Bengel FM, et al. Extent of cardiac sympathetic neuronal damage is determined by the area of ischemia in patients with acute coronary syndromes. *Circulation* 2000;101:2579–2585.

195. Stevens MJ, Raffel DM, Allman KC, et al. Cardiac sympathetic dysinnervation in diabetes: implications for enhanced cardiovascular risk. *Circulation* 1998;98:961–968.

196. Stevens M, Dayanikli F, Raffel D, et al. Scintigraphic assessment of regionalized defects in myocardial sympathetic innervation and blood flow regulation in diabetic patients with autonomic neuropathy. *J Am Coll Cardiol* 1998;31:1575–1584.

197. Stevens MJ, Raffel DM, Allman KC, et al. Regression and progression of cardiac sympathetic dysinnervation complicating diabetes: an assessment by C-11 hydroxyephedrine and positron emission tomography. *Metabolism* 1999;48:92–101.

198. DiCarli MF, Bianco-Batlles D, Landa ME, et al. Effects of autonomic neuropathy on coronary blood flow in patients with diabetes mellitus. *Circulation* 1999;100:813–819.

199. Ungerer M, Hartmann F, Karoglan M, et al. Regional in vivo and in vitro characterization of autonomic innervation in cardiomyopathic human heart. *Circulation* 1998;97:174–180.

200. Hartmann F, Ziegler S, Nekolla S, et al. Regional patterns of myocardial sympathetic denervation in dilated cardiomyopathy: an analysis using carbon-11 hydroxyephedrine and positron emission tomography. *Heart* 1999;81:262–270.

201. Syrota A. Positron emission tomography: evaluation of cardiac receptors. In: Marcus ML, et al., eds. *Cardiac imaging principles and practice: a companion of Braunwald's heart disease.* Philadelphia: WB Saunders, 1991:1256–1270.

202. Valette H, Syrota A, Merlet P. Use of PET radiopharmaceuticals to probe cardiac receptors. In: Schwaiger M, ed. *Cardiac positron emission tomography.* Boston: Kluwer, 1996:331–351.

203. Rosen SD, Boyd H, Rhodes CG, et al. Is overactivity of the sympathetic nervous system demonstrable in patients with syndrome X? *Circulation* 1995;92:I-652.

204. Wichter T, Schafers M, Rhodes CG, et al. Abnormalities of cardiac sympathetic innervation in arrhythmogenic right ventricular cardiomyopathy: quantitative assessment of presynaptic norepinephrine reuptake and postsynaptic beta-adrenergic receptor density with positron emission tomography. *Circulation* 2000;101:1552–1558.

205. Schafers M, Lerch H, Wichter T, et al. Cardiac sympathetic innervation in patients with idiopathic right ventricular outflow tract tachycardia. *J Am Coll Cardiol* 1998;32:181–186.

206. Schafers M, Dutka D, Rhodes CG, et al. Myocardial presynaptic and postsynaptic autonomic dysfunction in hypertrophic cardiomyopathy. *Circ Res* 1998;82:57–62.

207. Law MP, Osman S, Pike VW, et al. Evaluation of [11C]GB67, a novel radioligand for imaging myocardial alpha 1-adrenoceptors with positron emission tomography. *Eur J Nucl Med* 2000;27:7–17.

208. Bengel FM, Anton M, Avril N, et al. Uptake of radiolabeled 2'-fluoro-2'deoxy-5-iodo-1-beta-D-arabinofuranosyluracil in cardiac cells after adenoviral transfer of the herpes virus thymidine kinase gene (the cellular basis for cardiac gene imaging). *Circulation* 2000;102:948–950.

209. Carrel T, Jenni R, Haubold-Reuter S, et al. Improvement of severely reduced left ventricular function after surgical revascularization in patients with preoperative myocardial infarction. *Eur J Cardiothorac Surg* 1992;6:479–484.

210. Lucignani G, Paolini G, Landoni C, et al. Presurgical identification of hibernating myocardium by combined use of technetium-99m hexakis 2-methoxyisobutylisonitrile single photon emission tomography and fluorine-18 fluoro-2-deoxy-D-glucose positron emission tomography in patients with coronary artery disease. *Eur J Nucl Med* 1992;19:874–881.

211. Marwick T, MacIntyre W, Lafont A, et al. Metabolic responses of hibernating and infarcted myocardium to revascularization: a follow-up study of regional perfusion, function, and metabolism. *Circulation* 1992;85:1347–1353.

212. Tamaki N, Yonekura N, Yamashita K, et al. Value of rest-stress myocardial positron tomography using nitrogen-13 ammonia for the preoperative prediction of reversible asynergy. *J Nucl Med* 1989;30:1302–1310.

213. Tamaki N, Ohtani H, Yamashita K, et al. Metabolic activity in the areas of new fill-in after thallium-201 reinjection: comparison with positron emission tomography using fluorine-18-deoxyglucose. *J Nucl Med* 1991;32:673–678.

56

COMPUTED TOMOGRAPHY OF THE HEART

ROBERT DETRANO
J. JEFFREY CARR

▼▼ **ADDITIONAL ELECTRONIC TOPICS**

OVERVIEW

Cardiac computed tomography (CT), like echocardiography, provides image slices or tomograms of the anatomic features of the heart. These two modes of tomographic imaging complement each other. On the one hand, the natural echocardiographic contrast difference between fluid and solid tissues allows noninvasive visualization of intracavitary and endovascular lumina and even the visualization of detail in valve leaflets and occasionally the lumen of the left coronary artery. This distinction of blood and tissue would require injection of

R. Detrano: Department of Cardiology, South Bay Heart Watch, Harbor-UCLA Research and Education Institute, Torrance, California

J. J. Carr: Department of Public Health Sciences, Division of Radiological Sciences, Wake Forest University Baptist Medical Center, Winston-Salem, North Carolina

contrast with CT. On the other hand, the higher spatial resolution of CT allows visualization of coronary arteries both with and without contrast enhancement. The accentuated absorption of x-rays by elements of high atomic number such as calcium and iodine allows excellent visualization of small amounts of coronary calcium as well as the contrast-enhanced lumina of medium-sized coronary arteries. Figure 56.1 illustrates the major differences between these two types of imaging.

There are significant tradeoffs when comparing CT with ultrasound imaging. CT capable of accurately imaging the heart is relatively unavailable, often more expensive, and involves the use of ionizing radiation and often iodinated contrast injection. Without the latter, CT, like all radiographic imaging, cannot distinguish intracavitary and intraluminal blood from the muscular walls of vessels and cardiac chambers.

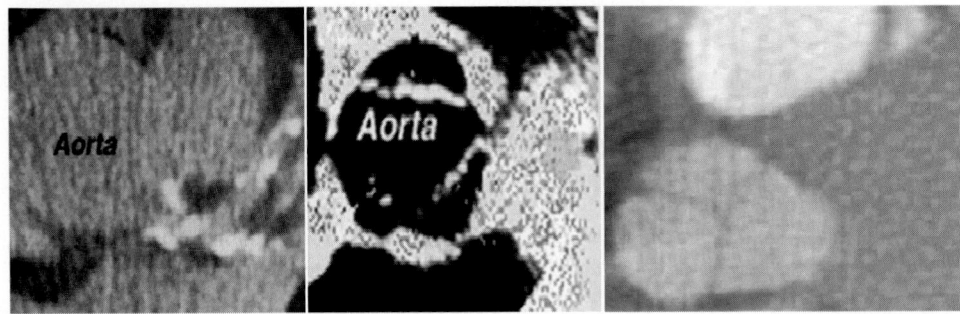

A–C

FIGURE 56.1 **A:** A computed tomographic (CT) scan at the level of the aortic valve. **B:** An echocardiogram at approximately the same anatomic location. **C:** A contrast-enhanced CT image of the aortic valve. The figure illustrates important differences between noncontrast CT, contrast CT, and echocardiography. The presence and severity of coronary calcium are easily seen in the left coronary artery in the computed tomogram on the left, whereas it is invisible in the echocardiogram. The distinction between valve leaflets and aortic wall from aortic blood pool can only be seen on the ultrasound image and the contrast-enhanced CT image. The periarterial fat is shown as a dark area around the left coronary artery on the CT image on the left, whereas this is not seen at all on the echo.

Echocardiography is capable of this distinction even without injections. ⚡ k32

This chapter presents all aspects of rapid CT scanning of the heart but emphasizes its most common use, which is, for better or worse, coronary calcium screening.

GLOSSARY

Calcium score: A mathematical calculation related to the amount of calcium determined by multiplying the area of calcified plaque by a weighting factor based on the CT number or Hounsfield unit of the calcified plaque. Weighted volume of calcium.

Spatial resolution: Quality of image as a function to resolve minute anatomic features.

Temporal resolution: Quality of image as a function of speed of acquisition.

Tomogram: Image slice of the body.

TECHNICAL ASPECTS

Scanning the Heart: A Technical Challenge

CT of the heart presents significant technical obstacles and dilemmas. The heart is far from quiet, and its continuous rhythmic displacement as well as even small degrees of respiratory motion cause great difficulty for imaging with standard CT techniques. Conventional scanners, whose exposure time exceeds one-half of a second, cannot possibly "freeze" this motion. More rapid scanning of the heart has been limited by the speed with which a single tomogram can be acquired. To better understand some of the advances that have allowed crisp images of cardiac anatomy and pathology, we have written this section.

Types of Computed Tomography Systems or Scanners

Two kinds of scanners are used to image the heart. Electron beam scanners use an x-ray source, which consists of a 210-degree arc ring of tungsten, and are activated by bombardment from a magnetically focused beam of electrons fired from an electron gun behind the scanner ring. For most scanning applications, it takes one-tenth of a second to complete a rotation of the electron beam using electron beam computed tomography (EBT) scanners. Subsecond, non–electron beam [multidetector computed tomography (MDCT)] scanners use a rapidly rotating x-ray tube and several rows of detectors, also rotating. The tube and detectors are fitted with slip rings that allow them to continuously move through multiple 360-degree rotations. Present versions complete a 360-degree rotation in approximately one-half of a second. These scanners' exposure times can be decreased to as little as 0.25 seconds by using only a portion of the 360-degree rotation. Further reduction is also possible but at the expense of increased radiation or less rapid acquisition of progression from one tomographic image to the next. For coronary calcium noncontrast scanning, the EBT scanner can acquire only one tomogram at a time; the MDCT scanner can acquire up to four tomograms at a time. Both the speed and the maximum number of tomograms are likely to increase for both types of scanners.

MDCT is also known as *multislice* and is an evolution from single-slice helical or spiral CT systems. The MDCT systems use a rotating x-ray tube and detectors with variable rotation times of less than 1 second. These scanners operate in two modes, helical and sequential, and it is somewhat misleading to call them *helical scanners*. Helical or spiral CT scanning refers not to a different type of scanner but rather to a different method for acquiring and

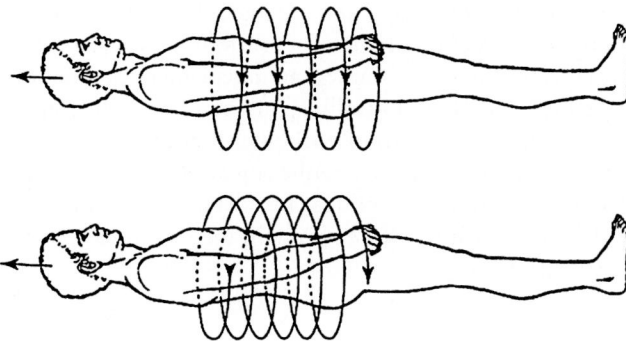

FIGURE 56.2 The top figure shows sequential scanning. The bottom figure shows helical scanning.

reconstructing images. When used normally, in sequential scanning mode, modern scanner tables move the patient through the scanner ring by a set increment of length (from 1 to 15 mm). Between table increments, the x-ray exposure occurs, during which the x-ray tube and detector array rotate slightly greater than a full 360 degrees. These exposures usually have a thickness (collimation) equal to the table increment. With a modern generation MDCT system, rather than a single 10-mm row of detectors, there is a detector array. The detector array allows the same 10-mm slice (x-ray beam collimation) to be divided into four channels or slices. So instead of one 10-mm slice, four 2.5-mm slices are obtained. Likewise, an eight-channel MDCT system could produce eight 1.25-mm slices. Thinner slices improve spatial resolution along the z-axis (head to foot).

Helical or spiral mode is possible secondary to the development of the slip-ring interconnect. This allows the x-ray tube and detectors to rotate continuously during image acquisition because no wires directly connect the rotating and stationary components of the system (i.e., no need to unwind the wires). With the gantry continuously rotating, the table moves the patient through the imaging plane at a predetermined speed. The relative speed of the gantry rotation table motion is the scan pitch. Figure 56.2 shows how both kinds of scanning work. The smooth rapid table motion or pitch in helical scanning allows complete coverage of the cardiac anatomy in 15 to 25 seconds. A disadvantage of this method in cardiac scanning, however, is an increase in radiation dose.

How Do Scanners Create Images?

All CT systems create images using the same basic principles. An x-ray source is used to create a filtered and collimated beam of x-ray photons, which irradiate the patient from a known point. On the other side of the patient, a detector array measures the x-ray photons, which exit the patient. The source and possibly the detector array rotate around the patient, providing different views or projections. These views fill a mathematical matrix referred to as

radon space. This information is then transformed through a filtered backprojection algorithm to create an x-ray attenuation map of the area or slice evaluated, which is generally recognized as the CT image.

Gating and Reconstruction

Gating refers to timing exposures to a point in the cardiac cycle when the heart is most still. EBT scanners have usually used 80% of the electrocardiographic RR interval for scanner triggering, although there are some more recent reports showing that earlier diastolic triggering might provide better images with less motion artifact (1–3). MDCT scanners usually trigger at 50% of the RR interval (4). *Reconstruction* refers to the computer calculations, which convert the digitally transformed data from the scanner's x-ray detectors into images of the heart and surrounding structures. ❦ k33

The array of digital numbers, when translated into tiny blocks of light with brightness proportional to their values, is the reconstructed image. Of course, this is an oversimplification of a more complex process, but we at least can see why the tomograms are called *computed*. Each individual tomogram can be thought of as a virtual slice of tissue consisting of blocks (voxels) containing numbers, each of which is proportional to the absorption of x-rays at that point and with a thickness and width determined by the reconstruction. Figure 56.3 shows a diagram of a tomogram.

Specific Problems with Specific Scanners

If time per scan were everything, the EBT scanners would be ahead of the pack. For at least a few years, the MDCT scanners will not be able to drive exposure times down to one-tenth of a second or better without sacrificing other important advantages they enjoy. Furthermore, it is unlikely that Imatron, the only company in the EBT business, will remain inactive. They are likely to further

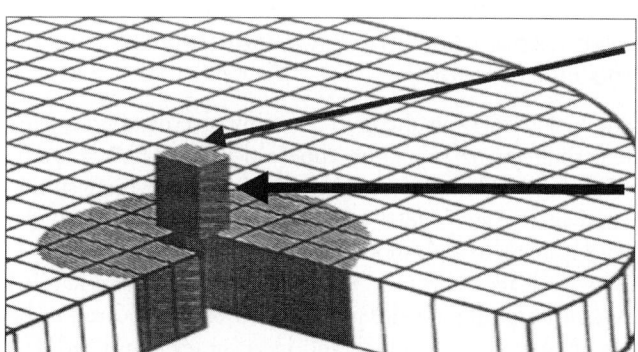

FIGURE 56.3 Each tomogram consists of voxels of given thickness (*thick arrow*) and width (*thin arrow*). One number between –1,000 and 2,000 represents each voxel.

decrease their exposure times and otherwise improve the quality of their images.

There are few carefully executed, head-to-head comparisons between the two scanner types. EBT scanners are still better for most cardiac applications. However, present EBT scanners have some distinct disadvantages, including excessive image noise, especially in obese patients. The limitation to only one or two detector rows is another concern. This limits the speed with which the entire heart can be imaged. Increased expense and difficult maintenance as well as relatively poor image quality for scanning other parts of the body are significant problems.

Noisy Images

When an x-ray beam encounters thick layers of tissue, absorption and scattering of x-ray photons within the tissue increase and thus fewer direct photons reach the detectors to record the image. Scattered x-ray photons result in noise. The signal-to-noise ratio is used as a measure of image quality. If the CT detector arrays record a high number of direct x-ray photons relative to scattered photons and other sources of noise within the CT system, then a clear and high-resolution image of acceptable signal-to-noise ratio will be obtained.

Current generation EBT scanners are unable to increase the number of x-ray photons without increasing image time. Thus, high levels of noise in the resulting images are observed, particularly for obese individuals. For this reason, EBT scanners cannot be used for subjects who weigh more than 300 lb. MDCT scanners usually have an upper limit of weight of at least 400 lb and have the added advantage of a variable tube current for obese subjects. The ability to increase tube current with patient size allows for image noise to be independent of patient size.

CLINICAL APPLICATIONS

Coronary Calcium: Historical Perspective

Other Modalities: Chest Radiography and Fluoroscopy

The first reports on the use of noninvasive fluoroscopy for detecting coronary calcium appeared in the 1960s (15,16) [▼ k34]. There was a surge of interest, which culminated in the late 1980s with a metaanalysis (17) and the development of two modifications, which increased sensitivity and accuracy (18,19). The metaanalysis concluded that although the sensitivity of fluoroscopy appeared to be low, its specificity was high and its accuracy compared well with most forms of stress testing. The most striking and encouraging finding was that of Margolis et al. (20), who followed a group of symptomatic adults who had under-

gone cardiac fluoroscopy and angiography and found that fluoroscopic calcium predicted a fourfold increase in future mortality and that calcium was an independent predictor of mortality even after controlling for extent of angiographic disease. Due to a dearth of economic pressure, and despite promising research results, neither medical centers nor professional societies gave serious consideration to the clinical application of cardiac fluoroscopy in the diagnosis of coronary heart disease.

Computed Tomography

CT scanners have been used since the 1970s. Scanners, like image intensifiers, are expensive. They serve for imaging multiple organs, both with and without contrast injections. Reinmuller and Lipton (21) in 1987 reported CT for coronary calcium to be more sensitive but less specific than fluoroscopy for predicting angiographic stenoses. Masuda et al. (22) and Timmins and Pinsk (23) also found CT to have increased sensitivity for stenoses, and Moore et al. (24) found that coronary calcium identified on CT scans predicted a worse outcome in symptomatic patients. The increased contrast resolution of CT is the reason for its expected increase in sensitivity. Localization of calcifications is also more accurate and easier with tomography than with projection imaging such as fluoroscopy.

Electron Beam Computed Tomography

Figure 56.4 shows an EBT scan, positive for coronary calcium. EBT scanners were introduced into the American market in the 1980s and represented a remarkable breakthrough in CT technology. The ability of EBT scanners to obtain rapid scan acquisition, as fast as 50 ms, makes them well suited for imaging the heart. To date, design tradeoffs to acquire these extremely high temporal resolution images have resulted in EBT not being widely accepted by the medical community for general CT imaging of the brain, liver, and other body parts.

Reports on their potential for imaging coronary calcifications began early with the papers of Tannenbaum and Kondos (25) and Agatston et al. (26). Tannenbaum and Kondos (25) were the first investigators to report the association of EBT coronary calcium with angiographic stenoses. Several other investigators (27–29) reported accuracies for predicting angiographic stenoses that are comparable with those of exercise testing. We know of one metaanalysis that shows encouraging results in this regard (30). Despite the fact that proponents of EBT frequently claim that it is far more accurate and useful for calcium assessment than either conventional CT or fluoroscopy, there have been few head-on comparisons. We believe that the accuracy of EBT exceeds that of other imaging modalities, but, in the case of multirow subsecond scanning, this difference in accuracy is modest or nonexistent (31,32).

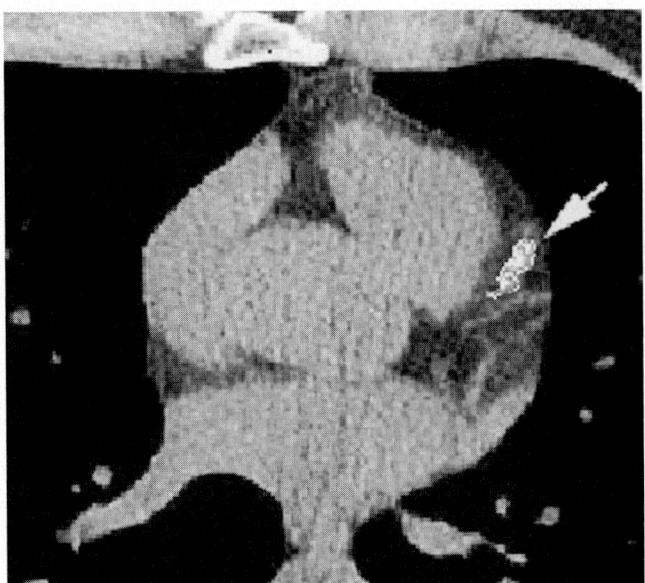

FIGURE 56.4 Tomogram from a study showing calcification in the left coronary artery (*arrow*).

After considering three possible clinical indications for calcium assessment using EBT, the American Heart Association concluded that there was a clear indication only in symptomatic adults with atypical chest pain (33). This was similar to the conclusions of the metaanalysis, published almost a decade earlier regarding cardiac fluoroscopy (17).

Some investigators have also done studies to determine the value of coronary calcium detected with this technique for predicting future coronary events in asymptomatic adults (34,35). These studies in asymptomatic subjects have received enormous attention and have produced widely divergent results and conclusions.

Measures of Coronary Calcium

All measures of coronary calcium depend on an inherent definition of a calcified lesion. Such definitions depend on two factors: a minimum brightness value (Hounsfield number) assigned to a pixel in the anatomic distribution of the coronary tree and a minimum number of adjacent or contiguous pixels that have that brightness value. The National Institutes of Health standard set by the Multi-ethnic Study of Atherosclerosis (MESA)/Coronary Artery Risk Development in Young Adults (CARDIA) CT committee is a brightness value of at least 130 Hounsfield units and four contiguous pixels using a 35-cm field of view.

The most popular measure of coronary calcium is the calcium score (26). This is a radiographic density-weighted volume of plaques whose pixel numbers exceed 130. A simpler and perhaps more reproducible measure is the calcium area or volume (26,36). The calcium volume is the total volume of all voxels with a Hounsfield number of at least 130. Callister et al. have developed an interpolated volume

scoring method, which smooths adjacent voxel numbers between image slices (36). They have found their method to be more reproducible, although this remains to be confirmed. Few reports have conclusively shown that any of the other measures are superior in accuracy and reproducibility when compared with the calcium score.

Prevalence

The prevalence of coronary calcium in asymptomatic as well as symptomatic persons is well known. Table 56.1 (26,37–39) shows the prevalence in young asymptomatic men and women of various ages. The prevalence in women lags behind that of men until well into the postmenopause period. The table shows the prevalence of coronary calcium in persons generally symptomatic and undergoing coronary angiography. These data thus indicate that the prevalence in symptomatic persons is generally higher than that in asymptomatic persons, and prevalence is age dependent. The prevalence in men is evidently higher than the prevalence in women. The lower prevalence of coronary calcium in those with myocardial infarction and negative coronary angiogram results is not shown in the table.

Reproducibility and Progression

Serial coronary calcium studies have been proposed to follow the progression of atherosclerosis. Such studies would be useful if the following conditions were met: (a) The progression of coronary calcium tracked the progression of unstable coronary plaque; as noted previously, the extent to which this is true is still a matter of debate; and (b) the measurement error, defined as the rescan percent variability, was much lower than the percent physiologic change over time.

Although coronary calcium is known to progress (40,41), the extent to which this progression tracks the progression of atherosclerotic plaque is unknown. Unfortunately, many who investigate temporal changes in calcium score over time have not considered that our understanding of the significance of atherosclerotic calcification is poor. A well-publicized retrospective nonrandomized review of sub-

TABLE 56.1 PREVALENCE OF CORONARY CALCIUM IN SYMPTOMATIC AND ASYMPTOMATIC ADULTS

Decade (yr)	Symptomatic (%) Men and women	Asymptomatic (%) Men	Asymptomatic (%) Women
30–40	26	21	11
40–50	43	44	28
50–60	81	70	50
60–70	83	84	73
70–80	—	94	89
>80	—	100	100

TABLE 56.2   RESCAN VARIABILITY IN FIVE STUDIES

Author	Year	No.	Variability (difference/mean; %)
Kajinami et al. (5)	1993	25	34
Bielak et al. (7)	1994	177	51
Shields et al. (42)	1995	50	38
Devries et al. (43)	1995	42	49
Wang et al. (3 mm slice) (6)	1996	72	29
Wang et al. (6 mm slice) (6)	1996	77	14

jects undergoing multiple scans showed decreased progression of calcification in a subgroup on effective lipid-lowering therapy (41).

Furthermore, the ability to track progression of calcium depends on the rescan variability compared with the expected rate of progression. If the former is much smaller than the latter, then progression within a year or two will be easy to detect in a single individual. If this is not true, it may take several years to be sure that progression is real and not due to measurement error.

The results of studies on reproducibility are listed in Table 56.2. Variability is seen to be at least 30% in most studies. Percent variability decreases rapidly for higher amounts of calcium. The reason for this is obvious because small calcium amounts can increase by 100% for spurious reasons.

Examination of age-dependent scores in cross-sectional data can most easily assess expected changes or progression over time. The approximate yearly increase in calcium score in such studies is between 20% and 35%. There are a few prospective studies showing similarly rapid progression of coronary calcium over time (40,41,44,45). Statistical arguments suggest that even with this rapid rate of progression, at least 4 years would have to pass before perceived changes in calcification could be judged to be significant in a single individual. This limitation on the clinical use of CT calcium assessments is similar to that seen for other types of vascular imaging such as coronary angiography (46). This drawback has far less effect on the utility of coronary calcium assessments for research studies when used in samples of at least 100 persons (47).

Coronary Calcium and Coronary Angiography

Available evidence suggests that a negative CT scan result for calcium does not completely exclude the presence of atherosclerotic plaque, but does imply a low likelihood of significant luminal obstruction. Most patients with angiographically normal coronary vessels have negative scan results and a low risk of coronary heart disease within 4 years after their scans. A positive scan result does indicate the presence of atherosclerotic plaque. Table 56.3 and refer-

ences 7, 28, 29, and 47 through 51 give the sensitivities and specificities of CT coronary calcium for predicting angiographic stenoses. Shemesh et al. (48) have found that infarct-related arteries are less likely to be heavily calcified than those not related to myocardial infarctions. These results remain to be confirmed.

All of these studies show that although sensitivity of coronary calcium for predicting coronary stenoses is high, specificity is low. This gives coronary calcium a high predictive value for ruling out but a low predictive value for identifying stenoses. It is on this basis that the American Heart Association writing group approved the use of coronary calcium for assessing patients with atypical chest pain (33). More recently, however, the combined American College of Cardiology/American Heart Association consensus panel took a more conservative stance on the same issue (52).

Screening and Predicting Events

This is an area that has generated much controversy and debate. The monograph by Morrison (53) contains an excellent definition of the purpose of screening for chronic diseases. "Screening for disease control can be defined as the examination of asymptomatic people in order to classify them as likely or not likely to have the disease that is the object of screening. . . . The goal of screening is to reduce morbidity and mortality from disease among the people screened by early treatment of the cases discovered."

There are two aspects of this definition that are unfortunately ignored during much of the debate regarding calcium screening. The first is that experiments to evaluate clinical screening should use asymptomatic research subjects. The second is implied in the phrase "reduce morbidity and mortality." If this goal cannot be achieved, then screening will not achieve its purpose and cannot be deemed effective. For example, cholesterol screening is effective only because lipoproteins are clinically effective targets for preventive therapy; mammographic screening for breast cancer and occult blood screening for colon cancer have been proven to be effective in certain groups, not solely because they predict clinical disease and mortality,

TABLE 56.3   RELATIONSHIP WITH CORONARY ANGIOGRAPHY

Author	No. of patients	Mean age (yr)	Sensitivity	Specificity
Breen et al. (28)	100	47	100	47
Fallavolita et al. (29)	106	44	85	45
Bielak et al. (7)	256	45	90	62
Devries et al. (49)	140	58	97	41
Rumberger et al. (50)	139	52	99	62
Budoff et al. (51)	710	58	95	44

but also because screening leads to a course of action proven to save lives.

Before we can endorse massive coronary calcium screening of the entire population, or even a subpopulation, of adults, we need to have a screening test that leads to effective preventive therapy when applied to asymptomatic persons. Thus, the test must predict clinical disease in asymptomatic persons in a way that allows therapeutically effective decisions to be made based on the results.

It is sometimes argued that coronary calcium measurements can be helpful in certain subsets of persons, based on risk factor status and specifically on lipoprotein levels. For example, some would aggressively treat a 45-year-old man with reductase inhibitors, angiotensin-converting enzyme inhibitors, and aspirin if his low-density lipoproteins were in the range between 100 and 160 and he had a coronary calcium score of 400 (well above the ninetieth percentile for age and gender). They would argue: "I know he has coronary disease. Therefore, he should be in a secondary prevention category, and I should treat him as if he had suffered a myocardial infarction." Logical though it seems, this argument has an important flaw. The flaw lies in the expanded definition of coronary heart disease from *clinical* to *preclinical* disease. A calcium score of 400 is simply not the same as a prior myocardial infarction. Those with prior infarctions have been proven to benefit from aggressive low-density lipoprotein lowering. Those with calcium scores of 400 may also receive such benefit, as the recent Air Force Coronary Artery Prevention Study (AFCAPS) has shown (54). However, even if a score of 400 in this person predicted a grave prognosis, we could not be sure that any benefit would be garnered from intervention.

One might argue, of course, that treatment could be justified based on high risk alone. If those with scores over 200 are more than ten times more likely to develop clinical disease, then one probably should not wait for a clinical trial of calcium screening to make a decision to treat. We would agree that if, indeed, there were conclusive proof of a large increased probability (at least eight times) of a morbid coronary event based on a coronary calcium score, treatment would be justified even in the absence of a corroborative clinical trial.

How well does coronary calcium predict coronary events? O'Malley et al. (55) have reviewed most of the literature on using CT calcium to predict future events in asymptomatic adults. Their results are summarized in Table 56.4. We see from the table that the relative risk of calcification varies from 1 to 22 with a weighted mean of 4. There seems to be general agreement that calcium predicts events. There is little agreement as to how well it can do this. Thus, the predictive value of coronary calcium for new cardiac events still remains to be determined. The National Heart, Lung and Blood Institute has sponsored a study called MESA that will examine this issue as one of its major hypotheses. MESA will use a cohort of 6,500 American adults who will undergo CT scanning and will be followed for coronary events for 7 years.

TABLE 56.4 RELATIVE RISKS OF CORONARY CALCIUM ACCORDING TO PUBLISHED PROGNOSTIC STUDIES

Author	Relative risk	95% Confidence interval
Detrano et al. (34)	2.3	1.2, 4.4
Agatston et al. (56)	16.9	1.0, 286.3
Arad et al. (35)	22.1	2.7, 179.0
Sullivan et al. (57)	1.0	0.3, 20.5
Raggi et al. (58)	7.2	2.5, 20.5
Overall	4.2	1.6, 11.3

Position of the Professional Societies

In 1996, the American Heart Association, at the persistent suggestion of the proponents of scanning, assembled a writing group on the application of EBT coronary calcium scanning. This group concluded that EBT had not yet been proven to be useful for screening asymptomatic subjects and that more research was needed (33).

Interestingly, this enormously expensive technology is the only one that has found a limited degree of acceptance and popularity in the medical community. Of the more than 40 EBT scanners in the United States, most are used almost exclusively for coronary artery calcium screening. This technology—not fluoroscopy, not conventional CT—has been the subject of not one, but three reviews by national consensus panels (33,52,59–61).

The application of calcium assessments has been confined largely to screening asymptomatic populations for whom there are only scanty supportive data. This use began long before the publication of any prognostic data and before most of the cross-sectional studies were reported. An estimated 60,000 Americans have been so screened.

Fortunately, the American Heart Association and the American College of Cardiology have taken responsible positions on this issue. In Table 56.5 we suggest the potential indications for which coronary calcium scanning should and should not be considered as indicated, based on the consensus documents published by the professional societies.

In this paradigm, a clinical examination including history, blood pressure measurement, and lipoproteins should always be used to determine the indication for a coronary calcium examination. General screening of asymptomatic adults should be discouraged, and coronary calcium studies should be restricted to those at intermediate risk who might benefit from aggressive risk factor modification and possibly to those with atypical chest pain.

Computed Tomographic Coronary Angiography

Medical and surgical management of coronary heart disease is in large part predicated on alterations in the lumen of the coronary arteries as demonstrated at coronary angiography. Although it is becoming clear that stenosis is only one

TABLE 56.5 INDICATIONS FOR CORONARY CALCIUM SCANNING

	Screening asymptomatic adults	Selected patients with intermediate risk [e.g., low-density lipoprotein (100–160, etc.)]	Diagnosis in those with chest pain	Prognostication in those with known coronary disease
Definitely indicated	–	–	–	–
Probably indicated	–	+	–	–
Possibly indicated	–	–	Atypical chest pain only	–

+, indicated; –, not indicated.

domain of a complex process, as detailed in other chapters, the presence and distribution of arterial diameter reduction remain important determinants of patient management.

Cardiac CT, like cardiac magnetic resonance imaging (MRI), can produce a four-dimensional image of the beating heart. Although cardiac MRI provides superior tissue contrast, velocity mapping, myocardial tagging, and kidney-friendly intravascular contrast agents, cardiac CT has several characteristics that, with continued technological advances, may make it a major and perhaps front-line technique for cardiac and coronary imaging. Several advancements in CT technology are driving the renewed interest in contrast-enhanced cardiac CT. These include continued evolution of EBT techniques using equipment with improved gating, detector arrays, and table motion. For helical CT systems, the development of 0.5-second gantry rotation time, the addition of cardiac gating, the development of four- and eight-slice detector arrays with sub–1-mm slice thickness and sophisticated multiphasic volumetric reconstruction algorithms are driving a renewed interest in contrast-enhanced cardiac CT. This section reviews current and developing techniques and application of contrast-enhanced CT in the heart.

Without the addition of an intravascular contrast agent, differentiation of the vessel wall from the vessel lumen is not possible in most instances with CT. This is due to the similar x-ray attenuation of blood and soft tissue. Cardiac CT is a four-dimensional multiplanar imaging technique. This multiplanar capability can provide quantitative information on vessel lumen, relatively irrespective of stenosis orientation, with a single acquisition (Fig. 56.5). In the next section we consider current technical aspects of contrast-enhanced CT imaging of the heart, review the published scientific literature, and conclude with areas of active research.

Computed Tomographic Angiography: Clinical Studies

Dr. Stephan Achenbach and colleagues have performed pioneering research in CT angiography with both EBT and MDCT. They have reviewed the ability of contrast-enhanced EBT to evaluate coronary artery bypass grafts (62), detect high-grade restenosis after percutaneous transluminal angioplasty (63), and determine patency of an infarct-related coronary vessel (64). They have also compared EBT

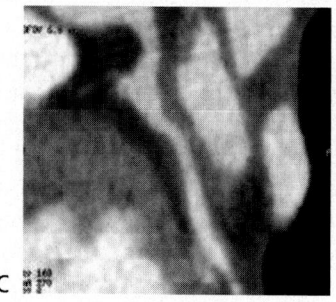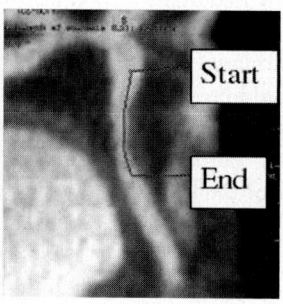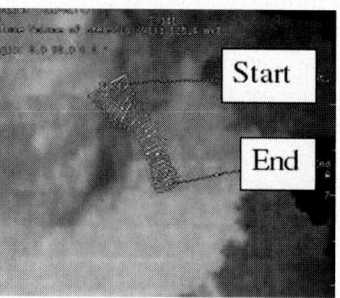

A–C

FIGURE 56.5 **A–C:** Contrast-enhanced computed tomographic coronary angiography. Left circumflex: curved reformatted image through the center of the lumen of the proximal left circumflex (segment 11) from a contrast-enhanced multidetector computed tomography study, helical acquisition with retrospective cardiac gating (General Electric Medical Systems Light-Speed Plus). Three-dimensional computer processing of the computed tomographic image data allows identification of the start and end points of various coronary segments with a potential stenosis **(B)** and determination of the central path of the vessel contrast column. From the central path, the orthogonal vessel cross-sectional area can automatically be determined and quantitative indices of stenosis measured from a wireframe representation **(C)**. Although there remain numerous challenges to validating techniques such as this for clinical application, they have the potential to provide quantitative information concerning coronary artery luminal dimensions noninvasively.

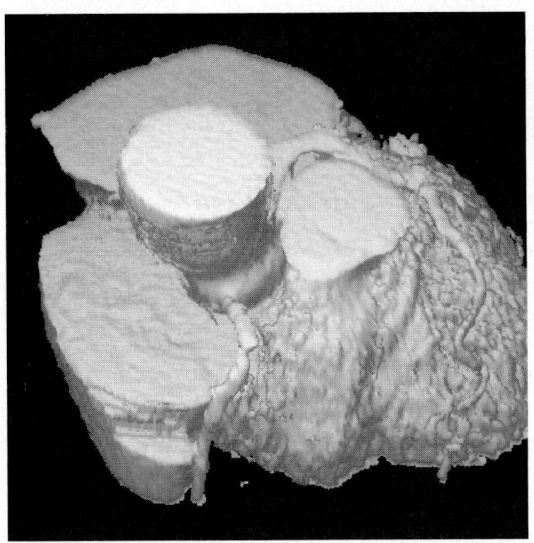
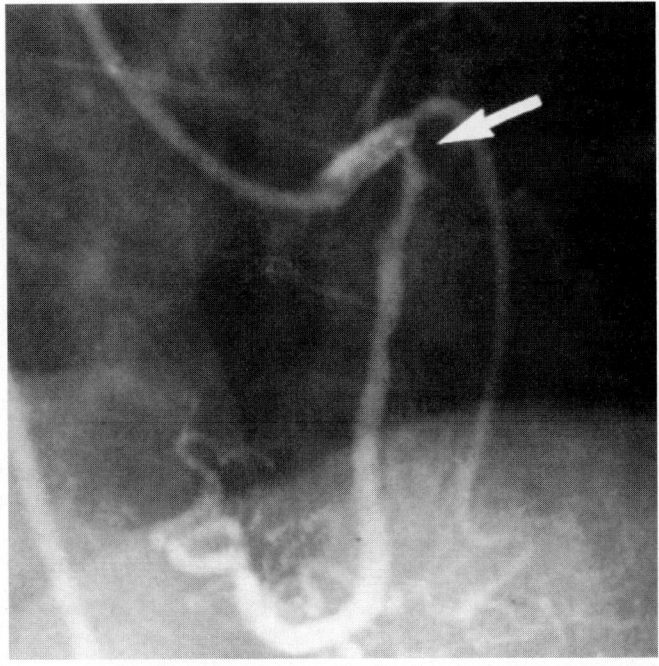

A

B

FIGURE 56.6 High-grade stenosis of proximal right coronary artery. Shaded surface display of a high-grade stenosis of the right coronary artery is demonstrated with contrast-enhanced cardiac computed tomography **(A)** (Imatron C150) and compared with stenosis (*arrow*) in the conventional coronary angiogram **(B)**. [Courtesy of S. Achenbach, Department of Internal Medicine II (Cardiology), University of Erlangen-Nuremberg.]

coronary angiography with catheter-based coronary angiography in a study of 125 patients (65,66). The study was a direct comparison of the proximal and middle segments of the major coronary arteries, using the American Heart Association reporting system with both EBT and conventional coronary angiography. In this study, 25% of coronary vessels could not be evaluated (124 of 500 vessels), mostly because of respiratory artifacts and coronary calcifications. The number of patients with none of the four major coronary arteries of sufficient quality to evaluate was 15%. After excluding the 124 vessels, which could not be evaluated, EBT angiography correctly categorized 69 of 75 (92%) coronary vessels as having high-grade stenoses or occlusions, and 282 of 301 (94%) vessels were normal or had stenoses of less than 75% reduction in vessel diameter as compared with the standard of conventional catheter-based angiography (Fig. 56.6).

The authors noted that the majority of missed stenoses (false-negative results) were located in the right and left circumflex coronary arteries, in the segments coursing perpendicular to the transverse imaging plane where the 3-mm slice thickness and volume averaging may be important factors. They concluded that when image quality is sufficient, EBT contrast-enhanced coronary angiography "may be useful to detect or rule out high-grade coronary-artery stenoses and occlusions."

Budoff and colleagues performed an additional study comparing EBT to conventional coronary angiography in 52 patients (67). They had similar high agreement between

the two techniques for identifying coronary stenosis and reported good agreement between observers with the technique (kappa, 0.86). They also noted technical difficulties in the right and left circumflex coronary arteries related to "cardiac and respiratory motion and poor electrocardiographic gating." ☜ k35

The continued rapid technological advancement of MDCT and EBT suggests that there will be further improvements in CT coronary angiography. Early efforts have demonstrated the feasibility of CT coronary angioscopy. In the near term, the development and introduction of MDCT systems with more than eight channels is likely. A 16-channel MDCT system could use the additional detector rows to improve temporal resolution, reduce breath-hold time, and reduce contrast dose. We will observe continued rapid advancement in CT for coronary angiography and a series of comparative studies evaluating these new CT techniques with existing measures of coronary heart disease.

Computed Tomographic Evaluation of Coronary Revascularization

Aortocoronary bypass grafts can be well demonstrated by modern CT techniques (Fig. 56.7). Through appropriate positioning of the imaging volume over the graft origin in the ascending aorta, the entire length of the graft can be imaged. When technically adequate studies are obtained, extremely high sensitivity and specificity for graft occlu-

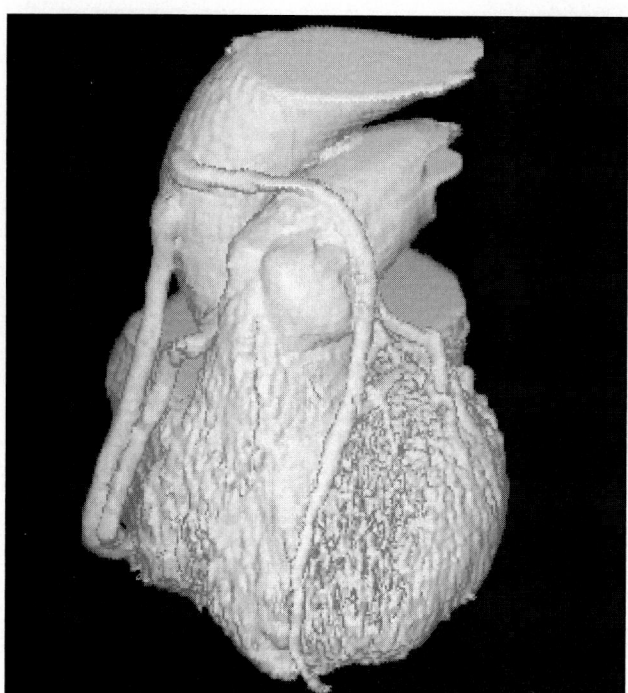

FIGURE 56.7 Patent aortocoronary vein grafts, patent (EBT Imatron C150). Two patent grafts are demonstrated in this three-dimensional shaded surface display. The more superior venous graft from the ventral aspect of the ascending aorta crosses the main pulmonary artery before anastomosis with the left anterior descending artery. The second vein graft courses alongside of the proximal right coronary before the anastomosis. [Courtesy of S. Achenbach, Department of Internal Medicine II (Cardiology), University of Erlangen-Nuremberg.]

sions and hemodynamically significant stenosis can be achieved (Fig. 56.8) (62). Problems remain regarding poor breath holding and improper positioning of the imaging volume, which results in the proximal aspect of the aorto-coronary graft not being imaged. Visualization of internal mammary grafts is often problematic. For all grafts, the presence of metallic surgical clips results in streak artifacts. These metallic artifacts typically prevent evaluation for stenosis at their location.

Coronary stents have become one of the mainstays of interventional cardiology. Cardiac-gated CT can accurately describe stent location. Flow through stents can be evaluated and occlusion assessed. However, the metal intrinsic to current generation stents prevents CT from imaging the stent interior (Fig. 56.9).

Pericardial Disease

The fat found on the surface of the heart and the surrounding air-filled lung provides natural contrast that permits easy identification of a normal pericardium. Thickening of the pericardium can easily be identified, and this technology surpasses any other in identifying chronic pericarditis, particularly when it is calcific (Fig. 56.10). CT is therefore

ideal for differentiating constrictive pericarditis from restrictive cardiomyopathy. The presence of normal pericardial thickness (i.e., 2 to 3 mm) excludes the diagnosis of constriction (76).

The tomographic format of CT makes it an excellent method to define primary and metastatic tumors of the pericardium. Extension into nearby mediastinal structures and to the lung can also be identified (77).

Congenital Heart Disease

Management of patients with congenital heart disease requires accurate information regarding structure and function of the cardiac chambers and great vessels. The traditional way of obtaining this has been with cardiac catheterization, and this remains the standard against which other imaging modalities are used in some institutions. Echocardiography is particularly useful and has replaced angiography to a great extent. There have been many reports of the use of CT as a modality to define abnormalities in structure and function of the heart. How-

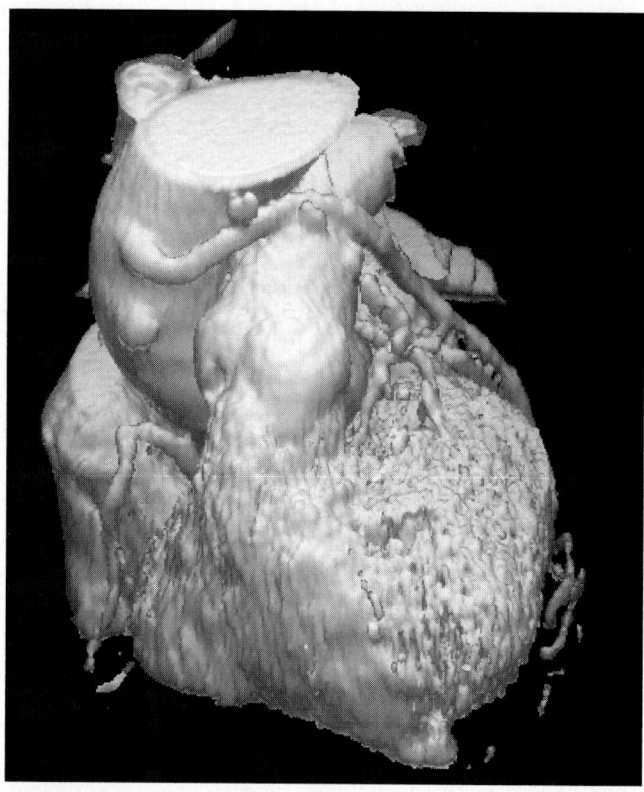

FIGURE 56.8 Aortocoronary vein graft occlusion (EBT Imatron C150). A patent aortocoronary graft to the left circumflex coronary is demonstrated. Note the proximal occlusion of the vein graft to the right coronary, which is identified as only a slight outpouching at the graft origin from the ascending aorta. [Courtesy of S. Achenbach, Department of Internal Medicine II (Cardiology), University of Erlangen-Nuremberg.]

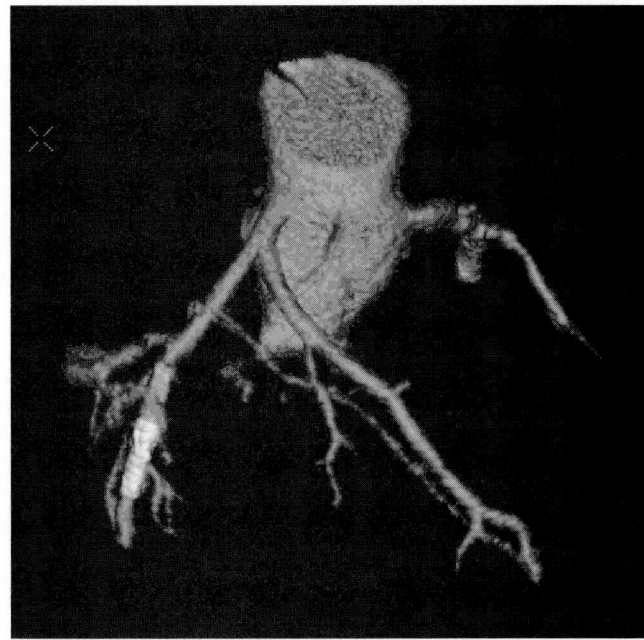

FIGURE 56.9 Coronary stent (General Electric LightSpeed). A metallic coronary stent is demonstrated in the left anterior descending coronary artery. Although contrast enhancement can be seen proximal and distal to the stent, the higher attenuation of the metallic stent prevents direct visualization of the stent interior in most cases with existing computed tomographic reconstruction techniques. (Courtesy of Drs. Geoffrey Rubin and Curtis Coulam, Stanford University.)

ever, the role of CT in this application remains largely supportive to angiography and perhaps even more so to echocardiography.

In some adults with congenital heart disease, the diagnostic information provided by transthoracic echocardiography is limited because of chest deformities and difficulties finding adequate imaging windows. In these cases, ancillary methods such as transesophageal echocardiography, MRI, and CT can be of great help. The choice of these modalities depends largely on local experience and availability. ⚜ k36

Specific problems for which rapid CT is indicated include determining the origin of the coronary arteries (78), visualization of the pulmonary arteries in cyanotic congenital heart disease (79), precise definition of aortic geometry in Marfan's disease (80), and partial or total anomalous pulmonary venous drainage (81). CT can also be used for visualization and assessment of patent ductus arteriosus (79,82) and aortic coarctation (83–85).

Aortic Disease

The thoracic aorta is an integral component of the cardiac CT examination and thoracic imaging in general. CT is the primary means of imaging the lung, thoracic trauma (blunt and penetrating), aneurysms, and aortic dissections (86). In the situation of an acute life-threatening event, CT can provide extensive information concerning the heart, aorta, and great vessels. In addition, during the same examina-

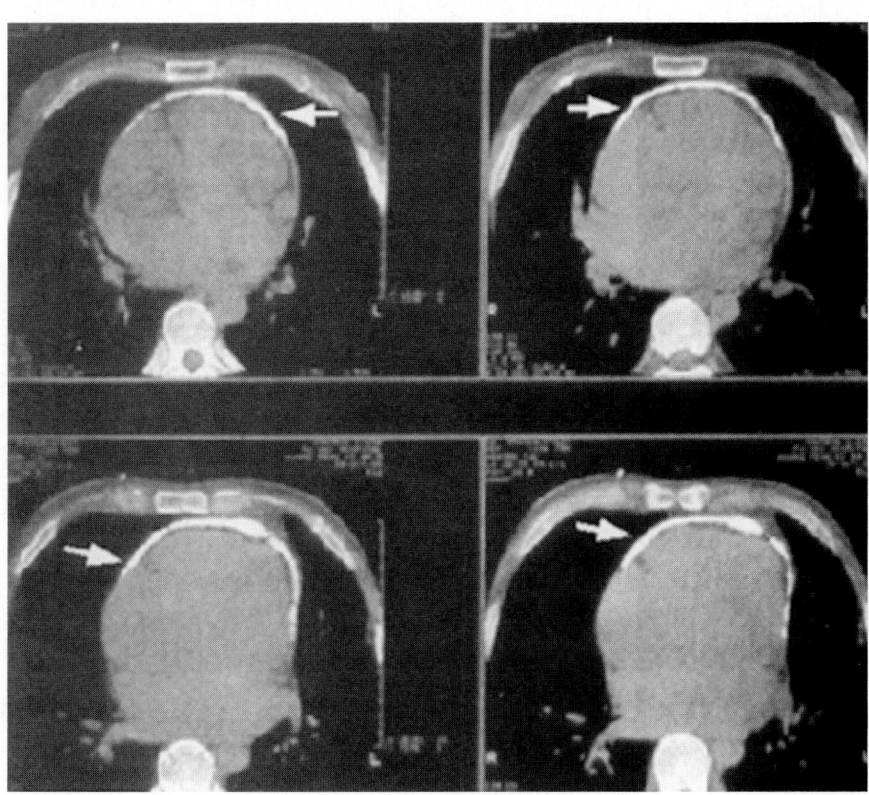

FIGURE 56.10 Thick, calcified pericardium is clearly demonstrated (*arrows*).

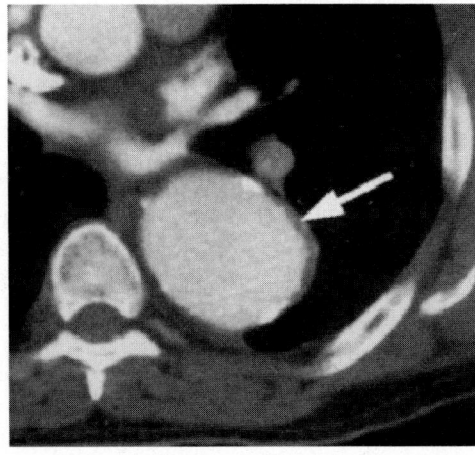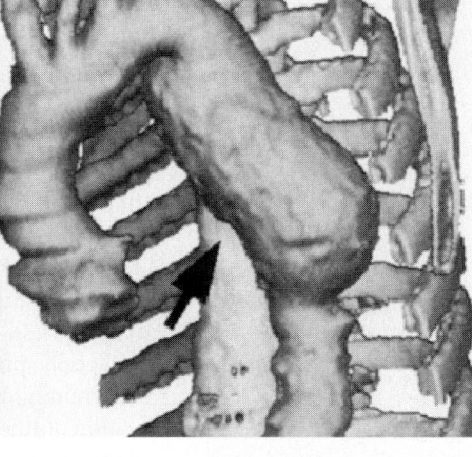

A,B

FIGURE 56.11 Descending thoracic aortic aneurysm. **A:** Image slice of atherosclerotic aneurysm (*arrow*). **B:** Three-dimensional reconstruction of thoracic aneurysm (Imatron C-150). Arrow points to large, cyndrical aortic aneurysm.

tion, the brain and spinal canal can be evaluated. The entire global CT examination (head, cervical spine, chest, abdomen, and pelvis) can be completed on modern MDCT systems in less than 15 minutes. These capabilities have made modern CT an indispensable tool in emergency departments and medical centers worldwide, and the development of the four-channel MDCT systems have further expanded these capabilities (87).

In the setting of blunt and penetrating trauma, CT of the chest can be extremely useful in diagnosis and as an aid to surgical management (86,88,89). Contrast CT can rapidly identify aortic tears, intramural hematoma, and dissection. In addition, the presence of mediastinal hematoma and other associated injuries can be assessed. These examinations are performed in critically ill patients who may require mechanical ventilation, invasive monitoring, intravenous infusion pumps, and cardiac pacing. The well-designed CT imaging suite is hospitable to life-support equipment, which can remain in the room and operational throughout the imaging procedure.

CT is playing an increasingly important role in the diagnosis and management of thoracic aortic pathology (90–92). Although MRI and transesophageal echocardiography can provide exquisite and unique information, the robust nature of CT often makes it the imaging modality of choice.

Contrast-enhanced CT can identify and classify aortic dissections and aortic aneurysms (Figs. 56.11 and 56.12) (93).

Advantages are the ability to image the entire aorta and beyond, demonstration of surrounding structures and organs, quantitative measures of aneurysm size and location, and a rapid examination time. Limitations are the negative effects of iodinated contrast on renal function, the rare adverse reactions to iodinated contrast, and the inability to directly measure blood flow. A current MDCT protocol for CT angiography provides high-resolution arterial phase images from the thoracic inlet to the femoral arteries. This coverage incorporates the entire aorta, as well as the organs of the chest, abdomen, and pelvis. Beyond classifying dissections as involving the ascending (Stanford type A) or descending (Stanford type B), CT can demonstrate associ-

ated findings critical to patient care such as mediastinal hematoma, pericardial effusions, pseudoaneurysm formation, and active extravasation of contrast from the aorta. Quantitative measurement of aneurysm size, location, and relation to branch vessels can be used for planning operative or intravascular repair and for monitoring postprocedure anatomy. The necessity for precise and quantitative measurements with CT has become more critical with the continued advancements in endovascular repair with stent grafts (94).

CONTROVERSIES AND PERSONAL PERSPECTIVES

To ensure efficacy and safety, national governments, including our own, have instituted regulatory agencies

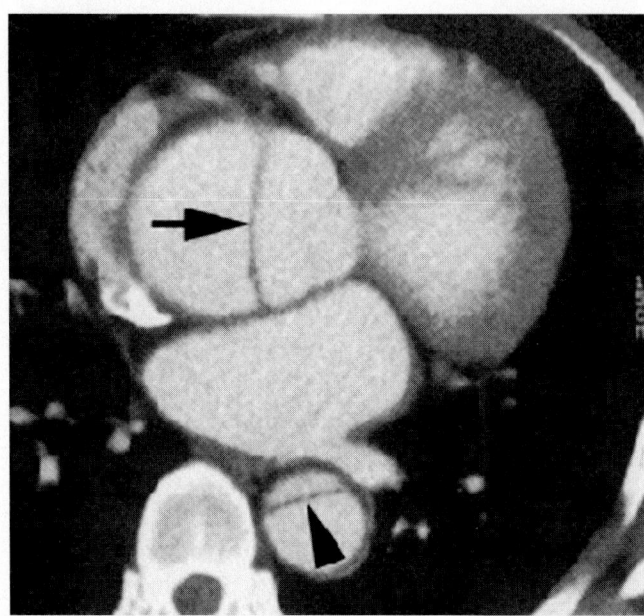

FIGURE 56.12 DeBakey type I or Stanford type A aortic dissection. Intimal flap is seen in both ascending and descending aorta (*arrows*) (Imatron C-150).

such as the Food and Drug Administration to ensure that research results and conclusions are accurate and appropriate. These measures are costly and something of a nuisance, but they protect the populace and the medical community from unscrupulous and evangelical crusades such as those of the laetrile enthusiasts of the 1960s. Much diagnostic testing has escaped from legal regulation (94). Doctors order and patients refer themselves for tests in order to discover hidden pathology and arrive at effective treatment. Much of this testing has questionable scientific validity.

During the 1990s, headlines appeared in the popular press regarding a new procedure for detecting heart disease and predicting heart attacks. At that time, there was no supportive scientific literature regarding the value of the new test, EBT, and for its stated purpose, to say nothing about its usefulness in improving outcomes.

Due to the initial popularity of the test, venture capital firms, small marketing operations, and university medical centers strapped for sources of income initiated and supported more coronary calcium screening projects. These grew into a kind of industry, organized by its strong bond to the, until relatively recently, unique manufacturer of CT equipment capable of performing this test. This industry promises to continue to mutate into other varieties of unproven radiographic self-diagnosis. Some coronary calcium screening centers already offer lung cancer screening and a few have expanded to "full body examinations," which proclaim themselves capable of finding multiple pathologies.

Participants in this new calcium screening industry compiled calcium score databases and followed participants for coronary events. These research subjects rarely knew they were a part of a study and were usually not asked to sign consent forms verifying that they had agreed to participate in the evaluation of an investigational test. In 1999, the calcium screeners founded a new society, The Society of Atherosclerosis Imagers. They state that this new organization is dedicated to unbiased research regarding all aspects of arterial imaging. However, in its initial years, the major focus of the society has been to attempt to validate the conclusions that its members have already accepted, i.e., that EBCT and only EBCT can be used to guide therapy for coronary atherosclerosis.

Greed is not the major factor motivating the new society or the spread of coronary calcium screening adventures. The primary leadership of the calcium screening industry are well meaning enthusiasts who believe that they are executing rigorous scientific research. Indeed, the coronary calcium screeners have made important contributions toward the understanding of subclinical atherosclerosis. However, they often design their research not around hypotheses that require proof, but instead around preconceived conclusions that are then engineered backward into manipulated analyses of specially selected data.

It is hoped that this chapter can provide some balance to the almost exclusive opinion that has been heard, not only in the professional journals but on radio advertisements and commercial Web sites. In our opinion, CT of the heart will have an important role in medicine. In order to realize that role, researchers and clinicians must base medical decisions on evidence rather than on marketing.

SUMMARY

Rapid cardiac CT has remained outside of the realm of commonly used imaging technologies for the past two decades. This is partly due to justified reluctance of the medical community to accept new concepts and to limitations in available technology. It is probably largely due to the relative unavailability of scanners with the rapid exposure times required to image the beating heart.

Only now is rapid CT finding its place in the armamentarium of imaging technologies. Its application to screening for subclinical heart disease has received a limited endorsement from the American College of Cardiology and American Heart Association. The newer technology of MDCT is less expensive, more available, and probably equally accurate for cardiac imaging. We estimate that there are approximately 300 MDCT scanners made by four manufacturers and located in the United States that are capable of imaging the heart if fitted with the proper software and operated by knowledgeable personnel.

This has stimulated greater interest in CT imaging of the heart among cardiologists and radiologists. The failure of MRI coronary angiography to produce adequate endoluminal images and the promise of this achievement from rapid CT has sparked a flurry of trials of CT angiography of the coronary arteries.

Accepted applications of this technology at this time include evaluating for the presence of subclinical atherosclerosis in those at intermediate risk, evaluation of certain congenital heart lesions when other methods are not available or fail to produce adequate images, evaluation of aortic dissection or other aortic pathology when other methods are not available or fail to produce adequate images, and evaluation of the patency of aortocoronary bypass grafts and stents. The *a priori* use of CT coronary angiography, although promising, still awaits an accepted niche in cardiac diagnosis.

We hope that some of the readers of this chapter will take sufficient interest in this exciting field to pioneer further research and development of this evolving technology.

ACKNOWLEDGMENT

The editorial assistance of Zephyr Detrano is deeply appreciated.

THE FUTURE

The recent history of CT coronary imaging has been unique in two ways.

First, until relatively recently, only one company produced equipment (EBCT) capable of obtaining accurate images of coronary calcium and of contrast-filled coronary lumina. Fortunately, several large medical imaging firms are now producing comparable equipment, which produces the same results at a reduced technical cost. This healthy industrial competition will lead not only to better images but also to more credible research.

Second, radiologists have largely rejected the accuracy of the older EBCT technology for scanning other organs or body parts due to high noise levels and other artifacts. Thus, once purchased, EBCT instruments must be used almost exclusively and extensively for coronary artery screening and CT angiography, or those responsible for the purchase must admit large fiscal mistakes. The advent of the newer MDCT scanning technology has obviated this problem in that these scanners can be shared between departments and have multiple approved uses.

These two features have stimulated the extreme positions taken by many in the coronary calcium screening industry that advocates therapeutic decisions based only on arbitrary thresholds of calcium score. This screening vogue is another American aberration soon to be cured by that even more American phenomenon, the free market.

MESA (47) will shed considerable light on the validity of coronary calcium screening. The results of MESA will determine whether a clinical trial similar to those that have proven the benefits of mammography is needed. If MESA shows powerful predictive values (relative risks greater than 8) for coronary events, then such a trial may not be necessary. However, if, on the other hand, the results of MESA are more modest, a decision as to whether or not such a trial is needed will have to be made.

REFERENCES

1. Wang Y, Vidan E, Bergman G. Cardiac motion of coronary arteries: variability in the rest period and implications for coronary MR angiography. *Radiology* 1999;213:751–758.

2. Mao S, Lu B, Oudiz RJ, et al. Coronary artery motion in electron beam tomography. *J Comput Assist Tomogr* 2000;24:253–255.

3. Achenbach S, Ropers D, Möhlenkamp S, et al. Variability of repeated coronary artery calcification measurements by electron beam tomography. *Am J Cardiol* 2001;87:210–213.

4. Becker CR, Knez A. Detection and quantification of coronary artery calcification with electron-beam and conventional CT. *Eur Radiol* 1999;9:620–624.

5. Kajinami K, Seki H, Takekoshi N, et al. Quantification of coronary artery calcification using ultrafast computed tomography: reproducibility of measurements. *Coronary Artery Dis* 1993;4:1103–1108.

6. Wang S, Detrano RC, Secci A, et al. Detection of coronary calcification with electron-beam computed tomography: evaluation of interexamination reproducibility and comparison of three image-acquisition protocols. *Am Heart J* 1996;132:550–558.

7. Bielak LF, Kaufmann RB, Moll PP, et al. Small lesions identified by electron beam computed tomographic exams of the heart: calcification or noise? *Radiology* 1994;192:631–636.

8. Doherty TM, Detrano RC. Coronary calcification: a new perspective on an old problem. *Calcif Tissue Int* 1994;54:224–230.

9. Fraser JD, Price PA. Lung, heart and kidney express high levels of mRNA for the vitamin K dependent gla protein. *J Biol Chem* 1988;263:11033–11036.

10. Cheng GC, Loree HM, Kamm RD, et al. Distribution of circumferential stress in ruptured and stable atherosclerotic lesions. *Circulation* 1993;87:1179–1187.

11. Lenck R. X-ray diagnosis of coronary atherosclerosis in vivo. *Fortschr Rontgenstr* 1927;35:1265.

12. Hobbe JE, Wright HH. Roentgenographic detection of coronary arteriosclerosis. *AJR Am J Roentgenol* 1950;63:50.

13. Souza AS, Bream PR. Chest film detection of coronary artery calcification. The value of the CAC triangle. *Radiology* 1978;129:7–10.

14. Kelley MJ, Newell JD. Chest radiography and cardiac fluoroscopy in cardiac disease. *Cardiol Clin* 1983;1:575.

15. Jorgens J, Blank N, Wilcox WA. Cinefluorographic detection and recording of within the heart. *Radiology* 1960;74:550–554.

16. Lieber A, Jorgens J. Cinefluorography of coronary artery calcifications. *AJR Am J Roentgenol* 1961;86:1063.

17. Gianrossi R, Detrano R, Colombo A, et al. Cardiac fluoroscopy for the diagnosis of coronary disease: a meta-analytic review. *Am Heart J* 1987;120:1179–1188.

18. Detrano R, Markovic D, Simpfendorfer C, et al. Digital subtraction fluoroscopy: a new method of detecting coronary calcifications with improved sensitivity for the prediction of coronary disease. *Circulation* 1990;71:827–832.

19. Molloi S, Detrano R, Ersahin A, et al. Quantification of coronary artery calcium by dual energy digital subtraction fluoroscopy. *Med Phys* 1991;18:295–299.

20. Margolis JR, Chen JT, Kong Y, et al. The diagnostic and prognostic significance of coronary artery calcification. *Radiology* 1980;137:609–616.

21. Reinmuller R, Lipton M. Detection of coronary artery calcification by computed tomography. *Dynam Cardiovasc Imaging* 1987;1:139–145.

22. Masuda Y, Naito S, Aoyagi Y, et al. Coronary artery calcification detected by CT. *Angiology* 1990;41:1037–1047.
23. Timmins ME, Pinsk R. The functional significance of calcification of the coronary arteries as detected on CT. *J Thorac Imaging* 1991;7:79–82.
24. Moore E, Greenberg RW, Merrick SH. Coronary artery calcification: significance of incidental detection on CT scans. *Radiology* 1989;172:711–716.
25. Tanenbaum SR, Kondos GT. Detection of calcific deposits in coronary arteries by ultrafast computed tomography and correlation with angiography. *Am J Cardiol* 1989;63:870–872.
26. Agatston AS, Janowitz WR, Hildner FJ, et al. Quantification of coronary artery calcium using ultrafast computed tomography. *J Am Coll Cardiol* 1990;15:827–832.
27. Detrano R, Hsiai T, Wang S, et al. Prognostic value of coronary calcification and angiographic stenoses in patients undergoing angiography. *J Am Coll Cardiol* 1996;27:285–290.
28. Breen JB, Sheedy PF, Schwartz RS, et al. Coronary artery calcification detected with ultrafast CT as an indication of coronary artery disease. *Radiology* 1992;185:435–439.
29. Fallavolita JA, Brody JS, et al. Fast computed tomography detection of coronary artery calcification in the diagnosis of coronary artery disease. *Circulation* 1994;89:285–289.
30. Nallamothu BK, Saint S, Bielak LF, et al. Electron-beam computed tomography in the diagnosis of coronary artery disease: a meta-analysis. *Arch Intern Med* 2001;161(6):833–838.
31. Becker CR, Knez A. Detection and quantification of coronary artery calcification with electron-beam and conventional CT. *Eur Radiol* 1999;9:620–624.
32. Carr JJ, Crouse JR, Goff DC, et al. Evaluation of sub-second gated helical CT for quantification of coronary artery calcium and comparison with electron beam CT. *AJR Am J Roentgenol* 2000;174:915–921.
33. Wexler L, Brundage B, Crouse J, et al. Coronary artery calcification: pathophysiology, epidemiology, imaging methods and clinical implications. A statement for health professionals from the American Heart Association. *Circulation* 1996;94:1175–1192.
34. Detrano RC, Wong ND, Doherty TM, et al. Coronary calcium does not accurately predict near-term coronary events in high risk adults. *Circulation* 1999;99:2633–2638.
35. Arad Y, Spadaro LA, Goodman K, et al. Predictive value of electron beam computed tomography of the coronary arteries. 19-month follow-up of 1173 asymptomatic subjects. *Circulation* 1996;93:1951–1953.
36. Callister TQ, Cooil B, Raya SP, et al. Coronary artery disease: improved reproducibility of calcium scoring with an electron-beam CT volumetric method. *Radiology* 1998;208:807–808.
37. Janowitz WR, Agatston AS, Kaplan G, et al. Differences in prevalence and extent of coronary artery calcium detected by ultrafast computed tomography in asymptomatic men and women. *Am J Cardiol* 1993;72:247–254.
38. Wong ND, Kouwabunpat D, Vo AN, et al. Coronary calcium and atherosclerosis by ultrafast computed tomography in asymptomatic men and women: relation to age and risk factors. *Am Heart J* 1994;127:422–430.
39. Wong ND, Vo A, Abrahamson D, et al. Detection of coronary artery calcium by ultrafast computed tomography and its relation to clinical evidence of coronary artery disease. *Am J Cardiol* 1994;73:223–225.
40. Budoff MJ, Lane KL, Bakhsheshi H, et al. Rates of progression of coronary calcium by electron beam tomography. *Am J Cardiol* 2000;86:8–11.
41. Callister TQ, Raggi P, Cooil B, et al. Effect of HMG-CoA reductase inhibitors on coronary artery disease as assessed by electron-beam computed tomography. *N Engl J Med* 1998;339:1972–1978.
42. Shields JP, Mielke CH, Rockwood TH, et al. Reliability of electron beam computed tomography to detect coronary artery calcification. *Am J Card Imaging* 1995;9:62–66.
43. Devries S, Wolfkiel C, Shah V, et al. Reproducibility of the measurement of coronary calcium with ultrafast computed tomography. *Am J Cardiol* 1995;75:973–975.
44. Wong ND, Teng W, Abrahamson D, et al. Noninvasive tracking of coronary atherosclerosis by electron beam computed tomography: rationale and design of the felodipine atherosclerosis prevention study (FAPS). *Am J Cardiol* 1995;76:1239–1242.
45. Maher JE, Bielak LF, Raz JA, et al. Progression of coronary artery calcification: a pilot study. *Mayo Clin Proc* 1999;74:347–355.
46. Zir LM. Observer variability in coronary angiography. *Int J Cardiol* 1983;3:171–173.
47. Multi-Ethnic Study of Atherosclerosis. NHLBI http://140.142.220.3/mesa/.
48. Shemesh J, Stroh CI, Tenenbaum A, et al. Comparison of coronary calcium in stable angina pectoris and in first acute myocardial infarction utilizing double helical computerized tomography. *Am J Cardiol* 1998;81:271–275.
49. DeVries S, Wolfkiel C, Fusman B, et al. Influence of age and gender on the presence of coronary calcium detected using ultrafast computed tomography. *J Am Coll Cardiol* 1995;25:76–82.
50. Rumberger J, Sheedy PF, Breen JF, et al. Electron beam computed tomography and coronary artery disease. Effect of sex on diagnosis. *Circulation* 1995;91:1363–1367.
51. Budoff MJ, Georgiou D, Brody A, et al. Ultrafast CT as a diagnostic modality in the detection of coronary artery disease: a multicenter study. *Circulation* 1996;93:898–894.
52. O'Rourke RA, Brundage BH, Froelicher VF, et al. American College of Cardiology/American Heart Association expert consensus document on electron-beam computed tomography for the diagnosis and prognosis of coronary artery disease. *Circulation* 2000;101:126–140.
53. Morrison A. *Screening in chronic disease.* New York: Oxford University Press, 1985:3.
54. Downs JR, Clearfield M, Weis S, et al. Primary prevention of acute coronary events with lovostatin in men and women with average cholesterol levels. *JAMA* 1998;279:1615–1622.
55. Agatston ASA, Janowitz WR, Kaplan GS, et al. Electron beam CT coronary calcium predicts future coronary events. *Circulation* 1996;94[Suppl]:I–360.
56. Hoff JA, Wolfkiel CJ, Chomka EV, et al. Can coronary events be predicted in asymptomatic individuals using electron beam tomography? *Circulation* 1996;94:I–33.
57. Raggi P, Callister TQ, Cooil B, et al. Identification of patients at increased risk of first unheralded acute myocar-

dial infarction by electron-beam computed tomography. *Circulation* 2000;101:850–855.

58. O'Malley PG, Taylor AJ, Jackson JL, et al. Prognostic value of coronary electron-beam computed tomography for coronary heart disease events in asymptomatic populations. *Am J Cardiol* 2000;85:945–948.

59. Potential value of ultrafast computed tomography to screen for coronary artery disease. Committee on Advanced Cardiac Imaging and Technology, Council on Clinical Cardiology, and Committee on Newer Imaging Modalities, Council on Cardiovascular Radiology, American Heart Association. *Circulation* 1993;87:2071.

60. O'Rourke RA. American College of Cardiology/American Heart Association expert consensus document on electron-beam computed tomography for the diagnosis and prognosis of coronary artery disease. *Am J Coll Cardiol* 2000;36:326–340.

61. Smith S, Greenland P, Grundy S. Prevention conference 5: beyond secondary prevention: identifying the high risk patient for coronary prevention. *Circulation* 2000;10:111–116.

62. Achenbach S, Moshage W, Ropers D, et al. Noninvasive, three-dimensional visualization of coronary artery bypass grafts by electron beam tomography. *Am J Cardiol* 1997;79:856–861.

63. Achenbach S, Moshage W, Bachmann K. Detection of high-grade restenosis after PTCA using contrast-enhanced electron beam CT. *Circulation* 1997;96:2785–2788.

64. Achenbach S, Ropers D, Regenfus M, et al. Contrast enhanced electron beam computed tomography to analyse the coronary arteries in patients after acute myocardial infarction. *Heart* 2000;84:489–493.

65. Achenbach S, Ulzheimer S, Baum U, et al. Noninvasive coronary angiography by retrospectively ECG-gated multislice spiral CT. *Circulation* 2000;102:2823–2828.

66. Achenbach S, Moshage W, Ropers D. Value of electron-beam CT for the noninvasive detection of high-grade coronary-artery stenoses and occlusions. *N Engl J Med* 1998;339:1964–1971.

67. Budoff MJ, Oudiz RJ, Zalace CP, et al. Intravenous three-dimensional coronary angiography using contrast enhanced electron beam computed tomography. *Am J Cardiol* 1999;83:840–845.

68. Bleiweis MS, Milliken JC, Baumgartner FJ, et al. Application of the ultrafast CT for diagnosis of perivalvular abscesses: surgical implications. *Chest* 1994;106:629–632.

69. Tomada H, Hoshiai M, Tagawa R, et al. Evolution of left atrial thrombus with computed tomography. *Am Heart J* 1980;100:306–310.

70. Helgason CM, Chomka E, Louie E, et al. The potential role for ultrafast cardiac computed tomography in patients with stroke. *Stroke* 1989;20:465–472.

71. Pietras RJ, Wolfkiel CJ, Veselik K. Validation of ultrafast computed tomographic left ventricular volume measurement. *Invest Radiol* 1991;26:28–34.

72. Roig E, Chomka EV, Castaner A, et al. Exercise ultrafast computed tomography for the detection of coronary artery disease. *J Am Coll Cardiol* 1989;13:1073–1081.

73. Lanzer P, Garrett J, Sievers R, et al. Quantitation of regional myocardial function by cine computed tomography: pharmacological changes in wall thickness. *J Am Coll Cardiol* 1986;8:682–692.

74. Budoff MJ, Shavelle DM, Lamont DH, et al. Usefulness of electron beam computed tomography scanning for distinguishing ischemic from nonischemic cardiomyopathy. *J Am Coll Cardiol* 1998;32:1173–1178.

75. Shemesh J, Tenenbaum A, Fisman EZ, et al. Coronary calcium as a reliable tool for differentiating ischemic from nonischemic cardiomyopathy. *Am J Cardiol* 1996;77:191–194.

76. Oren RM, Grover-McKay M, Stanford W, et al. Accurate preoperative diagnosis of pericardial constriction using cine computed tomography. *J Am Coll Cardiol* 1993;22:832–838.

77. Stanford W, Thompson BH. Cardiac masses and pericardial disease: imaging by electron-beam computed tomography. In: Skorton DJ, Schelbert HR, Braunwald E, eds. *Cardiac imaging: a companion to Braunwald's heart disease*, 2nd ed. Philadelphia: WB Saunders, 1996:863–871.

78. Liptom M, Coulden R. Valvular heart disease. *Radiol Clin North Am* 1999;37:319–339.

79. Taneja K, Sharma S, Kumar K, et al. *Cardiovasc Intervent Radiol* 1996;19:97–100.

80. Carrell T. Cardiovascular surgery in Marfan's syndrome. *Schweiz Med* 1997;127:992–1006.

81. Shinozaki H, Shimizu K, Anno H, et al. Total anomalous pulmonary venous drainage in an adult diagnosed with helical computed tomography. *Intern Med* 1997;36:912–916.

82. Sharma S, Mehta A, O'Donovan P. Computed tomography and magnetic resonance findings in long-standing patent ductus. *Angiology* 1996;47:393–398.

83. Pitlick P, Anthony C, More P, et al. Three dimensional visualization of the aorta by electron beam computed tomography and MRI. *Circulation* 1999;99:3086–3087.

84. Foster C, Kalbhen C, Demos T, et al. Aortobronchial fistula occurring after coarctation repair: findings on aortography, helical CT and CT angiography. *AJR Am J Roentgenol* 1987;171:401–402.

85. Becker C, Soppa C, Fink U, et al. Spiral CT angiography and 3D reconstruction in patients with aortic coarctation. *Eur Radiol* 1997;7:1473–1477.

86. Fishman JE. Imaging of blunt aortic and great vessel trauma. *J Thorac Imaging* 2000;15:97–103.

87. Rubin GD, Shiau MC, Leung AN, et al. Aorta and iliac arteries: single versus multiple detector-row helical CT angiography. *Radiology* 2000;215:670–676.

88. LeBlang SD, Dolich MO. Imaging of penetrating thoracic trauma. *J Thorac Imaging* 2000;15:128–135.

89. Zinck SE, Primack SL. Radiographic and CT findings in blunt chest trauma. *J Thorac Imaging* 2000;15:87–96.

90. Kouchoukos NT, Dougenis D. Surgery of the thoracic aorta. *N Engl J Med* 1997;336:1876–1888.

91. Rubin GD. Helical CT angiography of the thoracic aorta. *J Thorac Imaging* 1997;12:128–149.

92. Galla JD, Ergin MA, Lansman SL, et al. Identification of risk factors in patients undergoing thoracoabdominal aneurysm repair. *J Cardiac Surg* 12[Suppl]:292–299.

93. Semba CP, Kato N, Kee ST, et al. Acute rupture of the descending thoracic aorta: repair with use of endovascular stent-grafts. *J Vasc Int Radiol* 1997;8:337–342.

94. Black WC, Welch G. Advances in diagnostic imaging and overestimations of disease prevalence and the benefits of therapy. *N Engl J Med* 1993;38:1237–1243.

57

INTRAOPERATIVE ECHOCARDIOGRAPHY

WILLIAM J. STEWART

W. J. Stewart: Department of Cardiovascular Medicine, The Cleveland
Clinic Foundation, Cleveland, Ohio

▼ ADDITIONAL ELECTRONIC TOPICS

Historical Perspective k37;   Imaging Planes k38;   Goal-Oriented Study k39;   Idealizing Room and Loading Conditions k40;   Outcome Studies k41;   Postpump Assessment after Tricuspid Repair k42;   Postpump Intraoperative Echocardiography in Aortic Valve Repair k43;   Prepump Intraoperative Echocardiography in Homograft and Ross Procedures k44;   Postpump Echocardiography after Homograft Valve Replacement or Ross Procedure k45;   Prepump Intraoperative Echocardiography in Aortic Aneurysms k46;   Postpump Intraoperative Echocardiography k47;   Abscesses or Fistulas of the Heart k48;   Postpump Intraoperative Echocardiography k49;   Prepump Imaging in Congenital Heart Disease k50;   Changes in Surgery Based on Echocardiographic Findings k51;   Echocardiography in the Implantable Left Ventricular Assist Device k52;   Purposes and Indications for Intraoperative Echocardiography k53;   Diagnosis of Ischemia after Coronary Bypass k54;   Contrast Echocardiography in Coronary Bypass Surgery k55;   Determination of the Adequacy of Intravascular Volume k56;   Echocardiography of Diastolic Function and Ventricular Filling k57

OVERVIEW

Intraoperative echocardiography (IOE), mostly using transesophageal methods, provides an important means of assessing cardiac structure and function during cardiac and noncardiac operations (1,2,2a). IOE helps refine surgical plans immediately before cardiac surgery by defining the surgical mission and determining the severity and mechanism of the cardiac dysfunction. This provides the surgeon with an up-to-the-minute definition of the patient's anatomy and physiology, to help define or refine the objectives for surgery and to optimally plan repair of the dysfunctional valves, congenital abnormalities, coronary problems, and other disease. After surgery, the postpump IOE provides a safety net for immediately checking the success of the procedure at a time when further surgery can be performed (a second pump run) during the same thoracotomy. The frequency of changes in operative management varies directly with the difficulty of the procedure involved and is substantial for valve repair of various types, especially high for aortic valve repair, aortic homograft implantation, and myectomy for hypertrophic cardiomyopathy. This chapter describes the history, purposes, methodology, and effectiveness of IOE, as well as its impact on numerous types of surgeries. It is likely that IOE will contribute to the future development of innovative and emerging surgical procedures.

GLOSSARY

Contrast echocardiography: Imaging during injections to increase visualization of selected structures.

Epicardial echocardiography: Performed with the transducer placed directly on the surface of the heart during surgery.

Loading conditions: Factors related to intravascular volume and the pressures on the input and output sides of the heart.

Postpump: Refers to the IOE done after discontinuation of cardiopulmonary bypass.

Prepump: Refers to the IOE done before institution of cardiopulmonary bypass.

Second pump run: A second run of cardiopulmonary bypass for additional surgery done to correct residual problems after the initial surgery was thought to be sufficient.

Valve repair: Surgery to correct valve dysfunction using the native valve tissue, without removing or replacing the valve.

PREPUMP INTRAOPERATIVE ECHOCARDIOGRAPHY: GENERAL CONSIDERATIONS

Purposes

IOE before cardiopulmonary bypass (prepump) is useful in certain groups of patients undergoing cardiac surgery, for several important reasons. It provides an accurate way to determine the mechanism and severity of the problem requiring surgery (19). The prepump study is also helpful to obtain baseline information about an anesthetized patient that may be of better quality or reflect interval changes compared with preoperative studies.

Performed appropriately, echocardiography has the attribute of completeness, with its ability to diagnose the structure and function of all cardiac valves (19a) and chambers, even those that are not the primary problem mandating surgery. Dysfunction of other valves that is not treated effectively can lead to serious and potentially life-threatening complications and be mistaken for failure of the primary operation. This results from mistakes in the preoperative definition of the patient's problem or from changes that occur in the interval between workup and surgery. The prepump TEE often finds problems that were not detected on the preoperative evaluation, most commonly, a clot in the left atrial appendage or a patent foramen ovale.

A final purpose of the prepump IOE is to define methods of cannulation. This is particularly important when there is severe aortic atheroma, with its potential to embolize if disrupted by the operative process. It is also important in placement of intracardiac devices such as those used for port access surgery (19b). The prepump study has also been used to define optimal methods of cardioplegia administration (19c). For example, aortic regurgitation

(AR) of even moderate severity may limit the effectiveness of antegrade cardioplegia administration via the aortic root (20). Placement of a coronary sinus catheter for retrograde cardioplegia can also be confirmed by TEE (21,22).

Methods

Two methods of intraoperative imaging have been employed, TEE and epicardial echocardiography. TEE has substantial advantages in most situations, including the ability to monitor cardiac function without an echocardiographic transducer entering the sterile field or interrupting the surgical process. Posterior structures such as the atria and pulmonary veins are seen better with transesophageal echocardiography. ▼ k58

Record Keeping and Image Archival

A written record of the diagnoses made by TEE is an important part of the job of IOE. In addition, archiving images either by videotape or digital methods (35a) is important for comparison with previous and subsequent studies. Both of these issues are important when medical-legal issues regarding the operation are raised.

Indications for Intraoperative Echocardiography

The types of patients for whom intraoperative TEE is useful are detailed by the groups of disease states listed in this chapter. Thys et al. have published guidelines for perioperative echocardiography, delineating three categories: category I for those supported by strong evidence of clinical value for improving outcome; category II for applications supported by weaker evidence; and category III for applications that are uncertain to have clinical benefit (35b). This chapter discusses most of these indications in detail.

Outcome Studies for Prepump Intraoperative Echocardiography

One study by Chaliki et al. compared the prebypass TEE findings with surgical observations in a large group of 918 cases; TEE information was found to be quite reliable, showing discrepancies with operative findings in only 2.5% of cases (35c).

Several studies have determined the frequency with which the prepump IOE contributes to a change in surgical management. In several studies of mixed multiple groups of valvular lesions, prebypass imaging diagnosed unsuspected findings that changed the planned operation in 10.8% to 19.0% of patients (36,36a). In another study of 246 patients with ischemic mitral regurgitation (MR), prepump TEE resulted in a change in the operative plan with respect to the mitral valve in 27 patients (11%), involving less MR

than expected in 22 patients and more MR in five patients (34). In patients who come to the operating room in an emergent situation with unstable hemodynamics, the emergency intraoperative TEE has an even larger impact on clinical outcome, with new findings discovered in 80% of patients and an alteration of the planned surgical procedure in 23% (36b).

Ungerleider et al. (37) studied 328 patients before surgery for congenital heart disease and found that IOE played a role in surgical planning in 44% and discovered previously unappreciated details of anatomy in 18% of patients. Another author found a major problem on the prebypass echocardiogram that led to a change in plans in 6.7% (37a). In an early study of a mixed group of 426 consecutive patients with a mixture of valvular problems, our group found that 40 patients (9%) had a change in the operative mission based on the prepump IOE (unpublished data). In another study from our institution, Secknus et al. (38) evaluated 121 patients in whom prepump intraoperative TEE studies were performed to assess MR and the need for mitral repair; changes in operative plan occurred in 6.1%, mostly in cases in which less mitral disease was found than was expected on the basis of the preoperative workup.

Some findings, such as a thrombus in the left atrial appendage, should prompt operative removal. When this is found in a patient without mitral valve disease, removal may require bicaval rather than single-stage cannulation for the venous return to the heart-lung machine. However, it is not certain whether closure of the appendage should be recommended, as it remains at least partly open even after attempted closure in 36% of such cases (37b).

Click et al. from the Mayo Clinic reported a large series of 3,245 patients undergoing IOE, in whom new information was found before bypass in 15% of patients. This directly affected surgery in 14% of the patients. The most common new prepump finding was a patent foramen ovale, which was closed in the majority of patients (38a). The series by Click et al. is probably the most intensively reported large group of patients undergoing IOE. The important changes in plans included a decision to do something that had not been planned in 9.6% of the total, including a new decision to close a patent foramen ovale in 2.7%, to perform valvular surgery in 2.7%, and to remove a previously undiagnosed thrombus in 1.1% of the total. There were also decisions based on the prepump echocardiogram *not* to do something that had been planned in 3.9% of the total, which were mostly decisions not to do surgery on a valve for which the preoperative workup had indicated a need for surgery (3.6% of the total of 3,245 patients) (38a).

Another more recent study by Couture et al. found that prepump IOE led to a modification of planned surgical intervention in 30% of cases, with a frequency of 39% in complex surgical procedures, 19% in valvular surgery, and 10% in coronary artery bypass surgery (38b). Still another study of 5,016 cases by Mishra et al. found that prebypass imaging yielded unsuspected findings that either helped or modified the surgical plan in 12% of valve procedures and in 27% of coronary procedures (38c). ⚐ k59

POSTPUMP INTRAOPERATIVE ECHOCARDIOGRAPHY: GENERAL CONSIDERATIONS

Purposes

The primary purpose of echocardiography done after cardiopulmonary bypass (postpump) is to determine the success of the primary surgical mission. Like the prepump study, the postpump study should be goal oriented, examining the most important issues first (32a), with one modification. The postpump IOE should first evaluate the most vulnerable aspect of the surgery for immediate failure, which may be different from the primary indication for surgery. For example, in a patient with mitral stenosis with severe mitral calcification and functional tricuspid regurgitation (TR), the mitral replacement may be more important in the clinical improvement than tricuspid repair, but the most important problem to examine first on the postpump TEE study is the tricuspid repair, because the mitral prosthesis is less likely to have initial failure.

The postpump TEE is much more relevant if performed after establishing hemodynamic stability under conditions that match the ambulatory state, whereas misinformation can result from studies done during aberrant transient conditions early after coming off bypass. Imaging should be done before administration of protamine and removal of the arterial and venous cannulae, so that cardiopulmonary bypass can be reinstituted if problems are found. The exception to this is the patient with mild periprosthetic regurgitant jets found on postpump TEE, which have a tendency to improve after protamine is given (38e).

In some cases, the primary problem mandating surgery persists (e.g., residual valvular regurgitation after attempted repair of that valve). In occasional cases, new problems occur, such as new regurgitation of an additional valve not previously abnormal, or another complication. In general, we consider *no* valvular regurgitation to be the ideal result of surgery and mild (1+) regurgitation to be an acceptable outcome. Moderately severe or severe (3+ or 4+) are problematic and warrant a "second pump run" for further surgery during the same thoracotomy to correct the problem. In most cases of moderate (2+) regurgitation, further surgery is usually indicated, but the situation must be individualized, depending on the patient's age and overall condition. In such cases, we recommend careful, complete echocardiographic evaluation for a period of 5 to 10 minutes, without giving protamine or decannulating, during which time the hemodynamic conditions should be idealized and even provoked. Sometimes the regurgitation decreases in severity with recovery of ventricular function. In other cases, the regurgitation is obviously bad enough for further surgery. In many cases with moderate residual regurgitation, we find it useful to increase mean arterial pressure, observing the amount of regurgitation with this "afterload stress" echocardiogram. If the amount of MR or AR persists at a moderate (2+) level, or increases, the patient should probably undergo further surgery with a second pump run.

Numerous types of intraoperative provocation can be used to bring out postpump valvular dysfunction in cases in which the amount of residual problems is borderline or when loading conditions might otherwise lead to false reassurance. The most commonly used is the phenylephrine challenge, which is useful for borderline amounts of aortic and MR (39). Boluses of 100 µg of phenylephrine are given every 30 to 120 seconds to bring mean arterial pressure up to approximately 110 transiently. If moderate or more regurgitation results, consideration should be given to further surgery on that valve. Other types of provocation used in the operating room include isoproterenol for hypertrophic cardiomyopathy, intravascular volume challenge for any lesion, and partial pulmonary artery occlusion for TR. It is far better to know of a latent problem immediately in the operating room than to learn about it a day or a week after surgery.

Another purpose of postpump intraoperative imaging is to diagnose complications of surgery. These include iatrogenic problems generic to cardiac surgery, including outflow and inflow obstruction, aortic dissection at the site of aortic cannulation (38d), atrial septal defect, periprosthetic regurgitation, and intraoperative myocardial infarction. Definition of these cases by IOE allows a rational basis for pharmacologic management or for performing further surgery during the same thoracotomy.

The frequency of second pump runs overall is 5.4% of IOE studies in our series (19a), and it varies depending on the type of surgery performed and its complexity (Table 57.1). The procedures at highest risk of initial failure are myectomy for hypertrophic cardiomyopathy and aortic valve repair. Which surgery is most vulnerable to initial failure should be a factor in deciding which patients to invest resources for IOE and which problem to address first with the postpump study (16). Surprisingly, over the past 15 years, the frequency of second pump runs at our institution has essentially stayed the same, both overall and within each of the categories followed.

In the large study from the Mayo Clinic by Click et al., new information was found by IOE after bypass in 6% of the patients, resulting in a change in surgery or hemodynamic management in 4% of the total; it was highest in a selected group of patients with coronary artery bypass graft surgery (CABG), aortic surgery, and hypertrophic cardiomyopathy (38a). Michel-Cherqui et al. reported a frequency

TABLE 57.1 FREQUENCY OF SURGERIES STUDIED WITH INTRAOPERATIVE ECHOCARDIOGRAPHY AND SECOND PUMP RUNS PERFORMED (1984 TO 1996)

	Cases (no.)	Second pump runs (no.)	Second pump runs (%)
Total	9,826	531	5.4
Mitral repair	3,032	199	6.6
Aortic repair	516	74	14.1
Tricuspid repair	518	28	5.3
Congenital	681	39	5.7
Hypertrophic cardiomyopathy	232	42	17.9
Thoracic aneurysm	560	21	3.8

From Grimm RA, Stewart WJ. The role of intraoperative echocardiography in valve surgery. *Cardiol Clin* 1998;16:477–489, with permission.

of 2.5% of 203 cases in which immediate surgical intervention was required on account of the postpump TEE findings (36a).

The converse of these data is that the postpump study finds a satisfactory result with resolution of the initial problem in the majority (94% to 97%) of patients; this also provides a substantial benefit to the patient. When abnormal hemodynamic changes occur outside the operating room in the early postoperative period, the management team can be confident that the changes are not due to failure of the primary surgical mission if the postpump study has shown that it was accomplished.

Another purpose of the postpump study is to reassess ventricular function. It is important to document changes resulting from elimination of the primary surgical problem and to determine a new baseline for later comparison. However, early after cessation of cardiopulmonary bypass, LV function may be transiently depressed by residual effects of hyperkalemic cardioplegia or air embolization to the coronary bed. Finally, IOE can define the location and severity of intracardiac air to assist in its removal.

MITRAL VALVE REPAIR

In mitral valve dysfunction, IOE is particularly useful for determination of the mechanism of the problem, prediction of the methods that will be required for surgical repair, diagnosis of complications of repair, and assessment of the postrepair results of the surgery.

The prepump IOE has been found to change the operative plans in 6% to 17% of cases (36a,38). With both imaging and color Doppler, the mitral valve is investigated systematically by TEE using a short-axis view from the transverse transgastric window, and multiple midesophageal long-axis views (2,45b,45c). Most of the long-axis views help define *which leaflet* is involved. For examining which *portion* of the leaflet is most involved (Fig. 57.1), the best views are the short-axis transgastric view and the midesophageal intercommissural long-axis view. The latter

is obtained from the midesophageal window with the multiplane angle at approximately 60 degrees, with the plane parallel to the line between the mitral commissures.

Quantitating the severity of MR (a topic covered in Chapter 51) is accomplished using a weighted average of information from left atrial spatial mapping (31,46,47), proximal jet width (48), pulmonary vein pulsed Doppler (49), and proximal flow convergence information (50). It appears that TEE and epicardial echocardiography give relatively equivalent assessments in quantifying MR (51). Both are more sensitive than transthoracic echocardiography. As mentioned previously, hemodynamics in the operating room often include less intravascular volume and less afterload than the ambulatory state, which often decreases the amount of MR (51a).

Determining the Mechanism of Mitral Regurgitation from Leaflet Motion and Jet Direction

For determination of the mechanism of MR, IOE uses two-dimensional evaluation of leaflet motion and color flow Doppler evaluation of jet direction (19). Leaflet motion is separated into MR associated with excessive, normal, and restricted leaflet motion, a system derived from the surgical system used by Carpentier et al. (52). These leaflet motion groups, associated with jet direction characteristics, characterize the various mechanisms of MR (Table 57.2).

Each mechanism demands specific surgical techniques for optimal correction, and the feasibility of repair varies by the mechanism of regurgitation as defined by the preoperative echocardiogram (Table 57.3) (53) and by the etiology (54). In valves that are extensively calcified, fibrotic, or destroyed by endocarditis, repair is impossible. No matter what the mechanism of MR, almost all patients undergo annuloplasty as a component of the repair, in addition to the other surgical maneuvers, detailed in the following sections.

For *excessive* leaflet motion, the jet is deflected *away* from the most abnormal leaflet. The easiest type to repair is a flail or prolapsing posterior leaflet (Fig. 57.2), which most

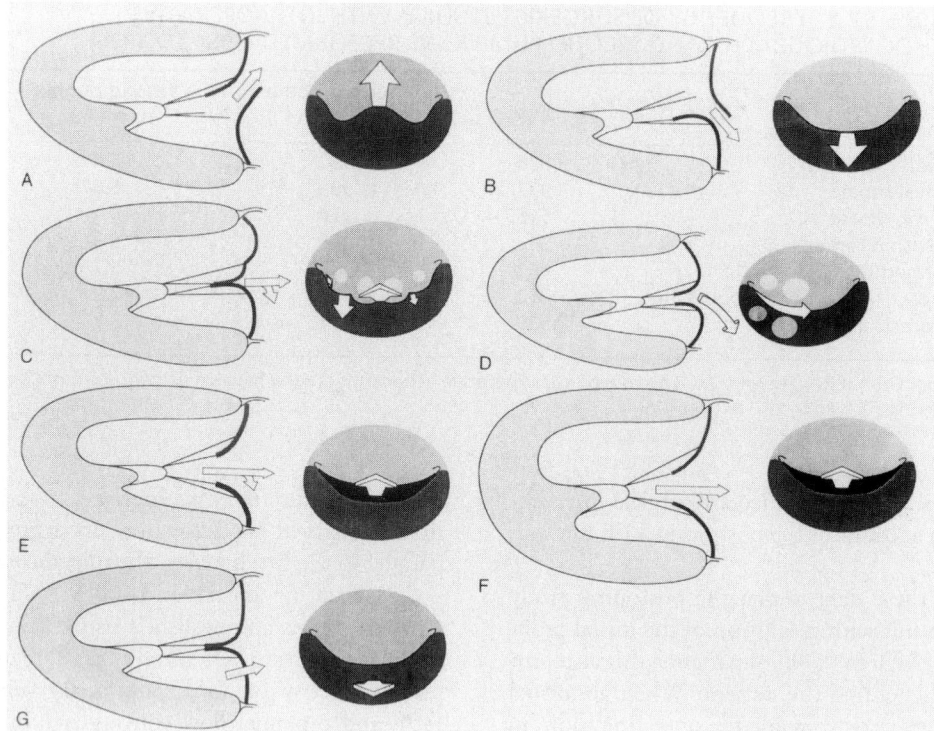

FIGURE 57.1 Mechanisms of mitral regurgitation, determined by echocardiographic assessment of leaflet motion and Doppler assessment of jet direction. Diagrams show long-axis views (left side of each pair) and short-axis views (right side of each pair). **A:** Posterior leaflet flail or prolapse with an anterior jet direction. **B:** Anterior leaflet flail or prolapse with a posterior jet direction. **C:** Bileaflet chordal elongation, flail, or prolapse with a central or posterior jet direction. **D:** Posteromedial papillary muscle infarction causing elongation or disruption of support to both leaflets at the commissure with a jet emanating from the medial commissure, directed posterolaterally. **E:** Leaflet restriction with a central or posterior jet direction. **F:** Ventricular-annular dilation displacing the papillary muscles outward with a central or posterior jet direction. **G:** Leaflet perforation with an eccentric location of the jet origin, originating from the leaflet body, away from the coaptation line. (From Stewart WJ, Currie PJ, Salcedo EE, et al. Evaluation of mitral leaflet motion by echocardiography and jet direction by Doppler color flow mapping to determine the mechanisms of mitral regurgitation. *J Am Coll Cardiol* 1992;20:1353–1361, with permission.)

TABLE 57.2   INFLUENCE OF JET MECHANISM AND CHARACTERISTICS ON SURGICAL PLANNING

Leaflet motion	Problem	Jet direction	Leaflet surgery	Annulus
Excessive				
	PL MVP	Anterior	Quad resection	Annuloplasty
	AL MVP	Posterior	Chordal transfer (chordal shortening, artificial chordae)	Annuloplasty
	Bileaflet MVP	Central[a]	Quad resection	Annuloplasty
	Papillary muscle rupture	Commissural	Papillary muscle reimplantation	Annuloplasty
	Commissural chordal rupture	Commissural	Suture commissure, chordal transfer	Annuloplasty
Normal				
	LVE, apical tethering	Central/posterior	None	Annuloplasty
	Perforation	Eccentric origin	Suture, patch	Annuloplasty
Restricted				
	Restricted leaflets	Central/posterior	OMC, débridement, division of fusion	Annuloplasty

AL, anterior leaflet; LVE, left ventricular enlargement; MVP, mitral valve prolapse; OMC, open mitral commissurotomy; PL, posterior leaflet.
[a]In bileaflet prolapse, jet direction reflects the most dominant problem; may be anteriorly directed with posterior greater than anterior prolapse, or posteriorly directed with anterior greater than posterior prolapse.

TABLE 57.3 PREDICTION OF THE FEASIBILITY OF REPAIR BASED ON THE PREOPERATIVE ECHOCARDIOGRAM

	No.	Feasibility of repair (%)	Initial failure of repair (second pump runs)
Excessive	222	82.9	4.4
Posterior	109	89.0	1.8
Anterior	49	61.2	8.2
Posterior and anterior	64	82.8	0
Restricted	140	35.7	10.0
Normal	65	84.6	0
Total	427	67.7	4.5

From Sun JP, Yang XS, Mayer EL, et al. Mitral valvular leaflet excursion by echo is a marker for the feasibility of repair and risk of failed repair. *Circulation* 1995;92:I-464(abst).

commonly involves the middle scallop and can be repaired in 89% of cases (55). The excessive leaflet motion is readily detected by two-dimensional echocardiography and the jet is deflected anteriorly, as assessed by color Doppler in the operating room before cardiopulmonary bypass. This problem is corrected by quadrilateral resection of the unsupported leaflet followed by suture closure of the gap (54).

By comparison, other types of MR are more difficult to repair. For example, it is feasible in 61% of cases to repair MR due to prolapse or flail of the anterior leaflet (Table 57.3). This is diagnosed by its characteristic posterior jet direction (19). Repair requires a surgical maneuver to provide chordae to the unsupported anterior leaflet, which can be done with chordal transfer, or less commonly with chordal shortening (54) or replacement with artificial chordae (56).

Repair of MR due to prolapse of both leaflets can usually be corrected by surgery only on the posterior leaflet, involving a quadrilateral resection, without anterior leaflet maneuvers (56a). However, when there is extensive destruction and flail of both leaflets, repair is feasible in only 41% of cases (55).

For MR due to *restricted* leaflet motion, the jet is directed *toward* the most abnormal leaflet. Most commonly the jet direction is posterior, with a fixed posterior leaflet, or central, from balanced bileaflet restriction. This occurs mostly from rheumatic mitral valve disease, and only 36% of cases can be repaired. In these patients, repair is more likely when there is a lower echocardiogram score, or "splitability index," an echocardiographic measure defined by four assessments, each on a scale of 1 to 4, of leaflet mobility, leaflet thickness, calcification, and subvalvular involve-

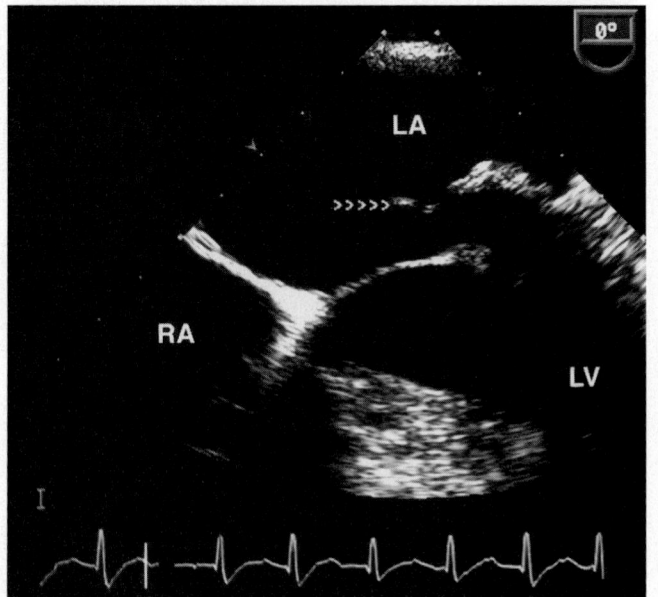
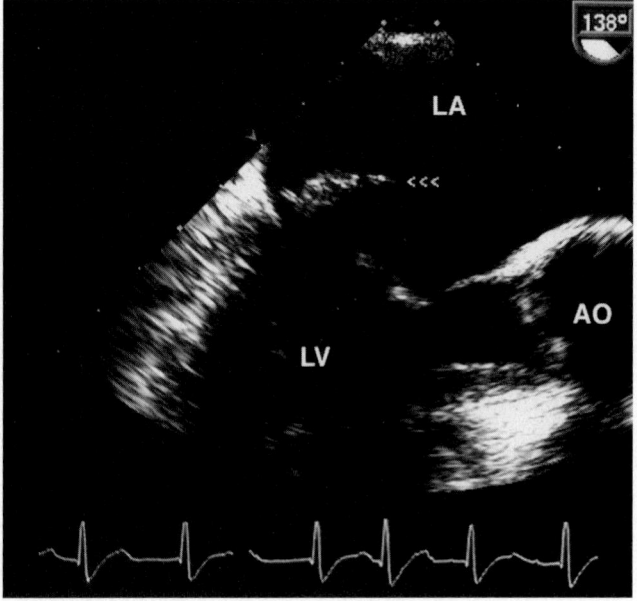

A   B

FIGURE 57.2 Posterior leaflet flail causing severe mitral regurgitation. **A:** Transverse midesophageal view (0 degrees) showing the flail posterior leaflet (*arrowheads*). **B:** Midesophageal long-axis (138 degrees) view showing the posterior leaflet flail (*arrowheads*). AO, aorta; LA, left atrium; LV, left ventricle; RA, right atrium. See also the transverse and long-axis color flow images showing the anteromedially directed jet of severe mitral regurgitation on the CD-ROM and online versions of this chapter.

ment, for a total score of up to 16 (57,58). Repair is more feasible in younger patients, but carries a greater risk of progressive disease and reoperation (59,60), likely due to more active fibrosis or recurrent valvulitis.

Patients with significant mitral stenosis with a low splitability index (not associated with calcification or extensive fibrosis) are usually candidates for percutaneous balloon valvotomy. In more recent years, the ones who come to surgery are those who are not suitable for balloon valvotomy, because they have a splitability index that is high (greater than 9) or concomitant MR. Therefore, most of the surgical repairs currently involve more extensive débridement, decalcification, and commissurotomy, as well as annuloplasty (60). When the echocardiography score (splitability index) is high, however, there is less likelihood of successful repair and more likely early failure of the repair (60a).

Patients with *normal* leaflets have a *central* (or sometimes posterior) jet direction. This type of MR is usually due to LV enlargement and dysfunction, which cause "relative restriction of normal leaflets" due to outward displacement of the papillary muscles, and therefore apical displacement of the coaptation line (61). This "apical tethering" results most commonly from ischemic MR (62). It is a misunderstood entity and really does not result from annular dilation, but rather from change in the shape of the LV (sphericalization), which makes the leaflet-chordal-papillary muscle length relatively short compared with the

increased distance outward to the LV walls. The mitral annulus in these patients also appears to have reduced cyclic variation in annular shape and area (62a). Paradoxically, repair is currently accomplished with an annuloplasty alone. This is feasible in 85% of patients (Table 57.3) but is associated with a significant rate of return of MR over months to years, mainly due to progression of LV dysfunction, often due to repeat infarction or volume overload.

Occasionally, patients with MR due to normal leaflets have a leaflet perforation or congenital cleft (62b). This can generally be sewn primarily or patched with a piece of pericardium, as long as there are no additional problems, such as disrupted leaflets or chordae from endocarditis. Of note, in patients with congenital cleft mitral valves, it is difficult to obtain a long-lasting repair, particularly in patients with Rastelli's type A or a divided inferior mitral leaflet.

Postpump Imaging and Second Pump Runs

After valve repair for MR, the vast majority of patients have a successful result, as defined previously and evidenced by the postpump IOE (Fig. 57.3). In the series from our institution, 6.6% of patients had problems discovered on the postpump TEE that warranted further surgery during the same thoracotomy (19a). ❤ k60

The mechanism of MR also affects the durability after repair for valvular regurgitation caused by degenerative dis-

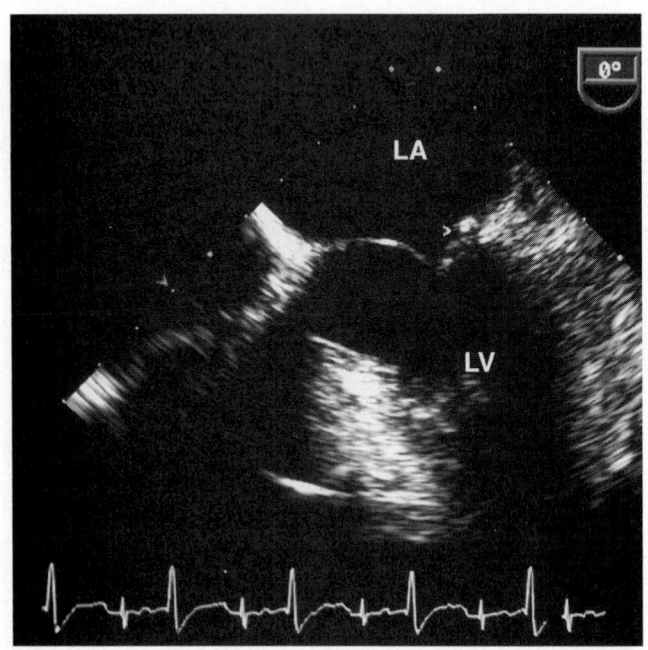 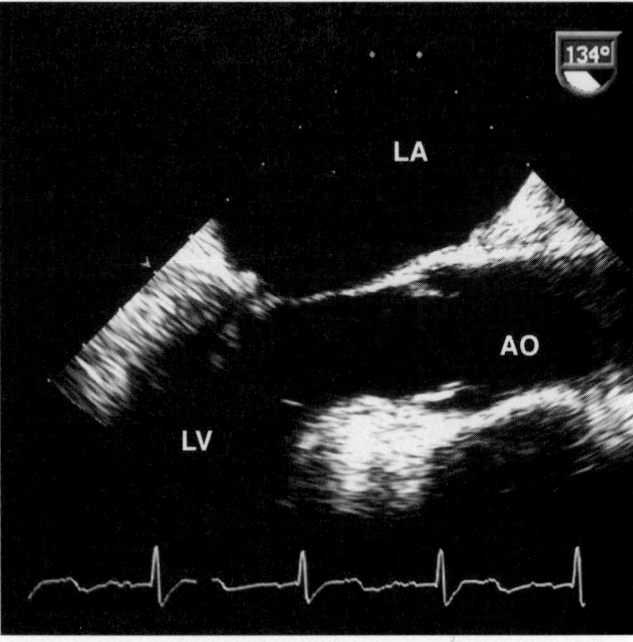

FIGURE 57.3 Postpump images after successful repair of mitral regurgitation from the same patient shown in Figure 57.2. **A:** Transverse (0 degrees) midesophageal four-chamber view showing no prolapse or flail. The annuloplasty is shown (*arrowhead*). **B:** Long-axis midesophageal view (134 degrees) showing no residual prolapse or flail. AO, aorta; LA, left atrium; LV, left ventricle. See also the color flow images showing only trivial mitral regurgitation after repair on the CD-ROM and online versions of this chapter.

ease. Durability is greatest after quadrangular resection and annuloplasty for posterior leaflet prolapse (45a).

TRICUSPID VALVE REPAIR

IOE is also useful in performing tricuspid valve repair. TR causing the need for tricuspid surgery arises most commonly due to left-sided congestive heart failure of any cause. Both intravascular volume overload and pulmonary hypertension can cause enlargement of the right ventricle, causing TR. In chronic conditions, the tricuspid annulus also dilates. Of patients having surgery for mitral or aortic valvular heart disease, tricuspid surgery is needed in approximately 25% (73). Over 93% of tricuspid surgery entails repair (74), in contrast to much lower percentages in other valves.

The tricuspid valve is assessed by TEE using a midesophageal four-chamber view at a 0-degree multiplane angle, a midesophageal 45-degree view at the level of the short axis of the aortic valve, a midesophageal 135-degree view at the level of the right atrium and tricuspid valve (*e*Fig. 57.3.1), and a transgastric view at 90 degrees showing the long axis of the right ventricle and right atrium. Additional value is obtained from deep transgastric views of the hepatic vein and inferior vena cava to detect systolic flow reversal using pulsed Doppler as an indicator of severe TR.

In doing the prepump IOE for tricuspid valve surgery, semiquantitative assessment of the amount of TR correlates with preoperative assessments (75,76). However, compared with other valves, the severity of TR is even more volatile and extremely dependent on loading conditions. Evaluating leaflet morphology such as prolapse or rheumatic leaflet restriction is important as the former may enhance and the latter may reduce the likelihood of successful repair. In addition, measurement of the maximum tricuspid annulus diameter may identify patients who need repair because the TR is less likely to resolve merely by fixing the left-sided valvular abnormalities (76).

AORTIC VALVE REPAIR

Compared with the past, when only bioprosthetic and mechanical prosthetic valve replacement was available, surgery for aortic valve disease has newly expanded options including aortic valve repair, homograft implantation, stentless bioprostheses, and Ross procedure. There are advantages and disadvantages of each option, but none of these is an ideal substitute for a normal native valve. Which surgery is best to use in each individual patient depends on the nature, etiology, and severity of the aortic valve dysfunction, and the clinical characteristics, age, and personal preferences of the patient. The prepump IOE has been found to change the operative plans in 15% of cases undergoing aortic valve surgery (38).

Aortic valve repair is applicable only to a small, highly selected subset of patients undergoing aortic valve surgery (85–87), particularly those with pure AR who are free of appreciable fibrosis or valvular thickening. Like mitral repair, this surgery demands the most from the echocardiographer and the surgeon, because of the necessity to understand the mechanism of the dysfunction. The prepump IOE is extremely useful in this group (88,89) to determine the mechanism and severity of regurgitation and the size of the aortic annulus and ascending aorta.

Determination of the Severity and Mechanism of Aortic Regurgitation

The severity of AR is judged intraoperatively from a weighted average of information from LV outflow tract spatial mapping (90), the flow convergence on the superior side of the regurgitant orifice, and the downstream events of descending aortic diastolic flow reversal (91) (see also Chapter 22). The proximal jet width in long-axis views and the jet area in short-axis views provide important and reliable criteria for severity (91a). Similar to MR, it is useful to separate the leaflet motion in AR into groups with normal, excessive, and restricted leaflet motion. Most patients with aortic valve disease have restricted leaflet motion resulting from degenerative and rheumatic etiologies. However, the vast majority of patients with AR has restricted leaflet motion, because of the predominance of degenerative, rheumatic, and fibrocalcific etiologies of aortic valve disease. These processes cause retraction of the leaflet size, leaving a central leak; 70% of patients have a central jet origin and direction (94). This type of aortic valve disease is not generally amenable to durable repair.

The primary group of patients in whom repair is feasible have noncalcified, nonstenotic valves with pure regurgitation resulting from aortic valve prolapse. Prolapse occurs most commonly in the settings of a congenital bicuspid aortic valve (Fig. 57.4) or a trileaflet valve with prolapse of one coronary cusp, usually the right. Prolapse of a trileaflet valve may result from leaflet fenestration or a congenital membranous ventricular septal defect (VSD) (92,93). In any of these categories, the regurgitation results from excessive length of the edge of the prolapsing leaflet, causing it to have a lower diastolic position. In 70% of patients with excessive leaflet motion, the jet is deflected to the opposite side of the LV outflow tract by the prolapsing leaflet (94). AR resulting from prolapse is surgically corrected using triangular resection of a small portion of the prolapsing leaflet, to adjust the length of the leaflet edge, causing its diastolic position to be at the same level as the opposing ones, thus promoting coaptation. In addition, pledgeted sutures at the commissures, a "commissuroplasty," bring the points of suspension of leaflets inward to improve coaptation (85,95).

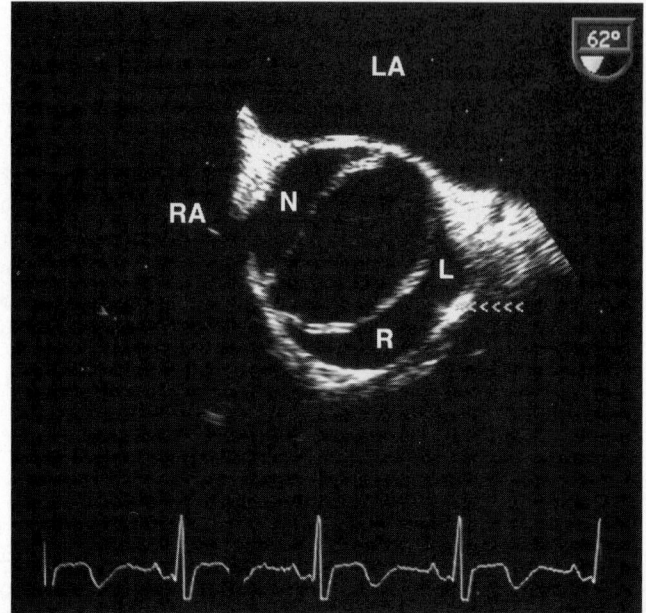

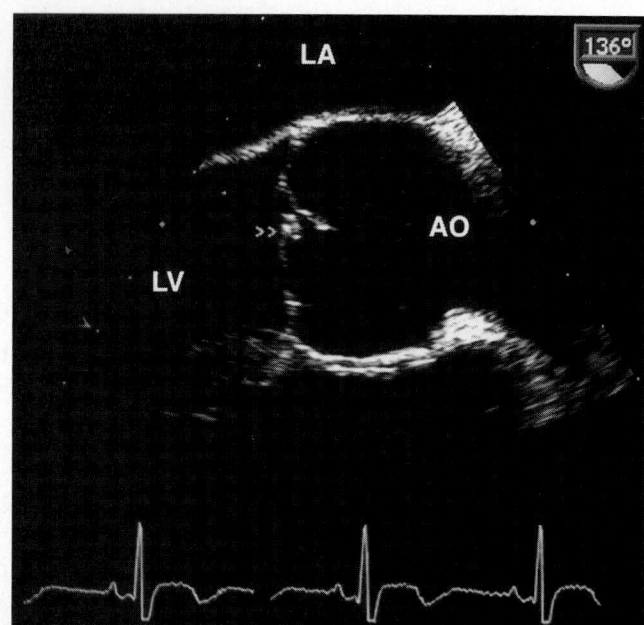

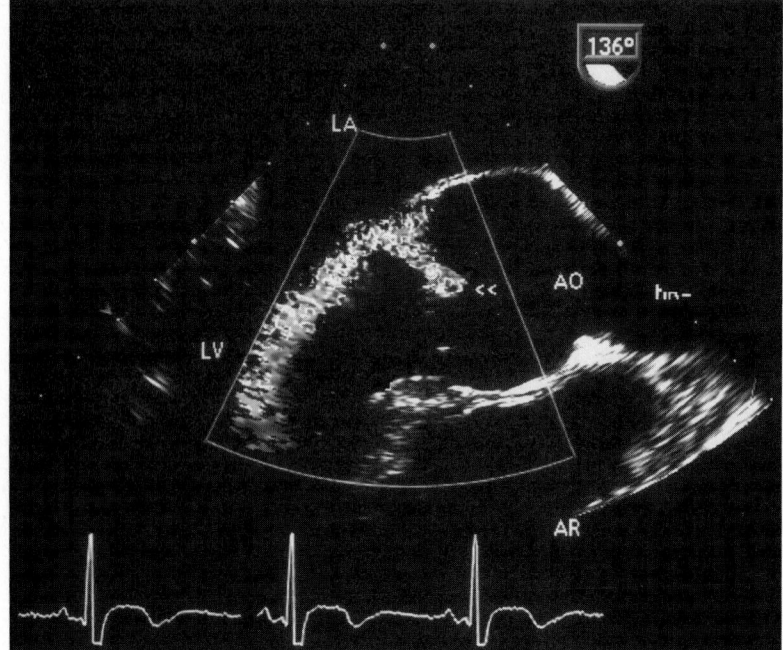

FIGURE 57.4 Aortic regurgitation amenable to valve repair. **A:** A short-axis, 62-degree, midesophageal view of the same patient, showing fusion of what would be the right (R) and left (L) cusps into a larger anterior cusp, compared with the posterior cusp, which would otherwise be the noncoronary (N) cusp. Arrowheads show the anterior raphe. **B:** Long-axis, 136-degree, midesophageal view of the aortic valve showing the aortic valve prolapse (*arrowheads*). **C:** Black and white copy of a color image in a long-axis view of the outflow tract, showing the posteriorly directed jet of aortic regurgitation emanating from the coaptation line (*arrowheads*) at the site of prolapse (*arrows*). AO, aorta; AR, aortic regurgitation; LA, left atrium; LV, left ventricle; RA, right atrium. See also the color flow images on the CD-ROM and online versions of this chapter, showing the posteriorly directed jet of aortic regurgitation in this entity before repair and the postpump images after successful repair of aortic regurgitation from the same patient showing trivial residual aortic regurgitation.

Repair can also be successful in certain patients with regurgitation from normal aortic leaflets. This type of AR has a central jet direction emanating from central failure of coaptation of a trileaflet valve. The regurgitation usually results from ascending aortic dilatation, because of outward displacement of the sinotubular ridge, causing "relative restriction of normal leaflets" similar to MR from LV dilatation, as detailed earlier in this chapter. AR from aortic dilatation is also repaired with a commissuroplasty. In certain cases, a structurally normal native aortic valve can be resuspended during surgery for conduit placement in patients with ascending aortic dilatation or aneurysm (96–97a).

In patients with restricted leaflets, for whom other options are available, repair is not the first choice of operation. When the clinical situation favors repair, such as in underdeveloped countries (98) for whom the cost of a prosthesis is unacceptable or anticoagulation is impossible, repair of this type of AR can be accomplished (99,100). Although the initial results are adequate, regurgitation redevelops quickly (101).

Another role for the prepump IOE in aortic valve disease is to look at the anatomy of the ascending aorta, especially the relative diameters in the long-axis view of the aortic annulus (at the hinge points of the aortic valve), and the sinotubular junction. Normally, these two measurements are approximately equal and roughly 19 to 23 mm. In bicuspid valves and other congenital aortic valve disease, the annular diameter is usually enlarged (approximately 26 to 32 mm). In patients who have central regurgitation with normal aortic leaflets, the diameter of the sinotubular junction is often larger than the annular diameter.

AORTIC HOMOGRAFTS, STENTLESS BIOPROSTHETIC VALVES, AND ROSS PROCEDURE

A case can be made for routine TEE (104) in the course of a standard aortic or mitral valve replacement, as it is unquestionably more sensitive for detection of prosthetic dysfunction than transthoracic echocardiography (105,106). However, because of limited resources and the low incidence of changes in operative management based on echocardiography, IOE is not performed routinely when a standard prosthesis is planned. IOE is useful in aortic valve replacements with a homograft (human valve) or pulmonary autograft (the patient's own pulmonic valve) (107). k61

AORTIC ANEURYSM SURGERY

With its rapidity and portability, TEE is extremely useful in the preoperative management of patients with aortic aneurysms and aortic dissection (116). By the time the patient comes to the operating room, in some cases a significant time interval has elapsed since the preoperative studies. Because the potential exists for interval progression or development of more complications, repeat evaluation in the operating room before surgery is often useful. TEE is also useful in transluminal endovascular stenting to repair thoracic aortic aneurysms, for navigating the graft placement and tailoring without intimal damage, and especially to assess perigraft leakage (116a) and graft kinking immediately after deployment (116b).

MASSES AND TUMORS OF THE HEART

The removal of a mass in the heart is also assisted substantially by the prepump and postpump use of TEE. Unexpected masses found during prepump IOE in a patient coming for surgery for something else are not uncommon. The most common is a thrombus in the left atrial appendage in a patient with atrial fibrillation or mitral valve disease. In suspected pulmonary emboli, epicardial echocardiography can be used to visualize the proximal right and left pulmonary arteries and pick out the exact location of thrombi (126a).

Some of the masses are tumors, of which most are benign and noncancerous. The most common tumor com-

ing to surgery is a myxoma, which most frequently is attached to the interatrial septum; however, they can be seen in the right atrium, in both atria, or in the ventricles. The presence of a mobile mass on a valve in a patient who is not infected is commonly a fibroelastoma, most commonly seen on the aortic side of the aortic valve. However, many fibroelastomas occur on valves that are thickened by other degenerative or fibrotic processes and are seen by TEE but not identified as being a tumor until the histology of the resected valve tissue is done (127a). k62

MYECTOMY FOR HYPERTROPHIC CARDIOMYOPATHY

For patients with surgical indications for myectomy, there is a particular need for IOE. This results from the variability of the location and extent of hypertrophy in patients with hypertrophic cardiomyopathy and the dynamic nature of the outflow tract obstruction. Echocardiography is an indispensable tool in planning and instituting effective surgical relief of the obstruction (128,129).

Prepump Echocardiography in Myectomy

Both transesophageal and epicardial echocardiography are useful in patients undergoing myectomy (Fig. 57.5). Either can define the location of hypertrophy and the location of the SAM. The location of the systolic contact of the mitral valve with the intraventricular septum and its distance from the aortic annular line in a long-axis view of the outflow tract are determined. This zone of SAM-septal contact is used as a guide to the best location for the myectomy. The surgeon must know the septal thickness in this region, to plan the extent of myectomy with the goal to resect all but approximately 1 cm of septal thickness at that location. It is also important to extend the myectomy beyond the zone of SAM-septal contact, especially in an apical direction. Measurement of the LV outflow tract velocity by continuous wave Doppler is also important during the prepump study, as a baseline for improvements that result from myectomy. k63

CONGENITAL HEART DISEASE

IOE is extremely useful in many types of congenital heart surgeries. Epicardial echocardiography has been traditionally used in a higher frequency of pediatric patients than adults, particularly in children smaller than appropriate for the available transesophageal probes (132,133). However, since the availability of the smaller pediatric TEE probes (133a,134), epicardial echocardiography has become much less common.

Ventilatory compromise is infrequent in small infants undergoing TEE examination and can be avoided by care-

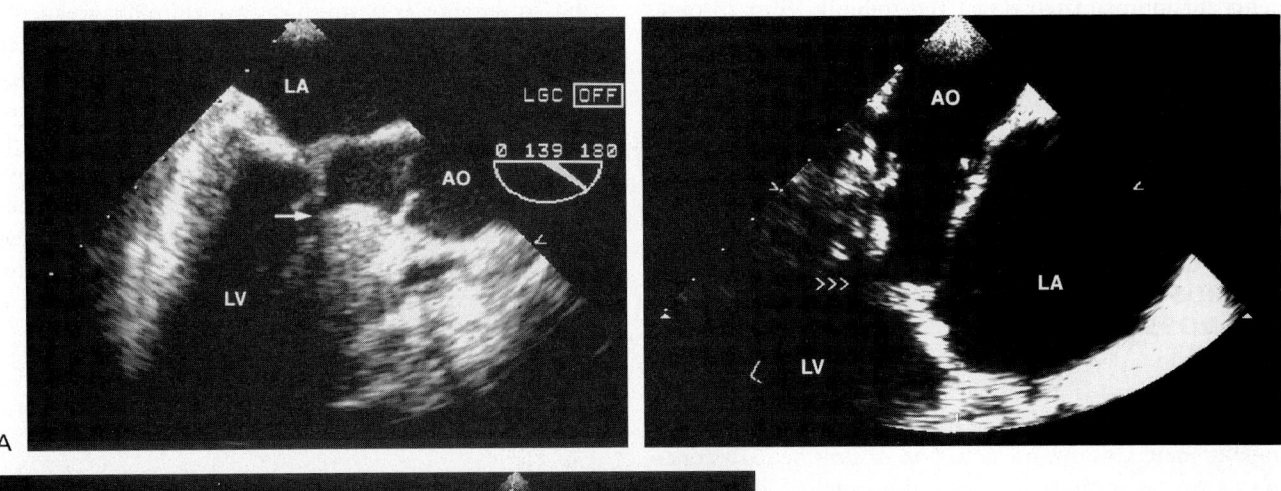

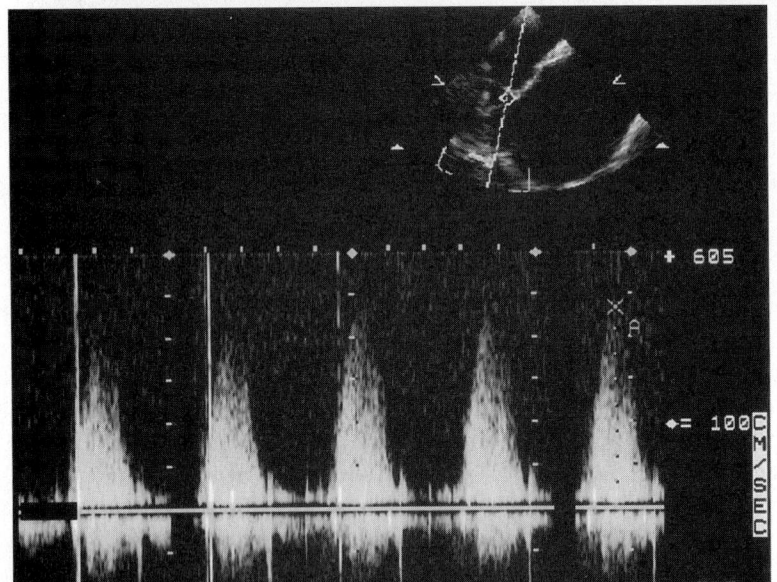

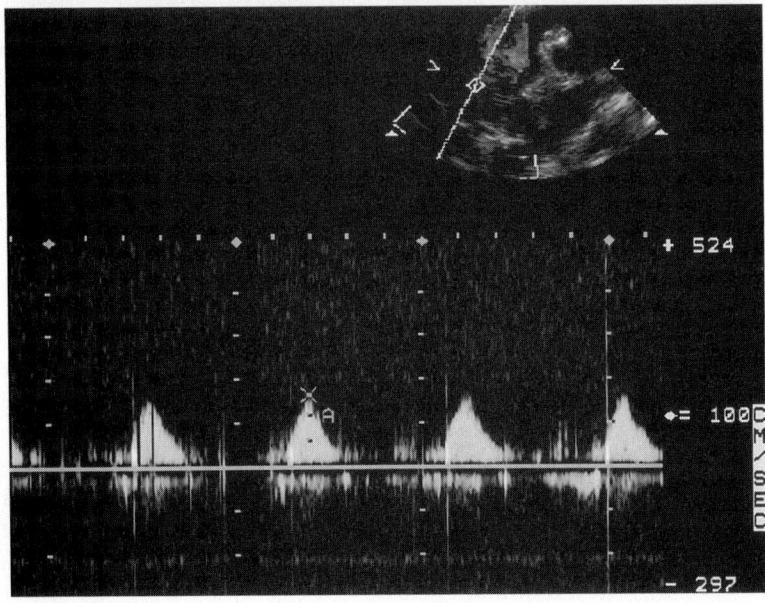

FIGURE 57.5 A patient with hypertrophic obstructive cardiomyopathy undergoing myectomy. **A:** A midesophageal image at a multiplane angle of 139 degrees showing the thick upper septum and the systolic anterior motion of the mitral valve touching the septum (*arrow*) causing dynamic outflow tract obstruction. See also the color flow images on a similar patient included on the CD-ROM and online versions of this chapter. **B:** An epicardial image taken from the aorta–superior vena cava transducer position, from which clean Doppler measurements of the outflow tract velocities can reliably be recorded. Arrowheads show the systolic anterior motion touching the septum. **C:** Prepump continuous wave Doppler recorded from an epicardial transducer, showing a 4.7 m per second maximum velocity (at the *X*, marked *A*), indicating a gradient of 88 mm Hg. **D:** Postpump continuous wave Doppler, showing a 1.7 per second maximum velocity (at the *X*, marked *A*), indicating an insignificant gradient of 12 mm Hg after myectomy. AO, aorta; LA, left atrium; LV, left ventricle.

ful ventilatory monitoring (134a). TEE is useful in this population to guide accurate placement of central venous catheters in congenital heart surgery patients (134b). However, esophagoscopy after intraoperative TEE shows minor traumatic abnormalities, particularly in patients weighing less than 9 kg, although no long-term feeding or swallowing difficulties were noted (134c).

Epicardial echocardiography may also be required in defining certain problems not easily visualized with TEE, such as abnormalities of the LV outflow tract (25) and right ventricular outflow tract (135), which are in the far field of TEE. Doubly committed subarterial VSD is particularly difficult to diagnose by TEE (136). For either epicardial echocardiography or TEE, a segmental approach to cardiac anatomy should be used, analyzing cardiac situs, atrioventricular connections, ventricular arterial connections, and expected anatomic variants. Using both color flow imaging and contrast imaging is more sensitive to detect shunts than is either one alone (137).

Postpump Imaging in Congenital Heart Disease

After congenital heart surgery, the postpump IOE provides an important safety net on the results of surgery. The most common problems found after congenital surgery are new or persistent valvular regurgitation or new or persistent obstruction of the right ventricular or LV outflow tract. The frequency of second pump runs at our institution is 5.7% (19a). In the largest series of 1,000 patients undergoing a wide spectrum of congenital heart surgery, Ungerleider et al. (143) reported that 44 patients (4.4%) underwent intraoperative revision of their repair during a second pump run based on echocardiographic findings, of which 39 had successful elimination of the problem.

In a study by Gussenhoven et al. (139), the postpump imaging information led to immediate further surgery during the same thoracotomy in 3% and to inotropic drug therapy in 2% of patients. In a cohort at the Mayo Clinic, postbypass biplane TEE led to immediate revision of the initial repair in 8.7% of cases (138). Sheil and Baines found moderate or severe residual defects in 11.0% of cases, with 5.3% of the total group returning to bypass for further surgery, with which most, 4.0% of the total group, achieved complete or adequate amelioration (140a). ❥ k64

DEFINING THE LOCATION AND SEVERITY OF AORTIC ATHEROMA

Of the complications that can occur after cardiac surgery, one of the most devastating is the phenomenon of atheroemboli. This can cause extensive microcapillary occlusion, with end-organ damage in the brain, liver, kidneys, spleen, and skin and is a common cause of perioperative death

(148). Diffuse atheroemboli produce the phenomenon of the "blue toe" syndrome (149). Despite that atherosclerotic lesions in the aorta are common in patients undergoing surgery for coronary or aortic atherosclerosis, observable events are surprisingly infrequent. Risk factors for clinical embolization include age, smoking, peripheral vascular disease, previous stroke, diabetes, and aortic knob calcification on chest radiographic films (151). Events are more common in patients who have larger atheromas of the thoracic aorta as defined by echocardiography (150)—as high as 15% in one series (151a).

Methods of Definition of Atheroma from Echocardiography

Echocardiography is one of the best ways of defining the location and presence of atheroma. The farther the atheroma protrudes into the lumen and the more mobile it is (*e*Fig. 57.5.2), the more likely that showers of atheroemboli will occur spontaneously (152) with a high risk of death (153). ❥ k65

It is clear that intraoperative aortic palpation is not sensitive to atheroma at risk for embolization (156). In fact, both manual palpation and TEE are inaccurate methods for detection of atheroma in the ascending aorta (156a). TEE is insensitive in the ascending aorta, probably because of far-field attenuation and because of the 2- to 4-cm blind spot anterior to the trachea (157). The ascending aorta is imaged best by epivascular echocardiography, using a high-frequency sector transducer or a linear array transducer (158,159). ❥ k66

MINIMALLY INVASIVE CARDIAC SURGERY

Surgical techniques have been developed in which certain cardiac surgical procedures can be performed through smaller incisions, avoiding a full midsternal thoracotomy (165,166) and avoiding some of the trauma of the traditional methods of cardiac surgery. These minimally invasive procedures have also been called less invasive operations, or sometimes "keyhole surgery." In some circumstances, there appear to be advantages, including fewer complications, less pain, less bleeding, less recovery time, and less in-hospital expense. However, numerous disadvantages occur, including the inability to directly visualize the anterior epicardial surface of the heart and the inability to lift the cardiac apex for needle evacuation of air. Another disadvantage is the additional cost of special equipment that enables the surgery or cardiopulmonary bypass to be accomplished with special methods.

Several varieties of minimally invasive procedures have been developed, including hemisternotomy, port access operations, videoscopic surgery, and off-pump coronary bypass. In our experience with approximately 1,700 hemisternotomy cases, most of which were single mitral or aortic valve procedures, less than 1% of surgeries begun using minimally invasive procedures have developed problems requiring conversion to a midsternal thoracotomy, using a larger incision. The bleeding rates, morbidity, length of stay, and hospital costs have all been lower than with use of a standard midsternal incision, and the reoperation rates are unchanged.

Purposes of Intraoperative Echocardiography in Minimally Invasive Surgery

In minimally invasive procedures, IOE is useful for determining ventricular filling, ventricular function, and the presence of intracardiac air. In addition, IOE is useful in delineating the exact cardiac pathology that requires surgery and excluding additional problems that the surgeon is otherwise unable to determine due to lack of exposure (167).

Intraoperative echocardiography can detect new wall motion abnormalities to define intraoperative myocardial ischemia, which is associated with reduced postoperative prognosis (167a). TEE has also been used in hemisternotomy cases to determine the precise location for "T'ing" off the sternotomy, rather than approximating the sternotomy site by physical examination and chest radiography (167b).

In port access procedures, TEE is useful for correct positioning of various devices, including the endopulmonary vent catheter, the coronary sinus retrograde cardioplegia catheter, the venous cannula, and the aortic balloon catheter (endoclamp) used for internal occlusion of the aorta. The latter is used to exclude the systemic circulation receiving pressurized cardiopulmonary flow without the trauma of external aortic cross-clamping, but the balloon must be monitored by TEE constantly during the procedure, as it can migrate up or down, affecting the endoaortic occlusion or even damaging the aortic valve (166a,167c). TEE is also used to visualize the coronary sinus for placement of the retrograde cardioplegia catheter, obviating the need for fluoroscopy (166b).

Coronary bypass surgery can be done off pump, which has been called *minimally invasive direct coronary bypass* or MIDCAB, which appears to be useful in some situations (167a). The distal coronary graft anastomosis is done using heart-stabilizing instruments. Proximal anastomoses are avoided if possible by the preferential use of *in situ* mammary arteries, sometimes with side branches or an additional venous jump graft off the mammary. However, to perform the distal anastomosis requires temporary occlusion of the coronary artery, which causes focal wall motion abnormalities as defined by TEE in two-thirds, most of which are transient. However, in approximately 10% of patients, the wall motion abnormality persists to the time of chest closure, in which case they are likely to be permanent, with higher levels of cardiac enzyme release, more ST-T changes on the electrocardiogram, and more clinical problems than patients in whom the wall motion abnormality resolves before chest closure (167f). Intraoperative contrast echocardiography has been used in off-pump CABG to assess flow and verify the patency of the coronary artery (167g), similar to the Allen's test. This can help to determine which graft to place first to cause the least ischemia.

Because they are done without aortic cross-clamping, both minimally invasive direct coronary bypass and port access techniques are excellent for management of patients with severe aortic atheroma, to avoid trauma to the ascending aorta and systemic embolization of debris. In a series of port access operations, the patient survival rate was 99%, the incidence of perioperative stroke was 1%, and the incidence of aortic dissection was 1% (19b), which are better statistics than historical controls in this population. ⚐ k67

TREATMENT OF SEVERE LEFT VENTRICULAR DYSFUNCTION

Several devices are useful for treatment of patients who are critically ill or in cardiogenic shock, including the ventricular assist device, the extracorporeal membrane oxygenator, and the intraaortic balloon pump. For patients who require these devices, echocardiography has a role in implantation, positioning, safety, and determination of the hemodynamic effects on the patient.

In patients with hypotension, mechanical causes including pericardial tamponade (176), occult valvular disease (177), and hypovolemia can be diagnosed by echocardiography. In patients with heart failure, echocardiography can also be influential in diagnosing the etiology. In cardiogenic shock patients, TEE can guide therapy and help adjust pharmacologic treatment. ⚐ k68

The temporary assist device is an external pump used in patients with severe left-sided heart failure to take over the mechanical function of the left side (LVAD) or the right side (right ventricular assist device) of the heart. A large cannula is placed into the left atrium to remove blood, oxygenate it, and pump it at systemic arterial pressure into an artery such as the ascending aorta or femoral artery (181). TEE can detect malfunction of the device (182,182a). It also may define resolution of transient cardiac abnormalities that may allow discontinuation of support (183), as well as complications such as intracardiac thrombi that can develop (184).

CORONARY ARTERY BYPASS SURGERY

Transesophageal Echocardiographic Anatomy Corresponding to Coronary Artery Distributions

It is important to understand the regional anatomy of each coronary artery bed with respect to the tomographic imaging planes available with TEE. Figure 57.6 shows a diagram of three midesophageal long-axis views and one transgastric short-axis view of the LV, coded for the distribution of each

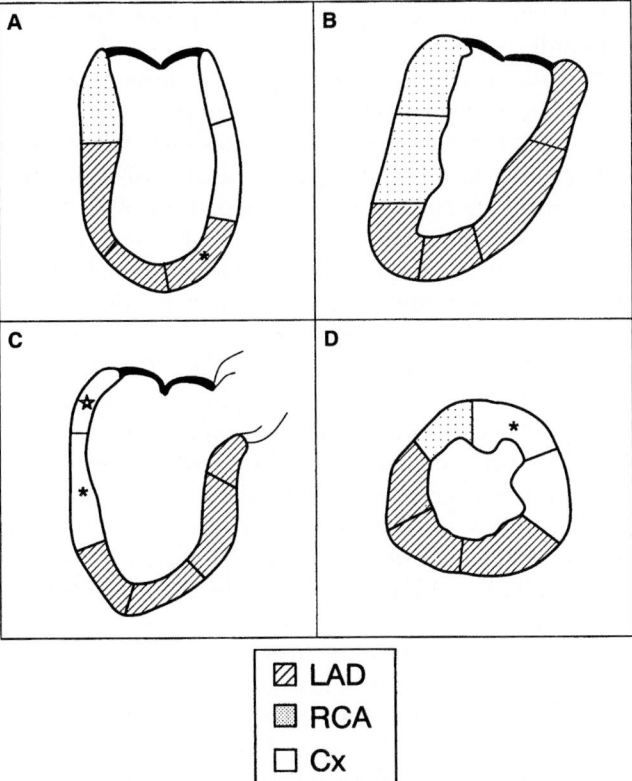

FIGURE 57.6 The four standard transesophageal echocardiographic monitoring views showing the distributions of the left anterior descending (*hatched*), right (*stippled*), and circumflex (*white*) artery territories. **A:** Basilar transverse (0 degrees) plane showing the septal (*left*) and lateral (*right*) walls from apex to base. **B:** Basilar 60-degree view showing the inferior (*left*) and anterior (*right*) walls. **C:** Basilar 120-degree plane showing the posterior (*left*) and anteroseptal (*right*) walls. **D:** Lower right transgastric short-axis view showing the midventricular segments of all six walls. The star and asterisks indicate segments that vary in their coronary artery supply depending on the dominance of the circulation.

coronary artery. These four views allow analysis of all 16 segments of the LV surface, composing the segmental model used by the American Society of Echocardiography. Obviously, the dominance of the right versus circumflex coronary artery supply determines which artery supplies the posterior segments of the heart. Other individual anatomic variations also affect, for example, whether the basilar posterior wall is perfused by the right or the circumflex coronary artery, whether the midseptum is perfused by the right or the left anterior descending artery, and whether the midlateral wall is perfused by the circumflex or the left anterior descending artery.

Methodology of Analysis of Left Ventricular Segmental Function

Similar to stress echocardiography, side-by-side simultaneous moving images in a gated loop format are best for qualitative assessment of subtle differences in segmental wall motion. It is useful to store standard cine loops in a digital format from

each of the four basic planes at baseline for later comparison. The methods of evaluating LV size, segmental function, and ischemia (see the section Decisions in Noncardiac Surgery Based on Intraoperative Echocardiography) for noncardiac surgery are equally applicable in coronary bypass patients.

IOE can also be useful in following improvement in LV systolic wall thickening after CABG. Wall thickening improves most in those segments with the abnormal preoperative function that had chronic ischemia or hibernation preoperatively (8,197). More immediate improvement is seen in severely abnormal, chronically underperfused segments than in mildly hypokinetic segments, presumably because of reversal of hibernation (198).

Before CABG, some have advocated evaluating segmental wall motion during an infusion in the operating room of 5 to 10 μg per kg per minute of dobutamine, to determine which walls would benefit the most from revascularization (193). Augmentation in response to low-dose dobutamine of a segment that has abnormal function at rest was predictive, in one published series, of sustained improvement of the segment after CABG (194).

DECISIONS IN NONCARDIAC SURGERY BASED ON INTRAOPERATIVE ECHOCARDIOGRAPHY

IOE is quite useful in patients undergoing noncardiac surgery. The purposes are to monitor development of myocardial ischemia, assess ventricular volume for fluid replacement, and define other cardiovascular abnormalities that affect hemodynamics and perioperative management. IOE is useful in a selected minority of noncardiac operations, particularly when the risk of problems is higher because of the type of surgery planned or the patient's underlying cardiac condition (211).

IOE is particularly useful in vascular surgery involving cross-clamping of the upper abdominal aorta (212) in which a sudden increase in afterload occurs, causing an increase in myocardial oxygen demand (213). During insertion of a cemented femoral hip prosthesis, there is a substantial incidence of new segmental wall motion abnormalities (214). TEE has also been used to determine the intraoperative occurrence of intrapulmonary shunting, presumably due to fat embolization, to help develop new cementing techniques during hip replacement (214b). Similarly, IOE benefits cases such as liver transplantation, in which a sudden or severe shift in intravascular volume status occurs. In operations done in the sitting position, intraoperative TEE can help detect venous air embolism (214a).

Detection of Myocardial Ischemia

Intraoperative TEE helps to determine the presence and severity of myocardial ischemia to facilitate pharmacologic treatment (215). In many circumstances, detection of segmental abnormalities due to ischemia is enabled by judicious use of simultaneous, side-by-side, gated cine loop displays, showing matched imaging planes before or after the onset or cessation of an abnormality. As a baseline at the beginning of each case, it is useful to store the standard LV views in a quad-screen format, including the transgastric short-axis view and midesophageal long-axis views at multiplane angles of 0, 60, and 120 degrees (Fig. 57.6). These are recalled for direct comparisons with later images at a time when ischemia or hypovolemia is clinically suspected or must be ruled out.

TEE detection of intraoperative myocardial ischemia has good concordance with, but is more sensitive than, electrocardiographic monitoring (215,216). Side-by-side cine loop comparisons are much more definitive than serial observation for qualitative diagnosis of new wall motion abnormalities and mild changes in blood volume (217). These may be quite subtle and difficult to see if viewed sequentially from tape playback. The detection of wall motion abnormalities has an intraobserver variation in only 5% of segments, whereas the interobserver variation is only 9% of segments (218).

However, one should be aware of the impact of plane orientation on apparent wall motion. Off-axis cuts can produce patterns that look similar to segmental wall motion abnormalities. In addition, false-negative assessments for ischemia are obtained if an inadequate number of imaging planes are assessed or side-by-side comparisons are not made with great care (219). One biplane TEE study found that 20% of segmental wall motion abnormalities were found by the transverse plane alone, 35% by the longitudinal plane alone, and 45% were detected in both planes (220).

In one study of patients at high risk of ischemia undergoing vascular surgery, alterations in ventricular wall motion were noted in almost 50% of patients, in whom 71% of the alterations were completely reversed by immediate and specific fluid and pharmacologic interventions without any evidence of permanent myocardial infarction (221). When acute segmental wall motion abnormalities persist to the conclusion of surgery, myocardial infarction is likely to have occurred (216) and postoperative intensive monitoring is mandatory.

CONTROVERSIES AND PERSONAL PERSPECTIVES

Anesthesiology versus Cardiology Qualifications: Who Should Do What in the Operating Room?

Various considerations are relevant to the question of who should perform IOE. Experience and training are more important than the specialty of the person doing the echocardiogram (237a).

Because the anesthesiologist is present during the entire case, he or she may naturally be the best person to do IOE for cardiac surgery, provided the individual has training and expertise in echocardiography. Because of their management role in surgery, the anesthesia team is also more likely than a cardiologist to use the TEE information to optimally manage the patient in surgery, especially when monitoring is the primary function. However, the anesthesiologist who is responsible for hemodynamic management is often busy doing just that, so it is best to have a second person do the echocardiography. The most crucial times to image the heart are also the times of most clinical instability, when the anesthesiologist needs to concentrate on patient management. Whether the second person who is doing TEE is from one specialty or the other, it is useful to have another experienced echocardiographer for backup when the TEE is primarily managed by the person who is also giving anesthesia.

In other respects, the cardiologist is the best person to do IOE, provided the geographic considerations make him or her available at the appropriate times. The people who are most current and skilled at performing diagnostic TEE studies, often the cardiologist who does them in the echocardiography laboratory, are likely to also provide the most reliable determinations for valvular problems, complex congenital heart disease, and other diagnostic determinations that are needed in surgery (238). However, most cardiologists are not consistently available for IOE, nor are they comfortable with the process or politics of the operating room. Many of the hemodynamic perturbations regarding cardiopulmonary bypass and anesthesia are unfamiliar to the cardiologist unless he or she has developed substantial experience in surgery.

In some cases, it works well for the surgeon to take the trouble to learn echocardiography and perform the IOE studies. The easiest method for many surgeons is to use epicardial echocardiography (28,239). This usually requires the presence of a separate person outside the sterile field, sometimes a sonographer, who operates the machine controls. One disadvantage of this is that the surgeon is therefore also the diagnostician and may be biased against finding fault with the procedure(s) he or she has just performed, in contrast to a separate person who can usually be more objective.

No matter what the specialty is from which a physician launches into IOE, the process requires education and experience in echocardiographic diagnosis and knowledge of ultrasound technology, image acquisition, interpretation, and clinical applications in the operating room environment (241,242). There is clearly a long learning curve (242a) to become an expert in echocardiography (243). Each of the potential contributors to the IOE team has a challenging learning curve, and who the

THE FUTURE

New technological and clinical developments are likely to be quickly applied to intraoperative diagnosis and treatment. Nowhere is successful clinical application of new techniques as likely to reap benefits in terms of quality, safety, and cost-effectiveness than in cardiac surgery. Innovations in cardiac surgery will undoubtedly continue to require the "safety net" of IOE. There is always a learning curve to a new practice and the potential for mistakes to occur. Therefore, IOE will probably be an important partner in future developments of new diagnostic and therapeutic techniques.

Three-Dimensional Echocardiography in the Operating Room

A technological innovation in cardiac ultrasound technology that is likely to achieve major steps in the near future is three-dimensional echocardiography (see Chapter 46). Three-dimensional echocardiography has already been studied preliminarily for its contribution to planning the surgical approach. With the capability to move the vantage point of viewing a three-dimensional data set to any angle or perspective, three-dimensional echocardiography has the potential to simulate surgical visualization of intracardiac anatomy and to dynamically represent intracardiac structure (248). This might be useful for planning surgery and evaluation of its probable results ahead of time by manipulating images to simulate various surgical options (e.g., determining the size and fit of implantable devices, valves, or other material). In addition to cardiac structure, the three-dimensional morphology of abnormal flow in the heart has also been studied (248c,248d).

Three-dimensional echocardiography may be particularly useful in certain types of surgeries. For valve surgery, it can provide new additional information not provided by two-dimensional echocardiography (248a). It is able to depict the shape, motion, and contour of the mitral annulus (62a,253). The size of prolapsing portions of the mitral valve correlate well between three-dimensional echocardiographic measurements and surgical findings (248b). For some types of congenital surgeries, it appears to add spatial comprehension (249,250). In congenital heart disease, three-dimensional echocardiography is particularly helpful in patients with VSDs (250a), especially doubly committed subarterial and restrictive VSDs and those associated with double inlet LV, as well as subaortic stenosis and supravalvar mitral membrane (251).

Three-dimensional echocardiography is also valuable in patients with cardiac tumors (252). It provides a better appreciation of the complex anatomy and aids in planning resection and deciding if curative surgery is feasible. The representations of cardiac anatomy are in some ways superior to standard intraoperative visualization in that they demonstrate the heart as a dynamic moving structure, as opposed to the empty, nonbeating heart the surgeon observes while the patient is on cardiopulmonary bypass (254).

Application to New Surgical Procedures

With the pace of developments in the field, it is likely that new cardiac surgery techniques will be developed. New practices have an inherent learning curve with the potential for mistakes to occur. Therefore, it is likely that IOE will be an important partner in future developments of new surgical techniques. For example, it is likely that IOE will contribute to the future development of procedures such as mitral homografts (255a), partial left ventriculectomy (255b), transmyocardial laser revascularization, complete correction of congenital heart disease, robotic and video-assisted thoracoscopic surgery (166a,167d), and autologous tissue valves (256), as well as numerous other emerging surgical innovations.

Intraoperative TEE is essential in video-assisted thoracoscopic surgery, which has already been successfully applied to surgical interruption of patent ductus arteriosus (167d) and mitral valve repair. In the latter, a computer-enhanced surgical telemanipulation system is used to robotically perform the surgery remotely from a surgical console; TEE found an inadequate repair in only one of ten patients, allowing further repair through an enlarged left thoracotomy (167e).

best person to do IOE is depends on the situation in each individual hospital.

Training and Credentialing for Intraoperative Echocardiography

Training for performance and interpretation of IOE has been the subject of some investigations and policy statements. The decisions required from intraoperative echocardiography make accuracy and reliability of diagnosis with this technique quite important. The educational goals for individuals desiring to develop competence in TEE in the operating room include a substantial amount of tutored learning and precepted performance of echocardiographic studies (241,241a). Participation in IOE without appropriate training appears to adversely affect the prevalence and detection of significant residual problems and the outcome of patients undergoing complex operations (243a). The Society of Cardiovascular Anesthesia and the American Society of Echocardiography have recognized the need for a policy that will likely lead to new recommendations for fellowship training programs in cardiovascular anesthesia. In addition, the accreditation of echocardiography laboratories and the availability of board certification in echocardiography may affect the requirements for performance of TEE and other advanced echocardiographic practice.

A major disparity between idealism and reality was pointed out in an interesting study of intraoperative TEE credentialing and performance (240). Based on a 1995 survey of practice patterns at 108 anesthesiology residency programs, of which 91% use intraoperative TEE, interpretations were rendered by anesthesiologists in 54% and by cardiologists in 46%. However, only 35% of anesthesiologists had formal echocardiography training in residency or fellowship, only 42% leave a formal interpretation on the chart, and only 43% bill specifically for performing TEE. Only 32% of programs reported that their institutions actually mandated formal credentials for performance of intraoperative TEE (240).

A decade ago, we instituted a training program in which a series of anesthesiology staff have each undertaken a 6-month fellowship for training in echocardiography, including a substantial time in the echocardiographic laboratory (242). Although this is not possible for most anesthesiologists who need to do IOE, an equivalent learning experience obtained on the job with available resources, such as a consulting cardiologist-echocardiographer, is necessary to achieve competence in this field (244).

It is important to maintain good records of IOE studies, including difficulties encountered with probe insertion (for medical-legal reasons) and a written chart report for *every* patient studied. An ongoing continuous quality improvement program should evaluate record keeping, accuracy, and quality of imaging, as judged by independent reviewers who should generate objective evidence of reviews performed (245,246).

Cost versus Efficacy

IOE involves finding the unexpected, monitoring for unanticipated problems, and imaging repeatedly to diagnose the change or lack of change expected from surgery. Despite the known frequencies of second pump runs in each type of surgery, it is not possible for the surgeon to predict the need for a revision based on his or her confidence in the repair. All of the patients who have had a second pump run were thought by the surgeon to have a good enough result to come off pump, but IOE revealed the need for operative revision.

When patients do return to the operating room later in their hospitalization for revision of a repair not fixed ini-

tially, the additional hospital costs are estimated to be much greater than for those whose repairs are revised during the initial thoracotomy ($94,000 vs. $21,000) (143). More important, many hidden costs arise in the patient whose initial surgery is unsuccessful, including additional hospitalizations for treatment of complications or reoperation.

Benson and Cahalan (247) performed a detailed cost-benefit analysis of IOE, being careful to keep estimates of direct and indirect costs liberal (high) and estimates of benefits conservative (low). They concluded that IOE results in a minimum savings of $600 per case for congenital heart surgery, $450 per case for valve repair surgery, and $150 per case for coronary bypass. Siwik et al. also looked at the cost-effectiveness of IOE in a series in which surgical therapy was altered by TEE findings in 3%, finding that the superior information reduced the need for additional postoperative studies in the intensive care setting (247a).

REFERENCES

1. Stewart WJ. Intraoperative echocardiography. In: Skorton D, ed. *Cardiac imaging—principles and practice.* Philadelphia: WB Saunders, 1996:566–581.
2. Griffin BP, Stewart WJ. Echocardiography in patient selection, operative planning, and intraoperative evaluation of mitral valve repair. In: Otto CM, ed. *The practice of clinical echocardiography.* Philadelphia: WB Saunders, 1997.
2a. Cahalan MK. *Intraoperative transesophageal echocardiography, an interactive text and atlas.* Philadelphia: Churchill Livingstone, 1996.
3. Johnson ML, Holmes JH, Spangler RD, et al. Usefulness of echocardiography in patients undergoing mitral valve surgery. *J Thorac Cardiovasc Surg* 1972;64:922–928.
4. Frazin L, Talano JV, Stephanides L. Esophageal echocardiography. *Circulation* 1975;54:102–104.
5. Hisanga K, Hisanaga A, Nagata K, et al. A new transesophageal real-time two-dimensional echocardiographic system using a flexible tube and its clinical application. *Proc Jpn Soc Ultrason Med* 1977;32:43–45.
6. Hanrath P, Kremer P, Langenstein BA. Transosophageale echokardiographie: ein neues verfahren zur dynamischen ventrikelfunktionsanalyse. *Dtsch Med Wochenschr* 1981;106:533.
7. Kremer P, Roizen MT, Gutman J, et al. Cardiac monitoring by transesophageal 2-D echocardiography during abdominal aortic aneurysmectomy. *Circulation* 1982;66:II-17(abst).
7a. Roizen MF, Beaupre PN, Alpert RA, et al. Monitoring with two dimensional transesophageal echocardiography. Comparison of myocardial function in patients undergoing supraceliac, suprarenal-infraceliac, or infrarenal aortic occlusion. *J Vasc Surg* 1984;1:300–305.
8. Topol EJ, Weiss JL, Guzman PA, et al. Immediate improvement of dysfunctional myocardial segments after coronary revascularization: detection by intraoperative transesophageal echocardiography. *J Am Coll Cardiol* 1984;4:1123–1134.

9. Goldman ME, Mindich BP, Teichholz LE, et al. Intraoperative contrast echocardiography to evaluate mitral valve operations. *J Am Coll Cardiol* 1984;4:1035–1040.

10. Takamoto S, Kyo S, Adachi H, et al. Intraoperative color flow mapping by real-time two-dimensional Doppler echocardiography for evaluation of valvular and congenital heart disease and vascular disease. *J Thorac Cardiovasc Surg* 1985;90:802–812.

11. Stewart WJ, Salcedo EE, Schiavone WA, et al. Intraoperative Doppler color flow mapping in valve conservation surgery. *Proc Tenth World Congress Cardiology* 1986:247(abst).

12. Maurer G, Czer LS, Chaux A. Intraoperative Doppler color flow mapping for assessment of valve repair for mitral regurgitation. *Am J Cardiol* 1987;60:333–338.

13. Stewart WJ, Currie PJ, Agler DA, et al. Intraoperative epicardial echocardiography: technique, imaging planes, and use in valve repair for mitral regurgitation. *Dynamic Cardiovasc Imaging* 1987;1:179–184.

14. DeBruijn NP, Clements FM, Kisslo JA. Intraoperative transesophageal color flow mapping: initial experience. *Anesth Analg* 1987;66:386–390.

15. Kyo S, Takamoto S, Matsumura M, et al. Immediate and early postoperative evaluation of results of cardiac surgery by transesophageal two-dimensional Doppler echocardiography. *Circulation* 1987;76:113–121.

16. Stewart WJ, Thomas JD, Klein AL, et al. Ten year trends in utilization of 6340 intraoperative echos. *Circulation* 1995;92:1–514(abst).

17. Omoto R, Kyo S, Matsumura M. Biplane color transesophageal Doppler echocardiography (color TEE): its advantages and limitations. *Int J Cardiac Imaging* 1989;4:57–59.

18. Roelandt JR, Thompson IR, Vletter WB. Multiplane transesophageal echocardiography: latest evolution in an imaging revolution. *J Am Soc Echocardiogr* 1992;5:361–369.

19. Stewart WJ, Currie PJ, Salcedo EE, et al. Evaluation of mitral leaflet motion by echocardiography and jet direction by Doppler color flow mapping to determine the mechanisms of mitral regurgitation. *J Am Coll Cardiol* 1992;20:1353–1361.

19a. Grimm RA, Stewart WJ. The role of intraoperative echocardiography in valve surgery. *Cardiol Clin* 1998;16:477–489.

19b. Reichenspurner H, Welz A, Gulielmos V, et al. Port-access cardiac surgery using endovascular cardiopulmonary bypass: theory, practice, and results. *J Cardiol Surg* 1998;13:275–280.

19c. Aronson S, Jacobsohn E, Savage R, et al. The influence of collateral flow on the antegrade and retrograde distribution of cardioplegia in patients with an occluded right coronary artery. *Anesthesiology* 1998;89:1099–1107.

20. Moisa RB, Zeldis SM, Alper SA, et al. Aortic regurgitation in coronary artery bypass grafting: implications for cardioplegia administration *Ann Thorac Surg* 1995;60:665–668.

21. Aldea GS, Connelly G, Fonger JD, et al. Directed atraumatic coronary sinus cannulation for retrograde cardioplegia administration. *Ann Thorac Surg* 1992;54:789–790.

22. Roth S, Aronson S. Placement of a right atrial air aspiration catheter guided by transesophageal echocardiography. *Anesthesiology* 1995;83:1359–1361.

23. Daniel WG, Erbel R, Kasper W, et al. Safety of transesophageal echocardiography. A multicenter survey of 10,419 examinations. *Circulation* 1991;83:817–821.

23a. Rousou JA, Tighe DA, Garb JL, et al. Risk of dysphagia after transesophageal echocardiography during cardiac operations. *Ann Thorac Surg* 2000;69:486–489.

24. Shintani H, Nakano S, Matsuda H, et al. Efficacy of transesophageal echocardiography as a perioperative monitor in patients undergoing cardiovascular surgery. Analysis of 149 consecutive studies. *J Cardiovasc Surg* 1990;31:564–570.

24a. Kallmeyer IJ, Collard CD, Fox JA, et al. The safety of intraoperative transesophageal echocardiography: a case series of 7200 cardiac surgical patients. *Anesth Analg* 2001;92:1126–1130.

25. Sreeram N, Sutherland GR, Bogers JJ, et al. Subaortic obstruction: intraoperative echocardiography as an adjunct to operation. *Ann Thorac Surg* 1990;50:579–585.

26. Stewart WJ, Schiavone WA, Salcedo EE, et al. Intraoperative Doppler echocardiography in hypertrophic cardiomyopathy: correlations with the obstructive gradient. *J Am Coll Cardiol* 1987;10:327–335.

27. Goldman ME, Fuster V, Guarino T, et al. Intraoperative echocardiography for the evaluation of valvular regurgitation: experience in 263 patients. *Circulation* 1986;74:1143–1149.

28. van Herwerden LA, Gussenhoven WJ, Roelandt J, et al. Intraoperative epicardial two-dimensional echocardiography. *Eur Heart J* 1986;7:386–395.

29. Seward JB, Khandheria BK, Freeman WK, et al. Multiplane transesophageal echocardiography: image orientation, examination technique, anatomic correlations, and clinical applications. *Mayo Clin Proc* 1993;68:523–551.

30. Cohen GI, Davison MB, Klein AL, et al. The frequency of acquisition and quality of images obtained by transesophageal echocardiography: a prospective study of 100 consecutive cases. *J Am Soc Echocardiogr* 1993;6:577–582.

30a. Shanewise JS, Cheung AT, Aronson S, et al. ASE/SCA guidelines for performing a comprehensive intraoperative multiplane transesophageal echocardiography examination: recommendations of the American Society of Echocardiography Council for Intraoperative Echocardiography and the Society of Cardiovascular Anesthesiologists Task Force for Certification in Perioperative Transesophageal Echocardiography. *J Am Soc Echocardiogr* 1999;12:884–900.

30b. Shanewise JS, Cheung AT, Aronson S, et al. ASE/SCA guidelines for performing a comprehensive intraoperative multiplane transesophageal echocardiography examination: recommendations of the American Society of Echocardiography Council for Intraoperative Echocardiography and the Society of Cardiovascular Anesthesiologists Task Force for Certification in Perioperative Transesophageal Echocardiography. *Anesth Analg* 1999;89:870–884.

31. Stewart WJ, Currie PJ, Salcedo EE, et al. Intraoperative Doppler color flow mapping for decision-making in valve repair for mitral regurgitation. Technique and results in 100 patients. *Circulation* 1990;81:556–566.

32. Klein AL, Stewart WJ, Cosgrove DM, et al. Intraoperative epicardial echocardiography: technique and imaging planes. *Echocardiography* 1990;7:241–251.

32a. Stewart W. Willie Sutton and the completeness and priorities of the ideal transesophageal echo exam. *Eur J Echocardiogr* 2001;3:1 (*in press*).

33. Bach DS, Deeb GM, Bolling SF. Accuracy of intraoperative transesophageal echocardiography for estimating the severity of functional mitral regurgitation. *Am J Cardiol* 1995;76:508–512.

34. Sheikh KH, Bengtson JR, Rankin JS, et al. Intraoperative transesophageal Doppler color flow imaging used to guide patient selection and operative treatment of ischemic mitral regurgitation. *Circulation* 1991;84:594–604.

35. Czer LS, Maurer G, Bolger AF, et al. Intraoperative evaluation of mitral regurgitation by Doppler color flow mapping. *Circulation* 1987;76:III-108–III-116.

35a. Lambert AS, Miller JP, Foster E, et al. The diagnostic validity of digitally captured intraoperative transesophageal echocardiography examinations compared with analog recordings: a pilot study. *J Am Soc Echocardiogr* 1999;12:974–980.

35b. Thys DM, Abel M, Bollen BA, et al. American Society of Anesthesiologists and the Society of Cardiovascular Anesthesiologists Task Force on Transesophageal Echocardiography. Practice guidelines for perioperative transesophageal echocardiography. *Anesthesiology* 1996;84:986.

35c. Chaliki HP, Click RL, Abel MD. Comparison of intraoperative transesophageal echocardiographic examinations with the operative findings: prospective review of 1918 cases. *J Am Soc Echocardiogr* 1999;12:237–240.

36. Sheikh KH, de Bruijn NP, Rankin JS, et al. The utility of transesophageal echocardiography and Doppler color flow imaging in patients undergoing cardiac valve surgery. *J Am Coll Cardiol* 1990;15:363–372.

36a. Michel-Cherqui M, Ceddaha A, Liu N, et al. Assessment of systematic use of intraoperative transesophageal echocardiography during cardiac surgery in adults: a prospective study of 203 patients. *J Cardiothorac Vasc Anesth* 2000;14:45–50.

36b. Brandt RR, Oh JK, Abel MD, et al. Role of emergency intraoperative transesophageal echocardiography. *J Am Soc Echocardiogr* 1998;11:972–977.

37. Ungerleider RM, Greeley WJ, Sheikh KH, et al. Routine use of intraoperative epicardial echocardiography and Doppler color flow imaging to guide and evaluate repair of congenital heart lesions. A prospective study. *J Thorac Cardiovasc Surg* 1990;100:297–309.

37a. Durongpisitkul K, Soongswang J, Sriyoschati S, et al. Utility of intraoperative transesophageal echocardiogram in congenital heart disease. *J Med Assoc Thai* 2000;83[Suppl 2]:S46–S53.

37b. Katz ES, Tsiamtsiouris T, Applebaum RM, et al. Surgical left atrial appendage ligation is frequently incomplete: a transesophageal echocardiographic study. *J Am Coll Cardiol* 2000;36:468–471.

38. Secknus MA, Klein AL, Smedira NG, et al. Does prepump intraoperative echocardiography change operative plans in mitral valve repair? *J Am Soc Echocardiogr* 1996;9:374.

38a. Click RL, Abel MD, Schaff HV. Intraoperative transesophageal echocardiography: 5-year prospective review of impact on surgical management. *Mayo Clin Proc* 2000;75:241–247.

38b. Couture P, Denault AY, McKenty S, et al. Impact of routine use of intraoperative transesophageal echocardiography during cardiac surgery. *Can J Anaesth* 2000;47:20–26.

38c. Mishra M, Chauhan R, Sharma KK, et al. Real-time intraoperative transesophageal echocardiography—how useful? Experience of 5,016 cases. *J Cardiothorac Vasc Anesth* 1998;12:625–632.

38d. Sakakibara Y, Matsuda K, Sato F, et al. Aortic dissection complicating cardiac surgery in a patient with calcified ascending aorta. *Jpn J Thorac Cardiovasc Surg* 1999;47:625–628.

38e. Morehead AJ, Firstenberg MS, Shiota T, et al. Intraoperative echocardiographic detection of regurgitant jets after valve replacement. *Ann Thorac Surg* 2000;69:135–139.

39. Akamatsu S, Terazawa E, Kagawa K, et al. Evaluation of intraoperative transesophageal echocardiography. *Jpn J Cardiol* 1991;26[Suppl]:103–108.

40. Reichert SL, Visser CA, Moulijn AC, et al. Intraoperative transesophageal color-coded Doppler echocardiography for evaluation of residual regurgitation after mitral valve repair. *J Thorac Cardiovasc Surg* 1990;100:756–761.

40a. Lee HR, Montenegro LM, Nicolson SC, et al. Usefulness of intraoperative transesophageal echocardiography in predicting the degree of mitral regurgitation secondary to atrioventricular defect in children. *Am J Cardiol* 1999;83:750–753.

41. Isada LR, Stewart WJ, Torelli J, et al. Morbidity and mortality is not affected by a second pump run for initially unsuccessful mitral valve repair. *J Am Soc Echocardiogr* 1992;5:318(abst).

42. Duran CM, Gometza B, Balasundaram S, et al. A feasibility study of valve repair in rheumatic mitral regurgitation. *Eur Heart J* 1991;12:34–38.

43. Leung JM, O'Kelly B, Browner WS, et al. Prognostic importance of postbypass regional wall-motion abnormalities in patients undergoing coronary artery bypass graft surgery. SPI Research Group. *Anesthesiology* 1989;71:16–25.

44. Fix J, Isada L, Cosgrove D, et al. Do patients with less than "echo-perfect" results from mitral valve repair by intraoperative echocardiography have a different outcome? *Circulation* 1993;88:II-39–II-48.

45. Stewart WJ, Secknus MA, Thomas JD, et al. Intraoperative echocardiography in the Ross procedure. *J Am Coll Cardiol* 1996;27:190A(abst).

45a. Gillinov AM, Cosgrove DM, Blackstone EH, et al. Durability of mitral valve repair for degenerative disease. *J Thorac Cardiovasc Surg* 1998;116:734–743.

45b. Shah PM, Raney AA, Duran CM, et al. Multiplane transesophageal echocardiography: a roadmap for mitral valve repair. *J Heart Valve Dis* 1999;8:625–629.

45c. Grewal KS, Malkowski MJ, Kramer CM, et al. Multiplane transesophageal echocardiographic identification of the involved scallop in patients with flail mitral valve leaflet: intraoperative correlation. *J Am Soc Echocardiogr* 1998;11:966–971.

45d. Casselman FP, Gillinov AM, Akhrass R, et al. Durability of repair of bicuspid aortic valve with leaflet prolapse. *Eur J Cardiothorac Surg* 1999;15:302–308.

46. Sadoshima J, Koyanagi S, Sugimachi M, et al. Evaluation of the severity of mitral regurgitation by transesophageal Doppler flow echocardiography. *Am Heart J* 1992;123:1245–1251.

47. Yoshida K, Yoshikawa J, Yamaura Y, et al. Assessment of mitral regurgitation by biplane transesophageal color Doppler flow mapping. *Circulation* 1990;82:1121–1126.

48. Tribouilloy C, Shen WF, Quere JP, et al. Assessment of severity of mitral regurgitation by measuring regurgitant jet width at its origin with transesophageal Doppler color flow imaging. *Circulation* 1992;85:1248–1253.

49. Klein AL, Stewart WJ, Bartlett J, et al. Effects of mitral regurgitation on pulmonary venous flow and left atrial pressure: an intraoperative transesophageal echocardiographic study. *J Am Coll Cardiol* 1992;20:1345–1352.

50. Pu M, Vandervoort PM, Griffin BP, et al. Quantification of mitral regurgitation by the proximal convergence method using transesophageal echocardiography. Clinical validation of a geometric correction for proximal flow constraint. *Circulation* 1995;92:2169–2177.

51. Kleinman JP, Czer LS, DeRobertis M, et al. A quantitative comparison of transesophageal and epicardial color Doppler echocardiography in the intraoperative assessment of mitral regurgitation. *Am J Cardiol* 1989;64:1168–1172.

51a. Grewal KS, Malkowski MJ, Piracha AR, et al. Effect of general anesthesia on the severity of mitral regurgitation by transesophageal echocardiography. *Am J Cardiol* 2000;85:199–203.

52. Carpentier A, Chauvaud S, Fabiani JN, et al. Reconstructive surgery of mitral valve incompetence: ten-year appraisal. *J Thorac Cardiovasc Surg* 1980;79:338–348.

53. Sun JP, Yang XS, Mayer EL, et al. Mitral valvular leaflet excursion by echo is a marker for the feasibility of repair and risk of failed repair. *Circulation* 1995;92:I-464(abst).

54. Cosgrove DM, Stewart WJ. Mitral valvuloplasty. *Curr Probl Cardiol* 1989;14:359–415.

55. Stewart WJ. Choosing the "golden moment" for operation in the era of valve repair for mitral regurgitation. *Learning Center Highlights* 1995;Summer:2–7.

56. Zussa C, Polesel T. Seven year experience with chordal replacement with expanded polytetrafluoroethylene in floppy mitral valve. *J Thorac Cardiovasc Surg* 1994;108:37–41.

56a. Cho L, Gillinov AM, Cosgrove DM, et al. Echocardiographic assessment of the mechanisms of correction of bileaflet prolapse causing mitral regurgitation with only posterior leaflet repair surgery. *Am J Cardiol* 2000;86:1349–1351.

57. Wilkins GT, Weyman AE, Abascal VM, et al. Percutaneous balloon dilation of the mitral valve: an analysis of echocardiographic variables related to outcome and the mechanism of dilatation. *Br Heart J* 1988;60:299–308.

58. Marwick TH, Torelli J, Obarski T, et al. Assessment of the mitral valve splitability score by transthoracic and transesophageal echocardiography. *Am J Cardiol* 1991;68:1106–1107.

59. Duran CM, Gometza B, Saad E. Valve repair in rheumatic mitral disease: an unsolved problem [review]. *J Cardiac Surg* 1994;9:282–285.

60. Duran CM, Gometza B, De Vol EB. Valve repair in rheumatic mitral disease. *Circulation* 1991;84:III-125–III-132.

60a. Longo M, Previti A, Morello M, et al. Usefulness of transesophageal echocardiography during open heart surgery of mitral stenosis. *J Cardiovasc Surg (Torino)* 2000;41:381–385.

61. Stewart WJ, Sun JP, Mayer E, et al. Mitral regurgitation with normal leaflets results from apical displacement of coaptation, not annular dilation. *Circulation* 1994;90:I-311(abst).

62. Rankin JS, Livesey SA, Smith LR, et al. Trends in the surgical treatment of ischemic mitral regurgitation: effects of mitral valve repair on hospital mortality [review]. *Semin Thorac Cardiovasc Surg* 1989;1:149–163.

62a. Kaplan SR, Bashein G, Sheehan FH, et al. Three-dimensional echocardiographic assessment of annular shape changes in the normal and regurgitant mitral valve. *Am Heart J* 2000;139:378–387.

62b. Suzuki K, Tatsuno K, Kikuchi T, et al. Predisposing factors of valve regurgitation in complete atrioventricular septal defect. *J Am Coll Cardiol* 1998;32:1449–1453.

63. Mihaileanu S, el AB, Acar C, et al. Intra-operative transoesophageal echocardiography after mitral repair—specific conditions and pitfalls. *Eur Heart J* 1991;12[Suppl]:26–29.

64. Freeman WK, Schaff HV, Khandheria BK, et al. Intraoperative evaluation of mitral valve regurgitation and repair by transesophageal echocardiography: incidence and significance of systolic anterior motion. *J Am Coll Cardiol* 1992;20:599–609.

64a. Muratori M, Berti M, Doria E, et al. Transesophageal echocardiography as predictor of mitral valve repair. *J Heart Valve Dis* 2001;10:65–71.

65. Stewart WJ, Salcedo EE, Cosgrove DM. The value of echocardiography in mitral valve repair. *Cleve Clin J Med* 1991;58:177–183.

66. Krenz HK, Mindich BP, Guarino T, et al. Sudden development of intraoperative left ventricular outflow obstruction: differential and mechanism. An intraoperative two-dimensional echocardiographic study. *J Cardiac Surg* 1990;5:93–101.

67. Lee KS, Stewart WJ, Lever HM, et al. Mechanism of outflow tract obstruction causing failed mitral valve repair. Anterior displacement of leaflet coaptation. *Circulation* 1993;88:II-24–II-29.

68. Webster PJ, Raper RF, Ross DE, et al. Pharmacologic abolition of severe mitral regurgitation associated with dynamic left ventricular outflow tract obstruction after mitral valve repair: confirmation by transesophageal echocardiography. *Am Heart J* 1993;126:480–483.

69. van Herwerden L, Fraser AG, Bos E. Left ventricular outflow tract obstruction after mitral valve repair assessed with intraoperative echocardiography: noninterventional treatment [letter]. *J Thorac Cardiovasc Surg* 1991;102:461–463.

70. Carpentier A. The sliding leaflet technique. *Le Club Mitrale Newsletter* 1988(August).

71. Jebara VA, Mihaileanu S, Acar C, et al. Left ventricular outflow tract obstruction after mitral valve repair. Results of the sliding leaflet technique. *Circulation* 1993;88:II-30–II-34.

72. Perier P, Hagen T, Stumpf J. Septal myectomy for left ventricular outflow tract obstruction after mitral valve repair. *Ann Thorac Surg* 1994;57:1328–1330.

73. Duran CM. Tricuspid valve surgery revisited. *J Cardiac Surg* 1994;9:242–247.

74. Prabhakar G, Kumar N, Gometza B, et al. Surgery for organic rheumatic disease of the tricuspid valve. *J Heart Valve Dis* 1993;2:561–566.

75. Tanaka M, Abe T, Hibi N. Intraoperative epicardial two-dimensional and pulsed Doppler echocardiography for assessing functional tricuspid regurgitation. *J Cardiol* 1990;20:349–358.

76. Czer LS, Maurer G, Bolger A, et al. Tricuspid valve repair. Operative and follow-up evaluation by Doppler color flow mapping. *J Thorac Cardiovasc Surg* 1989;98:101–110.

77. Popov LV, Solo'vev GM, Ivanov SP. Intraoperative echocardiography. *Sovetskaia Meditsina* 1989;1989:19–24.

78. Tanaka M, Abe T, Takashina Y, et al. Evaluation of secondary tricuspid regurgitation by intraoperative epicardial pulsed Doppler echocardiography. *Jpn J Cardiol* 1988;18:1083–1095.

79. Klein AL, Azzam SJ, Stewart WJ. Does intraoperative echocardiography prevent the development of tricuspid regurgitation during longterm follow-up for tricuspid valve repair surgery? *J Am Coll Cardiol* 1993;21:320A(abst).

80. Johnston SR, Freeman WK, Schaff HV, et al. Severe tricuspid regurgitation after mitral valve repair: diagnosis by intraoperative transesophageal echocardiography. *J Am Soc Echocardiogr* 1990;3:416–419.

80a. Bajzer CT, Stewart WJ, Cosgrove DM, et al. Tricuspid valve surgery and intraoperative echocardiography: factors affecting survival, clinical outcome, and echocardiographic success. *J Am Coll Cardiol* 1998;32:1023–1031.

81. McKay R, Ross DN. Primary repair and autotransplantation of cardiac valves. *Annu Rev Med* 1993;44:181–188.

82. Cook JW. Accurate adjustment of de Vega tricuspid annuloplasty using transesophageal echocardiography. *Ann Thorac Surg* 1994;58:570–572.

83. De Simone R, Lange R, Tanzeem A, et al. Adjustable De Vega tricuspid valve annuloplasty guided by transesophageal echocardiography. *Ann Thorac Surg* 1995;59:1272.

84. Melo JQ, Abecasis M, Neves J, et al. Atrioventricular valve repair using externally adjustable flexible rings. *J Thorac Cardiovasc Surg* 1995;110:1333–1336.

85. Cosgrove DM, Rosenkranz ER, Hendren WG, et al. Valvuloplasty for aortic insufficiency. *J Thorac Cardiovasc Surg* 1991;102:571–576.

86. Maurer I, Regensburger D, Bernhard A. Aortic valve reconstruction in Rubinstein-Taybi-syndrome: the valuable aid of transesophageal echocardiography. *J Cardiovasc Surg* 1991;32:327–329.

87. Pretre R, Faidutti B, Lerch R. Intraoperative TEE in aortic valve repair [Letter]. *Am Heart J* 1993;125:1822–1823.

88. Stewart WJ, Currie PJ, Salcedo EE, et al. Intraoperative echo in aortic valve repair. *Circulation* 1988;78:II-435(abst).

89. Currie PJ, Stewart WJ. Intraoperative echocardiography for surgical repair of the aortic valve and left ventricular outflow tract. *Echocardiography* 1990;7:273–288.

90. Rafferty T, Durkin MA, Sittig D, et al. Transesophageal color flow Doppler imaging for aortic insufficiency in patients having cardiac operations. *J Thorac Cardiovasc Surg* 1992;104:521–525.

91. Sutton DC, Kluger R, Ahmed SU, et al. Flow reversal in the descending aorta: a guide to intraoperative assessment of aortic regurgitation with transesophageal echocardiography. *J Thorac Cardiovasc Surg* 1994;108:576–582.

91a. Willett DL, Hall SA, Jessen ME, et al. Assessment of aortic regurgitation by transesophageal color Doppler imaging of the vena contracta: validation against an intraoperative aortic flow probe. *J Am Coll Cardiol* 2001;37:1450–1455.

92. Tee SD, Shiota T, Weintraub R, et al. Evaluation of ventricular septal defect by transesophageal echocardiography: intraoperative assessment. *Am Heart J* 1994;127:585–592.

93. Tatsuno K, Konno S, Ando M, et al. Pathogenic mechanisms of prolapsing aortic valve and aortic regurgitation associated with ventricular septal defect. *Circulation* 1973;48:1028–1037.

94. Cohen GI, Duffy CI, Klein AL, et al. Color Doppler determination of the mechanism of aortic regurgitation with surgical correlation. *J Am Soc Echocard* 1996;9:508–515.

95. Fraser C Jr, Wang N, Mee RB, et al. Repair of insufficient bicuspid aortic valves. *Ann Thorac Surg* 1994;58:386–390.

96. David TE. Aortic valve repair in patients with Marfan syndrome and ascending aorta aneurysms due to degenerative disease. *J Cardiac Surg* 1994;9:182–187.

97. David TE, Feindel CM, Bos J. Repair of the aortic valve in patients with aortic insufficiency and aortic root aneurysm. *J Thorac Cardiovasc Surg* 1995;109:345–351.

97a. Keane MG, Wiegers SE, Yang E, et al. Structural determinants of aortic regurgitation in type A dissection and the role of valvular resuspension as determined by intraoperative transesophageal echocardiography. *Am J Cardiol* 2000;85:604–610.

98. Duran CM, Gometza B, al-Halees Z. Non-prosthetic aortic valve surgery. *J Heart Valve Dis* 1994;3:439–444.

99. Baeza OR, Majid NK, Conroy DP, et al. Combined conventional mechanical and ultrasonic debridement for aortic valvular stenosis. *Ann Thorac Surg* 1992;54:62–67.

100. Duran C, Kumar N, Gometza B, et al. Indications and limitations of aortic valve reconstruction. *Ann Thorac Surg* 1991;52:447–453.

101. Duran CM, Gometza B. Aortic valve reconstruction in the young. *J Cardiac Surg* 1994;9:204–208.

102. Pretre R, Faidutti B, Lerch R. Intraoperative TEE in aortic valve repair. *Am Heart J* 1993;125:1822–1823.

103. Wang N, Stewart WJ, Rosenkranz ER, et al. Does intraoperative Doppler echocardiography reliably predict the durability of a repaired aortic valve? The American Heart Association, 67th Scientific Session, November 14–17, 1994, Dallas, Texas.

104. Deutsch HJ, Curtius JM, Leischik R, et al. Diagnostic value of transesophageal echocardiography in cardiac surgery. *Thorac Cardiovasc Surg* 1991;39:199–204.

105. Daniel WG, Mugge A, Grote J, et al. Comparison of transthoracic and transesophageal echocardiography for detection of abnormalities of prosthetic and bioprosthetic valves in the mitral and aortic positions. *Am J Cardiol* 1993;71:210–215.

106. Karalis DG, Chandrasekaran K, Ross JJ, et al. Single-plane transesophageal echocardiography for assessing

function of mechanical or bioprosthetic valves in the aortic valve position. *Am J Cardiol* 1992;69:1310–1315.

107. Bartzokis T, St GF, DiBiase A, et al. Freehand allograft aortic valve replacement and aortic root replacement. Utility of intraoperative echocardiography and Doppler color flow mapping. *J Thorac Cardiovasc Surg* 1991;101:545–553.

108. Petrou M, Wong K, Albertucci M, et al. Evaluation of unstented aortic homografts for the treatment of prosthetic aortic valve endocarditis. *Circulation* 1994;90:II-198–II-204.

108a. Doty JR, Salazar JD, Liddicoat JR, et al. Aortic valve replacement with cryopreserved aortic allograft: ten-year experience. *J Thorac Cardiovasc Surg* 1998;115:371–379.

108b. Pettersson G, Tingleff J, Joyce FS. Treatment of aortic valve endocarditis with the Ross operation. *Eur J Cardiothorac Surg* 1998;13:678–684.

108c. Bach DS. Echocardiographic assessment of stentless aortic bioprosthetic valves. *J Am Soc Echocardiogr* 2000;13:941–948.

109. O'Brien MF. Composite stentless xenograft for aortic valve replacement: clinical evaluation of function. *Ann Thorac Surg* 1995;60:S406–S409.

109a. Guarracino F, Zussa C, Polesel E, et al. Influence of transesophageal echocardiography on intraoperative decision making for Toronto stentless prosthetic valve implantation. *J Heart Valve Dis* 2001;10:31–34.

109b. Bach DS, LeMire MS, Eberhart D, et al. Impact of intraoperative post-pump aortic regurgitation with stentless aortic bioprostheses. *Semin Thorac Cardiovasc Surg* 1999;11[Suppl 1]:88–92.

110. Bolger AF, Bartzokis T, Miller DC. Intraoperative echocardiography and Doppler color flow mapping in freehand allograft aortic valve and root replacement. *Echocardiography* 1990;7:229–240.

110a. Fan CM, Liu X, Panidis JP, et al. Prediction of homograft aortic valve size by transthoracic and transesophageal two-dimensional echocardiography. *Echocardiography* 1997;14:345–348.

111. Kunzelman KS, Grande KJ, David TE, et al. Aortic root and valve relationships. Impact on surgical repair. *J Thorac Cardiovasc Surg* 1994;107:162–170.

112. Stewart WJ, Gillam L, Morehead AJ, et al. Impact of intraoperative echocardiography on homograft aortic valve surgery. *J Am Coll Cardiol* 1993;21:17A(abst).

113. al-Halees Z, Kumar N, Gallo R, et al. Pulmonary autograft for aortic valve replacement in rheumatic disease: a caveat. *Ann Thorac Surg* 1995;60:351.

114. Reddy VM, Rajasinghe HA, Teitel DF, et al. Aortoventriculoplasty with the pulmonary autograft: the "Ross-Konno" procedure. *J Thorac Cardiovasc Surg* 1996;111:158–165.

115. Rubay JE, Raphael D, Sluysmans T, et al. Aortic valve replacement with allograft/autograft: subcoronary versus intraluminal cylinder or root. *Ann Thorac Surg* 1995;60:S78–S82.

115a. Luciani GB, Casali G, Mazzucco A. Risk factors for coronary complications after stentless aortic root replacement. *Semin Thorac Cardiovasc Surg* 1999;11[Suppl 1]:126–132.

116. Erbel R, Oelert H, Meyer J, et al. Effect of medical and surgical therapy on aortic dissection evaluated by transesophageal echocardiography. Implications for prognosis and therapy. The European Cooperative Study Group on Echocardiography. *Circulation* 1993;87:1604–1615.

116a. Abe S, Ono S, Murata K, et al. Usefulness of transesophageal echocardiographic monitoring in transluminal endovascular stent-graft repair for thoracic aortic aneurysm. *Jpn Circ J* 2000;64:960–964.

116b. Orihashi K, Matsuura Y, Sueda T, et al. Echocardiography-assisted surgery in transaortic endovascular stent grafting: role of transesophageal echocardiography. *J Thorac Cardiovasc Surg* 2000;120:672–678.

117. Schippers OA, Gussenhoven WJ, van HL, et al. The role of intraoperative two-dimensional echocardiography in the assessment of thoracic aorta pathology. *Thorac Cardiovasc Surg* 1988;36:208–213.

118. San Roman JA, Vilacosta I, Castillo JA, et al. Role of transesophageal echocardiography in the assessment of patients with composite aortic grafts for therapy in acute aortic dissection. *Am J Cardiol* 1994;73:519–521.

119. Goldman ME, Guarino T, Mindich BP. Localization of aortic dissection intimal flap by intraoperative two-dimensional echocardiography. *J Am Coll Cardiol* 1985;6:1155–1159.

120. Simon P, Owen AN, Havel M, et al. Transesophageal echocardiography in the emergency surgical management of patients with aortic dissection. *J Thorac Cardiovasc Surg* 1992;103:1113–1117.

120a. Movsowitz HD, Levine RA, Hilgenberg AD, et al. Transesophageal echocardiographic description of the mechanisms of aortic regurgitation in acute type A aortic dissection: implications for aortic valve repair. *J Am Coll Cardiol* 2000;36:884–890.

121. Kusuhara K, Shiraishi S, Iwakura A. A new staged operation for extensive aortic aneurysm by means of the modified "elephant trunk" technique. *J Thorac Cardiovasc Surg* 1995;110:267–269.

122. Suto Y, Yasuda K, Shiiya N, et al. Stented elephant trunk procedure for an extensive aneurysm involving distal aortic arch and descending aorta. *J Thorac Cardiovasc Surg* 1996;112:1389–1390.

123. Daniel WG. Improvement in the diagnosis of abscesses associated with endocarditis by transesophageal echocardiography. *N Engl J Med* 1991;324:795–800.

124. Gonzales-Lavin L. The importance of the "jet lesion" in bacterial endocarditis involving the left heart: surgical considerations. *J Thorac Cardiovasc Surg* 1970;59:185–192.

125. Hendron W, Morris AS, Rosenkranz ER, et al. Mitral valve repair for bacterial endocarditis. *J Thorac Cardiovasc Surg* 1992;103:124–128.

126. Glazier JJ. Treatment of complicated prosthetic aortic valve endocarditis with annular abscess formation by homograft aortic root replacement. *J Am Coll Cardiol* 1991;17:1177–1182.

126a. Zlotnick AY, Lennon PF, Goldhaber SZ, et al. Intraoperative detection of pulmonary thromboemboli with epicardial echocardiography. *Chest* 1999;115:1749–1751.

127. Ross D. Allograft root replacement for prosthetic endocarditis. *J Cardiac Surg* 1990;5:5–11.

127a. Sun JP, Asher CR, Yang XS, et al. Clinical and echocardiographic characteristics of papillary fibroelastomas: a retrospective and prospective study in 162 patients. *Circulation* 2001;103:2687–2693.

127b. Dujardin KS, Click RL, Oh JK. The role of intraoperative transesophageal echocardiography in patients undergoing cardiac mass removal. *J Am Soc Echocardiogr* 2000;13:1080–1083.

127c. Sigman DB, Hasnain JU, Del Pizzo JJ, et al. Real-time transesophageal echocardiography for intraoperative surveillance of patients with renal cell carcinoma and vena caval extension undergoing radical nephrectomy. *J Urol* 1999;161:36–38.

127d. Sun JP, Asher CR, Xu Y, et al. Inferior vena caval masses identified by echocardiography. *Am J Cardiol* 1999;84:613–615.

128. Grigg LE, Wigle ED, Williams WG, et al. Transesophageal Doppler echocardiography in obstructive hypertrophic cardiomyopathy: clarification of pathophysiology and importance in intraoperative decision making. *J Am Coll Cardiol* 1992;20:42–52.

129. Marwick TH, Stewart WJ, Lever HM, et al. Benefits of intraoperative echocardiography in the surgical management of hypertrophic cardiomyopathy. *J Am Coll Cardiol* 1992;20:1066–1072.

130. Yock PG, Hatle L, Popp RL. Patterns and timing of Doppler-detected intracavitary and aortic flow in hypertrophic cardiomyopathy. *J Am Coll Cardiol* 1986;8:1047–1058.

131. Zhu WX, Oh JK, Kopecky SL, et al. Mitral regurgitation due to ruptured chordae tendineae in patients with hypertrophic obstructive cardiomyopathy. *J Am Coll Cardiol* 1992;20:242–247.

131a. Yu EH, Omran AS, Wigle ED, et al. Mitral regurgitation in hypertrophic obstructive cardiomyopathy: relationship to obstruction and relief with myectomy. *J Am Coll Cardiol* 2000;36:2219–2225.

132. Stevenson JG, Sorensen GK. Proper probe size for pediatric transesophageal echocardiography. *Am J Cardiol* 1993;72:491–492.

133. Lunn RJ, Oliver WJ, Hagler DJ, et al. Aortic compression by transesophageal echocardiographic probe in infants and children undergoing cardiac surgery. *Anesthesiology* 1992;77:587–590.

133a. Shiota T, Lewandowski R, Piel JE, et al. Micromultiplane transesophageal echocardiographic probe for intraoperative study of congenital heart disease repair in neonates, infants, children, and adults. *Am J Cardiol* 1999;83:292–295.

134. Shah PM, Stewart SD, Calalang CC, et al. Transesophageal echocardiography and the intraoperative management of pediatric congenital heart disease: initial experience with a pediatric esophageal 2D color flow echocardiographic probe. *J Cardiothorac Vasc Anesth* 1992;6:8–14.

134a. Andropoulos DB, Ayres NA, Stayer SA, et al. The effect of transesophageal echocardiography on ventilation in small infants undergoing cardiac surgery. *Anesth Analg* 2000;90:47–49.

134b. Andropoulos DB, Stayer SA, Bent ST, et al. A controlled study of transesophageal echocardiography to guide central venous catheter placement in congenital heart surgery patients. *Anesth Analg* 1999;89:65–70.

134c. Greene MA, Alexander JA, Knauf DG, et al. Endoscopic evaluation of the esophagus in infants and children immediately following intraoperative use of transesophageal echocardiography. *Chest* 1999;116:1247–1250.

135. Muhiudeen IA, Roberson DA, Silverman NH, et al. Intraoperative echocardiography for evaluation of congenital heart defects in infants and children. *Anesthesiology* 1992;76:165–172.

136. Muhiudeen IA, Roberson DA, Silverman NH, et al. Intraoperative echocardiography in infants and children with congenital cardiac shunt lesions: transesophageal versus epicardial echocardiography. *J Am Coll Cardiol* 1990;16:1687–1695.

137. Hagler DJ, Tajik AJ, Seward JB, et al. Intraoperative two-dimensional Doppler echocardiography. A preliminary study for congenital heart disease. *J Thorac Cardiovasc Surg* 1988;95:516–522.

138. O'Leary PW, Hagler DJ, Seward JB, et al. Biplane intraoperative transesophageal echocardiography in congenital heart disease. *Mayo Clin Proc* 1995;70:317–326.

139. Gussenhoven EJ, van HL, Roelandt J, et al. Intraoperative two-dimensional echocardiography in congenital heart disease. *J Am Coll Cardiol* 1987;9:565–572.

140. Stumper O, Sutherland GR, Sreeram N, et al. Role of intraoperative ultrasound examination in patients undergoing a Fontan-type procedure. *Br Heart J* 1991;65:204–210.

140a. Sheil ML, Baines DB. Intraoperative transoesophageal echocardiography for paediatric cardiac surgery—an audit of 200 cases. *Anaesth Intensive Care* 1999;27:591–595.

141. Stevenson JG, Sorensen GK, Stamm SJ, et al. Intraoperative transesophageal echocardiography of coronary artery fistulas. *Ann Thorac Surg* 1994;57:1217–1221.

142. van Son JA, Vander Woude JC, Cheng W, et al. Surgical closed atrial septotomy under transesophageal guidance. *Ann Thorac Surg* 1995;60:1403–1404.

143. Ungerleider RM, Kisslo JA, Greeley WJ, et al. Intraoperative echocardiography during congenital heart operations: experience from 1,000 cases. *Ann Thorac Surg* 1995;60:S539–S542.

143a. Kaushal SK, Radhakrishanan S, Dagar KS, et al. Significant intraoperative right ventricular outflow gradients after repair for tetralogy of Fallot: to revise or not to revise? *Ann Thorac Surg* 1999;68:1705–1712.

143b. Joyce JJ, Hwang EY, Wiles HB, et al. Reliability of intraoperative transesophageal echocardiography during tetralogy of Fallot repair. *Echocardiography* 2000;17:319–327.

144. Fyfe DA, Kline CH, Sade RM, et al. The utility of transesophageal echocardiography during and after Fontan operations in small children. *Am Heart J* 1991;122:1403–1415.

145. Wienecke M, Fyfe DA, Kline CH, et al. Comparison of intraoperative transesophageal echocardiography to epicardial imaging in children undergoing ventricular septal defect repair. *J Am Soc Echocardiogr* 1991;4:607–614.

146. Hsu YH, Santulli TJ, Wong AL, et al. Impact of intraoperative echocardiography on surgical management of congenital heart disease. *Am J Cardiol* 1991;67:1279–1283.

146a. Yang SG, Novello R, Nicolson S, et al. Evaluation of ventricular septal defect repair using intraoperative transesophageal echocardiography: frequency and significance of residual defects in infants and children. *Echocardiography* 2000;17:681–684.

147. Gussenhoven EJ, van HL, van SR, et al. Recognition of residual ventricular septal defect by intraoperative contrast echocardiography. *Eur Heart J* 1989;10:801–805.

148. Blauth CI, Cosgrove DM, Webb BW. Atheroembolism from the ascending aorta: an emerging problem in cardiac surgery. *J Thorac Cardiovasc Surg* 1992;103:1104–1112.

149. Kvilekval KH, Yunis JP, Mason RA, et al. After the blue toe: prognosis of noncardiac arterial embolization in the lower extremities. *J Vasc Surg* 1993;17:328–334.

150. Amarenco P, Cohen A, Tzourio C, et al. Atherosclerotic disease of the aortic arch and the risk of ischemic stroke. *N Engl J Med* 1994;331:1474–1479.

151. Barzilai B, Davila-Roman VG, Eaton MH, et al. Transesophageal echocardiography predicts successful withdrawal of ventricular assist devices. *J Thorac Cardiovasc Surg* 1992;104:1410–1416.

151a. Stern A, Tunick PA, Culliford AT, et al. Protruding aortic arch atheromas: risk of stroke during heart surgery with and without aortic arch endarterectomy. *Am Heart J* 1999;138:746–752.

152. Tunick PA, Rosenzweig BP, Katz ES, et al. High risk for vascular events in patients with protruding aortic atheromas: a prospective study. *J Am Coll Cardiol* 1994;23:1085–1090.

153. Montgomery DH, Ververis JJ, McGorisk G, et al. Natural history of severe atheromatous disease of the thoracic aorta: a transesophageal echocardiographic study. *J Am Coll Cardiol* 1996;27:95–101.

154. Katz ES, Tunick PA, Rusinek H, et al. Protruding aortic atheromas predict stroke in elderly patients undergoing cardiopulmonary bypass: experience with intraoperative transesophageal echocardiography. *J Am Coll Cardiol* 1992;20:70–77.

155. Newman MF, Wolman R, Kanchuger M, et al. Multicenter preoperative stroke risk index for patients undergoing coronary artery bypass graft surgery. Multicenter Study of Perioperative Ischemia (McSPI) Research Group. *Circulation* 1996;94[Suppl 9]:II-74–II-80.

155a. Matsuyama K, Goto T, Baba T, et al. Echocardiographic and pathological evaluation of atherosclerosis in the ascending aorta during coronary artery bypass grafting. *Anesth Analg* 2000;90:1262–1268.

156. Ribakove GH, Katz ES, Galloway AC, et al. Surgical implications of transesophageal echocardiography to grade the atheromatous aortic arch. *Ann Thorac Surg* 1992;53:758–761.

156a. Royse C, Royse A, Blake D, et al. Screening the thoracic aorta for atheroma: a comparison of manual palpation, transesophageal and epiaortic ultrasonography. *Ann Thorac Cardiovasc Surg* 1998;4:347–350.

157. Konstadt SN, Reich DL, Quintana C, et al. The ascending aorta: how much does transesophageal echocardiography see? *Anesth Analg* 1994;78:240–244.

158. Davila-Roman VG, Phillips KJ, Daily BB, et al. Intraoperative transesophageal echocardiography and epiaortic ultrasound for assessment of atherosclerosis of the thoracic aorta. *J Am Coll Cardiol* 1996;28:942–947.

159. Davila-Roman VG, Barzilai B, Wareing TH, et al. Atherosclerosis of the ascending aorta. Prevalence and role as an independent predictor of cerebrovascular events in cardiac patients. *Stroke* 1994;25:2010–2016.

160. Sabik JF, Lytle BW, McCarthy PM, et al. Axillary artery: an alternative site of arterial cannulation for patients with extensive aortic and peripheral vascular disease. *J Thorac Cardiovasc Surg* 1995;109:885–890.

161. Cosgrove DM. Management of the calcified aorta: an alternative method of occlusion. *Ann Thorac Surg* 1983;36:718–719.

162. Swanson SJ, Cohn LH. Excision of focal aortic arch atheroma using deep hypothermic circulatory arrest. *Ann Thorac Surg* 1995;60:457–458.

162a. Trehan N, Mishra M, Dhole S, et al. Significantly reduced incidence of stroke during coronary artery bypass grafting using transesophageal echocardiography. *Eur J Cardiothorac Surg* 1997;11:234–242.

163. Kouchoukos NT, Wareing TH, Daily BB, et al. Management of the severely atherosclerotic aorta during cardiac operations. *J Cardiac Surg* 1994;9:490–494.

164. Wareing TH, Davila-Roman VG, Barzilai B, et al. Management of the severely atherosclerotic ascending aorta during cardiac operations. A strategy for detection and treatment. *J Thorac Cardiovasc Surg* 1992;103:453–462.

165. Cosgrove DR, Sabik JF. Minimally invasive approach for aortic valve operations. *Ann Thorac Surg* 1996;62:596–597.

166. Acuff ET. Minimally invasive coronary bypass grafting. *Ann Thorac Surg* 1966;61:135–137.

166a. Mohr FW, Onnasch JF, Falk V, et al. The evolution of minimally invasive valve surgery—2 year experience. *Eur J Cardiothorac Surg* 1999;15:233–238.

166b. Applebaum RM, Cutler WM, Bhardwaj N, et al. Utility of transesophageal echocardiography during port-access minimally invasive cardiac surgery. *Am J Cardiol* 1998;82:183–188.

167. Secknus MA, Scalia GM, Asher CR, et al. Intraoperative transesophageal echocardiography in minimally invasive cardiac valve surgery. *Circulation* 1996;94:1–442.

167a. Kasliwal R, Mittal S, Shrivastava S, et al. Echocardiography in minimally invasive direct coronary artery bypass. *Echocardiography* 1999;16:603–610.

167b. Sardari FF, Schlunt ML, Applegate RL 2nd, et al. The use of transesophageal echocardiography to guide sternal division for cardiac operations via mini-sternotomy. *J Cardiol Surg* 1997;12:67–70.

167c. Schulze CJ, Wildhirt SM, Boehm DH, et al. Continuous transesophageal echocardiographic (TEE) monitoring during port-access trade mark cardiac surgery. *Heart Surg Forum* 1999;2:54–59.

167d. Ho AC, Tan PP, Yang MW, et al. The use of multiplane transesophageal echocardiography to evaluate residual patent ductus arteriosus during video-assisted thoracoscopy in adults. *Surg Endosc* 1999;13:975–979.

167e. Falk V, Autschbach R, Krakor R, et al. Computer-enhanced mitral valve surgery: toward a total endoscopic procedure. *Semin Thorac Cardiovasc Surg* 1999;11:244–249.

167f. Moisas VA, Mesquita CB, Campos O, et al. Importance of intraoperative transesophageal echocardiography during coronary artery surgery without cardiopulmonary bypass. *J Am Soc Echocardiogr* 1998;11:1139–1144.

167g. Aronson S, Albertucci M. Assessing flow during minimally invasive coronary artery bypass: an Allen's test equivalent. *Ann Thorac Surg* 1999;67:1173–1174.

168. Topol EJ, Humphrey LS, Borkon AM, et al. Value of intraoperative left ventricular microbubbles detected by transesophageal two-dimensional echocardiography in

predicting neurologic outcome after cardiac operations. *Am J Cardiol* 1985;56:773–775.

168a. Secknus MA, Asher CR, Scalia GM, et al. Intraoperative transesophageal echocardiography in minimally invasive cardiac valve surgery. *J Am Soc Echocardiogr* 1999;12:231–236.

169. Tingleff J, Joyce FS, Pettersson G. Intraoperative echocardiographic study of air embolism during cardiac operations. *Ann Thorac Surg* 1995;60:673–677.

170. Orihashi K, Matsuura Y, Hamanaka Y, et al. Retained intracardiac air in open heart operations examined by transesophageal echocardiography. *Ann Thorac Surg* 1993;55:1467–1471.

171. Orihashi K, Matsuura Y, Sueda T, et al. Pooled air in open heart operations examined by transesophageal echocardiography. *Ann Thorac Surg* 1996;61:1377–1380.

172. Obarski TP, Loop FD, Cosgrove DM, et al. Frequency of acute myocardial infarction in valve repairs versus valve replacement for pure mitral regurgitation. *Am J Cardiol* 1990;65:887–890.

173. Nishioka T, Friedman A, Cercek B, et al. Usefulness of transesophageal echocardiography for positioning the intraaortic balloon pump in the operating room. *Am J Cardiol* 1996;77:105–106.

174. Shanewise JS, Sadel SM. Intraoperative transesophageal echocardiography to assist the insertion and positioning of the intraaortic balloon pump. *Anesth Analg* 1994;79:577–580.

175. Orihashi K, Oka Y. Intraluminal projection of descending thoracic aorta and intraaortic balloon pump catheter examined by transesophageal echocardiography in patients undergoing coronary artery bypass surgery. *Hiroshima J Med Sci* 1991;40:119–126.

176. Reichert CL, Visser CA, Koolen JJ, et al. Transesophageal echocardiography in hypotensive patients after cardiac operations. Comparison with hemodynamic parameters. *J Thorac Cardiovasc Surg* 1992;104:321–326.

177. Goldman AP, Glover MU, Mick W, et al. Role of echocardiography/Doppler in cardiogenic shock: silent mitral regurgitation. *Ann Thorac Surg* 1991;52:296–299.

178. Haverich A, Albes JM, Fahrenkamp G, et al. Intraoperative echocardiography to detect and prevent tricuspid valve regurgitation after heart transplantation. *Eur J Cardiothorac Surg* 1991;5:41–45.

179. Polanco G, Jafri SM, Alam M, et al. Transesophageal echocardiographic findings in patients with orthotopic heart transplantation. *Chest* 1992;101:599–602.

180. Ritchie M, Waggoner AD, Davila-Roman VG, et al. Echocardiographic characterization of the improvement in right ventricular function in patients with severe pulmonary hypertension after single-lung transplantation. *J Am Coll Cardiol* 1993;22:1170–1174.

181. Frazier OH, Rose EA. Multicenter clinical evaluation of the HeartMate 1000 IP left ventricular assist device. *Ann Thorac Surg* 1992;53:1080–1090.

182. Pollock SG, Dent JM, Kaul S, et al. Diagnosis of ventricular assist device malfunction by transesophageal echocardiography. *Am Heart J* 1992;124:793–794.

182a. Scalia GM, McCarthy PM, Savage RM, et al. Clinical utility of echocardiography in the management of implantable ventricular assist devices. *J Am Soc Echocardiogr* 2000;13:754–763.

183. Scheinin SA, Radovancevic B, Ott DA, et al. Postcardiot-

omy LVAD support and transesophageal echocardiography in a child. *Ann Thorac Surg* 1993;55:529–531.

184. Muehrcke DD, McCarthy PM, Stewart RW, et al. Complications of extracorporeal life support systems using heparin-bound surfaces. The risk of intracardiac clot formation. *J Thorac Cardiovasc Surg* 1995;110:843–851.

185. McCarthy PM, Sabik JF. Implantable circulatory support devices as a bridge to heart transplantation [review]. *Semin Thorac Cardiovasc Surg* 1994;6:174–180.

186. Bryan AJ, Barzilai B, Kouchoukos NT. Transesophageal echocardiography and adult cardiac operations [review]. *Ann Thorac Surg* 1995;59:773–779.

187. McCarthy PM, Savage RM, Fraser CD. Hemodynamic and physiologic changes during support with an implantable left ventricular assist device. *J Thorac Cardiovasc Surg* 1995;109:409–418.

188. D'Ambra M. Is intraoperative echocardiography a useful monitor in the operating room? *Ann Thorac Surg* 1993;56:S83–S85.

189. Reeder GS. Identification and treatment of complications of myocardial infarction [review]. *Mayo Clin Proc* 1995;70:880–884.

190. Chirillo F, Cavarzerani A, Ius P, et al. Role of transthoracic, transesophageal, and transgastric two-dimensional and color Doppler echocardiography in the evaluation of mechanical complications of acute myocardial infarction. *Am J Cardiol* 1995;76:833–836.

191. Maurer G, Czer LS, Shah PK, et al. Assessment by Doppler color flow mapping of ventricular septal defect after acute myocardial infarction. *Am J Cardiol* 1989;64:668–671.

192. Manning WJ, Waksmonski CA, Boyle NG. Papillary muscle rupture complicating inferior myocardial infarction: identification with transesophageal echocardiography. *Am Heart J* 1995;129:191–193.

193. La Canna G, Alfieri O, Giubbini R, et al. Echocardiography during infusion of dobutamine for identification of reversible dysfunction in patients with chronic coronary artery disease. *J Am Coll Cardiol* 1994;23:617–626.

194. Voci P, Bilotta F, Caretta Q, et al. Low-dose dobutamine echocardiography predicts the early response of dysfunction myocardial segments to coronary artery bypass grafting. *Am Heart J* 1995;129:521–526.

195. Leung JM, Hollenberg M, O'Kelly BF, et al. Effects of steal-prone anatomy on intraoperative myocardial ischemia. The SPI Research Group. *J Am Coll Cardiol* 1992;20:1205–1212.

196. Leung JM, O'Kelly BF, Mangano DT. Relationship of regional wall motion abnormalities to hemodynamic indices of myocardial oxygen supply and demand in patients undergoing CABG surgery. *Anesthesiology* 1990;73:802–814.

197. Voci P, Bilotta F, Scibilia G, et al. Reversal of left ventricular dysfunction early after coronary artery bypass grafting *Cardiologia* 1992;37:105–111.

198. Simon P, Mohl W, Neumann F, et al. Effects of coronary artery bypass grafting on global and regional myocardial function. An intraoperative echocardiographic assessment. *J Thorac Cardiovasc Surg* 1992;104:40–45.

199. Simon P, Owen A, Neumann F, et al. Immediate effects of mammary artery revascularization versus saphenous vein on global and regional myocardial function: an intraopera-

tive echocardiographic assessment. *Thorac Cardiovasc Surg* 1991;3:228–232.

200. Savage RM, Lytle BW, Aronson S, et al. Intraoperative echocardiography is indicated in high-risk coronary artery bypass grafting. *Ann Thorac Surg* 1997;64:368–373.

201. Kabas JS, Kisslo J, Flick CL, et al. Intraoperative perfusion contrast echocardiography. Initial experience during coronary artery bypass grafting. *J Thorac Cardiovasc Surg* 1990;99:536–542.

202. Hirata N, Nakano S, Taniguchi K, et al. Assessment of regional and transmural myocardial perfusion by means of intraoperative myocardial contrast echocardiography during coronary artery bypass grafting. *J Thorac Cardiovasc Surg* 1992;104:1158–1166.

203. Keller MW, Spotnitz WD, Matthew TL, et al. Intraoperative assessment of regional myocardial perfusion using quantitative myocardial contrast echocardiography: an experimental evaluation. *J Am Coll Cardiol* 1990;16:1267–1279.

204. Villanueva FS, Spotnitz WD, Jayaweera AR, et al. On-line intraoperative quantitation of regional myocardial perfusion during coronary artery bypass graft operations with myocardial contrast two-dimensional echocardiography. *J Thorac Cardiovasc Surg* 1992;104:1524–1531.

205. Aronson S, Lee BK, Wiencek JG, et al. Assessment of myocardial perfusion during CABG surgery with two-dimensional transesophageal contrast echocardiography. *Anesthesiology* 1991;75:433–440.

206. Wei K, Le E, Bin JP, et al. Quantification of renal blood flow with contrast-enhanced ultrasound. *J Am Coll Cardiol* 2001;37:1135–1140.

207. Spotnitz WD, Matthew TL, Keller MW, et al. Intraoperative demonstration of coronary collateral flow using myocardial contrast two-dimensional echocardiography. *Am J Cardiol* 1990;65:1259–1261.

207a. Aronson S, Savage R, Toledano A, et al. Identifying the cause of left ventricular systolic dysfunction after coronary artery bypass surgery: the role of myocardial contrast echocardiography. *J Cardiothorac Vasc Anesth* 1998;12:512–518.

208. Zaroff J, Aronson S, Lee BK, et al. The relationship between immediate outcome after cardiac surgery, homogeneous cardioplegia delivery, and ejection fraction. *Chest* 1994;106:38–45.

209. Aronson S, Lee BK, Liddicoat JR, et al. Assessment of retrograde cardioplegia distribution using contrast echocardiography. *Ann Thorac Surg* 1991;52:810–814.

210. Spotnitz WD, Keller MW, Watson DD, et al. Success of internal mammary bypass grafting can be assessed intraoperatively using myocardial contrast echocardiography. *J Am Coll Cardiol* 1988;12:196–201.

211. Forrest JB, Rehder K, Cahalan MK, et al. Multicenter study of general anesthesia. III. Predictors of severe perioperative adverse outcomes. *Anesthesiology* 1992;76:3–15.

212. Roizen MF, Beaupre PN, Alpert RA, et al. Monitoring with two-dimensional transesophageal echocardiography. Comparison of myocardial function in patients undergoing supraceliac, suprarenal-infraceliac, or infrarenal aortic occlusion. *J Vasc Surg* 1984;1:300–305.

213. Gillespie DL, Connelly GP, Arkoff HM, et al. Left ventricular dysfunction during infrarenal abdominal aortic aneurysm repair. *Am J Surg* 1994;168:144–147.

214. Propst JW, Siegel LC, Schnittger I, et al. Segmental wall motion abnormalities in patients undergoing total hip replacement: correlations with intraoperative events. *Anesth Analg* 1993;77:743–749.

214a. Himmelseher S, Pfenninger E, Werner C. Intraoperative monitoring in neuroanesthesia: a national comparison between two surveys in Germany in 1991 and 1997. Scientific Neuroanesthesia Research Group of the German Society of Anesthesia and Intensive Care Medicine. *Anesth Analg* 2001;92:166–171.

214b. Koessler MJ, Fabiani R, Hamer H, et al. The clinical relevance of embolic events detected by transesophageal echocardiography during cemented total hip arthroplasty: a randomized clinical trial. *Anesth Analg* 2001;92:49–55.

215. Ellis JE, Shah MN, Briller JE, et al. A comparison of methods for the detection of myocardial ischemia during noncardiac surgery: automated ST-segment analysis systems, electrocardiography, and transesophageal echocardiography. *Anesth Analg* 1992;75:764–772.

216. Smith JS, Cahalan MK, Benefiel DJ, et al. Intraoperative detection of myocardial ischemia in high-risk patients: electrocardiography versus two-dimensional transesophageal echocardiography. *Circulation* 1985;72:1015–1021.

217. Reich DL, Konstadt SN, Nejat M, et al. Intraoperative transesophageal echocardiography for the detection of cardiac preload changes induced by transfusion and phlebotomy in pediatric patients. *Anesthesiology* 1993;79:10–15.

218. Deutsch HJ, Curtius JM, Leischik R, et al. Reproducibility of assessment of left-ventricular function using intraoperative transesophageal echocardiography. *Thorac Cardiovasc Surg* 1993;41:54–58.

219. Eisenberg MJ, London MJ, Leung JM, et al. Monitoring for myocardial ischemia during noncardiac surgery. A technology assessment of transesophageal echocardiography and 12-lead electrocardiography. The Study of Perioperative Ischemia Research Group. *JAMA* 1992;268:210–216.

220. Shah PM, Kyo S, Matsumura M, et al. Utility of biplane transesophageal echocardiography in left ventricular wall motion analysis. *J Cardiothorac Vasc Anesth* 1991;5:316–319.

221. Gewertz BL, Kremser PC, Zarins CK, et al. Transesophageal echocardiographic monitoring of myocardial ischemia during vascular surgery. *J Vasc Surg* 1987;5:607–613.

222. Cheung AT, Savino JS, Weiss SJ, et al. Echocardiographic and hemodynamic indexes of left ventricular preload in patients with normal and abnormal ventricular function. *Anesthesiology* 1994;81:376–387.

223. Leung JM, Levine EH. Left ventricular end-systolic cavity obliteration as an estimate of intraoperative hypovolemia. *Anesthesiology* 1994;81:1102–1109.

224. Coriat P, Vrillon M, Perel A, et al. A comparison of systolic blood pressure variations and echocardiographic estimates of end-diastolic left ventricular size in patients after aortic surgery. *Anesth Analg* 1994;78:46–53.

225. Thys DM, Hillel Z, Goldman ME, et al. A comparison of hemodynamic indices derived by invasive monitoring and two-dimensional echocardiography. *Anesthesiology* 1987;67:630–634.

226. Goertz AW, Lindner KH, Seefelder C, et al. Effect of phenylephrine bolus administration on global left ventricular

function in patients with coronary artery disease and patients with valvular aortic stenosis. *Anesthesiology* 1993;78:834–841.

227. Pu M, Griffin BP, Vandervoort PM, et al. Intraoperative validation of mitral inflow determination by transesophageal echocardiography: comparison of single-plane, biplane and thermodilution techniques. *J Am Coll Cardiol* 1995;26:1047–1053.

228. Darmon PL, Hillel Z, Mogtader A, et al. Cardiac output by transesophageal echocardiography using continuous-wave Doppler across the aortic valve. *Anesthesiology* 1994;80:796–805.

229. Stoddard MF, Prince CR, Ammash N, et al. Pulsed Doppler transesophageal echocardiographic determination of cardiac output in human beings: comparison with thermodilution technique. *Am Heart J* 1993;126:956–962.

230. Smith MD, MacPhail B, Harrison MR, et al. Value and limitations of transesophageal echocardiography in determination of left ventricular volumes and ejection fraction. *J Am Coll Cardiol* 1992;19:1213–1222.

231. Cahalan MK, Ionescu P, Melton H Jr, et al. Automated real-time analysis of intraoperative transesophageal echocardiograms. *Anesthesiology* 1993;78:477–485.

232. Perrino A Jr, Luther MA, O'Connor TZ, et al. Automated echocardiographic analysis. Examination of serial intraoperative measurements. *Anesthesiology* 1995;83:285–292.

233. Pinto FJ, Wranne B, St Goar FG, et al. Systemic venous flow during cardiac surgery examined by intraoperative transesophageal echocardiography. *Am J Cardiol* 1992;69:387–393.

234. Gorcsan JR, Diana P, Lee J, et al. Reversible diastolic dysfunction after successful coronary artery bypass surgery. Assessment by transesophageal Doppler echocardiography. *Chest* 1994;106:1364–1369.

235. Appleton CP, Hatle LK, Popp RL. Relation of transmitral flow velocity patterns to left ventricular diastolic function: new insights from a combined hemodynamic and Doppler echocardiographic study. *J Am Coll Cardiol* 1988;12:426–440.

236. Kuecherer HF, Muhiudeen IA, Kusumoto FM, et al. Estimation of mean left atrial pressure from transesophageal pulsed Doppler echocardiography of pulmonary venous flow. *Circulation* 1990;82:1127–1139.

237. Nishimura RA, Abel MD, Housmans PR, et al. Mitral flow velocity curves as a function of different loading conditions: evaluation by intraoperative transesophageal Doppler echocardiography. *J Am Soc Echocardiogr* 1989;2:79–87.

237a. Stevenson JG. Performance of intraoperative pediatric transesophageal echocardiography by anesthesiologists and echocardiographers: training and availability are more important than hats. *J Am Soc Echocardiogr* 1999;12:1013–1014.

238. Rice MJ, Sahn DJ. Transesophageal echocardiography for congenital heart disease: who, what, and when [Editorial]. *Mayo Clin Proc* 1995;70:401–402.

239. Ungerleider RM, Greeley WJ, Kanter RJ, et al. The learning curve for intraoperative echocardiography during congenital heart surgery. *Ann Thorac Surg* 1992;54:691–696.

240. Poterack KA. Who uses transesophageal echocardiography in the operating room? *Anesth Analg* 1995;80:454–458.

241. Pearlman AS, Gardin JM, Martin RP, et al. Guidelines for physician training in transesophageal echocardiography: recommendations of the American Society of Echocardiography Committee for Physician Training in Echocardiography. *J Am Soc Echocardiogr* 1992;5:187–194.

241a. Fyfe DA, Ritter SB, Snider AR, et al. Guidelines for transesophageal echocardiography in children. *J Am Soc Echocardiogr* 1992;5:640–644.

242. Savage RM, Licina MG, Koch CG, et al. Educational program for intraoperative transesophageal echocardiography. *Anesth Analg* 1995;81:399–403.

242a. Miller JP, Lambert AS, Shapiro WA, et al. The adequacy of basic intraoperative transesophageal echocardiography performed by experienced anesthesiologists. *Anesth Analg* 2001;92:1103–1110.

243. Picano E, Lattanzi F, Orlandini A, et al. Stress echocardiography and the human factor: the importance of being expert. *Am J Cardiol* 1991;17:666–669.

243a. Stevenson JG. Adherence to physician training guidelines for pediatric transesophageal echocardiography affects the outcome of patients undergoing repair of congenital cardiac defects. *J Am Soc Echocardiogr* 1999;12:165–172.

244. Cahalan MK, Foster E. Training in transesophageal echocardiography: In the lab or on the job? *Anesth Analg* 1995;81:217–218.

245. Rafferty T, LaMantia KR, Davis E, et al. Quality assurance for intraoperative transesophageal echocardiography monitoring: a report of 846 procedures. *Anesth Analg* 1993;76:228–232.

246. Kisslo J, Byrd BF, Geiser EA, et al. Recommendations for continuous quality improvement in echocardiography from the American Society of Echocardiography. *J Am Soc Echocardiogr* 1995;8:S1–S28.

247. Benson MJ, Cahalan MK. Cost-benefit analysis of transesophageal echocardiography in cardiac surgery. *Echocardiography* 1995;12:171–183.

247a. Siwik ES, Spector ML, Patel CR, et al. Costs and cost-effectiveness of routine transesophageal echocardiography in congenital heart surgery. *Am Heart J* 1999;138:771–776.

248. Delabays A, Sugeng L, Pandian NG, et al. Dynamic three-dimensional echocardiographic assessment of intracardiac blood flow jets. *Am J Cardiol* 1995;76:1053–1058.

248a. Abraham TP, Warner JG Jr, Kon ND, et al. Feasibility, accuracy, and incremental value of intraoperative three-dimensional transesophageal echocardiography in valve surgery. *Am J Cardiol* 1997;80:1577–1582.

248b. Chauvel C, Bogino E, Clerc P, et al. Usefulness of three-dimensional echocardiography for the evaluation of mitral valve prolapse: an intraoperative study. *J Heart Valve Dis* 2000;9:341–349.

248c. De Simone R, Glombitzo G, Vahl CF, et al. A new diagnostic procedure for assessing intracardiac flow disturbances in patients with heart valve disease. *Thorac Cardiovasc Surg* 1999;47:369–375.

248d. De Simone R, Glombitza G, Vahl CF. Three-dimensional color Doppler for assessing mitral regurgitation during valvuloplasty. *Eur J Cardiothorac Surg* 1999;15:127–133.

249. Marx GR, Fulton DR, Pandian NG, et al. Delineation of site, relative size and dynamic geometry of atrial septal

defects by real-time three-dimensional echocardiography. *J Am Coll Cardiol* 1995;25:482–490.

250. Vogel M, Ho SY, Buhlmeyer K, et al. Assessment of congenital heart defects by dynamic three-dimensional echocardiography: methods of data acquisition and clinical potential. *Acta Paediatr Suppl* 1995;410:34–39.

250a. Dall'Agata A, Cromme-Dijkhuis AH, Meijboom FJ, et al. Three-dimensional echocardiography enhances the assessment of ventricular septal defect. *Am J Cardiol* 1999;83:1576–1579.

251. Vogel M, Ho SY, Lincoln C, et al. Three-dimensional echocardiography can simulate intraoperative visualization of congenitally malformed hearts. *Ann Thorac Surg* 1995;60:1282–1288.

252. Borges AC, Witt C, Bartel T, et al. Preoperative two- and three-dimensional transesophageal echocardiographic assessment of heart tumors. *Ann Thorac Surg* 1996;61:1163–1167.

253. Pai RG, Tanimoto M, Jintapakorn W, et al. Volume-rendered three-dimensional dynamic anatomy of the mitral annulus using a transesophageal echocardiographic technique. *J Heart Valve Dis* 1995;4:623–627.

254. Schwartz SL, Cao QL, Azevedo J, et al. Simulation of intraoperative visualization of cardiac structures and study of dynamic surgical anatomy with real-time three-dimensional echocardiography. *Am J Cardiol* 1994;73:501–507.

255. Vrandecic MO, Fantini FA, Gontijo BF, et al. Surgical technique of implanting the stentless porcine mitral valve. *Ann Thorac Surg* 1995;60:S439–S442.

255a. Doty DB, Flores JH, Doty JR, et al. Mitral valve replacement with homograft. *Semin Thorac Cardiovasc Surg* 1999;11[Suppl 1]:191–193.

255b. Isomura T, Suma H, Horii T, et al. Partial left ventriculectomy, ventriculoplasty or valvular surgery for idiopathic dilated cardiomyopathy—the role of intra-operative echocardiography. *Eur J Cardiothorac Surg* 2000;17:239–245.

256. Gross C, Simon P, Mair R, et al. Autologous tissue cardiac valve for aortic valve replacement: technical aspects and early results. *Ann Thorac Surg* 1996;61:1759–1763.

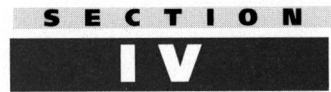

ELECTROPHYSIOLOGY AND PACING

ERIC N. PRYSTOWSKY

59

ELECTROCARDIOGRAPHY

ELENA B. SGARBOSSA
GALEN S. WAGNER

HISTORICAL PERSPECTIVE

The first demonstration of human cardiac activity was made during a congress of physiologists in London by Augustus Waller, who in May 1887 published the first single-lead electrocardiogram (ECG) (1). Waller recorded the electrical activity of the heart from a chest lead with a capillary electrometer (a glass tube filled with mercury) (2). When the electrometer was placed on the body's surface, the current was transmitted from the chest to the mercury column, which expanded or contracted. This movement could be observed only through a microscope and had to be projected onto photographic paper (*e*Fig. 59.0.1).

The pioneer of clinical electrocardiography, however, was Willem Einthoven. Einthoven had a background in physics and mathematics and had been present during Waller's demonstration (3). To refine Waller's concept, Einthoven worked in his laboratory in the Netherlands for several years, first with the electrometer and later with the string galvanometer (2). The galvanometer was an instrument developed in 1897 by Clément Ader for telegraphic transmissions. It reduced the distortion of the electrometer because it consisted of a thin wire extended between the poles of a magnet, but it still required the use of both a microscope and photographic paper. Einthoven presented his idea of applying the galvanometer to the recording of the cardiac electrical activity in 1903 (2). He also coined the term *elektrokardiogramm* in German (the dominant language at the time for scientific publications) and labeled the recorded waveforms P, Q, R, S, T, and U to differentiate them from the original—but incomplete—A, B, C, and D described by Waller. The selection of letters from the last part of the alphabet may have been related to a geometricians' convention at the time (which dictated that designations for curved lines should begin at the letter *P*) (2). Einthoven also described numerous abnormal findings and created the bipolar limb lead system known as *Einthoven's triangle* (2). ▼ 103

ANATOMIC REFERENCES

The position of the heart within the body determines the "view" of the cardiac electrical activity recorded from any ECG electrode on the body surface. When the patient is in the supine position, the heart is a conical structure that lies relatively horizontally with the atria at its base and the ventricles at its apex (14). Because the heart is rotated over its long axis, the right atrium and ventricle are more anterior than the left chambers, and the right and left sides of the heart are not aligned with the homonymous sides of the body (15,16). Thus, the interventricular septum is almost parallel with the frontal—not the sagittal—plane, and the left ventricular free wall (usually considered a lateral structure) includes nearly 300 degrees of the left ventricular circumference and faces superiorly, posteriorly, and inferiorly (14).

ELECTROCARDIOGRAPHIC RECORDING

The 12 Electrocardiographic Leads

Cardiac electrical activity is recorded through 12 surface leads designated I, II, III, aVR, aVL, aVF, V_1, V_2, V_3, V_4, V_5, and V_6. The electrodes that record the first six points are located on the limbs, whereas leads V_1 to V_6 are recorded from the chest (Fig. 59.1).

Leads I, II, and III were first used when Einthoven placed recording electrodes on both arms and the left leg to form an equilateral triangle. An additional electrode on the right leg was used for grounding. Leads I to III are bipolar because they record potential differences between two electrodes. For lead I, the left arm electrode is the positive pole and the right arm electrode is the negative pole. Lead II, with its positive pole on the left leg and its negative pole on the right arm, provides a view of the electrical activity along the long axis of the heart. Lead III has its positive pole on

E. B. Sgarbossa: Department of Cardiology, Rush-Presbyterian-St. Luke's Medical Center, Chicago, Illinois

G. S. Wagner: Department of Medicine, Duke University Medical Center, Durham, North Carolina

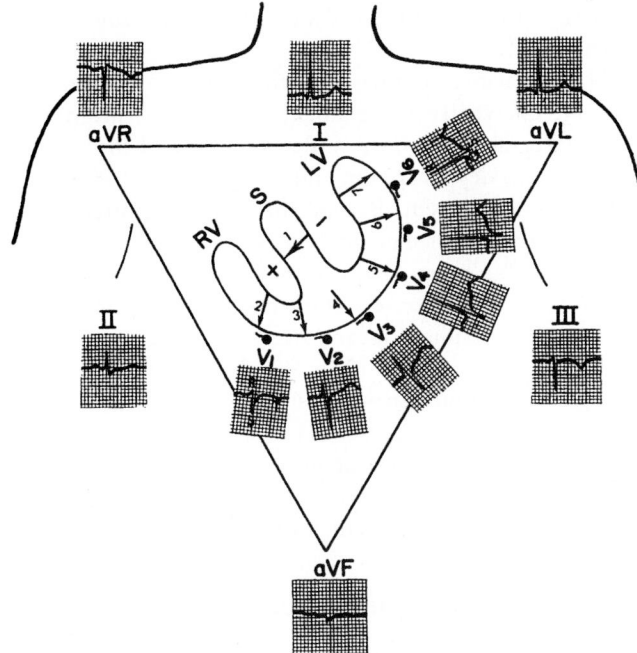

FIGURE 59.1 The standard 12 leads are shown with their recording sites. Both the frontal and the horizontal planes are depicted. Vectors 1 to 7 show the normal sequence of activation of the septum (S) and ventricles from the horizontal plane. LV, left ventricle; RV, right ventricle. (From Gazes PC, ed. *Clinical cardiology: a bedside approach.* Chicago: Year Book, 1983:39, with permission.)

the left leg and its negative pole on the left arm. Between leads I, II, and III are 60-degree angles. These wide viewing gaps are filled with the augmented unipolar (aV) leads aVR, aVL, and aVF, which record the electrical activity between the exploring limb electrode and a reference created by connecting the other two limb electrodes together through a 5,000-ohm resistor (Wilson's central terminal) (17). Lead aVF, for example, measures the potential difference between the left leg and the average of the potentials at the right and left arms. The addition of these three aV leads to the triaxial reference system in the frontal plane produces a hexaxial system, with the six leads separated by angles of only 30 degrees. The gap between leads I and II is filled by lead aVR, that between leads II and III by lead aVF, and that between leads III and I, by lead aVL. This provides a perspective of the frontal plane as illustrated in Figure 59.1. The limb leads are presented in the order I, II, III, aVR, aVL, and aVF, which spatially correspond to 0, 60, 120, −150, −30, and 90 degrees, respectively.

The last set of leads introduced into clinical practice were the six unipolar precordial leads (V_1 to V_6) (8). Augmentation is not necessary because the recording electrodes are close to the heart. Wilson's central terminal provides their negative poles, whereas the sites of the exploring electrodes are determined by bony landmarks on the anterior and left lateral aspects of the precordium (*e*Table 59.0.1, Fig. 59.2). The angles between the six transverse plane leads are slightly smaller than those between the six frontal plane

leads. Lead V_1 is located where the extension of the heart short axis (i.e., a perpendicular to the interatrial and interventricular septa) intersects with the precordial body surface. Because V_1 provides a right anterior to left posterior view, it distinguishes better between left and right cardiac electrical activity than does a lead providing a right lateral to left lateral view (such as lead I).

Special Leads

Some leads are not considered part of the standard ECG but are useful in specific circumstances. Posterior leads (V_7, V_8, and V_9) (*e*Table 59.0.1) increase the ECG sensitivity for injury in the posterior wall (21). Right precordial leads (V_3R, V_4R) (*e*Table 59.0.1) are particularly useful for the diagnosis of right ventricular infarcts and some congenital abnormalities (22). A routine use of the negative aVR (at 30 degrees) would add useful information to the standard ECG, and it would be less likely to be overlooked during routine ECG interpretation (23,24).

The P wave is not always seen distinctly in the 12-lead ECG, but it may be easily identified with the use of special leads. Distinct P waveforms can be seen by placing the right and left arm leads in various chest positions (if possible, parallel to the vector of atrial depolarization) while recording lead I (Lewis lead). Atrial activity can also be recorded semiinvasively from leads placed in the esophagus because the anterior wall of the esophagus lies against the left atrium. In patients with dual-chamber pacemakers, atrial electrograms can be recorded by telemetry from the pacing electrodes. In patients recovering from cardiac surgery, the placement of temporary epicardial pacing electrodes allows the direct recording of atrial activity.

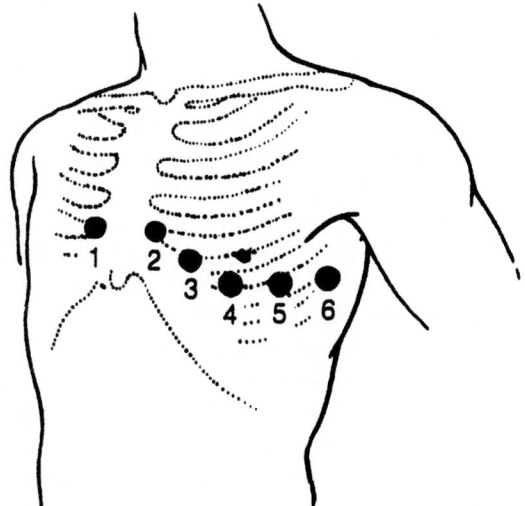

FIGURE 59.2 Location of the precordial lead electrodes. (From The electrocardiogram: fundamentals. In: Goldschlager N, Goldman MJ, eds. *Principles of clinical electrocardiography.* Stamford, CT: Appleton & Lange, 1989:1–10, with permission.)

Electrocardiograph Equipment

Electrocardiographs are calibrated to give a deflection of 10 mm per millivolt (this calibration is usually seen at the beginning or end of the ECG); thus, 1 mm equals 0.1 V. Electrocardiographic paper is graph paper divided in little squares of 1 mm each and larger squares of 5 mm each. The speed of the paper is standardized to 25 mm per second.

Commercial systems provide ECG programs with stereotyped methodologies of measurement. The only ECG limb leads that digital electrocardiographs record are leads I and II; the remaining limb leads are calculated in real time based on the Einthoven law (I + III = II) and using relationships derived from lead vectors for the aV leads. For the calculation of the electrical QRS axis, the entire QRS complex area is used. This is an advantage over the manual QRS-axis estimation, which is based mainly on R-wave measurements. ▾ 104

BASIC PRINCIPLES

Membrane Properties, Action Potential, and Cardiac Activation

Myocytes maintain a potential difference between the interior and the exterior of the cell of approximately –90 mV. This electrical transmembrane gradient depends on the chemical transmembrane gradient, which exists because the concentration of negative ions is higher inside the cell than outside. Such uneven distribution of ions is sustained by a sodium pump housed in the cell membrane (27). Electrical stimuli change the resting potential inside the cell from –90 mV to approximately +30 mV (*depolarization*), and the electrical activity recorded during this process is the *action potential*. Depolarization initiates the propagation of the impulse along both the interior and the exterior of the "polarized" membrane. Thus, the electrical front—which can be represented as a vector—flows from the positively charged (depolarized) to the negatively charged (resting) cells. The earliest ventricular activation occurs in the left side of the septum. The depolarization front then proceeds to the right side of the septum and to the anterior wall, following an inside-out course. Isolated myocytes from endocardium and epicardium have markedly different action potential shapes and durations. This is secondary to differences in the distribution of currents (and channel proteins) among different cardiac layers (28).

Electrical systole continues until the positively charged ions exit the cell, which causes *repolarization* (i.e., restitution of membrane polarity) (27). Atrial repolarization proceeds in the same direction as atrial depolarization, and thus the polarity of the repolarization waveform is opposite to that of depolarization. Ventricular repolarization, however, follows an inverted pattern. The process begins in the epicardium and ends in the endocardium, and therefore the polarity of the repolarization waveform is the same as that of depolarization.

This behavior is the basis for the concept of *ventricular gradient*. The ventricular gradient measures the magnitude of the integral between the QRS complex and the T wave (i.e., between depolarization and repolarization). If all ventricular action potentials had the same magnitude and duration, the ventricular gradient would be zero (29). In the mammalian heart, however, the duration of the repolarization forces is greater in some areas of the ventricles than in others. The resultant mean QRS vector and mean T vector form a narrow angle (27). Repolarization has not yet been mapped simultaneously in all layers of the human heart, but evidence suggests that the areas that depolarize last are the first in completing repolarization (30). The basis for this particular behavior is not known; theories regarding temperature or other gradients have been refuted.

Cardiac Impulse Formation and Conduction

The heart can be considered as a dipole with a positive and a negative charge. At any given time, cardiac cells are in various stages of activation (i.e., depolarization and repolarization). The formation (i.e., pacemaking) and timely conduction of an electrical impulse depends on strategically placed cardiac cells. These cells are arranged in nodes, bundles, and branching networks of fascicles (Purkinje cells). They lack contractile capability but are able to achieve spontaneous electrical impulse formation (act as pacemakers) and to alter the speed of electrical conduction. The intrinsic pacemaking rate is most rapid in the specialized cells in the sinus node (located in the right atrium) and slowest in the specialized cells in the ventricles. After leaving the sinus node, the wavefront travels through the right and left atria in a centrifugal manner. On arrival at the atrioventricular (AV) node, the impulse is delayed, which allows for a sequential, rather than simultaneous, contraction of the ventricles after the atria. The intraventricular conduction network includes the common bundle of His and its right and left bundle branches, proceeding along the septal surfaces to their respective ventricles. The left bundle branch is a diffuse structure that fans broadly over the ventricular septum toward the two papillary muscles of the mitral valve (31). Two divisions of the left bundle branch can usually be distinguished; they are called anterior and posterior but are indeed superior and inferior, respectively. Because the right bundle branch remains compact until it reaches the distal interventricular septal surface (where it branches into the septum and toward the lateral right ventricular wall), many authors consider that the intraventricular conduction system is trifascicular (32–34). These intraventricular conduction pathways are composed of Purkinje cells with specialized capabilities for both pacemaking and rapid conduction of electrical impulses. Purkinje fibers in turn branch into networks that extend

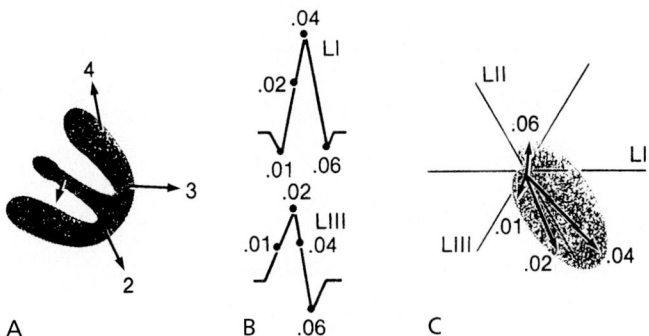

FIGURE 59.3 Correlation between the order of ventricular activation **(A)**, scalar electrocardiogram **(B)**, and vectorcardiogram **(C)**. **A:** The sequence of ventricular activation is represented by four instantaneous frontal plane vectors. **B:** The four vectors plotted on leads I and III at the appropriate time during inscription of the QRS. **C:** Each of the four vectors is derived in the frontal plane. A line joining the ends of the vectors results in a frontal plane QRS loop. L, lead. (From Fisch C. Electrocardiography and vectorcardiography. In: Braunwald E, ed. *Heart disease: a textbook of cardiovascular medicine,* 4th ed. Philadelphia: WB Saunders, 1992:116–160, with permission.)

just beneath the surface of the ventricular endocardium. Because the Purkinje system provides a specialized path for rapid activation, the entire ventricular mass can be depolarized in a short time—similar to the depolarization time in the atria, structures of much smaller mass. The impulses then proceed slowly from endocardium to epicardium throughout the right and left ventricles (35). The normal activation sequence begins at the midseptum, continues at the epicardial right ventricular wall near the apex, then at the lateral and basal left ventricle, and ends at the basal septum (Fig. 59.3).

Electrical Bases for Electrocardiography and Vectorcardiography

Differences in cardiac potentials of a single cardiac cell or a small group of cells do not produce enough current to be detected on the body surface. Electrical representation on the ECG depends on the activation of most of the atrial and ventricular masses. The depolarization process produces a relatively high-frequency ECG waveform, which varies according to the action potential properties, the spread of excitation, and the heart geometry. The earliest QRS complex is recorded in right precordial leads. Although depolarization persists, the ECG recording returns to baseline. Myocardial repolarization is then represented by a waveform of lower frequency, the T wave (36). Once the cells are in their resting state, the ECG records a flat baseline.

Only 10% to 15% of the ventricular activation process can be seen on the 12-lead ECG; the remaining activation forces cancel each other. The normal right ventricle, for example, has no representation on the ECG because its forces are obscured by the dipoles generated in the massive

left ventricle. The summation of all cardiac electrical forces can be represented with a single vector that originates at the center of the Einthoven triangle and whose arrowhead points to the positive pole. If all instantaneous single vectors were plotted consecutively, a vector loop would be formed in each of the three spatial planes (frontal, sagittal, and horizontal). Such recording constitutes a vectorcardiogram (Fig. 59.3). The vectorcardiogram integrates two surface leads out of three (named X, Y, and Z) in an orthogonal system and depicts a separate loop for each of the ECG components (P wave, QRS complex, T wave, and U wave). The advantage of the vectorcardiogram over the 12-lead ECG is that it provides information not only on magnitude and direction (i.e., positive or negative) of the signals but also on spatial orientation. ▼▼ 105

THE NORMAL ELECTROCARDIOGRAM

Overview of the Electrocardiographic Waveforms

Figure 59.4 depicts the waveforms of the normal ECG. ▼▼ 106

P Wave

The first part of the P wave represents the activation in the right atrium, and the middle and final sections of the P wave are recorded during left atrial activation. The normal P wave is rounded and upright in leads I and II and from V_2 to V_6. Its maximum amplitude is 0.25 mV in lead II (or 25% of the R wave) and its duration is 0.08 second. The P-wave axis is approximately 60 degrees. Because of the position of the right and left atria in the thorax, the activation front is directed first anteriorly and then posteriorly. Lead V_1 faces the right atrium; thus, the initial part of the P wave appears positive, whereas its terminal part appears negative.

Ta Segment

The Ta segment (or Ta wave) represents atrial repolarization. It may be seen in normal individuals but is more often obscured by the QRS complex and the early part of the ST segment. The orientation of the Ta wave is opposite that of the P wave. A normal but prominent Ta wave may mimic a pathologic Q wave by producing PR-segment depression.

PR Interval

The time from the onset of the P wave to the onset of the QRS complex constitutes the PR interval, whether the first wave in this complex is a Q or an R wave. The normal PR interval measures 0.12 to 0.22 second and it encompasses the time between the onset of atrial depolarization in the

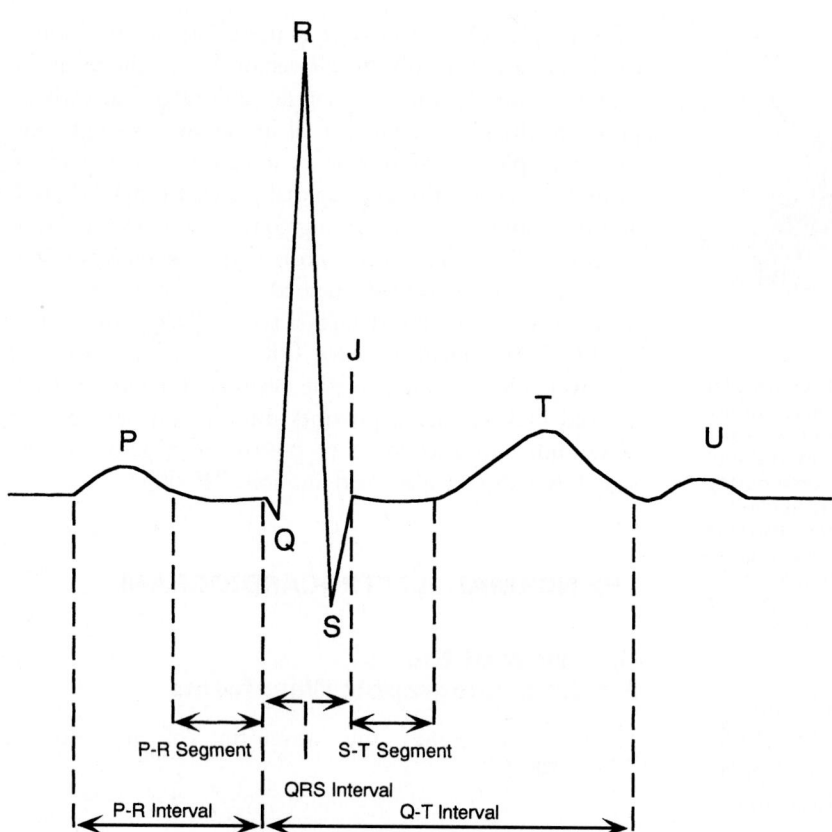

FIGURE 59.4 Waveforms and intervals of the electrocardiogram. (From Wagner GS, ed. *Marriott's practical electrocardiography,* 9th ed. Baltimore: Williams & Wilkins, 1994:13, with permission.)

myocardium adjacent to the sinus node and the onset of ventricular depolarization in the myocardium adjacent to the fibers of the Purkinje network.

A major portion of it is inscribed during the slow conduction through the AV node, which is under the influence of the autonomic nervous system. Normally, the PR interval increases with age and shortens with increasing heart rates during exercise or stress. This effect depends on higher sympathetic and lower vagal tones. Incremental atrial pacing at rest, however, *prolongs* the PR interval. The time from the end of the P wave to the onset of the QRS complex is called the PR *segment.*

Q Wave

A Q wave is a negative deflection at the onset of the QRS complex. It indicates that the net direction of early ventricular depolarization forces is oriented away from the positive axis of the lead in question, at least by 90 degrees. Normal septal activation results in a rapid 'q' wave in leads I, II, III, aVL, V_5, and V_6 (*e*Table 59.0.2). The presence of Q waves in leads V_1, V_2, and V_3 or the absence of small 'q' waves in leads V_5 and V_6 should be considered abnormal (41).

Positional factors may also result in the inscription of prominent but narrow Q waves. If the septal vector is horizontal, Q waves may appear in lead aVF; if the electrical axis is vertical, Q waves may be present in aVL. Precordial

lead electrodes misplaced in a high position may determine a pseudoinfarction pattern from the inscription of Q waves.

In right precordial leads, QR and QS complexes may be normal; they were found in 25% of subjects in V_6R, in 9.7% in V_5R, and in 2.4% in V_4R (42,43).

R Wave

The first positive wave of the QRS complex is the R wave, regardless of whether or not it is preceded by a Q wave. The second vector results in an R wave in leads II and III, and the third vector produces an R wave in leads I, II, III, aVL, aVF, V_5, and V_6. The precordial leads provide a panoramic view of cardiac electrical activity progressing from the right ventricle to the thicker left ventricle, and consequently the R wave increases its amplitude and duration from V_1 to V_4 or V_5. Normal subjects present an rS pattern in leads V_3R and V_4R (42). Larger R waves in V_5 and V_6 may indicate left ventricular enlargement.

The amplitude of the R wave in leads V_5 and V_6 varies directly with left ventricular dimension during exercise and also with variations in the distance of the left ventricle to the chest wall during positional changes (44). Reversal of the normal sequence with larger R waves in V_1 and V_2 can be produced by right ventricular enlargement.

When a second positive deflection occurs in any lead, it is called R'.

S Wave

A negative deflection after an R wave is an S wave. The third vector produces an S wave in leads aVr, V_1, V_2, V_3, and occasionally V_4. The S wave in the precordial leads is large in V_1, larger in V_2, and then progressively smaller from V_3 through V_6. As with the R wave, ventricular enlargement could alter this sequence. The last vector, directed superiorly and posteriorly, may result in a terminal S wave in leads I, V_5, and V_6. Leads V_4R and V_3R show an rS morphology in 80% of normal subjects (43).

Intrinsicoid Deflection

The time from the beginning of ventricular activation (onset of the QRS complex) to the point at which the impulse arrives under a particular electrode is called the *ventricular activation time*. The downward deflection that follows is the *intrinsicoid deflection*. By definition, the intrinsicoid deflection can only be measured in precordial leads, but some authors have applied this name to the turning point of the cardiac vector along the lead axis for the limb leads as well. For practical purposes, the "R peak time" is preferred as an estimate of the intrinsicoid deflection. It is measured from the onset of the QRS to the peak of the R wave or R' wave (*e*Fig. 59.4.1). The R peak time is 0.04 second or less in V_1 and V_2, and 0.05 second or less in V_5 and V_6 (45).

QRS Axis

The QRS axis can be manually determined in the frontal plane in three steps: (a) the lead with the equiphasic deflection (defined as positive and negative components of the QRS complex of similar amplitudes) is identified; (b) the lead that is perpendicular to the initial lead is identified; (c) if the predominant direction of the QRS complex in the lead identified in step (b) is positive, the axis is equal to the positive pole of that lead; if the direction is negative, the axis is equal to the negative pole of that lead. The normal electrical axis measures between −30 and +90 degrees (Fig. 59.5). QRS axes between 0 and −30 degrees are considered "left-axis deviation." 107

ST Segment

The ST segment represents the time period in which the ventricular myocardium remains depolarized. The term *ST segment* is used regardless of whether the final wave of the QRS complex is an R or an S wave. At its junction with the QRS (i.e., J point), the ST segment forms a nearly 90-degree angle and then proceeds horizontally until it curves gently into the T wave.

The ST segment is normally isoelectric with the PR and TP segments. Slight upsloping (particularly in leads V_1 to V_3 and in V_4R to V_3R), downsloping, or horizontal depression of the ST segment may occur as normal variants. The

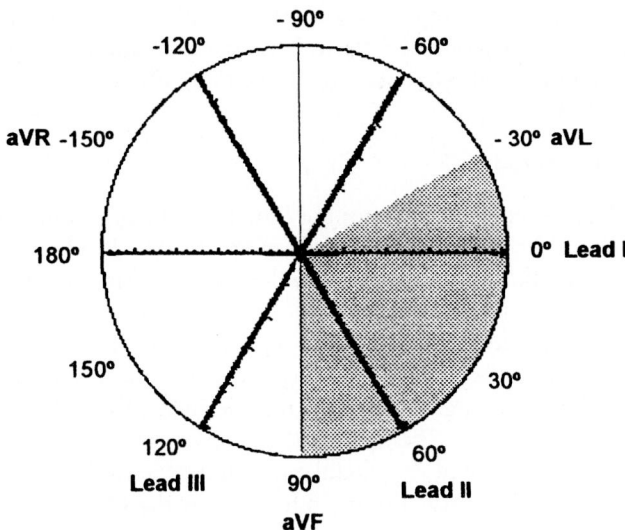

FIGURE 59.5 Frontal plane hexaxial reference system. The normal QRS axis in adults lies between −30 degree and +90 degrees (*area in gray*).

length and appearance of the ST segment are influenced by factors that alter the duration of ventricular activation, such as exercise or bundle branch block.

T Wave

The T wave represents exclusively uncancelled potential differences of ventricular repolarization; thus, it accounts for 8% or less of the total time-voltage product of the heart (46). The shape of the T wave is rounded but asymmetric, because the initial deflection is longer than the terminal deflection. The end of the T wave marks the completion of ventricular recovery, and it is not always easily identifiable. Slight "peaking" of the T wave is normal. The amplitude of the T wave does not normally exceed 0.5 mV in limb leads or 0.10 mV in precordial leads.

The direction of the T wave should be evaluated in relation to that of the QRS complex. The T wave is always positive in lead I, nearly always positive or isoelectric in lead II, and may have any polarity in leads III and aVF (27). In precordial leads the T wave is usually upright, except in 50% of women who present negative T waves in V_1.

U Wave

The U wave may be either absent or present as a small, rounded wave following the T wave. In a particular ECG lead, it shows the same direction as the T wave and it reaches approximately 10% of the amplitude of the latter. It is most prominent in leads V_2 through V_3. The origin of the U wave is uncertain. One theory attributes U-wave genesis to the repolarization of Purkinje fibers, and another to potentials generated during ventricular relaxation (47). Anatomic and electrophysiologic studies suggest that the U wave represents repolarization of the "M" cells, a population of subepicardial cells with unique activation properties, but this also has been questioned (48,49).

QT Interval

The QT interval measures the time from the beginning of the QRS complex until the end of the T wave. It estimates the duration of both ventricular depolarization and repolarization, but is mainly used as an estimate of ventricular recovery time. Repolarization measured as JT (i.e., the interval between the J point and the end of the T wave) is significantly longer in women than in men (316 ± 31 ms vs. 262 ± 31 ms). Presumably, QT intervals are also shorter in men because of the modulating effect of testosterone on repolarization (50). Ethnic differences in the QT interval have not been demonstrated (51).

The value of the information provided by the QT interval is often limited by the difficulty in identifying the end of the T wave. The terminal portion of the T wave may be isoelectric, or a U wave may merge with the T wave. According to Lepeschkin, if the interval between two peaks in a notched T wave is 150 msec or more, the second peak is a U wave (47). The onset of the U wave should be considered the approximate end of the QT interval. At faster heart rates, the P wave may merge with the T wave and create a TP junction. The end of the QT interval in this instance is measured at the onset of the P wave. Considering these inherent limitations, the fact that methods for QT measurement vary among investigators and that efforts for standardization have not succeeded is not surprising (52–54). Recommended techniques include measuring the QT interval in leads with an initial Q wave, in leads in which the T wave is most distinct, in lead II or in aVL—in which the U wave is usually isoelectric—and in leads in which the QT is longest (usually V_2 or V_3) (52,55,56). ❦ 108

Normal Variants

ECGs as screening tests are requested daily by clinicians, surgeons, and cardiologists for a number of purposes. A normal ECG is a good predictor of normal left ventricular function, and it greatly reduces the need to request an echocardiogram to assess systolic function (76).

RSR' Pattern in Lead V_1

An RSR' (or rSr') pattern in lead V_1 with a QRS duration of less than 0.12 second is present in 2.4% of normal persons (77). The R' wave may correspond to relatively late activation of the crista supraventricularis (78).

$S_1S_2S_3$ Pattern

The $S_1S_2S_3$ pattern has been observed in 20% of healthy subjects (77). The S waves in standard leads are inscribed when the terminal vector of the QRS complex originates in the outflow tract of the right ventricle or in the posterobasal septum and is directed rightward and superiorly. The typical $S_1S_2S_3$ pattern (with all S waves larger than their preceding R waves) is not as common as the case in which the amplitude of the S wave in lead I is smaller than that of the R wave.

Early Repolarization

Some individuals show marked (i.e., more than 0.1 mV) ST-segment elevation, which may be present in all precordial leads (79) (Fig. 59.6). Normal young men (particularly African-Americans) may have ST elevation of up to 0.4 mV in leads V_1 through V_3, mimicking acute myocardial infarction or pericarditis (80). Possible causes are early ventricular repolarization or a mild intraventricular conduction delay

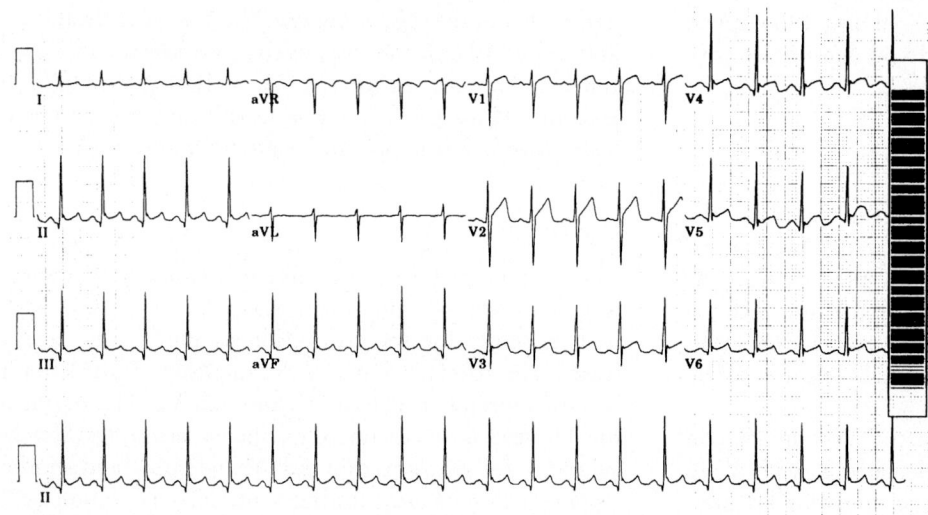

FIGURE 59.6 Electrocardiogram of patient with early repolarization and sinus tachycardia (19-year-old African-American woman). ST elevation is present in both inferior and precordial leads.

in the right ventricle. A distinct notching on the downstroke of the R wave, an upward concavity of the ST segment, and symmetric, prominent T waves may also be present (80). Early repolarization appears to be an independent marker of enhanced aerobic condition (81). 🏳 109

Unusual T Waves

Negative T waves, particularly in precordial leads (from V_6R to V_2, and sometimes through V_6) may be seen in young, usually African-American, vagotonic persons (87,88). These T waves may show intermittent changes in polarity, and in some cases follow a slightly elevated ST segment (early repolarization syndrome). Transient inverted T waves have been documented in normal subjects after meals (89) or after drinking cold water (90). Bifid T waves (i.e., T waves with two peaks different from a U wave) are present in 20% of children; their incidence decreases with age (91). Usually found in precordial leads, bifid T waves are more prevalent in V_1 and V_2 in younger groups, and shift toward V_5 and V_6 in older subjects. A likely mechanism producing bifid T waves is a delayed right ventricular repolarization; an asynchronous repolarization of the anterior and posterior walls would inscribe two separate peaks in the T wave. The probability of an underlying heart disease increases with age.

THE ABNORMAL ELECTROCARDIOGRAM

QRS-Axis Deviation

Although QRS axes between 0 degrees and –30 degrees are sometimes called "left-axis deviations," they are truly a normal variant. Severe left-axis deviations (QRS axes between –30 degrees and –90 degrees) are considered abnormal; yet they are found in 2% of healthy adults (77,98).

Although the term *left-axis deviation* is often used interchangeably with left anterior fascicular block (LAFB), isolated left superior displacement of the QRS axis may occur in the absence of LAFB (in inferior myocardial infarction and other disorders). In some patients, the extent of left-axis deviation varies over short periods of time. The significance of this finding is uncertain; it may result from conduction delays affecting selectively different groups of fibers in the fan-like anterior division of the left bundle branch (27).

P-Wave Abnormalities

Abnormalities of the P wave reflect disorders of atrial pressure or volume, or an anomalous origin of the cardiac impulse.

Right Atrial Abnormality

Right atrial enlargement has classically been diagnosed in the presence of (a) tall, peaked P waves in leads II, III, and aVF

(0.25 mV or more in lead II) ("P pulmonale"), (b) a P-wave axis of 75 degrees or more, and (c) a positive deflection of the P wave in V_1 or V_2 of 0.15 mV or more (99). The correlation of these ECG signs with anatomic findings is poor, however. The amplitude of the P wave may paradoxically decrease as right ventricular hypertrophy progresses. Also, P-wave signs have relatively low sensitivity to detect "pure" right atrial enlargement. In a population with low prevalence of coronary disease, no associated chronic obstructive pulmonary disease, and no left heart pathology, QRS changes in lead V_1 (R/S of 1 or more; presence of Q) in the absence of RBBB were as specific and much more sensitive than a P-wave height of 0.25 mV or more in lead II. In addition, ST depression of 0.05 mV or more in II or aVF [probably representing a prominent atrial repolarization (Ta) wave] was almost 100% specific (100).

Left Atrial Abnormality

Left atrial enlargement is characterized by (a) a notched P wave with a duration of 0.12 second or more ("P mitrale"), best observed in leads II and V_1, and (b) a wide terminal negative deflection in lead V_1 (0.1-mV amplitude per 0.4-second duration) (Fig. 59.7). The terminal force of the P wave correlates better with left atrial volume than with pressure, which may also explain the moderate correlation of the P terminal force with the left atrial weight (101). Interestingly, no characteristics of the P wave correlate with atrial size. The left atrial enlargement pattern indicates an intraatrial conduction disturbance, and thus the term *left atrial abnormality* is preferred (102).

The term *pseudo–P pulmonale* denotes a prominent P wave in inferior leads that is caused by left atrial rather than right atrial abnormality. Detailed examination of the P wave reveals that its terminal portion is increased, whereas the initial portion is normal. Participation of the left atrium in the genesis of the pseudo–P pulmonale is confirmed by identifying a marked negative terminal component of the P wave in V_1.

Biatrial Enlargement

Biatrial enlargement is characterized by tall P waves in lead II, and notched and broad P waves in leads I and II with a terminal negative deflection in V_1.

Ta Wave

Ta waves may be prominent in atrial hypertrophy or infarction and during pericarditis. In the presence of atrial enlargement the Ta wave is prolonged and may displace the ST segment, which appears depressed.

PR Interval

A short PR interval in the presence of a normal P-wave axis suggests an abnormally rapid conduction pathway within

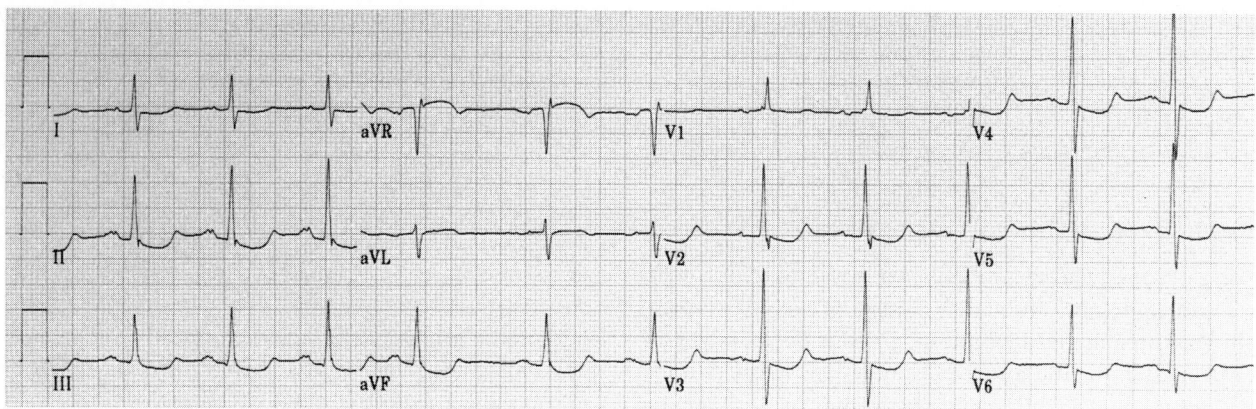

FIGURE 59.7 Left atrial abnormality. The P-wave duration is 0.125 second, and a prominent negative deflection is seen in V₁. Incomplete right bundle branch block and repolarization changes induced by digitalis are also present.

the AV node or in its surroundings (i.e., a bundle of cardiac muscle connecting atria and ventricles, bypassing the AV node). Early activation of the ventricular myocardium (ventricular preexcitation) creates the potential for electrical impulse reentry into the atria, producing a tachyarrhythmia (Wolff-Parkinson-White, or WPW, syndrome). When a short PR interval is accompanied by an abnormal P-wave direction, the site of impulse origin has moved from the sinus node to a position closer to the AV node.

A prolonged PR interval in the presence of a normal P-wave axis indicates a delay in impulse transmission at some point in the pathway between the atrial and ventricular myocardium. When a long PR interval is accompanied by an abnormal P-wave axis, the possibility that the P wave is associated with the preceding rather than the next QRS complex should be considered. This is a manifestation of retrograde activation from ventricles to atria, and the PR interval is usually longer than the preceding PR interval.

QRS Complex

Absence of R-wave progression from V₁ to V₅ may indicate left ventricular myocardial necrosis. The presence of notching and slurring of the QRS complex in the precordial leads is more sensitive than the presence of Q waves to detect anterior infarction, but is less specific (103). A rightward mediastinal shift in left pneumothorax may produce apparent loss of left precordial R waves (104). In dextrocardia, normal R-wave progression may be restored by recording leads V₁ to V₅R on the right side of the precordium.

Q Wave

Conditions associated with abnormal Q waves include myocardial infarction or injury, ventricular hypertrophy or dilatation, and intraventricular conduction disturbances (LBBB, ventricular pacing, and WPW syndrome). Less frequent causes of Q waves include infiltrative myocardial dis-

ease, chronic obstructive pulmonary disease (in precordial leads), acute pulmonary embolism (in lead aVF), pneumothorax, and misplacement of precordial electrodes (105).

ST Segment

Alterations of the ST segment include elevation and depression. The most important cause of ST-segment elevation is transmural injury. Outside the acute setting, ST elevation can be found in combination with other signs of remote or recent infarction and is associated with ventricular asynergy, and can be seen in other pseudoinfarction patterns (106). Depression of the ST segment occurs when myocardial ischemia is present and when ventricular repolarization is altered.

QT Interval

Causes of abnormal prolongation of the QT interval include myocardial ischemia, cardiomyopathies, hypokalemia, hypocalcemia, autonomic influences, drug effects, hypothermia, and congenital long QT syndrome. A prolonged QTc is a predictor of cardiovascular mortality even in the absence of overt heart disease (107).

T Wave

Abnormalities of the T wave (usually consisting of inverted T waves) are seen in a number of conditions. Although the T wave is a sensitive detector of repolarization differences over the myocardium, the magnitude of T-wave changes is not proportional to the extent of myocardium with repolarization abnormalities (27,30). Negative T waves are considered "primary" when the preceding sequence of ventricular depolarization is normal, and "secondary" when it is altered. Primary T waves often accompany ST-segment changes and are observed during myocardial ischemia, myocarditis, pericarditis, and mitral valve prolapse, and are induced by some drugs (phenothiazines, class Ia antiarrhythmic agents, and amiodarone hydrochloride). Postprandial status, a recent paroxysmal tachycardia, and the injection of contrast into coronary arteries all may induce primary T-wave abnormalities (27,30). Research has shown that the negative T waves that develop in infarct-related ECG leads shortly after thrombolysis may be powerful markers for improved 30-day survival, which calls into question the name "T-wave abnormality" (117). However, such T waves must be dynamic (i.e., revert to positive with time, exercise, or dobutamine hydrochloride treatment) to predict myocardial viability and favorable outcome (118,119).

Secondary T waves are those associated with bundle branch block, ventricular pacing, ventricular hypertrophy, cardiomyopathies (120), and WPW syndrome. ▼ 110

U Wave

Positive, prominent U waves are usually induced by hypokalemia (127), but they may also be seen in patients taking digitalis or quinidine and in patients with the congenital long QT syndrome. Negative U waves are highly specific for the presence of heart disease (128). The three most common conditions associated with negative U waves are systemic hypertension, valve regurgitation, and ischemic heart disease.

Electrical Alternans

Electrical alternans is defined as alternation of the QRS complex or T-wave morphology, usually in a 2:1 ratio (*e*Fig. 59.7.1). The PR interval or the ST segment is affected more rarely. Causes of this phenomenon include myocardial ischemia, ventricular dysfunction, rapid tachycardias, significant pericardial effusion, and acute pulmonary embolism (129,130). ▼ 111

VENTRICULAR HYPERTROPHY

Left Ventricular Hypertrophy

Left ventricular hypertrophy is a response to a pressure or volume overload. Because of the increase in myocardial mass, a longer time is required for the spread of the electrical activation from endocardium to epicardium. The intrinsicoid deflection, the R peak time, and the overall QRS duration are all prolonged (*e*Fig. 59.7.3). Because the thickness of the ventricular muscle correlates with the magnitude of the depolarization front, left ventricular hypertrophy exaggerates the normal ECG pattern of left ventricular predominance. An augmented mean QRS vector is oriented toward the left, posteriorly and superiorly, which thereby causes a positive deflection in leads I, II, aVL, V_5, and V_6. The precordial transitional zone is shifted to the left. An rS pattern

is usually observed in V_1 and V_2, although sometimes the initial 'r' wave disappears. ▼ 112

Left Ventricular Hypertrophy with Left Anterior Fascicular Block

Left ventricular hypertrophy superimposed on LAFB increases the S wave in lead III and the R or S wave (or both) in precordial leads. An index that includes these changes [i.e., (R + S) maximal precordial ≥3.0 mV + SIII] has 87% specificity and 96% sensitivity for left ventricular hypertrophy, with a positive predictive value of 89% and a negative predictive value of 95% (148).

Left Ventricular Hypertrophy with Right Bundle Branch Block

The presence of RBBB decreases the sensitivity of the ECG criteria for left ventricular hypertrophy, particularly for precordial signs. In nonobese patients with RBBB, a Sokolow index of 3.5 mV or above is 100% specific for left ventricular hypertrophy (149). Another useful sign when both disorders coexist is left atrial abnormality. The presence of a P-wave terminal force in lead V_1 increases the sensitivity for left ventricular hypertrophy to over 70%, with an approximate specificity of 80% (150). Each 0.1-mV increase in the P terminal force is associated with approximately 25 g of increase in left ventricular mass (151).

Right Ventricular Hypertrophy

Electrocardiographic Diagnosis of Right Ventricular Hypertrophy

Right ventricular hypertrophy is normal in the neonate because during fetal development resistance is greater in the pulmonary than in the systemic circulation. Hypertrophy of the right ventricle persists during the first months of life. The QRS axis measures 100 degrees or more, and the QRS complex is predominantly positive in lead V_1 and predominantly negative in V_6. Such a highly specific pattern for neonatal right ventricular hypertrophy can rarely be found later in life. In adults, changes in response to right pressure overload are less typical because the right ventricular mass must be sufficiently large to overcome the left forces (152). Initially, the QRS complex in lead V_1 loses its negative predominance and a late positive R' wave may appear. With moderate hypertrophy the initial QRS forces move anteriorly (increased R wave in V_1), and the terminal QRS forces move rightward (increased S wave in lead I). Marked hypertrophy results in a predominantly positive QRS complex in V_1; the R wave is greater than 0.7 mV, the R/S ratio is greater than 1, and the S wave is less than 0.2 mV (153,154). Repolarization of the right ventricular myocardium is delayed, which produces negativity of both the ST segment and the T wave (ventricular strain).

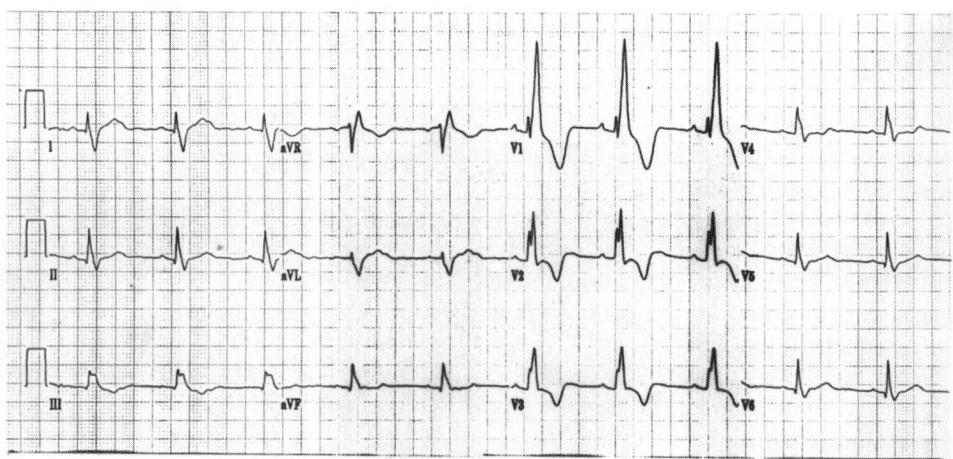

FIGURE 59.8 Right bundle branch block. The patient may also have right ventricular hypertrophy.

The ECG criteria have poor sensitivity for detecting right ventricular hypertrophy. Right-axis deviation of 110 degrees or more identifies only 12% of cases, and the sensitivity of R-wave amplitude and R/S ratio in V_1 is lower than 10%. The specificity of all the criteria is moderate (155).

BUNDLE BRANCH AND FASCICULAR BLOCKS

Electrocardiographic criteria for bundle branch and fascicular blocks [❦ 113] are listed in *e*Table 59.0.4.

Right Bundle Branch Block

The right ventricle contributes minimally to the normal QRS complex. Thus, RBBB produces little distortion during the time required for left ventricular activation; Figure 59.8 illustrates the slight changes of the early portion of the QRS complex contrasting with the marked distortion of its late portion. Late activation of the normal right ventricular myocardium via the spread of impulses from the left ventricle produces a late prominent R' wave in lead V_1 that follows the R wave produced by normal left-to-right activation of the septum. The presence of an RSR' configuration of the QRS complex is pivotal for the diagnosis of RBBB (*e*Table 59.0.4). However, this pattern may also be produced by a terminal conduction delay—vectorcardiographically dissimilar to either RBBB or LBBB—typical of posterior infarction (158). When the QRS duration is less than 0.12 second, the RSR' pattern may correspond to incomplete RBBB or a normal variant.

Fascicular Blocks

The anterior fascicle activates a portion of the left ventricle that is superior and to the left of that activated by the posterior fascicle. When both fascicles are intact, the impulse travels through them at the same time to depolarize the myocardium. The wavefronts from each fascicle then col-

lide near the end of ventricular depolarization. An interruption or delay of impulse conduction in one fascicle results in asynchronous activation of the left ventricle.

LAFB is common and benign; LPFB is rare (159). Fascicular blocks are often associated with coronary artery disease. In autopsy studies, the most frequent finding underlying LAFB is anterior infarction with proximal left anterior descending (LAD) artery occlusion. Posterior infarction, however, is not usually associated with LPFB; autopsy examination in LPFB shows massive infarct of the septum (compromising both the anterior and posterior areas) and widespread damage to the left bundle branch (160).

Left Anterior Fascicular Block

In epidemiologic surveys, LAFB is the most common conduction abnormality, perhaps because the left anterior fascicle is located in the outflow tract and in apposition to the aortic ring; this makes it susceptible to increases in intraventricular pressure and disorders of the aortic valve (161). The initial ventricular activation in LAFB spreads inferiorly and rightward via the left posterior fascicle (13). Block in the anterior fascicle removes the competition from activation directed superiorly and leftward, and Q waves appear in leads with the positive electrode on the left arm (I and aVL) (Fig. 59.9). The impulse arrives at the inferior and apical myocardium retrogradely from the posterior fascicle with a minimal delay that prolongs the QRS by 0.02 second. The remainder of the left anterior ventricular wall is activated in a superior, leftward, and counterclockwise direction. These terminal forces are first represented in lead aVL and then in aVR. Thus, the peak of the terminal R in lead aVL precedes the peak of the terminal R wave in a simultaneous lead aVR (*e*Fig. 59.9.1) (162). The R waves in leads I and aVL are prominent, and the large amplitude of the R wave in aVL may mimic left ventricular hypertrophy. Prominent S waves are seen in leads II, III, and aVF, causing a leftward shift of the QRS axis. This QRS-axis deviation is the major criterion for the diagnosis of LAFB

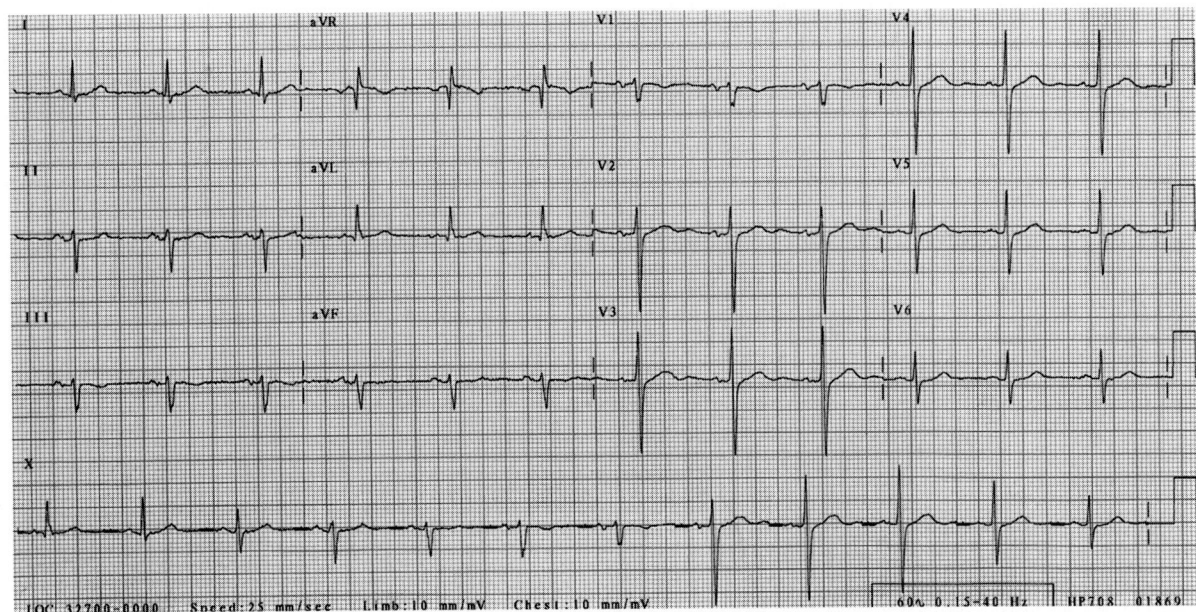

FIGURE 59.9 Left anterosuperior fascicular block. (From Wagner GS, ed. *Marriott's practical electrocardiography*, 9th ed. Baltimore: Williams & Wilkins, 1994:89, with permission.)

(*e*Table 59.0.4). The original QRS-axis criterion proposed by Rosenbaum (and adopted by the World Health Organization/International Society and Federation for Cardiology Task Force) of −45 degrees has been considered highly specific but rather insensitive to detect LAFB (45); other authors use −30 degrees.

The diagnosis of LAFB in the presence of inferior myocardial infarction is difficult because both entities produce left-axis deviation. In addition, inferior infarcts tend to produce a superior deviation of the initial depolarization forces, while LAFB directs them inferiorly, which thus counteracts the manifestations of inferior infarct. Warner and colleagues have proposed several criteria for the diagnosis of coexistent LAFB and inferior infarct, based on the correspondence of the QRS complex portions between simultaneous leads (162) (*e*Table 59.0.5, *e*Fig. 59.9.2).

Left Posterior Fascicular Block

LPFB is usually associated with RBBB; its isolated form is rare. Rosenbaum and colleagues attributed the low incidence of LPFB to the fact that the posterior fascicle is short and thick and it is the first group of fibers to depart from the bundle of His. The posterior fascicle may also be protected by its dual blood supply from the anterior and posterior descending coronary arteries and because it lies in the less turbulent left ventricular inflow tract (13).

Aside from its association with coronary artery disease, LPFB has also been identified in cardiomyopathies, aortic valve disease, and calcification of the left ventricular skeleton (163). The initial activation of the left ventricular free wall when the left posterior fascicle is blocked occurs via the left anterior fascicle (13). The excitation front is directed superiorly and leftward. No forces travel inferiorly or rightward, and thus Q waves appear in leads with the positive electrode on the left leg (leads II, III, and aVF). Next, the activation wave spreads over the remainder of the left ventricular free wall in an inferior and rightward direction. This produces prominent R waves in leads II, III, and aVF and prominent S waves in leads I and aVL, which cause a rightward shift of the QRS axis to at least +90 degrees (164) (*e*Fig. 59.9.3). The QRS duration is slightly prolonged (by 0.02 second). The diagnosis of LPFB can only be made in the absence of right ventricular hypertrophy, because this condition itself can produce an LPFB pattern.

Left Bundle Branch Block

LBBB produces marked distortion of the QRS complex (Fig. 59.10), and it may be caused by disease either in the main left bundle branch (predivisional) or in its fascicles (postdivisional). The presence of LBBB signs in a screening ECG correlates well with left ventricular systolic dysfunction (76).

The interventricular septum is normally activated from left to right. This produces an initial R wave in the right precordial leads and a Q wave in leads I and aVL as well as in the left precordial leads. During LBBB, the septum is activated from right to left. Initial Q waves are inscribed in the right precordial leads and the normal Q waves in V_5 and V_6 disappear. The ventricular activation front then proceeds from the left interventricular septum to the adjacent anterior superior and inferior walls, to the posterolateral free wall. This sequence of activation tends to produce

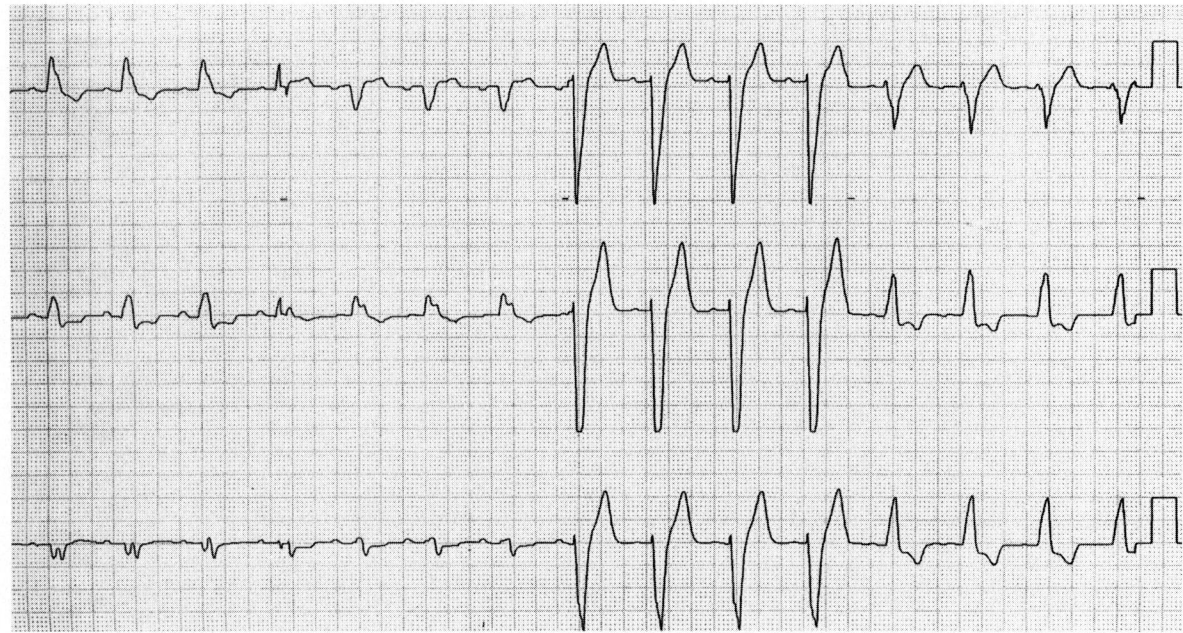

FIGURE 59.10 Uncomplicated left bundle branch block.

monophasic QRS complexes: QS in lead V$_1$ and R in leads I, aVL, and V$_6$.

LBBB is characterized by secondary repolarization changes of opposing polarity to that of the main QRS deflection. For leads with a predominantly negative QRS complex, this results in an ECG pattern of ST-segment elevation with positive T waves, similar to the current of injury of acute coronary occlusion. Uncomplicated LBBB thus resembles anterior wall myocardial infarction (Fig. 59.10), and when left-axis deviation is also present, the repolarization pattern mimics that of inferior infarct.

The most important differential diagnosis of LBBB is the QRS pattern of the "corrected" transposition of the great vessels. In this condition, the initial QRS force shows the same direction as in LBBB because propagation of the impulse is inverted, but the QRS duration is normal.

Trifascicular Blocks

Electrocardiographic documentation of trifascicular block during 1:1 AV conduction is rare and requires the presence of alternating RBBB and LBBB or fixed RBBB with alternating LAFB or LPFB (13). If both bundle branches are simultaneously affected by block, the ECG shows complete AV block. When the degree of block differs between the two bundle branches, ECG manifestations vary and include, for example, a shorter PR interval preceding either RBBB or LBBB, or a complete bundle branch block with prolonged PR interval (27). The combination of bifascicular block (RBBB + LAFB; RBBB + LPFB; or LBBB) with first-degree AV block on the surface ECG cannot be considered trifascicular block because the site of AV block can be either the AV node or the His-Purkinje system (178).

His bundle electrocardiography may be necessary to evaluate conduction in the remaining fascicle in symptomatic patients with bifascicular block.

ISCHEMIC HEART DISEASE

Myocardial Ischemia and Injury: General Electrophysiologic Principles

Myocardial ischemia results in two main electrophysiologic changes. First, myocytes partially depolarize and their membrane resting potential is reduced (i.e., becomes less negative). Second, the action potential duration and amplitude decrease. Local injury currents develop between ischemic and nonischemic cells that manifest in the ECG as ST-segment deviation toward the specifically involved area. During diastole, injury currents flow from ischemic to normal cells; during systole, injury currents flow in the opposite direction. Traditionally, ECG changes caused by an increase in myocardial metabolic demand or a decrease in coronary blood flow are called *ischemia* when changes affect only the T wave, and *injury* when changes affect the ST segment. Epicardial (or transmural) injury is characterized by ST-segment elevation and endocardial ("subendocardial") injury by ST-segment depression.

Electrocardiographic Ischemia (T-Wave Changes)

The first ECG change during transmural ischemia is the development of peaked, tall T waves; this usually precedes ST-segment elevation (181). The ischemic zone is electrically more negative than its surrounding myocardial area during the recovery phase. Thus, while ST elevation is still present or after it has subsided, the T waves become inverted in relation to the QRS complexes (*e*Fig. 59.10.3). Normally the angle between the directions of the QRS complexes and the T waves is less than 45 degrees in the frontal plane and less than 60 degrees in the horizontal plane. When the angles are increased, the presence of myocardial ischemia should be considered. The T-wave inversion may regress within minutes or persist for several months (27). These primary T-wave changes are not specific or sensitive for the diagnosis of myocardial ischemia (181).

For some patients with chest pain presenting to the emergency room, negative T waves may be the first electrocardiographic finding observed—perhaps because ST elevation has already subsided. Biochemical changes may indicate acute or subacute (i.e., non–Q wave) myocardial infarction. These negative T waves and those observed after documented ST-elevation infarction have been labeled "postischemic" (27). Yet negative T waves that appear soon after ST-elevation infarction seem to be predictors of improved survival (117). Thus, other factors aside from ischemia (e.g., reperfusion) possibly may have a role in the genesis of such T waves (181,182).

Electrocardiographic Injury (ST-Segment Changes)

Subendocardial Injury (ST-Segment Depression)

Ischemia secondary to an increased metabolic demand affects initially the subendocardium, the area most vulnerable to ischemic damage. Changes involve mainly the ST-T waveforms (and much less the QRS complex), because myocytes are less susceptible to ischemia during electrical depolarization than during electrical recovery. Diastolic injury currents produce TQ segment elevation in the surface ECG that results in apparent ST-segment depression, whereas systolic currents produce "true" ST-segment depression. Initial changes include a depression of the J point of at least 0.10 mV and a horizontal or downward sloping of the ST segment toward the T wave (*e*Fig. 59.10.4). The T wave may or may not be altered in the same direction as the ST segment. T-wave inversion may be secondary to ST depression (i.e., the T wave is "dragged" by the ST segment), or it may change as a direct manifestation of delayed repolarization in the ischemic myocardium.

The current of injury occurs at the time that the subendocardial cells complete their activation process, and therefore it affects the QRS complex. The QRS waveforms deviate in the same direction as the ST segment. This distortion affects the amplitude but not the duration of the QRS complex and alters its later part more than its initial part (183). The ST-segment depression of subendocardial injury resolves rapidly after removal of the cardiovascular stress. When the ST-segment depression persists in the absence of increased left ventricular workload, the diagnosis of subendocardial infarction should be considered.

Transmural or Epicardial Injury (ST-Segment Elevation)

Transmural injury is caused by interruption of the blood supply to the myocardium because of occlusion of one of the three coronary arteries or their branches. The first ECG change is tall, peaked T waves (181). Then the ST segment appears elevated in the ECG leads that face the ischemic area and may appear depressed in the opposite ECG leads.

One of the following criteria must be met for the diagnosis of transmural injury: (a) elevation of the origin of the ST segment at the J point of 0.10 mV or higher in two or more limb or precordial leads V_4 to V_6, or of 0.20 mV or higher in two or more precordial leads V_1 to V_3 (*e*Fig. 59.10.5, Fig. 59.11); or (b) depression of the origin of the ST segment at the J point of 0.10 mV or higher in two or more of leads V_1 to V_3, or ST-segment elevation greater than 0.10 mV in two or more of leads V_7 to V_9.

A highly specific marker of transmural injury is alternans of the ST segment. Electrical alternans consists of alternans of the degree of ST elevation and is secondary to variations in action potential duration or amplitude; alternating ST elevation and depression have not been reported (129).

Severe degrees of ischemia are associated with distortion of the later part of the QRS, which reverses after the acute phase (184). The ECG manifestations of transmural injury vary in duration. Those observed in patients during coronary angioplasty or in patients with coronary vasospasm disappear rapidly when the coronary occlusion is removed (171), whereas in patients with transmural injury secondary to coronary thrombosis they resolve gradually after spontaneous or therapeutic restoration of flow. When insufficient coronary blood flow persists after the myocardial metabolic reserves become depleted, the process of necrosis begins (185). In most patients, permanent new Q waves develop at some point after ST elevation or depression has occurred. In ECG leads in which rapid Q waves are normally present (*e*Table 59.0.2), they may become pathologically wide.

Acute Myocardial Infarction

The evolutionary changes during acute infarction include (a) ST elevation, often preceded by tall T waves, (b) abnormal Q waves, and (c) return of ST elevation to baseline with T-wave inversion. Tall or peaked T waves may be an early manifestation of transmural injury. The most typical change involves ST-segment elevation, which decreases significantly after the first 12 hours of chest pain (186) (Fig. 59.11). In some patients, multiple episodes of ST-segment elevation and resolution have been documented after thrombolytic therapy. A moderate ST elevation persists

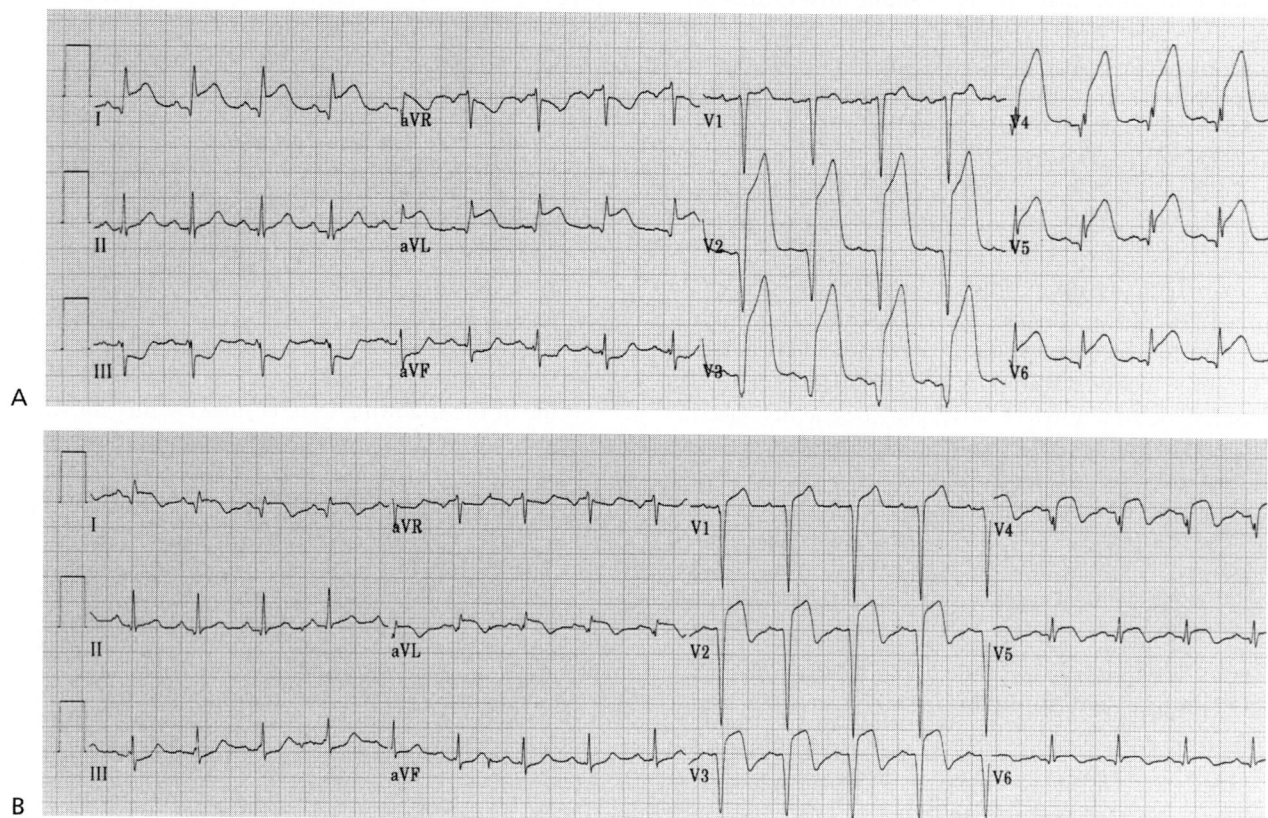

FIGURE 59.11 A: Acute anterior myocardial infarction, with ST elevation in precordial leads (day 1). The presence of ST elevation in leads I and aVL, plus ST depression in leads III and aVF, suggests proximal left anterior descending artery occlusion. **B:** Subacute anterior myocardial infarction (day 2). ST elevation is regressing, and negative T waves and new Q waves are developing.

usually for several days; when observed beyond 2 weeks of the acute event, it suggests ventricular aneurysm. If coronary reperfusion is rapidly achieved, negative T waves usually develop and Q waves do not.

CLINICAL VALUE OF THE ELECTROCARDIOGRAM DURING ACUTE MYOCARDIAL INFARCTION

The diagnostic accuracy of the ECG depends on the extent and location of transmural injury or necrosis. In general, the 12-lead ECG is specific but only moderately sensitive for detection of acute myocardial injury (187,188). Systematically recording leads V_4R, V_8, and V_9 (i.e., a 15-lead ECG) increases the probability of detecting ST elevation from 47% to 59%, with no decrease in specificity (22). The infarction descriptors *anterior*, *inferior*, and *lateral* have classically been attributed to occlusions of the LAD, right coronary artery (RCA), and circumflex artery (LCX), respectively. Other terms such as *apical*, *septal*, *high lateral*, and *posterior* are also in use. The 12-lead ECG is only moderately accurate in determining the anatomic location of acute infarction, however, and the correspondence of some

ECG terms with the pertinent site of infarction is rather poor (189). The ECG is most sensitive for detecting acute occlusion of the LAD and least sensitive for detecting involvement of the circumflex artery. Automated diagnoses of infarction (i.e., provided by the electrocardiographer) are specific but not sensitive; their most promising application is in the prehospital setting (190–192).

Acute Anterior/Anteroseptal/Anterolateral Infarction (Left Anterior Descending Artery Occlusion)

During acute anterior injury, V_2 is the most sensitive lead for recording ST elevation (sensitivity, 99%) and for identifying the culprit lesion in the LAD. Other powerful predictors of proximal LAD occlusion include ST elevation in aVL and concomitant ST depression in inferior leads (193,194) (Fig. 59.11). ST elevation that extends to leads I and aVL often coexists with inferior ST depression. The magnitude of ST depression in inferior leads correlates better with that of ST elevation in leads I and aVL than with the ST elevation of precordial leads. The maximal ST elevation is best recorded in V_2 as well as V_3 (195) (*e*Fig. 59.10.5; Fig. 59.11). Highly specific signs for occlusions at

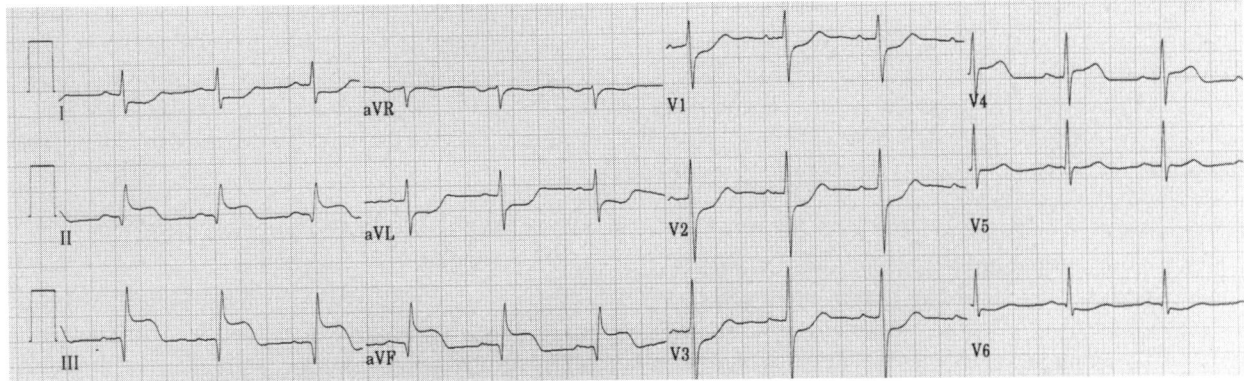

FIGURE 59.12 Acute inferior myocardial infarction. Transmural inferior injury is accompanied by ST-segment depression in leads I, aVL, and V_1 to V_3.

the level of the first septal perforator include ST elevation in aVR (196), disappearance of preexistent septal Q waves in lateral leads (197,198), and ST depression in V_5 (196).

Occasionally, ST elevation is also present in lead V_1. Lead V_1 captures electrical phenomena from the right paraseptal area, which is supplied by the septal branches of the LAD. In most patients the septum is additionally protected by a conal branch of the RCA (double circulation), and this explains why patients with anterior myocardial infarction usually have no ST elevation in V_1 (196). The presence of ST elevation in V_1 (*e*Fig. 59.10.5) correlates strongly with ST elevation in V_3R and predicts the less common anatomical scenario in which a small conal branch of the RCA does not reach the interventricular septum (199).

Acute Inferior Infarction (Right Coronary or Circumflex Artery Occlusion)

The typical ECG pattern of inferior infarction consists of ST-segment elevation in leads II, III, and aVF (Fig. 59.12). In 80% to 90% of cases the culprit lesion is in the RCA (200); the remainder of the patients have LCX occlusion.

Higher ST elevation in lead III than in lead II strongly suggests RCA occlusion (201,202). Because lead aVL faces the superior part of the left ventricle and directly opposes the inferior wall, ST-segment depression in aVL usually indicates RCA occlusion (sensitivity, 94%; specificity, 71%) (203). Precordial ST depression accompanying inferior injury is more likely to develop from LCX than from RCA occlusion (Fig. 59.13). Horizontal ST depression with initially negative then upright T waves in leads V_1 to V_3 or V_4 (Fig. 59.13) is associated with posterior wall motion abnormalities (204). Concomitant ST elevation in leads V_5 and V_6 also indicates posterolateral ischemia—triggered by either RCA or LCX occlusion (205). When this ST elevation is significant (more than 0.2 mV), it is likely a sign of infarction related to a "megaartery" (RCA or LCX), with a large ischemic burden (205).

Acute Lateral and Posterior Infarctions (Circumflex Artery Occlusion)

The vascular beds of the LCX show broad anatomic variability and supply a rather small ventricular area. This is why the

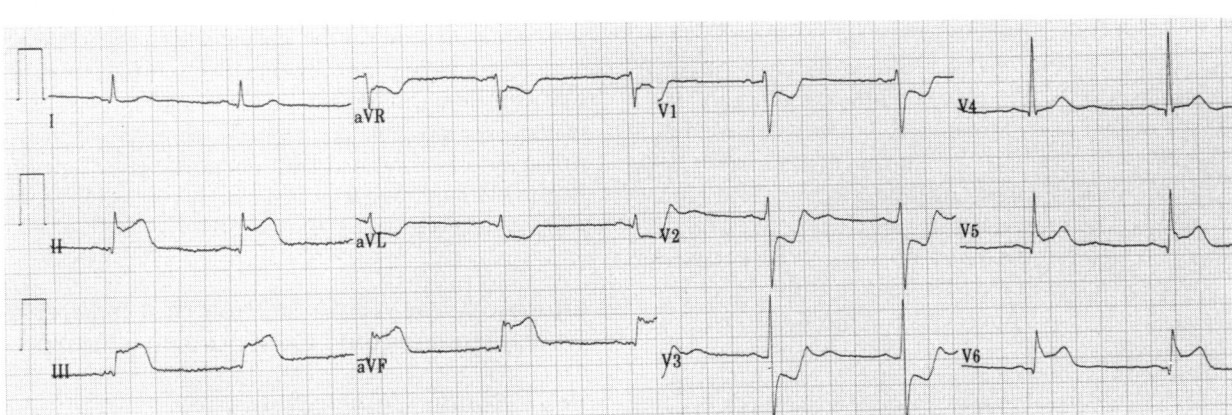

FIGURE 59.13 Acute inferior myocardial infarction produced by circumflex artery occlusion. ST elevation is present in leads V_5 and V_6 (suggesting "megaartery" occlusion), and ST depression with prominent U waves is seen in leads V_1 to V_3. The ST depression in aVL is unusual.

standard 12-lead ECG displays ST-segment elevation in less than half of cases of LCX occlusion. When present, ST elevation is more often seen in leads II, III, and aVF, followed by leads V_5, V_6, and aVL (206). In some cases, a concomitant ST depression is seen in leads V_1 to V_3 (Fig. 59.13).

One-third of patients with chest pain secondary to spontaneous LCX occlusion present with isolated ST depression. ST depression in V_1 and V_2 is a sensitive sign (203,206). Another one-third of patients present without any changes in the 12-lead ECG. In a study of 33 consecutively treated patients with LCX occlusion, however, ST elevation in V_7 through V_9 was always detected and was associated with posterior wall motion abnormalities (207). Leads V_7 to V_9 are more specific than precordial leads for detection of posterior infarction (84% vs. 57%), with similar sensitivity (approximately 80%) (208).

Acute Right Ventricular Infarction

Transmural injury of the right ventricle translates into ST-segment elevation of 0.1 mV or more in precordial leads. ST elevation in V_1 is highly specific for proximal RCA occlusion (202). In approximately 7% of patients, ST elevation extends to lead V_5, which suggests anterior infarction. This ST elevation decreases toward V_4, however, whereas in anterior injury from LAD occlusion, the ST segment is more elevated in V_2 and V_3 than in V_1 (209).

Right ventricular infarction is usually concurrent with infarcts of the inferior wall (eFig. 59.13.1). Half of patients with inferior injury have ST elevation in V_4R (sensitivity and predictive accuracy for right ventricular infarction are both 93%) (210). Isolated right ventricular infarction is rare and occurs mainly in patients with right ventricular hypertrophy (211).

ST-Segment Depression in Patients with Acute Coronary Syndromes

Isolated ST-Segment Depression

In a study of 136 patients presenting with isolated ST-segment depression in the 12-lead ECG, evolution to infarction was observed in 54% of cases. One-year mortality was high for patients both with and without infarction (212). In general, ST depression is associated with older age, multivessel or left main coronary artery disease, multiple infarctions, or poor left ventricular function (213,214). A common cause of primary ST depression is the subocclusion of the left main coronary artery, and the ECG frequently shows a combination of ST depression in leads I, II, and V_4 to V_6 with ST elevation in aVR. A sum of ST changes of 18 mm is 90% sensitive for left main artery disease (215). A maximum ST depression in leads V_2 and V_3, on the other hand, indicates LCX occlusion (specificity, 96%; sensitivity, 70%). Recognizing this is important,

because patients with isolated ST depression from LCX occlusion benefit from thrombolysis (216). Isolated ST depression in inferior leads may be caused by either inferior subendocardial ischemia or by a prominent atrial repolarization (Ta) wave during right atrial enlargement (100).

ST-Segment Depression Concomitant with ST Elevation

Many patients with acute chest pain present with "reciprocal" ST-segment depression, that is, ST depression concomitant with ST elevation in a different lead group. The mechanism underlying such ST depression is assumed to be mirroring, a phenomenon of electrical reflection of the transmural injury onto the opposite ventricular wall. The ST depression is captured by a lead placed at 180 degrees to the lead recording ST elevation, but the terms *reciprocal* and *mirror* are loosely applied to other recording points as well (217). For example, ST depression that is maximal in leads V_5 and V_6 may be related to acute ischemia of the right ventricle; it is the reciprocal of ST elevation in V_3R (181).

Another possible mechanism for ST depression is regional subendocardial ischemia or infarction. Although strictly speaking mirroring is also involved in the ST depression of subendocardial ischemia (because the ST elevation in the subendocardial layer is reflected onto the epicardial layer), most clinicians consider this ST depression "nonmirror" because it is a primary manifestation of artery occlusion, not secondary to ST elevation in a different territory (218). In patients with chest pain and predominant ST depression in any lead except aVR, ST depression of at least 0.4 mV is 97% specific (and 20% sensitive) for acute infarction (212). Several investigators have found that inferior ST depression during anterior injury is not accompanied by inferior ischemia (as assessed by perfusion imaging), which suggests that mirroring—rather than inferior subendocardial ischemia—is responsible for the ST depression (217,218). Over 85% of patients with ST depression in lead aVF have a culprit lesion in the proximal LAD. On the other hand, the significance of anterior ST depression accompanying inferior injury may depend on the leads involved. ST depression in leads V_1 through V_3 or I through aVL seems to correspond to mere mirroring, often from LCX occlusion. On the other hand, ST depression deeper in V_4 through V_6 than in V_1 through V_3 is associated with anterolateral or septal subendocardial injury from a severe lesion in the LAD or in the left main coronary artery (219) (Fig. 59.14).

Diagnosis of Acute Myocardial Infarction in the Presence of Confounding Factors

Right Bundle Branch Block

The diagnosis of evolving acute anterior infarction in patients with RBBB can be suspected when secondary T

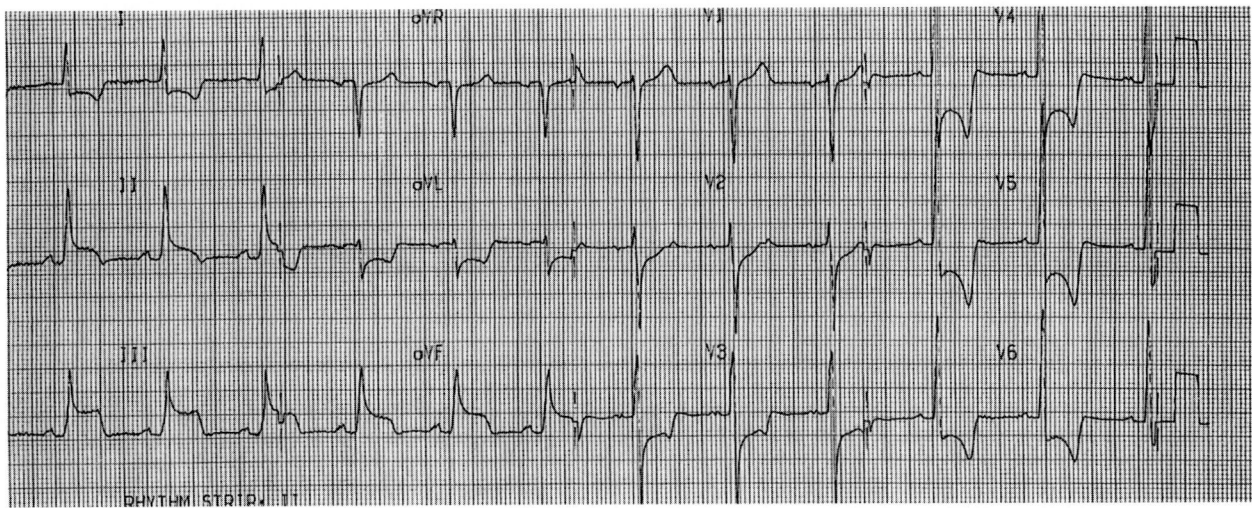

FIGURE 59.14 Electrocardiogram recorded in a patient with ST elevation in inferior leads from acute right coronary thrombosis. The concomitant precordial ST depression, maximum in V_3 to V_6, probably corresponds to concurrent subendocardial injury. (From Wagner GS, ed. *Marriott's practical electrocardiography*, 9th ed. Baltimore: Williams & Wilkins, 1994:140, with permission.)

waves (opposite to the QRS complex) in leads V_1 to V_3 or V_4 are replaced by T waves of concordant polarity with the QRS ("pseudonormalization"). ST elevation is often easily detected (Fig. 59.15).

Left Bundle Branch Block

In patients who present with acute chest pain and LBBB, ECG interpretation is difficult because the normal sequence of ventricular activation can be altered by both LBBB and acute myocardial injury. During either occlusion of a coronary artery by an angioplasty balloon or acute infarction, however, further ST-segment elevation does occur in LBBB (222–224). In a study that analyzed all published criteria for the diagnosis of acute infarction in the presence of LBBB, the ECGs of 131 patients who had LBBB and enzyme-confirmed acute infarction were compared with

131 ECGs of external controls who had chronic coronary artery disease and LBBB (*e*Table 59.0.6, Fig. 59.16). Criteria were validated in an independent sample of patients with acute coronary syndromes and LBBB. A scoring system suggested that a highly specific diagnosis of acute infarction could be made with a total score index of 3 points or higher (*e*Table 59.0.6). This score was associated with specificities of 90% or higher in both the derivation and the validation samples (225,226).

ESTABLISHED MYOCARDIAL INFARCTION

Q-Wave Infarction

Although the ST segment is still elevated during ongoing transmural injury, abnormal Q waves begin to develop as a

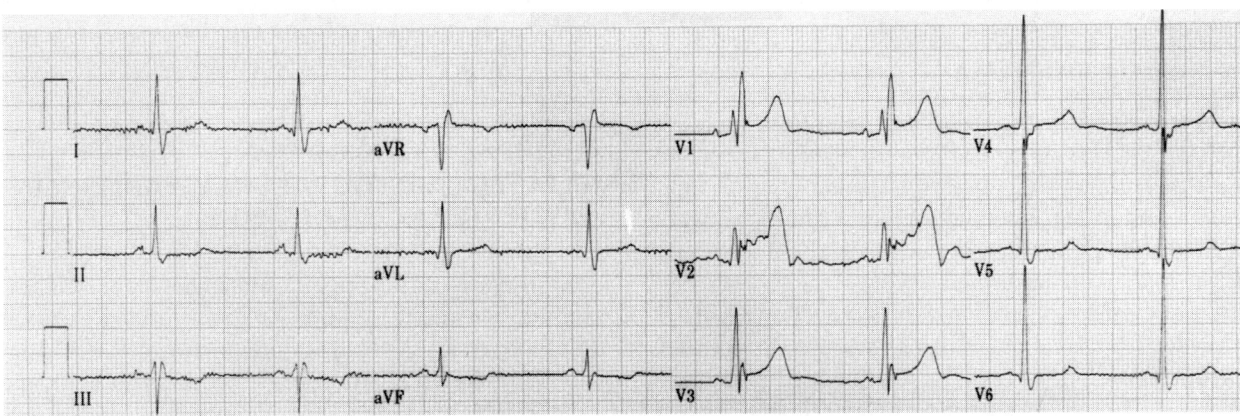

FIGURE 59.15 Acute anterior myocardial infarction with right bundle branch block (RBBB). Primary T waves have replaced the secondary T waves observed in RBBB.

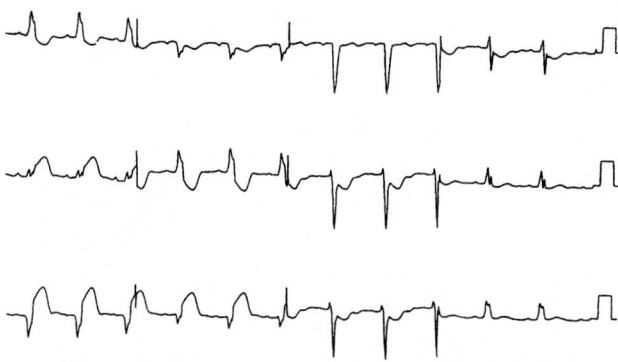

FIGURE 59.16 Electrocardiogram recorded in a patient with left bundle branch block and acute myocardial infarction. ST elevation greater than 0.3 mV is present in lead II (with concordant QRS polarity), ST elevation greater than 0.4 mV is present in leads III and aVF (with discordant QRS polarity), and ST depression is present in leads V_2 and V_3. (From Sgarbossa EB, Pinski SL, Barbagelata A, et al. Electrocardiographic diagnosis of evolving acute myocardial infarction in the presence of left bundle branch block. *N Engl J Med* 1996;334:481–487, with permission.)

consequence of both the loss of electrical forces in the necrotic area and the predominant effect of the resultant force directed away from the area (Fig. 59.11). The deviation of the ST segments may confound the capability to measure the amplitudes of the QRS waveforms. Pathologic Q waves are recorded from all myocardial regions that depolarize early during the cardiac cycle. The posterobasal area depolarizes late, which thereby produces a positive QRS waveform in the precordial leads opposing this zone (i.e., V_1 and V_2).

In most patients, necrotic Q waves persist indefinitely after the acute event, but in 15% to 30% of cases they disappear or become nonsignificant. These regression changes are similar for patients with anterior and inferior infarcts (234,235). Small, rapid 'r' waves may also result from recovery of electrical activity in a necrotic area when QS complexes developed immediately after the acute episode. The presence of an initial 'r' wave of less than 20 ms in lead V_2, for example, is an excellent discriminator between presence and absence of anterior infarction (236).

Non–Q-Wave Infarction

After an episode of cardiac chest pain, even if accompanied by biologic markers of cardiac necrosis, some patients do not develop pathologic Q waves. Only small 'q' waves or 'r' waves of diminished amplitude appear. The labeling of these alternative ECG changes as Q-wave or non–Q-wave infarctions varies among authors (237).

The most conspicuous changes of non–Q-wave infarction involve repolarization. Patients may present with ST elevation, depression, or both, or with isolated negative T waves (238). Early ECG changes cannot accurately predict evolution to non–Q-wave infarction. Also, approximately 9% of "non–Q-wave" infarctions result indeed from trans-

mural injury of the left inferoposterior wall. These patients present with isolated ST depression in leads V_1 to V_4. A distinctive feature of anterior non–Q-wave infarction is a downsloping ST depression (as opposed to a horizontal ST depression in posterior infarcts) with precordial T-wave inversion (181).

The underlying angiographic finding in many patients with non–Q-wave infarction is a recanalized vessel (239). When a culprit vessel is identified, in 60% of cases it is the circumflex (240). The absence of Q waves does not seem to correlate anatomically with nontransmural necrosis (241). The prognosis of non–Q-wave infarction among patients treated with thrombolysis is better than that of Q-wave infarction, and it is markedly predicted by the repolarization changes in the admission ECG (242). Changes restricted to the T wave predict much lower morbidity and mortality than changes consisting of ST depression (243–245).

Electrocardiogram during and after Thrombolysis

Thrombolytic therapy accelerates the ECG evolutionary changes of acute infarction. Early T-wave inversion and a rapid resolution of ST-segment elevation have been associated with patency of the infarct-related artery (244,245). Additional elevation of the ST segment within the first hour of thrombolytic therapy occurs in 59% of patients, usually preceding a subsequent rapid decline of the ST elevation (246). Reperfusion obtained through primary coronary angioplasty is associated with additional ST elevation in only 12% of cases (246). Achieving a steady-state ST deviation within 100 minutes of thrombolysis is highly sensitive and specific for patency of the infarct-related artery (247). The second most common electrocardiographic change during effective reperfusion is the presence of accelerated idioventricular rhythm (246).

Subsequent evolution of infarction after thrombolysis is characterized by decrease in R-wave amplitude and by Q-wave development of smaller magnitude than that observed among patients not receiving thrombolysis (248); non–Q-wave infarctions are also common (242).

CLINICAL VALUE OF THE ELECTROCARDIOGRAM IN ESTABLISHED MYOCARDIAL INFARCTION

Autopsy, echocardiographic, and angiographic studies have shown that the 12-lead ECG has a limited capability to diagnose established myocardial infarction (249,250). The accuracy of the ECG depends on both the location and size of the infarct, and may be hampered by the presence of intraventricular conduction defects, LAFB, Q-wave regression, multiple infarctions (e.g., an anterior infarct may

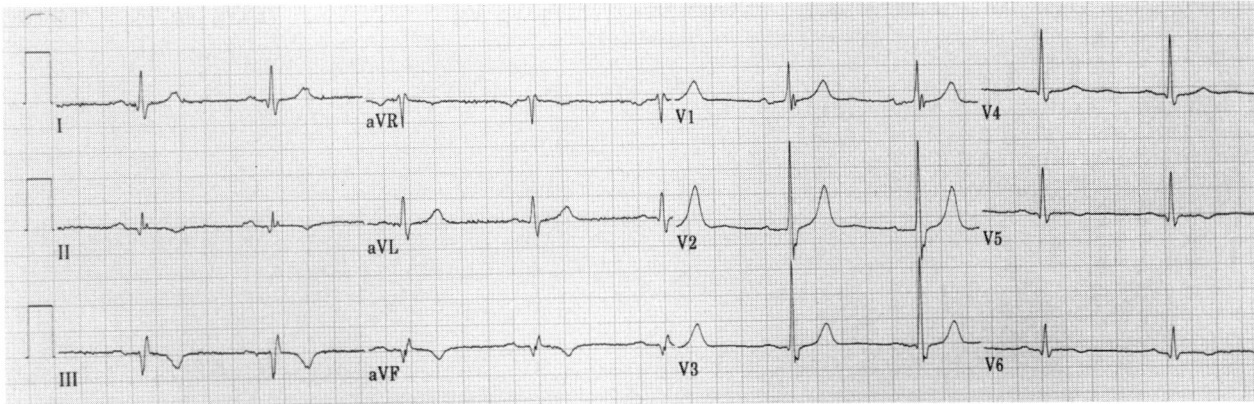

FIGURE 59.17 Inferoposterior infarction.

reduce tall R waves in V_1 and V_2 from a previous posterior infarct), and left ventricular hypertrophy.

Infarct Location

The presence of abnormal Q waves in two or more leads of a lead group permits the identification of the particular infarcted ventricular region (*e*Fig. 59.16.1). Studies of wall motion dynamics have suggested that the classic electrocardiographic designation of certain infarct areas may not be accurate. For example, abnormal Q waves in leads I, aVL, V_5, and V_6 are often associated with apical, rather than lateral, wall motion abnormalities in ventriculograms (251). Anteroseptal infarct has classically been defined by the presence of Q waves in leads V_1 to V_3 (252). Echocardiographic and angiographic examination of patients with ST-segment elevation in these leads, however, has shown anteroapical infarcts and normal septa (253,254). Anatomically defined septal infarcts result instead in disappearance of septal Q waves in inferior leads and in leads I, V_5, and V_6. These changes are preceded by ST depression in the same leads during the acute phase, or, if the infarction was inferoseptal, by precordial ST depression. Initial R waves may be reduced in V_1 to V_3 (198,255).

Prominent right precordial R waves have been classically attributed to posterior infarct (Fig. 59.17), which may be a misnomer, because the term *posterior* applies better to the thoracic wall facing these areas of the left ventricle than to the left ventricle itself. Prominent R waves in V_1 (duration 0.04 second or more, R/S greater than 1) are nearly 100% specific and have a 91% positive predictive value for basal *lateral* asynergy of the left ventricle (sensitivity, 36%) (256). Specificity and positive predictive value drop slightly for prominent R waves in V_2, but the sensitivity increases to 61%. Asynergy of adjacent inferior and lateral segments is common in these patients. Abnormal R waves in V_1 in patients with chest pain are 96% specific for circumflex artery occlusion (206), and in autopsy studies 50% of lateral infarctions are associated with tall precordial R waves (257). ▼▼ 114

ATRIAL INFARCTION

Atrial infarction is rarely recognized in the ECG. Atrial infarction is most unlikely in the absence of ventricular compromise, but it may occur in 1% to 17% of patients with acute myocardial infarction (270). The injury current affects atrial repolarization and results in elevation of the Ta wave with reciprocal changes in opposite leads. This produces displacement of the PR segment, better appreciated in patients with AV block (271).

PSEUDOINFARCTION PATTERNS

Conditions that suggest the ECG diagnosis of acute myocardial injury include severe hyperkalemia (Fig. 59.18), pericarditis, uncomplicated LBBB (Fig. 59.10), primary and secondary cardiac tumors (*e*Fig. 59.18.1), acute pulmonary embolism, and ventricular aneurysm (272–275).

The presence of myocardial necrosis with pathologic Q waves or decrease in R-wave amplitude may be mimicked by left ventricular hypertrophy, fascicular blocks, ventricular pre-excitation, infiltrative heart disease, lead misplacement, pulmonary emphysema, pleural effusion (276), and epicardial implantable defibrillator systems (277). LBBB and ventricular pacing may mimic the electrocardiographic appearance of either acute or remote myocardial infarction (278).

MISCELLANEOUS CAUSES OF ELECTROCARDIOGRAPHIC ABNORMALITIES

Acute Pericarditis

Early ECG abnormalities during acute pericarditis include diffuse ST-segment elevation and upright T waves. Because the myocardial area injured by the inflammation is only partially depolarized, new ST vectors develop, directed away from the ventricular cavity and toward the apical epi-

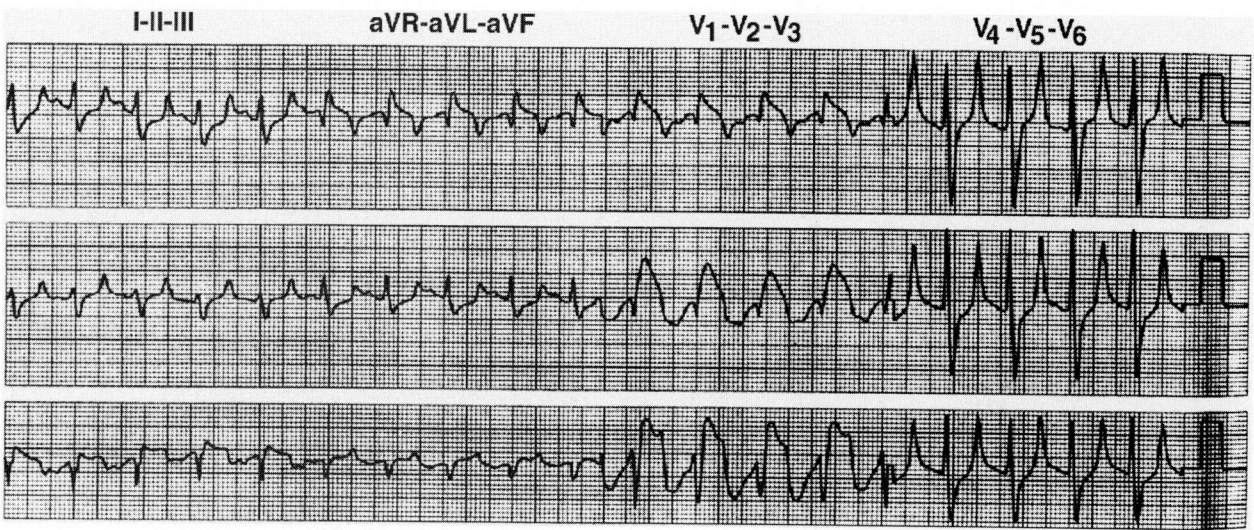

FIGURE 59.18 Pseudo–acute myocardial infarction mimicked by hyperkalemia. Peaked T waves are best seen in this case in leads V$_4$ to V$_6$. (From Kamimura M, Hancock W. Acute myocardial infarction in diabetic ketoacidosis. *Hosp Pract* 1992;27:28–30, with permission.)

cardium. Thus ST-segment elevation may be seen in all leads except aVR, which shows ST depression. Lead V$_1$ may also record ST depression because it faces the right atrium. Although the P wave is usually not affected, PR (STa)-segment depression may develop (80).

Acute pericarditis persists for 3 or 4 weeks. When the ST segment normalizes, the T waves become inverted. In some patients, the T-wave inversion may be the only documented ECG change. ▼ 115

Electrolyte Abnormalities

Because the cardiac action potential results from transmembrane ionic movements, changes in electrolyte concentration may alter cardiac depolarization, repolarization, and conduction properties.

Hypokalemia

Low plasma potassium levels are common in patients with acute myocardial infarction, after out-of-hospital cardiac arrest, and during treatment with diuretics. Hypokalemia prolongs repolarization. The initial ECG signs are T-wave flattening or inversion, ST-segment depression, and prominent U waves; the latter is the most characteristic change (27,127). As potassium levels decrease, the T wave fuses with the U wave, so that the ending of the QT interval is obscured (27).

More severe hypokalemia is manifested by a slight increase in the QRS complex and P-wave amplitudes and by prolongation of the PR interval. Ectopic atrial and ventricular beats are not unusual at potassium concentrations lower than 3.3 mEq per liter because automaticity is increased. Severe hypokalemia is associated with atrial tachycardia with block and with AV dissociation, and

finally with ventricular arrhythmias (torsades de pointes). Patients taking digitalis are especially prone to arrhythmias in the presence of hypokalemia.

Hypokalemia is often found in hypertensive patients treated with diuretics. In these patients, a positive Sokolow-Lyon index could represent a false-positive finding, as the index correlates better with hypokalemia than with left ventricular mass (279).

Hypercalcemia

A high concentration of calcium increases the excitability threshold and has an inotropic effect. Hyperkalemia shortens both the ST segment and the QT interval and prolongs the PR interval and the QRS complex. Severe hypercalcemia may be associated with second- or third-degree AV block (27).

Hypocalcemia

Hypocalcemia prolongs the ST segment and the QT interval. The duration of the ST segment is inversely related to the calcium blood level. The T wave remains relatively normal (27).

Hypothermia

The electrocardiographic changes of hypothermia include bradycardia, flattening of P waves, and prolongation of the PR, QRS, and QT intervals. Irregularities of the isoelectric line may be seen as a consequence of muscular tremor or atrial fibrillation. A typical sign—observed in approximately 80% of patients with hypothermia—is the appearance of a J wave. The J (or Osborn) wave is a deflection that distorts the QRS-ST junction and is more commonly observed in leads II, III, aVF, V$_5$, and V$_6$ (*e*Fig. 59.18.2).

The J wave disappears with normothermia. Prolonged QT intervals may persist after the body temperature and the QRS complex have normalized (280).

Drug Effects

Therapeutic or toxic cardiac effects of various medications may be detected on the ECG.

Digitalis

Digitalis accelerates ventricular repolarization, particularly in the subendocardium. This manifests on the ECG first by a T-wave flattening and by prominent U waves with a shorter QT interval. The most typical change, however, consists of a coved ST depression (Fig. 59.7). The T wave appears biphasic, with its first portion negative and merging with the ST segment. These repolarization changes do not correlate well with therapeutic or toxic blood levels of the drug.

Digitalis intoxication is often manifested by arrhythmias similar to those seen in severe hypokalemia (i.e., atrial tachycardia with block and AV dissociation). However, no particular arrhythmia is pathognomonic of digitalis intoxication (281).

Characteristics of digitalis-induced atrial tachycardia include atrial rate between 140 and 250 per minute, inferior-to-superior direction of atrial activation, and 2:1 AV block. During 2:1 AV conduction, the PP interval including a QRS complex is usually shorter than the one not including a QRS complex. This resembles the ventriculophasic arrhythmia of complete AV block and is probably caused by comparable changes in the autonomic tone during the cardiac cycle (281). Nonparoxysmal junctional tachycardia at a rate between 70 and 130 beats/min (generally with AV dissociation) is frequent (271).

Quinidine and Class Ia Antiarrhythmic Drugs

Quinidine blocks the fast sodium channel in the cell membrane, and it prolongs both the action potential duration and the repolarization. The effects of quinidine include narrowing and then inversion of the T waves, prominent U waves, and prolonged QT interval (282). Quinidine effects are exaggerated by the presence of digitalis. Prolongation of the QRS complex by 25% to 50%, AV block, ventricular arrhythmias (torsades de pointes), and sick sinus syndrome are toxic effects of quinidine. The psychotropic agents phenothiazines, tricyclic antidepressants, and lithium produce ECG changes similar to those of quinidine.

Propafenone and Class Ic Antiarrhythmic Drugs

Propafenone hydrochloride, flecainide acetate, and encainide prolong the AH and HV intervals and the atrial and ventric-

ular refractory periods. The QRS duration is increased. All class Ic drugs may induce ventricular arrhythmias (proarrhythmic effect). The JT interval is not prolonged.

The Transplanted Heart

Incomplete or complete RBBB is the most prevalent abnormality in transplanted patients, but it is unrelated to pre- or intratransplantation hemodynamic factors or to ischemia (283,284). The PR and QT intervals are shorter and the precordial transitional zone is displaced to the left in the transplanted patients in comparison with the last recorded ECGs in the donors. The shift in the transitional zone and the conduction delay of the right bundle would indicate a clockwise rotation of the heart on its vertical axis. The increased prevalence of RBBB during follow-up, however, may be associated with mildly increased pulmonary pressures (285).

Soon after transplantation, supraventricular arrhythmias are common and self-limited (284). The sudden appearance of first-degree AV block, however, should suggest acute cardiac rejection (286).

A curious finding soon after transplantation is that of remnant recipient atrial activity (*e*Fig. 59.18.3), which usually decreases with time (285). Modern surgical techniques, however, provide for a complete excision of the recipient atria, which will probably abolish their electrocardiographic manifestations in future transplant recipients.

Pulmonary Abnormalities

Acute Cor Pulmonale

The ECG changes in acute cor pulmonale (*e*Table 59.0.7) reflect acute pulmonary hypertension with dilatation of the right chambers and perhaps myocardial ischemia. The classic "right heart strain" patterns, $S_I Q_{III} T_{III}$ and $S_I Q_{III}$ (probably secondary to clockwise rotation), are not constant.

Several studies have found that the only ECG signs that are significantly more frequent among consecutively treated patients with confirmed acute pulmonary embolism than among those with suspected pulmonary embolism are sinus tachycardia and incomplete RBBB (287). A diagnosis of acute pulmonary embolism can be considered probable when three or more of these changes coexist in the admission ECG (288). Interestingly, the degree of right QRS-axis deviation, the presence of incomplete or complete RBBB, and the rate of sinus tachycardia correlate with the extent of embolization (289).

Pulmonary Emphysema

The overinflated lungs in pulmonary emphysema produce anatomic changes. The diaphragm is lowered and the cardiac electrical axis becomes more vertical and rotates clockwise. In the ECG, the most typical findings include prominent P waves [more than 0.25 mV; indeed, a P pulmonale predicts pulmonary emphysema or low diaphragm position better than it does right atrial enlargement (155)] and exaggerated atrial repolarization (Ta) waves producing more than 0.10 mV of ST-segment depression in inferior leads; a rightward shift of the QRS axis to 90 degrees or more in the frontal plane; decreased progression of the R-wave amplitudes in precordial leads; and low voltage of the QRS complexes, especially in the left precordial leads (290). 116

Misplacement of Electrocardiographic Leads

Misplacement of ECG leads is common. A study of 11,432 ECGs detected reversals involving the left arm and foot or adjacent precordial electrodes in 2% of the recordings (296). Estimates are that of the 300 million ECGs recorded annually in the world, approximately 6 million contain a lead reversal. The proportion may be higher when other combinations of lead reversals are considered.

Reversal of the Right and Left Arm Cables

When the electrodes attached to the arm cables are reversed, "lead I" shows negative P and T waves, and a predominantly negative QRS complex. "Lead II" is indeed lead III, and "lead aVR" is indeed lead aVL, and vice versa (297). Thus, the limb leads suggest the diagnosis of dextrocardia. The precordial leads, however, show the normal progression of R waves through V_6.

Reversal of Each Arm Cable with Its Corresponding Leg Cable

When the arm cables are switched with the leg cables, "lead I" shows a flat line that records the potential difference between both legs. "Lead II" is an inverted (upside-down) lead III, because the positive electrode is now in the left arm. "Lead III" mirrors its image, because the polarity of its two components is inverted. "Lead aVR" is a replica of "lead aVL," because both leads now record potentials derived from comparing each leg (aVF) with the same central terminal.

Misplacement of Precordial Lead Electrodes

In a prospective study in which precordial leads were deliberately misplaced, 2-cm changes in electrode position (too high or too low) resulted in significant ECG abnormalities (298). Variations included changes in R-wave amplitude, ST segments, Q waves, and the transition zone. The most important differential diagnosis when precordial lead electrodes are misplaced in a high position is anterior infarc-

tion, because QS complexes or low-voltage R waves may appear. The use of device-guided lead placement improves accuracy and reproducibility in interpretation of precordial waveforms (298).

HIGH-RESOLUTION ELECTROCARDIOGRAPHY

Standard recording techniques cannot detect low-amplitude bioelectric potentials from the body surface. Potentials generated by the His-Purkinje system and by depressed ventricular myocardium ("late potentials") are difficult to identify because their signals are smaller than the electrical noise produced by various sources (299). Two techniques have been developed to overcome this problem: (a) temporal averaging (usually referred to as "signal averaging"), which is applicable only to repetitive electrocardiographic signals; and (b) spatial averaging, which can record the His-Purkinje signal and late potentials on a beat-to-beat basis. Signal averaging (the most frequently used technique) can analyze potentials in either time domain, frequency domain, or a combination of both. Results of these analyses in patients with acute or remote myocardial infarction have shown an increased incidence of low-amplitude, high-frequency components within the QRS complex. These components are attributed to fragmentation of the depolarization front by fibrous tissue and to a decrease in electromotive force (300). The risk of ventricular arrhythmias in postinfarction patients and of cardiac death in patients with coronary artery disease or hypertrophic cardiomyopathy who have nonsustained ventricular tachycardia can be stratified on the basis of signal-averaging information (301). Although signal-averaged ECG is an interesting research tool, its clinical applications are currently limited.

BODY SURFACE MAPPING

Body surface mapping records cardiac electric events with numerous electrodes (from 16 to 200) and thus contributes additional information to that of the standard ECG. Cardiac field mapping provides details on the spatial and temporal sequence of cardiac excitation and recovery. Local intraventricular conduction disturbances, preexcitation, premature ventricular beats, and repolarization disorders can be precisely located (302). After a discriminant analysis of body torso maps derived from 120 leads in patients with various types of infarcts, the conclusion was that six torso sites accounted for a specificity of 96% and a sensitivity of 94%. Unfortunately, these sites did not coincide with any of the conventional 12-lead positions (303). Visual inspection of the ECG maps does not suffice for diagnostic purposes; sophisticated statistical and deterministic models are necessary. The difficulty in interpretation and the cumbersome recording and acquisition processes explain why the cost-effectiveness ratio for this technique is still unfavorable and confine it to the research arena.

CONTROVERSIES AND PERSONAL PERSPECTIVES

Proficiency and Accuracy in Electrocardiographic Recording and Interpretation

Perhaps because the ECG is widely available and easy to obtain, its recording and interpretation are regarded as minor tasks (92). The responsibility of ECG recording has shifted from physicians to nurses, technicians, or medical students, and cardiologists are rarely present at the time of a patient's initial evaluation. This is conducive to suboptimal ECG data collection. First, lead misplacements and noise are common (304). Second, in most acute clinical settings, only 12 ECG leads with few QRS complexes per lead are obtained. Special ECG leads and prolonged rhythm strips (other than in lead II) are underused in daily practice (305). The need to change the patient from the supine position or to use equipment beyond the standard provided with current ECG machines may be a deterrent to the addition of posterior or esophageal leads. Thus, acute myocardial infarctions, arrhythmias, and intermittent bundle branch block may remain inadequately documented.

In addition to these shortcomings of the ECG recording, interpretation may also be limited. The ever-increasing competition between electrocardiography and other procedures for the attention of the young physician may conspire against acquisition of a high level of individual competence in ECG principles and diagnosis (92). Even experienced physicians usually examine only 11 leads of the 12 available; lead aVR (and the information it may provide) is ignored (24).

The self-perception of proficiency in ECG interpretation may be overly optimistic. In a study of 100 consecutively treated cases of fatal myocardial infarction, 47% were missed throughout hospital evaluation (306). Residents in family practice programs missed acute infarctions in 21% of ECG recordings, and their expertise did not improve with the year of residence (307). General practitioners performed better in identifying normal ECGs (82% specificity) than in recognizing acute infarction (33% to 61% sensitivity) (308). Emergency physicians participating in a multicenter study classified as normal 41% of abnormal ST segments. Misreading was related to suboptimal triage and unnecessary cardiac care unit admissions (309). A study using electrocardiographer judgment as the gold standard found a 67% accuracy for family physicians versus a 91% accuracy for cardiologists (310). Because cardiologists perform better than internists (311), the specific medical training of the interpreter may play a role in diagnostic accuracy.

Although obvious ST-segment or Q-wave changes are absent in most cases of missed infarctions, approximately one-fourth of missed infarctions could be diagnosed with adequate competence in ECG reading (228,312). Fisch has suggested that the inevitable use of automated diagnoses "may be, in fact, an obstacle to the acquisition of ECG skills" (313).

Reproducibility

High variability within or between readers may put into question the validity of ECG analyses. Unfortunately, intra- and interobserver agreement rates are seldom tested or reported. Studies that systematically evaluated the reproducibility of ECG interpretations found approximately 80% intraobserver and 30% interobserver agreement rates (314–316). Discrepancies in ECG interpretation are related to the ECG waveform or interval under analysis, to variability in consecutive ECG recordings, and to the interpreter. For example, measurements of the ST segment are highly reproducible from beat to beat, but those of QT interval are not (59,226). The limb leads III, aVF, and aVL may be responsible for most intraobserver variation in the diagnosis of established infarction (314). For precordial recordings, variability is often a consequence of differences in lead placement (298). Day-to-day variability of the 12-lead ECG has been documented within normal persons and is associated with circadian influences and meal consumption (41). The role of expertise in the reproducibility of ECG interpretation is uncertain. At least among internal medicine residents, experience may be more important for intraobserver than for interobserver agreement; the latter rates may not improve after observers undergo training programs in electrocardiography (314). Comparative reproducibility between cardiologists and other physicians has been scrutinized only in limited settings and has been found to be acceptable (317).

Role of Computerized Electrocardiogram Interpretation

Computer-assisted ECG interpretation is now widely available. Ideally, automated measurements of ECG waveforms and intervals can significantly reduce physician time in ECG analysis while providing readings that are precise at the microvolt and millisecond level. In general, however, computer-derived intervals are longer than those determined visually. Reasons for the discrepancy include examination of multiple-lead versus single-lead measurements (in automated versus visual readings, respectively), and paper speed and amplification. Manual measurements performed with an amplification factor of 10 or 20 produce significantly wider intervals, similar to computer-derived results (45). Many computer programs apply longer-than-standard upper and lower normal limits for ECG intervals (e.g.,

THE FUTURE

The clinical use of the ECG has withstood the passage of time, and the contribution of ECG information to the care of cardiac patients remains unique. Despite the development of more sophisticated and expensive noninvasive diagnostic and prognostic techniques, the ECG is still the initial (and sometimes the only) test demonstrating cardiovascular abnormalities. Medical education must emphasize the value of the ECG, however. Systematic instruction and supervised practice in ECG diagnosis are fundamental to maintain proficiency in ECG interpretation.

Current emphasis in ECG research is on the study of dynamic patterns inherent in certain parameters (especially ventricular repolarization) with the aid of ambulatory recordings and newer, potent digital storage and analysis techniques. Correlation of findings from the ECG with those from emerging techniques such as electromechanical left ventricular mapping (which displays a color-coded map of the activation process) may help to further understanding of newly described ECG patterns (322).

Attempts to improve the resolution of standard electrocardiography have relied on an increase in the number of recording electrodes (body surface mapping) and on an improvement in the signal-to-noise ratio of the higher-frequency signals by averaging and filtering (signal-averaged ECG). Initial results with these techniques are promising, but their roles in clinical practice are still unclear.

The advent of effective myocardial reperfusion therapies has renewed the interest in the ECG manifestations of the acute ischemic syndromes. More recently, wireless technology is allowing the transmission of 12-lead ECG waveforms from remote locations to cardiologists' handheld computers. Because intraobserver agreement among cardiologists is high when interpreting both paper ECGs and their liquid-crystal–displayed counterparts, remote interpretation may become widely adopted and contribute to decreased time to treatment for patients in need of reperfusion or those with complex arrhythmias (26).

Overall, the standard 12-lead ECG will continue to expand in clinical importance and will remain an integral part of the evaluation of all cardiac patients, particularly those with ischemic heart disease or rhythm disturbances.

---

minimum PR = 130 ms; maximum QRS complex = 0.126 ms) (318). Additional limitations of computerized readings include minute-to-minute variability, inability to determine the anteroposterior direction of electrical forces, and discrepant measurements among programs (319–321). Automated diagnoses (e.g., "left ventricular hypertrophy") may be less reliable and accurate than automated raw measurements, because the rapid expansion of ECG digital technology during the 1980s outpaced most efforts to evaluate the quality of the product (53). Many diagnostic programs in electrocardiographs are now 25 years old (313). An investigation of commonly used ECG software found a variety of systematic errors. The accuracy rate for clinically validated ECG diagnoses of myocardial infarction or left ventricular hypertrophy was 70% for computer analysis versus 76% for visual readings by cardiologists (315,321).

Further refinement in automated ECG interpretation is expected in the near future. At present, computer-analyzed ECGs require overreading by an experienced cardiologist.

REFERENCES

1. Waller AD. A demonstration in man of electromotive changes accompanying the heart's beat. *J Physiol (Lond)* 1887;8:229–234.

2. Cooper JK. Electrocardiography 100 years ago. Origins, pioneers, and contributors. *N Engl J Med* 1986;315:461–464.

3. Shapiro E. The first textbook of electrocardiography. Thomas Lewis: clinical electrocardiography. *J Am Coll Cardiol* 1983;1:1160–1161.

4. Barker LF. Electrocardiography and phonocardiography: a collective review. *Bull Johns Hopkins Hosp* 1910;21:358–389.

5. Fleckenstein K. The early ECG in medical practice. *Med Instrum* 1984;18:191–192.

6. Surawicz B. Introduction: historical outline. In: *Electrophysiologic basis of ECG and cardiac arrhythmias*. Baltimore: Williams & Wilkins, 1995:3–12.

7. Kyle RA, Sampo MA. Frank Wilson. *JAMA* 1983;250:2680.

8. Wilson FN, Johnston FD, Rosenbaum F, et al. The precordial electrocardiogram. *Am Heart J* 1944;27:19–85.

9. Herrick JB. An intimate account of my early experience with coronary thrombosis. *Am Heart J* 1944;27:1–18.

10. Pardee HEB. An electrocardiographic sign of coronary artery obstruction. *Arch Intern Med* 1920;26:244–257.

11. Wilson FN. Disorders of the heartbeat and cardiac failure. *South Med J* 1936;29:397–400.

12. Barold SS, Fisch C, Schamroth L, et al. Richard Langendorf: 1908–1987. *Pacing Clin Electrophysiol* 1988;11:1242–1247.

13. Rosenbaum MB, Elizari MV, eds. *Frontiers of cardiac electrophysiology*. Boston: Martinus Nijhoff, 1983.

14. Grant RP. The relationship between the anatomic position of the heart and the electrocardiogram. A criticism of "unipolar" electrocardiography. *Circulation* 1953;7:890–902.

15. Mall FP. On the development of the human heart. *Am J Anat* 1912;13:249.

16. Rushmer RF. Functional anatomy and the control of the heart, part I. In: Rushmer RF, ed. *Cardiovascular dynamics.* Philadelphia: WB Saunders, 1976:76–104.

17. Goldberger E. A simple indifferent, electrocardiographic electrode of zero potential and a technique of obtaining augmented, unipolar, extremity leads. *Am Heart J* 1942;23:483.

18. Rautaharju PM. The inappropriateness of the commonly used augmentation and lead-recording sequence for ECG analysis. *Practical Cardiol* 1982;8:120–139.

19. Rautaharju PM, Warren J, Seale D, et al. Exploitation of the redundancy of the conventional limb lead electrocardiograms for prolongation of the record length. *J Electrocardiol* 1981;14:39–41.

20. Anderson ST, Pahlm O, Selvester RH, et al. Panoramic display of the orderly sequenced 12-lead ECG. *J Electrocardiol* 1994;27:347–352.

21. Khaw K, Moreyra AE, Tannenbaum AK, et al. Improved detection of posterior myocardial ischemia with the 15-lead electrocardiogram. *Am Heart J* 1999;138:934–940.

22. Zalenski RJ, Rydman RJ, Sloan EP, et al. Value of posterior and right ventricular leads in comparison to the standard 12-lead electrocardiogram in evaluation of ST segment elevation in suspected acute myocardial infarction. *Am J Cardiol* 1997;79:1579–1585.

23. Menown IBA, Adgey AAJ. Improving the ECG classification of inferior and lateral myocardial infarction by inversion of lead aVR. *Heart* 2000;83:657–660.

24. Pahlm US, Pahlm O, Wagner GS. The standard 11-lead ECG. Neglect of lead aVR in the classical limb lead display. *J Electrocardiol* 1996;29:270–274.

25. Bailey JJ, Berson AS, Garson A Jr, et al. Recommendations for standardization and specifications in automated electrocardiography: bandwidth and digital signal processing. A report for health professionals by an ad hoc writing group of the Committee on Electrocardiography and Cardiac Electrophysiology of the Council on Clinical Cardiology, American Heart Association. *Circulation* 1990;81:730–739.

26. Pettis KS, Savona MR, Leibrandt PN, et al. Evaluation of the efficacy of hand-held computer screens for cardiologists' interpretations of 12-lead electrocardiograms. *Am Heart J* 1999;138:765–770.

27. Surawicz B. *Electrophysiologic basis of ECG and cardiac arrhythmias.* Baltimore: Williams & Wilkins, 1995.

28. Antzelevitch C, Sicouri S, Lukas A, et al. Regional differences in the electrophysiology of ventricular cells: physiological and clinical implications. In: Zipes DP, Jalife J, eds. *Cardiac electrophysiology: from cell to bedside*, 2nd ed. Philadelphia: WB Saunders, 1995:228–245.

29. Wilson FN, Macleod AG, Barker PS. The T deflection of the electrocardiogram. *Trans Assoc Am Physicians* 1931; 46:29–38.

30. Franz MR, Bargheer K, Costard-Jäckle A, et al. Human ventricular repolarization and T wave genesis. *Prog Cardiovasc Dis* 1991;33:369–384.

31. Massing GK, James TN. Anatomical configuration of the His bundle and bundle branches in the human heart. *Circulation* 1976;53:609–621.

32. Rosenbaum MB, Elizari MV, Lazzari JO. *Los hemibloqueos.* Buenos Aires, Argentina: Paidos, 1968:442–464.

33. Uhley HN. Some controversy regarding the peripheral distribution of the conduction system. *Am J Cardiol* 1972;30:919–920.

34. Anderson RH, Ho SY, Wharton J, et al. Gross anatomy and microscopy of the conducting system. In: Mandel WJ, ed. *Cardiac arrhythmias. Their mechanisms, diagnosis, and management.* Philadelphia: JB Lippincott Co, 1995:13–54.

35. Scher AM. The sequence of ventricular excitation. *Am J Cardiol* 1964;14:287.

36. Franz MR, Bargheer K, Rafflenbeul W, et al. Monophasic action potential mapping in human subjects with normal electrocardiograms: direct evidence for the genesis of the T wave. *Circulation* 1987;75:379–386.

37. Chou TC. When is the vectorcardiogram superior to the scalar electrocardiogram? *J Am Coll Cardiol* 1986;8:791–799.

38. Barr, RC. Genesis of the electrocardiogram. In: Macfarlane PW, Lawrie TD, eds. *Comprehensive electrocardiology,* vol I. New York: Pergamon Press, 1989:139–147.

39. Wanderman KL, Loutaty G, Ovyshcher I, et al. Choice of electrocardiographic leads for recording the earliest QRS onset in noninvasive measurements. *Circulation* 1981;63: 933–937.

40. Surawicz B. Stretching the limits of the electrocardiogram's diagnostic utility. *J Am Coll Cardiol* 1998;32:483–485.

41. Macfarlane PW, Lawrie TD. The normal electrocardiogram and vectorcardiogram. In: Macfarlane PW, Lawrie TD, eds. *Comprehensive electrocardiology*, vol I. New York: Pergamon Press, 1989:451–452.

42. Morgera T, Alberti E, Silvestri F, et al. Right precordial ST and QRS changes in the diagnosis of right ventricular infarction. *Am Heart J* 1984;108:13–18.

43. Feola M, Ribichini F, Gallone G, et al. Analysis of right electrocardiographic leads in 195 normal subjects. *G Ital Cardiol* 1994;24:375–379.

44. Feldman T, Borow KM, Neumann A, et al. Relation of electrocardiographic R-wave amplitude to changes in left ventricular chamber size and position in normal subjects. *Am J Cardiol* 1985;55:1168–1174.

45. Willems JL, Robles De Medina EO, Bernard R, et al. Criteria for intraventricular conduction disturbances and pre-excitation. *J Am Coll Cardiol* 1985;5:1261–1275.

46. Burgess MJ, Millar K, Abildskov JA. Cancellation of electrocardiographic effects during ventricular recovery. *J Electrocardiol* 1969;2:101–107.

47. Lepeschkin E. The U wave of the electrocardiogram. *Mod Concept Cardiovasc Dis* 1969;38:39–45.

48. Antzelevitch C, Sicouri S. Clinical relevance of cardiac arrhythmias generated by afterdepolarizations. Role of M cells in the generation of U waves, triggered activity and torsade de pointes. *J Am Coll Cardiol* 1994;23:259–277.

49. Surawicz B. U wave: facts, hypotheses, misconceptions, and misnomers. *J Cardiovasc Electrophysiol* 1998;9:1117–1128.

50. Bidoggia H, Maciel JP, Capalozza N, et al. Sex differences on the electrocardiographic pattern of cardiac repolarization: possible role of testosterone. *Am Heart J* 2000;140:678–683.

51. Sgarbossa EB, Pinski SL, Williams D, et al. Comparison of QT intervals in African-Americans versus Caucasians. *Am J Cardiol* 2000;86:880–882.

52. Campbell RWF, Gardiner P, Amos PA, et al. Measurement of the QT interval. *Eur Heart J* 1985;6[Suppl D]:81–83.

53. The CSE Working Party. Recommendations for measurement standards in quantitative electrocardiography. *Eur Heart J* 1985;6:815–825.

54. Garson A Jr. How to measure the QT interval. What is normal? *Am J Cardiol* 1993;72:148–168.

55. Moss AJ. Measurement of the QT interval and the risk associated with QTc interval prolongation: a review. *Am J Cardiol* 1993;72:23B–25B.

56. Schamroth L. The QT interval. In: *An introduction to electrocardiography*. Oxford: Blackwell Scientific Publications, 1982:26–30.

57. Ahnve S. Errors in the visual determination of corrected QT (QTc) interval during acute myocardial infarction. *J Am Coll Cardiol* 1985;5:699–702.

58. Surawicz B, Knoebel S. Long QT: good, bad or indifferent? *J Am Coll Cardiol* 1984;4:398–413.

59. Kautzner J, Yi G, Camm AJ, et al. Short- and long-term reproducibility of QT, QTc, and QT dispersion measurement in healthy subjects. *Pacing Clin Electrophysiol* 1994;17:928–937.

60. Lepeschkin E, Surawicz B. The measurement of the QT-interval of the electrocardiogram. *Circulation* 1958;6:378–388.

61. Merri M, Benhorin J, Alberti M, et al. Electrocardiographic quantitation of ventricular repolarization. *Circulation* 1989;80:1301–1308.

62. Puddu PE, Bernard PM, Chaitman BR, et al. QT interval measurement by a computer assisted program: a potentially useful clinical parameter. *J Electrocardiol* 1982;15:15–22.

63. Bazett HC. An analysis of the time relations of electrocardiograms. *Heart* 1920;7:353–370.

64. Sarma JSM, Sarma RJ, Bilitch M, et al. An exponential formula for heart rate dependence of QT interval during exercise and cardiac pacing in humans: reevaluation of Bazett's formula. *Am J Cardiol* 1984;54:103–108.

65. Macfarlane PW, Lawrie TD, eds. *Comprehensive electrocardiology; theory and practice in health and disease*, vol 3. New York: Pergamon Press, 1989:1442.

66. Adams W. The normal duration of the electrocardiographic ventricular complex. *J Clin Invest* 1936;15:335–342.

67. Ashman R. The normal duration of the QT interval. *Am Heart J* 1942;23:522–534.

68. Rautaharju PM, Zhou SH, Wong S, et al. Functional characteristics of QT prediction formulas. The concepts of QT_{max} and QT rate sensitivity. *Computers Biomed Res* 1993;26:188–204.

69. Spodick DH, Rifkin R, Rajasingh MC. Effect of self-correlation on the relation between QT interval and cardiac cycle length. *Am Heart J* 1990;120:157–160.

70. Karjalainen J, Viitasalo M, Mäntäri M, et al. Relation between QT intervals and heart rates from 40 to 120 beats per minute in rest electrocardiograms of men and a simple method to adjust QT interval values. *J Am Coll Cardiol* 1994;23:1547–1553.

71. Laks MM. Long QT interval syndrome. A new look at an old electrocardiographic measurement. The power of the computer. *Circulation* 1990;82:1539–1541.

72. Higham PD, Campbell RWF. QT dispersion. *Br Heart J* 1994;71:508–510.

73. Fei L, Statters DJ, Camm AJ. QT-interval dispersion on 12-lead ECG in normal subjects: its reproducibility and relation to the T wave. *Am Heart J* 1994;127:1654–1655.

74. Sylvén JC, Horacek BM, Spencer CA, et al. QT interval variability on the body surface. *J Electrocardiol* 1984;17:179–188.

75. Krahn AD, Nguyen-Ho P, Klein GJ, et al. QT dispersion: an electrocardiographic derivative of QT prolongation. *Am Heart J* 2001;141:111–116.

76. Talreja D, Gruver C, Sklenar J, et al. Efficient utilization of echocardiography for the assessment of left ventricular systolic function. *Am Heart J* 2000;139:394–398.

77. Hiss RG, Lamb LE. Electrocardiographic findings in 122,043 individuals. *Circulation* 1962;25:947–961.

78. Chou TC. Normal electrocardiogram. In: Chou TE, ed. *Electrocardiography in clinical practice. Adult and pediatric.* Philadelphia: WB Saunders, 1996:3–22.

79. Brady WJ. Benign early repolarization: electrocardiographic manifestations and differentiation from other ST segment elevation syndromes. *Am J Emerg Med* 1998;16:592–597.

80. Spodick DH. Differential characteristics of the electrocardiogram in early repolarization and acute pericarditis. *N Engl J Med* 1976;295:523–526.

81. Haydar ZR, Brantley DA, Gittings NS, et al. Early repolarization: an electrocardiographic predictor of enhanced aerobic fitness. *Am J Cardiol* 2000;85:264–266.

82. Brugada P, Brugada J. Right bundle branch block, persistent ST segment elevation and sudden cardiac death: a distinct clinical and electrocardiographic syndrome. A multicenter report. *J Am Coll Cardiol* 1992;20:1391–1396.

83. Atarashi H, Ogawa S, Harumi K, et al. Characteristics of patients with right bundle branch block and ST segment elevation in right precordial leads. *Am J Cardiol* 1996;78:581–583.

84. Brugada J, Brugada P, Brugada R. El síndrome de Brugada y las miocardiopatías derechas como causa de muerte súbita. Diferencias y similitudes. *Rev Esp Cardiol* 2000;53:275–285.

85. Corrado D, Basso C, Buja G, et al. Right bundle branch block, right precordial ST segment elevation, and sudden death in young people. *Circulation* 2001;103:710–717.

86. Gussak I, Antzelevitch C. Early repolarization syndrome: clinical characteristics and possible cellular and ionic mechanisms. *J Electrocardiol* 2000;33:299–309.

87. Littman D. Abnormal electrocardiogram in the absence of demonstrable heart disease. *Am J Med* 1948;5:337.

88. Greene CE, Kelly JJ. Electrocardiogram of the healthy adult Negro. *Circulation* 1959;20:906–909.

89. Sears GA, Manning GW. Routine electrocardiography: postprandial T-wave changes. *Am Heart J* 1958;56:591–597.

90. Surawicz B. T wave abnormalities. In: Rosenbaum M, Elizari MV, eds. *Frontiers of electrocardiography*. Boston: Martinus Nijhoff, 1983:40–66.

91. Watanabe Y, Toda H, Nishimura M. Clinical electrocardiographic studies of bifid T waves. *Br Heart J* 1984;52:207–214.

92. Fisch C. Evolution of clinical electrocardiogram. *J Am Coll Cardiol* 1989;14:1127–1138.

93. Sackett DL, Haynes RB, Guyatt GH, et al. The selection of diagnostic tests. In: *Clinical epidemiology. A basic science for clinical medicine*, 2nd ed. Boston: Little, Brown and Company, 1991:51–68.

94. Hulley SB, Cummings SR. Planning the measurements: precision and accuracy. In: Hulley SB, Cummings SR, eds. *Designing clinical research*. Baltimore: Williams & Wilkins, 1988:31–41.

95. Rose G, Baxter PJ, Reid DD, et al. Prevalence and prognosis of electrocardiographic findings in middle aged men. *Br Heart J* 1978;40:636–643.

96. Sackett DL, Haynes RB, Guyatt GH, et al. The interpretation of diagnostic data. In: *Clinical epidemiology. A basic science for clinical medicine*, 2nd ed. Boston: Little, Brown and Company, 1991:69–152.

97. Shlipak MG, Lyons WL, Go AS, et al. Should the electrocardiogram be used to guide therapy for patients with left bundle-branch block and suspected myocardial infarction? *JAMA* 1999;281:714–719.

98. Ostrander LD Jr. Left axis deviation: prevalence, associated conditions, and prognosis. An epidemiologic study. *Ann Intern Med* 1971;75:23–28.

99. Kaplan JD, Evans T Jr, Foster E, et al. Evaluation of electrocardiographic criteria for right atrial enlargement by quantitative two-dimensional echocardiography. *J Am Coll Cardiol* 1994;23:747–752.

100. Sgarbossa EB, Pinski SL, Stevenson J, et al. Diagnosis of "true" right atrial enlargement: how useful are the classical ECG signs? *J Am Coll Cardiol* 2001;27[Suppl A]:115A.

101. Romhilt DW, Bove KE, Conradi S, et al. Morphologic significance of left atrial involvement. *Am Heart J* 1972;83:322–327.

102. Scott CC, Leier CV, Kilman JW, et al. The effect of atrial histology and dimension on P wave morphology. *J Electrocardiol* 1983;16:363–366.

103. Alpman A, Güldal M, Berkalp B, et al. Importance of notching and slurring of the resting QRS complex in the diagnosis of coronary artery disease. *J Electrocardiol* 1995;28:199–208.

104. Walston A, Brewer DL, Kitchens CS, et al. The electrocardiographic manifestations of spontaneous left pneumothorax. *Ann Intern Med* 1974;80:375–379.

105. Goldberger A. Normal and noninfarct Q waves. *Cardiol Clin* 1987;5:357–366.

106. Bär FW, Brugada P, Dassen WR, et al. Prognostic value of Q waves, R/S ratio, loss of R wave voltage, ST-T segment abnormalities, electrical axis, low voltage and notching: correlation of electrocardiogram and left ventriculogram. *J Am Coll Cardiol* 1984;4:17–27.

107. Schouten EG, Dekker JM, Meppelink P, et al. QT interval prolongation predicts cardiovascular mortality in an apparently healthy population. *Circulation* 1991;84:1516–1523.

108. Bijl M, Verheugt FW. Extreme QT prolongation solely due to reversible myocardial ischemia in single-vessel coronary disease. *Am Heart J* 1992;123:524–526.

109. Dritsas A, Sbarouni E, Gilligan D, et al. QT-interval abnormalities in hypertrophic cardiomyopathy. *Clin Cardiol* 1992;15:739–742.

110. Oka H, Mochio S, Sato K, et al. Correlation of altered QT interval and sympathetic nervous system dysfunction in diabetic autonomic neuropathy. *Eur Neurol* 1994;34:23–29.

111. Hanrahan JP, Choo PW, Carlson W, et al. Terfenadine-associated ventricular arrhythmias and QTc interval prolongation. A retrospective cohort comparison with other antihistamines among members of a health maintenance organization. *Ann Epidemiol* 1995;5:201–209.

112. Woosley RL. Drugs that prolong the QT interval and/or induce torsades de pointes. Available at: http://www.torsades.org. Accessed Nov. 13, 2001.

113. Moss AJ, Zareba W, Benhorin J, et al. ECG T-wave patterns in genetically distinct forms of the hereditary long QT syndrome. *Circulation* 1995;92:2929–2934.

114. Malfatto G, Beria G, Sala S, et al. Quantitative analysis of T wave abnormalities and their prognostic implications in the idiopathic QT syndrome. *J Am Coll Cardiol* 1994;23:296–301.

115. Rosenbaum MB, Acunzo RS. Pseudo 2:1 atrioventricular block and T wave alternans in long QT syndromes. *J Am Coll Cardiol* 1991;18:1363–1366.

116. Zareba W, Moss AJ, le Cessie S, et al. T wave alternans in idiopathic long QT syndrome. *J Am Coll Cardiol* 1994;23:1541–1546.

117. Sgarbossa EB, Meyer PM, Pinski SL, et al. Negative T waves shortly after ST-elevation acute myocardial infarction are a powerful marker for improved survival. *Am Heart J* 2000;140:385–394.

118. Mobilia G, Zanco P, Desideri A, et al. T wave normalization in infarct-related ECG leads during exercise testing for detection of residual viability: comparison in PET. *J Am Coll Cardiol* 1998;32:75–82.

119. Tamura A, Nagase K, Mikuriya Y, et al. Significance of spontaneous normalization of negative T waves in infarct-related leads during healing of anterior wall acute myocardial infarction. *Am J Cardiol* 1999;84:1341–1344.

120. Alfonso F, Nihoyannopoulos P, Stewart J, et al. Clinical significance of giant negative T waves in hypertrophic cardiomyopathy. *J Am Coll Cardiol* 1990;15:965–971.

121. Otrusinik R, Alpert M, Hamm CR, et al. Factors predicting coronary artery disease in patients with giant negative T waves. *Am J Cardiol* 2000;85:873–875.

122. Navarro-López F, Cinca J, Sanz G, et al. Isolated T wave alternans. *Am Heart J* 1978;95:369–373.

123. Bardají A, Vidal F, Richart C. T wave alternans associated with amiodarone. *J Electrocardiol* 1993;26:155–157.

124. Rosenbaum MB, Blanco HH, Elizari MV, et al. Electrotonic modulation of the T wave and cardiac memory. *Am J Cardiol* 1982;50:213–222.

125. Engel JR, Shah R, DePodesta LA, et al. T wave abnormalities of intermittent left bundle branch block. *Ann Intern Med* 1978;89:204–206.

126. Helguera ME, Pinski SL, Sterba R, et al. Memory T waves after radiofrequency ablation of accessory atrioventricular

connections in the WPW syndrome. *J Electrocardiol* 1994;27:243–249.

127. Reddy GV, Schamroth L, Schamroth CL. Tall and peaked U waves in hypokalemia. *Chest* 1987;91:605–607.

128. Kishida H, Cole JS, Surawicz B. Negative U wave: a highly specific but poorly understood sign of heart disease. *Am J Cardiol* 1982;49:2030–2036.

129. Surawicz B, Fisch C. Cardiac alternans: diverse mechanisms and clinical manifestations. *J Am Coll Cardiol* 1992;20:483–499.

130. Tighe DA, Chung EK, Park CH. Electric alternans associated with acute pulmonary embolism. *Am Heart J* 1994;128:188–190.

131. Devereux RB, Reichek N. Repolarization abnormalities of left ventricular hypertrophy. *J Electrocardiol* 1982;15:47.

132. Casale PN, Devereux RB, Kligfield P, et al. Electrocardiographic detection of left ventricular hypertrophy: development and prospective validation of improved criteria. *J Am Coll Cardiol* 1985;6:572–589.

133. Browne PJ, Shridhar S, Desser KB, et al. Hypertrophy or dilation? A vectorial analysis of echocardiographically determined left ventricular enlargement. *J Electrocardiol* 1978;11:117–122.

134. Romhilt DW, Bove KE, Norris RJ, et al. A critical appraisal of the electrocardiographic criteria for the diagnosis of left ventricular hypertrophy. *Circulation* 1969;40:185–195.

135. Okin PM, Roman MJ, Devereux RB, et al. Electrocardiographic identification of left ventricular mass by simple voltage-duration products. *J Am Coll Cardiol* 1995;25:417–423.

136. Devereux RB, Koren MJ, de Simone G, et al. Methods for detection of left ventricular hypertrophy: application to hypertensive heart disease. *Eur Heart J* 1993;14[Suppl D]:8–15.

137. Casale PN, Devereux RB, Alonso DR, et al. Improved sex-specific criteria of left ventricular hypertrophy for clinical and computer interpretation of electrocardiograms: validation with autopsy findings. *Circulation* 1987;75:565–572.

138. Schillaci G, Verdecchia P, Borgioni C, et al. Improved electrocardiographic diagnosis of left ventricular hypertrophy. *Am J Cardiol* 1994;74:714–719.

139. Okin PM, Roman MJ, Devereux RB, et al. Electrocardiographic identification of left ventricular hypertrophy: test performance in relation to definition of hypertrophy and presence of obesity. *J Am Coll Cardiol* 1996;27:124–131.

140. Mehta A, Jain AC, Mehta MC, et al. Usefulness of left atrial abnormality for predicting left ventricular hypertrophy in the presence of left bundle branch block. *Am J Cardiol* 2000;85:354–359.

141. Devereux RB, Casale PN, Eisenberg RR, et al. Electrocardiographic detection of left ventricular hypertrophy using echocardiogram determination of left ventricular mass as the reference standard: comparison of standard criteria, computer diagnosis and physician interpretation. *J Am Coll Cardiol* 1984;3:82–87.

142. Xie X, Liu K, Stamler J, et al. Ethnic differences in electrocardiographic left ventricular hypertrophy in young and middle-aged employed American men. *Am J Cardiol* 1994;73:564–567.

143. Pellicia A, Spataro A, Caselli G, et al. Absence of left ventricular wall thickening in athletes in intense power training. *Am J Cardiol* 1993;72:1048–1054.

144. Fragola PV, Colivicchi F, Fabrizi E, et al. Assessment of left ventricular hypertrophy in patients with essential hypertension. A rational basis for the electrocardiogram. *Am J Hypertens* 1993;6:164–169.

145. Xiao HB, Brecker SJD, Gibson DG. Relative effects of left ventricular mass and conduction disturbance on activation in patients with pathological left ventricular hypertrophy. *Br Heart J* 1994;71:548–553.

146. Klein RC, Vera Z, De Maria AN, et al. Electrocardiographic diagnosis of left ventricular hypertrophy in the presence of left bundle branch block. *Am Heart J* 1984;108:502–506.

147. Kafka H, Burggraf GW, Milliken JA. Electrocardiographic diagnosis of left ventricular hypertrophy in the presence of left bundle branch block: an echocardiographic study. *Am J Cardiol* 1985;55:103–106.

148. Gertsch M, Theler A, Foglia E. Electrocardiographic detection of left ventricular hypertrophy in the presence of left anterior fascicular block. *Am J Cardiol* 1988;61:1098–1101.

149. Vandenberg B, Sagar K, Paulsen W, et al. Electrocardiographic criteria for diagnosis of left ventricular hypertrophy in the presence of complete right bundle branch block. *Am J Cardiol* 1989;63:1080–1084.

150. Murphy ML, Thenabadu N, de Soyza N, et al. Left atrial abnormality as an electrocardiographic criterion for the diagnosis of left ventricular hypertrophy in the presence of right bundle branch block. *Am J Cardiol* 1983;52:381–383.

151. Mehta A, Jain AC, Morise AP, et al. Left atrial abnormality by electrocardiogram predicts left ventricular hypertrophy by echocardiography in the presence of right bundle branch block. *Clin Cardiol* 1998;21:109–114.

152. Selzer A. Approach to diagnosis. In: *Principles and practice of clinical cardiology*. Philadelphia: WB Saunders, 1983:7–13.

153. Sokolow M, Lyon TP. The ventricular complex in right ventricular hypertrophy as obtained by unipolar precordial and limb leads. *Am Heart J* 1949;38:273.

154. Myers GB, Klein HA, Stoffer BE. The electrocardiographic diagnosis of right ventricular hypertrophy. *Am Heart J* 1948;35:1.

155. Surawicz B. Electrocardiographic diagnosis of chamber enlargement. *J Am Coll Cardiol* 1986;8:711–724.

156. Pagnoni A, Goodwin JF. The cardiographic diagnosis of combined ventricular hypertrophy. *Br Heart J* 1952;14:451.

157. Das G. Left axis deviation: a spectrum of intraventricular conduction block. *Circulation* 1976;53:917–919.

158. Varriale P, Chryssos BE. The RSR' complex not related to right bundle branch block: diagnostic value as a sign of myocardial infarction scar. *Am Heart J* 1992;123:369–376.

159. Rosenbaum MB, Elizari MV, Lazzari JO. *The hemiblocks*. Oldsmar, FL: Tampa Tracings, 1970.

160. Davies MJ, Anderson RH, Becker AE. Pathology of bundle branch block. In: *The conduction system of the heart*. Boston: Butterworth, 1983:281–300.

161. Yano K, Peskoe SM, Rhoads GG, et al. Left axis deviation and left anterior hemiblock among 8,000 Japanese-American men. *Am J Cardiol* 1975;35:809–815.

162. Warner RA, Hill NE, Mookherjee S, et al. Improved electrocardiographic criteria for the diagnosis of left anterior hemiblock. *Am J Cardiol* 1983;51:718–722.

163. Demoulin JC, Kulbertus HE. Histopathologic correlates of left posterior fascicular block. *Am J Cardiol* 1979;44:1083–1088.

164. Rosenbaum MB. The hemiblocks: diagnostic criteria and clinical significance. *Mod Concepts Cardiovasc Dis* 1970;39:141–146.

165. Dhala A, González-Zuelgaray J, Deshpande S, et al. Unmasking the trifascicular left intraventricular conduction system by ablation of the right bundle branch. *Am J Cardiol* 1996;77:706–712.

166. Demoulin JC, Kulbertus HE. Histopathological examination of concept of left hemiblock. *Br Heart J* 1972;34:807–814.

167. Nakaya Y, Hiasa Y, Murayama Y, et al. Prominent anterior QRS force as a manifestation of left septal fascicular block. *J Electrocardiol* 1978;11:39–46.

168. Uhley H. The quadrifascicular nature of the peripheral conduction system in cardiac arrhythmias. In: Dreifus LS, Likoff W, eds. *Cardiac arrhythmias.* New York: Grune & Stratton, 1973:339–348.

169. Reiffel JA, Bigger JT. Pure anterior conduction delay: a variant "fascicular" defect. *J Electrocardiol* 1978;11:315–319.

170. Selvester RH, Wagner NB, Wagner GS. Ventricular excitation during percutaneous transluminal angioplasty of the left anterior descending coronary artery. *Am J Cardiol* 1988;62:1116–1121.

171. Wagner NB, Sevilla DC, Krucoff MK, et al. Transient alterations of the QRS complex and ST segment during percutaneous transluminal balloon angioplasty of the left anterior descending coronary artery. *Am J Cardiol* 1988;62:1038–1042.

172. Gambetta M, Childers RW. Rate-dependent right precordial Q waves: "septal focal block." *Am J Cardiol* 1973;32:196–201.

173. Dhingra RC, Amat-Y-Leon F, Wyndham C, et al. Significance of left axis deviation in patients with chronic left bundle branch block. *Am J Cardiol* 1978;42:551–556.

174. Schneider JF, Thomas HE, McNamara PM, et al. Clinical-electrocardiographic correlates of newly acquired left bundle branch block: the Framingham study. *Am J Cardiol* 1985;55:1332–1338.

175. Swiryn S, Abben R, Denes P, et al. Electrocardiographic determinants of axis during left bundle branch block: study in patients with intermittent left bundle branch block. *Am J Cardiol* 1980;46:53–58.

176. Fahy GJ, Pinski SL, Miller DP, et al. Natural history of isolated bundle branch block. *Am J Cardiol* 1996;77:1185–1190.

177. Freedman RA, Alderman EI, Sheffield LT, et al., and CASS investigators. Bundle branch block in patients with chronic coronary artery disease: angiographic correlates and prognostic significance. *J Am Coll Cardiol* 1987;10:73–80.

178. Barold SS. ACC/AHA guidelines for implantation of cardiac pacemakers: how accurate are the definitions of atrioventricular and intraventricular conduction blocks? *Pacing Clin Electrophysiol* 1993;16:1221–1225.

179. Chen CM, Damato AN. Contribution of His bundle recordings to aberrant intraventricular conduction. In: Rosenbaum MB, Elizari MV, eds. *Frontiers of cardiac electrophysiology.* Boston: Martinus Nijhoff, 1983:627–656.

180. Castellanos A, Sung RJ, Mendoza IJ, et al. Pseudo bundle branch block produced by premature impulses arising in the bundle branches. *Am J Cardiol* 1977;40:641–646.

181. Sclarovsky S, ed. *Electrocardiography of acute myocardial ischemic syndromes.* London: Martin Dunitz, 1999.

182. Figueras J, Cinca J, Gutiérrez L, et al. Prolonged angina pectoris and persistent negative T waves in the precordial leads: response to atrial pacing and to methoxamine-induced hypertension. *Am J Cardiol* 1983;51:1599–1607.

183. Wagner GS, Wagner NB. The 12-lead ECG and the extent of myocardium at risk of acute infarction: anatomic relationships among coronary, Purkinje, and myocardial anatomy. In: Califf, RM. *Acute coronary care in the thrombolytic era.* Chicago: Year Book, 1988:20–21.

184. Birnbaum Y, Maynard C, Wolfe S, et al. Terminal QRS distortion on admission is better than ST-segment measurements in predicting final infarct size and assessing the potential effect of thrombolytic therapy in anterior wall acute myocardial infarction. *Am J Cardiol* 1999;84:530–534.

185. Reimer KA, Ideker RE. Myocardial ischemia and infarction: anatomic and biochemical substrates for ischemic cell death and ventricular arrhythmias. *Hum Pathol* 1987;18:462–475.

186. Essen RV, Merx W, Effert S. Spontaneous course of ST-segment elevation in acute myocardial infarction. *Circulation* 1979;59:105–112.

187. Bren GB, Wasserman AG, Ross AM. The electrocardiogram in patients undergoing thrombolysis for myocardial infarction. *Circulation* 1987;76[Suppl II]:18–24.

188. Justis DL, Hession WT. Accuracy of 22-lead ECG analysis for diagnosis of acute myocardial infarction and coronary artery disease in the emergency department: a comparison with 12-lead ECG. *Ann Emerg Med* 1992;21:1–9.

189. Roberts WC, Gardin JM. Location of myocardial infarcts: a confusion of terms and definitions. *Am J Cardiol* 1978;42:868–872.

190. Elko PP, Weaver WD, Kudenchuk P, et al. The dilemma of sensitivity versus specificity in computer-interpreted acute myocardial infarction. *J Electrocardiol* 1992;24[Suppl]:2–7.

191. Cairns CB, Niemann JT, Selker HP, et al. Computerized version of the time-insensitive predictive instrument. *J Electrocardiol* 1992;24[Suppl]:46–49.

192. O'Rourke MF, Cook A, Carroll G, et al. Accuracy of a portable interpretive ECG machine in diagnosis of acute evolving myocardial infarction. *Aust N Z J Med* 1992;22:9–13.

193. Birnbaum Y, Sclarovsky S, Solodky A, et al. Prediction of the level of left anterior descending coronary artery obstruction during anterior wall acute myocardial infarction by the admission electrocardiogram. *Am J Cardiol* 1993;72:823–826.

194. Tamura A, Kataoka H, Mikuriya Y, et al. Inferior ST-segment depression as a useful marker for identifying proximal left anterior descending coronary artery occlusion during acute myocardial infarction. *Eur Heart J* 1995;16:1795–1799.

195. Aldrich HR, Hindman NB, Hinoara T, et al. Identification of optimal electrocardiographic leads for detecting acute epicardial injury in acute myocardial infarction. *Am J Cardiol* 1987;59:20–23.

196. Engelen DJ, Gorgels AP, Cheriex EC, et al. Value of the electrocardiogram in localizing the occlusion site in the left anterior descending coronary artery in acute myocardial infarction. *J Am Coll Cardiol* 1999;34:389–395.

197. Yotsukura M, Toyofuku M, Tajino K, et al. Clinical significance of the disappearance of septal Q waves after the onset of myocardial infarction: correlation with location of responsible coronary lesions. *J Electrocardiol* 1999;32:15–20.

198. Tamura A, Kataoka H, Mikuriya Y. Electrocardiographic findings in a patient with pure septal infarction. *Br Heart J* 1991;65:166–167.

199. Ben-Gal T, Sclarovsky S, Herz I, et al. Importance of the conal branch of the right coronary artery in patients with acute anterior wall myocardial infarction: electrocardiographic and angiographic correlation. *J Am Coll Cardiol* 1997;29:506–511.

200. Braat SH, Brugada P, Den Dulk K, et al. Value of lead V$_4$R for recognition of the infarct coronary in acute inferior myocardial infarction. *Am J Cardiol* 1984;53:1538–1541.

201. Herz I, Assali AR, Adler Y, et al. New electrocardiographic criteria for predicting either the right or left circumflex artery as the culprit coronary artery in inferior wall acute myocardial infarction. *Am J Cardiol* 1997;80:1343–1345.

202. Zimetbaum PJ, Krishnan S, Gold A, et al. Usefulness of ST-segment elevation in lead III exceeding that of lead II for identifying the location of the totally occluded coronary artery in inferior wall myocardial infarction. *Am J Cardiol* 1998;81:918–919.

203. Hasdai D, Birnbaum Y, Herz I, et al. ST segment depression in lateral limb leads in inferior wall acute myocardial infarction. Implications regarding the culprit artery and the site of obstruction. *Eur Heart J* 1995;16:1549–1553.

204. Porter A, Vaturi M, Adler Y, et al. Are there differences among patients with inferior acute myocardial infarction with ST depression in leads V$_2$ and V$_3$ and positive versus negative T waves in these leads on admission? *Cardiology* 1998;90:295–298.

205. Assali AR, Sclarovsky S, Herz I, et al. Comparison of patients with inferior wall acute myocardial infarction with versus without ST-segment elevation in leads V$_5$ and V$_6$. *Am J Cardiol* 1998;81:81–83.

206. Huey BL, Beller GA, Kaiser DL, et al. A comprehensive analysis of myocardial infarction due to left circumflex artery occlusion: comparison with infarction due to right coronary artery and left posterior descending artery occlusion. *J Am Coll Cardiol* 1988;12:1156–1166.

207. Boden WE, Kleiger RE, Gibson RS, et al., and the Diltiazem Reinfarction Study Group. Electrocardiographic evolution of posterior myocardial infarction: importance of early precordial ST-depression. *Am J Cardiol* 1987;59:782–787.

208. Matetzky S, Freimark D, Chouraqui P, et al. Significance of ST segment elevations in posterior chest leads (V$_7$ to V$_9$) in patients with acute inferior myocardial infarction: application for thrombolytic therapy. *J Am Coll Cardiol* 1998;31:506–511.

209. López-Sendon J, Coma-Canella I, Alcasena S, et al. Electrocardiographic findings in acute right ventricular infarction: sensitivity and specificity of electrocardiographic alterations in right precordial leads V$_4$R, V$_3$R, V$_1$, V$_2$, and V$_3$. *J Am Coll Cardiol* 1985;6:1273–1279.

210. Zehender M, Kasper W, Kauder E, et al. Right ventricular infarction as an independent predictor of prognosis after acute inferior myocardial infarction. *N Engl J Med* 1993;328:981–988.

211. Kopelman HA, Forman MB, Wilson H, et al. Right ventricular myocardial infarction in patients with chronic lung disease: possible role of right ventricular hypertrophy. *J Am Coll Cardiol* 1985;5:1302–1307.

212. Lee HS, Cross SJ, Rawles JM, et al. Patients with suspected myocardial infarction who present with ST depression. *Lancet* 1993;342:1204–1207.

213. Sgarbossa EB, Topol EJ. Semantic ambiguity, the "non-" nosology and myocardial infarction. *J Clin Epidemiol* 1994;47:441–446.

214. Maeda S. Different clinical implications for ST depression and T wave inversion in non-Q wave myocardial infarction. *J Cardiol* 1994;24:357–366.

215. Gorgels APM, Vos MA, Mulleneers R, et al. Value of the electrocardiogram in diagnosing the number of severely narrowed coronary arteries in rest angina pectoris. *Am J Cardiol* 1993;72:999–1003.

216. O'Keefe JH, Sayed-Taha K, Gibson W, et al. Do patients with left circumflex coronary artery-related acute myocardial infarction without ST-segment elevation benefit from reperfusion therapy? *Am J Cardiol* 1995;75:718–720.

217. Camara EJN, Chandra N, Ouyang P, et al. Reciprocal ST change in acute myocardial infarction. Assessment by electrocardiography and echocardiography. *J Am Coll Cardiol* 1983;2:251–257.

218. Tabbalat RA, Haft JI. Are reciprocal changes a consequence of "ischemia at a distance" or merely a benign electric phenomenon? A PTCA study. *Am Heart J* 1993;126:95–103.

219. Birnbaum Y, Wagner GS, Barbash GI, et al. Correlation of angiographic findings and right (V$_1$ to V$_3$) versus left (V$_4$ to V$_6$) precordial ST-segment depression in inferior wall acute myocardial infarction. *Am J Cardiol* 1999;15:83:143–148.

220. Davidson E, Weinberger I, Rotenberg Z, et al. Elevated serum creatine kinase levels: an early diagnostic sign of acute dissection of the aorta. *Arch Intern Med* 1988;148:2184–2186.

221. Weiss P, Weiss I, Zuber M, et al. How many patients with acute dissection of the thoracic aorta would erroneously receive thrombolytic therapy based on the electrocardiographic findings on admission? *Am J Cardiol* 1993;72:1329–1330.

222. Cannon A, Freedman B, Bailey BP, et al. ST-segment changes during transmural myocardial ischemia in chronic

left bundle branch block. *Am J Cardiol* 1989;64:1216–1217.

223. Stark KS, Krucoff MW, Schryver B, et al. Quantification of ST-segment changes during coronary angioplasty in patients with left bundle branch block. *Am J Cardiol* 1991;67:1219–1222.

224. Wackers FJ. Complete left bundle branch block: is the diagnosis of myocardial infarction possible? *Int J Cardiol* 1983;2:521–529.

225. Sgarbossa EB. Value of the ECG in suspected acute myocardial infarction with left bundle branch block. *J Electrocardiol* 2000;33[Suppl]:87–92.

226. Sgarbossa EB, Pinski SL, Barbagelata A, et al., for the GUSTO-I investigators. Electrocardiographic diagnosis of evolving acute myocardial infarction in the presence of left bundle branch block. *N Engl J Med* 1996;334:481–487.

227. Sgarbossa EB, Pinski SL, Gates KB, et al., for the GUSTO-I investigators. Electrocardiographic diagnosis of acute myocardial infarction in the presence of ventricular paced rhythm. *Am J Cardiol* 1996;77:423–424.

228. Zarling EJ, Sexton H, Milnor P Jr. Failure to diagnose acute myocardial infarction; the clinicopathologic experience at a large community hospital. *JAMA* 1983;250:1171–1181.

229. Gibler WB, Sayre MR, Levy RC, et al. Serial 12-lead electrocardiographic monitoring in patients presenting to the emergency department with chest pain. *J Electrocardiol* 1993;26[Suppl]:238–243.

230. Christian TF, Clements IP, Gibbons RJ. Noninvasive identification of myocardium at risk in patients with acute myocardial infarction and nondiagnostic electrocardiograms with technetium 99m sestamibi. *Circulation* 1991;83:1615–1620.

231. Caceres L, Cooke D, Zalenski R, et al. Myocardial infarction with an initially normal electrocardiogram. Angiographic findings. *Clin Cardiol* 1995;18:563–568.

232. Slater DK, Hlatky MA, Mark DB, et al. Outcome in suspected acute myocardial infarction with normal or minimally abnormal admission electrocardiographic findings. *Am J Cardiol* 1987;60:766–770.

233. Larsen GC, Griffith JL, Beshansky JR, et al. Electrocardiographic left ventricular hypertrophy in patients with suspected acute cardiac ischemia. Its influence on diagnosis, triage, and short-term prognosis. *J Gen Intern Med* 1994;9:666–673.

234. Takatsu F, Kawai S, Okada R, et al. The presence of small q waves and decreased precordial r waves indicates a small amount of fibrosis of the anterior myocardial wall. *J Electrocardiol* 1993;26:9–15.

235. Coll S, Betriu A, de Flores T, et al. Significance of Q-wave regression after transmural acute myocardial infarction. *Am J Cardiol* 1988;61:739–742.

236. Warner RA, Reger M, Hill NE, et al. Electrocardiographic criteria for the diagnosis of anterior myocardial infarction: importance of the duration of precordial R waves. *Am J Cardiol* 1983;52:690–692.

237. Sullivan W, Vlodaver Z, Tuna N, et al. Correlation of electrocardiographic and pathologic findings in healed myocardial infarction. *Am J Cardiol* 1978;42:724–732.

238. Ogawa H, Hiramori K, Haze K, et al. Classification of non-Q wave myocardial infarction according to electrocardiographic changes. *Br Heart J* 1985;54:473–478.

239. Park SE, Tani A, Minamino T, et al. Coronary angiographic features within 48 hours from onset of non-Q wave myocardial infarction with R wave regression and no ST segment depression. *Cardiology* 1990;77:121–129.

240. Chamorro H, Barquin I, Gómez P, et al. Angiographic findings in non-Q wave infarction and their relation to ST-T changes. *Rev Méd Chile* 1992;120:644–650.

241. Phibbs B. "Transmural" versus "subendocardial" myocardial infarction: an electrocardiographic myth. *J Am Coll Cardiol* 1983;1:561–564.

242. Barbagelata A, Califf RM, Sgarbossa EB, et al. Thrombolysis and Q-wave versus non-Q-wave first acute myocardial infarction: a GUSTO-I substudy. *J Am Coll Cardiol* 1997;29:770–777.

243. Poehlman JH, Silverman ME. Clinical characteristics, electrocardiographic and enzyme correlations, and long-term prognosis of patients with chest pain associated with ST depression and/or T wave inversion. *Am Heart J* 1980;99:173–180.

244. Richardson SG, Morton P, Murtaugh JG, et al. Relation of coronary arterial patency and left ventricular function to electrocardiographic changes after streptokinase treatment during acute myocardial infarction. *Am J Cardiol* 1988;61:961–965.

245. Oliva PB, Hammill SC, Edwards WD. Electrocardiographic diagnosis of postinfarction regional pericarditis: ancillary observations regarding the effect of reperfusion on the rapidity and amplitude of T-wave inversion after acute myocardial infarction. *Circulation* 1993;88:896–904.

246. Wehrens XHT, Doevendans PA, Oude Ophuis TJ, et al. A comparison of electrocardiographic changes during reperfusion of acute myocardial infarction by thrombolysis or percutaneous transluminal coronary angioplasty. *Am Heart J* 2000;139:430–436.

247. Krucoff MW, Green CE, Satler LF, et al. Noninvasive detection of coronary artery patency using continuous ST-segment monitoring. *Am J Cardiol* 1996;57:916–921.

248. Blanke H, Scheriff F, Karsch KR, et al. Electrocardiographic changes after streptokinase-induced recanalization in patients with acute left anterior descending artery obstruction. *Circulation* 1983;68:406–412.

249. Chou TC. Myocardial infarction, myocardial injury, and myocardial ischemia. In: Chou TE, ed. *Electrocardiography in clinical practice. Adult and pediatric.* Philadelphia: WB Saunders, 1996:121–213.

250. Sgarbossa EB, Birnbaum Y, Parrillo JE. Electrocardiographic diagnosis of acute myocardial infarction: current concepts for the clinician. *Am Heart J* 2001;141(4):507–517.

251. Warner RA. Recent advances in the diagnosis of myocardial infarction. *Cardiol Clin* 1987;5:381–392.

252. Rodriguez MI, Anselmi CA, Sodi-Pallares D. The electrocardiographic diagnosis of septal infarctions. *Am Heart J* 1953;45:524–544.

253. Shalev Y, Fogelman R, Oettinger M, et al. Does the electrocardiographic pattern of "anteroseptal" myocardial infarction correlate with the anatomic location of myocardial injury? *Am J Cardiol* 1995;75:763–766.

254. Dwyer EM Jr. The predictive accuracy of the electrocardiogram in identifying the presence and location of myo-

cardial infarction and coronary artery disease. *Ann N Y Acad Sci* 1990;601:67–76.

255. Boden WE, Bough EW, Korr KS, et al. Inferoseptal myocardial infarction: another cause of precordial ST-segment depression in transmural inferior wall myocardial infarction? *Am J Cardiol* 1984;54:1216–1223.

256. Bough EW, Boden WE, Korr KS, et al. Left ventricular asynergy in electrocardiographic "posterior" myocardial infarction. *J Am Coll Cardiol* 1984;4:209–215.

257. Ward RM, White RD, Ideker RE. Evaluation of a QRS scoring system for estimating myocardial infarct size. IV. Correlation with quantitative anatomic finds for posterolateral infarcts. *Am J Cardiol* 1984;53:706–714.

258. Bough EW, Korr KS. Prevalence and severity of circumflex coronary artery disease in electrocardiographic posterior myocardial infarction. *J Am Coll Cardiol* 1986;7:990–996.

259. Hoffman I, Mehta J, Helsenrath J, et al. Anterior conduction delay: a possible cause for prominent anterior QRS forces. *J Electrocardiol* 1976;9:15–21.

260. Brembilla-Perrot B, Terrier de la Chaise A, Isaaz K, et al. The tall R wave in lead V_1 in posterior myocardial infarction: a reciprocal sign or a His-Purkinje conduction disturbance? *Pacing Clin Electrophysiol* 1989;12:1650–1659.

261. Cárdenas M, Díaz del Río A, González Hermosillo JA, et al. El infarto agudo de miocardio del ventrículo derecho. En memoria de Ignacio Chávez. *Arch Inst Cardiol Mex* 1980;50:295–312.

262. Rhoads DV, Edwards JE, Pruitt RD. The electrocardiogram in the presence of myocardial infarction and intraventricular block of the left bundle branch block type. *Am Heart J* 1961;62:735–745.

263. Cabrera E, Friedland C. La onda de activación ventricular en el bloqueo de rama izquierda con infarto: un nuevo signo electrocardiográfico. *Arch Inst Cardiol Mex* 1953;23:441–447.

264. Hands ME, Cook EF, Stone PH, et al., and the MILIS Study Group. Electrocardiographic diagnosis of myocardial infarction in the presence of complete left bundle branch block. *Am Heart J* 1988;116:23–31.

265. Fesmire FM. ECG diagnosis of acute myocardial infarction in the presence of left bundle branch block in patients undergoing continuous ECG monitoring. *Ann Emerg Med* 1995;26:69–82.

266. Kafka W. The ECG and VCG diagnosis of infarction in pacer-dependent patients. *Pacing Clin Electrophysiol* 1985;8(Pt II):A-16.

267. Barold SS, Falkoff MD, Ong LS, et al. Electrocardiographic diagnosis of myocardial infarction during ventricular pacing. *Cardiol Clin* 1987;5:403–417.

268. Kindwall KE, Brown JP, Josephson ME. Predictive accuracy of criteria for chronic myocardial infarction in pacing-induced left bundle branch block. *Am J Cardiol* 1986;57:1255–1260.

269. Selvester RH, Wagner JO, Rubin HB. Quantitation of myocardial infarct size and location by electrocardiogram and vectorcardiogram. In: *Boerhave course in quantitation in cardiology*. New York: Marcel Dekker, 1979:417.

270. Gardin JM, Singer DH. Atrial infarction. Importance, diagnosis and localization. *Arch Intern Med* 1981;141:1345–1348.

271. Fisch C. Electrocardiography and vectorcardiography. In: Braunwald E, ed. *Heart disease. A textbook of cardiovascular medicine*. Philadelphia: WB Saunders, 1992:116–160.

272. Sweterlitsch EM, Murphy GW. Acute electrocardiographic pseudoinfarction pattern in the setting of diabetic ketoacidosis and severe hyperkalemia. *Am Heart J* 1996;132:1086–1089.

273. Kamimura M, Hancock W. Acute myocardial infarction in diabetic ketoacidosis. *Hosp Practice* 1992;27:28–30.

274. Houghton JL, Sinden JR, Gross CM. Acute presentation of pseudo myocardial infarction secondary to metastatic cancer. *Am J Med Sci* 1992;303:170–173.

275. Cassin M, Charmet P, Collazo R, et al. Electrocardiographic aspects simulating acute myocardial infarction in massive pulmonary embolism. *G Ital Cardiol* 1986;16:882–885.

276. Manthous CA, Schmidt GA. Pleural effusion masquerading as myocardial infarction. *Chest* 1993;103:1619–1621.

277. Osswald S, Roelke M, O'Nunain SS, et al. Electrocardiographic pseudo-infarct patterns after implantation of cardioverter-defibrillators. *Am Heart J* 1995;129:265–272.

278. Sgarbossa EB. Recent advances in the electrocardiographic diagnosis of myocardial infarction: left bundle branch block and pacing. *Pacing Clin Electrophysiol* 1996;19:1370–1379.

279. Maciejewska M, Dabrowska B. Influence of serum potassium on the electrocardiographic pattern of left ventricular hypertrophy in primary hyperaldosteronism. *Clin Cardiol* 1992;15:725–727.

280. Clements SD, Hurst JW. Diagnostic value of electrocardiographic abnormalities observed in subjects accidentally exposed to cold. *Am J Cardiol* 1972;29:729–734.

281. Vanagt EJ, Wellens HJJ. The electrocardiogram in digitalis intoxication. In: Wellens HJJ, ed. *What's new in electrocardiography*. Boston: Kluwer Academic Publishers, 1981:315–343.

282. Watanabe Y, Dreifus LS. Interactions of quinidine and potassium on atrioventricular transmission. *Circ Res* 1967;20:434–446.

283. Butman SM, Phibbs B, Wild J, et al. One heart, two bodies: insight from the transplanted heart and its new electrocardiogram. *Am J Cardiol* 1990;66:632–635.

284. Golshayan D, Seydoux C, Berguer DG, et al. Incidence and prognostic value of electrocardiographic abnormalities after heart transplantation. *Clin Cardiol* 1998;21:680–684.

285. Gao S, Hunt SA, Wiederhold V, et al. Characteristics of serial electrocardiograms in heart transplant recipients. *Am Heart J* 1991;122:771–774.

286. Calzolari V, Angelini A, Basso C, et al. Histologic findings in the conduction system after cardiac transplantation and correlation with electrocardiographic findings. *Am J Cardiol* 1999;84:756–759.

287. Rodger M, Makropoulos D, Turek M, et al. Diagnostic value of the electrocardiogram in suspected pulmonary embolism. *Am J Cardiol* 2000;86:807–809.

288. Sreeram N, Cheriex EC, Smeets JLRM, et al. Value of the 12-lead electrocardiogram at hospital admission in the diagnosis of pulmonary embolism. *Am J Cardiol* 1994;73:298–303.

289. Nielsen TT, Lund O, Ronne K, et al. Changing electrocardiographic findings in pulmonary embolism in relation to vascular obstruction. *Cardiology* 1989;76:274–284.

290. Phillips JH, Burch GE. Problems in the diagnosis of cor pulmonale. *Am Heart J* 1963;66:818–832.

291. Spodick DH, Hauger-Klevine JH, Tyler JM, et al. Electrocardiogram in pulmonary emphysema. *Am Rev Respir Dis* 1963;88:14.

292. Yamour BJ, Sridharan MR, Rice JF, et al. Electrocardiographic changes in cerebrovascular hemorrhage. *Am Heart J* 1980;99:294–300.

293. Hugenholtz PG. Electrocardiographic changes typical for central nervous system after right radical neck dissection. *Am Heart J* 1967;74:438–441.

294. Gould L, Gopalaswami C, Chandy F, et al. Electroconvulsive therapy-induced ECG changes simulating a myocardial infarction. *Arch Intern Med* 1983;143:1786–1787.

295. Koepp M, Schmidt D, Kern A. Electrocardiographic changes in patients with brain tumors. *Arch Neurol* 1995;52:152–155.

296. Hedén B, Ohlsson M, Holst H, et al. Detection of frequently overlooked electrocardiographic lead reversals using artificial neural networks. *Am J Cardiol* 1996;78:600–604.

297. Abdollah H, Milliken JA. Recognition of electrocardiographic left arm/left leg lead reversal. *Am J Cardiol* 1997;80:1247–1249.

298. Herman MV, Ingram DA, Levy JA, et al. Variability of electrocardiographic precordial lead placement: a method to improve accuracy and reliability. *Clin Cardiol* 1991;14:469–476.

299. El-Sheriff N. High-resolution electrocardiography. In: Moss AJ, Stern S, eds. *Noninvasive electrocardiology. Clinical aspects of Holter monitoring.* Philadelphia: WB Saunders, 1996:249–254.

300. Goldberger AL, Bhargava V, Froelicher V, et al. Effect of myocardial infarction on high frequency QRS potentials. *Circulation* 1981;64:34–42.

301. Kuchar DL, Rosenbaum DS. Noninvasive recording of late potentials: current state of the art. *Pacing Clin Electrophysiol* 1989;12:1538–1551.

302. Mirvis DM, ed. *Body surface electrocardiographic mapping.* Boston: Kluwer Academic Publishers, 1988.

303. Kornreich F, Montague TJ, Rautaharju PM. Identification of first acute Q-wave and non-Q wave myocardial infarction by multivariate analysis of body surface potential maps. *Circulation* 1991;84:2442–2253.

304. Laks M. The ECG bridge to the twenty-first century: progress report for 1997 and future directions. *J Electrocardiol* 1998;30[Suppl]:196–197.

305. Brady WJ, Hwang V, Sullivan R, et al. A comparison of 12- and 15-lead ECGs in ED chest pain patients: impact on diagnosis, therapy, and disposition. *Am J Emerg Med* 2000;18:239–243.

306. McCarthy BD, Beshansky JR, D'Agostino RB, et al. Missed diagnoses of acute myocardial infarction in the emergency department: results from a multicenter study. *Ann Emerg Med* 1993;22:579–582.

307. Sur DK, Kaye L, Mikus M, et al. Accuracy of electrocardiogram reading by family practice residents. *Fam Med* 2000;32:315–319.

308. McCrea WA, Saltisi S. Electrocardiogram interpretation in general practice: relevance to prehospital thrombolysis. *Br Heart J* 1993;70:219–225.

309. Jayes RL, Larsen GC, Beshansky JR, et al. Physician electrocardiogram reading in the emergency department. Accuracy and effect on triage decisions: findings from a multicenter study. *J Gen Intern Med* 1992;7:387–392.

310. Woolley D, Henck M, Luck J. Comparison of electrocardiogram interpretations by family physicians, a computer, and a cardiology service. *J Fam Pract* 1992;34:428–432.

311. Pryor WW, Blackhurst DW. Follow-up evaluation of computerized electrocardiographic interpretations: a comparison of cardiologists' vs internists' performance. *J S C Med Assoc* 1996;92:339–343.

312. Lee TH, Rouan GW, Weisberg MC, et al. Clinical characteristics and natural history of patients with acute myocardial infarction sent home from the emergency room. *Am J Cardiol* 1987;60:219–224.

313. Fisch C. Centennial of the string galvanometer and the electrocardiogram. *J Am Coll Cardiol* 2000;36:1737–1745.

314. Davies LG. Observer variation in reports on electrocardiograms. *Br Heart J* 1958;20:153–161.

315. Willems JL, Abreu-Lima C, Arnaud P, et al. The diagnostic performance of computer programs for the interpretation of electrocardiograms. *N Engl J Med* 1991;325:1767–1773.

316. Gjørup T, Helbæk H, Nielsen D, et al. Interpretation of the electrocardiogram in suspected myocardial infarction: a randomized controlled study of the effect of a training programme to reduce interobserver variation. *J Intern Med* 1992;231:407–412.

317. Sokolove PE, Sgarbossa EB, Wagner GS, et al. Interobserver agreement in the ECG diagnosis of acute myocardial infarction in the presence of left bundle branch block. *Acad Emerg Med* 1999;6:452–453.

318. Pipberger HV, Poblete PF, Pipberger HA. Computer analysis of ventricular conduction defects. *Adv Cardiol* 1975;14:242–248.

319. McLaughlin SC, Aitchison TC, Macfarlane PW. Improved repeatability of 12-lead ECG analysis using continuous scoring techniques. *J Electrocardiol* 1993;26[Suppl]:101–107.

320. Willems JL, Arnaud P, van Bemmel JH, et al. A reference database for multilead electro-cardiographic computer measurement programs. *J Am Coll Cardiol* 1987;10:1313–1321.

321. Willems JL, Arnaud P, van Bemmel JH, et al. Assessment of the performance of electro-cardiography computer programs with the use of a reference database. *Circulation* 1985;71:523–534.

322. Kornowski R, Leon MB. Left ventricular electromechanical mapping: current understanding and diagnostic potential. *Cathet Cardiovasc Interv* 1999;48:421–429.

ELECTROCARDIOGRAPHIC DIAGNOSIS
OF ARRHYTHMIAS

HEIN J. WELLENS

OVERVIEW

By using information provided by intracardiac recordings and programmed cardiac stimulation, diagnosing correctly the site of origin and the mechanism of an arrhythmia on a 12-lead electrocardiogram (ECG) has markedly improved in recent years. This chapter reviews how to use a 12-lead ECG in patients with supraventricular tachycardia (SVT), ventricular tachycardia (VT), and preexcitation.

A systematic approach to ECGs is essential for optimal interpretation. Correctly diagnosing an arrhythmia is important not only to prognosis and the selection of appropriate antiarrhythmic drugs, but also because of the possibility of completely curing an arrhythmia by radiofrequency catheter ablation.

INTRODUCTION AND HISTORY

This chapter is intended to serve as an introduction to the chapters in this textbook that cover supraventricular and ventricular arrhythmias (see Chapters 64–67). The ECG is a valuable tool to diagnose these arrhythmias, and the major features that differentiate key supraventricular and

ventricular arrhythmias are reviewed in this chapter. Although the chapters that follow provide an in-depth discussion of each arrhythmia, this chapter relies heavily on graphic examples to illustrate rapid and accurate diagnosis of these important rhythm disturbances.

The electrical impulse that is responsible for normal cardiac rhythm originates in the sinus node, spreads over the atrium, passes from atria to ventricles only by way of the atrioventricular (AV) node–His pathway, and spreads over the ventricles through the bundle branches and the Purkinje system. The ECG recording of this regularly occurring event characteristically shows a P-QRS-T complex with each of the components well defined as to its width, height, axis, and interrelation (Fig. 60.1).

Ventricular Preexcitation

In the normal heart, the AV node–His pathway is the only connection between the atria and the ventricles. However, some people are born with an extra connection between the atrium, AV node, and ventricle (1). Conduction over these pathways after a supraventricular beat results in earlier activation of the ventricle (*preexcitation*) than during conduction over the AV node–His pathway only. The most common type of preexcitation is caused by a direct connection between the atrium and ventricle. In this situation, described by Wolff et al. in 1930 (2), arrhythmias are often present.

H. J. Wellens: Department of Cardiology, The Interuniversity Cardiology Institute of The Netherlands, Utrecht, The Netherlands

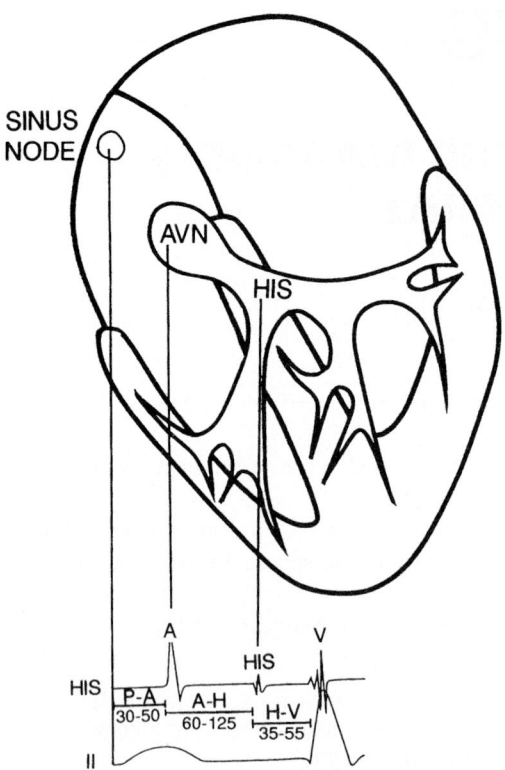

FIGURE 60.1 Time relations between the electrical activation of the different parts of the heart during sinus rhythm. A bundle of His electrogram and lead II are shown to illustrate the different time intervals. AVN, atrioventricular node.

Electrocardiogram in Preexcitation

When two AV pathways [the AV node–His pathway and the AV accessory pathway (AP)] are present, the conduction properties of the two pathways and the location of the AV AP determine the configuration of the QRS complex during sinus rhythm. This is shown in Figure 60.2. The typical picture of a short PR interval, a delta wave (representing ventricular activation over the AP) and a broad QRS complex, is present when there is a major contribution to ventricular activation by AV conduction over the AP. When contribution to ventricular activation over the AP is small because of the AP location or rapid transmission of the sinus impulse over the AV node, the ECG shows minimal changes pointing to ventricular preexcitation. Figure 60.3 illustrates a 12-lead ECG during sinus rhythm in the two situations shown in Figure 60.2.

As is discussed elsewhere (see Chapter 66), APs may not only be present as connections between atrium and ventricle, but also as fibers connecting the AV node with the ventricle (Mahaim fibers or nodoventricular fibers) (3) or the atrium with the bundle of His (atriofascicular fibers). It is also important to know that accessory connections may conduct anterogradely and retrogradely, only anterogradely, or only retrogradely. When conduction over the accessory

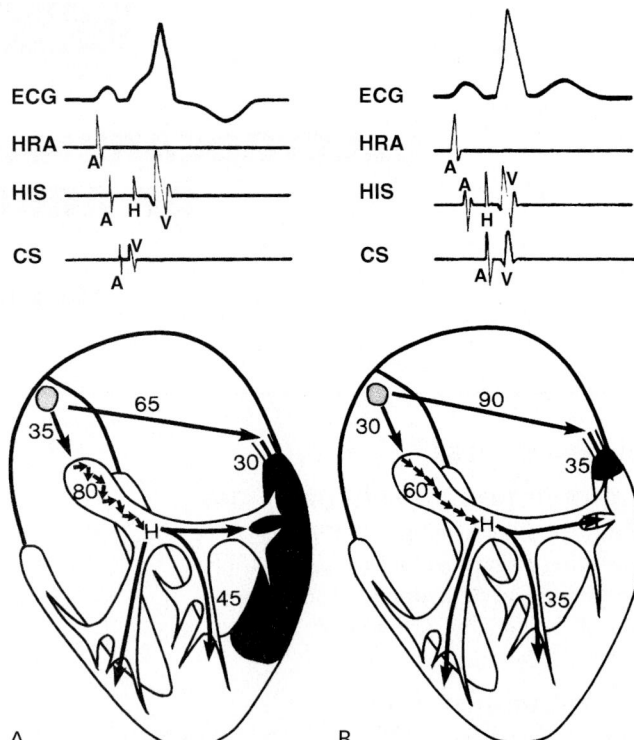

FIGURE 60.2 Factors determining the degree of ventricular preexcitation during sinus rhythm in a patient with Wolff-Parkinson-White (WPW) syndrome during sinus rhythm. The corresponding electrocardiographic (ECG) and intracavitary recordings from the high-right atrium (HRA), bundle of His region (HIS), and coronary sinus (CS) are shown in the upper part of the figure. In the heart in **A**, atrioventricular (AV) conduction time from the sinus node over the normal AV nodal–His pathway is 160 ms. The time required to travel from the sinus node to the atrial insertion of the AP is 65 ms, and the left-sided accessory pathway (AP) conduction time is 30 ms (total of 95 ms). Because of the shorter conduction time over the AP, an important part of the ventricle is preexcited, resulting in a short PR interval, a distinct delta wave, and a widened QRS complex. In the heart in **B**, there is longer conduction time from the sinus node to the atrial insertion of the AP, a longer conduction time over the AP itself, and a shorter conduction time over the AV node. Thus, the impulse arrives in the ventricles simultaneously through the AV node and the AP, producing a normal PR interval and a narrow QRS complex.

connection is possible only in the retrograde direction, the term *concealed accessory conduction* is used.

Localizing accessory connections is important, because it is possible to interrupt conduction in these connections by the application of radiofrequency energy. As is pointed out elsewhere, exact localization requires catheter mapping of cardiac activation. However, the ECG can be very useful in identifying the atrial and the ventricular ends of an accessory AV connection.

Figure 60.4 provides a schematic representation of the four zones of AV AP locations along the AV ring; Figure 60.5 gives representative examples. Although this is an oversimplification, it helps in understanding how to use the delta-wave axis (during preexcited sinus rhythm or preexcited tachycardia) or the P-wave axis [during tachy-

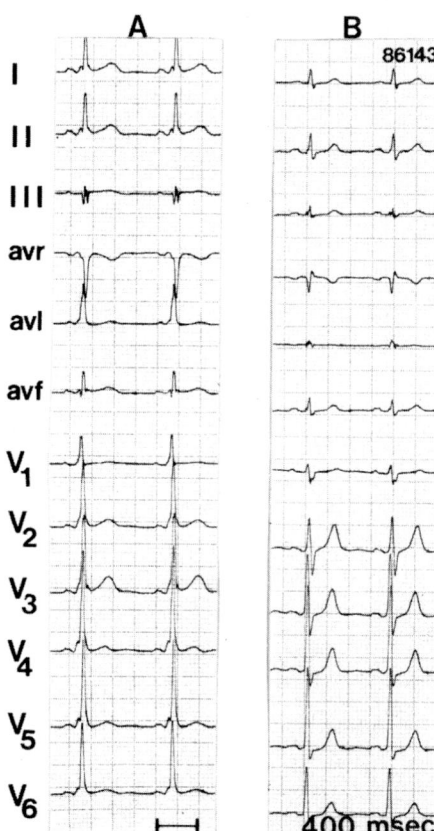

FIGURE 60.3 Electrocardiographic examples of the two diagrams shown in Figure 60.2. **A** and **B** in this figure correspond to **A** and **B**, respectively, in Figure 60.2. Note the prominent delta wave in **A**, indicating that a much larger area of the ventricle is preexcited than is shown in **B**.

cardias with ventriculoatrial (VA) conduction over the AV AP] for localizing the ventricular end and the atrial end of the AV AP.

Diagnosing an Arrhythmia

An arrhythmia is characterized on an ECG as a deviation from the normal sinus rhythm in rate [i.e., too fast (tachycardia) or too slow (bradycardia)], regularity (one or more heartbeats occurring earlier or later than expected), or a different pattern of activation of the cardiac muscle. These changes can be registered on the ECG, allowing clinicians not only to make the diagnosis of an arrhythmia but frequently to recognize its site of origin and mechanism. These aspects are important to prognosis and selection of therapy.

Normal sinus rhythm is regular or shows slight respiration-related rate changes, referred to as *sinus arrhythmias*. The rate of sinus rhythm is determined by several factors, such as activity of the autonomic nervous system (vagal vs. sympathetic stimulation), hormones, body temperature, and so forth. A sinus rate of greater than 100 beats/min is referred to as a *sinus tachycardia*; a sinus rate of less than 60 beats/min is known as a *sinus bradycardia*.

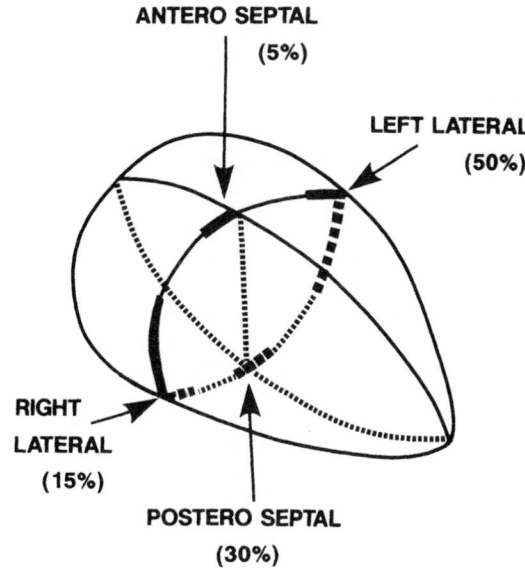

FIGURE 60.4 Frontal look at the heart, depicting the localization and incidence of the four most common types of accessory atrioventricular pathways. This drawing helps to explain how in the frontal plane the ventricular end (the delta wave) and the atrial end (the P wave during orthodromic circus-movement tachycardia) of the accessory pathway can be localized using the 12-lead electrocardiogram.

When impulse formation occurs outside the sinus node during a regular sinus rhythm, it is termed a *premature beat* if such impulse formation occurs earlier than the expected beat of the basic rhythm (Fig. 60.6); an *escape beat* refers to an impulse formation that occurs outside that of the basic rhythm and terminates an interval longer than the preceding basic rhythm (Fig. 60.7).

Premature or ectopic beats may arise anywhere in the heart. They may occur individually, two or three in a row [i.e., doublets (Fig. 60.6) or triplets], or continuously, resulting in a tachycardia.

When premature beats have a fixed time relation to the previous normal depolarization, they are referred to as *coupled* premature beats. If they have no fixed relation to normal beats but occur at fixed interectopic intervals, they may arise in a *parasystolic* focus (Fig. 60.8). Such a focus is completely or partially protected from other impulses. Partial protection may result in slight changes in interectopic intervals, known as *modulated parasystole* (4).

A tachycardia may show a regular or an irregular rhythm. The regularity or irregularity may be at the atrial level, at the ventricular level, or at both levels. When all complexes of a tachycardia show the same configuration, the tachycardia is termed a *monomorphic* tachycardia (Fig. 60.6). When the tachycardia complexes show marked differences in configuration, the tachycardia is referred to as a *polymorphic* tachycardia. If a tachycardia stops spontaneously within 30 seconds, it is defined as a *nonsustained* tachycardia; when the tachycardia persists for more than 30 seconds or does not stop spontaneously, it is termed a *sustained* tachycardia.

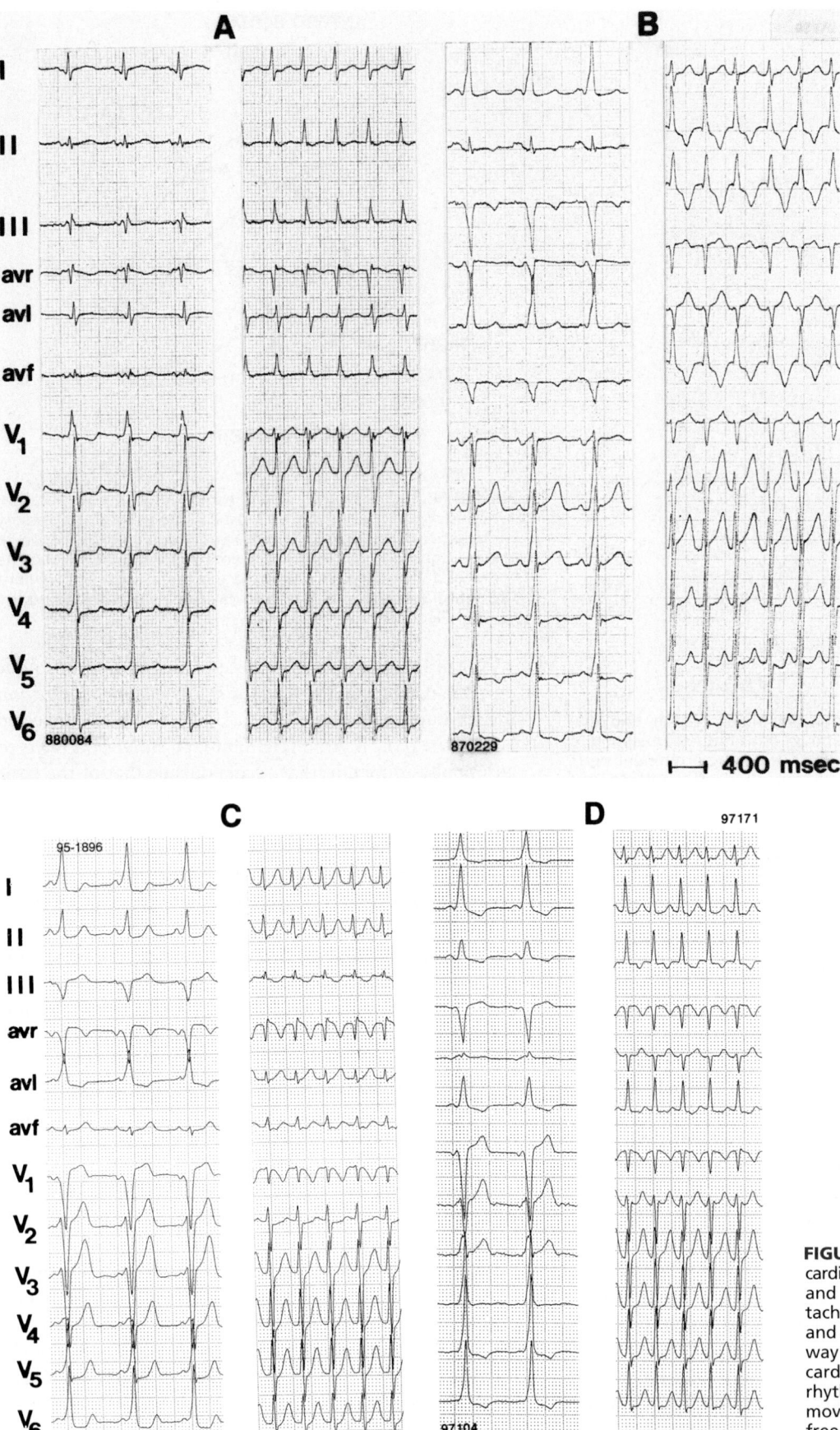

FIGURE 60.5 Twelve-lead electrocardiogram during sinus rhythm and orthodromic circus-movement tachycardia in a left free wall **(A)** and a posteroseptal accessory pathway (AP) **(B)**. Twelve-lead electrocardiogram is depicted during sinus rhythm and orthodromic circus-movement tachycardia in a right free wall **(C)** and anteroseptally located accessory pathway **(D)**.

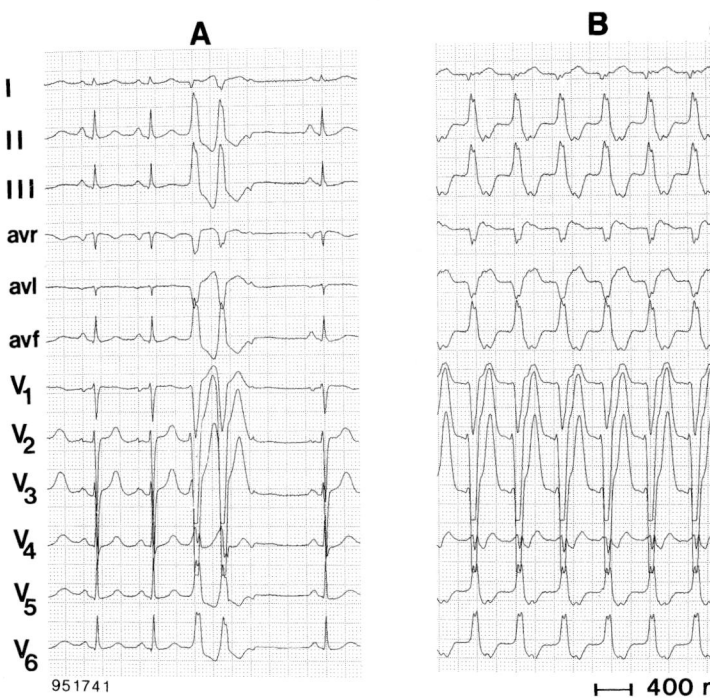

FIGURE 60.6 A: Two consecutive premature ventricular beats. The second one shows retrograde conduction to the atrium. **B:** A monomorphic ventricular tachycardia is present coming from the same area as the premature beats in **A** (the outflow tract of the right ventricle).

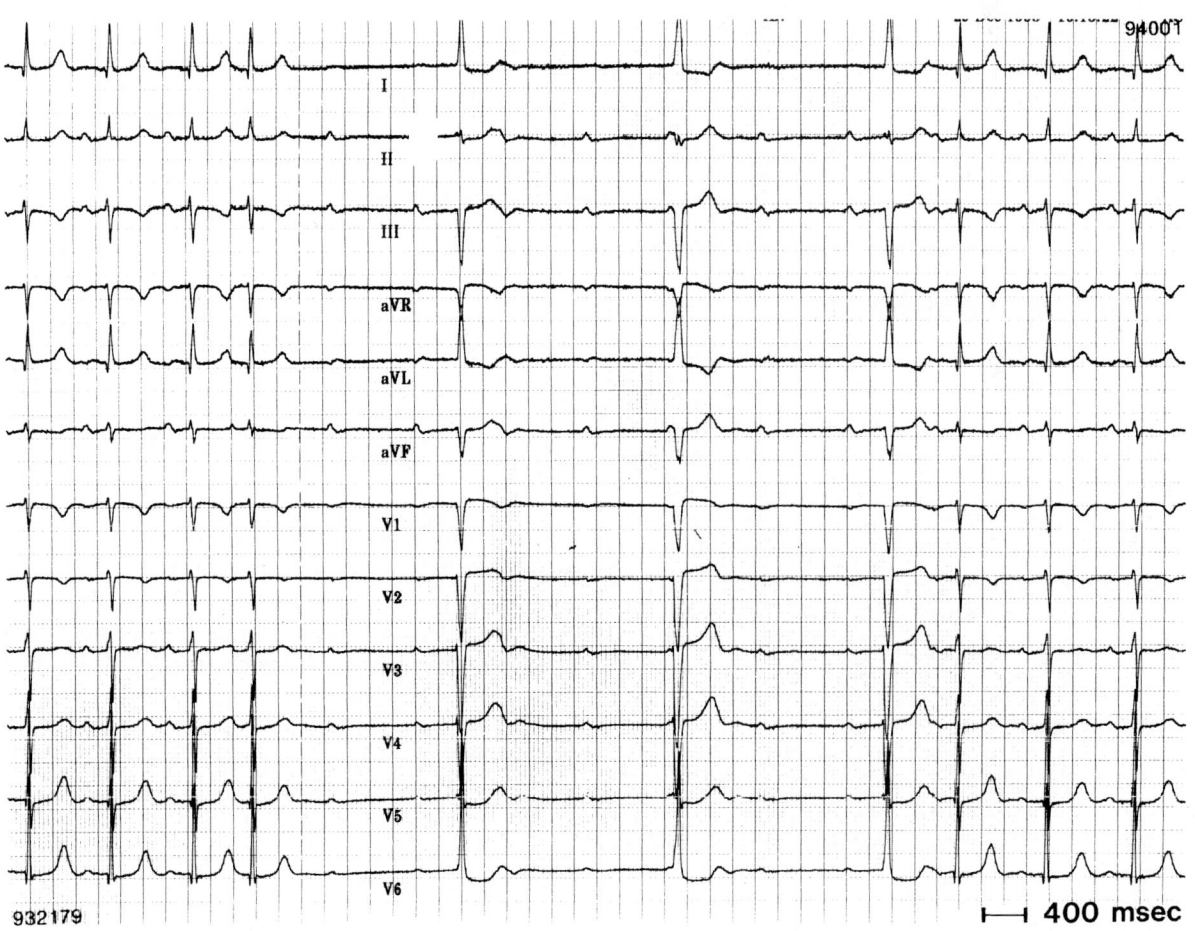

FIGURE 60.7 Escape beats terminating a pause that is longer than those of the QRS intervals of the preceding conducted sinus beats.

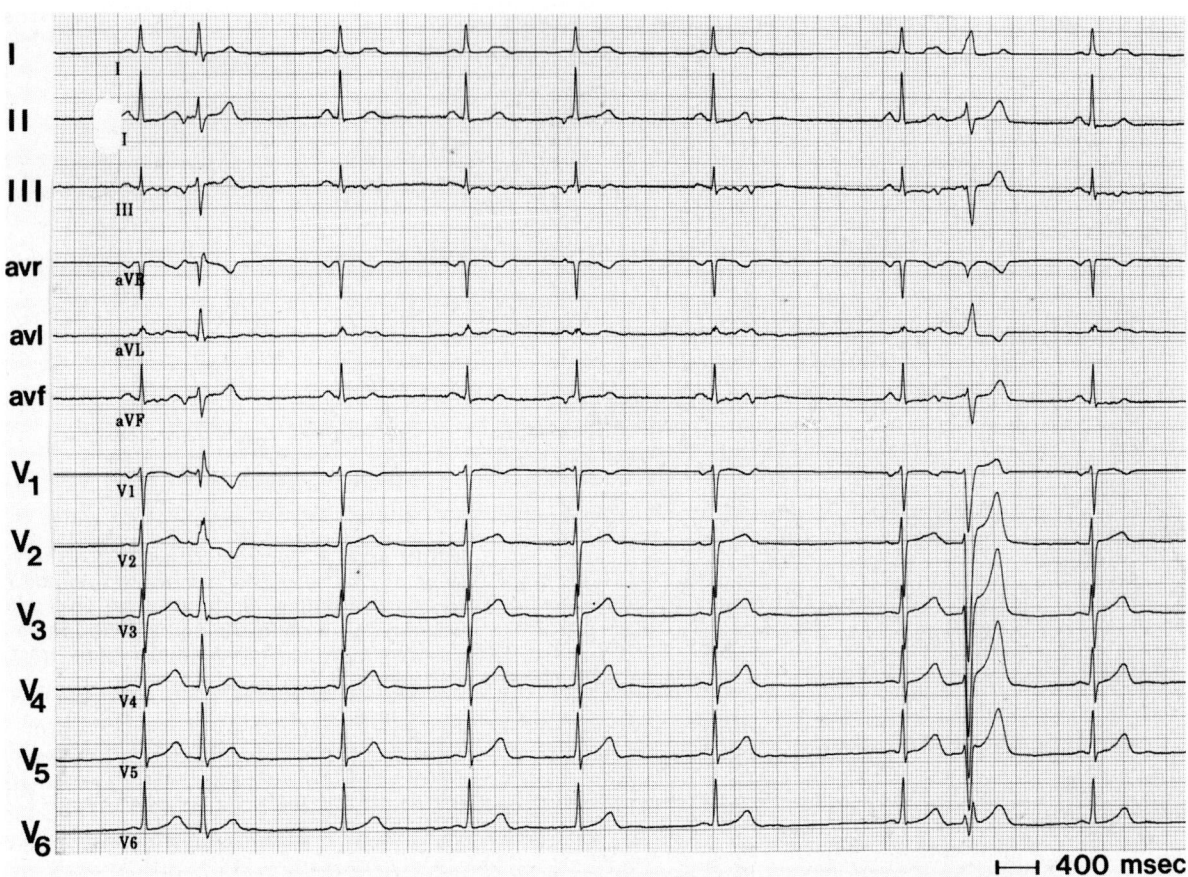

FIGURE 60.8 Atrial parasystole. Apart from sinus rhythm, there is ectopic impulse formation at the atrial level. Ectopic impulse formation is totally independent of the basic sinus rhythm. As shown, depending on the prematurity of the atrial ectopic beat, the QRS differs in configuration because of different degrees of aberrant conduction.

Site of Origin of an Arrhythmia

Arrhythmias may arise anywhere in the heart. For practical purposes, they are divided into those arising in the atrium, the AV nodal region, and the ventricle and those that use extra connections between the atrium and ventricle in their arrhythmic mechanism. Identification of the site of origin is based on (a) the relation between the P wave and QRS complex; (b) the width and configuration of the P wave, which indicate how the atria are activated during the arrhythmia; and (c) the width and configuration of the QRS complex, which indicate how the ventricles are activated during the arrhythmia.

Aberrant Conduction

Figure 60.8 illustrates the occurrence of *premature atrial beats* during sinus rhythm due to a parasystolic atrial focus. It should be noted that these beats occur earlier and have a P-wave configuration that differs from that of the P waves during sinus rhythm. Conduction of the premature atrial beat from atrium to ventricle depends on the prematurity of that beat. A very early atrial beat is not conducted to the ventricle because of refractoriness of the AV conduction system. When conducted to the ventricle, the QRS configuration of the premature atrial

beat depends on the time of arrival in the ventricle and, therefore, on the degree of refractoriness of the bundle branches. The amount of change (aberrancy) of the QRS complex following the premature atrial beat is related to the prematurity of that beat and the refractory state of the bundle branches, which, in turn, is related to the length of the RR interval that precedes the premature atrial complex (Fig. 60.8).

Aberrant conduction is quite common during the sudden rate change at the onset of an SVT, because the supraventricular impulse arrives at the bundle branches at such an early time that one of the bundle branches is still refractory (Fig. 60.9). The mechanism of aberrant conduction is thus termed a *phase 3–* or *tachycardia-dependent aberrancy*. Another cause of persistent aberrant conduction during SVT is retrograde invasion into one of the bundle branches (5). An example is given in Figure 60.10.

TACHYCARDIAS

Atrial Tachycardia

During atrial tachycardia, impulse formation is in the atrium, outside the sinus node. The P wave precedes the

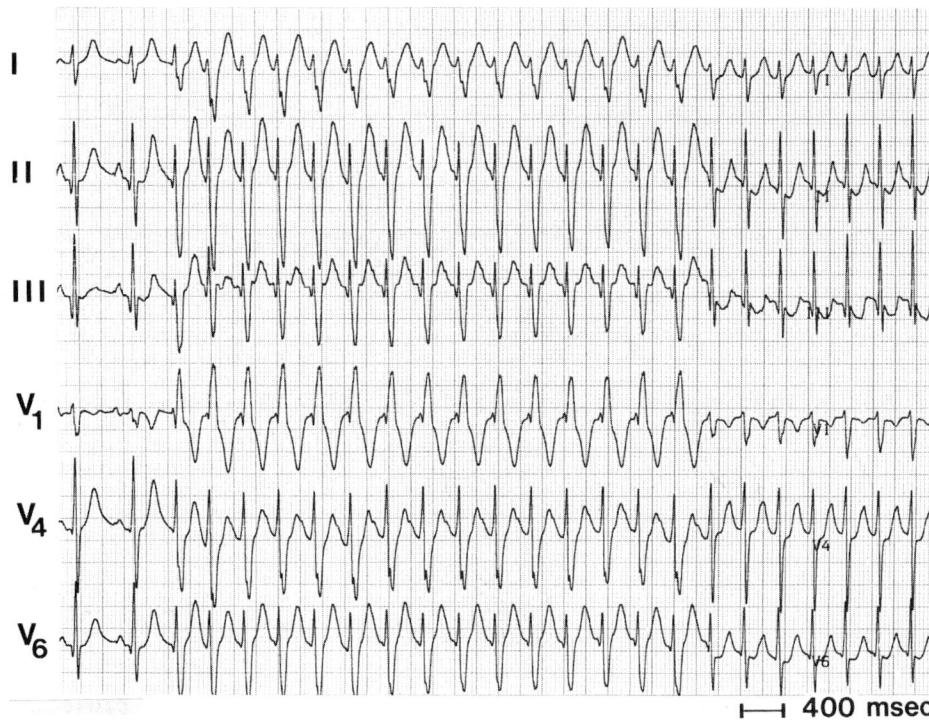

FIGURE 60.9 Aberrant conduction follows the onset of a supraventricular tachycardia (phase 3 aberrancy). Note that the right bundle branch block aberrancy disappears after 15 tachycardia complexes.

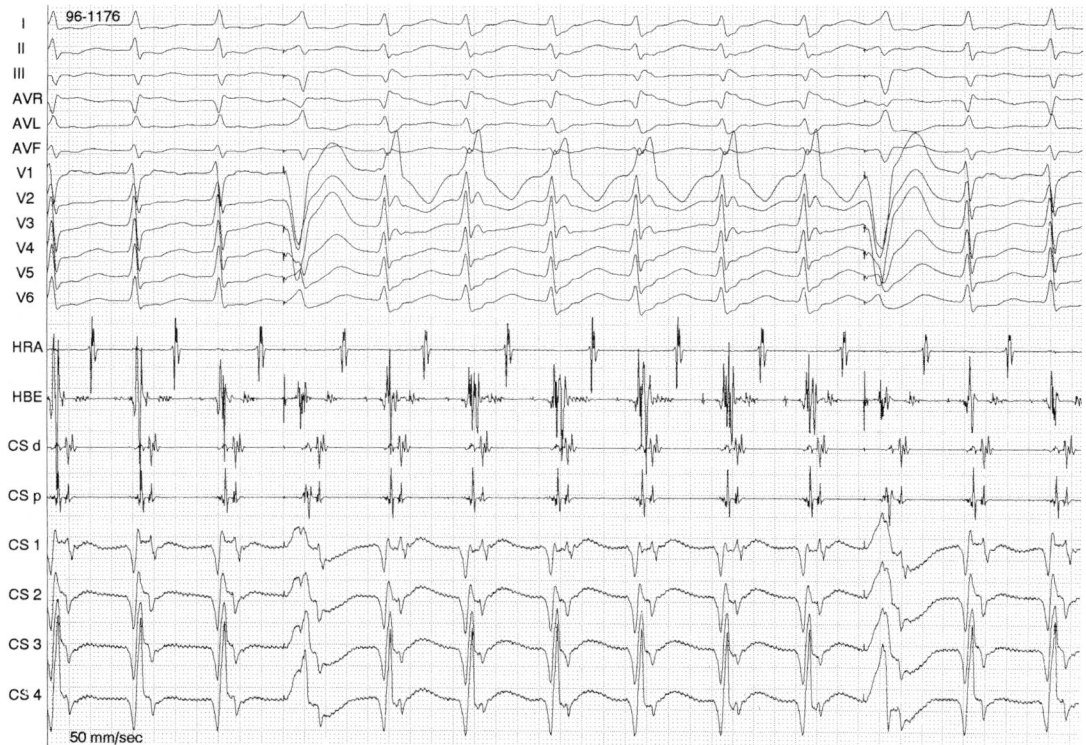

FIGURE 60.10 Supraventricular tachycardia with aberrant conduction due to retrograde invasion into the right bundle branch. Retrograde invasion was produced by an electrically induced right ventricular premature beat and persists until another induced right ventricular premature beat restores normal conduction over the right bundle branch. Apart from the 12-lead electrocardiogram, several intracardiac leads are shown. CS, coronary sinus; HBE, bundle of His electrogram; HRA, high-right atrium.

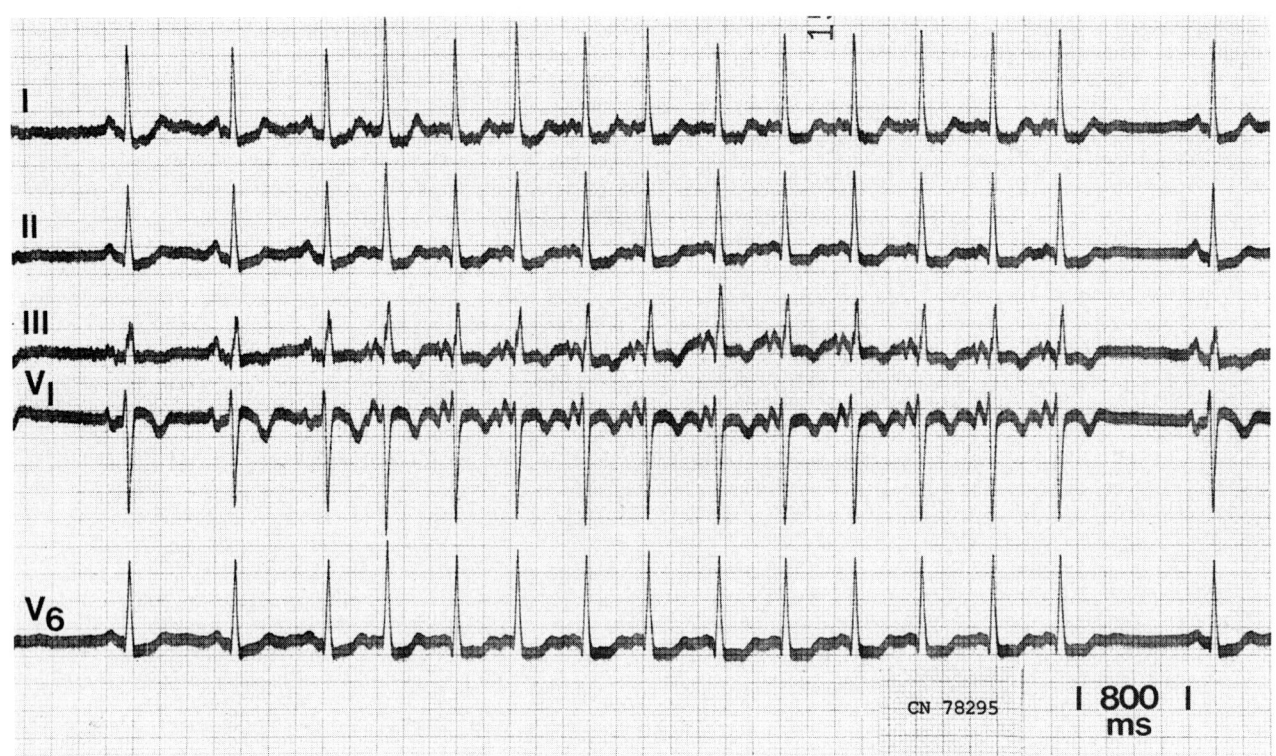

FIGURE 60.11 Paroxysmal atrial tachycardia. The tachycardia shown here starts after three sinus beats.

QRS complex. The polarity of the P wave indicates the site of origin in the atrium. Two types of atrial tachycardias must be distinguished. *Paroxysmal* atrial tachycardia is the most common and is characterized by a sudden onset and cessation of the arrhythmia (Fig. 60.11). A rare, but more serious, type of atrial tachycardia is a *permanent* or *incessant* atrial tachycardia, with the arrhythmia being present for more than 50% of the day (Fig. 60.12). In these patients, the rate of impulse formation in the atrium frequently increases during sympathetic stimulation (e.g., during exercise). Administration of antiarrhythmic drugs usually fails to prevent 1:1 AV conduction during exercise in these patients. The incessant nature of the arrhythmia and the difficulty in controlling the ventricular rate may lead to dilated (tachycardia-induced) cardiomyopathy (6). A fuller discussion of atrial tachycardia can be found in Chapter 65.

Atrial Flutter

Atrial flutter is typically characterized by a regular atrial rhythm, a rate of 250 to 350 beats/min, and an atrial activity with a sawtooth pattern. Identifying atrial activity during atrial flutter can be facilitated by carotid sinus massage (CSM) (Fig. 60.13). Depending on the pattern of atrial

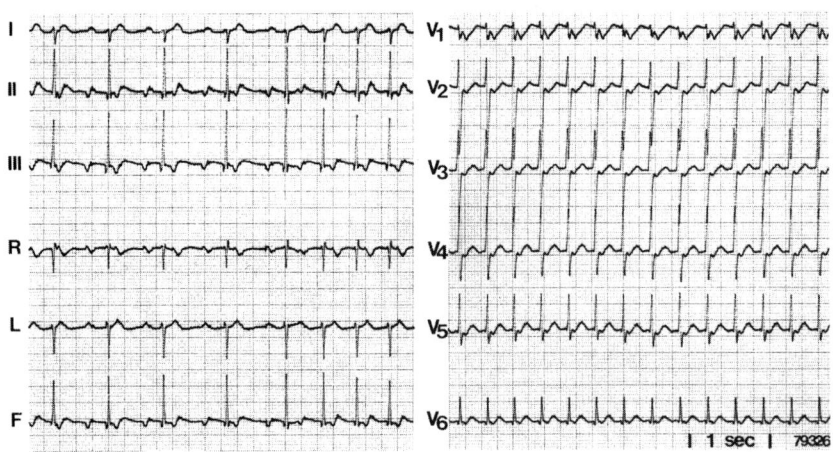

FIGURE 60.12 Incessant atrial tachycardia. Atrioventricular conduction of 2:1 is present in the left panel, changing into 1:1 atrioventricular conduction. The origin of the arrhythmia is low in the intraatrial septum.

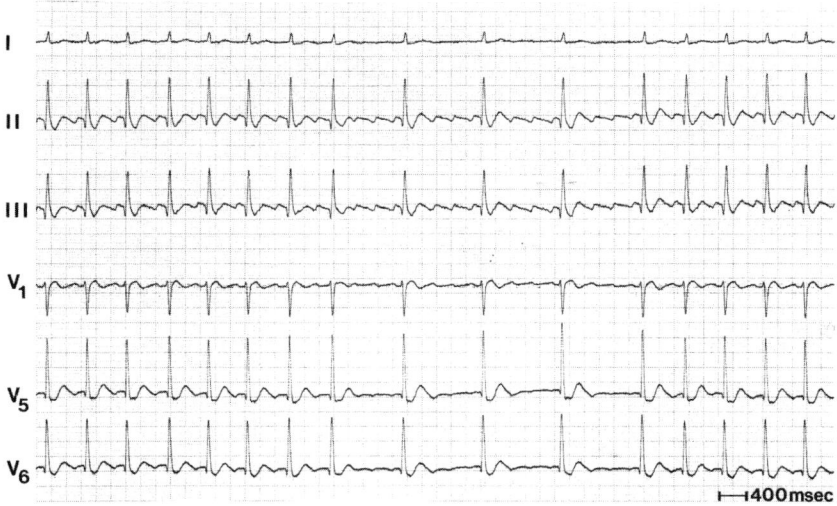

FIGURE 60.13 Atrial flutter. Shown here is an atrioventricular conduction of 2:1, changing in the middle to 4:1 atrioventricular conduction during carotid sinus massage.

activation during flutter, the shape and polarity of the flutter waves may differ. The ventricular rate during atrial flutter depends on the conduction characteristics of the AV conduction system and usually varies from a 2:1 AV relation to higher degrees of AV block. A fuller discussion of atrial flutter can be found in Chapter 65.

Atrial Fibrillation

During atrial fibrillation (AF) atrial activity is characteristically rapid, with a rate of 350 to 500 beats/min, and shows an irregular rhythm that varies continuously in shape (Fig. 60.14). Depending on the shape and duration of the fibrillatory waves, one can distinguish coarse from fine AF. The

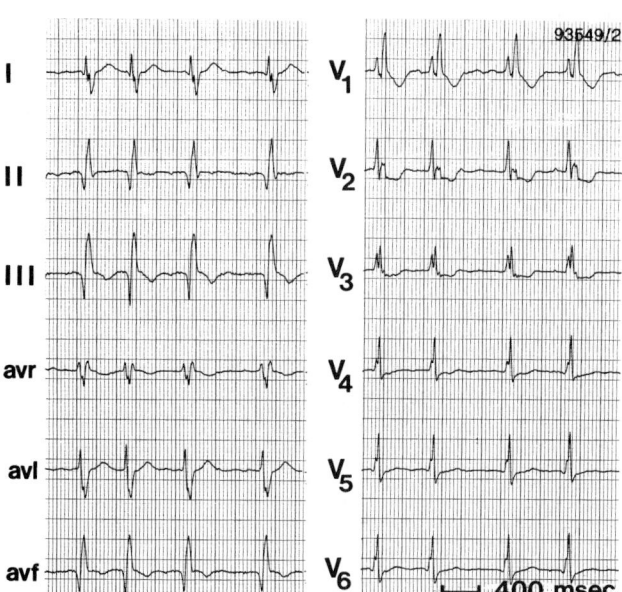

FIGURE 60.14 Atrial fibrillation. Characteristic of atrial fibrillation are the changes in atrial activation pattern and the irregularity of the RR intervals.

underlying mechanism cannot be identified by such ECG characteristics of AF. The ventricular rate during AF depends on the electrophysiologic properties of the AV conduction system. The refractory period of AV nodal and subnodal tissue and concealed conduction in the AV node determine the ventricular frequency during AF, which, in the absence of a refractory period prolonging drugs, is from 130 to 180 beats/min.

When two connections between the atrium and ventricle are present and are able to conduct the impulses from the atrium to the ventricle during preexcitation, the ventricular rate during AF relates to the duration of the refractory period of the two connections (7). When the AV AP has a short anterograde refractory period, a very high ventricular rate may occur during AF (Fig. 60.15). This high ventricular rate may deteriorate into ventricular fibrillation and may result in sudden cardiac death. The characteristic ECG feature of AF in the presence of ventricular preexcitation is a rapid, irregular ventricular rhythm with wide QRS complexes. The QRS configuration changes according to the contribution of the two AV pathways to ventricular activation. A fuller discussion of AF can be found in Chapter 64.

Tachycardias Located in the Atrioventricular Nodal Region

During these arrhythmias, there is usually 1:1 conduction from the AV nodal region to the atrium and to the ventricle (see Chapter 66), and because of the simultaneous activation of the atrium and the ventricle, the P waves are generally hidden within the QRS complex, or they may fall in the terminal part of the QRS complex, mimicking S waves in leads II, III, and aVF and a pseudo-incomplete right bundle branch block (RBBB) pattern in lead V_1 (Fig. 60.16); this is the *common* form of AV nodal tachycardia. The P wave rarely follows the QRS complex with an RP interval

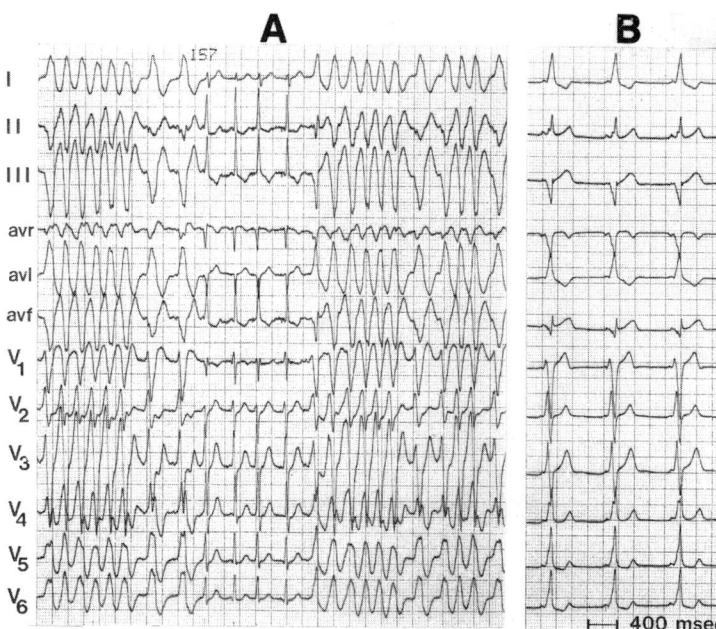

FIGURE 60.15 **A:** Atrial fibrillation in a patient with the Wolff-Parkinson-White syndrome. Note atrioventricular (AV) conduction over the accessory pathway (AP) on the left and right sides of the panel, with AV conduction over the AV node in the middle. As shown, the ventricular rate can become very high during AV conduction over the AP. **B:** Posteroseptal location of the AP is shown during sinus rhythm.

longer than the PR interval; this is an *uncommon form* of AV nodal tachycardia. In contrast to the common form of AV nodal tachycardia, the uncommon form is usually short lived and self-terminates within seconds to minutes.

Occasionally, 2:1 block develops between the AV node and the ventricle. The P wave typically is exactly in the middle between two QRS complexes. Because atrial activation starts low in the intraatrial septum, the P wave is narrow and negative in leads II, III, and aVF (Fig. 60.17). A

fuller discussion of these tachycardias can be found in Chapter 66.

Tachycardias Using Extra Connections between Atrium and Ventricle: Circus-Movement Tachycardia

The presence of more than one connection between the atrium and ventricle creates a possible pathway for a reentry

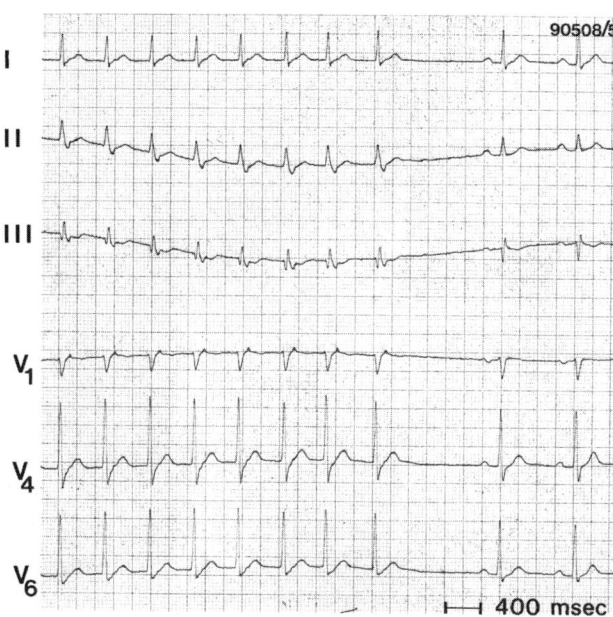

FIGURE 60.16 Common form of atrioventricular nodal tachycardia. Note the pseudo-S wave in leads II and III and the pseudo, incomplete right bundle branch block pattern in lead V₁ caused by the P wave during tachycardia.

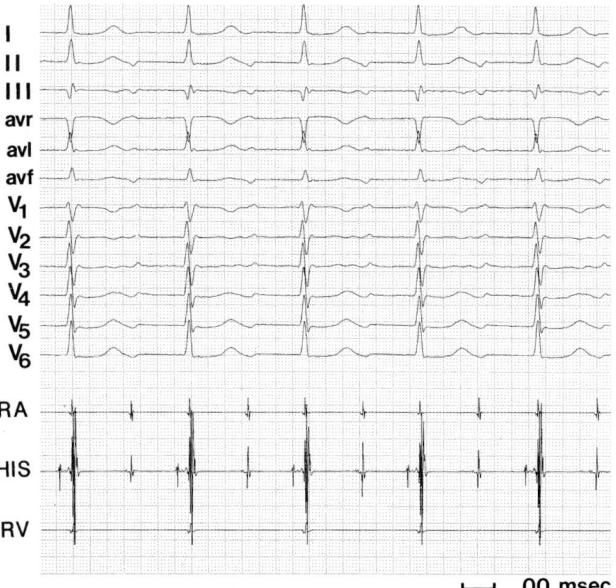

FIGURE 60.17 Atrioventricular (AV) nodal tachycardia with 2:1 block between the AV node and the ventricle and 1:1 conduction from the AV node to the atrium. As shown in the bundle of His recording (HIS), the 2:1 block is located in the distal part of the AV node. RA, right atrium; RV, right ventricle.

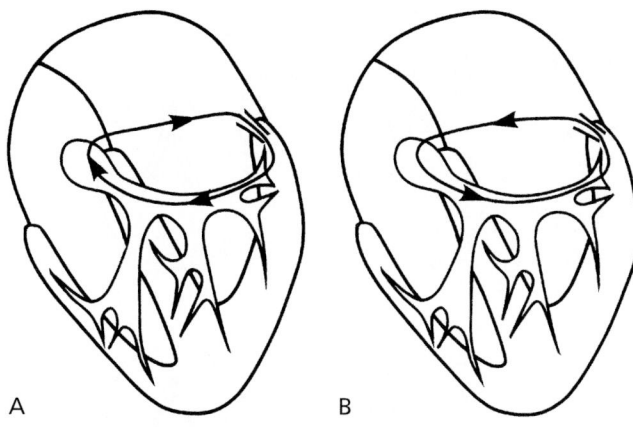

FIGURE 60.18 The two types of circus-movement tachycardias (CMT) in a patient with an accessory atrioventricular (AV) pathway. **A:** Orthodromic CMT with AV conduction over the AV node and ventricular conduction over the accessory pathway. **B:** CMT in the reverse direction—antidromic CMT.

circuit resulting in a tachycardia. During tachycardia, AV conduction occurs over one AV connection, and VA conduction occurs over the other. Depending on the pathway used for AV conduction, the tachycardia may show (a) a narrow QRS complex or a typical RBBB or left bundle branch block (LBBB) configuration when AV conduction occurs over the AV node–His pathway or (b) a preexcited QRS complex when AV conduction occurs over the accessory connection (Fig. 60.18).

In the first type of tachycardia, termed *orthodromic circus-movement tachycardia (CMT)*, the AP is the retrograde limb in the tachycardia circuit. If the AP rapidly conducts the impulse, a short RP interval results. Less frequently, an AP has slower conduction properties and the RP interval is long (Figs. 60.19 and 60.20). In the second type of tachycardia, referred to as an *antidromic CMT*, AV conduction occurs over the accessory connection, resulting in a wide QRS complex that shows pronounced slurring of its initial portion; such a wide QRS complex with pronounced slurring is due to ventricular activation starting outside the intraventricular conduction system (Fig. 60.21). VA conduction during this tachycardia may occur either by way of the His–AV node axis or by way of a second accessory connection. A fuller discussion of CMTs can be found in Chapter 65.

Additional Features That Are Helpful in Differentiating Supraventricular Tachycardias

Electrical Alternans

During a regular SVT, the QRS configuration and the T wave may alternate in height (Fig. 60.22). This phenomenon is more common in orthodromic CMT than in atrial or AV nodal tachycardia (8). It especially occurs during high rates of the tachycardia and can only be considered suggestive of orthodromic CMT when alternation occurs for longer than 5 seconds after the beginning of the tachycardia.

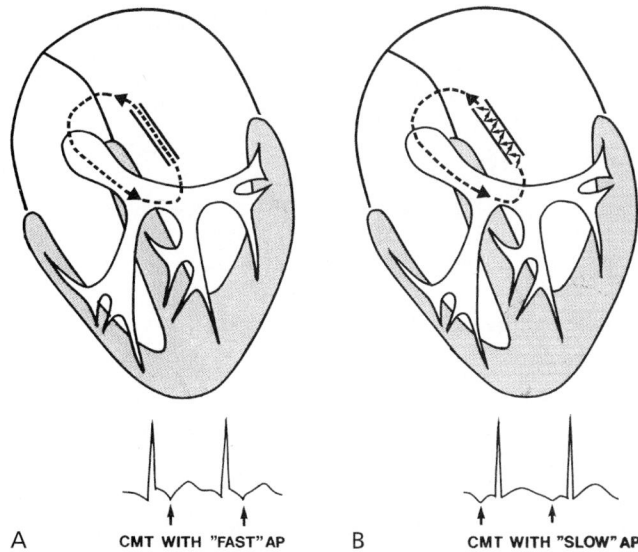

FIGURE 60.19 Two types of accessory pathways (AP) and their effect on the RP interval during circus-movement tachycardia (CMT). **A:** Rapidly conducting AP resulting in a short RP interval during orthodromic CMT. **B:** Slowly conducting AP leads to a long RP interval during tachycardia.

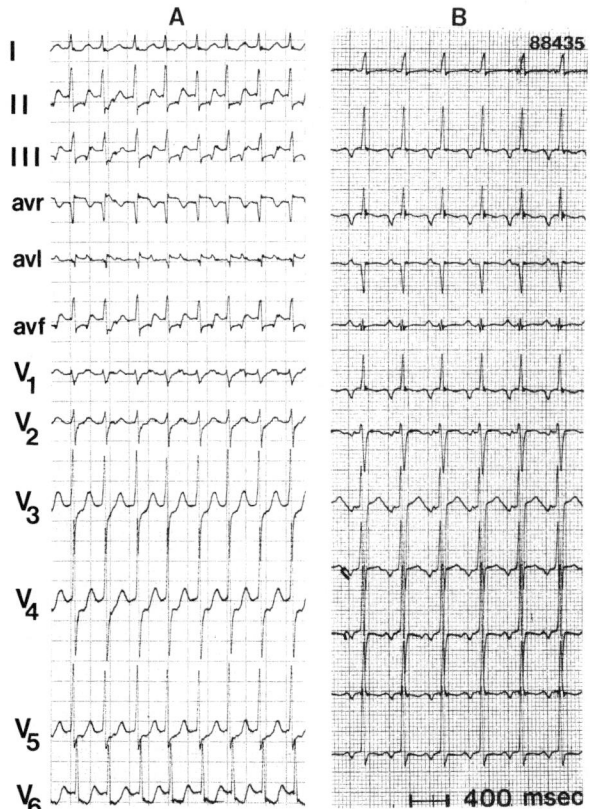

FIGURE 60.20 Examples of the two types of tachycardias for which the tachycardia circuit is shown in Figure 60.19. **A:** Ventriculoatrial conduction over the rapidly conducting accessory pathway. **B:** Conduction over a slowly conducting accessory pathway.

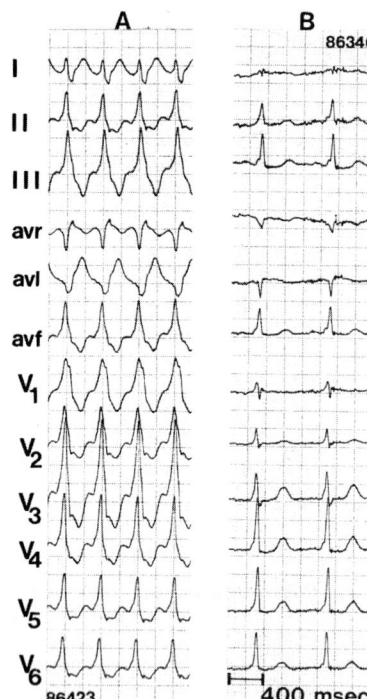

FIGURE 60.21 A: Antidromic circus-movement tachycardia with atrioventricular conduction over a left posterior accessory pathway. **B:** Same patient during sinus rhythm.

Effect of Bundle Branch Block on the Tachycardia Rate

When one of the bundle branches is incorporated into the tachycardia circuit, block in that bundle branch during tachycardia usually slows the tachycardia rate (9). As shown

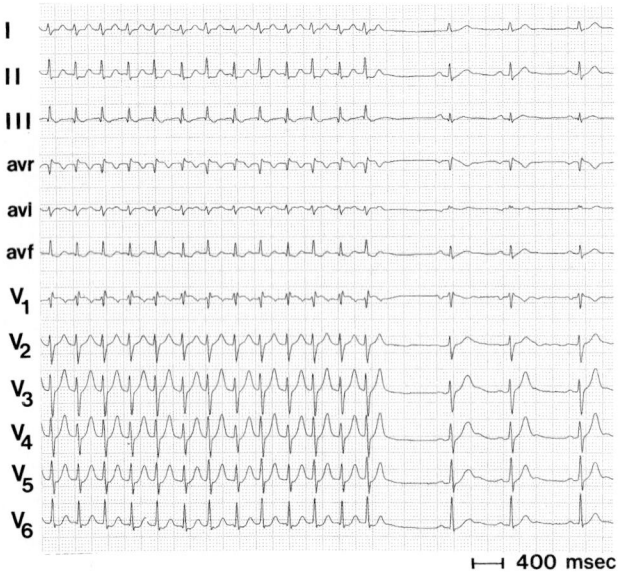

FIGURE 60.22 Electrical alternans of the QRS complex during a circus-movement tachycardia using a "concealed" atrioventricular accessory pathway. The tachycardia terminates when block occurs in the atrioventricular nodal part of the circuit.

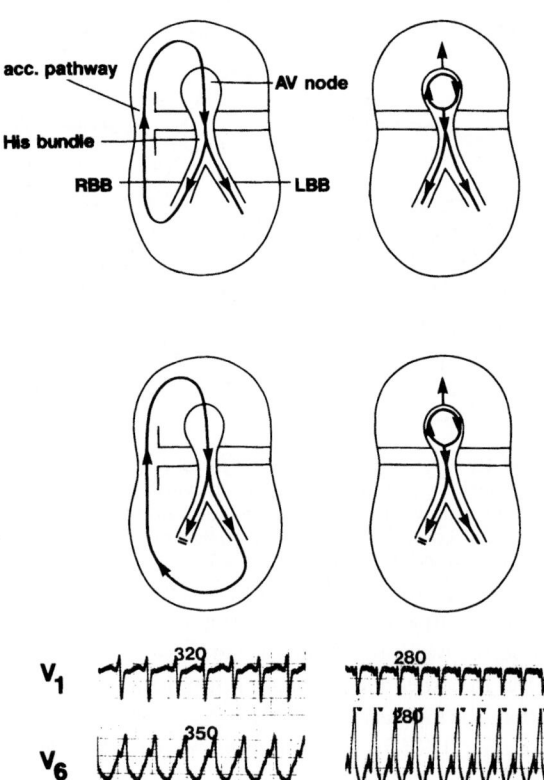

FIGURE 60.23 Effect of a bundle branch block during circus-movement tachycardia using an accessory (acc.) pathway that is on the same side of the heart as the bundle branch block. As shown, the circuit becomes longer when right bundle branch block (RBB) develops in a patient with a right-sided accessory pathway. Nothing happens to the tachycardia rate when bundle branch block develops during atrioventricular (AV) nodal reentrant tachycardia (measurements are in ms). LBB, left bundle branch block.

in Figures 60.23 and 60.24, this can only occur in orthodromic CMT.

Value of Carotid Sinus Massage

CSM can be very helpful in differentiating regular from irregular tachycardias. This is illustrated in Table 60.1. Table 60.2 summarizes the ECG features of the most common types of regular SVTs.

Wide QRS Tachycardia

Correctly identifying the site of origin of a wide QRS tachycardia is not only important to proper treatment of the arrhythmia but also to the prognosis. VT usually has a more ominous prognosis than does SVT.

Table 60.3 and Figure 60.25 illustrate the possible causes of a wide QRS tachycardia. To correctly diagnose such a tachycardia, it is essential to use a 12-lead ECG. This should be used systematically, checking for independent atrial and ventricular activity (AV dissociation) and

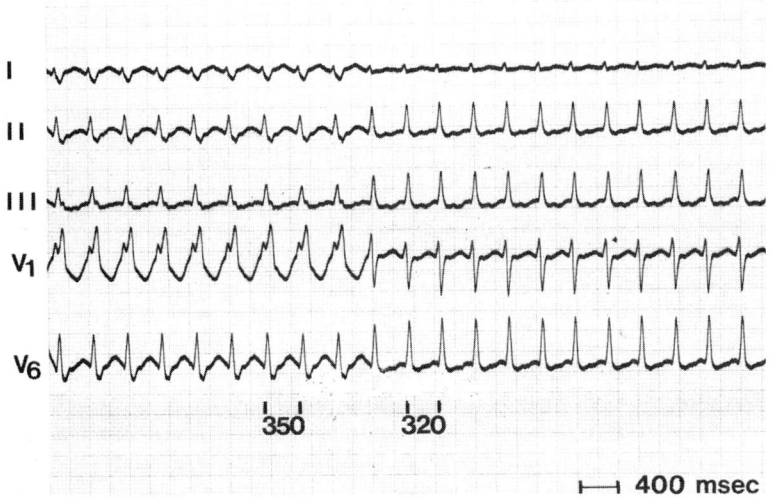

FIGURE 60.24 Example of rate change during right bundle branch block in a patient with an orthodromic circus-movement tachycardia using a right-sided accessory pathway. During right bundle branch block, the RR interval is 30 ms longer compared with the RR interval during nonaberrant conduction.

TABLE 60.1 EFFECT OF CAROTID SINUS MASSAGE ON SUPRAVENTRICULAR TACHYCARDIA

Type of supraventricular tachycardia	Effect of carotid sinus massage
Sinus tachycardia	Gradual and temporary slowing of the heart
Atrial tachycardia	
Paroxysmal	Cessation of tachycardia or no effect
Incessant	Temporary slowing of ventricular rate (because of AV block) or no effect
Atrial flutter	Temporary slowing of ventricular rate (because of AV block) or no effect
AVNRT	Cessation of tachycardia or no effect
CMT	Cessation of tachycardia or no effect

AV, atrioventricular; AVNRT, AV nodal reentry tachycardia; CMT, circus-movement tachycardia (using an AV accessory pathway and the AV node).

for characteristics of a QRS tachycardia such as its width, axis, and configuration.

Atrioventricular Dissociation

Independent atrial and ventricular activity during a wide QRS tachycardia has been correctly considered a hallmark of VT. However, during VT some form of VA conduction may be present, especially when the VT rate is relatively slow (10). When AV dissociation is present during VT, the atrial rate is usually slower than the ventricular rate, except in atrial tachycardia, atrial flutter, or AF. During VT, part or all of the ventricle may occasionally be activated by a supraventricular impulse (e.g., a sinus beat), which is conducted through the AV conduction system and arrives in the ventricle when the ventricle is partly or completely

TABLE 60.2 SUMMARY OF ELECTROCARDIOGRAPHIC FEATURES OF THE MOST COMMON TYPES OF REGULAR SUPRAVENTRICULAR TACHYCARDIAS

ECG signs	AT	CMT	AVNRT
AV block (spontaneous or by CSM)	If present, may not only be useful for diagnosing AT but also for differentiating atrial flutter (atrial rate >250/min) from AT	Rules out CMT	Unusual, but 2:1 block is possible
Electrical alternans	Rare	Common (especially at high tachycardia rates)	Rare
P-wave location in relation to QRS complex	Present between R waves; PR length varies with atrial site of origin and AV nodal conduction time	Present between R waves: RP <PR in fast AP, RP >PR in slow AP	Hidden in QRS or distorting the distal portion of the QRS
P polarity	Varies with the location of atrial impulse formation	Varies according to location of atrial-end AP	Always negative in leads II, III, and AVF
Aberrant conduction	Rare	Common	Rare

AP, accessory pathway; AT, atrial tachycardia; AV, atrioventricular; AVF, atrioventricular fibrillation; AVNRT, atrioventricular nodal reentry tachycardia; CMT, circus-movement tachycardia incorporating AP; CSM, carotid sinus massage; ECG, electrocardiogram.

TABLE 60.3 POSSIBLE CAUSES OF A WIDE QRS TACHYCARDIA

A supraventricular tachycardia (SVT) with preexisting or functional bundle branch block; this includes sinus tachycardia, atrial tachycardia, atrial flutter, atrial fibrillation, and atrioventricular (AV) nodal reentry tachycardia

Orthodromic circus-movement tachycardia (CMT) using the AV node in the anterograde direction and an accessory pathway (AP) in the retrograde direction with preexisting or functional bundle branch block

An SVT with conduction over an AP

Antidromic CMT using an AP in the anterograde direction and the AV node or another AP in the retrograde direction

A reentry tachycardia using a nodoventricular fiber in the anterograde direction and the bundle branch–His pathway or another AP in the retrograde direction

A ventricular tachycardia

---

excitable. This typically occurs when the VT rate is relatively slow. This phenomenon results in capture or fusion beats (Fig. 60.26).

Width of the QRS Complex

Absence or delay in RBB conduction during a supraventricular rhythm results in an RBBB configuration and a QRS complex with a width of 120 ms. When conduction in the LBB is blocked, the width of the QRS complex may become as long as 140 ms. These facts are of value in distinguishing an SVT from a VT. The wider the QRS complex, the more likely that the tachycardia is ventricular in origin. This is typically the case when ectopic ventricular impulse formation occurs in the free wall of the right or left ventricle and when activation of the two ventricles occurs sequentially rather than simultaneously. This finding prompted Wellens et al. (10) to evaluate the role of the width of the QRS complex in distinguishing an SVT from a VT complex. For several reasons, however, an SVT has a QRS width of greater than 140 ms. They include (a) SVT in the presence of BBB with additional intramyocardial conduction delay, (b) SVT with AV conduction over an AV, and (c) marked QRS widening during SVT because of the use of antiarrhythmic drugs that prolong intraventricular conduction.

VT may have a QRS width of less than 140 ms. Such is the case for VTs that originate in or close to the specific conduction system of the left ventricle (Fig. 60.27).

QRS Axis in the Frontal Plane

When impulse formation originates in the ventricle, the frontal plane axis is frequently abnormal. This axis depends on the site of origin of the VT. In 1976, Wellens et al. (10) observed that a frontal plane axis to the left of −30 degrees during tachycardia was suggestive of a VT. This observation still holds true in VT with an RBBB configuration but remains questionable in VT with an LBBB shape (11).

The etiology of VT with an LBBB shape is usually either (a) an anterior or inferoposterior scar from a previous myocardial infarction (MI) in or close to the interventricular septum, (b) an idiopathic VT arising from the outflow tract of the right ventricle, or (c) a VT in arrhythmogenic

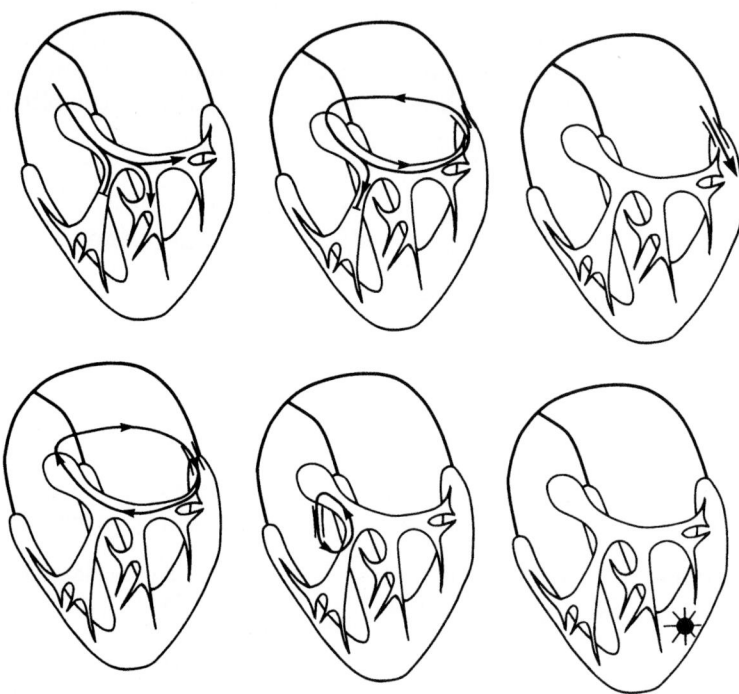

FIGURE 60.25 Six possible causes of a wide QRS tachycardia. See Table 60.3 for a full description.

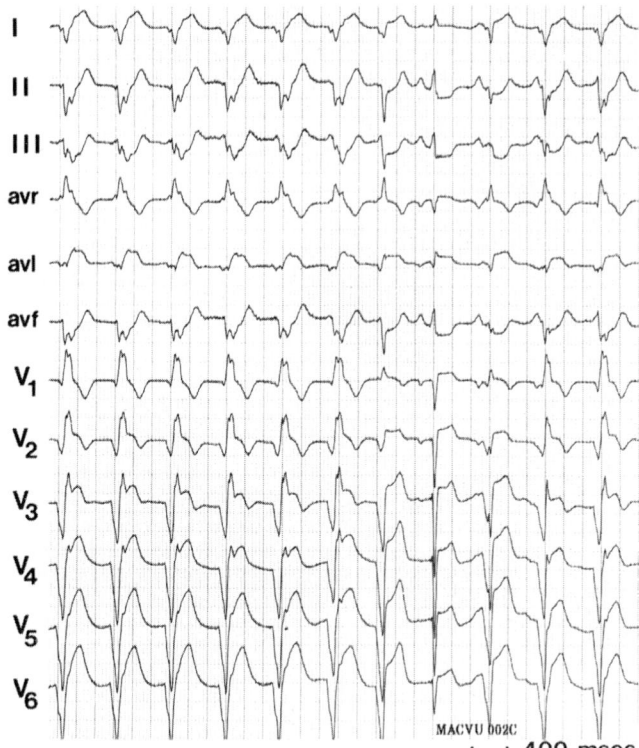

FIGURE 60.26 Ventricular tachycardia with a relatively slow rate, allowing the occurrence of capture and fusion beats. The tracing was recorded in a patient with a recent anterior wall myocardial infarction. Note the QR pattern in several leads during ventricular tachycardia.

right ventricular (RV) dysplasia. Whereas in the first and third etiologies the exit point of the VT and, therefore, of the QRS axis may vary, in idiopathic VT from the RV outflow tract the frontal plane axis is typically vertical or to the right. In general, in a patient with a wide LBBB-shaped tachycardia, marked left-axis deviation (i.e., to the left of –60 degrees) or marked right-axis deviation (i.e., to the right of +90 degrees) suggests a ventricular arrhythmia.

Configurational Characteristics of the QRS Complex

Right Bundle Branch Block–Shaped QRS Complex

In SVT with RBBB, leads V_1 and V_6 usually have a triphasic pattern (10,12). Lead V_1 has an rSR' pattern, with the initial r reflecting normal septal activation, the S wave reflecting left ventricular activation, and the R' wave reflecting delayed activation of the right ventricle. Lead V_6 shows a narrow q wave resulting from normal septal activation, an R wave representing left ventricular activation, and an S wave reflecting delayed RV activation. In lead V_6 the R:S ratio is typically greater than 1:1.

In VT with an RBBB shape, lead V_1 shows a monophasic or biphasic QRS complex (i.e., R, qr, rs). The presence of a deep S wave in lead V_6 with an R:S ratio of less than 1:1 supports a diagnosis of VT (10). This is typically the case when left-axis deviation is present. In the case of right-axis deviation, the R:S ratio in lead V_6 is usually greater than 1:1 (Fig. 60.28).

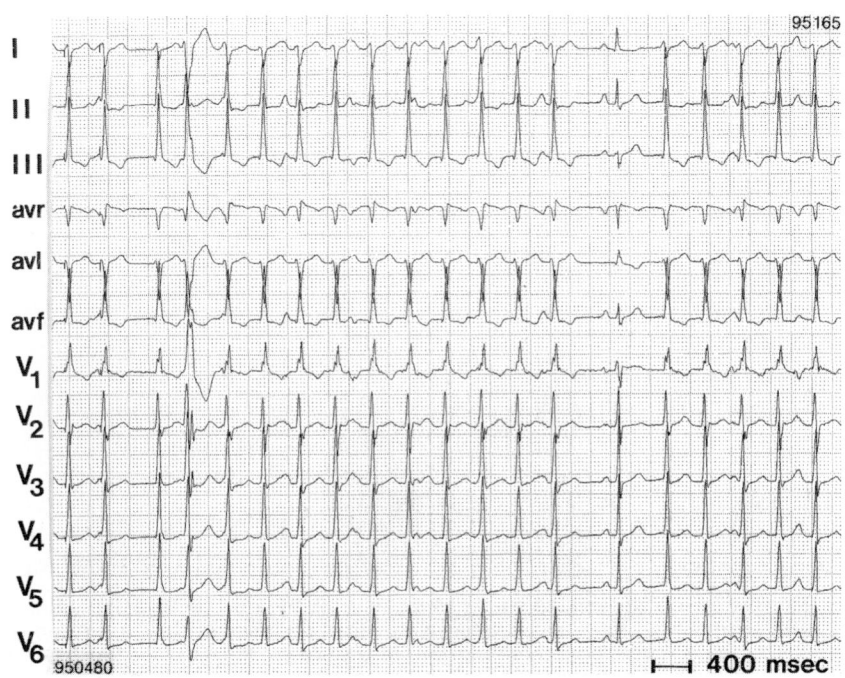

FIGURE 60.27 Idiopathic ventricular tachycardia arising in or close to the anterior fascicle of the left bundle branch. Note atrioventricular dissociation during ventricular tachycardia. Note also that the QRS width during ventricular tachycardia is only 120 ms.

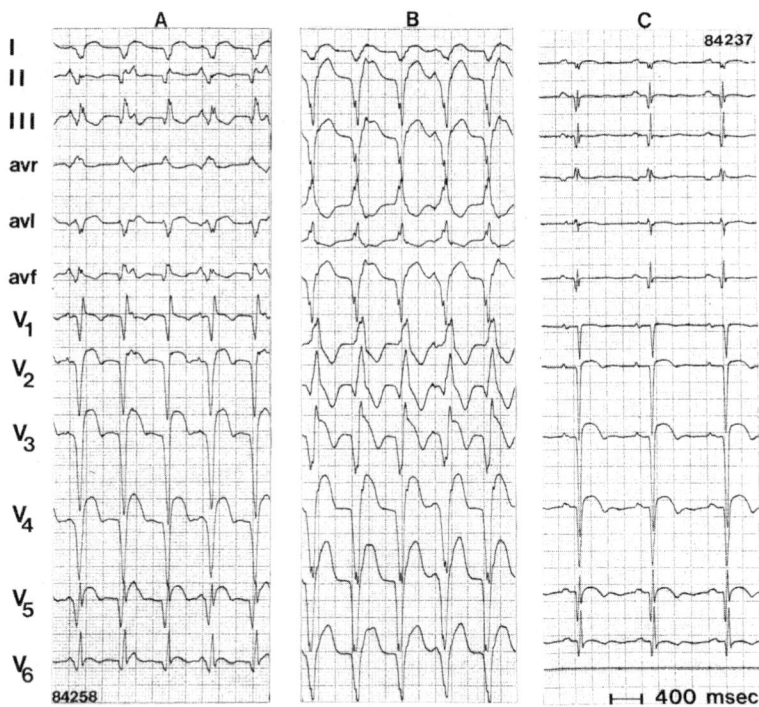

FIGURE 60.28 Two types of ventricular tachycardias in a patient with an old anteroseptal and apical myocardial infarction **(A)**. In **B** and **C**, a right bundle branch block pattern is present, with a QR and a monophasic R, respectively, in lead V₁. QRS negativity or positivity in lead V₆ is related to the frontal plane axis. A QS complex during left-axis deviation is shown in **B**, and a QR complex during right-axis deviation is shown in **C**. During ventricular tachycardia, atrioventricular dissociation is clearly present in **B** and in **C**.

Left Bundle Branch Block–Shaped QRS Complex

Leads V_1, V_2, and V_6 are the important ECG leads to use in distinguishing a VT from an SVT with LBBB (11). If an r wave is present in either lead V_1 or V_2, it is narrow (i.e., <0.04 second) in SVT with LBBB. Moreover, the downstroke of the S wave is fast, without slurring or notching, and the distance from the beginning of the QRS to the nadir of the S wave is 0.06 second or less. If in lead(s) V_1 or V_2, or both, the r wave is greater than 0.04 second and the downstroke of the S wave is slurred and delayed, a diagnosis of VT is likely (Fig. 60.29). A Q wave in lead V_6 is diagnostic of VT (11).

Concordant Pattern in the Precordial Leads

Leads V_1 through V_6 may all show positive or negative QRS complexes, referred to as *positive* and *negative concordancy*. Negative concordancy is diagnostic of VT (Fig. 60.30). Positive concordancy occurs not only in VT originating in the posterobasal area of the left ventricle but may also be seen in tachycardias with AV conduction over an AP inserting into the posterobasal left ventricle (Fig. 60.21).

Presence of Q Waves during Tachycardia

As a rule, QR complexes during a wide QRS tachycardia are highly suggestive of VT (Figs. 60.26, 60.28, 60.29) unless identical QR complexes are present in the same leads during sinus rhythm (13). However, Qr complexes may occur, although rarely, during tachycardia and sinus rhythm in the same leads in the presence of a bundle branch reentrant tachycardia (14) (Fig. 60.31). As is shown in Table 60.4, in patients with VT following MI,

approximately 40% have a QR complex in one or more of the ECG leads. QR complexes during VT typically occur in patients with a localized ventricular scar, as in

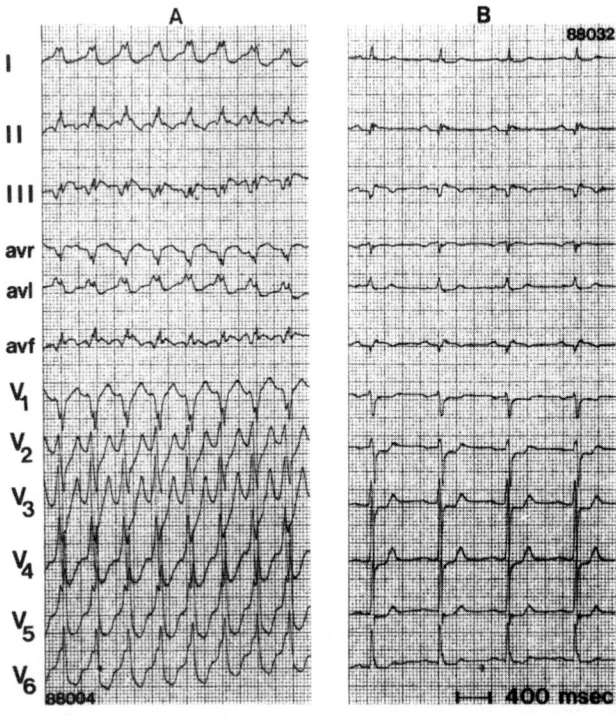

FIGURE 60.29 A: Ventricular tachycardia with a left bundle branch block shape. Note initial positivity of the QRS in lead V₁ (>0.04 second), slurring of the S wave in leads V₁ and V₂, and a distance from the beginning of the QRS to the nadir of the S wave of 120 ms in leads V₁ and V₂. **B:** An old inferior myocardial infarction.

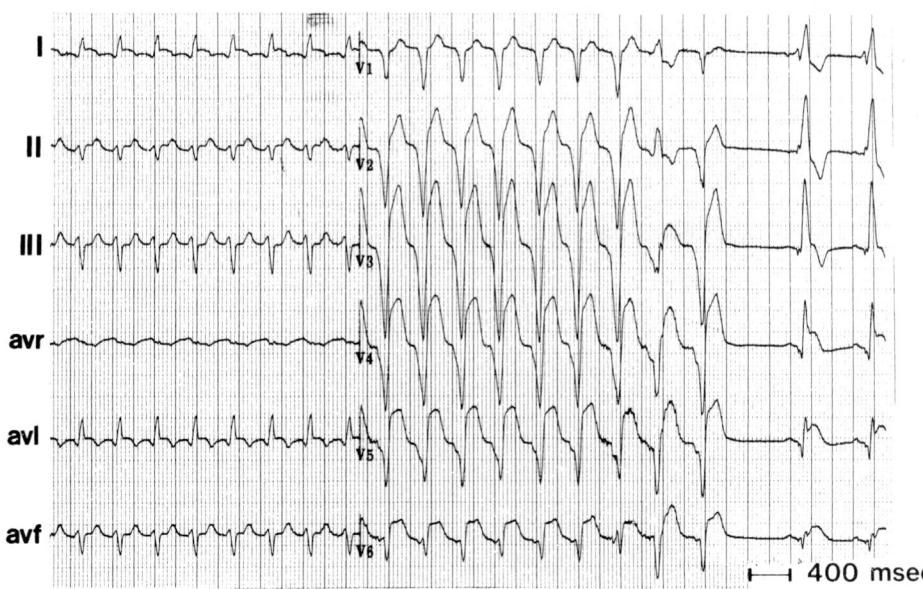

FIGURE 60.30 Ventricular tachycardia (VT) shows a negative concordant pattern in the precordial leads. This is diagnostic of VT. The QRS following termination of VT shows an old anteroapical myocardial infarction.

those with a previous MI or localized infiltrative or inflammatory myocardial disease.

Interval from Onset of QRS to Nadir of the S Wave in Precordial Leads

As already indicated in Left Bundle Branch Block–Shaped QRS Complex, the interval from the onset of QRS to the nadir of the S wave in precordial leads is increased in VT. Brugada et al. (15) have suggested that an RS interval of greater than 100 ms in one or more precordial leads is highly suggestive of VT. The clinician must be careful, however, because such a duration may occur in SVT with AV conduction over an AP, SVT during the administration of drugs that slow intraventricular conduction, and SVT with preexistent BBB, especially LBBB.

TABLE 60.4 INCIDENCE OF QR COMPLEXES IN PREVIOUS MYOCARDIAL INFARCTION AND THE CORRELATION BETWEEN QR PATTERN DURING VENTRICULAR TACHYCARDIA AND SITE OF MYOCARDIAL INFARCTION DURING SINUS RHYTHM

	LBBB morphology (n = 58) (%)	RBBB morphology (n = 75) (%)
Presence of a QR in any lead except aVR during VT	25/58 (43)	28/75 (37)
Correlation between the site of QR pattern during VT and site of myocardial infarction during sinus rhythm (in ≥1 lead)	21/25 (84)	20/28 (71)

LBBB, left bundle branch block; RBBB, right bundle branch block; VT, ventricular tachycardia.

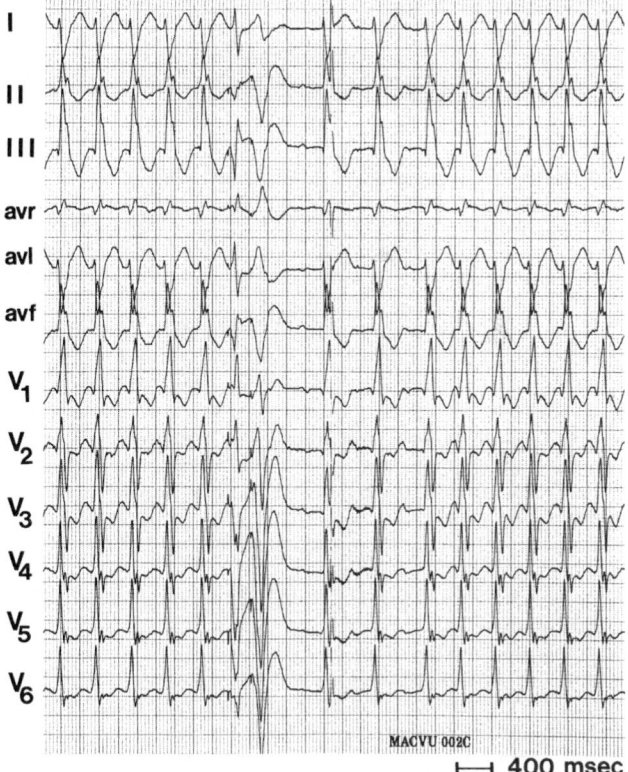

MACVU 002C

├──┤ 400 msec

FIGURE 60.31 Ventricular tachycardia based on bundle branch reentry. After two electrically induced premature ventricular beats, the tachycardia terminates in the middle of the recording. However, it resumes after three conducted sinus beats. QRS is identical during sinus rhythm and tachycardia. During electrophysiologic study, the tachycardia was found to be based on bundle branch reentry, with the right bundle branch as the retrograde pathway. The tachycardia was cured by radiofrequency ablation of the right bundle branch.

PRACTICAL APPROACH TO ELECTROCARDIOGRAPHIC ANALYSIS IN PATIENTS WITH WIDE QRS TACHYCARDIAS

It is essential to follow a systematic approach when analyz- ing ECGs in patients with wide QRS tachycardias. Table 60.5 reviews the different signs that should be systemati- cally checked for when analyzing a regular wide QRS tachycardia. Correctly diagnosing the tachycardia is imper- ative, because incorrectly diagnosing an SVT may lead to selecting inappropriate antiarrhythmic drugs and to delete- rious results (16,17). Such an error is one of the most fre- quent mistakes made in treating arrhythmias; hence, familiarity with the criteria described herein should almost invariably prevent such a misdiagnosis.

TABLE 60.5 VALUE AND LIMITATIONS OF SIGNS IN DIAGNOSING REGULAR WIDE QRS TACHYCARDIA

Atrioventricular (AV) dissociation suggests ventricular tachycardia (VT), but ventriculoatrial conduction may be present during VT.
A *QRS width* of >160 ms suggests VT, but one needs to rule out (a) preexistent bundle branch block [BBB, especially left BBB (LBBB)], (b) supraventricular tachycardia (SVT) with AV conduc- tion over an accessory pathway (AP), and (c) use of drugs that slow intraventricular conduction delay (class IA, IC, amiodarone).
Keep in mind: VT arising close to or in the intraventricular con- duction system may have a width of ≤140 ms.
Left-axis deviation (to the left of −30 degrees) suggests VT but is not helpful in (a) LBBB-shaped QRS, (b) SVT with conduction over a right-sided or posteroseptal AP, and (c) SVT during use of class IC drugs.
Right-axis deviation (to the right of +90 degrees) suggests VT in LBBB-shaped QRS.
QR complexes in leads other than aVR suggest VT unless the same QRS configuration is present in the same leads during sinus rhythm (unless bundle branch reentry is present).
Concordant pattern in precordial leads suggests VT, but positive concordancy may occur during SVT with AV conduction over a left posterior AP.
R-nadir S ≥100 ms in one or more precordial leads suggests VT but may be found in (a) SVT on drugs that slow intraventricu- lar conduction, (b) SVT with AV conduction over an AP, and (c) preexistent BBB (especially LBBB).
In the presence of capture or fusion beats, rule out (a) fusion with a contralateral premature ventricular beat and (b) fusion with a ventricular echo beat.

REFERENCES

1. Wellens HJ, Brugada P, Penn OC. The management of preexcitation syndromes. *JAMA* 1987;257:2325.
2. Wolff L, Parkinson J, White PD. Bundle-branch block with short PR interval in healthy young people prone to paroxysmal tachycardia. *Am Heart J* 1930;5:685.
3. Becker AE, Anderson RH, Durrer D, Wellens HJJ. The anatomic substrates of Wolff-Parkinson-White syndrome: a clinicopathological correlation in seven patients. *Circula- tion* 1978;57:870.
4. Moe GK, Jalife J, Mueller WJ, et al. A mathematical model of parasystole and its application to clinical arrhythmias. *Circulation* 1977;56:968.
5. Wellens HJJ, Ross DL, Farré J, Brugada P. Functional bundle-branch block during supraventricular tachycardia in man: observations on mechanisms and their incidence. In: Zipes D, Jalife J, eds. *Cardiac electrophysiology and arrhythmias.* New York: Grune & Stratton, 1985:435– 441.
6. Wellens HJ, Rodriguez LM, Smeets J, et al. Tachycardi- omyopathy in patients with supraventricular tachycardia with emphasis on atrial fibrillation. In: Olsson B, Allessie MA, Campbell RWF, eds. *Atrial fibrillation.* Armonk, NY: Futura Publishing, 1994:333–342.
7. Wellens HJ, Durrer D. Relation between refractory period of the accessory pathway and ventricular frequency during atrial fibrillation in patients with the Wolff-Parkinson- White syndrome. *Am J Cardiol* 1974;34:777.
8. Green M, Heddle B, Dassen W, et al. The value of QRS alternation in diagnosing the site of origin of narrow QRS supraventricular tachycardia. *Circulation* 1983;68:368.
9. Coumel PH, Attuel P. Reciprocating tachycardia in overt and latent preexcitation: influence of functional bundle- branch block on the rate of tachycardia. *Eur J Cardiol* 1974;1:423.
10. Wellens HJ, Bär FW, Lie KI. The value of the electrocar- diogram in the differential diagnosis of a tachycardia with a widened QRS complex. *Am J Med* 1978;64:27.
11. Kindwall E, Brown J, Josephson ME. Electrocardio- graphic criteria for ventricular tachycardia in wide QRS complex left bundle-branch block morphology tachycar- dia. *Am J Cardiol* 1988;61:1279.
12. Marriott HJ. Differential diagnosis of supraventricular and ventricular tachycardia. *Geriatrics* 1970;25:91.
13. Coumel P, Leclercq JF, Attuel P, Slama R. The QRS mor- phology in postmyocardial infarction ventricular tachycar-

dia: a study in 100 tracings compared with 70 cases of idiopathic ventricular tachycardia. *Eur Heart J* 1984;5:792.

14. Oreto G, Smeets J, Rodriguez LM, et al. Wide complex tachycardia with atrioventricular dissociation and QRS morphology identical to that of sinus rhythm: a manifestation of bundle-branch reentry. *Heart* 1996;76:541.

15. Brugada P, Brugada J, Mont L, et al. A new approach to the differential diagnosis of a regular tachycardia with a wide QRS complex. *Circulation* 1991;83:1649.

16. Dancy M, Camm AJ, Ward D. Misdiagnosis of chronic recurrent ventricular tachycardia. *Lancet* 1985;2:320.

17. Buxton AE, Marchlinski FE, Doherty JU. Hazards of intravenous verapamil for sustained ventricular tachycardia. *Am J Cardiol* 1987;59:1107.

BRADYCARDIAS: SINUS NODAL DYSFUNCTION AND ATRIOVENTRICULAR CONDUCTION DISTURBANCES

DEBORAH L. WOLBRETTE
GERALD V. NACCARELLI

OVERVIEW

Sinus nodal dysfunction and atrioventricular (AV) block account for the majority of significant bradyarrhythmias. In addition to structural abnormalities, drug effects and autonomic influences can cause sinus nodal dysfunction. Acquired AV block is most commonly caused by idiopathic fibrosis, acute myocardial infarction, or drug effects. Patients with asymptomatic sinus bradycardia or sinus pauses have a good prognosis and do not require treatment. On the other hand, those with tachycardia-bradycardia syndrome have a much worse prognosis, because of their risk of thromboembolic complications. Therefore, the aim of therapy is prevention of atrial fibrillation. Atrial pacing and anticoagulation can greatly reduce the incidence of stroke in this high-risk group. Once appropriate pacing has been

established for AV block, the prognosis is primarily dependent on the extent of the associated heart disease. The availability of dual-chamber and rate-responsive pacing has greatly improved the lifestyle and prognosis of symptomatic patients. In many instances, the challenge for physicians is documenting sinus nodal dysfunction or AV block in association with symptoms.

GLOSSARY

Acquired complete heart block: Third-degree AV block present as a result of some insult to the specialized conduction system, but not present at birth. Usually it is associated with block below the AV node.

Bifascicular block: Conduction delay in two fascicles; right bundle branch block with left anterior fascicular block, right bundle branch block with left posterior fascicular block, or left bundle branch block.

Congenital complete heart block: Third-degree AV block present from birth and seen as completely dissociated P

D. L. Wolbrette: Division of Cardiology, The Pennsylvania State University College of Medicine; and The Milton S. Hershey Medical Center, Hershey, Pennsylvania
G. V. Naccarelli: Division of Cardiology, The Pennsylvania State University College of Medicine, Hershey, Pennsylvania

waves and QRS complexes, each firing at their own pacemaker rate. The level of block is usually within the AV node.

Inappropriate sinus bradycardia: A sinus rate less than 60 beats/min, which is persistent and does not increase appropriately with exercise.

Sick sinus syndrome: See *tachycardia-bradycardia syndrome.*

Sinoatrial conduction time: An indirect measurement obtained during an electrophysiology study. Premature atrial extrastimuli are introduced at the high right atrium at progressively shorter intervals during sinus rhythm until atrial refractoriness is found. Calculations can then be made to estimate the conduction time.

Sinoatrial exit block: A period of asystole resulting from the generated sinus impulse not leaving the sinus nodal region, caused by delay in conduction or block.

Sinus arrest: Used interchangeably with the term *sinus pause.* A result of transient failure of impulse formation at the sinoatrial node during which time no P wave is seen.

Sinus nodal dysfunction: Any abnormality in sinus nodal function, including inappropriate sinus bradycardia, sinoatrial exit block, sinoatrial arrest, or alternating sinus bradycardia and atrial tachyarrhythmias. The term does not indicate a specific etiology or the presence of symptoms.

Sinus nodal recovery time: An indirect measurement obtained invasively by overdrive pacing of the sinus node. The interval between the last paced P wave and the first spontaneous atrial deflection is the sinus nodal recovery time.

Tachycardia-bradycardia syndrome: Frequently referred to as *sick sinus syndrome.* This common manifestation of sinus nodal dysfunction refers to intermittent sinus or junctional bradycardia alternating with atrial tachycardia (usually paroxysmal atrial fibrillation). Symptoms may result from either the bradycardia or the tachycardic phase.

Trifascicular block: Slowed conduction in all three fascicles; PR prolongation in addition to a bifascicular block.

Wenckebach periodicity: Type I second-degree AV block, demonstrating the following features: (a) progressive lengthening of the PR interval, (b) lengthening of the RR intervals at progressively decreasing increments, (c) a pause including the nonconducted P wave that is less than the sum of any two consecutively conducted beats, and (d) shortening of the PR interval postblock, compared with the PR interval just preceding the blocked cycle.

INTRODUCTION

Bradycardia is most commonly secondary to sinus nodal dysfunction. Bradyarrhythmias secondary to AV block at the level of the AV node or distal to the bundle of His also account for a large number of patients who have bradyarrhythmias. In this chapter, we review basic and anatomic concepts, clinical profiles, and therapeutic strategies relevant to the recognition and treatment of patients with bradyarrhythmias.

SINUS NODAL DYSFUNCTION

Electrocardiographic Features of Sinus Nodal Dysfunction

Inappropriate Sinus Bradycardia

Sinus bradycardia (sinus rate less than 60 beats/min) (Fig. 63.1) is considered inappropriate when it is persistent and does not increase appropriately with exercise. This arrhythmia should be distinguished from asymptomatic resting sinus bradycardia in young athletes and in normal adults during sleep (18,19). Chronotropic incompetence is not present in these individuals, as it is in patients with sinus nodal dysfunction.

Sinus Arrest

The terms *sinus arrest* (Fig. 63.2) and *sinus pause* are used interchangeably and are a result of the sinus node's principal pacemaker cells failing to fire. The pause is not an exact multiple of the preceding PP interval. Pauses greater than 3 seconds are rare in normal individuals and may or may not be associated with symptoms, but are usually caused by sinus nodal dysfunction (20,21). In contrast, asymptomatic pauses greater than 2 seconds (but less than 3 seconds) are seen in 11% of normal patients during 24-hour Holter monitoring and are especially common in trained athletes (22).

Chronic Atrial Fibrillation

The presence of chronic atrial fibrillation in a patient with a slow ventricular response not secondary to drug therapy is a sign of sinus nodal dysfunction. In some cases, cardioversion results in a long sinus pause before the appearance of sinus rhythm, or junctional escape rhythm. Although a combination of sinus nodal and AV conduction disease may be present in many instances, examples of rapid ventricular responses during atrial tachyarrhythmias can frequently be found.

Tachycardia-Bradycardia Syndrome

Tachycardia-bradycardia syndrome refers to the presence of intermittent sinus or junctional bradycardia alternating with atrial tachycardia (usually paroxysmal atrial fibrillation) in the same patient (Fig. 63.3). This condition, frequently referred to as *sick sinus syndrome*, is a common

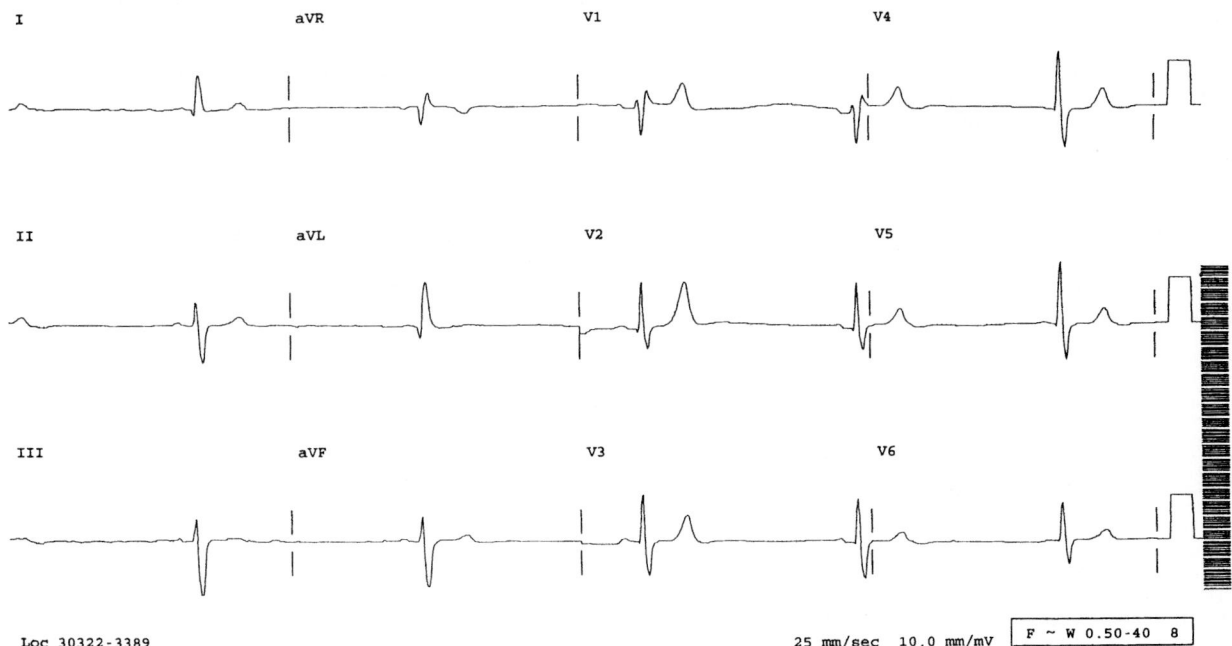

FIGURE 63.1 This electrocardiogram shows sinus bradycardia at a rate of 30 beats/min. Right bundle branch block and left anterior fascicular block are also present. aVF, augmented voltage unipolar left foot lead; aVL, augmented voltage unipolar left arm lead; aVR, augmented voltage unipolar right arm lead.

manifestation of sinus nodal dysfunction. The highest incidence of syncope associated with sinus nodal dysfunction probably occurs in this group (3). Syncope typically occurs secondary to a long sinus pause after the spontaneous termination of atrial fibrillation.

Pathophysiology

Intrinsic Sinus Nodal Dysfunction

Idiopathic degenerative disease is probably the most common cause of intrinsic sinus nodal dysfunction (Table 63.1). Pathologic studies have shown an increase in fibrous tissue in the area of the sinus node with age. Why some

individuals develop sinus nodal dysfunction whereas others do not, is not easily explained by fibrous tissue replacement only (23,24). Coronary artery disease may be responsible for one-third of cases of sinus nodal dysfunction. This estimation is based on a study by Shaw et al. (25), in which angiography was used to demonstrate the extent of coronary artery disease in the sinus nodal artery in patients with sinus nodal dysfunction. Transient slowing of the sinus rate, or sinus arrest, can complicate an acute myocardial infarction. This is usually seen with an acute inferior wall myocardial infarction, is caused by neural influences, and rarely persists (26). Cardiomyopathy, long-standing hypertension, infiltrative disorders, collagen vascular diseases, inflammatory processes, and surgical trauma can also result

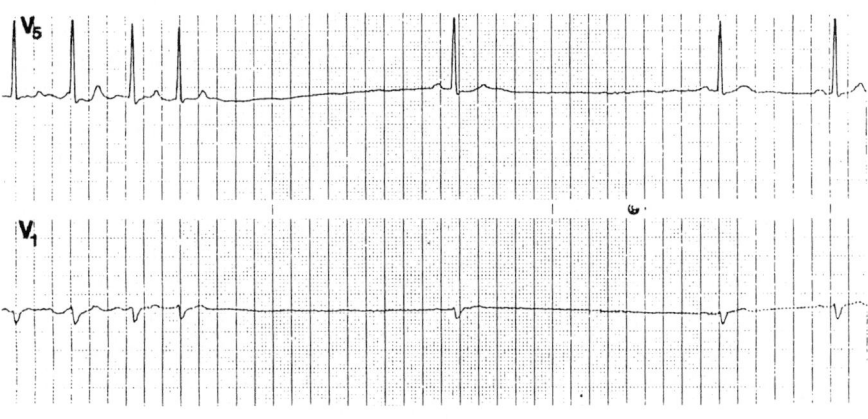

FIGURE 63.2 These rhythm strips of leads V₁ and V₅ were recorded simultaneously and depict sinus pauses of 3.0 and 2.8 seconds posttermination of atrial tachycardia.

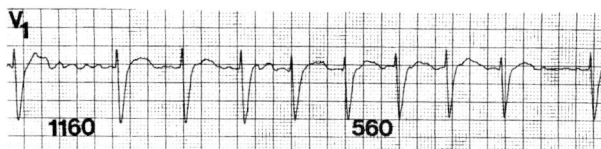

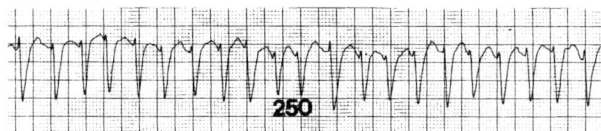

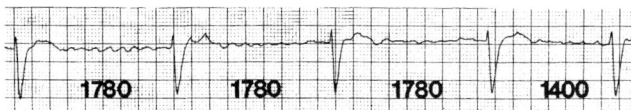

FIGURE 63.3 These three rhythm strips were obtained from the same patient at different times and illustrate the marked variability of heart rates in patients with tachycardia-bradycardia syndrome. The labeled cycle lengths are in milliseconds.

TABLE 63.1 CAUSES OF SINUS NODAL DYSFUNCTION

Intrinsic causes
　Idiopathic degenerative disease
　Coronary artery disease
　Cardiomyopathy
　Hypertension
　Infiltrative disorders (amyloidosis, hemochromatosis, tumors)
　Collagen vascular disease (scleroderma, lupus erythematosus)
　Inflammatory processes (myocarditis, pericarditis)
　Surgical trauma (orthotopic cardiac transplantation)
　Musculoskeletal disorders (myotonic dystrophy, Friedreich's ataxia)
　Congenital heart disease (postoperative or in absence of surgical correction)
Extrinsic causes
　Drug effects
　　Beta-blocking agents
　　Calcium channel blocking agents
　　Digoxin
　　Sympatholytic antihypertensives (clonidine, methyldopa, and reserpine)
　　Antiarrhythmic drugs
　　　Type IA (quinidine, procainamide, disopyramide)
　　　Type IC (flecainide, propafenone)
　　　Type III (sotalol, amiodarone)
　　Others (lithium, cimetidine, amitriptyline, phenytoin)
Autonomic influences
　Excessive vagal tone
　Carotid sinus syndrome
　Vasovagal syncope
　Well-trained athletes
Electrolyte abnormalities
　Hyperkalemia
　Hypercarbia
Endocrine disorders: hypothyroidism
Increased intracranial pressure
Hypothermia
Sepsis

in sinus nodal dysfunction. Orthotopic cardiac transplantation is associated with a high incidence of sinus nodal dysfunction in the donor heart. In an Austrian study with a series of 90 transplant patients, 45% were found to have sinus nodal dysfunction postoperatively, and 21% required permanent pacing. However, sudden death caused by donor sinus nodal dysfunction appears to be a rare occurrence in post–cardiac transplantation (27). The musculoskeletal disorders of myotonic dystrophy or Friedreich's ataxia are rare causes of sinus nodal dysfunction. A familial form of sinus nodal dysfunction accounts for a small number of cases (28).

In the pediatric population, most cases of sinus nodal dysfunction can be attributed to surgical trauma (see Chapter 70 for a further discussion of this subject). Most commonly associated with this complication is Mustard's procedure for transposition of the great arteries (29) and repair of atrial septal defects, especially of the sinus venosus type (30). Sinus nodal dysfunction can occur in children with congenital heart disease, such as secundum atrial defects, even though no surgery has been performed (31). In some children with sinus nodal dysfunction, no structural heart disease is known (32).

Extrinsic Sinus Nodal Dysfunction

In the absence of structural abnormalities, the predominant causes of sinus nodal dysfunction are drug effects and autonomic influences (Table 63.1). Drugs known to depress sinus nodal function include beta-blockers, calcium channel blockers, digoxin (33), and sympatholytic antihypertensives (e.g., clonidine, methyldopa, and reserpine) (34). Types IA, IC, and III antiarrhythmic drugs can depress

sinus nodal function (33) and, occasionally, may produce proarrhythmias in patients with sick sinus syndrome. Paroxysmal primary atrial tachycardias and pause-dependent ventricular tachycardia have been described (35,36). Other drugs reported to affect sinus nodal function include lithium, cimetidine, amitriptyline, and phenytoin (33).

Sinus nodal dysfunction may sometimes result from excessive vagal tone in individuals without intrinsic sinus nodal disease. The transient bradyarrhythmias produced can include marked sinus bradycardia, sinus pauses, or sinoatrial exit block (37,38). Autonomically induced asystole has been reported to occur rarely and may result in sudden death (39). Hypervagatonia can be seen in carotid sinus syndrome (*e*Fig. 63.3.1) and vasovagal syncope (*e*Fig. 63.3.2). Well-trained athletes with increased vagal tone may require some deconditioning to help prevent symptomatic bradyarrhythmias (40). Less common extrinsic causes of sinus nodal dysfunction include hyperkalemia, hypothyroidism, increased intracranial pressure, hypothermia, hypercarbia, and sepsis.

Clinical Profile

Incidence

Few data are available regarding the incidence of sinus nodal dysfunction in the general population. However, a Belgian study involving cardiac patients estimated the incidence in patients over 50 years of age to be 3 in 5,000 (41). Sinus nodal dysfunction affects men and women equally (42).

Symptoms

The symptoms reported by patients with sinus nodal dysfunction are varied, and many times nonspecific. Syncope and presyncope are the most frequent symptoms associated with significant bradycardia. Fatigue, angina, and shortness of breath can also be seen. Elderly patients may have the more subtle symptoms of gastrointestinal distress or change in mental status. Patients with tachycardia-bradycardia syndrome may only experience palpitations associated with the tachycardia or embolic events. Syncope in an individual with paroxysmal atrial fibrillation is classically associated with the long sinus pause at the spontaneous termination of the tachycardia. The intermittent nature of these symptoms makes documentation of the associated rhythm disturbance difficult at times. In other cases, marked sinus bradycardia and sinus pauses may be asymptomatic (6,42,43).

Diagnostic Techniques

Both noninvasive and invasive means of diagnosing sinus nodal dysfunction are available. Generally, the noninvasive methods of electrocardiographic (ECG) monitoring, exercise testing, and autonomic testing are used first. However, if symptoms are infrequent, invasive electrophysiologic testing may be pursued.

Noninvasive Testing

A 12-lead ECG needs to be obtained in the patient with syncope or near syncopal episodes. However, the diagnosis of sinus nodal dysfunction as the etiology of these symptoms is rarely made from the simple ECG. If symptoms are frequent, 24- or 48-hour ambulatory Holter monitoring can be useful. Documentation of symptoms in a diary by the patient while wearing the Holter monitor is essential for correlation of symptoms with the heart rhythm at the time. In some cases, the Holter monitor can exclude sinus nodal dysfunction as the cause of symptoms, if normal sinus rhythm is documented. In contrast, sinus pauses recorded may not be associated with symptoms. Several Holter monitor studies (21,44) have demonstrated the futility of treating asymptomatic pauses, even if 3 seconds

or longer. Most pauses, ranging from 2 to 15 seconds, were asymptomatic, and pacing did not benefit those without associated symptoms. The length of the pause correlated poorly with symptoms and prognosis.

A relatively newer diagnostic tool is the event recorder, or loop recorder, which is useful in patients whose symptoms occur infrequently. This device is used to record the heart rhythm only during symptoms. Later, the recorded ECG is sent transtelephonically by the patient to a central monitoring station.

Exercise testing is of limited value in diagnosing sinus nodal dysfunction. However, in some cases, it is useful in differentiating those patients with chronotropic incompetence from patients with resting bradycardia who demonstrate a normal heart rate increase with exercise. Certain patients with sinus nodal dysfunction and chronotropic incompetence exhibit abnormal heart rate responses to exercise. The increase in heart rate at each stage of exercise may be less than normal, with a plateau seen below the maximum predicted heart rate (adjusted for age). Other patients with sinus nodal dysfunction may achieve an appropriate peak heart rate during exercise but may have a slow heart rate acceleration in the initial stage or rapid deceleration of heart rate in the recovery stage. These abnormal chronotropic responses can help to identify the cause of exercise intolerance in some patients with sinus nodal dysfunction and can help to determine their pacemaker prescription (45,46).

Autonomic testing of the sinus node includes various pharmacologic interventions and maneuvers to test reflex responses. An abnormal response to carotid sinus massage (pause greater than 3 seconds) may indicate sinus nodal dysfunction (eFig. 63.3.3), but this response may also occur in asymptomatic elderly individuals (47). Heart rate response to Valsalva's maneuver (normally decreased) or upright tilt (normally increased) can also be used to verify that the autonomic nervous system is itself intact. The most commonly used pharmacologic intervention is used to determine the intrinsic heart rate. Complete autonomic blockade is accomplished by administering atropine, 0.04 mg per kg, and propranolol, 0.20 mg per kg. The resulting intrinsic heart rate represents the sinus nodal rate without autonomic influences. The normal intrinsic heart rate is age dependent and can be calculated using the following equation: intrinsic heart rate = $118.1 - (0.57 \times age)$ beats/min (48). A low intrinsic heart rate is consistent with abnormal intrinsic sinus nodal function. A normal intrinsic heart rate in a patient with known sinus nodal dysfunction suggests abnormal autonomic regulation.

Natural History

The natural history of sinus nodal dysfunction depends largely on the type of dysfunction and the presence of concomitant cardiovascular disease. The worst prognosis is associated with the tachycardia-bradycardia syndrome, whereas sinus bradycardia is much more benign. Those with sinus pauses have a prognosis intermediate to the other two types of sinus nodal dysfunction. These differing outlooks are most likely related to their relative risk for thromboembolic complications, probably the most important cause of death in this group. Because stroke is associated with atrial fibrillation, patients with sinus nodal dysfunction complicated by chronic or intermittent atrial fibrillation have an increased risk of embolization.

In a literature review by Sutton and Kenny (59), the incidence of new onset atrial fibrillation in patients with sinus nodal dysfunction was 5.2% per year. New atrial tachyarrhythmias occurred with less frequency in patients who were atrially paced (3.9%), compared with a greatly increased incidence of similar arrhythmias in those only ventricularly paced (22.3%). A more recent review (60) reported a weighted mean atrial fibrillation per year incidence of 6.8% for VVI pacing, compared with 2.6% (a 62.0% risk reduction) for dual-chamber pacing.

As noted previously, thromboembolic complications are a major cause of morbidity and mortality in patients with sinus nodal dysfunction. Sutton and Kenny's review found a 15.2% incidence of thromboembolism among unpaced patients with sinus nodal dysfunction. Those patients only ventricularly paced did not fare much better (13%). In contrast, atrially paced patients enjoyed a greatly decreased thromboembolic event incidence (1.6%) (59). In the future, increased use of atrial pacing and anticoagulation therapy should significantly reduce the incidence of stroke in high-risk patients with tachycardia-bradycardia syndrome. Several ongoing prospective trials are testing the hypothesis that physiologic pacing reduces the risk of cardiovascular death and stroke.

Of clinical interest is the incidence of concomitant AV nodal disease in patients with sinus nodal dysfunction. In the previously mentioned review (59), 17% of the patients had some degree of AV conduction system disease at the time of diagnosis of sinus nodal dysfunction. New AV conduction abnormalities developed at a rate of approximately 2.7% per year. These data indicate a low frequency and slow progression rate of AV conduction system disease in patients with sinus nodal dysfunction.

Principles of Management

Because of the broad range of symptoms associated with a variety of arrhythmia presentations in patients with sinus nodal dysfunction, treatment modalities must be individualized. For the patient with asymptomatic bradycardia or pauses and no atrial fibrillation, no treatment is necessary. In the case of symptomatic patients with sinus nodal dysfunction and atrial fibrillation, therapy depends on whether the symptoms are related to the tachycardia or bradycardia episodes. Depending on the etiology of the symptoms, drug therapy may be needed to control rapid ventricular response, pacing may be advised to prevent bradycardia, or both treatment modalities may be required. Ideally, if a patient with symptomatic bradycardia is on a drug known to depress sinus nodal function, the drug should be stopped. However, many times this is not possible, as the drug is needed for control of symptomatic tachycardia, ischemia, or hypertension. In these cases, permanent pacing may be required to allow continued use of the needed drug.

Sinus nodal dysfunction is currently the most common reported diagnosis for pacemaker implantation. However, once the decision to pace is made, choosing the optimal pacemaker prescription is essential to decrease stroke risk and improve quality of life. As discussed previously, a significant number of patients with sinus nodal dysfunction have concomitant atrial fibrillation or develop new atrial tachyarrhythmias after being diagnosed with sinus nodal dysfunction. Atrial pacing has been shown to greatly decrease the incidence of atrial fibrillation and thromboembolism in this population, whereas those who are only ventricularly paced have not seen a similar benefit (59). For those patients with sinus nodal dysfunction who have normal AV conduction, a single-chamber atrial pacemaker is a reasonable consideration. Of course, single-chamber ventricular pacing is still appropriate for individuals with sinus nodal dysfunction and chronic atrial fibrillation. The use of rate-adaptive pacing is important for improving exercise tolerance in single-chamber and dual-chamber pacing devices. Additionally, the development of the mode-switching feature in some dual-chamber devices allows for automatic mode change between DDDR and DDIR (or VVIR) in a patient with intermittent atrial tachyarrhythmias. The DDIR mode permits continued AV synchrony. However, because there is no atrial tracking, unwanted rapid ventricular pacing will not occur during atrial tachycardia. Guidelines for implantation of pacemakers in patients with sinus nodal dysfunction have been established by a task force from the American College of Cardiology and American Heart Association (*e*Table 63.1.1) (61).

As discussed previously, because of the high risk of thromboembolic events in patients with chronic or intermittent atrial fibrillation, anticoagulation with warfarin should be instituted in these patients. Warfarin has been clearly shown to be superior to placebo in the prevention of stroke in patients with atrial fibrillation (62). However, the role of aspirin therapy in this population is controversial (63). Patients with contraindications to warfarin or those with lone atrial fibrillation—defined as atrial fibrillation in the absence of underlying heart disease—may be considered candidates for aspirin therapy alone. For the other patients with atrial fibrillation, warfarin therapy to achieve an international normalized ratio between two and three is optimal to decrease stroke risk. A metaanalysis of the five major controlled trials of anticoagulation in atrial fibrillation has shown that patients at the highest risk for strokes are those with hypertension, recent congestive heart failure, or previous thromboembolism (64). The reader is referred to Chapter 64 for a more in-depth discussion of these anticoagulation issues.

ATRIOVENTRICULAR NODAL DYSFUNCTION

Electrocardiographic and Electrophysiologic Findings

Normal Atrioventricular Conduction

On the surface ECG, the PR interval is normally between 120 and 200 ms in duration. This interval reflects the conduction time from the high right atrium to the point of ventricular activation. To measure the different components of the conduction system that the PR interval includes, intracardiac tracings from the high right atrium and bundle of His region are needed (*e*Fig. 63.3.6). The PA interval—measured from the high right atrial electrogram to the low right atrial deflection in the bundle of His electrogram—gives an indirect approximation of the right atrial conduction time. The AH interval, measured from the low atrial to the bundle of His deflection, reflects conduction time through the AV node. The HV interval, measured from the bundle of His deflection to the earliest ventricular depolarization on the surface electrogram, represents the conduction time from the proximal bundle of His to the ventricular myocardium (82) (Table 63.2). The AH interval can vary greatly in an individual because of changes in sympathetic and parasympathetic tone. In contrast, the HV interval should remain constant, because this interval is not significantly affected by changes in autonomic tone.

First-Degree Atrioventricular Block

First-degree AV block on the surface ECG is seen as a PR interval >0.20 seconds in adults or >0.18 seconds in children. Each P wave is followed by a QRS complex with a constant, prolonged interval. Although the conduction delay can be anywhere along the system, the PR prolongation is usually caused by delay within the AV node (87% when the QRS complex is narrow). On the bundle of His electrogram, this would be seen as an AH interval >130 ms

TABLE 63.2 NORMAL CONDUCTION INTERVALS IN ADULTS

Type	Interval (ms)
PA	20–50
AH	50–140
HV	35–55
H	10–25

with a normal HV interval (*e*Fig. 63.3.7). In cases in which first-degree AV block is seen in the presence of a bundle branch block, a bundle of His electrogram is necessary to localize the site of block (83–85) (*e*Fig. 63.3.8). Infranodal conduction delay is present in 45% of these cases. A combination of delay within the AV node and in the His-Purkinje system must also be considered (86). In certain cases of congenital structural heart disease, such as Ebstein's anomaly of the tricuspid valve or endocardial cushion defects, intraatrial conduction delay can cause first-degree AV block. In addition, intra-Hisian conduction delay can cause first-degree AV block. On the bundle of His electrogram, a split His potential can be seen, resulting in a prolonged His potential, HV, and PR intervals (86). Dual AV nodal physiology can produce transient, abrupt, or alternating first-degree block caused by block in the fast AV nodal pathway (which is normally used), with conduction down the slow pathway instead. The change in the PR interval seen on the surface electrogram corresponds with a jump in the AH interval viewed on the bundle of His electrogram (87).

Second-Degree Atrioventricular Block

Type I

Type I second-degree AV block, or Wenckebach block, features on the surface electrogram progressive prolongation of the PR interval before failure of an atrial impulse to be conducted to the ventricles. The PR interval immediately postblock returns to its baseline interval, and the sequence begins again. Features of typical Wenckebach periodicity include the following (*e*Fig. 63.3.9):

- Progressive lengthening of the PR interval throughout the Wenckebach cycle
- Lengthening of the RR interval occurring at progressively decreasing increments, resulting in progressive shortening of the RR intervals
- A pause including the nonconducted P wave that is less than the sum of any two consecutively conducted beats
- Shortening of the PR interval postblock, compared with the PR interval just preceding the blocked cycle

Less than 50% of type I AV block cases follow this typical pattern (88). Atypical patterns are more likely found with longer Wenckebach periods, >6:5. Differentiating atypical from typical patterns, however, is of little clinical significance.

Wenckebach block is almost always within the AV node when a narrow QRS complex is present (88). Intra-Hisian block is the rare exception (89). When type I block is seen with a bundle branch block, the block is still more likely to be in the AV node, but it could also be localized below the bundle of His. A bundle of His electrogram would be needed to accurately identify the level of block. Wenckebach block in the AV node is characterized by progressive prolongation of the AH interval, until an atrial deflection is not followed by a bundle of His or ventricular deflection. In type I block secondary to block below the bundle of His, progressive prolongation of the HV interval is followed by an H deflection without an associated ventricular depolarization.

Type II

Type II, or Mobitz II, second-degree AV block is characterized on the surface electrogram by a constant PR interval, followed by sudden failure of a P wave to be conducted to the ventricles. The PP intervals remain constant, and the pause including the blocked P wave equals two PP intervals. Therefore, Mobitz II block should not be confused with a nonconducted premature atrial complex. Mobitz II block is usually associated with bundle branch block or bifascicular block. In a majority of these cases, the site of block is within or below the bundle of His (*e*Fig. 63.3.10) (84,86). When presumed Mobitz II block is seen in conjunction with a narrow QRS complex, Mobitz I with only minimal PR variation should be suspected. Only rarely is Mobitz II found with a narrow QRS complex and is caused by intra-Hisian block (90). The bundle of His electrogram is useful in verifying the site of the Mobitz II block. The blocked cycle features atrial and bundle of His deflections without a ventricular depolarization. The conducted beats usually show evidence of infranodal conduction system disease, with a prolonged HV interval, or even a split bundle of His potential (86).

2:1 Atrioventricular Block

Fixed 2:1 AV block poses a diagnostic dilemma because it is usually impossible to classify as type I or II block by a surface electrogram alone (*e*Fig. 63.3.11). A narrow QRS complex and recently seen Wenckebach block is highly suggestive of block at the AV nodal level. A 2:1 block associated with a wide QRS complex is likely infranodal, but it could still be at the level of the AV node. A definitive diagnosis can only be made with an intracardiac recording at the bundle of His region.

Nonconduction of two or more consecutive P waves when AV synchrony is otherwise maintained is sometimes termed *high-degree AV block*. The level of block can be at the AV node or the His-Purkinje system. When high-degree AV block is caused by block in the AV node, QRS complexes of the conducted beats are usually narrow. Wenckebach periodicity is also seen, and atropine administration produces 1:1 conduction. Features pointing toward block in the His-Purkinje system are conducted beats with bundle branch block and no improvement in block with atropine. Bundle of His recordings are sometimes needed to confirm the site of block.

Third-Degree Atrioventricular Block

Third-degree, or complete, AV block is seen on the surface electrogram as completely dissociated P waves and QRS complexes, each firing at their own pacemaker rate. The atrial impulse is never conducted to the ventricles, but different levels of block are possible. The level of block determines the QRS morphology along with the site and rate of the escape rhythm. Congenital complete heart block is characterized by a narrow QRS complex with an escape rate between 40 and 60 beats/min, which tends to increase with exercise or atropine. This is consistent with block within the AV node. Acquired complete heart block is usually associated with block in the His-Purkinje system, resulting in a wide QRS complex with an escape rate between 20 and 40 beats/min. The intracardiac electrogram shows bundle of His deflections consistently following the atrial electrograms, but the ventricular depolarization is completely dissociated from these. Block below the bundle of His is thus demonstrated. In contrast, complete heart block at the AV nodal level is seen on the intracardiac tracings as bundle of His potentials consistently preceding each ventricular depolarization. The atrial electrograms are dissociated from the HV complexes (*e*Fig. 63.3.12). The sinus rate is faster than the ventricular rate in patients with complete heart block. Data collected from patients with congenital complete heart block have showed the atrial rate to usually be age appropriate (92). It is important to note that complete antegrade AV block does not always predict retrograde (VA) conduction. Retrograde conduction may be intact in an individual with complete antegrade AV block (Fig. 63.1).

Pathophysiology

The term *AV block* denotes a delay or nonconduction of an atrial impulse to the ventricles when the AV junction is not physiologically refractory. Table 63.3 lists the majority of causes of AV block that have been identified. In each case, the abnormality may vary from a delay in conduction to intermittent or complete conduction failure.

Drug effects are a common cause of acquired AV block in adults. Digoxin and beta-blocking agents act indirectly on the AV node through their effect on the autonomic nervous system. Calcium channel blockers and other antiarrhythmic drugs, such as amiodarone, act directly to slow conduction in the AV node. Type I and III antiarrhythmic drugs can also affect conduction in the His-Purkinje system, resulting in infranodal block. Drugs that have a significant effect on blocking the sodium channels, such as flecainide, have the most effect on slowing conduction in the His-Purkinje system. When AV block occurs secondary to antiarrhythmic therapy, it is usually in cardiac patients with preexisting conduction abnormalities. Patients with normal conduction system function rarely develop complete heart block as a result of using antiarrhythmic agents.

Acute myocardial infarction is associated with varying degrees of AV block and is the most common cause of acquired complete AV block. Second- and third-degree AV

TABLE 63.3 CAUSES OF ATRIOVENTRICULAR BLOCK

Drug effects
  Digoxin
  Beta-blockers
  Certain calcium channel blockers
  Membrane-active antiarrhythmic drugs
Ischemic heart disease
  Acute myocardial infarction
  Chronic coronary artery disease
Idiopathic fibrosis of the conduction system
  Lenègre's disease
  Lev's disease
Congenital heart disease
  Congenital complete heart block
  Ostium primum atrial septal defect
  Transposition of the great vessels
  Maternal systemic lupus erythematosus
Calcific valvular disease
Cardiomyopathy
Infiltrative disease
  Amyloidosis
  Sarcoidosis
  Hemochromatosis
Infectious and inflammatory diseases
  Endocarditis
  Myocarditis (Chagas's disease, Lyme disease, rheumatic fever,
    tuberculosis, measles, mumps)
Collagen
  Vascular diseases (scleroderma, rheumatoid arthritis, Reiter's
    syndrome, systemic lupus erythematosus, ankylosing
    spondylitis, polymyositis)
Metabolic
  Hyperkalemia
  Hypermagnesemia
Endocrine: Addison's disease
Trauma
  Cardiac surgery
  Radiation
  Catheter trauma
  Catheter ablation
Tumors
  Mesothelioma
  Hodgkin's disease
  Malignant melanoma
  Rhabdomyosarcoma
Neurally mediated
  Carotid sinus syndrome
  Vasovagal syncope
Neuromyopathic disorders
  Myotonic muscular dystrophy
  Slowly progressive X-linked muscular dystrophy

blocks occur in up to 30% of patients presenting with acute myocardial infarction (93,94).

Abnormalities in AV nodal conduction are seen in 20% of patients hospitalized for acute inferior myocardial infarction (95), with the onset of block falling in a bimodal distribution (96,97). Eleven percent of those presenting in the first hour of symptoms are found to have second- or third-degree AV block (96). In contrast, the incidence of heart block is low in the second hour of symptoms. The majority of conduction abnormalities occur between 2 and 72 hours

(95,98). Because of the short duration of the early conduction abnormalities and their favorable response to atropine, an increase in vagal tone associated with acute inferior myocardial infarction is the probably etiology of this early phenomenon (99). Type I AV block occurring later in the course of an acute inferior myocardial infarction is less responsive to atropine and probably is associated with reversible ischemia of the AV node or the release of adenosine during acute infarction (100). In this setting, type I AV block rarely progresses to more advanced block and commonly resolves within 2 to 3 days of onset.

Type II AV block occurs in only 1% of patients with acute myocardial infarction, but it has a worse prognosis than type I block. It is associated with bundle branch infarction during an acute anterior myocardial infarction and frequently progresses to complete heart block.

Complete heart block can occur with either anterior or inferior acute myocardial infarction. The site of the block in inferior myocardial infarction is usually at the level of the AV node, resulting in a junctional escape rhythm with a rate of 50 to 60 beats/min and narrow QRS complex. The abnormality tends to be reversed with vagolytic drugs or exercise and usually resolves in several days. Complete heart block in the setting of acute anterior myocardial infarction is usually associated with infarction of the bundle branches (101,102). The escape rhythm is approximately 40 beats/min, with a wide QRS complex originating from the bundle branch and Purkinje's system. It is less likely to be reversible. In general, patients who develop either transient or irreversible AV block are older and have a larger area of damage associated with their acute myocardial infarction. Other markers seen in this group include high levels of cardiac enzymes, bundle branch block, right ventricular infarction, or left ventricular failure (93,103–106).

In addition to acute myocardial infarctions, chronic ischemic heart disease can result in persistent AV block (107). Transient AV block can occur not only during angina pectoris (108), but during episodes of Prinzmetal's variant angina (109).

The most common cause of acquired conduction system disease is progressive idiopathic fibrosis. Lev's disease (110) is a result of proximal bundle branch fibrosis. It is postulated as a hastening of the aging process by hypertension and arteriosclerosis of the blood vessels supplying the conduction system. Lenègre's disease (111) is a degenerative process occurring in a younger population and involving the more distal portions of the bundle branches.

Calcification of the aortic or mitral valve annulus can extend to the nearby conduction system and produce AV block (112,113). The incidence is more frequent with aortic than mitral stenosis. AV block can also result from a stenotic bicuspid aortic valve (114,115). Other causes of AV block include infiltrative cardiomyopathies such as amyloidosis (116), sarcoidosis (116,117), and hemochromatosis (118,119), as well as the collagen vascular diseases of scleroderma (120), rheumatoid arthritis (121), Reiter's syndrome (122), systemic lupus erythematosus (123), ankylosing spondylitis (124), and polymyositis (125).

Complete heart block occurs in 3% of cases of infective endocarditis, with the aortic valve being involved more frequently than the mitral valve (126,127). A variety of viral, bacterial, and parasitic etiologies of myocarditis result in varying degrees of AV block and include Lyme disease, rheumatic fever, Chagas's disease (128), tuberculosis, measles, and mumps. Transient AV block is the most frequently seen cardiac abnormality associated with Lyme disease. First-degree block is almost always observed in these cases, representing up to 8% of those infected. Complete heart block can develop in 50% of those with first-degree block, especially if the PR interval exceeds 0.30 seconds (129,130). Acute rheumatic fever almost invariably results in PR prolongation when carditis is present (131,132). Second-degree block occurs only occasionally, and progression to complete heart block is rare (133).

Cardiac surgery can be complicated by varying degrees of AV block caused by trauma and ischemic damage to the conduction system. Block is most frequently associated with aortic valve replacement (134). In the absence of myocardial infarction or a long ischemic time, block is rarely seen post–coronary artery bypass grafting. Repair of congenital heart defects in the region of the conduction system—such as endocardial cushion malformations, ventricular septal defects, and tricuspid valve abnormalities—can lead to transient or persistent AV block (see Chapter 70). The block is usually temporary and thought to be secondary to postoperative local inflammation. However, block can appear years later, usually in those who had transient block just after the operation (135).

Intracardiac catheter manipulation can inadvertently produce complete heart block, which is usually temporary. This can occur during a right-sided heart catheterization in a patient with preexisting left bundle branch block, or even during left ventricular angiography in a patient with previous right bundle branch block (136–138). Radiofrequency catheter ablation techniques are used to modify the AV nodal junction or to produce complete heart block in patients with supraventricular tachyarrhythmias that cannot be controlled by medical therapy alone (139). AV block can also complicate radiofrequency catheter ablation used to treat AV nodal reentrant tachycardia or AV reentrant tachycardia. The incidence of complete heart block complicating this procedure is low when performed by experienced operators and when the bundle of His region is avoided (140,141).

Other causes of acquired AV block include hyperkalemia (142), hypermagnesemia, Addison's disease (143), tumors that infiltrate the heart (144), and neuromyopathic disorders (145–147). Additionally, transient AV block can be seen with carotid sinus syndrome (*e*Fig. 63.3.13) (148) and vasovagal syncope (149).

Congenital complete AV block is thought to result from abnormal embryonic development of the AV node (150) and is thought to occur in 1 of every 25,000 live births (151). As the defect usually occurs proximal to the bundle of His, the QRS complex is narrow. This abnormality is found in otherwise structurally normal hearts in 50% of cases, whereas the rest have concurrent congenital heart disease (see Chapter 70) (152). Corrected transposition of the great vessels (153), ventricular septal defects, ostium primum atrial septal defects, and Ebstein's anomaly of the tricuspid valve (154) are all associated with AV nodal defects. Congenital complete heart block is also associated with collagen vascular disease in the mother, especially lupus erythematosus (155).

Clinical Profile

Incidence

PR prolongation, or first-degree AV block, is rarely found in young healthy adults, but the incidence increases with age and in those with heart disease. An epidemiologic study involving a large population of asymptomatic male pilots revealed PR intervals more than 0.2 seconds in only 0.52% (156). Two percent of adults over 20 years of age in Tecumseh, MI, were found to have a PR greater than or equal to 0.22 seconds (157). Both studies noted the PR interval to vary over time in young, healthy adults. Frequently in this population, the PR shortens with an increase in heart rate, suggesting vagal influence (156,157). Other epidemiologic surveys have shown a 5% incidence of first-degree AV block in men over 60 years of age and as high as 10% in older patients with cardiac disease (158,159).

In the large study of a population of healthy pilots, type II second-degree block was found to be extremely rare. In contrast, type I (Wenckebach) block can be seen in young athletes at rest and has been documented by ambulatory Holter monitoring in healthy teenagers during rest or sleep (160). Wenckebach periodicity in these settings disappears with exercise and should be considered a normal variant. On the other hand, in a population of patients with heart disease, the incidence of second-degree AV block (types I and II) was 2.7% (161).

Congenital complete heart block is estimated to occur in 1 of 15,000 to 25,000 live births, with a 60% female predominance (162,163). Acquired complete heart block is rarely seen in young individuals without heart disease (156). The highest incidence occurs in the seventh decade, and there is a 60% male predominance (164,165).

Symptoms

Individuals with first-degree AV block are asymptomatic. Symptoms of dizziness or syncope usually occur with acquired high-grade or complete AV block. With time, the majority of these patients experience a Stokes-Adams attack (166). Other symptoms can occur as a result of low cardiac output, including fatigue, congestive heart failure (166), dyspnea on exertion, angina, or even mental status changes.

Most children and adolescents with congenital complete heart block are asymptomatic, but some go on to develop symptoms later as adults. Those with concomitant structural heart disease, a wide QRS complex, long QT, or complete heart block discovered at an early age have an increased risk of developing symptoms, and some may die suddenly (167–169).

Diagnostic Techniques

Because the prognosis and the treatment differ in AV block depending on whether block is within the AV node or infranodal, determining the site of block is important. In many cases, this can be done noninvasively. As described previously, the QRS duration, PR intervals, and ventricular rate on the surface electrogram can provide important clues in localizing the level of block. Several noninvasive interventions may also prove helpful, such as vagal maneuvers, exercise, or administration of atropine. These methods take advantage of the differences in autonomic innervation of the AV node and His-Purkinje system. Whereas the AV node is richly innervated and highly responsive to both sympathetic and vagal stimuli, the His-Purkinje system is influenced minimally by the autonomic nervous system. Carotid sinus massage increases vagal tone and worsens AV nodal block. Exercise or atropine improves AV nodal conduction because of sympathetic stimulation. In contrast, carotid sinus massage improves infranodal block, whereas exercise and atropine worsen infranodal block because of the change in the rate of the impulses being conducted through the AV node.

Exercise testing is a useful tool to help confirm the level of block already suspected in second- or third-degree block caused by a narrow or wide QRS complex. Patients with presumed type I block or congenital complete heart block and a normal QRS complex usually enjoy an increased ventricular rate with exercise. On the other hand, patients with acquired complete heart block and a wide QRS complex usually show minimal or no increase in ventricular rate.

An electrophysiologic study is indicated in a patient with suspected high-grade AV block as the cause of syncope or presyncope, when documentation cannot be obtained noninvasively. In patients with coronary artery disease, it may be unclear whether symptoms are secondary to AV block or ventricular tachycardia; therefore, an electrophysiologic study can be useful in establishing the diagnosis. Some patients with known second- or third-degree block may benefit from an invasive study to localize the site of AV block to help determine therapy or assess prognosis. Once symptoms and AV block are correlated by ECG, further documentation by invasive studies is not required, unless

additional information, as discussed previously, is needed. Others who should not undergo electrophysiologic studies are asymptomatic patients with transient Wenckebach block associated with increased vagal tone.

The electrophysiology study allows analysis of the bundle of His electrogram, as well as atrial and ventricular pacing to look for conduction abnormalities and inducible ventricular tachycardia. The AH and HV intervals are measured from the bundle of His electrogram. A markedly prolonged HV interval greater than or equal to 100 ms is associated with a high incidence of progression to complete heart block (170). A His potential greater than or equal to 30 ms in duration or frankly split into two deflections is indicative of intra-Hisian conduction delay (*e*Fig. 63.3.14). When the bundle of His electrogram is observed during atrial pacing, the AH interval normally gradually lengthens until Wenckebach block is seen. The HV interval normally remains consistent, despite different pacing rates. Abnormal AV nodal conduction produces Wenckebach block at slower atrial-paced rates than what is normally seen (i.e., greater than 500 ms). To determine whether AV nodal disease is truly present or just under the influence of excessive vagal tone, atropine or isoproterenol is given to see if conduction improves. As discussed in the section Third-Degree Atrioventricular Block, infranodal block is present when the atrial deflection is followed by the bundle of His electrogram, but no ventricular depolarization is seen. Block below the bundle of His is abnormal, unless associated with short paced cycle lengths (350 m per second or less) (*e*Fig. 63.3.15) (171).

Natural History of Atrioventricular Blocks

The prognosis of any AV block is primarily dependent on the extent of the associated heart disease. First-degree AV block is usually benign and carries no increased mortality risk when seen as an isolated finding (157). However, first-degree AV block can be found in conjunction with bifascicular block or infranodal disease, therefore increasing the risk of progression to complete heart block.

Type I second-degree, or Wenckebach, AV block is generally benign, usually being transiently observed in the setting of acute inferior myocardial infarction or associated with increased vagal tone in healthy, athletic individuals. However, as with first-degree AV block, when type I AV block occurs in association with bifascicular or trifascicular block the risk of progression to complete heart block is significantly increased because of probable infranodal disease. Type II second-degree AV block, usually seen with bundle branch block, and associated with acute anterior myocardial infarction, carries a high risk of progression to advanced or complete AV block. The prognosis of 2:1 AV block depends on whether the site of block is within or below the AV node.

Before the availability of pacemakers, the prognosis for patients with symptomatic complete heart block was dismal, regardless of the extent of underlying heart disease. The 1-year survival rate after the first Adams-Stokes attack was less than 50% (172). Presently, once appropriate pacing therapy has been established, the prognosis depends on the underlying disease process (173). Patients who develop complete heart block as a result of an anterior myocardial infarction have a poor prognosis because of extensive cardiac damage. In contrast, those who develop complete heart block from idiopathic bundle branch fibrosis and who have no additional cardiac disease have a prognosis similar to those of similar age without heart block.

Congenital complete heart block generally carries a more favorable diagnosis than the acquired form when not associated with underlying heart disease. However, data have shown a significant risk of syncope, sudden death, and acquired mitral insufficiency in this group (174).

Principles of Management

Pacing is now the mainstay of treatment for symptomatic heart block. Medical therapy is only effective as a short-term emergency measure, until pacing can be accomplished. Before the availability of permanent pacing, drugs were used, but only because they were the only known therapies; no effective long-term medical therapy existed.

Before instituting permanent pacing, the possibility of a reversible cause of the heart block should be investigated (Table 63.3). Any offending drugs, such as digoxin, calcium channel blockers, or membrane-active antiarrhythmic drugs, should be withdrawn, if possible, to see if the block improves. Electrolyte abnormalities should also be looked for and then corrected. The possibility of infectious processes should be considered and then treated.

The key point in the decision to provide permanent pacing in AV block is the presence of symptoms. Intermittent block may make correlating bradycardia with symptoms difficult. However, once this is done, pacing should be instituted. Patients with complete heart block and syncope have clearly been shown to have improved survival with permanent pacing (175). Most patients with acquired complete heart block are symptomatic and require pacing. Patients with congenital complete heart block are more likely to be asymptomatic, but prophylactic pacemaker implantation is an appropriate consideration (174). Block in the AV node is less likely to be associated with slow ventricular rates, progression to complete heart block, and symptoms than is infranodal block.

The decision to pace is not always clear when dealing with the asymptomatic patient. However, investigation data and the American College of Cardiology/American Heart Association task force report (61) are helpful in providing some general guidelines (*e*Table 63.3.1). Permanent pacing is recommended in asymptomatic awake patients with documented pauses of greater than 3.0 seconds or a ventricular escape rhythm of less than 40 beats/min. When type II

second-degree heart block is found in an asymptomatic individual, an electrophysiologic study is warranted to determine if the block is infranodal. If this is the case, prophylactic pacing may be considered because of the high risk of progression to complete heart block (176). Permanent pacing is recommended in asymptomatic children with congenital heart block when found in association with a wide complex escape rhythm, complex congenital heart disease, ventricular dysfunction, or a long QT interval. Additionally, exercise intolerance, abrupt pauses in the intrinsic rate, and average ventricular rate inappropriate for the child's age are criteria for pacing in this population (*e*Table 63.3.2) (177–179). It is now recognized that dual-chamber pacing can be beneficial in some patients with marked first-degree AV block (>3.0 seconds) to reduce symptoms similar to pacemaker syndrome (180). Additionally, patients with left ventricular dysfunction and a long PR interval may see hemodynamic improvement once paced with a shorter AV delay. In both scenarios, improvement in symptoms, hemodynamics, or both should be documented with temporary AV pacing before the implantation of a permanent device (181).

Temporary pacing is sometimes required in patients with acute myocardial infarction (anterior more often than inferior wall). Patients with asymptomatic first-degree or type I second-degree block do not require pacing. However, patients with type II second-degree or complete heart block should be temporarily paced, even if asymptomatic.

If type II second-degree block or complete AV block persists once out of the periinfarct period, permanent pacing is indicated. Even if the type II or third-degree block was transient but associated with bundle branch block, studies suggest permanent pacing of the postmyocardial infarction patient improves long-term survival (182). In the setting of myocardial infarction, the criteria for permanent pacing depends less on the presence of symptoms (*e*Table 63.3.3). ⤐ 126

CONTROVERSIES AND PERSONAL PERSPECTIVES

The proper choice of the most appropriate, cost-effective pacemaker is often straightforward. A patient with chronic atrial fibrillation who needs a pacemaker should be prescribed a VVI or VVIR device. A patient with complete AV block and normal sinus node function should receive a dual-chamber device. In patients with chronotropic incompetence, a rate-responsive device should be prescribed. Because of technologic breakthroughs, industry continues to tempt physicians to use the smallest, newest, most sophisticated, dual-chamber, rate-responsive pacemakers in almost all patients, even though this approach may not be cost effective. *e*Table 63.3.6 lists current recommendations for optimal pacing modes recommended by the British Pacing and Electrophysiology Group (191).

THE FUTURE

Decreased pacemaker size along with software enhancements and increased battery longevity will help make the implantation and follow-up of pacemakers safer and more cost effective. Outcome studies will ultimately help us develop the most cost-effective and efficient strategies for prescribing and following pacemaker patients.

Many investigators propose that dual-chamber devices should be implanted in all patients who need pacemakers, unless the patient has chronic atrial fibrillation. This approach preserves AV synchrony under all scenarios except for paroxysms of atrial tachyarrhythmias. Retrospective studies have suggested that atrial-based pacing leads to fewer cases of chronic atrial fibrillation and thromboembolism and a possible reduction in mortality when compared with single-chamber ventricular pacing systems (60). In addition, dual-chamber systems minimize the occurrence of pacer syndrome, which can occur in 8% to 10% of patients with VVI pacemakers (192).

Antagonists of the previously mentioned position argue that these data are based on retrospective, uncontrolled trials. A metaanalysis of a large number of trials suggested that the data are not convincing for the superiority of dual-chamber pacing (60).

Several prospective trials are testing the hypothesis of the long-term superiority of dual-chamber or atrial-based pacing compared with single-chamber ventricular-based pacing. The Canadian Trial of Physiologic Pacing completed a 3-year follow-up of patients with sinus nodal dysfunction. Although the rate of atrial fibrillation was significantly lower in the physiologically paced group, more perioperative complications were noted caused by implantation of an atrial lead. The rate of cardiovascular death and stroke was similar in the two groups, as well as overall mortality and hospitalizations for heart failure (192). In a smaller Danish trial (193), a significant reduction in mortality was found with atrial pacing after 5.5 years, but not after only 3.3 years of follow-up. Therefore, the Canadian Trial of Physiologic Pacing investigators have elected to follow their cohort for an additional 3 years to see if a delayed benefit of physiologic over ventricular pacing occurs (194).

The results of the Pacemaker Selection in the Elderly Trial showed that patients with sinus nodal dysfunction—but not AV block—experienced improved quality of life and cardiovascular functional status with dual-chamber pacing as opposed to ventricular pacing (195). The Mode Selection Trial should help further define the benefits of dual-chamber versus single-chamber ventricular pacing in patients with sinus nodal dysfunction (196). The United Kingdom Pacing and Cardiovascular Events Trial is designed to answer the same question in elderly patients with high-degree AV block (197). Both studies have completed enrollment of 2,000 patients each and are now in their follow-up phases. The results of these trials, along with the extended follow-up Canadian Trial of Physiologic Pacing data, will likely provide the information needed for definitive evidence-based recommendations on pacemaker mode prescriptions (195).

REFERENCES

1. Laslett EE. Syncopal attacks with prolonged arrest of the whole heart. *QJM* 1908–1909;2:347–355.
2. Mackenzie J. *Diseases of the heart.* London: Oxford Medical Publications, 1913:370–379.
3. Short DS. The syndrome of alternating bradycardia and tachycardia. *Br Heart J* 1954;16:208–214.
4. Katz LN, Pick A. Part 1: The arrhythmias. In: *Clinical Electrocardiography.* Philadelphia: Lea & Febiger, 1956.
5. Lown B. Electrical reversion of cardiac arrhythmias. *Br Heart J* 1967;29:469–489.
6. Ferrer MI. The sick sinus syndrome in atrial disease. *JAMA* 1968;206:645–646.
7. Ferrer MI. The sick sinus syndrome. *Circulation* 1973;47:635–641.
8. Benditt DG, Benson DW Jr, Dunnigan A, et al. Drug therapy in sinus node dysfunction. In: Rapaport E, ed. *Cardiology update-1984.* New York: Elsevier, 1984:79–101.
9. Benditt DG, Sakaguchi S, Goldstein MA, et al. Sinus node dysfunction, pathophysiology, clinical features, evaluation, and treatment. In: Zipes DP, Jalife J, eds. *Cardiac electrophysiology: from cell to bedside.* 2nd ed. Philadelphia: WB Saunders, 1995:1215–1247.
10. Becker AE. Relation between structure and function of the sinus node: general comments. In: Bonke FI, ed. *The sinus node.* The Hague: Martinus Nijhoff, 1978:212–222.
11. Masson-Pevet M, Bleeker WK, Mackaay A, et al. Ultrastructural and functional aspects of the rabbit sinoatrial node. In: Bonke FI, ed. *The sinus node.* The Hague: Martinus Nijhoff, 1978:195–211.
12. Lu HH, Brooks CM. Intranodal shifts of pacemaker action. *Circulation* 1969;40:111–136.
13. Gomes JA, Winters SL. The origins of the sinus node pacemaker complex in man: demonstration of dominant and subsidiary foci. *J Am Coll Cardiol* 1987;9:45–52.
14. Strauss HC, Prystowsky EN, Scheinman MM. Sino-atrial and atrial electrogenesis. *Prog Cardiovasc Dis* 1977;19:385–404.
15. Bouman LN, Mackaay A, Bleeker WK, et al. Pacemaker shifts in the sinus node: effects of vagal stimulation, temper-

ature and reduction of extracellular calcium. In: Bonke FI, ed. *The sinus node.* The Hague: Nijhoff Medical Division, 1978:245–257.

16. Prystowsky EN, Grant AO, Wallace AG, et al. An analysis of the effects of acetylcholine on conduction and refractoriness in the rabbit sinus node. *Circ Res* 1979;44:112–120.

17. Asseman P, Reade R, Thery C. Catecholamine modulation of sinus node automaticity during complete sinoatrial block: demonstration by direct recording. *Am Heart J* 1992;124:780–781.

18. Brodksy M, Wu D, Denes P, et al. Arrhythmias documented by 24 hour continuous electrocardiographic monitoring in 50 male medical students without apparent heart disease. *Am J Cardiol* 1977;39:390–395.

19. Romano M, Clarizia M, Onofrio E, et al. Heart rate, PR, and QT intervals in normal children: a 24-hour Holter monitoring study. *Clin Cardiol* 1988;11:839–842.

20. Ector H, Rolies L, De Geest H. Dynamic electrocardiography and ventricular pauses of 3 seconds and more: etiology and therapeutic implications. *Pacing Clin Electrophysiol* 1983;6:548–551.

21. Hilgard J, Ezri MD, Denes P. Significance of ventricular pauses of three seconds or more detected on twenty-four–hour Holter recordings. *Am J Cardiol* 1985;55:1005–1008.

22. Viitasalo MT, Kala R, Eisalo A. Ambulatory electrocardiographic recording in endurance athletes. *Br Heart J* 1982;47:213–220.

23. Lev M. Aging changes in the human sinoatrial node. *J Gerontol* 1954;9:1–9.

24. Davies MJ, Pomerance A. Quantitative study of ageing changes in the human sinoatrial node and internodal tracts. *Br Heart J* 1972;34:150–152.

25. Shaw DB, Linker NJ, Heaver PA, et al. Chronic sinoatrial disorder (sick sinus syndrome): a possible result of cardiac ischaemia. *Br Heart J* 1987;58:598–607.

26. Rokseth R, Hatle L. Sinus arrest in acute myocardial infarction. *Br Heart J* 1971;33:639–642.

27. Heinz G, Hirschl M, Buxbaum P, et al. Sinus node dysfunction after orthotopic cardiac transplantation: postoperative incidence and long-term implications. *Pacing Clin Electrophysiol* 1992;15:731–737.

28. Caralis DG, Varghese PJ. Familial sinoatrial node dysfunction. Increased vagal tone a possible aetiology. *Br Heart J* 1976;38:951–956.

29. Gillette PC, Kugler JD, Garson A Jr, et al. Mechanisms of cardiac arrhythmias after the Mustard operation for transposition of the great arteries. *Am J Cardiol* 1980;45:1225–1230.

30. Young D. Later results of closure of secundum atrial septal defect in children. *Am J Cardiol* 1973;31:14–22.

31. Clark EB, Kugler JD. Preoperative secundum atrial septal defect with coexisting sinus node and atrioventricular node dysfunction. *Circulation* 1982;65:976–980.

32. Beder SD, Gillette PC, Garson A Jr, et al. Symptomatic sick sinus syndrome in children and adolescents as the only manifestation of cardiac abnormality or associated with unoperated congenital heart disease. *Am J Cardiol* 1983;51:1133–1136.

33. Benditt DG, Benson DW Jr, Dunnigan A, et al. Drug therapy in sinus node dysfunction. In: Rapaport E, ed. *Cardiology update.* New York: Elsevier, 1984:79–101.

34. Scheinman MM, Strauss HC, Evans GT, et al. Adverse effects of sympatholytic agents in patients with hypertension and sinus node dysfunction. *Am J Med* 1978;64:1013–1020.

35. Berns E, Rinkenberger RL, Jeang MK, et al. Efficacy and safety of flecainide acetate for atrial tachycardia or fibrillation. *Am J Cardiol* 1987;59:1337–1341.

36. Naccarelli GV, Dougherty AH, Berns E, et al. Assessment of antiarrhythmic drug efficacy in the treatment of supraventricular arrhythmias. *Am J Cardiol* 1986;58:31C–36C.

37. de Marneffe M, Gregoire JM, Waterschoote P, et al. Autonomic nervous system in relation to age in patients with and without sinus node disease. *Eur JCPE* 1992;2:44–52.

38. de Marneffe M, Jacobs P, Haardt R, Englert M. Variations of normal sinus node function in relation to age: role of autonomic influence. *Eur Heart J* 1986;7:662–672.

39. Milstein S, Buetikofer J, Lesser J, et al. Cardiac asystole: a manifestation of neurally mediated hypotension-bradycardia. *J Am Coll Cardiol* 1989;14:1626–1632.

40. Abdon NJ, Landin K, Johansson BW. Athlete's bradycardia as an embolising disorder? Symptomatic arrhythmias in patients aged less than 50 years. *Br Heart J* 1984;52:660–666.

41. Kulbertus HE, Leval-Rutten F, Mary L, et al. Sinus node recovery time in the elderly. *Br Heart J* 1975;37:420–425.

42. Rubenstein JJ, Schulman CL, Yurchak PM, et al. Clinical spectrum of the sick sinus syndrome. *Circulation* 1972;46:5–13.

43. Kaplan BM, Langendorf R, Lev M, et al. Tachycardia-bradycardia syndrome (so-called "sick sinus syndrome"): pathology, mechanisms and treatment. *Am J Cardiol* 1973;31:497–508.

44. Mazuz M, Friedman HS. Significance of prolonged electrocardiographic pauses in sinoatrial disease: sick sinus syndrome. *Am J Cardiol* 1983;52:485–489.

45. Benditt DG, Milstein S, Buetikofer J, et al. Sensor-triggered, rate-variable cardiac pacing: current technologies and clinical implications. *Ann Intern Med* 1987;107:714–724.

46. Holden W, McAnulty JH, Rahimtoola SH. Characterization of heart rate response to exercise in the sick sinus syndrome. *Br Heart J* 1978;40:923–930.

47. Peretz DI, Abdulla A. Management of cardioinhibitory hypersensitive carotid sinus syncope with permanent cardiac pacing—a 17-year prospective study. *Can J Cardiol* 1985;1:86–91.

48. Jose AD, Collison D. The normal range and determinants of the intrinsic heart rate in man. *Cardiovasc Res* 1970;4:160–167.

49. Mandel WJ, Hayakawa H, Allen HN, et al. Assessment of sinus node function in patients with the sick sinus syndrome. *Circulation* 1972;46:761–769.

50. Josephson ME. Sinus node function. In: Josephson ME, ed. *Clinical cardiac electrophysiology.* 2nd ed. Philadelphia: Lea & Febiger, 1993:83–84.

51. Reiffel JA, Gang E, Bigger JT Jr, et al. Sinus node recovery time related to paced cycle length in normals and patients with sinoatrial dysfunction. *Am Heart J* 1982;104:746–752.

52. Desai JM, Scheinman MM, Strauss HC, et al. Electrophysiologic effects on combined autonomic blockade in patients with sinus node disease. *Circulation* 1981;63:953–960.

53. Zipes DP, DiMarco JP, Gillette PC, et al. Guidelines for clinical intracardiac electrophysiological and catheter ablation procedures. A report of the American College of Cardiology/American Heart Association Task Force on Practice Guidelines (Committee on Clinical Intracardiac Electrophysiologic and Catheter Ablation Procedures). *JACC* 1995;26:555–573.

54. Strauss HC, Saroff AL, Bigger JT Jr, et al. Premature atrial stimulation as a key to the understanding of sinoatrial conduction in man. Presentation of data and critical review of the literature. *Circulation* 1973;47:86–93.

55. Narula OS, Shantha N, Vasquez M, et al. A new method for measurement of sinoatrial conduction time. *Circulation* 1978;58:706–714.

56. Reiffel JA, Gang E, Gliklich J, et al. The human sinus node electrogram: a transvenous catheter technique and a comparison of directly measured and indirectly estimated sinoatrial conduction time in adults. *Circulation* 1980;62:1324–1334.

57. Yee R, Strauss HC. Electrophysiologic mechanisms: sinus node dysfunction. *Circulation* 1987;75:12–18.

58. Kerr CR, Strauss HC. The measurement of sinus node refractoriness in man. *Circulation* 1983;68:1231–1237.

59. Sutton R, Kenny RA. The natural history of sick sinus syndrome. *Pacing Clin Electrophysiol* 1986;9:1110–1114.

60. Connolly SJ, Kerr C, Gent M, et al. Dual-chamber versus ventricular pacing: critical appraisal of current data. *Circulation* 1996;94:578–583.

61. Cheitlin MD, Conill A, Epstein AE, et al. ACC/AHA guidelines for implantation of cardiac pacemakers and antiarrhythmia devices. A report of the American College of Cardiology/American Heart Association task force on practice guidelines (Committee on Pacemaker Implantation). *JACC* 1998;31:1175–1209.

62. Stroke prevention in atrial fibrillation study: final results. *Circulation* 1991;84:527–539.

63. Stroke prevention in atrial fibrillation investigators. Warfarin versus aspirin for prevention of thromboembolism in atrial fibrillation: stroke prevention in atrial fibrillation II study. *Lancet* 1994;343:687–691.

64. The atrial fibrillator investigators. Risk factors for stroke and efficacy of antithrombotic therapy in atrial fibrillation: analysis of pooled data from five randomized controlled trials. *Arch Intern Med* 1994;154:1449–1457.

65. Adams R. *Dublin Hospital Report* 1827;4:353.

66. Stokes W. Dublin. *Q J Med Sci* 1846;2:73.

67. Wenckebach KF. Breitrage Zur Kenntis der Menschlichen Hertatigkeit. *Arch Anat Physiol (Physiol Abtheilung)* 1906;297–354.

68. Hay J. Bradycardia and cardiac arrhythmia produced by depression of certain functions of the heart. *Lancet* 1906;1:139–143.

69. Mobitz W. Uber die unvollstandige Storung der Erregungsuberleitung Zwischen Vorhof und Kammer des Menschlichen Herzens. *Z Gesamte Exp Med* 1924;41:180.

70. Damato AN, Lau SH, Helfant R, et al. A study of heart block in man using his bundle recordings. *Circulation* 1969;39:297–305.

71. Hecht HH, Kossmann CE, Childers RW, et al. Atrioventricular and intraventricular conduction. Revised nomenclature and concepts. *Am J Cardiol* 1973;31:232–244.

72. Janse MJ, van Capelli FJL, Anderson RH, et al. Electrophysiology and structure of the atrioventricular node of the isolated rabbit heart. In: Wellens HJJ, Lie KI, Janse MJ, eds. *The conduction system of the heart.* Leiden, The Netherlands: Stenfert Kroese, 1976:296.

73. Paes de Carvalho A, de Almeida DF. Spread of activity through the atrioventricular node. *Circ Res* 1960;8:801–809.

74. Anderson RH, Janse MJ, van Capelle FJ, et al. A combined morphological and electrophysiological study of the atrioventricular node of the rabbit heart. *Circ Res* 1974;35:909–922.

75. Scherlag BJ, Lazzara R, Helfant RH. Differentiation of "A-V junctional rhythms." *Circulation* 1973;48:304–312.

76. James TN. *Anatomy of the coronary arteries.* New York: Hoeber, Harper & Row, 1961.

77. James TN. Cardiac innervation: anatomic and pharmacologic relations. *Bull N Y Acad Sci* 1967;43:1041–1086.

78. Billman GE, Hoskins RS, Randall DC, et al. Selective vagal postganglionic innervation of the sinoatrial and atrioventricular nodes in the non-human primate. *J Auton Nerv Syst* 1989;26:27–36.

79. Imaizumi S, Mazgalev T, Dreifus LS, et al. Morphological and electrophysiological correlates of atrioventricular nodal response to increased vagal activity. *Circulation* 1990;82:951–964.

80. Massing GK, James TN. Anatomical configuration of the His bundle and bundle branches in the human heart. *Circulation* 1976;53:609–621.

81. Frink RJ, James TN. Normal blood supply to the human His bundle and proximal bundle branches. *Circulation* 1973;47:8–18.

82. Josephson ME. Electrophysiologic investigation: general concepts. In: Josephson ME, ed. *Clinical cardiac electrophysiology.* 2nd ed. Philadelphia: Lea & Febiger, 1993:26–30.

83. Rosen KM, Rahimtoola SH, Chuquimia R, et al. Electrophysiological significance of first degree atrioventricular block with intraventricular conduction disturbance. *Circulation* 1971;43:491–502.

84. Damato AN, Lau SH, Patton RD. A study of atrioventricular conduction in man using premature atrial stimulation and His bundle recordings. *Circulation* 1969;40:61–69.

85. Ranganathan N, Dhurandhar R, Phillips JH, et al. His bundle electrogram in bundle-branch block. *Circulation* 1972;45:282–294.

86. Pueck P, Grolleau R, Guimond C. Incidence of different types of AV block and their localization by His bundle recordings. In: Wellens HJJ, Lie KI, Janse NJ, eds. *The conduction system of the heart: structure, function and clinical implications.* Philadelphia: Lea & Febiger, 1976:467–484.

87. Rosen KM, Mehta A, Miller RA. Demonstration of dual atrioventricular nodal pathways in man. *Am J Cardiol* 1974;33:291–294.

88. Denes P, Levy L, Pick A, et al. The incidence of typical and atypical A-V Wenckebach periodicity. *Am Heart J* 1975;89:26–31.

89. Narula OS, Samet P. Wenckebach and Mobitz type II A-V block due to block within the His bundle and bundle branches. *Circulation* 1970;41:947–965.

90. Rosen KM. The contribution of His bundle recording to the understanding of cardiac conduction in man. *Circulation* 1971;43:961–966.

91. Pick A. AV dissociation: a proposal for a comprehensive classification and consistent terminology. *Am Heart J* 1963;66:147.

92. Kangos JJ, Griffiths SP, Blumenthal S. Congenital complete heart block. A classification and experience with 18 patients. *Am J Cardiol* 1967;20:632–638.

93. Tans AC, Lie KI, Durrer D. Clinical setting and prognostic significance of high degree atrioventricular block in acute inferior myocardial infarction: a study of 144 patients. *Am Heart J* 1980;99:4–8.

94. Berger PB, Ryan TJ. Inferior myocardial infarction. High-risk subgroups. *Circulation* 1990;81:401–411.

95. Meltzer LE, Cohen HE. The incidence of arrhythmias associated with acute myocardial infarction. In: Meltzer LE, Dunning AJ, eds. *Textbook of coronary care*. Amsterdam: Excerta Medica, 1972:197.

96. Adgey AA, Allen JD, Geddes JS, et al. Acute phase of myocardial infarction. *Lancet* 1971;2:501–504.

97. Sclarovsky S, Strasberg B, Hirshberg A, et al. Advanced early and late atrioventricular block in acute inferior wall myocardial infarction. *Am Heart J* 1984;108:19–24.

98. Lie KI, Duner D. Atrioventricular and intraventricular conduction disturbances in acute myocardial infarction: clinical aspects. In: Samet P, El-Sherif N, eds. *Cardiac pacing*. New York: Grune & Stratton, 1980:439.

99. Feigl D, Ashkenazy J, Kishon Y. Early and late atrioventricular block in acute inferior myocardial infarction. *J Am Coll Cardiol* 1984;4:35–38.

100. Clemo HF, Belardinelli L. Effect of adenosine on atrioventricular conduction. I: Site and characterization of adenosine action in the guinea pig atrioventricular node. *Circ Res* 1986;59:427–436.

101. Sutton R, Davies M. The conduction system in acute myocardial infarction complicated by heart block. *Circulation* 1968;38:987–992.

102. Hackel DB, Wagner G, Ratliff NB, et al. Anatomic studies of the cardiac conducting system in acute myocardial infarction. *Am Heart J* 1972;83:77–81.

103. Nicod P, Gilpin E, Dittrich H, et al. Long-term outcome in patients with inferior myocardial infarction and complete atrioventricular block. *J Am Coll Cardiol* 1988;12:589–594.

104. Mavric Z, Zaputovic L, Matana A, et al. Prognostic significance of complete atrioventricular block in patients with acute inferior myocardial infarction with and without right ventricular involvement. *Am Heart J* 1990;119:823–828.

105. Braat SH, de Zwaan C, Brugada P, et al. Right ventricular involvement with acute inferior wall myocardial infarction identifies high risk of developing atrioventricular nodal conduction disturbances. *Am Heart J* 1984;107:1183–1187.

106. Strasberg B, Pinchas A, Arditti A, et al. Left and right ventricular function in inferior acute myocardial infarction and significance of advanced atrioventricular block. *Am J Cardiol* 1984;54:985–987.

107. Ginks W, Sutton R, Siddons H, et al. Unsuspected coronary artery disease as cause of chronic atrioventricular block in middle age. *Br Heart J* 1980;44:699–702.

108. Chiche P, Haiat R, Steff P. Angina pectoris with syncope due to paroxysmal atrioventricular block: role of ischaemia: report of two cases. *Br Heart J* 1974;36:577–581.

109. Prinzmetal M, Kennamer R, Merliss R, et al. Angina pectoris. I: a variant form of angina pectoris; preliminary report. *Am J Med* 1959;27:375–388.

110. Lev M. The pathology of complete AV block. *Prog Cardiovasc Dis* 1964;6:317.

111. Lenegre J. Etiology and pathology of bilateral bundle block fibrosis in relation to complete heart block. *Prog Cardiovasc Dis* 1964;6:409.

112. Rytand DA, Lipsitch LS. Clinical aspects of calcification of mitral annulus. *Arch Intern Med* 1946;78:544.

113. Narula OS, Samet P. Predilection of elderly females for intra-His bundle (BH) blocks. *Circulation* 1974;50[Suppl]:195.

114. Ablaza SG, Blanco G, Maranhao V, et al. Calcific aortic valvular disease associated with complete heart block: case reports of successful correction. *Dis Chest* 1968;54:457–460.

115. Harris A, Sleight P, Drew CE. The diagnosis and treatment of aortic stenosis complicated by AV block. *Br Heart J* 1965;27:560.

116. Bharati S, Lev M, Denes P, et al. Infiltrative cardiomyopathy with conduction disease and ventricular arrhythmia: electrophysiologic and pathologic correlations. *Am J Cardiol* 1980;45:163–173.

117. Fawcett FJ, Goldberg MJ. Heart block resulting from myocardial sarcoidosis. *Br Heart J* 1974;36:220–223.

118. Schellhammer PF, Engle MA, Hagstrom JW. Histochemical studies of the myocardium and conduction system in acquired iron-storage disease. *Circulation* 1967;35:631–637.

119. Aronow WS, Meister L, Kent JR. Atrioventricular block in familial hemochromatosis treated by permanent synchronous pacemaker. *Arch Intern Med* 1969;123:433–435.

120. Kostis JB, Seibold JR, Turkevich D, et al. Prognostic importance of cardiac arrhythmias in systemic sclerosis. *Am J Med* 1988;84:1007–1015.

121. Ahern M, Lever JV, Cosh J. Complete heart block in rheumatoid arthritis. *Ann Rheum Dis* 1983;42:389–397.

122. Ruppert GB, Lindsay J, Barth WF. Cardiac conduction abnormalities in Reiter's syndrome. *Am J Med* 1982;73:335–340.

123. Bilazarian SD, Taylor AJ, Brezinski D, et al. High-grade atrioventricular heart block in an adult with systemic lupus erythematosus: the association of nuclear RNP (U1 RNP) antibodies, a case report, and review of the literature. *Arthritis Rheum* 1989;32:1170–1174.

124. Bergfeldt L. HLA-B27-associated rheumatic diseases with severe cardiac bradyarrhythmias: clinical features and prevalence in 223 men with permanent pacemakers. *Am J Med* 1983;75:210–215.

125. Kehoe RF, Bauernfeind R, Tommaso C, et al. Cardiac conduction defects in polymyositis: electrophysiologic studies in four patients. *Ann Intern Med* 1981;94:41–43.

126. Wang K, Gobel F, Gleason DF, et al. Complete heart block complicating bacterial endocarditis. *Circulation* 1972;46:939–947.

127. DiNubile MJ, Calderwood SB, Steinhaus DM, et al. Cardiac conduction abnormalities complicating native valve active infective endocarditis. *Am J Cardiol* 1986;58:1213–1217.

128. Hagar JM, Rahimtoola SH. Chagas' heart disease in the United States. *N Engl J Med* 1991;325:763–768.

129. Steere AC, Batsford WP, Weinberg M, et al. Lyme carditis: cardiac abnormalities in Lyme disease. *Ann Intern Med* 1980;93:8–16.

130. van der Linde MR, Crijns HJ, de Koning J, et al. Range of atrioventricular conduction disturbances in Lyme borreliosis: a report of four cases and review of other published reports. *Br Heart J* 1990;63:162–168.

131. Bland EF, Jones TD. Rheumatic fever and rheumatic heart disease. A twenty year report on 1000 patients followed since childhood. *Circulation* 1951;4:836–843.

132. Mirowski M, Rosenstein BJ, Marbowitz M. A comparison of atrioventricular conduction in normal children and in patients with rheumatic fever, glomerulonephritis, and acute febrile illnesses. *Pediatrics* 1964;33:334–340.

133. Wood P. *Diseases of the heart and circulation,* 3rd ed. Philadelphia: Lippincott, 1968:588.

134. Williams JF, Morrow AG, Braunwald E. The incidence and management of "medical" complications following cardiac operations. *Circulation* 1965;32:608–619.

135. Stevenson WG, Klitzner T, Perloff JK. Electrophysiologic abnormalities; natural occurrence and postoperative residua and sequelae. In: Perloff JK, Child JS, eds. *Congenital heart disease in adults.* Philadelphia: WB Saunders, 1991:259–295.

136. Thomas IR, Dalton BC, Lappas DG, et al. Right bundle-branch block and complete heart block caused by the Swan-Ganz catheter. *Anesthesiology* 1979;51:359–362.

137. Jacobson LB, Scheinman M. Catheter-induced intra-Hisian and intrafascicular block during recording of His bundle electrograms. *Circulation* 1974;49:579–584.

138. Kimbiris D, Dreifus LS, Linhart JW. Complete heart block occurring during cardiac catheterization in patients with preexisting bundle branch block. *Chest* 1974;65:95–97.

139. Williamson BD, Man KC, Daoud E, et al. Radiofrequency catheter modification of atrioventricular conduction to control the ventricular rate during atrial fibrillation. *N Engl J Med* 1994;331:944–945.

140. Hindricks G. The Multicentre European Radiofrequency Survey (MERFS): complications of radiofrequency catheter ablation of arrhythmias. *Eur Heart J* 1993;14:1644–1653.

141. Mitrani RD, Klein LS, Hackett FK, et al. Radiofrequency ablation for atrioventricular node reentrant tachycardia: comparison between fast (anterior) and slow (posterior) pathway ablation. *J Am Coll Cardiol* 1993;21:432–441.

142. Fisch C, Greenspan K, Edmands RE. Complete atrioventricular block due to potassium. *Circ Res* 1966;19:373–377.

143. Lown B, Arons WL, Ganong WF, et al. Adrenal steroids and auriculoventricular conduction. *Am Heart J* 1955;50:760–769.

144. Harvey WP. Clinical aspects of cardiac tumors. *Am J Cardiol* 1968;21:328–343.

145. Prystowsky EN, Pritchett EL, Roses AD, et al. The natural history of conduction system disease in myotonic muscular dystrophy as determined by serial electrophysiologic studies. *Circulation* 1979;60:1360–1364.

146. Perloff JK. Cardiac rhythm and conduction in Duchenne's muscular dystrophy: a prospective study of 20 patients. *J Am Coll Cardiol* 1984;3:1263–1268.

147. Zubair ul Hassan, Fastabend CP, Mohanty PK, et al. Atrioventricular block and supraventricular arrhythmias with X-

linked muscular dystrophy. *Circulation* 1979;60:1365–1369.

148. Almquist A, Gornick C, Benson W Jr, et al. Carotid sinus hypersensitivity: evaluation of the vasodepressor component. *Circulation* 1985;71:927–936.

149. Benditt DG, Goldstein MA, Adler S, et al. Neurally mediated syncopal syndromes: pathophysiology and clinical evaluation. In: Mandel WJ, ed. *Cardiac arrhythmias. Their mechanisms, diagnosis, and management.* Philadelphia: Lippincott, 1995:879–906.

150. Lev M. Pathogenesis of congenital atrioventricular block. *Prog Cardiovasc Dis* 1972;15:145–157.

151. McHenry MM, Cayler GC. Congenital complete heart block in newborns, infants, children and adults. *Med Times* 1969;97:113–123.

152. Nakamura FF, Nadas AS. Complete heart block in infants and children. *N Engl J Med* 1964;270:1261.

153. Gillette PC, Busch U, Mullins CE, et al. Electrophysiologic studies in patients with ventricular inversion and "corrected transposition." *Circulation* 1979;60:939–945.

154. Kastor JA, Goldreyer BN, Josephson ME, et al. Electrophysiologic characteristics of Ebstein's anomaly of the tricuspid valve. *Circulation* 1975;52:987–995.

155. Ross BA, Pinsky WW, Driscoll DJ. Complete atrioventricular block. In: Gillette PC, Garson A, eds. *Pediatric arrhythmias: electrophysiology and pacing.* Philadelphia: WB Saunders, 1990:306–316.

156. Johnson RL, Averill KH, Lamb LE. Electrocardiographic findings in 67,375 asymptomatic subjects. *Am J Cardiol* 1960;6:153–177.

157. Perlman LV, Ostrander LD Jr, Keller JB, et al. An epidemiologic study of first degree atrioventricular block in Tecumseh, Michigan. *Chest* 1971;59:40–46.

158. Fox TT, Weaver JC, Francis RL. Further studies on electrocardiographic changes in old age. *Geriatrics* 1948;3:35–41.

159. Rodstein M, Brown M, Wolloch L. First-degree atrioventricular heart block in the aged. *Geriatrics* 1968;23:159–165.

160. Dickinson DF, Scott O. Ambulatory electrocardiographic monitoring in 100 healthy teenage boys. *Br Heart J* 1984;51:179–183.

161. White PD. In: MacMillan D, ed. *Heart disease.* New York: Macmillan, 1951:933.

162. Michaelsson M, Engle MA. Congenital complete heart block: an international study of the natural history. *Cardiovasc Clin* 1972;4:85–101.

163. Perloff JK. The clinical recognition of congenital heart disease. In: Perloff JK, ed. *Congenital complete heart block.* Philadelphia: WB Saunders, 1987:49.

164. Penton GB, Miller H, Levine SA. Some clinical features of complete heart block. *Circulation* 1956;13:801–824.

165. Ide LW. The clinical aspects of complete auriculoventricular heart block: a clinical analysis of 71 cases. *Ann Intern Med* 1952;32:510–523.

166. Friedberg CK, Donoso E, Stein WG. Nonsurgical acquired heart block. *Ann N Y Acad Sci* 1964;111:835–847.

167. Esscher EB. Congenital complete heart block in adolescence and adult life: a follow-up study. *Eur Heart J* 1981;2:281–288.

168. Karpawich PP, Gillette PC, Garson A Jr, et al. Congenital complete atrioventricular block: clinical and electrophysio-

logic predictors of need for pacemaker insertion. *Am J Cardiol* 1981;48:1098–1102.

169. Camm AJ, Bexton RS. Congenital complete heart block. *Eur Heart J* 1984;5:115–117.

170. Scheinman MM, Peters RW, Sauve MJ, et al. Value of the H-Q interval in patients with bundle branch block and the role of prophylactic permanent pacing. *Am J Cardiol* 1982;50:1316–1322.

171. Damato AN, Varghese PJ, Caracta AR, et al. Functional 2:1 A-V block within the His-Purkinje system. Simulation of type II second-degree A-V block. *Circulation* 1973;47:534–542.

172. Katz LN, Pick A. Part I: The arrhythmias. In: *Clinical electrocardiography.* Philadelphia: Lea & Febiger, 1956:545.

173. Ginks W, Leatham A, Siddons H. Prognosis of patients paced for chronic atrioventricular block. *Br Heart J* 1979;41:633–636.

174. Michaelsson M, Jonzon A, Riesenfeld T. Isolated congenital complete atrioventricular block in adult life: a prospective study. *Circulation* 1995;92:442–449.

175. Donmoyer TL, DeSanctis RW, Austen WG. Experience with implantable pacemakers using myocardial electrodes in the management of heart block. *Ann Thorac Surg* 1967;3:218–227.

176. Dhingra RC, Denes P, Wu D, et al. The significance of second degree atrioventricular block and bundle branch block. Observations regarding site and type of block. *Circulation* 1974;49:638–646.

177. Pinsky WW, Gillette PC, Garson A Jr, et al. Diagnosis, management, and long-term results of patients with congenital complete atrioventricular block. *Pediatrics* 1982;69:728–733.

178. Dewey RC, Capeless MA, Levy AM. Use of ambulatory electrocardiographic monitoring to identify high-risk patients with congenital complete heart block. *N Engl J Med* 1987;316:835–839.

179. Serwer GA, Dorostkar PC. Pediatric pacing. In: Ellenbogen KA, Kay GN, Wilkoff BL, eds. *Clinical cardiac pacing.* Philadelphia: WB Saunders, 1995:706–731.

180. Barold SS. Indications for permanent cardiac pacing in first-degree AV block: class I, II, or III? *Pacing Clin Electrophysiol* 1996;19:747–751.

181. Brecker SJD, Xiao HB, Sparrow J, et al. Effects of dual chamber pacing with short atrioventricular delay in dilated cardiomyopathy. *Lancet* 1992;340:1308–1312.

182. Ritter WS, Atkins JM, Blomqvist CG, et al. Permanent pacing in patients with transient trifascicular block during acute myocardial infarction. *Am J Cardiol* 1976;38:205–208.

183. Newby KH, Pisan E, Krucoff MW, et al. Incidence and clinical relevance of the occurrence of bundle-branch block in patients treated with thrombolytic therapy. *Circulation* 1996;94:2424–2428.

184. McAnulty J, Rahimtoola S. Prognosis in bundle branch block. *Annu Rev Med* 1981;32:499–507.

185. Hiss RG, Lamb LE. Electrocardiographic findings in 122,043 individuals. *Circulation* 1962;25:947.

186. Smith RF, Jackson DH, Harthorne JW, et al. Acquired bundle branch block in a healthy population. *Am Heart J* 1970;80:746–751.

187. Rabkin SW, Mathewson FA, Tate RB. Natural history of left bundle-branch block. *Br Heart J* 1980;43:164–169.

188. Dhingra RC, Amat-Y-Leon F, Wyndham C, et al. Significance of left axis deviation in patients with chronic left bundle branch block. *Am J Cardiol* 1978;42:551–556.

189. Dhingra RC, Wyndham C, Bauernfeind R, et al. Significance of block distal to the His bundle induced by atrial pacing in patients with chronic bifascicular block. *Circulation* 1979;60:1455–1464.

190. Clarke M, Sutton R, Ward D, et al. Recommendations for pacemaker prescription for symptomatic bradycardia: report of a working party of the British Pacing and Electrophysiology Group. *Br Heart J* 1991;66:185–191.

191. Ausubel K, Furman S. The pacemaker syndrome. *Ann Intern Med* 1985;103:420–429.

192. Connolly SJ, Kerr CR, Gent M, et al. Effects of physiologic pacing versus ventricular pacing on the risk of stroke and death due to cardiovascular causes. Canadian Trial of Physiologic Pacing Investigators. *N Engl J Med* 2000;11:1385–1391.

193. Andersen HR, Nielsen JC, Thomsen PEB, et al. Long-term follow-up of patients from a randomized trial of atrial versus ventricular pacing for sick-sinus syndrome. *Lancet* 1997;350:1210–1216.

194. Gillis AM, Kerr CR. Whither physiologic pacing? Implications of CTOPP [editorial]. *PACE* 2000;23:1193–1196.

195. Lamas GA, Orav EJ, Stambler BS, et al. Pacemaker selection in the elderly investigators. Quality of life and clinical outcomes in elderly patients treated with ventricular pacing as compared with dual-chamber pacing. *N Engl J Med* 1998;338:1097–1104.

196. Lamas GA, Lee K, Sweeney M, et al. The Mode Selection Trial (MOST) in sinus node dysfunction: design, rationale, and baseline characteristics of the first 1000 patients. *Am Heart J* 2000;140:541–551.

197. Toff WD, Skehan JD, deBono DP, et al. The United Kingdom pacing and cardiovascular events (UKPACE) trial: United Kingdom Pacing and Cardiovascular Events. *Heart* 1997;78:221–223.

64

ATRIAL FIBRILLATION

ERIC N. PRYSTOWSKY
AMOS KATZ

▼▼ ADDITIONAL ELECTRONIC TOPICS

OVERVIEW

Atrial fibrillation is the most common sustained arrhythmia affecting humans. Pathology studies have found loss of atrial myocardium with fibrosis and fatty infiltration, but many similar changes can occur as a result of aging alone. Maintenance of atrial fibrillation likely depends on reentry, with multiple wavelets occurring simultaneously. The initiation of atrial fibrillation in many patients may be caused by a rapidly firing focus, often in the pulmonary vein(s). Although the atrial rate is rapid, typi-

cally greater than 300 beats/min, the ventricular response depends on atrioventricular (AV) node conduction properties and the level of autonomic tone. AV node conduction is facilitated by sympathetic tone and inhibited by parasympathetic tone. A variety of medical conditions are associated with atrial fibrillation, most frequently hypertension, coronary artery disease, and valvular heart disease. Many patients have idiopathic, or lone, atrial fibrillation. There are three major tenets of therapy: (a) restoration and maintenance of sinus rhythm, (b) ventricular rate control, and (c) prevention of thromboembolism. One or more of these may be indicated in a particular patient. Several antiarrhythmic agents are effective for restoring and maintaining sinus rhythm, and selection of a particular drug depends on many factors, including the presence and type of

E. N. Prystowsky: Electrophysiology Laboratory, The CARE Group, Indianapolis, Indiana

A. Katz: Department of Cardiology, Soroka University Medical Center, Beersheva, Israel

underlying heart disease, concomitant illnesses, and renal or hepatic dysfunction. Beta-adrenergic blockers and calcium channel blockers are more effective than digoxin in controlling ventricular response, although digoxin is the first-line treatment for patients who have congestive heart failure. In patients who have Wolff-Parkinson-White syndrome (WPW), intravenous procainamide or ibutilide is the preferred therapy for blocking conduction over the accessory pathway during atrial fibrillation, and digoxin, adenosine, beta-adrenergic blockers, and calcium channel blockers are contraindicated. In patients at high risk for thromboembolism, anticoagulation therapy using warfarin is recommended, aiming for an international normalized ratio (INR) of 2.0 to 3.0. Anticoagulation is also recommended for patients who are undergoing pharmacologic or electrical cardioversion, if atrial fibrillation has been present for at least 48 hours. Nonpharmacologic approaches to therapy include atrial pacing, radiofrequency catheter ablation, surgery, and implantable atrial defibrillators.

EPIDEMIOLOGY

Atrial fibrillation has a profound effect on morbidity and mortality among hundreds of thousands of patients and on health care costs in the United States (9). One report analyzed 3,806,000 patient hospital discharges in 1990 from 678 hospitals to determine the frequency with which arrhythmia was the principal diagnosis (10). Approximately 1.5% of all hospital discharges listed arrhythmia as a principal diagnosis, and atrial fibrillation accounted for nearly 35% of the arrhythmias noted. The epidemiology of atrial fibrillation has changed substantially since the early part of the twentieth century, primarily because of the dramatic decrease in rheumatic fever and the longer life span of the population (Table 64.1) (11–16). The patient populations evaluated in Table 64.1 differ substantially. For example, two studies included patients admitted through the emergency department (13,14), and one evaluated only outpatients (15). Regardless, it is obvious that rheumatic heart disease plays a relatively minor role in the current etiology of atrial fibrillation in the Western world, whereas

hypertension and, to a lesser extent, coronary artery disease currently are major etiologic factors in atrial fibrillation. The incidence of lone atrial fibrillation is quite variable and is influenced by the intensity of the diagnostic workup, the definition of *lone atrial fibrillation* used, and the patient population studied. Kannel and associates (12) reported a 31% incidence of lone atrial fibrillation, but some of their patients had obvious heart disease identified by an enlarged heart on chest radiography. Thus, these data are problematic. In contrast, Prystowsky and colleagues (15) studied only patients who had no known etiologic factors for atrial fibrillation and normal ventricular function identified by echocardiography. However, in their study, only outpatients were evaluated. It is clear that the prevalence and types of etiologic factors for atrial fibrillation depend on the setting in which atrial fibrillation is evaluated, including the country of origin. ▼ 137

Effect of Age and Gender

The prevalence of atrial fibrillation increases with age and is 0.5% for patients aged 50 to 59 years and 8.8% for those aged 80 to 89 years (17). Men are affected slightly more often than women. In the Framingham data, excluding individuals with rheumatic heart disease, the 2-year incidence of development of atrial fibrillation was 0.04% and 0.00% for men and women, respectively, aged 30 to 39 years, and 4.6% and 3.6%, respectively, for men and women aged 80 to 89 years (18). Thus, the number of patients who have atrial fibrillation will rise pari passu with the aging of the population. In the first two decades of life, atrial fibrillation is relatively rare (9). When it is found in patients in this age group, it is usually associated with heart disease or the presence of an accessory pathway.

PATHOLOGY

Pathology of the Atrium in Atrial Fibrillation

One study analyzed pathologic changes in the atria in 145 patients with atrial fibrillation (20). Etiologies were diverse

TABLE 64.1 ETIOLOGY OF ATRIAL FIBRILLATION

Author	Year	Country	Number of patients	Rheumatic heart disease (%)	Hypertensive heart disease (%)	Coronary heart disease (%)	Hyperthyroidism (%)	No heart disease (%)
Lewis (7)	1910	England	73	64	—	—	—	—
Parkinson and Campbell (11)	1930	England	200	22	24	—	14	9
Kannel et al. (12)[a]	1982	United States	98	18	48	10	—	31
Davidson et al. (13)[b]	1989	Israel	704	23	—	55	4	5
Lok and Lau (14)	1995	Hong Kong	291	11	29	25	6	29
Prystowsky et al. (15)[c]	1996	United States	285	4	56	19	11	35

[a]Some patients with no heart disease had cardiac stigmata.
[b]Atherosclerotic cardiovascular disease included hypertension.
[c]Consecutive series of outpatients only.

and included conditions such as rheumatic fever, hypertension, hyperthyroidism, and coronary artery disease. The hearts of 35 control subjects were compared with those of patients who had atrial fibrillation. No distinctions that would account for the atrial fibrillation were seen in the atria of the control subjects and those of patients with atrial fibrillation. Indeed, the author speculated that no specific histologic syndrome is associated with atrial fibrillation (20).

In another study, lesions of the sinus node were evaluated in the hearts of 65 patients (21). The anatomy of the sinus node was compared with clinical data in a blinded manner. The sinus node was obviously damaged in 15 patients, and an established arrhythmia, usually atrial fibrillation, was seen in 14 patients. The sinus node was not identified with certainty in one patient who had established atrial fibrillation. The sinus node was normal in 49 patients, and atrial fibrillation had been present in 5 patients. These data are interesting and important clinically, because it is well established that atrial fibrillation and sinus node dysfunction often occur in the same patient (this has been termed *tachycardia-bradycardia syndrome*). The common association in this study between sinus nodal damage and a clinical history of atrial fibrillation supports the idea that sick sinus syndrome is a panatrial disorder in many patients.

One of the most important pathologic studies of the atria of patients with atrial fibrillation was done by Davies and Pomerance (22). These authors analyzed the hearts of 100 patients with atrial fibrillation and subgrouped them into patients who had atrial fibrillation for less than 2 weeks before death and those who had atrial fibrillation for more than 1 month before death. Among patients who had long-term atrial fibrillation, cor pulmonale, rheumatic heart disease, and ischemic heart disease were the most frequently associated clinical conditions. In nearly 75% of cases of chronic atrial fibrillation, sinus node muscle loss, internodal tract muscle loss, and atrial dilatation of some degree were present. Notably, left atrial appendage thrombosis was identified in 46 patients with long-term atrial fibrillation, and cerebral infarction was identified in 19. However, only 3 of 19 patients with short-term fibrillation had left atrial thrombus, and only 1 patient with cerebral infarction. These authors offered an important hypothesis concerning the origin of pathologic changes in the atria. They stated that "while it is conventional to regard the fibrotic changes in the node and atria as the cause of atrial fibrillation, it is also possible that they result from the arrhythmia and consequent disordered function of the chamber" (22). This prescient observation supports the current belief that atrial fibrillation begets atrial fibrillation, therefore making it possible to retard or even prevent the development of permanent atrial fibrillation in some patients by maintaining sinus rhythm, which may beget sinus rhythm (see the section Therapy of Atrial Fibrillation.).

In recent studies involving patients with lone atrial fibrillation, atrial biopsies have shown histologic changes consistent with myocarditis (23), and high serum levels of antibodies against myosine heavy chains have been found (24). The pathophysiologic significance of these findings is unclear.

PATHOPHYSIOLOGY

Electrophysiologic Mechanism of Atrial Fibrillation

A wealth of data suggests that reentry is the primary mechanism of atrial fibrillation. An alternative theory, the ectopic focus theory, was championed by Scherf and coworkers (25,26). Using topical application of aconitine to the atria, several observations were made that appeared to indicate that there was a focal mechanism for atrial fibrillation. Aconitine could be applied to the appendix of the right or left atrium and yield arrhythmias that were similar in appearance. Clamping off the area of application from the rest of the atrium allowed the arrhythmia to continue in the area that was clamped off, but not in the rest of the atria. Similarly, cooling of the area on which aconitine had been applied terminated fibrillation. The experiments with aconitine suggested that atrial fibrillation depended on a single focus. However, atrial fibrillation induced by topical application of acetylcholine did not terminate when the area in which drug had been applied was cooled (26). The authors postulated that the AV node was able to maintain atrial fibrillation in this situation. These observations led to the supposition that an additional mechanism of atrial fibrillation existed, one with multiple (tachysystolic) foci.

The ectopic focus theory for atrial fibrillation was essentially smothered by the overwhelming weight of observations indicating that reentry is the mechanism of atrial fibrillation. However, recent observations made during intracardiac radiofrequency catheter ablation of atrial fibrillation have rekindled interest in the ectopic focus theory (27–29). These authors (27,28) were able to terminate atrial fibrillation with discrete applications of energy, primarily in the area of the pulmonary veins in the left atrium, although right atrial sites have also been identified (29). In such cases, it is likely that atrial fibrillation results from rapid, focal atrial tachycardia, a form of tachycardia-induced tachycardia (see the section Tachycardia-Induced Tachycardia). Thus, elimination of the primary inciting arrhythmia prevents the secondary arrhythmia. The pulmonary veins are most frequently the origin of these rapid atrial foci, and studies have confirmed that cardiac muscle extends onto the pulmonary veins in humans (30) and have found automaticity in an experimental model (31).

In a classic paper, Mines (32) demonstrated reentry in the myocardium. He used various experimental preparations and showed reciprocating rhythm in an AV preparation. In one experiment, using a tortoise heart, stimulation of one portion of the heart was followed by an orderly sequence of activation using the atrium and ventricle repeatedly without any further stimulation. He suggested that this mechanism was the cause of atrial fibrillation. Working independently, Garrey (33) performed innovative experiments that implicated reentry as the mechanism of fibrillation. He further proposed that persistence of fibrillation is directly proportional to the size of the tissue mass involved. Indeed, atrial fibrillation is relatively rare in children with normal-sized hearts (9).

A key development in our understanding of the mechanism of atrial fibrillation was the multiple wavelet hypothesis proposed by Moe and coauthors (34,35). They noted, "the grossly irregular wave front becomes fractionated as it divides about islets or strands of refractory tissue, and each of the daughter wavelets may now be considered as independent offspring. Such a wavelet may accelerate or decelerate as it encounters tissue in a more or less advanced state of recovery" (34). Thus, the larger the number of wavelets that present, the more likely it is that the arrhythmia will sustain. The number of wavelets depends on the atrial mass, the refractory period, and the conduction velocity of various areas of the atria. In essence, a large atrial mass with short refractory periods and conduction delay would yield increased wavelets and would present the most favorable situation for atrial fibrillation to be sustained. In the work of Moe and many other investigators, atrial fibrillation could only be sustained during constant vagal stimulation. This is consistent with Moe's hypothesis, because vagal stimulation shortens refractoriness in many atrial cells, a condition that should allow more wavelets to be present. A computer model of atrial fibrillation supported the multiple wavelet hypothesis (35).

Experimental validation of the multiple wavelet hypothesis was demonstrated by Allessie and colleagues (36). They analyzed the excitation of canine atria during induced atrial fibrillation with two egg-shaped multiple electrodes inserted into the cavities of the atria. Each electrode contained 480 recording electrodes, with an interelectrode distance of 3 mm. This enabled the first highly detailed activation sequencing of atrial fibrillation. As noted by other investigators, enhanced vagal tone was necessary for maintenance of atrial fibrillation, and infusions of acetylcholine were used for this purpose. Figure 64.1 demonstrates an arbitrary moment during atrial fibrillation and reveals seven wavelets (36). These reentrant wavelets were not stable, and over the course of time, various pathways of reentry could be demonstrated. When only three wavelets existed, there was a high chance that all would cease to exist, but when six wavelets were present, spontaneous termination of atrial fibrillation did not occur. ▼▼ 138

Traditionally, it has been thought that reentry requires a significant mass of tissue. The seminal work of Spach and associates (40,41) on conduction led to the understanding that anisotropic reentry is possible. Typically, propagation in the myocardium is faster in the longitudinal direction

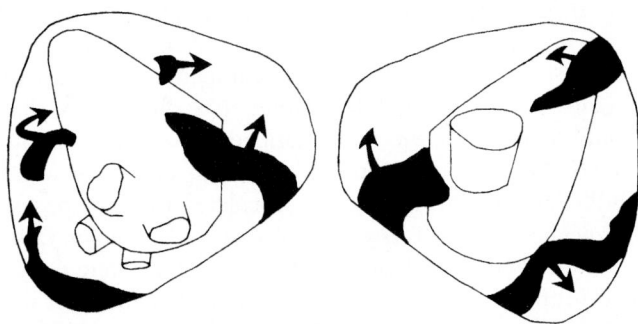

FIGURE 64.1 Canine atria with multiple propagating wavelets during sustained atrial fibrillation. Seven wavelets are present—three in the right atrium and four in the left atrium. The black contours mark the atrium that has been excited during the last 10 ms. (From Allessie MA, Lammers WJEP, Bonke FIM, et al. Experimental evaluation of Moe's multiple wavelet hypothesis of atrial fibrillation. In: Zipes DP, Jalife J, eds. *Cardiac arrhythmias.* New York: Grune & Stratton, 1985:265–276, with permission.)

than in the perpendicular direction, and this anisotropic propagation can be uniform or nonuniform. Nonuniform conduction is associated with decreased side-to-side electrical coupling between small groups of cells, which typically occurs with aging (40). During investigation of human atrial pectinate muscle bundles obtained at surgery, reentry was demonstrated in 1 to 2 mm areas (*e*Fig. 64.1.4). Even if the maintenance of reentry in atrial fibrillation requires the presence of multiple wavelets throughout the atria, this important observation may explain the initiation of atrial fibrillation in some circumstances, for example, in patients with tachycardia-induced tachycardia who have AV reentry, in which disorganization of the right atrium typically precedes that of the left atrium (Fig. 64.2) (42). An alternative mechanism for tachycardia-induced atrial fibrillation may be induction of a rapidly firing atrial focus, for example, in the superior right pulmonary vein, with initial activation observed at the right atrial recording site.

The mechanism of initiation of atrial fibrillation is not certain in most cases and likely is multifactorial. Even the example given in this chapter of tachycardia-induced tachycardia is merely descriptive, and the actual mechanism for induction of atrial fibrillation might be related to the tachycardia cycle length, to intrinsic atrial vulnerability, to contraction-excitation feedback, or to a combination of these factors (42). If reentry is assumed to be the mechanism of atrial fibrillation, initiation would require an area of conduction block and a wavelength of activation that is short enough to allow the reentrant circuit in the myocardium. The normal aging process results in anatomic changes likely to yield inhomogeneity in conduction that may create the milieu necessary for the development of reentry (19,40). These changes are likely magnified by the presence of certain disease processes, for example, those of coronary artery disease. Using high-density mapping of the left atrium of a rabbit, inhomogeneity in conduction was

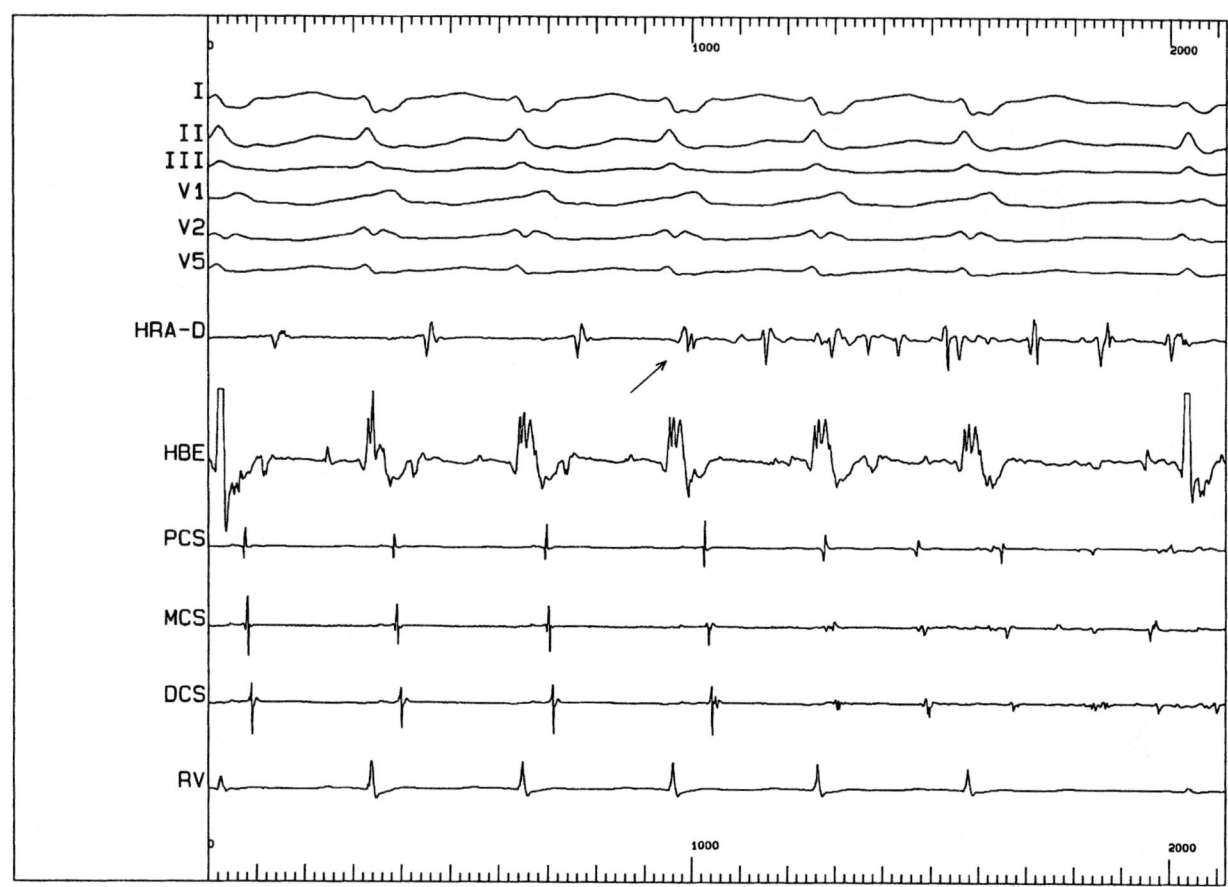

FIGURE 64.2 Patient with atrioventricular reentry using a left-sided accessory pathway in which atrioventricular reentry degenerates to atrial fibrillation. The arrow notes the earliest disorganization in the high right atrial electrogram, positioned near the junction of the right atrium and the superior vena cava. DCS, distal coronary sinus; HBE, bundle of His electrogram; HRA-D, high right atrium–distal; MCS, midcoronary sinus; PCS, proximal coronary sinus; RV, right ventricle.

found to be significantly increased by the presence of single close-coupled atrial premature complexes and further increased by the presence of multiple premature complexes (43). Of particular note was the marked inhomogeneity in conduction that occurred with rapid atrial pacing. The clinical counterpoint of this phenomenon is the presence on electrophysiologic study in humans of relatively frequent accidental initiation of atrial fibrillation during rapid atrial pacing, and the necessity that a relatively rapid rate of tachycardia be present for either AV or AV node reentry to initiate atrial fibrillation (42). ❦ 139

Tachycardia-Induced Atrial Cardiomyopathy

It has been recognized for several decades that a persistently fast ventricular rate secondary to supraventricular tachycardia can lead to ventricular cardiomyopathy, which is reversible if recognized in time. In fact, this is not an uncommon phenomenon in patients who present with atrial fibrillation and dilated cardiomyopathy. But might such a situation lead to tachycardia-induced atrial cardiomyopathy? It is not only possible, but probable, although this has not been

investigated in detail until recently (45). Notably, this concept was put forth in an earlier study on the pathology of atrial fibrillation, in which the authors suggested that the fibrotic changes in the sinus node and atria may be the result of atrial fibrillation rather than its cause (22). More recently, the effect of persistent atrial fibrillation on changes in atrial size was investigated in 15 patients who showed no evidence of significant structural or functional cardiac abnormalities other than atrial fibrillation (46). Normal left atrial size was among the inclusion criteria. During an average follow-up period of 20.6 months, mean left atrial volume increased from 45.2 to 64.1 cm³. Similarly, right atrial volume significantly increased, from 49.2 to 66.2 cm³. These changes in atrial size are consistent with the observation that atrial fibrillation begets atrial fibrillation. In another study, atrial size was evaluated at 6 months' follow-up after cardioversion in patients in whom sinus rhythm persisted and in patients in whom atrial fibrillation recurred (47). Importantly, in the 28 patients in whom sinus rhythm was maintained, left atrial volume decreased from 72.6 ± 15.1 to 58.5 ± 13.8 cm³ and right atrial volume decreased from 68.7 ± 14.6 to 58.6 ± 11.6 cm³

(p <.05). In contrast, atrial size did not change in patients in whom atrial fibrillation recurred. Thus, a window of opportunity appears to be present for reversal of the atrial dilatation that is often noted in association with atrial fibrillation. ❦ 140

Evidence for a tachycardia-induced atrial cardiomyopathy is supported further by echocardiographic observations before and after cardioversion (51,52). Using transesophageal echocardiography, left atrial appendage blood flow velocity and contractile function were assessed in patients with atrial fibrillation (52). The mean duration of atrial fibrillation was 49 months, and an inverse correlation was seen between the duration of the arrhythmia and left atrial appendage peak outflow velocities. Patients who spontaneously cardioverted to sinus rhythm had significantly greater left atrial appendage outflow velocities. The course of recovery of atrial systolic function after cardioversion was evaluated using transthoracic Doppler echocardiography (51). Within the first week after cardioversion, atrial mechanical function was greater in patients with atrial fibrillation of 2 weeks or less compared with those patients who had atrial fibrillation greater than 6 weeks in duration. Over the course of time, atrial mechanical function improved in all groups of patients. Thus, atrial mechanical function appeared to recover compared that measured before cardioversion, and the time to recovery was a function of the previous duration of atrial fibrillation. However, because atrial mechanical function before atrial fibrillation was unknown, the degree to which atrial mechanical function approached normal for individual patients remains unclear.

In summary, persistence of atrial fibrillation results in a cascade of electrical and anatomic changes in the atria that promote the persistence of atrial fibrillation. The result is perpetuation of atrial fibrillation and a decrease in atrial mechanical function secondary to tachycardia-induced atrial cardiomyopathy. If sinus rhythm is restored within a reasonable period of time, electrophysiologic changes appear to normalize, atrial size decreases, and restoration of atrial mechanical function occurs. These observations lend support to the idea that the negative downhill spiral in which atrial fibrillation begets atrial fibrillation can be arrested with sinus rhythm that perpetuates sinus rhythm. Two major questions remain unanswered: What duration of atrial fibrillation results in substantial irreversible changes, and can maintenance of sinus rhythm prevent the transition of intermittent atrial fibrillation to permanent atrial fibrillation? These are the subjects of future investigations.

Atrioventricular Conduction

In the absence of an accessory pathway, AV conduction occurs over the AV node during atrial fibrillation. The resultant ventricular rate depends on the intrinsic conduction and refractoriness of the AV node, the rate and organization of atrial inputs to the AV node, and the state of autonomic tone. The compact AV node is located anteriorly in the triangle of Koch (53). The compact AV node is surrounded by transitional cells with various microelectrode action potential characteristics. Maximal conduction slowing occurs predominantly in the zone of N cells in the AV node (53). There are two distinct atrial inputs to the AV node, anteriorly via the interatrial septum and posteriorly via the crista terminalis. Experiments in a rabbit AV nodal preparation demonstrated that propagation of impulses during atrial fibrillation through the AV node to the bundle of His was critically dependent on the relative timing of activation of septal inputs to the AV node at the crista terminalis and interatrial septum (54). Other investigators showed that the ventricular response also depended on atrial input frequency (55,56). Concealed conduction likely plays the predominant role in determining ventricular response during atrial fibrillation (55,57). Concealed conduction into the AV node occurs with atrial impulses that enter the AV node but do not conduct to the ventricle, leaving a wake of refractoriness that is encountered by subsequent impulses. The constant bombardment of atrial impulses into the AV node undoubtedly creates substantial and varying degrees of concealed conduction.

Alterations of autonomic tone can have profound effects on AV nodal conduction (58–60). Enhanced parasympathetic and sympathetic tone have negative and positive dromotropic effects, respectively, on AV nodal conduction. This can be seen in Figure 64.3, in which recordings of atrial fibrillation during the awake state and during sleep are shown. Note the substantial slowing of ventricular response, even with pauses, during sleep, a state in which there is heightened parasympathetic and decreased sympathetic tone.

Aberrant conduction commonly occurs during atrial fibrillation. It is important to distinguish aberrant conduction from ventricular ectopy, especially when repetitive wide QRS complexes occur. The refractoriness of the His-Purkinje tissue decreases as the heart rate increases (61). Thus, slower heart rates favor aberrancy. The gross irregularity of ventricular response during atrial fibrillation yields an abundance of RR cycle lengths, which statistically increases the chance for a long-short cycle length combination that will produce aberrant conduction. This phenomenon was described well by Gouaux and Ashman ("Ashman phenomenon") (62) and Lewis (63) and confirmed experimentally by Moe and coworkers (64). Figure 64.4 demonstrates an example of right bundle branch (RBB) block aberrancy during atrial flutter/fibrillation initiated during electrophysiologic study. RBB aberrancy results from the sudden lengthening of the preceding cycle length (long-short sequence), which prolongs RBB refractoriness. RBB block aberrancy is more common than left bundle branch block aberrancy, probably because the RBB has a longer refractory period at slower heart rates (65). To complicate matters further, it has been demonstrated that cycle lengths

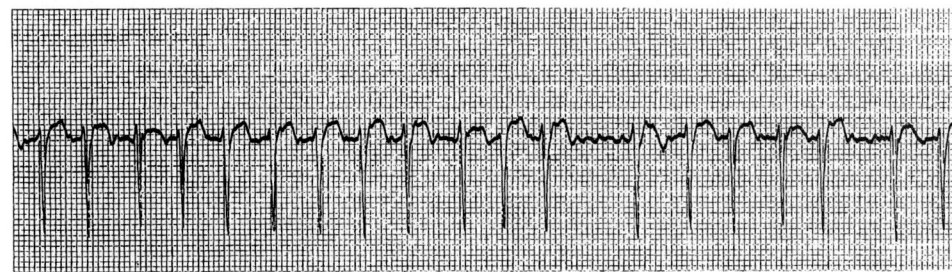

A

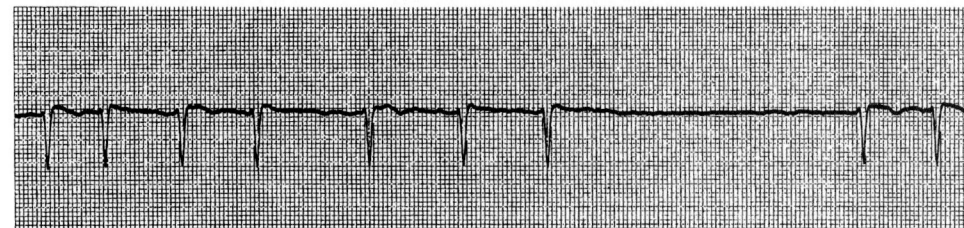

B

FIGURE 64.3 Effect of autonomic tone on atrioventricular node conduction during atrial fibrillation. **A:** Relatively rapid ventricular response during the awake state. **B:** Slow ventricular response recorded during sleep.

preceding the pause may also affect the chance for aberrancy after the pause (*e*Fig. 64.4.1) (66).

It is important to differentiate between aberrant ventricular conduction and ventricular tachycardia when repetitive wide QRS complexes occur during atrial fibrillation. This can usually be accomplished by careful analysis of the rhythm strip and application of certain guidelines (Table 64.2) (61,67,68). 141

The presence of a grossly irregular, very rapid ventricular response during atrial fibrillation is diagnostic of conduction over an accessory pathway, with rare exceptions (Fig. 64.5). At very fast heart rates, a tendency toward regularization of the RR intervals is present, but careful measurement always discloses definite irregularities. It would be rare for such rapid responses to result from conduction over the AV node, and the only other alternative is ventricular tachycardia. It is

axiomatic that rapid, irregular ventricular tachycardia is unstable and quickly degenerates into ventricular fibrillation. Thus, when a rapid, irregular wide QRS complex tachycardia is noted in a patient who has a reasonably stable hemodynamic state, preexcitation is the most likely diagnosis. The ability to conduct rapidly over an accessory pathway is determined primarily by the intrinsic conduction and refractory properties of the accessory pathway. However, as with AV node conduction, factors such as spatial and temporal characteristics of atrial wavefronts during atrial fibrillation, autonomic tone, and concealed conduction influence activation over the accessory pathway (70–72).

CLINICAL PROFILE

Associated Disease States

Atrial fibrillation has been reported to occur in patients with a wide variety of diseases, many of which are listed in Table 64.3. Why a particular disease results in atrial fibrillation is often unclear. In some cases—for example, hypertension—both occur with increased frequency in the elderly, and it is possible that a cause-and-effect relationship does not always exist. However, echocardiographic studies of left atrial function in patients who have hypertension

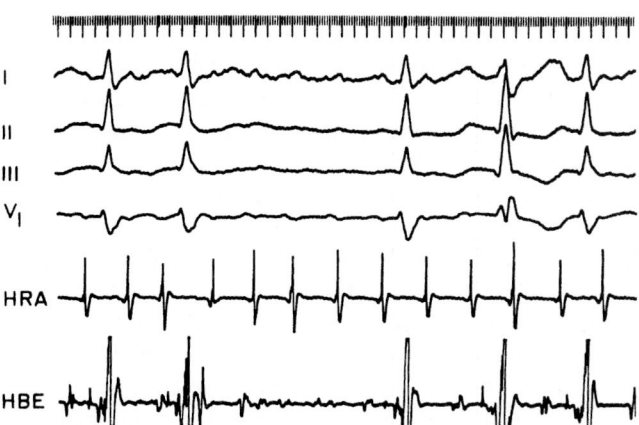

I

II

III

V₁

HRA

HBE

FIGURE 64.4 Right bundle branch block aberrancy caused by sudden lengthening of the preceding cycle length. See text for details. HBE, bundle of His electrogram; HRA, high right atrium. (From Prystowsky EN, Klein GJ. *Cardiac arrhythmias: an integrated approach for the clinician.* New York: McGraw-Hill, 1994, with permission.)

TABLE 64.2 FACTORS FAVORING ABERRANT VENTRICULAR CONDUCTION

Long-short cycle length sequence
Typical right bundle branch block
Relatively rapid ventricular rate
Lack of compensatory pause
Absence of bundle branch block with shorter cycle length without preceding pause
Normalization of QRS complexes with minimal change in cycle length

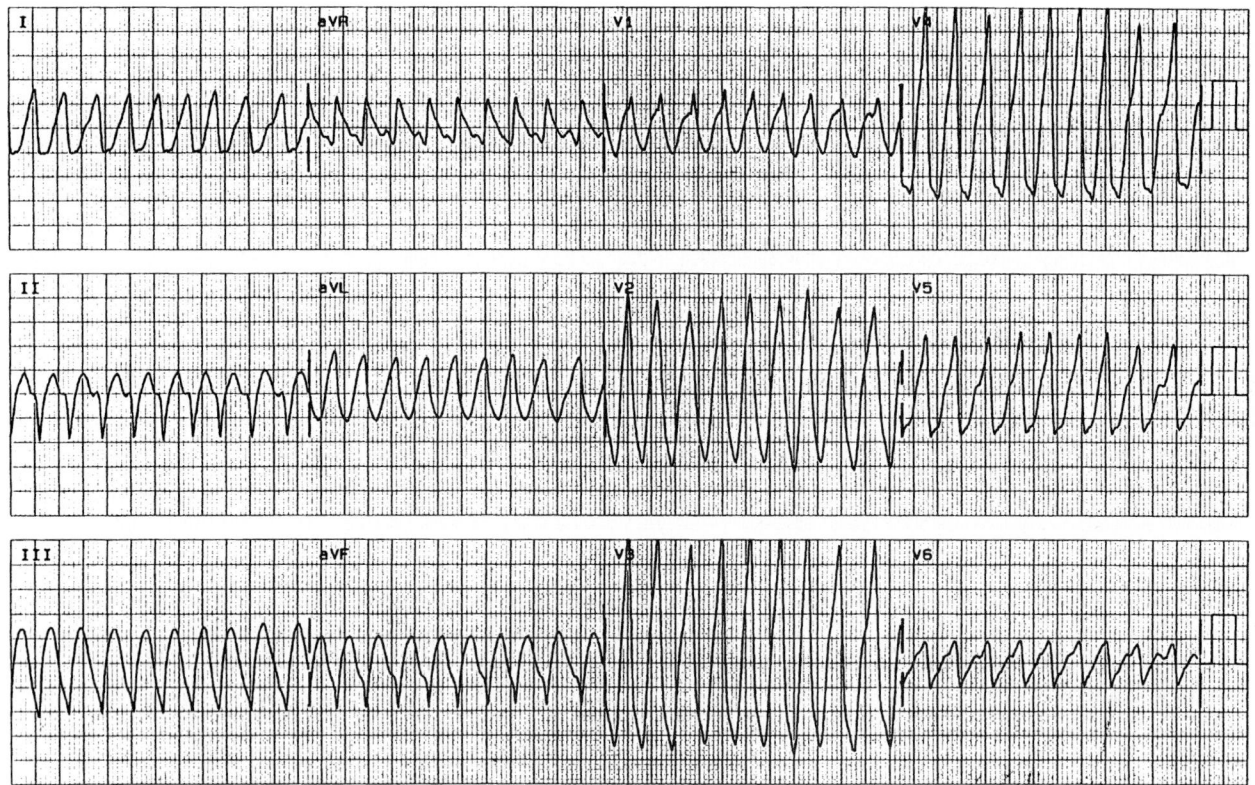

FIGURE 64.5 Twelve-lead electrocardiogram in a patient with ventricular preexcitation during atrial fibrillation who had a rapid preexcited ventricular response.

have demonstrated that patients with paroxysmal atrial fibrillation had left atrial enlargement and depression of atrial contractile function associated with an increased ventricular inflow during early diastole (81). It is unclear

TABLE 64.3 FACTORS ASSOCIATED WITH ATRIAL FIBRILLATION

Hypertension
Coronary heart disease
Cardiomyopathy
    Dilated
    Hypertrophic
Mitral valve disease
    Stenosis
    Regurgitation
Thyrotoxicosis
Sick sinus syndrome
Congenital heart disease
    Atrial septal defect
    Ebstein's anomaly
Cardiac surgery
Pericarditis
Tumors
Alcohol
Lung disease
Neurogenic
Tachycardia-induced tachycardia
Lone (idiopathic)

whether these changes cause or are the result of paroxysmal atrial fibrillation. In contrast, in patients with mitral valve disease with progressive enlargement of the atria, a pathophysiologic link between the disease state and the onset of atrial fibrillation is easier to understand.

Thyrotoxicosis

Thyroid hormone affects the circulatory system and myocardium (82). There is a decrease in total systemic vascular resistance, an increase in total blood volume, and a decrease in circulation time. This leads to an increase in preload and a reduction in afterload. There is also an increase in sinus rate and a reduction in the electrical threshold for excitation of the atrium. There appears to be an interaction between excess thyroid hormone and catecholamine action, including potentiation of catecholamine effect and an increased number of cardiac beta-adrenergic receptors (82). Atrial fibrillation is not uncommonly associated with thyrotoxicosis, is more frequent among men than among women, and increases with age. It occurs in more than 25% of patients aged 60 years or older, but it is rare in patients younger than 40 years. Although exclusion of occult thyrotoxicosis as a cause for atrial fibrillation is recommended, situations in which it is the cause are very uncommon. Notably, in one study, a low serum thyrotropin concentration in patients aged 60 years or older who show no evidence of hyperthyroidism was associated with a threefold higher risk of development of atrial fibrillation during a 10-year follow-up period (83). An increased risk of arterial thromboembolism is seen in association with thyrotoxicosis, mandating use of warfarin in patients with atrial fibrillation until a euthyroid state and sinus rhythm are achieved. The dose of warfarin necessary to maintain an INR of 2.0 to 3.0 may be smaller initially because of increased plasma clearance of vitamin K–dependent clotting factors, and a higher dose may be necessary as the thyroid hormone concentration decreases (82).

Congenital Heart Disease

Atrial fibrillation is relatively common in two forms of congenital heart disease in particular: atrial septal defect and Ebstein's anomaly. In patients with atrial septal defect, the incidence of atrial fibrillation is greater as patients age and has been reported to be more than 50% in a study involving patients aged 60 years or older (84). In general, the incidence of atrial fibrillation begins to increase in the fourth decade of life.

Ebstein's anomaly is commonly associated with atrial fibrillation, often at an early age (85). Atrial fibrillation may be caused by the underlying atrial dysfunction or, more commonly, may be a consequence of concomitant WPW. In patients who have WPW and AV reentry, atrial fibrillation is relatively common and most often secondary to degeneration of AV reentry into atrial fibrillation (42). Among patients who underwent surgical ablation of the accessory pathway and were followed up for 6.2 years, atrial fibrillation was documented in 42% of the patients before surgery, and this was reduced to 9% postoperatively (86). Thus, in patients with Ebstein's anomaly, the most significant etiologic factor for atrial fibrillation appears to be concomitant WPW.

Cardiac Surgery

Atrial fibrillation is the most frequent atrial arrhythmia noted after cardiac surgery. New atrial fibrillation develops in 25% to 50% of adult patients who undergo cardiac surgery (87). It is usually benign and self-limiting, but it may be associated with hemodynamic compromise, prolonged hospitalization, and embolic stroke (88). Patients most likely to develop atrial fibrillation are those with a history of atrial fibrillation before surgery who are in sinus rhythm initially after the operation (89).

Patients undergoing coronary artery bypass graft surgery are the group most likely to have a first episode of atrial fibrillation postoperatively. Development of atrial fibrillation is multifactorial, and several risk factors have been identified. Postoperative discontinuation of beta-adrenergic blockers that were taken regularly before surgery increases the risk of atrial fibrillation during the postoperative period; this complication can be expected in approximately 40% of patients in such a situation (90). Increased postoperative sympathetic activity demonstrated by elevated norepinephrine levels is associated with an increased risk of atrial fibrillation (91). Age is a major risk factor, and atrial fibrillation occurs in approximately 4% and 30% of patients aged less than 40 and 70 or more years, respectively, who are undergoing coronary artery bypass graft surgery (87). Other risk factors include chronic obstructive pulmonary disease, chronic renal disease, decreased postoperative serum magnesium level, history of paroxysmal atrial fibrillation, premature atrial complexes in the preoperative period, the presence of severe right coronary artery stenosis, and a history of congestive heart failure (91–94). The type of cardioplegia does not appear to correlate with the development of atrial fibrillation after cardiac operation (87,95). Notably, minimally invasive cardiac valve surgery may not reduce the incidence of postoperative atrial fibrillation (96).

Neurogenic

It has been known for decades that sustained atrial fibrillation is facilitated by increased parasympathetic tone. The atrial refractory period is decreased by acetylcholine, which shortens the wavelength, making it easier for atrial fibrillation to be sustained (44). Earlier investigators were aware of the profound influence of heightened vagal tone on atrial fibrillation (97–102). It was noted that rapid atrial stimulation in the presence of acetylcholine alone induced atrial fibrillation, and atrial fibrillation would continue in the absence of stimulation until the acetylcholine infusion was discontinued (100). Importantly, a nonuniform distribution of vagal effects on the refractoriness of the atrium has been found (102). In one study, right atrial refractoriness was determined at various sites before and during vagal stimulation (102). In the control state, atrial refractoriness differed by no more than 40 ms between sites. However, during vagal stimulation there was marked shortening of atrial refractoriness at some sites and minimal change at others. Because dispersion of refractoriness often promotes the development of reentry, this may be one mechanism by which heightened vagal tone facilitates the initiation of atrial fibrillation.

In some patients, atrial fibrillation occurs during enhancement of vagal tone. The patient's clinical history usually provides clues for this mechanism. For example, onset of atrial fibrillation during swallowing of a cold substance (e.g., ice cream or an ice cube) indicates that a vagal reflex may initiate atrial fibrillation. A specific syndrome of vagal atrial fibrillation has also been described (103), with occurrence at time of heightened vagal tone such as at night, during rest, or after consumption of food or alcohol. Reportedly, patients with vagal atrial fibrillation have an

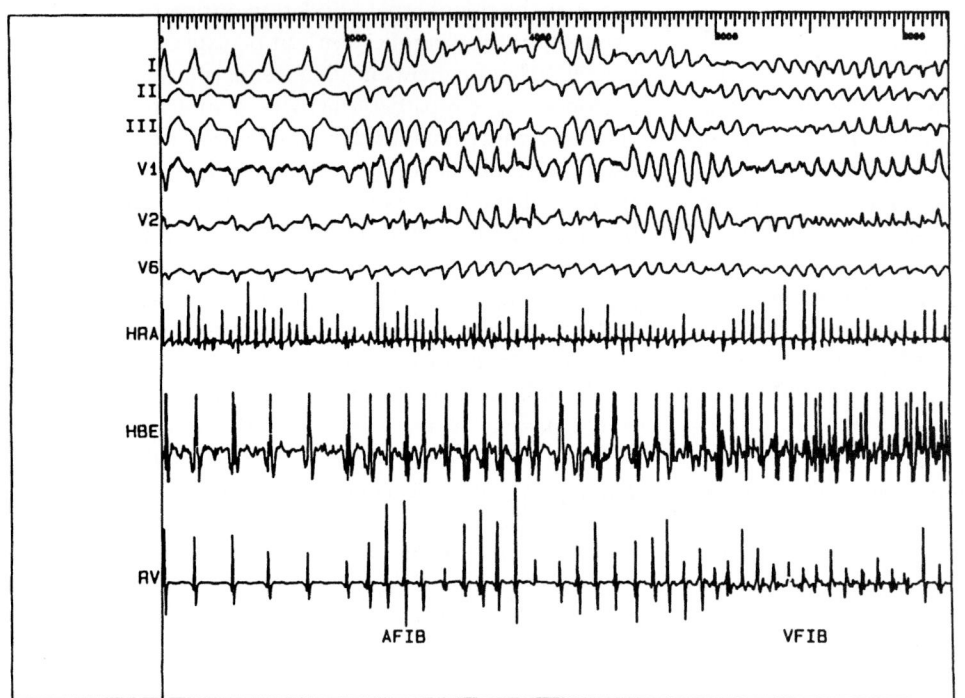

FIGURE 64.6 Atrial fibrillation in a patient with Wolff-Parkinson-White syndrome with degeneration from atrial fibrillation to ventricular fibrillation. AFIB, atrial fibrillation; HBE, bundle of His electrogram; HRA, high right atrium; RV, right ventricle; VFIB, ventricular fibrillation. (From Prystowsky EN, Knilans TK, Evans JJ. Diagnostic evaluation and treatment strategies for patients at risk for serious cardiac arrhythmias. II. Ventricular tachyarrhythmias and Wolff-Parkinson-White syndrome. *Mod Concepts Cardiovasc Dis* 1991;60: 55, with permission.)

increased number of attacks during therapy involving beta-blockers and digitalis (103). Although many patients relate a tendency towards increased episodes of atrial fibrillation during periods of presumed increased vagal tone, in our experience, it is rare for patients to have atrial fibrillation only during enhanced parasympathetic tone.

An adrenergic form of atrial fibrillation has also been described (103), with onset exclusively during the daytime hours and often preceded by emotional stress or exercise. In contrast to vagal atrial fibrillation, beta-adrenergic blockers are the treatment of choice.

Tachycardia-Induced Tachycardia

Tachycardia-induced tachycardia is a phenomenon in which one tachycardia degenerates into another tachycardia (42). A relatively common example is rapid ventricular tachycardia that degenerates into ventricular fibrillation. Several different tachycardias can degenerate into atrial fibrillation (42). Atrial flutter and atrial tachycardia are likely the most common causes of tachycardia-induced tachycardia that results in atrial fibrillation, but arrhythmias as diverse as ventricular tachycardia, AV node reentry, and AV reentry may also initiate atrial fibrillation (Fig. 64.2) (42,104–106). In WPW, transition of AV reentry into atrial fibrillation can produce dire consequences, with a rapid preexcited ventricular response that degenerates into ventricular fibrillation leading to sudden death (Fig. 64.6) (61,107–111). ▼ 142

Identification of the role of tachycardia-induced tachycardia as a mechanism for atrial fibrillation has important therapeutic implications. It presents an opportunity for the clinician to prevent further episodes of atrial fibrillation, not by treating atrial fibrillation itself, but by directing therapy at the initiating arrhythmia. The paradigm for this is ablation of an accessory pathway in a patient with AV reentry. Likewise, in patients who have atrial flutter predominantly with occasional episodes of atrial fibrillation, electrocardiographic confirmation that atrial fibrillation is caused by atrial flutter may allow cure using ablation of the atrial flutter reentrant circuit.

Lone (Idiopathic) Atrial Fibrillation

Certain patients have no clear etiologic factors that explain the presence of atrial fibrillation; in such patients, the condition is called *idiopathic* or *lone atrial fibrillation*. Our definition for lone atrial fibrillation is the absence of any potential etiologic factor and the lack of evidence of ventricular dysfunction on echocardiography (15). We do not use an age cutoff point to designate lone atrial fibrillation. The prevalence of lone atrial fibrillation depends on the population of patients studied, as demonstrated in Table 64.1.

Awareness of lone atrial fibrillation has existed for decades (7,11,119–123). Clearly, because normal atria do not spontaneously fibrillate, some anatomic or electrophysiologic milieu must allow emergence of atrial fibrillation in these patients. In some cases, autonomic perturbations may be the etiology and likely are transient in nature. In other patients, left atrial size is increased, even though ventricular function is normal, and these patients may have some unidentified anatomic pathophysiologic basis for atrial fibrillation (15). ❦ 143

Definition of Atrial Fibrillation

Traditionally, atrial fibrillation has been termed *paroxysmal* or *chronic atrial fibrillation*. However, no standardization regarding these terms has ever been achieved, and quite disparate time frames have been proposed for each category. A new classification has been proposed by the American College of Cardiology/American Heart Association/European Society of Cardiology Guidelines for the Management of patients with Atrial Fibrillation (131). Paroxysmal atrial fibrillation is self-terminating; persistent atrial fibrillation requires treatment for termination; in permanent atrial fibrillation, sinus rhythm cannot be restored, or the decision to avoid cardioversion has been made.

Symptoms of Atrial Fibrillation

Atrial fibrillation is associated with a diverse group of symptoms, palpitation being the most common (15,121,132). In one study that compared symptoms in patients with and without heart disease, palpitations occurred in 59% of patients with heart disease and in 77% of those with no heart disease (*p* <.002) (15). Other frequent symptoms were presyncope, fatigue, and dyspnea, and less common symptoms were chest pain and syncope. In a small group of patients, atrial fibrillation caused no symptoms. Care should be taken in ascribing a specific symptom to the actual occurrence of atrial fibrillation, because it is well documented that patients may have similar symptoms in the presence of sinus rhythm (132,133). Patients who experience dizziness, presyncope, or syncope may have associated carotid sinus hypersensitivity or neurally mediated syncope (134,135).

Why atrial fibrillation occurs at a particular point in time is unclear. In some patients, the onset may be related to a relative increase in parasympathetic tone, as demonstrated by an increased prevalence at night (136). Because patients with atrial fibrillation can have asymptomatic recurrences (137), it is possible that atrial fibrillation occurs even more frequently at night. In certain individuals, the reason for onset of atrial fibrillation is more obvious, for example, an alcoholic binge. For the majority of patients, no specific time of day, level of activity, or obvious inciting factor underlies each occurrence of atrial fibrillation, and initiation is likely multifactorial.

Echocardiography

An echocardiogram is an important test to obtain in patients with atrial fibrillation. It allows evaluation of atrial size, right and left ventricular function, and the presence of valvular lesions. Echocardiography, especially transesophageal echocardiography, has been valuable in investigating atrial function in patients with atrial fibrillation (45,51,52). Transesophageal echocardiography, but not transthoracic echocardiography, can provide valuable information on the presence of atrial thrombi, typically in the left atrial appendage (Fig. 64.7) (141–144). Atrial thrombi have been detected in as many as 15% of patients before cardioversion. Importantly, new thrombi can occur after successful cardioversion and may cause embolic events (142). Thus, at least two mechanisms are possible for thromboembolism after cardioversion: dislodgment of a preexisting thrombus and formation of a new thrombus after cardioversion.

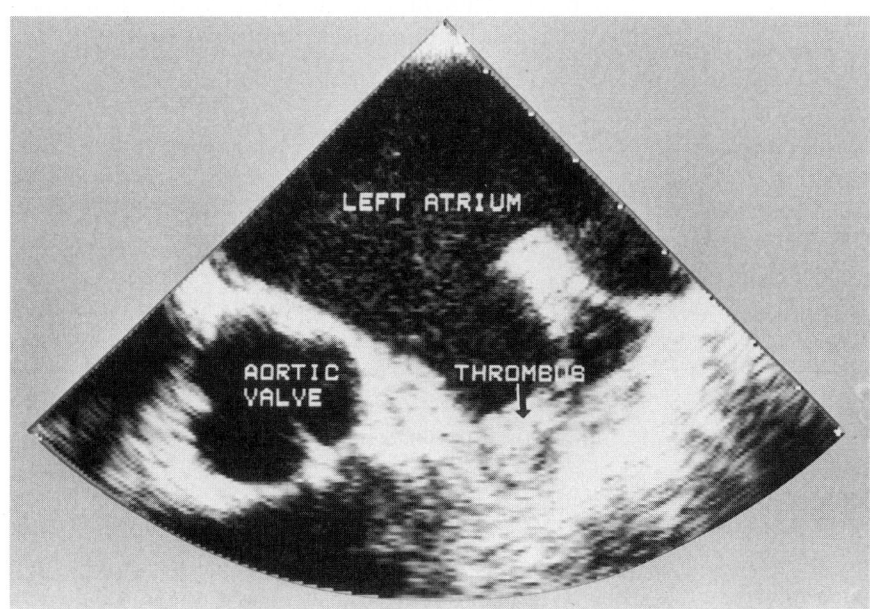

FIGURE 64.7 Transesophageal echocardiogram demonstrating left atrial appendage thrombus (*arrow*). (Courtesy of Drs. J. Bates and J. Steinmetz, the Care Group, St. Vincent Hospital, Indianapolis, IN.)

Wolff-Parkinson-White Syndrome

Atrial fibrillation in patients who have preexcitation can result in ventricular fibrillation and sudden cardiac death. This sequence of events occurs most commonly when a rapid preexcited ventricular response is present (Fig. 64.5), and degeneration to ventricular fibrillation may follow (Fig. 64.6). In our opinion, patients with ventricular preexcitation who have symptoms suggestive of tachycardia or documented arrhythmias should undergo electrophysiologic evaluation and, if indicated, endocardial catheter ablation of the accessory pathway (see Chapter 73). A more difficult situation exists for asymptomatic patients who have ventricular preexcitation during sinus rhythm (147). Some of these patients may be at risk for sudden cardiac death, although this is rarely the initial presentation of WPW. Because patients resuscitated from ventricular fibrillation invariably have a preexcited RR interval seen on electrophysiologic study during induced atrial fibrillation that is, at its shortest, less than 250 ms, the possibility for screening asymptomatic patients to detect those at risk for ventricular fibrillation exists (147). In general, we do not favor mass screening of asymptomatic patients who have ventricular preexcitation (147). Instead, we tend to screen patients who have a familial history of sudden death or tachycardia, patients who are considering competitive athletics, or individuals who are in certain occupations (e.g., airline pilots). See Chapter 66 for a more detailed discussion of this problem.

Hypertrophic Cardiomyopathy

Approximately 15% of patients with hypertrophic cardiomyopathy develop atrial fibrillation (148). In these individuals, atrial fibrillation can result in profound hemodynamic deterioration, leading to chest pain, presyncope, syncope, and even sudden cardiac death (148–150). In one retrospective study, the acute onset of atrial fibrillation resulted in deterioration by at least one New York Heart Association functional class in the majority of patients (148). Importantly, the mean values for maximal left ventricular wall thickness may be lower among patients with atrial fibrillation compared with those of patients with sinus rhythm (151). Thus, prediction of which patients are most likely to develop atrial fibrillation using analysis of ventricular wall thickness may not be possible. The weight of clinical data strongly suggests that efforts should be directed at maintaining sinus rhythm in these individuals, to avoid functional deterioration and the possibility of sudden cardiac death.

THERAPY OF ATRIAL FIBRILLATION: GENERAL PRINCIPLES

There are three potential therapeutic goals of treatment for patients with atrial fibrillation (Fig. 64.8) (152). These include restoration and maintenance of sinus rhythm, rate control during atrial fibrillation, and prevention of thromboembolism. The decision to try to maintain sinus rhythm rather than use

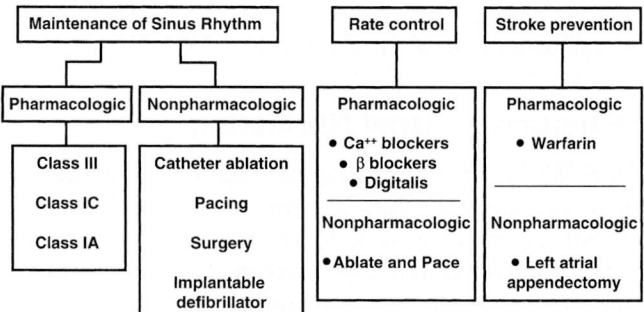

FIGURE 64.8 Therapeutic options in the treatment of patients with atrial fibrillation. See text for details. (From Prystowsky EN. Management of atrial fibrillation: therapeutic options and clinical decisions. *Am J Cardiol* 2000;85:3D–11D, with permission.)

ventricular rate control should be individual to each patient, based on analysis of the risk-benefit ratio for that individual. No large prospective, randomized clinical trials have demonstrated that either approach has a survival advantage. Advantages of sinus rhythm include amelioration of symptoms, possible retardation or prevention of the transition from intermittent to permanent atrial fibrillation, and a theoretical, though not proven, benefit in reduction of the risk for thromboembolic stroke. The primary risk is proarrhythmia, which can cause sudden death (153). The option of allowing atrial fibrillation to persist but controlling the ventricular response has the advantage of not exposing patients to the potential proarrhythmic effects of antiarrhythmic drugs. Two major disadvantages are continuation of symptoms in many patients, although symptoms may be lessened, and the absolute need for continued anticoagulation in patients at risk for thromboembolism. The longer a patient remains in atrial fibrillation, the greater are the chances that progressive electrophysiologic and anatomic atrial changes will occur, which over the course of time make it more difficult to maintain or even to restore sinus rhythm. Thus, the clinician should decide within a short period of time which approach is best for the patient.

PHARMACOLOGIC THERAPY

Use of Intravenous Agents to Restore Sinus Rhythm

Use of intravenous verapamil, digitalis, esmolol, or propranolol is not useful to terminate atrial fibrillation (9,154–156). An exception might be the use of beta-adrenergic blockers in patients after cardiac surgery. In general, drugs that alter atrial electrophysiologic properties are useful to terminate atrial fibrillation (Table 64.4) (9).

Procainamide

In one study, 9 of 21 patients converted to sinus rhythm while receiving procainamide at a mean dose of 13.3 ± 3.6 mg per kg (157). Notably, the left atrial diameter seen on

TABLE 64.4 ACUTE DRUG THERAPY (INTRAVENOUS) FOR ATRIAL FIBRILLATION

Drug	Dosage
To decrease ventricular response[a]	
Verapamil	5–10 mg i.v. over the course of 2 min; additional 3–10 mg i.v. every 4–6 h for rate control
Diltiazem	0.25 mg/kg i.v. over the course of 2 min; if response is inadequate, a second dose of 0.35 mg/kg over the course of 2 min may be given 15 min later; bolus may be followed with constant infusion of ≤10 mg/h for rate control.
Propranolol	1 mg/min i.v. to total dose of 0.15 mg/kg or 12 mg total; additional 1 mg doses as needed for control of heart rate
Esmolol	Initial load of 500 µg/kg/min i.v. for 1 min followed by 50 µg/kg/min for 4 min; if response inadequate, then repeat in 5 min with 500 µg/kg/min for 1 min and 100 µg/kg/min for 4 min; continue to titrate every 5 min until desired heart rate is reached; 50–200 µg/kg/min is usual maintenance dose
Digoxin	0.5–1.0 mg i.v., followed by 0.25 mg every 2–4 h, with total 24-h dose <1.5 mg
For pharmacologic conversion to sinus rhythm	
Procainamide	50 mg/min i.v. to total dose of 10–14 mg/kg
Ibutilide	1 mg i.v. over the course of 10 min; may repeat if atrial fibrillation is present after 20 min

[a]Avoid use of this agent in patients with ventricular preexcitation.

echocardiography was less than 4.0 cm in all patients who converted to sinus rhythm, whereas it was greater than 4.0 cm in all but one of the patients who did not convert. Further, the range of duration of atrial fibrillation among patients who converted was 2 hours to 1 day. In another investigation, patients who converted to sinus rhythm had a shorter mean duration of atrial fibrillation than did patients who did not convert (6 ± 7 days vs. 79 ± 88 days; p <.01) (158). Among patients with atrial fibrillation of less than 24 hours' duration, 92% were converted to sinus rhythm when intravenous flecainide was administered, compared with 65% who converted when intravenous procainamide was administered (159). Procainamide also appears to be useful in converting atrial fibrillation after cardiac surgery (160).

Ibutilide

Ibutilide prolongs refractoriness by enhancing an inward sodium current during the plateau, although it also may block outward potassium current (161). It may increase the QT interval, and torsades de pointes can occur with its use. It is effective for converting atrial fibrillation to sinus rhythm (162–164). The typical recommended dose is 1.0 mg administered over 10 minutes, which can be repeated if atrial fibrillation does not terminate during or within 10 minutes after the end of the initial infusion (163). The dosage can be adjusted downward for patients who weigh less than 60 kg. The conversion rate for atrial fibrillation in one study was

31%, and the success rate was higher among patients with shorter duration of atrial fibrillation (10 ± 13 days vs. 18 ± 15 days) (163). Further, conversion to sinus rhythm occurred in 67% of patients who had a left atrium of normal size compared with only 27% of patients who had an enlarged left atrium. Torsades de pointes may be associated with ibutilide infusion, but in almost all instances, it occurs either during infusion or within a few hours after termination of the final ibutilide infusion. Thus, administration of ibutilide, as well as procainamide, should be performed under circumstances in which resuscitative measures can be readily performed.

Amiodarone

Unlike oral amiodarone, minimal prolongation of the effective refractory period of the right atrium and right ventricle occurs shortly after administration of intravenous amiodarone (5 mg/kg) (165). In some studies, the effectiveness of intravenous amiodarone was similar to that of placebo in restoring sinus rhythm (166,167), whereas other studies suggest that amiodarone has a more beneficial effect (168). Oral quinidine is as effective or more effective in converting atrial fibrillation to sinus rhythm (169,170), but we rarely use it for this purpose because of the significant associated side effects. Intravenous amiodarone has the added effect of significantly slowing ventricular response. This can prove very useful when other agents, such as beta-adrenergic blockers and slow calcium channel blockers, are relatively contraindicated.

Flecainide, Propafenone, Sotalol, and Dofetilide

Intravenous flecainide, propafenone, and sotalol are not available for use in the United States. Intravenous flecainide is very effective in converting atrial fibrillation to sinus rhythm (159,167,171–173). Intravenous propafenone is useful in converting recent-onset atrial fibrillation to sinus rhythm, but it is ineffective in patients in whom atrial fibrillation has lasted many months (174,175). Intravenous sotalol is minimally effective in converting atrial fibrillation to sinus rhythm (176). Intravenous dofetilide, which prolongs refractoriness, appears to be useful in terminating atrial fibrillation (177–179).

Use of Oral Antiarrhythmic Agents for Restoration and Maintenance of Sinus Rhythm

A variety of antiarrhythmic drugs with disparate electrophysiologic actions can terminate or prevent atrial fibrillation. These include disopyramide, quinidine, procainamide, propafenone, flecainide, sotalol, dofetilide, amiodarone, and morizicine (180–204). A single oral loading dose of 300 to 600 mg of propafenone or 200 to 300 mg of flecainide is successful in restoring sinus rhythm in more than 50% of selected patients with recent-onset atrial fibrillation

(181,182). Few comparative studies exist that assess the efficacy of various agents in maintaining sinus rhythm during long-term follow-up. Overall, approximately 50% of patients maintain sinus rhythm for at least 6 months during antiarrhythmic therapy. Flecainide and propafenone appear to have equal efficacy (187). Quinidine is more useful than sotalol for conversion of atrial fibrillation to sinus rhythm (192), but the two drugs are equally effective in maintaining sinus rhythm (191). In one study, propafenone prevented atrial fibrillation more often than sotalol (193), but there was no difference between them in another investigation (190). Amiodarone is considered by some to be the most effective agent for drug-refractory recurrent atrial fibrillation, although few prospective comparative data are available (205). In small groups of patients, amiodarone prevented atrial fibrillation more often than quinidine or disopyramide (198,199). Amiodarone maintains sinus rhythm in nearly two-thirds of patients for up to 1 year follow-up (194–197). Typically, amiodarone has been associated with frequent side effects, some life-threatening (e.g., pulmonary toxicity). However, lower doses likely will decrease the risk of nuisance and serious side effects. In one study, in which amiodarone was administered at 600 mg daily for 4 weeks, approximately 16% of patients converted to sinus rhythm (197). During long-term therapy, the mean dose was 204 mg, and sinus rhythm was maintained in 53% of patients after 3 years with minimal serious side effects (197). The efficacy of antiarrhythmic drug therapy in maintaining sinus rhythm can be enhanced using a serial drug approach (206,207). Several large prospective trials have demonstrated the efficacy of dofetilide in maintaining sinus rhythm (202–204). Although procainamide is useful in preventing atrial fibrillation, in our opinion, its substantial side-effect profile precludes long-term use.

The efficacy of antiarrhythmic drug therapy should not be judged solely on the basis of whether atrial fibrillation recurs during follow-up (152). Preventing all episodes of atrial fibrillation over the course of years of treatment is exceedingly difficult. Therapeutic success should be based on the reduction in frequency and duration of symptomatic episodes of atrial fibrillation. For example, in a patient who has several episodes of atrial fibrillation weekly before treatment, recurrence of one or two short-lived episodes per year during drug therapy is an outstanding success. Recurrence of atrial fibrillation should not be equated with arrhythmias such as sustained ventricular tachycardia or ventricular fibrillation. An analogy can be made with treatment for angina or congestive heart failure. In both conditions, the need for occasional nitroglycerin use or an increase in diuretics, respectively, in patients who otherwise are well compensated is readily accepted.

Proarrhythmia

Proarrhythmia is the most serious side effect of antiarrhythmic drug therapy (9,153). Proarrhythmic events can be caused by tachyarrhythmias or bradyarrhythmias. Proarrhythmia caused by tachyarrhythmia is the most dangerous and life threatening, and torsades de pointes is the most frequently observed proarrhythmic event in this category (Fig. 64.9) (153). Torsades de pointes can occur during use of any drug that prolongs QT interval; amiodarone appears to have the lowest incidence among such agents. It has been postulated that early after-depolarizations initiate torsades de pointes (153). Conditions that favor early after-depolarizations are ventricular hypertrophy, slow heart rate, hypokalemia, and the presence of potassium channel blocking drugs (153), which commonly occur in patients with atrial fibrillation. Torsades de pointes is uncommon during atrial fibrillation in patients who have a relatively rapid ventricular response. It is more likely to emerge after restoration of sinus rhythm, with a resultant slower heart rate (153), which has been referred to as the "paradoxical risk of sinus rhythm for sudden cardiac death" (144). Other types of malignant ventricular arrhythmias can occur. Use of flecainide should be avoided in patients who have experienced myocardial infarction (208), and an enhanced mortality was reported among patients with atrial fibrillation and heart failure who were treated with drugs such as quinidine and procainamide (209). However, amiodarone and dofetilide do not appear to increase mortality in patients with congestive heart failure (202,210,211).

Bradyarrhythmias, including sinus nodal dysfunction and AV conduction disturbances, may also complicate antiarrhythmic drug therapy. One type of proarrhythmia, 1:1 AV conduction with conversion of atrial fibrillation to atrial flutter or tachycardia, is clearly preventable. This more frequently occurs with drugs such as propafenone and flecainide, which can markedly slow atrial tachycardia rates (9). It is important to prescribe concomitant AV nodal

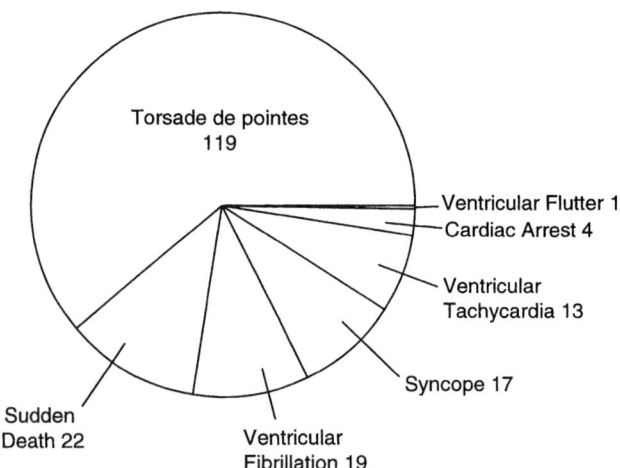

FIGURE 64.9 Types of proarrhythmic events (n = 195) occurring during drug therapy for supraventricular tachycardia. [Modified from Prystowsky EN. Proarrhythmia during drug treatment of supraventricular tachycardia: paradoxical risk of sinus rhythm for sudden death. *Am J Cardiol* 1996;78(8A):35–41.]

blocking agents to avoid this complication, especially for patients who are receiving propafenone or flecainide (152). Administration of concomitant AV nodal blocking agents is not necessary when sotalol or amiodarone is used, because both agents substantially decrease conduction through the AV node.

Antiarrhythmic Drug Selection

Reversible causes of atrial fibrillation (e.g., excess alcohol intake) should be considered and treated if possible. Correction of electrolyte abnormalities and cardiovascular problems such as heart failure need to be addressed before an antiarrhythmic agent is administered. Prophylactic drug therapy typically is not necessary for patients who have experienced a single detected episode of atrial fibrillation, or for patients who have infrequent, transient, and well-tolerated paroxysmal atrial fibrillation.

Every effort should be made to minimize the chance for proarrhythmia and other drug side effects. Antiarrhythmic drug therapy should be initiated in the hospital for patients who have heart disease, especially for patients with a history of congestive heart failure (9,152). Outpatient initiation of therapy appears to be reasonable for individuals who have normal QT intervals and no or minimal heart disease (9,131,152). Because no antiarrhythmic drug has been shown conclusively to be superior to other agents, selection of initial drug therapy is based more on avoidance of serious side effects than on predicted efficacy. Figure 64.10 shows our current scheme for choosing initial and subsequent antiarrhythmic agents to prevent atrial fibrillation. For patients who have lone atrial fibrillation, we prefer to use drugs that have minimal organ toxicity; initial choices are flecainide, propafenone, and sotalol. For patients who have congestive heart failure, amiodarone and dofetilide are our treatments of choice (202,210,211). Sotalol is our initial selection for patients who have coronary artery disease, because we prefer to use beta-adrenergic blockers for such individuals. Sotalol has both beta-adrenergic blocker and class III antiarrhythmic activity, and safety data are available for its use in such patients (212). Amiodarone and dofetilide also have safety data in patients after myocardial infarction (213–215). Patients with hypertension and left ventricular hypertrophy may be at increased risk for torsades de pointes, because hypertrophied ventricles appear more prone to develop early after-depolarizations (153). Thus, we prefer to start with flecainide or propafenone. If a patient has substantial left ventricular hypertrophy, use of flecainide and propafenone carries concerns about an increased proarrhythmic risk, and we prefer to use amiodarone.

Use of Drug Therapy to Control Ventricular Rate

In the absence of ventricular preexcitation, drugs that decrease conduction in the AV node are useful in control-

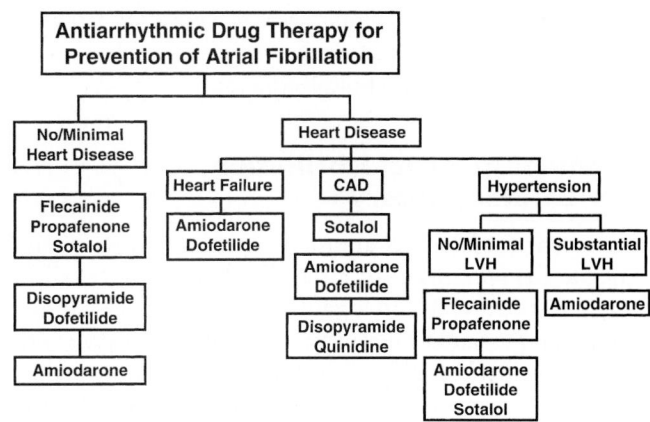

FIGURE 64.10 General scheme for selecting antiarrhythmic drug therapy for the prevention of atrial fibrillation. See text for details. CAD, coronary artery disease; LVH, left ventricular hypertrophy.

ling ventricular rate in patients who have atrial fibrillation (Table 64.4). It is very important to control ventricular rate, not only to decrease symptoms, but to prevent tachycardia-mediated cardiomyopathy (see the section Tachycardia-Induced Ventricular Cardiomyopathy). Drugs that depress conduction and prolong refractoriness in the AV node include digoxin, beta-adrenergic antagonists, and calcium channel blockers (9,155,156,216–223). Notably, the electrophysiologic effects of digoxin on the AV node are indirect and depend on an intact autonomic nervous system (224). Thus, whereas digoxin may slow ventricular response at rest, it is relatively ineffective in controlling the ventricular rate during exercise (220). Beta-adrenergic blockers and calcium channel blockers are preferred over digoxin for rate control in patients who have not experienced heart failure (9). Beta-adrenergic blockers are also recommended in situations in which sympathetic tone is increased, such as thyrotoxicosis (9). In patients who have congestive heart failure, digitalis is the first-line treatment (9). As noted previously, both sotalol and amiodarone may be used as monotherapy because they depress conduction through the AV node. In some patients, control of ventricular response can be facilitated with the use of combination drug therapy, for example, digoxin and a calcium channel blocker or a beta-adrenergic blocker. In this situation, rate control may be achieved without undue side effects. Preliminary data on the use of clonidine suggest that such agents may have a role in controlling ventricular response in patients who have atrial fibrillation (225).

In patients who have WPW, control of the rapid preexcited ventricular response requires the use of agents that depress conduction over the accessory pathway. In the acute setting, intravenous procainamide or ibutilide are the treatments of choice, unless the patient is unstable and requires urgent electrical cardioversion. The use of drugs such as digoxin, calcium channel blockers, beta-adrenergic blockers, and adenosine are contraindicated in this situation.

They do not block conduction over the accessory pathway and may accelerate the ventricular response, resulting in a potentially very unstable clinical situation.

Treatment of Atrial Fibrillation after Cardiac Surgery

Beta-adrenergic blockers are the best treatment currently available for prevention of atrial fibrillation after cardiac surgery (90,226–229). In a randomized, controlled study, sotalol demonstrated superiority to placebo in prevention of atrial fibrillation (230). Administration of intravenous amiodarone, 1 g per day for 2 days starting immediately after cardiac surgery, reduced the incidence of postoperative atrial fibrillation compared with placebo (231). Administration of oral amiodarone, starting at least 1 week before surgery, may also decrease postoperative atrial fibrillation (232).

The optimum approach to treating atrial fibrillation in the postoperative period is unclear. In most patients who experienced no preoperative atrial fibrillation, atrial fibrillation is a transient arrhythmia and typically is not a long-term problem (233). If simple measures such as administration of beta-adrenergic blockers do not prevent atrial fibrillation, additional therapy can be pursued to restore and maintain sinus rhythm or merely to control the ventricular response. In the latter situation, anticoagulation therapy should be started as soon as it is considered safe. The patient should be reevaluated 4 to 6 weeks after surgery.

PREVENTION OF THROMBOEMBOLISM

Prevention of stroke is key to the management of the condition of patients with atrial fibrillation (Fig. 64.8). A hypercoagulable state appears to exist in patients with atrial fibrillation (234,235). A high stroke risk has been well described for years in patients with atrial fibrillation and mitral stenosis or prosthetic mitral valves. Recently, several prospective multicenter, randomized clinical trials have conclusively demonstrated that warfarin is highly effective in reducing the incidence of ischemic stroke among patients with atrial fibrillation (eFig. 64.10.1) (9). Overall, a combined risk reduction of 68% is seen.

Independent predictors of thromboembolic risk have been identified (9,131). High-risk patients have a 5% to 7% or greater yearly risk of thromboembolism. High-risk variables from prospective trials include a history of hypertension, prior stroke or transient ischemic attack, diabetes, recent heart failure, and age greater than 65 years (9). Notably, paroxysmal atrial fibrillation has not been found to be an independent predictor of thromboembolic risk. Other studies have considered coronary artery disease to place a patient at high risk for stroke (131). At present, high-risk

patients who can receive anticoagulation therapy should be treated with warfarin, with the INR adjusted to between 2.0 and 3.0. Patients greater than 75 years old should be observed carefully, because bleeding complications increase in elderly patients. Patients with atrial fibrillation who have low risk for stroke may be treated with 325 mg of aspirin daily (9). Patients with lone atrial fibrillation who are less than 60 years old do not require specific therapy for prevention of thromboembolism. Some physicians prescribe aspirin to this group of patients, but few data are available to support this approach. Recent guidelines offer more detailed information (131).

Anticoagulation for Cardioversion

Electrical and pharmacologic cardioversion can result in thromboembolism (9). Prior anticoagulation appears to decrease the risk of emboli (9,45,236–239). In patients who have atrial fibrillation of unknown duration or duration greater than 48 hours, current recommendations are to administer warfarin for 3 weeks before and 4 weeks after cardioversion, maintaining an INR of 2.0 to 3.0 (9). In high-risk patients, warfarin therapy should be continued on a long-term basis after cardioversion. In an alternative approach, transesophageal echocardiography is used (9,131,141,144) (eFig. 64.10.2). The use of transesophageal echocardiography appears to offer an advantage to patients who are already hospitalized or in whom restoration of sinus rhythm is more urgent. However, the widespread use of this method for outpatient cardioversion cannot be supported at this time (45).

NONPHARMACOLOGIC THERAPY

Pharmacologic treatment has been used for decades for cardioversion and prevention of recurrent atrial fibrillation. Use of antiarrhythmic drugs is associated with substantial side effects and mortality in some groups of patients. Accordingly, it is not surprising that nonpharmacologic techniques for managing atrial fibrillation have been developed, including external and internal electrical cardioversion, atrial pacing methods to prevent atrial fibrillation, surgery, radiofrequency catheter ablation procedures, and use of implantable atrial defibrillators.

Electrical Cardioversion

Transthoracic Electrical Cardioversion

The technique of transthoracic direct current (DC) electrical cardioversion of atrial fibrillation was developed by Lown and associates (240). Lown (241) reported that "sinus rhythm was reinstated in 94% of the 456 episodes of atrial fibrillation." Although any patient who has atrial fibrillation may be a candidate for transthoracic DC cardioversion, certain characteristics predict immediate success and long-term maintenance of sinus rhythm. The best candidates are patients without mitral valve disease or a very large left atrium and patients who have atrial fibrillation of relatively short duration. Early echocardiographic studies suggested that there was minimal possibility of achieving or maintaining sinus rhythm when the anterior-posterior diameter of the left atrium was greater than 4.5 cm (242). In contrast, a recent randomized study showed that the size of the left atrium was not related to the success of cardioversion or to recurrence of atrial fibrillation (243). At present, no universally accepted threshold value for left atrial size or severity of mitral stenosis that would preclude attempts at cardioversion exists. It is our policy to attempt cardioversion at least once in most patients with atrial fibrillation in whom we think sinus rhythm would be preferable. Exceptions might be individuals known to have had atrial fibrillation for many years.

In patients undergoing transthoracic DC cardioversion, antiarrhythmic drugs are frequently used to maintain sinus rhythm (207). Drug therapy should be considered before use of cardioversion in patients with long-standing atrial fibrillation (e.g., more than 3 months), to lessen the chance of relapse into atrial fibrillation in the first few days after cardioversion. Digitalis therapy is not a contraindication to elective cardioversion, although it is customary to withhold digoxin on the day of cardioversion, a custom that is based on few scientific data. On the other hand, attempts to cardiovert arrhythmias associated with digitalis toxicity are hazardous and should be avoided (244). Concomitant antiarrhythmic drug therapy may increase energy requirements for successful cardioversion. In a nonrandomized series of 57 patients, flecainide was associated with a higher energy requirement than class Ia or III drugs, although overall success was similar in all groups (245).

Success of transthoracic DC cardioversion to restore sinus rhythm depends on several technical factors (246). The optimal electrode size is 12 to 13 cm in diameter. Initial electrode placement is right anterior–left posterior or left anterior–left posterior. If cardioversion with these electrode orientations is unsuccessful, a right anterior–apical electrode position can be tried. The clinician must be flexible and willing to try several electrode orientations. Application of firm pressure to the anterior electrode during full expiration may facilitate delivery of current to the heart. For most patients, we use an energy delivery of 360 J synchronized to the QRS complex for the first shock (246,247). Appropriate anesthesia is mandatory before shock delivery. If reversion to sinus rhythm is not achieved after multiple shocks have been given using various electrode positions, adjunctive measures can be used, such as higher energy levels (248), pretreatment with ibutilide (249), and internal cardioversion (250). More experience with transthoracic cardioversion using biphasic shocks will likely improve success of treatment at lower energies (251).

Catheter Ablation

Atrioventricular Block

For some patients who have permanent atrial fibrillation, drug therapy used to control ventricular response is either ineffective or not tolerated. An alternative approach is endocardial catheter ablation of the AV junction that results in complete heart block (265,266). Such patients require a permanent rate-responsive pacemaker. This technique can also be used for treatment of patients who have transient or persistent atrial fibrillation, in lieu of drugs that suppress AV node conduction. Improvement in exercise tolerance and quality of life has been demonstrated with this procedure (267). Radiofrequency catheter ablation is currently the method of choice for accomplishing these goals (see Chapter 73 for further details).

Surgery

The maze surgical procedure for treatment of atrial fibrillation was developed by Cox and associates (37). Multiple atrial incisions are made to direct sinus impulses through a path, or a "maze," to reach the AV node. The idea is to prevent formation of a critical mass of contiguous atrial tissue that would sustain atrial fibrillation. Further, at least some atrial contractility is maintained. The results of the maze operation have been promising. Alternative operations are the left atrial isolation technique, the "corridor" operation, and simple encircling of the pulmonary veins (275–277). However, surgery for atrial fibrillation as a primary indication has not gained much momentum and is infrequently used for this problem. We have found it useful for patients with atrial fibrillation who are undergoing other cardiac surgery. Because the left atrial appendage is the usual site of thrombus, we recommend removal of this structure in patients undergoing other cardiac surgery, especially if the patient has a history of atrial fibrillation.

CONTROVERSIES AND PERSONAL PERSPECTIVES

Sinus Rhythm versus Rate Control

A controversy currently exists regarding the relative merits of administering antiarrhythmic drugs to maintain sinus rhythm versus allowing atrial fibrillation to persist and using drugs to control ventricular rate. No large, randomized, prospective trials have demonstrated the superiority of either approach. Clearly, some patients do well with rate control only. For other patients, sinus rhythm must be

THE FUTURE

New and innovative approaches for the treatment of patients with atrial fibrillation are likely to emerge (278). Technological advances in catheter design and energy sources should facilitate a catheter-based approach to curing atrial fibrillation. This may be intracardiac or extracardiac (e.g., use of a thoracoscope). Antiarrhythmic drug development likely will target specific ionic channels in the atrium that do not involve the ventricles, improving efficacy and decreasing ventricular proarrhythmia. Novel cardiac pacing techniques may provide a nonpharmacologic alternative to prevention of atrial fibrillation. An implantable arrhythmia suppression device may be developed that will use subthreshold atrial stimulation to prevent emergence of atrial fibrillation (*e*Fig. 64.10.6) (279). An alternative new device, Tranquillity, will contain an implantable cardioverter-defibrillator/pacemaker/drug-delivery system (*e*Fig. 64.10.7) (280). This unit will have the capability of atrial and ventricular defibrillation and dual chamber pacing, and it can deliver one or more drugs through the atrial lead. It should manage any potential arrhythmic problem.

achieved to ameliorate symptoms. Sinus rhythm perpetuates sinus rhythm, which is the antithesis of atrial fibrillation begetting atrial fibrillation. Thus, if sinus rhythm can be maintained most of the time, it may be possible to prevent the anatomic and electrophysiologic abnormalities that result from atrial fibrillation. In our experience, if aggressive attempts are made to preserve sinus rhythm shortly after atrial fibrillation occurs, it is possible to prevent or markedly reduce atrial fibrillation recurrences in more than 60% of patients. With regard to the safety of antiarrhythmic drugs, we do not live in a risk-free environment, and it is impossible to guarantee a complete absence of proarrhythmic risk. However, with appropriate selection of antiarrhythmic agents, initiation of drug therapy in-hospital for patients at substantial risk for proarrhythmia, and careful follow-up, morbidity and mortality from proarrhythmia is 1% or less in our experience. For many patients, the risk is worth the gain.

Inpatient versus Outpatient Initiation of Therapy

Initiation of antiarrhythmic drugs to restore or maintain sinus rhythm can be performed on an inpatient or an outpatient basis. The risk of proarrhythmia is low, even among patients who have significant heart disease, and starting treatment in the hospital likely will not be cost-effective. Regardless, we feel that patients who have significant heart disease should be monitored during initiation of antiarrhythmic drug treatment, to identify any potential serious problems, especially proarrhythmia. However, patients who have paroxysmal atrial fibrillation with no or minimal heart disease may start antiarrhythmic drugs as outpatients. Before therapy is begun, normal electrolyte status should be confirmed. When an agent that prolongs the QT interval, such as sotalol, is prescribed, we begin with the lowest dose and obtain an electrocardiogram after 2 to 3 days before increasing the dose. This process is repeated until the desired dose is obtained. Event recorders might be used for this purpose. We have not had any significant problems with proarrhythmia using this approach. It is very important to advise patients about over-the-counter and prescription drugs that may interact with the antiarrhythmic agent. For example, antihistamines that may increase the QT interval should not be given to patients taking drugs that prolong the QT interval. We generally ask patients to call us before starting any new drug. When flecainide or propafenone is prescribed, beta-blockers or calcium channel blockers should be given initially to prevent atrial flutter with a 1:1 ventricular response.

ACKNOWLEDGMENTS

The authors thank Mrs. Mary Kay Franklin, for her superb secretarial assistance in the preparation of this chapter, and Mrs. Jane Gilmore, for her superb artwork.

REFERENCES

1. Rosner F, trans. and ed. *Maimonides' medical writings.* Haifa, Israel: The Maimonides Research Institute, 1989.
2. Stokes W. *The diseases of the heart and the aorta.* Dublin: Hodges and Smith, 1854.
3. Wenckebach KF. *Arrhythmia of the heart: a physiological and clinical study.* Edinburgh: William Green and Sons, 1904.
4. Cushny AR. On the interpretation of pulse-tracings. *J Exp Med* 1899;4:327–347.
5. Mackenzie J. The interpretation of the pulsations in the jugular veins. *Am J Med Sci* 1907;134:12–34.
6. Rothberger CJ, Winterberg H. Vorhofflimmern und Arrhythmia perpetua. *Wien Klin Wochenschr* 1909;22:839–844.
7. Lewis T. Auricular fibrillation and its relationship to clinical irregularity of the heart. *Heart* 1910;1:306–372.

8. Einthoven W. Le telecardiogramme. *Arch Internat Physiol* 1908;4:132–164.

9. Prystowsky EN, Benson DW, Fuster V, et al. Management of patients with atrial fibrillation: a statement for healthcare professionals from the subcommittee on electrocardiography and electrophysiology, American Heart Association. *Circulation* 1996;93:1262–1277.

10. Bialy D, Lehmann MH, Schumacher DN, et al. Hospitalization for arrhythmias in the United States: importance of atrial fibrillation. *J Am Coll Cardiol* 1992;19:41A.

11. Parkinson J, Campbell M. Paroxysmal auricular fibrillation: a record of two hundred patients. *QJM* 1930;67–100.

12. Kannel WB, Abbott RD, Savage DD, et al. Epidemiologic features of chronic atrial fibrillation: the Framingham study. *N Engl J Med* 1982;306:1018–1022.

13. Davidson E, Weinberger I, Rotenberg Z, et al. Atrial fibrillation: cause and time of onset. *Arch Intern Med* 1989;149:457–459.

14. Lok NS, Lau CP. Presentation and management of patients admitted with atrial fibrillation: a review of 291 cases in a regional hospital. *Int J Cardiol* 1995;48:271–278.

15. Prystowsky EN, Margiotti R, Fogel RI, et al. Atrial fibrillation with and without heart disease: clinical characteristics and proarrhythmia risk. *Circulation* 1996;94(8):I-191.

16. Godtfredsen J. Atrial fibrillation: cause and prognosis—a follow-up study of 1212 cases. In: Kulbertus HE, Olsson SB, Schlepper M, eds. *Atrial fibrillation*. Sweden: AB Hassle, 1982.

17. Wolf PA, Abbott RD, Kannel WB. Atrial fibrillation as an independent risk factor for stroke: the Framingham Study. *Stroke* 1991;22:983–988.

18. Wolf PA, Abbott RD, Kannel WB. Atrial fibrillation: a major contributor to stroke in the elderly. The Framingham Study. *Arch Intern Med* 1987;147:1561–1564.

19. Bharati S, Lev M. Histology of the normal and diseased atrium. In: Falk RH, Podrid PJ, eds. *Atrial fibrillation: mechanisms and management*. New York: Raven Press, 1992.

20. Yater WM. Pathologic changes in auricular fibrillation and in allied arrhythmias. *Arch Intern Med* 1929;43:808–838.

21. Hudson REB. The human pacemaker and its pathology. *Br Heart J* 1960;22:153–167.

22. Davies MJ, Pomerance A. Pathology of atrial fibrillation in man. *Br Heart J* 1972;34:520–525.

23. Frustaci A, Chimenti C, Bellocci F, et al. Histological substrate of atrial biopsies in patients with lone atrial fibrillation. *Circulation* 1997;96:1180–1184.

24. Maixent JM, Paganelli F, Scaglione J, et al. Antibodies against myosin in sera of patients with idiopathic paroxysmal atrial fibrillation. *J Cardiovasc Electrophysiol* 1998;9:612–617.

25. Scherf D, Romano FJ, Terranova R. Experimental studies on auricular flutter and auricular fibrillation. *Am Heart J* 1948;36:241.

26. Scherf D, Schaffer AI, Blumenfeld S. Mechanism of flutter and fibrillation. *Arch Intern Med* 1953;91:333–352.

27. Jais P, Haissaguerre M, Shah DC. A focal source of atrial fibrillation treated by discrete radiofrequency ablation. *Circulation* 1997;95:572–576.

28. Haissaguerre M, Jais P, Shah DC, et al. Spontaneous initiation of atrial fibrillation by ectopic beats originating in the pulmonary veins. *N Engl J Med* 1998;339:659–666.

29. Chen SA, Tai CT, Yu WC, et al. Right atrial focal atrial fibrillation: electrophysiologic characteristics and radiofrequency catheter ablation. *J Cardiovasc Electrophysiol* 1999;10:328–335.

30. Nathan H, Eliakim M. The junction between the left atrium and the pulmonary veins: an anatomic study of human hearts. *Circulation* 1966;34:412–422.

31. Cheung DW. Pulmonary vein as an ectopic focus in digitalis-induced arrhythmia. *Nature* 1981;294:582–584.

32. Mines GR. On dynamic equilibrium in the heart. *J Physiol* 1913;46:349–383.

33. Garrey WE. The nature of fibrillary contraction of the heart: its relation to tissue mass and form. *Am J Physiol* 1914;33:397–414.

34. Moe GK, Abildskov JA. Atrial fibrillation as a self-sustaining arrhythmia independent of focal discharge. *Am Heart J* 1959;58:59–70.

35. Moe GK, Rheinboldt WC, Abildskov JA. A computer model of atrial fibrillation. *Am Heart J* 1964;67:200–220.

36. Allessie MA, Lammers WJEP, Bonke FIM, et al. Experimental evaluation of Moe's multiple wavelet hypothesis of atrial fibrillation. In: Zipes DP, Jalife J, eds. *Cardiac arrhythmias*. New York: Grune & Stratton, 1985:265–276.

37. Cox JL, Canavan TE, Schuessler RB, et al. The surgical treatment of atrial fibrillation. II. Intraoperative electrophysiology mapping and description of the electrophysiologic basis of atrial flutter and atrial fibrillation. *J Thorac Cardiovasc Surg* 1991;101:406–426.

38. Konings KTS, Kirchhof CJ, Smeets JRLM, et al. High-density mapping of electrically induced atrial fibrillation in humans. *Circulation* 1994;89:1665–1680.

39. Morillo CA, Klein GJ, Jones DL, et al. Chronic rapid atrial pacing: structural, functional, and electrophysiological characteristics of a new model of sustained atrial fibrillation. *Circulation* 1995;91:1588–1595.

40. Spach MS, Boineau JP. Microfibrosis produces electrical load variations due to loss of side-to-side cell connections: a major mechanism of structural heart disease arrhythmias. *Pacing Clin Electrophysiol* 1997;20[Pt II]:397–413.

41. Spach MS, Dolber PC, Heidlage JF. Influence of the passive anisotropic properties on directional differences in propagation following modification of the sodium conductance in human atrial muscle: a model of reentry based on anisotropic discontinuous propagation. *Circ Res* 1988;62:811–832.

42. Prystowsky EN. Tachycardia-induced tachycardia: a mechanism of initiation of atrial fibrillation. In: DiMarco JP, Prystowsky EN, eds. *Atrial arrhythmias: state of the art*. Armonk, NY: Futura Publishing Co., 1995.

43. Lammers WJEP, Schalij MJ, Kirchhof CJ, et al. Quantification of spatial inhomogeneity in conduction and initiation of reentrant atrial arrhythmias. *Am J Physiol* 1990;259:H1254–H1263.

44. Allessie MA, Rensma PL, Lammers WJEP, et al. Length of excitation wave and susceptibility to reentrant atrial arrhythmias in normal conscious dogs. *Circ Res* 1988;62:395–410.

45. Prystowsky EN. Management of atrial fibrillation: simplicity surrounded by controversy. *Ann Intern Med* 1997;126:244–246.

46. Sanfilippo AJ, Abascal VM, Sheehan M, et al. Atrial

enlargement as a consequence of atrial fibrillation. *Circulation* 1990;82:792–797.

47. Gosselink AT, Grijns HJ, Hamer HPM, et al. Changes in left and right atrial size after cardioversion of atrial fibrillation: role of mitral valve disease. *J Am Coll Cardiol* 1993;22:1666–1672.

48. Wijiffels MC, Kirchhof CJ, Dorland R, et al. Atrial fibrillation begets atrial fibrillation: a study in awake chronically instrumented goats. *Circulation* 1995;92:1954–1968.

49. Daoud EG, Bogun F, Goyal R, et al. Effect of atrial fibrillation on atrial refractoriness in humans. *Circulation* 1996;94:1600–1606.

50. Yue L, Feng J, Gaspo R, et al. Ionic remodeling underlying action potential changes in a canine model of atrial fibrillation. *Circ Res* 1997;81:512–525.

51. Manning WJ, Silverman DI, Katz SE, et al. Impaired left atrial mechanical function after cardioversion: relation to the duration of atrial fibrillation. *J Am Coll Cardiol* 1994;23:1535–1540.

52. Mitusch R, Garbe M, Schmucker G, et al. Relation of left atrial appendage function to the duration and reversibility of nonvalvular atrial fibrillation. *Am J Cardiol* 1995;75:944–947.

53. Prystowsky EN. Atrioventricular node reentry: physiology and radiofrequency ablation. *Pacing Clin Electrophysiol* 1997;20[Pt II]:552–571.

54. Mazgalev T, Dreifus LS, Bianchi J, et al. Atrioventricular nodal conduction during atrial fibrillation in rabbit heart. *Am J Physiol* 1982;243:H754–H760.

55. Moe GK, Abildskov JA. Observations on the ventricular dysrhythmia associated with atrial fibrillation in the dog heart. *Circ Res* 1964;14:447–460.

56. Chorro FJ, Kirchhof CJ, Brugada J, et al. Ventricular response during irregular atrial pacing and atrial fibrillation. *Am J Physiol* 1990;259:H1015–H1021.

57. Langendorf R, Pick AL, Katz LN. Ventricular response in atrial fibrillation: role of concealed conduction in the AV junction. *Circulation* 1965;32:69–75.

58. Prystowsky EN, Page RL. Electrophysiology and autonomic influences of the human atrioventricular node. In: LS Dreifus, T Mazgalev, EL Michaelson, eds. *Electrophysiology of the sino-atrial and atrioventricular nodes.* New York: Alan R. Liss, 1988:259–277.

59. Page RL, Tang ASL, Prystowsky EN. Effect of continuous enhanced vagal tone on atrioventricular nodal and sinoatrial nodal function in humans. *Circ Res* 1991;68:1614–1620.

60. Page RL, Wharton JM, Prystowsky EN. Effect of continuous vagal enhancement on concealed conduction and refractoriness within the atrioventricular node. *Am J Cardiol* 1996;77:260–265.

61. Prystowsky EN, Klein GJ. *Cardiac arrhythmias: an integrated approach for the clinician.* New York: McGraw-Hill, 1994.

62. Gouaux JL, Ashman R. Auricular fibrillation with aberration simulating ventricular paroxysmal tachycardia. *Am Heart J* 1947;34:366–373.

63. Lewis T. *The mechanism and graphic registration of the heart beat,* 3rd ed. London: Shaw and Sons, 1925:256.

64. Moe GK, Mendez C, Han J. Aberrant A-V impulse propagation in the dog heart: a study of functional bundle branch block. *Circ Res* 1965;16:261.

65. Chilson DA, Zipes DP, Heger JJ. Functional bundle branch block: discordant response of right and left bundle branches to changes in heart rate. *Am J Cardiol* 1984;54(3):313–316.

66. Denker S, Shenasa M, Gilbert CJ, et al. Effects of abrupt changes in cycle length on refractoriness of the His-Purkinje system in man. *Circulation* 1983;67:60.

67. Pick A, Langendorf R. *Interpretation of complex arrhythmias.* Philadelphia: Lea and Febiger, 1979.

68. Pritchett ELC, Smith WM, Klein GJ, et al. The "compensatory pause" of atrial fibrillation. *Circulation* 1980;62:1021–1025.

69. Miles WM, Prystowsky EN. Alteration of human right bundle branch refractoriness by changes in atrial drive train duration. *Circulation* 1986;73:244–248.

70. Ong JJC, Cha YM, Kriett JM, et al. The relation between atrial fibrillation wavefront characteristics and accessory pathway conduction. *J Clin Invest* 1995;96:2284–2296.

71. Prystowsky EN, Pritchett ELC, Gallagher JJ. Concealed conduction preventing anterograde preexcitation syndrome. *Am J Cardiol* 1991;53:960–961.

72. Chen PS, Prystowsky EN. Role of concealed and supernormal conduction during atrial fibrillation in the preexcitation syndrome. *Am J Cardiol* 1991;68:1329–1334.

73. Phillips E, Levine SA. Auricular fibrillation without other evidence of heart disease: a cause of reversible heart failure. *Am J Med* 1949;7:478–489.

74. Packer DL, Bardy GH, Worley SJ, et al. Tachycardia-induced cardiomyopathy: a reversible form of left ventricular dysfunction. *Am J Cardiol* 1986;57:563–570.

75. Grogan M, Smith HC, Gersh BJ, et al. Left ventricular dysfunction due to atrial fibrillation in patients initially believed to have idiopathic dilated cardiomyopathy. *Am J Cardiol* 1992;69:1570–1573.

76. Keiny JR, Sacrez A, Facello A, et al. Increase in radionuclide left ventricular ejection fraction after cardioversion of chronic atrial fibrillation in idiopathic dilated cardiomyopathy. *Eur Heart J* 1992;13:1290–1295.

77. Rodriguez LM, Smeets JL, Xie B, et al. Improvement in left ventricular function by ablation of atrioventricular nodal conduction in selected patients with lone atrial fibrillation. *Am J Cardiol* 1993;72:1137–1141.

78. VanGelder IC, Crijns HJ, Blanksma PK, et al. Time course of hemodynamic changes and improvement of exercise tolerance after cardioversion of chronic atrial fibrillation unassociated with cardiac valve disease. *Am J Cardiol* 1993;72:560–566.

79. Brignole M, Gianfranchi L, Menozzi C, et al. Influence of atrioventricular junction radiofrequency ablation in patients with chronic atrial fibrillation and flutter on quality of life and cardiac performance. *Am J Cardiol* 1994;74:242–246.

80. Cobb FR, Blumenschein SD, Sealy WC, et al. Successful surgical interruption of the bundle of Kent in a patient with Wolff-Parkinson-White syndrome. *Circulation* 1968;38:1018.

81. Barbier P, Alioto G, Guazzi MD. Left atrial function and ventricular filling in hypertensive patients with paroxysmal atrial fibrillation. *J Am Coll Cardiol* 1994;24:165–170.

82. Woeber KA. Thyrotoxicosis and the heart. *N Engl J Med* 1992;327:94–98.

83. Sawin CT, Geller A, Wolf PA, et al. Low serum thyrotropin concentrations as a risk factor for atrial fibrillation in older persons. *N Engl J Med* 1994;331:1249–1252.

84. St John Sutton MG, Tajik AJ, McGoon DC. Atrial septal defect in patients ages 60 years or older: operative results and long-term postoperative follow-up. *Circulation* 1981;64:402–409.

85. Smith WM, Gallagher JJ, Ker CR, et al. The electrophysiologic basis and management of symptomatic recurrent tachycardia in patients with Ebstein's anomaly of the tricuspid valve. *Am J Cardiol* 1982;49:1223–1234.

86. Pressley JC, Wharton JM, Tang ASL, et al. Effect of Ebstein's anomaly outcome of surgically treated patients with Wolff-Parkinson-White syndrome. *Circulation* 1992;86:1147–1155.

87. Leitch JW, Thomason D, Baired DK, et al. The importance of age as a predictor of atrial fibrillation and flutter after coronary artery bypass grafting. *J Thorac Cardiovasc Surg* 1990;100:338–342.

88. Wong DH. Preoperative stroke. Part II. Cardiac surgery and cardiogenic embolic stroke. *Can J Anaesth* 1991;38:471–478.

89. Douglas PS, Hirshfeld JW, Edmunds LH. Clinical correlates of atrial tachyarrhythmias after valve replacement for aortic stenosis. *Circulation* 1985;72:II-159.

90. Matangi MF, Neutze JM, Graham KJ, et al. Arrhythmia prophylaxis after aorta-coronary bypass: the effect of mini-dose propranolol. *J Thorac Cardiovasc Surg* 1985;89:439.

91. Kalman JM, Munawar M, Howes LG, et al. Atrial fibrillation after coronary bypass grafting is associated with sympathetic activity. *Ann Thorac Surg* 1995;60:1709–1715.

92. Matthew JP, Parks R, Savino JS, et al. Atrial fibrillation following coronary artery bypass graft surgery: predictors, outcome and resources utilization. Multicenter study of perioperative research group. *JAMA* 1996;276:300–306.

93. Frost L, Christiansen EH, Molgaard H, et al. Frequent preoperative atrial premature complexes predicts atrial fibrillation after CABG surgery. *Circulation* 1996;94[Pt II]:1105.

94. Mendes LA, Connelly GP, McKenney PA, et al. Right coronary artery stenosis: an independent predictor of atrial fibrillation after coronary bypass surgery. *J Am Coll Cardiol* 1995;25:198–202.

95. Wandschneider W, Winter S, Thalmann M, et al. Crystalloid versus blood cardioplegia in coronary bypass surgery: a prospective, randomized, controlled study in 100 consecutive adults. *J Cardiovasc Surg Torino* 1994;35[6 Suppl 1]:85–89.

96. Asher CR, Chung K, Grimm RA, et al. Is the incidence of postoperative atrial fibrillation following cardiac valve surgery reduced by minimally invasive surgery? *Circulation* 1996;94[Pt I]:380.

97. Lewis T, Drury AN, Bulger HA. Observations upon flutter and fibrillation. Part VII. The effects of vagal stimulation. *Heart* 1921;8:141–170.

98. Nahum LH, Hoff HE. Production of auricular fibrillation by application of acetyl-B-methylcholine chloride to localized regions on the auricular surface. *Am J Physiol* 1940;129:428.

99. Scherf D, Chick FB. Abnormal cardiac rhythms caused by acetylcholine. *Circulation* 1951;3:764–769.

100. Burn JH, Williams EMV, Walker JM. The effects of acetylcholine in the heart-lung preparation including the production of auricular fibrillation. *J Physiol* 1995;128:277–293.

101. Loomis TA, Krop S. Auricular fibrillation induced and maintained in animals by acetylcholine or vagal stimulation. *Circ Res* 1955;3:390–396.

102. Alessi R, Nusynowitz M, Abildskov JA, et al. Nonuniform distribution of vagal effects on the atrial refractory period. *Am J Physiol* 1958;194:406–410.

103. Coumel P. Neurogenic and humoral influences of the autonomic nervous system in the determination of paroxysmal atrial fibrillation. In: Atteul P, Coumel P, Janse MJ, eds. *The atrium in health and disease.* Mount Kisco, NY: Futura Publishing Co., 1989:213–232.

104. Hurwitz JL, German LD, Packer DL, et al. Occurrence of atrial fibrillation in patients with paroxysmal supraventricular tachycardia due to atrioventricular nodal entry. *Pacing Clin Electrophysiol* 1990;13:705–710.

105. Campbell RWF, Smith RA, Gallagher JJ, et al. Atrial fibrillation in the preexcitation syndrome. *Am J Cardiol* 1977;40:515–520.

106. Sung RJ, Castellanos A, Mallon SM, et al. Mechanisms of spontaneous alteration between reciprocating tachycardia and atrial flutter-fibrillation in the Wolff-Parkinson-White syndrome. *Circulation* 1977;56:409–416.

107. Klein GJ, Bashore TM, Sellers TD, et al. Ventricular fibrillation in the Wolff-Parkinson-White syndrome. *N Engl J Med* 1979;301:1080–1085.

108. Fananapazir L, Packer DL, German LD, et al. Procainamide infusion test: Inability to identify patients with Wolff-Parkinson-White syndrome who are potentially at risk of sudden death. *Circulation* 1988;77:1291–1296.

109. Ahlinder S, Granath A, Holmer S, Mascher G. Wolff-Parkinson-White Syndrom med paroxysmalt Atrieflimmer overgaende i Ventrikelflimmer. *Nord Med* 1963;70:50.

110. Dreifus LS, Haiat R, Watanabe T, et al. Ventricular fibrillation: a possible mechanism of sudden death in patients with Wolff-Parkinson-White syndrome. *Circulation* 1971;43:520.

111. Prystowsky EN, Knilans TK, Evans JJ. Diagnostic evaluation and treatment strategies for patients at risk for serious cardiac arrhythmias. II. Ventricular tachyarrhythmias and Wolff-Parkinson-White syndrome. *Mod Concepts Cardiovasc Dis* 1991;60:55.

112. Wyndham CRC, Amat-y-Leon F, Wu D, et al. Effects of cycle length on atrial vulnerability. *Circulation* 1977;55:260–267.

113. Chen PS, Pressley JC, Tang ASL, et al. New observations on atrial fibrillation before and after surgical treatment in patients with the Wolff-Parkinson-White syndrome. *J Am Coll Cardiol* 1992;19:974–981.

114. Sharma AD, Klein GJ, Guiraudon GM, et al. Atrial fibrillation in patients with Wolff-Parkinson-White syndrome: incidence after surgical ablation of the accessory pathway. *Circulation* 1985;72:161–169.

115. Lab MJ. Contraction-excitation feedback in myocardium. *Circ Res* 1982;50:757–766.

116. Klein LS, Miles WM, Zipes DP. Effect of atrioventricular interval during pacing or reciprocating tachycardia on atrial size, pressure, and refractory period: contraction-

excitation feedback in human atrium. *Circulation* 1990;82:60–68.

117. Calkins H, El-Atassi R, Leon A, et al. Effect of the atrioventricular relationship on atrial refractoriness in humans. *Pacing Clin Electrophysiol* 1992;15:771–778.

118. Calkins H, El-Atassi R, Kalbfleisch S, et al. Effects of an acute increase in atrial pressure on atrial refractoriness in humans. *Pacing Clin Electrophysiol* 1092;15:1674–1680.

119. Gossage AM, Hicks JAB. On auricular fibrillation. *QJM* 1913;6:435–440.

120. Friedlander RD, Levine SA. Auricular fibrillation and flutter without evidence of organic heart disease. *N Engl J Med* 1934;211:624–629.

121. Brill IC. Auricular fibrillation: the present status with a review of the literature. *Ann Intern Med* 1937;10:1487–1502.

122. Hanson HH, Rutledge DI. Auricular fibrillation in normal hearts. *N Engl J Med* 1949;240:947–953.

123. Evans W, Swann P. Lone auricular fibrillation. *Br Heart J* 1954;16:189–194.

124. Kumagai K, Akimitsu S, Kawahira K, et al. Electrophysiological properties in chronic lone atrial fibrillation. *Circulation* 1981;84:1662–1668.

125. Misier ARR, Opthof T, Van Hemel NM, et al. Increased dispersion of "refractoriness" in patients with idiopathic paroxysmal atrial fibrillation. *J Am Coll Cardiol* 1992;19:1531–1535.

126. Elvan A, Wylie K, Zipes DP. Pacing-induced chronic atrial fibrillation impairs sinus node function in dogs: electrophysiological remodeling. *Circulation* 1996;94:2953–2960.

127. Brugada R, Tapscott T, Czernuszewicz GZ, et al. Identification of a genetic locus for familial atrial fibrillation. *N Engl J Med* 1997;336:905–911.

128. Kopecky SL, Gersh BJ, Phil D, et al. The natural history of lone atrial fibrillation: a population-based study over three decades. *N Engl J Med* 1987;317:669–674.

129. Davidson E, Rotenberg Z, Weinberger I, et al. Diagnosis and characteristics of lone atrial fibrillation. *Chest* 1989;95:1048–1050.

130. Brand FN, Abbott RD, Kannel WB, et al. Characteristics and prognosis of lone atrial fibrillation: 30-year follow-up in the Framingham Study. *JAMA* 1985;254:3449–3453.

131. Fuster V, Ryden LE, Asinger RW, et al. ACC/AHA/ESC guidelines for the management of patients with atrial fibrillation (in press, 2001).

132. Bhandari AK, Anderson JL, Gilbert EM, et al. Correlation of symptoms with occurrence of paroxysmal supraventricular tachycardia or atrial fibrillation: a transtelephonic monitoring study. Flecainide Supraventricular Tachycardia Study Group. *Am Heart J* 1992;124:381–386.

133. Fogel RI, Evans JJ, Prystowsky EN. Utility and cost of event recorders in the diagnosis of palpitations, presyncope and syncope. *Am J Cardiol* 1997;79:207–208.

134. Cicogna R, Mascioli G, Bonomi FG, et al. Carotid sinus hypersensitivity and syndrome in patients with chronic atrial fibrillation. *Pacing Clin Electrophysiol* 1994;17:1635–1640.

135. Brignole M, Gianfranchi L, Menozzi C, et al. Role of autonomic reflexes in syncope associated with paroxysmal atrial fibrillation. *J Am Coll Cardiol* 1993;22:1123–1129.

136. Rostagno C, Taddei T, Paladini B, et al. The onset of symptomatic atrial fibrillation and paroxysmal supraventricular tachycardia is characterized by different circadian rhythms. *Am J Cardiol* 1993;71:453–455.

137. Page RL, Wilkinson WE, Clair WK, et al. Asymptomatic arrhythmias in patients with symptomatic paroxysmal atrial fibrillation and paroxysmal supraventricular tachycardia. *Circulation* 1994;89:224–227.

138. Hewlett AW, Wilson FN. Coarse auricular fibrillation in man. *Intern Med* 1915;15:786–792.

139. Wells JL, Karp RB, Kouchoukos NT, et al. Characterization of atrial fibrillation in man: studies following open heart surgery. *Pacing Clin Electrophysiol* 1978;1:426–438.

140. Konings KT, Smeets JL, Penn OC, et al. Configuration of unipolar atrial electrograms during electrically induced atrial fibrillation in humans. *Circulation* 1997;95:1231–1241.

141. Manning WJ, Silverman DI, Keighley CS, et al. Transesophageal echocardiographically facilitated early cardioversion from atrial fibrillation using short-term anticoagulation: final results of a prospective 4.5-year study. *J Am Coll Cardiol* 1995;25:1354–1361.

142. Fatkin D, Kuchar DL, Thorburn CW, et al. Transesophageal echocardiography before and during direct current cardioversion of atrial fibrillation: evidence for "atrial stunning" as a mechanism of thromboembolic complications. *J Am Coll Cardiol* 1994;23:307–316.

143. Grimm RA, Stewart WJ, Maloney JD, et al. Impact of electrical cardioversion for atrial fibrillation on left atrial appendage function and spontaneous echo contrast: characterization by simultaneous transesophageal echocardiography. *J Am Coll Cardiol* 1993;22:1359–1366.

144. Klein AL, Grimm RA, Black IW, et al. Cardioversion guided by transesophageal echocardiography: the ACUTE Pilot Study. A randomized, controlled trial. *Ann Intern Med* 1997;126:200–209.

145. Fukunami M, Yamada T, Ohmori M, et al. Detection of patients at risk for paroxysmal atrial fibrillation during sinus rhythm by P wave–triggered signal-averaged electrocardiogram. *Circulation* 1991;83:162–169.

146. Steinberg JS, Zelenkofske S, Wong SC, et al. Value of the P-wave signal-averaged ECG for predicting atrial fibrillation after cardiac surgery. *Circulation* 1993;88:2618–2622.

147. Klein GJ, Prystowsky EN, Yee R, et al. Asymptomatic Wolff-Parkinson-White: should we intervene? *Circulation* 1989;80:1902–1905.

148. Robinson K, Frenneaux MP, Stockins B, et al. Atrial fibrillation in hypertrophic cardiomyopathy: a longitudinal study. *J Am Coll Cardiol* 1990;15:1279–1285.

149. Stafford WJ, Trohman RG, Bilsker M, et al. Cardiac arrest in an adolescent with atrial fibrillation and hypertrophic cardiomyopathy. *J Am Coll Cardiol* 1986;7:701–704.

150. Madariaga I, Carmona JR, Mateas FR, et al. Supraventricular arrhythmias as the cause of sudden death in hypertrophic cardiomyopathy. *Eur Heart J* 1994;15:134–137.

151. Spirito P, Lakatos E, Maron BJ. Degree of left ventricular hypertrophy in patients with hypertrophic cardiomyopathy and chronic atrial fibrillation. *Am J Cardiol* 1992;69:1217–1222.

152. Prystowsky EN. Management of atrial fibrillation: thera-

peutic options and clinical decisions. *Am J Cardiol* 2000;85:3D–11D.

153. Prystowsky EN. Proarrhythmia during drug treatment of supraventricular tachycardia: paradoxical risk of sinus rhythm for sudden death. *Am J Cardiol* 1996;78(8A):35–41.

154. Falk RH, Knowlton AA, Bernard SA, et al. Digoxin for converting recent-onset atrial fibrillation to sinus rhythm: a randomized, double-blinded trial. *Ann Intern Med* 1987;106:503–506.

155. Salerno DM, Dias VC, Kleiger RE, et al. Efficacy and safety of intravenous diltiazem for treatment of atrial fibrillation and atrial flutter: the Diltiazem-Atrial Fibrillation/Flutter Study Group. *Am J Cardiol* 1989;63:1046–1051.

156. Rinkenberger RL, Prystowsky EN, Heger JJ, et al. Effects of intravenous and chronic oral verapamil administration in patients with supraventricular tachyarrhythmias. *Circulation* 1980;62:996–1010.

157. Halpern SW, Ellrodt G, Singh BN, et al. Efficacy of intravenous procainamide infusion in converting atrial fibrillation to sinus rhythm: relation to left atrial size. *Br Heart J* 1980;44:589–595.

158. Fenster PE, Comess KA, Marsh R, et al. Conversion of atrial fibrillation to sinus rhythm by acute intravenous procainamide infusion. *Am Heart J* 1983;106:501–504.

159. Madrid AH, Moro C, Marin-Huerta E, et al. Comparison of flecainide and procainamide in cardioversion of atrial fibrillation. *Eur Heart J* 1993;14:1127–1131.

160. Hjelms E. Procainamide conversion of acute atrial fibrillation after open heart surgery compared with digoxin treatment. *Scand J Thorac Cardiovasc Surg* 1992;26:193–196.

161. Roden DM. Ibutilide and the treatment of atrial arrhythmias. *Circulation* 1996;94:1499–1502.

162. Ellenbogen KA, Stambler BS, Wood MA, et al. Efficacy of intravenous ibutilide for rapid termination of atrial fibrillation and atrial flutter: a dose-response study. *J Am Coll Cardiol* 1996;28:130–136.

163. Stambler BS, Wood MA, Ellenbogen KA, et al. Efficacy and safety of repeated intravenous doses of ibutilide for rapid conversion of atrial flutter or fibrillation. Ibutilide Repeat Dose Study Investigators. *Circulation* 1996;94:1613–1621.

164. Volgman AS, Carberry PA, Stambler B, et al. Conversion efficacy and safety of intravenous ibutilide compared with intravenous procainamide in patients with atrial flutter or fibrillation. *J Am Coll Cardiol* 1998;31:1414–1419.

165. Wellens HJJ, Brugada P, Abdollah H, et al. A comparison of the electrophysiologic effects of intravenous and oral amiodarone in the same patient. *Circulation* 1984;69(1):120–124.

166. Galve E, Rius T, Ballester R, et al. Intravenous amiodarone in treatment of recent-onset atrial fibrillation: results of a randomized, controlled study. *J Am Coll Cardiol* 1996;27:1079–1082.

167. Donovan KD, Power BM, Hockings BEF, et al. Intravenous flecainide versus amiodarone for recent-onset atrial fibrillation. *Am J Cardiol* 1995;75:693–697.

168. Faniel R, Schoenfeld PH. Efficacy of i.v. amiodarone in converting rapid atrial fibrillation and flutter to sinus rhythm in intensive care patients. *Eur Heart J* 1983;4:180–185.

169. McAlister HF, Luke RA, Whitlock RM, et al. Intravenous amiodarone bolus versus oral quinidine for atrial flutter and fibrillation after cardiac operations. *J Thorac Cardiovasc Surg* 1990;99:911–918.

170. Kerin NZ, Faitel K, Naini M. The efficacy of intravenous amiodarone for the conversion of chronic atrial fibrillation. *Arch Intern Med* 1996;156:49–53.

171. Borgeat A, Goy JJ, Maendly R, et al. Flecainide versus quinidine for conversion of atrial fibrillation to sinus rhythm. *Am J Cardiol* 1986;58:496–498.

172. Hellestrand KJ. Intravenous flecainide acetate for supraventricular tachycardias. *Am J Cardiol* 1988;62:16D–22D.

173. Suttorp MJ, Kingma JH, Jessurun ER, et al. The value of class IC antiarrhythmic drugs for acute conversion of paroxysmal atrial fibrillation or flutter to sinus rhythm. *J Am Coll Cardiol* 1990;16:1722–1727.

174. Bianconi L, Boccadamo R, Pappalardo A, et al. Effectiveness of intravenous propafenone for conversion of atrial fibrillation and flutter of recent onset. *Am J Cardiol* 1989;64:335–338.

175. Vita JA, Friedman PL, Cantillon C, et al. Efficacy of intravenous propafenone for the acute management of atrial fibrillation. *Am J Cardiol* 1989;63:1275–1278.

176. Sung RJ, Tan HL, Karagounis L, et al. Intravenous sotalol for the termination of supraventricular tachycardia and atrial fibrillation and flutter: a multicenter, randomized, double-blind, placebo-controlled study. The Sotalol Multicenter Study Group. *Am Heart J* 1995;129:739–748.

177. Falk RH, Pollak A, Singh SN, et al. Intravenous dofetilide, a class III antiarrhythmic agent, for the termination of sustained atrial fibrillation or flutter. *J Am Coll Cardiol* 1997;29:385–390.

178. Norgaard BL, Wachtell K, Christensen PD, et al. Efficacy and safety of intravenously administered dofetilide in acute termination of atrial fibrillation and flutter: a multicenter, randomized, double-blind, placebo-controlled trial. Danish Dofetilide in Atrial Fibrillation and Flutter Study Group. *Am Heart J* 1999;137:1062–1069.

179. Lindeboom JE, Kingma JH, Crijns HJ, et al. Efficacy and safety of intravenous dofetilide for rapid termination of atrial fibrillation and atrial flutter. *Am J Cardiol* 2000;85:1031–1033.

180. Sokolow M, Ball RE. Factors influencing conversion of chronic atrial fibrillation with special reference to serum quinidine concentration. *Circulation* 1956;14:568–583.

181. Capucci A, Boriani G, Botto GL, et al. Conversion of recent-onset atrial fibrillation by a single oral loading dose of propafenone or flecainide. *Am J Cardiol* 1994;74:503–505.

182. Botto GL, Bonini W, Broffoni T, et al. Conversion of recent onset atrial fibrillation with single loading oral dose of propafenone: is in-hospital admission absolutely necessary? *Pacing Clin Electrophysiol* 1996;19:1939–1943.

183. Coplen SE, Antman EM, Berline JA, et al. Efficacy and safety of quinidine therapy for maintenance of sinus rhythm after cardioversion: a meta-analysis of randomized control trials. *Circulation* 1990;82:1106–1116.

184. Hartel G, Louhija A, Konttinen A. Disopyramide in the prevention of recurrence of atrial fibrillation after electroconversion. *Clin Pharmacol Therapeut* 1974;15:551–555.

185. Anderson JL, Gilbert EM, Alpert BL, et al. Prevention of symptomatic recurrences of paroxysmal atrial fibrillation in patients initially tolerating antiarrhythmic therapy: a multicenter, double blind, crossover study of flecainide and placebo with transtelephonic monitoring. Flecainide Supraventricular Tachycardia Study Group. *Circulation* 1989;80:1157–1570.

186. Pritchett ELC, DaTorre SD, Platt ML, et al. Flecainide acetate treatment of paroxysmal supraventricular tachycardia and paroxysmal atrial fibrillation: dose-response studies. The Flecainide Supraventricular Tachycardia Study Group. *J Am Coll Cardiol* 1991;17:197–303.

187. Aliot E, Denjoy I. Comparison of the safety and efficacy of flecainide versus propafenone in hospital out-patients with symptomatic paroxysmal atrial fibrillation/flutter. *Am J Cardiol* 1996;77:66A–71A.

188. Antman EM, Beamer AD, Cantillon C, et al. Long-term oral propafenone therapy for suppression of refractory symptomatic atrial fibrillation and atrial flutter. *J Am Coll Cardiol* 1989;12:1005–1011.

189. Connoly SJ, Hoffert DL. Usefulness of propafenone for recurrent paroxysmal atrial fibrillation. *Am J Cardiol* 1989;63:817–819.

190. Reimold SC, Cantillon CO, Friedman PL, et al. Propafenone versus sotalol for suppression of recurrent symptomatic atrial fibrillation. *Am J Cardiol* 1993;71:558–563.

191. Juul-Moller S, Edvardsson N, Rehnqvist-Ahlberg N. Sotalol versus quinidine for the maintenance of sinus rhythm after direct current conversion of atrial fibrillation. *Circulation* 1990;82:1932–1939.

192. Hohnloser SF, Van de Loo A, Baedeker F. Efficacy and proarrhythmic hazards of pharmacologic cardioversion of atrial fibrillation: prospective comparison of sotalol versus quinidine. *J Am Coll Cardiol* 1995;26:852–858.

193. Bellandi F, Dabizzi RP, Niccoli L, et al. Propafenone and sotalol in the prevention of paroxysmal atrial fibrillation: long-term safety and efficacy study. *Curr Ther Res* 1995;56:1154–1168.

194. Horowitz LN, Spielman SR, Greenspan AM, et al. Use of amiodarone in the treatment of persistent and paroxysmal atrial fibrillation resistant to quinidine therapy. *J Am Coll Cardiol* 1985;6:1402–1407.

195. Gold RL, Haffajee CI, Chros G, et al. Amiodarone for refractory atrial fibrillation. *Am J Cardiol* 1986;57:124–127.

196. Brodsky MA, Allen BJ, Walker CJ, et al. Amiodarone for maintenance of sinus rhythm after conversion of atrial fibrillation in the setting of a dilated left atrium. *Am J Cardiol* 1987;60:572–574.

197. Gosselink AT, Crijns HJ, VanGelder IC, et al. Low-dose amiodarone for maintenance of sinus rhythm after cardioversion of atrial fibrillation or flutter. *JAMA* 1992;267:3289–3293.

198. Vitolo E, Tronci M, Larovere MT, et al. Amiodarone versus quinidine in the prophylaxis of atrial fibrillation. *Acta Cardiol* 1981;36:431–444.

199. Martin A, Benbow LJ, Leach C, et al. Comparison of amiodarone and disopyramide in the control of paroxysmal atrial fibrillation and atrial flutter (interim report).

200. Blevins RD, Kerin NZ, Benederet D, et al. Amiodarone in the management of refractory atrial fibrillation. *Arch Intern Med* 1987;147:1401–1404.

201. Geller JC, Geller M, Lott J, et al. Moricizine is effective and safe in patients with atrial fibrillation. *Circulation* 1995;92:I-774.

202. Torp-Pedersen C, Moller M, Bloch-Thomsen PE, et al. Dofetilide in patients with congestive heart failure and left ventricular dysfunction. Danish Investigations of Arrhythmia and Mortality on Dofetilide Study Group. *N Engl J Med* 1999;341:857–865.

203. Greenbaum RA, Campbell TJ, Channer KS, et al. Conversion of atrial fibrillation and maintenance of sinus rhythm by dofetilide. The EMERALD (European and Australian Multicenter Evaluative Research on Atrial Fibrillation Dofetilide) study. *Circulation* 1998;17[Suppl]:1633.

204. Singh SN, Berk M, Yellen L, et al. Efficacy and safety of oral dofetilide in maintaining sinus rhythm: 12 months follow-up results of SAFIRE-D. *Circulation* 1999;100:I-501(abst).

205. Roy D, Talajic M, Dorian P, et al. Amiodarone to prevent recurrence of atrial fibrillation. Canadian Trial of Atrial Fibrillation Investigators. *N Engl J Med* 2000;342:913–920.

206. Antman EM, Beamer AD, Cantillon C, et al. Therapy of refractory symptomatic atrial fibrillation and atrial flutter: a staged care approach with new antiarrhythmic drugs. *J Am Coll Cardiol* 1990;15:698–707.

207. Crijns HJ, VanGelder IC, VanGilst WH, et al. Serial antiarrhythmic drug treatment to maintain sinus rhythm after electrical cardioversion for chronic atrial fibrillation or atrial flutter. *Am J Cardiol* 1991;68:335–341.

208. Echt DS, Leibson PR, Mitchell LB, et al. Mortality and morbidity in patients receiving encainide, flecainide or placebo. The Cardiac Arrhythmia Suppression Trial. *N Engl J Med* 1991;324:781–788.

209. Flaker GC, Blackshear JL, McBride R, et al. Antiarrhythmic drug therapy and cardiac mortality in atrial fibrillation. The Stroke Prevention in Atrial Fibrillation Investigators. *J Am Coll Cardiol* 1992;20:527–532.

210. Singh SN, Fletcher RD, Fisher SG, et al. Amiodarone in patients with congestive heart failure and asymptomatic ventricular arrhythmia. The Survival Trial of Antiarrhythmic Therapy in Congestive Heart Failure. *N Engl J Med* 1995;333:77–82.

211. Doval HC, Nul DR, Grancelli HO, et al. Randomized trial of low-dose amiodarone in severe congestive heart failure. *Lancet* 1994;344:493–498.

212. Julian DG, Prescott RJ, Jackson FS, et al. Controlled trial of sotalol for one year after myocardial infarction. *Lancet* 1982;1:1142–1147.

213. Julian DG, Camm AJ, Frangin G, et al. Randomised trial of effect of amiodarone on mortality in patients with left ventricular dysfunction after recent myocardial infarction: EMIAT [published errata appear in *Lancet* 1997;349(9059):1180 and 1997;349(9067):1776]. European Myocardial Infarct Amiodarone Trial Investigators. *Lancet* 1997;349:667–674.

214. Cairns JA, Connolly SJ, Roberts R, et al. Randomised trial of outcome after myocardial infarction in patients with frequent or repetitive ventricular premature depolarisations: CAMIAT [published erratum appears in *Lancet* 1997;349(9067):1776]. Canadian Amiodarone Myocardial Infarction Arrhythmia Trial Investigators. *Lancet* 1997;349:675–682.

215. Kober L, Bloch Thomsen PE, Moller M, et al. Effect of dofetilide in patients with recent myocardial infarction and left-ventricular dysfunction: a randomised trial. *Lancet* 2000;356(9247):2052–2058.

216. Ellenbogen KA, Dias VC, Plumb VJ, et al. A placebo-controlled trial of continuous intravenous diltiazem infusion for 24-hour heart rate control during atrial fibrillation and atrial flutter: a multicenter study. *J Am Coll Cardiol* 1991;18:891–897.

217. Waxman JL, Myerburg RJ, Appel R, Sung RJ. Verapamil for control of ventricular rate in paroxysmal supraventricular tachycardia and atrial fibrillation or flutter: a double-blind randomized cross-over study. *Ann Intern Med* 1981;94:1–6.

218. Aronow WS, Landa D, Plasencia G, et al. Verapamil in atrial fibrillation and atrial flutter. *Clin Pharmacol Ther* 1979;26:578–583.

219. Anderson S, Blanski L, Byrd RC, et al. Comparison of the efficacy and safety of esmolol, a short-acting beta blocker, with placebo in the treatment of supraventricular tachyarrhythmias: the Esmolol vs. Placebo Multicenter Study Group. *Am Heart J* 1986;111:42–48.

220. David D, Segni ED, Klein HO, Kaplinsky E. Inefficacy of digitalis in the control of heart rate in patients with chronic atrial fibrillation: beneficial effect of an added beta adrenergic blocking agent. *Am J Cardiol* 1979;44:1378–1382.

221. DiBianco R, Morganroth J, Freitag JA, et al. Effects of nadolol on the spontaneous and exercise-provoked heart rate of patients with chronic atrial fibrillation receiving stable dosages of digoxin. *Am Heart J* 1984;109[Pt 2]:1121–1127.

222. Klein HO, Kaplinsky E. Digitalis and verapamil in atrial fibrillation and flutter: is verapamil now the preferred agent? *Drugs* 1986;31:185–197.

223. Roth A, Harrison E, Mitani G, et al. Efficacy and safety of medium- and high-dose diltiazem alone and in combination with digoxin for control of heart rate at rest and during exercise in patients with chronic atrial fibrillation. *Circulation* 1986;73:314–316.

224. Goodman DJ, Rossen RM, Cannom DS, et al. Effect of digoxin on atrioventricular conduction: studies in patients with and without cardiac autonomic innervation. *Circulation* 1975;51:251–256.

225. Roth A, Kaluski E, Felner S, et al. Clonidine for patients with rapid atrial fibrillation. *Ann Intern Med* 1992;116:388–390.

226. Rubin DA, Nieminiski KE, Reed GE, et al. Predictors, prevention, and long term prognosis of atrial fibrillation after coronary bypass graft operation. *J Thorac Cardiovasc Surg* 1987;94:331–339.

227. Silverman NA, Eright R, Levitsky S. Efficacy of low dose propranolol in preventing postoperative supraventricular tachyarrhythmias: a prospective, randomized study. *Ann Surg* 1982;196:194–200.

228. White HD, Elliott ChB, Antman MD, et al. Efficacy and safety of timolol for prevention of supraventricular tachyarrhythmias after coronary artery bypass surgery. *Circulation* 1984;70(3):479–484.

229. Daudon P, Corcos T, Gandjbakhch I, et al. Prevention of atrial fibrillation or flutter by acebutolol after coronary bypass grafting. *Am J Cardiol* 1986;58:933–936.

230. Gomes JA, Ip J, Santoni-Rugiu F, et al. Oral d,1 sotalol reduces the incidence of postoperative atrial fibrillation in coronary artery bypass surgery patients: a randomized, double-blind, placebo controlled study. *J Am Coll Cardiol* 1999;34:334–339.

231. Guarnieri T, Nolan S, Gottlieb SO, et al. Intravenous amiodarone for the prevention of atrial fibrillation after open heart surgery: the Amiodarone Reduction in Coronary Heart (ARCH) Trial. *J Am Coll Cardiol* 1999;34:343–347.

232. Daoud EG, Strickberger SA, Man KC, et al. Preoperative amiodarone as prophylaxis against atrial fibrillation after heart surgery. *N Engl J Med* 1997;337:1785–1791.

233. Kowey PR, Stebbins D, Igidbashian L, et al. Clinical outcome of patients who develop PAF after CABG surgery. *Pacing Clin Electrophysiol* 2001;24:191–193.

234. Heppell RM, Berkin KE, McLenachan JM, et al. Haemostatic and haemodynamic abnormalities associated with left atrial thrombosis in non-rheumatic atrial fibrillation. *Heart* 1997;77:407–411.

235. Sohara H, Amitani S, Kurose M, et al. Atrial fibrillation activates platelets and coagulation in a time-dependent manner; a study in patients with paroxysmal atrial fibrillation. *J Am Coll Cardiol* 1977;29:106–112.

236. Bjerkelund CJ, Orning OM. The efficacy of anticoagulant therapy in preventing embolism related to D.C. electrical conversion of atrial fibrillation. *Am J Cardiol* 1969;23:208–216.

237. Weinberg DM, Mancini J. Anticoagulation for cardioversion of atrial fibrillation. *Am J Cardiol* 1989;63:745–746.

238. Lip GYH. Hypercoagulability and haemodynamic abnormalities in atrial fibrillation. *Heart* 1997;77:395–396.

239. Heppell RM, Berkin KE, McLenachan JM, et al. Haemostatic and haemodynamic abnormalities associated with left atrial thrombosis in non-rheumatic atrial fibrillation. *Heart* 1997;77:407–411.

240. Lown B, Amarasingham R, Neuman J. New method for terminating cardiac arrhythmias: use of synchronized capacitor discharge. *JAMA* 1962;182:548.

241. Lown B. Electrical reversion of cardiac arrhythmias. *Br Heart J* 1967;29:469–489.

242. Henry WL, Morganroth J, Pearlman AS, et al. Relation between echocardiographically determined left atrial size and atrial fibrillation. *Circulation* 1976;53:273–279.

243. VanGelder IC, Crijns HJ, VanGilst WH, et al. Prediction of uneventful cardioversion and maintenance of sinus rhythm from direct-current electrical cardioversion of chronic atrial fibrillation and flutter. *Am J Cardiol* 1991;68:335–341.

244. Lown B, Krieger R, Williams J. Cardioversion and digitalis drugs: changed threshold to electrical shock in digitalized animals. *Circ Res* 1965;17:519–531.

245. Guarnieri T, Tomaselli G, Griffith LSC, et al. The interaction of antiarrhythmic drugs and the energy for cardioversion of chronic atrial fibrillation. *Pacing Clin Electrophysiol* 1991;14:1007–1012.

246. Prystowsky EN. Cardioversion of atrial fibrillation to sinus rhythm: who, when, how, and why? *Am J Cardiol* 2000;86:326–327.

247. Joglar JA, Haurdan MH, Ramaswamy K, et al. Initial energy for elective external cardioversion of persistent atrial fibrillation. *Am J Cardiol* 2000;86:348–350.

248. Saliba W, Juratli N, Chunk MK, et al. Higher energy synchronized external direct current cardioversion for refractory atrial fibrillation. *J Am Coll Cardiol* 1999;34:2031–2034.

249. Oral H, Souza JJ, Michaud GF, et al. Facilitating transthoracic cardioversion of atrial fibrillation with ibutilide pretreatment. *N Engl J Med* 1999;340:1849–1854.

250. Levy S, Laurie P, Dolla E, et al. A randomized comparison of external and internal cardioversion of chronic atrial fibrillation. *Circulation* 1992;86:1415–1420.

251. Mittal S, Ayati S, Stein KM, et al. Transthoracic cardioversion of atrial fibrillation: comparison of rectilinear biphasic versus damped sine wave monophasic shocks. *Circulation* 2000;101:1282–1287.

252. Mirowski M, Mower M, Langer A. Low-energy catheter cardioversion of atrial tachyarrhythmias. *Clin Res* 1974;22:290.

253. Levy S, Lacombe P, Cointe R, et al. High energy transcatheter cardioversion of chronic atrial fibrillation. *J Am Coll Cardiol* 1988;12:514–518.

254. Cooper RAS, Clif A, Smith WM, et al. Internal cardioversion of atrial fibrillation in sheep. *Circulation* 1993;87:1673–1686.

255. Baker BM, Botteron GW, Smith JM. Low-energy internal cardioversion for atrial fibrillation resistance to external cardioversion. *J Cardiovasc Electrophysiol* 1995;17:1058–1066.

256. Wharton JM, Johnson EE. Catheter based atrial defibrillation. *Pacing Clin Electrophysiol* 1994;17:1058–1066.

257. Muratroyed FD, Slade AK, Sopher SM, et al. Efficacy and tolerability of transvenous low energy cardioversion of paroxysmal atrial fibrillation in humans. *J Am Coll Cardiol* 1995;25:1347–1353.

258. Hesselson AB, Parsonnet V, Bernstein AD, et al. Deleterious effects of long-term single chamber ventricular pacing in patients with sick sinus syndrome: the hidden benefit of dual chamber pacing. *J Am Coll Cardiol* 1992;19:1542–1549.

259. Andersen HR, Thuesen L, Bagger JP, et al. Prospective randomized trial of atrial versus ventricular pacing in sick sinus syndrome. *Lancet* 1994;344:1523–1528.

260. Andersen HR, Nielsen JC, Thomsen PE, et al. Long-term follow-up of patients from a randomised trial of atrial versus ventricular pacing for sick-sinus syndrome. *Lancet* 1997;350:1210–1216.

261. Daubert C, Gras D, Berder Vleclercq C, et al. Permanent atrial resynchronization by synchronous bi-atrial pacing in the preventive treatment of atrial flutter associated with high degree intraatrial block. *Arch Mal Coeur Vaiss* 1994;87:1535–1546.

262. Gillis AM, Wyse DG, Connolly SJ, et al. Atrial pacing periablation for prevention of paroxysmal atrial fibrillation. *Circulation* 1999;99:2553–2558.

263. Fitts SM, Hill MR, Mehra R, et al. Design and implementation of the Dual Site Atrial Pacing to Prevent Atrial Fibrillation (DAPPAF) clinical trial. DAPPAF Phase 1 Investigators. *J Interv Cardiol Electrophysiol* 1998;2:139–144.

264. Delfaut P, Saksena S, Prakash A, et al. Long-term outcome of patients with drug-refractory atrial flutter and fibrillation after single- and dual-site right atrial pacing for

265. arrhythmia prevention. *J Am Coll Cardiol* 1998;32:1900–1908.

265. Scheinman MM, Morady F, Hess DS, et al. Catheter induced ablation of the atrioventricular junction to control refractory supraventricular arrhythmias. *JAMA* 1982;248:851–855.

266. Gallagher JJ, Svenson RH, Kasell JH, et al. Catheter technique for closed-chest ablation of the atrioventricular conduction system: a therapeutic alternative for the treatment of refractory supraventricular tachycardia. *N Engl J Med* 1982;306:194–200.

267. Kay GN, Bubien RS, Epstein AE, et al. Effect of catheter ablation of the atrioventricular junction on quality of life and exercise tolerance in paroxysmal atrial fibrillation. *Am J Cardiol* 1988;62:741–744.

268. Feld GK, Fleck RP, Fujimura O, et al. Control of rapid ventricular response by radiofrequency catheter modification of the atrioventricular node in patients with medically refractory atrial fibrillation. *Circulation* 1994;90:2299–2307.

269. Williamson B, Man KC, Daoud E, et al. Radiofrequency catheter modification of atrioventricular conduction to control the ventricular rate during atrial fibrillation. *N Engl J Med* 1994;331:910–917.

270. Swartz JF, Pelletsel G, Silvers J, et al. A catheter-based curative approach to atrial fibrillation in humans. *Circulation* 1994;90[Pt II]:I-335.

271. Jais P, Shah DC, Takahashi A, et al. Long-term follow-up after right atrial radiofrequency catheter treatment of paroxysmal atrial fibrillation. *Pacing Clin Electrophysiol* 1998;21:2533–2538.

272. Pappone C, Oreto G, Lamberti F, et al. Catheter ablation of paroxysmal atrial fibrillation using a 3D mapping system. *Circulation* 1999;100:1203–1208.

273. Natale A, Pisano E, Shewchik J, et al. First human experience with pulmonary vein isolation using a through-the-balloon circumferential ultrasound ablation system for recurrent atrial fibrillation. *Circulation* 2000;102:1879–1882.

274. Haissaguerre M, Shah DC, Jais P, et al. Electrophysiological breakthroughs from the left atrium to the pulmonary veins. *Circulation* 2000;102:2463–2465.

275. Williams JM, Ungerleider RM, Lofland GK, et al. Left atrial isolation: new technique for the treatment of supraventricular arrhythmias. *J Thorac Cardiovasc Surg* 1980;80:373–380.

276. Defauw JJ, Guiraudon GM, vanHemel NM, et al. Surgical therapy of paroxysmal atrial fibrillation with the corridor operation. *Ann Thorac Surg* 1992;53:564–571.

277. Hioki M, Ikeshita M, Iedokoro Y, et al. Successful combined operation for mitral stenosis and atrial fibrillation. *Ann Thorac Surg* 1993;55:776–778.

278. Lab MJ. Fibrillation, chaos and clinical control. *Nat Med* 1997;3:385–386.

279. Prystowsky EN. Future expectations of implantable cardioverter defibrillator therapy. *Pacing Clin Electrophysiol* 1995;18[Pt II]:609–615.

280. Prystowsky EN. Screening and therapy for patients with nonsustained ventricular tachycardia. *Am J Cardiol* 2000;86[Suppl]:34K–39K.

ATRIOVENTRICULAR NODAL–INDEPENDENT SUPRAVENTRICULAR TACHYCARDIAS

ALBERT L. WALDO
LEE A. BIBLO

A. L. Waldo: Department of Medicine, Case Western Reserve University School of Medicine, University Hospitals of Cleveland, Cleveland, Ohio
L. A. Biblo: Department of Medicine, Case Western Reserve University School of Medicine, MetroHealth Medical Center, Cleveland, Ohio

OVERVIEW

The clinical presentation of patients with atrioventricular (AV) nodal–independent arrhythmias is quite variable and may include nonspecific symptoms. The 12-lead electrocardiogram (ECG), 24-hour ambulatory ECG (Holter) monitor, and ECG event recorder usually establish the diagnosis. In addition, electrophysiologic studies have now become an important diagnostic tool, particularly with the emergence of effective nonpharmacologic therapies. In patients with frequent or incessant atrial arrhythmias, sustained rapid ventricular rates can lead to a tachycardia-mediated cardiomyopathy (CM) and congestive heart failure (CHF). Therefore, considerable caution should be exercised before attributing cardiac decompensation to worsening intrinsic myocardial disease in the presence of such an arrhythmia.

The management of atrial arrhythmias has improved due to a better understanding of the causative mechanisms. Most AV nodal–independent arrhythmias are due to reentry: atrial flutter, sinus-node reentry, and intraatrial reentrant tachycardia. However, AV nodal–independent arrhythmias may also occur due to automaticity or triggered activity. Regardless, acute treatment consists of obtaining prompt control of the ventricular rate and, if possible, restoring sinus rhythm.

A thorough characterization of the underlying cardiac substrate is usually indicated before embarking on long-term therapy. Catheter-ablation techniques provide the best hope of obtaining a permanent cure in most patients with these arrhythmias. Large clinical experiences now support the use of catheter ablation as primary therapy in symptomatic patients with atrial flutter, atrial tachycardia, and sinus-node reentry tachycardia. Alternative treatments consist of antiarrhythmic drugs to suppress recurrent symptomatic episodes, recognizing that occasional recurrences are common and do not represent drug failure.

INTRODUCTION

This chapter examines the AV nodal–independent tachycardias, with the exception of atrial fibrillation. This chapter deals principally with atrial flutter, the most common of these arrhythmias. The other arrhythmias discussed include atrial tachycardia, inappropriate sinus tachycardia, sinus node reentrant tachycardia, and multifocal atrial tachycardia (MAT).

Atrial tachyarrhythmias are associated with a wide spectrum of potential presentations, including palpitation, syncope, near-syncope, dyspnea, fatigue, malaise, and new or worsening CHF. Many, if not most, of these symptoms are primarily related to the associated rapid ventricular rate and the physiologic adaptation to that rapid rate. This is most fully discussed in the section on atrial flutter (see Atrial Flutter: Epidemiology and Clinical Significance), which serves as a reference for the other atrial tachyarrhythmias. Similarly, many, if not most, of the principles of treatment of atrial flutter apply to the other atrial tachyarrhythmias, particularly those due to a reentrant mechanism.

In the management of patients with an atrial tachyarrhythmia, identification of the mechanism of the atrial arrhythmia remains one of the cornerstones of successful therapy. Such an understanding now provides the opportunity for a definitive cure in many instances. However, providing successful therapy also mandates a careful evaluation of the patient, especially of the overall cardiac milieu. In many instances, non–AV nodal–dependent arrhythmias are associated with a cardiac substrate abnormality of consequence, such as ventricular hypertrophy, valvular heart disease, coronary artery disease, or left ventricular (LV) dysfunction. An assumption of this chapter is that the cardiac milieu must be adequately addressed as a necessary part of the treatment of atrial tachyarrhythmias.

Finally, regardless of the atrial tachyarrhythmia, if it is incessant or frequent and the ventricular response rate is rapid, a tachycardia-induced CM may result. Recognition of this possibility is particularly important, as primary therapy of this CM should be directed at the atrial tachyarrhythmia. An incessant, atrial tachyarrhythmia–induced dilated CM may be entirely reversible with correction of the tachyarrhythmia or control of the ventricular rate. In patients with preexisting heart disease, frequent or incessant atrial tachyarrhythmias may cause additional cardiac decompensation that may go unrecognized or may be incorrectly attributed to worsening of the underlying structural heart disease. This, too, should be improved or reversed with correction of the tachyarrhythmia or control of the ventricular rate.

ATRIAL FLUTTER

Potential Mechanisms

Mapping of atrial flutter in humans [156] began in the 1950s with the studies of Prinzmetal et al. (56). Photographic techniques with the heart exposed were used during thoracic surgery. Later, Wellens et al. (57) used sequential-site atrial epicardial mapping to study atrial flutter during human cardiac surgery. On the basis of these studies, both groups suggested that atrial flutter was due to a single focus firing rapidly. Pacing studies by Rosen et al. (58) of the human coronary sinus showed that a single focus firing rapidly could generate the classic clinical ECG of atrial flutter. Nevertheless, this mechanism has not been supported by numerous other mapping studies in humans that primarily have used electrode catheter techniques during electrophysiologic studies. As summarized by Rytand (59), initial and limited catheter mapping studies in the 1950s and 1960s suggested that atrial flutter was an intra-atrial reentrant rhythm. The mapping studies of Puech and colleagues (60,61) demonstrated that the entire duration of the atrial flutter cycle length may be explained by circus movement activation of the right atrium alone, with the impulse traveling up the septum and down the right atrial free wall.

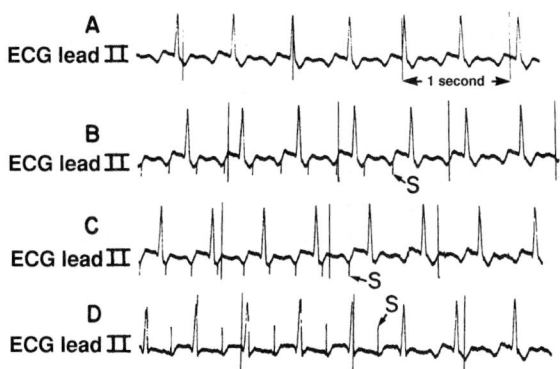

FIGURE 65.1 Electrocardiogram (ECG) lead II recorded during atrial flutter of an atrial cycle length of 264 ms **(A)** and at the end of 30 seconds of rapid atrial pacing from a high right atrial site at a cycle length of 254 ms **(B)**, at a cycle length of 242 ms **(C)**, and at a cycle length of 232 ms **(D)**. The atrial flutter was transiently entrained at each pacing rate. Note that when comparing the morphology of the atrial complexes during atrial pacing at each cycle length, especially that of the atrial complexes during atrial pacing in **D** with that in **A** and **B**, progressive fusion has occurred. Timelines are at 1-second intervals. S, stimulus artifact. (From Waldo AL, MacLean WAH, Karp RB, et al. Entrainment and interruption of atrial flutter with atrial pacing: studies in man following open-heart surgery. *Circulation* 1977;56:737–745, with permission.)

Demonstration of transient entrainment and interruption of atrial flutter in humans (62–64) provided additional strong evidence that atrial flutter was an intraatrial reentrant rhythm with an excitable gap (Fig. 65.1). Subsequent mapping studies, usually in concert with atrial pacing, have confirmed that the atrial flutter reentrant circuit is virtually always confined to the right atrium. Thus, the studies of Cosio et al. (65–67), Olshansky et al. (68,69), and Klein et al. (23) indicated that the reentrant circuit in typical atrial flutter in humans involved counterclockwise reentrant excitation in the right atrium in which the impulse traveled in a caudocranial direction in the interatrial septum and in a craniocaudal direction in the right atrial free wall. Atypical, or rare (uncommon), atrial flutter was shown to use the same reentrant circuit but in the opposite direction (70).

The studies of Cosio et al. (65–67) and Olshansky et al. (68,69) have also provided evidence that an area of slow conduction is present in the postero-inferior aspect of the right atrium. The central area of block around which the reentrant wavefront circulates likely includes an anatomic component and a functional component in the interatrial septum (65,66,70).

Catheter mapping techniques, including entrainment mapping, have localized the area of slow conduction in the reentrant circuit principally to an isthmus bounded by the coronary sinus ostium, the tricuspid annulus, inferior vena cava, and eustachian ridge (21,71–73). However, others have suggested that this atrial flutter isthmus is not an area of slow conduction during atrial flutter (74).

Exquisite anatomic and angiographic studies have examined the underlying milieu of the atrial flutter circuit.

Marked anatomic variations in the subeustachian isthmus are present in normal hearts. The arrangement of the subendothelial fibers in the isthmus recesses was unique among autopsy specimens (75,76). Furthermore, an angiographic study demonstrated that the inferior subeustachian isthmus is wider in patients with atrial flutter when compared with a control population (77). These studies demonstrate a strong anatomic contribution to the requisite atrial flutter reentrant circuit.

Mapping techniques have demonstrated the critical role of the region of the crista terminalis as one boundary for the reentrant circuit and the role of the tricuspid ring as another boundary of the reentrant circuit (71–73). Differences in the electrophysiologic properties of the crista terminalis have been identified in patients with atrial flutter (78,79). Specifically, transverse conduction block across the crista terminalis occurs at longer cycle lengths in patients with atrial flutter. This difference may in part explain the absence of atrial flutter in all individuals. But it remains clear that block, probably functional, in a region between the vena cavae is critical to establish stable atrial flutter. Nevertheless, a recent study (80) dismissed the role of the crista terminalis as a critical boundary for atrial flutter. A functional line of block was described in the postero-medial right atrium in the sinus venosa region. This was observed in 28 consecutive patients with atrial flutter. Additional mapping studies are needed to resolve this controversy.

Other locations can support an atrial flutter reentrant circuit and have been identified in humans. These atrial flutter circuits may or may not use the subeustachian isthmus. Locations include (a) the right atrial free wall, (b) the pulmonary veins in the left atrium, (c) nonpulmonary vein sites in the left atrium, (d) lower-loop reentry breaking through the crista terminalis and using the subeustachian isthmus, and (e) double-wave reentry using the usual right atrial flutter reentrant circuit. Better mapping data from studies in humans may well improve our understanding of the various reentrant circuits observed in humans and animals (81,82).

Furthermore, most instances of atrial flutter are preceded by a period of atrial fibrillation, usually brief, during which time the functional components of the atrial flutter reentrant circuit form (83). Anchoring of the multiple reentrant circuits seen in atrial fibrillation to components of the atrial flutter circuit likely explains the transition from atrial fibrillation to flutter. Conversely, breakdown of one or more functional components of the previously stable flutter circuit via crista terminalis breakthrough as seen in lower-loop reentry or via another boundary in the circuit likely explains the transition from atrial flutter to fibrillation.

Classification

In view of the new information about atrial flutter as well as the explosion of terms to describe it, the European Society of Cardiology/North American Society of Pacing and Electrophysiology Working Group has offered a new classification based on mechanism (Table 65.1). [⊀ 157] Any reentrant circuit which requires use of the atrial flutter (subeustachian) isthmus is called *typical atrial flutter*. Usually in typical atrial flutter, the reentrant circuit travels up the septum and down the right atrial free wall (Fig. 65.2A). Atrial flutter that uses the same circuit but in the opposite direction is called *reverse typical atrial flutter*. Lower-loop reentry atrial flutter (Fig. 65.2B) and double-wave reentry atrial

flutter (Fig. 65.2C) also use the subeustachian isthmus and thus are classified as types of typical atrial flutter (87,88).

At least 90% of atrial flutters fall into the typical category. Atrial flutter in which the reentrant circuit is confined to the left atrium is called *left atrial flutter*. Reentry around an incisional line of block in the rate range of atrial flutter is called *lesion atrial reentry*. All other forms of reentrant atrial tachycardia in the rate range of atrial flutter that are not described by the above are called *atypical atrial flutter*.

Diagnosis

Electrocardiogram

Atrial flutter usually can be diagnosed from the ECG. Whenever atrial flutter is suspected, the diagnosis should be clearly established before initiating therapy unless the patient is clinically very unstable. Atrial flutter waves in the ECG, particularly sawtooth atrial complexes in leads II, III, and aVF, remain the standard for diagnosis of atrial flutter (Fig. 65.3). Flutter waves appear as atrial complexes of con-

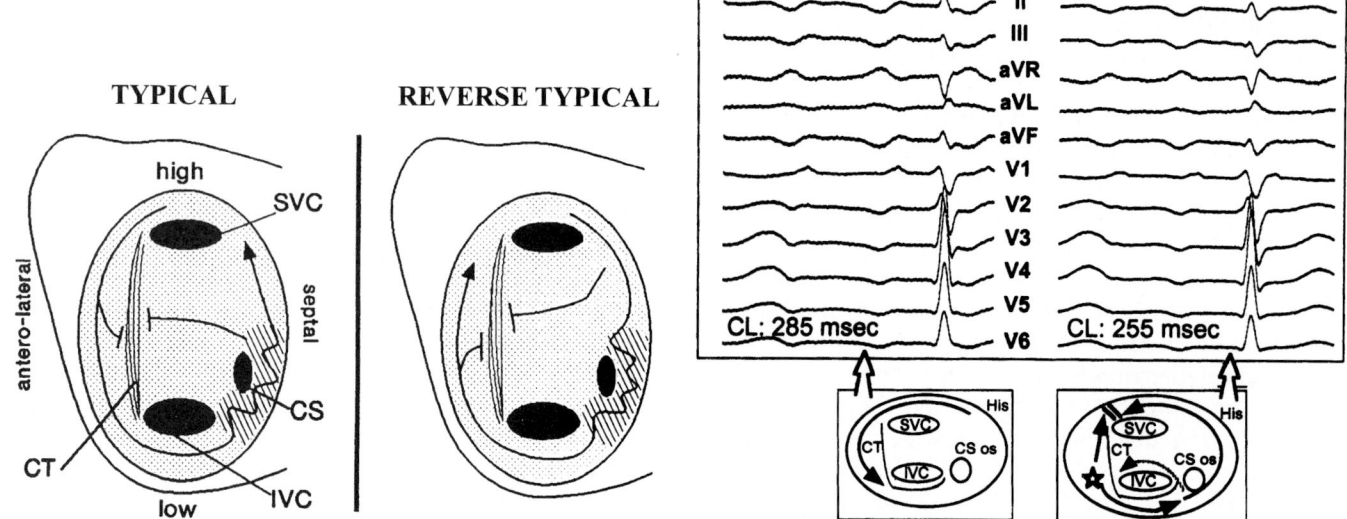

FIGURE 65.2 A: Schematic representation of typical and reverse typical atrial flutter circuits. The left anterior oblique view of the right atrium shows the endocardium through the tricuspid ring in a wide-angle perspective. The endocardium is shaded. The orifices of the superior and inferior caval veins (SVC and IVC) and coronary sinus (CS) are shown in black. The terminal crest (CT) is shown as a bundle of parallel lines linking the lateral aspects of the caval veins. The shaded area around the coronary sinus suggests the probable location of a slow conduction zone. Curved arrows indicate directions of activation. (Adapted from Cosio FG, Lopez-Gil M, Arribas F, Gonzalez HD. Mechanisms of induction of typical and reversed atrial flutter. *J Cardiovasc Electrophysiol* 1998;9:281–291.) **B:** Sustained spontaneous atrial flutter with two cycle lengths was observed in the same patient. Tracings on left show typical atrial flutter with a cycle length (CL) of 285 ms. Tracings on right show lower-loop reentry with a cycle length of 255 ms. Note the similar flutter wave morphologies despite different cycle lengths and different activation sequences, although there is a subtle difference in the terminal portion of the flutter waves in the inferior leads. Drawings depict the circuit anatomy. The hollow star delineates the breakthrough site, and the double line is the site of collision. His, His bundle. (Adapted from Cheng J, Cabeen WR, Scheinman MM. Right atrial flutter due to lower loop reentry, mechanism and anatomic substrates. *Circulation* 1999;99:1700–1705.) *(continued)*

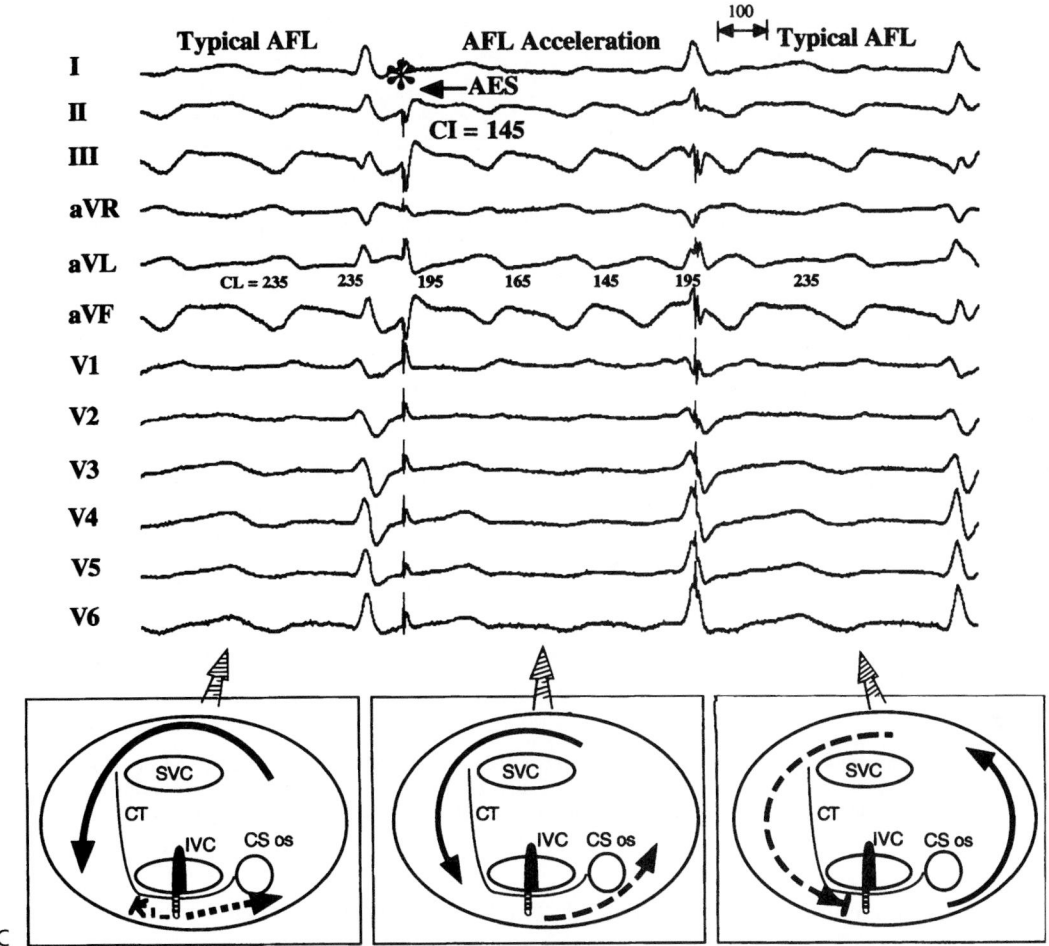

FIGURE 65.2 *Continued.* **C:** Critically timed atrial extrastimulus (AES) induced atrial flutter (AFL) acceleration. Surface 12-lead electrocardiogram showed P-wave morphology during AES-induced acceleration identical to that of flutter wave during spontaneous AFL. The accelerated flutter cycle length showed beat-to-beat variation (numbers are cycle length in milliseconds). The three diagrams schematically depict the positions of the activation wavefronts at induction, during, and at termination of double-wave reentry. Two wavefronts transiently are circulating in the typical AFL circuit and at the same time. Decremental conduction results in a cycle length greater than half the cycle length of the typical AFL circuit. (Adapted from Cheng J, Scheinmann MM. Acceleration of typical atrial flutter due to double-wave reentry induced by programmed electrical stimulation. *Circulation* 1998;97:1589–1596.)

stant morphology, polarity, and cycle length, with a rate ranging from 240 to 340 beats/min (85).

Typical and reverse typical atrial flutter can occur in the same patient at different times. Usually the reverse typical atrial flutter has a slower rate than the typical atrial flutter (Fig. 65.3.1). Atrial fibrillation with prominent (more than 0.2 mV) fibrillatory waves is often confused with atrial flutter (99). Care must be taken to ensure absolute regularity of atrial complexes before making a diagnosis of atrial flutter.

The atrial rate may be slower if the rhythm is present after therapy with antiarrhythmic drugs (i.e., class IA drugs, especially class IC drugs, moricizine, and amiodarone). If the ventricular response is half that of the atrial flutter rate, identifying the flutter waves on the ECG leads may be difficult due to temporal superimposition on other ECG deflections such as the QRS complex or the T wave.

As described in this section, the ventricular rate in atrial flutter is frequently 2:1 or 4:1 and is therefore regular. However, it may be irregular when there is variable AV conduction. Rarely, AV conduction may even be 1:1. The latter may be seen when an accessory AV connection is operative and may also be present in patients who have a very short PR interval during sinus rhythm. AV conduction may be enhanced during exertion, during therapy with catecholamines, or during administration of sympathomimetics for other underlying clinical problems. The ventricular response may paradoxically increase with slowing of the atrial flutter rate secondary to antiarrhythmic therapy (Fig. 65.4). ⚡ 158

Clinical Electrophysiologic Studies

For patients with paroxysms of tachycardia in whom atrial flutter is suspected but has yet to be documented, one of

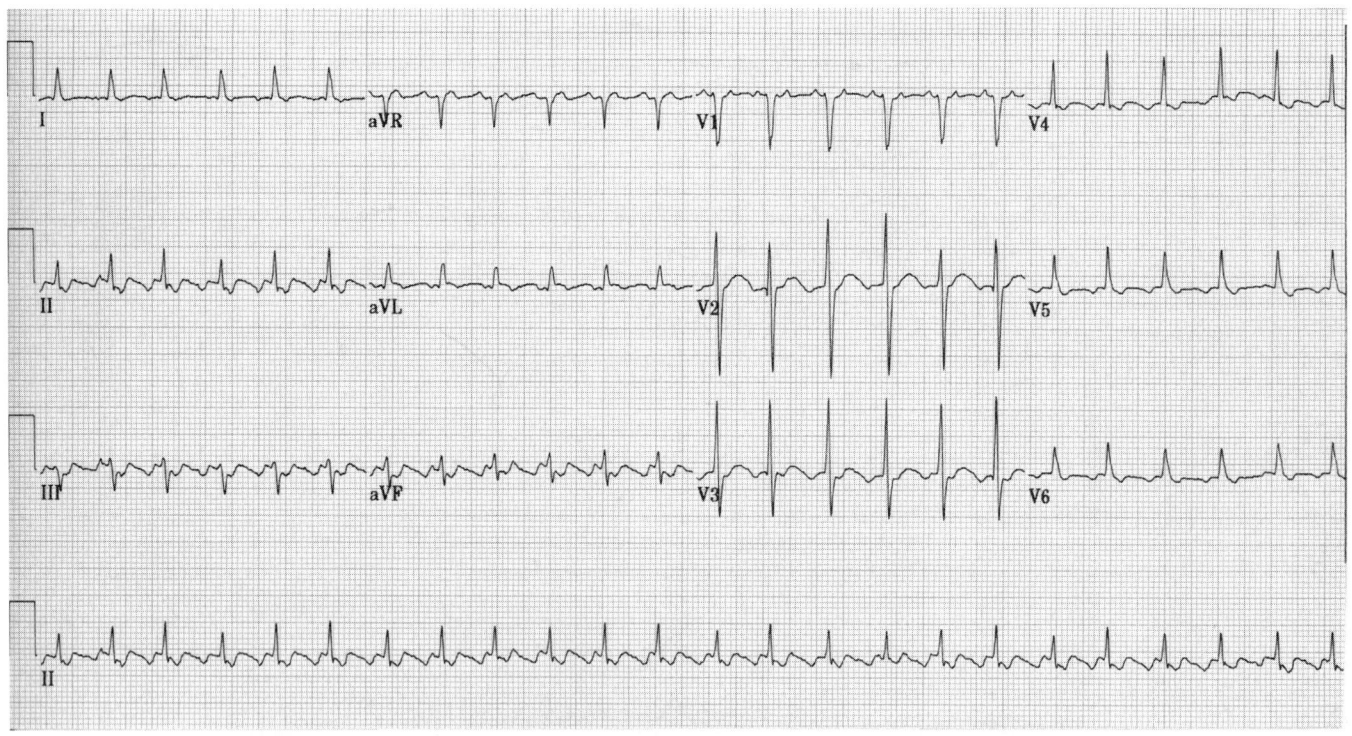

FIGURE 65.3 A 12-lead electrocardiogram of typical atrial flutter is shown. The atrial rate is 290 beats/min, and the ventricular rate is 145 beats/min; 2:1 atrioventricular conduction is present. Notice that the atrial activity is best seen in leads II, III, and aVF, but is barely perceptible in lead I.

several types of ECG monitoring is recommended. For most patients, particularly those with infrequent episodes of tachycardia, use of an event recorder is preferred to a 24-hour Holter monitor.

At present, electrophysiologic studies have become more important with the advent of catheter-based procedures to cure atrial flutter. Although no standards of programmed stimulation for the initiation of atrial flutter have evolved, the most reliable method is to pace the atria very rapidly to initiate atrial fibrillation and then await the evolution to atrial flutter (92). Initiation of atrial flutter by introducing premature atrial beats after a drive train is a much less reliable technique for inducing atrial flutter. Atrial pacing techniques may not reliably induce atrial flutter even in patients with a known history of atrial flutter.

Electrode catheter mapping studies (101) of atrial flutter are generally performed to help identify the location and type of the reentrant circuit. The mapping study must identify a vulnerable isthmus in the reentrant circuit that can be ablated to ensure success. In most patients with atrial flutter, such a location is thought to be the atrial flutter isthmus between the tricuspid valve orifice and the orifice of the inferior vena cava (19–21,71–73). However, as discussed previously, atrial flutter can operate independent of this isthmus (102,103). Techniques including entrainment mapping, electroanatomic mapping, and virtual electrode mapping play an important role in identifying the vulnerable isthmus.

Acute Treatment

Antiarrhythmic Drugs

When the diagnosis of atrial flutter is established, three acute nonablative options are available to restore sinus rhythm: (a) administer an antiarrhythmic drug, (b) initiate DC cardioversion, or (c) initiate rapid atrial pacing to interrupt atrial flutter. Treatment largely depends on the clinical status of the patient. In the past, the preferred option to interrupt atrial flutter was either DC cardioversion or rapid atrial pacing. However, the recent introduction of ibutilide provides another viable option, as use of that antiarrhythmic drug is associated with a 60% likelihood of converting recent onset atrial flutter to sinus rhythm (18). Antiarrhythmic drugs also may be used before initiating DC cardioversion or rapid atrial pacing for the following purposes:

1. To slow the ventricular response rate using a beta-blocker, a calcium channel blocker, digoxin, or some combination of these drugs
2. To enhance the efficacy of rapid atrial pacing in restoring sinus rhythm by using quinidine, procainamide, disopyramide, or ibutilide (104–106)
3. To enhance the likelihood that sinus rhythm will be maintained after effective DC cardioversion by using a class IA, class IC, or class III antiarrhythmic agent ⟍⟋ 159

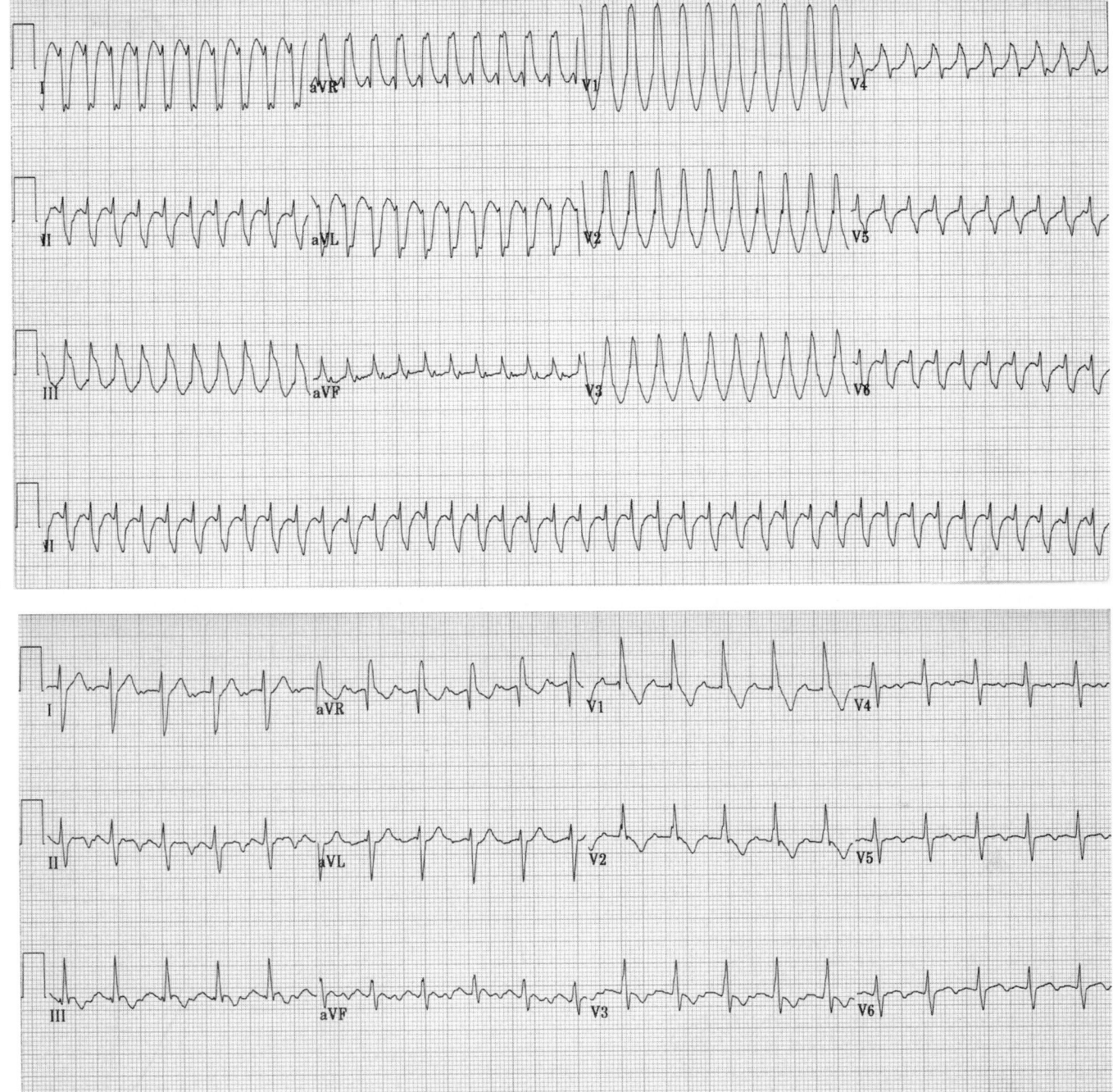

FIGURE 65.4 This patient presented 1 week after initiation of flecainide therapy for atrial flutter. **A** depicts 1:1 atrioventricular (AV) conduction. This was made possible by the slowing of the atrial rate (the pretherapy atrial rate was 300 beats/min with 2:1 AV conduction), now permitting 1:1 AV conduction, which "paradoxically" increased the ventricular rate. **B** was obtained 5 minutes later after therapy with esmolol, which decreased the ventricular response due to 2:1 AV conduction.

Direct Current Cardioversion/Rapid Atrial Pacing

Selecting DC cardioversion, atrial pacing, or antiarrhythmic drugs for acute treatment of atrial flutter depends on the clini-cal presentation of the patient and on both the clinical availability and ease of applying these techniques. DC cardioversion requires administration of an anesthetic agent. Therefore, this approach may be undesirable in patients who have recently eaten or in patients who have severe lung disease. These patients usually are best treated with antiarrhythmic drugs, rapid atrial pacing, or agents to slow the ventricular response rate. For patients with atrial flutter after open-heart surgery, the use of temporary atrial epicardial electrodes to perform rapid atrial pacing is clearly the treatment of choice (112,113).

Long-Term Treatment

Improvements in the efficacy of catheter-ablation techniques and the long-recognized difficulty in achieving adequate chronic suppression of atrial flutter with drugs have significantly altered the approach to long-term treatment of atrial flutter. In short, if in any patient atrial flutter is an important problem, characterization of the mechanism of atrial flutter followed by catheter ablation (cure) is now recommended.

Antiarrhythmic Drugs

For many years, standard therapy used the class IA antiarrhythmic agents (i.e., quinidine, procainamide, or disopyramide) to prevent recurrence. However, the type IC antiarrhythmic drugs, flecainide and propafenone, appear to be equally, if not more, effective than class IA drugs (15,16). Class IC agents are generally better tolerated and likely have less organ toxicity than class IA agents. Primarily because of serious adverse effects demonstrated in the Cardiac Arrhythmia Suppression Trial I (117), class IC agents should not be used in patients with underlying ischemic heart disease. This notion has generally been extrapolated to include underlying structural heart disease. However, class IC agents should be considered early on for long-term suppression in patients without structural heart disease.

Moricizine, a class I drug with A, B, and C properties, also may be effective in treating atrial flutter (118). The long-term data from the Cardiac Arrhythmia Suppression Trial II (119) suggested that moricizine and placebo were no different in terms of mortality. Thus, moricizine may be a good choice for patients with atrial flutter and coronary artery disease late (more than 6 months) after myocardial infarction. More data are required to establish efficacy in this clinical setting.

Class III antiarrhythmic agents may also be quite effective (16,17). When using sotalol, care must be taken to avoid QT interval prolongation beyond 500 ms (120) and precipitation of torsades de pointes. Amiodarone appears to be quite effective (17), but several toxicities make widespread use of this drug to treat atrial flutter problematic (121). In fact, several large placebo-controlled studies using low-dose amiodarone (200 mg per day) (although not in patients with atrial flutter) have demonstrated dropout rates as high as 45.0% (122) and 42.5% (123). Thus, using amiodarone as the first-choice drug should be limited to patients with depressed LV function (i.e., an ejection fraction of less than 25%). The safety and efficacy of several other new type III antiarrhythmic agents are currently being evaluated. Dofetilide has recently been marketed

for treatment of patients with atrial flutter and fibrillation. Recurrence rates of atrial arrhythmias were similar to sotalol. Like sotalol, caution with regard to QT prolongation and the hazard of torsades de pointes is warranted.

The overall perspective remains that atrial flutter is quite difficult to suppress with drug therapy. In fact, based on available long-term data, drug therapy offers a limited ability to maintain sinus rhythm without occasional to frequent recurrences, even when multiple agents are used (124). Thus, when evaluating drug therapy, an important measure of efficacy should be the frequency of recurrent atrial flutter rather than a single recurrent episode. For instance, recurrence only at long intervals (e.g., once or twice per year) should be classified as successful therapy.

Anticoagulants

The risk of stroke associated with atrial flutter is of concern. An early study (125) found neither evidence of atrial clot formation nor stroke associated with atrial flutter in a relatively small cohort of patients after open-heart surgery. No large prospective studies have been performed to confirm this finding in other patient populations. However, several recent studies (126–128) indicate that an increased risk of stroke is present in patients with atrial flutter.

Analysis of a Medicare cohort of 17,000 patients with atrial flutter (96) demonstrated a significant increase in the risk of stroke relative to a control population. This risk was concentrated entirely in those patients with atrial flutter who later experienced atrial fibrillation (Fig. 65.5). Unfortunately, no combination of clinical factors in this study could predict which patients with atrial flutter would develop atrial fibrilla-

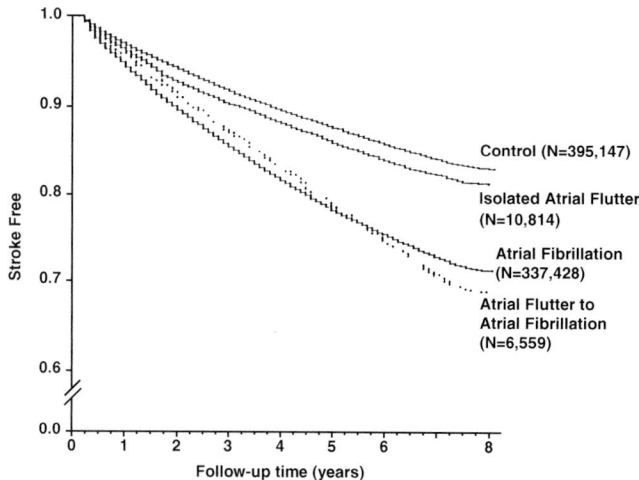

FIGURE 65.5 Medicare patients with an index hospitalization for atrial flutter were followed and compared with atrial fibrillation and control cohorts. The risk of stroke was concentrated almost entirely in the atrial flutter patients, who were rehospitalized at a later time with atrial fibrillation. (From Biblo LA, Yuan Z, Quan KJ, et al. Risk of stroke in patients with atrial flutter. *Am J Cardiol* 2001;87:346–349, with permission.)

tion. At present there is no consensus statement on the use of anticoagulation in patients with atrial flutter, whether it be acute, ablated, recurrent, or chronic. However, given the above studies, administering warfarin therapy to achieve an international normalized ratio of 2 to 3 is strongly recommended. Anticoagulation for the acute cardioversion of atrial flutter should require the same standards as used for the acute cardioversion of atrial fibrillation.

Catheter Ablation

Catheter ablation primarily uses radiofrequency energy delivered to selected portions of the heart by an electrode catheter. Initially, success in atrial flutter ablation was reportedly at 60% to 70%, with subsequent recurrence rates of approximately 50% (19,20). However, recent advances in both mapping and ablation techniques have improved efficacy rates to approximately 95%, with little subsequent risk of recurrence (129–131).

Catheter ablation first involves mapping the atria during atrial flutter to identify a critical isthmus of slow conduction in the atrial flutter reentrant circuit. When this area is identified, usually the atrial flutter isthmus, ablative energy is delivered to create a line of bidirectional block. This isthmus has irregular topography and therefore in some cases may be difficult to ablate successfully. In fact, it was believed that this was the principal cause of most ablation failures. However, combined pacing and mapping techniques have improved, allowing for the reliable determination of complete bidirectional conduction block in this region (132–135).

It must be emphasized that electrode catheter mapping and pacing are necessary not only to demonstrate the completeness of block in the atrial flutter isthmus, but also to confirm the critical participation of the atrial flutter isthmus. Although most types of atrial flutter are isthmus-dependent, atrial flutter can also be due to reentry in the right atrial free wall or in the left atrium. Finally, successful ablation of the atrial flutter reentrant circuit usually does not prevent the occurrence of atrial fibrillation (136,137).

Recently, a catheter ablation experience was reported in patients with left atrial flutter (138). Complete atrial mapping was used to identify a vulnerable isthmus for ablation. Variability was present in circuit locations; however, a left atrial "silent area" characterized most patients with this entity. The area of presumed atrial fibrosis appeared to create a lateral border, stabilizing rotation around the mitral valve.

Ablation has proven effective in lesion reentry atrial tachycardia, as well. In these patients, the lesion is often due to an atriotomy scar after a remote cardiac surgical procedure. Radiofrequency energy is used to extend the scar to a fixed anatomic border (often the tricuspid valve). Thus, rotation of the reentrant circuit around the scar is no longer possible, and the patient is cured of this tachycardia.

For patients in whom the atrial flutter is resistant to catheter ablation, reassessment of the mechanism of the atrial flutter must ensue. Entrainment techniques should be repeated to ensure the proper circuits and mechanisms have been delineated. Resistant atrial flutter (139) is often due to abnormalities in the atrial flutter isthmus region. Anatomic formations such as an unusually large isthmus or a deep, corrugated subeustachian pouch may be present. High-gain, low-noise signals are required to adequately record conduction gaps. Failure rates have declined greatly as a result of these careful and systematic approaches to atrial flutter ablation.

Summary

Atrial flutter is primarily due to reentrant excitation in the right atrium using the subeustachian isthmus. The 12-lead ECG remains the cornerstone for clinical diagnosis. Acute treatment requires control of the ventricular rate and, if possible, restoration of sinus rhythm. Antiarrhythmic drugs to suppress recurrent episodes of atrial flutter may prove useful but are now clearly second-tier therapy in symptomatic patients with atrial flutter. At present, catheter ablation provides a definitive cure, although atrial fibrillation may occur after a successful ablative procedure.

ATRIAL TACHYCARDIA

Background and Classification

The term *atrial tachycardia* encompasses several types of tachycardias that originate in the atria. In the past, classification schemes were largely descriptive and included terms such as *paroxysmal* or *incessant atrial tachycardia* and *atrial tachycardia with block*. Now the term *atrial tachycardia* refers to relatively regular arrhythmias that originate in the atria, do not require participation of the AV node for maintenance, and are neither atrial flutter nor atrial fibrillation. The subclassifications of atrial tachycardia are based on the mechanisms involved and include reentrant atrial tachycardia, ectopic automatic tachycardia, and triggered atrial tachycardia.

Mechanisms of Atrial Tachycardia

It is generally accepted that there are three different mechanisms responsible for atrial tachycardia: (a) intraatrial reentry, (b) ectopic automaticity, and (c) triggered activity due to delayed afterdepolarizations (DADs). Surprisingly, the details of the reentrant circuit in atrial tachycardia have not been well studied. Consequently, the characteristics of the reentrant circuit are not well delineated.

Atrial tachycardia due to an ectopic automatic focus also has not been well studied. The tachycardias described to date appear to be generated by a focus or foci that cluster around the crista terminalis in the right atrium and around the base of the pulmonary veins in the left atrium

(140,141). These tachycardias can be neither initiated nor terminated by atrial pacing.

Triggered activity as a mechanism of atrial tachycardia is thought to be due to DADs largely from digitalis toxicity, but catecholamines can also precipitate atrial tachycardia induced by this mechanism (142). DADs caused by catecholamines have been recorded in the canine heart by microelectrodes placed in atrial fibers of the mitral valve (143), in atrial fibers lining the coronary sinus (144), and in atrial fibers in the inferior right atrium (145). They have also been recorded in human hearts with CM (146).

A recent publication (147) has classified atrial tachycardias as focal or macroreentrant. Focal tachycardia was defined on the basis of (a) centrifugal activation pattern, (b) dissociation of nearly the entire right and left atria from the tachycardia with programmed atrial extra-stimuli, (c) and the absence of entrainment criteria. Macroreentry was defined if initiated or terminated with programmed stimulation and one of the following: (a) continuous electrical activity throughout the cardiac cycle with low-amplitude fractionated signals or (b) any of the entrainment criteria.

The focal versus macroreentrant classification is of benefit in the electrophysiology laboratory but cannot be directly extrapolated to "macroreentrant equals intraatrial reentry" and "focal equals triggered or automatic." Features consistent with automatic atrial tachycardia were failure to initiate or terminate with programmed stimulation, transient suppression with adenosine, and insensitivity to verapamil. Features consistent with triggered activity were repetitive monomorphic atrial tachycardia, initiation and termination with programmed stimulation, and sensitivity to adenosine and verapamil. Most, but not all, macroreentrant atrial tachycardias were insensitive to adenosine. Those macroreentrant tachycardias that terminated with adenosine were believed to use decremental tissue (outside the AV node).

A new mechanism has also recently been reported: lidocaine-sensitive atrial tachycardia (148). This report describes eight patients with a unique atrial arrhythmia that was suppressed by lidocaine. The arrhythmia could not be initiated or terminated with pacing, making reentry less likely. The arrhythmia occurred at slow heart rates and did not respond to verapamil, making DADs less likely. Overdrive suppression was absent, making automaticity unlikely. The authors speculate that early DAD-like activity in the atria may be responsible for this entity.

Epidemiology and Clinical Significance

The incidence of atrial tachycardia appears to increase with age, reportedly occurring in up to 13% of elderly patients (149–151). An increased incidence has been reported in patients with myocardial infarction (152,153), nonischemic heart disease (154,155), obstructive lung disease (156), serum electrolyte disorders, and drug toxicity, especially from digitalis (157,158). However, atrial tachycardia may occur in healthy

individuals (159,160), and nonsustained episodes have been noted in 2% of healthy young adults (161,162). Most episodes of atrial tachycardia are paroxysmal (usually due to reentry or triggered activity), but some may be incessant (usually due to enhanced automaticity) (163). In patients with incessant tachycardia, a tachycardia-induced CM may result.

Diagnosis

The initial diagnosis of atrial tachycardia is made by the atrial rate (usually 140 to 240 beats/min), on analysis of the 12-lead ECG. However, the range of both the atrial and the ventricular rates may overlap with that of AV nodal–dependent tachycardias and sinus tachycardia. Atrial tachycardia may be confused with atrial flutter if AV conduction is 2:1.

A standard way to determine the presence or absence of an AV nodal–independent atrial tachycardia is to demonstrate that with AV conduction block, the rhythm continues (Fig. 65.6). However, as seen from the following discussion, the confounding effects of many diagnostic interventions can make such differentiation quite difficult.

Intraatrial Reentry

In patients with reentrant atrial tachycardia, the rhythm generally can be induced by programmed electrical stimulation. During the arrhythmia, the criteria for either manifest or concealed entrainment usually can be demonstrated, and the interval between the initiating beat and the first beat of the atrial tachycardia is usually inversely related (165). These observations strongly suggest a reentrant mechanism.

As noted in this chapter, terminating a supraventricular tachycardia by a drug that causes transient conduction block (second-degree or third-degree) at the AV node generally would be expected to suggest a diagnosis of an underlying AV nodal–dependent reentrant tachycardia. However, in one reported study (165), adenosine terminated 24 of 27 ostensibly reentrant tachycardias, although in another study (167), in none of the five patients with intraatrial reentrant tachycardia did administration of adenosine affect the tachycardia. The different responses to adenosine observed in these two studies emphasize the need to characterize these rhythms more thoroughly. In any event, termination of an atrial tachyarrhythmia after intravenous administration of adenosine cannot be used per se to characterize the rhythm as AV nodal–dependent. The same seems to be true for beta-blockers, as their use terminated an ostensibly reentrant atrial tachycardia in 13 of 20 patients in one study (165), although they had no effect in three patients reported in another study (167).

Automatic Atrial Tachycardia

Automatic atrial tachycardia may be induced during treadmill testing or after administration of isoproterenol (165,167). Predictably, programmed atrial stimulation will

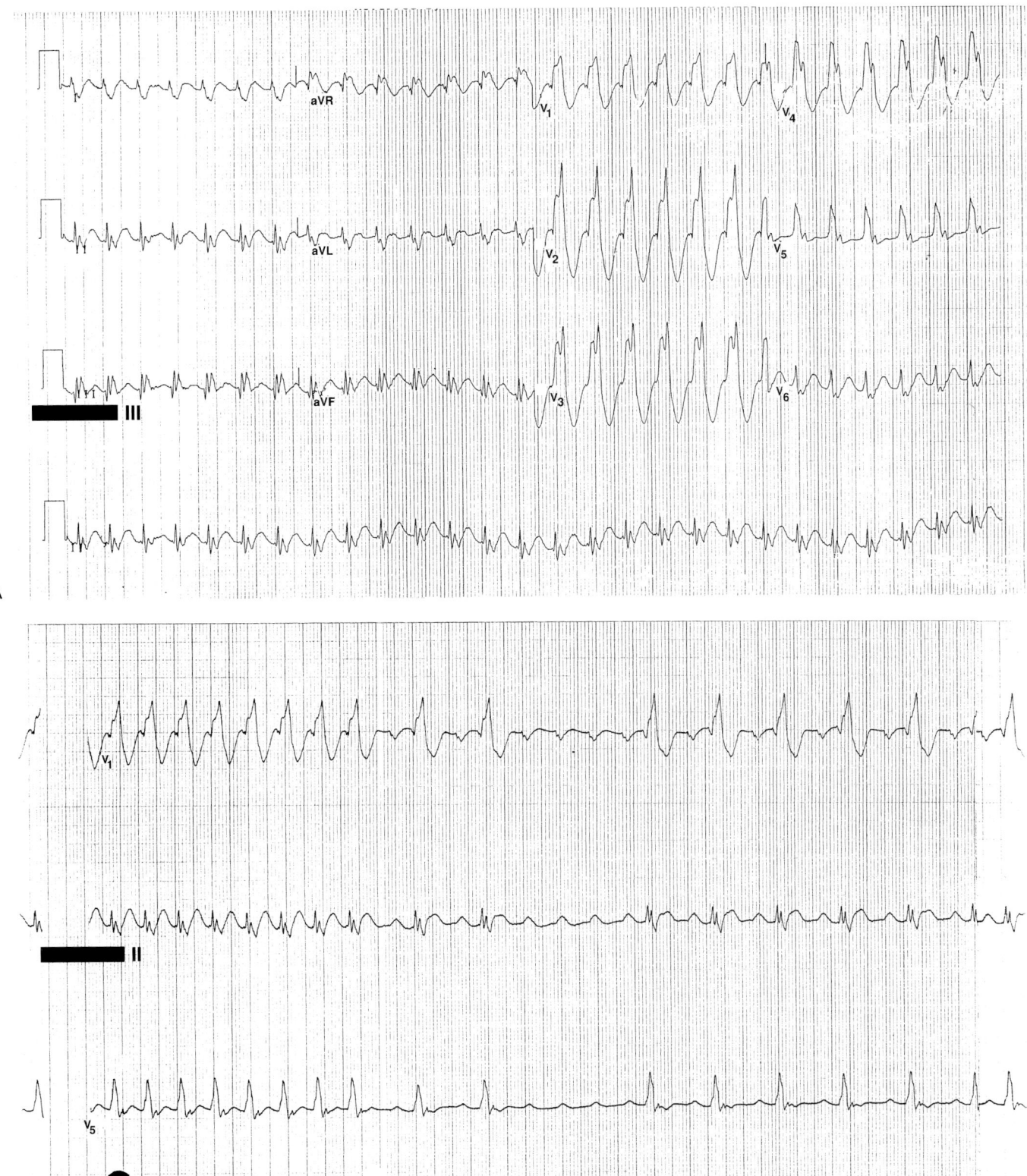

FIGURE 65.6 A: A 12-lead electrocardiogram was recorded in a 37-year-old man 29 years after repair of tetralogy of Fallot. The patient noted recurrent palpitation associated with lightheadedness. This 12-lead electrocardiogram documented a tachycardia in which the QRS complex morphology was quite similar to that recorded during sinus rhythm. No P waves could be readily identified. **B:** A Valsalva maneuver induced transient, high-degree atrioventricular block. The underlying atrial tachycardia (cycle length of 360 ms) was then easily demonstrated.

neither initiate nor terminate atrial tachycardia due to this mechanism (145). Propranolol has been shown to suppress putative automatic atrial tachycardias, but neither verapamil nor adenosine has been shown to do so. However, adenosine may transiently slow the atrial rate (165,167).

Triggered Atrial Tachycardia

Triggered atrial tachycardia can be initiated by rapid atrial pacing and has been shown to be cycle length–dependent (165). The onset of the arrhythmia induced by pacing is not pause-dependent. Because these rhythms can be caused by catecholamines, it should not be surprising that isoproterenol and treadmill testing may initiate this form of atrial tachycardia in some patients. Monophasic action potential recording may suggest DADs, and entrainment criteria should not be present. Verapamil and adenosine have been shown to terminate this form of atrial tachycardia.

Summary

The small number of published studies indicates the complexity of identifying the correct underlying mechanism of an atrial tachycardia. Invasive electrophysiologic studies have become an important tool in characterizing the mechanism of this arrhythmia. Induction by programmed stimulation with fulfillment of any of the criteria for entrainment lends support to a reentrant mechanism. The inability to induce or entrain the arrhythmia suggests, but does not prove, either an automatic or triggered mechanism. Thus, when programmed stimulation cannot induce the arrhythmia, successful termination with adenosine suggests a triggered etiology, whereas slowing of the arrhythmia by adenosine suggests an automatic mechanism. Additional insights can be garnered by mapping studies.

Treatment

Reentrant Atrial Tachycardia: Catheter Ablation

For reentrant atrial tachycardia, catheter ablation is now the primary therapy for symptomatic patients. However, radiofrequency ablation appears to be more challenging in these patients than in patients with atrial flutter because the location of the reentrant circuit is not as anatomically consistent as that in most patients with atrial flutter (141). Regardless, if a vulnerable isthmus in a reentrant circuit is found, ablation should prove effective. Reports on catheter ablation for reentrant atrial tachycardia have suggested a success rate of more than 75% (168,169).

Reentrant Atrial Tachycardia: Antiarrhythmic Drugs

Antiarrhythmic drug therapy for reentrant atrial tachycardia is similar to that for atrial flutter and atrial fibrillation. The important message is that overall efficacy as measured by simple recurrence is poor because this rhythm tends to recur in at least half of patients treated. The measure of drug efficacy should be the frequency of recurrence. Occasional arrhythmic recurrences may be quite acceptable in these patients because recurrences are rarely life-threatening and are usually well tolerated. Thus, should the arrhythmia recur and if it does not revert spontaneously, cardioversion to sinus rhythm should be considered. The patient should then be followed on the same antiarrhythmic regimen. When recurrences are too frequent or intolerable, the pharmacologic regimen should be changed. Finally, reentrant atrial tachycardia can be acutely treated with rapid atrial pacing techniques virtually identical to those used to treat atrial flutter.

Nonreentrant Atrial Tachycardia

Patients with nonreentrant atrial tachycardia who have minimal symptoms should be treated with either a beta-blocker or a calcium channel blocker. Automatic atrial tachycardia appears more responsive to beta-blockers, whereas triggered arrhythmias appear to respond best to calcium channel blockers. Extrapolation from acute studies suggests that such therapy is logical (Fig. 65.7). For patients in whom the tachycardia is due to digitalis toxicity, the dose of digitalis should either be stopped or reduced. In patients with clinically important symptomatic or incessant nonreentrant atrial tachycardia, catheter ablation is preferred. A combination of pace mapping, entrainment analyses, and identification of the earliest atrial activation site at electrophysiologic study are complementary methods to ensure an excellent ablative result. Long-term results are excellent (170).

Summary

Atrial tachycardia encompasses a wide spectrum of clinical presentations and mechanisms. Current classification schemes focus on mechanism. Therapy should be aggressive for those patients with significant symptoms, and whenever possible radiofrequency ablation is preferable. Despite the mechanistic heterogeneity of atrial tachycardia, radiofrequency catheter ablation is usually successful. Drug therapy remains an acceptable alternative for minimally symptomatic patients with an atrial tachyarrhythmia.

INAPPROPRIATE SINUS TACHYCARDIA

Background

Sinus tachycardia [⛌ 160] is usually the result of an appropriate reflex-controlled response. In adults, *sinus tachycardia* is defined as a rhythm originating from the sinus node at a rate of more than 100 beats/min. The normal maximum heart rate achieved by adults during strenuous exercise is rarely

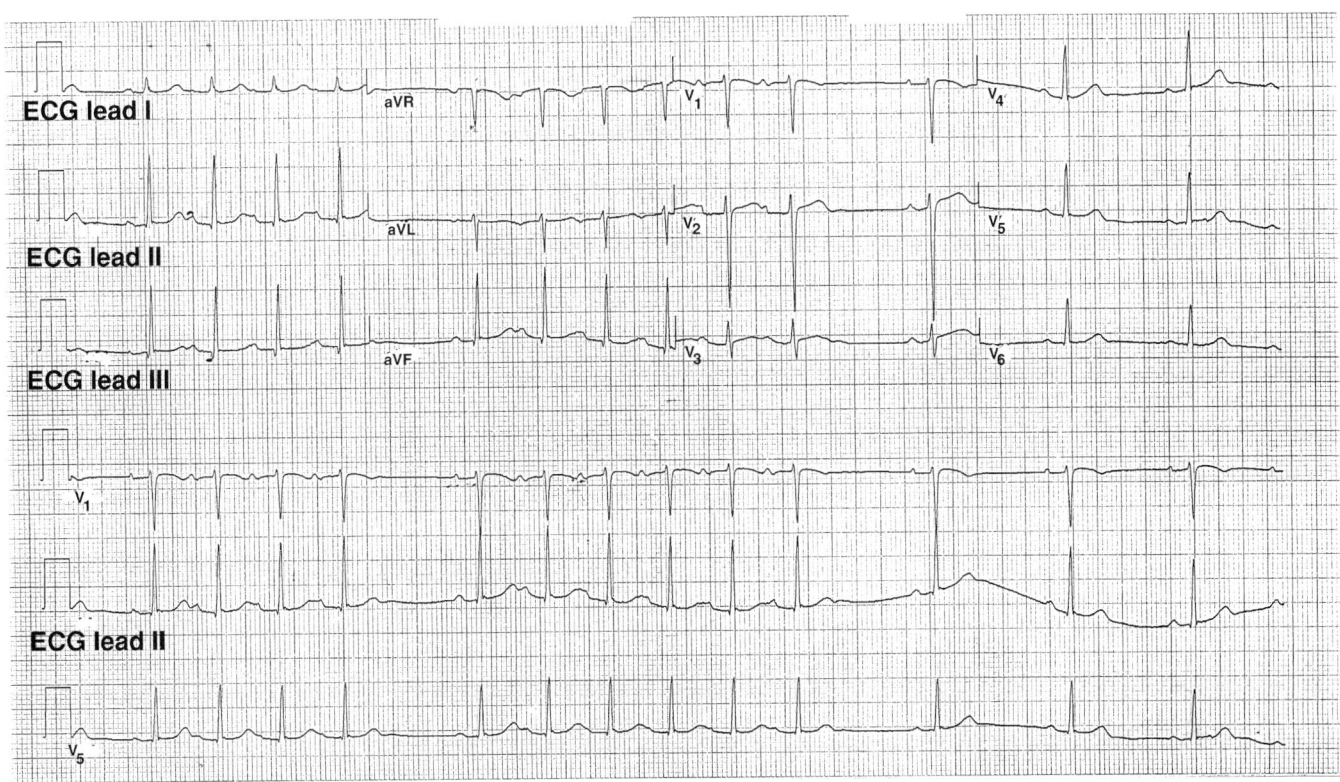

FIGURE 65.7 A 27-year-old woman complained of episodic palpitation. The 12-lead electrocardiogram (ECG) documented salvos of an atrial tachycardia. An echocardiogram was normal. At electrophysiologic study, an arrhythmia was not induced by programmed stimulation. Initial therapy with a beta-blocker proved ineffective, but subsequent therapy with diltiazem resulted in complete suppression of the arrhythmia.

more than 180 beats/min, and it can be calculated using the formula of 220 minus the patient's age (years). Sometimes during sinus tachycardia, the P-wave morphology in the ECG may change subtly compared with that during sinus rhythm. Such changes associated with rate are thought to represent a shift in the location of the dominant pacemaker cells in the sinus node area, with a consequent change in the initial excitation of the atrium. Treatment of appropriate sinus tachycardia rarely is directed at the sinus node pacemaker, but rather at the underlying trigger. Thus, management first focuses on identifying and then treating the underlying precipitant. A long list of potential causes of appropriate sinus tachycardia includes infection, hypotension, anemia, dehydration, hyperthyroidism, and pheochromocytoma.

In recent years, a syndrome originally called *nonparoxysmal sinus tachycardia* (172), but now called *inappropriate sinus tachycardia*, has been described (173). This entity is characterized by an incessant and symptomatic sinus tachycardia due to inappropriately enhanced automaticity of sinus node pacemaker cells.

Potential Mechanisms

There is only limited information available about the potential mechanisms of inappropriate sinus tachycardia

because only a small number of patients have been studied and reported. One study (172) in which inappropriate sinus tachycardia was defined as an atrial rate of more than 100 beats/min on all waking ECGs for 3 months with no demonstrable underlying cause described seven patients with this syndrome. Each patient underwent invasive electrophysiologic testing to exclude a reentrant arrhythmia. Based on resting heart rate responses to propranolol, excessive sympathetic tone was noted in two patients, and deficient resting vagal tone was noted in the other five patients. Three of the seven patients demonstrated an abnormal intrinsic heart rate. The P-wave morphology on the 12-lead ECG was normal.

Another study (173) described six patients with this syndrome. Inappropriate sinus tachycardia was defined as the following:

1. An atrial rate of 100 beats/min or more at rest or with minimal activity
2. A normal P-wave axis and morphology on 12-lead ECG during tachycardia
3. Absence of an underlying cause

The cardiovagal response in these patients as judged by the cold pressor test was blunted compared with that in normal patients. Hypersensitivity to isoproterenol was noted in all patients. A high intrinsic heart rate (mean of 129 beats/min) was noted in all patients after administration of intravenous propranolol and atropine. Based on the results of complete autonomic blockade, Morillo et al. (173) concluded that the major abnormality in this syndrome appears to be a primary sinus node abnormality exacerbated by autonomic dysfunction.

In still another study of 16 patients (174), the resting sinus rate was not significantly different from the resting heart rate after catheter ablation of the sinus node (85.5 ± 7.8 beats/min versus 79.0 ± 4.9 beats/min). However, the mean baseline measurement of intrinsic heart rate (118.6 ± 8.6 beats/min) was significantly higher than the mean predicted intrinsic heart rate (97.7 ± 1.7 beats/min; $p <.01$). However, the intrinsic heart rate was within normal range in five of the 11 patients who had a baseline measurement. Patients who underwent exercise treadmill tests had an inappropriate chronotropic response to a light workload (mean heart rate of 141.2 ± 5.1 beats/min after only 1.5 minutes of stage 1 of the Bruce protocol).

In summary, the mechanism of this entity is not well understood, and there is a clear need for improved understanding. It appears that inappropriate sinus tachycardia may be due to enhanced automaticity of sinus node pacemaker cells, a dysautonomia, or both. The dysautonomia appears to include beta-adrenergic hypersensitivity and depression of the efficient cardiovagal reflex, often superimposed on an abnormally high intrinsic heart rate.

Epidemiology and Clinical Significance

Patients with inappropriate sinus tachycardia usually are relatively young and have an abnormally high resting heart rate. This rate increases disproportionately with activity. Patients frequently are disabled by persistent palpitations, extreme dyspnea, chronic fatigue, and near syncope. It is noteworthy that patients frequently have been called neurotic. To date, many of the patients described with this syndrome have been health care employees. Patients reported to date (173,174) have been overwhelmingly female. The heart rate varies with activity but appears to be set 30 to 40 beats/min higher than normal. Surreptitious drug use and Munchausen syndrome must be excluded. During sinus tachycardia, stroke volume is maintained due to a complex interplay of neurohumoral reflexes and changes in peripheral resistance. Thus, in contrast to other atrial tachyarrhythmias, adverse hemodynamic findings are infrequently observed during sinus tachycardia despite rapid rates. Nevertheless, with sustained rapid ventricular rates, a dilated CM may evolve. Although no instances of an inappropriate sinus tachycardia–induced CM have been reported, we have treated one patient with inappropriate sinus tachycardia and an idiopathic CM. In this patient, LV ejection fraction improved from 44% to 67% after radiofrequency modification of the sinus node with associated normalization of the heart rate. The patient also

improved clinically from New York Heart Association class III heart failure to class I heart failure.

Diagnosis

To diagnose inappropriate sinus tachycardia, the following criteria should be satisfied:

1. The resting heart rate should be 100 beats/min or more or should increase to 100 beats/min or more with minimal exertion (e.g., when rising from the sitting position or when walking slowly).
2. The P-wave morphology and axis in the 12-lead ECG during the tachycardia should be quite similar or, better still, identical to that during sinus rhythm.
3. Secondary causes of sinus tachycardia (e.g., fever, anemia) should be excluded.
4. Symptoms of palpitation, presyncope, or both should be documented to be related to resting or easily provoked sinus tachycardia to differentiate inappropriate sinus tachycardia from severely deconditioned individuals who may otherwise fulfill the above criteria.

Additional testing should prove helpful. Thus, electrophysiologic testing should demonstrate that the tachyarrhythmia could not be initiated or terminated by atrial pacing techniques. In addition, atrial mapping should show that the tachycardia originates from the sinus node region. Producing autonomic blockade to identify the so-called intrinsic sinus rate may not prove helpful to diagnosis because approximately half of patients with this syndrome may have a normal intrinsic sinus rate, which supports the notion that this syndrome may have more than one etiology.

Treatment

Finding effective drug therapy for patients with this syndrome is often quite difficult. However, beta-blockers appear to be the most effective for ameliorating symptoms by normalizing heart rate. Effectiveness of therapy is best judged by serial 24-hour ambulatory ECGs (Holter monitor). Sinus node ablation or modification using radiofrequency energy and electrode catheter techniques recently has proven to be effective (174,175). Ablation of the sinus node appears to be more effective when guided by activation mapping (176) to identify the appropriate endocardial ablation sites. Successful sinus node ablation is often associated with a superior shift in the P-wave axis (Fig. 65.7.2). Long-term results vary considerably from institution to institution, with success in up to 66% of patients.

Summary

Inappropriate sinus tachycardia is a newly described entity that appears to be rare. The entity remains largely descriptive but may be due to a dysautonomia or a primary sinus node abnormality. Before initiating definitive therapy, the physician must carefully search for an underlying precipitant.

SINUS NODE REENTRANT TACHYCARDIA

Background

Sinus node reentrant tachycardia is believed to be due to reentry within the tissue in or near the sinus node. This tachycardia is characterized by an atrial rate of 105 to 150 beats/min and a P-wave morphology in the ECG similar to that of sinus rhythm (Fig. 65.8). Marked variation in cycle length during tachycardia is very common.

Mechanism

As is evident from its name, this rhythm is due to reentry involving the sinus node and perinodal tissue. It usually can be reproduced during electrophysiologic study using stan-

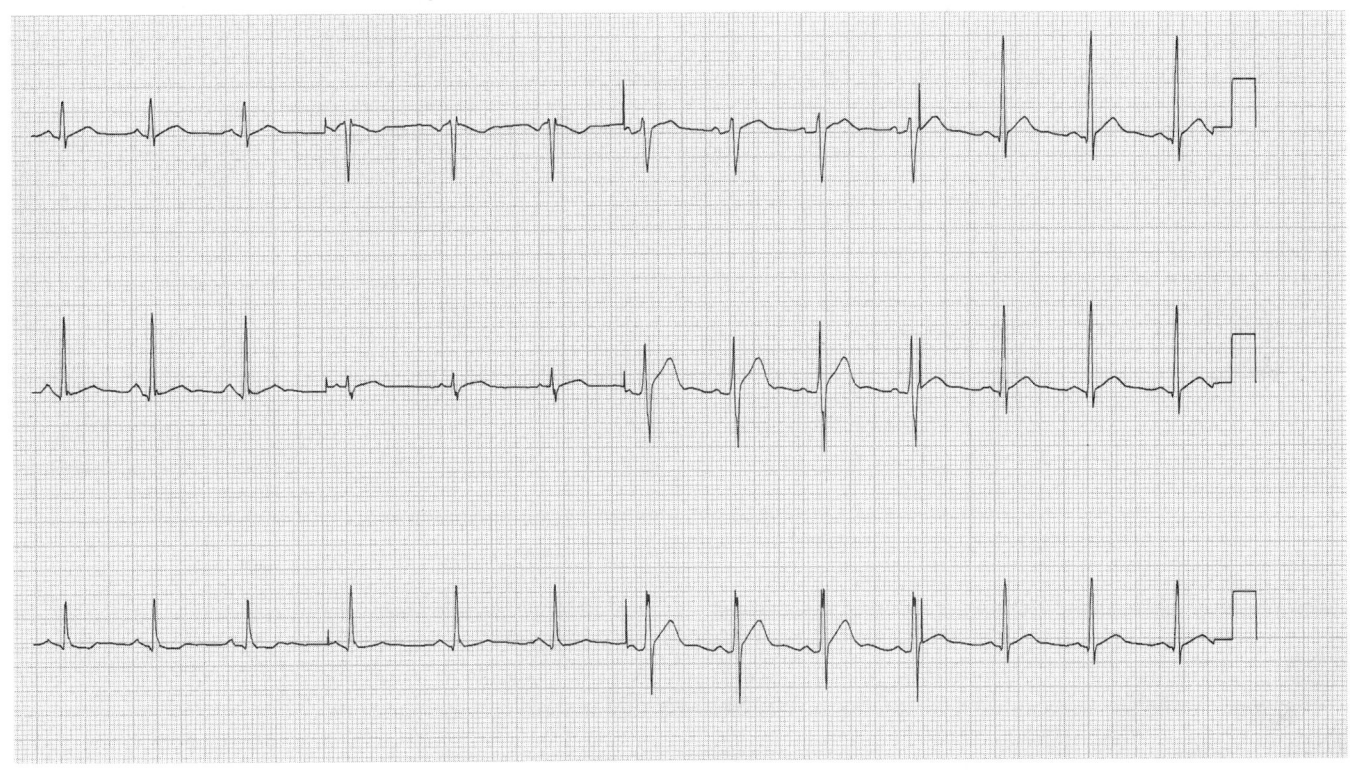

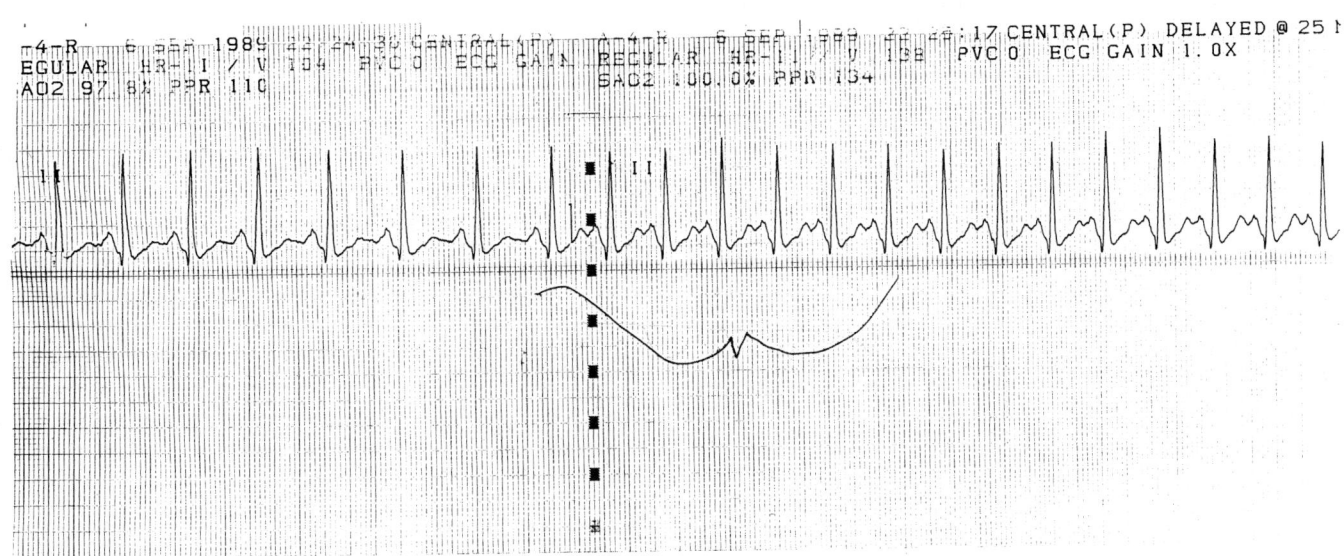

FIGURE 65.8 A: A 64-year-old man complained of episodic palpitation. A baseline 12-lead electrocardiogram (ECG) documented normal sinus rhythm. **B:** A telemetry strip documented the abrupt onset of tachycardia, which proved to be due to sinus node reentry. (*continued*)

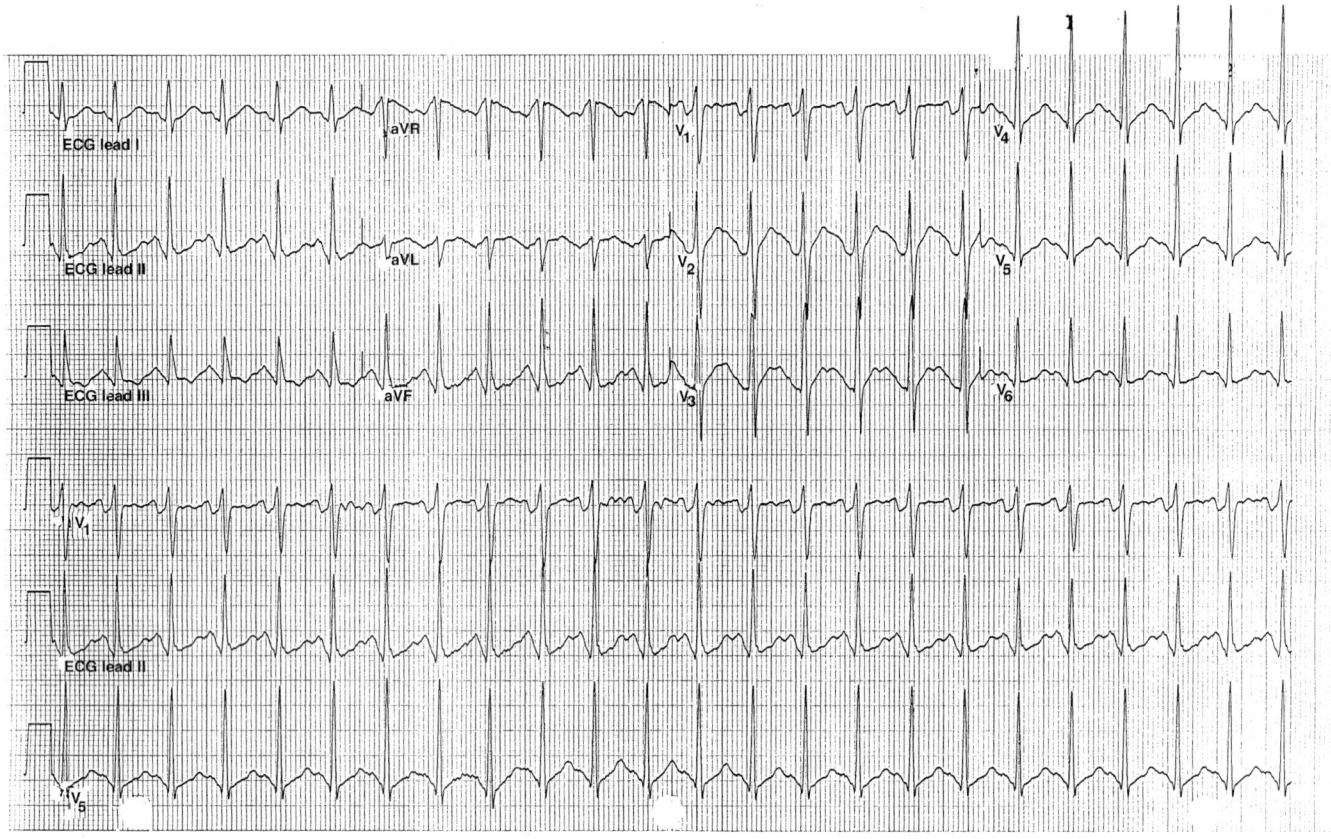

FIGURE 65.8 *Continued.* **C:** A 12-lead ECG obtained during palpitation showed that the P-wave morphology was quite similar to that on the baseline ECG.

dard programmed pacing techniques in the atria. Vagal maneuvers and administration of adenosine or verapamil terminate the arrhythmia (177). A noticeable association with coronary artery disease—specifically with inferior myocardial infarction—has led to speculation that ischemia or infarction in the sinus node area may provide the milieu for reentry.

Epidemiology and Clinical Significance

The majority of patients with sinus node reentrant tachycardia have structural heart disease. Sinus node reentry tachycardia can be associated with any of the classic symptoms associated with any tachycardia, including palpitation, dyspnea, near-syncope, or syncope (see Atrial Flutter: Epidemiology and Clinical Significance) (178,179). Although associated tachycardias have been believed to occur infrequently, one recent study noted one or two additional tachyarrhythmias (atrioventricular nodal reentrant tachycardia, atrioventricular reentrant tachycardia, bundle branch reentrant tachycardia, atrial tachycardia) in nine of 11 patients (179). In patients with prolonged, sustained sinus node reentrant tachycardia, dilated CM may result.

Diagnosis

The rhythm is characterized by rapid rates (usual range of 120 to 150 beats/min) in which the P-wave morphology in the 12-

lead ECG is virtually identical to that during sinus rhythm. Its spontaneous onset and offset are abrupt. The tachycardia behaves classically to interventions known to perturb or interrupt ordered reentrant rhythms. Thus, the tachycardia can be initiated or terminated with atrial pacing techniques; it can also be terminated with adenosine or with maneuvers that increase vagal tone. Mapping during electrophysiologic study demonstrates an atrial activation sequence similar to that of sinus rhythm.

Treatment

Intravenous adenosine and verapamil as well as vagal maneuvers have been used over the short term to terminate sustained episodes of sinus node reentry tachycardia. In several small series of studies, radiofrequency ablation of the sinus node region has been shown to prevent recurrence of sinus node reentrant tachycardia (180). Long-term drug therapy has not been systematically studied. However, digitalis, a calcium channel blocker, or a beta-blocker alone or in combination may prove effective.

Summary

Sinus node reentrant tachycardia is an infrequent tachyarrhythmia. Definitive therapy with catheter ablation should prove successful.

MULTIFOCAL ATRIAL TACHYCARDIA

Background

MAT remains largely a descriptive entity with a need for better characterization (181). MAT is usually diagnosed by ECG criteria that include an atrial rate of more than 100 beats/min with P waves of at least three distinct morphologies. Diagnosing MAT can be difficult. The chaotic nature of its P-wave morphology with varying AV intervals frequently may cause it to be confused with atrial fibrillation (Fig. 65.8.1).

Potential Mechanism(s)

The mechanism(s) underlying MAT remain unknown. Several reports have noted that MAT cannot be induced or initiated by programmed stimulation. Thus, reentry seems an unlikely mechanism. Anecdotal reports of successful treatment of MAT with calcium channel blockers or beta-blockers are consistent with both automatic and triggered mechanisms.

Epidemiology and Clinical Significance

MAT is often observed in patients with acute pulmonary disorders and associated hypoxia. Patients with MAT usually are acutely ill and often are receiving beta-agonists or theophylline preparations. As such, both beta-agonists and theophylline have been causally implicated. There are no data to support these observations as more than associations. Regardless, it seems reasonable to discontinue these agents in affected patients. Anecdotal reports have also noted an association of MAT with pulmonary embolism, coronary artery disease, CHF, and electrolyte disturbances.

Treatment

The therapeutic issues revolve around the extent to which the rapid ventricular response rate during MAT affects the clinical condition of the patient. If ventricular response can be controlled, which is usually difficult, MAT per se probably will not affect the patient's clinical course.

The basis for therapy should primarily be correction of the underlying pulmonary problem. DC cardioversion has not proved successful in patients with MAT. Only limited experience has been reported with use of standard antiarrhythmic drugs. Beta-blockers have been used successfully in selected patients. Precipitation of bronchospasm may be a potentially fatal complication when beta-blockers are used in acutely ill patients. Thus, short-acting beta$_1$-specific agents such as esmolol seem most appropriate for initial use. Calcium channel blockers have been used with limited success.

Beta-Blockers

Arsura et al. (182) compared both beta-blockers and calcium channel blockers in a blinded crossover study of patients with MAT. During this 22-month study, 16 of 79 consecutive patients with MAT were randomly assigned to placebo, verapamil, or metoprolol. Of the nonrandomized patients, unstable blood pressure and audible wheezing accounted for most of the exclusions. Patients were given either placebo or verapamil, 5 mg intravenously over 5 minutes, or metoprolol, 5 mg intravenously over 5 minutes. A statistically significant difference in the net decrease in heart rate was observed only when patients treated with metoprolol were compared with patients treated with placebo. Metoprolol-treated patients showed a decrease in heart rate of approximately 25%. Six of the study patients died during hospitalization. Unfortunately, this mortality does not differ from that reported in other studies. Although the data set is obviously small, Arsura et al. (182) cautiously concluded that in selected patients beta-blockers may play a role in the treatment of patients with MAT. It remains questionable whether antiarrhythmic drugs can affect outcome in this dramatically ill group of patients.

Calcium Channel Blockers

Salerno et al. (183) investigated the use of calcium channel blockers in treating patients with MAT. There has been concern regarding use of intravenous calcium channel blockers because of the potential of vasodilation-induced hypotension. Intravenous verapamil was administered at doses of up to 1 mg per minute to 16 consecutive patients with MAT. The mean heart rate decreased from 129 to 101 beats/min. Sinus rhythm was restored in eight patients. Patients who received pretreatment with calcium (1 g of calcium gluconate intravenously over 1 to 2 minutes) showed a systolic blood pressure drop of 11%. However, systolic blood pressure dropped by 27% in those patients who were not pretreated with calcium gluconate. No differences in antiarrhythmic efficacy were observed between the two groups. Salerno et al. (183) concluded that pretreatment with intravenous calcium gluconate was reasonable in patients receiving verapamil for MAT.

Nonpharmacologic Methods

A recent report (184) has advocated AV junction ablation and permanent pacing for those patients with refractory MAT. In this series, both improvement in quality of life and LV function was noted. Of note, right ventricular function did not improve. This study was not powered to examine mortality. Thus, this therapy should be reserved only for extremely symptomatic patients.

Summary

In summary, when precipitating causes of MAT have been corrected, specific drug therapy may be reasonable to help slow the ventricular rate. Although it appears logical that slowing of the ventricular rate would be desirable, there are no data supporting a meaningful change in outcome in

THE FUTURE

A more thorough understanding of the mechanisms of atrial arrhythmias has brought this field to the forefront of cardiology. More advances in understanding the underlying mechanism(s) of atrial arrhythmias will enable us to better target medications for specific rhythm disturbances. Advances in mapping techniques in the electrophysiology laboratory will further ensure more successful treatment of patients with atrial arrhythmias. Sophisticated mapping systems using a single intracavitary probe or thoracic multielectrode vests will facilitate identification of target sites for successful abla-

tion. A "Star Wars"-like atmosphere has occurred in the electrophysiology laboratory. More advanced systems will decrease the time needed for testing, the radiation exposure to patients and practitioners, and the complication rates to patients undergoing these procedures.

To date, with most atrial arrhythmias, the mechanistic approach has used whole organ physiology. However, a mechanistic approach emphasizing molecular genetics will evolve, and therapies analogous to those under way in patients with long QT syndrome will become commonplace.

these patients by such treatment. MAT remains a paraphenomenon. As such, therapy should not focus on the arrhythmia. The underlying cardiopulmonary substrate must be engaged therapeutically, with little emphasis placed on the arrhythmia.

CONTROVERSIES AND PERSONAL PERSPECTIVES

Clinical Presentation

A chronic or frequent atrial tachyarrhythmia can lead to ventricular dilatation and CHF. The full spectrum of symptoms associated with cardiac dysfunction is possible from pulmonary edema to a nonspecific cough. We believe that this syndrome, tachycardia-induced CM, is grossly unrecognized. Many nonischemic CMs may be entirely due to such an incessant arrhythmia. Equally important, frequent episodes of atrial tachyarrhythmias may exacerbate underlying cardiac disease, resulting in an exacerbation of symptoms and a worsening quality of life. We believe that many physicians attribute such a decompensation to the progression of underlying coronary disease, valve disease, and so forth. The possibility that the frequent arrhythmia is the culprit must be recognized and appropriately treated to ensure the best outcome for each patient. Not only must cardiologists recognize this possibility, but front-line physicians (e.g., internists and family practitioners) must screen for this diagnostic possibility as well.

Therapy

The traditional initial treatment for most AV nodal–independent atrial arrhythmias has been antiarrhythmic drugs. An increasing volume of data has confirmed an excessive mortality risk in those patients with structural heart disease

who have been treated with class IA or class III antiarrhythmic drugs. Thus, catheter ablation should assume a greater role as primary therapy for many atrial arrhythmias in these patients.

ACKNOWLEDGMENT

This chapter was supported in part by grant RO1 HL38408 from the National Institutes of Health, National Heart, Lung, and Blood Institute, Bethesda, Maryland.

REFERENCES

1. Jolly WA, Ritchie WJ. Auricular flutter and fibrillation. *Heart* 1911;2:177–221.
2. Lewis T. *Clinical disorders of the heart beat*, 4th ed. New York: Paul B. Hoeber, 1918:73–83.
3. Lewis T, Drury AN, Iliescu TT. A demonstration of circus movement in clinical flutter of the auricles. *Heart* 1921;8:341.
4. Waldo AL. Mechanisms of atrial fibrillation, atrial flutter, and ectopic atrial tachycardia: a brief review. *Circulation* 1987;75:37–40.
5. Waldo AL, MacLean WAH. *Diagnosis and treatment of arrhythmias following open-heart surgery: emphasis on the use of epicardial wire electrodes*. New York: Futura, 1980.
6. Waldo AL. Pathogenesis of atrial flutter. *J Cardiovasc Electrophysiol* 1998;9S:18–25.
7. Cosio FG, Lopez-Gil M, Arribas F, Gonzalez HD. Mechanisms of induction of typical and reversed atrial flutter. *J Cardiovasc Electrophysiol* 1998;9:281–291.
8. Morris JJ, Kong Y, North WC, et al. Experience with "cardioversion" of atrial fibrillation and flutter. *Am J Cardiol* 1964;14:94–100.
9. Castellanos A, Lemberg L, Gosselin A, et al. Evaluation of countershock treatment of atrial flutter. *Arch Intern Med* 1965;115:426–433.

10. Zipes DP. Management of cardiac arrhythmia: pharmacological, electrical, and surgical techniques. In: Braunwald E, ed. *Heart disease: a textbook of cardiovascular medicine*, 3rd ed. Philadelphia: WB Saunders 1988:621–657.

11. The Esmolol Research Group. Intravenous esmolol for the treatment of supraventricular tachyarrhythmia: results of a multicenter, baseline-controlled safety and efficacy study of 160 patients. *Am Heart J* 1986;112:498–505.

12. Plumb VJ, Karp RB, Kouchoukos NT, et al. Verapamil therapy of atrial fibrillation and atrial flutter following open heart surgery. *J Thorac Cardiovasc Surg* 1982;83:590–596.

13. Ellenbogen KA, Dias VC, Plumb VJ, et al. A placebo-controlled trial of continuous intravenous diltiazem infusion for 24-hour heart rate control during atrial fibrillation and atrial flutter: a multicenter study. *J Am Coll Cardiol* 1991;18:891–897.

14. Anderson JL, Gilbert EM, Alpert BL, et al., for the Flecainide Supraventricular Tachycardia Study Group. Prevention of symptomatic recurrences of paroxysmal atrial fibrillation in patients initially tolerating antiarrhythmic therapy: a multicenter, double-blind, cross over study of flecainide and placebo using transtelephonic monitoring. *Circulation* 1989;80:1557–1570.

15. Pritchett ELC, McCarthy EA, Wilkinson WE. Propafenone treatment of symptomatic paroxysmal supraventricular arrhythmias: a randomized, placebo-controlled, crossover trial in patients tolerating oral therapy. *Ann Intern Med* 1991;114:539–544.

16. Reimold SC, Cantillon CO, Friedman PL, Antman EM. Propafenone versus sotalol for suppression of recurrent symptomatic atrial fibrillation. *Am J Cardiol* 1993;71:558–563.

17. Gosselink ATM, Crijns HJGM, Van Gelder K, et al. Low-dose amiodarone for maintenance of sinus rhythm after cardioversion of atrial fibrillation or flutter. *JAMA* 1992;267:3289–3293.

18. Ellenbogen KA, Clemo HF, Stambler BS, et al. Efficacy of ibutilide for termination of atrial fibrillation and flutter. *Am J Cardiol* 1996;78S:42–45.

19. Saoudi N, Atallah G, Kirkorian G, et al. Catheter ablation of the atrial myocardium in human type I atrial flutter. *Circulation* 1990;81:762–771.

20. Cosio FG, Lopez-Gil M, Giocolea A, et al. Radiofrequency ablation of the inferior vena cava-tricuspid valve isthmus in common atrial flutter. *Am J Cardiol* 1993;71:705–709.

21. Feld GK, Fleck P, Cheng PS, et al. Radiofrequency catheter ablation for the treatment of human type I atrial flutter: identification of a critical zone in the reentrant circuit by endocardial mapping techniques. *Circulation* 1992;86:1233–1240.

22. Scheinman MM. Catheter techniques for ablation of supraventricular tachycardia. *N Engl J Med* 1989;320:460–461.

23. Klein GJ, Guiraudon GM, Sharma AD, et al. Demonstration of macroreentry and feasibility of operative therapy in the common type of atrial flutter. *Am J Cardiol* 1986;57:587–591.

24. Leitch JW, Klein GH, Yee R, Guiraudon GM. Sinus node-atrio-ventricular node isolation: long term results with the corridor operation for atrial fibrillation. *J Am Coll Cardiol* 1989;17:970–975.

25. Rosenblueth A, Garcia-Ramos J. Studies on flutter and fibrillation. II. The influence of artificial obstacles on experimental auricular flutter. *Am Heart J* 1947;33:677–684.

26. Frame LH, Page RL, Hoffman BF. Atrial reentry around an anatomic barrier with a partially refractory excitable gap: a canine model of atrial flutter. *Circ Res* 1986;58:495–511.

27. Frame LH, Page RL, Boyden PA, et al. Circus movement in the canine atrium around the tricuspid ring during experimental atrial flutter and during reentry in vivo. *Circulation* 1987;76:1155–1175.

28. Flinn CJ, Wolff GS, Dick M II, et al. Cardiac rhythm after the Mustard operation for complete transposition of the great arteries. *N Engl J Med* 1984;310:1625–1638.

29. Yamashita T, Inoue H, Nozaki A, et al. Role of anatomic architecture in sustained atrial reentry and double potentials. *Am Heart J* 1992;124:938–946.

30. Bink-Boelkens MT, Velvia H, van der Heide JJH, et al. Dysrhythmias after atrial surgery in children. *Am Heart J* 1983;106:125–130.

31. Feld GK, Shahandeh-Rad F. Mechanism of double potentials recorded during sustained atrial flutter in the canine right atrial crush-injury model. *Circulation* 1992;86:628–641.

32. Scherf D. Studies on auricular tachycardia caused by aconitine administration. *Proc Exp Biol Med* 1947;64:233–239.

33. Scherf D, Romano FJ, Terranova R. Experimental studies on auricular flutter and auricular fibrillation. *Am Heart J* 1958;36:241–251.

34. Kimura E, Kato K, Murao S, et al. Experimental studies on the mechanism of auricular flutter. *Tohoku J Exp Med* 1954;60:197–207.

35. Haissaguerre M, Shah DC, Jais P, et al. Spontaneous initiation of atrial fibrillation by ectopic beats originating in the pulmonary veins. *N Engl J Med* 1998;339:659–666.

36. Chen SA, Hsieh MH, Tai TC, et al. Initiation of atrial fibrillation by ectopic beats originating from the pulmonary veins: electrophysiological characteristics, pharmacological responses, and effects of radiofrequency ablation. *Circulation* 1999;100:1879–1886.

37. Allessie M, Lammers W, Smeets J, et al. Total mapping of atrial excitation during acetylcholine-induced atrial flutter and fibrillation in the isolated canine heart. In: Kulbertus HE, Olsson SB, Schlepper M, eds. *Atrial fibrillation.* Molndal, Sweden: AB Hassell, 1982:44–59.

38. Allessie MA, Lammers WJEP, Bonke FIM, Hollen J. Intra-atrial reentry as a mechanism for atrial flutter induced by acetylcholine in rapid pacing in the dog. *Circulation* 1984;70:123–135.

39. Boineau JP, Schuessler RB, Mooney CR, et al. Natural and evoked atrial flutter due to circus movement in dogs. *Am J Cardiol* 1980;45:1167–1181.

40. Boyden PA, Hoffman BF. The effects on atrial electrophysiology and structure of surgically induced right atrial enlargement in dogs. *Circ Res* 1981;49:1319–1331.

41. Boyden PA. Activation sequence during atrial flutter in dogs with surgically induced right atrial enlargement. I. Observations during sustained rhythms. *Circ Res* 1988;62:596–608.

42. Pagé P, Plumb VJ, Okumura K, et al. A new model of atrial flutter. *J Am Coll Cardiol* 1986;8:872–879.

43. Okumura K, Plumb VJ, Page PL, et al. Atrial activation sequence during atrial flutter in the canine pericarditis model and its effects on the polarity of the flutter wave in the electrocardiogram. *J Am Coll Cardiol* 1991;17:509–518.

44. Shimizu A, Nozaki A, Rudy Y, et al. Onset of induced atrial flutter in the canine pericarditis model. *J Am Coll Cardiol* 1991;17:1223–1234.

45. Shimizu A, Nozaki A, Rudy Y, et al. Multiplexing studies of effects of rapid atrial pacing on the area of slow conduction during atrial flutter in canine pericarditis model. *Circulation* 1991;83:983–994.

46. Ortiz J, Igarashi M, Gonzalez HX, et al. Mechanism of spontaneous termination of atrial flutter in the canine sterile pericarditis model. *Circulation* 1993;88:1866–1877.

47. Shimizu A, Nozaki A, Rudy Y, et al. Characterization of double potentials in a functionally determined reentrant circuit: multiplexing studies during interruption of atrial flutter in the canine pericarditis model. *J Am Coll Cardiol* 1993;22:2022–2032.

48. Ortiz J, Niwano S, Abe H, et al. Mapping the conversion of atrial flutter to atrial fibrillation and atrial fibrillation to atrial flutter: Insights into mechanism. *Circ Res* 1994;74:882–894.

49. Page PL, Hassanahzadeh H, Cardinal R. Transitions among atrial fibrillation, atrial flutter and sinus rhythm during procainamide infusion and vagal stimulation in dogs with sterile pericarditis. *Can J Physiol Pharmacol* 1991;69:15–24.

50. Schoels W, Gough WB, Ristivo M, et al. Circus movement atrial flutter in the canine sterile pericarditis model: activation patterns during initiation, termination, and sustained reentry in vivo. *Circ Res* 1990;67:35–50.

51. Schoels W, Offner B, Brachmann J, et al. Circus movement atrial flutter in the canine sterile pericarditis model. *J Am Coll Cardiol* 1994;23:799–808.

52. Uno K, Kumagai K, Khrestian C, et al. New insights into the mechanism of onset of the atrial flutter reentrant circuit in the canine sterile pericarditis model. *Circulation* 1996;94:I-352.

53. Shah D, Jais P, Takahashi A, et al. Dual-loop intra-atrial reentry in humans. *Circulation* 2000;101:631–639.

54. Kall JG, Rubenstein DS, Kopp DE, et al. Atypical atrial flutter originating in the right atrial free wall. *Circulation* 2000;101:270–279.

55. Cox JL, Canaven TE, Schuessler RB, et al. The surgical treatment of atrial fibrillation. II. Intraoperative electrophysiologic mapping and description of the electrophysiologic basis of atrial flutter and atrial fibrillation. *J Thorac Cardiovasc Surg* 1991;101:406–426.

56. Prinzmetal M, Corday E, Oblath RW, et al. Auricular flutter. *Am J Med* 1951;11:410–430.

57. Wellens HJJ, Janse MJ, van Dam RT, et al. Epicardial excitation of the atria in a patient with atrial flutter. *Br Heart J* 1971;33:233–237.

58. Rosen K, Lau SH, Damato AN. Simulation of atrial flutter by rapid coronary sinus pacing. *Am Heart J* 1969;78:635–642.

59. Rytand DA. The circus movement (entrapped circuit wave) hypothesis of atrial flutter. *Arch Intern Med* 1966;65:125–159.

60. Puech P. *L'Activite electrique auriculaire normale et pathologique.* Paris: Masson & Cie, 1956:214–240.

61. Puech P, Latour H, Grolleau R. Le flutter et ses limites. *Arch Mal Coeur* 1970;63:116–144.

62. Waldo AL, MacLean WAH, Karp RB, et al. Entrainment and interruption of atrial flutter with atrial pacing: studies in man following open-heart surgery. *Circulation* 1977;56:737–745.

63. Inoue H, Matsuo H, Takayanagi K, et al. Clinical and experimental studies of the effects of extrastimulation and rapid pacing on atrial flutter: evidence of macroreentry with an excitable gap. *Am J Cardiol* 1981;48:623–631.

64. Waldo AL, Plumb VJ, Henthorn RW. Observations on the mechanism of atrial flutter. In: Surawicz B, Reddy CP, Prystowsky EN, eds. *Tachycardias.* The Hague, The Netherlands: Martinus Nijhoff, 1984:213–229.

65. Cosio FG, Arribas F, Palacios J, et al. Fragmented electrograms and continuous electrical activity in atrial flutter. *Am J Cardiol* 1986;57:1309–1314.

66. Cosio FG, Arribas F, Barbero JM, et al. Validation of double-spike electrograms as markers of conduction delay or block in atrial flutter. *Am J Cardiol* 1988;61:775–780.

67. Cosio FG. Endocardial mapping of atrial flutter. In: Touboul P, Waldo AL, eds. *Atrial arrhythmias.* St. Louis: Mosby Year Book, 1990:229–240.

68. Olshansky B, Okumura K, Henthorn RW, et al. Characterization of double potentials in human atrial flutter: studies during transient entrainment. *J Am Coll Cardiol* 1990;15:833–841.

69. Olshansky B, Okumura K, Hess PG, et al. Demonstration of an area of slow conduction in human atrial flutter. *J Am Coll Cardiol* 1990;16:1639–1648.

70. Cosio FG, Goicolea A, Lopez-Gil M, et al. Atrial endocardial mapping in the rare form of atrial flutter. *Am J Cardiol* 1990;66:715–720.

71. Olgin JE, Kalman JM, Fitzpatrick AP, et al. Role of right atrial endocardial structures as barriers to conduction during human type I atrial flutter: activation and entrainment mapping guided by intracardiac echocardiography. *Circulation* 1995;92:1839–1848.

72. Kalman JM, Olgin JE, Saxon LA, et al. Activation and entrainment mapping defines the tricuspid annulus as the anterior boundary in atrial flutter. *Circulation* 1996;94:398–406.

73. Nakagawa H, Lazzara R, Khastgir T, et al. Role of the tricuspid annulus and the eustachian valve/ridge on atrial flutter: relevance to catheter ablation of the septal isthmus and a new technique for rapid identification of ablation success. *Circulation* 1996;94:407–424.

74. Kinder C, Kall J, Kopp D, et al. Conduction properties of the inferior vena cava—tricuspid annulus isthmus in patients with typical atrial flutter. *J Cardiovasc Electrophysiol* 1997;8:727–737.

75. Cabrera JA, Sanchez-Quinta D, Ho SY, et al. The architecture of the atrial musculature between the orifice of the inferior caval vein and the tricuspid valve: the anatomy of the isthmus. *J Cardiovasc Electrophysiol* 1998;9:1186–1195.

76. Waki K, Saito T, Becker AE. Right atrial flutter isthmus revisited: normal anatomy favors nonuniform anisotropic conduction. *J Cardiovasc Electrophysiol* 2000;11:90–94.

77. Cabrera JA, Sanchez-Quinta D, Ho SY, et al. Angiographic anatomy of the inferior right atrial isthmus in patients with and without history of common atrial flutter. *Circulation* 1999;99:3017–3023.

78. Arenal A, Almendral J, Alday JM, et al. Rate-dependent conduction block of the crista terminalis in patients with typical atrial flutter—influence on evaluation of cavotricuspid isthmus conduction block. *Circulation* 1999;99:2771–2778.

79. Tai CT, Chen SA, Chen YJ, et al. Conduction properties of the crista terminalis in patients with typical atrial flutter: basis for a line of block in the reentrant circuit. *J Cardiovasc Electrophysiol* 1998;9:811–819.

80. Friedman PA, Luria D, Fenton AM, et al. Global right atrial mapping of human atrial flutter: the presence of posteromedial (sinus venosa region) functional block and double potentials. A study in biplane fluoroscopy and intracardiac echocardiography. *Circulation* 2000;101:1568–1577.

81. Matsuo K, Tomita Y, Khrestian CM, et al. A new mechanism of sustained atrial fibrillation—studies in the sterile pericarditis model. *Circulation* 1998;98:I-209.

82. Skanes AC, Mandapati R, Berenfeld O, et al. Spatio-temporal periodicity during atrial fibrillation in the isolated sheep heart. *Circulation* 1998;98:1236–1248.

83. Shimizu A, Nozaki A, Rudy Y, et al. Onset of induced atrial flutter in the canine pericarditis model. *J Am Coll Cardiol* 1991;17:1223–1234.

84. Lewis T. Observations upon flutter and fibrillation. I. The regularity of clinical auricular flutter. *Heart* 1920;7:127–130.

85. Wells JL Jr, MacLean WAH, James TN, Waldo AL. Characterization of atrial flutter: studies in man after open-heart surgery using fixed atrial electrodes. *Circulation* 1979;60:665–673.

86. Puech P, Latour H, Grolleau R. Le flutter et ses limites. *Arch Mal Coeur* 1970;63:116–144.

87. Cheng J, Cabeen WR, Scheinman MM. Right atrial flutter due to lower loop reentry, mechanism and anatomic substrates. *Circulation* 1999;99:1700–1705.

88. Cheng J, Scheinmann MM. Acceleration of typical atrial flutter due to double-wave reentry induced by programmed electrical stimulation. *Circulation* 1998;97:1589–1596.

89. Bellet S. *Clinical disorders of the heart beat.* Philadelphia: Lea & Febiger, 1963:144–145.

90. Granada J, Uribe W, Chyour PH, et al. Incidence and predictors of atrial fibrillation in the general population. *J Am Coll Cardiol* 2000;36:2242–2246.

91. Waldo AL, Cooper TB. Spontaneous onset of type I atrial flutter in patients. *J Am Coll Cardiol* 1996;28:707–712.

92. Garson A Jr, Bink-Boelkens M, Hesslein PS, et al. Atrial flutter in the young: a collaborative study of 380 cases. *J Am Coll Cardiol* 1985;6:871–878.

93. Chan DP, Van Hare GF, Mackall JA, et al. Importance of atrial flutter isthmus in postoperative intra-atrial reentrant tachycardia. *Circulation* 2000;102:1283–1289.

94. Wu T, Yashima M, Xie F, et al. Role of pectinate muscle bundles in the generation and maintenance of intra-atrial reentry—potential implications for the mechanism of conversion between atrial fibrillation and atrial flutter. *Circ Res* 1998;83:448–462.

95. Roithinger FX, Lesh MD. What is the relationship of atrial flutter and fibrillation? *Pacing Clin Electrophysiol* 1999;22:643–654.

96. Biblo LA, Yuan Z, Quan KJ, et al. Risk of stroke in patients with atrial flutter. *Am J Cardiol* 2001;87:346–349.

97. Switzer D, Waldo A, Henthorn R. Hemodynamic effects of tachycardias. In: Saksena S, Goldschlager N, eds. *Electrical therapy for cardiac arrhythmias: supraventricular tachycardia.* Philadelphia: WB Saunders 1990:467–477.

98. Leitch JW, Klein GJ, Yee R, et al. Syncope associated with supraventricular tachycardia: an expression of tachycardia rate or vasomotor response? *Circulation* 1992;85:1064–1071.

99. Knight BP, Michaud GF, Strickberger SA, et al. Electrocardiographic differentiation of atrial flutter from atrial fibrillation by physicians. *J Electrocardiol* 1999;32:315–319.

100. Gatzoulis KA, Biblo LA, Waldo AL, et al. Atrial flutter causes pseudo late potentials on signal-averaged electrocardiogram. *Am J Cardiol* 1993;71:251–253.

101. Watson MM, Josephson ME. Atrial flutter. I. Electrophysiologic substrates and modes of initiation and termination. *Am J Cardiol* 1980;45:732–741.

102. Triedman JK, Saul JP, Weindling SN, et al. Radiofrequency ablation of intra-atrial reentrant tachycardia after surgical palliation of congenital heart disease. *Circulation* 1995;91:707–714.

103. Van Hare GF, Lesh MD, Ross BA, et al. Mapping and radiofrequency ablation of intraatrial reentrant tachycardia after the Senning or Mustard procedure for transposition of the great arteries. *Am J Cardiol* 1996;77:985–991.

104. Olshansky B, Okumura K, Hess PG, et al. Use of procainamide with rapid atrial pacing for successful conversion of atrial flutter to sinus rhythm. *J Am Coll Cardiol* 1988;11:359–364.

105. Camm J, Ward D, Spurrell R. Response of atrial flutter to overdrive atrial pacing and intravenous disopyramide phosphate singly and in combination. *Br Heart J* 1980;44:240.

106. Stambler BS, Wood MA, Ellenbogen KA. Comparative efficacy of intravenous ibutilide versus procainamide for enhancing termination of atrial flutter by overdrive pacing. *Am J Cardiol* 1996;77:960–966.

107. Kowey PR, Vanderlugt JI, Luderer JR. Safety and risk/benefit analysis of ibutilide for acute conversion of atrial fibrillation/flutter. *Am J Cardiol* 1996;78S:42–45.

108. Hellestrand KJ. Intravenous flecainide acetate for supraventricular tachycardias. *Am J Cardiol* 1988;62:16D–22D.

109. Suttorp MJ, Kingma JH, Jessuren ER, et al. The value of class IC antiarrhythmic drugs for acute conversion of paroxysmal atrial fibrillation or flutter to sinus rhythm. *J Am Coll Cardiol* 1990;16:1722–1727.

110. Capucci A, Lenzi T, Boriani G, et al. Effectiveness of loading oral flecainide for converting recent-onset atrial fibrillation to sinus rhythm in patients without organic heart disease or with only systemic hypertension. *Am J Cardiol* 1992;70:69–72.

111. Capucci A, Boriani G, Botto GL, et al. Conversion of recent-onset atrial fibrillation by a single oral loading dose of propafenone. *Am J Cardiol* 1994;74:503–505.

112. Waldo AL. Cardiac pacing: role in diagnosis and treatment of disorders of cardiac rhythm and conduction. In: Rosen MR, Hoffman BF, eds. *Cardiac therapy.* Boston: Martinus Nijhoff, 1983:299–336.

113. Plumb VJ, Karp RB, James TN, Waldo AL. Atrial excitability and conduction during rapid atrial pacing. *Circulation* 1981;63:1140–1149.

114. Benson DW, Sanford M, Dunnigan A, Benditt DG. Transesophageal atrial pacing threshold: role of interelectrode

spacing, pulse width and catheter insertion depth. *Am J Cardiol* 1984;53:63–67.

115. Waldo AL, MacLean WAH, Karp RB, et al. Continuous rapid atrial pacing to control recurrent or sustained supraventricular tachycardias following open-heart surgery. *Circulation* 1976;54:245–250.

116. Murgatroyd FD, Camm AJ. Atrial arrhythmias: who would be a candidate for an implantable atrial defibrillator? In: Waldo AL, Touboul P, eds. *Atrial flutter: advances in mechanisms and management.* Armonk, NY: Futura, 1996:427–438.

117. The Cardiac Arrhythmia Suppression Trial (CAST) Investigators. Effect of encainide and flecainide on mortality in a randomized trial of arrhythmia suppression after myocardial infarction. *N Engl J Med* 1989;321:406–412.

118. Geller JC, Geller M, Carlson MD, et al. Safety and efficacy of moricizine in the maintenance of sinus rhythm in patients with recurrent atrial fibrillation. *Am J Cardiol* 2001;87:172–177.

119. The Cardiac Arrhythmia Suppression Trial-II (CAST) Investigators. Effect of the antiarrhythmic agent moricizine on survival after myocardial infarction. *N Engl J Med* 1992;327:227–233.

120. MacNeil DJ, Davies RO, Deitchman D. Clinical safety profile of sotalol in the treatment of arrhythmias. *Am J Cardiol* 1993;72:44A–50A.

121. Podrid PJ. Amiodarone: reevaluation of an old drug. *Ann Intern Med* 1995;122:689–700.

122. Cairns JA, Connolly SJ, Roberts R, et al., for the Canadian Amiodarone Myocardial Infarction Arrhythmia Trial Investigators. Randomised trial of outcome after myocardial infarction in patients with frequent or repetitive ventricular premature depolarisations: CAMIAT. *Lancet* 1997;349:675–682.

123. Julian D, Camm AJ, Fangin G, et al., for the EMIAT Investigators. Effect of amiodarone on mortality in patients with left ventricular dysfunction after surviving a recent myocardial infarct. *Lancet* 1997;349:667–674.

124. Antman E, DiMarco J, Domanski MJ, et al., to the NHLBI Working Group on Atrial Fibrillation. Atrial fibrillation: current understandings and research imperative. *J Am Coll Cardiol* 1993;22:1830–1834.

125. Arnold AZ, Mick MJ, Mazurck RP, et al. Role of prophylactic anticoagulation for direct current cardioversion in patients with atrial fibrillation or atrial flutter. *J Am Coll Cardiol* 1992;19:851–855.

126. Lanzarotti CJ, Olshansky B. Thromboembolism in chronic atrial flutter: is the risk underestimated? *J Am Coll Cardiol* 1997;30:1506–1511.

127. Seidl K, Hauer B, Schwick NG, et al. Risk of thromboembolic events in patients with atrial flutter. *Am J Cardiol* 1998;82:580–583.

128. Wood KA, Eisenberg SJ, Kalman JM, et al. Risk of thromboembolism in chronic atrial flutter. *Am J Cardiol* 1997;79:1043–1047.

129. Fischer B, Haissaguerre M, Garrigues S, et al. Radiofrequency catheter ablation of common atrial flutter in 80 patients. *J Am Coll Cardiol* 1995;25:1365.

130. Miller JM, Cossu SF, Chmielewski IL, et al. Primary ablation of atrial flutter and atrial fibrillation. *Cardiol Clin* 1996;14:569–590.

131. Poty H, Saoudi N, Haissaguerre M, et al. Radiofrequency catheter ablation of atrial flutter. Further insights into the various types of isthmus block: application to ablation during sinus rhythm. *Circulation* 1996;94:3198–3203.

132. Shah DC, Takahashi A, Jaïs P, et al. Local electrogram-based criteria of cavotricuspid isthmus block. *J Cardiovasc Electrophysiol* 1999;10:662–669.

133. Yamabe H, Okumura K, Misumi I, et al. Role of bipolar electrogram polarity mapping in localizing recurrent conduction in the isthmus early and late after ablation of atrial flutter. *J Am Coll Cardiol* 1999;33:39–45.

134. Nabar A, Rodriguez LM, Timmermans C, et al. Isoproterenol to evaluate resumption of conduction after right atrial isthmus ablation in type I atrial flutter. *Circulation* 1999;99:3286–3291.

135. Willems S, Weiss C, Ventura R, et al. Catheter ablation of atrial flutter guided by electroanatomic mapping (CARTO): a randomized comparison to the conventional approach. *J Cardiovasc Electrophysiol* 2000;11:1223–1230.

136. Paydak H, Kall JG, Burke MC, et al. Atrial fibrillation after radiofrequency ablation of type I atrial flutter. Time to onset, determinants, and clinical course. *Circulation* 1998;98:315–322.

137. Touboul P, Saoudi N, Atallah G, et al. Catheter ablation for atrial flutter: current concepts and results. *J Cardiovasc Electrophysiol* 1992;3:641–652.

138. Jaïs P, Shah DC, Haïssaguerre M, et al. Mapping and ablation of left atrial flutters. *Circulation* 2000;101:2928–2934.

139. Shah DC, Haïssaguerre M, Jaïs P, et al. Atrial flutter: contemporary electrophysiology and catheter ablation. *Pacing Clin Electrophysiol* 1999;22:344–358.

140. Kalman JM, Olgin JE, Karch MR, et al. "Cristal tachycardias": Origin of right atrial tachycardias from the crista terminalis identified by intracardiac echocardiography. *J Am Coll Cardiol* 1998;31:451–459.

141. Callans DJ, Schwartzman D, Gottlieb CD, et al. Insights into the electrophysiology of atrial arrhythmias gained by the catheter ablation experience. Part II. Learning while burning. *J Cardiovasc Electrophysiol* 1995;6:229–243.

142. Waldo AL, Wit AL. Mechanism of cardiac arrhythmias and conduction disturbances. In: Schlant RC, Alexander RW, eds. *The heart*, 8th ed. New York: McGraw-Hill, 1994:659–704.

143. Wit AL, Cranefield PF. Triggered activity in cardiac muscle fibers of the simian mitral valve. *Circ Res* 1976;38:85–98.

144. Wit AL, Cranefield PF. Triggered and automatic activity in the canine coronary sinus. *Circ Res* 1977;41:435–445.

145. Rozanski GJ, Lipsius SL. Electrophysiology of functional subsidiary pacemakers in canine right atrium. *Am J Physiol* 1985;249:H594–H603.

146. Boyden PA, Tilley LP, Albala A, et al. Mechanisms for atrial arrhythmias associated with cardiomyopathy: a study of feline hearts with primary myocardial disease. *Circ Res* 1984;69:1036–1047.

147. Markowitz SM, Stein KM, Mittal S, et al. Differential effects of adenosine on focal and macroreentrant atrial tachycardia. *J Cardiovasc Electrophysiol* 1999;10:489–502.

148. Chiale PA, Franco A, Selva HO, et al. Lidocaine-sensitive atrial tachycardia. Lidocaine-sensitive, rate-related, repetitive atrial tachycardia: a new arrhythmogenic syndrome. *J Am Coll Cardiol* 2000;36:1637–1645.

149. Camm A, Evans K, Ward D, et al. The rhythm of the heart in active elderly subjects. *Am Heart J* 1980;99:598–603.

150. Fleig J, Kennedy H. Cardiac arrhythmias in a healthy elderly population. *Chest* 1982;81:302.

151. Rossi A. Twenty-four hour electrocardiographic study in the active very elderly. *Cardiology* 1987;74:159–166.

152. Cristal N, Szwarcberg J, Gueron M. Supraventricular arrhythmias in acute myocardial infarction. *Ann Intern Med* 1975;82:35–39.

153. Jewitt D, Raferty E, Balcon R, et al. Incidence and management of supraventricular arrhythmias after acute myocardial infarction. *Lancet* 1967;2:734–738.

154. Coumel P, Flammang D, Attuel P, et al. Sustained intraatrial reentrant tachycardia: electrophysiological study of 20 cases. *Cardiol Clin* 1979;2:167–178.

155. Lazzeroni E, Domeniencci S, Finardi A, et al. Severity of arrhythmias and extent of hypertrophy in hypertrophic cardiomyopathy. *Am Heart J* 1989;118:734–738.

156. Holford F, Mithoefer J. Cardiac arrhythmias in hospitalized patients with chronic obstructive pulmonary disease. *Am Rev Respir Dis* 1973;108:879–885.

157. Storstein O, Hansteen V, Hatle L, et al. Studies on digitalis. XIII. A prospective study of 649 patients on maintenance treatment with digitoxin. *Am Heart J* 1977;93:434–443.

158. Goren C, Denes P. The role of Holter monitoring in detecting digitalis-provoked arrhythmias. *Chest* 1981;79:555–558.

159. Sobotka P, Mayer J, Bauernfeind R, et al. Arrhythmias documented in 24-hour continuous ambulatory electrocardiographic monitoring in young women without apparent heart disease. *Am Heart J* 1981;101:753–759.

160. Brodsky M, Wu D, Denes P, et al. Arrhythmias documented by 24-hour continuous electrocardiographic monitoring in 50 male medical students without apparent heart disease. *Am J Cardiol* 1977;39:390–395.

161. Raferty E, Cashman P. Long-term recording of the electrocardiogram in a normal population. *Postgrad Med* 1976;52:32–37.

162. Talan D, Bauernfeind R, Ashley W, et al. Twenty-four hour continuous ECG recordings in long-distance runners. *Chest* 1982;82:19–24.

163. Wellens H, Brugada P. Mechanisms of supraventricular tachycardia. *Am J Cardiol* 1988;62:10D–15D.

164. Haines D, DiMarco J. Sustained intra-atrial reentrant tachycardia: clinical, electrocardiographic and electrophysiological characteristics and long-term follow-up. *J Am Coll Cardiol* 1990;15:1345–1354.

165. Chen SA, Chiang CE, Yang CJ, et al. Sustained atrial tachycardia in adult patients: electrophysiological characteristics, pharmacological response, possible mechanisms, and effects of radiofrequency ablation. *Circulation* 1994;90:1262–1278.

166. Mehta AV, Sanchez GR, Sacks EJ, et al. Ectopic automatic atrial tachycardia in children: clinical characteristics, management and follow-up. *J Am Coll Cardiol* 1988;11:379–385.

167. Englestein E, Lippman N, Stein K, et al. Mechanism-specific effects of adenosine on atrial tachycardia. *Circulation* 1994;89:2645–2654.

168. Poty H, Saoudi N, Haissaguerre M, et al. Radiofrequency catheter ablation of atrial tachycardias. *Am Heart J* 1996;131:481–489.

169. Baker BM, Lindsay BD, Bromberg BI, et al. Catheter ablation of clinical intraatrial reentrant tachycardias resulting from previous atrial surgery: localizing and transecting the critical isthmus. *J Am Coll Cardiol* 1996;28:411–417.

170. Chen CC, Tai CT, Chiang CE, et al. Atrial tachycardias originating from the atrial septum: electrophysiologic characteristics and radiofrequency ablation. *J Cardiovasc Electrophysiol* 2000;11:744–749.

171. MacLean WAH, Waldo AL, James TN. Formation and conduction of the cardiac electrical impulse. In: Yu PN, Goodwin JF, eds. *Progress in cardiology*. Philadelphia: Lea & Febiger, 1974:37–74.

172. Bauernfeind RA, Amat-Y-Leon F, Dhingra RC, et al. Chronic nonparoxysmal sinus tachycardia in otherwise healthy persons. *Ann Intern Med* 1979;91:702–710.

173. Morillo CA, Klein GJ, Thakur RK, et al. Mechanism of "inappropriate" sinus tachycardia. Role of sympathovagal balance. *Circulation* 1994;90:873–877.

174. Lee R, Kalman J, Fitzpatrick AP, et al. Radiofrequency catheter modification of the sinus node for "inappropriate" sinus tachycardia. *Circulation* 1995;92:2919–2928.

175. Waspe L, Chien W, Merillat JC, et al. Sinus node modification using radiofrequency current in a patient with persistent inappropriate sinus tachycardia. *Pacing Clin Electrophysiol* 1994;17:1569–1576.

176. Man KC, Knight B, Tse HF, et al. Radiofrequency catheter ablation of inappropriate sinus tachycardia guided by activation mapping. *J Am Coll Cardiol* 2000;35:451–457.

177. Gomes J, Hariman R, Kang P, et al. Sustained symptomatic sinus node reentrant tachycardia: incidence, clinical significance, electrophysiological observations, and the effects of antiarrhythmic agents. *J Am Coll Cardiol* 1985;5:45–57.

178. Narula OS. Sinus node reentry: a mechanism for supraventricular tachycardia. *Circulation* 1974;50:1114–1128.

179. Sanders W, Sorrentino R, Greenfield R, et al. Catheter ablation of sinoatrial node reentrant tachycardia. *J Am Coll Cardiol* 1994;23:926–934.

180. Gomes J, Mehta D, Langan M, et al. Sinus node reentrant tachycardia. *Pacing Clin Electrophysiol* 1995;18:1045–1057.

181. Scher D, Arsura E. Multifocal atrial tachycardia: mechanisms, clinical correlates, and treatment. *Am Heart J* 1989;118:574–580.

182. Arsura E, Lefkin A, Scher D, et al. A randomized, double-blind, placebo-controlled study of verapamil and metoprolol in treatment of multifocal atrial tachycardia. *Am J Med* 1988;85:519–524.

183. Salerno D, Anderson B, Sharkey P, Iber C. Intravenous verapamil for treatment of multifocal atrial tachycardia with and without calcium pretreatment. *Ann Intern Med* 1987;107:623–628.

184. Ueng KC, Lee SH, Wu DJ, et al. Radiofrequency catheter modification of atrioventricular junction in patients with COPD and medically refractory multifocal atrial tachycardia. *Chest* 2000;117:52–59.

66

ATRIOVENTRICULAR NODAL–DEPENDENT TACHYCARDIAS

THOMAS J. DRESING
ROBERT A. SCHWEIKERT
DOUGLAS L. PACKER

T. J. Dresing: Department of Cardiovascular Medicine, The Cleveland
Clinic Foundation, Cleveland, Ohio
R. A. Schweikert: Department of Cardiovascular Medicine, The Cleve-
land Clinic Foundation, Cleveland, Ohio
D. L. Packer: Division of Cardiovascular Diseases and Electrophysiol-
ogy, Mayo Clinic, Rochester, Minnesota

OVERVIEW

Atrioventricular (AV) nodal–dependent tachycardias
comprise a specific subgroup of rapid, regular supraventricular arrhythmias that critically depend on conduction
through the AV node for their perpetuation. The most

common are AV reentrant tachycardias that use an accessory pathway (AP) as the retrograde limb of the circuit and AV nodal reentrant tachycardia in which both anterograde and retrograde components of the reentrant substrate are within or near the compact portion of the AV node and neighboring bundle of His. The anatomic location around the mitral or tricuspid annulus of APs can be precisely identified at the time of electrophysiologic testing but can also be predicted with high accuracy based on the morphology of retrograde P waves during tachycardia or characteristic delta waves in those patients in whom these arrhythmias occur as a component of Wolff-Parkinson-White (WPW) syndrome. AV nodal–dependent tachycardias are typically initiated by premature atrial or ventricular extrastimuli and have reasonably specific characteristics that allow their differentiation. Although both are short RP tachycardias, AV reentrant tachycardia must have a ventriculoatrial (VA) or RP interval of at least 70 ms, whereas most AV nodal reentrant tachycardias have intervals of less than 60 ms, with retrograde P waves presenting as a pseudo-R wave in surface electrocardiogram (ECG) lead V_1 during tachycardia. In some patients with APs, a reversed-direction tachycardia with anterograde conduction through the AP may occur, producing a maximally preexcited QRS complex on the surface ECG. Some patients with WPW syndrome are at potential risk for atrial fibrillation degenerating into ventricular fibrillation. APs with unusual conduction characteristics contribute to the occurrence of preexcitation variants, including the permanent form of junctional reciprocating tachycardia and atriofascicular reentry. Because of their dependence on AV nodal conduction for their maintenance, AV nodal–dependent arrhythmias may be acutely terminated by vagal maneuvers or administration of adenosine or verapamil. Wide-complex tachycardias in these patients must be carefully approached without using drugs that accelerate AP conduction, which can lead to ventricular fibrillation. Both pharmacologic and nonpharmacologic therapies may be applied in the long term for managing patients with these arrhythmias. Drug therapy may be directed at the AV node, the AP, or the initiating atrial or ventricular extrastimuli. Ablative therapy has also emerged as the mainstay of nonpharmacologic treatment of these arrhythmias.

GLOSSARY

Anterior fibrous trigone: The region of convergent, dense, fibrous tissue of the posterior aortic and anterior mitral valve annuli.

Antidromic reciprocating tachycardia: A reversed-direction AV nodal–dependent tachycardia in which antero-

grade conduction occurs through the AP, whereas return retrograde atrial activation proceeds through the normal VA conduction system.

Atriofasciculoventricular Mahaim fiber: An atypical AP with AV node–like properties typically located in the anterior or anterolateral region of the tricuspid annulus. This pathway serves as a bridge between atrial and right bundle branch tissue.

Atriofasciculoventricular or "Mahaim" reentrant tachycardia: A preexcitation variant tachycardia that uses an atriofascicular fiber as its anterograde limb.

AV nodal reentrant tachycardia: An AV nodal–dependent tachycardia in which both anterograde and retrograde components of the reentrant substrate are located within or near the compact portion of the AV node.

AV nodal–dependent tachycardia: A tachycardia that critically depends on conduction through the AV node for its perpetuation.

AV reentrant tachycardia: An AV nodal–dependent tachycardia with the AV conduction system as the anterograde and the AP as the retrograde limb of the tachycardia circuit.

Concealed AP: AP with retrograde-only conduction existing without evidence of anterograde ventricular activation through that pathway.

Discontinuous conduction: Characteristic of dual AV nodal physiology in which a more than 50-ms abrupt prolongation of AV nodal conduction time occurs with a 10-ms decrease in the coupling time of an atrial premature complex (APC), producing anterograde conduction through the AV node.

Dual AV nodal physiology: Electrophysiologic manifestation of two AV nodal pathways with different anatomic and/or physiologic properties that serve as a substrate for AV nodal reentrant tachycardia.

Koch's triangle: A triangular space in the medial portion of the right atrium formed by the septal component of the tricuspid valve annulus, the coronary sinus orifice, and the tendon of Todaro. The AV node lies in the apex of this triangle.

Long RP tachycardia: Tachycardia with a retrograde P wave describing atrial activation occurring close to the succeeding QRS complex. These tachycardias have an RP interval that is more than 50% of the RR interval seen during tachycardia.

Permanent junctional reciprocating tachycardia (PJRT): Preexcitation variant in which retrograde atrial activation occurs through an AP with node-like or decremental electrical conduction properties. These long RP tachycardias may be incessant and show negative P waves in leads II, III, and aVF.

Preexcitation: Early ventricular activation before that proceeding through the normal AV conduction system, as seen in patients with APs.

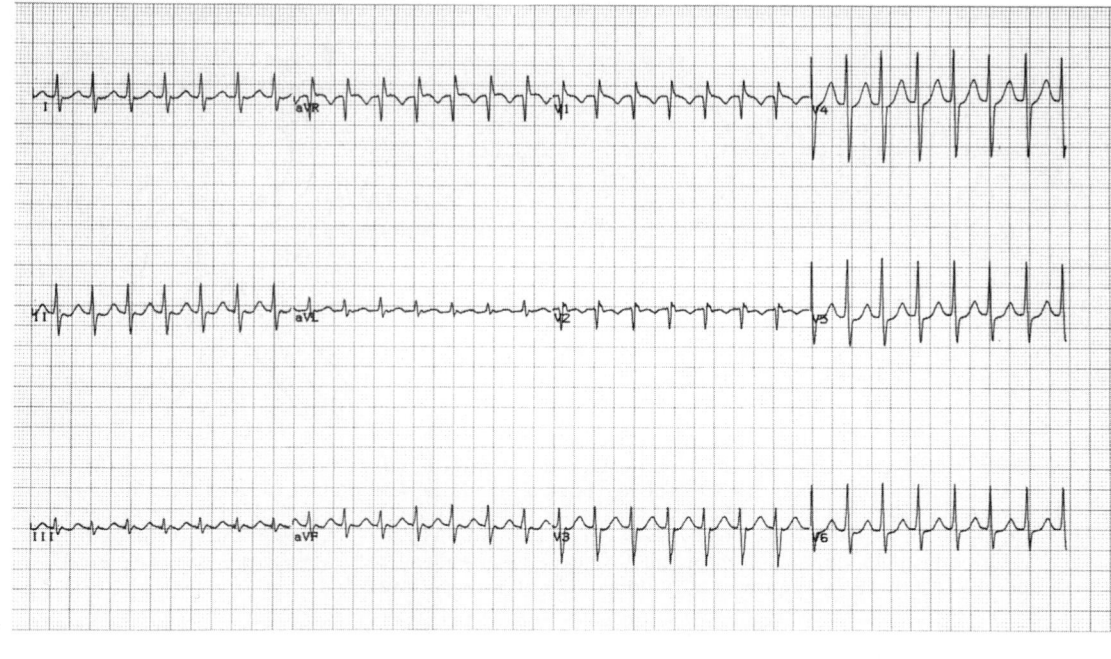

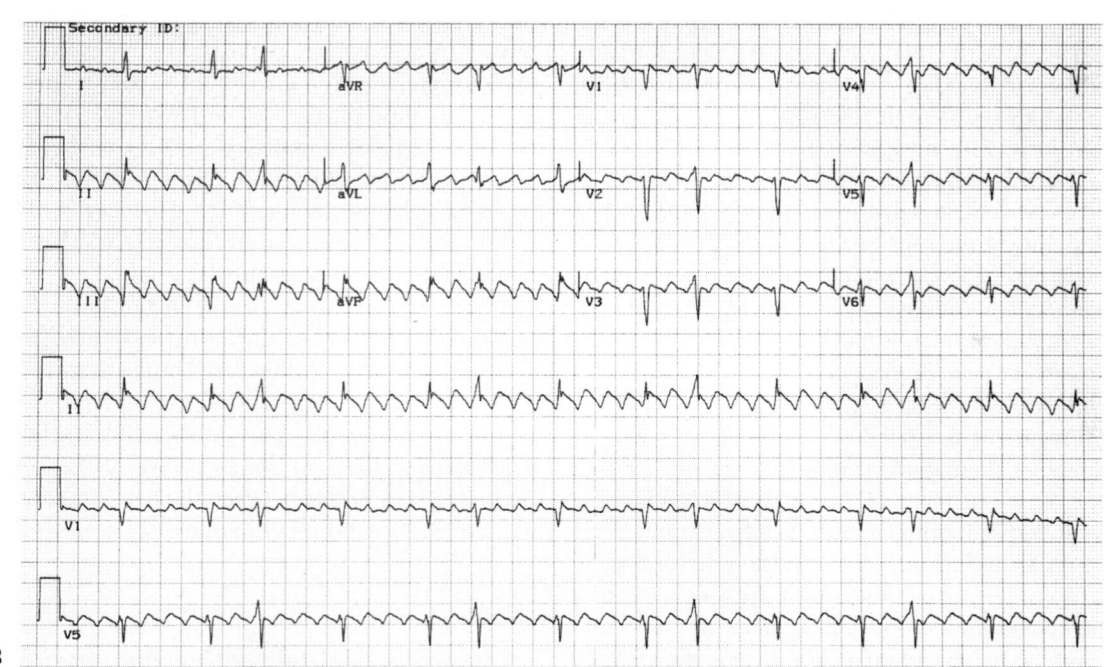

FIGURE 66.1 Electrocardiogram tracings from atrioventricular (AV) nodal–dependent and AV nodal–independent tachycardias. **A:** Narrow QRS complex tachycardia with a 1:1 AV relationship in a patient with an AV nodal reentrant tachycardia. **B:** Classic atrial flutter persisting despite variable AV block.

Short RP tachycardia: Tachycardia with a retrograde P wave describing atrial activation that occurs close to the preceding QRS complex. These tachycardias have an RP interval that is less than 50% of the RR interval seen during tachycardia.

VA interval: The VA interval beginning with the local ventricular activation and ending with earliest retrograde atrial activation. The surface ECG correlate is the RP interval from onset of the surface QRS to the retrograde P wave.

INTRODUCTION

AV nodal–dependent tachycardias comprise a specific subgroup of rapid, regular supraventricular arrhythmias that critically depend on conduction through the AV node for their perpetuation. These arrhythmias typically use the normal AV conduction system as the anterograde limb of the reentrant circuit and therefore present with a narrow QRS complex on the surface ECG, as shown in Figure 66.1.

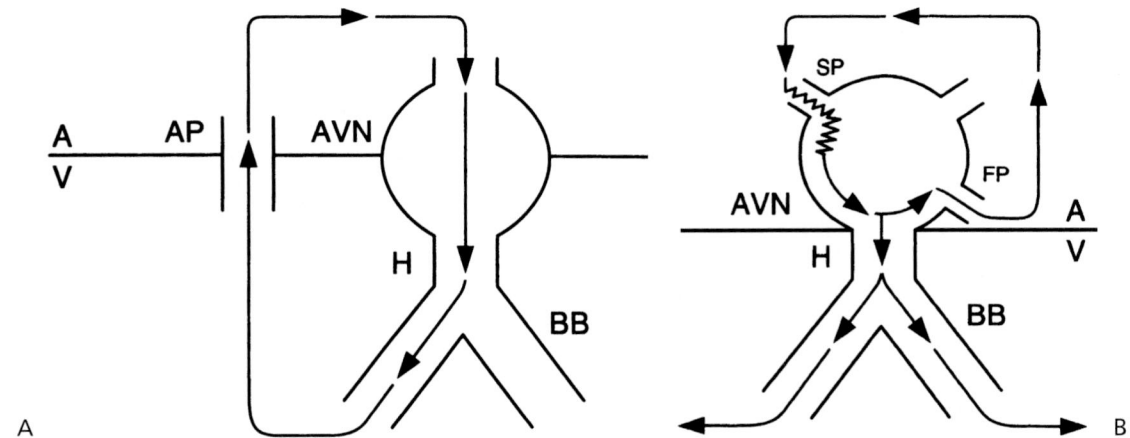

FIGURE 66.2 Mechanism of atrioventricular (AV) reentrant and AV nodal reentrant tachycardias. In both arrhythmias, the AV node serves as a mandatory component of the reentrant circuit. **A:** AV reentrant tachycardia in which the AP serves as the retrograde limb of the reentrant circuit. **B:** AV nodal reentrant tachycardia circuit with anterograde conduction through SP with return retrograde conduction through FP. AP, accessory pathway; AVN, atrioventricular node; BB, bundle branch; FP, fast pathway; H, bundle of His; SP, slow pathway.

Unlike atrial flutter or atrial tachycardias, which may continue despite the presence of high-grade AV block, AV nodal–dependent tachycardias are typically eliminated by vagal, drug, or nonpharmacologic interruption of AV nodal conduction. As such, with infrequent exceptions (e.g., AV nodal reentrant tachycardia with 2:1 A:V or V:A conduction), AV nodal–dependent tachycardias show a classic 1:1 AV relationship, unlike their AV nodal–independent counterparts that may have a 2:1 or more AV relationship, with or without these interventions (Fig. 66.1).

The most common of the AV nodal–dependent arrhythmias are AV reentrant tachycardias, in which an AP is used as the retrograde limb of the tachycardia circuit (Fig. 66.2), and AV nodal reentrant tachycardias (Fig. 66.2) in which both anterograde and retrograde components of the reentrant substrate are within or near the compact portion of the AV node and neighboring bundle of His. Some AV nodal–dependent arrhythmias, such as antidromic reciprocating tachycardias, less frequently use the AV conduction system as the retrograde component and an AP as the anterograde limb of the tachycardia circuit. Therefore, the QRS complex on the surface ECG during tachycardia is maximally preexcited.

ANATOMIC CONSIDERATIONS

Accessory Pathways

APs involved as the retrograde limb of the AV reentrant tachycardia circuit are formed by minute, electrically conducting muscle bundles that transverse the AV groove. These pathways establish a nonnodal avenue for AV or VA electrical propagation across the mitral and tricuspid annuli, which otherwise electrically isolate the atria from the ventricles. These fibers may cross the AV groove directly, proceed on an angle, or in some cases arborize with one or more branch points before insertion into either ventricular or atrial muscle (51–54). Whether atrial or ventricular muscle tissue comprises the AP remains unclear. The observation that APs follow Ebstein's malformation of the tricuspid valve to the anatomic left heart in patients with transposition of the great arteries suggests that the tissue is more likely to be of a ventricular origin.

With the exception of the region near the anterior fibrous trigone between the aortic and mitral valves, which is usually void of APs, these AV connections are distributed anywhere along the mitral or tricuspid annuli. As noted in Figure 66.3, surgical and catheter ablation studies have demonstrated that, on average, 55% of these AV connections serve as a bridge between the left atrium and ventricle in a free wall location. Furthermore, 25% are in the postero-

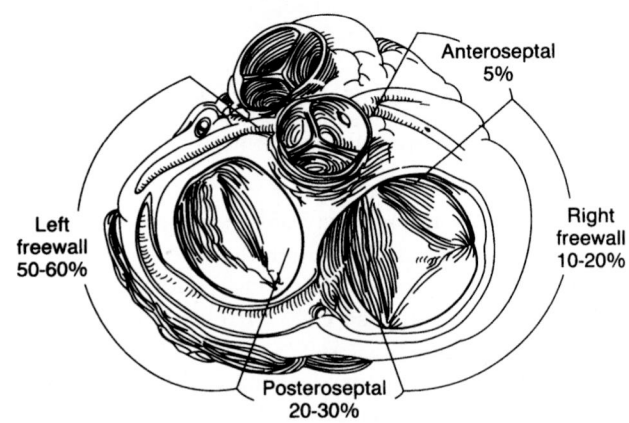

FIGURE 66.3 Distribution of accessory pathways (APs) around the mitral and tricuspid annuli. The left free wall position is the most common AP location.

septal region, 15% are in a right free wall location, and 5% are in the anteroseptal region (33,35–37,41,43–45,55). In addition, 7% to 15% of patients may have more than one AP (24,41,43–45,56–59). More recently, a unique AP involving a connection between the right atrial appendage and right ventricle has been described (60–63). This type of AP may be difficult to ablate with standard techniques endocardially, and successful catheter ablation with a percutaneous epicardial instrumentation approach has been described (61). ▼ 165

PHYSIOLOGIC MECHANISMS OF ATRIOVENTRICULAR NODAL–DEPENDENT TACHYCARDIAS

Tachycardia Initiation

AV nodal–dependent tachycardias require not only the appropriate anatomic substrate for reentry, but also an initiating event. In most cases, initiation is related to the occurrence of atrial or ventricular extrasystolic activity that conducts into and blocks in one of the anatomically distinct components of the reentrant circuit (19,68). An APC, for example, may enter and block within an AP capable of bidirectional conduction (Fig. 66.4). If ventricular activation occurs through the normal AV conduction system, followed by return retrograde atrial activation over the AP back toward the interatrial septum and the AV node, the reentrant circuit is completed. As such, both ventricular and atrial tissue are critical components of the reentrant

tachycardia circuit in this arrhythmia. Completing this circuit may be facilitated by delay within the AV node in response to the APC, allowing additional time for the AP to recover before the return impulse arrives at the ventricular end of the pathway (81). Isoproterenol or other adrenergic enhancement may be required to initiate tachycardia in those cases in which AV node conduction under baseline conditions precludes the onset of arrhythmia.

AV reentrant tachycardia can also be initiated by a ventricular premature complex (VPC) or pacing. Here, the initiating VPC typically blocks retrogradely in both sides of the His-Purkinje system, conducts to the atrium through the AP, and completes the circuit by reactivating the ventricles through the normal anterograde AV conduction system, as shown in Figure 66.4 (82,83).

Tachycardia Maintenance

Although ventricular activation occurs rapidly through the His-Purkinje system, the distance of the AP from the bundle of His region dictates that the time from onset of the surface QRS to the local atrial activation at the site of the pathway, referred to as the *VA interval*, must be at least 65 to 70 (64,84). For this reason, the ECG correlate of this VA interval, the "RP" interval, from the onset of the QRS complex to the P wave is usually more than 80 ms in duration. This specific VA activation time predicts that the inscription of the retrograde P wave will occur early in the ST segment or on the upslope of the T wave of the surface ECG, closer to the preceding than the succeeding QRS complex, as shown in Figure 66.5. If the RP interval is less

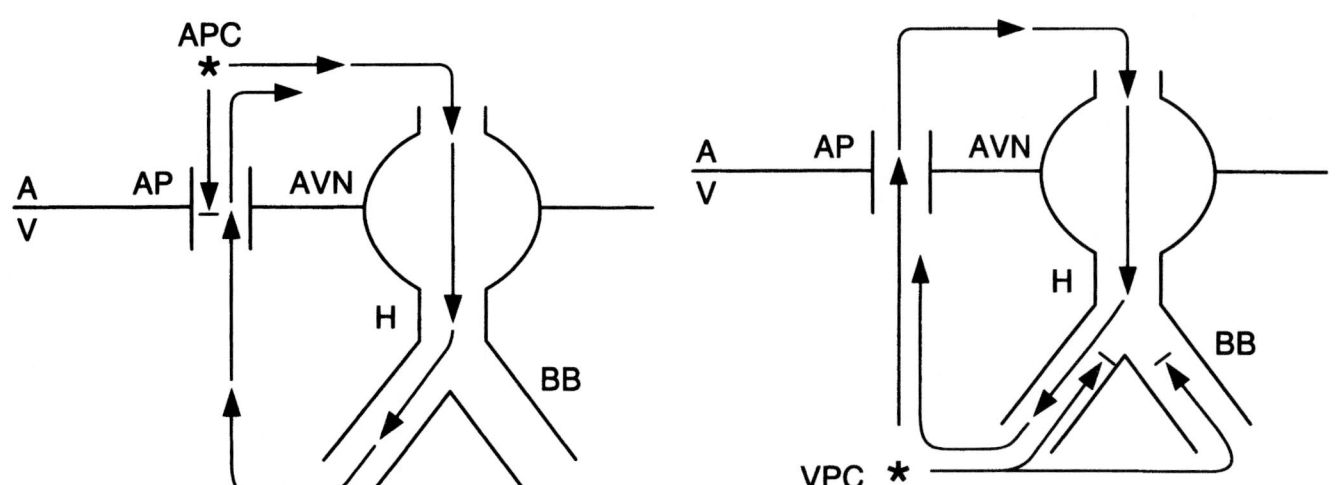

FIGURE 66.4 Initiation of atrioventricular (AV) reentrant tachycardia with an atrial premature complex (APC) or ventricular premature complex (VPC). **A:** APC that conducts into and blocks within the accessory pathway (AP). Additional conduction through the normal AV conduction system followed by return retrograde atrial activation through the AP leads to reentrant arrhythmia. **B:** Similar initiation with a VPC that first blocks retrogradely in both sides of the His-Purkinje system. Subsequent retrograde atrial activation through the AP with return conduction through the normal AV conduction system completes the reentrant circuit. AVN, atrioventricular node.

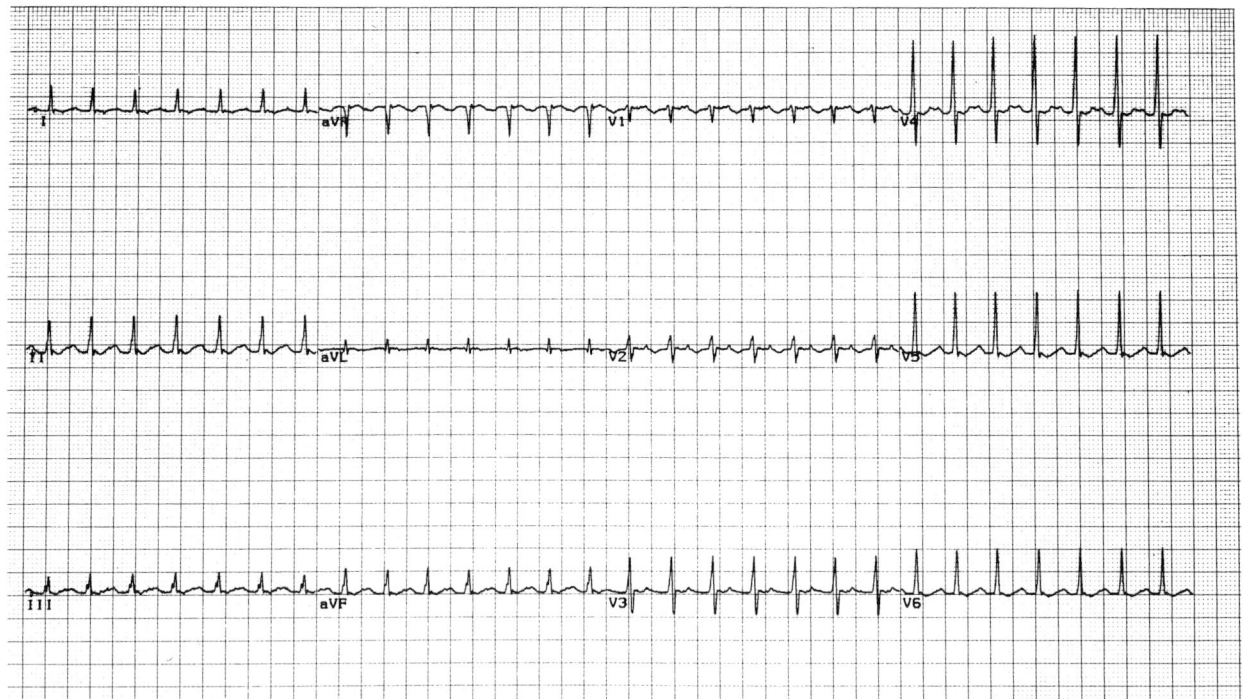

FIGURE 66.5 Narrow complex supraventricular tachycardia due to an atrioventricular reentrant mechanism. Note the retrograde P waves inscribed in the inferior and precordial ST segments and the short RP tachycardia appearance.

than 50% of the RR interval from one QRS complex to the next, the tachycardia is considered to be a short RP tachycardia (Fig. 66.6).

These VA or RP intervals during tachycardia typically use an AP and are relatively constant. An important exception to this is the more than 35-ms prolongation of the VA

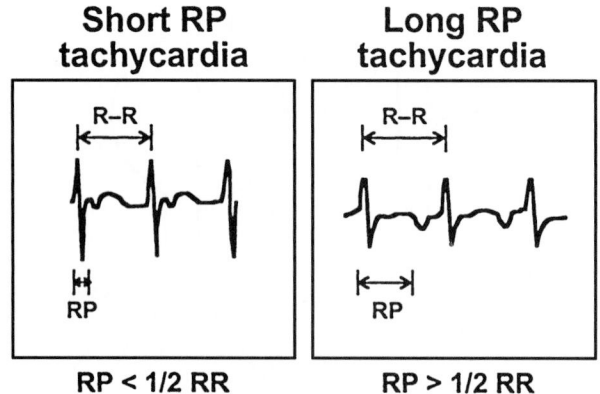

FIGURE 66.6 Classification of short and long RP tachycardias. The left panel shows a retrograde P wave in tachycardia that occurs closer to the preceding than succeeding QRS. Supraventricular arrhythmias with such an RP interval of less than 50% of the RR interval are designated "short" RP tachycardias. The right panel shows a retrograde P wave closer to the following QRS due to prolonged retrograde conduction time. An RP interval longer than 50% of the RR cycle length qualifies as a "long" RP tachycardia.

interval seen with the emergence of bundle branch block ipsilateral to the AP during the AV reentrant arrhythmia, as shown in *e*Figure 66.6.1 (85,86), because ventricular activation in the presence of bundle branch block must proceed through the contralateral bundle branch, with subsequent slower transseptal conduction and return propagation to the ventricular origin of the AP through ventricular muscle. For example, patients with left free wall pathways who develop left bundle branch block show classic prolongation of the VA interval during tachycardia. The alternative is true in patients with right free wall pathways who develop right bundle branch block. Unless this activation slowing is offset by reciprocal acceleration of conduction through the normal AV conduction system, the tachycardia in such patients is slowed. Conversely, acceleration of the tachycardia with abrupt resolution of bundle branch block, as seen on the surface ECG in *e*Figure 66.6.2, is virtually pathognomonic for an AP-related tachycardia. In contrast, patients with posteroseptal pathways show VA interval changes of 10 to 30 ms only with the emergence of left bundle branch block, whereas patients with anteroseptal pathways may develop a comparably limited VA interval change during onset of right bundle branch block (85).

An additional indication of an AP that is participating in a narrow QRS complex tachycardia that can be elucidated on electrophysiologic testing is based on the response to VPCs introduced during the tachycardia. An AP is present if a VPC introduced late in the tachycardia diastolic interval advances or preexcites retrograde atrial activation without changing the atrial activation sequence (87,88). As shown in *e*Figure 66.6.3, such advancement occurs through an AP, because the VPC cannot retrogradely penetrate the AV node or bundle of His, as the immediately preceding anterograde impulse during tachycardia placed these tissues into a state of refractoriness. Furthermore, termination of tachycardia by a premature impulse at a time when the bundle of His is refractory that does not produce retrograde atrial activation must occur within ventricular or His-Purkinje tissue, thus establishing such tissue as critical components of the reentrant circuit. This is even stronger evidence that narrow complex tachycardias critically depend on an AP as their retrograde limb (26–28).

Physiology of Preexcitation

When the AV reentrant tachycardia occurs in a patient with early or "preexcited" anterograde ventricular activation through the AP during normal sinus rhythm, a delta wave and a short PR interval are evident on the surface ECG (Fig. 66.7), and the criteria for WPW syndrome are met (8). The degree of accompanying preexcitation observed on a surface 12-lead ECG, however, depends on relative local ventricular activation proceeding through the normal AV conduction system versus that through the AP. This in turn depends on the relative time required for a propagating impulse from the sinus node to reach and traverse the AV node and His-Purkinje system or the AP (*e*Fig. 66.7.1). The additional activation time required to reach an AP well removed from the sinus node along the far left lateral region of the mitral annulus decreases the likelihood of expressing ventricular preexcitation during normal sinus rhythm with this pathway location. In the setting of increased sympathoadrenergic tone as that which accompanies exercise, ventricular activation through the normal AV conduction system is enhanced and can precede that which occurs

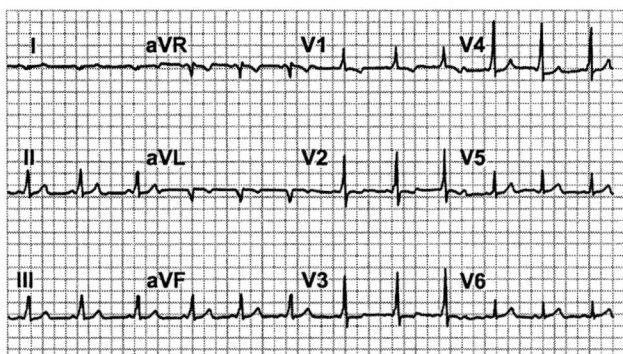

FIGURE 66.7 Electrocardiogram with ventricular preexcitation across a left free wall accessory pathway. Note the widened QRS complex with a slurred upstroke and a shortened PR interval consistent with a diagnosis of Wolff-Parkinson-White syndrome.

through the AP (*e*Fig. 66.7.1). During such circumstances, no or minimal ventricular preexcitation may be evident. At the other extreme, ventricular activation through the pathway, yielding moderate or marked preexcitation, may be more evident with pathways closer to the sinus node or in those conditions in which conduction through the AV node is slowed by intrinsic nodal factors, withdrawal of sympathetic tone, or heightened vagal tone (*e*Fig. 66.7.1). In some cases, the rapid intravenous (i.v.) administration of 6 to 12 mg of adenosine as a diagnostic maneuver exposes an anterograde AP by blocking or slowing AV node conduction (89,90). As such, the presence and degree of ventricular preexcitation in patients with WPW syndrome depend dynamically on a variety of different factors, chief of which is the autonomic modulation of the AV node.

The degree of preexcitation can also be enhanced with atrial pacing, as performed on electrophysiologic testing (28). With pacing directly over the AP, inherent intraatrial conduction delay from the sinus node to the atrial origin of the AP is eliminated. In addition, increments in rapid atrial pacing rates increase preexcitation by progressively slowing or decrementing conduction within the normal AV conduction system. The QRS complex thereby becomes more preexcited unless block in the AP occurs and the QRS complex narrows as conduction proceeds exclusively through the normal AV conduction system.

Preexcited Atrioventricular Nodal–Dependent Tachycardias

Although most AV nodal–dependent tachycardias use the AV conduction system as the anterograde limb of the tachycardia circuit, the reentrant circuit is reversed in the presence of antidromic reciprocating tachycardia, as seen in Figure 66.8. With this arrhythmia, the AV node is the requisite retrograde limb of the circuit, and ventricular activation proceeds through the AP, producing maximum QRS preexcitation (Fig. 66.9). This tachycardia can be induced on electrophysiologic testing in 6% to 8% of patients with an AP (55,91–93), although only 2% to 3% of patients clinically develop this arrhythmia (55,91,93).

AV nodal reentry with bystander conduction through a coexistent AP is a second preexcited AV nodal–dependent tachycardia. In this arrhythmia, perpetuation of the tachycardia depends on classic AV node reentry using anterograde and retrograde limbs found within or near the compact portion of the AV node. The wide or preexcited QRS morphology seen on ECG is due to concomitant ventricular activation through an AP. Ablation of the AP, although eliminating preexcitation, would not necessarily eliminate the tachycardia. Although AV nodal reentrant tachycardia may be seen in 10% to 20% of patients with an AP (94–97), concurrent anterograde conduction through an AP is seen in less than 2% of patients (96). When evaluating patients with these types of AV nodal–dependent

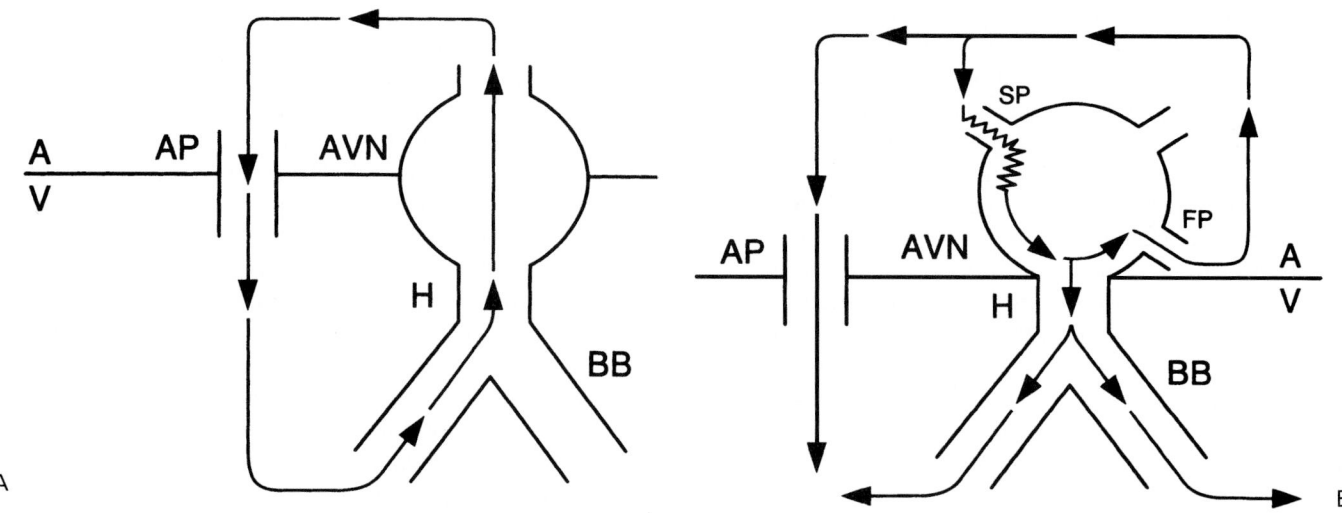

A

B

FIGURE 66.8 Mechanisms of preexcited atrioventricular (AV) nodal–dependent tachycardias. **A:** Antidromic reciprocating tachycardia with anterograde conduction through the accessory pathway (AP) and retrograde atrial activation through the normal ventriculoatrial conduction system. **B:** AV nodal reentry with a classic mechanism involving anterograde conduction through the slow pathway (SP) and retrograde or return atrial activation through the fast pathway (FP). Preexcitation occurs because of additional bystander conduction through the neighboring AP. AVN, atrioventricular node; BB, bundle branch; H, bundle of His.

tachycardias, alternative mechanisms of preexcited tachycardias such as any atrial tachycardia or flutter with ventricular activation through an AP should be considered. Well-defined criteria for differentiating these types of tachycardias from antidromic reciprocating tachycardia have been established (93,98).

CLINICAL PRESENTATION

General Considerations

Screening 12-lead ECG studies reveal that 1.0 to 1.5 in 1,000 patients demonstrate preexcitation. Population-based studies (106) have suggested that 50% to 60% of these patients show symptoms ranging from palpitations to syncope. In others, tachycardia may be accompanied by dyspnea, decreased exercise tolerance, chest pain or tightness, anxiety, dizziness, presyncope, or syncope. The latter is more likely in AV nodal reentrant tachycardia in which atrial and ventricular contractions accompanying respective electrical activation occur nearly simultaneously. Atrial contraction at the time of mitral valve closure may limit cardiac output and be accompanied by increases in right and left atrial pressure. These increases in turn may precipitate a posttachycardia diuresis due to release of atrial paracrine factors such as atrial natriuretic peptides. Of those patients with symptomatic arrhythmias, 85% have underlying AV reentrant tachycardias that use the AP as a retrograde limb (28,55,64). Only 2% to 3% of patients show clinical antidromic reciprocating tachycardia (93,107,108), whereas 30% to 40% of patients develop atrial fibrillation (55,64,109–112).

Unlike most ventricular tachycardias, which occur in patients with pump dysfunction, most AV nodal–dependent tachycardias occur in the absence of any other organic heart disease. Any underlying process that does occur, such as mitral valve prolapse or hypertrophic cardiomyopathy, is therefore a chance occurrence. The one exception is coexistent Ebstein's malformation of the tricuspid valve and an AP (55,64,95). Of those patients with APs reported in larger studies (113,114), 7% to 10% have this coexistent structural abnormality. This finding is of clinical importance because these patients typically have a higher prevalence of multiple APs and the success rate of RF ablation in patients with tricuspid valve abnormalities is lower.

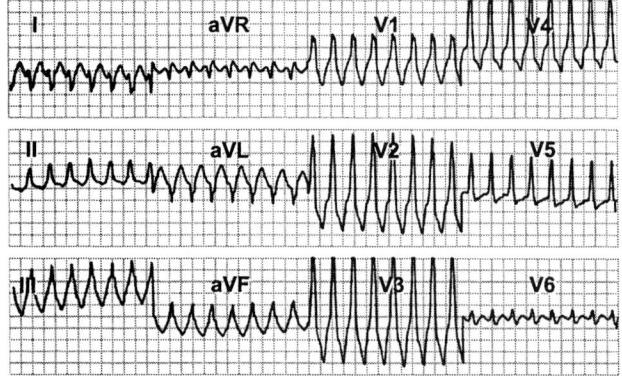

FIGURE 66.9 Antidromic reciprocating tachycardia with marked preexcitation. This electrocardiogram pattern occurs because of exclusive ventricular activation through the accessory pathway. Retrograde activation occurs through the normal ventriculoatrial conduction system.

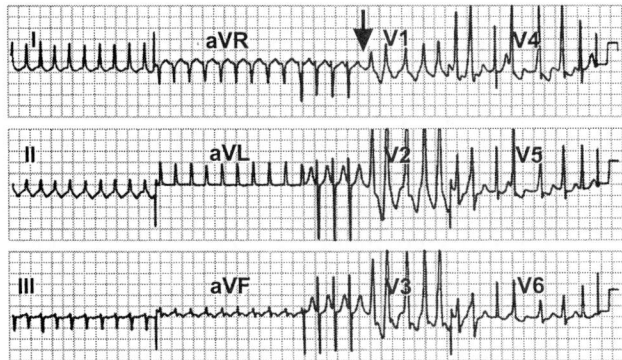

FIGURE 66.10 Atrial fibrillation with a rapid ventricular response rate during Wolff-Parkinson-White syndrome. Initial atrioventricular reentrant tachycardia degenerates into atrial fibrillation (*arrow*). The shortest RR interval in this case was 240 to 250 ms, which indicates an increased risk for sudden cardiac death.

Risk Stratification in Patients with Wolff-Parkinson-White Syndrome

Atrial fibrillation occurs in 30% to 40% of patients with WPW syndrome. Of greatest concern is the propensity of rapid conduction through the AP with accompanying risk for atrial fibrillation degenerating into ventricular fibrillation (Fig. 66.10). The degree of risk is related in part to the symptom status of the patient at the time of initial evaluation. In symptomatic patients from tertiary referral centers, the prevalence of patients with a history of aborted sudden cardiac death (SCD) is 2% to 11% (64,106,122). In contrast, population-based studies (106) demonstrate a lower incidence of SCD—0.0015 events per patient year, or approximately 0.15% per year—occurring exclusively in previously symptomatic individuals. Several other studies (106,120) have also shown that patients who are asymptomatic at the time of diagnosis are unlikely to suffer a subsequent cardiac arrest. This is related to relatively benign AP conduction capabilities in these patients (63,120,123).

A variety of testing methods have been proposed for stratifying the risk for atrial fibrillation degenerating into ventricular fibrillation, including ambulatory recordings, exercise testing, and the response to drugs. The most direct method of assessment is the actual induction of atrial fibrillation and determination of the propensity for rapid conduction as judged by the interval between consecutively preexcited QRS or "RR" complexes. Klein et al. (124) showed that those patients who survived a prior episode of ventricular fibrillation had the shortest preexcited RR intervals (i.e., less than 250 ms in duration) (*e*Fig. 66.10.1). Although this has been regarded as a highly sensitive marker for risk, it is of lower specificity. As such, the positive predictive value of this finding is only 20% over short-term follow-up. On the other hand, the shortest preexcited RR interval of more than 250 ms has a negative predictive value of more than 95%. Other indicators of risk include

an average RR interval during atrial fibrillation of 360 ms or less (125). A posteroseptal AP with accompanying rapid AV conduction capability and prior atrial fibrillation also suggests a higher risk (122,125).

Other findings on noninvasive testing, if present, indicate a lower risk for SCD. The demonstration of intermittent preexcitation on a 12-lead ECG or ambulatory monitor strip as shown in Figure 66.11 indicates the presence of precarious conduction through an AP (126). It must be noted, however, that the term *intermittent preexcitation* specifically denotes the *abrupt* loss of preexcitation from one beat to the next on a rhythm strip or ECG; it cannot be extended to include the loss of preexcitation on an ECG from one office visit to the next. Depending on the effect of autonomic tone on AV nodal conduction, ventricular activation may proceed exclusively through the normal AV conduction system, thus masking the anterograde conduction capability of the pathway on an ECG. The next ECG, if obtained at the time of heightened parasympathetic tone, alternatively may show increased preexcitation due to preferential ventricular activation through the pathway. This variability is of no predictive value and is of particular concern in patients with left free wall pathways in which the distance of the pathway from the sinus node decreases the chance of manifest preexcitation.

Exercise testing has also been proposed as a means of identifying patients with long AP refractoriness (127,128). Although several groups have shown that the *abrupt* loss of preexcitation during exercise (Fig. 66.12) is indicative of a low propensity for rapid conduction through an AP, this is an infrequent finding. Preexcitation more frequently disappears gradually during exercise because of enhanced conduction through the normal AV conduction system. Because of the low likelihood of an abrupt loss of preexcitation on exercise testing, persistent preexcitation during exercise testing is reasonably sensitive for identifying patients at risk for an untoward event. Unfortunately, the specificity for excluding those who are not at risk is less than 30%, which is substantially less than that of the shortest RR interval between two preexcited QRS complexes of 250 ms or less. Furthermore, the predictive accuracy of exercise testing is even lower than possible with the induction of atrial fibrillation (128).

Others have reported the use of drug testing measures to stratify risk. This is based on the presumption that the loss

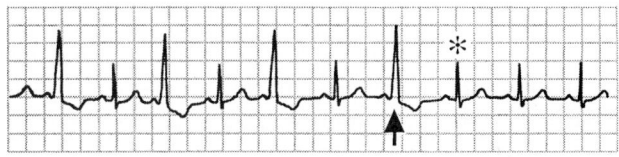

FIGURE 66.11 Rhythm strip showing intermittent preexcitation in a patient with Wolff-Parkinson-White syndrome. Both preexcited (*arrow*) and nonpreexcited (*asterisk*) QRS complexes are seen. Note the loss of QRS preexcitation from one beat to the next.

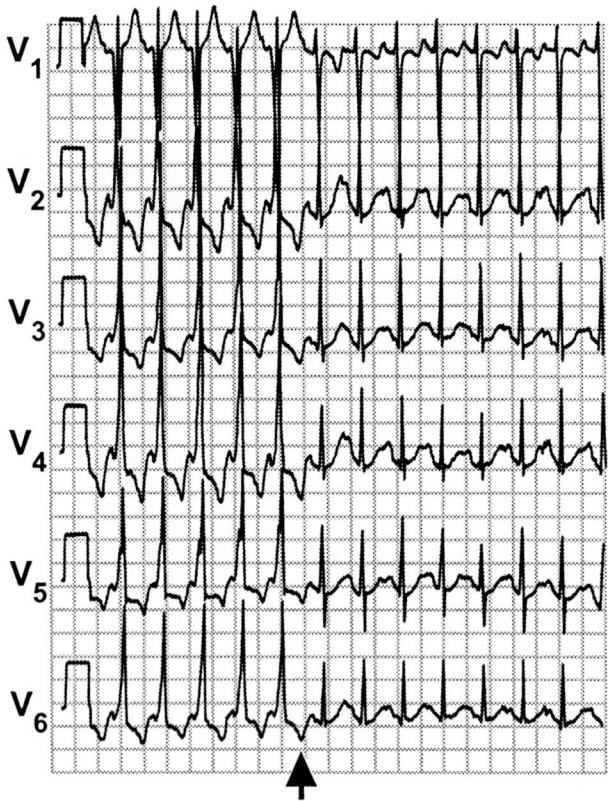

FIGURE 66.12 Electrocardiogram rhythm strip of leads V$_1$ to V$_6$ recorded during exercise in a patient with a left free wall accessory pathway. With an increasing workload, an abrupt loss of preexcitation (*arrow*) was seen. This indicates a low-risk pathway. Gradual loss of preexcitation accompanying exercise-induced enhancement of atrioventricular nodal conduction is of no prognostic significance.

of AP conduction with administration of an agent such as procainamide or ajmaline (129,130) indicates a low-risk pathway. Again, however, findings using such testing maneuvers appear to be falsely reassuring (28,128,130,131). In a previous report (130), the response to 10 to 12 mg per kg of procainamide in 56 patients with WPW syndrome failed to support infusion of this medication for establishing risk. Risk stratification is discussed in greater detail in other studies (28).

The most direct means of stratifying risk in symptomatic patients is initiation of atrial fibrillation. This can be performed in a relatively noninvasive way with atrial pacing using an esophageal lead (90,132,133). In those patients in whom risk stratification is important, this allows direct determination of risk at the level of ventricular response rate during atrial fibrillation. This is preferable to using surrogate indicators of risk available on ambulatory recordings or exercise testing or to the response to drugs that only indirectly predict pathway effective refractoriness or ventricular rates in atrial fibrillation.

Furthermore, the overall risk of an untoward event in an asymptomatic patient is clearly not zero but appears to be

sufficiently low that additional evaluation of asymptomatic individuals showing ventricular preexcitation on 12-lead ECG is unnecessary (134). The risks associated with drug or ablative therapy in these patients may be equal to or greater than the risks associated with an underlying AP. Potential exceptions to this include patients with a family history of SCD, competitive athletes, and patients with high-risk occupations whose performance may be unacceptably impaired by the unlikely occurrence of tachycardia or atrial fibrillation, with or without rapid ventricular response rates. In contrast, symptomatic patients, particularly those with a history of atrial fibrillation, are at higher risk for more rapid conduction through an AP during atrial fibrillation and warrant further evaluation (109,112,125).

PREEXCITATION VARIANTS

Unlike the more classic presentations seen in most patients with WPW syndrome, other individuals have arrhythmias related to atypical APs with distinctive anatomic and physiologic characteristics. The most common of these are PJRT and preexcited tachycardia related to atriofascicular fibers. The hallmark of these preexcitation variants is the presence of unusual APs that show node-like or decremental electrical conduction properties. Here, progressively slower conduction across the pathway occurs with faster stimulation rates.

PERMANENT JUNCTIONAL RECIPROCATING TACHYCARDIA

Most patients with PJRT have posteroseptal APs within 1 cm of the coronary sinus orifice (25,135,136), although free wall pathway locations have been described (136,137). Like more typical APs, these connections also participate as the retrograde limb of an AV nodal–dependent tachycardia. In addition to characteristic decremental conduction properties, these pathways also have a long circuitous route from ventricle to atrium, contributing to prolongation of retrograde conduction times (138,139). These pathways also appear to conduct in the retrograde direction only, although several instances of emergent anterograde conduction and more classic ventricular preexcitation have been reported after ablation of the normal AV conduction system (140). This suggests that preablation anterograde conduction into the pathway is blocked in part by retrogradely concealing penetration of impulses into the pathway from the ventricular end of the normal AV conduction system during sinus rhythm. Unlike typical reentrant tachycardias, this arrhythmia may occur spontaneously with alterations of the sinus rate without preceding APCs or VPCs. In such cases, return conduction through the AP and subsequent reactivation of the anterograde AV nodal limb of the circuit perpetuate the tachycardia (25,135).

Slow reverse VA conduction results in inscription of the retrograde P wave in late diastole or closer to the succeeding QRS than the preceding QRS, as shown in *e*Figure 66.12.1 (25,135). The finding of an RP interval of more than 50% of the RR tachycardia interval invokes the descriptor, long RP tachycardia. Because the low atrial septum is most frequently the first site of atrial activation, P waves during PJRT are typically negative in leads II, III, and aVF, indicating a low-to-high retrograde atrial activation sequence.

Many patients with this process develop rapid, nearly incessant, tachycardias, hence the designation PJRT. Because of the incessant nature of the tachycardia, the development of a tachycardia-induced cardiomyopathy (*e*Fig. 66.12.2) that resolves after elimination of the pathway is not uncommon (141). Other patients with this type of pathway show only frequent paroxysmal junctional reciprocating tachycardia.

Atriofascicular (Mahaim) Reentrant Tachycardias

Another type of tachycardia, referred to as *atriofascicular*, or *Mahaim, reentrant tachycardia*, is due to a similar decrementally conducting AP located in the right anterior or anterolateral aspect of the tricuspid annulus. When first described (142,143), these pathways were believed to originate in the upper portion of the AV node, with distal insertion in the ventricle or right bundle branch system. Electrophysiologic studies (144,145) have demonstrated more recently that the vast majority of patients with left bundle branch block left-axis deviation Mahaim tachycardias have pathways located several centimeters away from the AV node, as suggested in Figure 66.13. Local His-like potentials are usually seen when recording immediately over this pathway site. As with the normal AV node, conduction in these pathways is strongly altered by adenosine or verapamil. This pathway, which also shows progressively longer conduction times at faster pacing rates, inserts into the right bundle branch system (146), giving a left bundle branch block left-axis deviation QRS morphology on the surface ECG during tachycardia (*e*Fig. 66.13.1). In addition, small, sharp R waves are typically seen in lead V$_1$, and the transition from negative to positive QRS morphology seen in the precordial leads typically occurs after V$_4$ (108). Like antidromic reciprocating tachycardias, the VA conduction system serves as the retrograde limb of this circuit. Because of its left bundle branch block appearance, this arrhythmia must be differentiated from other tachycardias with a left bundle branch block morphology, such as any atrial or AV nodal–dependent tachycardia with bundle branch aberrancy, antidromic tachycardias using a right free wall AP, right ventricular tachycardia as seen in patients with arrhythmogenic right ventricular dysplasia, and bundle branch reentrant ventricular tachycardias.

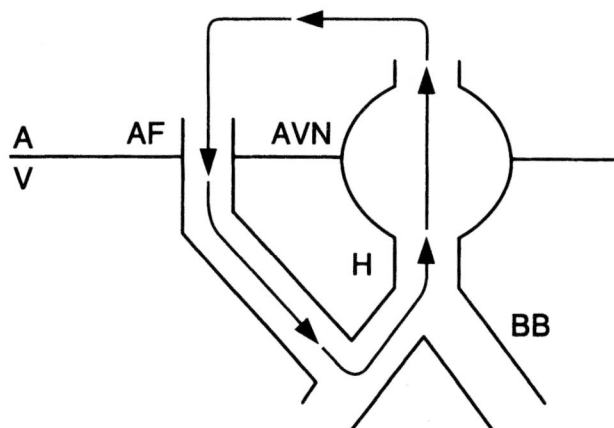

FIGURE 66.13 Mechanism of atriofascicular (AF) (Mahaim) reentrant tachycardias. Anterograde preexcitation typically occurs through a right anterolateral, decrementally conducting accessory pathway (AP) or AF pathway that inserts into the region of the right bundle branch (BB). Retrograde atrial activation occurs through the normal bundle of His (H) and atrioventricular (AV) node (AVN).

Fasciculoventricular Mahaim Fibers

A final variant of the preexcitation syndromes is created by a fasciculoventricular Mahaim fiber (64). Here, a conducting strand of tissue bypasses the distal component of the His-Purkinje system, resulting in earlier ventricular activation than expected through the normal His-Purkinje network. This is manifested at the time of electrophysiologic testing by a shortened HV interval recorded on the bundle of His electrogram. Unlike with atriofascicular fibers, bundle of His pacing fails to eliminate this preexcitation because pacing at these sites is upstream from the site of the bypassing fiber.

ATRIOVENTRICULAR NODAL OR JUNCTIONAL REENTRANT TACHYCARDIAS

Anatomic Considerations

The most common mechanism of AV nodal–dependent tachycardia is AV nodal or junctional reentry, as shown in Figure 66.14. Approximately 60% (147–149) of all narrow QRS complex SVTs seen in the clinical setting are due to reentry within at least two parallel components in or near the AV nodal portion of the normal AV conduction system. The precise anatomic construction of these pathways remains a subject of controversy, with debate centering on the existence of common pathways both at the entry and exit points of the AV conduction system. It had been accepted that two pathways with differing conduction properties were confined to the compact portion of the AV node, as shown in Figure 66.14. Recently other investigators have argued that at least a portion of the circuit lies outside the compact region of the AV node, as shown in Figure 66.2B (42,49,150,151). ▼ 166

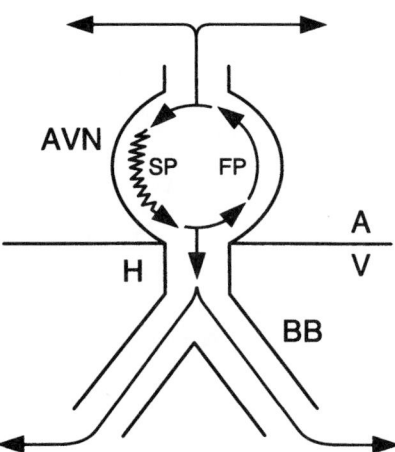

FIGURE 66.14 Microanatomy of atrioventricular (AV) nodal reentrant tachycardia. Here, dual physiologically or anatomically dissociated AV nodal pathways are confined to the compact portion of the AV node (AVN). Note the upper and lower final common pathways at the proximal and distal ends of the compact node. This is in contrast to the AV nodal reentrant circuit involving extranodal atrial tissue seen in Figure 66.2B, where the retrograde atrial activation proceeds through the fast pathway (FP), which exits near the distal portion of the compact AV node. A variable portion of the atrium is subsequently traversed by a reentrant impulse that then reenters the AV conduction system through a posterior slow pathway (SP). H, bundle of His.

Physiologic Mechanisms

Regardless of the anatomy of the circuit, pacing studies clearly demonstrate physiologically discontinuous, or longitudinally separate, conduction through the two or more components of the involved AV conduction system (10,11,16,150,159,160). During sinus rhythm, during slow atrial pacing, or with the introduction of late coupled APCs, AV conduction typically occurs through the faster of the dual functionally or anatomically distinct AV nodal pathways. Here, conduction times are short, and the PR interval inscribed on the surface ECG may be less than 140 ms. With faster pacing or with the introduction of progressively earlier APCs, a critical point of refractoriness or effective recovery time within the FP is reached. With subsequent decrements in the timing of the APC, AV conduction switches to the "slower" component of the dual AV conduction system, typically with a more than 50-ms prolongation of the AH interval conduction time through the AV node, as shown in *e*Figure 66.14.1. This jump from the FP to the SP over a 10-ms decrease in the APC coupling time produces a discontinuity in the plot of the trans-AV nodal conduction time or the AH interval given as a function of the timing of the premature impulse or A_1 to A_2 interval (*e*Fig. 66.14.2); hence, the descriptor, *discontinuous conduction*. Some patients may have several discontinuities, suggesting multiple SPs. Furthermore, the presence of such conduction may not, in and of itself, be "abnormal," because up to 70% of patients undergoing electrophysiologic testing who do not have clinical AV nodal reentrant

tachycardia reportedly have such anterograde or retrograde conduction discontinuities (161–163).

In 85% to 95% of patients, a slow/fast–type AV nodal–dependent tachycardia is seen in which the SP with the longest conduction time of the two AV nodal tracts comprises the anterograde limb of the reentrant circuit. This pathway is typically encountered in or near the posterior aspect of the compact portion of the AV node. Return or retrograde impulse propagation, as shown in *e*Figure 66.14.3, proceeds through the FP with a shorter conduction time located in the anterior and medial aspect of the compact portion of the AV node near the origin of the bundle of His. The inscription of a rapid electrogram deflection immediately after local atrial activation during sinus rhythm along the posterior aspect of the tricuspid annulus near the coronary sinus orifice has been shown to emanate from the SP. Similarly, a high-frequency deflection can also be observed before atrial activation during retrograde conduction through the SP (41). The exact origin of these potentials is unclear, however, as they may also result from the specific atrial architecture underlying the posteroseptal region (164–166).

In 3% to 20% of patients, the tachycardia circuit direction is reversed and a fast/slow or atypical type of AV nodal reentrant tachycardia is observed, as shown in *e*Figure 66.14.3 (16,167–171). In this case, anterograde conduction proceeds down the faster of the two pathways, with return activation through the SP. Given the potential of multiple SPs and therefore multiple discontinuities, the circuit involved in this atypical arrhythmia may not be the same as that involved in the slow/fast type of AV nodal reentrant tachycardia seen in the same patient. Furthermore, up to 9% of individuals also display a slow/slow type of AV nodal reentrant tachycardia in which both anterograde and retrograde conduction occurs through such multiple SPs (14,151,160,169,170,172).

Initiation of Tachycardia

AV nodal reentrant tachycardia is most frequently initiated when a critically timed APC blocks in the FP with longer refractoriness and conducts through the SP. If the impulse then returns retrogradely to the atria through the FP, which has since recovered from the anterogradely conducting and blocking APC, the reentrant circuit is completed. This is facilitated by the substantive delay within the SP, giving the FP sufficient time to recover from the original block created by the APC (10,81,159,173,174).

AV nodal reentrant tachycardia is initiated less frequently by a VPC that conducts to the atria through the retrograde FP but reenters with return conduction through the SP (175). This mechanism of initiation is also more common in atypical or fast/slow AV nodal reentrant tachycardia. In such cases, retrograde activation after the VPC proceeds through the slower AV nodal pathway, with return

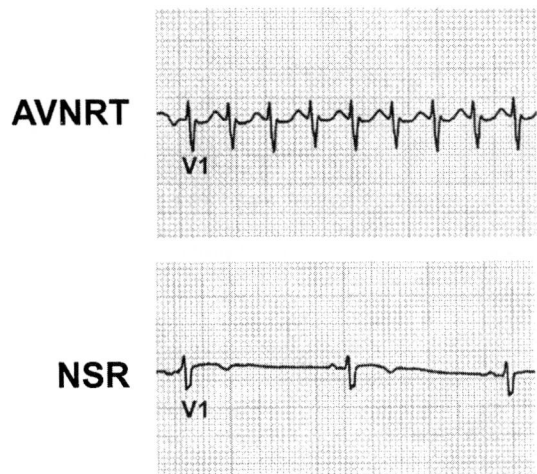

FIGURE 66.15 V₁ rhythm strips showing pseudo rSR' QRS configuration in a patient with atrioventricular nodal reentrant tachycardia (AVNRT). In the **upper panel**, the short ventriculoatrial conduction time during tachycardias results in inscription of the retrograde P wave at the end of the QRS complex, giving the "rSR prime" configuration. In the **lower panel**, normal sinus rhythm in the same lead shows resolution of that component. This is highly indicative of atrioventricular nodal reentry as the mechanism of the arrhythmia.

ventricular activation through the faster of the dual AV nodal physiologic or anatomic pathways.

Presentation on Electrocardiogram

Because return atrial activation and P-wave generation during typical AV nodal reentrant tachycardia is rapid, the earliest atrial deflection on the bundle of His electrogram during tachycardia is usually less than 60 ms (84). Although such a short VA interval excludes the possibility of a reentrant tachycardia using an AP, longer VA intervals do not eliminate the possibility of AV nodal reentrant tachycardias that use an SP as the retrograde limb of the reentrant circuit. As such, a short VA interval for diagnosing all AV nodal reentrant tachycardias is not completely sensitive, although its positive predictive value is very high.

Therefore, a retrograde P wave is inscribed within or at the end of the QRS complex or ECG. This dictates that this arrhythmia is a short RP tachycardia (46,84,149,176,177). If the P wave occurs at the end of the QRS complex on the surface 12-lead ECG, a pseudo–R-wave deflection in V₁ not present during normal sinus rhythm may be seen, as shown in Figure 66.15 (80,176,177). This is a highly sensitive and specific indicator of AV nodal reentry as the mechanism for a narrow QRS complex tachycardia (80,149,177).

In contrast, atypical AV nodal reentrant tachycardia with retrograde conduction through the SP, such as PJRT, inscribes its retrograde P wave later in the RR diastolic interval, more closely coupled to the following QRS complex (42,148,168,170). Thus, criteria for a long RP tachycardia are met. By virtue of the posteroseptal site of retrograde

atrial activation, retrograde P waves typically observed during this arrhythmia are negative in leads II, III, and aVF, again indicating a low-to-high atrial activation sequence.

This arrhythmia and PJRT must be distinguished from other long RP tachycardias (80,178). Sinus tachycardia, sinus node reentry, and a variety of atrial tachycardias in the absence of marked PR interval prolongation also show a close association between the P wave and the subsequent QRS complex. Given their AV nodal–independent mechanisms, these atrial tachycardias persist when higher-grade AV block occurs spontaneously or after vagal or drug interventions. Furthermore, many of these tachycardias show a high-to-low atrial activation sequence, unlike that seen with PJRT or atypical AV nodal reentry.

DIFFERENTIATING ATRIOVENTRICULAR NODE REENTRANT FROM ATRIOVENTRICULAR REENTRANT TACHYCARDIAS

Distinguishing AV reentrant from AV nodal or junctional reentrant narrow-complex tachycardias is important in planning therapeutic strategies for these tachycardias. An understanding of these aforementioned mechanisms provides the needed clues for such differentiation. It was once believed that both the tachycardia rate and the presence of QRS alternans were useful in establishing a diagnosis of AV reentrant tachycardia (149). Although AV reentrant tachycardias may be faster in some patients, the overlap in heart rates with these two mechanisms makes this factor unhelpful in establishing a diagnosis of AV reentrant tachycardia. Furthermore, the presence of QRS alternans, as shown in Figure 66.16, has since been shown to be a function of heart rate and not of the specific underlying mechanism (46).

The positions of the P wave and the RP intervals in tachycardia are more useful in distinguishing these two reentrant mechanisms (46,80,176,177). P waves inscribed

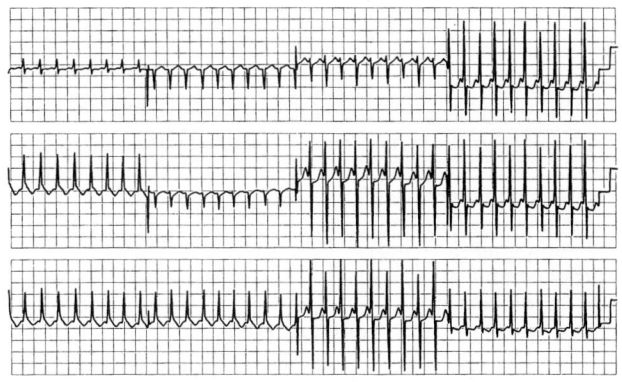

FIGURE 66.16 QRS alternans during reciprocating tachycardia. Note the alternating amplitude of the R wave in leads V₁ and V₄. This is a rate-related process and is not predictive of the underlying mechanism.

within the ST or T segments observed in AV reentry (46,68,149,176,179,180) contrast with the even shorter RP intervals and accompanying P waves producing the r' in lead V$_1$, which is highly predictive of an AV nodal reentrant mechanism (80,176,177). Obviously, in some cases the P waves are not obvious on the surface ECG, and recordings using an esophageal lead are required to determine the RP or VA interval. ✌ 167

Finally, it should be noted that 10% to 20% of patients with WPW syndrome also have AV nodal reentrant tachycardia with a narrow QRS morphology (94,96,97,162,181,182). Therefore, the presence of a narrow QRS SVT in a patient with WPW syndrome does not necessarily indicate AV reentrant tachycardia. In these patients, clarification of the precise mechanisms of arrhythmias requires more detailed electrophysiologic evaluation.

PRINCIPLES OF MANAGEMENT

Short-Term Therapy for Narrow Complex Tachycardias

The dependence of both AV reentrant and AV nodal reentrant tachycardias on AV nodal conduction has important implications for the short-term management of patients with these arrhythmias. As reviewed in Figure 66.17, the simplest approach to tachycardia termination takes advantage of vagal modulation of AV nodal conduction. In many patients, a Valsalva maneuver, carotid sinus massage, or application of ice water to the face will terminate the tachycardia by increasing vagal tone. If these approaches prove unsuccessful, the use of drugs with significant negative dromotropic effects on the AV node may also readily terminate either type of SVT. Adenosine, administered in a rapid bolus at an initial dosage of 6 mg i.v. (Fig. 66.18), will terminate 62% of tachycardias, whereas 91% of these tachy-

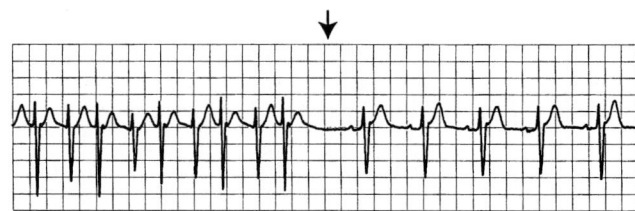

FIGURE 66.18 Termination of supraventricular tachycardia with adenosine. Twelve mg of adenosine given intravenously results in abrupt termination of narrow complex tachycardia in a patient with atrioventricular nodal reentry. Note the alternating tachycardia cycle lengths before termination.

cardias respond to 12 mg of adenosine from a peripheral i.v. site (183). Alternatively, 5 to 10 mg of i.v. verapamil will terminate up to 90% of tachycardias (184–186). The high success rate of these i.v. drugs has supplanted the use of edrophonium (a short-acting cholinesterase inhibitor), phenylephrine, or beta-blockers, which had been used at one time for this purpose. Although i.v. esmolol, a short-acting beta-blocker, may also be effective, accompanying hypotension has been reported (187). The use of these drugs or of vagal maneuvers is also useful to the diagnosis because the development of higher-grade AV nodal block during tachycardia, as shown in Figures 66.1 and 66.19, virtually excludes the presence of an AV nodal–dependent tachycardia. It should be noted that under rare circumstances AV nodal reentrant tachycardia may show 2:1 AV block due to physiologic impairment of infra-His conduction; however, this is unlikely to occur with vagal or drug interventions.

Intravenous flecainide, propafenone, sotalol, or amiodarone may also prove effective in restoring sinus rhythm, although these drugs may take longer to produce clinically relevant effects. Although i.v. ibutilide is effective in termi-

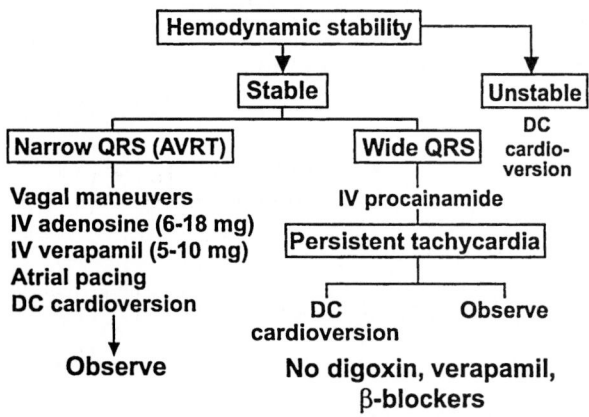

FIGURE 66.17 Algorithm for the acute management of patients with atrioventricular nodal–dependent tachycardias. AVRT, atrioventricular reentrant tachycardia; DC, direct current.

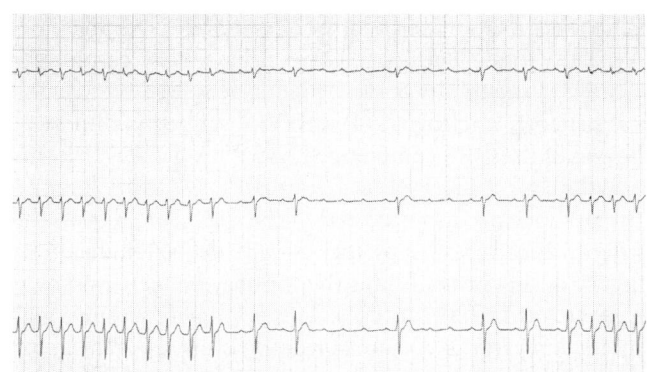

FIGURE 66.19 Effect of carotid sinus massage on atrioventricular conduction in a patient with an ectopic atrial tachycardia. On the left side of the figure, a narrow QRS complex tachycardia was observed with a 1:1 atrioventricular relationship, as seen in leads V$_1$ to V$_3$. With carotid sinus massage, high-grade atrioventricular nodal block, which readily discloses the continuing atrial tachycardia, appears as 1:1 conduction and resumes after resolution of the carotid sinus massage effect.

nating the acute onset of atrial fibrillation and its class III properties may effectively block AP conduction, the safety and efficacy of this agent for treating narrow, complex AV nodal–dependent tachycardia have not been established. The same is true for dofetilide and azimilide, which have been studied almost exclusively in atrial fibrillation and atrial flutter, the latter of which is not available in i.v. forms in the United States.

Nonpharmacologic therapies for patients with narrow, complex SVTs are also available to restore normal sinus rhythm. Atrial pacing using an esophageal lead positioned behind the atria proves routinely effective in terminating AV nodal–dependent tachycardia (38,188–190). With this approach, current strengths of 10 to 20 mA with pulse widths between 10 and 20 ms may be required. Although this approach is effective, it also produces some esophageal discomfort and can initiate atrial fibrillation. Administration of a low-energy direct current shock to stop tachycardia is an alternative, but it is rarely required, given the efficacy of pharmacologic and other nonpharmacologic measures.

Short-Term Management of Wide-Complex Tachycardias

The presence of a wide QRS complex tachycardia warrants careful consideration of several additional issues. Although the prolongation of the QRS complex may simply represent aberrancy accompanying an AV nodal–dependent tachycardia, the diagnosis of ventricular tachycardia should be carefully considered. The presence of underlying coronary artery disease or prior myocardial infarction has an accuracy of more than 90% in predicting a ventricular mechanism for wide-complex arrhythmias (191). These issues are reviewed in greater detail in Chapter 60. An additional mechanism of wide QRS tachycardia in patients with AV nodal–dependent arrhythmias is that of an antidromic reciprocating tachycardia that uses an AP as its anterograde limb, atrial fibrillation, or other atrial tachycardias with ventricular preexcitation through the accompanying pathway. Each of these arrhythmias should be manifest by their characteristic slurred upstroke delta waves seen in the first 40 ms of the wide QRS complex. During atrial fibrillation with a rapid ventricular response rate, however, the characteristic preexcited QRS pattern may be difficult to discern. Preexcitation may be most evident in the QRS complexes after the longest RR intervals during irregular tachycardias. Ventricular activation during atrial fibrillation in patients with multiple APs may proceed by several alternating avenues, thus mimicking torsades de pointes on a single rhythm strip. As with evaluation of any wide-complex arrhythmias, a surface 12-lead ECG is indispensable in correctly identifying the underlying mechanism.

The short-term treatment of wide-complex tachycardia first and foremost depends on the patient's underlying hemodynamic status. In the presence of hemodynamic compromise, direct current cardioversion after appropriate anesthesia is warranted. It is not uncommon for direct current cardioversion to require at least 200 J to restore normal sinus rhythm in patients with WPW syndrome and atrial fibrillation. In the presence of stable hemodynamics, several different i.v. antiarrhythmic agents are available. Intravenous procainamide has been most widely used for this purpose. This agent not only alters propagation through the APs, but it may also directly restore normal sinus rhythm. Use of beta-blockers (187,192–195) and lidocaine (192,196,197) is not effective for either purpose. Intravenous propafenone, flecainide, and sotalol are effective in both slowing the ventricular response rate during atrial fibrillation and restoring normal sinus rhythm in patients with APs. These drugs, however, are not commercially available in the United States. Intravenous amiodarone is also effective, although the time to conversion with this agent may be longer, and the overall conversion rate may be low. Intravenous ibutilide may also restore normal sinus rhythm, although its safety and efficacy in this setting have not been documented.

Several i.v. agents can also accelerate AV conduction through an AP, causing atrial fibrillation to degenerate into ventricular fibrillation. Digoxin, although slowing atrial fibrillation in some patients, clearly accelerates the ventricular response rate in others (198). This deterioration has also been described after use of i.v. verapamil (199–203). A similar reduction in the shortest RR interval during atrial fibrillation has also been observed after i.v., but not oral, diltiazem (13). This acceleration may be due to direct pathway effects, enhancement of peripheral sympathetic activity related to the precipitation of hypotension, or the reduction in retrograde concealment into the AP by generation of higher-grade AV nodal block. In the presence of atrial fibrillation in a patient with an anterogradely conducting AP, ventricular activation proceeds through the pathway or the normal AV conduction system. The latter avenue of propagation may be accompanied by impulse propagation across the ventricle in a reverse direction into the pathway. This retrograde penetration or concealment blocks ventricular activation proceeding anterogradely through the pathway because of impulse collision. This produces a net effect of slowing ventricular activation. Higher-grade AV nodal block can reduce this beneficial effect by withdrawing retrograde concealment. Ventricular fibrillation after adenosine administration in a patient with WPW syndrome and atrial fibrillation has also been reported (204). Because of this and the potential hemodynamic deterioration of ventricular tachycardia, these drugs should not be routinely used in patients with wide-complex tachycardias. This does not mean that their use is prohibited in patients with narrow QRS complex tachycardias, although the possibility of degeneration of such arrhythmias into atrial fibrillation dictates that facilities dealing with such unlikely transitions should be available.

Long-Term Therapy for Atrioventricular Nodal–Dependent Tachycardias

Drug Therapy

In selecting appropriate therapy for patients with supraventricular arrhythmias, several general principles should be carefully considered. The inherent risk for untoward events accompanying the target arrhythmia, as well as its impact on the patient's quality of life, must be carefully weighed against the anticipated treatment's efficacy and accompanying risks. Furthermore, the effectiveness and risks, including side effects, of a given strategy must be carefully compared with those of other treatment options. In the case of increased risk for SCD in symptomatic patients with WPW syndrome, aggressive evaluation and treatment are warranted. Here, the risks of intervention are likely to be small compared with the risks associated with the underlying arrhythmia. These patients are best treated with definitive ablative procedures. This is in part because of the relatively limited efficacy of antiarrhythmic therapy on AP conduction in those patients with the most rapid underlying conduction capabilities (205). This is a particularly true of class Ia antiarrhythmic agents.

In contrast, in the absence of a propensity for rapid anterograde conduction through an AP during atrial fibrillation or of marked neurologic symptoms, such as presyncope or syncope, the majority of AV nodal–dependent tachycardias are relatively benign. As such, therapy is warranted if prevention of symptomatic arrhythmia improves quality of life and can be accomplished without undue risk to the patient. The benefit of achieving such arrhythmic suppression must be weighed against possible side effects, the proarrhythmic risk from drug therapy, or complications from ablation. In those cases of single or infrequent tachycardia episodes with relatively mild symptoms, expectant observation without treatment or with sole use of vagal maneuvers to terminate tachycardia, where effective, may suffice. In such cases, ablative therapy is unnecessary. Patients with frequently recurring palpitations clearly related to an AV nodal–dependent tachycardia, those with problematic, associated cardiac or central nervous system symptoms, those in whom drugs are either ineffective or accompanied by side effects, or individuals facing lifetime medical therapy are best treated with catheter ablation. The exception to this approach is those patients in whom the risks associated with catheter ablation may be greater than the risk of the underlying arrhythmia. For example, patients with an AP located close to the normal AV conduction system in which the risk for high-grade or complete heart block is high may be better treated with medical therapy. Obviously, if such therapy proves ineffective or if

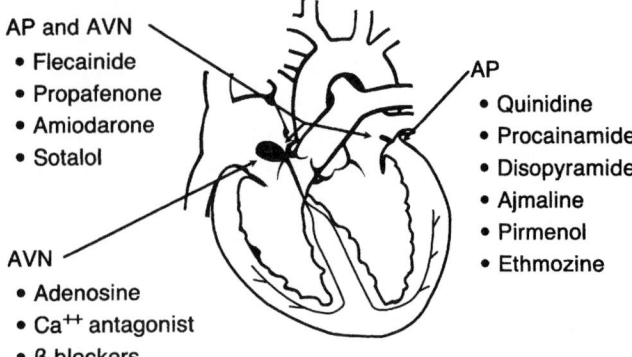

FIGURE 66.20 Antiarrhythmic drug effects in patients with Wolff-Parkinson-White syndrome. Shown here are drugs with exclusive accessory pathway (AP) effects, with exclusive atrioventricular nodal (AVN) actions, and with both AP- and AVN-modifying properties. Pharmacologic modulation of the fast pathway in AVN reentrant tachycardia is similar to that of an AP. The slow pathway behaves in a manner similar to that of AVN tissue.

the patient is at risk for SCD the potential complications of catheter ablation may be unavoidable to provide symptomatic relief and protection for the patient.

Other patients will benefit from the more readily available drug therapies. In the absence of anterograde preexcitation or atrial fibrillation, patients with AV reentrant tachycardia may be effectively managed using calcium channel blockers, such as verapamil or diltiazem (13,206–208), or any one of a number of beta-blockers (187,193) that target the AV node, as shown in Figure 66.20. The latter may be useful in those patients with exercise-related tachycardia. These agents are also effective in modifying conduction within the SP in AV nodal reentrant tachycardia and within the AP involved in PJRT or atriofascicular reentrant tachycardia. Efficacy rates of 40% to 50% in eliminating or significantly reducing the frequency of AV nodal–dependent tachyarrhythmias have been reported. Furthermore, the risk for proarrhythmia using these agents is very low and most of these drugs can be administered in single daily doses.

In contrast, class Ia agents such as quinidine (209,210), procainamide (209–211), or disopyramide (212,213) produce beneficial effects on the AP but not on the normal AV conduction system. Other class I agents such as propafenone (214–217), flecainide (218–222), and moricizine and class III drugs such as sotalol (223–226) and amiodarone (71,227–231) have demonstrable effects on both the AV conduction system and the AP (Fig. 66.20). Because the FP used as the retrograde limb of AV nodal reentrant tachycardia has many properties similar to those of APs, class I agents also produce beneficial effects on both the frequency and severity of this arrhythmia (208,232–236). Class Ic and class III drugs may also sufficiently modify the anterograde SP to reduce the occurrence of arrhythmias. These agents produce additional beneficial effects in patients with either type of AV nodal–dependent arrhythmia by reducing tachycardia-induced atrial or ventricular ectopy. Regardless of the specific underlying mechanism, the efficacy of these agents in treating AV nodal–dependent arrhythmia is 60% to 80% over short-term follow-up.

The choice of a specific membrane-active antiarrhythmic agent for use in patients with AV reentrant tachycardia depends on several factors. These include (a) the presence or absence of structural heart disease or other organ system problems; (b) the presence of preexcitation; and (c) the side effect profile of a given agent, including organ toxicity, negative inotropic effects, and propensity for proarrhythmias. In the absence of underlying heart disease, any one of the class Ic, III, or Ia drugs may be effective in managing AV reentrant tachycardias. Of these, flecainide, propafenone, disopyramide, and sotalol are less likely to produce organ toxicity or nuisance side effects. In this setting, the risk of a proarrhythmic event is low and ranges from 0.5% to 2.0%. In the presence of underlying heart disease, those agents such as disopyramide and flecainide, and to a lesser extent, propafenone and sotalol, that may have significant negative inotropic effects, should be used with caution, if at all. Although these agents are not absolutely contraindicated in patients with EFs of 30% to 45%, the presence of congestive heart failure should dictate an alternative choice of therapy. In the presence of congestive heart failure or prior myocardial infarction, amiodarone is least likely to produce a proarrhythmic effect. The risk for proarrhythmia with other class I and class III drugs may be as high as 5% to 8%, particularly with the class Ia agents producing significant QT interval prolongation in the presence of underlying heart disease. Specific drug therapy for these tachycardias and dosing strategies are reviewed in greater detail in other studies (26–28).

Nonpharmacologic Therapy: Radiofrequency Ablation

Although drug therapy was the mainstay of treatment for AV nodal–dependent tachycardias for many years, the advent and improvement of surgical techniques in the 1970s ushered in an era of nonpharmacologic therapy. Those patients with an AP who were at risk for SCD, those in whom antiarrhythmic therapy had failed because of inefficacy or side effects, or those patients who faced lifelong medical therapy were increasingly managed with surgical ablation. During the past 6 years, even this approach has been replaced by RF ablation. As described in greater detail in Chapter 73, success rates of 90% to 98% are routinely possible (41,43,44). A 5% to 8% recurrence rate of AP conduction nevertheless may occur (41,43,44). This ablative approach is accomplished at low risk, and the benefits to patients are achievable at lower cost and substantially less hospitalization and recovery times than are possible with

surgical ablation. Hence, RF ablation is a reasonable first-line modality in patients with recurrent arrhythmias. Again, potential exceptions to this approach are encountered in patients who are at higher risk for complete heart block due to pathways in close proximity to the AV conduction system or to other factors that increase the risks of invasive procedures.

In patients with AV nodal reentrant tachycardias, similar success rates are now possible with ablation of the SP or atrial approaches to that pathway, which lies posteriorly along the tricuspid annulus. The risk for heart block in these patients is 0.5% to 3.0%, depending to some extent on the experience of the operator and on the apparent SP location. This approach has virtually supplanted the alternative ablation of the FP, which has been accompanied by heart block rates of 5% to 25% (42,46,237,238).

CONTROVERSIES AND PERSONAL PERSPECTIVES

Risk Stratification in Patients with Asymptomatic Preexcitation

Although much of the physiology of the AV nodal–dependent arrhythmias has already been elucidated and management and treatment methods established, several areas of controversy remain. It is the opinion of the author (D.L.P.) that risk stratification in patients with asymptomatic preexcitation is not necessary, unless extenuating circumstances exist. Some clinicians, however, continue to be strong proponents of risk stratification in all patients. As discussed above, the likelihood of rapid conduction through an AP in the absence of symptoms is low; moreover, the risk of SCD has been shown in population-based studies to be very low. Still, the risk for an untoward event is not zero. On rare occasions, patients present with ventricular fibrillation as their first manifestation of WPW syndrome. As such, clinicians cannot give patients a blanket guarantee of freedom from untoward events over the long term. It is important that this uncertainty be discussed with patients to provide them with the necessary understanding needed to make informed decisions about proceeding with additional evaluation and treatment and any accompanying risks, if they are asymptomatic. If risk stratification is to be undertaken, it should be by direct initiation of atrial fibrillation and assessment of the ventricular response rate. Noninvasive methods are insufficiently predictive to be of any significant use. If rapid conduction through an AP is identified, the patient should have sufficient information to either accept the risks associated with such rapid conduction or the risks associated with ablation of the offending AP. When presented with the juxtaposition of the risks associated with no intervention versus those of catheter ablation, some patients may well opt for conservative follow-up. Others

THE FUTURE

Substantial progress has already been made in the area of AV nodal–dependent tachycardias. Excellent therapies are already available and have been applied successfully in thousands of patients. In the future, however, we will undoubtedly better define the cost-effectiveness of the various treatment modalities through outcome-based studies. A better understanding of the natural history of AV nodal–dependent arrhythmias will be forthcoming. Technology will be developed to facilitate noninvasive substrate localization and establishment of mechanisms. Nonfluoroscopic multisite mapping for creating three-dimensional maps of specific arrhythmias and improved energy sources and delivery techniques will also be forthcoming. With the anticipated progress during the next 5 to 10 years, it would not be surprising if arrhythmogenic substrate could be eliminated through energy delivery from the body surface.

---

may wish to face the risks of ablation immediately rather than confront continued pathway-related risks, no matter how low, over time.

Anatomy of Atrioventricular Nodal Reentrant Tachycardias

Another area of controversy is outlined previously in this chapter. Some clinicians argue that the circuit resides within the compact portion of the AV node. Others argue that at least a component of the reentrant circuit lies outside the compact region of the AV node. In the latter case, the SP is viewed as arising from atrial tissue, with insertion into the compact AV node. Given the various considerations on both sides of this argument, it seems most likely that an appreciable component of the reentrant circuit resides outside the AV node within atrial tissue. In fact the FP and SP may even be variable manifestations of anisotropic tissue architecture in the interatrial septum. It is therefore likely that the anterograde limb of the circuit is actually composed of both the atrial tissue inputs into the posterior region of the AV node and a component of AV nodal tissue itself. As such, successful SP ablation may simply mean that the atrial inputs into the AV node have been sufficiently modified to make onset of tachycardias unlikely.

Radiofrequency Ablation as First-Line Therapy for Atrioventricular Nodal–Dependent Tachycardia

Finally, in some quarters, the propriety of RF ablation as first-line treatment for AV nodal–dependent arrhythmias remains controversial. Some clinicians believe that patients with AV reentrant tachycardia in the absence of manifest preexcitation and those with AV nodal reentrant tachycardias should be managed with antiarrhythmic drugs that target the AV node. Ablative therapy is reasonable first-line therapy if (a) a patient faces lifelong medical therapy, (b) there is an arrhythmia refractory to previous medical treatment, (c) the patient is at risk for an untoward event, or (d) the patient resides in an area where medical therapy for tachycardia is less readily available. Again, the risks of this therapy must be weighed against the alternative of using membrane-active antiarrhythmic drugs. Although most of these agents are reasonably tolerated when appropriately administered, constitutional side effects and the risk of potentially lethal proarrhythmia remain a reality. In the hands of experienced interventionalists, the risks associated with ablation remain very low; moreover, ablation has the added advantage of curing the arrhythmia. RF catheter ablation of SVT has been shown to be cost-effective and improve quality of life for patients with WPW who survive cardiac arrest or who experience SVT or AF (239) and for highly symptomatic patients with AV nodal reentrant tachycardia or AV reentrant tachycardia using a concealed AP (240). Here again, patients should be informed of their options so they may participate in choosing an approach that best meets their needs.

CONCLUSIONS

Over the past 15 to 20 years, substantial progress has been made in the treatment of AV nodal–dependent tachycardias. This has been facilitated by the development of catheter-based electrophysiology study techniques that elucidate the underlying arrhythmic mechanisms, the development of better drugs for acute and chronic management, and the refinement of nonpharmacologic therapy such as RF catheter ablation for curing these arrhythmias. This progress has not only elucidated these arrhythmias, but has also provided the foundation for extrapolating these refinements to the more complicated AV nodal–independent atrial and ventricular tachycardias. An appreciation of these issues should improve the efficacy of therapies and reduce their risk in patients with AV nodal–dependent tachycardias.

REFERENCES

1. Kent A. Researches on the structure and function of the mammalian heart. *J Physiol* 1893;14:233–254.
2. Mines G. On dynamic equilibrium in the heart. *J Physiol* 1913;46:349–383.
3. Kent A. Observations on the auriculo-ventricular junction of the mammalian heart. *Q J Exp Physiol* 1913;7:193.
4. Mines G. On circulation excitation on heart muscles and their possible relation to tachycardia and fibrillation. *Trans R Soc Can* 1914;4:43.
5. Wolferth C, Wood F. The mechanism of production of short P-R intervals and prolonged QRS complexes in patients with presumably undamaged hearts: hypothesis of an accessory pathway of auriculo-ventricular conduction (bundles of Kent). *Am Heart J* 1933;8:297–311.
6. Cohn A, Fraser F. Paroxysmal tachycardia and the effect of stimulation of the vagus nerves by pressure. *Heart* 1913;5:93–107.
7. Wood F, Wolferth C, Geckler G. Histologic demonstration of accessory muscular connections between auricle and ventricle in a case of short PR interval and prolonged QRS complex. *Am Heart J* 1942:454–462.
8. Wolff L, Parkinson J, White P. Bundle-branch block with short PR interval in healthy young people prone to paroxysmal tachycardia. *Am Heart J* 1930;5:685–704.
9. Barker P, Wilson F, Johnston F. The mechanism of auricular paroxysmal tachycardia with alternation of cycle length. *Am Heart J* 1943;26:435–445.
10. Denes P, Wu D, Dhingra RC, et al. Demonstration of dual A-V nodal pathways in patients with paroxysmal supraventricular tachycardia. *Circulation* 1973;48:549–555.
11. Moe G. Physiological evidence for a dual AV nodal transmission system. *Circ Res* 1956;4:357–375.
12. Kistin A. Multiple pathways of conduction and reciprocal rhythm with interpolated ventricular premature systoles. *Am Heart J* 1963;65:162–179.
13. Shenasa M, Fromer M, Faugere G, et al. Efficacy and safety of intravenous and oral diltiazem for Wolff-Parkinson-White syndrome. *Am J Cardiol* 1987;59:301–306.
14. Sebag C, Chevalier P, Davy JM, et al. Triple antegrade nodal pathway in a patient with supraventricular paroxysmal tachycardia. *J Electrocardiol* 1986;19:85–90.
15. Swiryn S, Bauernfeind R, Palileo F, et al. Electrophysiologic study demonstrating triple antegrade AV nodal pathways in patients with spontaneous and/or induced supraventricular tachycardia. *Am Heart J* 1982;103:168–176.
16. Tai CT, Chen SA, Chiang CE, et al. Multiple anterograde atrioventricular node pathways in patients with atrioventricular node reentrant tachycardia. *J Am Coll Cardiol* 1996;28:725–731.
17. Dopirak M, Schaal S, Leier C. Triple A-V nodal pathways in man? *J Electrocardiol* 1980;13:185–188.
18. Kuck K, Kuch B, Bleifeld W. Multiple antegrade and retrograde AV nodal pathways: demonstration by multiple discontinuities in the AV nodal conduction curves and echo time intervals. *Pacing Clin Electrophysiol* 1984;7:656–662.
19. Durrer D, Schoo L, Schuilenburg RM, Wellens HJ. The role of premature beats in the initiation and the termination of supraventricular tachycardia in the Wolff-Parkinson-White syndrome. *Circulation* 1967;36:644–662.
20. Durrer D, Roos JP. Epicardial excitation of the ventricles in a patient with Wolff-Parkinson-White syndrome (type B). *Circulation* 1967;35:15–21.
21. Wellens HJ, Schuilenburg RM, Durrer D. Electrical stimulation of the heart in patients with Wolff-Parkinson-White syndrome, type A. *Circulation* 1971;43:99–114.
22. Wellens HJ, Durrer D. Patterns of ventriculo-atrial conduction in the Wolff-Parkinson-White syndrome. *Circulation* 1974;49:22–31.
23. Tonkin AM, Dugan FA, Svenson RH, et al. Coexistence of functional Kent and Mahaim-type tracts in the pre-excitation syndrome. Demonstration by catheter techniques and epicardial mapping. *Circulation* 1975;52:193–200.
24. Gallagher JJ, Sealy WC, Kasell J, Wallace AG. Multiple accessory pathways in patients with the pre-excitation syndrome. *Circulation* 1976;54:571–591.
25. Gallagher JJ, Sealy WC. The permanent form of junctional reciprocating tachycardia: further elucidation of the underlying mechanism. *Eur J Cardiol* 1978;8:413–430.
26. Prystowsky EN, Pritchett EL, Gallagher JJ. Concealed conduction preventing anterograde preexcitation in Wolff-Parkinson-White syndrome. *Am J Cardiol* 1984;53:960–961.
27. Prystowsky EN. Diagnosis and management of the preexcitation syndromes. *Curr Probl Cardiol* 1988;13:225–310.
28. Packer D, Prystowsky E. The Wolff-Parkinson-White syndrome: further progress in evaluation and treatment. *Prog Cardiol Vasc Dis* 1988;1:147–187.
29. Burchell HB, Frye RL, Anderson MW, McGoon DC. Atrioventricular and ventriculoatrial excitation in Wolff-Parkinson-White syndrome (type B). Temporary ablation at surgery. *Circulation* 1967;36:663–672.
30. Cobb FR, Blumenschein SD, Sealy WC, et al. Successful surgical interruption of the bundle of Kent in a patient with Wolff-Parkinson-White syndrome. *Circulation* 1968;38:1018–1029.
31. Sealy WC, Wallace AG. Surgical treatment of Wolff-Parkinson-White syndrome. *J Thorac Cardiovasc Surg* 1974;68:757–770.
32. Anselme F, Papageorgiou P, Monahan K, et al. Presence and significance of the left atrionodal connection during atrioventricular nodal reentrant tachycardia. *Am J Cardiol* 1999;83:1530–1536.
33. Cox JL, Gallagher JJ, Cain ME. Experience with 118 consecutive patients undergoing operation for the Wolff-Parkinson-White syndrome. *J Thorac Cardiovasc Surg* 1985;90:490–501.
34. Sealy WC. The Wolff-Parkinson-White syndrome and the beginnings of direct arrhythmia surgery. *Ann Thorac Surg* 1984;38:176–180.
35. Ott DA, Garson A, Cooley DA, McNamara DG. Definitive operation for refractory cardiac tachyarrhythmias in children. *J Thorac Cardiovasc Surg* 1985;90:681–689.
36. Guiraudon GM, Klein GJ, Sharma AD, et al. Surgery for Wolff-Parkinson-White syndrome: further experience with an epicardial approach. *Circulation* 1986;74:525–529.

37. Iwa T, Mitsui T, Misaki T, et al. Radical surgical cure of Wolff-Parkinson-White syndrome: the Kanazawa experience. *J Thorac Cardiovasc Surg* 1986;91:225–233.

38. Gallagher JJ, Svenson RH, Kasell JH, et al. Catheter technique for closed-chest ablation of the atrioventricular conduction system. *N Engl J Med* 1982;306:194–200.

39. Scheinman MM, Morady F, Hess DS, Gonzalez R. Catheter-induced ablation of the atrioventricular junction to control refractory supraventricular arrhythmias. *JAMA* 1982;248:851–855.

40. Borggrefe M, Budde T, Podczeck A, Breithardt G. High frequency alternating current ablation of an accessory pathway in humans. *J Am Coll Cardiol* 1987;10:576–582.

41. Jackman WM, Wang XZ, Friday KJ, et al. Catheter ablation of accessory atrioventricular pathways (Wolff-Parkinson-White syndrome) by radiofrequency current. *N Engl J Med* 1991;324:1605–1611.

42. Jackman WM, Beckman KJ, McClelland JH, et al. Treatment of supraventricular tachycardia due to atrioventricular nodal reentry, by radiofrequency catheter ablation of slow-pathway conduction. *N Engl J Med* 1992;327:313–318.

43. Calkins H, Langberg J, Sousa J, et al. Radiofrequency catheter ablation of accessory atrioventricular connections in 250 patients. Abbreviated therapeutic approach to Wolff-Parkinson-White syndrome. *Circulation* 1992;85:1337–1346.

44. Swartz JF, Tracy CM, Fletcher RD. Radiofrequency endocardial catheter ablation of accessory atrioventricular pathway atrial insertion sites. *Circulation* 1993;87:487–499.

45. Lesh MD, Van Hare GF, Schamp DJ, et al. Curative percutaneous catheter ablation using radiofrequency energy for accessory pathways in all locations: results in 100 consecutive patients. *J Am Coll Cardiol* 1992;19:1303–1309.

46. Kay GN, Epstein AE, Dailey SM, Plumb VJ. Selective radiofrequency ablation of the slow pathway for the treatment of atrioventricular nodal reentrant tachycardia. Evidence for involvement of perinodal myocardium within the reentrant circuit. *Circulation* 1992;85:1675–1688.

47. Becker AE, Anderson RH, Durrer D, Wellens HJ. The anatomical substrates of Wolff-Parkinson-White syndrome. A clinicopathologic correlation in seven patients. *Circulation* 1978;57:870–879.

48. Becker AE, Anderson RH. The Wolff-Parkinson-White syndrome and its anatomical substrates. *Anat Rec* 1981;201:169–177.

49. McGuire MA, Bourke JP, Robotin MC, et al. High resolution mapping of Koch's triangle using sixty electrodes in humans with atrioventricular junctional (AV nodal) reentrant tachycardia. *Circulation* 1993;88:2315–2328.

50. Dean JW, Ho SY, Rowland E, et al. Clinical anatomy of the atrioventricular junctions. *J Am Coll Cardiol* 1994;24:1725–1731.

51. Jackman WM, Friday KJ, Scherlag BJ, et al. Direct endocardial recording from an accessory atrioventricular pathway: localization of the site of block, effect of antiarrhythmic drugs, and attempt at nonsurgical ablation. *Circulation* 1983;68:906–916.

52. Jackman W, Friday K, Yeung-Lai-Wah J, et al. Accessory pathways: branching networks and tachycardia. *Circulation* 1985;72:III-270.

53. Jackman W, Yeung-Lai-Wah J, Friday K, et al. Tachycardias originating in accessory pathway networks mimicking atrial flutter and fibrillation. *J Am Coll Cardiol* 1986;7:6A.

54. Jackman WM, Friday KJ, Yeung-Lai-Wah JA, et al. New catheter technique for recording left free-wall accessory atrioventricular pathway activation. Identification of pathway fiber orientation. *Circulation* 1988;78:598–611.

55. Gallagher J, Sealy W, Cox J, et al. Results of surgery for preexcitation caused by accessory atrioventricular pathways in 267 consecutive cases. In: Josephson M, Wellens H, eds. *Tachycardia: mechanism, diagnosis and treatment.* Philadelphia: Lea & Febiger, 1984:259–269.

56. Wellens HJ, Brugada P, Heddle WF. Value of the 12 lead electrocardiogram in diagnosing type and mechanism of a tachycardia: a survey among 22 cardiologists. *J Am Coll Cardiol* 1984;4:176–179.

57. Heddle WF, Brugada P, Wellens HJ. Multiple circus movement tachycardias with multiple accessory pathways. *J Am Coll Cardiol* 1984;4:168–175.

58. Morady F, Scheinman MM, DiCarlo LA Jr, et al. Coexistent posteroseptal and right-sided atrioventricular bypass tracts. *J Am Coll Cardiol* 1985;5:640–646.

59. Colavita PG, Packer DL, Pressley JC, et al. Frequency, diagnosis and clinical characteristics of patients with multiple accessory atrioventricular pathways. *Am J Cardiol* 1987;59:601–606.

60. Goya M, Takahashi A, Nakagawa H, Iesaka Y. A case of catheter ablation of accessory atrioventricular connection between the right atrial appendage and right ventricle guided by a three-dimensional electroanatomic mapping system. *J Cardiovasc Electrophysiol* 1999;10:1112–1118.

61. Lam C, Schweikert R, Kanagaratnam L, Natale A. Radiofrequency ablation of a right atrial appendage-ventricular accessory pathway by transcutaneous epicardial instrumentation. *J Cardiovasc Electrophysiol* 2000;11:1170–1173.

62. Soejima K, Mitamura H, Miyazaki T, et al. Catheter ablation of accessory atrioventricular connection between right atrial appendage to right ventricle: a case report. *J Cardiovasc Electrophysiol* 1998;9:523–528.

63. Milstein S, Sharma AD, Klein GJ. Electrophysiologic profile of asymptomatic Wolff-Parkinson-White pattern. *Am J Cardiol* 1986;57:1097–1100.

64. Gallagher JJ, Pritchett EL, Sealy WC, et al. The preexcitation syndromes. *Prog Cardiovasc Dis* 1978;20:285–327.

65. De la Fuente D, Sasyniuk B, Moe GK. Conduction through a narrow isthmus in isolated canine atrial tissue. A model of the W-P-W syndrome. *Circulation* 1971;44:803–809.

66. Inoue H, Zipes DP. Conduction over an isthmus of atrial myocardium in vivo: a possible model of Wolff-Parkinson-White syndrome. *Circulation* 1987;76:637–647.

67. Cabo C, Pertsov AM, Baxter WT, et al. Wave-front curvature as a cause of slow conduction and block in isolated cardiac muscle. *Circ Res* 1994;75:1014–1028.

68. Prystowsky EN, Miles WM, Heger JJ, Zipes DP. Preexcitation syndromes. Mechanisms and management. *Med Clin North Am* 1984;68:831–893.

69. Klein GJ, Yee R, Sharma AD. Concealed conduction in accessory atrioventricular pathways: an important determi-

nant of the expression of arrhythmias in patients with Wolff-Parkinson-White syndrome. *Circulation* 1984;70:402–411.

70. Fujimura O, Kuo CS, Smith BA. Pre-excited RR intervals during atrial fibrillation in the Wolff-Parkinson-White syndrome: influence of the atrioventricular node refractory period. *J Am Coll Cardiol* 1991;18:1722–1726.

71. Rosenbaum F, Hecht H, Wilson F, et al. The potential variations of the thorax and the esophagus in anomalous atrioventricular excitation (Wolff-Parkinson-White syndrome). *Am Heart J* 1945;29:281–326.

72. Giraud F, Latour H, Peuch P, Roujon L. Les troubles de rhythme du syndrome de Wolff-Parkinson-White: analyze electrocardiographique endocavitaire. *Arch Mal Coeur* 1956;49:102.

73. Arruda MS, McClelland JH, Wang X, et al. Development and validation of an ECG algorithm for identifying accessory pathway ablation site in Wolff-Parkinson-White syndrome. *J Cardiovasc Electrophysiol* 1998;9:2–12.

74. Chiang CE, Chen SA, Teo WS, et al. An accurate stepwise electrocardiographic algorithm for localization of accessory pathways in patients with Wolff-Parkinson-White syndrome from a comprehensive analysis of delta waves and R/S ratio during sinus rhythm. *Am J Cardiol* 1995;76:40–46.

75. Fitzpatrick AP, Gonzales RP, Lesh MD, et al. New algorithm for the localization of accessory atrioventricular connections using a baseline electrocardiogram. *J Am Coll Cardiol* 1994;23:107–116.

76. Xie B, Heald SC, Bashir Y, et al. Localization of accessory pathways from the 12-lead electrocardiogram using a new algorithm. *Am J Cardiol* 1994;74:161–165.

77. Rodriguez LM, Smeets JL, de Chillou C, et al. The 12-lead electrocardiogram in midseptal, anteroseptal, posteroseptal and right free wall accessory pathways. *Am J Cardiol* 1993;72:1274–1280.

78. Lindsay BD, Crossen KJ, Cain ME. Concordance of distinguishing electrocardiographic features during sinus rhythm with the location of accessory pathways in the Wolff-Parkinson-White syndrome. *Am J Cardiol* 1987;59:1093–1102.

79. Garcia Civera R, Ferrero JA, Sanjuan R, et al. Retrograde P wave polarity in reciprocating tachycardia utilizing lateral bypass tracts. *Eur Heart J* 1980;1:137–145.

80. Tai CT, Chen SA, Chiang CE, et al. A new electrocardiographic algorithm using retrograde P waves for differentiating atrioventricular node reentrant tachycardia from atrioventricular reciprocating tachycardia mediated by concealed accessory pathway. *J Am Coll Cardiol* 1997;29:394–402.

81. Goldreyer BN, Damato AN. The essential role of atrioventricular conduction delay in the initiation of paroxysmal supraventricular tachycardia. *Circulation* 1971;43:679–687.

82. Akhtar M, Shenasa M, Schmidt DH. Role of retrograde His Purkinje block in the initiation of supraventricular tachycardia by ventricular premature stimulation in the Wolff-Parkinson-White syndrome. *J Clin Invest* 1981;67:1047–1055.

83. Akhtar M, Lehmann MH, Denker ST, et al. Electrophysiologic mechanisms of orthodromic tachycardia initiation during ventricular pacing in the Wolff-Parkinson-White syndrome. *J Am Coll Cardiol* 1987;9:89–100.

84. Benditt DG, Pritchett EL, Smith WM, Gallagher JJ. Ventriculoatrial intervals: diagnostic use in paroxysmal supraventricular tachycardia. *Ann Intern Med* 1979;91:161–166.

85. Kerr CR, Gallagher JJ, German LD. Changes in ventriculoatrial intervals with bundle branch block aberration during reciprocating tachycardia in patients with accessory atrioventricular pathways. *Circulation* 1982;66:196–201.

86. Pritchett EL, Tonkin AM, Dugan FA, et al. Ventriculoatrial conduction time during reciprocating tachycardia with intermittent bundle-branch block in Wolff-Parkinson-White syndrome. *Br Heart J* 1976;38:1058–1064.

87. Sellers TD Jr, Gallagher JJ, Cope GD, et al. Retrograde atrial preexcitation following premature ventricular beats during reciprocating tachycardia in the Wolff-Parkinson-White syndrome. *Eur J Cardiol* 1976;4:283–294.

88. Zipes DP, DeJoseph RL, Rothbaum DA. Unusual properties of accessory pathways. *Circulation* 1974;49:1200–1211.

89. Cohen TJ, Tucker KJ, Abbott JA, et al. Usefulness of adenosine in augmenting ventricular preexcitation for noninvasive localization of accessory pathways. *Am J Cardiol* 1992;69:1178–1185.

90. Canby RC, Horton RP, Kessler DJ, et al. Use of transesophageal atrial pacing with adenosine infusion to evaluate ventricular preexcitation. *Am J Cardiol* 1995;75:548–550.

91. Bardy GH, Packer DL, German LD, Gallagher JJ. Preexcited reciprocating tachycardia in patients with Wolff-Parkinson-White syndrome: incidence and mechanisms. *Circulation* 1984;70:377–391.

92. Atie J, Brugada P, Brugada J, et al. Clinical and electrophysiologic characteristics of patients with antidromic circus movement tachycardia in the Wolff-Parkinson-White syndrome. *Am J Cardiol* 1990;66:1082–1091.

93. Packer DL, Gallagher JJ, Prystowsky EN. Physiological substrate for antidromic reciprocating tachycardia. Prerequisite characteristics of the accessory pathway and atrioventricular conduction system. *Circulation* 1992;85:574–588.

94. Csanadi Z, Klein GJ, Yee R, et al. Effect of dual atrioventricular node pathways on atrioventricular reentrant tachycardia. *Circulation* 1995;91:2614–2618.

95. Smith WM, Gallagher JJ, Kerr CR, et al. The electrophysiologic basis and management of symptomatic recurrent tachycardia in patients with Ebstein's anomaly of the tricuspid valve. *Am J Cardiol* 1982;49:1223–1234.

96. Smith WM, Broughton A, Reiter MJ, et al. Bystander accessory pathway during AV node re-entrant tachycardia. *Pacing Clin Electrophysiol* 1983;6:537–547.

97. Sung RJ, Styperek JL. Electrophysiologic identification of dual atrioventricular nodal pathway conduction in patients with reciprocating tachycardia using anomalous bypass tracts. *Circulation* 1979;60:1464–1476.

98. Packer D, Prystowsky E. Anatomical and physiological substrate for antidromic reciprocating tachycardia. In: Zipes D, Jalife J, eds. *Cardiac electrophysiology: from cell to bedside.* Philadelphia: WB Saunders, 1995:655–665.

99. Wathen M, Klein G, Yee R, et al. Initiation of atrial fibrillation in the Wolff-Parkinson White syndrome: importance of the accessory pathway. *J Am Coll Cardiol* 1992;19:227A.

100. Waspe LE, Brodman R, Kim SG, Fisher JD. Susceptibility to atrial fibrillation and ventricular tachyarrhythmia in the Wolff-Parkinson-White syndrome: role of the accessory pathway. *Am Heart J* 1986;112:1141–1152.

101. Fujimura O, Klein GJ, Yee R, Sharma AD. Mode of onset of atrial fibrillation in the Wolff-Parkinson-White syndrome: how important is the accessory pathway? *J Am Coll Cardiol* 1990;15:1082–1086.

102. Borggrefe M, Seidl K, Shesana M, et al. Incidence of atrial fibrillation after successful radiofrequency ablation of accessory pathways. *J Am Coll Cardiol* 1992;19:27A.

103. Chen PS, Pressley JC, Tang AS, et al. New observations on atrial fibrillation before and after surgical treatment in patients with the Wolff-Parkinson-White syndrome. *J Am Coll Cardiol* 1992;19:974–981.

104. Haissaguerre M, Fischer B, Labbe T, et al. Frequency of recurrent atrial fibrillation after catheter ablation of overt accessory pathways. *Am J Cardiol* 1992;69:493–497.

105. Sharma AD, Klein GJ, Guiraudon GM, Milstein S. Atrial fibrillation in patients with Wolff-Parkinson-White syndrome: incidence after surgical ablation of the accessory pathway. *Circulation* 1985;72:161–169.

106. Munger TM, Packer DL, Hammill SC, et al. A population study of the natural history of Wolff-Parkinson-White syndrome in Olmsted County, Minnesota, 1953–1989. *Circulation* 1993;87:866–873.

107. Bardy GH, Fedor JM, German LD, et al. Surface electrocardiographic clues suggesting presence of a nodofascicular Mahaim fiber. *J Am Coll Cardiol* 1984;3:1161–1168.

108. Bardy G, Fedor J, Packer D, et al. ECG clues to the presence of a nodo-ventricular Mahaim fiber. *J Am Coll Cardiol* 1984;3:610.

109. de Chillou C, Rodriguez LM, Schlapfer J, et al. Clinical characteristics and electrophysiologic properties of atrioventricular accessory pathways: importance of the accessory pathway location. *J Am Coll Cardiol* 1992;20:666–671.

110. Bauernfeind RA, Wyndham CR, Swiryn SP, et al. Paroxysmal atrial fibrillation in the Wolff-Parkinson-White syndrome. *Am J Cardiol* 1981;47:562–569.

111. Campbell RW, Smith RA, Gallagher JJ, et al. Atrial fibrillation in the preexcitation syndrome. *Am J Cardiol* 1977;40:514–520.

112. Della Bella P, Brugada P, Talajic M, et al. Atrial fibrillation in patients with an accessory pathway: importance of the conduction properties of the accessory pathway. *J Am Coll Cardiol* 1991;17:1352–1356.

113. Cappato R, Schluter M, Weiss C, et al. Radiofrequency current catheter ablation of accessory atrioventricular pathways in Ebstein's anomaly. *Circulation* 1996;94:376–383.

114. Van Hare GF, Lesh MD, Stanger P. Radiofrequency catheter ablation of supraventricular arrhythmias in patients with congenital heart disease: results and technical considerations. *J Am Coll Cardiol* 1993;22:883–890.

115. Lundberg A. Paroxysmal atrial tachycardia in infancy: long-term follow-up study of 49 subjects. *Pediatrics* 1982;70:638–642.

116. Chen SA, Chiang CE, Tai CT, et al. Longitudinal clinical and electrophysiological assessment of patients with symptomatic Wolff-Parkinson-White syndrome and atrioventricular node reentrant tachycardia. *Circulation* 1996;93:2023–2032.

117. Orinious E. Studies on criteria, prognosis, and heredity. *Acta Med Scand Suppl* 1966;465:1.

118. Clair WK, Wilkinson WE, McCarthy EA, et al. Spontaneous occurrence of symptomatic paroxysmal atrial fibrillation and paroxysmal supraventricular tachycardia in untreated patients. *Circulation* 1993;87:1114–1122.

119. Guize L, Soria R, Chaouat JC, et al. [Prevalence and course of Wolf-Parkinson-White syndrome in a population of 138,048 subjects]. *Ann Med Interne (Paris)* 1985;136:474–478.

120. Leitch JW, Klein GJ, Yee R, Murdock C. Prognostic value of electrophysiology testing in asymptomatic patients with Wolff-Parkinson-White pattern. *Circulation* 1990;82:1718–1723.

121. Klein GJ, Yee R, Sharma AD. Longitudinal electrophysiologic assessment of asymptomatic patients with the Wolff-Parkinson-White electrocardiographic pattern. *N Engl J Med* 1989;320:1229–1233.

122. Timmermans C, Smeets JL, Rodriguez LM, et al. Aborted sudden death in the Wolff-Parkinson-White syndrome. *Am J Cardiol* 1995;76:492–494.

123. Leitch JW, Klein GJ, Yee R, et al. Syncope associated with supraventricular tachycardia. An expression of tachycardia rate or vasomotor response? *Circulation* 1992;85:1064–1071.

124. Klein GJ, Bashore TM, Sellers TD, et al. Ventricular fibrillation in the Wolff-Parkinson-White syndrome. *N Engl J Med* 1979;301:1080–1085.

125. Packer D, Pressley J, German L, Prystowsky E. Accuracy of invasive testing for direct identification of sudden death in the Wolff-Parkinson-White syndrome. *J Am Coll Cardiol* 1988;11:78A.

126. Klein GJ, Gulamhusein SS. Intermittent preexcitation in the Wolff-Parkinson-White syndrome. *Am J Cardiol* 1983;52:292–296.

127. Strasberg B, Ashley WW, Wyndham CR, et al. Treadmill exercise testing in the Wolff-Parkinson-White syndrome. *Am J Cardiol* 1980;45:742–748.

128. Sharma AD, Yee R, Guiraudon G, Klein GJ. Sensitivity and specificity of invasive and noninvasive testing for risk of sudden death in Wolff-Parkinson-White syndrome. *J Am Coll Cardiol* 1987;10:373–381.

129. Wellens HJ, Braat S, Brugada P, et al. Use of procainamide in patients with the Wolff-Parkinson-White syndrome to disclose a short refractory period of the accessory pathway. *Am J Cardiol* 1982;50:1087–1089.

130. Fananapazir L, Packer DL, German LD, et al. Procainamide infusion test: inability to identify patients with Wolff-Parkinson-White syndrome who are potentially at risk of sudden death. *Circulation* 1988;77:1291–1296.

131. Cavalli A, Maggioni A, Tusa M, Volpi A. Two false-negative responses to the ajmaline test in the Wolff-Parkinson-White syndrome. *Pacing Clin Electrophysiol* 1985;8:832–837.

132. Critelli G, Grassi G, Perticone F, et al. Transesophageal pacing for prognostic evaluation of preexcitation syndrome and assessment of protective therapy. *Am J Cardiol* 1983;51:513–518.

133. Drago F, Turchetta A, Calzolari A, et al. Detection of atrial vulnerability by transesophageal atrial pacing and the relation of symptoms in children with Wolff-Parkinson-White syndrome and in a symptomatic control group. *Am J Cardiol* 1994;74:400–401.

134. Klein GJ, Prystowsky EN, Yee R, et al. Asymptomatic Wolff-Parkinson-White. Should we intervene? *Circulation* 1989;80:1902–1905.

135. Coumel P, Cabrol C, Fabiato A, et al. Tachycardie permanente par rhythme reciproque. *Arch Mal du Coeur* 1967;60:1830–1867.

136. Gaita F, Haissaguerre M, Giustetto C, et al. Catheter ablation of permanent junctional reciprocating tachycardia with radiofrequency current. *J Am Coll Cardiol* 1995;25:648–654.

137. Ticho BS, Saul JP, Hulse JE, et al. Variable location of accessory pathways associated with the permanent form of junctional reciprocating tachycardia and confirmation with radiofrequency ablation. *Am J Cardiol* 1992;70:1559–1564.

138. Critelli G, Gallagher JJ, Thiene G, et al. Electrophysiologic and histopathologic correlations in a case of permanent form of reciprocating tachycardia. *Eur Heart J* 1985;6:130–137.

139. Critelli G, Gallagher JJ, Monda V, et al. Anatomic and electrophysiologic substrate of the permanent form of junctional reciprocating tachycardia. *J Am Coll Cardiol* 1984;4:601–610.

140. Critelli G, Perticone F, Coltorti F, et al. Antegrade slow bypass conduction after closed-chest ablation of the His bundle in permanent junctional reciprocating tachycardia. *Circulation* 1983;67:687–692.

141. Packer DL, Bardy GH, Worley SJ, et al. Tachycardia-induced cardiomyopathy: a reversible form of left ventricular dysfunction. *Am J Cardiol* 1986;57:563–570.

142. Gallagher JJ, Smith WM, Kasell JH, et al. Role of Mahaim fibers in cardiac arrhythmias in man. *Circulation* 1981;64:176–189.

143. Gillette PC, Garson A Jr, Cooley DA, McNamara DG. Prolonged and decremental antegrade conduction properties in right anterior accessory connections: wide QRS antidromic tachycardia of left bundle branch block pattern without Wolff-Parkinson-White configuration in sinus rhythm. *Am Heart J* 1982;103:66–74.

144. Tchou P, Lehmann MH, Jazayeri M, Akhtar M. Atriofascicular connection or a nodoventricular Mahaim fiber? Electrophysiologic elucidation of the pathway and associated reentrant circuit. *Circulation* 1988;77:837–848.

145. Klein GJ, Guiraudon GM, Kerr CR, et al. "Nodoventricular" accessory pathway: evidence for a distinct accessory atrioventricular pathway with atrioventricular node-like properties. *J Am Coll Cardiol* 1988;11:1035–1040.

146. Haissaguerre M, Cauchemez B, Marcus F, et al. Characteristics of the ventricular insertion sites of accessory pathways with anterograde decremental conduction properties. *Circulation* 1995;91:1077–1085.

147. Josephson ME. Paroxysmal supraventricular tachycardia: an electrophysiologic approach. *Am J Cardiol* 1978;41:1123–1126.

148. Wu D, Denes P, Amat-y-Leon F, et al. Clinical, electrocardiographic and electrophysiologic observations in patients with paroxysmal supraventricular tachycardia. *Am J Cardiol* 1978;41:1045–1051.

149. Bar FW, Brugada P, Dassen WR, Wellens HJ. Differential diagnosis of tachycardia with narrow QRS complex (shorter than 0.12 second). *Am J Cardiol* 1984;54:555–560.

150. Keim S, Werner P, Jazayeri M, et al. Localization of the fast and slow pathways in atrioventricular nodal reentrant tachycardia by intraoperative ice mapping. *Circulation* 1992;86:919–925.

151. Ross DL, Johnson DC, Denniss AR, et al. Curative surgery for atrioventricular junctional ("AV nodal") reentrant tachycardia. *J Am Coll Cardiol* 1985;6:1383–1392.

152. Wah J, Friday K, Sakurai M, et al. Is the His bundle part of the AV nodal reentry circuit? *Circulation* 1985;72:271.

153. Ko PT, Naccarelli GV, Gulamhusein S, et al. Atrioventricular dissociation during paroxysmal junctional tachycardia. *Pacing Clin Electrophysiol* 1981;4:670–678.

154. Otomo K, Beckman K, McClelland J, et al. Resetting response suggests the absence of an upper common pathway in slow/fast and presence in slow/slow atrioventricular nodal reentrant tachycardia. *Pacing Clin Electrophysiol* 1996;19:730.

155. Hwang C, Martin DJ, Goodman JS, et al. Atypical atrioventricular node reciprocating tachycardia masquerading as tachycardia using a left-sided accessory pathway. *J Am Coll Cardiol* 1997;30:218–225.

156. Sorbera C, Cohen M, Woolf P, Kalapatapu SR. Atrioventricular nodal reentry tachycardia: slow pathway ablation using the transseptal approach. *Pacing Clin Electrophysiol* 2000;23:1343–1349.

157. Jais P, Haissaguerre M, Shah DC, et al. Successful radiofrequency ablation of a slow atrioventricular nodal pathway on the left posterior atrial septum. *Pacing Clin Electrophysiol* 1999;22:525–527.

158. Inoue S, Becker AE. Posterior extensions of the human compact atrioventricular node: a neglected anatomic feature of potential clinical significance. *Circulation* 1998;97:188–193.

159. Akhtar M. Atrioventricular nodal reentrant tachycardia. *Med Clin North Am* 1984;68:819–830.

160. McGuire MA, Lau KC, Johnson DC, et al. Patients with two types of atrioventricular junctional (AV nodal) reentrant tachycardia. Evidence that a common pathway of nodal tissue is not present above the reentrant circuit. *Circulation* 1991;83:1232–1246.

161. Moulton K, Wang X, Xu Y, et al. High incidence of dual AV nodal pathway potentials in patients undergoing radiofrequency ablation of accessory pathways. *Circulation* 1990;82:III-319.

162. Hazlitt H, McClelland J, Wang X, et al. Prevalence of slow AV nodal pathway potentials in patients without AV nodal reentrant tachycardia. *J Am Coll Cardiol* 1993;21:281A.

163. Casta A, Wolff GS, Mehta AV, et al. Dual atrioventricular nodal pathways: a benign finding in arrhythmia-free children with heart disease. *Am J Cardiol* 1980;46:1013–1018.

164. de Bakker JM, Coronel R, McGuire MA, et al. Slow potentials in the atrioventricular junctional area of patients operated on for atrioventricular node tachycardias

and in isolated porcine hearts. *J Am Coll Cardiol* 1994;23:709–715.

165. McGuire MA, de Bakker JM, Vermeulen JT, et al. Origin and significance of double potentials near the atrioventricular node. Correlation of extracellular potentials, intracellular potentials, and histology. *Circulation* 1994;89:2351–2360.

166. McGuire MA, Yip AS, Lau KC, et al. Posterior ("atypical") atrioventricular junctional reentrant tachycardia. *Am J Cardiol* 1994;73:469–477.

167. Goldberger J, Brooks R, Kadish A. Physiology of "atypical" atrioventricular junctional reentrant tachycardia occurring following radiofrequency catheter modification of the atrioventricular node. *Pacing Clin Electrophysiol* 1992;15:2270–2282.

168. Sung RJ, Styperek JL, Myerburg RJ, Castellanos A. Initiation of two distinct forms of atrioventricular nodal reentrant tachycardia during programmed ventricular stimulation in man. *Am J Cardiol* 1978;42:404–415.

169. Lee MA, Morady F, Kadish A, et al. Catheter modification of the atrioventricular junction with radiofrequency energy for control of atrioventricular nodal reentry tachycardia. *Circulation* 1991;83:827–835.

170. Wu D, Denes P, Amat YLF, et al. An unusual variety of atrioventricular nodal re-entry due to retrograde dual atrioventricular nodal pathways. *Circulation* 1977;56:50–59.

171. Akhtar M, Damato AN, Ruskin JN, et al. Antegrade and retrograde conduction characteristics in three patterns of paroxysmal atrioventricular junctional reentrant tachycardia. *Am Heart J* 1978;95:22–42.

172. Baerman J, Wang X, Jackman W. Atrioventricular nodal reentry with an antegrade slow pathway and a retrograde slow pathway: clinical and electrophysiological properties. *J Am Coll Cardiol* 1991;17:197A.

173. Sung RJ, Chang MS, Chiang BN. Clinical electrophysiology of supraventricular tachycardia. *Cardiol Clin* 1983;1:225–251.

174. Brugada P, Wellens H. Electrophysiology, mechanisms, diagnosis, and treatment of paroxysmal recurrent atrioventricular nodal reentrant tachycardia. In: Surawicz B, Reddy CP, Prystowsky EN, eds. *Tachycardias*. Boston: Martinus Nijhoff, 1984.

175. Wu D, Kou HC, Yeh SJ, et al. Determinants of tachycardia induction using ventricular stimulation in dual pathway atrioventricular nodal reentrant tachycardia. *Am Heart J* 1984;108:44–55.

176. Farre J, Wellens H. The value of the electrocardiogram in diagnosing site or origin and mechanism of supraventricular tachycardia. In: Wellens H, Kulbertus H, eds. *What's new in electrocardiography*. The Hague, The Netherlands: Martinus Nijhoff, 1981:131–171.

177. Kalbfleisch S, El-Atassi R, Calkins H, et al. Differentiation of paroxysmal narrow QRS complex tachycardias using the 12-lead electrocardiogram. *J Am Coll Cardiol* 1993;21:85–89.

178. Brugada P, Farre J, Green M, et al. Observations in patients with supraventricular tachycardia having a P-R interval shorter than the R-P interval: differentiation between atrial tachycardia and reciprocating atrioventricular tachycardia using an accessory pathway with long conduction times. *Am Heart J* 1984;107:556–570.

179. Wellens H, Brugada P. Value of programmed stimulation of the heart in patients with the Wolff-Parkinson-White syndrome. In: Josephson M, Wellens H, eds. *Tachycardias: mechanisms, diagnosis and treatment*. Philadelphia: Lea & Febiger, 1981:199.

180. Ross DL, Uther JB. Diagnosis of concealed accessory pathways in supraventricular tachycardia. *Pacing Clin Electrophysiol* 1984;7:1069–1085.

181. Jazayeri M, Dhala A, Koch K. Atrioventricular nodal reentry in patients with accessory pathway: a suitable substrate for preexcited tachycardia. *Pacing Clin Electrophysiol* 1991;14:687.

182. Pritchett EL, Prystowsky EN, Benditt DG, Gallagher JJ. "Dual atrioventricular nodal pathways" in patients with Wolff-Parkinson-White syndrome. *Br Heart J* 1980;43:7–13.

183. diMarco JP, Sellers TD, Lerman BB, et al. Diagnostic and therapeutic use of adenosine in patients with supraventricular tachyarrhythmias. *J Am Coll Cardiol* 1985;6:417–425.

184. Akhtar M. Supraventricular tachycardias: electrophysiological mechanisms, diagnosis, and pharmacologic therapy. In: Josephson M, Wellens H, eds. *Tachycardias: mechanisms, diagnosis, treatment*. Philadelphia: Lea & Febiger, 1984:137.

185. Sung RJ, Elser B, McAllister RG, Jr. Intravenous verapamil for termination of re-entrant supraventricular tachycardias: intracardiac studies correlated with plasma verapamil concentrations. *Ann Intern Med* 1980;93:682–689.

186. Waxman HL, Myerburg RJ, Appel R, Sung RJ. Verapamil for control of ventricular rate in paroxysmal supraventricular tachycardia and atrial fibrillation or flutter: a double-blind randomized cross-over study. *Ann Intern Med* 1981;94:1–6.

187. Prystowsky E, Greer G, Packer D, et al. Beta blocker therapy in the Wolff-Parkinson-White syndrome. *Am J Cardiol* 1987;60:460–500.

188. Kerr CR, Gallagher JJ, Smith WM, et al. The induction of atrial flutter and fibrillation and the termination of atrial flutter by esophageal pacing. *Pacing Clin Electrophysiol* 1983;6:60–72.

189. Rhodes LA, Walsh EP, Saul JP. Programmed atrial stimulation via the esophagus for management of supraventricular arrhythmias in infants and children. *Am J Cardiol* 1994;74:353–356.

190. Gallagher JJ, Smith WM, Kasell J, et al. Use of the esophageal lead in the diagnosis of mechanisms of reciprocating supraventricular tachycardia. *Pacing Clin Electrophysiol* 1980;3:440–451.

191. Akhtar M, Shenasa M, Jazayeri M, et al. Wide QRS complex tachycardia. Reappraisal of a common clinical problem. *Ann Intern Med* 1988;109:905–912.

192. Barrett PA, Jordan JL, Mandel WJ, et al. The electrophysiologic effects of intravenous propranolol in the Wolff-Parkinson-White syndrome. *Am Heart J* 1979;98:213–224.

193. Denes P, Cummings JM, Simpson R, et al. Effects of propranolol on anomalous pathway refractoriness and circus movement tachycardias in patients with preexcitation. *Am J Cardiol* 1978;41:1061–1067.

194. Berkowitz WD, Wit AL, Lau SH, et al. The effects of propranolol on cardiac conduction. *Circulation* 1969;40:855–862.

195. Prystowsky EN, Jackman WM, Rinkenberger RL, et al. Effect of autonomic blockade on ventricular refractoriness and atrioventricular nodal conduction in humans. Evidence supporting a direct cholinergic action on ventricular muscle refractoriness. *Circ Res* 1981;49:511–518.

196. Akhtar M, Gilbert CJ, Shenasa M. Effect of lidocaine on atrioventricular response via the accessory pathway in patients with Wolff-Parkinson-White syndrome. *Circulation* 1981;63:435–441.

197. Rosen KM, Barwolf C, Ehsani A, Rahimtoola SH. Effects of lidocaine and propranolol on the normal and anomalous pathways in patients with preexcitation. *Am J Cardiol* 1972;30:801–809.

198. Sellers TD Jr, Bashore TM, Gallagher JJ. Digitalis in the pre-excitation syndrome. Analysis during atrial fibrillation. *Circulation* 1977;56:260–267.

199. Rinkenberger RL, Prystowsky EN, Heger JJ, et al. Effects of intravenous and chronic oral verapamil administration in patients with supraventricular tachyarrhythmias. *Circulation* 1980;62:996–1010.

200. McGovern B, Garan H, Ruskin JN. Precipitation of cardiac arrest by verapamil in patients with Wolff-Parkinson-White syndrome. *Ann Intern Med* 1986;104:791–794.

201. Gulamhusein S, Ko P, Klein GJ. Ventricular fibrillation following verapamil in the Wolff-Parkinson-White syndrome. *Am Heart J* 1983;106:145–147.

202. Jacob AS, Nielsen DH, Gianelly RE. Fatal ventricular fibrillation following verapamil in Wolff-Parkinson-White syndrome with atrial fibrillation. *Ann Emerg Med* 1985;14:159–160.

203. Rowland TW. Augmented ventricular rate following verapamil treatment for atrial fibrillation with Wolff-Parkinson-White syndrome. *Pediatrics* 1983;72:245–246.

204. Exner DV, Muzyka T, Gillis AM. Proarrhythmia in patients with the Wolff-Parkinson-White syndrome after standard doses of intravenous adenosine. *Ann Intern Med* 1995;122:351–352.

205. Wellens HJ, Bar FW, Dassen WR, et al. Effect of drugs in the Wolff-Parkinson-White syndrome. Importance of initial length of effective refractory period of the accessory pathway. *Am J Cardiol* 1980;46:665–669.

206. Harper RW, Whitford E, Middlebrook K, et al. Effects of verapamil on the electrophysiologic properties of the accessory pathway in patients with the Wolff-Parkinson-White syndrome. *Am J Cardiol* 1982;50:1323–1330.

207. Wellens HJ, Tan SL, Bar FW, et al. Effect of verapamil studied by programmed electrical stimulation of the heart in patients with paroxysmal re-entrant supraventricular tachycardia. *Br Heart J* 1977;39:1058–1066.

208. Shenasa M, Gilbert CJ, Schmidt DH, Akhtar M. Procainamide and retrograde atrioventricular nodal conduction in man. *Circulation* 1982;65:355–362.

209. Sellers TD Jr, Campbell RW, Bashore TM, Gallagher JJ. Effects of procainamide and quinidine sulfate in the Wolff-Parkinson-White syndrome. *Circulation* 1977;55:15–22.

210. Wellens HJ, Durrer D. Effect of procaine amide, quinidine, and ajmaline in the Wolff-Parkinson-White syndrome. *Circulation* 1974;50:114–120.

211. Mandel WJ, Laks MM, Obayashi K, et al. The Wolff-Parkinson-White syndrome: pharmacologic effects of procaine amide. *Am Heart J* 1975;90:744–754.

212. Kerr CR, Prystowsky EN, Smith WM, et al. Electrophysiologic effects of disopyramide phosphate in patients with Wolff-Parkinson-White syndrome. *Circulation* 1982;65:869–878.

213. Camm J, Ward D, Spurrell RA. The effect of intravenous disopyramide phosphate on recurrent paroxysmal tachycardias. *Br J Clin Pharmacol* 1979;8:441–449.

214. Breithardt G, Borggrefe M, Wiebringhaus E, Seipel L. Effect of propafenone in the Wolff-Parkinson-White syndrome: electrophysiologic findings and long-term follow-up. *Am J Cardiol* 1984;54:29D–39D.

215. Ludmer PL, McGowan NE, Antman EM, Friedman PL. Efficacy of propafenone in Wolff-Parkinson-White syndrome: electrophysiologic findings and long-term follow-up. *J Am Coll Cardiol* 1987;9:1357–1363.

216. Waleffe A, Mary-Rabine L, de Rijbel R, et al. Electrophysiological effects of propafenone studied with programmed electrical stimulation of the heart in patients with recurrent paroxysmal supraventricular tachycardia. *Eur Heart J* 1981;2:345–352.

217. Hammill SC, McLaran CJ, Wood DL, et al. Double-blind study of intravenous propafenone for paroxysmal supraventricular reentrant tachycardia. *J Am Coll Cardiol* 1987;9:1364–1368.

218. Neuss H, Buss J, Schlepper M, et al. Effects of flecainide on electrophysiological properties of accessory pathways in the Wolff-Parkinson-White syndrome. *Eur Heart J* 1983;4:347–353.

219. Ward DE, Jones S, Shinebourne EA. Use of flecainide acetate for refractory junctional tachycardias in children with the Wolff-Parkinson-White syndrome. *Am J Cardiol* 1986;57:787–790.

220. Hellestrand KJ, Nathan AW, Bexton RS, et al. Cardiac electrophysiologic effects of flecainide acetate for paroxysmal reentrant junctional tachycardias. *Am J Cardiol* 1983;51:770–776.

221. Kim S, Smith P, Lal R, Ruffy R. Treatment of atrial tachyarrhythmias and preexcitation syndrome with flecainide. *Circulation* 1986;74:II-102.

222. Olsson SB, Edvardsson N. Clinical electrophysiologic study of antiarrhythmic properties of flecainide: acute intraventricular delayed conduction and prolonged repolarization in regular paced and premature beats using intracardiac monophasic action potentials with programmed stimulation. *Am Heart J* 1981;102:864–871.

223. Kunze KP, Schluter M, Kuck KH. Sotalol in patients with Wolff-Parkinson-White syndrome. *Circulation* 1987;75:1050–1057.

224. Nathan AW, Hellestrand KJ, Bexton RS, et al. Electrophysiological effects of sotalol—just another beta blocker? *Br Heart J* 1982;47:515–520.

225. Touboul P, Atallah G, Kirkorian G, et al. Effect of intravenous sotalol in patients with accessory AV pathways. *Circulation* 1985;72:III-271.

226. Mitchell L, Wyse D, Duff H. Serial electrophysiological studies during dose ranging of sotalol in Wolff-Parkinson-White syndrome. *Circulation* 1985;72:III-170.

227. Wellens HJ, Lie KI, Bar FW, et al. Effect of amiodarone in the Wolff-Parkinson-White syndrome. *Am J Cardiol* 1976;38:189–194.

228. Rowland E, Krikler DM. Electrophysiological assessment of amiodarone in treatment of resistant supraventricular arrhythmias. *Br Heart J* 1980;44:82–90.

229. Brugada P, Wellens HJ. Effects of oral amiodarone on rate-dependent changes in refractoriness in patients with Wolff-Parkinson-White syndrome. *Am J Cardiol* 1985;56:863–866.

230. Kappenberger LJ, Fromer MA, Steinbrunn W, Shenasa M. Efficacy of amiodarone in the Wolff-Parkinson-White syndrome with rapid ventricular response via accessory pathway during atrial fibrillation. *Am J Cardiol* 1984;54:330–335.

231. Wellens HJ, Brugada P, Abdollah H, Dassen WR. A comparison of the electrophysiologic effects of intravenous and oral amiodarone in the same patient. *Circulation* 1984;69:120–124.

232. Bauernfeind RA, Wyndham CR, Dhingra RC, et al. Serial electrophysiologic testing of multiple drugs in patients with atrioventricular nodal reentrant paroxysmal tachycardia. *Circulation* 1980;62:1341–1349.

233. Wu D, Denes P, Bauernfeind R, et al. Effects of procainamide on atrioventricular nodal re-entrant paroxysmal tachycardia. *Circulation* 1978;57:1171–1179.

234. Naccarelli GV, Jackman WM, Akhtar M, et al. Efficacy and electrophysiologic effects of encainide for atrioventricular nodal reentrant tachycardia. *Am J Cardiol* 1988;62:31L–36L.

235. Wu D, Hung JS, Kuo CT, et al. Effects of quinidine on atrioventricular nodal reentrant paroxysmal tachycardia. *Circulation* 1981;64:823–831.

236. Swiryn S, Bauernfeind RA, Wyndham CR, et al. Effects of oral disopyramide phosphate on induction of paroxysmal supraventricular tachycardia. *Circulation* 1981;64:169–175.

237. Jazayeri MR, Hempe SL, Sra JS, et al. Selective transcatheter ablation of the fast and slow pathways using radiofrequency energy in patients with atrioventricular nodal reentrant tachycardia. *Circulation* 1992;85:1318–1328.

238. Tai CT, Chen SA, Chiang CE, et al. Electrophysiologic characteristics and radiofrequency catheter ablation in patients with multiple atrioventricular nodal reentry tachycardias. *Am J Cardiol* 1996;77:52–58.

239. Hogenhuis W, Stevens SK, Wang P, et al. Cost-effectiveness of radiofrequency ablation compared with other strategies in Wolff-Parkinson-White syndrome. *Circulation* 1993;88:II437–446.

240. Cheng CH, Sanders GD, Hlatky MA, et al. Cost-effectiveness of radiofrequency ablation for supraventricular tachycardia. *Ann Intern Med* 2000;133:864–876.

67

VENTRICULAR TACHYCARDIA

PATRICK J. TCHOU

▼⊿ ADDITIONAL ELECTRONIC TOPICS

OVERVIEW

Ventricular tachyarrhythmias are a major cause of sudden cardiac death, which makes up approximately 50% of all cardiac-related deaths. Most ventricular tachycardias are due to a reentrant mechanism but focal automatic as well as triggered automaticity play a role in certain types of ventricular tachycardias. The most common cause of ventricular tachycardia in the Western world is ischemic coronary artery disease. Both ischemia and the scarred tissue of old myocardial infarction can contribute to the initiation and sustainment of ventricular tachycardia in the setting of coronary artery disease. After a myocardial infarction, several clinical factors appear to indicate a high risk of spontaneous occurrence of

ventricular tachycardia or sudden death in a patient. Depressed left ventricular function, presence of nonsustained ventricular tachycardia, occurrence of syncope, presence of late potentials on the signal-averaged electrocardiogram (ECG), decreased heart rate variability, presence of microvolt T-wave alternans, and inducible sustained ventricular tachycardia during an electrophysiologic study are all predictors of this risk. Antiarrhythmic drug therapy is used infrequently as a primary therapy for sustained ventricular tachycardia in the setting of structural heart disease. When used, amiodarone and sotalol are the most common medications. The implantable cardioverter-defibrillator (ICD), especially with the improved technology that allows transvenous implantation of the electrode and pectoral implantation of a small generator, is the most reliable approach to reduce arrhythmic deaths. Catheter ablation is a modality that is useful for special circumstances.

P. J. Tchou: Department of Cardiovascular Medicine, The Cleveland Clinic Foundation, Cleveland, Ohio

Reentry using the His-Purkinje system is seen more often as the cause of sustained ventricular tachycardia in patients with nonischemic cardiomyopathy than in postmyocardial infarction patients. Recognition of this type of ventricular tachycardia is important because of the comparable ease of ablating this reentrant circuit when compared with ablation of myocardial scar–related ventricular tachycardia.

Both monomorphic and polymorphic types of tachycardias can occur in patients with otherwise structurally normal hearts. For the monomorphic varieties, radiofrequency catheter ablation in well-trained hands has a high success rate in eliminating the tachycardia. Long QT syndrome is a major cause of the polymorphic varieties. These tend to have a more malignant presentation, with syncope and sudden death. New genetic discoveries of the molecular defects associated with long QT syndrome can dramatically change our approach to treatment of this entity. The acquired form of polymorphic ventricular tachycardia associated with long QT is related to drug therapies and electrolyte imbalances that delay repolarization of the action potential and prolong the QT interval on the ECG. Treatment of these malignant arrhythmias is accomplished by removal of the offending drug, correction of electrolyte imbalance, and temporary pacing as needed.

A variety of inflammatory and infiltrative diseases can cause ventricular tachycardia. The most prominent are arrhythmogenic right ventricular dysplasia, sarcoidosis, acute myocarditis, muscular dystrophies, and Chagas' disease.

GLOSSARY

Delayed afterdepolarization (DAD): The normal action potential in the myocardium returns to the resting membrane potential after repolarization brought on by phase 3. Under abnormal conditions, which can be produced by digitalis toxicity and sympathetic stimulation, an oscillation of the transmembrane potential can occur after full repolarization, which can depolarize the membrane back up to threshold and cause repetitive generation of action potentials. These late depolarizations that occur after full repolarization of the transmembrane potential are called *delayed afterdepolarizations*.

Dispersion of refractoriness: The refractory period is the time after initiation of an action potential at a particular myocardial site during which another action potential cannot be elicited. *Dispersion of refractoriness* refers to the termination of refractory periods at different myocardial sites at varying times such that some areas of the myocardium may still be refractory, whereas others are ready for activation.

Early afterdepolarization: Early afterdepolarizations occur with membrane depolarization starting from the early portion of phase 3 of the action potential. Phase 3 is the repolarization phase driven mostly by potassium current. These early depolarizations take off from the early portion of phase 3. The onset of the afterdepolarizations

can bring repetitive firing of action potentials. Drugs and electrolyte changes that prolong the action potential duration have a tendency to activate these afterdepolarizations. They are called "early" afterdepolarizations to distinguish them from the "delayed" type, which are activated after full membrane repolarization.

Monomorphic ventricular tachycardia: Ventricular tachycardia in which the QRS morphology of each beat remains constant in any particular ECG lead. To make that assessment, it is best to compare QRS complexes that are 2 to 3 seconds apart rather than adjacent ones. Occasionally, the changes in QRS morphology may be quite subtle on a beat-to-beat basis. Over several beats, however, these subtle changes become quite obvious.

Polymorphic ventricular tachycardia: Ventricular tachycardia in which the QRS morphology of each sequential beat changes such that over multiple beats, the QRS morphology distinctly changes in at least one ECG lead. Furthermore, the QRS morphology of a polymorphic ventricular tachycardia continues to change over time. The demarcation between polymorphic ventricular tachycardia and ventricular fibrillation is unclear. In general, however, one can visually appreciate distinct initiation and termination of QRS complexes on the surface ECG in polymorphic ventricular tachycardia despite their changing morphologies, whereas that distinction cannot be appreciated during ventricular fibrillation.

QT prolongation: The QT interval changes in relationship to the heart rate, being longer at slower rates and faster at higher rates. Thus, an absolute value cannot be used to define a prolonged QT interval. The corrected QT interval is normalized to the heart rate and can be derived by the Bizet's formula, $QTc\ (ms) = QT\ (ms)/[RR\ (sec)]^{1/2}$, where RR is the cycle length of the heart rate measured in seconds. The upper limits of normal for the QTc is 440 ms.

Reentry: Propagation of a single action potential wavefront, or multiple simultaneous wavefronts, along a path or paths that allows reactivation of individual sites repetitively.

Sustained and nonsustained ventricular tachycardia: The demarcation of what constitutes sustained versus nonsustained ventricular tachycardia is somewhat arbitrary. In most literature describing induction of ventricular tachycardia during programmed ventricular stimulation, a sustained tachycardia is defined as one that lasts at least 30 seconds or one that caused significant hemodynamic compromise such that it needed termination by pacing or direct current cardioversion before 30 seconds. Tachycardias that terminate spontaneously in less than 30 seconds are considered nonsustained.

INTRODUCTION

The recognition of the underlying causes of ventricular tachycardia and the available options for treatment have dramatically changed since the early 1970s. Before that time, treatment of ventricular tachycardia was restricted to the use of a small number of antiarrhythmic medications that are now generally recognized as having limited efficacy in the treatment of most common forms of ventricular tachycardia. Although there was an appreciation of the association of ventricular tachycardia with various forms of cardiac disease, there was unclear understanding of the functional mechanisms and the microanatomic substrate responsible for these tachycardias. The last three decades have indeed seen a substantial growth in this understanding. With this understanding, there has also been a growth in the tools available to treat ventricular tachycardia and to prevent sudden cardiac death. Newer medications such as amiodarone and sotalol may have a higher efficacy rate than those available before them. The development of the ICD has dramatically altered the risk-versus-benefit analysis of using antiarrhythmic medications for the prevention of sudden cardiac death. Surgical resection and cryoablation of ventricular tachycardia sources, although not used frequently now, remains a viable option for treating ventricular tachycardia in special circumstances. Lastly, catheter ablation techniques together with enhanced mapping technologies have offered curative therapies that eliminate the substrate for tachycardia and could be all the therapy needed in some circumstances. Indeed, curative ablation therapies now offer perhaps the best option for treatment of monomorphic ventricular tachycardia in structurally normal hearts afflicting younger, otherwise healthy patients.

SIGNIFICANCE OF VENTRICULAR TACHYCARDIA

It is estimated that approximately half of the deaths due to cardiac diseases are sudden (1,2). Ambulatory ECG recordings of sudden deaths have indicated that these are mostly due to ventricular tachyarrhythmias (3,4). Thus, ventricular tachyarrhythmias are the immediate cause of a large number of deaths, estimated at approximately 300,000 annually in the United States. Death occurs through its interference with the cardiac pumping function.

ANATOMIC SUBSTRATE OF VENTRICULAR TACHYCARDIA RELATED TO ISCHEMIC MYOCARDIAL DISEASE

Because ischemic heart disease is still the most common cardiac disease in North America, ischemic myocardial scars remain the most common substrate for sustained monomorphic ventricular tachycardia. When arterial blood supply is interrupted to a portion of the ventricular myocardium, causing myocardial infarction, not all the muscle fibers die within that region. Especially within the suben-

docardial and subepicardial layers, surviving muscle fibers can be electrically active and may even generate normal-appearing action potentials. However, because of the interweaving of scar tissue within these muscle fibers, propagation of electrical impulses through this tissue may take a circuitous route. Cell-to-cell propagation may also be slowed due to a variety of factors associated with the scarring process and persistence of ischemia. Refractory periods within regions of surviving muscle in the scar may also be prolonged in comparison with the surrounding normal muscle. Recordings of electrical propagation in these scarred areas tend to show fractionated, low-amplitude, and prolonged signals. These properties form the basis of unidirectional block and slow conduction necessary for initiation and sustainment of a reentrant wavefront (10–12).

Risk Factors for Ventricular Tachyarrhythmia and Sudden Death in Ischemic Heart Disease

Patients who have experienced a myocardial infarction have the potential for reentrant ventricular tachycardia. Several clinical factors are useful for assessing the risk of experiencing sustained ventricular tachycardia. The probability that sustained ventricular tachycardia or sudden death would occur in a person after a myocardial infarction appears to be directly related to the size of the infarct and the consequent reduction in systolic ventricular function. Several reports have described a direct relationship between ventricular dysfunction and increased mortality rates in post–myocardial infarction patients (13,14). Sudden deaths make up a significant proportion of this mortality and are largely due to ventricular tachycardia and ventricular fibrillation. The extent of myocardial damage, as reflected by the patient's left ventricular ejection fraction and functional class, is probably the most important predictor of sudden arrhythmic deaths.

The occurrence of syncope, the presence of late potentials on a signal-averaged ECG, decreased heart rate variability, the presence of T-wave alternans, the occurrence of high-grade ventricular ectopy and nonsustained ventricular tachycardia, and the inducibility of sustained ventricular tachycardia during programmed ventricular stimulation are also predictors of mortality and occurrence of clinical sustained ventricular tachycardia (15–19). 170

Ischemia as a Cause of Ventricular Tachycardia

During ischemia, myocardial cells may undergo changes in their action potentials that could promote ventricular tachycardia. Depending on the degree of ischemia, refractoriness can be prolonged, action potentials can shorten, myocytes can become electrically uncoupled, or the cell can become electrically inert (43). Metabolic changes such as

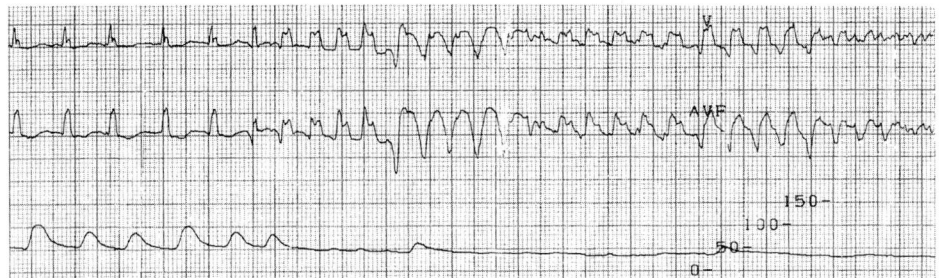

FIGURE 67.1 Polymorphic ventricular tachycardia related to cardiac ischemia. This figure illustrates the initiation of sustained polymorphic ventricular tachycardia resulting from ischemia without evidence of ST elevation. This polymorphic ventricular tachycardia should be distinguished from torsades de pointes (see Fig. 67.9). Note that the QT intervals were not prolonged, and initiation of polymorphic ventricular tachycardia was not preceded by a long RR interval.

increased extracellular potassium concentration and acidosis can further affect cellular electrical activation. Toxic lipid metabolites can accumulate in the ischemic area to provoke ventricular arrhythmias (44). The ventricular tachycardia seen during the acute ischemic event generally tends to be polymorphic ventricular tachycardia or ventricular fibrillation rather than a sustained monomorphic ventricular tachycardia. Marked ischemia can cause prolongation of the QT interval, usually associated with inversion of the T wave. QT interval prolongation, for example, can be seen during an acute myocardial infarction. However, myocardial ischemia may not prolong the QT interval. In fact, the presence of polymorphic ventricular tachycardia, sustained or nonsustained, in the absence of QT prolongation should be a clue that ischemia is likely to be an underlying cause (Fig. 67.1). Although nonischemic causes of polymorphic ventricular tachycardia can occur as described below, they are rare in comparison. Thus, high-grade coronary disease should be the first consideration in an adult patient with any coronary risk factor who manifests polymorphic ventricular tachycardia without QT prolongation. ❧ 171

Assessment of Risk after a Myocardial Infarction

The assessment of risk for ventricular tachycardia and sudden death in a patient after myocardial infarction is a multifactorial process. At the minimum this should include an assessment of left ventricular function and the presence of nonsustained runs of ventricular tachycardia on ECG monitoring. An assessment of any persistent ischemia either surrounding the infarct zone or in another portion of the myocardium unrelated to the infarct artery should be made. The use of a signal-averaged ECG may provide additional information to enhance or reduce the apparent risk of a particular patient. The other noninvasive tests such as heart rate variability and T-wave alternans, as discussed above, may prove to be good risk assessments. Those patients who appear to be at high risk as determined by the above noninvasive testing should undergo electrophysiologic testing. The inducibility of sustained ventricular tachycardia during an electrophysiologic study confirms the high risk, whereas the inability to induce sustained tachycardia suggests a lower risk.

Prevention and Treatment of Ventricular Tachycardia after Myocardial Infarction

As a general approach to the prevention of sustained ventricular tachyarrhythmia, patients who have an ischemic cardiomyopathy should have optimal therapy to relieve congestive heart failure and ischemia. The proper use of diuretics, potassium and perhaps magnesium supplements, angiotensin-converting enzyme inhibitors, beta-blockers, and digoxin as needed should form the basis of heart failure therapy. Significant ischemia should be relieved, where possible, by revascularization and minimized with drug therapies, especially beta-blockers. Beta-blockers and angiotensin-converting enzyme inhibitors in some studies have been shown to improve overall as well as arrhythmic mortality in this population (51–53).

With the possible exception of amiodarone, the use of antiarrhythmic medications has not improved or has worsened survival. Several clinical trials with amiodarone have demonstrated no detrimental effects and may, in selected subgroups, improve survival. ❧ 172

In contrast to the antiarrhythmic drug studies, two studies have now reported improved survival in high-risk post–myocardial infarction patients treated with an ICD. The Multicenter Automatic Defibrillator Implantation Trial demonstrated that patients with nonsustained ventricular tachycardia after a myocardial infarction who have left ventricular ejection fractions of 35% or less and who have inducible sustained ventricular tachycardia at electrophysiologic study are best treated with an ICD rather than with antiarrhythmic medications. The antiarrhythmic medication used in this trial consisted primarily of amiodarone (74%), with a small number of patients taking sotalol (7%). Patients treated with the implanted device had approximately one-half the mortality of the drug-treated

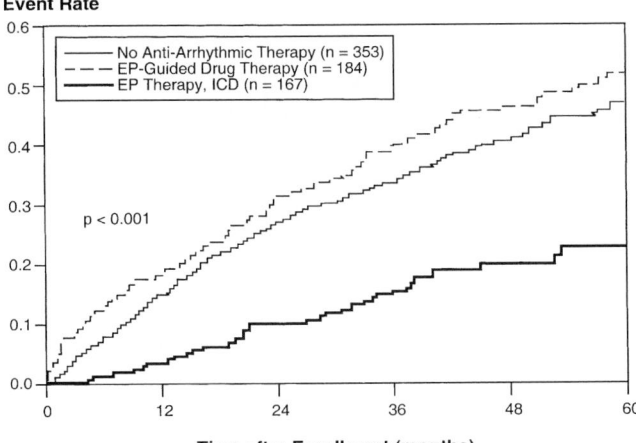

FIGURE 67.2 Survival of patients in the Multicenter Unsustained Tachycardia Trial: comparison of antiarrhythmic drug therapy, no therapy, and implantable cardioverter-defibrillator (ICD) therapy. The study enrolled post–myocardial infarction patients who had left ventricular ejection fraction of 40% or less and inducible sustained ventricular tachycardia during electrophysiology study. Patients who were treated with antiarrhythmic drugs had no better outcome than those who were not treated at all. Those treated with an ICD had significantly improved survival. EP, electrophysiologic. (From Buxton AE, Lee KL, Fisher JD, et al. A randomized study of the prevention of sudden death in patients with coronary artery disease. Multicenter Unsustained Tachycardia Trial Investigators. *N Engl J Med* 1999;341:1882, with permission.)

group (67). The Multicenter Unsustained Tachycardia Trial (MUSTT) enrolled 704 post–myocardial infarction patients with left ventricular ejection fractions of 40% or less who had nonsustained ventricular tachycardia on monitoring and inducible sustained ventricular tachycardia during electrophysiologic testing. In contrast to the Multicenter Automatic Defibrillator Implantation Trial, MUSTT contained a no-therapy arm. Antiarrhythmic treatment consisted of medications guided by the results of programmed ventricular stimulation or the ICD. Forty-six percent of the patients receiving therapy were given an ICD. The group of patients receiving the ICD had the best arrhythmic and all-cause mortality. Patients receiving antiarrhythmic drug therapy did no better than those who received no antiarrhythmic therapy (Fig. 67.2) (68). These two studies taken together have demonstrated that the particular group of patients characterized by prior myocardial infarction, reduced left ventricular ejection fraction, clinical nonsustained ventricular tachycardia, and inducible sustained ventricular tachycardia are at high risk for arrhythmic mortality and that treatment with an ICD results in lower arrhythmic and overall mortality.

Patients who have already experienced a clinical episode of sustained ventricular tachycardia or ventricular fibrillation are at the highest risk of recurrence (69). Unless one can clearly demonstrate that such an occurrence was associated with a reversible cause, a reliable therapeutic

approach should be used to minimize the risk of sudden death. The therapy of choice is now clearly the ICD. Publication of several studies have demonstrated that ICD therapy yields better survival outcomes in these patients when compared with antiarrhythmic drug therapy with sotalol or amiodarone. 173

An alternative to drug therapy of ventricular tachycardia associated with ischemic heart disease is catheter ablation. Current approaches mainly use radiofrequency energy. Success in eliminating a particular reentrant ventricular tachycardia is in the 50% to 70% range by most reports (77,78). At present, this technique is still mostly used as an adjunctive therapy for patients who have an ICD already but are having frequent or slow ventricular tachycardias that complicate device therapy.

Ischemic Ventricular Tachycardia Unrelated to Atherosclerotic Coronary Artery Disease

Although not related to atherosclerotic obstruction of the coronary arteries, several other causes of sudden death, presumably from ischemic polymorphic ventricular tachycardia and ventricular fibrillation, should be considered, especially in competitive athletes (79). Anomalous takeoff of the left coronary artery from the right coronary cusp or the right coronary artery from the left coronary cusp are potential, although rare, etiologies. Anatomically, this anomalous takeoff can result in compression of the artery, resulting in ischemia. Hypertrophic cardiomyopathy and other causes of myocardial hypertrophy such as aortic stenosis may also trigger ventricular fibrillation by an ischemic mechanism. Embolic occlusion of coronary arteries can also occur from blood clots or vegetations generated by endocarditis. Lastly, coronary spasm can induce ischemic polymorphic ventricular tachycardia and cardiac arrest (Fig. 67.3). In all these entities, the therapeutic approach is to prevent or alleviate the conditions leading to ischemia. Although medications may be helpful in cases such as coronary spasm, an ICD should be considered as back-up protection should medications fail to completely prevent ischemia.

VENTRICULAR TACHYCARDIA RELATED TO HIS-PURKINJE SYSTEM DISEASE

The His bundle and the bundle branches together with the Purkinje network and the myocardium form a potential reentrant pathway that could become the substrate for ventricular tachycardia. The ability of the normal His-Purkinje to generate reentrant beats during right ventricular premature stimulation was first described in the 1970s (80,81). It had been recognized that a stimulated right ventricular premature beat (V2) was frequently followed by another ventricular beat (V3) that had a QRS morphology similar to that

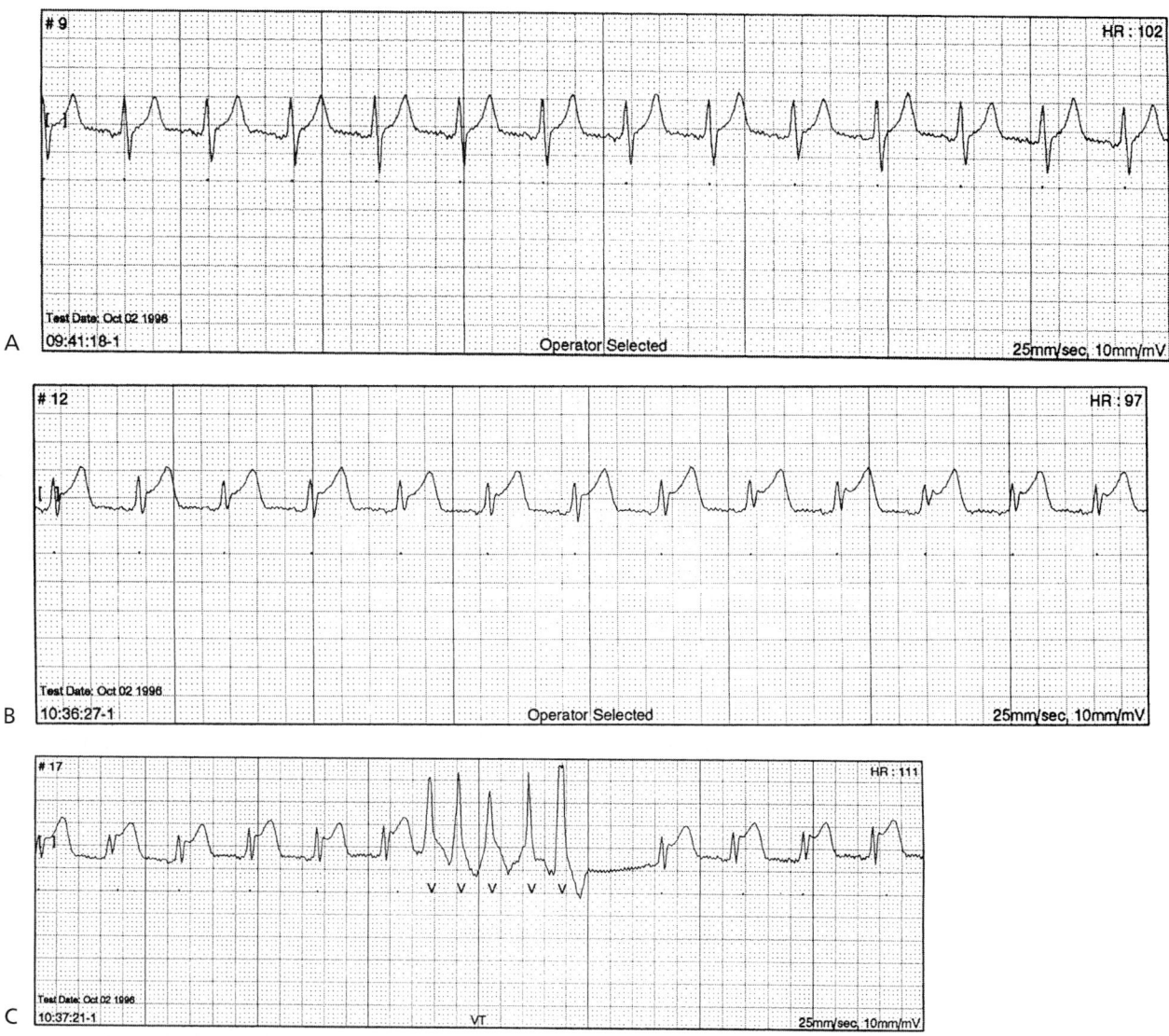

FIGURE 67.3 Polymorphic ventricular tachycardia related to coronary spasm. **A**, **B**, and **C** show Holter electrocardiographic tracings from a 38-year-old patient in the hospital after a cardiac arrest at home where ventricular fibrillation was documented. He had complained of chest pain just before the cardiac arrest. **A:** Baseline rhythm. **B:** Beginning of ST elevation. One minute later, the ST segments are markedly elevated **(C)**, accompanied by short nonsustained runs of polymorphic ventricular tachycardia. Cardiac catheterization in this patient showed minimal coronary disease, and the ischemic events were attributed to coronary spasm. Note that the QT intervals in Figure 67.2 and this figure are not prolonged. Although QT interval may prolong during acute ischemia, especially with T-wave inversion, it is not a common accompanying finding in ischemia-induced polymorphic ventricular tachycardia.

of V2. Akhtar and colleagues (80,81) demonstrated that the reentrant circuit of the V3 phenomenon involved the bundle branches as shown in *e*Figure 67.3.1. These reports were the first demonstration that the normal human His-Purkinje/myocardial system was capable of acting as a reentrant circuit. However, the electrophysiologic characteristics of the normal His-Purkinje system, fast conduction and long refractory periods, prevent sustainment of this reentrant process. When these normal electrophysiologic characteristics are altered by disease processes, however, this reentrant circuit can become the substrate for sustained tachycardia.

Several reports have defined the specific criteria useful in identifying the bundle branch reentrant mechanism in a ventricular tachycardia (82–85). In these reports, all patients had underlying His-Purkinje system disease as demonstrated by prolonged HV conduction time during sinus rhythm and the presence of intraventricular conduction defects on their surface 12-lead ECGs. Many had enlarged hearts due to various underlying cardiac diseases. However, there are reported cases in which isolated conduction system disease without other significant structural heart diseases can be the sole underlying cause of sustained bundle branch reentrant ventricular tachycardia (86). Myotonic dystrophy with its associated conduction system disease has been associated with bundle branch reentrant ventricular tachycardia (87). In the largest reported series (88), approximately half of the patients had nonischemic dilated cardiomyopathy; the other half had ischemic cardiac disease. However, when one looks at the frequency of bundle branch reentry as a mechanism of sustained tachycardia in these disease categories, the differences are quite striking. Bundle branch reentry can be the mechanism of tachycardia in 30% to 50% of patients with nonischemic dilated cardiomyopathy who have inducible sustained monomorphic ventricular tachycardia during programmed stimulation, although the incidence of inducing this tachycardia is no more than 5% to 6% in patients who have ischemic cardiac disease.

The tachycardia rate of bundle branch reentry tends to be fast, frequently above 200 beats/min. The most common clinical and laboratory-induced tachycardias have a left bundle branch block pattern (Fig. 67.4). Only isolated cases of right bundle branch block QRS morphologies have been reported. His-Purkinje system reentry generating a right bundle branch block QRS morphology on the surface ECG can also be due to fascicular reentry. 174

Although one can suspect the presence of bundle branch reentry as a mechanism of tachycardia based on clinical presentation and ECG characteristics, its diagnosis can be made only during a careful electrophysiologic study. Several studies have detailed the diagnostic criteria that have been summarized in a review of the topic (91).

The therapy of choice for this tachycardia is radiofrequency catheter ablation, usually of the right bundle branch (92,93). Left bundle ablation should be pursued only when there is a clear indication that antegrade conduction down the left bundle is not reliable. These patients frequently have an already depressed left ventricular function that can be further compromised with the development of complete left bundle branch block.

Long-term survival in these patients depends ultimately on the underlying cardiac disease and identification and appropriate treatment of other ventricular tachycardia. A report (94) of survival among 16 patients undergoing radiofrequency ablation of the right bundle and followed for a mean duration of 22 ± 10 months showed one sudden death and one death due to congestive heart failure. Three of those patients had ICDs, two of which were implanted before the ablation. Two patients underwent heart transplant during their follow-up.

MONOMORPHIC VENTRICULAR TACHYCARDIA IN AN OTHERWISE NORMALLY FUNCTIONING HEART

Primary electrophysiologic abnormalities of the heart can be associated with ventricular tachycardia with no hint of heart disease or dysfunction on the echocardiogram or the ECG during sinus rhythm. These ventricular tachycardias are sometimes referred to as "normal heart" ventricular tachycardias. It is important to recognize the source of these tachyarrhythmias, as some of them respond to calcium channel blockers and, thus, may mistakenly be called supraventricular tachycardia. Two distinct types of normal heart monomorphic ventricular tachycardias are described. One type originates from the outflow tract regions near the pulmonic and the aortic valves. On the 12-lead ECG, this tachycardia has a characteristic appearance of left bundle branch block and inferior axis (Fig. 67.5), a QRS morphology typically seen with outflow area pacing.

Several electrophysiologic characteristics of this tachycardia suggest that it originates from an automatic focus, perhaps related to delayed afterdepolarizations (94–96). The occurrence of the afterdepolarizations is enhanced by calcium loading and adrenergic stimulation (97–99). Clinically, these tachycardias can be exercise-induced or occur at other times of adrenergic stimulation. At times, these may manifest as frequent and virtually incessant ventricular premature beats to the extent that the patient may be in ventricular bigeminy constantly. A variation of the sustained tachycardia originating from the ventricular outflow region is the syndrome of repetitive monomorphic ventricular tachycardia. This syndrome is characterized by repetitive bursts of nonsustained ventricular tachycardia. These have

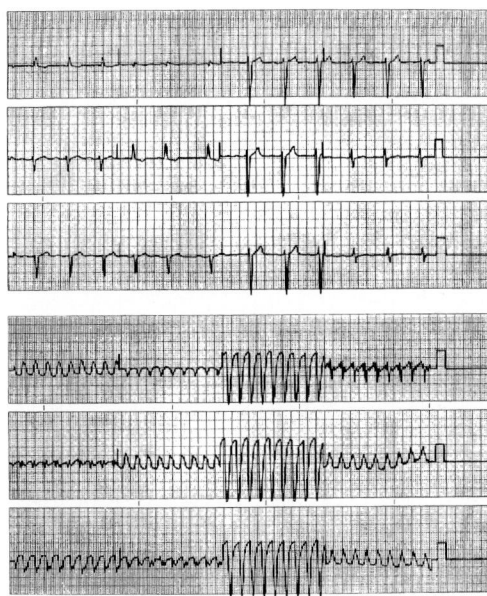

FIGURE 67.4 Electrocardiographic characteristics of a typical bundle branch reentrant ventricular tachycardia. This 12-lead electrocardiogram shows the typical characteristics of the common form of bundle branch reentrant ventricular tachycardia (*lower panel*). The anterior chest leads have a left bundle branch block QRS morphology with rapid downstroke of the S wave. The tachycardia is rapid. The QRS in sinus rhythm (*upper panel*) shows an intraventricular conduction defect of the left bundle branch type.

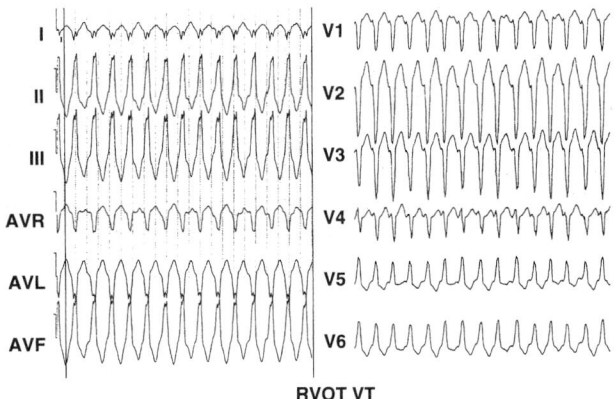

RVOT VT

FIGURE 67.5 Twelve-lead electrocardiogram of a ventricular outflow tachycardia (RVOT). The ventricular outflow tract tachycardia typically seen in structurally normal hearts has a characteristic QRS morphology that is similar to that seen with pacing at the pulmonic and aortic valve regions. The QRS has a left bundle branch block morphology with an inferior right axis. This QRS morphology is diagnostic for ventricular tachycardia (VT), as it is highly unusual for aberrant conduction to manifest this type of QRS.

also been shown to respond to calcium channel blockers, beta-blockers, as well as adenosine (100). Although the original descriptions suggested that the right ventricular outflow and the pulmonic valve area are the source of these ventricular tachycardias and premature ventricular complexes, more recent reports have found that the origin may also be located on the left side of the heart near the aortic valve (101,102). This type of ventricular tachycardia may respond to calcium channel blockers, beta-blockers, or a combination of both. However, they may also respond to a variety of antiarrhythmic agents, including type Ia and Ic agents. They may also be sensitive to adenosine, suggesting that cyclic adenosine monophosphate may function as an intracellular mediator (103,104).

Because of its focal nature, catheter ablation has an excellent chance of obtaining a cure when the tachycardia can be reproduced within the electrophysiologic study (105,106). Alternatively, drug therapy with verapamil, diltiazem (107), beta-blockers, or another antiarrhythmic agent may prevent clinical recurrence of this tachycardia. This ventricular tachycardia does not appear to associated with a progressive myopathy or other diseases of the heart except where it is incessant and could cause a tachycardia-mediated myopathy. The outflow-tract tachycardias should be distinguished from other right ventricular tachycardias that could be due to bundle branch reentry or to right ventricular dysplasia (see below).

A second type of normal heart ventricular tachycardia originates near the apex of the left ventricle. On the 12-lead ECG, this tachycardia has a typical right bundle branch block QRS morphology with a superior axis (Fig. 67.6). The earliest reports of this ventricular tachycardia described

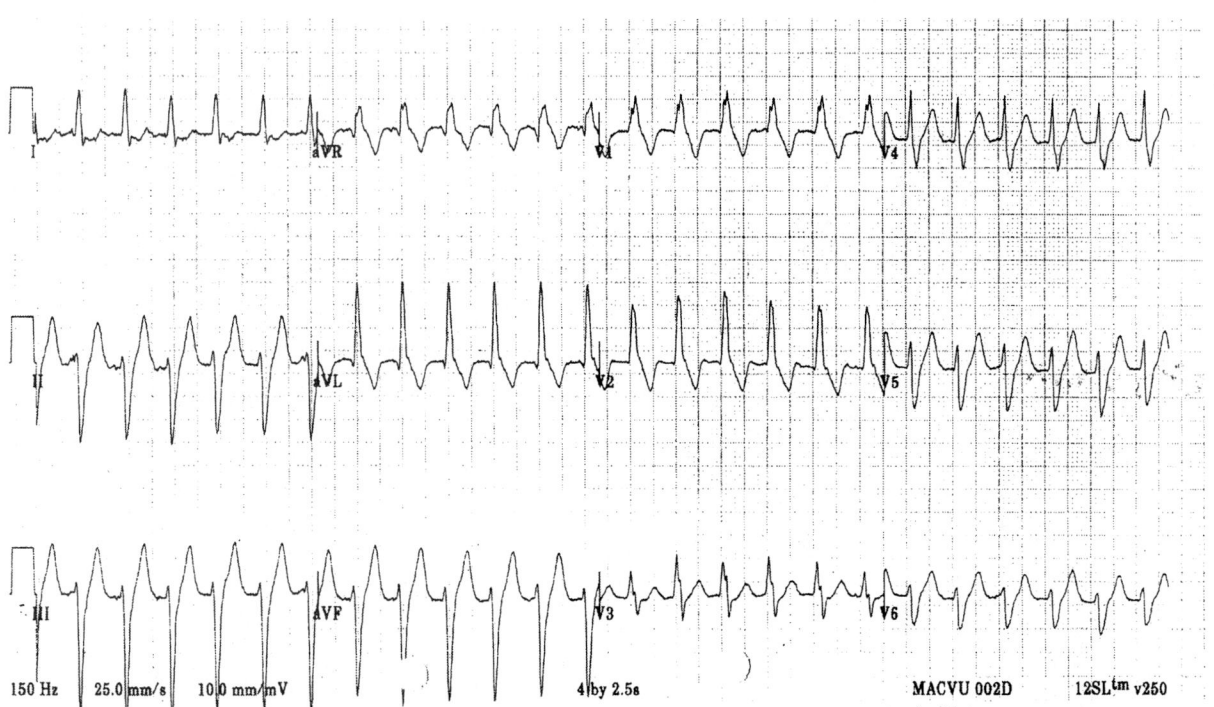

FIGURE 67.6 Ventricular tachycardia originating from the left ventricular apex in a structurally normal heart. The left ventricular origin of this ventricular tachycardia generates a typical right bundle branch block QRS morphology on the 12-lead electrocardiogram. Early ventricular activation occurs in the apical inferior septal region of the ventricle, giving the QRS a superior axis.

the typical response to verapamil treatment by slowing and terminating (108,109). However, other antiarrhythmic medications may also suppress it. The tachycardia originates from within the left-sided His-Purkinje system and has been described as a fascicular tachycardia in normal hearts (110). Success in ablating this tachycardia in competent hands is near 100%, and long-term survival after ablation is excellent (111). ◆▼ 175

Lastly, occasional monomorphic ventricular tachycardias are seen in normal hearts that do not necessarily fit into the two categories listed above. Some may originate in the left ventricle but do not have the typical QRS morphologies described above. Others are located at the mitral or tricuspid annulus. These tachycardias usually respond to type Ic agents such as flecainide, calcium channel blockers, or beta-blockers. They can also be treated with catheter ablation.

POLYMORPHIC VENTRICULAR TACHYCARDIA AND FIBRILLATION IN THE NORMAL HEART

Polymorphic ventricular tachycardia and ventricular fibrillation can also occur in the setting of a structurally normal heart. Whereas the monomorphic varieties typically do not present with syncope and cardiac arrest, the polymorphic varieties are more malignant and are associated with a high incidence of syncope and sudden death. These can be categorized into two general classes, those associated with prolonged QT intervals and abnormal-appearing T waves and those apparently unassociated with QT abnormality.

Jervell and Lange-Nielsen (114) reported in 1957 a family with congenitally deaf children, prolongation of the QT interval, and sudden death. Subsequent reports have demonstrated an autosomal recessive inheritance of this syndrome. Romano et al. (115) and Ward (116) subsequently reported familial clustering of sudden death and long QT without deafness. This more common form of long QT syndrome is inherited in an autosomal recessive pattern. In addition to these two reported inherited syndromes, there are occasional cases of new mutation causing this syndrome in a person who has no family history of such a genetic abnormality.

Recent advances in the genetics of long QT syndrome have revealed that they are associated with abnormalities of transmembrane ion channels causing the repolarization abnormality. Mutations associated with at least six genes coding for ion channel functions have been identified that cause clinical long QT syndrome. Within each gene or genetic locus, there can be multiple specific mutations that interfere the function of the ion channels. Each one of these mutations is usually seen in a particular family. The clinical long QT syndromes associated with these mutated genes or chromosomal loci have been named sequentially in order of their discovery, long QT syndrome 1 to long QT syndrome 6 (Table 67.1). ◆▼ 176

TABLE 67.1 GENETIC ABNORMALITIES ASSOCIATED WITH LONG QT SYNDROME

	Gene (alternate names)	Chromosome	Affected cardiac channel/current
LQT1	*KvLQT1 (KCNQ1)*	11	Potassium/I_{Ks}
LQT2	*HERG (KCNH2)*	7	Potassium/I_{Kr}
LQT3	*SCN5A*	3	Sodium/I_{Na^+}
LQT4	Not identified	4	Unknown
LQT5	*minK (KCNE1, IsK)*	21	Potassium/I_{Ks}
LQT6	*MiRP1 (KCNE2)*	21	Potassium/I_{Kr}

LQT, long QT syndrome.

Correlation of the genetic abnormality with ECG T-wave pattern has revealed characteristic patterns that seem to be associated with different forms of the long QT syndrome (Table 67.1). Moss et al. (125) have described three different ECG QT patterns associated with long QT syndrome 1, long QT syndrome 2, and long QT syndrome 3 (Fig. 67.7). These different types of long QT syndromes also appear to have different responses to heart rate acceleration. In long QT syndrome 3, increase in heart rate appears to markedly shorten the QT interval; such is not the case in long QT syndrome 2 (92). The different forms of long QT syndrome also respond differently to pharmacologic interventions aimed at shortening the QT interval. In long QT syndrome 2, in which the defect is in a delayed rectifier potassium channel, potassium loading appears to shorten the QT interval (126). On the other hand, in long QT syndrome 3, in which the defect is in the persistent opening of an abnormal sodium channel, mexiletine, a sodium channel blocker, appears to shorten the QT interval (92).

The greatest clinical concern with patients who have long QT syndrome is sudden death and syncope. Those patients who have already experienced such an event appear to be at the highest risk. Patients with long QT interval and first-degree family members who have experienced sudden death are also at significantly increased risk (127). Treatment of high-risk patients with the long QT syndrome may soon be undergoing a marked change as the molecular abnormalities associated with specific channel proteins are identified. Traditionally, the treatments have used beta-blockers (98), pacemakers (128), cervicothoracic sympathectomies (129), careful avoidance of drugs that could prolong the QT interval (Table 67.2), and ICDs. Sympathetic tone, especially when associated with sudden arousal, may be a potent stimulant for the development of polymorphic ventricular tachycardia in these patients. Beta-blockers serve to block this effect of sympathetic tone. Pacemakers can prevent bradycardia, which may be another trigger for polymorphic tachycardia. Left-sided sympathectomy may function in a similar manner as beta-blocker therapy but limits its effect to neurally mediated sympathetic stimulation of the heart. However, this approach is no longer used commonly. ICDs, of course, are intended as rescue devices

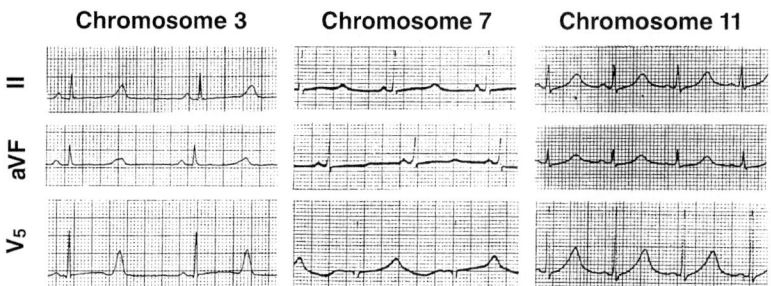

FIGURE 67.7 The QT abnormalities associated with long QT syndrome 1, long QT syndrome 2, and long QT syndrome 3. This figure shows some of the characteristic ST- and T-wave abnormalities associated with some of the long QT syndromes. The electrocardiogram in long QT syndrome 1, associated with an abnormality on chromosome 11, shows broad-based T waves with robust amplitudes. The T wave in long QT syndrome 2, associated with a genetic abnormality on chromosome 7, is also broad-based but tends to have lower amplitudes. Long QT syndrome 3, which comes from an abnormality on chromosome 3, shows a late-initiating and late-peaking T wave with a rather narrow base. (From Moss AJ, Zareba W, Benhorin J, et al. ECG T-wave patterns in genetically distinct forms of the hereditary long QT syndrome. *Circulation* 1995;92:2929, with permission.)

rather than prevention of the arrhythmia. With the pacing function available in current devices, ICDs could potentially perform a dual role of prevention as well as rescue. These traditional approaches, however, may be quickly changing. Recent advances in the understanding of the different manners in which long QT syndrome 3 and long QT syndrome 2 respond to heart rate acceleration, sodium channel blockers, potassium loading, and potassium channel openers, for example, may dramatically alter our approach to therapy and may provide a more rational approach to selection of the traditional therapies in conjunction with possible new pharmacologic approaches.

The occurrence of polymorphic ventricular tachycardia and fibrillation in the absence of prolonged QT interval,

cardiac ischemia, or marked metabolic abnormalities has been called *idiopathic ventricular fibrillation*. Three syndromes have been described and many isolated cases reported. Brugada and Brugada (130) reported a group of patients with recurrent polymorphic ventricular tachycardia leading to cardiac arrest who had characteristic ECG abnormalities during sinus rhythm. The precordial recordings in the standard 12-lead ECG showed ST elevation mimicking a right bundle branch block (Fig. 67.8). A genetic abnormality of the sodium channel has been identified with this syndrome (131). ▼ 177

DRUG-INDUCED MONOMORPHIC AND POLYMORPHIC VENTRICULAR TACHYCARDIA

Ventricular tachycardia can be seen in certain toxic or idiosyncratic reactions generated by drugs or electrolyte imbalances. Polymorphic ventricular tachycardia associated with drugs that prolong the QT interval is an example. The term "torsades de pointes" was coined by Dessertenne (139) to describe polymorphic ventricular tachycardia where the QRS axis appears to be twisting around a baseline. Torsades has been associated with a variety of antiarrhythmic drug therapies, electrolyte disturbances, and bradycardia due to heart block and hypothyroidism (140–143). A long cycle length, the pause, typically precedes the initiation of this arrhythmia (144) and appears to be a hallmark of drug-induced torsades de pointes (Fig. 67.9). This malignant arrhythmia frequently progresses to sustained ventricular fibrillation and cardiac arrest. Many of the drugs that produce marked QT prolongation in susceptible individuals appear to affect the *HERG*/I_{Kr} potassium repolarization current (145). Thus, a genetic predisposition is most likely present. When QT intervals prolong to 600 ms or when the QTc prolongs more than 500 ms, there is a significant incidence of torsades. Interestingly, amiodarone, although capa-

TABLE 67.2 DRUGS ASSOCIATED WITH QT PROLONGATION AND TORSADES DE POINTES

Antiarrhythmic medications
    Type Ia: quinidine, procainamide, disopyramide
    Type Ic: encainide (due to metabolites)
    Type III: sotalol, amiodarone, ibutilide, dofetilide, *N*-acetyl procainamide
    Type IV: bepridil
Antibiotics
    Erythromycin, trimethoprim-sulfamethoxazole, ketoconazole, pentamidine
Antihistamines
    Terfenadine, astemizole
Psychoactive compounds
    Phenothiazines, haloperidol, tricyclic and tetracyclic antidepressants
    Chloral hydrate
Miscellaneous
    Diuretics (hypokalemia and hypomagnesemia related)
    Probucol, cisapride
    Corticosteroids
    Organophosphate poisoning

Updated list on the World Wide Web: http://georgetowncert.org/qtdrugs_torsades.asp.

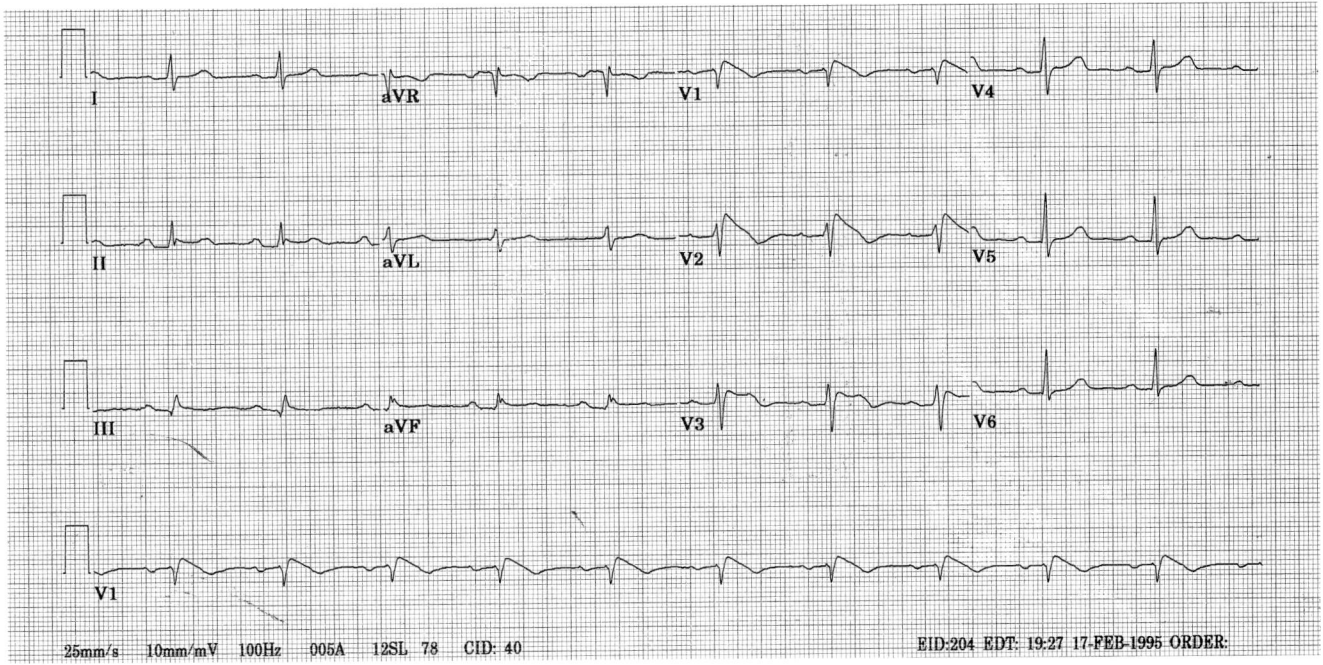

FIGURE 67.8 A 12-lead electrocardiogram from a patient with the Brugada syndrome. Note the ST elevation in the anterior chest leads, especially V1, which mimics the appearance of right bundle branch block. The ST segment slopes gently downward into the inverted T wave, giving the so-called saddleback appearance.

ble of prolonging the QT interval, appears to have a low incidence of causing torsades de pointes (146,147). Table 67.2 lists some of the medications and other conditions that have been shown to produce QT prolongation and torsades de pointes. The list of drugs that could cause QT prolongation and torsades de pointes, especially in patients with the prolonged QT syndrome, is frequently updated and can be obtained from the Georgetown Center for Education and Research on Therapeutics by accessing their Web page on the International Registry for Drug-Induced Arrhythmias (http://georgetowncert.org/qtdrugs_torsades.asp). Besides medications, hypokalemia, hypomagnesemia, hypocalce-

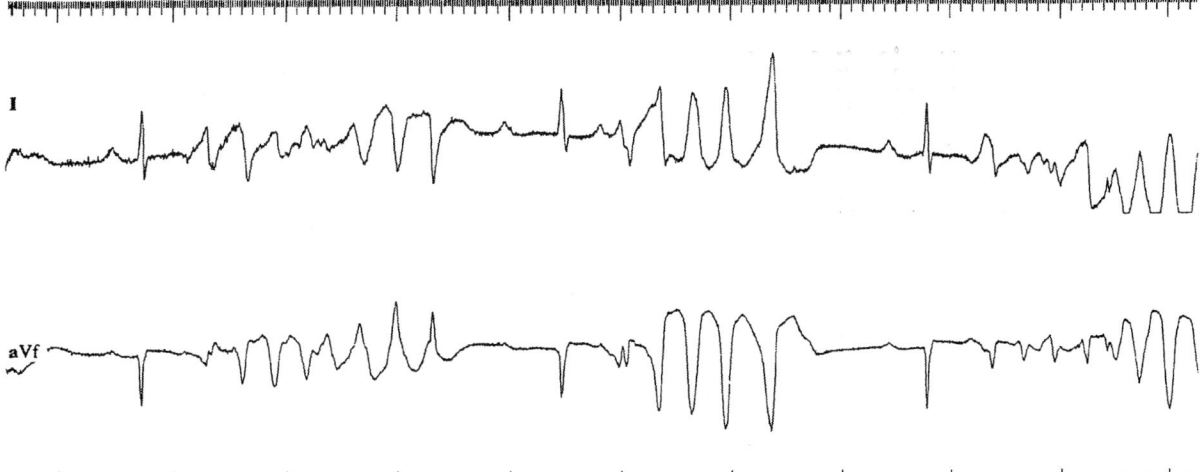

FIGURE 67.9 Typical characteristics of torsades de pointes. The initiation of the first ventricular ectopic beat of the tachycardia tends to occur after a pause. The QRS of this first beat initiates on the T wave, making it difficult to appreciate where the T wave ends. There is a beat-to-beat change in the QRS axis in a sinusoidal pattern. The rate of the tachycardia tends to be slower than the polymorphic ventricular tachycardia seen during cardiac ischemia, as shown in Figures 67.1 and 67.3.

mia, bradycardia associated with hypothyroidism, and heart block are also potential causes of torsades de pointes. Clinically, torsades de pointes appears to have a predilection for the female gender (148). The cause of this predilection is unclear but may be related to a protective effect of testosterone. ⌖ 178

Treatment of acquired torsades de pointes involves a two-pronged approach—acute therapy to prevent a cardiac arrest and removal of the offending factors generating the prolonged QT interval. Electrolyte levels, specifically those of potassium, magnesium, and calcium, should be checked and corrected to a normal range. Offending drugs should be stopped. Bradycardia due to sinus slowing or atrioventricular block should be corrected quickly with temporary pacing or isoproterenol infusion. Bringing the heart rate up to 100 beats/min is generally adequate to suppress the onset of polymorphic ventricular tachycardia. Intravenous magnesium has been found useful in acutely suppressing torsades de pointes, as it has been demonstrated to suppress early afterdepolarizations in experimental preparations (151). Two grams can be given over 10 to 15 minutes intravenously and repeated if needed. Raising the serum potassium level into the high normal range may also be helpful, as extracellular potassium is known to inhibit the potassium channel–blocking activity of antiarrhythmic drugs (152). These measures should be maintained until the etiologic factors can be removed. In the case of drugs, this may take several days or even longer if amiodarone is the offending agent.

Digitalis toxicity can also induce a ventricular tachycardia, although it is typically a monomorphic ventricular tachycardia. The mechanism by which digitalis causes ventricular tachycardia is through the generation of delayed afterdepolarizations. In experimental preparations, digitalis is one of the agents known to enhance DADs (153). The combination of digitalis toxicity and enhanced sympathetic tone may be a particularly potent stimulus for DADs. Rarely, digitalis toxicity can manifest as a bidirectional ventricular tachycardia. More commonly, it is monomorphic. Clinically, these often manifest as automatic fascicular tachycardias that respond to verapamil but not to adenosine. Because fascicular tachycardia can sometimes have a somewhat narrow QRS and because this tachycardia can respond to verapamil, it is sometimes misdiagnosed as supraventricular tachycardia (Fig. 67.10). Although the tachycardia will acutely respond to calcium channel blockers such as verapamil, the definitive therapy is to remove digoxin from the tissue through the infusion of digoxin antibody fragments.

In the case of drug-facilitated ventricular tachycardia, the underlying substrate such as a reentrant circuit within the scarred portion of the myocardium already exists and may even be able to sustain a reentrant tachycardia. However, the electrophysiologic characteristics of the circuit may make the tachycardia difficult to initiate and sustain.

In the presence of a drug that modifies these electrophysiologic characteristics, the tachycardia may become more easily initiated and sometimes can even become incessant. The most frequent cause of drug-facilitated ventricular tachycardia is antiarrhythmic medications that slow conduction of the action potential—that is, class I drugs with sodium channel–blocking activity. When such a drug causes frequent or incessant tachycardia, the best therapy is to discontinue the drug. However, clinical management of the patient may be difficult while the drug is being eliminated. Another cause of ventricular tachycardia in susceptible patients comes from the injection, ingestion, or inhalation of sympathomimetics or bronchodilators such as ephedrine (154) or terbutaline (155). Most likely, these patients have a sympathetic-mediated ventricular tachycardia as described above associated with structurally normal hearts. Under more intense sympathetic stimulation while receiving these drugs, the ventricular tachycardia may become sustained for the first time.

MISCELLANEOUS CAUSES OF VENTRICULAR TACHYCARDIA AND VENTRICULAR FIBRILLATION

Arrhythmogenic Right Ventricular Dysplasia

Arrhythmogenic right ventricular dysplasia, an entity first described in the 1970s and better characterized in the early 1980s (156), is a cardiomyopathy that begins in the right ventricle. It is characterized by right ventricle dilation, decreased contractile function, fatty infiltration and scarring of the myocardium, and ventricular tachycardia. The disease process is progressive and eventually affects the left ventricle as well (157,158). Ventricular tachycardia is frequently the first clinical presentation. The tachycardia is most likely reentrant in nature and arises from the right ventricle. Epicardial mappings have shown late potentials in the right ventricular free wall, and signal-averaged ECGs are generally positive for late potentials (159), both indicating that slow activation of parts of the myocardium occur as a result of the fatty infiltration and scarring of the myocardium. This slow conduction forms the substrate for reentry. ⌖ 179

Acute Myocarditis

Acute myocarditis has been associated with both polymorphic as well as monomorphic ventricular tachycardia. Conduction disturbances, ST-segment changes, and T-wave abnormalities can all be seen in acute myocarditis. Some authors have reported favorable responses to steroid therapy (175). Others have reported mixed results, in which ventricular arrhythmias persist even after resolution of acute

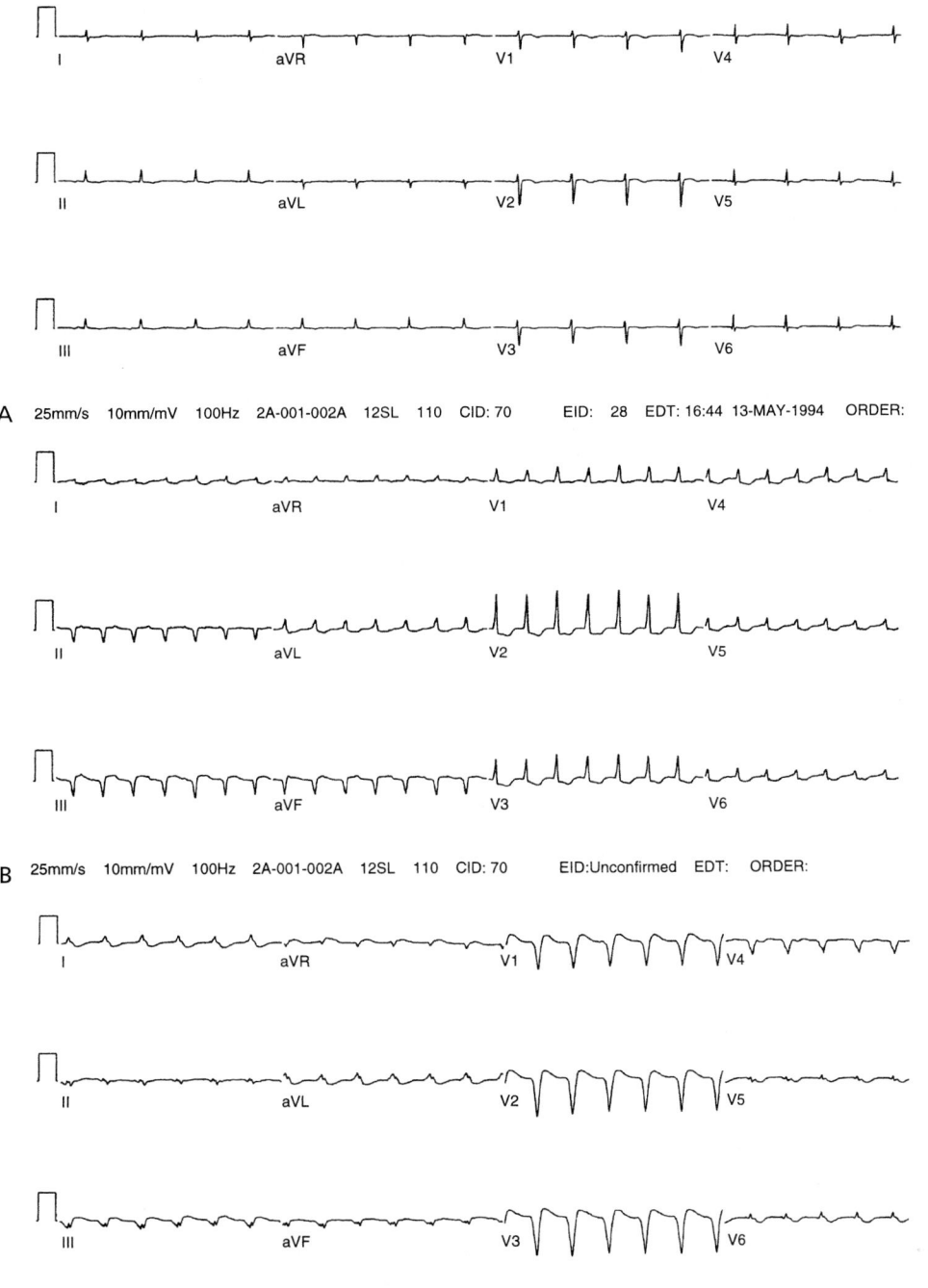

FIGURE 67.10 Ventricular tachycardia induced by digoxin toxicity. This figure illustrates ventricular tachycardia resulting from digoxin toxicity. This patient was in an intensive care unit as a result of acute exacerbation of chronic obstructive lung disease. Digoxin was being administered orally and intravenously because of episodes of atrial fibrillation. **A:** Sinus rhythm. **B,C:** Two different ventricular tachycardias that were initially mistaken for supraventricular tachycardias because of the relatively narrow QRS in **B** and the termination of these tachycardias with intravenous infusions of verapamil. The response of a tachycardia to verapamil cannot be used to indicate the involvement of the atrioventricular node in the tachycardia, as several forms of ventricular tachycardia can respond to this drug. At the time of occurrence of these ventricular tachycardias, the patient's digoxin level was higher than 5 ng per mL.

myocarditis after steroid therapy (176). A combination of antiarrhythmic drug therapy with an attempt at suppressing the inflammation with steroid therapy appears to be needed in these patients.

Muscular Dystrophies

Ventricular arrhythmia and conduction system disturbances have been associated with some of the muscular dystrophies. In particular, Duchenne's muscular dystrophy and myotonic dystrophy have a high incidence of ventricular arrhythmia and occasional sudden death (177,178). In both these entities, signal-averaged ECGs have shown late potentials consistent with delayed cardiac activation, probably originating from myocardium affected by the disease process (179,180). Whereas patients with Duchenne's dystrophy tend not to survive beyond the teenage years, patients with myotonic dystrophies generally survive well into adulthood. In myotonic dystrophy, conduction system disease is a prominent component of its myocardial involvement. This can lead to the development of bundle branch block as well as complete heart block. Besides ven-

THE FUTURE

Despite a number of unanswered and perhaps unanswerable questions, the direction in which therapy of ventricular tachycardia has moved in the past three decades indicates that it will have an exciting future. The development of preventive medicine aimed at eliminating the underlying disease processes that generate the substrate for ventricular tachycardia is already well under way for coronary artery disease. Similar preventive treatments may develop for the nonischemic cardiomyopathies. Treatment of congestive heart failure with better drugs, transplants, and mechanical hearts may considerably lessen if not eliminate the problem of arrhythmic sudden deaths in these patients. For those who are still at risk, the development of a very small ICD that is relatively inexpensive to insert will minimize the risk of sudden arrhythmic death at an acceptable cost. New mapping technologies that are now being explored combined with new ablation approaches perhaps using different energy sources will make catheter ablation of ventricular tachycardia a reliable and highly successful tool in selected patients. Lastly, the blossoming understanding of the molecular and genetic basis of certain syndromes such as long QT syndrome will allow the application of genetic cures or drug therapies targeted specifically at the molecular defects that promote ventricular arrhythmias and cause sudden deaths in these patients. Those advances would provide not only treatments but also an understanding of those physiologic properties that promote a stable rhythm as opposed to those that facilitate the development of lethal tachyarrhythmias.

tricular tachycardia originating from the affected myocardium, bundle branch reentry and fascicular reentry resulting from the conduction system disease have been reported in these patients (181).

Chagas' Disease

Chagas' disease, a chronic infection with the parasite *Trypanosoma cruzi*, causes a cardiomyopathy secondary to chronic multifocal myocarditis (182). Patients chronically infected with this agent can develop congestive heart failure, conduction system disease, and ventricular tachycardia. The signal-averaged ECG is frequently positive for late potentials in patients with ventricular tachycardia (183). There is a high incidence of sudden death among these patients, probably due to ventricular tachycardia, although complete heart block may contribute to some of these sudden deaths (184,185). Patients with more advanced congestive heart failure are at the highest risk for sudden death. Treatment includes drug eradication of the parasite, therapy for the congestive heart failure, antiarrhythmic drug therapy, pacemakers, and ICDs (186). Catheter ablation of ventricular tachycardia can be successful (187), although recurrence of tachycardia from other foci is frequent.

CONTROVERSIES AND PERSONAL PERSPECTIVES

Although the last 30 years have seen the development of a deeper understanding of the mechanisms of ventricular tachycardia and of several technologies for the treatment of ventricular tachycardia, the application of such technologies is frequently the subject of debate among physicians. With the publication of the Multicenter Unsustained Tachycardia Trial, extending the results of the Multicenter Automatic Defibrillator Implantation Trial, it is now generally accepted that high-risk patients with inducible sustained ventricular tachycardia form a group who are best treated with the ICD as opposed to currently available antiarrhythmic medications.

The use of the electrophysiology study, however, is a costly and invasive means of assessing increased risk for arrhythmic deaths in post–myocardial infarction patients. Whether less invasive means such as T-wave alternans, heart rate variability, and signal-averaged ECG may substitute as well are questions that remain to be answered. Furthermore, debate remains as to whether patients with decreased ventricular function, due to coronary disease or other processes, are all at a high enough risk for arrhythmic deaths to benefit from antiarrhythmic drug or ICD therapy. Several ongoing clinical trials may answer this question in the near future.

How to approach treatment to prevent sudden arrhythmic deaths among patients with nonischemic dilated cardiomyopathy is still undergoing debate. Besides ejection fraction, functional class, prior resuscitation from cardiac arrest, and perhaps the clinical occurrence of syncope, there are no other clinical factors that have a strong predictive value for arrhythmic deaths. Although the presence of nonsustained ventricular tachycardia appears to be associated with increased mortality (188,189), it is unclear whether this increase is due to sudden arrhythmic deaths (190) or if the predictive value of such a finding will be useful (191). Clinical studies have not demonstrated significant benefit of amiodarone in this population as a whole in preventing sudden death. Similarly, no studies exist on the use of ICD implantation. Yet, given the known increased risk of sudden death among these patients with poor ventricular function, should one consider ICD therapy because of its demonstrated ability to lower sudden death rates in other patients? Some would argue that such an approach is not justifiable until the extent to which life can be usefully prolonged by this approach has been demonstrated by clinical study. Clinical trials specifically aimed at this patient population may yield an answer to this question.

REFERENCES

1. Gillum RF. Sudden coronary deaths in the United States, 1980–1985. *Circulation* 1989;79:756–765.
2. *Report of the Working Group on Arteriosclerosis of the National Heart, Lung, and Blood Institute (Vol 2): patient oriented research-fundamental and applied, sudden cardiac death.* DHEW, NIH Publication 83-2035. Washington, D.C.: U.S. Government Printing Office, 1981:114–122.
3. Nickolic G, Bishop R, Singh J. Sudden death recorded during Holter monitoring. *Circulation* 1982;66:218–225.
4. Bayes de Luna, Coumel P, Leclerk J. Ambulatory sudden cardiac death: mechanisms of production of fatal arrhythmia on the basis of data from 157 cases. *Am Heart J* 1989;117:151–159.
5. Rosen MR. The relationship of delayed afterdepolarizations to arrhythmias in the intact heart. *Pacing Clin Electrophysiol* 1983;6:1151–1156.
6. Rosen MR, Danilo P Jr. Effects of tetrodotoxin, lidocaine, verapamil, and AHR-2666f on ouabain-induced delayed afterdepolarizations in canine Purkinje fibers. *Circ Res* 1980;46:117–124.
7. El-Sherif N, Bekheit SS, Henkin R. Quinidine-induced long QT interval and torsades de pointes: role of bradycardia-dependent early afterdepolarizations. *J Am Coll Cardiol* 1989;14:252.
8. Davidenko JM, Cohen L, Woodrow R, Antzelevitch C. Quinidine-induced action potential prolongation, early afterdepolarizations, and triggered activity in canine Purkinje fibers: effects of stimulation rate, potassium, and magnesium. *Circulation* 1989;79:674.
9. El-Sherif N, Zeiler RH, Craelius W, et al. QTU prolongation and polymorphic ventricular tachycardia due to bradycardia-dependent early afterdepolarizations. *Circ Res* 1988;63:286.
10. De Bakker JMT, van Capelle FJL, Janse MJ, et al. Reentry as a cause of ventricular tachycardia in patients with chronic ischemic heart disease: electrophysiologic and anatomic correlates. *Circulation* 1988;77:589.
11. Gardner PI, Ursell PVC, Fenoglio JJ Jr, et al. Electrophysiologic and anatomic basis for fractionated electrograms recorded from healed myocardial infarcts. *Circulation* 1985;72:596.
12. Spear JS, Michelson EL, Moore EN. Cellular electrophysiologic characteristics of chronically infarcted myocardium in dogs susceptible to sustained ventricular tachyarrhythmias. *J Am Coll Cardiol* 1983;14:1090.
13. Mukharji J, Rude RE, Pode WK, et al. Risk factors for sudden death after acute myocardial infarction: two-year follow up. *Am J Cardiol* 1984;54:31.
14. Bigger JT, Fleiss JL, Kleiger R, et al. The relationships among ventricular arrhythmias, left ventricular dysfunction, and mortality in the two years after myocardial infarction. *Circulation* 1984;69:250.
15. Gomes JA, Winters SL, Stewart D, et al. A new noninvasive index to predict sustained ventricular tachycardia and sudden death in the first year after myocardial infarction: based on signal-averaged electrocardiogram, radionuclide ejection fraction, and Holter monitoring. *J Am Coll Cardiol* 1987;10:348.
16. Middlekauff HR, Stevenson WG, Saxon LA. Prognosis after syncope: impact of left ventricular function. *Am Heart J* 1993;125:121–127.
17. Vismaara LA, Amsterdam BA, Mason DT. Relation of ventricular arrhythmias in the late-hospital phase of acute myocardial infarction to sudden death after hospital discharge. *Am J Med* 1975;59:6–12.
18. Ruberman W, Weinblatt M, Goldberg JD, et al. Ventricular premature complexes and sudden death after myocardial infarction. *Circulation* 1981;64:2297–2305.
19. Maggioni AP, Zuanetti G, Franzosi MG, et al. Prevalence and prognostic significance of ventricular arrhythmias after acute myocardial infarction in the fibrinolytic era. GISSI-2 results. *Circulation* 1993;87:312–322.
20. Rozanski JJ, Mortara D, Myerburg RJ, Castellanos A. Body surface detection of delayed depolarizations in patients with recurrent ventricular tachycardia and left ventricular aneurysm. *Circulation* 1981;63:1172–1178.
21. Simson MB. Use of signals in the terminal QRS complex to identify patients with ventricular tachycardia after myocardial infarction. *Circulation* 1981;64:235–242.
22. Breithardt G, Schwarzmaier M, Borggrefe M, et al. Prognostic significance of late ventricular potentials after acute myocardial infarction. *Eur Heart J* 1983;4:487–495.
23. Kuchar DL, Thorburn CW, Sammel NL. Prediction of serious arrhythmic events after myocardial infarction: signal-averaged electrocardiogram, Holter monitoring and radionuclide ventriculography. *J Am Coll Cardiol* 1987;9:531–538.
24. Denniss AR, Richards DA, Cody DV, et al. Prognostic significance of ventricular tachycardia and fibrillation induced at programmed stimulation and delayed potentials detected on the signal-averaged electrocardiograms of survivors of acute myocardial infarction. *Circulation* 1986;74:731–745.
25. Bigger JT, Fleiss JL, Rolnitzky LM, Steinman RC. The ability of several short-term measures of RR variability to predict mortality after myocardial infarction. *Circulation* 1993;88:927–934.
26. Makikallio TH, Huikuri HV, Hintze U, et al. Fractal analysis and time- and frequency-domain measures of heart rate variability as predictors of mortality in patients with heart failure. *Am J Cardiol* 2001;87:178–182.
27. Fauchier L, Babuty D, Cosnay P, Fauchier JP. Prognostic value of heart rate variability for sudden death and major arrhythmic events in patients with idiopathic dilated cardiomyopathy. *J Am Coll Cardiol* 1999;33:1203–1207.
28. Dekker JM, Crow RS, Folsom AR, et al. Low heart rate variability in a 2-minute rhythm strip predicts risk of cor-

onary heart disease and mortality from several causes: the ARIC Study. Atherosclerosis Risk In Communities. *Circulation* 2000;12:102:1239–1244.

29. Rosenbaum DS, Jackson LE, Smith JM, et al. Electrical alternans and vulnerability to ventricular arrhythmias. *N Engl J Med* 1994;330:235–241.

30. Pastore JM, Girouard SD, Laurita KR, et al. Mechanism linking T-wave alternans to the genesis of cardiac fibrillation. *Circulation* 199;99:1385–1394.

31. Pastore JM, Rosenbaum DS. Role of structural barriers in the mechanism of alternans-induced reentry. *Circ Res* 2000;87:1157–1163.

32. Ikeda T, Sakata T, Takami M, et al. Combined assessment of T-wave alternans and late potentials used to predict arrhythmic events after myocardial infarction. A prospective study. *J Am Coll Cardiol* 2000;35:722–730.

33. Gold MR, Bloomfield DM, Anderson KP, et al. A comparison of T-wave alternans, signal averaged electrocardiography and programmed ventricular stimulation for arrhythmia risk stratification. *J Am Coll Cardiol* 2000;36:2247–2253.

34. Uther JB, Richards DA, Denniss AR, Ross DL. The prognostic significance of programmed ventricular stimulation after myocardial infarction: a review. *Circulation* 1987;75:III161–168.

35. Brembilla-Perrot B, de la Chaise AT, Briancon S, et al. Programmed ventricular stimulation in survivors of acute myocardial infarction: long-term follow-up. *Int J Cardiol* 1995;49:55–65.

36. Bhandari AK, Widerhorn J, Sager PT, et al. Prognostic significance of programmed ventricular stimulation in patients surviving complicated acute myocardial infarction: a prospective study. *Am Heart J* 1992;124:87–96.

37. Kapoor W. Evaluation and outcome of patients with syncope. *Medicine* 1990;69:160–175.

38. Middlekauff HR, Stevenson WG, Saxon LA. Prognosis after syncope: impact of left ventricular function. *Am Heart J* 1993;125:121–127.

39. Olshansky B, Hahn EA, Hartz VL, et al. Clinical significance of syncope in the Electrophysiologic Study Versus Electrocardiographic Monitoring (ESVEM) Trial. The ESVEM Investigators. *Am Heart J* 1999;137:878–886.

40. Fonarow GC, Feliciano Z, Boyle NG, et al. Improved survival in patients with nonischemic advanced heart failure and syncope treated with an implantable cardioverter-defibrillator. *Am J Cardiol* 2000;85:981–985.

41. Link MS, Costeas XF, Griffith JL, et al. High incidence of appropriate implantable cardioverter-defibrillator therapy in patients with syncope of unknown etiology and inducible ventricular arrhythmias. *J Am Coll Cardiol* 1997;29:370–375.

42. Seidl K, Rameken M, Breunung S, et al. Diagnostic assessment of recurrent unexplained syncope with a new subcutaneously implantable loop recorder. Reveal-Investigators. *Europace* 2000;2:256–262.

43. Janse MJ, Kleber AG. Electrophysiological changes and ventricular arrhythmias in the early phase of regional myocardial ischemia. *Circ Res* 1981;49:1069–1081.

44. Corr PB, Gross RW, Sobel BE. Amphipathic metabolites and membrane dysfunction in ischemic myocardium. *Circ Res* 1984;55:135–154.

45. Zhang S, Skinner JL, Sims AL, et al. Three-dimensional mapping of spontaneous ventricular arrhythmias in a canine thrombotic coronary occlusion model. *J Cardiovasc Electrophysiol* 2000;11:762–772.

46. Simes RJ, Topol EJ, Holmes DR Jr, et al., for the GUSTO Investigators. Link between the angiographic substudy and mortality outcomes in a large randomized trial of myocardial reperfusion. Importance of early and complete infarct artery reperfusion. *Circulation* 1995;91:1923–1928.

47. Reiner JS, Lundergan CF, Rohrbeck SC, et al. The impact on left ventricular function of coronary reocclusion after successful thrombolysis for acute myocardial infarction. *J Am Coll Cardiol* 1994;23:13A.

48. White HD, Cross DB, Elliot JM, et al. Long term prognostic importance of patency of the infarct-related coronary artery after thrombolytic therapy for acute myocardial infarction. *Circulation* 1994;89:61–67.

49. Lamas GA, Flaker GC, Mitchell G, et al. Effect of infarct artery patency on prognosis after acute myocardial infarction. *Circulation* 1995;92:1101–1109.

50. Hohnloser SH, Franck P, Klingenheben T, et al. Open infarct artery, late potentials, and other prognostic factors in patients after acute myocardial infarction in the thrombolytic era. A prospective trial. *Circulation* 1994;90:1747–1756.

51. Held P. Effects of beta blockers on ventricular dysfunction after myocardial infarction: tolerability and survival effects. *Am J Cardiol* 1993;71:39C–44C.

52. Yosuf S, Peto R, Lewis J, Sleight P. Beta blockade during and after myocardial infarction: an overview of randomized trials. *Prog Cardiovasc Dis* 1985;27:335–363.

53. Cohn JN, Johnson G, Ziesche S, et al. A comparison of enalapril with hydralazine-isosorbide dinitrate in the treatment of chronic congestive heart failure. *N Engl J Med* 1991;325:303–310.

54. The Cardiac Arrhythmia Suppression Trial (CAST) Investigators. Preliminary report: effect of encainide and flecainide on mortality in a randomized trial of arrhythmia suppression after myocardial infarction. *N Engl J Med* 1989;321:406–412.

55. IMPACT Research Group. International Mexiletine and Placebo Antiarrhythmic Coronary Trial, I: report on arrhythmia and other findings. *J Am Coll Cardiol* 1984;4:1148–1163.

56. The Cardiac Arrhythmia Suppression Trial II Investigators. Effect of the antiarrhythmic agent moricizine on survival after myocardial infarction. *N Engl J Med* 1992;327:227–233.

57. Teo KK, Yusuf S, Furberg CD. Effects of prophylactic antiarrhythmic drug therapy in acute myocardial infarction: an overview of results from randomized controlled trials. *JAMA* 1993;270:1589–1595.

58. Waldo AL, Camm AJ, deRuyter H, et al. Effect of D-sotalol on mortality in patients with left ventricular dysfunction after recent and remote myocardial infarction. The SWORD Investigators. Survival With Oral D-Sotalol. *Lancet* 1996;348:7–12.

59. Camm AJ, Karam R, Pratt CM. The Azimilide Post-Infarct Survival Evaluation (ALIVE) Trial. *Am J Cardiol* 1998;81:35D–39D.

60. Greene HL. The CASCADE Study: randomized antiarrhythmic drug therapy in survivors of cardiac arrest in Seattle. CASCADE Investigators. *Am J Cardiol* 1993;72:70F–74F.

61. Singh SN, Fletcher RD, Fisher SG, et al. Amiodarone in patients with congestive heart failure and asymptomatic ventricular arrhythmia. Survival Trial of Antiarrhythmic Therapy in Congestive Heart Failure. *N Engl J Med* 1995;333:77–82.

62. Julian DG, Camm AJ, Frangin G, et al. Randomised trial of effect of amiodarone on mortality in patients with left-ventricular dysfunction after recent myocardial infarction: EMIAT. European Myocardial Infarct Amiodarone Trial Investigators. *Lancet* 1997;349:667–674.

63. Janse MJ, Malik M, Camm AJ, et al. Identification of post acute myocardial infarction patients with potential benefit from prophylactic treatment with amiodarone. A substudy of EMIAT (the European Myocardial Infarct Amiodarone Trial). *Eur Heart J* 1998;19:85–95.

64. Malik M, Camm AJ, Janse MJ, et al. Depressed heart rate variability identifies postinfarction patients who might benefit from prophylactic treatment with amiodarone: a substudy of EMIAT (The European Myocardial Infarct Amiodarone Trial). *J Am Coll Cardiol* 2000;35:1263–1275.

65. Cairns JA, Connolly SJ, Roberts R, Gent M. Randomised trial of outcome after myocardial infarction in patients with frequent or repetitive ventricular premature depolarisations: CAMIAT. Canadian Amiodarone Myocardial Infarction Arrhythmia Trial Investigators. *Lancet* 1997;349:675–682.

66. Boutitie F, Boissel JP, Connolly SJ, et al. Amiodarone interaction with beta-blockers: analysis of the merged EMIAT (European Myocardial Infarct Amiodarone Trial) and CAMIAT (Canadian Amiodarone Myocardial Infarction Trial) databases. The EMIAT and CAMIAT Investigators. *Circulation* 1999;99:2268–2275.

67. Moss AJ, Hall WJ, Cannom DS, et al., for the Multicenter Automatic Defibrillator Implantation Trial Investigators. Improved survival with an implanted defibrillator in patients with coronary disease at high risk for ventricular arrhythmia. *N Engl J Med* 1996;335:1933–1939.

68. Buxton AE, Lee KL, Fisher JD, et al. A randomized study of the prevention of sudden death in patients with coronary artery disease. Multicenter Unsustained Tachycardia Trial Investigators. *N Engl J Med* 1999;341:1882–1890.

69. Myerburg RJ, Kessler KM, Castellanos A. Sudden cardia death: structure, function and time-dependence of risk. *Circulation* 1992;85(suppl I):1–10.

70. The Antiarrhythmics versus Implantable Defibrillators (AVID) Investigators. A comparison of antiarrhythmic-drug therapy with implantable defibrillators in patients resuscitated from near-fatal ventricular arrhythmias. *N Engl J Med* 1997;337:1576–1583.

71. Connolly SJ, Gent M, Roberts RS, et al. Canadian implantable defibrillator study (CIDS): a randomized trial of the implantable cardioverter defibrillator against amiodarone. *Circulation* 2000;101:1297–1302.

72. Sheldon R, Connolly S, Krahn A, et al. Identification of patients most likely to benefit from implantable cardioverter-defibrillator therapy: the Canadian Implantable Defibrillator Study. *Circulation* 2000;101:1660–1664.

73. Connolly SJ, Hallstrom AP, Cappato R, et al. Meta-analysis of the implantable cardioverter defibrillator secondary prevention trials. AVID, CASH and CIDS studies. Antiarrhythmics vs Implantable Defibrillator study. Cardiac Arrest Study Hamburg. Canadian Implantable Defibrillator Study. *Eur Heart J* 2000;21:2071–2078.

74. Mason JW. A comparison of electrophysiologic testing with Holter monitoring to predict antiarrhythmic-drug efficacy for ventricular tachyarrhythmias. Electrophysiologic Study versus Electrocardiographic Monitoring Investigators. *N Engl J Med* 1993;329:445–451.

75. Prystowsky EN. Antiarrhythmic drug therapy as an adjunct or alternative to an implantable cardioverter defibrillator. *Pacing Clin Electrophysiol* 1992;15:678–680.

76. Dougherty AH. Interactions between antiarrhythmic drugs and implantable cardioverter-defibrillators. *Curr Opin Cardiol* 1996;11:2–8.

77. Kim YH, Sosa-Suarez G, Trouton TG, et al. Treatment of ventricular tachycardia by transcatheter radiofrequency ablation in patients with ischemic heart disease. *Circulation* 1994;89:1094–1102.

78. Stevenson WG, Khan H, Sager P, et al. Identification of reentry circuit sites during catheter mapping and radiofrequency ablation of ventricular tachycardia late after myocardial infarction. *Circulation* 1993;88:1647–1670.

79. Maron BJ, Epstein SE, Roberts WC. Causes of sudden death in competitive athletes. *J Am Coll Cardiol* 1986;7:204–214.

80. Akhtar M, Damato AN, Batsford WP, et al. Demonstration of reentry within the His-Purkinje system in man. *Circulation* 1974;50:1150.

81. Akhtar M, Gilbert CJ, Wolf FG, Schmidt DH. Reentry within the His-Purkinje system: elucidation of reentrant circuit using the right bundle and His bundle recordings. *Circulation* 1978;58:295.

82. Tchou P, Jazayeri M, Denker S, et al. Transcatheter electrical ablation of right bundle branch: a method of treating macroreentrant ventricular tachycardia attributed to bundle branch reentry. *Circulation* 1988;78:246.

83. Caceres J, Jazayeri M, McKinnie J, et al. Sustained bundle branch reentry as a mechanism of clinical tachycardia. *Circulation* 1989;79:256.

84. Cohen TJ, Chien WW, Lurie KG, et al. Radiofrequency catheter ablation for treatment of bundle branch reentrant ventricular tachycardia: results and long-term follow-up. *J Am Coll Cardiol* 1991;18:1767.

85. Chien WW, Scheinman MM, Cohen TJ, Lesh MD. Importance of recording the right bundle branch deflection in the diagnosis of His-Purkinje reentrant tachycardia. *Pacing Clin Electrophysiol* 1992;15:1015.

86. Blanck Z, Jazayeri M, Dhala A, et al. Bundle branch reentry: a mechanism of ventricular tachycardia in the absence of myocardial or valvular dysfunction. *J Am Coll Cardiol* 1993;22:1718.

87. Merino JL, Carmona JR, Fernandez-Lozano I, et al. Mechanisms of sustained ventricular tachycardia in myotonic dystrophy: implications for catheter ablation. *Circulation* 1998;98:541–546.

88. Blanck Z, Dhala A, Deshpande S, et al. Bundle branch reentrant ventricular tachycardia: cumulative experience in 48 patients. *J Cardiovasc Electrophysiol* 1993;4:253.

89. Mehdirad AA, Keim S, Rist K, et al. Asymmetry of retrograde conduction and reentry within the His-Purkinje system: a comparative analysis of left and right ventricular stimulation. *J Am Coll Cardiol* 1994;24:177.

90. Berger RD, Orias D, Kasper EK, Calkins H. Catheter ablation of coexistent bundle branch and interfascicular reentrant ventricular tachycardias. *J Cardiovasc Electrophysiol* 1996;7:341–347.

91. Tchou P, Mehdirad AA. Bundle branch reentry ventricular tachycardia. *Pacing Clin Electrophysiol* 1995;18:1427–1437.

92. Mehdirad AA, Keim S, Rist K, Tchou P. Long term clinical outcome of right bundle branch radiofrequency catheter ablation for treatment of bundle branch reentrant ventricular tachycardia. *Pacing Clin Electrophysiol* 199518:2135–2143.

93. Blanck Z, Deshpande S, Jazayeri MR, Akhtar M. Catheter ablation of the left bundle branch for the treatment of sustained bundle branch reentrant ventricular tachycardia. *J Cardiovasc Electrophysiol* 1995;6:40–43.

94. Sung RJ, Shen EN, Morady F, et al. Electrophysiologic mechanism of exercise-induced sustained ventricular tachycardia. *Am J Cardiol* 1983;51:525–530.

95. Sung RJ, Shapiro WA, Shen EN, et al. Effects of verapamil on ventricular tachycardias possibly caused by reentry, automaticity, and triggered activity. *J Clin Invest* 1983;72:350–360.

96. Sung RJ, Keung EC, Nguyen NX, Huycke EC. Effects of beta-adrenergic blockade on verapamil-responsive and verapamil-irresponsive sustained ventricular tachycardias. *J Clin Invest* 1988;81:688–699.

97. Kass RS, Lederer WJ, Tsien RW, Weingart R. Role of calcium ions in transient inward currents and aftercontractions induced by strophanthidin in cardiac Purkinje fibres. *J Physiol* 1978;281:187–208.

98. Kimmura S, Camerson JS, Kozlovskis PL, et al. Delayed afterdepolarizations and triggered activity induced in feline Purkinje fibers by alpha-adrenergic stimulation in the presence of elevated calcium. *Circulation* 1984;70:1074–1082.

99. Prior SG, Mantica M, Schwartz PJ. Delayed afterdepolarizations elicited in vivo by stellate ganglion stimulation. *Circulation* 1988;78:178–185.

100. Lerman BB, Stein K, Engelstein ED, et al. Mechanism of repetitive monomorphic ventricular tachycardia. *Circulation* 1995;92:421–429.

101. Hachiya H, Aonuma K, Yamauchi Y, et al. Electrocardiographic characteristics of left ventricular outflow tract tachycardia. *Pacing Clin Electrophysiol* 2000;23(11 Pt 2):1930–1934.

102. Kanagaratnam L, Tomassoni G, Schweikert R, et al. Ventricular tachycardias arising from the aortic sinus of Valsalva: an under-recognized variant of left outflow tract ventricular tachycardia. *J Am Coll Cardiol* 2001;37:1408–1414.

103. Lerman BB, Belardinelli L, West GA, et al. Adenosine-sensitive ventricular tachycardia: evidence suggesting cyclic AMP-mediated triggered activity. *Circulation* 1986;74:270–280.

104. Lerman B. Response of nonreentrant catecholamine-mediated ventricular tachycardia to endogenous adenosine and acetylcholine. Evidence of myocardial receptor-mediated effects. *Circulation* 1993;87:282–390.

105. Calkins H, Kalbfleisch SJ, el-Atassi R, et al. Relation between efficacy of radiofrequency catheter ablation and site of origin of idiopathic ventricular tachycardia. *Am J Cardiol* 1993;71:827–833.

106. Coggins DL, Lee RJ, Sweeney J, et al. Radiofrequency catheter ablation as a cure for idiopathic tachycardia of both left and right ventricular origin. *J Am Coll Cardiol* 1994;23:1333–1341.

107. Gill JS, Ward DE, Camm AJ. Comparison of verapamil and diltiazem in the suppression of idiopathic ventricular tachycardia. *Pacing Clin Electrophysiol* 1992;15:2122–2126.

108. Belhassen B, Rotmensch HH, Laniado S. Response of recurrent sustained ventricular tachycardia to verapamil. *Br Heart J* 1981;46:679–682.

109. Klein GJ, Millman PJ, Yee R. Recurrent ventricular tachycardia responsive to verapamil. *Pacing Clin Electrophysiol* 1984;7:938–948.

110. Ohe T, Shimomura K, Aihara N, et al. Idiopathic sustained left ventricular tachycardia: clinical and electrophysiologic characteristics. *Circulation* 1988;77:560–568.

111. Nakagawa H, Beckman KJ McClelland JH, et al. Radiofrequency catheter ablation of idiopathic left ventricular tachycardia guided by a Purkinje potential. *Circulation* 1993;88:2607–2617.

112. Okumura K, Yamabe H, Tsuchiya T, et al. Characteristics of slow conduction zone demonstrated during entrainment of idiopathic ventricular tachycardia of left ventricular origin. *Am J Cardiol* 1996;77:379–383.

113. Tsuchiya T, Okumura K, Honda T, et al. Significance of late diastolic potential preceding Purkinje potential in verapamil-sensitive idiopathic left ventricular tachycardia. *Circulation* 1999;99:2408–2413.

114. Jervell A, Lange-Nielsen F. Congenital deaf mutism, functional heart disease with prolongation of the QT interval, and sudden death. *Am Heart J* 1957;54:59–68.

115. Romano C, Gemme G, Pongiglione R. Aritmie cardiache rare dell'eta pediatrica. *Clin Pediatr* 1963;45:656–683.

116. Ward OC. A new familial cardiac syndrome in children. *J Irish Med Assoc* 1964;54:103–106.

117. Wang Q, Curran ME, Splawski I, et al. Positional cloning of a novel potassium channel gene: KVLQT1 mutations cause cardiac arrhythmias. *Nat Genet* 1996;12:17–23.

118. Schwartz PJ, Priori SG, Locati EH, et al. Long QT syndrome patients with mutations of the SCNA5 and HERG genes have differential responses to Na+ channel blockade and to increases in heart rate. Implications for gene-specific therapy. *Circulation* 1995;92:3381–3386.

119. Keating MT, Atkinson D, Dunn C, et al. Linkage of a cardiac arrhythmia, the long QT syndrome, and the Harvey ras-1 gene. *Science* 1991;252:704–706.

120. Hoorntje T, Alders M, van Tintelen P, et al. A homozygous premature truncation of the HERG protein: the human HERG knockout. *Circulation* 1999;100:1264–1267.

121. Jiang C, Atkinson D, Towbin JA, et al. Two long QT syndrome loci map to chromosomes 3 and 7 with evidence for further heterogeneity. *Nat Genet* 1994;8:141–147.

122. Wang Q, Shen J, Splawski I, et al. SCN5A mutations associated with an inherited cardiac arrhythmia, long QT syndrome. *Cell* 1995;80:805–811.

123. Schott JJ, Charpentier F, Peltier S, et al. Mapping of a gene for long QT syndrome to chromosome 4q25–27. *Am J Hum Genet* 1995;57:1114–1122.

124. Abbott GW, Sesti F, Splawski I, et al. MiRP1 forms IKr potassium channels with HERG, and is associated with cardiac arrhythmia. *Cell* 1999;97:175–187.

125. Moss AJ, Zareba W, Benhorin J, et al. ECG T-wave patterns in genetically distinct forms of the hereditary long QT syndrome. *Circulation* 1995;92:2929–2934.

126. Compton SJ, Lux RL, Ramsey MR, et al. Genetically defined therapy of inherited long QT syndrome. Correction of abnormal repolarization by potassium. *Circulation* 1996;94:1018–1022.

127. Moss AJ, Schwartz PJ, Crampton RS, et al. The long QT syndrome: prospective longitudinal study of 328 families. *Circulation* 1991;84:1136–1144.

128. Eldar M, Griffin JC, Abborr JA, et al. Permanent cardiac pacing in patients with the long QT syndrome. *J Am Coll Cardiol* 1987;10:600–607.

129. Schwartz PJ, Locati EH, Moss AJ, et al. Left cardiac sympathetic denervation in the therapy of congenital long QT syndrome: a worldwide report. *Circulation* 1991;84:503–511.

130. Brugada P, Brugada J. Right bundle branch block, persistent ST segment elevation and sudden cardiac death: a distinct clinical and electrocardiographic syndrome. A multicenter report. *J Am Coll Cardiol* 1992;20:1391–1396.

131. Chen Q, Kirsch GE, Zhang D, et al. Genetic basis and molecular mechanism for idiopathic ventricular fibrillation. *Nature* 1998;392:293–296.

132. Dumaine R, Towbin JA, Brugada P, et al. Ionic mechanisms responsible for the electrocardiographic phenotype of the Brugada syndrome are temperature dependent. *Circ Res* 1999;85:803–809.

133. Yan GX, Antzelevitch C. Cellular basis for the Brugada syndrome and other mechanisms of arrhythmogenesis associated with ST-segment elevation. *Circulation* 1999;100:1660–1666.

134. Bezzina C, Veldkamp MW, van Den Berg MP, et al. A single Na(+) channel mutation causing both long-QT and Brugada syndromes. *Circ Res* 1999;85:1206–1213.

135. Brugada R, Brugada J, Antzelevitch C, et al. Sodium channel blockers identify risk for sudden death in patients with ST-segment elevation and right bundle branch block but structurally normal hearts. *Circulation* 2000;101:510–515.

136. Hermida JS, Lemoine JL, Aoun FB, et al. Prevalence of the Brugada syndrome in an apparently healthy population. *Am J Cardiol* 2000;86:91–94.

137. Leenhardt A, Lucet V, Denjoy I, et al. Catecholaminergic polymorphic ventricular tachycardia in children. *Circulation* 1995;91:1512–1519.

138. Leenhardt A, Glaser E, Burguera M, et al. Short-coupled variant of torsades de pointes. A new electrocardiographic entity in the spectrum of idiopathic ventricular tachyarrhythmias. *Circulation* 1994;89:206–215.

139. Dessertenne F. La tachycardie ventriculaire a deux foyes oposes variables. *Arch Mal Coeur* 1966;59:263.

140. Keren A, Tzivoni D, Gavish D, et al. Etiology, warning signs and therapy of torsades de pointes. A study of 10 patients. *Circulation* 1981;64:1167–1174.

141. Singh BN, Gaarder TD, Kanegae T, et al. Liquid protein diets and torsades de pointes. *JAMA* 1978;240:115–119.

142. Ramee SR, White CJ, Svinarich JT, et al. Torsades de pointes and magnesium deficiency. *Am Heart J* 1985;109:164–167.

143. Smith WM, Gallagher JJ. "Les torsades de pointes": an unusual ventricular arrhythmia. *Ann Intern Med* 1980;93:578.

144. Locati EH, Maison-Blanche P, Dejode P, et al. Spontaneous sequences of onset of torsades de pointes in patients with acquired prolonged repolarization: quantitative analysis of Holter recordings. *J Am Coll Cardiol* 1995;25:1564–1575.

145. Witchel HJ, Hancox JC. Familial and acquired long QT syndrome and the cardiac rapid delayed rectifier potassium current. *Clin Exp Pharmacol Physiol* 2000;27:753–766.

146. Hohnloser SH, Klingenheben T, Singh BN. Amiodarone-associated proarrhythmic effects. A review with special reference to torsades de pointes tachycardia. *Ann Intern Med* 1994;121:529–535.

147. Sclarovsky S, Lewin RF, Kracoff O, et al. Amiodarone-induced polymorphous ventricular tachycardia. *Am Heart J* 1983;105:6–12.

148. Makkar RR, Fromm BS, Steinman RT, et al. Female gender as a risk factor for torsades de pointes associated with cardiovascular drugs. *JAMA* 1993;270:1590–1597.

149. Antzelevitch C, Sicouri S. Clinical relevance of cardiac arrhythmias generated by afterdepolarizations. Role of M cells in the generation of U waves, triggered activity and torsades de pointes. *J Am Coll Cardiol* 1994;23:259–277.

150. Hii JT, Wyse DG, Gillis AM, et al. Precordial QT interval dispersion as a marker of torsades de pointes. Disparate effects of class Ia antiarrhythmic drugs and amiodarone. *Circulation* 1992;86:1376–1382.

151. Kaseda S, Gilmour RF, Zipes DP. Depressant effect of magnesium on early afterdepolarizations and triggered activity induced by cesium, quinidine and 4-aminopyridine in canine cardiac Purkinje fibers. *Am Heart J* 1989;118:458.

152. Yang T, Roden DM. Extracellular potassium modulation of drug block of IKr. Implications for torsades de pointes and reverse use-dependence. *Circulation* 1996;93:407–411.

153. Ferrier GR, Saunders JH, Mendez C. A cellular mechanism for the generation of ventricular arrhythmias by acetylstrophanthidin. *Circ Res* 1973;32:600–609.

154. Murakawa T, Koh H, Tsubo T, et al. Two cases of circulatory failure after local infiltration of epinephrine during tonsillectomy. *Masui* 1998;47:955–962.

155. Banner AS, Sunderrajan EV, Agarwal MK, Addington WW. Arrhythmogenic effects of orally administered bronchodilators. *Arch Intern Med* 1979;139:434–437.

156. Marcus FI, Fontaine G, Guiraudon G, et al. Right ventricular dysplasia: a report of 24 cases. *Circulation* 1982;65:384–399.

157. Pinamonti B, Pagnan L, Bussani R, et al. Right ventricular dysplasia with biventricular involvement. *Circulation* 1998;98:1943–1945.

158. Nemec J, Edwards BS, Osborn MJ, Edwards WD. Arrhythmogenic right ventricular dysplasia masquerading as dilated cardiomyopathy. *Am J Cardiol* 1999;84:237–239.

159. Kinoshita O, Fontaine G, Rosas F, et al. Time- and frequency-domain analyses of the signal-averaged ECG in

patients with arrhythmogenic right ventricular dysplasia. *Circulation* 1995;91:715–721.

160. Solenthaler M, Ritter M, Candinas R, et al. Arrhythmogenic right ventricular dysplasia in identical twins. *Am J Cardiol* 1994;74:303–304.

161. Rampazzo A, Nava A, Erne P, et al. A new locus for arrhythmogenic right ventricular cardiomyopathy (ARVD2) maps to chromosome 1q42–q43. *Hum Mol Genet* 1995;4:2151–2154.

162. Rampazzo A, Nava A, Danieli GA, et al. The gene for arrhythmogenic right ventricular cardiomyopathy maps to chromosome 14q23–q24. *Hum Mol Genet* 1994;3:959–962.

163. Ahmad F, Li D, Karibe A, et al. Localization of a gene responsible for arrhythmogenic right ventricular dysplasia to chromosome 3p23. *Circulation* 1998;98:2791–2795.

164. McKoy G, Protonotarios N, Crosby A, et al. Identification of a deletion in plakoglobin in arrhythmogenic right ventricular cardiomyopathy with palmoplantar keratoderma and woolly hair (Naxos disease). *Lancet* 2000;355:2119–2124.

165. Daliento L, Turrini P, Nava A, et al. Arrhythmogenic right ventricular cardiomyopathy in young versus adult patients: similarities and differences. *J Am Coll Cardiol* 1995;25:655–664.

166. Peters S, Reil GH. Risk factors of cardiac arrest in arrhythmogenic right ventricular dysplasia. *Eur Heart J* 1995;16:77–80.

167. Wichter T, Borggrefe M, Haverkamp W, et al. Efficacy of antiarrhythmic drugs in patients with arrhythmogenic right ventricular disease. Results in patients with inducible and noninducible ventricular tachycardia. *Circulation* 1992;86:29–37.

168. Link MS, Wang PJ, Haugh CJ, et al. Arrhythmogenic right ventricular dysplasia: clinical results with implantable cardioverter defibrillators. *J Interv Card Electrophysiol* 1997;1:41–48.

169. Tavernier R, Gevaert S, De Sutter J, et al. Long term results of cardioverter-defibrillator implantation in patients with right ventricular dysplasia and malignant ventricular tachyarrhythmias. *Heart* 2001;85:53–56.

170. Shammas RL, Movahed A. Sarcoidosis of the heart. *Clin Cardiol* 1993;16:462–472.

171. Dupuis JM, Victor J, Furber A, et al. Value of magnetic resonance imaging in cardiac sarcoidosis. Apropos of a case. *Arch Mal Coeur* 1994;87:105–110.

172. Okamoto M, Hashimoto M, Sueda T, et al. Polymorphic ventricular tachycardia with cardiac sarcoidosis: treatment with low-dose metoprolol and cibenzoline. *Intern Med* 1994;33:296–299.

173. Winters SL, Cohen M, Greenberg S, et al. Sustained ventricular tachycardia associated with sarcoidosis: assessment of the underlying cardiac anatomy and the prospective utility of programmed ventricular stimulation, drug therapy and an implantable antitachycardia device. *J Am Coll Cardiol* 1991;18:937–943.

174. Paz HL, McCormick DJ, Kutalek SP, Patchefsky A. The automated implantable cardiac defibrillator. Prophylaxis in cardiac sarcoidosis. *Chest* 1994;106:1603–1607.

175. Ino T, Okubo M, Akimoto K, et al. Corticosteroid therapy for ventricular tachycardia in children with silent lymphocytic myocarditis. *J Pediatr* 1995;126:304–308.

176. Friedman RA, Kearney DL, Moak JP, et al. Persistence of ventricular arrhythmia after resolution of occult myocarditis in children and young adults. *J Am Coll Cardiol* 1994;24:780–783.

177. Yanagisawa A, Miyagawa M, Yotsukura M, et al. The prevalence and prognostic significance of arrhythmias in Duchenne type muscular dystrophy. *Am Heart J* 1992;124:1244–1250.

178. Hiromasa S, Ikeda T, Kubota K, et al. Ventricular tachycardia and sudden death in myotonic dystrophy. *Am Heart J* 1988;115:914–915.

179. Yotsukura M, Ishizuka T, Shimada T, Ishikawa K. Late potentials in progressive muscular dystrophy of the Duchenne type. *Am Heart J* 1991;121:1137–1142.

180. Milner MR, Hawley RJ, Jachim M, et al. Ventricular late potentials in myotonic dystrophy. *Ann Intern Med* 1991;115:607–613.

181. Berger RD, Orias D, Kasper EK, Calkins H. Catheter ablation of coexistent bundle branch and interfascicular reentrant ventricular tachycardias. *J Cardiovasc Electrophysiol* 1996;7:341–347.

182. Bellotti G, Bocchi EA, de Moraes AV, et al. In vivo detection of *Trypanosoma cruzi* antigens in hearts of patients with chronic Chagas' heart disease. *Am Heart J* 1996;131:301–307.

183. de Moraes AP, Moffa PJ, Sosa EA, et al. Signal-averaged electrocardiogram in chronic Chagas' heart disease. *Revista Paulista de Medicina* 1995;113:851–857.

184. Bestetti RB, Freitas OC, Muccillo G, Oliveira JS. Clinical and morphological characteristics associated with sudden cardiac death in patients with Chagas' disease. *Eur Heart J* 1993;14:1610–1614.

185. Elizari MV, Chiale PA. Cardiac arrhythmias in Chagas' heart disease. *J Cardiovasc Electrophysiol* 1993;4:596–608.

186. Rabinovich R, Muratore C, Iglesias R, et al. Time to first shock in implantable cardioverter defibrillator (ICD) patients with Chagas cardiomyopathy. *Pacing Clin Electrophysiol* 1999;22(1 Pt 2):202–205.

187. Tavora MZ, Mehta N, Silva RM, et al. Characteristics and identification of sites of chagasic ventricular tachycardia by endocardial mapping. *Arq Bras Cardiol* 1999;72:451–474.

188. Gradman A, Deedwania P, Cody R, et al., for the Captopril-Digoxin Study Group. Prediction of total morbidity and sudden death in mild to moderate heart failure. *J Am Coll Cardiol* 1989;14:564–570.

189. Hofman T, Meinertz T, Kasper W, et al. Mode of death in idiopathic dilated cardiomyopathy: a multivariate analysis of prognostic determinants. *Am Heart J* 1988;116:1455–1463.

190. Massie B, Francis G, Tandon P, et al., on behalf of the PROMISE Investigators. Asymptomatic ventricular arrhythmias do not identify patients with severe heart failure at risk for sudden death: results of the PROMISE trial. *J Am Coll Cardiol* 1993;21:459A.

191. Doval HC, Nul DR, Grancelli HO, et al., for the GESICA-GEMA Investigators. Nonsustained ventricular tachycardia in severe heart failure: independent marker of increased mortality due to sudden death. *Circulation* 1996;94:3198–3203.

69

CARDIOPULMONARY RESUSCITATION

JOSEPH P. ORNATO
MARY ANN PEBERDY

▼⊽ ADDITIONAL ELECTRONIC TOPICS

OVERVIEW

Closed-chest cardiopulmonary resuscitation (CPR), first described in 1960, circulates blood throughout the body by two different mechanisms: direct cardiac compression (the cardiac pump) and changes in intrathoracic pressure (the thoracic pump).

The most common victim of sudden, unexpected cardiac arrest is a male who is between 50 and 75 years of age and who has underlying coronary artery disease. The most common initial rhythm is pulseless ventricular tachycardia or ventricular fibrillation.

The most effective approach to resuscitation is to establish a strong chain of survival with early access, early CPR, early defibrillation, and early advanced cardiac life support. Public access to defibrillation is a promising new strategy for strengthening the early defibrillation link in the chain.

A variety of monitoring techniques can, and should, be used during clinical resuscitation.

There is little evidence that high-dose epinephrine is any better than standard 1-mg doses of epinephrine. Vasopressin is now considered to be an acceptable alternative for the first dose only in treating pulseless ventricular tachycardia or ventricular fibrillation in the adult. Sodium bicarbonate is of very limited value in most cardiac arrest cases, unless hyperkalemia is present or the patient has taken an overdose of a tricyclic antidepressant or barbiturates. Intravenous amiodarone is now the preferred antiarrhythmic agent for treating pulseless ventricular tachycardia or ven-

J. P. Ornato: Department of Emergency Medicine, Virginia Commonwealth University School of Medicine, Richmond, Virginia

M. A. Peberdy: Department of Internal Medicine, Virginia Commonwealth University School of Medicine, Richmond, Virginia

tricular fibrillation. Several promising new CPR techniques are currently undergoing clinical testing.

GLOSSARY

Automated external defibrillator (AED): A defibrillator that automatically determines the cardiac rhythm and advises rescuers of the need to defibrillate using voice prompts. Fully automated devices charge and deliver the defibrillation energy with no input from the user. Semiautomated devices prompt the user to defibrillate when ventricular fibrillation is detected by the device.

Chain of survival: A coordinated system for treating victims of cardiac arrest that provides early access to emergency medical services, early cardiopulmonary resuscitation (CPR), early defibrillation, and early advanced cardiac life support (ACLS).

High-dose epinephrine: Doses of epinephrine of greater than 1.0 mg in adults (typically 3 to 15 mg).

Public access defibrillation: The use of AEDs by laypersons.

Pulseless electrical activity (PEA): During cardiac arrest, an organized cardiac rhythm that does not generate a pulse. Previously known as electromechanical dissociation (EMD).

HISTORICAL PERSPECTIVE

Numerous and often barbaric methods to restore life to the newly deceased have been attempted for centuries (1). It was not until the last 50 years that the era of modern-day CPR was born. The field of resuscitation that exists as we enter the twenty-first century is an integrated science combining chest compression, ventilation, defibrillation, and pharmacotherapeutics with widespread use in both the prehospital and in-hospital arenas. Although it is difficult for us today to imagine these elements independently, that is precisely how they began.

Modern-Day Cardiopulmonary Resuscitation

The American Heart Association officially endorsed CPR in 1963 and developed a CPR committee. [▼ 193] In 1966 the National Research Council of the National Academy of Sciences brought together representatives from more than 30 organizations, such as the American Red Cross, and established official recommendations regarding standardized training and performance of CPR (12). Since then, the American Heart Association has hosted special conferences in 1973, 1979, 1985, 1992, and 2000 to establish consensus recommendations for resuscitation. Each of these conferences was followed by publication of educational documents that have been used worldwide to teach the science of resuscitation (13–38).

CLINICAL PROFILE OF SUDDEN, UNEXPECTED CARDIAC ARREST

Most episodes of sudden, unexpected cardiac arrest in adults occur in the home or workplace (83–86). The most common victim is a male who is between 50 and 75 years of age (83,85). The majority of these individuals has significant underlying structural heart disease such as coronary artery atherosclerosis, hypertension, left ventricular hypertrophy, and/or congestive heart failure (84,87–90).

Most cardiac arrests occur without an obvious immediate precipitant, although many families of cardiac arrest victims will report that the patient experienced a variety of nonspecific symptoms such as chest pain, dyspnea, fatigue, or malaise in the days preceding the event (84,87). On rare occasions, a dramatic emotional event can trigger cardiac arrest (91–95).

There is a definite circadian pattern to the onset of sudden, unexpected cardiac arrest. The incidence of cardiac arrest is lowest during sleep and begins to rise rapidly soon after awakening (96–98). Heart rate variability studies show that, at such times, vagal activity is relatively low and sympathetic activity is high, especially in patients with reduced left ventricular function (99).

In more than 80% of patients who develop out-of-hospital, primary cardiac arrest during ambulatory electrocardiographic monitoring, the initiating event is a ventricular tachyarrhythmia (ventricular tachycardia) degenerating rapidly to ventricular fibrillation in 62%, torsades de pointes in 13%, and "primary" ventricular fibrillation in 8% (100). Less than 70% of patients are in ventricular tachycardia or ventricular fibrillation by the time rescue personnel arrive on the scene [typically 5 to 10 minutes after the onset of collapse in most efficient emergency medical services (EMS) systems] (101). Most of the remaining patients (31%) are in a pulseless, bradycardic rhythm or asystole.

The outcome of field resuscitation is strongly influenced by the patient's initial cardiac rhythm. In one series of 352 consecutive out-of-hospital cardiac arrest patients, 67% of the patients with ventricular tachycardia and 23% of those who were initially in ventricular fibrillation survived to hospital discharge (102). None of the patients who presented with an initial bradyarrhythmia survived to hospital discharge. Similar observations have been made by others (103). One plausible hypothesis is that pulseless bradycardia or asystole may be a marker for a prolonged downtime interval or a more severe underlying disease process (104). Because ventricular tachyarrhythmias represent the most common, potentially treatable mechanism of sudden cardiac arrest in adults, the best in-hospital and out-of-hospital resuscitation programs have been designed to deliver rapid defibrillation to as many patients as possible.

PRINCIPLES OF MANAGEMENT

"Chain of Survival" Approach to Treatment

Survival from pulseless ventricular tachycardia or ventricular fibrillation is inversely related to the time interval between its onset and termination. Each minute that a patient remains in ventricular fibrillation, the odds of survival decrease by 7% to 10% (105). Survival is highest when CPR is started within the first 4 minutes of arrest and ACLS, including defibrillation and

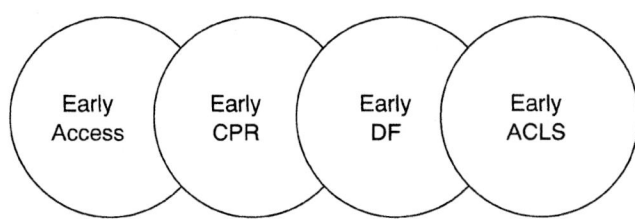

FIGURE 69.1 Chain of survival to optimize outcome from resuscitation. ACLS, advanced cardiac life support; CPR, cardiopulmonary resuscitation; DF, defibrillation.

drug therapy, is started within the first 8 minutes (106). The American Heart Association's Emergency Cardiovascular Care Committee and its Advanced Cardiovascular Life Support Subcommittee began to widely publicize the "chain of survival" concept in 1991. This symbolic phrase represents a sequence of

events that should occur in most cardiac arrest cases to maximize the odds of successful resuscitation (105). The steps include early recognition of the problem and activation of the EMS system by a bystander, early CPR, rapid provision of defibrillation for patients who need it, and ACLS (e.g., intubation, administration of medications). Schematically, this sequence can be depicted by a "chain of survival" (Fig. 69.1).

Algorithm Approach to Resuscitation

The American Heart Association's ACLS algorithms provide a "framework for dealing with the life-threatening cardiopulmonary emergencies in a logical sequence" (17,18). There are algorithms for initiating CPR (Fig. 69.2), treating patients with ventricular fibrillation or pulseless ventricular tachycardia (Fig. 69.3), bradycardia (Fig. 69.4), asystole

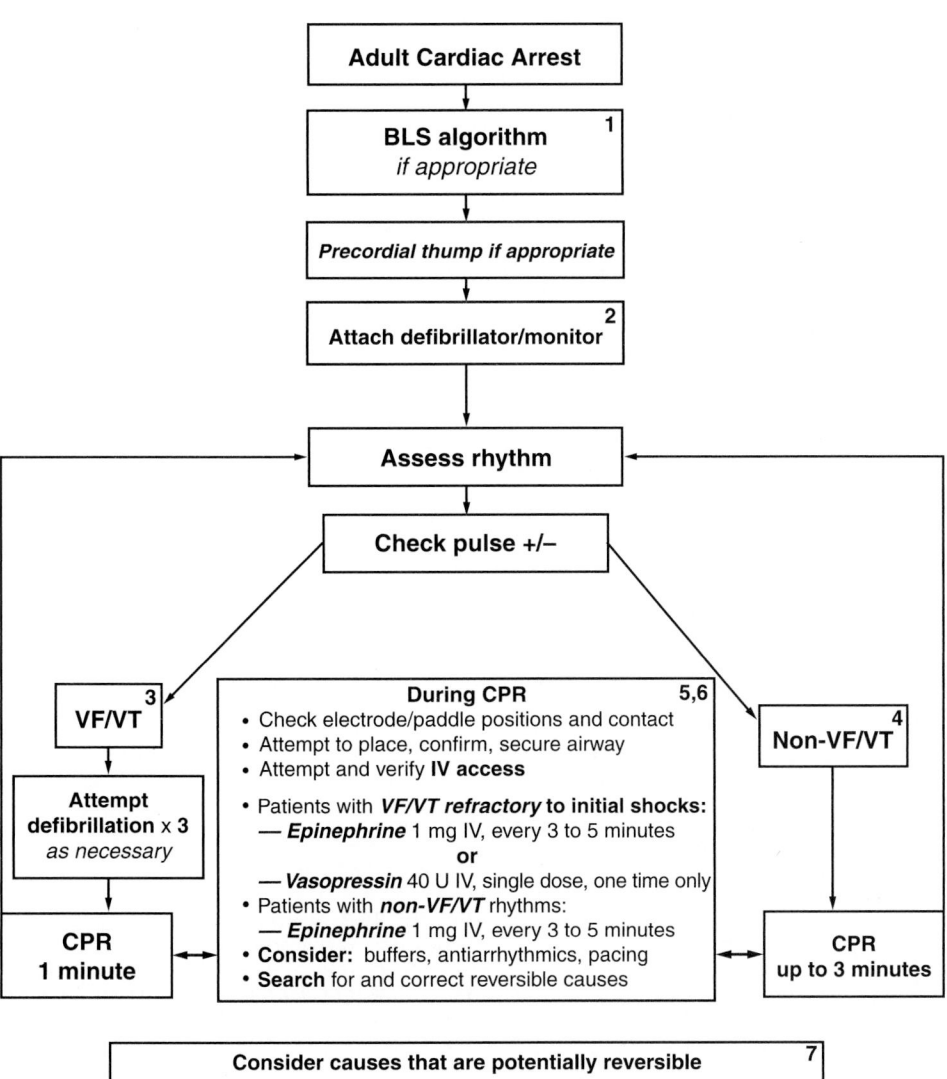

FIGURE 69.2 Comprehensive emergency cardiovascular care algorithm for cardiac arrest. ACS, acute coronary syndrome; BLS, basic life support; CPR, cardiopulmonary resuscitation; OD, overdose; VF/VT, ventricular fibrillation/ventricular tachycardia. (From *American Heart Association Guidelines.* 2000:I-144, with permission.)

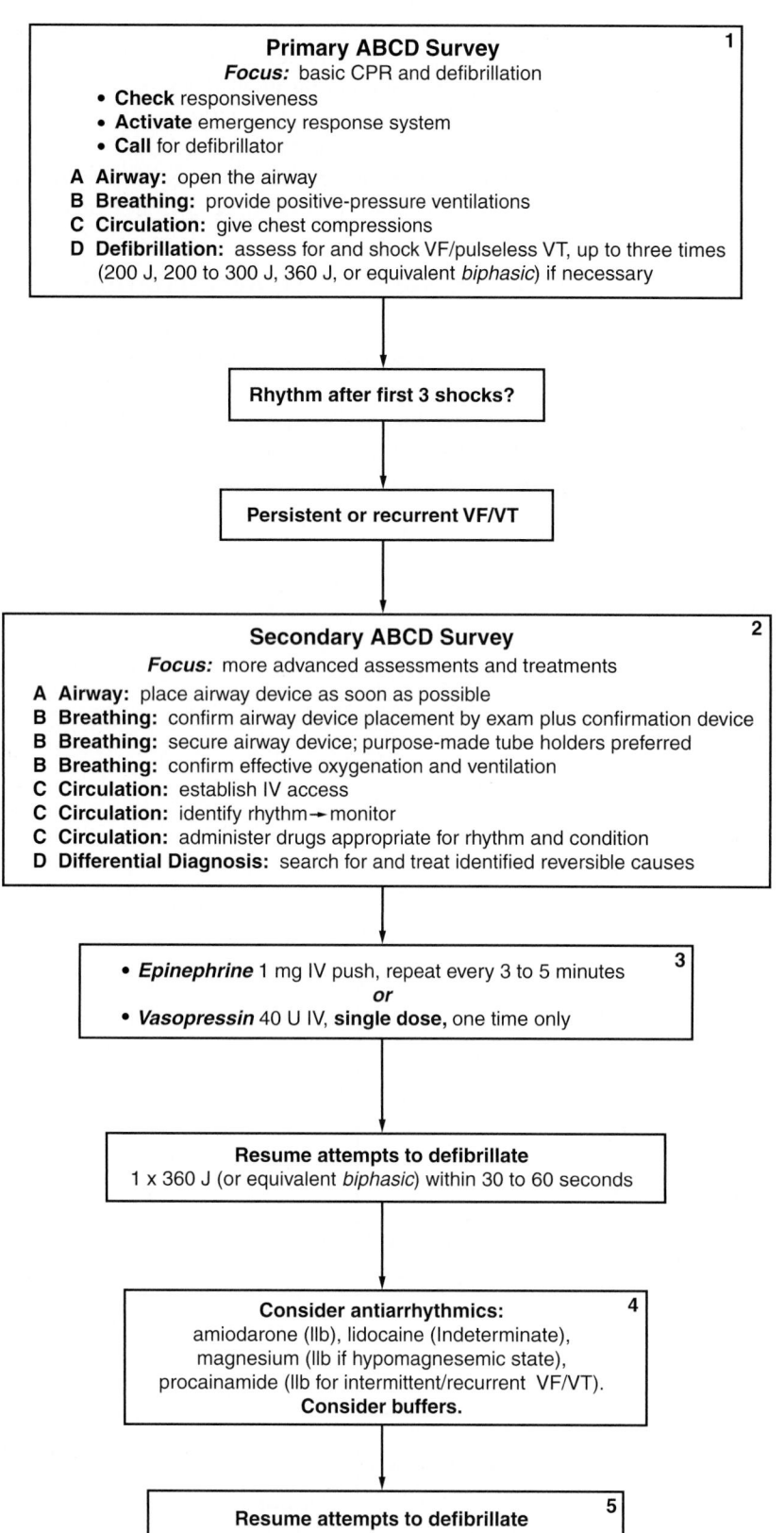

FIGURE 69.3 Ventricular fibrillation/pulseless ventricular tachycardia algorithm. CPR, cardiopulmonary resuscitation; VF, ventricular fibrillation; VT, ventricular tachycardia. (From *American Heart Association Guidelines*. 2000:I-147, with permission.)

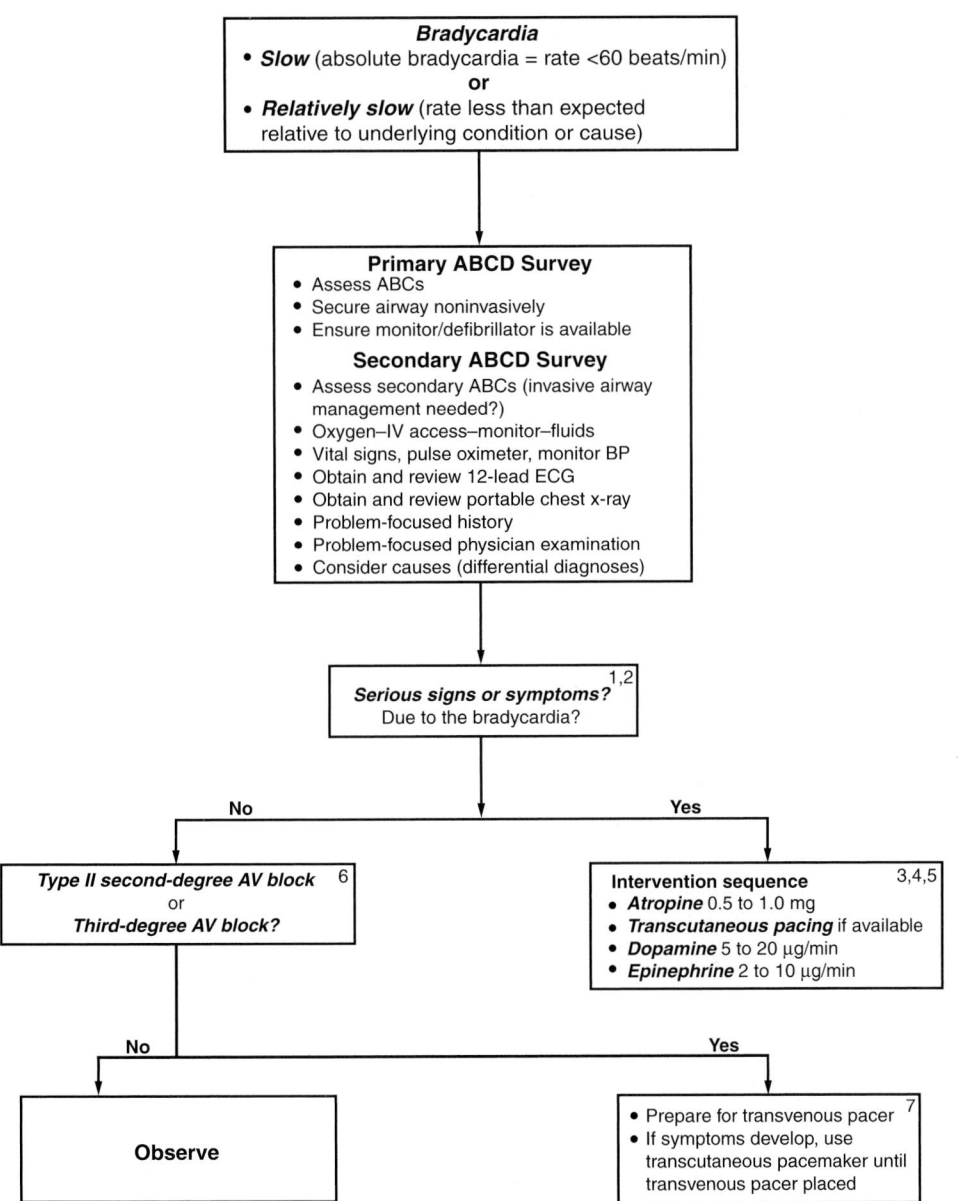

Bradycardia
- **Slow** (absolute bradycardia = rate <60 beats/min)

or

- **Relatively slow** (rate less than expected relative to underlying condition or cause)

Primary ABCD Survey
- Assess ABCs
- Secure airway noninvasively
- Ensure monitor/defibrillator is available

Secondary ABCD Survey
- Assess secondary ABCs (invasive airway management needed?)
- Oxygen–IV access–monitor–fluids
- Vital signs, pulse oximeter, monitor BP
- Obtain and review 12-lead ECG
- Obtain and review portable chest x-ray
- Problem-focused history
- Problem-focused physician examination
- Consider causes (differential diagnoses)

Serious signs or symptoms? [1,2]
Due to the bradycardia?

No

Type II second-degree AV block [6]

or

Third-degree AV block?

Yes

Intervention sequence [3,4,5]
- **Atropine** 0.5 to 1.0 mg
- **Transcutaneous pacing** if available
- **Dopamine** 5 to 20 µg/min
- **Epinephrine** 2 to 10 µg/min

No

Observe

Yes

- Prepare for transvenous pacer [7]
- If symptoms develop, use transcutaneous pacemaker until transvenous pacer placed

FIGURE 69.4 Symptomatic bradycardia algorithm. AV, atrioventricular; BP, blood pressure; ECG, electrocardiogram. (From *American Heart Association Guidelines*. 2000:I-156, with permission.)

(Fig. 69.5), or PEA (Fig. 69.6), which was formerly known as EMD. However, the algorithms are "not appropriate for every unique clinical circumstance, and the team leader must adapt them and the general ACLS principles when necessary." Resuscitation team leaders are encouraged to function as "thinking cooks" when applying these cookbook procedures.

Ventricular Fibrillation or Pulseless Ventricular Tachycardia

Electrical countershock is the treatment of choice for ventricular fibrillation and pulseless ventricular tachycardia. If three initial countershocks at increasing monophasic energies (200, 200 to 300, and 360 J), intubation, epinephrine, and a fourth countershock (360 J) fail to terminate the

arrhythmia (refractory ventricular fibrillation or ventricular tachycardia) or if, as in many cases, the arrhythmia rapidly recurs (recurrent ventricular fibrillation or ventricular tachycardia), antiarrhythmic drug therapy is indicated (17). There is increasing evidence that biphasic defibrillation waveforms using lower energy (typically 125 to 175 J) defibrillate successfully and are at least as effective as higher-energy, escalating monophasic waveforms (131–137). The American Heart Association now considers biphasic waveforms to be an acceptable alternative to the traditional escalating monophasic waveforms (17,138).

Pulseless Electrical Activity

PEA is present when there is organized electrical activity on the electrocardiogram but no effective circulation. There

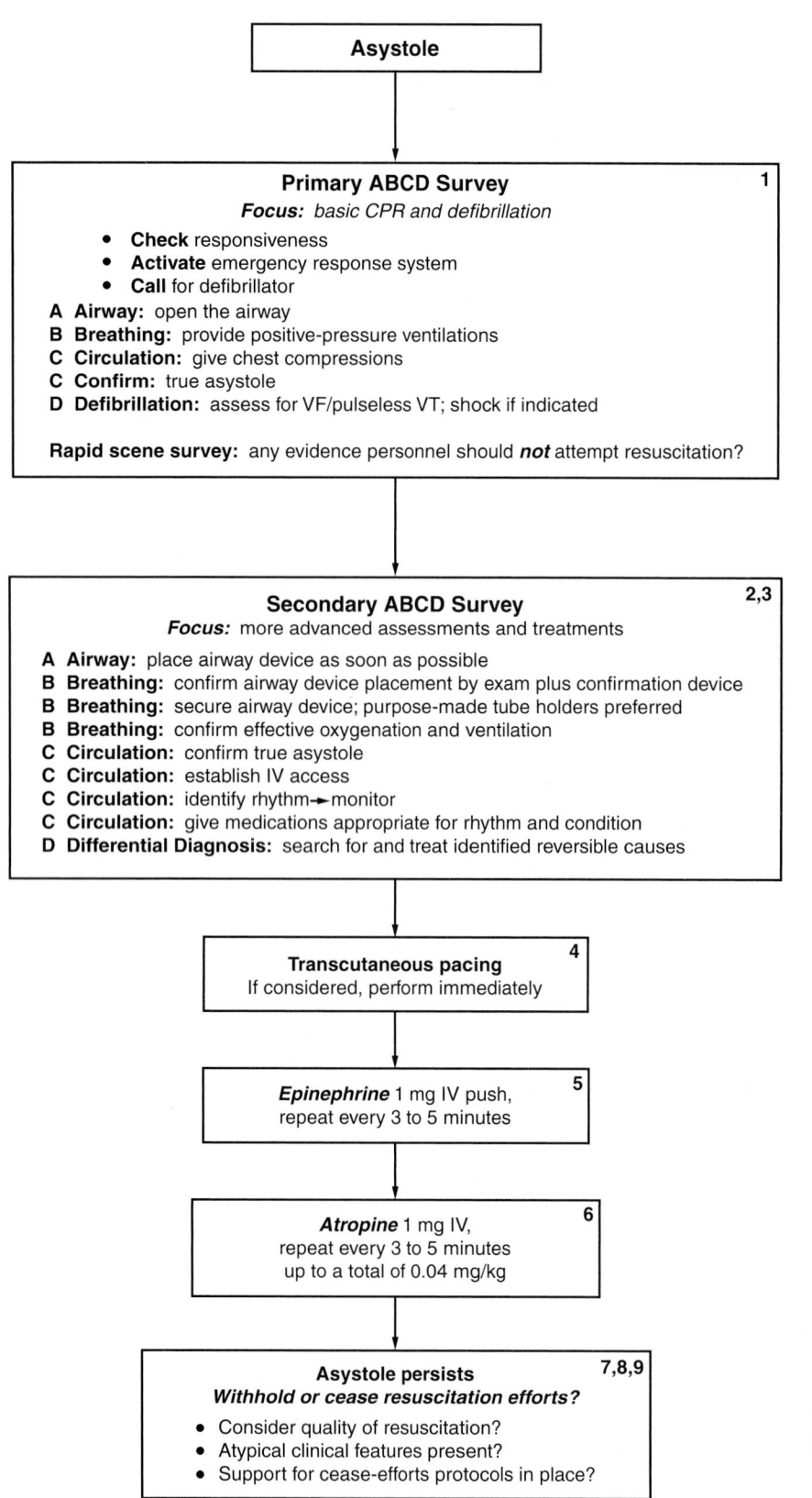

Asystole

↓

Primary ABCD Survey   1
Focus: basic CPR and defibrillation

- **Check** responsiveness
- **Activate** emergency response system
- **Call** for defibrillator

A **Airway:** open the airway
B **Breathing:** provide positive-pressure ventilations
C **Circulation:** give chest compressions
C **Confirm:** true asystole
D **Defibrillation:** assess for VF/pulseless VT; shock if indicated

Rapid scene survey: any evidence personnel should ***not*** attempt resuscitation?

↓

Secondary ABCD Survey   2,3
Focus: more advanced assessments and treatments

A **Airway:** place airway device as soon as possible
B **Breathing:** confirm airway device placement by exam plus confirmation device
B **Breathing:** secure airway device; purpose-made tube holders preferred
B **Breathing:** confirm effective oxygenation and ventilation
C **Circulation:** confirm true asystole
C **Circulation:** establish IV access
C **Circulation:** identify rhythm→monitor
C **Circulation:** give medications appropriate for rhythm and condition
D **Differential Diagnosis:** search for and treat identified reversible causes

↓

Transcutaneous pacing   4
If considered, perform immediately

↓

Epinephrine 1 mg IV push,   5
repeat every 3 to 5 minutes

↓

Atropine 1 mg IV,   6
repeat every 3 to 5 minutes
up to a total of 0.04 mg/kg

↓

Asystole persists   7,8,9
Withhold or cease resuscitation efforts?

- Consider quality of resuscitation?
- Atypical clinical features present?
- Support for cease-efforts protocols in place?

FIGURE 69.5 Asystole algorithm. CPR, cardiopulmonary resuscitation; VF, ventricular fibrillation; VT, ventricular tachycardia. (From *American Heart Association Guidelines*. 2000:I-153, with permission.)

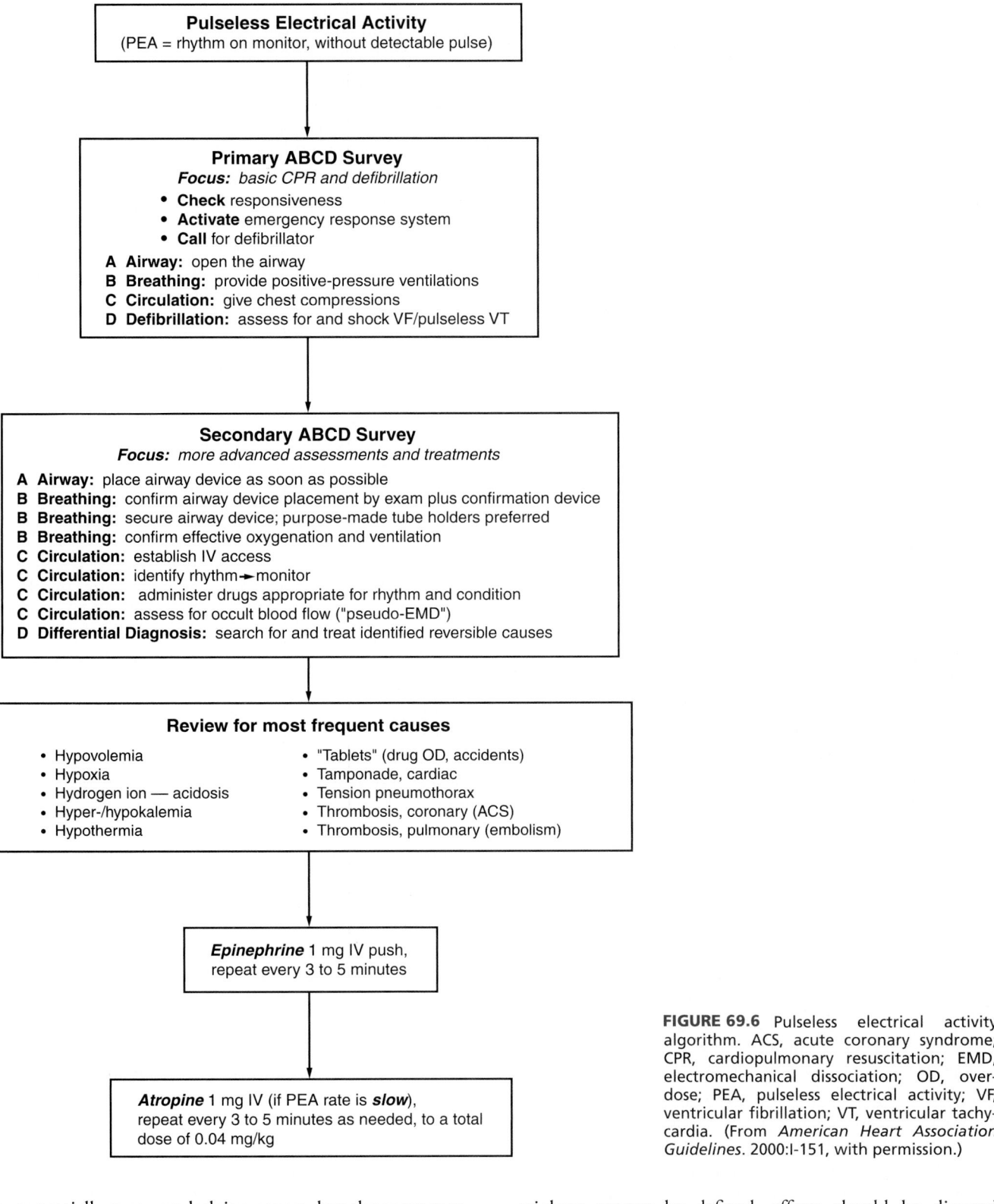

FIGURE 69.6 Pulseless electrical activity algorithm. ACS, acute coronary syndrome; CPR, cardiopulmonary resuscitation; EMD, electromechanical dissociation; OD, overdose; PEA, pulseless electrical activity; VF, ventricular fibrillation; VT, ventricular tachycardia. (From *American Heart Association Guidelines.* 2000:I-151, with permission.)

are potentially many underlying causes, but the most common denominator may involve myocardial ischemia and dysfunction due to intramyocardial increases in carbon dioxide (139). Prognosis is generally poor unless a discrete and treatable etiology for PEA can be discerned and corrected. Because of the poor prognosis when a correctable

etiology cannot be defined, efforts should be directed toward detecting causes such as hypovolemia, tension pneumothorax, and pericardial tamponade (17). Normal saline or Ringer's lactate solution should be infused rapidly if there is evidence of hypovolemia. Suspected pneumothorax or pericardial tamponade should be confirmed by needle aspiration of the chest or pericardium, respectively. If confirmed, more definitive surgical management (chest tube or thoracotomy) is usually required.

Scrutiny of the neck veins may be helpful in attempting to define an etiology for PEA. Most patients with cardiac arrest have high right-sided filling pressures and distended neck veins. When neck veins are not visible in this setting and PEA is present, hypovolemia should be suspected. In the "trauma" cardiac arrest victim (e.g., a patient with a gunshot wound of the chest), however, prominent neck veins should lead to the suspicion of pericardial tamponade or tension pneumothorax (140).

General measures such as (a) support of ventilation, (b) properly performed closed-chest compression, and (c) frequent doses of epinephrine to maintain arterial perfusion pressure and coronary and cerebral perfusion are recommended for treatment of PEA (17). Bradycardia may be treated with atropine. Although catecholamines are frequently given, there are no data to suggest a specific benefit (other than improvement in coronary and cerebral blood flow during closed-chest compression). Calcium chloride has not been shown to affect clinical survival in controlled trials (141,142). In addition, the pathologically high serum calcium levels caused by its administration (143,144) may exacerbate reperfusion injury (145).

If penetrating cardiac trauma is present, open-chest massage can be life saving (146). In other settings, open-chest massage is rarely of value, partly because it is usually initiated late after the onset of the arrest (147). Prehospital trauma victims who are pulseless and have asystole or agonal electrical cardiac activity (heart rate of less than 40 beats/min) have such a poor prognosis that some authors believe that they should be pronounced dead at the scene of injury (148).

Bradyasystole

Bradyasystole is one of the most common and least understood problems that can occur during resuscitation. For purposes of definition, *bradyasystole* refers to a cardiac rhythm that has a ventricular rate of below 60 beats/min in adults and/or periods of absent heart rhythm (asystole). Bradyasystolic states are clinical situations during which bradyasystole is the dominant heart rhythm.

Survival is poor (generally 1% to 3% or less), regardless of therapy for patients who present with bradyasystole. It is always important to exclude disconnection of a lead or monitor electrode before concluding that a "flatline" is the patient's rhythm. Because some patients with a flatline may have ventricular fibrillation (a rhythm more amenable to treatment) masquerading as asystole (149), the monitor lead configuration should be quickly switched to a second lead to confirm the diagnosis before treatment (17). Other general measures recommended for the treatment of bradyasystole include support of ventilation; properly performed

closed-chest compression; and frequent doses of epinephrine to maintain arterial perfusion pressure and coronary and cerebral perfusion (17).

Treatment with atropine sulfate may improve outcome in patients with bradyasystolic cardiac arrest that is due to excessive vagal stimulation, but atropine is less effective when asystole or pulseless idioventricular rhythms are the result of prolonged ischemia or mechanical injury in the myocardium (150).

For patients with bradyasystolic cardiac arrest, a 1-mg dose of atropine is administered intravenously and is repeated every 3 to 5 minutes if asystole persists. Three mg (0.04 mg per kg) given intravenously is a fully vagolytic dose in most patients (151). The administration of a total vagolytic dose of atropine should be reserved for patients with bradyasystolic cardiac arrest. ET atropine produces a rapid onset of action similar to that observed with intravenous injection. The recommended adult dose of atropine for ET administration is 1.0 to 2.0 mg diluted in 10 mL of sterile water or normal saline.

Pacing (transvenous, transthoracic, or transcutaneous) rarely influences survival in the unwitnessed cardiac arrest patient who is initially found with asystole or bradycardia without a pulse (152–154). However, pacing is extremely useful for bradycardic patients with a pulse and in selected patients in whom a pacemaker can be placed immediately after the development of the conduction disturbance (153,154). In such cases, a precordial thump can also stimulate ventricular complexes and a pulse ("fist pacing") (155).

Endogenous adenosine released during myocardial hypoxia and ischemia relaxes vascular smooth muscle, decreases atrial and ventricular contractility, depresses pacemaker automaticity, and impairs atrioventricular conduction (156). The cellular electrophysiologic effects of adenosine can be competitively antagonized by methylxanthines but not by atropine. A specific adenosine antagonist (BW-A1433U) has been shown to reverse and prevent postdefibrillation bradyasystole and hemodynamic depression in a domestic pig model (157).

Aminophylline, a competitive nonspecific adenosine antagonist, has been shown to restore cardiac electrical activity within 30 seconds in 12 of 15 in-hospital, bradysystolic cardiac arrest patients who were refractory to atropine and epinephrine (158). Other anecdotal case reports seem to indicate that adenosine blockade may restore normal sinus rhythm in some bradyasystole patients who do not respond to conventional therapy (159). In a relatively small, randomized, prospective clinical trial on adults with asystole refractory to epinephrine and atropine, there was a trend toward improved return of spontaneous circulation (ROSC) in patients who received aminophylline versus placebo, but the results did not reach statistical significance (160). Forty-five patients were assigned to the placebo group, and 37 received aminophylline. Nine of 45 controls (20%; 95% confidence interval, 10% to 35%) achieved

ROSC compared with 10 of 37 (27%; 95% confidence interval, 14% to 44%) in the aminophylline group. Although further clinical research will be necessary to determine the potential value of adenosine blockade for bradyasystolic cardiac arrest, it is clear that these agents should not be used when ventricular fibrillation is present because they may make it more difficult to terminate this arrhythmia (161).

CONTROVERSIES AND PERSONAL PERSPECTIVES

Need for Mouth-to-Mouth Ventilation during the First Few Minutes of Cardiopulmonary Resuscitation

In the United States, debate continues about the need to provide artificial ventilation during the first few minutes of CPR because of fear of contracting infectious diseases. Surveys of CPR instructors and other health care providers indicate great reluctance on the part of many rescuers to perform mouth-to-mouth ventilation on strangers (120,245–252).

It is not clear that it is necessary to provide mouth-to-mouth ventilation for the first several minutes of resuscitation as long as chest compression is performed and the airway is patent. Chandra et al. (253) assessed the time course of change in arterial blood gases during resuscitation in a canine experimental model during ventricular fibrillation. The dogs had no ET tube in place during CPR and received only chest compression (no ventilation). Prearrest arterial pH, carbon dioxide partial pressure (PCO_2), and oxygen saturation were 7.39 ± 0.02, 27.0 ± 1.5 mm Hg, and 97% ± 11.5%, respectively. After 4 minutes of chest compression alone, the corresponding values were 7.39 ± 0.03, 24.3 ± 3.1 mm Hg, and 93.9% ± 3.0%. Mean minute ventilation during the fourth minute of CPR, measured with a face mask pneumotachometer, was 5.2 ± 1.1 L per minute. These findings suggest that, in the dog model of witnessed arrest, chest compression alone during CPR can maintain adequate gas exchange to sustain the oxygen saturation above 90% for at least 4 minutes. These findings appear to be confirmed by the observation that survival from cardiac arrest is almost as good in humans when bystanders perform only chest compressions as occurs when bystanders perform both chest compressions and mouth-to-mouth ventilation (119). Some investigators believe that mouth-to-mouth ventilation may not be essential during the first few minutes of CPR because chest compression alone with a patent airway generates a reasonable minute ventilation and the quantity of oxygen needed is reduced significantly during low blood flow states (249). Some investigators have even questioned whether mouth-to-mouth ventilation with exhaled gas containing as much as 4% carbon dioxide and less oxygen than air might even have adverse effects during CPR (248).

The American Heart Association recommends that rescuers perform mouth-to-mouth ventilation along with chest compressions because clinical data indicate that this combination results in the highest rate of neurologically intact survival (38,119). If rescuers are unwilling to perform mouth-to-mouth ventilation, bystanders should activate the EMS system immediately and initiate chest compressions (38).

In a recent prospective clinical trial in Seattle, telephone EMS dispatchers gave bystanders at the scene of apparent cardiac arrest instructions to perform chest compressions alone or chest compression plus mouth-to-mouth ventilation (254). Data were analyzed for 241 patients randomly assigned to receive chest compression alone and 279 assigned to chest compression plus mouth-to-mouth ventilation. Complete instructions were delivered in 62% of episodes for the group receiving chest compression plus mouth-to-mouth ventilation and 81% of episodes for the group receiving chest compression alone ($p = .005$). Instructions for compression required 1.4 minutes less to complete than instructions for compression plus mouth-to-mouth ventilation. Survival to hospital discharge was better among patients assigned to chest compression alone than among those assigned to chest compression plus mouth-to-mouth ventilation (14.6% vs. 10.4%), but the difference was not statistically significant ($p = .18$). The authors concluded that the outcome after CPR with chest compression alone is similar to that after chest compression with mouth-to-mouth ventilation, and chest compression alone may be the preferred approach for bystanders inexperienced in CPR.

Spontaneous agonal respirations often contribute to respiratory exchange of gases. In one case series, agonal respirations occurred in 40% of 445 out-of-hospital cardiac arrests (255). Agonal respirations were present in 46% of arrests caused by a cardiac etiology compared with 32% in other etiologies ($p < .01$). Fifty-five percent of witnessed arrest patients had agonal activity compared with 16% of unwitnessed arrest patients ($p < .001$). Agonal respirations occurred in 56% of arrests due to ventricular fibrillation compared with 34% of cases with a non–ventricular fibrillation rhythm ($p < .001$). Twenty-seven percent of patients with agonal respirations were discharged alive compared with 9% without them ($p < .001$). These findings suggest that there is a high incidence of agonal respiratory activity associated with out-of-hospital cardiac arrest, and the presence of agonal respirations appears to be associated with increased survival.

It is important to point out that assisted ventilation, particularly when performed with supplemental oxygen through a properly inserted ET tube, is clearly beneficial during CPR if resuscitation efforts continue beyond the first few minutes (246). Until the airway is protected by a properly inserted and secured ET tube, each mouth-to-mouth or bag-valve-mask ventilation must be delivered with a slow inspiratory flow rate to allow adequate time for lung inflation and to prevent gastric insufflation (38). This is necessary because the lungs become very stiff during resuscitation due to decreased compliance (256). Forceful efforts to inflate the lungs rapidly will only result in elevation of the pharyngeal pressure effect, which will be transmitted down the esophagus to the esophageal-gastric sphincter, causing it to open and allow passage of air into the stomach (257).

Is There a Need for "High-Dose" Epinephrine during Resuscitation?

Epinephrine, an endogenous catecholamine with both alpha- and beta-adrenergic activity, is the vasopressor of choice for use during resuscitation. Epinephrine's potent alpha$_1$- and alpha$_2$-adrenergic effects improve cerebral blood flow by preventing arterial collapse and by increasing peripheral vasoconstriction (163,166–170,258,259). Epinephrine also enhances CPP, which is the major determinant of the ROSC after cardiac arrest (164,167,260). An aortic diastolic blood pressure of 30 to 40 mm Hg markedly improves survival during resuscitation in animal models (64,164,167,171,173,217,260–264). Restoration of myocardial blood flow facilitates the resynthesis of high-energy phosphates within myocardial mitochondria and enhances cellular viability and contractile force. However, the increased myocardial blood flow is at least partially antagonized by the increased myocardial oxygen consumption caused by epinephrine's beta-adrenergic actions (265,266).

The optimal dose of epinephrine to augment aortic diastolic blood pressure in humans during closed-chest compression is unknown. The American Heart Association currently recommends a 1.0-mg dose based on studies in dogs weighing approximately 20 kg (17). In a 70-kg male, the current recommendations provide only 7.5 to 15 µg per kg of epinephrine every 5 minutes.

Some studies have concluded that dosages of more than 15 µg per kg may be required during closed-chest CPR in animal models. Kosnik et al. showed that a dose of epinephrine of 15 µg per kg (the upper range of the recommended human dose) did not maintain an aortic diastolic blood pressure above 40 mm Hg during closed-chest compression in dogs (267). Larger doses (45, 75, and 150 µg per kg) effectively raised aortic diastolic blood pressure. High-dose (10 µg per kg) constant infusions of epinephrine have been shown to significantly increase aortic diastolic blood pressure and coronary blood flow during closed-chest compression in dogs (268). Epinephrine (0.02, 0.2, and 2.0 mg per kg) also produced significant dose-dependent improvement in regional myocardial and cerebral blood flow during closed-chest compression in animal models (269–276). Preliminary data in humans suggested a similar dose dependence with respect to aortic blood pressure (277).

From these studies it appeared that higher doses of epinephrine might be required in adult humans to improve hemodynamics and to achieve successful resuscitation. Anecdotal case series and retrospective studies published in the late 1980s and early 1990s (277–281) set the stage for prospective randomized clinical trials. Unfortunately, none of these trials has shown any convincing evidence that higher doses of epinephrine than those which are used customarily (1 mg) are associated with any better survival to hospital discharge in adults or children (232,282–290).

Could higher doses of epinephrine be of value to some subgroups of patients and harmful to others? One of the high-dose epinephrine trials showed a threefold increase in hospital discharge rates in patients presenting with EMD and asystole when treated with 5.0 mg versus 1.0 mg of epinephrine as the initial dose, but this difference did not reach statistical significance (285). Another study showed that patients older than 65 years and those in ventricular fibrillation did better with standard doses of epinephrine (284). However, additional clinical trials have failed to show benefit from the use of high versus standard doses of epinephrine in adults (288,290,291) or in children (282,289).

Most of the patients who survive cardiac arrest respond to early defibrillation and never receive epinephrine. What percent of those who do not respond are salvageable is unclear. However, because patients who are defibrillated did not qualify for these clinical trials, the survival rates of patients studied were low regardless of the dosage of epinephrine. Of some comfort is the fact that these trials did not demonstrate significant harm from higher doses of epinephrine. These studies emphasize the importance of the "standard" early interventions: airway management, chest compression, and rapid defibrillation. They suggest that epinephrine (whether at low or high dosages) as well as other late interventions represent a last desperate effort to resuscitate individuals who have a very poor chance for survival.

Based on available clinical data, the American Heart Association continues to recommend an intravenous epinephrine dosage of 1 mg (10 mL of a 1:10,000 solution) every 3 to 5 minutes during resuscitation in adults (30). If the dose is given by peripheral injection, it should be followed by a 20-mL flush of intravenous fluid to ensure drug delivery into the central compartment. Higher doses of epinephrine are not recommended for routine use but can be considered if 1-mg doses fail.

The recommended pediatric epinephrine dosage for bradycardia, asystolic, or pulseless arrest is 0.01 mg per kg (0.1 mL per kg of a 1:10,000 solution) by the intravenous or intraosseous route or 0.1 mg per kg (0.1 mL per kg of a 1:1,000 solution) by the ET route (17). Repeated doses are recommended every 3 to 5 minutes for ongoing arrest. The same dose of epinephrine is recommended for second and subsequent doses for unresponsive asystolic and pulseless arrest, but higher doses of epinephrine (0.1 to 0.2 mg per kg; 0.1 to 0.2 mL per kg of a 1:1,000 solution) by any intravascular route may be considered. If high-dose epinephrine is used, extra care should be taken to avoid dosing errors because two different dilutions of epinephrine are needed. The recommended pediatric ET dosage of epinephrine is 0.1 mg per kg (0.1 mL per kg of a 1:1,000 solution).

Intracardiac administration should be used only during open cardiac compression or when other routes of administration are unavailable. Intracardiac injections increase the risk of coronary artery laceration, cardiac tamponade, and pneumothorax and cause interruption of external chest compression and ventilation.

During cardiac arrest, epinephrine also may be administered by continuous intravenous infusion. The dose should be comparable to the standard intravenous dose of epinephrine (1 mg every 3 to 5 minutes). This is accomplished by adding 1 mg of epinephrine hydrochloride to 250 mL of normal saline or dextrose 5% in water (D5W) to run at 1 μg per minute and increased to 3 to 4 μg per minute (30). A continuous infusion of epinephrine should be administered by central venous access to reduce the risk of extravasation and to ensure good bioavailability.

Autooxidation of catecholamines and related sympathomimetic compounds is pH-dependent. Contact of epinephrine with other drugs that have an alkaline pH (e.g., sodium bicarbonate) can cause autooxidation, but the reaction rate is too slow to be clinically important when epinephrine is given by bolus injection or when it is infused rapidly. Epinephrine should not be added to infusion bags or bottles that contain alkaline solutions.

Use of Vasopressin during Resuscitation

Vasopressin produces significantly higher CPP and myocardial blood flow than epinephrine during closed-chest CPR in a pig model of ventricular fibrillation (292) and in humans during CPR (293). Both vasopressin and adrenocorticotropin concentrations are higher during CPR in patients in whom resuscitation is successful compared with those in whom it fails (294). Because of these observations, there has been considerable interest in the use of vasopressin for supporting CPP during CPR in humans.

In a small, blinded, randomized clinical study, 40 patients with out-of-hospital ventricular fibrillation resistant to electrical defibrillation were treated with either epinephrine (1 mg intravenously; $n = 20$) or vasopressin (40 U intravenously; $n = 20$) during resuscitation (295). Seven (35%) patients in the epinephrine group and 14 (70%) in the vasopressin group survived to hospital admission ($p = .06$). At 24 hours, four (20%) epinephrine-treated patients and 12 (60%) vasopressin-treated patients were alive ($p = .02$). Three (15%) patients in the epinephrine group and eight (40%) in the vasopressin group survived to hospital discharge ($p = .16$). Neurologic outcomes were similar in both groups.

The *American Heart Association Guidelines* considers vasopressin to be an effective vasopressor and recommends it as an alternative to epinephrine for the treatment of adult shock refractory ventricular fibrillation cardiac arrest (30). Although vasopressin may also be effective in patients with asystole or PEA, data were insufficient to recommend the use of vasopressin for these conditions in the latest *Guidelines* recommendations. The recommended dosage is 40 units intravenously in place of the first dose of epinephrine in the pulseless ventricular tachycardia/ventricular fibrillation algorithm. Although its pharmacokinetics are not fully understood yet, it is generally believed that this single dose should last approximately 10 to 20 minutes, after which epinephrine should be resumed if ROSC has not occurred.

It is not clear whether vasopressin should be used at all in children or infants. Unfortunately, vasopressin was less effective than epinephrine in a piglet model of prolonged asphyxial cardiac arrest (296). At this time, the American Heart Association does not recommend the use of vasopressin in infants or children because data are inadequate to evaluate its efficacy and safety (21).

Use of Buffers during Resuscitation

The marked fall in cardiac output during closed-chest compression critically reduces tissue oxygen delivery. Cells shift to anaerobic metabolism, gradual building up lactic acid as a waste product (297–300). During anaerobic metabolism, the carbon dioxide concentration increases rapidly inside cells. Anoxic arrest of the heart causes a progressive increase in the concentration of PCO_2 inside heart muscle cells that may reach very high levels (90 to 475 mm Hg) (301). Above an intramyocardial PCO_2 of approximately 475 mm Hg, PEA is present, and the heart cannot be resuscitated (301). Intracellular carbon dioxide eventually diffuses into capillary blood and returns to the heart and lungs in venous blood.

Central (mixed) venous blood during closed-chest compression is acidotic (pH of approximately 7.15) and hypercarbic ($PaCO_2$ of approximately 74 mm Hg) (216). With hyperventilation, carbon dioxide is removed as blood flows through the lungs. Accordingly, arterial blood is less acidotic. Arterial blood pH during well-performed closed-chest compression is usually normal, slightly acidotic, or mildly alkalotic (152,154–156,216,300,302,303). Arterial blood can be slightly alkalotic while the venous blood is acidotic because pulmonary blood flow is only a fourth to a third of normal amount during closed-chest compression (this phenomenon has been termed the *venous paradox*) (216). It is, in fact, not a paradox but part of normal physiology that occurs when anaerobic metabolism is required (e.g., during strenuous exercise), at which time the intramyocardial pH is much closer to the venous than the arterial pH.

Severe arterial acidosis during closed-chest compression is usually due to inadequate ventilation (304). The best solution is usually to improve the technique of closed-chest compression and to increase ventilation, if possible. If severe acidosis is present despite hyperventilation, correct intubation, and properly performed external chest compression, an alternate method for providing assisted circulation (e.g., open-chest compressions or venoarterial bypass) may need to be considered.

In the past, administration of sodium bicarbonate was recommended during closed-chest compression because of the belief that bicarbonate would buffer the H+ ion produced during anaerobic metabolism. However, sodium bicarbonate itself contains a high concentration of carbon dioxide (260 to 280 mm Hg) (305). In plasma, the carbon dioxide is released and diffuses into cells more rapidly than HCO_3^-, causing a paradoxical rise in intracellular PCO_2 and a fall in intracellular pH. The increases in intracellular PCO_2 in heart muscle cells decrease cardiac contractility, cardiac output, and blood pressure (306,307). Paradoxical acidosis of cerebrospinal fluid also can occur after the use of sodium bicarbonate (308) and may be responsible for prolonged confusion after a successful resuscitation as the venous acidosis increases. Sodium bicarbonate causes other potentially harmful effects, including hyperosmolality, alkalemia, and sodium overload.

At present, there are no convincing data proving treatment with sodium bicarbonate is of benefit during closed-chest compression and it does not improve survival in experimental animals (166,309–311). Sodium bicarbonate should not be given during a routine cardiac arrest because it provides minimal, if any, benefit and adds significant risk. If used at all, bicarbonate should not be used until proven interventions such as defibrillation, cardiac compression, support of ventilation including intubation, and pharmacologic therapies such as epinephrine and antiarrhythmic agents have been used (17). If used, the initial dose of sodium bicarbonate is 1 mEq per kg. No more than half of the original dose should be given every 10 minutes thereafter.

Measurement of arterial pH during closed-chest compression is rarely helpful because of the markedly reduced cardiac output and the venous paradox in pH. $PETCO_2$ will increase in keeping with the delivered load of carbon dioxide and will no longer reflect pulmonary perfusion (312). Ready-to-use, prefilled injection syringes containing 8.4% sodium bicarbonate (50 mEq per 50 mL) are recommended for use during CPR. The administration of sodium bicarbonate may help to buffer hydrogen ions washed out after reestablishment of spontaneous circulation. In this situation, the use of bicarbonate should be guided by arterial blood gas measurement. However, bicarbonate in this situation may still depress cardiac function (313,314). In certain circumstances, such as patients with preexisting metabolic acidosis, hyperkalemia, or tricyclic or phenobarbital overdose, bicarbonate is beneficial. Sodium bicarbonate can be administered by continuous infusion when the therapeutic goal is gradual correction of acidosis or alkalin-

ization of blood (i.e., tricyclic antidepressant overdose) or urine (e.g., barbiturate overdose). A 5% sodium bicarbonate solution (297.5 mEq per 500 mL) can be used to administer a sodium bicarbonate infusion. The infusion rate should be guided by arterial blood gas monitoring. Avoid attempting to completely correct the base deficit to minimize the risk of alkalosis.

Alternate buffer agents have not yet been shown to improve survival during cardiac resuscitation. Tromethamine (THAM) (TRIS buffer) is a potent amine buffer that actively binds H+ ions. It combines with carbonic acid, increasing the amount of bicarbonate anion available. THAM penetrates into cells and may neutralize acidic ions in the intracellular fluid. In dogs, THAM corrects the metabolic acidosis that occurs during cardiac arrest (315). Anecdotal reports suggest that THAM may be of value during prolonged cardiac resuscitations in humans (316), but more research is needed. Dichloroacetate reduces the serum lactate concentration by stimulating pyruvate dehydrogenase, the enzyme that catalyzes the rate-limiting step in the oxidation of lactate to pyruvate (317). It is a safe and effective adjunct for the treatment of patients with lactic acidosis but does not affect intramyocardial pH during closed-chest compression in experimental animals (303).

In a recent Scandinavian study, 502 adults with asystole or ventricular fibrillation with failure of the first defibrillation attempt were entered into a prospective, randomized, double-blind, controlled trial comparing the use of a combination buffer agent (Tribonat, containing 250 mL of a sodium bicarbonate-THAM-acetate-phosphate mixture with a buffering capacity of 500 mmol per L) and 250 mL of 0.9% saline placebo (318). Eighty-seven patients (36%) receiving buffer were admitted to the hospital, and 24 (10%) were discharged from the hospital alive versus 92 (36%) and 35 (14%) receiving saline (no significant difference between groups). Thus, this landmark clinical trial lends further evidence to the belief that buffer therapy does not improve patient outcome from routine cardiac arrest.

Use of Antiarrhythmic Drugs for Refractory Ventricular Fibrillation

Frequently used agents for treatment of refractory ventricular fibrillation or pulseless ventricular tachycardia include lidocaine, bretylium tosylate, procainamide, beta blockers, magnesium sulfate, and intravenous amiodarone. With the exception of intravenous amiodarone, there are no randomized controlled clinical trial data confirming whether any of the other agents are any better than just repeated electrical countershocks.

The American Heart Association considers lidocaine to be acceptable therapy for pulseless ventricular tachycardia/ventricular fibrillation that persists after defibrillation and administration of a vasopressor agent (epinephrine or vasopressin). The primary basis for this recommendation is historical precedent and no evidence of significant harm (31). An initial dose of 1.0 to 1.5 mg per kg is suggested. For refractory ventricular fibrillation and pulseless ventricular tachycardia, an additional bolus of 0.5 to 0.75 mg per kg can be given over 3 to 5 minutes if necessary. The total dose should not exceed 3 mg per kg (or more than 200 to 300 mg during a 1-hour period). Administration of antiarrhythmic agents after ROSC is controversial, but it is common to initiate a lidocaine intravenous infusion at a rate of 1 to 4 mg per minute. Recurrence of ventricular tachyarrhythmias during a constant infusion should be treated with a small bolus dose (0.5 mg per kg) and an increase in the infusion rate in incremental doses (maximal infusion rate of 4 mg per minute). The dosage should be reduced and/or blood levels monitored if the patient remains on lidocaine for 24 hours or more because the half-life of the drug increases after 24 to 48 hours of continuous therapy.

Bretylium is a class 3 antiarrhythmic that increases myocardial electrical stability by elevating the ventricular fibrillation threshold and by reducing the disparity in action potential duration and refractory periods between ischemic and nonischemic myocardium. Nowak et al. (319) reported a higher rate of successful resuscitation when bretylium was used (35%) than after placebo (6%) alone in prehospital cardiac arrest victims but their retrospective analysis left substantial questions concerning the comparability of the groups. Other studies also support the efficacy of bretylium for prehospital ventricular fibrillation (320,321). However, no difference in clinical outcome has been observed in prospective randomized studies comparing bretylium and lidocaine for the treatment of prehospital ventricular fibrillation using intravenous doses of bretylium (0.5 to 1.0 g) and lidocaine (100 to 200 mg) (322) or bretylium (10 to 30 mg per kg) and lidocaine (2 to 3 mg per kg) (320). Neither study found a significant difference in the incidence of conversion from ventricular fibrillation and tachycardia to a more organized rhythm or survival. Bretylium is presently unavailable due to a shortage of substrate to manufacture the agent. It has been removed from the American Heart Association treatment algorithms and guidelines because of its high incidence of side effects, the availability of other equally effective alternatives, and limited availability (31).

Procainamide, a class 1A antiarrhythmic agent, is a presynaptic ganglionic blocker; it vasodilates and induces modest negative inotropic effects, especially in patients with left ventricular dysfunction. Procainamide-induced hypotension is most pronounced after rapid intravenous injection or when high plasma concentrations of procainamide are present.

During resuscitation, procainamide is usually given by infusion at 20 mg per minute until the tachyarrhythmia is suppressed, hypotension and/or QRS prolongation by 50% from its original duration has occurred, or 17 mg per kg has been given (31). Bolus administration can result in significant hypotension and toxicity. In urgent situations, up to 50 mg per minute can be given up to a total of 17 mg per kg. The maintenance infusion dosage of procainamide is 1 to 4 mg per minute. Blood levels should be monitored in renal failure patients or in those receiving more than a 3-mg-per-minute intravenous infusion for more than 24 hours.

Occasionally, ventricular fibrillation or ventricular tachycardia without a pulse will remain refractory to, or will recur incessantly, despite repeated electrical countershocks and conventional pharmacologic treatment. In such cases, additional treatment options should be considered. The use of intravenous beta-blockers, traditionally with intravenous propranolol (1 mg every 5 minutes intravenously up to a total dose of 0.1 mg per kg) or esmolol, is worthy of consideration.

Underlying metabolic derangements should also be sought and corrected. Arterial hypoxemia should be reversed or minimized by ET intubation and ventilation with 100% oxygen. Acidosis is best prevented (or treated) during closed-chest compression by optimizing CPR techniques to improve blood flow and hyperventilation. Electrolyte abnormalities are common during resuscitation, either as primary disturbances that may have triggered the arrest or as secondary phenomena due to intracellular shifts and therapeutic interventions; such electrolyte abnormalities should be corrected if present.

Resuscitation from refractory ventricular fibrillation is less likely to be successful if hypokalemia and/or hypomagnesemia are present. Hypokalemia is common in cardiac patients and occurs in 23% to 40% of individuals treated with thiazide diuretics (323). When loop and thiazide diuretics are used in combination, the incidence approaches 100% (323,324). Hypokalemia can trigger ventricular fibrillation in experimental animal models and in patients with heart disease (especially acute myocardial infarction) (324,325). Hypokalemia is also common (up to 50%) in survivors of out-of-hospital ventricular fibrillation (326,327). Hypokalemia after resuscitation may be due to a shift in the distribution of potassium between the extracellular and intracellular space induced by metabolic events during resuscitation. Many patients (55% in one study) have predisposing risk factors for the development of hypokalemia before cardiac arrest (327).

Hypokalemia in the patient with cardiac arrest and refractory ventricular fibrillation must be treated aggressively. Guidelines for potassium replacement that are acceptable in the less emergent clinical circumstance may be inadequate to correct hypokalemia in a timely fashion during cardiac arrest (328). One regimen that has been suggested includes administration of 10 mEq of potassium chloride diluted in 50 mL D5W over 20 minutes. This dose can be repeated as necessary while rechecking serum levels.

Hypomagnesemia should be corrected if present because it can precipitate ventricular fibrillation in experimental models in association with hypokalemia and can hinder the replenishment of intracellular potassium (329,330). Magnesium sulfate is no longer recommended for routine management of pulseless ventricular tachycardia or ventricular fibrillation unless hypomagnesemia is suspected or present or the patient has torsades de pointes because two clinical in-hospital trials have not shown benefit (31,331,332).

For acute administration during ventricular tachycardia or fibrillation with known or suspected hypomagnesemia or for torsades de pointes, 1 or 2 g of magnesium sulfate (2 to 4 mL of a 50% solution) is diluted in 50 to 100 mL of D5W and administered over 5 to 60 minutes. Caution should be used when magnesium is administered to safeguard against clinically significant hypotension or asystole. A 24-hour magnesium infusion (8 g of magnesium sulfate in 500 mL D5W at eight drops per minute) should be considered in patients with documented magnesium deficiency. Magnesium toxicity is rare, but side effects from rapid administration include flushing, sweating, mild bradycardia, and hypotension. Hypermagnesemia can produce depressed reflexes, flaccid paralysis, circulatory collapse, respiratory paralysis, or diarrhea.

Other treatment strategies can also be used in managing incessantly refractory or recurrent ventricular fibrillation or pulseless ventricular tachycardia. The possibility that there has been a proarrhythmic drug effect that may be exacerbating the arrhythmia must be considered. Proarrhythmic drug effects, hypokalemia, and/or hypomagnesemia can induce ventricular arrhythmias such as torsades de pointes. Torsades de pointes should be treated by stopping medications known to prolong the QT interval and correcting any electrolyte abnormalities. Other interventions can be tried, including administration of magnesium sulfate or the use of pacing or other forms of overdrive suppression (including the cautious use of isoproterenol if there are no contraindications) (333).

There has been considerable interest in the use of intravenous amiodarone to treat patients with recurrent arrhythmias (334–344). Despite prolonged resuscitative efforts before the administration of intravenous amiodarone, 11 of 12 patients with refractory ventricular tachyarrhythmias responded, and eight left the hospital alive (334). In one recent double-blind clinical trial, 302 patients with refractory hemodynamically destabilizing ventricular tachycardia or ventricular fibrillation were randomly assigned to therapy with intravenous bretylium (4.7 g) or intravenous amiodarone administered in a high dose (1.8 g) or a low dose (0.2 g). The arrhythmia event rate during the first 48 hours of therapy showed comparable efficacy between bretylium and high-dose (1,000 mg per 24 hours) amiodarone, and both bretylium and high-dose amiodarone were better than low-dose (125 mg per 24 hours) amiodarone. Overall mortality in the 48-hour double-blind period was 13.6% and was not significantly different among the three treatment groups. Significantly more patients treated with bretylium had hypotension compared with the two amiodarone groups. It was concluded that bretylium and amiodarone have comparable efficacy for the treatment of highly malignant ventricular arrhythmias. Bretylium use, however, may be limited by a high incidence of hypotension.

In a recent randomized controlled clinical prehospital trial conducted on 504 cardiac arrest patients with recurrent and/or refractory ventricular tachyarrhythmias, the administration of a single 300-mg bolus of intravenous amiodarone at the time of the first intravenous epinephrine administration resulted in 26% greater survival to hospital admission compared with standard ACLS therapy (345,346). There was no significant difference between the amiodarone and placebo groups in the duration of the resuscitation attempt (42 ± 16.4 and 43 ± 16.3 minutes, respectively), the number of shocks delivered (4 ± 3 and 6 ± 5), or the proportion of patients who required additional antiarrhythmic drugs after the administration of the study drug (66% and 73%). More patients in the amiodarone group than in the placebo group had hypotension (59% vs. 48%, $p = .04$) or bradycardia (41% vs. 25%, $p = .004$) after receiving the study drug. These side effects usually respond readily to therapy (volume infusion and vasopressors; atropine and/or electrical pacing). Recipients of amiodarone were more likely to survive to hospital admission (44% vs. 34% of the placebo group; $p = .03$). The adjusted odds ratio for survival to admission to the hospital in the amiodarone group as compared with the placebo group was 1.6 (95% confidence interval of 1.1 to 2.4; $p = .02$). The trial did not have sufficient statistical power to detect differences in survival to hospital discharge, which differed only slightly between the two groups.

The manufacturer adds polysorbate 80 to the intravenous amiodarone preparation to keep the latter in solution (amiodarone is relatively insoluble in water). Because diluent is a "soapy" compound, it can create bubbles if the vial is shaken before the amiodarone is drawn up into the syringe. It is recommended that the vial not be shaken. The bubbling phenomenon can usually be kept to a minimum by drawing up the drug with a large needle (18 gauge or larger). If bubbles do appear in the syringe, it should be held vertically as it is being injected into the intravenous tubing, and the bubbles should not be injected into the patient.

The American Heart Association currently recommends the use of amiodarone after defibrillation and a vasopressor (either epinephrine or vasopressin) in cardiac arrest with persistent or recurrent pulseless ventricular tachycardia or ventricular fibrillation (31). In this setting, it is usually administered as a 300-mg rapid infusion diluted to 20 to 30 mL with saline or D5W. Supplementary doses of 150 mg by rapid infusion can be given for recurrent or refractory pulseless ventricular tachycardia or ventricular fibrillation up to a maximum dosage of 2,000 mg for 24 hours (31,346). For patients not in cardiac arrest, intravenous amiodarone is usually diluted and administered as 150 mg over 10 minutes followed by a 1-mg-per-minute infusion for 6 hours, and then 0.6 mg per minute.

U.S. Food and Drug Administration Issues of Informed Consent

Most clinical trials that involve research on emergency patients who cannot give prospective informed consent (including all resuscitation research) have been halted in the United States by a regulatory moratorium. The issues and problems surrounding the ban were of concern to federal regulators and many researchers for several years. In May 1993, the U.S. Food and Drug Administration (FDA) prematurely terminated a clinical resuscitation trial involving a comparison of the Ambu CardioPump (Ambu Inc., Denmark) and standard CPR because the FDA believed that the device involved "significant risk" to the subjects and that there were no means for the subjects to give informed consent to participate in the trial (347,348).

Widespread public attention became focused on the issue in May 1994 when a congressional subcommittee questioned whether existing laws and regulations governing the FDA and the U.S. Department of Health and Human Services (DHHS)/National Institutes of Health permit inclusion of unconscious human subjects who cannot give informed consent in clinical trials dealing with emergency medical conditions. The subcommittee charged these two federal agencies with the task of working together with other interested parties to develop consistent guidelines that local institutional review boards (IRBs) can follow to permit such research.

Until the congressional hearing, investigators in the United States customarily conducted such research by receiving a waiver of informed consent from their IRB or by using the method known as "deferred consent" (349). In retrospect, IRBs have creatively interpreted and adapted prevailing rules to permit such research.

FDA regulations require informed consent in all clinical trials over which they have jurisdiction. The FDA regulations permit an "emergency exception" to this requirement for immediate, one-time use of an investigational device or drug for compassionate use to a single individual when (a) a patient is confronted by a life-threatening situation necessitating the investigational use of the drug or device; (b) informed consent cannot be obtained from the patient because of an inability to communicate with, or to obtain legally effective consent from, the patient; (c) time is insufficient to obtain consent from the patient's legal representative; and (d) no alternative method of approved or generally recognized therapy is available that provides an equal or greater likelihood of saving the patient's life.

The DHHS also has jurisdiction over the conduct of research in humans by means of its Office for Protection from Research Risks. This agency oversees research in humans by a different set of rules and regulations than that of the FDA. DHHS regulations do not contain an emergency exception. However, they provide a mechanism for waiver or alteration of informed consent when (a) the research involves no more than "minimal risk" to the subjects; (b) the waiver or alteration will not adversely affect the rights and welfare of the subjects; and (c) the research could not practicably be carried out without the waiver or alteration. Whenever appropriate, the subjects will be provided with additional pertinent information after participation.

"Minimal risk" is defined in the DHHS regulations by the following test: "[T]he probability and magnitude of harm or discomfort anticipated in the research are not greater in and of themselves than those ordinarily encountered in daily life or during the performance of routine physical or psychological examinations or tests." No resuscitation technique (standard or experimental) would pass this test of "minimal risk."

Thus, neither the FDA nor the DHHS rules and regulations provide a legal means for IRBs to approve emergency medical research in humans where it is impossible to obtain informed consent. On October 25, 1994, the Coalition Conference of Acute Resuscitation and Critical Care Researchers was held in Washington, D.C., to discuss informed consent in emergency research. Representatives from more than 20 organizations worked diligently to explore the issues and produced consensus recommendations for resolving some of the difficult issues that surround emergency medical research.

These recommendations and many other ideas were presented and discussed at the FDA/National Institutes of Health Public Forum on Informed Consent in Clinical Research Conducted in Emergency Circumstances, held in Bethesda, Maryland, January 9–10, 1995. Although this was not a consensus conference, the discussion appeared to indicate that legislative change is needed to give the FDA and the DHHS a common set of tools that will make it legal for them to oversee the conduct of legitimate, ethical, scientifically sound emergency care research. The next step is to translate the consensus statement drafted at the October meeting and ideas emanating from the Bethesda conference into legislative language and to introduce a congressional bill that will correct the deficiencies in the existing rules and regulations.

In the meantime, the only clinical resuscitation trials that are permitted in the United States are in-hospital studies in which potential cardiac arrest victims are approached and give their informed consent to participate in the trial if, by chance, they should experience a cardiac arrest during their hospitalization. Such a process has been used successfully before (80,350) but may require the screening of hundreds of potential individuals for every subject enrolled in the trial. Such a procedure is expensive and time-consuming. More important, it may result in a biased sample of patients.

Clearly, these have sobering implications for resuscitation research in the United States and throughout the world. The issue is not whether such research is morally, ethically, scientifically necessary and justifiable. These are, of course, absolute prerequisites. The real question is whether each country's laws, rules, and regulations explicitly permit emergency medical research when subjects cannot give informed consent. The FDA and the DHHS have recently released new rules that are intended to allow at least limited resumption of resuscitation research in humans.

Unfortunately, initial experience with these new rules has been problematic. In the first 4 years of the new FDA/DHHS rules, no prospective resuscitation drug or device trials have been completed or initiated successfully in the United States. In fact, several trials have been abandoned because of the expense and difficulty of complying with the new regulations (351–353). The American College of Cardiology has recently convened a Bethesda Conference on Emergency Cardiac Care that, in part, discussed problems with the waiver of informed consent procedures and proposed potential solutions (354).

New Experimental Cardiopulmonary Resuscitation Techniques

Investigators have begun to exploit the physiologic opportunities afforded by understanding the mechanisms of blood flow during CPR in an attempt to overcome the hemodynamic shortcomings of conventional chest compression. Standard chest compression of the sternum to a depth of 1.5 to 2.0 in. at a rate of 80 per minute as recommended by the American Heart Association produces only about one-fourth to one-third of the normal cardiac output and less than half of the normal arterial perfusion pressure (14,221). This is usually inadequate to generate the 25 to 35 mm Hg aortic diastolic pressure needed to restart the arrested heart (184,262).

Applying higher compression force to displace the sternum farther than the 1.5 to 2.0 in. recommended by the American Heart Association can improve arterial systolic pressure and cardiac output significantly (179). However, there is a practical limit to the amount of extra force that can be applied safely without causing physical injury to the chest and underlying structures. Computer modeling indicates that substantially greater force is required to generate adequate coronary and cerebral pressure and flow than that which can be provided safely by conventional sternal compression (355).

Circumferential Compression Cardiopulmonary Resuscitation

Circumferential application of force to the chest using a pneumatic vest can generate enough intrathoracic pressure to provide virtually normal systemic arterial pressure and flow in animals and humans during cardiac arrest (356–359). The device looks like a large blood pressure cuff that

is wrapped around the patient's thorax. It contains a bladder that can be inflated and deflated in cycles by a pneumatic pump. Compression duration, inflation pressure, and rate are all controlled by the device. Typical inflation pressure is 250 mm Hg, and the chest compression rate is 60 per minute. A small positive pressure is maintained between the chest and the vest to provide a tight fit between the two, but the device totally deflates during ventilation to provide for chest expansion. The total force applied to the chest with "vest CPR" is much greater than that which can be applied safely with conventional CPR. Despite this, "vest CPR" is much less traumatic than standard CPR because it distributes force over a much larger surface area (the entire chest).

When the pneumatic vest was applied to 29 patients who repeatedly did not respond to conventional CPR, defibrillation, and drug therapy for 42 ± 16 minutes, vest CPR increased the peak aortic pressure from 78 ± 26 mm Hg to 138 ± 28 mm Hg (p <.001) and the CPP from 15 ± 8 mm Hg to 23 ± 11 mm Hg (p <.003) (358). Despite prolonged unsuccessful manual CPR, spontaneous circulation returned with vest CPR in 4 of the 29 patients. An additional 34 patients were randomly assigned to undergo vest CPR (17 patients) or continued manual CPR (17 patients) after initial manual CPR (mean duration, 11 ± 4 minutes) was unsuccessful. Spontaneous circulation returned in eight of the 17 patients who underwent vest CPR as compared with only three of the 17 patients who received continued manual CPR (p = .14) (358). More patients in the vest CPR group than in the manual CPR group were alive 6 hours after attempted resuscitation (six of 17 vs. one of 17) and 24 hours after attempted resuscitation (three of 17 vs. one of 17), but none survived to leave the hospital.

Despite the fact that preliminary experience with the pneumatic vest has been encouraging, clinical trials using the device early in resuscitation have been halted due to the difficulties with the FDA/DHHS process of obtaining a waiver of informed consent (352). Alternative mechanical methods for providing circumferential chest compression using less energy than that required by a pneumatic device are being explored. Although the device is not presently FDA-approved or marketed in the United States, the American Heart Association considers vest CPR to be an acceptable alternative to standard CPR in-hospital or during ambulance transport (32).

Active Compression-Decompression Cardiopulmonary Resuscitation

Active compression-decompression CPR (ACD-CPR) is similar to conventional CPR, but it also provides negative intrathoracic pressure during the relaxation phase using a device that resembles a toilet plunger (*e*Fig 69.0.3). ACD-CPR is performed with a suction-cup device called the *Ambu CardioPump*.

The ACD-CPR device consists of three parts: (a) a neoprene suction cup, (b) a plastic circular handle with an undercut handgrip, and (c) a force gauge. The gauge can be calibrated to a fixed depth, which usually is similar to standard CPR (1.5 to 2.0 in.). To ensure proper function by the operator, the decompression force is also measured up to −30 pounds by the gauge. The device is positioned at the midsternum in alignment with the nipples.

Initial studies on ACD-CPR in both experimental animal models and human subjects late after cardiac arrest have demonstrated improved cardiopulmonary hemodynamics when compared with standard manual CPR (54,55,58,360–362). In one clinical study, conventional CPR was compared with ACD-CPR in 21 patients undergoing routine induction of ventricular fibrillation as part of a transvenous lead cardioverter/defibrillator implantation procedure (360). Mean CPP was increased throughout the entire CPR cycle with ACD-CPR (compression of 21.5 ± 9.0 mm Hg; decompression of 21.9 ± 8.7 mm Hg) compared with conventional CPR (compression of 17.9 ± 8.2 mm Hg; decompression of 18.5 ± 6.9 mm Hg; $p < .02$ and $p < .02$, respectively). Unfortunately, despite promising initial clinical results (347), several recent randomized clinical trials have not shown any superiority of ACD-CPR over conventional CPR (363–366). However, one trial conducted in Paris has reported benefit in short-term survival with this technique (367).

The American Heart Association considers ACD-CPR to be an acceptable alternative to standard CPR when rescue personnel adequately trained in use of the device are available (32); however, the device is not FDA approved for sale in the United States.

Interposed Abdominal Compression

Interposed abdominal compression CPR (IAC-CPR) (*e*Fig 69.0.4), also known as *abdominal counterpulsation CPR*, attempts to mimic intraaortic balloon counterpulsation. Two rescuers are needed to perform this technique: One rescuer compresses the sternum, and the other rescuer interposes abdominal compressions between each chest compression. Several investigators have demonstrated improvements in coronary perfusion, carotid and cerebral blood flows, and augmented venous return using IAC-CPR compared with standard CPR (59,61,71).

An early prehospital clinical trial in the mid-1980s failed to demonstrate any improvement in survival when IAC-CPR was compared with conventional CPR (368). Recently, IAC-CPR has been shown to improve survival in 143 consecutive patients experiencing in-hospital cardiac arrest with an initial arrest rhythm of asystole or EMD (78). Patients were randomized to receive either IAC-CPR or conventional CPR. The rate of ROSC was significantly higher in the group receiving IAC-CPR compared with the group receiving conventional CPR (49% vs. 28%, $p = .01$).

At 24 hours, there were significantly more patients alive in the IAC-CPR group than in the conventional CPR group (33% vs. 13%, $p = .009$). No complications were demonstrated in a small subset of patients who died and underwent autopsy.

Similar findings were noted in another randomized clinical trial involving 135 resuscitation attempts in 103 patients (80). The rate of ROSC was significantly greater in the group receiving IAC-CPR compared with the group receiving conventional CPR (51% vs. 27%, $p = .007$). At hospital discharge, a significantly greater proportion of patients were alive in the IAC-CPR group than in the conventional CPR group (25% vs. 7%, $p = .02$). Eight (17%) of 48 patients who received IAC-CPR survived to hospital discharge neurologically intact compared with only three (6%) of 55 patients from the conventional CPR group (not significant). Thus, IAC-CPR appears to be a promising technique that may improve survival in selected cardiac arrest patients. The American Heart Association recommends the use of IAC-CPR for in-hospital resuscitation as an alternative to standard CPR whenever sufficient personnel trained in the technique are available (32).

Other Cardiopulmonary Resuscitation Techniques

A number of other interesting CPR techniques have been evaluated recently. Some of these techniques have been unequivocally shown to be of little or no clinical value. For example, the use of abdominal binding with a pneumatic antishock garment (also known as *military antishock trousers*, or *MAST*) during resuscitation does not improve survival even though it increases mean arterial pressure (369). The problem is that it raises central venous pressure by the same amount as the increase in arterial pressure, thus failing to increase the CPP. Similarly, simultaneous compression-ventilation CPR has been shown to decrease survival from cardiac arrest compared with conventional CPR, perhaps by causing collapse of arteries exiting the thorax and/or by creating significant barotrauma (370,371).

On the other hand, "cough" CPR has been shown to be of value in experimental animals and in clinical use (40,372–375). At the onset of lethal arrhythmias such as asystole, profound bradycardia, ventricular tachycardia, or fibrillation, coughing may assist in maintaining consciousness and an adequate systolic blood pressure. In some cases, it may also play a role in terminating the arrhythmia. The simplicity and effectiveness of this technique warrant its consideration for greater clinical use by health care providers. Similarly, "high-impulse CPR" using a rapid downstroke velocity may, in some circumstances, improve blood flow by transferring greater energy into the thorax and, perhaps, by enhancing the "cardiac pump" mechanism (44,45).

An impedance threshold valve has been developed to enhance the return of blood to the thorax during the chest

THE FUTURE

Better understanding of the mechanisms responsible for blood flow during closed-chest compression is leading to new CPR devices and techniques. It is highly probable that one or more of these innovations will result in significant improvement in the likelihood of successful resuscitation. If this occurs, the greatest challenge will be to better define from a medical and ethical perspective who should, or should not, receive such intervention. In addition, there will likely be much broader implementation of public access defibrillation.

decompression phase (376). This new device enhances negative intrathoracic pressure during chest wall recoil or the decompression phase, leading to improved vital organ perfusion during both standard CPR and ACD-CPR (376–381). With ACD-CPR, addition of the impedance threshold valve results in sustained diastolic pressures of more than 55 mm Hg in patients in cardiac arrest. The new valve shows promise for patients in asystole or shock refractory ventricular fibrillation, when enhanced return of blood flow to the chest is needed to "prime the pump." The American Heart Association considers this device to be acceptable as an adjunct to be used with ACD-CPR (32).

Public Access Defibrillation

Another innovative idea is termed "public access defibrillation," so named because the intent is to have non–health care citizens perform early defibrillation. So far, early attempts to train family members of high-risk patients or community workers in the use of AEDs have met with variable success. For example, Eisenberg et al. trained family members of 59 patients who had survived out-of-hospital cardiac arrest in King County, Washington (382). Only six of the ten cardiac arrests that occurred in these patients were defibrillated successfully, and only one patient survived for a few months and sustained new neurologic impairment.

In contrast, Swenson et al. reported three successful resuscitations out of five cardiac arrests in 48 patients whose families had been trained to use an AED (383). More encouraging results have been obtained when community first responders have been trained to use automated defibrillators. For example, 160 security officers were trained to use these devices at Vancouver's World Expo 1986. Five cardiac arrests occurred among the 22.1 million visitors. Security personnel applied the AED correctly in all cases. In two cases, the initial rhythm was ventricular fibrillation. and defibrillation was successful. Both patients had a pulse and were regaining consciousness by the time EMS personnel arrived on the scene (384). Other experimental approaches to rapid defibrillation in the workplace include use on commercial aircraft, airports, British rail stations, oil platforms in the North Sea, electricity plants, casinos, passenger cruise ships, and merchant marine vessels (385–391).

In Las Vegas casinos, security officers were trained and equipped to use AEDs on suspected cardiac arrest victims (388). AEDs were placed in the casinos at strategic locations to permit rapid defibrillation in 3 minutes or less from collapse. Out of 105 patients whose initial cardiac rhythm was ventricular fibrillation, 56 (53%) survived to hospital discharge. Among the 90 patients whose collapse was witnessed (86%), the clinically relevant time intervals were a mean (± standard deviation) of 3.5 ± 2.9 minutes from collapse to attachment of the defibrillator, 4.4 ± 2.9 minutes from collapse to the delivery of the first defibrillation shock, and 9.8 ± 4.3 minutes from collapse to the arrival of the paramedics. The survival rate was 74% for patients who received their first defibrillation no later than 3 minutes after a witnessed collapse and 49% for those who received their first defibrillation after more than 3 minutes.

AEDs are also becoming common on commercial aircraft (389–392). American Airlines was the first U.S. carrier to deploy this technology. In a recent report on the carrier's experience, American Airlines reported that AEDs were attached to 200 patients (191 on the aircraft and nine in the terminal), including 99 with documented loss of consciousness. Electrocardiographic data were available for 185 patients. A shock was advised in all 14 patients who had electrocardiographically documented ventricular fibrillation, and no shock was advised in the remaining patients (sensitivity and specificity of the defibrillator in identifying ventricular fibrillation of 100%). The first shock successfully defibrillated the heart in 13 patients (defibrillation was withheld in one case at the family's request). The rate of survival to discharge from the hospital after shock with the AED was 40%. A total of 36 patients either died or were resuscitated after cardiac arrest. No complications arose from use of the AED as a monitor in conscious passengers.

The National Heart, Lung, and Blood Institute and the American Heart Association are encouraging research into the safety, efficacy, and potential cost-benefit of this interesting concept (393–397). A multicenter, prospective, randomized, controlled clinical trial is currently under way to further assess the safety, efficacy, and cost-benefit of more widespread use of AEDs by trained laypersons in a public setting (397).

REFERENCES

1. Hermreck AS. A history of cardiopulmonary resuscitation. *Am J Surg* 1988;156:430–436.
2. Gordon AS, Raymon F, Sadove M, Ivy AC. Manual artificial respiration. *JAMA* 1950;14:1447–1452.
3. Wright-St Clair RE. The development of resuscitation. *N Z Med J* 1985;8:339–341.
4. Dill DB. Symposium on mouth-to-mouth resuscitation (expired air inflation). *Council Med Phys* 1958;167:317–319.
5. Roth N. First stammering of the heart: Ludwig's kymograph. *Med Instrum* 1978;13:226.
6. McWilliam JA. Cardiac failure and sudden death. *BMJ* 1889;5:6–8.
7. Beck CS. Prevost and Battelli. *Ariz Med* 1965;22:691–694.
8. Kouwenhoven WB, Hooker RD. Resuscitation by countershock. *Electr Engin* 1922:475–477.
9. Zoll PM, Linenthal AJ, Gibson W, et al. Termination of ventricular fibrillation in man by externally applied electrical countershock. *N Engl J Med* 1956;254:727–732.
10. Jude JR, Kouwenhoven WB, Knickerbocker GG. External cardiac resuscitation. *Monogr Surg Sci* 1964;1:59–117.
11. Jude JR, Kouwenhoven WB, Knickerbocker GG. Closed chest cardiac massage. *JAMA* 1960;173:1064–1067.
12. Ad hoc committee on cardiopulmonary resuscitation of the Division of Medical Sciences National Academy of Sciences—National Research Council. Cardiopulmonary resuscitation. *JAMA* 1966;198:372–379.
13. American Heart Association Emergency Cardiac Care Committee. Guidelines for cardiopulmonary resuscitation (CPR) and emergency cardiac care (ECC). *JAMA* 1992;268:2171–2295.
14. American Heart Association. Standards and guidelines for cardiopulmonary resuscitation (CPR) and emergency cardiac care (ECC). *JAMA* 1986;255:2841–3044.
15. American Heart Association. Standards and guidelines for cardiopulmonary resuscitation (CPR) and emergency cardiac care (ECC). *JAMA* 1980;244:453–509.
16. American Heart Association. Standards for cardiopulmonary resuscitation (CPR) and emergency cardiac care (ECC). *JAMA* 1974;227:833–868.
17. The American Heart Association in collaboration with the International Liaison Committee on Resuscitation. Guidelines 2000 for cardiopulmonary resuscitation and emergency cardiovascular care. Part 6: advanced cardiovascular life support: 7C: a guide to the International ACLS algorithms. *Circulation* 2000;102:I142–157.
18. The American Heart Association in collaboration with the International Liaison Committee on Resuscitation. Guidelines 2000 for cardiopulmonary resuscitation and emergency cardiovascular care. Part 6: advanced cardiovascular life support: 7B: understanding the algorithm approach to ACLS. *Circulation* 2000;102:I140–141.
19. The American Heart Association in collaboration with the International Liaison Committee on Resuscitation. Guidelines 2000 for cardiopulmonary resuscitation and emergency cardiovascular care. Part 12: from science to survival: strengthening the chain of survival in every community. *Circulation* 2000;102:I358–370.
20. The American Heart Association in collaboration with the International Liaison Committee on Resuscitation. Guidelines 2000 for cardiopulmonary resuscitation and emergency cardiovascular care. Part 11: neonatal resuscitation. *Circulation* 2000;102:I343–357.
21. The American Heart Association in collaboration with the International Liaison Committee on Resuscitation. Guidelines 2000 for cardiopulmonary resuscitation and emergency cardiovascular care. Part 10: pediatric advanced life support. *Circulation* 2000;102:I291–342.
22. The American Heart Association in collaboration with the International Liaison Committee on Resuscitation. Guidelines 2000 for cardiopulmonary resuscitation and emergency cardiovascular care. Part 9: pediatric basic life support. *Circulation* 2000;102:I253–290.
23. The American Heart Association in collaboration with the International Liaison Committee on Resuscitation. Guidelines 2000 for cardiopulmonary resuscitation and emergency cardiovascular care. Part 8: advanced challenges in resuscitation: section 3: special challenges in ECC. *Circulation* 2000;102:I229–252.
24. The American Heart Association in collaboration with the International Liaison Committee on Resuscitation. Guidelines 2000 for cardiopulmonary resuscitation and emergency cardiovascular care. Part 8: advanced challenges in resuscitation: section 2: toxicology in ECC. *Circulation* 2000;102:I223–228.
25. The American Heart Association in collaboration with the International Liaison Committee on Resuscitation. Guidelines 2000 for cardiopulmonary resuscitation and emergency cardiovascular care. Part 8: advanced challenges in resuscitation: section 1: life-threatening electrolyte abnormalities. *Circulation* 2000;102:I217–222.
26. The American Heart Association in collaboration with the International Liaison Committee on Resuscitation. Guidelines 2000 for cardiopulmonary resuscitation and emergency cardiovascular care. Part 7: the era of reperfusion: section 2: acute stroke. *Circulation* 2000;102:I204–216.
27. The American Heart Association in collaboration with the International Liaison Committee on Resuscitation. Guidelines 2000 for cardiopulmonary resuscitation and emergency cardiovascular care. Part 7: the era of reperfusion: section 1: acute coronary syndromes (acute myocardial infarction). *Circulation* 2000;102:I172–203.
28. The American Heart Association in collaboration with the International Liaison Committee on Resuscitation. Guidelines 2000 for cardiopulmonary resuscitation and emergency cardiovascular care. Part 6: advanced cardiovascular life support: section 8: postresuscitation care. *Circulation* 2000;102:I166–171.
29. The American Heart Association in collaboration with the International Liaison Committee on Resuscitation. Guidelines 2000 for cardiopulmonary resuscitation and emergency cardiovascular care. Part 6: advanced cardiovascular life support: section 7: algorithm approach to ACLS emergencies: section 7A: principles and practice of ACLS. *Circulation* 2000;102:I136–139.
30. The American Heart Association in collaboration with the International Liaison Committee on Resuscitation. Guide-

lines 2000 for cardiopulmonary resuscitation and emergency cardiovascular care. Part 6: advanced cardiovascular life support: section 6: pharmacology II: agents to optimize cardiac output and blood pressure. *Circulation* 2000;102:I129–135.

31. The American Heart Association in collaboration with the International Liaison Committee on Resuscitation. Guidelines 2000 for cardiopulmonary resuscitation and emergency cardiovascular care. Part 6: advanced cardiovascular life support: section 5: pharmacology I: agents for arrhythmias. *Circulation* 2000;102:I112–128.

32. The American Heart Association in collaboration with the International Liaison Committee on Resuscitation. Guidelines 2000 for cardiopulmonary resuscitation and emergency cardiovascular care. Part 6: advanced cardiovascular life support: section 4: devices to assist circulation. *Circulation* 2000;102:I105–111.

33. The American Heart Association in collaboration with the International Liaison Committee on Resuscitation. Guidelines 2000 for cardiopulmonary resuscitation and emergency cardiovascular care. Part 6: advanced cardiovascular life support: section 3: adjuncts for oxygenation, ventilation and airway control. *Circulation* 2000;102:I95–104.

34. The American Heart Association in collaboration with the International Liaison Committee on Resuscitation. Guidelines 2000 for cardiopulmonary resuscitation and emergency cardiovascular care. Part 6: advanced cardiovascular life support: section 2: defibrillation. *Circulation* 2000;102:I90–94.

35. The American Heart Association in collaboration with the International Liaison Committee on Resuscitation. Guidelines 2000 for cardiopulmonary resuscitation and emergency cardiovascular care. Part 6: advanced cardiovascular life support: section 1: introduction to ACLS 2000: overview of recommended changes in ACLS from the guidelines 2000 conference. *Circulation* 2000;102:I86–89.

36. The American Heart Association in collaboration with the International Liaison Committee on Resuscitation. Guidelines 2000 for cardiopulmonary resuscitation and emergency cardiovascular care. Part 5: new guidelines for first aid. *Circulation* 2000;102:I77–85.

37. The American Heart Association in collaboration with the International Liaison Committee on Resuscitation. Guidelines 2000 for cardiopulmonary resuscitation and emergency cardiovascular care. Part 4: the automated external defibrillator: key link in the chain of survival. *Circulation* 2000;102:I60–76.

38. The American Heart Association in collaboration with the International Liaison Committee on Resuscitation. Guidelines 2000 for cardiopulmonary resuscitation and emergency cardiovascular care. Part 3: adult basic life support. *Circulation* 2000;102:I22–59.

39. Criley JM, Blaufuss AH, Kissel GL. Self-induced form of cardiopulmonary resuscitation. *JAMA* 1976;236:1246–1250.

40. Niemann JT, Rosborough JP, Ung S, et al. Cough CPR. Documentation of systemic perfusion in man and in an experimental model: a "window" to the mechanism of blood flow in external CPR. *Crit Care Med* 1980;8:141–146.

41. Halperin HR, Brower R, Weisfeldt ML, et al. Air trapping in the lungs during cardiopulmonary resuscitation in dogs. A mechanism for generating changes in intrathoracic pressure. *Circ Res* 1989;65:946–954.

42. Weisfeldt ML, Halperin HR. Cardiopulmonary resuscitation: beyond cardiac massage. *Circulation* 1986;74:443–448.

43. Fisher J, Vaghaiwalla F, Tsitlik J, et al. Determinants and clinical significance of jugular venous valve competence. *Circulation* 1982;65:188.

44. Maier GW, Newton JR Jr, Wolfe JA, et al. The influence of manual chest compression rate on hemodynamic support during cardiac arrest: high-impulse cardiopulmonary resuscitation. *Circulation* 1986;74[6 Pt 2]:IV51–59.

45. Feneley MP, Maier GW, Gaynor JW, et al. Sequence of mitral valve motion and transmitral blood flow during manual cardiopulmonary resuscitation in dogs. *Circulation* 1987;76:363–375.

46. Wolfe JA, Maier GW, Newton JR Jr, et al. Physiologic determinants of coronary blood flow during external cardiac massage. *J Thorac Cardiovasc Surg* 1988;95:523–532.

47. Deshmukh HG, Weil MH, Rackow EC, et al. Echocardiographic observations during cardiopulmonary resuscitation: a preliminary report. *Crit Care Med* 1985;13:904–906.

48. Porter TR, Ornato JP, Guard CS, et al. Transesophageal echocardiography to assess mitral valve function and flow during cardiopulmonary resuscitation. *Am J Cardiol* 1992;70:1056–1060.

49. Pell ACH, Guly LM, Sutherland YR, et al. Mechanism of closed chest cardiopulmonary resuscitation investigated by transoesophageal echocardiography. *J Accid Emerg Med* 1994;11:139–143.

50. Kuhn C, Juchems R, Frese W. Transoesophageal echocardiography during cardiopulmonary resuscitation in man: proof of the cardiac pump theory? *Intensiv Notfallbehandl* 1994;19:1–7.

51. Halperin HR, Tsitlik JE, Guerci AD, et al. Determinants of blood flow to vital organs during cardiopulmonary resuscitation in dogs. *Circulation* 1986;73:539–550.

52. Ornato JP, Gonzalez ER, Garnett AR, et al. Effect of cardiopulmonary resuscitation compression rate on end-tidal carbon dioxide concentration and arterial pressure in man. *Crit Care Med* 1988;16:241–245.

53. Tucker KJ, Redberg RF, Schiller NB, Cohen TJ. Active compression-decompression resuscitation: analysis of transmitral flow and left ventricular volume by transesophageal echocardiography in humans. Cardiopulmonary Resuscitation Working Group. *J Am Coll Cardiol* 1993;22:1485–1493.

54. Chang MW, Coffeen P, Lurie KG, et al. Active compression-decompression CPR improves vital organ perfusion in a dog model of ventricular fibrillation. *Chest* 1994;106:1250–1259.

55. Tucker KJ, Idris A. Clinical and laboratory investigations of active compression-decompression cardiopulmonary resuscitation. *Resuscitation* 1994;28:1–7.

56. Lurie KG. Active compression-decompression CPR: a progress report. *Resuscitation* 1994;28:115–122.

57. Cohen TJ, Tucker KJ, Lurie KG, et al. Active compression-decompression. A new method of cardiopulmonary resuscitation. *JAMA* 1992;267:2916–2923.

58. Lindner KH, Pfenninger EG, Lurie KG, et al. Effects of active compression-decompression resuscitation on myocardial and cerebral blood flow in pigs. *Circulation* 1993;88:1254–1263.

59. Einagle V, Bertrand F, Wise RA, et al. Interposed abdominal compressions and carotid blood flow during cardiopulmonary resuscitation. Support for a thoracoabdominal unit. *Chest* 1988;93:1206–1212.

60. Babbs CF, Tacker WA Jr. Cardiopulmonary resuscitation with interposed abdominal compression. *Circulation* 1986;74[6 Pt 2]:IV37–41.

61. McDonald JL. Effect of interposed abdominal compression during CPR on central arterial and venous pressures. *Am J Emerg Med* 1985;3:156–159.

62. Hoekstra OS, Van Lambalgen AA, Groeneveld ABJ, et al. Abdominal compressions increase vital organ perfusion during CPR in dogs: relation with efficacy of thoracic compressions. *Ann Emerg Med* 1995;25:375–385.

63. Babbs CF, Blevins WE. Abdominal binding and counterpulsation in cardiopulmonary resuscitation. *Crit Care Clin* 1986;2:319–332.

64. Kern KB, Carter AB, Showen RL, et al. Twenty-four hour survival in a canine model of cardiac arrest comparing three methods of manual cardiopulmonary resuscitation. *J Am Coll Cardiol* 1986;7:859–867.

65. Babbs CF, Thelander K. Theoretically optimal duty cycles for chest and abdominal compression during external cardiopulmonary resuscitation. *Acad Emerg Med* 1995;2:698–707.

66. Hoekstra OS, van Lambalgen AA, Groeneveld AB, et al. Abdominal compressions increase vital organ perfusion during CPR in dogs: relation with efficacy of thoracic compressions. *Ann Emerg Med* 1995;25:375–385.

67. Babbs CF. The evolution of abdominal compression in cardiopulmonary resuscitation. *Acad Emerg Med* 1994;1:469–477.

68. Hillman H. Abdominal pumping. *Acad Emerg Med* 1994;1:478–481.

69. Ward KR. Possible reasons for the variability of human responses to IAC-CPR. *Acad Emerg Med* 1994;1:482–489.

70. Sack JB, Kesselbrenner MB. Hemodynamics, survival benefits, and complications of interposed abdominal compression during cardiopulmonary resuscitation. *Acad Emerg Med* 1994;1:490–497.

71. Adams CP, Martin GB, Rivers EP, et al. Hemodynamics of interposed abdominal compression during human cardiopulmonary resuscitation. *Acad Emerg Med* 1994;1:498–502.

72. Tucker KJ, Savitt MA, Idris A, Redberg RF. Cardiopulmonary resuscitation. Historical perspectives, physiology, and future directions. *Arch Intern Med* 1994;154:2141–2150.

73. Inchiosa MA Jr, Frost EA. Interposed abdominal compression-CPR: which patients are benefited? Why? *Circulation* 1994;90:1113–1114.

74. Babbs CF, Sack JB, Kern KB. Interposed abdominal compression as an adjunct to cardiopulmonary resuscitation. *Am Heart J* 1994;127:412–421.

75. Babbs CF. Interposed abdominal compression-cardiopulmonary resuscitation: are we missing the mark in clinical trials? *Am Heart J* 1993;126:1035–1041.

76. Salgo IS. Interposed abdominal compression—cardiopulmonary resuscitation. *Circulation* 1993;88:806–807.

77. Babbs CF. Interposed abdominal compression-CPR: a case study in cardiac arrest research. *Ann Emerg Med* 1993;22:24–32.

78. Sack JB, Kesselbrenner MB, Jarrad A. Interposed abdominal compression-cardiopulmonary resuscitation and resuscitation outcome during asystole and electromechanical dissociation. *Circulation* 1992;86:1692–1700.

79. Babbs CF. Interposed abdominal compression-CPR. Low technology for the clinical armamentarium. *Circulation* 1992;86:2011–2012.

80. Sack JB, Kesselbrenner MB, Bregman D. Survival from in-hospital cardiac arrest with interposed abdominal counterpulsation during cardiopulmonary resuscitation. *JAMA* 1992;267:379–385.

81. Barranco F, Lesmes A, Irles JA, et al. Cardiopulmonary resuscitation with simultaneous chest and abdominal compression: comparative study in humans. *Resuscitation* 1990;20:67–77.

82. Lindner KH, Ahnefeld FW, Bowdler IM. Cardiopulmonary resuscitation with interposed abdominal compression after asphyxial or fibrillatory cardiac arrest in pigs. *Anesthesiology* 1990;72:675–681.

83. Bossaert L, Van Hoeyweghen R. Bystander cardiopulmonary resuscitation (CPR) in out-of-hospital cardiac arrest. *Resuscitation* 1989;17:S55–69.

84. Cobb LA, Hallstrom AP. Community-based cardiopulmonary resuscitation: what have we learned? *Ann N Y Acad Sci* 1982;382:330–342.

85. Litwin PE, Eisenberg MS, Hallstrom AP, Cummins RO. The location of collapse and its effect on survival from cardiac arrest. *Ann Emerg Med* 1987;16:787–791.

86. Dracup K, Heaney DM, Taylor SE, et al. Can family members of high-risk cardiac patients learn cardiopulmonary resuscitation? *Arch Intern Med* 1989;149:61–64.

87. Cobb LA, Werner JA, Trobaugh GB. Sudden cardiac death. I. A decade's experience with out-of-hospital resuscitation. *Mod Concepts Cardiovasc Dis* 1980;49:31.

88. Messerli FH, Soria F. Hypertension, left ventricular hypertrophy, ventricular ectopy, and sudden death. *Am J Med* 1992;93(2A):21S–26S.

89. Jimenez RA, Myerburg RJ. Sudden cardiac death. Magnitude of the problem, substrate/trigger interaction, and populations at high risk. *Cardiol Clin* 1993;11:1–9.

90. Fornes P, Lecomte D, Nicolas G. [Sudden coronary death outside of hospital—a comparative autopsy study of subjects with and without previous cardiovascular diseases]. *Arch Mal Coeur Vaiss* 1994;87:319–324.

91. Cas LD, Metra M, Nodari S, et al. Stress and ischemic heart disease. *Cardiologia* 1993;38[12 Suppl 1]:415–425.

92. Kaada B. An emotional trigger mechanism for sudden infant death. *Arch Dis Child* 1991;66:274.

93. Bairey CN, Krantz DS, Rozanski A. Mental stress as an acute trigger of ischemic left ventricular dysfunction and blood pressure elevation in coronary artery disease. *Am J Cardiol* 1990;66):28G–31G.

94. Adler SR. Refugee stress and folk belief: Hmong sudden deaths. *Soc Sci Med* 1995;40:1623–1629.

95. Leor J, Poole WK, Kloner RA. Sudden cardiac death triggered by an earthquake. *N Engl J Med* 1996;334:413–419.

96. Muller JE, Abela GS, Nesto RW, Tofler GH. Triggers, acute risk factors and vulnerable plaques: the lexicon of a new frontier. *J Am Coll Cardiol* 1994;23:809–813.

97. Arntz HR, Willich SN, Stern R, et al. Circadian variation of cardiopulmonary disease onset in the general population: an emergency care system perspective from Berlin. *Ann Emerg Med* 1994;23:281–285.

98. Willich SN. Epidemiologic studies demonstrating increased morning incidence of sudden cardiac death. *Am J Cardiol* 1990;66:15G–17G.

99. Hohnloser SH, Klingenheben T. Insights into the pathogenesis of sudden cardiac death from analysis of circadian fluctuations of potential triggering factors. *Pacing Clin Electrophysiol* 1994;17:428–433.

100. Bayes de Luna A, Coumel P, Leclercq JF. Ambulatory sudden cardiac death: mechanisms of production of fatal arrhythmia on the basis of data from 157 cases. *Am Heart J* 1989;117:151–159.

101. Myerburg RJ, Conde CA, Sung RJ, et al. Clinical, electrophysiologic and hemodynamic profile of patients resuscitated from prehospital cardiac arrest. *Am J Med* 1980;68:568–576.

102. Weaver WD, Cobb LA, Hallstrom AP, et al. Factors influencing survival after out-of-hospital cardiac arrest. *J Am Coll Cardiol* 1986;7:754.

103. Hinkle LE, Argyros DC, Hayes JC, et al. Pathogenesis of an unexpected sudden death: role of early cycle ventricular contractions. *Am J Cardiol* 1977;39:873.

104. Schaffer WA, Cobb LA. Recurrent ventricular fibrillation and modes of death in survivors of out-of-hospital ventricular fibrillation. *N Engl J Med* 1975;293:259–262.

105. Cummins RO, Ornato JP, Thies WH, Pepe PE. Improving survival from sudden cardiac arrest: the "chain of survival" concept. A statement for health professionals from the Advanced Cardiac Life Support Subcommittee and the Emergency Cardiac Care Committee, American Heart Association. *Circulation* 1991;83:1832–1847.

106. Eisenberg MS, Bergner L, Hallstrom A. Cardiac resuscitation in the community. Importance of rapid provision and implications for program planning. *JAMA* 1979;241:1905–1907.

107. Walters G, Gluckman F. Planning a pre-hospital cardiac resuscitation programme: an analysis of community and system factors in London. *J R Coll Physicians Lond* 1989;23:107.

108. Stults KR. Phone first. *J Emerg Med Services* 1987;12:78.

109. Mayron R, Long RS, Ruiz E. The 911 emergency telephone number: impact on emergency medical systems access in a metropolitan area. *Am J Emerg Med* 1984;2:491–493.

110. Hunt RC, Allison EJJ, Yates JGI. The need for improved emergency medical services in Pitt County. *N C Med J* 1986;47:39–42.

111. Hunt RC, McCabe JB, Hamilton GC, Krohmer JR. Influence of emergency medical services systems and prehospital defibrillation on survival of sudden cardiac death victims. *Am J Emerg Med* 1989;7:68–82.

112. Murphy RJ, Luepker RV, Jacobs DRJ, et al. Citizen cardiopulmonary resuscitation training and use in a metropolitan area: the Minnesota Heart Survey. *Am J Public Health* 1984;74:513–515.

113. Selby ML, Kautz JA, Moore TJ, et al. Indicators of response to a mass media CPR recruitment campaign. *Am J Public Health* 1982;72:1039.

114. Mandel LP, Cobb LA. CPR training in the community. *Ann Emerg Med* 1985;14:669–671.

115. Gombeski WRJ, Effron DM, Ramirez AG, Moore TJ. Impact on retention: comparison of two CPR training programs. *Am J Public Health* 1982;72:849–852.

116. Muelleman RL, Ornato JP. Factors affecting the likelihood that cardiopulmonary resuscitation (CPR) will be used by trained rescuers. *Nebr Med J* 1985;70:172–177.

117. Goldberg RJ. Physicians and CPR training in high-risk family members. *Am J Public Health* 1987;77:671–672.

118. Bossaert L, Van Hoeyweghen R, The Cerebral Resuscitation Study Group. Evaluation of cardiopulmonary resuscitation (CPR) techniques. *Resuscitation* 1989;17:S99–109.

119. Van Hoeyweghen RJ, Bossaert LL, Mullie A, et al. Quality and efficiency of bystander CPR. Belgian Cerebral Resuscitation Study Group. *Resuscitation* 1993;26:47–52.

120. Ornato JP, Hallagan LF, McMahon SB, et al. Attitudes of BCLS instructors about mouth-to-mouth resuscitation during the AIDS epidemic. *Ann Emerg Med* 1990;19:151–156.

121. Cobb LA, Fahrenbruch CE, Walsh TR, et al. Influence of cardiopulmonary resuscitation prior to defibrillation in patients with out-of-hospital ventricular fibrillation. *JAMA* 1999;281:1182–1188.

122. Van Camp SP, Peterson RA. Cardiovascular complications of outpatient cardiac rehabilitation programs. *JAMA* 1986;256:1160–1163.

123. Haskell WL. Cardiovascular complications during exercise training in cardiac patients. *Circulation* 1978;57:920.

124. Hossack KF, Hartwig R. Cardiac arrest associated with supervised cardiac rehabilitation. *J Cardiac Rehab* 1982;2:402.

125. Ornato JP, McNeill SE, Craren EJ, Nelson NM. Limitation on effectiveness of rapid defibrillation by emergency medical technicians in a rural setting. *Ann Emerg Med* 1984;13:1096–1099.

126. Eisenberg MS, Copass MK, Hallstrom AP, et al. Treatment of out-of-hospital cardiac arrest with rapid defibrillation by emergency medical technicians. *N Engl J Med* 1980;302:1379–1383.

127. Kerber RE. Statement on early defibrillation from the Emergency Cardiac Care Committee, American Heart Association. *Circulation* 1991;83:2233.

128. Kaye W, Mancini ME, Giuliano KK, et al. Strengthening the in hospital chain of survival with rapid defibrillation by first responders using automated external defibrillators: training and retention issues. *Ann Emerg Med* 1995;25:163–168.

129. Barnes TA, Aufderheide TP, Mathews, et al. Clinical practice guidelines for resuscitation in acute care hospitals. *Respir Care* 1995;40:346–363.

130. Ornato JP, Racht EM, Fitch JJ, Berry JF. The need for ALS in urban and suburban EMS systems. *Ann Emerg Med* 1990;19:1469–1470.

131. Schneider T, Martens PR, Paschen H, et al. Multicenter, randomized, controlled trial of 150-J biphasic shocks compared with 200- to 360-J monophasic shocks in the resuscitation of out-of-hospital cardiac arrest victims. *Circulation* 2000;102:1780–1787.

132. Gliner BE, White RD. Electrocardiographic evaluation of defibrillation shocks delivered to out-of-hospital sudden cardiac arrest patients. *Resuscitation* 1999;41:133–144.

133. Gliner BE, Jorgenson DB, Poole JE, et al. Treatment of out-of-hospital cardiac arrest with a low-energy impedance-compensating biphasic waveform automatic external defibrillator. The LIFE Investigators. *Biomed Instrum Technol* 1998;32:631–644.

134. White RD. Early out-of-hospital experience with an impedance-compensating low-energy biphasic waveform automatic external defibrillator. *J Interv Card Electrophysiol* 1997;1:203–208; discussion 209–210.

135. Poole JE, White RD, Kanz KG, et al. Low-energy impedance-compensating biphasic waveforms terminate ventricular fibrillation at high rates in victims of out-of-hospital cardiac arrest. LIFE Investigators. *J Cardiovasc Electrophysiol* 1997;8:1373–1385.

136. Bardy GH, Marchlinski FE, Sharma AD, et al. Multicenter comparison of truncated biphasic shocks and standard damped sine wave monophasic shocks for transthoracic ventricular defibrillation. Transthoracic Investigators. *Circulation* 1996;94:2507–2514.

137. Bardy GH, Ivey TD, Allen MD, et al. A prospective randomized evaluation of biphasic versus monophasic waveform pulses on defibrillation efficacy in humans. *J Am Coll Cardiol* 1989;14:728–733.

138. Cummins RO, Hazinski MF, Kerber RE, et al. Low-energy biphasic waveform defibrillation: evidence-based review applied to emergency cardiovascular care guidelines: a statement for healthcare professionals from the American Heart Association Committee on Emergency Cardiovascular Care and the Subcommittees on Basic Life Support, Advanced Cardiac Life Support, and Pediatric Resuscitation. *Circulation* 1998;97:1654–1667.

139. Ewy GA. Defining electromechanical dissociation. *Ann Emerg Med* 1984;13:830–832.

140. Ornato JP. Special resuscitation situations: near drowning, traumatic injury, electric shock, and hypothermia. *Circulation* 1986;74:IV23–26.

141. Harrison EE, Amey BD. Use of calcium in electromechanical dissociation. *Ann Emerg Med* 1984;13:944–945.

142. Stueven H, Thompson BM, Aprahamian C, et al. Use of calcium in prehospital cardiac arrest. *Ann Emerg Med* 1983;12:136–139.

143. Dembo DH. Calcium in advanced life support. *Crit Care Med* 1981;9:358–359.

144. Carlon GC, Howland WS, Kahn RC, et al. Calcium chloride administration in normocalcemic critically ill patients. *Crit Care Med* 1980;8:209–212.

145. Schanne FAX, Kane AB, Young EE, Farber JL. Calcium dependence of toxic cell death: a final common pathway. *Science* 1979;206:700–702.

146. Bodai BI, Smith JPT, Ward RE, et al. Emergency thoracotomy in the management of trauma. A review. *JAMA* 1983;249:1891–1896.

147. Paradis NA, Martin GB, Rivers EP. Use of open chest cardiopulmonary resuscitation after failure of standard closed chest CPR: illustrative cases. *Resuscitation* 1992;24:61–71.

148. Battistella FD, Nugent W, Owings JT, Anderson JT. Field triage of the pulseless trauma patient. *Arch Surg* 1999;134:742–745; discussion 745–746.

149. Ewy GA, Dahl CF, Zimmerman M, et al. Ventricular fibrillation masquerading as ventricular standstill. *Crit Care Med* 1981;9:841–844.

150. Iseri LT, Humphrey SB, Siner EJ. Prehospital bradyasystolic cardiac arrest. *Ann Intern Med* 1978;88:741–745.

151. O'Rourke GW, Greene NM. Autonomic blockade and the resting heart rate in man. *Am Heart J* 1970;80:469–474.

152. Ornato JP, Carveth WL, Windle JR. Pacemaker insertion for prehospital bradyasystolic cardiac arrest. *Ann Emerg Med* 1984;13:101–103.

153. Zoll PM, Zoll RH, Falk RH, et al. External noninvasive temporary cardiac pacing. *Circulation* 1985;71:937–944.

154. Falk RH, Jacobs L, Sinclair A, et al. External non-invasive cardiac pacing in out-of-hospital cardiac arrest. *Crit Care Med* 1983;11:779–782.

155. Tucker KJ, Shaburihvili TS, Gedevanishvili AT. Manual external (fist) pacing during high-degree atrioventricular block: a lifesaving intervention. *Am J Emerg Med* 1995;13:53–54.

156. Belardinelli L, Linden J, Berne RM. The cardiac effects of adenosine. *Prog Cardiovasc Dis* 1989;32:73–97.

157. Clemo HF, Belardinelli L. Effect of adenosine on atrioventricular conduction. I. Site and characterization of adenosine action in the guinea pig atrioventricular node. *Circ Res* 1986;59:427–436.

158. Viskin S, Belhassen B, Roth A, et al. Aminophylline for bradyasystolic cardiac arrest refractory to atropine and epinephrine. *Ann Intern Med* 1993;118:279–281.

159. Gareis R, Stork T, Mockel M, et al. Theophylline in rhythm asystole and pulseless bradyarrhythmia. *Intensivmed Notf Med* 1995;32:147–154.

160. Mader TJ, Smithline HA, Gibson P. Aminophylline in undifferentiated out-of-hospital asystolic cardiac arrest. *Resuscitation* 1999;41:39–45.

161. Littmann L, Ashline PT, Hayes WJ, et al. Aminophylline fails to improve the outcome of cardiopulmonary resuscitation from prolonged ventricular fibrillation: a placebo-controlled, randomized, blinded experimental study. *J Am Coll Cardiol* 1994;23:1708–1714.

162. Kovach AGB, Sandor P. Cerebral blood flow and brain function during hypotension and shock. *Annu Rev Physiol* 1976;38:571.

163. Michael JR, Guerci AD, Koehler RC, et al. Mechanisms by which epinephrine augments cerebral and myocardial perfusion during cardiopulmonary resuscitation in dogs. *Circulation* 1984;69:822–835.

164. Crile G, Dolley DH. An experimental research into the resuscitation of dogs killed by anesthetics and asphyxia. *J Exp Med* 1906;8:713–725.

165. Crile GW. Preliminary note on a method of resuscitation of apparently recently dead animals. *Cleveland Med J* 1903;2:35.

166. Redding JS, Pearson JW. Resuscitation from ventricular fibrillation. *JAMA* 1969;203:255–260.

167. Pearson JW, Redding JS. Influence of peripheral vascular tone on cardiac resuscitation. *Anesth Analg* 1967;46:746–752.

168. Pearson JW, Redding JS. Peripheral vascular tone in cardiac resuscitation. *Anesth Analg* 1965;44:746–762.

169. Pearson JW, Redding JS. The role of epinephrine in cardiac resuscitation. *Anesth Analg* 1963;42:599–606.

170. Pearson JW, Redding JS. Epinephrine in cardiac resuscitation. *Am Heart J* 1963;66:210–214.

171. Kern KB, Ewy GA, Voorhees WD, et al. Myocardial perfusion pressure: a predictor of 24-hour survival during prolonged cardiac arrest in dogs. *Resuscitation* 1988;16:241–250.

172. Niemann JT. Differences in cerebral and myocardial perfusion during closed-chest resuscitation. *Ann Emerg Med* 1984;13:849–853.

173. Sanders AB, Ewy GA, Taft TV. Prognostic and therapeutic importance of the aortic diastolic pressure in resuscitation from cardiac arrest. *Crit Care Med* 1984;12:871–873.

174. Paradis NA, Martin GB, Rivers EP, et al. Coronary perfusion pressure and the return of spontaneous circulation in human cardiopulmonary resuscitation. *JAMA* 1990;263:1106–1113.

175. Ralston SH, Voorhees WD, Babbs CF. Intrapulmonary epinephrine during prolonged cardiopulmonary resuscitation: improved regional blood flow and resuscitation in dogs. *Ann Emerg Med* 1984;13:79–86.

176. Grunau CFV. Doppler ultrasound monitoring of systemic blood flow during CPR. *JACEP* 1978;1978:180–185.

177. Taylor GJ, Tucker WM, Greene HL, et al. Importance of prolonged compression during cardiopulmonary resuscitation in man. *N Engl J Med* 1977;296:1515–1517.

178. McDonald JL. Systolic and mean arterial pressures during manual and mechanical CPR in humans. *Ann Emerg Med* 1982;11:292–295.

179. Ornato JP, Levine RL, Young DS, et al. The effect of applied chest compression force on systemic arterial pressure and end-tidal carbon dioxide concentration during CPR in human beings. *Ann Emerg Med* 1989;18:732–737.

180. Chandra NC, Tsitlik JE, Halperin HR, et al. Observations of hemodynamics during human cardiopulmonary resuscitation. *Crit Care Med* 1990;18:929–934.

181. Sanders AB, Oble M, Ewy GA. Coronary perfusion pressure during cardiopulmonary resuscitation. *Am J Emerg Med* 1985;3:11–14.

182. Swenson RD, Weaver WD, Niskanen RA, et al. Hemodynamics in humans during conventional and experimental methods of cardiopulmonary resuscitation. *Circulation* 1988;78:630–639.

183. Gonzalez ER, Ornato JP, Garnett AR, et al. Dose-dependent vasopressor response to epinephrine during CPR in human beings *Ann Emerg Med* 1989;18:920–926.

184. Paradis NA, Martin GB, Goetting MG, et al. Aortic pressure during human cardiac arrest. Identification of pseudo-electromechanical dissociation. *Chest* 1992;101:123–128.

185. Thomsen JE, Stenlund RR, Rowe GG. Intracardiac pressures during closed-chest cardiac massage. *JAMA* 1968;205:116–118.

186. Paradis NA, Martin GB, Goetting MG, et al. Simultaneous aortic, jugular bulb, and right atrial pressures during cardiopulmonary resuscitation in humans. Insights into mechanisms. *Circulation* 1989;80:361–368.

187. Chandra N, Guerci A, Weisfeldt ML, et al. Contrasts between intrathoracic pressures during external chest compression and cardiac massage. *Crit Care Med* 1981;9:789–792.

188. Rudikoff MT, Maughan WL, Effron M, et al. Mechanism of blood flow during cardiopulmonary resuscitation. *Circulation* 1980;61:345–352.

189. Newton JR Jr, Glower DD, Wolfe JA, et al. A physiologic comparison of external cardiac massage techniques. *J Thorac Cardiovasc Surg* 1988;95:892–901.

190. Ornato JP, Ryschon TW, Gonzalez ER, Bredthauer JL. Rapid change in pulmonary vascular hemodynamics with pulmonary edema during cardiopulmonary resuscitation. *Am J Emerg Med* 1985;3:137–142.

191. Dohi S, Ujike Y, Nishikawa T, Miyabe M. Pulmonary hemodynamics during external cardiac massage in humans. *Jpn Heart J* 1982;31:222–228.

192. Dohi S. Post-cardiopulmonary resuscitation pulmonary edema. *Crit Care Med* 1983;11:434–437.

193. Paidipaty BBT, Kyff J, Vaughn S, Puri VK. Pulmonary artery catheterization and hemodynamic monitoring after cardiopulmonary resuscitation. *Acute Care* 1984;10:189–193.

194. Nagel EL, Fine EG, Krischer JP, et al. Complications of CPR. *Crit Care Med* 1981;9:424.

195. Ward KR, Yealy DM. End-tidal carbon dioxide monitoring in emergency medicine, Part 1: Basic principles. *Acad Emerg Med* 1998;5:628–636.

196. Ward KR, Yealy DM. End-tidal carbon dioxide monitoring in emergency medicine, Part 2: clinical applications. *Acad Emerg Med* 1998;5:637–646.

197. Ornato JP, Garnett AR, Glauser FL. Relationship between cardiac output and the end-tidal carbon dioxide tension. *Ann Emerg Med* 1990;19:1104–1106.

198. Phan CQ, Tremper KK, Lee SE, et al. Noninvasive monitoring of carbon dioxide: a comparison of the partial pressure of transcutaneous and end-tidal carbon dioxide with the partial pressure of arterial carbon dioxide. *J Clin Monit* 1987;3:149–154.

199. Goldberg JS, Rawle PR, Zehnder JL, Sladen RN. Colorimetric end-tidal carbon dioxide monitoring for tracheal intubation. *Anesth Analg* 1990;70:191–194.

200. Strunin L, Williams T. The FEF end-tidal carbon dioxide detector. *Anesthesiology* 1989;71:621–622.

201. MacLeod BA, Heller MB, Gerard J, et al. Verification of endotracheal tube placement with colorimetric end-tidal CO_2 detection. *Ann Emerg Med* 1991;20:267–270.

202. Menegazzi JJ, Heller MB. Endotracheal tube confirmation with colorimetric CO_2 detectors. *Anesth Analg* 1990;71:440–446.

203. Ornato JP, Shipley JB, Racht EM, et al. Multicenter study of a portable, hand-size, colorimetric end-tidal carbon dioxide detection device. *Ann Emerg Med* 1992;21:518–523.

204. Garnett AR, Gervin CA, Gervin AS. Capnographic waveforms in esophageal intubation: effect of carbonated beverages. *Ann Emerg Med* 1989;18:387–390.

205. MacKenzie GJ, Taylor SH. Haemodynamic effects of external cardiac compression. *Lancet* 1964;1:1342–1345.

206. Del Guercio LRM, Feins NR, Cohn JD, et al. Comparison of blood flow during external and internal cardiac massage in man. *Circulation* 1965;31[Suppl 1]:171–180.

207. Del Guercio LRM, Coomaraswamy RP, State D. Cardiac output and other hemodynamic variables during external cardiac massage in man. *N Engl J Med* 1963;269:1398–1404.

208. Garnett AR, Ornato JP, Gonzalez ER, Johnson EB. End-tidal carbon dioxide monitoring during cardiopulmonary resuscitation. *JAMA* 1987;257:512–515.

209. Falk JL, Rackow EC, Weil MH. End-tidal carbon dioxide concentration during cardiopulmonary resuscitation. *N Engl J Med* 1988;318:607–611.

210. Gudipati CV, Weil MH, Bisera J, et al. Expired carbon dioxide: a noninvasive monitor of cardiopulmonary resuscitation. *Circulation* 1988;77:234–239.

211. Weil MH, Bisera J, Trevino RP, et al. Cardiac output and end tidal carbon dioxide. *Crit Care Med* 1985;13:907–909.

212. Kalenda Z. The capnogram as a guide to the efficacy of cardiac massage. *Resuscitation* 1978;6:259–263.

213. Sanders AB, Atlas M, Ewy GA, et al. Expired PCO_2 as an index of coronary perfusion pressure. *Am J Emerg Med* 1985;3:147–149.

214. Kern KB, Sanders AB, Voorhees WD, et al. Changes in expired end-tidal carbon dioxide during cardiopulmonary resuscitation in dogs: a prognostic guide for resuscitation efforts. *J Am Coll Cardiol* 1989;13:1184–1189.

215. Sanders AB, Kern KB, Otto CW, et al. End-tidal carbon dioxide monitoring during cardiopulmonary resuscitation. A prognostic indicator for survival. *JAMA* 1989;262:1347–1351.

216. Weil MH, Rackow EC, Trevino R, et al. Difference in acid-base state between venous and arterial blood during cardiopulmonary resuscitation. *N Engl J Med* 1986;315:153–156.

217. Chase PB, Kern KB, Sanders AB, et al. Effects of graded doses of epinephrine on both noninvasive and invasive measures of myocardial perfusion and blood flow during cardiopulmonary resuscitation. *Crit Care Med* 1993;21:413–419.

218. Angelos MG, DeBehnke DJ. Epinephrine-mediated changes in carbon dioxide tension during reperfusion of ventricular fibrillation in a canine model. *Crit Care Med* 1995;23:925–930.

219. Callaham M, Barton C, Matthay M. Effect of epinephrine on the ability of end-tidal carbon dioxide readings to predict initial resuscitation from cardiac arrest. *Crit Care Med* 1992;20:337–343.

220. Chopin C, Fesard P, Mangalaboyi J, et al. Use of capnography in diagnosis of pulmonary embolism during acute respiratory failure of chronic obstructive pulmonary disease. *Crit Care Med* 1990;18:353–357.

221. Ornato JP. Hemodynamic monitoring during CPR. *Ann Emerg Med* 1993;22:289–295.

222. Klausner JM, Lelcuk S, Gutman M, et al. Expired carbon dioxide: a noninvasive monitor of cardiopulmonary resuscitation. *Circulation* 1988;77:234–239.

223. Domsky M, Wilson RF, Heins J. Intraoperative end-tidal carbon dioxide values and derived calculations correlated with outcome: prognosis and capnography. *Crit Care Med* 1995;23:1497–1503.

224. Asplin BR, White RD. Prognostic value of end-tidal carbon dioxide pressures during out-of-hospital cardiac arrest. *Ann Emerg Med* 1995;25:756–761.

225. Cantineau JP, Lambert Y, Merckx P, et al. End-tidal carbon dioxide during cardiopulmonary resuscitation in humans presenting mostly with asystole: a predictor of outcome. *Crit Care Med* 1996;24:791–796.

226. von Planta M, von Planta I, Bisera J, Weil MH. Determinants of survival in cardiopulmonary resuscitation. *Med Klin* 1990;85:181–186, 228.

227. Herschman Z, Lorbert J, Rahal W, Wilson RF. End-tidal CO_2 and prognosis. *Crit Care Med* 1996;24:1093.

228. Levine RL, Wayne MA, Miller CC. End-tidal carbon dioxide and outcome of out-of-hospital cardiac arrest. *N Engl J Med* 1997;337:301–306.

229. Martin GB, Gentile NT, Paradis NA, et al. Effect of epinephrine on end-tidal carbon dioxide monitoring during CPR. *Ann Emerg Med* 1990;19:396–398.

230. Lindner KH, Ahnefeld FW, Bowdler IM, Prengel AW. Influence of epinephrine on systemic, myocardial, and cerebral acid-base status during cardiopulmonary resuscitation. *Anesthesiology* 1991;74:333–339.

231. Cantineau JP, Merckx P, Lambert Y, et al. Effect of epinephrine on end-tidal carbon dioxide pressure during pre-hospital cardiopulmonary resuscitation. *Am J Emerg Med* 1994;12:267–270.

232. Berg RA, Otto CW, Kern KB, et al. High-dose epinephrine results in greater early mortality after resuscitation from prolonged cardiac arrest in pigs: a prospective, randomized study. *Crit Care Med* 1994;22:282–290.

233. Werner JA, Greene HL, Janko CL, Cobb LA. Two-dimensional echocardiography during CPR in man: implications regarding the mechanism of blood flow. *Crit Care Med* 1981;9:375–376.

234. Werner JA, Greene HL, Janko CL, Cobb LA. Visualization of cardiac valve motion in man during external chest compression using two-dimensional echocardiography: implications regarding the mechanism of blood flow. *Circulation* 1981;63:1417–1421.

235. Higano ST, Oh JK, Ewy GA, Seward JB. The mechanism of blood flow during closed chest cardiac massage in humans: transesophageal echocardiographic observations (see comments). *Mayo Clin Proc* 1990;65:1432–1440.

236. Hackl W, Simon P, Mauritz W, Steinbereithner K. Echocardiographic assessment of mitral valve function during mechanical cardiopulmonary resuscitation in pigs. *Anesth Analg* 1990;70:350–356.

237. Halperin HR, Weiss JL, Guerci AD, et al. Cyclic elevation of intrathoracic pressure can close the mitral valve during cardiac arrest in dogs. *Circulation* 1988;78:754–760.

238. Deshmukh HG, Weil MH, Gudipati CV, et al. Mechanism of blood flow generated by precordial compression during CPR. I. Studies on closed chest precordial compression. *Chest* 1989;95:1092–1099.

239. Rich S, Wix HL, Shapiro EP. Clinical assessment of heart chamber size and valve motion during cardiopulmonary resuscitation by two-dimensional echocardiography. *Am Heart J* 1981;102:368–373.

240. Ma MH, Huang GT, Wang SM, et al. Aortic valve disruption and regurgitation complicating CPR detected by transesophageal echocardiography. *Am J Emerg Med* 1994;12:601–602.

241. Nomura T, Shinzawa M, Hashimoto K, et al. Usefulness of transesophageal echocardiography in a case of cardiac arrest during anesthesia. *Anesth Resusc* 1994;30:243–246.

242. Ma MH, Hwang JJ, Lai LP, et al. Transesophageal echocardiographic assessment of mitral valve position and pulmonary venous flow during cardiopulmonary resuscitation in humans. *Circulation* 1995;92:854–861.

243. Pell AC, Guly UM, Sutherland GR, et al. Mechanism of closed chest cardiopulmonary resuscitation investigated by transoesophageal echocardiography. *J Accid Emerg Med* 1994;11:139–143.

244. Redberg RF, Tucker K, Schiller NB. Transesophageal echocardiography during cardiopulmonary resuscitation. *Cardiol Clin* 1993;11:529–535.

245. Ornato JP. Should bystanders perform mouth-to-mouth ventilation during resuscitation? *Chest* 1994;106:1641–1642.

246. Idris AH. Is mouth-to-mouth ventilation necessary for successful resuscitation? *Chest* 1995;108:1490–1491.

247. Locke CJ, Berg RA, Sanders AB, et al. Bystander cardiopulmonary resuscitation: concerns about mouth-to-mouth contact. *Arch Intern Med* 1995;155:938–943.

248. Wenzel V, Idris AH, Banner MJ, et al. The composition of gas given by mouth-to-mouth ventilation during CPR. *Chest* 1994;106:1806–1810.

249. Idris AH. Reassessing the need for ventilation during CPR. *Ann Emerg Med* 1996;27:569–575.

250. Safar P. Initiation of closed-chest cardiopulmonary resuscitation basic life support. A personal history. *Resuscitation* 1989;18:7–20.

251. Lawrence PJ, Sivaneswaran N. Ventilation during cardiopulmonary resuscitation: which method? *Med J Aust* 1985;143:443–446.

252. Brenner BE, Kauffmann J. Response to cardiac arrests in a hospital setting: delays in ventilation. *Resuscitation* 1996;31:17–23.

253. Chandra NC, Gruben KG, Tsitlik JE, et al. Observations of ventilation during resuscitation in a canine model. *Circulation* 1994;90:3070–3075.

254. Hallstrom A, Cobb L, Johnson E, Copass M. Cardiopulmonary resuscitation by chest compression alone or with mouth-to-mouth ventilation. *N Engl J Med* 2000;342:1546–1553.

255. Clark JJ, Larsen MP, Culley LL, et al. Incidence of agonal respirations in sudden cardiac arrest. *Ann Emerg Med* 1992;21:1464–1467.

256. Ornato JP, Bryson BB, Donovan PJ, et al. Measurement of ventilation during cardiopulmonary resuscitation. *Crit Care Med* 1983;11:79–82.

257. Melker RJ. Recommendations for ventilation during cardiopulmonary resuscitation: time for change? *Crit Care Med* 1985;13:882–883.

258. Koehler RC, Michael JR, Guerci AD, et al. Beneficial effect of epinephrine infusion on cerebral and myocardial blood flow during CPR. *Ann Emerg Med* 1985;14:744–749.

259. Otto CW, Yakaitas RW. The role of epinephrine in CPR: a reappraisal. *Ann Emerg Med* 1984;13:840–843.

260. White RD. Defining the pressure needs of the fibrillating heart during prolonged arrest: identification and application. *Ann Emerg Med* 1985;14:587–588.

261. Niemann JT, Criley JM, Rosborough JP, et al. Predictive indices of successful cardiac resuscitation after prolonged arrest and experimental cardiopulmonary resuscitation. *Ann Emerg Med* 1985;14:521–528.

262. Sanders AB, Ogle M, Ewy GA. Coronary perfusion pressure during cardiopulmonary resuscitation. *Am J Emerg Med* 1985;3:11–14.

263. Raessler KL, Kern KB, Sanders AB, et al. Aortic and right atrial systolic pressures during cardiopulmonary resuscitation: a potential indicator of the mechanism of blood flow. *Am Heart J* 1988;115:1021–1029.

264. Lindner KH, Ahnefeld FW, Bowdler IM. The effect of epinephrine on hemodynamics, acid-base status and potassium during spontaneous circulation and cardiopulmonary resuscitation. *Resuscitation* 1988;16:251–261.

265. Ditchey RV, Lindenfeld J. Failure of epinephrine to improve the balance between myocardial oxygen supply and demand during closed-chest resuscitation in dogs. *Circulation* 1988;78:382–389.

266. Ditchey RV, Goto Y, Lindenfeld J. Myocardial oxygen requirements during experimental cardiopulmonary resuscitation. *Cardiovasc Res* 1992;26:791–797.

267. Kosnik JW, Jackson RE, Keats S, et al. Dose-related response of centrally administered epinephrine on the change in aortic diastolic pressure during closed-chest massage in dogs. *Ann Emerg Med* 1985;14:204–208.

268. Livesy JJ, Follette DM, Fey KH, et al. Optimizing myocardial supply/demand balance with alpha-adrenergic drugs during cardiopulmonary resuscitation. *J Thorac Cardiovasc Surg* 1978;76:244.

269. Brown CG, Birinyi F, Werman HA, et al. The comparative effects of epinephrine versus phenylephrine on regional cerebral blood flow during cardiopulmonary resuscitation. *Resuscitation* 1986;14:171–183.

270. Jackson RE, Joyce K, Danosi SF, et al. Blood flow in the cerebral cortex during cardiac resuscitation in dogs. *Ann Emerg Med* 1984;13:657–659.

271. Brown CG, Davis EA, Werman HA, Hamlin RL. Methoxamine versus epinephrine on regional cerebral blood flow during cardiopulmonary resuscitation. *Crit Care Med* 1987;15:682–686.

272. Brown CG, Werman HA, Davis EA, et al. The effects of graded doses of epinephrine on regional myocardial blood flow during cardiopulmonary resuscitation in swine. *Circulation* 1987;75:491–497.

273. Brown CG, Werman HA, Davis EA, et al. Comparative effect of graded doses of epinephrine on regional brain blood flow during CPR in a swine model. *Ann Emerg Med* 1986;15:1138–1144.

274. Brown CG, Werman HA. Adrenergic agonists during cardiopulmonary resuscitation. *Resuscitation* 1990;19:1–16.

275. Brown CG, Katz SE, Werman HA, et al. The effect of epinephrine versus methoxamine on regional myocardial blood flow and defibrillation rates following a prolonged cardiorespiratory arrest in a swine model. *Am J Emerg Med* 1987;5:362–369.

276. Brown CG, Robinson LA, Jenkins J, et al. The effect of

norepinephrine versus epinephrine on regional cerebral blood flow during cardiopulmonary resuscitation. *Am J Emerg Med* 1989;7:278–282.

277. Gonzalez ER, Ornato JP, Levine RL. Vasopressor effect of epinephrine with and without dopamine during cardiopulmonary resuscitation. *Drug Intell Clin Pharm* 1988;22:868–872.

278. Callaham M. Epinephrine doses in cardiac arrest: is it time to outgrow the orthodoxy of ACLS? *Ann Emerg Med* 1989;18:1011.

279. Paradis NA, Koscove EM. Epinephrine in cardiac arrest: a critical review. *Ann Emerg Med* 1990;19:1288–1301.

280. Koscove EM, Paradis NA. Successful resuscitation from cardiac arrest using high-dose epinephrine therapy. Report of two cases. *JAMA* 1988;259:3031–3034.

281. Gonzalez ER, Ornato JP. The dose of epinephrine during cardiopulmonary resuscitation in humans: what should it be? *DICP* 1991;25:773–777.

282. Dieckmann RA, Vardis R. High-dose epinephrine in pediatric out-of-hospital cardiopulmonary arrest. *Pediatrics* 1995;95:901–913.

283. Lipman J, Wilson W, Kobilski S, et al. High-dose adrenaline in adult in-hospital asystolic cardiopulmonary resuscitation: a double-blind randomised trial. *Anaesth Intensive Care* 1993;21:192–196.

284. Callaham M, Madsen CD, Barton CW, et al. A randomized clinical trial of high-dose epinephrine and norepinephrine vs standard-dose epinephrine in prehospital cardiac arrest *JAMA* 1992;268:2667–2672.

285. Lindner KH, Ahnefeld FW, Prengel AW. Comparison of standard and high-dose adrenaline in the resuscitation of asystole and electromechanical dissociation. *Acta Anaesthesiol Scand* 1991;35:253–256.

286. Stiell IG, Hebert PC, Weitzman BN, et al. A study of high-dose epinephrine in human CPR. *N Engl J Med* 1992;327:1047–1050.

287. Brown CG, Martin DR, Pepe PE, et al. A comparison of standard dose epinephrine and high dose epinephrine in cardiac arrest outside the hospital. *N Engl J Med* 1992;327:1051–1055.

288. Choux C, Gueugniaud PY, Barbieux A, et al. Standard doses versus repeated high doses of epinephrine in cardiac arrest outside the hospital. *Resuscitation* 1995;29:3–9.

289. Carpenter TC, Stenmark KR. High-dose epinephrine is not superior to standard-dose epinephrine in pediatric in-hospital cardiopulmonary arrest. *Pediatrics* 1997;99:403–408.

290. Gueugniaud PY, Mols P, Goldstein P, et al. A comparison of repeated high doses and repeated standard doses of epinephrine for cardiac arrest outside the hospital. European Epinephrine Study Group (see comments). *N Engl J Med* 1998;339:1595–1601.

291. Sherman BW, Munger MA, Foulke GE, et al. High-dose versus standard-dose epinephrine treatment of cardiac arrest after failure of standard therapy. *Pharmacotherapy* 1997;17:242–247.

292. Lindner KH, Prengel AW, Pfenninger EG, et al. Vasopressin improves vital organ blood flow during closed-chest cardiopulmonary resuscitation in pigs. *Circulation* 1995;91:215–221.

293. Morris DC, Dereczyk BE, Grzybowski M, et al. Vasopressin can increase coronary perfusion pressure during human cardiopulmonary resuscitation. *Acad Emerg Med* 1997;4:878–883.

294. Lindner KH, Haak T, Keller A, et al. Release of endogenous vasopressors during and after cardiopulmonary resuscitation. *Heart* 1996;75:145–150.

295. Lindner KH, Dirks B, Strohmenger HU, et al. Randomised comparison of epinephrine and vasopressin in patients with out-of-hospital ventricular fibrillation. *Lancet* 1997;349:535–537.

296. Voeckel WG, Lurie KG, Lindner KH, et al. Comparison of epinephrine and vasopressin in a pediatric porcine model of asphyxial cardiac arrest (abstract). *Circulation* 1999;100[Suppl I]:I-316.

297. Weil MH, Trevino RP, Rackow EC. Sodium bicarbonate during CPR. Does it help or hinder? *Chest* 1985;88:487.

298. Weil MH, Ruiz CE, Michaels S, Rackow EC. Acid-base determinants of survival after cardiopulmonary resuscitation. *Crit Care Med* 1985;13:888–892.

299. Bishop RL, Weisfeldt ML. Sodium bicarbonate administration during cardiac arrest. *JAMA* 1976;235:506–509.

300. Grundler W, Weil MH, Yamaguchi M, et al. The paradox of venous acidosis and arterial alkalosis during CPR. *Chest* 1984;86:282.

301. MacGregor DC, Wilson GJ, Holmes DE, et al. Intramyocardial carbon dioxide tension: a guide to the safe period of anoxic arrest of the heart. *J Thorac Cardiovasc Surg* 1974;68:101–107.

302. Jaffe AS. New and old paradoxes. Acidosis and cardiopulmonary resuscitation. *Circulation* 1989;80:1079–1083.

303. Kette F, Weil MH, von Planta M, et al. Buffer agents do not reverse intramyocardial acidosis during cardiac resuscitation. *Circulation* 1990;81:1660–1666.

304. Ornato JP, Gonzalez ER, Coyne MR, et al. Arterial pH in out-of-hospital cardiac arrest: response time as a determinant of acidosis. *Am J Emerg Med* 1985;3:498–502.

305. Niemann JT, Rosborough JP. Effects of acidemia and sodium bicarbonate therapy in advanced cardiac life support. *Ann Emerg Med* 1984;13:781–784.

306. Clancy RL, Cingolani HE, Taylor RR, et al. Influence of sodium bicarbonate on myocardial performance. *Am J Physiol* 1967;212:917–923.

307. Graf H, Leach W, Arieff AI. Evidence for a detrimental effect of bicarbonate therapy in hypoxic lactic acidosis. *Science* 1985;227:754–756.

308. Berenyi KJ, Wolk M, Killip T. Cerebrospinal fluid acidosis complicating therapy of experimental cardiopulmonary arrest. *Circulation* 1975;52:319–324.

309. Redding JS, Pearson JW. Metabolic acidosis: a factor in cardiac resuscitation. *South Med J* 1967;60:926–932.

310. Yakaitas RW, Thomas JD, Mahaffey JE. Influence of pH and hypoxia on the success of defibrillation. *Crit Care Med* 1975;3:139–142.

311. Guerci AD, Chandra N, Johnson E, et al. Failure of sodium bicarbonate to improve resuscitation from ventricular fibrillation in dogs. *Circulation* 1986;74[6 Pt 2]:IV75–79.

312. Gazmuri RJ, von Planta M, Weil MH, Rackow EC. Cardiac effects of carbon dioxide-consuming and carbon

dioxide-generating buffers during cardiopulmonary resuscitation. *J Am Coll Cardiol* 1990;15:482–490.

313. Bersin RM, Chatterjee K, Arieff AI. Metabolic and hemodynamic consequences of sodium bicarbonate administration in patients with heart disease. *Am J Med* 1989;87:7–14.

314. Cooper DJ, Walley KR, Wiggs BR, Russell JA. Bicarbonate does not improve hemodynamics in critically ill patients who have lactic acidosis. A prospective, controlled clinical study. *Ann Intern Med* 1990;112:492–498.

315. Minuck M, Sharma GP, Minuck M, Sharma GP. Comparison of THAM and sodium bicarbonate in resuscitation of the heart after ventricular fibrillation in dogs. *Anesth Analg* 1977;56:38–45.

316. Lee WH, Darby TD, Aldinger EE, et al. Use of THAM in the management of refractory cardiac arrest. *Am J Surg* 1962;28:87–89.

317. Stacpoole PW, Harman EM, Curry SH, et al. Treatment of lactic acidosis with dichloroacetate. *N Engl J Med* 1983;309:390–396.

318. Dybvik T, Strand T, Steen PA. Buffer therapy during out-of-hospital cardiopulmonary resuscitation. *Resuscitation* 1995;29:89–95.

319. Nowak RM, Bodnar TJ, Dronen S, et al. Bretylium tosylate as initial treatment for cardiopulmonary arrest: a randomized comparison with placebo. *Ann Emerg Med* 1981;10:404–407.

320. Olson DW, Thompson BM, Darin JC, et al. A randomized comparison study of bretylium tosylate and lidocaine in resuscitation of patients from out-of-hospital ventricular fibrillation in a paramedic system. *Ann Emerg Med* 1984;13:807–810.

321. Harrison EE, Amey BD. The use of bretylium in prehospital ventricular fibrillation. *Am J Emerg Med* 1983;1:1–6.

322. Haynes RE, Chinn TL, Copass MK, et al. Comparison of bretylium tosylate and lidocaine in management of out-of-hospital ventricular fibrillation: a randomized clinical trial. *Am J Cardiol* 1981;48:353–356.

323. Morgan DB, Davidson C. Hypokalemia and diuretics: an analysis of publications. *BMJ* 1980;280:905–909.

324. Hollifield JW. Potassium and magnesium abnormalities: diuretics and arrhythmias in hypertension. *Am J Med* 1984;77:28–32.

325. Nordrehaug JE, von der Lippe G. Hypokalemia and ventricular fibrillation in acute myocardial infarction. *Br Heart J* 1983;50:525–529.

326. Thompson RG, Cobb LA. Hypokalemia after resuscitation from out-of-hospital ventricular fibrillation. *JAMA* 1982;248:2860–2863.

327. Ornato JP, Gonzalez ER, Starke H, et al. Incidence and causes of hypokalemia associated with cardiac resuscitation. *Am J Emerg Med* 1985;3:503–506.

328. Ornato JP, Gonzalez ER. Refractory ventricular fibrillation. *Emerg Decisions* 1986;4:35–41.

329. Vobruba V, Cerna O. The role of magnesium in acute condition. *Cesko-Slov Pediatr* 1995;50:33–35.

330. Craddock L, Miller B, Clifton G, et al. Resuscitation from prolonged cardiac arrest with high-dose intravenous magnesium sulfate. *J Emerg Med* 1991;9:469–476.

331. Thel MC, Armstrong AL, McNulty SE, et al. Randomised trial of magnesium in in-hospital cardiac arrest. Duke

Internal Medicine Housestaff. *Lancet* 1997;350:1272–1276.

332. Miller B, Craddock L, Hoffenberg S, et al. Pilot study of intravenous magnesium sulfate in refractory cardiac arrest: safety data and recommendations for future studies. *Resuscitation* 1995;30:3–14.

333. Kowey PR, Engel TR. Overdrive pacing for ventricular tachyarrhythmias: a reassessment. *Ann Intern Med* 1983;99:651–656.

334. Williams ML, Woelfel A, Cascio WE, et al. Intravenous amiodarone during prolonged resuscitation from cardiac arrest. *Ann Intern Med* 1989;110:839–842.

335. Perry JC, Fenrich AL, Hulse JE, et al. Pediatric use of intravenous amiodarone: efficacy and safety in critically ill patients from a multicenter protocol. *J Am Coll Cardiol* 1996;27:1246–1250.

336. Pohlgeers A, Villafane J. Ventricular fibrillation in two infants treated with amiodarone hydrochloride. *Pediatr Cardiol* 1995;16:82–84.

337. Levine JH, Massumi A, Scheinman MM, et al. Intravenous amiodarone for recurrent sustained hypotensive ventricular tachyarrhythmias. Intravenous Amiodarone Multicenter Trial Group. *J Am Coll Cardiol* 1996;27:67–75.

338. Scheinman MM. Parenteral antiarrhythmic drug therapy in ventricular tachycardia/ventricular fibrillation: evolving role of class III agents—focus on amiodarone. *J Cardiovasc Electrophysiol* 1995;6(10 Pt 2):914–919.

339. Naccarelli GV, Jalal S. Intravenous amiodarone. Another option in the acute management of sustained ventricular tachyarrhythmias (editorial; comment). *Med Lett Drugs Ther* 1995;37:114–115.

340. Kojima S, Wu ST, Wikman-Coffelt J, Parmley WW. Acute amiodarone terminates ventricular fibrillation by modifying cellular Ca++ homeostasis in isolated perfused rat hearts. *J Pharmacol Exp Ther* 1995;275:254–262.

341. Anastasiou-Nana MI, Nanas JN, Nanas SN, et al. Effects of amiodarone on refractory ventricular fibrillation in acute myocardial infarction: experimental study. *J Am Coll Cardiol* 1994;23:253–258.

342. Kowey PR, Levine JH, Herre JM, et al. Randomized, double-blind comparison of intravenous amiodarone and bretylium in the treatment of patients with recurrent, hemodynamically destabilizing ventricular tachycardia or fibrillation. The Intravenous Amiodarone Multicenter Investigators Group. *Circulation* 1995;92:3255–3263.

343. Scheinman MM, Levine JH, Cannom DS, et al. Dose-ranging study of intravenous amiodarone in patients with life-threatening ventricular tachyarrhythmias. The Intravenous Amiodarone Multicenter Investigators Group. *Circulation* 1995;92:3264–3272.

344. Jaffe AS. The use of antiarrhythmics in advanced cardiac life support. *Ann Emerg Med* 1993;22:307–316.

345. Kudenchuk PJ, Cobb LA, Copass MK, et al. Amiodarone for resuscitation after out-of-hospital cardiac arrest due to ventricular fibrillation. *N Engl J Med* 1999;341:871–878.

346. Gonzalez ER, Kannewurf BS, Ornato JP. Intravenous amiodarone for ventricular arrhythmias: overview and clinical use. *Resuscitation* 1998;39:33–42.

347. Lurie KG, Shultz JJ, Callaham ML, et al. Evaluation of

active compression-decompression CPR in victims of out-of-hospital cardiac arrest. *JAMA* 1994;271:1405–1411.

348. Olson CM. The letter or the spirit: consent for research in CPR. *JAMA* 1994;271:1445–1447.

349. Abramson NS. Deferred consent: use in clinical resuscitation research. *Ann Emerg Med* 1990;19:781–784.

350. Sack JB, Kesselbrenner MB, Bregman D. Survival from in-hospital cardiac arrest with interposed abdominal counterpulsation during cardiopulmonary resuscitation. *JAMA* 1992;267:379–385.

351. Lurie KG, Benditt D. Regulated to death: the matter of informed consent for human experimentation in emergency resuscitation research. *Pacing Clin Electrophysiol* 1995;18:1443–1447.

352. Kremers MS, Whisnant DR, Lowder LS, Gregg L. Initial experience using the Food and Drug administration guidelines for emergency research without consent. *Ann Emerg Med* 1999;33:224–229.

353. Kowey P, Ornato J. Resuscitation research and emergency waiver of informed consent. *Resuscitation* 2000;47:307–310.

354. Passamani ER, Weisfeldt ML. 31st Bethesda Conference. Emergency Cardiac Care. Task force 3: special aspects of research conduct in the emergency setting: waiver of informed consent. *J Am Coll Cardiol* 2000;35:862–880.

355. Talley DB, Ornato JP, Clarke AM. Computer-aided characterization and optimization of the Thumper compression waveform in closed-chest CPR. *Biomed Instrum Technol* 1990;24:283–288.

356. Halperin HR, Guerci AD, Chandra N, et al. Vest inflation without simultaneous ventilation during cardiac arrest in dogs: improved survival from prolonged cardiopulmonary resuscitation. *Circulation* 1986;74:1407–1415.

357. Halperin HR, Weisfeldt ML. New approaches to CPR. Four hands, a plunger, or a vest. *JAMA* 1992;267:2940–2941.

358. Halperin HR, Tsitlik JE, Gelfand M, et al. A preliminary study of cardiopulmonary resuscitation by circumferential compression of the chest with use of a pneumatic vest. *N Engl J Med* 1993;329:762–768.

359. Halperin HR, Chandra NC, Levin HR, et al. Newer methods of improving blood flow during CPR. *Ann Emerg Med* 1996;27:553–562.

360. Shultz JJ, Coffeen P, Sweeney M, et al. Evaluation of standard and active compression-decompression CPR in an acute human model of ventricular fibrillation. *Circulation* 1994;89:684–693.

361. Tucker KJ, Khan J, Idris A, Savitt MA. The biphasic mechanism of blood flow during cardiopulmonary resuscitation: a physiologic comparison of active compression-decompression and high-impulse manual external cardiac massage. *Ann Emerg Med* 1994;24:895–906.

362. Orliaguet GA, Carli PA, Rozenberg A, et al. End-tidal carbon dioxide during out-of-hospital cardiac arrest resuscitation: comparison of active compression-decompression and standard CPR. *Ann Emerg Med* 1995;25:48–51.

363. Luiz T, Ellinger K, Denz C. Active compression-decompression cardiopulmonary resuscitation does not improve survival in patients with prehospital cardiac arrest in a physician-manned emergency medical system. *J Cardiothorac Vasc Anesth* 1996;10:178–186.

364. Stiell IG, Hebert PC, Wells GA, et al. The Ontario trial of active compression-decompression cardiopulmonary resuscitation for in-hospital and prehospital cardiac arrest. *JAMA* 1996;275:1417–1423.

365. Schwab TM, Callaham ML, Madsen CD, Utecht TA. A randomized clinical trial of active compression-decompression CPR vs standard CPR in out-of-hospital cardiac arrest in two cities. *JAMA* 1995;273:1261–1268.

366. Lurie KG, Shultz JJ, Callaham ML, et al. Evaluation of active compression-decompression CPR in victims of out-of-hospital cardiac arrest. *JAMA* 1994;271:1405–1411.

367. Plaisance P, Adnet F, Vicaut E, et al. Benefit of active compression-decompression cardiopulmonary resuscitation as a prehospital advanced cardiac life support. A randomized multicenter study. *Circulation* 1997;95:955–961.

368. Mateer JR, Stueven HA, Thompson BM, et al. Pre-hospital IAC-CPR versus standard CPR: paramedic resuscitation of cardiac arrests. *Am J Emerg Med* 1985;3:143–146.

369. Mahoney BD, Mirick MJ. Efficacy of pneumatic trousers in refractory prehospital cardiopulmonary arrest. *Ann Emerg Med* 1983;12:8–12.

370. Hou SH, Lue HC, Chu SH. Comparison of conventional and simultaneous compression-ventilation cardiopulmonary resuscitation in piglets. *Jpn Circ J* 1994;58:426–432.

371. Krischer JP, Fine EG, Weisfeldt ML, et al. Comparison of prehospital conventional and simultaneous compression-ventilation cardiopulmonary resuscitation. *Crit Care Med* 1989;17:1263–1269.

372. Schultz DD, Olivas GS. The use of cough cardiopulmonary resuscitation in clinical practice. *Heart Lung* 1986;15:273–282.

373. Miller B, Lesnefsky E, Heyborne T, et al. Cough-cardiopulmonary resuscitation in the cardiac catheterization laboratory: hemodynamics during an episode of prolonged hypotensive ventricular tachycardia. *Cathet Cardiovasc Diagn* 1989;18:168–171.

374. Miller B, Cohen A, Serio A, Bettock D. Hemodynamics of cough cardiopulmonary resuscitation in a patient with sustained torsades de pointes/ventricular flutter. *J Emerg Med* 1994;12:627–632.

375. Niemann JT, Rosborough JP, Niskanen RA, et al. Mechanical "cough" cardiopulmonary resuscitation during cardiac arrest in dogs. *Am J Cardiol* 1985;55:199–204.

376. Lurie KG, Coffeen P, Shultz J, et al. Improving active compression-decompression cardiopulmonary resuscitation with an inspiratory impedance valve. *Circulation* 1995;91:1629–1632.

377. Lurie KG. Recent advances in mechanical methods of cardiopulmonary resuscitation. *Acta Anaesthesiol Scand Suppl* 1997;111:49–52.

378. Plaisance P, Lurie KG, Payen D. Inspiratory impedance during active compression-decompression cardiopulmonary resuscitation: a randomized evaluation in patients in cardiac arrest. *Circulation* 2000;101:989–994.

379. Lurie K, Voelckel W, Plaisance P, et al. Use of an inspiratory impedance threshold valve during cardiopulmonary resuscitation: a progress report. *Resuscitation* 2000;44:219–230.

380. Lurie K, Zielinski T, McKnite S, Sukhum P. Improving the efficiency of cardiopulmonary resuscitation with an inspiratory impedance threshold valve. *Crit Care Med* 2000;28:N207–209.

381. Lurie KG, Mulligan KA, McKnite S, et al. Optimizing standard cardiopulmonary resuscitation with an inspiratory impedance threshold valve. *Chest* 1998;113:1084–1090.

382. Eisenberg MS, Moore J, Cummins RO, et al. Use of the automatic external defibrillator in homes of survivors of out-of-hospital ventricular fibrillation. *Am J Cardiol* 1989;63:443–446.

383. Swenson RD, Hill DL, Martin JS, et al. Automatic external defibrillators used by family members to treat cardiac arrest. *Circulation* 1987;76[Suppl IV]:IV-463.

384. Weaver WD, Sutherland K, Wirkus MJ, Bachman R. Emergency medical care requirements for large public assemblies and a new strategy for managing cardiac arrest in this setting. *Ann Emerg Med* 1989;18:155–160.

385. Chadda KD, Kammerer RJ, Kuphal J, Miller K. Successful defibrillation in the industrial, recreational, and corporate settings by laypersons. *Circulation* 1987;76[Suppl IV]:IV-12.

386. Wilson BD, Graton MC, Overton J, Watson W. Unexpected ALS procedures on non-emergency ambulance calls: the value of a single tier system. *Prehosp Disaster Med* 1991;6:382.

387. Cummins RO. From concept to standard-of-care? Review of the clinical experience with automated external defibrillators. *Ann Emerg Med* 1989;18:1269–1275.

388. Valenzuela TD, Roe DJ, Nichol G, et al. Outcomes of rapid defibrillation by security officers after cardiac arrest in casinos. *N Engl J Med* 2000;343:1206–1209.

389. Page RL, Joglar JA, Kowal RC, et al. Use of automated external defibrillators by a U.S. airline. *N Engl J Med* 2000;343:1210–1216.

390. Donaldson E, Pearn J. First aid in the air. *Aust N Z J Surg* 1996;66:431–434.

391. O'Rourke MF, Donaldson E, Geddes JS. An airline cardiac arrest program. *Circulation* 1997;96:2849–2853.

392. Glazer I. Airline use of automatic external defibrillator: shocking developments. *Aviat Space Environ Med* 2000;71:556.

393. Weisfeldt ML, Kerber RE, McGoldrick RP, et al. Public access defibrillation: a statement for healthcare professionals from the American Heart Association Task Force on Automatic External Defibrillation. *Circulation* 1995;92:2763.

394. Weisfeldt ML, Kerber RE, McGoldrick RP, et al. American Heart Association Report on the Public Access Defibrillation Conference, December 8–10, 1994. *Circulation* 1995;92:2740–2747.

395. Nichol G, Hallstrom AP, Kerber R, et al. American Heart Association report on the second public access defibrillation conference, April 17–19, 1997. *Circulation* 1998;97:1309–1314.

396. Kern KB. Public access defibrillation: a review. *Heart* 1998;80:402–404.

397. Ornato JP, Hankins DG. Public-access defibrillation. *Prehosp Emerg Care* 1999;3:297–302.

SYNCOPE

DAVID G. BENDITT

OVERVIEW

Syncope—a syndrome of relatively limited duration with subsequent spontaneous recovery and characterized by the sudden loss of consciousness and postural tone—is a common medical problem and an important cause of emergency department visits and hospital admissions (1–10). It has been estimated that approximately one-third of individuals experience a syncopal episode during their lifetime (10). Susceptibility to syncope increases in association with advancing age and increasing infirmity (10,11). Thus, in the Framingham experience (10), the prevalence of "isolated" syncope (i.e., syncope in the absence of apparent neurologic or cardiovascular disease) increased from 8 in 1,000 person-examinations in the 35- to 44-year-old age group to approximately 40 in 1,000 person-examinations in the >75-year-old age group. However, in a presumably more infirm population (i.e., elderly individuals confined to long-term care institutions), Lipsitz et al. (11) reported an annual incidence of syncope as high as 6%.

Apart from first syncopal events, approximately 35% of syncope patients experience recurrences within 3 years of follow-up (10–13). A history of recurrent syncope at the

time of initial presentation—especially if the recurrences have been spread over a relatively long period—is a strong predictor of future recurrences (12,13). In one report, more than five lifetime syncope recurrences were associated with a 50% chance of recurrence in the following year (12).

PATHOPHYSIOLOGY

Cerebral perfusion is critically dependent on systemic arterial pressure. [▼ 194] Thus, factors that diminish systemic arterial pressure (e.g., decreased cardiac output or peripheral vascular resistance) may impair cerebral perfusion. In syncope patients, decreased venous filling is often a major factor in triggering a reduced cardiac output. Excessive pooling of blood in dependent parts of the body or diminished blood volume predisposes the patient to syncope. Impaired cardiac output may also be the result of tachyarrhythmias or bradyarrhythmias, especially in the setting of left ventricular dysfunction, valvular heart disease, volume depletion, or abnormal vascular reactivity. In terms of vascular resistance, inadequate vasoconstriction or inappropriate vasodilatation may contribute to syncope by undermining cerebral perfusion pressure. In fact, inappropriate vasodilatation is the main cause of fainting in reflex syncopal syndromes. Vasodi-

D. G. Benditt: Department of Medicine/Cardiology, University of Minnesota Medical School—Minneapolis, Minneapolis, Minnesota

latation resulting in diminished cerebral perfusion also can contribute to lightheadedness and syncope in association with thermal stress (e.g., hot environments, excessive exercise). Impaired capacity to increase vascular resistance adequately during upright posture is critical in orthostatic hypotension, syncope associated with use of vasoactive drugs, and patients with autonomic neuropathies (14–18). Cerebral hypoperfusion may also result from an abnormally high cerebral vascular resistance (e.g., due to low carbon dioxide tension in hyperventilation syndromes).

CLASSIFICATION OF THE CAUSES OF SYNCOPE

The classification of the causes of syncope is found in Table 71.1.

TABLE 71.1 SYNCOPE: DIAGNOSTIC CLASSIFICATION

Neurally mediated reflex syncope
  Vasovagal faint
  Carotid sinus syncope
  Cough/swallow syncope and related disorders
  Gastrointestinal, pelvic, or urologic origin (swallowing, defecation, postmicturition)
Orthostatic syncope
  Primary autonomic failure
  Secondary autonomic failure (e.g., diabetic and alcoholic neuropathy, drug effects)
Cardiac arrhythmias as primary cause of syncope
  Sinus node dysfunction (including bradycardia/tachycardia syndrome)
  Atrioventricular conduction system disease
  Paroxysmal supraventricular tachycardias
  Paroxysmal ventricular tachycardia (including torsades de pointes)
  Implanted pacing system malfunction, pacemaker syndrome
Structural cardiovascular or cardiopulmonary disease
  Cardiac valvular disease/ischemia
  Acute myocardial infarction
  Obstructive cardiomyopathy
  Subclavian steal syndrome
  Pericardial disease/tamponade
  Pulmonary embolus
  Primary pulmonary hypertension
Cerebrovascular causes
  Obstructive vascular disease
    Intracerebral steal
Miscellaneous impaired consciousness: syncope mimics
  Metabolic/endocrine disturbances
    Hyperventilation (hypocapnia)
    Hypoglycemia
    Volume depletion (Addison's disease, pheochromocytoma)
    Hypoxemia
  Psychiatric disorders
    Panic attacks
    Hysteria
  Central nervous system substrates
    Seizure disorders
    Subarachnoid hemorrhage
    Narcolepsy
    Hydrocephalus

TABLE 71.2 NEURALLY MEDIATED SYNCOPAL SYNDROMES

Emotional syncope (common or vasovagal faint, malignant vasovagal faint)
Carotid sinus syncope
Gastrointestinal stimulation
  Swallow syncope, defecation syncope
Micturition syncope
Cough syncope
Sneeze syncope
Glossopharyngeal neuralgia
Airway stimulation
Raised intrathoracic pressure
  Brass or wind instrument playing, weightlifting

Neurally Mediated Reflex Syncopal Syndromes

The neurally mediated syncopal syndromes (Table 71.2) comprise a variety of pathophysiologically related conditions. For the most part, clinical distinctions are based on the source of the "trigger" for the episodes (e.g., pain, carotid sinus stimulation, cough, micturition). In this regard, the presumed triggering neural signals may arise within the central nervous system (CNS) itself (e.g., syncope associated with fear or anxiety), or from any of a number of peripheral "receptors" that respond to stimuli of various types (e.g., mechanical, chemical, painful). The nature of these receptors is perhaps best understood in carotid sinus syncope and postmicturition syncope. In carotid sinus syndrome, the afferent aspect of the reflex loop typically is believed to arise from stimulation of autonomic receptors in the cervical region. However, it now seems likely that, to trigger the syndrome, carotid sinus stimulation may need to interact with the failure of parallel CNS inputs from the ipsilateral neck muscles (19). In typical vasovagal syncope (Fig. 71.1), the location and nature of the trigger sites are usually less certain. Cardiac mechanoreceptors, along with other central mechanoreceptors and chemoreceptors, appear to contribute to the afferent neural traffic (20–26). 195

Orthostatic Syncope

Orthostatic syncope is often termed *postural hypotension* or *orthostatic hypotension* (Table 71.3). Volume depletion (often iatrogenic) (22,23,27–34) or neurologic disturbances of vascular control due to concomitant disease are the most frequent causes of orthostatic syncope. In certain cases, however, patients may manifest a form of primary autonomic failure with inadequate reflex adaptations to upright posture. 196

Cardiac Arrhythmias as Primary Causes of Syncope

Among syncope patients with underlying congenital or acquired structural heart disease, a primary cardiac arrhyth-

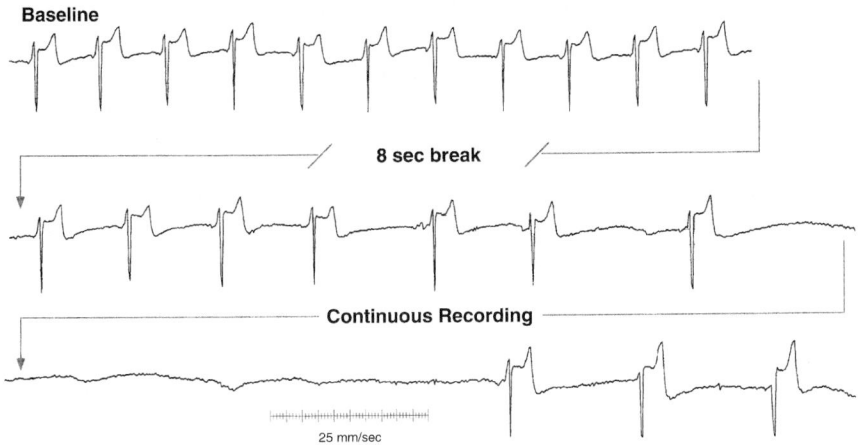

Baseline

8 sec break

Continuous Recording

25 mm/sec

FIGURE 71.1 Recording from an in-hospital electrocardiogram monitor illustrating brady-cardia associated with a spontaneous vasovagal faint accompanying an abrupt hemorrhage after an invasive cardiac procedure.

mia is probably the most common cause of symptoms. Primary cardiac arrhythmias encompass those rhythm disturbances associated with intrinsic cardiac disease, accessory conduction pathways, or other structural abnormalities (e.g. congenital anomalies, postoperative disturbances), as well as disturbances due to proarrhythmic effects of cardioactive drugs (e.g., cardiac glycosides, positive inotropic agents, antiarrhythmic drugs).

The basis for syncope is readily apparent in patients with long periods of severe bradycardia or cardiac asystole in the setting of sinus node dysfunction or atrioventricular (AV) conduction disease. The same is true in individuals with extremely rapid tachyarrhythmias. However, in many cases,

TABLE 71.3 SYNCOPE OF ORTHOSTATIC ORIGIN: A CLASSIFICATION OF CAUSES

Primary autonomic failure
  Pure autonomic failure
  Autonomic failure with multiple system atrophy
  Parkinson's disease with autonomic failure
Secondary autonomic failure
  Diabetes mellitus
  Volume/fluid depletion
  Autoimmune acute and subacute dysautonomias (e.g., Guillain-Barré syndrome, myasthenia gravis)
  Autonomic neuropathy associated with malignancies
  Metabolic diseases (e.g., porphyria, Fabry's disease)
  Central nervous system infections (e.g., syphilis, Chagas disease)
  Hypothalamic and midbrain lesions/tumors (e.g., craniopharyngioma)
  Spinal cord lesions/tumors
Drug/toxin-induced autonomic failure
  Alcohol
  Diuretics
  Sedatives/tranquilizers: phenothiazines, barbiturates
  Vasodilators (e.g., peripheral and central sympatholytic agents)
  Angiotensin-converting enzyme inhibitors
  Tricyclic antidepressants

Modified from Bannister R, ed. *Autonomic failure. A textbook of clinical disorders of the autonomic nervous system.* Oxford: Oxford University Press, 1988.

hypotension is multifactorial; it is dependent on the interaction between heart rate, ventricular function, central volume status, and peripheral vascular reactivity. In this regard, assessment of response to upright posture (i.e., tilt-table testing during induced or spontaneous arrhythmia) may be crucial in understanding the hemodynamic impact of arrhythmias (35).

Structural Cardiovascular or Cardiopulmonary Disease

Cardiac arrhythmias are the most frequent causes of syncope in patients with structural cardiac disease. However, other hemodynamic disturbances may also be responsible for symptomatic hypotension. Acute myocardial ischemia or infarction is probably the most important of these disturbances (36,37). In this setting, the basis of the faint is multifactorial; it is, in part, dependent on neural reflex effects leading to inadequate peripheral vascular compensatory response. Similarly, syncope associated with aortic stenosis or hypertrophic obstructive cardiomyopathy (HOCM) is due not only to mechanical obstruction, but also to neurally mediated inappropriate vascular responsiveness (38–40). Prosthetic valve disorders also require consideration as causes of syncope in patients who have previously undergone such surgery.

Noncardiac cardiovascular structural disturbances may also be associated with syncope. For instance, in subclavian steal syndrome, dizziness and syncope may develop during upper extremity exercise in association with ipsilateral stenosis of the subclavian artery near its origin. Syncope also is associated with pulmonary hypertension and acute pulmonary embolism. In these latter conditions, the basis for the faint encompasses reduced blood flow, diminished oxygenation, and neural reflex vascular disturbances.

Cerebrovascular Syncope

Transient global diminution of cerebral nutrient flow is, for the most part, a necessary requirement for development of syncope. However, it is exceedingly rare for this diminution to occur solely as a result of cerebrovascular disease (i.e., in the absence of a cardiac arrhythmia, orthostatic stress, or other precipitating factor). One example in which cerebrovascular disease could cause transient loss of consciousness without global disturbance of nutrient supply is in intracerebral vascular "steal." In this case, diversion of blood flow away from regions of the brain controlling wakefulness is presumed to be the basis for syncope. Currently, establishing such a diagnosis in the clinic is, essentially, impossible.

Miscellaneous Nonsyncopal Conditions Associated with Impaired Consciousness

In most circumstances, metabolic disturbances of sufficient severity to cause loss of consciousness are not typically transient and self-correcting. Consequently, the clinical picture is not that of true syncope. However, impaired consciousness associated with metabolic and endocrine disturbances does occur. The presumed pathophysiology of this condition is a disturbance of cerebral nutrient availability (e.g., marked hypoglycemia), a major perturbation of acid/base or electrolyte environment, or both. Hyperventilation of presumably psychogenic origin, with consequent marked reduction of the partial pressure of carbon dioxide and reduced cerebral blood flow due to vasospasm, is probably the only relatively common problem in this class.

In regard to more well-established primary neurologic diseases (e.g., aneurysms, tumors, seizure disorders), episodes of loss of consciousness are, once again, usually not true syncope. Nevertheless, making a clinical diagnostic distinction can prove challenging. Astatic or akinetic seizures are particularly difficult to distinguish from syncope (41). Drop attacks may also be included in this category. The basis of drop attacks remains unclear, but because loss of consciousness is not an issue, these attacks are excluded from the category of true syncope.

The pathophysiology of psychiatric disturbances (e.g., somatization disorders) known to mimic syncope (see the section Psychiatric Disorders) is poorly understood. For the most part, these disturbances do not result in true syncopal events. However, patients manifesting such disturbances may have a greater tendency to be subject to the emotional faint or other forms of neurally mediated syncope (see the section Neurally Mediated Reflex Syncopal Syndromes). Additionally, these patients may be prescribed certain medications that increase syncope risk (e.g., phenothiazines, tricyclics).

GENERAL CLINICAL CONSIDERATIONS IN THE EVALUATION OF SYNCOPE

In the clinical evaluation of the syncope patient, the principal goal is to establish an accurate diagnosis; only after a definitive diagnosis is made can an appropriate treatment strategy be embarked on. Given the numerous causes of syncope and the unpredictable nature of syncopal events, achieving this goal is difficult, and special testing is often essential (Fig. 71.2). This is especially true when symptoms are recurrent. However, even solitary syncopal events may warrant such steps when risks to the patient or public may be excessive (e.g., syncope associated with substantial physical injury or motor vehicle accident, syncope in individuals with high-risk occupations such as pilots, commercial truck drivers, or competitive athletes). ▾▾ 197

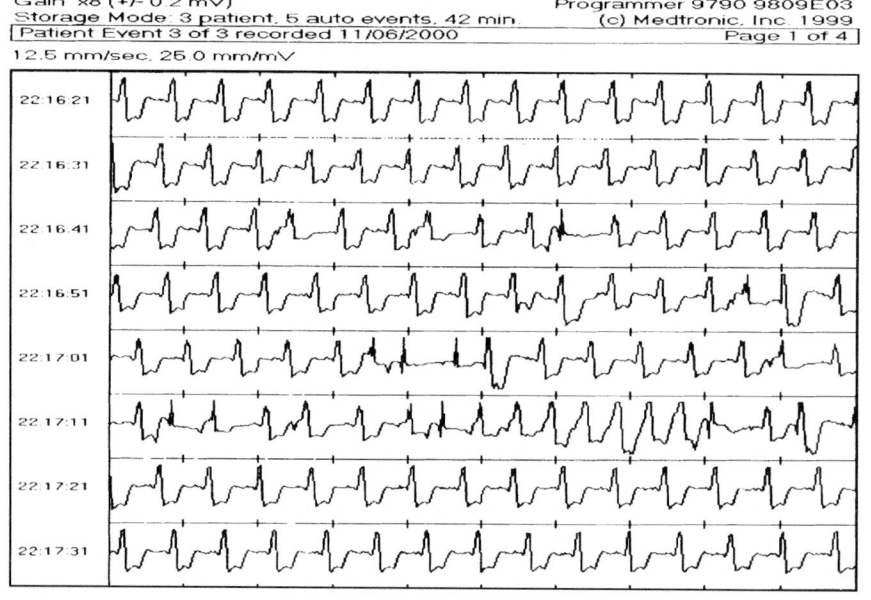

FIGURE 71.2 Recording from an implantable loop recorder. Patient complained of lightheadedness but had no symptoms of rapid heart action. The recording illustrates a wide-QRS nonsustained tachycardia suggestive of nonsustained ventricular tachycardia.

SPECIFIC CONDITIONS

Neurally Mediated Syncopal Syndromes

Syncope of neurally mediated reflex origin encompasses vasovagal syncope, carotid sinus syndrome, and other, much less frequent forms of neurally mediated syncope (e.g., cough, deglutition, and micturition syncope) (Table 71.2). The electrophysiologic and hemodynamic picture associated with a neurally mediated syncopal event may be quite variable (43). Most patients present a mixed vasodepressor and cardioinhibitory response (43–48).

Vasovagal syncope may be triggered by any of a variety of situational factors. Some of these factors are unpleasant sights (e.g., sight of blood), pain, and extreme emotion. Common venues for fainting are churches, hospitals, queues, and restaurants. In many, but not all, cases, this type of faint is easy to diagnose because a clear history of preceding dizziness, together with other typical phenomena, is obtained (49). The patient may report feelings of lack of air, a change in breathing pattern, sweating, loss of hearing, and nausea before partial or total loss of consciousness. Pallor is a common physical finding in association with these faints, and witnesses to the event should be queried directly in regard to their recollection of this finding. During the recovery phase, there is rapid return of orientation. However, fatigue, weakness, nausea, and headache may last from minutes to hours. Often, in older individuals, warning symptoms may be brief or nonexistent, thereby complicating establishment of the diagnosis. In such cases, syncope may occur without apparent warning. Such an outcome often results in falls and physical injury—presentations difficult to distinguish by history alone from syncope complicating conduction disturbances of the heart. This variant of the vasovagal faint has been termed *malignant vasovagal syndrome* (50).

In instances in which vasovagal syncope is suspected by clinical history but in which uncertainty remains, tilt-table testing diagnostic techniques have been of value (23,45–54). Tilt-table testing has a specificity of approximately 90%, a reproducibility in the short term of 80% to 90%, and a reproducibility in the longer term (i.e., more than 1 year) of approximately 60% (54). Tilt-table testing is the only investigation that provides the opportunity to precipitate a typical attack under the eyes of the investigator and allows the victim to confirm the associated symptoms. A recent American College of Cardiology expert consensus document addresses the role of tilt-table testing and appropriate laboratory protocols (54).

Carotid sinus syndrome is probably the second most common form of the neurally mediated syncopal syndromes (55–58). In this setting, syncope often presents without warning (i.e., absence of premonitory symptoms). Although rare, a history suggesting that head movements trigger dizziness or syncope supports this diagnosis. As a rule, the condition almost exclusively afflicts older people, especially men.

In clinical practice, carotid sinus syndrome is often overlooked. The reasons for this include failure to perform carotid sinus massage routinely in syncope patients or failure to record blood pressure and heart rate responses when carotid massage is undertaken. As in other forms of neurally mediated reflex syncope, vasodepressor and cardioinhibitory features participate in most cases of carotid sinus syncope. In the absence of adequate arterial pressure measurements, a clinically important vasodepressor response may be missed. ⚑ 198

Among the other forms of neurally mediated reflex syncope, postmicturition syncope, swallow syncope, and cough syncope are probably the next most frequent. The remaining conditions (Table 71.2) are only rarely encountered.

Orthostatic Syncope

Presyncopal or syncopal symptoms associated with abrupt assumption of upright posture are common occurrences (Table 71.3). Elderly persons, less physically fit individuals, or patients who are, for whatever reason, dehydrated or volume depleted are at greatest risk for orthostatic syncope. Iatrogenic factors such as excessive diuresis or overly aggressive use of certain antihypertensive agents are important contributors. Environmental factors (e.g., excessive heat), complications associated with certain medical conditions (e.g., hemorrhage), or diseases (e.g., diabetes insipidus, adrenal insufficiency) may also play a role in specific cases. Patients previously diagnosed with idiopathic orthostatic hypotension may be considered to be manifesting autonomic dysfunctions; these dysfunctions may be primary neurologic disturbances (e.g., pure autonomic failure) or secondary to other diseases or drug effects.

In general medical practice, specific primary autonomic nervous system dysfunctions leading to disturbances of vascular control are considered to be relatively infrequent causes of syncope. Nevertheless, as the broad spectrum of these disturbances and their potentially subtle manifestations become more widely appreciated by physicians, these diagnoses will be made more often (41,59–62). More commonly, neuropathies associated with chronic diseases (e.g., diabetes) or toxic agents (e.g., alcohol) are the source of the problem. ⚑ 199

In a review of 155 patients referred for assessment of suspected orthostatic hypotension, Low et al. (63) found that among the most severely affected symptomatic patients (n = 90; mean age, 64 years), pure autonomic failure accounted for 33%, multisystem atrophy accounted for 26%, and autonomic/diabetic neuropathy accounted for 31%. The most frequently reported symptoms in these individuals were lightheadedness (88%), weakness or tiredness (72%), cognitive difficulties (47%), blurred vision (47%), tremulousness (38%), and vertigo (37%). The prominence of fatigue and weakness has raised the as-yet-unsettled issue regarding the possible relationship between these conditions and so-called "chronic fatigue syndrome" (64). Patients with postural orthostatic tachycardia syndrome, on the other hand, tended to be symptomatic during upright posture but did not typically manifest sufficient hypotension to result in syncope or marked hypotension.

The clinical evaluation of orthostatic hypotension is facilitated by the availability of tilt-table testing facilities. However, tilt-table test results, as in the case of vasovagal syncope, are affected by various factors such as the volume status of the patient, temperature, and chronobiologic issues. Consequently, the diagnosis of the various forms of autonomic failure using tilt-table testing and other autonomic testing procedures (63,65,66) require a level of experience that is available in relatively few centers. A relatively abrupt drop in systolic pressure of ≥50 mm Hg is probably diagnostic, but it is better supported by the concomitant development of symptoms.

Cardiac Arrhythmias as Primary Causes of Syncope

Arrhythmias due to intrinsic conduction system disturbances—usually acquired but occasionally congenital—are important causes of syncope. However, it is often difficult to substantiate the relationship between syncope and a suspected arrhythmia in free-living individuals (e.g., by ambulatory electrocardiographic monitoring) due to the unpredictable occurrence of symptomatic events. Thus, implantable long-term loop recorders are becoming more widely applied. In some cases, invasive electrophysiologic testing may be indicated.

Sinus node dysfunction—commonly termed *sick sinus syndrome*—encompasses an array of sinus node and atrial arrhythmias that result in persistent or intermittent periods of inappropriate slow or fast beating of the heart (67–72). The electrocardiographic manifestations of sinus node dysfunction include sinus bradycardia, sinus pauses, sinoatrial exit block, inexcitable atrium, and chronotropic incompetence, as well as various atrial tachyarrhythmias—principally, atrial fibrillation or atrial flutter (Fig. 71.3). For the most part, sinus node dysfunction is closely associated with underlying fibrosis or chamber enlargement. However, extrinsic factors (e.g., autonomic nervous system influences, cardioactive drugs) are also frequent contributors. Of these factors, drug-induced disturbances are, clinically, the most important (69–71). ☟ m01

Sinus node dysfunction patients, in large part due to their age and tendency to harbor coexisting diseases (especially cardiovascular disorders), are also susceptible to loss-of-consciousness spells that may not be due to primary arrhythmias. Orthostatic syncope, thromboembolism, myocardial ischemia, and new onset seizure disturbances are important considerations. In the past (i.e., before more widespread use of anticoagulation), it is notable that thromboembolism was the principal factor accounting for

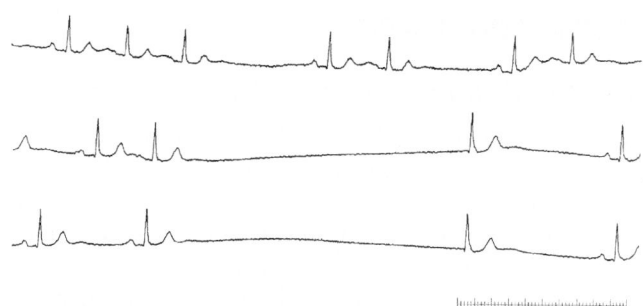

FIGURE 71.3 Symptomatic sinus pauses of varying duration recorded during ambulatory electrocardiogram monitoring in a 70-year-old woman with recurrent dizziness.

the excess morbidity and mortality in sinus node dysfunction patients (69,73–75).

Atrioventricular Conduction Disturbances

Acquired disturbances of AV conduction are most often associated with syncopal symptoms. Progressive idiopathic fibrosis of the cardiac conduction system is the most common cause of acquired conduction system disease with AV block (76,77). Acute myocardial infarction is also associated with the various forms of AV block and is another common cause of acquired complete AV block. Chronic ischemic and valvular heart disease, complications associated with cardiac surgical procedures, and administration of various antiarrhythmic drugs are other potential contributors.

Drug effects also deserve special consideration because they are a particularly common and potentially reversible cause of AV conduction disturbances (69,78,79). Cardiac glycosides, beta-blockers, and calcium-channel blockers are, perhaps, the most widely recognized drugs in this regard. Antiarrhythmic drugs may act directly, as well as through effects on the autonomic nervous system, to alter conduction in the AV node. At usual doses, however, antiarrhythmic drugs are rarely associated with *de novo* development of complete AV block. Patients with preexisting infranodal conduction system disease are at highest risk. Once again, however, syncope in this setting cannot be assumed to be bradycardic in origin because drug-induced tachycardias (i.e., the proarrhythmic effects of antiarrhythmic drugs) are also a consideration in this situation. Torsades de pointes is the most important example of this type of tachycardia. ☟ m02

In general, the risk for syncope or dizziness is greatest at onset of AV block, before "warm-up" of a subsidiary rhythm (Fig. 71.4). Thereafter, the ventricular rhythm often stabilizes and may average 35 to 40 beats/min in acquired third degree AV block. In fixed complete AV block, syncope may occur as a result of the unreliability of subsidiary pacemakers or of the inability of the heart-rate–limited circulation to provide sufficient cerebral blood flow during periods of exercise or stress. In both cases, the close

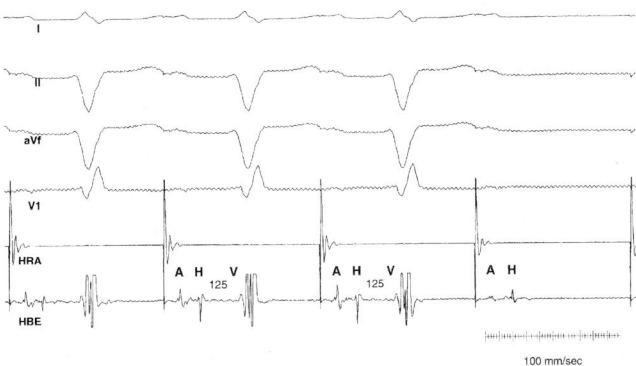

FIGURE 71.4 Electrocardiogram and intracardiac recordings illustrating a prolonged HV interval and infra-His block (Mobitz II) in a patient undergoing electrophysiologic evaluation for recurrent syncope of unknown cause. HBE, bundle of His electrogram; HRA, high rate atrium.

association with severe underlying heart disease also raises concern regarding tachyarrhythmia-induced syncope, including increased proarrhythmia risk in patients treated with antiarrhythmic drugs.

Traditionally, congenital complete AV block has been accorded a more benign prognosis than that accorded to acquired AV block (84,85). The site of block in patients with congenital AV block is typically at the level of the AV node. Generally, the QRS complexes are narrow, and the block usually is associated with a reasonable subsidiary rhythm, which tends to increase in rate with exercise. Recently, however, concern has been raised regarding the supposedly benign natural history of congenital AV block (86), and further evaluation of this issue is needed. In the meantime, syncope and dizziness, along with exertional intolerance, are accepted indications for pacing in these patients.

Bifascicular conduction system disease is a relatively common electrocardiographic finding. However, in most cases, progression to more severe forms of AV block is slow. Susceptibility to higher-grade block (i.e., blocks that may be long enough to cause syncope) increases the longer the HV interval is, particularly for HV ≥100 ms (87–89). However, once again, it should be borne in mind that syncope in patients with evident conduction system disease may not be solely the result of bradyarrhythmias. VT is a concern in these cases because of the usual presence of significant underlying heart disease.

Supraventricular and Ventricular Tachyarrhythmias

Supraventricular tachyarrhythmias have been reported to be the causes of syncope in approximately 15% of patients referred for electrophysiologic evaluation (6). When syncope does occur, it is typically at the onset of an arrhythmic episode and before adequate peripheral vascular compensation can occur. A number of factors determine whether syncope or dizziness occurs in patients with SVT, including the tachycardia rate, the volume status and posture of the patient at onset of the arrhythmia, the presence of associated valvular, left ventricular, or pulmonary vascular disease, the mechanism of the arrhythmia, and the integrity of reflex peripheral vascular compensation. Additionally, it has come to be recognized that neural reflex responsiveness may be less efficient in individuals susceptible to syncope with SVT (90).

Electrophysiologic testing in SVT patients offers the possibility of obtaining direct evidence of the role played by the arrhythmia in the patient's symptoms. However, to document symptomatic hypotension, it may be necessary to induce the arrhythmia with the patient in the head-up posture on a tilt table.

Sustained VT has been reported to be the cause of syncope in up to 20% of syncope patients referred for electrophysiologic testing (6). This diagnosis is of particular concern in the setting of underlying structural heart disease or long-QT syndrome (congenital or acquired). In regard to VT susceptibility, a detailed medical history should be supplemented with assessment of the status of underlying cardiac disease. In this regard, an echocardiographic study is adequate in most cases, but other imaging modalities—including angiography—may be required as well. Although the utility of a signal-averaged electrocardiogram (ECG) is controversial, it may be an appropriate consideration in individuals with ischemic heart disease in whom VT is a concern. If the signal-averaged ECG is normal, the likelihood that VT is the cause of syncope is low (91,92).

Nonsustained ventricular tachycardia (NSVT) remains a difficult dilemma for physicians evaluating syncope patients. NSVT is a common finding during ambulatory electrocardiographic monitoring in patients with structural heart disease. Consequently, finding NSVT in a syncope patient usually is not helpful in the absence of concomitant symptoms (Fig. 71.2). Similarly, induced NSVT during electrophysiologic testing, especially if polymorphic, is not a reliable diagnostic finding. However, if reproducible periods of hypotensive NSVT are easily inducible, and there is no other apparent explanation for syncope, it is probably prudent to proceed with pharmacologic or device prophylaxis. The Multicenter Unsustained Tachycardia Trial data, although not directly focused on a syncope population, seem to provide additional support for this argument (93). ▼ m03

Structural Cardiovascular or Cardiopulmonary Disease

Apart from cardiac arrhythmias, the most common cause of syncope attributable to left ventricular disease is acute myocardial ischemia or infarction. Other relatively common acute medical conditions associated with syncope include pulmonary embolism and pericardial tamponade. The basis of syncope in all of these conditions is multifactorial, including the hemodynamic impact of the specific lesion and neurally mediated reflex effects.

Syncope may also occur in conditions in which there is fixed or dynamic obstruction to left ventricular outflow (e.g., aortic stenosis, HOCM). In such cases, symptoms often are provoked by physical exertion but may also develop if an otherwise benign arrhythmia should occur (e.g., atrial fibrillation). In part, the basis for the faint may be inadequate blood flow due to the mechanical obstruction. However, especially in the case of valvular aortic stenosis, ventricular mechanoreceptor-mediated bradycardia and vasodilatation are thought to be important contributors (38). ⌖ m04

Cerebrovascular Causes of Syncope

Cerebrovascular disease, including severe carotid artery disease, rarely causes syncope. Occasionally, however, transient disturbances of cerebrovascular blood flow may initiate a true syncopal spell. For example, arterial entrapment with intermittent obstruction of posterior circulation vessels can occur in conjunction with cervical spine disease. In such cases, any concomitant problems with the anterior circulatory supply may result in syncope.

Migraine may be associated with syncope. In such cases, extracranial vascular spasm may trigger neural reflex syncope, although cerebrovascular spasm might also occur. In any case, historical features of migraine and migraine susceptibility usually are sufficient to distinguish the diagnosis. Finally, symptoms secondary to cerebrovascular disease may be referred for evaluation as a syncopal episode. In particular, transient ischemic attacks due to vertebrobasilar disease may mimic syncope (41,59). In such cases, there are usually concomitant findings (e.g., vertiginous complaints, ocular disturbances, or speech problems) not typically encountered in the syncope patient.

Miscellaneous Causes of Impaired Consciousness: Syncope Mimics

Metabolic and Endocrine Disturbances

Metabolic and endocrine disturbances are more often responsible for confusional states or behavioral disturbances, rather than true syncope. However, it may be difficult to make a clear-cut distinction between such symptoms and syncope by medical history alone. One potentially useful distinguishing feature is that, unlike true syncope, conditions such as diabetic coma and severe hypoxia or hypercapnia do not resolve without active therapeutic intervention. In the case of syncope due to psychogenic hyperventilation, tilt-table testing may prove helpful for reproducing the event and permitting its documentation by blood gas analysis of arterial samples obtained from a previously placed indwelling catheter.

Psychiatric Disorders

Syncope may be mimicked by anxiety attacks, hysteria, or other psychiatric disturbances. Anxiety attacks are frequently associated with hyperventilation and hypocapnia. Hysteria, however, tends to be characterized by its "drama" because it can occur in the presence of onlookers and is not associated with marked alterations of heart rate, systemic pressure, or skin color.

Central Nervous System Causes

In Kapoor's extensive review of more than 400 patients presenting with syncope, only a few were found to have abnormal neurologic studies (9). Typically, any diagnostic confusion is due to the fact that these conditions may result in a clinical picture, at least from a lay viewpoint, that may be mistaken for syncope. However, the differences are usually clearly distinguishable by careful history taking and neurologic physical examination.

Seizures may be mistaken for syncope, and vice versa (7,9,41,59,97). In some patients, temporal lobe seizures may so closely mimic or induce neurally mediated reflex bradycardia and hypotension, that differentiation from true syncope is difficult. Astatic or akinetic seizures are characterized by the patient slumping to the ground—or, if the patient is supine, by a period of muscular hypotonia—combined with unresponsiveness (41,59). However, these conditions are uncommon. More often, a careful history permits differentiation of seizures from true syncope. ⌖ m05

Cataplexy, an uncommon condition characterized by abrupt onset of generalized muscle weakness, can be confused with syncope. As in the case of vasovagal syncope, symptoms may be triggered by emotional reactions or surprise. A narcoleptic sleep may follow. Cataplexy generally can be distinguished from syncope because the patient can be aroused. Electroencephalographic findings compatible with rapid eye movement sleep differentiate the narcoleptic state from a postictal event.

Drop attacks refer to a poorly defined condition in which abrupt loss of postural tone occurs but consciousness is generally preserved. The etiology of these attacks is unknown. In certain cases, drop attacks appear to be associated with atherosclerotic cerebrovascular disease, especially within the vertebrobasilar system, and are presumed to be the result of transient nutrient insufficiency to corticospinal tracts, which results in sudden atonia in the lower extremities (41). The dramatic clinical presentation of a fall often leads to syncope being the initial diagnosis.

MANAGEMENT: DIAGNOSIS AND TREATMENT

Strategy for Diagnostic Evaluation of the Syncope Patient

The goal of diagnostic testing in syncope patients is to obtain a sufficiently strong correlation between syncopal symptoms and detected abnormalities to permit confident statement of the cause of the faint, an accurate assessment of prognosis, and initiation of an appropriate treatment plan.

A detailed medical history—with particular attention to bystander observations—and a thorough physical examination may lead the physician to suspect the basis for syncope. However, unless these findings are classic, it is usually necessary to undertake selected diagnostic studies to establish the etiology with a greater degree of certainty. In all cases, testing should be carefully targeted. The ordering of routine hematologic and biochemical screens is not productive. Similarly, routine application of specialized neurologic studies (e.g., computed tomography, magnetic resonance imaging) has a low yield (9). A practicable strategy for the syncope evaluation is depicted in Fig. 71.5. As a rule, the first step—apart from excluding a history of seizure disorder—is differentiation of individuals with normal cardiovascular status from those with evident cardiac or cardiovascular disease. Usually, physical examination and echocardiographic assessment is sufficient for this purpose, although exercise testing should also be undertaken if syncope occurred with exertion or if ischemic heart disease is suspected.

In the absence of structural heart disease, tilt-table testing is usually the next diagnostic step. On the other hand, in patients with abnormal cardiac findings, functional studies of the structural disturbance (e.g., hemodynamic, angiographic) and evaluation of susceptibility to tachyarrhythmias and bradyarrhythmias by conventional electrophysiologic testing is appropriate. In patients with demonstrable vascular disease, appropriate studies to assess the hemodynamic significance of observed arrhythmias (e.g., ultrasound) are needed. Thereafter, tilt-table testing should follow if the diagnosis remains in doubt. In only a few instances should special neurologic studies be elected as an initial step.

Specific Diagnostic Testing

Electrocardiographic Recordings

Electrocardiographic documentation during a spontaneous syncopal event is usually a high priority, because cardiac arrhythmias are so frequently the cause of syncope. In this regard, the 12-lead ECG is usually too brief to identify or exclude an arrhythmic cause. However, on occasion, findings such as ventricular preexcitation (e.g., Wolff-Parkinson-White syndrome) or QT interval prolongation suggest a potential mechanism. Other relatively common findings such as sinus bradycardia, ventricular ectopic beats, bundle branch block, or even NSVT often are not particularly helpful. Similarly, exercise testing is usually of limited utility in the evaluation of syncope, unless the events are clearly exertionally related by history. Only in rare instances does exercise testing uncover certain helpful findings [e.g., rate-dependent AV block, exertionally related tachyarrhythmias, severe degrees of chronotropic incompetence, excessively rapid heart rate deceleration after exercise, or the exercise-associated variant of neurally mediated syncope (98–100)]. For the most part, obtaining ECG documentation during spontaneous symptoms—if feasible at all—necessitates an extended period of cardiac monitoring using Holter monitors or event recorders. The latter systems can be used in a continuous-loop mode for patients whose symptoms preclude responding appropriately when the episode begins. Recently, the introduction of implantable loop recorders (Reveal, Medtronic, Inc., Minneapolis, MN) has added a powerful new diagnostic tool. The ability of these devices to be programmed for automatic storage of rhythm strips in which heart rates fall outside a predetermined range is particularly advantageous (101).

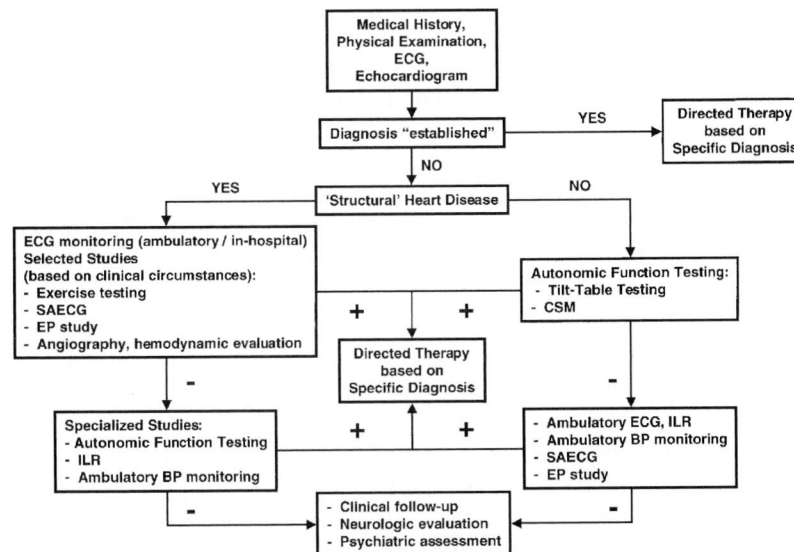

FIGURE 71.5 A proposed strategy for syncope evaluation. BP, blood pressure; CSM, carotid sinus massage; ECG, electrocardiogram; EP, electrophysiologic; ILR, implantable loop recorder; SAECG, signal-averaged electrocardiogram.

As a rule, if ambulatory ECG monitoring is successful in providing a symptom-arrhythmia correlation, the need for additional diagnostic testing may be diminished but not necessarily eliminated. For example, documentation of symptomatic bradycardia does not exclude the possibility of a neurally mediated etiology in which a concomitant vasodepressor element could complicate treatment.

Echocardiography and Vascular Ultrasound

Echocardiography rarely provides a definitive basis for syncope. Nevertheless, the echocardiogram has become essential for assessment of underlying structural heart disease. Furthermore, echocardiographic findings may be suggestive of a basis for syncope if evidence is obtained for HOCM, atrial myxoma, severe valvular aortic stenosis, or anomalous origin of one or more coronary arteries. Ultrasound techniques also are appropriately used to assess vascular disturbances detected on physical examination when these disturbances are deemed potential contributors to syncope. Thus, assessment of the carotid and subclavian systems may be an appropriate step in selected individuals.

Invasive Electrophysiologic Testing

In general, invasive electrophysiologic testing is useful for defining potential arrhythmic causes of syncope in individuals with underlying structural heart disease, including conduction system disturbances and the various forms of preexcitation syndromes. This is especially true when tachyarrhythmias are at fault. On the other hand, such testing is less successful among patients without apparent structural substrate for arrhythmia (5,6,102–104). For example, in one report (6), electrophysiologic testing was deemed to provide a diagnosis in 56% of all patients. However, the testing was clearly more successful in patients with evident structural cardiac disease (71%) than in patients without such disease (36%).

As with any test, care must be taken in interpreting findings of invasive electrophysiologic studies. This seems to be particularly a concern when evaluating potential bradyarrhythmic causes of syncope. In this regard, Fujimura et al. (105) undertook such studies in patients in whom bradyarrhythmias were known to be the cause of syncope; there were 21 syncopal patients with known symptomatic AV block or sinus pauses. Electrophysiologic testing only correctly identified three of eight patients with documented sinus pauses (sensitivity 37.5%) and 2 of 13 patients with documented AV block (sensitivity 15.4%). On the other hand, other abnormalities not known to have occurred spontaneously were often induced during electrophysiologic study. Tilt-table testing was not carried out in these patients; had it been undertaken, the additional findings may have been helpful in placing the apparently "false positive" electrophysiologic findings in perspective.

Head-Up Tilt-Table Testing

The importance of identifying susceptibility to vasovagal reactions in syncope patients is readily evident, given the frequency with which vasovagal syncope appears to be responsible for patient symptoms. To date, the head-up tilt-table test is the only diagnostic tool subjected to sufficient clinical scrutiny to assess its effectiveness in this setting.

Several reports have provided strong evidence that the symptomatic hypotension-bradycardia associated with a positive head-up tilt-table test is comparable to the spontaneous neurally mediated vasovagal syncope (106–111). Furthermore, tilt-table testing, especially when undertaken in the absence of provocative pharmacologic agents, appears to discriminate between symptomatic patients and asymptomatic control subjects with a level of precision considered acceptable for other clinically useful medical testing procedures (51–54). ⋎ m06

The response to upright tilt-table testing in patients with suspected neurally mediated syncope differs from the response observed in syncope patients in whom other diagnostic studies have provided a firm basis for symptoms. For example, Fitzpatrick et al. (113) found that 60-degree upright tilt reproduced symptoms in 53 of 71 patients (75%) with unexplained syncope; 40 patients exhibited both hypotension and bradycardia, whereas 13 subjects manifested primarily a vasodepressor response. As a result of this and many other studies, head-up tilt-table testing has become a key component of the diagnostic strategy in patients suspected of having neurally mediated syncope.

Combined Electrophysiologic and Tilt-Table Studies in Syncope

The addition of tilt-table testing to electrophysiologic testing has substantially enhanced diagnostic capabilities in syncope patients. For example, Sra et al. (102) reported results of electrophysiologic testing in conjunction with head-up tilt-table testing in 86 consecutive patients referred for evaluation of unexplained syncope. Electrophysiologic testing was abnormal in 29 patients (34%), with the majority of these (21 patients) having inducible sustained monomorphic VT. The remainder comprised inducible SVTs (five patients), sinus node dysfunction (one patient), and conduction system disease (two patients). Among the remaining patients, head-up tilt-table testing proved positive in 34 cases (40%), whereas 23 patients (26%) remained undiagnosed. During follow-up, syncope recurrence occurred in approximately 13% of patients. Importantly, however, syncope recurrence in patients in whom treatment was directed by electrophysiologic testing or tilt-table testing seemed to be highly associated with discontinuation of recommended therapies.

A further evaluation of the combined use of electrophysiologic testing and head-up tilt-table testing in the assessment of syncope is provided in the report by Fitzpatrick et al. (51). Among 322 syncope patients evaluated between 1984 and 1988, conventional electrophysiologic testing provided a basis for syncope in 229 of 322 cases (71%), with 93 patients having a normal electrophysiologic study. In terms of abnormal electrophysiologic findings, AV conduction disease was diagnosed in 34% of patients, sinus node dysfunction in 21%, carotid sinus syndrome in 10%, and inducible sustained tachyarrhythmias in 6%. As noted above, in the 93 patients with normal conventional electrophysiologic studies, tilt-table testing was undertaken in 71 cases; the testing reproduced syncope consistent with a vasovagal mechanism in 53 of these cases (75%).

Carotid Sinus Massage

The technique for undertaking carotid sinus massage and the interpretation of the test has been previously discussed. In general, the test has proved very safe; however, care should be exercised in using this test in patients with carotid bruits or prior strokes.

Neurologic Studies

Conventional neurologic laboratory studies (e.g., electroencephalogram, computed tomography of the head, and magnetic resonance imaging) have had a relatively low yield in the syncope patient. Consequently, these studies should be restricted to situations in which other clinical observations suggest organic nervous system disease (see the section Central Nervous System Causes). On the other hand, given the importance of orthostatic causes of syncope, tilt-table testing and other tests of autonomic function play an increasingly important role.

Treatment

Neurally Mediated Syncopal Syndromes

In the case of neurally mediated syncopal syndromes, treatment strategies remain in evolution. Specific treatment should, when possible, be directed at relieving apparent trigger factors. Thus, alleviating or suppressing the cause of cough in cough syncope or treating esophageal abnormalities in swallow syncope are desirable approaches. However, in conditions such as carotid sinus syncope and vasovagal syncope, comparable approaches usually are not available. Therefore, in carotid sinus syncope, cardiac pacing has become a primary treatment modality—recognizing that, in many instances, additional consideration must be given to the concomitant vasodepressor element of the syndrome.

In the case of vasovagal syncope, the mainstay in treatment is education and reassurance. This approach proves most effective when there is a prodrome of sufficient duration to permit the patient to take suitable evasive action. Patients whose symptoms demand more than mere reassurance are those whose attacks have minimal or no prodrome (especially if they have had resulting injury), those who cannot be taught to abort attacks, and those whose attacks are complicated by seizure-like activity or incontinence. Of particular concern are patients with high-risk occupations or avocations in which syncope might lead to injury to themselves or others (e.g., pilots, commercial drivers, window washers, swimmers).

In patients in whom a more aggressive treatment strategy is needed, volume expanders (e.g., increased dietary salt and electrolyte intake with salt tablets or fluids such as sports drinks) or moderate exercise training appear to be among the safest initial approaches. Additionally, in highly motivated patients with recurrent vasovagal symptoms, the prescription of progressively prolonged periods of exposure to still upright posture (i.e., tilt training) may be beneficial (115,116). Beyond these measures, a variety of pharmacologic approaches have been proposed, but few randomized clinical studies are available to confirm their utility. In this regard, beta-adrenergic blocking drugs, disopyramide, and vasoconstrictor agents [e.g., midodrine (117,118)] are the principal agents. Other drugs that appear to be useful in selected cases are serotonin-reuptake inhibitors (119,120).

Cardiac pacing has proved highly successful in carotid sinus syndrome when bradycardia has been documented (121). Currently, dual-chamber pacing is widely acknowledged to be the treatment of choice in all but the mildest forms of carotid sinus syndrome. Single-chamber atrial pacing is contraindicated due to the propensity for these patients to exhibit paroxysmal high-grade AV block during the episodes. Clinical experience with pacing in vasovagal syncope and other forms of neurally mediated syncope has been more limited than in carotid sinus syncope (122–126). However, the effectiveness of pacing in selected highly symptomatic patients with recurrent vasovagal faints has been supported by findings of two important multicenter randomized controlled trials (124,125). ❦ m07

Orthostatic Syncope

In orthostatic syncope, the mainstay of treatment is avoidance or removal (to the extent possible) of drugs that aggravate volume status (e.g., diuretics) and vasoconstriction (e.g., vasodilators). The desire is to favor expansion of central circulating volume. To this end, certain pharmacologic approaches are well accepted; specifically, administration of increased salt in the diet or use of salt-retaining steroids (e.g., principally fludrocortisone) is usually the first step (117–120). Additional benefit has been reported with the use of erythropoietin, but it is not widely used for this indication. A second element in the treatment strategy of orthostatic syncope is reduction of the tendency for central volume to be displaced to the lower extremities with upright posture. To this end, physical training (e.g., tilt training, aerobic exercise) and directly and indirectly acting vasoconstrictors have been used. In regard to drugs, clonidine has been reported to be helpful, but there appears to be little ongoing enthusiasm for its use. Of greatest current interest is midodrine—an agent that has prominent venoconstrictive properties (117,118). Physical maneuvers such as the use of counter-pressure clothing (e.g., fitted stockings, abdominal compression devices) can be helpful. Unfortunately, fitted clothing is often uncomfortable, especially in hot climates, and exposes the patient to even worse symptoms when removed. In some cases, support stockings contain latex, thereby opening the door to latex allergy. ❦ m08

Primary Cardiac Arrhythmias

The appropriate treatment of patients in whom tachyarrhythmias or bradyarrhythmias are the cause of syncope is relatively well understood. Patients in whom the correlation between syncope and bradycardia is well defined do well with cardiac pacemaker therapy (130–149). However, other factors are often important in the treatment decision process. For instance, in the case of individuals with sinus node dysfunction, optimal selection of treatment necessitates consideration of not only the culprit arrhythmic disturbance, but also the effects of drugs on sinus node and AV conduction properties and on ventricular function and proarrhythmic tendency. Additionally, current indications for and available modes of cardiac pacing and the role of anticoagulation must be incorporated into the overall treatment strategy. Finally, bundle of His ablation with placement of a permanent cardiac pacemaker remains an important tool in treatment of selected sinus node dysfunction patients who are symptomatic due to rapid ventricular rates during atrial fibrillation (131). ❦ m09

In patients with syncope resulting from paroxysmal SVTs, drug and transcatheter ablation treatment options can be highly effective, although the former is often preferable, if available.

Many paroxysmal supraventricular tachyarrhythmias can be adequately controlled by conventional antiarrhythmic drug treatment. Beta-adrenergic blockers or calcium-channel blockers may be effective alone or, if necessary, in combination with class I antiarrhythmics—particularly class IC drugs such as flecainide and propafenone. Sotalol may also be used effectively, although there is greater concern regarding QT interval prolongation and its potential proarrhythmic consequences. However, long-term drug treatment is not readily maintained in many patients due to side-effects, issues of compliance, and, occasionally, expense. Transcatheter ablation has become a reasonable and highly effective treatment option (137,138). In the case of paroxysmal reentrant SVT

associated with syncope, transcatheter ablation is probably the treatment of choice. For the most part, implantable devices for treatment of SVTs recently have been out of favor. However, the role of devices in difficult-to-control conditions may be making a resurgence with the availability of atrial implantable defibrillators and improved antitachycardia pacing systems (e.g., AT500, Medtronic, Inc., Minneapolis, MN). ❦ m10

In the case of syncope due to VT, underlying heart disease—especially left ventricular dysfunction—of varying severity is usually present. The latter also increases the proarrhythmic risk associated with antiarrhythmic drug therapy, especially with class I agents. Consequently, pharmacologic therapeutic strategies often involve early consideration of class III agents, principally sotalol or amiodarone, but also dofetilide to an increasing extent. However, given the difficulty of assuring effective prophylaxis in this apparently high-risk patient population (94–96,104), in many cases, the use of implantable cardioverter-defibrillators (ICDs) has become an important element of the overall treatment plan. In this context, Middlekauff et al. (95) noted that among patients with severe left ventricular dysfunction, the presence of a history of syncope was accompanied by a worrisome 1-year mortality (65% vs. 25% in comparable patients without syncope) and a greater tendency to sudden death (45% of deaths vs. 12% in comparable patients).

Currently, ablation techniques are appropriate first choices in patients with right ventricular outflow tract tachycardia and bundle branch reentry tachycardia. The future may bring more extensive use of such techniques into the treatment of a broader range of VT patients (144–146).

Structural Cardiovascular or Cardiopulmonary Disease

In cases of structural cardiovascular or cardiopulmonary disease, syncope is often only one of several possible types of symptoms being experienced by the patient with underlying structural disease. In such cases, treatment is best directed at amelioration of the specific structural lesion or its consequences. Thus, in syncope associated with myocardial ischemia, pharmacologic therapy or revascularization is clearly the appropriate strategy. If successful, syncope susceptibility—whether the result of tachyarrhythmias, bradyarrhythmias, or neural reflex effects—is reduced. Similarly, when syncope is closely associated with surgically addressable lesions (e.g., valvular aortic stenosis, pericardial disease, atrial myxoma, congenital cardiac anomaly), a direct, corrective approach is often feasible. On the other hand, when syncope is caused by certain difficult-to-treat conditions (e.g., primary pulmonary hypertension or restrictive cardiomyopathy), it is often impossible to ameliorate the underlying problem adequately. Even modifying outflow gradients in HOCM is not readily achieved surgically. In HOCM, the effectiveness of standard pharmacologic therapies remain uncertain (147,148); consequently, despite ongoing controversy, recent success with cardiac pacing techniques offers considerable promise to symptomatic individuals (149).

Cerebrovascular Causes

Treatment of cerebrovascular causes of syncope are critically dependent on an accurate diagnosis. Imaging studies and neurologic or neurosurgical consultation assistance should be sought. For the most part, cerebrovascular disease rarely accounts for syncope; consequently, its evaluation is generally a low priority in the absence of new neurologic signs or other nervous system symptoms. On the other hand, the possibility of such a cause should not be completely ignored. For example, arterial entrapment in conjunction with cervical spine disease is correctable but so rare that it is almost never considered.

Miscellaneous Disturbances

Syncope-like states occurring in the setting of conditions such as diabetic coma or severe hypoxia or hypercapnia obviously require addressing the underlying problem. True syncope is rarely, if ever, solely caused by these conditions. Syncope due to psychogenic hyperventilation is the most important to consider and, over the long haul, challenging to treat. Psychiatric assistance is essential in such cases. Pharmacotherapy, counseling, and biofeedback may be needed in combination.

Recognition of temporal lobe seizures, akinetic seizures, and drop attacks requires considerable clinical acumen, appropriate laboratory testing, and expert neurologic consultation. The first two conditions are controllable with antiepileptic medications, whereas drop attacks have proven difficult to control. Migraine is far more common, and, while an infrequent cause of syncope, pharmacologic treatment is highly effective.

Syncope accompanying anxiety attacks and hysteria can prove to be a chronically recurring problem. A psychiatric diagnosis for symptoms has to be considered carefully before the "label" is applied. Subtle disturbances of autonomic control may be overlooked in this setting.

CONTROVERSIES AND PERSONAL PERSPECTIVES

Despite the strides that have been taken in the assessment of the syncope patient, many aspects of this multifaceted problem remain to be settled. This is particularly true in the management of patients with neurally mediated syncope. For example, although tilt-table testing is generally accepted as the "gold standard" in terms of confirming susceptibility to vasovagal syncope, its role in the assessment of treatment effectiveness continues to be controversial. In my view, the effectiveness of pharmacologic management of syncope patients cannot be reliably predicted by tilt-table testing. However, other treatment techniques such as tilt training may be able to take advantage of the laboratory's ability to assess tolerance to upright posture. Why there should be a difference between the usefulness of tilt-table testing in assessing physical maneuvers as opposed to that of pharmacologic interventions is certainly not obvious, and I cannot claim any scientific basis for this opinion; time will tell whether it is valid.

In regard to treatment of neurally mediated syncopal syndromes, progress has been made since publication of the last edition of this book. Specifically, tilt training has become an important addition to the armamentarium and should be used in preference to drug treatments in most vasovagal fainters. Furthermore, there are now two multicenter randomized trials supporting the value of cardiac pacing in patients with frequently recurrent vasovagal syncope. On the other hand, the evaluation of pharmacologic therapies remains generally disappointing. There are as yet no large randomized drug treatment trials to report.

Still uncertain is the point at which patients with syncope should be referred for specialty evaluation. It continues to be my view that this referral is warranted if any of the following are present: (a) episodes are recurrent (i.e., >2 within a 1-year period); (b) there is evidence of underlying structural heart or cardiovascular disease; (c) physical injury has occurred; (d) the patient is at risk of economic loss (e.g., job loss); (e) the public is at risk due to his or her occupation (e.g., pilot, bus driver); or (f) the patient or his or her family indicates alarm regarding possible recurrences. The establishment of practice guidelines addressing these and related issues is essential in assuring that all syncope patients receive optimal care.

Recently, trends in medical care reimbursement in the United States and other countries have not been favorable to the introduction and study of new technologies. In the case of the syncope evaluation, large insurers (e.g., Medicare, Blue Cross–Blue Shield) continue to attempt to save money in the short-term by denying payment or compensating at miniscule levels for techniques such as tilt-table testing, despite substantial literature documenting its value. The ability to clarify diagnoses and address new therapies is a long-term economic saving that these insurers have tended to ignore. Hopefully, concerted efforts by physician-investigators, practitioners, and professional organizations ultimately will overcome this shortsightedness.

Finally, a recent "crisis" in the United States has surrounded the disappearance of isoproterenol from the marketplace. This drug has multiple uses in the electrophysiologic laboratory, but it has been particularly important in tilt-table testing. It appears that the principal supplier has had manufacturing problems, and the relatively limited income derived from the drug does not seem to merit the supplier's making the necessary investment to clear this up. Despite the fact that this may be a sound, if somewhat ruthless, business deci-

THE FUTURE

In recent years, considerable progress has been made in understanding the causes of syncope and the relative frequency with which each class of causes occurs. However, important diagnostic dilemmas remain. Most important, we continue to be limited in our ability to undertake long-term diagnostic monitoring in syncope patients. In this regard, the development of easy-to-use implantable electrocardiographic loop recorders (e.g., Reveal Plus, Medtronic, Inc., Minneapolis, MN) has been important. However, documenting electrocardiography is only part of the problem. Next-generation devices must focus on some assessment of systemic pressure recording. Furthermore, by using wireless communication from implantable devices, it should be possible to effect more rapid recognition of symptomatic rhythm and blood pressure problems, thereby permitting more efficient resolution of potentially hazardous conditions.

Syncope is a multifaceted disorder involving many organ systems. The most important and least understood of these systems is the CNS. In particular, the role of the CNS in neurally mediated syncope, syncope associated with orthostatic hypotension, and the dysautonomias remains a mystery. Future studies need to be directed at better understanding the multiple neurotransmitters and neural pathways associated with these disorders. Studies should address the molecular and genetic factors leading to the apparent increased susceptibility certain individuals exhibit with respect to these forms of syncope. Development of an understanding of these topics will have important implications in terms of the treatment of individuals and, in the most severe cases, the appropriate direction for advice regarding prognosis and family counseling.

sion, physicians—and especially electrophysiologists—should make every effort to encourage the development of means by which "niche" agents can be made available to the marketplace. In the meantime, perhaps we can avoid the use of other products from suppliers who place their economic advantage ahead of patient needs.

SUMMARY

Prevention of recurrent syncope is critically dependent on establishing the basis for symptoms in each patient. The principal diagnostic step is differentiation of individuals with normal cardiovascular status from those with evident structural disease. In the former, assuming that the medical history or physical examination has not identified another system problem, tilt-table testing should be undertaken. In the latter group of patients, a functional assessment of the suspected structural disturbance and evaluation of susceptibility to tachyarrhythmias and bradyarrhythmias by conventional electrophysiologic testing are appropriate at an early stage. Tilt-table testing should follow if the diagnosis remains in doubt. In only a few instances should special neurologic studies be selected as an initial step. In all cases, the ultimate objective is to obtain a sufficiently strong correlation between the syncopal symptoms and detected abnormalities to permit an accurate assessment of prognosis and initiation of an appropriate treatment plan.

In cases in which structural cardiac or vascular disturbances or primary cardiac arrhythmias are determined to have caused syncope, therapy is relatively well defined. On the other hand, whereas considerable progress is being made, the treatment of neurally mediated reflex syncope, orthostatic syncope, and various neurologic and psychiatric conditions that can mimic syncope is less well established.

ACKNOWLEDGMENTS

The author would like to thank Wendy Markuson and Barry L. S. Detloff for assistance in preparation of the manuscript.

REFERENCES

1. Day SC, Cook EF, Funkenstein H, et al. Evaluation and outcome of emergency room patients with transient loss of consciousness. *Am J Med* 1982;72:15–23.
2. Silverstein MD, Singer DE, Mulley AG, et al. Patients with syncope admitted to medical intensive care units. *JAMA* 1982;248:1185–1189.
3. Gendelman HE, Linzer M, Gabelman M, et al. Syncope in a general hospital population. *N Y State J Med* 1983;83:116–165.
4. Martin GJ, Adams SL, Martin HG, et al. Prospective evaluation of syncope. *Ann Emerg Med* 1984;13:499–504.
5. Kudenchuk PJ, McAnulty JH. Syncope: evaluation and treatment. *Mod Conc Cardiovasc Dis* 1985;54:25–29.
6. Camm AJ, Lau CP. Syncope of undetermined origin: diagnosis and management. *Prog in Cardiol* 1988;1:139–156.
7. Ross RT. *Syncope*. London: WB Saunders, 1988.
8. Wayne HH. Syncope: physiological considerations and an analysis of the clinical characteristics in 510 patients. *Am J Med* 1961;30:418–438.

9. Kapoor W. Evaluation and outcome of patients with syncope. *Medicine* 1990;69:160–175.

10. Savage DD, Corwin L, McGee DL, et al. Epidemiologic features of isolated syncope: the Framingham Study. *Stroke* 1985;16:626–629.

11. Lipsitz LA, Pluchino FC, Wei JY, et al. Syncope in an elderly institutionalised population: prevalence, incidence and associated risk. *Q J Med* 1985;55:45–54.

12. Sheldon R, Rose S, Flanagan P, et al. Risk factors for syncope recurrence after a positive tilt-table test in patients with syncope. *Circulation* 1996;93:973–981.

13. Nyman J, Krahn A, Bland P, et al. The costs of recurrent syncope of unknown origin in elderly patients. *PACE* 1999;22:1386–1394.

14. McHenry LC, Fazekas JF, Sullivan JF. Cerebral hemodynamics of syncope. *Am J Med Sci* 1961;214:173–178.

15. Gibson GE, Pulsinelli W, Blass JP, et al. Brain dysfunction in mild to moderate hypoxia. *Am J Med* 1981;70:1247–1254.

16. Rowell LB. *Human cardiovascular control*. Oxford: Oxford University Press, 1993.

17. Hainsworth R. Syncope and fainting: classification and pathophysiological basis. In: Mathias CJ, Bannister R, eds. *Autonomic failure. A textbook of clinical disorders of the autonomic nervous system*, 4th ed. Oxford, Oxford University Press, 1999:428–436.

18. Smit AAJ, Halliwill JR, Low PA, et al. Topical review. Pathophysiological basis of orthostatic hypotension in autonomic failure. *J Physiol* 1999;519:1–10.

19. Tea SH, Mansourati J, L'Heveder G, et al. New insights into the pathophysiology of carotid sinus syndrome. *Circulation* 1996;93:1411–1416.

20. Sharpey-Schafer EP, Hayter CJ, Barlow ED. Mechanism of acute hypotension from fear and nausea. *BMJ* 1958;2:878–880.

21. Thoren P. Role of cardiac C fibres in cardiovascular control. *Rev Physiol Biochem Pharmacol* 1979;86:1–94.

22. Oberg B, Thoren P. Increased activity in left ventricular receptors during hemorrhage or occlusion of caval veins in the cat. A possible cause of the vaso-vagal reaction. *Acta Physiol Scand* 1972;85:164–173.

23. Benditt DG, Goldstein MA, Adler S, et al. Neurally mediated syncopal syndromes: pathophysiology and clinical evaluation. In: Mandel WJ, ed. *Cardiac arrhythmias*, 3rd ed. Philadelphia: JB Lippincott Co, 1995:879–906.

24. Scherrer U, Vissing S, Morgan BJ, et al. Vasovagal syncope after infusion of a vasodilator in a heart-transplant recipient. *N Engl J Med* 1990;322:602–604.

25. Fitzpatrick AP, Banner N, Cheng A, et al. Vasovagal syncope may occur after orthotopic heart transplantation. *J Am Coll Cardiol* 1993;21:1132–1137.

26. Morgan-Hughes NJ, Kenny RA, Scott CD, et al. Vasodepressor reactions after orthotopic cardiac transplantation: relationship to reinnervation status. *Clin Autonom Res* 1994;4:125–129.

27. Barcroft H, Edholm OG. On the vasodilatation in human skeletal muscle during posthemorrhagic fainting. *J Physiol (Lond)* 1945;104:161–175.

28. Barcroft H, Edholm OG, McMichael J, et al. Posthaemorrhagic fainting. *Lancet* 1944;1:489–491.

29. Barcroft H, Edholm OG. On the vasodilatation in human skeletal muscle during posthemorrhagic fainting. *J Physiol (Lond)* 1945;104:161–175.

30. Oberg B, White S. The role of vagal cardiac nerves and arterial baroreceptors in the circulatory adjustments to hemorrhage in the cat. *Acta Physiol Scand* 1970;80:395–403.

31. Oberg B, Thoren P. Increased activity in vagal cardiac afferents correlated to the appearance of reflex bradycardia during severe hemorrhage in cats. *Acta Physiol Scand* 1970;80:22A–23A.

32. Secher NH, Sander-Jensen K, Werner C, et al. Bradycardia, a severe but reversible hypovolemic shock in man. *Circ Shock* 1984;14:267–274.

33. Morita H, Vatner SF. Effects of hemorrhage on renal nerve activity in conscious dogs. *Circ Res* 1985;57:788–793.

34. Secher NH, Jensen KS, Werner J, et al. Vagal slowing of the heart during hemorrhage: observations from 20 consecutive hypotensive patients. *BMJ* 1986;292:365–366.

35. Hammill SC, Holmes DR, Wood DL, et al. Electrophysiologic testing in the upright position: Improved evaluation of patients with rhythm disturbances using a tilt table. *J Am Coll Cardiol* 1984;4:65–71.

36. Pathy MS. Clinical presentation of myocardial infarction in the elderly. *Br Heart J* 1967;29:190–199.

37. Dixon MS, Thomas P, Sheridon DJ. Syncope is the presentation of unstable angina. *Int J Cardiol* 1988;19:125–129.

38. Johnson AM. Aortic stenosis, sudden death, and the left ventricular baroreceptors. *Br Heart J* 1971;33:1–5.

39. Lombard JT, Selzer A. Valvular aortic stenosis. *Ann Intern Med* 1987;106:292–298.

40. Atwood JE, Kawanishi S, Myers J, et al. Exercise testing in patients with aortic stenosis. *Chest* 1988;93:1083–1087.

41. Sulg IA. Differential diagnosis in syncope and epilepsy. Clinical neurophysiological and cardiological aspects. In: Refsum H, Sulg IA, Rasmussen K, eds. *Heart and brain, brain and heart*. Berlin: Springer-Verlag, 1989:202–221.

42. Alboni P, Dinelli M. Bettiol K, et al. What is the value of clinical history in establishing the cause of syncope? In: Raviele A, ed. *Cardiac arrhythmias*, Vol. 1. Milan, Italy: Springer-Verlag, 2000:419–422.

43. Sutton R, Petersen M, Brignole M, et al. Proposed classification for tilt induced vasovagal syncope. *Eur J Cardiac Pacing Electrophysiol* 1992;2:180–183.

44. Almquist A, Gornick C, Benson DW Jr, et al. Carotid sinus hypersensitivity: evaluation of the vasodepressor component. *Circulation* 1985;71:927–936.

45. Kenny RA, Bayliss J, Ingram A, et al. Head up tilt: a useful test for investigating unexplained syncope. *Lancet* 1986;1:1352–1354.

46. Abi-Samra F, Maloney JD, Fouad-Tarazi FM, et al. The usefulness of head-up tilt testing and hemodynamic investigations in the workup of syncope of unknown origin. *PACE* 1988;11:1202–1214.

47. Almquist A, Goldenberg IF, Milstein S, et al. Provocation of bradycardia and hypotension by isoproterenol and upright posture in patients with unexplained syncope. *N Engl J Med* 1989;320:346–351.

48. Benditt DG, Lurie KG, Adler SW, et al. Rationale and methodology of head-up tilt table testing for evaluation of neurally mediated (cardioneurogenic) syncope. In: Zipes DP, Jalife J, eds. *Cardiac electrophysiology. From cell to bedside*, 2nd ed. Philadelphia: WB Saunders, 1995:1115–1128.

49. Sutton R, Petersen MEV. The clinical spectrum of neurocardiogenic syncope. *J Cardiovasc Electrophysiol* 1995;6:569–576.

50. Fitzpatrick A, Theodorakis G, Vardas P, et al. The incidence of malignant vasovagal syndrome in patients with recurrent syncope. *Eur Heart J* 1991;12:389–394.

51. Fitzpatrick A, Theodorakis G, Vardas P, et al. Methodology of head-up tilt testing in patients with unexplained syncope. *J Am Coll Cardiol* 1991;17:125–130.

52. Benditt DG, Sakaguchi S, Shultz JJ, et al. Syncope. Diagnostic considerations and the role of tilt table testing. *Cardiol Rev* 1993;1:146–156.

53. Kapoor WN, Smith M, Miller NL. Upright tilt testing in evaluating syncope: a comprehensive literature review. *Am J Med* 1994;97:78–88.

54. Benditt DG, Ferguson DW, Grubb BP, et al. Tilt table testing for assessing syncope. American College of Cardiology. *J Am Coll Cardiol* 1996;28(1):263–275.

55. Morley CA, Sutton R. Carotid sinus syncope. *Int J Cardiol* 1984;6:287–293.

56. Brignole M, Menozzi C, Gianfranchi L, et al. Neurally mediated syncope detected by carotid sinus massage and head-up tilt test in sick sinus syndrome. *Am J Cardiol* 1991;68:1032–1036.

57. Imholz BP, Settels JJ, van der Meiracker AH, et al. Noninvasive continuous finger blood pressure measurement during orthostatic stress compared to intra-arterial pressure. *Cardiovasc Res* 1990;24:214–221.

58. Petersen MEV, Williams TR, Sutton R. A comparison of non-invasive continuous finger blood pressure measurement (Finapres) with intra-arterial pressure during prolonged head-up tilt. *Eur Heart J* 1995;16:1647–1654.

59. Hoefnagels WA, Padberg GW, Overweg J, et al. Syncope or seizure? The diagnostic value of the EEG and hyperventilation test in transient loss of consciousness. *J Neurol Neurosurg Psychiatry* 1991;54:953–956.

60. Bannister R. Chronic autonomic failure with postural hypotension. *Lancet* 1979;2:404–406.

61. Hopkins A, Neville B, Bannister R. Autonomic neuropathy of acute onset. *Lancet* 1974;1:769–771.

62. Edmonds ME, Sturrock RD. Autonomic neuropathy in the Guillain-Barré syndrome. *BMJ* 1979;2:668-670.

63. Low PA, Opfer-Gherking TL, McPhee BR, et al. Prospective evaluation of clinical characteristics of orthostatic hypotension. *Mayo Clin Proc* 1995;70:617–622.

64. Rowe P, Bou-Holaigah I, Kan J, et al. Is neurally mediated hypotension an unrecognized cause of chronic fatigue. *Lancet* 1995;345:623–624.

65. Low PA. Autonomic nervous system function. *J Clin Neurophys* 1993;10:14–27.

66. Weiling W, van Lieshout JJ. Investigation and treatment of autonomic circulatory failure. *Curr Opinion Neurol Neurosurg* 1993;6:537–543.

67. Rubenstein JJ, Schulman CL, Yurchak PM, et al. Clinical spectrum of the sick sinus syndrome. *Circulation* 1972;6:5–13.

68. Kaplan BM, Langendorf R, Lev M, et al. Tachycardia-bradycardia syndrome (so-called "sick sinus syndrome"). *Am J Cardiol* 1973;26:497–508.

69. Benditt DG, Sakaguchi S, Goldstein MA, et al. Sinus node dysfunction: Pathophysiology, clinical features, evaluation and treatment. In: Zipes DP, Jalife J, eds. *Cardiac electrophysiology. From cell to bedside*, 2nd ed. Philadelphia: WB Saunders, 1995:1215–1246.

70. Scheinman MM, Strauss HC, Evans GT, et al. Adverse effects of sympatholytic agents in patients with hypertension and sinus node dysfunction. *Am J Med* 1978;64:1013–1020.

71. Linker NJ, Camm AJ. Drug effects on the sinus node. A clinical perspective. *Cardiovasc Drugs Ther* 1988;2:165–170.

72. Sutton R, Perrins EJ. Neurological manifestations of the sick sinus syndrome. In: Busse EW, ed. *Cerebral manifestations of episodic cardiac dysrhythmias*. Amsterdam: Excerpta Medica, 1979:174–181.

73. Sutton R, Kenny R-A. The natural history of sick sinus syndrome. *PACE* 1986;9:1110–1114.

74. Skagen K, Hansen JF. The long-term prognosis for patients with sinoatrial block treated with permanent pacemaker. *Acta Med Scand* 1975;199:13–15.

75. Sasaki S, Shimotori M, Akahane K, et al. Long-term follow-up of patients with sick sinus syndrome: a comparison of clinical aspects among unpaced, ventricular inhibited paced, and physiologically paced groups. *PACE* 1988;11:1575–1583.

76. Lev M. The pathology of atrioventricular block. *Cardiovasc Clin* 1972;4:159–186.

77. Lev M, Bharati S. Atrioventricular and intraventricular conduction system disease. *Arch Int Med* 1975;135:405–410.

78. van Mechelen R, Segers A, Hagemeijer F. Serial electrophysiologic studies after single chamber atrial pacemaker implantation in patients with symptomatic sinus node dysfunction. *Eur Heart J* 1984;5:628–636.

79. Kocovic DZ, Friedman PL. Atrioventricular nodal block. In: PJ Podrid, PR Kowey, eds. *Cardiac arrhythmias. Mechanisms, diagnosis, and management*. Baltimore: Williams & Wilkins, 1995:1039–1050.

80. Ausubel K, Furman S. The pacemaker syndrome. *Ann Intern Med* 1985;103:420–429.

81. Ellenbogen K, Wood MA, Stambler B. Pacemaker syndrome: clinical, hemodynamic, and neurohumoral features. In: Barold SS, Mugica J, eds. *New perspectives in cardiac pacing*, Vol. 3. Mount Kisco, NY: Futura Publishing Co, 1993:85–112.

82. Rowe JC, White PD. Complete heart block: a follow-up study. *Ann Intern Med* 1958;49:260–270.

83. Penton GB, Miller H, Levine SA. Some clinical features of complete heart block. *Circulation* 1956;13:801–824.

84. Michaelson M, Engle MA. Congenital complete heart block: an international study of the natural history. *Cardiovasc Clin* 1972;4:86–101.

85. Pordon CM, Moodie DJ. Adults with congenital complete heart block: 25-year follow-up. *Clev Clinic J Med* 1992;59:587–590.

86. Michaelsson M, Jonzon A, Riesenfeld T. Isolated congenital complete atrioventricular block in adult life. *Circulation* 1995;92:442–449.

87. Dhingra RC, Denes P, Wu D, et al. Syncope in patients with chronic bifascicular block. *Ann Intern Med* 1974;81:302–306.

88. Scheinman MM, Peters RW, Sauve MJ, et al. Value of H-Q interval in patients with bundle branch block and the role of

prophylactic permanent pacing. *Am J Cardiol* 1982;50:1316–1322.

89. Dhingra RC, Amat y Leon F, Pouget M, et al. Infranodal block. Diagnosis, clinical significance and management. *Med Clin North Am* 1976;60:175–192.

90. Leitch JW, Klein GJ, Yee R, et al. Syncope associated with supraventricular tachycardia: An expression of tachycardia or vasomotor response. *Circulation* 1992;85:1064–1071.

91. Simson MB. Signal-averaged electrocardiography. In: Zipes DP, Jalife J, eds. *Cardiac electrophysiology. From cell to bedside*, 2nd ed. Philadelphia: WB Saunders, 1995:1038–1048.

92. Kuchar DL, Thorburn CW, Sammel NL. Signal-averaged electrocardiogram for evaluation of recurrent syncope. *Am J Cardiol* 1986;58:949–953.

93. Buxton AE, Lee KL, Fisher JD, et al., for the Multicenter Unsustained Tachycardia Trial Investigators. *N Engl J Med* 1999;341:1882–1890.

94. Swerdlow CD, Winkle RA, Mason JW. Determinants of survival in patients with ventricular tachyarrhythmias. *N Engl J Med* 1983;308:1436–1442.

95. Middlekauff HR, Stevenson WG, Stevenson LW, et al. Syncope in advanced heart failure: High risk of sudden death regardless of origin of syncope. *J Am Coll Cardiol* 1993;21:110–116.

96. Middlekauff HR, Stevenson WG, Saxon LA. Prognosis after syncope: Impact of left ventricular function. *Am Heart J* 1993;125:121–127.

97. Grubb BP, Gerard G, Rousch K, et al. Differentiation of convulsive syncope and epilepsy with head-up tilt testing. *Ann Intern Med* 1991;115:871–876.

98. Grubb BP, Temesy-Armos PN, Samoil D, et al. Tilt table testing in the evaluation and management of athletes with recurrent exercise-induced syncope. *Med Sci Sports Exerc* 1993;25:24–28.

99. Sakaguchi S, Shultz J, Remole C, et al. Syncope associated with exercise, a manifestation of neurally mediated syncope. *Am J Cardiol* 1995;75:476–481.

100. Calkins H, Seifert M, Morady F. Clinical presentation and long term follow-up of athletes with exercise-induced vasodepressor syncope. *Am Heart J* 1995;129:1159–1164.

101. Krahn A, Klein GJ, Yee R, et al. Use of an extended monitoring strategy in patients with problematic syncope. *Circulation* 1999;99:406–410.

102. Sra JS, Anderson AJ, Sheikh SH, et al. Unexplained syncope evaluated by electrophysiologic studies and head-up tilt testing. *Ann Intern Med* 1991;114:1013–1019.

103. Morady F, Shen E, Schwartz A, et al. Long-term follow-up of patients with recurrent unexplained syncope evaluated by electrophysiologic testing. *J Am Coll Cardiol* 1983;2:1053–1059.

104. Bass EB, Elson JJ, Fogoros RN, et al. Long-term prognosis of patients undergoing electrophysiologic studies for syncope of unknown origin. *Am J Cardiol* 1988;62:1186–1191.

105. Fujimura O, Yee R, Klein GJ, et al. The diagnostic sensitivity of electrophysiologic testing in patients with syncope caused by bradycardia. *N Engl J Med* 1989;321:1703–1707.

106. Fitzpatrick A, Williams T, Ahmed R, et al. Echocardiographic and endocrine changes during vasovagal syncope induced by prolonged head-up tilt. *Eur J Cardiac Pacing Electrophysiol* 1992;2:121–128.

107. Benditt DG, Lurie KG, Adler SW, et al. Rationale and methodology of head-up tilt table testing for evaluation of neurally mediated (cardioneurogenic) syncope. In: Zipes DP, Jalife J, eds. *Cardiac electrophysiology. From cell to bedside*, 2nd ed. Philadelphia: WB Saunders, 1995:115–1128.

108. van Lieshout JJ, Wieling W, Karemaker JM, et al. The vasovagal response. *Clin Sci* 1991;81:575–586.

109. Chen M-Y, Goldenberg IF, Milstein S, et al. Cardiac electrophysiologic and hemodynamic correlates of neurally mediated syncope. *Am J Cardiol* 1989;63:66–72.

110. Chosy JJ, Graham DT. Catecholamines in vasovagal fainting. *J Psychosom Res* 1965;9:189–194.

111. Sander-Jensen K, Secher NH, Astrup A, et al. Hypotension induced by passive head-up tilt: endocrine and circulatory mechanisms. *Am J Physiol* 1986;251:R742–R748.

112. de Mey C, Enterling D. Assessment of the hemodynamic responses to single passive head-up tilt by non-invasive methods in normotensive subjects. *Methods Find Exp Clin Pharmacol* 1986;8:449–457.

113. Fitzpatrick A, Theodorakis G, Vardas P, et al. The incidence of malignant vasovagal syndrome in patients with recurrent syncope. *Eur Heart J* 1991;12:389–394.

114. Natale A, Akhtar M, Jazayeri M, et al. Provocation of hypotension during head-up tilt testing in subjects with no history of syncope or presyncope. *Circulation* 1995;92:54–58.

115. Ector H, Reybrouck T, Heidbuchel H, et al. Tilt training: a new treatment for recurrent neurocardiogenic syncope or severe orthostatic intolerance. *PACE* 1998;21:193–196.

116. Di Girolamo E, Di Iorio C, Leonzio L, et al. Usefulness of a tilt training program for the prevention of refractory neurocardiogenic syncope in adolescents. A controlled study. *Circulation* 1999;100:1798–1801.

117. Sra J, Maglio C, Biehl M, et al. Efficacy of midodrine hydrochloride in neurocardiogenic syncope refractory to standard therapy. *J Cardiovasc Electrophysiol* 1997;8:42–46.

118. Benditt DG, Wilbert L, Fahy G, et al. Midodrine for treatment of vasovagal syncope. In: Raviele A, ed. *Cardiac arrhythmias*, Vol. 1. Milan, Italy: Springer-Verlag, 2000:463–468.

119. Grubb BP, Wolfe D, Samoil D, et al. Usefulness of fluoxetine hydrochloride for prevention of resistant upright tilt induced syncope. *PACE* 1993;16:458–464.

120. Kosinski D, Grubb BP, Temesy-Armos PN. The use of serotonin re-uptake inhibitors in the treatment of neurally mediated cardiovascular disorders. *J Serotonin Res* 1994;1:85–90.

121. Benditt DG, Remole S, Asso A, et al. Cardiac pacing for carotid sinus syndrome and vasovagal syncope. In: Barold SS, Mugica J, eds. *New perspectives in cardiac pacing*, Vol. 3. Mount Kisco, NY: Futura Publishing Co, 1993:15–28.

122. Benditt DG, Peterson M, Lurie K, et al. Cardiac pacing for prevention of recurrent vasovagal syncope. *Ann Intern Med* 1995;122:204–209.

123. Benditt DG. Cardiac pacing for prevention of vasovagal syncope [editorial]. *J Am Coll Cardiol* 1999;33:21–23.

124. Connolly SJ, Sheldon R, Roberts RS, et al. The North American Vasovagal Pacemaker Study (VPS). A randomized trial of permanent cardiac pacing for the prevention of vasovagal syncope. *J Am Coll Cardiol* 1999;33:16–20.

125. Sutton R, Brignole M, Menozzi C, et al., for the VASIS investigators. Dual-chamber pacing is efficacious in treat-

ment of neurally mediated tilt-positive cardioinhibitory syncope. Pacemaker versus no therapy: a multicentre randomized study. *Circulation* 2000;102:294–299.

126. Petersen MEV, Chamberlain-Webber R, Fitzpatrick AP, et al. Permanent pacing for cardioinhibitory malignant vasovagal syndrome. *Br Heart J* 1994;71:274–281.

127. Bannister R, Mathias C. Management of postural hypotension. In: Bannister R, ed. *Autonomic failure. A textbook of clinical disorders of the autonomic nervous system.* Oxford: Oxford University Press, 1988:569–595.

128. Ten Harkel ADJ, van Lieshout JJ, Wieling W. Treatment of orthostatic hypotension with sleeping in the head-up tilt position, alone and in combination with fludrocortisone. *J Int Med* 1992;232:139–145.

129. Weiling W, van Lieshout JJ, van Leeuwen AM. Physical maneuvers that reduce postural hypotension in autonomic failure. *Clin Autonom Res* 1993;3:57–65.

130. Rattes MF, Klein GJ, Sharma AD, et al. Efficacy of empirical cardiac pacing in syncope of unknown cause. *Can Med Assoc J* 1989;140:381–385.

131. Scheinman MM, Evans-Bell T, and the Executive Committee of the Percutaneous Cardiac Mapping and Ablation Registry. Catheter ablation of the atrioventricular junction: a report of the percutaneous mapping and ablation registry. *Circulation* 1984;70:1024–1029.

132. Rosenqvist M, Brandt J, Schuller H. Atrial versus ventricular pacing in sinus node disease: A treatment comparison study. *Am Heart J* 1986;111:292–297.

133. Stangl K, Wirtzfeld A, Seitz K, et al. Atrial stimulation (AAI): long-term follow-up of 110 patients. In: Belhassen B, Feldman S, Copperman Y, eds. *Cardiac pacing and electrophysiology. Proceedings of the 8th World Symposium on Cardiac Pacing and Electrophysiology.* Jerusalem: R & L Creative Communications, 1987:283–285.

134. Rosenqvist M, Brandt J, Schuller H. Long-term pacing in sick sinus node disease: effects of stimulation mode on cardiovascular morbidity and mortality. *Am Heart J* 1988;116:16–22.

135. Andersen HR, Thuesen L, Bagger JP, et al. Prospective randomized trial of atrial versus ventricular pacing in sick-sinus syndrome. *Lancet* 1994;344:1523–1528.

136. Laupacis A, Albers G, Dalen J, et al. Antithrombotic therapy in atrial fibrillation. *Chest* 1995;108:352S–359S.

137. Jackman WM, Wang W, Friday K, et al. Catheter ablation of accessory atrioventricular pathways (Wolff-Parkinson-White syndrome) by radiofrequency current. *N Engl J Med* 1991;324:1605–1611.

138. Naccarelli GV, Dougherty AH, Jalal S, et al. Paroxysmal supraventricular tachycardia: Comparative role of therapeutic methods—drugs, devices, and ablation. In: Saksena S, Luderitz B, eds. *Interventional electrophysiology. A textbook,* 2nd ed. Armonk, NY: Futura Publishing Co, 1996:461–470.

139. Cox JL. The surgical treatment of atrial fibrillation IV. Surgical technique. *J Thorac Cardiovasc Surg* 1991;101:5884–5892.

140. Cox JL, Boineau JP, Schuessler RB, et al. Modifications of the MAZE procedure for atrial flutter and atrial fibrillation: I—rationale and surgical results. *J Thorac Cardiovasc Surg* 1995;110:473–484.

141. Haissaguerre M, Gencel L, Fischer B, et al. Successful catheter ablation of atrial fibrillation. *J Cardiovasc Electrophysiol* 1994;5:1045–1052.

142. Haissaguerre M, Jais P, Shah DC, et al. Spontaneous initiation of atrial fibrillation by ectopic beats originating in the pulmonary veins. *N Engl J Med* 1998;339:659–666.

143. Chen SA, Tai CT, Hsieh MH, et al. Radiofrequency catheter ablation of atrial fibrillation initiated by spontaneous ectopic beats. *Europace* 2000;2:99–105.

144. Morady F, Harvey M, Kalbfleisch SJ, et al. Radiofrequency catheter ablation of ventricular tachycardia in patients with coronary artery disease. *Circulation* 1993;87:363–372.

145. Stevenson WG, Khan H, Sager P, et al. Identification of reentry circuit sites during catheter mapping and radiofrequency ablation of ventricular tachycardia late after myocardial infarction. *Circulation* 1993;88:1647–1670.

146. Borgreffe M, Chen X, Hindricks G, et al. Catheter ablation of ventricular tachycardia in patients with heart disease. In: Zipes DP, ed. *Catheter ablation of arrhythmias.* Armonk, NY: Futura Publishing Co, 1994:277–308.

147. McKenna WJ, Deanfield J, Faruqui A, et al. Prognosis in hypertrophic cardiomyopathy: role of age and clinical electrocardiographic and hemodynamic features. *Am J Cardiol* 1981;47:532–538.

148. Maron BJ, Roberts WC, Epstein SE. Sudden death in hypertrophic cardiomyopathy: A profile of 78 patients. *Circulation* 1982;65:1388–1394.

149. McAreavey D, Epstein ND, Fananapazir L. Dual chamber pacing is effective therapy for hypertrophic cardiomyopathy patients with provocable LV outflow tract obstruction and symptoms refractory to medical therapy [abstract]. *J Am Coll Cardiol* 1994;23:11.

CATHETER ABLATION THERAPY FOR ARRHYTHMIAS

DAVID E. HAINES

▼▼ **ADDITIONAL ELECTRONIC TOPICS**

Cellular Effects of Radiofrequency Ablation m11;   Complications of Catheter Ablation m12

OVERVIEW

The rationale behind ablative therapy is that, for any arrhythmia, there exists a critical anatomic substrate that allows propagation of that arrhythmia. If that substrate is irreversibly damaged or destroyed, then the arrhythmia should no longer occur spontaneously or with provocation.

A number of methods of catheter ablation have been attempted experimentally and clinically, but radiofrequency catheter ablation has emerged as the safest and most effective modality.

Radiofrequency energy heats myocardium by the passage of the radiofrequency electrical current through the tissue, resulting in resistive tissue heating.

Deeper tissue heating results in larger lesions. Larger electrodes, higher temperatures, and very high-power deliveries coupled with irrigated or cooled tip catheters increase lesion size.

Radiofrequency ablative lesions are thermally mediated. Temperatures exceeding 50°C result in breakdown of the sarcolemmal membrane and cell death.

The mechanisms of paroxysmal supraventricular tachycardia are varied and include atrioventricular (AV) reciprocating tachycardia, AV nodal reentrant tachycardia, atrial fibrillation, atrial flutter, and atrial tachycardia of focal automatic or reentrant mechanisms.

Catheter ablation of accessory pathways responsible for the Wolff-Parkinson-White syndrome and AV reciprocating tachycardias may be accomplished at either the atrial or ventricular insertion sites of the pathway with a high (greater than 95% at experienced centers) success rate.

Catheter modification of the AV node is highly successful in eliminating AV nodal reentrant tachycardia. In most cases, ablation in the low septal region results in elimination or marked modification of the slow AV nodal pathway and prevents tachycardia recurrence.

D. E. Haines: Cardiovascular Division, University of Virginia Health System, Charlottesville, Virginia

Atrial flutter is a macroreentrant rhythm that travels around the tricuspid valve annulus and through the isthmus between the valve and the inferior vena caval inlet. A linear ablative lesion placed across this isthmus results in successful ablation of the atrial flutter. However, concomitant atrial fibrillation is not altered by this ablation and will likely recur unless additional therapy is prescribed.

Atrial fibrillation may have a reentrant mechanism or, particularly in patients with frequent paroxysmal atrial fibrillation and normal atrial size, may originate from rapid firing from a pulmonary vein focus.

Ablation of focal origins of atrial fibrillation initiation is moderately successful in eliminating this arrhythmia in highly selected patients.

Common atrial fibrillation has a reentrant mechanism. Cure with ablation usually requires successful creation of long transmural continuous linear lesions in left and right atria. This has been difficult to achieve with catheter-based technologies.

Ventricular tachycardia may be idiopathic or caused by the presence of underlying structural heart disease.

Idiopathic ventricular tachycardia from the right ventricle is usually focal in origin, with a likely mechanism of abnormal automaticity or triggered activity. It may be ablated with a high likelihood of success.

Ventricular tachycardia in the setting of structural heart disease is usually caused by a reentrant mechanism in regions of patchy fibrosis. Ablation may be accomplished at sites within the zone of slowed electrical conduction that is identified with techniques such as activation and entrainment mapping.

GLOSSARY

Accessory pathway: An anomalous bridge of electrically conducting tissue between the atrium and ventricle, which is responsible for Wolff-Parkinson-White syndrome and AV reciprocating tachycardias, also known as a *bundle of Kent* or *bypass tract*.

Activation mapping: Multipoint electrogram acquisition during ongoing tachycardia demonstrates sites where the local electrical activity precedes the onset of the surface QRS complex. These sites represent exit points from the slow conduction zone for reentrant tachycardias or sites of arrhythmia origin for automatic or triggered tachycardias.

AV nodal modification: (a) Ablation of the slow AV nodal pathway to treat AV nodal reentrant tachycardia; (b) nonspecific ablation of the AV node to impair anterograde conduction and decrease the ventricular response rate to atrial fibrillation.

Coagulum: When boiling occurs at the electrode tip, coagulated protein from tissue and blood adhere to the tip of the electrode.

Convective cooling: The process by which thermal energy is removed by circulating blood flow through the heart.

Dispersive electrode: An electrode with a large surface area that is placed in contact with the patient's skin (usually with electrically conductive gel) to complete the electrical circuit during ablation with radiofrequency electrical current.

Electrical impedance: The resistance and capacitance of the radiofrequency electrical circuit, including the electronic components, conducting wires, point of conduction between the ablation electrode and the heart, tissue between the heart and the skin, and junction between the skin and the dispersive electrode.

Entrainment mapping: Pacing slightly faster than ongoing reentrant ventricular tachycardia from various sites in the ventricle. When one is in or near the slow conduction zone, the morphology of the resulting complex matches the tachycardia morphology exactly, and the time from the stimulus to the QRS complex is prolonged (concealed entrainment).

Impedance rise: If boiling and coagulum adherence occur, the available surface area for radiofrequency current conduction decreases, resulting in a sudden increase in system impedance.

Pace mapping: During sinus rhythm, pacing is performed from a variety of ventricular sites. For ventricular tachycardias of focal origin, the electrocardiograms during pacing should be almost identical to those during tachycardia if the pacing site is in close proximity to the arrhythmia origin.

Radiofrequency energy: High-frequency alternating electrical current; when passed through a resistive medium, it creates heat.

Slow and fast AV nodal pathways: The AV node has multiple atrial inputs that have varying properties, including conduction time. In typical AV nodal reentrant tachycardia, electrical activation travels anterograde down a slowly conducting AV nodal pathway and retrograde up a fast conducting pathway.

Tricuspid-inferior vena cava isthmus: The narrow anatomic region between the tricuspid annulus and the inferior vena caval orifice in the right atrium through which atrial flutter reentrant circuits conduct. This is the usual site targeted for atrial flutter ablation.

Ventricular preexcitation: Pattern seen on surface electrocardiograms characterized by delta waves (slurred QRS upstrokes) and resulting from the presence of an accessory pathway that conducts in an anterograde fashion. Wolff-Parkinson-White syndrome is the most common form of preexcitation syndrome.

Ventricular tachycardia slow conduction zone: Region in the border zone of scar in the ventricle bounded by areas of anatomic or physiologic conduction block, which has a slow conduction velocity. Conduction through this region accounts for the diastolic period of electrical silence on the surface electrocardiogram during ongoing reentrant ventricular tachycardia.

Volume heating: Heating from radiofrequency energy or other energy source that is direct and not a result of heat conduction from a contiguous region of heated tissue.

INTRODUCTION

Ablative therapy for the management of arrhythmias is based on the observation that most arrhythmias arise from a focal origin or are critically dependent on conduction through a defined anatomic structure. If those critical regions are irreversibly damaged or destroyed, then the arrhythmia should no longer occur spontaneously or with provocation. Traditionally, ablation was performed with open surgical techniques. It was discovered, however, that focal endocardial injury could also be achieved by a controlled delivery of destructive energy through a catheter. In the past decade, catheter designs have evolved to improve site access dramatically, and our knowledge and understanding of the anatomy of the heart and the sources of arrhythmia origin have significantly expanded. In response to this progress, the indications for catheter ablation have continued to broaden, and it is now the therapy of choice for a number of arrhythmias.

HISTORY OF CATHETER ABLATION

The concept of ablative therapy for the treatment of arrhythmias was well established in the surgical literature throughout the 1970s. Since the original description of the surgical division of an accessory pathway by Sealy et al. in 1969 (1), there have been several reports of surgical treatment of the Wolff-Parkinson-White syndrome (2,3) and ventricular tachycardia (4,5). In these series, the concept of curative ablative therapy was proved. However, the obvious limitation to this approach was that an open thoracotomy and, in most cases, cardiopulmonary bypass were required. Although researchers were pursuing a variety of approaches to decrease surgical morbidity and mortality, it was not thought possible to eliminate these arrhythmic substrates without direct visualization.

In 1979, a complication of transthoracic cardioversion was reported. Catheters had been placed for recording in the bundle of His position, and multiple direct current (DC) shocks were administered transthoracically to terminate an episode of ventricular tachycardia. At the conclusion of the cardioversion, complete heart block was observed. It was hypothesized that shunting of defibrillator current through the His bundle catheter caused irreversible damage to the AV conduction system (6). After this report, Scheinman et al. (7) and Gallagher et al. (8) published the first series of catheter ablation of the AV junction in patients with atrial fibrillation and a rapid ventricular response rate that could not be con-

trolled with drugs. In these cases, high-voltage DC electrical energy was intentionally delivered between the tip of an electrode catheter placed contiguous to the bundle of His and a dispersive patch electrode placed on the skin. The field of catheter ablation was born. ➤ m13

The modern era of radiofrequency catheter ablation was entered with the first report of successful catheter ablation of an accessory pathway with high-frequency alternating (radiofrequency) electrical current by Borggrefe et al. (20). Based on the important work of Jackman, Kuck, Haissaguerre, Morady, and others, the correlations between electrographic patterns, anatomic locations of accessory pathways, and access to those sites with ablation catheters were elucidated (21–23). Success rates exceeding 90% were reported by investigators in the treatment of paroxysmal supraventricular tachycardia (24–26). In the present day, experienced operators achieve greater than 95% success rates in the ablation of these patients. The indications for radiofrequency catheter ablation continue to expand, and it has become a dominant therapeutic modality for many varieties of symptomatic tachycardia.

BIOPHYSICS OF RADIOFREQUENCY CATHETER ABLATION

Radiofrequency electrical energy is employed to create thermal lesions in the heart. The frequencies generally employed are 300 to 1,000 kHz. It is important to note that, although this energy is similar to that employed for broadcast radio, the radiofrequency energy is electrically conducted, not radiated, during catheter ablation. The radiofrequency current is similar to low-frequency alternating current or DC with regard to its ability to heat tissue and create a lesion, but it oscillates so rapidly that cardiac and skeletal muscles are not stimulated, thereby avoiding induction of arrhythmias and decreasing the pain perceived by the patient. As the electrical current passes through the myocardium, the energy dissipates as heat. Direct resistive myocardial heating (volume heating) is proportional to the radiofrequency power density (or the square of the current density) that decreases in proportion to the fourth power of the distance from the electrode. Therefore, most of the volume heating occurs within the first 2 mm of depth from the electrode (17). Heating to deeper tissue layers occurs by heat conduction from the region of volume heating.

The radiofrequency current is generally delivered in a unipolar fashion between the tip of the ablation electrode and a dispersive electrode applied to the patient's skin. Because the surface area of the ablation electrode is much smaller than that of the dispersive electrode, the current density is higher at the ablation site, and heating occurs preferentially at that site (*e*Fig. 73.0.1). If, however, ablation is performed with a high-amplitude current and skin contact by the dispersive electrode is poor, it is possible to cause

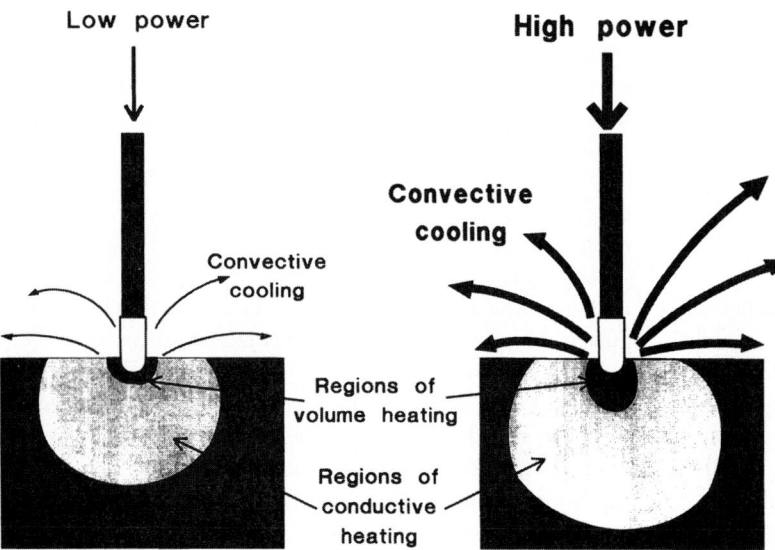

FIGURE 73.1 Schematic representation of two conditions during radiofrequency catheter ablation. The left panel depicts conventional conditions with a moderate degree of convective cooling. A low magnitude of radiofrequency power is applied to achieve heating at the electrode-tissue interface. This results in a small depth of volume heating and a moderate depth of conductive heating that create the final pathologic lesion. The right panel depicts radiofrequency ablation in the setting of increased convective cooling, either by active tip cooling with perfused or circulating saline or by unstable catheter-tissue contact. A high magnitude of radiofrequency power is applied, but the electrode-tissue interface does not exceed 100°C because of convective dissipation of heat at the tissue surface. The higher-applied power results in a greater depth of volume heating and a larger overall lesion size.

skin burns. The geometry of the radiofrequency current field is defined by the geometry of the ablation electrode and is relatively uniform in the region of volume heating. Thus, the position of the dispersive electrode has little effect on the geometry of the resulting lesion. ❦ m14

The dominant factor opposing effective heating of myocardium is the convective cooling from the circulating blood pool. If the catheter position is not stable, or if it is positioned in a region of high blood flow, the magnitude of convective cooling is increased (33). Efficiency of energy delivery to the tissue may vary from approximately 70% to 10% *in vivo*. The effects of convective cooling have been exploited to increase the size of catheter ablative lesions. To eliminate the risk of overheating at the electrode-tissue contact point but increase the magnitude of power delivery and the depth of volume heating, investigators have employed porous-tipped electrodes for open irrigation of the electrode tip (34) or closed irrigation systems for electrode tip cooling (Fig. 73.1) (35). Nakagawa et al. achieved temperatures of 95° ± 9°C at depths of 3.5 mm and lesion dimensions of 10 ± 1 mm depth by 14 ± 2 mm diameter with ablation through an irrigated-tip electrode in a superfused canine thigh muscle preparation. However, superheating within the tissue with a resulting sudden explosive release of the expanding steam to the surface (the so-called pop lesion) was observed in 7.5% of the ablations (34). Thus, increasing power delivery and convective cooling may create large lesions, but lesion production is somewhat difficult to control.

Because the success of radiofrequency catheter ablation in the clinical setting is sometimes limited by the relatively small size of the lesion, attempts have been made to increase the size of those lesions reliably and safely. One approach to this end is to increase the size and surface area of the electrode. The radiofrequency power needs to be increased comparably in order to achieve a similar current density and temperature at the electrode-tissue interface, and the result

is a greater depth of volume heating and a larger lesion (18). The introduction of the larger 4-mm ablation electrode was an important factor in the improved success rates of present-day catheter ablation (35). Investigators are continuing to pursue novel electrode geometries for special applications of radiofrequency catheter ablation (36).

MECHANISMS OF MYOCARDIAL INJURY CAUSED BY RADIOFREQUENCY CATHETER ABLATION

It is likely that the major mechanism of tissue injury from radiofrequency catheter ablation is thermal. Heating of the myocardium occurs reproducibly during radiofrequency energy delivery, and the association of clinical effect and temperature measured at the electrode-catheter interface has been established. Experimentally, lesions created from a radiofrequency or microwave source have a reliable isotherm of irreversible tissue injury of 52° to 55°C (37). In the clinical setting, successful ablations were associated with a mean temperature measured at the electrode-tissue interface of 62° ± 15°C (38). During ablation of the AV junction, the reversible physiologic effect of an accelerated junctional rhythm was observed at temperatures of 51° ± 4°C, whereas temperatures of 58° ± 6°C were required to achieve heart block (39). Clinical effects of radiofrequency ablation have been observed with electrode tip temperatures of less than 40°C (40), indicating that the electrical effects of radiofrequency current may alter tissue properties as well.

Tissue Effects of Radiofrequency Catheter Ablation

Changes in myocardial tissue are apparent immediately on completion of the radiofrequency lesion. Pallor of the central zone of the lesion is attributable to myoglobin denaturation with an associated color change. Some volume loss in the central region of lesion formation is apparent as evidenced by a slight deformation at the point of catheter contact. Fibrin usually adheres to the endocardial surface and, if a temperature of 100°C has been exceeded, adherent char and thrombus are often apparent. On sectioning, the central portion of the lesion shows desiccation, with a surrounding region of hemorrhagic tissue, then normal appearing tissue (*e*Fig. 73.1.1) (41,42). The histology of an acute lesion shows typical coagulation necrosis with basophilic stippling consistent with intracellular calcium overload. Immediately surrounding the central lesion is a region of hemorrhage and acute monocellular and neutrophilic inflammation. The progressive changes seen in the evolution of a radiofrequency lesion are typical of healing after any acute injury. Within 2 months of the ablation, the lesions show fibrosis, granulation tissue, chronic inflammatory infiltrates, and significant volume contraction (41). The lesion border is well demarcated from the surrounding viable myocardium without evidence of patchy fibrosis. This likely accounts for the absence of proarrhythmia side effects of radiofrequency catheter ablation. Because of the high-velocity blood flow within the epicardial coronary arteries, these vessels are continuously cooled and are spared from injury despite nearby delivery of radiofrequency energy (43). However, high radiofrequency power delivery in small hearts, such as in pediatric patients, may potentially cause coronary arterial injury, so caution is warranted (44). ❧ m15

ABLATION OF SPECIFIC SUPRAVENTRICULAR ARRHYTHMIAS

Accessory Pathway–Mediated Arrhythmias

A giant step forward was achieved with the first successful catheter ablations of accessory pathways (20). Before the catheter ablation era, patients with Wolff-Parkinson-White syndrome and concealed accessory pathways frequently required open surgical ablation of their extranodal pathways. The ability to map precisely the location of accessory pathways and deliver a precise ablative lesion with radiofrequency energy not only proved to be a valuable therapeutic modality, but also greatly enhanced the understanding of the physiologic and anatomic correlates of this relatively common abnormality. Important preliminary work by Jackman et al. identified electrogram patterns that correlated precisely with accessory pathway insertions in the atria and ventricles (21). The ultimate validation of the origin of these potentials arrived when small, discrete radiofrequency lesions placed at those locations resulted in elimination of both anterograde and retrograde accessory pathway conduction (*e*Fig. 73.1.2) (24–26,53). It has been

proposed that the pathways frequently follow a slanting course with separation of atrial and ventricular insertion points by 4 ± 30 mm, and that they may be composed of multiple closely spaced fibers (21). The majority of accessory pathways has a discrete and narrow ventricular and atrial insertion. The presence of occasional branching accessory pathway insertions may be assumed in cases in which accessory pathway conduction is modified but not blocked by one lesion, and then is blocked by a second application of energy at a second discrete site. The high success rate of radiofrequency catheter ablation delivered from the endocardial approach implies that most pathways are situated closely to the endocardial surface. However, a small proportion of left free wall accessory pathways (1% to 4%) can only be ablated successfully from the epicardial approach via the coronary sinus and probably represent true epicardial pathways (54).

The successful catheter ablation of accessory pathways is directly related to the skill and experience of the operator (55). Careful mapping of the accessory pathway atrial and ventricular insertion points before any radiofrequency energy delivery greatly enhances the efficiency of the ablation procedure and minimizes the risk of distortion of local electrograms by poorly placed ablative lesions. In patients with manifest ventricular preexcitation (Wolff-Parkinson-White syndrome), mapping is best performed in the anterograde direction during sinus or atrial-paced rhythm. The local ventricular activation recorded from the mapping and ablation catheter should precede the onset of the delta wave on the surface electrocardiogram by at least 10 ms (optimally an interval of at least 20 ms should be pursued), and the electrographic pattern should be stable, indicating stable catheter-tissue contact (Fig. 73.2). An excellent ablation site shows the presence of a high-frequency accessory pathway potential immediately preceding the local ventricular activation and a relatively short atrial-to-ventricular electrographic interval (56,57). This latter finding, however, should not be used to guide ablation catheter positioning, because parallel activation of atrium and ventricle distal to the insertion point of the accessory pathway may result in short AV times, but late ventricular electrogram timing relative to the delta wave onset.

In cases in which the accessory pathway is concealed (absent anterograde but intact retrograde conduction), mapping of retrograde activation during ventricular pacing or ongoing orthodromic AV reciprocating tachycardia must be pursued. Some patients do not tolerate the prolonged periods of sustained tachycardia necessary for complete mapping, and the former approach must be employed. Discrimination between retrograde AV nodal conduction and conduction up the accessory pathway may be enhanced by pacing near the pathway's ventricular insertion site. The atrial insertion of the accessory pathway is determined by identifying the site with the shortest interval between the reference ventricular electrogram and the local atrial activa-

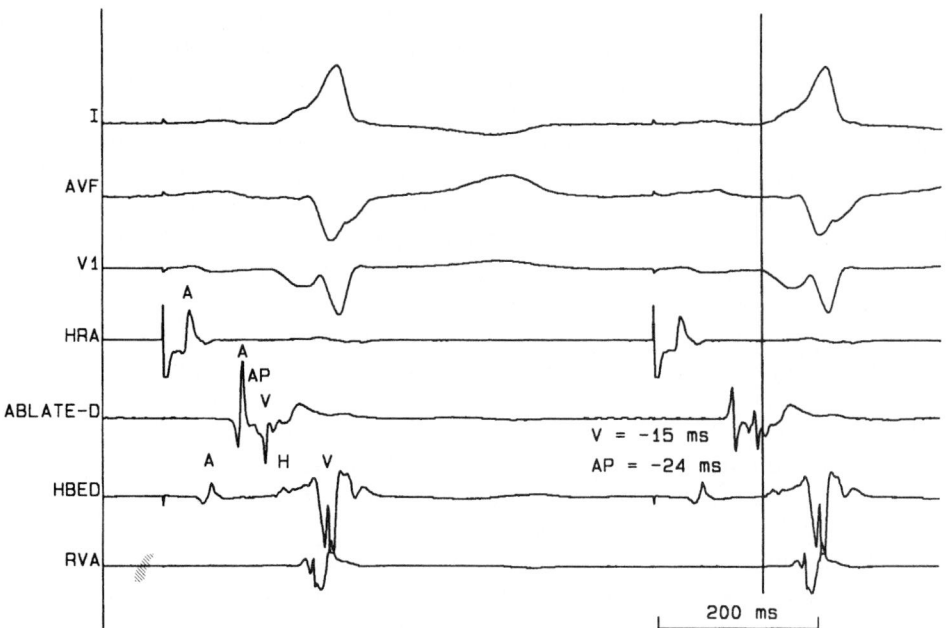

FIGURE 73.2 Surface electrocardiogram tracings I, aVF, and V$_1$, and intracardiac recordings from the high right atrium (HRA), distal ablation catheter bipole (ABLATE-D), the distal bundle of His bipole (HBED), and the right ventricular apex (RVA) in a patient with the Wolff-Parkinson-White syndrome. The vertical line indicates the onset of the delta wave on the surface electrocardiogram. The recording from the ablation electrode shows a discrete atrial (A) and ventricular (V) potential with an interposed high-frequency negative deflection that arises from the accessory pathway (AP). The local AP activation precedes the delta wave onset by 24 ms, and the local ventricular activation precedes the delta wave by 15 ms. H, bundle of His.

tion from the mapping and ablation electrode. One must be cautious not to confuse late components of the local ventricular electrogram as early atrial signals. As with anterograde mapping, the presence of a local high-frequency accessory pathway potential is an excellent marker for successful ablation sites. ✌ m16

The anatomic courses of slowly and decrementally conducting accessory pathways that activate the ventricle with a left bundle branch block configuration (previously referred to as *Mahaim's pathways*) have been demonstrated to commonly originate from the right atrial free wall. Discrete pathway potentials may be mapped from the tricuspid annulus, along the right ventricular endocardial surface to arborized insertions into the right bundle branch. Application of radiofrequency energy along this course successfully ablates the pathways and prevents further AV reciprocating tachycardia (64,67,68).

A number of large clinical series of radiofrequency catheter ablations of accessory pathways have been published with excellent overall results (Table 73.1). Presently, experienced electrophysiology laboratories routinely achieve acute procedure success rates in the ablation of accessory pathways of greater than 95%, with recurrence rates of less than 5%. The procedure duration and fluoroscopic exposure have shortened dramatically with increasing knowledge and experience in this field. Accordingly, the indications for catheter ablation of accessory pathways have broadened to include all patients with symptomatic arrhythmias who are refractory to suppressive drug therapy or who prefer a drug-free lifestyle (69). Although there is little rationale for performing catheter ablation on patients with asymptomatic ventricular preexcitation, this may be pursued on occasion in patients with high-risk or special occupations (such as commercial airline

pilots) in whom a single arrhythmic occurrence could have serious consequences.

Atrioventricular Nodal Reentry

The AV node is located anatomically within the triangle of Koch, which is bounded by the tricuspid annulus, the tendon of Todaro, and the coronary sinus os. The compact AV node is located at the apex of the triangle and makes its transition with nodal-His cells to the common bundle of His. Spreading throughout the remainder of Koch's triangle are atrial transitional cells (atrial-nodal cells) and atrial myocytes. The mechanism of AV nodal reentrant tachycardia is reentrant, using a slowly conducting and a fast conducting pathway in the AV node. The typical form of this arrhythmia has anterograde slow and retrograde fast conduction, whereas the atypical form has the opposite conduction sequence or employs two separate slow pathways for the two limbs of the reentrant circuit. Before the era of catheter ablation, it was commonly hypothesized that the entire reentry circuit was within the compact AV node. However, that notion was challenged by the observation that surgical dissection of the perinodal region successfully eliminated the tachycardia (70). Anatomic study of the AV nodal region has demonstrated the presence of multiple anatomic insertions of atrial myocardium into the transitional cells of the AV nodal region (71). It is currently proposed that these pathways participate as separate pathways in AV nodal reentrant tachycardia. Typically, the atrial insertion of the slowly conducting pathway is located at the inferior-posterior extent of the triangle of Koch, near the coronary sinus os (72). The fast conducting pathway (which is thought to account for "normal" anterograde AV nodal conduction in most cases) is located in the anterior-

TABLE 73.1 CLINICAL RESULTS OF RADIOFREQUENCY CATHETER ABLATION OF PATIENTS WITH WOLFF-PARKINSON-WHITE SYNDROME OR ATRIOVENTRICULAR RECIPROCATING TACHYCARDIA CAUSED BY CONCEALED ACCESSORY PATHWAYS

Authors	Year	No. of patients	Location of pathways	Acute success (%)	Complication rate (%)	Recurrence rate (%)
Jackman et al. (24)	1991	166	All	99	3	9
Calkins et al. (25)	1991	56	All	93	2	2
Schluter et al. (53)	1991	92	All	86	3	3
Calkins et al. (55)	1999	500	All	93	3[a]	8
Kay et al. (26)	1993	363	All	95	1	—
Swartz et al. (60)	1993	114	LFW	95	2	9
Lesh et al. (62)	1993	106	LFW	96	8	3
Deshpande et al. (61)	1994	100	LFW	100	6	7
Schluter and Kuck (65)	1992	12	Anteroseptal	100	0	8
Haissaguerre et al. (64)	1994	8	Anteroseptal	100	0	8
Xie et al. (63)	1994	48	Posteroseptal	92	4	—
Dhala et al. (66)	1994	50	Posteroseptal	100	6	12

LFW, left free wall.
[a]Total major complication rate for all patients, including atrioventricular nodal modification, accessory pathway ablation, and atrioventricular nodal ablation.

superior region of the triangle, close to the compact node (*e*Fig. 73.2.1). It is likely that part of the atrium participates in the reentrant circuit, but this point is unproved and somewhat controversial.

Attempts have been made to map the slow pathway region and develop electrophysiologic criteria to identify the optimal site for selective slow pathway ablation. A pattern of double atrial potentials and late atrial activity is often observed along the tricuspid annulus at the base of the triangle of Koch from sites at which the slow pathway may be successfully ablated. It has been suggested that the late atrial potentials may represent slow pathway activation (73). Careful studies comparing the local electrophysiology and histopathology of canine and porcine hearts indicate that late atrial potentials may be attributed to asynchronous activation of the coronary sinus septum and the atrial tissue between the os and tricuspid valve, or to simultaneous activation of superficial transitional AV nodal tissue and a contiguous layer of atrial tissue along the tricuspid annulus (74). Microelectrode impalements in the region of slow potentials have demonstrated action potentials with AV node characteristics (75). This electrographic pattern may represent conduction through the slowly conducting AV nodal pathway but more likely originates from the distal extent of the compact AV node.

Initially, the fast pathway was targeted for ablation, but lower success rates and high rates of symptomatic heart block have led most operators away from this approach and toward slow pathway ablation (76). The technique for slow pathway ablation involves positioning the catheter in the inferior-posterior position of the triangle of Koch at a site where a typical pattern of slow pathway potentials is observed (*e*Fig. 73.2.2). Subsequent catheter movement can be anatomically (77) or map guided (73). Similar success rates and complication rates between the two

approaches have been observed (78). During radiofrequency energy delivery at successful sites, one may observe an accelerated junctional rhythm and 1:1 junctional to atrial conduction. The earliest site of retrograde atrial activation in this setting is superior to the tendon of Todaro, suggesting that the automaticity arises distal to the ablation site with conduction through the compact AV node and retrograde up the fast pathway (79).

The clinical success rates for catheter ablation of AV nodal reentrant tachycardia that have been generally reported are high (greater than 95%), and the complication rates low (less than 2%). The results of more recent clinical series are shown in Table 73.2. The major complication that has been reported in conjunction with this procedure is symptomatic heart block, with a prevalence of 0% to 4%. The lower prevalence of heart block in later clinical series compared with earlier may be attributable to an increased use of the posterior (slow pathway) approach, an increased understanding of the electrophysiology and anatomy of the AV nodal region, and improved skills of the individual operators (80). Aside from careful stepwise manipulation and positioning of the catheter, the most useful approach to prevent anterograde heart block is to terminate power delivery if there is evidence of loss of retrograde 1:1 conduction from a junctional tachycardia to the atrium via the fast pathway, because this implies that there is evolving injury to the compact AV node (80). Faster rates of junctional tachycardia have been observed in patients with anterograde heart block versus those without it (cycle length 363 ± 44 ms vs. 558 ± 116 ms, respectively) (81), because accelerated junctional rhythm implies proximity to the compact AV node (82). Some patients show evidence of impaired anterograde conduction before the ablation procedure. Although this may suggest the presence of fast pathway pathology, slow pathway ablation may still be pur-

TABLE 73.2 CLINICAL RESULTS OF RADIOFREQUENCY CATHETER ABLATION OF PATIENTS WITH ATRIOVENTRICULAR NODAL REENTRANT TACHYCARDIA

Author	Year	No. of patients	Primary approach[a]	Acute success (%)	Heart block (%)	Other complications (%)	Recurrence rate (%)
Jackman et al. (73)	1992	80	SP	99	1[b]	1.3	0
Jazayeri et al. (77)	1992	49	FP/SP	98	4[c]	0	4[d]
Kay et al. (85)	1992	34	SP	100	3[b]	6	9
Langberg et al. (76)	1993	127	FP	87	7[c]	0	15
Wu et al. (86)	1993	100	FP/SP	97	3[c]	—	1
Lindsay et al. (87)	1993	59	SP	100	2[b]	0	2
Baker et al. (84)	1994	143	SP	99	4[c]	—	7
Manolis et al. (88)	1994	55	SP	100	0	0	13
Kottkamp et al. (89)	1995	53	FP	96	0	0	6
Calkins et al. (55)	1999	373	SP	97	1	3[e]	5

FP, fast pathway; SP, slow pathway.
[a]Cross overs from slow to fast pathway ablation approach reported in 0% to 10% of slow pathway ablations.
[b]Heart block occurred during slow pathway ablation (either as primary approach or after cross-over).
[c]Heart block occurred during fast pathway ablation (either as primary approach or after cross-over).
[d]Tachycardia induced at electrophysiologic study.
[e]Total major complication rate for all patients, including atrioventricular nodal modification, accessory pathway ablation, and atrioventricular nodal ablation.

sued with a low risk of complete heart block (83). The reported recurrence rates of AV nodal reentrant tachycardia after initial successful AV nodal modification procedures are 2% to 15%. The majority of recurrences are reported within the first 2 months of the procedure. Some authors have found an association between persisting dual AV nodal physiology (presence of single AV nodal echo beats or evidence of a shift in anterograde conduction from a fast to a slow pathway) and late clinical recurrence of tachycardia (84), but this is in contrast to the experience of other operators who have not observed that association (85,86). The common practice among most operators is to terminate the ablation procedure once tachycardia can no longer be initiated at baseline or during infusion of isoproterenol and to accept the presence of persisting but impaired slow pathway function.

Atrial Flutter

It has been observed that the dominant activation wavefront during atrial flutter is cranial to caudal along the lateral atrial wall, and caudal to cranial up the septum. Cosio et al. originally determined that the mechanism of this rhythm was macroreentry using the tricuspid annulus as an anatomic barrier. It was hypothesized that the difference between "typical" type I atrial flutter and "atypical" type I atrial flutter was that the former had reentrant activation sequence in a counterclockwise direction around the tricuspid valve in the frontal plane (viewed from apex to base), whereas the latter had a clockwise activation pattern (Fig. 73.3). Cosio et al. also observed that the necessary prerequisite for this arrhythmia was a region of physiologic conduction block between the posterior and lateral atrial walls (90). Without this region of block, the reentrant wavefront would conduct rapidly from the septum around the poste-

rior wall of the atrium and render the lateral wall of the atrium refractory, thus preventing propagation of the subsequent reentrant wavefront. Subsequent mapping studies in humans using intracardiac ultrasound and careful entrainment mapping techniques have demonstrated physiologic conduction block in the posteromedial (sinus venosa) region of the right atrium during atrial flutter (91).

Understanding the path of reentry of atrial flutter led researchers to identify critical sites of conduction that would be amenable to catheter ablation in order to cure this arrhythmia (92,93). Cosio et al. pioneered the present-day approach of anatomically guided catheter ablation of atrial flutter. They reasoned that the reentrant circuit should always uses the subeustachian isthmus between the inferior vena cava orifice and the tricuspid annulus as a requisite limb of the reentrant circuit. They then demonstrated that a line of radiofrequency ablative lesions traversing this isthmus was successful in terminating atrial flutter (94). ▼ m17

The results of clinical series are presented in Table 73.3. The acute success rate of this procedure now exceeds 90% when performed by experienced operators, and the late atrial flutter recurrence rate is 10% to 20%. Confirmation of bidirectional block of electrical conduction through the isthmus between the tricuspid valve and inferior vena cava has been demonstrated to be an important criterion for the procedure's success. Despite successful termination and prevention of reinduction of atrial flutter by ablative lesions, some patients still have residual conduction through the isthmus that can result in clinical arrhythmia recurrence (*e*Fig. 73.3.1) (99,100). Success rates may also be improved with the use of irrigated-tip ablation catheters (101). Despite successful ablation of atrial flutter, the patient will likely have clinical recurrence of atrial fibrillation or type II atrial flutter if these arrhythmias were observed clinically

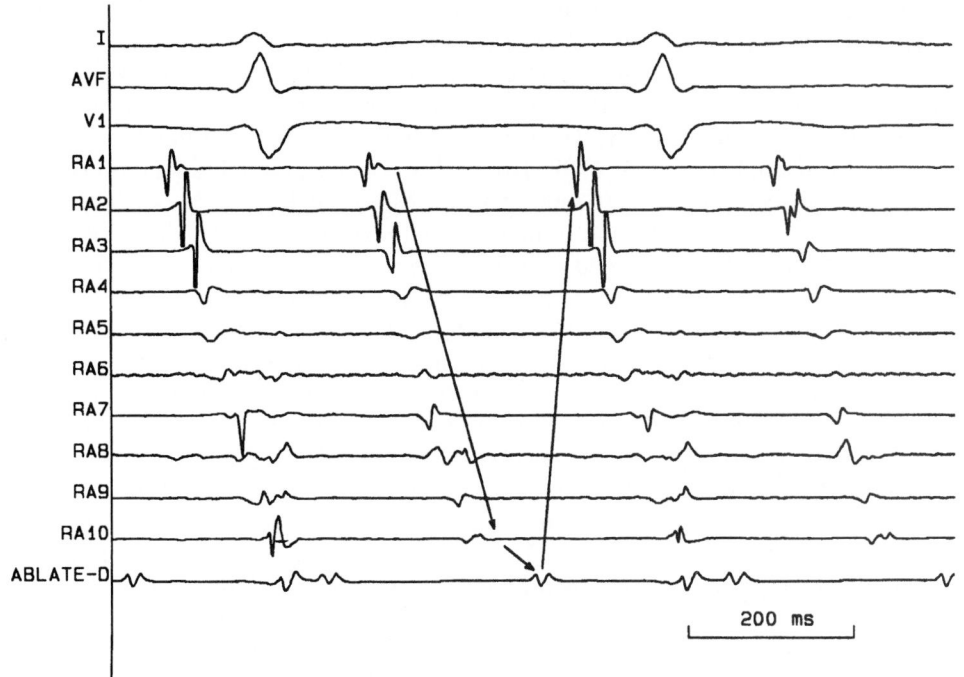

FIGURE 73.3 Surface electrocardiogram tracings I, aVF, and V$_1$, and intracardiac recordings from ten bipolar recording pairs (RA1 to RA10) positioned around the tricuspid annulus. RA1 is located on the low interatrial septum, RA3 is on the high septum, RA7 is on the high lateral wall, and RA10 is on the low atrial wall. The distal bipole of the ablation catheter (ABLATE-D) is positioned at the tricuspid-inferior vena cava isthmus. The arrows demonstrate the pattern of activation during ongoing atrial flutter. This is an example of typical "counterclockwise" atrial flutter in that the pattern of activation (viewing the heart from apex to base) rotates in that direction.

before the ablation procedure (98,102–104). After initiation of antiarrhythmic drugs, particularly type 1C agents, some patients with atrial fibrillation or a combination of atrial fibrillation and atrial flutter convert to pure type I atrial flutter. In these cases, a combination of drug and atrial flutter ablation therapy may be effective in preventing arrhythmia recurrence (105).

Atrial Fibrillation: Palliative Therapy

Atrial fibrillation is the most common sustained arrhythmia in the world, with a reported prevalence of 1.9% for patients under 65 years of age, and 5% to 6% for the population of patients over age 65 (107). The morbidity and mortality of this arrhythmia may be attributed primarily to three factors: the propensity of the fibrillating atria for thrombus formation with the sequelae of systemic thromboembolism including stroke; the loss of atrial systolic function as a contributor to ventricular filling; and the irregular and rapid ventricular rate response leading to symptoms of palpitations and reduction of diastolic filling time. Therefore, the two main strategies for management of patients with atrial fibrillation are maintenance of sinus rhythm with suppressive antiarrhythmic agents or rate control and anticoagulation. If the latter strategy is pursued, warfarin anticoagulation can significantly reduce (but not eliminate) the risk of thromboembolism. Symptomatic palpitations may be reduced with appropriate use of digitalis, beta-sympathetic blockers, or calcium channel blockers. Unfortunately, these drugs are often poorly tolerated, and

TABLE 73.3 CLINICAL RESULTS OF RADIOFREQUENCY CATHETER ABLATION OF PATIENTS WITH ATRIAL FLUTTER

						Recurrence rate (%)	
Author	Year	No. of patients	Acute success (%)	Isthmus block confirmed	Complication rate (%)	Atrial flutter	Atrial fibrillation
Feld et al. (93)	1992	12	83	No	0	17	0
Cosio et al. (94)	1993	9	78	No	0	0	9
Poty et al. (99)	1995	12	100	Yes	—	8	—
Philippon et al. (103)	1995	59	90	No	—	9	26
Fischer et al. (106)	1995	80	90	No	8	17	5
Cauchemez et al. (100)	1996	20	100	Yes	—	15	5
Paydak et al. (104)	1998	110	98	Yes[a]	—	5	25
Chen et al. (96)	1999	39	100	Yes	0	5	—
Heidbuchel et al. (98)	2000	100	99	Yes	1	0	30

[a]Isthmus block confirmed in a subgroup of 90 patients.

because the AV nodal blocking action of digitalis is mediated through central vagotonic effects, the ventricular response rate to atrial fibrillation increases dramatically in settings of spontaneous vagolysis (such as exercise). Frequently, adequate doses of AV nodal blocking agents result in symptomatic bradycardia, requiring pacemaker implantation. Therefore, nonpharmacologic means of rate control are sometimes required.

The palliative ablative procedures that are available for the treatment of atrial fibrillation are AV junctional ablation and AV nodal modification. The goal of AV junctional ablation is to interrupt completely the AV conduction with an ablative lesion placed in the vicinity of the compact AV node. In most cases, the patient has a slow but tolerable junctional escape rhythm after AV junctional ablation, which arises from the low compact AV node or high bundle of His region, immediately distal to the site of ablation. This escape rhythm is usually adequate to prevent hemodynamic embarrassment, but not adequate to maintain a normal heart rate at rest or with activity. Therefore, permanent pacemaker implantation is always required. Selection of a single-chamber rate-responsive ventricular pacemaker is appropriate for patients who are in chronic atrial fibrillation. Patients with paroxysmal atrial fibrillation benefit most from implantation of a dual-chamber rate-responsive pacemaker with mode-switching capabilities. These devices maintain AV synchrony when the patient is in sinus rhythm, thus avoiding symptoms of pacemaker syndrome. After atrial fibrillation onset, the device automatically recognizes the atrial tachycardia and effectively converts from a dual-chamber to a single-chamber pacing mode, which prevents the pacemaker from tracking the atrium and pacing the ventricle at a high rate (eFig. 73.3.2).

The goal of AV nodal *modification* procedures is to damage but not destroy all AV nodal conduction. In the ideal case, the patient has adequate basal rates, but the rapid heart-rate acceleration exercise is prevented. It is important to note that the atria continue to fibrillate after AV junctional ablation or modification despite excellent heart-rate control and resolution of the patient's symptoms. Therefore, the patient is still at risk for thromboembolic events, and ongoing treatment with warfarin is recommended. ◥◢ m18

Atrial Fibrillation: Curative Therapy

The understanding of the pathophysiology of atrial fibrillation has advanced considerably in recent years. The long-standing hypothesis of atrial fibrillation has been that multiple wavelets of reentrant atrial activity conduct throughout both atria, and that reactivation of new wavelets of reentry perpetuate this arrhythmia. Factors that promote the formation and increase the number of wavelets have been associated with clinical atrial fibrillation propagation (115,116). An alternative hypothesis of reentrant atrial fibrillation propagation is that a dominant rotor of atrial

reentrant activation drives the arrhythmia and the remaining atrium is passively activated (117). The regions of dominant periodic electrical activity measured in experimental atrial fibrillation have a characteristic frequency of 7 to 10 Hz, corresponding to atrial rates of 400 to 600 beats/min. In 1997, Jais et al. made the groundbreaking observation that some patients had atrial fibrillation on the basis of rapid firing of arrhythmogenic foci (118). These foci were found to arise predominantly from the pulmonary veins, and some patients had two or more focal sources of arrhythmia origin (119,120). Patients with atrial fibrillation of focal origin tend to be younger, have multiple brief paroxysms of arrhythmia, and most commonly have normal hearts. However, a continuum probably exists between these patients and those with persistent atrial fibrillation, structural heart disease, and a reentrant mechanism of atrial fibrillation. It is likely that patients with minimal to moderate heart disease and recurrent episodes of atrial fibrillation that are prolonged or persistent have focal initiation of their arrhythmia with reentrant propagation.

Atrial fibrillation that is dependent on reentrant propagation requires a minimal geographic region for the maintenance of the driving wavelets or rotor. If lines of anatomic conduction block are placed such that this critical circuit size cannot be achieved, then the fibrillation cannot propagate. This was the theoretical basis of the surgical maze procedure (121). It was hypothesized that similar long linear atrial lesions could be achieved by catheter ablation. Experimental studies have demonstrated that multiple linear lesions in the right and left atria can prolong atrial fibrillation cycle length and, ultimately, terminate this ongoing arrhythmia (eFig. 73.3.3) (122). The first cases of linear atrial fibrillation ablation in patients were reported by Swartz et al., who employed a technique of dragging a typical 4-mm tip ablation electrode on multiple lines along the atrial wall during ongoing radiofrequency energy delivery. Chronic atrial fibrillation could be successfully terminated in the majority of cases, but over one-half of the patients had arrhythmia recurrence and required at least a second ablation session. In addition, significant complications including stroke were observed (123). Haissaguerre et al. employed a multiple-ring electrode catheter that, when positioned tangentially to the atrial walls, allowed sequential multiple electrode radiofrequency energy delivery and achieved long linear lesions. In his series of 45 patients with drug-refractory paroxysmal atrial fibrillation, a staged procedure was performed with linear ablation, focal atrial tachycardia ablation, or both in the right, left, or both atria. Success, defined as less than one symptomatic episode of 6 hours' duration in 3 months with or without additional suppressive antiarrhythmic drug therapy, was achieved in 21 patients (47%) (124).

Linear atrial ablation can be accomplished by a point-to-point technique, a "drag" approach, or with multiple electrode side-contact catheters. At this time, the lines that are targeted are anatomically determined. Most investigators agree that some approach to isolate the pulmonary veins and a tricuspid-caval isthmus lesion is important for procedure success. Other lesion locations that are of potential value include a lesion that connects the encircling pulmonary vein lesions to the mitral annulus, a lesion extending anteriorly from the pulmonary vein lesions to Bachmann's bundle, a vertical intercaval lesion in the right atrium, and a vertical right or left septal lesion. Although a pattern of transition from disorganized to organized atrial fibrillation has been described as a favorable observation in the modification of atrial fibrillation wavelet conduction, most present-day linear ablation procedures are anatomically guided, not map guided. Because the relationship of the linear lesions to anatomic structures and the contact between the catheter and tissue are important factors in procedure success, advanced imaging modalities such as intracardiac echocardiography have been useful tools in this procedure (125).

Reported series of linear atrial ablation have employed a variety of techniques and tools to achieve continuous and transmural linear lesions (Table 73.4). Comparison among trials is difficult for a variety of reasons. The patients studied likely include a mix of both focal and reentrant mechanisms. The ablation targets vary among right atrial, left atrial, and biatrial procedures. The definitions of procedure success may or may not include concomitant suppressive antiarrhythmic drug therapy. Finally, the follow-up durations of all the studies are relatively short. Some common themes in linear ablation are emerging. Many investigators have concluded that ablation in the right atrium alone has a low success rate, and in most cases left atrial or biatrial ablation is required. A consequence of creation of incomplete lesions is arrhythmia exacerbation (proarrhythmia) caused

by the production of scar-related left atrial "flutter" (126). The complexity and long duration of these procedures may increase their complication rate relative to standard catheter ablation procedures. The field of linear atrial ablation is still evolving, but available data suggest that transcatheter approaches achieve a far lower success rate than that observed with open surgical procedures such as the maze operation. This outcome is most likely caused by residual gaps in linear ablation lines from the catheter-based approaches that allow for the continued propagation of reentrant atrial fibrillation wavelets (127). As the technology of catheter-based linear ablation improves, success rates may ultimately approach those of the open surgical procedure. Alternatively, minimally invasive surgical maze procedures may supplant the catheter approaches if high success rates can be achieved with minimal surgical morbidity.

Identification of a focal mechanism of atrial fibrillation initiation led to advances in curative therapy for atrial fibrillation in selected patients. It was initially described by Jais et al. that foci of rapid electrical firing could trigger atrial fibrillation (118). Follow-up studies from the same group in a larger series (119), as well as studies from Chen et al. (120), confirmed that focal atrial fibrillation is a significant clinical entity and is very treatable by limited catheter ablation techniques. The majority of triggering foci for atrial fibrillation arises from the sleeve of muscular tissue that extends from the left atrial body into the pulmonary veins. The average extension of these muscle fibers into the vein is greater for the superior pulmonary veins (30 to 40 mm) than the inferior pulmonary veins (15 to 20 mm) (120). Although mapping studies indicate that they are truly focal in nature (135), the precise mechanism of these beats (microreentrant, automatic, or triggered) has not been clearly defined. In many cases, the focal activity is

TABLE 73.4 CLINICAL RESULTS OF LINEAR ATRIAL ABLATION OF PATIENTS WITH ATRIAL FIBRILLATION

Author	Year	No. of patients	Structural heart disease (%)	Paroxysmal atrial fibrillation (%)	Right atrial/left atrial ablation	Percent cured (no antiarrhythmic drugs)	Percent improved (with antiarrhythmic drugs)	Compli-cation rate (%)	Follow-up duration (mo)
Haissaguerre et al. (124)	1996	45	29	100	45/10	18	47	—	11 ± 4
Gaita et al. (128)	1998	16	0	50	16/0	25	56	0	—
Maloney et al. (129)	1998	15	53	0	15/15	20	60	26	18 ± 10
Garg et al. (130)	1999	12	33	67	12/0	9	67	9	21.3 ± 11.2
Pappone et al. (131)	1999	27	7	100	27/0	44	71	4	10.5 ± 3.0
Ernst et al. (132)	1999	45	0	82	44/13	4	—	11	—
Natale et al. (133)	2000	18	11	100	18/0	28	50	11	22 ± 11
Haines et al. (134)	2000	23	61	74	23/23	22	48	26	8 ± 12

TABLE 73.5 CLINICAL RESULTS OF FOCAL ATRIAL ABLATION OF PATIENTS WITH PAROXYSMAL ATRIAL FIBRILLATION

Author	Year	No. of patients	No. of foci ablated per patient	Structural heart disease (%)	Percent cured (no antiarrhythmic drugs)	Percent multiple procedures	Complication rate (%)	Follow-up duration (mo)
Haissaguerre et al. (119)	1998	45	1.5	31	62	56	0	8 ± 6
Chen et al. (120)	1999	79	1.5	42	86	9	6[a]	6 ± 2
Lau et al. (139)	1999	7[b]	1.0	0	86	0	0	—
Haissaguerre et al. (140)	2000	90	2.2	19	71	54	6	8 ± 5
Natale et al. (138)	2000	15	3.1	40	60	0	27	9 ± 2
University of Virginia series[c]	2001	43	1.3	12	72	10	7	9 ± 5

[a]Forty-two percent of patients had angiographic pulmonary stenosis, of whom 3% were symptomatic.
[b]Three of seven patients had persistent atrial fibrillation.
[c]Consecutive patients undergoing intracardiac echocardiographically guided focal atrial fibrillation ablation at the University of Virginia Health Sciences Center.

increased by adrenergic stimulation or rapid pacing and blocked by beta-adrenergic blocking drugs and calcium channel blockers (120), suggesting triggered activity as the most likely arrhythmia mechanism. The reason for the clustering of triggering foci in the pulmonary veins is unknown at this time. Other less prevalent sites of origin of triggering foci include the ligament of Marshall (a remnant of the left superior vena cava on the posterior left atrium) (136), the crista terminalis in the right atrium, and the superior vena cava (137). ➴ m19

The early clinical series of pulmonary vein ablation are listed in Table 73.5. Acute success rates of this procedure are high (greater than 95%), but overall success rates are much lower (60% to 86%). There are several possible explanations for the high recurrence rate of atrial fibrillation observed after this procedure. First, the sensitivity of provocative maneuvers for initiating focal trigger activity is limited in some patients. Thus, despite successful ablation of all apparent triggering foci at the time of the procedure, some quiescent foci may emerge later. The more focal sites of origin identified, the lower the procedural success rates (140). Second, the triggering foci can be variable in their activity and can "turn off" coincident with catheter manipulation. Thus, the appearance of successful ablation can be achieved acutely with late recurrence due to reactivation of the focus. Finally, if a pulmonary vein isolation technique is employed, the line of ablation required to isolate the vein may range from 1 to 4 cm in length. Any recovery of conduction along the line of ablation results in conduction of the rapid atrial impulses from the targeted vein. Complications in focal atrial fibrillation ablation include all those related to all catheter ablation procedures. In addition, the unique complication of pulmonary vein stenosis may occur if ablation powers and temperatures are not limited (120,141). Also, the risk of systemic thromboembolism is probably higher than that observed with other left-sided ablation procedures because of the increased instrumenta-

tion and longer procedure duration, but the exact prevalence of this complication is not known.

The ultimate success of atrial fibrillation ablation will rest with the development of the ablation tools and further understanding of the pathophysiology of this arrhythmia in different patient subsets. Ultimately, the proof of its value will depend on its ability to eliminate symptoms, restore normal left atrial mechanical activity, and prevent late thromboembolic complications.

Other Atrial Arrhythmias

Tachycardias that arise from the sinus node region include sinoatrial reentrant tachycardia and "inappropriate" sinus tachycardia. The former is characterized by its paroxysmal nature, the ability to initiate and terminate the rhythm with programmed atrial stimulation, and a P-wave morphology and intraatrial activation sequence that are indistinguishable from normal sinus rhythm. This is an uncommon arrhythmia and therefore the experience with ablative therapy is somewhat limited. It typically has its origin in the high atrial region at the junction between the atrium and superior vena cava in the classical sinus node anatomic region. The optimal site of ablation may be identified by searching for the earliest site of atrial activation relative to the P-wave onset. Ablation in this region results in termination of the tachycardia and frequently results in a slight shift of sinus node activation to a lower site along the crista terminalis (142,143). Although most patients have normal sinus node function postablation, sinus node dysfunction requiring pacemaker implantation is a potential risk. The reported clinical series are limited, but include one description of 11 patients who were identified out of a cohort of 343 consecutive patients referred for electrophysiologic evaluation of supraventricular tachycardia. Nine of the 11 patients had additional tachycardia mechanisms identified. Radiofrequency catheter ablation was successful in all ten patients in whom it was attempted, and no complications were noted (143).

Inappropriate sinus tachycardia is similar in P-wave morphology and atrial activation sequence to sinoatrial reentry and normal sinus rhythm, but does not follow a paroxysmal pattern and sometimes occurs incessantly. Patients with this arrhythmia have an exaggerated heart-rate response to minor physiologic stresses and often have heart rates greater than 100 beats/min at rest. It is important to confirm that patients presenting with apparent inappropriate sinus tachycardia do not have the postural orthostatic tachycardia syndrome (144). These patients have a marked compensatory sinus tachycardia because of failure of peripheral autonomic vascular response to orthostatic stress. "Successful" sinus node ablation in these patients may result in crippling hypotension. For patients with true inappropriate sinus tachycardia, catheter ablation has been successfully performed by targeting a relatively broad region of the superior crista terminalis for radiofrequency energy delivery (*e*Fig. 73.3.4). Lee et al. used intracardiac echocardiography to assist catheter positioning and were able to achieve complete sinus node ablation in four of four patients, and successful arrhythmia modification (defined as a 25% reduction in sinus rate) in 12 of 12 patients (145). However, permanent atrial pacing was required in two patients, arrhythmias recurred in short-term follow-up in two patients, and two patients had significant procedural complications (transient superior vena cava syndrome and phrenic nerve injury). Thus, catheter ablation for inappropriate sinus tachycardia may be useful in the management of these challenging patients, but it should not be considered as first-line therapy.

Atrial tachycardia is a rhythm that may originate from either the left or right atrium and may be caused by reentry or triggered or abnormal automaticity. In the right atrium, it commonly arises from the crista terminalis, although its origin may also be low atrial septum or right atrial appendage. In the left atrium, the arrhythmia origin is most often from the origins of the pulmonary veins. Surface electrocardiography can be useful to determine the arrhythmia site of origin. A positive or biphasic P wave in surface lead aVL suggests a right atrial origin, whereas a positive P wave in V_1 and a negative P wave in aVL imply a left atrial arrhythmia origin (146). Because the right pulmonary veins are located posterior and rightward from the right atrial septum, the surface P-wave morphology can sometimes be inaccurate in predicting the arrhythmia site of origin. Mapping of atrial tachycardia is best achieved with activation mapping to identify local atrial activity before onset of the surface P wave, pace mapping to identify a site where the paced P wave is identical to the spontaneous tachycardia P wave, and paced activation sequence mapping where the relative activation timing from multiple atrial recording sites is identical between pacing and spontaneous tachycardia. Using this approach, Tracy et al. successfully ablated

eight of ten patients, one of whom had multiple foci. Two patients had clinical recurrence, and one was successfully reablated (147).

ABLATION OF SPECIFIC VENTRICULAR ARRHYTHMIAS

Idiopathic Ventricular Tachycardia

Patients with structurally normal hearts may have ventricular tachycardia with a variety of underlying arrhythmia mechanisms. Idiopathic ventricular tachycardia most commonly arises from the right ventricle in the outflow tract below the pulmonic valve. These arrhythmias tend to fall into two main categories. Repetitive monomorphic ventricular tachycardia is characterized by multiple repeating bursts of nonsustained ventricular tachycardia and high-density premature ventricular beats. These arrhythmias may be increased in the setting of catecholamine stress, but frequently are suppressed in the setting of catecholamine-induced increases in sinus rate. It is hypothesized that the mechanism for repetitive monomorphic ventricular tachycardia is abnormal automaticity (148). Catecholamine-sensitive ventricular tachycardia may be nonsustained or sustained. Because these arrhythmias are catecholamine sensitive, they are frequently exercise induced. They should terminate in response to intravenous adenosine or verapamil bolus infusions. It is hypothesized that the mechanism for these arrhythmias is triggered automaticity. The typical features of these arrhythmias on 12-lead electrocardiograms include a left bundle branch block morphology, an inferior frontal plane axis, and a relatively isoelectric complex in surface lead (149,150). Idiopathic ventricular tachycardia of left ventricular origin is typically a reentrant tachycardia that uses Purkinje's network as part of its reentrant circuit. The site of slowed conduction in the reentry circuit has not been well characterized, but it is typically sensitive to verapamil and not to adenosine (151,152). This feature allows for differentiation of this arrhythmia from the rare left ventricular form of adenosine-sensitive left ventricular tachycardia that has a presumed triggered automatic mechanism (45). As anticipated, idiopathic left ventricular tachycardias have a right bundle branch block morphology on the surface 12-lead electrocardiography. ⌖ m20

The reported clinical success rate of catheter ablation of idiopathic ventricular tachycardia is 76% to 100% and generally greater than 90% for those arrhythmias arising from the right ventricular outflow tract (Table 73.6). The reported complications with this procedure have been infrequent. Two cases of pericardial effusion (one requiring pericardiocentesis) were observed in a series of 44 patients undergoing radiofrequency ablation of ventricular tachycardia in the right and left ventricles (161). One case of catheter-induced mitral

TABLE 73.6   CLINICAL RESULTS OF RADIOFREQUENCY CATHETER ABLATION OF PATIENTS WITH IDIOPATHIC VENTRICULAR TACHYCARDIA

Author	Year	No. of patients	Ventricular tachycardia location	Acute success (%)	Complication rate (%)	Recurrence rate (%)
Klein et al. (153)	1992	16	RVOT	100	0	6
Calkins et al. (154)	1993	18	RVOT (10)[a] RV (5)[a] LV (5)[a]	72	0	0
Wilber et al. (149)	1993	7	RVOT	100	0	0
Nakagawa et al. (155)	1993	8	LV	100	13	13
Wen et al. (156)	1997	7	LV	100	—	0
Peeters et al. (158)	1999	19	RVOT (10) LV (9)	89	5	12
Tsuchiya et al. (159)	1999	16	LV	100	—	0

LV, left ventricle; RV, right ventricle (excluding outflow tract); RVOT, right ventricular outflow tract.
[a]Two tachycardias identified in each of two patients.

regurgitation has been reported as a consequence of catheter manipulation in the left ventricle (155).

Reentrant Ventricular Tachycardia with Structural Heart Disease

Patients with structural heart disease have varying degrees of fibrosis interspersed among bundles of surviving myocardial bundles. The most common arrhythmogenic substrate among patients with reentrant ventricular tachycardia is chronic ischemic heart disease. The central portion of a complete transmural scar from prior infarction is commonly electrically inactive, but some broad wavefronts of slowed conduction can occur across this region in a thin surviving endocardial layer (162). The border zone of the scar is extremely heterogeneous, making it an ideal substrate for reentry. A typical reentrant circuit uses these small myocardial bundles at the scar border zone as regions of slowed conduction (163). Conduction through these regions accounts for the isoelectric period between QRS complexes on surface electrocardiography, particularly with slower tachycardias. The return circuit is complex and uses the surrounding myocardium on one or both sides of the central conduction zone, thereby creating a circular or a figure-eight conduction pattern (164,165). In patients with posterior scars, the central conduction zone is often the isthmus between the scar and the mitral valve annulus (166). The slow conduction zone is characterized by a zigzag activation sequence through regions of patchy fibrosis. Most of the conduction delay is seen at the site of conduction from one fiber to another perpendicular to the fiber orientation (167).

The precise courses of the reentrant wavefronts in the ventricular tachycardias of patients with nonischemic myopathies are not well understood. Diffuse regions of fibrosis mingling with normal or hypertrophied myocytes are typically observed and create a substrate for reentrant rhythms (168). However, the diffuse nature of the structural abnormalities allows for dynamic changes in the reentrant circuits

beat to beat and makes these patients more prone to polymorphic ventricular tachycardias. An interesting variant of ventricular tachycardia found predominantly in patients with dilated cardiomyopathy is bundle branch reentrant tachycardia. This is a macroreentrant tachycardia that uses one limb of the bundle branches in an anterograde fashion and another limb in a retrograde fashion (167). It is important to recognize this arrhythmia mechanism because bundle branch reentrant tachycardia is easily treated by ablation of the right or left bundle branch (170,171). Unfortunately, many of these patients have concomitant ventricular tachycardias of myocardial origin that require treatment despite elimination of the bundle branch reentry.

The critical zone for propagation of ventricular tachycardia is located in the septum or left ventricular free wall in most patients with reentrant ventricular tachycardia and structural heart disease. The one notable exception is ventricular tachycardia in patients with arrhythmogenic right ventricular dysplasia. A clinical presentation of a patient with normal left ventricular size and function and a tachycardia with a left bundle branch block morphology might suggest the diagnosis of idiopathic ventricular tachycardia. Careful evaluation of these patients with high-quality echocardiography of the right ventricle or contrast cine right ventriculography is necessary to identify those rare cases of right ventricular dysplasia (172). Mapping and entrainment studies of ventricular tachycardia in these patients have demonstrated that the common locations of the reentrant circuit sites were around the tricuspid annulus and in the right ventricular outflow tract (173). Of interest, a cohort of patients undergoing repeated attempted ablation of ventricular tachycardia arising from the right ventricular outflow tract underwent magnetic resonance imaging scanning. Despite normal right ventricular size and function and the presumptive diagnosis of idiopathic focal ventricular tachycardia, 65% of these selected patients had evidence of fatty deposition, wall thinning, or dyskinesis (174). ▼ m21

The clinical series of radiofrequency catheter ablation of reentrant ventricular tachycardia are small and comprise a highly selected subset of patients. Because patients must be able to tolerate their tachycardia hemodynamically to allow for mapping, patients with rapid, life-threatening tachycardias are not included in these series. The mean cycle lengths of the tachycardias in the reported clinical series of ablations were greater than 350 ms (less than 171 beats/min), and the patients undergoing ablative therapy made up only 10% to 20% of the overall ventricular tachycardia population. The results of the largest clinical series are summarized in Table 73.7. The reported success rates on the suppression of "clinical" tachycardias with radiofrequency catheter ablation range from 64% to 81%. Patients frequently have "nonclinical" tachycardias, defined as sustained monomorphic ventricular tachycardias with morphologies that have never been observed to occur spontaneously in the clinical setting but that can be induced by programmed ventricular stimulation. In these cases, adjunctive therapy with an implantable defibrillator is usually warranted. An expanding indication for ventricular tachycardia ablation is for patients in whom an implantable defibrillator has been previously implanted, but who are now suffering frequent or incessant runs of slower ventricular tachycardia, resulting in multiple device discharges. Radiofrequency catheter ablation can successfully palliate a significant number of these patients (187,190).

An uncommon but important subset of patients with ventricular tachycardia are those with bundle branch reentrant tachycardia. This is a macroreentrant rhythm most commonly found in patients with dilated cardiomyopathy and conduction system disease. The reentrant wavefront uses one bundle branch in an anterograde fashion and one bundle branch for retrograde conduction. It is a rapid, potentially life-threatening rhythm found in as many as 5% of patients with ventricular tachycardia (192) and is readily treatable with catheter ablation. Bundle branch reentrant tachycardia may be identified by the presence of a bundle of His deflection that precedes each ventricular depolarization and shows identical beat-to-beat variability as the subsequent ventricular beats. In typical cases in which the right bundle branch is one limb of the circuit, the ablation catheter is positioned across the tricuspid valve beyond the common bundle of His, and the right bundle branch is selectively ablated. Using this approach, bundle branch reentrant tachycardia was successfully ablated in 42 of 42 patients in one clinical series (193). However, the presence of other concomitant ventricular tachycardias and underlying myopathic disease portends a poor prognosis even with successful ablation. In the previously mentioned studies, 23 of 42 patients died during the 16-month follow-up, and 13 of these died suddenly.

CONTROVERSIES AND PERSONAL PERSPECTIVES

In the last 15 years, radiofrequency catheter ablation has become a dominant modality in the treatment of a number of symptomatic arrhythmias. The popularity of catheter ablation is due in large part to the extremely low complication rate observed by practitioners. The major factor that has limited the number and severity of complications is that the volume of injury produced by radiofrequency catheter ablation is small. Thus, small lesions are associated with minimal endocardial disruption, a low prevalence of significant thrombus formation, a low rate of transmural injury with left ventricular lesions (which eliminates the risk of free wall rupture and significant ablation-induced ventricular dysfunction), and rare prevalence of coronary arterial injury, even though most accessory pathway ablations are performed in close proximity to the epicardial coronary arteries. However, with small lesions come higher skill requirements for target selection. In addition, some targets are inaccessible because of their location deep within the myocardium away from the endocardial plane. For these reasons, investigators have been working to increase dramatically the size of ablative lesions by using novel catheter designs and new energy sources. As the depth and volume of myocardial injury increase with catheter ablation, it is likely that the complications will increase as well. The lingering effects of this injury in young people may not be realized for decades when they present with premature coronary artery disease. Intramural superheating and sudden "popping" result in crater-like lesions with a small but real risk of free wall perforation.

The popularity of catheter ablation therapy may be attributed to the observation that it has been curative in the majority of cases, and the procedure-related morbidity and mortality have been extremely low. Thus, the indications for catheter ablation have continued to broaden. In fact, the majority of patients presenting for catheter ablation of paroxysmal supraventricular tachycardia at the University of Virginia has never failed drug therapy but simply desires a drug-free lifestyle. Although it is often an appropriate decision to subject an otherwise healthy patient to the risk of an invasive procedure if one can eliminate the requirement of lifelong drug therapy, not all patients with arrhythmias amenable to catheter ablation should undergo this therapy. It is still appropriate to pursue vagal maneuvers and medical therapy with AV nodal blocking drugs before performing interventional therapy. Although a supraventricular tachycardia may cause significant symptoms, it is not a life-threatening arrhythmia.

Most arrhythmia experts will agree that symptomatic patients with the Wolff-Parkinson-White syndrome should undergo diagnostic electrophysiologic testing to determine if they have an increased risk of fatal arrhythmias. Because the main morbidity of catheter ablation is caused by the placement of multiple diagnostic catheters in the heart, it is common practice to proceed with ablation of the accessory pathway even if it is determined to be low risk. The approach toward asymptomatic patients with evidence of ventricular preexcitation on the electrocardiogram is some-

TABLE 73.7 CLINICAL RESULTS OF RADIOFREQUENCY CATHETER ABLATION OF PATIENTS WITH VENTRICULAR TACHYCARDIA IN PATIENTS WITH STRUCTURAL HEART DISEASE

Author	Year	No. of patients	No. of ventricular tachycardias per patient	Ventricular tachycardia cycle length (ms)	Success rate (%) All ventricular tachycardias	Success rate (%) Clinical ventricular tachycardias	Complication rate (%)	Follow-up duration (mo)	Ventricular tachycardia recurrence (%)	Late survival (%)	Patients with AAD Rx (%)	Patients with ICD Rx (%)
Stevenson et al. (181)	1993	15	2.1	—	—	66	0	8.7	0	80	67	7
Morady et al. (184)	1993	15	1.3	438 ± 82	—	73	0	9.1	18	100	93	20
Gursoy et al. (185)	1993	14	1.1	357 ± 56	—	57	—	9	13	—	7	50
Kim et al. (186)	1994	21	1.1	445 ± 52	43	81	0	13.2	31	95	57	43
Strickberger et al. (187)	1997	21	2.2	455 ± 93	—	76	5	11.8	43	90	—	100
Rothman et al. (188)	1997	35	3.0	345 ± 74	31	86	11	14.1	34	80	23	51
Callans et al. (189)	1998	66	1.2	406 ± 63	35	71	4	—	—	—	—	—
Stevenson et al. (190)	1998	52	3.6	433 ± 108	40	71	10	18	33	70	59	45
Calkins et al. (191)	2000	146	3.1	—	41	75	8	8	46	75	66	79

AAD Rx, concomitant therapy with suppressive antiarrhythmic drug therapy; ICD Rx, concomitant therapy with an implantable cardioverter defibrillator.

what variable. The natural history of these patients suggests that no evaluation or therapy is needed until and unless they develop symptoms. However, a potential for dangerous arrhythmias may exist in pediatric patients who have yet to present with clinical arrhythmias. Thus, there is some rationale for studying and ablating pediatric Wolff-Parkinson-White patients.

The field of curative atrial fibrillation ablation is advancing rapidly. The outcomes of catheter ablation for atrial fibrillation with a focal mechanism are good enough that many practitioners are offering this as a clinically indicated procedure. Presently, there is significant variability among laboratories as to the techniques employed and the patient selection criteria. Thus, determining the best approach to employ has been difficult. It is clear that this procedure is becoming more anatomically guided. It is hoped that with development of the tools for this procedure, procedure times will decrease and success rates will increase. Presently, patients with frequent bursts of self-terminating atrial fibrillation and atrial tachycardia and normal hearts should be strongly considered for ablative therapy. Patients with structural heart disease and longer, less frequent atrial fibrillation episodes should probably only be considered for curative catheter ablation as a final alternative to AV junctional ablation and pacemaker implantation. Linear ablation is presently investigational only and should not be considered as an alternative to drug therapy. Highly motivated patients who have failed multiple drug trials are appropriate candidates for this procedure, but it must be acknowledged that the risks of the procedure may ultimately outweigh its benefits.

Catheter ablation for the treatment of ventricular tachycardia in patients with structural heart disease has not emerged as a dominant modality. In fact, most practitioners employ catheter ablation as a palliative therapy only, because almost all patients with ventricular tachycardia and ischemic cardiomyopathy have multiple tachycardia morphologies. Therefore, although one can often modify or eliminate the clinical tachycardia, a number of different (usually faster) tachycardias with morphologies not previously seen can be induced with programmed ventricular stimulation. Each investigator and practitioner may choose to define clinically significant tachycardia and procedure success differently. Therefore, it is not clear when, if ever, it is appropriate to leave a patient without any antiarrhythmic therapy after a successful catheter ablation when one or more nonclinical tachycardias could still be induced. In these cases, patients at the University of Virginia almost uniformly receive an implantable cardioverter defibrillator if one is not already in place. Similarly, catheter ablation is rarely offered as first-line therapy for patients with reentrant ventricular tachycardia and structural heart disease.

Advanced mapping systems and more extensive ablation techniques may improve ablation results over time for a variety of arrhythmias. Clearly, many of the mapping systems can recreate the anatomic relationships and create improved electroanatomic correlations. Some systems provide global mapping information on individual beats, whereas others require point-to-point data acquisition from multiple points. One feature is common among all mapping systems: Procedure cost is increased. In addition, some systems require placement of additional large-diameter mapping catheters into the chamber being mapped, increasing the potential for catheter-related complications. The risk-benefit relationship for advanced mapping systems and the impact of the added procedural cost have not been fully explored, but their use is probably of benefit in select cases.

The number of catheter ablation procedures increased exponentially in the years for which survey data are available. This has been associated with a dramatic growth in the number of practitioners who perform catheter ablation procedures. Curative catheter ablation is cost-effective, and expansion of case numbers has not been held in check by financial disincentives, because reimbursement by third-party payers has not been restricted. The proliferation of catheter ablation procedures may be associated with some undesirable phenomena, including inappropriate self-referral for invasive catheter ablation procedures and performance of catheter ablation procedures by inadequately trained and inexperienced operators. The number of catheter ablation procedures required for adequate training and maintenance of skills has not been determined, but it is proposed that trainees have experience with at least 75 cases as primary operators, and practitioners maintain a volume of at least 50 cases per year in order to be certified to perform catheter ablation procedures. These numerical guidelines will undoubtedly trigger outraged cries of "restraint of trade," but ultimately the patients and the field of interventional electrophysiology will benefit. The most important criteria for selecting a physician and laboratory to whom a patient should be referred are the chronologic and numerical experience of the primary operator and laboratory staff in catheter ablation procedures. Operators with limited experience may achieve excellent outcomes through careful patient selection, but may be inadequately prepared to diagnose and treat unusual arrhythmia variants.

Catheter ablation of supraventricular and ventricular arrhythmias has advanced rapidly and is now a widely accepted modality of therapy for symptomatic arrhythmias, along with drugs and devices. The tools for ablation are continuing to improve, thereby increasing procedure efficacy and decreasing the risk of complications. This has resulted and will continue to result in expanding indications for ablative therapy. Although the opportunity to cure a patient suffering from an arrhythmia is extremely attractive, one must be vigilant to present all aspects of the risks and benefits to the patient. It is inappropriate to treat an electrocardiographic abnormality in an asymptomatic patient with a potentially morbid intervention. Similarly, if easy, well-tolerated medical therapy is effective in suppressing an arrhythmia, one should not be compelled to send

THE FUTURE

Curative catheter ablation of common forms of supraventricular tachycardia has exceeded most expectations with regard to both safety and efficacy. Although catheter designs and ablation techniques may evolve, it is likely that the overall outcome statistics will not change significantly. The main frontiers remaining in catheter ablation are curative therapy for atrial fibrillation and reentrant ventricular tachycardia. A wide variety of ablation tools are being developed for atrial fibrillation ablation. More important, selective linear atrial ablation will help us understand the pathophysiol-ogy of this complex arrhythmia and direct us to the optimal ablation targets to achieve arrhythmia cure. Reentrant ventricular tachycardia is often hemodynamically unstable, precluding prolonged periods of mapping. New mapping tools will allow for rapid ablation site selection. Because ablation targets are frequently mid-myocardial or subepicardial, larger and deeper lesions than can be created with conventional radiofrequency energy ablation will be required for procedure success. Future innovative catheter designs and new ablation energy sources may solve this present limitation.

the patient for catheter ablation. More intensive catheter ablative therapies such as curative atrial fibrillation ablation have lower success rates, higher complication rates, and unclear long-term benefits. Patients need to be well informed of these issues before undergoing these interventions. Ultimately, if the patient understands and is willing to accept the small but real risks associated with the procedure in order to achieve improved arrhythmia control or arrhythmia cure, then catheter ablation should be pursued.

REFERENCES

1. Sealy WC, Hattler BG Jr, Blumenschein SD, et al. Surgical treatment of Wolff-Parkinson-White syndrome. *Ann Thorac Surg* 1969;8:1–11.
2. Guiraudon GM, Klein GJ, Sharma AD, et al. Surgery for Wolff-Parkinson-White syndrome: further experience with an epicardial approach. *Circulation* 1986;74:525–529.
3. Cox JL, Gallagher JJ, Cain ME. Experience with 118 consecutive patients undergoing operation for the Wolff-Parkinson-White syndrome. *J Thorac Cardiovasc Surg* 1985;90:490–501.
4. Horowitz LN, Harken AH, Kastor JA, et al. Ventricular resection guided by epicardial and endocardial mapping for treatment of recurrent ventricular tachycardia. *N Engl J Med* 1980;302:589–593.
5. Haines DE, Lerman BB, Kron IL, et al. Surgical ablation of ventricular tachycardia with sequential map-guided subendocardial resection: electrophysiologic assessment and long-term follow-up. *Circulation* 1988;77:131–141.
6. Vedel J, Frank R, Fontaine G, et al. Bloc auriculo-ventriculaire intra-Hisien définitif induit au cours d'une exploration endoventriculaire droite. *Arch Mal Coeur* 1979;72:107–112.
7. Scheinman MM, Morady F, Hess DS, et al. Catheter-induced ablation of the atrioventricular junction to control refractory supraventricular arrhythmias. *JAMA* 1982;248:851–855.
8. Gallagher JJ, Svenson RH, Kasell JH, et al. Catheter tech-nique for closed-chest ablation of the atrioventricular conduction system. *N Engl J Med* 1982;306:194–200.
9. Weber H, Schmitz L. Catheter technique for closed-chest ablation of an accessory pathway. *N Engl J Med* 1983;308:654.
10. Morady F, Scheinman MM. Transvenous catheter ablation of a posteroseptal accessory pathway in a patient with the Wolff-Parkinson-White syndrome. *N Engl J Med* 1984;310:705–707.
11. Warin JF, Haissaguerre M, Lemetayer P, et al. Catheter ablation of accessory pathways with a direct approach. Results in 35 patients. *Circulation* 1988;78:800–815.
12. Belhassen B, Miller HI, Geller E, et al. Transcatheter electrical shock ablation of ventricular tachycardia. *J Am Coll Cardiol* 1986;7:1347–1355.
13. Borggrefe M, Breithardt G, Podczeck A. Catheter ablation of ventricular tachycardia using defibrillator pulses: electrophysiological findings and long-term results. *Eur Heart J* 1989;10:591–601.
14. Evans GT Jr, Scheinman MM, Scheinman MM, et al. The Percutaneous Cardiac Mapping and Ablation Registry: final summary of results. *Pacing Clin Electrophysiol* 1988;11:1621–1626.
15. Huang SK, Jordan N, Graham A. Closed-chest catheter desiccation of atrioventricular junction using radiofrequency energy—a new method of catheter ablation. *Circulation* 1985;72:111–389.
16. Wittkampf FH, Hauer RN, Robles de Medina EO. Control of radiofrequency lesion size by power regulation. *Circulation* 1989;80:962–968.
17. Haines DE, Watson DD. Tissue heating during radiofrequency catheter ablation: a thermodynamic model and observations in isolated perfused and superfused canine right ventricular free wall. *Pacing Clin Electrophysiol* 1989;12:962–976.
18. Haines DE, Watson DD, Verow AF. Electrode radius predicts lesion radius during radiofrequency energy heating. Validation of a proposed thermodynamic model. *Circ Res* 1990;67:124–129.
19. Jackman WM, Wang XZ, Friday KJ, et al. Catheter abla-

tion of atrioventricular junction using radiofrequency current in 17 patients. Comparison of standard and large-tip catheter electrodes. *Circulation* 1991;83:1562–1576.

20. Borggrefe M, Budde T, Podczeck A, et al. High frequency alternating current ablation of an accessory pathway in humans. *J Am Coll Cardiol* 1987;10:576–582.

21. Jackman WM, Friday KJ, Yeung-Lai-Wah JA, et al. New catheter technique for recording left free-wall accessory atrioventricular pathway activation. Identification of pathway fiber orientation. *Circulation* 1988;78:598–611.

22. Jackman WM, Kuck, Naccarelli GV, et al. Radiofrequency current directed across the mitral anulus with a bipolar epicardial-endocardial catheter electrode configuration. *Circulation* 1988;78:1288–1298.

23. Haissaguerre M, Fischer B, Warin JF, et al. Electrogram patterns predictive of successful radiofrequency catheter ablation of accessory pathways. *Pacing Clin Electrophysiol* 1992;15:2138–2145.

24. Jackman WM, Wang X, Friday KJ, et al. Catheter ablation of accessory atrioventricular pathways (Wolff-Parkinson-White syndrome) by radiofrequency current. *N Engl J Med* 1991;324:1605–1611.

25. Calkins H, Sousa J, el-Atassi R, et al. Diagnosis and cure of the Wolff-Parkinson-White syndrome or paroxysmal supraventricular tachycardias during a single electrophysiologic test. *N Engl J Med* 1991;324:1612–1618.

26. Kay GN, Epstein AE, Dailey SM, et al. Role of radiofrequency ablation in the management of supraventricular arrhythmias: experience in 760 consecutive patients. *J Cardiovasc Electrophysiol* 1993;4:371–389.

27. Nath S, DiMarco JP, Gallop RG, et al. Effects of dispersive electrode position and surface area on electrical parameters and temperature during radiofrequency catheter ablation. *Am J Cardiol* 1996;77:765–767.

28. Wittkampf FH, Hauer RN, Robles de Medina EO. Control of radiofrequency lesion size by power regulation. *Circulation* 1989;80:962–968.

29. Haines DE, Verow AF. Observations on electrode-tissue interface temperature and effect on electrical impedance during radiofrequency ablation of ventricular myocardium. *Circulation* 1990;82:1034–1038.

30. Ring ME, Huang SK, Gorman G, et al. Determinants of impedance rise during catheter ablation of bovine myocardium with radiofrequency energy. *Pacing Clin Electrophysiol* 1989;12:1502–1513.

31. Wittkampf FH, Simmers TA, Hauer RN, et al. Myocardial temperature response during radiofrequency catheter ablation. *Pacing Clin Electrophysiol* 1995;18:307–317.

32. Wittkampf FH, Nakagawa H, Yamanashi WS, et al. Thermal latency in radiofrequency ablation. *Circulation* 1996;93:1083–1086.

33. Haines DE. Determinants of lesion size during radiofrequency catheter ablation: the role of electrode-tissue contact pressure and duration of energy delivery. *J Cardiovasc Electrophysiol* 1991;2:509–515.

34. Nakagawa H, Yamanashi WS, Pitha JV, et al. Comparison of *in vivo* tissue temperature profile and lesion geometry for radiofrequency ablation with a saline-irrigated electrode versus temperature control in a canine thigh muscle preparation. *Circulation* 1995;91:2264–2273.

35. Jackman WM, Wang XZ, Friday KJ, et al. Catheter ablation of atrioventricular junction using radiofrequency current in 17 patients. Comparison of standard and large-tip catheter electrodes. *Circulation* 1991;83:1562–1576.

36. Langberg JJ, Gallagher M, Strickberger SA, et al. Temperature-guided radiofrequency catheter ablation with very large distal electrodes. *Circulation* 1993;88:245–249.

37. Whayne JG, Nath S, Haines DE. Microwave catheter ablation of myocardium in vitro. Assessment of the characteristics of tissue heating and injury. *Circulation* 1994;89:2390–2395.

38. Langberg JJ, Calkins H, el-Atassi R, et al. Temperature monitoring during radiofrequency catheter ablation of accessory pathways. *Circulation* 1992;86:1469–1474.

39. Nath S, DiMarco JP, Mounsey JP, et al. Correlation of temperature and pathophysiological effect during radiofrequency catheter ablation of the AV junction. *Circulation* 1995;92:1188–1192.

40. Tracy LM, Moore HJ, Solomon AJ, et al. Thermistor guided radiofrequency ablation of atrial insertion sites in patients with accessory pathways. *Pacing Clin Electrophysiol* 1995;18:2001–2007.

41. Huang SK, Bharati S, Lev M, et al. Electrophysiologic and histologic observations of chronic atrioventricular block induced by closed-chest catheter desiccation with radiofrequency energy. *Pacing Clin Electrophysiol* 1987;10:805–816.

42. Huang SK, Bharati S, Graham AR, et al. Closed chest catheter desiccation of the atrioventricular junction using radiofrequency energy—a new method of catheter ablation. *J Am Coll Cardiol* 1987;9:349–358.

43. Solomon AJ, Tracy CM, Swartz JF, et al. Effect on coronary artery anatomy of radiofrequency catheter ablation of atrial insertion sites of accessory pathways. *J Am Coll Cardiol* 1993;21:1440–1444.

44. Bokenkamp R, Wibbelt G, Sturm M, et al. Effects of intracardiac radiofrequency current application on coronary artery vessels in young pigs. *J Cardiovasc Electrophysiol* 2000;11:565–571.

45. DeLacey WA, Nath S, Haines DE, et al. Adenosine and verapamil-sensitive ventricular tachycardia originating from the left ventricle: radiofrequency catheter ablation. *Pacing Clin Electrophysiol* 1992;15:2240–2244.

46. Nath S, Whayne JG, Kaul S, et al. Effects of radiofrequency catheter ablation on regional myocardial blood flow: possible mechanism for late electrophysiological outcome. *Circulation* 1994;89:2667–2672.

47. Nath S, Redick JA, Whayne JG, et al. Ultrastructural observations in the myocardium beyond the region of acute coagulation necrosis following radiofrequency catheter ablation. *J Cardiovasc Electrophysiol* 1994;5:838–845.

48. Nath S, Lynch C III, Whayne JG, et al. Cellular electrophysiologic effects of hyperthermia on isolated guinea pig papillary muscle: implications for catheter ablation. *Circulation* 1993;88:1826–1833.

49. Simmers TA, De Bakker JM, Wittkampf FH, et al. Effects of heating on impulse propagation in superfused canine myocardium. *J Am Coll Cardiol* 1995;25:457–464.

50. Everett TH, Nath S, Lynch C, et al. Calcium overload as the mechanism of acute hyperthermic myocardial injury

during radiofrequency catheter ablation. *J Cardiovasc Electrophysiol* 2001;12:563–569.

51. Chang DC. Cell poration and cell fusion using an oscillating electric field. *Biophys J* 1989;56:641–652.

52. Jones JL, Jones RE, Balasky G. Microlesion formation in myocardial cells by high-intensity electric field stimulation. *Am J Physiol* 1987;253:H480–H486.

53. Schluter M, Geiger M, Siebels J, et al. Catheter ablation using radiofrequency current to cure symptomatic patients with tachyarrhythmias related to an accessory atrioventricular pathway. *Circulation* 1991;84:1644–1661.

54. Morady F, Strickberger A, Man KC, et al. Reasons for prolonged or failed attempts at radiofrequency catheter ablation of accessory pathways. *J Am Coll Cardiol* 1996;27:683–689.

55. Calkins H, Yong P, Miller JM, et al. Catheter ablation of accessory pathways, atrioventricular nodal reentrant tachycardia, and the atrioventricular junction: final results of a prospective, multicenter clinical trial. *Circulation* 1999;99:262–270.

56. Calkins H, Kim YN, Schmaltz S, et al. Electrogram criteria for identification of appropriate target sites for radiofrequency catheter ablation of accessory atrioventricular connections. *Circulation* 1992;85:565–573.

57. Bashir Y, Heald SC, Katritsis D, et al. Radiofrequency ablation of accessory atrioventricular pathways: predictive value of local electrogram characteristics for the identification of successful target sites. *Br Heart J* 1993;69:315–321.

58. Hindricks G, Kottkamp H, Chen X, et al. Localization and radiofrequency catheter ablation of left-sided accessory pathways during atrial fibrillation: feasibility and electrogram criteria for identification of appropriate target sites. *J Am Coll Cardiol* 1995;25:444–451.

59. Barlow MA, Klein GJ, Simpson CS, et al. Unipolar electrogram characteristics predictive of successful radiofrequency catheter ablation of accessory pathways. *J Cardiovasc Electrophysiol* 2000;11:146–154.

60. Swartz JF, Tracy CM, Fletcher RD. Radiofrequency endocardial catheter ablation of accessory atrioventricular pathway atrial insertion sites. *Circulation* 1993;87:487–499.

61. Deshpande SS, Bremner S, Sra JS, et al. Ablation of left free-wall accessory pathways using radiofrequency energy at the atrial insertion site: transseptal versus transaortic approach. *J Cardiovasc Electrophysiol* 1994;5:219–231.

62. Lesh MD, Van Hare GF, Scheinman MM, et al. Comparison of the retrograde and transseptal methods for ablation of left free wall accessory pathways. *J Am Coll Cardiol* 1993;22:542–549.

63. Xie B, Heald SC, Bashir Y, et al. Radiofrequency catheter ablation of septal accessory atrioventricular pathways. *Br Heart J* 1994;72:281–284.

64. Haissaguerre M, Marcus F, Poquet F, et al. Electrocardiographic characteristics and catheter ablation of parahissian accessory pathways. *Circulation* 1994;90:1124–1128.

65. Schluter M, Kuck KH. Catheter ablation from right atrium of anteroseptal accessory pathways using radiofrequency current. *J Am Coll Cardiol* 1992;19:663–670.

66. Dhala AA, Deshpande SS, Bremner S, et al. Transcatheter ablation of posteroseptal accessory pathways using a venous approach and radiofrequency energy. *Circulation* 1994;90:1799–1810.

67. Haissaguerre M, Cauchemez B, Marcus F, et al. Characteristics of the ventricular insertion sites of accessory pathways with anterograde decremental conduction properties. *Circulation* 1995;91:1077–1085.

68. McClelland JH, Wang X, Beckman KJ, et al. Radiofrequency catheter ablation of right atriofascicular (Mahaim) accessory pathways guided by accessory pathway activation potentials. *Circulation* 1994;89:2655–2666.

69. Zipes DP, DiMarco JP, Gillette PC, et al. Guidelines for clinical intracardiac electrophysiological and catheter ablation procedures. A report of the American College of Cardiology/American Heart Association Task Force on Practice Guidelines (Committee on Clinical Intracardiac Electrophysiologic and Catheter Ablation Procedures), developed in collaboration with the North American Society of Pacing and Electrophysiology. *J Am Coll Cardiol* 1995;26:555–573.

70. Guiraudon GM, Klein GJ, Sharma AD, et al. Skeletonization of the atrioventricular node for AV node reentrant tachycardia: experience with 32 patients. *Ann Thorac Surg* 1990;49:565–572.

71. Anderson RH, Janse MJ, van Capelle FJ, et al. A combined morphological and electrophysiological study of the atrioventricular node of the rabbit heart. *Circ Res* 1974;35:909–922.

72. Inoue S, Becker AE, Riccardi R, et al. Interruption of the inferior extension of the compact atrioventricular node underlies successful radio frequency ablation of atrioventricular nodal reentrant tachycardia. *J Intervent Card Electrophys* 1999;3:273–277.

73. Jackman WM, Beckman KJ, McClelland JH, et al. Treatment of supraventricular tachycardia due to atrioventricular nodal reentry by radiofrequency catheter ablation of slow-pathway conduction. *N Engl J Med* 1992;327:313–318.

74. McGuire MA, de Bakker JM, Vermeulen JT, et al. Origin and significance of double potentials near the atrioventricular node. Correlation of extracellular potentials, intracellular potentials, and histology. *Circulation* 1994;89:2351–2360.

75. de Bakker JM, Coronel R, McGuire MA, et al. Slow potentials in the atrioventricular junctional area of patients operated on for atrioventricular node tachycardias and in isolated porcine. *J Am Coll Cardiol* 1994;23:709–715.

76. Langberg JJ, Harvey M, Calkins H, et al. Titration of power output during radiofrequency catheter ablation of atrioventricular nodal reentrant tachycardia. *Pacing Clin Electrophysiol* 1993;16:465–470.

77. Jazayeri MR, Hempe SL, Sra JS, et al. Selective transcatheter ablation of the fast and slow pathways using radiofrequency energy in patients with atrioventricular nodal reentrant tachycardia. *Circulation* 1992;85:1318–1328.

78. Kalbfleisch SJ, Strickberger SA, Williamson B, et al. Randomized comparison of anatomic and electrogram mapping approaches to ablation of the slow pathway of atrioventricular node reentrant tachycardia. *J Am Coll Cardiol* 1994;23:716–723.

79. Thakur RK, Klein GJ, Yee R, et al. Junctional tachycardia: a useful marker during radiofrequency ablation for atrioventricular node reentrant tachycardia. *J Am Coll Cardiol* 1993;22:1706–1710.

80. Mitrani RD, Klein LS, Hackett FK, et al. Radiofrequency ablation for atrioventricular node tachycardia: comparison between fast (anterior) and slow (posterior) pathway ablation. *J Am Coll Cardiol* 1993;21:432–441.

81. Jentzer JH, Goyal R, Williamson BD, et al. Analysis of junctional ectopy during radiofrequency ablation of the slow pathway in patients with atrioventricular nodal reentrant tachycardia. *Circulation* 1994;90:2820–2826.

82. Hsieh MH, Chen SA, Tai CT, et al. Absence of junctional rhythm during successful slow-pathway ablation in patients with atrioventricular nodal reentrant tachycardia. *Circulation* 1998;98:2296–2300.

83. Sra JS, Jazayeri MR, Blanck Z, et al. Slow pathway ablation in patients with atrioventricular node reentrant tachycardia and a prolonged PR interval. *J Am Coll Cardiol* 1994;24:1064–1068.

84. Baker JH II, Plumb VJ, Epstein AE, et al. Predictors of recurrent atrioventricular nodal reentry after selective slow pathway ablation. *Am J Cardiol* 1994;73:765–769.

85. Kay GN, Epstein AE, Dailey SM, et al. Selective radiofrequency ablation of the slow pathway for the treatment of atrioventricular nodal reentrant tachycardia. *Circulation* 1992;85:1675–1685.

86. Wu D, Yeh SJ, Wang CC, et al. A simple technique for selective radiofrequency ablation of the slow pathway in atrioventricular node reentrant tachycardia. *J Am Coll Cardiol* 1993;21:1612–1621.

87. Lindsay BD, Chung MK, Gamache MC, et al. Therapeutic end points for the treatment of atrioventricular node reentrant tachycardia by catheter-guided radiofrequency current. *J Am Coll Cardiol* 1993;22:733–740.

88. Manolis AS, Wang PJ, Estes NA. Radiofrequency ablation of slow pathway in patients with atrioventricular nodal reentrant tachycardia. Do arrhythmia recurrences correlate with persistent slow pathway conduction or site of successful ablation? *Circulation* 1994;90:2815–2819.

89. Kottkamp H, Hindricks G, Willems S, et al. An anatomically and electrogram-guided stepwise approach for effective and safe catheter ablation of the fast pathway for elimination of atrioventricular node reentrant tachycardia. *J Am Coll Cardiol* 1995;25:974–981.

90. Cosio FG, Goicolea A, Lopez-Gil M, et al. Atrial endocardial mapping in the rare form of atrial flutter. *Am J Cardiol* 1990;66:715–720.

91. Friedman PA, Luria D, Fenton AM, et al. Global right atrial mapping of human atrial flutter: the presence of posteromedial (sinus venosa region) functional block and double potentials: a study in biplane fluoroscopy and intracardiac echocardiography. *Circulation* 2000;101:1568–1577.

92. Saoudi N, Atallah G, Kirkorian G, et al. Catheter ablation of the atrial myocardium in human type I atrial flutter. *Circulation* 1990;81:762–771.

93. Feld GK, Fleck RP, Chen PS, et al. Radiofrequency catheter ablation for the treatment of human type 1 atrial flutter. Identification of a critical zone in the reentrant circuit by endocardial mapping techniques. *Circulation* 1992;86:1233–1240.

94. Cosio FG, Lopez-Gil M, Goicolea A, et al. Radiofrequency ablation of the inferior vena cava-tricuspid valve isthmus in common atrial flutter. *Am J Cardiol* 1993;71:705–709.

95. Takahashi A, Shah DC, Jais P, et al. Partial cavotricuspid isthmus block before ablation in patients with typical atrial flutter. *J Am Coll Cardiol* 1999;33:1996–2002.

96. Chen J, de Chillou C, Basiouny T, et al. Cavotricuspid isthmus mapping to assess bidirectional block during common atrial flutter radiofrequency ablation. *Circulation* 1999;100:2507–2513.

97. Yamabe H, Okumura K, Misumi I. Role of bipolar electrogram polarity mapping in localizing recurrent conduction in the isthmus early and late after ablation of atrial flutter. *J Am Coll Cardiol* 1999;33:39–45.

98. Heidbuchel H, Willems R, van Rensburg H, et al. Right atrial angiographic evaluation of the posterior isthmus: relevance for ablation of typical atrial flutter. *Circulation* 2000;101:2178–2184.

99. Poty H, Saoudi N, Abdel Aziz, et al. Radiofrequency catheter ablation of type 1 atrial flutter: prediction of late success by electrophysiological criteria. *Circulation* 1995;92:1389–1392.

100. Cauchemez B, Haissaguerre M, Fischer B, et al. Electrophysiological effects of catheter ablation of inferior vena cava-tricuspid annulus isthmus in common atrial flutter. *Circulation* 1996;93:284–294.

101. Jais P, Haissaguerre M, Shah DC, et al. Successful irrigated-tip catheter ablation of atrial flutter resistant to conventional radiofrequency ablation. *Circulation* 1998;98:835–838.

102. Nath S, Mounsey JP, Haines DE, et al. Predictors of acute and long-term success after radiofrequency catheter ablation of type 1 atrial flutter. *Am J Cardiol* 1995;76:604–606.

103. Philippon F, Plumb VJ, Epstein AE, et al. The risk of atrial fibrillation following radiofrequency catheter ablation of atrial flutter. *Circulation* 1995;92:430–435.

104. Paydak H, Kall JG, Burke MC, et al. Atrial fibrillation after radiofrequency ablation of type I atrial flutter: time to onset, determinants, and clinical course. *Circulation* 1998;98:315–322.

105. Schumacher B, Jung W, Lewalter T, et al. Radiofrequency ablation of atrial flutter due to administration of class IC antiarrhythmic drugs for atrial fibrillation. *Am J Cardiol* 1999;83:710–713.

106. Fischer B, Haissaguerre M, Garrigues S, et al. Radiofrequency catheter ablation of common atrial flutter in 80 patients. *J Am Coll Cardiol* 1995;25:1365–1372.

107. Kannel WB, Abbott RD, Savage DD, et al. Epidemiologic features of chronic atrial fibrillation: the Framingham study. *N Engl J Med* 1982;306:1018–1022.

108. Kalbfleisch SJ, Williamson B, Man KC, et al. A randomized comparison of the right- and left-sided approaches to ablation of the atrioventricular junction. *Am J Cardiol* 1993;72:1406–1410.

109. Nath S, DiMarco JP, Mounsey JP, et al. Correlation of temperature and pathophysiological effect during radiofre-

quency catheter ablation of the atrioventricular junction. *Circulation* 1995;92:1194–2092.

110. Yeung-Lai-Wah JA, Alison JF, Lonergan L, et al. High success rate of atrioventricular node ablation with radiofrequency energy. *J Am Coll Cardiol* 1991;18:1753–1758.

111. Brignole M, Gianfranchi L, Menozzi C, et al. Influence of atrioventricular junction radiofrequency ablation in patients with chronic atrial fibrillation and flutter on quality of life and cardiac performance. *Am J Cardiol* 1994;74:242–246.

112. Rodriguez LM, Smeets JL, Xie B, et al. Improvement in left ventricular function by ablation of atrioventricular nodal conduction in selected patients with lone atrial fibrillation. *Am J Cardiol* 1993;72:1137–1141.

113. Feld GK, Fleck RP, Fujimura O, et al. Control of rapid ventricular response by radiofrequency catheter modification of the atrioventricular node in patients with medically refractory atrial fibrillation. *Circulation* 1994;90:2299–2307.

114. Williamson BD, Man KC, Daoud E, et al. Radiofrequency catheter modification of atrioventricular conduction to control the ventricular rate during atrial fibrillation. *N Engl J Med* 1994;331:910–917.

115. Konings KT, Kirchhof CJ, Smeets JR, et al. High-density mapping of electrically induced atrial fibrillation in humans. *Circulation* 1994;89:1665–1680.

116. Smeets JL, Allessie MA, Lammers WJ, et al. The wavelength of the cardiac impulse and reentrant arrhythmias in isolated rabbit atrium: the role of heart rate, autonomic transmitters, temperature, and potassium. *Circ Res* 1986;58:96–108.

117. Mandapati R, Skanes A, Chen J, et al. Stable microreentrant sources as a mechanism of atrial fibrillation in the isolated sheep heart. *Circulation* 2000;101:194–199.

118. Jais P, Haissaguerre M, Shah DC, et al. A focal source of atrial fibrillation treated by discrete radiofrequency ablation. *Circulation* 1997;95:572–756.

119. Haissaguerre M, Jais P, Shah DC, et al. Spontaneous initiation of atrial fibrillation by ectopic beats originating in the pulmonary veins. *N Engl J Med* 1998;339:659–666.

120. Chen SA, Hsieh MH, Tai CT, et al. Initiation of atrial fibrillation by ectopic beats originating from the pulmonary veins: electrophysiological characteristics, pharmacological responses, and effects of radiofrequency ablation. *Circulation* 1999;100:1879–1886.

121. Cox JL, Boineau JP, Schuessler RB, et al. Five-year experience with the maze procedure for atrial fibrillation. *Ann Thorac Surg* 1993;56:814–823.

122. Mitchell MA, McRury ID, Haines DE. Linear atrial ablations in a canine model of chronic atrial fibrillation: morphological and electrophysiological observations. *Circulation* 1998;97:1176–1185.

123. Swartz JF, Pellersels G, Silvers J, et al. A catheter-based curative approach to atrial fibrillation in humans [abst]. *Circulation* 1994;90:1–335.

124. Haissaguerre M, Jais P, Shah DC, et al. Right and left atrial radiofrequency catheter therapy of paroxysmal atrial fibrillation. *J Cardiovasc Electrophysiol* 1996;7:1132–1144.

125. Epstein LM, Mitchell MA, Smith TW, et al. Comparative study of fluoroscopy and intracardiac echocardiographic

126. Jais P, Shah DC, Haissaguerre M, et al. Mapping and ablation of left atrial flutters. *Circulation* 2000;101:2928–2934.

127. Mitchell MA, McRury ID, Everett TH, et al. Morphological and physiological characteristics of discontinuous linear atrial ablations during atrial pacing and atrial fibrillation. *J Cardiovasc Electrophys* 1999;10:378–386.

128. Gaita F, Riccardi R, Calo L, et al. Atrial mapping and radiofrequency catheter ablation in patients with idiopathic atrial fibrillation. Electrophysiological findings and ablation results. *Circulation* 1998;97:2136–2145.

129. Maloney JD, Milner L, Barold S, et al. Two-staged biatrial linear and focal ablation to restore sinus rhythm in patients with refractory chronic atrial fibrillation: procedure experience and follow-up beyond 1 year. *PACE* 1998;21:2527–2532.

130. Garg A, Finneran W, Mollerus M, et al. Right atrial compartmentalization using radiofrequency catheter ablation for management of patients with refractory atrial fibrillation. *J Cardiovasc Electrophysiol* 1999;10:763–771.

131. Pappone C, Oreto G, Lamberti F, et al. Catheter ablation of paroxysmal atrial fibrillation using a 3D mapping system. *Circulation* 1999;100:1203–1208.

132. Ernst S, Schluter M, Ouyang F, et al. Modification of the substrate for maintenance of idiopathic human atrial fibrillation: efficacy of radiofrequency ablation using nonfluoroscopic catheter guidance. *Circulation* 1999;100:2085–2092.

133. Natale A, Leonelli F, Beheiry S, et al. Catheter ablation approach on the right side only for paroxysmal atrial fibrillation therapy: long-term results. *PACE* 2000;23:224–233.

134. Haines DE, Hummel JD, Kalbfleisch SJ, et al. Bi-atrial linear ablation with the multiple electrode catheter ablation (MECA) system in patients with atrial fibrillation. *PACE* 2000;23:II-567.

135. Mangrum JM, Haines DE, DiMarco JP, et al. Elimination of focal atrial fibrillation with a single radiofrequency ablation: use of a basket catheter in a pulmonary vein for computerized activation sequence mapping. *J Cardiovasc Electrophys* 2000;11:1159–1164.

136. Hwang C, Wu TJ, Doshi RN, et al. Vein of marshall cannulation for the analysis of electrical activity in patients with focal atrial fibrillation. *Circulation* 2000;101:1503–1505.

137. Tsai CF, Tai CT, Hsieh MH, et al. Initiation of atrial fibrillation by ectopic beats originating from the superior vena cava: electrophysiological characteristics and results of radiofrequency ablation. *Circulation* 2000;102:67–74.

138. Natale A, Pisano E, Shewchik J, et al. First human experience with pulmonary vein isolation using a through-the-balloon circumferential ultrasound ablation system for recurrent atrial fibrillation. *Circulation* 2000;102:1879–1882.

139. Lau CP, Tse HF, Ayers GM. Defibrillation-guided radiofrequency ablation of atrial fibrillation secondary to an atrial focus. *J Am Coll Cardiol* 1999;33:1217–1226.

140. Haissaguerre M, Jais P, Shah DC, et al. Electrophysiological end point for catheter ablation of atrial fibrillation ini-

tiated from multiple pulmonary venous foci. *Circulation* 2000;101:1409–1417.

141. Robbins IM, Colvin EV, Doyle TP, et al. Pulmonary vein stenosis after catheter ablation of atrial fibrillation. *Circulation* 1998;98:1769–1775.

142. Sanders WE Jr, Sorrentino RA, Greenfield RA, et al. Catheter ablation of sinoatrial node reentrant tachycardia. *J Am Coll Cardiol* 1994;23:926–934.

143. Kay GN, Chong F, Epstein AE, et al. Radiofrequency ablation for treatment of primary atrial tachycardias. *J Am Coll Cardiol* 1993;21:901–909.

144. Grubb BP, Kosinski DJ, Boehm K, et al. The postural orthostatic tachycardia syndrome: a neurocardiogenic variant identified during head-up tilt table testing. *Pacing Clin Electrophysiol* 1997;20:2205–2212.

145. Lee RJ, Kalman JM, Fitzpatrick AP, et al. Radiofrequency catheter modification of the sinus node for "inappropriate" sinus tachycardia. *Circulation* 1995;92:2919–2928.

146. Tang CW, Scheinman MM, Van Hare GF, et al. Use of P wave configuration during atrial tachycardia to predict site of origin. *J Am Coll Cardiol* 1995;26:1315–1324.

147. Tracy CM, Swartz JF, Fletcher RD, et al. Radiofrequency catheter ablation of ectopic atrial tachycardia using paced activation sequence mapping. *J Am Coll Cardiol* 1993;21:910–917.

148. Rahilly GT, Prystowsky EN, Zipes DP, et al. Clinical and electrophysiologic findings in patients with repetitive monomorphic ventricular tachycardia and otherwise normal electrocardiogram. *Am J Cardiol* 1982;50:459–468.

149. Wilber DJ, Baerman J, Olshansky B, et al. Adenosine-sensitive ventricular tachycardia: clinical characteristics and response to catheter ablation. *Circulation* 1993;87:126–134.

150. Lerman BB, Belardinelli L, West GA, et al. Adenosine-sensitive ventricular tachycardia: evidence suggesting cyclic AMP-mediated triggered activity. *Circulation* 1986;74:270–280.

151. Ohe T, Shimomura K, Aihara N, et al. Idiopathic sustained left ventricular tachycardia: clinical and electrophysiologic characteristics. *Circulation* 1994;77:560–568.

152. Okumura K, Matsuyama K, Miyagi H, et al. Entrainment of idiopathic ventricular tachycardia of left ventricular origin with evidence for reentry with an area of slow conduction and effect of verapamil. *Am J Cardiol* 1994;62:727–732.

153. Klein LS, Shih HT, Hackett FK, et al. Radiofrequency catheter ablation of ventricular tachycardia in patients without structural heart disease. *Circulation* 1992;85:1666–1674.

154. Calkins H, Kalbfleisch SJ, el-Atassi R, et al. Relation between efficacy of radiofrequency catheter ablation and site of origin of idiopathic ventricular tachycardia. *Am J Cardiol* 1993;71:827–833.

155. Nakagawa H, Beckman KJ, McClelland JH, et al. Radiofrequency catheter ablation of idiopathic left ventricular tachycardia guided by a Purkinje potential. *Circulation* 1993;94:2607–2617.

156. Wen MS, Yeh SJ, Wang CC, et al. Successful radiofrequency ablation of idiopathic left ventricular tachycardia at a site away from the tachycardia exit. *J Am Coll Cardiol* 1997;30:1024–1031.

157. Kamakura S, Shimizu W, Matsuo K, et al. Localization of optimal ablation site of idiopathic ventricular tachycardia from right and left ventricular outflow tract by body surface ECG. *Circulation* 1998;98:1525–1533.

158. Peeters HA, SippensGroenewegen A, Wever EF, et al. Clinical application of an integrated 3-phase mapping technique for localization of the site of origin of idiopathic ventricular tachycardia. *Circulation* 1999;99:1300–1311.

159. Tsuchiya T, Okumura K, Honda T, et al. Significance of late diastolic potential preceding Purkinje potential in verapamil-sensitive idiopathic left ventricular tachycardia. *Circulation* 1999;99:2408–2413.

160. de Bakker JM, Hauer RN, Simmers TA. Activation mapping: unipolar versus bipolar recording. In: Zipes DP, Jalife, eds. *Cardiac electrophysiology: from cell to bedside.* Philadelphia: WB Saunders, 1995:1068–1078.

161. Klein LS, Miles WM, Mitrani RD, et al. Ablation of ventricular tachycardia in patients with structurally normal hearts. In: Zipes DP, Jalife, eds. *Cardiac electrophysiology: from cell to bedside.* Philadelphia: WB Saunders, 1995:1518–1523.

162. Downar E, Kimber S, Harris L, et al. Endocardial mapping of ventricular tachycardia in the intact human heart. II. Evidence for multiuse reentry in a functional sheet of surviving myocardium. *J Am Coll Cardiol* 1992;20:869–878.

163. de Bakker JM, Coronel R, Tasseron S, et al. Ventricular tachycardia in the infarcted, Langendorff-perfused human heart: role of the arrangement of surviving cardiac fibers. *J Am Coll Cardiol* 1990;15:1594.

164. Harris L, Downar E, Mickleborough L, et al. Activation sequence of ventricular tachycardia: endocardial and epicardial mapping studies in the human ventricle. *J Am Coll Cardiol* 1987;10:1040–1047.

165. Downar E, Saito J, Doig JC, et al. Endocardial mapping of ventricular tachycardia in the intact human ventricle. III. Evidence of multiuse reentry with spontaneous and induced block in portions of reentrant path complex. *J Am Coll Cardiol* 1995;25:1591–1600.

166. Wilber DJ, Kopp DE, Glascock DN, et al. Catheter ablation of the mitral isthmus for ventricular tachycardia associated with inferior infarction. *Circulation* 1995;92:3481–3489.

167. de Bakker JM, van Capelle FJ, Janse MJ, et al. Slow conduction in the infarcted human heart. "Zigzag" course of activation. *Circulation* 1993;94:915–926.

168. de Bakker JM, van Capelle FJ, Janse MJ, et al. Fractionated electrograms in dilated cardiomyopathy: origin and relation to abnormal conduction. *J Am Coll Cardiol* 1996;27:1071–1078.

169. Caceres J, Jazayeri M, McKinnie J, et al. Sustained bundle branch reentry as a mechanism of clinical tachycardia. *Circulation* 1989;84:256–270.

170. Tchou P, Jazayeri M, Denker S, et al. Transcatheter electrical ablation of right bundle branch: a method of treating macroreentrant ventricular tachycardia attributed to bundle branch reentry. *Circulation* 1994;78:246–257.

171. Cohen TJ, Chien WW, Lurie KG, et al. Radiofrequency catheter ablation for treatment of bundle branch reentrant ventricular tachycardia: results and long-term follow-up. *J Am Coll Cardiol* 1991;18:1767–1773.

172. Marcus FI, Fontaine G. Arrhythmogenic right ventricular dysplasia/cardiomyopathy: a review. *Pacing Clin Electrophysiol* 1995;18:1298–1314.

173. Ellison KE, Friedman PL, Ganz LI, Stevenson WG. Entrainment mapping and radiofrequency catheter ablation of ventricular tachycardia in right ventricular dysplasia. *J Am Coll Cardiol* 1998;32:724–728.

174. Globits S, Kreiner G, Frank H, et al. Significance of morphological abnormalities detected by MRI in patients undergoing successful ablation of right ventricular outflow tract tachycardia. *Circulation* 1997;96:2633–2640.

175. Stevenson WG, Delacretaz E, Friedman PL, et al. Identification and ablation of macroreentrant ventricular tachycardia with the CARTO electroanatomical mapping system. *Pacing Clin Electrophys* 1998;21:1448–1456.

176. Greenspon AJ, Hsu SS, Datorre S. Successful radiofrequency catheter ablation of sustained ventricular tachycardia postmyocardial infarction in man guided by a multielectrode "basket" catheter. *J Cardiovasc Electrophys* 1997;8:565–570.

177. Strickberger SA, Knight BP, Michaud GF, et al. Mapping and ablation of ventricular tachycardia guided by virtual electrograms using a noncontact, computerized mapping system. *J Am Coll Cardiol* 2000;35:414–421.

178. Pogwizd SM, Hoyt RH, Saffitz JE, et al. Reentrant and focal mechanisms underlying ventricular tachycardia in the human heart. *Circulation* 1992;86:1872–1887.

179. Weber H, Enders S, Keiditisch E. Percutaneous Nd:YAG laser coagulation of ventricular myocardium in dogs using a special electrode laser catheter. *Pacing Clin Electrophysiol* 1989;12:899–910.

180. He DS, Zimmer JE, Hynynen K, et al. Application of ultrasound energy for intracardiac ablation of arrhythmias. *Eur Heart J* 1995;16:961–966.

181. Stevenson WG, Khan H, Sager P, et al. Identification of reentry circuit sites during catheter mapping and radiofrequency ablation of ventricular tachycardia late after myocardial infarction. *Circulation* 1993;88:1647–1670.

182. Bogun F, Bahu M, Knight BP, et al. Comparison of effective and ineffective target sites that demonstrate concealed entrainment in patients with coronary artery disease undergoing radiofrequency ablation of ventricular tachycardia. *Circulation* 1997;95:183–190.

183. El-Shalakany A, Hadjis T, Papageorgiou P, et al. Entrainment/mapping criteria for the prediction of termination of ventricular tachycardia by single radiofrequency lesion in patients with coronary artery disease. *Circulation* 1999;99:2283–2289.

184. Morady F, Harvey M, Kalbfleisch SJ, et al. Radiofrequency catheter ablation of ventricular tachycardia in patients with coronary artery disease. *Circulation* 1993;87:363–372.

185. Gursoy S, Chiladakis I, Kuck KH. First lessons from radiofrequency catheter ablation in patients with ventricular tachycardia. *Pacing Clin Electrophysiol* 1993;16:687–691.

186. Kim YH, Sosa-Suarez G, Trouton TG, et al. Treatment of ventricular tachycardia by transcatheter radiofrequency ablation in patients with ischemic heart disease. *Circulation* 1994;89:1094–1102.

187. Strickberger SA, Man KC, Daoud EG, et al. A prospective evaluation of catheter ablation of ventricular tachycardia as adjuvant therapy in patients with coronary artery disease and an implantable cardioverter-defibrillator. *Circulation* 1997;96:1525–1531.

188. Rothman SA, Hsia HH, Cossu SF, et al. Radiofrequency catheter ablation of postinfarction ventricular tachycardia: long-term success and the significance of inducible nonclinical arrhythmias. *Circulation* 1997;96:3499–3508.

189. Callans DJ, Zado E, Sarter BH, et al. Efficacy of radiofrequency catheter ablation for ventricular tachycardia in healed myocardial infarction. *Am J Cardiol* 1998;82:429–432.

190. Stevenson WG, Friedman PL, Kocovic D, et al. Radiofrequency catheter ablation of ventricular tachycardia after myocardial infarction. *Circulation* 1998;98:308–314.

191. Calkins H, Epstein A, Packer D, et al. Catheter ablation of ventricular tachycardia in patients with structural heart disease using cooled radiofrequency energy: results of a prospective multicenter study. Cooled RF Multi Center Investigators Group. *J Am Coll Cardiol* 2000;35:1905–1914.

192. Cohen TJ, Chien WW, Lurie KG, et al. Radiofrequency catheter ablation for treatment of bundle branch reentrant ventricular tachycardia: results and long-term follow-up. *J Am Coll Cardiol* 1991;18:1767–1773.

193. Blanck Z, Dhala A, Deshpande S, et al. Bundle branch reentrant ventricular tachycardia: cumulative experience in 48 patients. *J Cardiovasc Electrophysiol* 1993;4:253–262.

194. Scheinman MM. NASPE Survey on Catheter Ablation. *Pacing Clin Electrophysiol* 1995;18:1474–1478.

195. Danford DA, Kugler JD, Deal B, et al. The learning curve for radiofrequency ablation of tachyarrhythmias in pediatric patients. *Am J Cardiol* 1995;75:587–590.

196. Rosenheck S, Rose M, Sharon Z, et al. The ongoing influence of staff training on the performance of radiofrequency catheter ablation. *Pacing Clin Electrophysiol* 1997;20:1312–1317.

197. Thakur RK, Klein GJ, Yee R, et al. Complications of radiofrequency catheter ablation: a review. *Can J Cardiol* 1994;10:885–889.

198. Hindricks G. The Multicentre European Radiofrequency Survey (MERFS): complications of radiofrequency catheter ablation of arrhythmias. *Eur Heart J* 1993;14:1644–1653.

199. Chen SA, Chiang CE, Tai CT, et al. Complications of diagnostic electrophysiologic studies and radiofrequency catheter ablation in patients with tachyarrhythmias: an eight-year survey of 3,966 consecutive procedures in a tertiary referral center. *Am J Cardiol* 1996;77:41–46.

200. Calkins H, Niklason L, Sousa J, et al. Radiation exposure during radiofrequency catheter ablation of accessory atrioventricular connections. *Circulation* 1991;84:2376–2382.

PACEMAKERS

DAVID L. HAYES

⚡ ADDITIONAL ELECTRONIC TOPICS

Historical Perspective m22; Neurocardiogenic Syncope m23; Temperature Sensors m24; Other Sensors m25; Dual-Sensor Combinations m26; Effect of Pacing Mode on Morbidity and Mortality m27; Programming of Energy (Pulse Width and Voltage Amplitude) m28; Refractory Periods m29; Atrioventricular Interval m30; Ventricular Safety Pacing m31; Differential Atrioventricular Interval m32; Rate-Variable or Rate-Adaptive Atrioventricular Interval m33; Mode Switching m34; Programming Goals of Rate Adaptation m35; Loose Set-Screw Connection m36; Retained Lead Fragments m37; Pacemaker Allergy m38; Limitations Following Pacemaker Implantation m39; Temporary Pacemaker Placement m40; Management of Temporary Pacemakers m41; Esophageal Pacing m42

D. L. Hayes: Department of Medicine, Mayo Medical School; and Division of Cardiovascular Diseases and Internal Medicine, Mayo Clinic, Rochester, Minnesota

OVERVIEW

When pacemaker implantation is being considered, the clinician should be able to document that implantation is justified and the pacemaker will benefit the patient clinically.

This is valuable for long-term care of the patient and subsequent pacing needs as well as for purposes of reimbursement.

The selection of the pacing mode should be based on the immediate needs of the patient and the potential long-term benefit of specific pacing modes. When determining the most appropriate pacing mode for a patient, the clinician should consider the patient's activity level, need for atrioventricular (AV) synchrony, need for chronotropic support, and associated medical conditions. When choosing a pacemaker, remember that rate-adaptive pacing technology allows, for most patients, restoration of a near normal chronotropic response.

Potential interference from outside electrical sources is always of concern to both the patient with a pacemaker and referring physicians. The most common sources of electromagnetic interference for permanent pacemakers are found in a hospital environment (e.g., electrocautery, cardioversion, and magnetic resonance imaging).

The utilization and sophistication of permanent pacemakers have increased steadily since the first pacemaker implantation in 1958 (*e*Fig. 74.0.1) (1,2). Initially, pacemakers were indicated only for the prevention of Stokes-Adams attacks, but the indications have broadened as the technology has advanced. According to the estimates of four manufacturers, there were 152,909 primary pacemaker implantations (571 per million population) in 1997 and 37,946 pacemaker pulse generator replacements (3). Despite the continued sophistication and, at times, complexities of permanent pacemakers, they have become such a mainstay of therapy that it is imperative for clinical cardiologists to have a working knowledge of these devices.

GLOSSARY

AAI/AAIR: Single-chamber atrial pacing modes, with *R* noting the capability of rate adaptation.

Blanking period: Temporary disabling of pacemaker-sensing amplifiers following the delivery of an output pulse. This prevents inappropriate sensing of residual energy from the pacemaker output pulse and, in dual-chamber pacemakers, prevents sensing of pacemaker output pulses or intrinsic events in the chamber other than that in which the event occurs.

DDD/DDDR: Dual-chamber pacing modes, with *R* noting the capability of rate adaptation.

Electromagnetic interference: Any strong source of electromagnetic interference potentially could interfere with the pacemaker and alter its function.

Functional pacing abnormalities (e.g., functional undersensing or functional failure to capture): Failure to sense or capture that is appropriate because of imposed pacemaker refractory periods or myocardial refractoriness due to a previous intrinsic atrial or ventricular event.

Mode switch: Capability of a dual-chamber pacemaker to switch automatically from an atrial-tracking (P synchronous) mode to a non–atrial-tracking mode in the presence of an atrial rhythm that the pacemaker determines to be pathologic. When the atrial rhythm meets the criteria for a physiologic rhythm, the mode switches back to an atrial-tracking mode.

Postventricular atrial refractory period: The period during which the atrial-sensing circuit is refractory following a sensed ventricular event. The purpose of this is to avoid sensing retrograde atrial activity that could initiate an endless-loop tachycardia.

Total atrial refractory period: The period during which the atrial channel of a dual-chamber or VDD pacemaker ignores intrinsic atrial activity or other activity sensed on the atrial-sensing circuit.

Ventricular safety pacing: Delivery of a ventricular output pulse, following atrial pacing, if a signal is sensed by the ventricular channel during the early portion of the AV interval (AVI). This is used to ensure that ventricular depolarization occurs if the sensed event was something other than an intrinsic ventricular depolarization.

VVI/VVIR: Single-chamber ventricular pacing modes, with *R* noting the capability of rate adaptation.

PACEMAKER NOMENCLATURE

A three-letter code describing the basic function of the various pacing systems was first proposed in 1974 by a combined task force from the American College of Cardiology and the American Heart Association (ACC/AHA) (10). Since then, the responsibility for periodically updating the code has been assumed by the North American Society of Pacing and Electrophysiology and the British Pacing and Electrophysiology Group. The code is designated by the NBG code for pacing nomenclature (11) (Table 74.1). The code has five positions, but the fifth position is rarely used. It is a generic code and does not describe specific or unique functional characteristics of each device.

The first position reflects the chamber or chambers in which stimulation occurs: A, atrium; V, ventricle; and D, dual chamber; or both A and V.

The second position refers to the chamber or chambers in which sensing occurs. The letters are the same as those for the first position. (Manufacturers also use *S* in both the first and second positions to indicate that the device is capable of pacing only a single cardiac chamber.)

The third position refers to the mode of sensing, or how the pacemaker responds to a sensed event. An *I* indicates that a sensed event inhibits the output pulse and causes the pacemaker to recycle for one or more timing cycles. *T* means that an output pulse is triggered in response to a sensed event. *D* means that both T and I responses may occur. This designation is restricted to dual-chamber sys-

TABLE 74.1 NBG CODE

Position[a]	I	II	III	IV	V
Category	Chamber(s) paced	Chamber(s) sensed	Response to sensing	Programmability, rate modulation	Antitachyarrhythmia function(s)
	O = None	O = None	O = None	O = None	O = None
	A = Atrium	A = Atrium	T = Triggered	P = Simple programmable	P = Pacing (antitachyarrhythmia)
	V = Ventricle	V = Ventricle	I = Inhibited	M = Multiprogrammable	S = Shock
	D = Dual (A + V)	D = Dual (A + V)	D = Dual (T + I)	C = Communicating	D = Dual (P + S)
Manufacturer's designation only	S = Single (A or V)	S = Single (A or V)		R = Rate modulation	

[a]Positions I through III are used exclusively for antibradyarrhythmia function.
From Bernstein AD, Camm AJ, Fletcher RD, et al. The NASPE/BPEG generic pacemaker code for antibradyarrhythmia and adaptive-rate pacing and antitachyarrhythmia devices. *Pacing Clin Electrophysiol* 1987;10:794–799, with permission of Futura.

tems. An event sensed in the atrium inhibits the atrial output but triggers a ventricular output. Unlike a single-chamber–triggered mode (VVT or AAT), in which an output pulse is triggered immediately on sensing, there is a delay between the sensed atrial event and the triggered ventricular output to mimic the normal PR interval. If a native ventricular signal or R wave is sensed, it inhibits the ventricular output and possibly even the atrial output, depending on where sensing occurs.

The fourth position of the code reflects both programmability and rate modulation. An *R* in the fourth position indicates that the pacemaker incorporates a sensor to control the rate independently of intrinsic cardiac activity. From a practical standpoint, R is the only indicator commonly used in the fourth position. Other indicators are described in Table 74.1.

The fifth position is restricted to antitachycardia functions and is rarely used.

INDICATIONS FOR CARDIAC PACING

According to the criteria established by a joint committee of the ACC/AHA, the indications for pacing are divided into three categories: generally indicated, may be indicated, and not indicated (12,13). The clinician prescribing permanent pacing systems should be aware of the published indications and the controversies regarding the indications. Although some indications for permanent pacing are relatively certain or unambiguous, others require considerable expertise and judgment.

The clinical need for pacing and appropriate objective data, such as electrocardiographic tracings, must be documented clearly in the patient's medical record to ensure reimbursement by Medicare or third-party payers.

Indications are considered here for the categories of acquired AV block, congenital AV block, chronic bifascicular and trifascicular block, sinus node dysfunction, and neurocardiogenic syndromes. Potential hemodynamic indications for permanent pacing are discussed separately.

Acquired Atrioventricular Block

Traditionally, AV block is classified into first-, second-, and third-degree (or complete) heart block. Alternatively, it can be defined anatomically as supra-, intra-, or infra-Hisian. If the QRS is wide, there is a greater probability that the conduction disturbance is infra-Hisian. Most commonly, acquired AV block is idiopathic and related to aging, but it has many potential causes (Table 74.2). The indications for permanent pacing in acquired AV block are listed in Table 74.3.

Indications for permanent pacing for AV block that occurs with myocardial infarction are more controversial. Generally, a pacemaker is considered to be indicated if complete AV block, Mobitz II block, or bilateral or alternating bundle branch block persists longer than 72 hours after the acute event. Some clinicians would consider new and persistent bifascicular block an indication for pacing, and others would consider pacing for a new left anterior or left posterior hemiblock alone.

Congenital Complete Heart Block

Although some controversy remains about when patients with congenital complete heart block should have pacing, the tendency now is to provide pacing to these patients earlier.

In pediatric patients, pacemaker implantation is recommended for the following indications: congestive heart failure, average heart rate less than 50 beats/min in an awake infant, history of syncope or presyncope, significant ventricular ectopy, or exercise intolerance (14). Prophylactic pacemaker implantation is generally considered appropriate in adults, even if asymptomatic, because of a high incidence of unpredictable syncope with significant mortality from initial attacks, a gradual decrease in heart rate, and a high

TABLE 74.2 ACQUIRED ATRIOVENTRICULAR BLOCK: DIFFERENTIAL DIAGNOSIS

Idiopathic (senescent) atrioventricular block
Coronary artery disease
Calcific valvular disease
Postoperative/traumatic
Atrioventricular node ablation
Therapeutic radiation of the chest
Infectious[a]
   Syphilis
   Diphtheria
   Chagas' disease
   Tuberculosis
   Toxoplasmosis
   Viral myocarditis (Epstein-Barr, varicella, and so forth)
   Infective endocarditis
Collagen-vascular
   Rheumatoid arthritis
   Scleroderma
   Dermatomyositis
   Ankylosing spondylitis
   Polyarteritis nodosa
   Systemic lupus erythematosus
   Marfan's syndrome
Infiltrative
   Sarcoidosis
   Amyloidosis
   Hemochromatosis
   Malignancy (lymphomatous or solid tumor)
Neuromuscular
   Progressive external ophthalmoplegia (Kearns-Sayre syndrome)
   Myotonic muscular dystrophy
   Peroneal muscular atrophy (Charcot-Marie-Tooth)
   Scapuloperoneal syndrome
   Limb-girdle dystrophy
Drug effect
   Digoxin
   Beta-blockers
   Calcium-blocking agents
   Amiodarone
   Procainamide
   Class IC agents: propafenone, encainide, flecainide
   Paclitaxel

[a]Lyme disease may require temporary cardiac pacing. Lyme disease is not an indication for permanent pacing.

incidence of acquired mitral insufficiency (15). This author recommends permanent pacing in all adults with congenital complete heart block.

Chronic Bifascicular or Trifascicular Block

If the bifascicular or trifascicular block is associated with symptoms or transient complete heart block, pacing is clearly indicated. If the bifascicular or trifascicular block is associated with high-grade AV block without symptoms, pacing is also indicated. An important class II ACC/AHA indication is the probable necessity for pacing in a patient with bifascicular or trifascicular block and syncope that cannot be attributed to any other cause. If fascicular block is noted in an asymptomatic patient, pacing is not indicated (16).

Sinus Node Dysfunction

Tachycardia-bradycardia syndrome, sick sinus syndrome, symptomatic sinus bradycardia, sinus arrest and sinus pauses, and chronotropic incompetence are all variants of sinus node dysfunction and the terms are often used synonymously. The definition of bradycardia varies, but it generally is accepted to be rates less than 40 beats/min during waking hours. There is disagreement about the absolute cycle length at which treatment should be required. Although every patient needs to be considered individually, most clinicians would agree that sinus pauses of 3 seconds during waking hours should be considered abnormal and may warrant pacing. Pauses that occur during sleep are more difficult to categorize. Because of vagal influences, many healthy persons may have pauses significantly longer than 3 seconds during sleep and, in the absence of symptoms or rhythm disturbances during waking hours, should not require treatment. Permanent pacing should be considered for any patient who has symptomatic bradyarrhythmias when the cause of the bradyarrhythmia is not reversible (Table 74.4).

TABLE 74.3 INDICATIONS IN ATRIOVENTRICULAR BLOCK

Degree	Pacemaker necessary	Pacemaker probably necessary	Pacemaker not necessary
Third	Symptomatic congenital CHB Acquired symptomatic CHB Atrial fibrillation with CHB Acquired asymptomatic CHB		
Second	Symptomatic type I Symptomatic type II	Asymptomatic type II Asymptomatic type I at intra-His or infra-His levels[a]	Asymptomatic type I at supra-His (atrioventricular nodal) level
First			Asymptomatic or symptomatic[a]

CHB, complete heart block.
[a]Data from Campbell RW. Chronic Mobitz type I second degree atrioventricular block. Has its importance been underestimated? [Editorial]. *Br Heart J* 1985;53:585–586.

TABLE 74.4 INDICATIONS FOR PERMANENT PACING IN SINUS NODE DYSFUNCTION

Pacemaker necessary	Pacemaker probably necessary	Pacemaker not necessary
Symptomatic bradycardia Symptomatic sinus bradycardia due to long-term drug therapy of a type and dose for which there is no accepted alternative	Symptomatic patients with sinus node dysfunction with documented rates of <40 beats/min without a clear-cut association between significant symptoms and the bradycardia	Asymptomatic sinus node dysfunction

Permanent pacing for patients with sinus node dysfunction after myocardial infarction is reserved for those who have symptoms. If drug therapy results in symptomatic bradycardia, criteria for permanent pacing should follow the guidelines given for sinus node dysfunction in Table 74.4.

NONBRADYARRHYTHMIC INDICATIONS FOR PACING

Hypertrophic Obstructive Cardiomyopathy

Dual-chamber pacing has been proposed as a therapeutic modality for patients with severe, symptomatic hypertrophic obstructive cardiomyopathy (27–30). Several investigators have reported a significant decrease in the left ventricular outflow tract gradient and symptomatic improvement in patients with hypertrophic obstructive cardiomyopathy after implantation of a dual-chamber pacemaker (Fig. 74.1).

It has been recognized that AV timing is critical if optimal hemodynamic improvement is to be achieved (31). Although some patients with hypertrophic obstructive cardiomyopathy have optimal improvement with a very short AVI, others may have hemodynamic deterioration if the AVI is too short. Also, it has been recognized that depolarization of the ventricle must occur via the pacemaker. Some have advocated AV nodal ablation to ensure paced ventricular depolarization if rapid intrinsic AV nodal conduction prevents total ventricular depolarization via the pacing stimulus (32).

In the Pacing in Cardiomyopathy study, a multicenter, randomized, cross-over study, dual-chamber pacing resulted in a 50% decrease of the left ventricular outflow tract gradient, a 21% increase in exercise duration, and improvement in New York Heart Association (NYHA) functional class compared with baseline status (33). When clinical variables, including chest pain, dyspnea, and subjective health status, were compared between DDD and backup AAI pacing, the difference was not significant, again suggesting an important placebo effect (eFig. 74.1.1).

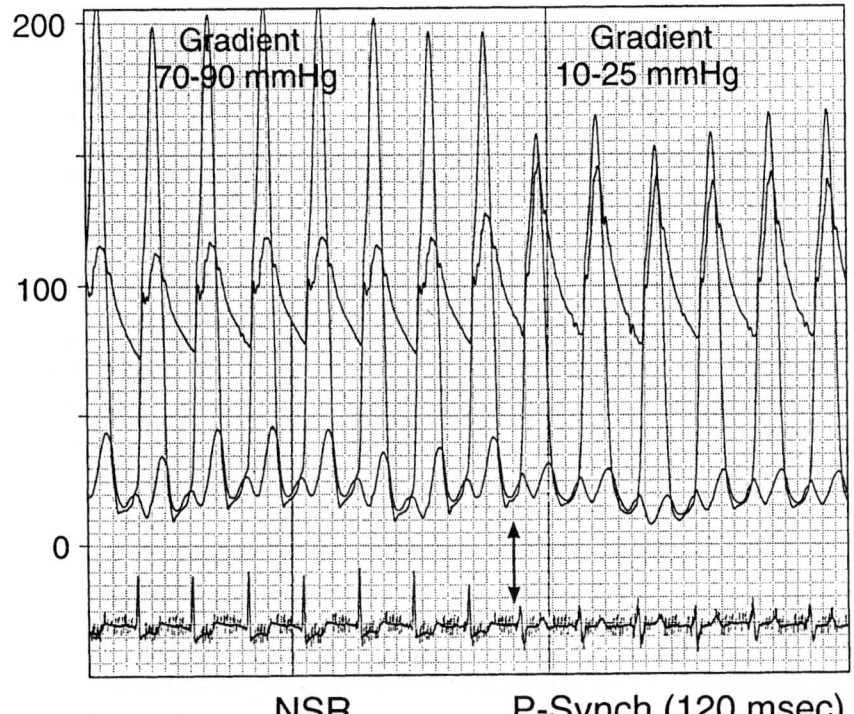

FIGURE 74.1 Hemodynamic tracing demonstrating left ventricular outflow gradient reduction during a temporary pacing study. During normal sinus rhythm (NSR), the patient exhibits marked left ventricular outflow obstruction, with a gradient of 70 to 90 mm Hg. With initiation of P-synchronous pacing at an AV interval of 120 ms, the gradient is decreased to 10 to 25 mm Hg. (From Symanski JD, Nishimura RA. The use of pacemakers in the treatment of cardiomyopathies. *Curr Probl Cardiol* 1996;21:385–443, with permission of Mosby.)

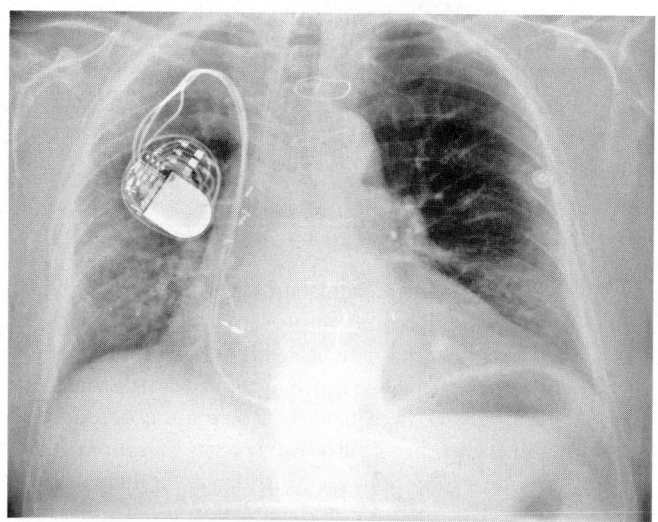
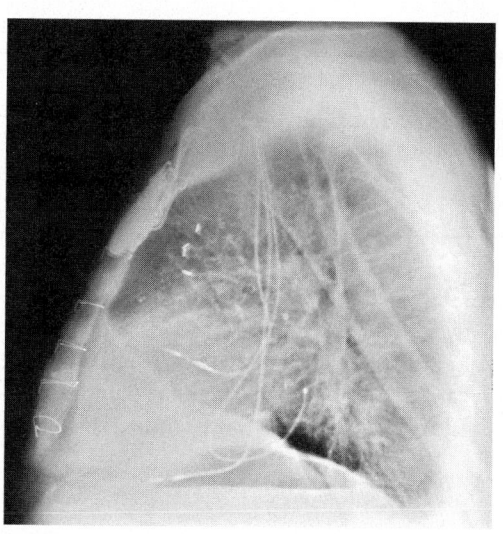

FIGURE 74.2 Postero-anterior **(A)** and lateral **(B)** chest radiographs demonstrating a ventricular lead that courses posteriorly in the coronary sinus and into a cardiac vein, probably a tributary of the posterior cardiac vein. From the postero-anterior view alone, this determination cannot be made. (From Hayes DL, Zipes DP. Cardiac pacemakers and cardioverter-defibrillators. In: Braunwald E, Zipes DP, Libby P, eds. *Heart disease: a textbook of cardiovascular medicine*, 6th ed. Philadelphia: WB Saunders, 2001:775–814, with permission.)

In another randomized, double-blinded, cross-over study, the Multicenter Study of Pacing Therapy for Hypertrophic Cardiomyopathy trial, no significant differences were evident with randomization between pacing and no pacing, either subjectively or objectively, when exercise capacity, quality-of-life score, treadmill exercise time, and peak oxygen consumption were compared (34). The investigators concluded that pacing should not be regarded as a primary treatment for hypertrophic obstructive cardiomyopathy, and subjective benefit without objective evidence of improvement should be interpreted cautiously.

Currently, pacing for the treatment of medically refractory hypertrophic obstructive cardiomyopathy is a class IIb indication by the ACC/AHA guidelines (2).

Dilated Cardiomyopathy

Dual-chamber pacing has been reported to be effective in the treatment of selected patients with dilated cardiomyopathy of idiopathic or ischemic cause (35).

Treatment of idiopathic dilated cardiomyopathy with short AVI DDD pacing was first reported by Hochleitner et al. (36). They treated 16 patients with idiopathic dilated cardiomyopathy refractory to pharmacologic therapy who were in NYHA functional class III or IV. These authors reported marked improvement in NYHA functional class and a decrease in mortality over that expected at 1 year. ⬇ m43

The mechanism by which standard dual-chamber permanent pacing may produce improvement probably is due to optimization of AV synchrony (38). However, standard dual-chamber pacing resulted in improvement in only a

limited number of patients (39–41). Subsequently, it was hypothesized that, in addition to the need for optimization of AV synchrony, the correction of intraventricular conduction disturbances might result in clinical improvement. Ventricular dyssynchrony is common among the heart failure population and has been associated with paradoxical septal wall motion, decreased left ventricular pressure, prolonged duration of mitral regurgitation, and decreased diastolic filling times in patients with left bundle branch block.

Biventricular or left ventricular pacing may counter the decreased septal contribution to stroke volume caused by late left ventricular activation occurring as the septum has begun repolarizing and help to increase the ejection fraction (Fig. 74.2).

To date, the data have been promising (42), but randomized prospective trials are needed to prove the efficacy and safety of cardiac resynchronization. An early nonrandomized trial, InSync, demonstrated improvement in 6-minute walking, quality of life, and NYHA functional class. Randomized trials that have demonstrated similar outcomes include Pacing Therapy in Congestive Heart Failure (43) and MUSTIC (Multisite Stimulation in Cardiomyopathies) (44).

Pacing for the Prevention of Atrial Fibrillation

There is considerable interest in the potential prevention of recurrent atrial tachyarrhythmias by dual-site or alternate-site atrial pacing (45–47). The proposed mechanism of this technique is to decrease the refractoriness of dispersion of the atrium by simultaneously depolarizing both left and right atria. Early applications of dual-site atrial pacing have had some success, and this has significant promise.

The optimal method of pacing for prevention of atrial fibrillation has not been established, but it should be determined by the numerous trials that are being conducted. Techniques include dual-site or alternate-site pacing, with the alternate site usually being an atrial septal position.

SELECTION OF THE APPROPRIATE PACING MODE

In selecting the optimal pacing mode, the patient's overall physical condition, associated medical problems, exercise capacity, and chronotropic response to exercise must be considered in conjunction with the underlying rhythm disturbance (48). Table 74.5 describes clinical applications of various pacing modes in three classifications: conduction

TABLE 74.5 INDICATIONS FOR VARIOUS PACING MODES

Mode	Generally agreed on indications	Controversial indications	Contraindicated
VVI	Atrial fibrillation with symptomatic bradycardia in CC patient.	Symptomatic bradycardia in the patient with associated terminal illness or other medical conditions from which recovery is not anticipated and pacing is life-sustaining only	Patients with known pacemaker syndrome or hemodynamic deterioration with ventricular pacing at the time of implant. CI patient who will benefit from rate response. Patients with hemodynamic need for dual-chamber pacing.
VVIR	Fixed atrial arrhythmias (atrial fibrillation or flutter) with symptomatic bradycardia in CI patient.	As for VVI	As for VVI.
AAI	Symptomatic bradycardia as a result of sinus node dysfunction in the otherwise CC patient and when AV conduction can be proven normal.		Sinus node dysfunction with associated AV block either demonstrated spontaneously or during preimplant testing; when adequate atrial sensing cannot be attained.
AAIR	Symptomatic bradycardia as a result of sinus node dysfunction in the CI patient and when AV conduction can be proven normal.		As for AAI.
VDD[a]	Congenital AV block. AV block when sinus node function can be proven normal.		Sinus node dysfunction. AV block when accompanied by sinus node dysfunction. When adequate atrial sensing cannot be attained. AV block when accompanied by paroxysmal supraventricular tachycardias.
VDDR[b]	—	—	—
DVI[c]	—	—	Chronotropic incompetence in the patient with a demonstrated need or improvement with rate responsiveness.
DDI	Need for dual-chamber pacing in the presence of significant PSVT in the CC patient.	Sinus node dysfunction in the absence of AV block in the presence of significant PSVT in the CC patient	
DDIR[d]	AV block and sinus node dysfunction in the CI patient in the presence of significant PSVT.	Sinus node dysfunction without AV block in the CI patient in the presence of significant PSVT	
DDD	AV block and sinus node dysfunction in the CC patient. Need for AV synchrony (i.e., to maximize cardiac output) in CC active patients. Previous pacemaker syndrome.	For any rhythm disturbance when atrial sensing and capture are possible for the potential purpose of minimizing future atrial fibrillation and improved morbidity and survival	Presence of chronic atrial fibrillation, atrial flutter, or giant inexcitable atrium. When adequate atrial sensing cannot be attained.
DDDR	AV block and sinus node dysfunction in the CI patient.	As for DDD	As for DDD.

AV, atrioventricular; CC, chronotropically competent (the ability to achieve an appropriate heart rate for a given physiologic activity); CI, chronotropically incompetent (the inability to achieve an appropriate heart rate for a given physiologic activity); PSVT, paroxysmal supraventricular tachycardia.
[a]VDD as a stand-alone pacing mode (i.e., a pacemaker capable of VDD as the only dual-chamber mode of operation) is currently used primarily as a single-lead VDD system. If a dual-lead system is implanted, then the capability of DDD pacing is desirable.
[b]In current single-lead VDDR pacemakers, P-wave tracking occurs as long as the sinus rate is appropriate. However, in the presence of sinus bradycardia or chronotropic incompetence, the pacemaker operates in the VVIR mode.
[c]DVI as a stand-alone pacing mode (i.e., a pacemaker capable of DVI as the only dual-chamber mode of operation) is obsolete. All primary uses of this mode should be considered individually.
[d]DDIR is being supplanted by DDD or DDDR pacemakers with the capability of mode-switching (i.e., the pacemaker automatically reprograms to a mode incapable of tracking the atrial rhythm in the presence of an atrial rhythm that the pacemaker classifies as a pathologic rhythm). When the pacemaker recognizes the atrial rhythm as being physiologic, the pacemaker reprograms to the previously programmed mode.

disorders for which a given pacing mode is indicated, those for which a given pacing mode is controversial, and those for which a given pacing mode is contraindicated.

It is difficult to comprehend completely the advantages and disadvantages of each of the pacing modes unless the timing cycle of each mode is also understood. Single-chamber–triggered pacing (AAT and VVT) releases an output pulse every time a native event is sensed. This feature increases the current drain on the battery, which accelerates its rate of depletion, and deforms the native signal, thus compromising interpretation of the electrocardiogram. However, it can serve as an excellent marker for the site of sensing within an intrinsic complex and can prevent inappropriate inhibition from oversensing when the patient does not have a stable native escape rhythm. Also, it can be used for noninvasive electrophysiologic studies, with the already implanted pacemaker tracking chest wall stimuli created by a programmable stimulator.

Ventricular-inhibited (VVI) pacing incorporates sensing on the ventricular channel, and pacemaker output is inhibited by a sensed ventricular event (Fig. 74.3). VVI pacemakers are refractory for a period after a paced or sensed ventricular event, the *ventricular refractory period*. Any ventricular event occurring within this period is not sensed and does not reset the ventricular timer.

Worldwide, VVI pacing is the most commonly used pacing mode. Although VVI pacing protects the patient from lethal bradycardias, it has significant limitations in that it does not restore or maintain AV synchrony or provide rate responsiveness in patients with chronotropic incompetence. Also, some patients with VVI pacing experience symptomatic hemodynamic deterioration with ventricular pacing (49,50). Adverse hemodynamics associated with a normally functioning pacing system that result in overt symptoms or limit the patient's ability to achieve optimal functional status are referred to as *pacemaker syn-*

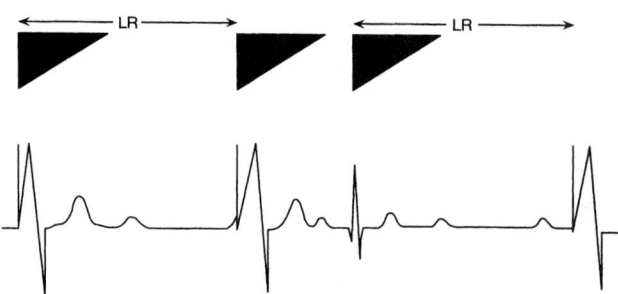

FIGURE 74.3 The VVI timing cycle consists of a defined lower rate (LR) limit and a ventricular refractory period (*black triangle*). When the LR limit timer is complete, a pacing artifact is delivered in the absence of a sensed intrinsic ventricular event. If an intrinsic QRS occurs, the LR limit timer is started from that point. A ventricular refractory period begins with any sensed or paced ventricular activity. (From Hayes DL, Levine PA. Pacemaker timing cycles. In: Ellenbogen KA, ed. *Cardiac pacing*. Boston: Blackwell Scientific, 1992:263–308, with permission.)

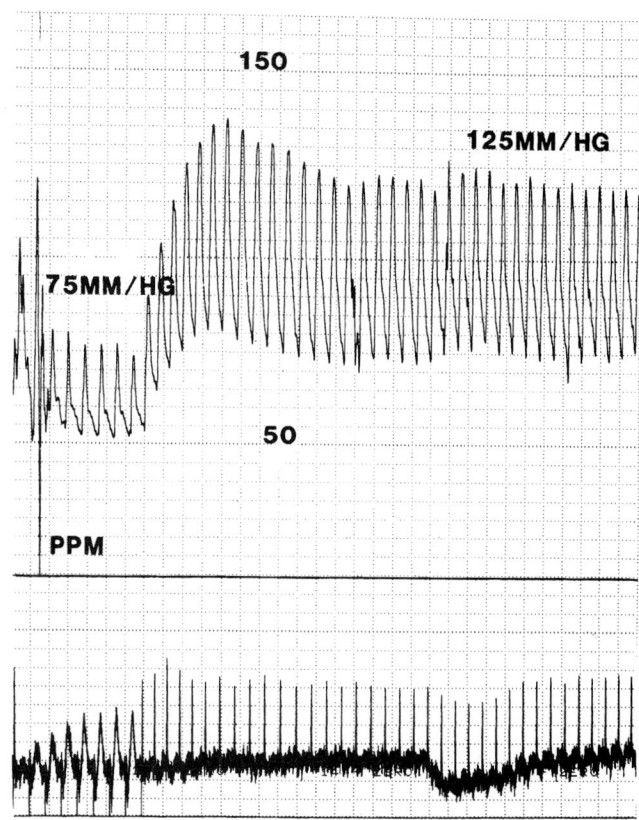

FIGURE 74.4 Hemodynamic tracing of a patient with pacemaker syndrome. In the initial portion of the tracing, there is ventricular pacing, with a systolic arterial pressure of approximately 75 mm Hg. The patient's intrinsic sinus rhythm inhibits ventricular pacing, and the arterial systolic pressure increases to approximately 125 mm Hg. PPM, pulses per minute. (From Hayes DL, Holmes DR Jr. Hemodynamics of cardiac pacing. In: Furman S, Hayes DL, Holmes DR Jr. *A practice of cardiac pacing*, 3rd ed. Mount Kisco, NY: Futura, 1993:195–218, with permission.)

drome (Fig. 74.4). Pacemaker syndrome was recognized initially with ventricular (VVI) pacing, but it may occur with any pacing mode if there is AV dissociation. The incidence of pacemaker syndrome is difficult to determine and depends on how the syndrome is defined. If the definition is restricted to patients with clinical limitations during any pacing mode that results in AV dissociation, the incidence, as estimated in an older review by Ausubel and Furman (49), is probably in the range of 7% to 10% of patients with VVI pacing. In a study by Heldman et al. (50), patients with DDD pacemakers who were randomly assigned to DDD or VVI pacing mode for 1 week and subsequently to the alternate mode completed questionnaires comparing 16 symptoms experienced during each pacing mode. Some degree of pacemaker syndrome was thought to be present in 83% of those studied. The most common symptoms reported were shortness of breath, dizziness, fatigue, pulsations in the neck or abdomen, cough, and apprehension. It can be concluded from this study that if patients with VVI pacing have some basis for comparison, they may be more aware of symptoms with VVI pacing.

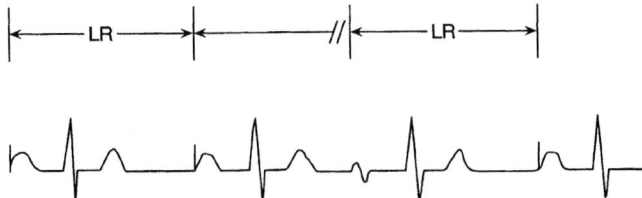

FIGURE 74.5 The AAI timing cycle consists of a defined lower rate (LR) limit and an atrial refractory period. When the LR limit timer is complete, a pacing artifact is delivered in the atrium in the absence of a sensed atrial event. If an intrinsic P wave occurs, the LR limit timer is started from that point. An atrial refractory period begins with any sensed or paced atrial activity. (From Hayes DL, Levine PA. Pacemaker timing cycles. In: Ellenbogen KA, ed. *Cardiac pacing.* Boston: Blackwell Scientific, 1992:263–308, with permission.)

Atrial-inhibited (AAI) pacing incorporates the same timing cycles, with the obvious difference that pacing and sensing occur from the atrium, and pacemaker output is inhibited by a sensed atrial event (Fig. 74.5). An atrial-paced or sensed event initiates a refractory period during which nothing is sensed by the pacemaker. Confusion can arise when multiple ventricular events occur while there is atrial pacing. For example, in addition to the intrinsic QRS that occurs in response to the paced atrial beat, if a premature ventricular beat follows, it does not inhibit an atrial pacing artifact from being delivered. When the atrial timing cycle ends, the atrial pacing artifact is delivered regardless of ventricular events, because an AAI pacemaker should not sense anything in the ventricle. The single exception to this rule is far-field sensing; that is, the ventricular signal is large enough to be sensed inappropriately by the atrial lead. In this situation, the atrial timing cycle is reset. Sometimes, this anomaly can be corrected by making the atrial channel less sensitive or by lengthening the refractory period.

AAI pacing is appropriate for patients with sinus node dysfunction. The obvious disadvantage of atrial pacing is lack of ventricular support should AV block occur. If the patient with sinus node dysfunction is evaluated carefully for the presence of AV nodal disease at the time of pacemaker implantation, the occurrence of clinically significant AV nodal disease is low, 2% per year (51). The evaluation before the use of an AAI system should include incremental atrial pacing at the time of pacemaker implant. Although criteria vary among institutions and implanting physicians, adult patients should be capable of one-to-one AV nodal conduction to rates of 120 to 140 beats/min.

AV sequential, ventricular-inhibited pacing (DVI) is rarely used as the preimplantation pacing mode of choice. By definition, DVI provides pacing in both the atrium and the ventricle (D), but provides sensing only in the ventricle (V). The pacemaker is inhibited and reset by sensed ventricular activity, but it ignores all intrinsic atrial complexes. ♥ m44

Atrial synchronous (P-tracking) pacemakers (VDD) pace only in the ventricle, sense in both the atrium and ventricle, and respond both by inhibition of ventricular output by intrinsic ventricular activity and by ventricular tracking of P waves. The VDD mode also has become increasingly available as a single-lead pacing system. In this system, a single lead is capable of pacing in the ventricle in response to sensing atrial activity by way of a remote electrode situated on the intraatrial portion of the ventricular pacing lead (53).

A sensed atrial event initiates the AVI. If an intrinsic ventricular event occurs before the termination of the AVI, ventricular output is inhibited and the lower rate timing cycle is reset (Fig. 74.6). If a paced ventricular beat occurs at the end of the AVI, this beat resets the lower rate. If no atrial event occurs, the pacemaker escapes with a paced ventricular event at the lower rate limit (i.e., the pacemaker displays VVI activity in the absence of a sensed atrial event).

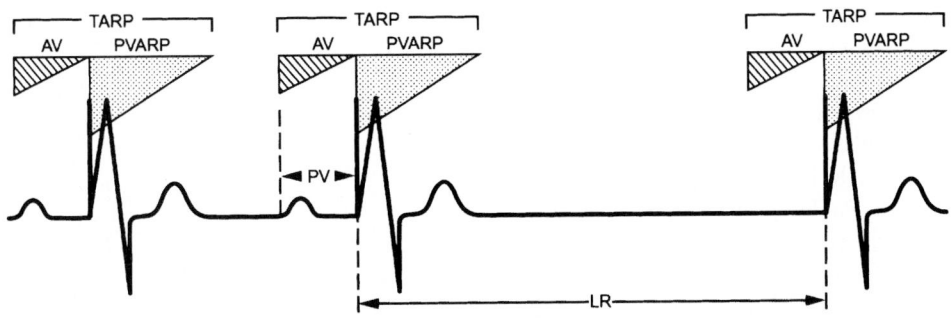

FIGURE 74.6 The timing cycle of VDD consists of a lower rate (LR) limit, an atrioventricular (AV) interval, a ventricular refractory period, a postventricular atrial refractory period (PVARP), and an upper rate limit. A sensed P wave initiates the AV interval (during this interval, the atrial-sensing channel is refractory). At the end of the AV interval, a ventricular pacing artifact is delivered if no intrinsic ventricular activity has been sensed (i.e., P-wave tracking). Ventricular activity, paced or sensed, initiates the PVARP and the ventriculoatrial interval (the LR limit interval minus the AV interval). If no P-wave activity occurs, the pacemaker escapes with a ventricular pacing artifact at the LR limit. PV, postventricular; TARP, total atrial refractory period. (From Hayes DL, Zipes DP. Cardiac pacemakers and cardioverter-defibrillators. In: Braunwald E, Zipes DP, Libby P, eds. *Heart disease: a textbook of cardiovascular medicine*, 6th ed. Philadelphia: WB Saunders, 2001:775–814, with permission.)

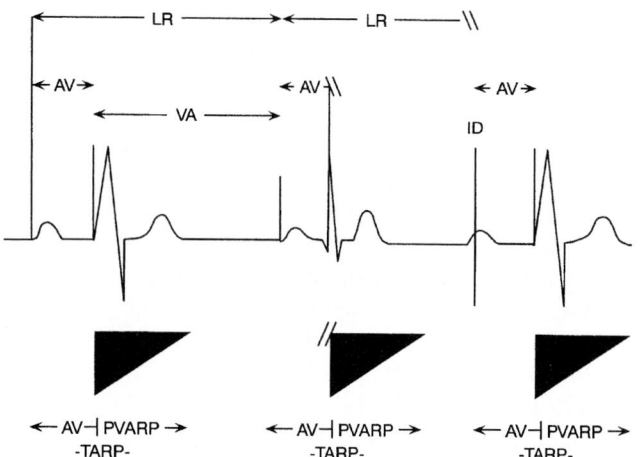

FIGURE 74.7 The timing cycle in DDD consists of a lower rate (LR) limit, an atrioventricular (AV) interval, a postventricular atrial refractory period (PVARP), and an upper rate limit. The AV interval and PVARP together constitute the total atrial refractory period (TARP). There are four variations of the DDD timing cycle. If intrinsic atrial and ventricular activity occurs before the LR limit times out, both channels are inhibited and no pacing occurs. If no intrinsic atrial or ventricular activity occurs, there is AV sequential pacing (first sequence). If no atrial activity is sensed before the ventriculoatrial (VA) interval is completed, an atrial pacing artifact is delivered, which initiates the AV interval. If intrinsic ventricular activity occurs before the termination of the AV interval, the ventricular output from the pacemaker is inhibited [i.e., atrial pacing (second sequence)]. If a P wave is sensed before the VA interval is completed, output from the atrial channel is inhibited. The AV interval is initiated, and if no ventricular activity is sensed before the AV interval terminates, a ventricular pacing artifact is delivered [i.e., P-synchronous pacing (third sequence)]. ID, intrinsic deflection. (From Hayes DL, Levine PA. Pacemaker timing cycles. In: Ellenbogen KA, ed. *Cardiac pacing.* Boston: Blackwell Scientific, 1992:263–308, with permission.)

VDD pacing may be appropriate for patients who have normal sinus node function and conduction disease of the AV node.

Dual-chamber pacing and sensing with inhibition and tracking (DDD) are reasonably easy to comprehend. The basic timing circuit associated with lower rate pacing is divided into two sections: the ventriculoatrial (VA) interval and the AVI. The AVI may be defined by AV sequential pacing, initiated (a) by pacing, with subsequent intrinsic ventricular conduction, or (b) by a native P wave, with subsequent ventricular pacing (Fig. 74.7). The total atrial refractory period, which consists of the AVI and the postventricular atrial refractory period (PVARP), defines the maximal tracking rate of the pacemaker.

In summary, four different rhythms can occur as a result of normal DDD function: (a) normal sinus rhythm, (b) atrial pacing, (c) AV sequential pacing, and (d) P-synchronous pacing. The DDD pacing mode is most appropriate for patients with normal sinus node function and AV block. Some consider DDD pacing the mode of choice in neurocardiogenic syndromes with symptomatic cardioinhibition.

DDD pacing has limitations in patients with sinus node dysfunction. P-synchronous pacing is not possible in the presence of chronic atrial fibrillation or in patients with a paralyzed or nonexcitable atrium. Also, DDD pacing is not able to restore rate response in a patient with chronotropic incompetence (a patient in whom atrial rate is unable to increase appropriately with exercise). In a patient with chronotropic incompetence, DDD pacing is suboptimal because rate responsiveness is not restored.

INDICATIONS FOR RATE-ADAPTIVE PACEMAKERS

Single-chamber rate-adaptive pacing modes (AAIR, VVIR) have timing cycles that are not significantly different from those of their non–rate-adaptive counterparts. The difference lies in the potential variability of the paced rate (Fig. 74.8). Depending on the sensor incorporated and the level of exertion of the patient, the basic interval is shorter than the programmed lower rate limit. Shortening requires that an upper rate limit be programmed to define the absolute shortest cycle length allowable.

VVIR pacing, like VVI, is contraindicated if ventricular pacing results in retrograde (VA) conduction, a decrease in blood pressure, or both. VVIR pacing should not be used as an excuse to forego attempts at placing an atrial lead in a patient who is undergoing pacemaker implantation, has normal sinus node function, and would benefit from rate-adaptive pacing. If the sinus node is intact, P-synchronous pacing should still be considered the optimal rate-adaptive parameter and be used when possible.

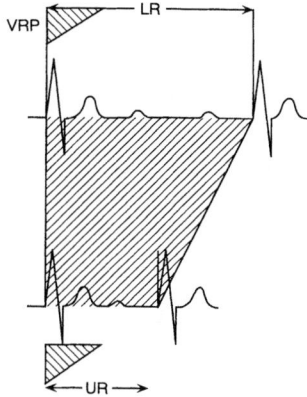

FIGURE 74.8 The VVIR timing cycle consists of a lower rate (LR) limit, an upper rate (UR) limit, and a ventricular refractory period (VRP) (*triangle*). As indicated by sensor activity, the VV cycle length shortens accordingly. (The striped area represents the range of sensor-driven VV cycle lengths.) In most VVIR pacemakers, the VRP remains fixed despite the changing VV cycle length. In selected VVIR pacemakers, the VRP shortens as the cycle length shortens. (From Hayes DL, Levine PA. Pacemaker timing cycles. In: Ellenbogen KA, ed. *Cardiac pacing.* Boston: Blackwell Scientific, 1992:263–308, with permission.)

AAIR pacing can be considered in patients with sinus node dysfunction and normal AV node function, because this mode restores rate responsiveness and maintains AV synchrony. If AAIR pacing is contemplated, normal AV node conduction must first be determined as discussed previously for AAI pacing. ❧ m45

CHOOSING THE PACEMAKER SYSTEM HARDWARE

After the appropriate pacing mode has been selected, the actual pacemaker must be selected. The advising physician or the one performing the implantation should select a pacemaker that provides the specific features needed for the patient. It is imperative that the physician responsible for following the patient be completely familiar with the pacemaker implanted.

Lead selection should also be individualized. This requires a thorough knowledge of the available leads as well as the performance records of specific models (54,55).

Selecting the Appropriate Sensor for Rate-Adaptive Pacing

To classify sensors on the basis of their response to physiologic variables, Rossi (56) divided them into five orders (*e*Table 74.5.1). A variety of sensors appropriate for rate-adaptive pacing have been developed and are shown in *e*Figure 74.8.3 as end points of some physiologic response.

Activity Sensors

Currently, activity-controlled pacing with vibration detection (piezoelectric crystal or accelerometer) is the most widely used form of rate adaptation, because it is simple, easy to apply clinically, and rapid in onset of rate response (57,58).

The main difference between the piezoelectric crystal sensor and the accelerometer is that the crystal senses vibration from up and down motion and the accelerometer also senses anterior and posterior motion (*e*Fig. 74.8.4). Some investigators (57,58) have shown that with accelerometer-based pacemakers, heart-rate response tends to be more physiologic and less responsive to local pressure and tapping than with piezoelectric crystal-based pacemakers.

Subsequent variations of activity sensors have included a gravitational sensor able to discriminate changes in vertical gravitational acceleration (59) and to measure electrical signals from a moving magnetic ball (60).

Minute-Ventilation Sensors

Minute volume (respiratory rate multiplied by tidal volume) has an excellent correlation with metabolic demand.

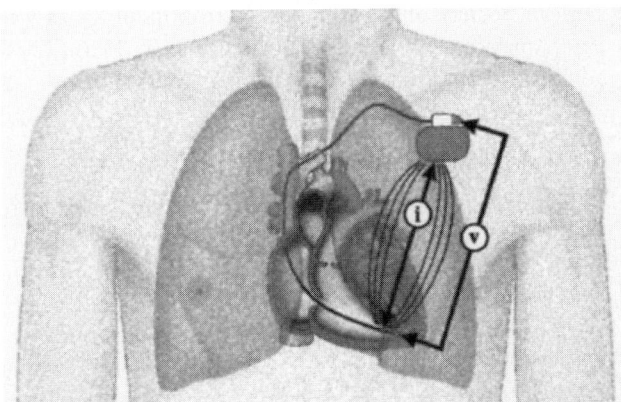

FIGURE 74.9 The mV sensor signal for rate change is derived by measuring the changes in transthoracic impedance. Ohm's law, R = V/I. (Courtesy of Guidant Inc., St. Paul, MN.)

In a rate-adaptive pacing system, minute volume is measured by emitting a small charge of known current from the pacemaker and measuring the resulting voltage at the lead tip (61) (Fig. 74.9). When both current and voltage are known, transthoracic impedance can be measured between the ring electrode and the pacemaker can. Because transthoracic impedance varies with respiration and its amplitude varies with tidal volume, the impedance measurement can be used to determine respiratory rate and tidal volume. A pacing algorithm uses the minute-volume measurements to alter pacing rate (62). Long-term reliability of the minute-volume sensor has been excellent (63), and this sensor is increasingly being used.

Stimulus-T or QT-Sensing Pacemaker

The interval from the onset of a paced QRS complex to the end of the T wave has been used for rate adaptation for many years (64,65). This *stimulus-T interval* is affected by autonomic activity and heart rate. This relationship allows measurement of the stimulus-T interval to be used for rate adaptation. The QT-sensing rate-adaptive pacing system has been successful clinically. Response characteristics of this sensor make it a reasonable partner for activity sensors in dual-sensor systems.

Many other sensors have been incorporated, with varied success, in rate-adaptive pacing sensors. Other variables that have been used for rate-adaptive pacing include temperature, preejection interval, dP/dT, paced depolarization integral, and mixed venous oxygen saturation. These are discussed in the accompanying CD-ROM and in the online version of this text.

PACEMAKER IMPLANTATION

Guidelines for appropriate training for pacemaker implantation and follow-up have been established by the North

American Society of Pacing and Electrophysiology as well as the American College of Cardiology (105,106). These guidelines are summarized in *e*Table 74.5.3. ▼ m46

Implantation Measurements

The position of the pacing leads must be tested acutely to establish that myocardial stimulation and sensing of intrinsic cardiac electrical activity are adequate and reliable. Stimulation threshold may be defined as the smallest amount of electrical activity that produces consistent myocardial capture outside the refractory period. The threshold may be affected by several factors, including the duration of the stimulus (pulse width), type of electrode and its age, site of stimulation, electrolyte status, and state of the myocardium.

The threshold, acute or chronic, is described in terms of voltage or current (milliampere) requirements for capture. Acceptable values for ventricular stimulation thresholds should be 1.0 V or less at a pulse width of 0.5 ms. The acceptable values for atrial pacing thresholds should certainly be less than 1.5 V at a pulse width of 0.5 ms, and with the atrial leads available currently, the threshold usually should be less than 1.0 V. Acute impedance measurements can range from 300 to 1,500 Ω, depending on the type of lead used.

The thresholds increase shortly after implantation and then usually decrease, reaching a stable value at approximately 6 weeks after implantation (113). The early increase in threshold is thought to be due to an inflammatory reaction at the electrode–myocardial interface. This reaction is minimized with leads capable of steroid elution (114,115).

Although the threshold for stimulation is described in terms of voltage and current, it is equally important that the pulse duration (the amount of time a given amount of energy is delivered) is also known. The shortest duration of an electrical impulse that produces consistent capture (at a constant pulse amplitude) represents the threshold of stimulation as a function of pulse duration. The strength-duration curve can be generated by comparing stimulation thresholds at various pulse widths (Fig. 74.10). This measurement is particularly important because the proper adjustment of pulse duration and output voltage allows long-term pacing with maximal conservation of energy.

The lead impedance, or resistance to current flow, is determined by Ohm's law: $R = E/I$, in which E is voltage, I is current in milliamperes, and R is resistance in ohms. By simultaneously measuring voltage and the resultant current, the resistance can easily be calculated by transposing the equation. Average impedance tends to decrease slightly after initial implantation of the lead and then stabilizes. In the absence of lead complications or myocardial abnormalities, the long-term values for impedance tend to remain constant and do not differ significantly from the original value. Measurement of lead impedance is equally important at the time of pacemaker replacement in determining the integrity of the pacing lead.

Postimplantation Management

The length of time the patient is kept in the hospital after pacemaker implantation varies considerably among institutions. Many physicians who perform implantation allow patients who are not pacemaker dependent to ambulate the evening of the procedure, with dismissal the following morning. The patient's condition is usually monitored to assess normalcy of pacing in the immediate postimplantation period. Before dismissal, thresholds are documented and the pacemaker is programmed to its final settings. If a rate-adaptive pacemaker has been implanted, informal exer-

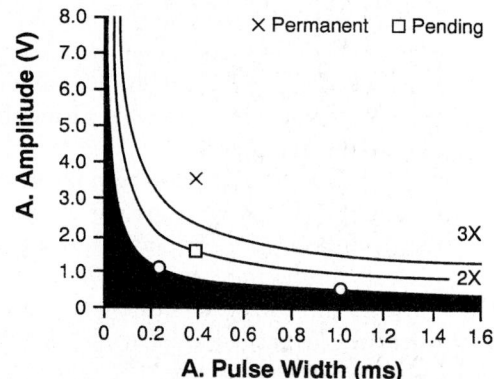

Pending Values Provide:		
Safety Margin of	2.0	
Estimated battery life of 78 months		
	Pending	**Permanent**
Atrial Amplitude	1.50 V	3.50 V
Atrial Pulse Width	0.40 ms	0.40 ms
Threshold Points:	0.50 V, 1.00 ms	
	1.00 V, 0.25 ms	

FIGURE 74.10 Atrial strength-duration threshold curve generated by the pacemaker programmer. The voltage amplitude is represented on the *y*-axis and the pulse width in milliseconds on the *x*-axis. The shaded area of the graph represents amplitude/pulse width combinations that would not allow successful capture or depolarization. The upper two curves represent output combinations that would result in two times and three times safety margin (i.e., areas above the capture threshold), which is represented by the lowermost of the three curves and the open circles. The X is the pacemaker-derived suggested point of permanent programming, in this example, 3.5 V and 0.4-ms pulse width.

cise is performed the morning after implantation and the rate-responsive parameters are adjusted to the needs of the patient. Pacemaker-dependent patients may be kept in the hospital one night. When the patient's pacemaker reaches battery depletion indicators, replacement is performed as an outpatient procedure.

Many physicians now perform initial pacemaker implantation as an outpatient procedure. Some perform outpatient implantation only in non–pacemaker-dependent patients, whereas others do not consider dependency status. Possibly, ambulatory pacemaker implantation with outpatient follow-up the next day may become the more usual approach (116).

PACEMAKER PROGRAMMING

All currently available pacemakers have some degree of programmability. In most markets, the simplest single-chamber pacemaker available is capable of rate, pulse width, voltage amplitude, sensitivity, refractory period, and polarity programmability. An attempt is being made to automatize many programmable features to allow optimal programming at all times. Programmable options that are available in many current pacemakers are listed in Table 74.6.

PACEMAKER COMPLICATIONS

Complications can occur directly from the implantation technique or from failure of a component of the pacing system (125). Many complications are related directly to the experience of the physician performing the implantation.

Implant-Related Complications

Most patients undergoing pacemaker implantation have some discomfort at the site of the incision in the early postoperative period, and mild analgesics may be required. Mild ecchymoses around the incision are common.

Access to the subclavian vein, commonly used for implantation of an endocardial pacemaker lead, is usually accomplished by subclavian vein puncture with a modified Seldinger technique. Because of the relationship of the subclavian vein with the apex of the lung, traumatic pneumothorax and hemopneumothorax are always possible when a subclavian puncture technique is used. Hemothorax can be caused by laceration of the subclavian artery and hemopneumothorax by laceration of the lung and subclavian artery. ⚐ m47

Hematoma Formation

Because local ecchymoses are common after pacemaker implantation, a small or large ecchymosis that is not expanding is treated with observation only. Discrete hematoma formation at the site must be managed on the basis of its secondary consequences. Aspiration or evacuation of the hematoma should be considered only if there is continued bleeding or potential compromise of the suture line or skin integrity or if pain from the hematoma cannot be managed with analgesics.

To avoid hematoma formation, patients should have a normal prothrombin time before pacemaker implantation, and heparin administration should have been discontinued long enough to allow a normal partial thromboplastin time. Ideally, the patient should not recently have taken aspirin or other platelet-inhibitory drugs. For patients who have been receiving platelet-inhibitory drugs, hemostasis during implantation is often quite difficult. Careful attention to hemostasis before closure of the incision should prevent complications in most patients taking platelet-inhibitory drugs.

For patients who require therapeutic anticoagulation, a 48-hour delay after implantation is ideal before resuming full heparinization. If heparinization is started in less than 48 hours, bleeding may be minimized by avoiding a bolus dose and beginning with a maintenance dose only. Warfarin (Coumadin) usually can be administered safely 24 hours after implantation, but 48 hours is preferable if it does not compromise the patient's condition. Warfarin treatment should be started at the patient's maintenance dose and not at the higher doses that would be used to initiate therapy. The absolute timing for reinstitution of anticoagulant therapy varies from patient to patient. Anticoagulation at greater than therapeutic levels can result in late hematoma formation.

Arterial Lead Puncture and Cannulation

Introduction of the lead(s) into the subclavian artery, the aorta, and the left ventricle usually is readily recognized because of the pulsatile flow of saturated blood. If this is recognized promptly and the needle removed, it is unlikely that a problem will occur. Hemothorax may occur if the artery is lacerated, but this is an extremely rare complication. However, entry into the artery may not be recognized because of desaturation of the arterial blood, making it appear venous, or because of loss of pulsatile arterial flow due to hypotension or diminution of the arterial pulse pressure. Once the lead is within the great arteries, its passage into the left ventricle is as easy as passage into the right ventricle via the venous system.

Usually, entry into the artery can be recognized fluoroscopically as passage into the left ventricle, as viewed in the anteroposterior projection, and is significantly medial to the entry into the right ventricle. If a lateral view is used, a right ventricular lead will be anterior (i.e., posterior to the sternum), and a left ventricular lead will be in the posterior aspect of the heart.

TABLE 74.6 POTENTIAL PROGRAMMABLE OPTIONS

Mode
  Preset or programmed response (paced or sensed, and inhibited or triggered) from a pacemaker in the presence or absence of intrinsic cardiac events

Lower rate limit
  Preset or programmed rate at which a pacemaker will emit an output pulse in the absence of intrinsic cardiac activity

Ventricular refractory period
  An interval of the pacemaker timing cycle following a sensed or paced ventricular event during which the ventricular sensing channel is totally or partially unresponsive to incoming signals

Pulse width (atrial, ventricular, or both)
  Duration, in milliseconds, over which the output is delivered

Pulse amplitude (atrial, ventricular, or both)
  Magnitude of the voltage or amperage level reached during a pacemaker output pulse, usually expressed in volts or milliamperes

Sensitivity (atrial, ventricular, or both)
  Ability to sense an intrinsic electrical signal, which depends on the amplitude, slew rate, and frequency of the signal

Polarity
  In electrical circuits, the sign (positive or negative) of one point relative to another; in pacing, the stimulating electrode typically is the cathode, which has negative polarity to the indifferent electrode (anode)

Single-chamber hysteresis
  Extension of the escape interval after a sensed intrinsic event

Circadian lower rate limit
  Reduces the lower rate limit during sleeping hours

Maximum pacing rate
  DDDR pacemakers have one or two programmable upper rates. Some DDDR devices have a single upper rate limit that indicates the maximum sensor-indicated rate that can be reached and the MTR is defined by the TARP. Other devices have independently programmable MTR and maximum sensor rates, but the MTR is still defined by the TARP.

Mode switch
  Capability of a dual-chamber pacemaker to automatically switch from an atrial tracking (P-synchronous) mode to a non–atrial-tracking mode in the presence of an atrial rhythm that the pacemaker determines to be pathologic. When the atrial rhythm meets the criteria for a physiologic rhythm, the mode switches back to an atrial tracking mode.

Upper rate limit options
  Fallback: An upper rate response in which the ventricular-paced rate decelerates to, and is maintained at, a programmable fall-back rate that is lower than the original programmed MTR. Fall-back mechanisms vary among pacemakers.

Rate-smoothing: Prevents atrial- or ventricular-paced rate from changing by more than a programmed percentage from one cardiac cycle to the next. This prevents large cycle-to-cycle intervals that can be seen at the upper rate limit or during rapid acceleration of atrial rate.

AVI
  Period between the initiation of the paced or sensed atrial event and the delivery of a consecutive ventricular output pulse

Differential AVI
  Feature that permits a longer AVI after a paced atrial event than after a sensed AVI. In some pacemakers this differential is fixed and in others it is programmable.

Rate-adaptive AVI
  Feature that shortens the AVI as the heart rate increases. AVI shortening may be linear or stepwise.

PVARP
  The portion of the timing cycle during which the atrial channel is refractory following a paced or sensed ventricular event

PVARP extension
  An extension of the PVARP following a sensed premature ventricular contraction, as defined by the pacemaker. This feature is designed to prevent sensing of retrograde P waves and to prevent the potential initiation of a PMT.

PMT algorithms
  Features designed to prevent initiation of continuation of a PMT

Blanking period
  Temporary disabling of pacemaker-sensing amplifiers following the delivery of an output pulse. This prevents inappropriate sensing of residual energy from the pacemaker output pulse and, in dual-chamber pacemakers, prevents sensing of pacemaker output pulses or intrinsic events in the chamber other than that in which the event occurs.

Ventricular safety pacing
  Delivery of a ventricular output pulse, following atrial pacing, if a signal is sensed by the ventricular channel during the early portion of the AVI. This is used to ensure that ventricular depolarization occurs if the sensed event was something other than an intrinsic ventricular depolarization.

Rate adaptation
  In a rate-adaptive pacemaker, the capability of the pacemaker to arbitrate between the patient's intrinsic rate and the sensor-determined rate
  Rate adaptation can be programmed on or off

Rate-adaptive sensor variables
  Programmable features that determine the response of the sensor that drives rate adaptation

AVI, atrioventricular interval; MTR, maximum tracking (P-synchronous) rate; PMT, pacemaker-mediated tachycardia; PVARP, postventricular atrial refractory period; TARP, total atrial refractory period.

In right ventricular pacing, the electrocardiogram shows a left bundle branch block pattern, and during left ventricular pacing, it shows a right bundle branch block pattern.

A pacing lead may also be placed in the left ventricle by passing it across an unsuspected atrial or ventricular septal defect. In patients with a ventricular septal defect, endocardial pacing should be avoided because small emboli potentially could cross the ventricular septal defect, causing symptoms in the arterial circulation. ▼ m48

Lead Perforation

Ventricular perforation may be asymptomatic. The only sign may be a rising stimulation threshold. In other patients, the signs may include (a) right bundle branch block pattern from a lead placed in the left ventricle (depending on lead position, it is also possible to see this pattern when the lead is within the right ventricular cavity); (b) contraction of intercostal muscle or the diaphragm; (c) friction rub after implantation; and (d) pericarditis, pericardial effusion, or cardiac tamponade.

Ventricular perforation may be suggested by radiographic, electrocardiographic, and echocardiographic findings. After the perforation has been identified, lead withdrawal and repositioning usually are uncomplicated and rarely result in pericardial bleeding or tamponade.

If the patient has mild symptoms or signs compatible with lead perforation (e.g., pericardial pain, friction rub) but a persistent perforation cannot be identified, it is reasonable to observe the patient. If the symptoms or signs resolve over 24 to 48 hours, it probably will not be necessary to reposition the lead. If an echocardiogram shows a small pericardial effusion but no definite perforation, serial echocardiograms should be performed to confirm that the effusion is not hemodynamically significant or enlarging.

Lead Damage

Leads may be damaged acutely by sharp instruments or by the stylets. Such damage is infrequently recognized, and the true frequency with which it occurs is unknown.

Venous Thrombosis

Partial or silent inconsequential thrombosis following transvenous lead placement is not uncommon and usually is clinically insignificant. Such partial or silent thrombosis may limit venous access at the time of pacing system revision (eFig. 74.10.3) (127).

If thrombosis involves the superior vena cava, axillary vein, or area around the pacemaker lead in the right atrium or right ventricle, several problems can develop, including occlusion of the superior vena cava and superior vena cava syndrome; thrombosis of the superior vena cava, right atrium, or right ventricle, with hemodynamic compromise or pulmonary embolism; or symptomatic thrombosis of the subclavian vein, with an edematous, painful upper extremity.

Lead Fracture

Lead fractures most often occur adjacent to the pacemaker or near the site of venous access (i.e., at a stress point). Although uncommon, direct trauma may damage the pacing lead. If a bipolar lead fractures and the pacemaker is polarity programmable, it may be possible to restore pacing by reprogramming to the unipolar configuration. This is a short-term solution and should not be a substitute for replacing the lead.

Lead Insulation Defect

Insulation defects and conductor fractures may be caused by crush injury, specifically at the costoclavicular space, when the lead is placed via the subclavian puncture technique. In bipolar coaxial leads, the insulation defect often occurs internally (i.e., the layer of insulation between coils) as opposed to an external, outer surface insulation defect. ⚑ m49

Exit Block

The most commonly accepted clinical definition of exit block is high pacing thresholds, often progressive, that cannot be explained on the basis of radiographic dislodgment or perforation. (If normal thresholds are achieved and maintained after the lead has been repositioned, then the term *exit block* does not apply.) Exit block is uncommon and appears to represent an abnormality at the interface of myocardial tissue and the electrode. Steroid-eluting leads are often effective in preventing exit block.

Lead Dislodgment

Active and passive fixation mechanisms common to current pacing leads have significantly decreased the incidence of lead dislodgment. Dislodgment has been classified by some as *macrodislodgment* and *microdislodgment*. Macrodislodgment is evident radiographically, and microdislodgment is not. Adequate lead position is assessed by postero-anterior and lateral chest radiographs. It must be remembered that on chest radiographs, lead placement may appear excellent in patients with microdislodgment.

Pacemaker-Related Arrhythmias

Supraventricular and ventricular arrhythmias are often encountered during pacemaker implantation and are usually inconsequential.

*Tip extrasystole*s may be seen in the early postimplantation period. These are ventricular complexes with morphology similar to that of the paced beats, because they originate at the same site as the paced beats but are not preceded by a pacemaker stimulus (Fig. 74.11). Tip extrasystoles occur most often during the first 24 to 48 hours after implantation and usually resolve spontaneously. Rarely is it necessary to suppress tip extrasystoles pharmacologically.

Runaway pacemaker describes a sudden increase in pacing rate caused by circuit malfunction. This phenomenon is rare with current pacemakers. In more recent years, the rare reports of runaway pacemaker have usually described it as a complication of pacemaker exposure to therapeutic radiation, with subsequent circuit damage (128).

Pacing either cardiac chamber could induce rhythm disturbances if pacing occurred during a vulnerable portion of the cardiac cycle. This could happen with asynchronous pacing (VOO, AOO, DOO) if a pacing stimulus occurred during the vulnerable portion following intrinsic depolarization. From a practical standpoint,

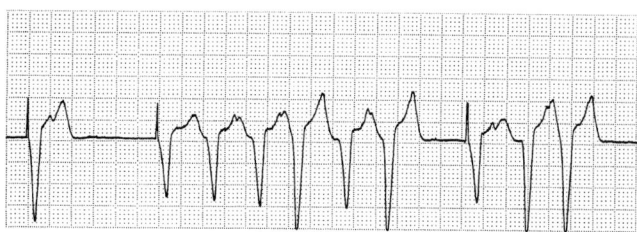

FIGURE 74.11 Electrocardiographic tracing from a patient with a newly implanted dual-chamber pacemaker. The paced beats are followed by ventricular complexes of similar morphology. The patient had not displayed ventricular ectopy before implantation, and the tip extrasystoles had resolved the morning after implantation.

induction of atrial or ventricular arrhythmias during asynchronous pacing is uncommon. Historically, the induction of atrial rhythm disturbances was seen with DVI pacing, which allowed atrial pacing but not atrial sensing, and ventricular rhythm disturbances were described with VAT pacing, which allowed ventricular pacing but not ventricular sensing.

Endless-loop tachycardia is another well-recognized pacemaker-related rhythm disturbance (see previous discussion). In the presence of intact VA conduction, any event that uncouples AV synchrony may allow retrograde atrial activation. (The most common stimulus for VA conduction is a premature ventricular contraction.) If the atrium is refractory at the time of VA conduction, the atrium will be depolarized and the atrial depolarization will initiate the AVI. Paced ventricular depolarization may once again result in VA conduction, establishing a reentrant or endless-loop tachycardia (117).

Extracardiac Stimulation

Extracardiac stimulation usually involves the diaphragm or pectoral muscle. Diaphragmatic stimulation may be due to direct stimulation of the diaphragm (usually stimulation of the left hemidiaphragm) or stimulation of the phrenic nerve (usually stimulation of the right hemidiaphragm). At the time of implantation, if any extracardiac stimulation is noted when pacing at 10 V, the pacing lead should be repositioned. Because this usually is tested with the patient supine, it does not eliminate the possibility of diaphragmatic stimulation when the patient is upright. Diaphragmatic stimulation occurring during the early postimplantation period may be due to either microdislodgment or macrodislodgment of the pacing lead. (Although perforation of the myocardium by the pacing lead may result in diaphragmatic pacing, perforation is uncommon.) Stimulation may be minimized or alleviated by decreasing the voltage output or pulse width, or both. (An adequate pacing margin of safety must be maintained after decreasing the output parameters.) Local muscle stimulation occurs more often with unipolar than with bipolar

pacemakers and usually is noted in the early postimplantation period. ▼ m50

Erosion

Erosion is an uncommon complication that usually occurs because of an indolent infection. With the small size of current pacemakers, it is unlikely that erosion is due to insufficient pocket size, but this is possible. ▼ m51

Pacemaker System Infection

The incidence of infection after pacemaker implantation should be less than 2% and, in most series, has been less than 1%. Careful attention to surgical details and sterile procedures are paramount in avoiding infection of the pacemaker site. Prophylactic antibiotic therapy before implantation and in the immediate postoperative period is controversial (130). Most studies have not shown any significant difference in the rate of infection between patients who have had prophylactic antibiotic treatment and those who have not. Irrigation of the pacemaker pocket with an antibiotic solution at the time of implantation probably is more important in preventing infection.

Pacemaker infection must be recognized and treated properly. It may appear as local inflammation and abscess formation in the area of the pacemaker pocket, as erosion of part of the pacing system through the skin with secondary infection, or as fever associated with positive findings on blood culture, with or without a focus of infection elsewhere. The most common clinical presentation is infection around the generator; septicemia is an uncommon mode of presentation. Early infections usually are caused by *Staphylococcus aureus*, are aggressive, and are often associated with fever and systemic symptoms. Late infections commonly are caused by *Staphylococcus epidermidis* and usually are more indolent, without fever or systemic manifestation. Treatment for both organisms requires removal of the entire infected pacing system, pacemaker and leads. Many other organisms have been reported in pacemaker system infections. ▼ m52

Lead Extraction

A detailed description of extraction techniques is beyond the scope of this textbook, but these techniques include various approaches: simple traction, locking stylet/telescoping sheaths with countertraction, laser-assisted extraction, electrodessication-assisted extraction, and open surgical techniques (133,134).

TROUBLESHOOTING ELECTROCARDIOGRAPHIC ABNORMALITIES

Electrocardiographic abnormalities in a patient with pacing can be grouped broadly into failure to capture, failure to

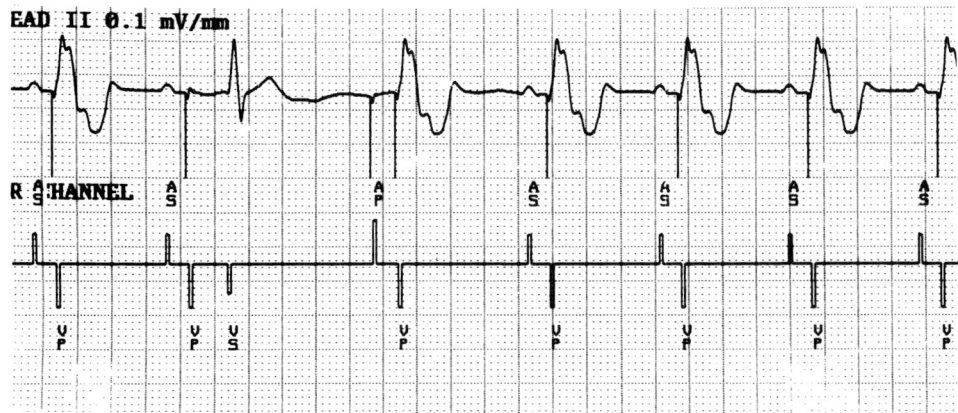

FIGURE 74.12 Electrocardiographic tracing from a patient with a DDD pacemaker. The second ventricular pacing artifact fails to result in ventricular depolarization, failure to capture, and is followed by an intrinsic ventricular escape beat after a PR interval of approximately 300 ms. AP, atrial-paced event; AS, atrial-sensed event; VP, ventricular-paced event; VS, ventricular-sensed event.

output, undersensing, oversensing, and inappropriate rate change (136,137).

Failure to capture indicates that a pacing artifact is present without subsequent cardiac depolarization (Fig. 74.12). The differential diagnosis for failure to capture includes the following items:

- High thresholds with an inadequately programmed output
- Partial conductor coil fracture
- Insulation defect
- Lead dislodgment or perforation
- Impending total battery depletion
- Functional noncapture
- Poor or incompatible connection at connector block
- Circuit failure
- Air in pocket (unipolar pacemaker)
- Increased thresholds due to drugs or metabolic abnormality

Failure to output is sometimes used synonymously with *failure to capture*, but this is not appropriate. Failure to output is often due to oversensing and inhibition of output, but it also can be due to true failure to output from the pacemaker or circuit interruption such that the electrical signal cannot reach the heart (Fig. 74.13). The differential diagnosis for failure to output includes the following items:

- Circuit failure
- Complete or intermittent conductor coil fracture
- Intermittently or permanently loose set screw
- Internal insulation failure (bipolar lead)
- Oversensing any noncardiac activity
- Total battery depletion
- Lack of anodal connector contact (examples include unipolar lead in bipolar generator, bipolar lead in a pace-

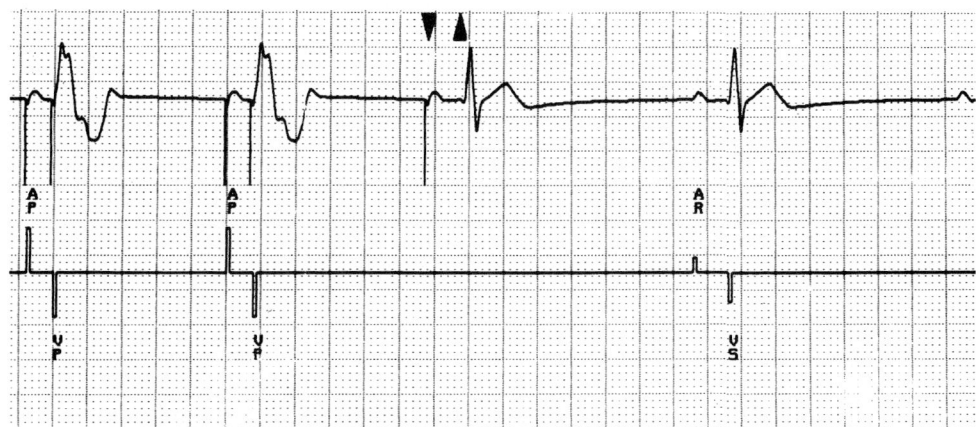

FIGURE 74.13 Electrocardiographic tracing from a patient with a DDD pacemaker with a lower rate of 55 beats/min. The tracing begins with atrioventricular (AV) sequential pacing for two cycles. The next atrial pacing artifact results in atrial capture but is not followed by a ventricular pacing artifact at the programmed AV interval. (The programmed AV interval can be determined from the two initial paced cycles.) Following the intrinsic ventricular beat is a pause of 1,520 ms, which is greater than the programmed lower rate of 55 beats/min, or 1,090 ms. The first event that is recognized by the pacemaker is a P wave, which is designated as an atrial beat that occurs within a refractory period (AR). Whatever extrinsic, noncardiac event that has been oversensed has initiated a refractory period(s), because there is no evidence of any intrinsic cardiac event that has initiated the refractory period. AP, atrial-paced event; VP, ventricular-paced event; VS, ventricular-sensed event.

maker programmed unipolar, air in the pocket of a unipolar device, unipolar pacemaker not in the pocket)
■ Cross talk

The differential diagnoses of failure to capture and failure to output overlap. For example, electrocardiographic manifestations of a conductor coil fracture may include failure to capture due to significant leakage of current at the incomplete fracture site, leaving inadequate current to result in stimulation. Nonetheless, the pacemaker stimuli may appear. Alternatively, escaping current may be sensed by the pacemaker and inhibit pacemaker output. If the conductor coil is completely fractured, rendering the circuit incomplete, no pacemaker output will be detected on the electrocardiogram. Also, secondary sensing abnormalities may be noted.

Insulation defects may also present with oversensing and failure to output or with failure to capture, although the most common presentation of insulation failure is sensing abnormalities.

As the pacemaker battery reaches the end stages of depletion, either failure to capture due to dropping voltage output or failure to output due to total battery depletion may be seen. This degree of battery depletion could and should be avoided with appropriate pacemaker follow-up.

Apparent failure to capture will be noted if a pacemaker stimulus occurs during the refractory period of a spontaneous beat. This is referred to as *functional noncapture.*

Sensing abnormalities can be divided into true abnormalities, including undersensing (failure to recognize normal intrinsic cardiac activity; Fig. 74.14), oversensing (see Fig. 74.13), unexpected sensing of intrinsic or extrinsic electrical signals, and functional sensing abnormalities. The differential diagnosis for undersensing includes the following items:

■ Morphology of intrinsic event different from that measured at implantation
■ Lead dislodgment or poor lead positioning
■ Lead insulation failure
■ Circuit failure
■ Magnet application
■ Malfunction of reed switch
■ Electromagnetic interference
■ Battery depletion

Most commonly, true undersensing is due to lead dislodgment or inadequate initial lead placement. Sensing abnormalities commonly are due to insulation defects and uncommonly to intermittent conductor fracture.

Occasionally, a normally functioning pacing system fails to detect atrial or ventricular extrasystoles. The intrinsic events measured at the time of implantation generate an electrogram at the electrode tip. If an extrasystole is occurring elsewhere in the heart, the sensing vector would be different from that of the normal intrinsic beat and the resulting voltage generated may not be great enough to be sensed by the pacemaker. This cannot be anticipated unless extrasystoles of the same morphology occur during implantation and can be measured. It is reasonable to attempt reprogramming the sensitivity to allow sensing of extrasystoles, but if this is unsuccessful, it is rarely, if ever, necessary to reposition the lead for this abnormality.

Functional undersensing is present when an intrinsic cardiac event is not sensed because it falls within a programmed refractory period (136). For example, if an intrinsic atrial event occurs within the PVARP, the event

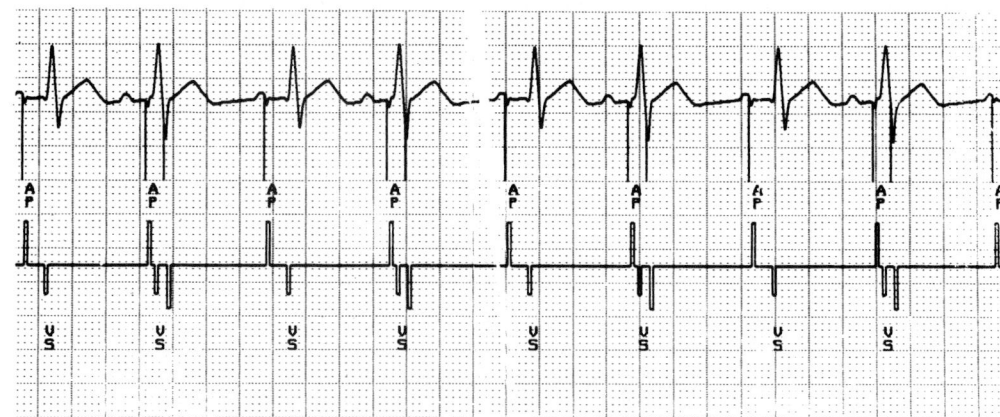

FIGURE 74.14 Electrocardiographic tracing from a patient with a DDD pacemaker programmed to a lower rate of 85 beats/min. There is atrial failure to sense throughout the tracing. The arrow indicates an atrial-paced event (AP) that occurs immediately after an intrinsic atrial event and does not represent failure to capture but functional noncapture. When atrioventricular sequential pacing does occur, the atrioventricular interval is approximately 100 ms. This represents ventricular safety pacing that occurs because the intrinsic ventricular beat is occurring in the cross talk–sensing window. VS, ventricular-sensed event.

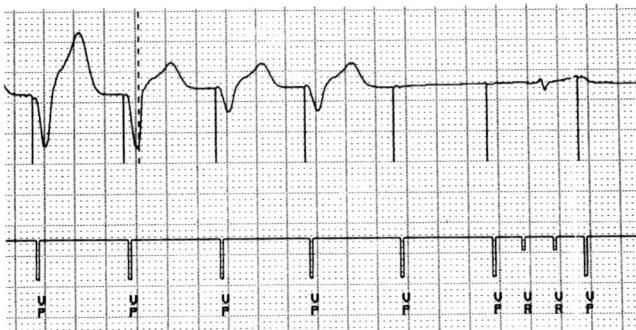

FIGURE 74.15 Electrocardiographic tracing from a patient with a VVI pacemaker. The first two complexes represent fully paced ventricular depolarizations. The third and fourth events result in different paced morphology and represent fusion beats. This is followed by failure to capture and a single ventricular escape. VP, ventricular-paced event.

will not and should not be sensed. However, if the timing cycle is not understood thoroughly, it may appear as though there is true undersensing.

Fusion and *pseudofusion* beats occur as a result of superimposition of an ineffective pacemaker stimulus on a spontaneously occurring P wave or QRS complex (Fig. 75.15). Fusion is present when the morphology of the cardiac event is a hybrid of the intrinsic morphology and the paced morphology. Pseudofusion is present when the pacemaker artifact occurs late enough that the intrinsic morphology is not deformed. It usually is the consequence of pacemaker discharge during the refractory period of atrial or ventricular activity before sufficient intracardiac voltage is generated to activate the sensing circuit. This would be expected to occur when the pacing rate and the intrinsic rate are similar. Pseudofusion beats also may be the result of the delayed arrival of ventricular activity in a VVI system because of intraventricular conduction abnormalities at the site of the sensing electrodes.

Every pacing mode has a defined lower rate limit, and dual-chamber pacemakers, as well as rate-adaptive pacemakers, also require a defined upper rate limit. One must be familiar with the timing cycle of a particular pacing mode as well as any idiosyncrasies of the specific pacemaker to determine whether the paced rate is appropriate. There are multiple causes of a paced rate that appear to be different from the programmed rate. The differential diagnosis includes the following items:

- Circuit failure
- Battery failure
- Magnet application
- Hysteresis (Fig. 74.16)
- Cross talk
- Undocumented reprogramming of the pacemaker
- Oversensing
- Runaway
- Malfunction of the electrocardiographic recording equipment, alteration in paper speed

Drugs may affect sensing and pacing thresholds and result in electrocardiographic abnormalities (136). Although many drugs have been reported to affect pacing thresholds, the class IC agents are the only drugs that commonly cause a problem. Encainide, flecainide, propafenone, and moricizine have the potential to increase pacing thresholds. If these drugs are administered to a patient with a pacemaker, treatment should be monitored for an increase in pacing threshold. Class IC agents also have been reported to cause sensing abnormalities.

Electrolyte and metabolic abnormalities may also affect pacing and sensing thresholds. Hyperkalemia is the electrolyte abnormality that most commonly causes clinically significant problems, but severe acidosis or alkalosis, hypercarbia, severe hyperglycemia, hypoxemia, and myxedema should also be considered (136).

PACEMAKER DIAGNOSTICS

Various diagnostic functions are available in many current generation pacemakers and can be extremely helpful during pacemaker troubleshooting. Diagnostic capabilities vary widely from pacemaker to pacemaker (e.g., real-time telemetry of programmed parameters and battery status, lead impedance, electrograms, annotated electrocardiograms, histograms, or long-term recordings of rate variations, or a combination of these). A full discussion of this topic is beyond the scope of this textbook, but outstanding summaries of pacemaker diagnostics are available (138).

ELECTROMAGNETIC INTERFERENCE

Electromagnetic interference can be defined as any signal, biologic or nonbiologic, occurring within a frequency spec-

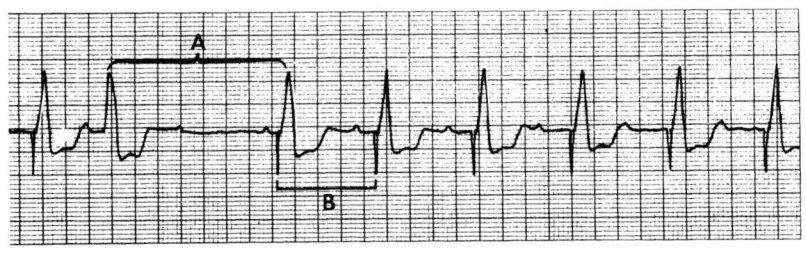

FIGURE 74.16 Electrocardiographic tracing from a patient with a VVI pacemaker programmed to a lower rate of 60 beats/min and hysteresis rate of 40 beats/min. The longer cycle (A) follows an intrinsic ventricular beat. The shorter cycle (B) represents the programmed lower rate of 60 beats/min (1,000 ms). (From Hayes DL. Pacemaker electrocardiography. In: Furman S, Hayes DL, Holmes DR Jr, eds. *A practice of cardiac pacing*, 3rd ed. Mount Kisco, NY: Futura, 1993:309–359, with permission.)

TABLE 74.7 SOURCES OF ELECTROMAGNETIC INTERFERENCE IN THE HOSPITAL ENVIRONMENT

Electrocautery/cardiovascular/defibrillation
Magnetic resonance imaging
Lithotripsy
Radiofrequency ablation
Electroshock therapy
Diathermy

trum that may be detected by the sensing circuitry of the pacemaker. Electromagnetic interference can result in rate alteration, sensing abnormalities, magnet mode response, or reprogramming.

Biologic signals that may be responsible for oversensing include T waves, myopotential interference, afterpotential delay, and P waves. Isoelectric extrasystoles may give the appearance of oversensing (136,137).

Although there are many potential nonbiologic sources of electromagnetic interference, few sources of electromagnetic interference are truly a threat to patients with a pacemaker. Hospital sources of potentially significant electromagnetic interference are listed in Table 74.7. The effects of electrocautery and guidelines for cardioversion and defibrillation in the patient with a pacemaker are given in Table 74.8. There are additional potential nonbiologic sources of electromagnetic interference and oversensing that are listed in eTable 74.8.1 (139).

Electromagnetic interference during the last portion of the refractory period of a pacemaker, the *noise-sampling period*, can disable the demand function of the pacemaker and cause reversion to a fixed-rate mode for one cycle, creating the impression of undersensing.

Currently, there is considerable interest in cellular telephones (140) and antitheft devices (141) as potential sources of electromagnetic interference. The information available suggests that analog cellular telephones are safe for patients with pacemakers. Digital cellular telephones have a greater potential for electromagnetic interference, and pacemaker-dependent patients who use a telephone with digital technology should exercise caution. If the patient avoids having the telephone over the pacemaker, either from random motion of the telephone or from carrying the activated telephone in a breast pocket over

TABLE 74.8 EFFECTS OF ELECTROCAUTERY

Reprogramming
Permanent damage to the pulse generator
Pacemaker inhibition
Reversion to a fall-back mode, noise reversion mode, or electrical reset
Myocardial thermal damage
Cardioversion/defibrillation of the pacemaker patient
    Ideally place paddles in the anterior-posterior position
    Try to keep paddles at least 4 in. from the pulse generator
    Have the appropriate pacemaker programmer available
    Interrogate the pacemaker following the procedure

the pacemaker, it is unlikely that any adverse clinical event will occur; however, research is being conducted on this question.

Antitheft devices also potentially can interfere with pacemakers (142–144). Patients with a pacemaker or an implantable cardioverter defibrillator (ICD) should be aware of electronic equipment for surveillance of articles and should avoid leaning on or lingering near such devices. If the patient passes through the equipment at a normal pace, adverse effects are unlikely. Any patient who feels unusual in any way when near electronic surveillance equipment should move away.

Hospital sources of potentially significant electromagnetic interference are electrocautery, cardioversion, defibrillation, magnetic resonance imaging, lithotripsy, radiofrequency ablation, electroshock therapy, and diathermy. The most important aspect of pacemaker or ICD care after exposure to any of these sources of electromagnetic interference is to reassess the device to be certain that the programmed parameters have not been changed.

Frequently, the question is asked about how to manage a patient with a pacemaker or ICD during a surgical procedure, given the potential effects of electrocautery and guidelines for cardioversion and defibrillation. Routine interrogation of the device and deactivation of ICD therapy should be performed before the operation. After the operation, the device should be reinterrogated and ICD therapy reinitiated. (During the time ICD therapy is off, the patient must be monitored.) For pacemaker-dependent patients, it is reasonable to program the pacemaker to an asynchronous pacing mode, VOO or DOO, or to achieve the same effect by placing a magnet over the pacemaker throughout the procedure. The potential effects of electrocautery are myocardial thermal damage, reprogramming, permanent damage to the pulse generator, pacemaker inhibition, and reversion to a fallback mode, noise reversion mode, or electrical reset.

FOLLOW-UP OF PATIENTS WITH PACEMAKERS

After the pacemaker has been implanted, the physician who performed the procedure or the institution where it was performed should assume responsibility for or arrange follow-up. Follow-up may be performed at the institution or at several commercial pacemaker follow-up centers.

There are several follow-up requirements (16,145). Although many centers have specific follow-up routines, the exact timing and location of follow-up, as well as programming routines, need to be established by the individual center to best meet its needs and institutional capabilities. The following requirements are included:

- Initial programming and optimization of rate response for all rate-adaptive pacemakers should be done.
- In-clinic follow-up should be done at 2 to 4 months to reassess energy output needs: Increase output if safety

margin is inadequate, and decrease output to increase pacemaker longevity when appropriate. At the same follow-up visit, rate-adaptive parameters should be reassessed. Special attention also should be given to the incision and pacemaker pocket.

■ Routine follow-up should assess battery status. In the United States, most patients have transtelephonic follow-up. The approved Medicare schedule for transtelephonic monitoring is more frequent than that followed by some centers. Regular transtelephonic follow-up should occur every 3 months until the first sign of battery depletion indicators (i.e., change in magnet rate or widening of pulse width), at which time the patient begins calling monthly until elective replacement indicators are reached; this has been shown to be an effective and safe follow-up schedule. Routine transtelephonic transmissions should include electrocardiographic monitoring with and without a magnet. Ideally, these records should be stored and available for retrieval for subsequent comparison should questions arise about change in pacemaker function.

■ All patients should be reevaluated in the clinic setting at least once annually. Depending on the individual center's transtelephonic schedule, the center may prefer to have the patient assessed in the clinic more frequently. ❦ m53

TEMPORARY PACING

Familiarity with temporary cardiac pacing is essential for those involved in permanent cardiac pacing and the treatment of patients in coronary care units and postoperative units. Knowledge of the indications, techniques, and routes of implantation, postinsertion management, and risk-benefit ratio for each patient is required for safe, reliable pacing.

Temporary pacing may be used for diagnostic or therapeutic purposes (146). Most commonly, it is used for short-term management of symptomatic bradycardias, either as a bridge to permanent pacing or for self-limited bradycardias (e.g., bradyarrhythmias associated with Lyme disease).

The indications for temporary pacing include both bradycardia and tachycardia (Table 74.9). There are two general categories: (a) patients with symptomatic bradycardia, and (b) patients with asymptomatic bradycardia or conduction defects. The decision to proceed with temporary pacing depends on assessment of the risk of development of symptomatic bradycardia. With the advent of reliable and readily available external temporary pacing, it is less common to place a temporary transvenous pacemaker in patients with asymptomatic conduction disturbances.

TABLE 74.9 INDICATIONS FOR TEMPORARY PACING

Third-degree atrioventricular block
  Symptomatic congenital complete heart block
  Symptomatic acquired complete heart block
  Postoperative symptomatic complete heart block
Symptomatic second-degree atrioventricular block
Acute myocardial infarction with:
  Symptomatic bradycardia
  Complete heart block
  New bundle branch block with transient complete heart block[a]
  Alternating bundle branch block[a]
Sinus node dysfunction
  Symptomatic bradyarrhythmias
Tachycardia, prevention or treatment
  Bradycardia-dependent arrhythmias
  Long QT syndrome with ventricular arrhythmias

[a]If asymptomatic, could consider observation and readily available external pacing. Transvenous temporary pacing only if external pacing is required.

CONTROVERSIES AND PERSONAL PERSPECTIVES

Controversies regarding the effect of pacing mode on morbidity and mortality continue. It was hoped that the publication of the CTOPP trial would bring some closure to the controversy, but it did not (104). With CTOPP failing to show a difference in mortality but a decreased incidence of atrial fibrillation with physiologic pacing, we now need to wait for longer follow-up of this population and for other trials that are under way.

Biventricular or left ventricular pacing for subjective and objective improvement in patients with congestive heart failure remains controversial but is becoming less so. With the publication of several randomized trials that have demonstrated clinical improvement, the controversy is no longer about whether pacing may be of benefit in a subset of this patient population but about the selection of patients and the optimal pacing site(s).

ICD therapy is discussed in Chapter 75. However, ICDs with extensive dual-chamber pacing capabilities are gaining widespread acceptance, and increasingly the clinical disciplines of cardiac pacing and cardiac defibrillation overlap.

Continued automaticity of permanent pacemakers undoubtedly will lead to better optimization of implanted devices and provide patients greater benefit from devices that previously may not have been tailored optimally to their needs.

Overall, permanent pacing was one of the remarkable success stories of the twentieth century. Having entered the twenty-first century, there are no signs that continued improvements in pacing therapy are slowing.

THE FUTURE

With the next decade, permanent pacemakers will continue to become more sophisticated, with automatic functions being the most prominent refinement. Also, dual-sensor rate-adaptive pacemakers will increasingly be accepted.

Prospective information is still limited about the effect of pacing mode on survival, but this information will become available within the next 2 to 3 years. The results of these prospective studies likely will support the results of retrospective studies, which consistently have shown lower morbidity and mortality with atrial-based pacing systems.

Biventricular and left ventricular pacing will gain increasing acceptance for the treatment of congestive heart failure, but it is too early to speculate whether either one may be used for patients with asymptomatic left ventricular dysfunction and an intraventricular conduction delay. If coronary lead placement becomes increasingly easier and reliable with the development of better leads and placement techniques, it could replace standard right ventricular apical pacing if a hemodynamic advantage can be shown. Pacing for the prevention of atrial fibrillation will also gain acceptance. A combination of alternate atrial pacing sites, either septal or left atrial pacing via the coronary sinus, with pacing algorithms that respond to premature atrial contraction will be the most likely successful application.

REFERENCES

1. Bernstein AD, Parsonnet V. World survey on cardiac pacing: United States 1993. *Reblampa* 1995;8:135–137.
2. Silverman BG, Gross TP, Kaczmarek RG, et al. The epidemiology of pacemaker implantation in the United States. *Public Health Rep* 1995;110:42–46.
3. Bernstein AD, Parsonnet V. Survey of cardiac pacing and implanted defibrillator practice patterns in the United States in 1977. *Pacing Clin Electrophysiol* 2001;24:842–855.
4. Elmqvist R, Landegren J, Pettersson SO, et al. Artificial pacemaker for treatment of Adams-Stokes syndrome and slow heart rate. *Am Heart J* 1963;65:731–748.
5. Furman S, Schwedel JB. An intracardiac pacemaker for Stokes-Adams seizures. *N Engl J Med* 1959;261:943–948.
6. Greatbatch W, Chardack WM. A transistorized implantable pacemaker for the long-term correction of complete A-V block. *NEREM Record* 1959;1:8–9.
7. Stephenson SE Jr, Edwards WH, Jolly PC, et al. Physiologic P-wave cardiac stimulator. *J Thorac Cardiovasc Surg* 1959;38:604–609.
8. Nathan DA, Center S, Wu CY, et al. An implantable, synchronous pacemaker for the long-term correction of complete heart block. *Circulation* 1963;11:362–367.
9. Irnich W, Parsonnet V, Myers GH. Compendium of pacemaker technology. Introduction and historical review. *Pacing Clin Electrophysiol* 1978;1:371–374.
10. Parsonnet V, Furman S, Smyth NP. Implantable cardiac pacemakers status report and resource guideline. Pacemaker Study Group. *Circulation* 1974;50:A21–A35.
11. Bernstein AD, Camm AJ, Fletcher RD, et al. The NASPE/BPEG generic pacemaker code for antibradyarrhythmia and adaptive-rate pacing and antitachyarrhythmia devices. *Pacing Clin Electrophysiol* 1987;10:794–799.
12. Dreifus LS, Fisch C, Griffin JC, et al. Guidelines for implantation of cardiac pacemakers and antiarrhythmia devices. A report of the American College of Cardiology/American Heart Association Task Force on Assessment of Diagnostic and Therapeutic Cardiovascular Procedures (Committee on Pacemaker Implantation). *J Am Coll Cardiol* 1991;18:1–13.
13. Report of a working party of the British Pacing and Electrophysiology Group. Recommendations for pacemaker prescription for symptomatic bradycardia. *Br Heart J* 1991;66:185–191.
14. Serwer GA, Dorostkar PC. Pediatric pacing. In: Ellenbogen KA, Kay GN, Wilkoff BL, eds. *Clinical cardiac pacing.* Philadelphia: WB Saunders, 1995:706–734.
15. Michaelsson M, Jonzon A, Riesenfeld T. Isolated congenital complete atrioventricular block in adult life. A prospective study. *Circulation* 1995;92:442–449.
16. Hayes DL, Osborn MJ. Antibradycardia devices. In: Giuliani ER, Gersh BJ, McGoon MD, et al., eds. *Mayo Clinic practice of cardiology*, 3rd ed. St. Louis: Mosby, 1996:909–976.
17. Benditt DG, Remole S, Asso A, et al. Cardiac pacing for carotid sinus syndrome and vasovagal syncope. In: Barold SS, Mugica J, eds. *New perspectives in cardiac pacing*, 3rd ed. Mount Kisco, NY: Futura Publishing, 1993:15–28.
18. Abi-Samra F, Maloney JD, Fouad-Tarazi FM, et al. The usefulness of head-up tilt testing and hemodynamic investigations in the workup of syncope of unknown origin. *Pacing Clin Electrophysiol* 1988;11:1202–1214.
19. Fabian WH, Benditt DG, Lurie KG. Neurally mediated syncope. *Curr Treat Options Cardiovasc Med* 1999;1:137–144.
20. Almquist A, Goldenberg IF, Milstein S, et al. Provocation of bradycardia and hypotension by isoproterenol and upright posture in patients with unexplained syncope. *N Engl J Med* 1989;320:346–351.
21. Fitzpatrick A, Theodorakis G, Ahmed R, et al. Dual chamber pacing aborts vasovagal syncope induced by head-up 60 degrees tilt. *Pacing Clin Electrophysiol* 1991;14:13–19.

22. Connolly SJ, Sheldon R, Roberts RS, et al. The North American Vasovagal Pacemaker Study (VPS). A randomized trial of permanent cardiac pacing for the prevention of vasovagal syncope. *J Am Coll Cardiol* 1999;33:16–20.

23. Brignole M, Menozzi C, Lolli G, et al. Long-term outcome of paced and nonpaced patients with severe carotid sinus syndrome. *Am J Cardiol* 1992;69:1039–1043.

24. Benditt DG, Petersen M, Lurie KG, et al. Cardiac pacing for prevention of recurrent vasovagal syncope. *Ann Intern Med* 1995;122:204–209.

25. Sheldon R. Pacing to prevent vasovagal syncope. *Cardiol Clin* 2000;18:81–93.

26. Vasovagal Syncope International Study. Is dual-chamber pacing efficacious in treatment of neurally-mediated tilt positive cardioinhibitory syncope? Pacemaker vs no therapy: a multicentre randomised study. *Eur J Cardiac Pacing Electrophysiol* 1993;3:169–172.

27. Glikson M, Espinosa RE, Hayes DL. Expanding indications for permanent pacemakers. *Ann Intern Med* 1995;123:443–451.

28. Fananapazir L, Cannon RO III, Tripodi D, et al. Impact of dual-chamber permanent pacing in patients with obstructive hypertrophic cardiomyopathy with symptoms refractory to verapamil and beta-adrenergic blocker therapy. *Circulation* 1992;85:2149–2161.

29. Fananapazir L, Epstein ND, Curiel RV, et al. Long-term results of dual-chamber (DDD) pacing in obstructive hypertrophic cardiomyopathy. Evidence for progressive symptomatic and hemodynamic improvement and reduction of left ventricular hypertrophy. *Circulation* 1994;90:2731–2742.

30. Sorajja P, Elliott PM, McKenna WJ. Pacing in hypertrophic cardiomyopathy. *Cardiol Clin* 2000;18:67–79.

31. Nishimura RA, Hayes DL, Ilstrup DM, et al. Effect of dual-chamber pacing on systolic and diastolic function in patients with hypertrophic cardiomyopathy. Acute Doppler echocardiographic and catheterization hemodynamic study. *J Am Coll Cardiol* 1996;27:421–430.

32. Jeanrenaud X, Goy JJ, Kappenberger L. Effects of dual-chamber pacing in hypertrophic obstructive cardiomyopathy. *Lancet* 1992;339:1318–1323.

33. Kappenberger L, Linde C, Daubert C, et al. Pacing in hypertrophic obstructive cardiomyopathy. A randomized crossover study. PIC Study Group. *Eur Heart J* 1997;18:1249–1256.

34. Maron BJ, Nishimura RA, McKenna WJ, et al. Assessment of permanent dual-chamber pacing as a treatment for drug-refractory symptomatic patients with obstructive hypertrophic cardiomyopathy. A randomized, double-blind, crossover study (M-PATHY). *Circulation* 1999;99:2927–2933.

35. Peters RW, Gold MR. Pacing for patients with congestive heart failure and dilated cardiomyopathy. *Cardiol Clin* 2000;18:55–66.

36. Hochleitner M, Hortnagl H, Ng CK, et al. Usefulness of physiologic dual-chamber pacing in drug-resistant idiopathic dilated cardiomyopathy. *Am J Cardiol* 1990;66:198–202.

37. Hochleitner M, Hortnagl H, Fridrich L, et al. Long-term efficacy of physiologic dual-chamber pacing in the treatment of end-stage idiopathic dilated cardiomyopathy. *Am J Cardiol* 1992;70:1320–1325.

38. Nishimura RA, Hayes DL, Holmes DR Jr, et al. Mechanism of hemodynamic improvement by dual-chamber pacing for severe left ventricular dysfunction: an acute Doppler and catheterization hemodynamic study. *J Am Coll Cardiol* 1995;25:281–288.

39. Gold MR, Feliciano Z, Gottlieb SS, et al. Dual-chamber pacing with a short atrioventricular delay in congestive heart failure: a randomized study. *J Am Coll Cardiol* 1995;26:967–973.

40. Linde C, Gadler F, Edner M, et al. Results of atrioventricular synchronous pacing with optimized delay in patients with severe congestive heart failure. *Am J Cardiol* 1995;75:919–923.

41. Innes D, Leitch JW, Fletcher PJ. VDD pacing at short atrioventricular intervals does not improve cardiac output in patients with dilated heart failure. *Pacing Clin Electrophysiol* 1994;17:959–965.

42. Leclercq C, Cazeau S, Ritter P, et al. A pilot experience with permanent biventricular pacing to treat advanced heart failure. *Am Heart J* 2000;140:862–870.

43. Auricchio A, Stellbrink C, Block M, et al. Effect of pacing chamber and atrioventricular delay on acute systolic function of paced patients with congestive heart failure. Pacing Therapies for Congestive Heart Failure Study Group and Guidant Congestive Heart Failure Research. *Circulation* 1999;99:2993–3001.

44. Cazeau S, Leclercq C, Lavergne T, et al. Effects of multisite biventricular pacing in patients with heart failure and intraventricular conduction delay. *N Engl J Med* 2001;344:873–880.

45. Daubert C, Mabo P, Berder V, et al. Atrial tachyarrhythmias associated with high degree interatrial conduction block: prevention by permanent atrial resynchronisation. *Eur J Cardiac Pacing Electrophysiol* 1994;1[Suppl 3]:35–44.

46. Saksena S, Prakash A, Hill M, et al. Prevention of recurrent atrial fibrillation with chronic dual-site right atrial pacing. *J Am Coll Cardiol* 1996;28:687–694.

47. Daubert JC, Mabo P, Berder V, et al. Atrial flutter and interatrial conduction block: preventive role of biatrial synchronous pacing? In: Waldo AL, Touboul P, eds. *Atrial flutter: advances in mechanisms and management.* Armonk, NY: Futura Publishing, 1996:331–346.

48. Kusumoto FM, Goldschlager N. Cardiac pacing. *N Engl J Med* 1996;334:89–97.

49. Ausubel K, Furman S. The pacemaker syndrome. *Ann Intern Med* 1985;103:420–429.

50. Heldman D, Mulvihill D, Nguyen H, et al. True incidence of pacemaker syndrome. *Pacing Clin Electrophysiol* 1990;13:1742–1750.

51. Hayes DL, Furman S. Stability of AV conduction in sick sinus node syndrome patients with implanted atrial pacemakers. *Am Heart J* 1984;107:644–647.

52. Irwin M, Harris L, Cameron D, et al. DDI pacing: indications, expectations, and follow-up. *Pacing Clin Electrophysiol* 1994;17:274–279.

53. Lau CP, Tai YT, Leung SK, et al. Long-term stability of P wave sensing in single lead VDDR pacing: clinical versus

subclinical atrial undersensing. *Pacing Clin Electrophysiol* 1994;17:1849–1853.

54. Mugica J. Importance of a systematic long-term follow-up to guide the choice of pacemaker electrodes: the experience of a single center with 18,132 leads. *Pacing Clin Electrophysiol* 1994;17:1995–2000.

55. Mond HG, Helland JR. Engineering and clinical aspects of pacing leads. In: Ellenbogen KA, Kay GN, Wilkoff BL, eds. *Clinical cardiac pacing.* Philadelphia: WB Saunders, 1995:69–90.

56. Rossi P. Rate-responsive pacing: biosensor reliability and physiological sensitivity. *Pacing Clin Electrophysiol* 1987;10:454–466.

57. Alt E, Millerhagen JO, Heemels J-P. Accelerometers. In: Ellenbogen KA, Kay GN, Wilkoff BL, eds. *Clinical cardiac pacing.* Philadelphia: WB Saunders, 1995:267–276.

58. Benditt DG, Duncan JL. Activity-sensing, rate-adaptive pacemakers. In: Ellenbogen KA, Kay GN, Wilkoff BL, eds. *Clinical cardiac pacing.* Philadelphia: WB Saunders, 1995:167–186.

59. Bongiorni MG, Soldati E, Arena G, et al. Multicenter clinical evaluation of a new SSIR pacemaker. *Pacing Clin Electrophysiol* 1992;15:1798–1803.

60. Faerastrand S, Ohm OJ. Clinical study of a new activity sensor for rate adaptive pacing controlled by electrical signals generated by the kinetic energy of a moving magnetic ball. *Pacing Clin Electrophysiol* 1994;17:1944–1949.

61. Nappholtz T, Valenta H, Maloney J, et al. Electrode configurations for a respiratory impedance measurement suitable for rate responsive pacing. *Pacing Clin Electrophysiol* 1986;9:960–964.

62. Slade AK, Pee S, Jones S, et al. New algorithms to increase the initial rate response in a minute volume rate adaptive pacemaker. *Pacing Clin Electrophysiol* 1994;17:1960–1965.

63. Li H, Neubauer SA, Hayes DL. Follow-up of a minute ventilation rate adaptive pacemaker. *Pacing Clin Electrophysiol* 1992;15:1826–1829.

64. Benditt DG, Mianulli M, Lurie K, et al. Multiple-sensor systems for physiologic cardiac pacing. *Ann Intern Med* 1994;121:960–968.

65. Connelly DT, Rickards AF. The evoked QT interval. In: Ellenbogen KA, Kay GN, Wilkoff BL, eds. *Clinical cardiac pacing.* Philadelphia: WB Saunders, 1995:250–257.

66. Jolgren D, Fearnot N, Geddes L. A rate-responsive pacemaker controlled by right ventricular blood temperature. *Pacing Clin Electrophysiol* 1984;7:794–801.

67. Chirife R. Physiological principles of a new method for rate responsive pacing using the pre-ejection interval. *Pacing Clin Electrophysiol* 1988;11:1545–1554.

68. Salo R, O'Donoghue S, Platia EV. The use of intracardiac impedance-based indicators to optimize pacing rate. In: Ellenbogen KA, Kay GN, Wilkoff BL, eds. *Clinical cardiac pacing.* Philadelphia: WB Saunders, 1995:234–249.

69. Kay GN, Philippon F, Bubien RS, et al. Rate modulated pacing based on right ventricular dP/dt: quantitative analysis of chronotropic response. *Pacing Clin Electrophysiol* 1994;17:1344–1354.

70. Yee R, Bennett TD. Rate-adaptive pacing controlled by dynamic right ventricular pressure (dP/dtmax). In: Ellen-

bogen KA, Kay GN, Wilkoff BL, eds. *Clinical cardiac pacing.* Philadelphia: WB Saunders, 1995:212–218.

71. Kay GN, Bornzin GA. Rate-modulated pacing controlled by mixed venous oxygen saturation. In: Ellenbogen KA, Kay GN, Wilkoff BL, eds. *Clinical cardiac pacing.* Philadelphia: WB Saunders, 1995:187–200.

72. Callaghan F, Vollmann W, Livingston A, et al. The ventricular depolarization gradient: effects of exercise, pacing rate, epinephrine, and intrinsic heart rate control on the right ventricular evoked response. *Pacing Clin Electrophysiol* 1989;12:1115–1130.

73. Singer I, Callaghan FJ. Evoked potentials as a sensor for rate-adaptive pacing. In: Ellenbogen KA, Kay GN, Wilkoff BL, eds. *Clinical cardiac pacing.* Philadelphia: WB Saunders, 1995:258–266.

74. Lau CP. *Rate adaptive cardiac pacing: single and dual chamber.* Mount Kisco, NY: Futura Publishing, 1993:137–146.

75. Israel CW, Hohnloser SH. Current status of dual-sensor pacemaker systems for correction of chronotropic incompetence. *Am J Cardiol* 2000;86[Suppl 1]:K86–K94.

76. Tang CY, Kerr CR, Connolly SJ. Clinical trials of pacing mode selection. *Cardiol Clin* 2000;18:1–23.

77. Charles RG. Prospective randomized trials on pacing mode: what have we learned? *Am J Cardiol* 2000;86[Suppl 1]:K116–K118.

78. Rosenqvist M, Brandt J, Schuller H. Long-term pacing in sinus node disease: effects of stimulation mode on cardiovascular morbidity and mortality. *Am Heart J* 1988;116:16–22.

79. Alpert MA, Curtis JJ, Sanfelippo JF, et al. Comparative survival following permanent ventricular and dual-chamber pacing for patients with chronic symptomatic sinus node dysfunction with and without congestive heart failure. *Am Heart J* 1987;113:958–965.

80. Bianconi L, Boccadamo R, Di Florio A, et al. Atrial versus ventricular stimulation in sick sinus syndrome: effects on morbidity and mortality. *Pacing Clin Electrophysiol* 1989;12:1236[abstract].

81. Feuer JM, Shandling AH, Messenger JC. Influence of cardiac pacing mode on the long-term development of atrial fibrillation. *Am J Cardiol* 1989;64:1376–1379.

82. Grimm W, Langenfeld H, Maisch B, et al. Symptoms, cardiovascular risk profile and spontaneous ECG in paced patients: a five-year follow-up study. *Pacing Clin Electrophysiol* 1990;13:2086–2090.

83. Hayes DL, Espinosa RE, Neubauer SA, et al. Association of atrial fibrillation, pacing mode, and survival following pacemaker implantation. *Pacing Clin Electrophysiol* 1993;16:1115[abstract].

84. Hesselson AB, Parsonnet V, Bernstein AD, et al. Deleterious effects of long-term single-chamber ventricular pacing in patients with sick sinus syndrome: the hidden benefits of dual-chamber pacing. *J Am Coll Cardiol* 1992;19:1542–1549.

85. Kosakai Y, Ohe T, Kamakura S, et al. Long term follow-up of incidence of embolism in sick sinus syndrome after pacing. *Pacing Clin Electrophysiol* 1991;14:680[abstract].

86. Langenfeld H, Grimm W, Maisch B, et al. Atrial fibrillation and embolic complications in paced patients. *Pacing Clin Electrophysiol* 1988;11:1667–1672.

87. Markewitz A, Schad N, Hemmer W, et al. What is the most appropriate stimulation mode in patients with sinus node dysfunction? *Pacing Clin Electrophysiol* 1986;9:1115–1120.

88. Nürnberg M, Frohner K, Podczeck A, et al. Is VVI pacing more dangerous than AV-sequential pacing in patients with sick sinus syndrome? *Pacing Clin Electrophysiol* 1991;14:674[abstract].

89. Santini M, Alexidou G, Ansalone G, et al. Relation of prognosis in sick sinus syndrome to age, conduction defects and modes of permanent cardiac pacing. *Am J Cardiol* 1990;65:729–735.

90. Santamauro M, Pappone C, Damiano M, et al. Single and dual chamber pacing influence on patients' survival. In: Adornato E, Galassi A, eds. *How to approach cardiac arrhythmias in 1994. Proceedings of the IVth Southern Symposium on Cardiac Pacing*, Vol. 2. Rome: Edizioni Ligi Pozzi, 1994:148–154.

91. Sasaki Y, Furihata A, Suyama K, et al. Comparison between ventricular inhibited pacing and physiologic pacing in sick sinus syndrome. *Am J Cardiol* 1991;67:771–774.

92. Sethi KK, Bajaj V, Mohan JC, et al. Comparison of atrial and VVI pacing modes in symptomatic sinus node dysfunction without associated tachyarrhythmias. *Ind Heart J* 1990;42:143–147.

93. Stangl K, Seitz K, Wirtzfeld A, et al. Differences between atrial single chamber pacing (AAI) and ventricular single chamber pacing (VVI) with respect to prognosis and antiarrhythmic effect in patients with sick sinus syndrome. *Pacing Clin Electrophysiol* 1990;13:2080–2085.

94. Sutton R, Kenny RA. VVI versus AAI or dual chamber pacing in sick sinus syndrome. In: Santini M, Pistolese M, Alliegro A, eds. *Progress in clinical pacing*. Rome: Centro Editorial Pubblicitario Italiano, 1986:253–265.

95. van Erckelens F, Sigmund M, Lambertz H, et al. Atrial fibrillation in rate responsive, DDD- and VVI-pacing: incidence, time of onset, influencing factors. *Pacing Clin Electrophysiol* 1990;13:1194[abstract].

96. Witte J, von Knorre GH, Volkmann HJ, et al. Survival rate in patients with sick sinus syndrome in AAI/DDD vs. VVI pacing. In: Santini M, Pistolese M, Alliegro A, eds. *Progress in clinical pacing*. Mount Kisco, NY: Futura Media Services, 1993:175–177.

97. Zanini R, Facchinetti AI, Gallo G, et al. Morbidity and mortality of patients with sinus node disease: comparative effects of atrial and ventricular pacing. *Pacing Clin Electrophysiol* 1990;13:2076–2079.

98. Barold SS, Santini M. Natural history of sick sinus syndrome after pacemaker implantation. In: Barold SS, Mugica J, eds. *New perspectives in cardiac pacing*, 3rd ed. Mount Kisco, NY: Futura Publishing, 1993:169–211.

99. Lamas GA, Pashos C, Normand SL, et al. Natural history of sick sinus syndrome (SSS) following pacemaker implantation. *Eur J Cardiac Pacing Electrophysiol* 1994;4:34[abstract].

100. Lamas GA, Estes NM III, Schneller S, et al. Does dual chamber or atrial pacing prevent atrial fibrillation? The need for a randomized controlled trial. *Pacing Clin Electrophysiol* 1992;15:1109–1113.

101. Andersen HR, Thuesen L, Bagger JP, et al. Prospective randomised trial of atrial versus ventricular pacing in sick-sinus syndrome. *Lancet* 1994;344:1523–1528.

102. Andersen HR, Nielsen JC, Thomsen PE, et al. Long-term follow-up of patients from a randomised trial of atrial versus ventricular pacing for sick-sinus syndrome. *Lancet* 1997;350:1210–1216.

103. Lamas G, Stambler B, Mittelman R, et al. Clinical events following DDDR vs VVIR pacing: results of a prospective trial. *Pacing Clin Electrophysiol* 1996;19:619[abstract].

104. Connolly SJ, Kerr CR, Gent M, et al. Effects of physiologic pacing versus ventricular pacing on the risk of stroke and death due to cardiovascular causes. Canadian Trial of Physiologic Pacing Investigators. *N Engl J Med* 2000;342:1385–1391.

105. Hayes DL, Naccarelli GV, Furman S, et al. Report of the NASPE Policy Conference training requirements for permanent pacemaker selection, implantation, and follow-up. North American Society of Pacing and Electrophysiology. *Pacing Clin Electrophysiol* 1994;17:6–12.

106. Josephson ME, Maloney JD, Barold SS, et al. Guidelines for training in adult cardiovascular medicine. Core Cardiology Training Symposium (COCATS). Task Force 6: training in specialized electrophysiology, cardiac pacing and arrhythmia management. *J Am Coll Cardiol* 1995;25:23–26.

107. Hayes DL. Implantation techniques. In: Hayes DL, Lloyd MA, Friedman PA, eds. *Cardiac pacing and defibrillation: a clinical approach*. Armonk, NY: Futura Publishing, 2000:159–200.

108. Leclercq C, Gras D, Le Helloco A, et al. Hemodynamic importance of preserving the normal sequence of ventricular activation in permanent cardiac pacing. *Am Heart J* 1995;129:1133–1141.

109. Guidici MC, Thornburg GA, Buck DL, et al. Permanent right ventricular outflow tract pacing improves cardiac output: comparison with apical placement in 58 patients. *Eur J Cardiac Pacing Electrophysiol* 1994;4:80[abstract].

110. Gadler F, Linde C, Juhlin-Dannfeldt A, et al. Influence of right ventricular pacing site on left ventricular outflow tract obstruction in patients with hypertrophic obstructive cardiomyopathy. *J Am Coll Cardiol* 1996;27:1219–1224.

111. Foster AH, Gold MR, McLaughlin JS. Acute hemodynamic effects of atrio-biventricular pacing in humans. *Ann Thorac Surg* 1995;59:294–300.

112. Cazeau S, Ritter P, Bakdach S, et al. Four chamber pacing in dilated cardiomyopathy. *Pacing Clin Electrophysiol* 1994;17:1974–1979.

113. Platia EV, Brinker JA. Time course of transvenous pacemaker stimulation impedance, capture threshold, and electrogram amplitude. *Pacing Clin Electrophysiol* 1986;9:620–625.

114. Hayes DL, Broadbent JC, Holmes DR Jr, et al. Steroid-tipped leads: one year follow-up. In: Aubert AE, Ector H, eds. *Pacemaker leads: Proceedings of the International Symposium on Pacemaker Leads, Leuven, Belgium, September 5–7, 1984*. Amsterdam: Elsevier, 1985:317–322.

115. Crossley GH, Brinker JA, Reynolds D, et al. Steroid elution improves the stimulation threshold in an active-fixation atrial permanent pacing lead. A randomized, controlled study. Model 4068 investigators. *Circulation* 1995;92:2935–2939.

116. Irwin ME, Gulamhusein SS, Senaratne MP, et al. Out-

comes of an ambulatory cardiac pacing program: indications, risks, benefits, and outcomes. *Pacing Clin Electrophysiol* 1994;17:2027–2031.

117. Hayes DL. Endless-loop tachycardia: the problem has been solved? In: Barold SS, Mugica J, eds. *New perspectives in cardiac pacing.* Mount Kisco, NY: Futura, 1988:375–386.

118. Rees M, Haennel RG, Black WR, et al. Effect of rate-adapting atrioventricular delay on stroke volume and cardiac output during atrial synchronous pacing. *Can J Cardiol* 1990;6:445–452.

119. Daubert C, Ritter P, Mabo P, et al. Rate modulation of the AV delay in DDD pacing. In: Santini M, Pistolese M, Alliegro A, eds. *Proceedings of the International Symposium on Progress in Clinical Pacing: Rome, Italy, 5–8 December 1990.* New York: Elsevier, 1990:415–430.

120. Chirife R. Proposal of a method for automatic optimization of left heart atrioventricular interval applicable to DDD pacemakers. *Pacing Clin Electrophysiol* 1995;18:49–56.

121. Lau CP, Tai YT, Fong PC, et al. Atrial arrhythmia management with sensor controlled atrial refractory period and automatic mode switching in patients with minute ventilation sensing dual chamber rate adaptive pacemakers. *Pacing Clin Electrophysiol* 1992;15:1504–1514.

122. Provenier F, Jordaens L, Verstraeten T, et al. The "automatic mode switch" function in successive generations of minute ventilation sensing dual chamber rate responsive pacemakers. *Pacing Clin Electrophysiol* 1994;17:1913–1919.

123. Wilkoff BL. Cardiac chronotropic responsiveness. In: Ellenbogen KA, Kay GN, Wilkoff BL, eds. *Clinical cardiac pacing.* Philadelphia: WB Saunders, 1995:432–446.

124. Hayes DL, Von Feldt L, Higano ST. Standardized informal exercise testing for programming rate adaptive pacemakers. *Pacing Clin Electrophysiol* 1991;14:1772–1776.

125. Hayes DL. Pacemaker complications. In: Furman S, Hayes DL, Holmes DR Jr, eds. *A practice of cardiac pacing,* 3rd ed. Mount Kisco, NY: Futura, 1993:537–569.

126. Higano ST, Hayes DL, Spittell PC. Facilitation of the subclavian-introducer technique with contrast venography. *Pacing Clin Electrophysiol* 1990;13:681–684.

127. Spittell PC, Hayes DL. Venous complications after insertion of a transvenous pacemaker. *Mayo Clinic Proc* 1992;67:258–265.

128. Souliman SK, Christie J. Pacemaker failure induced by radiotherapy. *Pacing Clin Electrophysiol* 1994;17:270–273.

129. Griffith MJ, Mounsey JP, Bexton RS, et al. Mechanical, but not infective, pacemaker erosion may be successfully managed by reimplantation of pacemakers. *Br Heart J* 1994;71:202–205.

130. Mounsey JP, Griffith MJ, Tynan M, et al. Antibiotic prophylaxis in permanent pacemaker implantation: a prospective randomised trial. *Br Heart J* 1994;72:339–343.

131. Lewis AB, Hayes DL, Holmes DR Jr, et al. Update on infections involving permanent pacemakers. Characterization and management. *J Thorac Cardiovasc Surg* 1985;89:758–763.

132. Furman S, Behrens M, Andrews C, et al. Retained pacemaker leads. *J Thorac Cardiovasc Surg* 1987;94:770–772.

133. Smith HJ, Fearnot NE, Byrd CL, et al. Five-years experience with intravascular lead extraction. U.S. Lead Extraction Database. *Pacing Clin Electrophysiol* 1994;17:2016–2020.

134. Love CJ, Wilkoff BL, Byrd CL, et al. Recommendations for extraction of chronically implanted transvenous pacing and defibrillator leads: indications, facilities, training. North American Society of Pacing and Electrophysiology Lead Extraction Conference Faculty. *Pacing Clin Electrophysiol* 2000;23:544–551.

135. Abdallah HI, Balsara RK, O'Riordan AC. Pacemaker contact sensitivity: clinical recognition and management. *Ann Thorac Surg* 1994;57:1017–1018.

136. Love CJ, Hayes DL. Evaluation of pacemaker malfunction. In: Ellenbogen KA, Kay GN, Wilkoff BL, eds. *Clinical cardiac pacing.* Philadelphia: WB Saunders, 1995:656–683.

137. Hayes DL. Pacemaker electrocardiography. In: Furman S, Hayes DL, Holmes DR Jr, eds. *A practice of cardiac pacing,* 2nd ed. Mount Kisco, NY: Futura, 1989:289–321.

138. Levine PA, Sanders R, Markowitz HT. Pacemaker diagnostics: measured data, event marker, electrogram, and event counter telemetry. In: Ellenbogen KA, Kay GN, Wilkoff BL, eds. *Clinical cardiac pacing.* Philadelphia: WB Saunders, 1995:639–655.

139. Telectronics: electromagnetic interference and the pacemaker patient. *Technical Notes* May 1991;110.

140. Hayes DL, Carrillo RG, Findlay GK, et al. State of the science: pacemaker and defibrillator interference from wireless communication devices. *Pacing Clin Electrophysiol* 1996;19:1419–1430.

141. Lucas EH, Johnson D, McElroy BP. The effects of electronic article surveillance systems on permanent cardiac pacemakers: an in vitro study. *Pacing Clin Electrophysiol* 1994;17:2021–2026.

142. McIvor ME. Electronic article surveillance systems and pacemakers: a perspective on advising patients. *Cardiovasc Rev Rep* 1999;20:216–222.

143. Santucci PA, Haw J, Trohman RG, et al. Interference with an implantable defibrillator by an electronic antitheft-surveillance device. *N Engl J Med* 1998;339:1371–1374.

144. Groh WJ, Silka MJ, Oliver RP, et al. Use of implantable cardioverter-defibrillators in the congenital long QT syndrome. *Am J Cardiol* 1996;78:703–706.

145. Goldschlager N, Ludmer P, Creamer C. Follow-up of the paced outpatient. In: Ellenbogen KA, Kay GN, Wilkoff BL, eds. *Clinical cardiac pacing.* Philadelphia: WB Saunders, 1995:780–808.

146. Hayes DL, Holmes DR Jr. Temporary cardiac pacing. In: Furman S, Hayes DL, Holmes DR Jr, eds. *A practice of cardiac pacing,* 3rd ed. Mount Kisco, NY: Futura, 1993:231–260.

147. Deal BJ. Esophageal pacing. In: Ellenbogen KA, Kay GN, Wilkoff BL, eds. *Clinical cardiac pacing.* Philadelphia: WB Saunders, 1995:701–705.

IMPLANTABLE CARDIOVERTER-DEFIBRILLATORS

SERGIO L. PINSKI
PENG-SHENG CHEN

▼▼ *ADDITIONAL ELECTRONIC TOPICS*

Historical Perspective m54;   Ventricular Fibrillation m55;   Cost-Effectiveness of the Implantable Cardioverter-Defibrillator m56

OVERVIEW

Randomized controlled trials have demonstrated the superiority of the implantable cardioverter-defibrillator (ICD) over antiarrhythmic drug treatment in patients with serious ventricular arrhythmias. At the same time, technological advances have made ICDs small, easy to implant, and very versatile. The surgical mortality rate has dropped to less than 1%. Antitachycardia pacing allows for the painless termination of many episodes of sustained monomorphic ventricular tachycardia (VT), whereas defibrillation shocks are needed for more rapid or polymorphic VT or for ventricular fibrillation (VF). However, complications including lead failure, infection, spurious shocks for supraventricular tachyarrhythmias, and psychological morbidity still occur. In the next few years, ongoing randomized studies will clarify the role of ICDs in the management of larger populations at risk for

sudden cardiac death. These trials will assess not only the impact of ICDs on overall survival, but also their effects on quality of life and their cost-effectiveness. If these studies show positive results, ICDs will become the preeminent clinical tool for the prevention of sudden cardiac death. Future technological developments will continue to improve the performance of ICDs, expand their therapeutic capabilities for treatment of heart failure and supraventricular arrhythmias, and reduce complications associated with their use.

GLOSSARY

Biphasic waveform: Shock waveform that consists of two phases of opposite polarity.
Dedicated bipolar: Defibrillator lead in which sensing of the depolarization signal and pacing are delivered between a distal-tip electrode and a closely positioned ring electrode, neither of which participates in the defibrillation pathway.
Defibrillation threshold: Minimal shock strength that terminates induced VF during implant or follow-up testing.

S. L. Pinski: Section of Cardiology, Rush Medical College of Rush University, Rush-Presbyterian-St. Luke's Medical Center, Chicago, Illinois
P. Chen: Department of Medicine/Cardiology, Cedars Sinai Medical Center, Los Angeles, California

Detection enhancements: Optional programmable criteria (e.g., sudden onset or rate stability) used to increase the specificity of detection algorithms for VT.

Integrated bipolar: Defibrillator lead in which sensing of the depolarization signal and pacing are delivered between a distal-tip electrode and a more proximal defibrillation coil that is part of the defibrillation pathway.

Upper limit of vulnerability: Shock strength at and above which VF is not induced, even when the shock is delivered during the ventricular vulnerable period.

CURRENT STATUS OF IMPLANTABLE CARDIOVERTER-DEFIBRILLATOR TECHNOLOGY

ICD systems consist of two main components: the pulse generator, which harbors the electronic circuitry, power sources, and memory; and the lead electrode system that interfaces with the heart (6). Among the important components of ICD generators, the microprocessor orchestrates the interplay between the various subsections of the system. The read-only memory contains instructions that determine the general functional characteristics of the device, and individualized programming and diagnostic information are stored in random access memory. Lithium/silver vanadium oxide batteries provide the power source. The predicted longevity of current generators varies between 5 and 9 years, depending on the model and the frequency of activation. The pacing and high-output sections convert the 3 to 10 V provided by the batteries into device discharges that range from less than 1 V (for pacing) to 750 V (for defibrillation). The circuitry for delivering pacing pulses is similar to that found in standard bradycardia pacemakers, and high-voltage pulses are provided by capacitors. Batteries and capacitors consume two-thirds of the volume of current devices. The sense amplifier section adapts continually to the intracardiac ventricular depolarization signal, which may vary dramatically in amplitude (i.e., from sinus rhythm to VF) while avoiding significant signal drop and oversensing of T waves or extracardiac interference. This adaptation is achieved by adjusting either the gain or the sensing threshold. The communications section allows the ICD to exchange information with the dedicated programmer. ❤ m57

ELECTROPHYSIOLOGIC MECHANISMS

Ventricular Defibrillation

Defibrillation is best described as a dose-response phenomenon that can be depicted with a sigmoidal curve of energy versus probability of success (14). Construction of a probability-of-success curve in patients is impractical, because it requires at least 20 to 30 fibrillation-defibrillation trials. Determination of the defibrillation threshold (i.e., the lowest

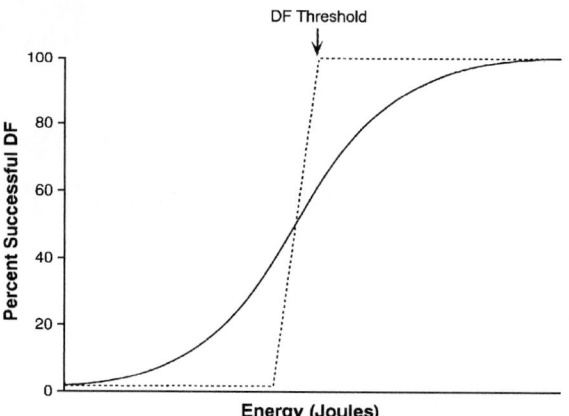

FIGURE 75.1 Comparison of defibrillation (DF) probability-of-success curve and DF threshold concepts. A probability-of-success curve implies a dose-response relationship in which increasing energies are associated with a higher percentage of success, whereas a DF threshold implies a clear-cut distinction between effective and ineffective energies. (Reproduced from Davy JM, Fain ES, Dorian P, et al. The relationship between successful defibrillation and delivered energy in open-chest dogs: reappraisal of the "defibrillation threshold" concept. *Am Heart J* 1987;113:77–84, with permission from Mosby–Year Book.)

energy that successfully terminates VF) is clinically more applicable (15). The defibrillation threshold determined by clinical protocols generally identifies energies with 50% to 75% probability of success (Fig. 75.1). ❤ m58

The type of defibrillation waveform and the surface area, impedance, and geometry of the defibrillation electrodes are crucial determinants of the energy requirements for defibrillation; clinical variables are less important (30). The ICDs currently in use deliver biphasic shocks (i.e., the pulse has two phases of opposite polarity). This waveform markedly decreases the energy requirements for defibrillation in comparison with the earlier monophasic waveform (31). However, identification of the optimal waveform remains elusive. Variables that influence the efficiency of the biphasic waveform are the duration and relative amplitude of each phase (32), and capacitance (32,33). With current ICD systems, a high defibrillation threshold (i.e., ≥23 J) is more likely to occur in patients with idiopathic dilated cardiomyopathy (as opposed to coronary artery disease) and in patients taking amiodarone or other antiarrhythmic drugs with sodium channel blockade activity (34).

CLINICAL TRIALS OF THE IMPLANTABLE CARDIOVERTER-DEFIBRILLATOR

Recent trials have examined the role of the ICD in secondary prevention of sudden cardiac death (i.e., in patients who have already had a clinical episode of life-threatening ventricular arrhythmia) and primary prevention of sudden cardiac death (i.e., in patients at high risk for this outcome

TABLE 75.1 COMPLETED RANDOMIZED TRIALS OF THE IMPLANTABLE CARDIOVERTER-DEFIBRILLATOR (ICD)

Study	Control intervention	Population	Findings
Antiarrhythmics versus Implantable Defibrillator Trial (AVID)	Amiodarone or sotalol	Cardiac arrest survivor *or* syncopal ventricular tachycardia *or* symptomatic sustained ventricular tachycardia with left ventricular ejection fraction ≤0.40	Significant improvement in overall survival with ICDs.
Canadian Implantable Defibrillator Study (CIDS)	Amiodarone	Cardiac arrest survivor *or* syncopal ventricular tachycardia *or* symptomatic sustained ventricular tachycardia with left ventricular ejection fraction ≤0.35 *or* syncope and inducible ventricular tachycardia	Nonsignificant improvement in overall survival with ICDs.
Cardiac Arrest Study—Hamburg (CASH)	Propafenone, metoprolol, or amiodarone	Cardiac arrest survivor	Nonsignificant improvement in overall survival with ICDs.
Multicenter Automatic Implantable Defibrillator Trial (MADIT)	Conventional therapy	Prior myocardial infarction *and* left ventricular ejection fraction ≤0.35 *and* nonsustained ventricular tachycardia *and* inducible ventricular tachycardia *and not* suppressible with intravenous procainamide	Significant improvement in overall survival with ICDs.
Coronary Artery Bypass Graft–Implantable Cardioverter-Defibrillator Study (CABG Patch)	None	Coronary bypass surgery *and* left ventricular ejection fraction ≤0.35 *and* positive signal-averaged electrocardiogram	No difference in overall survival.
Multicenter Unsustained Tachycardia Trial (MUSTT)	None	Previous myocardial infarction *and* left ventricular ejection fraction ≤0.40 *and* asymptomatic, unsustained ventricular tachycardia *and* inducible ventricular tachycardia	Significant improvement in overall survival in patients randomly assigned to electrophysiologically guided therapy. All the benefit in this arm occurred in patients who received ICDs.
Amiodarone versus Implantable Cardioverter-Defibrillator Randomized Trial (AMIOVIRT)	Amiodarone	Nonischemic cardiomyopathy *and* left ventricular ejection fraction <0.35 *and* asymptomatic nonsustained ventricular tachycardia	No difference in overall survival.

who have not yet experienced a serious arrhythmic event) (Table 75.1 and Fig. 75.2).

Secondary Prevention of Sudden Death

Despite the unquestionable efficacy of the ICD in terminating VF and preventing sudden death, competing causes of death in ICD recipients (e.g., heart failure) may limit the overall survival benefit (35). Early nonrandomized studies suggested the superiority of the ICD over antiarrhythmic drugs in patients who had life-threatening ventricular arrhythmias (36), but the presence of selection bias, the use of controversial end points, and a lack of adequate controls limited the applicability of their implications. After controlled studies demonstrated an increase in the mortality rate with class I or pure class III antiarrhythmic drugs, only amiodarone (37) and sotalol (38) remained viable alternative therapies for ventricular arrhythmias. Well-powered randomized controlled trials were needed to assess the impact of the ICD on survival of patients with life-threatening ventricular arrhythmias.

The Antiarrhythmics versus Implantable Defibrillators Trial (AVID) (39) studied 1,016 patients with VF, sus-

tained VT with syncope, or sustained VT with serious symptoms and left ventricular ejection fraction ≤0.40 that was not believed to be secondary to correctable or reversible causes. Patients were randomly assigned to receive an ICD or antiarrhythmic drugs (empiric amiodarone or guided sotalol). The study essentially compared the ICD to amiodarone, because only 2.6% of patients randomized to the antiarrhythmic drug limb were discharged on sotalol. ICD patients had better survival throughout the course of the study (unadjusted survival at 1 year, 89% among patients with ICD vs. 82% among patients treated with amiodarone, and at 3 years, 75% vs. 61%; p <.02). The corresponding reductions in mortality rates in the ICD group were 39% and 31% at 1 and 3 years, respectively. The ICD significantly decreased the incidence of cardiac arrhythmic death but had no effect on nonarrhythmic deaths (40). No significant differences were seen in the benefit conferred by ICD therapy among prespecified subgroups categorized according to age, degree of left ventricular dysfunction, presence of coronary artery disease, or presenting rhythm. More patients in the ICD group were treated with beta-blockers, but adjusting for this imbal-

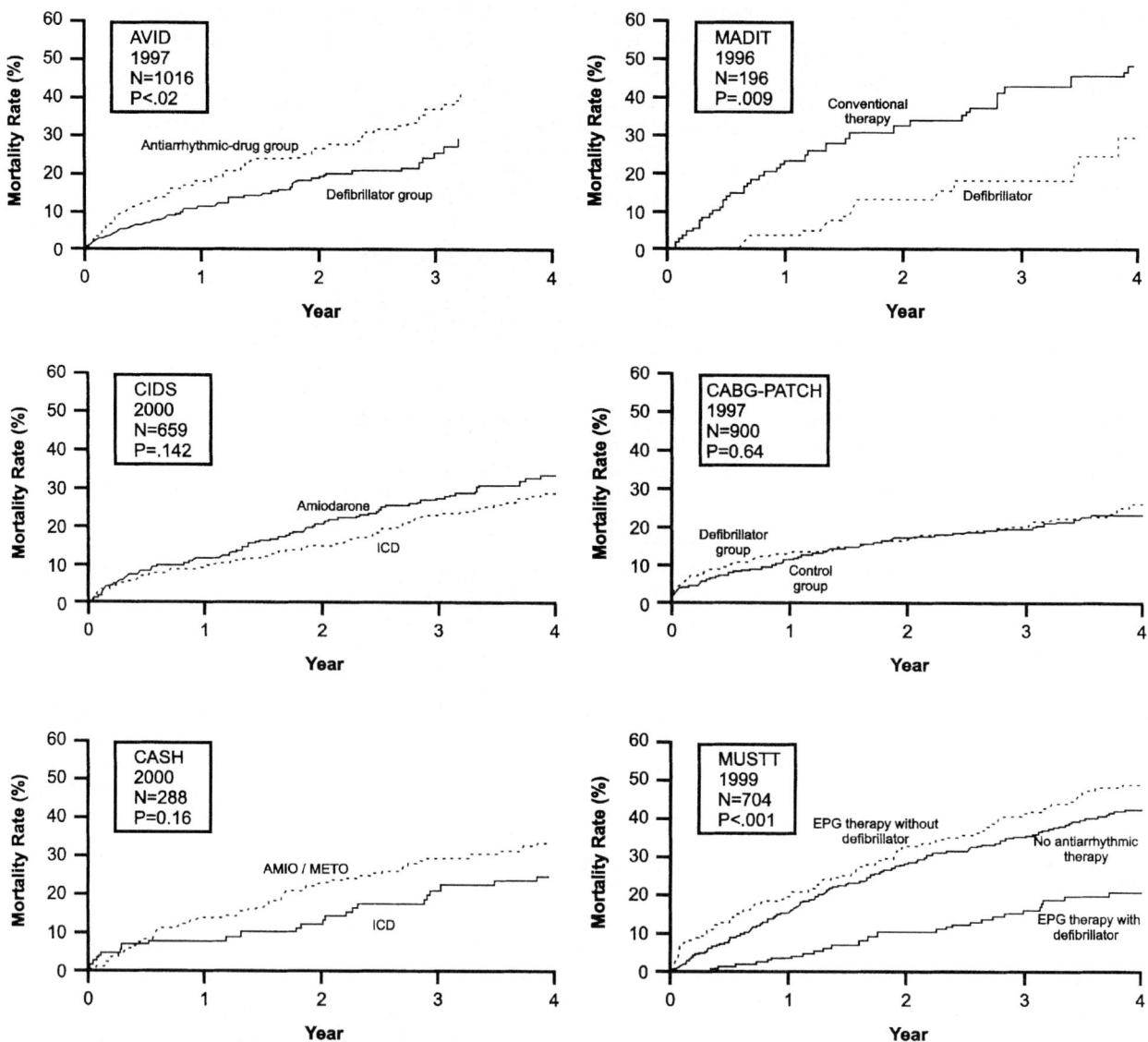

FIGURE 75.2 Plots of actuarial total mortality rate end points for published multicenter controlled trials involving use of implantable cardioverter-defibrillators. The mortality rates and follow-up periods have been normalized for each study so that the control and intervention mortality rates can be compared. The legends show year of publication, total number of patients enrolled, and two-tailed *p* value for each study. AMIO, amiodarone; AVID, Antiarrhythmics versus Implantable Defibrillators Trial; CABG Patch, Coronary Artery Bypass Graft–Implantable Cardioverter-Defibrillator Study; CASH, Cardiac Arrest Study—Hamburg; CIDS, Canadian Implantable Defibrillator Study; EPG, electrophysiologic; MADIT, Multicenter Automatic Defibrillator Implantation Trial; METO, metoprolol; MUSTT, Multicenter Unsustained Tachycardia Trial.

ance did not change the estimate of the mortality rate reduction attributable to the ICD. Several design features of this study, including the enrollment of a wide spectrum of patients with little evidence of selection biases [as supported by a concomitant comprehensive registry (41)], the almost exclusive use of transvenous defibrillators, and the comparison of ICD use against the best available antiarrhythmic drug therapy, make extrapolation of its findings to clinical practice valid. ▼ m59

The Canadian Implantable Defibrillator Study (CIDS) (43) included 659 patients who had been resuscitated after

cardiac arrest or who had syncopal VT, presyncopal VT with a heart rate <150 beats/min or accompanied by left ventricular ejection fraction <0.36, or unmonitored syncope with subsequent spontaneous or inducible VT. Patients were randomly assigned to receive ICD implantation or treatment with empiric amiodarone. The 3-year mortality rate was 25% in the group who received ICD and 30% in the group being treated with amiodarone. A nonsignificant reduction in the risk of death was observed with the ICD, from 10.2% per year to 8.3% per year (relative risk reduction, 19.7%; 95% confidence interval, −7.7%

to 40%; *p* = .142). A nonsignificant reduction in the risk of arrhythmic death was observed, from 4.5% per year to 3.0% per year (relative risk reduction, 32.8%; 95% confidence interval, −7.2% to 57.8%; *p* = .094). ❖ m60

Primary Prevention of Sudden Death

Sudden cardiac death represents a major public health challenge that requires continuing development of new, multi-faceted approaches for primary prevention. Use of the ICD is a potentially useful intervention, but the expense and invasiveness involved make accurate identification of candidates imperative. Efficient interventions require methods of identifying higher-risk clusters within the lower-risk subgroups (45). Target populations considered for prophylactic ICD implantation include patients with various combinations of left ventricular dysfunction, congestive heart failure, complex ventricular ectopy, late potentials on signal-averaged electrocardiography, depressed heart-rate variability, exercise-induced microvoltage T-wave alternans, and inducibility of VT at electrophysiologic study.

The Multicenter Automatic Defibrillator Implantation Trial (MADIT) (46) examined the efficacy of the ICD versus conventional therapy for prolonging survival in 196 patients with prior myocardial infarction, left ventricular ejection fraction ≤0.35, spontaneous nonsustained VT, and inducible VT not suppressed by intravenous procainamide at electrophysiologic study. Amiodarone was the most frequently used therapy in the group of patients receiving conventional therapy. ICD patients had better survival throughout the course of the study (actuarial survival at 1 year, 97% among patients who had ICDs vs. 77% among patients receiving conventional therapy; at 3 years: 83% vs. 56%; *p* <.009). This translated into a 54% reduction in death from all causes. More patients in the ICD group were treated with beta-blockers (26% vs. 8% 1 month after enrollment; 27% vs. 5% at last contact). Separate analyses revealed no evidence that antiarrhythmic medications, including amiodarone and beta-blockers, other cardiac medications being given 1 month after enrollment, or any of 11 preselected baseline variables had a meaningful influence on the magnitude of the ICD effect.

The Multicenter Unsustained Tachycardia Trial (47) was a randomized, controlled trial that tested the hypothesis that electrophysiologically guided antiarrhythmic therapy would reduce the risk of sudden death among patients with coronary artery disease, a left ventricular ejection fraction ≤0.40, and asymptomatic, unsustained VT. A total of 704 such patients in whom sustained ventricular tachyarrhythmias were induced by programmed stimulation were randomly assigned to receive either antiarrhythmic therapy, including drugs or use of ICDs (as indicated by the results of electrophysiologic testing), or no antiarrhythmic therapy. The 5-year incidence of the primary end point of cardiac arrest or death from arrhythmia was 25% among patients who

received electrophysiologically guided therapy and 32% among those assigned to receive no antiarrhythmic therapy (relative risk, 0.73; 95% confidence interval, 0.53–0.99; relative risk reduction, 27%). The 5-year estimates of overall mortality rates were 42% and 48%, respectively (relative risk, 0.80; 95% confidence interval, 0.64–1.01). All the observed benefit occurred in patients who were given ICDs before discharge after failure to identify an effective drug during serial electropharmacologic testing. The risk of cardiac arrest or death from arrhythmia among the patients who received treatment with ICDs was significantly lower than that among the patients discharged without ICDs (relative risk, 0.24; 95% confidence interval, 0.13–0.45; *p* <.001). Neither the rate of cardiac arrest or death from arrhythmia nor the overall mortality rate was lower among patients who were assigned to electrophysiologically guided therapy and treated with antiarrhythmic drugs than among the patients who were assigned to no antiarrhythmic therapy.

The Coronary Artery Bypass Graft–Implantable Cardioverter-Defibrillator Study (CABG Patch) (48) randomly assigned 900 patients with left ventricular ejection fraction ≤0.35 and late-potentials on signal-averaged electrocardiography who were scheduled for coronary bypass surgery to treatment with ICD (implanted at the time of bypass surgery) or to no antiarrhythmic treatment. The study was halted prematurely after an average follow-up of 32 months when interim analysis showed no difference between the treatment groups (hazard ratio, 1.07; 95% confidence interval, 0.81–1.42). ❖ m61

INDICATIONS AND CONTRAINDICATIONS FOR USE OF THE IMPLANTED CARDIOVERTER-DEFIBRILLATOR

Indications for ICDs are evolving as technology improves and results from clinical trials are incorporated into clinical practice (Table 75.2) (57). ICDs should be considered first-line therapy for patients who have survived episodes of cardiac arrest or hemodynamically significant sustained VT that is not caused by reversible causes and for patients who have coronary artery disease, left ventricular dysfunction, and nonsustained VT and in whom sustained ventricular tachyarrhythmias can be induced during electrophysiologic testing.

Although most ICD recipients involved in clinical trials had coronary artery disease or idiopathic dilated cardiomyopathy, growing evidence from nonrandomized trials suggests that patients with other forms of cardiomyopathy and primary electrical disorders may benefit from use of ICDs. In a retrospective multicenter study of 128 patients with hypertrophic cardiomyopathy who were judged to be at high risk for sudden death, the rate of appropriate ICD discharge was 7% per year. The study suggested that VT or VF is the principal mechanism of sudden death in patients with hypertrophic cardiomyopathy, and that the ICD has

TABLE 75.2 CURRENT INDICATIONS FOR IMPLANTABLE CARDIOVERTER-DEFIBRILLATOR IMPLANTATION[a]

Secondary prevention
Patients with at least one clinical episode of ventricular fibrillation or hemodynamically significant ventricular tachycardia without reversible, correctable cause
Patients with unexplained syncope and inducible sustained ventricular tachycardia on electrophysiologic study
Patients with structural heart disease and sustained monomorphic ventricular tachycardia, regardless of hemodynamic tolerance[b]
Patients with idiopathic dilated cardiomyopathy and unexplained syncope despite electrophysiologic testing[b]

Primary prevention
Patients with coronary artery disease, at least moderate left ventricular dysfunction, spontaneous nonsustained ventricular tachycardia, and inducible sustained ventricular tachycardia
Patients with familial or inherited conditions who have a high risk for life-threatening ventricular tachyarrhythmias such as long-QT syndrome or hypertrophic cardiomyopathy[b]

[a]Several other indications are being evaluated in ongoing randomized studies.
[b]Experts may differ regarding the appropriateness of implantable cardioverter-defibrillator therapy in these patients.

an important role in its prevention (58). Some experts recommend ICD implantation (in conjunction with treatment with beta-blockers) as a fail-safe back-up therapy in high-risk patients who have congenital long-QT syndrome, especially those who have experienced an aborted cardiac arrest (59). Use of the ICD is also indicated in patients with idiopathic VF, including those with Brugada syndrome (60). Children who have life-threatening ventricular arrhythmia can also be successfully treated with ICDs (61).

Patients with syncope of undetermined origin and inducible sustained VT have a high incidence of appropriate defibrillator discharge (62,63) and also appear to benefit from ICD implantation. Patients with unexplained syncope, nonischemic dilated cardiomyopathy, and negative results of electrophysiologic examination have also been considered as candidates for ICD implantation because of the difficulties in risk-stratification. In a small series of 14 such patients, the incidence of appropriate shocks was high (50%) and similar to the rate observed in patients with idiopathic cardiomyopathy who were resuscitated from cardiac arrest (64). Other series have reported a lower (but not negligible) incidence of appropriate ICD intervention (65). Another retrospective analysis reported improved survival in patients who had nonischemic cardiomyopathy and unexplained syncope and were treated with ICDs (66). On the basis of this observational evidence, ICD implantation appears reasonable in this group of patients after other causes of syncope have been ruled out.

The role of the ICD in patients who have structural heart disease and present with nonsyncopal sustained monomorphic VT is unclear. Such patients had a low risk

of sudden death in nonrandomized observational studies of antiarrhythmic drug therapy (67). On the other hand, a relatively high incidence of shocks for rapid, potentially life-threatening ventricular arrhythmias has been reported in a selected population of patients with stable VT who were treated with ICDs (68) (*e*Fig. 75.2.1). Furthermore, among 3,559 patients enrolled in the AVID registry who had documented sustained ventricular tachyarrhythmias, the hemodynamic impact of the index arrhythmia did not influence overall survival (69). Until more information is gathered, we believe that use of the ICD should be strongly considered in all patients who have structural heart disease and sustained VT. Catheter ablation of the tachycardia circuit(s) is another potentially curative option in these patients (70), but we believe it should, for now, be reserved as adjunctive therapy in patients who have ICDs and frequently recurring VT (71).

ICDs should not be implanted in patients whose ventricular tachyarrhythmias have been triggered by acute ischemia or infarction, correctable toxic or metabolic factors, or atrial fibrillation in the Wolff-Parkinson-White syndrome. The assessment of the reversibility of ventricular tachyarrhythmias in patients who have myocardial ischemia or severe coronary disease but not acute infarction is difficult and often inaccurate. Coronary artery disease was present in 81.5% of 270 patients in the AVID Registry who were thought to have VT or VF due to transient or correctable causes. Revascularization was performed in approximately one-half of the patients, and most of them were discharged without specific antiarrhythmic treatment. Actuarial 3-year survival was only 71% (lower than the 73% observed in patients in the same registry who had VT thought to be from uncorrectable causes) (41). The decision to perform surgical or percutaneous revascularization in patients with life-threatening ventricular arrhythmias should be based on grounds similar to those used in other clinical settings (e.g., presence of large areas of viable, ischemic myocardium). Observational studies suggest that the prognosis is good with revascularization alone in patients who have VF and normal left ventricular function, but arrhythmias frequently recur in patients who have left ventricular dysfunction or who present with VT. The value of using programmed ventricular stimulation after the revascularization procedure has been debated (72,73).

Patients with very frequent VT or VF that is not responsive to drugs, ablation, or antitachycardia pacing should not receive ICDs, because such arrhythmias would trigger frequent shock therapy. The low morbidity of current ICD implant techniques has made surgical or medical contraindications less relevant than in the past. However, patients who have terminal illness or a life expectancy of less than 6 to 12 months are not good candidates for ICD implantation. Patients awaiting cardiac transplantation have a high incidence of sudden death, but the use of the ICD as a "bridge" to transplantation remains controversial (74).

CLINICAL MANAGEMENT OF PATIENTS WITH IMPLANTABLE CARDIOVERTER-DEFIBRILLATORS

Implantation

ICDs are implanted via the subclavian, axillary, or cephalic veins. [▼ m62] A right ventricular lead is used for sensing and pacing. Shocks are delivered between a coil in this lead and the case of the generator. Leads incorporating a second coil at the level of the superior vena cava are often preferred, because the resulting bidirectional shocking vector improves the efficiency of defibrillation (79). Defibrillators capable of dual-chamber pacing require an additional pacing lead in the right atrium (*e*Fig. 75.2.2). Some ICDs can also deliver electrical therapy for atrial tachyarrhythmias, including cardioversion shocks for atrial fibrillation (80). This can be achieved with conventional systems that include a coil electrode in the superior vena cava (81). However, the lowest atrial fibrillation cardioversion thresholds are achieved when a coil electrode is added in the coronary sinus (82). Newer units that provide resynchronization therapy for heart failure (i.e., biventricular pacing) require insertion of an additional lead into a coronary vein to achieve left ventricular capture (83) (Fig. 75.3).

The generator is implanted in a subcutaneous pocket in the pectoral area, although a submuscular plane is of value in patients who have a thin layer of subcutaneous tissue (84). The left side is preferred because of the smoother venous route to the heart and the more favorable shocking vector (85). Intraoperative testing is performed to establish appropriate pacing thresholds and adequate sensing during sinus rhythm and VF (86). The system's defibrillation capabilities are also tested, and the shocking lead configuration is optimized. In many institutions, this is accomplished by determining the ventricular defibrillation threshold (i.e., the minimal energy that terminates induced VF) (15), which is usually between 5 and 15 J. This ensures an adequate safety margin for defibrillation in most cases, because the maximum output of currently available ICDs ranges between 26 and 38 J (*e*Fig. 75.3.1). A safety margin can also be established by step-down protocols that do not require a failed shock. ▼ m63

The operative mortality rate after implantation of ICDs is less than 1% (89). Most patients can be discharged to their homes on the same day or the next day after surgery. Complications are similar to those accompanying pacemaker implantation and include pneumothorax, hemothorax, cardiac perforation, pericardial tamponade, pocket hematoma (90), lead dislodgment, skin erosion, venous thrombosis, and frozen shoulder (91). Infection occurs in

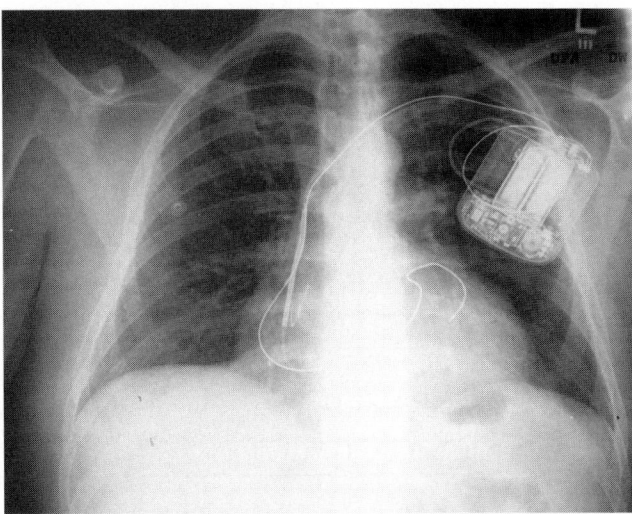

FIGURE 75.3 Posteroanterior chest radiograph after implantation of a triple-chamber implantable cardioverter-defibrillator capable of biventricular pacing. In addition to the atrial and defibrillation leads, a unipolar pacing lead was advanced via the coronary sinus into the middle segment of the anterior interventricular coronary vein.

up to 2% of patients (92). Complete system removal and intravenous antibiotic therapy are generally needed to cure infection (93). Percutaneous extraction of chronic defibrillator leads is technically challenging, but it can be performed at low risk by trained operators equipped with specially designed tools (94). A large-bore (16 French) excimer laser sheath is particularly useful (95). ▼ m64

Programming

The therapeutic target of ICD therapy should be the complete prevention of sudden death and syncope due to ventricular tachyarrhythmias using only sporadic delivery of high-energy shocks. Antitachycardia pacing is useful mostly for monomorphic VTs with rates lower than 200 beats/min (97). For these tachycardias, pacing and low-energy cardioversion both have a success rate of approximately 80% and have a similar risk of tachycardia acceleration (98). Antitachycardia pacing has the advantages of much better patient tolerance, lower energy consumption, and lack of atrial proarrhythmia (Fig. 75.4 and *e*Fig. 75.4.1).

VF can be successfully treated only with a defibrillation shock. Charging to approximately 30 J (700 V) takes 5 to 13 seconds, depending on the model and battery status of the ICD (99). A first shock energy ≥30 J, however, is not universally necessary. Programming of the initial energy at 5 J above the upper limit of vulnerability (100) or at twice the defibrillation threshold when it is <15 J (101) still results in almost 100% successful conversion of spontaneous arrhythmia episodes during follow-up. The shorter charge time decreases the risk of arrhythmia-induced syncope. If the first shock fails, the device will recharge and

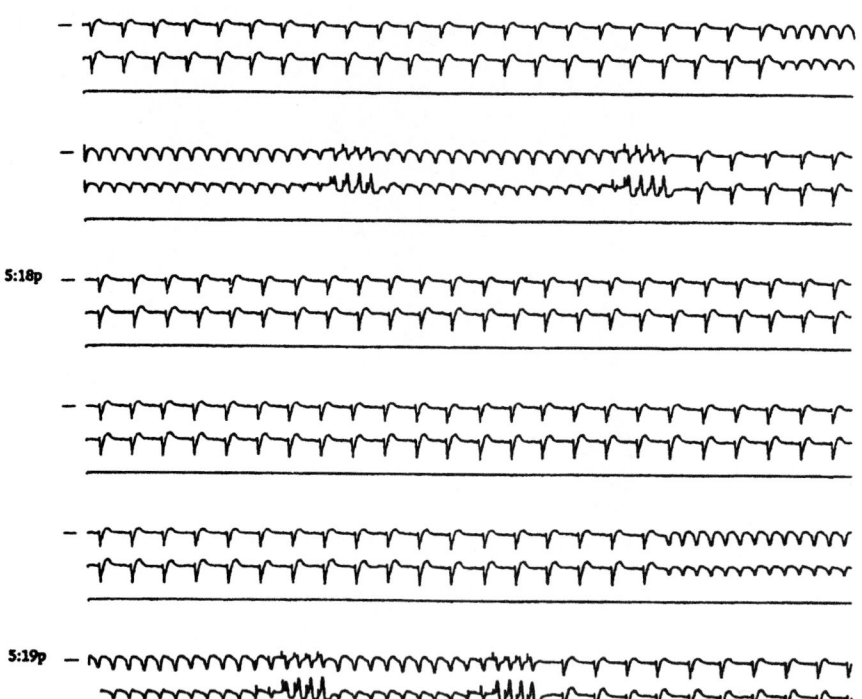

FIGURE 75.4 Antitachycardia pacing. Holter monitor shows that during a 2-minute period, two episodes of monomorphic ventricular tachycardia were converted by the scanning antitachycardia pacing algorithm (both in the second attempt). The patient remained asymptomatic. (Reproduced from Pinski SL, Simmons TW, Maloney JD. Troubleshooting antitachycardia pacing in patients with defibrillators. In: Estes NAM, Wang P, Manolis A, eds. *Implantable cardioverter-defibrillators: a comprehensive textbook.* New York: Marcel Dekker, 1994:445–477, with permission.)

deliver up to five additional high-output shocks. Spontaneous episodes of de novo VF are not common, even in patients with a history of this arrhythmia (102). Most episodes begin as fast monomorphic VT, which the ICD detects and cardioverts before it has an opportunity to spontaneously degenerate into fibrillation.

ICDs recognize ventricular tachyarrhythmias based on programmable rate and duration criteria. Assuming correct sensing of the cardiac depolarization signal, this ensures 100% sensitivity for tachycardias above the programmed cutoff rate, but the specificity may be poor (103). Underdetection of tachycardias is uncommon when adequate sensing has been demonstrated during implantation. With some integrated bipolar leads, underdetection of VF has occurred after a failed shock. Increasing the distance between the distal tip and coil has largely averted this problem (104).

Failure to discriminate between supraventricular and ventricular tachyarrhythmias results in clinically inappropriate ICD interventions. Many of these spurious interventions can be avoided by adequate device programming. The cutoff rate for tachycardia detection should ideally be programmed to be higher than the patient's maximal exercise-induced sinus rate. However, in many patients (more frequently in those on antiarrhythmic drugs), the sinus and VT rates overlap. Detection enhancements can be programmed that will improve the accuracy of arrhythmia diagnosis. The sudden onset criterion helps to discriminate between sinus tachycardia and VT, and the rate stability criterion is useful in rejecting atrial fibrillation with a rapid ventricular response (105). Morphology criteria assess the

differences (e.g., width) in the intracardiac QRS electrogram between beats of supraventricular and ventricular origin. The incorporation of these enhancements into the detection algorithms represents a trade-off between sensitivity and specificity; a perfectly specific algorithm may fail to detect some episodes of hemodynamically significant VT (106,107). However, empiric enabling of conservative discrimination criteria is safe and effective in reducing the occurrence of inappropriate shocks (108). In some devices, a programmable sustained high rate criterion overrides the other enhancement criteria and allows therapy delivery for persistent tachycardia episodes that did not fulfill enhancement criteria. Dual-chamber ICDs can achieve better discrimination between ventricular and supraventricular arrhythmias by incorporating information that originates in the atrium into the detection algorithms (109) (Fig. 75.5 and eFig. 75.5.1). However, the diagnostic performance of these devices is algorithm dependent, and in some cases, it may not surpass that of single-chamber devices with optimal programming (110). ▼ m65

Follow-Up and Long-Term Complications

Follow-up of ICD patients is best carried out in a focused device clinic (117). Routine follow-up should include taking a careful history with regard to interim symptoms of tachyarrhythmias and ICD discharges; device interrogation (including real-time telemetry of battery status and retrieval of diagnostic data from the memory) (eFigs. 75.5.3 and 75.5.4); and determination of pacing and sensing thresholds. Radiologic examination can demonstrate lead dis-

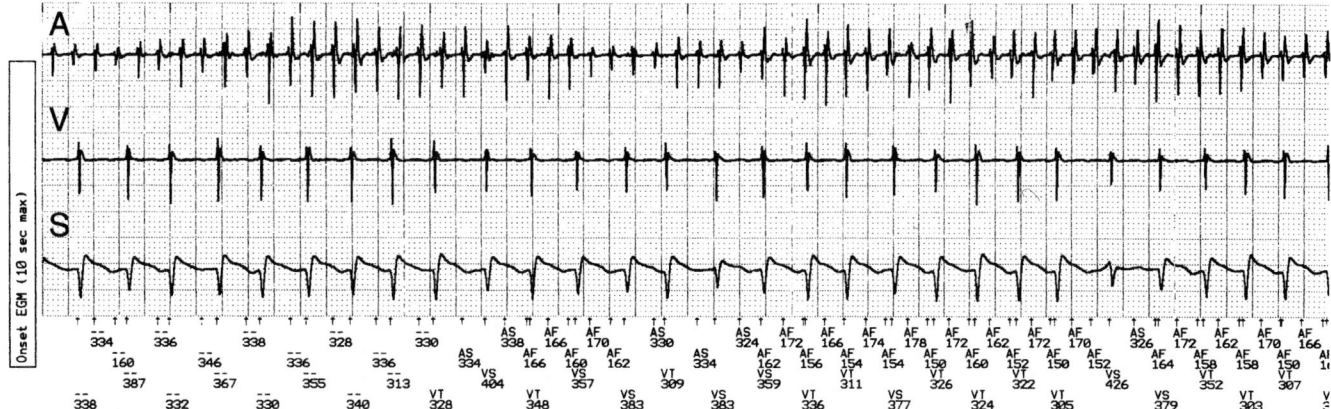

FIGURE 75.5 Accurate rejection of atrial fibrillation with rapid ventricular response by a dual-chamber implantable cardioverter-defibrillator. Stored atrial (A), ventricular (V), and shocking lead (S) electrograms (EGMs) show a very rapid atrial rate (approximately 350 beats per minute) and an irregular ventricular rate of approximately 165 beats per minute. Despite the fact that the ventricular rate was within the programmed ventricular tachycardia detection window, the device interpreted the fast atrial rate and the slower and irregular ventricular rate as representing atrial fibrillation and appropriately withheld intervention.

placement or migration but is less useful for the identification of lead fractures (118). Routine predischarge noninvasive arrhythmia induction in the electrophysiology laboratory is no longer recommended (119). It should be selectively performed when satisfactory testing is not achieved during implantation or when treatment with antiarrhythmic drugs that can decrease defibrillation efficacy is added during follow-up (120). The relative merits of empiric programming of detection and therapeutic algorithms (121) for VT versus fine-tuning based on the results of noninvasive arrhythmia induction are not clear (122). ▼▼ m66

Complete withdrawal of antiarrhythmic drugs is a desirable (but not always attainable) goal in patients with ICDs (129). Indications for concomitant antiarrhythmic drug therapy include suppression of frequently recurring ventricular arrhythmias that trigger device intervention, suppression of supraventricular arrhythmias, and slowing of VT to avoid syncope and facilitate pace termination. In a double-blind, placebo-controlled study of 302 patients, sotalol was significantly effective in reducing the incidence of death from any cause or the delivery of a first shock for any reason (including appropriate and inappropriate shocks) (130). In a smaller study of 70 patients with ICDs, metoprolol was significantly more effective than sotalol in preventing recurrences of ventricular tachyarrhythmias (131). Amiodarone is also used often to decrease the incidence of shocks, although definitive controlled data regarding its efficacy for this indication are lacking. Treatment with amiodarone seems to decrease the incidence of shocks compared with treatment with class I drugs (124,132). Potentially significant interactions between antiarrhythmic drugs and ICD systems include dose-dependent increases in defibrillation [lidocaine (133), procainamide, flecainide,

and amiodarone (134)] or pacing (flecainide) energy requirements; slowing of VT rate below the programmed cutoff (135); and increases in latency or conduction time leading to double counting, reduced efficacy of antitachycardia pacing, and proarrhythmic effects.

Long-term complications are not uncommon during ICD therapy. Transvenous defibrillator leads have a relatively high structural failure rate (e.g., conductor fracture or insulation cracking) causing spurious shocks (delivered or aborted), undersensing, or loss of pacing capture and requiring operative lead replacement (91,136). The incidence of lead failure may be higher when subclavian puncture is used for venous access (137). Rarer hardware problems include inadvertent device inactivation by electromagnetic fields, premature battery depletion, random component failure, and twiddler's syndrome.

Even with dual-chamber discrimination algorithms, some supraventricular tachyarrhythmias are detected as ventricular, resulting in spurious shocks (138). The incidence of spurious shocks is higher (>20% of patients) with single-chamber ICDs, especially when they are left at nominal programming settings (89). In patients with spurious shocks, reprogramming of detection criteria to increase specificity should be attempted first. It is often necessary to add pharmacologic therapy to reduce the sinus rate, prevent recurrences of paroxysmal atrial tachyarrhythmias, or slow AV conduction. Catheter ablation may also be considered.

Quality of Life

Most patients adapt well to living with the ICD, in a process described as "securing life through technology acceptance" (139). Studies examining quality of life measured before and after ICD implantation have showed unchanged or improved quality-of-life scores after implantation (140,141). Common concerns in ICD patients include fear of shocks, fear of device malfunction, fear of public shocks and embarrassment, and altered body image (142). Younger patients worry about the need for repeat surgeries, the cosmetic appearance of the device and the scar, and risks during pregnancy (143). However, ICD implantation is compatible with subsequent normal pregnancy and delivery (144).

Experiencing an ICD shock can be frightening. Most patients perceive ICD shocks as quite uncomfortable, comparing them with a jolt from an electric socket or a kick in the chest. Fewer than 15% of patients lose consciousness during the lag between arrhythmia onset and device discharge (145). Patients who receive multiple shocks have higher levels of anxiety, anger, and depression (146,147). A few patients develop adjustment disorders specific to the ICD, such as anticipatory anxiety with secondary panic reaction and phobia, imaginary shocks, and defibrillator dependence, abuse or withdrawal (148). Patient support groups provide a valuable opportunity for dissemination of relevant information, alleviation of anxiety, and promotion of a positive attitude toward device therapy (149). Psychotherapeutic counseling, behavioral therapies (150), and psychotropic medication may be required. Some antidepressant and antipsychotic drugs have proarrhythmic effects similar to those of antiarrhythmic drugs and should be used with caution in patients with ICDs.

Safety issues arise frequently during the follow-up of patients with ICDs. Most of these patients are able to exercise safely when appropriate clinical guidelines are provided (151). The ability to drive is an important determinant of quality of life; however, although prohibition from driving is a major inconvenience, safety must be the most important consideration. Arrhythmia-induced impairment of consciousness during driving could harm the patient or others. ◥ m67

Most U.S. states do not have specific laws governing driving by ICD patients. A joint statement by the American Heart Association and the North American Society of Pacing and Electrophysiology (154) advised that patients who had ICDs implanted for sustained ventricular tachyarrhythmias refrain from private driving for 6 months after implantation and for 6 months after each subsequent shock. [In survivors of VT or VF, the risk of arrhythmia recurrence is higher soon after an index event and decreases to <0.7% per month after the seventh month (155).] Noncommercial driving should not be restricted in patients who receive ICDs for prophylactic indications. Commercial driving should be prohibited entirely in ICD patients. Slightly different recommendations have been issued by the Working Groups on Cardiac Pacing and Arrhythmias of the European Society of Cardiology (156). These restrictions could represent a hardship, especially for patients with sporadic nonsyncopal arrhythmias that trigger single shocks that do not warrant pharmacologic suppression, who may

display low compliance (157). Many ICD patients resume driving early, against physician recommendations, but they tend to drive only when absolutely necessary, avoiding rush hour, highways, and night driving (158). ◥ m68

Patients frequently ask about the risks of electromagnetic radiation sources they may encounter during daily life (161). Microwave ovens represent no hazard. When traveling, patients should notify airport security personnel that they have an ICD. It is not dangerous to walk through the security gate as instructed, although it may detect the metal device. A quick pass of the hand-held weapon detector is innocuous, but prolonged exposure to its magnetic field should be avoided. Cellular telephones are unlikely to interact deleteriously with ICDs. However, it has been recommended that patients not carry or place cellular telephones within 15 cm (6 in.) of an ICD, to minimize risks. Walking through electronic antitheft devices at a normal pace has no consequences, but prolonged exposure can result in pacing inhibition, spurious shocks, or both (162).

Management of Emergencies

Guidelines for the management of medical emergencies in ICD patients have been published (163,164). Patients with ICDs should carry identification cards with information about the manufacturer, model, and lead system of the ICD and a 24-hour emergency contact telephone number. An overpenetrated radiograph including the generator permits identification of the model by a radiopaque identifier. During emergencies, placement of a magnet on top of the device when the specific programmer is not readily available can temporarily disable recognition and treatment of tachyarrhythmias. The magnetic field closes a reed switch in the generator circuit, triggering a response that differs among models. In general, tachyarrhythmia recognition and treatment is disabled as long as the magnet remains close to the generator. Pacing is not affected. ◥ m69

Multiple defibrillator discharges within a short period require prompt attention (eFig. 75.5.5). Multiple shocks can be a manifestation of ICD system failure; can result in significant battery drainage, leading to premature depletion; and may produce psychological morbidity. Accurate diagnosis is needed for correct management (eTable 75.2.1). Initial evaluation of patients with multiple ICD shocks should be performed in a setting in which electrocardiographic monitoring and advanced cardiac resuscitation are possible. The device should be interrogated as soon as possible. Detailed event logging and storage of interval-by-interval cycle length data and intracardiac electrograms of detected tachyarrhythmias facilitate the diagnosis. Electrical storm (i.e., frequently recurring VT or VF) occurs in 10% of patients (166). Patients with electrical storm should be admitted to an intensive care unit. Sympathetic blockade and intravenous amiodarone are often effective in treating this condition (167). If spurious firing is documented, the ICD should be deactivated and the patient placed under continuous electrocardiographic monitoring. Consultation with the cardiac electrophysiologist is required for definitive treatment (reprogramming or hardware revision). The ICD should be reactivated only after the condition that triggered the spurious shocks is controlled.

Many diagnostic and therapeutic procedures involve sources of electromagnetic radiation that could affect ICD function (161). Possible effects include cessation or intermittent delivery of antibradycardia pacing, inadvertent delivery of antitachycardia therapy, resetting of programmed parameters, and damage to the pulse generator, the tissues interfacing with the electrodes, or both. Most diagnostic and therapeutic maneuvers, including electrosurgery, shock wave lithotripsy (168), electroconvulsive therapy (169), and most imaging methods, can be safely performed under continuous electrocardiographic monitoring in ICD patients. Trained personnel should be readily available to deactivate the device before the procedure and to reactivate it and confirm that it is operating appropriately afterward. Magnetic resonance imaging is contraindicated in ICD patients because of the very strong electromagnetic fields involved.

CONTROVERSIES AND PERSONAL PERSPECTIVES

Knowledge about basic electrophysiologic mechanisms is accumulating rapidly. However, despite advances in the understanding of the structure and function of cardiac ion channels (177), the electrophysiologic heterogeneity of myocardial cells (178), and the fundamental mechanisms of reentry (179), clinical applications remain scarce (180,181). The development of widely effective and safe gene (182), pharmacologic, or ablative therapies for ventricular arrhythmias is not likely in the foreseeable future. In the long run, the best strategy for preventing sudden cardiac death will be the prevention of coronary artery disease and its sequelae. We believe that, in the meantime, ICDs will become a key clinical tool in the fight against sudden death.

During the next decade, progress in ICD therapy will occur on both the clinical and technological fronts. Primary prevention trials will identify additional populations who will benefit from ICD implantation. Current validated indications restrict prophylactic use to patients with previous myocardial infarction and are based on inducibility of VT at invasive electrophysiologic study. Identification of ICD candidates with other substrates and with noninvasive methods could greatly expand the application of this therapy. If that is the case, the cost-effectiveness of ICDs will be very carefully scrutinized. In view of the potential allocation of scarce resources to diverse therapies and populations, society will have to decide the extent to which ICDs should be used.

Two avenues have been proposed to improve cost-effectiveness: more refined risk-stratification (183) (cost-effectiveness should be most favorable in patients at high risk for sudden death but at low risk of dying from competing causes) and reduced costs. It is quite apparent that not all patients with ventricular tachyarrhythmias have the same prognosis (69). The pooled AVID/CIDS/CASH analysis showed significantly higher benefit in patients with severe left ventricular dysfunction (44). The CIDS investigators devised a clinical prediction rule to identify patients likely to benefit from ICD therapy that included two or three of the following: age ≥70 years, left ventricular ejection fraction ≤0.35, and New York Heart Association class III or IV (184). However, post hoc prediction rules should not be accepted without prospective validation. When the same rule was applied to the AVID population, it lacked discriminatory power (185). It is likely that the relationship between severity of heart disease and benefit from ICD has an inverted U shape. Patients with severe (but not end-stage) heart disease should benefit the most, but patients with severe heart failure and those with almost normal heart function will benefit less. However, specific thresholds for identifying patients who will not benefit are unlikely. Furthermore, patients who have life-threatening ventricular arrhythmias but mild structural heart disease have a low risk of dying from competing causes, and a survival benefit should be apparent with longer follow-up.

It has been speculated that manufacturers could make prophylactic ICD therapy more cost-attractive by making stripped-down devices available (i.e., single-chamber shock-only units capable of delivering only a limited number of shocks and with shorter longevity) at a significant discount. However, we foresee strong resistance from clinicians in the United States to implanting suboptimal hardware that could require premature replacement in at least some patients. The approach may be more viable in countries with centralized financing of health care.

Paradoxically, the ICD may help to develop safe and effective pharmacologic therapies by providing a safety net in randomized clinical trials of new antiarrhythmic drugs (186). Advances in storage, retrieval, and accurate interpretation of ICD electrograms may allow the use of an ICD end point as a clinical surrogate for sudden death. However, the extent to which the results of data on antiarrhythmic drug efficacy and safety acquired in the context of an ICD endpoint trial might be extrapolated to patients not using the device is controversial.

The debate over whether surgical or medical practitioners should be providers of ICD therapy has been largely settled, and, at least in the United States, cardiac electrophysiologists now perform most implants (187). However, because of the broadly accepted indications and the ease of implantation, the debate has now shifted within the cardiology community as cardiologists without spe-

THE FUTURE

ICD technology will continue to evolve. The next generation of devices will be smaller, owing to improvements in battery and capacitor technology and optimization of shock waveforms and electrodes. Emphasis will be placed on decreasing the complexity of programming, device interrogation, and patient monitoring during routine patient follow-up. The addition of sensors to assess the hemodynamic impact of tachyarrhythmias will further refine therapy delivery and eradicate spurious device interventions. Continuous monitoring for myocardial ischemia (192), subtle hemodynamic decompensation (193), and electrical instability (194) will be feasible. The device could warn the patient, automatically transmit data to a Web-based server accessible by authorized health care staff, and then initiate corrective action. The capability to intervene before an arrhythmia occurs is particularly desirable (195).

Future research should produce reliable methods of predicting impending VT or VF. VF may be a form of deterministic chaos whose development is compatible with the quasiperiodic route seen in fluid dynamics (196). Potential preventive interventions include multisite pacing (197,198), pacing algorithms aimed at the suppression of long-short cardiac cycle sequences (199), subthreshold stimulation of arrhythmogenic tissues exploiting the phenomenon of cardiac inhibition (200), and the timely infusion of antiarrhythmic or antiadrenergic agents via a venous port. Specific pacing algorithms also have the potential to prevent atrial fibrillation. During the next decade, we will witness the culmination of the evolution of the ICD from a "shock-box" to a smart, multimodal monitoring, communications, and therapeutic unit.

cific electrophysiology training have begun to indicate ICD treatment, implant the devices, and follow up after implantation in some institutions (188). The body of knowledge and the experience for such practices have been promulgated by professional organizations, and the implementation of ICD therapy by unqualified practitioners should be viewed with great concern. For example, training guidelines for ICD implantation from the American College of Cardiology require that a clinician perform 20 procedures as the primary operator, and they also consider the maintenance of established competence critical (189). For pacemaker implantation, inexperience (e.g., performance of fewer than 12 implants per year) is the main determinant of surgical complications (190), and a similar association can be expected for ICDs. The availability of systems with very different capabilities, from the simple single-chamber unit to the complex combined atrioventricular defibrillators or triple-chamber units that provide resynchronization therapy, makes understanding the value and limitations of these devices in relation to the individual patient's needs crucial.

The increasing versatility of the devices has made programming and troubleshooting complicated and time-consuming. The untrained physician who is a "casual" follower of ICDs may rely excessively on the expertise of manufacturer representatives to determine appropriate device function. This practice is questionable on both medical and ethical grounds and cannot guarantee optimal results (191). As stated by professional organizations, cardiac electrophysiologists should prescribe the type of ICD, be involved in the implant, and provide follow-up care of ICD patients (57).

REFERENCES

1. Mirowski M, Mower MM. The automatic implantable defibrillator: some historical notes. In: Brugada P, Wellens HJJ, eds. *Cardiac arrhythmias: where to go from here?* Mount Kisco, NY: Futura Publishing, 1987:655–661.
2. Kastor JA. Michel Mirowski and the automatic implantable defibrillator. *Am J Cardiol* 1989;63:977–982; 1121–1126.
3. Lown B, Axelrod P. Implanted standby defibrillators. *Circulation* 1972;46:637–639.
4. Mirowski M, Reid PR, Mower MM, et al. Termination of malignant ventricular arrhythmias with an implanted automatic defibrillator in human beings. *N Engl J Med* 1980;303:322–324.
5. Saksena S, Parsonnet V. Implantation of a cardioverter/defibrillator without thoracotomy using a triple electrode system. *JAMA* 1988;259:69–72.
6. Kroll MW, Lehmann MH, eds. *Implantable cardioverter-defibrillator therapy: the engineering-clinical interface.* Norwell, MA: Kluwer Academic Publishers, 1996.
7. Lang DJ, Heil JE, Hahn SJ, et al. Implantable cardioverter defibrillator lead technology: improved performance and lower defibrillation thresholds. *Pacing Clin Electrophysiol* 1995;18:548–559.
8. Menz V, Schwartzman D, Drachman D, et al. Recording of pacing stimulus artifacts by endovascular defibrillation lead systems: comparison of true and integrated bipolar circuits. *J Interv Card Electrophysiol* 1998;2:269–272.
9. Fye WB. Ventricular fibrillation and defibrillation: historical perspectives with emphasis on the contributions of John MacWilliam, Carl Wiggers, and William Kouwenhoven. *Circulation* 1985;71:858–865.
10. Wiggers CJ. The mechanism and nature of ventricular fibrillation. *Am Heart J* 1940;20:399–412.
11. Chen P-S, Wolf P, Dixon EG, et al. Mechanism of ventricu-

lar vulnerability to single premature stimuli in open chest dogs. *Circ Res* 1988;62:1191–1209.

12. Bonometti C, Hwang C, Hough D, et al. Interaction between strong electrical stimulation and reentrant wavefronts in canine ventricular fibrillation. *Circ Res* 1995;77:407–416.

13. Lee JJ, Kamjoo K, Hough D, et al. Reentrant wave fronts in Wiggers' stage II ventricular fibrillation: characteristics and mechanisms of termination and spontaneous regeneration. *Circ Res* 1996;78:660–675.

14. Davy JM, Fain ES, Dorian P, et al. The relationship between successful defibrillation and delivered energy in open-chest dogs: reappraisal of the "defibrillation threshold" concept. *Am Heart J* 1987;113:77–84.

15. Singer I, Lang D. The defibrillation threshold. In: Kroll MW, Lehmann MH, eds. *Implantable cardioverter-defibrillator therapy: the engineering-clinical interface.* Norwell, MA: Kluwer Academic Publishers, 1997:89–129.

16. Chen P-S, Wolf P, Claydon FJ, et al. The potential gradient field created by epicardial defibrillation electrodes in dogs. *Circulation* 1986;74:626–636.

17. Roth BJ, Krassowska W. The induction of reentry in cardiac tissue. The missing link: how electrical fields alter transmembrane potential. *Chaos* 1998;8:221–233.

18. Dillon SM. Synchronized repolarization after defibrillation shocks: a possible component of the defibrillation process demonstrated by optical recordings in rabbit heart. *Circulation* 1992;85:1865–1878.

19. Efimov IR, Gray RA, Roth BJ. Virtual electrodes and deexcitation: new insights into fibrillation induction and defibrillation. *J Cardiovasc Electrophysiol* 2000;11:339–353.

20. Chen P-S, Shibata N, Wolf P, et al. Activation during ventricular defibrillation in open-chest dogs: evidence of complete cessation and regeneration of ventricular fibrillation after unsuccessful shocks. *J Clin Invest* 1986;77:810–823.

21. Zhou X, Daubert JP, Wolf PD, et al. Epicardial mapping of ventricular defibrillation with monophasic and biphasic shocks in dogs. *Circ Res* 1993;72:145–160.

22. Chen P-S, Wolf PD, Melnick SD, et al. Comparison of activation during ventricular fibrillation and following unsuccessful defibrillation shocks in open chest dogs. *Circ Res* 1990;66:1544–1560.

23. Cha Y-M, Peters BB, Chen P-S. The effects of lidocaine on the vulnerable period during ventricular fibrillation. *J Cardiovasc Electrophysiol* 1994;5:571–580.

24. Zipes DP, Fischer J, King RM, et al. Termination of ventricular fibrillation in dogs by depolarizing a critical amount of myocardium. *Am J Cardiol* 1975;36:37–44.

25. Chen P-S, Swerdlow CD, Hwang C, et al. Current concepts of ventricular defibrillation. *J Cardiovasc Electrophysiol* 1998;84:553–562.

26. Chen P-S, Shibata N, Dixon EG, et al. Comparison of the defibrillation threshold and the upper limit of ventricular vulnerability. *Circulation* 1986;73:1022–1028.

27. Chen P-S, Feld GK, Kriett JM, et al. Relation between upper limit of vulnerability and defibrillation threshold in humans. *Circulation* 1993;88:186–192.

28. Hwang C, Fan W, Chen P-S. Recurrent appearance of protective zones after an unsuccessful defibrillation shock. *Am J Physiol* 1996;4:H1491–H1497.

29. Ideker RE, Hillsley RE, Wharton JM. Shock strength for the implantable defibrillator: can you have too much of a good thing? *Pacing Clin Electrophysiol* 1992;15:841–844.

30. Hillsley RE, Wharton JM, Cates AW, et al. Why do some patients have high defibrillation thresholds at defibrillator implantation? Answers from basic research. *Pacing Clin Electrophysiol* 1994;17:222–239.

31. Block M, Hammel D, Böcker D, et al. A prospective randomized cross-over comparison of mono- and biphasic defibrillation using nonthoracotomy lead configurations in humans. *J Cardiovasc Electrophysiol* 1994;5:581–590.

32. Swerdlow CD, Fan W, Brewer JE. Charge-burping theory correctly predicts optimal ratios of phase duration for biphasic defibrillation waveforms. *Circulation* 1996;94:2278–2284.

33. Swerdlow CD, Kass RM, Chen P, et al. Effect of capacitor size and pathway resistance on defibrillation threshold for implantable defibrillators. *Circulation* 1994;90:1840–1846.

34. Oral H, Gold MR, Patel S, et al. Clinical predictors of a high implant defibrillation threshold in patients with a transvenous biphasic active-can ICD. *Circulation* 2000;102[Supp1]:II-439(abst).

35. Connolly SJ, Yusuf S. Evaluation of the implantable cardioverter-defibrillator in survivors of cardiac arrest: the need for randomized trials. *Am J Cardiol* 1992;69:959–962.

36. Saksena S, Madan N, Lewis C. Implantable cardioverter-defibrillators are preferable to drugs as primary therapy in sustained ventricular tachyarrhythmias. *Prog Cardiovasc Dis* 1996;38:445–454.

37. The CASCADE Investigators. Cardiac Arrest in Seattle: Conventional versus Amiodarone Drug Evaluation (The CASCADE Study). *Am J Cardiol* 1991;67:578–584.

38. Mason JW. A comparison of seven antiarrhythmic drugs in patients with ventricular tachyarrhythmias. Electrophysiologic Study versus Electrocardiographic Monitoring Investigators. *N Engl J Med* 1993;329:452–458.

39. The Antiarrhythmics versus Implantable Defibrillators (AVID) Investigators. A comparison of antiarrhythmic-drug therapy with implantable defibrillators in patients resuscitated from near-fatal ventricular arrhythmias. *N Engl J Med* 1997;337:1576–1583.

40. The AVID Investigators. Causes of death in the Antiarrhythmics Versus Implantable Defibrillators (AVID) Trial. *J Am Coll Cardiol* 1999;34:1552–1559.

41. Anderson JL, Hallstrom AP, Epstein AE, et al. Design and results of the Antiarrhythmics vs. Implantable Defibrillators (AVID) Registry. The AVID Investigators. *Circulation* 1999;99:1692–1699.

42. Kuck KH, Cappato R, Siebels J, et al. Randomized comparison of antiarrhythmic drug therapy with implantable defibrillators in patients resuscitated from cardiac arrest: the Cardiac Arrest Study Hamburg. *Circulation* 2000;102:748–754.

43. Connolly SJ, Gent M, Roberts RS, et al. Canadian implantable defibrillator study (CIDS): a randomized trial of the implantable cardioverter defibrillator against amiodarone. *Circulation* 2000;101:1297–1302.

44. Connolly SJ, Hallstrom AP, Cappato R, et al. Meta-analysis of the implantable cardioverter defibrillator secondary prevention trials. *Eur Heart J* 2000;21:2071–2078.

45. Myerburg RJ, Kessler KM, Castellanos A. Sudden cardiac death: structure function, and time-dependence of risk. *Circulation* 1992; 85[Suppl I]:I2–I10.

46. Moss AJ, Hall WJ, Cannom DS, et al. Improved survival with an implanted defibrillator in patients with coronary disease at high risk for ventricular arrhythmia. *N Engl J Med* 1996;335:1933–1940.

47. Buxton AE, Lee KL, Fisher JD, et al. A randomized study of the prevention of sudden death in patients with coronary artery disease [erratum appears in *N Engl J Med* 2000;342:1300]. *N Engl J Med* 1999;341:1882–1890.

48. Bigger JT Jr. Prophylactic use of implanted cardiac defibrillators in patients at risk for ventricular arrhythmias after coronary artery bypass graft surgery. Coronary Artery Bypass Graft (CABG) Patch Trial Investigators. *N Engl J Med* 1997;337:1569–1575.

49. Strickberger SA. Presented at the 73rd American Heart Association Scientific Sessions, New Orleans, LA, November 2000.

50. Bigger JT Jr, Whang W, Rottman JN, et al. Mechanisms of death in the CABG Patch trial: a randomized trial of implantable cardiac defibrillator prophylaxis in patients at high risk of death after coronary artery bypass graft surgery. *Circulation* 1999;99:1416–1421.

51. Moss AJ, Cannom DS, Daubert JP. Multicenter Automatic Defibrillator Implantation Trial II (MADIT II): design and clinical protocol. *Ann Noninvasive Electrocardiol* 1999;4:83–91.

52. Raviele A, Bongiorni MG, Brignole M, et al. Which strategy is "best" after myocardial infarction? The Beta-Blocker Strategy plus Implantable Cardioverter Defibrillator Trial: rationale and study design. *Am J Cardiol* 1999;83:104D–111D.

53. Hohnloser SH, Connolly SJ, Kuck KH, et al. The Defibrillator in Acute Myocardial Infarction Trial (DINAMIT): study protocol. *Am Heart J* 2000;140:735–739.

54. Bardy GH. The Sudden Cardiac Death–Heart Failure Trial (SCD-HeFT). In: Woosley RL, Singh SN, eds. *Arrhythmia treatment and therapy: evaluation of clinical trial evidence.* Marcel Dekker, New York, 2000:323–342.

55. Bristow MR, Feldman AM, Saxon LA, et al. Heart failure management using implantable devices for ventricular resynchronization: Comparison of Medical Therapy, Pacing, and Defibrillation in Chronic Heart Failure (COMPANION) trial. COMPANION Steering Committee and COMPANION Clinical Investigators. *J Card Fail* 2000;6:276–285.

56. Kadish A, Quigg R, Schaechter A, et al. Defibrillators in nonischemic cardiomyopathy treatment evaluation. *Pacing Clin Electrophysiol* 2000;23:338–343.

57. Gregoratos G, Cheitlin MD, Conill A, et al. ACC/AHA guidelines for implantation of cardiac pacemakers and antiarrhythmia devices: a report of the American College of Cardiology/American Heart Association Task Force on Practice Guidelines (Committee on Pacemaker Implantation). *J Am Coll Cardiol* 1998;31:1175–1209.

58. Maron BJ, Shen WK, Link MS, et al. Efficacy of implantable cardioverter-defibrillators for the prevention of sudden death in patients with hypertrophic cardiomyopathy. *N Engl J Med* 2000;342:365–373.

59. Moss AJ, Zareba W, Hall WJ, et al. Effectiveness and limitations of beta-blocker therapy in congenital long-QT syndrome. *Circulation* 2000;101:616–623.

60. Gussak I, Antzelevitch C, Bjerregaard P, et al. The Brugada syndrome: clinical, electrophysiologic and genetic aspects. *J Am Coll Cardiol* 1999;33:5–15.

61. Silka MJ, Kron J, Dunnigan A, et al. Sudden cardiac death and the use of implantable cardioverter-defibrillator in pediatric patients. *Circulation* 1993;87:800–807.

62. Link MS, Costeas XF, Griffith JL, et al. High incidence of appropriate implantable cardioverter-defibrillator therapy in patients with syncope of unknown etiology and inducible ventricular arrhythmias. *J Am Coll Cardiol* 1997;29:370–375.

63. Menon V, Steinberg JS, Akiyama T, et al. Implantable cardioverter defibrillator discharge rates in patients with unexplained syncope, structural heart disease, and inducible ventricular tachycardia at electrophysiologic study. *Clin Cardiol* 2000;23:195–200.

64. Knight BP, Goyal R, Pelosi F, et al. Outcome of patients with nonischemic dilated cardiomyopathy and unexplained syncope treated with an implantable defibrillator. *J Am Coll Cardiol* 1999;33:1964–1970.

65. Santucci PA, Bredikis AJ, Pinski SL, et al. Low incidence of ICD shocks in patients with cardiomyopathy and syncope associated with nondiagnostic electrophysiology study. *Pacing Clin Electrophysiol* 1999;22:801(abst).

66. Fonarow GC, Feliciano Z, Boyle NG, et al. Improved survival in patients with nonischemic advanced heart failure and syncope treated with an implantable cardioverter-defibrillator. *Am J Cardiol* 2000;85:981–985.

67. Sarter BH, Finkle JK, Gerszten RE, et al. What is the risk of sudden cardiac death in patients presenting with hemodynamically stable sustained ventricular tachycardia after myocardial infarction? *J Am Coll Cardiol* 1996;28:122–129.

68. Böcker D, Block M, Isbruch F, et al. Benefits of treatment with implantable cardioverter-defibrillators in patients with stable ventricular tachycardia. *Br Heart J* 1995;73:158–163.

69. Pinski SL, Yao Q, Epstein AA, et al. Determinants of outcome in patients with sustained ventricular tachyarrhythmias: The Antiarrhythmics versus Implantable Defibrillators (AVID) Study Registry. *Am Heart J* 2000;139:804–813.

70. Rothman SA, Hsia HH, Cossu SF, et al. Radiofrequency catheter ablation of postinfarction ventricular tachycardia: long-term success and the significance of inducible nonclinical arrhythmias. *Circulation* 1997;96:3499–3508.

71. Strickberger SA, Man KC, Daoud EG, et al. A prospective evaluation of catheter ablation of ventricular tachycardia as adjuvant therapy in patients with coronary artery disease and an implantable cardioverter-defibrillator. *Circulation* 1997;96:1525–1531.

72. Pinski SL, Mick MJ, Arnold AZ, et al. Retrospective analysis of patients undergoing one- or two-stage strategies for myocardial revascularization and implantable cardioverter-defibrillator implantation. *Pacing Clin Electrophysiol* 1991;14:1138–1147.

73. Daoud EG, Niebauer M, Kou WH, et al. Incidence of implantable defibrillator discharges after coronary revascularization in survivors of ischemic sudden cardiac death. *Am Heart J* 1995;130:277–280.

74. Schmidinger H. The implantable cardioverter defibrillator as a "bridge to transplant": a viable clinical strategy? *Am J Cardiol* 1999;83:151D–157D.

75. Strickberger SA, Hummel JD, Daoud E, et al. Implantation by electrophysiologists of 100 consecutive cardioverter defibrillators with nonthoracotomy lead systems. *Circulation* 1994;90:868–872.

76. Strickberger SA, Niebauer M, Man KC, et al. Comparison of implantation of nonthoracotomy defibrillators in the operating room versus the electrophysiology laboratory. *Am J Cardiol* 1995;75:255–257.

77. Pacifico A, Cedillo-Salazar FR, Nasir N Jr, et al. Conscious sedation with combined hypnotic agents for implantation of implantable cardioverter-defibrillators. *J Am Coll Cardiol* 1997;30:769–773.

78. Stix G, Anvari A, Podesser B, et al. Local anaesthesia versus general anaesthesia for cardioverter-defibrillator implantation. *Wien Klin Wochenschr* 1999;111:406–409.

79. Gold MR, Olsovsky MR, DeGroot PJ, et al. Optimization of transvenous coil position for active can defibrillation thresholds. *J Cardiovasc Electrophysiol* 2000;11:25–29.

80. Jung W, Wolpert C, Esmailzadeh B, et al. Clinical experience with implantable atrial and combined atrioventricular defibrillators. *J Interv Card Electrophysiol* 2000;4[Suppl 1]:185–195.

81. Cooklin M, Olsovsky MR, Brockman RG, et al. Atrial defibrillation with a transvenous lead: a randomized comparison of active can shocking pathways. *J Am Coll Cardiol* 1999;34:358–362.

82. Ayers GM. New concepts in atrial defibrillation. *J Interv Card Electrophysiol* 2000;4[Suppl 1]:155–161.

83. Pürerfellner H, Nesser HJ, Winter S, et al. Transvenous left ventricular lead implantation with the EASYTRAK lead system: the European experience. *Am J Cardiol* 2000;86:157K–164K.

84. Manolis AS, Chiladakis J, Vassilikos V, et al. Pectoral cardioverter defibrillators: comparison of prepectoral and submuscular implantation techniques. *Pacing Clin Electrophysiol* 1999;22:469–478.

85. Epstein AE, Kay GN, Plumb VJ, et al. Elevated defibrillation threshold when right-sided venous access is used for nonthoracotomy implantable defibrillator lead implantation. *J Cardiovasc Electrophysiol* 1995;6:979–986.

86. Ellenbogen KA, Wood MA, Stambler BS, et al. Measurement of ventricular electrogram amplitude during intraoperative induction of ventricular tachyarrhythmias. *Am J Cardiol* 1992;70:1017–1022.

87. Runsio M, Bergfeldt L, Brodin LA, et al. Left ventricular function after repeated episodes of ventricular fibrillation and defibrillation assessed by transoesophageal echocardiography. *Eur Heart J* 1997;18:124–131.

88. Hwang C, Swerdlow CD, Kass RM, et al. Upper limit of vulnerability reliably predicts the defibrillation threshold in humans. *Circulation* 1994;90:2308–2314.

89. Rosenqvist M, Beyer T, Block M, et al. Adverse events with transvenous implantable cardioverter-defibrillators: a prospective multicenter study [erratum appears in *Circulation* 1998;98:2647]. *Circulation* 1998;98:663–670.

90. Michaud GF, Pelosi F Jr, Noble MD, et al. A randomized trial comparing heparin initiation 6 h or 24 h after pacemaker or defibrillator implantation. *J Am Coll Cardiol* 2000;35:1915–1918.

91. Kron J, Herre J, Graham Renfroe E, et al. Lead- and device-related complications in the Antiarrhythmics Versus Implantable Defibrillators Trial. *Am Heart J* 2001;141:92–98.

92. O'Nunain S, Perez I, Roelke M, et al. The treatment of patients with infected implantable cardioverter-defibrillator systems. *J Thorac Cardiovasc Surg* 1997;73:121–129.

93. Chua JD, Wilkoff BL, Lee I, et al. Diagnosis and management of infections involving implantable electrophysiologic cardiac devices. *Ann Intern Med* 2000;133:604–608.

94. Love CJ, Wilkoff BL, Byrd CL, et al. Recommendations for extraction of chronically implanted transvenous pacing and defibrillator leads: indications, facilities, training. *Pacing Clin Electrophysiol* 2000;23:544–551.

95. Epstein LM, Byrd CL, Wilkoff BL, et al. Initial experience with larger laser sheaths for the removal of transvenous pacemaker and implantable defibrillator leads. *Circulation* 1999;100:516–525.

96. Spotnitz HM, Herre JM, Raza ST, et al. Effect of implantable cardioverter-defibrillator implantation on surgical morbidity in the CABG Patch Trial. *Circulation* 1998;98[19 Suppl]:II77–II80.

97. Rosenqvist M. Antitachycardia pacing: which patients and which methods? *Am J Cardiol* 1996;78(5A):92–97.

98. Bardy GH, Poole JE, Kudenchuck PJ, et al. A prospective randomized repeat-crossover comparison of antitachycardia pacing with low-energy cardioversion. *Circulation* 1993;87:1889–1896.

99. Mann DE, Kelly PA, Robertson AD, et al. Significant differences in charge times among currently available implantable cardioverter defibrillators. *Pacing Clin Electrophysiol* 1999;22:903–907.

100. Swerdlow CD, Peter CT, Kass RM, et al. Programming of implantable cardioverter-defibrillators on the basis of the upper limit of vulnerability. *Circulation* 1997;95:1497–1504.

101. Neuzner J, Liebrich A, Jung J, et al. Safety and efficacy of implantable defibrillator therapy with programmed shock energy at twice the augmented step-down defibrillation threshold: results of the prospective, randomized, multicenter Low-Energy Endotak Trial. *Am J Cardiol* 1999;83:34D–39D.

102. Raitt MH, Dolack GL, Kudenchuk PJ, et al. Ventricular arrhythmias detected after transvenous defibrillator implantation in patients with a clinical history of only ventricular fibrillation: implications for use of implantable defibrillator. *Circulation* 1995;91:1996–2001.

103. Reiter MJ, Mann DE. Sensing and tachyarrhythmia detection problems in patients with implantable cardioverter defibrillators. *J Cardiovasc Electrophysiol* 1996;7:542–558.

104. Natale A, Sra J, Axtell K, et al. Undetected ventricular fibrillation in transvenous implantable cardioverter-defibrillators: prospective comparison of different lead system–device combinations. *Circulation* 1996;93:91–98.

105. Swerdlow CD, Chen P-S, Kass RM, et al. Discrimination of ventricular tachycardia from sinus tachycardia and atrial fibrillation in a tiered-therapy cardioverter-defibrillator. *J Am Coll Cardiol* 1994;23:1342–1355.

106. Swerdlow CD, Ahern T, Chen P-S, et al. Underdetection of ventricular tachycardia by algorithms to enhance specificity

in a tiered-therapy cardioverter-defibrillator. *J Am Coll Cardiol* 1994;24:416–424.

107. Unterberg C, Stevens J, Vollmann D, et al. Long-term clinical experience with the EGM width detection criterion for differentiation of supraventricular and ventricular tachycardia in patients with implantable cardioverter defibrillators. *Pacing Clin Electrophysiol* 2000;23:1611–1617.

108. Weber M, Böcker D, Bansch D, et al. Efficacy and safety of the initial use of stability and onset criteria in implantable cardioverter defibrillators. *J Cardiovasc Electrophysiol* 1999;10:145–153.

109. Nair M, Saoudi N, Kroiss D, et al. Automatic arrhythmia identification using analysis of the atrioventricular association: application to a new generation of implantable defibrillators. *Circulation* 1997;95:967–973.

110. Kuhlkamp V, Dornberger V, Mewis C, et al. Clinical experience with the new detection algorithms for atrial fibrillation of a defibrillator with dual chamber pacing and sensing. *J Cardiovasc Electrophysiol* 1999;10:905–915.

111. Higgins SL, Williams SK, Pak JP, et al. Indications for implantation of a dual-chamber pacemaker combined with an implantable cardioverter-defibrillator. *Am J Cardiol* 1998;81:1360–1362.

112. Best PJM, Hayes DL, Stanton MS. The potential usage of dual chamber pacing in patients with implantable cardioverter-defibrillators. *Pacing Clin Electrophysiol* 1999;22:79–85.

113. Jung W, Lüderitz B. Should all candidates for ICD therapy receive a dual-chamber system? *J Interv Card Electrophysiol* 1999;3:203–206.

114. Pinski SL, Trohman RG. Permanent pacing via implantable defibrillators. *Pacing Clin Electrophysiol* 2000;23:1667–1682.

115. Pinski SL, Fahy GJ. The proarrhythmic potential of implantable defibrillators. *Circulation* 1995;92:1651–1664.

116. Olatidoye AG, Verroneau J, Kluger J. Mechanisms of syncope in implantable cardioverter-defibrillator recipients who receive device therapies. *Am J Cardiol* 1998;82:1372–1376.

117. Wilbur SL, Marchlinski FE. Implantable cardioverter-defibrillator follow-up: what everyone needs to know. *Cardiol Rev* 1999;7:176–190.

118. Drucker EA, Brooks R, Garan H, et al. Malfunction of implantable cardioverter-defibrillators placed by a nonthoracotomy approach: frequency of malfunction and value of chest radiography in determining cause. *AJR Am J Roentgenol* 1995;165:275–279.

119. Lurie KG, Iskos D, Fetter J, et al. Prehospital discharge defibrillation testing in ICD recipients: a prospective study based on cost analysis. *Pacing Clin Electrophysiol* 1999;22[1 Pt 2]:192–196.

120. Brunn J, Bocker D, Weber M, et al. Is there a need for routine testing of ICD defibrillation capacity? Results from more than 1000 studies. *Eur Heart J* 2000;21:162–169.

121. Schaumann A, von zur Mühlen F, Herse B, et al. Empirical versus tested antitachycardia pacing in implantable cardioverter defibrillators: a prospective study including 200 patients. *Circulation* 1998;97:66–74.

122. Pinski SL, Simmons TW, Maloney JD. Troubleshooting antitachycardia pacing in patients with defibrillators. In: Estes NAM, Wang P, Manolis A, eds. *Implantable cardio-*

123. Reiter MJ, Fain ES, Senelly KM, et al. Predictors of device activation for ventricular arrhythmias and survival in patients with implantable pacemaker/defibrillators. *Pacing Clin Electrophysiol* 1994;17:1487–1498.

124. Grimm W, Flores BT, Marchlinski FE. Shock occurrence and survival in 241 patients with implantable cardioverter-defibrillator therapy. *Circulation* 1993;87:1880–1888.

125. Englund A, Behrens S, Wegscheider K, et al. Circadian variation of malignant ventricular arrhythmias in patients with ischemic and nonischemic heart disease after cardioverter defibrillator implantation. *J Am Coll Cardiol* 1999;34:1560–1568.

126. Pacifico A, Ferlic LL, Cedillo-Salazar FR, et al. Shocks as predictors of survival in patients with implantable cardioverter-defibrillators. *J Am Coll Cardiol* 1999;34:204–210.

127. Exner DV, Pinski SL, Wyse DG, et al. Electrical storm presages nonsudden death: the Antiarrhythmics Versus Implantable Defibrillators (AVID) Trial. *Circulation* 2001;103:2066–2071.

128. Bänsch D, Böcker D, Brunn J, et al. Clusters of ventricular tachycardias signify impaired survival in patients with idiopathic dilated cardiomyopathy and implantable cardioverter defibrillators. *J Am Coll Cardiol* 2000;36:566–573.

129. Page RL. Effects of antiarrhythmic medication on implantable cardioverter-defibrillator function. *Am J Cardiol* 2000;85:1481–1485.

130. Pacifico A, Hohnloser SH, Williams JH, et al. Prevention of implantable-defibrillator shocks by treatment with sotalol. D,L-Sotalol Implantable Cardioverter-Defibrillator Study Group. *N Engl J Med* 1999;340:1855–1862.

131. Seidl K, Hauer B, Schwick NG, et al. Comparison of metoprolol and sotalol in preventing ventricular tachyarrhythmias after the implantation of a cardioverter/defibrillator. *Am J Cardiol* 1998;82:744–748.

132. Dolack GL. Clinical predictors of implantable cardioverter-defibrillator shocks (results of the CASCADE trial). Cardiac Arrest in Seattle, Conventional versus Amiodarone Drug Evaluation. *Am J Cardiol* 1994;73:237–241.

133. Echt DS, Gremillion ST, Lee JT, et al. Effects of procainamide and lidocaine on defibrillation energy requirements in patients receiving implantable cardioverter defibrillator devices. *J Cardiovasc Electrophysiol* 1994;5:752–760.

134. Pelosi F Jr, Oral H, Kim MH, et al. Effect of chronic amiodarone therapy on defibrillation energy requirements in humans. *J Cardiovasc Electrophysiol* 2000;11:736–740.

135. Bänsch D, Castrucci M, Bocker D, et al. Ventricular tachycardias above the initially programmed tachycardia detection interval in patients with implantable cardioverter-defibrillators: incidence, prediction and significance. *J Am Coll Cardiol* 2000;36:557–565.

136. Lawton JS, Wood MA, Gilligan DM, et al. Implantable transvenous cardioverter-defibrillator leads: the dark side. *Pacing Clin Electrophysiol* 1996;19:1273–1278.

137. Roelke M, O'Nunain SS, Osswald S, et al. Subclavian crush syndrome complicating transvenous cardioverter defibrillator systems. *Pacing Clin Electrophysiol* 1995;18:973–979.

138. Dijkman B, Wellens HJ. Dual chamber arrhythmia detection in the implantable cardioverter defibrillator. *J Cardiovasc Electrophysiol* 2000;11:1105–1115.

verter-defibrillators: a comprehensive textbook. New York: Marcel Dekker, 1994:445–477.

139. Burke LJ. Securing life through technology acceptance: the first six months after transvenous internal cardioverter defibrillator implantation. *Heart Lung* 1996;25:352–366.

140. May CD, Smith PR, Murdock CJ, et al. The impact of the implantable cardioverter defibrillator on quality-of-life. *Pacing Clin Electrophysiol* 1995;18:1411–1418.

141. Bainger EM, Fernsler JI. Perceived quality of life before and after implantation of an internal cardioverter defibrillator. *Am J Crit Care* 1995;4:36–43.

142. Sears SF Jr, Todaro JF, Lewis TS, et al. Examining the psychosocial impact of implantable cardioverter defibrillators: a literature review. *Clin Cardiol* 1999;22:481–489.

143. Bolles Vitale M, Funk M. Quality of life in younger persons with an implantable cardioverter defibrillator. *Dimens Crit Care Nurs* 1995;14:100–111.

144. Natale A, Davidson T, Geiger MJ, et al. Implantable cardioverter-defibrillators and pregnancy: a safe combination? *Circulation* 1997;96:2808–2812.

145. Bänsch D, Brunn J, Castrucci M, et al. Syncope in patients with implantable cardioverter-defibrillator: incidence, prediction and implications for driving restrictions. *J Am Coll Cardiol* 1998;31:608–615.

146. Dougherty CM. Psychological reactions and family adjustment in shock versus no shock groups after implantation of internal cardioverter defibrillator. *Heart Lung* 1995;24:281–291.

147. Bourke JP, Turkington D, Thomas G, et al. Florid psychopathology in patients receiving shocks from implantable cardioverter-defibrillators. *Heart* 1997;78:581–583.

148. Fricchione GL, Vlay LC, Vlay SC. Cardiac psychiatry and the management of malignant ventricular arrhythmias with the internal cardioverter-defibrillator. *Am Heart J* 1994;128:1050–1059.

149. Badger JM, Morris PLP. Observations of a support group for automatic implantable cardioverter-defibrillator recipients and their spouses. *Heart Lung* 1989;18:238–243.

150. Kohn CS, Petrucci RJ, Baessler C, et al. The effect of psychological intervention on patients' long-term adjustment to the ICD: a prospective study. *Pacing Clin Electrophysiol* 2000;23:450–456.

151. Lampman RM, Knight BP. Prescribing exercise training for patients with defibrillators. *Am J Phys Med Rehabil* 2000;79:292–297.

152. Assessment of the cardiac patient for fitness to drive. *Can J Cardiol* 1992;8:406–411.

153. Curtis AB, Conti JB, Tucker KJ, et al. Motor vehicle accidents in patients with an implantable cardioverter-defibrillator. *J Am Coll Cardiol* 1995;26:180–184.

154. Epstein AE, Miles WM, Benditt DG, et al. Personal and public safety issues related to arrhythmias that may affect consciousness: implications for regulations and physician recommendations. A medical/scientific statement from the American Heart Association and the North American Society of Pacing and Electrophysiology. *Circulation* 1996;94:1147–1166.

155. Larsen GC, Stupey MR, Walance CG, et al. Recurrent cardiac events in survivors of ventricular fibrillation or tachycardia: implications for driving restrictions. *JAMA* 1994;271:1335–1339.

156. Jung W, Anderson M, Camm AJ, et al. Recommendations for driving of patients with implantable cardioverter-defibrillators. *Eur Heart J* 1997;18:1210–1219.

157. Beauregard LA, Barnard PW, Russo AM, et al. Perceived and actual risks of driving in patients with arrhythmia control devices. *Arch Intern Med* 1995;155:609–613.

158. Conti JB, Woodard DA, Tucker KJ, et al. Modification of patient driving behavior after implantation of a cardioverter defibrillator. *Pacing Clin Electrophysiol* 1997;20:2200–2204.

159. Porter MT, Pinski SL, Haw J, et al. Determinants of employment status after ICD implantation. *Circulation* 1998;98:I693 (abst).

160. Kalbfleisch KR, Lehmann MH, Steinman RT, et al. Reemployment following implantation of the automatic implantable cardioverter defibrillator. *Am J Cardiol* 1989;64:199–202.

161. Pinski SL, Trohman RG. Interference with cardiac pacing. *Cardiol Clin* 2000;18:219–239.

162. Groh WJ, Boschee SA, Engelstein ED, et al. Interactions between electronic article surveillance systems and implantable cardioverter-defibrillators. *Circulation* 1999;100:387–392.

163. Pinski SL, Trohman RG. Implantable cardioverter-defibrillators: implications for the non-electrophysiologist. *Ann Intern Med* 1995;122:770–777.

164. Pinski SL. Emergencies related to implantable antiarrhythmia devices. *Crit Care Med* 2000;28[10 Suppl]:N174–N180.

165. Peters W, Kowallik P, Reisberg M, et al. Body surface potentials during discharge of the implantable cardioverter-defibrillator. *J Cardiovasc Electrophysiol* 1998;9:491–497.

166. Credner SC, Klingenheben T, Mauss O, et al. Electrical storm in patients with transvenous implantable cardioverter-defibrillators: incidence, management and prognostic implications. *J Am Coll Cardiol* 1998;32:1909–1915.

167. Nademanee K, Taylor R, Bailey WE, et al. Treating electrical storm: sympathetic blockade versus advanced cardiac life support-guided therapy. *Circulation* 2000;102:742–747.

168. Chung MK, Streem SB, Ching E, et al. Effects of extracorporeal shock wave lithotripsy on tiered therapy implantable cardioverter defibrillators. *Pacing Clin Electrophysiol* 1999;22:738–742.

169. Goldberg RJ, Badger JM. Major depressive disorder in patients with the implantable cardioverter defibrillator: two cases treated with ECT. *Psychosomatics* 1993;34:273–277.

170. Stanton MS, Bell GK. Economic outcomes of implantable cardioverter-defibrillators [published erratum appears in *Circulation* 2000;101:2872]. *Circulation* 2000;101:1067–1074.

171. Owens DK, Sanders GD, Harris RA, et al. Cost-effectiveness of implantable cardioverter-defibrillators relative to amiodarone for prevention of sudden cardiac death. *Ann Intern Med* 1997;126:1–12.

172. Wever EF, Hauer RN, Schrijvers G, et al. Cost-effectiveness of implantable defibrillator as first-choice therapy versus electrophysiologically guided tiered strategy in postinfarct sudden death survivors: a randomized study. *Circulation* 1996;93:489–496.

173. Mushlin AI, Hall WJ, Zwanziger J, et al. The cost-effectiveness of automatic implantable cardiac defibrillators: results from MADIT. *Circulation* 1998;97:2129–2135.

174. O'Brien BJ, Connolly SJ, Goeree R, et al. Cost-effectiveness

of the implantable cardioverter-defibrillator: results from the Canadian Implantable Defibrillator Study (CIDS). *Circulation* 2001;103:1416–1421.

175. Dolack GL, Poole JE, Kudenchuk PJ, et al. Management of ventricular fibrillation with transvenous defibrillators without baseline electrophysiologic testing or antiarrhythmic drugs. *J Cardiovasc Electrophysiol* 1996;7:197–202.

176. Fahy GJ, Sgarbossa EB, Tchou PJ, et al. Hospital readmission in patients treated with tiered-therapy implantable defibrillators. *Circulation* 1996;94:1350–1356.

177. Nerbonne JM. Molecular basis of functional voltage-gated K+ channel diversity in the mammalian myocardium. *J Physiol* 2000;525(Pt 2):285–298.

178. Antzelevitch C, Yan GX, Shimizu W, et al. Electrical heterogeneity, the ECG and cardiac arrhythmias. In: Zipes DP, Jalife J, eds. *Cardiac electrophysiology: from cell to bedside.* 3rd ed. Philadelphia: WB Saunders, 2000:222–238.

179. Karagueuzian HS, Chen PS. Graded response and restitution hypotheses of ventricular vulnerability to fibrillation: insights into the mechanism of initiation of fibrillation. *J Electrocardiol* 1999;32[Suppl]:87–91.

180. Garfinkel A, Kim YH, Voroshilovsky O, et al. Preventing ventricular fibrillation by flattening cardiac restitution. *Proc Natl Acad Sci U S A* 2000;97:6061–6066.

181. Schwartz PJ, Priori SG, Locati EH, et al. Long QT syndrome patients with mutations of the SCN5A and HERG genes have differential responses to Na+ channel blockade and to increases in heart rate: implications for gene-specific therapy. *Circulation* 1995;92:3381–3386.

182. Kevin Donahue J, Heldman AW, Fraser H, et al. Focal modification of electrical conduction in the heart by viral gene transfer. *Nat Med* 2000;6:1395–1398.

183. Moss AJ. Implantable cardioverter defibrillator therapy: the sickest patients benefit the most. *Circulation* 2000;101:1638–1640.

184. Sheldon R, Connolly S, Krahn A, et al. Identification of patients most likely to benefit from implantable cardioverter-defibrillator therapy: the Canadian Implantable Defibrillator Study. *Circulation* 2000;101:1660–1664.

185. Exner DV, Sheldon RS, Pinski SL, et al. Do baseline characteristics accurately discriminate between patients likely versus unlikely to benefit from implantable defibrillator therapy? Evaluation of the Canadian Implantable Defibrillator Study implantable cardioverter defibrillatory efficacy score in the Antiarrhythmics Versus Implantable Defibrillators Trial. *Am Heart J* 2001;141:99–104.

186. Pratt CM, Camm AJ, Bigger JT Jr, et al. Evaluation of antiarrhythmic drug efficacy in patients with an ICD: unlimited potential or replete with complexity and problems? *J Cardiovasc Electrophysiol* 1999;10:1534–1549.

187. Parsonnet V, Bernstein AD, Neglia D. Nonthoracotomy ICD implantation: lessons to be learned from permanent pacemaker implantation. *Pacing Clin Electrophysiol* 1995;18:1597–1600.

188. Saksena S. Clinical practice patterns in implantable rhythm management device therapy: new players and new norms. *Pacing Clin Electrophysiol* 1999;22:814–815.

189. Josephson ME, Maloney JD, Barold SS, et al. Task Force 6: training in specialized electrophysiology, cardiac pacing, and arrhythmia management. *J Am Coll Cardiol* 1995;25:23–26.

190. Parsonnet V, Bernstein AD, Lindsay BD. Pacemaker-implantation complication rates: an analysis of some contributing factors. *J Am Coll Cardiol* 1989;13:917–921.

191. Schoenfeld MH. Quality assurance in cardiac electrophysiology and pacing: a brief synopsis. *Pacing Clin Electrophysiol* 1994;17:267–269.

192. Zehender M, Faber T, Grom A, et al. Continuous monitoring of acute myocardial ischemia by the implantable cardioverter defibrillator. *Am Heart J* 1994;127:1057–1063.

193. Steinhaus DM, Lemery R, Bresnahan DR Jr, et al. Initial experience with an implantable hemodynamic monitor. *Circulation* 1996;93:745–752.

194. Pruvot E, Thonet G, Vesin JM, et al. Heart rate dynamics at the onset of ventricular tachyarrhythmias as retrieved from implantable cardioverter-defibrillators in patients with coronary artery disease. *Circulation* 2000;101:2398–2404.

195. Prystowsky EN. Future expectations of implantable cardioverter defibrillator therapy. *Pacing Clin Electrophysiol* 1995;18:609–615.

196. Weiss JN, Garfinkel A, Karagueuzian HS, et al. Chaos and the transition to ventricular fibrillation: a new approach to antiarrhythmic drug evaluation. *Circulation* 1999;99:2819–2826.

197. Higgins SL, Yong P, Sheck D, et al. Biventricular pacing diminishes the need for implantable cardioverter defibrillator therapy. *J Am Coll Cardiol* 2000;36:824–827.

198. Okishige K, Ohkubo T, Goseki Y, et al. Experimental study of the effects of multi-site sequential ventricular pacing on the prophylaxis of ventricular fibrillation. *Jpn Heart J* 2000;41:193–204.

199. Viskin S, Glikson M, Fish R, et al. Rate smoothing with cardiac pacing for preventing torsade de pointes. *Am J Cardiol* 2000;86:K111–K115.

200. Prystowsky EN, Zipes DP. Inhibition in the human heart. *Circulation* 1983;68:381–386.

77

CLINICAL ASSESSMENT OF THE AUTONOMIC NERVOUS SYSTEM

CHRISTOPHER R. COLE
MICHAEL S. LAUER
J. THOMAS BIGGER

▼ ADDITIONAL ELECTRONIC TOPICS

   C. R. Cole: Department of Cardiovascular Medicine, The Cleveland Clinic Foundation, Cleveland, Ohio
   M. S. Lauer: Department of Cardiovascular Medicine, The Cleveland Clinic Foundation, Cleveland, Ohio
   J. T. Bigger: Department of Medicine, Columbia University College of Physicians and Surgeons, New York, New York

OVERVIEW

Disturbances of autonomic nervous system function are thought to contribute significantly to risk of ventricular arrhythmias and sudden death in patients with coronary heart disease and other cardiac diseases.

Excessive activity of the sympathetic nervous system promotes malignant ventricular arrhythmias.

The parasympathetic nervous system antagonizes sympathetically mediated malignant ventricular arrhythmias and therefore is considered to have a major protective effect against sudden death.

The autonomic nervous system can be assessed in humans by measuring RR variability, baroreflex sensitivity (BRS), or heart-rate changes during and immediately after exercise.

High-frequency (HF) cyclic fluctuations of RR intervals reflect vagal modulation of RR intervals linked to breathing.

Low-frequency (LF) cyclic fluctuations of RR intervals reflect modulation of RR intervals by baroreflexes and other cardiovascular control mechanisms.

The physiologic mechanisms responsible for ultra-low-frequency fluctuations in RR intervals are not established, but the renin-angiotensin system may be partly responsible.

Low BRS indicates inadequate vagal response to fluctuations in arterial blood pressure and results in sympathetic dominance.

Low values of RR-interval variability or BRS predict cardiac death and sustained ventricular arrhythmias.

LF or ultra-low-frequency fluctuations are the best measures of RR variability for predicting cardiac death or arrhythmic events.

RR-interval variability or BRS has a strong and independent relationship with cardiac death, sudden cardiac death, and sustained ventricular arrhythmias in coronary heart disease.

RR variability and BRS can be combined with other risk predictors [e.g., left ventricular ejection fraction (LVEF) or ventricular arrhythmias] to improve predictive accuracy for cardiac death or arrhythmic events.

Beta-blockers may improve autonomic balance; it is conceivable that in this way they improve survival in patients with coronary heart disease and chronic heart failure.

Abnormalities of autonomic nervous system function can be easily detected by measuring heart rates during and after exercise. A failure of heart rate to rise appropriately during exercise ("chronotropic incompetence") as well as a failure of heart rate to fall quickly after exercise ("impaired heart-rate recovery") are powerful, independent, and easily measured predictors of all-cause mortality.

GLOSSARY

Autoregression: A parametric statistical algorithm for resolving a complex signal into its component frequencies.

Baroreflex sensitivity: The magnitude of increase in RR intervals when systolic blood pressure increases.

Chronotropic incompetence: A failure of heart rate to rise appropriately during exercise. Chronotropic incompetence is predictive of increased mortality.

Chronotropic index: A marker of chronotropic response to exercise calculated as [(exercise heart rate) − (resting heart rate)]/[(220 − age) − (resting heart rate)]. It can also be considered as the proportion of heart-rate reserve used at peak exercise. A chronotropic index less than 0.8 at peak exercise is abnormal.

E:I ratio: Ratio of maximum RR interval during expiration to the minimum RR interval during inspiration.

Fourier transform: A nonparametric mathematical algorithm for resolving a complex signal into its component frequencies.

Heart-rate recovery (HRR): The parasympathetically mediated return toward baseline of heart rate immediately after exercise. An abnormal 1-minute HRR is less than 12. An abnormal HRR is a powerful predictor of all-cause mortality.

Heart-rate variability (HRV): Periodic fluctuations of heart rate. See *RR-interval variability*.

NN interval: Difference between adjacent normal QRS complexes.

Power spectrum: Plot of power (energy) versus frequency of a complex signal composed of oscillations at multiple frequencies.

RR interval: Difference between adjacent QRS complexes.

RR-interval variability: The periodic fluctuations of RR intervals. Information about the general health of the heart, the prognosis, and the propensity toward malignant ventricular arrhythmias may be determined from analysis of these fluctuations.

INTRODUCTION

A large body of clinical and experimental evidence indicates an important role for the autonomic nervous system in the triggering or sustaining of malignant ventricular arrhythmias. Experimentally, sympathetic stimulation reduces ventricular refractoriness and fibrillation threshold and promotes arrhythmias; it also promotes afterdepolarizations and triggered activity. Vagal stimulation opposes these effects, prolonging ventricular refractoriness and reducing the effects of adrenergic stimulation. The antiarrhythmic effects of vagal activity are much more pronounced when adrenergic activity is increased. Normally, afferent nerve impulses from the arterial baroreceptors to the brain cause inhibition of the sympathetic outflow, while increasing efferent parasympathetic activity. Lowered BRS can lead to increased sympathetic drive with decreased vagal activity, a situation promoting ventricular arrhythmias, particularly during myocardial ischemia.

There are several noninvasive or minimally invasive ways to evaluate the autonomic nervous system in intact humans. This chapter discusses three of these approaches: RR-interval variability from continuous electrocardiographic (ECG) recordings, BRS, and heart-rate changes during and immediately after exercise. RR variability measurements provide a low-cost, widely available method for assessing the status of the parasympathetic nervous system in humans and for predicting cardiovascular events, especially cardiac death and sustained ventricular arrhythmias in coronary heart disease patients. BRS also is useful for predicting cardiac death and sustained ventricular arrhythmias after myocardial infarction and adds prognostic information to RR variability.

Chronotropic incompetence during exercise and HRR immediately after exercise are important and easily obtained autonomic markers. Chronotropic incompetence may reflect excess resting sympathetic activity, and HRR reflects parasympathetic reactivation after exercise. Both have been shown to be predictive of cardiac and all-cause mortality. This chapter focuses on the mechanistic association between changes in autonomic function and sustained ventricular arrhythmias or death, and on the clinical use of the RR variability, BRS, and exercise heart-rate responses.

PHYSIOLOGIC AND PATHOPHYSIOLOGIC EFFECTS OF THE AUTONOMIC NERVOUS SYSTEM ON THE HEART

Sympathetic Nervous System and Cardiac Arrhythmias

There is a vast literature that documents an important role for the sympathetic nervous system in the genesis of cardiac arrhythmias (49–54). Some of the proarrhythmic effects of increased cardiac sympathetic nervous activity can be attributed to adverse effects of tachycardia and some to heterogeneity of ventricular repolarization during intense sympathetic nervous activity. Stimulation of the hypothalamus and other areas that increase sympathetic nervous system activity cause cardiac arrhythmias, including ventricular fibrillation (VF) in healthy animals (55). Also, interruption of central pathways that inhibit sympathetic nervous system activity causes cardiac arrhythmias (56,57). Experimental situations that evoke anger or fear also can evoke cardiac arrhythmias in intact animals (58). In all of these settings, cardiac arrhythmias can be prevented by pretreatment with beta-adrenergic blockade. When the myocardium is "sensitized" to cardiac arrhythmias by acute myocardial ischemia or drug toxicity (e.g., digitalis toxicity, cocaine, or certain anesthetics), the probability of VF during increased sympathetic nervous system activity is increased substantially. ᐅ m93

Antiarrhythmic Effects of the Parasympathetic Nervous System

The parasympathetic nervous system has pronounced antiarrhythmic properties by reducing heart rate and by coun-

teracting the proarrhythmic effects of sympathetic nervous system activity (66). The antiarrhythmic benefit of increased parasympathetic activity is especially evident when the sympathetic nervous system plays a role in the arrhythmic activity. There are three clinical methods for quantifying parasympathetic nervous system modulation of cardiac activity: BRS, RR variability, and HRR. A number of experimental studies have attempted to define the value of these markers for assessing parasympathetic activity and for evaluating the risk of VF.

Baroreflex Sensitivity Predicts Ischemic Ventricular Fibrillation

The predictive value of BRS for ischemic VF was suggested by a series of elegant studies in an experimental model of sudden cardiac death (67–70). Thirty days after left anterior descending coronary artery ligation, conscious dogs with healed anterior myocardial infarctions were subjected to transient circumflex coronary artery occlusions while running on a treadmill to increase heart rate and sympathetic nervous system activity. Of 192 dogs subjected to transient ischemia during exercise, 55% developed VF during exercise and ischemia and 45% did not (69). Dogs susceptible to VF showed a substantial increase in heart rate during ischemia before the onset of VF, whereas dogs resistant to VF showed a decrease in heart rate.

In this model of sudden cardiac death, ischemic VF can be predicted with considerable accuracy by measuring BRS (69). Dogs with a lower BRS had a much higher chance of VF during the exercise ischemia challenge (*e*Fig. 77.0.1). Unexpectedly, dogs susceptible to VF during exercise ischemia after experimental myocardial infarction already had a lower BRS before coronary artery ligation. There were large differences in BRS among healthy dogs, and those with the lowest values of BRS before myocardial infarction were most susceptible to VF after myocardial infarction when challenged with myocardial ischemia and sympathetic activation (69). This finding suggests that individuals at high risk of arrhythmic events after myocardial infarction can be identified and treated before infarction occurs. In dogs, 6 weeks of daily exercise training substantially increased BRS and markedly reduced the likelihood of VF during exercise ischemia (68). Exercise also might benefit coronary heart disease patients at high risk of VF.

Vagal stimulation prevented susceptible dogs from developing VF during the exercise ischemia test (71). Part of the vagal protection was due to the decrease in heart rate and part to other factors.

RR-Interval Variability Predicts Ischemic Ventricular Fibrillation

RR variability has been studied in the same dog model of sudden cardiac death that showed the value of BRS as a predictor of arrhythmic events. The study was done on dogs to test the hypothesis that low values of RR variability would predict which dogs would develop VF when challenged by exercise ischemia 1 month after myocardial infarction (72).

Immediately after infarction, RR variability decreased substantially in all dogs, but the time course of recovery of RR variability was different for dogs that were resistant and those that were susceptible to VF. In resistant dogs, RR variability recovered to pre–myocardial infarction levels within 10 days, whereas susceptible dogs had persistent attenuation of RR variability throughout the 30 days after myocardial infarction (73). Decreased RR variability 30 days after myocardial infarction had 88% sensitivity and 80% specificity for predicting VF. No sham-operated animals developed VF (72).

Chronotropic Incompetence May Reflect Baseline Sympathetic Overload

The heart-rate response to exercise can yield important prognostic information for the clinician. In the healthy individual, heart rate increases during exercise to an age-related maximum heart rate. There is a wide individual variation in peak heart rates obtained, but the maximum heart rate declines uniformly with advancing age. Age-predicted peak heart rate is commonly estimated using the formula 220 minus age. A commonly used definition of chronotropic incompetence is failure to reach 85% of the age-predicted peak heart rate, but other investigators have suggested the use of the chronotropic index as a better marker of chronotropic incompetence (22,23). ▼ m94

The chronotropic response to exercise has been demonstrated to be an important predictor of mortality (19,20,22,24,25,81,82). The mechanisms to explain this finding are not entirely clear, but it may be that a blunted chronotropic response is indicative of a baseline sympathetic overload (83). There is evidence to suggest that individuals with a blunted chronotropic response to exercise have a postsynaptic desensitization to beta-adrenergic receptor stimulation (83). Colucci et al. demonstrated that heart failure patients with blunted chronotropic responses had similar increments of change of norepinephrine levels from resting to peak exercise but much higher baseline levels when compared with healthy controls (83). When isoproterenol was infused the heart rate increased less in heart failure patients than in healthy controls. These data suggest that although individuals with chronotropic incompetence have an increase in sympathetic activity to maximum levels, they are unable to attain higher heart rates due to an increased baseline sympathetic level along with a decreased sensitivity to further sympathetic stimulation, leading to a blunting of the heart-rate response. This situation is analogous to an automobile that is "out of tune." Gasoline use during idling is increased, but the car is unable to increase speed by much in response to increased gasoline delivery.

Heart-Rate Recovery Reflects Parasympathetic Reactivation

The increase in heart rate during exercise is due to the combination of parasympathetic withdrawal and sympathetic activation, whereas the recovery of heart rate back toward baseline is due to the reverse (30,42,45,46,48,74,84–86). What is less well understood is the relative contributions and timing of parasympathetic and sympathetic activity during recovery. To address this question, Imai et al. (31) measured HRR in three groups of individuals: healthy controls, trained athletes, and heart failure patients. They studied postexercise HRR under two different conditions: after parasympathetic blockade with atropine and after sympathetic blockade with propranolol. Across all groups, the decrease in heart rate during the first 30 seconds of recovery was markedly prolonged following atropine administration but not with beta-blockade. This effect was less pronounced at 2 minutes. Crouse et al. (47), Maciel et al. (46), and Perini et al. (48) obtained similar results. These findings suggest that HRR during the first minute of recovery is due almost exclusively to parasympathetic activity.

Two additional observations provide evidence that early HRR is a marker of parasympathetic activity. First, Imai et al. (31) demonstrated that HRR was accentuated in athletes, but blunted in patients with heart failure. Other investigators have also noted an increased HRR in trained individuals (87) and a decreased HRR in poorly fit persons (88). The link between these findings and the autonomic nervous system may be established by nearly identical changes in RR variability. There are data that show RR variability is decreased in poorly fit individuals and those with heart failure (89) and may be increased through exercise training (90). Arai et al. (45) found an increase in the HF power, which reflects parasympathetic activity, during early recovery that was more pronounced in individuals with higher fitness levels. Based on these studies, it may be hypothesized that parasympathetic activity is the link between fitness level and HRR.

A second observation is that HRR is known to be faster in children than in adults (87,91). A study by Ohuchi et al. (92) may shed light on this finding. They measured both HRR and RR variability in children and adults after exercise. The children had significantly higher log HF power than adults during recovery, corresponding to increased parasympathetic activity. There was a strong correlation between HRR and log HF power (*e*Fig. 77.0.2), thus linking the two together and providing additional evidence that HRR in early recovery is primarily a function of the parasympathetic nervous system.

TABLE 77.1 DEFINITIONS FOR TIME AND FREQUENCY DOMAIN MEASURES OF HEART PERIOD VARIABILITY[a]

Variable	Units	Definition
Time domain–statistical measures		
Night–day difference	Millisecond	Difference between the average of all the normal RR intervals at night (24:00 to 05:00) and the average of all the normal RR intervals during the day (07:30 to 21:30)
SDNN	Millisecond	Standard deviation of all normal RR intervals in the entire 24-h ECG recording
SDANN	Millisecond	Standard deviation of the average normal RR intervals for all 288 5-min segments of a 24-h ECG recording (each average is weighted by the fraction of the 5 min that has normal RR intervals)
ASDNN	Millisecond	Average of the standard deviations of normal RR intervals for all 288 5-min segments of a 24-h ECG recording
r-MSSD	Millisecond	Root mean square successive difference, the square root of the mean of the squared differences between adjacent normal RR intervals over the entire 24-h ECG recording
pNN50	Percent	Percent of differences between adjacent normal RR intervals that are greater than 50 ms computed over the entire 24-h ECG recording
NN50	None	Number of adjacent normal RR intervals that are greater than 50 ms counted over the entire 24-h ECG recording
Time domain–geometric measures		
Heart-rate variability triangular index	None	Total number of NN intervals divided by the number of NN intervals in the modal bin of a histogram of all NN intervals with a bin width of 7.8125 ms (for a sampling rate of 128/sec)
TINN	Millisecond	Baseline width of the minimum square difference triangular interpolation of the highest peak of the histogram of all NN intervals
Frequency domain measures		
Total power	Square milliseconds	The energy in the heart period power spectrum up to 0.40 Hz
Ultra low-frequency power	Square milliseconds	The energy in the heart period power spectrum up to 0.0033 Hz
Very low-frequency power	Square milliseconds	The energy in the heart period power spectrum between 0.0033 and 0.04 Hz
Low-frequency power	Square milliseconds	The energy in the heart period power spectrum between 0.04 and 0.15 Hz
High-frequency power	Square milliseconds	The energy in the heart period power spectrum between 0.15 and 0.40 Hz
Low-frequency to high-frequency ratio	None	The ratio of low- to high-frequency power
α	None	Slope of log(power) on log(frequency) between 0.01 and 0.0001 Hz on a log-log plot

ASDNN, average standard deviation of normal to normal intervals in 5-minute intervals calculated over 24 hours; ECG, electrocardiography; NN, normal to normal intervals; NN50, number of times that successive RR intervals differed by greater than 50 ms in a 24-hour period; pNN50, proportion of differences between successive normal to normal intervals that are greater than 50 ms; r-MSSD, square root of the mean squared successive differences of normal to normal intervals; SDANN, standard deviation of the average normal to normal intervals for the 288 5-minute intervals in a 24-hour continuous electrocardiographic recording; SDNN, standard deviation of normal to normal intervals over a 24-hour period.
[a]The physiologic interpretation of these measures of RR variability is given in the text.
From Jiang W, Hayano J, Coleman ER, et al. Relation of cardiovascular responses to mental stress and cardiac vagal activity in coronary artery disease. *Am J Cardiol* 1993;72:551–554, with permission.

MEASUREMENT OF RR-INTERVAL VARIABILITY AND BAROREFLEX SENSITIVITY

Measurement of RR Variability

Variation in RR intervals can be measured by many methods; these methods can be categorized as time domain measures or frequency domain measures (93). Table 77.1 lists the commonly used measures of RR-interval variability. Every frequency domain measure of RR variability has an equivalent time domain measure (*e*Table 77.1.1). The physiologic correlates of RR variability are discussed later (see Frequency Domain Measures of RR Variability).

Time Domain Measures of RR Variability

Time domain measures of RR variability can be used to summarize information about either short-term or long-term variation in RR intervals, and a large number of measures have been proposed. These measures attempt to estimate the influence of nervous and humoral influences on the sinus node so they usually exclude RR intervals caused by ectopic (nonsinus) beats. In a continuous ECG recording, each R wave (QRS complex) is detected and labeled as normal (N) or abnormal. The series of NN intervals is used to calculate time domain measures, which may be expressed directly as NN intervals or as instantaneous heart rate.

Statistical Measures

From a series of NN intervals, various statistical measures are calculated (93,94). Most often the NN series is recorded for an entire 24-hour period or for a short period, typically 5 minutes or 1 hour. Some of the commonly used time domain measures are summarized in Table 77.1. A commonly used and useful measure of RR variability is SDNN. This measure summarizes all sources of variation in NN intervals over the period of calculation. The longer the recording for an individual, the greater is the magnitude of SDNN. If the SDNN is calculated on an interval substantially different from 24 hours, this should always be stated clearly because the values cannot be compared with standard 24-hour values. A common time domain measure of long-term (slow) variation in NN intervals is the standard deviation of the average NN intervals for the 288 5-minute intervals in a 24-hour continuous ECG recording (SDANN). A common time domain measure of short-term (fast) variation in NN intervals is the average standard deviation of NN intervals in 5-minute intervals calculated over 24 hours (ASDNN). SDANN measures fluctuations in NN intervals with cycles longer than 5 minutes, and ASDNN measures fluctuations with cycles shorter than 5 minutes.

Geometric Methods

Geometric patterns have been used to quantify long-term RR variability (93,95). The 24-hour NN interval time series is plotted as a frequency distribution of NN intervals, and then summary measures are calculated to describe it. HRV triangular index and the triangular interpolation of NN intervals (TINN) are two geometric measures that have been used to describe the frequency histogram of NN intervals over a 24-hour period. These measures are determined by finding the length of the base of a triangle that best fits the frequency histogram (93). ▼ m95

Frequency Domain Measures of RR Variability

Five-Minute Power Spectra

The Task Force on Heart Rate Variability of the European Society of Cardiology and the North American Society of Pacing and Electrophysiology recommended that power spectral analysis of 5-minute ECG recordings be used to assess autonomic physiology and pharmacology (93). Frequencies between 0.0033 and 0.40 Hz can be estimated from a 5-minute ECG recording. Figure 77.1A shows a 5-minute power spectrum in a healthy person lying supine. Two "peaks" are present in the 5-minute power spectrum: HF power in the frequency range 0.15 to 0.40 Hz and LF power in the frequency range 0.04 to 0.15 Hz. The power spectral density usually is expressed as absolute units of power (square milliseconds), but may be expressed in normalized units (Fig. 77.2). Normalized units can be used to emphasize the reciprocal action of the parasympathetic and

sympathetic limbs of the autonomic nervous system and to minimize the effect of changes in total power on the values of LF and HF components (97). HF power reflects modulation of efferent parasympathetic (vagal) activity by ventilation (respiratory sinus arrhythmia). LF power reflects modulation of efferent parasympathetic (vagal) and efferent sympathetic nervous system activity by baroreflex activity. It should be emphasized that the amplitude of LF or HF power reflects modulation of sinus node firing rate, not the average level of parasympathetic or sympathetic tone (13,98). Note that the amplitude of LF power is greater than HF power in a healthy person resting in the supine position. The LF/HF ratio is used as an index of vagosympathetic balance (15).

The energy between 0.0033 and 0.04 Hz is called *very low-frequency power*; the physiologic correlates of very low-frequency power are not known, but the power in this range can be influenced substantially by physical activity (99).

USE OF AUTONOMIC MARKERS TO PREDICT DEATH OR ARRHYTHMIC EVENTS

Clinical Use of RR Variability for Assessment of Risk

In the opinion of the Task Force on Heart Rate Variability, there were two proven clinical uses of RR variability: (a) to predict risk of cardiac death or arrhythmic events after acute myocardial infarction, and (b) to detect and quantify autonomic neuropathy in diabetes mellitus (93). In the following sections of this chapter, we review some of the studies that have established RR variability as a predictor of cardiac death after acute myocardial infarction and in chronic coronary heart disease. Both time and frequency domain measures have been used to predict mortality, and nonfatal arrhythmic events in coronary heart disease. The measures most often used for this purpose include SDNN, SDANN, HRV triangular index, total power, ultra-low-frequency power, LF power, and power law regression parameters (Table 77.1).

Prediction of Hospital Mortality after Myocardial Infarction Using the Variance of 30 RR Intervals

In 1978, Wolf et al. published the first report of an association between RR variability and prognosis (16). These workers studied 176 patients admitted to hospital for acute myocardial infarction to evaluate the relationship between RR variability and in-hospital mortality. A 60-second ECG recording was made on the day of admission to the coronary care unit, and the variance of 30 consecutive RR intervals was calculated for each patient. Wolf et al. arbitrarily dichotomized their group using a variance of 1,000 ms^2; 73 patients (42%) had a variance greater than or equal to 1,000 ms^2, and 103 patients (59%) had a variance less than

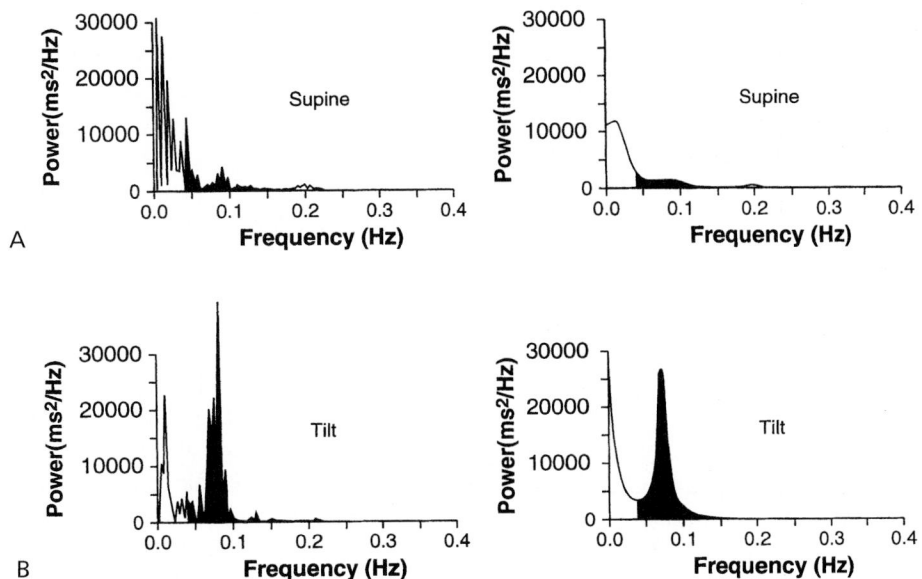

FIGURE 77.1 A,B: Power spectral analysis of RR-interval time series. The left panels show fast Fourier transform (FFT) analysis of two 5-minute recordings of RR intervals. The left panel of **A** shows the FFT of a recording made supine and resting; the left panel of **B** shows the FFT of a recording made during 60-degree head-up tilt. The right panels show the results of autoregression analysis of the same two 5-minute recordings. The autoregressive algorithm smooths the data, but gives almost identical areas under the curves as the FFT algorithm in the frequency bands of interest. In the supine recording, there is a peak at approximately 0.20 Hz in the high-frequency (HF) power band, and a peak at approximately 0.08 Hz in the low-frequency (LF) power band. More than one-half the power is in the very low-frequency power band. Both methods show a decrease in HF power and a marked increase in LF power during head-up tilt. (From Bigger JT Jr. RR variability to evaluate autonomic physiology and pharmacology and to predict cardiovascular outcomes in humans. In: Zipes DP, ed. *Cardiac arrhythmias: from cell to bedside.* Philadelphia: WB Saunders, 1995:1151–1170, with permission.)

1,000 ms^2 (*e*Table 77.1.2). Patients with RR variance less than 1,000 ms^2 were more likely to have anterior myocardial infarction, a Norris index greater than or equal to 10, low values for average RR interval, and admission to hospital longer after onset of chest pain.

The study by Wolf et al. showed that RR variability, estimated from a short ECG recording on the day of myocardial infarction, predicted mortality over the next 9 to 14 days (16). The hospital mortality of patients with RR variance less than 1,000 ms^2 was 15.5% compared with 4.1% for patients with RR variance greater than or equal to 1,000 ms^2. After adjusting for average RR interval and location of the infarct, low RR variance was still significantly associated with higher mortality.

Prediction of Long-Term Mortality after Acute Myocardial Infarction Using Time Domain Measures of RR Variability

In 1987, Kleiger et al. (17) reported that SDNN, measured at the time of hospital discharge after myocardial infarction, predicted death during the subsequent 2 to 4 years. They performed baseline studies on a group of 808 patients with acute myocardial infarction and then followed them an average of 31 months. Twenty-four-hour ECG record-

ings were done 11 ± 3 days after acute myocardial infarction. SDNN was calculated for the 24-hour period, and a value of 50 ms was chosen arbitrarily to dichotomize their group into 125 patients (16%) with low values and 683 patients (84%) with high values. During 2 to 4 years of follow-up, 127 deaths occurred (Fig. 77.3). The mortality of patients with an SDNN less than 50 ms was 34% compared with a 12% mortality in patients with an SDNN greater than or equal to 50 ms, a relative risk of 2.8 (95% confidence interval, 2.0 to 3.8). SDNN predicted mortality independently of other risk predictors such as LVEF or ventricular arrhythmias. ⚡ m96

Prediction of Long-Term Mortality after Acute Myocardial Infarction Using Frequency Domain Measures of RR Variability

Power Spectral Measures of RR Variability Measured over a Five-Minute Interval

Bigger et al. studied 715 patients 2 weeks after myocardial infarction and showed that short-term power spectral measures of RR variability (calculated from 5 minutes of normal RR-interval data) predict all-cause mortality or arrhythmic death (119). From continuous 24-hour ECG recordings, two 5-minute segments were selected for analy-

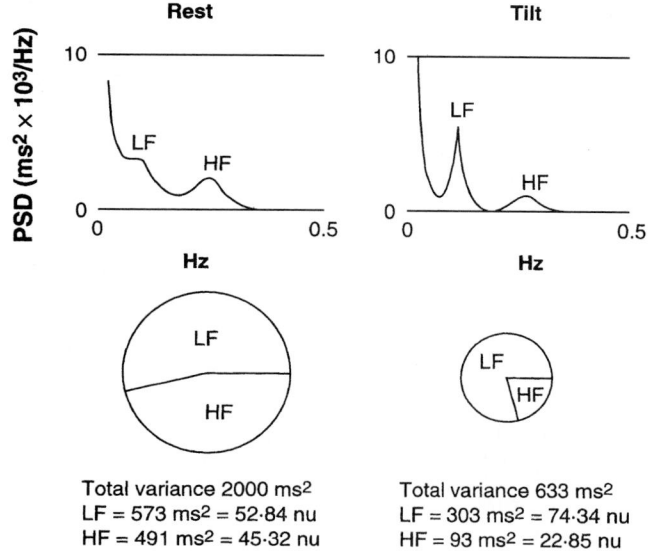

Total variance 2000 ms²
LF = 573 ms² = 52·84 nu
HF = 491 ms² = 45·32 nu

Total variance 633 ms²
LF = 303 ms² = 74·34 nu
HF = 93 ms² = 22·85 nu

FIGURE 77.2 Use of normalized units to interpret spectral analysis (autoregressive model) of RR-interval variability in a healthy subject. The recording on the left was made while the subject was resting in the supine position; the recording on the right was made during 90-degree head-up tilt. At rest, low-frequency (LF) and high-frequency (HF) power have a similar magnitude, whereas during the head-up tilt, LF power is much greater than HF power. Total variance is markedly reduced during tilting, so both LF power and HF power are diminished when expressed in absolute units. The use of normalized units (nu) clearly indicates the altered relation between the two spectral components induced by tilting. The pie charts show the absolute power of the two components (represented by the area of the circles) as well as the relative distribution of LF and HF power. The LF/HF ratio also quantifies the relative distribution of LF and HF power. These changes in the normalized units and LF/HF ratio are interpreted as a decrease in parasympathetic modulation and an increase in sympathetic modulation of RR intervals. PSD, power spectral density. (From Malliani A, Lombardi F, Pagani M. Power spectrum analysis of heart rate variability: a tool to explore neural regulatory mechanisms. *Br Heart J* 1994;71:1–2, with permission.)

sis, one from the 8 a.m. to 4 p.m. interval, and one from the 12 midnight to 5 a.m. interval. The former corresponds to the time interval during which short-term measures of RR variability would most likely be obtained. The latter simulates the conditions that exist when patients have an ECG recorded while lying quietly in a laboratory. Four frequency domain measures were calculated from the daytime and nighttime 5-minute intervals: (a) very low-frequency power; (b) LF power; (c) HF power; and (d) LF/HF ratio. Mean power spectral values from 5-minute periods during the day and night were similar to 24-hour values, and the correlations between short segment values and 24-hour values were strong (most correlations were greater than or equal to 0.75). Power spectral measures of RR variability, obtained from 5-minute ECG recordings, were excellent predictors of all-cause, cardiac, and arrhythmic mortality. Patients with low values were two to four times as likely to die over an average follow-up of 31 months than were patients with high values.

Short-Term Fractal Scaling Exponent (α_1) and Mortality after Myocardial Infarction

Huikuri et al. studied several nonlinear dynamic measures of RR variability in a 446-patient subgroup from the Danish Investigations of Arrhythmia and Mortality on Dofetilide in Survivors of Acute Myocardial Infarction (DIAMOND-MI) trial with acute myocardial infarction and LVEF less than 0.36 (120). Time, frequency, and fractal measures of RR-interval variability were related to deaths during 2 years of follow-up. The reduced short-term fractal scaling exponent, α_1, was the strongest predictor of total mortality (n = 114), arrhythmic death (n = 75), and nonarrhythmic cardiac death (n = 28) (relative risk, 3.0; 95% confidence interval, 2.5 to 4.2). The short-term scaling exponent, α_1, remained a significant predictor of death after statistical adjustment for age, New York Heart Association functional class, ejection fraction, and use of cardiac medications.

RR Variability Identifies Patients with Left Ventricular Dysfunction Who Benefit from Amiodarone Treatment

A prospective substudy of the European Myocardial Infarction Amiodarone Trial (EMIAT) tested the hypothesis that patients with recent myocardial infarctions, LVEF less than 0.41, and reduced RR variability would benefit from amiodarone treatment (121). The rationale for this substudy was

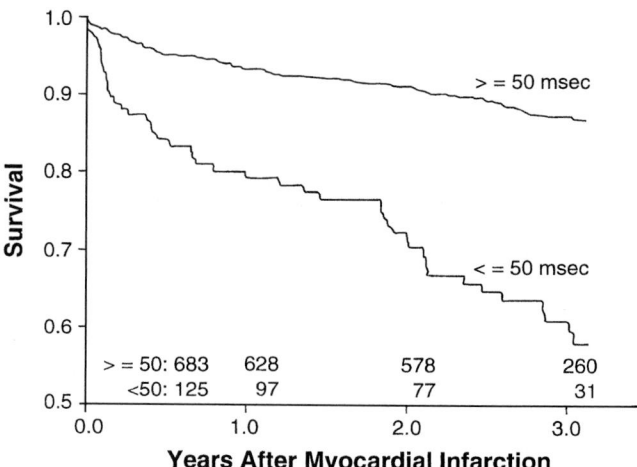

FIGURE 77.3 Survival as a function of the 24-hour standard deviation of normal RR intervals in 808 patients with myocardial infarction. Time after myocardial infarction is plotted on the *x*-axis; proportion surviving is plotted on the *y*-axis. (Adapted from data published in Kleiger RE, Miller JP, Bigger JT Jr, et al. Decreased heart rate variability and its association with increased mortality after acute myocardial infarction. *Am J Cardiol* 1987;59:256–262. This figure was first published as Figure 19.6 in Bigger JT Jr, Rottman JN. Spectral analysis of RR variability. In: Podrid PJ, Kowey PR, eds. *Cardiac arrhythmia. Mechanisms, diagnosis, and management.* Baltimore: Williams & Wilkins, 1995:280–298, with permission.)

that RR variability predicts more specifically arrhythmic than nonarrhythmic death; therefore, such a group would benefit from amiodarone.

In EMIAT, 1,216 patients (82%) had RR variability index calculated from 24-hour Holter recordings. The substudy consisted of the 363 (30%) patients who had an HRV index less than 21 units. In placebo-treated patients, those with reduced RR variability had a substantially higher mortality than patients with preserved RR variability (22.8% vs. 9.5%, p <.05). In the substudy, there was a 23% reduction in all-cause mortality in those treated with amiodarone (22.8% vs. 17.5%, p = .24) and a 66% reduction in cardiac mortality (12.8% vs. 4.4%, p <.01). The efficacy of amiodarone in patients with reduced RR variability was further evaluated in a number of patient categories. The benefit of amiodarone was large in patients with reduced RR variability and a resting heart rate greater than or equal to 75 beats/min; this subgroup had 29.0% mortality when treated with placebo compared with 19.3% when treated with amiodarone, a 33.7% reduction in mortality (p = .075). The EMIAT substudy is the first to demonstrate that RR variability can select a group of patients with autonomic dysfunction that will benefit from prophylactic amiodarone therapy.

RR Variability to Assess Prognosis in Patients with Heart Failure

Patients with heart failure often have autonomic dysfunction. The United Kingdom Heart Failure Evaluation and Assessment of Risk Trial prospectively evaluated the predictive value of RR variability in 433 patients with heart failure followed for 482 ± 161 days (128). SDNN was only weakly related to LVEF (r = 0.12). SDNN was a strong predictor of mortality: 6% of the patients had an SDNN less than 50 ms with an annual mortality of 51%, 32% had an SDNN of 50 to 100 ms with an annual mortality of 13%, and 62% had an SDNN greater than 100 ms with an annual mortality of 6%.

Significance of Low RR Variability in the Elderly

In 1948, a sample of 5,209 residents of Framingham, MA, was selected to undergo biennial examinations in a prospective study (129). In the eighteenth examination cycle (1983 to 1985), 1,028 2-hour Holter recordings were made during routine clinic examinations of 1,825 surviving participants (130). ▼ m97

A 1 SD decrement in natural log-transformed LF power was associated with a relative risk (hazard ratio) of 1.87 (95% confidence interval, 1.55 to 2.26). After statistical adjustment for age, sex, and clinical risk factors (history of myocardial infarction, heart failure, diuretic use, and frequent or complex ventricular premature complexes), the relative risk was 1.70. These results indicate that reduced RR variability predicts mortality in a population-based sample of elderly subjects.

Significance of Low RR Variability in Patients Referred for 24-Hour Holter Recordings

Algra et al. conducted a retrospective case control study to determine whether a disturbance of autonomic nervous system activity may play a role in sudden cardiac death (131). All 6,693 consecutive patients who had 24-hour Holter ECG recordings in four Rotterdam hospitals between August 1, 1980, and December 31, 1984, were included.

The indications for the 24-hour ECG recordings were evaluation of palpitations, dizziness, syncope, or angina pectoris, 65%; evaluation of risk after myocardial infarction, 10%; evaluation of antiarrhythmic therapy, 8%; and search for a cardiac cause of transient cerebral events, 7%. Seventy-five percent of the recordings were done in outpatients. Patients were excluded for unanalyzable Holter recordings and for frequent supraventricular arrhythmias, leaving approximately 5,500 patients. During a 2-year follow-up period, 193 sudden cardiac deaths (less than 1 hour) occurred.

Three time domain measures of RR variability were used in the Rotterdam study: (a) pNN50; (b) short-term variation (mean over 24 hours of per minute standard deviations of RR intervals); and (c) long-term variation (standard deviation over 24 hours of per minute means of RR intervals). Although the latter two measures are unorthodox, the measure of short-term variation is similar to ASDNN or LF power, and the measure of long-term variation is similar to SDANN or ultra low-frequency power. Patients with low values for these three measures of RR variability had a higher relative risk of experiencing sudden cardiac death in 2 years of follow-up. The relative risks were pNN50, 1.8; short-term variation, 3.0; and long-term variation, 2.7. This study showed that RR variability had predictive value in a consecutive, heterogeneous group of patients referred to a Holter laboratory.

How to Interpret and Use RR-Variability Reports from Commercial Holter Systems

Most commercial Holter systems provide some measures of RR variability. The calculation of statistical measures of RR variability is straightforward if ectopic complexes are correctly measured. For example, measurements of SDNN made by commercial systems are comparable with those made with research systems. Power spectral measures of RR variability in most commercial systems have not been validated against research systems that establish their predictive value for cardiac death or sustained arrhythmias. Betablocker therapy increases RR variability somewhat in patients with recent myocardial infarctions and is known to improve survival. A careful evaluation for the sources of risk is recommended for patients with low values for RR variability after myocardial infarction, and beta-blocker therapy should be instituted if there is no contraindication.

Summary of RR Variability in Coronary Heart Disease

RR variability has proven to be a remarkably effective predictor of death and arrhythmic events after acute myocardial infarction and in chronic coronary heart disease. RR variability is a better predictor than LVEF or ventricular arrhythmias. Both time and frequency domain measures of RR variability measured during 5-minute or 24-hour ECG recordings predict deaths after myocardial infarction. RR variability predicts death of all causes, cardiac death, arrhythmic death, and also nonfatal sustained arrhythmias. However, RR variability, measured soon after acute myocardial infarction, does not predict recurrent infarction. Combined with other risk predictors, RR variability has a positive predictive accuracy up to 50%. RR variability is readily available in commercial Holter equipment and is inexpensive. The EMIAT substudy indicates that patients with left ventricular dysfunction and low RR variability benefit from prophylactic amiodarone therapy.

Clinical Use of Baroreflex Sensitivity for Assessment of Risk in Coronary Heart Disease

Autonomic Tone and Reflexes after Myocardial Infarction Study

Based on the strong experimental evidence that BRS predicted ischemic VF, and encouraging evidence from small clinical studies, ATRAMI, a large epidemiologic study, was launched in 1991 (114). ATRAMI was designed to definitively assess the predictive value of BRS after myocardial infarction and to determine how the predictive value of BRS ranked with RR variability, LVEF, and ventricular premature complexes. A total of 1,284 patients were enrolled 6 to 28 days after myocardial infarction, had BRS measured, and were followed for greater than or equal to 12 months. The primary end point was cardiac death or nonfatal cardiac arrest.

The a priori hypotheses were that a BRS less than 3.0 ms per mm Hg would predict higher cardiac mortality and that it would add predictive power to that of SDNN less than 70 ms. The strength of association of BRS and SDNN with cardiac death and cardiac arrest with and without adjusting for LVEF and ventricular premature complexes was estimated using a Cox regression model.

The average age in ATRAMI was 57 ± 10 years and their risk was relatively low, as indicated by the mean LVEF of 0.49 ± 0.12. The average BRS for the group was 7.2 ± 4.6 ms per mm Hg and the average SDNN was 108 ± 35 ms; 17%

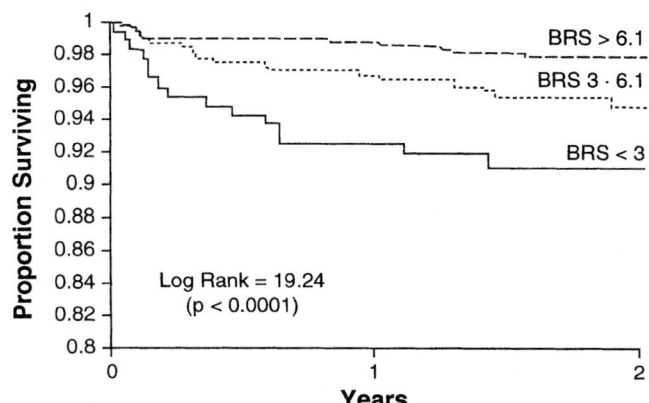

FIGURE 77.4 The ability of baroreflex sensitivity (BRS) to predict cardiac death (n = 44) or cardiac arrest (n = 5) after myocardial infarction in 1,182 patients who participated in the Autonomic Tone and Reflexes after Myocardial Infarction study and had BRS measured by the phenylephrine method. Patients were divided into three groups: 179 patients below the fifteenth percentile (BRS less than 3.0 ms per mm Hg), 414 patients from the fifteenth percentile to the median value (BRS 3.0 to 6.1 ms per mm Hg), and 589 patients above the median value (BRS greater than 6.1 ms per mm Hg). The p value refers to differences in the event rates among the three groups. [From La Rovere MT, Bigger JT Jr, Marcus FI, et al. Baroreflex sensitivity and heart rate variability in the prediction of total cardiac mortality after myocardial infarction. The results of ATRAMI (Autonomic Tone and Reflexes After Myocardial Infarction). *Lancet* 1998;351:478–484, with permission.]

of the patients had greater than or equal to 10 ventricular premature complexes per hour. Patients with depressed BRS or SDNN were older, were more frequently women, and had more ventricular premature complexes and lower LVEFs.

During a mean follow-up of 21 ± 8 months, cardiac death or cardiac arrest occurred in 49 patients (3.9%) (Fig. 77.4). Two-year mortality was 9% among patients with BRS less than 3 ms per mm Hg compared with 2% in patients with BRS less than or equal to 3.0 (vs. *p* <.0001), definitively establishing the predictive value of this autonomic marker. Similarly, patients with SDNN less than 70 ms had a 10% mortality compared with 2% in those with SDNN less than or equal to 70 ms (*p* <.0001), thus confirming the predictive value of SDNN. The relative risk of patients with BRS values less than 3.0 ms per mm Hg or SDNN values less than 70 ms remained strong even after adjusting for LVEF and ventricular premature complexes. BRS and SDNN both had relative risks of approximately 3.0 for cardiac death or cardiac arrest.

Patients with depressed BRS and depressed SDNN had a 1-year mortality of 15% versus 1% (*p* <.0001), a relative risk of 10.9, indicating that BRS adds significantly to the predictive value of SDNN. Similarly, BRS or SDNN combined with LVEF improved predictive accuracy for cardiac mortality and cardiac arrest. When LVEF less than 0.35 was combined with an SDNN less than 70 ms, the relative risk was 7.4 (95% confidence interval, 3.1 to 17.8), and when it was combined with a BRS less than 3.0 ms per mm

Hg, the relative risk was 11.9 (95% confidence interval, 5.1 to 27.4). This large prospective study provides definitive evidence that BRS is a strong and independent predictor of death after myocardial infarction. Moreover, BRS adds significantly to the predictive value of SDNN.

Clinical Use of Heart-Rate Responses to Exercise to Predict Death

Chronotropic Incompetence as a Prognostic Marker

Increase in heart-rate rise during exercise is a prognostic marker for coronary events and all-cause mortality (19,20,22,24,25,81,82). Lauer et al. examined 1,575 men from the Framingham Offspring Study who underwent exercise testing and classified their heart-rate response to exercise using three different criteria: (a) failure to reach 85% of the age-predicted maximum heart rate; (b) change in heart rate from rest to peak exercise; and (c) the percentage of the heart-rate reserve used during exercise (chronotropic response index) (22). After almost 8 years of follow-up, 55 deaths and 95 new cases of coronary artery disease accumulated. All three markers predicted total mortality and coronary artery disease. After adjustment for confounding factors, the chronotropic response index emerged as the strongest predictor of mortality.

Although chronotropic response is predictive of coronary artery disease (81), it is independent of ischemia (24,25) and coronary artery plaque burden (82). Lauer et al. studied 2,953 patients undergoing stress thallium testing to assess the interaction between ischemic response and chronotropic response (25). Failure to achieve 85% of age-predicted maximum heart rate or a low chronotropic index was predictive of all-cause mortality outcomes even after adjusting for myocardial ischemia and other risk factors. The independence of chronotropic response from coronary artery disease was confirmed by Dresing et al. in an angiographic study (82). They looked at a cohort of patients who had undergone both exercise testing and angiography. Coronary artery plaque burden was assessed using the Duke Prognostic Weight Score. Chronotropic response remained predictive of death even after adjustment for severity of coronary artery disease. In fact, although angiographic severity of coronary disease was associated with risk of death in univariate analyses, once the chronotropic response to exercise was considered the angiographic findings had no independent predictive value.

Heart-Rate Recovery as a Prognostic Marker

Although used as a marker of physical fitness for many years, the use of HRR as a prognostic marker is a relatively recent development. In the first study to look at the predictive potential of HRR, Cole et al. (35) followed 2,428

adults who underwent symptom-limited exercise testing and single photon emission computed tomographic thallium imaging. Patients exercised to peak workload and then continued to walk at 2.4 km (1.5 miles) per hour at a grade of 2.5% for at least 2 minutes into recovery. HRR was defined as the decrease in heart rate from peak exercise to 1 minute of recovery.

$$\text{HRR} = \text{Heart rate}_{\text{Peak}} - \text{Heart rate}_{\text{1-Minute Recovery}}$$

An abnormal value for HRR was determined by finding the maximal value for the log-rank chi-square test statistic for all possible cutoff points between the tenth and ninetieth percentiles for the study cohort. This turned out to be less than 12 beats/min. The median value for HRR was 17 beats/min, with a range from the twenty-fifth to the seventy-fifth percentile of 12 to 23 beats/min. An abnormal value was found in 26% of the population.

During 6 years of follow-up, there were 213 deaths from all causes. A low value of HRR (less than 12 beats/min) was highly predictive of mortality, with a relative risk of 4.0 (mortality at 6 years, 19% vs. 5%, $p < .001$) (Fig. 77.5). Even after adjusting for age, fitness level, and thallium perfusion defects, HRR remained predictive of death. These data suggest that an abnormal HRR is independent of cardiac ischemia. When both an abnormal HRR and thallium perfusion defects were present, the mortality was markedly increased, with a relative risk of 7.8 (mortality at 6 years, 31% vs. 4%, $p < .001$). Abnormal HRR has also been demonstrated in a large population of healthy young adults undergoing routine submaximal exercise testing (138). More than 5,000 healthy adults enrolled in the Lipid Research Clinics Prevalence Study, with no known heart disease, were followed 12 years after near maximal exercise treadmill testing. Abnormal HRR was defined as less than a 42-beat fall in

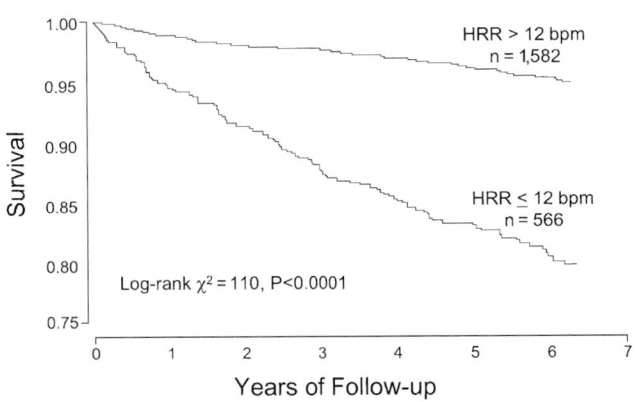

FIGURE 77.5 Kaplan-Meier plot relating heart-rate recovery (HRR) to all-cause mortality. (From Cole CR, Lauer MS. Exercise testing and risk assessment. In: Foody JM, ed. Preventive cardiology. Totowa, NJ: Humana Press, 2001, with permission. Based on data from Cole CR, Blackstone EH, Pashkow FJ, et al. Heart-rate recovery immediately after exercise as a predictor of mortality. *N Engl J Med* 1999;341:1351–1357.)

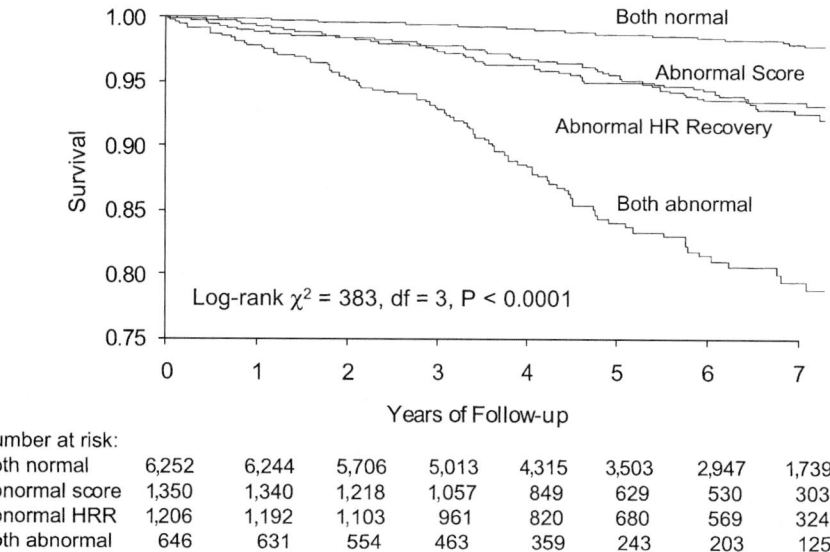

FIGURE 77.6 Kaplan-Meier survival curves according to heart rate (HR), heart-rate recovery (HRR), and treadmill exercise score. (From Nishime EO, Cole CR, Blackstone EH, et al. Heart rate recovery and treadmill exercise score as predictors of mortality in patients referred for exercise ECG. *JAMA* 2000;284: 1392–1398, with permission.)

heart rate 2 minutes into recovery. Those with abnormal HRR were at increased risk for cardiac deaths (4% vs. 1%) and for all-cause mortality (10% vs. 4%).

There were important similarities and differences between this study and the prior study. First, the population studied was younger and at lower risk for heart disease at baseline. Second, the tests were not true maximal exercise tests but were stopped when the subjects achieved 85% to 90% of age-predicted maximum heart rate. Third, there was no cool-down period, and the subjects went directly from maximum exercise to a seated position. Last, heart rate during recovery was not measured until 2 minutes had elapsed and thus could not be directly compared with the prior study. Despite these differences, HRR was a strong, independent predictor of mortality in both populations.

To better understand the interactions that HRR has with other exercise-derived predictors of outcome, we studied HRR and the Duke treadmill exercise score in a population of 9,454 patients who underwent symptom-limited exercise ECG testing (139). The Duke treadmill exercise score incorporates exercise duration and ST-segment deviation and symptoms and has been validated as a predictor of mortality (140). Patients were divided into low-, intermediate-, or high-risk groups based on their treadmill exercise scores. For HRR a cutoff value of 12 beats/min or less after 1 minute of recovery was called an abnormal response. The primary end point was all-cause mortality.

In 5 years of follow-up, there were 312 deaths. Either an abnormal HRR or an intermediate- or high-risk treadmill exercise score predicted a fourfold increase in mortality (Fig. 77.6). If both the treadmill exercise score and HRR were normal the 5-year mortality was only 2%, but if both were abnormal mortality increased to 14%. There was no interaction between the two predictors. These findings demonstrate that HRR adds important informa-

tion to the interpretation of the exercise test in addition to standard predictors.

CONTROVERSIES AND PERSONAL PERSPECTIVES

There is little controversy about the value of RR variability or BRS for predicting cardiac death or arrhythmic events in coronary heart disease. This new knowledge should be put to use more frequently and incorporated into practice guidelines. RR variability and BRS have positive predictive accuracy as good as any other risk predictor in coronary heart disease. After myocardial infarction, patients who have values of RR variability and BRS below the critical high-risk cut points have double the risk of cardiac death or an arrhythmic event, even if they have a good ejection fraction and lack ventricular arrhythmias. Furthermore, when combined with LVEF, ventricular arrhythmia frequency, or both, they substantially improve positive predictive accuracy and identify groups at very high risk.

The controversies with respect to diagnostic use of RR variability and BRS are when to measure these variables and what to do for patients who have critically low values for RR variability or BRS. Given what we know about the role of the autonomic nervous system in the pathophysiology of coronary heart disease, it is reasonable to measure RR variability, BRS, or both in patients with previous myocardial infarction. RR variability and BRS are best measured 6 to 21 days or greater than or equal to 3 months after myocardial infarction. Between 3 and 12 weeks, RR variability is increasing as recovery from infarction proceeds and the values are more difficult to interpret. Many commercial Holter systems provide measurements of RR variability, making these measurements easily accessible and inexpensive. Although the RR variability measures provided by various

THE FUTURE

The future will bring a clearer understanding about the physiologic systems that determine cyclic fluctuations in RR intervals. This knowledge will increase our ability to interpret alterations in RR variability in disease states or during drug therapy and to react to them appropriately. Further research will provide information on the role that the autonomic nervous system plays in cardiac death and establish treatments that target the autonomic nervous system to decrease cardiac death in patients with coronary artery disease.

We still have much to learn about how physiologic control systems determine the fluctuations of heart rate that we quantify and use diagnostically. In the future, we will learn more about the physiologic systems that determine cyclic fluctuations in RR intervals and heart-rate changes. This knowledge will increase our ability to interpret these alterations in disease states or during drug therapy and to react to them appropriately.

The predictive value of RR variability and BRS is established for death and arrhythmic events in coronary heart disease. However, the predictive value of these measures of autonomic nervous system activity for death and other important cardiovascular outcomes is yet to be firmly established for other cardiac diseases. This is an important task for the future.

Sudden cardiac death remains one of our biggest public health problems. Most out-of-hospital cardiac arrests occur in persons with coronary heart disease and are due to VF. The low salvage rate for out-of-hospital cardiac arrest motivates attempts to predict this event and to prevent it. In the 1990s, the predictive value of RR variability and BRS was established for cardiac death in coronary heart disease. These findings suggest that the autonomic nervous system is intimately involved in the pathogenesis of cardiac deaths, presumably by arrhythmic mechanisms. However, it is possible that RR variability and BRS are not responsible for cardiac death, but

reflect other factors that are. It remains to be proven that the autonomic nervous system plays a major causal role in cardiac death. To establish a causal role for the autonomic nervous system, a treatment that increases RR variability and BRS must be shown to decrease cardiac death in patients with coronary heart disease. The EMIAT substudy demonstrated that amiodarone prophylaxis in patients with recent myocardial infarction and LVEF less than 0.41 was beneficial for patients who had low RR variability, but not for patients with normal RR variability. Defibrillators in Acute Myocardial Infarction Trial (DINAMIT) is recruiting patients who have reduced LVEF and low RR variability and randomizing them to implantable cardioverter-defibrillator (ICD) prophylaxis or no antiarrhythmic therapy (121).

At the present time, ICDs are the dominant treatment for coronary heart disease patients who survive out-of-hospital cardiac arrest, and beta-adrenergic blocking drugs are the dominant therapy for those at risk, but who have not had a sustained ventricular tachyarrhythmia. The dominance of implantable defibrillator therapy for cardiac arrest survivors is based several randomized trials that show ICD therapy to be superior to amiodarone therapy in patients who have survived a spontaneous cardiac arrest. For patients at risk who have not yet had a sustained ventricular arrhythmia, it remains to be proven that RR variability or BRS will predict the deaths that can be prevented by ICDs. ICD prophylaxis should be restricted in clinical practice to groups that have been shown in randomized controlled trials to benefit. The value of RR variability and BRS for identifying patients who will benefit from ICD prophylaxis is being studied in ongoing trials (e.g., DINAMIT). Also, it will be possible to conduct randomized trials of drug prophylaxis to prevent sudden cardiac death in patients who have had an ICD implant (142); before ICDs, such trials would have been unethical.

commercial Holter systems vary, many of the measures are equivalent and can be used interchangeably (eTable 77.1.1). Thus, nearly every commercial Holter system provides one or more useful measure(s) of RR variability. Equipment to measure BRS is not widely available at the present time. However, equipment is likely to become more widely available over the coming years now that measurement of BRS has been shown to be useful and safe.

Patients categorized as high risk based on their RR variability, BRS values, or both should be evaluated carefully for reversible risk. Also, these patients should be treated

with drugs proven to decrease postinfarction risk (e.g., aspirin, statins, and beta-adrenergic blocking drugs). Beta-adrenergic blocking drugs are known to be safe and effective for preventing cardiac deaths after myocardial infarction. By blocking peripheral beta-receptors, beta-adrenergic blocking drugs decrease the adverse cardiovascular effects of the sympathetic nervous system. By blocking beta-receptors in the central nervous system, beta-adrenergic blocking drugs also increase parasympathetic activity. These effects of beta-adrenergic blocking drugs increase RR variability and BRS.

Many physicians do not prescribe beta-blockers for low-risk patients with recent myocardial infarctions (i.e., patients with good left ventricular function, no ventricular arrhythmias, and a negative exercise test result). However, among such "low-risk" patients, there are some whose risk is identified only by critically low values of RR variability or BRS. These patients also should be treated with beta-adrenergic blocking drugs. Patients who have an LVEF less than 0.41 and low RR variability should be considered for prophylactic amiodarone.

The recognition that heart-rate changes during and immediately after exercise are both correlated with autonomic function and with long-term mortality now means that the exercise stress laboratory is a venue for easy, inexpensive, and prognostically meaningful assessment of autonomic disturbances. As with HRV, it might be argued that since the pathophysiology and treatment of exercise heart-rate abnormalities are not known, no practical clinical value exists. We believe that this is not the case. By combining exercise heart-rate responses with other exercise test measures, it is simple to identify a large number of very low risk patients, for whom conservative management can be confidently recommended. Although the optimal treatment of patients with abnormal heart-rate dynamics is not known, these patients can be identified as being at increased risk and therefore it is reasonable to aggressively manage all correctable disturbances for which there is evidence of benefit, such as elevated low-density lipoprotein cholesterol in the setting of known coronary disease or aggressive reduction of elevated blood pressure.

Several questions remain to be answered about HRR. The optimal time to measure the recovery rate has not been well defined. One-minute recovery heart rate has been used successfully in two studies and is also routinely measured in most exercise laboratories. However, 2-minute recovery is also predictive of outcome and may be an alternative. It is also possible that a shorter HRR, such as 30-second recovery (31), may be a better predictor of death. A cool-down period following exercise is currently routinely used except in certain situations such as stress echocardiography. HRR for the use or nonuse of different cool-down periods still needs to be defined. Last, it is unclear if HRR is a modifiable risk factor. It is possible that exercise may increase HRR (141) as may pharmacologic intervention, but this currently is unknown.

Currently, we recommend that all individuals undergoing exercise testing have 1-minute HRR measured during a cool-down period and the findings reported in the results. For those individuals whose heart rates fail to decrease by more than 12 beats/min an abnormal HRR should be reported and they should be considered at higher risk for death. Their other risk factors should be optimized, but there is no need to proceed to heart catheterization based solely on an abnormal HRR. There are no current recommendations regarding exercise or medications for an abnormal HRR.

ACKNOWLEDGMENTS

Supported in part by NIH Grants HL-41552, HL-48120, HL-48159, and HC-95184, from the National Heart, Lung, and Blood Institute, Bethesda, MD, and RR-00645 from the Research Resources Administration, NIH; and by funds from the Brugher Foundation, The Dana Foundation, and Mrs. Adelaide Segerman, New York, NY.

REFERENCES

1. Ludwig C. Beitrage zur Kenntniss des Enflusses der respirations bewegungen auf den Blutlauf im Aortensysteme. *Arch Anat Physiol* 1847;13:242–302.
2. Anrep G, Pascual W, Rossler R. Respiratory variations of the heart rate. IIC. The central mechanism of the respiratory arrhythmia and the inter-relations between the central and reflex mechanisms. *Proc R Soc (Lond)* 1936;119B:218–230.
3. Anrep G, Pascual W, Rossler R. Respiratory variations of the heart rate. IC. The reflex mechanism of the respiratory arrhythmia. *Proc R Soc (Lond)* 1936;119B:191–217.
4. Katona PG, Poitras JW, Barnett GO, et al. Cardiac vagal efferent activity and heart period in the carotid sinus reflex. *Am J Physiol* 1970;218:1030–1037.
5. Katona PG, Jih F. Respiratory sinus arrhythmia: noninvasive measure of parasympathetic cardiac control. *J Appl Physiol* 1975;39:801–805.
6. Fouad FM, Tarazi RC, Ferrario CM, et al. Assessment of parasympathetic control of heart rate by a noninvasive method. *Am J Physiol* 1984;246:H838–842.
7. Hirsch JA, Bishop B. Respiratory sinus arrhythmia in humans: how breathing pattern modulates heart rate. *Am J Physiol* 1981;241:H620–629.
8. Eckberg DL. Human sinus arrhythmia as an index of vagal cardiac outflow. *J Appl Physiol* 1983;54:961–966.
9. Bennett T, Farquhar IK, Hosking DJ, et al. Assessment of methods for estimating autonomic nervous control of the heart in patients with diabetes mellitus. *Diabetes* 1978;27:1167–1174.
10. Smith SA. Reduced sinus arrhythmia in diabetic autonomic neuropathy: diagnostic value of an age-related normal range. *BMJ* 1982;285:1599–1601.
11. Ewing DJ, Martyn CN, Young RJ, et al. The value of cardiovascular autonomic function tests: 10 years experience in diabetes. *Diabetes Care* 1985;8:491–498.
12. Ewing DJ, Clarke BF. Diagnosis and management of diabetic autonomic neuropathy. *BMJ* 1982;285:916–918.
13. Akselrod S, Gordon D, Ubel FA, et al. Power spectrum analysis of heart rate fluctuation: a quantitative probe of beat-to-beat cardiovascular control. *Science* 1981;213:220–222.
14. Pomeranz B, Macaulay RJ, Caudill MA, et al. Assessment of autonomic function in humans by heart rate spectral analysis. *Am J Physiol* 1985;248:H151–153.
15. Pagani M, Lombardi F, Guzzetti S, et al. Power spectral analysis of heart rate and arterial pressure variabilities as a marker of sympathovagal interaction in man and conscious dog. *Circ Res* 1986;59:178–193.

16. Wolf M, Varigos G, Hunt D, et al. Sinus arrhythmia in acute myocardial infarction. *Med J Aust* 1978;2:52–53.

17. Kleiger RE, Miller JP, Bigger JT Jr, et al. Decreased heart rate variability and its association with increased mortality after acute myocardial infarction. *Am J Cardiol* 1987;59:256–262.

18. Hinkle LE Jr, Carver ST, Plakun A. Slow heart rates and increased risk of cardiac death in middle-aged men. *Arch Intern Med* 1972;129:732–748.

19. Ellestad MH. Chronotropic incompetence. The implications of heart rate response to exercise (compensatory parasympathetic hyperactivity?) [editorial; comment]. *Circulation* 1996;93:1485–1487.

20. Ellestad MH, Wan MK. Predictive implications of stress testing. Follow-up of 2700 subjects after maximum treadmill stress testing. *Circulation* 1975;51:363–369.

21. Ladenheim ML, Pollock BH, Rozanski A, et al. Extent and severity of myocardial hypoperfusion as predictors of prognosis in patients with suspected coronary artery disease. *J Am Coll Cardiol* 1986;7:464–471.

22. Lauer MS, Okin PM, Larson MG, et al. Impaired heart rate response to graded exercise. Prognostic implications of chronotropic incompetence in the Framingham Heart Study. *Circulation* 1996;93:1520–1526.

23. Lauer MS, Pashkow FJ, Larson MG, et al. Association of cigarette smoking with chronotropic incompetence and prognosis in the Framingham Heart Study. *Circulation* 1997;96:897–903.

24. Lauer MS, Mehta R, Pashkow FJ, et al. Association of chronotropic incompetence with echocardiographic ischemia and prognosis. *J Am Coll Cardiol* 1998;32:1280–1286.

25. Lauer MS, Francis GS, Okin PM, et al. Impaired chronotropic response to exercise stress testing as a predictor of mortality. *JAMA* 1999;281:524–529.

26. Cotton FS, Dill DB. On the relation between the heart rate during exercise and that of the immediate post-exercise period. *Am J Physiol* 1935;111:554–556.

27. Johnson RE, Brouha L, Darling RC. A test of physical fitness for strenuous exertion. *Rev Can Bio* 1942;1:491–503.

28. Herxheimer H. Heart rate recovery from severe exercise. *J Appl Physiol* 1948;1:279–284.

29. Cardus D, Spencer WA. Recovery time of heart frequency in healthy men: its relation to age and physical condition. *Arch Phys Med Rehabil* 1967;48:71–77.

30. Pierpont GL, Stolpman DR, Gornick CC. Heart rate recovery post-exercise as an index of parasympathetic activity. *J Auton Nerv Syst* 2000;80:169–174.

31. Imai K, Sato H, Hori M, et al. Vagally mediated heart rate recovery after exercise is accelerated in athletes but blunted in patients with chronic heart failure. *J Am Coll Cardiol* 1994;24:1529–1535.

32. Gettman LR. Fitness testing. In: American College of Sports Medicine, ed. *Resource manual for guidelines for exercise testing and prescription.* Philadelphia: Lea & Febiger, 1989.

33. Golding LA, Myers CR, Sinning WE, eds. *Y's way to physical fitness*, 3rd ed. Champaign, IL: Human Kinetics Publishers, 1989.

34. Cowell JM, Montgomery AC, Talashek M. Cardiovascular risk stability: from grade school to high school. *J Pediatr Health Care* 1992;6:349–354.

35. Cole CR, Blackstone EH, Pashkow FJ, et al. Heart-rate recovery immediately after exercise as a predictor of mortality. *N Engl J Med* 1999;341:1351–1357.

36. Jose AD, Taylor RR. Autonomic blockade by propranolol and atropine to study intrinsic myocardial function in man. *J Clin Invest* 1969;48:2019–2031.

37. Wallin BG, Sundlof G. A quantitative study of muscle nerve sympathetic activity in resting normotensive and hypertensive subjects. *Hypertension* 1979;1:67–77.

38. Hjemdahl P, Fagius J, Freyschuss U, et al. Muscle sympathetic activity and norepinephrine release during mental challenge in humans. *Am J Physiol* 1989;257:E654–664.

39. Pagani M, Furlan R, Pizzinelli P, et al. Spectral analysis of R-R and arterial pressure variabilities to assess sympathovagal interaction during mental stress in humans. *J Hypertens Suppl* 1989;7:S14–15.

40. Pagani M, Mazzuero G, Ferrari A, et al. Sympathovagal interaction during mental stress. A study using spectral analysis of heart rate variability in healthy control subjects and patients with a prior myocardial infarction. *Circulation* 1991;83[4 Suppl]:II43–II51.

41. Jiang W, Hayano J, Coleman ER, et al. Relation of cardiovascular responses to mental stress and cardiac vagal activity in coronary artery disease. *Am J Cardiol* 1993;72:551–554.

42. Robinson SM, Epstein SE, Beiser GD, et al. Control of heart rate by the autonomic nervous system. *Circ Res* 1966;29:400–411.

43. Yamamoto Y, Hughson RL. Coarse-graining spectral analysis: new method for studying heart rate variability. *J Appl Physiol* 1991;71:1143–1150.

44. Wallin BG, Fagius J. Peripheral sympathetic neural activity in conscious humans. *Annu Rev Physiol* 1988;50:565–576.

45. Arai Y, Saul JP, Albrecht P, et al. Modulation of cardiac autonomic activity during and immediately after exercise. *Am J Physiol* 1989;256:H132–141.

46. Maciel BC, Gallo L Jr, Marin Neto JA, et al. Autonomic nervous control of the heart rate during dynamic exercise in normal man. *Clin Sci* 1986;71:457–460.

47. Crouse SF, Sterling J, Tolson H, et al. The effect of beta-adrenergic blockade on heart rate recovery from exercise. *J Cardiopulmon Rehab* 1989;9:202–206.

48. Perini R, Orizio C, Comande A, et al. Plasma norepinephrine and heart rate dynamics during recovery from submaximal exercise in man. *Eur J Appl Physiol* 1989;58:879–883.

49. Schwartz PJ, Brown AM, Malliani A, et al., eds. *Neural mechanisms in cardiac arrhythmias.* New York: Raven Press, 1978.

50. Lown B, Verrier RL. Neural activity and ventricular fibrillation. *N Engl J Med* 1976;294:1165–1170.

51. Zipes DP, Barber MJ, Takahashi N, et al. Influence of the autonomic nervous system on the genesis of cardiac arrhythmias. *Pacing Clin Electrophysiol* 1983;6:1210–1220.

52. Corr PB, Yamada KA, Witkowski FX. Mechanisms controlling cardiac autonomic function and their relation to

arrhythmogenesis. In: Fozzard HA, Jennings RB, Haber E, et al., eds. *The heart and cardiovascular system. Vol. II.* New York: Raven Press, 1986:1343–1403.

53. Levy MN, Schwartz PJ, eds. *Vagal control of the heart: experimental basis and clinical implications.* Armonk, NY: Futura Publishing, 1994.

54. Schwartz PJ, Zipes DP. Autonomic modulation of cardiac arrhythmias. In: Zipes DP, Jalife J, eds. *Cardiac electrophysiology from cell to bedside,* 3rd ed. Philadelphia: WB Saunders, 2000:300–314.

55. Hockman CH, Mauck HP Jr, Hoff EC. ECG changes resulting from cerebral stimulation. II. A spectrum of ventricular arrhythmias of sympathetic origin. *Am Heart J* 1966;71:695–700.

56. Skinner JE, Reed JC. Blockade of frontocortical-brain stem pathway prevents ventricular fibrillation of ischemic heart. *Am J Physiol* 1981;240:H156–163.

57. Carpeggiani C, Landisman C, Montaron MF, et al. Cryoblockade in limbic brain (amygdala) prevents or delays ventricular fibrillation after coronary artery occlusion in psychologically stressed pigs. *Circ Res* 1992;70:600–606.

58. Verrier RL, Lown B. Behavioral stress and cardiac arrhythmias. *Annu Rev Physiol* 1984;46:155–176.

59. Schwartz PJ, Pagani M, Lombardi F, et al. A cardiocardiac sympathovagal reflex in the cat. *Circ Res* 1973;32:215–220.

60. Malliani A, Recordati G, Schwartz PJ. Nervous activity of afferent cardiac sympathetic fibres with atrial and ventricular endings. *J Physiol (Lond)* 1973;229:457–469.

61. Cascio WE, Johnson TA, Gettes LS. Electrophysiologic changes in ischemic ventricular myocardium: I. Influence of ionic, metabolic, and energetic changes. *J Cardiovasc Electrophysiol* 1995;6:1039–1062.

62. Barber MJ, Mueller TM, Henry DP, et al. Transmural myocardial infarction in the dog produces sympathectomy in noninfarcted myocardium. *Circulation* 1983;67:787–796.

63. Esperer HD, Bentrup A, Geller JC. Decreased heart rate variability in the early postinfarction period correlates with the extent of myocardial sympathetic denervation. *PACE* 1997;20:1090.

64. Takahashi N, Barber MJ, Zipes DP. Efferent vagal innervation of canine ventricle. *Am J Physiol* 1985;248:H89–97.

65. Barber MJ, Mueller TM, Davies BG, et al. Interruption of sympathetic and vagal-mediated afferent responses by transmural myocardial infarction. *Circulation* 1985;72:623–631.

66. De Ferrari GM, Vanoli E, Schwartz PJ. Vagal activity and ventricular fibrillation. In: Levy MN, Schwartz PJ, eds. *Vagal control of the heart: experimental basis and clinical implications.* Armonk, NY: Futura Publishing, 1994:613–636.

67. Billman GE, Schwartz PJ, Stone HL. Baroreceptor reflex control of heart rate: a predictor of sudden cardiac death. *Circulation* 1982;66:874–880.

68. Billman GE, Schwartz PJ, Stone HL. The effects of daily exercise on susceptibility to sudden cardiac death. *Circulation* 1984;69:1182–1189.

69. Schwartz PJ, Vanoli E, Stramba-Badiale M, et al. Autonomic mechanisms and sudden death. New insights from

analysis of baroreceptor reflexes in conscious dogs with and without a myocardial infarction. *Circulation* 1988;78:969–979.

70. Schwartz PJ, Billman GE, Stone HL. Autonomic mechanisms in ventricular fibrillation induced by myocardial ischemia during exercise in dogs with healed myocardial infarction. An experimental preparation for sudden cardiac death. *Circulation* 1984;69:790–800.

71. Vanoli E, De Ferrari GM, Stramba-Badiale M, et al. Vagal stimulation and prevention of sudden death in conscious dogs with a healed myocardial infarction. *Circ Res* 1991;68:1471–1481.

72. Hull SS Jr, Evans AR, Vanoli E, et al. Heart rate variability before and after myocardial infarction in conscious dogs at high and low risk of sudden death. *J Am Coll Cardiol* 1990;16:978–985.

73. Adamson PB, Huang MH, Vanoli E, et al. Unexpected interaction between beta-adrenergic blockade and heart rate variability before and after myocardial infarction. A longitudinal study in dogs at high and low risk for sudden death [see comments]. *Circulation* 1994;90:976–982.

74. Hammond HK, Froelicher VF. Normal and abnormal heart rate responses to exercise. *Prog Cardiovasc Dis* 1985;27:271–296.

75. Paffenbarger RS, Hale WE. Work activity and coronary heart mortality. *N Engl J Med* 1975;292:545–550.

76. Willich SN, Lewis M, Lowel H, et al. Physical exertion as a trigger of acute myocardial infarction. Triggers and Mechanisms of Myocardial Infarction Study Group [see comments]. *N Engl J Med* 1993;329:1684–1690.

77. Mittleman MA, Maclure M, Tofler GH, et al. Triggering of acute myocardial infarction by heavy physical exertion. Protection against triggering by regular exertion. Determinants of Myocardial Infarction Onset Study Investigators [see comments]. *N Engl J Med* 1993;329:1677–1683.

78. Dyer AR, Persky V, Stamler J, et al. Heart rate as a prognostic factor for coronary heart disease and mortality: findings in three Chicago epidemiologic studies. *Am J Epidemiol* 1980;112:736–749.

79. Wilkoff BL, Miller RE. Exercise testing for chronotropic assessment. *Cardiol Clin* 1992;10:705–717.

80. Okin PM, Lauer MS, Kligfield P. Chronotropic response to exercise. Improved performance of ST-segment depression criteria after adjustment for heart rate reserve. *Circulation* 1996;94:3226–3231.

81. Brener SJ, Pashkow FJ, Harvey SA, et al. Chronotropic response to exercise predicts angiographic severity in patients with suspected or stable coronary artery disease. *Am J Cardiol* 1995;76:1228–1232.

82. Dresing TJ, Blackstone EH, Pashkow FJ, et al. Usefulness of impaired chronotropic response to exercise as a predictor of mortality, independent of the severity of coronary artery disease. *Am J Cardiol* 2000;86:602–609.

83. Colucci WS, Ribeiro JP, Rocco MB, et al. Impaired chronotropic response to exercise in patients with congestive heart failure. Role of postsynaptic beta-adrenergic desensitization. *Circulation* 1989;80:314–323.

84. Linnarsson D. Dynamics of pulmonary gas exchange and heart rate changes at start and end of exercise. *Acta Physiol Scand Suppl* 1974;415:1–68.

85. Savin WM, Davidson DM, Haskell WL. Autonomic contribution to heart rate recovery from exercise in humans. *J Appl Physiol* 1982;53:1572–1575.

86. Victor RG, Seals DR, Mark AL. Differential control of heart rate and sympathetic nerve activity during dynamic exercise. Insight from intraneural recordings in humans. *J Clin Invest* 1987;79:508–516.

87. Darr KC, Bassett DR, Morgan BJ, et al. Effects of age and training status on heart rate recovery after peak exercise. *Am J Physiol* 1988;254:H340–H343.

88. Koike A, Hiroe M, Marumo F. Delayed kinetics of oxygen uptake during recovery after exercise in cardiac patients. *Medicine & Science in Sports & Exercise* 1998;30:185–189.

89. Tulppo MP, Makikallio TH, Seppanen T, et al. Vagal modulation of heart rate during exercise: effects of age and physical fitness. *Am J Physiol* 1998;274:H424–429.

90. Hull SS Jr, Vanoli E, Adamson PB, et al. Exercise training confers anticipatory protection from sudden death during acute myocardial ischemia. *Circulation* 1994;89:548–552.

91. Baraldi E, Cooper DM, Zanconato S, et al. Heart rate recovery from 1 minute of exercise in children and adults. *Pediatr Res* 1991;29:575–579.

92. Ohuchi H, Suzuki H, Yasuda K, et al. Heart rate recovery after exercise and cardiac autonomic nervous activity in children. *Pediatr Res* 2000;47:329–335.

93. Heart rate variability: standards of measurement, physiological interpretation and clinical use. Task Force of the European Society of Cardiology and the North American Society of Pacing and Electrophysiology. *Circulation* 1996;93:1043–1065.

94. Bigger JT Jr, Fleiss JL, Steinman RC, et al. Correlations among time and frequency domain measures of heart period variability two weeks after acute myocardial infarction. *Am J Cardiol* 1992;69:891–898.

95. Malik M. Geometrical methods for heart rate variability assessment. In: Malik M, Camm AJ, eds. *Heart rate variability*. Armonk, NY: Futura Publishing, 1995:47–61.

96. Rottman JN, Steinman RC, Albrecht P, et al. Efficient estimation of the heart period power spectrum suitable for physiologic or pharmacologic studies. *Am J Cardiol* 1990;66:1522–1524.

97. Malliani A, Lombardi F, Pagani M. Power spectrum analysis of heart rate variability: a tool to explore neural regulatory mechanisms [editorial]. *Br Heart J* 1994;71:1–2.

98. Malik M, Camm AJ. Components of heart rate variability—what they really mean and what we really measure [editorial]. *Am J Cardiol* 1993;72:821–822.

99. Casadei B, Cochrane S, Johnston J, et al. Pitfalls in the interpretation of spectral analysis of the heart rate variability during exercise in humans. *Acta Physiol Scand* 1995;153:125–131.

100. Fallen EL, Kamath MV, Ghista DN. Power spectrum of heart rate variability: a non-invasive test of integrated neurocardiac function. *Clin Invest Med* 1988;11:331–340.

101. Bigger JT Jr, Fleiss JL, Steinman RC, et al. Frequency domain measures of heart period variability and mortality after myocardial infarction. *Circulation* 1992;85:164–171.

102. Saul JP, Albrecht P, Berger RD, et al. Analysis of long term heart rate variability: methods, 1/f scaling and implications. *Computers in Cardiology* 1987;14:419–422.

103. Bigger JT Jr, Steinman RC, Rolnitzky LM, et al. Power law behavior of RR-interval variability in healthy middle-aged persons, patients with recent acute myocardial infarction, and patients with heart transplants. *Circulation* 1996;93:2142–2151.

104. Goldberger AL, West BJ. Applications of nonlinear dynamics to clinical cardiology. *Ann N Y Acad Sci* 1987;504:195–213.

105. Goldberger AL. Nonlinear dynamics, fractals and chaos: applications to cardiac electrophysiology. *Ann Biomed Eng* 1990;18:195–198.

106. Skinner JE, Carpeggiani C, Landisman CE, et al. Correlation dimension of heartbeat intervals is reduced in conscious pigs by myocardial ischemia. *Circ Res* 1991;68:966–976.

107. Peng CK, Havlin S, Stanley HE, et al. Quantification of scaling exponents and crossover phenomena in nonstationary heart beat time series. *Chaos* 1995;5:82–87.

108. Bigger JT Jr, Fleiss JL, Steinman RC, et al. RR variability in healthy, middle-aged persons compared with patients with chronic coronary heart disease or recent acute myocardial infarction. *Circulation* 1995;91:1936–1943.

109. Smyth HS, Sleight P, Pickering GW. Reflex regulation of arterial pressure during sleep in man. A quantitative method of assessing baroreflex sensitivity. *Circ Res* 1969;24:109–121.

110. Gribbin B, Pickering TG, Sleight P, et al. Effect of age and high blood pressure on baroreflex sensitivity in man. *Circ Res* 1971;29:424–431.

111. Adamopoulos S, Piepoli M, McCance A, et al. Comparison of different methods for assessing sympathovagal balance in chronic congestive heart failure secondary to coronary artery disease. *Am J Cardiol* 1992;70:1576–1582.

112. Parati G, Frattola A, Omboni S, et al. Analysis of heart rate and blood pressure variability in the assessment of autonomic regulation in arterial hypertension. *Clin Sci (Colch)* 1996;91[Suppl]:129–132.

113. Imholz BP, van Montfrans GA, Settels JJ, et al. Continuous non-invasive blood pressure monitoring: reliability of Finapres device during the Valsalva manoeuvre. *Cardiovasc Res* 1988;22:390–397.

114. La Rovere MT, Bigger JT Jr., Marcus FI, et al. Baroreflex sensitivity and heart-rate variability in prediction of total cardiac mortality after myocardial infarction. ATRAMI (Autonomic Tone and Reflexes After Myocardial Infarction) Investigators. *Lancet* 1998;351:478–484.

115. Robbe HW, Mulder LJ, Ruddel H, et al. Assessment of baroreceptor reflex sensitivity by means of spectral analysis. *Hypertension* 1987;10:538–543.

116. Pagani M, Somers V, Furlan R, et al. Changes in autonomic regulation induced by physical training in mild hypertension. *Hypertension* 1988;12:600–610.

117. Farrell TG, Bashir Y, Cripps T, et al. Risk stratification for arrhythmic events in postinfarction patients based on heart rate variability, ambulatory electrocardiographic variables and the signal-averaged electrocardiogram. *J Am Coll Cardiol* 1991;18:687–697.

118. Katz A, Liberty IF, Porath A, et al. A simple bedside test of 1-minute heart rate variability during deep breathing as a prognostic index after myocardial infarction. *Am Heart J* 1999;138:32–38.

119. Bigger JT, Fleiss JL, Rolnitzky LM, et al. The ability of several short-term measures of RR variability to predict mortality after myocardial infarction. *Circulation* 1993;88:927–934.

120. Huikuri HV, Makikallio TH, Peng CK, et al. Fractal correlation properties of R-R interval dynamics and mortality in patients with depressed left ventricular function after an acute myocardial infarction. *Circulation* 2000;101:47–53.

121. Malik M, Camm AJ, Janse MJ, et al. Depressed heart rate variability identifies postinfarction patients who might benefit from prophylactic treatment with amiodarone: a substudy of EMIAT (The European Myocardial Infarct Amiodarone Trial). *J Am Coll Cardiol* 2000;35:1263–1275.

122. Bigger JT Jr, Fleiss JL, Rolnitzky LM, et al. Time course of recovery of heart period variability after myocardial infarction. *J Am Coll Cardiol* 1991;18:1643–1649.

123. Bigger JT Jr, La Rovere MT, Steinman RC, et al. Comparison of baroreflex sensitivity and heart period variability after myocardial infarction. *J Am Coll Cardiol* 1989;14:1511–1518.

124. Flapan AD, Wright RA, Nolan J, et al. Differing patterns of cardiac parasympathetic activity and their evolution in selected patients with a first myocardial infarction. *J Am Coll Cardiol* 1993;21:926–931.

125. Bigger JT Jr, Fleiss JL, Rolnitzky LM, et al. Frequency domain measures of heart period variability to assess risk late after myocardial infarction [published erratum appears in *J Am Coll Cardiol* 1993;21:1537]. *J Am Coll Cardiol* 1993;21:729–736.

126. Liao D, Barnes RW, Chambless LE, et al. Age, race, and sex differences in autonomic cardiac function measured by spectral analysis of heart rate variability—the ARIC study. Atherosclerosis Risk in Communities. *Am J Cardiol* 1995;76:906–912.

127. Singh JP, Larson MG, O'Donnell CJ, et al. Heritability of heart rate variability: the Framingham Heart Study. *Circulation* 1999;99:2251–2254.

128. Nolan J, Batin PD, Andrews R, et al. Prospective study of heart rate variability and mortality in chronic heart failure: results of the United Kingdom heart failure evaluation and assessment of risk trial (UK-heart). *Circulation* 1998;98: 1510–1516.

129. Dawber TR, Meadors GF, Moore FE. Epidemiologic approaches to heart disease: the Framingham study. *Am J Public Health* 1951;41:279–286.

130. Tsuji H, Venditti FJ Jr, Manders ES, et al. Reduced heart rate variability and mortality risk in an elderly cohort. The Framingham Heart Study. *Circulation* 1994;90:878–883.

131. Algra A, Tijssen JG, Roelandt JR, et al. Heart rate variability from 24-hour electrocardiography and the 2-year risk for sudden death. *Circulation* 1993;88:180–185.

132. La Rovere MT, Specchia G, Mortara A, et al. Baroreflex sensitivity, clinical correlates, and cardiovascular mortality among patients with a first myocardial infarction. A prospective study. *Circulation* 1988;78:816–824.

133. Farrell TG, Odemuyiwa O, Bashir Y, et al. Prognostic value of baroreflex sensitivity testing after acute myocardial infarction. *Br Heart J* 1992;67:129–137.

134. Mortara A, Specchia G, La Rovere MT, et al. Patency of infarct-related artery. Effect of restoration of anterograde flow on vagal reflexes. ATRAMI (Automatic Tone and Reflexes After Myocardial Infarction) Investigators. *Circulation* 1996;93:1114–1122.

135. Hohnloser SH, Klingenheben T, van de Loo A, et al. Reflex versus tonic vagal activity as a prognostic parameter in patients with sustained ventricular tachycardia or ventricular fibrillation. *Circulation* 1994;89:1068–1073.

136. De Ferrari GM, Landolina M, Mantica M, et al. Baroreflex sensitivity, but not heart rate variability, is reduced in patients with life-threatening ventricular arrhythmias long after myocardial infarction. *Am Heart J* 1995;130:473–480.

137. Bonaduce D, Petretta M, Piscione F, et al. Influence of reversible segmental left ventricular dysfunction on heart period variability in patients with one-vessel coronary artery disease. *J Am Coll Cardiol* 1994;24:399–405.

138. Cole CR, Foody JM, Blackstone EH, et al. Heart rate recovery after submaximal exercise testing as a predictor of mortality in a cardiovascularly healthy cohort. *Ann Intern Med* 2000;132:552–555.

139. Nishime EO, Cole CR, Blackstone EH, et al. Heart rate recovery and treadmill exercise score as predictors of mortality in patients referred for exercise ECG. *JAMA* 2000;284:1392–1398.

140. Mark DB, Shaw L, Harrell FE Jr, et al. Prognostic value of a treadmill exercise score in outpatients with suspected coronary artery disease. *N Engl J Med* 1991;325:849–853.

141. Hagberg JM, Hickson RC, Ehsani AA, et al. Faster adjustment to and recovery from submaximal exercise in the trained state. *J Appl Physiol* 1980;48:218–224.

142. Pratt CM, Camm AJ, Bigger JT, et al. Evaluation of antiarrhythmic drug efficacy in patients with an ICD. Unlimited potential or replete with complexity and problems? *Eur Heart J* 1999;20:1538–1552.

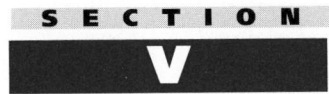

SECTION V

INVASIVE CARDIOLOGY AND SURGICAL TECHNIQUES

ERIC J. TOPOL

CORONARY ANGIOGRAPHY

DEEPAK L. BHATT
FREDERICK A. HEUPLER, JR.

OVERVIEW

Coronary angiography remains the clinical gold standard for the diagnosis of coronary artery disease. Approximately 2 million procedures are performed annually in the United States. More than 60% of cardiologists in the United States perform coronary angiography as part of their practice (1). Because it is an invasive procedure with potentially serious risks, it should be performed only by well-trained individuals when an appropriate clinical indication exists. Physicians who perform coronary angiography must clearly understand its limitations and possess a firm grasp of the fundamental technical aspects of catheterization (2). From gaining arterial access to obtaining adequate images of the coronary arteries, angiographers must obtain and maintain a specific set of skills.

GLOSSARY

Caudal projection: Radiographic view with the image intensifier pointing to the inferior surface of the heart.
Conus artery: A branch that variably arises either from the right coronary artery or in close proximity to it and perfuses the right ventricular outflow tract.
Cranial projection: Radiographic view with the image intensifier pointing to the superior surface of the heart.
Crux: The intersection of the atrioventricular groove and the interatrial and interventricular septa on the inferior aspect of the heart.
Damping: Blunting of a recording of the arterial pressure waveform.

D. L. Bhatt: Department of Cardiovascular Medicine, The Cleveland Clinic Foundation, Cleveland, Ohio
F. A. Heupler, Jr.: Department of Cardiovascular Medicine, The Cleveland Clinic Foundation, Cleveland, Ohio

Diagonal artery: A branch of the left anterior descending artery that perfuses the left ventricular free wall.

Dominance: Refers to the vessel, either the right coronary artery or the left circumflex artery, that supplies the posterior part of the heart; codominance refers to the situation in which both arteries provide circulation to the posterior heart.

Image intensifier: The portion of the catheterization laboratory imaging equipment that increases the brightness of images produced by x-rays.

Internal mammary artery (IMA): An artery that runs from the subclavian artery down the chest wall, which can be harvested for use as a surgical conduit for bypass grafting; sometimes called the *internal thoracic artery*.

Left anterior descending (LAD) artery: The artery that supplies the anterior surface of the heart.

Left anterior oblique (LAO) projection: Radiographic view with the image intensifier on the left side of the patient.

Left circumflex artery (LCx): The artery that supplies blood to the lateral aspect of the heart.

Left main (LM) coronary artery: The short artery that divides into the left anterior descending artery and the left circumflex artery (and sometimes the ramus intermedius) and supplies most of the left side of the heart.

Marginal artery: A branch (acute marginal) of the right coronary artery that supplies the right ventricle; also, a branch (obtuse marginal) of the left circumflex, sometimes referred to as a *lateral branch*.

Posterior descending artery (PDA): The branch of the right coronary artery, or occasionally the left circumflex artery, that provides blood flow to the posterior aspect of the interventricular septum.

Ramus intermedius (RI): A branch of the left main artery that supplies the lateral wall of the left ventricle.

Right anterior oblique (RAO) projection: Radiographic view with the image intensifier on the right of the patient.

Right coronary artery (RCA): The artery that supplies blood to the right side of the heart and usually to the posterior aspect of the left ventricle.

Saphenous vein graft: A surgical conduit harvested from the legs, used to reroute blood from the aorta to the coronary arteries.

Scatter: Dispersion of radiation as it passes through the body; it is the source of most of the radiation exposure to the operator.

Ventricularization: Distortion of the recorded arterial pressure waveform such that the diastolic component is blunted, simulating a left ventricular pressure tracing.

GENERAL PRINCIPLES OF CORONARY ANGIOGRAPHY

Historical Perspective

The first selective coronary angiogram was performed in 1958 by Dr. F. Mason Sones, Jr., a cardiologist at The Cleveland Clinic Foundation (3). Quite accidentally, the catheter positioned in the aorta for an angiogram to assess aortic insufficiency dove into the RCA, and an image was obtained before it was fully realized what had occurred. Although the patient's heart rate slowed down transiently, there were no other untoward effects, and the era of selective coronary angiography was born. When Dr. Sones and Dr. Earl K. Shirey published their results of more than 1,000 procedures in 1962, interest in coronary angiography surged. Coronary angiography as a diagnostic tool blossomed with Dr. René Favaloro's description in 1968 of his pioneering work in performing saphenous vein coronary artery bypass grafting at The Cleveland Clinic.

Radiologists played an important role in the development of catheterization techniques in the early 1960s. New preformed catheter designs, such as those by Dr. Melvin Judkins and Dr. Kurt Amplatz, enabled selective angiography to be performed with greater ease than was previously possible with the Sones catheters. Additionally, percutaneous approaches were also now possible, and arterial cutdowns were no longer required. Improvements in radiographic imaging concomitantly led to better image quality. After Dr. Andreas Grüntzig introduced percutaneous coronary angioplasty in 1977, cardiologists were able to make the transition from being diagnosticians to becoming endovascular surgeons.

Coronary Artery Anatomy

Normal Anatomy

The LM coronary artery originates from the left sinus of Valsalva and usually bifurcates into the LAD, which supplies the left ventricle's anterior surface, and the LCx, which supplies the lateral aspect of the left ventricle (Fig. 78.1). The LAD traverses the anterior interventricular groove, giving rise to septal perforating branches to supply the interventricular septum and to diagonal branches that supply the anterolateral wall. It then bifurcates distally and tapers out as a "whale's tail" at the cardiac apex, although sometimes it "wraps around" the apex to supply part of the inferior wall. The LCx courses along the left atrioventricular groove and provides small atrial branches to the left atrium and marginal branches that supply the lateral wall of the left ventricle. The marginal branches are sometimes referred to as *lateral branches*, with the first marginal branch called the *high lateral* and subsequent lateral branches referred to as *lateral* or *posterolateral branches*. Occasionally, the LM coronary artery trifurcates to give rise also to a ramus intermedius branch that supplies the high lateral wall of the left ventricle.

The RCA originates from the right sinus at a slightly more caudal level than the LM coronary artery and supplies the right ventricle and the inferior aspect of the left ventricle (Fig. 78.2). It traverses the right atrioventricular groove

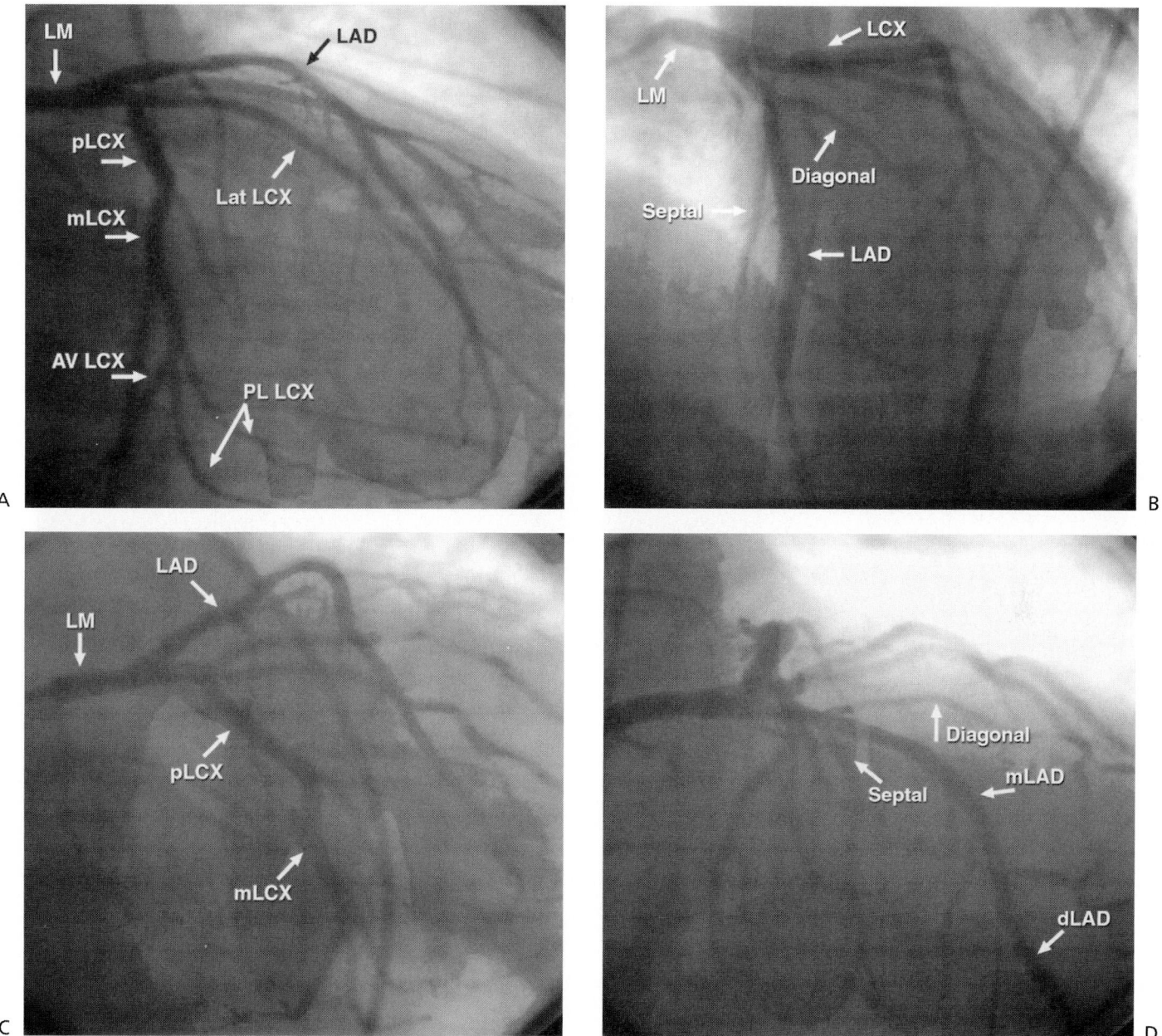

FIGURE 78.1 Normal left coronary artery with segments labeled. **A:** Shallow right anterior oblique (RAO) caudal projection. **B:** Left anterior oblique cranial projection. **C:** Posteroanterior caudal projection. **D:** RAO cranial projection. AV, atrioventricular continuation of the left circumflex artery; dLAD, distal left anterior descending artery; Lat LCX, lateral branch of the left circumflex artery; LM, left main coronary artery; mLAD, mid-left anterior descending artery; mLCX, mid-left circumflex artery; PL, posterolateral branch of the left circumflex artery; pLAD, proximal left anterior descending artery; pLCX, proximal left circumflex artery.

and provides small branches to the right atrium and marginal branches to the right ventricle. Approximately 60% of the time, the RCA atrial branches supply the sinus node; otherwise, the LCx atrial branches serve this function. Approximately 50% of the time, the first branch of the RCA is a conus branch, supplying the right ventricular outflow tract; the remainder of the time, the conus branch originates separately from an ostium near the RCA ostium. The dominant artery is generally defined as the one that provides the PDA to supply the posterior wall. In approximately 85% of patients, the RCA is dominant, with the remainder of patients having either a dominant LCx or a codominant RCA and LCx. The PDA of the RCA (or the LCx) courses along the inferior interventricular groove, providing septal perforators, a feature that may aid in its identification and differentiation from the posterolateral segment of the RCA (or LCx), which gives off branches to the posterior ventricle. More than 90% of the time, the

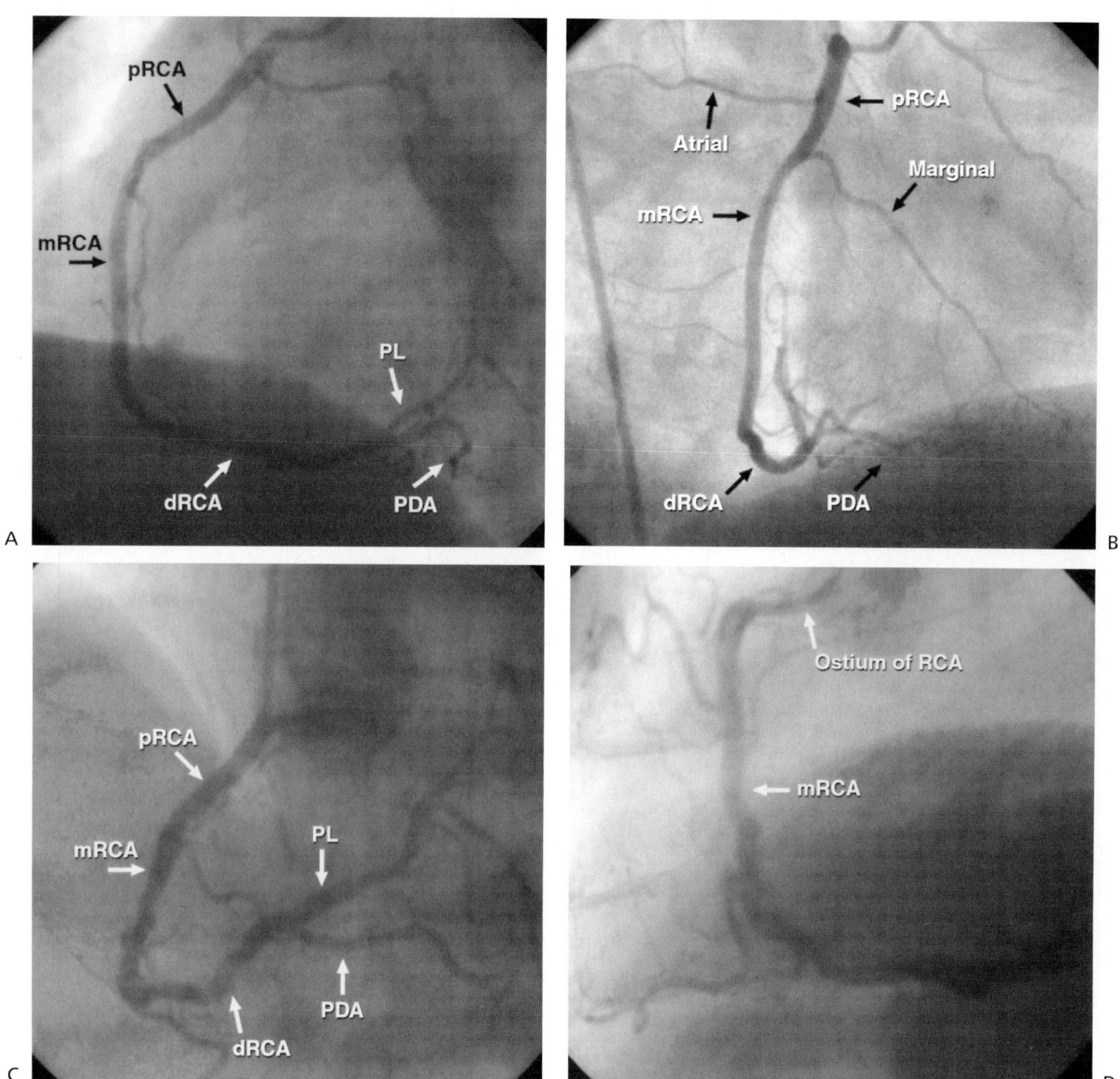

FIGURE 78.2 Normal right coronary artery with segments labeled. **A:** Left anterior oblique projection. **B:** Right anterior oblique projection. **C:** Posteroanterior cranial projection. **D:** Lateral projection. dRCA, distal right coronary artery; mRCA, mid-right coronary artery; PDA, posterior descending artery branch; PL, posterolateral branch of the right coronary artery; pRCA, proximal right coronary artery.

artery to the atrioventricular node originates from the atrioventricular branch of the RCA as it passes through the crux.

Lesion Assessment

An important component of coronary angiography is the description of coronary artery stenoses. Historically, lesions of at least 70% diameter stenosis of a coronary artery (50%

diameter stenosis of the LM coronary artery) are considered hemodynamically significant. For the purposes of many research studies, 50% or greater stenosis constitutes significant coronary artery disease. However, the realization that the majority of myocardial infarctions are due to stenoses of less than 50% severity underscores the importance of the identification of milder degrees of atherosclerosis. Thus, the term *clean coronary arteries* is best avoided, because the absence of hemodynamically significant lesions does not preclude plaque rupture and a future ischemic event.

In addition to the percent diameter stenosis, the morphology and length of the lesion are important and should be described. The presence of calcification, angulation, eccentricity, or ulceration should be noted, because these characteristics may have an impact on the ability to perform percutaneous intervention (15) (*e*Fig. 78.2.5). Any angiographically apparent thrombus should be mentioned (*e*Fig. 78.2.6). However, the absence of thrombus on an angiogram does not mean that none is present, because angiography is a relatively crude method to detect thrombus (16). The size of the vessel should also be described, because lesions in vessels that are smaller than 1.5 mm usually do not warrant bypass surgery or angioplasty. Lesion size can be estimated by comparison with the size of the catheter. A 6-French (Fr) catheter is approximately 2 mm in external diameter (0.33 mm per Fr size). Automated quantitative coronary analysis is now commonly available and can be used to quantitate stenosis severity and length with more consistency than visual estimation (17). ▼ n14

Indications for Coronary Angiography

Coronary angiography is indicated when there is a need for delineation of coronary artery anatomy. The ACC has published guidelines to assist the clinician in appropriate use of this invasive procedure (59) (Table 78.1). Indications are listed as class I when there is general consensus that angiography is indicated, class II when there is a divergence of opinion, and class III when there is consensus that angiography should not be performed. The guidelines are useful as a starting point for discussion about evidence supporting angiography for specific indications. In a patient with anginal chest discomfort and evidence of ischemia on a functional study, coronary angiography may reveal a stenosis that is amenable to angioplasty or coronary artery bypass surgery (class I). In a patient with an acute coronary syndrome, angiography is given a class II indication. However, emerging evidence supports an invasive approach in the initial evaluation of patients with acute coronary syndromes (60,61). The development of pharmacologic adjuncts, such as the glycoprotein IIb/IIIa inhibitors, has enhanced the safety of percutaneous intervention and broadened the indications for cardiac catheterization. Thus, the ACC guidelines provide a framework for the practice of evidence-based medicine but do not substitute for clinical judgment, and they do not necessarily incorporate the most current research.

Contraindications to Coronary Angiography

The only absolute contraindication to coronary angiography is patient refusal. According to the ACC classification, indications that are labeled as class III are actually situa-

TABLE 78.1 INDICATIONS FOR CORONARY ANGIOGRAPHY

Class	Indications
I	Unstable angina/ACS, refractory to medical therapy or with high/intermediate risk features
	Suspected Prinzmetal's angina
	As a plan to proceed with primary PCI for ST-elevation MI
	Cardiogenic shock due to acute MI
	Recurrent ischemia after ST-elevation MI
	Persistent chest pain after fibrinolysis
	Abnormal stress test after fibrinolysis
	CCS class III or IV angina with inadequate response to medical therapy
	Abnormal stress test with high-risk features
	Sudden cardiac death or ventricular arrhythmia with no obvious cause
	Congestive heart failure with angina or ischemia
	Patient requiring valve surgery or repair of a congenital defect, with angina
	Suspected stent thrombosis
	Recurrent angina within 9 mo of PCI
	Before repair of a mechanical complication of MI
	Planned vascular surgery with angina or positive stress test
II	Unstable angina/ACS controlled with medical therapy
	Acute ST-elevation MI after fibrinolysis when it appears that reperfusion has not occurred, to perform rescue PCI
	CCS class III or IV angina that improves to CCS class I or II with medical therapy
	Abnormal stress test without high-risk features
	Worsening ischemia on noninvasive testing
	CCS class I or II angina that is intolerant or unresponsive to medication
	Yearly angiography after cardiac transplantation
	Perioperative MI
III	Patient refusing revascularization
	Patient not a candidate for revascularization due to medical comorbidities
	Within 24 h of fibrinolysis with no evidence of ischemia
	Screening of asymptomatic patients

ACS, acute coronary syndrome; CCS, Canadian Cardiovascular Society; MI, myocardial infarction; PCI, percutaneous coronary intervention. Data adapted from Scanlon PJ, Faxon DP, Audet AM, et al. ACC/AHA guidelines for coronary angiography. A report of the American College of Cardiology/American Heart Association Task Force on practice guidelines (Committee on Coronary Angiography). Developed in collaboration with the Society for Cardiac Angiography and Interventions. *J Am Coll Cardiol* 1999;33:1756–1824, with permission.

tions in which coronary angiography is contraindicated (Table 78.1). Common sense supports these recommendations. Additional relative contraindications are shown in Table 78.2. It should be emphasized that *relative* contraindications imply that in certain urgent clinical circumstances, proceeding with angiography may be appropriate, although caution must be exercised.

Operator Proficiency

The ACC has set minimum training requirements for the performance of diagnostic angiography. During cardiology

TABLE 78.2   RELATIVE CONTRAINDICATIONS TO CORONARY ANGIOGRAPHY

Renal insufficiency
Bleeding diathesis or active bleeding
Fever or active infection
Aortic valve vegetation
Anemia
Severe dye allergy
Metabolic abnormalities
  Hyperkalemia
  Hypokalemia
Digitalis toxicity
Uncontrolled hypertension
Decompensated heart failure
Uncontrolled tachyarrhythmia
Untreated high-grade heart block

fellowship, each trainee must perform 300 diagnostic coronary angiograms while serving as the primary operator on 200. Operator and institutional procedure volumes are linked to outcomes in the catheterization laboratory (62). After training is completed, a minimum yearly volume of 150 diagnostic catheterizations per year for each angiographer has been recommended, although more recently the number has been revised to 100 (63). It is desirable to have cardiac surgical backup nearby (64). Although nonphysicians may assist in coronary angiography, they should not function as independent operators (65). Additionally, performance standards for cardiac catheterization laboratories have been established. Principally, this involves monitoring of procedural outcomes to ensure that some degree of internal review of complications occurs (66,67).

Informed Consent

The risks, benefits, and alternatives to coronary angiography should be discussed with the patient and also the family, if possible. Specifically, the risk of death, stroke, myocardial infarction, renal failure, or emergency coronary bypass surgery should be discussed. Notation of this discussion should be made in the medical record to satisfy the legal requirements for "informed consent." In particular, consideration should be given for noninvasive assessment of coronary artery disease, if this can be substituted for initial diagnostic angiography. A discussion about percutaneous intervention and its greater level of risk should also occur at this time. Separate informed consent should be obtained for this procedure, because many patients who undergo diagnostic angiography proceed to angioplasty at the same setting.

Preprocedural Medication

Aspirin, 325 mg, should be given to eligible patients before the procedure in case an angioplasty is necessary. If the probability of percutaneous intervention seems high, a loading dose of clopidogrel, 300 mg, can also be given. Metformin (Glucophage) should be discontinued on the day of the procedure, because this medication may cause lactic acidosis if renal failure results from the procedure and if metformin is continued after the onset of renal failure (68). Warfarin should be stopped before the procedure if possible until the international normalized ratio is less than 1.8. If anticoagulation is essential, warfarin can be stopped several days before the anticipated procedure, and subcutaneous injections of the low-molecular-weight heparin, enoxaparin (1 mg per kg b.i.d.), can be substituted; the dose of enoxaparin can then be withheld the morning of the procedure.

TECHNICAL ASPECTS OF CARDIAC CATHETERIZATION

Technique

Cardiac catheterization involves multiple sequential steps, each fraught with potential hazards. The first step is gaining arterial access. After this, coronary angiography is performed. Next, left ventriculography and measurement of left ventricular pressures can be done. Aortography and imaging of the cerebral or peripheral vasculature can also be performed. Sterile surgical technique should be maintained throughout the procedure (88). This includes proper preparation of the access site with hair removal and skin cleaning and sterile draping. The operator should wear a surgical cap, gown, shoe covers, and facial mask.

Femoral Arterial Access

The most common form of arterial access for cardiac catheterization in the United States is femoral cannulation. Typically, an 18-gauge, hollow beveled needle is used. Fluoroscopy should be used to facilitate puncture of the common femoral artery at the appropriate level. Rupp et al. (89) identified the target site as 1 cm lateral to the most medial cortex of the femoral head as seen on an anteroposterior (AP) projection (Fig. 78.3). This increases the likelihood of infrainguinal puncture as well as the ability to compress the puncture site against the femoral head after sheath removal. Puncture of the artery more cranially may be associated with a greater risk of retroperitoneal hemorrhage, whereas a more caudal puncture is associated with arterial entry below the femoral artery bifurcation and with pseudoaneurysm formation (*e*Fig. 78.3.1). Use of the skin crease to determine the arterial entry site may be misleading, especially in the obese, in whom the skin crease is often well below the desired point of entry.

    The angle of entry of the needle is critical, with 30 to 45 degrees being the optimal range. A greater degree of angulation may cause problems during sheath insertion, leading to

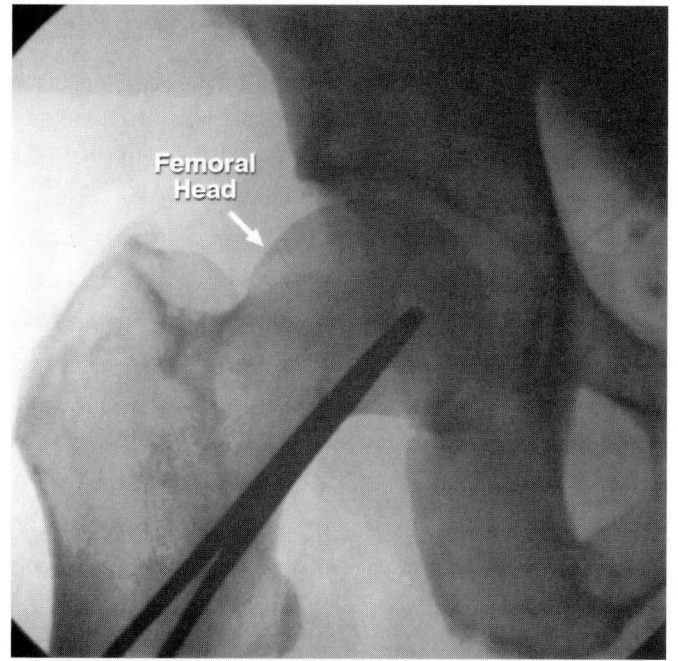

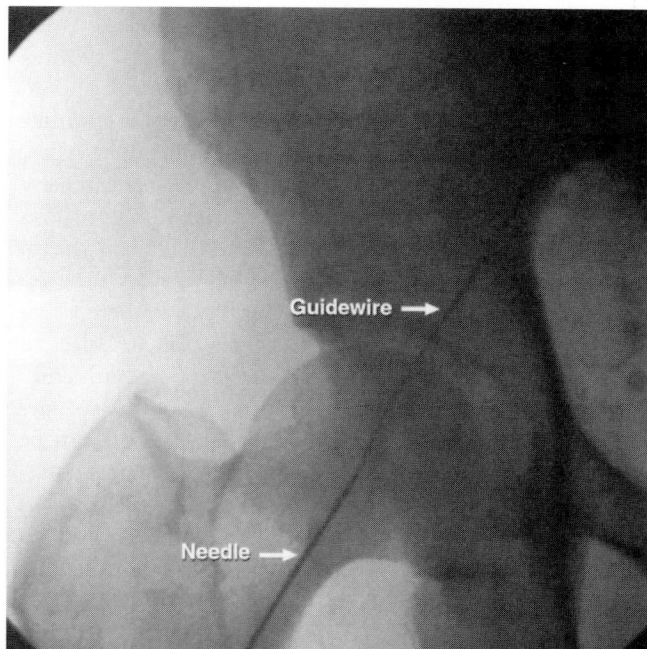

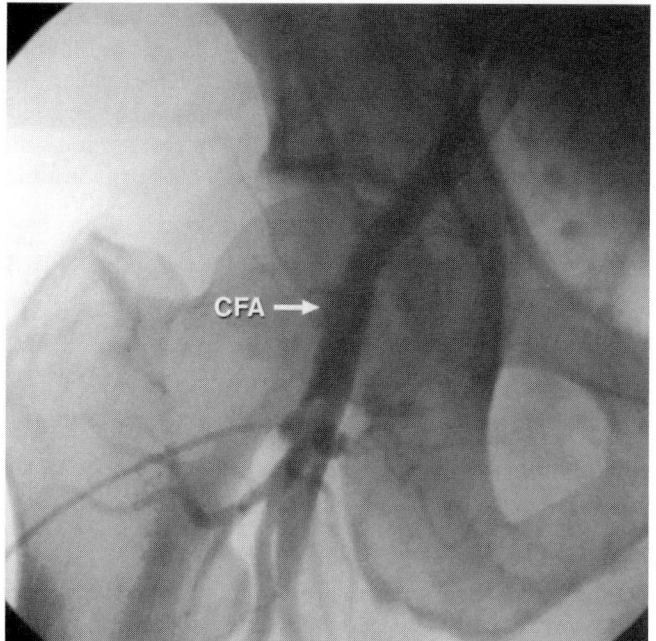

FIGURE 78.3 A: Fluoroscopic landmark for femoral artery cannulation in posteroanterior projection, marked with a hemostat. **B:** Cannulation of femoral artery and passage of guidewire. **C:** Angiogram shows the right common femoral artery and its relation to the femoral head in a posteroanterior projection. CFA, common femoral artery.

sheath kinking. Pulsatile blood flow should be obtained once the artery is effectively cannulated. Weaker degrees of blood flow could be due to subintimal position of the needle bevel or an awkward angle of the needle, with bevel abutting the vessel wall. In these situations, gentle manipulation of the needle backward or forward, or a slight change in angulation (usually a shallower angle), usually restores blood flow. In the presence of marked hypotension or severe peripheral vascular disease, blood return may not be brisk. In cases in which the pulse is not palpable, the Smart Needle, a flow needle attached to a Doppler probe, can be used to generate acoustic signals of arterial flow and facilitate

puncture of the artery (90). It is helpful to use this device a few times in healthy arteries with a strong pulse before trying it for the first time on a nonpalpable one. It is relatively easy to puncture the posterior wall of the artery with this approach. Fluoroscopy can be used to locate the medial border of the femoral head, and this facilitates locating the artery. Often, with extensive peripheral vascular disease, fluoroscopic calcification is present in the vessel wall, further helping to identify the approximate location for needle entry. Old peripheral bypass grafts may also be calcified.

Once the artery is cannulated with the needle and pulsatile flow is obtained, a guidewire is passed through the needle. If resistance is encountered, fluoroscopy should be used to ensure that the wire tip is free, and undetected subintimal wire advancement is not occurring. The wire should follow a pathway to the anatomic left of the spine, unlike with venous cannulation, in which the wire follows the inferior vena cava to the right of the spine. With extensive vessel calcification or extensive scar tissue from previous procedures, resistance may be encountered during sheath advancement. Use of a small dilator, followed by progressively larger dilators, as well as a stiff wire, such as an Amplatz wire, may facilitate placement of the desired sheath size. This same technique can be used to enter Dacron grafts if they are at least 2 months old. After successful sheath placement, a blood pressure should be obtained and recorded from the sheath sidearm and correlated with the blood pressure cuff measurement. This allows detection of any aortoiliac disease, and it provides accurate documentation of the patient's arterial pressure.

Catheter Selection

The size of the catheter is largely a matter of physician choice and the size of the coronary arteries to be visualized; 6-Fr diagnostic catheters are commonly used. They provide good opacification, with easy manual injections of contrast. A 5-Fr system creates a smaller hole at the arterial access site, but adequate coronary artery opacification may be more challenging for the operator because "streaming" (incomplete mixing of contrast and blood) may occur, resulting in over- or underestimation of stenosis severity. A 4-Fr system can be used, in particular from the radial artery, but, again, coronary opacification and catheter manipulation may be problems. In certain circumstances, larger catheter sizes, up to 8 Fr, may be desirable, although this warrants a femoral approach or a brachial artery cutdown approach. If a patient has large coronary arteries or ectasia, it may be necessary to use one of the larger-bore catheters. This is also true of vein grafts, which may be quite large. Similarly, in any condition that leads to a state of increased coronary flow, such as aortic stenosis, aortic insufficiency, hypertrophic ventricular enlargement, dialysis, or tachycardia, better opacification may occur with a larger-bore catheter.

The initial catheter selected is the Judkins Left 4 (JL4) for the images of the left coronary system. The Judkins Right 4 (JR4) is next used to obtain images of the RCA. The size of the initial catheters selected depends on the aortic root. If there is a dilated aortic root or a large person, a JL5 or JR5 may be necessary. Similarly, if the aortic root is small, a JL3.5 or JR3.5 may be necessary. From the left brachial or radial artery, the standard Judkins catheters are usually adequate. However, from the right arm, multipurpose or Amplatz-type catheters are most useful. In an average-sized aorta, an AL2 is often the correct size for the LM, and an AL1 or AL2 is often appropriate for the RCA. Amplatz catheters are particularly useful if the origin of LM or RCA is more anterior, posterior,

or superior than usual in the aorta. The multipurpose-A catheter is well suited for coronary artery ostia that have an inferiorly directed takeoff. Amplatz catheters are more likely than Judkins catheters to lead to ostial dissection due to their ability to engage the coronary arteries deeply. This risk can be minimized by rotating the catheter counterclockwise before disengaging from the artery.

Left Coronary Artery

LM coronary artery disease is a serious finding that mandates proceeding with extreme caution. Clues to its presence include heavy calcification of the ostium. A stress test that demonstrates marked hypotension with exercise is another red flag. Damping or ventricularization of the pressure waveform on catheter engagement raises the possibility of LM coronary artery stenosis. Alternatively, the catheter may not be coaxial to the LM coronary artery, and slight withdrawal of the catheter tip should relieve damping in this situation; forceful contrast injection through a damped, noncoaxial catheter tip pointed upward into the LM coronary artery may lead to dissection. A contrast injection in the left coronary cusp is a reasonable first step to define the ostium of the LM coronary artery. An AP view or a shallow RAO caudal view may be useful to evaluate for mid- and distal LM coronary artery stenosis. A shallow LAO or LAO cranial view is usually best to visualize ostial LM stenosis. As soon as significant LM disease is identified, nonionic contrast should be used for the rest of the angiography. Limited injections of the left and right coronary arteries should be performed, sufficient to identify other stenoses and delineate surgical targets. A left ventriculogram should usually not be performed in the presence of severe LM coronary artery stenosis, because the contrast load and depression in cardiac contractility may prove fatal. If the patient is hemodynamically unstable, consideration should be given to intraaortic balloon pump placement.

Initial engagement of the LM coronary artery is performed in the 30-degree LAO position. If the JL4 catheter does not line up coaxially with the LM coronary artery, slight counterclockwise rotation should move the catheter tip anteriorly and engage it. If this does not work, gentle clockwise rotation, which moves the catheter posteriorly, can be applied. In a dilated aorta, the "elbow" of the JL4 catheter curve does not rest on the aortic wall, and clockwise rotation is necessary to move the catheter tip anteriorly in the aorta. Also, in the dilated aorta, larger-sized catheters such as a JL5 or JL6 may be necessary.

If Amplatz catheters are being used to engage the LM coronary artery, these are pushed down into the left cusp, with the catheter tip pointing upward until the engagement is accomplished. The catheter is then withdrawn slightly, which causes the catheter to advance into the LM coronary artery. To disengage, the catheter is advanced slightly and gently rotated counterclockwise out of the LM coronary artery. Although the JL catheters typically find the LM coronary artery with little manipulation, the Amplatz catheters are particularly useful when the orientation of this artery is unusual or anomalous. However, particular care must be used with Amplatz catheters, as the motions that are used to engage and disengage are the opposite of the Judkins catheters.

Isolated LM coronary artery disease occurs rarely (94). When there appears to be no other significant coronary artery disease, consideration should be given to LM coronary artery spasm, and intracoronary nitroglycerin should be administered before repeat angiography. Alternatively, the LM artery may just taper, and IVUS is particularly useful to document whether angiographic narrowing is due to vessel tapering or to atheroma. Additionally, whenever ostial LAD or ostial LCx stenosis, or both, are present, the index of suspicion for distal LM coronary artery stenosis should fall, and further views should be obtained to exclude this possibility.

In the setting of separate ostia of the LAD and LCx, an LAO caudal view may be particularly helpful. If the catheter first engages the LAD, a larger catheter is often necessary for the engagement of the LCx, such as upsizing from a JL4 to a JL5, with clockwise rotation applied to the catheter. Alternatively, if the LCx is first engaged with the catheter, a shorter catheter is usually necessary to engage the LAD selectively, such as downsizing from a JL4 to a JL3.5, with counterclockwise rotation applied.

Several additional views of the left coronary artery should be obtained after the LM coronary artery has been evaluated. The AP cranial view is useful for evaluating the midportion of the LAD. Additional LAO or RAO cranial views may help further evaluate the mid-LAD, as well as separate the diagonal branches of the LAD, allowing the ostia to be imaged. The lateral view may further delineate the mid-LAD. The AP caudal view is useful for evaluating the body of the LCx, as well as the marginal-branch ostia. Added shallow LAO or RAO angulation may further maximize this view. For a ramus intermedius branch, an LAO caudal view is most useful to evaluate the ostium. An LAO cranial view is also useful for displaying a left-sided PDA.

Right Coronary Artery

In the 30-degree LAO projection, the JR4 is advanced to the aortic valve level and slowly withdrawn approximately 2 cm while clockwise rotation is applied to rotate the catheter anteriorly to the right sinus of Valsalva. Then the catheter should sit in the RCA ostium. If this maneuver does not work, the RCA ostium can be approached from slightly above its expected level, with clockwise rotation being applied to the catheter. With ostial disease of the RCA, if damping occurs with the catheter, it may sometimes be helpful to use a larger-sized catheter, which is less likely to engage the artery deeply. Usually, two or three views of the RCA are obtained. The LAO view is useful to evaluate the proximal and mid-RCA. The AP view with 30-degree cra-

nial angulation is often the best for evaluating the RCA bifurcation and ostia of the PDA and posterolateral branches. A shallow RAO view is useful to lay out the entire PDA. In the RAO view, the marginal branches point to the patient's left, and the atrial branches point to the patient's right; thus, this view is useful in differentiating atrial and marginal branches that may be overlapped in an LAO view. The lateral view may be useful to evaluate the mid-RCA and the ostia of RV marginal branches. If significant LM coronary artery disease has been identified, a single view of the RCA, probably an LAO cranial to identify any needed surgical targets, may be sufficient for planning bypass surgery.

Surgical Bypass Grafts

If left ventriculography is performed, opacification of vein grafts is sometimes observed. [⊻ n15] Perhaps more useful is observation of the contraction pattern of the left ventricle. For example, if the anterior wall is completely normal but the LAD is occluded and no patent graft has been found that supplies the LAD territory, it is highly likely that a graft has been overlooked.

Left Ventriculography

Even with the refinement of several noninvasive measures, ventriculography remains a useful modality to assess left ventricular function. Before left ventriculography is performed, an assessment of LVEDP should be made with the pigtail catheter. If the pressure is markedly elevated, sublingual nitroglycerin should be administered until the pressure is reduced. If LVEDP remains elevated (e.g., LVEDP >30 mm Hg), consideration should be given to aborting the left ventriculogram.

The 30-degree RAO is the usual view for left ventriculography, although biplane ventriculography with an additional LAO or LAO cranial view may be preferable in some cases, if available. If mitral regurgitation is known to be present and an assessment of severity is required, 50 to 60 mL of dye should be used to opacify the left atrium (96). Care must be taken in positioning the catheter and ensuring that it is free, such that it does not trigger premature ventricular contractions or entwine the mitral valve apparatus, thereby artificially causing mitral regurgitation. The LAO cranial is the optimal view for a muscular ventricular septal defect, and the left lateral view is optimal for a membranous ventricular septal defect. The LAO cranial is also useful to assess for left ventricular outflow obstruction in patients with hypertrophic cardiomyopathy (*e*Fig. 78.3.5). ⊻ n16

Postprocedural Care

The angiographic images should be reviewed and a plan formulated in the catheterization laboratory. Once it is certain that all necessary information has been obtained from the angiogram, the sheath can be pulled. If heparin was administered for a diagnostic coronary angiogram (e.g., when a radial/brachial approach was used or cerebral angiography was performed), an activated clotting time or activated partial thromboplastin time should be checked before the sheath is pulled. If the activated clotting time is less than 160 seconds or the activated partial thromboplastin time is under 45 seconds, the sheath can be pulled and manual pressure applied for several minutes until hemostasis is obtained. Direct compression of the artery a few fingerbreadths above the needle insertion site in the skin (above the estimated arterial entry site) with the pads of the fingertips is the most reliable method to obtain hemostasis and should be the initial approach if a closure device is not used. After a few minutes of direct manual pressure, a C-clamp can be positioned appropriately, although the patient must still be monitored. A FemoStop is an alternative to the C-clamp, but some care must be taken to ensure correct positioning over the artery. Use of smaller-sized sheaths may greatly decrease the time to ambulation. With the use of 5-Fr sheaths, ambulation has been demonstrated to be safe after 2 hours of bed rest.

Closure devices are increasingly used to obtain hemostasis. It is recommended that an oblique angiogram be performed through the sidearm of the sheath to determine the sheath insertion site. Additionally, vessel size and the presence of any plaque may be noted. If it appears that the sheath is in the bifurcation of the common femoral artery, manual pressure is best applied. If the sheath is placed in the profunda femoris or the superficial femoral artery, or if there is atherosclerotic plaque at the insertion site, it may be best not to use any closure device. Vessels of 4 mm or less in size are not well suited to current closure devices. If a slight degree of blood oozing from the skin occurs, a 10-mL solution of lidocaine hydrochloride 1% and epinephrine 1:100,000 can be injected into the skin tract.   n17

After radial artery catheterization, if the radial pulse is lost but the hand is otherwise asymptomatic (and the ulnar supply is adequate), there is no cause for action. With loss of the brachial or radial pulse after brachial artery catheterization, vascular surgical consultation ought to be obtained. Loss of distal pulses after femoral catheterization should also prompt surgical consultation or lower extremity angiography. In patients with extensive peripheral vascular disease, if pressure is being applied to the femoral catheterization site, particular care must be given to the distal extremity to ensure that ischemia is not occurring; this is best accomplished with direct visualization of the distal extremity (i.e., the foot should not be covered up with a sheet).

Elective diagnostic coronary angiography has been transformed into an outpatient procedure in most circumstances. This appears to be a safe development. However, there are patients for whom outpatient catheterization is not appropriate. Individuals with severe aortic stenosis or LM coronary artery disease should be monitored for a more extended period, as should patients who are at risk of developing renal failure. Similarly, patients with severely impaired left ventricular function or unstable coronary artery disease should remain for observation. Individuals who live alone and have no one to watch them should be monitored overnight.

Before discharge, patients should be told to notify their physician if they subsequently have any sudden drop-off in urine quantity. Any pain or swelling at the site of the catheterization should also prompt emergency care. Patients should be counseled to avoid driving for a day to allow sedation to wear off and heavy lifting for at least 2 days to allow the catheterization site to heal. Warfarin, if necessary, can be reinitiated the night of the procedure. If more immediate anticoagulation with heparin is desired, this can be started a few hours after the sheath is removed, or immediately if a closure device is used. If metformin was given, this can be resumed after 2 days if renal function appears stable.

Complications and Management

Major complications are unusual after cardiac catheterization, but the operator must be familiar with them. An analysis of 59,792 patients documented the frequency of major complications with cardiac catheterization and coronary angiography (Table 78.3). Although that analysis is somewhat old, the numbers have not changed significantly, although older, sicker patients are being catheterized. Death occurs in approximately 1 in 1,000 cases. Patients with severe LM coronary artery stenosis or critical aortic stenosis are at particularly high risk. Myocardial infarction occurs in approximately 1 in 2,000 cases; stroke occurs in

TABLE 78.3 INCIDENCE OF COMPLICATIONS WITH CARDIAC CATHETERIZATION AND CORONARY ANGIOGRAPHY

Complication	Percent
Death	0.11
Myocardial infarction	0.05
Stroke	0.07
Arrhythmia	0.38
Vascular complications	0.43
Contrast reaction	0.37
Hemodynamic complications	0.26
Perforation of cardiac chamber	0.03
Other complications	0.28
Total	**1.70**

Adapted from Noto TJ Jr, Johnson LW, Krone R, et al. Cardiac catheterization 1990: a report of the Registry of the Society for Cardiac Angiography and Interventions (SCA&I). *Cathet Cardiovasc Diagn* 1991;24:75–83, with permission.

approximately 1 in 1,000 cases. Thus, a major complication of death, myocardial infarction, or stroke occurs in about 1 of 500 cases.

Hypotension and Bradycardia

Vasovagal reactions may occur, especially with initial arterial access or sheath removal. Patients should be instructed not to hold their breath, because breath-holding may predispose to a vagal reaction. Hypotension in the catheterization laboratory may be catastrophic in certain circumstances, and prompt treatment may be lifesaving. Norepinephrine (Levophed) should be administered to reverse rapidly hypotension that is due to vasovagal reactions. Dopamine is often used in catheterization laboratories; however, this is not the ideal initial agent for serious hypotension, because it takes a period of time for blood levels to reach a level at which the pressor effect occurs. At the initial low serum concentrations, dopamine acts primarily as a renal and splanchnic vasodilator and may transiently decrease blood pressure. Therefore, norepinephrine, not dopamine, is the agent of choice for prompt treatment of hypotension. Epinephrine is the treatment of choice for hypotension secondary to an anaphylactoid reaction. For hypotension that is unresponsive to i.v. fluids and vasopressors, placement of a Swan-Ganz catheter and an intraaortic balloon pump should be considered. With the availability of the lower profile 8-Fr intraaortic balloon pump systems, a balloon pump can often be placed through an existing sheath.

Atropine, 1.0 mg i.v., should be administered for symptomatic bradycardia. Additionally, if bradycardia occurs with injections of ionic contrast, nonionic contrast should be substituted. Furthermore, if the bradycardia occurs with RCA injection, the minimum amount of dye to ensure opacification should be used. For sustained and symptomatic bradycardia, a transvenous pacemaker should be placed.

Vascular Complications

Bleeding from the arterial cannulation site with development of a hematoma is a risk of angiography. Retroperitoneal bleeding can be particularly sinister due to the difficulty in making the diagnosis. Although symptoms such as inguinal or abdominal tenderness, femoral neuropathy, and back pain may be clues to retroperitoneal hemorrhage, hypotension with a falling hemoglobin may be the only manifestation and, if undetected, may lead to death. An abdominal CT scan can confirm the diagnosis (107). The risk of vascular complications is increased in patients who are receiving anticoagulation at the time of angiography (108). Female gender, obesity, and advanced age are other risk factors for groin complications. Color

duplex ultrasound is the preferred mode of assessing groin complications (109). Pseudoaneurysm and arteriovenous fistula formation are additional risks. When pseudoaneurysms are less than 3 cm in size, conservative management usually results in spontaneous closure (110). Although ultrasound-guided compression of pseudoaneurysm and arteriovenous fistula has become commonly used, surgical therapy is still necessary in a significant minority of cases, especially when anticoagulation is being administered (111). A newer method of ultrasound-guided thrombin injection has been described for the management of pseudoaneurysms that develop after catheterization (112). The success rate with this method is high, even in patients who are receiving anticoagulation, and, in experienced hands, this should likely be the first approach tried before consideration of surgical repair. Endovascular techniques have also been used successfully to treat pseudoaneurysm and arteriovenous fistula (113).

CONTROVERSIES AND PERSONAL PERSPECTIVES

Numerous critics of coronary angiography decry the overuse of this invasive procedure. Certainly, overuse may be a problem, especially given patient demand in fee-for-service health-care systems. Improved noninvasive screening techniques may diminish the need for angiography as a diagnostic tool in the future. As magnetic resonance imaging continues to improve, it may one day replace coronary angiography as a diagnostic tool for suspected coronary artery disease. Alternatively, newer modalities such as CT scanning may identify a larger number of people who need coronary angiography for more definitive delineation of coronary anatomy. Furthermore, percutaneous coronary intervention continues to grow as a revascularization method, necessitating coronary angiography to define stenoses. The aging of the population will further increase the need for coronary angiography. Additionally, emerging evidence suggests that an invasive strategy incorporating angiography is the ideal approach to patients with acute coronary syndromes (60,61). Individuals with unstable angina who are treated with aggressive catheterization strategies in the United States fare better than their more conservatively treated counterparts in Canada (114). For patients with acute ST-segment elevation myocardial infarction, an invasive approach, including percutaneous intervention, where available, leads to better outcomes than pharmacologic therapy (115–117). If a patient with acute myocardial infarction is in cardiogenic shock, an initial invasive approach may be lifesaving (118). Thus, the prominence of coronary angiography is likely to grow, as a diagnostic tool and as a prelude to percutaneous intervention.

THE FUTURE

Although the future of coronary angiography remains bright, limitations will be placed on who actually performs it. As minimum volume standards become more widely accepted and separate certification examinations are developed, coronary angiography will become part of a discrete invasive subspecialty within cardiology. The evolution and refinement of arterial closure devices will continue, allowing an even greater proportion of cases to be performed on an outpatient basis. Older patients with a greater degree of medical comorbidities, as in the very elderly, will undergo coronary angiography at much higher rates. Further refinements in imaging, through magnetic resonance and CT, will likely reduce radiation exposure to the operator, enhance image quality, and ultimately yield "noninvasive" coronary angiography using an i.v. injection of a contrast agent. Real-time three-dimensional reconstruction of coronary arteries will become feasible. Potentially, hybrid imaging technologies will enable the identification of vulnerable atherosclerotic plaque, the veritable "holy grail" of diagnostic angiography. Thus, although coronary angiography will probably continue to evolve, it will remain central to the evaluation of coronary artery disease.

REFERENCES

1. Vetrovec GW. Optimal performance of diagnostic coronary angiography. In: Pepine CJ, Nissen SE, eds. *CathSAP*. Bethesda, MD: ACC, 1999;5:3–19.
2. Pepine CJ, Babb JD, Brinker JA, et al. Guidelines for training in adult cardiovascular medicine. Core Cardiology Training Symposium (COCATS). Task Force 3: training in cardiac catheterization and interventional cardiology. *J Am Coll Cardiol* 1995;25:14–16.
3. Fye WB. *American cardiology: the history of a specialty and its college*. Baltimore: The Johns Hopkins University Press, 1996.
4. Yamanaka O, Hobbs RE. Coronary artery anomalies in 126,595 patients undergoing coronary arteriography. *Cathet Cardiovasc Diagn* 1990;21:28–40.
5. Hobbs RE, Millit HD, Raghavan PV, et al. Coronary artery fistulae: a 10-year review. *Cleve Clin Q* 1982;49:191–197.
6. Tuzcu EM, Moodie DS, Chambers JL, et al. Congenital heart diseases associated with coronary artery anomalies. *Cleve Clin J Med* 1990;57:147–152.
7. Hobbs RE, Millit HD, Raghavan PV, et al. Congenital coronary artery anomalies: clinical and therapeutic implications. *Cardiovasc Clin* 1981;12:43–58.
8. Kramer JR, Kitazume H, Proudfit WL, Sones FM Jr. Clinical significance of isolated coronary bridges: benign and frequent condition involving the left anterior descending artery. *Am Heart J* 1982;103:283–288.
9. Kostis JB, Moreyra AE, Natarajan N, et al. The pathophysiology and diverse etiology of septal perforator compression. *Circulation* 1979;59:913–919.
10. Haager PK, Schwarz ER, vom Dahl J, et al. Long term angiographic and clinical follow up in patients with stent implantation for symptomatic myocardial bridging. *Heart* 2000;84:403–408.
11. Prendergast BD, Kerr F, Starkey IR. Normalisation of abnormal coronary fractional flow reserve associated with myocardial bridging using an intracoronary stent. *Heart* 2000;83:705–707.
12. Klues HG, Schwarz ER, vom Dahl J, et al. Disturbed intracoronary hemodynamics in myocardial bridging: early normalization by intracoronary stent placement. *Circulation* 1997;96:2905–2913.
13. Stables RH, Knight CJ, McNeill JG, Sigwart U. Coronary stenting in the management of myocardial ischaemia caused by muscle bridging. *Br Heart J* 1995;74:90–92.
14. Green CE, Kelley MJ, Higgins CB, Bookstein JJ. Acquired coronary-to-bronchial artery communication: a possible cause of coronary steal. *Cathet Cardiovasc Diagn* 1981;7:191–196.
15. Ellis SG, Guetta V, Miller D, et al. Relation between lesion characteristics and risk with percutaneous intervention in the stent and glycoprotein IIb/IIIa era: an analysis of results from 10,907 lesions and proposal for new classification scheme. *Circulation* 1999;100:1971–1976.
16. Lincoff AM, Popma JJ, Ellis SG, et al. Abrupt vessel closure complicating coronary angioplasty: clinical, angiographic and therapeutic profile. *J Am Coll Cardiol* 1992;19:926–935.
17. Ellis SG, Pinto IM, McGillem MJ, et al. Accuracy and reproducibility of quantitative coronary arteriography using 6 and 8 French catheters with cine angiographic acquisition. *Cathet Cardiovasc Diagn* 1991;22:52–55.
18. Ellis SG, Vandormael MG, Cowley MJ, et al. Coronary morphologic and clinical determinants of procedural outcome with angioplasty for multivessel coronary disease. Implications for patient selection. Multivessel Angioplasty Prognosis Study Group. *Circulation* 1990;82:1193–1202.
19. Kastrati A, Schomig A, Elezi S, et al. Prognostic value of the modified American College of Cardiology/American Heart Association stenosis morphology classification for long-term angiographic and clinical outcome after coronary stent placement. *Circulation* 1999;100:1285–1290.
20. Bhatt DL, Patel VB, Robbins MA, et al. Effect of coronary morphology and vessel size on the benefit of abciximab with stenting. *Circulation* 1999;100:I-857.
21. The Thrombolysis in Myocardial Infarction (TIMI) trial. Phase I findings. TIMI Study Group. *N Engl J Med* 1985;312:932-936.

22. Ellis SG, Topol EJ, George BS, et al. Recurrent ischemia without warning. Analysis of risk factors for in-hospital ischemic events following successful thrombolysis with intravenous tissue plasminogen activator. *Circulation* 1989;80:1159–1165.

23. Gibson CM, Cannon CP, Daley WL, et al. TIMI frame count: a quantitative method of assessing coronary artery flow. *Circulation* 1996;93:879–888.

24. Gibson CM, Murphy SA, Rizzo MJ, et al. Relationship between TIMI frame count and clinical outcomes after thrombolytic administration. Thrombolysis in Myocardial Infarction (TIMI) study group. *Circulation* 1999;99:1945–1950.

25. Bhatt DL, Ellis SG, Ivanc TB, et al. Corrected TIMI frame count does not predict 30-day adverse outcomes after reperfusion therapy for acute myocardial infarction. *Am Heart J* 1999;138:785–790.

26. Gibson CM, Cannon CP, Murphy SA, et al. Relationship of TIMI myocardial perfusion grade to mortality after administration of thrombolytic drugs. *Circulation* 2000;101:125–130.

27. Topol EJ, Nissen SE. Our preoccupation with coronary luminology. The dissociation between clinical and angiographic findings in ischemic heart disease. *Circulation* 1995;92:2333–2342.

28. Glagov S, Weisenberg E, Zarins CK, et al. Compensatory enlargement of human atherosclerotic coronary arteries. *N Engl J Med* 1987;316:1371–1375.

29. Heupler FA Jr. Syndrome of symptomatic coronary arterial spasm with nearly normal coronary arteriograms. *Am J Cardiol* 1980;45:873–881.

30. Bott-Silverman C, Heupler FA Jr, Yiannikas J. Variant angina: comparison of patients with and without fixed severe coronary artery disease. *Am J Cardiol* 1984;54:1173–1175.

31. Bott-Silverman C, Heupler FA Jr. Natural history of pure coronary artery spasm in patients treated medically. *J Am Coll Cardiol* 1983;2:200–205.

32. Heupler FA Jr, Proudfit WL, Razavi M, et al. Ergonovine maleate provocative test for coronary arterial spasm. *Am J Cardiol* 1978;41:631–640.

33. Heupler FA Jr. Provocative testing for coronary arterial spasm: risk, method and rationale. *Am J Cardiol* 1980; 46:335–337.

34. Heupler FA Jr, Proudfit WL. Nifedipine therapy for refractory coronary arterial spasm. *Am J Cardiol* 1979; 44:798–803.

35. Williams MJ, Restieaux NJ, Low CJ. Myocardial infarction in young people with normal coronary arteries. *Heart* 1998;79:191–194.

36. Basso C, Morgagni GL, Thiene G. Spontaneous coronary artery dissection: a neglected cause of acute myocardial ischaemia and sudden death. *Heart* 1996;75:451–454.

37. Almahmeed WA, Haykowski M, Boone J, et al. Spontaneous coronary artery dissection in young women. *Cathet Cardiovasc Diagn* 1996;37:201–205.

38. Sherrid MV, Mieres J, Mogtader A, et al. Onset during exercise of spontaneous coronary artery dissection and sudden death. Occurrence in a trained athlete: case report and review of prior cases. *Chest* 1995;108:284–287.

39. Bucciarelli E, Fratini D, Gilardi G, Affronti G. Spontaneous dissecting aneurysm of coronary artery in a pregnant woman at term. *Pathol Res Pract* 1998;194:137–139.

40. Greenblatt JM, Kochar GS, Albornoz MA. Multivessel spontaneous coronary artery dissection in a patient with severe systolic hypertension: a possible association. A case report. *Angiology* 1999;50:509–513.

41. Masuda T, Akiyama H, Kurosawa T, Ohwada T. Long-term follow-up of coronary artery dissection due to blunt chest trauma with spontaneous healing in a young woman. *Intensive Care Med* 1996;22:450–452.

42. Chu KH, Menapace FJ, Blankenship JC, et al. Polyarteritis nodosa presenting as acute myocardial infarction with coronary dissection. *Cathet Cardiovasc Diagn* 1998;44:320–324.

43. Elming H, Kober L. Spontaneous coronary artery dissection. Case report and literature review. *Scand Cardiovasc J* 1999;33:175–179.

44. Vale PR, Baron DW. Coronary artery stenting for spontaneous coronary artery dissection: a case report and review of the literature. *Cathet Cardiovasc Diagn* 1998;45:280–286.

45. Kearney P, Singh H, Hutter J, et al. Spontaneous coronary artery dissection: a report of three cases and review of the literature. *Postgrad Med J* 1993;69:940–945.

46. Koller PT, Cliffe CM, Ridley DJ. Immunosuppressive therapy for peripartum-type spontaneous coronary artery dissection: case report and review. *Clin Cardiol* 1998; 21:40–46.

47. Borczuk AC, van Hoeven KH, Factor SM. Review and hypothesis: the eosinophil and peripartum heart disease (myocarditis and coronary artery dissection)—coincidence or pathogenetic significance? *Cardiovasc Res* 1997;33:527–532.

48. Ge J, Haude M, Gorge G, et al. Silent healing of spontaneous plaque disruption demonstrated by intracoronary ultrasound. *Eur Heart J* 1995;16:1149–1151.

49. Sorrell VL, Davis MJ, Bove AA. Current knowledge and significance of coronary artery ectasia: a chronologic review of the literature, recommendations for treatment, possible etiologies, and future considerations. *Clin Cardiol* 1998;21:157–160.

50. Syed M, Lesch M. Coronary artery aneurysm: a review. *Prog Cardiovasc Dis* 1997;40:77–84.

51. Shapira OM, Shemin RJ. Aneurysmal coronary artery disease. Atherosclerotic coronary artery ectasia or adult mucocutaneous lymph node syndrome (Kawasaki's disease)? *Chest* 1997;111:796–799.

52. Rowley AH, Shulman ST. Kawasaki syndrome. *Clin Microbiol Rev* 1998;11:405–414.

53. Kato H, Sugimura T, Akagi T, et al. Long-term consequences of Kawasaki disease. A 10- to 21-year follow-up study of 594 patients. *Circulation* 1996;94:1379–1385.

54. Fukushige J, Takahashi N, Ueda K, et al. Long-term outcome of coronary abnormalities in patients after Kawasaki disease. *Pediatr Cardiol* 1996;17:71–76.

55. Pongratz G, Gansser R, Bachmann K, et al. Myocardial infarction in an adult resulting from coronary aneurysms previously documented in childhood after an acute episode of Kawasaki's disease. *Eur Heart J* 1994;15:1002–1004.

56. Osevala MA, Heleotis TL, DeJene BA. Successful treatment of a ruptured mycotic coronary artery aneurysm. *Ann Thorac Surg* 1999;67:1780–1782.

57. von Rotz F, Niederhauser U, Straumann E, et al. Myocardial infarction caused by a large coronary artery aneurysm. *Ann Thorac Surg* 2000;69:1568–1569.

58. Leung AW, Wong P, Wu CW, et al. Left main coronary artery aneurysm: sealing by stent graft and long-term follow-up. *Catheter Cardiovasc Interv* 2000;51:205–209.

59. Scanlon PJ, Faxon DP, Audet AM, et al. ACC/AHA guidelines for coronary angiography. A report of the American College of Cardiology/American Heart Association Task Force on practice guidelines (Committee on Coronary Angiography). Developed in collaboration with the Society for Cardiac Angiography and Interventions. *J Am Coll Cardiol* 1999;33:1756–1824.

60. Invasive compared with non-invasive treatment in unstable coronary-artery disease: FRISC II prospective randomised multicentre study. FRagmin and Fast Revascularisation during InStability in Coronary artery disease Investigators. *Lancet* 1999;354:708–715.

61. Cannon CP. TACTICS-TIMI 18. Presented at the American Heart Association Annual Meeting, New Orleans, 2000.

62. Ellis SG, Weintraub W, Holmes D, et al. Relation of operator volume and experience to procedural outcome of percutaneous coronary revascularization at hospitals with high interventional volumes. *Circulation* 1997;95:2479–2484.

63. Laboratory Performance Standards Committee. Guidelines for professional staff privileges in the cardiac catheterization laboratory. *Cathet Cardiovasc Diagn* 1990;21:203–204.

64. Pepine CJ, Allen HD, Bashore TM, et al. ACC/AHA guidelines for cardiac catheterization and cardiac catheterization laboratories. American College of Cardiology/American Heart Association Ad Hoc Task Force on Cardiac Catheterization. *Circulation* 1991;84:2213–2247.

65. Marshall D, Chambers CE, Heupler F Jr. Performance of adult cardiac catheterization: nonphysicians should not function as independent operators—a position statement. *Catheter Cardiovasc Interv* 1999;48:167–169.

66. Heupler FA Jr, Chambers CE, Dear WE, et al. Guidelines for internal peer review in the cardiac catheterization laboratory. Laboratory Performance Standards Committee, Society for Cardiac Angiography and Interventions. *Cathet Cardiovasc Diagn* 1997;40:21–32.

67. Heupler FA Jr, al-Hani AJ, Dear WE. Guidelines for continuous quality improvement in the cardiac catheterization laboratory. Laboratory Performance Standards Committee of the Society for Cardiac Angiography and Interventions. *Cathet Cardiovasc Diagn* 1993;30:191–200.

68. Heupler FA Jr. Guidelines for performing angiography in patients taking metformin. Members of the Laboratory Performance Standards Committee of the Society for Cardiac Angiography and Interventions. *Cathet Cardiovasc Diagn* 1998;43:121–123.

69. Holmes DR Jr, Wondrow MA, Bell MR, et al. Cine film replacement: digital archival requirements and remaining obstacles. *Cathet Cardiovasc Diagn* 1998;44:346–356; discussion 357.

69a. Balter S, Heupler FA, Lin PP, Wondrow MH. A new tool for benchmarking cardiovascular fluoroscopes. *Cathet Cardiovasc Interv* 2001;52:67–72.

70. Matthai WH Jr, Kussmaul WG 3rd, Krol J, et al. A comparison of low- with high-osmolality contrast agents in cardiac angiography. Identification of criteria for selective use. *Circulation* 1994;89:291–301.

71. Grines CL, Schreiber TL, Savas V, et al. A randomized trial of low osmolar ionic versus nonionic contrast media in patients with myocardial infarction or unstable angina undergoing percutaneous transluminal coronary angioplasty. *J Am Coll Cardiol* 1996;27:1381–1386.

72. Moliterno DJ, Topol EJ. Another step toward resolving the contrast controversy. *J Am Coll Cardiol* 1996;27:1387–1389.

73. Davidson CJ, Laskey WK, Hermiller JB, et al. Randomized trial of contrast media utilization in high-risk PTCA: the COURT trial. *Circulation* 2000;101:2172–2177.

74. Hirshfeld JW Jr, Laskey W, Martin JL, et al. Hemodynamic changes induced by cardiac angiography with ioxaglate: comparison with diatrizoate. *J Am Coll Cardiol* 1983;2:954–957.

75. Conn JJ, Sebastian MJ, Deam D, et al. A prospective study of the effect of nonionic contrast media on thyroid function. *Thyroid* 1996;6:107–110.

76. Kussmaul WG 3rd, Mishra JP, Matthai WH, Hirshfeld JW Jr. Complications of cardiac angiography using low- or high-osmolality contrast agents in patients with left main coronary stenosis. *Cathet Cardiovasc Diagn* 1997;42:376–379.

77. Parfrey PS, Griffiths SM, Barrett BJ, et al. Contrast material–induced renal failure in patients with diabetes mellitus, renal insufficiency, or both. A prospective controlled study. *N Engl J Med* 1989;320:143–149.

78. Rudnick MR, Goldfarb S, Wexler L, et al. Nephrotoxicity of ionic and nonionic contrast media in 1196 patients: a randomized trial. The Iohexol Cooperative Study. *Kidney Int* 1995;47:254–261.

79. Solomon R, Werner C, Mann D, et al. Effects of saline, mannitol, and furosemide to prevent acute decreases in renal function induced by radiocontrast agents. *N Engl J Med* 1994;331:1416–1420.

80. Stevens MA, McCullough PA, Tobin KJ, et al. A prospective randomized trial of prevention measures in patients at high risk for contrast nephropathy: results of the P.R.I.N.C.E. study. Prevention of Radiocontrast Induced Nephropathy Clinical Evaluation. *J Am Coll Cardiol* 1999;33:403–411.

81. Tepel M, van der Giet M, Schwarzfeld C, et al. Prevention of radiographic-contrast-agent–induced reductions in renal function by acetylcysteine. *N Engl J Med* 2000;343:180–184.

82. Cigarroa RG, Lange RA, Williams RH, Hillis LD. Dosing of contrast material to prevent contrast nephropathy in patients with renal disease. *Am J Med* 1989;86:649–652.

83. Manske CL, Sprafka JM, Strony JT, Wang Y. Contrast nephropathy in azotemic diabetic patients undergoing coronary angiography. *Am J Med* 1990;89:615–620.

84. Lasser EC, Berry CC, Talner LB, et al. Pretreatment with corticosteroids to alleviate reactions to intravenous contrast material. *N Engl J Med* 1987;317:845–849.

85. Goss JE, Chambers CE, Heupler FA Jr. Systemic anaphylactoid reactions to iodinated contrast media during cardiac catheterization procedures: guidelines for prevention, diagnosis, and treatment. Laboratory Performance Standards Committee of the Society for Cardiac Angiography and Interventions. *Cathet Cardiovasc Diagn* 1995;34:99–104; discussion 105.

86. Pedersen SH, Svaland MG, Reiss AL, Andrew E. Late allergy-like reactions following vascular administration of radiography contrast media. *Acta Radiol* 1998;39:344–348.

87. Courvoisier S, Bircher AJ. Delayed-type hypersensitivity to a nonionic, radiopaque contrast medium. *Allergy* 1998;53:1221–1224.

88. Heupler FJ, Heisler M, Keys TF, Serkey J. Infection prevention guidelines for cardiac catheterization laboratories. Society for Cardiac Angiography and Interventions Laboratory Performance Standards Committee. *Cathet Cardiovasc Diagn* 1992;25:260–263.

89. Rupp SB, Vogelzang RL, Nemcek AA Jr, Yungbluth MM. Relationship of the inguinal ligament to pelvic radiographic landmarks: anatomic correlation and its role in femoral arteriography. *J Vasc Interv Radiol* 1993;4:409–413.

90. Criado FJ, Abdul-Khoudoud O, Wellons E. Complications and troubleshooting. In: White RA, Fogarty TJ, eds. *Peripheral endovascular interventions*, 2nd ed. New York: Springer-Verlag, 1999:445–454.

91. Bhatt DL. Left heart catheterization. In: Marso SP, Griffin BP, Topol EJ, eds. *Manual of cardiovascular medicine.* Philadelphia: Lippincott Williams & Wilkins, 1999:700–721.

92. Green CE. *Coronary cinematography.* Philadelphia: Lippincott–Raven Publishers, 1996.

93. Boucher RA, Myler RK, Clark DA, Stertzer SH. Coronary angiography and angioplasty. *Cathet Cardiovasc Diagn* 1988;14:269–285.

94. Kapadia SR, Martin GV, Flores JR, et al. Isolated left main trunk stenosis: how common is it? Accepted for presentation at ACC 2001. *J Am Coll Cardiol* 2001;37:375A.

95. Mendelsohn FO, Yadav JS. *Management of atherosclerotic carotid disease: medical, surgical, and interventional aspects.* London: ReMEDICA, 2000.

96. Carabello BA. Valvular heart disease. In: Pepine CJ, Nissen SE, eds. *CathSAP.* Bethesda, MD: ACC, 1999.

97. Penn MS, Smedira N, Lytle B, Brener SJ. Does coronary angiography before emergency aortic surgery affect in-hospital mortality? *J Am Coll Cardiol* 2000;35:889–894.

98. Carere RG, Webb JG, Ahmed T, Dodek AA. Initial experience using Prostar: a new device for percutaneous suture-mediated closure of arterial puncture sites. *Cathet Cardiovasc Diagn* 1996;37:367–372.

99. Kulick DL, Rediker DE. Use of the Perclose device in the brachial artery after coronary intervention. *Catheter Cardiovasc Interv* 1999;46:111–112.

100. Ward SR, Casale P, Raymond R, et al. Efficacy and safety of a hemostatic puncture closure device with early ambulation after coronary angiography. Angio-Seal investigators. *Am J Cardiol* 1998;81:569–572.

101. Warren BS, Warren SG, Miller SD. Predictors of complications and learning curve using the Angio-Seal closure device following interventional and diagnostic catheterization. *Cathet Cardiovasc Interv* 1999;48:162–166.

102. Foran JP, Patel D, Brookes J, Wainwright RJ. Early mobilisation after percutaneous cardiac catheterisation using collagen plug (VasoSeal) haemostasis. *Br Heart J* 1993;69:424–429.

103. Chamberlin JR, Lardi AB, McKeever LS, et al. Use of vascular sealing devices (VasoSeal and Perclose) versus assisted manual compression (FemoStop) in transcatheter coronary interventions requiring abciximab (ReoPro). *Cathet Cardiovasc Interv* 1999;47:143–147; discussion 148.

104. Cura FA, Kapadia SR, L'Allier PL, et al. Safety of femoral closure devices after percutaneous coronary interventions in the era of glycoprotein IIb/IIIa platelet blockade. *Am J Cardiol* 2000;86:780–782, A9.

105. Sesana M, Vaghetti M, Albiero R, et al. Effectiveness and complications of vascular access closure devices after interventional procedures. *J Invasive Cardiol* 2000;12:395–399.

106. Noto TJ Jr, Johnson LW, Krone R, et al. Cardiac catheterization 1990: a report of the Registry of the Society for Cardiac Angiography and Interventions (SCA&I). *Cathet Cardiovasc Diagn* 1991;24:75–83.

107. Sreeram S, Lumsden AB, Miller JS, et al. Retroperitoneal hematoma following femoral arterial catheterization: a serious and often fatal complication. *Am Surg* 1993;59:94–98.

108. Omoigui NA, Califf RM, Pieper K, et al. Peripheral vascular complications in the Coronary Angioplasty versus Excisional Atherectomy Trial (CAVEAT-I). *J Am Coll Cardiol* 1995;26:922–930.

109. Paulson EK, Kliewer MA, Hertzberg BS, et al. Color Doppler sonography of groin complications following femoral artery catheterization. *AJR Am J Roentgenol* 1995;165:439–444.

110. Toursarkissian B, Allen BT, Petrinec D, et al. Spontaneous closure of selected iatrogenic pseudoaneurysms and arteriovenous fistulae. *J Vasc Surg* 1997;25:803–808; discussion 808–809.

111. Cox GS, Young JR, Gray BR, et al. Ultrasound-guided compression repair of postcatheterization pseudoaneurysms: results of treatment in one hundred cases. *J Vasc Surg* 1994;19:683–686.

112. La Perna L, Olin JW, Goines D, et al. Ultrasound-guided thrombin injection for the treatment of postcatheterization pseudoaneurysms. *Circulation* 2000;102:2391–2395.

113. Waigand J, Uhlich F, Gross CM, et al. Percutaneous treatment of pseudoaneurysms and arteriovenous fistulas after invasive vascular procedures. *Cathet Cardiovasc Interv* 1999;47:157–164.

114. Fu Y, Chang WC, Mark D, et al. Canadian-American differences in the management of acute coronary syndromes in the GUSTO IIb trial: one-year follow-up of patients without ST-segment elevation. *Circulation* 2000;102:1375–1381.

115. Grines CL, Browne KF, Marco J, et al. A comparison of immediate angioplasty with thrombolytic therapy for acute myocardial infarction. The Primary Angioplasty in Myocardial Infarction Study Group. *N Engl J Med* 1993;328:673–679.

116. Madsen JK, Grande P, Saunamaki K, et al. Danish multi-

center randomized study of invasive versus conservative treatment in patients with inducible ischemia after thrombolysis in acute myocardial infarction (DANAMI). Danish trial in acute myocardial infarction. *Circulation* 1997;96:748–755.

117. A clinical trial comparing primary coronary angioplasty with tissue plasminogen activator for acute myocardial infarction. The Global Use of Strategies to Open Occluded Coronary Arteries in Acute Coronary Syndromes (GUSTO IIb) angioplasty substudy investigators. *N Engl J Med* 1997;336:1621–1628.

118. Hochman JS, Sleeper LA, Webb JG, et al. Early revascularization in acute myocardial infarction complicated by cardiogenic shock. SHOCK investigators. Should we emergently revascularize occluded coronaries for cardiogenic shock. *N Engl J Med* 1999;341:625–634.

CARDIAC CATHETERIZATION AND HEMODYNAMIC ASSESSMENT

RICHARD A. LANGE
L. DAVID HILLIS

INDICATIONS AND CONTRAINDICATIONS

Diagnostic cardiac catheterization is appropriate in several circumstances. First, it is indicated to confirm or exclude the presence of a condition already suspected from the history, physical examination, or noninvasive evaluation. In such a circumstance, it allows one both to establish the presence and to assess the severity of cardiac disease. Second, catheterization is indicated to clarify a confusing or obscure clinical picture in a patient whose clinical findings and noninvasive data are inconclusive. Third, catheterization is performed in some patients for whom corrective cardiac surgery is contemplated to confirm the suspected abnormality and to exclude associated abnormalities that might require the surgeon's attention.

Fourth, catheterization is occasionally performed purely as a research procedure.

Therapeutic catheterization is appropriate in several circumstances. Percutaneous coronary revascularization (e.g., angioplasty, directional or rotational atherectomy, or endovascular stenting) may be indicated in the patient with symptomatic atherosclerotic coronary artery disease whose coronary anatomy is suitable for the procedure. Valvuloplasty is indicated in the subject with symptomatic isolated pulmonic stenosis, and it is an acceptable alternative to surgery in the patient with mitral stenosis or aortic stenosis in whom valvular anatomy is suitable and surgery is believed to offer an unfavorable risk-benefit ratio, due, for example, to advanced age or comorbid medical conditions (i.e., chronic pulmonary, hepatic, or renal disease or an underlying malignancy).

Catheterization is absolutely contraindicated if a mentally competent individual does not consent. It is relatively contraindicated if an intercurrent condition exists that, if corrected, would improve the safety of the procedure (*e*Table 79.0.2).

R. A. Lange: Department of Internal Medicine, University of Texas Southwestern Medical Center at Dallas, Dallas, Texas

L. D. Hillis: Department of Internal Medicine, University of Texas Southwestern Medical Center at Dallas, Dallas, Texas

RISKS AND COMPLICATIONS

As cardiac catheterization has been more frequently performed, the incidence of complications has diminished (*e*Table 79.0.3). However, even in skilled hands, the procedure is not without risk (1–4). The overall incidence of a major complication (death, myocardial infarction, or cerebrovascular accident) during or within 24 hours of diagnostic catheterization is 0.2% to 0.3%. Of these major complications, death during or within 24 hours of the procedure occurs in 0.1% to 0.2% of patients. Such deaths may be caused by perforation of the heart or great vessels, cardiac arrhythmias, acute myocardial infarction, or anaphylaxis to radiographic contrast material. Individuals with an increased risk of death include those with (a) advanced (older than 70 years) or very young (younger than 1 year) age, (b) marked functional impairment (class IV angina or heart failure), (c) severe left ventricular dysfunction or coronary artery disease (particularly left main disease), (d) severe valvular disease, (e) severe comorbid medical conditions (i.e., renal, hepatic, or pulmonary disease), or (f) history of an allergy to radiographic contrast material. Patients with significant left main coronary artery stenosis have a substantially greater risk of periprocedural death (2.8%) compared with those without left main coronary artery stenosis (0.1%) (5,6).

Myocardial infarction during or immediately after diagnostic catheterization occurs in approximately 0.07% of patients, but most are small and uncomplicated. Cerebrovascular accidents in the pericatheterization period may be (a) embolic (from the arterial catheter, guidewire, left ventricular or atrial thrombus, or dislodged atherosclerotic plaque) or (b) thrombotic (i.e., existence of previous extensive cerebrovascular disease that, in association with the hemodynamic alterations induced by arteriography, leads to inadequate cerebral perfusion).

Numerous minor complications may cause morbidity but exert no effect on mortality. Local vascular complications occur in 0.5% to 1.5% of patients. The incidence is similar for the brachial and femoral approaches and somewhat higher for the radial approach. After arterial catheterization by the brachial or radial approach, thrombosis, dissection, intimal flap formation, or subintimal hemorrhage may compromise blood flow to the hand or arm, and the patient may require thrombectomy or surgical exploration after catheterization. With the percutaneous femoral approach, hemorrhage, hematoma formation, or both at the arterial puncture site are the most common problems and, if severe, may require limited surgical exploration. Arteriovenous (AV) fistulae or pseudoaneurysm formation may occur, especially if protracted bleeding at the puncture site occurs after sheath removal, as may result from inadequate compression of the femoral vessel, insertion of large sheaths, severe systemic arterial hypertension, prolonged heparinization, or administration of thrombolytic or antiplatelet agents. Less commonly, femoral arterial thrombosis occurs, which requires urgent thrombectomy. Compression by a large hematoma or groin clamp may cause local nerve damage. Local infection may occur at the site of catheter entrance and manipulation, but this can usually be treated effectively with meticulous wound care and antibiotics.

The injection of radiographic contrast material commonly causes nausea and vomiting as well as a transient decrease in systemic arterial pressure. Occasionally, such injections are associated with allergic reactions of varying severity, and a rare individual has anaphylaxis. Only 15% of individuals with a known allergy to contrast material have another adverse reaction with repeat administration, and most of these are minor (urticaria, nausea, vomiting) (7). In the vast majority of patients with a history of contrast allergy, angiography can be performed safely; however, premedication with glucocorticosteroids and antihistamines as well as use of a nonionic contrast agent are usually recommended. The endocardial injection of contrast material during ventriculography (so-called endocardial staining) may cause ventricular irritability. Finally, use of excessive quantities of radiographic contrast material may result in renal insufficiency, which is usually transient. This is particularly likely to occur in patients with preexisting renal dysfunction and diabetes mellitus, and its occurrence can be minimized by (a) limiting the amount of contrast material used during catheterization based on the patient's body surface area and baseline serum creatinine (8), and (b) administering sufficient oral and intravenous fluids after catheterization to ensure that the osmotic diuresis caused by the hyperosmolar contrast material does not induce intravascular volume depletion.

HEMODYNAMIC MEASUREMENTS

Cardiac Output

The role of the heart is to deliver an adequate quantity of oxygenated blood to the body. This flow of blood is known as the *CO* and is expressed in liters per minute. Since the magnitude of CO is proportional to body surface area, one person may be compared with another by means of the cardiac index (i.e., the CO adjusted for body surface area). The normal cardiac index is 2.6 to 4.2 L per minute per m^2 of body surface area (Table 79.1). The two commonly used methods of measuring CO are the Fick method and the indicator dilution technique. The latter can be performed by thermodilution or the injection of indocyanine green.

Fick Method

The measurement of CO by the Fick method is based on the hypothesis that the uptake or release of a substance by an organ is the product of the blood flow to that organ and

TABLE 79.1 NORMAL HEMODYNAMIC VALUES

Flows	
Cardiac index (L/min/m²)	2.6–4.2
Stroke volume index (mL/m²)	35–55
Pressures (mm Hg)	
Aorta/systemic artery	
Peak systolic/end diastolic	100–140/60–90
Mean	70–105
Left ventricle	
Peak systolic/end diastolic	100–140/3–12
Left atrium (pulmonary capillary wedge)	
Mean	1–10
'a' wave	3–15
'v' wave	3–15
Pulmonary artery	
Peak systolic/end diastolic	16–30/0–8
Mean	10–16
Right ventricle	
Peak systolic/end diastolic	16–30/0–8
Right atrium	
Mean	0–8
'a' wave	2–10
'v' wave	2–10
Resistances	
Systemic vascular resistance	
Wood units	10–20
Dynes-sec-cm⁻⁵	770–1500
Pulmonary vascular resistance	
Wood units	0.25–1.50
Dynes-sec-cm⁻⁵	20–120
Oxygen consumption (mL/min/m²)	110–150
AVo₂ difference (mL/dL)	3.0–4.5

AV, arteriovenous.

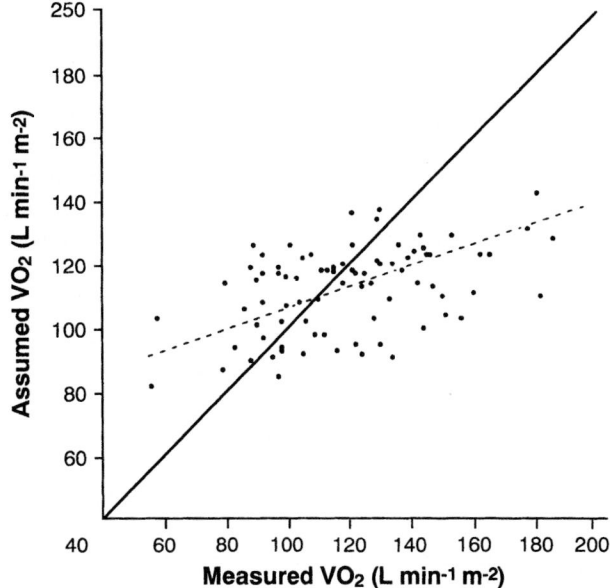

FIGURE 79.1 Comparison of measured (*x*-axis) and assumed (*y*-axis) oxygen consumption (Vo₂), with the latter derived from a formula. The relationship between the measured and assumed oxygen consumptions is poor. (From Kendrick AH, West J, Papouchado M, et al. Direct Fick cardiac output: are assumed values of oxygen consumption acceptable? *Eur Heart J* 1988;9:337–342, with permission.)

the regional AV concentration difference of the substance (15). To measure CO in humans, this principle is applied to the lungs, and the substance measured is oxygen (O_2). By measuring the amount of O_2 extracted from inspired air by the lungs and the AVO_2 difference across the lungs, pulmonary blood flow may be calculated. Because pulmonary blood flow is similar to systemic blood flow in most people, the Fick method allows one to measure systemic blood flow. The Fick formula for the calculation of CO is:

$$CO \ (L/min) = \frac{O_2 \ consumption \ (mL/min)}{AVO_2 \ difference \ across \ the \ lungs \ (mL/L)}$$

The normal O_2 consumption index (O_2 consumption per m² of body surface) is 110 to 150 mL per minute per m² (Table 79.1) (16). In general, the O_2 consumption is higher for men than women and decreases gradually with age. It increases with hyperthyroidism, hyperthermia, and exercise, whereas it decreases with hypothyroidism and hypothermia. In many laboratories, the O_2 consumption is estimated from a nomogram, formula, or table. However, studies (17) have demonstrated a poor relationship between estimated and measured O_2 consumption (Fig. 79.1), in part because of the wide range of values among patients (*e*Fig. 79.1.1) (16).

Thus, to determine CO accurately via the Fick method, O_2 consumption should be measured directly. ▼ n34

Determining the AVO_2 difference across the lungs requires that blood from the vessels entering and draining the lungs (i.e., the pulmonary artery and vein) be analyzed for O_2 content. Since the O_2 content of pulmonary venous blood is similar to that of systemic arterial blood (provided that a right-to-left shunt is not present), systemic and pulmonary arterial samples are usually obtained for the Fick determination of CO. The O_2 content of pulmonary and systemic arterial blood may be measured directly or calculated from the O_2 saturation of the blood and its hemoglobin (Hgb) concentration: O_2 content = Hgb (in g per 100 mL) × 1.36 (mL O_2 per g Hgb) × saturation, where 1.36 is the maximum O_2-carrying capacity of 1 g of Hgb. The normal AVO_2 difference is 3.0 to 4.5 vol percent (mL O_2 per dL of blood). The following is an example of the Fick calculation of CO: (a) O_2 consumption = 250 mL per minute; (b) Hgb = 14 g per dL; (c) systemic arterial O_2 saturation = 0.95 (95%); (d) pulmonary arterial O_2 saturation = 0.65 (65%); and (e) 10 = dL per L (conversion factor).

$$CO = \frac{250}{(14)(1.36)(10)(0.95) - (14)(1.36)(10)(0.65)}$$

$$= 4.38 \ L \ per \ minute$$

The Fick method has several potential sources of error (19). First, an incomplete collection of expired air causes an underestimation of O_2 consumption, leading to the calculation of a falsely low value for CO. This is the most common source of error. Second, incorrect timing of the collection of expired air leads to an inaccurate estimate of O_2 consumption. Third, analysis of the Douglas bag contents should be performed soon after its collection, since air may diffuse in or out of the bag if a substantial delay between collection and analysis is allowed to occur. Fourth, with commercially available polarographic systems, determination of the fractional content of oxygen or carbon dioxide may be inaccurate if the gas sensors are not calibrated regularly and correctly. Fifth, spectrophotometric determination of the O_2 saturations may be inaccurate if certain substances, such as indocyanine green, have been introduced into the blood. Finally, the mixed venous blood sample must, indeed, be *mixed venous*. It is generally obtained from the pulmonary artery; it must not be partially contaminated by pulmonary capillary wedge blood or left-to-right shunted blood.

The average error in determining O_2 consumption is approximately 6%, and that for AVO_2 difference is 5%. When the AVO_2 saturation difference is small, errors in measurement are magnified. Therefore, the Fick method is most accurate in the patient with a low CO (i.e., one with a relatively wide AVO_2 saturation difference) and least accurate in one with a high CO (i.e., one with a relatively narrow AVO_2 saturation difference) (Table 79.2).

Indicator Dilution Technique

The indicator dilution technique is based on the principle that the volume of fluid within a container can be determined if one adds a known quantity of indicator to the fluid and then measures the concentration of the indicator after it has completely mixed with the fluid. To determine CO, a known amount of indicator is injected into the circulation and allowed to mix completely in the blood, after which its concentration is measured over time. A time-concentration curve is generated (Fig. 79.2), and a minicomputer calculates the area of the inscribed curve.

The indicator most often used to measure CO is cold saline or 5% dextrose in water. A balloon-tipped flow-directed polyvinyl chloride catheter with a thermistor at its tip and an opening 25 to 30 cm proximal to the tip is inserted into a vein and advanced to the pulmonary artery, so that the proximal opening is located in the venae cavae or right atrium, and the thermistor is in the pulmonary artery. Five to 10 mL of iced fluid is injected into the proximal port, and the change in temperature at the thermistor is recorded (20,21). CO via the thermodilution method is calculated with a computer via the equation:

$$CO = \frac{(T_B - T_I)(vol)(60)(1.10)(0.825)}{\int \Delta T_B(t)dt}$$

in which T_B = body temperature, T_I = temperature of the injectate, vol = volume of the injectate (in milliliters), 60 = number of seconds in 1 minute, and 1.10 = ratio of the products of specific heat and gravity for normal saline and blood; 0.825 is an empiric factor that accounts for the warming of injectate within the catheter. The denominator of the equation is the integral of the change in blood temperature during the injection of cold and is reflected by the area of the inscribed curve (Fig. 79.2). The thermodilution technique is relatively inexpensive, easy to perform, widely available, and does not require arterial sampling or blood withdrawal. In most patients, it accurately determines pulmonary blood flow, which (in the absence of intracardiac shunting) is similar to systemic blood flow. However, certain conditions may render the results of the thermodilution technique unreliable, including (a) tricuspid or pulmonic regurgitation (22) and (b) intracardiac shunting (Table 79.2).

Indocyanine green, an easily detectable, water-soluble, nontoxic substance, can also be used for the indicator dilution measurement of CO (23). To do so, (a) a known concentration (5 to 10 mg) of indicator must be injected; (b) there must be complete mixing of the indocyanine green between the sites of injection and sampling; and (c) there must be no metabolism or disappearance of the indicator between the sites of injection and sampling. In most catheterization laboratories that use this method, CO is measured by injecting indocyanine green into the pulmonary artery as blood is withdrawn at a constant rate from a systemic artery through an optical densitometer (Fig. 79.2). The lungs, left atrium, and left ventricle act as

TABLE 79.2 METHODS FOR DETERMINING CARDIAC OUTPUT AND CONDITIONS IN WHICH THEY ARE MOST (OR LEAST) RELIABLE

Method	Most reliable	Least reliable
Fick	Low cardiac output	High cardiac output
Thermodilu-tion	High cardiac output	Pulmonic regurgitation
		Tricuspid regurgitation
		Intracardiac shunting
Indocyanine green	High cardiac output	Aortic regurgitation
		Mitral regurgitation
		Low cardiac output
		Intracardiac shunting
Angiographic	Normal-shaped ventricle	Extensive segmental wall motion abnormalities
		Dilated ventricle
		Aortic regurgitation[a]
		Mitral regurgitation[a]

[a]In these circumstances, angiographic output is greater than forward cardiac output (see text).

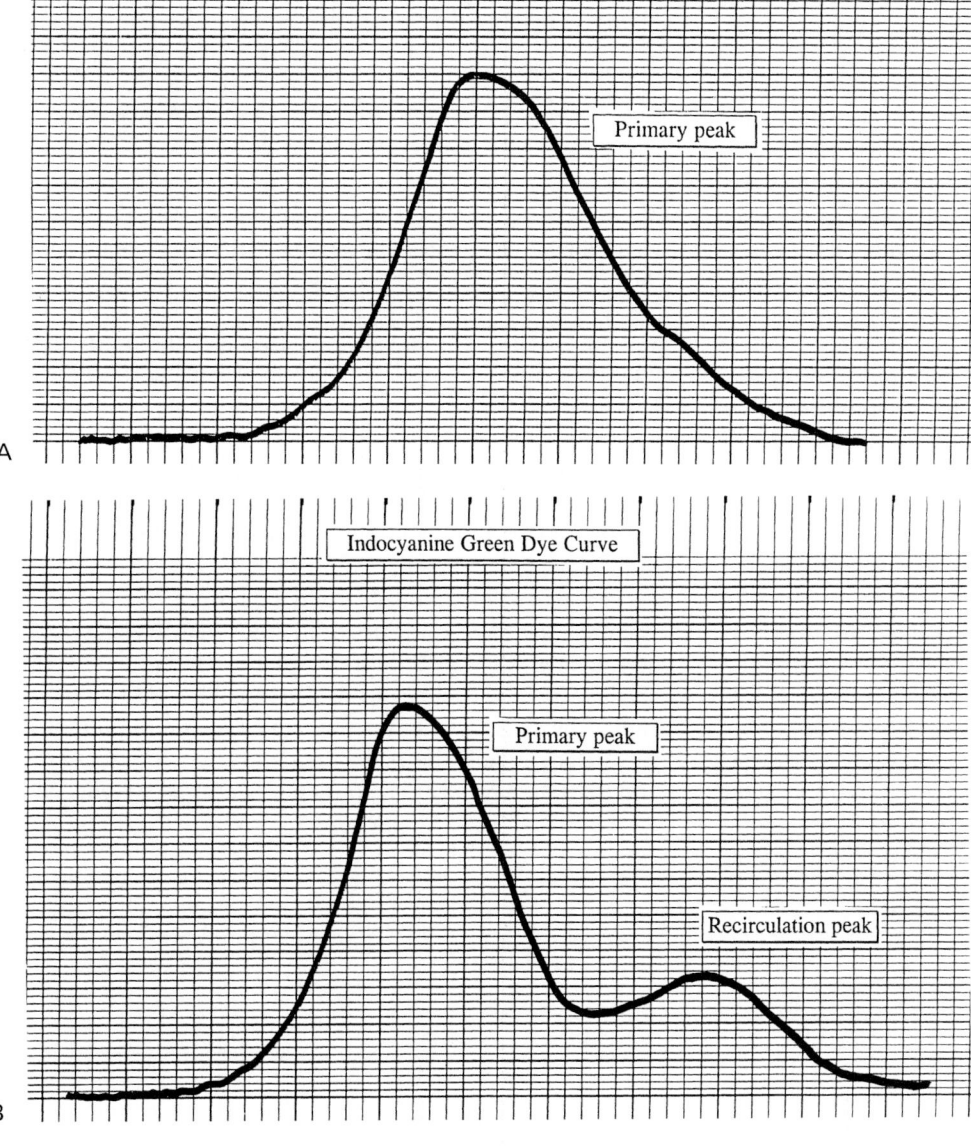

FIGURE 79.2 Time-activity curves for the indicator dilution technique for determining cardiac output: thermodilution **(A)** and indocyanine green **(B)**. With indocyanine green, a primary peak and a recirculation peak are present, whereas with thermodilution, only a primary peak is observed.

adequate mixing sites, and there is no degradation of indocyanine green between the pulmonary and systemic arteries. The calculation of CO by the indicator dilution technique is usually done by a minicomputer, which establishes that the downslope of the inscribed curve is exponential. It then computes the area inscribed by the curve, excluding the recirculation peak. The results obtained with this method compare favorably with those of other techniques for measuring CO, but it may provide inaccurate results in circumstances in which the recirculation peak cannot be easily separated from the primary peak (e.g., low CO) or when one of the valves between

the site of injection and sampling (i.e., mitral or aortic) is regurgitant (Table 79.2). ❧ n35

Angiographic Technique

From the left ventriculogram, one can determine the volume of blood ejected with each heart beat (stroke volume) and then multiply it by heart rate, yielding the angiographic CO. In patients with mitral or aortic regurgitation, a portion of the blood ejected from the left ventricle regurgitates into the left atrium or ventricle and does not enter the systemic circulation. In these patients, the angiographic

CO exceeds the forward output. The measurement of CO by the angiographic method is potentially erroneous in patients with extensive segmental wall motion abnormalities or misshapen ventricles, in whom the determination of stroke volume may be inaccurate (Table 79.2).

Pressure Waveforms

Right atrial systole follows the P wave of the electrocardiogram and produces the 'a' wave of the right atrial pressure tracing (Fig. 79.3). With atrial relaxation, there is a decline in the pressure, which is known as the *'x' descent*. This descent may be interrupted by a slight upward deflection, the 'c' wave, due to tricuspid valve closure. Filling of the right atrium from the venous circulation and retrograde movement of the tricuspid valve annulus during right ventricular systole produce the 'v' wave, which follows the QRS complex on the electrocardiogram. When the tricuspid valve opens, blood from the right atrium empties into the right ventricle, and the right atrial pressure declines, producing the 'y' descent. During diastole, the right ventricular and right atrial pressures are equal if tricuspid stenosis is absent. Typically, the peak 'a' wave, 'v' wave, and mean right atrial pressures are reported. In the normal right atrium, the peak 'a' wave is higher than the peak 'v' wave pressure.

In the right ventricular pressure tracing, atrial systole produces an 'a' wave, which occurs after the P wave of the electrocardiogram (Fig. 79.4). Right ventricular systole follows the QRS complex of the electrocardiogram and gives rise to the rapidly increasing systolic pressure waveform. With ventricular relaxation, the pressure waveform declines and reaches a nadir, after which continuous filling of the chamber from the right atrium causes a slow, steady rise in

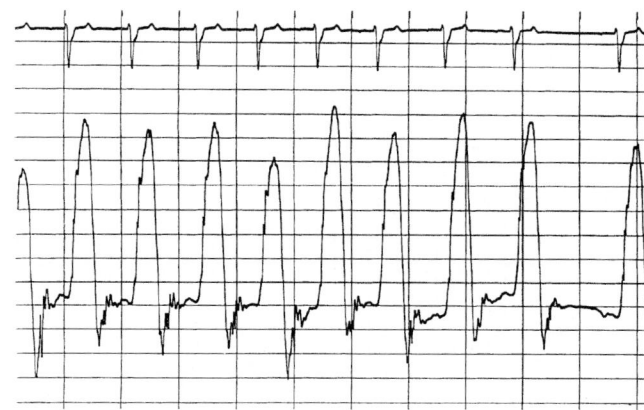

FIGURE 79.4 Simultaneous surface electrocardiogram and right ventricular pressure recordings. The right ventricular peak systolic pressure averages 45 mm Hg, and the end diastolic pressure (measured at the R-wave peak of the QRS complex) averages 16 mm Hg. The distance between each horizontal line represents 4 mm Hg, and the distance between each vertical time line represents 1 second.

the pressure waveform. The peak systolic and end diastolic (measured at the peak of the QRS complex of the electrocardiogram) right ventricular pressures are usually reported. Similar pressures are reported for the left ventricle.

The normal pulmonary arterial pressure consists of a systolic wave that coincides with right ventricular systole and follows the QRS complex of the electrocardiogram (Fig. 79.5). The decline of this pressure wave may be interrupted by a notch, the incisura, which is due to pulmonic valve closure, and the nadir of the decline represents the end diastolic pressure. The pulmonary arterial systolic, end

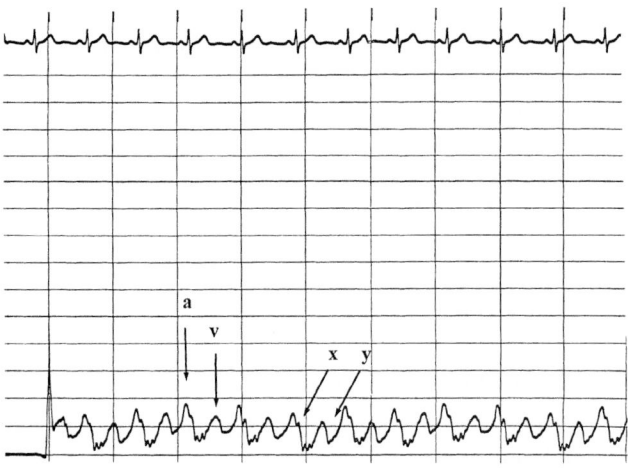

FIGURE 79.3 Typical pressure tracings from the right atrium. There is an 'a' wave, 'x' descent, 'v' wave, and 'y' descent, which correlate with right atrial systole, relaxation, filling, and emptying, respectively. The distance between each horizontal line represents 4 mm Hg, and the distance between each vertical time line represents 1 second.

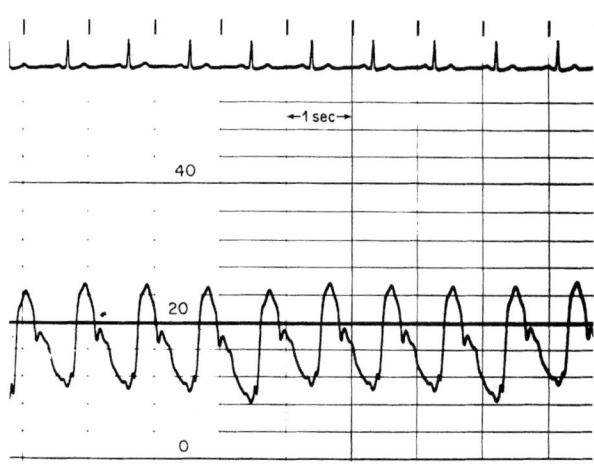

FIGURE 79.5 Simultaneous surface electrocardiogram and pulmonary arterial pressure tracings. The pulmonary arterial pressure averages 25/10 mm Hg, and the incisura, caused by closure of the pulmonic valve, is evident on the downslope of the pressure contour. The distance between each horizontal line represents 4 mm Hg, and the distance between each vertical time line represents 1 second. (From Willard JE, Lange RA, Hillis LD. Cardiac catheterization. In: Kloner RA, ed. *The guide to cardiology*, 3rd ed. New York: Wiley, 1995:145–164, with permission.)

diastolic, and mean pressures are usually reported. Similar pressures are reported for the aorta and peripheral arteries.

When a catheter is advanced to the pulmonary capillary wedge position and its position confirmed oximetrically (by aspirating blood with an O_2 saturation greater than 95%), the pressure waveform obtained is a transmitted left atrial pressure (Fig. 79.6). The configuration of the waveform is similar to a right atrial pressure, in that there is an 'a' wave, 'x' descent, 'v' wave, and 'y' descent, which correlate with left atrial systole, relaxation, filling, and emptying, respectively. In the left atrium, however, the peak 'v' wave pressure is typically higher than the peak 'a' wave pressure. Transmission of the left atrial pressure through the pulmonary vasculature usually causes modest distortion of the pressure waveform (*e*Fig. 79.6.1). To obtain the most accurate representation of left atrial pressure, the pulmonary capillary wedge pressure should be measured through a stiff catheter with a large lumen (26). Time is required for transmission of the left atrial pressure through the pulmonary vasculature. Thus, if left atrial and pulmonary capillary wedge pressures are recorded simultaneously, a 50- to 100-ms time difference is noted, with the pulmonary wedge pressure occurring later.

In addition to the recording of pressures from each of the cardiac chambers, it is important that the pressures from certain chambers be examined simultaneously to confirm or exclude the presence of valvular abnormalities (26,27). Thus, left ventricular and left atrial (or pulmonary capillary wedge) pressures should be recorded simultaneously to ascertain if mitral stenosis is present (*e*Fig. 79.6.2 and Fig. 79.7). Likewise, the left ventricular and

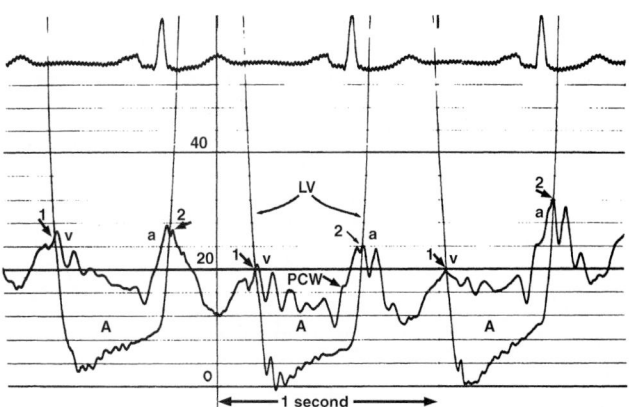

FIGURE 79.7 Simultaneous recording of left ventricular (LV) and pulmonary capillary wedge (PCW) pressures in a patient with severe mitral stenosis. Throughout diastole (from points 1 to 2), there is a pressure gradient (A) between the LV and PCW pressures. This patient had a cardiac output of 3,740 mL per minute and a heart rate of 68 beats/min. The mean diastolic filling period was 0.49 seconds per beat, and the mean pressure gradient was 13 mm Hg. Using Gorlin's equation, the mitral valve area is:

$$\frac{3,740 / (68)(0.49)}{(38)(\sqrt{13})} = 0.8 \text{ cm}^2$$

(From Willard JE, Lange RA, Hillis LD. Cardiac catheterization. In: Kloner RA, ed. *The guide to cardiology*, 3rd ed. New York: Wiley, 1995:145–164, with permission.)

systemic arterial pressures should be displayed concurrently to evaluate the presence or absence of left ventricular outflow tract obstruction (*e*Fig. 79.7.1 and Fig. 79.8). The recording of intracardiac and peripheral vascular pressures may demonstrate hemodynamic findings consistent with valvular regurgitation. For instance, large regurgitant waves in the pulmonary capillary wedge tracing may be indicative of mitral regurgitation or other causes of left atrial pressure or volume overload (Fig. 79.9) (28). Conversely, a wide peripheral arterial pulse pressure in conjunction with a greatly elevated left ventricular end diastolic pressure is suggestive of aortic regurgitation. In short, both the absolute level and the qualitative configuration of the intracardiac and peripheral vascular pressures are important in the diagnosis and quantitation of valvular heart disease. The normal intracardiac and peripheral vascular flows, pressures, and resistances are listed in Table 79.1.

Vascular Resistance

The resistance of a vascular bed is calculated by dividing the pressure gradient across the bed by the flow through it. Thus,

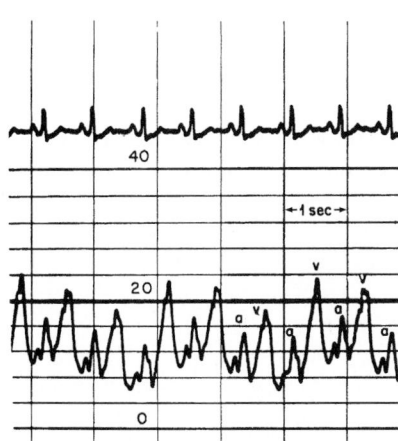

FIGURE 79.6 Pulmonary capillary wedge pressure tracing obtained through a stiff, large-lumen catheter, the position of which was confirmed oximetrically. Like the right atrial pressure tracing, there is an 'a' wave and 'v' wave, which correlate with atrial systole and filling, respectively. The distance between each horizontal line represents 4 mm Hg, and the distance between each vertical time line represents 1 second. (From Willard JE, Lange RA, Hillis LD. Cardiac catheterization. In: Kloner RA, ed. *The guide to cardiology*, 3rd ed. New York: Wiley, 1995:145–164, with permission.)

$$\text{Systemic vascular resistance} = \frac{\text{mean systemic arterial pressure} - \text{mean right atrial pressure}}{\text{systemic blood flow}}$$

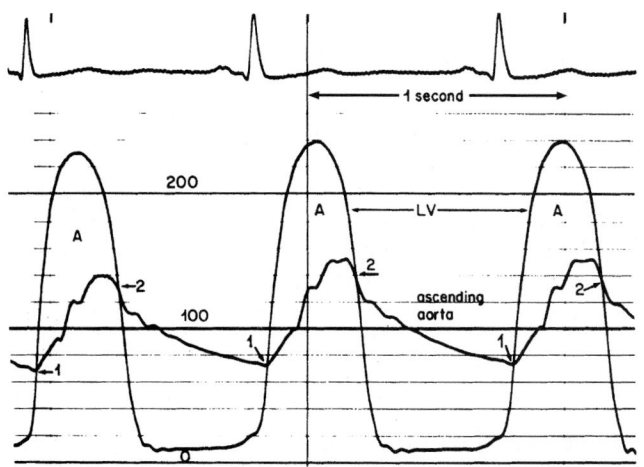

FIGURE 79.8 Simultaneous recording of left ventricular (LV) and ascending aortic pressures in a patient with severe aortic stenosis. Throughout systole, there is a pressure gradient (A) between the LV and ascending aorta. The patient had a cardiac output of 3,350 mL per minute and a heart rate of 62 beats/min. The systolic ejection period (between points 1 and 2) was 0.36 seconds per beat, and the mean systolic pressure gradient was 83 mm Hg. Thus, the aortic valve area was:

$$\frac{3,350/(62)(0.36)}{44.5(\sqrt{83})} = 0.4 \text{ cm}^2$$

(From Willard JE, Lange RA, Hillis LD. Cardiac catheterization. In: Kloner RA, ed. *The guide to cardiology*, 3rd ed. New York: Wiley, 1995:145–164, with permission.)

and

$$\text{Pulmonary vascular resistance} = \frac{\text{mean pulmonary artery pressure} - \text{mean pulmonary vein pressure}}{\text{pulmonary blood flow}}$$

Since pulmonary venous pressure is not usually measured, left atrial or pulmonary capillary wedge pressure is substituted for it. Resistances are expressed in (a) resistance units (mm Hg per L per minute), (b) dynes-second-cm^{-5} (resis-

tance units × 80), or (c) Wood units (resistance units × body surface area in m^2). The normal values for vascular resistances are displayed in Table 79.1.

An increased systemic vascular resistance is usually present in patients with systemic arterial hypertension. It may also be seen in the patient with a reduced forward CO and compensatory arteriolar vasoconstriction. In turn, a reduced systemic vascular resistance may be present in the patient with an inappropriately increased CO, the causes of which include AV fistula, severe anemia, high fever, sepsis, and thyrotoxicosis. An elevated pulmonary vascular resistance may be caused by primary lung disease, Eisenmenger's syndrome (alterations in the pulmonary vasculature in response to increased pulmonary flow and pressure), and a greatly elevated pulmonary venous pressure due to left-sided myocardial or valvular dysfunction or both.

ASSESSMENT OF VALVULAR HEART DISEASE

Valvular Stenosis

Through the application of standard fluid dynamic principles, the resistance to blood flow through a stenotic valve can be expressed as an effective valve orifice area (29). The data required for the calculation of a valve area may be obtained during cardiac catheterization. Specifically, the pressures on either side of a stenotic valve and the flow across it must be known. The Gorlin's equation is then used to calculate the valve area:

$$\text{Valve area} = \frac{\text{CO}/(\text{DFP or SEP})(\text{heart rate})}{(\text{constant})\sqrt{\text{mean pressure gradient}}}$$

where DFP is diastolic filling period and SEP is systolic ejection period. If an atrioventricular valve (mitral or tricuspid) is being evaluated, the diastolic filling period is used; if the aortic or pulmonic valve is involved, the systolic ejection period is used. The filling periods and transvalvular

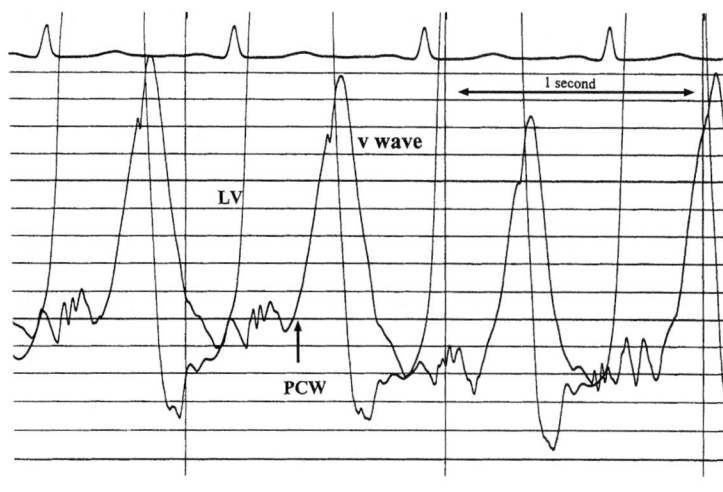

FIGURE 79.9 Simultaneous recording of left ventricular (LV) and pulmonary capillary wedge (PCW) pressures from a patient with severe mitral regurgitation. The PCW pressure tracing demonstrates large regurgitant 'v' waves.

gradient are measured from pressure tracings obtained simultaneously from either side of the stenotic valve. The constant used is 38.0 for the mitral valve and 44.5 for the other valves. The mean pressure gradient is the average gradient throughout systole (for aortic and pulmonic valves) or diastole (for mitral or tricuspid valves).

The normal mitral valve orifice area is 4 to 6 cm^2, and substantial stenosis may occur before a pressure gradient appears. A mitral valve with an effective orifice area less than 1.0 cm^2 is considered severely stenotic (Fig. 79.7); 1.1 to less than 1.5 cm^2, moderately stenotic; and 1.6 to less than 2.0 cm^2, mildly stenotic. A valve area greater than 2.0 cm^2 is not necessarily normal, but does not usually constitute a hemodynamically significant obstruction to flow. The normal aortic valve has a cross-sectional area of 3 to 4 cm^2, but hemodynamically important aortic stenosis does not develop until the valve orifice area falls below 1.1 to 1.3 cm^2. Specifically, an aortic valve with an effective orifice area less than 0.7 cm^2 is severely stenotic (Fig. 79.8); 0.8 to 1.0 cm^2, moderately stenotic; and 1.1 to 1.3 cm^2, mildly stenotic. The normal pulmonic valve has a cross-sectional area similar to the aortic valve. Although Gorlin's equation can be applied to the pulmonic valve, by convention the severity of stenosis is based on the peak right ventricular systolic pressure. Pulmonic stenosis with a right ventricular peak systolic pressure of 25 to less than 50 mm Hg is termed mild; 50 to less than 100 mm Hg, moderate; and greater than 100 mm Hg, severe. Finally, the tricuspid valve is large, with a normal orifice area of 6 to 10 cm^2. The assessment of the severity of tricuspid stenosis is most accurate when right atrial and right ventricular pressures are recorded simultaneously. Patients with a tricuspid valve area less than 3.0 cm^2 in the presence of medically refractory right-sided heart failure should be considered for appropriate mechanical intervention (i.e., balloon valvuloplasty, open commissurotomy, or valve replacement).

It is essential that all the variables used to calculate a valve area (CO, systolic ejection period or diastolic filling period, heart rate, and pressure gradient) be measured in close temporal proximity to one another and with the patient in a hemodynamically stable state. Great care must be exercised in the acquisition of these data, since the decision for operative intervention is based on the calculated valve area.

Valvular Regurgitation

The presence and severity of mitral regurgitation may be evaluated qualitatively by observing the amount of radiographic contrast material that regurgitates into the left atrium during left ventricular systole on a standard left ventriculogram (eFig. 79.9.1). The magnitude of regurgitation is estimated as trivial (1+), mild (2+), moderate (3+), or severe (4+) (see Left Ventriculography, later in this chapter). To obtain a quantitative assessment of the severity of mitral regurgitation, one can calculate the volume of blood that regurgitates from the left ventricle into the left atrium per minute (so-called regurgitant volume) by measuring the difference between the angiographic CO (determined by left ventriculography) and the forward CO (determined by the Fick method or thermodilution). The regurgitant fraction is the percentage of the total angiographic output that regurgitates into the left atrium: It is the quotient of the regurgitant volume and the angiographic output. Typically, valvular regurgitation with a regurgitant fraction 0.6 or greater is severe; 0.40 to 0.59, moderate; 0.20 to 0.39, mild; and less than 0.20, trivial.

The presence and severity of aortic regurgitation may be evaluated qualitatively by observing the amount of radiographic contrast material that regurgitates into the left ventricle during ventricular diastole by aortography; it is also graded as trivial (1+), mild (2+), moderate (3+), or severe (4+) (see Aortography, later in this chapter). As with mitral regurgitation, a quantitative assessment of the severity of aortic regurgitation can be obtained by calculating the regurgitant volume and fraction.

ASSESSMENT OF INTRACARDIAC SHUNTING

Left-to-Right Shunting

In the patient with known or suspected congenital heart disease, as well as the subject with unexplained heart failure, cardiac catheterization may be performed to assess the presence, location, and magnitude of intracardiac shunting. To accomplish this, several techniques may be used (Table 79.3) (30).

TABLE 79.3 COMPARISON OF METHODS TO DETECT, LOCALIZE, AND QUANTIFY INTRACARDIAC LEFT-TO-RIGHT SHUNTING

Method	Able to localize?	Able to quantify?	Minimal Qp/Qs reliably detected
Oximetry	Yes	Yes	1.5–1.9 at level of atrium 1.3–1.5 at level of ventricle 1.3 at level of great vessels
Indocyanine green	No	Yes	1.35
Angiography	Yes	No	Unknown

Oximetric Assessment

The oximetric detection and localization of intracardiac left-to-right shunting is based on the principle that oxygenated blood shunted from the left side to the right side of the heart causes an abnormal increase ("step up") in the oxygen content or saturation of blood in the chamber into which shunting occurs. To detect the presence and site of the left-to-right shunt, multiple blood samples are obtained from the pulmonary artery, right ventricle, right atrium, and venae cavae, and the oxygen content or saturation of each sample is evaluated for evidence of such a step up. An abnormal step up is present when the right atrial oxygen content is greater than 1.9 mL per dL higher than that of the venae cavae; the right ventricular oxygen content is greater than 0.9 mL per dL higher than that of the right atrium; or the pulmonary arterial oxygen content is greater than 0.5 mL per dL higher than that of the right ventricle (31,32). The oxygen content of blood can be measured directly or calculated from the saturation [saturation × hemoglobin (gram per deciliter) × 1.36 mL O_2 per g of hemoglobin].

The oximetric quantitation of shunting is accomplished by calculating pulmonic (Qp) and systemic (Qs) blood flows according to the Fick principle, where:

$$Qp \text{ (L per minute)} = \frac{\text{Oxygen consumption (mL per minute)}}{\text{AV oxygen content difference across the lungs (mL per L)}}$$

and

$$Qs \text{ (L per minute)} = \frac{\text{Oxygen consumption (mL per minute)}}{\text{AV oxygen content difference across the body (mL per L)}}$$

The AV oxygen content difference across the lungs is the difference in oxygen contents between pulmonary arterial and venous blood. The AV oxygen content across the body is the difference in oxygen contents between systemic arterial and mixed venous blood, with the latter obtained from the chamber immediately before (proximal to) the site of shunting. For example, if a ventricular septal defect is present, the mixed venous chamber is the right atrium; if a patent ductus arteriosus is present, the mixed venous chamber is the right ventricle. An example of the calculations for a patient with an intracardiac left-to-right shunt is presented in Table 79.4.

The oximetric determination of intracardiac left-to-right shunting is highly specific but relatively insensitive, in that an oximetric assessment reliably demonstrates the presence of a moderate or large shunt but may fail to detect a small one (Table 79.3) (30).

Indocyanine Green Assessment

As described previously, when a bolus of indocyanine green is introduced into a right-sided heart chamber and its concentration measured in systemic arterial blood, a concentration-time curve is inscribed, which is characterized by a primary peak and a recirculation peak. In the patient with left-to-right intracardiac shunting, the inscribed curve demonstrates prominent early recirculation (*e*Fig. 79.9.2) due to indocyanine green's rapid recirculation to the systemic arterial system through the intracardiac shunt. Since the area of the inscribed recirculation curve is proportional to shunt flow, the magnitude of shunting can be calculated with this technique (33,34). Although this method cannot identify the site of left-to-right shunting, it can detect shunts with a Qp/Qs as small as 1.35; thus, it is somewhat more sensitive than oximetry (35).

TABLE 79.4 OXIMETRIC ASSESSMENT OF THE PRESENCE, SITE, AND SIZE OF LEFT-TO-RIGHT INTRACARDIAC SHUNTING IN A PATIENT WITH A VENTRICULAR SEPTAL DEFECT[a]

Chamber	O_2 saturation (%)	O_2 content (mL/dL)	O_2 content difference (mL/dL)
Venae cavae	65	13.1	0.4
Right atrium	67	13.5	2.2
Right ventricle	78	15.7	0.2
Pulmonary artery	79	15.9	
Systemic artery	97		

Site of O_2 step up = right ventricle   Mixed venous chamber = right atrium

$$Qp = \frac{250 \text{ mL/min}}{(0.97 - 0.79)(15 \text{ g/dL})(1.36 \text{ mL } O_2/\text{g hemoglobin})(10 \text{ dL/L})} = 6.81 \text{ L/min}$$

$$Qs = \frac{250 \text{ mL/min}}{(0.97 - 0.67)(15 \text{ g/dL})(1.36 \text{ mL } O_2/\text{g hemoglobin})(10 \text{ dL/L})} = 4.08 \text{ L/min}$$

[a]Measured oxygen consumption = 250 mL per minute. Hemoglobin = 15 g per dL. Qp/Qs ratio = 6.81/4.08 = 1.7.

Angiographic Assessment

When radiographic contrast material is introduced into a left-sided chamber during angiography in a subject with left-to-right intracardiac shunting, its movement into a right-sided chamber may be visualized. The reliability of any angiographic technique for detecting or localizing intracardiac left-to-right shunting depends on the location of the defect and the obliquity in which the angiogram is performed. Left-sided angiography may be used to detect and localize certain kinds of intracardiac left-to-right shunts. For example, the interventricular septum may be visualized by performing left ventriculography in a 40- to 50-degree left anterior oblique projection, allowing the diagnosis of a ventricular septal defect. A communication between the thoracic aorta and the pulmonary artery (i.e., patent ductus arteriosus or aortopulmonary window) may be identified by performing aortography in the left anterior oblique or left lateral projections. In contradistinction, atrial septal defects and anomalous pulmonary venous drainage are difficult to visualize angiographically. Although angiography can detect and localize certain intracardiac left-to-right shunts, it cannot measure the magnitude of shunting.

Right-to-Left Shunting

In the patient with right-to-left intracardiac shunting, passage of unoxygenated blood from the venous circulation to the systemic circulation results in arterial desaturation (less than 95%). When desaturation is due to other conditions (i.e., a ventilation-perfusion mismatch or hypoventilation), it is corrected when 100% oxygen is administered, whereas this does not happen when the arterial desaturation is due to right-to-left shunting. Thus, demonstration of a systemic arterial oxygen saturation less than 95% that does not correct with the administration of 100% oxygen (via face mask) is consistent with right-to-left intracardiac shunting.

ANGIOGRAPHY

Left Ventriculography

Cineangiocardiography of the left ventricle allows one to assess (a) global and segmental left ventricular function, (b) left ventricular volumes and ejection fraction, and (c) the presence and severity of mitral regurgitation. To achieve adequate opacification, a large bolus of radiographic contrast material must be delivered to the left ventricle over a short period of time. In the normal adult, 40 to 60 mL of contrast material is injected over 3 to 4 seconds; thus, 10 to 20 mL are injected per second. As the contrast material is injected into the left ventricle, cineangiography is performed. Ventriculography may be performed in two projections (biplane) or more commonly in one projection (single plane), which is usually performed in the 30-degree right

anterior oblique projection. If biplane cineangiographic equipment is available, two projections, 90 degrees apart in obliquity (60-degree left anterior oblique and 30-degree right anterior oblique), are performed (*e*Fig. 79.9.3).

A variety of catheters may be used for left ventriculography, but all have certain features in common. First, the catheter should be of sufficient size so that a high-pressure injection of contrast material does not cause it to recoil, with resultant ventricular ectopy. Second, the catheter should be designed so that the jet of injected contrast material exits a series of side holes rather than just an end hole; as a result, the chance of a high-pressure jet of contrast material being injected into the endocardium (endocardial staining) is minimized. Finally, although the angiographic catheter should have multiple side holes for the injection of contrast material, these holes should be confined to the distal 2 to 3 cm of the catheter to avoid contrast injection into both the left ventricle and the ascending aorta.

Left ventriculography allows for calculation of left ventricular volumes and ejection fraction using a standard area-length formula (36–38). End diastolic and end systolic volumes are measured; from these, left ventricular stroke volume is derived (end diastolic volume minus end systolic volume), and ejection fraction is calculated (stroke volume divided by end diastolic volume). The normal values for left ventricular volumes and ejection fraction are displayed in *e*Table 79.4.1. In addition to the calculation of left ventricular volumes, segmental wall motion may be assessed. A segment of the left ventricular wall with reduced systolic motion is said to be *hypokinetic*; a segment that does not move during ventricular contraction is *akinetic*; and one that moves paradoxically during ventricular systole is termed *dyskinetic*. Finally, the presence and severity of mitral regurgitation may be evaluated qualitatively during sinus beats as trivial (1+), mild (2+), moderate (3+), or severe (4+): (a) with 1+, contrast material enters the left atrium during systole and clears with each beat; (b) with 2+, contrast opacification of the left atrium does not clear with each beat and is less dense than the left ventricle; (c) with 3+, opacification of the left atrium is equal to that of the left ventricle; and (d) with 4+, the presence of one of three findings is observed—opacification of the left atrium greater than that of the left ventricle, opacification of the left atrium in one systolic ejection period, or the presence of contrast material in a pulmonary vein.

Right Ventriculography

Cineangiography of the right ventricle allows one to assess global right ventricular function as well as the presence and severity of tricuspid regurgitation. Right ventriculography may be performed in single or biplane projections. Single plane right ventriculography is usually performed in a 30-degree right anterior oblique projection. If biplane angiography is available, a 60-degree left anterior oblique projection is also performed. To achieve adequate opacification, a bolus of 24 to 36 mL of radiographic contrast is injected over 2 seconds as cineangiography is performed. The presence and severity of tricuspid regurgitation may be qualitatively evaluated in a manner similar to mitral regurgitation: trivial (1+), mild (2+), moderate (3+), or severe (4+). There are no reliable methods for the quantitative assessment of right ventricular volumes or ejection fraction by ventriculography.

Aortography

Aortography is performed with the rapid injection of a large amount of radiographic contrast material into the aorta. A proximal aortogram is performed to assess the competency of the aortic valve, to evaluate the anatomy of the proximal aorta and large vessels that supply the head and neck, and occasionally to assess the presence of bypass graft anastomoses that have been difficult or impossible to cannulate selectively. In turn, a distal aortogram is performed to assess the presence of vascular abnormalities (e.g., aneurysm, dissection, intraluminal thrombus, coarctation). The catheters used for aortography are similar to those used for left ventriculography. For proximal aortography, 50 to 60 mL of contrast material is injected over 2.0 to 2.5 seconds and filmed either by cineangiography or rapid cut film angiography. The standard proximal aortogram is filmed in a 45- to 60-degree left anterior oblique projection. The severity of aortic regurgitation may be qualitatively evaluated during sinus beats as trivial (1+), mild (2+), moderate (3+), or severe (4+): (a) with 1+, contrast material enters the left ventricle during diastole and clears with each beat; (b) with 2+, contrast opacification of the left ventricle does not clear with each beat and is less dense than the ascending aorta; (c) with 3+, opacification of the left ventricle is equal to that of the aorta; and (d) with 4+, opacification of the left ventricle is greater than that of the aorta, or the left ventricle is opacified in one diastolic filling period (39).

Pulmonary Angiography

Pulmonary angiography is performed primarily to confirm or to exclude the presence of pulmonary emboli (40,41). A large-bore angiographic catheter is advanced from a systemic vein to the main pulmonary artery and is positioned so that it does not recoil into the right ventricle during the injection of contrast material, with resultant ventricular irritability. A large amount of contrast material (40 to 60 mL) is injected over 2 to 3 seconds. During the injection, cineangiography or rapid cut film angiography is performed.

If injection into the main pulmonary artery does not provide a definitive diagnosis, subselective injections are made into those segments of lung where the suspicion of

pulmonary emboli is highest. These injections can be made with either a small power injection through the same angiographic catheter or a hand injection through a balloon-tipped catheter. ☞ n36

CONTROVERSIES AND PERSONAL PERSPECTIVES

There is considerable controversy regarding the value and safety of right-sided heart catheterization. In many centers, right-sided heart catheterization is performed routinely in conjunction with coronary angiography. In those with proper indications (*e*Table 79.4.2), it may provide valuable diagnostic and prognostic information, which influences therapy in 35% to 55% of cases (42). In contrast, right-sided heart catheterization seldom provides information that influences patient management in the absence of these indications (43). In these individuals, therefore, it should not be performed routinely.

When performed by physicians experienced with the technique, right-sided heart catheterization is extremely safe. Over the past two decades, we have performed over 4,700 right-sided heart catheterizations with a stiff large-lumen (e.g., No. 8 Fr Goodale Lubin) catheter with no major complications (i.e., infection, hemorrhage, perforation, or death) and only one (0.02%) minor complication (femoral vein thrombosis).

An observational study (44) suggested that routine right-sided heart catheterization in critically ill patients is associated with an increased mortality. In such patients, physicians with limited catheterization experience often place an indwelling flow-directed pulmonary artery catheter. Complications associated with such indwelling catheters (i.e., pulmonary arterial perforation, sepsis, bacterial endocarditis, and large vein thrombosis) and placement by less experienced operators may account for the observed increased mortality. Some (45) have recommended a moratorium on routine right-sided heart catheterization in critically ill patients until properly conducted, randomized trials have assessed its utility and safety.

In our opinion, right-sided heart catheterization should not be performed in critically ill patients unless done so (a) by a physician experienced with the technique, (b) in a patient with a clear indication, or (c) for training purposes.

Likewise, left-sided heart catheterization should be performed only for a proper indication (*e*Table 79.4.3) and in a facility capable of handling complications. Free-standing or mobile catheterization facilities without immediately available hospital and surgical support are ill equipped to handle serious catheterization-related complications. Patients with unstable symptoms or clinical features suggestive of an increased risk for cardiac or vascular complications (Table 79.1) should undergo catheterization in an inpatient setting (46).

THE FUTURE

Cardiac catheterization plays a central role in the diagnostic evaluation of the patient with suspected or known cardiac disease, and it offers percutaneous therapeutic possibilities in many individuals. Over the next decade, the indications for therapeutic catheterization (e.g., percutaneous coronary revascularization, endoluminal stenting, and intracardiac defect closure) will continue to increase as the techniques, equipment, and operator skill improve.

REFERENCES

1. Wyman RM, Safian RD, Portway V, et al. Current complications of diagnostic and therapeutic cardiac catheterization. *J Am Coll Cardiol* 1988;12:1400–1406.
2. Johnson LW, Krone R. Cardiac catheterization 1991: a report of the Registry of the Society for Cardiac Angiography and Interventions (SCA&I). *Cathet Cardiovasc Diagn* 1993;28:219–220.
3. Kennedy JW, the Registry Committee of the Society for Cardiac Angiography. Symposium on catheterization complications. Complications associated with cardiac catheterization and angiography. *Cathet Cardiovasc Diagn* 1982;8:5–11.
4. Gersh BJ, Kronmal RA, Frye RL, et al. Coronary arteriography and coronary artery bypass surgery: morbidity and mortality in patients ages 65 years or older. *Circulation* 1983;67:483–491.
5. Gordon PR, Abrams C, Gash AK, et al. Pericatheterization risk factors in left main coronary artery stenosis. *Am J Cardiol* 1987;59:1080–1083.
6. Boehrer JD, Lange RA, Willard JE, et al. Markedly increased periprocedure mortality of cardiac catheterization in patients with severe narrowing of the left main coronary artery. *Am J Cardiol* 1992;70:1388–1390.
7. Brogan WC, Lange RA, Hillis LD. Contrast agents for catheterization: conceptions and misconceptions. *Am Heart J* 1991;122:1129–1235.
8. Cigarroa RG, Lange RA, Williams RH, et al. Dosing of contrast material to prevent contrast nephropathy in patients with renal disease. *Am J Med* 1989;86:649–651.
9. Sones FM Jr, Shirey EK. Cine coronary arteriography. *Mod Concepts Cardiovasc Dis* 1962;31:735–738.
10. Judkins MP. Percutaneous transfemoral selective coronary arteriography. *Radiol Clin North Am* 1968;6:467–492.
11. Roelke W, Smith AJ, Palacios IF. The technique and safety of transseptal left heart catheterization: the Massachusetts General Hospital experience with 1,279 procedures. *Cathet Cardiovasc Diagn* 1994;32:332–339.
12. Morgan JM, Gray HH, Gelder C, et al. Left heart catheterization by direct ventricular puncture: withstanding the test of time. *Cathet Cardiovasc Diagn* 1989;16:87–90.
13. Baraldi-Junkins C, Levin HR, Kasper EK, et al. Complications of endomyocardial biopsy in heart transplant patients. *J Heart Lung Transpl* 1993;12:63–67.
14. Fitchett DH, Forbes C, Guerraty J. Repeated endomyocardial biopsy causing coronary artery-right ventricular fistula after cardiac transplantation. *Am J Cardiol* 1988;62:829–831.
15. Fick A. Uber die Messung des Blutquantums in den Herzventriken. *Phys-med Ges Wurzburg* July 9, 1870.
16. Dehmer GJ, Firth BG, Hillis LD. Oxygen consumption in adult patients during cardiac catheterization. *Clin Cardiol* 1982;5:436–440.
17. Kendrick AH, West J, Papouchado M, et al. Direct Fick cardiac output: are assumed values of oxygen consumption acceptable? *Eur Heart J* 1988;9:337–342.
18. Lange RA, Dehmer GJ, Wells PJ, et al. Measurement of oxygen consumption and cardiac output: limitations of the metabolic rate meter. *Am J Cardiol* 1989;64:783–786.
19. Hillis LD, Firth BG, Winniford MD. Analysis of factors affecting the variability of Fick versus indicator dilution measurements of cardiac output. *Am J Cardiol* 1985;56:764–768.
20. Branthwaite MA, Bradley RD. Measurement of cardiac output by thermal dilution in man. *J Appl Physiol* 1968;24:434–438.
21. Forrester JS, Ganz W, Diamond G, et al. Thermodilution cardiac output determination with a single flow-directed catheter. *Am Heart J* 1972;83:306–311.
22. Cigarroa RG, Lange RA, Williams RH, et al. Underestimation of cardiac output by thermodilution in patients with tricuspid regurgitation. *Am J Med* 1989;86:417–420.
23. Hamilton WF, Moore JW, Kinsman JM, et al. Studies on the circulation. IV. Further analysis of the injection method, and of changes in hemodynamics under physiological and pathological conditions. *Am J Physiol* 1932;99:534–551.
24. Hillis LD, Firth BG, Winniford MD. Comparison of thermodilution and indocyanine green dye in low cardiac output or left-sided regurgitation. *Am J Cardiol* 1986;57:1201–1202.
25. Swan HJC, Ganz W, Forrester J, et al. Catheterization of the heart in man with use of a flow-directed balloon-tipped catheter. *N Engl J Med* 1970;283:447–451.
26. Lange RA, Moore DM, Cigarroa RG, et al. Use of pulmonary capillary wedge pressure to assess severity of mitral stenosis: is true left atrial pressure needed in this condition? *J Am Coll Cardiol* 1989;13:825–829.
27. Brogan WC, Lange RA, Hillis LD. Accuracy of various methods of measuring the transvalvular pressure gradient in aortic stenosis. *Am Heart J* 1992;123:948–953.
28. Snyder RW, Glamann DB, Lange RA, et al. Predictive value of prominent pulmonary arterial wedge *v* waves in assessing the presence and severity of mitral regurgitation. *Am J Cardiol* 1994;73:568–570.
29. Gorlin R, Gorlin SG. Hydraulic formula for calculation of the area of the stenotic mitral valve, other cardiac valves, and central circulatory shunts. I. *Am Heart J* 1951;41:1–29.
30. Boehrer JD, Lange RA, Willard JE, et al. Advantages and lim-

itations of methods to detect, localize, and quantitate intra-cardiac left-to-right shunting. *Am Heart J* 1992;124:448–455.

31. Dexter L, Haynes FW, Burwell CS, et al. Studies of congenital heart disease. II. The pressure and oxygen content of blood in the right auricle, right ventricle, and pulmonary artery in control patients, with observations on the oxygen saturation and source of pulmonary "capillary" blood. *J Clin Invest* 1947;26:554–560.

32. Hillis LD, Firth BG, Winniford MD. Variability of right-sided cardiac oxygen saturations in adults with and without left-to-right intracardiac shunting. *Am J Cardiol* 1986;58:129–132.

33. Carter SA, Bajec DF, Yannicelli E, et al. Estimation of left-to-right shunt from arterial dilution curves. *J Lab Clin Med* 1960;55:77–88.

34. Hillis LD, Winniford MD, Jackson JA, et al. Measurements of left-to-right intracardiac shunting in adults: oximetric versus indicator dilution techniques. *Cathet Cardiovasc Diagn* 1985;11:467–472.

35. Niggemann EH, Ma PTS, Sunnergren KP, et al. Detection of intracardiac left-to-right shunting in adults: a prospective analysis of the variability of the standard indocyanine green technique in patients without shunting. *Am J Cardiol* 1987;60:355–357.

36. Dodge HT, Sandler H. Baxley WA, et al. Usefulness and limitations of radiographic methods for determining left ventricular volume. *Am J Cardiol* 1966;18:10–24.

37. Kennedy JW, Trenholme SE, Kasser IS. Left ventricular volume and mass from single-plane cineangiocardiogram. A comparison of anteroposterior and right anterior oblique methods. *Am Heart J* 1970;80:343–352.

38. Hillis LD, Winniford MD, Dehmer GJ, et al. Left ventricular volumes by single-plane cineangiography: in vivo validation of the Kennedy regression equation. *Am J Cardiol* 1984;53:1159–1163.

39. Croft CH, Lipscomb K, Mathis K, et al. Limitations of qualitative angiographic grading in aortic or mitral regurgitation. *Am J Cardiol* 1984;53:1593–1598.

40. Sasahara AA, Stein M, Simon M, et al. Pulmonary angiography in the diagnosis of thromboembolic disease. *N Engl J Med* 1964;270:1075–1081.

41. Dalen JE, Brooks HL, Johnson LW, et al. Pulmonary angiography in acute pulmonary embolism: indications, techniques, and results in 367 patients. *Am Heart J* 1971;81:175–185.

42. Coles NA, Hibberd M, Russell M, et al. Potential impact of pulmonary artery catheter placement on short-term management decisions in the medical intensive care unit. *Am Heart J* 1993;126:815–819.

43. Shanes JG, Stein MA, Dierenfeldt BJ, et al. The value of routine right heart catheterization in patients undergoing coronary arteriography. *Am Heart J* 1987;113:1261–1263.

44. Connors AF, Speroff T, Dawson NV, et al. The effectiveness of right heart catheterization in the initial care of critically ill patients. *JAMA* 1996;276:889–897.

45. Dalen JA, Bone RC. Is it time to pull the pulmonary artery catheter? *JAMA* 1996;276:916–918.

46. American College of Cardiology/American Heart Association Ad Hoc Task Force on Cardiac Catheterization. ACC/AHA Guidelines for cardiac catheterization and cardiac catheterization laboratories. *J Am Coll Cardiol* 1991;18:1149–1182.

PERCUTANEOUS CORONARY INTERVENTION

BERNHARD MEIER

▼▼ ADDITIONAL ELECTRONIC TOPICS

Assistants n37;   Material n38;   Radiographic Equipment n39;   Monitoring Equipment n40;   Balloon Catheter n41;   Guiding Catheter n42;   Guidewire n43;   Accessories n44;   Technique n45;   Angiographic Indications n46;   Lesion Location and Morphology n47;   Need for Emergency Coronary Bypass Surgery n48;   Coronary Dissection n49;   Coronary Thrombosis n50;   Coronary Spasm n51;   No-(Re)Flow Phenomenon n52;   Elderly Patients n53;   Diabetic Patients n54;   Poor Left Ventricular Function n55;   Chronic Total Coronary Occlusion n56;   Single- and Multivessel Disease n57;   Proximal Left Anterior Descending Coronary Artery n58;   Left Main Stem n59;   Ostial, Small, Long Diffuse, or Calcified Lesions n60;   Comparison with Alternative Therapies n61;   Rehabilitation n62;   Economic Aspects n63

OVERVIEW

Percutaneous coronary intervention (PCI), traditionally known as *percutaneous transluminal coronary angioplasty* (PTCA), has emerged, predominantly as balloon angioplasty, in its first 20 years as the most common major medical intervention.

It is performed under local anesthesia, occasionally even as an outpatient procedure. For optimal performance, it requires state-of-the-art radiographic and dilatation equipment as well as a properly trained operator with an experienced crew.

It works best for single-vessel disease, but it may also be of great value for double-vessel disease and for selected triple-vessel disease, particularly in patients who are old, fragile, or have had prior coronary artery bypass grafting (CABG). It plays a dominant role in the treatment of acute myocardial infarction.

The major drawbacks are low success rates in old and long chronic total coronary occlusions, fatal outcomes in approximately 1%, acute ischemic complications in approximately 5%, and clinically significant restenosis within the first months in approximately 20% of cases. Its strong points are a greater than 90% success rate, the possibility for the patients to immediately return to a normal life, the repeatability of the procedure, and the paucity of complications after the first 24 hours or of recurrences after the first 6 months. Stents have proved to be an important complement to PCI. Although unequivocally required in less than one-half the lesions, routine stenting and even direct stenting are about to become the standard approach.

The current focus in related research is on technical advances in the crossing of chronic total coronary occlusions and on improved antiplatelet and antithrombin therapy to reduce acute occlusions. The restenosis problem, already ameliorated by stenting, is about to be further curbed by brachytherapy and drug-eluting stent coatings.

B. Meier: Cardiovascular Department, University Hospital, Bern, Switzerland

GLOSSARY

Ad hoc: Performed during diagnostic catheterization.
Culprit lesion: Lesion responsible for current event or predominant symptoms.
Fr: French, diameter unit for equipment, 1 Fr = 0.33 mm.
Guidewire: Wire over which to advance balloon catheter.
Guiding catheter: Catheter through which to introduce balloon catheter into coronary artery.
Monorail: Catheter type with side exit for guidewire in distal portion.

HISTORICAL PERSPECTIVE

Coronary balloon angioplasty is an offspring of transluminal angioplasty of peripheral arteries initiated by Dotter and Judkins in 1964 (1). Their method of dilating stenoses by successively introducing a coaxial double catheter with a diameter of 8 Fr (2.7 mm) and 12 Fr (3.7 mm), respectively, was crude. It required an access hole with a diameter equal to the target lumen. The surgically oriented care system for peripheral artery disease in the United States further impeded the development of the method. In Germany, angiology, an important subspecialty of internal medicine, provided fertile soil for such a technique.

Gruentzig had introduced the Dotter method at the University Hospital in Zurich in 1971, inspired by Zeitler from Germany. For several years, he experimented with different balloon types (2). In 1974, he performed the first balloon angioplasty in a peripheral artery using a form-constant polyvinyl chloride balloon in Zurich (3). In 1975, Gruentzig presented the double-lumen balloon catheter, which was introduced over a guidewire (4). In 1976, he presented a poster at the American Heart Association meeting in Miami demonstrating the feasibility of coronary balloon angioplasty in dogs. In 1977, the coronary dilatation balloon was used by Gruentzig in Zurich in a patient for the first time (5).

On March 22, 1976, in Zurich, a first PTCA attempt had been aborted by Gruentzig. It occurred as a last resort procedure in a patient with inoperable end-stage coronary artery disease and failed because the coronary ostium could not be engaged with the guiding catheter introduced through the arm because of iliac artery disease. On May 9, 1977, the first intraoperative balloon angioplasty procedure was performed in San Francisco jointly by Gruentzig, Myler, and Hanna, a cardiac surgeon. On September 16, 1977, in Zurich, a 38-year-old man with a single discrete stenosis of the left anterior descending coronary artery (LAD) became the first patient to undergo PTCA, or PCI as it is currently referred to (5). As the fellow in charge, I have followed the patient since. He has remained free of complications and recurrence for longer than 20 years, a living triumph of the method (6).

Primary success in the first 50 patients in Zurich was 64% without mortality. Emergency bypass operation was required in 14%, and infarction occurred in 6% (7,8).

In 1986, the Monorail principle (9) facilitated the use of guidewires (10). The shortened segment riding on the guidewire simplified exchanges over a standard length wire.

After the first clinical use of a coronary stent on March 28, 1986, by Puel in Toulouse (11), the pattern of PCI changed. The stent, first a rare and then a common ally of the balloon, matured to its Siamese twin, much in contrast to the balloon's many other short-lived companions and alternatives.

Twenty-four years after the birth of PCI, the method is thriving in spite of a tight medico-economic situation. With more than 1 million procedures performed yearly worldwide, it tops the list of major medical interventions.

In its first two decades, PCI has withstood the scrutiny of local and global peer review. It has been analyzed in numerous single-institution and multicenter registries. It has been subjected to a flurry of well-focused and meticulously monitored randomized studies. It has seen its indications expanded and then cropped again. It has turned out far from perfect but likable and extremely useful, just as Gruentzig had presaged.

MECHANISM

Dissection of intima and media, usually in thin areas of the plaque or adjacent to it, and dilatation of the vessel circumference (Fig. 80.1) constitute the key mechanisms for the luminal gain achieved by PCI (12–14). A stent prevents elastic recoil and keeps loose intimal flaps or plaque components out of the way. Reendothelialization commonly smoothes the rough surface within a few weeks. Yet, in unstented lesions together with constrictive remodeling (15), it may also cause restenosis.

PROCEDURE

Personnel

Primary Operator

Table 80.1 represents a reasonable compromise for a minimum curriculum to independence, considering the training facilities available and the general standard of practicing interventional cardiologists. For maintenance of skill, 50 to 75 cases per year are required. Such a low figure is only acceptable in case of a more active training period in the past and an experienced interventional environment (peers and team) as support.

Surgical Standby

A surgical standby under the same roof remains the ideal setting. However, coronary angioplasty without in-house surgery is a valid option to foster ad hoc procedures and to avoid waiting periods. The risk for myocardium and life

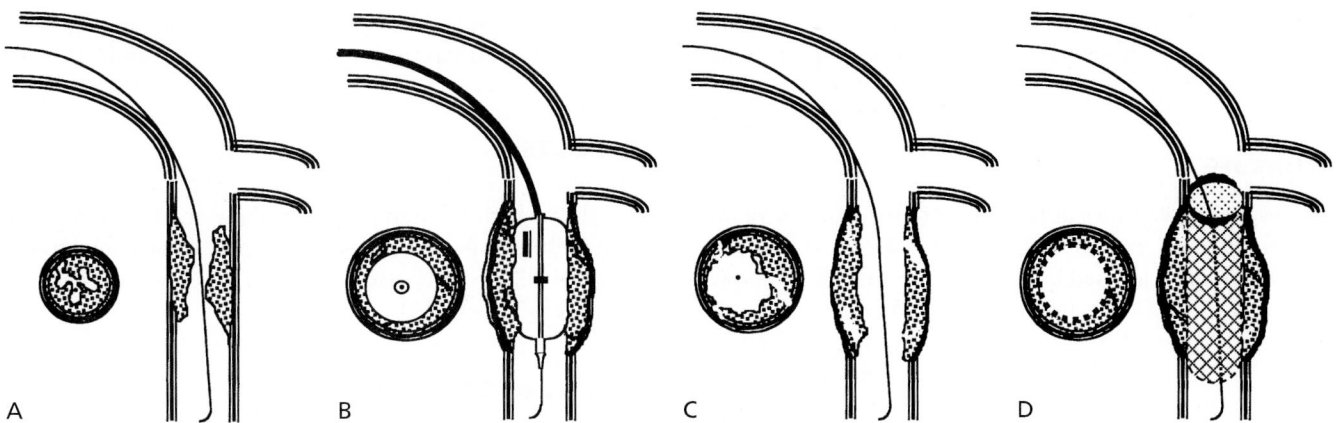

FIGURE 80.1 Schematic diagram of the primary mechanisms of balloon angioplasty and stenting. The initial gain in lumen derives from vessel dilatation and rearrangement of the noncompressible parts of the plaque made possible by an intimal dissection **(A–C)**. A stent avoids recoil and tacks flaps to the wall **(D)**.

during typical PCI procedures is low (Fig. 80.2), lower than the risk of cardiac events during an extended waiting period (16).

There are important precautions for PCI without in-house surgery. There should be no local legal objections, and the respective operators should be particularly well trained, the case selection adapted, the patient informed, and the institution fully equipped for advanced resuscitation and intensive care.

Adjunctive Drug Therapy

Platelet inhibitors have to be administered at the latest at the inception of the procedure. Acetylsalicylic acid is standard except for unequivocal allergy. Clopidogrel, a thienopyridine interfering with glycoprotein IIb/IIIa receptors by reducing adenosine diphosphate activation, is advocated in addition in case of stenting. Its role in plain balloon angioplasty remains to be examined.

Intravenous direct glycoprotein IIb/IIIa receptor blockers (abciximab, tirofiban, or eptifibatide) have proved efficacious in large trials (18–21). Abciximab reduces death

and myocardial infarction as well as the need for subsequent myocardial revascularization (*e*Fig. 80.2.1).

Heparin is part of the standard regimen. Doses employed vary without a clear-cut clinical difference between a bolus of 5,000 or 20,000 U (22). Low-molecular-weight heparin has not yet been tested in the setting of catheter interventions. Direct thrombin antagonists (hirudin, hirulog, and so forth) have yet to show clinical superiority to heparin worth their expense.

The original contrast medium diatrizoate (ionic, high osmolar) has been largely abandoned in favor of nonionic

TABLE 80.1 MINIMUM CURRICULUM OF INTERVENTIONAL CARDIOLOGISTS BEFORE INDEPENDENCE

General (internal) medicine (yr)	2
Clinical cardiology (yr)	3
Invasive cardiology (yr)	0.5
Diagnostic catheterization (cases)	
As assistant	50
As operator	100
Interventional cardiology (yr)	1
Therapeutic catheterization (percutaneous coronary intervention) (cases)	
As assistant	50
As operator	50
Practical courses	1

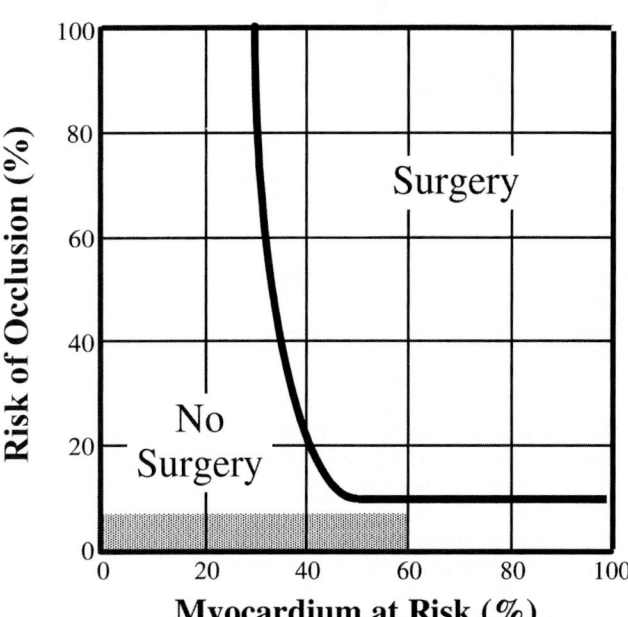

FIGURE 80.2 Chart to estimate the need for emergency bypass surgery at any stage of percutaneous coronary intervention. The hatched area encompasses the typical percutaneous coronary intervention indications and risks in the era of stents and glycoprotein IIb/IIIa antagonists. It lies outside of the area where (emergency) surgery appears beneficial.

agents for comfort reasons. Ioxaglate (ionic, low osmolar) is an alternative sharing an anticoagulant property with diatrizoate.

Aftercare

The level of surveillance after the procedure depends on the clinical situation and the result of PCI. ECG monitoring for a few hours is advised but not indispensable for the routine case (23). Any bleeding from the puncture site should be carefully assessed. Chest pain should prompt an immediate ECG for comparison with the baseline tracing. Patients with nonabating chest pain should be monitored for arrhythmia and reinvestigated by catheterization.

Hospital discharge of uncomplicated cases is usually the morning after the intervention. A control ECG before discharge should be standard, and cardiac enzymes should be checked in case of problems. The value of a stress test before discharge is controversial. It is safe but rarely performed.

INDICATIONS

The steady increase of yearly PCI cases was mainly due to an earlier invasive diagnosis of coronary artery disease in addition to a more aggressive attitude with elderly patients. The share of multivessel PCI did not increase over the 1990s in Europe (24) (eFig. 80.2.2) or Canada (25) despite stents. Many patients undergoing PCI today would have been treated medically a decade ago. Three-vessel disease of the major branches, however, has largely remained the domain of CABG.

Clinical Indications

Clinical indications and contraindications are listed in Table 80.2. They have to be customized to patients and situations, which requires experience. They are met by the

TABLE 80.2 CLINICAL INDICATIONS AND CONTRAINDICATIONS

Indications
  Acute myocardial infarction
  Angina (stable or unstable)
  Angina equivalent (arrhythmia, dyspnea, dizziness, and so forth)
  Objective signs of reversible ischemia
  Resting electrocardiogram
  Stress test
  Stress echocardiography
  Holter monitoring
  Scintigraphy
  Positron emission tomography
Contraindications
  Rapidly terminal cardiac or other disease (exception: uncontrollable angina)
  Prolonged cardiogenic shock after myocardial infarction

vast majority of patients undergoing coronary angiography. Age is not as important for PCI as it is for CABG.

RESULTS

Results of high-volume providers show an edge over those of occasional operators (34,35). Hence, the recommended volume of 200 yearly cases per center is being challenged by some as too small (35).

Impact of Stenting

Among the various mechanical additions or alternatives to balloon angioplasty, only the stent has stood the test of time (11,36). Stenting does not complicate the procedure, some difficulties in negotiating the stent notwithstanding (compared with a naked balloon, slightly stiffer). Stenting yields an immediate result that is appealing to the eyes of the operator and the patient.

The initial problems with stent thrombosis have largely been overcome with a two-pronged antiplatelet regimen (acetylsalicylic acid and a thienopyridine). However, subacute stent thrombosis remains a concern (37) (eFig. 80.2.3). The stent showed its real potential more where it was least expected, in the prevention of restenosis (38,39). Albeit highly effective in remedying impending occlusion due to obstructive dissection, routine stenting loses the advantage on balloon angioplasty over the first few weeks due to the occurrence of subacute thromboses virtually unknown to balloon angioplasty. Elective stenting has either the same or a higher (sub)acute event rate when compared with balloon angioplasty and provisional stenting. This holds true for all comers (38), diabetic patients (19), restenoses (40), small vessels (41), long lesions (42), chronic occlusions (43), LAD stenoses (44), saphenous vein grafts (45), unstable angina, or acute infarctions (46).

The Optimal PTCA versus Primary Stenting-1 trial (47) appears to make clear that elective stenting, performed as direct stenting according to the Doppler Endpoint Balloon Angioplasty Trial Europe-II (39), is the way to go. Provisional (conditional) stenting seems to require intravascular ultrasound as a cumbersome and costly additional decisional tool to remain competitive (48). Yet the sole effect of elective stenting is that a reintervention is spared for every tenth stent implanted. Some of these reinterventions may be operator driven because a patient may be taken back for an additional intervention more readily if no stent had been implanted the first time, not to forget that an in-stent restenosis tends to be more intricate to treat than an unstented restenosis. The risk of acute occlusion in the first hours after balloon angioplasty is not really eliminated but rather deferred to the first days and weeks by stenting. Some of these stent problems fail to be brought to the attention of the operator. This makes them more dangerous, but, para-

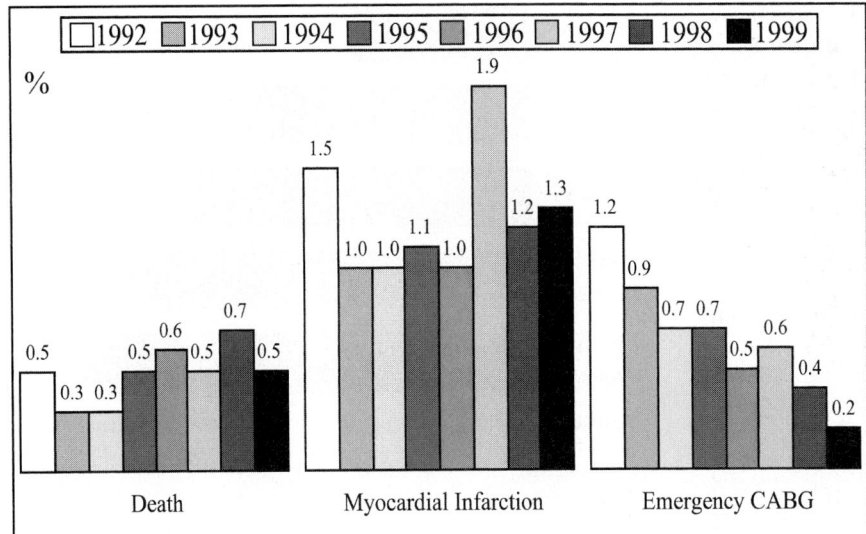

FIGURE 80.3 Evolution of adverse events in the European registry (some underreporting likely). Based on almost 500,000 percutaneous coronary intervention cases reported per year, there was no clear trend in terms of mortality or infarction rate since 1992 despite a marked increase of stenting. The reduction in need for emergency coronary artery bypass grafting (CABG) was a continuation of a trend that started 20 years ago. Yet there is an impact of stenting for the final reduction below 1%.

doxically, enhances the benefit of stenting as perceived by the operator.

The outcome of balloon angioplasty is reliably stable for decades if not for life after a few hours of risk for acute closure and a few months of risk for restenosis. Before stents were available, approximately 70% of dilated lesions never had an acute problem or a restenosis (perfect outcome impossible to improve on). Stenting all patients means ignoring the 70% of patients whose result can be jeopardized but not improved by a stent for the benefit of the 30% with potential for improvement. Admittedly, it is impossible to accurately predict to which group the dilated lesion of the patient will belong. Yet, experienced operators do have clues and apply them to the benefit of the patient. A stenting rate of 50% to 70% could well be the trademark of an accomplished and astute interventional cardiologist.

Complications

The threat of a major acute complication haunts the operator more than the possibility of recurrence but is talked about less.

Mortality

In-hospital mortality after PCI ranges from virtually naught in young patients with single-vessel disease (49) to approximately 70% in patients with cardiogenic shock after myocardial infarction (50). Overall, it lies below 2% (51) and has remained stable during the period of general adoption of stenting (Fig. 80.3) (24,25). Mortality reduction was achieved in randomized studies with PCI compared with fibrinolysis in acute infarction (52), with stenting in conjunction with abciximab (19), with abciximab in mixed PCI cases at 3

years (pooled studies), and with PCI rather than conservative treatment in unstable angina (53).

Myocardial Infarction

The incidence of PCI-induced myocardial infarction varies widely according to definitions used. Yet it has remained fairly stable over time (Fig. 80.3) (24,25). It is estimated that approximately 8% of patients show a creatine kinase release of greater than three times the upper limit of normal after PCI (54). This alone may be relevant to long-term outcome (54,55) [e.g., by doubling cardiac mortality from 5% to 10% over 1 year (56) and from 10% to 20% over 5 to 10 years (54,57)]. ✸ n64

Coronary Perforation or Rupture

Coronary perforation at the site of the lesion with a guidewire may not be rare, especially during recanalization attempts of chronic total occlusions. It is innocuous unless the perforation is enlarged by the balloon catheter. Distal perforations with hydrophilic guidewires represent a new hazard. They occur silently and perhaps multiply while balloons or stents are being introduced with the operator ignoring the wire tip (often outside the visible frame). They have a reduced tendency to seal spontaneously because the walls of normal peripheral vessels are thin.

Low blood pressure in the wake of a PCI involving a hydrophilic guidewire evokes suspicion of tamponade.

Coronary rupture by subintimal or oversized balloon inflation or debulking devices is a rare but serious complication with a mortality of approximately 10% (66). Coronary ruptures can be acutely plugged with a balloon inflation. This may permanently cover the defect with a tissue flap and solve the problem. Implantation of a (covered) stent at the ruptured site or sacrifice of the vessel by embolization or exclusion (covered stent in main vessel at bifurcation) are further options short of surgery (67). Cardiac tamponade is always first treated by pericardiocentesis. The aspirated blood may be reinjected into a vein to avoid anemia.

Results with Special Indications

Unstable Angina

Unstable angina hints at the severity of the culprit lesion, but it does not necessarily inform about the extent of coronary artery disease.

PCI of the unstable plaque (fissured atheroma with partial thrombosis) engenders more acute occlusions than routine PCI. The stent and new antiaggregant or antithrombotic agents have improved on this (19,20,63). Pretreatment with abciximab (19) or eptifibatide (76) is recommended before stenting and the ideal time for PCI appears early (77). Postponing PCI carries the risk of an intercurrent infarction while increasing cost (53).

A preliminary risk assessment is recommended according to *e*Figure 80.3.5.

Acute Myocardial Infarction

Ongoing infarction is one of the most pressing and rewarding indications for PCI. Mortality is beneficially influenced when compared with fibrinolysis (52). Although coronary flow may be restored somewhat later with direct PCI than with fibrinolysis, particularly if the latter is aided by the dethrombotic effect of a glycoprotein IIb/IIIa antagonist (Fig. 80.4) (87–89), reperfusion is more complete and the underlying stenosis has simultaneously been taken care of (Fig. 80.5). PCI facilitated by a glycoprotein IIb/IIIa antagonist, a fibrinolytic agent, or both appears therefore as the ideal approach.

PCI for acute myocardial infarction [▼ n65] is an exception in many respects. It dictates an ad hoc procedure and, for most, imposes restriction to the culprit vessel in

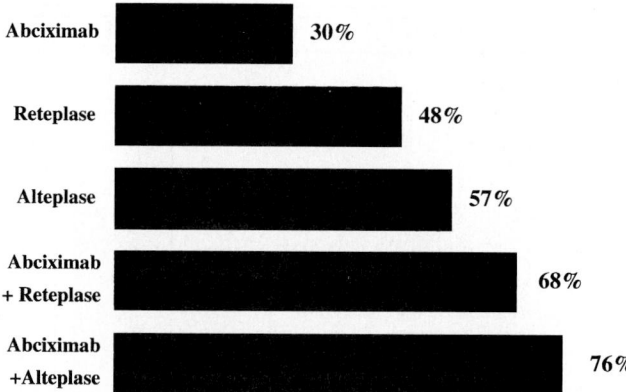

FIGURE 80.4 Flow restoration at 90 minutes by thrombolytic drugs for acute infarction. The combination of abciximab with reteplase (87,88) or alteplase (89) yields the highest patency rates.

multivessel disease. Although it carries a higher overall complication rate than elective PCI, it has a smaller potential to harm. The major complication of PCI, abrupt closure of the lesion, is relatively innocuous when starting with an occluded vessel.

There are data warranting stenting for all cases with PCI for infarction. Although acute results are not improved, reinterventions are reduced (Fig. 80.6) (46,90). However, the stent increases no-reflow problems and side branch occlusions. Both damage myocardium; a later restenosis does not. An experienced interventional cardiologist knows to select cases not to stent (good result with crisp flow after balloon dilatation). Direct stenting is not attractive, as the extent of the lesion cannot be anticipated in totally occluded arteries.

PCI for cardiogenic shock is warranted unless the shock is too advanced or too long-standing or the patient is old (50,91). In 2000, a percutaneous left ventricular assist device was introduced that may aid these patients as a bridge to recovery or transplantation.

PCI should be done acutely for myocardial infarction if it can be performed within the hour. Otherwise (or perhaps

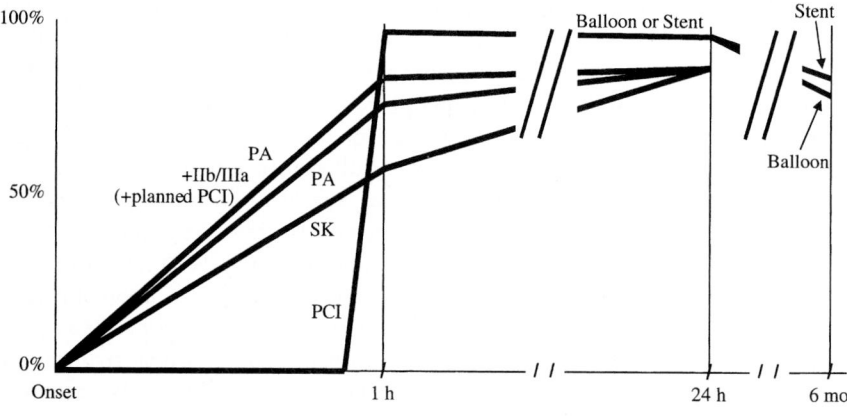

FIGURE 80.5 Percentage of normal coronary flow over time with primary percutaneous coronary intervention (PCI) or (facilitated) systemic fibrinolysis for treatment of acute myocardial infarction. The goal is to stay as high and as far to the left as possible. Up to 1 hour, the combination of a plasminogen activator (PA) with a glycoprotein IIb/IIIa antagonist (IIb/IIIa) is preferable to PA alone or to streptokinase (SK). Meanwhile, immediate percutaneous coronary intervention should be readied. The stent is clearly superior to the balloon only during follow-up that is depicted up to 6 months.

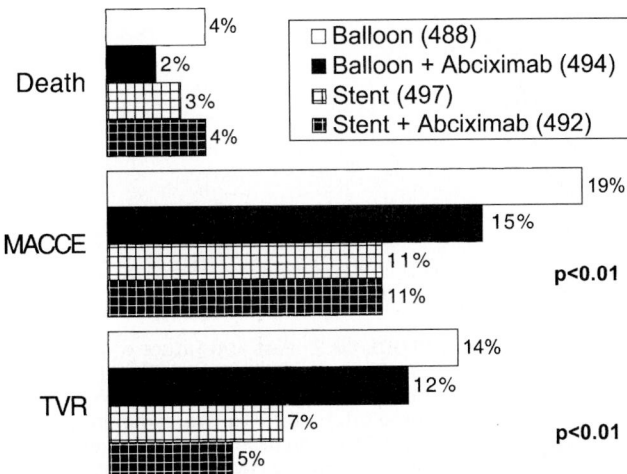

FIGURE 80.6 Randomized trial comparing balloon angioplasty for acute infarction to stenting with or without abciximab. At 6 months, there was an advantage of stenting over balloon angioplasty irrespective of the use of abciximab. It was significant only for target vessel revascularization (TVR) and remained so when major adverse cardiac and cerebral events (MACCE) were pooled. (From Stone GW. Stenting and IIb/IIIa receptor blockade in acute myocardial infarction: an introduction to the CADILLAC trial. *J Invasive Cardiol* 1998;10:36B–47B.)

in any case) modern fibrinolysis, preferably supported by a glycoprotein IIb/IIIa antagonist, should be initiated and PCI treatment appended if feasible. Only sizable infarctions (greater than or equal to three ECG leads with ST elevation) qualify for fibrinolysis or PCI.

CONTROVERSIES AND PERSONAL PERSPECTIVES

Several issues of PCI cannot be solved based on evidence and remain highly subjective and thus controversial. They have to be seen in the light of variable geographic, economic, temperamental, and philosophical backgrounds and are also subject to change as time goes by. It is difficult to deal with such topics in a way applicable to all situations, everywhere, and at any time.

The question of where PCI should be performed and by whom has been iteratively debated with high emotions. A high-volume operator working at a high-volume institution, backed up by a high-volume cardiac surgical program, is the ideal setting. However, this means that the population with coronary artery disease will have to converge at the few megacenters to receive PCI under scientifically optimal circumstances. Approximately one center for 2

million people will suffice. It will perform between 2,000 and 4,000 PCIs per year with five to ten primary operators. The operators will not be assisted by doctors because those would decrease quality while learning the trade, spread out, and dilute the high-volume scenario. Interventional cardiologists would be trained exclusively to replace retiring operators and to meet the growing demand for procedures.

But will the patients like that? Many of them prefer get the treatment at their local hospital by their familiar cardiologist. There, they find their way around. There, they know people and people come to visit. Most patients do not care so much about the theoretic variance in the quality of PCI. First, they are unable to grasp the subtle differences, and, second, most PCI results are good, anyhow, even with low-volume teams. Referring doctors like to deal with angioplasty operators they know personally, rather than sending their patients to an anonymous "superinstitution." Smaller communities can use the business involved, too. Concentration of the facilities to PCI "hubs" hurts their economy and keeps away investors and settlers.

When respected authorities, let alone governments, set regulations, they should honor these facts to a reasonable degree. It seems unwise to set limits that "outlaw" a substantial number of current operators. It is unlikely that they will abandon their practice, as that jeopardizes their professional existence. Nevertheless, guidelines should be clear regarding what is preferable, and reasonable minimal standards must be set.

Indications for PCI are another topic in which science and the "real world" diverge. Data show that the risk of coronary lesions is related to the extent of ischemia they produce. Scientifically, one could deduct that it is unethical to dilate lesions for which objective proof of ischemia or at least hemodynamic significance is lacking. Yet, this disregards patients with lesions that at the time of an "objectively unwarranted" PCI were not significant in terms of ischemia but that would have caused an infarction under conservative treatment while waiting for them to attain a hemodynamically significant degree.

Admittedly, it is currently impossible to predict these exceptions, but it is equally impossible to predict with accuracy which lesion will adhere to the rules. Moreover, it is customary in many centers around the globe to include the eventuality of an unanticipated spontaneous occlusion of the lesion when pondering a PCI indication. Imposing a different approach with costly assessment of the functional significance of the stenosis or the instability of the plaque is difficult to enforce and may not be to the benefit of the patients overall.

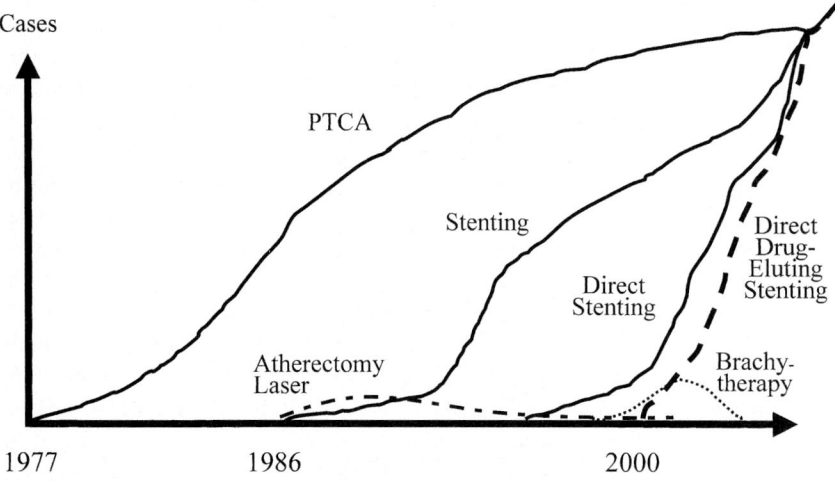

FIGURE 80.7 Past and future of percutaneous coronary intervention. The increase in cases may regain momentum once direct drug-eluting stenting has completely taken over. PTCA, percutaneous transluminal coronary angioplasty. (Modified from ideas of M. E. Bertrand and P. W. Serruys.)

THE FUTURE

PCI is currently one of the dominant assets of modern health care. It engenders abundant medical literature, occupies a significant segment of medical education programs, and is a remarkable economic factor. It produces gigantic costs but also tax revenue. It creates income, jobs, and career opportunities for countless people. It unequivocally benefits well-being and perhaps even longevity of the elder generations of industrialized countries.

Figure 80.7 reflects the past and the future of technical aspects. Stenting will be the rule before long. The approach will be direct stenting to save time and spare the predilatation balloon. The stents will be drug eluting, which will not complicate the procedure or the logistics. New gimmicks will come and go as before, but the balloon-mounted stent will reign.

The immediate future of balloon angioplasty is bright because coronary artery disease will remain the number one health problem of industrialized countries for quite some time and become increasingly prevalent in the rest of the world. It is bright because further improving technologies will expand the role of PCI for this disease, especially for its early, and perhaps for its very late, stage. The disease is increasingly discovered and documented at the early stage, and the general aging of the population creates a growing need for PCI at that end of the spectrum.

On the other hand, economic constraints increasingly frustrate those capable and willing to perform the procedure. Quality assurance activities take up more and more of the time of the interventional cardiologist. Finally, primary prevention will succeed in drastically reducing the need for PCI in middle age, stripping it of its coveted role as the most important intervention in modern medicine for people in their "best years." Then again, there is nothing wrong with this.

REFERENCES

1. Dotter CT, Judkins MP. Transluminal treatment of arteriosclerotic obstruction: description of a new technic and a preliminary report of its application. *Circulation* 1964;3:654–670.
2. King III SB. Angioplasty from bench to bedside to bench. *Circulation* 1996;93:1621–1629.
3. Grüntzig A, Hopff H. Perkutane Rekanalisation chronischer arterieller Verschlüsse mit einem neuen Dilatationskatheter. *Dtsch Med Wochenschr* 1974;99:2502–2505.
4. Grüntzig A. Die perkutane Rekanalisation chronischer arterieller Verschlüsse (Dotter–Prinzip) mit einem neuen doppellumigen Dilatationskatheter. *Fortschr Röntgenstr* 1976;124:80–86.
5. Hurst JW. The first coronary angioplasty as described by Andreas Gruentzig. *Am J Cardiol* 1986;57:185–186.
6. Meier B. The first patient to undergo coronary angioplasty—23-year follow-up. *N Engl J Med* 2001;344:144–145.
7. Grüntzig A. Transluminal dilatation of coronary-artery stenosis. *Lancet* 1978;1:263.
8. Grüntzig AR, Senning Å, Siegenthaler WE. Nonoperative dilatation of coronary-artery stenosis. Percutaneous transluminal coronary angioplasty. *N Engl J Med* 1979;301:61–68.

9. Finci L, Meier B, Roy P, et al. Clinical experience with the Monorail balloon catheter for coronary angioplasty. *Cathet Cardiovasc Diagn* 1988;14:206–212.

10. Gruentzig AR, Meier B. Current status of dilatation catheters and guiding systems. *Am J Cardiol* 1984;53:92C–93C.

11. Puel J, Joffre F, Rousseau H, et al. Endo-prothèses coronariennes auto-expansives dans la prévention des resténoses après angioplastie transluminale. *Arch Mal Coeur* 1987;8:1311–1312.

12. Block PC. Mechanism of transluminal angioplasty. *Am J Cardiol* 1984;53:69C–71C.

13. Waller BF. Crackers, brakers, stretchers, drillers, scrapers, shavers, burners, welders, and melters—the future treatment of atherosclerotic coronary artery disease? A clinical-morphologic assessment. *J Am Coll Cardiol* 1989;13:969–987.

14. Farb A, Virmani R, Atkinson JB, et al. Plaque morphology and pathologic changes in arteries from patients dying after coronary balloon angioplasty. *J Am Coll Cardiol* 1990;16:1421–1429.

15. Mintz GS, Popma JJ, Pichard AD. Arterial remodeling after coronary angioplasty: a serial intravascular ultrasound study. *Circulation* 1996;94:35–43.

16. Meier B. Surgical standby for percutaneous intervention. In: Topol E, ed. *Textbook of interventional cardiology*. Philadelphia: WB Saunders, 1998:466–474.

17. Meier B, Bonzel T, Heyndrickx G, et al. Recommendations for training and quality control in coronary angioplasty. *Eur Heart J* 1996;17:1477–1481.

18. The EPIC Investigators. Use of a monoclonal antibody directed against the platelet glycoprotein IIb/IIIa receptor in high-risk coronary angioplasty. *N Engl J Med* 1994;330:956–961.

19. Topol EJ, Mark DB, Lincoff AM, et al. Outcomes at 1 year and economic implications of platelet glycoprotein IIb/IIIa blockade in patients undergoing coronary stenting: results from a multicentre randomised trial. *Lancet* 1999;354:2019–2024.

20. Lincoff AM, Califf RM, Topol EJ. Platelet glycoprotein IIb/IIIa receptor blockade in coronary artery disease. *J Am Coll Cardiol* 2000;35:1103–1115.

21. Bhatt DL, Topol EJ. Current role of platelet glycoprotein IIb/IIIa inhibitors in acute coronary syndromes. *JAMA* 2000;284:1549–1558.

22. Vainer J, Fleisch M, Gunnes P, et al. Low-dose heparin for routine coronary angioplasty and stenting. *Am J Cardiol* 1996;78:964–966.

23. Li JM, Camenzind E, Meier B, et al. In-hospital monitoring after coronary angioplasty. *J Intervent Cardiol* 1994;7:229–235.

24. Maier W, Windecker S, Boersma E, et al. Evolution of percutaneous transluminal coronary angioplasty in Europe from 1992 to 1996. *Eur Heart J* 2001;22:1733–1740.

25. Rankin JM, Spinelli JJ, Carere RG, et al. Improved clinical outcome after widespread use of coronary-artery stenting in Canada. *N Engl J Med* 1999;341:1957–1965.

26. Faxon DP, Vogel R, W Y, and the NHLBI PTCA Registry Investigators. Value of visual versus central quantitative measurements of angiographic success after percutaneous

27. Di Mario C, Gil PR, De Feyter PJ, et al. Utilization of translesional hemodynamics: comparison of pressure and flow methods in stenosis assessment in patients with coronary artery disease. *Cathet Cardiovasc Diagn* 1996;38:189–201.

28. Pijls NHJ, De Bruyne B, Peels K, et al. Measurement of fractional flow reserve to assess the functional severity of coronary-artery stenoses. *N Engl J Med* 1996;334:1703–1708.

29. Emanuelsson H. Future challenges to coronary angioplasty: perspectives on intracoronary imaging and physiology. *J Intern Med* 1995;238:111–119.

30. Meier B, Ramamurthy S. Plaque sealing by coronary angioplasty. *Cathet Cardiovasc Diagn* 1995;36:295–297.

31. Weissberg PL, Clesham GJ, Bennett MR. Is vascular smooth muscle cell proliferation beneficial? *Lancet* 1996;347:305–307.

32. Kern MJ, Meier B. Evaluation of the culprit plaque and physiological significance of coronary atherosclerotic narrowings. *Circulation* 2001;103:3142–3149.

33. Bittl JA. Advances in coronary angioplasty. *N Engl J Med* 1996;335:1290–1302.

34. Jollis JG, Peterson ED, DeLong ER, et al. The relation between the volume of coronary angioplasty procedures at hospitals treating Medicare beneficiaries and short-term mortality. *N Engl J Med* 1994;331:1625–1629.

35. Kimmel SE, Berlin JA, Laskey WK. The relationship between coronary angioplasty procedure volume and major complications. *JAMA* 1995;274:1137–1142.

36. Meier B. New devices for coronary angioplasty: the emperor's new clothes revisited. *Am J Med* 1995;98:429–431.

37. Urban P, Macaya C, Rupprecht HJ, et al. Randomized evaluation of anticoagulation versus antiplatelet therapy after coronary stent implantation in high-risk patients: the multicenter aspirin and ticlopidine trial after intracoronary stenting (MATTIS). *Circulation* 1998;98:2126–2132.

38. Serruys PW, van Hout B, Bonnier H, et al. Randomised comparison of implantation of heparin-coated stents with balloon angioplasty in selected patients with coronary artery disease (Benestent II). *Lancet* 1998;352:673–681.

39. Serruys PW, de Bruyne B, Carlier S, et al. Randomized comparison of primary stenting and provisional balloon angioplasty guided by flow velocity measurement. *Circulation* 2000;102:2930–2937.

40. Erbel R, Haude M, Hopp HW, et al. Coronary-artery stenting compared with balloon angioplasty for restenosis after initial balloon angioplasty. *N Engl J Med* 1998;339:1672–1678.

41. Kastrati A, Schomig A, Dirschinger J, et al. A randomized trial comparing stenting with balloon angioplasty in small vessels in patients with symptomatic coronary artery disease. *Circulation* 2000;102:2593–2598.

42. Advance Trial. 2001 (*submitted*).

43. Buller CE, Dzavik V, Carere RG, et al. Primary stenting versus balloon angioplasty in occluded coronary arteries: the Total Occlusion Study of Canada (TOSCA). *Circulation* 1999;100:236–242.

44. Versaci F, Gaspardone A, Tomai F, et al. A comparison of coronary-artery stenting with angioplasty for isolated

stenosis of the proximal left anterior descending coronary artery. *N Engl J Med* 1997;336:817–822.

45. Savage MP, Douglas JS, Fischman DL, et al. Stent placement compared with balloon angioplasty for obstructed coronary bypass grafts. Saphenous Vein De Novo Trial Investigators. *N Engl J Med* 1997;337:740–747.

46. Mattos LA, Grines CL, Cox D, et al. A comparative analysis of primary stenting and optimal balloon coronary angioplasty in acute myocardial infarction. Six month results from the STENT PAMI trial. *Arq Bras Cardiol* 2000;75:508–514.

47. Weaver WD, Reisman MA, Griffin JJ, et al. Optimum percutaneous transluminal coronary angioplasty compared with routine stent strategy trial (OPUS-1): a randomised trial. *Lancet* 2000;355:2199–2203.

48. Di Mario C, Moses JW, Anderson TJ, et al. Randomized comparison of elective stent implantation and coronary balloon angioplasty guided by online quantitative angiography and intracoronary doppler. *Circulation* 2000;102:2938–2944.

49. Mehan VK, Urban P, Dorsaz PA, et al. Coronary angioplasty in the young: procedural results and late outcome. *J Invas Cardiol* 1994;6:202–208.

50. Urban P, Stauffer JC, Bleed D, et al. A randomized evaluation of early revascularization to treat shock complicating acute myocardial infarction. The (Swiss) Multicenter Trial of Angioplasty for Shock-(S)MASH. *Eur Heart J* 1999;20:1030–1038.

51. Williams DO, Holubkov R, Yeh W, et al. Percutaneous coronary intervention in the current era compared with 1985–1986: the National Heart, Lung, and Blood Institute registries. *Circulation* 2000;102:2945–2951.

52. The Global Use of Strategies to Open Occluded Coronary Arteries in Acute Coronary Syndromes (GUSTO IIb) Angioplasty Substudy Investigators. A clinical trial comparing primary coronary angioplasty with tissue plasminogen activator for acute myocardial infarction. The Global Use of Strategies to Open Occluded Coronary Arteries in Acute Coronary Syndromes (GUSTO IIb) Angioplasty Substudy Investigators. *N Engl J Med* 1997;336:1621–1628.

53. Wallentin L, Lagerqvist B, Husted S, et al. Outcome at 1 year after an invasive compared with a non-invasive strategy in unstable coronary-artery disease: the FRISC II invasive randomised trial. FRISC II Investigators. Fast Revascularisation during Instability in Coronary artery disease. *Lancet* 2000;356:9–16.

54. Abdelmeguid AE, Topol EJ. The myth of the myocardial "infarctlet" during percutaneous coronary revascularization procedures. *Circulation* 1996;94:3369–3375.

55. Danchin N, Abdelmeguid AE, Topol EJ. Significance of CK values after coronary angioplasty. *Circulation* 1996;93:397–398.

56. Waksman R, Ghazzal ZM, Baim DS, et al. Myocardial infarction as a complication of new interventional devices. *Am J Cardiol* 1996;78:751–756.

57. Abdelmeguid AE, Topol EJ, Whitlow PL, et al. Significance of mild transient release of creatine kinase-MB fraction after percutaneous coronary interventions. *Circulation* 1996;94:1528–1536.

58. Meier B, Gruentzig AR, King SB, et al. Risk of side branch occlusion during coronary angioplasty. *Am J Cardiol* 1984;53:10–14.

59. Aliabadi D, Tilli FV, Bowers TR, et al. Incidence and angiographic predictors of side branch occlusion following high-pressure intracoronary stenting. *Am J Cardiol* 1997;80:994–997.

60. Delacrétaz E, Meier B. Use of coronary angioplasty, bypass surgery, and conservative therapy for treatment of coronary artery disease over the past decade. *Eur Heart J* 1998;19:1042–1046.

61. De Feyter PJ, Van den Brand M, Jaarman G, et al. Acute coronary artery occlusion during and after percutaneous transluminal coronary angioplasty. Frequency, prediction, clinical course, management, and follow-up. *Circulation* 1991;83:927–936.

62. Neuhaus KL, Zeymer U. Prevention and management of thrombotic complications during coronary interventions. Combination therapy with antithrombins, antiplatelets, and/or thrombolytics: risks and benefits. *Eur Heart J* 1995;16:63–67.

63. Topol EJ. Novel antithrombotic approaches to coronary artery disease. *Am J Cardiol* 1995;75:27B–33B.

64. Simoons ML, Deckers JW. New directions in anticoagulant and antiplatelet treatment. *Br Heart J* 1995;74:337–340.

65. Baim DS, Carrozza JP Jr. Understanding the no-reflow problem. *Cathet Cardiovasc Diagn* 1996;39:7–8.

66. Ajluni SC, Glazier S, Blankenship L, et al. Perforations after percutaneous coronary interventions: clinical, angiographic, and therapeutic observations. *Cathet Cardiovasc Diagn* 1994;32:206–212.

67. Dorros G, Jain A, Kumar K, et al. Management of coronary artery rupture: covered stent or microcoil embolization. *Cathet Cardiovasc Diagn* 1995;36:148–155.

68. Simons LA. Epidemiologic considerations in cardiovascular diseases in the elderly: international comparisons and trends. *Am J Cardiol* 1989;63:5H–8H.

69. O'Keefe JH Jr, Sutton MB, McCallister BD, et al. Coronary angioplasty versus bypass surgery in patients greater than 70 years old matched for ventricular function. *J Am Coll Cardiol* 1994;24:425–430.

70. Kip KE, Faxon DP, Detre KM, et al. Coronary angioplasty in diabetic patients: the National Heart, Lung, and Blood Institute Percutaneous Transluminal Coronary Angioplasty Registry. *Circulation* 1996;94:1818–1825.

71. Detre KM, Guo P, Holubkov R, et al. Coronary revascularization in diabetic patients: a comparison of the randomized and observational components of the Bypass Angioplasty Revascularization Investigation (BARI). *Circulation* 1999;99:633–640.

72. The BARI Investigators. Seven-year outcome in the Bypass Angioplasty Revascularization Investigation (BARI) by treatment and diabetic status. *J Am Coll Cardiol* 2000;35:1122–1129.

73. Weintraub WS, Stein B, Kosinski A, et al. Outcome of coronary bypass surgery versus coronary angioplasty in diabetic patients with multivessel coronary artery disease. *J Am Coll Cardiol* 1998;31:10–19.

74. Goldberg S, Savage MP, Fischman DL. The interventional cardiologist and the diabetic patient. Have we pushed the

envelope too far or not far enough? *Circulation* 1996;94:1804–1806.

75. Aronson D, Bloomgarden Z, Rayfield EJ. Potential mechanisms promoting restenosis in diabetic patients. *J Am Coll Cardiol* 1996;27:528–535.

76. The ESPRIT Investigators. Enhanced suppression of the platelet IIb/IIIa receptor with Integrilin therapy. *Lancet* 2000;356:2037–2044.

77. Cannon CP, Weintraub WS, Demopoulos LA, et al. Comparison of early invasive and conservative strategies in patients with unstable coronary syndromes treated with the glycoprotein IIb/IIIa inhibitor tirofiban. *N Engl J Med* 2001;344:1879–1887.

78. Meyer J, Merx W, Schmitz H, et al. Percutaneous transluminal coronary angioplasty after intracoronary streptokinase in evolving acute myocardial infarction. *Circulation* 1982;66:905–913.

79. Serruys PW, Wijns W, Van den Brand M, et al. Is transluminal coronary angioplasty mandatory after successful thrombolysis? Quantitative coronary angiographic study. *Br Heart J* 1983;50:257–265.

80. O'Neill W, Timmis GC, Bourdillon PD, et al. A prospective randomized clinical trial of intracoronary streptokinase versus coronary angioplasty for acute myocardial infarction. *N Engl J Med* 1986;314:812–818.

81. Simoons ML, Arnold AER, Betriu A, et al. Thrombolysis with rt-PA in acute myocardial infarction: no beneficial effects of immediate PTCA. *Lancet* 1988;1:197–203.

82. Topol EJ, Califf RM, George BS, et al. A randomized trial of immediate versus delayed elective angioplasty after intravenous tissue plasminogen activator in acute myocardial infarction. *N Engl J Med* 1987;317:581–588.

83. Grines CL, Browne KF, Marco J, et al. A comparison of immediate angioplasty with thrombolytic therapy for acute myocardial infarction. *N Engl J Med* 1993;328:673–679.

84. Zijlstra F, de Boer MJ, Hoorntje JC, et al. A comparison of immediate coronary angioplasty with intravenous streptokinase in acute myocardial infarction. *N Engl J Med* 1993;328:680–684.

85. Gibbons RJ, Holmes DR, Reeder GS, et al. Immediate angioplasty compared with the administration of a thrombolytic agent followed by conservative treatment for myocardial infarction. *N Engl J Med* 1993;328:685–691.

86. Meier B. Balloon angioplasty for acute myocardial infarction. Was it buried alive? *Circulation* 1990;82:2243–2245.

87. Antman EM, Gibson CM, de Lemos JA, et al. Combination reperfusion therapy with abciximab and reduced dose reteplase: results from TIMI 14. *Eur Heart J* 2000;21:1944–1953.

88. Herrmann HC, Moliterno DJ, Ohman EM, et al. Facilitation of early percutaneous coronary intervention after reteplase with or without abciximab in acute myocardial infarction: results from the SPEED (GUSTO-4 Pilot) trial. *J Am Coll Cardiol* 2000;36:1489–1496.

89. Campbell KR, Ohman EM, Cantor W, et al. The use of glycoprotein IIb/IIIa inhibitor therapy in acute ST-segment elevation myocardial infarction: current practice and future trends. *Am J Cardiol* 2000;85:32C–38C.

90. Stone GW. Stenting and IIb/IIIa receptor blockade in acute myocardial infarction: an introduction to the CADILLAC trial. *J Invasive Cardiol* 1998;10:36B–47B.

91. Hochman JS, Sleeper LA, White HD, et al. One-year survival following early revascularization for cardiogenic shock. *JAMA* 2001;285:190–192.

92. Kern MJ, Aguirre F, Bach R, et al. Augmentation of coronary blood flow by intra-aortic balloon pumping in patients after coronary angioplasty. *Circulation* 1993;87:500–511.

93. Shawl FA, Quyyumi AA, Bajaj S, et al. Percutaneous cardiopulmonary bypass-supported coronary angioplasty in patients with unstable angina pectoris or myocardial infarction and left ventricular ejection fraction < or = 25%. *Am J Cardiol* 1996;77:14–19.

94. Delacrétaz E, Meier B. Therapeutic strategy with total coronary artery occlusions. *Am J Cardiol* 1997;79:185–187.

95. Puma JA, Sketch MH Jr, Tcheng JE, et al. Percutaneous revascularization of chronic coronary occlusions: an overview. *J Am Coll Cardiol* 1995;26:1–11.

96. Moles VP, Meier B, Urban P, et al. Instantaneous recruitment of reversed coronary collaterals that had been dormant for six years. *Cathet Cardiovasc Diagn* 1992;26:148–151.

97. Danchin N, Angioï M, Cador R, et al. Effect of late percutaneous angioplastic recanalization of total coronary artery occlusion on left ventricular remodeling, ejection fraction, and regional wall motion. *Am J Cardiol* 1996;78:729–735.

98. Finci L, Meier B, Favre J, et al. Long-term results of successful and failed angioplasty for chronic total coronary arterial occlusion. *Am J Cardiol* 1990;66:660–662.

99. Ivanhoe RJ, Weintraub WS, Douglas JS Jr, et al. Percutaneous transluminal coronary angioplasty of chronic total occlusions: primary success, restenosis, and long-term clinical follow-up. *Circulation* 1992;85:106–115.

100. Bell MR, Berger PB, Bresnahan JF, et al. Initial and long-term outcome of 354 patients after coronary balloon angioplasty of total coronary artery occlusions. *Circulation* 1992;85:1003–1011.

101. Horie H, Takahashi M, Minai K, et al. Long-term beneficial effect of late reperfusion for acute anterior myocardial infarction with percutaneous transluminal coronary angioplasty. *Circulation* 1998;98:2377–2382.

102. Weintraub WS, King SB, III, Douglas JS Jr, et al. Percutaneous transluminal coronary angioplasty as a first revascularization procedure in single-, double- and triple-vessel coronary artery disease. *J Am Coll Cardiol* 1995;26:142–151.

103. Ten Berg JM, Gin MTJ, Ernst SMPG, et al. Ten-year follow-up of percutaneous transluminal coronary angioplasty for proximal left anterior coronary artery stenosis in 351 patients. *J Am Coll Cardiol* 1996;28:82–88.

104. Goy JJ, Eeckhout E, Burnand B, et al. Coronary angioplasty versus left internal mammary artery grafting for isolated proximal left anterior descending artery stenosis. *Lancet* 1994;343:1449–1453.

105. Goy JJ, Kaufmann U, Goy-Eggenberger D, et al. A prospective randomized trial comparing stenting to internal mammary artery grafting for proximal, isolated de novo left anterior coronary artery stenosis: the SIMA trial. Stenting vs Internal Mammary Artery. *Mayo Clin Proc* 2000;75:1116–1123.

106. Cremer JT, Wittwer T, Boning A, et al. Minimally invasive coronary artery revascularization on the beating heart. *Ann Thorac Surg* 2000;69:1787–1791.

107. O'Keefe JH Jr, Hartzler GO, Rutherford BD, et al. Left main coronary angioplasty: early and late results of 127 acute and elective procedures. *Am J Cardiol* 1989;64:144–147.

108. Miketic S, Carlsson J, Neuhaus KL, et al. Percutaneous transluminal coronary angioplasty of left main stenosis—results of the German PTCA registry. *Z Kardiol* 2000;89:508–512.

109. Briguori C, Nishida T, Adamian M, et al. Coronary stenting versus balloon angioplasty in small coronary artery with complex lesions. *Catheter Cardiovasc Intervent* 2000;50:390–397.

110. Park S, Lee CW, Hong M, et al. Randomized comparison of coronary stenting with optimal balloon angioplasty for treatment of lesions in small coronary arteries. *Eur Heart J* 2000;21:1785–1789.

111. Hueb WA, Bellotti G, Almeida De Oliveira S, et al. The medicine, angioplasty or surgery study (MASS): a prospective, randomized trial of medical therapy, balloon angioplasty or bypass surgery for single proximal left anterior descending artery stenoses. *J Am Coll Cardiol* 1995;26:1600–1605.

112. Hartigan PM, Giacomini JC, Folland ED, et al. Two- to three-year follow-up of patients with single-vessel coronary artery disease randomized to PTCA or medical therapy (results of a VA cooperative study). Veterans Affairs Cooperative Studies Program ACME Investigators. Angioplasty Compared to Medicine. *Am J Cardiol* 1998;82:1445–1450.

113. The RITA-2 (Randomised Intervention Treatment of Angina) trial participants. Coronary angioplasty versus medical therapy for angina. *Lancet* 1997;350:461–468.

114. Boden WE, O'Rourke RA, Crawford MH, et al. Outcomes in patients with acute non-Q-wave myocardial infarction randomly assigned to an invasive as compared with a conservative management strategy. Veterans Affairs non-Q-wave infarction strategies in hospital (VANQWISH) trial investigators. *N Engl J Med* 1998;338:1785–1792.

115. Pitt B, Waters D, Brown WV, et al. Aggressive lipid-lowering therapy compared with angioplasty in stable coronary artery disease. *N Engl J Med* 1999;341:70–76.

116. Bech GJ, De Bruyne B, Pijls NH, et al. Fractional flow reserve to determine the appropriateness of angioplasty in moderate coronary stenosis: a randomized trial. *Circulation* 2001;103:2928–2934.

117. RITA trial participants. Coronary angioplasty versus coronary artery bypass surgery: the Randomised Intervention Treatment of Angina (RITA) trial. *Lancet* 1993;341:573–580.

118. King III SB, Lembo NJ, Weintraub WS, et al. A randomized trial comparing coronary angioplasty with coronary bypass surgery. Emory Angioplasty versus Surgery Trial (EAST). *N Engl J Med* 1994;331:1044–1050.

119. CABRI Trial Participants. First-year results of CABRI (coronary angioplasty versus bypass revascularisation investigation). *Lancet* 1995;346:1179–1184.

120. Rodriguez A, Boullon F, Perez Balino N, et al. Argentine randomized trial of percutaneous transluminal coronary angioplasty versus coronary artery bypass surgery in multi-vessel disease (ERACI): in-hospital results and 1-year follow-up. *J Am Coll Cardiol* 1993;22:1060–1067.

121. Hamm CW, Reimers J, Ischinger T, et al. A randomized study of coronary angioplasty compared with bypass surgery in patients with symptomatic multivessel coronary disease. German Angioplasty Bypass Surgery Investigation (GABI). *N Engl J Med* 1994;331:1037–1043.

122. Serruys PW, Unger F, van Hout BA, et al. The ARTS study (Arterial Revascularization Therapies Study). *Semin Intervent Cardiol* 1999;4:209–219.

123. SOS Trial. 2001 (*submitted*).

124. Simoons ML. Myocardial revascularization—bypass surgery or angioplasty? *N Engl J Med* 1996;335:275–277.

125. Bhatt DL, Marso SP, Lincoff AM, et al. Abciximab reduces mortality in diabetics following percutaneous coronary intervention. *J Am Coll Cardiol* 2000;35:922–928.

126. Pocock SJ, Henderson RA, Seed P, et al. Quality of life, employment status, and anginal symptoms after coronary angioplasty or bypass surgery. 3-year follow-up in the Randomized Intervention Treatment of Angina (RITA) Trial. *Circulation* 1996;94:135–142.

127. Heidenreich PA, Chou TM, Amidon TM, et al. Impact of the operating physician on costs of percutaneous transluminal coronary angioplasty. *Am J Cardiol* 1996;77:1169–1173.

128. Nino CL, Freed M, Blankenship L, et al. Procedural cost of new interventional devices. *Am J Cardiol* 1994;74:1165–1166.

129. Lincoff AM, Mark DB, Tcheng JE, et al. Economic assessment of platelet glycoprotein IIb/IIIa receptor blockade with abciximab and low-dose heparin during percutaneous coronary revascularization: results from the EPILOG randomized trial. Evaluation in PTCA to improve long-term outcome with abciximab GP IIb/IIIa blockade. *Circulation* 2000;102:2923–2929.

130. Sculpher MJ, Seed P, Henderson RA, et al. Health service costs of coronary angioplasty and coronary artery bypass surgery: the Randomised Intervention Treatment of Angina (RITA) trial. *Lancet* 1994;344:927–930.

131. Rodriguez A, Mele E, Peyregne E, et al. Three-year follow-up of the Argentine randomized trial of percutaneous transluminal coronary angioplasty versus coronary artery bypass surgery in multivessel disease (ERACI). *J Am Coll Cardiol* 1996;27:1178–1184.

132. Weintraub WS, Mauldin PD, Becker E, et al. A comparison of the costs of and quality of life after coronary angioplasty or coronary surgery for multivessel coronary artery disease: results from the Emory Angioplasty Versus Surgery Trial (EAST). *Circulation* 1995;92:2831–2840.

133. Hlatky MA. Analysis of costs associated with CABG and PTCA. *Ann Thorac Surg* 1996;61:S30–S32.

134. Weintraub WS, Becker ER, Mauldin PD, et al. Costs of revascularization over eight years in the randomized and eligible patients in the Emory Angioplasty versus Surgery Trial (EAST). *Am J Cardiol* 2000;86:747–752.

135. Bull DA, Neumayer LA, Stringham JC, et al. Coronary artery bypass grafting with cardiopulmonary bypass versus off-pump cardiopulmonary bypass grafting: does eliminating the pump reduce morbidity and cost? *Ann Thorac Surg* 2001;71:170–173.

NEW TECHNIQUES IN INTERVENTIONAL CARDIOLOGY: RADIATION, EMBOLI PROTECTION, AND THERAPEUTIC ANGIOGENESIS

JUDAH WEINBERGER
A. MICHAEL LINCOFF
JEFFREY J. POPMA

▼▼ ADDITIONAL ELECTRONIC TOPICS

Stent-Based Beta Implants n66;   Emboli Protection: Pathophysiology n67;   Percutaneous Methods of Myocardial Revascularization: Other Methods n68

RADIATION

Studies of restenosis have identified at least four mechanisms that contribute to luminal narrowing. These include elastic recoil of the artery, local thrombus formation, neointimal formation, and vascular remodeling (1–5). The relative contribution of these processes in humans is variable, with poststent restenosis dominated by neointimal hyperplasia and postballoon angioplasty restenosis primarily attributable to elastic recoil and negative remodeling of the target arterial segment (4).

The reduction of neointimal proliferation has been the primary target of experimental and clinical restenosis efforts.

J. Weinberger: Department of Medicine, New York-Presbyterian Hospital, New York, New York
A. M. Lincoff: Experimental Interventional Laboratory; and Department of Cardiovascular Medicine, The Cleveland Clinic Foundation, Cleveland, Ohio
J. J. Popma: Cardiovascular Division, Brigham and Women's Hospital, Boston, Massachusetts

The predominant cell type in the neointima has a smooth muscle phenotype; however, a significant amount of extracellular matrix is elaborated to form the bulk of the neointimal mass. More recent studies have suggested probucol (6) and tranilast (7) may both reduce restenosis rates in certain settings, although each compound has significant limitations.

Attempts to minimize elastic recoil and remodeling using permanently deployed metallic stents have led to a decrease in restenosis rates in carefully controlled clinical trials (8,9). Even in these trials, however, the mass of neointimal tissue seen as a consequence of stent implantation is greater than the neointimal tissue seen in response to balloon angioplasty (10). Furthermore, stents are commonly used to treat lesions that deviate significantly from "ideal" lesions, as defined by these large studies. Multiple stents, newer stent designs, and intentional oversizing of stents are all associated with higher restenosis rates.

There is a long history of clinical use of ionizing radiation, both diagnostic and therapeutic. Fluoroscopic studies use x-rays in the 60- to 100-keV range; keloids, pterygia, cerebral arteriovenous malformations, heterotopic bone formation, and thyroid hyperplasia are all "benign" proliferative processes that are safely and successfully treated with ionizing radiation from external photon sources (gamma or x-rays) or systemic administration of a beta-emitting radioisotope (11). Radiation doses required to destroy function in mature nondividing cells are greater than doses required to stop the proliferative activity of dividing cells (12). Because the mass of neointima is thought to be generated by proliferating cells, therapeutic radiation treatments for prevention of restenosis have been initially studied in animal models.

Ionizing radiation, from x-rays, gamma rays, or beta particles, causes cell death at appropriate doses. Gamma radiation from an endovascular iridium-192 (^{192}I) source was first shown to inhibit intimal hyperplasia as a result of mechanical injury to the aorta of rabbits over 30 years ago (13). With the advent of clinical percutaneous revascularization several decades later, the use of ionizing radiation was extended to prevention of neointimal responses consequent to balloon-induced coronary injury using intravascular radiation sources (14–17). These observations were subsequently confirmed and extended by a number of groups, most notably in regard to the efficacy of beta sources of radiation in preventing experimental neointimal hyperplasia (18,19).

Clinical trials subsequently examined the effects of beta and gamma brachytherapy in treating patients with in-stent restenosis, as well as to prevent restenosis in percutaneous treatment of *de novo* coronary lesions. The initial studies suggested the expected magnitude of inhibition of subsequent restenosis events available using radiation. In addition, several surprising findings from the early rounds of clinical studies modified the technique and management of patients undergoing brachytherapy. Two important issues raised in these studies include an apparent prolonged susceptibility to stent thrombosis in patients undergoing new stent implantation at the time of brachytherapy, and the arterial response at the edges of the radiated field. This section reviews the basic science and the preclinical and clinical studies leading to release of this addition to the interventional armamentarium.

Characteristics of Radiation

The effects of a given activity (*e*Table 81.0.1) of a gamma or beta source on tissue vary dramatically. This difference stems from the differences in the dose of ionizing radiation absorbed from the energetic photons of gamma sources compared with the far more effective beta-mediated local energy absorption. Similar considerations account for differences in shielding requirements necessary for safe delivery of radiation.

Radiation dose is a measure of the amount of energy from a source of ionizing radiation deposited in a mass of a particular material. The dose of radiation absorbed by a tissue determines the biologic effect of that radiation. Dose depends on the type of radiation (e.g., beta, gamma, or neutrons), the amount of radiation, and properties of the absorbing material itself. Absorbed dose is measured in units of rad or gray, and effective and equivalent doses in rem or sievert (*e*Table 81.0.1). The relevant properties of isotopes currently in use or being studied are listed in *e*Table 81.0.2.

Biologic Considerations

Ionizing radiation may interact with individual cells via direct ionization of DNA or other critical molecules, or indirectly by ionizing water molecules to form free radicals, which themselves are freely diffusible and can damage chromosomal DNA or critical membrane sites.

In general, the radiation dose necessary to destroy the function of a differentiated cell, such as a smooth muscle cell or endothelial cell, is far greater than the dose of radiation necessary to prevent cell division. Most lethally irradiated cells die during the mitotic process (12). It is unclear what, if any, the relative contribution of apoptosis is to postirradiation cell death seen in the arterial wall.

In radiotherapy of parenchymal organs, injury to capillaries and arterioles of normal parenchyma accounts for the majority of delayed effects of radiation. Experimental studies of large arteries (greater than 100 μm in diameter) have revealed that these vessels are less sensitive to radiation than smaller caliber vessels. Rarely, arterial perforation may occur. Large veins appear to be even more resistant to radiation than corresponding size arteries (20). ❦ n69

Preclinical Studies

A number of approaches to delivery of radiation to an arterial segment in the hope of preventing luminal compromise by neointimal tissue have been studied in various animal models. Broadly, these approaches can be categorized as external radiation source therapies, endovascular radiation delivery from a removable source (termed *brachytherapy*), or stent-based permanent radioisotope-coated stents. Intravascular radiation sources minimize the volume of tissue irradiated compared with external sources and should minimize the late complications due to unintended collateral irradiation of surrounding tissues. ❦ n70

Late Effects

The administration of significant doses of therapeutic radiation has been associated with a vasculopathy, which affects vessels in the radiated region (40). In parenchymal organ radiation, the principal effect of radiation injury to blood vessels is at the level of the capillaries and arterioles. The effects on large arteries, such as the epicardial coronary arteries, analyzed in retrospective studies of patients who have received radiation for thoracic neoplasms, appear to be dose-related and inversely related to the age

TABLE 81.1 SELECTED BRACHYTHERAPY TRIALS

Trial (reference)	Patient population	Source	No. of Patients		Binary restenosis rate (%)
Gamma sources					
Venezuela (163)	Open label, *de novo* PTCA	^{192}Ir	21	—	27
SCRIPPS (41)	Single-center, double-blind restenosis	^{192}Ir	55	54	17
GAMMA-1 (44)	Multicenter, double-blind, in-stent restenosis	^{192}Ir	252	56.3	34.2
WRIST (164)	Single-center, double-blind, in-stent restenosis	^{192}Ir	130	60.7	22
GAMMA-2	Multicenter, high-dose, in-stent restenosis	^{192}Ir	125		33.7
Beta sources					
GENEVA (165)	Open label, *de novo* PTCA	^{90}Y	15	—	
BERT (166)	Open label, *de novo* PTCA	Sr/^{90}Y	23	—	15
PREVENT (48)	Open label, *de novo* PTCA/stent	^{32}P	80	50	22
BRIE	Open label, *de novo* PTCA	Sr/^{90}Y	150		
Verin et al. (167)	Multicenter, dose-finding, *de novo* PTCA	^{32}P	160	—	8.3
CURE (168)	Open label, native PTCA or stent	^{188}Re	47	—	21.2
BETA WRIST (43)	Registry, single-center, in-stent restenosis	^{90}Y	50	—	22
INHIBIT	Multicenter, double-blind, in-stent restenosis	^{32}P	320	52	26
START (45)	Multicenter, double-blind, in-stent restenosis	Sr/^{90}Y	476	45	28.8

^{192}Ir, iridium-192; ^{32}P, phosphorus-32; PTCA, percutaneous transluminal coronary angioplasty; Sr, strontium; ^{90}Y, yttrium-90.

of the patient at the time of irradiation (23). The earliest evidence of coronary disease appears 5 years after radiation. These data are derived from studies of patients who have received fractionated doses of radiation and have had the entire heart in the radiated field. The long-term effects of single-dose (as opposed to fractionated dose) radiation of the magnitude suggested by the animal trials are not known. It is clear, however, that the risk of late complication, such as myocardial infarction or pericarditis, is related to the volume of radiated tissue (12). The late risk of radiation to the arterial wall is thus minimized when the volume of treated tissue is small, as with treatment by endovascular sources.

Clinical Studies

In-Stent Restenosis

The clinical utility of brachytherapy has been best studied for patients with in-stent restenosis, although some data exist for treatment of *de novo* lesions following native coronary angioplasty or stent placement. Animal studies initially suggested a prominent antiproliferative effect in irradiated arterial segments. Because in-stent restenosis is primarily a problem related to neointimal proliferation, with minimal vascular recoil or remodeling, the greatest benefit from radiation was hypothesized to occur in this patient population. A number of significant double-blind clinical trials using gamma sources [Scripps Coronary Radiation to Inhibit Proliferation Post Stenting (SCRIPPS) (41,42), Washington Radiation for In-Stent Restenosis Trial (WRIST) (43), GAMMA-1 (44)] and a beta source [Sr-90 Treatment of Angiographic Restenosis Trial (START) (45) and Intimal Hyperplasia Inhibition with

Beta In-Stent Trial (INHIBIT)] have been reported to show striking efficacy in preventing restenosis for patients with established in-stent restenosis (Table 81.1). SCRIPPS 3-year follow-up, reported from the most recent SCRIPPS study (42), provides evidence for continued clinical benefit for at least 3 years (*e*Fig. 81.0.1).

The GAMMA-1 study represents the first large, placebo-controlled, multicenter study of gamma irradiation to treat in-stent restenosis with a maximum lesion length of 45 mm. The primary end point of this study, a composite of death, myocardial infarction, or the need for repeated revascularization of the target lesion during the 9-month follow-up, occurred in 43.8% of the placebo-treated patients compared with 28.2% of the radiated patients (*p* <.02). The entire benefit conferred by radiation was a diminished need to revascularize. This study underlined the problems of late stent thrombosis occurring when a stent was newly implanted in the freshly radiated arterial segment (*vide infra*). These late thrombotic events only occurred after discontinuation of either ticlopidine or clopidogrel antiplatelet therapy.

INHIBIT was a prospective, placebo-controlled, double-blind, multicenter study of 332 patients with in-stent restenosis and maximum lesion length of 47 mm, randomized to receive 20 Gy at 1 mm into the vessel wall, from a centered ^{32}P beta-emitting wire source at the time of percutaneous revascularization. The primary end point from which this study was powered was 9-month angiographic binary restenosis. There was a 33% reduction in the frequency of 9-month major adverse cardiac events (MACE), defined as death, Q-wave myocardial infarction, or target vessel revascularization, in the brachytherapy group (*p* <.037), due exclusively to a decrease in the rate of target vessel revascularization from 31% to 20%. There were three different antiplatelet regimens used during this trial, to minimize the concurrently appreciated risk of late thrombosis (*vide infra*).

Prolonged "Subacute" Thrombosis

Several concerns were raised by these and other early clinical trials. One predictable effect of intravascular radiation was impairment of the wound-healing response consequent to arterial injury. Indeed, intravascular ultrasound studies of coronary arteries that underwent balloon angioplasty had evidence of unhealed dissections at 6 months post–*de novo* balloon angioplasty (46). An important clinical correlate of the inhibition of the healing response is a prolongation of the course of the normal stent-healing process. Indeed, late (post–30 day) acute thromboses occurred in patients treated with brachytherapy plus either angioplasty or new stent implantation, when given standard 30-day ticlopidine/clopidogrel plus aspirin antithrombotic therapy (47). A pooled analysis of the gamma radiation trials—GAMMA-1, SCRIPPS, and WRIST—suggests a late thrombosis rate as high as 6%, particularly in patients in whom new stents were implanted in the radiated arterial segment. Preliminary evidence from trials using prolonged antiplatelet regimes (clopidogrel for greater than 3 months) suggests a marked reduction in this complication. However, it is notable that there are reports of late sudden stent thrombosis greater than 1 year after stent implantation (48), and alternative mechanisms, such as late positive vascular remodeling with stent dehiscence, may be responsible for these events.

Edge Effects

An additional problem noted first in studies of radioactive stent implants (34) (*e*Fig. 81.0.2) is increased frequency of the occurrence of restenosis at one or both edges of the radiated field. Initially thought to be limited to radioactive stents, these events have now been seen with nonradioactive stents and with edge effects seen with removable-source brachytherapy treatments. There is significant speculation as to the cause of these observations or if these findings are even radiation related. We initially demonstrated a proliferative effect of low-dose radiation together with balloon coronary injury in a porcine model (39). Careful analysis has suggested that these edge effects may represent a "geographic miss" of radiation with regard to the zone of instrumented coronary artery (49). Alternatively, plaque shifting may account for the appearance of "new" lesions at the edge of the instrumented segment (50). A multicenter dose-finding study using ^{90}Y, a beta emitter, in which compulsive attention was directed to minimizing geometric miss, reported both a low incidence of core angiography laboratory detection of this technical problem and a notable lack of edge effects (51), together with late loss index of only 0.04 in balloon-treated *de novo* lesions. Typical late-loss indices for balloon-treated arteries are 0.50 to 0.60, depending on the prevalence of diabetics in the study. This suggests that geographic miss and the consequent propensity for edge effects may be significantly abated with careful attention to registering adequate doses of radiation throughout the instrumented segment of the coronary artery. It is important to note that the instrumented segment of the vessel is almost always significantly larger than the initially defined target lesion.

De Novo Lesions

Evidence for efficacy of brachytherapy in *de novo* lesions is less compelling and rests on small open-label groups of patients. A large, international, multicenter, double-blind, placebo-controlled trial using Sr/^{90}Y beta sources together with angioplasty to treat *de novo* coronary stenoses (Beta-Cardiac Cath) is scheduled to be reported later in 2001. The future investigation of brachytherapy clearly lies in defining high-risk subsets, such as long lesions, small-caliber reference vessels, diabetics, or chronic occlusions, which might benefit from *de novo* brachytherapy at the time of initial revascularization.

Durability of Restenosis Benefit

Radiation biologists have noted that the expected durability of the restenosis inhibition effects engendered by radiation depends on the proliferative capacity of the residual cells capable of producing the restenotic mass. In fact, theoretical studies have suggested that at the doses used currently, a recurrence of restenosis might be expected to occur at approximately 3 years. There is still a relative paucity of data regarding the durability of the brachytherapy. It is noteworthy that even after 18 months after gamma radiation, Teirstein and colleagues (42) report continued MACE events in the radiated group. In the radioactive stent population, these stents appear to simply delay rather than permanently inhibit restenosis. The ultimate value of this therapy will depend on long-term outcome studies.

Beta versus Gamma Radiation Sources

Substantial differences in handling and dwell times are required for these two classes of sources. Based on physical considerations, beta sources are more easily shielded, deposit a greater fraction of their emitted energy locally, and provide less collateral dose to nontarget tissues than do gamma sources. Because the efficiency of beta energy deposition is greater than comparable gamma sources, the intraarterial dwell time for a brachytherapy treatment for beta sources is generally substantially shorter than for available gamma sources. Because of the steep slope of their energy fall-off curve, beta-emitting isotopes obligate larger luminal and endothelial cell doses than do beta sources. The majority of the large clinical studies to date has reported on the efficacy of ^{192}I, a gamma emitter. More recently, two multicenter studies using beta sources to treat in-stent restenosis [Sr-90 Treatment of Angiographic Restenosis Trial (Sr/^{90}Y) and INHIBIT (P32)], have been announced (Table 81.1). Both studies featured significant reduction of restenosis rates and clinical event rates. The disparity between the clinical evidence for the two sorts of systems appears to be narrowing; however, no direct head-to-head clinical trial has been performed.

Delivery Systems

Currently, three systems have European CE (Conformité Européene) marks, and two of these systems have received marketing approval in the United States by the Food and Drug Administration. The Cordis Checkmate System is based on a ribbon source containing encapsulated ^{192}I gamma sources delivered via a manually operated afterloader device, which deposits the sources in a dedicated, noncentered catheter. Additional shielding is placed around the patient during the dwell time, and typically all personnel leave the room to minimize exposure to the source. Typical dwell times are 15 to 30 minutes per site treated. A variety of source train lengths are available, minimizing the necessity for stepped application. The Novoste Beta-Cath Catheterization Laboratory System is based on small canisters containing Sr/^{90}Y, which are delivered hydraulically down a dedicated, noncentered catheter. A single source length is currently available, allowing treatment of a 20 mm long arterial segment. The Guidant Galileo System, available for routine clinical use only in Europe, is based on an 0.018-in. ^{32}P beta-emitting source wire that is delivered to a dedicated spiral perfusion balloon using an automated remote afterloader. The latter two systems have typical dwell times of less than 5 minutes per treatment site. In the United States, the only currently approved indication for coronary brachytherapy is for the treatment of in-stent restenosis. Treatment of an adjacent site in the artery to ensure adequate margins of therapy by moving the source to another site and a second brachytherapy treatment are not approved.

Controversies and Personal Perspectives

Coronary brachytherapy is at the early stages of clinical adoption as a significant treatment modality for in-stent restenosis. Significant improvements in intermediate-term clinical event rates and secondary restenosis rates have been demonstrated using a variety of radiation sources and radiation delivery systems. The role of brachytherapy for preventing restenosis when *de novo* lesions undergo percutaneous revascularization remains to be defined. It is likely that certain anatomic and clinical subgroups (e.g., long lesions, small-diameter vessels, diabetics, and possibly vein graft lesions) might benefit from primary brachytherapy treatment at the time of initial intervention. The duration of antiplatelet therapy remains a controversial question. The most feared complication of coronary brachytherapy is "delayed subacute thrombosis," which has occurred as late as 18 months after

treatment. Clarification of an optimal duration and regimen of antiplatelet therapy becomes even more critical as stents are implanted into newly radiated segments of coronary arteries. Finally, the utility of brachytherapy relative to newly evolving technologies, such as drug-eluting stents (55) and alternative energy therapies (e.g., sonotherapy), will be closely scrutinized in the ensuing several years.

EMBOLI PROTECTION

Microembolization has traditionally been regarded as a relatively infrequent contributor to the major complications of percutaneous arterial revascularization or coronary acute ischemic syndromes. Although limited autopsy series demonstrate embolization of plaque and thrombotic material into the microcirculation of some patients with unstable angina or myocardial infarction who die suddenly (56), it is occlusion of the epicardial vessel that has been thought to be the important culprit leading to myocardial ischemia and infarction. Similarly, angiographically apparent distal embolization during coronary balloon or device intervention is uncommonly observed (typically in less than 2% of cases) and is usually confined to procedures performed in degenerated bypass grafts or in the presence of intraluminal thrombus, suggesting that abrupt closure of the target epicardial coronary vessel is the most frequent cause of periprocedural myocardial necrosis. In the cerebrovascular and peripheral circulations, however, emboli play a more conspicuous role in the pathogenesis of spontaneous stroke and systemic arterial ischemic events. The availability of new imaging techniques that allow demonstration of microembolization in living patients, such as myocardial contrast echocardiography, transcranial Doppler, and magnetic resonance imaging, has enhanced our appreciation of the frequency and importance of microvascular obstruction in arterial disease states and revascularization procedures. With this understanding has come the recognition that some of the clinical benefit derived from pharmacologic agents intended to treat the epicardial atherosclerotic plaque may in fact be related to suppression of distal embolization. Most recently, devices have been specifically designed to protect the microvasculature from embolization during revascularization procedures.

Clinical Evidence

Microembolization may be a relatively frequent event among patients with acute coronary ischemic syndromes or after percutaneous coronary intervention. In a series of 32 patients dying within 3 weeks of undergoing balloon angioplasty or receiving thrombolytic therapy for acute myocardial infarction, thrombotic or atheromatous emboli were observed on autopsy in 26 (81%) (58). Without the pathologic confirmation afforded by postmortem examination, however, the occurrence of microembolization in clinical practice can only be inferred from surrogate measurements, and the frequency and consequences of this event are likely underappreciated.

"Reperfusion" therapy for acute ST-elevation myocardial infarction is directed at restoration of infarct vessel patency, based on the paradigm that recanalization of the epicardial artery translates into improved tissue-level perfusion. A dissociation may exist, however, between epicardial artery patency and the quality of myocardial reperfusion. In a pioneering study, Ito and associates (59) described 39 patients with anterior myocardial infarction in whom myocardial contrast echocardiography demonstrated absence of tissue-level reflow in 23%, despite restoration of infarct artery patency; patients without microcirculatory reflow had significantly less recovery of left ventricular function than those in whom myocardial perfusion had been achieved. Subsequent series using contrast echocardiography (60) or magnetic resonance imaging (61) confirmed the absence of microcirculatory reflow in 25% to 37% of patients following coronary recanalization, a finding that was correlated with larger infarct size, adverse remodeling, and more frequent cardiovascular complications. More recently, Gibson and colleagues have established an angiographic index of quality of myocardial reperfusion, demonstrating that mortality is lowest among patients with normalization of both epicardial artery and tissue-level blood flow following fibrinolytic therapy for acute myocardial infarction (62). Similarly, among patients undergoing primary angioplasty or stenting for acute infarction, inadequate myocardial reperfusion despite restoration of infarct vessel patency has been associated with substantially diminished mortality benefit (63). The dissociation between epicardial and microcirculatory reperfusion may in part explain why long-term mortality with primary stenting has tended to be higher than with balloon angioplasty, despite the consistent reduction in restenosis achieved with stents (64).

Embolization, visualized angiographically as a new filling defect or "cutoff" in a distal vessel, has been reported to complicate 1% to 2% of percutaneous coronary revascularization procedures. Additionally, however, "slow-reflow" or "no-reflow" phenomena may also occur in 6% or more of patients undergoing coronary intervention, characterized by profound reduction in epicardial antero-grade coronary flow without evidence of vessel dissection, thrombosis, or embolization (65,66). This angiographic observation likely represents diffuse embolization and obstruction of the distal microvasculature and appears to be most frequent with revascularization of saphenous vein grafts, during acute coronary syndromes, in the presence of coronary thrombus, or with ablative device technologies (66–68). Using sensitive techniques such as technetium-99m sestamibi scintigraphy, regional myocardial hypoperfusion has been observed in as many as 87% of patients undergoing rotational atherectomy (69). The no-reflow phenomenon has been consistently associated with an increased risk for periprocedural death or myocardial infarction (66,68).

Assessment of postprocedural myocardial enzyme release (creatine kinase MB fraction or troponin) provides further insight into the prevalence of microembolization during coronary revascularization. In published reports in which enzyme determinations were made according to a systematic schedule in all patients, postprocedural rates of myocardial infarction have typically been in the range of 8% to 12% (70–73). Yet only a minority of these enzyme elevations can be attributed to recognized complications during the angioplasty procedure, such as target vessel or side branch closure; consequently, reported infarction rates are only 2% to 5% in studies in which enzymes were measured only in patients suspected of having an event (74–77). Distal microembolization represents the likely cause of many of the "silent" or unsuspected myocardial infarctions following coronary intervention. These events are clinically important in that a number of studies have demonstrated that patients who experience myocardial infarctions during and after coronary intervention are at significantly greater risk for late cardiac death than those who do not (78–83).

Balloon angioplasty and stenting of extracranial carotid stenoses appear to provide long-term results similar to those of surgical endarterectomy with regard to patency and stroke prevention (84). An important potential limitation of this technique, however, is dislodgement and embolization of atherosclerotic and thrombotic fragments from the carotid plaque, which may be associated with transient or permanent neurologic sequelae. Embolic load during percutaneous carotid revascularization appears to be greater than with endarterectomy (85). Plaque fragments in experimental models range in size as large as 1 mm in greatest dimension, with evidence of neuronal ischemia following embolization to the brain of particles as small as 200 µm (86). During percutaneous carotid revascularization procedures in humans, embolization of particulate material can be documented by transcranial Doppler in virtually all patients, with the maximum number of emboli signals occurring during stent deployment and balloon inflation (87).

The most compelling evidence for the ubiquitous nature of arterial microembolization during percutaneous revascularization derives from the clinical experience using distal emboli protection devices (see Mechanical Approaches to Embolization, later in this chapter). Aspirated blood or filter contents from these devices demonstrate the presence of grossly visible or microscopic embolic material in the majority of cases following stenting of carotid arteries, saphenous vein grafts, and even native coronary vessels (88). Examination of retrieved debris reveals atherosclerotic, thrombotic, and calcific particles, ranging in size as large as 2 mm or more.

Pharmacologic Approaches to Embolization

Pharmacologic approaches to prevent or treat embolization have focused primarily on vasodilators or antithrombotic agents. Vasodilators are intended to enhance clearance of microparticulate debris from the vasculature or counteract the adverse effect of vasoconstrictive mediators released from upstream plaque. Antithrombotic agents are used to enhance endogenous dissolution of thrombotic emboli, as well as to prevent amplification of the cascade of platelet activation and thrombus formation in the microvasculature. Clinical results with potent antiplatelet agents appear to be particularly promising. ❧ n71

There are substantial data to suggest that part of the clinical benefit derived from intravenous platelet glycoprotein IIb/IIIa inhibitors may be through improvements in microvascular perfusion. Several randomized placebo-controlled trials have demonstrated unequivocally that administration of these agents during and after coronary intervention reduces the risk of death, myocardial infarction, or emergency repeat revascularization over 30 days by as much as 50% (93). The predominant adverse event prevented by this therapy is periprocedural myocardial infarction; as discussed previously, these infarctions are usually not associated with recognized complications in the epicardial artery but may often be due instead to microembolization. ❧ n72

The most compelling evidence for an effect of glycoprotein IIb/IIIa blockade on microembolization is derived from studies using imaging techniques or end points that directly assess the quality of myocardial perfusion. During rotational atherectomy, regional myocardial hypoperfusion representing diffuse microembolization was detected by Tc-99m sestamibi scintigraphy in only 33% versus 87% of patients who did or did not receive adjunctive abciximab, respectively (69). In an important mechanistic study, Neumann and colleagues randomized 200 patients with acute myocardial infarction to abciximab or conventional therapy during stenting. Despite restoration of normal epicardial artery flow by stenting in virtually all patients in both treatment groups, patients who had received abciximab had improved tissue-level perfusion as measured by Doppler peak flow velocity in the infarct-related artery or improvements in regional and global left ventricular function (97). Similarly, improvements in myocardial perfusion and coronary flow reserve have been observed during elective stenting with the glycoprotein IIb/IIIa antagonist eptifibatide (97a). Outside of the setting of percutaneous revascularization, abciximab appears to improve myocardial reperfusion during fibrinolytic therapy for acute myocardial infarction. Among a subgroup of patients who had achieved normal epicardial artery flow 90 minutes after administration of various combinations of tissue-type plasminogen activator

and abciximab in a dose-ranging study, treatment with abciximab plus half-dose tissue-type plasminogen activator was associated with a substantially higher rate of complete ST-segment resolution than was tissue-type plasminogen activator alone (69% vs. 44%, respectively, *p* = .0004) (98).

Mechanical Approaches to Embolization

In an initial feasibility report, no embolic events or ischemic complications occurred during stenting of degenerated saphenous vein grafts in 15 patients using the Guardwire Balloon Protection System (100) [❧ n73]. During the subsequent multicenter phase II registry experience of 106 patients treated for vein graft stenosis, the in-hospital MACE rate of 4.9% was approximately 70% lower than for historic controls. The efficacy of this device for saphenous vein graft interventions was convincingly demonstrated in a randomized controlled trial of 555 patients. The PercuSurge system was successfully deployed in 93% of cases; rates of in-hospital MACE were reduced from 17.3% to 8.8% (*p* = .001), myocardial infarction from 16.5% to 8.4%, and no-reflow from 8.0% to 3.4% (99a). Preliminary experience with this device during stenting of native coronary vessels for acute myocardial infarction produced similarly favorable results: Normal myocardial perfusion was achieved in 55% of patients, compared with only 19% to 28% of patients who had undergone stenting for acute infarction without emboli protection in previous trials (101). The Guardwire system has also been used successfully in several pilot studies of carotid stenting, with recovery of particulate material ranging in size from 50.0 μm to 1.6 mm. Approximately 5% of patients were intolerant of the occlusion balloon, however, developing transient neurologic symptoms immediately or at some point during the procedure. The number of embolic signals on transcranial Doppler was reduced by 65% to 80% as compared with unprotected carotid stenting, and rates of neurologic complications (stroke or transient ischemic attack) compared favorably with historic controls. ❧ n74

Controversies and Personal Perspectives

It remains unclear in which settings emboli protection will provide the most clinical benefit. It seems likely that there will be an unequivocal indication for these techniques in the setting of carotid artery stenting, in which the consequences of distal embolization to the brain can be most catastrophic. For myocardial revascularization, certain high-risk settings are also likely to mandate an antiembolic approach. Degenerated saphenous vein grafts or thrombotic native coronary lesions have proven to be particularly difficult problems from the standpoint of embolization during percutaneous revascularization, with only marginal progress achieved with a variety of ablative devices or pharmacologic therapies. For routine percutaneous revascularization of native coronary stenoses, however, the indications for antiembolic devices will be less straightforward. Certainly, embolic debris seems to be a ubiquitous consequence of coronary intervention, even in "simple" native lesions, but the magnitude of risk for clinical consequences from such embolization remains incompletely defined, particularly relative to the potential risk of complications associated with the antiemboli devices.

What is the best approach to antiembolic therapy? There are compelling clinical data that glycoprotein IIb/IIIa inhibitors are indicated in all patients undergoing coronary intervention, but will the availability of distal protection devices render pharmacologic therapy unnecessary in many cases? I suspect this will not be so, as potent antithrombotic agents also affect other mechanisms leading to periprocedural complications as well as provide sustained suppression of embolization after a protection device has been removed. Thus, a combination of both pharmacologic and mechanical approaches will likely prove most beneficial. Which type of device, occlusion versus filter, will be the most efficacious? Although occlusion balloons may capture smaller particles, I anticipate that filters will gain more widespread acceptance due to better patient tolerance and stenosis visualization.

THERAPEUTIC ANGIOGENESIS

Despite the advances in percutaneous and surgical revascularization methods, a limited number of patients have severe ischemia but are poor candidates for conventional revascularization (105). Few options are available for these patients using conventional approaches, and the disability resulting from severe limiting angina is substantial. One potential strategy for "no options" patients is creation of new blood vessel channels in the region of ischemia or therapeutic angiogenesis.

New blood vessel growth may occur as a result of vasculogenesis, arteriogenesis, or angiogenesis (106). Although vasculogenesis is the process responsible for the growth of new blood vessels during embryonic development, its role in the formation of new blood vessels in adults is not known (106). Arteriogenesis involves the formation of new blood vessels that have a fully developed tunica media and may be manifest by the development of new collateral branches in patients with peripheral vascular disease (106). Angiogenesis relates to the development of a new blood vessel that lack a tunica media, such as capillary formation in wound healing (106). It is highly likely that neorevascularization that will benefit patients with no options results from arteriogenesis, and to a lesser extent, angiogenesis. Although the precise stimuli for therapeutic angiogenesis is not known, it likely relates to the combination of chronic ischemia and inflammation

and propagation of a cascade of events that induce proliferative, chemotactic, and inflammatory factors (106).

Mechanical Approaches

Both surgical and percutaneous approaches have been used to improve regional blood flow to the ischemic myocardium by injuring the myocardium using laser energy, radiofrequency ablation, or direct myocardial injections. Each of these approaches has substantial differences with respect to the depth of myocardial injury, the laser–tissue interactions, the presence or absence of guidance, and the number of channels created. These differences may have a profound effect on the results of clinical studies in patients with refractory CAD.

Mechanism of Benefit

Three mechanisms of clinical benefit of transmyocardial revascularization (TMR) have been proposed. The first relates to the creation of channels within the myocardium to enhance blood flow into the ischemic area, although pathologic studies have demonstrated that these channels close soon after their creation (107–110). A second potential explanation relates to denervation of cardiac nerve fibers that cause angina (111,112). This mechanism may explain why some patients experience immediate relief after myocardial revascularization. The most likely mechanism of benefit of myocardial revascularization relates to the stimulation of neorevascularization that improves blood supply to the ischemic myocardium (113,114).

Surgical Transmyocardial Revascularization

TMR by the creation of transmural left ventricular conduits using CO_2 laser was first reported in 12 patients with refractory angina in 1988 (115). Since then, over 3,000 patients have been treated with TMR using the CO_2 laser (116,117) or holmium:yttrium-aluminum-garnet (YAG) laser (118,119). Registry series demonstrated a marked improvement in Canadian Cardiovascular Society (CCS) angina class in these patients (116–118) and late clinical benefits after TMR has been sustained up to 5 years. One series of 78 patients treated with the CO_2 laser reported a greater than two CCS class improvement in angina status in 68% of patients 5 years after the procedure, and 17% of patients had no angina (120). Some series have also demonstrated improvements in myocardial perfusion as assessed by thallium scintigraphy (121,122) and positron emission tomographic scanning (116). The effect on left ventricular function has been variable (123,124).

Early series of TMR were associated with 5% to 9% perioperative mortality (125); overall morbidity was also high, with a 19% incidence of myocardial infarction, 52% incidence of cardiac ischemia, and a 35% incidence of noncardiac morbidity (126). Patients with adequate myocardial supply to at least one region of the heart through a native coronary artery or patent bypass graft have markedly reduced perioperative mortality (127). Patients with severe, refractory unstable angina also have a high mortality (128). More recent mortality with appropriate patient selection of patients undergoing TMR ranges from 1% to 2% (128).

Four randomized trials have been performed in patients with refractory angina randomly assigned to TMR or continued medical therapy (117,118) (*e*Table 81.1.1). The first of these studies randomly assigned 200 patients with CCS class III or IV angina that was refractory to medical therapy to treatment with TMR with a CO_2 laser (Heart Laser, PLC Medical Systems, Franklin, MA) or to continued medical therapy (117). In patients assigned to TMR, transmural channels approximately 1 mm in diameter were created with a single pulse of the CO_2 laser (peak power, 850 W) through the left ventricle (117). One channel was created per square centimeter of myocardial surface, resulting in approximately 36 channels per patient (117). Angina had improved by at least two CCS classes in 72% of patients assigned to TMR compared with 13% in those assigned to medical therapy at 12-month follow-up (p <.001) (117). Myocardial perfusion improved by 20% in the TMR group but worsened by 27% in patients treated with conventional therapy (p = .002) (117). The perioperative mortality was 3% with TMR, but survival was not different in the two groups at follow-up (117).

The second randomized trial of TMR assigned 275 patients with CCS class IV angina that was not amenable to surgical or percutaneous revascularization to TMR or to continued medical therapy (118). TMR was performed using a 20-W pulsed holmium laser (Eclipse Surgical Technologies, Sunnyvale, CA). The laser was calibrated to deliver 6 to 8 W per pulse, and the energy was delivered at a rate of 5 pulses per second. Channels were placed every square centimeter, and an average of 39 channels was created per patient. An improvement in two CCS angina classes was found in 76% of patients receiving TMR compared with 32% of patients assigned to continued medical therapy at 1-year follow-up (p <.001) (118). Patients treated with TMR also had a higher rates of freedom from late cardiac events (54% compared with 31% in medically treated patients; p <.001) and cardiac-related hospitalization (61% vs. 33% in medically treated patients; p <.001) (118). Exercise tolerance and quality-of-life scores were also better in patients treated with TMR. The perioperative mortality was 5%. There were no differences in myocardial perfusion or overall survival in the two groups (118). Two additional randomized trials demonstrated similar findings (124,129).

In aggregate, these studies demonstrate a dramatic improvement in symptoms resulting from TMR in patients with medically refractory angina. In some cases, the improvement in symptoms was associated with documented improvements in myocardial perfusion in the regions treated with TMR. The high (1% to 9%) periprocedural mortality seen in some of these studies appears to be lower in those patients who have adequate myocardial perfusion through a

native coronary or arterial or venous conduit to one myocardial zone or in those patients with stable angina.

A limited number of studies has evaluated the incremental benefit of TMR performed in conjunction with conventional coronary artery bypass grafting (CABG) in patients with suboptimal surgical anatomy. Preliminary reports suggested that perioperative and late mortality and the need for postoperative left ventricular support were reduced using the combined approach (130,131). A synergistic angiogenic effect of TMR and administration of vascular endothelial growth factor (VEGF) was reported in one preclinical study (132). Whether this effect can also be demonstrated in patients with refractory CAD is the subject of ongoing study.

Percutaneous Methods of Myocardial Revascularization

Percutaneous approaches to myocardial revascularization have been developed, varying by the laser source, delivery catheter types, and use of guidance to direct placement of the laser channels (*e*Table 81.1.2). These methods are less invasive, can be performed from the femoral access, and have a lower periprocedural mortality than surgical approaches to myocardial revascularization. In contrast to the full-thickness myocardial channel produced with TMR, percutaneous myocardial revascularization results in partial-thickness myocardial channels, generally ranging from 3 to 5 mm in depth. Three percutaneous myocardial revascularization systems have been evaluated.

Percutaneous Transmyocardial Myocardial Revascularization

A fluoroscopically guided percutaneous system for myocardial revascularization was developed for use in patients with medically refractory angina. The percutaneous transmyocardial myocardial revascularization (PTMR) technique uses a 5- or 7-cm steerable PTMR catheter (Eclipse Surgical Technologies, Sunnyvale, CA) that is positioned in the left ventricular cavity (133). A SlimFlex laser fiber is introduced and advanced under fluoroscopy to the left ventricular apex, deflected to the myocardial region to undergo laser ablation (133). The laser delivers 3.5 W through the 1-mm-diameter optical fiber in a series of three sequential pulses. The laser channels were spaced 1 cm apart and an average of 15 to 20 channels were created per patients (133).

A pilot study reported clinical benefit in 27 patients treated with the fluoroscopically guided Eclipse holmium:YAG laser system; an average of 17 channels were formed for each patient (133). Mean CCS functional class fell from 3.6 to 0.6 by 30 days after the procedure (133). There were no procedure-related deaths, pericardial effusions, or perforations. A subsequent randomized trial compared the clinical outcomes of 335 patients with CCS class III or IV angina assigned to treatment with PTMR or continued medical therapy (134). An average of 19 channels were placed per patient in those assigned to PTMR. There was one death and five (3%) cases of cardiac tamponade. There was a significant (p = .001) improvement in angina status and exercise time in those patients treated with PTMR compared with medical therapy. An improvement in angina by two or more CCS classes was achieved in 35% of patients treated with PTMR compared with 15% in those treated with conventional medical therapy (133).

Percutaneous Myocardial Revascularization

Another holmium:YAG laser system has been developed as an alternative method of myocardial revascularization in patients with medically refractory disease. The percutaneous myocardial revascularization (PMR) system (Cardio-Genesis Corporation, Sunnyvale, CA) consists of a 9-Fr coaxial catheter system used to deliver an optical fiber coupled to a holmium:YAG laser (135). The optical fiber, capped with a 1.75-mm lens and four nitinol pedals 3 mm from the tip to prevent full-thickness advancement during laser stimulation, was advanced through the catheter until it made contact with the endocardial surface. Each laser channel was created with four laser pulses of 2 J, and the laser channels are separated by at least 1 cm.

A phase I pilot study reported improved clinical outcomes in 34 patients with severe CAD not amenable to revascularization treated with the fluoroscopically guided CardioGenesis holmium:YAG system (136). PMR was successfully performed in all cases (136). An average of 11 channels were created per patient, and there was one death early after PMR due to a myocardial infarction in an untreated region (136). There was a significant improvement in CCS angina class from 3.0 at baseline to 1-, 3-, and 6-month follow-up. Although there was also a significant increase in exercise time, there was no improvement in myocardial perfusion found to the regions treated with PMR (136).

The Potential Angina Class Improvement from Intramyocardial Channels Trial evaluated the effect of PMR compared with medical therapy in 221 patient with medically refractory angina. Exercise tolerance at 12 months had increased by a median of 89 seconds in patients treated with PTMR compared with 12.5 seconds in patients treated with medical therapy only (135). CCS angina class improved by two or more classes in 34.1% of patients treated with PTMR compared with 12.0% of those patients treated with medical therapy. Angina scores were similarly improved in patients who received PTMR.

Direct Myocardial Revascularization

A third system uses electromechanical mapping to localize the region of myocardium treated with the Biosense Webster Holmium:YAG laser system (137). The Biosense system uses a navigational control at the tip that uses magnetic field emitters and local sensors to determine the precise location of the position of the tip of the catheter. At the conclusion of the left ventricular mapping, an 8-Fr laser catheter is advanced into the left ventricle. The laser source is a pulsed holmium:YAG laser integrated with a 300-µm fiber (LaserStar, Biosense Webster, Diamond-Barr, CA). A single laser pulse (2 J per pulse) is fired perpendicular to the endocardial surface to create 0.5- to 1.0-mm-diameter channels to a depth of 3 to 5 mm. Between 10 and 25 laser pulses are created and successive laser channels are kept greater than 5 mm between successive laser ablation zones.

In a pilot series of 77 patients with chronically refractory angina, percutaneous direct myocardial revascularization (DMR) was performed using left ventricular electromechanical guidance, delivering approximately 26 channels per patient (137). Major cardiac events occurred in 2.6% of patients; one patient required a postprocedural pericardiocentesis. Exercise duration after DMR increased from 387 seconds at baseline to 454 seconds at 30 days to 479 seconds at 6 months' follow-up. CCS angina class decreased from 3.3 at baseline to 2.0 at 6 months' follow-up (137). There were no improvements in the treated zones with dual-isotope scintigraphy at 1 or 6 months after therapy (137).

The DMR in Regeneration of Endomyocardial Channels Trial (DIRECT) evaluated the effect of DMR in 298 "no options" patients with medically refractory angina randomized to receive high-dose DMW (20 to 25 channels per zone), low-dose DMR (10 to 15 channels per zone), or a sham procedure in which the laser was positioned but not fired (138). Patients remained blinded to treatment. MACE at 30 days were more common in patients treated with low-dose or high-dose DMR than placebo patients (p = .014). All patients improved their exercise duration, but there were no incremental benefits in patients treated with low-dose or high-dose DMR (138). The frequency of class III or IV angina was reduced from 100% to approximately 40% in all three groups. All other quality-of-life measurements showed similar improvements in all groups.

Growth Factor Administration

Although a number of potential angiogenic agents have been identified to enhance the natural process of collateral development, only two growth factors, fibroblastic growth factor (FGF) and VEGF, have been developed for clinical use in patients with refractory ischemia. These agents have been developed using both protein-based and gene-based strategies, administered by intravenous, intracoronary, intramyocardial, and intrapericardial delivery. Given the potential that therapeutic angiogenesis may stimulate vascular growth, it should not be used in patients with unstable angina or accelerated atherosclerosis, proliferative retinopathy, or suspected or confirmed malignancy.

Fibroblast Growth Factor

FGF is a member of a family of nine heparin-binding growth factors that stimulate cells of mesenchymal origin

(139). FGF promotes angiogenesis by exerting its action on the endothelial cells (140), and a number of experimental studies have demonstrated the angiogenic effect of FGF (141–143) (*e*Table 81.1.3).

Fibroblast Growth Factor-1

The first clinical use of FGF-1 was reported in 20 patients who underwent direct intramyocardial injection of FGF-1, 0.01 mg per kg, at the time of CABG in the region of the left internal mammary artery to the left anterior descending artery anastomosis (144). Repeat angiography performed 12 weeks later demonstrated a pronounced accumulation of contrast medium in the region of the anastomosis, suggesting new blood vessel growth in FGF-1–treated patients (144).

A subsequent phase I randomized, double-blinded, placebo-controlled study of 24 patients undergoing CABG evaluated the effect of direct intramyocardial administration of basic FGF (bFGF) (142). Patients were assigned to treatment with placebo or 10 or 100 µg bFGF delivered into ischemic myocardium via sustained-release heparin-alginate microcapsules (142). Stress nuclear perfusion imaging at baseline and 3 months after CABG showed a trend toward worsening of perfusion in the placebo group and a significant improvement in the 100-µg bFGF group ($p = .01$) (142).

Fibroblast Growth Factor-2

Intracoronary recombinant human fibroblast growth factor-2 (rhFGF-2; Chiron Corporation, South San Francisco, CA) was administered as a single 20-minute infusion in a phase I, open-label, dose-escalating study of 52 subjects with advanced CAD (145). A single dose of rhFGF-2 (0.33 to 48.0 µg per kg) was associated with a significant decrease in angina class, increase in exercise tolerance, and improvement in regional left ventricular function and perfusion by quantitative magnetic resonance imaging and radionuclide scintigraphy (145). Adverse effects included transient renal dysfunction and hypotension with higher dose infusions (145).

A subsequent phase II FGF-2 Initiating Revascularization Support Trial compared the efficacy of placebo and three doses (0.3, 3.0, or 30.0 µg per kg) of intracoronary administration of FGF-2 in 337 patients with severe CAD (146). After 3 months, the treatment group had an increase in exercise duration of 65 seconds compared with 45 seconds in placebo-treated patients (p = not significant). Patients older than 63 years showed a significant improvement in exercise duration associated with rhFGF-2 therapy. Although there were also no differences in quality-of-life measurement or CCS angina class, patients with the severest symptoms had the greatest improvement in angina as a result of therapy. At 180 days, exercise tolerance remained similar in placebo and treatment arms (147).

The Therapeutic Angiogenesis with FGF-2 for Intermittent Claudication Trial evaluated the safety and efficacy of intraarterial injection of FGF-2 in a randomized, placebo-controlled, dose-finding phase II study of patients with severe intermittent claudication (148,149). Patients were given placebo, a "single dose" of 30 µg per kg of FGF-2 by intraarterial infusion in both legs at day 1, or a "double bolus" of 30 µg per kg of FGF-2 by intraarterial infusion rFGF-2 in both legs at day 1 and day 30 (149). Single-dose FGF-2 resulted in a significant ($p = .026$) improvement in the primary end point, peak walking time at 90 days, although the change in peak walking time at 90 days was not different in patients receiving a double bolus compared with those receiving placebo. By 180 days, however, there were no differences among the groups, due to a large increase in peak walking time in the placebo group (148).

Recombinant Adenovirus 5 Fibroblast Growth Factor-4

Genetic delivery of angiogenic proteins may result in higher retention rates within the myocardium when given by intracoronary injection than protein infusions. The phase I/II, dose escalation Adenovirus Gene Therapy (AGENT) trial compared the safety and efficacy of an intracoronary infusion of recombinant adenovirus 5 FGF-4 (Ad5 FGF-4; Collateral Therapeutics, San Diego, CA) in 79 patients with class II or III angina (150). Patients were randomly assigned to placebo or to one of five escalating doses of Ad5 FGF-4 (ranging from 3.2×10^8 to 3.2×10^{10} viral particles) injected into the left or right coronary artery (150). Preliminary results reported that patients who received active therapy had a greater increase in exercise time than those receiving placebo (150), although there was a substantial improvement in placebo-treated patients. There were no adverse effects in patients during the Ad5 FGF-4 infusion. Although these results are encouraging, the sample size is small and larger studies are needed. A phase III pivotal efficacy trial is planned.

Vascular Endothelial Growth Factor

VEGF is an endothelial cell-specific mitogen that has been implicated as another potent angiogenic agent (151). Endothelial responses to VEGF include proliferation, production of proteases such as plasminogen activators and collagenases that promote capillary bed formation, and triggering migration of monocytes (151).

VEGF has been studied by numerous investigators in various *in vitro* and *in vivo* animal models (152,153). In addition to these favorable responses that promoted angiogenesis, VEGF has also been shown to be a mediator of proliferative retinopathy, age-related macular degeneration, rheumatoid arthritis, and in the formation of atherosclerotic plaque (151). VEGF has also been shown to promote the release of nitric oxide, resulting in clinical hypotension if given in high doses.

A recombinant human VEGF (rhVEGF) phase I clinical study of 14 patients who received an intracoronary infusion of low-dose rhVEGF (Genzyme, South San Francisco, CA)

(0.005 and 0.017 µg per kg) or high-dose rhVEGF (0.05 and 0.167 µg per kg) over 20 minutes demonstrated improved myocardial perfusion in a dose-dependent fashion (154) (*e*Table 81.1.4). The VEGF in Ischemia for Vascular Angiogenesis (VIVA) Trial, a phase II, double-blinded, placebo-controlled trial, randomly assigned 178 patients who were poor candidates for conventional revascularization to treatment with placebo, low-dose (17 µg per kg per min), or high-dose (50 µg per kg per min) intracoronary rhVEGF infusion over 20 minutes followed by a 4-hour intravenous rhVEGF infusion at 3, 6, and 9 days (155). All groups had a similar increase in exercise time, Canadian class angina, and quality of life at 60 days (155,156). At 120 days, the improvement in the placebo group became diminished and the high-dose infusion continued to improved, resulting in a significant improvement in CCS angina class ($p = .04$) and a trend toward improvement in exercise time ($p = .17$) in patients treated with high-dose rhVEGF compared with placebo. In a subset analysis of 107 patients who were followed for an additional 8 months, placebo-treated patients continued to worsen, whereas patients receiving high-dose rhVEGF continued to have significant improvement. The occurrence of 1-year death, myocardial infarction, revascularization, or cancer was lower in patients treated with high-dose rhVEGF (11.8%) compared with patients treated with placebo (31.6%) ($p < .04$) (156).

Naked Plasmid DNA Encoding the Vascular Endothelial Growth Factor–165 Gene

A phase I clinical trial demonstrated the safety of naked plasmid DNA encoding the VEGF-165 gene (Vascular Genetics, Research Triangle Park, NC) injected directly into the myocardium of patients via a minithoracotomy (157,158). Angina episodes requiring nitroglycerin therapy were reduced in most patients, and exercise tolerance improved significantly after gene transfer (158,159).

Using another approach, direct intramyocardial administration of the naked plasmid VEGF-165 was achieved using a specially designed delivery catheter that uses electromechanical mapping to localize the region of myocardial injection (160). In this series, 13 consecutive patients treated with a direct intramyocardial injection of VEGF-165 and single-photon sestamibi examinations were used to assess improvements in perfusion over a 60-day follow-up period (160). Partial or complete resolution of perfusion defects seen on the sestamibi scan were improved during the follow-up period. Improvements in the electromechanical mapping profiles were also noted.

Adenovirus Gene Transfer Vascular Endothelial Growth Factor 121.10

A phase I study used a gene-therapy strategy used an E1-E3-adenovirus (Ad) gene transfer vector expressing VEGF121 cDNA (Ad$_{GV}$VEGF121.10) (GenVec, Inc., Gaithersburg,

MD) to induce therapeutic angiogenesis in 21 patients with symptomatic CAD (161). Ad$_{GV}$VEGF121.10 was administered to 15 patients as an adjunct to CABG and to six patients as sole therapy via a minithoracotomy. There was no evidence of toxicity related to the administration of the agent or vector. All patients reported an improvement in their angina class, and patients who received Ad$_{GV}$VEGF121.10 as sole therapy reported an increase in exercise duration in most cases (161). These effects were sustained 6 months after the procedure (162).

Candidates for Therapeutic Angiogenesis

Patients who have no options for conventional revascularization may either have a single long-standing occlusion of a proximal vessel that subtends a large amount of myocardium or have undergone one or more prior CABG surgeries, with occlusion or stenoses saphenous vein grafts in association with native CAD that is poorly suited for conventional revascularization. It is estimated that patients with no options account for approximately 4% to 12% of those undergoing coronary arteriography (105). A larger percentage of patients (20% to 30%) have incomplete revascularization due to unsuitable coronary anatomy after conventional revascularization. These patients may also be amenable to alternative approaches targeted at increasing perfusion to ischemic tissues.

It is understandable that an aggressive approach to new blood vessel formation is needed in these patients, as these individuals are "resistant" to physiologic angiogenesis that results in extensive collateral formation in some patients with long-standing occlusion (106). Resistance to therapeutic angiogenesis may occur as a result of medications, with hypercholesterolemia, smoking, and diabetes, among other factors (106).

Because of the potential that therapeutic angiogenesis may be associated with some untoward effects, patients with cancer, diabetic retinopathy, unstable angina, or protein nephropathy have not been included in studies assessing the efficacy of angiogenesis (106).

Controversies and Personal Perspectives

Patients who have refractory angina but are poor candidates for revascularization still have few options for symptom relief. Although the use of systemic and local delivery of growth factors and surgical laser revascularization to promote angiogenesis remains an active area of investigation, the clinical results obtained with these therapies have been somewhat disappointing to date. Adjunct surgical TMR appears to be the best approach to the patient who undergoes CABG but has important residual ischemic zones, and isolated TMR may also benefit patients who require symptom relief from refractory ischemia in zones not amenable to revascularization. It appears that percutaneous approaches

THE FUTURE

The immediate future will see a refinement in the technology for distal protection devices, with improved flexibility, lower profiles, and reduced risk for vessel injury. The optimal device will be one that can be placed beyond distal lesions in tortuous vessels without interfering substantially with the interventional procedure itself. Clinical investigation will be directed at establishing the optimal clinical and anatomic indications for antiemboli devices, as well as critically assessing the potential complementarity between the pharmacologic and mechanical approaches.

Continued evolution of the molecular approaches to angiogenesis will likely be the next frontier for patients with refractory CAD and no options. The encouraging preliminary results of the AGENT trial require confirmation in a larger phase III trial that will measure clinical end points in a larger number of patients. Direct intramyocardial injection of growth factors using fluoroscopically or electromechanically guided injection systems may allow more precise delivery of protein-based and gene-based factors into the ischemic myocardium. It is likely that new imaging modalities, such as functional magnetic resonance imaging, may also provide a more sensitive index to assessing the therapeutic effect of angiogenesis.

---

may not provide a sufficient extent of injury to promote angiogenesis. The DIRECT trial also emphasized the importance of blinding of the treatment method to patients and their physicians, as the placebo effect may be a powerful stimulus for symptom relief in these patients. Early clinical trial results from intracoronary and intravenous protein and gene-based approaches to angiogenesis have also failed to identify a truly viable approach for the majority of patients with refractory ischemia, although more investigation is needed.

REFERENCES

1. Glagov S, Weisenberg E, Zarins CK, et al. Compensatory enlargement of human atherosclerotic coronary arteries. *N Engl J Med* 1987;316:1371–1375.
2. Libby P, Schwartz D, Brogi E, et al. A cascade model for restenosis. A special case of atherosclerosis progression. *Circulation* 1992;86:III47–III52.
3. Casscells W, Engler D, Willerson JT. Mechanisms of restenosis. *Tex Heart Inst J* 1994;21:68–77.
4. Mintz GS, Popma JJ, Pichard AD, et al. Arterial remodeling after coronary angioplasty: a serial intravascular ultrasound study. *Circulation* 1996;94:35–43.
5. Topol EJ, Califf RM, Weisman HF, et al. Randomised trial of coronary intervention with antibody against platelet IIb/IIIa integrin for reduction of clinical restenosis: results at six months. The EPIC Investigators. *Lancet* 1994;343:881–886.
6. Tardif J-C, Cote G, Lesperance J, et al. Probucol and multivitamins in the prevention of restenosis after coronary angioplasty. *N Engl J Med* 1997;337:365–372.
7. Tamai H, Katoh O, Suzuki S, et al. Impact of tranilast on restenosis after coronary angioplasty: tranilast restenosis following angioplasty trial (TREAT). *Am Heart J* 1999;138:968–975.
8. Fischman DL, Leon MB, Baim DS, et al. A randomized comparison of coronary-stent placement and balloon angioplasty in the treatment of coronary artery disease. Stent Restenosis Study Investigators. *N Engl J Med* 1994;331:496–501.
9. Serruys PW, de Jaegere JP, Kiemeneij F, et al. A comparison of balloon-expandable-stent implantation with balloon angioplasty in patients with coronary artery disease. Benestent Study Group. *N Engl J Med* 1994;331:489–495.
10. Mintz GS, Popma JJ, Hong MK, et al. Intravascular ultrasound to discern device-specific effects and mechanisms of restenosis. *Am J Cardiol* 1996;78:18–22.
11. Bomford CK, Kunkler IH, Sheriff SB. Non-malignant disorders. In: Bomford CK, Kunkler IH, Sherriff SB, et al., eds. *Walter and Miller's textbook of radiotherapy: radiation physics, therapy, and oncology*, 5th ed. Edinburgh, UK: Churchill Livingstone, 1993:521–526.
12. Hall EJ. Dose-response relationships for normal tissues. In: *Radiobiology for the radiologist*. Philadelphia: Lippincott, 1994:45–74.
13. Friedman M, Felton L, Byers S. The antiatherogenic effects of Ir192 upon the cholesterol-fed rabbit. *J Clin Invest* 1964;43:185–192.
14. Wiedermann J, Marboe C, Amols H, et al. Intracoronary irradiation markedly reduces restenosis after balloon angioplasty in a porcine model. *Circulation* 1993;86:I-655.
15. Wiedermann JG, Marboe C, Amols H, et al. Intracoronary irradiation: minimal effective dose for prevention of restenosis in swine. *Circulation* 1994;90:I-59.
16. Wiedermann JG, Marboe C, Amols H, et al. Intracoronary irradiation markedly reduces restenosis after balloon angioplasty in a porcine model. *J Am Coll Cardiol* 1994;23:1491–1498.
17. Wiedermann JG, Marboe C, Amols H, et al. Intracoronary irradiation markedly reduces restenosis after balloon angioplasty in a porcine model: six month follow-up. *Circulation* 1994;90:I-652.
18. Waksman R, Robinson KA, Crocker IR, et al. Intracoronary low-dose beta-irradiation inhibits neointima forma-

tion after coronary artery balloon injury in the swine restenosis model. *Circulation* 1995;92:3025–3031.

19. Verin V, Popowski Y, Urban P, et al. Intra-arterial beta irradiation prevents neointimal hyperplasia in a hypercholesterolemic rabbit restenosis model. *Circulation* 1995;92:2284–2290.

20. Mazur W, Ali MN, Khan MM, et al. High dose rate intracoronary radiation for inhibition of neointimal formation in the stented and balloon-injured porcine models of restenosis: angiographic, morphometric, and histopathologic analyses. *Int J Radiat Oncol Biol Phys* 1996;36:777–788.

21. Boivin JF, Hutchison GB, Lubin JH, et al. Coronary artery disease mortality in patients treated for Hodgkin's disease. *Cancer* 1992;69:1241–1247.

22. Rutqvist LE, Lax I, Fornander T, et al. Cardiovascular mortality in a randomized trial of adjuvant radiation therapy versus surgery alone in primary breast cancer. *Int J Radiat Oncol Biol Phys* 1992;22:887–896.

23. Hancock SL, Donaldson SS, Hoppe RT. Cardiac disease following treatment of Hodgkin's disease in children and adolescents. *J Clin Oncol* 1993;11:1208–1215.

24. Shimotakahara S, Mayberg MR. Gamma irradiation inhibits neointimal hyperplasia in rats after arterial injury. *Stroke* 1994;25:424–428.

25. Waksman R, Robinson KA, Crocker IR, et al. Endovascular low-dose irradiation inhibits neointima formation after coronary artery balloon injury in swine. A possible role for radiation therapy in restenosis prevention. *Circulation* 1995;91:1533–1539.

26. Waksman R, Robinson KA, Crocker IR, et al. Intracoronary radiation before stent implantation inhibits neointima formation in stented porcine coronary arteries. *Circulation* 1995;92:1383–1386.

27. Laird JR, Carter AJ, Kufs WM, et al. Inhibition of neointimal proliferation with low-dose irradiation from a beta-particle-emitting stent. *Circulation* 1996;93:529–536.

28. Hehrlein C, Gollan C, Donges K, et al. Low-dose radioactive endovascular stents prevent smooth muscle cell proliferation and neointimal hyperplasia in rabbits. *Circulation* 1995;92:1570–1575.

29. Hehrlein C, Stintz M, Kinscherf R, et al. Pure beta-particle-emitting stents inhibit neointima formation in rabbits. *Circulation* 1996;93:641–651.

30. Eigler N, Whiting J, Makkar R, et al. Effects of β+ emitting V48 ACT-One nitinol stent on neointimal proliferation in pig coronary arteries. *J Am Coll Cardiol* 1997;29:237A.

31. Taylor AJ, Gorman PD, Hudak C, et al. The 90-day coronary vascular response to (90)Y-beta particle-emitting stents in the canine model. *Int J Radiat Oncol Biol Phys* 2000;46:1019–1024.

32. Taylor AJ, Gorman PD, Farb A, et al. Long-term coronary vascular response to 32P β-particle-emitting stents in a canine model. *Circulation* 1999;100:351.

33. Albiero R, Adamian M, Kobayashi N, et al. Short- and intermediate-term results of (32)P radioactive beta-emitting stent implantation in patients with coronary artery disease: the Milan Dose-Response Study. *Circulation* 2000;101:18–26.

34. Albiero R, Nishida T, Adamian M, et al. Edge restenosis

35. after implantation of high activity (32)P radioactive beta-emitting stents. *Circulation* 2000;101:2454–2457.

35. Wiedermann JG, Marboe C, Amols H, et al. Intracoronary irradiation markedly reduces neointimal proliferation after balloon angioplasty in swine: persistent benefit at 6-month follow-up. *J Am Coll Cardiol* 1995;25:1451–1456.

36. Waksman R, Robinson KA, Crocker IR, et al. Intracoronary radiation before stent implantation inhibits neointima formation in stented porcine coronary arteries. *Circulation* 1995;92:1383–1386.

37. Weinberger J. Solution-applied beta-emitting radioisotope (SABER) system. In: Waksman R, Serruys P, eds. *Handbook of vascular brachytherapy*. London: Martin Dunitz, 1998:33–40.

38. Makkar R, Whiting J, Li A, et al. Effects of β-emitting 188Re balloon in stented porcine coronary arteries: an angiographic, intravascular ultrasound, and histomorphometric study. *Circulation* 2000;102:3117–3351.

39. Weinberger J, Amols H, Ennis RD, et al. Intracoronary irradiation: dose response for the prevention of restenosis in swine. *Int J Radiat Oncol Biol Phys* 1996;36:767–775.

40. Fajardo LF. Radiation injury to blood vessels. In: Waksman R, King SB, Crocker IR, et al., eds. *Vascular brachytherapy*. Veenendaal, The Netherlands: Nucleotron, 1996:66–74.

41. Teirstein P, Massullo V, Jani S, et al. Catheter-based radiotherapy to inhibit restenosis after coronary stenting. *N Engl J Med* 1997;336:1697–1703.

42. Teirstein PS, Massullo V, Jani S, et al. Three-year clinical and angiographic follow-up after intracoronary radiation: results of a randomized clinical trial. *Circulation* 2000;101:360–365.

43. Waksman R, Bhargava B, White L, et al. Intracoronary beta-radiation therapy inhibits recurrence of in-stent restenosis. *Circulation* 2000;101:1895–1898.

44. Leon MB, Teirstein PS, Moses JW, et al. Localized intracoronary gamma-radiation therapy to inhibit the recurrence of restenosis after stenting. *N Engl J Med* 2001;344:250–256.

45. Popma J. Late clinical and angiographic outcomes after use of Sr-90/Y-90 beta radiation for the treatment of in-stent restenosis: results from the Sr-90 treatment of angiographic restenosis (START) trial. *J Am Coll Cardiol* 2000;36:311–312.

46. Meerkin D, Tardif JC, Crocker IR, et al. Effects of intracoronary beta-radiation therapy after coronary angioplasty: an intravascular ultrasound study. *Circulation* 1999;99:1660–1665.

47. Costa MA, Sabat M, van der Giessen WJ, et al. Late coronary occlusion after intracoronary brachytherapy. *Circulation* 1999;100:789–792.

48. Raizner AE, Oesterle SN, Waksman R, et al. Inhibition of restenosis with beta-emitting radiotherapy: report of the Proliferation Reduction with Vascular Energy Trial (PREVENT). *Circulation* 2000;102:951–958.

49. Sabate M, Costa MA, Kozuma K, et al. Geographic miss: a cause of treatment failure in radio-oncology applied to intracoronary radiation therapy. *Circulation* 2000;101:2467–2471.

50. Kim H, Cottin Y, Lansky A, et al. Edge stenosis and geo-

graphical miss after intracoronary gamma radiation therapy for in-stent restenosis. *Am J Cardiol* 2000;86:22.

51. Erbel R, Verin V, Popowski Y, et al. Intracoronary beta-irradiation to reduce restenosis after balloon angioplasty: results of a multicenter European dose-finding study. *Circulation* 1999;100:S801.

52. Carter AJ, Laird JR, Bailey LR, et al. Effects of endovascular radiation from a beta-particle-emitting stent in a porcine coronary restenosis model. A dose-response study. *Circulation* 1996;94:2364–2368.

53. Wardeh AJ, Kay IP, Sabate M, et al. β-Particle-emitting radioactive stent implantation. A safety and feasibility study. *Circulation* 1999;100:1684–1689.

54. Kay IP, Wardeh AJ, Kozuma K, et al. Radioactive stents delay but do not prevent in-stent neointimal hyperplasia. *Circulation* 2001;103:351.

55. Sousa JE, Costa MA, Abizaid A, et al. Lack of neointimal proliferation after implantation of Sirolimus-coated stents in human coronary arteries: a quantitative coronary angiography and three-dimensional intravascular ultrasound study. *Circulation* 2001;103:192–195.

56. Falk E. Unstable angina with fatal outcome: dynamic coronary thrombosis leading to infarction and/or sudden death. Autopsy evidence of recurrent mural thrombosis with peripheral embolization culminating in total vascular occlusion. *Circulation* 1985;71:699–708.

57. Erbel R, Heusch G. Coronary microembolization. *J Am Coll Cardiol* 2000;36:22–24.

58. Saber RS, Edwards WD, Bailey KR, et al. Coronary embolization after balloon angioplasty of thrombolytic therapy: an autopsy study of 32 cases. *J Am Coll Cardiol* 1993;22:1283–1288.

59. Ito H, Tomooka T, Sakai N, et al. Lack of myocardial perfusion immediately after successful thrombolysis. A predictor of poor recovery of left ventricular function in anterior myocardial infarction. *Circulation* 1992;85:1699–1705.

60. Ito H, Maruyama A, Iwakura K, et al. Clinical implications of the "no reflow" phenomenon. A predictor of complications and left ventricular remodeling in reperfused anterior wall myocardial infarction. *Circulation* 1996;93:223–228.

61. Wu KC, Zerhouni EA, Judd RM, et al. Prognostic significance of microvascular obstruction by magnetic resonance imaging in patients with acute myocardial infarction. *Circulation* 1998;97:765–772.

62. Gibson CM, Cannon CP, Murphy SA, et al. Relationship of TIMI myocardial perfusion grade to mortality after administration of thrombolytic drugs. *Circulation* 2000;101:125–130.

63. Stone GW, Lansky AJ, Mehran R, et al. Beyond TIMI-3 flow: the importance of restored myocardial perfusion for survival in high risk patients undergoing primary or rescue PTCA (abstr). *J Am Coll Cardiol* 2000;35:403A.

64. Grines CL, Cos DA, Stone GW, et al. Stent PAMI: 12 month results and predictors of mortality (abstr). *J Am Coll Cardiol* 2000;35:402A.

65. Piana RN, Pak GY, Moscucci M, et al. Incidence and treatment of "no reflow" after percutaneous coronary intervention. *Circulation* 1994;89:2514–2518.

66. Leopold JA, Berger CJ, Cupples LA, et al. No-reflow dur-

ing coronary intervention: observations and implications. *Circulation* 2000;102:II-644(abst).

67. Abbo KM, Dooris M, Glazier S, et al. Features and outcome of no-reflow after percutaneous coronary intervention. *Am J Cardiol* 1995;75:778–782.

68. Resnic FS, Lee MKY, Wainstein M, et al. No-reflow is an independent predictor of death and myocardial infarction after percutaneous coronary intervention. *Am J Cardiol* 2000;86:2I(abst).

69. Koch K-C, vom Dahl J, Kleinhans E, et al. Influence of a platelet GP IIb/IIIa receptor antagonist on myocardial hypoperfusion during rotational atherectomy as assessed by myocardial Tc-99m sestamibi scintigraphy. *J Am Coll Cardiol* 1999;33:998–1004.

70. EPIC Investigators. Use of a monoclonal antibody directed against the platelet glycoprotein IIb/IIIa receptor in high-risk coronary angioplasty. *N Engl J Med* 1994;330:956–961.

71. EPILOG Investigators. Platelet glycoprotein IIb/IIIa blockade with abciximab with low-dose heparin during percutaneous coronary revascularization. *N Engl J Med* 1997;336:1689–1696.

72. EPISTENT Investigators. Randomised placebo-controlled and balloon-angioplasty-controlled trial to assess safety of coronary stenting with use of platelet glycoprotein IIb/IIIa blockade. *Lancet* 1998;352:87–92.

73. IMPACT II Investigators. Randomized placebo-controlled trial of effect of eptifibatide on complications of percutaneous coronary intervention: IMPACT II. *Lancet* 1997;349:1422–1428.

74. Bittl JA, Strony J, Brinker JA, et al. Treatment with bivalirudin (Hirulog) as compared with heparin during coronary angioplasty for unstable or postinfarction angina. *N Engl J Med* 1995;333:764–769.

75. Serruys PW, Herrman J-PR, Simon R, et al. A comparison of hirudin with heparin in the prevention of restenosis after coronary angioplasty. *N Engl J Med* 1995;333:757–763.

76. Weintraub WS, Boccuzzi SJ, Klein L, et al. Lack of effect of lovastatin on restenosis after coronary angioplasty. *N Engl J Med* 1994;331:1331–1337.

77. RESTORE Investigators. Effects of platelet glycoprotein IIb/IIIa blockade with tirofiban on adverse cardiac events in patients with unstable angina or acute myocardial infarction undergoing coronary angioplasty. *Circulation* 1997;96:1445–1453.

78. Abdelmeguid AE, Topol EJ, Whitlow PL, et al. Significance of mild transient release of creatine kinase–MB fraction after percutaneous coronary intervention. *Circulation* 1996;94:1528–1536.

79. Kugelmass AD, Cohen CJ, Moscucci M, et al. Elevation in creatine kinase myocardial isoform following otherwise successful directional coronary atherectomy and stenting. *Am J Cardiol* 1994;74:748–754.

80. Kong TQ, Davidson CJ, Meyers SN, et al. Prognostic implication of creatine kinase elevation following elective coronary artery interventions. *JAMA* 1997;277:461–466.

81. Topol EJ, Ferguson JJ, Weisman HF, et al. Long-term protection from myocardial ischemic events in a randomized trial of brief integrin β3 blockade with percutaneous coronary intervention. *JAMA* 1997;278:479–484.

82. Lincoff AM, Tcheng JE, Califf RM, et al. Sustained suppression of ischemic complications of coronary intervention by platelet GP IIb/IIIa blockade with abciximab: one year outcome in the EPILOG trial. *Circulation* 1999;99:1951–1958.

83. Tardiff B, Califf R, Tcheng J, et al. Clinical outcomes after detection of elevated cardiac enzymes in patients undergoing percutaneous intervention. *J Am Coll Cardiol* 1999;33:88–96.

84. Yadav JS, Roubin GS, Iyer S, et al. Elective stenting of the extracranial carotid arteries. *Circulation* 1997;99:376–381.

85. Crawley F, Stygall J, Lunn S, et al. Comparison of microembolism detected by transcranial Doppler and neuropsychological sequelae of carotid surgery and percutaneous transluminal angioplasty. *Stroke* 2000;31:1329–1334.

86. Rapp JH, Pan XM, Sharp FR, et al. Atheroemboli to the brain: size threshold for causing acute neuronal death. *J Vasc Surg* 2000;32:68–76.

87. Al-Mubarak N, Roubin GS, New GS, et al. Does distal balloon occlusion during carotid artery stenting reduce microembolization? *Circulation* 2000;102:II-475(abst).

88. Gerckens U, Mueller R, Soblik S, et al. Prevention of distal embolization during interventions in CABG and native coronary lesions using a new protection filter device. *J Am Coll Cardiol* 2000;35:10A(abst).

89. Taniyama Y, Ito H, Iwakura K, et al. Beneficial effect of intracoronary verapamil on microvascular and myocardial salvage in patients with acute myocardial infarction. *J Am Coll Cardiol* 1997;33:654–660.

90. Ely SW, Berne RM. Protective effects of adenosine in myocardial ischemia. *Circulation* 1992;85:893–904.

91. Marzilli M, Orsini E, Maraccini P, et al. Beneficial effects of intracoronary adenosine as an adjunct to primary angioplasty in acute myocardial infarction. *Circulation* 2000;101:2154–2159.

92. Mahaffey KW, Puma JA, Barbagelata A, et al. Adenosine as an adjunct to thrombolytic therapy for acute myocardial infarction. *J Am Coll Cardiol* 1999;34:1711–1720.

93. Lincoff AM, Califf RM, Topol EJ. Platelet glycoprotein IIb/IIIa blockade in coronary artery disease. *J Am Coll Cardiol* 2000;35:1103–1115.

94. Lefkovits J, Blankenship JC, Anderson KM, et al. Increased risk of non-Q wave myocardial infarction after directional atherectomy is platelet dependent: evidence from the EPIC trial. Evaluation of c7E3 for the Prevention of Ischemic Complications trial. *J Am Coll Cardiol* 1996;28:849–855.

95. Sullebarger JT, Dalton RD, Nasser A, et al. Adjunctive abciximab improves outcomes during recanalization of totally occluded saphenous vein grafts using transluminal extraction atherectomy. *Cathet Cardiovasc Intervent* 1999;46:107–110.

96. Mak KH, Challapalli R, Eisenberg MJ, et al. Effect of platelet glycoprotein IIb/IIIa receptor inhibition on distal embolization during percutaneous revascularization of aortocoronary saphenous vein grafts. *Am J Cardiol* 1997;80:985–988.

97. Neumann FJ, Blasini R, Schmitt C, et al. Effect of glycoprotein IIb/IIIa receptor blockade on recovery of coronary flow and left ventricular function after the placement of coronary artery stents in acute myocardial infarction. *Circulation* 1999;98:2695–2701.

97a. Gibsom CM, Cohen DJ, Cohen EA, et al. Eptifibatide improves coronary flow reserve following stent placement: an ESPRIT substudy. *Circulation* 2000;102:II–366(abst).

98. de Lemos JA, Antman EM, Gibson CM, et al. Abciximab improves both epicardial flow and myocardial reperfusion in ST-elevation myocardial infarction: observations from the TIMI 14 trial. *Circulation* 2000;101:239–243.

99. Theron J, Raymond J, Casasco A, et al. Percutaneous angioplast of atherosclerotic and postsurgical stenosis of carotid arteries. *Am J Neuroradiol* 1987;8:495–500.

99a. Baim D. SAFER Trial. Presentation at Transcatheter Cardiovascular Therapeutics Meeting. Washington: September 2000.

100. Carlino M, De Gregorio J, Di Mario C, et al. Prevention of distal embolization during saphenous vein graft lesion angioplasty: experience with a new temporary occlusion and aspiration system. *Circulation* 1999;99:3221–3223.

101. Sutsch G, Amann FW, Murphy SA, et al. Impact of embolization protection on angiographic parameters in percutaneous coronary intervention with stenting in acute myocardial infarction. *Am J Cardiol* 2000;86:8I(abst).

102. Parodi JC, Bates MC, Schonholz C, et al. International multi-center Parodi Anti-Emboli System Study: preliminary results. *Am J Cardiol* 2000;86:34I(abst).

103. Bonnier H, Eberli FR, Schrader R, et al. The TRAP vascular filtration system: initial European experience in saphenous vein graft interventions. *Am J Cardiol* 2000;86:33I(abst).

104. Grube E, Gerckens U, McColl M, et al. A feasibility study of a new distal protection device for use during coronary artery, saphenous vein graft, and carotid artery interventions. *Am J Cardiol* 2000;86:33I(abst).

105. Mukherjee D, Bhatt D, Roe M. Direct myocardial revascularization and angiogenesis: how many patients might be eligible? *Am J Cardiol* 1999;84:598–600.

106. Simons M, Bonow R, Chronos N, et al. Clinical trials in coronary angiogenesis. Issues, problems, consensus: an expert panel summary. *Circulation* 2000;102:73–86.

107. Hardy R, Bove K, James F, et al. A histologic study of laser-induced transmyocardial channels. *Lasers Surg Med* 1987;6:563–573.

108. Burkhoff D, Fisher P, Apfelbaum M, et al. Histologic appearance of transmyocardial laser channels after 4 1/2 weeks. *Ann Thorac Surg* 1996;61:1532–1534.

109. Fisher P, Khomoto T, DeRosa C, et al. Histologic analysis of transmyocardial channels: comparison of CO_2 and holmium:YAG lasers. *Ann Thorac Surg* 1997;64:466–472.

110. Kohmoto T, Fisher P, Gu A, et al. Physiology, histology, and 2-week morphology of acute transmyocardial channels made with a CO_2 laser. *Ann Thorac Surg* 1997;63:1275–1283.

111. Al-Sheikh T, Allen K, Straka S, et al. Cardiac sympathetic denervation after transmyocardial laser revascularization. *Circulation* 1999;100:135–140.

112. Kwong K, Kanellopoulos G, Nickols J, et al. Transmyocardial laser treatment denervates canine myocardium. *J Thorac Cardiovasc Surg* 1997;114:883–990.

113. Krabatsch T, Schaper F, Leder C, et al. Histologic findings after transmyocardial revascularization. *J Cardiac Surg* 1996;11:326–331.

114. Yamamoto N, Kohmoto T, Gu A, et al. Angiogenesis is enhanced in ischemic canine myocardium by transmyocar-

dial laser revascularization. *J Am Coll Cardiol* 1998;31:1426–1433.

115. Mirhoseini M, Shelgikar S, Cayton M. New concepts in revascularization of the myocardium. *Ann Thorac Surg* 1988;45:415–420.

116. Cooley D, Frazier O, Kadipasaoglu K, et al. Transmyocardial laser revascularization: clinical experience with twelve month follow-up. *J Thorac Cardiovasc Surg* 1996;111:791–797.

117. Frazier O, March R, Horvath K. Transmyocardial revascularization with a carbon dioxide laser in patients with end-stage coronary artery disease. *N Engl J Med* 1999;341:1021–1028.

118. Allen K, Dowling R, Fudge T, et al. Comparison of transmyocardial revascularization with medical therapy in patients with refractory angina. *N Engl J Med* 1999;341:1029–1036.

119. Horvath K. Clinical studies of TMR with the CO_2 laser. *J Clin Laser Med Surg* 1997;15:281–285.

120. Horvath K, Aranki S, Cohn L, et al. Sustained angina relief five years after transmyocardial revascularization with a CO_2 laser. *Circulation* 2000;102:II-765.

121. Horvath K, Mannting F, Cummings N, et al. Transmyocardial laser revascularization: operative techniques and clinical results at two years. *J Thorac Cardiovasc Surg* 1996;111:1047–1053.

122. Triggiani M, Marchetto G, Alfieri O. Refractory angina despite patent coronary artery bypass grafts: treatment with transmyocardial laser revascularization and scintigraphic evidence of improved myocardial perfusion. *G Ital Cardiol* 1999;29:72–75.

123. March R, Macioch J, Donoghue J, et al. Transmyocardial laser revascularization preserves segmental left ventricular contractile reserve: a blinded echocardiographic evaluation. *Circulation* 1997;96:I-585–586.

124. Burkhoff D, Schmidt S, Schulman S, et al. Transmyocardial laser revascularization compared with continued medical therapy for treatment of refractory angina pectoris: a prospective randomised trial. *Lancet* 1999;354:885–890.

125. Horvath K, Cohn L, Cooley D, et al. Transmyocardial laser revascularization: results of a multicenter trial with transmyocardial laser revascularization used as sole therapy for end-stage coronary artery disease. *J Thorac Cardiovasc Surg* 1997;113:653–654.

126. Brinker J. A tunnel at the end of the light. *J Am Coll Cardiol* 1999;34:1671–1674.

127. Burkhoff D, Wesley M, Resar J, et al. Factors correlating with risk of mortality after transmyocardial revascularization. *J Am Coll Cardiol* 1999;34:55–61.

128. Frazier O, March R, Horvath K. Transmyocardial laser revascularization [letter]. *N Engl J Med* 2000;342:436–438.

129. Schofield P, Sharples L, Caine N, et al. Transmyocardial laser revascularization in patients with refractory angina: a randomised controlled trial. *Lancet* 1999;353:519–524.

130. Frazier O, Boyce S, Griffith B, et al. Transmyocardial revascularization using a synchronized CO_2 laser as adjunct to coronary artery bypass grafting: results of a prospective, randomized, multicenter trial with 12-month follow-up. *Circulation* 1999;100:I-240.

131. Allen K, Dowling R, DelRossi A. Transmyocardial laser revascularization combined with coronary artery bypass grafting: a multicenter, blinded, prospective, randomized controlled trial. *J Thorac Cardiovasc Surg* 2001 (*in press*).

132. Sayeed-Shah U, Mann M, Martin J, et al. Complete reversal of ischemic wall motion abnormalities by combined use of gene therapy with transmyocardial laser revascularization. *J Thorac Cardiovasc Surg* 1998;116:763–769.

133. Shawl F, Domanski M, Kaul U, et al. Procedural results and early clinical outcome of percutaneous transluminal myocardial revascularization. *Am J Cardiol* 1999;83:498–501.

134. Whitlow PJ. Results of the randomized PTMR trial. J Am Coll Cardiol Late Breaking Clinical Trials; 2000.

135. Oesterle S, Sanborn T, Resar J, et al. Percutaneous transmyocardial laser revascularization for severe angina: the PACIFIC randomised trial. *Lancet* 2000;356:1705–1710.

136. Lauer B, Junghans U, Stahl F, et al. Catheter-based percutaneous myocardial laser revascularization in patients with end-stage coronary artery disease. *J Am Coll Cardiol* 1999;34:1663–1670.

137. Kornowski R, Baim D, Moses J, et al. Short- and intermediate term clinical outcomes from direct myocardial laser revascularization guided by Biosense left ventricular electromechanical mapping. *Circulation* 2000;102:1120–1125.

138. Leon M, Baim D, Kuntz R. The DIRECT trial. *J Am Coll Cardiol* 2000;35.

139. Goncalves LM. Fibroblast growth factor-mediated angiogenesis for the treatment of ischemia. Lessons learned from experimental models and early human experience. *Rev Port Cardiol* 1998;17:II11–20.

140. Fujita M, Ikemoto M, Kishishita M, et al. Elevated basic fibroblast growth factor in pericardial fluid of patients with unstable angina. *Circulation* 1996;94:610–613.

141. Banai S, Jaklitsch MT. Effects of acidic fibroblast growth factor on normal and ischemic myocardium. *Circ Res* 1991;69:76–85.

142. Laham R, Sellke F, Edelman E, et al. Local perivascular delivery of basic fibroblast growth factor in patients undergoing coronary bypass surgery. Results of a phase I randomized, double blind, placebo-controlled trial. *Circulation* 1999;100:1865–1971.

143. Laham R, Rezaee M, Post M, et al. Intrapericardial delivery of fibroblast growth factor-2 induces neovascularization in a porcine model of chronic myocardial ischemia. *J Pharmacol Exp Ther* 2000;292:795–802.

144. Schumacher B, Pecher P, von Specht B, et al. Induction of neoangiogenesis with basic fibroblast growth factor: technique and early results. *Circulation* 1998;97:645–650.

145. Laham R, Chronos N, Pike M. Intracoronary basic fibroblast growth factor (FGF-2) in patients with severe ischemic heart disease: results of a phase I open label dose escalating study. *J Am Coll Cardiol* 2001 (*in press*).

146. Chronos N. FIRST Results. American College of Cardiology Meeting. Late Breaking Clinical Trials. *J Am Coll Cardiol* 2000.

147. Williams L. The 180-day FIRST results. In: American Heart Association conference on therapeutic angiogenesis and myocardial laser revascularization, Santa Fe, NM, 2001.

148. Williams L. The TRAFFIC trial results. In: American Heart Association conference on therapeutic angiogenesis and myocardial laser revascularization. Santa Fe, NM, 2001.

149. Lederman R. Therapeutic angiogenesis with FGF-2 for intermittent claudication (TRAFFIC Trial). In: American College of Cardiology, Late Breaking Clinical Trials. Orlando, FL. *J Am Coll Cardiol* 2001.

150. Grines C. Adenovirus GENe Therapy (AGENT) trial results. In: American College of Cardiology, Late Breaking Clinical Trials. Orlando, FL. *J Am Coll Cardiol* 2001.

151. Henry T, Abraham J. Review of preclinical and clinical results with vascular endothelial growth factors for therapeutic angiogenesis. *Curr Intervent Cardiol Rep* 2000;2:228–241.

152. Banai S, Shweiki D, Pinson A, et al. Upregulation of vascular endothelial growth factor expression induced by myocardial ischaemia: implications for coronary angiogenesis. *Cardiovasc Res* 1994;28:1176–1179.

153. Banai S, Jaklitsch MT, Shou M, et al. Angiogenic-induced enhancement of collateral blood flow to ischemic myocardium by vascular endothelial growth factor in dogs. *Circulation* 1994;89:2183–2189.

154. Hendel R, Henry T, Rocha-Singh K, et al. Effect of intracoronary recombinant human vascular endothelial growth factor on myocardial perfusion. Evidence for a dose-dependent effect. *Circulation* 2000;101:118–131.

155. Henry TD, Annex BH, Azrin MA, et al. Final results of the VIVA Trial in rhVEGF for human therapeutic angiogenesis. *Circulation* 1999;100:I-476.

156. Henry TD, Annex BH, Azrin MA, et al. One year results of the VIVA trial of rhVEGF for human therapeutic angiogenesis. *Circulation* 2000;101.

157. Losordo D, Vale P, Symes J, et al. Gene therapy for myocardial angiogenesis. Initial clinical results with direct myocardial injection of phVEGF165 as sole therapy for myocardial ischemia. *Circulation* 1998;98:2800–2804.

158. Symes J, Losordo D, Vale P, et al. Gene therapy with vascular endothelial growth factor for inoperable coronary artery disease. *Ann Thorac Surg* 1999;68:830–837.

159. Vale PR, Milliken CE, Tkebuchava T, et al. Catheter-based gene transfer of VEGF utilizing electromechanical LV mapping accomplishes therapeutic angiogenesis: preclinical studies in swine. *Circulation* 1999;100:I-512.

160. Vale PR, Losordo D, Milliken CE, et al. Left ventricular electromechanical mapping to assess efficacy of phVEGF165 gene transfer for therapeutic angiogenesis in chronic myocardial ischemia. *Circulation* 2000;102:965–974.

161. Rosengart T, Lee L, Patel S, et al. Angiogenesis gene therapy. Phase I assessment of direct intramyocardial administration of an adenovirus vector expressing VWGF121 cDNA to individuals with clinically significant severe coronary artery disease. *Circulation* 1999;100:469–474.

162. Rosengart T, Lee L, Patel S, et al. Six-month assessment of a phase I trial of angiogenic gene therapy for the treatment of coronary artery disease using a direct intramyocardial administration of an adenovirus vector expressing the VEGF121 cDNA. *Ann Surg* 1999;230:466–472.

163. Condado J, Waksman R, Gurdiel OG, et al. Long-term angiographic and clinical outcome after percutaneous transluminal coronary angioplasty and intracoronary irradiation therapy in humans. *Circulation* 1997;96:727–732.

164. Waksman R, White RL, Chan RC, et al. Intracoronary gamma-radiation therapy after angioplasty inhibits recurrence in patients with in-stent restenosis. *Circulation* 2000;101:2165–2171.

165. Verin V, Urban P, Popowski Y, et al. Feasibility of intracoronary beta-irradiation to reduce restenosis after balloon angioplasty. A clinical pilot study. *Circulation* 1997;95:1138–1144.

166. King SB 3rd, Williams DO, Chougule P, et al. Endovascular beta-radiation to reduce restenosis after coronary balloon angioplasty: results of the beta energy restenosis trial (BERT). *Circulation* 1998;97:2025–2030.

167. Verin V, Popowski Y, de Bruyne B, et al. Endoluminal beta-radiation therapy for the prevention of coronary restenosis after balloon angioplasty. *N Engl J Med* 2001;344:243–249.

168. Weinberger J, Schiff PB, Trichter F, et al. Results of the Columbia Safety and Feasibility (CURE) trial of liquid radioisotopes for coronary vascular brachytherapy. *Circulation* 1999;100:I-75.

CORONARY ARTERY BYPASS SURGERY

A. MARC GILLINOV
FLOYD D. LOOP

HISTORICAL PERSPECTIVE

Evolution of Direct Coronary Artery Surgery

Now in its fourth decade, surgical myocardial revascularization has benefited millions of patients. Excellent early and late results are attributable to improvements in technology rather than selection of lower-risk patients. The surgical achievements relate to advances in myocardial protection, use of arterial conduits for bypass grafting, and postoperative intensive care management. The original coronary artery bypass operation as popularized by Favaloro (1) and Johnson and colleagues (2) and performed earlier by Garret and colleagues (3) involved aortocoronary saphenous vein grafts. Later, after surgeons acquired the necessary technical expertise, internal thoracic arteries (4) and other arterial conduits were successfully used. Anesthesiologists deserve a large part of the credit for advances in myocardial protection, intraoperative stabilization, and intensive care management. Improvements in anesthetic agents, afterload reduction, and ventilation management have contributed to reduction of complications, shorter hospitalization, and lower cost.

SELECTION OF CANDIDATES FOR SURGERY

Current Indications

Advanced age affects selection for surgical procedures and has stimulated risk assessment. At age 70, clinically detectable coronary atherosclerosis occurs in 15% of men and 9% of women; by age 80, this figure rises to 20% in both sexes. In addition, increasing age is associated with increas-

A. M. Gillinov: Department of Thoracic and Cardiovascular Surgery, The Cleveland Clinic Foundation, Cleveland, Ohio
F. D. Loop: The Cleveland Clinic Foundation, Cleveland, Ohio

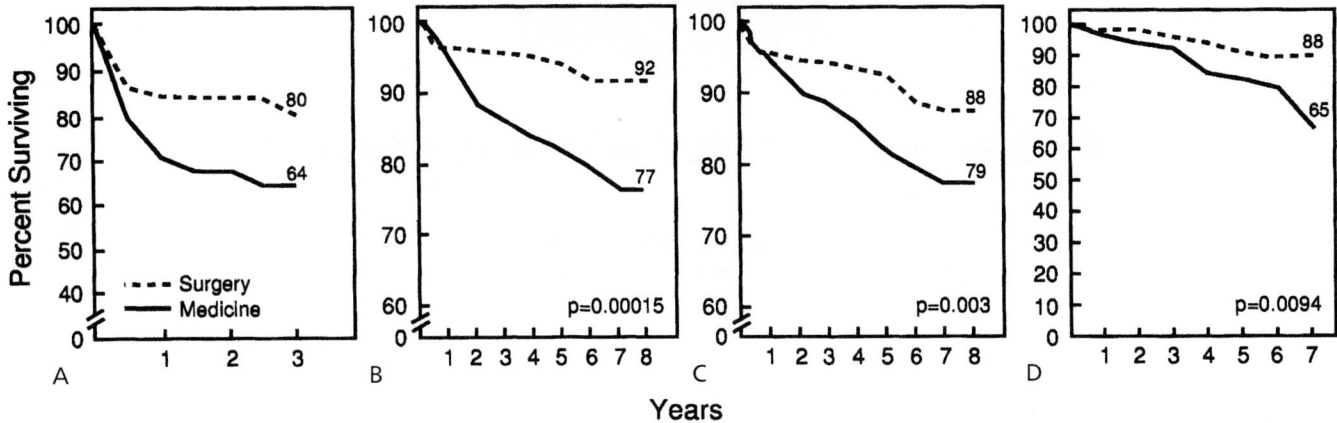

FIGURE 82.1 Survival from published randomized trials comparing coronary artery bypass surgery with medical treatment. **A:** The original Veterans Administration Coronary Arterial Disease Study, which randomly allocated 113 patients with severe left main coronary narrowing to medical or surgical treatment from 1970 to 1974. The 3-year survival was 80% for surgery and 64% for medicine. **B:** Long-term results of two- and three-vessel disease patients from the European Coronary Surgery Study Group are depicted in this panel. Actuarial survival curves for three-vessel disease patients who had an 8-year survival of 92% for surgery and 77% for medicine (*p* = .00015). **C:** In the subgroup of patients with more than 50% narrowing in the proximal third of the anterior descending coronary artery, there was a highly significant difference in favor of surgery in both two- and three-vessel disease subsets. **D:** Seven-year cumulative survival rates for surgery and medical patients from the randomized trial of the coronary artery surgery study. The surgical survival of 88% was significantly better (*p* = .012) than medical treatment when the left ventricular ejection fraction was under 0.50. (Data from Takaro T, Hultgren HN, Lipton MJ, et al. The VA Cooperative randomized study of surgery for coronary arterial occlusive disease II. Subgroup with significant left main lesions. *Circulation* 1976;54[Suppl III]:III107–III117; European Coronary Surgery Study Group. Long-term results of prospective randomised study of coronary artery bypass surgery in stable angina pectoris. *Lancet* 1982;2;1173–1180; and Passamani E, Davis KB, Gillespie MJ, et al. A randomized trial of coronary artery bypass surgery: survival of patients with a low ejection fraction. *N Engl J Med* 1985;312:1665–1671.)

ing prevalence of diabetes, peripheral vascular and cerebrovascular disease, cardiac dysfunction, and left main narrowing (5). ⍣ n94

Given that the patient is an acceptable candidate based on clinical characteristics and evidence of myocardial ischemia, the next important step is coronary arteriography. The location(s) of myocardial jeopardy influences the decision about the type of revascularization. Left main and proximal anterior descending narrowing of 50% or more of lumen diameter impacts the prognosis for adverse events and death more than lesions in other arteries. Patients with angina or ischemia and two-vessel coronary atherosclerosis with a proximal anterior descending lesion or proximal three-vessel disease should be considered for surgery (10). When viable myocardium is demonstrated, poor left ventricular function is not a contraindication to surgery, provided the target vessels are graftable.

Lessons from Clinical Trials

The lessons learned from clinical trials of coronary bypass surgery compared with medical treatment and with angioplasty are the bases for selection of the surgical candidate. In low-risk patients (i.e., those with marginal lesions and no ischemia or with narrowing in small branch coronary

arteries) medical treatment is effective. Coronary bypass surgery is indicated for patients with multivessel disease and is most appropriate in patients with left main and proximal anterior descending lesions as part of a complicated atherosclerotic pattern (Fig. 82.1) (11–14). As left ventricular performance worsens, survival with surgical treatment tends to be better than that with medical treatment (15). Angioplasty may yield equivalent results in single-vessel and selected two-vessel disease in the intermediate term, but more complicated atherosclerotic plaques and calcification in diffuse coronary atherosclerosis make standard balloon angioplasty less effective. In calcified vessels, rotational atherectomy combined with balloon angioplasty has been successful, as well as atherectomy performed before stent placement. Stents have reduced but not eliminated the restenosis problem.

Selected Subsets

Acute Ischemic Syndromes

Acute ischemic syndromes include the spectrum from unstable angina to myocardial infarction. Unstable angina is a broadly interpreted condition. New and progressive angina may be categorized as unstable, but a stricter definition includes pain at rest with electrocardiographic evidence of ischemia (29). Most such patients can be stabilized, but approximately 10% experience myocardial infarction. Necropsy studies indicate that unstable angina patients frequently have severe coronary atherosclerosis. A ruptured atherosclerotic plaque has been linked to persistent instability. Refractory unstable angina may lead to early coronary arteriography and intervention. Multivessel graftable coronary atherosclerosis is an indication for coronary bypass surgery, preferably when the patient is stable. Operations in the face of acute symptoms, especially with ischemic electrocardiographic change, are associated with a higher perioperative myocardial infarction rate and associated risk (30).

Reports on emergency surgery for acute myocardial infarction demonstrated good intermediate-term results (31); however, thrombolytic therapy and angioplasty have largely supplanted emergency surgery. Today, emergency coronary bypass surgery is generally reserved for patients who have severe left main coronary atherosclerosis, who fail angioplasty intervention, or who have mechanical defects. The greatest decrease in risks for operative mortality and perioperative myocardial infarction occurs within 48 hours of infarction, and there is little to be gained by delaying surgery longer (32). Patients with non–Q-wave infarction may, with appropriate indications, undergo bypass surgery with relative safety at any time. ▼ n95

Ischemic Mitral Regurgitation

In ischemic mitral regurgitation, the mitral leaflets and chordae are normal, and the regurgitation is a consequence of ischemic disease of the myocardium. Although published classification schemes for this entity are confusing, classification by mechanism of mitral valve dysfunction is straightforward. Some patients have transient mitral regurgitation caused by intermittent ischemia. In such patients, mitral regurgitation is relieved by revascularization alone. In most cases, however, ischemic mitral regurgitation can be corrected only by mitral valve repair or replacement. In such cases, ischemic mitral regurgitation has one of three causes: (a) ruptured papillary muscle, (b) infarcted but unruptured papillary muscle, and (c) functional ischemic mitral regurgitation (43). Patients with a ruptured papillary muscle usually present with acute pulmonary edema and require urgent surgery. Patients with an infarcted but unruptured papillary muscle generally have a fibrotic, elongated papillary muscle. This causes leaflet prolapse and mitral regurgitation. The majority of patients with ischemic mitral regurgitation has functional ischemic mitral regurgitation. In such patients, alterations in ventricular and annular geometry produce restricted leaflet motion and a jet of mitral regurgitation that is frequently central or eccentric.

Surgical treatment of ischemic mitral regurgitation consists of mitral valve repair or replacement, generally with concomitant coronary artery bypass grafting. In most patients, there is a survival advantage to mitral valve repair over mitral valve replacement (43). When mitral valve replacement is performed, the subvalvular apparatus should be preserved. Hospital mortality is 10% to 20%, and 5-year survival is approximately 50% (43). These unfavorable results are attributable to left ventricular dysfunction in this subset of patients.

Coronary Artery Aneurysms

Ectasia and Kawasaki disease exhibit aneurysmal coronary arterial changes. The term *ectasia* denotes a diffuse ballooning of the coronary artery probably related to atherosclerosis, although some of these cases may be traced to past Kawasaki disease. Kawasaki coronary artery disease (also known as *mucocutaneous lymph node syndrome*) is a self-limited vasculitis of unknown etiology, occurring in children younger than 5 years of age and more commonly in males (44). Asian children are seven times more susceptible than non-Asians. The pathology is aneurysm formation, which may manifest itself 20 years or more after the acute illness. In many patients, obstructions develop at the aneurysm site. Coronary artery bypass surgery is indicated for multiple coronary artery narrowing and ischemia (45). Many of these patients are young, and extended internal thoracic artery bypass grafting is a better alternative than vein grafts, both for long-term patency and for reduction of late cardiac death. Excision of coronary artery aneurysms is rarely indicated.

Reduced Left Ventricular Function

Poor left ventricular function is defined as a left ventricular ejection fraction of less than 0.30. Coronary bypass surgery may be indicated when such patients have angina or demonstrable ischemia coupled with critical lesions and bypassable vessels (46,47). Reversal of hibernating myocardium may be dramatic with adequate revascularization. Patients with heart failure only and poor ventricular function are rarely candidates for isolated revascularization, although selected patients may require bypass combined with ventricular aneurysmectomy. In addition to the clinical presentation, coronary pathoanatomy, and evidence of ischemia, identification of myocardial viability is important in assessing surgical candidacy of patients with impaired left ventricular function. Between 25% and 40% of patients with coronary atherosclerosis and left ventricular global dysfunction show improved contraction after revascularization. The physiologic markers used to demonstrate contractile reserve include positron emission tomographic imaging in which enhanced fluorine 18-fluorodeoxyglucose is measured relative to myocardial blood flow, thallium single-photon emission computed tomography, and dobutamine

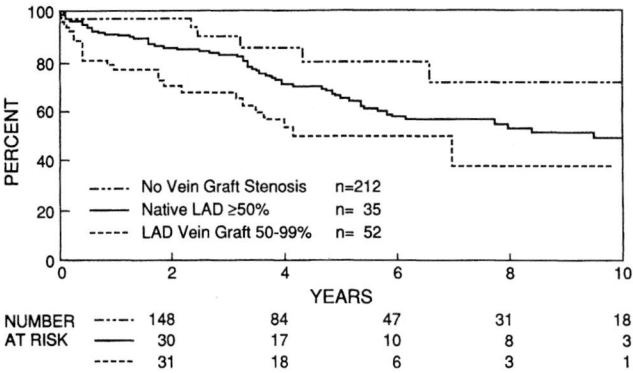

FIGURE 82.2 Patients with late stenoses and vein grafts to the anterior descending coronary artery have worse survival compared to that of either patients with native coronary anterior descending or patients with no stenotic vein grafts. LAD, left anterior descending. (From Lytle BW, Loop FD, Taylor PC, et al. Vein graft disease: the clinical impact of stenoses in saphenous vein bypass grafts to coronary arteries. *J Thorac Cardiovasc Surg* 1992;103:831–840, with permission.)

echocardiography. Each method has its proponents (see Chapters 47, 50, and 52) (48). ❦ n96

Coronary Reoperation

Reoperation may be required for recurring symptoms (ischemia) and angiographic evidence of vein graft atherosclerosis, progressive coronary atherosclerosis, or both. Late stenosis in an anterior descending vein graft predicts a higher death and event rate than late stenosis in vein grafts to other coronary arteries and is an indication for further revascularization (Fig. 82.2) (72). For appropriately selected patients, coronary artery reoperation offers improved longevity compared with medical treatment (73).

In the presence of severe diffuse coronary atherosclerosis, most patients with vein graft atherosclerosis are better served by reoperation than by catheter interventions. The exceptions are fibrous lesions or intimal hyperplasia causing graft stenosis that occurs within 18 to 36 months after the first operation. In selected cases, an isolated vein graft with a discrete lesion may be well suited for percutaneous revascularization. In general, however, angioplasty of saphenous vein grafts with or without stenting has a high rate of complications and unsatisfactory late results (74,75).

The method of revascularization hinges on the age of the graft, the location of the stenosis, the status of left ventricular performance, and overall clinical characteristics. After coronary artery surgery, four arteriographic situations warrant consideration for angioplasty or stenting: (a) progressive atherosclerosis in nonbypassed major coronary arteries when bypass grafts to other major vessels are patent; (b) distal anastomotic stricture that is less than 3 years old; (c) saphenous vein graft lesions less than 3 years old; and (d) native vessel narrowing distal to an open graft accessible via a fully

patent, nondiseased graft (76). Angioplasty or stenting of early vein graft lesions or for progressive coronary artery stenoses is more successful than intraluminal dilatation of late vein graft atherosclerosis.

SURGICAL PRINCIPLES

Basic Strategies

The design of the operation is based on estimated risk and a review of revascularization techniques, including availability and type of bypass conduit. The objective is to provide safe, durable, and complete revascularization with a low probability of complications. Same-day admission is safe and cost-effective and avoids at least 1 day of hospitalization (89,90). Patients may continue on beta-blockers, calcium channel blockers, antihypertensives, and nitrate therapy until the day of surgery. Aspirin should be discontinued 7 to 10 days before elective surgery. We use pulmonary artery catheters in all patients (approximately $35 total cost) to monitor hemodynamic changes and to facilitate management. An increasing number of patients have heparin-induced platelet antibodies preoperatively due to prior heparin exposure (91). These patients are at risk for thrombotic complications with additional heparin exposure.

Conduits in Coronary Bypass Surgery

Vein grafts develop endothelial proliferation as soon as they are placed in arterial circulation and after a few years tend to develop atherosclerosis with thrombus formation. Low- or regular-dose aspirin therapy may prevent platelet thrombi, the release of platelet mediators, and consequent platelet aggregation in vein grafts (106). Dipyridamole has antithrombotic and vasodilating capabilities, but the addition of dipyridamole to aspirin does not improve vein graft patency (107). Also, compared with aspirin, oral anticoagulants do not improve patency. Aspirin that is begun early postoperatively and continued indefinitely does not prevent atheroma formation. Reports on serial postoperative angiograms from Montreal (108) and from The Cleveland Clinic (109) are complemented by an angiographic investigation of 1,388 Canadian military personnel operated on in the 1970s (110), in which approximately 5,000 bypass grafts were reexamined by angiography at 1 year, 5 years, and 15 years or more after surgery. These latter results are the latest available and concur with the classic studies from Montreal and Cleveland. Vein graft patency was 88% early and 81%, 75%, and 50% at 1, 5, and 15 years or more. Approximately half of the grafts showed luminal defects at 5 years, and 81% had lumen irregularities at 15 years or more (Fig. 82.3).

Vein graft atherosclerosis is characterized by diffuse involvement of the venous conduit, circumferential atheroma instability, and fragility (111). Vein graft atheroscle-

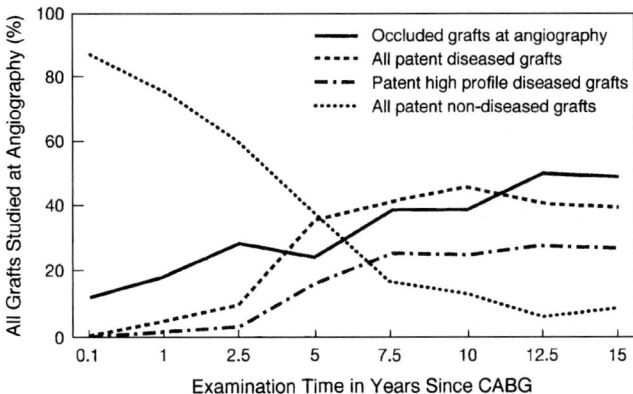

FIGURE 82.3 The latest and longest serial study of aortocoronary vein grafts has classified vein grafts through angiographic findings. High-profile lumen irregularities are defined as more than 59% graft stenosis. Note that the rate of vein graft occlusion progresses after 25 years. Vein graft occlusion rate was 2.1% per year after the first postoperative study. CABG, coronary artery bypass surgery. (From Fitzgibbon GM, Kafka HP, Leach AJ, et al. Coronary bypass graft fate and patient outcome: angiographic follow up of 5,065 grafts related to survival and reoperation in 1,388 patients during 25 years. *J Am Coll Cardiol* 1996;28:616–626, with permission.)

sis begins as a deposition of foam cells followed by plaque formation that varies in extent of fibrosis, lipid deposition, thrombosis, and even calcification. Late thrombosis is a frequent cause of graft closure and may form slowly or suddenly after plaque rupture (112).

In diffuse native-vessel atherosclerosis wherein the artery is completely obstructed or exhibits diffuse distal involvement, coronary endarterectomy may be performed to improve arterial runoff (113,114). Endarterectomy is rarely successful in small arteries that have been completely occluded for a long time. Anterior descending endarterectomy requires an extended arteriotomy to clean out all side branches, whereas a right coronary endarterectomy is accomplished by a distal arteriotomy and dissection of the plaque from the two main branches. It is generally concluded that there is a higher rate of perioperative infarction after endarterectomy and that vein graft patency is slightly lower in endarterectomized arteries.

In the past 15 years, the internal thoracic artery graft has displaced the saphenous vein graft as the conduit of choice. There are three reasons for this change: (a) lower hospital mortality (115), (b) higher long-term patency rate (116), and (c) favorable effect on longevity (116,117). Even in patients with diffuse multisystem atherosclerosis, the internal thoracic artery is rarely affected by atherosclerosis. Metabolism in the arterial wall confers immunity compared with the more inert saphenous vein, which is prone to atherosclerotic degeneration. Coronary arteries narrowed an estimated 50% or more may be grafted with an internal thoracic artery; progression of the proximal native lesion is less after internal thoracic artery grafting than with vein grafts (118). This conduit used in young patients with Kawasaki disease has also

shown growth on serial angiography (119). Competitive flow from a major coronary artery not critically narrowed may account for the infrequent internal thoracic artery "string sign" (120) on postoperative angiograms. Whether an internal thoracic artery graft with this diffuse narrowing will progress to subsequent graft closure or reopen later is not known. However, this no-flow situation was reexamined by temporary occlusion of the recipient coronary artery with a percutaneous transluminal coronary angioplasty balloon (121). The internal thoracic artery with a demonstrable string sign reopened, showing anatomic patency. Therefore, it appears that the string sign may be a reaction to reduced demand and not an intrinsic problem.

Whenever feasible, the internal thoracic artery should be the conduit of choice for anterior descending and other major arteries that supply large regions of myocardium (117,122). This recommendation is particularly important for the anterior descending artery, because severe proximal stenosis in this vessel has greater prognostic importance than stenoses elsewhere in major coronary arteries except for the left main coronary artery (123). n97

The internal thoracic artery used for anterior descending grafting has consistently shown patency of greater than 90% 10 to 15 years postoperatively. Early anastomotic stenosis may be treated by angioplasty with good results (125). Late occlusions occur infrequently from progressive native-vessel atherosclerosis beyond the distal anastomosis. Rarely, a subclavian steal may occur when the proximal subclavian artery narrows or occludes proximally and blood flows from the coronary circulation retrograde through the internal thoracic artery into the distal subclavian distribution.

Increasing use of bilateral internal thoracic artery grafts has expanded arterial grafting further. Free (126), sequential, and Y or T grafts (127) increase versatility by extending graft length and by avoiding the crossing of the midline. Long-term patency of free grafts is 69% to 77%, whereas patencies of sequential and Y or T grafts are consistently 90% or greater. One series of free grafts demonstrated a 95% patency in 40 free right internal thoracic artery grafts studied an average of 40 months postoperatively (128). A study of more than 10,000 patients having primary coronary artery bypass grafting at The Cleveland Clinic has demonstrated that two internal thoracic arteries are better than one (129). This study concluded that patients who received two internal thoracic artery grafts had decreased risks of death, reoperation, and angioplasty. Although this result held for all patient subgroups, further analysis revealed that in high-risk patients, the benefit of two internal thoracic artery grafts on freedom from intervention was eroded considerably by death (130). The conclusions of these large studies support the use of bilateral internal thoracic artery grafting in most patients having primary coronary artery bypass grafting.

Some of the previous concerns about infection related to internal thoracic artery grafting have been dispelled by better

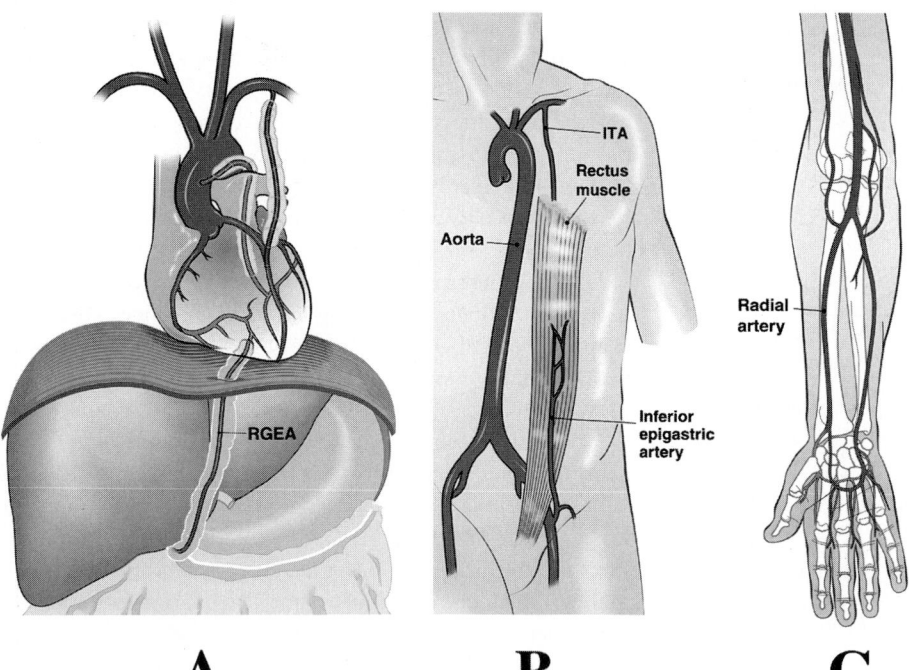

A   **B**   **C**

FIGURE 82.4 A: The gastroepiploic artery is mobilized from the greater curvature of the stomach and generally brought anterior to the liver through the diaphragm and grafted to one of the two branches of the right coronary artery. The conduit is small and prone to spasm. Using it to graft a large coronary artery may result in hypoperfusion. **B:** The inferior epigastric artery lies behind each rectus muscle and is removed through a midline incision. This conduit is used infrequently today but may be advantageous as a Y graft sewn proximally to an arterial conduit and distally to a secondary target. **C:** The radial artery is removed with its venae comitantes. Today, it is the second arterial graft of choice after both internal thoracic arteries, and it may be used as an aortocoronary graft or attached as a Y graft. ITA, internal thoracic artery; RGEA, right gastroepiploic artery.

techniques of internal thoracic artery dissection and wound closure. Bilateral internal thoracic artery grafting is still associated with a higher wound infection rate in diabetic patients (131). Nevertheless, the sternal blood supply in patients with diabetes is not reduced, compared with nondiabetics. Wound complications may be minimized by good surgical techniques, including a minimum of electrocautery, short operating time, blood conservation, and meticulous wound closure. Diabetes is not a contraindication to use one or both internal thoracic arteries as bypass grafts.

The gastroepiploic artery (Fig. 82.4A) may be used for revascularization of right coronary artery branches and, less frequently, the circumflex branches or the anterior descending (132,133). In addition, using the gastroepiploic artery as a composite graft by attaching it to a segment of radial artery allows grafting of two or three coronary arteries with gastroepiploic inflow (134). Previous laparotomy and severe obesity complicate procurement of this artery. The patency reported from the largest series is 80% at 5 years and 62% at 10 years (135). Once the gastroepiploic artery is perfectly anastomosed to a coronary artery with tight proximal stenosis and good runoff, late patency is good and new stenosis in both the gastroepiploic artery trunk and the anastomotic site was uncommon. The severity of the stenosis of the target artery should be high because retrograde coronary artery–to–gastroepiploic artery flow may occur if the native vessel narrowing is modest.

The inferior epigastric artery (Fig. 82.4B), generally 10 to 12 cm in length, is located behind the rectus muscle. This artery is generally used as a Y or T graft and is often connected to secondary targets such as branch vessels (136). The intermediate-term patency of the inferior epi-

gastric artery graft is lower (75%) than that reported for pedicled internal thoracic artery grafts. Today, it is probably the least frequently used arterial conduit (137).

The radial artery (Fig. 82.4C) has enjoyed widespread resurgence after early reports that showed a high incidence of spasm leading to focal intimal hyperplasia (138,139). Improved results in the current era have been attributed to improved harvesting technique and use of calcium channel blockers or other vasodilators to prevent perioperative spasm of the graft (139). Patients with radial artery grafts are treated today with calcium antagonists and postoperative use of aspirin. ✌ n98

REOPERATION

A number of factors influence the rate of reoperation; the single greatest determinant is the type of conduit used in the first operation. Patients with only vein grafts have a much higher and earlier reoperation rate than do patients with one or more arterial grafts. Other factors that increase the probability of reoperation include young age at the first operation, incomplete revascularization, one- or two-vessel grafting initially, and good left ventricular function. Young age, less extensive coronary disease, and normal ventricular function are markers of a good prognosis, which allows the patient to survive to eventual reoperation. The cumulative incidence of reoperation was 3% 5 years after the original surgery, 10% at 10 years, and 30% at 15 years (149).

In the past 10 years, the evolution of catheter intervention techniques has reduced the number of reoperation candidates, although the effects of angioplasty, atherectomy, and stents are not fully elucidated. Patients who are protected by patent grafts but who require native-vessel dilatation or early catheter manipulation after the original bypass operation tend to be referred for catheter intervention, whereas patients at higher risk with diffuse graft atherosclerosis or compromised left ventricular function tend to be referred for surgery rather than for angioplasty (150).

The most frequent indication for reoperation is vein graft atherosclerosis. Atherosclerosis in an anterior descending saphenous vein graft is associated with a particularly poor prognosis (72). We recommend strong consideration for reoperation in those cases. Lesions in old saphenous vein grafts are friable and are not treated consistently well by catheter intervention techniques; the restenosis rate is upward of 50% to 70%. Stenting probably results in less restenosis than does angioplasty, but stent implantation in vein grafts has not been associated with a particularly good 5-year clinical outcome, with high event rates due to infarction, repeat surgery, and repeat angioplasty (151,152). Directional, rotational, and transluminal extraction catheter atherectomy used in atherosclerotic vein grafts have been shown to cause more distal embolization than conventional angioplasty (153).

The hospital mortality for second operations is less than 5% in centers reporting large series (149,154). Emergency surgery, poor left ventricular performance, older age, and female gender influence higher in-hospital mortality. Manipulation of old vein grafts at reoperation may cause atheroembolism and myocardial infarction. Ideally, vein grafts should be replaced with arterial grafts; however, there is a risk of hypoperfusion when large patent but atherosclerotic vein grafts are replaced with *in situ* internal thoracic artery grafts. Adequacy of perfusion depends on the size of the vessel and the arterial runoff and the size of the left ventricular region perfused. In older patients, re-replacement with saphenous veins generally suffices, but younger patients should have every consideration for arterial grafting for the most critical areas of ischemia. The use of an internal thoracic artery graft at the first operation does not increase the risk of reoperation, and the use of an internal thoracic artery graft at reoperation does not increase hospital mortality or morbidity (155).

MINIMALLY INVASIVE CORONARY ARTERY BYPASS SURGERY

Off-Pump Coronary Artery Bypass Grafting

The most dramatic change in coronary artery surgery during the last decade has been the resurgence of coronary artery bypass grafting on the beating heart. Off-pump approaches to coronary artery bypass grafting seek to eliminate morbidity and mortality associated with cardiopulmo-

nary bypass, hasten patient recovery, and reduce cost. Initial widespread use of off-pump techniques was limited to revascularization of the left anterior descending coronary artery using the left internal thoracic artery via a small left anterior thoracotomy, so-called minimally invasive direct coronary artery bypass grafting (MIDCAB). Although technically difficult, this procedure is feasible and provides optimal revascularization of the left anterior descending coronary artery. Early concerns over graft patency using this procedure have been answered, and early patency generally exceeds 95% (176–179). In addition, nonocclusive early angiographic abnormalities frequently disappear during the first postoperative year (176,179). Long-term patency with this approach is superior to that attained with angioplasty (180). 🔻 n99

Although there is no demonstrable benefit in survival with MIDCAB when compared with on-pump coronary artery bypass grafting, there is some suggestion that this approach may decrease morbidity in the most seriously ill patients (186). Postoperative atrial fibrillation remains a problem with this approach (187). Costs associated with MIDCAB are less than those for standard on-pump surgery and similar to those for percutaneous coronary interventions (188–190).

Technological improvements in coronary artery stabilization and surgical advances in coronary artery exposure have enabled widespread application of multivessel off-pump coronary artery bypass grafting. Using current techniques, virtually all patients are candidates for multivessel off-pump coronary artery bypass grafting. This procedure is performed through a sternotomy but without cardiopulmonary bypass. Aortic manipulation is limited to a single application of a clamp to perform proximal anastomoses. All coronary artery targets are accessible, and conduits used may include all arterial and venous grafts used for on-pump surgery.

As with MIDCAB, the question of anastomotic patency with multivessel off-pump coronary artery bypass grafting has been answered. Studies performed before the advent of modern coronary stabilizer platforms suggested reduced anastomotic quality (191). However, in a large prospective study that involved postoperative catheterization of all patients, Puskas et al. found graft patency after off-pump surgery comparable to that documented after on-pump surgery (192). Long-term patency results are not yet available, however. 🔻 o01

Although there are suggestions that off-pump surgery reduces hospital mortality in the elderly and sick (193,194), a survival advantage to this approach remains speculative (195). Nevertheless, there are several advantages to multivessel off-pump coronary artery bypass grafting when compared with conventional on-pump surgery. These include decreased cardiac damage (196), decreased inotrope requirement (196), decreased blood loss (194,197), decreased inflammation and infection (198), and decreased hospital length of stay (194,199). Most important, there appears to be decreased neurologic damage, as demonstrated by decreased cerebral edema (200), decreased cerebral micro-emboli (201,202), decreased serum S-100 protein (202), and decreased neurocognitive dysfunction (202). Nearly all patients experience some neurocognitive dysfunction after cardiopulmonary bypass. Occasionally, patients develop a temporary confusional state, termed "pump head." Reduction of neurologic insults, coupled with the other aforementioned advantages, tends to result in reduced hospital costs for off-pump surgery as compared with on-pump surgery (188,203). However, atrial fibrillation still occurs with high frequency after off-pump surgery (204).

LATE RESULTS

Coronary artery surgery has been influenced by randomized clinical trials that were initiated during the 1970s (Fig. 82.1). Surgery has provided improved longevity in subsets of patients with left main narrowing, proximal two- and three-vessel disease (with proximal anterior descending stenosis), and multivessel disease combined with compromised left ventricular function.

The Coronary Artery Surgery Study registry followed approximately 7,000 patients operated on from 1974 to 1977. After 4 to 6 postoperative years, patients with multivessel disease and poor left ventricular function (226), patients with three-vessel disease with proximal arterial stenoses (227), patients with multivessel disease with severe angina or mild angina (228,229), and patients 65 years of age or older (230) all showed an improved survival with surgery compared with patients who received medical treatment. The disparity in the survival outcomes of the two groups widened with increasing left ventricular dysfunction (i.e., poor left ventricular function adversely affected medically treated patients more than it did surgical patients). The myocardial infarction–free survival was improved by coronary bypass surgery rather than medical treatment in patients with severe angina and in patients with mild angina (231).

Most studies show a 5-year survival rate of 90% to 95%, 10-year, 80% to 90%, and 15-year, 65% to 75% (232). Completeness of revascularization is a strong univariate and multivariate predictor of survival (233). A metaanalysis of the major clinical trials of surgery versus medical treatment indicates that surgery produced lower mortality at 5, 7, and 10 years. In pooled data from all major randomized trials of bypass surgery, Yusuf and colleagues (234) reported a risk reduction of 39% at 5 years in the bypass surgery group despite a crossover rate from medical therapy of 23%. The best differentiation in favor of surgery occurred in patients with left main and three-vessel disease with left ventricular dysfunction; however, patients with focal proximal three-vessel disease with normal left ventricular function and patients with proximal anterior descending disease also

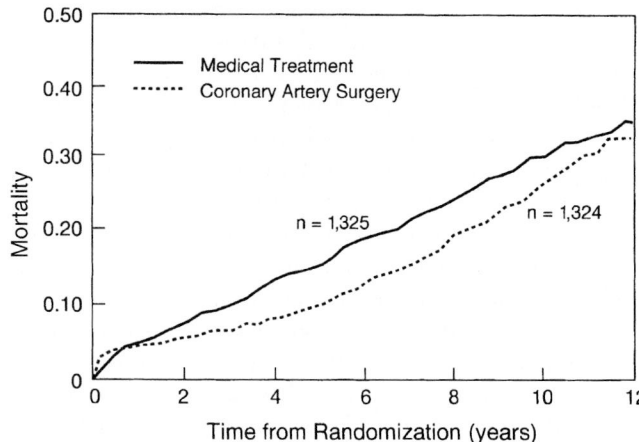

FIGURE 82.5 Results from a metaanalysis of seven randomized trials that have compared coronary artery bypass surgery with initial medical therapy. The risk reduction favored coronary surgery at 5 years, 39%; 7 years, 32%; and 10 years, 17%. The mortality curves are shown for each treatment group. The coronary artery surgery patients had significantly lower mortality than the medical group at all years surveyed. The risk reduction was greatest among left main disease patients than in those with three-vessel or one- or two-vessel disease (odds ratio at 5 years, 0.32, 0.58, and 0.77, respectively). (From Yusuf S, Zucker D, Peduzzi P, et al. Effect of coronary artery bypass graft surgery on survival: overview of 10-year results from randomised trials by the Coronary Artery Bypass Graft Surgery Trialists Collaboration. *Lancet* 1994;344:563–570, with permission.)

showed higher survival with surgery than with medical treatment (Fig. 82.5).

In 15-year studies, it has been shown that performance of the left internal thoracic artery graft to the anterior descending is a more important predictor of survival than progression of native coronary atherosclerosis (Fig. 82.6) (117). Patients who received internal thoracic artery grafting at either the first or the second operation fare significantly better than those who had vein grafts. Because internal thoracic artery grafting to the anterior descending is the single most important determinant of survival and event-free survival, it should not be withheld from any group of patients. The only relative contraindications were noted earlier.

Coronary atherosclerosis is a highly degenerative disease, and after the fifth year, the number of angina-free patients becomes progressively less due to native coronary and conduit atherosclerosis. Typical results show 1-, 5-, and 10-year angina-free survival of 98%, 92%, and 81%, respectively (235). Recurring angina relates also to hypertension, diabetes, obesity, and other comorbidities. By the tenth to twelfth year, approximately half of the patients originally angina-free remain so. Late angina correlates with type of conduit, hyperlipidemia, and hypertension (236).

Continued cigarette smoking after surgery is the greatest determinant of early vein graft thrombosis (237). Smokers are at higher risk of myocardial infarction and reoperation compared with patients who stop smoking. Patients who

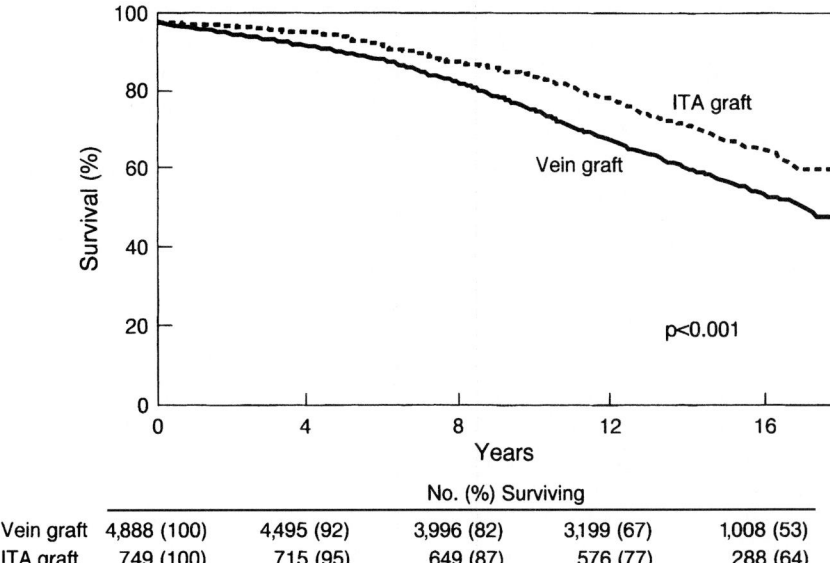

		No. (%) Surviving			
Vein graft	4,888 (100)	4,495 (92)	3,996 (82)	3,199 (67)	1,008 (53)
ITA graft	749 (100)	715 (95)	649 (87)	576 (77)	288 (64)

FIGURE 82.6 Actuarial survival up to 18 years comparing cohorts of patients with internal thoracic artery (ITA) bypass grafts and those with vein grafts. After 5 postoperative years, the differences in survival favor patients with ITA grafting and consistently reach statistical significance. (From Cameron A, Davis KB, Green G, et al. Coronary bypass surgery with internal-thoracic-artery grafts—effects on survival over a 15-year period. *N Engl J Med* 1996;334:216–219.)

continued to smoke 1 year after surgery had more than twice the risk for myocardial infarction and reoperation compared with patients who stopped smoking before surgery. Patients who were still smoking 5 years after surgery had even greater risk for myocardial infarction and reoperation and had a higher rate of recurring angina pectoris compared with patients who stopped smoking before surgery and patients who never smoked (238).

These and other older reports do not reflect the trend toward arterial grafting, nor do they compare surgery with current catheterization interventions. In general, the highest-risk patients (defined by severity of angina, extent of coronary artery disease, and left ventricular dysfunction) showed higher survival with surgery than with medical treatment. Lower-risk patients (mildly symptomatic, less extensive coronary atherosclerosis, and normal or near normal left ventricular function) showed less differentiation from medical treatment, although approximately 40% eventually underwent surgery over a 10-year period (239).

COMPARISON WITH ANGIOPLASTY AND STENTING

The nine major randomized trials comparing angioplasty and bypass surgery have shown no significant differences in intermediate-term mortality (240–244). However, the cardiac event rates, notably additional revascularization procedures and recurring angina, favor bypass surgery for multivessel disease. Patients in these trials were selected by the feasibility of either angioplasty or surgery, which excluded patients with left main narrowing, those with totally obstructed major vessels, and those with previous revascularization. Thus, these trials enrolled approximately 5% of multivessel coronary atherosclerosis revascularization

candidates. Application of conclusions from these studies to all patients with multivessel coronary artery disease is problematic. Patients in the randomized angioplasty/surgery trials have tended to be of low risk; less than 10% had significant impairment of left ventricular function. Approximately half had one- or two-vessel disease, and thus those enrolled in these trials were not among those for whom a benefit from bypass surgery had previously been documented.

Most trials found that there were no differences in early mortality or combined end point of death and nonfatal myocardial infarction comparing surgery with angioplasty, but they did show repeat revascularization was more common by several-fold in patients receiving initial angioplasty (241–244). The angina relief, which favored surgery, abated as early as the third year, and the costs of the therapies were equivalent by the third to fifth year (241–244).

The Bypass Angioplasty Revascularization Investigation (BARI), the largest clinical trial with the longest follow-up, demonstrated improved survival for surgery patients at 7-year follow-up (245). This difference could be explained by the patients with treated diabetes, for whom estimates of 7-year survival were 76.4% for surgery and 55.7% for angioplasty. Among nondiabetics, survival was similar by assigned treatment (86.4% for surgery, 86.8% for angioplasty). The angioplasty group had substantially higher subsequent revascularization rates than the surgery group (59.7% vs. 13.1%). Of patients initially randomized to angioplasty, 35.5% had bypass surgery over the next 8 years.

The BARI finding that treated diabetics with multivessel coronary artery disease have excess mortality with an initial treatment strategy of angioplasty has been challenged (246,247). It is clear that diabetes is an independent risk factor for death with both strategies of revascularization (245,247,248). However, careful analysis of the BARI results (245,246) and recent reports from other studies support a strategy of initial bypass surgery in treated diabetics with multivessel disease (248–251).

BARI investigators analyzed medical care costs and quality of life (252). Initially, the mean cost of angioplasty was 65% of that of surgery ($21,113 vs. $32,347; $p < .001$), but after 5 years, the difference narrowed to only 5% ($56,225 vs. $58,889; $p = .047$). The cost differences favored angioplasty for two-vessel but not three-vessel disease. Surgery was especially cost-effective in diabetic patients. In the first 3 years, surgery, more so than angioplasty, was associated with improved physical function (253).

In the largest study examining death and revascularization after surgery or angioplasty, New York's surgery and angioplasty registries were used to identify nearly 30,000 people undergoing each treatment (254). Patients with single-vessel disease not involving the left anterior descending coronary artery had improved survival with angioplasty. Patients with proximal left anterior descending coronary artery disease had better 3-year survival with surgery regardless of the number of coronary vessels diseased. Also, patients with three-vessel disease had better 3-year survival with surgery than with angioplasty. These results, which reflect clinicians' decision making rather than enrollment in a randomized trial, support an initial strategy of surgery in patients with proximal left anterior descending coronary artery disease or three-vessel disease.

Other studies of one-vessel disease are noteworthy. Patients with single proximal left anterior descending stenoses were randomized to medicine, angioplasty, or surgery (255). All interventions resulted in symptom relief; however, the incidence of totally asymptomatic patients was 32% for the medically treated patients, 82% after angioplasty, and 98% after surgery. An internal thoracic

artery graft to the anterior descending was associated with greater event-free probability at 3 years than was either angioplasty or medical treatment. Another study of one-vessel anterior descending revascularization found that 86% of surgically revascularized patients and 43% of angioplasty patients were free of adverse events after a mean follow-up of 2.5 years (256). Recent 5-year results of a randomized study support this, with 62% of angioplasty patients and 91% of surgery patients free of repeat revascularization (257). In each of these studies, there was no difference in cardiac death or myocardial infarction rate between surgery and angioplasty. In a study comparing different treatment modalities for isolated left anterior descending coronary artery disease, at a mean follow-up of 27 months repeat revascularization was necessary in 30% of patients having percutaneous transluminal coronary angioplasty, 24% of patients having percutaneous transluminal coronary angioplasty with stent, and 5% of patients having surgery with a left internal mammary artery (258).

Finally, a comprehensive prospective nonrandomized treatment comparison was conducted from 1984 to 1990 on 9,263 patients referred to cardiac catheterization at Duke University (Fig. 82.7) (259). In patients with three-vessel coronary atherosclerosis, coronary artery surgery provided a consistent 5-year survival advantage over angioplasty and medical treatment. For less severe coronary disease (i.e., some two- and one-vessel disease), there was a trend toward a relative survival advantage of angioplasty over medical treatment.

How angioplasty alters the natural history of coronary arthrosclerosis depends on the selection criteria for balloon intervention. Using Rand appropriateness selection criteria, the acute success rate for angioplasty was significantly less

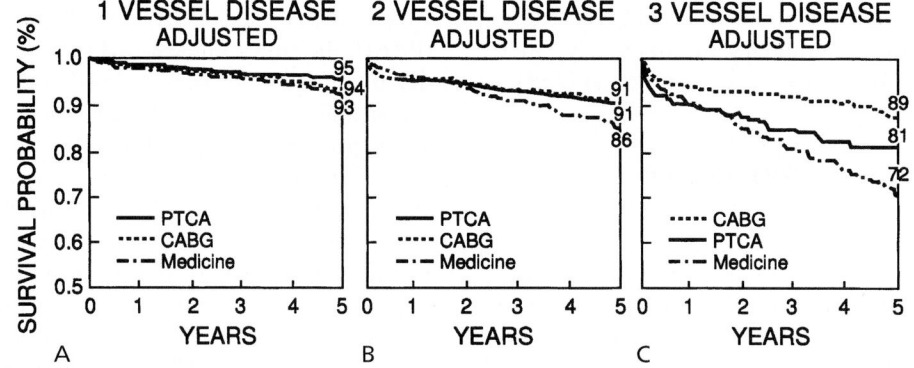

FIGURE 82.7 Survival curves for one-, two-, and three-vessel disease showing adjusted comparisons of angioplasty [percutaneous transluminal coronary angioplasty (PTCA)], coronary artery surgery [coronary artery bypass surgery (CABG)], and medicine. **A:** For one-vessel disease, there is a slight but insignificant trend toward higher survival in the angioplasty group: PTCA, 95%; CABG, 93%; medicine, 94%. **B:** Patients with two-vessel disease showed adjusted 5-year survivals of PTCA, 91%; CABG, 91%; medicine, 86%. **C:** In three-vessel disease, CABG was superior to medicine and PTCA: CABG, 89%; PTCA, 81%; medicine, 72%. (From Mark DB, Nelson CL, Califf RM, et al. Continuing evolution of therapy for coronary artery disease: initial results from the era of coronary angioplasty. *Circulation* 1994;89:2015–2025, with permission.)

TABLE 82.1 DIFFERENCES BETWEEN CORONARY ANGIOPLASTY AND SURGERY

Coronary artery bypass grafting		Percutaneous transluminal coronary angioplasty	
Advantages	Disadvantages	Advantages	Disadvantages
Established differences			
Results in more complete revascularization	Involves major surgery (possible perioperative problems)	Major surgery avoided in 70% of patients (at 5 yr)	Results in less complete revascularization
Provides excellent relief of angina	Requires longer hospitalization and high initial costs	Associated with shorter hospitalization and lower initial costs	Angina may recur
			Associated with more subsequent procedures
Possible differences			
Possibly better long-term survival	Associated with more early infarctions	Associated with fewer periprocedural infarctions	Possibly poorer long-term survival

From Simoons ML. Myocardial revascularization—bypass surgery or angioplasty? *N Engl J Med* 1996;335:275–277, with permission.

in patients who have "necessary" revascularization compared with patients undergoing angioplasty for "uncertain" revascularization criteria. Patients undergoing angioplasty for "necessary" indications had a significantly different 5-year survival (97.8%) compared with patients who had unsuccessful, "necessary" angioplasty (85.5%). In patients classified as having "uncertain" criteria, there was no difference in survival between successful and unsuccessful cases (94.8% vs. 94.4%) (260).

Conclusions from the medical literature may be summarized as follows. Patients who have moderate to high risk of death or cardiac events, including those with diffuse multivessel disease, are generally better off with surgery because of the high restenosis rate of angioplasty and its less consistent results. For patients who qualify for angioplasty, approximately two-thirds will avoid subsequent revascularization, including surgery within the first 3 to 5 years. In multivessel disease patients selected by angioplasty criteria, coronary bypass surgery and angioplasty have similar mortalities up to the first 7 years postprocedure. Surgery offers more complete revascularization because of the greater ability to graft totally obstructed coronary arteries; however, the morbidity is higher and hospitalization is longer. Excepting restenosis, the intermediate term after angioplasty has shown a high rate of revascularization, a higher rate of recurring angina, more use of antianginal drugs, and a trend toward higher mortality compared with surgery for multivessel disease (Table 82.1).

Randomized trials comparing coronary artery surgery to angioplasty with stenting are under way (261,262). It is clear that coronary stent implantation reduces the restenosis rate associated with angioplasty in favorable lesions (263,264). Initial results of the Arterial Revascularization Therapies Study and the Stent or Surgery trials are encouraging for multivessel stenting compared with bypass surgery, but only 1-year follow-up has been reported. The

addition of platelet glycoprotein-IIb/IIIa blockade to percutaneous coronary interventions has also had an important impact (265–267). As long-term results of coronary stenting become available and results of randomized trials are published, it will be important to remember that clinical results in selected patients may not apply to all patients with multivessel coronary artery disease.

CONTROVERSIES AND PERSONAL PERSPECTIVES

Coronary artery revascularization is changing at an increasingly rapid pace. In the past 30 years, the operation has advanced to provide more complete revascularization, more durable conduits, and a positive effect on later survival and incidence of cardiac events. The heterogeneity of coronary atherosclerosis pathoanatomy and patient characteristics has made clinical trials difficult to design and generally not applicable to the population of patients regularly seen in practice.

Early clinical trials that compared medical and surgical treatment of unstable angina showed that conservative treatment of patients with repeated attacks of angina that ultimately required coronary artery surgery resulted in more cost than a strategy of early surgery under stable conditions. The same will be found when repeated catheter-based interventions culminate in coronary artery surgery.

In the past decade, the number of percutaneous revascularization procedures have eclipsed the number of coronary bypass procedures. Percutaneous coronary intervention has a secure place in the armamentarium of revascularization. However, there remain the problems of restenosis in stents and after angiography, the inability to approach chronic occlusions in most patients, and addressing diffuse multivessel disease.

THE FUTURE

Cardiac surgery offers a large menu of arterial conduits that can be used to provide consistent high-quality, long-lasting, biologically better conduits that are affected only by distal progression of native atherosclerosis. The whole field is moving rapidly toward minimally invasive techniques that will compete effectively for revascularization of complicated proximal anterior descending or ostial stenosis, which is often difficult to dilate or stent with consistently good results. In addition, off-pump surgery is likely to reduce the morbidity and mortality of multivessel coronary artery bypass grafting, particularly in patients with multiple comorbidities. In the near future, vein grafts, even in older patients, will be supplanted by all arterial grafting performed through small ports. Virtually every subset of coronary atherosclerosis patients in whom myocardial jeopardy and ischemia of large regions are conclusively demonstrated deserves consideration for coronary bypass surgery. In each of these subsets—even in patients with advanced age, previous coronary artery surgery, and poor ventricular function—the results have consistently shown advantages for patients receiving internal thoracic artery grafting for the anterior descending artery. More recent evidence suggests advantages of expanded arterial grafting for younger patients.

REFERENCES

1. Favaloro RG. Saphenous vein autograft replacement of severe segmental coronary artery occlusion: operative technique. *Ann Thorac Surg* 1968;5:334–339.
2. Johnson WD, Flemma RJ, Lepley D Jr, Ellison EH. Extended treatment of severe coronary artery disease: a total surgical approach. *Ann Surg* 1969;170:460–470.
3. Garrett HE, Dennis EW, DeBakey ME. Aortocoronary bypass with saphenous vein graft: seven year follow up. *JAMA* 1973;223:792–794.
4. Green GE. Internal mammary artery to coronary artery anastomosis: three year experience with 165 patients. *Ann Thorac Surg* 1972;14:260–271.
5. Keller NM, Feit F. Coronary artery disease in the geriatric population. *Prog Cardiovasc Dis* 1996;38:407–418.
6. Peterson ED, Cowper PA, Jollis JG, et al. Outcomes of coronary artery bypass graft surgery in 24,461 patients aged 80 years or older. *Circulation* 1995;92:II85–II91.
7. Wei JY. Age and the cardiovascular system. *N Engl J Med* 1992;327:1735–1739.
8. Frye RL, Gibbons RJ, Schaff HV, et al. Treatment of coronary artery disease. *J Am Coll Cardiol* 1989;13:957–968.
9. Loop FD, Lytle BW, Cosgrove DM, et al. Coronary artery bypass graft surgery in the elderly: indications and outcome. *Cleve Clin J Med* 1988;55:23–34.
10. Kirklin JW, Akins CW, Blackstone EH, et al. ACC/AHA guidelines and indicators for coronary artery bypass graft surgery: a report of the American College of Cardiology/American Heart Association Task Force on Assessment of Diagnostic and Therapeutic Cardiovascular Procedures (Subcommittee on Coronary Artery Bypass Graft Surgery). *Circulation* 1991;83:1125–1173.
11. Varnauskas E. Twelve year follow up of survival in the randomized European Coronary Surgery Study. *N Engl J Med* 1988;319:332–337.
12. Takaro T, Hultgren HN, Lipton MJ, et al. The VA Cooperative randomized study of surgery for coronary arterial occlusive disease II. Subgroup with significant left main lesions. *Circulation* 1976;54[Suppl III]:III107–III117.
13. European Coronary Surgery Study Group. Long-term results of prospective randomised study of coronary artery bypass surgery in stable angina pectoris. *Lancet* 1982;2;1173–1180.
14. Passamani E, Davis KB, Gillespie MJ, et al. A randomized trial of coronary artery bypass surgery: survival of patients with a low ejection fraction. *N Engl J Med* 1985;312:1665–1671.
15. The Veterans Administration Coronary Artery Bypass Surgery Cooperative Study Group. Eleven-year survival in the Veterans Administration randomized trial of coronary bypass surgery for stable angina. *N Engl J Med* 1984;311:1333–1339.
16. Mangano DT, Goldman L. Preoperative assessment of patients with known or suspected coronary disease. *N Engl J Med* 1995;333:1750–1756.
17. Eagle KA, Brundage BH, Chaitman BR, et al. Guidelines for perioperative cardiovascular evaluation for noncardiac surgery: Report of the American College of Cardiology/American Heart Association Task Force on Practice Guidelines (Committee on Perioperative Cardiovascular Evaluation for Noncardiac Surgery). *J Am Coll Cardiol* 1996;27:910–948.
18. Lytle BW, Kramer JR, Golding LR, et al. Young adults with coronary atherosclerosis: 10-year results of surgical myocardial revascularization. *J Am Coll Cardiol* 1984;4:445–453.
19. French JK, Scott DS, Whitlock RM, et al. Late outcome after coronary artery bypass graft surgery in patients <40 years old. *Circulation* 1995;92[Suppl II]:II14–II19.
20. Calafiore AM, de Giammarco G, Losiani N, et al. Composite arterial conduits for a wider arterial myocardial revascularization. *Ann Thorac Surg* 1994;58:185–190.
21. Rahimtoola SH. The hibernating myocardium. *Am Heart J* 1989;117:211–221.
22. Braunwald E, Kloner RA. The stunned myocardium: prolonged, postischemic ventricular dysfunction. *Circulation* 1982;66:1146–1149.

23. Martinez RR, Bennett J, Eikman EA, et al. Comparison of nitroglycerin magnetic resonance imaging with dobutamine echocardiography for predicting recovery of function after revascularization. *Am J Cardiol* 2000;85:1250–1252.

24. Loop FD, Effler DB, Navia JA, et al. Aneurysms of the left ventricle: survival and results of a ten-year surgical experience. *Ann Surg* 1973;178:399–405.

25. Loop FD, Effler DB, Webster JS, Groves LK. Posterior ventricular aneurysms: etiologic factors and results of surgical treatment. *N Engl J Med* 1973;288:237–239.

26. Shapira OM, Davidoff R, Hilkert RJ, et al. Repair of left ventricular aneurysm: long-term results of linear repair versus endoaneurysmorrhaphy. *Ann Thorac Surg* 1997;63:701–705.

27. Dor V, Sabatier M, Di Donato M, et al. Late hemodynamic results after left ventricular patch repair associated with coronary grafting in patients with postinfarction akinetic or dyskinetic aneurysm of the left ventricle. *J Thorac Cardiovasc Surg* 1995;110:1291–1301.

28. Grossi EA, Chinitz LA, Galloway AC, et al. Endoventricular remodeling of left ventricular aneurysm: functional, clinical and electrophysiological results. *Circulation* 1995;92[Suppl II]:II98–II100.

29. Braunwald E, Mark DB, Jones RJ, et al. Unstable angina: diagnosis and management. In: *Clinical practice guideline*, number 10. Rockville, MD: U.S. Department of Health and Human Services, 1994. Agency for Health Care Policy and Research publication 940602.

30. Golding LR, Loop FD, Sheldon WC, et al. Emergency revascularization for unstable angina. *Circulation* 1978;58:1163–1166.

31. DeWood MA, Notske RN, Berg R Jr, et al. Medical and surgical management of early Q wave myocardial infarction, I: effects of surgical reperfusion on survival, recurrent myocardial infarction, sudden death and functional class at 10 or more years of follow-up. *J Am Coll Cardiol* 1989;14:65–77.

32. Braxton JH, Hammond GL, Letsou GV, et al. Optimal timing of coronary artery bypass graft surgery after acute myocardial infarction. *Circulation* 1995;92[Suppl II]:II66–II68.

33. Every NR, Maynard C, Cochran RP, et al. Characteristics, management, and outcome of patients with acute myocardial infarction treated with bypass surgery. *Circulation* 1996;94[Suppl II]:II81–II86.

34. DeWood MA, Leonard J, Grunwald RP, et al. Medical and surgical management of early Q wave myocardial infarction, II: effects on mortality and global and regional left ventricular function at 10 or more years of follow-up. *J Am Coll Cardiol* 1989;14:78–90.

35. Kelly P, Ruskin JN, Vlahakes GJ, et al. Surgical coronary revascularization in survivors of prehospital cardiac arrest: its effect on inducible ventricular arrhythmias and long-term survival. *J Am Coll Cardiol* 1990;15:267–273.

36. Allen BS, Buckberg GD, Fontan FM, et al. Superiority of controlled surgical reperfusion versus percutaneous transluminal coronary angioplasty in acute coronary occlusion. *J Thorac Cardiovasc Surg* 1993;105:864–884.

37. Reddy SG, Roberts WC. Frequency of rupture of the left ventricular free wall or ventricular septum among

necropsy cases of fatal acute myocardial infarction since introduction of coronary care units. *Am J Cardiol* 1989;63:906–911.

38. Cox FF, Morshius WJ, Plokker HW, et al. Early mortality after surgical repair of postinfarction ventricular septal rupture: importance of rupture location. *Ann Thorac Surg* 1996;61:1752–1758.

39. Lijoi A, Scarano F, Parodi E, et al. Subacute left ventricular free wall rupture complicating acute myocardial infarction. *J Cardiovasc Surg* 1996;37:627–630.

40. Schwarz CD, Punzengruber C, Ng CK, et al. Clinical presentation of rupture of the left-ventricular free wall after myocardial infarction: report of five cases with successful surgical repair. *Thorac Cardiovasc Surg* 1996;44:71–75.

41. Daggett WM. Surgical technique for early repair of posterior ventricular septal rupture. *J Thorac Cardiovasc Surg* 1982;84:306–312.

42. David TE, Dale L, Sun Z. Postinfarction ventricular septal rupture: repair by endocardial patch with infarct exclusion. *J Thorac Cardiovasc Surg* 1995;110:1315–1322.

43. Gillinov AM, Wierup PN, Blackstone EH, et al. Repair is preferable to replacement for ischemic mitral regurgitation. *J Thorac Cardiovasc Surg* 2001 (*in press*).

44. Kato H, ed. *Kawasaki disease: proceedings of the 5th International Kawasaki Disease Symposium*. Amsterdam: Elsevier, 1995.

45. Kitamura S, Kameda Y, Seki T, et al. Long-term outcome of myocardial revascularization in patients with Kawasaki coronary artery disease: a multicenter cooperative study. *J Thorac Cardiovasc Surg* 1994;107:663–674.

46. Vanoverschelde JL, Gerber BL, D'Hondt AM, et al. Preoperative selection of patients with severely impaired left ventricular function for coronary revascularization. *Circulation* 1995;92[Suppl]:II37–II44.

47. Kaul TK, Agnihotri AK, Fields BL, et al. Coronary artery bypass grafting in patients with an ejection fraction of twenty percent or less. *J Thorac Cardiovasc Surg* 1996;111:1001–1012.

48. Bonow RO. Identification of viable myocardium. *Circulation* 1996;94:2674–2680.

49. Carpentier A, Chachques JC, Acar C, et al. Dynamic cardiomyoplasty at seven years. *J Thorac Cardiovasc Surg* 1993;106:42–54.

50. Lange R, Sack FU, Voss B, et al. Dynamic cardiomyoplasty: indications, surgical technique, and results. *Thorac Cardiovasc Surg* 1995;43:243–251.

51. Furnary AP, Jessup M, Moreira LF. Multicenter trial of dynamic cardiomyoplasty for chronic heart failure. *J Am Coll Cardiol* 1996;28:1175–1180.

52. Paul SD, Eagle KA, Kuntz KM, et al. Concordance of preoperative clinical risk with angiographic severity of coronary artery disease in patients undergoing vascular surgery. *Circulation* 1996;94:1561–1566.

53. Hertzer NR, Loop FD. Combined carotid and coronary artery disease. *ACC Curr J Rev* 1995;4:45–48.

54. North American Symptomatic Carotid Endarterectomy Trial Collaborators. Beneficial effect of carotid endarterectomy in symptomatic patients with high-grade carotid stenosis. *N Engl J Med* 1991;325:445–453.

55. European Carotid Surgery Trialists' Collaborative Group.

Endarterectomy for moderate symptomatic carotid stenosis: interim results from the MRC European Carotid Surgery Trial. *Lancet* 1996;347:1591–1593.

56. Executive Committee for the Asymptomatic Carotid Atherosclerosis Study. Endarterectomy for asymptomatic carotid artery stenosis. *JAMA* 1995;273:1421–1428.

57. Hertzer NR, O'Hara PJ, Mascha EJ, et al. Early outcome assessment for 2228 consecutive carotid endarterectomy procedures: The Cleveland Clinic experience from 1989 to 1995. *J Vasc Surg* 1997;26:1–10.

58. Trachiotis GD, Pfister AJ. Management strategy for simultaneous carotid endarterectomy and coronary revascularization. *Ann Thorac Surg* 1997;64:1013–1018.

59. Renton S, Hornick P, Taylor KM, et al. Rational approach to combined carotid and ischaemic heart disease. *Br J Surg* 1997;84:1503–1510.

60. Hines GL, Scott WC, Schubach SL, et al. Prophylactic carotid endarterectomy in patients with high-grade carotid stenosis undergoing coronary bypass: does it decrease the incidence of perioperative stroke? *Ann Vasc Surg* 1997;12:23–27.

61. Terramani TT, Rowe VL, Hood DB, et al. Combined carotid endarterectomy and coronary artery bypass grafting in asymptomatic carotid artery stenosis. *Am Surg* 1998;64:993–997.

62. Palerme LP, Hill AB, Obrand D, Steinmetz OK. Is Canadian cardiac surgeons' management of asymptomatic carotid artery stenosis at coronary artery bypass supported by the literature? A surgery and a critical appraisal of the literature. *Canadian J Surg* 2000;43:93–103.

63. Yadav JS, Roubin GS, Iyer S, et al. Elective stenting of the extracranial carotid arteries. *Circulation* 1997;95:376–381.

64. Wholey MH, Wholey M, Bergeron P, et al. Current global status of carotid artery stent placement. *Cathet Cardiovasc Diagn* 1998;44:1–6.

65. Beeba HG, Kritpracha B. Carotid stenting versus carotid endarterectomy: update on the controversy. *Semin Vasc Surg* 1998;11:46–51.

66. Wholey MH, Wholey MH, Eles G. Cervical carotid artery stent placement. *Semin Interv Cardiol* 1998;3:105–115.

67. Waigand J, Gross CM, Uhlich F, et al. Elective stenting of carotid artery stenosis in patients with severe coronary artery disease. *Eur Heart J* 1998;19:1365–1370.

68. Kleikamp G, Schnepper U, Korfer R. Coronary artery and aortic valve disease as a long term sequel of mediastinal and thoracic irradiation. *J Thorac Cardiovasc Surg* 1997;45:27–31.

69. Cosgrove DM, Stewart WJ. Mitral valvuloplasty. *Curr Probl Cardiol* 1989;14:353–416.

70. Flameng WJ, Herijgers P, Szecsi J, et al. Determinants of early and late results of combined valve operations and coronary artery bypass grafting. *Ann Thorac Surg* 1996;61:621–628.

71. Odell JA, Mullany CJ, Schaff HV, et al. Aortic valve replacement after previous coronary artery bypass grafting. *Ann Thorac Surg* 1996;62:1424–1430.

72. Lytle BW, Loop FD, Taylor PC, et al. Vein graft disease: the clinical impact of stenoses in saphenous vein bypass grafts to coronary arteries. *J Thorac Cardiovasc Surg* 1992;103:831–840.

73. Lytle BW, Loop FD, Taylor PC, et al. The effect of coronary reoperation on the survival of patients with stenoses in saphenous vein bypass grafts to coronary arteries. *J Thorac Cardiovasc Surg* 1993;105:605–614.

74. Savage MP, Douglas JS Jr, Fischman DL, et al. and Saphenous Vein De Novo Trial Investigators. Stent placement compared with balloon angioplasty for obstructed coronary bypass grafts. *N Engl J Med* 1997;337:740–747.

75. Choussat R, Black AJ, Bossi I, et al. Long-term clinical outcome after endoluminal reconstruction of diffusely degenerated saphenous vein grafts with less-shortening wall stents. *J Am Coll Cardiol* 2000;36:387–394.

76. Platko WP, Hollman J, Whitlow PL, et al. Percutaneous transluminal angioplasty of saphenous vein graft stenosis: long-term follow-up. *J Am Coll Cardiol* 1989;14:1645–1650.

77. Higgins TL, Estafanous FG, Loop FD, et al. Stratification of morbidity and mortality outcome by preoperative risk factors in coronary artery bypass patients: a clinical severity score. *JAMA* 1992;267:2344–2348.

78. Parsonnet V, Dean D, Bernstein AD. A method of uniform stratification of risk for evaluating the results of surgery in acquired adult heart disease. *Circulation* 1989;79:3–12.

79. Hannan EL, Kilburn H, O'Donnell JF, et al. Adult open heart surgery in New York State: an analysis of risk factors and hospital mortality rates. *JAMA* 1990;264:2768–2774.

80. O'Connor GT, Plume SK, Olmstead EM. Multivariate prediction of in-hospital mortality associated with coronary artery bypass graft surgery: Northern New England Cardiovascular Disease Study Group. *Circulation* 1992;85:2111–2118.

81. Fisher LD, Kennedy JW, Davis KB, et al. Association of sex, physical size, and operative mortality after coronary artery bypass in the Coronary Artery Surgery Study (CASS). *J Thorac Cardiovasc Surg* 1982;84:334–341.

82. Loop FD, Golding LR, MacMillan JP, et al. Coronary artery surgery in women compared with men: analyses of risks and long-term results. *J Am Coll Cardiol* 1983;1:383–390.

83. O'Connor GT, Morton JR, Diehl MJ, et al. Differences between men and women in hospital mortality associated with coronary artery bypass graft surgery: Northern New England Cardiovascular Disease Study Group. *Circulation* 1993;88:2104–2110.

84. Christakis GT, Weisel RD, Buth KJ, et al. Is body size the cause of poor outcomes of coronary artery bypass operations in women? *J Thorac Cardiovasc Surg* 1995;110:134–158.

85. Kurlansky PA, Dorman MJ, Galbut DL, et al. Bilateral internal mammary artery grafting in women: a 21-year experience. *Ann Thorac Surg* 1996;62:63–69.

86. Newman MF, Wolman R, Kanchuger M, et al. Multicenter preoperative stroke risk index for patients undergoing coronary artery bypass graft surgery. *Circulation* 1996;94[Suppl II]:II74–II80.

87. Higgins TL, Estafanous FG, Loop FD, et al. An ICU admission score for predicting morbidity and mortality

risk after coronary artery bypass surgery. *Ann Thorac Surg* 1997;64:1050–1058.

88. Estafanous FG, Loop FD, Higgins TL, et al. Increased risk and decreased morbidity in coronary artery surgery between 1986 and 1994. *Ann Thorac Surg* 1998;65:383–389.

89. Loop F, Christiansen EK, Lister JL, et al. A strategy for cost containment in coronary surgery. *JAMA* 1983;250:63–66.

90. Arom KV, Emery RW, Petersen RJ, Schwartz M. Patient characteristics, safety, and benefits of same-day admission for coronary artery bypass grafting. *Ann Thorac Surg* 1996;61:1136–1140.

91. Bauer TL, Arepally G, Konkle BA. Prevalence of heparin-associated antibodies without thrombosis in patients undergoing cardiopulmonary bypass surgery. *Circulation* 1997;95:1242–1246.

92. Cosgrove DM, Loop FD, Lytle BW, et al. Determinants of blood utilization during myocardial revascularization. *Ann Thorac Surg* 1985;40:380–384.

93. Mossad E, Estafanous F. Blood use in cardiac surgery and the limitations of hemodilution. *Curr Opin Cardiol* 1995;10:584–590.

94. Bashein G, Nessly ML, Rice AL, et al. Preoperative aspirin therapy and reoperation for bleeding after coronary artery bypass surgery. *Arch Intern Med* 1991;151:89–93.

95. Cosgrove DM III, Heric B, Lytle BW, et al. Aprotinin therapy for reoperative myocardial revascularization: a placebo-controlled study. *Ann Thorac Surg* 1992;54:1031–1038.

96. Lemmer JH, Dilling EW, Morton JR, et al. Aprotinin for primary coronary artery bypass grafting: a multicenter trial of three dose regimens. *Ann Thorac Surg* 1996;62:1659–1668.

97. Dietrich W, Spath P, Ebell A, Richter JA. Prevalence of anaphylactic reactions to aprotinin: analysis of two hundred forty-eight reexposures to aprotinin in heart operations. *J Thorac Cardiovasc Surg* 1997;113:194–201.

98. Daily PO, Lamphere JA, Dembitsky WP, et al. Effect of prophylactic epsilon-aminocaproic acid on blood loss and transfusion requirements in patients undergoing first-time coronary artery surgery bypass grafting: a randomized, prospective, double-blind study. *J Thorac Cardiovasc Surg* 1994;108:99–106.

99. VanderSalm TJ, Kaur S, Lancey RA, et al. Reduction of bleeding after heart operations through the prophylactic use of epsilon-aminocaproic acid. *J Thorac Cardiovasc Surg* 1996;112:1098–1107.

100. Kjaergard HK, Fairbrother JE. Controlled clinical studies of fibrin sealant in cardiothoracic surgery—a review (review). *Eur J Cardiothorac Surg* 1996;10:727–733.

101. Buckberg GD. Studies of controlled reperfusion after ischemia: a series of experimental and clinical observations from the Division of Thoracic Surgery, UCLA School of Medicine. *J Thorac Cardiovasc Surg* 1986;92:483–648.

102. Blauth CI, Cosgrove DM, Webb BW, et al. Atheroembolism from the ascending aorta: an emerging problem in cardiac surgery. *J Thorac Cardiovasc Surg* 1992;103:1104–1112.

103. Loop FD, Higgins TL, Panda R, et al. Myocardial protection during cardiac operations: decreased morbidity and lower cost with blood cardioplegia and coronary sinus perfusion. *J Thorac Cardiovasc Surg* 1992;104:608–618.

104. Moncada S, Higgs EA. The L-arginine–nitric oxide pathway. *N Engl J Med* 1993;329:2002–2012.

105. Gross SS, Wolin MS. Nitric oxide: pathophysiological mechanisms. *Annu Rev Physiol* 1995;57:737–769.

106. Chesebro JH, Fuster V, Elveback LR, et al. Effect of dipyridamole and aspirin on late vein-graft patency after coronary bypass operations. *N Engl J Med* 1984;310:209–214.

107. van der Meer, Hillege HL, Koostra GJ, et al. Prevention of one-year vein-graft occlusion after aortocoronary-bypass surgery: a comparison of low-dose aspirin, low-dose aspirin plus dipyridamole, and oral anticoagulants. *Lancet* 1993;342:257–264.

108. Campeau L, Enjalbert M, Lesperance J, et al. The relation of risk factors to the development of atherosclerosis in saphenous-vein bypass grafts and the progression of disease in the native circulation: a study 10 years after aortocoronary bypass surgery. *N Engl J Med* 1984;311:1329–1332.

109. Lytle BW, Loop FD, Cosgrove DM, et al. Long-term (5 to 12 years) serial studies of internal mammary artery and saphenous vein coronary bypass grafts. *J Thorac Cardiovasc Surg* 1985;89:248–258.

110. Fitzgibbon GM, Kafka HP, Leach AJ, et al. Coronary bypass graft fate and patient outcome: angiographic follow-up of 5,065 grafts related to survival and reoperation in 1,388 patients during 25 years. *J Am Coll Cardiol* 1996;28:616–626.

111. Bryan AJ, Angelini GD. The biology of saphenous vein graft occlusion: etiology and strategies for prevention. *Curr Opin Cardiol* 1994;9:641–649.

112. Bourassa MG. Fate of venous grafts: the past, the present and the future. *J Am Coll Cardiol* 1991;17:1081–1083.

113. Brenowitz JB, Kayser DL, Johnson WD. Results of coronary artery endarterectomy and reconstruction. *J Thorac Cardiovasc Surg* 1988;95:1–10.

114. Djalilian AR, Shumway SJ. Adjunctive coronary endarterectomy: improved safety in modern cardiac surgery. *Ann Thorac Surg* 1995;60:1749–1754.

115. Edwards FH, Clark RE, Schwartz M. Impact of internal mammary artery conduits on operative mortality in coronary revascularization. *Ann Thorac Surg* 1994;57:27–32.

116. Loop FD, Lytle BW, Cosgrove DM, et al. Influence of the internal mammary artery graft on 10-year survival and other cardiac events. *N Engl J Med* 1986;314:1–6.

117. Cameron A, Davis KB, Green G, Schaff HV. Coronary bypass surgery with internal-thoracic-artery grafts—effects on survival over a 15-year period. *N Engl J Med* 1996;334:216–219.

118. Cosgrove DM, Loop FD, Saunders CR, et al. Should coronary arteries with less than fifty percent stenosis be bypassed? *J Thorac Cardiovasc Surg* 1981;82:520–530.

119. Kitamura S, Seki T, Kawachi K, et al. Excellent patency and growth potential of internal mammary artery grafts in pediatric coronary bypass surgery: new evidence for a "live" conduit. *Circulation* 1989;78[Suppl I]:I29–I39.

120. Siebenmann R, Egloff L, Hirzel H, et al. The internal thoracic mammary artery "string phenomenon": analysis of 10 cases. *Eur J Cardiothorac Surg* 1993;7:235–238.

121. Kitamura S, Kawachi K, Seki T, et al. Angiographic demonstration of no-flow anatomical patency of internal tho-

racic–coronary artery bypass grafts. *Ann Thorac Surg* 1992;53:156–159.

122. Loop FD. Internal-thoracic-artery grafts: biologically better coronary arteries [editorial]. *N Engl J Med* 1996;334:263–265.

123. Klein LW, Weintraub WS, Agarwal JB, et al. Prognostic significance of severe narrowing of the proximal portion of the left anterior descending coronary artery. *Am J Cardiol* 1986;58:42–46.

124. Carrel T, Kujawski T, Zund G, et al. The internal mammary artery malperfusion syndrome: incidence, treatment and angiographic verification. *Eur J Cardiothorac Surg* 1995;9:190–197.

125. Ishizaka N, Ishizaka Y, Ikari Y, et al. Initial and subsequent angiographic outcome of percutaneous transluminal angioplasty performed on internal mammary artery grafts. *Br Heart J* 1995;74:615–619.

126. Loop FD, Lytle BW, Cosgrove DM, et al. Free (aorta-coronary) internal mammary artery graft: late results. *J Thorac Cardiovasc Surg* 1986;92:827–831.

127. Tector AJ, Amundsen S, Schmahl TM, et al. Total revascularization with T grafts. *Ann Thorac Surg* 1994;57:33–39.

128. Tatoulis J, Buxton BF, Fuller JR. Results of 1454 free right internal thoracic artery–coronary artery grafts. *Ann Thorac Surg* (in press).

129. Lytle BW, Blackstone EH, Loop FD, et al. Two internal thoracic artery grafts are better than one. *J Thorac Cardiovasc Surg* 1999;117:855–872.

130. Blackstone EH, Lytle BW. Competing risks after coronary bypass surgery: the influence of death on reintervention. *J Thorac Cardiovasc Surg* 2000;119:1221–1232.

131. Loop FD, Lytle BW, Cosgrove DM, et al. Sternal wound complications after isolated coronary artery bypass grafting: early and late mortality, morbidity, and cost of care. *Ann Thorac Surg* 1990;49:179–187.

132. Pym J, Brown P, Pearson M, Parker J. Right gastroepiploic-to-coronary artery bypass: the first decade of use. *Circulation* 1995;92:II45–II49.

133. Suma H, Amano A, Horii T, et al. Gastroepiploic artery graft in 400 patients. *Eur J Cardiothorac Surg* 1996;10:6–11.

134. Sato T, Isomura T, Suma H, et al. Coronary artery bypass grafting with gastroepiploic artery composite graft. *Ann Thorac Surg* 2000;69:65–69.

135. Suma H, Isomura T, Horii T, Sato T. Late angiographic result of using the right gastroepiploic artery as a graft. *J Thorac Cardiovasc Surg* 2000;120:496–498.

136. Puig LB, Ciongolli W, Cividanes GV, et al. Inferior epigastric artery as a free graft for myocardial revascularization. *J Thorac Cardiovasc Surg* 1990;99:251–255.

137. Suma H. Arterial grafts in coronary bypass surgery. *Ann Thorac Cardiovasc Surg* 1999;5:141–145.

138. Acar C, Jebara VA, Portoghese M, et al. Revival of the radial artery for coronary bypass grafting. *Ann Thorac Surg* 1992;54:652–660.

139. Parolari A, Rubini P, Alamanni F, et al. The radial artery: which place in coronary operation? *Ann Thorac Surg* 2000;69:1288–1294.

140. He T, Yang C. Comparative study on calcium channel antagonists in the human radial artery: clinical implications. *J Thorac Cardiovasc Surg* 2000;119:94–100.

141. Bond BR, Zellner JL, Dorman H, et al. Differential effects of calcium channel antagonists in the amelioration of radial artery vasospasm. *Ann Thorac Surg* 2000;69:1035–1041.

142. Reyes AT, Frame R, Brodman RF. Technique for harvesting the radial artery as a coronary artery bypass graft. *Ann Thorac Surg* 1995;59:118–126.

143. Calafiore AM, DiGiammarco G, Teodori G. Radial artery and inferior epigastric artery in composite grafts: improved midterm angiographic results. *Ann Thorac Surg* 1995;60:517–524.

144. Possati GF, Gaudino M, Alessandrini F, et al. Midterm clinical and angiographic results of radial artery grafts used for myocardial revascularization. *J Thorac Cardiovasc Surg* 1998;116:1015–1021.

145. Acar C, Ramshey A, Pagny JY, et al. The radial artery for coronary artery bypass grafting: clinical and angiographic results at five years. *J Thorac Cardiovasc Surg* 1998;116:901–909.

146. Bhan A, Gupta V, Choudhary SK, et al. Radial artery in CABG: could the early results be comparable to internal mammary artery graft? *Ann Thorac Surg* 1999;67:1631–1636.

147. Borger MA, Cohen G, Buth KJ, et al. Multiple arterial grafts. Radial versus right internal thoracic arteries. *Circulation* 1998;98:II-7–II-14.

148. Tashiro T, Nakamura K, Iwakuma A, et al. Inverted T graft: novel technique using composite radial and internal thoracic arteries. *Ann Thorac Surg* 1999;67:629–631.

149. Loop FD, Lytle BW, Cosgrove DM, et al. Reoperation for coronary atherosclerosis: changing practice in 2509 consecutive patients. *Ann Surg* 1990;212:378–386.

150. Brener SJ, Loop FD, Lytle BW, et al. A profile of candidates for repeat myocardial revascularization: implications for selection of treatment. *J Thorac Cardiovasc Surg* 1997;114:153–161.

151. Holmes DR, Garrett KN, Isner JM, et al. Effect of subintimal resection on initial outcome and restenosis for native coronary lesions and saphenous vein graft disease treated by directional coronary atherectomy—a report from the CAVEAT I and II investigators. *J Am Coll Cardiol* 1996;28:645–651.

152. de Jaegere PP, van Domburg RT, de Feyter PJ, et al. Long-term clinical outcome after stent implantation in saphenous vein grafts. *J Am Coll Cardiol* 1996;28:89–96.

153. Lefkovits J, Holmes DR, Califf RM, et al. Predictors and sequelae of distal embolization during saphenous vein graft intervention from the CAVEAT-II trial: Coronary Angioplasty Versus Excisional Atherectomy Trial. *Circulation* 1995;92:734–740.

154. Weintraub WS, Jones EL, Craver JM, et al. In-hospital and long-term outcome after reoperative coronary artery bypass graft surgery. *Circulation* 1995;92:II50–II57.

155. Lytle BW, McElroy D, McCarthy P, et al. Influence of arterial coronary bypass grafts on the mortality in coronary reoperations. *J Thorac Cardiovasc Surg* 1994;107:675–683.

156. Frazier OH, Cooley DA, Kadipasaoglu KA, et al. Myocardial revascularization with laser: preliminary findings. *Circulation* 1995;92[Suppl II]:II58–II65.

157. Burkhoff D, Schmidt S, Schulman P, et al., for the ATLANTIC Investigators. Transmyocardial laser revascu-

larisation compared with continued medical therapy for treatment of refractory angina pectoris: a prospective randomised trial. *Lancet* 1999;354:885–890.

158. Lange RA, Hills LD. Editorial. Transmyocardial laser revascularization. *N Engl J Med* 1999;341:1075–1076.

159. Aaberge L, Nordstrand K, Dragsund M, et al. Transmyocardial revascularization with CO_2 laser in patients with refractory angina pectoris. *J Am Coll Cardiol* 2000;35:1170–1177.

160. March RJ. Transmyocardial laser revascularization with the CO_2 laser: one year results of a randomized, controlled trial. *Semin Thorac Cardiovasc Surg* 1999;11:12–18.

161. Horvath KA, Cohn LH, Cooley DA, et al. Transmyocardial laser revascularization: results of a multicenter trial with transmyocardial laser revascularization used as sole therapy for end-stage coronary artery disease. *J Thorac Cardiovasc Surg* 1997;113:645–654.

162. Burns SM, Sharples LD, Tait S, et al. The transmyocardial laser revascularization international registry report. *Eur Heart J* 1999;20:31–37.

163. Hughes GC, Landolfo KP, Lowe JE, et al. Perioperative morbidity and mortality after transmyocardial laser revascularization: incidence and risk factors for adverse events. *J Am Coll Cardiol* 1999;33:1021–1026.

164. Lauer B, Junghans U, Stahl F, et al. Catheter-based percutaneous myocardial laser revascularization in patients with end-stage coronary artery disease. *J Am Coll Cardiol* 1999;34:1663–1670.

165. Allen KB, Dowling RD, DelRossi AJ, et al. Transmyocardial laser revascularization combined with coronary artery bypass grafting: a multicenter, blinded, prospective, randomized, controlled trial. *J Thorac Cardiovasc Surg* 2000;119:540–549.

166. Trehan N, Mishra M, Bapna R, et al. Transmyocardial laser revascularization combined with coronary artery bypass grafting without cardiopulmonary bypass. *Eur J Cardiothorac Surg* 1997;12:276–284.

167. Sigel JE, Abramovich CM, Lytle BW, Ratliff NB. Transmyocardial laser revascularization: three sequential autopsy cases. *J Thorac Cardiovasc Surg* 1998;115:1381–1385.

168. Chu VF, Giaid A, Kuang J, et al. Angiogenesis in transmyocardial revascularization: comparison of laser versus mechanical punctures. *Ann Thorac Surg* 1999;68:301–308.

169. Horvath KA, Chiu E, Maun DC, et al. Up-regulation of vascular endothelial growth factor mRNA and angiogenesis after transmyocardial laser revascularization. *Ann Thorac Surg* 1999;68:825–829.

170. Sinnaeve P, Varenne O, Collen D, et al. Gene therapy in the cardiovascular system: an update. *Cardiovasc Res* 1999;44:498–506.

171. Hamawy AH, Lee LY, Crystal RG, Rosengart TK. Cardiac angiogenesis and gene therapy: a strategy for myocardial revascularization. *Curr Opin Cardiol* 1999;14:515–522.

172. Losordo DW, Vale PR, Isner JM. Gene therapy for myocardial angiogenesis. *Am Heart J* 1999;138:S132–S141.

173. Rosengart TK, Lee LY, Patel SR, et al. Angiogenesis gene therapy. Phase I assessment of direct intramyocardial administration of an adenovirus vector expressing VEGF121 cDNA to individuals with clinically significant severe coronary artery disease. *Circulation* 1999;100:468–474.

174. Rosengart TK, Lee LY, Patel SR, et al. Six-month assessment of a phase I trial of angiogenic gene therapy for the treatment of coronary artery disease using direct intramyocardial administration of an adenovirus vector expressing the VEGF121 cDNA. *Ann Surg* 1999;230:466–472.

175. Symes JF, Losordo DW, Vale PR, et al. Gene therapy with vascular endothelial growth factor for inoperable coronary artery disease. *Ann Thorac Surg* 1999;68:830–837.

176. Diegeler A, Matin M, Kayser S, et al. Angiographic results after minimally invasive coronary bypass grafting using the minimally invasive direct coronary bypass grafting (MIDCAB) approach. *Eur J Cardiothorac Surg* 1999;15:680–684.

177. Cremer J, Mügge A, Wittwer T, et al. Early angiographic results after revascularization by minimally invasive direct coronary artery bypass (MIDCAB). *Eur J Cardiothorac Surg* 1999;15:383–388.

178. Diegeler A, Spyrantis N, Matin M, et al. The revival of surgical treatment for isolated proximal high grade LAD lesions by minimally invasive coronary artery bypass grafting. *Eur J Cardiothorac Surg* 2000;17:501–504.

179. Mack MJ, Magovern JA, Acuff TA, et al. Results of graft patency by immediate angiography in minimally invasive coronary artery surgery. *Ann Thorac Surg* 1999;68:383–390.

180. Mariani MA, Boonstra PW, Grandjean JG, et al. Minimally invasive coronary artery bypass grafting versus coronary angioplasty for isolated type C stenosis of the left anterior descending artery. *J Thorac Cardiovasc Surg* 1997;114:434–439.

181. Izzat MB, Yim APC, Mehta D, et al. Staged minimally invasive direct coronary artery bypass and percutaneous angioplasty for multivessel coronary artery disease. *Int J Cardiol* 1997;62:S105–S109.

182. Wittwer T, Cremer J, Boonstra P, et al. Myocardial hybrid revascularisation with minimally invasive direct coronary artery bypass grafting combined with coronary angioplasty: preliminary results of a multicentre study. *Heart* 2000;83:58–63.

183. Lewis BS, Porat E, Halon DA, et al. Same-day combined coronary angioplasty and minimally invasive coronary surgery. *Am J Cardiol* 1999;84:1246–1247.

184. Zenati M, Cohen HA, Griffith BP. Alternative approach to multivessel coronary disease with integrated coronary revascularization. *J Thorac Cardiovasc Surg* 1999;177:439–446.

185. Cohen HA, Zenati M, Smith AJC, et al. Feasibility of combined percutaneous transluminal angioplasty and minimally invasive direct coronary artery bypass in patients with multivessel coronary artery disease. *Circulation* 1998;90:1048–1050.

186. Izzat MB, Yim APC, El-Zufari MH. Minimally invasive left anterior descending coronary artery revascularisation in high-risk patients with three-vessel disease. *Ann Thorac Cardiovasc Surg* 1998;4:205–208.

187. Siebert J, Rogowski J, Jagielak D, et al. Atrial fibrillation after coronary artery bypass grafting without cardiopulmonary bypass. *Eur J Cardiothorac Surg* 2000;17:520–523.

188. Reichenspurner H, Boehm D, Detter C, et al. Economic evaluation of different minimally invasive procedures for the treatment of coronary artery disease. *Eur J Cardiothorac Surg* 1999;16:S76–S79.

189. King RC, Reece TB, Hurst JL, et al. Minimally invasive coronary artery bypass grafting decreases hospital stay and cost. *Ann Surg* 1997;225:805–811.

190. Doty JR, Fonger JD, Nicholson CF, et al. Cost analysis of current therapies for limited coronary artery revascularization. *Circulation* 1997;96[Suppl II]:II-16–II-20.

191. Gundry SR, Romano MA, Shattuck OH, et al. Seven-year follow-up of coronary artery bypasses performed with and without cardiopulmonary bypass. *J Thorac Cardiovasc Surg* 1998;115:1273–1278.

192. Puskas JD, Thourani VH, Marshall JF, et al. Clinical outcomes, angiographic patency, and resource utilization in 200 consecutive off-pump coronary bypass patients. *Ann Thorac Surg* 2001;71:1477–1483.

193. Stamou SC, Pfister AJ, Dangas G, et al. Beating heart versus conventional single-vessel reoperative coronary artery bypass. *Ann Thorac Surg* 2000;69:1383–1397.

194. Koutlas TC, Elbeery JR, Williams M, et al. Myocardial revascularization in the elderly using beating heart coronary artery bypass surgery. *Ann Thorac Surg* 2000;69:1042–1047.

195. Svennevig JL. Off-pump vs on-pump surgery. *Scand Cardiovasc J* 2000;34:7–11.

196. Ascione R, Lloyd CT, Gomes WJ, et al. Beating versus arrested heart revascularization: evaluation of myocardial function in a prospective randomized study. *Eur J Cardiothorac Surg* 1999;15:685–690.

197. Kshettry VR, Flavin TF, Emery RW, et al. Does multivessel, off-pump coronary artery bypass reduce postoperative morbidity? *Ann Thorac Surg* 2000;69:1725–1731.

198. Ascione R, Lloyd CT, Underwood MJ, et al. Inflammatory response after coronary revascularization with or without cardiopulmonary bypass. *Ann Thorac Surg* 2000;69:1198–1204.

199. Boyd WD, Desai ND, Del Rizzo DF, et al. Off-pump surgery decreases postoperative complications and resource utilization in the elderly. *Ann Thorac Surg* 1999;68:1490–1493.

200. Anderson RE, Li TQ, Hindmarsh T, et al. Increased extracellular brain water after coronary artery bypass grafting is avoided by off-pump surgery. *J Cardiothorac Vasc Anesth* 1999;13:689–702.

201. BhaskerRao B, VanHimbergen D, Edmonds Jr HL, et al. Evidence for improved cerebral function after minimally invasive bypass surgery. *J Card Surg* 1998;13:27–31.

202. Diegeler A, Hirsch R, Schneider F, et al. Neuromonitoring and neurocognitive outcome in off-pump versus conventional coronary bypass operation. *Ann Thorac Surg* 2000; 69:1162–1166.

203. Arom KV, Emery RW, Flavin TF, Petersen RJ. Cost-effectiveness of minimally invasive coronary artery bypass surgery. *Ann Thorac Surg* 1999;68:1562–1566.

204. Stamou SC, Dangas G, Hill PC, et al. Atrial fibrillation after beating heart surgery. *Am J Cardiol* 2000;86:64–67.

205. Galloway AC, Ribakove GH, Grossi EA, et al. Port-access coronary artery bypass grafting: technical considerations and results. *J Card Surg* 1998;13:281–285.

206. Galloway AC, Shemin RJ, Glower DD, et al. First report of the port access international registry. *Ann Thorac Surg* 1999;67:51–58.

207. Groh MA, Sutherland SE, Burton III HG, et al. Port-access coronary artery bypass grafting: technique and comparative results. *Ann Thorac Surg* 1999;68:1506–1508.

208. Grossi EA, Groh MA, Lefrak EA, et al. Results of a prospective multicenter study on port-access coronary bypass grafting. *Ann Thorac Surg* 1999;68:1475–1477.

209. Watson DR, Duff SB. The clinical and financial impact of port-access coronary revascularization. *Eur J Cardiothorac Surg* 1999;16[Suppl 1]:S103–S106.

210. Falk V, Diegeler A, Walther T, et al. Total endoscopic computer enhanced coronary artery bypass grafting. *Eur J Cardiothorac Surg* 2000;17:38–45.

211. Damiano Jr RJ, Ehrman WJ, Ducko CT, et al. Initial United States clinical trial of robotically assisted endoscopic coronary artery bypass grafting. *J Thorac Cardiovasc Surg* 2000;119:77–82.

212. Gundry SR, Black K, Izutani H. Sutureless coronary artery bypass with biologic glued anastomoses: preliminary in vivo and in vitro results. *J Thorac Cardiovasc Surg* 2000;120:473–477.

213. Lazar HL, Fitzgerald C, Gross S, et al. Determinants of length of stay after coronary artery bypass graft surgery. *Circulation* 1995;92[Suppl II]:II20–II24.

214. Engelman RM, Rousou JA, Flack JE, et al. Fast-track recovery of the coronary bypass patient. *Ann Thorac Surg* 1994;58:1742–1746.

215. Moulton MJ, Creswell LL, Mackey ME, et al. Reexploration for bleeding is a risk factor for adverse outcomes after cardiac operations. *J Thorac Cardiovasc Surg* 1996;111:1037–1046.

216. Hornick P, Smith PL, Taylor KM. Cerebral complications after coronary bypass grafting. *Curr Opin Cardiol* 1994;9:670–679.

217. Kronzon I, Tunick PA. Atheromatous disease of the thoracic aorta: pathologic and clinical implications. *Ann Intern Med* 1997;126:629–637.

218. Roach GW, Kanchuger M, Mangano CM, et al. Adverse cerebral outcomes after coronary bypass surgery. *N Engl J Med* 1996;335:1857–1863.

219. Aranki SF, Shaw DP, Adams DH, et al. Predictors of atrial fibrillation after coronary artery surgery: current trends and impact on hospital resources. *Circulation* 1996;94:390–397.

220. Castillo CF, Harringer W, Warshaw AL, et al. Risk factors for pancreatic cellular injury after cardiopulmonary bypass. *N Engl J Med* 1991;325:382–387.

221. Hannah EL, Kilburn H Jr, Racz M, et al. Improving the outcomes of coronary artery bypass surgery in New York State. *JAMA* 1994;271:761–766.

222. *A consumer guide in coronary artery bypass graft surgery, III: 1992 Data.* Harrisburg, PA: Pennsylvania Health Care Cost Containment Council, 1994.

223. O'Connor GT, Plume SK, Olmstead EM, et al. A regional intervention to improve the hospital mortality associated with coronary artery bypass graft surgery. *JAMA* 1996;275:841–846.

224. Omoigui MA, Miller DP, Brown KJ, et al. Outmigration for coronary bypass surgery in an era of public dissemination of clinical outcomes. *Circulation* 1996;93:27–33.

225. Ghali WA, Ash AS, Hall RE, Moskowitz MA. Statewide quality improvement initiatives and mortality after cardiac surgery. *JAMA* 1997;277:379–382.

226. Alderman EL, Fisher LD, Litwin P, et al. Results of coronary artery surgery in patients with poor left ventricular function (CASS). *Circulation* 1983;68:785–795.

227. Mock MB, Fisher L, Killip T, et al. The natural history of nonoperated patients with ischemic heart disease: the CASS experience. In: Hammermeister KE, ed. *Coronary bypass surgery: the late results.* New York: Praeger Publishers, 1983:83–97.

228. Myers WO, Schaff HV, Gersh BJ, et al. Improved survival of surgically treated patients with triple vessel coronary artery disease and severe angina pectoris: a report from the Coronary Artery Surgery Study (CASS) registry. *J Thorac Cardiovasc Surg* 1989;97:487–495.

229. Myers WO, Gersh BJ, Fisher LD, et al. Medical versus early surgical therapy in patients with triple-vessel disease and mild angina pectoris: a CASS registry study of survival. *Ann Thorac Surg* 1987;44:471–486.

230. Gersh BJ, Kronmal RA, Frye RI, et al. Coronary arteriography and coronary artery bypass surgery: morbidity and mortality in patients ages 65 years or older—a report from the Coronary Artery Surgery Study. *Circulation* 1983;67:483–491.

231. Myers WO, Schaff HV, Fisher LD, et al. Time to first new myocardial infarction in patients with severe angina and three-vessel disease comparing medical and early surgical therapy: a CASS registry study of survival. *J Thorac Cardiovasc Surg* 1988;95:382–389.

232. Rahimtoola SH, Fessler CL, Grunkemeier GL, Starr A. Survival 15 to 20 years after coronary bypass surgery for angina. *J Am Coll Cardiol* 1993;21:151–157.

233. Jones EL, Weintraub WS. Importance of completeness of revascularization during long-term followup after coronary artery surgery. *J Thorac Cardiovasc Surg* 1996;112:227–237.

234. Yusuf S, Zucker D, Peduzzi P, et al. Effect of coronary artery bypass graft surgery on survival: overview of 10-year results from randomised trials by the Coronary Artery Bypass Graft Surgery Trialists Collaboration. *Lancet* 1994;344:563–570.

235. Sergeant P, Lesaffre E, Flameng W, et al. The return of clinically evident ischemia after coronary artery bypass grafting. *Eur J Cardiothorac Surg* 1991;5:447–457.

236. Risum O, Abdelnoor M, Svennevig JL, et al. Risk factors of recurrent angina pectoris and of nonfatal myocardial infarction after coronary artery bypass surgery. *Eur J Cardiothorac Surg* 1996;10:173–188.

237. Solymoss BC, Nadeau P, Millette D, Campeau L. Late thrombosis of saphenous vein coronary bypass grafts related to risk factors. *Circulation* 1988;78[Suppl 1]:140–143.

238. Voors AA, van Brussel BL, Plokker HW, et al. Smoking and cardiac events after venous coronary bypass surgery. *Circulation* 1996;93:42–47.

239. Alderman EL, Bourassa MG, Coyhen LS, et al. Ten-year follow-up of survival and myocardial infarction in the randomized Coronary Artery Surgery Study. *Circulation* 1990;82:1629–1646.

240. Moliterno DJ, Elliott JM. Randomized trials of myocardial revascularization. *Curr Probl Cardiol* 1995;20:1–90.

241. Währborg P. Percutaneous transluminal coronary angioplasty or coronary artery bypass grafting for coronary artery disease? *Scand Cardiovasc J* 1997;31:201–211.

242. Solomon AJ, Gersh BJ. Management of chronic stable angina: medical therapy, percutaneous transluminal coronary angioplasty, and coronary artery bypass graft surgery. *Ann Int Med* 1998;128:216–223.

243. Levine GN, Ali N. The role of percutaneous revascularization in the treatment of ischemic heart disease. *Chest* 1997;112:805–821.

244. Shemin RJ. Randomized studies of coronary artery bypass grafting vs. medical or percutaneous catheter-based revascularization: a review. *Adv Card Surg* 1999;11:1–34.

245. The BARI Investigators. Seven-year outcome in the Bypass Angioplasty Revascularization Investigation (BARI) by treatment and diabetic status. *J Am Coll Cardiol* 2000;35:1122–1129.

246. Kelsey SF. Patients with diabetes did better with coronary bypass graft surgery than with percutaneous transluminal coronary angioplasty: was this BARI finding real? *Am Heart J* 1999;138:S387–S393.

247. Barsness GW, Peterson ED, Ohman EM, et al. Relationship between diabetes mellitus and long-term survival after coronary bypass and angioplasty. *Circulation* 1997;96:2551–2556.

248. O'Keefe JH, Blackstone EH, Sergeant P, et al. The optimal mode of coronary revascularization for diabetics. *Eur J Cardiothorac Surg* 1998;19:1696–1703.

249. King III SB, Kosinski AS, Guyton RA, et al., for the Emory Angioplasty Versus Surgery Trial (EAST) Investigators. Eight-year mortality in the Emory Angioplasty Versus Surgery Trial (EAST). *J Am Coll Cardiol* 2000;35:1116–1121.

250. Weintraub WS, Stein B, Kosinski A, et al. Outcome of coronary bypass surgery versus coronary angioplasty in diabetic patients with multivessel coronary artery disease. *J Am Coll Cardiol* 1998;31:10–19.

251. Detre KM, Lombardero MS, Brooks MM, et al., for the Bypass Angioplasty Revascularization Investigation Investigators. The effect of previous coronary artery bypass surgery on the prognosis of patients with diabetes who have acute myocardial infarction. *N Engl J Med* 2000;342:989–997.

252. Hlatky MA, Rogers WJ, Johnstone I, et al. Economic and quality of life outcomes after randomization to coronary angioplasty or coronary bypass surgery: a sub-study of the Bypass Angioplasty Revascularization Investigation. *N Engl J Med* 1997;336:92–99.

253. Hlatky MA, Rogers WJ, Johnstone I, et al., for the Bypass Angioplasty Revascularization Investigation (BARI) Investigators. Medical care costs and quality of life after randomization to coronary angioplasty or coronary bypass surgery. *N Engl J Med* 1997;336:92–99.

254. Hannan EL, Racz MJ, McCallister BD, et al. A comparison of three-year survival after coronary artery bypass graft surgery and percutaneous transluminal coronary angioplasty. *J Am Coll Cardiol* 1999;33:63–72.

255. Hueb WA, Bellotti G, deOliveira SA, et al. The Medicine, Angioplasty or Surgery Study (MASS): a prospective, randomized trial of medical therapy, balloon angioplasty or bypass surgery for single proximal left anterior descending artery stenoses. *J Am Coll Cardiol* 1995;26:1660–1665.

256. Goy JJ, Eeckhout E, Burnand B, et al. Coronary angioplasty versus left internal mammary artery grafting for isolated proximal left anterior descending artery stenosis. *Lancet* 1994;343:1449–1453.

257. Goy JJ, Eeckhout E, Moret C, et al. Five-year outcome in patients with isolated proximal left anterior descending coronary artery stenosis treated by angioplasty or left internal mammary artery grafting. A prospective trial. *Circulation* 1999;99:3255–3259.

258. O'Keefe Jr JH, Kreamer TR, et al. Isolated left anterior descending coronary artery disease. Percutaneous transluminal coronary angioplasty versus stenting versus left internal mammary artery bypass grafting. *Circulation* 1999;100[Suppl II]:II-114–II-118.

259. Mark DB, Nelson CL, Califf RM, et al. Continuing evolution of therapy for coronary artery disease: initial results from the era of coronary angioplasty. *Circulation* 1994;89:2015–2025.

260. Kadel C. Die Bewertung von Indikationen zur PTCA. *Herz* 1996;21:347–358.

261. Stables RH, on behalf of the SoS Trial Steering Committee and Investigators. Design of the "Stent or Surgery" trial (SoS): a randomized controlled trial to compare coronary artery bypass grafting with percutaneous transluminal coronary angioplasty and primary stent implantation in patients with multi-vessel coronary artery disease. *Semin Interv Cardiol* 1999;4:201–207.

262. Serruys PW, Unger F, van Hout BA, et al., on behalf of the ARTS study-group. The ARTS study (Arterial Revascularization Therapies Study). *Semin Interv Cardiol* 1999;4:209–219.

263. Nobuyoshi M, Kimura T. Editorial comment. Intracoronary stenting: where we are, where are we going? *Cathet Cardiovasc Diagn* 1998;43:17–18.

264. Hannan EL, Racz MJ, Arani DT, et al. A comparison of short- and long-term outcomes for balloon angioplasty and coronary stent placement. *J Am Coll Cardiol* 2000;36:395–403.

265. The EPISTENT Investigators. Randomised placebo-controlled and balloon-angioplasty-controlled trial to assess safety of coronary stenting with use of platelet glycoprotein-IIb/IIIa blockade. *Lancet* 1998;352:87–92.

266. Serruys PW, van Hout B, Bonnier H, et al., for the Benestent Study Group. Randomised comparison of implantation of heparin-coated stents with balloon angioplasty in selected patients with coronary artery disease (Benestent II). *Lancet* 1998;352:673–681.

267. Lincoff AM, Tcheng JE, Califf RM, et al., for the EPILOG Investigators. Sustained suppression of ischemic complications of coronary intervention by platelet GP IIb/IIIa blockade with abciximab: one-year outcome in the EPILOG trial. *Circulation* 1999;99:1951–1958.

268. Fuster V, Gotto AM Jr, Libby P, et al. Pathogenesis of coronary disease: the biologic role of risk factors. *J Am Coll Cardiol* 1996;27:964–976.

269. Azen SP, Mack WJ, Cashin-Hemphill L, et al. Progression of coronary artery disease predicts clinical coronary events: long-term follow-up from the Cholesterol Lowering Atherosclerosis Study. *Circulation* 1996;93:34–41.

270. Brown BG, Zhao XQ, Sacco DE, et al. Lipid lowering and plaque regression: new insights into prevention of plaque disruption and clinical events in coronary disease. *Circulation* 1993;87:1781–1791.

271. MAAS Investigators. Effect of simvastatin on coronary atheroma: the Multicentre Antiatheroma Study (MAAS). *Lancet* 1994;344:633–638.

272. Superko HR, Kraus RM. Coronary artery disease regression. Convincing evidence for the benefit of aggressive lipoprotein management. *Circulation* 1994;90:1056–1069.

273. Brown G, Albers JJ, Fisher LD, et al. Regression of coronary artery disease as a result of intensive lipid-lowering therapy in men with high levels of apolipoprotein B. *N Engl J Med* 1990;323:1289–1298.

274. Law MR, Wald NJ, Thompson SG. By how much and how quickly does reduction in serum cholesterol concentration lower risk of ischaemic heart disease? *BMJ* 1994;308:367–372.

275. Law MR, Wald NJ, Thompson SG. Systemic underestimation of association between serum cholesterol concentration and ischaemic heart disease in observational studies: data from the BUPA study. *BMJ* 1994;308:363–366.

276. Scandinavian Simvastatin Survival Study Group. Randomised trial of cholesterol lowering in 4444 patients with coronary heart disease: the Scandinavian Simvastatin Survival Study (4S). *Lancet* 1994;344:1383–1389.

277. Sacks FM, Pfeffer MA, Moye LA, et al. The effect of pravastatin on coronary events after myocardial infarction in patients with average cholesterol levels. *N Engl J Med* 1996;335:1001–1009.

278. Post Coronary Artery Bypass Graft Trial Investigators. The effect of aggressive lowering of low-density lipoproteins and cholesterol levels and low-dose anticoagulation on obstructive changes in saphenous-vein coronary-artery bypass grafts. *N Engl J Med* 1997;336:153–162.

279. Cummings SR, Rubin SM, Oster G. The cost-effectiveness of counseling smokers to quit. *JAMA* 1989;261:75–79.

RESTENOSIS: EPIDEMIOLOGY AND TREATMENT

DAVID J. MOLITERNO
ERIC J. TOPOL

OVERVIEW

Percutaneous coronary revascularization is an increasingly attractive alternative to medical therapy and surgical revascularization for coronary artery disease. The leading drawback continues to be the occurrence of restenosis within 6 months. The epidemiology of restenosis after balloon angioplasty has been studied in many clinical trials, and several predictors of restenosis have been consistently identified: diabetes mellitus, unstable angina, preprocedural and postprocedural minimum lumen diameter, chronic occlusions, lesion length, reference vessel diameter, ostial

stenoses, and lesions in saphenous vein grafts. The mechanisms of restenosis include a combination of vessel recoil, vascular remodeling, thrombus transformation, and neointimal proliferation. As indicated by intravascular ultrasonography, remodeling is the predominant mechanism after balloon angioplasty and neointimal hyperplasia dominates in in-stent restenosis. Substantial progress has been made over the past 5 years in lowering the rate of restenosis as vessel recoil and remodeling have been nearly eliminated by the use of intracoronary stents.

Restenosis occurs in one-fourth to one-third of patients within 3 to 6 months of percutaneous revascularization. Most patients with restenosis have symptom recurrence, whereas the minority have silent restenosis, and myocardial infarction is rare. Symptom status alone has weak predictive value for stenosis recurrence, so the optimal method of evaluation is stress myocardial imaging studies. For prophylaxis

D. J. Moliterno: Department of Cardiovascular Medicine, The Cleveland Clinic, Cleveland, Ohio

E. J. Topol: Department of Cardiovascular Medicine, The Cleveland Clinic Foundation, Cleveland, Ohio

of restenosis, numerous pharmacologic therapies, including antithrombotics, vasodilators, lipid-lowering agents, and growth factor inhibitors, have been tested but have failed. Likewise, use of several atherectomy catheters (rotational, directional, laser) has been studied, again without consistent improvement noted in the occurrence of restenosis.

Now stents are commonly used to safely maximize post-procedural lumen diameter and decrease the incidence of angiographically identified restenosis and the need for target vessel revascularization. Compared to balloon angioplasty, intracoronary stent placement has been shown to improve the rate of restenosis in nearly all patients and for nearly all lesion subsets. On the other hand, a new disorder, in-stent restenosis, has been created, although it is less common than restenosis after balloon angioplasty. The neointimal proliferation produced by stents has required the development of agents, techniques, and equipment to address it when vessel renarrowing occurs. Radiation and cell-cycle inhibitors hold the current promise in treating in-stent restenosis.

HISTORICAL PERSPECTIVE

As percutaneous coronary revascularization has evolved over the past 25 years, it has become an increasingly attractive alternative to medical therapy and surgical revascularization for coronary artery disease. During this time most of the advancement in the field of interventional cardiology has been to make the procedure safer and more immediately successful while expanding the treatment to progressively more complex coronary arterial lesions. The leading drawback to percutaneous coronary intervention (PCI) has been and continues to be the recurrence of stenosis within 6 months, or restenosis. Among the first 169 patients in whom percutaneous transluminal coronary angioplasty (PTCA, balloon angioplasty) was performed by Gruentzig in Zurich, 31% of those undergoing repeat angiography at 6 months were noted to have recurrence of stenosis (1).

Currently, well over 1 million percutaneous coronary interventions are performed each year throughout the world (2–5). The majority of these procedures is performed in the United States and Western Europe, and the rate on both sides of the Atlantic continues to nearly double every 5 to 8 years (Fig. 83.1). Of these angioplasty cases, approximately one-fourth involve lesions previously treated by PCI. In the United States alone, restenosis still occurs in approximately 150,000 patients annually, which translates into over $3 billion of medical expenditures (6). With an increasing number of PCI procedures performed each year, the absolute number of patients who will be affected by restenosis will rise until successful treatments to prevent restenosis are discovered and implemented.

Historically, early reports of restenosis showed a broad range in the incidence and prevalence of restenosis. This

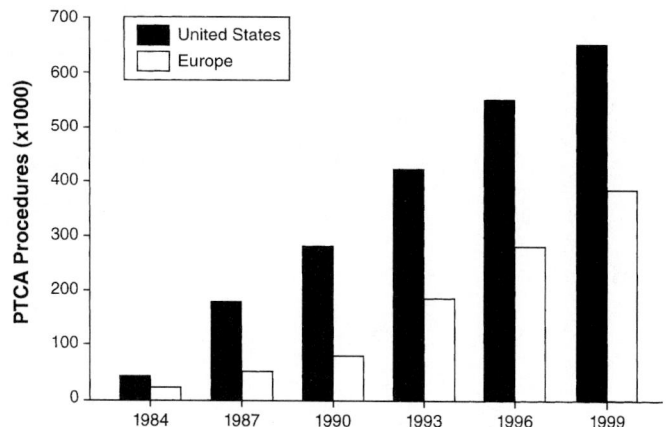

FIGURE 83.1 The number of percutaneous revascularization procedures performed in Europe and the United States has steadily increased over time, and well over 1 million procedures are now carried out each year worldwide. PTCA, percutaneous transluminal coronary angioplasty. (Data from Gruentzig AR, King SD, Schlumpf M, et al. Long-term follow-up after percutaneous transluminal coronary angioplasty: the early Zurich experience. *N Engl J Med* 1987;316:1127–1132; Bittl JA. Advances in coronary angioplasty. *N Engl J Med* 1996;335:1290–1302; Windecker S, Maier-Rudolph W, Bonzel T, et al. Interventional cardiology in Europe 1995. *Eur Heart J* 1999;20:484–495; and American Heart Association. 2001 heart and stroke statistical update. Available at: http://www.americanheart.org/statistics/index.html. Accessed September 4, 2001.)

occurred because a number of arbitrary definitions existed for angiographically determined restenosis, and many early clinical studies were small and their results were confounded by problems of incomplete revascularization, withdrawal bias, and limited follow-up. Finally, the technique and technology of percutaneous revascularization have continually evolved, which perhaps limits assessments of restenosis to snapshots in time, rather than providing a dynamic perspective. This chapter reviews issues involved in the epidemiology of restenosis and contemporary efforts to prevent restenosis after coronary intervention.

PATHOPHYSIOLOGY

The response of the vessel to coronary interventions is complex (Figs. 83.2 and 83.3) (7)—with injury to the intima and media likely occurring in all patients during angioplasty, even if to a small extent—and is detailed in Chapter 105 (8). Briefly, restenosis can be broadly divided into three interrelated facets: vessel wall recoil and remodeling, thrombus formation and organization, and neointimal growth. Studies report that many patients (15% to 65%) have a 10% or greater increase in the diameter of stenosis within 2 days of balloon angioplasty (9–14), and some patients (10%) have a substantial early renarrowing (more than 50% acute loss) (10). This vessel wall recoil may represent elastic rebound of the arterial wall or plaque, abnormal vasoconstriction, the presence of a thrombus, or a combi-

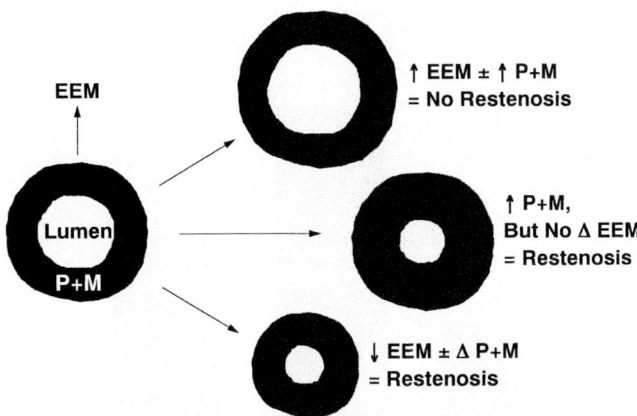

FIGURE 83.2 Restenosis can occur by several interrelated mechanisms. As shown in the schematic of the "doughnut and the hole," neointimal proliferation can decrease lumen area by increasing the plaque plus media (P+M) cross-sectional area. If the overall vessel area (external elastic membrane, or EEM) increases adequately (compensatory arterial dilatation or favorable arterial remodeling), no restenosis will occur. Alternatively, if (a) neointimal growth is excessive, (b) arterial remodeling is inadequate, or (c) negative arterial remodeling (arterial contracture) occurs, then restenosis ensues. ↑, increase; ↓, decrease; Δ, change. (Adapted from Mintz G, Popma J, Pichard A, et al. Arterial remodeling after coronary angioplasty: a serial intravascular ultrasound study. *Circulation* 1996;94:35–43, with permission.)

nation of these factors. Regardless of the underlying mechanism, this very early vessel wall response affects the likelihood of subsequent restenosis. Vessel wall remodeling also occurs over the long term, and the vessel may adaptively enlarge (positive remodeling) in response to atherosclerosis or may shrink (negative remodeling) in response to the trauma of angioplasty (Fig. 83.2) (15–17). ▼ o23

Presentation of Restenosis

The interrelated mechanisms of restenosis can translate into an anatomically or physiologically important stenosis recurrence. Depending on the predominant mechanism and its severity, as well as on characteristics of the index lesion, the timing and presentation of symptoms may vary. Restenosis can be categorized or defined angiographically or clinically, or it may be silent (asymptomatic).

Timing

Three events may occur after angioplasty that can produce symptom recurrence referable to the treated lesion. The first, elastic recoil, occurs within minutes to hours after PTCA but usually does not cause symptoms. The second, abrupt vessel closure, occurs minutes to days after angioplasty in several percent of patients and produces recurrent angina or acute infarction. Finally, over the weeks to months after PTCA, restenosis due to neointimal growth and remodeling may occur. To study the time course of restenosis, Nobuyoshi and colleagues performed sequential angiography in

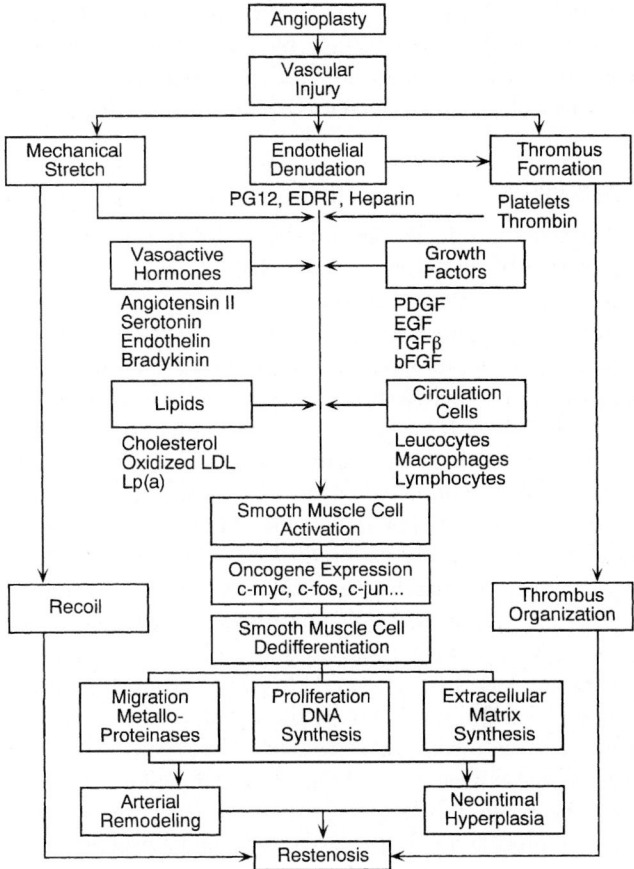

FIGURE 83.3 Pathophysiologic mechanisms of restenosis after percutaneous revascularization. After balloon angioplasty, recoil occurs followed by activation of growth factors and smooth muscle cell proliferation. These lead to vessel contracture or negative remodeling in some patients. After intracoronary stent placement, the majority of lumen loss is from neointimal hyperplasia. In most cases, the mechanisms of restenosis are likely interrelated. bFGF, basic fibroblast growth factor; EDRF, endothelium-derived relaxing factor; EGF, epidermal growth factor; LDL, low-density lipoprotein; Lp(a), lipoprotein(a); PDGF, platelet-derived growth factor; PGI₂, prostacyclin; TGF-β, transforming growth factor-β.

229 patients at 24 hours, 1 month, 3 months, 6 months, and 1 year after balloon angioplasty (10). An appreciable loss (more than 0.5 mm) in lumen diameter was detected in 15% of patients at 24 hours, consistent with lesion recoil or thrombus formation. In approximately one-half of these patients, the loss proceeded to restenosis. In the interval from 1 day to 1 month, most lesions remained unchanged or regressed, with a mean improvement in lumen diameter. During this same period, few patients (12%) were classified as having restenosis. The actuarial patient rate of restenosis increased markedly (from 12% to 43%) between 1 and 3 months, and increased only modestly thereafter (*e*Fig. 83.3.3A). This and other studies using serial angiography (*e*Fig. 83.3.3B) (37) make it evident that the majority of restenosis occurs within the first 3 months after balloon angioplasty and that restenosis after 3 to 6 months is rare

(10,38,39). The time course for restenosis after intracoronary stent implantation is later by 1 to 3 months. Regardless, most patients who are free of restenosis at 6 to 8 months will have continued success for the index lesion.

Symptoms

Because restenotic lesions usually develop gradually, the recurrence of symptoms or inducible ischemia also occurs gradually over weeks to months. Although soft *de novo* lesions may rupture abruptly, causing vessel occlusion, infarction, and in some cases death, fibromuscular restenotic lesions rarely present as acute infarction (2% or fewer cases) or death (1% or fewer cases) (40–42). Rather, the majority of patients with symptomatic restenosis experience the return of their typical angina or its equivalent. The safety of restenosis was seen even among angioplasty patients at high risk for ischemic events in the Evaluation of Chimeric Monoclonal 7E3 for the Prevention of Ischemic Complications (EPIC) trial (43). At 6-month follow-up, of the 549 patients who received placebo and had no clinical event during the first 30 days, only 2.0% had myocardial infarction and 1.7% died. Although these data are from patients both with and without restenosis, Weintraub et al. (44) have reported similar results among 3,363 patients followed for 6 years. In this large cohort, those with and without angiographically identified restenosis had an annual rate of death of approximately 1.0%, and the annual rate of myocardial infarction was 2.5% and 2.0% for these groups, respectively. Among all patients undergoing intracoronary stent placement, approximately 2% die between 30 days and 1 year (45,46). ▼ o24

Angiographically Identified Restenosis

Beyond furnishing an estimate of percent diameter stenosis, quantitative angiography is able to provide a number of indices related to the MLD of the coronary lumen. [▼ o25] These indices (Fig. 83.4) can be helpful in understanding the mechanics of restenosis and the effect of different technologies on restenosis. The immediate gain in MLD is simply the final postprocedural MLD obtained with percutaneous revascularization minus the preprocedural MLD. Immediate gain is usually smallest for balloon angioplasty (0.7 to 1.0 mm), intermediate for rotational atherectomy (1.0 to 1.5 mm) and directional atherectomy (1.5 to 2.0 mm), and largest for intracoronary stent placement (1.5 to 2.5 mm). The late loss is the MLD at follow-up angiography minus the final postprocedural MLD. Late loss is proportional to immediate gain, so that it is greatest after stent placement and directional atherectomy, and least after balloon angioplasty. This device "taxing" is a result of the marked reparative response of the vessel wall (i.e., aggressive neointimal proliferation) to deep injury or need for extensive reendothelialization. The net gain is the follow-up MLD minus the preprocedural MLD. Because the

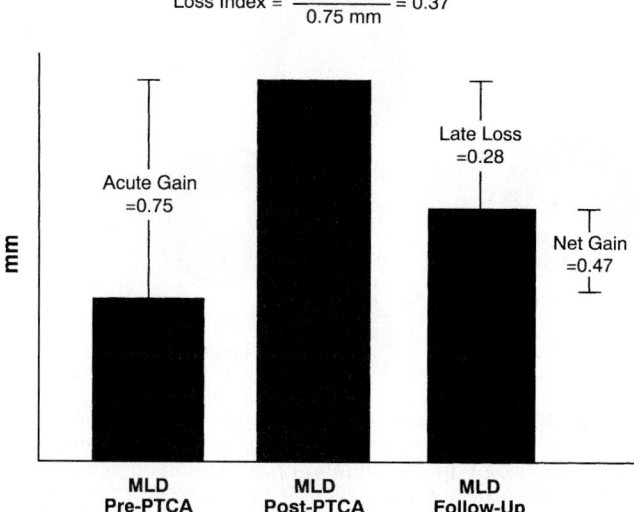

FIGURE 83.4 Indices measured and calculated during serial quantitative coronary angiography. The immediate gain is the change in minimum lumen diameter (MLD) from baseline to immediately after angioplasty. The late loss is the measured difference between the immediately postprocedure MLD and that measured at 6-month follow-up. Net gain is the difference between the follow-up MLD and the baseline MLD (immediate gain minus late loss). The loss index or "tax rate" refers to the fraction or percentage of early gain that is ultimately lost (late loss minute immediate gain). PTCA, percutaneous transluminal coronary angioplasty.

immediate gain is so large with intracoronary stents and the late loss is moderate, the net gain is greatest with stents (approximately 1 mm). In limited series directional atherectomy has shown a net gain similar to stent placement, although in other studies has demonstrated a net gain only slightly better than that with balloon angioplasty. Balloon angioplasty and rotational and laser atherectomy usually result in a similarly moderate net gain. Finally, an important concept is the loss index, which is the late loss divided by the immediate gain and represents a "device taxing" for restenosis. The loss index is higher for new device technologies than for balloon angioplasty but may be intermediate for stents (Fig. 83.5, *e*Table 83.0.2) (45,67–77). If indeed the loss index is similar for different technologies and levels of aggressiveness that achieve the largest immediate gain, the theory that obtaining the largest lumen possible will give the best long-term result might hold true. This theory, called "bigger is better," has been advanced and is discussed in the section on Procedure-Related Factors.

When data are pooled from 15 clinical trials (70,71,73,78–89) that defined restenosis as stenosis of 50% of luminal diameter or more and included a total of over 8,000 patients (Table 83.1), the rate of angiographically determined restenosis is found to average 40% with routine balloon angioplasty. The highest reported restenosis rate in this group (53%) is from the Coronary Angioplasty Versus Excisional Atherectomy Trial (CAVEAT), in which the angiographic core laboratory reported data from

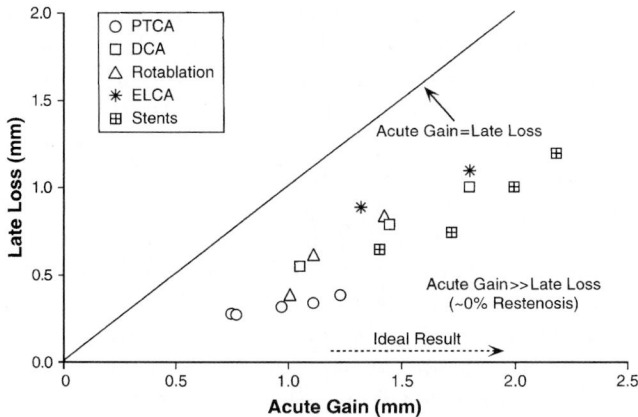

FIGURE 83.5 The loss index for angioplasty and new device technologies is represented as the relationship of late loss to immediate gain. Balloon angioplasty has the lowest loss index but produces a relatively smaller immediate gain. New technologies such as atherectomy produce a large immediate gain but have the highest loss index. Intracoronary stents also produce a large immediate gain with an intermediate loss index and, thus, a more favorable restenosis rate. The ideal revascularization procedure would produce a large immediate gain and have a low loss index. (Data are from eTable 83.0.2.) DCA, directional coronary atherectomy; ELCA, excimer laser coronary angioplasty; PTCA, percutaneous transluminal coronary angioplasty.

the angiographic view demonstrating the severest stenosis, that is, the "worst view" method. Other angiographic trials have used the average of stenosis severity from several views, and this may artifactually lower the reported rate of angiographically identified restenosis. Also, more recent studies using more aggressive angioplasty techniques to obtain an optimally large final lumen diameter and relying on stenting in the case of important dissections report the lowest angiographically determined restenosis rates. The Balloon versus Optimal Atherectomy Trial (BOAT) (87) was conducted 3 years after CAVEAT and compared directional coronary atherectomy to PTCA using a more aggressive approach for both techniques. In the PTCA group, the final residual stenosis was 28%, compared to 36% in CAVEAT. Restenosis in the BOAT angioplasty cohort was 25% lower than that in CAVEAT (40% vs. 53%), and a substantial number of BOAT patients required intracoronary stents. Similarly, the Belgian-Netherlands Stent II (BENESTENT-II) trial (90) reported the lowest rate of angiographically determined restenosis for balloon angioplasty of any large-scale trial, nearly 35% lower than reported in the Belgian-Netherlands Stent I (BENESTENT-

TABLE 83.1 RATES OF ANGIOGRAPHICALLY IDENTIFIED RESTENOSIS

Study	Year	n	Treatment	6-Month restenosis rate (%)
Balloon angioplasty				
Raizner et al. (78)	1988	539	Prostacyclin	47
Schwartz et al. (79)	1988	625	ASA-dipyridamole	39
Ellis et al. (80)	1989	416	Intravenous heparin sodium	39
M-HEART (81)	1990	1,235	Corticosteroid	43
Franzen et al. (82)	1990	329	Fish oil	35
Knudtson et al. (83)	1990	494	Prostacyclin	30
CAVEAT (73)	1993	500	PTCA vs. DCA	57
BENESTENT (71)	1994	257	PTCA vs. stent	32
STRESS (70)	1994	202	PTCA vs. stent	42
Weintraub et al. (84)	1994	404	Lovastatin	41
MHEART II (85)	1995	752	Thromboxane antagonist	45
MARCATOR (86)	1995	1,436	Cilazapril	36
BOAT (87)	1996	492	PTCA vs. DCA	40
BENESTENT-II (88)	1996	410	PTCA vs. stent	21
START (89)	1999	223	PTCA vs. stent	37
Pooled		*8,314*		*40*
Intracoronary stent				
BENESTENT (71)	1994	259	PTCA vs. stent	22
STRESS (70)	1994	205	PTCA vs. stent	32
BENESTENT-II (88)	1998	413	PTCA vs. stent	16
START (89)	1999	229	PTCA vs. stent	22
CrossFlex (91)	1999	209	PTCA vs. stent	16
Kastrati et al. (92)	2000	731	Gold vs. steel Inflow stent	44
ASCENT (93)	2001	1,040	Multi-Link vs. Palmaz-Schatz stent	19
vom Dahl et al. (94)	2001	204	Gold vs. steel Inflow stent	30
NIRVANA (95)	2001	849	NIR vs. Palmaz-Schatz stent	21
Pooled		*4,139*		*25*

ASA, aspirin; ASCENT, ACS MultiLink Stent Clinical Equivalence in *De Novo* Lesions Trial; BENESTENT, Belgian-Netherlands Stent trial; BOAT, Balloon versus Optimal Atherectomy Trial; CAVEAT, Coronary Angioplasty Versus Excisional Atherectomy Trial; DCA, directional coronary atherectomy; MARCATOR, Multicenter American Research Trial with Cilazapril after Angioplasty to Prevent Transluminal Coronary Obstruction and Restenosis; M-HEART, Multi-Hospital Eastern Atlantic Restenosis Trial; NIRVANA, NIR Vascular Advanced North American Trial; PTCA, percutaneous transluminal coronary angioplasty; START, [90]Sr Treatment of Angiographic Restenosis Trial; STRESS, Stent Restenosis Study.

I) trial (21% vs. 32%) (71). This is likely attributable to more aggressive balloon dilation.

When data are pooled from many trials studying intracoronary stents (70,71,88,89,91–95) (Table 83.1), the average 6-month angiographically determined restenosis rate is 25%. These data encompass both early and more contemporary stent designs. Early stent trial data were from studies used to approve the stent design. Because of this, cases were selected and the target lesions were "ideal" for stent placement. A more recent large study reported by Kastrati and colleagues examined 2,944 consecutively treated patients divided into subgroups with simple and complex coronary lesions. Among those with simple lesions (n = 898), the rate of angiographically determined restenosis was 25%, whereas among those with complex lesions (rated B2 and C according to the classification system of the American College of Cardiology and American Heart Association; n = 2,046), the restenosis rate was 33% (45).

Clinically Apparent Restenosis

Restenosis occurs to some extent in all individuals after coronary interventions. Given that the extent of angiographic renarrowing after balloon angioplasty follows a near normal (gaussian) distribution (*e*Fig. 83.5.1) (38,68), all angiographic definitions of restenosis are arbitrary unless they are linked to physiologic or clinically relevant parameters. The clinical return of a significant coronary stenosis most often presents as recurrent angina or a positive result on a stress test. The range of reported rates for chest pain recurrence within 6 months after angioplasty is vast: 25% to 93% (40,96), with an average rate of approximately 50% from pooled data (56). When combined with results of angiographic follow-up, this clinical information becomes difficult to interpret. The proportion of patients presenting with recurrent chest pain who have restenosis demonstrable at angiography ranges from 48% to 92% (56). The average positive predictive value of symptoms alone, therefore, is approximately 60%.

Because symptoms are a weak end point or marker of restenosis, "clinical" restenosis could be defined as a clinically serious cardiac event likely related to restenosis. This would include myocardial infarction, cardiac-related death, or revascularization of the target vessel by repeat percutaneous intervention or bypass surgery. Broader definitions of clinical restenosis include a positive stress test result in the territory of the target vessel. Most contemporary clinical PCI trials use a composite end point including target vessel revascularization, myocardial infarction, and death. For example, in the placebo group in the EPIC trial, the late (1- to 6-month) rate of repeat revascularization (18.4%), when hierarchically combined with the rates for myocardial infarction (2.4%) and death (1.8%), produced a composite clinical event rate of approximately 20%. This rate increased to 35% when early postangioplasty events (1 month or less), which are likely related to poor initial outcome rather than restenosis,

were included. This same composite rate from immediately postprocedure to 6-month follow-up for the placebo cohort in the Evaluation of PTCA to Improve Long-term Outcomes by c7E3 Glycoprotein Receptor Blockade (EPILOG) trial (97) was 26%. This one-fourth reduction in overall clinically apparent restenosis between the EPIC and EPILOG trials is reflected by an 18% lower target vessel revascularization in EPILOG (Fig. 83.6) and likely indicates a more aggressive revascularization strategy because 14% of the placebo group required intracoronary stents to be placed. More recently, the Evaluation of Platelet IIb/IIIa Inhibitor for Stenting Trial (EPISTENT) reported an approximately 10% rate of target vessel revascularization among patients receiving an intracoronary stent (i.e., roughly half of the patients in the EPIC trial). This reemphasizes the continued change in rates of clinically apparent restenosis in contemporary practice with more aggressive percutaneous revascularization strategies. Thus, given the different ways of estimating clinical restenosis, reported rates in some studies may be as low as 10% if only target vessel revascularization is considered, 30% if all ischemic and revascularization events are considered, or over 50% if any chest pain recurrence is included.

NONINVASIVE METHODS FOR CLINICAL EVALUATION OF RESTENOSIS

Because the presence of symptoms is an unreliable marker for restenosis after angioplasty, results of noninvasive cardiac stress tests have been studied by a number of investigators. The attractions of noninvasive tests over repeat angiography include a more favorable procedural cost, time requirement, and risk. When reviewing trials assessing restenosis, one should remember that, to study the accuracy of noninvasive testing, a high percentage of follow-up angiograms are needed to avoid selection bias. In addition, as newer noninvasive modalities have been developed over the past decade that have improved sensitivity and specificity for detecting myocardial ischemia, the angioplasty cases being undertaken have become more complex and often involve multivessel disease, so that the possibility arises of incomplete revascularization or multiple potential sites of restenosis. Early in the evolution of coronary angioplasty, many patients were followed by routine treadmill testing. This test was soon coupled with nuclear scintigraphy, stress echocardiography, or positron emission tomography (PET).

Additional Noninvasive Methods

Several additional nuclear and nonnuclear imaging modalities, such as PET, isonitrile imaging, and stress echocardiography, have been studied more recently to determine their predictive ability for restenosis. Each of these modalities provides unique information or benefit. For example, by using different isotopes, PET studies can quantitate regional myocardial metabo-

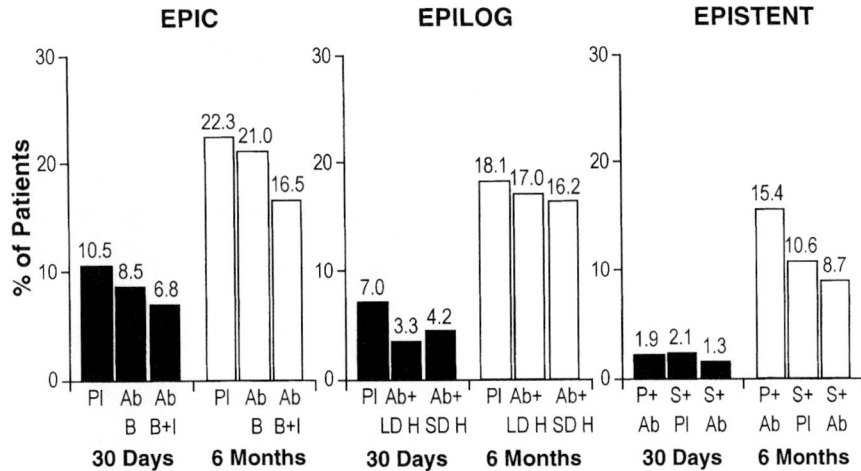

FIGURE 83.6 Target vessel revascularizations (urgent and nonurgent) performed by 30 days and by 6 months in the Evaluation of Chimeric Monoclonal 7E3 for the Prevention of Ischemic Complications (EPIC) trial, the Evaluation of PTCA to Improve Long-term Outcomes by c7E3 Glycoprotein Receptor Blockade (EPILOG) trial, and the Evaluation of Platelet IIb/IIIa Inhibitor for Stenting Trial (EPISTENT). The EPILOG trial, which involved many of the same investigators as the EPIC trial, showed a reduced occurrence in target vessel revascularization compared with the latter. This may be due to evolution of a more aggressive angioplasty technique with bail-out stenting when needed. Likewise, a further reduction in target vessel revascularization was seen in EPISTENT with routine use of intracoronary stents. Ab, abciximab; B, bolus; B+I, bolus plus infusion; LD H, low-dose heparin; P, percutaneous transluminal coronary angioplasty; Pl, placebo; S, stent; SD H, standard-dose heparin.

lism as well as perfusion, whereas isonitrile imaging or stress echocardiography can provide assessment of myocardial perfusion and wall motion. Several studies of exercise or pharmacologic stress echocardiography have been completed (106,112–115). Using supine bicycle stress echocardiography to detect restenosis in 80 patients with 129 treated sites, Hecht et al. (113) reported a sensitivity and specificity of 87% and 95%, respectively, for this test. This high sensitivity may be due, in part, to the high rate of restenosis (56%) and incomplete revascularization (32%) among patients in the study group. Overall, the positive predictive value and negative predictive value for stress echocardiography in over 500 patients are 84% and 76%, respectively (*e*Table 83.1.3).

In summary, the predictive accuracy of symptom occurrence for restenosis is, at best, moderate and is not significantly improved by the use of exercise electrocardiography. The addition of imaging by nuclear scintigraphy or echocardiography increases both the positive and negative predictive value of testing to approximately 80%. SPECT imaging with thallium or technetium-99m sestamibi have respectably high accuracy, and more recent data show stress echocardiography to be similarly accurate. These are the leading choices for noninvasive assessment of restenosis. Testing is most reliable between 1 and 5 months after revascularization.

CLINICAL PROFILE

Although no favorable variable has been identified that assures freedom from restenosis, and none has been identi-

fied that makes restenosis inevitable, several factors clearly influence the likelihood of restenosis. A large number of clinical, anatomic, and procedural variables have been associated with restenosis in various studies. Many of these observations, however, were from retrospective or small prospective studies, so some findings have been inconsistent. Large pharmacologic or device trials with high rates of angiographic follow-up have been most helpful. Importantly, many factors that were shown to be associated with restenosis after balloon angioplasty are no longer predictive of restenosis in the stent era. Table 83.2 lists factors reported to be associated with restenosis. Factors that have been independent predictors in multivariable modeling or consistently associated in many balloon angioplasty studies are printed in italics, as are similar factors for stent procedures. Factors associated with stenosis recurrence can be categorized as related to the patient, to the lesion, or to the procedure.

Patient-Related Factors

Patient characteristics (e.g., age, race, gender, etc.) obviously have the same effect for all coronary lesions within the given individual. Weintraub et al. (117) showed that the leading predictor of restenosis for a particular lesion among patients undergoing multisite angioplasty was the occurrence of restenosis at the other treated sites. The list of patient-related variables considered in predictive models of restenosis is extensive and includes demographic characteristics, medications, concomitant medical diseases, serologic

TABLE 83.2 CHARACTERISTICS ASSOCIATED WITH RESTENOSIS

After balloon angioplasty[a]	After stent placement
Patient characteristics	
ACE-D genotype	ACE-D genotype
Advanced age	Arterial hypertension
Diabetes mellitus	*Diabetes mellitus*
End-stage renal disease	Prior restenosis
Hypercholesterolemia	Tobacco use
Male gender	
Multivessel coronary artery disease	
Prior myocardial infarction	
Tobacco use	
Unstable angina	
Variant angina	
Lesion characteristics	
Angle >45 degrees	*Baseline percentage stenosis or MLD*
Balloon to artery ratio	
Baseline percentage stenosis or MLD	Chronic total occlusions
Bifurcation stenosis	*Long lesions*
Calcification	*Vessel diameter*
Chronic total occlusions	Saphenous vein grafts
Collateral vessels	
Location in left anterior descending artery	
Long length	
Ostial location	
Proximal location	
Recurrence in <3 mo	
Saphenous vein grafts	
Thrombus	
Vessel diameter	
Procedural characteristics	
Abrupt closure	Multiple stents
Balloon inflation time	*Final percentage stenosis or MLD*
Dissection	
Final percentage stenosis or MLD	Stent design
	Stent material (gold)
Residual gradient	Lumen cross-sectional area

MLD, minimal lumen diameter.
Note: Factors listed in italics are those that have been consistently reported to be associated with restenosis or were independent predictors in large-scale reports.
[a]Includes nonstent cases such as atherectomy followed by balloon angioplasty.

markers, and genetic polymorphisms. Large-scale clinical trials of restenosis have not revealed any consistent age-, race-, or gender-related patterns. At this time, only two patient-related risk factors have certain effects on restenosis: diabetes mellitus and unstable angina pectoris.

Diabetes Mellitus

Just as diabetes is a strong risk factor for atherosclerotic heart disease, with insulin dependency producing a higher risk, so too is diabetes an important risk factor for restenosis. This association was found first in early NHLBI PTCA Registry data (47), and a series of subsequent reports (120–122) demonstrated the relative risk of restenosis among patients with diabetes to be approximately 1.3 compared with that of patients without diabetes. Although the exact degree of risk for patient groups with type I and type II diabetes is uncertain, several studies have shown insulin-dependent diabetes to be associated more often with restenosis (123,124). Other investigations have examined this association with restenosis by studying glycosylated hemoglobin levels, insulin levels, or microalbuminuria. Regardless, the mechanisms leading to restenosis among diabetic patients are multiple (125–144) (Table 83.3) and vary in effect between those with type I and type II diabetes and among patients with type II diabetes depending on insulin use (145,146). High glucose concentrations and the presence of advanced glycosylation end products inhibit endothelial cell function in several ways, including by decreasing production of endothelium-derived relaxing factor and prostacyclin, and by retarding cellular replication during reendothelialization (Table 83.3). Because the process of endothelial cell regeneration at the site of vessel wall injury is slowed, the triggers of intimal hyperplasia linger, which may explain the greater neoproliferative response of diabetic patients (124,147). In an animal model of restenosis, Van Belle et al. demonstrated a reduction of in-stent intimal formation and restenosis by accelerating endothelialization with local delivery of vascular endothelial growth factor (148).

Platelets are known to exist more frequently in an activated state in diabetic patients despite clinical absence of vascular inflammation or injury (137). Similarly, in patients with diabetes, platelets have been shown to be more adhesive and aggregable when stimulated. These and other

TABLE 83.3 POSSIBLE MECHANISMS BY WHICH DIABETES AFFECTS RESTENOSIS

Endothelial dysfunction
↓ Endothelium-derived relaxing factor (EDRF) (131,144)
↓ Prostacyclin (133,138)
↓ Endothelial cell replication (134,140)
↑ Endothelin-1 production (126,135)
↑ Platelet-derived growth factor (PDGF) (128)
Heightened platelet activity
↑ Number of activated platelets (137)
↑ Platelet adhesiveness (141)
↑ Platelet aggregability (140)
↑ Thromboxane A_2 synthesis (139,140)
↑ PDGF (140)
↑ Fibrinogen levels (132)
Increased growth factors
↓ EDRF (125,136)
↑ PDGF (142)
↑ Insulin-like growth factor-1 (129,130)
↑ Endothelin-1 (125)
↑ Fibroblast growth factor (127)
↑ Transforming growth factor-β (143)

↑, increasing; ↓, decreasing.

hypercoagulable features of diabetic patients (Table 83.3) likely contribute to the restenosis process. Finally, the endothelial and platelet abnormalities of diabetic patients allow growth factor promotion. The normally functioning endothelium and platelets serve to inhibit or suppress medial smooth muscle cell growth, and derangements in these systems enhance expression of mitogens such as PDGF, TGF-β, and bFGF (Table 83.3). Because of these multiple mechanisms leading to restenosis, the contemporary approach to treating patients with diabetes is aggressive.

The NHLBI presented a national health alert based on the findings of the Bypass Angioplasty Revascularization Investigation (BARI) study (149) showing patients with diabetes to have a worse 5-year survival rate after multivessel angioplasty than after bypass surgery (66% vs. 81%), perhaps in part due to late or silent restenosis. On the other hand, the survival curves for diabetic patients treated by angioplasty or bypass surgery in BARI separate slowly over a several-year period, so that restenosis is unlikely to be a primary explanation for the survival difference. A survival difference between diabetic patients undergoing percutaneous revascularization and those undergoing surgical revascularization has not been reported by any other prospective clinical trial (150) nor was this observed in the BARI registry of approximately 2,000 patients. A multicenter database encompassing nearly 16,000 patients undergoing a first revascularization also showed patients with diabetes to have a worse outcome after angioplasty than after bypass surgery, but on multivariable analysis of survival, no interaction of revascularization type and diabetes was present (151). Beyond balloon angioplasty, studies of directional, rotational, and laser atherectomy have shown diabetic patients to experience restenosis more often than nondiabetic patients.

The use of intracoronary stents has not ameliorated the effect of diabetes on restenosis. Combined data from four separate reports including nearly 3,300 patients (123,152–154) showed that angiographically identified restenosis occurred in 35% of diabetic patients and 23% of nondiabetic patients when contemporary stenting methods were used. Patients with diabetes were also more likely to undergo target vessel revascularization by 6-month follow-up than were nondiabetic patients (22% vs. 15%). Kastrati et al. reported diabetes to be a leading independent risk for restenosis in multivariable modeling based on data from over 4,500 consecutive patients. Diabetes was associated with an increase in rate of angiographically apparent stenosis from 31% to 35% and an odds ratio of 1.21 (155). Similarly, after directional atherectomy, diabetic patients in CAVEAT-I had greater late loss and restenosis than nondiabetic patients (156). That patients with diabetes have greater late loss after angioplasty, atherectomy, and stenting reemphasizes the biologic effects of diabetes. Using serial intravascular ultrasonography, Kornowski et al. (157) showed that the late loss after angioplasty among diabetic patients was due to exaggerated intimal hyperplasia. Interestingly, in EPISTENT, the combination of intracoronary stent placement and platelet glycoprotein IIb/IIIa inhibition did lead to clinically and angiographically determined restenosis rates that were low and similar among patients with and without diabetes (158). The rate of target vessel revascularization at 6 months was 8.1% and 8.8% for patients with and without diabetes, respectively (Fig. 83.7). Aside from this report, most data support the concept that, even with aggressive revascularization strategies, diabetic patients have restenosis and recurrent ischemic events more often than nondiabetic patients.

Unstable Angina

Like diabetes, unstable angina has been consistently associated with restenosis, especially when unstable angina is defined as pain at rest or accompanied by ischemic changes in the electrocardiogram. Because unstable angina defined in this way is often associated with thrombus-containing coronary lesions, the view that restenosis occurs acutely from clot

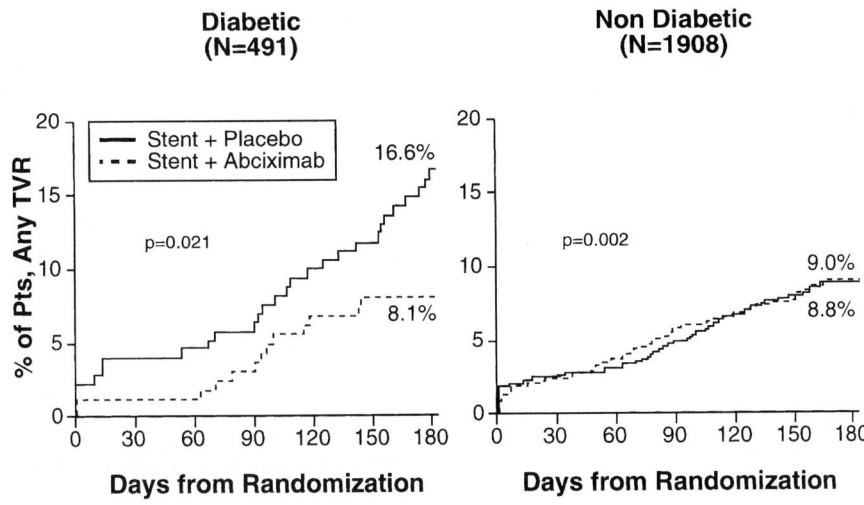

FIGURE 83.7 Kaplan-Meier distribution curves for the likelihood of restenosis among diabetic and nondiabetic patients in the Evaluation of Platelet IIb/IIIa Inhibitor for Stenting Trial (EPISTENT). As seen in previous stent trials, diabetic patients had a higher rate of target vessel revascularization (TVR) than did nondiabetic patients. In contrast, diabetic patients receiving abciximab during intracoronary stent placement had a low 6-month rate of target vessel revascularization similar to that of nondiabetic patients.

propagation and chronically from clot transformation is plausible. Over the hours to days after angioplasty in the setting of a ruptured plaque, thrombus may propagate and organize to cause a substantial loss in lumen diameter. Thrombin present within the clot facilitates the release and heightened activity of several mitogens, including PDGF and bFGF, thereby promoting cellular proliferation and clot transformation into a neointimal thickening. The contents of the underlying plaque in unstable angina may also directly promote restenosis. Moreno and colleagues (159) studied 50 atherectomy specimens from patients with unstable angina. By careful immunocytochemical study of the tissue removed, they were able to demonstrate that lesions with subsequent restenosis had twice as large an area of macrophage-rich tissue within the plaque. In the lesions studied, the number of macrophages present was the only independent predictor for restenosis by logistic regression analysis. Macrophages are known to be increased in plaques from patients with unstable angina (160), and they release cytokines, metalloproteinases, and growth factors that may lead to neointimal growth and constrictive scarring of the adventitia.

Clinically, several trials have reported an increased occurrence of restenosis among patients with new-onset angina (less than 2 months) (47,54), accelerating angina (161), or rest angina (162). The degree of symptom instability appears to be directly proportional to the subsequent event rate. Taken together, these and other balloon angioplasty trials (163) suggest that the relative risk of restenosis in those with unstable angina is 1.2 to 1.4 times higher than in patients with no or stable angina. Among patients receiving an intracoronary stent, unstable angina has not been consistently associated with restenosis.

Genetics of Restenosis

Coronary artery disease and stenosis recurrence after PTCA are likely complex processes involving multiple genes as well as interactions with many nongenetic factors. Consid-

ering balloon angioplasty cases, Berger and colleagues performed a retrospective analysis of 144 treated lesions in 113 patients and found the rate of restenosis to be 35% among patients with a history of restenosis at a different coronary site and 27% among patients without such a history (177). This observed difference did not reach statistical significance in this report but has reached significance in several others (117,178), and these findings suggest that a history of restenosis at one site increases the likelihood of restenosis at future sites. Some data also suggest that patients undergoing multivessel PTCA have a patient-specific risk of restenosis that is separate from lesion-related factors (117). Considering this concept in the stent era, Kastrati and colleagues analyzed a series of 3,370 consecutively treated patients, more than 80% of whom had follow-up angiography at 6 months. Using a multivariate model for restenosis, they found that 12% of the predictive value for restenosis was patient specific. The remaining factors were lesion related (54%) or procedure related (34%) (179). Obviously, genetic determinants of restenosis could explain some of the patient-related factors. Indeed, examining the distribution of angiographically determined stenosis diameter 6 months after stent placement, Schömig et al. (180) showed the frequency distribution curves to be bimodal, which suggests two different populations with different propensities for restenosis (Fig. 83.8).

Several genomic studies have assessed the relationship between restenosis and a particular gene, locus, or combination of genes, including the angiotensin-converting enzyme (ACE) gene, HLA-C locus Cw1, apolipoprotein E (apoE) genes (181), and platelet glycoprotein IIb/IIIa polymorphisms. Experimental studies support the hypothesis that the renin-angiotensin system plays a role in the pathogenesis of restenosis (182), and ACE inhibitors have been shown to prevent neointimal thickening after angioplasty in animal models. In humans, the presence of the ACE deletion (ACE-D) allele is associated with higher tissue and plasma levels of ACE and has been identified as a potential risk factor for myocar-

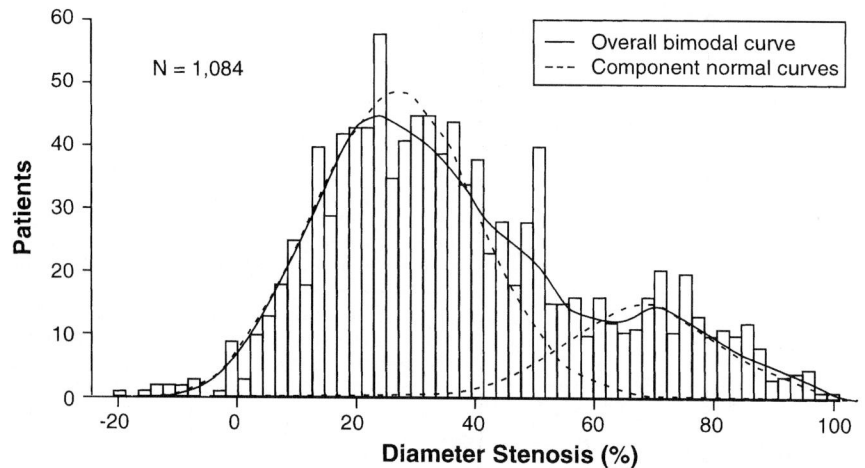

FIGURE 83.8 Distribution of percentage diameter of stenosis at follow-up angiography for 1,084 patients receiving an intracoronary stent. The overall curve appears bimodal, which suggests the existence of two separate populations or components of the normal curve. These two populations appear to have divergent propensities for restenosis, which implies a genetic or populational basis for restenosis. (From Kastrati A, Dirschinger J, Schömig A. Genetic risk factors and restenosis after percutaneous coronary interventions. *Herz* 2000;25:34–46.)

dial infarction (183). In 1993 Ohishi et al. (184) reported presence of this ACE deletion to be a potent genetic risk factor for coronary restenosis. In this relatively small study of patients undergoing emergency angioplasty for acute myocardial infarction, the investigators found a greater likelihood of angiographically identified restenosis among those with the ACE-D allele. Subsequent studies have not been consistent. Hamon et al. (185) studied 118 consecutively treated patients with single-vessel coronary artery disease after successful angioplasty. In this quantitative study, the ACE gene polymorphism had no influence or association with angiographically apparent restenosis. A similar negative finding was reported by Samani et al. (186) for 233 patients in the Subcutaneous Heparin Angioplasty Restenosis Prevention study.

Table 83.4 summarizes studies assessing the ACE polymorphism as it relates to angiographically determined restenosis (184–191). When data were pooled for 640 patients after balloon angioplasty, the odds ratio for restenosis for patients with the deletion genotype was 1.3 relative to patients with the insertion genotype. When this relationship was assessed among patients after coronary stenting, the odds ratio was 1.2 (95% confidence interval, 0.9 to 1.5). Important, however, is the wide variability in odds ratios among studies. This is likely due to the small sample size in most studies. As can be seen, the larger studies found the smaller odds ratios, and their results suggest no or minimal effect of ACE genotype. Addressing this issue, Koch et al. (190) prospectively studied 1,850 consecutively treated patients undergoing stent implantation. The ACE-DD genotype was not associated with angiographically apparent restenosis at 6 months (odds ratio of 0.9), nor did this genotype influence 1-year clinical outcome. In summary, the likely contribution of the ACE-deletion genotype alone to restenosis is minor. ◥ o26

Lesion-Related Factors

Vessel

In general, saphenous vein grafts have a substantially higher rate of restenosis than native coronary arteries after balloon angioplasty and somewhat higher rates after stent placement. In the M-HEART study of 510 patients with angiographic follow-up, the highest restenosis rate (68%) was found for saphenous vein graft lesions (212). Within saphenous vein grafts, stenoses tend to recur more commonly for lesions at the proximal anastomosis or in the shaft of the conduit, although data remain limited (213,214). More recent data on saphenous vein graft intervention suggest that the predictors of restenosis are more similar to those for native coronary vessels (i.e., vessel size, residual MLD, lesion ulceration) than previously considered (215). In a randomized trial in which 220 patients with vein graft stenoses were treated with either balloon angioplasty or stent placement, the 6-month restenosis rates were 46% for the group undergoing angioplasty and 37% for the group given stents (216). For native coronary arteries, the highest rate of restenosis after balloon angioplasty has been for the left anterior descending artery (LAD). M-HEART investigators reported restenosis in 45% of LAD lesions (Fig. 83.9), compared with 31% and 32% for lesions of the left circumflex artery and right coronary artery, respectively. Considering 3,736 lesions from several large-scale trials, Foley et al. (217) found only location in the LAD to independently predict a greater loss and smaller MLD at follow-up. Similarly, Wein-

TABLE 83.4 ACE-DD POLYMORPHISM AND RESTENOSIS

Study	Year	n[a]	DD vs. II odds ratio (95% CI)
Balloon angioplasty			
Ohishi et al. (184)	1993	82	5.6 (1.6–19.8)
Samani et al. (186)	1995	233	0.8 (0.4–1.7)
Hamon et al. (185)	1995	118	0.9 (0.3–2.7)
van Bockxmeer et al. (187)	1995	207	1.8 (0.8–3.9)
Pooled		*640*	*1.3 (0.9–2.1)*
Stent			
Amant et al. (188)	1997	158	2.6 (0.8–9.1)
Ribichini et al. (169)	1998	176	16.9 (2.2–132)
Koch et al. (190)	2000	1,556	0.9 (0.7–1.3)
Gürlek et al. (191)	2000	158	6.3 (1.8–22.1)
Pooled		*1,890*	*1.2 (0.9–1.6)*

ACE, angiotensin-converting enzyme; CI, confidence interval; DD, homozygosity for ACE gene deletion; II, homozygosity for ACE gene insertion.
[a]Total study size.

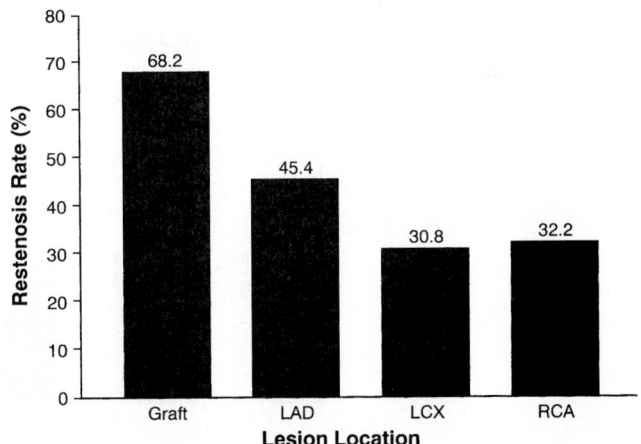

FIGURE 83.9 The vessel treated was found to be an independent predictor for restenosis for 598 treated sites in the Multi-Hospital Eastern Atlantic Restenosis Trial (chi-square *p* value for vessel = .003). The height of each column represents the restenosis rate for each group of segregated lesions. Graft, saphenous vein graft conduit; LAD, left anterior descending artery; LCX, left circumflex artery; RCA, right coronary artery. (Adapted from Hirshfeld JWJ, Schwartz JS, Jugo R, et al. Restenosis after coronary angioplasty: a multivariate statistical model to relate lesion and procedure variables to restenosis. *J Am Coll Cardiol* 1991;18:647–656, with permission.)

traub and colleagues (218) showed LAD location to be among the highest independent predictors of restenosis among 11,337 patients. The mechanism of increased restenosis after balloon angioplasty of the LAD is uncertain. Speculations include the possibility that the LAD may be undertreated because it is usually the largest coronary segment on which intervention is performed, and it has more recoil because of its course along the muscular interventricular septum.

Placement of intracoronary stents likely minimizes the effect of the LAD predisposition toward restenosis, because in the Stent Restenosis Study (STRESS) the restenosis rate for stented LAD lesions was similar to that for the other coronary arteries (70). Phillips et al. (219) suggested that LAD location lowered restenosis for patients receiving an intracoronary stent, which is a plausible tenet because larger vessel size is associated with lower restenosis rates. Two separate and sizable reports have since shown that LAD location is not a predictor of restenosis with intracoronary stent placement. The pooled data from BENESTENT-I, BENESTENT-II, and Multicenter Ultrasound Stenting in Coronaries (MUSIC) studies gathered by Serruys et al. (220) showed vessel size and residual diameter of stenosis alone to be the best predictors of restenosis, whereas Schömig and colleagues (155) found no independent predictive value from LAD lesion location.

Vessel Size

Several large-scale studies have reported an inverse relationship between vessel size and restenosis. Separating reference vessel diameters into quartiles, the M-HEART investigators found the restenosis rate to decrease from 44% to 36% after balloon angioplasty when vessel size was greater than 2.9 mm (Fig. 83.10). Likewise, vessel diameter was one of the few variables found independently to predict restenosis in MARCATOR (86). Foley and colleagues pooled data from several large pharmacologic trials of restenosis to assess the influence of vessel size on restenosis using quantitative coronary angiography (217). Lesions from over 3,000 patients were systematically studied and, by multiple linear regression analysis, increasing coronary vessel size was noted independently to predict decreasing late lumen loss and increasing MLD. The investigators concluded that the maxim "Bigger is better" (referring to a larger postprocedural lumen) should be modified to "Bigger vessels have a better outcome." In the large registry report from Emory University (218), the odds ratio for restenosis was 0.86 per 1-mm increase in vessel size.

Considering the effect of vessel size on restenosis after coronary artery stenting, Kastrati and colleagues (155) have shown this to be the strongest predictor (Figs. 83.10 and 83.11) in a series of 4,510 consecutively treated patients. Vessel size accounted for 34% of all predictive value, and the risk of restenosis for a vessel of 2.7 mm was 79% higher than for a vessel of 3.4 mm. In a separate report from this group, in which 2,602 patients were systematically studied with quantitative coronary angiography and long-term follow-up, similar results were found. Vessel size was divided into terciles (less than 2.8 mm, 2.8 to 3.2 mm, and larger than 3.2 mm), and vessel size was highly significantly linked with angiographically apparent restenosis (39%, 28%, and 20% for the

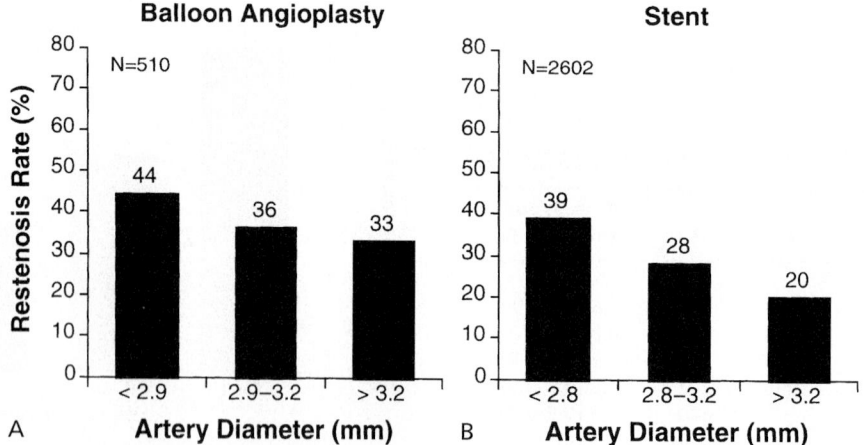

FIGURE 83.10 A: Separating reference vessel diameters into quartiles, Multi-Hospital Eastern Atlantic Restenosis Trial investigators found the restenosis rate to decrease from 44% to 36% when vessel size was larger than 2.9 mm by angiography. This inverse relationship of vessel size to restenosis has also been observed in other large-scale nonstent studies. **B:** Elezi and colleagues reported a similar pattern of restenosis in relation to vessel size among 2,602 stent patients. Vessel size is a leading predictor of restenosis regardless of method used. The benefit of stent placement over balloon angioplasty with regard to restenosis is likely lost for vessel diameters below 2.8 mm. (Adapted from Hirshfeld JWJ, Schwartz JS, Jugo R, et al. Restenosis after coronary angioplasty: a multivariate statistical model to relate lesion and procedure variables to restenosis. *J Am Coll Cardiol* 1991;18:647–656; and from Elezi S, Kastrati A, Neumann F-J, et al. Vessel size and long-term outcome after coronary stent placement. *Circulation* 1998;98:1875–1880, with permission.)

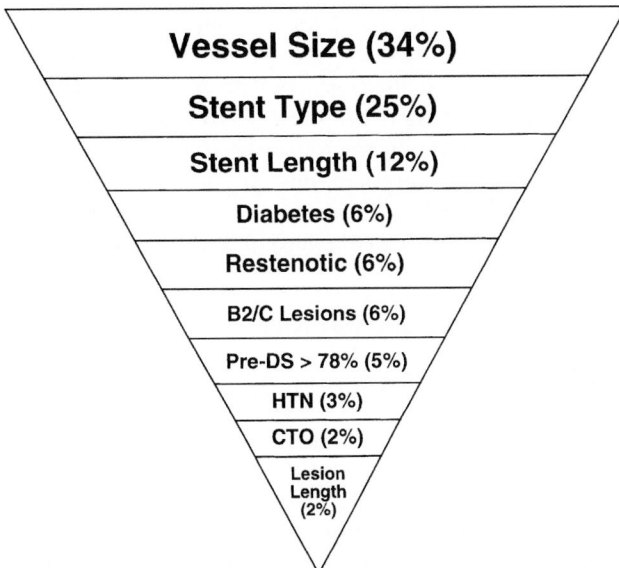

FIGURE 83.11 Pyramid of predictive factors affecting restenosis among 4,510 consecutively treated patients undergoing coronary stent placement. Percentages represent the amount of the restenosis in the model that was accounted for by the individual predictive factors. Vessel diameter and stent length accounted for nearly half of all predictive value for restenosis. CTO, chronic total occlusion; DS, diameter stenosis; HTN, hypertension. (Data from Kastrati A, Mehilli J, Dirschlinger J, et al. Restenosis after coronary stent placement of various stent types. *Am J Cardiol* 2001;87:34–39.)

terciles, respectively) (*p* <.001) (Fig. 83.10). Interestingly, for each size tercile, the late lumen loss was similar (1.1 mm), and two associated covariates affected restenosis: namely, diabetes and lesion complexity (227). As mentioned earlier, the pooled BENESTENT-MUSIC data sets (220) systematically showed vessel size and postprocedural diameter stenosis to be the best predictors of restenosis.

Preprocedural Percent Diameter Stenosis

The preprocedural and postprocedural lesion severity or MLD has been shown to be a leading and independent predictor of stenosis recurrence in nearly every large-scale clinical study of restenosis, regardless of the revascularization device used. For example, in the CARPORT study (68), in which quantitative coronary angiography was performed on over 600 lesions before and 6 months after successful balloon angioplasty, the preprocedural MLD was directly correlated with the late loss in lumen diameter at follow-up. Specifically, as the preprocedural MLD decreased by 40%, the late loss in lumen diameter increased by nearly 70%. A similar association was also noted by the M-HEART investigators (212), who reported an increased rate of restenosis from 25% to 40% as pre-PTCA stenosis severity surpassed 73% (Fig. 83.12). Likewise, among patients receiving an intracoronary stent, preprocedural stenosis greater than 78% lumen diameter has been shown to be an independent predictor of angiographically identified restenosis (Fig. 83.11) (155). The complex interrelationship between preprocedural MLD, lumen gain, late loss, and follow-up MLD was also studied by Foley et al. (217) using the combined quantitative coronary angiography data set from several trials. In brief, the investigators showed, using mathematical models, that although smaller MLDs were associated with greater initial gain, this gain was associated with proportionally more late loss, so that larger preprocedural MLD was directly correlated with a more favorable long-term result.

Lesion Length

Long lesion length has been associated with an increased rate of restenosis in several large, prospective clinical trials (161,212,228). Bourassa et al. (161), categorizing lesions in

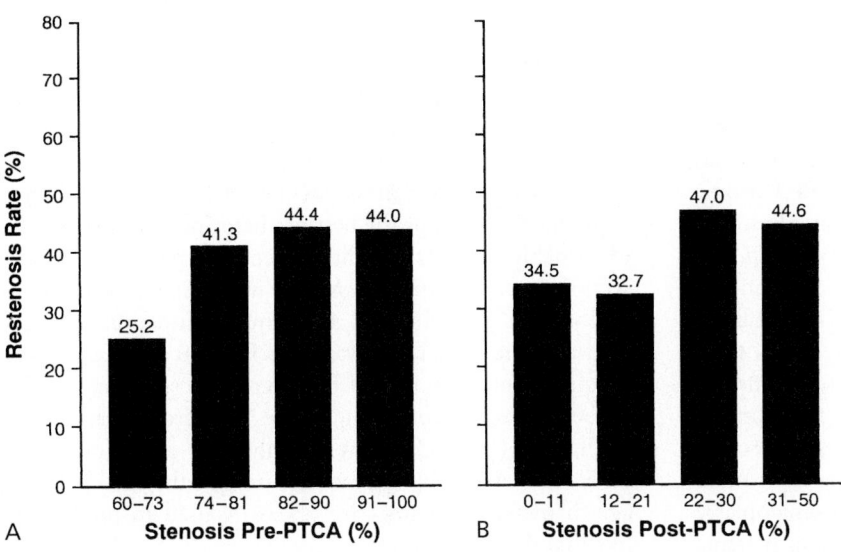

A   B

FIGURE 83.12 Relation of preprocedural **(A)** and postprocedural **(B)** stenosis severity on restenosis for 598 treated sites. In both panels, the height of each column represents the restenosis rate for each group of segregated lesions. Preprocedural stenosis severity was observed to be strongly associated with restenosis (*p* = .004), with higher restenosis rates for lesions with greater than 73% lumen diameter narrowing. Similarly, the postprocedural stenosis severity was independently associated with restenosis (*p* = .022), with a higher incidence of restenosis for lesions with a residual narrowing of more than 21%. PTCA, percutaneous transluminal coronary angioplasty. (Adapted from Hirshfeld JWJ, Schwartz JS, Jugo R, et al. Restenosis after coronary angioplasty: a multivariate statistical model to relate lesion and procedure variables to restenosis. *J Am Coll Cardiol* 1991;18:647–656, with permission.)

a binary fashion, reported an increase in restenosis rate from 38% to 52% for lesions greater than 10 mm long. Others have divided lesion lengths into percentiles and have reported increased restenosis for lengths longer than 4.6 mm (212) to 6.8 mm (228). Long lesions, in addition to representing greater atherosclerotic burden at the treatment site and requiring a more extensive revascularization, are associated with diffuse coronary artery disease in general. Although it is not easily quantitated, more diffuse disease such as seen in diabetic patients and those with chronic renal insufficiency has a greater restenosis potential. Intracoronary stents placed in long lesions have also been associated with an increased occurrence of restenosis. Kastrati et al. (155) reported rates of restenosis to increase from 32% to 36% for lesions longer than 10 mm. Hamasaki et al. (229) reported an increase from 20% to 31% for lesions 15 mm or longer. Yokoi et al. (230) studied several different types of stents placed in lesions longer than 20 mm and reported restenosis rates of 35% to 56%.

Degree of Occlusion

PTCA of chronically occluded coronary arteries has been estimated to comprise 10% of the total number of coronary interventions (231). The initial success rate of PTCA is lower and the incidence of restenosis is higher in cases of chronic occlusion, especially for vessels occluded 3 months or more (232). Combined data from several studies show that the recurrence of angina pectoris within months of successful balloon angioplasty of chronic occlusions is roughly 40% (233–237), whereas the rate of angiographically identified restenosis is over 60% (232,235–240). In the MARCATOR study, 139 patients were followed after successful angioplasty of a total occlusion and compared with 1,295 patients treated for a subtotal stenosis. The rate of angiographically demonstrated restenosis was not dissimilar in the two groups (49% in the chronic occlusion group and 42% in the subtotal stenosis group; *p* = .119), although complete vessel occlusion at follow-up was present in 19% and 7%, respectively (*p* >.001) (241). On the basis of these findings, intracoronary stent placement after successful balloon angioplasty has been advocated. The first randomized study of balloon angioplasty versus intracoronary stent placement, the Stenting in Chronic Coronary Occlusions trial, enrolled 119 patients. Restenosis occurred in 74% of the balloon angioplasty group, but in only 32% of the stent group (*p* <.001). Reocclusion was also lower in the stent group (12%) than in the balloon angioplasty group (26%). Several studies have since reported restenosis rates for stented chronic occlusions ranging from 19% to 52% depending on the rate of angiographic follow-up (238,239,242,243). In nearly every study, the rate of reocclusion and restenosis has been more favorable with stenting than with balloon angioplasty alone, yet these rates remain higher than among patients without preprocedural complete occlusions (244). Schömig and colleagues reported the rate of restenosis after coronary stent placement to increase from 33% to 48% when a chronic total occlusion was present (155). The reason for the higher predilection for restenosis among treated complete occlusions is uncertain, but these lesions may contain the highest plaque burden (i.e., the smallest possible MLD) and many have recently contained an active thrombus.

Procedure-Related Factors

Postprocedural or Residual Diameter of Stenosis

As does the severity of preprocedural stenosis, the extent of residual stenosis after successful PTCA strongly predicts restenosis. In the M-HEART study (212), the percentage of stenosis immediately after PTCA was separated into quartiles, and lesions with residual stenosis of more than 21% had a significantly higher restenosis rate than did those with a post-PTCA stenosis of 21% or less (Fig. 83.12). Similar results of reduced restenosis in the setting of least residual stenosis were reported by Bourassa et al. (161), who found that postangioplasty stenosis of 30% or more of luminal diameter was associated with a restenosis rate of 40%, compared to 28% for segments with residual stenosis of less than 30%. These studies, along with statistical models of restenosis (39), have given rise to the concept of maximizing immediate gain (i.e., the gain in lumen diameter from baseline to immediately after PTCA), or the "bigger is better" concept. Kuntz et al. (39) compared models of restenosis after balloon angioplasty, stenting, and directional atherectomy. They concluded that the loss index (late loss divided by immediate gain) was the same for all device strategies and that therefore the immediate result (procedural stenosis) was what determined the late outcome. Challenging this view, Foley and others have studied large databases of quantitative angiographic results and demonstrated different device "taxing," with more favorable angiographic profiles found for dilating devices (balloons and stents) than for debulking procedures (atherectomy). Their findings suggest that restenosis is not only influenced strongly by vessel size and lumen gain, but also by the technique used to achieve the larger lumen (Fig. 83.5). Aside from measures obtained by quantitative angiography, perhaps the best predictor of angiographically identifiable restenosis is the percent postprocedural cross-sectional narrowing as assessed by intravascular ultrasonography (IVUS) (245). In examining numerous clinical, angiographic, and IVUS variables for 360 coronary artery lesions, Mintz et al. found IVUS cross-sectional narrowing to be the most consistent single predictor of restenosis (245,246) (Fig. 83.13). Clinically, the angiographically determined parameters of vessel size and the final percentage diameter of stenosis are primarily used to predict the likelihood of restenosis.

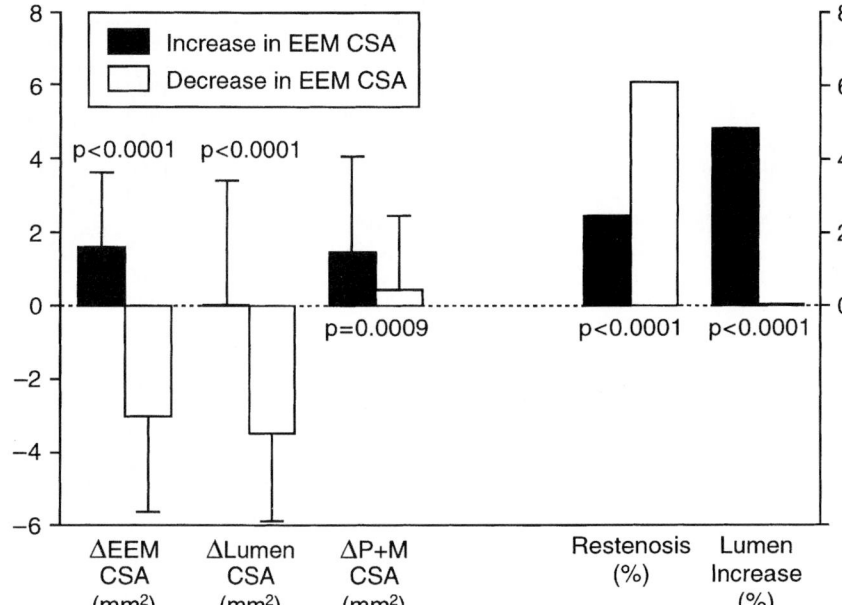

FIGURE 83.13 When numerous clinical, angiographic, and intravascular ultrasonographic variables were considered, cross-sectional narrowing as measured by ultrasonography was found to be the most consistent single predictor of restenosis. During serial study, 22% of lesions showed an increase in overall vessel size (increased external elastic membrane, or EEM, area), whereas the remainder showed a decrease. Lesions with an increased EEM had lower rates of angiographically identified restenosis than those with a decreased EEM (26% vs. 62%). Δ, change; CSA, cross-sectional area; P+M, plaque plus media. (From Mintz G, Popma J, Pichard A, et al. Intravascular ultrasound predictors of restenosis after percutaneous transcatheter coronary revascularization. *J Am Coll Cardiol* 1996;27:1678–1687, with permission.)

PRINCIPLES OF MANAGEMENT

When the epidemiology of restenosis is pulled together, a framework for monitoring the patient after successful angioplasty can be established. One might begin by considering the patient-, lesion-, and procedure-related factors associated with the angioplasty. Factors consistently identified as risks for restenosis after balloon angioplasty include the presence of diabetes mellitus, the presence of unstable angina, lesion location in saphenous vein grafts, lesion location in the ostium of the major epicardial arteries, long (diffuse) lesions, small vessel size, and greater severity of preprocedural and postprocedural stenosis. In the stent era, the factors consistently associated with increased rates of restenosis include the presence of diabetes, small vessel size, and larger residual diameter of stenosis (Table 83.2). Because the process of restenosis is complete within 3 to 6 months after angioplasty, clinical follow-up should take place during this interval. Depending on the patient's initial symptoms, extent of myocardium at risk, and associated comorbidities, a tailored level of treatment aggressiveness can be established. For example, a patient initially presenting with predictable exertional angina and a small area of myocardium at risk might be followed for symptoms alone if the underlying ventricular function and overall health are good. In contrast, patients with atypical or unpredictable ischemia, a large area of myocardium at risk, or important comorbidities such as depressed ventricular function should routinely undergo stress cardiac imaging in the early months after angioplasty. Many interventional cardiologists perform cardiac stress testing for all asymptomatic patients even though most patients with restenosis have recurrent angina and not infarction.

Given the poor predictive value of symptom status alone and the invasive nature of repeat angiography, this is not unreasonable. In choosing a cardiac stress test, simultaneous imaging with nuclear scintigraphy or echocardiography is worthwhile as demonstrated in *e*Table 83.1.3. If the baseline stress test results were positive and accurately located the ischemic territory, repeat testing with that particular imaging modality is logical. The positive predictive value of imaging cardiac stress testing averages approximately 80%, and this has been considered acceptable for most patients. When stress testing is believed to be unreliable and the amount of myocardium at risk is large (e.g., with ostial lesions in LAD or left-dominant left circumflex artery systems), angiography should be performed to be certain restenosis has not occurred. The need for routine or serial angiography in clinical practice is infrequent.

For patients who develop restenosis, several treatment options are available, including repeat percutaneous revascularization, which has a similar short-term and long-term success rate as with *de novo* lesions (*e*Table 83.4.1). Intracoronary stent placement is a prudent option for lesions not previously treated with a stent, provided the anatomy is suitable. Most patients with single-vessel restenosis undergo a second angioplasty, whereas patients with restenosis in multiple vessels may undergo percutaneous or surgical revascularization. When all patients initially treated by PTCA for multivessel disease are considered, slightly more of those with restenosis undergo a repeat angioplasty than undergo coronary artery bypass grafting. In the BARI study, nearly 70% of the cohort randomly assigned to undergo PTCA avoided surgery at 5-year follow-up (149).

Restenosis within stents is an increasing occurrence owing to the dramatic increase in stent use. In-stent reste-

TABLE 83.5 ANIMAL STUDIES AND CLINICAL TRIALS OF AGENTS TO PREVENT RESTENOSIS

Agent	Animal study	Year	n	Clinical trial	Year	n
Heparin sodium	Clowes et al. (27)	1983	61	Ellis et al. (80)	1989	416
Low-molecular-weight heparin	Buchwald et al. (250)	1992	18	Faxon et al. (251)	1992	459
Aspirin	Völker et al. (252)	1990	18	Thornton et al. (253)	1984	248
Dipyridamole	Ingerman-Wojenski et al. (254)	1988	44	Schwartz et al. (79)	1988	249
Warfarin sodium	August et al. (255)	1980	60	Urban et al. (256)	1988	77
Thromboxane antagonist	Yabe et al. (257)	1989	33	CARPORT (170)	1991	697
Angiopeptin	Eriksen et al. (258)	1993	112	Kent et al. (259)	1993	1,246
Fish oil	Dehmer et al. (260)	1988	82	Grigg et al. (261)	1989	108
Lovastatin	Sahni et al. (262)	1991	157	Lovastatin Restenosis trial (84)	1994	404
Calcium channel blocker	Unverdorben et al. (264)	1993	189	Whitworth et al. (265)	1986	241
ACE inhibitor	Powell et al. (266)	1989	127	MARCATOR (86)	1995	1,436
Colchicine	Currier et al. (267)	1989	24	CART (268)	1989	79
Corticosteroids	Villa et al. (269)	1994	39	Pepine et al. (81)	1990	915

ACE, angiotensin-converting enzyme; CARPORT, Coronary Artery Restenosis Prevention on Repeated Thromboxane-Antagonism; CART, Colchicine Angioplasty Restenosis Trial; MARCATOR, Multicenter American Research Trial with Cilazapril after Angioplasty to Prevent Transluminal Coronary Obstruction and Restenosis.

nosis usually is a diffuse proliferation of neointima (30,35), and the optimal interventional treatment is uncertain. Balloon angioplasty, perfusion balloon angioplasty, atherectomy (rotational and laser), and stent-within-stent approaches have all been tried. For focal restenotic lesions, the rate of second restenosis is 30% to 40%, whereas for diffuse restenotic lesions it is roughly 70% (36). The mainstay of current treatment is balloon angioplasty with or without intracoronary brachytherapy (local radiation). This is reviewed in the section In-Stent Restenosis.

As with most medical treatments, the best strategy for restenosis is prevention. Numerous basic scientific and clinical investigations using a wide variety of therapeutic agents (247–249) have been conducted in search of an inhibitor of restenosis. By using animal models for preclinical testing on targets of restenosis, the biology of restenosis has been advanced, although the clinical impact remains limited.

CLINICAL PREVENTION TRIALS: PHARMACOLOGIC

Many different therapeutic agents have been tested in an attempt to find a treatment that can inhibit the development of restenosis (247–249). Although thousands of patients have been enrolled in over 50 clinical trials over the past 20 years, no large-scale study has produced a pharmacologic therapy to suppress restenosis. Many animal studies targeting factors from thrombin to thromboxane, microtubules to calcium channels, and prostacyclin to platelets (i.e., factors associated with thrombus formation and cellular proliferation) have engendered hope of producing a meaningful reduction in restenosis, but these findings have been discounted by negative results from human studies, as displayed in Table 83.5 (27,79,81,83,84,86,170,250–269). Given the mechanisms of restenosis, most studies have spe-

cifically targeted a factor associated with thrombus formation, vascular remodeling, or neointimal growth. An important point to be remembered when reviewing these many trials is that restenosis after balloon angioplasty is primarily a result of vessel wall remodeling as opposed to neointimal formation, and that in balloon angioplasty trials many of these agents were used in an attempt to influence neointimal proliferation.

Strategies Targeting Thrombus Formation

Antiplatelet Agents

Because platelet functions (adhesion, aggregation, and release of vasoactive, mitogenic, and chemoattractant factors) are central to thrombus formation and the vascular response to injury, they are logical targets to limit restenosis. Virtually all percutaneous revascularization procedures are performed in the setting of antiplatelet therapy to prevent acute ischemic complications, although none of these therapies has shown a clear effect on angiographically identified restenosis. Aspirin, dipyridamole, thienopyridines, thromboxane antagonists, and prostacyclin analogs each has shown some promise in animal models of restenosis, although none has produced clinical benefit (Table 83.6). The most potent antiplatelet therapy, that using glycoprotein IIb/IIIa antagonists, has been studied in animal models and in several large-scale clinical trials. Animal models of restenosis demonstrated a reduction in neointimal development through blocking of either the platelet glycoprotein IIb/IIIa ($\alpha_{IIb}\beta_3$) or vitronectin receptor ($\alpha_v\beta_3$) (270,271). Matsuno et al. (270) postulated that this effect was due both to an early event such as inhibited secretion of PDGF and to a late event, possibly the interference of the smooth muscle cell $\alpha_v\beta_3$ receptor.

By using a glycoprotein IIb/IIIa inhibitor, chimeric 7E3 Fab, and blocking the final common pathway for platelet

TABLE 83.6 CLINICAL TRIALS EVALUATING THE USE OF ANTITHROMBOTIC AGENTS TO LIMIT ANGIOGRAPHICALLY IDENTIFIED RESTENOSIS

Study	Year	n	No. (%) with angio-graphic follow-up	Agent(s) and dose	Definition of restenosis	Restenosis rate (%) Agent(s)	Placebo or control	Odds ratio
Aspirin								
White	1987	157	111 (71)	ASA, 990 mg/DIP, 225 mg	≥70% steno-sis[a,b]	18	20	
Schwartz et al. (79)	1988	376	249 (66)	ASA, 900 mg/DIP, 225 mg	≥50% stenosis[b]	38	39	
Thornton et al. (253)	1984	248	179 (72)	ASA, 325 mg	Loss of 50% gain[a]	27	36	
Ticlopidine hydrochloride								
White	1987	157	119 (76)	Ticlopidine, 750 mg	≥70% steno-sis[a,b]	29	20	
Kitazume	1988	189	189 (100)	Ticlopidine, 200 mg	≥50% steno-sis[a]	27	38	
Bertrand	1990	266	244 (92)	Ticlopidine, 200 mg	Loss of 50% gain[a]	50	41	
Anticoagulants								
Thornton et al. (253)	1984	248	178 (72)	Warfarin sodium, target PT	Loss of 50% gain[a]	36	27	
Urban et al. (256)	1988	110	85 (77)	Warfarin sodium, INR	≥50% stenosis[a]	29	37	
Ellis et al. (80)	1989	416	259 (61)	Heparin sodium, target aPTT	≥50% stenosis[b]	41	37	
Faxon et al. (280)	1994	458	394 (86)	Enoxaparin sodium, 40 mg	Loss of 50% gain[b]	52	51	
Brack et al. (279)	1995	339	299 (88)	Heparin sodium s.c. × 4 mo	Loss of 50% gain[b]	39	48	
Karsch et al. (283)	1996	625	514 (84)	Reviparin s.c. × 4 wk	Loss of 50% gain[b]	34	33	
Kiesz et al. (284)	2001	100	99 (99)	Enoxaparin sodium local	≥50% stenosis[b]	10	24	

aPTT, activated partial thromboplastin time; ASA, aspirin; DIP, dipyridamole; INR, international normalized ratio; PT, prothrombin time.
Note: Trials were included if they enrolled ≥100 patients and completed ≥60% angiographic follow-up.
[a]Visual assessment.
[b]Quantitative angiography.

aggregation, the EPIC (272) investigators showed the incidence of acute ischemic complications during high-risk angioplasty to be substantially reduced. At 6-month follow-up, clinically apparent restenosis was also reduced (43), but this was primarily due to a reduction in myocardial infarction. Since then, several trials have completed 6-month follow-up on patients randomly assigned to receive platelet IIb/IIIa antagonists or placebo. The Integrilin to Manage Platelet Aggregation and Coronary Thrombosis II trial, Randomized Efficacy Study of Tirofiban for Clinical Outcomes and Restenosis, EPILOG study, and Chimeric 7E3 Antiplatelet in Unstable Angina Refractory to Standard Treatment trial studied eptifibatide (Integrilin), tirofiban hydrochloride, and abciximab. Pooling of results for these 12,305 patients showed no significant reduction in target vessel revascularization at 6-month follow-up for patients given active treatment versus those receiving placebo (18.6% vs. 20.2%) (43,273–275), and no difference was seen in quantitative angiographic or neointimal tissue vol-ume (276). The only potential exception may be for diabetic patients who received an intracoronary stent and were given abciximab, as observed in the Evaluation of Platelet IIb/IIIa Inhibitor for Stenting Trial (158) (Fig. 83.7), although this result is not confirmed in other studies.

Anticoagulants

In addition to containing activated platelets, a thrombus at the site of injury can act as a bioabsorbable matrix and also serve as a reservoir of active thrombin. Therapy with warfarin sodium, a broad-spectrum anticoagulant, did not reduce restenosis in an early angiographic study (256) but did reduce target vessel revascularization in a more recent trial of 1,058 patients (277). More specific inhibitors, such as the antithrombins heparin sodium, low-molecular-weight heparin, hirudin, and bivalirudin, have also been studied. Beyond being an anticoagulant, heparin inhibits smooth muscle cell proliferation and migration. Several small randomized trials of heparin versus placebo unfortunately showed no salutary effect on restenosis (80,278) after nonstent procedures. Long-term heparin administration (twice-daily subcutaneous injections for 4 months) also did not favorably affect angiographic or clinical outcome (279). Low-molecular-weight (fractionated) heparin has a longer half-life than unfractionated heparin, is a more potent factor X_a inhibitor, and has been studied in several balloon angioplasty trials (280–282). Restenosis was not reduced in any of these trials, even when therapy extended for weeks postprocedure (283). More recently, a small study (n = 100) was performed using some contemporary practices: implantation of intracoronary stents, local drug delivery versus systemic administration, and therapy with low-molecular-weight heparin versus unfractionated heparin. This study, the Polish-American Local Lovenox NIR Assessment study (284), randomly assigned patients to receive locally delivered enoxaparin sodium or systemic unfractionated heparin for stent placement. At 6-month follow-up, restenosis was found in 10% of the group receiving enoxaparin versus 24% of the group given systemic heparin. Late lumen loss and target vessel revascularization were also improved by local enoxaparin delivery.

Finally, more potent antithrombins that do not require antithrombin as a cofactor (hirudin, bivalirudin, and argatroban) have been studied. The trial Hirudin in a European Trial versus Heparin in the Prevention of Restenosis after PTCA randomly assigned 1,141 patients to receive heparin during the PTCA procedure and in 24-hour infusion, hirudin during the procedure and in 24-hour infusion, or hirudin during the procedure, in 24-hour infusion, and in 3 days of subcutaneous therapy (285). Early ischemic events were reduced by the use of hirudin, but no difference in late outcome related to restenosis was observed. Similarly, the Hirulog Angioplasty Study (286) randomly assigned 4,098 patients undergoing angioplasty to receive either Hirulog (bivalirudin) or heparin. At 6 months the rate of repeat revascularization was similar for the two groups (22.9% and 23.9%). These data reveal no reduction in restenosis with anticoagulant therapies even when administered for days to weeks after angioplasty.

Antiproliferative Agents

Immunosuppressant and Antiinflammatory Agents

The antiproliferative agents are the current hopes for reducing restenosis in the contemporary stent era. Previously tested in patients undergoing balloon angioplasty, several immunosuppressive and antimitogenic agents showed encouraging results in animal studies without demonstrating success in human trials. Corticosteroids were among the first classes of agents studied because of their known clinical effects on suppression of inflammatory response to

injury and reduction in the production of smooth muscle mitogens. Specifically, corticosteroids suppress monocyte-lymphocyte interaction and lymphocyte proliferation, perhaps by decreasing platelet and macrophage-derived growth factor expression (298,299). Pepine et al. (81) performed the largest corticosteroid-angioplasty study, randomly assigning 915 patients to receive 1 g methylprednisolone or placebo the day before angioplasty. Six-month angiographic follow-up in 71% of those with successful angioplasty showed a nearly identical per-lesion restenosis rate for steroid-treated patients (40%) and placebo-treated patients (39%). Colchicine, which acts by binding to tubulin and disrupting spindle formation during cell division and inhibiting collagen formation (300,301), produced a dose-dependent reduction in neointimal formation in animal models. In clinical trials in which colchicine was used in tolerable doses alone (268,302,303), however, it was ineffective in preventing restenosis.

Finally, tranilast is an antiinflammatory agent that suppresses macrophages and fibroblasts, inhibits smooth muscle cell migration induced by PDGF, inhibits collagen synthesis in vascular smooth muscle cells, and is used to prevent keloid formation. Tranilast was initially tested in the Tranilast Restenosis Following Angioplasty Trial. Two hundred fifty-five patients were randomly assigned to receive 600 mg of tranilast, 300 mg of tranilast, or placebo for 3 months. The rate of angiographically determined restenosis for these groups at 3 months was 18%, 39%, and 39%, respectively (304). The largest clinical trial ever performed in interventional cardiology—the Prevention of Restenosis with Tranilast and Its Outcomes trial—tested the use of tranilast among 11,500 PCI patients. Tranilast was administered (300 or 450 mg twice daily) for 1 or 3 months after stent or nonstent procedures to treat *de novo* or restenotic lesions. The primary end point was the 9-month composite of death, myocardial infarction, or ischemia-driven target vessel revascularization. A 2,000-patient angiographic substudy was also performed (305).

Growth Factor Inhibitors

Trapidil

As listed in Table 83.3, several growth factors, including PDGF, bFGF, insulin-like growth factor-1, TGF-β, and EGF have been implicated in the hyperproliferative response after vascular injury. In addition to nonspecific immunosuppressant and antiinflammatory agents, specific antagonists to these growth factors have been studied in prevention of restenosis. Trapidil is a PDGF inhibitor that significantly reduces neointimal formation in animal models of restenosis (306). A small randomized clinical trial of trapidil showed a significant reduction in restenosis (from 42% to 19%) at 6 months (307). This finding was substantiated by the Studio Trapidil versus Aspirin nella Restenosi Coronarica trial (308), a multicenter, double-blind, randomized study of trapidil versus aspirin involving 305 patients. The occurrence of angiographically identified restenosis was reduced by 40% (*e*Table 83.6.1). Another study randomly assigned 97 stent patients to receive ticlopidine hydrochloride plus aspirin or ticlopidine plus trapidil (309). At 6 months, no difference was seen in angiographically determined restenosis (approximately 29% for all groups). These small studies are encouraging and indicate that further investigation is warranted.

Angiopeptin

The most widely studied growth hormone antagonist in restenosis prophylaxis is angiopeptin, a synthetic analog of somatostatin. Angiopeptin acts on the pituitary gland to reduce growth hormone secretion and may limit release of insulin-like growth factor-1 (310). In animal models of vascular injury, administration of angiopeptin before or during angioplasty reduced neointimal growth (258,311,312). Clinical results, however, have been inconsistent (259,313,314). Two trials, one using low-dose angiopeptin and the other high-dose angiopeptin, included nearly 1,400 patients and performed angiographic follow-up but showed no reduction in restenosis (259,314). Questions remain as to whether a more prolonged dosing of angiopeptin is needed to affect neointimal growth. A small placebo-controlled study in which angiopeptin was administered for hours after PTCA demonstrated angiographically determined and clinically determined restenosis rates that were 70% lower and 26% lower, respectively, with angiopeptin treatment. These discrepant findings indicate the need for further study before large-scale efforts are repeated.

Cilostazol

Acting as an antiplatelet agent by increasing levels of cyclic adenosine monophosphate, cilostazol is also an antiproliferative agent that inhibits smooth muscle cell growth by blocking synthesis of DNA. Sekiya and colleagues (315) randomly assigned 126 stent patients to receive placebo, probucol, cilostazol, or the combination of probucol and cilostazol. Drug treatment began 5 days before coronary intervention and continued until 6-month angiographic follow-up. At follow-up, restenosis was found in 32% of patients receiving the placebo, 17% of those given probucol, 13% of those getting cilostazol, and 10% of those receiving both probucol and cilostazol. Among 211 balloon angioplasty patients randomly assigned to receive either 3 months of cilostazol (200 mg per day) or a control regimen, the rate of angiographically identified restenosis at 3 months was lowered from 40% to 18% by cilostazol (316). In two more recent studies, 409 patients and 130 patients undergoing stent implantation were randomly assigned to receive either aspirin plus ticlopidine or aspirin plus cilostazol. The larger of the trials, by Park et al. (317), showed no reduction in restenosis at 6-month follow-up angiography among patients receiving cilostazol compared with those

given ticlopidine (restenosis rates of 27% vs. 23%, respectively), although the smaller trial, conducted by Kozuma and colleagues (318), reported a halving of angiographically identified restenosis and target vessel revascularization rates at late follow-up among patients receiving cilostazol. Together, these trials included nearly 900 patients and showed a substantial (40%) reduction in relative risk of angiographically determined restenosis with cilostazol (32% vs. 19%).

Paclitaxel

Paclitaxel (Taxol) is a microtubule-stabilizing drug that reduces cellular functions such as migration and proliferation, which makes it a potent cytotoxic antitumor agent. Animal models of restenosis have shown delivery of paclitaxel via local catheters to be associated with reduced neointimal proliferation and increased vessel size (319). Because paclitaxel is a potent agent, local delivery is key. Linking the molecule in a polymer fashion to a stent, stent sleeve, or biodegradable stent is an option being tested (320,321). Preliminary reports of a small number of early clinical cases have reported zero restenosis rates. Although the results seem overly promising, several larger-scale clinical trials are already under way in Europe, Asia, and North America.

Rapamycin

Sirolimus (Rapamune) is a macrocyclic lactone with antibiotic, immunosuppressive, and antiproliferative actions. It is approved for use as prophylaxis for renal transplant rejection. Biologically it induces cell-cycle arrest and affects proliferation and migration of smooth muscle cells. It has been shown in animal models of restenosis to substantially reduce neointimal thickening after vascular injury (322). Sousa and colleagues (323) reported quantitative angiographic and three-dimensional intravascular ultrasonographic data on 30 patients who received sirolimus-coated stents. At 4-month follow-up, the in-stent late loss was negligible (approximately 0.1 mm) and the diameter of stenosis was virtually unchanged (approximately 5%). These remarkable results have prompted several moderate-sized (400-patient) studies in Europe and the United States, including the Rapamycin-Eluding versus Plain Polymer Stents trial and the Sirolimus-coated BX Velocity Balloon-Expandable Stent trial.

CLINICAL TRIALS: TECHNOLOGIES

Atherectomy

As mentioned previously, the leading predictor of angiographically determined restenosis is the postprocedural or residual stenosis diameter. Most new technologies in interventional cardiology, such as the atherectomy devices, have targeted debulking of coronary artery lesions to produce the largest postprocedural lumen possible. Each new technology brings the hope of reducing restenosis or treating specific lesion subsets better than can balloon angioplasty. The directional coronary atherectomy (DCA) catheter allows shaving and extraction of atheroma and enables the production of a larger lumen and net gain. Data from the DCA registry and from two large multicenter trials, CAVEAT (73) and the Canadian Coronary Atherectomy Trial (74), demonstrated this; however, in combination, these studies report similar restenosis rates for DCA and balloon angioplasty. The BOAT study compared balloon angioplasty to "optimal" DCA. In BOAT, atherectomy produced larger immediate and net gain, and the rate of angiographically identified restenosis at the specific enrolling centers able to perform optimal atherectomy (15% mean residual stenosis) was lower for DCA (32%) than for balloon angioplasty alone (40%) (87). This occurred without an increase in "major" adverse events, although patients undergoing DCA were nearly three times more likely to have a significant periprocedural rise in levels of myocardial muscle creatine kinase isoenzyme. Target vessel revascularization rates at 6-month and 1-year follow-up were similar for the groups undergoing PTCA and optimal DCA.

Excimer laser and rotational atherectomy have been assessed in the Excimer Laser Rotational Atherectomy Balloon Angioplasty Complications study (77), the Study to Determine Rotablator and Transluminal Angioplasty Strategy, the Amsterdam Rotterdam (AMRO) trial (343), and the Comparison of Balloon Angioplasty versus Rotational Atherectomy in Complex Coronary Lesions study (67). Compared with balloon angioplasty, these atherectomy devices used to debulk the lesion before balloon dilation have yielded higher procedural success rates and greater immediate gain. No significant outcome differences have been found during clinical or angiographic follow-up, however, with restenosis rates approximating 50% in all treatment groups in each trial. Like DCA, these debulking devices facilitate balloon angioplasty but cause a greater late lumen loss, or device taxing, which implies that remodeling and neointimal proliferation are not favorably reduced.

Intracoronary Stents

Stent Placement Compared with Balloon Angioplasty

The increasingly popular intracoronary stents address restenosis from the perspective of plaque persistence, recoil, and remodeling (Fig. 83.3) by compressing the plaque and scaffolding the vessel lumen to safely maximize diameter. Early stent registry data indicated that restenosis rates were similar to those with balloon angioplasty unless the lesion treated was "ideal," in other words, was a short, *de novo* lesion in a vessel 3 mm or more in diameter. With

this in mind, two randomized trials of stent implantation versus stand-alone balloon angioplasty in *de novo* native coronary artery lesions were undertaken: the BENESTENT trial (71,344,345) and the STRESS trial (344,346). The BENESTENT investigators reported a restenosis rate of 22% in the stent group and 32% in the balloon angioplasty group. A decreased incidence of cardiac events—mainly repeat percutaneous coronary revascularization—was noted for the stent group at 6-month follow-up. The STRESS trial (70) also demonstrated an absolute 10% lower occurrence of restenosis among subjects receiving a Palmaz-Schatz coronary stent than among those undergoing balloon angioplasty (32% and 42%, respectively). Similarly, at 8-month follow-up, the STRESS stent group had a better event-free survival and had undergone fewer revascularization procedures. Comparison of angiographically determined restenosis rates in past balloon angioplasty trials and in more recent stent trials confirms this 10% to 15% lower rate of restenosis after stent implantation (Table 83.1).

Since completion of the BENESTENT and STRESS trials, many other stent-versus-angioplasty trials have been performed (Table 83.1) to assess the effect of contemporary stenting techniques (high-pressure deployment, IVUS, reduced anticoagulation), characteristics of patient and clinical subgroups (presence of diabetes or acute myocardial infarction), features of specific lesions (restenotic lesions, chronic occlusions, long lesions), and new stent designs. Although restenosis rates have been somewhat lowered with more aggressive balloon angioplasty, intracoronary stenting has proven superior in nearly every study. In BENESTENT-II, for example, in which aggressive balloon angioplasty was tested against placement of heparin-coated stents with high-pressure delivery, the restenosis rate after angioplasty was only 31%, but the rate was an impressively low 16% in the stent group. Other studies using different stents or more contemporary practices than in STRESS-I and BENESTENT-I confirm this impressively low restenosis rate (347).

Important points to be remembered regarding restenosis in the current stent era include the exception in which stent placement has not been proven superior to balloon angioplasty—in small vessels. Several studies showed comparable rates of restenosis for balloon angioplasty and stent placement when vessel size was 2.8 mm or less (155). For small vessels, the rate of restenosis approximates 40% regardless of treatment assignment. In addition, the rates of restenosis initially published for nearly all stent designs were for ideal lesions, and large-scale observational studies have reported higher overall rates than in those trials used to gain U.S. Food and Drug Administration approval of particular stent designs. In summary, target vessel revascularization rates in contemporary stent practice can approximate the single digits (i.e., less than 10%). When angiographically determined restenosis is considered, the rates increase to 20% to

25%, and when the nonideal end of the spectrum is included, this rate may double.

In-Stent Restenosis

With the exponential increase in stent use over the past few years and the increased rate of percutaneous revascularization overall, in-stent restenosis has become a new epidemic in medicine. Angiographically identified restenosis (stenosis of 50% or more lumen diameter) occurs in one of four stent patients, and repeat revascularization of the target lesion is needed in roughly 10% of patients receiving an intracoronary stent. Because stents stimulate more neointimal proliferation than other interventional methods (balloon angioplasty and atherectomy), antiproliferation strategies are the main therapeutic consideration. Results of the conventional mechanical treatment of in-stent restenosis using balloon angioplasty, cutting balloon angioplasty, repeat stenting, or atherectomy have been disappointing, with recurrent rates of restenosis averaging 30% to 50% for focal disease and approximately 70% for diffuse in-stent restenosis (348–351). Current treatment options include gamma and beta radiation, and antiproliferative drugs are being studied.

Vascular Brachytherapy for In-Stent Restenosis

Gamma and beta radiotherapy have been studied for the treatment of in-stent restenosis over the past several years. Radiation is emitted during the spontaneous decay of the nuclei of certain elements. This radiation can be gamma radiation (electromagnetic energy carried by photons, which may penetrate more than 10 mm of human tissue) or beta particles (electrons carrying a wide range of energy levels and traveling 2 to 3 mm in human tissue). By affect-

ing DNA in the actively dividing cells in the vascular media and intima, brachytherapy inhibits smooth muscle proliferation and neointima formation. Isotopes studied for clinical brachytherapy include iridium-192 (Ir-192, gamma emitter), phosphorus-32 (P-32, beta emitter), strontium-90 (Sr-90, beta emitter), yttrium-90 (Y-90, beta emitter), and rhenium-188 (Re-188, beta emitter). Three types of radiation delivery systems have been tested: balloon-filled catheters, radioactive stents, and catheter-based delivery of radioactive seeds. Only the last one has been examined in randomized clinical trials and approved by U.S. Food and Drug Administration.

Gamma Radiation

Several randomized clinical trials have reported the efficacy of Ir-192 gamma radiation in preventing restenosis in patients with in-stent restenosis (352–355) (Fig. 83.14). Teirstein and colleagues have reported the 1-year and 3-year results of the Scripps Coronary Radiation to Inhibit Proliferation Post-Stenting trial, which randomly assigned 55 patients with restenosis (both in-stent restenosis and post-PTCA restenosis) to receive gamma radiation or placebo after undergoing a successful angioplasty procedure. Late luminal loss was significantly lower in the Ir-192–treated group than in the placebo group (1.85 ± 0.89 mm vs. 2.43 ± 0.78 mm, $p = .02$) in the first year of follow-up, and adverse ischemic events remained lower at 3 years (352) (Table 83.7). In the GAMMA-1 trial (353) Ir-192 was administered after a successful PTCA and was associated with less target lesion revascularization (24% vs. 42%; $p < .01$) (Fig. 83.14) and less binary angiographically determined restenosis (32% vs. 55%; $p = .01$) than was delivery of a placebo. In the Gamma Washington Radiation for In-Stent Restenosis Trial (WRIST), patients who were assigned to receive ^{192}Ir also had less target lesion revascu-

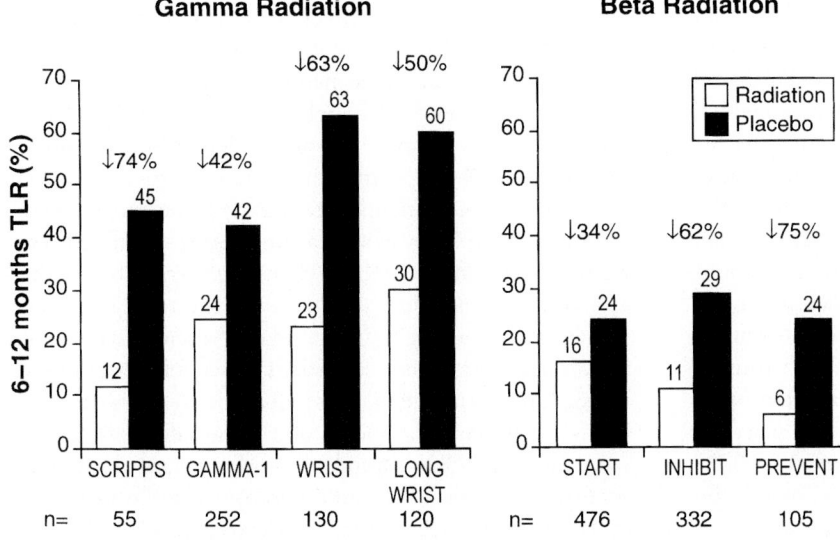

FIGURE 83.14 Rates of target lesion revascularization (TLR) after intracoronary brachytherapy for in-stent restenosis. Compared with results after placebo administration, target vessel revascularization was relatively reduced by 43% to 74% after gamma radiation therapy and by 34% to 63% after beta radiation at 6 to 12 months of follow-up. INHIBIT, Intimal Hyperplasia Inhibition with Beta In-stent Trial; PREVENT, Proliferation Reduction with Vascular Energy Trial; SCRIPPS, Scripps Coronary Radiation to Inhibit Proliferation Post-Stenting trial; START, ^{90}Sr Treatment of Angiographic Restenosis Trial; WRIST, Washington Radiation for In-stent Restenosis Trial.

TABLE 83.7 CLINICAL TRIALS OF INTRACORONARY RADIATION FOR TREATMENT OF IN-STENT RESTENOSIS

Study	n	Dosimetry	Follow-up period (mo)	MACE (%) Radiation	MACE (%) Control	p Value
Gamma radiation (Ir-192)						
SCRIPPS (352)	55	8–30 Gy, IVUS guidance	12	15	48	.01
			39	23	55	.01
GAMMA-1 (353)	252	8–30 Gy, IVUS guidance	9	28	44	.02
WRIST (354)	130	15 Gy, 2 mm from the source	12[a]	35	68	<.001
LONG WRIST (355)	120	15 Gy, 2.0 mm from the source	12	38	62	.01
Beta radiation (Y-90, Sr-90, P-32)						
START (358)	476	Sr-90/Y-90: 16–20 Gy, 2.0 mm from center	8	18	26	.039
INHIBIT (357)	332	P-32: 20 Gy, 1 mm from center	9	22	33	.037
PREVENT (356)	105	P-32: 16–24 Gy, 1 mm in artery wall	12	16	24	NS

INHIBIT, Intimal Hyperplasia Inhibition with Beta In-stent Trial; Ir-192, iridium-192; IVUS, intravascular ultrasonography; MACE, major adverse cardiovascular events (death, myocardial infarction, target lesion revascularization); NS, not significant; P-32, phosphorus-32; PREVENT, Proliferation Reduction with Vascular Energy Trial; SCRIPPS, Scripps Coronary Radiation to Inhibit Proliferation Post-Stenting trial; St-90, strontium-90; START, [90]Sr Treatment of Angiographic Restenosis Trial; WRIST, Washington Radiation for In-stent Restenosis Trial; Y-90, yttrium-90.
[a]Death, myocardial infarction, target lesion revascularization.

larization (23% vs. 63%; *p* <.001) (Fig. 83.14) and less angiographically identified restenosis (19% vs. 58%; *p* = .001) than did those in the placebo group at 6 months. For long lesions (mean stent length 70 mm), the Long WRIST study reported a 50% reduction of target lesion revascularization (*p* = .001) (Fig. 83.14). A significant reduction in the composite of death, myocardial infarction, and target vessel revascularization was noted in each study at 6-month to 1-year follow-up (352–355) (Table 83.7).

Beta Radiation

Initially studied as an adjunctive treatment to prevent restenosis in *de novo* lesions in native coronary arteries, beta radiation has been demonstrated to effectively lower recurrent stenosis after PCI for in-stent stenosis (356–358). The Beta WRIST (359), a registry of Y-90 beta radiation in treating in-stent restenosis, first reported the safety of Y-90 administration. At 6 months, target lesion revascularization was 26%, which compared favorably with the previous results of the placebo cohort in Gamma WRIST. The Sr-90 Treatment of Angiographic Restenosis Trial (358), in which 476 patients were randomly assigned to undergo either Sr-90 brachytherapy or a placebo procedure for in-stent restenosis, demonstrated a marked reduction in favor of the group receiving beta radiation in both clinically determined restenosis (Sr-90 24% vs. placebo 34%; risk reduction, 34%; *p* = .008) and angiographically determined restenosis (Sr-90 14% vs. placebo 42%; *p* <.001) at 8 months (356,358,359) (Table 83.7; Fig. 83.14). The Intimal Hyperplasia Inhibition with Beta In-stent Trial is a moderately sized (332-patient) multicenter, randomized, placebo-controlled trial that has preliminarily observed a 63% reduction in target vessel revascularization (11% for the radiation group vs. 29% for the placebo group) at 8

months through treatment with a P-32 beta radiation source (Table 83.7; Fig. 83.14).

Parallel to the development of catheter-based brachytherapy, stent-based brachytherapy using a beta-emitting P-32 radiation source has been investigated (360,361). Advantages of this technique include the fact that it does not require the presence of radiation oncologists, additional shielding in the catheterization laboratory, or particular additional equipment. Although in-stent restenosis is essentially eliminated, stent-edge hyperplasia due to the stimulating effect of low-dose radiation (geographic miss) and balloon injury is a major limitation of this technique.

Late Restenosis and Late Thrombosis

Although intracoronary radiotherapy has been proven to attenuate restenosis overall, its effects are not always consistent or curative. At the extremes of outcomes are patients who have divergent late effects of either thrombosis (perhaps due to inadequate reendothelialization) or restenosis (possibly from paradoxical neointimal stimulation of adjacent vessel segment), although such occurrences are infrequent. In the Scripps Coronary Radiation to Inhibit Proliferation Post-Stenting trial, late luminal loss was observed in some patients between the 6-month and 3-year follow-up. This suggests that a time course–modified restenosis model may be needed when considering brachytherapy. Although not reported in any of the trials mentioned earlier, mitotic changes (carcinoma) or aneurysmal changes in coronary arteries are potential late sequelae, and observing such potential events may require many years of follow-up. More important concern about the safety of radiation was raised when late thrombosis and myocardial infarction occurred months after radiotherapy. After intracoronary radiation, endothelial repair is delayed due to the same inhibiting effect of radiation in attenuating tissue proliferation. Late thrombosis is thought to be due either to delayed reendothelialization of stents or to late positive arterial remodeling that causes separation of the stent from the arterial wall. The reduction in the composite primary end points with radiation therapy in these clinical trials is driven mainly by the reduction in target vessel revascularization. For example, in GAMMA-1 (353) a trend was seen in the ^{192}Ir arm toward increased death (3.1% vs. 0.8% for the placebo arm; $p = .17$) and increased myocardial infarction (4.6% vs. 2.5% in the placebo arm; $p = .09$) at 9 months. When data for the brachytherapy trials are combined, late thrombosis is found to occur in 9.1% of the radiation-treated group versus 1.2% of the placebo group ($p <.0001$). By multivariate logistic regression analysis, new stent implantation and long lesions were found to be the major predictors of late thrombosis. Current recommendations, therefore, include either the avoidance of new stent placement or long-term therapy with thienopyridine. The GAMMA-V and Plavix WRIST registries are intended to study the efficacy of a 6-month course of clopidogrel bisulfate and aspirin for prevention of subacute thrombosis after Ir-192 radiotherapy (362). In beta radiation trials, prolonged clopidogrel and aspirin therapy (3 to 6 months) was associated with low (less than 2%) incidence of late thrombosis (357,358).

CONTROVERSIES AND PERSONAL PERSPECTIVES

Despite extensive basic scientific and clinical research, the epidemiology, prophylactic measures, and treatment of restenosis after angioplasty are still surrounded by controversy. For example, for many years the working hypothesis of restenosis pathophysiology focused on neointimal hyperplasia. Thus, pharmacologic and mechanical therapies targeted thrombus formation, intimal dissection, and smooth muscle cell proliferation in keeping with this hyperplastic paradigm. Subsequent histologic investigations in animal models (363) and serial intravascular ultrasonographic data from clinical studies (18), however, suggested that the majority of lumen loss after balloon angioplasty was due to negative arterial remodeling or vessel contracture, not neointimal growth. These new findings may explain why some final lumen diameters have been reported to increase in the months after angioplasty, whereas in other cases lumen diameters remain the same or restenosis develops (Fig. 83.2) (38). They would also explain why early pharmacologic therapies did not improve restenosis after balloon angioplasty. Hence, reevaluation of those therapies that limited neointimal growth but were not successful in halting the remodeling-induced restenosis of balloon angioplasty is reasonable. Used in association with intracoronary stents, these agents may prove to be particularly useful.

Agents for which results currently appear hopeful include probucol, cilostazol, paclitaxel, and rapamycin.

Although the effect of remodeling was being elucidated in the balloon angioplasty population, intracoronary stent placement increased in frequency to become the leading procedure, and in-stent restenosis is almost entirely due to neointimal hyperplasia. This has necessarily led to reevaluation of the epidemiology of restenosis. Regarding predictors of restenosis, most of the previously described anatomic and demographic risk factors still apply to contemporary balloon angioplasty procedures. On the other hand, data on intracoronary stents show that these well-entrenched restenosis predictors have decreased in importance (Table 83.2). For example, unstable angina, chronic total occlusion, vessel treated, and lesion length—all strong predictors of restenosis after balloon angioplasty—have little or no predictive value for restenosis after stent placement.

The rapid replacement of balloon angioplasty by intracoronary stent placement has also introduced several other important controversies. First, despite several focused studies comparing balloon angioplasty to stent placement, much of the rush to use stents in the interventional laboratory has not been evidence based. For example, although few controlled data are available, stents are being placed in gradually smaller vessels, in longer lesions, and in lesions already containing a restenotic stent. Although these practices may be the treatment of choice in the future, current practice remains ahead of prospectively collected evidence and technology. Several studies are continuing to elucidate when a "stent-like" result obtained with balloon angioplasty or other techniques alone provides a restenosis rate similar to that achieved with stent placement.

A second area of current interest created by the rapid flux of stent use includes both the prophylaxis and treatment of in-stent restenosis. Despite the relatively low rate of restenosis within stents, the actual number of patients with in-stent restenosis now exceeds the number with non-stent restenosis. For the prophylaxis of in-stent restenosis, radiation therapy and use of platelet glycoprotein IIb/IIIa inhibitors continue to be studied. Because diabetic patients account for approximately 20% of all patients undergoing intervention, the suggestion that abciximab may reduce target vessel revascularization among diabetic patients needs to be further explored. The 6-month data from the Do Tirofiban and ReoPro Give Similar Efficacy Outcome Trial (364) and Enhanced Supresion of the Platelet IIb/IIIa Receptor with Integrilin Therapy (365) trials may give additional insight. Administration of gamma and beta radiation has proven successful in attenuating recurrent in-stent restenosis. Data must accumulate before the factors that predict benefit from radiation therapy can be understood (366). Likewise, one hopes that the several unattractive features of radiation delivery and safety will be improved. Although controversies do abound, the future will undoubtedly continue to supply new pharmacologic and

THE FUTURE

With new information regarding the mechanisms of restenosis and the application of strategies to limit recurrence of stenosis, the future for interventional cardiology is bright. The spectrum of patients and coronary anatomy that can be successfully treated with percutaneous revascularization will continue to broaden. At the same time, the occurrence of restenosis should be further reduced as novel techniques and agents, such as intracoronary stents incorporating radiation or antiproliferative agents, are applied.

mechanical therapies targeting restenosis. Given the complex and interrelated mechanisms of restenosis, a combination of therapies will most likely provide the optimal preventive strategy.

REFERENCES

1. Gruentzig AR, King SD, Schlumpf M, et al. Long-term follow-up after percutaneous transluminal coronary angioplasty. The early Zurich experience. *N Engl J Med* 1987;316:1127–1132.
2. Bittl J. Advances in coronary angioplasty. *N Engl J Med* 1996;335:1290–1302.
3. Windecker S, Maier-Rudolph W, Bonzel T, et al. Interventional cardiology in Europe 1995. *Eur Heart J* 1999;20:484–495.
4. U.S. Department of Health and Human Services. Detailed diagnoses and procedures, National Hospital Discharge Survey, 1993. *Vital Health Stat 13* 1995;121:95–1783.
5. American Heart Association. 2001 heart and stroke statistical update. Available at: http://www.americanheart.org/statistics/index.html, 29–31. Accessed September 4, 2001. Can be downloaded at http://www.americanheart.org/statistics/pdf/HSSTATS2001_1.0.pdf.
6. Topol E, Ellis S, Cosgrove D, et al. Analysis of coronary angioplasty practice in the United States with an insurance-claims data base. *Circulation* 1993;87:1489–1497.
7. Forrester JS, Fishbein M, Helfant R, et al. A paradigm for restenosis based on cell biology: clues for the development of new preventive therapies. *J Am Coll Cardiol* 1991;17:758–769.
8. Rensing BJ, Hermans WRM, Beatt KJ, et al. Quantitative angiographic assessment of elastic recoil after percutaneous transluminal coronary angioplasty. *Am J Cardiol* 1990;66:1039–1044.
9. Sanders M. Angiographic changes thirty minutes following percutaneous transluminal coronary angioplasty. *Angiology* 1985;36:419–424.
10. Nobuyoshi M, Kimura T, Nosaka H, et al. Restenosis after successful percutaneous transluminal coronary angioplasty: serial angiographic follow-up of 229 patients. *J Am Coll Cardiol* 1988;12:616–623.
11. Preisack M, Athanasiadis A, Voelker W, et al. Early luminal deterioration following successful percutaneous transluminal coronary angioplasty: frequency, prediction, and clinical implications. *Eur Heart J* 1994;15:739–746.
12. Rodriguez A, Santaera O, Larribeau M, et al. Early decrease in minimal luminal diameter after successful percutaneous transluminal coronary angioplasty predicts late restenosis. *Am J Cardiol* 1993;71:1391–1395.
13. Rodriguez A, Santaera O, Larribeau M, et al. Coronary stenting decreases restenosis in lesions with early loss in luminal diameter 24 hours after successful PTCA. *Circulation* 1995;91:1397–1402.
14. Daniel W, Pirwitz M, Willard J, et al. Incidence and treatment of elastic recoil occurring in the 15 minutes following successful percutaneous transluminal coronary angioplasty. *Am J Cardiol* 1996;78:253–259.
15. Glagov S, Weisenberg E, Zarins C, et al. Compensatory enlargement of human atherosclerotic coronary arteries. *N Engl J Med* 1987;316:1371–1375.
16. McPherson D, Sirna S, Hiratzka L, et al. Coronary arterial remodeling studied by high-frequency epicardial echocardiography: an early compensatory mechanism in patients with obstructive coronary atherosclerosis. *J Am Coll Cardiol* 1991;17:79–86.
17. Mehta V, Jorgensen M, Raizner A, et al. Spontaneous regression of restenosis: an angiographic study. *J Am Coll Cardiol* 1995;26:696–702.
18. Mintz G, Popma J, Pichard A, et al. Arterial remodeling after coronary angioplasty: a serial intravascular ultrasound study. *Circulation* 1996;94:35–43.
19. den Heijer P, van Dijk R, Hillege H, et al. Serial angioscopic and angiographic observations during the first hour after successful coronary angioplasty: a preamble to a multicenter trial addressing angioscopic markers for restenosis. *Am Heart J* 1994;128:656–663.
20. Uchida Y, Hasegawa K, Kawamura K, et al. Angioscopic observation of the coronary luminal changes induced by percutaneous transluminal coronary angioplasty. *Am Heart J* 1989;117:769–776.
21. Fukami MH, Salganicoff L. Human platelet storage organelles. *Thromb Haemost* 1977;38:963–970.
22. Holmsen H. Secretable storage pools in platelets. *Annu Rev Med* 1979;30:119–134.
23. Le Breton H, Plow E, Topol E. Role of platelets in restenosis after percutaneous coronary revascularization. *J Am Coll Cardiol* 1996;28:1643–1651.
24. Lindner V, Reidy M. Expression of basic fibroblast growth factor and its receptor by smooth muscle cells and endothelium in injured rat arteries. An en face study. *Circ Res* 1993;73:589–595.
25. Shimokawa H, Ito A, Fukumoto Y, et al. Chronic treat-

ment with interleukin-1b induces coronary intimal lesions and vasospastic responses in pigs in vivo. *J Clin Invest* 1996;97:769–776.

26. Schwartz RS, Holmes D Jr, Topol E. The restenosis paradigm revisited: an alternative proposal for cellular mechanisms. *J Am Coll Cardiol* 1992;20:1284–1293.

27. Clowes AW, Reidy MA, Clowes MM. Kinetics of cellular proliferation after arterial injury. I. Smooth muscle growth in the absence of endothelium. *Lab Invest* 1983;49:327–333.

28. Nobuyoshi M, Kimura T, Ohishi H, et al. Restenosis after percutaneous transluminal coronary angioplasty: pathologic observations in 20 patients. *J Am Coll Cardiol* 1991;17:433–439.

29. Garratt K, Edwards W, Kaufmann U, et al. Differential histopathology of primary atherosclerotic and restenotic lesions in coronary arteries and saphenous vein bypass grafts: analysis of tissue obtained from 73 patients by directional atherectomy. *J Am Coll Cardiol* 1991;17:442–448.

30. Hoffman R, Mintz G, Dussaillant G, et al. Patterns and mechanisms of in-stent restenosis: a serial intravascular ultrasound study. *Circulation* 1996;94:1247–1254.

31. Schwartz RS, Huber KC, Murphy JG, et al. Restenosis and the proportional neointimal response to coronary artery injury: results in a porcine model. *J Am Coll Cardiol* 1992;19:267–274.

32. Karas S, Gravanis M, Santoian E, et al. Coronary intimal proliferation after balloon injury and stenting in swine: an animal model of restenosis. *J Am Coll Cardiol* 1992;20:467–474.

33. Gordon P, Gibson C, Cohen D, et al. Mechanisms of restenosis and redilation within coronary stents: quantitative angiographic assessment. *J Am Coll Cardiol* 1993;21:1166–1174.

34. Serruys P, Strauss B, Beatt K, et al. Angiographic follow-up after placement of self-expanding coronary-artery stent. *N Engl J Med* 1991;324:13–17.

35. Dussaillant G, Mintz G, Pichard A, et al. Small stent size and intimal hyperplasia contribute to restenosis: a volumetric intravascular ultrasound analysis. *Am J Cardiol* 1995;26:720–724.

36. Yokoi H, Kimura T, Nobuyoshi M. Palmaz-Shatz coronary stent restenosis: pattern and management. *J Am Coll Cardiol* 1994;23:117A.

37. Serruys PW, Luijten HE, Beatt KJ, et al. Incidence of restenosis after successful coronary angioplasty: a time-related phenomenon. *Circulation* 1988;77:361–371.

38. Kuntz RE, Safian RD, Levine MJ, et al. Novel approach to the analysis of restenosis after the use of three new coronary devices. *J Am Coll Cardiol* 1992;19:1493–1499.

39. Kuntz R, Gibson C, Nobuyoshi M, et al. Generalized model of restenosis after conventional balloon angioplasty, stenting and directional atherectomy. *J Am Coll Cardiol* 1993;21:15–25.

40. Piessens J, Stammen F, Desmet W, et al. Immediate and 6 month follow-up results of coronary angioplasty for restenosis: analysis of factors predicting recurrent clinical restenosis. *Am Heart J* 1993;126:565–570.

41. Holmes DJ, Topol E, Califf R, et al. A multicenter, randomized trial of coronary angioplasty versus directional angio-

plasty for patients with saphenous vein bypass graft lesions. CAVEAT-II investigators. *Circulation* 1995;91(7):1966–1974.

42. Roubin GS, Douglas JS Jr, King SB III, et al. Influence of balloon size on initial success, acute complications, and restenosis after percutaneous transluminal coronary angioplasty. A prospective randomized study. *Circulation* 1988;78:557–565.

43. Topol E, Califf R, Weisman H, et al. Randomised trial of coronary intervention with antibody against platelet IIb/IIIa integrin for the reduction of clinical restenosis: results at six months. *Lancet* 1994;343:881–886.

44. Weintraub WS, Ghazzal ZM, Douglas J Jr, et al. Long-term clinical follow-up in patients with angiographic restudy after successful angioplasty. *Circulation* 1993;87:831–840.

45. Kastrati A, Schömig A, Elezi S, et al. Prognostic value of the modified American College of Cardiology/American Heart Association stenosis morphology classification for long-term angiographic and clinical outcome after coronary stent placement. *Circulation* 1999;100:1285–1290.

46. Topol E, Mark D, Lincoff A, et al. Outcomes at 1 year and economic implications of platelet glycoprotein IIb/IIIa blockade in patients undergoing coronary stenting: results from a multicentre randomised trial. EPISTENT investigators. *Lancet* 2000;355:2019–2024.

47. Holmes DRJ, Vlietstra RE, Smith HC, et al. Restenosis after percutaneous transluminal coronary angioplasty (PTCA): a report from the PTCA registry of the National Heart, Lung, and Blood Institute. *Am J Cardiol* 1984;53:77C–81C.

48. Levine S, Ewels C, Rosing D, et al. Coronary angioplasty: clinical and angiographic follow-up. *Am J Cardiol* 1985;55:673–676.

49. Popma JJ, van den Berg EK, Dehmer GJ. Long-term outcome of patients with symptomatic restenosis after percutaneous transluminal coronary angioplasty. *Am J Cardiol* 1988;62:1298–1299.

50. Vetrovec G, DiSciascio G, Hugo R, et al. Comparative clinical and angiographic findings in patients with symptomatic and asymptomatic restenosis following angioplasty. *J Am Coll Cardiol* 1990;15:59A(abstr).

51. Hernandez RA, Macaya C, Iniguez A, et al. Midterm outcome of patients with asymptomatic restenosis after coronary balloon angioplasty. *J Am Coll Cardiol* 1992;19:1402–1409.

52. Bengtson JR, Mark DB, Honan MB, et al. Detection of restenosis after elective percutaneous transluminal coronary angioplasty using the exercise treadmill test. *Am J Cardiol* 1990;65:28–34.

53. Mata L, Bosch X, David P, et al. Clinical and angiographic assessment 6 months after double vessel percutaneous coronary angioplasty. *J Am Coll Cardiol* 1985;6:1239–1244.

54. Leimgruber PP, Roubin GS, Hollman J, et al. Restenosis after successful coronary angioplasty in patients with single-vessel disease. *Circulation* 1986;73:710–717.

55. Joelson J, Most A, Williams D. Angiographic findings when chest pain recurs after successful percutaneous transluminal angioplasty. *Am J Cardiol* 1987;60:792–795.

56. Hillegass WB, Ohman EM, Califf RM. Restenosis: the clinical issues. In: Topol EJ, ed. *Textbook of interventional*

cardiology, 2nd ed. Philadelphia: WB Saunders, 1993:415–435.

57. Serruys PW, Rensing BJ, Hermans WRM, et al. Definition of restenosis after percutaneous transluminal coronary angioplasty: a quickly evolving concept. *J Interv Card* 1991;4:265–276.

58. Vlodaver Z, French R, van Tassel R, et al. Correlation of the antemortem coronary arteriogram and the postmortem specimen. *Circulation* 1973;47:162–169.

59. Grondin C, Dysda I, Pasternac A, et al. Discrepancies between cineangiographic and postmortem findings in patients with coronary revascularization. *Circulation* 1974;49:703–708.

60. Arnett E, Isner J, Redwood D, et al. Coronary narrowings in coronary heart disease: comparison of cineangiographic and necropsy findings. *Ann Intern Med* 1979;91:350–358.

61. Fisher L, Judkins M, Lesperance J, et al. Reproducibility of coronary arteriographic readings in the Coronary Artery Surgery Study (CASS). *Cathet Cardiovasc Diagn* 1982;8:565–575.

62. Zir L, Miller S, Dinsmore R, et al. Interobserver variability in coronary angiography. *Circulation* 1976;53:627–632.

63. Galbraith J, Murphy M, Desoyza N. Coronary angiogram interpretation: interobserver variability. *JAMA* 1981;240:2053–2059.

64. Topol E, Nissen S. Our preoccupation with coronary luminology: the dissociation between clinical and angiographic findings in ischemic heart disease. *Circulation* 1995;92:2333–2342.

65. Lincoff A, Keeler G, Berdan L, et al. "Worst view" angiographic analysis in CAVEAT provided a "worse case" scenario of restenosis rates and vessel luminal diameters. *Circulation* 1994;90:I-60.

66. Escaned J, Baptista J, Di Mario C, et al. Significance of automated stenosis detection during quantitative angiography: insights gained from intracoronary ultrasound imaging. *Circulation* 1996;94:966–972.

67. Dill T, Dietz U, Hamm C, et al. A randomized comparison of balloon angioplasty versus rotational atherectomy in complex coronary lesions (COBRA study). *Eur Heart J* 2000;21:1759–1766.

68. Rensing B, Hermans W, Deckers J, et al. Lumen narrowing after percutaneous transluminal coronary balloon angioplasty follows a near Gaussian distribution: a quantitative angiographic study in 1,445 successfully dilated lesions. *J Am Coll Cardiol* 1992;19:939–945.

69. The MERCATOR study group. Does the new angiotensin converting enzyme inhibitor cilazapril prevent restenosis after percutaneous transluminal coronary angioplasty? Results of the MERCATOR study: a multicenter, randomized, double-blind placebo-controlled trial. *Circulation* 1992;86:100–110.

70. Fischman D, Leon M, Baim D, et al. A randomized comparison of coronary-stent placement and balloon angioplasty in the treatment of coronary artery disease. *N Engl J Med* 1994;331:496–501.

71. Serruys P, de Jaegere P, Kiemeniej F, et al. A comparison of balloon-expandable-stent implantation with balloon angioplasty in patients with coronary artery disease. *N Engl J Med* 1994;331:489–495.

72. Popma JJ, De Cesare NB, Pinkerton CA, et al. Quantitative analysis of factors influencing late lumen loss and restenosis after directional coronary atherectomy. *Am J Cardiol* 1993;71:552–557.

73. Topol EJ, Leya F, Pinkerton CA, et al. A comparison of directional atherectomy with coronary angioplasty in patients with coronary artery disease. The CAVEAT study group. *N Engl J Med* 1993;329:221–227.

74. Adelman A, Cohen E, Kimball B, et al. A comparison of directional atherectomy with balloon angioplasty for lesions of the left anterior descending artery. *N Engl J Med* 1993;329:228–233.

75. Ellis S, Savage M, Fischman D, et al. Restenosis after placement of Palmaz-Schatz stents in native coronary arteries. Initial results of a multicenter experience. *Circulation* 1992;86:1836–1844.

76. Bittl J, Sanborne T. Excimer laser-facilitated coronary angioplasty. Relative risk analysis of acute and follow-up results in 200 patients. *Circulation* 1992;86:71–80.

77. Reifart N, Vandormael M, Krajcar M, et al. Randomized comparison of angioplasty of complex coronary lesions at a single center: excimer laser, rotational atherectomy, and balloon angioplasty comparison (ERBAC) study. *Circulation* 1997;96:91–98.

78. Raizner A, Hollman J, Abukhalil J, et al. Ciprostene for restenosis revisited: quantitative analysis of angiograms. *J Am Coll Cardiol* 1993;21:321A.

79. Schwartz L, Bourassa MG, Lesperance J, et al. Aspirin and dipyridamole in the prevention of restenosis after percutaneous transluminal coronary angioplasty. *N Engl J Med* 1988;318:1714–1719.

80. Ellis SG, Roubin GS, Wilentz J, et al. Effect of 18- to 24-hour heparin administration for prevention of restenosis after complicated coronary angioplasty. *Am Heart J* 1989;117:777–782.

81. Pepine CJ, Hirshfeld JW, MacDonald RG, et al. A controlled trial of corticosteroids to prevent restenosis after coronary angioplasty. *Circulation* 1990;81:1753–1761.

82. Franzen D, Schannwell M, Oette K, et al. A prospective, randomized, and double-blind trial on the effect of fish oil on the incidence of restenosis following PTCA. *Cathet Cardiovasc Diagn* 1993;28:301–310.

83. Knudtson ML, Flintoft VF, Roth DL, et al. Effect of short-term prostacyclin administration on restenosis after percutaneous transluminal coronary angioplasty. *J Am Coll Cardiol* 1990;15:691–697.

84. Weintraub W, Boccuzzi S, Klein J, et al. Lack of effect of lovastatin on restenosis after coronary angioplasty. Lovastatin restenosis study group. *N Engl J Med* 1994;331:1331–1337.

85. Savage MP, Goldberg S, Bove AA, et al. Effect of thromboxane A_2 blockade on clinical outcome and restenosis after successful coronary angioplasty: Multi-Hospital Eastern Atlantic Restenosis Trial (M-HEART II). *Circulation* 1995;92:3194–3200.

86. Faxon D, on behalf of the MARCATOR study group. Effect of high dose angiotensin-converting enzyme inhibition on restenosis: final results of the MARCATOR study, a multicenter, double-blind, placebo-controlled trial of cilazapril. *J Am Coll Cardiol* 1995;25:362–369.

87. Baim DS, Cutlip DE, Sharma SK, et al. Final results of the Balloon vs. Optimal Atherectomy Trial (BOAT). *Circulation* 1998;97:322–331.

88. Serruys P, van Hout B, Bonnier H, et al. Randomized comparison of implantation with heparin-coated stents with balloon angioplasty in selected patients with coronary artery disease (BENESTENT II). *Lancet* 1998;352: 673–681.

89. Betriu A, Masotti M, Serra A, et al. Randomized comparison of coronary stent implantation and balloon angioplasty in the treatment of de novo coronary artery lesions (START). *J Am Coll Cardiol* 1999;34:1498–1506.

90. Serruys PW, van Hout B, Bonnier H, et al. Randomised comparison of implantation of heparin-coated stents with balloon angioplasty in selected patients with coronary artery disease (BENESTENT II). *Lancet* 1998;352:673–681.

91. Park S, Park S, Lee C, et al. Immediate results and late clinical outcomes after new CrossFlex coronary stent implantation. *Am J Cardiol* 1999;83:502–506.

92. Kastrati A, Schömig A, Dirschinger J, et al. Increased risk of restenosis after placement of gold-coated stents. Results of a randomized trial comparing gold-coated with uncoated steel stents in patients with coronary artery disease. *Circulation* 2000;101:2478–2483.

93. Baim D, Cutlip D, Midei M, et al. Final results of a randomized trial comparing the Multi-Link stent with the Palmaz-Schatz stent for narrowings in native coronary arteries. ASCENT investigators. ACS Multi-Link stent clinical equivalence in de novo lesions trial. *Am J Cardiol* 2001;87:157–162.

94. vom Dahl J, Haager P, Grube E, et al. Gold coating of coronary stents increases neointimal proliferation following stent implantation: a prospective randomized multicenter trial with quantitative intravascular ultrasound at 6 months. *J Am Coll Cardiol* 2001;37:73A.

95. Baim D, Cutlip D, O'Shaughnessy C, et al. Final results of a randomized trial comparing the NIR stent to the Palmaz-Schatz stent for narrowings in native coronary arteries. NIRVANA investigators. NIR Vascular Advanced North American. *Am J Cardiol* 2001;87:152–156.

96. Simonton C, Mark D, Hinohara T, et al. Late restenosis after coronary angioplasty for acute myocardial infarction: comparison with elective coronary angioplasty. *J Am Coll Cardiol* 1988;11:698–705.

97. The EPILOG Investigators. Platelet glycoprotein IIb/IIIa receptor blockade and low-dose heparin during percutaneous coronary revascularization. *N Engl J Med* 1997;336:1689–1696.

98. Korzick D, Underwood D, Simpfendorfer C. Early exercise testing following percutaneous transluminal coronary angioplasty. *Cleve Clin J Med* 1990;57:53–56.

99. Balady G, Leitschuh M, Jacobs A, et al. Safety and clinical use of exercise testing one to three days after percutaneous transluminal coronary angioplasty. *Am J Cardiol* 1992;69:1259–1264.

100. Wijns W, Serruys PW, Reiber JHC, et al. Early detection of restenosis after successful percutaneous transluminal coronary angioplasty by exercise-redistribution thallium scintigraphy. *Am J Cardiol* 1985;55:357–361.

101. El-Tamimi H, Davies GJ, Hackett D, et al. Very early prediction of restenosis after successful coronary angioplasty: anatomic and functional assessment. *J Am Coll Cardiol* 1990;15:259–264.

102. Hillegass W, Ancukiewicz M, Bengston J, et al. Does follow-up exercise testing predict restenosis after successful angioplasty? *Circulation* 1992;86[Suppl I]:I-137.

103. Honan M, Bengston J, Pryor D, et al. Exercise treadmill testing is a poor predictor of anatomic restenosis after angioplasty for acute myocardial infarction. *Circulation* 1989;80:1585–1594.

104. O'Keefe JH Jr, Lapeyre AC III, Holmes DR Jr, et al. Usefulness of early radionuclide angiography for identifying low-risk patients for late restenosis after percutaneous transluminal coronary angioplasty. *Am J Cardiol* 1988;61:51–54.

105. Coma-Canella I, Daza N, Orbe L. Detection of restenosis with dobutamine stress test after coronary angioplasty. *Am Heart J* 1992;124:1196–1204.

106. Pirelli S, Danzi GB, Alberti A, et al. Comparison of usefulness of high-dose dipyridamole echocardiography and exercise electrocardiography for detection of asymptomatic restenosis after coronary angioplasty. *Am J Cardiol* 1991;67:1335–1338.

107. DePuey EG, Leatherman LL, Leachman RD, et al. Restenosis after transluminal coronary angioplasty detected with exercise-gated radionuclide ventriculography. *J Am Coll Cardiol* 1984;4:1103–1113.

108. Hardoff R, Shefer A, Gips S, et al. Predicting late restenosis after coronary angioplasty by very early (12 to 24 h) thallium-102 scintigraphy: implications with regard to mechanisms of late coronary restenosis. *J Am Coll Cardiol* 1990;15:1486–1492.

109. Breisblatt WM, Weiland FL, Spaccavento LJ. Stress thallium-201 imaging after coronary angioplasty predicts restenosis and recurrent symptoms. *J Am Coll Cardiol* 1988;12:1199–1204.

110. Hecht H, Shaw R, Bruce T, et al. Usefulness of tomographic thallium-201 imaging for detection of restenosis after percutaneous transluminal coronary angioplasty. *Am J Cardiol* 1990;66:1314–1318.

111. Marie P, Danchin N, Karcher G, et al. Usefulness of exercise SPECT-thallium to detect asymptomatic restenosis in patients who had angina before coronary angioplasty. *Am Heart J* 1993;126:571–577.

112. Aboul-Enein H, Bengtson J, Adams D, et al. Effect of the degree of effort on exercise echocardiography for the detection of restenosis after coronary angioplasty. *Am Heart J* 1991;122:430–437.

113. Hecht H, DeBord L, Shaw R, et al. Usefulness of supine bicycle stress echocardiography for detection of restenosis after percutaneous transluminal coronary angioplasty. *Am J Cardiol* 1993;71:293–296.

114. Heinle S, Lieberman E, Ancukiewicz M, et al. Usefulness of dobutamine echocardiography for detecting restenosis after percutaneous transluminal coronary angioplasty. *Am J Cardiol* 1993;72:1220–1225.

115. Takeuchi M, Miura Y, Toyokawa T, et al. The comparative diagnostic value of dobutamine stress echocardiography and thallium stress tomography for detecting restenosis

after coronary angioplasty. *J Am Soc Echocardiogr* 1995;8:696–702.

116. Manyari D, Knudtson M, Kloiber R, et al. Sequential thallium-201 myocardial perfusion studies after successful percutaneous transluminal coronary angioplasty: delayed resolution of exercise-induced scintigraphic abnormalities. *Circulation* 1988;77:86–95.

117. Weintraub W, Brown C, Liberman H, et al. Effect of restenosis at one previously dilated coronary site on the probability of restenosis at another previously dilated coronary site. *Am J Cardiol* 1993;72:1107–1113.

118. MacDonald RG, Henderson MA, Hirshfeld JW, et al. Patient-related variables and restenosis after percutaneous transluminal coronary angioplasty—a report from the M-HEART group. *Am J Cardiol* 1990;66:926–931.

119. Arora RR, Konrad K, Badhwar K, et al. Restenosis after transluminal coronary angioplasty: a risk factor analysis. *Cathet Cardiovasc Diagn* 1990;19:17–22.

120. Lambert M, Bonan R, Cote G, et al. Multiple coronary angioplasty: a model to discriminate systemic and procedural factors related to restenosis. *J Am Coll Cardiol* 1988;12:310–344.

121. Carrozza J, Kuntz R, Fishman R, et al. Restenosis after arterial injury caused by coronary stenting in patients with diabetes mellitus. *Ann Intern Med* 1993;118:344–350.

122. Myler RK, Shaw RE, Stertzer SH, et al. Recurrence after coronary angioplasty. *Cathet Cardiovasc Diagn* 1987;13:77–86.

123. Abizaid A, Mehran R, Bucher T, et al. Does diabetes influence clinical recurrence after coronary stent implantation? *J Am Coll Cardiol* 1997;29.

124. Aronson D, Bloomgarden Z, Rayfield E. Potential mechanisms promoting restenosis in diabetic patients. *J Am Coll Cardiol* 1996;27:528–535.

125. Fuster V, Badimon L, Badimon J, et al. The pathogenesis of coronary artery disease and the acute coronary syndromes. *N Engl J Med* 1992;326:310–318.

126. Takahashi K, Ghatei M, Lam H, et al. Elevated plasma endothelin in patients with diabetes mellitus. *Diabetologia* 1990;33:306–310.

127. McClain D, Paterson A, Roos M, et al. Glucose and glucosamine regulate growth factor gene expression in vascular smooth muscle cells. *Proc Natl Acad Sci U S A* 1992;89:8150–8154.

128. Scott-Burden T, Schini V, Elizondo E, et al. Platelet-derived growth factor suppresses and fibroblast growth factor enhances cytokine-induced production of nitric oxide by cultured smooth muscle cells: effects on cell proliferation. *Circ Res* 1992;71:1088–1100.

129. Banskota N, Taub R, Zellner K, et al. Insulin, insulin-like growth factor I and platelet-derived growth factor interact additively in the induction of protooncogene c-myc and cellular proliferation in cultured bovine aortic smooth muscle cells. *Mol Endocrinol* 1989;3:1183–1190.

130. Merimee T, Zapf J, Froesch E. Insulin-like growth factors. Studies in diabetics with and without retinopathy. *N Engl J Med* 1983;309:527–530.

131. Cohen R. Dysfunction of vascular endothelium in diabetes mellitus. *Circulation* 1993;87:V67–V76.

132. De Feo P, Gaisano M, Haymond M. Differential effects of insulin deficiency on albumin and fibrinogen synthesis in humans. *J Clin Invest* 1991;88:833–840.

133. Inoguchi T, Umeda F, Ono H, et al. Abnormality in prostacyclin stimulatory activity in sera from diabetics. *Metabolism* 1989;38:837–842.

134. Lorenzi M, Cagliero E, Toldeo S. Glucose toxicity for human endothelial cells in culture. Delayed replication, disturbed cell cycle, and accelerated death. *Diabetes* 1985;34:621–627.

135. Oliver F, de la Rubia G, Feenr E, et al. Stimulation of endothelin-1 gene expression by insulin in endothelial cells. *J Biol Chem* 1991;266:23251–23256.

136. Scott-Burden T, Vanhoutte P. The endothelium as a regulator of vascular smooth muscle proliferation. *Circulation* 1993;87:V51–V55.

137. Tschöpe D, Esser J, Schwippert B, et al. Large platelets circulate in an activated state in diabetes mellitus. *Semin Thromb Hemost* 1991;17:433–439.

138. Umeda F, Inoguchi T, Nawata H. Reduced stimulatory activity on prostacyclin production by cultured endothelial cells from serum of aged diabetic patients. *Atherosclerosis* 1989;75:61–66.

139. Davi G, Catalano I, Averna M, et al. Thromboxane biosynthesis and platelet function in type II diabetes mellitus. *N Engl J Med* 1990;322:1769–1774.

140. Winoccur P. Platelet abnormalities in diabetes mellitus. *Diabetes* 1992;41:26–31.

141. Winoccur P, Richardson M, Kinlough-Rathbone R. Continued platelet interaction with de-endothelialized aortae associated with slower re-endothelialization and more extensive intimal hyperplasia in spontaneously diabetic BB Wistar rats. *Int J Exp Pathol* 1993;74:603–613.

142. Walker L, Bowen-Pope D, Ross R, et al. Production of platelet-like growth factor–like molecules by cultured arterial smooth muscle cells accompanies proliferation after arterial injury. *Proc Natl Acad Sci U S A* 1986;83:7311–7315.

143. Yamamato T, Nakamura T, Noble N, et al. Expression of transforming growth factor β is elevated in human and experimental diabetic nephropathy. *Proc Natl Acad Sci U S A* 1993;90:1814–1818.

144. Johnstone M, Creager S, Scales K, et al. Impaired endothelium-dependent vasodilation in patients with insulin-dependent diabetes mellitus. *Circulation* 1993;88:2510–2516.

145. Sobel B. Restenosis in diabetic patients: is hyperinsulinemia the culprit? *Circulation* 1996;94:3004–3005.

146. Aronson D. Restenosis in diabetic patients: is hyperinsulinemia the culprit? *Circulation* 1996;94:3003–3004.

147. Ip JH, Fuster V, Israel D, et al. The role of platelets, thrombin and hyperplasia in restenosis after coronary angioplasty. *J Am Coll Cardiol* 1991;17:77B–88B.

148. Van Belle E, Maillard L, Tio F, et al. Accelerated endothelialization by local delivery of recombinant human VEGF reduces in-stent intimal formation. *J Am Coll Cardiol* 1997;29:77A.

149. The Bypass Angioplasty Revascularization Investigation (BARI) Investigators. Comparison of coronary bypass surgery with angioplasty in patients with multivessel disease. *N Engl J Med* 1996;335:217–225.

150. Frantz E, Pfautsch P, Möddel S, et al. No excess mortality after coronary angioplasty in diabetic patients with multivessel disease after prior bypass surgery. *J Am Coll Cardiol* 1997;29:455A.

151. O'Keefe J Jr, McCallister B, Blackstone E, et al. Is diabetes per se responsible for worse outcome after angioplasty than bypass surgery among diabetics? *J Am Coll Cardiol* 1997;29:181A.

152. Elezi S, Schühlen H, Wehinger A, et al. Stent placement in diabetic versus non-diabetic patients. Six-month angiographic follow-up. *J Am Coll Cardiol* 1997;29:188A.

153. Tilli F, Aliabadi D, Bowers T, et al. Optimal coronary stenting in diabetics: a viable percutaneous alternative to cardiac surgery. *J Am Coll Cardiol* 1997;29:455A.

154. Yokoi H, Nosaka H, Kimura T, et al. Coronary stenting in diabetic patients: early and follow-up results. *J Am Coll Cardiol* 1997;29:455A.

155. Kastrati A, Mehilli J, Dirschlinger J, et al. Restenosis after coronary placement of various stent types. *Am J Cardiol* 2001;87:34–39.

156. Levine G, Jacobs A, Keeler G, et al. Impact of diabetes mellitus on percutaneous revascularization (CAVEAT-I). *Am J Cardiol* 1997;79:748–755.

157. Kornowski R, Mintz G, Kent K, et al. Increased restenosis in diabetes mellitus after coronary interventions is due to exaggerated intimal hyperplasia. A serial intravascular ultrasound study. *Circulation* 1997;95:1366–1369.

158. Marso S, Lincoff A, Ellis S, et al. Optimizing the percutaneous interventional outcomes for patients with diabetes mellitus: results of the EPISTENT (Evaluation of Platelet IIb/IIIa Inhibitor for Stenting Trial) diabetic substudy. *Circulation* 1999;100:2477–2484.

159. Moreno P, Berenardi V, López-Cuéllar J, et al. Macrophage infiltration predicts restenosis after coronary intervention in patients with unstable angina. *Circulation* 1996;94:3098–3102.

160. Moreno P, Falk E, Palacios I, et al. Macrophage infiltration in acute coronary syndromes: implications for plaque rupture. *Circulation* 1994;90:775–778.

161. Bourassa MG, Lesperance J, Eastwood C, et al. Clinical, physiologic, anatomic, and procedural factors predictive of restenosis after percutaneous transluminal coronary angioplasty. *J Am Coll Cardiol* 1991;18:368–376.

162. Rupprecht HJ, Brennecke R, Bernhard G, et al. Analysis of risk factors for restenosis after PTCA. *Cathet Cardiovasc Diagn* 1990;19:151–159.

163. Umans V, de Feyter P, Deckers J, et al. Acute and long-term outcome of directional coronary atherectomy for stable and unstable angina. *Am J Cardiol* 1994;74:641–646.

164. Reis GJ, Kuntz RE, Silverman DI, et al. Effects of serum lipid levels on restenosis after coronary angioplasty. *Am J Cardiol* 1991;68:1431–1435.

165. Raizner AE, Oesterle SN, Waksman R, et al. Inhibition of restenosis with beta-emitting radiotherapy. Report of the Proliferation Reduction with Vascular Energy Trial (PREVENT). *Circulation* 2000;102:951–958.

166. Desmarais R, Sarembock I, Ayers C, et al. Elevated serum lipoprotein[a] is a risk factor for clinical recurrence after coronary balloon angioplasty. *Circulation* 1995;91:1403–1409.

167. Chiarugi L, Prisco D, Antonucci E, et al. Lipoprotein (a) and anticardiolipin antibodies are risk factors for clinically relevant restenosis after elective balloon percutaneous transluminal coronary angioplasty. *Atherosclerosis* 2001;154:129–135.

168. Rozenman Y, Gilon D, Welber S, et al. Plasma lipoproteins are not related to restenosis after successful coronary angioplasty. *Am J Cardiol* 1993;72:1206–1207.

169. Ribichini F, Steffenino G, Dellavalle A, et al. Plasma lipoprotein (a) is not a predictor for restenosis after elective high-pressure elective coronary stenting. *Circulation* 1998;98:1172–1177.

170. Serruys PW, Rutsch W, Heyndricks GR, et al. Prevention of restenosis after percutaneous transluminal coronary angioplasty with thromboxane A_2-receptor blockade—a randomized, double-blind, placebo-controlled trial. *Circulation* 1991;84:1568–1580.

171. Serruys PW, Klein W, Tijssen JPG, et al. Evaluation of ketanserin in the prevention of restenosis after percutaneous transluminal coronary angioplasty. A multicenter randomized double-blind placebo-controlled trial. *Circulation* 1993;88:1588–1601.

172. Violaris A, Melkert R, Serruys P. Influence of serum cholesterol and cholesterol subfractions on restenosis after successful angioplasty. *Circulation* 1994;90:2267–2279.

173. Yamamoto H, Imazu M, Yamabe T, et al. Risk factors for restenosis after percutaneous transluminal coronary angioplasty: role of lipoprotein[a]. *Am Heart J* 1995;130:1168–1173.

174. Miyata M, Biro S, Arima S, et al. High serum concentration of lipoprotein(a) is a risk factor for restenosis after percutaneous transluminal coronary angioplasty in Japanese patients with single-vessel disease. *Am Heart J* 1996;132:269–273.

175. Cooke T, Sheahan R, Foley D, et al. Lipoprotein[a] in restenosis after percutaneous transluminal coronary angioplasty and coronary artery disease. *Circulation* 1994;89:1593–1598.

176. Wehinger A, Walter H, Zitzmann E, et al. Influence of hyperlipidemia on restenosis after coronary artery stent implantation. *J Am Coll Cardiol* 1997;29:47A.

177. Berger PB, Bell MR, Holmes DR, et al. Effect of restenosis after an earlier angioplasty at another coronary site on the frequency of restenosis after a subsequent coronary angioplasty. *Am J Cardiol* 1992;69:1086–1089.

178. Bresee SJ, Jacobs AK, Gareber GR, et al. Prior restenosis predicts restenosis after coronary angioplasty of a new significant narrowing. *Am J Cardiol* 1991;68:1158–1162.

179. Kastrati A, Dirschinger J, Schömig A. Genetic risk factors and restenosis after percutaneous coronary interventions. *Herz* 2000;25:34–46.

180. Schömig A, Kastrati A, Elezi S, et al. Bimodal distribution of angiographic measures of restenosis six months after coronary stent placement. *Circulation* 1997;96:3880–3887.

181. Watanabe Y, Yamada N, Yokoi H, et al. Relationship between HLA-C locus and restenosis after coronary artery balloon angioplasty. *JAMA* 1997;277:983–984.

182. Huber K, Schwartz R, Edwards W, et al. Effects of angiotensin converting enzyme inhibition on neointimal prolif-

eration in a porcine coronary injury model. *Am Heart J* 1993;125:695–701.

183. Cambien F, Poirier O, Lecerf L, et al. Deletion polymorphism in the gene for angiotensin-converting enzyme is a potent risk factor for myocardial infarction. *Nature* 1992;359:641–644.

184. Ohishi M, Fujii K, Minamino T, et al. A potent genetic risk factor for restenosis [Letter]. *Nat Genet* 1993:324–325.

185. Hamon M, Bauters C, Amant C, et al. Relation between the deletion polymorphism of the angiotensin-converting enzyme gene and late luminal narrowing after coronary angioplasty. *Circulation* 1995;92:296–299.

186. Samani N, Martin D, Brack M, et al. Insertion/deletion polymorphism in the angiotensin-converting enzyme gene and risk of restenosis after coronary angioplasty. *Lancet* 1995;345:1013–1016.

187. van Bockxmeer F, Mamotte C, Gibbons F, et al. Angiotensin-converting enzyme and apolipoprotein E genotypes and restenosis after coronary angioplasty. *Circulation* 1995;92:2066–2071.

188. Amant C, Bauters C, Bodart J, et al. D allele of the angiotensin I–converting enzyme is a major risk factor for restenosis after coronary stenting. *Circulation* 1997;96:56–60.

189. Ribichini F, Steffenino G, Dellavalle A, et al. Plasma activity and insertion/deletion polymorphism of angiotensin I–converting enzyme: a major risk factor and a marker of risk for coronary stent restenosis. *Circulation* 1998;97:147–154.

190. Koch W, Kastrati A, Mehilli J, et al. Insertion/deletion polymorphism of the angiotensin I–Converting enzyme gene is not associated with restenosis after coronary stent placement. *Circulation* 2000;102:197–202.

191. Gürlek A, Gülec S, Karabulut H, et al. Relation between the insertion/deletion polymorphism of the angiotensin I converting enzyme gene and restenosis after coronary stenting. *J Cardiovasc Risk* 2000;7:403–407.

192. Meier B, King SB III, Gruentzig AR, et al. Repeat coronary angioplasty. *J Am Coll Cardiol* 1984;4:463–466.

193. Quigley PJ, Hlatky MA, Hinohara T, et al. Repeat percutaneous transluminal coronary angioplasty and predictors of recurrent restenosis. *Am J Cardiol* 1989;63:409–414.

194. Williams DO, Gruentzig AR, Kent KM, et al. Efficacy of repeat percutaneous transluminal coronary angioplasty for coronary restenosis. *Am J Cardiol* 1984;53:32–35C.

195. Rapold HJ, David PR, Val PG, et al. Restenosis and its determinants in first and repeat coronary angioplasty. *Eur Heart J* 1987;8:575–586.

196. Bauters C, Lablanche J, McFadden E, et al. Clinical characteristics and angiographic follow-up of patients undergoing early or late repeat dilation for a first restenosis. *J Am Coll Cardiol* 1992;20:845–848.

197. Bauters C, McFadden E, Lablanche J, et al. Restenosis rate after multiple percutaneous transluminal coronary angioplasty procedures at the same site. A quantitative angiographic study in consecutive patients undergoing a third angioplasty procedure for a second restenosis. *Circulation* 1993;88:969–974.

198. Weintraub WS, Ghazzal ZMB, Douglas JS, et al. Initial management and long-term clinical outcome of restenosis after initially successful percutaneous transluminal coronary angioplasty. *Am J Cardiol* 1992;70:47–55.

199. Weintraub W, Agarwal S, Hoffmeister J, et al. Examination of restenosis sites in patients with restenosis in one of two previously dilated coronary artery narrowings. *Am J Cardiol* 1993;71:867–869.

200. Teirstein PS, Hoover CA, Ligon RW, et al. Repeat coronary angioplasty: efficacy of a third angioplasty for a second restenosis. *J Am Coll Cardiol* 1989;13:291–296.

201. Tan K, Sulke N, Taub N, et al. Efficacy of a third coronary angioplasty for a second restenosis: short-term results, long-term follow up, and correlates of a third restenosis. *Br Heart J* 1995;73:327–333.

202. Glazier JJ, Varricchione TR, Ryan TJ, et al. Outcome in patients with recurrent restenosis after percutaneous transluminal balloon angioplasty. *Br Heart J* 1989;61:485–488.

203. Dimas AP, Grigera F, Arora RR, et al. Repeat coronary angioplasty as treatment for restenosis. *J Am Coll Cardiol* 1992;19:1310–1314.

204. Joly P, Bonan R, Palisaitas D, et al. Treatment of recurrent restenosis with repeat percutaneous transluminal angioplasty. *Am J Cardiol* 1988;68:906–908.

205. Colombo A, Ferraro M, Itoh A, et al. Results of coronary stenting for restenosis. *J Am Coll Cardiol* 1996;28:830–836.

206. Kitazume H, Ichiro K, Iwama T, et al. Repeat coronary angioplasty as the treatment of choice for restenosis. *Am Heart J* 1996;132:711–715.

207. Abi-Mansour P, Whitworth HB, Hoffmeister J, et al. Initial and late outcome after a third coronary angioplasty (PTCA) for recurrent native coronary artery restenosis. *Circulation* 1985;72:III–141.

208. Bauters C, Lablanche J, Leroy F, et al. Traitement d'une première resténose par nouvelle angioplastie: résultats immédiats et suivi angiographique à 6 mois. *Arch Mal Coeur Vaiss* 1992;85:1515–1520.

209. Mittal S, Weiss D, Hirshfeld J Jr, et al. Restenotic lesions have a worse outcome after stenting. *Circulation* 1996;94:I-331.

210. Hong M, Kent K, Satler L, et al. Are long-term results different when stents are used in de novo versus restenotic lesions? *Circulation* 1996;94:I-331.

211. Lablanche J-M, Danchin N, Grollier G, et al. Factors predictive of restenosis after stent implantation managed by ticlopidine and aspirin. *Circulation* 1996;94:I-256.

212. Hirshfeld JWJ, Schwartz JS, Jugo R, et al. Restenosis after coronary angioplasty: a multivariate statistical model to relate lesion and procedure variables to restenosis. *J Am Coll Cardiol* 1991;18:647–656.

213. Platko W, Hollman J, Whitlow P, et al. Percutaneous transluminal angioplasty of saphenous vein graft stenosis: long-term follow-up. *J Am Coll Cardiol* 1989;14:1645–1650.

214. Block P, Cowley M, Kaltenbach M, et al. Percutaneous angioplasty of stenoses of bypass grafts or bypass graft anastomotic sites. *Am J Cardiol* 1984;53:666–668.

215. Fischman D, Savage M, Bailey S, et al. Predictors of restenosis after saphenous vein graft interventions. *Circulation* 1996;94:I-621.

216. Savage M, Douglas J, Fischman D, et al. Stent placement compared with balloon angioplasty for obstructed coronary bypass grafts. Saphenous Vein De novo Trial investigators. *N Engl J Med* 1997;337:740–747.

217. Foley D, Melkert R, Serruys P. Influence of coronary vessel size on renarrowing process and late angiographic outcome after successful balloon angioplasty. *Circulation* 1994;90:1239–1251.
218. Weintraub W, Douglas J, Ghazzal Z, et al. Evaluation and prediction of clinical restenosis. *Circulation* 1996;94:I-90.
219. Phillips P, Segovia J, Alfonso F, et al. Advantages of stents in the most proximal left anterior descending coronary artery. *Am Heart J* 1998;135:719–725.
220. Serruys P, Kay P, Disco C, et al. Periprocedural quantitative coronary angiography after Palmaz-Schatz stent implantation predicts the restenosis rate at six months. *J Am Coll Cardiol* 1999;34:1067–1074.
221. Piovaccari G, Fattori R, Marzocchi A, et al. Percutaneous transluminal coronary angioplasty of the very proximal left anterior descending artery lesions: immediate results and follow-up. *Int J Cardiol* 1991;30:151–155.
222. Boehrer J, Ellis S, Pieper K, et al. Directional atherectomy versus balloon angioplasty for coronary ostial and nonostial left anterior descending coronary artery lesions: results from a randomized multicenter trial. *J Am Coll Cardiol* 1995;25:1380–1386.
223. Whitworth H, Pilcher G, Roubin G, et al. Do proximal lesions involving the origin of the left anterior descending artery (LAD) have a higher restenosis rate after coronary angioplasty (PTCA)? *Circulation* 1985;72:III-398.
224. Topol E, Ellis S, Fishman J, et al. Multicenter study of percutaneous transluminal angioplasty for right coronary artery ostial stenosis. *J Am Coll Cardiol* 1987;9:1214–1218.
225. Mathias D, Fishman Mooney J, Lange H, et al. Frequency of success and complications of coronary angioplasty of a stenosis at the ostium of a branch vessel. *Am J Cardiol* 1991;67:491–495.
226. Ellis S, Roubin G, King S III, et al. Importance of stenosis morphology in the estimation of restenosis risk after elective percutaneous transluminal coronary angioplasty. *Am J Cardiol* 1989;63:30–34.
227. Elezi S, Kastrati A, Neumann F-J, et al. Vessel size and long-term outcome after coronary stent placement. *Circulation* 1998;98:1875–1880.
228. Rensing BJ, Hermans WRM, Vos J, et al. Luminal narrowing after percutaneous transluminal coronary angioplasty. *Circulation* 1993;88:975–985.
229. Hamasaki N, Nosaka H, Kimura T, et al. Influence of lesion length on late angiographic outcome and restenotic process after successful stent implantation. *J Am Coll Cardiol* 1997;29:239A.
230. Yokoi H, Nobuyoshi M, Nosaka H, et al. Coronary stenting for long lesions (lesion length >20 mm) in native coronary arteries: comparison of three different types of stent. *Circulation* 1996;94:I-685.
231. Laarman G, Plante S, de Feyter PJ. PTCA of chronically occluded coronary arteries. *Am Heart J* 1990;119:1153–1160.
232. Meier B. Total coronary occlusion: a different animal. *J Am Coll Cardiol* 1991;17:50B–57B.
233. Kereiakes D, Selmon M, McAuley B, et al. Angioplasty in total coronary artery occlusion: experience in 76 consecutive patients. *J Am Coll Cardiol* 1985;6:526–533.
234. Safian R, McCabe C, Sipperly M, et al. Initial success and long-term follow-up of percutaneous transluminal coronary angioplasty in chronic total occlusions versus conventional stenoses. *Am J Cardiol* 1988;61:23–28G.
235. Clark D, Wexman M, Murphy M, et al. Factors predicting recurrence in patients who have had angioplasty of total occluded vessels. *J Am Coll Cardiol* 1986;7:20A.
236. DiSciascio G, Vetrovec G, Cowley M, et al. Early and late outcome of percutaneous transluminal coronary angioplasty for subacute and chronic total coronary occlusion. *Am Heart J* 1986;111:833–839.
237. Melchior J, Meier B, Urban P, et al. Percutaneous transluminal coronary angioplasty for chronic total coronary arterial occlusion. *Am J Cardiol* 1987;59:535–538.
238. Nienaber C, Fratz S, Lund G, et al. Primary stent placement or balloon angioplasty for chronic coronary occlusions: a matched pair analysis of 100 patients. *Circulation* 1996;94:I-686.
239. Etsuo T, Osamu K, Masanobu F, et al. Impact of coronary stenting on PTCA of chronic coronary total occlusions. *Circulation* 1996;94:I-249.
240. Cerisier A, Isaaz K, Dacosta A, et al. Prevention of reocclusion after successful balloon PTCA of totally occluded coronary arteries: a prospective randomized pilot-study comparing ticlopidine-aspirin association with aspirin alone. *J Am Coll Cardiol* 1997;29:395A.
241. Berger P, Holmes D Jr, Ohman E, et al. Restenosis, reocclusion and adverse cardiovascular events after successful angioplasty of occluded versus nonoccluded coronary arteries. *J Am Coll Cardiol* 1996;27:1–7.
242. Mathey D, Seidensticker A, Rau T, et al. Chronic coronary artery occlusion: reduction of restenosis- and reocclusion-rates by stent treatment. *J Am Coll Cardiol* 1997;29:396A.
243. Suttrop M, Mast E, Plokker H, et al. Primary coronary stenting after successful balloon angioplasty of chronic total occlusions: a single-center experience. *Circulation* 1996;94:I-687.
244. Elezi S, Schühlen H, Hausleiter J, et al. Six-month angiographic follow-up after stenting of chronic total coronary occlusions. *J Am Coll Cardiol* 1997;29:16A.
245. Mintz G, Popma J, Pichard A, et al. Intravascular ultrasound predictors of restenosis after percutaneous transcatheter coronary revascularization. *J Am Coll Cardiol* 1996;27:1678–1687.
246. The GUIDE trial investigators. IVUS-determined predictors of restenosis in PTCA and DCA: an interim report from the GUIDE trial, phase II. *Circulation* 1994;90:I-23.
247. Paranandi S, Topol E. Contemporary clinical trials of restenosis. *J Invasive Cardiol* 1994;6:109–124.
248. Franklin S, Faxon D. Pharmacologic prevention of restenosis after coronary angioplasty: review of the randomized clinical trials. *Coron Artery Dis* 1993;4:232–242.
249. Gruberg L, Waksman R, Satler L, et al. Novel approaches for the prevention of restenosis. *Exp Opin Invest Drugs* 2000;9:2555–2578.
250. Buchwald A, Unterberg C, Nebendahl K, et al. Low-molecular-weight heparin reduces neointimal proliferation after coronary stent implantation in hypercholesterolemic minipigs. *Circulation* 1992;86:531–537.

251. Faxon DP, Spiro T, Minor S, et al. Enoxaparin a low molecular weight heparin in the prevention of restenosis after angioplasty: result of a double blind randomized trial. *J Am Coll Cardiol* 1992;19:258A.

252. Völker W, Faber V. Aspirin reduces the growth of medial and neointimal thickenings in balloon-injured rat carotid arteries. *Stroke* 1990;21:IV44–45.

253. Thornton MA, Gruentzig AR, Hollman J, et al. Coumadin and aspirin in prevention of recurrence after transluminal coronary angioplasty: a randomized study. *Circulation* 1984;69:721–727.

254. Ingerman-Wojenski C, Silver M. Model system to study the interaction of platelets with damaged arterial wall. II. Inhibition of smooth muscle cell proliferation by dipyridamole and AH-P719. *Exp Mol Pathol* 1988;48:116–134.

255. August D, Tilson M. Modification of myointimal response to arterial injury: effects of aspirin and warfarin. *Surg Forum* 1980;31:337–338.

256. Urban P, Buller N, Fox F, et al. Lack of effect of warfarin on the restenosis rate or on clinical outcome after balloon coronary angioplasty. *Br Heart J* 1988;60:485–488.

257. Yabe Y, Okamoto K, Oosawa H, et al. A thromboxane A$_2$ synthetase inhibitor prevents restenosis after PTCA. *Circulation* 1989;80:II-260.

258. Eriksen UH, Amtorp O, Bagger JP, et al. Continuous angiopeptin infusion reduces coronary restenosis following balloon angioplasty. *Circulation* 1993;88:I-594.

259. Kent K, Williams D, Cassagneau B, et al. Double blind, controlled trial of the effect of angiopeptin on coronary restenosis following balloon angioplasty. *Circulation* 1993;88:I-506.

260. Dehmer GJ, Popma JJ, van den Berg EK, et al. Reduction in the rate of early stenosis after coronary angioplasty by a diet supplemented with n-3 fatty acids. *N Engl J Med* 1988;319:733–740.

261. Grigg LE, Kay TWH, Valentine PA, et al. Determinants of restenosis and lack of effect of dietary supplementation with eicosapentaenoic acid on the incidence of coronary artery stenosis after angioplasty. *J Am Coll Cardiol* 1989;13:665–672.

262. Sahni R, Maniet AR, Voci G, et al. Prevention of restenosis by lovastatin after successful coronary angioplasty. *Am Heart J* 1991;121:1600–1608.

263. Raizner A, Hollman J, Demke D, et al., and the Ciprostene Investigators. Beneficial effects of ciprostene in PTCA: a multicenter, randomized, controlled trial. *Circulation* 1988;78:II-290.

264. Unverdorben M, Kunkel B, Leucht M, et al. Reduction of restenosis after PTCA by diltiazem? *Circulation* 1992;86:I-53.

265. Whitworth HB, Roubin GS, Hollman J, et al. Effect of nifedipine on recurrent stenosis after percutaneous transluminal coronary angioplasty. *J Am Coll Cardiol* 1986;8:1271–1276.

266. Powell JS, Clozel JP, Muller RKM, et al. Inhibitors of angiotensin-converting enzyme prevent myointimal proliferation after vascular injury. *Science* 1989;245:186–188.

267. Currier JP, Pow TK, Minihan AC, et al. Colchicine inhibits restenosis after iliac angioplasty in the atherosclerotic rabbit. *Circulation* 1989;80:II-66.

268. Grines CL, Rizik T, Levine A, et al. Colchicine angioplasty restenosis trial (CART). *Circulation* 1989;84:II-365.

269. Villa A, Guzman L, Weilam C, et al. Local delivery of dexamethasone for prevention of neointimal proliferation in a rat model of balloon angioplasty. *J Clin Invest* 1994;93:1243–1249.

270. Matsuno H, Stassen J, Vermylen J, et al. Inhibition of integrin function by a cyclic RGD-containing peptide prevents neointima formation. *Circulation* 1994;90:2203–2206.

271. Choi E, Engel L, Callow A, et al. Inhibition of neointimal hyperplasia by blocking $\alpha_v\beta_3$ integrin with a small peptide antagonist. *J Vasc Surg* 1994;19:125–134.

272. The EPIC investigators. Use of a monoclonal antibody directed against the platelet glycoprotein IIb/IIIa receptor in high-risk coronary angioplasty. *N Engl J Med* 1994;330:956–961.

273. Lincoff A, Tcheng J, Ellis S, et al. Randomized trial of platelet glycoprotein IIb/IIIa inhibition with Integrelin for prevention of restenosis following coronary intervention: the IMPACT-II angiographic substudy. *Circulation* 1995;92:I-607.

274. Tcheng J, Lincoff A, Sigmon K, et al. Platelet glycoprotein IIb/IIIa inhibition with Integrelin during percutaneous coronary intervention: the IMPACT-II trial. *Circulation* 1995;92:I-545.

275. The RESTORE Investigators. Effects of platelet glycoprotein IIb/IIIa blockade with tirofiban on adverse cardiac events in patients with unstable angina or acute myocardial infarction undergoing coronary angioplasty. Randomized Efficacy Study of Tirofiban for Outcomes and Restenosis. *Circulation* 1997;96:1445–1453.

276. The ERASER investigators. Acute platelet inhibition with abciximab does not reduce in-stent restenosis (ERASER study). *Circulation* 1999;100:799–806.

277. ten Berg J, Kelder J, Suttorp M, et al. Effect of coumarins started before coronary angioplasty on acute complications and long-term follow-up. A randomized trial. *Circulation* 2000;102:386–391.

278. Lehman K, Doris RJ, Feuer JM, et al. Paradoxical increase in restenosis rate with chronic heparin use: final results of a randomized trial. *J Am Coll Cardiol* 1991;17:181A.

279. Brack M, Ray S, Chauhan A, et al. The subcutaneous heparin and angioplasty restenosis prevention (SHARP) trial. *J Am Coll Cardiol* 1995;26:947–954.

280. Faxon D, Spiro T, Minor S, et al. Low molecular weight heparin in the prevention of restenosis after angioplasty: results of Enoxaparin Restenosis (ERA) trial. *Circulation* 1994;90:908–914.

281. Cairns J, Gill J, Morton B, et al. Fish oils and low-molecular-weight heparin for the reduction of restenosis after percutaneous transluminal coronary angioplasty. The EMPAR study. *Circulation* 1996;94:1553–1560.

282. Lablanche J-M. Low molecular weight heparin in the prevention of restenosis after coronary angioplasty: results of the FACT study. *J Am Coll Cardiol* 1995;25:226A.

283. Karsch K, Preisack M, Baildon R, et al. Low molecular weight heparin (Reviparin) in percutaneous transluminal coronary angioplasty: results of a randomized, double-blind, unfractionated heparin and placebo-controlled,

multicenter trial (REDUCE trial). *J Am Coll Cardiol* 1996;28:1437–1443.

284. Kiesz R, Buszman P, Martin J, et al. Local delivery of enoxaparin to decrease restenosis after stenting: results of initial multicenter trial. Polish-American Local Lovenox NIR Assessment Study (the POLONIA study). *Circulation* 2001;103:26–31.

285. Serruys P, Herrman J-P, Simon R, et al. A comparison of hirudin with heparin in the prevention of restenosis after coronary angioplasty. *N Engl J Med* 1995;333:757–763.

286. Bittl J, Strony J, Brinker J, et al. Treatment with bivalirudin (Hirulog) as compared with heparin during coronary angioplasty for unstable or postinfarction angina. *N Engl J Med* 1995;333:764–769.

287. Feldman R, Bengston J, Pryor D, et al. Use of a thromboxane A$_2$ receptor blocker to reduce adverse clinical events after coronary angioplasty. *J Am Coll Cardiol* 1992;19:259A.

288. Gershlick A, Spriggins D, Davies S, et al. Failure of epoprostenol (prostacyclin PGI$_2$) to inhibit platelet aggregation and to prevent restenosis after coronary angioplasty: results of a randomised placebo controlled trial. *Br Heart J* 1994;71:7–15.

289. Nemececk G, Coughlin S, Handley D, et al. Stimulation of aortic smooth muscle cell mitogenesis by serotonin. *Proc Natl Acad Sci U S A* 1986;83:674–678.

290. Aalto M, Kulonen E. Effects of serotonin, indomethacin and other antirheumatic drugs on the synthesis of collagen and other proteins in granulation tissue slices. *Biochem Pharmacol* 1972;21:2835–2840.

291. Ardissino D, Barberis P, De Servi S, et al. Abnormal coronary vasoconstriction as a predictor of restenosis after successful coronary angioplasty in patients with unstable angina pectoris. *N Engl J Med* 1991;325:1053–1057.

292. Ardissino D, Di Somma S, Kubica J, et al. Influence of elastic recoil on restenosis after successful coronary angioplasty in unstable angina pectoris. *Am J Cardiol* 1993;71:659–663.

293. Hoberg E, Schwary F, Schömig A, et al. Prevention of restenosis by verapamil. The verapamil angioplasty study (VAS). *Circulation* 1990;82:III-428.

294. Dens J, Desmet W, Coussement P, et al. Usefulness of nisoldipine for prevention of restenosis after percutaneous transluminal coronary angioplasty (results of the NICOLE study). *Am J Cardiol* 2001;87:28–33.

295. Hillegass W, Ohman E, Leimburger J, et al. A meta-analysis of randomized trials of calcium antagonists to reduce restenosis after coronary angioplasty. *Am J Cardiol* 1994;73:835–839.

296. Naftilan AJ, Pratt RE, Dayau VJ. Induction of platelet derived growth factor A chain and C-myc expression by angiotensin II in culture rat vascular smooth muscle cells. *J Clin Invest* 1989;83:1419–1424.

297. Desmet W, Vrolix M, De Scheeder I, et al. Angiotensin-converting enzyme inhibition with fosinopril sodium in the prevention of restenosis after coronary angioplasty. *Circulation* 1994;89:385–392.

298. Berk BC, Gordon JB, Alexander RW. Pharmacologic roles of heparin and glucocorticoids to prevent restenosis after coronary angioplasty. *J Am Coll Cardiol* 1991;17:111B–117B.

299. Stone GW, Rutherford BD, McConahay DR, et al. A randomized trial of corticosteroids for the prevention of restenosis in 102 patients undergoing repeat coronary angioplasty. *Cathet Cardiovasc Diagn* 1989;18:227–231.

300. Soppitt G, Mitchell J. The effect of colchicine on human platelet behavior. *J Atheroscler Res* 1969;10:247–252.

301. Ehelich H. Microtubules in transcellular movement of procollagen. *Nature* 1972;238:257–260.

302. O'Keefe JHJ, McCallister BD, Bateman TM, et al. Ineffectiveness of colchicine for the prevention of restenosis after coronary angioplasty. *J Am Coll Cardiol* 1992;19:1597–1600.

303. Freed M, Safian R, O'Neill W, et al. Combination of lovastatin, enalapril, and colchicine does not prevent restenosis after percutaneous transluminal coronary angioplasty. *Am Heart J* 1995;76:1185–1188.

304. Tamai H, Katoh O, Suzuki S, et al. Impact of tranilast on restenosis after coronary angioplasty: Tranilast Restenosis Following Angioplasty Trial (TREAT). *Am Heart J* 1999;138:968–975.

305. Holmes D, Fitzgerald P, Goldberg S, et al. The PRESTO (Prevention of Restenosis with Tranilast and Its Outcomes) protocol: a double-blind, placebo-controlled trial. *Am Heart J* 2000;139:23–31.

306. Liu M, Roubin G, Robinson K, et al. Trapidil in preventing restenosis after balloon angioplasty in the atherosclerotic rabbit. *Circulation* 1990;81:1089–1093.

307. Okamoto S, Inden M, Setsuda M, et al. Effects of trapidil (triazolopyrimidine), a platelet-derived growth factor antagonist, in preventing restenosis after percutaneous transluminal coronary angioplasty. *Am Heart J* 1992;123:1439–1444.

308. Maresta A, Balducelli M, Cantini L, et al. Trapidil (triazolopyrimidine), a platelet-derived growth factor antagonist, reduces restenosis after percutaneous transluminal angioplasty. Results of the randomized, double-blind STARC study. *Circulation* 1994;90:2710–2715.

309. Galassi A, Tamburino C, Nicosia A, et al. A randomized trial of trapidil (triazolopyrimidine), a platelet-derived growth factor antagonist, versus aspirin in prevention of angiographic restenosis after coronary artery Palmaz-Schatz stent implantation. *Cathet Cardiovasc Interv* 1999;46:162–168.

310. Fingerle J, Faulmuller A, Muller G, et al. Pituitary factors in blood plasma are necessary for smooth muscle cell proliferation in response to injury in vivo. *Arterioscler Thromb* 1992;12:1488–1495.

311. Santoian E, Schneider J, Gravanis M, et al. Angiopeptin inhibits intimal hyperplasia after angioplasty in porcine coronary arteries. *Circulation* 1993;88:11–14.

312. Howell M, Trowbridge R, Foegh M. Effects of delayed angiopeptin treatment on myointima hyperplasia following angioplasty. *J Am Coll Cardiol* 1991;17:181A.

313. Eriksen UH, Amtorp O, Bagger JP, et al. Randomized double-blind Scandinavian trial of angiopeptin versus placebo for the prevention of clinical events and restenosis after coronary balloon angioplasty. *Am Heart J* 1995;130:1–8.

314. Emanuelsson H, Beatt K, Bagger J, et al. Long-term effects of angiopeptin treatment in coronary angioplasty. *Circulation* 1995;91:1689–1696.

315. Sekiya M, Funada J, Watanabe K, et al. Effects of probucol and cilostazol alone and in combination on the frequency of poststenting restenosis. *Am J Cardiol* 1998;82:144–147.

316. Tsuchikane E, Fukuhara A, Kobayashi T, et al. Impact of cilostazol on restenosis after percutaneous coronary balloon angioplasty. *Circulation* 1999;100:21–26.

317. Park S, Lee C, Kim H, et al. Effects of cilostazol on angiographic restenosis after coronary stent placement. *Am J Cardiol* 2000;86:499–503.

318. Kozuma K, Hara K, Yamasaki M, et al. Effects of cilostazol on late lumen loss and repeat revascularization after Palmaz-Schatz coronary stent implantation. *Am Heart J* 2001;141:124–130.

319. Herdeg C, Oberhoff M, Baumbach A, et al. Local paclitaxel delivery for the prevention of restenosis: biological effects and efficacy in vivo. *J Am Coll Cardiol* 2000;35:1969–1976.

320. Lincoff A, Topol E, Ellis S. Local drug delivery for the prevention of restenosis: fact, fancy, and future. *Circulation* 1994;90:2070–2084.

321. Tamai H, Igaki K, Kyo E, et al. Initial and 6-month results of biodegradable poly-l-lactic acid coronary stents in humans. *Circulation* 2000;102:399–404.

322. Gallo R, Padurean A, Jayaraman T, et al. Inhibition of intimal thickening after balloon angioplasty in porcine coronary arteries by targeting regulators of the cell cycle. *Circulation* 1999;99:2164–2170.

323. Sousa J, Costa M, Abizaid A, et al. Lack of neointimal proliferation after implantation of sirolimus-coated stents in human coronary arteries: a quantitative coronary angiography and three-dimensional intravascular ultrasound study. *Circulation* 2001;103:192–195.

324. Hamon M, Bauters C, McFadden N, et al. Restenosis after coronary angioplasty. *Eur Heart J* 1995;16:33–48.

325. Simons M, Edelman E, DeKeyser J-L, et al. Antisense c-myb oligonucleotides inhibit intimal arterial smooth muscle cell accumulation in vivo. *Nature* 1992;359:67–70.

326. Roque F, Belardi J, Rodriguez A, et al. Safety trial of intracoronary administration of c-myc antisense in patients undergoing percutaneous transluminal coronary angioplasty. *Eur Heart J* 1995;16:424.

327. Knapp H, Reilly I, Alessandrini P, et al. In vivo indexes of platelet and vascular function during fish-oil administration in patients with atherosclerosis. *N Engl J Med* 1986;314:937–942.

328. Dehmer GJ. Omega-3 fatty acids. In: Topol EJ, ed. *Textbook of interventional cardiology*, 2nd ed. Philadelphia: WB Saunders, 1993:112–136.

329. Kromhout D, Bosschieter E, de Lezenne Coulander C. The inverse relationship between fish consumption and 20-year mortality from coronary heart disease. *N Engl J Med* 1985;312:1205–1209.

330. Bairati I, Roy L, Meyer F. Double-blind, randomized, controlled trial of fish oil supplements in prevention of recurrence of stenosis after coronary angioplasty. *Circulation* 1992;85:950–956.

331. Milner MR, Gallino RA, Leffingwell A, et al. Usefulness of fish oil supplements in preventing clinical evidence of restenosis after percutaneous transluminal coronary angioplasty. *Am J Cardiol* 1989;64:294–299.

332. Nye ER, Ilsley CD, Ablett MB, et al. Effect on eicosapentaenoic acid on restenosis rate, clinical course and blood lipids in patients after percutaneous transluminal coronary angioplasty. *Aust N Z J Med* 1990;20:549–552.

333. Slack JD, Pinkerton CA, van Tasse J, et al. Can oral fish oil supplement minimize restenosis after percutaneous transluminal coronary angioplasty? *J Am Coll Cardiol* 1987;9:64A.

334. Leaf A, Jorgensen MB, Jacobs AK, et al. Do fish oils prevent restenosis after coronary angioplasty? *Circulation* 1994;90:2248–2257.

335. Constantinescu DE, Banka VS, Tulenko TN. Lovastatin inhibits proliferation of arterial smooth muscle and endothelial cells. Indication in atherosclerosis and prevention of restenosis. *Eur Heart J* 1992;13:82.

336. Serruys P, Foley D, Jackson G, et al. A randomized placebo-controlled trial of fluvastatin for prevention of restenosis after successful coronary balloon angioplasty; final results of the fluvastatin angiographic restenosis (FLARE) trial. *Eur Heart J* 1999;20:58–69.

337. Walter D, Schachinger V, Elsner M, et al. Effect of statin therapy on restenosis after coronary stent implantation. *Am J Cardiol* 2000;85:962–968.

338. Godfried S, Deckelbaum L. Natural antioxidants and restenosis after percutaneous transluminal coronary angioplasty. *Am Heart J* 1995;129:203–210.

339. Lafont A, Chai Y-C, Cornhill J, et al. Effect of alpha-tocopherol on restenosis after angioplasty in a model of experimental atherosclerosis. *J Clin Invest* 1995;95:1108–1125.

340. Schneider J, Berk B, Gravanis M, et al. Probucol decreases neointimal formation in a swine model of coronary artery balloon injury. *Circulation* 1993;88:628–637.

341. Tardif J, Côté G, Lespérance J, et al. Prevention of restenosis by pre- and post-PTCA probucol therapy: a randomized clinical trial. *Circulation* 1996;94:I-91.

342. Watanabe K, Sekiya S, Miyagawa M, et al. Preventive effects of probucol on restenosis after percutaneous transluminal coronary angioplasty. *Am Heart J* 1996;132:23–29.

343. Foley D, Appelman Y, Piek J. Comparison of angiographic restenosis propensity of excimer laser coronary angioplasty (ELCA) and balloon angioplasty (BA) in the Amsterdam Rotterdam (AMRO) trial. *Circulation* 1995;92:I-477.

344. Ferguson JI. Meeting highlights. 15th Congress of the European Society of Cardiology. *Circulation* 1993;88:2491–2492.

345. Serruys PW, Macaya C, de Jaegere P, et al. Interim analysis of the BENESTENT-trial. *Circulation* 1993;88:I-594.

346. Schatz RA, Penn IM, Baim DS, et al. Stent restenosis study (STRESS): analysis of in-hospital results. *Circulation* 1993;88:I-594.

347. Versaci F, Gaspardone A, Tomai F, et al. A comparison of coronary-artery stenting with angioplasty for isolated stenosis of the proximal left anterior descending coronary artery. *N Engl J Med* 1997;336:817–822.

348. Hoffmann R, Mintz G. Coronary in-stent restenosis—predictors, treatment and prevention. *Eur Heart J* 2000;21:1739–1749.

349. Giri S, Shigenori I, Lansky A, et al. Clinical and angiographic outcome in the laser angioplasty for restenotic

stents (LARS) multicenter registry. *Cathet Cardiovasc Interv* 2001;52:24–34.

350. Mintz G, Hoffmann R, Mehran R, et al. In-stent restenosis: the Washington Hospital Center experience. *Am J Cardiol* 1998;81:7E–13E.

351. Mehran R, Dangas G, Mints G, et al. Treatment of in-stent restenosis with excimer laser coronary angioplasty versus rotational atherectomy. Comparative mechanisms and results. *Circulation* 2000;101:2484–2489.

352. Teirstein P, Massullo V, Jani S, et al. Three-year clinical and angiographic follow-up after intracoronary radiation. Results of a randomized clinical trial. *Circulation* 2000;101:360–365.

353. Leon M, Teirstein P, Moses J, et al. Localized intracoronary gamma-radiation therapy to inhibit the recurrence of restenosis after stenting. *N Engl J Med* 2001;344:250–256.

354. Waksman R, White R, Chan R, et al. Intracoronary γ-radiation therapy after angioplasty inhibits recurrence in patients with in-stent restenosis. *Circulation* 2000;101:2165–2171.

355. Waksman R. The Washington Radiation for In-stent Restenosis Trial for Long Lesions: (LONG WRIST). Paper presented at: 49th Annual Scientific Session of the American College of Cardiology; March 2000; Anaheim, CA.

356. Raizner A, Oesterle S, Waksman R, et al. Inhibition of restenosis with β-emitting radiotherapy. Report of the Proliferation Reduction with Vascular Energy Trial (PREVENT). *Circulation* 2000;102:951–958.

357. Waksman R. Intimal hyperplasia inhibition with beta in-stent trial (INHIBIT). Paper presented at: American Heart Association Scientific Session; November 2000; New Orleans, LA.

358. Popma J. Late clinical and angiographic outcomes after use of ^{90}Sr/^{90}Y beta radiation for the treatment of in-stent restenosis: results from the ^{90}Sr treatment of angiographic restenosis (START) trial. Paper presented at: American College of Cardiology 49th Annual Scientific Session; March 2000; Anaheim, CA.

359. Waksman R, Bhargava B, White L, et al. Intracoronary β-radiation therapy inhibits recurrence of in-stent restenosis. *Circulation* 2000;101:1895–1898.

360. Albiero R, Adamian M, Kobayashi N, et al. Short- and intermediate-term results of ^{32}P radioactive β-emitting stent implantation in patients with coronary artery disease. The Milan dose-response study. *Circulation* 2000;101:18–26.

361. Serruys P, Kay I. I like the candy, I hate the wrapper: the (32)P radioactive stent. *Circulation* 2000;101:3–7.

362. Waksman R, Ajani A, Kim H, et al. Is 6 months of Plavix enough to prevent late total occlusion after gamma radiation for in-stent restenosis? *J Am Coll Cardiol* 2001;37:14A.

363. Post M, Borst C, Kuntz R. The relative importance of arterial remodeling compared with intimal hyperplasia in lumen renarrowing after balloon angioplasty: a study in the normal rabbit and the hypercholesterolemic Yucatan micropig. *Circulation* 1994;89:2816–2821.

364. Moliterno D, Topol E. A direct comparison of tirofiban and abciximab during percutaneous coronary revascularization and stent placement: rationale and design of the TARGET study. *Am Heart J* 2000;140:722–726.

365. The ESPRIT investigators. Novel dosing regimen of eptifibatide in planned coronary stent implantation (ESPRIT): a randomised, placebo-controlled trial. *Lancet* 2000;356:2037–2044.

366. Ahmed J, Mintz G, Waksman R, et al. Serial intravascular ultrasound analysis of the impact of lesion length on the efficacy of intracoronary gamma-irradiation for preventing recurrent in-stent restenosis. *Circulation* 2001;103:188–191.

367. Azpitarte J, Tercedor L, Melgares R, et al. The value of exercise electrocardiography testing in the identification of coronary restenosis: a probability analysis. *Int J Cardiol* 1995;48:239–247.

368. Bellamy C, Schofield P, Faragher E, et al. Can supplementation of diet with omega-3 polyunsaturated fatty acids reduce coronary angioplasty restenosis rate? *Eur Heart J* 1992;13:1626–1631.

369. Crouse L, Vacek J, Beauchamp G, et al. Use of exercise electrocardiography to evaluate patients after coronary angioplasty. *Am J Cardiol* 1996;78:1163–1166.

370. Daida H, Lee YJ, Yokoi H, et al. Prevention of restenosis after percutaneous transluminal coronary angioplasty by reducing lipoprotein(a) levels with low-density lipoprotein apheresis. Low-Density Lipoprotein Apheresis Angioplasty Restenosis Trial (L-ART) Group. *Am J Cardiol* 1994;73:1037–1040.

371. Desmet W, De Scheerder I, Piessens J. Limited value of exercise testing in the detection of silent restenosis after successful coronary angioplasty. *Am Heart J* 1995;129:452–459.

372. Ernst SM, Hillebrand FA, Klein B, et al. The value of exercise tests in the follow-up of patients who underwent transluminal coronary angioplasty. *Int J Cardiol* 1985;7:267–279.

373. Hoffmann R, Kleinhans E, Lambertz H, et al. Transesophageal pacing echocardiography for detection of restenosis after percutaneous transluminal coronary angioplasty. *Eur Heart J* 1994;15:823–831.

374. Jain A, Mahmarian JJ, Borges-Neto S, et al. Clinical significance of perfusion defects by thallium-201 single photon emission computed tomography following oral dipyridamole early after coronary angioplasty. *J Am Coll Cardiol* 1988;11:970–976.

375. Kaul U, Sanghvi S, Bahl V, et al. Fish oil supplements for prevention of restenosis after coronary angioplasty. *Int J Cardiol* 1992;1:87–93.

376. Milan E, Zoccarato O, Terzi A, et al. Technetium-99m-sestamibi SPECT to detect restenosis after successful percutaneous coronary angioplasty. *J Nucl Med* 1996;37:1300–1305.

377. O'Keefe JJ, Giorgi L, Hartzler G, et al. Effects of diltiazem on complications and restenosis after coronary angioplasty. *Am J Cardiol* 1991;67:373–376.

378. O'Keefe JJ, Stone G, McCallister BJ, et al. Lovastatin plus probucol for prevention of restenosis after percutaneous transluminal coronary angioplasty. *Am J Cardiol* 1996;77:649–652.

379. Reis GJ, Boucher TM, Sipperly ME, et al. Randomised trial of fish oil for prevention of restenosis after coronary angioplasty. *Lancet* 1989;2:177–181.

380. Roth A, Miller HI, Keren G, et al. Detection of restenosis following percutaneous coronary angioplasty in single-vessel coronary artery disease: the value of clinical assessment and exercise tolerance testing. *Cardiology* 1994;84:106–113.

381. Scholl JM, Chaitman BR, David PR, et al. Exercise electrocardiography and myocardial scintigraphy in the serial evaluation of the results of percutaneous transluminal coronary angioplasty. *Circulation* 1982;66:380–390.

382. The Multicenter European Research Trial with Cilazapril after Angioplasty to Prevent Transluminal Coronary Obstruction and Restenosis (MERCATOR) Study Group. Does the new angiotensin converting enzyme inhibitor cilazapril prevent restenosis after percutaneous transluminal coronary angioplasty? Results of the MERCATOR Study: a multicenter, randomized, double-blind placebo-controlled trial. *Circulation* 1992;86:100–110.

383. Yui Y, Kawai C, Hosoda S. Pravastatin (mevalotin) restenosis trial after percutaneous transluminal coronary angioplasty. Cholesterol reduction rate determines the restenosis rate. *Ann N Y Acad Sci* 1995;748:208–216.

APPROACHES TO THE PATIENT
WITH PRIOR BYPASS SURGERY

JOHN S. DOUGLAS, JR.

OVERVIEW

The important issues in the postbypass patient who has recurrent angina or ischemia are providing relief of symptoms and ischemia with the least morbidity and cost and doing it in a manner that provides durable benefit. It takes considerable judgment to make the best decision in these patients because there are frequently many options, most of which have substantial baggage (complications and short-term benefit).

HISTORICAL PERSPECTIVE

Advent and Maturation of Surgical Revascularization

As was later true of percutaneous transluminal coronary angioplasty (PTCA) (1–3), surgical coronary revascularization began more than 30 years ago with attempts to revascularize a single coronary artery. The result of these efforts was a dramatic change in cardiologic practice as surgical

techniques adequate to palliate multivessel obstructive disease evolved. Within a decade, the growth of coronary bypass surgery was exponential (Fig. 84.1). Hundreds of thousands of patients were operated on annually, creating a large population of several million postbypass patients in the United States alone. Owing to the progressive nature of the atherosclerotic process and the limited durability of venous conduits and in spite of widespread use of arterial grafts and antiplatelet agents, recurrent ischemia after surgical revascularization is a problem all cardiologists face with increasing frequency. Recurrence of angina in the first year alone was reported in 24% of patients in the Coronary Artery Surgery Study (4), and by the fifth postoperative year, almost one-half of the broad spectrum of postoperative patients have recurrent symptoms (4–6).

Recurrent angina sufficient to require reoperation occurred in 12% to 15% of patients within one decade of a first coronary operation at Emory University and at The Cleveland Clinic, and by the twelfth to fifteenth year, 30% required reoperation (7,8). Reoperative coronary surgery when compared with initial operation proved to be more costly, two to three times more likely to lead to in-hospital death or myocardial infarction (MI), and less

J. S. Douglas, Jr.: Department of Medicine, Interventional Cardiology, Emory University Hospital, Atlanta, Georgia

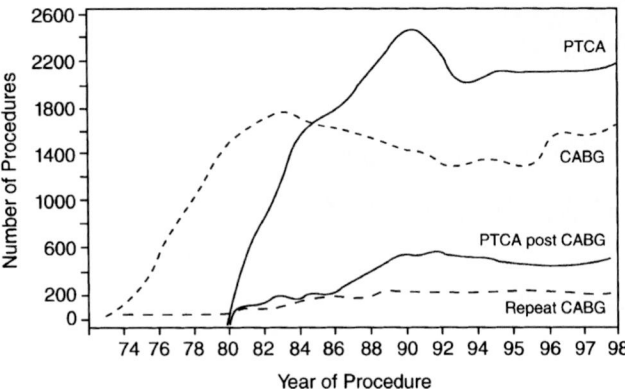

FIGURE 84.1 Coronary artery revascularization procedures at Emory University Hospitals from 1973 to 1998. CABG, coronary artery bypass grafting; PTCA, percutaneous transluminal coronary angioplasty.

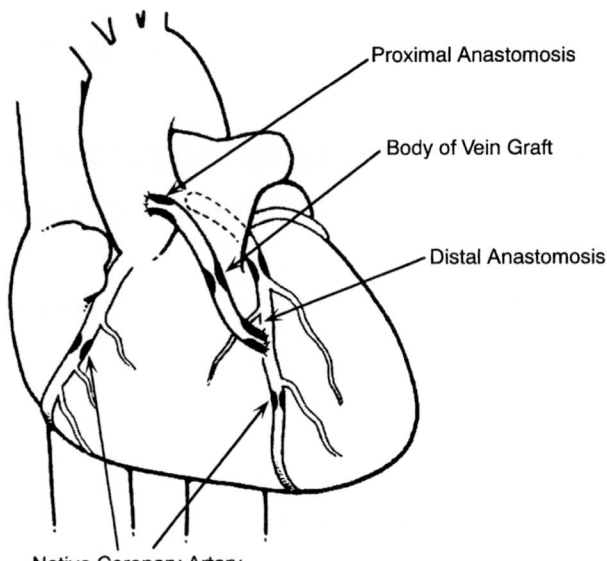

FIGURE 84.2 Targets for percutaneous coronary intervention include saphenous vein grafts and native coronary artery sites in unbypassed and bypassed vessels. In addition, internal mammary artery, radial, subclavian, innominate, and gastroepiploic artery grafts are potential targets. (Adapted from Douglas JS Jr, Gruentzig AR, King SB III, et al. Percutaneous transluminal coronary angioplasty in patients with prior coronary bypass surgery. *J Am Coll Cardiol* 1983;2:745–754, with permission.)

effective in achieving angina relief (7,9–11). Among 2,030 patients who underwent reoperation at Emory University, in-hospital mortality was 7.0% (4.6% younger than 60 years, 8.2% aged 60 to 69, 10.0% 70 years or older). Five- and 10-year survival was 76% and 55%, respectively (10). Reported outcome data confined to patients who underwent reoperation in the 1990s confirmed the high operative mortality noted previously (7.4%) and reported a higher rate of Q-wave infarction, a longer length of stay, and higher costs than initial operations (11). The increase in complications and reduced efficacy of reoperative coronary surgery are probably related to the more extensive disease present, the requirement to use second-line venous conduits in many cases, and the technically more difficult and operator-dependent nature of reoperative heart surgery.

Percutaneous Intervention Postbypass

Percutaneous catheter revascularization in patients who had prior coronary bypass surgery (Fig. 84.2) was first described by Gruentzig, who treated eight patients, six successfully, among the first 50 patients he reported. Seven of the eight postbypass patients had angioplasty of saphenous vein graft (SVG) lesions, and three of five treated successfully had recurrences, leading Gruentzig to make the following insightful comments based on such limited observations: "The different kind of disease may explain the high incidence of recurrence in graft stenosis. Further experience will show whether we should eliminate this lesion from consideration" (12).

Among the first 1,116 patients treated with coronary angioplasty in the National Heart, Lung, and Blood Institute PTCA Registry, 62 patients had had previous bypass surgery. The in-hospital mortality in these patients, 8.1%, was significantly higher than in patients without prior surgery, 0.7%, causing concern about the safety of the procedure in this group of patients (13). The early experience at

Emory University was reassuring, however; 116 patients were treated with no procedural death, three emergency operations, and one Q-wave MI (Fig. 84.2). One late death occurred during an 8.3-month mean follow-up. Gruentzig's observation of higher restenosis rates for SVGs was reaffirmed for mid- and proximal graft sites, but an acceptable restenosis rate for distal anastomosis lesions of 18% (4 of 22) was first reported (Fig. 84.3) as well as the initial report of attempted internal mammary artery (IMA) graft angioplasty (14). In subsequent experience with more than 34,000 coronary angioplasty procedures at Emory University, a history of prior bypass surgery was not associated with increased risk of death or Q-wave MI and was negatively correlated with need for in-hospital coronary artery bypass graft (CABG) surgery (15).

Percutaneous coronary intervention (PCI) became a less invasive revascularization alternative for many symptomatic postbypass patients (Fig. 84.1), including an increasing number who, because of contraindications (pulmonary and renal failure, old age, malignancy), were not candidates for reoperative coronary artery surgery. Patients with patent arterial grafts that would be jeopardized by reoperation, patients with relatively small amounts of ischemic, symptom-producing myocardium, and patients with no available venous or arterial conduits for grafts underwent percutaneous revascularization at an acceptable risk. At many centers, patients with prior bypass surgery account for up to 25% of the PCI procedures performed (Fig. 84.1). ▼ o33

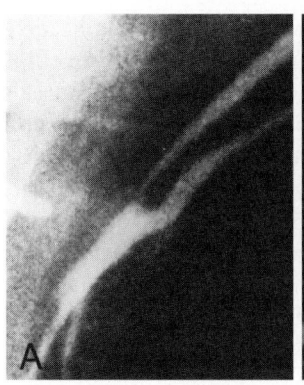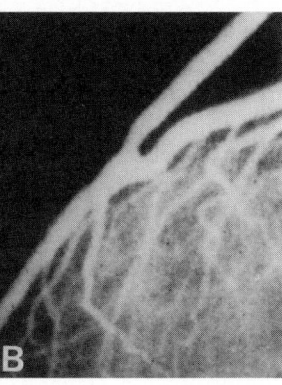

FIGURE 84.3 A 57-year-old man underwent saphenous vein bypass grafting to the distal left anterior descending (LAD) artery in July 1981; coronary arteriography a few months later **(A)** revealed high-grade stenosis at the junction of the saphenous vein graft to the LAD artery (left lateral view). Percutaneous transluminal coronary angioplasty was successful (residual stenosis, 13%), and recatheterization 9 months later showed a widely patent anastomosis **(B)**. The patient subsequently remained completely asymptomatic, and at last follow-up 19 years later (July 2000), he had a negative stress thallium scan result. (From Douglas JS Jr, Gruentzig AR, King SB III, et al. Percutaneous transluminal coronary angioplasty in patients with prior coronary bypass surgery. *J Am Coll Cardiol* 1983;2:745–754, with permission.)

ANATOMIC CONSIDERATIONS

Among the anatomic factors influencing revascularization decisions (Table 84.1), the status of the left anterior descending coronary artery (LAD) and its graft is paramount. Placement of an IMA, a conduit immune to atherosclerosis, as a graft to the LAD has been shown to enhance survival and reduce ischemic events 10 to as long as 20 years later (17–19). In a patient with a patent IMA graft to the LAD, reoperative surgery to treat non-LAD ischemia has been reported to offer no survival benefit (20,21), may jeopardize the arterial graft, and, in our experience and others, more frequently leads to percutaneous intervention. Multivessel involvement, small number of patent grafts, severe vein graft disease (especially if to LAD), and a damaged left ventricle are factors more likely to lead to reoperative surgery (22,23).

PATHOPHYSIOLOGY: BASIS FOR RECURRENT ISCHEMIA

Incomplete Revascularization

In many patients, complete surgical revascularization was not achieved due to the presence of distal coronary disease, whereas less common causes include the following: an inadequate amount of venous or arterial conduit, inadequate conduit lumen due to small vessel size (IMA especially) or injury, intramyocardial location of target coronary vessel, placement of grafts to the wrong coronary artery or to a coronary vein, creating an arterial venous fistula (24), use of an IMA in the presence of significant stenosis of the subclavian or innominate arteries (25,26), or coronary steal phenomenon attributed to large arterial graft side branches (27), a cause that has been questioned (28). Intentional incomplete surgical revascularization is an increasingly frequent phenomenon in patients selected for "beating heart" operations because of the technical difficulty of bypassing posteriorly located coronary arteries. In some patients, this strategy has resulted in subsequent percutaneous revascularization because of inadequate relief of symptoms. In others, incomplete surgical revascularization has been dealt with up front with adjunctive percutaneous revascularization during the same hospitalization, the so-called hybrid approach. In addition to less complete revascularization with beating heart surgery, there is some evidence that less precise anastomoses may compromise graft patency, especially in the surgical learning curve (see Venous Graft Attrition and Arterial Graft Compromise, later in this chapter).

Loss of Revascularization Benefit

Venous Graft Attrition

In patients with recurrent ischemia and infarction after bypass surgery, stenosis, occlusion, or both stenosis and occlusion of SVGs is the most common cause of venous graft attrition (6,21,29–40). Thrombotic occlusion related to surgical technical problems or slow graft flow secondary

TABLE 84.1 ANATOMIC FACTORS INFLUENCING REVASCULARIZATION DECISIONS IN POSTBYPASS PATIENTS

Often leads to percutaneous transluminal coronary angioplasty	Often leads to coronary artery bypass grafting
Patent arterial graft (especially left anterior descending coronary artery)	Diseased saphenous vein graft to left anterior descending
≥2 patent grafts	Bulky saphenous vein graft atheroma
1–3 culprit lesions	>3 culprit lesions
Difficult surgical access	Multiple saphenous vein graft lesions
Mediastinal scarring secondary to radiation, infection, or pericarditis	Available arterial conduits
Prior muscle transfer closure of unhealed sternotomy	Ejection fraction 25% to 35%
Posterior lateral target vessel	
Inadequate conduits	
Near normal left ventricle	
Future cardiac surgery anticipated	
In situ prosthetic valve	
Mild to moderate aortic or mitral valve disease	

to a small or compromised distal coronary arterial bed results in closure of 10% to 15% of SVGs within the first month (29–31), and even with aspirin therapy, 7% of vein grafts were shown to be occluded by 9 days, with up to 17% of patients having a closed graft at that time (29). Subsequently 15% to 20% of vein grafts occlude by 1 year, 1% to 2% per year from years 1 to 6, and 4% per year from 6 to 10 years after surgery (*e*Fig. 84.3.1) (29–31,41). After 10 years, a minority of vein grafts were free of significant occlusion disease (32,45). ♥ o34

Native Coronary Artery Progression

Worsening of native coronary artery disease after bypass surgery has been reported in approximately 5% of patients annually (52–54). Frequency of disease progression at native vessel sites at 5 years was reported as follows: proximal to graft insertion (70%), unbypassed artery (15%), and distal to graft insertion (0%) (55). Loop and colleagues noted that progression of disease distal to grafts was uncommon and that at 2 years progression of disease proximal to grafts was more common for SVG than for IMA grafts (67% vs. 39%) (18). Progression of native coronary disease proximal to grafts has implications for coronary intervention when graft disease or occlusion occurs and is an important cause of ischemia due to poor perfusion of side branches (such as diagonal coronary arteries).

Arterial Graft Compromise

Although numerous publications attest to the excellent long-term patency of arterial grafts, several hundred patients have been reported who required IMA, radial artery, or subclavian artery intervention (25–27,56–62). In most instances IMA interventions were needed for anastomotic lesions, but proximal and midgraft sites have been treated (see Arterial Graft Intervention). The technical difficulty of performing an anastomosis in beating heart surgery probably accounts for more anastomotic problems after this type of surgery.

PRINCIPLES OF MANAGEMENT

Preventive Measures

Patients who have had coronary bypass surgery are at substantial risk for subsequent cardiac events related in large part to progressive arteriosclerosis. Recurrence of angina, angiographic progressions of vein graft atheroma, and pathologic changes at autopsy have been correlated with increased serum lipids and smoking, and lipid lowering has been shown to be beneficial (4,9,41,48,66–68). Given the increased effectiveness of current strategies for lipid lowering and smoking cessation, and reduced cardiac events that

accrue, an aggressive approach to risk factor modification is mandatory in all postbypass patients. An aggressive lipid-lowering strategy resulted in a 30% reduction in revascularization (*p* = .0006) and a 24% reduction in a composite clinical end point (*p* = .001) during 7.5 years of follow-up in the post-CABG trial (67,68). The place of more aggressive antiplatelet therapy in the post-CABG patient is not clear, but more recently reported mortality benefits with clopidogrel are provocative and suggest that the use of this or other adjunctive agents may become routine in the future (69).

Treatment of Ischemia in the Postoperative Patient

Patients with recurrent symptoms or signs of ischemia after bypass surgery constitute an extremely heterogeneous group (Fig. 84.2). Treatment strategies must be based on a careful analysis of multiple factors (many angiographically based) including anatomic factors (Table 84.1), the likelihood of a successful percutaneous intervention, risk of complications, probability of long-term symptomatic benefit, and resource consumption compared with other viable options (7,14,70–75). Patient preferences must be considered since reinterventions are common with percutaneous intervention in postbypass patients, occurring in approximately 50% of patients at 5 years (72). In the postbypass patient, the ability to effect ischemia relief percutaneously is influenced by the time that has lapsed since surgery, the type of conduit (SVG vs. native vessel vs. IMA graft), and location of the stenotic segment.

Native Coronary Intervention

Results of Native Coronary Intervention

The procedural outcome of angioplasty for native coronary intervention after CABG was reported for the first 372 such patients treated at Emory in 1987 (74). Most were men (81%), and 78% had multivessel disease. Angiographic success was achieved in 91%, and in-hospital complications were infrequent: mortality, 0.3%; Q-wave MI, 2%; non–Q-wave infarction, 4%; bypass surgery, 6%. At Mid-America Heart Institute, 1,543 postbypass patients underwent angioplasty of native coronary arteries; 21% were older than 70 years, 47% had unstable angina, and 74% had triple-vessel disease. Angiographic success was 94%, in-hospital mortality 0.8%, Q-wave MI 1.5%, and emergency bypass surgery 1.0% (75). At Emory University between 1980 and 1995, 2,246 postbypass patients underwent coronary intervention of native arteries with favorable outcome: procedural success 89%, in-hospital mortality 1%, Q-wave MI 1%, non–Q-wave infarction 4% (creatine kinase greater than three times normal), and emergency or elective surgery 2.8%. Although the definitions of outcomes were slightly different in these series, the overall procedural results were favorable, with a trend toward less need for in-hospital bypass surgery for failed percutaneous intervention. These outcomes were largely that of conventional balloon angioplasty. The Mayo Clinic experience with 937 post-CABG patients treated between 1995 and 1998 reflected a dramatic increase in stent use to 76% of patients and a reduction in use of atherectomy and laser strategies. Patients who underwent interventions in native vessels were younger, more likely female, had less severe coronary disease (70), and had a more favorable long-term outlook than those who underwent venous bypass graft intervention (71).

Saphenous Vein Graft Intervention

Results of Saphenous Vein Graft Intervention

A number of reports have described the results of balloon angioplasty in SVG disease (*e*Table 84.1.1) (14,99–118), indicating that in selected patients success rates of approximately 90% were achieved with mortality of approximately 1%, Q-wave MI of less than 2%, and in-hospital CABG in approximately 2% of patients. Many of these patients had relatively favorable anatomy with focal lesions free of obvious thrombus. Non–Q-wave MI, the most frequent complication, occurred in 78 (13%) of 599 patients at Emory University (105). The length of time since surgery was an important predictor of restenosis (less than 6 months, 32%; 6 months to 1 year, 43%; 1 to 5 years, 61%; and 64% for those older than 5 years, $p < .02$) as was the location of the lesion (proximal anastomosis, 68%; midgraft, 61%; distal anastomosis, 45%; $p < .06$). The lowest restenosis rate, 22%, was noted for lesions that occurred at the distal anastomosis within 1 year of surgery, and these patients had excellent event-free survival (Fig. 84.3). ▼ o35

Stenting of SVGs, which has become the dominant percutaneous strategy, was carried out for more than a decade, initially with mixed results. The first vein graft implantations were with the Wallstent (Schneider, Zurich, Switzerland) (119), and subsequent reports (Table 84.2) indicated a 99% to 100% deployment success rate, a 4% to 10% rate of early thrombosis, and restenosis in 34% to 47% (125–130). In follow-up of 62 patients with 93 stents (90% were Wallstents) out to 5.9 years (median, 2.5 years), there was a

TABLE 84.2 RESULTS OF STENTING OF AORTOCORONARY SAPHENOUS VEIN GRAFTS (SVG): SELECTED REPORTS OF GREATER THAN OR EQUAL TO 50 PATIENTS

Author (yr)	Reference	Implantation success (%)	Early thrombosis (%)	Coronary artery bypass grafting (%)	Death (%)	Acute myocardial infarction (%)	Restenosis (%)
Palmaz-Schatz							
Pomerantz et al. (1992)	119	83/84 (99)	0	0	0	10	36
Carrozza et al. (1992)	120	84/84 (100)	0	0	0	8	—
Fenton et al. (1994)	122	196/198 (99)	0.5	—	—	—	34
Piana et al. (1994)	121	147/150 (98)	1	0	1	7.3	17
Wong et al. (1995)	123	571/589 (97)	1.4	0.9	1.7	0.3	30
Savage et al. (1997)	124	105/108 (97)	1	2	2	4	36
Wallstent							
de Scheerder et al. (1992)	125	69/69 (100)	10	0	1.5	7	47
Strauss et al. (1992)	126	145/145 (100)	8	—	—	—	34
de Jaegere et al.[a] (1996)	127	92/93 (99)	4	5	3	3	—
Wiktor							
Fortuna et al. (1993)	128	101/101 (100)	2	1	1	3	—
Hanekamp et al. (2000)	148	77/78 (99)	—	—	—	—	22
Various stents							
Safian et al. (1998)	59						
Palmaz-Schatz		101/101 (100)	—	—	—	—	32
Wallstent		109/114 (95)	—	—	—	—	13
Wallstent (SVG >4 mm)		197/207 (95)	—	—	—	—	39
Le May et al. (1999)	131	103/106 (98)	0	0	0	—	—
Dharmadhikari (2000)	140						
Covered stents		30	—	3	0	0	Revascularization, 20
Noncovered stents		125	—	0	0	8.8	Revascularization, 28
Baldus et al.[b] (2000)	141	108/109 (99)	0.9	0	0	1	26
Nishida et al. (2000)	178	97/101 (96)	—	2	1	10.9	Target vessel revascularization, 21

[a]Ninety percent Wallstents.
[b]All covered stents.

high cardiac event rate: 8% died, 23% had MI, 20% underwent bypass surgery, and 23% underwent angioplasty. The estimated 5-year survival and event-free survival rates were 83% ± 5% and 30% ± 7% (127). Of potential importance is the fact that optimal Wallstent expansion with high-pressure balloons was not routinely used in the reported patients.

The largest experience in vein graft stenting has been with the Palmaz-Schatz stent (Johnson & Johnson Interventional Systems) (Table 84.2). Deployment success rates were high, and in-hospital complications were low, including a lower rate of stent thrombosis than was observed in native coronary artery use at that time. Six-month restenosis rates in the Multicenter U.S. Palmaz-Schatz Registry were a surprisingly low 18% for *de novo* lesions and 46% for restenotic lesions. The 12-month actuarial event-free survival was 76% (123). When used in the treatment of aortoostial vein graft disease in 29 patients, stents proved effective with 100% deployment success, and at 11 months, 24 (82%) were free of death, MI, and repeat revascularization (131). In a report of 20 patients who underwent stenting of aortoostial lesions, seven (35%) restenosed (132).

The first randomized multicenter comparison of the use of balloon angioplasty and stents in SVGs (the SAVED trial) was carried out with the Palmaz-Schatz coronary stent in 215 patients with focal *de novo* stenosis (124). Patients were excluded who had MI within 7 days, thrombus, ejection fraction less than 25%, and contraindications to coumadin anticoagulation. Graft age (mean, 10 years), lesion characteristics, and patient characteristics in the balloon (n = 107) and stent (n = 108) groups were similar except for an increased incidence of diabetes in the balloon group (36% vs. 23%, p = .03). In the stent group, 105 (97%) had successful stent deployment, two patients were treated with balloon angioplasty alone, and one with bypass surgery. In the balloon group, 96 patients (90%) were treated with balloons, seven (7%) received bailout stenting, two had bypass surgery, and two were treated medically. Procedural technical success (less than 50% stenosis with assigned therapy) was therefore higher with stenting (95% vs. 75%, p <.001). In-hospital complications of death, Q-wave MI, bypass surgery, and abrupt closure were similar, but there was a trend toward more non–Q-wave infarctions in the balloon group (7% vs. 2%, p = .10), and more stent patients required transfusions (10% vs. 1%, p = .003). At 6 months, restenosis occurred in 36% of stent patients versus 47% of balloon patients (p = .11) (Fig. 84.4A), and the minimal luminal diameter of stent patients was significantly larger (1.75 vs. 1.47 mm, p = .05) (Fig. 84.4B) as was the net gain in lumen diameter (0.87 vs. 0.52 mm, p = .015). Cumulative cardiac events (death, Q-wave MI, non–Q-wave infarction, CABG, and repeat PTCA) were significantly less frequent in stent patients (26% vs. 38%, p = .05) (Fig. 84.4C). A number of single-center and multicenter observational reports of stenting in SVGs have been reported (Table 84.2).

In one of the most recent publications, 106 consecutive patients who underwent SVG stenting at the Ottawa Heart Institute were reported; in-hospital success was 98%, and before discharge, no patient died, required bypass surgery, or had repeat PCI of the same graft (131). With complete follow-up at a median of 18 months, only 44% experienced event-free survival emphasizing the high late event rate after SVG stent implantation (15% died, 17% had MI, 20% had repeat CABG, and 37% had repeat PCI). Factors that have been reported to have the strongest predictive value for late adverse events after SVG stenting include unstable angina, diabetes, previous PTCA, and number of stents (132).

Several other studies of contemporary SVG stenting indicated that even with mostly single-lesion, single-stent procedures, the incidence of clinically important myocardial necrosis (creatine kinase greater than three times normal) was approximately 20%. In the Reduced Anti-coagulation Vein Graft Study, 22% of patients had Q-wave or non–Q-wave MI (133), and in more than 400 patients treated in two high-volume centers from 1995 to 1997, 17% had creatine kinase MB greater than three times normal, and among these patients the 30-day mortality was 14% (134). As the lesion complexity, length, and plaque volume increased, so did the rate of myonecrosis and procedure risks (93). Procedural MI also affected long-term outcomes. In a study of 1,056 consecutive SVG PCI procedures, procedural creatine kinase MB elevation was the strongest independent predictor of late mortality (135). A heightened appreciation of the importance of atheroembolic MI in SVG PCI dovetailed with the development of strategies for distal protection generating enormous interest in its potential for improving outcomes of SVG PCI (136). Webb and colleagues, using the PercuSurge system (distal occlusion balloon and aspiration, Medtronic-AVE, Santa Rosa, CA) in 45 patients, reported aspiration of atherosclerotic debris in more than 80% of patients and an MI rate of less than 4% (137). Carlino et al. used this device in 15 patients with degenerated SVGs with no evidence of atheroembolic infarction (138). In a randomized trial comparing SVG PCI outcomes with and without PercuSurge (SAFER trial) in 551 patients, in-hospital major adverse cardiac events were reduced by 50% (17.3% to 8.8%, p <.001) with distal protection (139). Q-wave MI was reduced from 2.2% to 1.1%, and non–Q-wave MI from 14.4% to 7.3%. It seems likely that some form of distal protection will be used in many, perhaps all, SVG PCI procedures in the future. Other strategies currently being evaluated include the use of filters to catch atherosclerotic debris liberated during PCI procedures and using covered stents to trap debris, excluding it from the circulation. Both of these strategies avoid the need to routinely occlude blood flow in the SVG for several minutes. Randomized trials are currently testing these approaches. Observational reports of the use of a polytetrafluoroethylene (PTFE)-covered stent in SVG PCI by Colombo and colleagues suggested that both immediate

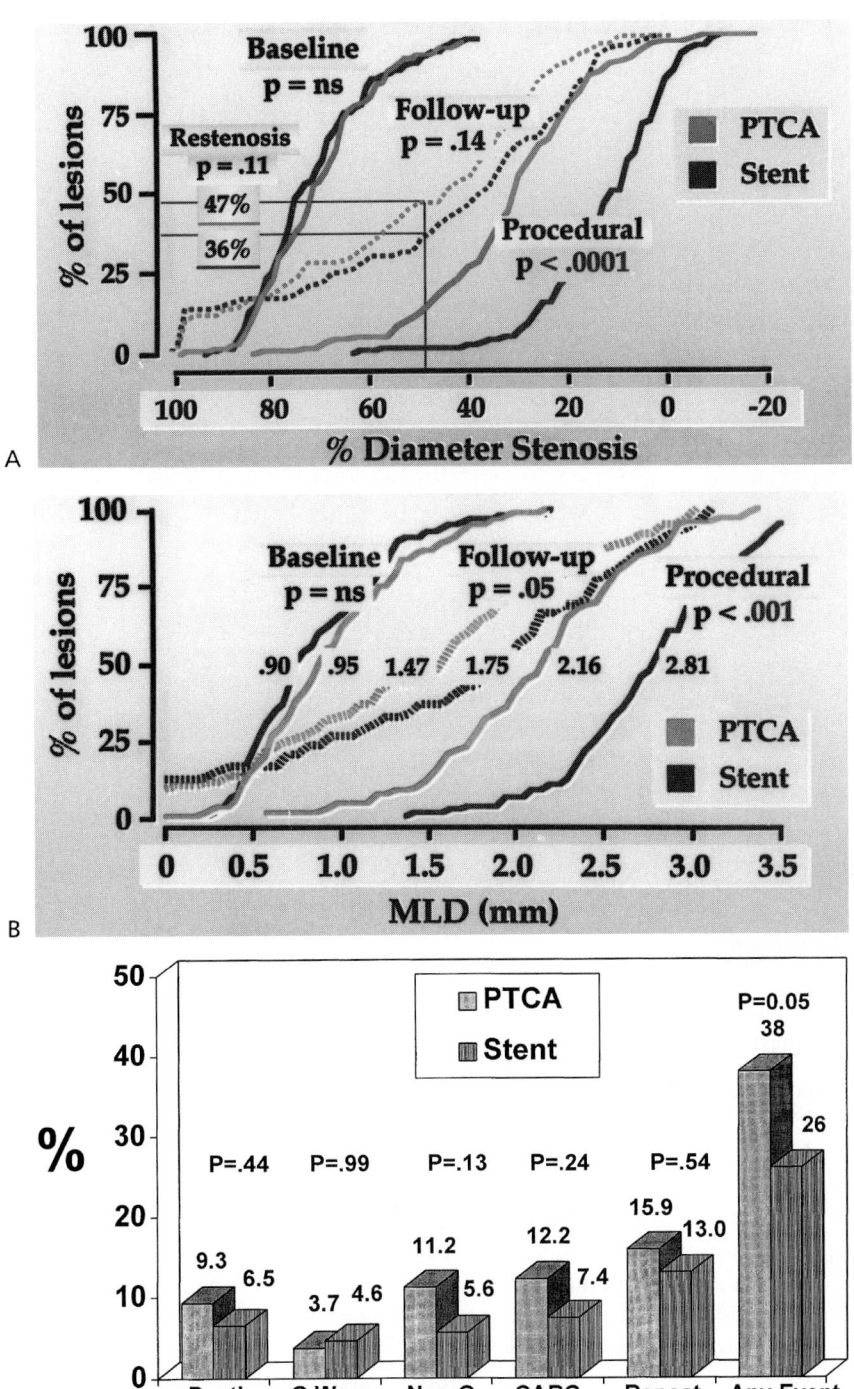

FIGURE 84.4 A: Cumulative frequency of percent diameter stenosis determined by quantitative coronary angiography before, immediately after, and at 6 months after stent or balloon angioplasty in the Stent Versus Angioplasty in Saphenous Vein Graft (SAVED) trial. **B:** Cumulative frequency of minimal luminal diameter (MLD) before, immediately after, and 6 months after stenting or balloon angioplasty in the SAVED trial. **C:** Major cardiac events experienced by patients 6 months after randomization to balloon angioplasty or stent in the SAVED trial. CABG, coronary artery bypass grafting; MI, myocardial infarction; ns, not significant; PTCA, percutaneous transluminal coronary angioplasty.

and long-term outcomes were better than with conventional stents or balloon angioplasty (140) (Fig. 84.5). In a multicenter study Baldus et al. reported 6-month outcomes from 109 consecutive patients who received PTFE-covered stents for *de novo* stenoses in SVG, noting periprocedural increase in creatine kinase MB in 5%, angiographic evidence of in-stent restenosis in 8%, vessel occlusion in 9%, and an 8% mortality (141). In five consecutive patients who received a PTFE-covered stent in

one SVG and a conventional stent in another SVG, Baldus et al. reported that four of five conventional stents developed restenosis, but all five covered stents remained patent, with only a 9% decrease in lumen diameter at 5 months (142). A variety of filter devices also appear promising for "distal protection" in SVG procedures (136,143,144). In an initial experience with a porous membrane filter (80- to 100-μm holes) mounted in a 0.014 PTCA wire and supported by a nitinol basket, it was possible to successfully

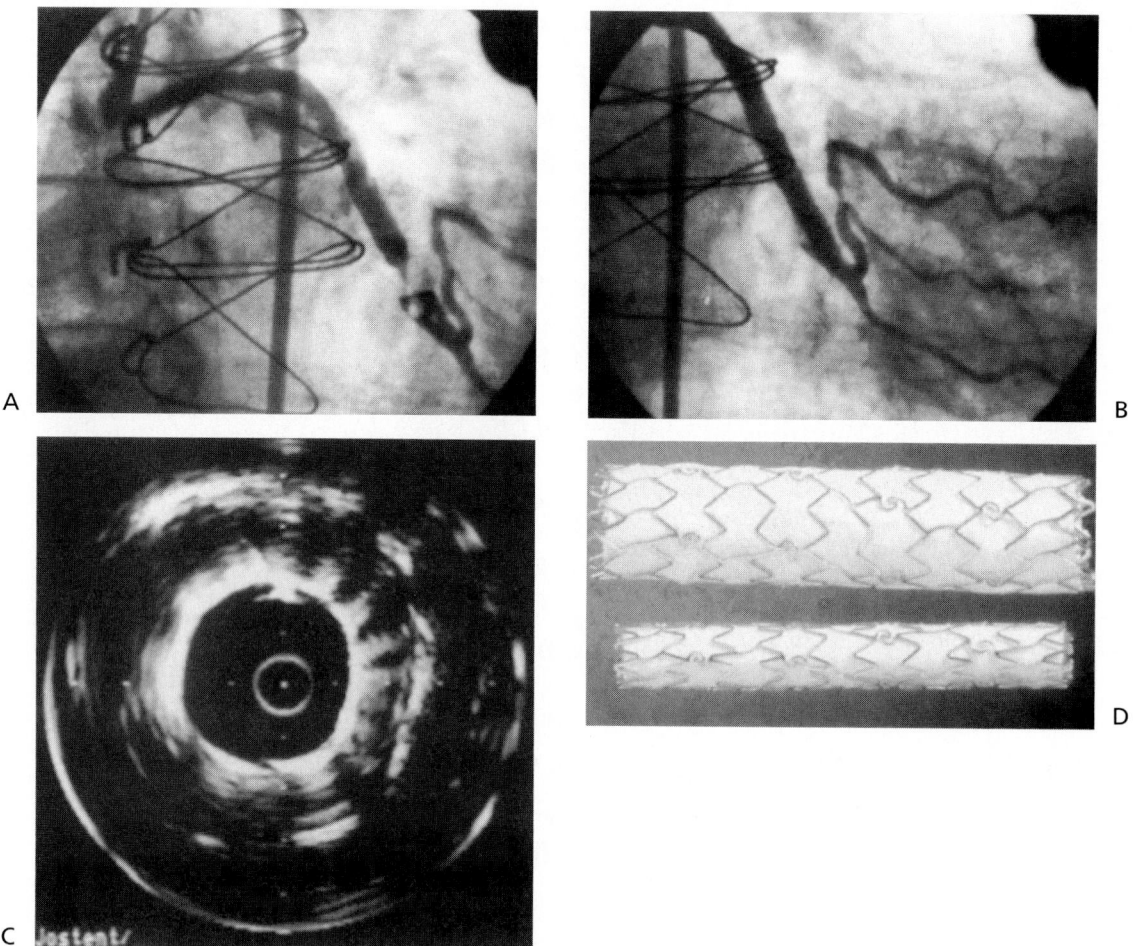

FIGURE 84.5 Severely diseased saphenous vein graft with large filling defect consistent with thrombus **(A)** successfully treated **(B)** with a 4.0- by 16.0-mm Jostent coronary stent graft (Jomed, Rangendingen, Germany), a polytetrafluoroethylene-covered stent. Intravascular ultrasound revealed a widely patent site **(C)**. (Courtesy of Dr. Fausto Feres.) **D:** Jostent coronary stent graft. (From Douglas JS Jr. Diffuse saphenous vein graft disease. In: Ellis SG, Holmes DR, eds. *Strategic approaches in coronary intervention*, 2nd ed. Philadelphia: Lippincott Williams & Wilkins, 2000:355, with permission.)

deploy the filter in 23 of 24 patients, and no in-hospital death, MI, or CABG occurred; one patient experienced a small creatine kinase elevation, and visible debris was removed in more than 80% of patients (144) (*e*Fig. 84.5.1).

The large amount of atheroembolic debris filtered or aspirated during SVG stent procedures (137,139,144) provides insight into the failure of IIb/IIIa platelet receptor inhibitors to reduce periprocedural ischemic events during SVG PCI. Ellis et al. found degenerated SVG to be the only lesion type not to benefit from abciximab when data from the Evaluation of c7E3 for the Prevention of Ischemic Complications (EPIC) trial and the Evaluation of PTCA to Improve Long-Term Outcome with Abciximab GPIIb/IIIa Receptor Blockade (EPILOG) trial were pooled (145). Similarly when data from five trials [EPIC, EPILOG, Evaluation of Platelet IIb/IIIa Inhibitor for Stenting (EPIS-TENT), Integrelin to Minimize Platelet Aggregation and Coronary Thrombosis in Stenting II (IMPACT II), and

Platelet Glycoprotein IIb/IIIa in Unstable Angina: Receptor Suppression Using Integrilin Therapy (PURSUIT)] totaling 627 patients with SVG PCI and The Cleveland Clinic registry of 278 patients with SVG PCI were analyzed, there was no benefit from IIb/IIIa inhibitors or stents with respect to 30-day outcome, and a trend was present toward increased MI with stenting ($p = .09$) (146,147). The lack of any acute benefit with SVG stent deployment is consistent with the SAVED trial (124) and the VENEST-ENT Study (148), each of which randomized patients to balloon angioplasty or stent implantation and demonstrated an improved major adverse cardiac event-free survival at 6 months, but no early difference in major adverse cardiac events.

The transluminal extraction catheter (Interventional Technologies, San Diego, CA) and the rheolytic thrombectomy catheter (Angiojet; Possis Medical, Inc., Minneapolis, MN) have been used for the treatment of

TABLE 84.3 RESULTS OF INTERNAL MAMMARY ARTERY GRAFT PERCUTANEOUS CORONARY INTERVENTION: SELECTED SERIES

Author (yr)	Reference	No. of patients	Success	Complications	Restenosis
Webb et al. (1990)	106	18	12	1 dissection and coronary artery bypass graft	—
Dimas et al. (1991)	56	31	28	2 dissections	1
Sketch et al. (1992)	57	14	13	—	1
Shimshak et al. (1988)	58	26	24	3 dissections	1
Hill et al. (1989)	25	11	9	0	2
Shimshak et al. (1991)	60	86	81	1 Q-wave myocardial infarction	4 late deaths
Hearne et al. (1995)	176	68	60	2 dissections	9 (19%)
Ishizaka et al. (1995)	177	46	34	1 spasm	30%
Gruberg et al. (2000)	61	174	168	1 death, 1 coronary artery bypass graft, 15 non–Q-wave myocardial infarction	1-yr target lesion revascularization, 7.4%

thrombus-associated lesions in SVGs (81–84,116) (*e*Fig. 84.3.7). Although both devices were shown to be relatively effective in clearing thrombus from the treatment site as judged by angioscopy (83,149), distal embolization remained a problem, occurring in 15% with transluminal extraction catheters, associated with a 36% mortality (150), and resulting in non–Q wave in 27% with the Angiojet (151,152).

Recanalizing totally occluded SVGs not in the setting of acute MI has tempted interventional cardiologists for years in spite of low long-term patency and significant procedural complications (91,92,153–162). In a multicenter trial of 107 patients with total vein graft occlusion who received an intragraft infusion of thrombolytic agent for a mean of 25 hours, 74 (69%) achieved initial patency. Adverse acute events included MI (22.0%), emergency CABG (4.0%), stroke (3.0%), transfusion (19.0%), and death (6.5%) (161). Of 40 patients who underwent recatheterization at 6 months, 16 had a patent graft. In a single-center report of 77 consecutive patients with intervention to occluded vein graft, angiographic success was achieved in 71%, 5% died, and 8% underwent bypass surgery within 30 days (162). Three-year survival, event-free survival, and freedom from severe angina were not different in patients with angiographic success and failure. Whether new strategies of mechanical thrombectomy or ultrasound thrombolysis will alter the risk-benefit relationship in these difficult patients remains unclear.

On a brighter note, intravascular radiation for the prevention of recurrence of restenosis yielded promising results in the Washington Radiation for In-Stent Restenosis Trial for Saphenous Vein Grafts. This was a double-blind, randomized trial in 120 patients with diffuse in-stent restenosis (less than 47 mm in length) in SVGs, which compared iridium-192 versus placebo. Of the first 78 patients who completed 6-month angiographic evaluation, 48 (62%) had restenosis, 14 (29%) from the radiation arm and 34 (71%) from the placebo group (163). It is, therefore, anticipated that the final results of Washington Radiation for In-Stent Restenosis Trial for Saphenous

Vein Grafts will demonstrate effectiveness of intravascular radiation in this setting.

Arterial Graft Intervention

Results of Arterial Graft Intervention

Procedural success in IMA graft intervention was approximately 90% and highly dependent on the presence of excessive graft tortuosity and lesion location (Table 84.3). The most common complication was dissection, which occurred in 3.5%, rarely resulting in infarction or bypass surgery. In a published report of 68 consecutive patients, angiographic follow-up at a mean interval of 8 months was available in 78% of successful procedures. Restenosis occurred in 15% (6 of 40) of distal anastomotic sites and 43% (3 of 7) in the midportion of the graft (176). At a mean follow-up of 14 months, 76% of patients had class I or II angina, and event-free survival was 86%. The favorable results at the distal anastomosis parallel those of vein graft lesions at that site (176–179). Gruberg et al. reported outcomes in 174 consecutive patients, 63% with anastomotic lesions treated predominantly with balloon angioplasty (116 of 128, 91%), whereas ostial lesions were treated more frequently with stents (11 of 16, 69%) (61). Procedural success was 97% and 1-year target lesion revascularization was 7.4%. Long-term results of radial and gastroepiploic artery graft intervention have not been reported.

CONTROVERSIES AND PERSONAL PERSPECTIVES

Value of Saphenous Vein Graft Intervention

After successful SVG intervention, there is a high cardiac event rate for most patient subgroups. Distal anastomotic lesions are an exception. The restenotic process in vein grafts does not plateau as it does in native coronary arteries, and mild to moderate nontarget vein graft lesions are associated with recurrent ischemic events in approximately one-

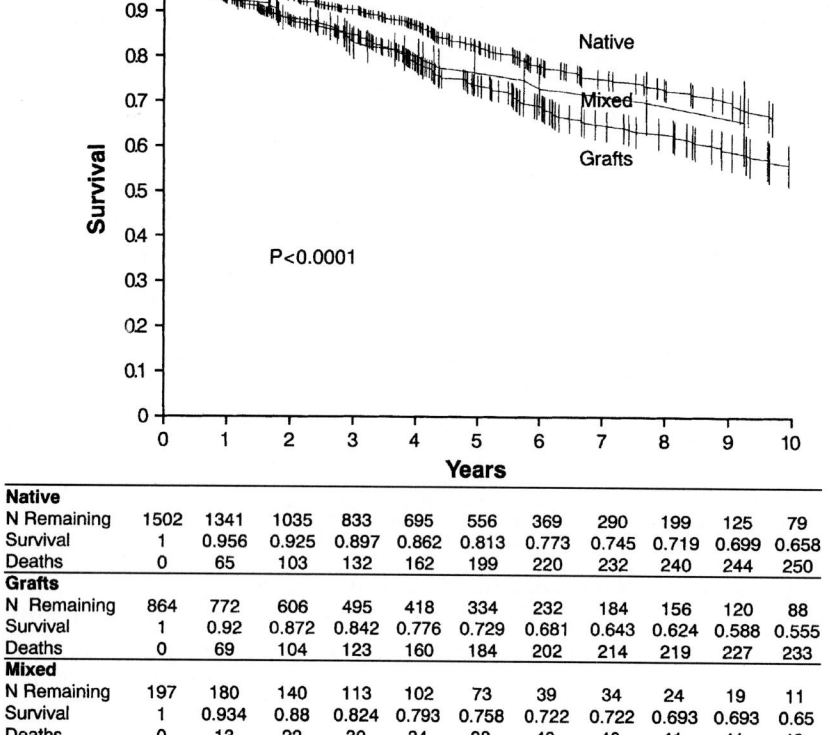

Native											
N Remaining	1502	1341	1035	833	695	556	369	290	199	125	79
Survival	1	0.956	0.925	0.897	0.862	0.813	0.773	0.745	0.719	0.699	0.658
Deaths	0	65	103	132	162	199	220	232	240	244	250
Grafts											
N Remaining	864	772	606	495	418	334	232	184	156	120	88
Survival	1	0.92	0.872	0.842	0.776	0.729	0.681	0.643	0.624	0.588	0.555
Deaths	0	69	104	123	160	184	202	214	219	227	233
Mixed											
N Remaining	197	180	140	113	102	73	39	34	24	19	11
Survival	1	0.934	0.88	0.824	0.793	0.758	0.722	0.722	0.693	0.693	0.65
Deaths	0	13	22	30	34	38	40	40	41	41	42

FIGURE 84.6 Ten-year survival of postbypass patients who underwent percutaneous coronary intervention of a native coronary artery (native), saphenous vein grafts (grafts), or both (mixed) at Emory University Hospitals (Kaplan-Meier method).

third of patients (51). Even with careful selection of patients, emphasizing focal disease and absence of thrombus as was the case in the SAVED trial, the 6-month major cardiac event rate was 26% for SVG stenting, and restenosis occurred in almost 40% of patients (124). At Emory, 5-year event-free survival for vein graft intervention was 31% (105), and survival was less favorable than that with native coronary intervention (Fig. 84.6). If one moves from these relatively ideal candidates to the treatment of diffuse vein graft disease, recent total occlusions, or even to chronic occlusions, the prospects for long-term patency and clinical stability diminish, while the acute risk of thromboembolic MI and bleeding and costs escalate. Although continued study is needed to develop methods to prolong the functional life of degenerating venous grafts, day-to-day appli-

cation of percutaneous strategies to these difficult problems must be done with caution.

Repeat Interventions

Andreas Gruentzig envisioned coronary angioplasty as a strategy that could be used over the years to prevent patients from moving from low-risk categories (nil or single-vessel disease) to high-risk coronary disease. In the postbypass patient, percutaneous intervention is more often performed in an attempt to control symptoms and preserve quality of life. If the patient can be palliated safely by repeat interventions, even for periods as short as a year, this may be reasonable (179,180). However, thoughtful cost-conscious consideration of risks and benefits and of resource consumption must take place.

THE FUTURE

In the next decade, there will be an increasing number of postbypass patients who have begun to have recurrent angina requiring hospitalization. Because of the enormous cost, morbidity, and impracticality of surgical revascularization, it will be important to palliate these patients by percutaneous means as much as possible. We

expect improved technology (especially better, coated, and covered stents) to help, but a major problem is the inadequacy of strategies to treat old, degenerated SVGs. Perhaps with the development of reliable methods of distal protection, techniques to renew (pave?) old grafts and prevent restenosis will evolve.

REFERENCES

1. Gruentzig A. Transluminal dilatation of coronary artery stenosis. *Lancet* 1978;1:263.
2. Hurst JW. History of cardiac catheterization. In: King SB III, Douglas JS Jr, eds. *Coronary arteriography and angioplasty.* New York: McGraw-Hill, 1985:1–9.
3. King SB III. Angioplasty from bench to bedside to bench. *Circulation* 1996;93:1621–1629.
4. Cameron AAC, David KB, Rodgers WJ. Recurrence of angina after coronary artery bypass surgery: predictors and prognosis (CASS Registry). *J Am Coll Cardiol* 1995;26:895–899.
5. Laird-Meeter K, Ten Katen HJ, Brower RW, et al. Angina pectoris, one to 10 years after aorto-coronary bypass surgery. *Eur Heart J* 1983;4:678–686.
6. Campeau L, Lesperance J, Hermann J, et al. Loss of the improvement of angina between 1 and 7 years after aorto-coronary bypass surgery. *Circulation* 1979;60:1.
7. Loop FD, Lytle BW, Cosgrove DM, et al. Reoperation for coronary atherosclerosis. *Ann Surg* 1990;212:378–386.
8. Weintraub WS, Jones EL, Craver JM, et al. Incidence of repeat revascularization after coronary bypass surgery. *J Am Coll Cardiol* 1992;19:98A.
9. Lytle BW, Loop FD, Cosgrove DM. Fifteen hundred coronary reoperations: results and determinants of early and late survival. *J Thorac Cardiovasc Surg* 1987;93:847–857.
10. Weintraub WS, Jones EL, Craver JM, et al. In-hospital and long-term outcome after reoperative coronary artery bypass graft surgery. *Circulation* 1995;92[Suppl II]:II-50–II-57.
11. Jurkovitz C, Jones EL, Craver JM, et al. Update on reoperative coronary bypass surgery; results from the 1990's. *Circulation* 2000;102[Suppl II]:II-555.
12. Gruentzig AR, Senning A, Siegenthaler WE. Nonoperative dilatation of coronary artery stenosis: percutaneous transluminal coronary angioplasty. *N Engl J Med* 1979;303:61–68.
13. Mock MB, Kent KM, Bentivoglio LG. The National Heart, Lung, and Blood Institute percutaneous transluminal coronary angioplasty registry: the first 1116 cases. In: Kaltenbach M, Gruentzig A, Rentrop K, et al., eds. *Transluminal coronary angioplasty and intracoronary thrombolysis. Coronary heart disease, IV.* New York: Springer-Verlag, 1982:11–19.
14. Douglas JS Jr, Gruentzig AR, King SB III, et al. Percutaneous transluminal coronary angioplasty in patients with prior coronary bypass surgery. *J Am Coll Cardiol* 1983;2:745–754.
15. Douglas JS, Ghazzal ZMB, Morris DC, et al. Twenty years of angioplasty at Emory University. *Circulation* 2000;102[Suppl II]:II-753.
16. Weintraub WS, Mauldin PD, Becker E, et al. Cost vs. outcome for redo coronary surgery vs. coronary angioplasty for clinical recurrence after coronary surgery. *J Am Coll Cardiol* 1996;27[Suppl A]:318A.
17. Cameron A, Davis KB, Green G, et al. Coronary bypass surgery with internal-thoracic-artery grafts—effects on survival over a 15-year period. *N Engl J Med* 1996;334:216–219.
18. Loop FD. Internal-thoracic-artery grafts. *N Engl J Med* 1996;334:263–265.
19. Cameron AAC, Green GE, Brogno DA, et al. Internal thoracic artery grafts: 20-year clinical follow-up. *J Am Coll Cardiol* 1995;25:188–192.
20. Lytle BW, Loop FD, Taylor PC, et al. The effect of coronary reoperation on the survival of patients with stenoses in saphenous vein to coronary bypass grafts. *J Thorac Cardiovasc Surg* 1993;105:605–614.
21. Lytle BW. The clinical impact of the atherosclerotic saphenous vein to coronary artery bypass grafts. *Semin Thorac Cardiovasc Surg* 1994;6:81–86.
22. Brener SJ, Ellis SG, Dykstra DM, et al. Determinants of the key decision for prior CABG patients facing need for repeat revascularization: PTCA or CABG? *J Am Coll Cardiol* 1996;27[Suppl A]:45A.
23. Choussat R, Black A, Bossi IM, et al. Diffusely diseased saphenous vein grafts implanted to the left anterior descending coronary artery. What is the best treatment strategy? *Circulation* 2000;102[Suppl II]:II-680.
24. Calkins JB Jr, Talley JD, Kim NH. Iatrogenic aorto-coronary venous fistula as a complication of coronary artery bypass surgery: patient report and review of literature. *Cathet Cardiovasc Diagn* 1996;37:55–59.
25. Hill DM, McAuley BJ, Sheehan DJ, et al. Percutaneous transluminal angioplasty of internal mammary artery bypass grafts. *J Am Coll Cardiol* 1989;13:221A.
26. Belz M, Marshall JJ, Cowley MJ, et al. Subclavian balloon angioplasty in the management of the coronary-subclavian steal syndrome. *Cathet Cardiovasc Diagn* 1992;25:161–163.
27. Ishizaka N, Ikari Y, Seaki F, et al. Repeat embolization of the side branch of the internal mammary artery graft by gelatin sponge particles and micro cells. *Cathet Cardiovasc Diagn* 1995;34:245–249.
28. Kern MJ, Bach RG, Donohue TJ, et al. Part XIII: role of large pectoralis branch artery in flow through a patent left internal mammary artery conduit. *Cathet Cardiovasc Diagn* 1995;34:240–244.
29. Goldman S, Copeland J, Moritz T, et al. Starting aspirin therapy after operation: effects on early graft patency. *Circulation* 1991;84:520–525.
30. Tan E, van der Meer J, de Kam PF, et al. Worse clinical outcome but similar graft patency in women versus men one year after coronary artery bypass surgery owing to an excess of risk factors in women. *J Am Coll Cardiol* 1999;34:1760–1768.
31. Fitzgibbon GM, Leach AJ, Kafka HP, et al. Coronary bypass graft fate: long-term angiographic study. *J Am Coll Cardiol* 1991;17:1075–1080.
32. Bourassa MG, Enjalbert M, Campeau L, et al. Progression of atherosclerosis in coronary arteries and bypass grafts: ten years later. *Am J Cardiol* 1984;53:102C.
33. Chen L, Theroux P, Lesperance J, et al. Angiographic features in vein grafts versus in ungrafted coronary arteries in patients with unstable angina and previous bypass surgery. *J Am Coll Cardiol* 1996;27[Suppl A]:333A.
34. Maynard C, Weaver WD, Litwin P, et al. Acute myocardial infarction and prior coronary artery surgery in the Myocardial Infarction Triage and Intervention Registry:

patient characteristics, treatment, and outcome. *Coronary Artery Dis* 1991;2:443–448.

35. Stone GW, Brodie BR, Griffin JJ, et al. Clinical and angiographic outcome in patients with previous coronary artery bypass graft surgery treated with primary balloon angioplasty for acute myocardial infarction. *J Am Coll Cardiol* 2000;35:605–611.

36. Little WC, Gwinn NS, Burrows MT, et al. Cause of acute myocardial infarction late after successful coronary artery bypass grafting. *Am J Cardiol* 1990;65:808–810.

37. Grines CL, Booth DC, Nissen SE, et al. Mechanism of acute myocardial infarction in patients with prior coronary artery bypass grafting and therapeutic implications. *Am J Cardiol* 1990;65:1292–1296.

38. Kavanaugh KM, Topol EJ. Acute intervention during myocardial infarction in patients with prior coronary bypass surgery. *Am J Cardiol* 1990;65:924–926.

39. Kleiman NS, Berman DA, Gaston WR, et al. Early intravenous thrombolytic therapy for acute myocardial infarction in patients with prior coronary artery bypass grafts. *Am J Cardiol* 1989;63:102–104.

40. Kahn JK, Rutherford BD, McConahay DR, et al. Usefulness of angioplasty during acute myocardial infarction in patients with prior coronary artery bypass grafting. *Am J Cardiol* 1990;65:698–702.

41. Lawrie GM, Morris GC Jr, Earle N, et al. Factors affecting patency of 3682 aorto-coronary vein grafts up to 20 years after operation. *J Am Coll Cardiol* 1996;27[Suppl A]:45A.

42. Bulkley BH, Hutchins GM. Pathology of coronary artery bypass graft surgery. *Arch Pathol* 1978;102:273–280.

43. Spray TL, Roberts WC. Changes in saphenous veins used as aortocoronary bypass grafts. *Am Heart J* 1997;94:500–516.

44. Smith SH, Geer JC. Morphology of saphenous vein–coronary artery bypass grafts: seven to 116 months after surgery. *Arch Pathol Lab Med* 1983;107:13–18.

45. Moore GW, Hutchins GM. Coronary artery bypass grafts in 109 autopsied patients: statistical analyses of graft and anastomosis patency and regional myocardial injury. *JAMA* 1981;246:1785–1789.

46. Mautner SL, Mautner GC, Hunsberger SA, et al. Comparison of composition of atherosclerotic plaques in saphenous veins used as aortocoronary bypass conduits with plaques in native coronary arteries in same men. *Am J Cardiol* 1992;70:1378–1380.

47. Waller BF, Tothbaum DA, Gorfinkel HJ, et al. Morphologic observations after percutaneous transluminal balloon angioplasty of early and late aortocoronary saphenous vein bypass grafts. *J Am Coll Cardiol* 1984;4:784–792.

48. Neitzel GF, Barboriak JJ, Pintar K, et al. Atherosclerosis in aortocoronary bypass grafts: morphologic study and risk factor analysis 6 to 12 years after surgery. *Arteriosclerosis* 1986;6:594–600.

49. Walts AE, Fishbein MC, Sustaita H, et al. Ruptured atheromatous plaques in saphenous vein coronary artery bypass grafts: a mechanism of acute, thrombotic late graft occlusion. *Circulation* 1982;65:197.

50. Tilli FV, Kaplan BM, Safian RD, et al. Angioscopic plaque friability: a new risk factor for procedural complications following saphenous vein graft interventions. *J Am Coll Cardiol* 1996;27[Suppl A]:364A.

51. Ellis SG, Brener S, De Luca S, et al. Late myocardial ischemic events after saphenous vein graft intervention—importance of initially "non-significant" vein graft lesions. *Am J Cardiol* 1997;79:1460–1464.

52. Palac RT, Hwang MH, Meadows WR, et al. Progression of coronary artery disease in medically and surgically treated patients 5 years after randomization. *Circulation* 1981;64:II-17.

53. Hwang MH, Meadows WR, Palac RT, et al. Progression of native coronary artery disease at 10 years: insights from a randomized study of medical versus surgical therapy for angina. *J Am Coll Cardiol* 1990;16:1066–1070.

54. Frick MH, Valle M, Harjola PT. Progression of coronary artery disease in randomized medical and surgical patients over a 5-year angiographic follow-up. *Am J Cardiol* 1983;52:681.

55. Hair D, Antonescu A, Ishimori T, et al. Does coronary artery bypass surgery cause native vessel occlusion? *J Am Coll Cardiol* 1996;27[Suppl A]:92A.

56. Dimas AP, Arora RR, Whitlow PL, et al. Percutaneous transluminal angioplasty involving internal mammary artery grafts. *Am Heart J* 1991;122:423–429.

57. Sketch MH, Quigley PG, Perez JA, et al. Angiographic follow-up after internal mammary artery graft angioplasty. *Am J Cardiol* 1992;70:401–403.

58. Shimshak TM, Giorgi LV, Johnson WL, et al. Application of percutaneous transluminal coronary angioplasty to the internal mammary artery graft. *J Am Coll Cardiol* 1988;12:1205–1214.

59. Safian RD, Kaplan B, Schreiber T, et al. Interim results of the Wallstent endoprosthesis in saphenous vein graft trial. *Circulation* 1998;98:I-662.

60. Shimshak TM, Rutherford BD, McConahay DR, et al. PTCA of internal mammary artery (IMA) grafts procedural results and late follow-up. *Circulation* 1991;84[Suppl II]:II-590.

61. Gruberg L, Dangas G, Mehran R, et al. Percutaneous revascularization of the internal mammary artery graft: short- and long-term outcomes. *J Am Coll Cardiol* 2000;35:944–948.

62. Kollar A, Simonton CA, Thomley AM, et al. Balloon angioplasty of the internal mammary artery trunk for early postoperative ischemia: a case report. *Cathet Cardiovasc Diagn* 1996;37:49–51.

63. Cutlip DE, Dauerman HL, Carrozza JP. Recurrent ischemia within thirty days of coronary artery bypass surgery: angiographic findings and outcome of percutaneous revascularization. *Circulation* 1996;94[Suppl I]:I-249.

64. Reifart N, Haase J, Storger H, et al. Interventional standby for cardiac surgery. *Circulation* 1996;94[Suppl I]:I86.

65. Coronary Artery Surgery Study (CASS) and Their Associates. A randomized trial of coronary artery bypass: quality of life in patients randomly assigned to treatment groups. *Circulation* 1983;68:951–956.

66. Knatterud GL, Rosenberg Y, Campeau L, et al. Long term effects on clinical outcomes of aggressive lowering of low density lipoprotein cholesterol levels and low dose anticoagulation in the post coronary artery bypass graft trial. *Circulation* 2000;102:157–165.

67. Domanski MJ, Borkowf CB, Campeau L, et al. Prognostic factors for atherosclerosis progression in saphenous vein grafts. The Post Coronary Artery Bypass Grafts (Post-CABG) Trial. *J Am Coll Cardiol* 2000;36:1877–1883.

68. Waters DD, Azar RR. Post scripts from the Post Coronary Artery Bypass Graft Trial. *Circulation* 2000;102:144–146.

69. Bhatt DL, Chew DP, Hirsch AT, et al. Superiority of clopidogrel versus aspirin in patients with prior cardiac surgery. *Circulation* 2001;103:363–368.

70. Mathew V, Clavell AL, Lennon RJ, et al. Percutaneous coronary interventions in patients with prior coronary bypass surgery: changes in patient characteristics and outcome during two decades. *Am J Med* 2000;108:127–135.

71. Mathew V, Berger PB, Lennon RK, et al. Comparison of percutaneous interventions for unstable angina in patients with and without previous coronary artery bypass grafting. *Am J Cardiol* 2000;86:931–937.

72. Frantz E, Sauer HU, Pfautsch P, et al. Angioplasty for recurrent ischemia after coronary artery bypass grafting predicts highest reintervention need, but lowest mortality at follow-up. *Circulation* 1995;92[Suppl I]:I-178.

73. Kahn JK, Hartzler GO. Retrograde coronary angioplasty of isolated arterial segments through saphenous vein bypass grafts. *Cathet Cardiovasc Diagn* 1990;20:88–93.

74. Douglas JS Jr, King SB III, Roubin GS, et al. Native coronary artery angioplasty in patients with previous coronary bypass surgery: update of in-hospital and long-term results. *Circulation* 1987;76[Suppl IV]:IV-465.

75. Miranda CP, Rutherford BD, McConahay DR, et al. Elective PTCA in post-bypass patients: comparison between those undergoing native artery dilatations and those undergoing bypass graft dilatations. *Circulation* 1992;86:I-457.

76. Savage MP, Fischman DL, Douglas JS, et al. The dark side of high pressure stent deployment. *J Am Coll Cardiol* 1997;29[Suppl A]:368A.

77. Rechavia E, Litvack F, Macko G, et al. Stent implantation of saphenous vein graft aorto-ostial lesions in patients with unstable ischemic syndromes: immediate angiographic results and long-term clinical outcome. *J Am Coll Cardiol* 1995;25:866–870.

78. Rocha-Singh K, Morris N, Wong SC, et al. Coronary stenting for treatment of ostial stenoses of native coronary arteries or aortocoronary saphenous venous grafts. *Am J Cardiol* 1995;75:26–29.

79. Amed JM, Hong MK, Mehran R, et al. Comparison of debulking followed by stenting versus stenting alone for aorto-ostial lesions: immediate and one-year clinical outcomes. *J Am Coll Cardiol* 2000;35:1560–1568.

80. Thomas WJ, Cowley MJ, Vetrovec GW, et al. Effectiveness of rotational atherectomy in aortocoronary saphenous vein grafts. *Am J Cardiol* 2000;86:88–91.

81. Ramee SR, Baim DS, Popma JJ, et al. A randomized, prospective, multi-center study comparing intracoronary urokinase to rheolytic thrombectomy with the POSSIS Angioget catheter for intracoronary thrombus: final results of the VeGAS 2 Trial. *Circulation* 1998;98[Suppl I]:I-86.

82. Drasler WJ, Jenson ML, Wilson GJ, et al. Rheolytic catheter for percutaneous removal of thrombus. *Radiology* 1992;182:263–267.

83. Rodes J, Bilodeau L, Bonan R, et al. Angioscopic evaluation of thrombus removal by the Possis Angiojet thrombectomy catheter. *Cathet Cardiovasc Diagn* 1998;43:338–343.

84. Meany TB, Leon MB, Kramer BL, et al. Transluminal extraction catheter for the treatment of diseased saphenous vein grafts: a multicenter experience. *Cathet Cardiovasc Diagn* 1995;34:112–120.

85. Chapekis AT, George BS, Candela RJ. Rapid thrombus dissolution by continuous infusion of urokinase through an intracoronary perfusion wire before and following PTCA: results in native coronaries and patent saphenous vein grafts. *Cathet Cardiovasc Diagn* 1991;23:89–92.

86. Cundey PE, Whitlock RR, Norman J, et al. Prolonged intragraft urokinase with a new infusion wire: improved short-term results. *Cathet Cardiovasc Diagn* 1997;31:150–152.

87. Denardo SJ, Morris NB, Rocha-Singh KJ, et al. Safety and efficacy of extended urokinase infusion plus stent deployment for treatment of obstructed, older saphenous vein grafts. *Am J Cardiol* 1995;76:776–780.

88. McKay RG. Site-specific, catheter-based thrombolysis: a new technique for treating intracoronary thrombus and thrombus-containing stenosis. *J Invas Cardiol* 1995;7:36E–43E.

89. Mitchel JF, Fram DB, Palme DF, et al. Enhanced intracoronary thrombolysis with urokinase using a novel, local drug delivery system. *Circulation* 1995;91:785–793.

90. Barsness GW, Buller CE, Ohman EM, et al. Reduced thrombus burden in saphenous vein grafts with abciximab given through a local delivery catheter. *Circulation* 1998;98[Suppl I]:I-354.

91. Holmes DR, Berger PB. Percutaneous revascularization of occluded vein grafts. Is it still a temptation to be resisted? *Circulation* 1999;99:8–11.

92. Rosenschein U, Gaul G, Erbel R, et al. Percutaneous transluminal therapy of occluded saphenous vein grafts. Can the challenge be met with ultrasound thrombolysis? *Circulation* 1999;99:26–29.

93. Liu MW, Douglas JS Jr, King SB III, et al. Angiographic predictors of coronary embolization in the PTCA of vein graft lesions. *Circulation* 1989;80:II-172.

94. Piana RN, Paik GY, Moscucci M, et al. Incidence and treatment of "no-reflow" after percutaneous coronary intervention. *Circulation* 1994;89:2514–2518.

95. Turi ZG. The periangioplasty polypharmacy: a role for diltiazem? *Cathet Cardiovasc Diagn* 1995;35:292–293.

96. Marzilli M, Marraccini P, Gliozheni E, et al. Intracoronary adenosine as an adjunct to combined use of primary angioplasty in acute myocardial infarction: beneficial effects on angiographically assessed no-reflow. *J Am Coll Cardiol* 1996;27[Suppl A]:81A.

97. Hillegrass WB, Dean NA, Liano L, et al. Treatment of no-reflow and impaired flow with the nitric oxide donor nitroprusside following percutaneous coronary interventions: initial human clinical experience. *J Am Coll Cardiol* 2001;37:1335–1343.

98. Bhatt DL, Topol EJ. Percutaneous coronary intervention for patients with prior bypass surgery: therapy in evolution. *Am J Med* 2000;108:176–177.

99. Douglas J, Robinson K, Schlumpf M. Percutaneous transluminal angioplasty in aortocoronary venous graft

stenoses: immediate results and complications. *Circulation* 1986;74:II-281.

100. Cote G, Myler RK, Stertzer SH, et al. Percutaneous transluminal angioplasty of stenotic coronary artery bypass grafts: 5 years' experience. *J Am Coll Cardiol* 1987;9:8–17.

101. Dorros G, Lewin RF, Mathiak LM, et al. Percutaneous transluminal coronary angioplasty in patients with two or more previous coronary artery bypass graft operations. *Am J Cardiol* 1988;61:1243–1247.

102. Reed DC, Beller GA, Nygaard TW, et al. The clinical efficacy and scintigraphic evaluation of post-coronary bypass patients undergoing percutaneous transluminal coronary angioplasty for recurrent angina pectoris. *Am Heart J* 1989;117:60.

103. Platko WP, Hollman J, Whitlow PL, et al. Percutaneous transluminal angioplasty of saphenous vein graft stenosis: long-term follow-up. *J Am Coll Cardiol* 1989;7:1645–1650.

104. Plokker HW, Meester BH, Serruys PW. The Dutch experience in percutaneous transluminal angioplasty of narrowed saphenous veins used for aortocoronary arterial bypass. *Am J Cardiol* 1991;67:361–366.

105. Douglas JS Jr, Weintraub WS, Liberman HA, et al. Update of saphenous graft (SVG) angioplasty: restenosis and long-term outcome. *Circulation* 1991;84:II-249.

106. Webb JG, Myler RF, Shaw RE, et al. Coronary angioplasty after coronary bypass surgery: initial results and late outcome in 422 patients. *J Am Coll Cardiol* 1990;16:812–820.

107. Reeves F, Bonan R, Cote G, et al. Long-term angiographic follow-up after angioplasty of venous coronary bypass grafts. *Am Heart J* 1991;122:620–627.

108. Morrison DA, Crowley ST, Veerakul G, et al. Percutaneous transluminal angioplasty of saphenous vein grafts for medically refractory unstable angina. *J Am Coll Cardiol* 1994;23:1066–1070.

109. Douglas JS Jr, Weintraub WS, King SB III. Changing perspectives in vein graft angioplasty. *J Am Coll Cardiol* 1995;25[Suppl A]:78A.

110. De Feyter PJ, Van Suylen R, de Jaegere PPT, et al. Balloon angioplasty for the treatment of lesions in saphenous vein bypass grafts. *J Am Coll Cardiol* 1993;21:1539–1549.

111. Holmes DR, Topol EJ, Califf RM, et al. A multicenter, randomized trial of coronary angioplasty versus directional atherectomy for patients with saphenous vein graft lesions. *Circulation* 1995;91:1966–1974.

112. Lefkovits J, Holmes DR, Califf RM, et al. Predictors and sequelae of distal embolization during saphenous vein graft intervention from the CAVEAT-II Trial. *Circulation* 1995;92:734–740.

113. Wong SC, Popma JJ, Hong MK, et al. Procedural results and long-term clinical outcome in aorto-ostial saphenous vein graft lesions after new device angioplasty. *J Am Coll Cardiol* 1995;25[Suppl A]:394A.

114. Waksman R, Weintraub WS, Ghazzal ZMB, et al. Acute and long-term outcome of narrowed saphenous vein bypass graft: a comparison of treatment with Palmaz-Schatz stent, directional coronary atherectomy and balloon angioplasty. *Am Heart J* 1997;134:274–278.

115. Bittl JA, Sanborn TA, Yardley DE, et al. Predictors of outcome of percutaneous excimer laser coronary angioplasty of saphenous vein bypass graft lesions. *Am J Cardiol* 1994;74:144–148.

116. Hong MK, Wong SC, Popma JJ, et al. Favorable results of debulking followed by immediate adjunct stent therapy for high risk saphenous vein graft lesions. *J Am Coll Cardiol* 1996;27[Suppl A]:A179.

117. Deckelbaum LI, Natarjan K, Bittl JA, et al. Effect of intracoronary saline infusion on dissection during excimer laser coronary angioplasty: a randomized trial. *J Am Coll Cardiol* 1995;26:1264–1269.

118. Pinkerton CA, Slack JD, Orr CM, et al. Percutaneous transluminal angioplasty in patients with prior myocardial revascularization surgery. *Am J Cardiol* 1988;61:15G–22G.

119. Pomerantz RM, Kuntz RE, Carroza J, et al. Acute and long-term outcome of narrowed saphenous vein grafts treated with endoluminal stenting and directional atherectomy. *Am J Cardiol* 1992;70:161–167.

120. Carrozza JP, Kuntz RE, Levine MJ, et al. Angiographic and clinical outcome of intracoronary stenting: immediate and long-term results from a large single-center experience. *J Am Coll Cardiol* 1992;20:328–337.

121. Piana RN, Moscucci M, Cohen DJ, et al. Palmaz-Schatz stenting for treatment of focal vein graft stenosis: immediate results and long-term outcome. *J Am Coll Cardiol* 1994;23:1296–1304.

122. Fenton SH, Fischman DL, Savage MP, et al. Long-term angiographic and clinical outcome after implantation of balloon-expandable stents in aortocoronary saphenous vein grafts. *Am J Cardiol* 1994;74:1187–1191.

123. Wong SC, Baim DS, Schatz RA, et al. Acute results and late outcomes after stent implantation in saphenous vein graft lesions: the multicenter USA Palmaz-Schatz stent experience. *J Am Coll Cardiol* 1995;26:704–712.

124. Savage MP, Douglas JS Jr, Fischman DL, et al. A randomized trial of coronary stenting and balloon angioplasty in the treatment of aortocoronary saphenous vein bypass graft disease. *N Engl J Med* 1997;337:740–747.

125. de Scheerder JK, Strauss BH, De Feyter PJ, et al. Stenting of venous bypass grafts: a new treatment modality of patients who are poor candidates for reintervention. *Am Heart J* 1992;23:1296–1304.

126. Strauss BH, Serruys PW, Bertrand ME, et al. Qualitative angiographic follow-up of the coronary Wallstent in native vessel bypass grafts. *Am J Cardiol* 1992;69:475–481.

127. de Jaegere PP, Van Domburg RT, De Feyter PJ, et al. Long-term clinical outcome after stent implantation in saphenous vein grafts. *J Am Coll Cardiol* 1996;28:89–96.

128. Fortuna R, Heuser RR, Garrat KN, et al. Wiktor intracoronary stent: experience in the first 101 graft patients. *Circulation* 1993;88[Suppl I]:I-308.

129. Colombo, Itoh A, Hall P, et al. Implantation of the Wallstent for diffuse lesions in native coronary arteries and venous bypass grafts without subsequent anticoagulation. *J Am Coll Cardiol* 1996;91:53A.

130. Eeckhout E, Kappenberger L, Goy J. Stents for intracoronary placement: current status and future directions. *J Am Coll Cardiol* 1996;27:757–765.

131. Le May MR, Labinaz M, Marquis JF, et al. Predictors of long-term outcome after stent implantation in a saphenous vein graft. *Am J Cardiol* 1999;83:681–686.

132. Ahmed JM, Dangas GD, Mehran R, et al. Clinical, angiographic and intravascular ultrasound predictors of target vessel revascularization and late cardiac events after stent implantation in saphenous vein grafts. *J Am Coll Cardiol* 2001;37[Suppl A]:20A.

133. Leon MB, Ellis SG, Moses J, et al. Interim report from the reduced anticoagulation vein graft stent (RAVES) study. *Circulation* 1996;94[Suppl I]:I-683.

134. Kalon KL, Carrozza JP, Popma JJ, et al. Creatine-kinase MB isoform (CK-MB) elevations following single vessel percutaneous revascularization of saphenous vein grafts. *Circulation* 1998;98[Suppl I]:I-353.

135. Hong MK, Mehran R, Dangas G, et al. Creatine kinase-MB enzyme elevation following successful saphenous vein graft intervention is associated with late mortality. *Circulation* 1999;100:2400–2405.

136. Topol EJ, Yadav JS. Recognition of the importance of embolization in atherosclerotic vascular disease. *Circulation* 2000;101:570–580.

137. Webb JG, Carere RG, Virmani R, et al. Retrieval and analysis of particulate debris following saphenous vein graft intervention. *J Am Coll Cardiol* 1999;34:461–467.

138. Carlino M, De Gregorio J, Di Mario C, et al. Prevention of distal embolization during saphenous vein graft lesion angioplasty. Experience with a new temporary occlusion and aspiration system. *Circulation* 1999;99:3221–3223.

139. Baim DS. SAFER Trial results, oral presentation at Transcatheter Therapeutic Meeting, October 2000, Washington, DC.

140. Dharmadhikari A, Di Mario C, Tzifos V, et al. Comparison of procedural and one-year outcome with only balloon angioplasty, covered stents, and non-covered stents in saphenous vein grafts. *J Am Coll Cardiol* 2000;35[Suppl A]:26A.

141. Baldus S, Koster R, Elsner M, et al. Treatment of aortocoronary vein graft lesions with membrane-covered stents. A multicenter surveillance trial. *Circulation* 2000;102:2024–2027.

142. Baldus S, Koster R, Reimers J, et al. Membrane-covered stents: a new treatment strategy for saphenous vein graft lesions. *Cathet Cardiovasc Intervent* 2001;53:1–4.

143. Gerckens U, Mueller R, Rowold S, et al. The filter wire: first evaluation of a new protection catheter device for distal embolization in native coronary arteries and SVG's. *J Am Coll Cardiol* 2001;37[Suppl A]:34A.

144. Gerckens U, Mueller R, Soblik S, et al. Prevention of distal embolization during interventions in CABG and native coronary lesions using a new protection filter device. *J Am Coll Cardiol* 2000;35[Suppl A]:10A.

145. Ellis SG, Lincoff AM, Miller D, et al. Reduction in complications of angioplasty with abciximab occurs largely independently of baseline lesion morphology. *J Am Coll Cardiol* 1998;32:1619–1623.

146. Roffi M, Chan A, Chew DP, et al. Stents and glycoprotein IIb/IIIa inhibitors do not improve 30-day outcome in bypass graft percutaneous interventions: a retrospective registry-based analysis. *J Am Coll Cardiol* 2001;37[Suppl A]:77A.

147. Roffi M, Bhatt DL, Mukherjee D, et al. Stents and glycoprotein IIb/IIIa blockade have no salutary effect on 30-day outcome following percutaneous interventions of coronary bypass grafts. *J Am Coll Cardiol* 2001;37[Suppl A]:68A.

148. Hanekamp CEE, Koolen JJ, Den Heyer P, et al. A randomized comparison between balloon angioplasty and elective stent implantation in venous bypass grafts: the VENESTENT study. *J Am Coll Cardiol* 2000;35[Suppl A]:9A.

149. Annex BH, Larkin TJ, O'Neill WW, et al. Evaluation of thrombus removal by transluminal extraction coronary atherectomy by percutaneous coronary angioscopy. *Am J Cardiol* 1994;74:606–609.

150. Moses JW, Teirstein PS, Sketch MH Jr, et al. Angiographic determinants of risk and outcome of coronary embolus and myocardial infarction (MI) with the transluminal extraction catheter (TEC): a report from the New Approaches to Coronary Intervention (NACI) Registry. *J Am Coll Cardiol* 1994;74:220A.

151. Ramee SR, Schatz RA, Carrozza JR, et al. Results of the VeGAS I pilot study of the Possis coronary Angiojet thrombectomy catheter. *Circulation* 1996;94:3622.

152. Whisanant BK, Baim DS, Kuntz, et al. Rheolytic thrombectomy with the Possis Angiojet: technical considerations and initial clinical experience. *J Invas Cardiol* 1999;11:421–426.

153. De Feyter PJ, Serruys P, Van Den Brand M, et al. Percutaneous transluminal angioplasty of a totally occluded bypass graft: a challenge that should be resisted. *Am J Cardiol* 1989;64:88–90.

154. Gurley JC, MacPhail BS. Acute myocardial infarction due to thrombolytic reperfusion of chronically occluded saphenous vein coronary bypass grafts. *Am J Cardiol* 1991;68:274–275.

155. McKeever LS, Hartman JR, Bufalino VJ, et al. Acute myocardial infarction complicating recanalization of aortocoronary bypass grafts with urokinase therapy. *Am J Cardiol* 1989;64:683–685.

156. Bedotto JB, Rutherford BD, Hartzler GO. Intramyocardial hemorrhage due to prolonged intracoronary infusion of urokinase into a totally occluded saphenous vein bypass graft. *Cathet Cardiovasc Diagn* 1992;25:52–56.

157. Blankenship JC, Modesto TA, Madigan NP. Acute myocardial infarction complicating urokinase infusion for total saphenous vein graft occlusion. *Cathet Cardiovasc Diagn* 1993;28:39–43.

158. Taylor MA, Santoian EC, Ali J, et al. Intracerebral hemorrhage complicating urokinase infusion into an occluded aortocoronary bypass graft. *Cathet Cardiovasc Diagn* 1994;31:206–210.

159. Kaplan BM, Safian RD, Goldstein JA, et al. Efficacy of angioscopy in determining the effectiveness of intracoronary urokinase and TEC atherectomy thrombus removal from an occluded saphenous vein graft before stent implantation. *Cathet Cardiovasc Diagn* 1995;36:335–337.

160. Glazier JJ, Bauer HH, Kiernan FJ, et al. Recanalization of totally occluded saphenous vein grafts using local urokinase delivery with the Dispatch catheter. *Cathet Cardiovasc Diagn* 1995;36:326–332.

161. Hartmann JR, McKeever LS, O'Neill WW, et al. Recanalization of chronically occluded aortocoronary saphenous vein bypass grafts with long-term, low dose direct infusion

of urokinase (ROBUST): a serial trial. *J Am Coll Cardiol* 1996;27:60–66.

162. Berger PB, Bell MR, Simari R, et al. Immediate and long-term clinical outcome in patients undergoing angioplasty of occluded vein grafts. *J Am Coll Cardiol* 1996;76[Suppl A]:180A.

163. Waksman R. Intracoronary gamma radiation for in-stent restenosis in saphenous vein grafts. A multi-center randomized clinical study—SVG WRIST. Late Breaking Trials. 50th Annual Scientific Session of the American College of Cardiology 2001, Orlando, FL.

164. Brown RIG, Gilligan L, Penn IM, et al. Right internal mammary artery graft angioplasty through a right brachial artery approach using a new custom guide catheter: a case report. *Cathet Cardiovasc Diagn* 1992;25:42–45.

165. Ernst S, Bal E, Plokker T, et al. Percutaneous balloon angioplasty (PBA) of a left subclavian artery stenosis or occlusion to establish adequate flow through the left internal mammary artery for coronary bypass purposes. *Circulation* 1991;84:II-591.

166. Shapira S, Braun S, Puram B, et al. Percutaneous transluminal angioplasty of proximal subclavian artery stenosis after left internal mammary to left anterior descending artery bypass surgery. *J Am Coll Cardiol* 1991;18:1120–1123.

167. Kugelmass AD, Kim D, Kuntz RE, et al. Endoluminal stenting of a subclavian artery stenosis to treat ischemia in the distribution of a patent left internal mammary graft. *Cathet Cardiovasc Diagn* 1994;33:175–177.

168. Sullivan TM, Bacharach JM, Childs MB. PTA and primary stenting of the subclavian and innominate arteries. *Circulation* 1995;92[Suppl I]:I-383.

169. Kumar K, Dorros G, Bates MC, et al. Primary stent deployment in occlusive subclavian artery disease. *Cathet Cardiovasc Diagn* 1995;34:281–285.

170. Galli M, Goldberg SL, Zerboni S, et al. Balloon expandable stent implantation after iatrogenic arterial dissection of the left subclavian artery. *Cathet Cardiovasc Diagn* 1995;35:355–357.

171. Almagor Y, Thomas J, Colombo A. Balloon expandable stent implantation of a stenosis at the origin of the left internal mammary artery graft. *Cathet Cardiovasc Diagn* 1991;24:256–258.

172. Bajaj RK, Roubin GS. Intravascular stenting of the right internal mammary artery. *Cathet Cardiovasc Diagn* 1991;24:252–255.

173. Miller RM, Knox M. Patient tolerance of ioxaglate and iopamidol in internal mammary artery arteriography. *Cathet Cardiovasc Diagn* 1992;25:31–34.

174. Stratienko AA, Ginsberg R, Schatz RA, et al. Technique for shortening angioplasty guide catheter length when therapeutic catheter fails to reach target stenosis. *Cathet Cardiovasc Diagn* 1993;30:331–333.

175. Isshiki T, Yamaguchi T, Tamura T, et al. Percutaneous angioplasty of stenosed gastroepiploic artery grafts. *J Am Coll Cardiol* 1993;22:727.

176. Hearne SE, Wilson JS, Harrington J, et al. Angiographic and clinical follow-up after internal mammary artery graft angioplasty: a 9-year experience. *J Am Coll Cardiol* 1995;25[Suppl A]:139A.

177. Ishizaka N, Ishizaka Y, Ikari Y, et al. Initial and subsequent angiographic outcome of percutaneous transluminal angioplasty performed on internal mammary artery grafts. *Br Heart J* 1995;74:615–619.

178. Nishida T, Colombo A, Briguori C, et al. Contemporary percutaneous treatment of saphenous vein graft stenosis: immediate and late outcomes. *J Invas Cardiol* 2000;12:505–512.

179. Douglas JS Jr. Percutaneous strategies for the management of angina pectoris after bypass surgery. In: Ventrovec GW, Carabello BA, eds. *Invasive cardiology: current diagnostic and therapeutic issues.* Armonk, NY: Futura Publishing, 1996:489.

180. Lehmann KG, Maas AC, Van Domberg R, et al. Repeat interventions as a long-term treatment strategy in the management of progressive coronary artery disease. *J Am Coll Cardiol* 1996;27:1398–1405.

VALVULOPLASTY

ALEC SYLVAIN VAHANIAN

▼ ADDITIONAL ELECTRONIC TOPICS
Percutaneous Aortic Valvuloplasty: Mechanisms o36

OVERVIEW

Fifteen years of experience with percutaneous valve dilatation for acquired valve stenoses have shown the following:

- Percutaneous mitral valvuloplasty is an effective treatment in a wide range of patients with mitral stenosis. Its risk is low when it is performed by experienced teams, and follow-up at more than 10 years demonstrates excellent durability of the procedure. The prediction of immediate and midterm results is multifactorial and based on clinical and anatomic variables.
- Percutaneous aortic valvuloplasty for degenerative calcified aortic stenosis provides short-term palliation of symptoms at the cost of high periprocedural risk. Its role is in question.
- Percutaneous tricuspid or multivalve dilatation is used in exceptional cases.
- Percutaneous dilatation of a bioprosthesis has no future.

A. S. Vahanian: Department of Cardiology, Bichat Hospital, Paris, France

HISTORICAL PERSPECTIVE

Until the early 1980s, surgery was the only possible treatment for severe valvular stenoses; thereafter a new alternative appeared: percutaneous balloon valvuloplasty.

The first to perform balloon valvuloplasty as an alternative to surgery in the treatment of mitral stenosis was K. Inoue in 1982 during open-heart surgery. The initial report of percutaneous balloon valvuloplasty was published in 1984 (1); most subsequent reports concerning the technique have been published since 1986. As was to be expected from earlier experience with closed surgical commissurotomy, the good immediate and midterm results obtained during this period led to increasing worldwide use of the technique, which became the second most important in the field of interventional cardiology.

In the field of aortic stenosis, percutaneous valvuloplasty was used for the first time by Cribier et al. in 1985 in an elderly patient with severe calcific aortic stenosis (2). Despite great initial enthusiasm related to encouraging preliminary immediate reports, the technique has largely lost favor because of the lack of midterm benefit, and today it has a very limited role, if any.

Percutaneous balloon valvuloplasty is therefore still a recent innovation that, despite marked changes in practice during the first decade of its use, will continue to be refined and subjected to long-term surveillance.

This chapter deals with percutaneous balloon valvuloplasty for acquired valvular stenoses in the fields of mitral stenosis, aortic stenosis, and the less frequent lesions of tricuspid, bioprosthesis, and multivalve stenoses.

PERCUTANEOUS MITRAL VALVULOPLASTY

Rheumatic fever continues to be endemic in developing countries where mitral stenosis is the most common valve disease. Although the prevalence of rheumatic heart disease has greatly decreased in Western countries, it continues to represent an important clinical entity because of out-migration from developing countries and the presence of restenosis after previous surgical commissurotomy (3).

Mechanisms

Balloon dilatation acts in the same way as surgical commissurotomy by opening the fused commissures (4); therefore, a more appropriate term for the procedure is probably *percutaneous mitral commissurotomy* rather than *percutaneous mitral valvuloplasty*. Balloons are also able to enlarge the valve area by fracturing nodular deposits in patients with calcified valves (5).

Technique

The techniques and devices used have varied over time and from group to group.

Approaches

At the present time, two approaches are used: transarterial and transvenous.

The *transvenous* or *antegrade approach* is the most widely used. Transseptal catheterization, which allows access to the left atrium, is the first step in the procedure and one of the most crucial. It is performed through the femoral vein or, in exceptional circumstances, through the jugular vein (6).

The *retrograde approach* using transseptal catheterization, described by Babic, has now been abandoned. In the retrograde technique without transseptal catheterization (*e*Fig. 86.0.1) described by Stefanadis (7), the balloon is introduced through the femoral artery or, less frequently, the brachial artery. [▼ o37] Knowledge of this approach does provide an alternative in the rare cases in which use of the transseptal approach is contraindicated.

Devices

Currently, two main techniques are used: balloon commissurotomy [▼ o38] and metallic commissurotomy.

Balloons

The Inoue technique (Fig. 86.1) was the first to be developed (1,12–14). The Inoue balloon, made of nylon and rubber micromesh, is self-positioning and pressure extensible. Because the balloon has three distinct parts, each with a specific elasticity, each part can be inflated sequentially. This sequence allows fast and stable positioning across the valve. The Inoue balloon comes in four sizes (24, 26, 28, and 30 mm), and each is pressure dependent, so that its diameter can be varied by up to 4 mm as required by circumstances. ▼ o39

Metallic Dilator

In the late 1990s, Cribier introduced the metallic commissurotomy (Fig. 86.2), which uses a device similar to the Tubb dilator used during closed commissurotomy (20). [▼ o40] The potential advantage of the metallic commissurotomy is that the dilator is reusable, which reduces the cost of the procedure.

Monitoring of the Procedure and Assessment of Immediate Results

Two means are used to assess immediate results in the catheterization laboratory: hemodynamics and echocardiography. Although echocardiography may be difficult to perform in the catheterization laboratory for logistic reasons, it provides essential information. ▼ o41

The following criteria have been proposed for the desired end point of the procedure: (a) mitral valve area greater than 1 cm^2 per square meter of body surface area, (b) complete opening of at least one commissure, or (c) appearance or increment of regurgitation greater than 1 in the Sellers 0 to 4 classification. ▼ o42

The strong predictive value of the quality of the immediate results for long-term outcome stresses the importance of a careful evaluation of the immediate results. After the procedure, the most accurate evaluation of valve area is provided by echocardiography (26). ▼ o43

Immediate Results

The technique of mitral valvuloplasty has now been evaluated in several thousand patients with different clinical conditions and valve anatomy (7,10–12,14,21,28–33).

Hemodynamics

The results shown in Table 86.1 demonstrate the efficacy of mitral valvuloplasty, which usually provides an increase of over 100% in valve area.

The improvement in valve function results in an immediate decrease in left atrial pressure and a slight increase in cardiac index. A gradual decrease in pulmonary arterial pressure and pulmonary vascular resistances is seen. High

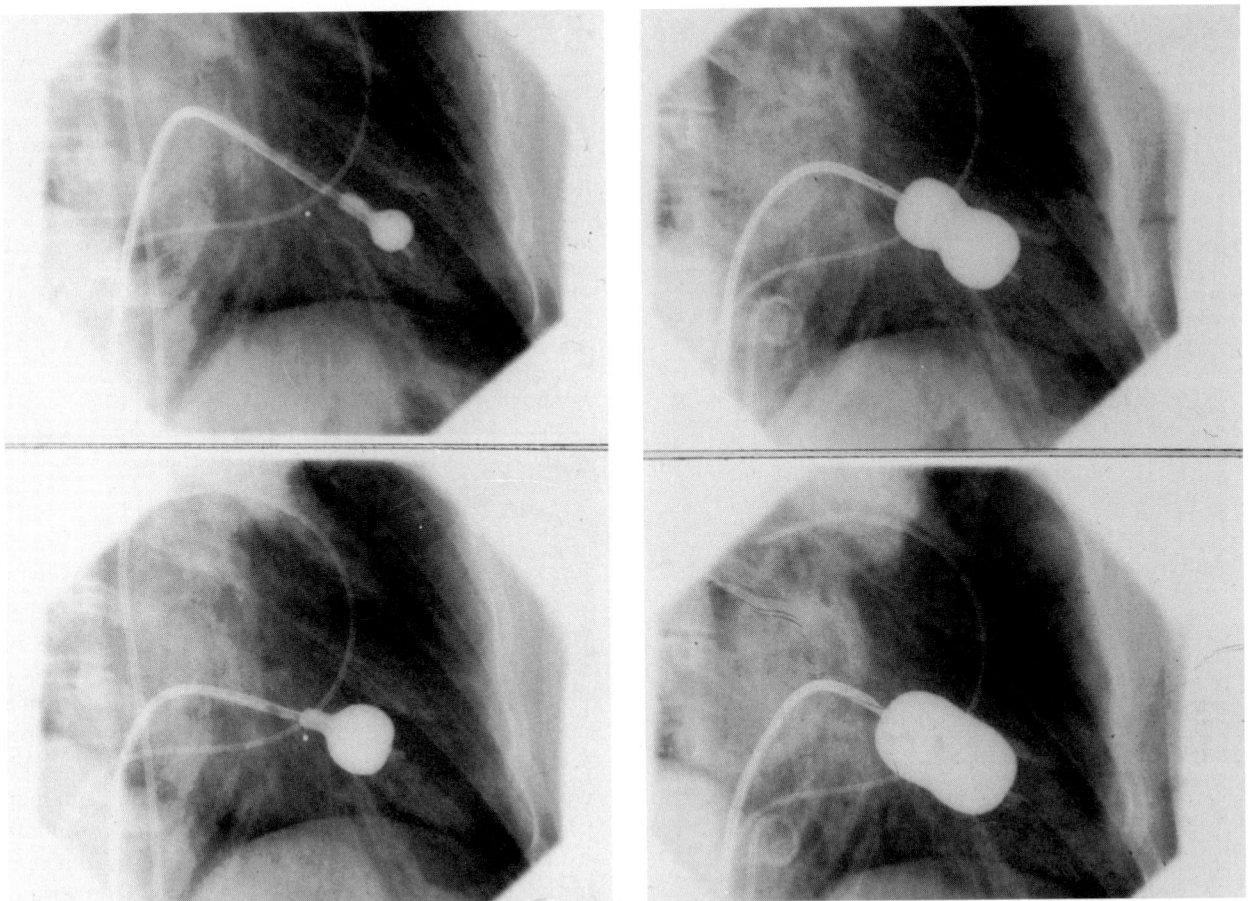

A   B

FIGURE 86.1 Mitral valvuloplasty: Inoue technique. **A:** Inflation of the distal portion of the balloon, which is thereafter pulled back and anchored at the mitral valve. **B:** Subsequent inflation of the proximal and middle portions of the balloon. At full inflation, the waist of the balloon in its midportion has disappeared.

pulmonary vascular resistances continue to decrease over the first 24 hours after the procedure and decrease further later in the absence of restenosis (34). ⚡ o44

Failures

The failure rates range from 1% to 17% (7,14,21,28–33). Most failures occurred in the early part of the investigators' experience. Others were due to unfavorable anatomy, such as severe left atrial enlargement or cardiothoracic deformity.

Risks

Procedural mortality ranges from 0% to 3% in most series (18,28–33,43) (Table 86.2). The main causes of death are left ventricular perforation or the poor general condition of the patient. The incidence of hemopericardium varies from 0.5% to 12%. Pericardial hemorrhage may be related to transseptal catheterization or to apex perforation by the guidewires or the balloon itself when exaggerated movement occurs. Embolism is encountered in 0.5% to 5% of

cases. It is rarely the cause of permanent incapacitation and even more rarely of death. Embolism may be cerebral or coronary in location, and it may be due to fibrinothrombotic material from a thrombus that was preexistent or developed during the procedure (44), less frequently to gas, and very seldom to calcium. In most cases, the degree of mitral regurgitation remains stable or increases slightly after valvuloplasty. In a few cases, however, the degree of mitral regurgitation may decrease. Severe mitral regurgitation is rare; its frequency ranges from 2% to 19% (45–49). Surgical findings (46–48) have shown that it is related to noncommissural leaflet tearing, which is often associated with chordal rupture. In these cases, one or both commissures are often too tightly fused to be split. Severe mitral regurgitation may also be due to excessive commissural splitting or, in very rare cases, rupture of a papillary muscle. In the majority of cases, severe mitral regurgitation occurred in patients with unfavorable anatomy. The suggestion has been made that the development of severe mitral regurgitation after percutaneous mitral commissurotomy depends more on the distribution of morphologic changes than on

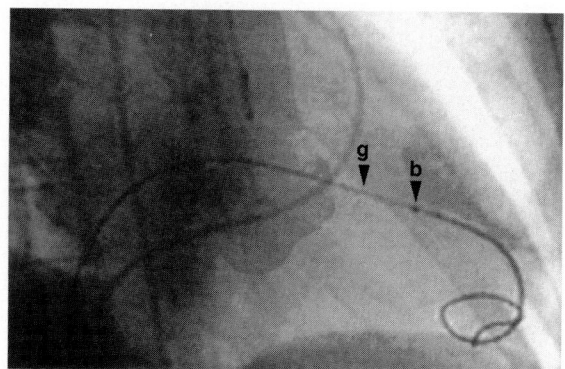

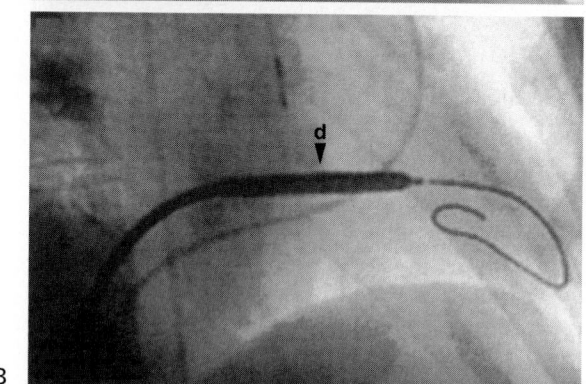

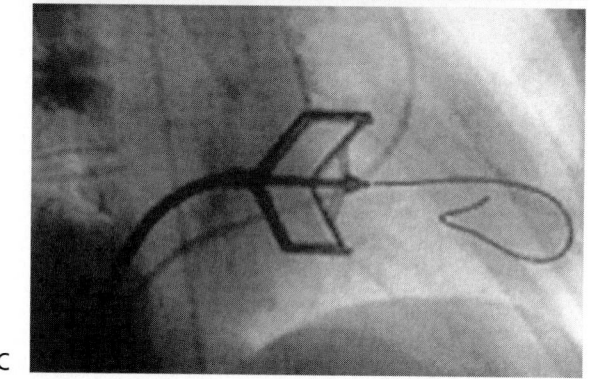

FIGURE 86.2 Percutaneous metallic commissurotomy. **A:** Guidewire (g) is placed in left ventricle after transseptal catheterization. Metallic bead (b) is positioned at midventricle, beyond mitral valve. **B:** After dilation of septal puncture site, device is pushed over guidewire and metallic dilator (d) is positioned across mitral valve. Metallic bead is placed in contact with distal end of dilator. **C:** Commissurotomy is performed by opening dilator to its maximum extent of 40 mm. (Adapted from Cribier A, Eltchaninoff H, Koning R, et al. Percutaneous mechanical mitral commissurotomy with a newly designed metallic valvotome: immediate results of the initial experience in 153 patients. *Circulation* 1999;99:793–799.)

their severity (5,49). Severe mitral regurgitation may be well tolerated, but more often it is not, and surgery on a scheduled basis is necessary. In most cases, valve replacement is required because of the severity of the underlying valve disease. Conservative surgery has been successfully performed in cases of less severe valve deformity (47). The frequency of atrial septal defect reported after valvuloplasty varies from 10% to 90% depending on the technique used

TABLE 86.1   VALVE AREA AFTER PERCUTANEOUS MITRAL VALVULOPLASTY (PMV)

Study	Number	Valve area (cm²)	
		Before PMV	After PMV
Tuzcu et al. (10)	311	0.9	2
Ben Farhat et al. (29)	463	1	2.1
Arora et al. (30)	600	0.75	2.2
Chen and Cheng (31)	4,832	1.1	2.1
NHLBI (32)	738	1	2
Iung et al. (33)	1,514	1.1	2
Stefanadis et al. (7)	893	1	2.1
Cribier et al. (21)	882	0.9	2.1
Bonhoeffer et al. (11)	153	0.7	2

NHLBI, National Heart, Lung, and Blood Institute.

for its detection (50,51). These shunts are usually small. Right to left shunts can occur on rare occasions in patients with elevated right heart pressures and pulmonary hypertension (52). The incidence of transient, complete heart block is 1.5%, and it seldom requires implantation of a permanent pacemaker (53). After the transvenous approach, vascular complications are the exception. Finally, endocarditis is extremely rare (54). Although urgent surgery (within 24 hours) is seldom needed for complications, it may be required for massive hemopericardium resulting from left ventricular perforation intractable to treatment by pericardiocentesis or, less frequently, for severe mitral regurgitation leading to hemodynamic collapse or refractory pulmonary edema (47).

Predictors of Immediate Results

The results from multicenter studies (21,31,55) and large single-center studies (29,30,33), which include a wide population of patients with varied characteristics, enable us to identify predictors of the results to be identified and the strength of these predictors to be evaluated.

Evaluation of the immediate results is based mainly on anatomic criteria. The definition of good immediate results varies from series to series. The two definitions usually used are a final valve area larger than 1.5 cm² and an increase in valve area of at least 25%, or a final valve area larger than 1.5 cm² without mitral regurgitation greater than 2/4.

Valve anatomy was initially considered (56,57) to be the main predictor of the results, but later it appeared to be only a relative predictor (33,55,58,59). In fact, prediction of results is multifactorial (33,57). Several studies have shown that, in addition to morphologic factors, preoperative variables such as age, history of surgical commissurotomy, functional class, small mitral valve area, presence of mitral regurgitation before valvuloplasty, atrial fibrillation, high pulmonary artery pressure, and presence of severe tricuspid regurgitation, as well as procedural factors such as

TABLE 86.2 MAJOR COMPLICATIONS OF MITRAL VALVULOPLASTY

Study	Number	Mortality (%)	Hemopericardium (%)	Embolism (%)	Severe mitral regurgitation (%)
Tuzcu et al. (10)	311	1.7	—	—	8.7 (>2+ increase)
Ben Farhat et al. (29)	463	0.4	0.7	2	4.6
Arora et al. (30)	600	1	1.3	0.5	1
Chen and Cheng (31)	4,832	0.12	0.8	0.5	1.4
NHLBI (32)	738	3	4	3	3
Iung et al. (33)	1,514	0.4	0.3	0.3	3.4
Stefanadis et al. (7)	893	0.3	0	0	3.1
Cribier et al. (21)	882	NA	1.4	NA	2.1

NA, not available; NHLBI, National Heart, Lung, and Blood Institute.

balloon type and size, are all independent predictors of the immediate results. ♥ o45

Long-Term Results

Data from follow-up at more than 10 years can now be analyzed. In clinical terms, which are the most widely used, the overall long-term results of valvuloplasty are good in a large population of patients comprising a variety of patient subsets (61–70) (Table 86.3). As shown for surgical commissurotomy (71–73), late outcome after valvuloplasty differs according to the quality of the immediate results (Fig. 86.3).

When the immediate results are unsatisfactory, patients experience only transient or no functional improvement. In these cases, late symptomatic deterioration may be related to lasting poor initial results. In cases of severe mitral regurgitation, the prognosis after surgical commissurotomy or balloon valvuloplasty is usually poor, with lack of improvement in symptoms and secondary objective deterioration; surgical treatment is usually undertaken during the following months. In cases of insufficient initial opening, delayed surgery is usually performed when the extracardiac conditions allow. Here, valve replacement is necessary in almost all cases because of the unfavorable valve anatomy responsible for the initial poor results. In some patients, however, moderate initial improvement in valve function provides functional improvement for several years, although such patients must be carefully followed to allow for a timely operation.

Conversely, if valvuloplasty is initially successful, then survival rates are excellent, functional improvement occurs in the majority of cases, and the need for secondary surgery is infrequent (69). When clinical deterioration occurs in these patients, it is late and mainly related to mitral restenosis.

Determining the incidence of restenosis by echocardiography is compromised by the absence of a uniform definition. It has generally been defined as a loss of more than 50% of the initial gain with a valve area less than 1.5 cm². After a successful procedure, the incidence of echographically identified restenosis is usually low, ranging from 2% to 40% at time intervals of 3 to 5 years (29,31,68,69,74,75). The possibility of repeating valvuloplasty in cases of recurrent mitral stenosis is one of the potentials of this nonsurgical procedure. Repeated valvuloplasty can be proposed if recurrent stenosis leads to symptoms, if it occurs several years after an initially successful procedure, and if the predominant mechanism of restenosis is commissural refusion. ♥ o46

Predictors of Long-Term Results

Prediction of long-term results is also multifactorial (62–69,78,79) and is based on clinical variables such as age; valve anatomy as assessed by different echocardiography scores [one study has shown the negative prognostic value of the presence of commissural calcification (80)]; factors related to the evolutional stage of the disease, that is, a higher New York Heart Association class before valvuloplasty; history of

TABLE 86.3 FOLLOW-UP AFTER MITRAL VALVULOPLASTY

Study	Number	Mean age (yr)	Length of follow-up (yr)	Survival (%)	Freedom from operation (%)	NYHA class I/II (%)
Stefanadis et al. (7)	441	44	9	—	—	75
Meneveau et al. (67)	532	54	7.5	83	—	52
Hernandez et al. (68)	561	53	7	95	84	69
Iung et al. (69)	1,024	49	10	85	61	56
Orrange et al. (65)	132	44	7	95	65	—

NYHA, New York Heart Association.

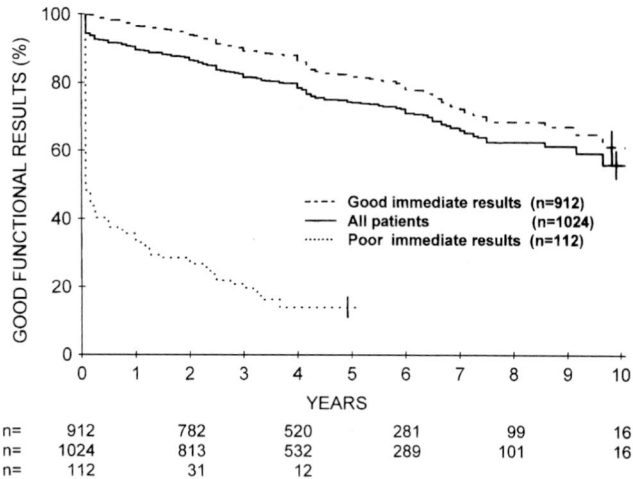

FIGURE 86.3 Long-term results of mitral valvuloplasty. "Good functional results" refers to survival considering cardiovascular-related deaths with no need for mitral surgery or repeat dilatation and in New York Heart Association functional class I or II. (Adapted from Iung B, Garbarz E, Michaud P, et al. Late results of percutaneous mitral commissurotomy in a series of 1024 patients: analysis of late clinical deterioration: frequency, anatomic findings, and predictive factors. *Circulation* 1999;99:3272–3278.)

previous commissurotomy; severe tricuspid regurgitation; cardiomegaly; atrial fibrillation; high pulmonary vascular resistances; and the results of the procedure, that is, final valve area, final gradient, and degree of regurgitation. The quality of the late results is generally considered as independent of the technique used (69). 🐦 o47

Despite interpatient variability, the degree of mitral regurgitation generally remains stable or slightly decreases during follow-up (46,48,51). Atrial septal defects are likely to close over time in the majority of cases because of reduction in the interatrial pressure gradient. The persistence of shunts is related to their magnitude or to unsatisfactory relief of the valve obstruction (81). Finally, clinical series of surgical and balloon commissurotomy suggest that intervention reduces the risk of embolism even if it does not eliminate it (69,82).

Indications

The decision to perform valvuloplasty must be based on both clinical and anatomic variables.

Clinical Variables

Clinical evaluation of patients concentrates mainly on functional disability and the alternative risk with surgery.

For symptomatic patients, the indication for valvuloplasty is perfectly clear. Truly asymptomatic patients, however, are not usually candidates for the procedure because of the small but definite risk inherent in the technique. For patients in the latter group, balloon commissurotomy may

be considered in the following cases: patients at high risk of thromboembolism, for example, patients with a previous history of embolism or with heavy spontaneous contrast in the left atrium; and patients with recurrent atrial arrhythmias. Pulmonary hypertension is an adverse prognostic indicator, and patients with pulmonary hypertension are likely to become symptomatic in the near future. Guidelines recommend balloon valvuloplasty for patients with systolic pulmonary pressures higher than 50 mm Hg at rest or 60 mm Hg on exercise (83). Finally, balloon valvuloplasty can be considered for patients requiring major extracardiac surgery or to allow for pregnancy.

Valvuloplasty is the only solution when surgery is contraindicated. It is also preferable to surgery, at least as a first attempt, in patients with an increased risk for surgery of cardiac origin, as in patients with restenosis after surgical commissurotomy. Available data show that the results of the procedure are good in such cases, even if slightly less satisfactory than those obtained in patients without previous surgery (33,84–86). This suggests that valvuloplasty may well postpone reoperation in selected patients, provided anatomy is still suitable and restenosis is due mainly to commissural refusion. The same reasoning applies in cases of patients who have undergone aortic valve replacement. Preliminary reports have suggested that valvuloplasty can be performed safely and effectively in patients with pulmonary hypertension (87). In cases of coexistence of mitral stenosis and moderate aortic valve disease (88), balloon valvuloplasty can be performed as a means of postponing the inevitable later surgical treatment of both valves.

In Western countries, many patients with mitral stenosis have concomitant noncardiac disease, which may also increase the risk of surgery. Valvuloplasty can be performed as a lifesaving procedure in critically ill patients (89–91)—as the sole treatment in case of absolute contraindication to surgery or as a bridge to surgery in the other cases. In elderly patients, valvuloplasty results in moderate but significant improvement in valve function at an acceptable risk, although subsequent functional deterioration is frequent (92–94). In such cases valvuloplasty may be an effective treatment in patients with favorable characteristics. It is also a useful palliative procedure for those who are unsuitable for surgery. In pregnant patients the procedure is efficacious in terms of improving the mother's hemodynamic status; it is also well tolerated by the fetus if performed after the twentieth week. Due to the ever-present risk of complication, use of valvuloplasty should be limited to patients who remain symptomatic despite appropriate other treatment (95–97).

Anatomic Aspects

The assessment of anatomy has several aims with respect to establishing indications and prognostic considerations. Assuring that no anatomic contraindications exist to use of the technique is very critical (Table 86.4). 🐦 o48

TABLE 86.4 CONTRAINDICATIONS FOR MITRAL VALVULOPLASTY

Left atrial thrombosis
Mitral regurgitation greater than 2/4
Massive or bicommissural calcification
Severe aortic valve disease, or severe tricuspid stenosis + regurgitation associated with mitral stenosis
Severe concomitant coronary artery disease requiring bypass surgery

For prognostic purposes, echocardiographic assessment allows the classification of patients into anatomic groups with a view to predicting the results. Most investigators use the Wilkins score (Table 86.5) for categorization, whereas others, such as our group, use a more general assessment of valve anatomy (Table 86.6). [✍ o49] More recently, scores that take into account the uneven distribution of the anatomic deformities of the leaflets or the commissural area have been developed (49,99). Preliminary results for their use are promising (100,101) but disputed (102); therefore, further studies are needed to determine their exact value (*e*Table 86.6.1).

Thus, even if it is not the sole criterion, anatomy is a simple and practical way of selecting patients for valvuloplasty. In patients with good anatomy—that is, pliable

TABLE 86.5 ANATOMIC CLASSIFICATION OF THE MITRAL VALVE (MASSACHUSETTS GENERAL HOSPITAL, BOSTON): ECHOCARDIOGRAPHIC EXAMINATION

Leaflet mobility
1. Valve is highly mobile, with restriction of only the leaflet tips.
2. Midportion and base of leaflets have reduced mobility.
3. Valve leaflets move forward in diastole mainly at the base.
4. No or minimal forward movement of the leaflets occurs in diastole.

Valvular thickening
1. Leaflets near normal (4–5 mm).
2. Midleaflet thickening, marked thickening of the margins.
3. Thickening extending through the entire leaflets (5–8 mm).
4. Marked thickening of all leaflet tissue (>8–10 mm).

Subvalvular thickening
1. Minimal thickening of chordal structures just below the valve.
2. Thickening of chordae extending up to one-third of chordal length.
3. Thickening extending to the distal third of the chordae.
4. Extensive thickening and shortening of all chordae extending down to the papillary muscle.

Valvular calcification
1. A single area of increased echo brightness.
2. Scattered areas of brightness confined to leaflet margins.
3. Brightness extending into the midportion of leaflets.
4. Extensive brightness through most of the leaflet tissue.

Note: The final score is found by adding the scores for each of the components.
From Wilkins GT, Gillam LD, Weyman AE, et al. Percutaneous balloon dilatation of the mitral valve: an analysis of echocardiographic variables related to outcome and the mechanism of dilatation. *Br Heart J* 1988;60:299–308.

TABLE 86.6 ANATOMIC CLASSIFICATION OF THE MITRAL VALVE

Echocardiographic group	Mitral valve anatomy
Group 1	Pliable noncalcified anterior mitral leaflet and mild subvalvular disease (i.e., thin chordae ≥10 mm long)
Group 2	Pliable noncalcified anterior mitral leaflet and severe subvalvular disease (i.e., thickened chordae <10 mm long)
Group 3	Calcification of mitral valve of any extent, as assessed by fluoroscopy, any condition of subvalvular apparatus

From Iung B, Cormier B, Ducimetiere P, et al. Immediate results of percutaneous mitral commissurotomy. *Circulation* 1996;94:2124–2130.

valves and moderate subvalvular disease (echocardiographic score of 8 or less)—results of valvuloplasty are generally excellent. Results of several randomized studies with follow-up comparing valvuloplasty and surgical commissurotomy are available (103–105). They show that valvuloplasty is at least comparable to surgical commissurotomy as regards immediate and long-term results and is no doubt more comfortable for the patient. Valvuloplasty would thus appear to be the procedure of choice for these patients, provided that it is affordable. In addition, if restenosis occurs, patients treated by valvuloplasty could undergo repeat balloon procedures or surgery without the difficulties and inherent risk resulting from pericardial adhesions and chest wall scarring (*e*Table 86.6.2).

On the other hand, much remains to be done in refining the indications for valvuloplasty in other patients, especially those with unfavorable anatomy (106–109), who are more common in Western countries. For this group, some favor immediate surgery because of the less satisfying results of valvuloplasty, whereas others prefer valvuloplasty as an initial treatment for selected candidates and reserve surgery for cases in which this treatment fails.

PERCUTANEOUS AORTIC VALVULOPLASTY

As reviewed in Chapter 22, Aortic Valve Disease, severe degenerative calcified aortic stenosis is the most frequent valve disease in Western countries, which accounts for the initial interest in its potential treatment by interventional cardiology.

Technique

Approaches

The femoral retrograde approach is most frequently used (115,116). After placement of an introducer sheath, the aortic valve is crossed (*e*Fig. 86.3.1); this represents the most difficult technical part of the procedure. Then, a stiff wire is inserted into the apex of the left ventricle to stabilize the balloon during inflation (115–117).

The alternative is the anterograde approach, which necessitates a transseptal catheterization. This latter technique is a difficult procedure but constitutes a recourse in case of inaccessibility of the femoral approach (117).

Balloons

Valvuloplasty is performed with balloons from 15 mm to 25 mm in diameter, from 3 cm to 5 cm in length, and of variable form: conventional, bifoil, trefoil, or, more recently, double size, which has the advantage of a low profile. ▼ o50

Monitoring of the Procedure and Assessment of Immediate Results

Methods for evaluating immediate results during the procedure include the monitoring of the transaortic gradient and cardiac output, which enables repeated calculation of the valve area. Nevertheless, because of the hemodynamic instability of the patient during the procedure and very early loss in valve area after the procedure, the most viable method is measurement of the valve area by Doppler echocardiography in the days after the procedure (118). Aortography before and after the procedure evaluates any change in the degree of aortic incompetence.

Immediate Results

The technique has been used in several hundred patients, and the results from single-center (115–117) and multicenter registries (119) can be evaluated. The series reported concern essentially aortic stenosis in older subjects. Any analysis of the results must take into account the severity of the cardiac disease and comorbidities found in such an aged population.

Hemodynamics

Immediately after the procedure the transvalvular pressure gradient is reduced; cardiac output is little modified. Over-all, percutaneous aortic valvuloplasty (PAV) reduces tight stenosis to moderate stenosis with a final area between 0.7 and 1.1 cm^2 (115–118,120,121). These results are clearly inferior to those obtained with a valvular prosthesis, which usually provides a valve area over 1.5 cm^2 (*e*Table 86.6.3).

Risks

Mortality and morbidity of the procedure are high (115–117,119–124) (Table 86.7). Hospital mortality varies from 3.5% to 13.5%, and 20% to 25% of the patients have at least one serious complication within the first 24 hours. The most frequent complications are vascular complications at the puncture site, which necessitate an intervention in nearly half of the cases. Ventricular perforations are responsible for tamponade. Acute aortic incompetence is rare. Embolic complications are also rare. Two complications are exceptional but can be fatal: mitral regurgitation and the rupture of the aortic ring.

Predictors of Immediate Results

The immediate outcome is linked to the clinical status of the patient (age, New York Heart Association class, and presence of congestive heart failure) or to procedural complications. Depressed left ventricular function, low cardiac output, and the existence of diffuse coronary lesions are all important covariates associated with worse outcome (115,120,124). Finally, a final valve area smaller than 0.7 cm^2 carries a negative prognosis (124).

Long-Term Results

Despite a relatively modest improvement in valve function, a degree of functional improvement is commonly noted during the first weeks or months. This is of short duration, however. PAV seems to improve survival rates at 1 year and especially improves the quality of life. The benefit decreases, however, and finally disappears after 2 years (115,124–128) (Table 86.8). In selected patients, an aortic valve replacement has been subsequently performed with good results (129); on the other hand, the prognosis of the

TABLE 86.7 IMMEDIATE COMPLICATIONS OF AORTIC VALVULOPLASTY

	NHBLI (119) (n = 674)	Mansfield registry (121) (n = 492)	Cribier et al. (115) (n = 363)	Safian et al. (120) (n = 170)
Hospital mortality (%)	10	7.5	4	3.5
Tamponade (%)	1.5	1.8	1	1.8
Severe aortic regurgitation (%)	1	1	0	1.2
Stroke (%)	3	2.2	1.4	0
Myocardial infarction (%)	2	0.2	0.3	0.6
Vascular events[a] (%)	7	5.5	5	10

NHLBI, National Heart, Lung, and Blood Institute.
[a]Vascular events requiring surgical treatment.

TABLE 86.8 RESULTS OF CLINICAL FOLLOW-UP AFTER AORTIC VALVULOPLASTY

Study	n	Survival (%)				Survival without reintervention (%)			
		1 yr	2 yr	3 yr	5 yr	1 yr	2 yr	3 yr	5 yr
Lieberman et al. (127)	165	60	48	35	—	40	19	6	—
Otto et al. (128)	674	55	35	23	—	—	—	—	—
Bernard et al. (136)	46	75	47	—	33	70	25	—	7

other patients is particularly poor (129–131) (Fig. 86.4). Overall, the opinion is now that PAV alone does not change the natural course of the disease (132). These poor long-term results are mainly due to the clinical status of the patients and to the moderate and transient improvement in valve function obtained by PAV.

Indications

In practice, [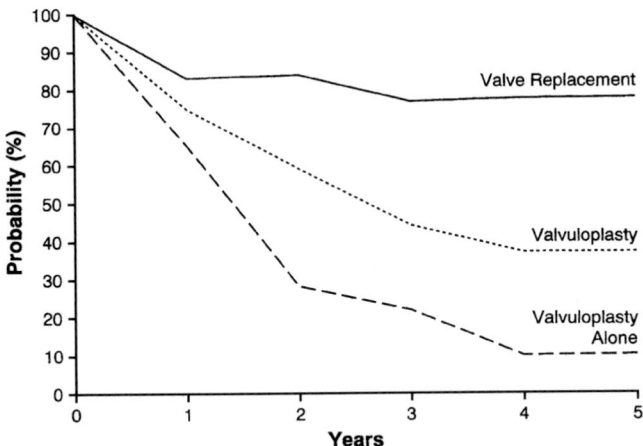 o51] aortic valve replacement is the treatment of choice for symptomatic patients with tight aortic stenosis. Valvuloplasty can be considered only in the following circumstances:

- For critically ill patients with cardiogenic shock with multivisceral failure. Good midterm results have been obtained in limited series if surgical intervention was possible secondarily (137). For this group of patients, valvuloplasty can be considered a bridge to surgery, permitting the secondary operation with less risk.
- For patients with severe, poorly tolerated aortic stenosis who require significant emergency noncardiac surgery.
- For patients who have an absolute, but not life-threatening, short-term contraindication to surgery and have a significant functional disability.
- For patients who refuse surgery.

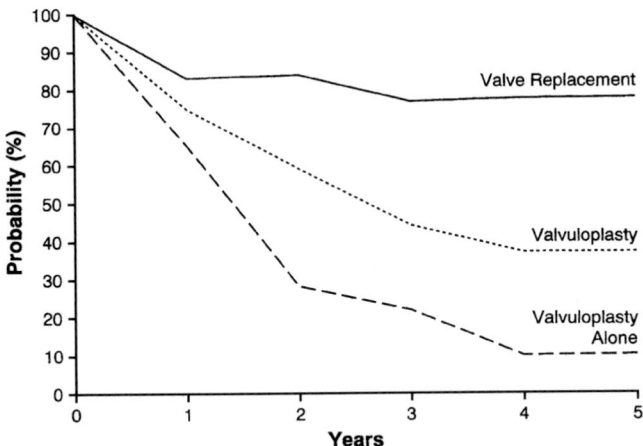

FIGURE 86.4 Long-term survival rate after aortic valve replacement or balloon valvuloplasty. (From Bernard Y, Etievent J, Mourand JL, et al. Long-term results of percutaneous aortic valvuloplasty compared with aortic replacement in patients older than 75 years. *J Am Coll Cardiol* 1992;20:796–801.)

OTHER PERCUTANEOUS VALVE DILATATIONS

Unlike percutaneous valvuloplasty for mitral and aortic stenosis, other applications of percutaneous valve dilatation have been used only sparingly. The few interventions performed show that the procedures are feasible, but the cases are insufficient in number to allow evaluation of results and establishment of indications.

Percutaneous Tricuspid Valvuloplasty

The indications of tricuspid valvuloplasty are rare. The procedure is reserved for symptomatic patients presenting with tight tricuspid stenosis, pure or associated with mild regurgitation (138–140). In all other cases in which the tricuspid stenosis is accompanied by significant or moderate regurgitation, or is associated with another valvular disease necessitating surgical treatment, the treatment must be surgery.

Percutaneous Dilatation of Bioprostheses

Anatomic findings and experimental dilatations lead one to conclude that dilatations of bioprostheses do not produce good results (141–146). They may give rise to severe immediate complications at the level of the left heart (145) and give poor midterm results in the tricuspid position. Percutaneous dilatation may in certain rare cases be performed as a palliative treatment for stenotic degeneration of a bioprosthesis in the tricuspid position (146–148).

Multiple Dilatations

Actual experience allows one to say only that multiple dilatations are technically feasible in selected patients (149–151). One application that might be imagined in the field of rheumatic pathology is in cases of contraindication to surgery or high surgical risk, such as during pregnancy.

Percutaneous Valve Dilatation and Coronary Angioplasty

Because of the aging of the population in Western countries, the association of calcified aortic stenosis and coronary pathology is frequently encountered; however, the association of a tight mitral stenosis and obstructive coronary lesions is observed much less frequently. Few cases of percutaneous valve dilatations for calcified aortic stenosis and coronary angioplasty in either one or two sessions have been reported (152). In addition, a single case was reported in which dilation for mitral stenosis and coronary angioplasty with stent placement was performed with success (153). The rarity of the indications for aortic dilatation suggests that such a combined procedure has little practical application.

CONTROVERSIES AND PERSONAL PERSPECTIVES

Mitral valvuloplasty is the valvuloplasty technique used most frequently, if not exclusively (154). Because of the good results that have been obtained with mitral valvuloplasty, currently this technique has an important place in the treatment of mitral stenosis. The main objects of controversy and the main questions still to be solved concern economic aspects, the technique itself, and the respective indications for treatment by balloon valvuloplasty or surgery.

Further developments of the technique depend on the possibilities for application in countries where mitral stenosis is endemic and where means are lacking. In such countries, limitations in finances restrict the use of the Inoue balloon or leads to its reuse, with the attendant risks. With this in mind, the price of the devices must be reduced by making them reusable, as with the metallic commissurotome, or by simplifying them, as with the Multi-Track system.

Regarding the choice of technique, the Inoue technique has become the most popular in the world and has been used in more than 30,000 patients with good and reproducible results. The experience with the metallic commissurotome is only preliminary and almost exclusively reported by the promoter of the method. Comparison of the respective merits of this new technique and the Inoue technique requires accumulation of further data concerning the metallic commissurotome and randomized comparisons of the two techniques. In the author's opinion, the efficacy, safety, and applicability of the Inoue technique are clearly established, whereas those of the metallic commissurotome are yet to be fully proven. This new device is unlikely to replace the Inoue balloon in Western countries because safety is probably decreased and the technique is more demanding. On the other hand, a potential exists for the application of the metallic commissurotome in developing countries.

The considerable simplification resulting from use of the Inoue balloon could lead to a false sense of security in the application of the technique and should not overshadow the importance of training. In the author's opinion, performance of percutaneous valvuloplasty should be restricted to groups whose experience with transseptal catheterization has been positive and who have been able to carry out an adequate number of procedures and thus improve their technical performance and ability to select patients. This recommendation carries even more weight in Western countries, where mitral stenosis is infrequent. In particular, valvuloplasty should be performed only in centers with sufficient experience, in cases where patients have minimal symptoms, during pregnancy, or in cases of cardiothoracic deformity. The decision to perform valvuloplasty also depends on the results of surgery at the institution concerned. The potential for valve repair in case of traumatic regurgitation is an important incentive in favor of performing valvuloplasty at an earlier stage of the disease.

The debate on how best to perform the technique must not overshadow other, probably more important matters such as the selection of candidates. Regarding indications, no problems are presented in cases in which surgery is contraindicated or for "ideal candidates," such as young adults (155) with favorable characteristics. On the other hand, much remains to be done in refining the indications for other patients, especially those with minimal symptoms and those with unfavorable anatomy (156).

The level of evidence for performing valvuloplasty in asymptomatic patients is low because no data exist comparing the results of valvuloplasty and medical therapy for such patients. For these patients, the goal is not to prolong life or to decrease symptoms but rather to prevent thromboembolism. The efficacy of valvuloplasty for the specific problem of embolism is not established, but the different findings previously mentioned consistently show the beneficial effect of valvuloplasty on the causes of thromboembolism: intensity of left atrial echocardiographic contrast, size of the atrium, left atrial function, and coagulation activity in the left atrium. No direct evidence exists that valvuloplasty reduces the incidence of atrial fibrillation, even if its favorable influence on predictors of atrial fibrillation, such as atrial size or degree of obstruction, seems to indicate that this is indeed the case. In such patients, valvuloplasty should be performed only by experienced interventionists and when valve anatomy is favorable, in which case a safe and successful procedure can be expected.

Among patients with less favorable valve anatomy (echocardiographic score higher than 8) as a result of extensive subvalvular disease or mild valve calcification, the comparison between the results of valvuloplasty and of surgery is much more difficult. Unfortunately, no randomized study has been performed examining this issue, and comparison of the results of balloon commissurotomy with those of surgical series is difficult due to differences in the patient populations and the fact that the surgical alternative can include surgical commissurotomy, in practice seldom, and also valve replacement in most cases. Valve replacement has its drawbacks: namely, operative mortality, particularly in the elderly, and prosthesis-related complications whose cumulative incidence compromises late outcome, particularly in young patients who are most exposed to the risk of long-term deterioration.

The indications in this subgroup of patients must take into account their heterogeneity with respect to anatomy, especially the extent and location of calcification. The clinical status is even more vital because this subgroup includes patients in good clinical condition and others who are not surgical candidates because of an associated comorbid condition. For this group of patients, an individualistic approach is favored that allows for the multifactorial nature of prediction (Fig. 86.5). The possibility of good results in poor candidates cannot be excluded; consequently, wider indications are proposed for valvuloplasty as an initial treatment in selected patients. Current opinion is that surgery can be considered the treatment of choice in patients with bicommissural or heavy calcification. On the other hand, in the author's opinion, balloon valvuloplasty can be attempted as a first approach in patients with extensive lesions of the subvalvular apparatus or moderate or unicommissural calcification, the more so because their clinical status argues in favor of this. Surgery should be considered reasonably early after unsatisfactory results or secondary deterioration. Extending knowledge regarding this group requires evaluation of new anatomic scores that may be developed in the future using new echocardiographic methods such as three-dimensional imaging (157), predictive models that take into account the multifactorial aspect of the prediction, and, ideally, the conduct of randomized studies on an "intent-to-treat" basis that compare balloon valvuloplasty with surgery. Such studies should include follow-up and should simultaneously be cost-effective.

In addition, no consensus has been reached regarding indication for valvuloplasty in patients with left atrial thrombosis located in the left atrial appendage and in patients with moderate stenosis.

A number of small series have reported that valvuloplasty is feasible for patients with thrombosis localized in the left atrial appendage (158,159). However, these studies have not satisfactorily shown that even use of the Inoue technique under transesophageal echocardiographic guidance precludes a risk of embolism. In such cases, the indications for valvuloplasty are limited to patients with contraindications to surgery or those without urgent need for intervention, when oral anticoagulation can be given for at least 2 months and provided a new transesophageal echocardiographic examination shows the disappearance of the thrombus.

The suggestion has been made that valvuloplasty be performed in patients with moderate stenosis in the hope of delaying the natural course of the disease (160). These patients are usually candidates for medical treatment, however, and the risks of valvuloplasty probably outweigh the benefits. To define a threshold of valve area above which valvuloplasty should not be performed is somewhat arbitrary because, besides measuring valve area, one must take into account functional disability and pulmonary pressures at rest and on exercise. The author's current practice is usu-

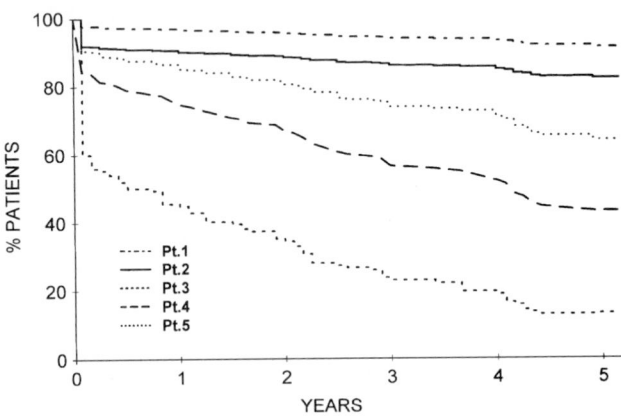

FIGURE 86.5 Multifactorial nature of the prediction of the results of mitral valvuloplasty. Predicted probability of good immediate results (valve area at least 1.5 cm² without regurgitation, Seller's grade greater than 2) and good late functional results [survival with no intervention and in New York Heart Association (NYHA) class I or II] according to patient characteristics. Values are given for a procedure using an Inoue balloon with an effective balloon dilating area of at least 5.5 cm² (i.e., a final diameter greater than or equal to 27 mm). Pt. 1, less than 50 years, NYHA class II, sinus rhythm, calcium grade I, valve area 1.25 to 1.5 cm²; Pt. 2, less than 50 years, NYHA class II, sinus rhythm, calcium grade 2, valve area 1 to 1.25 cm²; Pt. 3, 50 to 70 years, NYHA class III, sinus rhythm, calcium grade 2, valve area 1.25 to 1.5 cm²; Pt. 4, 50 to 70 years, NYHA class III, atrial fibrillation, calcium grade 2, valve area 1.25 to 1.5 cm²; Pt. 5, at least 70 years, NYHA class III, atrial fibrillation, calcium grade 3, valve area 0.75 to 1 cm². (Adapted from Iung B, Garbarz E, Doutrelant L, et al. Late results of percutaneous mitral commissurotomy for calcific mitral stenosis. *Am J Cardiol* 2000;85:1308–1314.)

ally to avoid valvuloplasty in patients with a valve area over 1.5 cm² or greater than 1 cm² per square meter of body surface area for unusually large patients.

Finally, the comparison between percutaneous valvuloplasty and surgery in the future will need to include minimally invasive surgery. In comparison with traditional surgery, these new techniques seem promising from an aesthetic point of view, because they lower potential risk by obviating or limiting the sternotomy, and because they use new videoscopic techniques. Few patients have so far been treated in this way, however, and data are still insufficient to evaluate the efficacy and the safety of the method; moreover, the expectation is that such methods will be reserved for surgeons of wide experience in the field of conservative surgery.

The question today is whether aortic valvuloplasty still really has a place (161,162). Most groups have abandoned the technique, but others see some role for it, albeit a very limited one. The remaining indication is mainly cardiogenic shock, with multivisceral failure if secondary operation is not definitely contraindicated. The use of valvuloplasty to treat rheumatic aortic stenosis should be better evaluated, however, because this might ultimately be an attractive application of the method.

Other percutaneous valve dilatation techniques will probably be used in exceptional cases in tricuspid stenosis

THE FUTURE

After nearly 15 years of extensive clinical evaluation, the technique of percutaneous valve dilatation, which for practical purposes can be summed up as percutaneous mitral valvuloplasty, is now here to stay. This is because of its proven efficacy in the treatment of mitral stenosis as a substitute for surgical commissurotomy (164) and as a complement to valve replacement.

or multiple valve disease. Percutaneous dilatation of bioprostheses seems to have no future.

Publication of a report of the first case of percutaneous valve replacement leaves the door open for the future (163).

REFERENCES

1. Inoue K, Owaki T, Nakamura T, et al. Clinical application of transvenous mitral commissurotomy by a new balloon catheter. *J Thorac Cardiovasc Surg* 1984;87:394–402.
2. Cribier A, Savin T, Saoudi N, et al. Percutaneous transluminal valvuloplasty of acquired aortic stenosis in elderly patients: an alternative to valve replacement? *Lancet* 1986;11:63–67.
3. Carroll JD, Feldman T. Percutaneous mitral balloon valvotomy and the new demographics of mitral stenosis. *JAMA* 1993;270:1731–1736.
4. Block PC, Palacios IF, Jacobs ML, et al. Mechanism of percutaneous mitral valvotomy. *Am J Cardiol* 1987;59:178–179.
5. Reifart N, Nowak B, Baykut D, et al. Experimental balloon valvuloplasty of fibrotic and calcific mitral valves. *Circulation* 1990;81:1105–1111.
6. Joseph G, Rajendiran G, Rajpal KA, et al. Transjugular approach to concurrent mitral-aortic and mitral-tricuspid balloon valvuloplasty. *Cathet Cardiovasc Interv* 2000;49:335–341.
7. Stefanadis CI, Stratos CG, Lambrou SG, et al. Accomplishments and perspectives with retrograde nontransseptal balloon mitral valvuloplasty. *J Interv Cardiol* 2000;13:269–280.
8. Zaibag M, Al Kasab S, Ribeiro PA, et al. Percutaneous double balloon mitral valvotomy for rheumatic mitral valve stenosis. *Lancet* 1986;i:757–761.
9. Vahanian A, Michel PL, Cormier B, et al. Results of percutaneous mitral commissurotomy in 200 patients. *Am J Cardiol* 1989;63:847–852.
10. Tuzcu EM, Block PC, Palacios IF, et al. Comparison of early versus late experience with percutaneous mitral balloon valvuloplasty. *J Am Coll Cardiol* 1991;17:1121–1124.
11. Bonhoeffer P, Hausse A, Yonga G. Technique and results of percutaneous mitral valvuloplasty with the multi-track system. *J Interv Cardiol* 2000:13:263–269.
12. Inoue K, Hung JS. Percutaneous transvenous mitral commissurotomy: the Far East experience. In: Topol EJ, ed. *Textbook of interventional cardiology.* Philadelphia: WB Saunders, 1994:1226–1243.
13. Feldman T, Herrmann HC, Inoue K. Technique of percutaneous transvenous mitral commissurotomy using the Inoue balloon catheter. *Cathet Cardiovasc Diagn* 1994;2:26–34.
14. Vahanian A, Cormier B, Iung B. Percutaneous transvenous mitral commissurotomy using the Inoue balloon: international experience. *Cathet Cardiovasc Diagn* 1994;2:8–15.
15. Rihal CS, Holmes DR. Percutaneous balloon mitral valvuloplasty: issues involved in comparing techniques. *Cathet Cardiovasc Diagn* 1994;2:35–41.
16. Gupta S, Schiele F, Xu C, et al. Simplified percutaneous mitral valvuloplasty with the Inoue balloon. *Eur Heart J* 1998;19:610–616.
17. Kang DH, Park SW, Song JK, et al. Long-term clinical and echocardiographic outcome of percutaneous mitral valvuloplasty: randomized comparison of Inoue and double-balloon techniques. *J Am Coll Cardiol* 2000;35:169–175.
18. Roth BR, Block PC, Palacios IF. Predictors of increased mitral regurgitation after percutaneous mitral balloon valvotomy. *Cathet Cardiovasc Diagn* 1990;20:17–21.
19. Chen C, Wang X, Wang Y, et al. Value of two-dimensional echocardiography in selecting patients and balloon sizes for percutaneous balloon mitral valvuloplasty. *J Am Coll Cardiol* 1989;14:1651–1658.
20. Cribier A, Eltchaninoff H, Koning R, et al. Percutaneous mechanical mitral commissurotomy with a newly designed metallic valvotome: immediate results of the initial experience in 153 patients. *Circulation* 1999;99:793–799.
21. Cribier A, Eltchaninoff H, Carlot R. Percutaneous mechanical mitral commissurotomy with the metallic valvotome: detailed technical aspect and overview of the results of the multicenter registry 882 patients. *J Interv Cardiol* 2000;13:255–262.
22. Park SH, Kim MA, Hyon MS. The advantages of on-line transesophageal echocardiography guide during percutaneous balloon mitral valvuloplasty. *J Am Soc Echocardiogr* 2000;13:26–34.
23. Cafri C, de la Guardia B, Barasch E, et al. Transseptal puncture guided by intracardiac echocardiography during percutaneous transvenous mitral commissurotomy in patients with distorted anatomy of the fossa ovalis. *Cathet Cardiovasc Interv* 2000;50:463–467.
24. Thomas JD, Weyman AE. Doppler mitral half-time: a clinical tool in search of theoretical justification. *J Am Coll Cardiol* 1987;10:923–929.

25. Hildick-Smith DJ, Taylor GJ, Shapiro LN. Inoue balloon mitral valvuloplasty: long-term clinical and echocardiographic follow-up of a predominantly unfavorable population. *Eur Heart J* 2000;21:1690–1697.
26. Palacios IG. What is the gold standard to measure mitral valve area post-mitral balloon valvuloplasty? *Cathet Cardiovasc Diagn* 1994;33:315–316.
27. Nakatani S, Nagata S, Beppu S, et al. Acute reduction of mitral valve area after percutaneous balloon mitral valvuloplasty: assessment with Doppler continuity equation method. *Am Heart J* 1991;121:770–775.
28. Cheng TO. Percutaneous balloon mitral valvuloplasty: are Chinese and Western experiences comparable? *Cathet Cardiovasc Diagn* 1994;31:23–28.
29. Ben Farhat M, Betbout F, Gamra H, et al. Results of percutaneous double-balloon mitral commissurotomy in one medical center in Tunisia. *Am J Cardiol* 1995;76:1266–1270.
30. Arora R, Singh Kalra G, Ramachandra Murty GS, et al. Percutaneous transatrial mitral commissurotomy: immediate and intermediate results. *J Am Coll Cardiol* 1994;23:1327–1332.
31. Chen CR, Cheng TO. Percutaneous balloon mitral valvuloplasty by the Inoue technique: a multicenter study of 4832 patients in China. *Am Heart J* 1995;129:1197–1202.
32. The National Heart, Lung, and Blood Institute Balloon Valvuloplasty Registry. Complications and mortality of percutaneous balloon mitral commissurotomy. *Circulation* 1992;85:2014–2024.
33. Iung B, Cormier B, Ducimetiere P, et al. Immediate results of percutaneous mitral commissurotomy. *Circulation* 1996;94:2124–2130.
34. Levine MJ, Weinstein JS, Diver DJ, et al. Progressive improvement in pulmonary vascular resistance after percutaneous mitral valvuloplasty. *Circulation* 1989;79:1061–1067.
35. Marzo KP, Herrmann HC, Mancini DM. Effect of balloon mitral valvuloplasty on exercise capacity, ventilation and skeletal muscle oxygenation. *J Am Coll Cardiol* 1993;21:856–865.
36. Tanabe Y, Oshima M, Suzuki M, et al. Determinants of delayed improvement in exercise capacity after percutaneous transvenous mitral commissurotomy. *Am Heart J* 2000;139:889–894.
37. Burger W, Kneissl GD, Kober G, et al. Effect of balloon valvuloplasty for mitral stenosis on right ventricular function. *Am J Cardiol* 1993;71:994–996.
38. Goto S, Handa S, Akaishi M, et al. Left ventricular ejection performance in mitral stenosis, and effects of successful percutaneous mitral commissurotomy. *Am J Cardiol* 1992;69:233–237.
39. Stefanadis C, Dernellis J, Stratos C, et al. Effects of balloon mitral valvuloplasty on left atrial function in mitral stenosis as assessed by pressure-area relation. *J Am Coll Cardiol* 1998;32:159–168.
40. Porte JM, Cormier B, Iung B, et al. Early assessment by transesophageal echocardiography of left atrial appendage function after percutaneous mitral commissurotomy. *Am J Cardiol* 1996;77:72–76.
41. Cormier B, Vahanian A, Iung B, et al. Influence of percutaneous mitral commissurotomy on left atrial spontaneous contrast of mitral stenosis. *Am J Cardiol* 1993;71:842–847.
42. Zaki A, Salama M, El Masry M, et al. Immediate effect of balloon valvuloplasty on hemostatic changes in mitral stenosis. *Am J Cardiol* 2000;85:370–375.
43. Harrison KJ, Wilson JS, Hearne SE, et al. Complications related to percutaneous transvenous mitral commissurotomy. *Cathet Cardiovasc Diagn* 1994;2:52–60.
44. Lee KS, Tuzcu ME, Elliott JM, et al. Development of left atrial thrombus following attempted percutaneous mitral valvuloplasty. *Cathet Cardiovasc Diagn* 1994;33:345–348.
45. Essop MR, Wisenbaugh T, Skoularigis J, et al. Mitral regurgitation following mitral balloon valvotomy: differing mechanisms for severe versus mild-to-moderate lesions. *Circulation* 1991;84:1669–1679.
46. Herrmann HC, Lima JAC, Feldman T, et al. Mechanisms and outcome of severe mitral regurgitation after Inoue balloon valvuloplasty. *J Am Coll Cardiol* 1993;27:783–789.
47. Acar C, Jebara VA, Grare PH, et al. Traumatic mitral insufficiency following percutaneous mitral dilation: anatomic lesions and surgical implications. *Eur J Cardiothorac Surg* 1992;6:660–664.
48. Hernandez R, Macaya C, Benuelos C, et al. Predictors, mechanisms and outcome of severe mitral regurgitation complicating percutaneous mitral valvotomy with the Inoue balloon. *Am J Cardiol* 1993;70:1169–1174.
49. Padial LR, Freitas N, Sagie A, et al. Echocardiography can predict which patients will develop severe mitral regurgitation after percutaneous mitral valvulotomy. *J Am Coll Cardiol* 1996;27:1225–1231.
50. Cequier A, Bonan R, Dyrda I, et al. Atrial shunting after percutaneous mitral valvuloplasty. *Circulation* 1990;81:1190–1197.
51. Porte JM, Cormier B, Iung B, et al. Intérêt de l'échographie transoesophagienne dans le suivi des commissurotomies mitrales percutanées réussies. *Arch Mal Coeur Vaiss* 1994;87:211–218.
52. Goldberg N, Roman CF, Do Cha S, et al. Right to left interatrial shunting following balloon mitral valvuloplasty. *Cathet Cardiovasc Diagn* 1989;16:133–135.
53. Carlson MD, Palacios I, Thomas JD, et al. Cardiac conduction abnormalities during percutaneous balloon mitral or aortic valvotomy. *Circulation* 1989;79:1197–1203.
54. Moriyama Y, Toyohira H, Saigenji H, et al. Infective mitral valve endocarditis after percutaneous transvenous mitral commissurotomy. *Eur J Cardiothorac Surg* 1995;9:111–112.
55. The National Heart, Lung and Blood Institute Balloon Valvuloplasty Registry participants. Multicenter experience with balloon mitral commissurotomy: NHLBI Balloon Valvuloplasty Registry report on immediate and 30-day follow-up results. *Circulation* 1992;85:448–461.
56. Wilkins GT, Gillam LD, Weyman AE, et al. Percutaneous balloon dilatation of the mitral valve: an analysis of echocardiographic variables related to outcome and the mechanism of dilatation. *Br Heart J* 1988;60:299–308.
57. Abascal V, Wilkins GT, O'Shea JP, et al. Prediction of successful outcome in 130 patients undergoing percutaneous balloon mitral valvotomy. *Circulation* 1990;82:448–456.

58. Herrmann HC, Ramaswamy K, Isner JM, et al. Factors influencing immediate results, complications, and short-term follow-up status after Inoue balloon mitral valvotomy: a North-American multicenter study. *Am Heart J* 1992;124:160–166.

59. Feldman T, Carroll JD, Isner JM, et al. Effect of valve deformity on results and mitral regurgitation after Inoue balloon commissurotomy. *Circulation* 1992;85:180–187.

60. Nair M, Agarwala R, Kalra GS, et al. Can mitral regurgitation after balloon dilatation of the mitral valve be predicted? *Br Heart J* 1992;67:442–444.

61. Zaibag M, Ribeiro PA, Kasab S, et al. One year follow-up after percutaneous double balloon mitral valvotomy. *Am J Cardiol* 1989;63:126–127.

62. Cohen DJ, Kuntz RE, Gordon SPF, et al. Predictors of long-term outcome after percutaneous balloon mitral valvuloplasty. *N Engl J Med* 1992;327:1329–1335.

63. Pan M, Medina A, Lezo JJ, et al. Factors determining late success after mitral balloon valvulotomy. *Am J Cardiol* 1993;71:1181–1186.

64. Palacios IF, Tuzcu ME, Weyman AE, et al. Clinical follow-up of patients undergoing percutaneous mitral balloon valvotomy. *Circulation* 1995;91:671–676.

65. Orrange S, Kawanishi D, Lopez B, et al. Actuarial outcome after catheter balloon commissurotomy in patients with mitral stenosis. *Circulation* 1997;95:382–389.

66. Stefanadis C, Stratos C, Lambrou S, et al. Retrograde non-transseptal balloon mitral valvuloplasty: immediate results and intermediate long-term outcome in 441 cases—a multi-centre experience. *J Am Coll Cardiol* 1998;32:1009–1016.

67. Meneveau N, Schiele F, Seronde MF, et al. Predictors of event-free survival after percutaneous mitral commissurotomy. *Heart* 1998;80:359–364.

68. Hernandez R, Bañuelos C, Alfonso F, et al. Long-term clinical and echocardiographic follow-up after percutaneous mitral valvuloplasty with the Inoue balloon. *Circulation* 1999;99:1580–1586.

69. Iung B, Garbarz E, Michaud P, et al. Late results of percutaneous mitral commissurotomy in a series of 1024 patients: analysis of late clinical deterioration: frequency, anatomic findings, and predictive factors. *Circulation* 1999;99:3272–3278.

70. Chen CR, Cheng T, Chen JY, et al. Long-term results of percutaneous balloon mitral valvuloplasty for mitral stenosis: a follow-up study to 11 years in 202 patients. *Cathet Cardiovasc Diagn* 1998;43:132–139.

71. Smith WM, Neutze JM, Baratt-Boyes BG, et al. Open mitral valvotomy: effect of preoperative factors on result. *J Thorac Cardiovasc Surg* 1981;82:738–751.

72. John S, Bashi VV, Jairap PS, et al. Closed mitral valvotomy: early results and long-term follow-up of 3274 consecutive patients. *Circulation* 1983;68:891–896.

73. Rihal CS, Schaff H, Frye RL, et al. Long-term follow-up of patients undergoing closed transventricular mitral commissurotomy: a useful surrogate for percutaneous balloon mitral valvuloplasty? *J Am Coll Cardiol* 1992;20:781–786.

74. Desideri A, Vanderperren O, Serra A, et al. Long-term (9 to 33 months) echocardiographic follow-up after successful percutaneous mitral commissurotomy. *Am J Cardiol* 1992;69:1602–1606.

75. Thomas MR, Monaghan MJ, Michalis LK, et al. Echocardiographic restenosis after successful balloon dilatation of the mitral valve with the Inoue balloon: experience of a United Kingdom centre. *Br Heart J* 1993;69:418–423.

76. Iung B, Garbarz E, Michaud P, et al. Immediate and mid-term results of repeat percutaneous mitral commissurotomy for restenosis following earlier percutaneous mitral commissurotomy. *Eur Heart J* 2000;21:1683–1690.

77. Pathan AZ, Mahdi NA, Leon MN, et al. Is redo percutaneous mitral balloon valvuloplasty (PMV) indicated in patients with post-PMV mitral restenosis? *J Am Coll Cardiol* 1999;34:49–54.

78. Langerveld J, Thijs Plokker HW, Ernst SMPG, et al. Predictors of clinical events or restenosis during follow-up after percutaneous mitral balloon valvotomy. *Eur Heart J* 1999;20:519–526.

79. Leon MN, Harrell LC, Simosa HF, et al. Mitral balloon valvotomy for patients with mitral stenosis in atrial fibrillation. Immediate and long-term results. *J Am Coll Cardiol* 1999;34:1145–1152.

80. Cannan CR, Nishimura RA, Reeder GS, et al. Echocardiographic assessment of commissural calcium: a simple predictor of outcome after percutaneous mitral balloon valvotomy. *J Am Coll Cardiol* 1997;29:175–180.

81. Sadaniantz A, Luttmann C, Shulman RS, et al. Acquired Lutembacher syndrome or mitral stenosis and acquired atrial septal defect after transseptal mitral valvuloplasty. *Cathet Cardiovasc Diagn* 1990;21:7–9.

82. Wang A, Pulsipher M, Harrison JK, et al. Predictors and significance of atrial rhythm before and six months after percutaneous balloon mitral commissurotomy. *Am J Cardiol* 1999;83:125–128.

83. ACC/AHA Guidelines for the management of patients with valvular heart disease. A report of the American College of Cardiology/American Heart Association. Task Force on Practice Guidelines (Committee on Management of Patients with Valvular Heart Disease). *J Am Coll Cardiol* 1998;32:1486–1588.

84. Serra A, Bonan R, Lefevre T, et al. Balloon mitral commissurotomy for mitral restenosis after surgical commissurotomy. *Am J Cardiol* 1993;71:1311–1315.

85. Jang IK, Block PC, Newell JB, et al. Percutaneous mitral balloon valvotomy for recurrent mitral stenosis after surgical commissurotomy. *Am J Cardiol* 1995;75:601–605.

86. Iung B, Garbarz E, Michaud P. Percutaneous mitral commissurotomy for restenosis after surgical commissurotomy: late efficacy and implications for patient selection. *J Am Coll Cardiol* 2000;35:1295–1302.

87. Alfonso F, Macaya C, Hernandez R, et al. Percutaneous mitral valvuloplasty with severe pulmonary artery hypertension. *Am J Cardiol* 1993;72:325–330.

88. Chen CR, Cheng TO, Chen JY, et al. Percutaneous balloon mitral valvuloplasty for mitral stenosis with and without associated aortic regurgitation. *Am Heart J* 1993;125:128–137.

89. Shaw TRD, McAreavey D, Essop AR, et al. Percutaneous balloon dilatation of mitral valve in patients who were unsuitable for surgical treatment. *Br Heart J* 1992;67:454–459.

90. Wu JJ, Chern MS, Yeh KH, et al. Urgent/emergent percutaneous transvenous mitral commissurotomy. *Cathet Cardiovasc Diagn* 1994;31:18–22.

91. Goldman J, Slade A, Clague J. Cardiogenic shock to mitral stenosis treated by balloon mitral valvuloplasty. *Cathet Cardiovasc Diag* 1998;43:195–197.

92. Tuzcu EM, Block PC, Griffin BP, et al. Immediate and long-term outcome of percutaneous mitral valvotomy in patients 65 years and older. *Circulation* 1992;85:963–971.

93. Iung B, Cormier B, Farah B, et al. Percutaneous mitral commissurotomy in the elderly. *Eur Heart J* 1995;16:1092–1099.

94. Sutaria N, Elder AT, Shaw TRD. Long term outcome of percutaneous mitral balloon valvotomy in patients aged 70 and over. *Heart* 2000;83:433–438.

95. Iung B, Cormier B, Elias J, et al. Usefulness of percutaneous balloon commissurotomy for mitral stenosis during pregnancy. *Am J Cardiol* 1994;73:398–400.

96. Presbitero P, Prever SB, Brusca A. Interventional cardiology in pregnancy. *Eur Heart J* 1996;17:182–188.

97. Mangione JA, Lourenco RM, Souza dos Santo E, et al. Long-term follow-up of pregnant women after percutaneous mitral valvuloplasty. *Cathet Cardiovasc Interv* 2000;50:413–417.

98. Sagie A, Schwammenthal E, John B, et al. Significant tricuspid regurgitation is a marker for adverse outcome in patients undergoing percutaneous balloon mitral valvuloplasty. *J Am Coll Cardiol* 1994;24:696–702.

99. Fatkin D, Roy P, Morgan JJ, et al. Percutaneous balloon mitral valvotomy with the Inoue single balloon catheter: commissural morphology as a determination of outcome. *J Am Coll Cardiol* 1993;21:390–397.

100. Mezilis ME, Salame MY, Oakly DG. Predicting mitral regurgitation following percutaneous mitral valvotomy with the Inoue balloon: comparison of two echocardiographic scoring systems. *Clin Cardiol* 1999;22:453–458.

101. Padial LR, Abascal VM, Moreno PR, et al. Echocardiography can predict the development of severe mitral regurgitation after percutaneous mitral valvuloplasty by the Inoue technique. *Am J Cardiol* 1999;83:1210–1213.

102. Sutaria N, Northridge DB, Shaw TRD. Significance of commissural calcification on outcome of mitral balloon valvotomy. *Heart* 2000;84:398–402.

103. Turi ZG, Reyes VP, Soma Raju B, et al. Percutaneous balloon surgical closed commissurotomy for mitral stenosis. *Circulation* 1991;83:1179–1185.

104. Reyes VP, Raju BS, Wynne J, et al. Percutaneous balloon valvuloplasty compared with open surgical commissurotomy for mitral stenosis. *N Engl J Med* 1994;331:961–967.

105. Ben Farhat M, Ayari M, Maatouk F. Percutaneous balloon versus surgical closed and open mitral commissurotomy: seven-year follow-up results of a randomized trial. *Circulation* 1998;97:245–250.

106. Tuzcu ME, Block PC, Griffin B, et al. Percutaneous mitral balloon valvotomy in patients with calcific mitral stenosis: immediate and long-term outcome. *J Am Coll Cardiol* 1994;23:1604–1609.

107. Ping Zhang H, Allen JW, Lau FYK, et al. Immediate and late outcome of percutaneous balloon mitral valvotomy in patients with significantly calcified valves. *Am Heart J* 1995;129:501–506.

108. Post JR, Feldman T, Isner J, et al. Inoue balloon mitral valvotomy in patients with severe valvular and subvalvular deformity. *J Am Coll Cardiol* 1995;25:1129–1136.

109. Iung B, Garbarz E, Doutrelant L, et al. Late results of percutaneous mitral commissurotomy for calcific mitral stenosis. *Am J Cardiol* 2000;85:1308–1314.

110. Safian RD, Mandell VS, Thurer RE, et al. Post-mortem and intra-operative balloon valvuloplasty of calcific aortic stenosis in elderly patients: mechanisms of successful dilatation. *J Am Coll Cardiol* 1987;9:665–670.

111. Robicsek F, Harbold NB. Limited value of balloon dilatation in calcified aortic stenosis in adults: direct observations during open heart surgery. *Am J Cardiol* 1987;60:857–864.

112. Fedman T, Glagou S, Caroll JD. Restenosis following successful balloon valvuloplasty: bone formation in aortic valve leaflets. *Cathet Cardiovasc Diagn* 1993;29:1–7.

113. Van Den Brand M, Essed CES, Di Mario C. Histological changes in aortic valve after balloon dilatation: evidence for a delayed process. *Br Heart J* 1993;70:445–449.

114. Ribeiro PA, Al Zaibag M, Rajendran V. Double balloon aortic valvotomy for rheumatic aortic stenosis: *in vitro* studies. *Eur Heart J* 1989;10:417–423.

115. Cribier A, Gerber LI, Letac B. Aortic valvuloplasty. In: Topol EJ, ed. *Update 3. Textbook of interventional cardiology.* Philadelphia: WB Saunders, 1992:43–58.

116. Acar J, Vahanian A, Slama M, et al. Treatment of calcified aortic stenosis: surgery or percutaneous transluminal aortic valvuloplasty. *Eur Heart J* 1988;9[Suppl E]:163–168.

117. Block PC, Palacios IF. Comparison of hemodynamic results of anterograde versus retrograde percutaneous balloon aortic valvuloplasty. *Am J Cardiol* 1987;60:659–662.

118. Nishimura RA, Holmes DR Jr, Reeders GS, et al. Doppler evaluation of results of percutaneous aortic balloon valvuloplasty in calcific aortic stenosis. *Circulation* 1988;78:791–799.

119. NHLBI Balloon Registry participants. Percutaneous balloon aortic valvuloplasty. Acute and 30-day follow-up results in 674 patients from the NHBLI Balloon Valvuloplasty Registry. *Circulation* 1991;84:2383–2387.

120. Safian RD, Berman AD, Diver DJ, et al. Balloon aortic valvuloplasty in 170 consecutive patients. *N Engl J Med* 1988;319:125–130.

121. McKay R. Mansfield Scientific Registry experience. Overview of acute hemodynamic results and procedural complications. *J Am Coll Cardiol* 1991;17:485–491.

122. Holmes DR Jr, Nishimura RA, Reeder GS. Mansfield Scientific Registry experience. In-hospital mortality after balloon aortic valvuloplasty: frequency and associated factors. *J Am Coll Cardiol* 1991;17:189–192.

123. Isner JM. Mansfield Scientific Registry experience. Acute catastrophic complications of balloon aortic valvuloplasty. *J Am Coll Cardiol* 1991;17:1436–1444.

124. Block PC, Palacios IF. Aortic and mitral balloon valvuloplasty: the United States experience. In: Topol EJ, ed. *Textbook of interventional cardiology.* Philadelphia: WB Saunders, 1994:1189–1205.

125. Block PC, Palacios IF. Clinical and hemodynamic follow-up after percutaneous aortic valvuloplasty in the elderly. *Am J Cardiol* 1988;62:760–763.

126. O'Neill WW. Mansfield Scientific Registry experience. Predictors of long term survival after percutaneous aortic valvuloplasty: Report of the Mansfield Valvuloplasty Registry. *J Am Coll Cardiol* 1991;17:193–198.

127. Lieberman EB, Bashore TM, Hermiller JB, et al. Balloon aortic valvuloplasty in adults: failure of procedure to improve long-term survival. *J Am Coll Cardiol* 1995;26:1522–1528.

128. Otto CM, Mickel MC, Kennedy W, et al. Three-year outcome after balloon aortic valvuloplasty: insights into prognosis of valvular aortic stenosis. *Circulation* 1994;89:642–650.

129. Lieberman EB, Wilson JS, Harnisai JK, et al. Aortic valve

replacement in adult after balloon aortic valvuloplasty. *Circulation* 1994;90:II-205–II-208.

130. Ferguson JJ, Garza RA. Mansfield Scientific Registry experience. Efficacy of multiple balloon aortic valvuloplasty procedures. *J Am Coll Cardiol* 1991;17:1430–1435.

131. Bashore TM, Davidson CJ. Mansfield Scientific Registry experience. Follow-up recatheterization after balloon aortic valvuloplasty. *J Am Coll Cardiol* 1991;17:1188–1195.

132. O'Keefe JTL Jr, Vliesta RE, Bailey KR, et al. Natural history of candidates for balloon aortic valvuloplasty. *Mayo Clin Proc* 1987;62:986–991.

133. Cormier B, Luxereau P, Bloch C, et al. Prognosis and long term results of surgically treated aortic stenosis with or without insufficiency. *Eur Heart J* 1988;9[Suppl E]:113–120.

134. Culliford AT, Galloway AC, Colvin SB, et al. Aortic valve replacement for aortic stenosis in persons aged 80 years and over. *Am J Cardiol* 1991;67:1256–1260.

135. Freeman WK, Schaff HV, O'Brien PC, et al. Cardiac surgery in octogenarians: perioperative outcome and clinical follow-up. *J Am Coll Cardiol* 1991;18:29–35.

136. Bernard Y, Etievent J, Mourand JL, et al. Long-term results of percutaneous aortic valvuloplasty compared with aortic replacement in patients more than 75 years old. *J Am Coll Cardiol* 1992;20:796–801.

137. Moreno PR, Ik-Kyung Jang, Newell JB, et al. The role of percutaneous aortic balloon valvuloplasty in patients with cardiogenic shock and critical aortic stenosis. *J Am Coll Cardiol* 1994;23:1071–1075.

138. Bourdillon PDV, Hookman LD, Morris SN, et al. Percutaneous balloon valvuloplasty for tricuspid stenosis: hemodynamic and pathological findings. *Am Heart J* 1989;117:492–495.

139. Goldenberg I, Pedersen W, Olson J, et al. Percutaneous double balloon valvuloplasty for severe tricuspid stenosis. *Am Heart J* 1989;118:417–419.

140. Shaw TRD. The Inoue balloon for dilatation of the tricuspid valve: a modified over-the-wire approach. *Br Heart J* 1992;67:263–265.

141. Waller BF, McKay C, Vanassel J. Catheter balloon valvuloplasty of stenotic porcine bioprosthetic valves. Part I: anatomic considerations. *Clin Cardiol* 1991;14:686–691.

142. Waller BF, McKay C, Vanassel J, et al. Catheter balloon valvuloplasty of stenotic porcine bioprosthetic valves. Part II: mechanisms, complications, and recommendations for clinical use. *Clin Cardiol* 1991;764–772.

143. Orbe LC, Sobrino N, Mate I, et al. Effectiveness of balloon percutaneous valvuloplasty for stenotic bioprosthetic valves in different positions. *Am J Cardiol* 1991;68:1719–1721.

144. McKay C, Waller BF, Hong R, et al. Problems encountered with catheter balloon valvuloplasty of bioprosthetic aortic valves. *Am Heart J* 1988;115:463–465.

145. Lin PJ, Chang JP, Chu JJ, et al. Balloon valvuloplasty is contraindicated in stenotic mitral bioprosthesis. *Am Heart J* 1994;127:724–726.

146. Chow WH, Cheung KL, Tai YT, et al. Successful percutaneous balloon valvuloplasty of a stenotic tricuspid bioprosthesis. *Am Heart J* 1990;119:666–668.

147. Slama MS, Drieu LH, Malergue MC, et al. Percutaneous double balloon valvuloplasty for stenosis bioprostheses in

the tricuspid valve position: a report of 2 cases. *Cathet Cardiovasc Diagn* 1993;28:142–148.

148. Block PC, Smalling R, Owing RM. Percutaneous double balloon valvotomy for bioprosthetic tricuspid stenosis. *Cathet Cardiovasc Diagn* 1994;33:342–344.

149. Savas V, Grines CL, O'Neill W. Percutaneous triple-valve balloon valvuloplasty in a pregnant woman. *Cathet Cardiovasc Diagn* 1991;24:288–294.

150. Berman AD, Weinstein JS, Safian RD, et al. Combined aortic and mitral balloon valvuloplasty in patients with mitral aortic and mitral valve stenosis: results in six cases. *J Am Coll Cardiol* 1988;1213–1218.

151. Sobrino N, Calvo Orbe L, Merino JL. Percutaneous balloon valvuloplasty for concurrent mitral, aortic, and tricuspid rheumatic stenosis. *Eur Heart J* 1995;16:711–713.

152. Vandermael M, Deligonul V, Gabliani G, et al. Percutaneous balloon valvuloplasty and coronary angioplasty for the treatment of calcific aortic stenosis and obstructive coronary disease in an elderly patient. *Cathet Cardiovasc Diagn* 1988;14:49–52.

153. Rothlisberger C, Kaufmann U, Meyer B. Combined percutaneous balloon mitral valvotomy and coronary angioplasty with stent implantation. *Cathet Cardiovasc Diagn* 1995;35:183–185.

154. Meyer BJ, Meier B, Bonzelt T, et al. Interventional cardiology in Europe 1993. *Eur Heart J* 1996;17:1318–1328.

155. Rothlisberger C, Essop MR, Skudicky D, et al. Results of percutaneous balloon mitral valvotomy in young adults. *Am J Cardiol* 1991;72:73–77.

156. Lau KW, Hung JS, Ding ZP, et al. Controversies in balloon mitral valvuloplasty: the when (timing for intervention), what (choice of valve), and how (selection of technique). *Cathet Cardiovasc Diagn* 1995;35:91–100.

157. Binder TM, Rosenhek R, Porenta G, et al. Improved assessment of mitral valve stenosis by volumetric real-time three-dimensional echocardiography. *J Am Coll Cardiol* 2000;36:1355–1361.

158. Hung JS, Lin FC, Chiang CW. Successful percutaneous transvenous catheter balloon mitral commissurotomy after warfarin therapy and resolution of left atrial thrombus. *Am J Cardiol* 1989;64:126–128.

159. Chen WJ, Chen MF, Liau CS, et al. Safety of percutaneous transvenous balloon mitral commissurotomy in patients with mitral stenosis and thrombus in the left atrial appendage. *Am J Cardiol* 1992;70:117–119.

160. Pan M, Medina A, Suarey de Lejo J, et al. Balloon valvuloplasty for mild mitral stenosis. *Cathet Cardiovasc Diagn* 1991;24:1–5.

161. Serruys PW, Luitjen HE, Beatt KJ, et al. Percutaneous valvuloplasty for calcific aortic stenosis: a treatment "sinecure"? *Eur Heart J* 1988;9:782–794.

162. Rahimtoola SH. Catheter balloon valvuloplasty for severe calcific aortic stenosis: a limited role. *J Am Coll Cardiol* 1994;203:1076–1078.

163. Bonhoeffer P, Boudjemline Y, Saliba Z, et al. Percutaneous replacement of pulmonary valve in a right-ventricle to pulmonary-artery prosthetic conduit with valve dysfunction. *Lancet* 2000;356:1403–1405.

164. Palacios I. Farewell to surgical mitral commissurotomy for many patients. *Circulation* 1998;97:223–226.

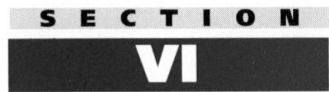

HEART FAILURE AND TRANSPLANTATION

JAMES B. YOUNG

PATHOPHYSIOLOGY OF THE HEART FAILURE CLINICAL SYNDROME

GARY S. FRANCIS

OVERVIEW

Heart failure continues to emerge as an enormous public health problem in the new millennium. The aging population continues to grow around the world, and the incidence of heart failure continues to climb commensurate with the graying of the world population. It is estimated that 10% of patients older than 75 years have heart failure. Because it is a syndrome and not a specific disease, heart failure has many forms and faces. This has led to persistent controversy and lack of agreement regarding the definition. The confusion

G. S. Francis: Department of Cardiovascular Medicine, Coronary Intensive Care Unit, The Cleveland Clinic Foundation, Cleveland, Ohio

regarding the definition stems in part from the differences between historical bedside observations (e.g., cardiomegaly, third heart sound gallop, rales, fluid retention, oliguria, breathlessness, and fatigue) and elaborations emanating from careful laboratory exercises performed from 1950 to 2000 (e.g., measurement of contractile abnormalities, isolated papillary muscle function, identification of key molecular abnormalities). The clinical definition of *heart failure*, a syndrome readily diagnosed by a careful history and physical examination, is considered in very broad terms to be an abnormality of the heart with a characteristic pattern of hemodynamic and neuroendocrine responses. The clinical picture is dominated by secondary organ abnormalities in the lungs (shortness of breath), the kidneys (salt and water retention), and the skeletal muscles (fatigue), but the central problem is always in the heart. The syndrome of heart failure is the expression of the final common pathway by which many etiologic factors can damage the heart, including acute myocardial infarction, inflammatory myocarditis, gene mutations with abnormal contractile function, valvular heart disease, severe undertreated hypertension, and so forth. Virtually any form of heart disease can culminate in the syndrome of heart failure.

We now understand that chronic systolic heart failure is often characterized by progressive remodeling of the left ventricular (LV) chamber. The other three chambers are also frequently involved and can progressively dilate as well. The LV becomes larger and more spherical over months to years, obligating a reduction in LV ejection fraction. The process of remodeling is highly complex and is addressed in detail later in this chapter. However, the remodeling process is central to the pathophysiology of heart failure and is now the prime target for two major effective forms of treatment—angiotensin-converting enzyme (ACE) inhibitors and beta-adrenergic blockers. The observation by clinicians that treatment designed to block various neuroendocrine responses can result in inhibition and, in some cases, reversal of LV remodeling has been an epiphany. Although there are many gaps in our knowledge of pathophysiology, especially in cellular biology, we are beginning to recognize complex but coherent patterns that develop in the pathogenesis of heart failure. The purpose of this chapter is to feature the most current thinking as it relates to the pathophysiology.

DIAGNOSIS AND EVALUATION OF HEART FAILURE

History and Physical Examination

Perhaps the most predominant symptom of heart failure is breathlessness. The medical term for breathlessness, *dyspnea*, is the awareness by the patient of increased respiratory effort. This may occur at rest or with minimal physical activity. The patient is aware of an uncomfortable sensation, not being able to get enough air. It is somewhat surprising that to this day the mechanism of dyspnea is poorly understood. In patients with acute pulmonary edema, hypoxemia probably contributes to the sensation of dyspnea. However, patients with more chronic forms of heart failure have dyspnea that bears no direct relationship to hypoxemia, elevated pulmonary capillary wedge pressure, or other central hemodynamics (46). Likewise, the level of dyspnea is not related in a simple manner to dead space inhalation. It is likely that chronic shortness of breath at rest or with minimal activity is due to multiple peripheral mechanisms, including fatigue of the respiratory muscles, increased physiologic dead space, reduced pulmonary compliance, increased airway resistance,

endothelial dysfunction, abnormal skeletal muscle metabolism, and perhaps signals from the pulmonary J receptors and respiratory muscles (48,49).

Orthopnea and paroxysmal nocturnal dyspnea occur in the more advanced stages of heart failure. Neither orthopnea nor paroxysmal nocturnal dyspnea is specific for heart failure and can occur in other conditions. Patients with more advanced and chronic heart failure frequently have Cheyne-Stokes respirations. This type of periodic breathing in patients with heart failure, characterized by repeated episodes of apnea and hypopnea during sleep, is associated with severe nocturnal arterial blood saturation. It also carries a poor prognosis (50) and is correlated with an elevated pulmonary capillary wedge pressure (51). Central sleep apnea is common in patients with heart failure (52) and may be related to enhanced sensitivity to carbon dioxide (53). Continuous positive airway pressure improves cardiac function in patients with heart failure who demonstrate Cheyne-Stokes respiration or central sleep apnea (54). Coughing and wheezing can also occur in patients with heart failure and may be the predominant symptoms.

The second cardinal feature of heart failure is chronic fatigue. Fatigue is also a very nonspecific symptom and, like dyspnea, is rather poorly understood. In the past, fatigue was attributed to low cardiac output, but we now know that the mechanism is far more complex. Drugs that improve blood flow to exercising muscles in heart failure do not necessarily improve exercise tolerance or reduce fatigue (55,56). It is likely that abnormalities of skeletal muscle histology and biochemistry contribute to poor exercise tolerance and chronic fatigue (57–60).

Circulatory congestion is responsible for many of the physical signs of heart failure. Occasionally patients with new-onset heart failure present with severe right-upper-quadrant pain and abdominal fullness. This may be accompanied by nausea and vomiting and is probably due to engorgement of the liver and bowel from high venous pressure. Rarely, heart failure can even present as an acute surgical abdomen. However, peripheral edema and pulmonary rales are not invariably present in heart failure, even when cardiac filling pressure is markedly increased (61).

The physical findings in heart failure span the spectrum from very unimpressive to highly remarkable. In the current era of loop diuretics and ACE inhibitor therapy, patients frequently have an absence of the traditional findings, such as pulmonary rales, gallop rhythm, hepatomegaly, ascites, and peripheral edema. Even jugular venous distention may be absent in the face of severe LV dysfunction if the patient is well compensated. On the contrary, the presence of neck vein distention, a third heart sound, pulmonary rales, and peripheral edema is highly characteristic of the syndrome of heart failure. During the sequential follow-up of patients in the clinic over time, particular attention should be focused on examination of venous pressure. Sequential examination of the patient is most impor-

TABLE 88.1 RECOMMENDED TESTS FOR PATIENTS WITH SIGNS OR SYMPTOMS OF HEART FAILURE

Test recommendation	Finding	Suspected diagnosis
Electrocardiogram	Acute ST-T–wave changes	Myocardial ischemia
	Atrial fibrillation, other tachy-arrhythmia	Thyroid disease or heart failure due to rapid ventricular rate
	Bradyarrhythmias rate	Heart failure due to low heart rate
	Previous myocardial infarction (e.g., Q waves) left ventricular performance	Heart failure due to reduced contractile tissue
	Low voltage	Pericardial effusion
	Left ventricular hypertrophy	Diastolic dysfunction
Complete blood cell count	Anemia	Heart failure due to or aggravated by decreased oxygen-carrying capacity
Urinalysis	Proteinuria	Nephrotic syndrome
	Red blood cells or cellular casts	Glomerulonephritis
Serum creatinine	Elevated failure	Volume overload due to renal dysfunction
Serum albumin	Decreased	Increased extravascular volume due to hypoalbuminemia
T4 and TSH (obtain only if atrial fibrillation, evidence of thyroid disease, or patient age >65 yr)	Abnormal T4 or TSH	Heart failure due to or aggravated by hypo/hyperthyroidism

TSH, thyroid-stimulating hormone.
From Konstam M, Dracup K, Baker D, et al. *Heart failure: management of patients with left-ventricular systolic dysfunction. Quick reference guide for clinicians No. 11.* AHCPR Publication No. 94-0613. Rockville, MD: Agency for Health Care Policy and Research, Public Health Service, U.S. Department of Human Services, June 1994, with permission.

tant, and examination of the neck veins is perhaps the single most useful physical finding. The presence or absence of venous distention is also most helpful in determining the dose of diuretic therapy.

The cardiac examination itself should be carried out with the patient in both the supine and the left lateral decubitus position. Often the cardiac apex impulse is displaced and sustained. A third heart sound gallop, when present, may be palpable. Patients with heart failure frequently have a murmur of mitral regurgitation that radiates to the axilla. Tricuspid regurgitation is also common in patients with heart failure, although sometimes more difficult to auscultate.

Routine Laboratory Tests

A number of routine laboratory tests useful in the evaluation of patients with heart failure are suggested in Table 88.1. Evaluation of a new patient with heart failure should also include a chest x-ray to assess the size of the heart and the pulmonary vascular markings. Occasionally the cardiac silhouette is normal in size, which should signal the possibility of pure diastolic heart failure. Enlargement of the cardiac silhouette can be due to either right, left, or biventricular enlargement. Heart failure is characterized by roentgenographic perihilar engorgement of the pulmonary vasculature with cephalization of lung vascular markings. Pleural effusions may be present and are more likely to occur on the right.

The cornerstone of evaluation remains the echocardiogram. Every new patient with heart failure should have an echocardiogram performed with Doppler interrogation to assess LV size, cardiac performance, as well as valvular architecture and function. The echocardiogram can be used to distinguish systolic from diastolic heart failure. It is also useful in diagnosing pericardial effusion, hypertrophic cardiomyopathy, regional wall motion abnormalities, and unsuspected valvular heart disease.

Although the radionuclide ventriculography can provide very precise information regarding ejection fraction, most laboratories prefer to use echocardiographic data because they provide a more comprehensive observation, are simpler to obtain, and are less costly. The use of transthoracic Doppler is also helpful. The features of both echocardiography and radionuclide left ventriculography are compared in Table 88.2.

The electrocardiogram continues to be useful in the evaluation of new patients with heart failure. It is inexpensive and provides information about the rhythm and conduction of the heart. The presence of old myocardial infarction, LV hypertrophy, left atrial enlargement, and underlying ischemic heart disease can also be suggested by a careful examination of the 12-lead electrocardiogram. Patients with advanced heart failure frequently have arrhythmias, which are usually diagnosed by simple electrocardiography. The presence of new atrial fibrillation on the electrocardiogram may provide a clue as to why a patient may have suffered acute decompensation. Approximately 20% to 30% of patients with heart failure have atrial fibrillation. In general, the electrocardiogram remains part of the standard initial evaluation but is probably not indicated for routine follow-up visits.

TABLE 88.2 ECHOCARDIOGRAPHY AND RADIONUCLIDE VENTRICULOGRAPHY COMPARED IN EVALUATION OF LEFT VENTRICULAR PERFORMANCE

Test	Advantages	Disadvantages
Echocardiogram	Permits concomitant assessment of valvular disease, left ventricular hypertrophy, and left atrial size	Difficult to perform in patients with lung disease
	Less expensive than radionuclide ventriculography in most areas	Usually only semiquantitative estimate of ejection fraction provided
	Able to detect pericardial effusion and ventricular thrombus	Technically inadequate in up to 18% of patients under optimal circumstances
	More generally available	
Radionuclide ventriculogram	More precise and reliable measurement of ejection fraction	Requires venipuncture and radiation exposure
	Better assessment of right ventricular function	Limited assessment of valvular heart disease and left ventricular hypertrophy

From Konstam M, Dracup K, Baker D, et al. *Heart failure: management of patients with left-ventricular systolic dysfunction. Quick reference guide for clinicians No. 11.* AHCPR Publication No. 94-0613. Rockville, MD: Agency for Health Care Policy and Research, Public Health Service, U.S. Department of Human Services, June 1994, with permission.

All new patients should have a complete blood count and urinalysis, serum electrolytes, blood urea nitrogen, serum creatinine, blood glucose, and, in some cases, an assay for thyroid-stimulating hormone. Measurement of the levels of plasma norepinephrine, plasma ANF, and PRA, although increased in patients with heart failure, is not considered routine or clinically necessary. Plasma neurohormone levels are primarily research tools. This may change with the emerging data on BNP (31–33). This peptide tracks with LV filling pressure and is an excellent tool to aid in the diagnosis of heart failure. It may also be useful in confirming vague physical findings, making decisions about hospital admission, and determining the response to therapy (62,63). The availability of a quantitative bedside "point-of-care" kit may facilitate the use of BNP for the diagnosis of heart failure.

FACTORS KNOWN TO PRECIPITATE HEART FAILURE

Chronic heart failure is characterized by a waxing and waning of the signs and symptoms of circulatory congestion, sometimes culminating in severe pump dysfunction leading to death. It now seems apparent that approximately one-third to one-half of patients die suddenly and unexpectedly from a presumed arrhythmic death, whereas remaining patients appear to die from progressive pump dysfunction. However, recent experience with clinical trials has suggested that this distinction with regard to the mechanism of death in patients with heart failure is not a simple matter (93). Nevertheless, an undulating course characterized as compensation and decompensation is familiar to all physicians who care for these patients on a long-term basis. When patients acutely deteriorate, specific reasons for this acute deterioration should always be explored (Table 88.3).

Among the causes of acute decompensation of previously stable heart failure is the syndrome of acute myocardial ischemia. Although classic angina pectoris is not usually a prominent feature of patients with heart failure, we now know that approximately half or more patients with heart failure harbor severe underlying coronary artery disease. It is important to consider this etiologic factor when seeing patients with heart failure and acute decompensation. A 12-lead electrocardiogram should always be performed and compared with previous electrocardiograms. If there is any evidence for acute myocardial ischemia, patients should be considered for hospitalization, and acute myocardial infarction should be excluded. The importance of acute coronary events as a trigger for sudden death in patients with heart failure has likely been underappreciated (94).

Superimposed infections are well known to provide the nidus for acute decompensation. Even so-called simple viral illnesses can present a severe stress to the already compromised cardiovascular system of patients with advanced heart failure. Bronchial pneumonia is still a common cause of death in patients with chronic heart failure, and any

TABLE 88.3 CAUSES OF ACUTE DECOMPENSATION OF CHRONIC HEART FAILURE

Acute myocardial ischemia
Uncorrected high blood pressure
Obesity
Superimposed infection
Atrial fibrillation and other arrhythmias
Excessive alcohol consumption
Endocrine abnormalities (e.g., diabetes mellitus, hyperthyroidism, hypothyroidism)
Negative inotropic drugs (e.g., verapamil, nifedipine, diltiazem, beta-adrenergic blockers)
Nonsteroidal antiinflammatory drugs
Treatment and Na+ noncompliance; lack of information given to patient about diet, medications, etc.

infectious process occurring in the setting of decompensated heart failure may well be an indication for hospitalization and more aggressive therapy.

The onset of atrial fibrillation is well known to precipitate decompensation of previously stable heart failure. Although it is still not entirely clear if atrial fibrillation predicts an overall worse prognosis, ample anecdotal experience would suggest that the onset of new atrial fibrillation is often accompanied by worsening heart failure. With the loss of atrial contribution, cardiac output may be further reduced. Additionally, an excess ventricular response to the atrial fibrillation and inadequate filling of the left ventricle can both be contributory factors toward acute decompensation. When the atrial fibrillation is of 48 hours or more in duration, chronic anticoagulation with warfarin is usually indicated. Aggressive attempts toward restoration of normal sinus rhythm are sometimes in order, including the need for hospitalization and electrical cardioversion. In some cases, atrial fibrillation becomes chronic and is resistant to preventive antiarrhythmic therapy. In such cases, control of the heart rate may be the best strategy for the patient's well-being. Although digoxin has long been used to control heart rate in this setting, it may not be particularly effective in patients with heart failure who demonstrate excessive sympathetic activity. Agents with negative inotropic properties, such as beta-adrenergic blockers and diltiazem, are sometimes required as adjunctive therapy to digitalis. Low-dose amiodarone is sometimes highly effective in preventing recurrent atrial fibrillation in patients with advanced heart failure. A rapid ventricular response to atrial fibrillation that is sustained can cause heart failure, and atrioventricular node ablation should be considered in such patients (95).

Patients who acutely decompensate should always be queried on the excessive use of alcohol. Many patients are unfamiliar with the concept of alcoholic cardiomyopathy and need intensive education with regard to potential detrimental effects of alcohol in the setting of advanced heart failure. For patients with severe heart failure, it is probably prudent to recommend complete abstinence, although recently this has been called into question (96). It should be remembered that there is an epidemiologic link between chronic alcohol use and systemic hypertension, a situation to be clearly avoided in the patient with advanced heart failure. Patients with chronic alcoholism may have a tendency early to have abnormal ejection with a dilated ventricle, LV hypertrophy, and impaired LV relaxation (97).

Poorly controlled diabetes mellitus, hyperthyroidism, or hypothyroidism can all lead to acute decompensation of heart failure. Signs and symptoms of hypothyroidism can be difficult to elicit and/or can even be masked by episodes of depression and chronic fatigue. Poorly controlled diabetes mellitus can lead to substantial abnormalities in fluid and electrolyte balance and must always be aggressively corrected. In each case of acute decompensation of heart failure, possible endocrine or metabolic causes should be pursued.

Perhaps one of the commonest causes of worsening heart failure is noncompliance with drug therapy and dietary indiscretion. In general, medication compliance is approximately 75% in patients with heart failure, somewhat better than with hypertension. Nevertheless, patients must continually be educated about their medications and the need to take them on a regular basis. The importance of diet should be continually stressed. The most common cause for "diuretic resistance" is excessive dietary sodium, which can easily go unnoticed by the patient.

It is extremely important that the physician caring for the patient with heart failure be aware of the patient's full medication repertoire, including prescribed drugs and over-the-counter agents. Medications that are knowingly associated with negative inotropy, such as the first-generation calcium channel blockers and beta-adrenergic blockers, should be reduced or sometimes discontinued in the face of worsening heart failure. Nonsteroidal antiinflammatory agents are frequently a cause of excessive sodium and water retention and may offset the use of potent loop diuretics. Patients with advanced heart failure should be discouraged from using either prescribed or over-the-counter nonsteroidal antiinflammatory drugs. Such agents are well known to be associated with hemodynamic compromise (98).

MECHANISMS OF LEFT VENTRICULAR DYSFUNCTION

Abnormalities of Chamber Function

Heart failure is a very common clinical syndrome, but the pathophysiologic factors that affect chamber function vary considerably among patients. In my experience, coronary artery disease remains the most common cause of heart failure, although systemic hypertension continues to be the most common risk factor for heart failure in the Framingham studies (119). Differences between clinical trial patients and population-based cohorts may explain such differences, as well as difficulties with defining heart failure. Dilated cardiomyopathy and valvular heart disease also continue to be common causes of chronic heart failure.

The fundamental abnormality of the heart in the syndrome of heart failure is a diminished ability of the failing muscle to develop force and shorten at a given velocity and at specified loading conditions. The decreased velocity of shortening is conceptually related to the observed decrease in the maximal rate of force development. In general, there is little or no change in the passive length–tension relations of isolated failing heart muscle. Despite this, there can be dramatic changes in the passive pressure–volume relationship of the intact ventricle. Another elastic property of the heart muscle, the series elastic element, also does not appear to be grossly changed in the failing heart muscle. However, the failing left ventricle is exquisitely sensitive to afterload conditions (Fig. 88.1).

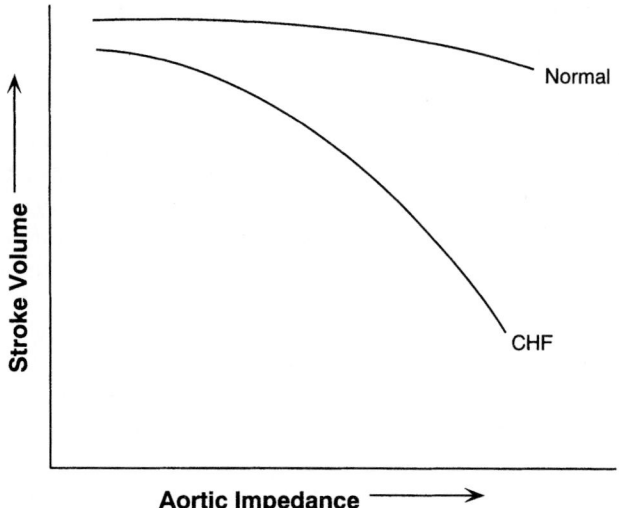

FIGURE 88.1 A hallmark of heart failure is the exquisite sensitivity of the left ventricle to an afterload stress. As impedance to ejection is raised, there is an impressive reduction in left ventricular performance. CHF, congestive heart failure.

To improve myocardial performance, several compensatory mechanisms are activated. One of these (previously discussed briefly) is the Frank-Starling mechanism, in which an increased preload enhances contractile force. The relationship between muscle length and the development of tension in cardiac muscle represents the basis of Starling's law of the heart. The dependence of the development of tension on muscle length arises from several observations, the most important of which is length-dependent activation of cardiac myofibrils by calcium. This effect is believed to be due to a change in the calcium sensitivity of the myofibrils. The failing heart does not generate a normal increase in force development when preload is enhanced (Fig. 88.2). Thus, Starling's mechanism fails to improve myocardial performance as much as normally expected in the failing heart (120). This becomes apparent clinically when it is noted that diuretic treatment, which reduces preload, is not necessarily accompanied by a diminishment in stroke volume. Experimentally, it has also been noted that the Frank-Starling mechanism is exhausted in dogs with rapid pacing–induced chronic dilation (121). In these animals, the application of an acute volume load fails to elicit a further increase in cardiac output or stroke volume, further substantiating a reduction in the Frank-Starling mechanism. Difference in the length-dependent force development in the failing heart may be due to either a change of calcium sensitivity in the myofibrils or an altered amount of calcium supplied to the myofibrils. Because contractile proteins are basically unchanged in severe heart failure, alterations in filament-regulatory proteins such as troponin T or troponin I and other isoform changes may play some role (122).

It seems extraordinary that despite decades of investigations into the mechanism of heart failure, there still is not a coherent understanding of the precise sequence of events whereby LV performance is progressively diminished. Undoubtedly, multiple mechanisms are operative, including abnormalities of phenotypic gene expression, as yet imprecisely understood metabolic changes, and critically important peripheral adaptations, including activation of various neurohormones. The complexities inherent in the syndrome of heart failure make it unlikely that any single therapy is likely to emerge as solely effective. Current therapeutic strategies using polypharmacy to treat heart failure are consistent with this observation.

LEFT VENTRICULAR REMODELING

Ventricular remodeling is an alteration in the contour or volume of the ventricular cavity that is not attributed to

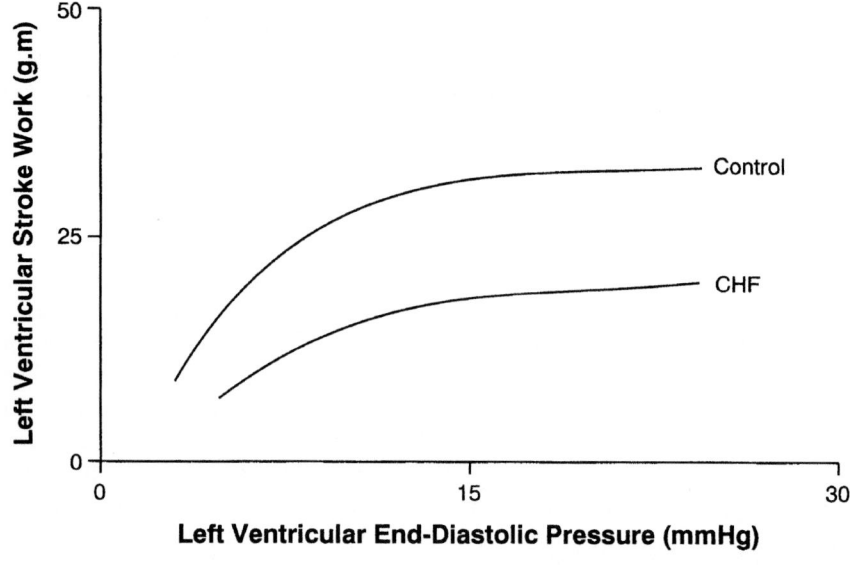

FIGURE 88.2 The Frank-Starling mechanism is altered in heart failure. The failing ventricle is unable to respond to an increase in preload with a normal increase in left ventricular stroke work. CHF, congestive heart failure.

acute changes in distending pressure (123). Cardiomegaly occurs and leads to a dilated and thinned-out left ventricle, a common but very complex finding in patients with congestive heart failure. The mechanism whereby LV remodeling occurs has been the subject of intensive study during the past decade (124,125). Multiple mechanisms drive this process, including myocyte loss, replacement scarring, and reactive growth mechanisms in the remaining viable cells. Although the early sequence of events at the molecular level are still not unraveled, much clinical and experimental data support the old concept that ventricular dilatation after myocardial infarction is a most accurate predictor of an unfavorable long-term prognosis (126,127).

The classic setting of LV remodeling occurs after an acute myocardial infarction. The infarcted territory may exhibit abnormal contraction patterns during systole, and this may ultimately lead to a progressive alteration in the shape of the ventricle. Although many investigators have suggested that LV remodeling represents an adaptive process serving to preserve stroke volume and cardiac output, it is now clear that the enlargement process has very deleterious long-term effects (123). With acute myocardial infarction, the extent of LV remodeling is very dependent on the size of the infarction as well as the location and depth of the acute myocardial injury. Immediately after myocardial infarction, sometimes within hours, there can be "infarct expansion," which is an important complication and is associated with increased mortality. Infarct expansion is caused by acute dilatation and thinning of the area of infarction that is not explained by additional myocardial necrosis (128). Although the process of infarct expansion is still incompletely understood, it is believed that wall thinning occurs due to slippage between myocyte bundles as well as loss of intracellular space (129). This process can be detected clinically by echocardiogram and is more common in patients experiencing acute transmural infarction of the anterior apical left ventricle (130). In long-term studies, it is the extent of LV end systolic volume that has the most important prognostic power, even more so than the extent of underlying coronary artery disease.

Mechanisms of Progressive Left Ventricular Remodeling

Unlike infarct expansion, LV remodeling is the slowly progressive increment in volume of the heart that occurs over a prolonged period after acute myocardial injury (*e*Fig. 88.2.1) (131). Stroke volume may be preserved by augmenting cavity size, but this occurs at a significant cost. According to the Laplace principle, LV enlargement is accompanied by an increase in wall stress. Wall stress then serves as a stimulus for compensatory myocardial hypertrophy. In addition to mechanical stresses that drive the remodeling process, there are probably also important neuroendocrine signals that act in an autocrine or a paracrine

TABLE 88.4 FACTORS THAT CONTRIBUTE TO LEFT VENTRICULAR REMODELING

Neurohormones and cytokines
Increased left ventricular volume and pressure
Myocardial cell elongation
Replacement and reactive collagen deposition (i.e., increased collagen turnover)
Myocyte slippage secondary to dissolution of collagen struts
Apoptosis
Necrosis
Myocardial infarct expansion
Dilation and reshaping of left ventricle

fashion to augment myocardial cellular hypertrophy (132–135). Experimentally, and in human dilated ventricles, it is now clear that cardiac myocytes increase in length shortly after acute myocardial injury (136,137). This increase in the length of the myocyte cell is largely due to so-called eccentric hypertrophy, or an increase in the number of sarcomeres in series. A suggestion has been made that the elongated cell is structurally inadequate and may contribute to the heart failure syndrome (138), although direct proof in support of this hypothesis is still lacking. Factors that contribute to LV remodeling are shown in Table 88.4.

Patency of the infarct-related artery is also important in protecting against LV enlargement (139,140). The presence of antegrade blood flow through the infarct-related artery, either by collaterals or by reperfusion therapy, tends to protect against the development of LV wall motion abnormalities and progressive dilatation of the left ventricle (141–143). o68

NEUROENDOCRINE ABNORMALITIES

It has been known for many years that heart failure is characterized by activation of a number of neuroendocrine systems (Table 88.5) (12,14). Activation of neurohormones in heart failure has long been considered to be an "adaptive" process, perhaps a response to a fall in cardiac output and an attempt to maintain blood pressure. The perceived threat to circulatory homeostasis is similar to that of volume depletion, even though blood volume is usually increased in patients with heart failure. The sympathetic nervous system is activated, there is activation of the systemic renin-angiotensin-aldosterone system, and in many patients there is a release of AVP. The extent of neuroendocrine activations varies widely from patient to patient, but in general there appears to be a gradual incremental change during the evolution from LV dysfunction to overt heart failure (21) (Fig. 88.3). For many years, and to some extent still today, there has been a serious question as to whether these neuroendocrine changes represent simple markers (epiphenomena) or whether they actually contribute to the pathogenesis of the heart failure syndrome. In all likelihood, neuroendocrine activation makes an important con-

TABLE 88.5 NEUROENDOCRINE FACTORS KNOWN TO BE INCREASED IN PATIENTS WITH HEART FAILURE

Norepinephrine	Endothelin
Epinephrine	Beta-endorphins
Renin activity	Calcitonin gene–related peptide
Angiotensin II	Growth hormone
Aldosterone	Cortisol
Arginine vasopressin	Tumor necrosis factor-α
Neuropeptide Y	Neurokinin A
Vasoactive intestinal peptide	Substance P
Prostaglandins	Adrenomedullin
Atrial natriuretic factor	Brain natriuretic peptide

tribution to the pathogenesis of heart failure. This statement is based on the fact that activation occurs very early in the course of the illness, even in the asymptomatic stage (21), and therapies designed to block neuroendocrine activation, such as ACE inhibitors and beta-adrenergic blockers, have had a favorable effect on the natural history of the illness (160).

It is generally believed that a number of vasopressor/sodium-retaining peptides or hormones dominate the end stages of heart failure. These include norepinephrine (marked activation of the sympathetic nervous system), angiotensin II and aldosterone, AVP, and endothelin. There are also counterregulatory vasodilators/natriuretic peptides that are released in a presumed attempt to offset excessive peripheral vasoconstriction and salt and water retention. These natriuretic peptides include ANF, BNP, and adrenomedullin. Prostaglandins are also increased, at least locally within the kidney, to maintain homeostasis of renal blood flow and intraglomerular hydraulic pressure. On balance, however, there appears in most cases a dominance of

heightened peripheral vascular resistance with sodium and water retention. In all likelihood, the increase in ventricular afterload, coupled with the inability to normally excrete salt and water, contributes importantly to worsening pump failure and circulatory congestion.

The mechanisms responsible for neuroendocrine activation in the syndrome of heart failure have been the subject of numerous studies. It is still unclear how the sympathetic nervous system is activated, although some investigators have suggested that altered reflex control mechanisms are at least partly responsible for excessive sympathetic drive. However, the fundamental signals that are responsible for altered reflex control mechanisms and the incremental change in sympathetic activity remain poorly understood. This lack of insight has impaired, to some extent, our therapeutic attempts to directly block neuroendocrine activation, forcing therapists to rely on drugs that inhibit neuroendocrine responses.

Abnormalities of the Sympathetic Nervous System

There is now direct evidence that increased central sympathetic nerve outflow occurs in patients with heart failure and is associated with an increase in plasma norepinephrine (20). In general, the greater the activation of the sympathetic nervous system, the worse the prognosis (*e*Fig. 88.3.1). A single resting venous blood sample of plasma norepinephrine concentration provides a better guide to prognosis than many of the other commonly measured indexes of cardiac performance (18,166). Because hemodynamic abnormalities do not correlate well with levels of plasma norepinephrine, a direct causal link between heightened sympathetic activity

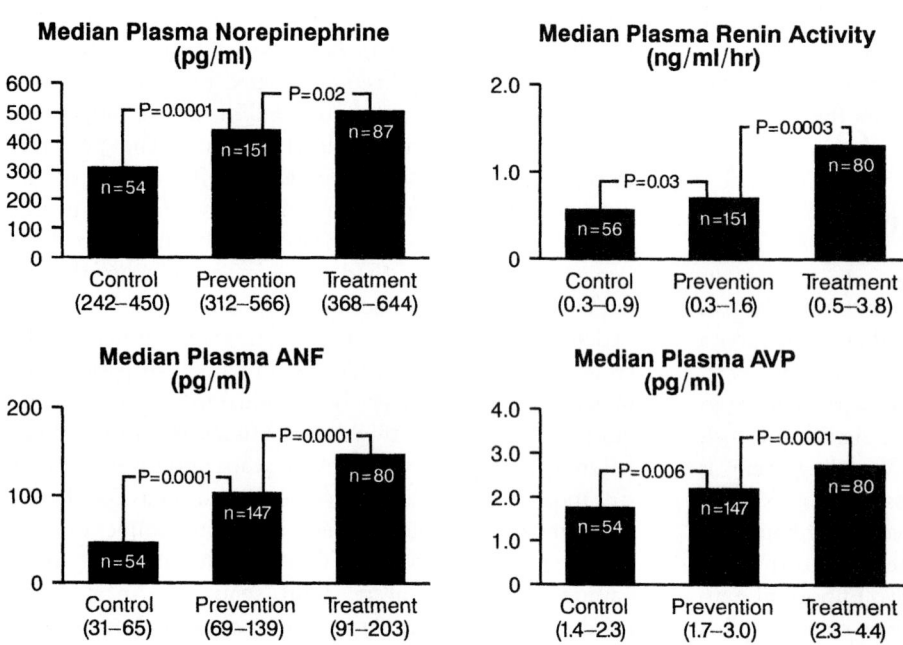

FIGURE 88.3 Data from the Studies of Left Ventricular Dysfunction substudy of baseline neurohormones. There is a progressive incremental rise in neurohormones as patients pass from the asymptomatic left ventricular dysfunction phase (prevention) to overt heart failure (treatment), suggesting that neurohormone activation may precede the onset of symptomatic heart failure. ANF, atrial natriuretic factor; AVP, arginine vasopressin. (From Francis GS, Benedict C, Johnstone DE, et al. Comparison of neuroendocrine activation in patients with left ventricular dysfunction with and without congestive heart failure. *Circulation* 1990;82:1724–1729, and the American Heart Association, with permission.)

and LV dysfunction has been difficult to substantiate. Moreover, there is a relatively loose correlation between plasma norepinephrine and PRA, suggesting that the two systems are independently activated in heart failure (167). However, it is well known that sympathetic stimulation may be one factor contributing to renin release.

It is now believed that both increased neuronal release of norepinephrine and decreased efficiency of neuronal norepinephrine reuptake contribute to decreased cardiac adrenergic drive in congestive heart failure (168). Diminished norepinephrine stores in the failing heart are likely due to chronically increased norepinephrine turnover and reduced efficiency of norepinephrine reuptake in storage. In the short term, the adrenergic nervous system is important in supporting the failing circulation in patients with heart failure. However, in the long term, excessive sympathetic activity is likely making a major contribution to progressive LV dysfunction. It is well known that high levels of catecholamines are directly toxic to the myocardium (169,170). Cardiac norepinephrine spillover rate is perhaps the single most powerful prognostic neuroendocrine marker for patients destined to do poorly (171). It is the marked increase in norepinephrine spillover from the heart, or excessive sympathetic nerve firing, that is the dominant mechanism of heightened sympathetic activity, rather than faulty neuronal reuptake of norepinephrine (172). Adrenal medullary activity is also increased in patients with heart failure leading to increased plasma epinephrine concentrations, particularly toward the end stages of the disease. The fact that skin sympathetic nerve activity (in contrast to muscle sympathetic nerve activity) is not increased in heart failure supports the concept that altered reflex systems (which have nonuniform effects on muscle and skin sympathetic activity) may underlie much of the sympathoexcitation found in patients with heart failure (173). There is also increased central nervous system turnover of both norepinephrine and epinephrine in patients with heart failure (174), perhaps related to epinephrine neurons in the brain. The fact that norepinephrine kinetics return to normal after heart transplantation would suggest that many of the abnormalities of the sympathetic nervous system in heart failure are functional and to some extent reversible (175).

It is now believed that excessive sympathetic drive to the heart in patients with heart failure is responsible for downregulation of the beta$_1$-receptor and perhaps uncoupling of the beta$_2$-receptor (118). Isolated papillary muscles from pretransplant patients have been demonstrated to be nearly devoid of membrane beta-adrenergic receptors but respond normally to calcium. It has been hypothesized that receptor downregulation of the beta$_1$-receptor and uncoupling of the beta$_2$-receptor is more likely due to excessive local concentrations of norepinephrine and not due to high circulating levels of catecholamines.

The fact that excessive sympathetic stimulation has been repeatedly demonstrated in patients with heart failure and

that patients respond to agents that knowingly inhibit excessive neuroendocrine activity would support the contention that neurohormonal activation is a critical factor in the pathogenesis of heart failure. These observations have stimulated a change in thinking away from drugs designed to have direct positive inotropic effects to those that secondarily improve cardiac function via inhibition of the sympathetic nervous system and the renin-angiotensin-aldosterone system.

Renin-Angiotensin-Aldosterone System

As with the sympathetic nervous system, it has been known for many years that the renin-angiotensin-aldosterone system is activated in patients with heart failure (Fig. 88.4) (7,12,14,176). Unlike the sympathetic nervous system, activation of the renin-angiotensin-aldosterone system is less obvious in patients with minimally symptomatic LV dysfunction (21). However, as heart failure progresses, there are profound incremental changes in circulating renin, angiotensin II, and aldosterone (177,178). Moreover, there are now substantial data to support the concept of a tissue renin-angiotensin-aldosterone system, which may play a critical role in both myocardial and vascular remodeling (179,180). A number of factors are responsible for the release of renin (Table 88.6). Decreased perfusion to the

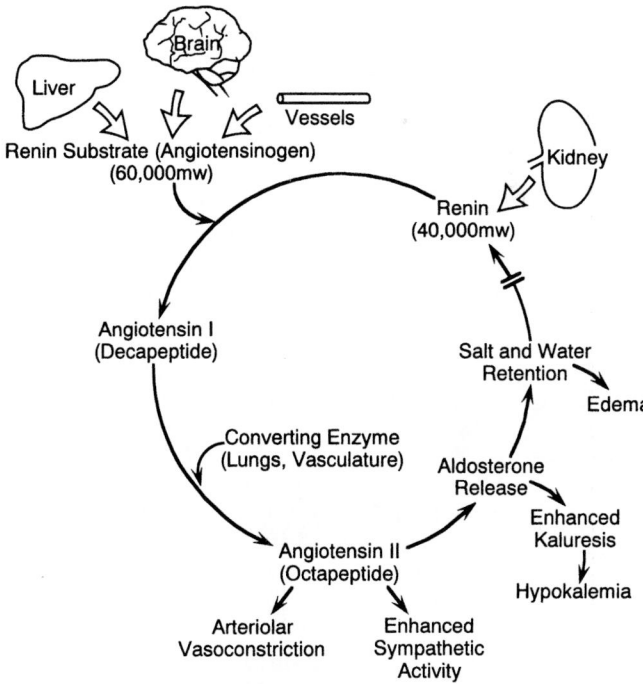

FIGURE 88.4 The circulating renin-angiotensin-aldosterone system. Angiotensinogen and renin produce a small decapeptide, angiotensin I, which is cleaved to angiotensin II by a converting enzyme. Angiotensin II, in turn, causes vasoconstriction, enhanced sympathetic nervous system activity, and aldosterone release. Increased salt and water retention expands circulating volume, which normally reduces renin release.

TABLE 88.6 FACTORS THAT RELEASE RENIN

Renal artery baroreceptor activity
Renal hypoperfusion
Hyponatremic perfusate to the macula densa
Volume contraction secondary to diuretics and salt restriction
Stimulation of beta-adrenergic receptors in the kidney

kidney with an accompanying reduction in the renal tubular concentrations of sodium and chloride ions in the macula densa can activate the renin-angiotensin-aldosterone system. Increased activity of the sympathetic nervous system is also a potent stimulus for renin-angiotensin-aldosterone system activation. The institution of a low-sodium diet, vasodilator therapy, and diuretics are all known to further activate the renin-angiotensin system.

Angiotensin II is known to be a potent vasoconstrictor substance and also acts on the adrenal cortex to release aldosterone, a mineralocorticoid with potent sodium retentive properties (Fig. 88.5). Hypokalemia and hypomagnesemia often occur in the setting of heart failure, in part induced by the use of powerful diuretics. The combination of excessive adrenergic nervous system drive and hypokalemia is believed to predispose patients to lethal cardiac arrhythmias, from which nearly 30% to 50% of patients with severe heart failure die suddenly. The effectiveness of ACE inhibitors is in part related to their ability to block excessive angiotensin II activity, thus reducing some of the pathoexcitatory drive and diminishing the hypokalemic and hypomagnesemic effects of aldosterone in the kidney. Converting enzyme inhibitor therapy also increases local concentrations of bradykinin, which in principle may have antiremodeling effects on the heart and contribute to vasodilation. Both excessive adrenergic nervous system activity and an overly active renin-angiotensin-aldosterone system are believed to contribute to progressive remodeling of the left ventricle and may form the underpinnings of the important transition from myocardial hypertrophy to myocardial failure. The precise molecular and cellular abnormalities that are operative in this important transition have yet to be elucidated.

Atrial Natriuretic Factor

ANF is a naturally occurring hormone that has been demonstrated to be increased in several pathologic states, including hypertension and heart failure (26). Several different molecular forms of ANF have been isolated, but it is alpha-ANF that represents the major circulating form in humans. Synthesis of ANF occurs predominantly in the atria, where right atrial stretch appears to be an important stimulus for release. The peptide has also been identified in several other tissues, including ventricular myocardium. It is now known that the ANF gene is not expressed fully until late in embryonic life and after birth. However, there is heightened expression of the ANF gene in ventricular myocardium during hypertrophy and cardiomyopathy (209). It is believed that the reemergence of the fetal capacity to synthesize ANF in the setting of ventricular overload in hypertrophy represents an adaptive response to maintain volume homeostasis in response to the failing circulation. As with many other neuropeptides, ANF is progressively released into the circulation during the transition from asymptomatic LV dysfunction to overt heart failure (21). The peptide has vasodilatory

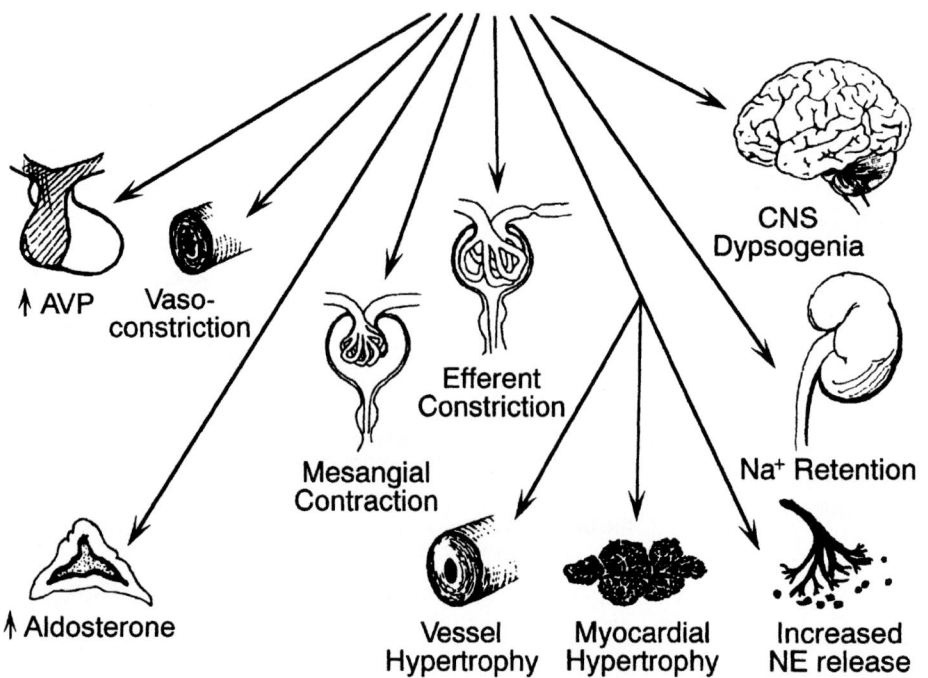

FIGURE 88.5 Angiotensin II has a vast array of biologic activities. These include release of arginine vasopressin (AVP) from the posterior pituitary, peripheral arteriole vasoconstriction, release of aldosterone from the adrenal cortex, mesangial contraction, constriction of the efferent glomerular arterioles, vascular hypertrophy, myocardial hypertrophy, facilitation of norepinephrine (NE) release from sympathetic neurons, sodium retention, and thirst sensation. CNS, central nervous system. (From Francis GS. The relationship of the sympathetic nervous system and the renin-angiotensin system in congestive heart failure. *Am Heart J* 1989;118:642–648, with permission.)

properties and can thereby potentially improve cardiac function. It also may inhibit aldosterone secretion in patients with heart failure (210). Although it is a potent natriuretic, the renal effects of ANF appear to be attenuated during progressive heart failure. NEPs, which are highly concentrated in the proximal tubule brush border of the kidney, are responsible for degradation of ANF. This concept has driven the development of NEP inhibitors, some of which are hybrid molecules that include ACE inhibitors, of which omapatrilat is now in clinical trials for treatment of hypertension and heart failure.

In addition to the cardiovascular, renal, and neuroendocrine effects of ANF, the peptide may also have a moderating effect on cell growth (211). Unlike vasoconstrictor peptides, which tend to increase afterload, promote cell growth, and promote retention of salt and water, ANF appears to have important vasodilator properties, may be antigrowth *in vitro*, and has the ability to attenuate neuroendocrine activation and promote natriuresis. It is therefore part of a counterregulatory system that to some extent offsets excessive sympathetic nervous system and renin-angiotensin system activity. Although ANF has not itself become established as a therapeutic drug for heart failure, NEP inhibitors are potentially very important therapy for heart failure and hypertension, particularly when combined with ACE inhibitors (212).

Brain Natriuretic Peptide and C-Type Natriuretic Peptide

BNP was first isolated from the brains of pigs and forms a peptide family with ANF that is involved in the regulation of blood pressure and fluid volume (213). Plasma levels of BNP mainly reflect the degree of LV overload, and the secretion patterns of ANF and BNP vary with underlying cardiac disorders. BNP has been isolated from both brain and heart, whereas C-type natriuretic peptide is purified from porcine brain (214,215). Like ANF, both CNP and BNP can elicit vasorelaxant activity. All three natriuretic peptides share a common structural motif consisting of a 17-amino-acid loop formed by an intermolecular disulfide linkage bridge. When BNP is infused into humans with heart failure, urine volume significantly increases, excretion of sodium is enhanced, and plasma levels of BNP are increased (216). As with ANF, BNP causes a decrease in plasma aldosterone concentrations. Hemodynamic changes with BNP include an increase in heart rate, a decrease in blood pressure, as well as reduction in pulmonary capillary wedge pressure with little or no change in stroke volume index (217). Nesiritide, a human synthetic BNP, is currently approved as an infusion therapy for acute heart failure (218,219). Like ANF, BNP appears to be predominantly synthesized and secreted from the heart. BNP infusion also causes beneficial hemodynamic and neuroendocrine effects during exercise in patients with diastolic heart failure (220). It has been suggested that BNP, when persistently elevated, is a marker for poor long-term prognosis after acute myocardial infarction (184) and may serve as an important marker for ventricular dysfunction and myocardial hypertrophy. Perhaps the most exciting development is the use of BNP as a diagnostic marker for elevated LV filling pressures (31–33) and the potential to use bedside kits to quantitatively measure the response of circulating BNP to therapy. If successful, this strategy may obviate the need for invasive monitoring in some patients.

DISTURBANCES OF SALT AND WATER CONTROL

It has been understood by generations of physicians that heart failure is characterized by excessive sodium and water retention, but the mechanisms that underlie this observation continue to be elusive. It is unlikely that any single mechanism accounts for the maintenance of normal sodium balance. Patients with very severe heart failure have glomerular filtration reduced to approximately one-half of normal and renal blood flow reduced to approximately one-fifth of normal, suggesting that there is a considerable diversion of blood away from the kidney. As a result of the lowered filtration rate, a smaller quantity of sodium is probably delivered to the renal tubular cells. However, glomerular filtration rate is not invariably reduced in patients with heart failure, and its preservation is dependent by activation of the renin-angiotensin system (246).

Vasoconstriction and sodium retention are appropriate responses to loss of circulating volume. In heart failure, the kidney is responding to a perceived loss of extracellular fluid and plasma volume. The kidney, therefore, is not the culprit, but the victim. Glomerular filtration may be maintained by the vasoconstrictor effects of angiotensin II on glomerular efferent arterials. In the later stages of heart failure, salt and water retention are enhanced due to the effects of aldosterone and angiotensin II on the kidney. In some cases, vasopressin is released, leading to further reabsorption of free water. Eventually, heightened systemic resistance, circulatory congestion, edema, and hyponatremia become clinically manifested.

The primary signal that the kidney receives to initiate salt and water retention has remained elusive. It is not known what initiates the signal, nor is it understood where the signal is processed. Early studies by Barger observed that sodium excretion alterations are detected even in the mildest forms of experimental heart failure, before venous pressure is even changed (247). Abnormalities of cardiac output may not necessarily precede the increase in salt and water retention. These findings would suggest that sodium excretion abnormalities occur very early in the syndrome of heart failure, perhaps before there is a major reduction in maximal LV performance (248). Clearly, a reduction in cardiac output alone is not sufficient to cause sodium retention.

One of the major determinants of sodium retention is activation of the renin-angiotensin system. But there is only a rough correlation among hemodynamic measurements, the renin-angiotensin system, and urinary sodium excretion in patients with heart failure. Undoubtedly, neural and humoral pathways involve physical adjustments in renal microvascular hemodynamics, tubule fluid composition, flow rate, and tubular ion gradients, but these interactions are highly complex and difficult to precisely characterize (249).

Despite the lack of a penetrating understanding of how the initiation of salt and water retention occurs in heart failure, it does seem rather clear that the kidney perceives, in some way, a threat to the arterial blood pressure. There is a very consistent response to this perceived threat, with activation of baroreceptor reflexes, increases in sympathetic nervous system activity, and enhanced activity of the renin-angiotensin-aldosterone system. Ultimately, the increase in sympathetic nervous system activity may be coupled to reduced renal blood flow, thus leading to the nonosmotic release of vasopressin and other neurohormones. The net effect of these changes is an expansion of the extracellular volume, which helps to maintain blood pressure. Increased blood volume, in turn, acts as a negative feedback message to reduce the renin-angiotensin-aldosterone response, thus accounting for some of the observed heterogeneity in the renin-angiotensin-aldosterone system in patients with early heart failure.

To some extent, the expanded blood volume and intracardiac pressures lead to counterregulatory steps, including the release of ANF and other natriuretic peptides that have important endogenous natriuretic and vasodilator properties. However, the effects of the various natriuretic peptides on the kidney seem to be diminished as the syndrome of heart failure progresses. Ultimately, the effects of the natriuretic peptides are overwhelmed by opposing influences, and the overall effect is one of salt and water retention. It seems fortunate for the patient that our knowledge of how to treat salt and water retention has probably surpassed our understanding of the fundamental mechanisms that cause edema formation (250).

ABNORMALITIES OF THE PERIPHERAL CIRCULATION

It is now recognized that the maladaptive changes in the peripheral vasculature and skeletal muscle of patients with heart failure are largely responsible for symptoms of exercise intolerance. In the peripheral vasculature, impaired vasodilator capacity results from enhanced vessel wall stiffness, endothelial dysfunction, and other structural abnormalities. Blood vessels of patients with heart failure are generally more vasoconstricted. Initially, the vasoconstriction is minimal and somewhat selective as the body strives to redistribute blood flow between organs to maintain cir-

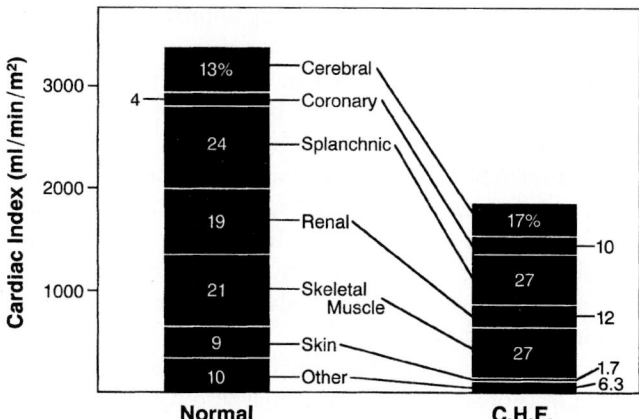

FIGURE 88.6 Cardiac output at rest. The normal distribution of cardiac index and the distribution of flow in heart failure. Renal and skin blood flow are markedly reduced in heart failure, whereas flow to the brain, heart, splanchnic bed, and skeletal muscles is preserved. CHF, congestive heart failure. (From Zelis R, Nellis SH, Longhurst J, et al. Abnormalities in the regional circulations accompanying congestive heart failure. *Prog Cardiovasc Dis* 1975;18:181–199, with permission.)

culatory efficiency (Fig. 88.6) (251). However, over time, vasoconstriction becomes excessive in an attempt to protect blood pressure. Only the coronary and cerebral circulations are spared. The vasoconstriction ultimately becomes inappropriate and increases aortic impedance, thus placing a further burden on the already failing heart.

Although the cause of the heightened vasoconstrictor tone in heart failure is not entirely clear, it appears to be related to increased circulating catecholamines, particularly norepinephrine, as well as to other vasoconstrictors, including angiotensin II, vasopressin, and possibly endothelin. The abnormal redistribution of blood flow that occurs at rest is accentuated by exercise in patients with heart failure (251). Maximum metabolic vasodilation is significantly reduced. The increased sodium content of the vessels accounts for some of the vascular stiffness observed in heart failure. There is also heightened venous tone. Ultimately, the limited arteriolar dilator capacity results in a relative skeletal muscle hypoxia that may, through a reflex arc, lead to further sympathetic tone.

Although the increase in vascular resistance in heart failure is obvious, it is only partially explained by neurogenic and humoral stimuli. More recently, interest has focused on endothelial function, which is well known to be impaired in heart failure (252). Endogenous NO is known to be increased in patients with heart failure (253,254) and correlates with the severity of the syndrome as measured by the New York Heart Association functional class (255). It is believed that increased NO production in heart failure may compensate to some extent for the excessive vasoconstrictor adaptation. Despite an elevated basal release of NO and its role in depressing cardiac function, there is evidence to suggest that the peripheral vasculature has impaired release of

NO on stimulation, which may play a role in inadequate vasodilator responses to exercise (256). In support of this hypothesis, there are data to suggest that oral L-arginine, when given in a supplemental fashion to patients with heart failure, has a beneficial effect by increasing forearm blood flow, improving the distances as walked during the 6-minute walk test, and improving quality of life as measured by a questionnaire (257). Dysfunction of the endothelium may persist and worsen as heart failure progresses, as evidenced by diminished vasodilator responses to acetylcholine and attenuated hyperemic responses to exercise and ischemia, both of which are largely endothelium-dependent. Of interest, heart transplantation results in some reversal of impaired vasodilation, but it is delayed and incomplete (258).

In summary, congestive heart failure is characterized by abnormal peripheral vascular blood flow distribution with diminished hepatic, renal, and limb flow. The changes in peripheral blood flow are proportional and linearly related to the reduction in cardiac output. Vascular resistance is increased and is related to circulating catecholamines, angiotensin II, and AVP. Additionally, there appears to be significant impairment of NO release due to endothelial dysfunction, which probably accounts for some of the exercise intolerance noted in patients with heart failure. A generalized inability to maximally dilate a response to various stimuli characterizes the abnormal circulatory response, which may be corrected to some extent by medical therapy and heart transplantation.

EXERCISE INTOLERANCE IN HEART FAILURE

One of the hallmarks of the syndrome of heart failure is exercise intolerance. Although exercise tolerance is associated with LV systolic dysfunction, numerous studies have suggested that the extent of LV dysfunction bears little correlation to it (259–263). Moreover, it has been demonstrated that short-term administration of positive inotropic agents and vasodilators, which acutely improve LV performance, do not improve maximal exercise capacity in patients with heart failure (264). Even agents that are knowingly effective for the long-term therapy of heart failure, such as ACE inhibitors, have failed to consistently demonstrate improvement in exercise tolerance. The reasons for this are not entirely understood but may be related to inadequate methodology. The maximal exercise test may not be very representative of the daily activities of patients suffering from advanced heart failure (264). Maximal exercise testing is also somewhat subjective in that motivational factors and the experience of the operator/investigator can influence the end point. Because of this, the anaerobic threshold may be a more objective end point, but it is sometimes difficult to demonstrate, even with sophisticated gas exchange techniques. The simple 6-minute walk test is highly correlated to overall prognosis and seems to be emerging as an important measurement of exercise tolerance (265).

Maximal oxygen consumption is characterized by a plateau in oxygen uptake despite an increasing work rate (64). It is highly reproducible in normal subjects but can be difficult to determine in patients with advanced heart failure. The regional distribution of cardiac output during exercise is regulated by a complex interaction between the sympathetic nervous system, regional vasoactive factors including metaboreceptors, and endothelial-derived vasoactive substances including NO. The extent of widening of the arteriovenous oxygen difference is determined by increasing oxygen extraction in the exercising skeletal muscles. This in turn is somewhat dependent on capillary density, the number of open capillaries, and the transit time of the red blood cells through the capillaries. These complexities, coupled to the notorious difficulty in making accurate measurements during maximal exercise, have made it difficult to understand the precise mechanism of exercise intolerance in patients with heart failure.

In contrast to normal subjects, patients with heart failure do not achieve a plateau in oxygen uptake at the end of exercise. Rather, a "peak" oxygen uptake is determined in patients with heart failure that can be somewhat less reproducible. Whereas normal subjects distribute close to 90% of their total output to exercising skeletal muscle during maximal exercise, patients with heart failure distribute only 50% to 60% of the total cardiac output to exercising muscle. It has been presumed that the maximum caliber of the resistance arterioles is decreased in patients with heart failure due to changes in structure or perhaps vascular remodeling. When blood flow is chronically reduced, as occurs in advanced heart failure, the maximal vasodilator capacity of the peripheral circulation is markedly diminished through a complex sequence of events. These events include neurohormonal activation, diminished endothelial function related to impaired synthesis of NO, increased synthesis of endothelin, and possibly activation of cytokines and local factors that may further reduce arteriolar diameter. Patients with heart failure compensate for the reduced perfusion by widening their arteriovenous oxygen difference. Complete oxygen extraction can occur in the exercising skeletal muscle beds of patients with heart failure. This compensatory increase in oxygen extraction by skeletal muscles is similar to that observed in highly trained athletes. The mechanism of hyperextraction of oxygen is not understood very well. Unlike in well-trained athletes, increased capillary density has not been observed in patients with heart failure. In fact, there may well be diffuse atrophy of the lower extremities with diminished oxidative skeletal muscle fibers and oxidative enzyme content. This paradox remains poorly explained.

The exercise response in heart failure is very complex. Pump function is poorly related to exercise tolerance. Factors in the peripheral musculature, not the central hemodynamics, largely determine shortness of breath and fatigue. These peripheral factors include endothelial function, vasodilator capacity, distribution of cardiac output, heightened chemoreceptor and ergoreceptor sensitivity, skeletal muscle histology, and oxidative enzyme activity. Minute ventilation is markedly increased. There is a higher ventilation for any given carbon dioxide production (VE/VCO_2 slope), which reflects the severity of heart failure and the prognosis. Enhanced ergoreflexes and chemoreceptor responses drive hyperventilation and heightened sympathetic outflow, leading to increased peripheral resistance and a decrease in muscle perfusion.

Reduced muscle endurance can be improved with chronic exercise training in patients with heart failure (266–268). Although drugs such as ACE inhibitors may not improve maximal exercise tolerance in patients with heart failure, they can redistribute blood flow to the skeletal muscles during exercise and thereby improve submaximal exercise tolerance. Changes in skeletal muscle structure and function in heart failure may be related in part to deconditioning (266). Therefore, it is reasonable to recommend that all patients with heart failure continue to be physically active, at least with regard to isotonic activity. On the other hand, isometric activities such as work against gravity, are to be discouraged, because such activities impose an immediate afterload stress on the left ventricle. Reduced physical activity alone, however, does not easily explain the genesis of the skeletal muscle changes observed in heart failure (269). Clearly, we still have much to learn regarding the problem of exercise intolerance in heart failure.

CONTROVERSIES AND PERSONAL PERSPECTIVES

Heart failure remains a problem of growing magnitude in the Western world. It primarily afflicts the older population and is a major drain on scarce medical resources. Although great strides have been made in the past two decades regarding the management of this complex syndrome, much work remains to be done (274–277).

Heart failure is a prime example whereby a clearer understanding of the basic pathophysiology has led to highly specific therapies that are uniformly effective, such as ACE inhibitors and beta-adrenergic blockers. As we delve further into the neuroendocrine and cytokine disturbances in the syndrome, it becomes clear that other potential therapeutic targets are worth developing. Over the years there has been a rather direct course away from drugs designed to stimulate the inotropic state to agents that block excessive neuroendocrine activation pathways. In the future, we can look forward to drugs that are designed to more specifically inhibit the sympathetic nervous system, perhaps through mechanisms other than beta-adrenergic blockade. Drugs designed to block specific ET_A receptors

have recently become available in an oral form (278). Preliminary data would suggest that endothelin blockers may have a primary role in the management of patients with heart failure by causing both a reduction in systemic vascular resistance and by stimulating vasodilator counterregulatory mechanisms. Augmentation of these vasodilator counterregulatory mechanisms is also possible through hybrid molecules that contain both NEP inhibitors and ACE inhibitors. Short-term infusion of peptides such as BNP may also find a role.

It will be useful, perhaps, to clinically screen for asymptomatic LV enlargement. Identification of markers in such patients might enable the early introduction of pharmaceutical interdiction. It is also possible that surgical reduction of a markedly expanded LV cavity will prove to be a valuable adjunct form of therapy. If cell dropout via apoptosis is found to be a dominant mechanism in the transition of LV dilation to overt heart failure, research in this arena may allow for the development of agents that block TNF-α receptor activity, thereby reducing iNOS synthase and blocking apoptosis. Until such agents are available, it is perhaps important to recognize that most cases of heart failure are due to coronary artery disease and hypertension. Many of the consequences of long-term high blood pressure can now be prevented with early identification and aggressive treatment. All physicians need to recognize that LV hypertrophy is a powerful risk factor for heart failure and premature death and should be prevented or controlled when possible. Although the prevention of coronary artery disease is still not fully within our grasp, identification and aggressive control of risk factors are now certainly possible. In the long run, it is through the prevention of heart failure that measurable strides will be made in curbing what is now described as an emerging epidemic. Despite obvious progress, many controversies and uncertainties remain. The role of anticoagulation, especially aspirin, is still debated. The role of myocardial reperfusion on outcome is not entirely clear. The role and costs of polypharmacy remain a challenge. Controversy and uncertainty remain the driving force behind additional study, however, and will continue to serve us well.

CONCLUSIONS

Heart failure is a complex disorder that is still rather poorly understood. An index event occurs, such as acute myocardial infarction or onset of cardiomyopathy, and a host of "adaptations" are staged. Abnormal LV function from any cause appears to stimulate the release of a number of neurohormones and cytokines in an attempt to provide presumed circulatory homeostasis. However, over time neuroendocrine and cytokine activity may become highly maladaptive, contributing to LV remodeling, heightened systemic vascular resistance, and ultimately, worsening heart failure (*e*Fig.

THE FUTURE

Heart failure is a common and highly disabling clinical syndrome. Although advancements have been made in our understanding of the pathogenesis and management of this complex disorder, we are still lacking substantial information regarding fundamental abnormalities, particularly at the cellular level. The mechanisms whereby neurohormones are activated and released are still not explained, but we have the means to abrogate their excessive activity. The underlying myocyte contractile abnormalities that occur on a molecular level are still poorly defined. The precise mechanism leading to exercise intolerance is still debated. Despite these misgivings, it is likely that continued research at both the basic and clinical level will afford clinicians the opportunity to better understand and manage this common clinical syndrome, provided there is sufficient support for basic science as well as clinical investigation. It is likely we will be able to better screen for heart failure via biochemical markers such as BNP, thereby initiating therapy at an earlier stage and thus preventing onset of the full-blown syndrome.

88.6.1). To date, the most impressive long-term effective therapy has been designed to limit excessive neuroendocrine activation, and this is likely where future and more imaginative therapies will also reside.

REFERENCES

1. Hope JA. *Treatise on the diseases of the heart and great vessels.* London: William Kidd, 1832.
2. Starling EH. On the absorption of fluids from the connective tissue spaces. *J Physiol* 1896;312–326.
3. Mackenzie J. *Diseases of the heart,* 3rd ed. Oxford: Oxford Medical Publications, 1913.
4. Starr I, Rawson AJ. Role of the "static blood pressure" in abnormal increments of venous pressure, especially in heart failure. I. Theoretical studies on an improved circulation schema whose pumps obey Starling's law. *Am J Med Sci* 1940;199:27–39.
5. Starr I. Role of the "static blood pressure" in abnormal increments of venous pressure, especially heart failure. II. Clinical and experimental studies. *Am J Med Sci* 1940;199:40–55.
6. Warren JV, Stead EA Jr. Fluid dynamics in chronic congestive heart failure. *Arch Intern Med* 1944;73:138–147.
7. Merrill AJ. Edema and decreased renal blood flow in patients with chronic congestive heart failure: evidence of "forward failure" as the primary cause of edema. *J Clin Invest* 1946;25:389–400.
8. Hickman JB, Cargill WH. Effect of exercise cardiac output and pulmonary arterial pressure in normal persons and in patients with cardiovascular disease and pulmonary emphysema. *J Clin Invest* 1948;27:10–23.
9. Barger AC. The pathogenesis of sodium retention in congestive cardiac failure. *Metabolism* 1956;5:480–489.
10. Watkins L Jr, Burton JA, Haber E, et al. The renin-aldosterone system in congestive failure in conscious dogs. *J Clin Invest* 1976;57:1606–1607.
11. Chidsey CA, Harrison DC, Braunwald E. Augmentation of the plasma norepinephrine response to exercise in patients with congestive heart. *N Engl J Med* 1962;267:650–654.
12. Laragh JH. Hormones and the pathogenesis of congestive heart failure: vasopressin, aldosterone, and angiotensin II. *Circulation* 1962;25:1015–1023.
13. Gaffney TE, Braunwald E. Importance of the adrenergic nervous system in the support of circulatory function in patients with congestive heart failure. *Am J Med* 1963;34:320–324.
14. Genest J, Granger P, DeChamplain J, Boucher R. Endocrine factors in congestive heart failure. *Am J Cardiol* 1968;22:35–42.
15. Burch GE. The role of the central nervous system in chronic congestive heart failure. *Am Heart J* 1978;95:255–261.
16. Thomas JA, Marks BH. Plasma norepinephrine in congestive heart failure. *Am J Cardiol* 1978;41:233–243.
17. Levine TB, Francis GS, Goldsmith SR, et al. Activity of the sympathetic nervous system and renin-angiotensin system assessed by plasma hormone levels and their relation to hemodynamic abnormalities in congestive heart failure. *Am J Cardiol* 1982;49:1659–1666.
18. Cohn JN, Levine B, Olivari MT, et al. Plasma norepinephrine as a guide to prognosis in patients with chronic congestive heart failure. *N Engl J Med* 1984;311:819–823.
19. Francis GS, Goldsmith SR, Levine TB, et al. The neurohumoral axis in congestive heart failure. *Ann Intern Med* 1984;101:370–377.
20. Leimbach WN, Wallin BG, Victor RG, et al. Direct evidence from intraneural recordings for increased central sympathetic outflow in patients with heart failure. *Circulation* 1986;73:913–919.
21. Francis GS, Benedict C, Johnstone DE, et al. Comparison of neuroendocrine activation in patients with left ventricular dysfunction with and without congestive heart failure. *Circulation* 1990;82:1724–1729.
22. Goldsmith SR, Francis GS, Cowley AW, et al. Increased plasma arginine vasopressin levels in patients with congestive heart failure. *J Am Coll Cardiol* 1993;1:1385–1390.
23. Wei C-M, Lerman A, Rodeheffer RJ, et al. Endothelin in human congestive heart failure. *Circulation* 1994;89:1580–1586.
24. Harris P. Evolution and the cardiac patient. *Cardiovasc Res* 1983;17:3–22.
25. Harris P. Congestive cardiac failure: central role of the arterial blood pressure. *Br Heart J* 1987;58:190–203.

26. Burnett JC, Kao PC, Hu DC, et al. Atrial natriuretic peptide elevation in congestive heart failure in the human. *Science* 1986;231:1145–1147.

27. Peterson TS, Benjamin BA. The heart and control of renal excretion: neural and endocrine mechanisms. *FASEB J* 1992;6:2923–2932.

28. Christensen G. Release of atrial natriuretic factor. *Scand J Clin Lab Invest* 1993;53:91–100.

29. Wei C-M, Heublein DM, Perrella MA, et al. Natriuretic peptide system in human heart failure. *Circulation* 1993;88:1004–1009.

30. Butler GC, Senn BL, Floras JS. Influence of atrial natriuretic factor on spontaneous baroreflex sensitivity for heart rate in humans. *Hypertension* 1995;25:1167–1171.

31. McDonagh TA, Morrison CE, Lawrence A, et al. Symptomatic and asymptomatic left-ventricular systolic dysfunction in an urban population. *Lancet* 1997;350:829–833.

32. Cowie MR, Struthers AD, Wood DA, et al. Value of natriuretic peptides in assessment of patients with possible new heart failure in primary care. *Lancet* 1997;350:1347–1351.

33. McDonagh TA, Robb SD, Murdoch DR, et al. Biochemical detection of left-ventricular systolic dysfunction. *Lancet* 1998;351:9–13.

34. Harlan WR, Oberman A, Grimm R, Rosati RA. Chronic congestive heart failure in coronary artery disease: clinical criteria. *Ann Intern Med* 1977;86:133–138.

35. Marantz PR, Tobin JN, Wassertheil-Smoller S, et al. The relationship between left ventricular systolic function and congestive heart failure diagnosed by clinical criteria. *Circulation* 1988;77:607–612.

36. Francis GS, Archer SL. Diagnosis and management of acute congestive heart failure in the intensive care unit. *J Intens Care Med* 1989;4:84–92.

37. Cody RJ, Torre S, Clark M, Pondolfino K. Age-related hemodynamic, renal, and hormonal differences among patients with congestive heart failure. *Arch Intern Med* 1989;149:1023–1028.

38. Topol EJ, Traill TA, Fortuin NJ. Hypertensive hypertrophic cardiomyopathy in the elderly. *N Engl J Med* 1985;312:277–283.

39. Goldsmith SR, Dick C. Differentiating systolic from diastolic heart failure: pathophysiologic and therapeutic considerations. *Am J Med* 1993;95:645–655.

40. Vasan RS, Larson MG, Benjamin EJ, et al. Congestive heart failure in subjects with normal versus reduced left ventricular ejection fraction. *J Am Coll Cardiol* 1999;33:1948–1955.

41. Vasan RS, Levy D. Defining diastolic heart failure. *Circulation* 2000;101:2118–2121.

42. Cohen GI, Pietrolungo JF, Thomas JD, Klein AL. A practical guide to assessment of ventricular diastolic function using Doppler echocardiography. *J Am Coll Cardiol* 1996;27:1753–1760.

43. Grossman W. Defining diastolic dysfunction. *Circulation* 2000;101:2020–2021.

44. Bonow RO, Udelson JE. Left ventricular diastolic dysfunction as a cause of congestive heart failure. *Ann Intern Med* 1992;117:502–510.

45. Matter CM, Mandivnov L, Kaufmann PA, et al. Effect of NO donors on LV diastolic function in patients with severe pressure-overload hypertrophy. *Circulation* 1999;99:2396–2401.

46. Lipkin DP, Canepa-Anson R, Stephens MR, Poole-Wilson PA. Factors determining symptoms in heart failure: comparison of fast and slow exercise tests. *Br Heart J* 1986;55:439–445.

47. Eichna LW. The George E. Brown Memorial Lecture. Circulatory congestion and heart failure. *Circulation* 1960;22:864–886.

48. Myers J, Froelicher VF. Hemodynamic determinants of exercise capacity in chronic heart failure. *Ann Intern Med* 1991;115:377–386.

49. Myers J, Salleh A, Buchanan N, et al. Ventilatory mechanisms of exercise intolerance in chronic heart failure. *Am Heart Fail* 1992;124:7–10.

50. Lanfranchi PA, Brahiroli A, Bosimini E, et al. Prognostic value of nocturnal Cheyne-Stokes respiration in chronic heart failure. *Circulation* 1999;99:1435–1440.

51. Solin P, Bergin P, Richardson M, et al. Influence of pulmonary capillary wedge pressure on central apnea in heart failure. *Circulation* 1999;99:1574–1579.

52. Javaheri S, Parker TJ, Liming JD, et al. Sleep apnea in 81 ambulatory male patients with stable heart failure. *Circulation* 1998;97:2154–2159.

53. Javaheri S. A mechanism of central sleep apnea in patients with heart failure. *N Engl J Med* 1999;341:949–954.

54. Sin DD, Logan AG, Fitzgerald FS, et al. Effects of continuous positive airway pressure on cardiovascular outcomes in heart failure patients with and without Cheyne-Stokes respiration. *Circulation* 2000;102:61–66.

55. Wilson JR, Martin JL, Ferraro N, Weber KT. Effect of hydralazine on perfusion and metabolism in the leg during upright bicycle exercise in patients with heart failure. *Circulation* 1983;68:425–432.

56. LeJemtel TH, Sonnenblick EH. Should the failing heart be stimulated? (editorial). *N Engl J Med* 1984;310:1384–1385.

57. Massie BM. Exercise tolerance in congestive heart failure. *Am J Med* 1988;84:75–82.

58. Wilson JR. Exercise intolerance in heart failure. *Circulation* 1995;91:559–561.

59. Chati Z, Zannad F, Jeandel C, et al. Physical deconditioning may be a mechanism for the skeletal muscle energy phosphate metabolism abnormalities in chronic heart failure. *Am Heart J* 1996;131:560–566.

60. Massie BM, Simonini A, Sahgal P, et al. Relation of systemic and local muscle exercise capacity to skeletal muscle characteristics in men with congestive heart failure. *J Am Coll Cardiol* 1996;27:140–145.

61. Stevenson LW, Perloff JK. The limited reliability of physical signs for estimating hemodynamics in chronic heart failure. *JAMA* 1989;261:884–888.

62. Omland T, Aakvaag A, Bonarjee VVS, et al. Plasma brain natriuretic peptide as an indicator of left ventricular systolic function and long-term survival after acute myocardial infarction. *Circulation* 1996;93:1963–1969.

63. Tsutamoto T, Wada A, Maeda K, et al. Attenuation of compensation of endogenous cardiac natriuretic peptide system in chronic heart failure. *Circulation* 1997;96:509–516.

64. Weber KT, Kinasewitz GT, Janicki JS, Fishman AP. Oxygen utilization and ventilation during exercise in patients with chronic cardiac failure. *Circulation* 1982;65:1213–1223.

65. Aaronson KD, Mancini DM. Is percentage of predicted maxi-

mal exercise oxygen consumption a better predictor of survival than peak exercise oxygen consumption for patients with severe heart failure? *J Heart Lung Transplant* 1995;14:981–989.

66. Tristani FE, Hughes CV, Archibald DG, et al. Safety of graded symptom-limited exercise testing in patients with congestive heart failure. *Circulation* 1987;76:VI-54.

67. Mancini DM, Eisen H, Kussmaul W, et al. Value of peak exercise oxygen consumption for optimal timing of cardiac transplantation in ambulatory patients with heart failure. *Circulation* 1991;83:778–786.

68. ACC/AHA Task Force. Guidelines for the evaluation and management of heart failure. *J Am Coll Cardiol* 1995; 26:1376–1398.

69. Stevenson LW, Tillisch JH, Hamilton M, et al. Importance of hemodynamic responses to therapy in predicting survival with ejection fraction of 20% or less secondary to ischemic or nonischemic dilated cardiomyopathy. *Am J Cardiol* 1990;66:1348–1354.

70. Braunwald E, Kloner RA. The stunned myocardium: prolonged, postischemic ventricular dysfunction. *Circulation* 1982;66:1146–1149.

71. Becker LC, Levine JH, DiPaula AF, et al. Reversal of dysfunction in postischemic stunned myocardium by epinephrine and postextrasystolic potentiation. *J Am Coll Cardiol* 1986;7:580–589.

72. Dilsizian V, Bonow RO. Current diagnostic techniques of assessing myocardial viability in patients with hibernating and stunned myocardium. *Circulation* 1993;87:1–20.

73. Bounous EP, Mark DB, Pollock BG, et al. Surgical survival benefits for coronary disease patients with left ventricular dysfunction. *Circulation* 1988;78:I-151–I-157.

74. Sanchez JA, Smith CR, Drusin RE, et al. High-risk reparative surgery. *Circulation* 1990;82:IV-302–IV-305.

75. Louie HW, Laks H, Milgalter E, et al. Ischemic cardiomyopathy. *Circulation* 1991;84:III-290–III-295.

76. Elefteriades JA, Tolis G, Levi E, et al. Coronary artery bypass grafting in severe left ventricular dysfunction: excellent survival with improved ejection fraction and functional state. *J Am Coll Cardiol* 1993;22:1411–1417.

77. Kiat H, Berman DS, Maddahi J, et al. Late reversibility of tomographic myocardial thallium-201 defects: an accurate marker of myocardial viability. *J Am Coll Cardiol* 1988;12:1456–1463.

78. Dilsizian V, Rocco TP, Freedman NMT, et al. Enhanced detection of ischemic but viable myocardium by the reinjection of thallium after stress-redistribution imaging. *N Engl J Med* 1990;323:141–146.

79. Dilsizian V, Smeltzer WR, Freedman NMT, et al. Thallium reinjection after stress-redistribution imaging. *Circulation* 1991;83:1247–1255.

80. Dilsizian V, Perrone-Filardi P, Arrighi JA, et al. Concordance and discordance between stress-redistribution-reinjection and rest-redistribution thallium imaging for assessing viable myocardium. *Circulation* 1993;88:941–952.

81. Ragosta M, Beller GA, Watson DD, et al. Quantitative planar rest-redistribution 201Tl imaging in detection of myocardial viability and prediction of improvement in left ventricular function after coronary bypass surgery in patients with severely depressed left ventricular function. *Circulation* 1993;87:1630–1641.

82. Udelson JE, Coleman PS, Metherall J, et al. Predicting recovery of severe regional ventricular dysfunction. *Circulation* 1994;89:2552–2561.

83. Kauffman GJ, Boyne TS, Watson DD, et al. Comparison of rest thallium-201 imaging and rest technetium-99m sestamibi imaging for assessment of myocardial viability in patients with coronary artery disease and severe left ventricular dysfunction. *J Am Coll Cardiol* 1996;27:1592–1597.

84. Tillisch J, Brunken R, Marshall R, et al. Reversibility of cardiac wall-motion abnormalities predicted by positron tomography. *N Engl J Med* 1986;314:884–888.

85. Brunken R, Schwaiger M, Grover-McKay M, et al. Positron emission tomography detects tissue metabolic activity in myocardial segments with persistent thallium perfusion defects. *J Am Coll Cardiol* 1987;10:557–567.

86. Di Carli MF, Asgarzadie F, Schelbert HR, et al. Quantitative relation between myocardial viability and improvement in heart failure symptoms after revascularization in patients with ischemic cardiomyopathy. *Circulation* 1995;92:3436–3444.

87. Conversano A, Walsh JF, Geltman EM, et al. Delineation of myocardial stunning and hibernation by positron emission tomography in advanced coronary artery disease. *Am Heart J* 1996;131:440–450.

88. Mody FV, Brunken RC, Stevenson LW, et al. Differentiating cardiomyopathy of coronary artery disease from nonischemic dilated cardiomyopathy utilizing positron emission tomography. *J Am Coll Cardiol* 1991;17:373–383.

89. Foster E, O'Kelly B, LaPidus A, et al. Segmental analysis of resting echocardiographic function and stress scintigraphic perfusion: implications for myocardial viability. *Am Heart J* 1995;129:7–14.

90. Haque T, Furukawa T, Takahashi M, Kinoshita M. Identification of hibernating myocardium by dobutamine stress echocardiography: comparison with thallium-201 reinjection imaging. *Am Heart J* 1995;130:553–563.

91. Meluzin J, Cigarroa CG, Brickner ME, et al. Dobutamine echocardiography in predicting improvement in global left ventricular systolic function after coronary bypass or angioplasty in patients with healed myocardial infarct. *Am J Cardiol* 1995;76:877–880.

92. Arnese M, Cornel JA, Salustri A, et al. Prediction of improvement of regional left ventricular function after surgical revascularization. *Circulation* 1995;91:2748–2752.

92a. Hillenbrand HB, Kim RJ, Parker MA, et al. Early assessment of myocardial salvage by contrast-enhanced magnetic resonance imaging. *Circulation* 2000;102:1678–1683.

92b. Kim RJ, Wu E, Rafael A, et al. The use of contrast-enhanced magnetic resonance imaging to identify reversible myocardial dysfunction. *N Engl J Med* 2000;343:1445–1453.

93. Lauer MS, Blackstone EH, Young JB, et al. Cause of death in clinical research: time for a reassessment? *J Am Coll Cardiol* 1999;34:618–620.

94. Uretsky BF, Thygesen K, Armstrong, et al. Acute coronary findings at autopsy in heart failure patients with sudden death. *Circulation* 2000;102:611–616.

95. Redfield MM, Kay GN, Jenkins LS, et al. Tachycardia-related cardiomyopathy. *Mayo Clin Proc* 2000;75:790–795.

96. Cooper HA, Exner DV, Domanski MJ, et al. Light-to-moderate alcohol consumption and prognosis in patient

with left ventricular systolic dysfunction. *J Am Coll Cardiol* 2000;35:1753–1759.

97. Lazarevic AM, Nakatani S, Neskovic AN, et al. Early changes in left ventricular function in chronic asymptomatic alcoholics: relation to the duration of heavy drinking. *J Am Coll Cardiol* 2000;35:1599–1606.

98. Dzau VJ, Packer M, Lilly LS, et al. Prostaglandins in severe congestive heart failure. *N Engl J Med* 1984;310:347–352.

99. Arai M, Matsui H, Periasamy M. Sarcoplasmic reticulum gene expression in cardiac hypertrophy and heart failure. *Circ Res* 1994;74:555–564.

100. Movsesian MA, Karimi M, Green K, Jones LR. Ca^{2+}-transporting ATPase, phospholamban, and calsequestrin levels in nonfailing and failing human myocardium. *Circulation* 1994;90:653–657.

101. D'Agnolo A, Luciani GB, Mazzucco A, et al. Contractile properties and Ca^{2+} release activity of the sarcoplasmic reticulum in dilated cardiomyopathy. *Circulation* 1992;85:518–525.

102. Meyer M, Schillinger W, Pieske B, et al. Alterations of sarcoplasmic reticulum proteins in failing human dilated cardiomyopathy. *Circulation* 1995;92:778–784.

103. Brillantes A-M, Allen P, Takahashi T, et al. Differences in cardiac calcium release channel (ryanodine receptor) expression in myocardium from patients with end-stage heart failure caused by ischemic versus dilated cardiomyopathy. *Circ Res* 1992;71:18–26.

104. Vatner DE, Sato N, Kiuchi K, et al. Decrease in myocardial ryanodine receptors and altered excitation-contraction coupling early in the development of heart failure. *Circulation* 1994;90:1423–1430.

105. Mercadier J-J, Lompre A-M, Duc P, et al. Altered sarcoplasmic reticulum Ca^{2+}-ATPase gene expression in the human ventricle during end-stage heart failure. *J Clin Invest* 1990;85:305–309.

106. Movsesian MA, Bristow MR, Krall J. Ca^{2+} uptake by cardiac sarcoplasmic reticulum from patients with idiopathic dilated cardiomyopathy. *Circ Res* 1989;65:1141–1144.

107. Studer R, Reinecke H, Bilger J, et al. Gene expression of the cardiac Na^+-Ca^{2+} exchanger in end-stage human heart failure. *Circ Res* 1994;75:443–453.

108. Norgaard A, Bagger JP, Bjerregaard P, et al. Relation of left ventricular function and Na, K-pump concentration in suspected idiopathic dilated cardiomyopathy. *Am J Cardiol* 1988;61:1312–1315.

109. Morgan JP, Erny RE, Allen PD, et al. Abnormal intracellular calcium handling, a major cause of systolic and diastolic dysfunction in ventricular myocardium from patients with heart failure. *Circulation* 1990;81:III-21–III-32.

110. Beuckelmann DJ, Nabauer M, Kruger C, Erdmann E. Altered diastolic $[Ca^{2+}]_i$ handling in human ventricular myocytes from patients with terminal heart failure. *Am Heart J* 1995;129:684–689.

111. Feldman MD, Copelas L, Gwathmey JK, et al. Deficient production of cyclic AMP: pharmacologic evidence of an important cause of contractile dysfunction in patients with end-stage heart failure. *Circulation* 1987;75:331–339.

112. Davies CH, Davia K, Bennett JG, et al. Reduced contraction and altered frequency response of isolated ventricular myocytes from patients with heart failure. *Circulation* 1995;92:2540–2549.

113. Gwathmey JK, Copelas L, MacKinnon R, et al. Abnormal intracellular calcium handling in myocardium from patients with end-stage heart failure. *Circ Res* 1987;61:70–76.

114. Katz AM. Cardiomyopathy of overload. *N Engl J Med* 1990;322:100–110.

115. McLenachan JM, Henderson E, Morris KI, Dargie HJ. Ventricular arrhythmias in patients with hypertensive left ventricular hypertrophy. *N Engl J Med* 1987;317:787–792.

116. Weber KR, Brilla CG. Pathological hypertrophy and cardiac interstitium. *Circulation* 1991;83:1849–1865.

117. Bristow MR, Ginsburg R, Minobe W, et al. Decreased catecholamine sensitivity and beta-adrenergic-receptor density in failing human hearts. *N Engl J Med* 1982;307:205–211.

118. Bristow MR, Port JD, Sandoval AB, et al. Beta-adrenergic-receptor pathways in the failing human heart. *Heart Failure* 1989;5:77–90.

119. Levy D, Larson MG, Vasan RS, et al. The progression from hypertension to congestive heart failure. *JAMA* 1996;275:1557–1562.

120. Schwinger RHG, Bohm M, Koch A, et al. The failing human heart is unable to use the Frank-Starling mechanism. *Circ Res* 1994;74:959–969.

121. Komamura K, Shannon RP, Ihara R, et al. Exhaustion of Frank-Starling mechanism in conscious dogs with heart failure. *Am J Physiol* 1993;265:H1119–H1131.

122. Kitsis RN, Scheuer J. Functional significance of alterations in cardiac contractile protein isoforms. *Clin Cardiol* 1996;19:9–18.

123. Pfeffer MA, Braunwald E. Ventricular remodeling after myocardial infarction. *Circulation* 1990;81:1161–1172.

124. Cohn JN, Ferrari R, Sharpe N, et al. Cardiac remodeling—concepts and clinical implications: a consensus paper from an international forum on cardiac remodeling. *J Am Coll Cardiol* 2000;35:569–582.

125. St. John Sutton MG, Sharpe N. Left ventricular remodeling after myocardial infarction. *Circulation* 2000;101:2981–2988.

126. Hammermeister KE, DeRouen TA, Dodge HT. Variables predictive of survival in patients with coronary disease: selection by univariate and multivariate analysis from the clinical electrocardiographic, exercise, arteriographic, and quantitative angiographic evaluations. *Circulation* 1979;59:421–430.

127. White HD, Norris RM, Brown MA, et al. Left ventricular end-systolic volume as the major determinant of survival after recovery from myocardial infarction. *Circulation* 1987;76:44–51.

128. Weisman HF, Bush DE, Mannisi JA, et al. Cellular mechanisms of myocardial infarct expansion. *Circulation* 1988;78:186–201.

129. Eaton LW, Bulkley BH. Expansion of acute myocardial infarction: its relationship to infarct morphology in a canine model. *Circ Res* 1981;49:80–88.

130. Eaton LW, Weiss JL, Garrison JB, Bulkley BH. Regional cardiac dilatation after acute myocardial infarction: recognition by two-dimensional echocardiography. *N Engl J Med* 1979;300:57–62.

131. McKay RG, Pfeffer MA, Pasternak RC, et al. Left ventricular remodeling after myocardial infarction: a corollary to infarct expansion. *Circulation* 1986;74:693–702.

132. Francis GS, McDonald KM. Left ventricular hypertrophy:

an initial response to myocardial injury. *Am J Cardiol* 1992;69:3G–9G.

133. Francis GS, McDonald KM, Cohn JN. Neurohumoral activation in preclinical heart failure. *Circulation* 1993;87:IV-90–IV-96.

134. Francis GS, Carlyle WC. Hypothetical pathways of cardiac myocyte hypertrophy: response to myocardial injury. *Eur Heart J* 1993;14:49–56.

135. Francis GS, Chu C. Post-infarction myocardial remodeling: why does it happen? *Eur Heart J* 1995;16:31–36.

136. Anversa P, Li P, Zhang X, et al. Ischaemic myocardial injury and ventricular remodelling. *Cardiovasc Res* 1993; 27:145–157.

137. Beltrami CA, Finato N, Rocco M, et al. Structural basis of end-stage heart failure in ischemic cardiomyopathy in humans. *Circulation* 1994;89:151–163.

138. Gerdes AM, Capasso JM. Structural remodeling and mechanical dysfunction of cardiac myocytes in heart failure. *J Mol Cell Cardiol* 1995;27:849–856.

139. Kim CB, Braunwald E. Potential benefits of late reperfusion of infarcted myocardium. *Circulation* 1993;88:2426–2436.

140. Brown EJ, Swinford RD, Gadde P, Lillis O. Acute effects of delayed reperfusion on myocardial infarct shape and left ventricular volume: a potential mechanism of additional benefits from thrombolytic therapy. *J Am Coll Cardiol* 1991;17:1641–1650.

141. Hirayama A, Adachi T, Asada S, et al. Late reperfusion for acute myocardial infarction limits the dilatation of left ventricle without the reduction of infarct size. *Circulation* 1993;88:2565–2574.

142. Lamas GA, Flaker GC, Mitchell G, et al. Effect of infarct artery patency on prognosis after acute myocardial infarction. *Circulation* 1995;92:1101–1109.

143. Popvic AD, Neskovic AN, Babic R, et al. Independent impact of thrombolytic therapy and vessel patency on left ventricular dilation after myocardial infarction. *Circulation* 1994;90:800–807.

144. Linzbach AJ. Heart failure from the point of view of quantitative anatomy. *Am J Cardiol* 1960;5:370–382.

145. Gerdes AM, Kellerman SE, Moore JA, et al. Structural remodeling of cardiac myocytes in patients with ischemic cardiomyopathy. *Circulation* 1992;86:426–430.

146. Engler RL, Gottlieb RA, Burelson KO, et al. Myocyte cell death by apoptosis during reperfusion (abstract 5). *Circulation* 1993;88[Suppl 1].

147. Katz AM. Cardiac interstitium in health and disease: the fibrillar collagen network. *J Am Coll Cardiol* 1989;13:1637–1652.

148. Morgan HE, Baker KM. Cardiac hypertrophy. Mechanical, neural and endocrine dependence. *Circulation* 1991;83:13–25.

149. Pfeffer MA, Lamas GA, Vaughan DE, et al. Effect of captopril on progressive ventricular dilatation after anterior myocardial infarction. *N Engl J Med* 1988;319:8–86.

150. Konstam MA, Kronenberg MW, Rousseau MR, et al. Effects of the angiotensin converting enzyme inhibitor enalapril on the long-term progression of left ventricular dilatation in patients with asymptomatic systolic dysfunction. *Circulation* 1993;88:2277–2283.

151. St. John Sutton M, Pfeffer MA, Plappert T, et al. Quantitative two-dimensional echocardiographic measurements

are major predictors of adverse cardiovascular events after acute myocardial infarction. *Circulation* 1994;89:68–75.

152. Greenberg B, Quinones MA, Koilpillaie C, et al. Effects of long-term enalapril therapy on cardiac structure and function in patients with left ventricular dysfunction. *Circulation* 1995;91:2573–2581.

153. Van Gilst WH, Kingma H, Peels KH, et al. Which patient benefits from early angiotensin-converting enzyme inhibition after myocardial infarction? *J Am Coll Cardiol* 1996;28:114–121.

154. McDonald KM, Francis GS, Matthews J, et al. Long-term oral nitrate therapy prevents chronic ventricular remodeling in dog. *J Am Coll Cardiol* 1993;21:514–522.

155. Jugdutt BI, Warnica JW. Intravenous nitroglycerin therapy to limit myocardial infarct size, expansion, and complications. *Circulation* 1988;78:906–919.

156. Garg UC, Hassid A. Nitric oxide-generating vasodilators and 8-bromo-cyclic guanosine monophosphate inhibit mitogenesis and proliferation of cultured rat vascular smooth muscle cells. *J Clin Invest* 1989;83:1774–1777.

157. Hall SA, Cigarroa CG, Marcoux L, et al. Time course of improvement in left ventricular function, mass and geometry in patients with congestive heart failure treated with beta-adrenergic blockade. *J Am Coll Cardiol* 1995;25:1154–1161.

158. Australia/New Zealand Heart Failure Research Collaborative Group. Randomized, placebo-controlled trial of carvedilol in patients with congestive heart failure due to ischaemic heart disease. *Lancet* 1997;349:375–380.

159. Doughty RN, Whalley GA, Gamble G, et al. Left ventricular remodeling with carvedilol inpatients with congestive heart failure due to ischemic heart disease. *J Am Coll Cardiol* 1997;29:1060–1066.

160. Eichhorn EJ, Bristow MR. Medical therapy can improve the biological properties of the chronically failing heart. *Circulation* 1996;94:2285–2296.

161. Senior R, Basu S, Kinsey C, et al. Carvedilol prevents remodeling in patients with left ventricular dysfunction after acute myocardial infarction. *Am Heart J* 1999;137:646–652.

162. Bristow PM, Cohn JN, Colucci WS, et al. The effect of carvedilol on morbidity and mortality in patients with chronic heart failure. *N Engl J Med* 1996;23:1349–1355.

163. Bristow MR, Gilbert Em, Abraham WT, et al. Carvedilol produces dose-related improvements in left ventricular function and survival in subjects with chronic heart failure. *Circulation* 1996;94:2807–2816.

164. CIBIS II Investigators and committees. The cardiac insufficiency bisoprolol study II (CIBIS II): a randomized trial. *Lancet* 1999;353:9–13.

165. MERIT-HF Study Group. Effect of metoprolol CR/XL in chronic heart failure: metoprolol CR/XL randomized intervention trial in congestive heart failure (MERIT HF). *Lancet* 1999;353:2001–2007.

166. Rector TS, Olivari MT, Levine TB, et al. Predicting survival for an individual with congestive heart failure using the plasma norepinephrine concentration. *Am Heart J* 1987;114:148–152.

167. Francis GS, Goldsmith SR, Cohn JN. Relationship of exercise capacity to resting left ventricular performance and basal plasma norepinephrine levels in patients with congestive heart failure. *Am Heart J* 1982;104:725–731.

168. Eisenhofer G, Friberg P, Rundqvist B, et al. Cardiac sympathetic nerve function in congestive heart failure. *Circulation* 1996;93:1667–1676.

169. Jiang JP, Downing SE. Catecholamine cardiomyopathy: review and analysis of pathogenetic mechanisms. *Yale J Biol Med* 1990;63:581–591.

170. Mann DL, Kent RL, Parsons B, Cooper G. Adrenergic effects of the biology of the adult mammalian cardiocyte. *Circulation* 1992;85:790–804.

171. Kaye DM, Lefkovits J, Jennings GL, et al. Adverse consequences of high sympathetic nervous activity in the failing human heart. *J Am Coll Cardiol* 1995;26:1257–1263.

172. Meredith IT, Eisenhofer G, Lambert GW. Cardiac sympathetic nervous activity in congestive heart failure. *Circulation* 1993;88:136–145.

173. Middlekauff HR, Hamilton MA, Stevenson LW, Mark AL. Independent control of skin and muscle sympathetic nerve activity in patients with heart failure. *Circulation* 1994;90:1794–1798.

174. Lambert GW, Kaye DM, Lefkovits J, et al. Increased central nervous system monoamine neurotransmitter turnover and its association with sympathetic nervous activity in treated heart failure patients. *Circulation* 1995;92:1813–1818.

175. Rundqvist B, Elam M, Eisenhofer G, Friberb P. Normalization of total body and regional sympathetic hyperactivity in heart failure after heart transplantation. *J Heart Lung Transplant* 1996;15:516–526.

176. Brown JJ, Davies DL, Johnson VW, et al. Renin relationships in congestive cardiac failure, treated and untreated. *Am Heart J* 1970;80:329–342.

177. Curtiss C, Cohn JN, Vrobel T, Franciosa JA. Role of the renin-angiotensin system in the systemic vasoconstriction of chronic congestive heart failure. *Circulation* 1978;58:763–776.

178. Anand IS, Ferrari R, Kalra GS, et al. Edema of cardiac origin. *Circulation* 1989;80:299–305.

179. Lindpaintner K, Ganten D. The cardiac renin-angiotensin system. *Circ Res* 1991;68:905–921.

180. Grinstaed WC, Young JB. The myocardial renin-angiotensin system: existence, importance, and clinical implications. *Am Heart J* 1992;123:1039–1045.

181. Goldsmith SR. Vasopressin as vasopressor. *Am J Med* 1987;82:1213–1219.

182. Goldsmith SR, Dodge D. Response of plasma vasopressin to ethanol in congestive heart failure. *Am J Cardiol* 1985;55:1354–1357.

183. Liard J-F. Peripheral vasodilatation induced by a vasopressin analogue with selective V_2-agonism in dogs. *Am Physiol Soc* 1989;256:H1621–H1626.

184. Tagawa T, Imaizumi T, Shiramoto M, et al. V2 receptor-mediated vasodilation in healthy humans. *J Cardiovasc Pharmacol* 1995;25:387–392.

185. Nicod P, Waeber B, Bussien J-P, et al. Acute hemodynamic effect of a vascular antagonist of vasopressin in patients with congestive heart failure. *Am J Cardiol* 1985;55:1043–1047.

186. Creager MA, Faxon DP, Cutler SS, et al. Contribution of vasopressin to vasoconstriction in patients with congestive heart failure: comparison with the renin-angiotensin system and the sympathetic nervous system. *J Am Coll Cardiol* 1986;7:758–765.

187. Yanagisawa M, Kurihara H, Kimura S, et al. A novel potent vasoconstrictor peptide produced by vascular endothelial cells. *Nature* 1988;332:411–415.

188. Levin ER. Endothelins. *N Engl J Med* 1995;333:356–363.

189. Kurihara Y, Kurihara H, Suzuki H, et al. Elevated blood pressure and craniofacial abnormalities in mice deficient in endothelin-1. *Nature* 1994;368:703–710.

190. Ito H, Hiroe M, Hirata Y, et al. Endothelin ET_A receptor antagonist blocks cardiac hypertrophy provoked by hemodynamic overload. *Circulation* 1994;89:2198–2203.

191. Kaddoura S, Firth JD, Boheler KR, et al. Endothelin-1 is involved in norepinephrine-induced ventricular hypertrophy in vivo. *Circulation* 1996;93:2068–2079.

192. Marguilies KB, Hildebrand FL, Lerman A, et al. Increased endothelin in experimental heart failure. *Circulation* 1990;82:2226–2230.

193. Hiroe M, Hirata Y, Fujita N, et al. Plasma endothelin-1 levels in idiopathic dilated cardiomyopathy. *Am J Cardiol* 1991;68:1114–1115.

194. Rodeheffer RJ, Lerman A, Heublein D, Burnett JC. Increased plasma concentrations of endothelin in congestive heart failure in humans. *Mayo Clin Proc* 1992;67:719–724.

195. Lerman A, Kubo SH, Tschumperlin LK, Burnett JC. Plasma endothelin concentrations in humans with end-stage heart failure and after heart transplantation. *J Am Coll Cardiol* 1992;20:849–853.

196. Stewart DJ, Cernacek P, Costello KB, Rouleau JL. Elevated endothelin-1 in heart failure and loss of normal response to postural change. *Circulation* 1992;85:510–517.

197. McMurray JJ, Ray SG, Abdullah I, et al. Plasma endothelin in chronic heart failure. *Circulation* 1992;85:1374–1379.

198. Lerman A, Hildegrand FL, Aarhus LL, Burnett JC. Endothelin has biological actions at pathophysiological concentrations. *Circulation* 1991;83:1808–1814.

199. Sugedn PH, Bogoyevitch MA. Endothelin-1-dependent signaling pathways in the myocardium. *Trends Cardiovasc Med* 1996;6:87–94.

200. Colucci WS. Myocardial endothelin. Does it play a role in myocardial failure? *Circulation* 1996;93:1069–1072.

201. Abassi Z, Golomb E, Keiser HR. Neutral endopeptidase inhibition increases the urinary excretion and plasma levels of endothelin. *Metabolism* 1992;41:683–685.

202. Abassi ZA, Tate JE, Golomb, Keiser HR. Role of neutral endopeptidase in the metabolism of endothelin. *Hypertension* 1992;20:89–95.

203. Grantham JA, Schirger JA, Wennberg PW, et al. Modulation of functionally active endothelin-converting enzyme by chronic neutral endopeptidase inhibition in experimental atherosclerosis. *Circulation* 2000;101:1976–1981.

204. Kiowski W, Sutsch G, Hunziker P, et al. Evidence of endothelin-1-mediated vasoconstriction in severe chronic heart failure. *Lancet* 1995;346:732–736.

205. Benigni A, Remuzzi G. Endothelin antagonists. *Lancet* 1999;353:133–138.

206. Spieker LE, Mitrovic V, Noll G, et al. Acute hemodynamic and neurohumoral effects of selective ET_A receptor blockade in patients with congestive heart failure. *J Am Coll Cardiol* 2000;35:1745–1752.

207. Givertz MM, Colucci WS, LeJemtel TH, et al. Acute endothelin A receptor blockade causes selective pulmonary vasodilation in patients with chronic heart failure. *Circulation* 2000;101:2922–2927.

208. Sakai S, Miyauchi T, Yamaguchi I, et al. Long-term endothelin receptor antagonist administration improves alteration in expression of various cardiac genes in failing myocardium of rats with heart failure. *Circulation* 2000;101:2849–2853.

209. Taemura G, Fujiwara H, Horike K, et al. Ventricular expression of atrial natriuretic polypeptide and its relations with hemodynamics and histology in dilated human hearts. *Circulation* 1989;80:1137–1147.

210. Cody RJ, Atlas SA, Laragh JH, et al. Atrial natriuretic factor in normal subjects and heart failure patients. *J Clin Invest* 1986;78:1362–1374.

211. Itoh H, Pratt RE, Dzau VJ. Atrial natriuretic polypeptide inhibits hypertrophy of vascular smooth muscle cells. *J Clin Invest* 1990;86:1690–1697.

212. McClean DR, Ikram H, Garlick AH, et al. The clinical, cardiac, renal, arterial and neurohormonal effects of omapatrilat, a vasopeptidase inhibitor, in patients with chronic heart failure. *J Am Coll Cardiol* 2000;36:479–486.

213. Wei C-M, Heublein DM, Perrella MA, et al. Natriuretic peptide system in human heart failure. *Circulation* 1993;88:1004–1009.

214. Levin ER. Natriuretic peptide C-receptor: more than a clearance receptor. *Am J Physiol* 1993;264:E483–E489.

215. Davidson NC, Barr CS, Struthers AD. C-type natriuretic peptide. *Circulation* 1996;93:1155–1159.

216. Yoshimura M, Yasue H, Morita E, et al. Hemodynamic, renal and hormonal responses to brain natriuretic peptide infusion in patients with congestive heart failure. *Circulation* 1991;84:1581–1588.

217. Clarkson PBM, Wheelen NM, MacFadyen RJ, et al. Effects of brain natriuretic peptide on exercise hemodynamics and neurohormones in isolated diastolic heart failure. *Circulation* 1996;93:2037–2042.

218. Mills RM, LeJemtel TH, Horton DP, et al. Sustained hemodynamic effects of an infusion of nesiritide (human b-type natriuretic peptide) in heart failure. *J Am Coll Cardiol* 1999;34:155–162.

219. Colucci WS, Elkayam U, Horton DP, et al. Intravenous nesiritide, a natriuretic peptide, in the treatment of decompensated congestive heart failure. *N Engl J Med* 2000;343:246–253.

220. Omland T, Aakvaag A, Bonarjee VVS, et al. Plasma brain natriuretic peptide as an indicator of left ventricular systolic function and long-term survival after acute myocardial infarction. *Circulation* 1996;93:1962–1969.

221. Giustina A, Lorusso R, Borghetti V, et al. Impaired spontaneous growth hormone secretion in severe dilated cardiomyopathy. *Am Heart J* 1996;131:620–622.

222. Fazio S, Sabatini D, Capaldo B, et al. A preliminary study of growth hormone in the treatment of dilated cardiomyopathy. *N Engl J Med* 1996;334:809–814.

223. Yang R, Bunting S, Gillett N, et al. Growth hormone improves cardiac performance in experimental heart failure. *Circulation* 1995;92:262–267.

224. Duerr RL, McKirnan MD, Gim RD, et al. Cardiovascular effects of insulin-like growth factor-1 and growth hormone in chronic left ventricular failure in the rat. *Circulation* 1996;93:2188–2196.

225. Duerr RL, Huang S, Miraliakbar HR, et al. Insulin-like growth factor-1 enhances ventricular hypertrophy and function during the onset of experimental cardiac failure. *J Clin Invest* 1995;95:619–627.

226. Torre-Amione G, Kapadia S, Lee J, et al. Tumor necrosis factor-alpha and tumor necrosis factor receptors in the failing human heart. *Circulation* 1996;93:704–711.

227. Gurevitch J, Frolkis I, Yuhas Y, et al. Tumor necrosis factor-alpha is released from the isolated heart undergoing ischemia and reperfusion. *J Am Coll Cardiol* 1996;28:247–252.

228. Doyama K, Fujiwara H, Fukimoto M, et al. Tumour necrosis factor is expressed in cardiac tissue of patients with heart failure. *Int J Card* 1996;54:217–225.

229. Habib FM, Springall DR, Davies GJ, et al. Tumor necrosis factor and inducible nitric oxide synthase in dilated cardiomyopathy. *Lancet* 1996;347:1151–1155.

230. Smith CA, Farrah T, Goodwin RG. The TNF receptor superfamily of cellular and viral proteins: activation, costimulation, and death. *Cell* 1994;76:959–962.

231. Levine B, Kalman J, Mayer L, et al. Elevated circulating levels of tumor necrosis factor in severe chronic heart failure. *N Engl J Med* 1990;323:236–241.

232. McMurray J, Abdullah I, Dargie HJ, Shapiro D. Increased concentrations of tumour necrosis factor in "cachectic" patients with severe chronic heart failure. *Br Heart J* 1991;66:356–358.

233. Ferrari R, Bachetti T, Confortini R, et al. Tumor necrosis factor soluble receptors in patients with various degrees of congestive heart failure. *Circulation* 1995;92:1479–1486.

234. Feldman AM, Combes AL, Wagner D, et al. The role of tumor necrosis factor in the pathophysiology of heart failure. *J Am Coll Cardiol* 2000;35:537–544.

235. Jougasaki M, Wei C-M, McKinley LJ, Burnett JC. Elevation of circulation and ventricular adrenomedullin in human congestive heart failure. *Circulation* 1995;92:286–289.

236. Kobayashi K, Kitamura K, Etoh T, et al. Increased plasma adrenomedullin levels in chronic congestive heart failure. *Am Heart J* 1996;131:994–998.

237. Hirsch AT, Dzau VJ, Creager MA. Baroreceptor function in congestive heart failure: effect on neurohumoral activation and regional vascular resistance. *Circulation* 1987;75[Suppl IV]:IV-36.

238. Thames MD, Kinugawa T, Smith ML, Dibner-Dunlap ME. Abnormalities of baroreflex control in heart failure. *J Am Coll Cardiol* 1993;22:56A–60A.

239. Eckberg DL, Drabinsky M, Braunwald E. Defective cardiac parasympathetic control in patients with heart disease. *N Engl J Med* 1971;265:877–883.

240. Levine TB, Francis GS, Goldsmith ST, Cohn JN. The neurohumoral and hemodynamic response to orthostatic tilt in patients with congestive heart failure. *Circulation* 1983;67:1070–1075.

241. Zucker IH, Wang W, Brandle M. Baroreflex abnormalities in congestive heart failure. *NIPS* 1993;8:87–90.

242. Creager MA, Creager SJ. Arterial baroreflex regulation of blood pressure in patients with congestive heart failure. *J Am Coll Cardiol* 1994;23:401–405.

243. Zucker IH, Wang W, Brandle M, et al. Neural regulation of sympathetic nerve activity in heart failure. *Prog Cardiovasc Dis* 1995;37:397–414.

244. Wang W, Han H-Y, Zucker IH. Depressed baroreflex in heart failure is not due to structural change in carotid sinus nerve fibers. *J Auton Nerv Syst* 1996;57:101–108.

245. Ellenbogen KA, Mohanty PK, Szentpetery S, Thames MD. Arterial baroreflex abnormalities in heart failure. *Circulation* 1989;79:51–58.

246. Packer M, Lee W-H, Kessler PD. Preservation of glomerular filtration rate in human heart failure by activation of the renin-angiotensin system. *Circulation* 1986;74:766–774.

247. Barger AC. The pathogenesis of sodium retention in congestive heart failure. *Metabolism* 1956;5:480–489.

248. Hostetter TH, Pfeffer JM, Pfeffer MA, et al. Cardiorenal hemodynamics and sodium excretion in rats with myocardial infarction. *Am J Physiol* 1983;245:H98–H103.

249. Skorecki KL, Brenner BM. Body fluid homeostasis in congestive heart failure and cirrhosis with ascites. *Am J Med* 1982;72:323–338.

250. Francis GS. Sodium and water excretion in heart failure: efficacy of treatment has surpassed knowledge of pathophysiology. *Ann Intern Med* 1986;105:272.

251. Zelis R, Nellis SH, Longhurst J, et al. Abnormalities in the regional circulations accompanying congestive heart failure. *Prog Cardiovasc Dis* 1975;18:181–199.

252. Drexler H, Hayoz D, Munzel T, et al. Endothelial function in chronic congestive heart failure. *Am J Cardiol* 1992;69:1596–1601.

253. Habib F, Dutka D, Crossman D, et al. Enhanced basal nitric oxide production in heart failure: another failed counter-regulatory vasodilator mechanism? *Lancet* 1994;344:371–373.

254. Winlaw DS, Smythe GS, Keogh AM, et al. Increased nitric oxide production in heart failure. *Lancet* 1994;344:373–374.

255. Hickey M, Fraser IS. Nitric oxide production and heart failure (letter). *Lancet* 1995;345:390–391.

256. Gilligan DM, Panza JA, Kilcoyne CM, et al. Contribution of endothelium-derived nitric oxide to exercise-induced vasodilation. *Circulation* 1994;90:2853–2858.

257. Rector RS, Bank AJ, Mullen KA, et al. Randomized, double-blind, placebo-controlled study of supplemental oral L-arginine in patients with heart failure. *Circulation* 1996;93:2135–2141.

258. Sinoway LI, Minotti JR, Davis D, et al. Delayed reversal of impaired vasodilation in congestive heart failure after heart transplantation. *Am J Cardiol* 1988;61:1076–1079.

259. Franciosa JA, Ziesche S, Wilen M. Functional capacity of patients with chronic left ventricular failure. *Am J Med* 1979;67:460–466.

260. Benge W, Litchfield RL, Marcus ML. Exercise capacity in patients with severe left ventricular dysfunction. *Circulation* 1980;61:955–959.

261. Franciosa JA, Park M, Levine TB. Lack of correlation between exercise capacity and indexes of resting left ventricular performance in heart failure. *Am J Cardiol* 1981;47:33–39.

262. Litchfield RL, Kerber RE, Benge W, et al. Normal exercise capacity in patients with severe left ventricular dysfunction: compensatory mechanisms. *Circulation* 1982;66:129–134.

263. Wilson JR, Martin JL, Ferraro N, Weber KT. Effect of hydralazine on perfusion and metabolism in the leg during upright bicycle exercise in patients with heart failure. *Circulation* 1983;68:425–432.

264. Francis GS, Rector TS. Maximal exercise tolerance as a therapeutic end point in heart failure—are we relying on the right measure? *Am J Cardiol* 1994;73:304–306.

265. Bittner V, Weiner DH, Yusuf S, et al. Prediction of mortality and morbidity with a 6-minute walk test in patients with left ventricular dysfunction. *JAMA* 1993;270:1702–1707.

266. Sullivan MJ, Higginbotham MB, Cobb FR. Exercise training in patients with severe left ventricular dysfunction. *Circulation* 1988;78:506–515.

267. Coats AJS, Adamopoulos S, Radaelli A, et al. Controlled trial of physical training in chronic heart failure. *Circulation* 1992;85:2119–2131.

268. Keteyian SJ, Levine AB, Brawner CA, et al. Exercise training in patients with heart failure. *Ann Intern Med* 1996;124:1051–1057.

269. Simonini A, Long CS, Dudley GA, et al. Heart failure in rats causes changes in skeletal muscle morphology and gene expression that are not explained by reduced activity. *Circ Res* 1996;79:128–136.

270. Haywood GA, Tsao PS, von der Leyen HE, et al. Expression of inducible nitric oxide synthase in human heart failure. *Circulation* 1996;93:1087–1094.

271. Hare JM, Loh E, Creager MA, Colucci WS. Nitric oxide inhibits the positive inotropic response to beta-adrenergic stimulation in humans with left ventricular dysfunction. *Circulation* 1995;92:2198–2203.

272. Bocchi EA, Bacal F, Auler JOC, et al. Inhaled nitric oxide leading to pulmonary edema in stable severe heart failure. *Am J Cardiol* 1994;74:70–72.

273. Tartaglia LA, Ayres TM, Wong GHW, Goeddel DV. A novel domain within the 55 kd TNF receptor signals cell death. *Cell* 1993;74:845–853.

274. Atherton JJ, Moore TD, Lele SS, et al. Diastolic ventricular interaction in chronic heart failure. *Lancet* 1997;349:1720–1724.

275. deBono D. Diastolic ventricular interaction: Starling (and Bernheim) revisited. *Lancet* 1997;349:1712.

276. Vasan RS, Larson MG, Benjamin EJ, et al. Left ventricular dilatation and the risk of congestive heart failure in people without myocardial infarction. *N Engl J Med* 1997;336:1650–1655.

277. Poole-Wilson PA. Predictions of heart failure—an art aided by technology. *N Engl J Med* 1997;336:1381–1382.

278. Love MP, McMurray JJV. Endothelin in heart failure: a promising therapeutic target? *Heart* 1997;77:93–94.

HEALTH CARE IMPACT
OF HEART FAILURE

RANDALL C. STARLING

▼⫙ ADDITIONAL ELECTRONIC TOPICS

Reasons for Increasing Prevalence of Heart Failure o69;   Severity of Heart Failure and Resource Use o70;   Heart Failure Guidelines o71;   Cardiac Transplantation and Alternatives o72;   Risk Factors and High-Risk Patients o73

OVERVIEW

Congestive heart failure is an increasing, global epidemic, particularly in the elderly, that results in significant health care expenditure, disability, and mortality. Coronary artery disease, hypertension, and diabetes mellitus are the major etiologic risk factors. Ironically, advances in the treatment of coronary artery disease and acute ischemic syndromes, which have saved lives, have resulted in a growing population of survivors with left ventricular dysfunction destined to develop the heart failure syndrome. Preventive measures that have evolved over the last 25 years, including hypertension management, have not reduced the incidence of heart failure. Congestive heart failure is the leading indication for hospitalization in the United States for patients older than 65 years. The majority of health care dollars spent on heart failure is for inpatient care. Heart failure is a chronic disease amenable to an intensive multidisciplinary care model (disease management program) designed to prevent hospital admissions through patient education, focused outpatient initiatives, and adherence to management guidelines that should enhance

cost effectiveness and improve quality of life. Patients with advanced heart failure represent approximately 10% of the total heart failure population, have the highest short-term mortality, and consume the greatest percentage of resources (labor and dollars). Regionalized centers with expertise in the management of advanced heart failure patients (through pharmacotherapy, circulatory support devices, surgical procedures, and transplantation) are necessary to deliver sophisticated care for this expanding population.

INTRODUCTION

Fifty years ago, chronic heart failure was considered primarily an edematous disorder. Hypertension and valvular heart disease were the most frequent predisposing causes (1). Physicians attempted to control pulmonary and peripheral congestion with diuretic therapy. Heart failure was a slowly progressive disease until patients succumbed with biventricular failure, anasarca, and renal insufficiency. Today, symptomatic heart failure is most often characterized by effort intolerance (dyspnea) and fatigue. ▼⫙ o74

Heart failure is a chronic disease that may evolve over years and progress from minimal to severe impairment.

R. C. Starling: Department of Cardiovascular Medicine, Section of Heart Failure and Cardiac Transplant Medicine, The Cleveland Clinic, Cleveland, Ohio

Successful heart failure management requires lifestyle modifications and impinges on the activities and lives of family members and caregivers as well. Patients may live a limited but reasonable lifestyle for years. Most are disabled, however, and thus are not productive members of society. Aside from the economic burden from a health care resources standpoint, the disability and long-term nature of the condition that limit a patient's ability to be gainfully employed are significant. The components of cost to be considered from a public health perspective include hospitalization costs, outpatient care costs, and disability costs (11). Management of a chronic disease requires a multidisciplinary continuum of care designed to improve quality of life, reduce hospitalizations, and decrease costs (12,13). Thus, heart failure is not an isolated encounter, such as acute pharyngitis or bacterial pneumonia. Rather, it is an "epic of care," and patients, their families, and health care providers must develop relationships. Optimal outcomes can be achieved when physicians have the expertise to care for the patient through the various phases of his or her illness, effect lifestyle changes through education, and use a multidisciplinary team for effective chronic disease management (14).

EPIDEMIOLOGY

Heart failure is a widespread epidemic affecting 2 to 4 million Americans and nearly 15 million people worldwide (10,15,16). The American Heart Association estimated that, in 2001, 4.7 million Americans were alive with congestive heart failure (11). Although mortality rates are declining for cardiovascular disease in the United States, hospitalizations for heart failure have increased substantially (17). In 1990, more than 700,000 hospital discharges had heart failure as the primary diagnosis in the United States (15). This represents a fourfold increase since 1971. Hospital discharges of patients with congestive heart failure in the United States rose from 377,000 in 1979 to 978,000 in 1998, a 155% increase (11). In 1990, there were 708,000 new heart failure patients and 280,000 deaths, which represents a net increase of 428,000 patients or a 12% growth per year (18). Estimates are that approximately one-half of patients with heart failure are age 65 years or older. ✔ o75

The crude incidence (unadjusted for age) ranges from one to five cases per 1,000 population per year and increases sharply with advancing age to as high as 40 cases per 1,000 population over age 75 years in some studies (20). An indication of the incidence of heart failure in the United States can be obtained from the Framingham study and the Framingham Offspring Study, which represent a population of over 10,000 (15). The incidence of heart failure rises with age in both men and women, as shown in Figure 89.1. In the Framingham study, the annual inci-

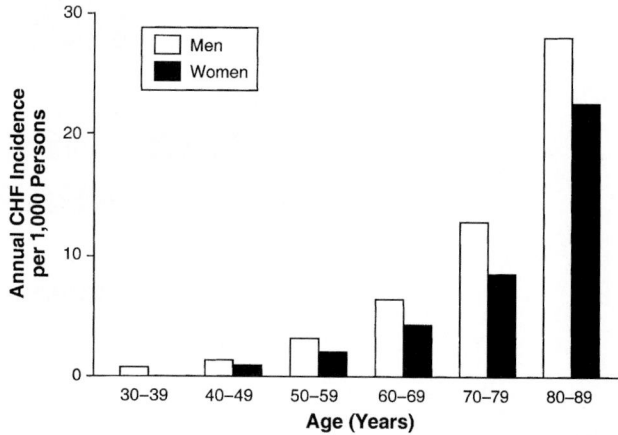

FIGURE 89.1 The annual incidence of congestive heart failure (CHF) among subjects in the Framingham Heart Study, shown by age in decades for men and women. (Adapted from Ho KKL, Pinsky JL, Kannel WB, et al. The epidemiology of heart failure: the Framingham study. *J Am Coll Cardiol* 1993;22[Suppl A]:6A–13A, with permission.)

dence increased from 3 per 1,000 in men aged 50 to 59 to 27 per 1,000 in men aged 80 to 89 years, and from 2 per 1,000 in women aged 50 to 59 to 22 per 1,000 in women aged 80 to 89 years. The incidence of congestive heart failure after adjustment for age is one-third lower in women than in men. Crude prevalence, unadjusted for age, ranges from 3 to 20 cases per 1,000 and, for those older than 65 years, from 30 to 130 cases per 1,000 population (20). Based on the increasing age of the U.S. population, estimates are that the prevalence of congestive heart failure will nearly double to 5.7 million cases by the year 2030 (21).

Etiologic Risk Factors

The prevalence of certain causes of and risk factors for congestive heart failure among Framingham Heart Study subjects is shown in Figure 89.2. The Framingham study documented the relative risk for the development of heart failure in the presence of specific risk factors, including hypertension, hypercholesterolemia, cigarette smoking, electrocardiographically identified left ventricular hypertrophy, and diabetes mellitus, in a population-based cohort study (15). Among 331 men and 321 women in the Framingham study who developed congestive heart failure during follow-up, hypertension and coronary artery disease were the two most common preexisting conditions (15). Only 11% of men and 15% of women had no antecedent history of coronary artery disease or hypertension. Interestingly, in the 40-year period from 1948 to 1988, the age-adjusted prevalence of coronary disease in men with new congestive heart failure increased by 46% per calendar decade (*p* <.05). However, the age-adjusted prevalence of coronary heart disease among all males in the Framingham Heart Study decreased by 8% per calendar decade (*p* <.05) (15).

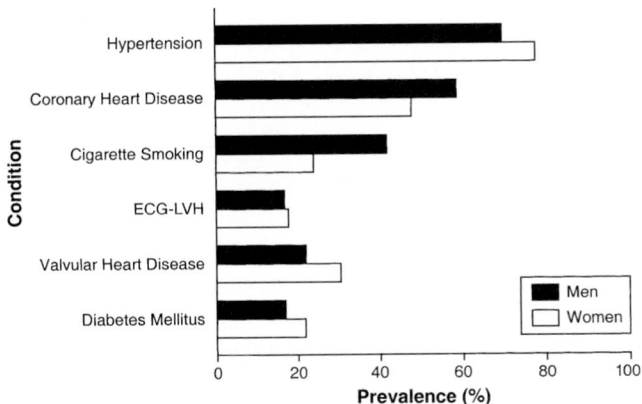

FIGURE 89.2 Prevalence of causes and risk factors for the development of congestive heart failure by gender in the Framingham Heart Study cohort. ECG-LVH, electrocardiographically identified left ventricular hypertrophy. [Adapted from Ho KKL, Pinsky JL, Kannel WB, et al. The epidemiology of heart failure: the Framingham study. *J Am Coll Cardiol* 1993;22(Suppl A):6A–13A, with permission.]

The incidence of heart failure is twice as high in persons with hypertension, and the incidence can be stratified based on severity of hypertension as shown in Figure 89.3 (2). Similarly, when followed prospectively, persons with a history of prior myocardial infarction are found to have a five-fold greater incidence of heart failure over a 5-year period (2) (Fig. 89.4).

Mortality

Although a significant decline in mortality due to coronary heart disease and hypertension has occurred over the past 40

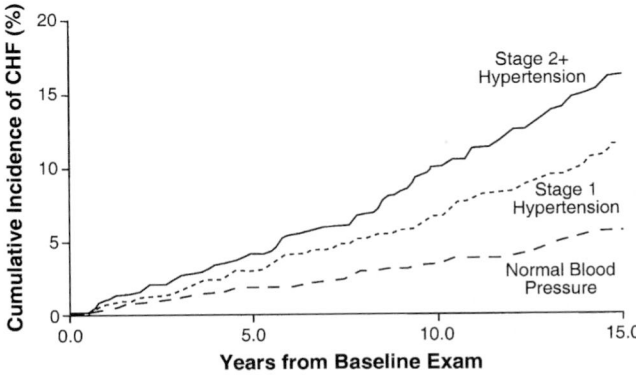

FIGURE 89.3 Incidence of congestive heart failure (CHF) in men and women aged 50 to 79 years by hypertension status. Stage 1 hypertension is defined as systolic blood pressure of 140 to 159 mm Hg or diastolic blood pressure of 90 to 99 mm Hg in people not receiving antihypertensive medication; stage 2 or higher hypertension is defined as systolic blood pressure of 160 or greater, diastolic blood pressure of 100 or greater, or current use of antihypertensive medication. (Adapted from National Heart, Lung and Blood Institute. Congestive heart failure in the United States: a new epidemic. Bethesda, MD: U.S. Department of Health and Human Services, 1996.)

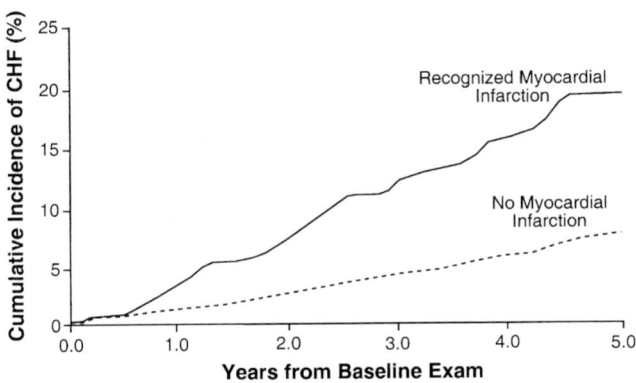

FIGURE 89.4 Incidence of congestive heart failure (CHF) by myocardial infarction status. (Adapted from National Heart, Lung and Blood Institute. *Congestive heart failure in the United States: a new epidemic.* Bethesda, MD: U.S. Department of Health and Human Services, 1996.)

years, no significant decline was observed in age-adjusted mortality in patients diagnosed with congestive heart failure in the Framingham cohort (15). Heart failure remains a lethal condition, with 5-year survival rates of less than 40% from the time of diagnosis, as shown in Figure 89.5. Data obtained from the National Center for Health Statistics in 1988 show that 267,356 deaths due to heart failure occurred. At all ages, the death rates from heart failure are greater for the African-America population, as shown in Figure 89.6, and the mortality rate from heart failure increases precipitously after age 65 years (15). Since 1968, the incidence of heart failure as the primary cause of death has increased four-fold (15). The most dismal prognosis for patients with severe symptoms [New York Heart Association (NYHA) class IV] and coronary artery disease was a survival rate of 43% and 18% at 1 and 3 years, respectively (22). Patients with dilated, nonischemic cardiomyopathy who are symptomatic with medical therapy have a better prognosis than patients with underlying coronary artery disease (22). ▼ o76

Hospitalization Rates

Congestive heart failure represents America's largest diagnosis-related group, with an annual inpatient volume of more than 600,000, almost double the number of all other cardiovascular disorders (21). As the U.S. population ages, heart failure is a rapidly increasing indication for hospitalization, as depicted in Figure 89.7 (17). A sharp increase in the rates of hospital admission for heart failure in the elderly cohort older than 65 years was observed from 1972 to 1990, with the rate tripling from 55 per 10,000 to more than 150 per 10,000 population (17). The National Hospital Discharge Survey, which analyzed data from 1973 to 1986, identified a dramatic increase in hospital discharges for congestive heart failure in the population older than 74 years (23). Data for persons aged 35 to 54 years showed a significant gender and race differential (nonwhite men and

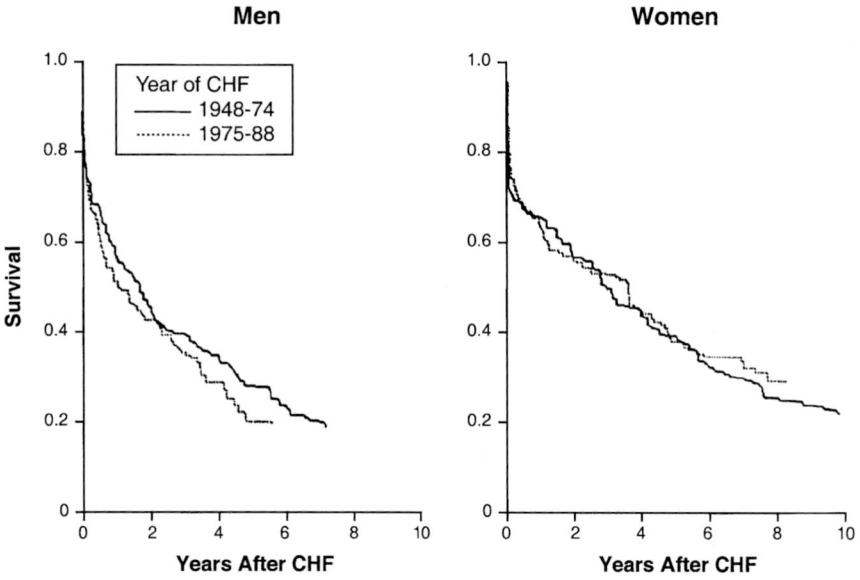

FIGURE 89.5 Age-adjusted survival rates by calendar year after the first diagnosis of congestive heart failure (CHF) for men and women in the Framingham Heart Study. No significant change in survival over 40 years of follow-up was found despite a considerable decline in coronary artery disease mortality. [Adapted from Kannel WG, Ho K, Thom T. Changing epidemiological features of cardiac failure. *Br Heart J* 1994;72(Suppl 2):S3–S9, with permission.]

white men have the highest hospitalization rates). With advancing age, however, the gender and race differential for hospitalization attributable to heart failure disappears (23). Overall, since 1971, a fourfold increase has occurred in hospital admissions for which congestive heart failure was the primary diagnosis, rising from 165,000 to 722,000 in 1990 (17). In 1997, 957,000 Americans were discharged from short-stay hospitals with a primary diagnosis of heart failure; of these, 79% were age 65 and older (11).

ECONOMICS AND THE HEALTH CARE IMPACT OF HEART FAILURE

Medical economics and heart failure are reviewed in Chapter 42. Health care reform in the United States has led to

the reexamining, restructuring, and reengineering of all aspects of health care delivery in America. Because congestive heart failure represents the number one public health problem in cardiovascular medicine, its economic impact is tremendous. Projections attempting to estimate the total health care costs of heart failure are performed using indirect measures, extrapolations, and assumptions. Statistics, including those from the National Disease and Therapeutics Index, National Hospital Discharge Survey, and National Ambulatory Medical Care Survey, are used (18,24). Recent estimates of total annual health care expenditures for heart failure in America have ranged from $10.3 billion to $37.8 billion (18,24). The disparity of these figures demonstrates the unavailability of accurate economic data, but the cost to American society per year is at least $10 billion and may be as high as $40 billion. The

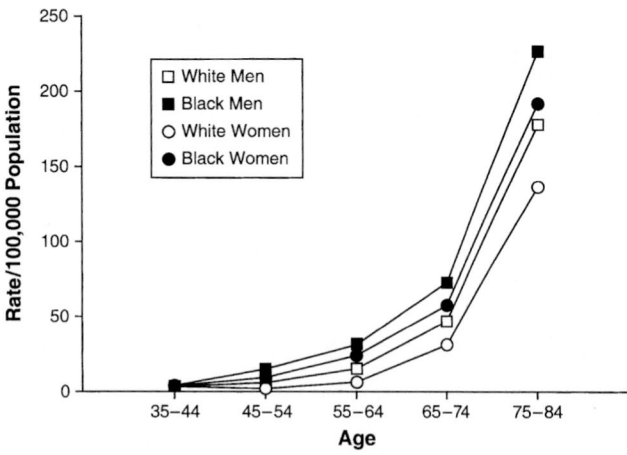

FIGURE 89.6 U.S. heart failure death rate in 1988 by age, gender, and race. Compiled from data from the National Center for Health Statistics. [Adapted from Kannel WG, Ho K, Thom T. Changing epidemiological features of cardiac failure. *Br Heart J* 1994;72(Suppl 2):S3–S9, with permission.]

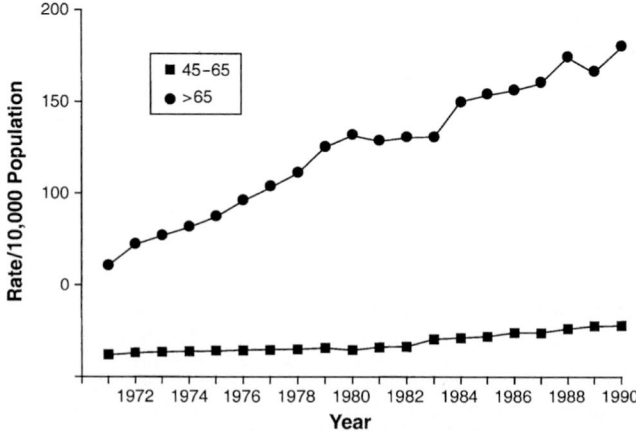

FIGURE 89.7 Hospital admissions per 10,000 population per year for congestive heart failure in the United States. [Adapted from Kannel WG, Ho K, Thom T. Changing epidemiological features of cardiac failure. *Br Heart J* 1994;72(Suppl 2):S3–S9, with permission.]

American Heart Association estimated $21.0 billion for direct and indirect costs of congestive heart failure in the United States in 2001 (11). The breakdown included: $14.3 billion for hospital and nursing home care, $1.5 billion for physician and professional services, $1.6 billion for medications, $1.5 billion for home health care, and $1.6 billion for lost productivity and mortality. Hence, 68% of the total expense is for inpatient care, very similar to the estimates for inpatient care (73% and 62%) in the other two reports cited earlier (18,24). Considering the rates of hospitalization (including readmissions) for heart failure, the fact that 1% to 2% of total health care expenditures is consumed by treatment of heart failure in a number of industrialized countries is not surprising (9) (*e*Fig. 89.0.2). Actual health care expenditures for treatment of heart failure can only be estimated. All estimates assume the accuracy of discharge summaries, death certificates, prescription use, and physician surveys in coding heart failure events. ▼ o77

ECONOMIC IMPACT OF PHARMACOTHERAPY

ACEIs reduce mortality, progression of symptomatic disease, and hospitalizations in patients with symptomatic and asymptomatic left ventricular dysfunction (34,35). In the Studies of Left Ventricular Dysfunction (SOLVD) treatment trial, a 26% reduction in risk of death or hospitalizations for heart failure was seen among patients treated with enalapril maleate (34). In the SOLVD prevention trial, which enrolled asymptomatic patients with left ventricular systolic dysfunction, enalapril-treated patients experienced a 36% risk reduction for first hospitalizations and a 44% risk reduction for multiple hospitalizations for heart failure (35). Based on results of published randomized trials with hydralazine hydrochloride/isosorbide dinitrate and enalapril, the incremental cost-effectiveness ratio per year of life saved was calculated (36). The cost per year of life saved is an additional $5,600 for a patient receiving hydralazine and isosorbide and an additional $9,700 for a patient receiving enalapril above the costs for patients receiving no vasodilator therapy (Table 89.1). In comparison, when this modeling technique is used, the cost for a year of life saved by treatment of moderate hypertension is $25,000 and for a year of "useful life saved" by renal dialysis is $35,000 (36). A study in the United Kingdom found that only 17% of patients with heart failure were prescribed ACEIs by their general practitioner (37). In the United States, surveys have indicated that cardiologists are more likely to prescribe ACEIs than are general practitioners and internists (38). Furthermore, "heart failure specialty cardiologists" are more likely to use the documented efficacious dosage of studied drugs and to avoid concomitant use of potentially deleterious medications. ▼ o78

ECONOMIC STRATEGIES FOR TREATMENT OF HEART FAILURE

Principles

Imperative for effective treatment is correctly diagnosing the heart disease and, hence, facilitating definition of the best therapy. Already acknowledged was the fact that heart failure specialists believe that many patients receive suboptimal pharmacotherapy. Perhaps more problematic is the failure to recognize and apply an effective surgical or medical treatment. Regional heart failure centers evaluate many patients referred for consideration of heart transplantation (54). Only approximately 30% of patients referred are listed for transplantation initially. Treatable forms of heart failure must be identified. The expert opinion of a heart failure specialist may often identify an appropriate treatment other than cardiac transplantation. Examples would include the treatment of an arrhythmia that leads to improvement in ventricular function, successful surgical revascularization of a patient with hibernating myocardium, and careful observation of a patient with new-onset dilated cardiomyopathy who ultimately has spontaneous improvement in ventricular function. Transplantation in these situations would be medically inappropriate and expensive and would deprive another patient of a potential donor organ. A positive spin-off of the creation of regional heart failure/transplantation centers has been the exposure of referred patients to heart failure specialists who can make definitive diagnostic and treatment plans (55). These observations are most relevant to patients with advanced heart failure, who have the highest short-term mortality. Patients with stable NYHA class I or II heart failure are generally cared for very appropriately by the primary care physician or general cardiologist. Patients with problematic refractory heart failure may benefit from evaluation by a heart failure specialist (14).

Educational Programs

The heart failure guidelines stress the importance of education in the treatment of heart failure. Education must extend beyond the patient to the family members and care providers who assist in the necessary dietary and lifestyle modifications (42,58). Educational initiatives improve quality of life for the patient and prevent hospitalization. Hence, the cost-savings potential is tremendous. Educational interventions designed to improve dietary compliance and reduce hospital admissions in heart failure patients have been found to be highly successful (59,60). A physician-supervised, nurse-managed, home care program for heart failure management that implemented pharmacologic and dietary therapy with frequent monitoring via telephone contact was conducted in northern California (59). Three generic problems in the outpatient management of heart failure were addressed: cognitive (what to do), execu-

TABLE 89.1 COST EFFECTIVENESS OF PHARMACOLOGIC AGENTS FOR THE TREATMENT OF HEART FAILURE

Study and yr	Data extraction	Therapeutic agent(s)	Clinical outcomes	Cost outcomes	Comments
Paul et al. 1994	V-HeFT I V-HeFT II SOLVD	Enalapril maleate, hydralazine hydrochloride/ isosorbide dini-trate	V-HeFT I: 34% reduction in mortality with hydralazine/isosorbide V-HeFT II: 28% reduction in mortality with enal-april SOLVD: 10% reduction in mortality with enalapril, fewer HF admissions	Compared with stan-dard therapy: Hydralazine/isosorbide: $5,600/yr of life saved Enalapril: $9,700/yr of life saved	Assumptions: Therapy continued for 10 yr; benefits linear over time; discount rate: 5%/ yr; estimated cost for HF admissions: $6,750; sensi-tivity analysis: little effect
Butler and Fletcher 1996	SOLVD	Enalapril	16% mortality reduc-tion, increased sur-vival by 1.68–1.80 mo, decreased HF admis-sion	Net savings of $171–$252/patient treated with enalapril; worst-case scenario: $21,735/ yr of life saved	Assumptions: 4-yr treatment period; $622/HF admission; dis-count rate: 5%/yr
Kleber 1994	Munich MHFT	Captopril	59% reduction in HF pro-gression	Total costs "almost identical" with cap-topril and placebo	Modest increase in cost for stable patients; cost sav-ing for patients with pro-gressive HF
Tsevat et al. 1995	SAVE	Captopril	19% mortality reduc-tion, 22% reduction in HF admissions, 25% reduction in MIs	Cost per QALY ranged from $60,800 to $3,700 for patients aged 50–80 if benefit ceased after 4 yr	If benefits persist beyond 4 yr, CE ratio improves in younger patients; sensi-tivity analysis: CE ratio always favorable for patients 60–80 yr
Ward et al. 1995	PROVED RADIANCE	Digoxin	PROVED: 50% reduction in HF exacerbations RADIANCE: 77% reduc-tion in HF exacerbations	Continuation of digoxin therapy saved $338/patient	Withdrawal studies; sensi-tivity analysis: digoxin is cost saving if incidence of toxic effects is <33%/yr
Delea et al. 1999	U.S. Carvedilol Heart Fail-ure Trials	Carvedilol	65% mortality reduc-tion, 27% reduction in CV admissions	Incremental CE; ratio of $12,800 to $29,500/ life-year saved	Projected lifetime costs based on limited or sus-tained benefits of therapy
Marius-Nunez et al. 1996	Michael Reese Hos-pital, Chi-cago, IL	Milrinone lactate, dobutamine hydrochloride	55% reduction in admis-sions, 72% reduction in hospital days	86% reduction in inpa-tient expenditures	Not a formal cost analysis, effect on mortality unknown

CE, cost effectiveness; CV, cardiovascular; HF, heart failure; MHFT, Mild Heart Failure Trial; MIs, myocardial infarctions; PROVED, Prospective Ran-domized Study of Ventricular Failure and Efficacy of Digoxin trial; QALY, quality-adjusted life-year; RADIANCE, Randomized Assessment of Digoxin and Inhibitors of Angiotensin Converting Enzyme trial; SAVE, Survival and Ventricular Enlargement trial; SOLVD, Studies of Left Ventric-ular Dysfunction treatment trial; V-HeFT, Veterans Administration Heart Failure Trial.

tive (who should do it), and organizational (when and where it should be done). Consensus guidelines (of the American College of Cardiology/American Heart Associa-tion consensus report and Agency for Health Care Policy and Research) were embedded in the clinical algorithms. The nurse-manager was responsible for obtaining essential information from the patient and laboratory and carrying out the therapeutic program. Fifty-one patients with mod-erate to severe heart failure were followed for over 4 months, and hospitalization rates for heart failure declined significantly by 87%. Other key findings included a reduc-tion in dietary sodium by 38% and a significant increase in dosages of lisinopril and hydralazine (59). Although this was not a randomized trial, nonetheless it emphasizes the health care impact of adherence to heart failure guidelines and dietary and educational programs in the management of heart failure. Eight studies (Table 89.2) without a phar-

macologic component have shown the benefit of multidis-ciplinary education-based therapy for heart failure (7).

Management of Chronic Disease

Disease management programs are designed to reduce net costs and improve patient outcomes. The primary care model includes a primary care physician as the gatekeeper. Medical care is scheduled and episodic, and the focus is on reducing specialist referrals. In contrast, the chronic care model emphasizes more liberal access to specialized physi-cian and nursing care, disease management, patient moni-toring and proactive interventions, and reduction of acute hospital admissions. Disease management is a concept aimed at patient populations with a discrete clinical prob-lem and proposes that tertiary care provided by specialists can be more cost effective and of higher quality than care

TABLE 89.2 COST EFFECTIVENESS OF NONPHARMACOLOGIC INTERVENTIONS FOR THE TREATMENT OF HEART FAILURE

Study and yr	Study design	No. of patients	Intervention	Duration of follow-up	Results	Comments
Studies without a pharmacologic component						
Cintron et al. 1983	Observational: preintervention and postintervention	15	Nurse-practitioner–based clinic with physician referral as needed, average of 18 clinic visits/yr	24 mo[a]	61% reduction in hospitalizations, 85% reduction in hospital days, cost reduction of $8,000/patient/yr	Mean age, 65 yr; NYHA class III–IV; improved patient satisfaction
Rich et al. 1993	Randomized pilot study	98	Nurse-directed team with patient education, dietary counseling, social services, home care, telephone follow-up	90 d	27% reduction in readmission, 25% reduction in hospital days	All patients aged ≥70 yr; mean NYHA class, 2.8
Lasater 1996	Observational: preintervention and postintervention	8	Nurse-managed heart failure clinic with access to physician, dietitian, and social worker	6 mo	14% reduction in readmissions, 25% reduction in hospital days	No information provided on patient population
Kostis et al. 1994	Randomized parallel groups	20	Exercise, cognitive therapy, stress management, dietary counseling	12 wk	Improved exercise tolerance; reduced anxiety, depression; enhanced weight loss	Age range, 54–77 yr; digoxin group and placebo group as controls
Kornowski et al. 1995	Observation: preintervention and postintervention	42	Intensive home care, surveillance by internist and paramedical team, at least 1 visit/wk	1 yr	62% reduction in hospitalizations, 77% reduction in hospital days, 72% reduction in CV admissions, improved ability to perform activities of daily living	Mean age, 78 yr; NYHA class III–IV
Rich et al. 1995	Randomized clinical trial	282	Nurse-directed team with patient education, dietary counseling, social services, home care, telephone follow-up	90 d	44% reduction in readmission, 56% reduction in HF admissions, improved quality of life, improved compliance, cost reduction of $460/patient	Mean age, 79 yr; high-risk population; benefits persisted up to 1 yr
Stewart et al. 1999	Randomized clinical trial	97	Single home visit by nurse and pharmacist 1 wk after discharge	18 mo	50% reduction in admissions, 46% reduction in mortality, 52% reduction in hospital costs	Mean age, 75 yr; NYHA class II–III; high-risk population
Dennis et al. 1996	Retrospective chart review	24	Home health nurse, teaching, clinical assessments	90 d	36% fewer readmissions for patients receiving home care	Mean age, 71 yr
Studies with a pharmacologic component						
West et al. 1997	Observational: preintervention and postintervention	51	Physician-supervised, nurse-mediated, home-based system with frequent telephone contacts targeting medication dosing, compliance, activities, symptom status	138 ± 44 d[b]	74% reduction in hospitalization; 87% reduction in HF admissions; fewer office and ED visits; improved symptoms, quality of life, exercise tolerance; improved ACEI dosing and salt restriction	Mean age, 66 yr; NYHA class I–II, 60%; class III–IV, 40%; initial clinic visit, subsequent follow-up by telephone
Fonarow et al. 1997	Observational: preintervention and postintervention	214	Comprehensive management by HF/transplant team, including diet, exercise, teaching, medication	6 mo	35% reduction in hospitalizations, improved NYHA class and exercise tolerance, improved medication dosing, cost reduction of $9,800/patient	Mean age, 52 yr; NYHA class III–IV

ACEI, angiotensin-converting enzyme inhibitor; CV, cardiovascular; ED, emergency department; HF, heart failure; NYHA, New York Heart Association.
[a]Mean.
[b]Mean ± standard deviation.

THE FUTURE

Potential economic strategies to face the epidemic of heart failure should include the following initiatives: (a) targeted reduction of inpatient costs, (b) investment in outpatient care and development of chronic disease management programs for heart failure, (c) prevention of admissions (more important than reduction in length of stay), (d) concentration of efforts and resources on high-risk patients (those with a history of frequent readmissions), (e) use of specialized heart failure treatment providers (physicians, nurses, dietitians, rehabilitation specialists), and (f) provisions for extensive patient education. The establishment and implementation of regional specialized heart failure centers should include the following to help achieve these initiatives: (a) detailed patient evaluation to stage disease and ensure appropriate diagnosis and treatment, (b) close patient monitoring at intervals tailored to the individual patient's needs (direct and telephone or electronic contact), (c) immediate access of patients to heart failure team staff and timely responses to patient crises, and (d) comprehensive and continuing patient education concerning heart failure. Regional heart failure centers will provide expertise in the medical and surgical management of heart failure (54,70). Surgical therapy [high-risk standard cardiac surgical procedures, transplantation, connection to mechanical circulatory assist devices, ventricular remodeling procedures (partial left ventriculec-

tomy, Dor procedure, Acorn device, Myosplint), transmyocardial laser revascularization, etc.] has become an essential component and now extends far beyond transplantation. Increasing numbers of high-risk patients will benefit from standard surgical procedures, with a safety net of mechanical support and transplantation available at specialized heart failure centers.

Developing and perfecting a health care delivery system for heart failure should help achieve these goals and result in improved survival, better quality of life, and reduction in cost. Primary prevention is the solution to the challenge. Secondary prevention strategies to alleviate morbidity should be an immediate focus, however, to reduce the economic burden of this devastating epidemic.

The development of health care delivery systems incorporating specialized heart failure centers with systemwide disease management programs will provide the infrastructure to achieve cost-effective improved clinical outcomes for the rapidly expanding heart failure patient population. Efforts and resources will be concentrated on high-risk patients so that overall costs are reduced. Increased emphasis on education of patients and care providers is required. The role of the heart failure nurse-practitioner will expand in heart failure patient management. Emphasis will continue to be on primary prevention as the seminal solution to the increasing cost of heart failure management.

---

given in the primary care setting (61). Heart failure is a specific clinical condition that is amenable to treatment by means of a disease management program using specialized physicians and intensive nursing and education programs (14,21,59). A typical heart failure disease management program consists of inpatient consultation and care, treatment at an outpatient heart failure clinic, cardiac home care, and compliance monitoring (62). ▼ o79

CONTROVERSIES AND PERSONAL PERSPECTIVES

Many heart failure patients are treated suboptimally with pharmacotherapy and receive medical regimens that do not comply with published guidelines for heart failure management (41,44,45). A U.S. survey showed that cardiologists are more likely to prescribe ACEIs than are general practitioners and internists (38). Furthermore, a survey comparing the practice patterns of cardiologists and heart failure specialists showed general conformity but concluded that a portion of

heart failure patients may be managed more optimally by heart failure specialists (64). The conclusion was that the improved outcomes observed in heart failure clinics was attributable to the optimal management provided by cardiologists with additional experience in treating heart failure.

These observations indicate that specialist care is cost effective and improves outcomes. Efforts to contain health care costs have attempted to limit patients' access to specialists, including cardiologists. As discussed previously, the experience of the cardiologist has been shown to be linked to the outcome of patients after cardiac transplantation (48). Few data are currently available to prove that heart failure specialists provide superior care for heart failure patients. An observational study at a single institution showed that hospitalized heart failure patients cared for by a cardiologist were sicker, had a longer length of stay, and underwent more diagnostic studies; however, the incidence of 6-month readmission was lower than that for patients cared for by generalists (65). An analysis of all New York State hospital discharges in heart failure cases (44,296 patients) in 1995 showed that 23% received care from cardiologists, 63% from internists, 11% from family physicians, and 3% from other physicians (66). Care by cardiologists was not associated with longer stay or higher hospital charges, a result that belies the tenet that specialist care is more costly. Conclusions cannot be drawn at present, but the question of who should deliver care to heart failure patients in a manner that is cost effective while maintaining good-quality outcomes requires investigation. Patients with advanced heart failure represent a subpopulation for which specialist treatment seems clearly justified, and the multidisciplinary care model of disease management appears cost effective with superior clinical outcomes.

The a priori end point in most randomized heart failure trials is mortality. Pharmacologic agents that improve quality of life and reduce hospitalizations but increase mortality are unlikely to obtain approval from the U.S. Food and Drug Administration. Initial reports on the use of outpatient dobutamine hydrochloride therapy showed that functional class improved significantly, but mortality was high in this uncontrolled study (67). Outpatient inotropic therapy appears to be cost effective and is reimbursed by many third-party payers despite the lack of randomized trials showing efficacy or a U.S. Food and Drug Administration–approved indication. An uncontrolled study followed 36 patients with intractable heart failure on intermittent inotropic therapy for a mean duration of 294 days (68). The number of emergency room visits, hospital admissions, and days hospitalized all decreased significantly compared to the pretreatment period, and no adverse events were reported. The results of a randomized controlled study evaluating the use of weekly milrinone lactate infusions in treating refractory heart failure over 6 months of follow-up [Randomized Outpatient Assessment of Milrinone Efficacy in Heart Failure (ROME) trial] remain unpublished. No conclusions or projections can be drawn from these uncontrolled studies; nonetheless, many heart failure clinics with outpatient infusion programs have been established throughout the United States. Outpatient inotropic infusions are likely vastly overused in patients who could be readily managed by experienced heart failure specialists with conventional oral medications (69). Outpatient inotropic infusions administered as palliative treatment for refractory heart failure in patients who are not candidates for transplantation may facilitate a return to the home setting with an improved quality of life. In a fatal chronic illness such as heart failure, the quality-of-life benefits of a therapy must be considered, as they may outweigh any mortality effects.

REFERENCES

1. Garg R, Packer M, Pitt B, et al. Heart failure in the 1990s: evolution of a major public health problem in cardiovascular medicine. *J Am Coll Cardiol* 1993;22[Suppl A]:3A–5A.

2. National Heart, Lung and Blood Institute. Congestive heart failure in the United States: a new epidemic. Bethesda, MD: US Department of Health and Human Services, 1996.

3. Shepherd J, Cobbe SM, Ford I, et al., for the West of Scotland Coronary Prevention Study Group. Prevention of coronary heart disease with pravastatin in men with hypercholesterolemia. *N Engl J Med* 1995;333:1301–1307.

4. Kostis JB, Davis BR, Cutte J, et al. Prevention of heart failure by antihypertensive drug treatment in older persons with isolated systolic hypertension. *JAMA* 1997;278:212–216.

5. Pfeffer MA, Braunwald E, Moye LA, et al. Effect of captopril on mortality and morbidity in patients with left ventricular dysfunction after myocardial infarction: results of the survival and ventricular enlargement trial. *N Engl J Med* 1992;327:669–677.

6. Kupersmith J, Holmes-Rovner M, Hogan A, et al. Cost-effectiveness analysis in heart disease, part I: general principles. *Prog Cardiovasc Dis* 1994;37:161–184.

7. Rich MW, Nease RF. Cost-effectiveness analysis in clinical practice: the case of heart failure. *Arch Intern Med* 1999;159:1690–1700.

8. Kleber FX. The economics of heart failure. *J R Soc Med* 1996;89:9–12.

9. McMurray JJ, Stewart S. Epidemiology, aetiology, and prognosis of heart failure. *Heart* 2000;83:596–602.

10. Eriksson H. Heart failure: a growing public health problem. *J Intern Med* 1995;237:135–141.

11. American Heart Association. *2001 heart and stroke statistical update: economic cost of cardiovascular diseases.* Dallas, TX: American Heart Association, 2001.

12. Stewart S, Marley JE, Horowitz JD. Effects of a multidisciplinary, home-based intervention on unplanned readmissions and survival among patients with chronic congestive heart failure: a randomised controlled study. *Lancet* 1999;354:1077–1083.

13. Rich MW. Multidisciplinary interventions for the management of heart failure: where do we stand? *Am Heart J* 1999;138:599–601.

14. Albert NM, Young JB. Heart failure disease management: a team approach. *Cleve Clin J Med* 2001;68:53–62.

15. Ho KKL, Pinsky JL, Kannel WB, et al. The epidemiology of heart failure: the Framingham study. *J Am Coll Cardiol* 1993;22:[Suppl A]:6A–13A.

16. Kannel WB, Belanger AJ. Epidemiology of heart failure. *Am Heart J* 1991;121:951–957.

17. Kannel WB, Ho K, Thom T. Changing epidemiological features of cardiac failure. *Br Heart J* 1994;72[Suppl 2]:S3–S9.

18. O'Connell JB, Bristow MR. Economic impact of heart failure in the United States: time for a different approach. *J Heart Lung Transplant* 1993;13:S107–S112.

19. Marantz PR, Tobin JN, Wassertheil-Smoller S, et al. The relationship between left ventricular systolic function and congestive heart failure diagnosed by clinical criteria. *Circulation* 1988;77:607–612.

20. Cowie MR, Mosterd A, Wood DA, et al. The epidemiology of heart failure. *Eur Heart J* 1997;18:208–225.

21. Field JL. *Beyond four walls: research summary for clinicians*

and administrators on CHF management. Washington, DC: Cardiology Preeminence Round Table, Advisory Board Company, 1994.

22. Smith WM. Epidemiology of congestive heart failure. *Am J Cardiol* 1985;55[Suppl A]:3A–8A.

23. Ghali JK, Cooper R, Ford E. Trends in hospitalization rates for heart failure in the United States, 1973–1986. *Arch Intern Med* 1990;150:769–773.

24. Parmley WW. Cost-effective cardiology: cost-effective management of heart failure. *Clin Cardiol* 1996;19:240–242.

25. Rich MW, Beckham V, Wittenberg C, et al. A multidisciplinary intervention to prevent the readmission of elderly patients with congestive heart failure. *N Engl J Med* 1995;333:1190–1195.

26. Mudge GH, Goldstein S, Addonizio LJ, et al. 24th Bethesda conference: cardiac transplantation. Task Force 3: recipient guidelines/prioritization. *J Am Coll Cardiol* 1993;22:21–31.

27. Michalsen A, Konig MA, Thimme W. Preventable causative factors leading to hospital admission with decompensated heart failure. *Heart* 1998;80:437–441.

28. Cohn JN. The management of chronic heart failure. *N Engl J Med* 1996;335:490–498.

29. Anderson GF, Steinberg EP. Hospital readmission in the Medicare population. *N Engl J Med* 1984;311:1349–1353.

30. Ashton CM, Kuykendall DH, Johnson ML, et al. The association between the quality of inpatient care and early readmission. *Ann Intern Med* 1995;122:415–421.

31. Lee TH, Hamilton MA, Stevenson LW, et al. Impact of left ventricular cavity size on survival in advanced heart failure. *Am J Cardiol* 1993;72:672–676.

32. Mancini DM, Eisen H, Kussmaul W, et al. Value of peak exercise oxygen consumption for optimal timing of cardiac transplantation in ambulatory patients with heart failure. *Circulation* 1991;83:778–786.

33. Cleland JGF. Health economic consequences of the pharmacological treatment of heart failure. *Eur Heart J* 1998;19[Suppl P]:32–39.

34. Studies of Left Ventricular Dysfunction investigators. Effect of enalapril on survival in patients with reduced left ventricular ejection fractions and congestive heart failure. *N Engl J Med* 1991;325:293–302.

35. Studies of Left Ventricular Dysfunction investigators. Effect of enalapril on mortality and the development of heart failure in asymptomatic patients with reduced left ventricular ejection fractions. *N Engl J Med* 1992;327:685–691.

36. Paul SD, Kuntz KM, Eagle KA, et al. Cost and effectiveness of angiotensin converting enzyme inhibition in patients with congestive heart failure. *Arch Intern Med* 1994;154:1143–1149.

37. Clarke KW, Gray D, Hampton JR. Evidence of inadequate investigation and treatment of patients with heart failure. *Br Heart J* 1994;71:584–587.

38. Edep ME, Shah NB, Tateo IM, et al. Differences between primary care physicians and cardiologists in management of congestive heart failure: relation to practice guidelines. *J Am Coll Cardiol* 1997;30(2):518–526.

39. Packer M, Bristow MR, Cohn JN, et al. The effect of carvedilol on morbidity and mortality in patients with chronic heart failure. U.S. Carvedilol Heart Failure Study Group. *N Engl J Med* 1996;334:1349–1355.

40. Ward RE, Gheorghiade M, Young JB, et al. Economic outcomes of withdrawal of digoxin therapy in adult patients with stable congestive heart failure. *J Am Coll Cardiol* 1995;26:93–101.

41. Baker DW, Konstam MA, Bottorff M, et al. Management of heart failure I: pharmacologic treatment. *JAMA* 1994;272:1361–1366.

42. Dracup K, Baker DW, Dunbar SB, et al. Management of heart failure II: counseling, education and lifestyle modifications. *JAMA* 1994;272:1442–1446.

43. Guidelines for the evaluation and management of heart failure. ACC/AHA Task Force. *J Am Coll Cardiol* 1995;26:1376–1398.

44. Consensus recommendations for the management of chronic heart failure. On behalf of the membership of the advisory council to improve outcomes nationwide in heart failure. *Am J Cardiol* 1999;83(2A):1A–38A.

45. Heart Failure Society of America Practice Guidelines. HFSA guidelines for the management of patients with heart failure due to left ventricular systolic dysfunction: pharmacological approaches. *Congestive Heart Failure* 2000;4:11–39.

46. Starling RC. The heart failure pandemic: changing patterns, costs, and treatment strategies. *Cleve Clin J Med* 1998;65:351–358.

47. Renlund DG, Bristow MR, Lybbert MR, et al. Medicare-designated centers for cardiac transplantation. *N Engl J Med* 1987;316:873–876.

48. Laffel GL, Barnett A, Finkelstein S, et al. The relation between experience and outcome in heart transplantation. *N Engl J Med* 1992;327:1220–1225.

49. Hosenpud JD, Breen TJ, Edwards EB, et al. The effect of transplant center volume on cardiac transplant outcome. *JAMA* 1994;271:1844–1849.

50. Evans RW. Socioeconomic aspects of heart transplantation. *Curr Opin Cardiol* 1995;10:169–179.

51. O'Connell JB, Gunnar RM, Evans RW, et al. Task force 1: organization of heart transplantation in the U.S. *J Am Coll Cardiol* 1993;22:8–14.

52. Starling RC, Goormastic M, Leier C, et al., for the Ohio Organ Transplant Consortium. Maturation of heart transplantation in Ohio: evolving outcomes and changing economics. In: *Proceedings of the 15th Annual Meeting, American Society of Transplant Physicians.* Thorofare, NJ: American Society of Transplant Physicians, 1996:127.

53. Starling RC, McCarthy PM, Buda T, et al. Results of partial left ventriculectomy for dilated cardiomyopathy: hemodynamic, clinical and echocardiographic observations. *J Am Coll Cardiol* 2000;36:2098–2103.

54. Abraham WT, Bristow MR. Specialized centers for heart failure management. *Circulation* 1997;96:2755–2757.

55. Fonarow GC, Stevenson LW, Walden JA. Impact of a comprehensive management program on hospital readmission and functional status of patients with advanced heart failure. *J Am Coll Cardiol* 1997;30:725–732.

56. Krumholz HM, Chen YT, Vaccarino V, et al. Predictors of readmission among elderly survivors of admission with heart failure. *Am Heart J* 2000;139:72–77.

57. Kornowski R, Zeeli D, Averbuch M, et al. Intensive home-care surveillance prevents hospitalization and improves morbidity rates among elderly patients with severe congestive heart failure. *Am Heart J* 1995;129:762–766.

58. Chin MH, Goldman L. Correlates of early hospital readmission or death in patients with congestive heart failure. *Am J Cardiol* 1997;79:1640–1644.

59. West JA, Miller NH, Parker KM, et al. A comprehensive management system for heart failure improves clinical outcomes and reduces medical resource utilization. *Am J Cardiol* 1997;79:58–63.

60. Rosenberg SG. Patient education leads to better care for heart patients. *Health Serv Mental Health Admin Health Rep* 1971;Suppl A:793–802.

61. Schulman KA, Mark DB, Califf RM. Outcomes and costs within a disease management program for advanced congestive heart failure. *Am Heart J* 1998;135(6 Pt 2):S285–S292.

62. Knox D, Mischke L. Implementing a congestive heart failure disease management program to decrease length of stay and cost. *J Cardiovasc Nurs* 1999;14;55–74.

63. Keteyian SJ, Levine AB, Brawner CA, et al. Exercise training in patients with heart failure: a randomized, controlled trial. *Ann Intern Med* 1996;124:1051–1057.

64. Bello D, Shah NB, Edep ME, et al. Self-reported differences between cardiologists and heart failure specialists in the management of chronic heart failure. *Am Heart J* 1999;138:100–107.

65. Reis SE, Holubkov R, Edmundowicz D, et al. Treatment of patients admitted to the hospital with congestive heart failure: specialty-related disparities in practice patterns and outcomes. *J Am Coll Cardiol* 1997;30:733–738.

66. Philbin EF, Jenkins PL. Differences between patients with heart failure treated by cardiologists, internists, family physicians, and other physicians: analysis of a large, statewide database. *Am Heart J* 2000;139;491–496.

67. Applefeld MM, Newman KA, Sutton FJ, et al. Outpatient dobutamine and dopamine infusions in the management of chronic heart failure: clinical experience in 21 patients. *Am Heart J* 1987;114:589–595.

68. Marius-Nunez AL, Heaney L, Fernandez RN, et al. Intermittent inotropic therapy in an outpatient setting: a cost-effective therapeutic modality in patients with refractory heart failure. *Am Heart J* 1996;132:805–808.

69. Leier CV, Binkley PF. Parenteral inotropic support for advanced congestive heart failure. *Prog Cardiovasc Dis* 1998;41:207–224.

70. Hanumanthu S, Butler J, Chomsky D, et al. Effect of a heart failure program on hospitalization frequency and exercise tolerance. *Circulation* 1997;96:2842–2848.

CARDIOMYOPATHY AND MYOCARDIAL FAILURE

SUZANNE R. LUTTON
NORMAN B. RATLIFF
JAMES B. YOUNG

▼▼ *ADDITIONAL ELECTRONIC TOPICS*

Historical Perspective o80;   Idiopathic Dilated Cardiomyopathy: Pathophysiology o81;   Hypertrophic Cardiomyopathy: Clinical Profile and Management o82;   Arrhythmogenic Right Ventricular Cardiomyopathy: Prevalence and Background o83;   Arrhythmogenic Right Ventricular Cardiomyopathy: Pathophysiology o84;   Noncompacted Myocardium o85;   Human Immunodeficiency Virus o86;   Human Immunodeficiency Virus: Background and Prevalence o87;   Human Immunodeficiency Virus: Pathophysiology o88;   Human Immunodeficiency Virus: Clinical Profile and Management o89;   Anderson-Fabry's Disease o90;   Selenium Deficiency o91;   Thiamine Deficiency (Beriberi) o92;   Carnitine Deficiency o93;   Amyloidosis: Clinical Profile and Management o94;   Erb's Limb-Girdle Dystrophy o95;   Myotonic Dystrophy o96;   Alcoholic Cardiomyopathy o97;   Alcoholic Cardiomyopathy: Background and Prevalence o98;   Alcoholic Cardiomyopathy: Pathology o99;   Alcoholic Cardiomyopathy: Clinical Profile and Management p01;   Cocaine p02;   Irradiation p03;   Chloroquine Cardiomyopathy p04;   Peripartum Cardiomyopathy: Clinical Profile and Management p05

S. R. Lutton: Diagnostic Cardiology Associates, Youngstown, Ohio
N. B. Ratliff: Department of Anatomic Pathology, The Cleveland Clinic Foundation, Cleveland, Ohio
J. B. Young: Department of Medicine, Kaufman Center for Heart Failure, The Cleveland Clinic Foundation, Cleveland, Ohio

OVERVIEW

The current World Health Organization definition and classification of cardiomyopathy have been revised to reflect the recent insight gained into the pathogenesis of the heart muscle disorders. Cardiomyopathies are categorized into dilated, restrictive, hypertrophic, and unclassified based on the predominant pathophysiologic characteristics. A new category has been added to include right ventricular abnormalities. The disorders that are associated with systemic or certain cardiac diseases are called *specific heart muscle diseases* and include, for example, ischemic cardiomyopathy, diabetic cardiomyopathy, and alcoholic cardiomyopathy. Dilated cardiomyopathy (DCM) is characterized by myocyte hypertrophy and ventricular chamber dilation with diminution of systolic function. This is the most common of the cardiomyopathies. Hypertrophic cardiomyopathy (HCM) is a syndrome that results in heart failure due to left ventricular outflow tract obstruction, diastolic cardiac dysfunction, global cardiac ischemia, dysrhythmias, and sudden cardiac death syndrome in a setting of hyperactive autonomic states. Myocardial hypertrophy and mitral valve abnormalities are gross characteristics of the difficulty with myocardial histology, revealing cellular hypertrophy and disarray with substantive interstitial fibrosis. Inheritance is seemingly in an autosomal dominant fashion, due to mutations in multiple and different contractile protein genes. Restrictive cardiomyopathy is a primarily diastolic disorder, with impairment of ventricular relaxation and filling, usually resulting from an infiltrative or fibrotic process. The myocyte and its surrounding interstitium can be affected. Arrhythmogenic right ventricular cardiomyopathy (ARVC) is a fascinating disorder that primarily involves the right ventricle and may be the result of uncontrolled apoptosis. The unclassified cardiomyopathy category includes disorders such as fibroelastosis, noncompacted myocardium, and systolic dysfunction with minimal dilation. These diseases either have features that overlap the other classifications or do not readily fit any category. Ischemic cardiomyopathy is a common disorder, and one of the most important aspects of its management is identifying areas of viable, but not contracting, myocardium and restoring adequate blood flow if possible. A cardiomyopathy that is associated with infection with the human immunodeficiency virus (HIV) has many possible mechanisms; gaining a better understanding of them will improve treatment of this cardiomyopathy and others. This disorder will certainly be encountered with increasing frequency in the future. Identification of toxins that are associated with left ventricular dysfunction is important because often, if the offending agent is withdrawn, ventricular function returns to near normal levels. Finally, peripartum cardiomyopathy occurs in young women in the last trimester of pregnancy or shortly after delivery. Because its signs and symptoms may resemble some of the normal findings in pregnancy, awareness is key. No reliable methods are available to predict which patients will improve and which will progressively deteriorate. The identification of the etiology of any patient who presents with cardiomyopathy is very important, because specific treatment may reverse cardiac dysfunction. Endomyocardial biopsy is indicated in select situations: to diagnose a specific disease, as part of a clinical trial, to differentiate between restrictive and constrictive disorders, and to monitor anthracycline toxicity. Routine biopsies for idiopathic DCM are of little benefit. Future directions in the diagnosis and management of cardiomyopathies include elucidating genetic and molecular mechanisms and examining the roles of proinflammatory cytokines and apoptosis in the pathogenesis of heart failure.

DILATED CARDIOMYOPATHY

DCM is characterized by ventricular remodeling that produces chamber dilation, with normal or decreased wall thickness, and diminution in systolic function (Fig. 90.1). The impairment of systolic function can involve the left, right, or both ventricles, with the ejection fraction traditionally being defined as less than 40% (6). Although the total mass of the heart is increased, the ratio of left ventricular volume to ventricular wall thickness is much greater than for patients with HCM or diastolic dysfunction due to hypertensive heart disease (7). This eccentric hypertrophy provides a unifying concept for many different disease processes, ultimately resulting in dilation of the heart. It is important to note that remodeling of this sort is caused by diseases that are, for the most part, distinct from those causing hypertrophic and restrictive cardiomyopathy, problems that generally do not result in chamber dilation. Myocardial remodeling is associated with altered hemodynamics characterized by diminished ejection fraction, reduced stroke volume, increased chamber volumes, and, therefore, increased chamber pressures. This triggers the multiple neurohormonal aberrations that are characteristic of the heart failure milieu.

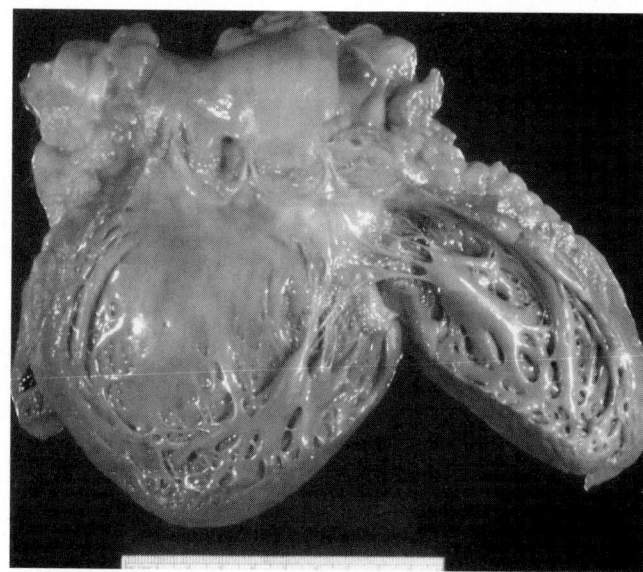

FIGURE 90.1 Dilated cardiomyopathy. The cardiomegaly, globular shape of the heart, dilated ventricular chambers, and flattened trabeculae, which are characteristic of this disease, are all evident in this photograph. No significant endocardial fibrosis is present.

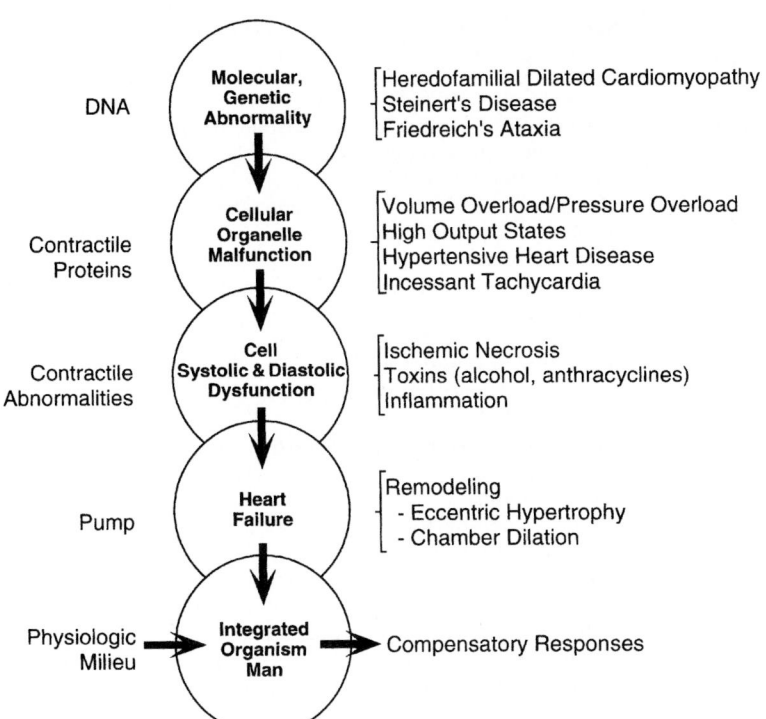

DNA — Molecular, Genetic Abnormality — [Heredofamilial Dilated Cardiomyopathy / Steinert's Disease / Friedreich's Ataxia]

Contractile Proteins — Cellular Organelle Malfunction — [Volume Overload/Pressure Overload / High Output States / Hypertensive Heart Disease / Incessant Tachycardia]

Contractile Abnormalities — Cell Systolic & Diastolic Dysfunction — [Ischemic Necrosis / Toxins (alcohol, anthracyclines) / Inflammation]

Pump — Heart Failure — [Remodeling / - Eccentric Hypertrophy / - Chamber Dilation]

Physiologic Milieu — Integrated Organism Man — Compensatory Responses

FIGURE 90.2 The milieu of dilated cardiomyopathy from molecular biodynamics to a clinical syndrome.

Often, if the toxic or injurious agent can be identified and removed before a cell mortality program is triggered (apoptosis), further detrimental chamber remodeling can be blocked and systolic function returned to a more normal state. However, DCMs generally pass through an early and late evolutionary period. The stages parallel pathophysiologic events triggered by whatever myocardial insult initiated the heart failure process in the first place. At some point, injury produces myocyte and myocardial dysfunction that antedates clinically apparent disease. As progression occurs and decompensation develops, symptoms begin to appear that are characteristic of heart failure in general. Cardiac and extracardiac signs and symptoms that are disease specific may provide insight to the etiology of the heart failure and cardiomyopathy. If the process is not interdicted, later stages will appear and manifest with profound eccentric hypertrophy and, ultimately, marked reduction in systemic flows accompanying elevation of intracardiac pressures. Figure 90.2 conceptually presents the relationship of the heart failure clinical syndrome to molecular and organspecific physiology.

DCM was previously referred to as *congestive cardiomyopathy*; however, this term is no longer applied because congestion is not consistently present, particularly in the milder and earlier stages or after therapy. DCM is the most common of the cardiomyopathies, comprising more than 90% of all cases that are referred to specialized centers (8), and represents the end result of more than 50 distinct diseases (9,10). When diagnosing DCM, it is important to review the major etiologic and pathophysiologic classes that are responsible for this disorder, as detailed in *e*Table 90.0.2. By and large,

DCMs include those that can be familial or genetic in origin, secondary to infection or inflammation, toxic substance exposure, metabolic derangements, and idiopathic. Examples of genetic disorders that cause cardiomyopathies include Friedreich's ataxia, myotonic dystrophy, Duchenne's muscular dystrophy, and certain mitochondrial dysfunction syndromes. DCM can also be ischemic in origin, particularly when microvascular disease complicating diabetes mellitus is present. A category sometimes referred to as *hyperergopathic* DCM includes heart failure caused by high cardiac output states as noted with certain vitamin deficiencies (beriberi), thyrotoxicosis (particularly Graves' disease), severe anemia, arteriovenous fistulae, osteitis deformans (Paget's disease), chronic liver disease with cirrhosis (intrahepatic arteriovenous shunts), pregnancy, and hypernephroma. Hypertensive heart disease, valvular insufficiency or stenosis, and incessant tachycardia are also examples of DCM due to an "overworked" ventricle (11). Pathogenic factors to consider when evaluating patients with DCM are the potential for substance abuse (alcohol and cocaine in particular), coronary artery disease or atherosclerotic risk factors, family history of DCM, presence of systemic arterial hypertension, history compatible with significant viral illness, presence of diabetes mellitus, cardiotoxin exposure (anthracyclines, for example), malnutrition, and valvular heart disease.

Some progress has been made in characterizing the molecular genetics of DCM (12,13). Perhaps as many as 30% of DCM cases are inherited or familial, with a significant percentage of the remaining being acquired as alluded to above. Inherited forms of DCM may have autosomal dominant, autosomal recessive, X-linked, or mitochondrial transmission, and, to date, genes for X-linked DCM and autosomal dominant DCM have been mapped with genetic heterogeneity documented. The genes for two X-linked cardiomyopathies have been identified, specifically, the dystrophin gene, also responsible for Duchenne's and Becker's muscular dystrophy, and G4.5 in Barth's syndrome, which is X-linked cardioskeletal myopathy with neutropenia and aciduria. Dystrophin is a large cytoskeletal protein that is noted in myocyte sarcolemma. The protein attaches at its N-terminal domain to F-actin in the sarcolemma matrix region and to the dystrophin-associated glycoprotein complex at its C-terminal domain. Although the protein encoded by the G4.5 gene has been identified and referred to as *Tafazzin*, its function is not presently known. Autosomal dominant DCM genes have been noted at six different loci, with "pure" DCM localized to 1q32, 2p31, 9q13, and 10q21–10q23, in contrast to DCM, with conduction defects that have been mapped to 1p1, 1q1, and 3p22–3p25 (12). Mutations in cardiac actin located on chromosome 15q14 have also been identified. Indeed, it has been suggested that DCM is, ultimately, a consequence of defective transmission of force in cardiac myocytes that leads to heart failure.

Idiopathic Dilated Cardiomyopathy

Background and Prevalence

Idiopathic DCM is a primary global myocardial disorder of unknown cause. Because it is the pathophysiologic model for other specific DCMs, this section focuses on the idiopathic type, with distinguishing characteristics of other specific disorders discussed subsequently. Idiopathic DCM alone accounts for 36 cases per 100,000 population, 10,000 deaths in the United States per year (14,15), and approximately 25% of all cases of cardiomyopathy.

Clinical Profile and Management

Most patients initially present with signs and symptoms of fluid overload or low cardiac output. Usually, by the time of diagnosis, they have severe ventricular dysfunction and New York Heart Association (NYHA) class III and IV symptoms (22). Chest pain is surprisingly common and affects up to 35% of patients with normal coronaries (22,23). This angina, in part, may be because of limited coronary vascular reserve (24). The electrocardiogram (ECG) may complicate the picture by having unexplained Q waves, and this has led to the term *pseudoinfarction*. Occasionally, patients present with more right- than left-sided heart failure symptoms, mesenteric congestion more than pulmonary edema, which can be mistaken for a gastrointestinal disorder. Arrhythmias and sudden death are common and may occur at any level of dysfunction and disability. Pulmonary and systemic thromboembolism

TABLE 90.1 PREDICTORS OF POOR OUTCOME IN DILATED CARDIOMYOPATHY

Ventricular size and functioning
  Increased left ventricular end diastolic volume
  Increased right ventricular end diastolic volume
  Low ejection fraction
  Decreased ventricular mass-volume ratio
  Global rather than segmental wall motion abnormalities
Clinical features
  New York Heart Association class IV symptoms
  Older age
  Male sex
  History of syncope
  Right-sided heart failure symptoms
  Persistent S_3
  Symptomatic ventricular tachycardia
Laboratory tests
  Hyponatremia
  Increased norepinephrine levels
  Increased atrial natriuretic factor
  Hyperreninemia
Hemodynamic monitoring
  Pulmonary capillary wedge pressure >20 mm Hg
  Cardiac index <2.5 L/min/m²
  Systemic hypotension
  Pulmonary hypertension
  Elevated central venous pressure
Cardiac tests
  Chest x-ray–increased cardiothoracic ratio
  Electrocardiographic–1- or 2-degree atrioventricular blocks,
    left bundle branch block
  Stress test–maximal systemic oxygen uptake <10–12 mL/kg
  Endomyocardial biopsy–loss of intracellular myofilaments

occur at a variable rate of approximately 1% to 6% per year without anticoagulation (25,26). It is difficult to predict the natural history of idiopathic DCM, and in the past the average 5-year survival rate was approximately 50% (27). With the increasingly aggressive use of ACE inhibitors and other therapies, survival has improved. Predictors of poor outcome are listed in Table 90.1 and parallel prognostic indicators for adverse events in patients with heart failure generally. Various ventricular size and function parameters, laboratory tests, clinical features, and cardiac studies may all be helpful in assessing prognosis. Chapters 91 and 92 discuss in full detail the treatment of acute and chronic heart failure. Management options include supportive therapy (diet, sodium, toxin and fluid restriction, exercise, etc.), medications (diuretics, digoxin, ACE inhibitors, angiotensin II receptor blockers, inotropes, anticoagulants, antiarrhythmics, and beta-blockers), ventricular assist devices, and novel surgical procedures (cardiomyoplasty, mitral and tricuspid valve repair, and partial left ventriculectomy and cardiac transplantation).

Hyperergasic Dilated Cardiomyopathy

Hyperergasia refers to an increased or excessive functional activity. Hyperergasic or hyperergopathic cardiomyopathy is cardiac remodeling and heart failure that develop secondary to chronically increased myocardial workload. This cardiomyopathy of overwork produces all of the characteristics of DCM. It is this process that is important, additionally, in settings such as acute myocardial infarction whereby well-perfused and remaining healthy myocytes are forced to tote greater workloads to compensate for the loss of neighboring contractile elements and maintain reasonable cardiac output. Situations that produce increased chronic workload with resultant myocardial hypertrophy and dilation include incessant tachycardias, high-output states that accompany anemia, thyrotoxicosis, beriberi, arteriovenous fistulae, cirrhosis of the liver, osteitis deformans, pregnancy, hypernephroma, and hypertensive heart disease. Valvular stenoses that produce significant afterload increase (aortic stenosis and pulmonic stenosis, for example) or valvular insufficiency with volume overload (aortic regurgitation and mitral regurgitation) are examples of hyperergopathic cardiomyopathies. Diagnosis and treatment of these conditions focus on the clinical link between heart failure and each of these specific disease processes. It is important to diagnose this condition because some of the most gratifying treatment responses in heart failure patients are associated with eliminating the primary process that causes the cardiomyopathy and heart failure in the first place. For example, complete normalization of profoundly depressed cardiac contractile activity has been well described after control of tachycardia, resolution of anemia, and repair of arteriovenous fistulae.

HYPERTROPHIC CARDIOMYOPATHY

Prevalence and Background

HCM is addressed in detail in Chapter 29. However, it is important to consider some of the contrasts between hypertrophic, dilated, and restrictive cardiomyopathies (28). The contemporary definition of HCM focuses on the fact that this disorder is characterized by disproportionate and remarkable left, and sometimes right, ventricular hypertrophy. Typically, the septum is more involved than the free left ventricular wall, although on occasion the hypertrophy can be completely concentric in nature (Fig. 90.3). HCM, which may develop at any age, is associated with marked left ventricular volume reduction, and systolic left ventricular outflow tract gradients are common. Up to 70% of cases have a familial pattern of occurrence, with autosomal dominant inheritance.

Pathophysiology

Some reports have emphasized that variable degrees of myocyte ultrastructural, myofibrillar, and muscle bundle

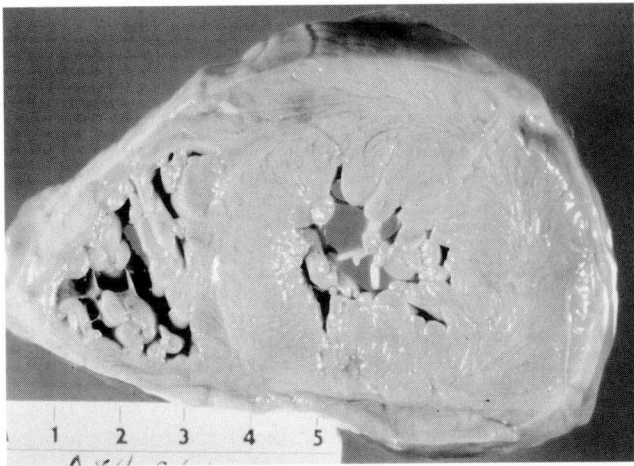

FIGURE 90.3 Severe concentric left ventricular hypertrophy: The left ventricle and interventricular septum are severely and concentrically hypertrophied, with a marked reduction in the size of the ventricular cavity.

disorganization can be detected, often with substantial degrees of interstitial fibrosis (28–31) (Fig. 90.4). Identification of specific gene mutations associated with HCM has led to the suggestion that the severity of hypertrophy is associated with cardiac troponin t-gene mutations and also mutations at the loci that are responsible for alpha-tropomyosin formation. Intense study of the molecular biodynamics and genetic characteristics of this syndrome is now under way. It is likely that many genetic abnormalities are associated with this pathologic hypertrophy. Indeed, HCM can be a component of many inheritable disease states, such as Noonan's syndrome, Friedreich's ataxia, Fabry's disease, and Hunter's and Hurler's syndromes.

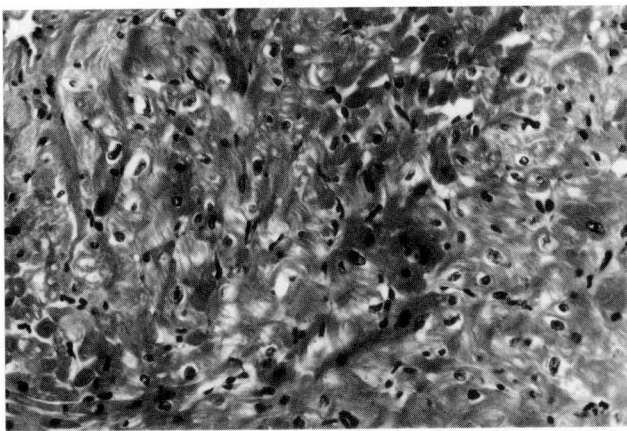

FIGURE 90.4 Hypertrophic cardiomyopathy: In this light micrograph, the myocyte disarray, characteristic of hypertrophic obstructive cardiomyopathy, is evident.

RESTRICTIVE CARDIOMYOPATHY

The restrictive cardiomyopathies, sometimes referred to as *nondilated, nonhypertrophic cardiomyopathies*, are described in Chapter 26. Several points deserve reiteration to aid in understanding specific restrictive disorders, as well as to contrast this myopathy with the others. Generally, this is the least common of the major myopathies and is characterized by a normal or only slightly enlarged heart, decreased diastolic volumes, and, early in the disease, normal systolic function. The main pathologic disorder is one of impaired diastolic functioning, resulting from decreased ventricular compliance and filling. This dysfunction may result from a process that involves, primarily, the endocardium, myocardium, or both. The most commonly encountered myocardial disorders are amyloid heart disease and idiopathic myocardial fibrosis, which are fully discussed in the sections Idiopathic Myocardial Fibrosis and Amyloidosis. Other specific myocardial forms include metabolic storage disorders such as Fabry's disease and hemochromatosis, sarcoid heart disease, radiation fibrosis, and various tumor infiltrations, many of which are also addressed under the section Specific Cardiomyopathies. The endocardial disorders, less common in the United States, include entities such as endomyocardial fibrosis, Löffler's endocardial fibrosis (endocarditis parietalis fibroplastica), and, even more rarely, endocardial fibroelastosis. Endocardial fibroelastosis is typically placed in the unclassified cardiomyopathy category. Another restrictive cardiomyopathy is frequently encountered after cardiac transplantation (32). Immediately after transplant and for up to a year, restrictive hemodynamics may exist. Later on, restriction is associated with acute and with chronic rejection (33). Restrictive cardiomyopathy should be considered when patients present with signs and symptoms of myocardial failure but normal cardiac size. Frequently, right-sided findings of increased jugular venous pressure, ascites, and peripheral edema predominate, although left-sided failure does occur. The differential diagnosis includes constrictive pericarditis, which is a more readily treatable condition. Echocardiography and right heart catheterization may help differentiate these disorders. The hemodynamic findings usually demonstrate elevation of left and right ventricular end diastolic pressures, and a characteristic early ventricular diastolic dip and rapid rise to a plateau (square-root sign). Early diastolic pressure typically does not fall to 0 mm Hg, however. Endomyocardial biopsy should also be considered if other historical and physical clues to the diagnosis are not present. The treatment of restrictive cardiomyopathy is also reviewed in Chapter 26 and generally remains quite unsatisfactory.

Idiopathic Myocardial Fibrosis

Idiopathic myocardial fibrosis results in a restrictive physiology; however, no specific histopathologic changes are present to account for the extensive fibrosis (34). Grossly, the heart is increased in weight, with normal ventricular cavity size and wall thickness. By light microscopy, there is patchy endocardial and interstitial fibrosis that ranges from mild to quite severe. The disorder is frequently associated with distal skeletal myopathies, atrioventricular blocks, and possibly an autosomal dominant inheritance. It may occur in children or adults but carries a worse prognosis in children. No specific therapy is present, except that heart blocks frequently necessitate pacemaker insertion. Atrial fibrillation is readily controlled with digoxin. Some have proposed that the etiology of this disorder is related to an abnormality in a calcium-dependent phase of cardiac relaxation. Therefore, calcium antagonists may have a role in therapy, but this has yet to be proven.

Endomyocardial Fibrosis

Endomyocardial fibrosis, also known as *tropical eosinophilic endomyocardial fibrosis*, is common in South and Central America and tropical and subtropical Africa. Surprisingly, it accounts for 15% to 25% of the cardiac deaths in equatorial Africa (35). Endomyocardial fibrosis is characterized by thickening and scarring of the endocardium (Fig. 90.5), which can be so extensive that the ventricular cavity is obliterated. Thrombi may overlie these lesions, increasing the risk of thromboembolism. Frequently, the subendocardial myocardium is also affected. In 50% of cases, the left and the right ventricles are involved, whereas another 40% of cases have lesions isolated to the left ventricle. The mitral and tricuspid valves may become fibrotic as well, leading to

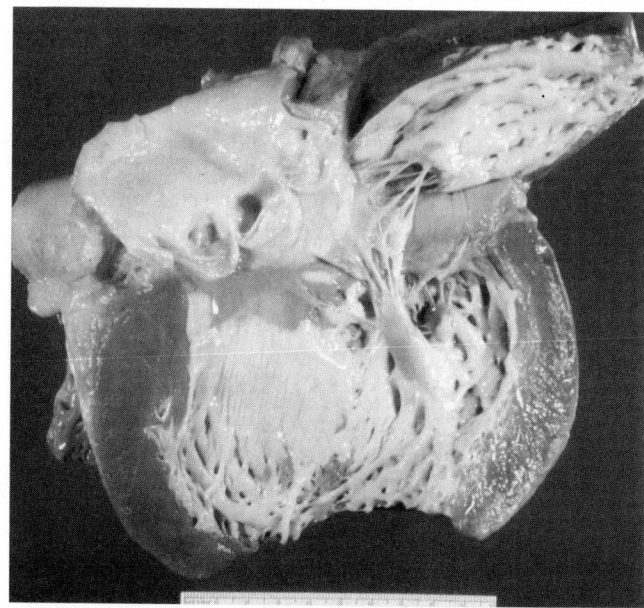

FIGURE 90.5 Endocardial fibrosis. The left ventricle is markedly dilated and hypertrophied. The endocardium, including the papillary muscles, is covered by thick, white, shiny, fibrotic endocardium.

TABLE 90.2 CRITERIA FOR THE DIAGNOSIS OF ARRHYTHMOGENIC RIGHT VENTRICULAR CARDIOMYOPATHY[a]

Category	Major criteria	Minor criteria
Global and/or regional dysfunction and structural alterations	Severe dilatation and reduction of RV ejection Localized RV aneurysms (akinetic or dyskinetic areas with diastolic building) Severe segmental dilatation of the RV	Mild global RV dilatation and/or EF reduction with normal LV Mild segmental dilatation of the RV Regional RV hypokinesia
Tissue characterization of walls	Fibrofatty replacement of myocardium on endomyocardial biopsy	—
Repolarization abnormalities	—	Inverted T waves in right precordial leads (V_2 and V_3)[b]
Depolarization/conduction abnormalities	Epsilon waves or localized prolongation (>110 ms) of the QRS complex in right precordial leads (V_1–V_3)	Late potentials on signal-averaged ECG
Arrhythmias	—	LBBB-type ventricular tachycardia (sustained and nonsustained) Frequent ventricular extrasystoles (>1,000/24 h)
Family history	Familial disease confirmed at autopsy or surgery	Family history of premature sudden death (<35) due to suspected RV dysplasia Family history (clinical diagnosis based on present criteria)

ECG, electrocardiogram; EF, ejection fraction; LBBB, left bundle branch block; LV, left ventricle; RV, right ventricle.
[a]The diagnosis of arrhythmogenic right ventricular myocardium is based on meeting two major, one major plus two minor, or four minor criteria as outlined in the table. These criteria are based on the known structural and functional abnormalities of the right ventricle, family history, and repolarization/depolarization and electrical conduction disturbances.
[b]Patient must be >12 yr old; in the absence of right bundle branch block.
From McKenna WJ, Thiene G, Nava A, et al. Diagnosis of arrhythmogenic right ventricular dysplasia/cardiomyopathy. *Br Heart J* 1994;71:215–218.

valvular regurgitation. Many believe that this disease is a form of, if not the same as, Löffler's endocardial fibrosis, perhaps at a different stage (36,37). Although the overall prognosis is poor, palliative treatment with surgical endocardiectomy and valvular repair/replacement may alleviate some symptoms (38).

Löffler's Endocardial Fibrosis

Löffler's endocardial fibrosis is also associated with eosinophilia, giving it its other names: eosinophilic cardiomyopathy and nontropical eosinophilic endomyocardial fibrosis. The severity of cardiac dysfunction seems to parallel the degree and duration of the eosinophilia, leading to the belief that the eosinophil itself is responsible for the dysfunction. Compared to normal eosinophils, the cells in endocardial fibrosis have fewer granules and contain vacuoles and may represent an abnormal cell line producing a type of autoimmune disorder (39). The contents of the intracytoplasmic granules of the eosinophils can cause direct myocardial necrosis. It has also been observed that the eosinophils bind immunoglobulin G and increase peroxidase, which can have further direct toxic effects. The cardiac manifestations of this eosinophilic disorder are similar, if not identical to, those produced by eosinophilic leukemia and the eosinophilia-myalgia syndrome, which has been associated with tryptophan. Treatment with corticosteroids and cytotoxic agents (hydroxyurea) can improve symptoms and survival (40).

RIGHT VENTRICULAR CARDIOMYOPATHY

Arrhythmogenic Right Ventricular Cardiomyopathy

Clinical Profile and Management

Because of the difficulties and risks of obtaining tissue to confirm the diagnosis of ARVC, as well as inaccuracies in assessing right ventricular structure and function with many of the noninvasive tests, a task force from the European Society of Cardiology and the International Society and Federation of Cardiology met and released criteria to assist in this process. The diagnosis can be made by meeting any of the following: two major criteria, one major plus two minor, or four minor criteria (57) (Table 90.2). These criteria are based on the clinical manifestations of the disease, family history, endomyocardial biopsy, and electrophysiologic abnormalities. Other diagnoses can mimic ARVC: atrial septal defects, abnormal pulmonary venous return, congenital absence of the left pericardium, Ebstein's anomaly, right ventricular outflow tract tachycardia, and pulmonic insufficiency.

Severe ventricular dysrhythmias and, less frequently, supraventricular dysrhythmias are a common presentation for ARVC. Patients may also present with right heart failure, asymptomatic cardiomegaly, syncope, or sudden death syndrome. Polymorphic ventricular tachycardia originating from the right ventricle, with a left bundle branch morphology, is often associated with exertion. In patients who have ventricular tachycardia, the signal-averaged ECG is almost always abnormal, with a very long duration of the low-amplitude signals (58). Premature death results from right-sided congestive heart failure or sudden death. In fact, ARVC is one of the most common causes of juvenile sudden death.

The clinical course of ARVC is unknown, and patients may live to be quite old, whereas others die in early childhood. Treatment of ARVC is aimed at the specific manifestations of the disease. The ventricular dysrhythmias can be treated with antiarrhythmics such as amiodarone and sotalol but may be quite refractory. Radiofrequency ablation of severe refractory tachycardias may be successful, although it is possible to have recurrence of the dysrhythmias but from a different area within the right ventricle. Not uncommonly, automatic cardioverter defibrillators are necessary. Because of conduction abnormalities, pacemakers may be required. Right-sided heart failure should be treated with sodium restriction, diuretics, digoxin, and afterload reducers. Cardiac transplantation also has been successfully performed for this syndrome. In the future, the identification of ARVC carriers by linkage analysis in affected families (50) may allow for earlier treatment with more standard therapies such as automatic defibrillators or even with the administration of agents that can prevent further apoptosis.

Uhl's Anomaly

Prevalence and Background

Uhl's anomaly, first described in 1952, is similar to ARVC (59). It is rare, tends to occur in infancy and early childhood, and has a more equal male-female sex distribution. Primarily, it affects the right ventricle but has much more extensive loss of the myocytes, with severe dilatation. Unlike ARVC, which tends to be focal and episodic in nature, Uhl's anomaly is an incessant disease that frequently results in complete destruction of the entire ventricle.

Pathophysiology

In Uhl's anomaly, the entire right ventricular wall can be paper thin, with apposition of the endocardium to the epicardium, explaining its other moniker: parchment heart. Apoptosis has been described in Uhl's anomaly (60,61). At birth, when the pressure in the right ventricle decreases with pulmonary flow, appropriate apoptosis may occur as fewer myocytes are needed. Uhl's anomaly may represent a case in which the triggering signals for apoptosis do not stop or for some other reason escape appropriate regulation. Indeed, massive apoptosis has been reported in other systems, including the central nervous system and bone marrow (62,63).

Clinical Profile and Management

The manifestations of Uhl's anomaly are quite similar to those of ARVC and include right heart failure, supraventricular and ventricular dysrhythmias, and conduction abnormalities. The right-sided failure tends to be more common and severe. The treatment of Uhl's anomaly is the same as for ARVC. Unfortunately, because of the progressive, more extensive nature of this disease, patients tend to be refractory to treatment. Cardiac transplantation has been successfully performed in these cases, but the timing of listing for transplant can be exceedingly difficult because there is a high risk of sudden cardiac death on the one hand and patients who live for several years with ventricular dysrhythmias on the other. Many investigators have contemplated whether Uhl's anomaly and ARVC are the same or different entities (64–66). It is best explained, at this time, that they share the common pathogenesis of apoptosis, but they remain separate clinical diseases.

UNCLASSIFIED CARDIOMYOPATHIES

Endocardial Fibroelastosis

Endocardial fibroelastosis is an abnormal thickening of the endocardium of the left ventricle and aortic and mitral valves. It occurs in infancy and early childhood. The fibrosis leads to decreased compliance of the myocardium and diastolic dysfunction. Typically, a DCM occurs frequently with significant mitral regurgitation, but a restrictive cardiomyopathy can also occur. The exact genetic defect has not been identified; autosomal recessive, autosomal dominant, and X-linked recessive patterns of inheritance have been reported. The X-linked forms demonstrate mitochondrial abnormalities that are similar to those of Barth's syndrome. Endocardial fibroelastosis has also been associated with tissue carnitine deficiency (67), and there is evidence that it may be related to a defect in the plasma membrane carnitine transporter (68). Other theories of its pathogenesis include inadequate subendocardial blood flow, pre- or postnatal inflammation, and infections. The diagnosis is one of exclusion, with diseases such as hypertrophic obstructive cardiomyopathy, myocarditis, anomalous pulmonary origin of the left coronary artery, and glycogen storage diseases needing to be ruled out. The ECG frequently shows features of left ventricular hypertrophy, with occasional pseudoinfarction patterns and atrioventricular block. The echocardiogram is remarkable for dense echoes along the left ventricular endocardium. The treatment consists of prolonged administration of digoxin. In one study, up to 74% of children were cured, with the remainder having either persistent ventricular dysfunction or dying. Prolonged treatment with high doses of digoxin seemed to be a determining prognostic factor, with relapses demonstrated with cessation of therapy (69). Cardiac transplantation has been successful in select cases.

Mitochondrial Cardiomyopathy

Mitochondrial cardiomyopathy is defined as ventricular dysfunction caused by mitochondrial DNA mutations, which are maternally inherited. These mutations are not limited to the heart mitochondria and may also be demonstrated throughout the liver, kidney, pancreas, central nervous system, skeletal muscles, and thyroid gland. The mitochondria are typically irregular, vary in size, and have a very abnormal cristae structure (Fig. 90.6). Within the myocardium, there may be focal fibrosis and myofibrillar disarray, closely resembling idiopathic HCM. Mitochondrial cardiomyopathy may also present with signs, symptoms, and features of DCM. Progressive hypertrophy and dilation of the heart with cardiac dysrhythmias are characteristics of these mitochondrial abnormalities. DNA defects frequently result in cytochrome c oxidase deficiency and abnormalities in the mitochondrial respiratory chain. Research is active in identifying these mutations by endomyocardial biopsy (77). Several systemic diseases are associated with mitochondrial dysfunction. For example, the MELAS syndrome (*m*itochondrial *e*ncephalopathy, *l*actic *a*cidosis, and *s*troke-like episodes) is complicated by cardiomyopathy and generalized microangiopathic occlusive disease.

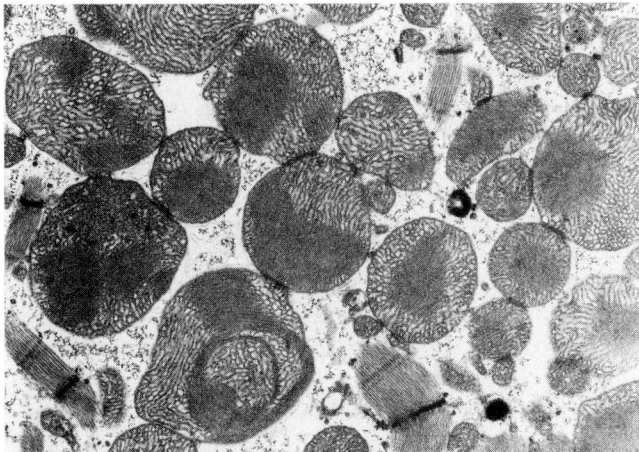

FIGURE 90.6 Mitochondrial myopathy. In this electron micrograph, the bizarre mitochondria, which are characteristic of a mitochondrial myopathy, are evident. All of the mitochondria illustrated here are abnormal. The normal mitochondria in a myocyte are filamentous and branching with regular cristae. The mitochondria in this myopathy are predominantly spherical. The extreme variation in size and structure of the cristae is distinctly abnormal. Within individual mitochondria, two distinct conformations of cristae can be seen. One of the mitochondria has ring-shaped cristae. Other abnormalities, too numerous to illustrate, were noted in this patient.

Systolic Dysfunction with Minimal Dilatation

Patients with DCM have ventricular dysfunction with enlarged ventricles. However, there is an entity in which ventricular dysfunction that is similar to DMC occurs but with minimal or no dilation (78). Furthermore, there are no signs of restrictive physiology to suggest that it is a restrictive or early HCM. This variant of DCM is termed *mildly dilated congestive cardiomyopathy* (MDCM) or *systolic dysfunction with minimal dilatation cardiomyopathy*. MDCM is defined as end-stage heart failure of unknown etiology (NYHA class IV), with an ejection fraction of less than 30%, without significant ventricular dilation (<15% above the normal range of ventricular size for body surface area) (79). Additionally, the ventricular hemodynamic waveforms should not suggest restriction, such as with an early diastolic dip and plateau. MDCM can be differentiated from early stages of DCM, because early DCM does not have severe dysfunction clinically by echocardiogram or with right heart catheterization. On endomyocardial biopsy, the light microscopic findings demonstrate myocyte hypertrophy, bizarre-shaped nuclei, and interstitial fibrosis. Little to no myofibrillar loss occurs by electron microscopy, despite severe ventricular impairment. This preservation of myofibrils may explain the lack of dilation. Vitamin and nutritional element deficiencies must be ruled out before this diagnosis can be made, because these processes can cause profound reduction in systolic performance with preserved heart size as well. The etiology of this disorder is unknown; however, a positive family history of DCM can frequently be elicited. The prognosis overall is similar to that of DCM, but it appears more related to the hemodynamic impairment than to ventricular size. This is in contrast to DCM, in which increasing ventricular size denotes a poorer survival. For this reason, cardiac transplant should be considered if congestive symptoms persist after medical therapy.

SPECIFIC CARDIOMYOPATHIES

Ischemic

Ischemic cardiomyopathy, defined as an ejection fraction of less than 40%, with multifocal wall motion abnormalities due to coronary artery diseases, is the most common DCM in the United States (Figs. 90.7 and 90.8). It carries with it significant disability and mortality. In the past, a 5-year survival rate of only approximately 40% has been reported (80). Adequate perfusion of the myocardium is essential for appropriate cellular aerobic respiration, and heart failure due to ischemic cardiomyopathy is caused by at least four distinct mechanisms. The predominant mechanism is ischemic necrosis, owing to myocardial infarction (81). It is vital to determine the amount of stunned myocardium in

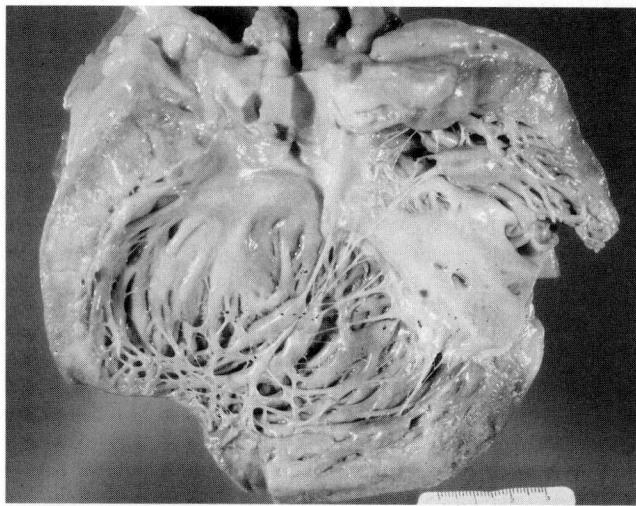

FIGURE 90.7 Ischemic cardiomyopathy. Photograph shows a heart that has been sectioned through the mitral and aortic valves, exposing the left ventricle. The heart is dilated, round, and globular, with an overall appearance much like that of an idiopathic dilated cardiomyopathy. However, in the cut surfaces of the left ventricle, visible here, the extensive white scar tissue of remote myocardial infarcts can be appreciated.

these ischemic cardiomyopathy patients, particularly in the periinfarction phase, as well as the extent of hibernating tissue, because they may play significant roles in contractile dysfunction (82). Stunned and hibernating myocardial tissue are viable, with potential for improvement in functioning with better perfusion. Differentiation of ischemia, scar, and hibernating myocardial tissue is discussed fully in Chapters 50 and 55 and includes methods such as positron

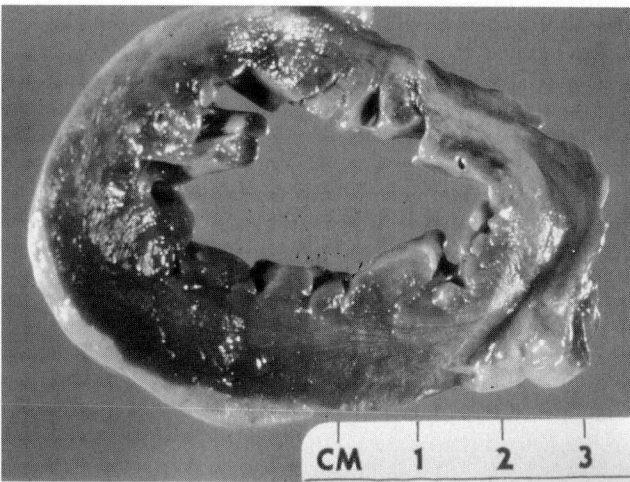

FIGURE 90.8 Ischemic cardiomyopathy. In this cross section from a heart with a remote myocardial infarct, many of the features of ischemic cardiomyopathy are demonstrated. A remote infarct is at the top of the picture. The portion of the left ventricular wall involved by this transmural infarct is notably thinner than the remainder of the ventricle, reflecting stretching and distention of the infarcted area. The left ventricular cavity is substantially enlarged, a reflection of the overall dilatation of the left ventricle.

emission tomography, dobutamine and myocardial contrast echocardiography, and rest-redistribution thallium-201 scintigraphy (83). The final mechanism of ischemia that causes cardiomyopathy is related to pathologic remodeling after acute myocardial infarction. Nonischemic myocytes are subjected to increased workloads as infarcted cardiac tissue drops out of the contractile scene. Pathologic hypertrophy is induced in these remaining myocytes, as well as other molecular biodynamic characteristics of remodeling. Additional important factors include the development of ventricular aneurysm, dysrhythmias, and mitral regurgitation from papillary muscle ischemia and dysfunction. It is the combination of these factors that contributes to progression from normal cardiac function to cardiac dilation and heart failure.

This characterization of ischemic cardiomyopathy is more generally related to the traditional large-vessel epicardial coronary artery disease that is seen in most patients with atherosclerotic heart disease. However, diffuse small-vessel atherosclerosis can also produce ischemic-related malfunction of the cardiac myocyte. Indeed, the cardiomyopathy of diabetes mellitus may be due, in part, to epicardial vessel disease as well as diffuse, small-vessel subendocardial atherosclerosis. Syndrome X, systemic lupus erythematosus, and other autoimmune chronic inflammatory disease states produce, on occasion, similar findings. The allograft arteriopathy noted in patients after cardiac transplantation is also an example of diffuse small-vessel coronary artery disease that can produce myocyte contractile dysfunction that leads to cardiac remodeling and heart failure. These diseases are difficult to address because of the limited ability to restore adequate myocardial perfusion. **Ⅴ** p06

Valvular

Valvular cardiomyopathy is a hyperergopathic DCM produced by valvular defects of numerous etiologies, discussed in Chapters 21 through 24. Typically, defects that produce volume-overloaded states (regurgitation) are more likely to cause cardiomyopathy than are lesions associated with pressure overload (valvular stenosis). The etiologies of valvular cardiomyopathy have changed considerably over the past several decades. The aggressive treatment of rheumatic fever and the earlier and more successful valvular repairs and replacements being performed are leading to a decreased incidence of more common causes. Further, the identification of nonrheumatic disorders are increasing the documented frequency of other problems. The clinical presentation of valvular cardiomyopathy is similar to that of any of the other dilated cardiomyopathies. The prominent signs and symptoms of failure depend on what valve or valves are dysfunctional and on what side of the heart they are located. It may be difficult to evaluate fully the severity of some disorders when myocardial dysfunction is present. For example, the degree of aortic stenosis can be underestimated by echocardiography, because the ventricle may be too weak to generate a large gradient across the valve. The use of dobutamine may help to clarify this. Another area in which physicians frequently struggle is mitral regurgitation in the setting of a very dilated ventricle. Unless a good history is available, it may be difficult to ascertain whether the insufficiency caused the dilation and dysfunction or whether the regurgitation is a result of ventricular dilation with stretching of the annulus. Medical treatment is the same as with the other DCMs. Frequently, the issue of corrective valvular surgery in the setting of severe myocardial dysfunction is raised, with the hope of promoting myocardial recovery if the lesion is fixed. For instance, attempts at reducing mitral regurgitation have been performed in patients with severe cardiomyopathy, either as an isolated surgery or in conjunction with partial left ventriculectomy, with some symptomatic success and at least early improvement in certain cases (84,85).

Hypertensive

Hypertensive cardiomyopathy is discussed in detail in Chapter 5.

Obesity

Obesity is recognized as a specific separate disorder that can result in a cardiomyopathy. This is a condition distinct from other entities that can cause heart failure and are also associated with obesity, such as hypertension, coronary atherosclerosis, sleep apnea, and diabetes. It is believed that the severity of the cardiomyopathy is associated with the duration and the severity of the obesity and initially is a type of high-output failure. Obesity cardiomyopathy results in systolic and diastolic dysfunction, left ventricular hypertrophy, and elevations in left ventricular filling pressure. Substantial weight loss has been correlated with improvement in the ventricular function.

Inflammatory

Inflammatory cardiomyopathies are addressed specifically in Chapter 93. They are generally divided into idiopathic, autoimmune, and infectious categories and are listed in Table 90.3. The cardiomyopathies that are associated with systemic autoimmune disorders include the collagen-vascular disease syndromes and many of the mixed connective tissue diseases. Numerous viral infections are associated with DCM, including viral (enterovirus, adenovirus and cytomegalovirus, Coxsackie), rickettsial, bacterial (diphtheria), mycobacterial, fungal, parasitic (toxoplasmosis, trichinosis, Chagas' disease), and spirochetal (see Chapter 39). One particular cardiomyopathy, associated with HIV, warrants further mention here because it will, unfortunately, be encountered more and more frequently in clinical practice.

TABLE 90.3 CAUSES OF INFLAMMATORY CARDIOMYOPATHY

Idiopathic
Autoimmune
Collagen-vascular and mixed connective tissue diseases
   Churg-Strauss syndrome
   Systemic lupus erythematosus
   Polyarteritis nodosa
   Progressive systemic sclerosis
Infectious
Bacterial
Fungal
Parasitic
   Schistosomiasis
   Trichinosis
   Toxoplasmosis
   Trypanosoma cruzi
Rickettsial
   Leptospirosis
Spirochetal
Viral
   Adenovirus
   Coxsackie virus
   Cytomegalovirus
   Echovirus
   Human immunodeficiency virus

Tachycardia Induced

One of the more important cardiomyopathies is that related to chronic tachyarrhythmia. In many senses this form of cardiomyopathy is a classic hyperergasic cardiomyopathy. If substantive ventricular dysfunction and heart failure are due to this difficulty, response to treatment can be gratifying. Severe dropsical states can resolve quickly, for example, by simply slowing the ventricular heart-rate response in patients with heart failure due to rapid atrial fibrillation. In fact, William Withering's (110) description of patients who are likely to respond to his foxglove herbal tea therapy were characterized as having pale countenances with weak, thready, and irregular pulses accompanying their dropsical state. It is very likely, in retrospect, that these individuals had atrial fibrillation with rapid ventricular response rates. Although ventricular and atrial tachycardias are very common in patients with heart failure, whether or not they are the primary etiology of the difficulty or simply an added complication that contributes to decompensation varies from patient to patient. This is of little consequence, however, because control of dysrhythmia, with slowing of the heart rate, is mandatory in either circumstance. Further, it is often difficult to know whether tachyarrhythmias that are seen in heart failure patients caused or are the result of ventricular chamber dilatation, hypertrophy, and heart failure. Indeed, in 1913, Gossage and Braxton Hicks (111) first suggested that atrial fibrillation might have been the etiology of left ventricular dilation and hypertrophy. This report did not, however, document reversal of the cardiac remodeling with control of the "auricular fibrillation." Many reports in the 1930s and 1940s did, however, describe resolution of congestive heart failure syndromes after termination of atrial fibrillation and cardioversion to normal sinus rhythm (112–114). Because atrial fibrillation frequently complicates hypertension and coronary heart disease, with both difficulties also contributing to ventricular dysfunction and possibly precipitating heart failure, it is difficult to determine precisely the degree of contribution that the dysrhythmia is making to the cardiomyopathy in some patients. On the other hand, descriptions of heart failure syndromes associated with reentrant atrial tachyarrhythmias with resolution of the syndrome after control of the arrhythmia are convincing that heart rate alone contributes to contractile dysfunction (115–117). As electrophysiologic techniques became more sophisticated and pathophysiologic clarification of atrial tachycardias emerged, it became even more apparent that rapid heart rates alone could cause heart failure and cardiomyopathy. Restoration of systolic function, manifest by normalization of ejection fraction, has been reported for accessory pathway–reciprocating tachycardias (118,119) and atrial ventricular nodal reentry tachyarrhythmia (120,121). In children, control of incessant ventricular tachycardia has also been noted to reverse dilated myopathic ventricles (122,123).

In an attempt to mimic tachycardia-induced heart failure clinically, an experimental model was proposed by Whipple et al. (124) in 1962 that demonstrated that cardiomyopathy could be produced in large mammals if the heart was stimulated to incessantly beat very fast. Furthermore, this model of low-output biventricular failure demonstrated that termination of the pacing stimulation with slowing of the heart rate reversed the heart failure syndrome. Tachycardia-pacing animal models of heart failure have been invaluable during characterization of heart failure syndromes in general. Overall, they have served to stress the importance of controlling tachycardia in managing clinical heart failure (125). The reasons for the development of ergopathic myocyte contractile impairment in patients with incessant tachyarrhythmias or rapid pacing–induced cardiomyopathy are complicated. Decompensation of cardiac performance may be due to myocardial energy depletion or impaired energy use, regional ischemia (usually subendocardial), abnormalities of myocyte organelle calcium flux, and acute leading to chronic cardiac myocyte and interstitial matrix remodeling. Chronic tachy-pacing in animals has been demonstrated in some studies to reduce creatine, phosphocreatine, and adenosine trisphosphate (126). Furthermore, mitochondrial structural injury and functional abnormalities have been noted. Particularly intriguing is the observation that altered subendocardial-subepicardial blood flow ratios impair coronary flow reserve states when tachycardia is induced in animals and might contribute to myocyte dysfunction by promoting a relative ischemic setting. This is an important observation because many patients have concomitant coronary heart disease or

substantive hypertension-induced left ventricular hypertrophy and could be quite susceptible to myocardial flow changes. A considerable amount of attention has focused on abnormalities of calcium channel activity and sarcoplasmic reticulum calcium transport in paced heart failure models. The downregulation of calcium cycling, which ultimately decreases availability of this ion to the myocyte contractile machinery, may be a unifying hypothesis to explain the failure that develops in this syndrome. Observations of myocyte hypertrophy and extracellular matrix deposition with resultant stiffening could explain the more chronic abnormalities noted in paced cardiac models. Collectively, these pathophysiologic effects translate into low cardiac output and, ultimately, high cardiac filling pressures with dilatation and hypertrophy of the heart. Concomitant aberration in neurohumoral characteristics of the clinical heart failure syndrome subsequently occurs. ◆ p07

Metabolic

Many metabolic disorders are known to induce myocardial dysfunction and can be categorized into endocrine, familial storage disease and infiltrations, deficiency states and nutritional disorders, and amyloidosis. Endocrine diseases, such as adrenocortical insufficiency, thyrotoxicosis, hypothyroidism, acromegaly, and pheochromocytoma, are covered in detail in the endocrine section of Chapter 35. Because diabetes mellitus and diabetic heart disease are so frequently encountered, they are further explored here. Additionally, amyloidosis and its unique nature deserve additional description.

Diabetic

Heart failure in the setting of diabetes is multifactorial and can be due to epicardial atherosclerotic coronary artery disease, small-vessel subendocardial disease, or the diabetes itself (127). Patients with diabetes mellitus are well known to be prone to silent myocardial ischemia and infarction. Furthermore, hypertension often complicates diabetes and can also contribute to the detrimental remodeling of the heart. It is disturbing to note that almost half of asymptomatic diabetics experience a reduction in left ventricular ejection fraction during stress.

The hearts of diabetic patients at autopsy demonstrate the characteristic findings of DCM, with widespread regions of myocardial fibrosis, intimal proliferation of small myocardial arterioles, and accumulation of interstitial glycoprotein and collagen, all leading to decreased ventricular compliance and contractility (128). In laboratory animals, alterations in myocytes occurred before any damage to the intramural arteries, suggesting other derangements in cellular metabolism (129). It has been presumed that some of the resultant dysfunction may be related to abnormal processing of lipids and decreased lysosomal activity (130).

Many additional theories have been postulated and explored to explain the ventricular failure, including the possible role of increased circulating catecholamines (131). It has also been observed that the concentration of collagen increases when diabetes is poorly controlled (132), and other studies have documented improvement in left ventricular functioning and reversal of biochemical abnormalities with the administration of insulin (133). In addition to the more standard treatments for DCM, tighter control of glucose levels may be beneficial to cardiac functioning in diabetics. Finally, the chronic addition of propionyl-L-carnitine to the diets of diabetic rats in one study overcame the induced myocardial dysfunction (134), raising the potential of testing this treatment in humans.

Familial Storage Disease and Infiltrations

Many of the familial storage diseases and infiltrations cause various substances to be deposited within the myocardium, either intracellularly (frequently interfering with cellular metabolism and functioning) or extracellularly (resulting in a restrictive cardiomyopathy). Many of these disorders, such as Hurler's syndrome, Niemann-Pick disease, Hand-Schüller-Christian disease, and Morquio-Ullrich disease, are more fully reviewed in the neurology section of Chapter 35. A few of the more understood and common disorders are further discussed here.

Hemochromatosis

Hemochromatosis is a metabolic storage disorder, associated with HLA-A3 and HLA-B14 autosomal recessive inheritance, leading to iron deposition in the sarcoplasmic reticulum of many organs (Fig. 90.9). It results clinically in the classic description of the bronzed diabetic with heart failure due to skin, pancreatic, and cardiac iron deposition. The cardiac deposits tend to be in the subepicardial and subendocardial regions and in the papillary muscles. Cardiac hemochromatosis may present as either a restrictive cardiomyopathy early on or, more commonly, a dilated one, with impressively enlarged ventricles. In addition to the iron deposition, an interstitial fibrosis that is unrelated to the degree of iron overload may occur independently. Endomyocardial biopsy is useful in demonstrating the iron deposits and important in establishing the diagnosis because the most common form of death in hemochromatosis is cardiac. Treatment consists of repeated phlebotomy or possibly chelation therapy, with the cardiomyopathy often reversible when the iron load is decreased.

Refsum's Syndrome

Refsum's syndrome is an autosomal recessive disorder caused by the absence of the enzyme alpha-hydroxylase, which metabolizes dietary phytol and phytanic acid. This

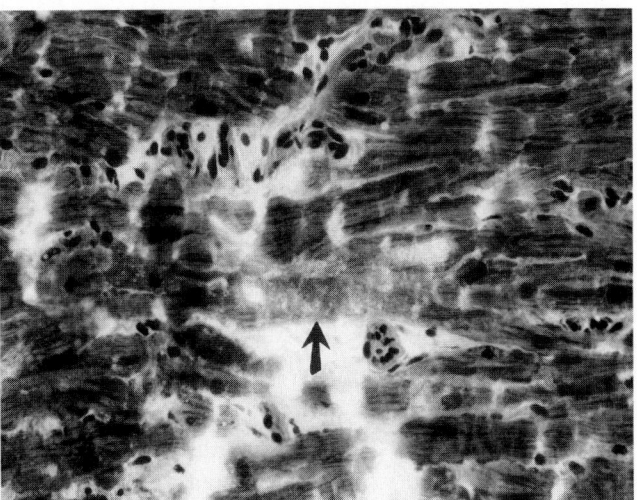

FIGURE 90.9 Cardiac hemochromatosis. This longitudinal light microscopic section of myocardium has been stained for iron. It has been specially stained blue for iron, but in black and white print all of the dark material seen within the myocytes is iron, with one large aggregate of iron in the center (*arrow*). This particular area does not have any overlying cardiac structures and appears lighter than other iron-laden areas in this picture. In the normal heart, there should be virtually no stainable iron.

results in an accumulation of intracellular phytanic acid. The syndrome is characterized by cerebellar ataxia, peripheral neuropathies, retinitis pigmentosa, and cardiac disorders. A cardiomyopathy may result and can be either dilated or hypertrophic, depending on the stage of the disease. Wide-ranging conduction disturbances may occur, as well as dysrhythmias and sudden cardiac death. Current treatment consists of dietary modifications. Plasmapheresis has been shown to remove the accumulated phytanic acid.

Amyloidosis

Background and Prevalence

Amyloid restrictive cardiomyopathy is caused by the abnormal deposition of various proteins into the interstitium of the myocardium. The four general categories of amyloid heart disease are primary systemic, secondary, familial or hereditary, and senile. These are summarized in Table 90.4. Primary systemic amyloidosis is also known as *myeloma-associated* or *amyloid AL*. It is caused by the uncontrolled production of an amyloid protein subunit, the ammonia terminal portion of an immunoglobulin light chain (kappa or lambda), from a monoclonal population of plasma cells. It is usually, but not always, the consequence of multiple myeloma, is more common in men, and rarely presents before age 30. Secondary amyloidosis results from the production of a nonimmunoglobulin protein, termed *AA*. It is frequently encountered with chronic inflammatory disorders, such as rheumatoid arthritis, tuberculosis, and Crohn's disease, and in familial Mediterranean fever. Familial and hereditary cardiac amyloidosis consists of six differ-

TABLE 90.4 CLASSIFICATION OF AMYLOIDOSIS

Name	Designation	Other names	Amyloid deposit
Primary	AL	Myeloma-associated, idiopathic[a]	Immunoglobulin light chain, kappa or lambda
Secondary	AA	Associated with other inflammatory disorders, familial Mediterranean fever	Nonimmunoglobulin protein A
Familial	AF	Hereditary	Transthyretin
Senile	SSA	Senile systemic amyloid	Transthyretin

[a]This term is outdated and should no longer be used.

ent forms. They result from the production of amyloid AF, a prealbumin protein component known as transthyretin. They are autosomally dominant disorders, unlike familial Mediterranean fever, which is autosomal recessive. Senile cardiac amyloid, also known as *amyloid SSA*, is also due to the production of an abnormal transthyretin and is seen in older individuals (147). The three forms of this disorder are amyloid IAA, which only affects the atria; senile systemic amyloidosis, which may involve other organs; and a third form that is limited to the aorta. Each of the four main categories of amyloid heart disease has varying degrees of cardiac involvement, clinical significance, and survival rates. For instance, cardiac failure is the most common cause of death in primary amyloidosis. At autopsy, nearly 100% of systemic amyloid cases have demonstrable cardiac infiltration, although only 25% to 33% have clinically apparent disease (148,149). In contrast, fewer than 10% of secondary amyloid cases are associated with clinically significant cardiac derangement. Even when present, the deposits are typically small and perivascular in location and do not result in considerable ventricular dysfunction. Familial amyloidosis rarely has cardiac involvement, and then only very late in the disease. Senile amyloidosis is much more variable than the other types. Almost all individuals over the age of 60 have scattered deposits of amyloid in locations such as the aorta, and one-fourth have some cardiac infiltration (150). This ranges from small atrial deposits to extensive ventricular involvement with severe congestive failure. The survival with senile amyloidosis is much longer than with primary amyloid. In one study, the median survival was 60.0 months and 5.5 months, respectively, from the time of diagnosis (151).

Pathophysiology

The myocardium in amyloidosis is usually firm, thickened, and noncompliant, with the amyloid being present extracellularly. The deposits occur in the interstitium in a pericellular or focal nodular pattern and can result in systolic and diastolic impairment (Figs. 90.10 and 90.11). Nodular deposits and thick perimyocyte layers of amyloid are associated with shorter survival (152). Mild atrial enlargement is generally present, usually without significant ventricular dilatation. Besides the myocardial infiltration, there can also be deposition in the papillary muscles, the sinoatrial

and atrioventricular nodes, the bundle branches, and the endocardium. Amyloidosis can incite focal thickening of all four valves, especially the mitral; however, it rarely interferes with overall valve function and competence. Finally, the intramural arteries and veins can contain deposits in the media and adventitia, occasionally compromising blood flow. Rarely, deposits can also occur directly in the lumen of the vessels. The different types of amyloid vary in their vascular encroachment. Only 4% of senile amyloidosis has vascular involvement, whereas it is found in up to 90% of primary amyloid cases (153).

General System Diseases

The connective tissue and collagen-vascular disorders, such as systemic lupus erythematosus, polyarteritis nodosa, and rheumatoid arthritis, are covered in Chapter 35E. A few entities warrant additional description.

Sarcoidosis

Sarcoidosis is a systemic disease that is typified by noncaseating granulomas infiltrating the lungs, skin, and reticuloendothelial system. Cardiac sarcoidosis results in a restrictive

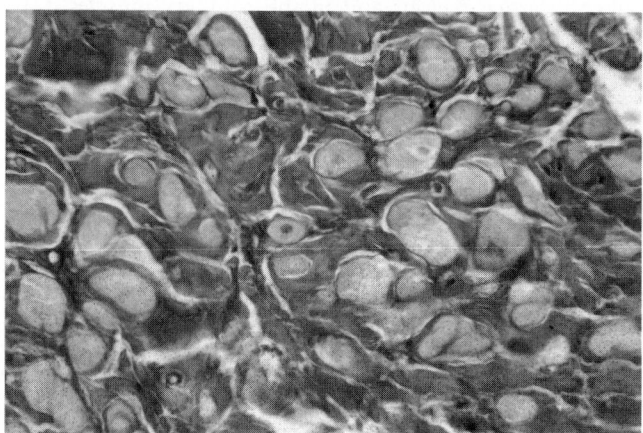

FIGURE 90.10 Cardiac amyloid. Light microscopic section from an endomyocardial biopsy stained with sulfonated alcian blue. Although the color cannot be appreciated, the myocytes are the lighter-shaded cells. The darker-colored amyloid closely surrounds each myocyte and isolates it.

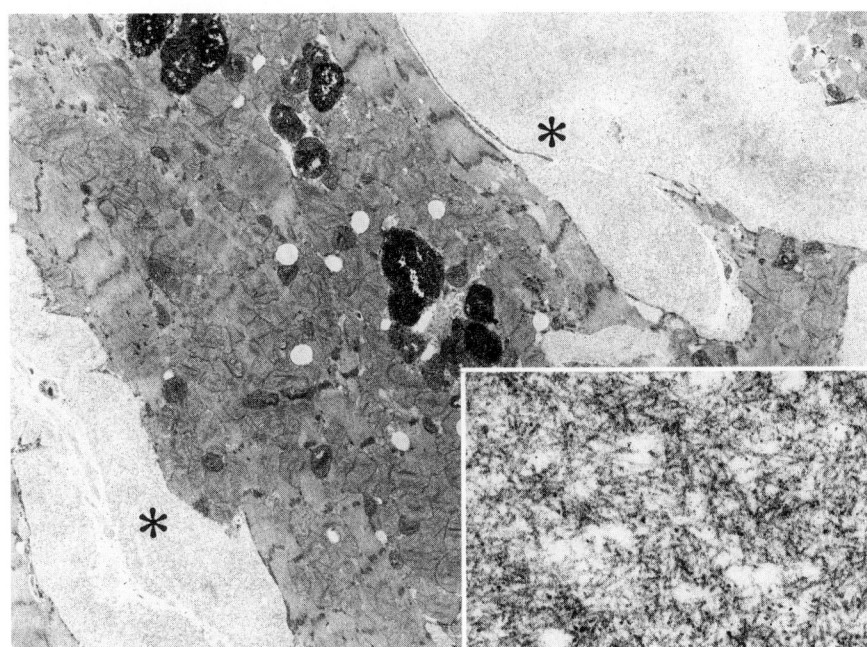

FIGURE 90.11 Amyloid. Electron micrograph showing a dense accumulation on amyloid fibrils (*asterisks*) hugging the myocyte. **Inset:** At high magnification, 10-nm nonbranching straight filaments, which are characteristic of amyloid, are revealed.

cardiomyopathy, although rarely it more closely resembles a DCM. Interstitial lymphocytic inflammation and fibrosis may be present, in addition to the myocardial granulomas, which early on cause diastolic dysfunction but preserve systolic function. Later on, further fibrosis and infiltration can lead to systolic impairment as well. Cardiac sarcoid is often present with systemic sarcoidosis but clinically remains silent approximately 95% of the time (166). The initial cardiac presentation may be with high-degree atrioventricular blocks, syncope, or sudden cardiac death. Gallium-67, thallium-201, and Tc-99m–pyrophosphate myocardial imaging have been useful in localizing segmental myocardial involvement (167,168). Endomyocardial sampling can be helpful in confirming the diagnosis; however, the false-negative rate is high, even when numerous pieces are obtained. One explanation for this is that the granulomas have a predilection for the basal and free wall portions of the myocardium, areas where sampling does not usually occur. The cardiac granulomas occasionally respond to treatment with steroids. Pacemakers may help with symptomatic conduction disturbances.

Scleroderma

The cardiac manifestations of scleroderma include a slowly progressive fibrosis that involves the pericardium, myocardial interstitium, and conduction system. Small-vessel coronary artery disease may also occur. These patients can present with either dilated or restrictive cardiomyopathies.

Muscular Dystrophies

Many cases of DCM are familial (169). Pedigree analysis of families with suspected heredofamilial cardiomyopathy suggest a polygenic inheritance pattern, which in turn suggests

that environmental factors such as infections or other toxins play a role in precipitating the detrimental remodeling process. A variety of neuromuscular diseases are associated with cardiomyopathy as part of their syndrome complex. Disorders of oxidative phosphorylation have been identified that are associated with these neuromuscular disorders (170), and linkage analysis has demonstrated that these difficulties are related to DNA mutations of mitochondrial protein function. Many of the muscular dystrophies and neuromuscular disorders are covered in Chapter 35D.

Duchenne's Muscular Dystrophy

Duchenne's muscular dystrophy, also known as *pseudohypertrophic muscular dystrophy*, is an X-linked, proximal muscle dystrophic disease that is frequently associated with cardiac involvement manifesting as DCM (166). Indeed, death usually results either from respiratory infection due to cardiorespiratory failure or from the development of congestive heart failure with sudden cardiac death syndrome. Specific point mutations have been identified for this particular muscular dystrophy, and sometimes a DCM may be the only manifestation of the dystrophin gene mutation (171). Becker-type muscular dystrophy, similar to Duchenne's, is also X-linked recessive in inheritance. Its onset is later in life, but it is slowly progressive once it manifests signs and symptoms.

Neuromuscular Disorders

X-Linked Cardioskeletal Myopathy

Barth's syndrome is an X-linked recessive condition characterized by cardiomyopathy, accompanied by a variety of neuromuscular abnormalities (proportionate short stature) and recurrent neutropenia (173). Some patients exhibit carnitine deficiency, although this is an inconsistent finding. Contrary to most cardiomyopathies, this syndrome tends to improve with age. It is proposed that the primary defect in this disorder rests in the mitochondrial electron transport chain (174).

Friedreich's Ataxia

Friedreich's ataxia is a spinocerebellar degenerative disorder that has an autosomal recessive form of inheritance, with the genetic defect located to chromosome 9. It is characterized by a broad-based gait, impaired vibration, position and joint sense, dysarthria, pes cavus, and incoordination. Childhood onset has a high likelihood of also developing diabetes, although the reasons for this are unclear (175). Interestingly, Friedreich's ataxia is commonly associated with HCM, either with concentric or asymmetric left ventricular hypertrophy (176). More rarely, this neuromuscular syndrome can present as a DCM, with myocardial fibrosis, at times apparently transformed from an initially hypertrophic ventricle. Death from cardiac origin occurs in 5% of cases. Histologic findings include diffuse interstitial fibrosis, myocellular hypertrophy, and necrosis. Abnormalities of large and small coronary arteries can also occur. One theory of the etiology of the dysfunction suggests that myocardial calcium overload may have a role. Verapamil treatment, effective with other forms of HCM, has had no effect on patients with established hypertrophy (177).

Sensitivity and Toxic Reactions

A variety of toxins can cause myocyte injury, with subsequent dysfunction leading to actual cell death with fibrotic replacement or, simply, more transient contractile dysfunction. *e*Table 90.4.1 lists many cardiotoxic agents that have been reported to cause heart muscle disease. Discontinuing some of these drugs has led to substantive improvement in cardiac function on occasion. Specific examples of this include lithium, phenothiazines, and tricyclic antidepressants. One should always be particularly sensitive to the possibility that these drugs are producing cardiomyopathy in patients who receive them for psychiatric conditions. Some other specific toxins are discussed in the following sections.

Anthracycline-Induced Cardiomyopathy

Chronic anthracycline toxic cardiomyopathy is a dose-dependent DCM that is seen after therapy with agents such as doxorubicin (190). It is believed that anthracyclines cause myocyte cell death by increasing oxygen-derived free radical molecules, activating platelets, increasing histamine secretion, and producing C-13 hydroxymetabolites. This ultimately inhibits enzymatic activity within the sarcoplastic reticulum, mitochondria, and sarcolemma such that

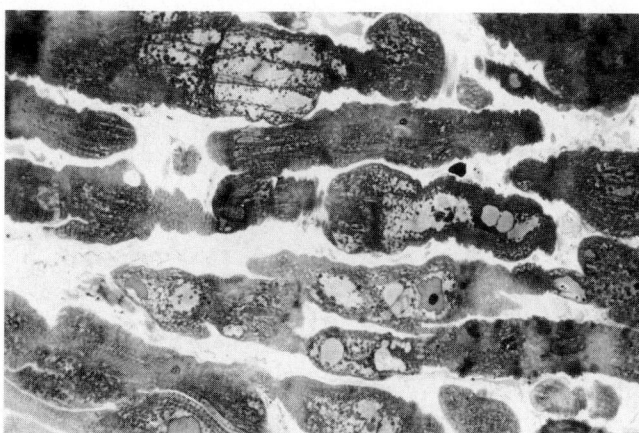

FIGURE 90.12 Severe doxorubicin cardiotoxicity. This light micrograph of a semithin plastic section illustrates the swollen sarcoplasmic reticulum, appearing as cytoplasmic vacuoles by light microscopy, and the loss of contractile elements.

energy production by adenosine triphosphate cleavage is altered. Doxorubicin can cause the release of TNF-α and interleukin-2, which may create further toxicity. Myocyte destruction is associated with characteristic histopathologic findings, and this is one of the cardiomyopathies that is readily diagnosed by specific electron microscopic changes noted at the time of endomyocardial biopsy sample analysis (191) (Figs. 90.12 and 90.13). Evaluation of anthracycline cardiotoxicity requires semithin (1 to 2 μ) plastic sections with electron microscopy to ensure an adequate evaluation of the severity of cardiotoxicity. Therefore, it is essential that this information be conveyed to the pathologist before the endomyocardial biopsy specimens reach the histology laboratory. Doxorubicin has been associated with this cardiomyopathy, with cumulative doses under 400 mg per m^2 having a trivial incidence, but dose levels over 700 mg per m^2 have resulted in a nearly 20% incidence of cardiomyop-

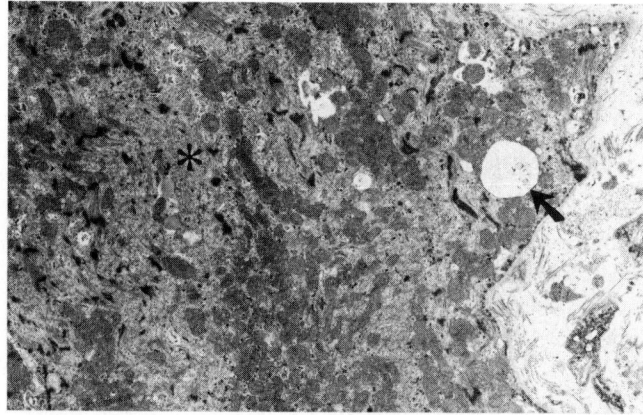

FIGURE 90.13 Doxorubicin cardiotoxicity. This electron micrograph illustrates the dilation of the sarcoplasmic reticulum (*arrow*) and the loss of contractile elements (*asterisk*), which are characteristic of doxorubicin cardiotoxicity.

athy. Why some patients who receive very low doses of doxo-rubicin still get cardiomyopathy and others who receive extraordinarily high doses do not remains unclear. Some of the risk factors identified for the development of toxicity include higher rates of administration and a history of previous cardiac irradiation. Patients can present either acutely or several years after exposure to this chemotherapeutic agent. Most patients who are exposed to this drug have a determination of the baseline ejection fraction with serial studies performed to follow ventricular performance indexes during treatment. Some data suggest that using continuous infusion of doxorubicin rather than bolus dosing, coadministering antioxidants or free radical scavengers, or treating patients with concomitant beta-adrenergic or calcium channel blocking drugs reduces the incidence of anthracycline cardiotoxicity. Unfortunately, this form of DCM does not usually improve with time.

Peripartum Cardiomyopathy

Background and Prevalence

Peripartum DCM is defined as left ventricular systolic dysfunction without other apparent causes or underlying heart disease, occurring in the peripartum period. The onset must occur during the last month of pregnancy or within the first 5 months after delivery, although it is most common (75%) during the first 2 months postpartum (205). Because of differences in precisely defining this cardiomyopathy and aggressiveness in searching out other causes, the incidence has been reported to be anywhere between 1 in 1,300 to 1 in 15,000 pregnancies (206–208). Several risk factors have been identified, including twin pregnancy, age greater than 30, multiparity, a family history of peripartum cardiomyopathy, African descent, and prolonged therapy with tocolytic agents. The natural history differs from other forms of DCM. If recovery is going to occur, there is usually some sign of improvement within the first 6 weeks. Approximately 50% of patients spontaneously recover, usually in the first 6 months, with improvement after that time unlikely. The initial severity of heart failure or ventricular dysfunction is not predictive of long-term outcome (209). Death or deterioration to the point of requiring transplantation occurs in 25% to 50% of patients (210). Progressive congestive heart failure, dysrhythmias, and embolic events are the usual immediate causes of death. However, identifying patients who are likely to improve is not usually possible. A notable exception: In one small report, women who appeared to have peripartum cardiomyopathy associated with prolonged β-sympathomimetic tocolysis had full recovery (211).

Pathophysiology

The actual mechanism that causes ventricular dysfunction remains unknown, although several explanations have been offered. Numerous series have reported a higher incidence of myocarditis diagnosed by endomyocardial biopsy compared to idiopathic DCM (212–215). The cases of confirmed myocarditis may represent one of two distinct possibilities. It may be that these patients should not be labeled as having peripartum cardiomyopathy at all but rather an inflammatory cardiomyopathy. Indeed, in one study, the incidence of myocarditis by biopsy with "peripartum cardiomyopathy" did not differ from age- and sex-controlled matches that had idiopathic DCM (216). Alternatively, cases in which myocarditis is not confirmed by biopsy may represent a false-negative test. Diagnostic tissue may not have been obtained either because of insufficient tissue sampling or because the timing of the biopsy was not during the acute phase when inflammation was present. To some extent, perhaps all peripartum cardiomyopathies represent a pregnancy-induced, abnormal, immune-mediated response with myocarditis. It is known that T-cell suppressor activity is decreased during pregnancy. This may make patients more susceptible to certain viral infections such as Coxsackie virus, or perhaps maternal exposure to fetal or placental antigens may result in the production of antibodies that cross-react with the myocardium.

CONTROVERSIES AND PERSONAL PERSPECTIVES

Even with the most recent revisions in the World Health Organization classification scheme of cardiomyopathy, it remains difficult to categorize certain disease states. At times there can be overlap because of changing ventricle characteristics. For example, hypertensive cardiomyopathy may initially best fit classification as an HCM, but when end-stage dilation occurs, it may be better defined as a DCM. Similarly, a patient may present with numerous risk factors that, alone or in combination, could be responsible for the ventricular dysfunction. Consider, for instance, how a gentleman who had diabetes, coronary artery disease, and hypertension would be classified if he were found to have an ejection fraction of 30% and a mildly dilated ventricle. Further complicating the issue would be a history of a flu-like illness with fever developing 2 months before presentation with a low ejection fraction.

When such a patient presents with signs and symptoms that are suggestive of ventricular dysfunction, one of the first steps in devising a management plan is obtaining an accurate diagnosis. With the desire to provide exemplary care, while at the same time maintaining cost effectiveness, the provider must choose tests carefully. One should not overlook the importance of a detailed history and physical examination, which can often provide insight into the disease process. Specifically important is looking for onset and duration history, a positive family history of heart failure, evidence of systemic diseases, and a history of other illnesses or toxin exposure. If a specific cardiomyopathy is suggested, the evaluation usually proceeds along a fairly demarcated path. However, when an illness appears obscure, idiopathic in origin, or due to a number of different possibilities, one must decide critically which of the multiple tests will lead one to a more definite diagnosis. A rational approach is imperative. Echocardiography is extremely helpful and can, for example, determine which chambers are involved (and to what degree), differentiate a focal from a global process, determine if the major dysfunction is systolic or diastolic, and detect valvular abnormalities. It is the single most important test to obtain, because it is necessary to determine a cardiomyopathy etiology that might respond to medical or surgical therapies or elimination of toxins. These patients with heart failure usually have a gratifying response, with, at times, dramatic reversal of their failure syndrome. Stopping ethanol consumption in the face of alcoholic cardiomyopathy, for example, can effect substantial improvement in ventricular function in more than 50% of patients. If a DCM is present, often a viral myocarditis is suspected. It is tempting to order large panels of acute and convalescent viral titers; however, the clinician should refrain from doing so because it is extremely expensive and the tests' conclusiveness is questionable. (Consider the current general public incidence of cytomegalovirus or Epstein-Barr virus seroconversion evidence.) Further, patient management would not generally change. The question of whether to perform right ventricular endomyocardial biopsy for a diagnosis frequently arises. Currently, if a specific disease process is strongly suggested and cannot be diagnosed by a less invasive manner, a biopsy is reasonable. *e*Table 90.4.3 lists some specific cardiomyopathies that can be diagnosed by biopsy. A second reason for biopsy is to monitor the effects of anthracycline cardiotoxicity, guiding further chemotherapy. Third, if a patient will be participating in a randomized trial to evaluate a specific therapeutic intervention, a biopsy might be useful to document entry criteria. The Intervention in Myocarditis and Acute Cardiomyopathy with Intravenous Immunoglobulin (IMAC) multicenter trial is such a study (see below). Fourth, in patients in whom it is unclear, after other noninvasive studies, that a restrictive process (as opposed to constrictive pathology) is responsible for the syndrome, the prognosis and treatment can be considerably different. Routine endomyocardial biopsy in patients with idiopathic DCM serves little purpose.

The treatment of cardiomyopathy is covered in Chapters 91 and 92; however, one area that remains unsettled regards diseases for which transplantation may not be indicated because of an increased likelihood of primary disease recurrence in the transplanted heart. Although early- and intermediate-term follow-up reports of patients with cardiac amyloid indicated that transplantation could be successfully performed (227–229), long-term results suggest a high incidence of failure due to recurrent amyloid

(230,231). Transplantation in sarcoidosis, when other end-organ involvement is present, is also unwise. When the only manifestation of sarcoid is cardiac infiltration, transplantation has been performed and can be successful (232). It is, however, possible to have recurrence of noncaseating granulomas in the heart in as short a time as 6 months (233). Inflammatory cardiac conditions, such as lymphocytic myocarditis, may have an increased incidence of rejection after heart transplant as compared with control groups, and they may have a significantly higher mortality. Although this diagnosis does not represent an absolute contraindication to transplant, this therapy should be considered with caution.

Importantly, in a controlled trial of intravenous immunoglobulin in recent-onset DCM (234), 62 patients with recent onset (less than 6 months of symptoms) of DCM and left ventricular ejection fraction of less than 40% were randomized to receive 2 g per kg intravenous immunoglobulin or placebo. The mean age of the group was 43.0 ± 12.3 years, with 37 men and 25 women participating. All underwent an endomyocardial biopsy before randomization, which revealed cellular inflammation (lymphocytic myocarditis) in 16%. The primary outcome was change in left ventricular ejection fraction at 6 and 12 months after randomization, with the ejection fraction improving from 25% to 41% at 6 months ($p < .001$) and 42% ($p < .001$ vs. baseline) at 12 months. The increase was the same for patients who received intravenous immunoglobulin and placebo. Overall, 56% of patients at 1 year had an increase in ejection fraction of greater than 10% from study entry, and 36% normalized their ejection fraction (greater than 50%). The transplant-free survival rate was 92% at 1 year and 88% at 2 years. Thus, the IMAC trial suggests that for patients with recent-onset DCM, intravenous immunoglobulin does not augment the improvement in left ventricular ejection fraction and, as an overall cohort, ejection fraction is likely to improve significantly during follow-up, with short-term prognosis remaining favorable in patients who meet this trial's entry criteria. The debate about treating these patients will likely continue.

Further highlighting the issues is the European Study of Epidemiology and Treatment of Cardiac Inflammatory Diseases (ESETCID) (235). Initial epidemiologic results have been published from this registry. By adding immunohistochemical parameters, the World Heart Federation Task Force for the Definition of Acute and Chronic Myocarditis expanded the light microscopy "Dallas" criteria of myocarditis, referred to in previous sections. Polymerase chain reaction molecular biologic techniques and *in situ* hybridization have improved our understanding of the underlying etiologic and pathophysiologic mechanisms in inflammatory heart disease. Because of this, patients in ESETCID are screened not only for infiltrating cells but for the presence of persisting viral genomes and, specifically, footprints of enterovirus, cytomegalovirus, and adenovirus. ESET-

THE FUTURE

Every day, new insight is gained in all areas of basic research addressing the pathophysiology of cardiomyopathy. Clarification and elucidation of genetic and molecular biodynamic mechanisms that are important to the development of cardiomyopathy are anticipated. The time when recognition of genetic markers that can identify susceptible or asymptomatic patients, thereby allowing preventive and early-treatment strategies to be instituted, is rapidly approaching. Clinical trials are under way that examine the role of various humors, including proinflammatory cytokines (TNF-α, interleukin-1, interleukin-6) and nitric oxide, in the cardiomyopathic process and may allow identification of new, specific treatment modalities such as anticytokine agents and antioxidants. Likewise, the use of cell transplants and gene-vector therapy is actively being pursued. Finally, we are entering a new era of examining mechanisms that mediate apoptosis. Inappropriate apoptosis has been associated with arrhythmogenic right ventricular cardiomyopathy, and already more than 30 inducers of programmed cell death have been discovered. Apoptosis in end-stage heart failure, for example, has been suggested to be the result of TNF-α exposure, amyloidosis, incessant tachycardia syndromes, pressure overload states, ischemia-reperfusion injuries, hypertension, situations with increased mechanical stretch, and chemotherapeutic and radiation injuries (236–243).

CID investigated endomyocardial biopsies from 3,055 patients but could find an ongoing inflammatory process in the heart in only approximately 17%. Of these patients, only 182 showed a reduced ejection fraction below 45%, fulfilling the entrance criteria for the ESETCID trial. The observations suggest that in symptomatic patients, inflammatory heart disease muscle has to be considered regardless of left ventricular function and that endomyocardial biopsy can in fact be an important tool for diagnosis. However, virus could be detected in only approximately 12% of patients (enterovirus in 2%, cytomegalovirus in 5%, and adenovirus in 4%). This exercise was the first epidemiologic study to demonstrate that viral persistence may contribute to the pathogenesis of inflammatory heart muscle disease and that in chronic myocarditis, viral persistence occurs in a small percentage of patients compared to previous studies that were performed on highly selected individuals. The implications of this study are that, perhaps, more specific viral treatment therapeutics will be useful in the future to attenuate ventricular function deterioration.

REFERENCES

1. Krehl L. Beitrag zur Kentniss der idiopathischen Herzmuskelerkrankungen. *Dtsch Arch Klin Med* 1891;48:414–431.
2. Bridgen W. Uncommon myocardial diseases: the non-coronary cardiomyopathies. *Lancet* 1957;2:1179–1184.
3. Report of the WHO/ISFC task force on the definition and classification of cardiomyopathies. *Br Heart J* 1980;44:672–673.
4. Giles TD. A perspective on nosology and incidence of cardiomyopathy. In: Giles TD, Sanders GE, eds. *Cardiomyopathy.* Littleton, MA: PSG Publishing, 1988.
5. Report of the 1995 World Health Organization/International Society and Federation of Cardiology task force on the definition and classification of cardiomyopathies. *Circulation* 1996;93:841–842.
6. Feild BJ, Baxley WA, Russell Jr RO, et al. Left ventricular function and hypertrophy in cardiomyopathy with depressed ejection fraction. *Circulation* 1973;47:1022–1031.
7. Goodwin JF. Cardiac function in primary myocardial disorders. *BMJ* 1964;1:1527–1533, 1595–1597.
8. Bristow MR, O'Connell JB. Myocardial diseases. In: Kelley WN, ed. *Textbook of internal medicine,* 3rd ed. Philadelphia: JB Lippincott Co, 1997:398–405.
9. Johnson RA, Palacios I. Dilated cardiomyopathies of the adult (Pt 1). *N Engl J Med* 1982;307:1051–1058.
10. Johnson RA, Palacios I. Dilated cardiomyopathies of the adult (Pt 2). *N Engl J Med* 1982;307:1119–1126.
11. Giles T. Dilated cardiomyopathy. In: Poole-Wilson PA, Colucci WS, Massie BM, et al., eds. *Heart failure: scientific principles and clinical practice.* New York: Churchill Livingstone, 1997:401–422.
12. Priori SG, Barhanin J, Hauer RN, et al. Genetic and molecular basis of cardiac arrhythmias: impact on clinical management (Pts I and II) [Review]. *Circulation* 1999;99(4):518–528.
13. Priori SG, Barhanin J, Hauer RN, et al. Genetic and molecular basis of cardiac arrhythmias: impact on clinical management (Pt III) [Review]. *Circulation* 1999;99(5):674–681.
14. Gillum RF. Idiopathic cardiomyopathy in the United States, 1970–1982. *Am Heart J* 1986;111:752–755.
15. Codd MB, Sugrue DD, Gersh BJ, Melton LJ III. Epidemiology of idiopathic dilated and hypertrophic cardiomyopathy: a population-based study in Olmstead County, Minnesota, 1975–1984. *Circulation* 1989;80:564–572.
16. Dec GW, Fuster V. Idiopathic dilated cardiomyopathy. *N Engl J Med* 1994;331:1564–1575.
17. Raynolds MV, Bristow MR, Bush EW, et al. Angiotensin-converting enzyme DD genotype in patients with ischemic or idiopathic dilated cardiomyopathy. *Lancet* 1993;342:1073–1075.

18. Carlquist JF, Menlove RL, Murray MB, et al. HLA class II (DR and DQ) antigen associations in idiopathic dilated cardiomyopathy: validation study and meta-analysis of published HLA association studies. *Circulation* 1992;83:515–522.

19. Towbin JA, Hejtmancik JF, Brink P, et al. X-linked dilated cardiomyopathy: molecular genetic evidence of linkage to the Duchenne muscular dystrophy (dystrophin) gene at the Xp21 locus. *Circulation* 1993;87:1854–1865.

20. Grasso M, Arbustini E, Silini E, et al. Search for coxsackievirus B3 RNA in idiopathic dilated cardiomyopathy using gene amplification by polymerase chain reaction. *Am J Cardiol* 1992;69:658–664.

21. Olsen EGJ. The pathology of cardiomyopathies: a critical analysis. *Am Heart J* 1979; 98:385–392.

22. Sugrue DD, Rodeheffer RJ, Codd MB, et al. The clinical course of idiopathic dilated cardiomyopathy: a population-based study. *Ann Intern Med* 1992;117:117–123.

23. Komajda M, Jais JP, Reeves F, et al. Factors predicting mortality in idiopathic dilated cardiomyopathy. *Eur Heart J* 1990;11:824–831.

24. Cannon III RO, Cunnion RE, Parrillo JE, et al. Dynamic limitation of coronary vasodilator reserve in patients with dilated cardiomyopathy and chest pain. *J Am Coll Cardiol* 1987;10:1190–1200.

25. Fuster V, Gersh BJ, Giuliani ER, et al. The natural history of idiopathic dilated cardiomyopathy. *Am J Cardiol* 1981;47:525–531.

26. Baker DW, Wright EF. Management of heart failure, IV: anticoagulation for patients with heart failure due to left ventricular systolic dysfunction. *JAMA* 1994;272:1614–1618.

27. Packer M, O'Connor CM, Ghali JK, et al., for the Prospective Randomized Amlodipine Survival Evaluation Study Group (PRAISE). Effect of amlodipine on morbidity and mortality in severe chronic heart failure. *N Engl J Med* 1996;335:1107–1114.

28. Maron B, Epstein S. Hypertrophic cardiomyopathy: a discussion of nomenclature. *Am J Cardiol* 1979;43:1242–1244.

29. Teare D. Asymmetrical hypertrophy of the heart in young adults. *Br Heart J* 1958;20:1–8.

30. Davies JM. The current status of myocardial disarray in hypertrophic cardiomyopathy [Editorial]. *Br Heart J* 1984;51:361–363.

31. Ferrans VJ, Morrow AG, Roberts WC. Myocardial ultrastructure in idiopathic hypertrophic subaortic stenosis: a study of operatively excised left ventricular outflow tract muscle in 14 patients. *Circulation* 1972;45:769–792.

32. Young JB, Leon CA, Short HD, et al. Evolution of hemodynamics after orthotopic heart and heart-lung transplantation: early restrictive patterns persisting in occult fashion. *J Heart Lung Transplant* 1987;6:34–43.

33. Valentine HA, Fowler MB, Hunt SA, et al. Changes in Doppler echocardiographic indexes of left ventricular function as potential markers of acute cardiac rejection. *Circulation* 1987;76[Suppl V]:V86–V92.

34. McManus BM, Bren GB, Robertson EA. Hemodynamic cardiac constriction without anatomic myocardial restriction or pericardial constriction. *Am Heart J* 1981;102:134–136.

35. Goodwin JF. Cardiomyopathies and specific heart muscle diseases: definitions, terminology, classifications and new and old approaches. *Postgrad Med J* 1992;68[Suppl 1]:S3–S6.

36. Spry CJ. Eosinophils in eosinophilic endomyocardial disease. *Postgrad Med J* 1986;62:609–613.

37. Fauci AS, Harley JB, Roberts WC, et al. The idiopathic hypereosinophilic syndrome: clinical, pathophysiologic, and therapeutic considerations. *Ann Intern Med* 1982;97:78–92.

38. Moraes CR, Buffolo E, Lima R, et al. Surgical treatment of endomyocardial fibrosis. *J Thorac Cardiovasc Surg* 1983;85:738–745.

39. Spry CJ, Tai PC. Studies on blood eosinophilia: 11 patients with Löeffler's cardiomyopathy. *Clin Exp Immunol* 1976;24:423–434.

40. Parillo JE, Borer JS, Henry WC, et al. The cardiovascular manifestations of the hypereosinophilic syndrome: prospective study of 26 patients, with review of the literature. *Am J Med* 1979;67:572–582.

41. Marcus FI, Fontaine GH, Guiraudon G, et al. Right ventricular dysplasia: a report of 24 adult cases. *Circulation* 1982;65:384–398.

42. Manyari D, Klein G, Gulamhusein S. Arrhythmogenic right ventricular dysplasia: generalized cardiomyopathy? *Circulation* 1983;68:251–257.

43. Webb J, Kerr C, Huckell V, et al. Left ventricular abnormalities in arrhythmogenic right ventricular dysplasia. *Am Heart J* 1986;58:568–570.

44. Pinamonti B, Sinagra G, Salvi A, et al. Left ventricular involvement in right ventricular dysplasia. *Am Heart J* 1992;123:711–724.

45. Thiene G, Nava A, Angelini A, et al. Anatomoclinical aspects of arrhythmogenic right ventricular cardiomyopathy. In: Baroldi G, Camerini F, Goodwin JF, eds. *Advances in cardiomyopathies*. Berlin: Springer-Verlag, 1990:397–408.

46. Angelini A, Thiene G, Boffa GM, et al. Endomyocardial biopsy in right ventricular cardiomyopathy. *Int J Cardiol* 1993;40:274–282.

47. Ricci C, Longo R, Pagnan L, et al. Magnetic resonance imaging in right ventricular dysplasia. *Am J Cardiol* 1992;70:1589–1585.

48. Marcus FL, Fontaine G. Arrhythmogenic right ventricular dysplasia/cardiomyopathy: a review. *Pacing Clin Electrophysiol* 1995;18:1298–1314.

49. Auffermann W, Wichter T, Breithardt G, et al. Arrhythmogenic right ventricular disease: MR imaging versus angiography. *AJR Am J Roentgenol* 1993;161:549–555.

50. Nava A, Thiene G, Canciani B, et al. Familial occurrence of right ventricular dysplasia: a study involving nine families. *J Am Coll Cardiol* 1988;12:1222–1228.

51. Rampazzo A, Nava A, Erne P, et al. A new locus for arrhythmogenic right ventricular cardiomyopathy (ARVD2) maps to chromosome 1q42-q43. *Hum Mol Genet* 1995;4:2151–2154.

52. Rampazzo A, Nava A, Danieli GA, et al. The gene for arrhythmogenic right ventricular cardiomyopathy maps to chromosome 14q23-q24. *Hum Mol Genet* 1994;3:959–962.

53. Severini GM, Krajinovic M, Pinamoni B, et al. A new locus for arrhythmogenic right ventricular dysplasia on the long arm of chromosome 14. *Genomics* 1996;31:193–200.

54. Mallat Z, Tedgui A, Fontaliran F, et al. Evidence of apoptosis in arrhythmogenic right ventricular dysplasia. *N Engl J Med* 1996;335:1190–1196.

55. Duvall E, Wyllie AH, Morris RG. Macrophage recognition of cells undergoing programmed cell death (apoptosis). *Immunology* 1985;56:351–358.

56. Nicholson DW, Ali A, Thornberry NA, et al. Identification and inhibition of the ICE/CED-3 protease necessary for mammalian apoptosis. *Nature* 1995;376:37–43.

57. McKenna WJ, Thiene G, Nava A, et al. Diagnosis of arrhythmogenic right ventricular dysplasia/cardiomyopathy. *Br Heart J* 1994;71:215–218.

58. Oselladore L, Nava A, Buja G, et al. Signal-average electrocardiography in familial form of arrhythmogenic right ventricular cardiomyopathy. *Am J Cardiol* 1995;75:1038–1041.

59. Uhl HSM. A previously undescribed congenital malformation of the heart: almost total absence of the myocardium of the right ventricle. *Bull Johns Hopkins Hosp* 1972;91:197–209.

60. James TN, Nichols MM, Sapire DW, et al. Complete heart block and fatal right ventricular failure in an infant. *Circulation* 1996;93:1588–1600.

61. James TN. Normal and abnormal consequences of apoptosis as a possible cause of gradual development of complete heart block and fatal arrhythmias associated with absence of the AV node, the sinus node and the internodal pathways. *Circulation* 1994;90:556–573.

62. Motoyama N, Wand F, Roth KA, et al. Massive cell death of immature hematopoietic cells and neurons in Bcl-x-deficient mice. *Science* 1995;267:1506–1510.

63. Raza A, Gezer S, Mundle S, et al. Apoptosis in bone marrow biopsy samples involving stromal and hematopoietic cells in 50 patients with myelodysplastic syndromes. *Blood* 1995;86:268–276.

64. Gerlis LM, Schmidt-Ott SC, Ho SY, Anderson RH. Dysplastic conditions of the right ventricular myocardium: Uhl's anomaly versus arrhythmogenic right ventricular dysplasia. *Br Heart J* 1993;69:142–150.

65. Marcus FI. Is arrhythmogenic right ventricular dysplasia, Uhl's anomaly, and right ventricular outflow tract tachycardia a spectrum of the same disease? *Cardiol Rev* 1997;5:25–29.

66. Gaffney FA, Nicod P, Lin JC, Rude RE. Noninvasive recognition of the parchment right ventricle (Uhl's anomaly arrhythmogenic right ventricular dysplasia) syndrome. *Clin Cardiol* 1983;6:235–242.

67. Tripp ME, Katcher ML, Peters HA, et al. Systemic carnitine deficiency presenting as familial endocardial fibroelastosis: a treatable cardiomyopathy. *N Engl J Med* 1981;305:385–390.

68. Bennett MJ, Hale DE, Pollitt RJ, et al. Endocardial fibroelastosis and primary carnitine deficiency due to a defect in the plasma membrane carnitine transporter. *Clin Cardiol* 1996;19:243–246.

69. Jarrar M, Vaksmann G, Godart F, et al. Natural history and prognostic factors in primary endocardial fibroelastosis in infants. *Arch Mal Coeur Vaiss* 1994;86:653–656.

70. Chin TK, Perloff JK, Williams RG, et al. Isolated noncompaction of left ventricular myocardium: a study of eight cases. *Circulation* 1990;82:507–513.

71. Dusek J, Ostadal B, Duskova M. Postnatal persistence of spongy myocardium with embryonic blood supply. *Arch Pathol Lab Med* 1975;99:312–371.

72. Oechslin EN, Harrison DA, Connelly MS, et al. Mode of death in adults with congenital heart disease. *Am J Cardiol* 2000;86:1111–1116.

73. Jenni R, Goebel N, Tartini R, et al. Persisting myocardial sinusoids of both ventricles as an isolated anatomical finding. *Cardiovasc Intervent Radiol* 1986;9:127–131.

74. Hook S, Ratliff NB, Rosenkranz E, Sterba R. Isolated non-compaction of the ventricular myocardium. *Pediatr Cardiol* 1996;17:43–45.

75. Oechslin EN, Jost CH, Rojas JR, et al. Long-term follow-up of 34 adults with isolated left ventricular noncompaction: a distinct cardiomyopathy with poor prognosis. *J Am Coll Cardiol* 2000;36(2):493–500.

76. Junga G, Kneifel S, Von Smekal A, et al. Myocardial ischaemia in children with isolated ventricular non-compaction. *Eur Heart J* 1999;20(12):910–916.

77. Rustin P, Chretien D, Bourgeron T, et al. Investigation of respiratory chain activity in the human heart. *Biochem Med Metab Biol* 1993;50:120–126.

78. Keren A, Billingham ME, Weintraub D, et al. Mildly dilated congestive cardiomyopathy. *Circulation* 1985;72:302–309.

79. Keren A, Gottlieb S, Tzivoni D, et al. Mildly dilated congestive cardiomyopathy: use of prospective diagnostic criteria and description of the clinical course without heart transplantation. *Circulation* 1990;81:506–517.

80. Manley JC, King JF, Zeft HJ, Johnson WD. The "bad" left ventricle: results of coronary surgery and effect on late survival. *J Thorac Cardiovasc Surg* 1976;72:841–848.

81. Burch GE, Giles TD. Ischemic cardiomyopathy: diagnostic, pathophysiologic and therapeutic considerations. *Cardiovasc Clin* 1972;4:203–220.

82. Braunwald E, Kloner RA. The stunned myocardium: prolonged, postischemic ventricular dysfunction. *Circulation* 1982;66:1146–1149.

83. Nagueh SF, Vaduganathan P, Ali N, et al. Identification of hibernating myocardium: comparative accuracy of myocardial contrast echocardiography, rest-redistribution thallium-201 tomography and dobutamine echocardiography. *J Am Coll Cardiol* 1997;29:985–993.

84. Bolling SF, Deeb M, Brunsting LA, Bach DS. Surgery for acquired heart disease. *J Thorac Cardiovasc Surg* 1995;109:676–683.

85. Scalia PM, McCarthy PM, Starling RC. Intra-operative echocardiography in left ventricular remodeling surgery. *J Am Coll Cardiol* 1997;29[Suppl A]:66A.

86. Autran BR, Gorin I, Lerbowitch M. AIDS in a Haitian woman with cardiac Kaposi's sarcoma and Whipple's disease. *Lancet* 1983;1:767–768.

87. Cohen IS, Anderson DW, Viemani R, et al. Congestive cardiomyopathy in association with the acquired immunodeficiency syndrome. *N Engl J Med* 1986;315:628–630.

88. Kaul S, Fishbein MC, Siegel RJ. Cardiac manifestations of acquired immune deficiency syndrome: a 1991 update. *Am Heart J* 1991;122:535–544.

89. Francis CK. Cardiac involvement in AIDS. *Curr Probl Cardiol* 1990;10:569–639.

90. Reilly JM, Cunnion RE, Anderson DW, et al. Frequency of myocarditis, left ventricular dysfunction and ventricular tachycardia in the acquired immune deficiency syndrome. *Am J Cardiol* 1988;62:789–793.

91. Anderson DW, Virmani R, Reilly JM, et al. Prevalent myocarditis at necropsy in the acquired immunodeficiency syndrome. *J Am Coll Cardiol* 1988;11:792–799.

92. Anderson DW, Virmani R. Emerging patterns of heart disease in human immunodeficiency virus infection. *Hum Pathol* 1990;21:253–259.

93. Currie PF, Jacob AJ, Foreman AR, et al. Heart muscle disease related to HIV infection: prognostic implications. *BMJ* 1994;309:1605–1607.

94. DeCastro S, Migliau G, Silvestri A, et al. Heart involvement in AIDS: a prospective study during various stages of the disease. *Eur Heart J* 1992;13:1452–1459.

95. Herskowitz A, Ansari A, Neumann D, et al. Cardiomyopathy in acquired immunodeficiency syndrome: evidence for autoimmunity. *Circulation* 1989;80[Suppl II]:IIB-322(abst).

96. Domanski MJ, Sloas MM, Follmann DA, et al. Effect of zidovudine and didanosine treatment on heart function in children infected with human immunodeficiency virus. *J Pediatr* 1995;127:137–146.

97. Odeh M. Tumor necrosis factor-alpha as a myocardial depressant substance. *Int J Cardiol* 1993;42:231–238.

98. Hegewisch S, Weh HJ, Hossfeld DK. TNF-induced cardiomyopathy. *Lancet* 1990;335:294–295.

99. Odeh M. AIDS and dilated cardiomyopathy. *Postgrad Med J* 1995;71:59.

100. De Belder AJ, Radomski MW, Why HJ, et al. Nitric oxide synthase activities in human myocardium. *Lancet* 1993;341:84–85.

101. Grody WW, Cheng L, Lewis W. Infection of the heart by the human immunodeficiency virus. *Am J Cardiol* 1990;66:203–206.

102. Calabrese LH, Proffitt MR, Yen-Lieberman B, et al. Congestive cardiomyopathy and illness related to the acquired immunodeficiency syndrome (AIDS) associated with isolation of retrovirus from myocardium. *Ann Intern Med* 1987;108:691–692.

103. Ho DD, Pomerantz RJ, Kaplan JC. Pathogenesis of infection with human immunodeficiency virus. *N Engl J Med* 1987;317:278–286.

104. Dworkin BM, Antonecchia PP, Smith F, et al. Reduced cardiac selenium content in the acquired immunodeficiency syndrome. *JPEN* 1989;13:644–647.

105. Dworkin BM. Selenium deficiency in HIV infection and the acquired immunodeficiency syndrome (AIDS). *Chem Biol Interact* 1994;91:181–186.

106. Segal BH, Factor SM. Myocardial risk factors other than human immunodeficiency virus infection may contribute to histologic cardiomyopathic changes in acquired immune deficiency syndrome. *Mod Pathol* 1993;6:560–564.

107. van Hoeven KH, Segal B, Factor SM. AIDS cardiomyopathy: first rule out other myocardial risk factors. *Int J Cardiol* 1990;29:35–37.

108. Kavanaugh-McHugh AL, Ruff A, Perlman E, et al. Selenium deficiency and cardiomyopathy in acquired immunodeficiency syndrome. *JPEN* 1991;15:347–349.

109. Levy WS, Varghese PJ, Anderson DW, et al. Myocarditis diagnosed by endomyocardial biopsy in human immunodeficiency virus infection with cardiac dysfunction. *Am J Cardiol* 1988;62:658–659.

110. Withering W. *An account of the foxglove, and some of its medical uses: with practical remarks on dropsy and other disease.* London: Robinson and Paternoster-Row, 1785.

111. Gossage AM, Braxton Hicks JA. On auricular fibrillation. *Q J M* 1913;6:435–440.

112. Parkinson J, Campbell M. Paroxysmal auricular fibrillation: a record of two hundred patients. *Q J M* 1930;24:67–100.

113. Brill IC. Auricular fibrillation with congestive failure and no evidence of organic heart disease. *Am Heart J* 1937;13:175–182.

114. Phillips E, Levine SA. Auricular fibrillation without other evidence of heart disease: a cause of reversible heart failure. *Am J Med* 1949;7:478–489.

115. Shachnow N, Spellman S, Rubin I. Persistent supraventricular tachycardia: case report with review of the literature. *Circulation* 1954;10:232–236.

116. Morgan CL, Nadas AS. Chronic ectopic tachycardia in infancy and childhood. *Am Heart J* 1964;67:617–627.

117. Keane JF, Plauth WH, Nadas AS. Chronic ectopic tachycardia of infancy and childhood. *Am Heart J* 1972;84:748–757.

118. McLaran CJ, Gersh BJ, Sugrue DD, et al. Tachycardia induced myocardial dysfunction: a reversible phenomenon? *Br Heart J* 1985;53:323–327.

119. Cruz FE, Cheriex EC, Smeets JL, et al. Reversibility of tachycardia-induced cardiomyopathy after cure of incessant supraventricular tachycardia. *J Am Coll Cardiol* 1990;16:739–744.

120. Rosenqvist M, Lee MA, Moulinier L, et al. Long-term follow-up of patients after transcatheter direct current ablation of the atrioventricular junction. *J Am Coll Cardiol* 1990;16:1467–1474.

121. Corey WA, Markel ML, Hoit BD, Walsh RA. Regression of a dilated cardiomyopathy after radiofrequency ablation of incessant supraventricular tachycardia. *Am Heart J* 1993;126:1469–1473.

122. Kugler JD, Baisch SD, Cheatham JP, et al. Improvement of left ventricular dysfunction after control of persistent tachycardia. *J Pediatr* 1984;105:543–548.

123. Fyfe DA, Gillette PC, Crawford FJ, Kline CH. Resolution of dilated cardiomyopathy after surgical ablation of ventricular tachycardia in a child. *J Am Coll Cardiol* 1987;9:231–234.

124. Whipple GH, Sheffield LT, Woodman EG, et al. Reversible congestive heart failure due to chronic rapid stimulation of the normal heart. *Proc N Engl Cardiovasc Soc* 1962;20:39–40.

125. Moe GW, Stopps TP, Howard RJ, Armstrong PW. Early recovery from heart failure: insights into the pathogenesis of experimental chronic pacing-induced heart failure. *J Lab Clin Med* 1988;112:426–432.

126. Shinbane JS, Wood MA, Jensen DN, et al. Tachycardia-

induced cardiomyopathy: a review of animal models and clinical studies. *J Am Coll Cardiol* 1997;29:709–715.

127. Starling MR. Does a clinically definable diabetic cardiomyopathy exist? *J Am Coll Cardiol* 1990;15:1518–1520.

128. Regan TJ, Wu CF, Yeh CK, et al. Myocardial composition and function in diabetes: the effects of chronic insulin use. *Circ Res* 1981;49:1268–1277.

129. Giacomelli F, Wiener J. Primary myocardial disease in the diabetic mouse: an ultrastructural study. *Lab Invest* 1979;40:460–473.

130. Giacomelli F, Skazo L, Wiener J. Lysosomal enzymes in experimental diabetic cardiomyopathy. *Clin Biochem* 1980;13:227–231.

131. Ganguly PK, Pierce GN, Dhalla NS. Diabetic cardiomyopathy: membrane dysfunction and therapeutic strategies. *J Appl Cardiol* 1987;2:323.

132. Baandrup U, Ledet T, Rasch R. Experimental diabetic cardiomyopathy preventable by insulin treatment. *Lab Invest* 1981;46:169–173.

133. Schaible TF, Malhotra A, Bauman WA, et al. Left ventricular function after chronic insulin treatment in diabetic and normal rats. *J Mol Cell Cardiol* 1983;15:445–458.

134. Pasini E, Comini L, Ferrari R, et al. Effect of propionyl-L-carnitine on experimental induced cardiomyopathy in rats. *Am J Cardiovasc Pathol* 1992;4:216–222.

135. Sakuraba H, Yanagawa Y, Igarashi T, et al. Cardiovascular manifestations in Fabry's disease: a high incidence of mitral valve prolapse in hemizygotes and heterozygotes. *Clin Genet* 1986;29:276–283.

136. Okumiya T, Sakuraba H. Fabry's disease (alpha-galactosidase deficiency). *Nippon Rinsho* 1995;53:2952–2959.

137. Sakuraba H. Molecular genetics of inherited metabolic disease: its application to the investigation of pathogenesis and the diagnosis of Fabry disease. *Rinsho Byori* 1994;42:628–635.

138. Ishii S, Kase R, Sakuraba H, Suzuki Y. Characterization of a mutant alpha-galactosidase gene product for the late-onset cardiac form of Fabry disease. *Biochem Biophys Res Commun* 1993;197:1585–1589.

139. Ogawa T, Kawai M, Matsui T, et al. Vasospastic angina in a patient with Fabry's disease who showed normal coronary angiographic findings. *Jap Circ* 1996;60:315–318.

140. Colucci WS, Lorell BH, Schoen FJ, et al. Hypertrophic obstructive cardiomyopathy due to Fabry's disease. *N Engl J Med* 1982;307:926–928.

141. Matsui S, Murakami E, Takekoshi N, et al. Myocardial tissue characterization by magnetic resonance imaging in Fabry's disease. *Am Heart J* 1989;117:472–474.

142. Kramer W, Thormann J, Mueller K, Frenzel H. Progressive cardiac involvement by Fabry's disease despite successful renal allotransplantation. *Int J Cardiol* 1985;7:72–75.

143. Medin JA, Tudor M, Simovitch R, et al. Correction in trans for Fabry disease: expression, secretion and uptake of alpha-galactosidase A in patient-derived cells driven by a high-titer recombinant retroviral vector. *Proc Natl Acad Sci U S A* 1996;93:7917–7922.

144. Akbarian M, Yankopoulos NA, Abelmann WH. Hemodynamic studies in beriberi heart disease. *Am J Med* 1966;41:197–212.

145. Waber LJ, Valle D, Neill C, et al. Carnitine deficiency presenting as familial cardiomyopathy: a treatable defect in carnitine transport. *J Pediatr* 1982;101:700–705.

146. Tripp ME, Katcher ML, Peters HA, et al. Systemic carnitine deficiency presenting as familial endocardial fibroelastosis: a treatable cardiomyopathy. *N Engl J Med* 1984;310:142–148.

147. Cornwell GG III, Westermark P, Natvig JB, Murdoch W. Senile cardiac amyloid: evidence that fibrils contain a protein immunologically related to prealbumin. *Immunology* 1981;44:447–452.

148. Gertz MA, Kyle RA. Primary systemic amyloidosis: a diagnostic primer. *Mayo Clin Proc* 1989;64:1505–1519.

149. Falk RH. Cardiac amyloidosis. In: Zipes DP, Rowlands DJ, eds. *Progress in cardiology.* Philadelphia: Lea & Febiger, 1988:143–155.

150. Pomerance A. Senile cardiac amyloidosis. *Br Heart J* 1965;27:711–718.

151. Kyle RA, Spittell PC, Gertz MA, et al. The premortem recognition of systemic senile amyloidosis with cardiac involvement. *Am J Med* 1996;101:395–400.

152. Arbustini E, Merlini G, Gavazzi A, et al. Cardiac immunocyte-derived (AL) amyloidosis: an endomyocardial biopsy study in 11 patients. *Am Heart J* 1995;130:528–536.

153. Smith TJ, Kyle RA, Lie JT. Clinical significance of histopathologic patterns of cardiac amyloidosis. *Mayo Clin Proc* 1984;59:547–555.

154. Narang R, Chopra P, Wasir HS. Cardiac amyloidosis presenting as ischemic heart disease: a case report and review of literature. *Cardiology* 1993;82:294–300.

155. Tei C, Dujardin KS, Hodge DO, et al. Doppler index combining systolic and diastolic myocardial performance: clinical value in cardiac amyloidosis. *J Am Coll Cardiol* 1996;28:658–664.

156. Fournier C, Grimon G, Rinaldi JP, et al. Usefulness of technetium-99m pyrophosphate myocardial scintigraphy in amyloid polyneuropathy and correlation with echocardiography. *Am J Cardiol* 1993;72:854–857.

157. Gertz MA, Skinner M, Connors LH, et al. Selective binding of nifedipine to amyloid fibrils. *Am J Cardiol* 1985;55:1646.

158. Matsouka H, Hamada M, Honda T, et al. Precise assessment of myocardial damage associated with secondary cardiomyopathies by use of Gd-DTPA-enhanced magnetic resonance imaging. *Angiology* 1993;44:945–950.

159. Pollak A, Falk RH. Left ventricular systolic dysfunction precipitated by verapamil in cardiac amyloidosis. *Chest* 1993;104:618–620.

160. Gertz MA, Falk RH, Skinner M, et al. Worsening of congestive heart failure in amyloid heart disease treated by calcium channel-blocking agents. *Am J Cardiol* 1985;55:1645.

161. Griffiths BE, Hughes P, Dowdle R, Stephens MR. Cardiac amyloidosis with asymmetrical septal hypertrophy and deterioration after nifedipine. *Thorax* 1982;37:711–712.

162. Rubinow A, Skinner M, Cohen AS. Digoxin sensitivity in amyloid cardiomyopathy. *Circulation* 1981;63:1285–1288.

163. Cassidy JT. Cardiac amyloidosis: two cases with digitalis sensitivity. *Ann Intern Med* 1961;55:989–994.

164. Comenzo RL, Vosburgh E, Simms RW, et al. Dose-intensive melphalan with blood stem cell support for the treat-

ment of AL amyloidosis: one-year follow-up in five patients. *Blood* 1996;88:2801–2806.

165. Young JB. Potential for the recurrence of original disease in transplanted hearts. *Transplant Immunol Lett* 1996;12:3,8–9.

166. Perry A, Vuitch F. Causes of death in patients with sarcoidosis: a morphologic study of 38 autopsies with clinicopathologic correlations. *Arch Pathol Lab Med* 1995;119:167–172.

167. Bulkley BH, Rouleau JR, Whitaker JQ, et al. The use of ^{201}thallium for myocardial perfusion imaging in sarcoid heart disease. *Chest* 1977;72:27–32.

168. Forman MB, Sandler MP, Sacks GA, et al. Radionuclide imaging in myocardial sarcoidosis: demonstration of myocardial uptake of technetium pyrophosphate^{99m} and gallium. *Chest* 1983;83:578–580.

169. McKenna WJ. Clinical genetics of dilated cardiomyopathy. *Herz* 1994;19:91–96.

170. Remes AM, Hassinen IE, Ikaheimo MJ, et al. Mitochondrial DNA deletions in dilated cardiomyopathy: a clinical study employing endomyocardial sampling. *J Am Coll Cardiol* 1994;23:935–942.

171. Mirabella M, Servidei S, Manfredi G, et al. Cardiomyopathy may be the only clinical manifestation in female carriers of Duchenne muscular dystrophy. *Neurology* 1993;43:2342–2345.

172. Kawashima S, Ueno M, Kondo T, et al. Marked cardiac involvement limb girdle muscular dystrophy. *Am J Med Sci* 1990;299:411–414.

173. Ades LC, Gedeon AK, Wilson MJ, et al. Barth syndrome. Clinical features and confirmation of gene localization to distal Xq28. *Am J Med Genet* 1993;45:327–334.

174. Christodoulou J, McInnes RR, Jay V, et al. Barth syndrome: clinical observations and genetic linkage studies. *Am J Med Genet* 1994;50:255–264.

175. De Michele G, Di Maio L, Filla A, et al. Childhood onset of Friedreich's ataxia: a clinical and genetic study of 36 cases. *Neuropediatrics* 1996;27:3–7.

176. Gunal N, Saraclar M, Ozkutlu S, et al. Heart disease in Friedreich's ataxia: a clinical and echocardiographic study. *Acta Pediatr Jpn* 1996;38:308–311.

177. Casazza F, Ferrari F, Finocchiaro G. Echocardiographic evaluation of verapamil in Friedreich's ataxia. *Br Heart J* 1986;55:400–404.

178. Wood GB. *A treatise on the practice of medicine*, 4th ed. Philadelphia: JB Lippincott Co., 1855.

179. McCall D. Alcohol and the cardiovascular system. *Curr Probl Cardiol* 1987;12:349–414.

180. Regan TJ. Alcoholic and cardiomyopathy. *Prog Cardiovasc Dis* 1984;28:141–152.

181. Moushmoush B, Abi-Mansour P. Alcohol and the heart. The long-term effects of alcohol on the cardiovascular system. *Arch Intern Med* 1991;151:36–42.

182. Walsh TK, Vacek JL. Ethanol and heart disease: an underestimated contributing factor. *Postgrad Med* 1986;79:60–75.

183. Schwarz F, Mall G, Zebe H, et al. Determinants of survival in patients with congestive cardiomyopathy: quantitative morphologic findings and left ventricular hemodynamics. *Circulation* 1984;70:923–928.

184. Kinney EL, Wright RJ, Caldwell JW. Risk factors in alcoholic cardiomyopathy. *Angiology* 1989;40:270–275.

185. Ratliff NB, McMahon JT. *Unpublished observation.*

186. Urbano-Marquez A, Estruch R, Navarro-Lopez F, et al. The effects of alcoholism on skeletal and cardiac muscle. *N Engl J Med* 1989;320:409–415.

187. Guarnieri T, Lakatta EG. Mechanism of myocardial contractile depression by clinical concentrations of ethanol: a study in ferret papillary muscles. *J Clin Invest* 1990;85:1462–1467.

188. Mørlgaard H, Kristensen BØ, Baandrup U. Importance of abstention from alcohol in alcoholic heart disease. *Int J Cardiol* 1990;26:373–375.

189. Pavan D, Nicolosi GL, Lestuzzi C, et al. Normalization of variables of left ventricular function in patients with alcoholic cardiomyopathy after cessation of excessive alcohol intake: an echocardiographic study. *Eur Heart J* 1987;8:535–540.

190. Shan K, Lincoff M, Young JB. Anthracycline-induced cardiotoxicity. *Ann Intern Med* 1996;125:47–58.

191. Billingam ME, Bristow MR. Endomyocardial biopsy for cardiac monitoring of patients receiving anthracyclines. In: Fenoglio JJ, ed. *Endomyocardial biopsy: techniques and application.* Boca Raton, FL: CRC Press, 1982:66–77.

192. Isner JM, Estes III NAM, Thompson PD, et al. Acute cardiac events temporally related to cocaine use. *N Engl J Med* 1986;315:1438–1443.

193. Karch RA, Billingham ME. The pathology and etiology of cocaine-induced heart disease. *Arch Pathol Lab Med* 1988;112:225–230.

194. Ikaheimo MJ, Niemela KO, Linnaluoto MM, et al. Early cardiac changes related to radiation therapy. *Am J Cardiol* 1985;56:943–946.

195. Totterman KG, Pesonen E, Siltanen P. Radiation-related chronic heart disease. *Chest* 1983;83:875–878.

196. Taymor-Luria H, Kohn K, Pasternak RC. Radiation heart disease. *J Cardiovasc Surg* 1983;8:113.

197. Fajardo LF, Stewart JR. Pathogenesis of radiation-induced myocardial fibrosis. *Lab Invest* 1973;29:244–257.

198. Schultz-Hector S, Balz K. Radiation-induced loss of endothelial alkaline phosphatase activity and development of myocardial degeneration: an ultrastructural study. *Lab Invest* 1994;71:252–260.

199. Warda M, Khan A, Massumi A, et al. Radiation-induced valvular dysfunction. *J Am Coll Cardiol* 1983;2:180–185.

200. Simon EB, Ling J, Mendizabal RC, Midawell J. Radiation-induced coronary artery disease. *Am Heart J* 1984;108:1032–1034.

201. Merrill J, Greco Fa, Zimbler H. Adriamycin and radiation: synergistic cardiotoxicity. *Ann Intern Med* 1975;82:122–123.

202. Hancock SL, Tucker MA, Hoppe RT. Factors affecting late mortality from heart disease after treatment of Hodgkin's disease. *JAMA* 1993;270:1949–1955.

203. Estes ML, Ewing-Wilson D, Chou SM, et al. Chloroquine neuromyotoxicity: clinical and pathologic perspective. *Am J Med* 1987;82:447–455.

204. Ratliff NB, Estes ML, Myles JL, et al. The diagnosis of chloroquine cardiomyopathy by endomyocardial biopsy. *N Engl J Med* 1987;316:191–193.

205. Pearson GD, Veille JC, Rahimtoola S, et al. Peripartum cardiomyopathy: National Heart, Lung, and Blood Insti-

tute and Office of Rare Diseases (National Institutes of Health) workshop recommendations and review. *JAMA* 2000;283:1183–1188.

206. Cunningham FG, Pritchard JA, Hankins GD, et al. Peripartum heart failure: idiopathic cardiomyopathy or compounding cardiovascular events? *Obstet Gynecol* 1986;67:157–168.

207. Pierce JA, Price BO, Joyce JW. Familial occurrence of postpartal heart failure. *Arch Intern Med* 1963;111:651–655.

208. Veille JC. Peripartum cardiomyopathies: a review. *Am J Obstet Gynecol* 1984;148:805–818.

209. Cole P, Cook F, Plappert T, et al. Longitudinal changes in left ventricular architecture and function in peripartum cardiomyopathy. *Am J Cardiol* 1987;60:871–876.

210. Demakis JG, Rahimtoola SH, Sutton GC, et al. Natural course of peripartum cardiomyopathy. *Circulation* 1971; 44:1053–1061.

211. Lampert MB, Hibbard J, Weinert L, et al. Peripartum heart failure associated with prolonged tocolytic therapy. *Am J Obstet Gynecol* 1993;168:493–495.

212. O'Connell JB, Costanzo-Nordin MR, Subramanian R, et al. Peripartum cardiomyopathy: clinical, hemodynamic, histologic, and prognostic characteristics. *J Am Coll Cardiol* 1986;8:52–56.

213. Melvin KR, Richardson PJ, Osen EGJ, et al. Peripartum cardiomyopathy due to myocarditis. *N Engl J Med* 1982;307:731–734.

214. Midei MG, DeMent SH, Feldman AM, et al. Peripartum myocarditis and cardiomyopathy. *Circulation* 1990;81:922–928.

215. Herskowitz A, Cambell S, Deckers J, et al. Demographic features and prevalence of idiopathic myocarditis in patients undergoing endomyocardial biopsy. *Am J Cardiol* 1993;71:982–986.

216. Rizeq MN, Rickenbacher PR, Fowler MB, Billingham ME. Incidence of myocarditis in peripartum cardiomyopathy. *Am J Cardiol* 1994;74:474–477.

217. Tomaru A, Goto Y, Miura S, et al. Two cases of peripartum cardiomyopathy. *J Cardiol* 1995;25:43–49.

218. Walsh JJ, Burch GE, Black WC, et al. Idiopathic myocardiopathy of the puerperium: postpartal heart disease. *Circulation* 1965;32:19–31.

219. Wulsch JJ, Burch GE. Postpartal heart disease. *Arch Intern Med* 1961;108:817–823.

220. Rutherford SE, Phelan JP. Thromboembolic disease in pregnancy. *Clin Perinatol* 1986;13:719–739.

221. Hovsepian PG, Ganzel B, Sohi GS, et al. Peripartum cardiomyopathy treated with a left ventricular assist device as a bridge to cardiac transplantation. *South Med J* 1989;82:527–529.

222. Lewis R, Mabie WC, Burlew B, et al. Biventricular assist device as a bridge to cardiac transplantation in the treatment of peripartum cardiomyopathy. *South Med J* 1997;90:955–958.

223. Bozkurt B, Villaneuva FS, Holubkov R, et al. Intravenous immune globulin in the therapy of peripartum cardiomyopathy. *J Am Coll Cardiol* 1999;34:177–180.

224. Elkayam U, Ostrzega EL, Shotan A. Peripartum cardiomyopathy. In: Gleicher N, ed. *Principles and practice of medical therapy in pregnancy*, 2nd ed. Norwalk, CT: Appleton & Lange, 1992.

225. Lampert MB, Weinert L, Hibbard J, et al. Contractile reserve in patients with peripartum cardiomyopathy and recovered left ventricular function. *J Am Coll Cardiol* 1994;23:428A(abst).

226. De Belder AJ, Radomski MW, Why HJ, et al. Myocardial calcium-independent nitric oxide synthase activity is present in dilated cardiomyopathy, myocarditis, and postpartum cardiomyopathy but not in ischaemic or valvular heart disease. *Br Heart J* 1995;74:426–430.

227. Cameron JS. Glomerulonephritis in renal transplants. *Transplantation* 1982;34:237–245.

228. Cameron JS. Recurrent primary disease and *de novo* nephritis following renal transplantation. *Pediatr Nephrol* 1991;5:412–421.

229. Cameron JS. Recurrent disease in renal allografts. *Kidney Int* 1993;44[Suppl 43]:S91–S94.

230. Mathew TH. Recurrence of disease following renal transplantation. *Am J Kidney Dis* 1988;12:85–96.

231. Gagnadoux MF, Niaudet P, Broyer M. Non-immunological risk factors in paediatric renal transplantation. *Pediatr Nephrol* 1993;7:89–95.

232. Dantal J, Giral M, Hoormant M, Soulillou JP. Glomerulonephritis recurrences after kidney transplantation. *Curr Opin Nephrol Hyper* 1995;4:146–154.

233. Cameron JS. In: Tilney N, ed. *Transplantation biology: cellular and molecular aspects*. New York: Lippincott–Raven Publishers, 1996:619–662.

234. Olivetti G, Abbi R, Quaini F, et al. Apoptosis in the failing human heart. *N Engl J Med* 1997;336:1131–1141.

235. Hufnagel G, Pankuweit S, Richter A, et al. The European Study of Epidemiology and Treatment of Cardiac Inflammatory Diseases (ESETCID). First epidemiological results. *Herz* 2000;25(3):279–285.

236. Thompson CB. Apoptosis in the pathogenesis and treatment of disease. *Science* 1995;267:1456–1461.

237. Weinberg SL. Apoptosis: the good and the bad—possible therapeutic implications. *Clin Cardiol* 1999;22:383–384.

238. Williams RS. Apoptosis in heart failure. *N Engl J Med* 1999;341:759–760.

239. Anversa P. Myocyte death in the pathological heart. *Circ Res* 2000;86:121–124.

240. Kang PM, Izumo S. Apoptosis and heart failure. A critical review of the literature. *Circ Res* 2000;86:1107–1113.

241. Springer CJ, Niculescu-Duraz I. Prodrug-activating systems in suicide gene therapy. *J Clin Invest* 2000;105:1161–1167.

242. Nakamura T, Veda Y, Juan Y, et al. Fas-mediated apoptosis in Adriamycin-induced cardiomyopathy in rats. *Circulation* 2000;102:572–578.

243. McNamara DM, Holubkov R, Starling RC, et al. Controlled trial of intravenous immune globulin in recent-onset dilated cardiomyopathy. *Circulation* 2001;103:2254–2259.

ACUTE HEART FAILURE MANAGEMENT

GARRIE J. HAAS
JAMES B. YOUNG

OVERVIEW

Acute heart failure is a complex syndrome that is often a direct result of myocardial systolic dysfunction caused by underlying ischemia or infarction. Although atherosclerotic heart disease is the most common cause of acute heart failure in Western societies, a broad spectrum of other potential causes exists, including such diverse conditions as acute valvular abnormalities, pericardial disease, acute myocarditis, and pulmonary embolism. The management of acute heart failure requires rapid identification of the underlying mechanism, with specific treatment directed at reversing the associated abnormal pathophysiologic state. The support of patients while the diagnostic evaluation is pursued can range from therapy with intravenous nitrates and diuretics to full pharmacologic support with combinations of inotropic, vasodilator, and vasopressor agents. In complicated situations, hemodynamic monitoring is essential. In circumstances in which a reparable lesion has been identified or in which cardiac transplantation is considered an option, mechanical circulatory support may be required until definitive treatment can be instituted. Because of the complexity and diverse nature of the acute heart failure syndrome, treatment must be individualized.

The ultimate success of acute heart failure management depends heavily on the rapid institution of effective pharmacologic support to relieve symptoms and reverse hemodynamic derangement with simultaneous pursuit of definitive diagnostic studies. The inability to identify or correct an underlying lesion or condition is associated with significant short-term mortality.

INTRODUCTION

The syndrome of acute heart failure represents a true medical emergency that warrants an expedient diagnostic and thera-

G. J. Haas: Heart Failure Disease Management Program, Mid Ohio Cardiology Consultants, Riverside Methodist Hospital, Columbus, Ohio
J. B. Young: Kaufman Center for Heart Failure, The Cleveland Clinic Foundation, Cleveland, Ohio

peutic approach by the clinician. If appropriate treatment is not instituted within a reasonable period of time, irreversible cardiac decompensation may ensue, leading to a progressive syndrome of shock, multiorgan failure, and death. The complexity of acute heart failure and the diversity of its potential causes make a precise definition difficult. But in clinical practice, it is generally recognized when symptoms develop within hours to days in patients without a history of cardiac decompensation (1). A history of previous treatment for heart disease may be elicited, however, because many patients will have experienced symptoms (i.e., angina, exertional dyspnea) related to myocardial ischemia. In fact, atherosclerotic heart disease and the complications of myocardial ischemia and infarction are the most common causes of acute heart failure in Western societies. A multitude of other potential causes must also be considered, however, including acute valvular dysfunction, pericardial disease, acute myocarditis with left ventricular dysfunction, uncontrolled severe hypertension, and pulmonary embolism (Table 91.1). Many of the conditions resulting in acute heart failure may be definitively treated, which results in a favorable impact on the patient's short- and long-term course. Although the majority of patients presenting with acute heart failure suffer from some degree of myocardial systolic dysfunction, diastolic heart failure with preserved systolic function may also occur in those with underlying restrictive or hypertrophic myocardial diseases. When acute pulmonary edema is the presenting problem, consideration must also be given to possible noncardiac causes. A brief history and directed physical examination, electrocardiogram, and possibly echocardiography usually suffice to differentiate cardiogenic from noncardiogenic pulmonary edema.

Guidelines published by a task force of the American College of Cardiology and American Heart Association have categorized presentations of acute heart failure into three major clinical groups: acute cardiogenic pulmonary edema, cardiogenic shock, and acute decompensation of chronic left heart failure (2). Treatment strategies differ for these groups, but in general, rapid evaluation, diagnosis, and therapy are imperative. The 1-year mortality rate for patients presenting with acute pulmonary edema may exceed 50% when an underlying lesion or condition is not defined and treated

(3). In certain life-threatening conditions, such as acute ischemic myocardial injury or complications thereof (i.e., acute valvular regurgitation, ventricular septal defect, cardiac tamponade), immediate evaluation and specific, directed therapy are indicated for stabilization and treatment of the acute heart failure syndrome. In these emergency situations, definitive therapy should not be delayed by prolonged efforts to achieve a stabler clinical situation. Without correction of the underlying lesion, such efforts are often unsuccessful and commonly result in further clinical deterioration with the development of irreversible myocardial dysfunction. When the disorder precipitating acute heart failure does not appear to be one requiring urgent therapy, definitive diagnostic studies and consideration for specific forms of therapy can be delayed until clinical and hemodynamic stabilization have been achieved. In patients with decompensated chronic heart failure, an urgent diagnostic evaluation is often unnecessary because the underlying cause of myocardial dysfunction is usually known.

This chapter focuses on patients presenting with predominantly acute systolic heart failure. Because management strategies differ for different clinical groups across the spectrum of acute heart failure (e.g., acute myocardial infarction is managed differently from acute valvular insufficiency or right ventricular infarction), specific therapeutic principles for the treatment of patients presenting within the major clinical subsets of acute cardiogenic pulmonary edema, cardiogenic shock, and decompensated chronic heart failure are addressed. Individualization of the therapeutic strategy is always necessary. The standard intravenous pharmacologic agents used to manage acute heart failure are discussed in detail, as are some of the more promising investigational drugs currently being evaluated in clinical trials. For those situations in which pharmacologic stabilization of the patient is not achieved, selection criteria for mechanical support are reviewed. The initial assessment of the patient with acute heart failure is reviewed with an emphasis toward disease-specific treatment. One must recognize that the evaluation process (determination of cause) and the initial management and stabilization of the patient occur nearly simultaneously.

TABLE 91.1   MAJOR CAUSES OF ACUTE HEART FAILURE

Myocardial ischemia or infarction
Complications of myocardial infarction
    Acute mitral regurgitation (papillary muscle rupture)
    Ventricular septal rupture
    Cardiac free wall rupture and pericardial tamponade
Acute valvular catastrophe (mitral or aortic)
Severe, poorly controlled hypertension
Myocarditis
Sustained cardiac arrhythmias
Acute pulmonary embolism
Decompensation of chronic heart failure or cardiomyopathy
Acute aortic dissection with myocardial ischemia or infarction

PATHOPHYSIOLOGY AND CLINICAL PRESENTATION OF ACUTE HEART FAILURE

Acute left ventricular failure usually occurs as a result or complication of coronary artery disease, valvular disease, or, less commonly, primary myocardial disease such as myocarditis. An acute exacerbation of chronic heart failure or cardiomyopathy may also manifest as pulmonary edema and cardiogenic shock. The majority of patients presenting with acute heart failure has suffered significant injury to or ischemia of the myocardium, producing a substantial degree of regional and global myocardial systolic and diastolic dysfunction. This leads to a progressive deterioration in central hemodynamics that usually results in elevated left ventricular filling pressures and a variable reduction in stroke volume and cardiac output with subsequent circulatory failure. Often concomitant valvular dysfunction secondary to increased ventricular volumes and annular distention is found, which further exacerbates the hemodynamic abnormality (6). If immediate intervention with the goal of stabilizing the patient and definitively treating the underlying condition is not pursued, progressive left ventricular dysfunction and hemodynamic compromise may ensue.

Acute Cardiogenic Pulmonary Edema

The accumulation of extravascular fluid in the pulmonary interstitium or alveolar space resulting in pulmonary edema is caused by an imbalance in the equilibrium that normally exists between the opposing hydrostatic and oncotic forces of the pulmonary capillaries and the pulmonary interstitium (Starling forces). Under normal conditions, the balance of forces favors a continuous transudation of fluid from the capillaries to the interstitial space of approximately 500 mL per day, which is removed by the lymphatics (7). If the pulmonary capillary wedge pressure (PCWP) acutely exceeds 20 to 25 mm Hg, as may occur in acute left ventricular dysfunction, the increase in capillary hydrostatic pressure results in increased filtration of fluid and protein across the vascular endothelium, which leads to interstitial or alveolar pulmonary edema (7). As a result, the patient experiences breathlessness and increased work of breathing due to a drop in pulmonary compliance and hypoxia. ▼ p14

When evaluating acute pulmonary edema, one must always be aware of noncardiac causes that are seen in the clinical setting of normal to low PCWP and most often result from injury to the alveolar-capillary membrane due to any of a number of reasons (7,11). Edema formation by this mechanism often occurs more rapidly and to a greater degree than cardiogenic pulmonary edema.

Cardiogenic Shock

The often catastrophic condition of cardiogenic shock (see Chapter 19) is usually the result of myocardial damage resulting either from a single acute event or as the culmination of multiple events resulting in extensive (greater than 40%) ischemic myocardial injury. Cardiogenic shock most commonly occurs as a consequence of left ventricular dysfunction resulting from coronary occlusion. Data from the SHOCK (Should We Emergently Revascularize Occluded Coronaries for Cardiogenic Shock?) Trial Registry identified predominant left ventricular failure as the cause of shock in 78.5% of all cases (12). Complications of myocardial infarction, including severe mitral regurgitation and ventricular septal rupture, were identified as the primary cause of shock in 6.9% and 3.9% of cases, respectively (12).

Several additional cardiovascular causes may also produce cardiogenic shock, including acute myocarditis, primary valvular catastrophe, and acute decompensation of end-stage cardiomyopathy (13). The shock syndrome may also result from predominant right ventricular infarction, which generally has a better prognosis than shock due to left ventricular failure and is treated primarily with volume resuscitation and inotropic support.

The incidence of cardiogenic shock in patients suffering acute myocardial infarction is approximately 7.5% (14,15). The cardiogenic shock syndrome is often accompanied by severe hypotension with diminished pulse pressure and tachycardia, low cardiac output, and signs and symptoms of reduced tissue and organ perfusion, including renal dysfunction, cool and clammy extremities, lethargy and confusion due to cerebral hypoperfusion, and metabolic acidosis resulting from elevated blood lactate levels. In the absence of prompt reperfusion and pharmacologic or mechanical support to correct the profound hemodynamic derangement associated with shock, progressive deterioration will occur, resulting in a high probability of continued cardiac dysfunction and circulatory failure (Fig. 91.1) (13). Although significant progress has been made in the short-term support of the cardiovascular system in shock, if the ischemic myocardium is not reperfused, the mortality rate remains high and in excess of 70% (14,16). In the SHOCK Trial Registry, in-hospital mortality was approximately 60% in patients with shock after myocardial infarction (12).

The neurohormonal compensatory mechanisms activated to acutely support the cardiovascular system in shock are similar to those activated in chronic heart failure (see Chapter 88). As shown in Figure 91.1, a dramatic and often acute reduction in cardiac output leads to the perception that intravascular volume is reduced. Baroreceptor inactivation results in increased sympathetic tone with consequent vasoconstriction and increased heart rate and myocardial contractility. Diminished renal perfusion causes activation of the renin-angiotensin-aldosterone axis, which causes further vasoconstriction (mediated by angiotensin II) and sodium and water reabsorption mediated by elevated aldosterone levels. Hypotension induces the central release of antidiuretic hormone, which serves to further increase renal water resorption and intravascular volume. Peripheral autoregulation and local production of vasoactive metabolites cause redistribution of blood flow away from skin, intestines, and skeletal muscle in favor of the brain, heart, and kidneys (13). These compensatory mechanisms may support the cardiovascular system for a brief period of time, but without appropriate intervention, they are soon overwhelmed, which results in continued hypoperfusion and myocardial dysfunction. Pharmacologic intervention is directed toward supporting the blood pressure and systemic perfusion with inotropic and possibly vasopressor therapy. If an adequate systemic blood pressure can be sustained, vasodilators may also be considered in an attempt to lower filling pressures and decrease pul-

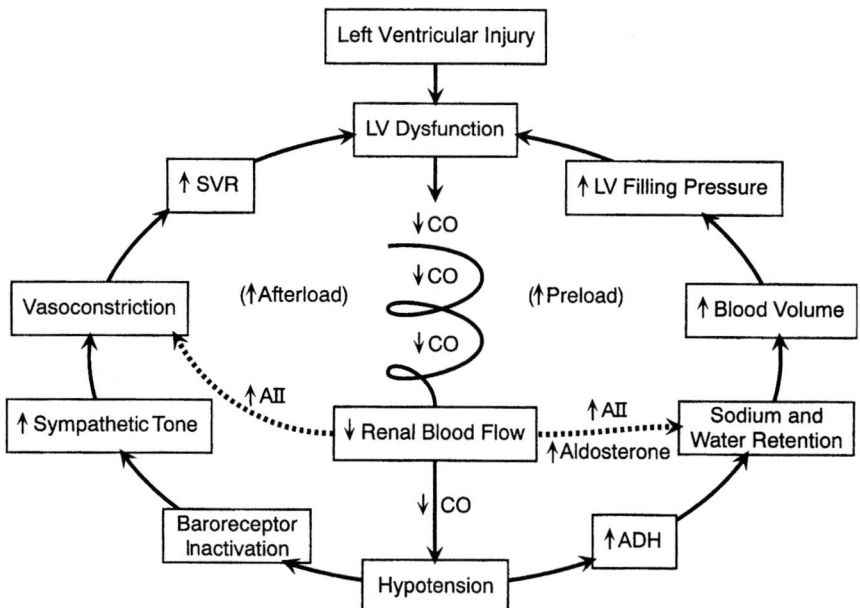

FIGURE 91.1 Depicted are the factors in cardiogenic shock perpetuating continued left ventricular (LV) dysfunction and progressive deterioration in cardiac output (CO). As CO falls, renal blood flow is reduced, which thus activates the renin-angiotensin-aldosterone system. Angiotensin II (AII) directly results in vasoconstriction and indirectly increases blood volume by enhancing aldosterone release. Hypotension resulting from a further fall in CO activates the central nervous system release of antidiuretic hormone (ADH). Inactivation of baroreceptors enhances sympathetic tone and vasoconstriction. As CO, renal blood flow, and hypotension remain reduced, preload and afterload continue to increase, which leads to further LV dysfunction. ↑, increased; ↓, decreased; SVR, systemic vascular resistance.

monary congestion and valvular regurgitation. Mechanical support will likely be necessary to allow for definitive diagnostic studies and therapeutic interventions.

Acute Decompensation of Chronic Heart Failure

Acute decompensation and clinical deterioration in a patient with previously documented chronic heart failure represent a different pathophysiologic state than the acute heart failure syndrome in patients without prior left ventricular dysfunction. These patients have a marked reduction in left ventricular systolic function at baseline due to a previous substantial injury to the myocardium. In approximately 50% of cases, the underlying disease is ischemic in etiology. In the remainder, a variety of causes may be identified, such as valvular disease or longstanding hypertension. The majority of cases of nonischemic chronic heart failure, however, is idiopathic (17). The typical patient with chronic heart failure is likely receiving some rational combination of oral therapy (angiotensin-converting enzyme inhibitors, beta-blockers, aldosterone antagonists, vasodilators, diuretics, digoxin) in an attempt to maintain stability and adequate functional capacity. Despite this treatment, however, these patients generally have mild to moderate symptoms of heart failure and exhibit some degree of total volume overload even in the compensated state. Left ventricular wall stress, because of left ventricular dilatation, is usually elevated, and compensatory neurohormonal mechanisms are activated (see Chapter 88). When acute decompensation occurs, these baseline abnormalities become further deranged. This is in contrast to the patient without significant myocardial dysfunction who suffers an acute insult to the myocardium leading to acute heart failure. Before the precipitating event, these patients generally have normal heart size and total body volume and do not exhibit baseline neurohormonal perturbation.

Table 91.2 outlines some of the important clinical and pathophysiologic characteristics of acute and chronic heart failure (18). Patients with decompensated chronic heart failure usually present with low output and congestive symptoms. They may describe worsening exertional dyspnea or dyspnea at rest, orthopnea, paroxysmal nocturnal dyspnea, and fatigue. Findings of the physical examination often reflect volume overload with peripheral edema and jugular venous distention. Pulmonary rales may be present but are certainly not as impressive as in the patient with acute myocardial injury and pulmonary edema. In fact, pulmonary findings may be relatively unremarkable in cases of decompensated chronic heart failure even when cardiac filling pressure is markedly elevated. A gallop rhythm and murmur of mitral regurgitation are typically audible, and the cardiac impulse is enlarged, sustained, and laterally displaced (8). Again, this is in contrast to the findings in acute pulmonary edema, in which cardiac size is usually normal and mitral regurgitation is less audible due to rapid equilibration of pressures between the left ventricle and normal left atrium. ❦ p15

PHARMACOTHERAPEUTICS OF ACUTE HEART FAILURE

Goal of Acute Pharmacologic Therapy

The objectives of the pharmacologic management of acute heart failure are to relieve disabling symptoms and discomfort rapidly, to reverse hemodynamic derangement, to preserve myocardial blood flow and energetics, and to stabilize the patient while further definitive diagnostic evaluation and therapy are pursued. Acute intravenous therapy is directed toward improving overall ventricular performance by favorably affecting the major determinants of ventricular func-

TABLE 91.2 COMPARISON OF ACUTE AND CHRONIC HEART FAILURE

Feature	Acute heart failure	Decompensated chronic heart failure	Stable chronic heart failure
Symptom severity	Marked	Marked	Mild to moderate
Pulmonary edema	Frequent	Frequent	Rare
Peripheral edema	Rare	Frequent	Frequent
Weight gain	None to mild	Marked	Frequent
Total body volume	No change or mildly increased	Markedly increased	Increased
Cardiomegaly	Uncommon	Usual	Common
Left ventricular systolic function	Hypo-, normo-, or hypercontractile	Reduced	Markedly reduced
Wall stress	Elevated	Markedly elevated	Elevated
Activation of sympathetic nervous system	Marked	Marked	Mild to marked
Activation of RAAS	Acutely abnormal	Marked	Mild to marked
Acute ischemia	Common	Occasional	Rare
Hyperventilative crisis	Common	Occasional	Rare
Reparable, remediable causative lesions[a]	Common	Occasional	Occasional

RAAS, renin-angiotensin-aldosterone system.
[a]Coronary thrombosis, acute mitral regurgitation, etc.
From Leier CV. Unstable heart failure. In: Colucci WS, ed. *Heart failure: cardiac function and dysfunction.* St. Louis: Mosby, 1995:9.2–9.15; and Braunwald E, ed. *Atlas of heart disease*, vol 4, with permission.

tion, including ventricular preload, afterload, and myocardial contractility. Acute intravenous pharmacologic support merely serves as a bridge to a more definitive treatment (i.e., myocardial revascularization, valve replacement) in most situations of acute heart failure and therefore should be viewed as a temporary means of support. The medications commonly used to stabilize the patient presenting with acute heart failure are usually administered intravenously, exhibit pharmacokinetic properties that allow for rapid titration to hemodynamic effect, and have a short plasma half-life so that any untoward effect can be quickly terminated. The medications commonly used to initially support the patient with acute heart failure are discussed in detail.

Acute Vasodilator Therapy

Nitroglycerin

Nitroglycerin is often effective in the early management of acute heart failure. The major hemodynamic effect of nitrates is to evoke a reduction in ventricular filling pressure and volume by increasing venous capacitance through venodilation (19–29). This shifts central blood volume to the venous capacitance vessels, which causes a decrease in pulmonary congestion and often a dramatic improvement in the symptoms of breathlessness associated with acute heart failure and elevated ventricular filling pressures. This vasodilating action is mediated through relaxation of vascular smooth muscle resulting primarily from a nitrate-induced production of *S*-nitrosothiols, which cause an increase in intracellular cyclic guanosine monophosphate (30,31). Nitrates may also elicit vasodilation by other mechanisms, including stimulation of the endothelial production and release of prostacyclin or prostaglandin E (32–34). Although these agents are predominantly considered for venodilation, higher doses of nitrates produce arterial

dilatation and therefore reduce systemic vascular resistance (SVR) and ventricular impedance (35). ❦ p16

Nitrates are effective therapy in the urgent treatment of acute heart failure, acute cardiogenic pulmonary edema, and acute decompensation of chronic heart failure (21,42–47). Nitroglycerin therapy can generally be instituted rapidly when it is evident that pulmonary congestion is present and therefore preload reduction is desired. Intravenous nitroglycerin is the preparation most commonly used. However, sublingual tablets and lingual-buccal spray may occasionally be used until an intravenous preparation is available to be infused (48,49). Sublingual nitrates have rapid onset of action (3 to 6 minutes) and can be administered in 0.4- to 0.8-mg doses every 5 to 10 minutes as necessary to reduce the severe dyspnea and elevated ventricular filling pressures commonly associated with acute heart failure, particularly if myocardial dysfunction is secondary to ischemia or infarction. A 0.4-mg sublingual tablet given every 4 to 5 minutes is approximately equivalent to a 1.5-μg-per-kg-per-minute continuous infusion (50). The sublingual preparation is often used at the authors' institution to reverse high pulmonary artery pressures in patients with chronic heart failure who are undergoing transplant evaluation (51). Therefore, its potency should not be underestimated.

Intravenous nitroglycerin (typically starting at a dosage of 0.2 μg per kg per minute) may be rapidly titrated upward in increments of 0.1 to 0.2 μg per kg per minute to improve symptoms and reduce pulmonary and systemic venous pressures and resistance, ventricular filling pressures, and, to a variable degree, SVR. As noted previously, however, the ability of nitrates to augment stroke volume and cardiac output by decreasing left ventricular afterload is often dose dependent and usually requires an initial intravenous dosage of at least 0.4 μg per kg per minute (21). One must also consider the propensity for the development of pharmacodynamic tolerance during continuous intravenous infusions, which necessitates an intermittent increase in dose to maintain the desired hemodynamic effect (52). ☛ p17

Nitroprusside

Sodium nitroprusside is a powerful venous and arterial vasodilator with potent afterload-reducing properties (54). It is the agent most frequently used early in the treatment of acute heart failure, particularly when a rapid and substantial reduction in SVR is necessary. Common clinical conditions for which it is used include complications of myocardial infarction such as acute mitral regurgitation secondary to papillary muscle dysfunction or rupture, ventricular septal defect, and acute aortic regurgitation. Nitroprusside relaxes arterial and venous smooth muscle via the production of nitric oxide and nitrosothiols, which leads to an increase in cyclic guanosine monophosphate and smooth muscle relaxation (23). As with nitroglycerin, nitroprusside causes preload reduction by diminishing heightened venous tone and increasing venous capacitance with a concomitant shift in central blood volume to the periphery (24). This causes a reduction in right ventricular pressure and volume. Unique to nitroprusside is its rapid and powerful effect on afterload. This agent reduces the major components of aortic impedance (mean and hydraulic vascular load), which results in an improved and often dramatic increase in forward stroke volume and cardiac output with reductions in left ventricular filling pressure, volume, and valvular regurgitation (19,21,24,55–58). Fortunately, this decrease in afterload occurs without major changes in aortic pressure (56). ☛ p18

The most common serious adverse effect of nitroprusside administration in acute heart failure is systemic hypotension (54,62,66). One should be particularly cautious when initiating nitroprusside therapy in a patient with ischemia or infarction and a systolic arterial pressure of less than 100 mm Hg. An increase in heart rate during the infusion is an ominous finding and usually presages hypotension. This typically occurs when stroke volume has not increased appropriately, often because of ongoing or worsening ischemia, valvular regurgitation, and inadequate cardiac reserve. A reduction or cessation of the nitroprusside infusion is usually warranted. Alternatively, the addi-

tion of a positive inotropic agent such as dobutamine hydrochloride is often advantageous and may allow for the continuation of nitroprusside. Such a combination is commonly used to stabilize particularly severe, low-output heart failure until more definitive therapy can be instituted (see the section Combination Pharmacologic Therapy later in this chapter). When systemic hypotension and poor peripheral perfusion are present at the outset, nitroprusside should generally be avoided as initial treatment. ☛ p19

Positive Inotropic Therapy

Dobutamine

Dobutamine hydrochloride is a synthetic catecholamine and positive inotropic agent that is useful in the acute management of systolic heart failure associated with systemic hypoperfusion. Along with intravenous diuretics, it is used commonly in patients with acute decompensation of chronic heart failure or myocardial infarction presenting with pulmonary congestion and low cardiac output symptoms. Dobutamine exists as a racemic mixture of dextro- and levoisomers, which are potent beta- and alpha-adrenergic agonists, respectively (67). Therefore, dobutamine produces its positive inotropic effect via stimulation of myocardial $beta_1$ and probably $alpha_1$ receptors (68). Theoretically, the opposing forces of $alpha_1$ and $beta_2$ stimulation on the peripheral vasculature should result in a negligible change in vascular resistance. Binkley and colleagues have shown, however, that in a total-artificial-heart model, dobutamine improves ventricular performance through direct modulation of arterial and venous tone (69). Dobutamine also has a favorable effect on aortic impedance, which allows for more efficient transfer of ventricular work and energy into stroke volume, cardiac output, and systemic perfusion. This maximizes the blood volume ejected by the ventricle for any augmentation in myocardial contractility (70,71). This is in contrast to the inotropic/vasopressor agent dopamine hydrochloride, which does not decrease aortic impedance and therefore limits the amount of blood ejected for any given increase in contractility (70,71) (Table 91.3). These differences in ventricular-vascular coupling explain why dobu-

TABLE 91.3 SYSTEMIC VASCULAR PROFILES OF DOBUTAMINE AND DOPAMINE IN HEART FAILURE

	Dobutamine hydrochloride	Dopamine hydrochloride
Systemic vascular resistance	↓	→ or ↑
Characteristic aortic impedance	↓	→ or ↑
Ventricular-vascular coupling	↑Systolic ejection ↑Stroke volume ↑Cardiac output	→ or ↓Ejection ↑Systemic blood pressure
Transfer of ventricular work-energy	Systemic blood flow	Systemic pressure

↑, increased; ↓, decreased; →, unchanged.
Adapted from Leier CV. Positive inotropic therapy: an update and new agents. *Curr Probl Cardiol* 1996;21:538, with permission.

tamine augments cardiac output and improves ventricular performance whereas dopamine, at moderate to high doses, is a vasopressor and ultimately worsens cardiac function in heart failure (71–73) (Fig. 91.2, *e*Fig. 91.2.1). Thus, these inotropic and vascular effects of dobutamine account for its favorable hemodynamic profile in acute heart failure. Dobutamine increases stroke volume and cardiac output, reduces ventricular volume and mitral regurgitant fraction, and lowers left ventricular diastolic pressure without producing a significant increase in heart rate (72,74). This cardiocirculatory response to dobutamine results from its potent inotropic and substantial vasodilator effects, which are linearly related to dose and plasma concentration (74,75). 🖛 p20

Milrinone

Milrinone lactate, a bipyridine analog of amrinone, is a second-generation phosphodiesterase inhibitor that exhibits both direct inotropic and vasodilator properties (71,76,84). Milrinone is approved by the U.S. Food and Drug Administration (FDA) for parenteral use in the treatment of congestive heart failure. The parent compound, amrinone, is also available parenterally but because of its substantial side-effect profile and weak inotropic properties, it has largely been supplanted by milrinone. 🖛 p21

The acute hemodynamic effects of milrinone in patients with chronic heart failure have been well described (85–89). The hemodynamic profile is one that would be expected from a drug with potent inotropic and balanced vasodilator properties. Once therapeutic plasma levels are achieved, milrinone elicits a reduction in right and left ventricular filling pressures and increases cardiac output without producing significant changes in the heart rate–blood pressure product. Because of its potent vasodilator properties, however, milrinone has the potential to worsen preexisting systemic hypotension. A reduction in pulmonary vascular resistance is usually observed and is primarily secondary to the reduction in left ventricular filling pressure rather than a direct pulmonary vasodilator effect. Even though milrinone may be expected to increase MVO_2 via its direct positive inotropic effect, its substantial vasodilator properties usually offset any detrimental increase in MVO_2 (87). This favorable effect is further enhanced by mild coronary vasodilatation (90). Compared with dobutamine, milrinone tends to evoke a greater reduction in left ventricular filling pressure and SVR while producing an equivalent increase in cardiac output (88) (Fig. 91.3). For the same reduction in SVR, milrinone produces a greater increase in stroke work index than nitroprusside, which reflects its additional inotropic properties (88,89). 🖛 p22

Vasopressor Therapy

Dopamine

Dopamine hydrochloride is a drug that exhibits complex pharmacologic properties. This agent mediates its effects through either direct activation or indirect activation (via norepinephrine release) of multiple pre- and postsynaptic receptors (93,94). Receptors that are activated are extremely sensitive to dopamine concentration, and this contributes further to the complexity of drug administration (94). The positive inotropic and chronotropic effect of dopamine is mediated through activation of postsynaptic myocardial beta$_1$ receptors. This effect is most evident clinically at dosages greater than 5 µg per kg per minute. At low doses, the primary effect of dopamine is one of vascular relaxation and sodium excretion by stimulation of specific dopaminergic receptors located postsynaptically on vascular smooth muscle cells (primarily in renal and mesenteric vascular beds) and renal tubular cells (95,96). Dopamine receptors may also be found in cerebral, coronary, skeletal muscle, and cutaneous vessels (93). Low-dose dopamine (0.5 to 2.0 µg per kg per minute) is often used to treat patients with heart failure and renal insufficiency to selectively activate renal dopaminergic receptors, induce renal vasodilatation and improve renal blood flow, and provoke natriuresis (97). As the dopamine dosage is progressively increased above 5 µg per kg per minute, postsynaptic alpha$_1$ and alpha$_2$ receptors are activated, and this mediates vasoconstriction and produces blood pressure elevation. 🖛 p23

To summarize, dopamine is the drug of choice in acute heart failure when significant hypotension is present despite adequate intravascular volume and ventricular filling pressures. In addition to evoking peripheral vasoconstriction and elevating blood pressure, it also has the unique property of enhancing renal blood flow through dopaminergic receptor activation, although this effect is probably negligible at doses in excess of 10.0 to 12.5 µg per kg per minute. Because of undesirable effects on myocardial function and hemodynamics, dopamine at high doses should be used only until more effective and definitive treatment is available.

Norepinephrine and Epinephrine

Norepinephrine is a potent alpha-adrenergic agonist that also possesses mild beta$_1$-agonist properties. It elicits a cardiovascular vasopressor response through dose-related vasoconstriction (76,103,104). This drug is not used for positive inotropic therapy because any increase in myocardial contractility is offset by increased afterload. During norepinephrine infusion, the combination of high preload and afterload markedly increases MVO_2 to the point at which the myocardial oxygen demand to supply ratio is threatened (76). Its primary indication in acute heart failure is to improve blood pressure and coronary perfusion in the setting of shock and persistent hypotension when dopamine and dobutamine are ineffective.

Norepinephrine can be infused starting at a rate of 0.02 to 0.04 µg per kg per minute and the dose can be advanced every 10 to 15 minutes until the desired blood pressure response is achieved (76). The target blood pressure should be that which is considered minimally acceptable in the

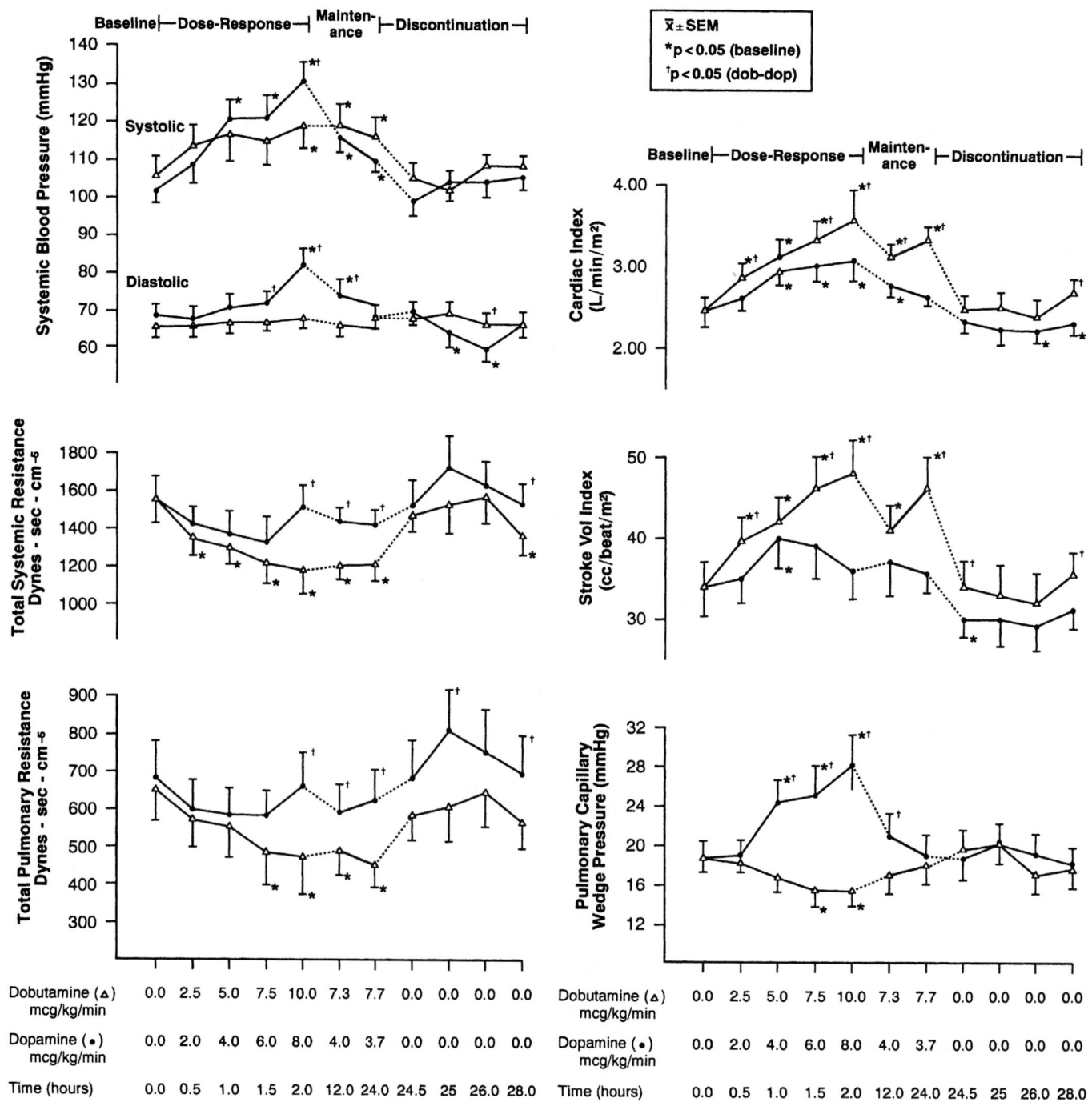

FIGURE 91.2 Comparison of dopamine hydrochloride (*filled circles*) and dobutamine hydrochloride (*open triangles*) on central hemodynamics in patients with low-output congestive heart failure. Infusions for both medications followed a baseline period, with titration of each drug to peak effect. The maximal dosage of dobutamine was 10 μg per kg per minute and of dopamine was 8 μg per kg per minute. The data illustrate that dopamine given at infusion rates that exceed 2 to 4 μg per kg per minute does not have a favorable effect on total systemic vascular resistance. This results in a reduction in stroke volume and cardiac index compared to those of dobutamine. Dopamine at moderate dosages also increases pulmonary capillary wedge pressure. Dobutamine produces a mild increase in systemic blood pressure, with reduction in total systemic resistance and improvement in cardiac filling pressure and cardiac index. SEM, standard error of the mean. (From Leier CV, Heban PT, Huss P, et al. Comparative systemic and regional hemodynamic effects of dopamine and dobutamine in patients with cardiomyopathic heart failure. *Circulation* 1978;58:466–475, with permission.)

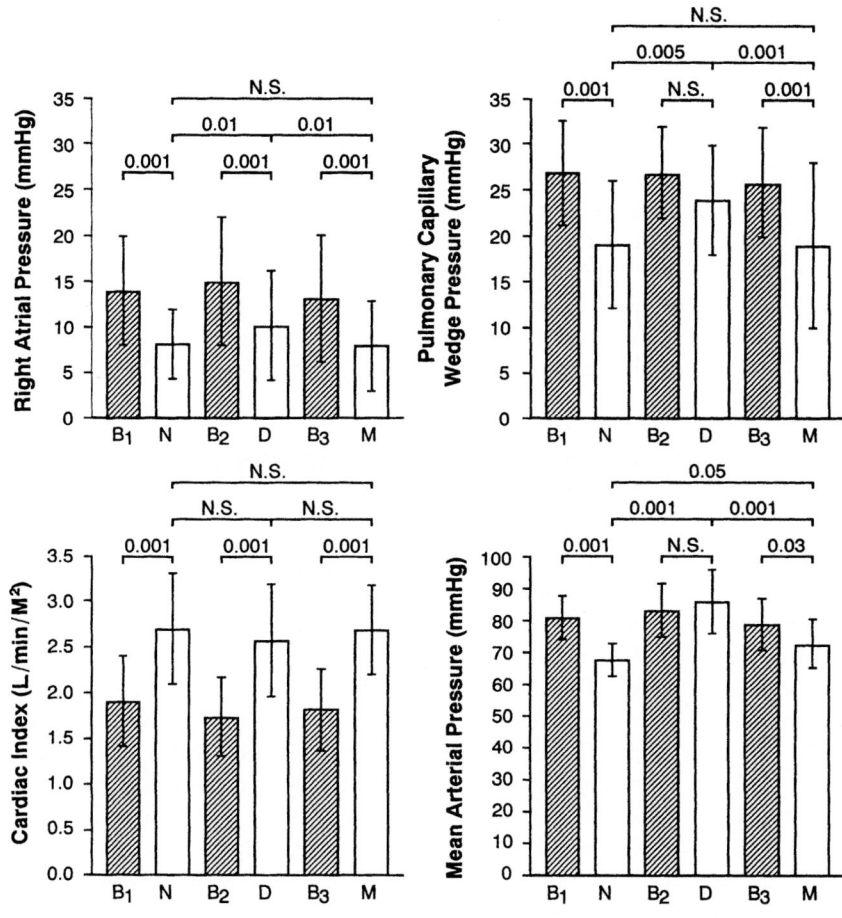

FIGURE 91.3 Effects of sodium nitroprusside (N), dobutamine hydrochloride (D), and milrinone lactate (M) on cardiac index, mean arterial pressure, right atrial pressure, and pulmonary capillary wedge pressure in patients with severe heart failure (B_1, B_2, and B_3 = baseline measurements). At dosages evoking a similar increase in cardiac index, all agents significantly reduced right atrial pressure, with nitroprusside and milrinone also producing a significant reduction in mean arterial pressure compared to baseline. The effect of milrinone and nitroprusside on pulmonary capillary wedge pressure was greater than that observed with dobutamine. N.S., not significant. (Adapted from Monrad ES, Baim DS, Smith HS, et al. Milrinone, dobutamine, and nitroprusside: comparative effects on hemodynamics and myocardial energetics in patients with severe congestive heart failure. *Circulation* 1986; 73[Suppl III]:168–174.)

individual patient to maintain adequate coronary perfusion and avoid serious side effects. Dopamine or dobutamine may be used in combination with norepinephrine to allow for lower dosing.

Epinephrine, like norepinephrine, is a catecholamine with potent alpha- and beta-agonist properties. Unlike norepinephrine, epinephrine also exhibits mild beta$_2$-agonist properties, which offsets some of the alpha effect and thereby mildly reduces its pressor response in comparison to norepinephrine (105). Epinephrine may be used in intensive care units for hemodynamic support in patients with severe heart failure and shock. It may be used in conjunction with other catecholamine inotropic and pressor drugs. Infusions of 0.1 to 1.0 µg per minute are commonly used. ⚑ p24

Diuretic Therapy

Intravenous furosemide is the loop diuretic most commonly used to treat the patient presenting with acute heart failure and pulmonary congestion. The major objective of diuretic therapy in this circumstance is to decrease excessive lung water through natriuresis and diuresis with a reduction in intravascular volume. Intravenous administration is necessary to rapidly achieve adequate furosemide levels at its site of action, the renal tubules.

The most important effect of furosemide in the acute management of heart failure probably relates to its substantial hemodynamic effects. Although both vasodilator and vasoconstrictor properties have been attributed to intravenous furosemide (108–111), most data support the view that furosemide evokes a reduction in cardiac filling pressures, and this likely results from an early vasodilator effect. A vasoconstrictor effect with reduction in cardiac output has also been reported, however, and may be a consequence of diuretic-induced neurohormonal activation (110,111). Furosemide, by decreasing systemic and pulmonary venoconstriction, has been shown to reduce left ventricular filling pressure in acute heart failure associated with myocardial infarction (112,113).

Diuretic therapy must be used judiciously in acute heart failure secondary to myocardial infarction because intravascular and total body volume is usually normal (Table 91.2). Excessive diuresis can result in hypotension with progression of myocardial ischemia by further compromise of coronary perfusion. In fact, subgroup analysis of data from two large post–myocardial infarction treatment trials suggests that diuretic therapy may be detrimental in this patient population (114,115).

The effective dosage of intravenous furosemide is variable but is usually in the range of 20 to 40 mg in the patient not previously receiving diuretic therapy and exhibiting normal renal function. On the other hand, patients with acute decompensation of chronic heart failure often present with substantial volume overload and usually require much larger dosages to achieve an adequate diuresis. This is because of prior chronic oral diuretic use and activation of renal compensatory mechanisms to counteract natriuresis in the chronic heart failure milieu. In patients exhibiting volume overload and diuretic resistance, a continuous infusion of furosemide (5 to 20 mg per hour) may prove advantageous (50,116). An attempt to enhance renal perfusion by increasing cardiac output (with dobutamine or nitroprusside) or by reducing renal vascular resistance (with low-dose dopamine) should also be considered. In patients with massive volume overload unresponsive to these therapeutic maneuvers, ultrafiltration may be effective (117).

Combination Pharmacologic Therapy

The use of multiple agents to support the failing circulation may provide certain advantages over treatment with a single agent (76,118). This is because acute heart failure or acute decompensation of chronic heart failure is associated with several hemodynamic abnormalities that cannot be entirely addressed by a single drug. The administration of an inotrope treats systolic dysfunction by improving contractility and stroke volume, but cardiac filling pressures and SVR (and associated valvular regurgitation) may not be substantively altered. A pure vasodilator alone may not be sufficient to support the circulation, and in fact may be detrimental when myocardial contractility is severely diminished and systemic blood pressure is unacceptably low. Using only a vasopressor drug to raise blood pressure in a patient with hypotension would increase afterload, ventricular wall stress, and filling pressures, which would inhibit the desired increase in cardiac output and potentially worsen ischemia.

Several combinations of intravenous drugs are theoretically appealing in the setting of severe acute heart failure. The simultaneous administration of dobutamine and a vasodilator such as nitroglycerin or nitroprusside augments stroke volume and lowers cardiac filling pressures more effectively than either agent alone (119,120). This combination is particularly useful in treating patients with cardiogenic shock resulting from a complication of myocardial infarction such as ventricular septal or papillary muscle rupture. As noted previously, the phosphodiesterase inhibitors also offer the advantage of potent vasodilation and positive inotropy; unfortunately, their pharmacokinetics and long half-life make these agents less than ideal in managing acute, unstable heart failure (71,76).

Using dobutamine (a beta-agonist), and milrinone (a phosphodiesterase inhibitor) simultaneously also offers possible advantages (85,118,121,122). The rationale behind this approach is based on the different mechanisms by which these drugs increase inotropy. Both agents, by different and complementary mechanisms, increase inotropy by

elevating cAMP levels in cardiomyocytes (71,76,89). Studies in patients with stable heart failure have shown an added effect of combination therapy on major hemodynamic parameters (122) (Fig. 91.4).

Dobutamine plus low-dose dopamine is one of the most commonly used combinations. The goal of this therapy is to achieve the inotropic effect of dobutamine with the concomitant renal vasodilator effect of low-dose dopamine (72,84,118). This combination is usually considered for the patient exhibiting marginal urine output and poor responsiveness to diuretics despite seemingly adequate central hemodynamics and systemic blood pressure. ❦ p25

HEMODYNAMIC MONITORING IN ACUTE HEART FAILURE

Catheterization with a flow-directed thermodilution pulmonary artery catheter (Swan-Ganz catheter) is often indicated for optimal management of acute heart failure. Although hemodynamic monitoring is rarely necessary in uncomplicated cases of acute pulmonary edema, it is often helpful in the patient who does not respond initially to standard therapy (usually nitroglycerin and diuretics) and is vital in managing those with persistent hypotension and preshock or shock syndromes (2) (Table 91.4). These patients have evidence of hypoperfusion on examination, including a narrow pulse pressure, cool skin, reduced urine output, and mental obtundation. Continuous assessment of cardiac output and ventricular filling pressure is essential to appropriately guide and determine the effectiveness of pharmacologic therapy or assess the need for mechanical support. Other indications for hemodynamic monitoring include acute heart failure in which volume status is in question and pulmonary edema in which a cardiac cause has not been definitely determined (2,142,143). As discussed previously, some patients presenting with acute cardiogenic pulmonary edema may have only mild elevation of PCWP. This is typically a result of reduced plasma volume from extravasation of water outside of the pulmonary capillaries further complicated by diuretic therapy. Hemodynamic monitoring may also be diagnostically helpful in further defining the severity of hemodynamic compromise due to specific lesions or conditions such as pericardial tamponade, right ventricular infarction, ventricular septal rupture, or circulatory collapse secondary to various shock syndromes (Table 91.5) (143). ❦ p26

GENERAL APPROACH TO THE MANAGEMENT OF ACUTE HEART FAILURE

Acute Cardiogenic Pulmonary Edema

The patient presenting with acute pulmonary edema is often in great distress, and the diagnosis is usually not in

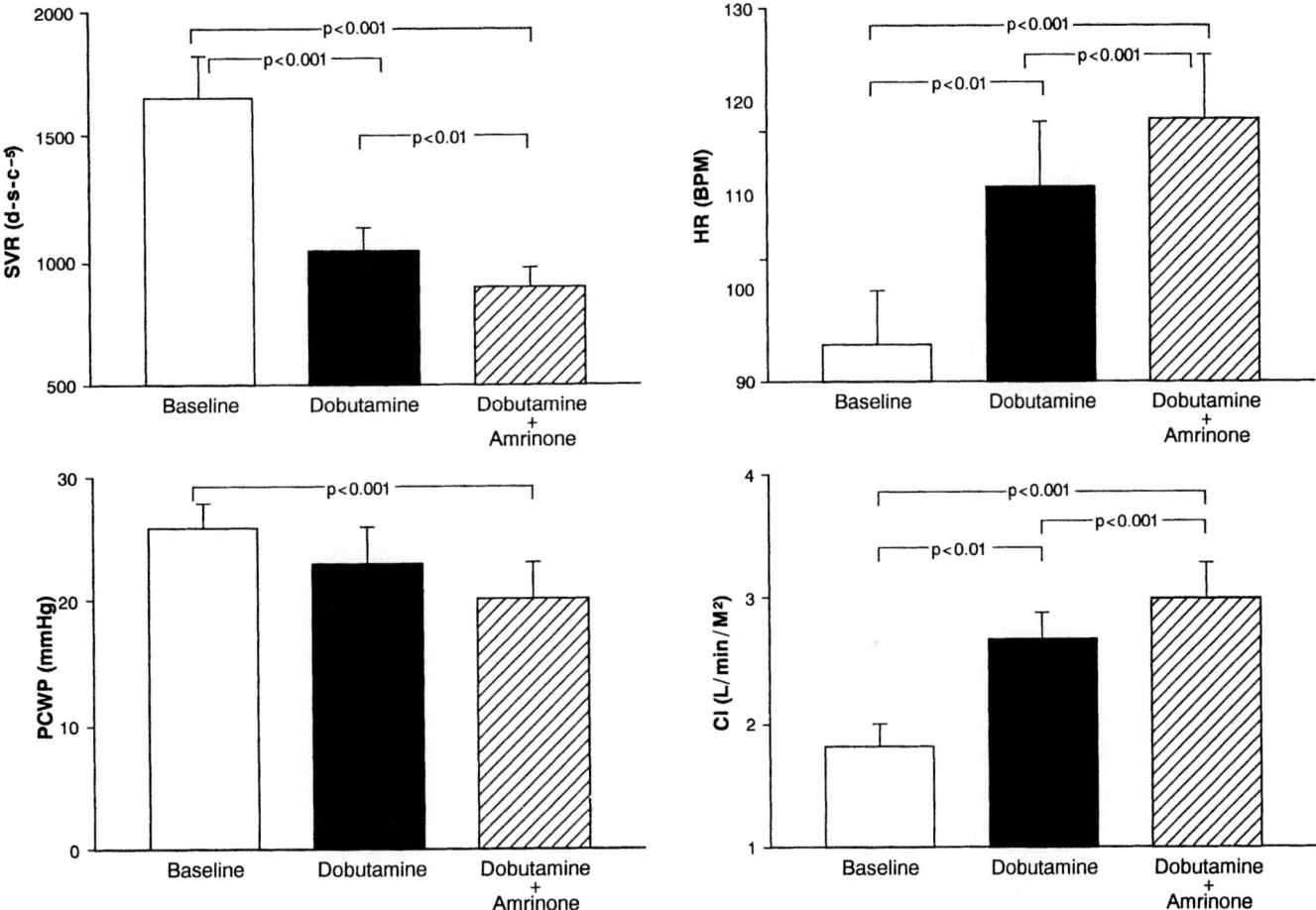

FIGURE 91.4 Effects of dobutamine hydrochloride and amrinone in ten patients with severe congestive heart failure. Dobutamine at peak dose increases cardiac index and reduces pulmonary wedge pressure (PCWP) and systemic vascular resistance (SVR). Dobutamine also increases heart rate (HR) above baseline. The addition of amrinone to dobutamine results in further augmentation in cardiac index (CI) and reduction in pulmonary wedge and SVR. Amrinone added to dobutamine further elevates the HR. (Modified from Uretsky BF, Lawless CE, Verbalis JG, et al. Combined therapy with dobutamine and amrinone in severe heart failure. *Chest* 1987;92:657–662.)

question because of the dramatic nature of the clinical presentation. Although the ultimate management strategy is dictated by the precipitating factor or factors causing pulmonary edema, initial therapy must be guided by the early clinical findings until a definitive diagnostic evaluation can be completed. As mentioned previously, the evaluation for

TABLE 91.4 INDICATIONS FOR PULMONARY ARTERY CATHETERIZATION AND HEMODYNAMIC MONITORING IN ACUTE HEART FAILURE

Acute pulmonary edema
  After poor response to initial treatment
  To exclude noncardiogenic pulmonary edema
Cardiogenic shock or preshock syndrome not responsive to initial fluid challenge
Acute decompensation of chronic heart failure (to allow tailored therapy)
Questionable volume status

precipitating factors and the initial therapeutic intervention usually occur simultaneously.

The management strategy for the patient with acute cardiogenic pulmonary edema is outlined in Table 91.6. Nitroglycerin, administered by the sublingual route, is a rational first step in the treatment of most patients (2). This preload-reducing agent, which can be administered every 5 minutes, often relieves a significant amount of the sensation of breathlessness and can provide a bridge for preparation of the patient for further treatment and diagnostic procedures. Sublingual nitroglycerin is an effective means of immediately reducing preload and afterload until the intravenous preparation can be infused (49,51). If afterload reduction is the most important objective, as in a patient with pulmonary edema, acute valvular insufficiency, or hypertension, or if the response to nitroglycerin is suboptimal, nitroprusside should be substituted or added for its balanced vasodilator effect. An indwelling arterial catheter for continuous monitoring of systemic blood pressure is

TABLE 91.5   COMMON HEMODYNAMIC PATTERNS IN LOW CARDIAC OUTPUT STATES

	CO	RAP	PAP	PCWP	SVR	$S\bar{v}o_2$
Acute pulmonary edema	Variable	→	Variable	Variable	Variable	Variable
Cardiogenic shock	↓	↑	↑ or →	↑ or →	↑↑	↓↓
Decompensated heart failure	↓	↑	↑↑	↑↑	↑	↓
Acute right ventricular failure	↑	↑↑	→ or ↓	→ or ↓	↑	↓
Massive pulmonary embolism	↓	↑	↑	→	↑	↓
Acute aortic/mitral valve insufficiency	↓	→	↑	↑↑	↑	↓
Tamponade	↓	↑[a]	↑[a]	↑[a]	↑	↓
Hypovolemic shock	↓	↓	↓	↓	↑	↓

↑, increased; →, normal; ↓, decreased; ↑↑, markedly increased; ↓↓, markedly decreased; CO, cardiac output; PAP, pulmonary artery pressure; PCWP, pulmonary capillary wedge pressure; RAP, right atrial pressure; $S\bar{v}o_2$, mixed venous oxygen saturation; SVR, systemic vascular resistance.
[a]Equalization of pressures is characteristic.

optimal but not mandatory for initiation of treatment. Intravenous furosemide should also be administered early in the clinical course but with care to avoid overdiuresis. In acute heart failure, intravascular volume is often normal or low; judicious diuretic therapy is useful primarily for its early vasodilator effect (108–110). The patient's failure to respond within a reasonable period to these measures should warrant strong consideration of hemodynamic monitoring and the addition of inotropic therapy (Table 91.4; also see the section Cardiogenic Shock and Decompensated Heart Failure).

In the acute setting, patients with pulmonary edema may also benefit from morphine sulfate 2 to 6 mg given intravenously (50). This medication may have an immediate hemodynamic effect through its preload-reducing properties. It may also alleviate anxiety and blunt the catecholamine response to the acute illness. Caution must be used, however, in patients with evidence of respiratory or metabolic acidosis or in those with significant underlying obstructive lung disease. ❦ p27

TABLE 91.6   INITIAL MANAGEMENT OF ACUTE CARDIOGENIC PULMONARY EDEMA

Sublingual nitroglycerin
    0.4 mg every 5 min
Intravenous nitroglycerin
    Start at 0.2 to 0.4 µg/kg/min
Intravenous furosemide
    20 to 40 mg i.v.
    Follow volume status closely
Sodium nitroprusside if further afterload reduction required
Supplemental oxygen/mechanical ventilation as guided by arterial blood gas analysis
Consider intravenous morphine sulfate (2 to 6 mg) if no pulmonary contraindication
Electrocardiogram
    Exclude myocardial infarction
Echocardiography
    Evaluate ventricular function, valvular status
Proceed with urgent coronary angiography if reperfusion therapy indicated

Cardiogenic Shock and Decompensated Heart Failure

Patients with acute unstable heart failure (preshock or shock syndromes) require an expedient diagnostic evaluation and therapeutic plan. They usually exhibit severe cardiac dysfunction and hemodynamic compromise, and often present with symptoms and signs of organ hypoperfusion (cyanosis, cool extremities, altered mentation) (13). If the high mortality associated with this syndrome is to be avoided, a rapid diagnostic evaluation and institution of supportive therapy (pharmacologic and mechanical) is necessary.

In patients with acute decompensation of chronic heart failure, the underlying heart disease is often known. In this setting, the therapeutic strategy incorporates a search for factors precipitating acute decompensation. Patients are usually receiving standard medical therapy for chronic heart failure, and a reparable lesion is less likely to be identified. Nevertheless, one must always consider the possibility of correctable ischemic myocardial dysfunction if a prior assessment for coronary artery disease has not been performed.

When cardiogenic shock occurs or when standard therapy fails to stabilize decompensated chronic heart failure, hemodynamic monitoring to guide pharmacologic support is essential (142,143,145). In addition, hemodynamic evaluation, along with the physical examination and echocardiography, can assist in the identification of common shock syndromes requiring specific forms of therapy (e.g., right ventricular infarction) (143,152) (Table 91.5).

Figure 91.5 provides a general approach to the selection of specific intravenous pharmacologic agents based on hemodynamic profile. The initial therapeutic decision is influenced primarily by systemic arterial pressure. Although the optimal systolic or mean arterial pressure for the individual patient is variable, a systolic arterial pressure of less than 80 to 85 mm Hg would be classified as significant hypotension when accompanied by evidence of organ hypoperfusion, such as renal dysfunction and altered central nervous system activity. When this clinical situation presents, arterial pressure must be rapidly aug-

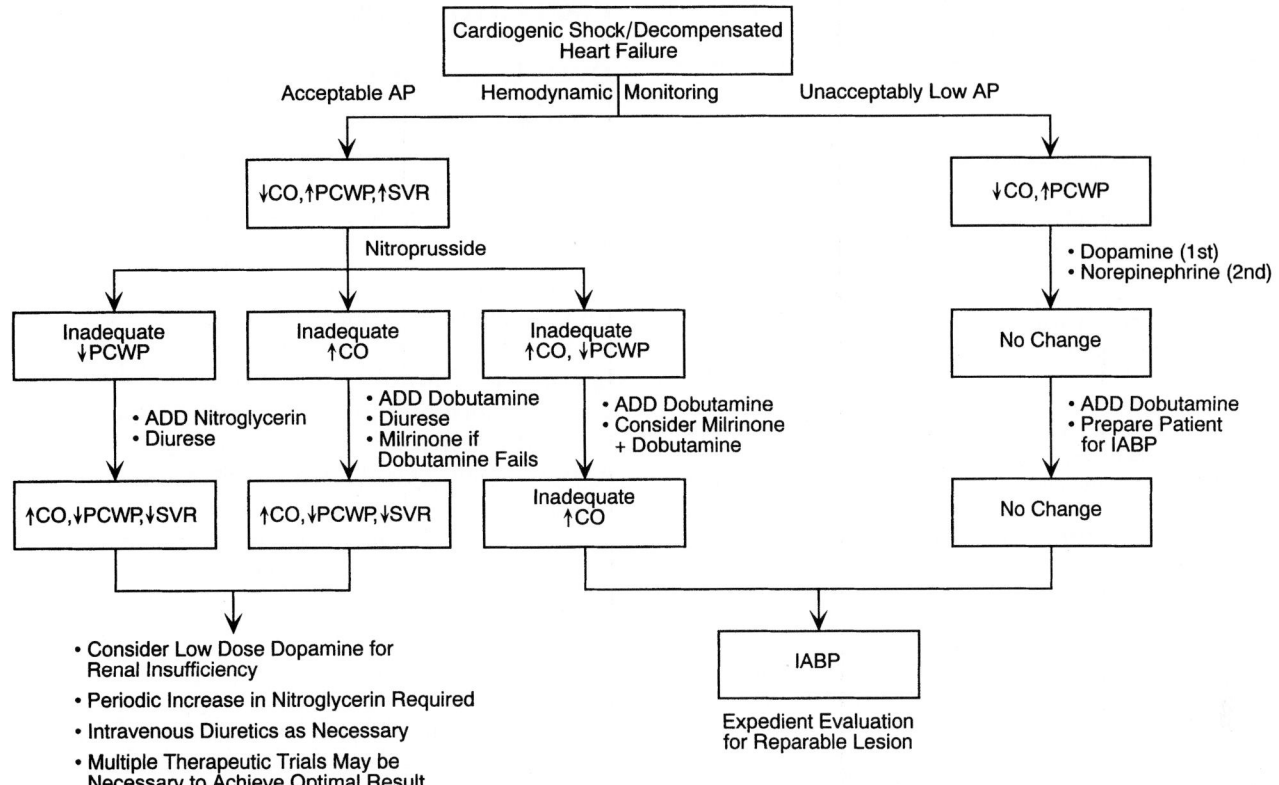

FIGURE 91.5 Algorithm for hemodynamics-directed pharmacologic support of cardiogenic shock and decompensated heart failure. ↑, increased; ↓, decreased; AP, arterial pressure; CO, cardiac output; IABP, intraaortic balloon pump; PCWP, pulmonary capillary wedge pressure; SVR, systemic vascular resistance.

mented to the level at which myocardial perfusion is not jeopardized. General hemodynamic goals would include increasing the cardiac index above 2.2 L per minute per m², reducing the PCWP below 20 mm Hg (15 mm Hg or less in chronic heart failure), maintaining SVR at 1,000 to 1,200 dynes per second per cm⁵, and reducing right atrial pressure to 7 mm Hg or less (Table 91.7) (153). For the individual patient, these goals will vary depending on the nature and acuteness of the cardiac dysfunction. The optimal PCWP would be the lowest pressure that can be maintained without a preload-related decline in systolic arterial pressure or cardiac index. In dilated cardiomyopathy and severe systolic dysfunction, stroke volume is primarily afterload-dependent and is affected minimally by manipulation of preload (19,154). Therefore, relatively normal PCWP can be targeted (147). The optimal SVR would be the lowest that one could achieve while maintaining adequate systemic perfusion.

When significant systemic hypotension is present, therapy with vasopressor doses of dopamine (more than 5 μg per kg per minute) should be used (99,100). Failure to achieve an acceptable blood pressure response with high-dose dopamine would warrant consideration of switching to another vasopressor, such as norepinephrine or vasopressin, or adding dobutamine (71,76). In either case,

preparations should be made for proceeding to mechanical assistance if appropriate (see the section Circulatory Support Devices). In refractory hypotension and shock, the mortality is extremely high if a surgically correctable lesion is not identified or if mechanical support (as a bridge to transplantation) is not an option (2).

Unstable or decompensated heart failure with low cardiac output but acceptable arterial pressure may initially be treated with nitroprusside to augment stroke volume and reduce the quantity of valvular regurgitation (19,21). A failure to augment cardiac output with this approach would warrant consideration of dobutamine or milrinone to enhance inotropy and vasodilation (71,74,79,86,87,89,118). If cardiac output increases appropriately with nitroprusside but left ventricular filling pressure remains elevated, then nitroglycerin can be added for further preload reduction (21,26,28,29). If both cardiac output and PCWP remain unacceptable, the option of changing to or adding milrinone should be considered (86,88,118,121). Other therapeutic considerations would include the addition of low-dose dopamine to augment renal blood flow, frequent assessment of volume status and appropriate intravenous diuretic administration, and upward titration of intravenous nitroglycerin when hemodynamic tolerance develops (52,95–97,108,110,116).

TABLE 91.7 HEMODYNAMICS-DIRECTED PROTOCOL FOR TREATMENT OF DECOMPENSATED HEART FAILURE

General hemodynamic goals
Right atrial pressure ≤7 mm Hg
Pulmonary capillary wedge pressure (PCWP) ≤15 mm Hg
Systemic vascular resistance (SVR) 1,000 to 1,200 dynes/sec/cm⁵
Cardiac index (CI) >2.5 L/min/m²
"Optimum" systolic or mean blood pressure (BP) is the lowest pressure that adequately supports renal function and central nervous system activity without significant orthostatic symptoms (systolic BP generally >80 to 90 mm Hg).

Patient-specific hemodynamic goals
"Optimum filling pressure" (PCWP): lowest PCWP that can be maintained without preload-related decline in systolic BP and/or CI. A higher PCWP (18 to 20 mm Hg) is usually required in acute myocardial injury.
"Optimum afterload" (SVR): lowest SVR that leads to reasonable CI while maintaining adequate systolic BP (generally >80 mm Hg) and renal perfusion (urine output >0.5 mL/kg/h).

Specific intravenous pharmacologic therapy
Sodium nitroprusside
Begin when combined preload and afterload reduction is most important hemodynamic goal.
Start at 0.1 to 0.2 µg/kg/min.
Titrate upward by 0.2 µg/kg/min at 3- to 5-min intervals.
Target hemodynamics (see General hemodynamic goals).
Hemodynamic effects resolve rapidly when infusion stopped.
Nitroglycerin
Begin when preload reduction is primarily desired.
Start at 0.2 to 0.3 µg/kg/min.
Titrate at 3- to 5-min intervals.
Be aware of tolerance.
Target hemodynamics (see General hemodynamic goals).
Effects resolve rapidly when infusion stopped.
Dobutamine hydrochloride
Begin when both inotropic and vasodilating effects desired but inotropic effects most important.
Start at 2.5 µg/kg/min.
Attempt to keep dosage at <15 µg/kg/min; avoid significant tachycardia.
Consider adding low-dose dopamine hydrochloride or milrinone lactate to assist with augmenting renal perfusion and/or achieving hemodynamic end points.
Hemodynamic effects resolve over minutes to hours when infusion stopped, but benefits occasionally persist longer.
Milrinone lactate
Begin when both vasodilating and inotropic effects desired.
Dosage range is 0.375 to 0.75 µg/kg/min (usual is 0.5 µg/kg/min).
Target hemodynamics (see General hemodynamic goals).
Excessive hypotension with loading dose; avoid loading in acute heart failure.
Prolonged hemodynamic effects after drug is stopped.

The approach to the pharmacologic support of the patient with cardiogenic shock or severely decompensated heart failure must be individualized. Evaluation of multiple clinical variables is often necessary for appropriate drug selection. Even then, several therapeutic trials may be required. When pharmacologic support obviously will not be sufficient to avoid progressive circulatory failure, then mechanical assistance must be considered.

CIRCULATORY SUPPORT DEVICES

Overview of Available Devices

In cardiology, few situations are as dramatic as observing the successful use of circulatory-support-device technology in an individual about to succumb to acute heart failure with cardiogenic shock and devastating hemodynamic profiles. A wide spectrum of mechanical circulatory assistance devices is now available and can provide extended hemodynamic support for patients showing acute deterioration while awaiting definitive therapy (see Chapter 95). Implantable ventricular assist devices successfully provide extended support for patients hemodynamically deteriorating to the degree that they are unlikely to survive until transplantation. This observation served as a major impetus for the successful development of many circulatory support systems (155–157). Many types of ventricular assist devices have also been used as a bridge to recovery. In select individuals suffering shock after acute myocardial infarction or myocarditis, timely insertion of mechanical support can allow for recovery of the injured heart so that primary responsibility for hemodynamic support can ultimately once again be carried by the heart. Indeed, relieving pressure and stress-load burdens from the injured myocardium might be therapeutic in and of itself. ☙ p28

Patient Selection

Table 91.8 summarizes many considerations that come into play when ventricular assist devices or other circulatory-support machinery is considered for the individual patient. Devices capable of being used as a short-term bridge to cardiac transplantation can be singled out. Devices used to "bail out" a patient from acute shock (such as might occur after myocardial infarction) or used for a more subacute insertion in a patient with "preterminal" heart failure and hemodynamics are in this category. Furthermore, some patients undergo device insertion with the idea of bridging to recovery. These patients are those likely to be suffering acute inflammatory conditions of the heart or shock syndromes rooted in difficulties with stunned or hibernating myocardium. The reality and implications of using ventricular-assist-device insertion long term as an alternative to cardiac transplantation are just beginning to be explored. Obviously, mechanical circulatory support and, more specifically, ventricular-assist-device insertion, attenuates the multifactorial difficulties apparent in circulatory decompensation. Pump dynamics are important, as is flow. That ventricular-assist-device insertion can dramatically reverse the neurohumoral perturbation characteristic of heart failure states has been elegantly demonstrated. These devices are capable of returning catecholamine levels, for example, to near normal (159).

Indications for emergency mechanical support vary. Patients with long-standing heart failure deteriorate more

TABLE 91.8 CONSIDERATIONS FOR VENTRICULAR-ASSIST DEVICE INSERTION IN CASES OF ADVANCED HEART FAILURE

Patient selection
  Short-term bridge to heart transplantation
  Acute insertion: bailout from acute shock (after myocardial infarction)
  Subacute insertion: insertion in patients with "preterminal" heart failure
  Short-term bridge to recovery
  Long-term alternative to transplantation
Ventricular-assist device interdiction of circulatory decompensation
  Pump dynamics
  Flow dynamics
  Impact on neural-humoral perturbation
Troublesome circumstances
  Small patient size
  Cachexia
  Infection (particularly sepsis)
  Fixed pulmonary hypertension
  Substantive right heart failure
  Significant hepatic or renal dysfunction
  Malignant tachyarrhythmias (atrial and ventricular)
  Hypercoagulable states
  Consumption coagulopathy
  Acute/chronic pulmonary emboli
Challenging acute clinical situations
  Myocardial infarction with shock
  Cardiac arrest with ongoing cardiopulmonary resuscitation
  Failure to wean from cardiopulmonary bypass after open heart surgery

slowly than those with the recent onset of ventricular dysfunction, but patients with both acute and chronic heart failure can be saved with this technology. One must remember that exacerbation of chronic heart failure frequently reverses after aggressive adjustment of tailored medication and resolution of concomitant difficulties such as acute ischemia or infection (145). Such patients do not require mechanical circulatory support. In general, the indication for the use of circulatory-support devices is evidence of critical organ hypoperfusion despite aggressive and adequate medication therapies, including infusion of inotropic drugs such as milrinone and dobutamine, as previously discussed. ▼ p29

Contraindications to circulatory-support-device insertion relate largely to device choice and therapeutic goal. For implantable left ventricular assist devices, technical contraindications include a body surface area less than 1.5 m² or greater than 2.5 m² or a weight greater than 150% of the patient's ideal body weight. Currently, most implantable devices are large and will not fit into very small patients. Obese patients can have problems with percutaneous access sites and are at higher risk for comorbid events such as pulmonary embolism. A highly calcified aorta, particularly at the proposed site of outflow conduit anastomoses, can be problematic, as can substantive aortic insufficiency. Presence of a prosthetic aortic valve is considered to be a contraindi-

cation to ventricular-assist-device insertion because frequently the aortic valve closes permanently as blood is pumped during diastole into the ventricular assist device. This sets the stage for thromboembolism. Some device controllers that regulate the circulatory pressure/electrocardiography/device interphase react adversely in electrical fields in which pacemakers or defibrillating units are present. Therefore, pacemaker dependence or presence of an implanted defibrillating device may be a contraindication to the use of certain ventricular assist devices. Certainly, the inability to deliver long-term anticoagulation therapy to a patient is also cause for great concern. As suggested, hemodynamic contraindications to device insertion might include significant right heart failure as reflected by right atrial pressures higher than 20 mm Hg despite aggressive medical therapy. Likewise, patients with a PCWP below 15 mm Hg and a cardiac index of more than 2 L per minute per m² without the use of parenteral inotropes represent a population that might, although very sick, do reasonably well without insertion of a circulatory support device. ▼ p30

CONTROVERSIES AND PERSONAL PERSPECTIVES

The complexity and significant mortality associated with the acute heart failure syndrome have served to generate a broad spectrum of potential therapeutic modalities, as has been discussed. Potent intravenous vasodilator and inotropic drugs, designed to correct specific hemodynamic abnormalities, are now available for use alone, or in combination, to support patients with acute pulmonary edema as well as those with severe cardiac dysfunction and cardiogenic shock. New drug therapies targeting more specific hemodynamic and neurohormonal perturbations are promising. Advancements in medical technology have improved the ability to monitor and evaluate continuously the patient with severe hemodynamic compromise so that medical therapy can be appropriately tailored. For those not responding to aggressive pharmacologic management, short- and long-term mechanical assist devices can now be used to support the sickest of patients until further therapeutic options are explored. These advances in the ability to treat and support the patient with acute heart failure allow for a more thorough and aggressive diagnostic evaluation in many instances. As emphasized throughout this chapter, the finding of a treatable condition has important prognostic implications, and the ability to uncover a reparable lesion in an individual with heart failure continues to improve. The continued advancements in reperfusion strategies (thrombolysis, angioplasty, antithrombotic therapy) as well as improved outcome after high-risk coronary bypass surgery provides a means potentially to avoid irreversible myocardial injury and its sequela of severe heart failure. These therapeutic options also offer some encouragement

THE FUTURE

Although a decade has passed since the introduction of a new pharmacologic treatment for the management of acute heart failure, important progress has been made recently toward the development of novel, more directed, and perhaps safer therapies. As with the pharmacologic approach for treating chronic heart failure, the treatment of acute hemodynamic compromise may also follow the neurohormonal paradigm. One or more drugs directed toward specific neurohormonal abnormalities of acute heart failure likely will be approved in the near future. Certainly, the continued development of aggressive myocardial reperfusion strategies will be important for the majority who present with acute ischemia and infarction to minimize ventricular remodeling and left ventricular dysfunction. Advances toward smaller, totally implantable mechanical devices will also continue.

that the high mortality of cardiogenic shock may be favorably altered in the future. Various reperfusion strategies continue to undergo clinical investigation.

The advances in technological support and treatment options for acute heart failure, however, have not simplified its management. The significance of the initial clinical assessment and treatment plan cannot be overemphasized. Due to the complexity and diverse nature of the acute heart failure syndrome, diagnostic and therapeutic strategies must be individualized and a "cookbook" approach to pharmacologic therapy or other modes of support cannot be advocated. Certainly, the patient presenting with acute pulmonary edema and hypertension is treated differently from the patient with a large anterior myocardial infarction presenting with congestion and hypotension. Within these two extremes lies a great diversity of acute heart failure presentations, each with subtle differences requiring a different diagnostic and therapeutic approach. Therefore, the basics of patient care cannot be ignored but must be used in conjunction with advanced monitoring capabilities.

The algorithm for the pharmacologic management of heart failure presented in this chapter should be viewed as a generalized approach to therapy in which various treatment trials may be necessary. Even when one uses specific drugs with known hemodynamic profiles, close observation and monitoring are essential because the response of a given patient is not always predictable. For example, dobutamine administration is often avoided in the setting of myocardial ischemia and marginal cardiac output because of the perceived potential for inducing worsening ischemia and myocardial dysfunction or arrhythmia, or both. As has been discussed, dobutamine may also evoke hemodynamic effects that are favorable, even in the setting of ongoing ischemia. Some individuals, however, experience untoward effects if the drug is not judiciously administered. (For instance, one should not administer dobutamine to those with normal or low left ventricular filling pressures, and rapid titration or initiation at a dosage greater than 5 µg per kg per minute should also generally be avoided.) The identification of an excessive heart-rate response during dobutamine titration would also identify the patient with marginal cardiac reserve and potential for adverse effects. Therefore, repeated clinical evaluation in conjunction with appropriate medication adjustment is necessary.

Hemodynamic monitoring should be used in concert with, but should not replace, the overall clinical assessment. Unfortunately, major alterations in therapy based solely on hemodynamic parameters are often seen in intensive care settings. For example, a cardiac index of 2.2 L per minute per m² might lead to an increase in inotropic therapy even though no evidence of organ hypoperfusion otherwise exists. This pharmacologic manipulation based only on hemodynamics without account taken of other important clinical variables is often not necessary and potentially detrimental.

At the other end of the spectrum are patients who continue to exhibit clinical deterioration despite maximal pharmacologic support. In this scenario an early decision to proceed with mechanical assistance is imperative. Failure to recognize this and proceed to mechanical assistance in an expedient manner, unfortunately, is common. Often, excessive delays are incurred in an attempt to stabilize a condition that is clearly unstable and nonresponsive to medical therapy. The greater the delay when significant organ hypoperfusion is evident, the less effective mechanical support will be, and this translates into fewer definitive therapeutic options. At the present time, options primarily include surgical approaches such as coronary bypass surgery, valvular repair or replacement, and cardiac transplantation.

A tremendous amount of progress has occurred in the management of acute heart failure over recent years, particularly with respect to mechanical circulatory support systems that can bridge patients from devastating hemodynamic decompensation to more clinically acceptable stages. The beginning of the century is an exciting time in which smaller and more reliable devices with fewer complications will become available for implantation. Even then, individualization of therapy and careful, repeated clinical assessment will be important.

REFERENCES

1. Chatterjee K, Hutchison SJ, Chou TM. Acute ischemic heart failure: pathophysiology and management. In: Poole-Wilson P, Colucci W, Chatterjee K, et al., eds. *Heart failure: scientific principles and clinical practice.* New York: Churchill Livingstone, 1996:523–549.

2. Guidelines for the evaluation and management of heart failure. American College of Cardiology/American Heart Association Task Force on Practice Guidelines (Committee on Evaluation and Management of Heart Failure). *J Am Coll Cardiol* 1995;26:1376–1398.

3. Goldberger JJ, Peled HB, Stroh JA, et al. Prognostic factors in acute pulmonary edema. *Arch Intern Med* 1986;146:489–493.

4. Tuttle RR, Mills J. Dobutamine: development of a new catecholamine to selectively increase cardiac contractility. *Circ Res* 1975;36:185–196.

5. Pagani FD, Lynch W, Swaniker F, et al. Extracorporeal life support to left ventricular assist device bridge to transplant: a strategy to optimize survival and resource utilization. *Circulation* 1999;100(19)[Suppl]:II-206–II-210.

6. Rosario LB, Stevenson LW, Solomon SD, et al. The mechanism of decrease in dynamic mitral regurgitation during heart failure treatment: importance of reduction in the regurgitant orifice size. *J Am Coll Cardiol* 1998;32:1819–1824.

7. Goldstein RA, Passmore JM. Hemodynamic support of the critically-ill patient. In: Dantzker DR, ed. *Cardiopulmonary critical care.* Philadelphia: WB Saunders, 1991:407–436.

8. Young JB. Assessment of heart failure. In: Colucci WS, ed. *Heart failure: cardiac function and dysfunction.* St. Louis: Mosby, 1995:7.2–8.1. Braunwald E, ed. *Atlas of heart disease,* vol 4.

9. Forrester JS, Diamond G, Chatterjee K, et al. Medical therapy of acute myocardial infarction by application of hemodynamic subsets (part I). *N Engl J Med* 1976;295:1356–1362.

10. McHugh TJ, Forrester JS, Adler L, et al. Pulmonary vascular congestion in acute myocardial infarction: hemodynamic and radiologic correlations. *Ann Intern Med* 1972;76:29–33.

11. Kloner RA, Fowler MB, Dzau V. The guide to cardiology: heart failure. *Congestive Heart Failure* 1996;2:17–34.

12. Hochman JS, Buller CE, Sleeper LA, et al. Cardiogenic shock complicating acute myocardial infarction—etiologies, management, and outcome: a report from the SHOCK trial registry. *J Am Coll Cardiol* 2000;36:1063–1070.

13. Califf RM, Bengtson JR. Cardiogenic shock. *N Engl J Med* 1994;330:1724–1730.

14. Goldberg RJ, Gore JM, Alpert JS, et al. Cardiogenic shock after myocardial infarction: incidence and mortality from a community-wide perspective, 1975 to 1988. *N Engl J Med* 1991;325:1117–1122.

15. The GUSTO investigators. An international randomized trial comparing four thrombolytic strategies for acute myocardial infarction. *N Engl J Med* 1993;329:673–682.

16. Bates ER, Topol EJ. Limitations of thrombolytic therapy for acute myocardial infarction complicated by congestive heart failure and cardiogenic shock. *J Am Coll Cardiol* 1991;18:1077–1084.

17. Teerlink JR, Goldhaber SZ, Pfeffer MA. An overview of contemporary etiologies of congestive heart failure. *Am J Cardiol* 1991;121:1852–1853.

18. Leier CV. Unstable heart failure. In: Colucci WS, ed. *Heart failure: cardiac function and dysfunction.* St. Louis: Mosby, 1995:9.2–9.15. Braunwald E, ed. *Atlas of heart disease,* vol 4.

19. Haas GJ, Leier CV. Vasodilator therapy for congestive heart failure (non-ACE inhibition). In: Hosenpud JD, Greenberg BH, eds. *Congestive heart failure: pathophysiology, differential diagnosis and comprehensive approach to therapy.* New York: Springer-Verlag, 1994:400–454.

20. Delius W, Enghoff E. Studies of the central and peripheral hemodynamic effects of amyl nitrate in patients with aortic insufficiency. *Circulation* 1970;42:787–796.

21. Leier CV, Bambach D, Thompson MJ, et al. Central and regional hemodynamic effects of intravenous isosorbide dinitrate, nitroglycerin, and nitroprusside in patients with congestive heart failure. *Am J Cardiol* 1981;48:1115–1123.

22. Leier CV, Magorien RD, Desch CE, et al. Hydralazine and isosorbide dinitrate: comparative central and regional hemodynamic effects when administered alone or in combination. *Circulation* 1981;63:102–109.

23. Tsai SC, Adamik R, Manganiello VC, et al. Effects of nitroprusside and nitroglycerin on cGMP content and PGI$_2$ formation in aorta and vena cava. *Biochem Pharmacol* 1989;38:61–65.

24. Miller RR, Vismara LA, Williams DO, et al. Pharmacological mechanisms for left ventricular unloading in clinical congestive heart failure. *Circ Res* 1976;39:127–133.

25. Leier CV, Magorien RD, Boudoulas H, et al. The effect of vasodilator therapy on systolic and diastolic time intervals in congestive heart failure. *Chest* 1982;81:723–729.

26. Flaherty JT. Comparison of intravenous nitroglycerin and sodium nitroprusside in acute myocardial infarction. *Am J Med* 1983;74(6B):53–60.

27. Packer M. New perspectives on therapeutic application of nitrates as vasodilator agents for severe chronic heart failure. *Am J Med* 1983;74(6B):61–72.

28. Cohn JN. Nitrates for congestive heart failure. *Am J Cardiol* 1985;56:19A–23A.

29. Cohn JN. Role of nitrates in congestive heart failure. *Am J Cardiol* 1987;60:39H–43H.

30. Needleman P, Jakschik B, Johnson EM. Sulfhydryl requirement for relaxation of vascular smooth muscle. *J Pharmacol Exp Ther* 1973;187:324–331.

31. Ignarro LJ, Lippton H, Edwards JC, et al. Mechanism of vascular smooth muscle relaxation by organic nitrates, nitrites, nitroprusside, and nitric oxide: evidence for the involvement of *S*-nitrosothiols as active intermediates. *J Pharmacol Exp Ther* 1981;218:739–749.

32. Levin RI, Jaffe EA, Weksler BB, et al. Nitroglycerin stimulates synthesis of prostacyclin by cultured human endothelial cells. *J Clin Invest* 1981;67:762–769.

33. DeCaterina R, Dorso CR, Tack-Goldman K, et al. Nitrates and endothelial prostacyclin production: studies *in vitro. Circulation* 1985;71:176–182.

34. Morcillio E, Reid PR, Dubin N, et al. Myocardial prostaglandin E release by nitroglycerin and modification by indomethacin. *Am J Cardiol* 1980;45:53–57.

35. Keren G, Katz S, Gage J, et al. Effect of isometric exercise on cardiac performance and mitral regurgitation in patients with severe congestive heart failure. *Am Heart J* 1989;118:973–979.

36. Elkayam U, Roth A, Kumar A, et al. Hemodynamic and volumetric effects of venodilation with nitroglycerin in chronic mitral regurgitation. *Am J Cardiol* 1987;60:1106–1111.

37. Unverferth DV, Magorien RD, Lewis RP, et al. The role of subendocardial ischemia in perpetuating myocardial failure in patients with nonischemic congestive cardiomyopathy. *Am Heart J* 1983;105:176–179.

38. Dupuis J, Lalonde G, Lebeau R, et al. Sustained beneficial effect of a seventy-two hour intravenous infusion of nitroglycerin in patients with severe chronic congestive heart failure. *Am Heart J* 1990;120:625–637.

39. Lavine SJ, Campbell CA, et al. Effect of nitroglycerin-induced reduction of left ventricular filling pressure on diastolic filling in acute dilated heart failure. *J Am Coll Cardiol* 1989;14:233–241.

40. Ludbrook PR, Byrne JD, Kurnik PB, et al. Influence of reduction of preload and afterload by nitroglycerin on left ventricular diastolic pressure-volume relation and relaxation in man. *Circulation* 1977;56:937–943.

41. Amende I, Simon R, Hood WP, et al. Effects of nitroglycerin on left ventricular diastolic properties in man. *Z Kardiol* 1983;72[Suppl 3]:62–65.

42. Armstrong PW, Armstrong JA, Marks GS. Pharmacokinetic-hemodynamic studies of intravenous nitroglycerin in congestive heart failure. *Circulation* 1980;62:160–166.

43. Mantle JA, Russell RO, Moraski RE, et al. Isosorbide dinitrate for the relief of severe heart failure after myocardial infarction. *Am J Cardiol* 1976;37:263–268.

44. Flaherty JT, Reid PR, Kelly DT, et al. Intravenous nitroglycerin in acute myocardial infarction. *Circulation* 1975;51:132–139.

45. Ar.nstrong PW, Walker DC, Burton JR, et al. Vasodilator therapy in acute myocardial infarction: a comparison of sodium nitroprusside and nitroglycerin. *Circulation* 1975;52:1118–1122.

46. Flaherty JT, Come PC, Baird MG, et al. Effects of intravenous nitroglycerin on left ventricular function and ST segment changes in acute myocardial infarction. *Br Heart J* 1976;38:612–621.

47. Cintron GB, Glasser SP, Weston BA, et al. Effect of intravenous isosorbide dinitrate versus nitroglycerin on elevated pulmonary arterial-wedge pressure during acute myocardial infarction. *Am J Cardiol* 1988;61:21–25.

48. Baxter RH, Tait CM, McGuinness JB. Vasodilator therapy in acute myocardial infarction: use of sublingual isosorbide dinitrate. *Br Heart J* 1977;39:1067–1070.

49. Bussmann WD, Schupp D. Effects of sublingual nitroglycerin in emergency treatment of severe pulmonary edema. *Am J Cardiol* 1978;41:931–936.

50. Stevenson LW, Colucci WS. Management of patients hospitalized with heart failure. In: Smith WT, ed. *Cardiovascular therapeutics: a companion to Braunwald's heart disease.* Philadelphia: WB Saunders, 1996:199–209.

51. Dunlap S, Starling RC, Haas GJ. Simplified assessment of pulmonary hypertension in heart transplant candidates. *J Am Coll Cardiol* 1996:144A(abstr).

52. Elkayam U, Kulick D, McIntosh N, et al. Incidence of early tolerance to hemodynamic effects of continuous infusion of nitroglycerin in patients with coronary artery disease and heart failure. *Circulation* 1987;76:577–584.

53. Magrini F, Niarchos AP. Ineffectiveness of sublingual nitroglycerin in acute left ventricular failure in the presence of massive peripheral edema. *Am J Cardiol* 1980;45:841–847.

54. Cohn JN, Burke LP. Nitroprusside. *Ann Intern Med* 1979;91:752–757.

55. Laskey WK, Kussmaul WG. Arterial wave reflection in heart failure. *Circulation* 1987;75:711–722.

56. Pepine CJ, Nichols WW, Curry RC Jr, et al. Aortic input impedance during nitroprusside infusion. *J Clin Invest* 1979;64:643–654.

57. Merillon JP, Fontenier G, Lerallut JF, et al. Aortic input impedance in heart failure: comparison with normal subjects and its changes during vasodilator therapy. *Eur Heart J* 1984;5:447–455.

58. Yin FC, Guzman PA, Brin KP, et al. Effect of nitroprusside on hydraulic vascular loads on the right and left ventricle of patients with heart failure. *Circulation* 1983;67:1330–1339.

59. Miller RR, Vismara LA, Zelis R, et al. Clinical use of sodium nitroprusside in chronic ischemic heart disease. *Circulation* 1975;51:328–336.

60. Hasenfuss G, Holubarsch C, Heiss W, et al. Myocardial energetics in patients with dilated cardiomyopathy. *Circulation* 1989;80:51–64.

61. Powers ER, Reison DS, Berke A, et al. The effect of nitroprusside on coronary and systemic hemodynamics in patients with severe congestive heart failure. *Circulation* 1982;66:II-211(abstr).

62. Mann T, Cohn PF, Holman BL, et al. Effect of nitroprusside on regional myocardial blood flow in coronary artery disease. *Circulation* 1978;57:732–738.

63. Simkus GJ, Fitchett DH. Radial artery pressure measurements may be a poor guide to the beneficial effects of nitroprusside on left ventricular systolic pressure in congestive heart failure. *Am J Cardiol* 1990;66:323–326.

64. duCailar J, Mathier-Daude JC, Kienlen J, et al. Blood and urinary cyanide concentrations during long-term sodium nitroprusside infusions. *Anesthesiology* 1979;51:363–364.

65. Vesey CJ, Cole PV. Blood cyanide and thiocyanate concentrations produced by long-term therapy with sodium nitroprusside. *Br J Anaesth* 1985;57:148–155.

66. Chiariello M, Gold HK, Leinbach RC, et al. Comparison between the effects of nitroprusside and nitroglycerin on ischemic injury during acute myocardial infarction. *Circulation* 1976;54:766–773.

67. Ruffolo RR Jr, Spradlin TA, Pollack GD, et al. Alpha and beta adrenergic effects of the stereoisomers of dobutamine. *J Pharmacol Exp Ther* 1981;219:447–452.

68. Schumann HJ, Wagner J, Knorr A, et al. Demonstration in human atrial preparations of alpha-adrenoceptors mediating positive inotropic effects. *Naunyn Schmiedebergs Arch Pharmacol* 1978;302:333–336.

69. Binkley PF, Murray KD, Watson KM, et al. Dobutamine increases cardiac output of the total artificial heart: implica-

tions for vascular contribution of inotropic agents to augmented ventricular function. *Circulation* 1991;84:1210–1215.

70. Binkley PF, VanFossen DB, Haas GJ, et al. Increased ventricular contractility is not sufficient for effective positive inotropic intervention. *Am J Physiol* 1996;271:H1635–H1642.

71. Leier CV. Positive inotropic therapy: an update and new agents. *Curr Probl Cardiol* 1996;21:521–581.

72. Leier CV, Heban P, Huss P, et al. Comparative systemic and regional hemodynamic effects of dopamine and dobutamine in patients with cardiomyopathic heart failure. *Circulation* 1978;58:466–475.

73. Loeb HS, Bredakis J, Gunnar RM. Superiority of dobutamine over dopamine for augmentation of cardiac output in patients with chronic low output cardiac failure. *Circulation* 1977;55:375–381.

74. Keren G, Laniado S, Sonnenblick EH, et al. Dynamics of functional mitral regurgitation during dobutamine therapy in patients with severe congestive heart failure: a Doppler echocardiographic study. *Am Heart J* 1989;118:748–753.

75. Leier CV, Unverferth DV, Kates RE. The relationship between plasma dobutamine concentrations and cardiovascular responses in cardiac failure. *Am J Med* 1979;66:238–242.

76. Leier CV. Acute inotropic support: intravenously administered positive inotropic drugs. In: Leier CV, ed. *Cardiotonic drugs: a clinical review.* New York: Marcel Dekker, 1991:63–105.

77. Boudoulas H, Rittgers SE, Lewis RP, et al. Changes in diastolic time with various pharmacologic agents: implications for myocardial perfusion. *Circulation* 1979;60:164–169.

78. Dubois-Rande JL, Merlet P, Duval-Moulin AM, et al. Coronary vasodilating action of dobutamine in patients with idiopathic dilated cardiomyopathy. *Am Heart J* 1983;105:176–181.

79. Vatner SF, McRitchie RJ, Braunwald E. Effects of dobutamine on left ventricular performance, coronary dynamics, and distribution of cardiac output in conscious dogs. *J Clin Invest* 1974;53:1265–1273.

80. Bendersky R, Chatterjee K, Parmley WW, et al. Dobutamine in chronic ischemic heart failure: alterations in left ventricular function and coronary hemodynamics. *Am J Cardiol* 1981;48:554–558.

81. Pozen RG, DiBianco R, Katz RJ, et al. Myocardial metabolic and hemodynamic effects of dobutamine in heart failure complicating coronary artery disease. *Circulation* 1981;63:1279–1285.

82. Gillespie TA, Ambos HD, Sobel BE, et al. Effects of dobutamine in patients with acute myocardial infarction. *Am J Cardiol* 1977;39:588–594.

83. Bianchi C, Diaz R, Gonzales C, et al. Effects of dobutamine on atrioventricular conduction. *Am Heart J* 1975;90:474–478.

84. Feldman AM, Massie BM. Positive inotropic therapy. In: Poole-Wilson P, Colucci W, Chatterjee K, et al., eds. *Heart failure: scientific principles and clinical practice.* New York: Churchill Livingstone, 1996:701–718.

85. Colucci WS, Denniss AR, Leatherman GF, et al. Intracoronary infusion of dobutamine to patients with and without severe congestive heart failure: dose-response relationships, correlation with circulating catecholamines and effect of phosphodiesterase inhibition. *J Clin Invest* 1988;81:1103–1110.

86. Simonton CA, Chatterjee K, Cody RJ, et al. Milrinone in congestive heart failure: acute and chronic hemodynamic and clinical evaluation. *J Am Coll Cardiol* 1985;6:453–459.

87. Grose R, Strain J, Greenberg M, et al. Systemic and coronary effects of intravenous milrinone and dobutamine in congestive heart failure. *J Am Coll Cardiol* 1986;7:1107–1113.

88. Monrad ES, Baim DS, Smith HS, et al. Milrinone, dobutamine, and nitroprusside: comparative effects on hemodynamics and myocardial energetics in patients with severe congestive heart failure. *Circulation* 1986;73[Suppl III]:III-168–III-174.

89. Jaski BE, Fifer M, Wright RF, et al. Positive inotropic and vasodilator actions of milrinone in patients with severe congestive heart failure. *J Clin Invest* 1985;75:643–649.

90. Monrad ES, Baim DS, Smith HS, et al. Effects of milrinone on coronary hemodynamics and myocardial energetics in patients with congestive heart failure. *Circulation* 1985;71:972–979.

91. Lowes BD, Simon MA, Tsvetkova TO, et al. Inotropes in the beta blocker era. *Clin Cardiol* 2000;23[Suppl III]:III-11–III-16.

92. Sigmund M, Jakob H, Becker H, et al. Effects of metoprolol on myocardial beta-adrenoreceptors and G alpha i-proteins in patients with CHF. *Eur J Clin Pharmacol* 1996;51:127–132.

93. Goldberg LI. Cardiovascular and renal actions of dopamine: potential clinical application. *Pharmacol Rev* 1972;241:1–29.

94. McDonald RH, Goldberg LI. Analysis of the cardiovascular effects of dopamine in the dog. *J Pharmacol Exp Ther* 1963;140:60.

95. Lee MR. Dopamine and the kidney. *Clin Sci* 1982;62:439–448.

96. Lokhandwala MF, Barrett RJ. Cardiovascular dopamine receptors: physiological, pharmacological, and therapeutic implications. *J Auton Pharmacol* 1982;3:189–215.

97. Beregovich J, Bianchi C, Rubler S, et al. Dose-related hemodynamic and renal effects of dopamine in congestive heart failure. *Am Heart J* 1974;87:550–557.

98. Stoof JC, Kebabian JW. Two dopamine receptors: biochemistry, physiology, and pharmacology. *Life Sci* 1984;35:2281–2296.

99. Loeb HS, Winslow EBJ, Rahimtoola SH, et al. Acute hemodynamic effects of dopamine in patients with shock. *Circulation* 1971;44:163–173.

100. Holzer J, Karliner JS, O'Rourke RA, et al. Effectiveness of dopamine in patients with cardiogenic shock. *Am J Cardiol* 1973;32:79–84.

101. Brooks HL, Stein PD, Matson JL, et al. Dopamine-induced alterations in coronary hemodynamics in dogs. *Circ Res* 1969;24:699–704.

102. Toda N, Goldberg LI. Effects of dopamine on isolated canine coronary arteries. *Cardiovasc Res* 1975;9:384–389.

103. Cohn JN. Comparative cardiovascular effects of tyramine, ephedrine, and norepinephrine in man. *Circ Res* 1965;16:174.

104. Mueller H, Ayres SM, Giannelli S, et al. Effect of isoproterenol, L-norepinephrine, and intra-aortic counterpulsation on hemodynamics, and myocardial metabolism in shock following acute myocardial infarction. *Circulation* 1972;45:335–351.

105. The American Heart Association in collaboration with the International Liaison Committee on Resuscitation (ILCOR). Agents to optimize cardiac output and blood pressure. *Circulation* 2000;102[Suppl I]:I-129–I-135.

106. Wenzel V, Lindner KH, Augenstein S. Vasopressin combined with epinephrine decreases cerebral perfusion compared with vasopressin alone during CPR in pigs. *Stroke* 1998;29:1467–1468.

107. Oyama H, Suzuki Y, Satoh S. Role of nitric oxide in the cerebral vasodilatory responses to vasopressin and oxytocin in dogs. *J Cereb Blood Flow Metab* 1993;13:285–290.

108. Cody RJ. Clinical trials of diuretic therapy in heart failure: research directions and clinical considerations. *J Am Coll Cardiol* 1993;22[Suppl A]:165A–171A.

109. Lal S, Murtagw JG, Pollock AM, et al. Acute hemodynamic effects of furosemide in patients with normal and raised left atrial pressures. *Br Heart J* 1969;31:711–717.

110. Ikram H, Chan W, Espiner EA, et al. Hemodynamic and hormone response to acute and chronic furosemide therapy in congestive heart failure. *Clin Sci* 1980;59:443–449.

111. Francis GS, Siegel RM, Goldsmith SR, et al. Acute vasoconstrictor response to intravenous furosemide in patients with chronic congestive heart failure. *Ann Intern Med* 1985;103:1–6.

112. Dikshit K, Vyden JK, Forrester JS, et al. Renal and extrarenal hemodynamic effects of furosemide in congestive heart failure after myocardial infarction. *N Engl J Med* 1973;288:124–128.

113. Taylor SH. Diuretics in post-infarction heart failure. *Cardiovasc Drugs Ther* 1993;7:5–9.

114. Acute Infarction Ramipril Efficiency (AIRE) study investigators. Effect of ramipril on mortality and morbidity of survivors of acute myocardial infarction with clinical evidence of heart failure. *Lancet* 1993;342:821–828.

115. Bourassa MG, Gurne O, Bangdiwala SI, et al. Natural history and patterns of current practice in heart failure: the Studies of Left Ventricular Dysfunction (SOLVD) investigators. *J Am Coll Cardiol* 1993;22[Suppl A]:14A–19A.

116. Dormans TP, VanMeyel JJ, Gerlag PG, et al. Diuretic efficacy of high dose furosemide in severe heart failure: bolus injection versus continuous infusion. *J Am Coll Cardiol* 1996;28:376–382.

117. Agostoni PG, Marenzi GC, Pepi M, et al. Isolated ultrafiltration in moderate congestive heart failure. *J Am Coll Cardiol* 1993;21:424–431.

118. Uretsky BF, Hua J. Combined intravenous pharmacotherapy in the treatment of patients with decompensated congestive heart failure. *Am Heart J* 1991;121:1879–1885.

119. Miller RR, Palomo AR, Brandon TA, et al. Combined vasodilator and inotropic therapy of heart failure: experimental and clinical concepts. *Am Heart J* 1981;102:500–508.

120. Awan NA, Evanson MK, Needham KE, et al. Effect of combined nitroglycerin and dobutamine in left ventricular dysfunction. *Am Heart J* 1983;106:35–40.

121. Gage J, Rutman H, Lucido D, et al. Additive effects of dobutamine and amrinone on myocardial contractility and ventricular performance in patients with severe heart failure. *Circulation* 1986;74:367–373.

122. Uretsky BF, Lawless CE, Verbalis JG, et al. Combined therapy with dobutamine and amrinone in severe heart failure. *Chest* 1987;92:657–662.

123. Hasenfuss G, Pieske B, Castell M, et al. Influence of the novel inotropic agent levosimendan on isometric tension and calcium cycling in failing human myocardium. *Circulation* 1998;98:2141–2147.

124. Haikala H, Nissinen E, Etemadzadeh E, et al. Troponin C-mediated calcium sensitization induced by levosimendan does not impair relaxation. *J Cardiovasc Pharmacol* 1995;25:794–801.

125. Movesian MA. Beta-adrenergic receptor agonists and cyclic nucleotide phosphodiesterase inhibitors: shifting the focus from inotropy to cyclic adenosine monophosphate. *J Am Coll Cardiol* 1999;34:318–324.

126. Slawsky MT, Colucci WS, Gottlieb SS, et al. Acute hemodynamic and clinical effects of levosimendan in patients with severe heart failure. *Circulation* 2000;102:2222–2227.

127. Yokoshiki H, Katsube Y, Sunagawa M, et al. Levosimendan, a novel calcium sensitizer, activates the glibenclamide-sensitive potassium channel in rat arterial myocytes. *Eur J Pharmacol* 1997;333:249–259.

128. Packer M, Nieminen MS, Hasenfuss G, et al. Effect of intravenous levosimendan, a calcium sensitizer, on the survival of hospitalized patients with heart failure. *Circulation* 1999;100[Suppl I]:I-646(abstr).

129. Leier CV, Binkley PF. Parenteral inotropic support for advanced congestive heart failure. *Prog Cardiovasc Dis* 1998;41:207–224.

130. Feldman A, Pak PH, Wu CC, et al. Acute cardiovascular effects of OPC-18790 in patients with congestive heart failure. *Circulation* 1996;93:474–483.

131. Kanda H, Yokoto M, Ishihara H, et al. A novel inotropic vasodilator, OPC-18790, reduces myocardial oxygen consumption and improves mechanical efficiency with congestive heart failure. *Am Heart J* 1996;132:361–368.

132. Semeniuk LM, Belenkie I, Tyberg JV. Acute cardiovascular effects of toborinone on vascular capacitance and conductance in experimental heart failure. *Circulation* 1998;98:58–63.

133. Cody RJ. Hormonal alterations in heart failure. In: Hosenpud JD, Greenberg BH, eds. *Congestive heart failure: pathophysiology, diagnosis, and comprehensive approach to management.* Philadelphia: Lippincott Williams & Wilkins, 2000:199–212.

134. Marcus LS, Hart D, Packer M, et al. Hemodynamic and renal excretory effects of human brain natriuretic peptide infusion in patients with congestive heart failure. *Circulation* 1996;94:3184–3189.

135. Hobbs RE, Miller LW, Bott-Silverman C, et al. Hemodynamic effects of a single intravenous injection of synthetic human brain natriuretic peptide in patients with heart

failure secondary to ischemic or idiopathic dilated cardiomyopathy. *Am J Cardiol* 1996;78:891–901.

136. Mills RM, LeJemtel TH, Horton DP, et al. Sustained hemodynamic effects of an infusion of nesiritide (human b-type natriuretic peptide) in heart failure. *J Am Coll Cardiol* 1999;34:155–162.

137. Colucci WS, Elkayam U, Horton DP, et al. Intravenous nesiritide, a natriuretic peptide, in the treatment of decompensated congestive heart failure. *N Engl J Med* 2000;343:246–253.

138. Cody RJ, Haas GJ, Binkley PF, et al. Plasma endothelin correlates with the extent of pulmonary hypertension in patients with chronic congestive heart failure. *Circulation* 1992;85:504–509.

139. Cody RJ, Haas GJ, Binkley PF. Endothelin as a vasoconstrictor substance in congestive heart failure. *Heart Failure* 1992;8:135–141.

140. Clozel M, Ramuz H, Clozel JP, et al. Pharmacology of tezosentan, a new endothelin receptor antagonist designed for parenteral use. *J Pharm Exp Ther* 1999;290:840–846.

141. Torre-Amione G, Young JB, Durand JB, et al. Hemodynamic effects of tezosentan, an intravenous dual endothelin receptor antagonist, in patients with chronic heart failure. *Circulation* 2001;103:973–980.

142. Haas GJ, Leier CV. Invasive cardiovascular testing in chronic congestive heart failure. *Crit Care Med* 1990;18:S1–S4.

143. Vincent JL. Hemodynamic monitoring: pharmacologic therapy and arrhythmia management in acute congestive heart failure. In: Hosenpud JD, Greenberg BH, eds. *Congestive heart failure: pathophysiology, differential diagnosis, and comprehensive approaches to therapy.* New York: Springer-Verlag, 1994:509–521.

144. Edwards JD. Practical application of oxygen transport principles. *Crit Care Med* 1990;18:S45–S48.

145. Stevenson LW, Dracup KA, Tillisch JH. Efficacy of medical therapy tailored for severe congestive heart failure in patients transferred for urgent cardiac transplantation. *Am J Cardiol* 1989;63:461–464.

146. Crexells C, Chatterjee K, Forrester JS, et al. Optimal level of filling pressure in the left side of the heart in acute myocardial infarction. *N Engl J Med* 1973;289:1263–1266.

147. Stevenson LW, Tillisch JH. Maintenance of cardiac output with normal filling pressures in dilated heart failure. *Circulation* 1986;74:1303–1308.

148. Mavric Z, Zaputovic L, Zagar D, et al. Usefulness of blood lactate as a predictor of shock development in acute myocardial infarction. *Am J Cardiol* 1991;67:565–568.

149. Weil MW, Afifi AA. Experimental and clinical studies on lactate and pyruvate as indicators of acute circulatory failure. *Circulation* 1970;16:989–1001.

150. Connors AFJ, Speroff T, Dawson NV, et al. for the SUPPORT investigators. The effectiveness of right heart catheterization in the initial care of critically ill patients. *JAMA* 1996;276:889–897.

151. Hague WA, Boehmer J, Clemson BS, et al. Hemodynamic effects of supplemental oxygen administration in congestive heart failure. *J Am Coll Cardiol* 1996;27:353–357.

152. Cohn JN, Guiha NH, Broder MI, et al. Right ventricular infarction: clinical and hemodynamic features. *Am J Cardiol* 1974;33:209–214.

153. Stevenson LW. Tailored therapy before transplantation for treatment of advanced heart failure: effective use of vasodilators and diuretics. *J Heart Lung Transplant* 1991;10:468–476.

154. Cohn JN, Franciosa JA. Vasodilator therapy of cardiac failure. *N Engl J Med* 1977;297:27–31.

155. Consensus conference report. Mechanical cardiac support 2000: current applications and future trial design. *J Am Coll Cardiol* 2001;37:340–370.

156. Levin HR, Chen JM, Oz MC, et al. Potential of left ventricular–assist devices as outpatient therapy while awaiting transplantation. *Ann Thorac Surg* 1994;58:1515–1520.

157. McCarthy PM, Sabik JF. Implantable circulatory support devices as a bridge to heart transplantation. *Semin Thorac Cardiovasc Surg* 1994;6(3):174–180.

158. Mehta SM, Aufiero TX, Pae WE, et al. Combined registry for the clinical use of mechanical ventricular assist pumps and the total artificial heart in conjunction with heart transplantation: sixth official report—1994. *J Heart Lung Transplant* 1995;14:585–593.

159. James KB, McCarthy PM, Thomas JD, et al. Effect of the implantable left ventricular–assist device on neuroendocrine activation in heart failure. *Circulation* 1995;92[Suppl II]:191–195.

160. Stevenson LW, Belil D, Grover-McKay M, et al. Effects of afterload reduction on left ventricular volume and mitral regurgitation in severe congestive heart failure. *Am J Cardiol* 1987;60:654–658.

161. Loisance DY, Deleuze PH, Houel R, et al. Pharmacologic bridge to cardiac transplantation: current limitations. *Ann Thorac Surg* 1993;55:310–313.

CHRONIC HEART FAILURE MANAGEMENT

JAMES B. YOUNG

▼▼ ADDITIONAL ELECTRONIC TOPICS

Positive Inotropic Agents p31;   Newer Inotropic Agents p32;   Direct-Acting Vasodilators p33;   Beta-Adrenergic Blocking Agents p34

OVERVIEW

Treatment of heart failure is a challenging task that depends on making the proper diagnosis, staging the syndrome severity, and choosing interventions that are likely to diminish suffering while decreasing an exceptionally high mortality. Contemporary insight into the pathophysiology of heart failure has set the stage for designing and implementing a large number of clinical trials, whose results give guidance when planning medical therapies and surgical adventures. No longer is treatment of heart failure the simple dispensation of a diuretic and digitalis preparation. Therapies are now very complicated, and an appreciation of

J. B. Young: Department of Medicine, Kaufman Center for Heart Failure, The Cleveland Clinic Foundation, Cleveland, Ohio

the sometimes subtle nuances of the heart failure syndrome is mandatory if greater strides are to be made with treatment paradigms. Medications for heart failure have evolved from diuretics to digoxin to vasodilators to angiotensin-converting enzyme (ACE) inhibitors to angiotensin II receptor blockers to beta-adrenergic receptor blockers, and they have included a vast variety of drug combinations. A greater focus has more recently been placed on surgical treatment of heart failure. Implantable arrhythmia management devices and biventricular cardiac resynchronizing pacemakers are presently undergoing intense study. Equally important has been clarification of therapeutic strategies that have proved detrimental in heart failure patients, such as use of certain inotropic and antiarrhythmic agents. Much can be done today to ameliorate heart failure's devastating natural course, and familiarity with treatment options is essential. We are now seeing another paradigm shift occurring in heart failure treatment: the early diagnosis of cardiac failure such that "preventive" strategies can be implemented in an attempt to forestall ventricular function deterioration and manifest congestive heart failure. Furthermore, it is now well established that use of agents capable of countermanding the complicated neurohumoral cascade characteristic of heart failure (ACE inhibitors and beta-blockers) is the primary focus when considering therapeutic options. Greater understanding of the molecular dynamics, humoral perturbation, and circulatory insufficiency characteristic of heart failure will lead to even newer and more radical heart failure treatments.

HISTORICAL PERSPECTIVES ON THE TREATMENT OF HEART FAILURE

Evolution of Heart Failure Therapies Related to Pathophysiologic Insight

Treating patients with heart failure is no longer the simple matter of prescribing concoctions of digitalis and primitive diuretics. Largely because of insight gained from well-designed and meticulously performed clinical trials undertaken to define better strategies with new drugs, therapeutic schemes have become very complicated. Substantive evolution of treatment paradigms has occurred (Table 92.1). Therapies have moved from crude attempts to relieve dropsy toward the amelioration of hemodynamic and, subsequently, neurohormonal perturbation characteristic of the syndrome (1–3). Today, strategies that block or ameliorate adverse remodeling seem most important (4–6). Future treatment paradigms will shift toward attenuation of inflammatory processes important in the pathophysiology of heart failure and toward blocking, at the molecular signaling level, necrotic or apoptotic events that lead to cell death. A wide array of surgical, electrophysiologic, and pharmacologic treatment options are now available, and prescribing safe and effective therapies requires a sophisticated understanding of the etiology and pathophysiology of the syndrome as well as drug effects, arrhythmia management, and anticipated surgical results. ▼ p35

Prescription Practice in Heart Failure

To set the stage for contemporary heart failure treatment recommendations, it is important to mark more recent practice patterns (43–48). Studies of Left Ventricular Dysfunction (SOLVD) and the Studies of Patients Intolerant to Converting Enzyme inhibitors (SPICE) trial registries were two of the most extensive evaluations of patterns of medication use in patients with heart failure (44,47) undertaken to date. They are important data sets to review because they document the change in prescription practice with regard to heart failure over the last decade. In SOLVD, drug use

TABLE 92.1 PROGRESS OF UNDERSTANDING OF HEART FAILURE RELATED TO THERAPIES

Heart failure is a dropsical condition.
  Lymphatic drainage tubes
  Primitive diuretic therapies
  Foxglove tea
Heart failure is central cardiac pump inadequacy.
  Cardiac glycoside preparations
  Alternative inotropic therapies
  Cardiac transplantation
  Mechanical ventricular assist devices and total artificial hearts
Heart failure is caused by decompensated ventricular hypertrophy.
  Antihypertensive therapy
  Surgical repair of valvular defects
Heart failure is circulatory dysfunction.
  Vasodilator therapy
Heart failure is an endocrinopathy.
  Angiotensin-converting enzyme inhibitor therapy
  Angiotensin II receptor blockade
  Beta-blocker use
Heart failure is a fever.
  Development of cytokine-modulating agents
Heart failure is a complicated milieu of pump dysfunction, myocardial remodeling, humoral perturbation, and subsequent circulatory insufficiency.
  Angiotensin-converting enzyme inhibitor therapy
Digoxin therapy
Diuretic therapy
Beta-blocker therapy
Surgical therapies (revascularization, remodeling, valve repair, transplantation)

was analyzed in almost 6,000 patients participating in a registry running concurrently with the two SOLVD clinical trials from 1986 through 1989. The SOLVD Registry comprised a broad spectrum of patients with heart failure, including some with predominantly diastolic dysfunction. Drug use was determined in a population cross-section manner at the time patients were identified as having "heart failure." Almost three-fourths of the patients were evaluated during a hospitalization. The median number of cardiovascular drugs used per patient was four (Fig. 92.1), with diuretics taken by 62%, digitalis by 45%, ACE inhibitors by 32%, calcium channel blockers by 36%, antiarrhythmics (nonamiodarone) by 22%, and beta-blockers by 18%. At that time (data were compiled between January 1988 and February 1989), only 18% were on the combination of ACE inhibitor, diuretic, and digitalis. Stratification for diagnosis, heart failure symptoms, and ejection fraction demonstrated that triple-drug therapy (digitalis, diuretic, and ACE inhibitor) was common only in patients with ejection fraction less than 20% and several concomitant signs or symptoms of heart failure. "Preventive" strategies in individuals with a few symptoms did not appear to be common practice. Older patients were taking diuretics frequently (73% of patients older than 70 years).

The SPICE Trial Registry was designed to evaluate heart failure treatment practices, and, more specifically, determine the incidence of ACE inhibitor intolerance in an

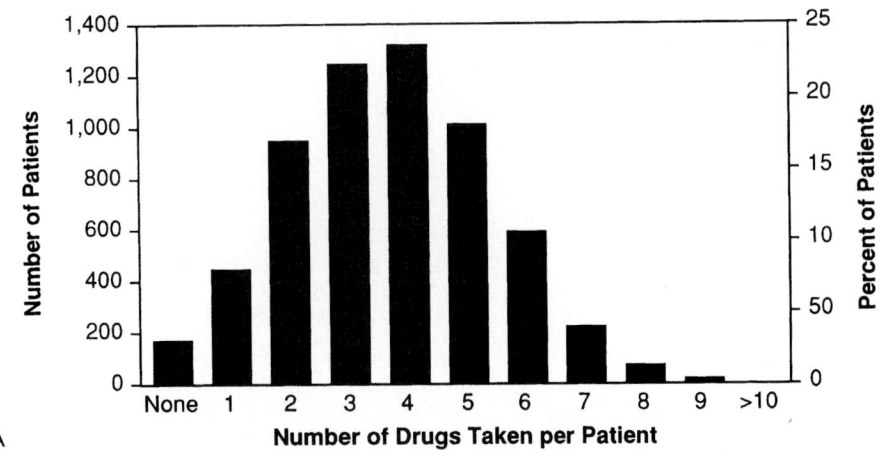

A

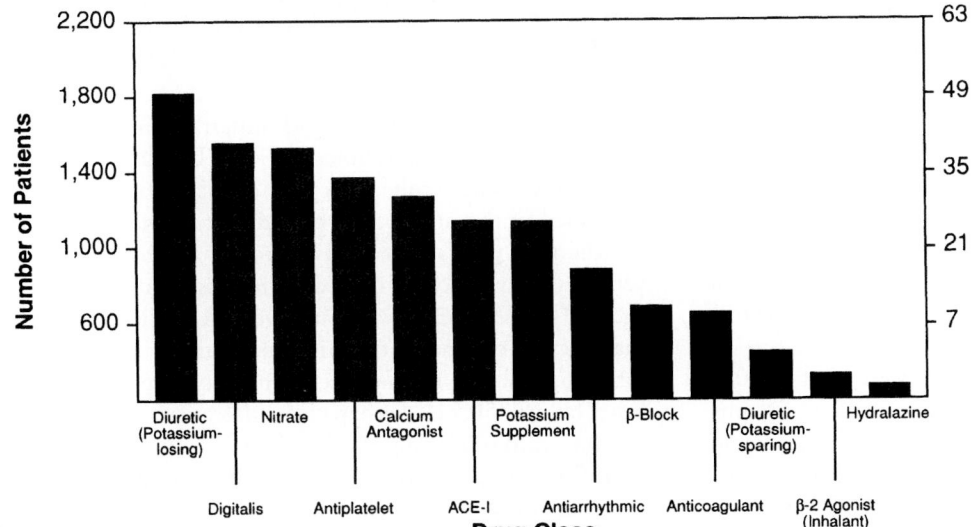

B

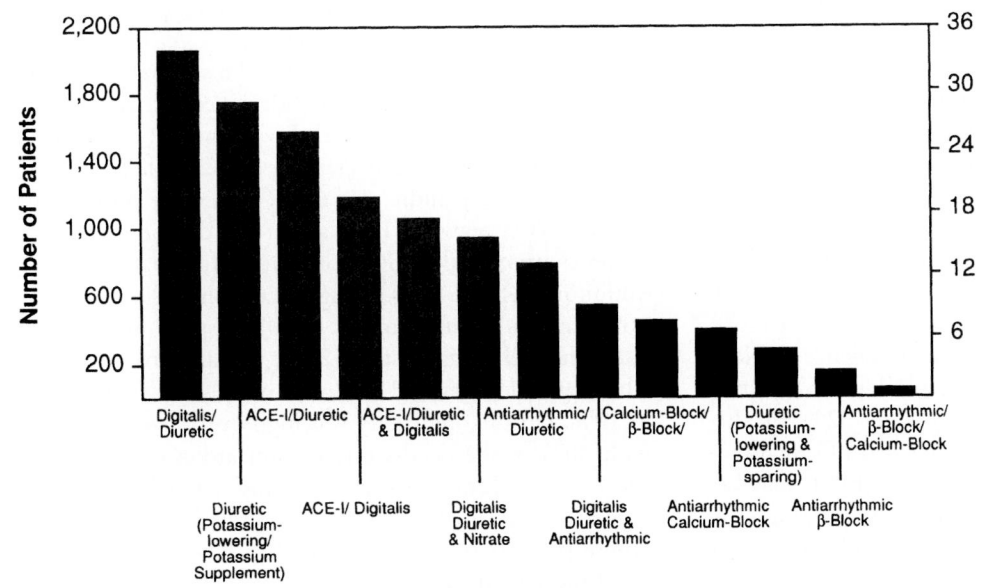

C

FIGURE 92.1 Data from 5,999 patients in the Studies of Left Ventricular Dysfunction (SOLVD) Registry indicated that the median number of cardiac drugs taken per patient with heart failure was four **(A)**. The rank-order histographic plot of drugs most commonly used by registry participants **(B)** and the most common drug combinations **(C)**. These data were compiled in 1988 and, therefore, represent the prescription practice to which we should compare contemporaneous habits. In 1988, more calcium antagonists were used than angiotensin-converting enzyme (ACE-I) inhibitors in patients with heart failure, and antiarrhythmic therapies (generally Vaughn Williams class I agents) were noted in approximately one-fifth of patients. Triple therapy (i.e., ACE inhibitor, diuretic, and digitalis) were used in less than 20% of patients with heart failure at that time. [Modified from Young JB, Weiner DH, Yusuf S, et al. Patterns of medication use in patients with heart failure: a report from the registry of Studies of Left Ventricular Dysfunction (SOLVD). *South Med J* 1994;88:514–523.]

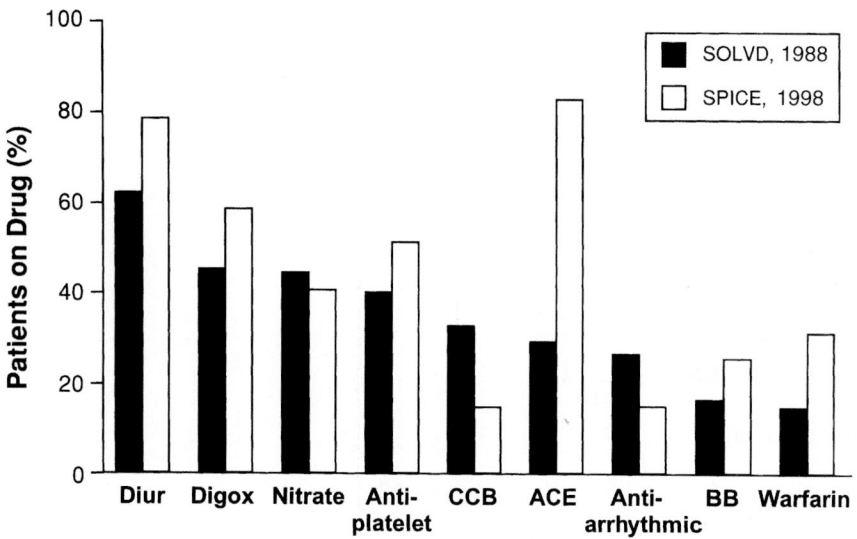

FIGURE 92.2 Comparison of Studies of Left Ventricular Dysfunction (SOLVD) Registry medication use (1988) to the Studies of Patients Intolerant to Converting Enzyme Inhibitors (SPICE) Registry (1998). More angiotensin-converting enzyme (ACE) inhibitors and beta-blockers (BB) are used today, with fewer calcium channel blocker (CCB) and class I antiarrhythmic medications prescribed. Nonetheless, optimal treatment prescription practices have not generally been met. Digox, digoxin; Diur, diuretics.

"optimal" practice situation (48). Between 1996 and 1997, study centers located in eight American and European countries retrospectively reviewed the medical records of 100 consecutive patients with heart failure and an ejection fraction less than or equal to 35%. There were 9,580 subjects studied, and the mean age was 66 years with 26% women and a median ejection fraction of 27%. Ischemic heart disease was the primary cause of the heart failure in 63% of the population. ACE inhibitors were used in 80% of the patients, and this likely represents an ideal circumstance because the study was conducted at largely academic medical centers with education and interests in this issue. The most common reason for not using ACE inhibitors was intolerance, and of these patients, 80% were said to be intolerant because of cough. Figure 92.2 compares the use of medications, generally, in the SPICE and SOLVD Registries, giving insight into the changing prescription practices in heart failure evolving over the last decade. The difference in the prevalence of ACE inhibitors was the most obvious difference, with 30% of the SOLVD Registry population on these agents compared with 80% in SPICE. This likely reflects the acceptance of clinical trial results into day-to-day clinical practice. Other descriptive differences between the groups merit commentary as well. The higher use of diuretics among SPICE Registry patients may reflect more advanced heart failure symptoms as the prevalence of New York Heart Association (NYHA) class III or IV in the SPICE Registry was 43% compared with 32% in the SOLVD Treatment Trial and 17% in the SOLVD Registry. The increase in the use of beta-blockers in SPICE may be related to the growing acceptance of the important role these agents play in ameliorating perturbed neurohormonal activation in patients with heart failure. Of course, today, it is known that these agents are essential. The increase in the use of digoxin and warfarin in the SPICE Registry probably relates to the higher prevalence of atrial fibrillation (27% vs. 14% in the SOLVD Registry). Interestingly, the use of

calcium channel antagonists and antiarrhythmic drugs in SPICE was less than that noted in SOLVD. This is not surprising given the results of several clinical trials that were published in the intervening period that showed increased mortality in post–myocardial infarction patients with left ventricular dysfunction treated with class I antiarrhythmic agents (49). As well, several intervening studies suggested that calcium channel antagonists (particularly short-acting dihydropyridines) may increase mortality in patients with heart failure (50,51). Perhaps the differences in the use of certain cardiovascular medications as noted in the SOLVD-SPICE Registry comparison indicate that so-called evidence-based medicine has had an effect on routine clinical practice (52).

It is accepted today that congestive heart failure patients should be treated with combinations of ACE inhibitors, diuretics, and digoxin (22,53–59). This should be compared with patterns of practice identified by the Clinical Quality Improvement Network Investigators (45). Perhaps giving a more real world assessment of ACE inhibitor use in heart failure, this audit of 4,606 consecutive hospitalized patient charts between 1992 and 1993 demonstrated that diuretics were used in 86% of heart failure patients, ACE inhibitors in 53%, long-acting nitrates in 49%, digoxin in 46%, potassium supplements in 40%, aspirin in 36%, calcium channel antagonists in 20%, warfarin in 17%, beta-adrenergic blockers in 15%, and magnesium supplements in 10%. Hospital mortality was high in this cohort (19%), with 30% of the deaths due to noncardiovascular causes. More data accumulated in 1994 and 1995 in Ohio also suggest that ACE inhibitors are underused in at-risk heart failure patients (46). The Ohio Peer Review Project analyzed the records of 760 patients in 21 hospitals admitted with a principal diagnosis of congestive heart failure. In those having objective measurements of left ventricular ejection fraction less than 40%, with serum creatinine less than 3.0 mg per dL, serum potassium less than 5.5 mEq per L, and systolic blood pressure greater than 90 mm Hg (n = 381), an assessment of admission and discharge medications was made with respect to ACE inhibitor use. Patients in both rural (n = 280) and urban (n = 480) hospitals were evaluated. Mean patient age was approximately 75 years, and 55% were men. In cases eligible for ACE inhibitors at hospital discharge, 16% were said to have contraindications to ACE inhibitors at hospital admission. No difference with respect to hospital type or location was noted with respect to ACE inhibitor use. Although only 37.7% of patients with documented systolic dysfunction were on ACE inhibitors at admission, 73% were prescribed this drug class at discharge.

Now that beta-blockers are also considered important adjuncts to a heart failure patient's polypharmacy protocol, new approaches to educating care givers and patients about the importance of compliance with consensus statement recommendations are needed. Perhaps implementation of heart failure disease management protocols will be helpful (58,59). Although the observations regarding the increasing number of heart failure patients being treated with ACE inhibitors is reassuring in some senses, it is obvious that a large cohort of patients who would likely benefit from this class of drugs is not being so treated. Also troublesome is the fact that patients were often noted to be on medication doses lower than those generally used in the ACE inhibitor heart failure trials. What dose of beta-blocker and ACE inhibitor to prescribe to patients with heart failure has become contentious, with some suggesting that aggressive dosing of these drugs is best, whereas others are content to see patients simply on, at the least, the combination of any dose of the agents (60,61).

CREATING A CHRONIC HEART FAILURE MANAGEMENT STRATEGY

Therapeutic Philosophy

Figure 92.3 links an overview of heart failure therapy to prevention and treatment strategies. [▼ p36] Besides ameliorating symptoms with tailored therapeutic programs, identifying individuals with insidious hemodynamic and hormonal perturbation early on is critical so that therapy can be given early in the syndrome's course to prevent development of symptomatic heart failure. It is imperative that treatment of asymptomatic ventricular dysfunction begin early to interdict harmful remodeling. Obviously, treatment strategies are designed to ameliorate symptoms when present, maintain functional capacity at maximal levels, keep patients out of the hospital, reduce mortality, and reverse remodeling.

Table 92.2 summarizes important questions to ask when designing protocols for patients with chronic heart failure (62,63). Does the patient actually suffer from heart failure

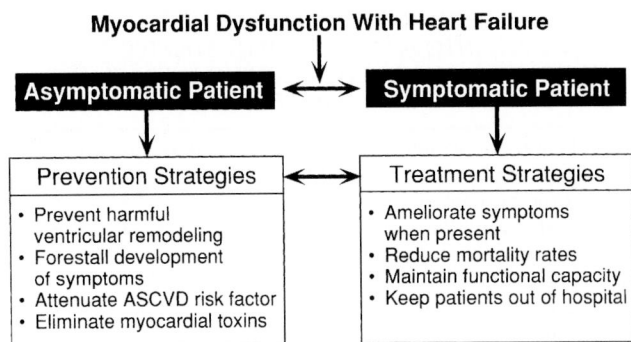

FIGURE 92.3 This diagram emphasizes the importance of a philosophy of heart failure therapy that focuses on practices revolving around *prevention* strategies for the asymptomatic patient and *treatment* strategies for the symptomatic patient. Obviously, one would like to identify myocardial dysfunction in asymptomatic or minimally symptomatic individuals early on so that intervention has the greatest likelihood of preventing ventricular function deterioration and subsequent symptoms. When symptoms are present, treatment protocols should move patients into an asymptomatic position. ASCVD, arteriosclerotic cardiovascular disease.

and are symptoms or physical findings related to this difficulty? Many patients with weakness, fatigue, dyspnea, and dropsical states do not have heart failure. Furthermore, patients with heart failure may present with these symptoms and physical findings, but the symptoms are related to ancillary comorbidities rather than cardiac dysfunction. What is the etiology of the syndrome? This question forces consideration of diseases that can be treated and eliminated or, at the least, ameliorated, such that progression of the heart failure milieu is halted. Following this is questioning what evaluation is needed to confirm the diagnosis and stage the syndrome severity. Indeed, it is important to note what precipitated the patient's deterioration. Frequently, medication noncompliance, excessive sodium or fluid consumption, worsening ischemic syndromes, atrial and ventricular arrhythmias, intercurrent infection, uncontrolled chronic obstructive pulmonary disease, diabetes mellitus, and hypertension plunge patients into the realm of symptomatic congestive heart failure. Staging the syndrome severity is critical to answering the question of what a patient's short- and long-term prognosis might be. A question that often goes unasked is whether the patient takes medications that can be detrimental in the heart failure setting, such as nonsteroidal antiinflammatory agents, certain calcium channel blockers, and Vaughn Williams class I antiarrhythmic drugs. Obviously, designing a treatment protocol is intimately linked to the question of how the patient should be treated acutely as well as chronically (22,53,57,72–76). Often, we neglect social factors that play a significant role in morbidity, and we should always ask what social support mechanisms that can be considered adjunctive nonpharmacologic treatments are available to the patient (73). Again, it is critical to remember that patients with heart failure have varied clinical presentations

TABLE 92.2 INTEGRATION OF DIAGNOSTIC EVALUATION INTO A MANAGEMENT STRATEGY: QUESTIONS TO ASK WHEN DESIGNING THERAPEUTIC PROTOCOLS FOR CHRONIC HEART FAILURE PATIENTS

Does the patient actually suffer from heart failure, and are presenting symptoms or physical findings related to this difficulty?

What is the etiology of the syndrome?

What evaluation is needed to confirm diagnosis, clarify etiology, and stage syndrome severity?

What precipitated the patient's deterioration?

How severe is the heart failure syndrome, and what are the patient's short- and long-term prognoses?

Is the patient on medications that are potentially detrimental in the heart failure milieu?

How should the patient be treated acutely?

How should the patient be treated chronically?

Can the precipitating disease process be cured, or can the state of heart failure be ameliorated?

What social factors played a role in morbidity, and what social support mechanisms should be considered as adjunctive therapeutic measures?

Guidelines for Heart Failure Patient Evaluation and Management

The Agency for Health Care Policy and Research (AHCPR) published the first guidelines for evaluating and treating heart failure patients in 1994 (72–76). Subsequently, guidelines have emerged from several groups as our knowledge base increased (see Table 92.3 for a listing). Diagnosis and treatment algorithms subsequently have been based largely on experience gained during the performance of carefully controlled clinical trials evaluating a variety of strategies. These trials are subsequently reviewed. In general, a well-constructed practice guideline specifies the types of professionals involved in developing the guideline, defines the methods of primary evidence analysis, and provides a grading of one sort or another to characterize the strength of data the recommendations are based on. There are several problems with clinical practice guidelines, however. Generally, the guidelines do not emphasize the importance of risk stratification with regard to syndrome severity (particularly in asymptomatic or minimally symptomatic patients and more advanced, decompensated patients), and, therefore, largely ignore the issue of tailoring therapies to patients in the mildly or severely ill categories. Furthermore, guidelines cannot possibly address all relevant clinical situations (76). Often, consensus cannot be reached because evidence is not always available regarding certain therapeutic strategies. Guideline development can be a slow, politically charged, and ponderous process with guidelines being slow to respond to new knowledge and therapies. It is also difficult

TABLE 92.3 CLINICAL HEART FAILURE GUIDELINES

Guidelines	Year published
U.S. Department of Health and Human Services, Agency for Health Care Policy and Research (Clinical Practice Guideline no. 11, publication 94-0612)	1994
American College of Cardiology/American Heart Association Guidelines for the Evaluation and Management of Heart Failure (*Circulation* 1995;92:2764)	1995
World Health Organization Heart Failure Guidelines (*J Card Fail* 1996;2:153)	1996
European Society of Cardiology Heart Failure Guidelines (*Eur Heart J* 1997;18:736)	1997
ACTION Heart Failure Treatment Guidelines [*Am J Cardiol* 1999;83(2A):1]	1999
Heart Failure Society of America Guidelines for the Management of Heart Failure (*J Card Fail* 1999;5:358)	1999

to educate clinicians regarding guidelines, and many practitioners perceive guidelines as being intrusive and excessively regulatory. Nonetheless, practice guidelines are, arguably, the best method of defining treatment practices that continuing quality improvement programs can use to grade any health care provider's practice.

The commonest themes of all of these guidelines are summarized in Table 92.4. All guidelines support an aggressive approach to diagnosing and treating patients with active ischemia and left ventricular dysfunction. The guidelines are unanimous in recommending ACE inhibitors in all patients with left ventricular systolic dysfunction. The more recent guidelines address use of beta-blockers in stable patients with mild to moderate heart failure symptoms and no significant congestion. All guidelines suggest avoiding agents with incomplete benefit-risk profiles and reminding clinicians about diagnosing and treating underlying and precipitating difficulties. Furthermore, most of the guidelines emphasize the importance of prescribing nonpharmacologic therapy such as exercise and salt and fluid restriction while

TABLE 92.4 MOST COMMON THEMES OF HEART FAILURE GUIDELINES

Identify and aggressively treat ischemia in patients with heart failure (revascularization)

Use angiotensin-converting enzyme inhibitors in all tolerant patients with left ventricular systolic dysfunction

Use beta-blockers in stable patients with mild to moderate symptoms and no significant congestion

Avoid agents with incomplete benefit-risk profiles

Diagnose and address underlying and precipitating disorders

Prescribe nonpharmacologic therapies

    Exercise

    Salt and fluid restriction

Educate patient, family, and care givers

as they move from asymptomatic cardiac dysfunction to symptomatic heart failure. Complicating this issue further is the fact that patients make this transition over highly variable time intervals.

addressing patient education about heart failure. Largely ignored in present guidelines are patients with congestive heart failure but preserved left ventricular systolic function and management of advanced heart failure (particularly the acutely decompensated chronic heart failure patient who requires hospitalization and the terminal "hospice-type" patient with heart failure). ⌖ p37

CLINICAL TRIAL INSIGHTS

Certainly, clinical trials cannot answer all questions about heart failure therapeutics. Anecdotal experience as well as more detailed, but small, uncontrolled experimental paradigms can offer guidance. Clinical trials performed in heart failure cohorts are limited by certain design difficulties. There is a tremendous winnowing of patients screened for these studies, for example, and it is not unusual to see a 10:1 or 20:1 ratio of patient screening to trial entry. Figures 92.4 and 92.5 depict mortality end points in a variety of clinical heart failure trials and emphasize, by reviewing placebo group death rates, the tremendous heterogeneity of populations included in the trials. To be successful, clinical trials require that specific questions be asked in well-characterized and relatively homogeneous patient populations; therefore, the most challenging patient to manage (the aged patient, female in particular, with multiple comorbidities) is often not allowed into clinical trials. Unfortunately, there is a large underrepresentation of women, minority races, the elderly, and youth in clinical trials. Furthermore, end points used to evaluate potentially beneficial or detrimental treatment strategies are sometimes imprecise or not necessarily clinically relevant. Another difficulty is that the studies are performed on varying "background" pharmacotherapeutic strategies. It is extremely important to assess clinical trials with respect to their analyzed end points and the power with which the study was designed to answer the questions asked. It must be emphasized that the success of a clinical trial is not rooted solely in demonstration of a positive result. Trials that do not support a priori hypotheses are sometimes more important than those that do because they can clarify what should be done in these populations as well as strategies that should not be pursued.

Despite these issues, the clinical trial remains an excellent method for fashioning rational protocols and identifying their cost effectiveness by exploring schemes that are effective, neutral, or detrimental with respect to endpoint impact. Because of the multiple drugs heart failure patients take and the complicated interrelationship of comorbidities, it is important to create algorithms that include only advantageous strategies. Those that are neutral or disadvantageous should be avoided.

*e*Table 92.4.1 lists select clinical trials that provide important insight into treatment of patients with a wide range of heart failure. Highlighting a few specific trials

allows the stage to be set for proffering contemporary heart failure treatment recommendations. The first Veterans Administration Cooperative Vasodilator Heart Failure Trial (V-HeFT-I) (77) was made up of men with moderate congestive heart failure and was a landmark study because it was the first to suggest that vasodilators beneficially affected mortality in patients with congestive heart failure. At the time it was performed, the trial was controversial because conventional wisdom dictated that diuretics and inotropic agents were the most logical approach to congestive heart failure. Insight into detrimental ventricular remodeling in heart failure was not great at that time, but the beneficial effects of direct-acting vasodilators, such as hydralazine and isosorbide dinitrate, on cardiac output and ventricular filling pressures gave rise to the so-called hemodynamic hypothesis of heart failure therapy and led to the design of V-HeFT-I. Specifically, this hypothesis speculated that drugs that lowered impedance to ventricular ejection, with subsequent reduction of diastolic pressures and augmentation of forward flow (or reduction of venous blood return after venodilation with nitrates), was beneficial and decreased mortality and morbidity. This study was also important because it demonstrated disparity among vasodilating drugs. Although the combination of hydralazine and isosorbide dinitrate, prescribed in addition to digoxin and a diuretic, arguably improved morbidity and mortality (the study was relatively small, and its statistical analysis has been criticized), V-HeFT-I showed that the peripherally acting alpha-adrenergic blocking agent prazosin, known to effectively reduce both preload and afterload in heart failure, was no better than placebo. Thus, the conclusion was reached that all vasodilators may not be alike with respect to long-term morbidity and mortality effects. Since V-HeFT-I, we have seen drugs that improve heart failure hemodynamics significantly but produce higher mortality in clinical trials (67–82) (*e*Table 92.4.1).

The Cooperative Scandinavian Enalapril Survival Study (CONSENSUS) (83) used an agent that was not only an effective vasodilating antihypertensive drug but one that also blocked certain neurohormonal characteristics of heart failure and demonstrated a profound mortality reduction in severely ill heart failure patients (NYHA class IV). The dramatic CONSENSUS results supported yet a new hypothesis in the treatment of heart failure: the *neurohumoral interdiction hypothesis*. Clinical benefit with respect to mortality reduction could be achieved by blocking certain aspects of neurohormonal compensatory systems characteristic of heart failure, and, specifically, the renin-angiotensin-aldosterone cascade.

Subsequently, V-HeFT-II (84) compared the combination of hydralazine and isosorbide dinitrate to the ACE inhibitor enalapril and demonstrated that enalapril effected greater mortality reduction than did the direct-acting vasodilator combination. This raised the question of whether agents primarily blocking humoral factors were bet-

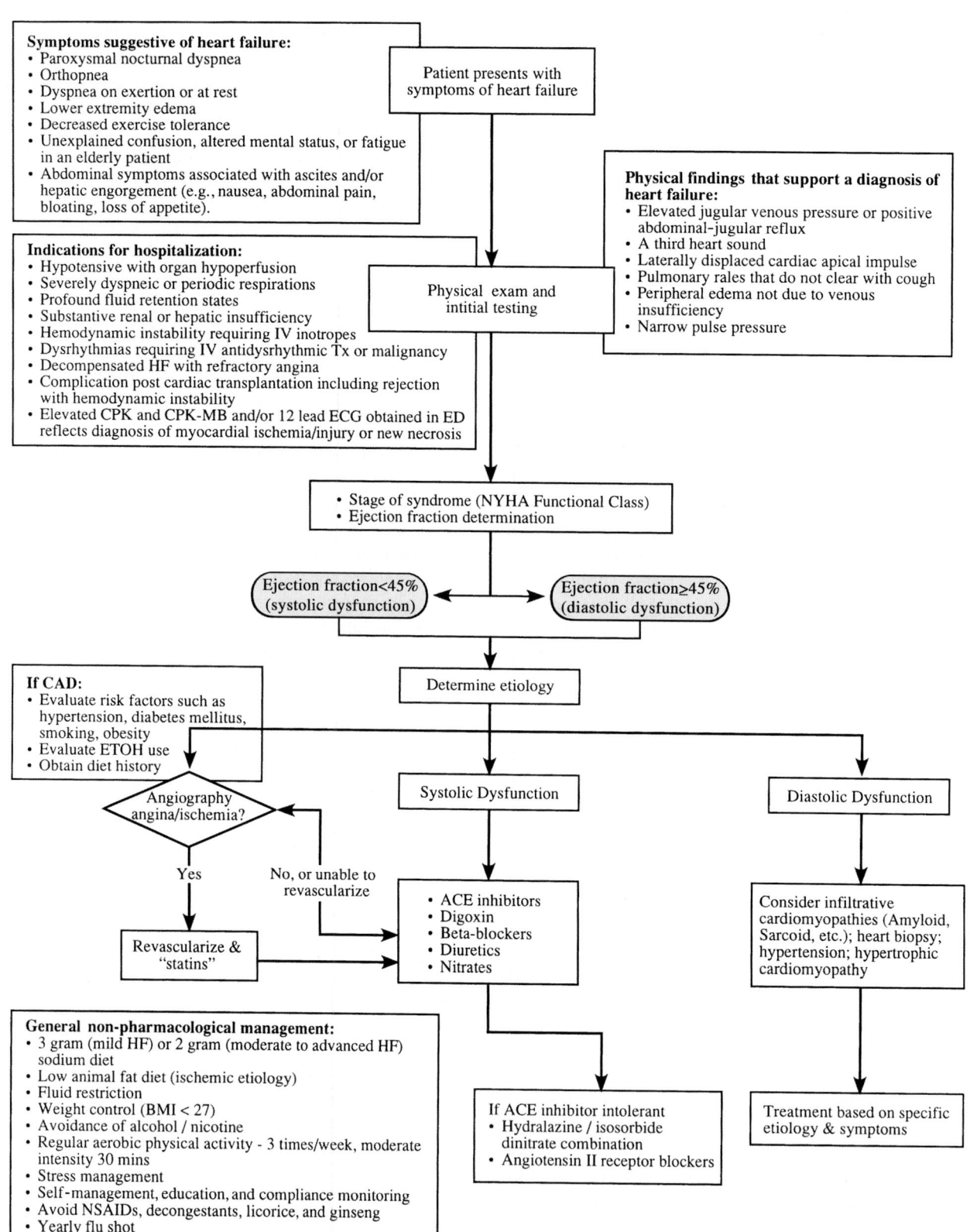

FIGURE 92.4 An algorithm for diagnosis and pharmacologic management of heart failure (HF) patients that focuses largely on symptomatic out-of-hospital patients with suspected congestive HF. In these patients, initiating diuretic, angiotensin-converting enzyme (ACE) inhibitor therapy, and beta-blockers is initially recommended, with addition of digoxin and other vasodilating agents suggested for cases with persistent symptomatology. BMI, body mass index; CAD, coronary artery disease; CPK-MB, creatine phosphokinase-MB; ECG, electrocardiography; ED, emergency department; ETOH, ethanol; NSAIDs, nonsteroidal antiinflammatory drugs; NYHA, New York Heart Association; Tx, treatment.

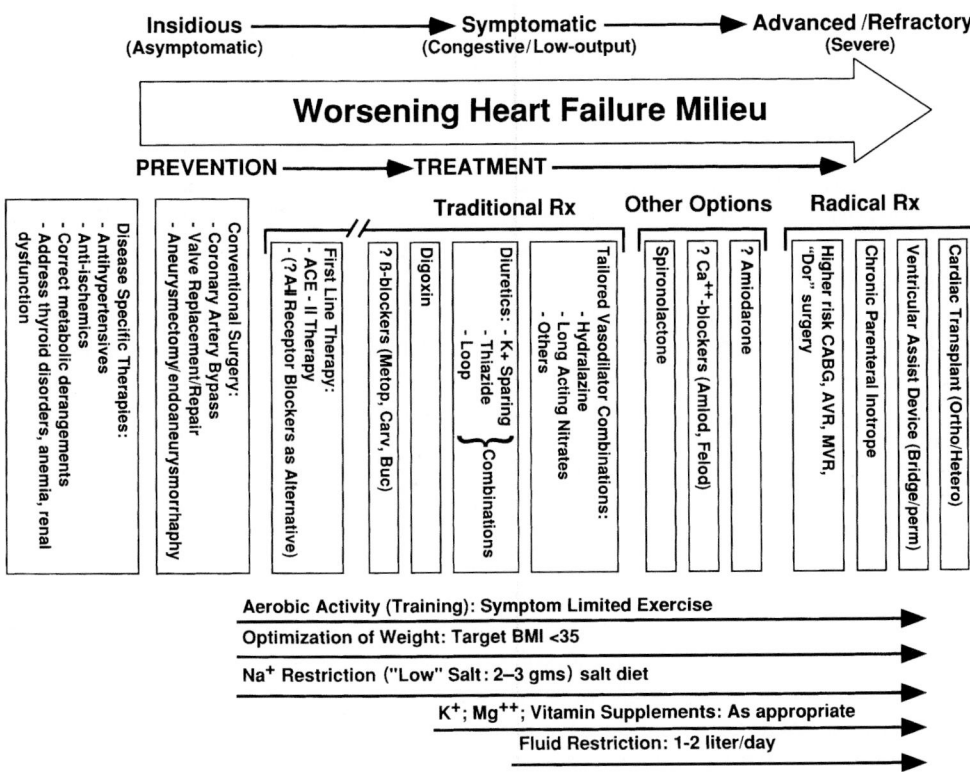

FIGURE 92.5 This figure graphically plots a scheme for tailoring therapies to individual heart failure patients. It is based on the fact that treatments change as the heart failure milieu worsens. Preventive strategies are recommended for individuals with insidious and asymptomatic or minimally symptomatic heart failure, with treatment strategies accelerating in intensity as congestive or low-output states worsen. At the root of all treatment protocols, however, is disease-specific therapy. Also important is a variety of lifestyle changes, including aerobic activity training, optimization of weight, and dietary restriction of salt use. ACE, angiotensin-converting enzyme inhibitor; AVR, aortic valve replacement; BMI, body mass index; CABG, coronary artery bypass grafting; MVR, mitral valve replacement.

ter in heart failure than those with only hemodynamic actions. It is logical that both types of drugs might be important. The syndrome stage in any given patient may have great bearing on outcome with respect to drugs chosen, but this is not entirely clear now. It is interesting to note that the combination of direct-acting vasodilators and ACE inhibitors might be even more effective, but this has not directly been addressed. Some information from the Prospect of Randomized Amlodipine Survival Evaluation (PRAISE) (85) and the V-HeFT-III (86) provide insight into this hypothesis. PRAISE demonstrated mortality reduction, but only in patients with no coronary heart disease. Amlodipine was prescribed as adjunctive therapy to ACE inhibitors and digoxin. V-HeFT-III was a 2-by-2 factorially designed protocol that studied the combination of felodipine, digoxin, and placebo on a background of angiotensin-converting therapy. In this study, felodipine demonstrated no benefit in any group, but harm was not suggested either. PRAISE and V-HeFT-III are also important because they focus on calcium channel blockers in heart failure, which are generally found to be detrimental in this setting. Studies performed with first- and second-generation calcium antagonists usually showed increased morbidity and mortality when prescribed in a heart failure milieu.

The SOLVD program (87,88) evaluated enalapril in asymptomatic or minimally symptomatic patients (the prevention trial) (87) and in patients with mild to moderate congestive heart failure (the treatment trial) (88). Baseline medications generally included diuretics and digoxin. In patients with ejection fraction less than 35% and symptom-

atic heart failure, enalapril significantly reduced mortality, morbidity, and, importantly, major ischemic events, such as acute myocardial infarction or hospital admission for unstable angina. In fact, the reduction in major ischemic events was more impressive than reduction of any other single morbid event, including hospitalization for heart failure. The SOLVD prevention trial demonstrated significant decrement in the combined end point of congestive heart failure morbidity (hospital admission for heart failure) and mortality. This trial was the first to suggest that a preventive intervention strategy with ACE inhibitors could attenuate progression toward clinically manifest heart failure when used as first-line drug therapy in asymptomatic or minimally symptomatic patients with systolic left ventricular dysfunction. Observations from SOLVD shift the paradigm of therapy from simply a diuretic and digoxin prescription, begun when patients develop congestive heart failure, to instituting ACE inhibitor therapy first even in noncongested, asymptomatic, or minimally symptomatic patients.

In an attempt to finally put to rest the controversy surrounding digoxin use in heart failure, the Digoxin Investigators Group (DIG) Trial (89) followed 7,788 patients with congestive heart failure for 5 years. DIG suggested that digoxin did not significantly affect mortality one way or another but substantially diminished the likelihood that patients would develop worsening heart failure requiring hospitalization. The DIG Trial was performed on a background of diuretic and ACE inhibitor and thus supports the contention that triple therapy is likely the best strategy in congestive heart failure patients. An important result was that a large subset of patients having only diastolic dysfunction with congestive heart failure also saw substantive benefits with digoxin. Some have suggested that a subset analysis in this trial increased risk of "arrhythmic death," but this conclusion may not be completely justified.

The Survival and Ventricular Enlargement Trial (90) demonstrated that captopril improved survival, functional status, and reduced repeat myocardial infarction rate compared with placebo when this ACE inhibitor was begun the first week after acute myocardial infarction when left ventricular systolic dysfunction in the absence of substantive congestion (ejection fraction less than 40%) was observed. Several other clinical trials after acute myocardial infarction (91–94) (*e*Fig. 92.5.1) have confirmed that ACE inhibitors begun shortly after the event were associated with significant benefit when either asymptomatic systolic left ventricular dysfunction or mild clinical congestive heart failure was present. Captopril, ramipril, zofenopril, and trandolapril, therefore, have been used in this setting, and it is suggested that long-term benefit accrues when a variety of ACE inhibitors are used. Furthermore, several "megatrials" of ACE inhibitors after myocardial infarction conclude that ACE inhibitors given routinely after myocardial infarction (i.e., irrespective of presence or absence of left ventricular systolic dysfunction or congestive heart failure) produce short-term reduction in mortality. The International Study of Infarct Survival IV (95) and Gruppo Italiano Della Infarto Miocardial III trial (96) included patients with a wide spectrum of ejection fractions. Their positive findings suggested that early administration of ACE inhibitors would translate more generally into postinfarct benefit.

Although small clinical trials attempting to evaluate beneficial effects of beta-blockers in heart failure had been published with disparate results, the Metoprolol in Dilated Cardiomyopathy (97) study was the first larger-scale trial to resolve some of the controversy about this strategy. The beta$_1$-selective beta-blocker metoprolol versus placebo was studied in dilated cardiomyopathy patients. Compared with placebo, patients in the active drug limb had improved symptoms with a decrement in the combined end point of survival and need for heart transplant. Many design issues were raised, however, such as the reasonability of including heart transplant as an end point. Although conclusions were tenuous, the observations added some support to the growing portfolio of heart failure therapy benefits with beta-blockers. Subsequently, the Prospective Randomized Evaluation of Carvedilol on Symptoms and Exercise (98) and the Multicenter Oral Carvedilol Heart Failure Assessment (99) trials were completed. These studies demonstrated improvement in patients with mild to moderate heart failure receiving this beta-blocker and vasodilator on top of digoxin, diuretic, and ACE inhibitors. More interesting was the pooled analysis of four large carvedilol treatment protocols, which indicated that mortality was reduced substantially (100). More recently, other studies with different beta-blockers support the contention that these agents should be used, albeit carefully, in patients with heart failure. Cardiac Insufficiency Bisoprolol Studies I and II using bisoprolol (101–103) and Metoprolol CR/XL Randomized Intervention Trial in Heart Failure (104) using sustained-release metoprolol (104) were also positive beta-blocker studies. The Randomized Evaluation of Strategies for Left Ventricular Dysfunction (RESOLVD) study has also been completed, and one aspect of this clinical trial evaluated the effects of sustained-release metoprolol in an aggressive heart failure protocol in which an angiotensin II receptor antagonist (candesartan) and the beta-blocker were added to ACE inhibitors and other heart failure medications (generally diuretics and digoxin) (105). Although not a mortality trial by design, when added to ACE inhibitors, angiotensin II receptor antagonists, or both, the use of metoprolol improved ventricular function, reduced activation of the renin-angiotensin system, and resulted in fewer deaths. Perhaps the most ill heart failure patients yet studied with beta-blockers were in the Carvedilol Prospective Randomized Cumulative Survival Trial (COPERNICUS) (106–108). This mortality endpoint study extended observations of benefit noted in prior trials with carvedilol to more ill NYHA class IV patients. This study did not, however, include patients who could not reach some degree of compensation (euvolemic at trial entry). Nonetheless, COPERNICUS markedly broadened the patient population likely to benefit from these agents, demonstrating that, when carefully titrated, even very ill individuals could tolerate beta-blockers. Interestingly, in the Beta-blocker Evaluation and Survival Trial (BEST), bucindolol, a nonselective beta-adrenergic blocker with mild vasodilating properties, did not show significant overall survival benefit in a demographically diverse group of patients with NYHA class III and IV congestive heart failure (109). Perhaps important was the fact that in BEST the point estimate of mortality reduction favored bucindolol, but the confidence intervals were wide and not statistically significant compared with placebo, yet when white participants only were included in the analysis, benefits were noted (107). In the United States, then, two beta-adrenergic blocking drugs now have approval by the Food and Drug Administration for use in heart failure patients, carvedilol (Coreg) and long-acting metoprolol (Toprol XL).

Antiarrhythmic drugs have not generally fared well in clinical trials evaluating their effects in heart failure patients (27,28,110–120). This has been tremendously disappointing. Many patients with substantive ventricular dysfunction have malignant or potentially malignant ventricular arrhythmias. Furthermore, sudden cardiac death (frequently presumed due to ventricular tachycardia and fibrillation) often accounts for this difficulty. It seems logical that efforts to eliminate these arrhythmias should translate into mortality reduction. Many agents studied are potent with respect to elimination of ventricular dysrhythmia. The Cardiac Arrhythmia Suppression Trial (113,114,120) studied encainide, flecainide, and moricizine post–myocardial infarction in patients with multiple premature ventricular contractions and, generally, left ventricular dysfunction. Indeed, in many senses, the patient population resembled the populations of several other trials (90–93). This study was terminated prematurely, however, because of excessive mortality in the treatment groups. All three drugs seemed to exhibit detriment more than benefit when used routinely in post–myocardial infarction patients with ventricular arrhythmias. The Survival with Oral D-Sotalol (115) trial evaluated the effect of D-sotalol on mortality in patients after recent and remote myocardial infarction [again, populations similar to several other trials, including SOLVD (87,88,90–93)] with ejection fraction less than 40%. This trial was stopped prematurely because of excessive treatment group mortality. Even with an antiarrhythmic agent with only pure potassium channel blocking effects, adverse outcome has been demonstrated. Amiodarone may be, arguably, the one exception to this observation. The Group Study of Heart Failure in Argentina (121) was a placebo-controlled (but unblinded) study of amiodarone in moderate to severe congestive heart failure having mortality end points. Mortality was significantly reduced in the amiodarone group compared with placebo (42% vs. 53%), which suggested that amiodarone could be used safely in congestive heart failure patients and might provide benefit. The European Myocardial Infarction Amiodarone Trial (122) randomized patients 5 to 21 days after myocardial infarction who had an ejection fraction less than 40% and evaluated total mortality as a primary end point. Although the primary end point was not affected by amiodarone, the combined end point of presumed arrhythmic death and resuscitated cardiac arrest was reduced slightly. The Canadian Myocardial Infarction Amiodarone Trial (123,124) evaluated patients 6 to 45 days after myocardial infarction and had no ejection fraction entry criteria, but electrocardiographic ventricular arrhythmias, for combined end points of arrhythmic death or resuscitated ventricular fibrillation. All-cause mortality and cardiac mortality were secondary end points. Although this study demonstrated that amiodarone reduces the incidence of ventricular fibrillation or arrhythmic death among survivors of acute myocardial infarction having frequent or repetitive ventricular premature depolarizations, 42% of the treatment group had stopped the drug by year 2 because of toxicity. The Canadian Myocardial Infarction Amiodarone Trial was not a heart failure trial, per se, but many of its subjects had left ventricular dysfunction. Concern has been raised about making strong conclusions from end points such as "presumed" ventricular tachyarrhythmic death and, therefore, use of amiodarone routinely in heart failure patients is still open to question (125). The Congestive Heart Failure Survival Trial of Antiarrhythmic Therapy (126) studied amiodarone versus placebo in congestive heart failure patients generally who had ten premature ventricular contractions per hour on ambulatory monitoring. Amiodarone in this study did not improve survival compared with placebo. Thus, the routine use of amio-

darone in patients with heart failure, whether it be manifest as congestive heart failure or left ventricular dysfunction after myocardial infarction, remains highly controversial. Furthermore, it is an expensive therapy in both cost and toxicity. Two large studies of the newest available antiarrhythmic drug, dofetilide, Danish Investigations of Arrhythmia and Mortality on Dofetilide—Congestive Heart Failure (127) and Danish Investigations of Arrhythmia and Mortality on Dofetilide—Myocardial Infarction (128), have now been published. Both trials were primary mortality endpoint studies with the heart failure study assessing mortality in symptomatic congestive heart failure patients with severe left ventricular dysfunction and the myocardial infarction study randomizing patients with severe left ventricular dysfunction after an acute infarct. The heart failure study did show that dofetilide decreased heart failure hospitalizations and converted atrial fibrillation more frequently but with a significant incidence of torsades de pointes in the antiarrhythmic group. In patients with severe left ventricular dysfunction and recent myocardial infarction, treatment with dofetilide did not decrease all-cause mortality, cardiac mortality, or total arrhythmic deaths. However, dofetilide was effective in treating atrial fibrillation and atrial flutter.

Other mortality endpoint heart failure trials have suggested that intervention with certain drugs might actually increase mortality. Studies of flosequinan, milrinone, and prostacyclin (Flolan) are examples. These studies include the Prospective Randomized Flosequinan on Longevity Evaluation (80), the Prospective Randomized Milrinone Survival Evaluation (81), the Xamoterol in Severe Heart Failure (Xamoterol-CHF) (129), and the Flolan International Randomized Survival Trial (78). Milrinone is a potent phosphodiesterase inhibitor demonstrating both inotropic and vasodilating properties. It is an effective drug when used parenterally in acute heart failure patients and may, in fact, be helpful during treatment of chronic and refractory heart failure when given in either chronic or pulsed parenteral infusion fashion (130). However, chronic oral treatment with this drug increased mortality (131). Flosequinan is also likely an "inodilator," exhibiting inotropic and vasodilating properties, yet it demonstrated increased mortality. Prostacyclin is quite different from phosphodiesterase inhibitors in action and, specifically, does not elicit inotropic effects. Prostacyclin is a potent pulmonary and peripheral arteriolar dilator, yet it was associated with higher mortality than placebo when given chronically to severely ill heart failure patients.

Again, although not a heart failure trial per se, the Multicenter Diltiazem Reinfarction Trial (132) was important because of its demonstration that diltiazem, when routinely administered after myocardial infarction, significantly increased adverse cardiac events in patients with heart failure. Generally, results with calcium channel blocking agents in heart failure have been disappointing, particularly post infarct.

More recently, the Vesnarinone Survival Trial (82) demonstrated a 24% increase in total mortality with the 60-mg dose of vesnarinone ($p <.05$) and a 12% mortality increase with the 30-mg dose (p = not significant). This should be counterposed to a previous vesnarinone study that indicated that this drug reduced mortality substantially at the 60-mg dose, whereas 120 mg increased death rates (133). The lower vesnarinone doses do not, for the most part, produce clinically measurable inotropic or hemodynamic changes in heart failure. Vesnarinone is an interesting proposed heart failure therapy because it may interdict the inflammatory (cytokine or tumor necrosis factor) components of heart failure. Observations are incomplete at this time, but the disparity between outcomes noted in two well-designed, well-controlled, compulsively performed mortality endpoint clinical trials is troubling. One wonders whether vesnarinone may have specific beneficial effects in only a well-defined subset patient population that is yet to be characterized.

Studies with calcium channel blockers generally have demonstrated increased morbidity and mortality in heart failure. PRAISE I and II and V-HeFT-III are the only clinical trials to date that suggest that specific calcium channel blocking agents (amlodipine and felodipine) might not carry such concerns for heart failure patients (134,135). The calcium channel blocker mibefradil studied in Mortality Assessment in Congestive Heart Failure I actually increased morbidity. This drug is no longer available (136).

Other pharmacologic approaches in heart failure have been studied including the use of human growth hormone, but concern has been raised about the induction of ventricular hypertrophy and diastolic dysfunction with this agent (137). Spironolactone proved quite efficacious in the Randomized Aldactone Evaluation Study trial when added to diuretics, digoxin, and ACE inhibitors in NYHA class II and III patients (138).

*e*Figure 92.5.2 graphically presents selected mortality endpoint clinical trials that have greatly shaped our philosophy regarding best approaches to the patients with heart failure. The figure is arranged so that all of the trials are comparable with respect to total mortality end points and length of patient follow-up. These trials were well performed and therefore provide credible information regarding therapeutic algorithms. Important to note is the fact that a wide spectrum of placebo mortality can be observed, implying that different patient populations have been studied. It is also likely that, over time, patient management strategies have improved more generally.

SPECIFIC THERAPIES FOR CHRONIC HEART FAILURE

It is important to reemphasize that the principles of chronic heart failure therapeutics are rooted in making the appropriate diagnosis, staging the syndrome (different therapies

are warranted for asymptomatic vs. symptomatic patients), addressing diseases causing or precipitating the difficulty, and using strategies that prevent disease progression (e.g., appropriate treatment of hypertension and atherosclerotic cardiovascular risk factors). Patient counseling and general education of family and home care givers is also important but is often ignored.

Suggested Topics for Patient, Family, and Care Giver Education

Table 92.5 presents topics for patient, family, and care giver education and counseling that have been modified from the

TABLE 92.5 SUGGESTED TOPICS FOR PATIENT, FAMILY, AND CARE GIVER EDUCATION AND COUNSELING

General counseling
   Explanation of heart failure and the reason for symptoms
   Cause or probable cause of heart failure
   Expected symptoms
   Symptoms of worsening heart failure
   What to do if symptoms worsen
   Self-monitoring with daily weights, blood pressure, pulse rate, blood sugar (in diabetics)
   Explanation of treatment or care plan
   Clarification of patient's responsibilities
   Importance of cessation of tobacco use
   Role of family members or other care givers in the treatment or care plan
   Availability and value of qualified local support group
   Importance of obtaining vaccinations against influenza and *Pneumococcus*
Prognosis
   Life expectancy
   Advance directives
   Advice for family members in the event of cardiac arrest
Activity recommendations
   Cardiac rehabilitation programs with supervised exercise protocols
   Recreations, leisure, and work activity
   Exercise
   Sex, sexual difficulties, and coping strategies
Dietary recommendations
   Sodium restriction
   Avoidance of excessive fluid intake
   Alcohol restriction, if appropriate
   Low-animal-fat diet, if appropriate
Medications
   Effects of medications on quality of life and survival
   Dosing of drugs
   Likely side effects and what to do if they occur
   Coping mechanisms for complicated medical regimens
Importance of compliance with treatment or care plan
   Methods to ensure medications taken timely
   Provision of forms to record medications taken
   Pulse rate, blood pressure, weight charts

Modified from Konstam M, Dracup K, Baker D, et al. *Heart failure: evaluation and care of patient with left-ventricular systolic dysfunction. Clinical practice guideline.* AHCPR publication no. 94-0612. Rockville, MD: Agency for Health Care Policy and Research, U.S. Department of Health and Human Services, 1994.

AHCPR guidelines (72,73). Central to therapy is an explanation to the patient of heart failure and the reason for symptoms, if the patient is symptomatic. Discussion of the cause or probable cause of heart failure is important, as are expected symptoms, symptoms that herald worsening heart failure, and strategies to pursue if symptoms worsen. Instruction with regard to self-monitoring of daily weights, blood pressure, pulse rate, and blood sugar in diabetics is helpful. Explicit explanation of treatment and care plans is important to gain acceptance of therapeutic strategies. One should be specific when discussing patient responsibilities with regard to cessation of tobacco and alcohol use, salt restriction, and fluid intake reduction. The important role of family members or other care givers in the treatment plan should be stressed. Atherosclerotic risk factor intervention is essential, as is the need for obtaining vaccinations at appropriate intervals against influenza and pneumococcal disease. Prognosis should be frankly discussed, and advanced directives elicited when appropriate. This is particularly important for those patients suffering with advanced or end-stage heart failure. Advice should be given to family members with regard to resuscitation efforts should sudden cardiac death syndrome occur. Activity recommendations need to focus on benefits of exercise-based cardiac rehabilitation programs. Recreational, leisure, work, and exercise activities can be frankly addressed, and patients should be encouraged to perform aerobic activities that are symptom limited. Exercise should not necessarily be banned in patients with heart failure. Generally, patients "can do what they can, and can't do what they can't." Dietary recommendations are essential and focus on restriction of salt and excessive fluid intake. Alcohol might be proscribed in certain situations. The effects of medications on quality of life and survival should be frankly addressed, and schemes designed to optimize compliance with treatment and care plans are important. One must emphasize the necessity of taking medications in timely fashion, and it is good practice to provide forms to record medication consumption, pulse rate, blood pressure, and daily weights so that the patient can take an active part in the therapeutic program. One should not ignore the importance of education with regard to atherosclerotic cardiovascular disease risk factor modification. Because ischemic heart disease is the major reason for patients developing heart failure, it makes sense to halt progression of atherosclerosis.

Surgical Therapeutics

When appropriate, surgical therapies can provide dramatic symptomatic relief in patients with congestive heart failure (53,72,74,139). Particularly important is identifying individuals who might benefit from coronary revascularization with percutaneous coronary interventional strategies or coronary artery bypass surgery (74,140,141). ▼ p38

Relatively recently, an innovative surgical procedure has been proposed as an additional treatment option for select patients with advanced heart failure (142). Partial left ventriculectomy (or volume reduction surgery) in patients with severely dilated hearts due to cardiomyopathy may make some patients better. Ventricular remodeling involves removal of a wedge of cardiac tissue from the enlarged heart to relieve myocardial wall stress and reshape the cardiac chamber. This operation is usually performed concomitantly with attempts to reduce mitral and tricuspid valve leakage. However, outcomes after this procedure were not optimal, with only one-third of patients seeing long-term improvements. The operation has largely been abandoned (143,144). On the other hand, resection of myocardial scar tissue or aneurysm formation after myocardial infarction appears to be a more rational procedure in the sense that patients undergoing this later remodeling operation have myocardial scar tissue removed rather than actual muscle (145). More traditional left ventricular aneurysmectomy is effective in select ischemic heart disease patients with significant focal dyskinesia of the left ventricle (particularly when mitral regurgitation is present and substantive). Cardiac transplantation can play an extraordinarily dramatic role in truly end-stage patients without contraindications to this operation. The problem is that donor organ supply is inadequate, and, at best, only 2,000 to 3,000 of these operations can be performed annually around the world. Dynamic cardiomyoplasty is a procedure that involves mobilization of a latissimus dorsi muscle into the chest, wrapping the heart, and then training the skeletal muscle to become fatigue resistant with an electrical stimulating device that is coupled to a pacemaker (146–148). Anecdotal experience suggests that this procedure can effect symptomatic improvement in some class II and III patients and has an acceptable mortality risk. Unfortunately, the cardiac myostimulating device is no longer available. Other even more innovative surgeries include the insertion of a variety of endomyocardial splinting devices and epicardial wraps designed to extrinsically reshape the heart into a more normal configuration. Clinical trials are ongoing with the so-called MyoSplint and Acorn devices (145).

Pharmacotherapeutic Approaches

Figure 92.5 presents an overview algorithm for drug management of patients with heart failure. Again, drug therapy needs to be linked to staging the heart failure syndrome severity and determining whether the problem is due to left ventricular systolic dysfunction or so-called diastolic dysfunction (meaning, generally, that the left ventricular systolic ejection fraction is greater than approximately 45%). At the core of therapy for systolic dysfunction are ACE inhibitors, with digoxin and diuretics added when congestive heart failure is present. Beta-blockers are also critical drugs to use, generally added to the triple-therapy core. Long-acting nitrate preparations may be important for dyspnea relief. If an ACE inhibitor cannot be used because of intolerance or undesirable pharmacologic effects, one should consider the combination of hydralazine and isosorbide dinitrate or, alternatively, angiotensin II receptor blocking agents. As has been repeatedly emphasized, if coronary artery disease is present, consideration of revascularization is important. In patients with atherosclerosis generally, use of lipid-lowering drugs should also be considered. For patients with diastolic dysfunction, treatment options are less well defined. In individuals with congestive heart failure but relative preservation of left ventricular systolic function, one should first attempt to make a diagnosis of an infiltrative cardiomyopathy and base treatment on symptoms. Perhaps the most important drugs in diastolic dysfunction are nitrates and vasodilating agents, with diuretics used to control fluid retention states, but this is contentious. *e*Table 92.5.1 lists alternatives to diuretics, beta-blockers, and ACE inhibitors that might be useful in patients with hypertension or high normal blood pressure who have heart failure associated with either systolic or diastolic left ventricular dysfunction.

Specific Strategies

Diuretics

Long the mainstay of congestive heart failure treatment, diuretics continue to play an important role (136). It is essential, however, that their utility be placed into proper perspective. Diuretics, for example, have never been studied in large-scale mortality trials in patients with heart failure but no overt congestion. There is no question that they are essential agents to relieve the volume-overload states associated with congestive heart failure, but congestion is not necessarily always present in the majority of patients with heart failure. Furthermore, patients may develop congestive states that resolve with pulsed or intermittent diuretic therapy (163,164). As can be seen in *e*Table 92.5.2, substantive difficulties are possible, including hyponatremia, hypokalemia, metabolic alkalosis, and increased uric acid levels, setting the stage for overt gout or worsening renal function. Carbohydrate metabolism is frequently disturbed, with resultant hyperglycemia, insulin resistance, decreased insulin secretion, and nonketotic hyperosmolar states. Lipid perturbation is also a problem, but its significance is not well understood. Diuretic-specific side effects include the ototoxicity of furosemide, gynecomastia, and galactorrhea with spironolactone, metabolic acidosis caused by carbonic anhydrase inhibitors, and hyperkalemia caused by potassium-sparing diuretics, such as triamterene, spironolactone, and amiloride. When treating congestive heart failure, generally the least toxic drug (thiazides, such as hydrochlorothiazide or chlorthalidone) is prescribed in the lowest dose necessary to induce effective diuresis (*e*Table 92.5.3). As congestion worsens, longer-acting loop diuretics (such as furosemide, bumetanide, or torsemide) are prescribed.

Occasionally, for particularly refractory edematous states, combinations of diuretic classes may be necessary. It should be emphasized that failure to mobilize salt and water is often due to inadequate sodium and fluid restriction, particularly in individuals recently diuresed and at risk of rebound sodium retention. Ensuring low sodium consumption is essential to success with these compounds. Acute resistance is generally overcome with an increased single diuretic dose. Chronic resistance can be addressed with the coadministration of thiazide or potassium-sparing diuretics with a loop diuretic. Using combinations of agents active at different points of the nephron is essential. From a pharmacokinetic standpoint, overcoming diuretic resistance by simply increasing diuretic dose is important. Altered bioavailability may account for some aspects of diuretic resistance, and there are different absorption kinetics associated with furosemide, bumetanide, and torsemide. Switching among these oral loop diuretics may be helpful. Alternatively, giving diuretics intravenously may accomplish the same end point.

It must be remembered that by reducing blood volume, diuretics lower cardiac filling pressures, with subsequent reduction in wall stress, pulmonary edema, and peripheral congestion. All these effects are advantageous, but reduction in plasma volume might adversely activate the renin-angiotensin-aldosterone and sympathetic nervous systems, paradoxically promoting further sodium and water retention while increasing impedance to left ventricular ejection. This effect could eventually contribute to the progression of heart failure remodeling. For this reason, diuretic therapy alone is not justified during heart failure treatment. The one exception might be the use of diuretics for treatment of hypertension (165,166). Long-term studies assessing major disease-specific outcomes in hypertensive patients receiving diuretics have demonstrated reduction in the incidence of stroke, congestive heart failure, coronary disease, and total mortality. This should be contrasted to outcomes noted with calcium channel blockers, which are meager with respect to similar benefits in hypertensives. Beta-blocker therapy in hypertensive patients is also effective in preventing stroke and congestive heart failure. When used primarily as antihypertensive agents or as adjuncts to control blood pressure, diuretics likely provide substantial benefits (166). Still, compulsive attention to the serum electrolyte profile is necessary. ▼ p39

Angiotensin-Converting Enzyme Inhibitors

As might be anticipated from reviewing heart failure clinical trials (*e*Table 92.4.1 and Figs. 92.1 and 92.2), ACE inhibitors have now assumed the role of first-line drug in patients with heart failure. The reason for this is their multifactorial benefits, including interdiction of the renin-angiotensin-aldosterone system and balanced arterial and venous vasodilation. Significantly, a broad spectrum of heart failure patients have been studied with respect to ACE inhibitor use. Clinical trials that included asymptomatic patients with systolic left ventricular dysfunction (e.g., SOLVD prevention trial) (87) as well as extremely ill NYHA class IV congestive heart failure patients (e.g., CONSENSUS) (83) justify their use in such a wide spectrum. Every effort must be made to get patients with heart failure on a drug of this class at a proper dose. *e*Table 92.5.3 lists selective ACE inhibitors that have been evaluated extensively with mortality endpoint clinical trials so that the proper target dosages can be defined. It is important to remember that many smaller double-blind, placebo-controlled clinical trials have demonstrated the ability of ACE inhibitors to relieve dyspnea, improve exercise tolerance, and decrease the incidence of hospitalization for patients with mild to moderate heart failure. Furthermore, these drugs appear to prevent development of symptomatic congestive heart failure in many patients with asymptomatic left ventricular systolic dysfunction. In patients without symptoms, ACE inhibitors should be considered first-line drug therapy (even as monotherapy), with digoxin, diuretics, and possibly beta-blockers becoming important additive components as congestive symptoms develop. Although the beneficial effects of ACE inhibitors are likely related to "class" actions, regulatory labeling has been based on the types of clinical trials performed. For example, some agents have been suggested as useful in the postinfarct setting, and others have been given labeling approbation for mortality as well as morbidity reduction in heart failure patients. *e*Table 92.5.4 describes a reasonable ACE I dose-titration sequence for hospitalized patients. The prescription of these drugs in dosages similar to those used during clinical trial performance and in similar patient populations appears to be important (144). It has been suggested, for example, that underdosing of captopril is common. This may be fueled by fear of causing unacceptable reduction in blood pressure or worsening renal function. As discussed previously, defining optimal blood pressure in patients with ventricular dysfunction and heart failure is a contentious issue, and no precise target pressure can easily be identified. It appears, however, that the lowest blood pressure a patient can tolerate without significant orthostatic symptoms or renal dysfunction is the best in any specific clinical setting. *e*Table 92.5.4 proposes a schema for initiating ACE inhibitor therapy when patients are hospitalized with substantive congestive states. This schema is based on using the shorter-acting agent captopril acutely and avoiding it during aggressive diuretic administration. Although low doses are used initially, higher doses should be mandated (171). After patients have been exposed to the short-acting drug, switching to a longer-acting preparation such as enalapril or lisinopril seems reasonable so that compliance can be increased by decreasing multiple dosing points. Reasonable target dosages are 150 mg daily for captopril, 20 mg daily for enalapril, and 20 mg for lisinopril. Patients who are at

risk for developing orthostatic hypotension after ACE inhibitor exposure include those with hyponatremia, azotemia, volume depletion, and orthostatic dizziness or syncope (172,173). Problems can be avoided with simple dosage adjustment techniques or reduction of aggressive diuretic therapies. It is important to remember ACE inhibitors are likely more important than diuretics in the heart failure patient long term, and therefore, when congestive states are relieved, it is more appropriate to sacrifice diuretic administration so that ACE inhibitors can be begun or maintained rather than continuing high diuretic dosages (or continuing diuretics at all). Still, ACE inhibitors can be challenging to administer. In the SOLVD study analysis of adverse effects of enalapril in 6,797 patients (double-blinded and placebo-controlled) followed over a 40-month average period, 28% of participants randomized to drug compared with 16% in the placebo group reported side effects (172). Enalapril use was associated with a higher rate of orthostatic hypotension (15% vs. 7%), azotemia (4% vs. 2%), cough (5% vs. 2%), fatigue (6% vs. 4%), and hyperkalemia (1.2% vs. 0.4%). All these observations were statistically significant. Angioedema occurred in 0.4% of patients exposed to the ACE inhibitor. Side effects resulted in discontinuation of blinded therapy in 15% of the treatment group compared with 9% in the placebo group. One must put the benefits of ACE inhibitors in perspective, however, and stopping the drug for a mild but troublesome cough might not be in the best long-term interests of the heart failure patient.

More recently, attention has been directed toward the question of differential effects of drugs based on race. Indeed, African-American patients with heart failure seemingly have a worse prognosis than Caucasians. To address this issue with respect to ACE inhibitors, an analysis of the SOLVD database has been published (174). Using a matched cohort design in which up to four white patients were matched with each black patient, a total of 1,196 white patients were compared with 800 black patients. The average duration of follow-up was approximately 34 months. The black and white patients had similar demographic and clinical characteristics, but the black patients had higher rates of death from any cause (12 vs. 10 per 100 person-years of follow-up) and of hospitalization for heart failure (13 vs. 8 per 100 person-years of follow-up). Despite similar doses of drug in the two groups, enalapril therapy, as compared with placebo, was associated with a 44% reduction (95% confidence interval, 27% to 57%) in the risk of hospitalization for heart failure among the white patients (*p* <.001), but with no significant reduction among black patients (*p* = .74). At 1 year, enalapril therapy was associated with significant reductions from baseline and systolic blood pressure and diastolic blood pressure among the white but not among the black patients. No significant change in the risk of death was observed in association with enalapril therapy in either group. The conclusion of this study was that enalapril therapy is associated with a significant reduction in the risk of hospitalization for heart failure among white patients with left ventricular dysfunction, but not among similar black patients. It is important, however, to note that this observation simply underscores the need for additional research on the efficacy of therapies for heart failure in black patients. It does not mean that ACE inhibitors should not be prescribed in this cohort. Furthermore, it must be pointed out that this was a retrospective analysis that was not prespecified. Furthermore, this type of observation has not been recapitulated with at least one beta-blocker, carvedilol, in clinical trials (see Beta-Adrenergic Blocking Agents, later in this chapter).

Angiotensin II Receptor Blockers

An alternative to ACE inhibitors might be a specific angiotensin II receptor antagonist (146,147). Such drugs might induce similar benefits to those observed in heart failure patients on ACE inhibitors, without some of the side effects seen with these agents (172,173,176). On the other hand, these compounds do not affect potentially beneficial cyclooxygenase pathways, which are activated by ACE inhibitors (176). Small clinical trials have demonstrated that the first commercially available angiotensin II receptor blocking agent, losartan, when given to patients with symptomatic heart failure, produced beneficial hemodynamic effects in the short term as well as after 12 weeks of therapy (173). There was a dose-related response, with 50 mg daily of losartan effecting the most significant changes, but higher doses likely not helpful. Hemodynamic effects are similar to ACE inhibitors with respect to reducing preload and afterload and increasing cardiac output. Furthermore, these agents are effective in preventing left ventricular hypertrophy in animals.

The first large-scale clinical trial with mortality endpoint data to give some insight into use of specific angiotensin II receptor blockade in patients with heart failure was the Evaluation of Losartan in the Elderly study (177,178). This multicenter, international clinical trial was a prospective, double-blind, randomized, parallel-group, captopril-controlled study performed in 722 ACE I–naïve patients (1:1 group randomization) age 65 years or older (66% older than 70 years) with mild to moderately symptomatic heart failure (primarily NYHA class II and III) and left ventricular ejection fraction of 40% or less. Mean ejection fraction was approximately 30%, and patients primarily had heart failure due to coronary heart disease (68%). The primary end point was development of renal dysfunction after drug titration, defined as an increase in serum creatinine by 0.3 mg per dL from baseline. Secondary end points were combined mortality from all causes and heart failure hospitalization and mortality and hospitalizations for heart failure individually. Tertiary end points included drug tolerability and focused on symptomatic hypotension, potassium

increase (greater than 0.5 mmol per L), cough, or other side effects prompting drug discontinuation. Drug administration protocol gives some insight into losartan dosing. After a 2-week placebo run-in, patients received either captopril (6.25 mg titrated to 12.5 mg, 25 mg, and then 50 mg three times daily) or losartan (12.5 mg titrated to 25 mg and then 50 mg daily). Dose increases generally occurred at 7-day intervals, as tolerated. Patients were followed for 48 weeks. The incidence of persistent renal dysfunction was the same (10.5%) in losartan and captopril cohorts. Losartan did appear to be better tolerated in this trial, with 27 patients stopping captopril because of dysgeusia, rash, or angioneurotic edema compared with none in the losartan group. It is interesting that the secondary mortality end point (composite of death and heart failure hospital admissions) demonstrated less all-cause mortality in the losartan group. This benefit was observed early and persisted throughout the 48-week observation period. This study prompted the Evaluation of Losartan in the Elderly II trial, which was a larger clinical trial having mortality as the primary end point (179,180). In contrast to Evaluation of Losartan in the Elderly trial, the second trial had no beneficial effect on mortality according to initial data analysis.

Still, the hypothesis that angiotensin II receptor antagonists might be beneficial in heart failure is intriguing because ACE activity may not be completely suppressed by traditional ACE I therapy because angiotensin II can also be formed by non-ACE or tissue chymase-dependent pathways (181–183). The more complete blockade of angiotensin II activity is theoretically more beneficial, but one reason to think these drugs might not be as effective as ACE I in heart failure is their lack of effect on bradykinin. As alluded to previously, bradykinin actions seem related to nitric oxide, and prostacyclin release, which may mediate vasodilation, is thought to be beneficial in these patients. On the other hand, bradykinin might account for some of the ACE I adverse reactions, such as cough, angioneurotic edema, and dysgeusia (173,175). Losartan could therefore provide more complete blockade of the tissue-active ACE systems without increasing bradykinin, which, in addition to being associated with certain mediators of vasodilation, can also precipitate norepinephrine spill.

Other studies addressing angiotensin II receptor blocking drugs in heart failure include the RESOLVD, Valsartan Heart Failure Trial, and Candesartan in Heart Failure—Assessment of Reduction in Mortality and Morbidity projects. RESOLVD focused on candesartan and was a double-blind (pilot) study (with 768 patients) in which congestive heart failure patients were randomized to candesartan in several doses, candesartan plus enalapril, or enalapril, for a mean of 43 weeks with exercise tolerance, ventricular function, quality of life, neurohormone levels, and tolerability of drug treatment protocol as end points (184). No differences were noted in exercise, functional class, or quality of life measurements, but left ventricular volumes decreased with natriuretic peptide and aldosterone levels significantly lower with the combination of an ACE inhibitor and angiotensin II receptor blocking drug. Perhaps more important was the fact that candesartan was as effective, safe, and tolerable as enalapril in congestive heart failure patients, with seemingly more beneficial effects when the drugs were combined than when used alone.

A second RESOLVD report details the addition of long-acting metoprolol to ACE inhibitors and candesartan (105). In this portion of the RESOLVD pilot program, metoprolol-CR was given in double-blind factorial designed fashion after the initial uptitration of candesartan or enalapril or their combination in 426 patients. The primary reason for this trial was to determine tolerability of extensive neurohormonal blockade with the combination of an ACE inhibitor, angiotensin II receptor blocker, and beta-blocker. No differences in exercise, functional class, or quality of life were noted between any of the groups, but significant improvement of left ventricular systolic function and attenuation of detrimental remodeling with a greater decrease of angiotensin II and renin levels was noted when metoprolol was added. Particularly impressive was the reduction in heart size and improvement in left ventricular systolic dysfunction in the group receiving an ACE inhibitor, candesartan, and the beta-blocker metoprolol.

Exploring the potential for added benefit with an angiotensin II receptor blocking drug was the Valsartan Heart Failure Trial (185). This study was a double-blind, placebo-controlled multicenter clinical trial of valsartan generally added onto an ACE inhibitor (92% of patients concomitantly on ACE inhibitors) with approximately 35% of the population on beta-blockers. All-cause mortality and combined mortality and morbidity were end points in this trial of over 5,000 patients. Results were preliminarily reported at the November 2000 American Heart Association meeting. This was the largest angiotensin II receptor blocking drug trial reported to date, and no mortality reduction was noted. Patients were, however, less likely to be hospitalized for worsening congestive heart failure when taking valsartan. Interestingly, perhaps there was an adverse interaction with patients on both ACE inhibitors and beta-blockers when valsartan was added. This is somewhat at odds with the previously summarized RESOLVD beta-blocker observations. We will have to await further clarification of this issue.

Perhaps the Candesartan in Heart Failure—Assessment of Reduction in Mortality and Morbidity program will help resolve some of these issues (186). Candesartan in Heart Failure—Assessment of Reduction in Mortality and Morbidity is actually three independent international parallel placebo-controlled mortality endpoint trials of candesartan in patients with congestive heart failure. The first trial of over 2,300 patients is in patients with left ventricular systolic ejection fraction less than 40% and treated with concomitant ACE inhibitors. The second trial is in patients with a similar degree of left ventricular systolic dysfunction

but deemed "ACE intolerant." Almost 2,000 patients will be entered into this trial. Finally, a third trial of over 2,500 patients will evaluate candesartan in individuals with congestive heart failure and ejection fraction greater than 40%. This program obviously will be testing the angiotensin II receptor blocking agent candesartan across the broad spectrum of chronic congestive heart failure and is the only ongoing trial of these agents evaluating this strategy in ACE-intolerant and "diastolic dysfunction" heart failure patients.

Calcium Channel Antagonists

Calcium channel blockers, as a group, are an example of agents that may create significant problems in patients with heart failure. Although these drugs are very effective in lowering systemic vascular resistance, they generally have negative inotropic effects. Granted, newer drugs in this class seem to have less negative inotropic activity and more potent selective peripheral vasodilatory effects. Still, to date, no sustaining symptomatic or mortality benefit, overall, has been demonstrated for these drugs when used in patients with congestive heart failure. At best, effects seem to be neutral for a few select compounds (amlodipine and felodipine) (85,86). Indeed, in patients who have had acute myocardial infarction complicated by left ventricular systolic dysfunction, calcium channel blockers have proved detrimental more often than not, with a greater chance of adverse effects seen in patients randomized to drugs such as nifedipine and diltiazem. Because patients with heart failure frequently have concomitant ischemic heart disease or hypertension, calcium channel blockers are frequently found as therapies in heart failure patients. Indeed, in the late 1980s, more patients in the SOLVD registry were on calcium channel blockers than on ACE inhibitors (47). Although this has changed somewhat more recently, it has been suggested that significant numbers of patients with heart failure (probably around 20%) are still taking these drugs. This strategy might best be reassessed on an individual patient basis. In the patient with heart failure, for example, control of hypertension with ACE inhibitors, diuretics, beta-blockers, angiotensin II receptor blockers, or other agents summarized in Table 92.6 may be preferred strategies. Treatment of angina pectoris with nitrates can be considered a substitute for treatment with calcium channel blockers. It should also be emphasized that, although ACE inhibitors are not acutely antiischemic in their actions, clinical trials have consistently demonstrated long-term diminution in major atherosclerotic heart disease end points (187,188). Patients with heart failure and angina pectoris should have aggressive attempts at percutaneous or surgical revascularization or medication therapies refocused on long-acting nitrates and beta-blockers.

To date, amlodipine (85) and felodipine (86) have been the only two agents studied with reasonably designed clinical trials to suggest no detriment with the drugs. Because of

TABLE 92.6 COMMON PITFALLS IN THE TREATMENT OF HEART FAILURE: FACTORS PREDISPOSING TO HEART FAILURE DECOMPENSATION

Inadequate syndrome recognition
   Symptoms unrelated to cardiac dysfunction
   Treating late in the course of the illness
Ignoring underlying disease state
   Not correcting areas of reversible myocardial ischemia
   Not considering patients for standard (although higher risk) surgical procedures, such as valve repair or replacement or aneurysmectomy
   Unrecognized hypothyroidism or hyperthyroidism
   Poorly controlled diabetes mellitus
   Inadequate control of hypertension
   Not treating dyslipidemia
   Not treating chronic obstructive pulmonary disease
   Not considering possibility of cardiac metastasis in malignancies
Not recognizing or not treating certain comorbidities
   Intercurrent infections uncontrolled
   Hypoventilation (sleep apnea syndromes) not addressed
Patient-related difficulties
   Poor compliance with drug treatment protocols
   Inadequate salt and water restriction
   Excessive alcohol consumption
   Cigarette smoking
   Ponderosity
   Cardiovascular deconditioning
Pharmacotherapeutic issues
   Inadequate ACE inhibitor therapy (or drug not begun)
   Not trying beta-blocker
   Suboptimal doses of vasodilators, ACE inhibitors, beta-blockers
   Ineffective diuretic prescription
   Excessive diuresis
   Discontinuation of digoxin in stable congestive heart failure patients
   Downtitration of ACE inhibitor instead of diuretics for hypotension or azotemia
   Concomitant use of potentially harmful medications (certain antiarrhythmics, nonsteroidal antiinflammatory drugs, beta-blockers, or calcium channel antagonists in certain circumstances)
Other treatment concerns and pitfalls
   Administration of anthracyclines
   Not evaluating, correcting, or controlling atrial fibrillation
   Inappropriate drug treatment of certain ventricular arrhythmias
   Not considering pacemaker therapies for chronotropic incompetence (or "cardiac resynchronization")
   Not preventing or treating hypokalemia, hypomagnesemia, hyponatremia
   Salt or fluid administration parenteral or orthostatic hypotension or hyponatremia
   Failure to use hemodynamic monitoring to resolve confusing or challenging situations

ACE, angiotensin-converting enzyme.

the importance of this issue, details of these two studies should be reviewed. The PRAISE (74) trial randomly assigned 1,153 patients with severe chronic congestive heart failure (NYHA class III or IV) and ejection fraction less than 30% to either placebo or amlodipine for 6 to 33 months, while their usual therapy (digoxin, diuretics, and ACE inhibitors) was continued. Prerandomization stratification occurred based on a diagnosis of ischemic versus nonischemic heart disease etiology. Primary end point was all-cause mortality and hospitalization for major cardiovascular events. The primary end point was reached in 42% of placebo and 39% of the amlodipine group, an insignificant 9% reduction in the combined mortality and morbidity events ($p = .07$). In coronary artery disease patients, there was no difference between the amlodipine and placebo groups in the occurrence of a prior end point. On the other hand, among patients with nonischemic heart failure, amlodipine reduced the combined risk of fatal and nonfatal events by 31% ($p = .04$) and the risk of death by 46% ($p < .001$). Amlodipine, therefore, did not increase cardiovascular morbidity or mortality in patients with symptomatic and relatively severe heart failure and may actually decrease mortality in patients with nonischemic dilated cardiomyopathy. PRAISE II is critically evaluating this specific issue. V-HeFT-III (75) studied 451 male patients with NYHA class II or III symptoms, with chest radiographic cardiothoracic ratio greater than 0.66, echocardiographic left ventricular internal diastolic diameter greater than 2.7 cm per m², and ejection fraction less than 45%. Background therapy was enalapril. Patients were randomized in factorial fashion to digoxin or placebo and then to felodipine or placebo. The cohort mean age was 63 years, approximately 53% had coronary heart disease accounting for their heart failure, and the mean ejection fraction was 30%. At the end of the 18-month follow-up period, total mortality was 31 deaths in the felodipine and 29 in the placebo groups ($p = NS$). Cardiovascular mortality also was not significantly different. Subgroup (coronary artery disease vs. nonischemic, NYHA class II or III, ejection fraction greater or less than 30%, norepinephrine levels, exercise time, or digoxin use) mortality risk ratios did not suggest that any particular set was benefited or harmed by felodipine. At the 27-week follow-up point, ejection fraction was significantly increased by felodipine compared with placebo, as was exercise time. The group on felodipine noted a decrease in atrial natriuretic peptide levels compared with placebo. In the early dosing phase, felodipine seemed associated with worsening heart failure. Conclusions from this trial are that felodipine, in ACE inhibitor–treated patients with mild to moderate heart failure, improves left ventricular function and certain humoral factors but does not produce any apparent effect on long-term morbidity or mortality. Although the small number of deaths in V-HeFT-III does not exclude an increase or decrease of mortality from felodipine, the overall experience suggests that this drug may be safe when used for other indications in mild to moderate heart failure. Still, this conclusion has to be balanced by the fact that these other conditions are usually hypertension or angina pectoris. There are many alternative strategies. It is interesting that the observations in V-HeFT-III were somewhat discordant with those of PRAISE in that no mortality benefit was seen in nonischemic veteran patients. Possible explanations for this difference include the fact that PRAISE enrolled NYHA class III and IV patients, whereas V-HeFT-III enrolled class II and III subjects and turned out to be underpowered with respect to mortality end points (too few events occurred). Other explanations might be that the nonischemic stratification scheme was flawed (no stress test was done in PRAISE to exclude ischemia, and neither study required coronary angiography). Alternatively, one could postulate that the PRAISE subgroup finding was a chance occurrence or that amlodipine really is quite different from felodipine.

Antiarrhythmic Drugs and Implantable Defibrillating Devices

One of the more difficult issues to address in patients with heart failure is how to treat arrhythmia. The incidence of atrial and ventricular dysrhythmia in this patient population is high, and the temptation to use antiarrhythmic drugs is great. As indicated, class I antiarrhythmic agents are problematic in patients exhibiting clinical heart failure, particularly in the setting of an acute myocardial infarction. As reviewed, the Cardiac Arrhythmia Suppression Trial and Survival with Oral D-Sotalol trials (*e*Table 92.4.1) indicated that encainide, flecainide, moricizine, and D-sotalol actually increased mortality. These observations are troublesome because the patient at highest risk of sudden cardiac death seems to be the individual who would benefit most from arrhythmia control. However, this is also the patient likely to have proarrhythmic events associated with antiarrhythmic drug prescription. Indeed, there is a fairly clear-cut relationship between ejection fraction and antiarrhythmic drug efficacy, as well as a direct relationship between heart failure severity and adverse proarrhythmic effects with most compounds. The lower the ejection fraction, the less likely potent antiarrhythmic drugs are to control potentially malignant arrhythmias. Beta-blockers and amiodarone may be possible exceptions to this generalization, but clinical trials have produced disparate results. Amiodarone use is, indeed, more controversial (197–201). Amiodarone does seem to be a valuable adjunct during therapy for atrial fibrillation. Unfortunately, amiodarone is expensive and sometimes poorly tolerated, with toxicities that include pulmonary fibrosis, thyroid function disorders, and photosensitization syndromes. It is intriguing, however, to note that low-dose amiodarone may be better tolerated and still have apparently beneficial hemodynamic effects (199). Indeed, any beneficial effects amiodarone may have in the heart failure syndrome might be independent of antiarrhythmic drug action.

Because antiarrhythmic drug therapy has been so problematic in the heart failure patient, use of implantable electronic arrhythmic termination devices may be preferable in patients with potentially malignant ventricular arrhythmias

and heart failure. Still, however, it should be realized that many patients who have these devices continue to be on antiarrhythmic therapies. A relatively recently completed clinical trial has given some insight into this issue. The Multicenter Automatic Defibrillator Implantation Trial (202) was a randomized trial of defibrillating devices versus conventional therapy in post–myocardial infarction patients with ejection fraction less than 35%, nonsustained ventricular tachycardia, and then nonsuppressible ventricular tachycardia at the time of electrophysiologic study. This trial suggested that device implantation led to better survival in this high-risk atherosclerotic cardiovascular disease population with ventricular dysfunction and heart failure. Beta-blockers and amiodarone use did not appear to have a significant effect on the risk reduction ratio in patients assigned to the device group.

Several additional clinical trials have prospectively evaluated the value of antiarrhythmic drugs or defibrillating devices in a setting of ischemic heart failure (coronary heart disease with an ejection fraction of less than 40%) and ventricular tachycardia. Three secondary prevention trials have suggested that an implantable cardioverter defibrillator was superior to antiarrhythmic drugs (generally amiodarone) in reducing mortality. Some have argued that the major benefit of implantable defibrillating devices occurred in those with lower ejection fractions. The Antiarrhythmics vs. Implantable Defibrillators Trial (203), the Canadian Implantable Defibrillator Study (204), and Cardiac Arrest Study—Hamburg trial (205) were secondary prevention trials and should be compared with the Multicenter Automatic Defibrillator Implantation Trial discussed previously and an additional primary prevention trial, Multicenter Unsustained Tachycardia Trial (206).

These observations provide an alternative strategy for treatment of selective patients with heart failure and life-threatening arrhythmias. It must be emphasized that often the best treatment of ventricular arrhythmias in the heart failure milieu is careful attention to relieving the congestive state and optimizing ventricular performance with vasodilators, diuretics, and ACE inhibitors. Correction of fluid balance and electrolyte disorders may be quite helpful. Addressing atrial fibrillation in heart failure is also sometimes critical to improving patients' symptoms. Obviously, care must be taken in these patients to ensure that risk of thromboembolism is as low as possible with anticoagulants. Because of the known adverse outcome of heart failure patients treated with Vaughn Williams class I antiarrhythmic drugs, consideration of the relative risk of using quinidine, procainide, and other similar agents is challenging.

Indeed, it should be emphasized that the American College of Cardiology/American Heart Association guidelines regarding heart failure therapeutics caution against aggressive pharmacologic or mechanical treatment of asymptomatic ventricular arrhythmias (53). To consider either pharmacologic strategies or implantation of arrhythmia-termination devices, patients should have significantly symptomatic ventricular tachycardia (not simply palpitations) or an episode of syncope or sudden cardiac death syndrome.

Ventricular Resynchronization

Because patients with heart failure, systolic left ventricular dysfunction, and wide QRS complexes have dyssynergic contractility, using multisite atrial right and left ventricular pacing strategies has been proposed. So-called biventricular cardiac resynchronization pacing for heart failure is being actively studied, with some trials focusing solely on resynchronization pacing for severe congestive heart failure [Multicenter InSync Randomization Clinical Evaluation (North America); *e*Table 92.4.1], whereas others include defibrillator insertion or antiarrhythmic therapies (Sudden Cardiac Death–Heart Failure Trial, Multicenter InSync Randomization Clinical Evaluation Implantable Cardioverter Defibrillator; *e*Table 92.4.1). Some trials are secondary prevention studies (secondary prevention with heart failure treatment) or primary sudden cardiac death prevention (primary sudden cardiac death prevention with heart failure therapy). Completion of these studies will clarify best strategies regarding defibrillator implantation or coupling defibrillator implantation to resynchronization pacing therapeutics. More recently published data do, however, suggest that patient quality of life and exercise capacity are improved with resynchronization mode pacing. The Multisite Stimulation Cardiomyopathy Trial was the first such study to be reported (207). Particularly interesting is the fact that patients appear to have reduction in mitral regurgitation when undergoing biventricular pacing.

Anticoagulants

Routine anticoagulation in patients with heart failure may not be necessary (75). Patients with substantive congestive heart failure frequently have significant hepatic congestion, and, because of this, anticoagulation can be difficult to achieve safely. Furthermore, with the large number of drugs taken by patients with heart failure (Figs. 92.1 and 92.2), an important tenet is to continue only those medications with demonstrated effectiveness. This practice helps ensure compliance with drug treatment regimens. Routine anticoagulation in heart failure patients has never been convincingly demonstrated to be beneficial in well-designed clinical trials despite the fact that heart failure patients have relative hypercoagulable states (208). Some studies have suggested a lower incidence of pulmonary and peripheral emboli in patients on warfarin (209), but, on the whole, the data are not overwhelmingly persuasive. It may be prudent to anticoagulate heart failure patients with a history of systemic or pulmonary embolism or when left or right ventricular thrombi are noted on echocardiography. Certainly, atrial fibrillation is a clear-cut indication for careful anticoagulation. Candidates for anticoagulation should be monitored carefully, with a goal of achieving an international normalization ratio for prothrombin times of 2 to 4.

PITFALLS IN TREATING HEART FAILURE

Table 92.6 lists many of the common pitfalls that trap clinicians when evaluating and treating heart failure patients. Inadequate recognition of the syndrome, or symptoms that are related not to cardiac dysfunction but to other conditions, makes any therapeutic adventure a challenge. Starting late in a patient's disease course makes failure to beneficially affect long-term morbidity and mortality more likely. A focus on preventive therapeutics is necessary. Ignoring the patient's underlying disease state and focusing only on symptomatic elements of heart failure sets the stage for recurring difficulties. Granted, some disease processes, such as advanced ischemic heart disease, are difficult to ameliorate. However, it is a mistake to not consider therapies to reverse myocardial ischemia. Obviously, unrecognized hyperthyroidism, hypothyroidism, poorly controlled diabetes mellitus, and inadequate control of hypertension contribute to making the heart failure state worse. Atrial arrhythmias can be quite problematic, and an attempt should be made, if at all possible, to keep patients in normal sinus rhythm. Chronotropic incompetence or certain arrhythmias might respond to pacemaker therapy. Inadequate salt and water restriction sets the stage for hyponatremia, hypokalemia, and dropsical states despite aggressive diuretic use. Excessive alcohol consumption, particularly in patients with dilated cardiomyopathy, is likely harmful and can contribute to worsening heart failure states. Concomitant use of potentially harmful medications (such as Vaughn Williams class I antiarrhythmic drugs and nonsteroidal antiinflammatory agents) might be part of a therapeutic protocol and should be stopped, if possible. Excessive intravascular volume depletion with diuretics can be counterproductive by producing orthostatic symptoms and further activating adverse neurohumoral factors important in the pathophysiology of heart failure. On the opposite side of this spectrum is ineffective diuretic prescription, which does not mobilize fluid adequately: diuretic doses that are too low, combinations that are not rational (e.g., combining two loop diuretics, such as furosemide and torsemide), or failure to switch from oral to parenteral diuretic administration when necessary. Use of inadequate ACE inhibitor doses or failure to start ACE inhibitor therapy is a major difficulty. Every attempt should be made to get patients on target ACE inhibitor doses, and, rather than sacrificing the ACE inhibitor in an aggressively diuresed patient, the diuretic dose should be decreased. Likewise, use of suboptimal doses of vasodilators because of "relative hypotension" can produce a clinical scenario in which high afterload negatively affects cardiac systolic performance.

Sometimes we see the reflex prescription of parenteral salt solutions for orthostatic hypotension or hyponatremia. A cycle of aggressive diuretic administration, low blood pressure, parenteral fluid administration, then congestion often develops in hospitalized patients, and this is counterproductive to appropriate long-term therapy. Only patients with shock and clear-cut intravascular volume depletion should have volume-expanding fluids administered. It is best to allow hyponatremia to correct on its own, with salt and water restriction and, possibly, concomitant parenteral loop diuretic administration. Orthostatic hypotension generally responds to bed rest with a reduction in diuretics or, possibly, vasodilators. When the situation becomes confusing and volume status is difficult to clinically assess, failure to use hemodynamic monitoring simply perpetuates the inability to resolve the challenging situation. Ponderosity with cardiovascular deconditioning and poorly compliant patients are difficult situations, but sometimes aggressive counseling and cardiac rehabilitation programs help to ameliorate these challenges. Because of the cytokine liberation that infections produce, not recognizing or treating intercurrent infections in patients with heart failure allows the syndrome to worsen. Furthermore, some difficulties, such as hypoventilation sleep apnea syndromes, when treated with theophylline preparations or nocturnal positive pressure breathing devices, dramatically improve the heart failure syndrome. This is particularly the case in individuals with pulmonary hypertension and right-sided heart failure.

CONSIDERATIONS DURING IMPLEMENTATION OF HEART FAILURE TREATMENT GUIDELINES

Table 92.7 summarizes important issues to consider when initiating heart failure therapy. Assuming that the proper diagnosis has been made, etiology identified, and precipitating causes of clinical decompensation eliminated, clinicians can strive to create effective therapeutic programs. With regard to institution of ACE inhibitor therapy, one must assess and intermittently reassess volume status if unacceptable hypotension or azotemia is present. Decreasing ACE inhibitor dose or adjusting the use of diuretic therapies often allows uptitration of the ACE inhibitor so that optimal doses can be taken. One should use a target dose strategy. These ACE inhibitor doses were chosen for evaluation in the many clinical trials carried out in heart failure populations. When patients are hyponatremic, ACE inhibitor–naïve, azotemic, or have

TABLE 92.7 ISSUES TO CONSIDER WHEN INITIATING HEART FAILURE THERAPY

ACE inhibitor therapy	Vasodilator therapy	Diuretic therapy	Digoxin therapy	Beta-blocker therapy
Reassess volume if unacceptable decreased blood pressure or increased blood urea nitrogen-creatinine ratio; if patient volume depleted, hold ACE inhibitor dose at that which is tolerated and decrease diuretic. Use "target" dose strategy to achieve ACE inhibitor doses used in clinical trial protocols. Adding long-acting dinitrate or mononitrate preparations often helps control dyspnea syndromes. Slow the uptitration protocol when patient is hyponatremic, ACE inhibitor naive, azotemic, or recently aggressively diuresed. Monitoring and therapy for Mg^{2+} <1.8 mg/dL, K^+ <3.5 or >5.5 mEq/dL, Na^+ <135 mEq/dL, creatinine >3.0 mg/dL. Monitor for rash, angioneurotic edema, severe cough (harsh involuntary bark in the absence of congestion), worsening renal function.	Particularly useful with elevated blood pressure and in settings of mitral regurgitation. Pulmonary hypertension may respond to long-acting nitrate therapy. Nitrate patches should not be used in continuous fashion. Patients with paroxysmal nocturnal dyspnea may benefit greatly from long-acting nitrates at bedtime.	Use in the congested patients. Consider pulsed or intermittent therapy. Elderly require lower doses. Start with lowest effective dose. Combine different classes for added effect. Monitoring and therapy for Mg^{2+} <1.8 mg/dL, K^+ <3.5 or >5.5 mEq/dL, Na^+ <135 mEq/dL, creatinine >3.0 mg/dL. Couple with Na^+ and free water restriction. Watch for hyponatremia. Rapid diuresis will require electrolyte replenishment.	Use low doses. Obtain digoxin level if renal function deteriorates or toxicity suspected (nausea, anorexia, confusion, visual disturbances, arrhythmia). Serial of frequent digoxin levels not necessary. Hypokalemia enhances toxicity. Monitoring and therapy for Mg^{2+} <1.8 mg/dL, K^+ <3.5 or >5.5 mEq/dL, Na^+ <135 mEq/dL, creatinine >3.0 mg/dL.	Strongly consider post–myocardial infarction and all stable congestive heart failure. Start when patient not congested. Nonselective agents with vasodilating effects may be preferred (but this is not yet clear). Metoprolol is $beta_1$-selective agent used frequently. Start with low doses and titrate slowly to target over many weeks (carvedilol, 6.25 mg q.d. to 25–50 mg b.i.d.; metoprolol, 12.5 mg q.d. to 100 mg b.i.d. or 200 mg q.d.). Short-term, many deteriorate; but long-term patients generally improve.

ACE, angiotensin-converting enzyme.

recently been diuresed aggressively, slow upward titration of drug after starting with low doses is reasonable. Serum magnesium levels should be kept above 1.8 mg per dL, potassium levels between 3.5 and 5.5 mEq per dL, sodium greater than 135 mEq per L, and creatinine greater than 3.0 mg per dL if at all possible. Administering magnesium often helps to control hypokalemia. One should monitor patients for development of rash, angioneurotic edema, worsening renal function, and severe cough, which can be blamed on the ACE inhibitor use. This troublesome cough is frequently described as a harsh involuntary bark in the absence of congestion. One must be cautious about the inappropriate discontinuation of the ACE inhibitor, however, because many patients cough due to pulmonary hypertension, pulmonary congestion, or chronic obstructive pulmonary disease that accompanies the heart failure syndrome. It may be inappropriate to discontinue the ACE inhibitor for the latter reasons. Rather, attention to ameliorating these difficulties seems more appropriate. Often, when patients are told of the importance of ACE inhibitor effects, they are willing to continue taking these drugs. Some have proposed substituting angiotensin II receptor blocking drugs, such as losartan, for ACE inhibitor–intolerant patients.

When initiating diuretic therapy as part of the treatment algorithm, make certain that the focus is on either congestion or hypertension. Consider the use of pulsed or intermittent diuretic therapy, use lower doses in elderly patients, and, generally, start with the lowest effective dose of the class chosen. For more intense diuresis, consider combinations of different classes of diuretics. Strive for substantive sodium and free water restriction, and monitor serum solutes to keep the magnesium, potassium, and sodium greater than 135 mEq and creatinine levels reasonable. Remember that thiazide and thiazide-type diuretics and the combination of thiazide diuretics with a loop diuretic can precipitate hyponatremia easily. This is generally the case when free water and sodium consumption is excessive. Again, sodium and water restriction is important to prevent this difficulty. Also important is the fact that a rapid diuresis generally requires electrolyte replenishment.

When digoxin is prescribed for heart failure, it should be used in lower doses than previously suggested. Frequent digoxin levels are not necessary. Serum concentration should be determined if the heart failure syndrome worsens, if absorption problems or patient noncompliance are suspected, if renal function deteriorates, or if toxicity is possible. As with ACE inhibitor and diuretic therapy, it is important to monitor patients intermittently for serum magnesium, potassium, sodium, and creatinine levels.

The use of non–ACE inhibitor vasodilator therapy in heart failure patients can be particularly useful when the systemic blood pressure is elevated (sometimes despite ACE inhibitors) and in the setting of mitral regurgitation. Of course, the combination of hydralazine and isosorbide dinitrate is more frequently used because this combination was the first to suggest that mortality could be attenuated in heart failure populations with vasoactive compounds. When used as mortality-reducing therapies, the drugs should be combined. Pulmonary hypertension often responds nicely to long-acting nitrate therapy. One should be careful to administer these drugs in a fashion that does not produce continuous serum levels of nitrate such that tachyphylaxis might occur. Often, troublesome paroxysmal nocturnal dyspnea or orthopnea improves greatly when chronic long-acting nitrates are administered at bedtime.

Major issues to consider when initiating beta-blocker therapy include considering them in every patient who has had an acute myocardial infarction, particularly in combination with an ACE inhibitor when left ventricular systolic dysfunction is present. Beta-blocker therapy should be begun when patients are stable and not overtly congested. Some suggest that nonselective agents with vasodilating effects (e.g., carvedilol) are preferred. Still, metoprolol is one beta$_1$-selective agent used frequently in heart failure settings, including post–myocardial infarction left ventricular systolic dysfunction. Therapy should be begun with low drug doses and a titration time period of many weeks.

STRATEGIES TO CONSIDER WHEN CONGESTION PERSISTS DESPITE OPTIMIZED MEDICAL THERAPY

*e*Table 92.7.1 addresses several strategies to consider when there is apparent failure of chronic oral outpatient treatments. One should review the pitfalls listed in Table 92.6 in an attempt to identify ancillary or extraneous issues that might account for this decompensation and then move toward the strategies outlined. Of course, many patients simply have progression of their disease.

Placing pulmonary artery catheters and objectively measuring hemodynamics is at the root of clarifying confusing or challenging situations. With objective flow and pressure measurements, as well as the frequent determination of mixed venous oxygen saturation, tailoring therapeutics to each patient's clinical situation becomes possible. Parenteral vasodilator therapy (generally nitroglycerin and nitroprusside) alone or in combination with inotrope infusion (usually dobutamine or milrinone) can be dramatically effective. Continuous diuretic infusions, generally with a loop diuretic, such as furosemide, are an alternative strategy to consider in the patient with refractory edema. Although controversial, infusion of dopaminergic or so-called renal doses of dopamine (less than 5 μg per kg per minute) has been said to be helpful in patients refractory to diuretics and in those with worsening renal function. When substantive dropsy persists despite all of these recommendations, hemofiltration ultrafiltration, or, possibly, peritoneal dialysis frequently removes substantial quantities of volume and improves the patient's symptoms rather dramatically.

TREATMENT OF ADVANCED OR REFRACTORY HEART FAILURE

*e*Table 92.7.1 lists options to consider for the patient with advanced heart failure. In patients who have progressive and steadily worsening heart failure syndromes, therapeutic tracks become narrowed, but many still exist. When all attempts fail to create an adequate pharmacotherapeutic program that is successful in keeping patients symptom free over the long term, parenteral drug infusion protocols (which generally use dobutamine, dopamine, or milrinone or sometimes combinations of these drugs) can dramatically reduce symptoms. There is a suggestion, however, that these infusion therapies actually increase mortality. One must weigh carefully the risks and benefits of this approach. It may be an entirely acceptable trade-off in the truly end-stage patient suffering greatly from refractory congestive states. Furthermore, the necessity of indwelling central venous catheter line access creates many challenges with respect to provision of skilled care givers and provision of support for administering the drugs. Obviously, infections and catheter malfunction are major difficulties. Whether chronic infusion of these drugs is necessary, or if they can be given in pulsed parenteral fashion once weekly or monthly over shorter periods (6 to 24 hours), is not known. Also unknown is the best strategy to attempt long-term drug weaning. One practice is to infuse these drugs continuously for a 4- to 6-week period and then attempt to wean as an outpatient over several days or weeks.

One should always consider higher-risk standard operative or percutaneous coronary interventional procedures in the patient with advanced heart failure. Although they are not always options, some patients with substantive ischemia or repairable valvular heart lesions have responded rather dramatically. Coronary artery bypass graft surgery, mitral and aortic valve repair or replacement, left ventricular aneurysmectomy, and endoaneurysmorrhaphy can all be effective options. Percutaneous transluminal coronary angioplasty also likely plays a role when objective evidence of ischemic myocardium related to target coronary lesions is apparent. The main challenge is to identify patients with viable and salvageable myocardium, who are likely to benefit from procedures of this sort. Individuals with extensive scarring of their ventricles may not be the best candidates. Several alternative operative approaches are currently being evaluated. These include dynamic cardiomyoplasty, ventricular remodeling surgery, ventricular assist devices, and total artificial heart implantation. ❦ p40

SUMMARY OF APPROACH TO HEART FAILURE THERAPEUTICS

Table 92.8 summarizes a rational approach to heart failure therapeutics. Tailored therapeutic protocols are based on the progression of patients from insidious to symptomatic to advanced or refractory heart failure settings. It relates the philosophy of prevention to treatment strategies. Also important is the coupling of efforts to address underlying diseases with medication prescription and lifestyle issues, which include increased aerobic activity, optimization of weight, dietary restriction of sodium and fluid, and appropriate vitamin and electrolyte supplementation.

TABLE 92.8 SUMMARY OF APPROACH TO HEART FAILURE THERAPEUTICS

Make appropriate diagnosis.
　Dyspnea, edema, and rales do not always mean congestive heart failure.
Stage syndrome severity.
　Discover asymptomatic left ventricular systolic dysfunction.
　Heart failure does not always mean *congestive* heart failure present.
　Therapeutics of heart failure varies with severity of syndrome.
Treat underlying diseases.
　Address etiology of myocardial dysfunction (particularly hypertension and ischemia syndromes).
　Eliminate exacerbating factors.
　Consider surgical options (bypass surgery, valve repair, and so forth).
Stop potentially detrimental drugs or those of unproven benefit.
　Antiarrhythmic agents (especially Vaughn Williams class I).
　Calcium channel blockers (especially first-generation class).
　Tricyclic antidepressants.
　Nonsteroidal antiinflammatory agents.
　Nasal decongestants.
　Beta-blockers in certain settings.
　Rosiglitazone/piaglitazone.
　Anticoagulants.
Begin therapeutic regimens with proven efficacy.
　Drugs to prevent functional deterioration.
　　ACE inhibitors.
　　Beta-blockers.
　Drugs to reduce mortality.
　　ACE inhibitors.
　　Hydralazine/isosorbide dinitrate.
　　Beta-blockers.
　Drugs to control symptoms.
　　Diuretics.
　　Digoxin.
　　ACE inhibitors.
　　Hydralazine/isosorbide dinitrate.
　　Beta-blockers.
　　Angiotensin II receptor blockers.
Prescribe rational polypharmacy.
　Fewest drugs possible.
　Doses designed to produce fewest side effects possible.
　Program designed to ensure compliance.
　Consider cost of drugs used.
Refer for supervised cardiac rehabilitation classes and aerobic exercise training.
　Avoid physical inactivity.
　Nonaerobic weight training likely should be discouraged.

ACE, angiotensin-converting enzyme.

THE FUTURE

Emerging pharmacotherapeutic strategies will likely influence the direction heart failure treatment paradigms take in the future. Preliminary reports using growth hormone in patients with substantive left ventricular dysfunction are intriguing (210). Administration of this humor might beneficially remodel the heart. On the other hand, growth hormone might induce undesired levels of interstitial matrix deposition that results in diastolic dysfunction and unnatural myocyte hypertrophy. Endothelin has been recognized as a paracrine humor important in increasing vascular bed resistance. Endothelin-blocking agents are being studied with respect to their hemodynamic, humoral, and clinical effectiveness (211–213). A variety of natriuretic peptides have been identified and found useful in characterizing severity of heart failure as well as having some potential therapeutic benefits (214). B-type natriuretic peptide blood concentration measurement now available as a "point of care" test appears to be a sensitive and specific test to diagnose congestive heart failure in the urgent care setting (215). Indeed, this test may become the "CBC" of heart failure as it has been shown to reliably predict the presence or absence of left ventricular dysfunction on echocardiography. This test may be an excellent screening tool for left ventricular dysfunction and may preclude the need for echocardiography in many patients (216). Furthermore, in patients admitted with decompensated congestive heart failure, changes in B-type natriuretic peptide levels during treatment are strong predictors of mortality and morbidity and have been successfully used to guide treatment of patients admitted for decompensated congestive heart failure (217). B-type natriuretic peptide produced by recombinant DNA techniques is now available for parenteral infusion in severe congestive heart failure (218). With the realization that heart failure has inflammatory elements characterizing the milieu, methods to attenuate cytokine trafficking with antibodies or anticytokine agents may prove beneficial. Intriguing studies are ongoing to clarify this issue (19). Simple, durable, and reliable permanent ventricular assist device pumps will become available and will be used as both alternative treatments versus transplantation or bridges to recovery with subsequent pump removal (145). Myoblast implants (219,220) may serve a similar purpose. Even more futuristic is the likelihood that therapies can be designed to interdict the apoptotic signaling loops at a molecular biodynamic level. This would be the ultimate in reversing adverse remodeling (221–228).

Making an appropriate diagnosis is paramount, as is staging the heart failure syndrome severity. Stopping potentially detrimental drugs, or those of unproved benefit, is as important as beginning appropriate therapeutic regimens designed to prevent functional deterioration, reduce mortality, or control symptoms when symptomatic heart failure (particularly congestive heart failure) is present. Underlying these important principles is the concept that rational polypharmacy is mandatory because these patients are on multiple drugs and combinations of drugs. The fewest drugs possible should be prescribed and dispensed in such a way that the fewest side effects appear and compliance can be high. Finally, the period is over in which chronic bed rest is an important component of heart failure therapy. It is likely that the medications used today achieve the same results of yesteryear's bed rest prescriptions. We now know it is quite important that patients with all except the severest end stage of heart failure attempt to exercise aerobically. Patients with heart failure should be referred to supervised cardiac rehabilitation programs, if at all possible, to become schooled in aerobic training exercises. This is an adjunctive opportunity for more general patient education as well.

CONTROVERSIES AND PERSONAL PERSPECTIVES

Obviously, individuals frequently managing patients with heart failure have had different experiences and interpret anecdotal or clinical trial data in many ways. Controversy exists. It should be apparent from the foregoing discussion that heart failure treatment protocols are broad and complex. This is because the syndrome is, in fact, a difficult milieu. Much has been learned about designing heart failure treatment protocols, but perhaps most important is the necessity of beginning early in the difficulty to prevent deterioration to advanced stages. Therefore, tailoring therapeutics to each individual's particular clinical situation seems most important. ACE inhibitors are now first-line treatment for heart failure. Beta-blockers have emerged as rational options, and an argument is even made that they provide greater opportunity for benefits than ACE inhibitors. Still, it is apparent that despite the fact that ACE inhibitors and beta-blockers are now considered first-line therapy, they are frequently not prescribed, are underdosed, or prematurely discontinued. Whether angiotensin II receptor blocking agents are effective substitutes for ACE inhibitors in intolerant patients or, more generally, better than ACE inhibitors is not yet known, although initial data are encouraging. Combining these two drug classes is an intriguing thought. It seems that beta-blocker benefits are most notable over the long term and that, during the short term, patients frequently feel worse. Many argue that digoxin should be prescribed in all congestive heart failure patients for morbidity reduction, and that triple therapy with digoxin, diuretics, and ACE inhibitors is the best basic heart failure treatment protocol in those with congestive states. Antiarrhythmics should be avoided if at all possible, particularly Vaughn Williams class I antiarrhythmic drugs. Alternative strategies might include arrhythmia ablation techniques, implantation of electronic arrhythmia-terminating devices, and, possibly, amiodarone. Amiodarone is one antiarrhythmic agent that may actually be beneficial in some heart failure patients, and it is possible that the toxicity of this drug can be controlled with prescription of much lower doses. Cardiac resynchronization with multisite pacing is emerging as an attractive strategy.

It is not clear if chronic parenteral inotrope infusion reduces end-stage heart failure morbidity and mortality, although most believe that symptoms are substantively reduced at the cost of higher sudden cardiac death rates. Arguably, chronic parenteral inotropic infusion is preferred to intermittent or periodic pulsed infusions. In general, positive inotropic drugs that do not ameliorate adverse neurohormonal profiles seem detrimental to long-term prognosis in heart failure patients, although they may attenuate morbidity. Diuretics should only be used in congestive states or as an antihypertensive agent. It seems that we pay inadequate attention to electrolyte and solute replenishment in many heart failure patients. Furthermore, aerobic exercise is good for heart failure patients, not detrimental, and should be encouraged.

REFERENCES

1. Armstrong PW, Moe CW. Medical advances in the treatment of congestive heart failure. *Circulation* 1993;88:2941–2952.
2. Young JB, Pratt CM. Hemodynamic and hormonal alterations in patients with heart failure: toward a contemporary definition of heart failure. *Semin Nephrol* 1994;10:427–440.
3. Harris P. The problem of defining heart failure. *Cardiovasc Drugs Ther* 1994;8:447–452.
4. Chatterjee K. Heart failure therapy in evolution. *Circulation* 1996;94:2689–2693.
5. Cohn JN. The management of chronic heart failure. *N Engl J Med* 1996;335:490–498.
6. Young JB. Contemporary management of patients with heart failure. *Med Clin North Am* 1995;79:1171–1191.
7. Withering W. *An account of the foxglove, and some of its medical uses: with practical remarks on dropsy and other diseases.* London: Robinson and Paternoster-Row, 1785.
8. Sydenham T. A treatise of the gout and dropsy. In: *The works of Thomas Sydenham, M.D., on acute and chronic diseases.* Vol II. London: Robinson, Otridge, Hayes and Newbery, 1683.
9. Corvisart-Desmarret JN. *Essay on the organic diseases of the heart.* Paris, 1812.
10. Flint A. *A treatise on the principles and practice of medicine,* 4th ed. Philadelphia: Henry C. Lea, 1873.
11. Mackenzie J. *Diseases of the heart.* London, 1910.
12. Burch GE, Walsh JJ, Black WC. Value of prolonged bed rest in management of cardiomegaly. *JAMA* 1963;183:81–87.
13. Fishberg A. *Heart disease.* Philadelphia: WB Saunders, 1937.
14. Friedberg CK. *Diseases of the heart,* 2nd ed. Philadelphia: WB Saunders, 1956.
15. Moulopoulos SD, Topaz SR, Kolff WJ. Extracorporeal assistance to the circulation and intraaortic balloon pumping. *Trans Am Soc Artif Intern Organs* 1962;8:36–41.
16. Lillehei CW, Leng MJ, DeWall RA, et al. Resection of myocardial aneurysms after infarction during temporary cardiopulmonary bypass. *Circulation* 1962;26:206–216.
17. Lown B, Amarasingham R, Neuman J. New method for terminating cardiac arrhythmias: use of synchronized capacitor discharge. *JAMA* 1962;182:548–555.
18. Barnard CN. A human cardiac transplant: an interim report of a successful operation performed at Grote Schurr Hospital, Capetown. *S Afr Med J* 1967;41:1271–1278.
19. Cohn JN. Vasodilator therapy: implications in myocardial infarction and congestive heart failure. *Am Heart J* 1982;103:773–778.
20. Young JB. Evolving concepts in the treatment of heart failure: should new inotropic agents carry promise or paranoia? *Pharmacotherapy* 1996;16:78S–74S.
21. Hurst J, Logue RB, Schlant RC, et al., eds. *The heart, arteries and veins,* 4th ed. New York: McGraw-Hill, 1978.
22. Baker DW, Konstam MA, Bottorff M, et al. Management of heart failure: I. Pharmacologic treatment. *JAMA* 1994;272:1361–1366.
23. Garg R, Yusuf S. Overview of randomized trials of angiotensin-converting enzyme inhibitors on mortality and morbidity in patients with heart failure. *JAMA* 1995;18:1450–1455.
24. Young JB. Angiotensin-converting enzyme inhibitors in heart failure: new strategies justified by recent clinical trials. *Int J Cardiol* 1994;43:151–163.
25. Curfman GD. Inotropic therapy for heart failure: an unfulfilled promise. *N Engl J Med* 1991;325:1509–1510.
26. Niebauer J, Coats AJ. Treating chronic heart failure: time to take stock. *Lancet* 1997;349:966–967.
27. Pratt CM, Eaton T, Francis M, et al. The inverse relationship between baseline left ventricular ejection fraction and outcome of antiarrhythmic therapy: a dangerous imbalance in the risk-benefit ratio. *Am Heart J* 1989;118:433–440.
28. Stevenson WG, Stevenson LW, Middlekauff HR, et al. Sudden death prevention in patients with advanced ventricular dysfunction. *Circulation* 1993;88:2953–2961.
29. Packer M. End of the oldest controversy in medicine: are we ready to conclude the debate on digitalis? *N Engl J Med* 1997;336:575–576.

30. Smith TW. Digoxin in heart failure. *N Engl J Med* 1993;329:51–53.

31. Young JB. Do digitalis glycosides still have a role in congestive heart failure? *Cardiol Clin* 1994;25:51–61.

32. Pfeffer MA, Stevenson LW. Beta adrenergic blockers and survival in heart failure. *N Engl J Med* 1996;334:1396–1397.

33. Doughty RN, Sharpe N, MacMahon S. Effects of beta-blocker therapy on mortality in patients with heart failure: a systematic overview of randomized controlled trials. *Eur Heart J* 1987;18:560–565.

34. Eichhorn E, Bristow MR. Practical guidelines for initiating beta adrenergic blockade in patients with chronic heart failure. *Am J Cardiol* 1997;79:794–798.

35. Haber HL, Simek CL, Gimple LW, et al. Why do patients with congestive heart failure tolerate the initiation of β-blocker therapy? *Circulation* 1993;88:1610–1619.

36. Kelly RA, Smith TW. Cytokines and cardiac contractile function. *Circulation* 1997;95:778–781.

37. Levine B, Kalman J, Mayer L, et al. Elevated circulating levels of tumor necrosis factor in severe chronic heart failure. *N Engl J Med* 1990;323:236–241.

38. Asanoi H, Kameyama T, Ishizaka S, et al. Energetically optimal left ventricular pressure for the failing human heart. *Circulation* 1996;93:67–73.

39. Torre-Amione G, Kapadia S, Benedict G, et al. Proinflammatory cytokine levels in patients with depressed left ventricular ejection fraction: a report from the studies of left ventricular dysfunction (SOLVD). *J Am Coll Cardiol* 1996;27:1201–1206.

40. Torre-Amione G, Kapadia S, Lee J, et al. Expression of tumor necrosis factor alpha and tumor necrosis factor receptors in the failing human heart. *Circulation* 1996;93:704–711.

41. Young J. Cardiac transplantation and other surgical treatment of advanced heart failure. In: DeBakey ME, Gotto AM, eds. *The new living heart,* 2nd ed. New York: David McKay, 1997.

42. Oz MC, Argensiano M, Catanese KA, et al. Bridge experience with long-term implantable left ventricular assist devices: are they an alternative to transplantation? *Circulation* 1997;95:1844–1852.

43. Hlatky MA, Fleg JL, Hinton PC, et al. Physician practice in the management of congestive heart failure. *J Am Coll Cardiol* 1986;8:966–970.

44. Bourassa MG, Gurn O, Bangdiwala SI, et al., for the SOLVD Investigators. Natural history and patterns of current practice in heart failure patients. *J Am Coll Cardiol* 1993;22[Suppl A]:14A–19A.

45. Clinical Quality Improvement Network Investigators. Mortality risk and patterns of practice in 4606 acute care patients with congestive heart failure. The relative importance of age, sex, and medical therapy. *Arch Intern Med* 1996;156:1669–1673.

46. *Ohio heart failure project report.* Westerville, OH: Peer Review Systems, Inc., 1995.

47. Young JB, Weiner DH, Yusuf S, et al. Patterns of medication use in patients with heart failure: a report from the registry of Studies of Left Ventricular Dysfunction (SOLVD). *South Med J* 1994;88:514–523.

48. Contemporary management of patients with left ventricular systolic dysfunction: results from the Study of Patients Intolerant of Converting Enzyme Inhibitors (SPICE) Registry. *Eur Heart J* 1999;20:1182–1190.

49. Epstein AC, Hallstrom AP, Rogers WJ, et al. Mortality following ventricular arrhythmia suppression by encainide, flecainide, and moricizine after myocardial infarction. The original design concept of the Cardiac Arrhythmia Suppression Trial (CAST). *JAMA* 1993;270:2451–2455.

50. Anonymous. The effect of diltiazem on mortality and reinfarction after myocardial infarction. The Multicenter Postinfarction Trial Research Group. *N Engl J Med* 1988;319:385–392.

51. Furberg CD, Psaty BM, Meyer JV. Nifedipine. Dose related increase in mortality in patients with coronary heart disease. *Circulation* 1995;92:1326–1331.

52. Lamas GA, Pfeffer MA, Hamm P, et al. Do the results of randomized clinical trials of cardiovascular drugs influence medical practice? The SAVE investigators. *N Engl J Med* 1992;327:241–247.

53. Guidelines for the evaluation and management of heart failure. Report of the American College of Cardiology/American Heart Association Task Force on Practice Guidelines (Committee on Evaluation and Management of Heart Failure). *J Am Coll Cardiol* 1995;26:1376–1398.

54. Nozba MM, Boskis B, Bristow M, et al. WHO concise guide to the management of heart failure. *J Cardiac Failure* 1996;2:153–155.

55. The Task Force of the Working Group on Heart Failure of the European Society of Cardiology. The treatment of heart failure. *Eur Heart J* 1997;18:736–753.

56. Packer M, Cohn JN. ACTION heart failure treatment guidelines. *Am J Cardiol* 1999;83(2A):1.

57. Adams KA. Heart Failure Society of America guidelines for the treatment of heart failure. *J Card Fail* 2000;5:356.

58. Young JB, Mills RM. *Clinical management of heart failure.* Caddo, OK: Professional Communications, 2001.

59. Young JB, Lang R, Albert N. *Guidelines for heart failure: clinical practice guideline and provider desk reference.* Cleveland, OH: The Cleveland Clinic Foundation, Office of Clinical Effectiveness and I. H. Page Center for Health Outcomes Research, 2000.

60. Packer M, Poole-Wilson PA, Armstrong PW, et al. Comparative effects of low and high doses of the angiotensin-converting enzyme inhibitor lisinopril on morbidity and mortality in chronic heart failure. ATLAS Study Group. *Circulation* 1999;100:2312–2318.

61. Young JB. Angiotensin converting enzyme inhibitors and cytokines in heart failure: dose and effect? *J Am Coll Cardiol* 1999;34:2068–2071.

62. Young JB. Assessment of heart failure. In: Colucci WS, Braunwald E, eds. *Heart failure: cardiac function and dysfunction. Atlas of heart diseases.* Philadelphia: 1994;7.1–7.20.

63. Young JB, Farmer JA. The diagnostic evaluation of patients with heart failure. In: Hosenpud JD, Greenberg GH, eds. *Congestive heart failure: pathophysiology, diagnosis, and comprehensive approach to management.* New York: Springer-Verlag, 1994:597–622.

64. Grinstead WC, Young JB. The myocardial renin-angiotensive system: existence, importance, and clinical implications. *Am Heart J* 1992;123:1040–1045.

65. Izumo S, Nadal-Ginard B, Mahdavi V. Proto-oncogene induction and reprogramming of cardiac gene expression produced by pressure overload. *Proc Natl Acad Sci U S A* 1988;85:339–343.

66. Katz AM. Cardiomyopathy of overload: a major determinant of prognosis in congestive heart failure. *N Engl J Med* 1990;322:100–110.

67. Ross JJ. Afterload mismatch and preload reserve: a conceptual framework for the analysis of ventricular function. *Prog Cardiovasc Dis* 1976;18:255–264.

68. Weber KT. Cardiac interstitium in health and disease: remodeling of the fibrillar collagen matrix. *J Am Coll Cardiol* 1989;137:1637–1652.

69. Weber KT, Brilla CG. Pathological hypertrophy and the cardiac interstitium: fibrosis and the renin-angiotensin-aldosterone system. *Circulation* 1990;83:1840–1865.

70. Leier CV. Regional blood flow in human congestive heart failure. *Am Heart J* 1992;124:726–738.

71. Cotsamire DL, Unverferth DV, Leier CV. The relationship between drug-induced changes in central and regional hemodynamics in congestive heart failure. *Canadian J Cardiol* 1986;2:272–277.

72. Konstam M, Dracup K, Baker D, et al. *Heart failure: evaluation and care of patient with left-ventricular systolic dysfunction. Clinical practice guideline.* AHCPR publication No. 94-0612 (abstract). Rockville, MD: Agency for Health Care Policy and Research, Public Health Service, U.S. Department of Health and Human Services, June 1994.

73. Dracup K, Baker DW, Dunbar SB, et al. Management of heart failure. II. Counseling, education, and lifestyle modifications. *JAMA* 1994;272:1442–1446.

74. Baker DW, Jones R, Hodges J, et al. Management of heart failure. III. The role of revascularization in the treatment of patients with moderate or severe left ventricular systolic dysfunction. *JAMA* 1994;272:1528–1534.

75. Baker DW, Wright RF. Management of heart failure. IV. Anticoagulation for patients with heart failure due to left ventricular systolic dysfunction. *JAMA* 1994;272:1614–1618.

76. Parmley WW. Clinical practice guidelines. Does the cookbook have enough recipes? *JAMA* 1994;272:1374–1375.

77. Cohn JN, Archibald DG, Ziesche S, et al. Effect of vasodilator therapy on mortality in chronic congestive heart failure: results of a Veterans Administration Cooperative Study (V-Heft I). *N Engl J Med* 1986;314:1547–1552.

78. Califf RM, Adams K, McKenna W, et al. A randomized controlled trial of epoprostenol therapy for severe congestive heart failure: the Flolan International Randomized Survival Trial (FIRST). *Am Heart J* 1997;134:44–59.

79. Hampton JR, van Veldhuisen DJ, Kleber FX, et al. For the Second Prospective Randomised Study of Ibopamine on Mortality and Efficacy (PRIME II) Investigators. Randomised study of effect of ibopamine on survival in patients with advanced severe heart failure. *Lancet* 1997;349:971.

80. PROFILE Investigators Group. Prospective randomized flosequinan longevity evaluation. *Circulation* 1993;88[Suppl I]:1–301(abst).

81. Packer M, Carver JR, Rodeheffer RJ, et al., for the PROMISE Study Research Group. Effect of oral milrinone on mortality in severe chronic heart failure. *N Engl J Med* 1991;325:1468–1475.

82. Feldman A, Young JB, Bourge R, et al., for the VesT Investigators. Pittsburgh, PA, Minneapolis, MN. Mechanism of increased mortality from vesnarinone in the severe heart failure trial (VesT). *J Am Coll Cardiol* 1997;29[Suppl A]:64A.

83. CONSENSUS Trial Study Group. Effects of enalapril on mortality in severe congestive heart failure: results of the Cooperative North Scandinavian Enalapril Survival Study (CONSENSUS). *N Engl J Med* 1987;316:1429–1435.

84. Cohn JN, Johnson G, Ziesche S, et al. A comparison of enalapril with hydralazine-isosorbide dinitrate in the treatment of chronic congestive heart failure (VeHEFT-II). *N Engl J Med* 1991;325:303–310.

85. Packer M, O'Connor CM, Ghali JK, et al., for the Prospective Randomized Amlodipine Survival Evaluation Study Group (PRAISE). Effect of amlodipine on morbidity and mortality in severe chronic heart failure. *N Engl J Med* 1996;335:1107–1114.

86. Cohn JN, Ziesche S, Smith R, et al. Effect of the calcium antagonist felodipine as supplementary vasodilator therapy in patients with chronic heart failure treated with enalapril. V-Heft III. *Circulation* 1997;96:856–863.

87. SOLVD Investigators. Effect of enalapril on mortality and the development of heart failure in asymptomatic patients with reduced left ventricular ejection fractions. *N Engl J Med* 1992;327:685–691.

88. SOLVD Investigators. Effect of enalapril on survival in patients with reduced left ventricular ejection fractions and congestive heart failure. *N Engl J Med* 1991;325:293–302.

89. Digitalis Investigation Group. The effect of digoxin on mortality and morbidity in patients with heart failure. *N Engl J Med* 1997;336:525–533.

90. Pfeffer MA, Braunwald E, Moy LA, et al., on behalf of the SAVE Investigators. Effect of captopril on mortality and morbidity in patients with ventricular dysfunction after myocardial infarction. Results of the survival and ventricular enlargement trial. *N Engl J Med* 1992;327:669–677.

91. Acute Infarction Ramipril Efficacy (AIRE) Study Investigators. Effect of ramipril on mortality and morbidity of survivors of acute myocardial infarction with clinical evidence of heart failure. *Lancet* 1993;342:821–828.

92. Ambrosioni E, Borghi C, Magnani B, for the Survival of Myocardial Infarction Long-Term Evaluation (SMILE) Study Investigators. *N Engl J Med* 1995;332:80–85.

93. Kober L, Torp-Pedersen C, Carlsen JE, for the Trandolapril Cardiac Evaluation (TRACE) Study Group. *N Engl J Med* 1995;333:1670–1676.

94. Hall AS, Murray GD, Ball SG. On behalf of the AIREX Study Investigators. Follow-up study of patients randomly allocated ramipril or placebo for heart failure after acute myocardial infarction: AIRE Extension (AIREX) Study. *Lancet* 1997;349:1493–1497.

95. ISIS-IV. A randomized factorial trial assessing early oral captopril, oral mononitrate, and intravenous magnesium sulfate in 58,000 patients with suspected acute myocardial infarction (Fourth International Study of Infarct Survival). *Lancet* 1995;345:669–685.

96. GISSI-3. Effects of lisinopril and transdermal glyceryl trinitrate singly and together on 6 week mortality and ventricular function after myocardial infarction. *Curr Opin Cardiol* 1997;12:407–417.

97. Wangstein F, Bristow MR, Snedberg K, et al. For the metoprolol in dilated cardiomyopathy (MDC) trial study group. Beneficial effects of metoprolol in idiopathic dilated cardiomyopathy. *Lancet* 1993;342:1441–1446.

98. Packer M, Colucci WS, Sackner-Bernstein JD, et al., for the PRECISE Study Group. Double-blind, placebo controlled study of the effects of carvedilol in patients with moderate to severe heart failure. The PRECISE Trial. *Circulation* 1996;94:2793–2799.

99. Bristow MR, Gilbert EM, Abraham WT, et al. For the MOCHA Investigators. Carvedilol produces dose-related improvements in left ventricular function and survival in subjects with chronic heart failure. *Circulation* 1996;94:2807–2816.

100. Packer M, Bristow MR, Cohn JN, et al., for the U.S. Carvedilol Heart Failure Study Group. The effect of carvedilol on morbidity and mortality in patients with chronic heart failure. *N Engl J Med* 1996;334:1349–1355.

101. CIBIS investigators. A randomized trial of beta blockade in heart failure; the Cardiac Insufficiency Bisoprolol Study (CIBIS). *Circulation* 1994;90:1765–1773.

102. CIBIS II investigators. The Cardiac Insufficiency Bisoprolol II (CIBIS II) Study. *Lancet* 1999;353:9–12.

103. Krumholz HM. Beta blockers for mild to moderate heart failure. *Lancet* 1999;353:2–3.

104. Hjalmarson A, Goldstein S, Fagerberg B, et al. Effects of controlled release metoprolol on total mortality, hospitalizations, and well-being in patients with heart failure. The metoprolol CR/XL Randomized Intervention Trial in Congestive Heart Failure (Merit-HF). *JAMA* 2000;283:1295–1302.

105. The RESOLVED Investigators. Effects of metoprolol CR in patients with ischemic and dilated cardiomyopathy. The Randomized Evaluation of Strategies for Left Ventricular Dysfunction Pilot Study. *Circulation* 2000;101:378–384.

106. Packer M, Coates AJS, Fowler MB, et al. Effect of carvedilol on survival in severe chronic heart failure. *N Engl J Med* 2001;344:1651–1658.

107. Braunwald E. Expanding indications for beta blockers. *N Engl J Med* 2001;344:1711–1712.

108. Eichhorn EJ, Bristow MR. Commentary: the Carvedilol Prospective Randomized Cumulative Survival (COPERNICUS) trial. *Curr Control Trials Cardiovasc Med* 2001; 2:20–23.

109. The Beta Blocker Evaluation of Survival Trial Investigators. A trial of the beta blocker bucindolol in patients with advanced chronic heart failure. *N Engl J Med* 2001; 344:1659–1667.

110. Friedman PL, Stevenson WG. Unsustained ventricular tachycardia—to treat or not to treat? *N Engl J Med* 1996;335:1984–1985.

111. Teo KK, Yusuf S, Furburg CD. Effects of prophylactic antiarrhythmic drug therapy in acute myocardial infarction: an overview of results from randomized controlled clinical trials. *JAMA* 1993;270:1589–1595.

112. Hennekens CH, Albert CM, Godfried SL, et al. Adjunctive drug therapy after acute myocardial infarction—evidence from clinical trials. *N Engl J Med* 1996;335:1660–1667.

113. CAST Investigators. Preliminary Report: special report: effect of encainide and flecainide on mortality in a randomized trial of arrhythmia suppression after myocardial infarction. *N Engl J Med* 1989;321:406.

114. Cardiac Arrhythmia Suppression Trial II Investigators. Effect of the antiarrhythmic agent moricizine on survival after myocardial infarction. *N Engl J Med* 1992;327:227–333.

115. Waldo AL, Camm AJ, deRuyter H, et al., for the SWORD Investigators. Effect of D-sotalol on mortality in patients with left ventricular dysfunction after recent and remote myocardial infarction. *Lancet* 1996;348:7–12.

116. Pratt CM, Francis M, Mahler S, et al. The natural history of benign and potentially malignant ventricular arrhythmias with special reference to nonsustained ventricular tachycardia. *Am Heart J* 1988;116:897–903.

117. Pratt CM, Podrid PJ, Seals AA, et al. Effects of Ethmozine (moricizine HCL) on ventricular function using echocardiographic, hemodynamic and radionuclide assessments. *Am J Cardiol* 1987;60:73.

118. Seals AA, English L, Leon CA, et al. Hemodynamic effects of moricizine at rest and during supine bicycle exercise: results in patients with ventricular tachycardia and left ventricular dysfunction. *Am Heart J* 1986;112:36–43.

119. Seals AA, Haider R, Leon C, et al. Antiarrhythmic efficacy and hemodynamic effects of cibenzoline in patients with nonsustained ventricular tachycardia and left ventricular dysfunction. *Circulation* 1987;75:800–808.

120. Hallstrom A, Pratt CM, Greene HL, et al., for the Cardiac Arrhythmia Suppression Trial Investigators: relations between heart failure, ejection fraction, arrhythmia suppression and mortality: analysis of the Cardiac Arrhythmia Suppression Trial. *J Am Coll Cardiol* 1995;25:1250–1270.

121. Doval HC, Nul DR, Grancelli HO, et al. For Grupo de Estudio de la Insuficiencia Cardiaca en Argentina. Randomized trial of low dose amiodarone in severe congestive heart failure (GESICA). *Lancet* 1994;344:493–498.

122. Julian DG, Camm AJ, Frangin G, et al. Randomized trial of effect of amiodarone on mortality in patients with left ventricular dysfunction after recent myocardial infarction: EMIAT. *Lancet* 1997;349:667–674.

123. Cairns JA, Conolly SJ, Roberts R, et al. Randomized trial of outcome after myocardial infarction in patients with frequent or repetitive ventricular premature depolarizations. CAMIAT. *Lancet* 1997;349:675–682.

124. Cairns JA, Connolly SJ, Roberts RS, et al. Canadian Amiodarone Myocardial Infarction Arrhythmia Trial (CAMIAT): rationale and protocol. *Am J Cardiol* 1993;72:87F–94F.

125. Gottlieb SS. Dead is dead; artifical definitions are no substitute. *Lancet* 1997;349:662–663.

126. Singh SN, Fletcher RD, Gross Fisher S, et al., for the Survival Trial of Antiarrhythmic Therapy in Congestive Heart Failure. Veterans Affairs Anti-arrhythmia in Heart Failure trial. *N Engl J Med* 1995;333:77–82.

127. Kober L, Block-Thompsen PE, Moller M, et al. Effect of dofetilide in patients with recent myocardial infarction

and left ventricular dysfunction: a randomized trial. *Lancet* 2000;356:2052–2058.

128. Torp-Pederson C, Moller M, Block-Thomsen PE, et al. Dofetilide in patients with congestive heart failure and left ventricular dysfunction. Danish Investigations of Arrhythmia and Mortality on Dofetilide Study Group. *N Engl J Med* 1999;334:857–865.

129. Xamoterol in Severe Heart Failure Study Group. Xamoterol in severe heart failure. *Lancet* 1990;336:1–6.

130. Marius-Nunez AL, Heaney RN, Fernandez RN, et al. Intermittent inotropic therapy in an outpatient setting: a cost-effective therapeutic modality in patients with refractory heart failure. *Am Heart J* 1996;132:805–808.

131. Packer M. Effects of phosphodiesterase inhibitors on survival of patients with chronic congestive heart failure. *Am J Cardiol* 1989;63:41A–45A.

132. Multicenter Diltiazem Postinfarction Trial Research Group (MDPII). The effect of diltiazem on mortality and reinfarction after myocardial infarction. *N Engl J Med* 1988;319:385–392.

133. Feldman AM, Bristow MR, Parmley WW, et al. Effects of vesnarinone on morbidity and mortality in patients with heart failure: Vesnarinone Study Group. *N Engl Med* 1993;329:149–155.

134. Packer M, O'Conner CM, Ghali JK, et al. Effect of amlodipine on morbidity and mortality in severe chronic heart failure. Prospective Randomized Amlodipine Survival Evaluation Study Group. *N Engl J Med* 1996;335:1107–1114.

135. Cohn JN, Johnson G, Ziesche S, et al. Effect of the calcium antagonist felodipine as supplementary vasodilator therapy in patients with chronic heart failure treated with enalapril; VeHeft III. *Circulation* 1997;96:856–863.

136. Levine TB, Bernik PJ, Caspi A, et al. Effect of mibefradil, a T-type calcium channel blocker, on morbidity and mortality in moderate to severe congestive heart failure: the MACH-1 study. Mortality Assessment in Congestive Heart Failure Trial. *Circulation* 2000;1001:758–764.

137. Loh E, Swain JL. Growth hormone for heart failure: cause for cautious optimism. *N Engl J Med* 1996;334:856–857.

138. Pitt B, Zannad F, Remme WJ, et al. The effect of spironolactone on morbidity and mortality in patients with severe heart failure. Randomized Aldactone Evaluation Study Investigators. *N Engl J Med* 1999;341:709–717.

139. Pagley PR, Beller GA, Watson DD, et al. Improved outcome after coronary bypass surgery in patients with ischemic cardiomyopathy and residual myocardial viability. *Circulation* 1997;96:793–800.

140. Alderman EL, Fisher LD, Liturin P, et al. Results of coronary artery surgery in patients with poor left ventricular function (CASS). *Circulation* 1983;68:785–795.

141. European Coronary Surgery Study Group. Long-term results of prospective randomized study of coronary artery bypass surgery in stable angina pectoris. *Lancet* 1982;2:1173–1180.

142. Starling RC, Young JB, Scalia GM, et al. Preliminary observations with ventricular remodeling surgery for refractory congestive heart failure. *J Am Coll Cardiol* 1997;29:2A–64A.

143. Starling RC, McCarthy PM, Buda T, et al. Results of partial left ventriculectomy for dilated cardiomyopathy:

hemodynamic, clinical, and echocardiographic observations. *J Am Coll Cardiol* 2000;36:2098–2103.

144. Franco-Cereceda A, McCarthy P, Blackstone EH, et al. Partial left ventriculectomy for dilated cardiomyopathy: is this an alternative to transplantation? *J Thorac Cardiovasc Surg* 2001;121:879–893.

145. Masters RG. *Surgical options for the treatment of heart failure.* Boston: Kluwer, 1999.

146. Furnary AP, Jessupp M, Moreira LF. For the American Cardiomyoplasty Group. Multicenter trial of dynamic cardiomyoplasty for chronic heart failure. *J Am Coll Cardiol* 1996;28:1175–1180.

147. Leier CV. Cardiomyoplasty: is it time to wrap it up? *J Am Coll Cardiol* 1996;28:1181–1182.

148. Young JB, Kirklin J, for the C-SMART Investigators. Cardiomyoplasty Skeletal Muscle Assist Randomized Trial: 6 month results. *Circulation* 1999;100:i514.

149. van Veldhuisen DJ, Pieter A, de Graeff, et al. Value of digoxin in heart failure and sinus rhythm: new features of an old drug? *J Am Coll Cardiol* 1996;28:813–819.

150. Uretsky BF, Young JB, Shahidi FE, et al. Randomized study assessing the effect of digoxin withdrawal in patients with mild to moderate chronic congestive heart failure: results of the PROVED trial: PROVED Investigative Group. *J Am Coll Cardiol* 1993;22:955–962.

151. Packer M, Gheorghiade M, Young JB, et al., on behalf of the RADIANCE Study. Withdrawal of digoxin from patients with chronic heart failure treated with angiotensin-converting-enzyme inhibitors. *N Engl J Med* 1993;329:1–7.

152. Moss AJ, Davis HT, Conard DL, et al. Digitalis-associated cardiac mortality after myocardial infarction. *Circulation* 1981;64:1150–1156.

153. Ryan TJ, Bailey KR, McCabe CH, et al. The effects of digitalis on survival in high-risk patients with coronary artery disease. The Coronary Artery Surgery Study (CASS). *Circulation* 1983;67:735–742.

154. Madsen EB, Gilpin E, Henning H, et al. Prognostic importance of digitalis after acute myocardial infarction. *J Am Coll Cardiol* 1984;3:681–689.

155. Bigger JT, Fleiss JL, Rolnitzky LM, et al. Effect of digitalis on survival after acute myocardial infarction. *Am J Cardiol* 1985;55:623–630.

156. Byington R, Goldstein S, for the BHAT Research Group. Association of digitalis therapy with mortality in survivors of acute myocardial infarction: observations in the Beta-blocker Heart Attack Trial. *J Am Coll Cardiol* 1985;6:976–982.

157. Mueller JE, Turi ZG, Stone PH, et al., and the MILIS Study Group. Digoxin therapy and mortality after myocardial infarction. *N Engl J Med* 1986;3114:265–271.

158. Redfors A. Plasma digoxin concentration: its relation to digoxin dosage and clinical effects in patients with atrial fibrillation. *Br Heart J* 1972;34:383–391.

159. Slatton ML, Irani WN, Hall SA, et al. Does digoxin provide additional hemodynamic and autonomic benefit at higher doses in patients with mild to moderate heart failure and normal sinus rhythm? *J Am Coll Cardiol* 1997;29:1206–1213.

160. Young JB, Gheorghiade M, Packer M, et al. On behalf of the PROVED and RADIANCE investigators: Are low

serum levels of digoxin effective in chronic heart failure? Evidence challenging the accepted guidelines for a therapeutic serum level of the drug. *J Am Coll Cardiol* 1993;21[Suppl A]:378A.

161. Niebauer J, Coats JS. Treating chronic heart failure: time to take stock. *Lancet* 1997;349:966–967.

162. Pagel PS, Haikala H, Pentikainen PJ, et al. Pharmacology of levosimendan: a new myofilament calcium sensitizer. *Cardiovasc Drug Rev* 1996;14:286–316.

163. Rodkey SM, Young JB. The cardiovascular use of diuretics. *Cardiology Clinics: Annual of Drug Therapy* 1997;1:63–80.

164. Grinstead WC, Francis MJ, Marks GF, et al. Discontinuation of chronic diuretic therapy in stable heart failure patients. *Am J Cardiol* 1994;73:881–886.

165. Psaty BM, Smith NL, Siscovick DS, et al. Health outcomes associated with antihypertensive therapies used as first-line agents. *JAMA* 1997;277:739–745.

166. Kostis JB, Davis BR, Cutler J. Prevention of heart failure by antihypertensive drug treatment in older persons with isolated systolic hypertension. *JAMA* 1997;278:212–216.

167. Cohn JN. Efficacy of vasodilators in the treatment of heart failure. *J Am Coll Cardiol* 1993;22[Suppl A]:135A–138A.

168. Abrams J. Beneficial actions of nitrates in cardiovascular disease. *Am J Cardiol* 1996;77:31c–37c.

169. Elkayam U. Prevention of nitrate tolerance with concomitant administration of hydralazine. *Can J Cardiol* 1996;12:17c–21c.

170. Elkayam U, Roth A, Mehra A, et al. Randomized study to evaluate the relation between oral isosorbide dinitrate dosing interval and the development of early tolerance to its effect on left ventricular filling pressure in patients with chronic heart failure. *Circulation* 1991;84:2090–2098.

171. Packer M. Do angiotensin-converting enzyme inhibitors prolong life in patients with heart failure treated in clinical practice? *J Am Coll Cardiol* 1996;28:1323–1327.

172. Kostis JB, Shelton MS, Gosselin G, et al. Adverse effects of enalapril in the studies of left ventricular dysfunction (SOLVD). *Am Heart J* 1996;131:350–355.

173. Crozier I, Ikram H, Awan N, et al., for the Losartan Hemodynamic Study Group. Losartan in heart failure: hemodynamic effects and tolerability. *Circulation* 1995;91:691–697.

174. Exner DV, Dries DL, Domanski MJ, et al. Lesser response to angiotensin-converting enzyme inhibitor therapy in black as compared with white patients with left ventricular dysfunction. *N Engl J Med* 2001;344:1351–1357.

175. Goodfriend TL, Elliott ME, Catt KJ. Angiotensin receptors and their antagonists. *N Engl J Med* 1996;334:1649–1654.

176. Gavras I. Bradykinin-mediated effects of ACE-inhibition. *Kidney Int* 1992;42:1020–1029.

177. Pitt B, Chong P, Timmmermans P. Angiotensin II receptor antagonists in heart failure: rationale and design of the Evaluation of Losartan in the Elderly (ELITE) trial. *Cardiovasc Drug Ther* 1995;9:693–700.

178. Pitt B, Segal R, Martinez FA, et al. Randomized trial of losartan versus captopril in patients over 65 with heart failure (Evaluation of Losartan in the Elderly Study, ELITE). *Lancet* 1997;349:747–752.

179. Pitt B, Poole-Wilson P, Segal R, et al. Effects of losartan versus captopril on mortality in patients with symptomatic heart failure. Design of ELITE-II. *J Card Fail* 1999;5:146–154.

180. Farquharson CAJ, Struthers AD. Angiotensin-II receptor blockers in chronic heart failure—not as ELITE as expected! *J Renin-Angiotensin-Aldosterone Sys* 2000;1:21–22.

181. Hirsch AT, Talsness CE, Schunkert H, et al. Tissue-specific activation of cardiac angiotensin converting enzyme in experimental heart failure. *Circ Res* 1991;69:475–482.

182. Miura S, Ideisha M, Sakai T, et al. Angiotensin-II formation by an alternative pathway during exercise in humans. *J Hypertension* 1994;12:1177–1181.

183. Urata H, Kinoshita A, Misono KS, et al. Identification of a highly specific chymase as the major angiotensin-II forming enzyme in the human chymase. *J Biol Chem* 1990;265:58–59.

184. McKelvie RS, Yusuf S, Pericak D, et al. Comparison of candesartan, enalapril, and their combination in congestive heart failure: Randomized Evaluation of Strategies for Left Ventricular Dysfunction (RESOLVD) pilot study. *Circulation* 1999;100:1056–1064.

185. Cohn JN, Tognoni G, Glazer RD, et al. Rationale and design of the Valsartan Heart Failure Trial: a large, multinational trial to assess the effects of valsartan, and angiotensin-II receptor blocker, on morbidity and mortality in chronic congestive heart failure. *J Cardiac Fail* 1999;5:155–160.

186. Swedberg K, Pfeffer M, Granger C, et al. Candesartan in Heart failure—Assessment of Reduction in Morbidity and mortality (CHARM): rationale and design. *J Cardiac Fail* 1999;5:276–282.

187. Young JB. Reduction of ischemic events with angiotensin-converting enzyme inhibitors: lessons and controversy emerging from recent clinical trials. *Cardiovasc Drugs Ther* 1995;9:89–102.

188. Young JB. Angiotensin-converting enzyme inhibitors and ischemic heart disease. *Coron Artery Dis* 1995;6:272–280.

189. Swedberg K, Hjalmarson A, Waagstein F, et al. Prolongation of survival in congestive cardiomyopathy by beta-receptor blockade. *Lancet* 1979;1:1374–1376.

190. CIBIS Investigators and Committees. A randomized trial of β-blockade in heart failure: the Cardiac Insufficiency Bisoprolol Study (CIBIS). *Circulation* 1994;90:1765–1773.

191. Beta-blocker Evaluation of Survival Trial (BEST). *Can we reduce CHF mortality?* Lecture program. New York: Bioscience Communications, 1996.

192. Beta-Blocker Heart Attack Trial Research Group. A randomized trial of propanolol in patients with acute myocardial infarction. Mortality results. *JAMA* 1982;247:1707–1714.

193. Pedersen TR, and the Norwegian Multicenter Study Group. Six-year follow-up of the Norwegian multicenter study on timolol after acute myocardial infarction. *N Engl J Med* 1985;313:1055–1058.

194. Yancy CW, Fowler MB, Colucci WS, et al. Race and the response to adrenergic blockade with carvedilol in patients with chronic heart failure. *N Engl J Med* 2001;344:1358–1365.

195. Wood AJJ. Racial differences in the response to drugs—pointers to genetic differences. *N Engl J Med* 2001;344:1393–1395.

195a. Packer M, Antonopoulos GV, Berlin JA, et al. Comparative effects of carvedilol and metoprolol on left ventricular ejection fraction in heart failure: results of a meta-analysis. *Am Heart J* 2001;141:899–907.

196. Adams KF. Which beta blocker for heart failure? *Am Heart J* 2001;141:884–888.

197. Ceremuzynski L, Leczar E, Krzeminska-Pakula M, et al. Effect of amiodarone on mortality after myocardial infarction: a double-blind, placebo-controlled pilot study. *J Am Coll Cardiol* 1992;20:1056–1062.

198. Hamer AWF, Arkles LB, Johns JA. Beneficial effects of low dose amiodarone in patients with congestive heart failure: a placebo-controlled trial. *J Am Coll Cardiol* 1989;14:1768–1774.

199. Mahmarian JJ, Smart FW, Moy LA, et al. Exploring the minimal dose of amiodarone with antiarrhythmic and hemodynamic activity. *Am J Cardiol* 1994;74:681–686.

200. Podrid PJ. Amiodarone: re-evaluation of an old drug. *Ann Intern Med* 1995;122:689–700.

201. Silver MJ, Young JB, Topol EJ. Amiodarone in congestive heart failure. *N Engl J Med* 1995;333:1639.

202. Moss AJ, Hall WJ, Cannom DS, et al., for the Multicenter Automatic Defibrillator Implantation Trial Investigators (MADIT). Improved survival with an implanted defibrillator in patients with coronary disease at high risk for ventricular arrhythmias. *N Engl J Med* 1996;335:1933–1940.

203. Antiarrhythmics Versus Implantable Defibrillators Trial investigators. A comparison of antiarrhythmic drug therapy with implantable defibrillators in patients resuscitated from near-fatal ventricular arrhythmias. *N Engl J Med* 1997;337:1576–1583.

204. Connolly SJ, Gent M, Roberts RS, et al. Canadian Implantable Defibrillator Study (CIDS): a randomized trial of the implantable cardioverter defibrillator against amiodarone. *Circulation* 2000;101:1297–1302.

205. Kuck KH, Cappato R, Siebels J, et al. Randomized comparison of antiarrhythmic drug therapy with implantable defibrillators in patients resuscitated from cardiac arrest: the Cardiac Arrest Study, Hamburg. *Circulation* 2000;102:748–754.

206. Buxton AE, Lee KL, Di Carlo L, et al. Electrophysiologic testing to identify patients with coronary artery disease who are at risk for sudden death. Multicenter Unsustained Tachycardia Trial investigators (MUTT). *N Engl J Med* 2000;342:1937–1945.

207. Cazeau S, LeClerq C, Lavergne T, et al. Effects of Multisite biventricular pacing in patients with heart failure and intraventricular conduction delay. *N Engl J Med* 2001;344:873–880.

208. Jafri SM, Mammen EF, Masura J, et al. Effects of warfarin on markers of hypercoagulability in patients with heart failure. *Am Heart J* 1997;134:27–36.

209. Jafri SM, Cleland J, Massie B. Is there a role for warfarin or aspirin therapy in heart failure? *Heart Failure Rev* 1997;1:271–276.

210. Fazio S, Sabatini D, Capaldo B, et al. A preliminary study of growth hormone in the treatment of dilated cardiomyopathy. *N Engl J Med* 1996;334:809–814.

211. Kubo SH, Rector TS, Bank AJ, et al. Endothelium-dependent vasodilation is attenuated in patients with heart failure. *Circulation* 1991;84:1589–1596.

212. Treasure CB, Alexander RW. The dysfunctional endothelium in heart failure. *J Am Coll Cardiol* 1993;22:129A–134A.

213. Cohn JN, Bristow MR, Chien KR, et al. Report of the National Heart, Lung, and Blood Institute Special Emphasis Panel on Heart Failure Research. *Circulation* 1997;95:766–770.

214. Cody RJ. Atrial natriuretic factor in edematous disorders. *Annu Rev Med* 1990;41:377–382.

215. Dao Q, Krishnaswamy P, Kazanegra R, et al. Utility of B-type natriuretic peptide in the diagnosis of congestive heart failure in an urgent care setting. *J Am Coll Cardiol* 2001;37:379–385.

216. Maisel AS, Koon J, Krishnaswamy P, et al. Utility of B-natriuretic peptide as a rapid, point-of-care test for surviving patients undergoing echocardiography to determine left ventricular dysfunction. *Am Heart J* 2001;141:367–374.

217. Cheng V, Kazanegra R, Garcia A, et al. A rapid bedside test for B-type peptide predicts treatment outcomes in patients admitted for decompensated heart failure. A pilot study. *J Am Coll Cardiol* 2001;37:386–391.

218. Young J, Warner-Stevenson L, Abraham WT, et al. Rationale and design of the VMAC trial: vasodilation in the management of acute congestive heart failure. *J Cardiac Fail* 200;6:48.

219. Murray CE, Wiseman RW, Schwartz SM, et al. Skeletal myoblast transplantation for repair of myocardial necrosis. *J Clin Invest* 1996;98:2512–2523.

220. Menasche P, Hagege AA, Scorsin M, et al. Myoblast transplantation for heart failure. *Lancet* 2001;357:279–280.

221. Colucci WS. Apoptosis in the heart. *N Engl J Med* 1996;335:1224–1226.

222. Lenfant C. Fixing the failing heart. *Circulation* 1997;95:771–772.

223. Mallat Z, Tedgui A, Fontaliran F, et al. Evidence of apoptosis in arrhythmogenic right ventricular dysplasia. *N Engl J Med* 1996;335:1190–1196.

224. Narula J, Haider N, Virmani R, et al. Apoptosis in myocytes in end-stage heart failure. *N Engl J Med* 1996;335:1182–1189.

225. Sharov VG, Sabbah HN, Shimoyama H, et al. Evidence of cardiocyte apoptosis in myocardium of dogs with chronic heart failure. *Am J Pathol* 1996;148:141–149.

226. Olivetti G, Abbi R, Quaini F, et al. Apoptosis in the failing human heart. *N Engl J Med* 1997;336:1131–1141.

227. Assessment of Treatment with Lisinopril (ATLAS) Study Group. *Clinical Trial Operations Manual*, 1990.

228. Massie BM, Berk MR, Brozena SC, et al. Can further benefit be achieved by adding flosequinan to patients with congestive heart failure who remain symptomatic on diuretic, digoxin, and an angiotensin converting enzyme inhibitor? Results of the flosequinan-ACE inhibitor trial (FACET). *Circulation* 1993;88:492–501.

93

DIAGNOSIS AND MEDICAL TREATMENT OF INFLAMMATORY CARDIOMYOPATHY

DENNIS M. MCNAMARA

OVERVIEW

Myocardial inflammation underlies cardiac dysfunction in a wide spectrum of disorders, from lymphocytic myocarditis (1,2) to idiopathic dilated cardiomyopathy (IDC) (3). Animal models and clinical studies support viral etiologies in the majority of cases, although specific infectious agents are documented in only a fraction. Therapy remains supportive, because, despite this inflammatory pathogenesis and scores of anecdotal series that suggest a therapeutic role for immunosuppression, controlled trials have consistently failed to demonstrate clinical benefit (4–6). Endomyocardial biopsy, once widely used for diagnosis, is currently not recommended for the majority of cases given the absence of specific biopsy-guided therapies (7). Giant-cell myocarditis remains one exception, as biopsy confirmation of this aggressive disorder may assist in therapeutic decisions, including the consideration of immunosuppressive therapy (8). The potential future role for immune modulatory therapy remains an intense area of investigation.

INTRODUCTION

Primary dilated cardiomyopathy or IDC is a leading cause of congestive heart failure in the United States, particularly among young people (9). Although cardiac inflammation is postulated as an important early pathologic event, signs of systemic inflammation are rarely seen at presentation. Myocarditis, an often suspected but infrequently diagnosed disorder of primary cardiac inflammation, is believed to be an early precursor of IDC (10). Whether these two diagnoses are distinct entities or merely separate time points in a pathologic progression remains a matter of significant controversy. Over the last two decades, the search for mecha-

D. M. McNamara: Department of Medicine, Cardiovascular Institute, University of Pittsburgh Medical Center, Pittsburgh, Pennsylvania

nistic-based therapies for primary dilated cardiomyopathy has focused on the inflammatory pathogenesis. This current intensive period of investigation can be seen as the culmination of nearly two centuries of broad clinical interests in this common and mysterious form of cardiac disease.

INFLAMMATORY CARDIOMYOPATHY: TERMINOLOGY AND CLINICAL SUBSETS

With the increasing use of endomyocardial biopsy for diagnosis, the term *myocarditis* gradually became synonymous with left ventricular (LV) dysfunction with histologic evidence of cellular inflammation. Indeed, as recently as 1995, the World Health Organization task force defined *inflammatory cardiomyopathy* as "myocarditis in association with myocardial dysfunction. Myocarditis is an inflammatory disease of the myocardium and is diagnosed by established histologic, immunologic, and immunohistochemical criteria" (19). In the current age in which biopsy data are infrequently obtained, reliance on histologically defined criteria may be impractical. From the standpoint of clinical practice, myocarditis can be defined more simply and literally as inflammation of the myocardium or heart muscle as assessed by a number of clinical criteria.

The risk of broadened clinical criteria remains that the pathologic and clinical distinction between inflammatory myocarditis and IDC can become somewhat obscured. As stated by eminent cardiac pathologist Michael Davies, "Cardiomyopathy and myocarditis are terms used with an expectation that they are generally understood. In practice, once their definition is attempted, difficulties emerge and their meaning seems less clear" (20). In its broadest definition, *inflammatory cardiomyopathy* includes a heterogeneous set of disorders in which myocardial inflammation plays the primary role in the pathogenesis of cardiac dysfunction. This heterogeneous grouping can be subdivided into more distinct subsets based on the clinical setting of presentation (e.g., pregnancy) or diagnostic histopathology (Table 93.1).

For many patients with the clinical syndrome of myocarditis, endomyocardial biopsy is either not obtained or is uninformative. Approximately 30% to 40% (6,21,22) of

TABLE 93.1 INFLAMMATORY CARDIOMYOPATHY: CLINICAL SUBSETS

Myocarditis
  Biopsy defined: lymphocytic, eosinophilic
  Clinically defined
Giant-cell myocarditis
Systemic autoimmune disorders with myocarditis
  Systemic lupus erythematosus
  Polymyositis
  Sarcoid
Peripartum cardiomyopathy
Subsets of idiopathic dilated cardiomyopathy

patients with new-onset, unexplained LV dysfunction have dramatic recovery of systolic function during subsequent follow-up. Myocarditis is the suspected etiology for most cases; however, this conclusion is generally only reached retrospectively. Only a fraction of patients who undergo biopsy have evidence of cellular myocardial inflammation (6).

Among those patients with biopsy evidence of cellular inflammation, most are classified as having "lymphocytic myocarditis" based on lymphocyte predominance in the myocardial cellular infiltrates (23). An eosinophilic predominance can be seen in myocarditis that is associated with an allergic reaction or with peripheral eosinophilia (24–27). Although lymphocytic myocarditis is seen in roughly 10% of biopsied patients (5), only 1% to 2% are diagnosed with giant-cell myocarditis, defined by the presence of multinucleated giant cells in the myocardium (28). The distinction between this disorder and lymphocytic myocarditis is critically important, as giant-cell myocarditis is a much more aggressive pathologic process with a distinct natural history (8,28).

Myocarditis can also be seen as part of systemic autoimmune disorders such as sarcoidosis (29) or systemic lupus erythematosus (30). These disorders are defined by their respective systemic syndromes in terms of their clinical course and treatment. The histologic appearance of myocarditis as part of a systemic disorder is similar to that seen in isolated myocarditis. The granulomas of cardiac sarcoid in particular can be difficult to distinguish from its histologic mimic, giant-cell myocarditis (31).

IDC may be the most common form of "inflammatory" heart disease despite the fact that IDC endomyocardial biopsy is generally uninformative (3). Peripartum cardiomyopathy, the form of primary dilated cardiomyopathy that is seen as a complication of pregnancy, also likely has an inflammatory pathogenesis, and cellular inflammation is frequently seen on endomyocardial biopsy (32).

PREVALENCE

The prevalence of primary "idiopathic" dilated cardiomyopathy has been estimated at 0.4 per 1,000, with an annual incidence of 0.08 per 1,000 (33). This correlates to approximately 120,000 cases within the United States alone, with 24,000 new cases each year. The prevalence of histologic myocarditis, defined specifically as cellular inflammation on endomyocardial biopsy, varies widely in published series (Table 93.2) but can be best estimated from multicenter studies at approximately 10% to 20% of patients with new-onset IDC (5,6,34). The MTT noted biopsies that were positive for inflammation in only 10% of 2,233 screened patients (5). In a similar fashion, the ongoing European Study of Epidemiology and Treatment of Cardiac Inflammatory Diseases has reported positive biopsies in 17.2% of the first 3,055 patients screened (34). Evidence of myo-

TABLE 93.2 PREVALENCE OF MYOCARDITIS IN PUBLISHED SERIES

Author (reference)	Years	Percent with positive biopsy	Patient group
Dec et al. (21)	1975–1983	67 (18/27)	Recent-onset cardiomyopathy with <6 mo of symptoms
Parillo et al. (4)	1982–1988	38 (38/102)	Patients referred to the National Institutes of Health for randomized trial of prednisone in idiopathic dilated cardiomyopathy
Mason et al. (5)	1986–1989	10 (214/2,233)	Patients screened for the Myocarditis Treatment Trial
McCarthy et al. (162)	1984–1997	14 (252/1,757)	Large single-center series from Johns Hopkins
McNamara et al. (6)	1996–1998	16 (10/62)	All recent-onset dilated cardiomyopathy enrolled in the IMAC trial
Drucker et al. (122)	1985–1991	51 (20/39)	Children referred with the clinical syndrome of suspected myocarditis
Midei et al. (82)	1983–1988	78 (14/18)	Patients with peripartum cardiomyopathy from a single center, Johns Hopkins
Bozkurt et al. (124)	1990–1998	9 (1/11)	Patients with peripartum cardiomyopathy from a single center, University of Pittsburgh

From Feldman AM, McNamara D. Myocarditis. *N Engl J Med* 2000;343:1388–1398, with permission.

carditis may be found in 1% to 9% of routine autopsy cases (35–37) and up to 20% of those that are performed for unexplained sudden cardiac death in young people (38). Although autopsy series and multicenter trials provide estimates for myocarditis with major cardiac consequences (LV dysfunction or sudden death), most cases of myocarditis are likely self-limited and never present to medical attention. The true prevalence of these subacute forms of myocarditis is difficult to determine, as is their role in initiating the pathway that leads to IDC.

IMMUNOPATHOLOGY OF PROGRESSION

Whether virally initiated, peripartum, or idiopathic, the most common histologic appearance of myocardial cellular inflammation, lymphocytic myocarditis, is indistinguishable from the appearance of acute allograft rejection in the transplanted heart (95), with a predominance of T-lymphocytes. In murine models, whether the initial immune response is self-limited or results in progressive inflammation and cardiomyopathy is strain dependent (96), supporting a strong role of genetic background in determining outcome. In clinical studies, specific human leukocyte antigen genotypes appear to confer an increased risk of the development of dilated cardiomyopathy (97), suggesting that genetic susceptibility may be equally important in the human perpetuation of immune-mediated injury. Genetic predisposition to autoimmune pathology may be particularly important in giant-cell myocarditis, as a high percentage of patients who present with this disorder also have previously had other autoimmune diseases such as thyroiditis and colitis (8). Perpetuation of myocardial inflammatory disease requires not only antigenic similarity of myocardial and viral peptides, but also a genetic "background" that facilitates the continuation of the pathologic immune response (98,99).

Increasing evidence over the last decade points toward myocardial expression of cytokines in general and TNF-α in particular as being important driving forces in the develop-

ment of the end-stage cardiomyopathy phenotype (100,101). Myocardial expression and plasma levels of TNF-α and IL-6 increase as functional status worsens (102,103). The explanted heart from patients who are undergoing transplantation frequently demonstrates inflammatory myocardial infiltrates (104), even in those with coronary artery disease as the primary etiology of their heart failure. This demonstrates that in the end-stage ischemic heart, expression of inflammatory mediators can elicit cellular infiltration of the myocardium and contribute to the decline in cardiac function. The role of myocardial cytokine expression in the progression of heart failure from the compensated to the end-stage phenotype has broadened our appreciation of the inflammatory nature of chronic heart failure and led many investigators to focus efforts at immune modulation on chronic or end-stage disease (105,106). ❦ p46

IMMUNOSUPPRESSIVE AND IMMUNE MODULATORY THERAPIES: LESSONS FROM CLINICAL TRIALS

The immune hypothesis for the progression of myocarditis to dilated cardiomyopathy has led to intense clinical interests over the years in improving ventricular function by blunting or modulating the pathologic aspects of the immune response. The challenge in studying the impact of therapeutic interventions in this disorder has been the clinical heterogeneity and a high spontaneous recovery rate in small subsets of patients. In addition, given the relative infrequency of patients who present with myocarditis and LV dysfunction, single-center anecdotal series are generally quite small, and a multicenter format is required to evaluate therapeutic interventions. Three major prospective randomized trials of immune suppression or modulation have been reported over the last decade, and all three controlled studies failed to confirm the therapeutic benefits that were suggested by anecdotal reports (4–6) (Table 93.3). ❦ p47

Recruitment for the MTT was challenging due to the strict biopsy criteria. Local pathologists found evidence of

TABLE 93.3 RANDOMIZED CLINICAL TRIALS OF IMMUNE MODULATION IN MYOCARDITIS AND DILATED CARDIOMYOPATHY

Author (reference)	Agent studied	No. randomized	Primary outcome measure	Result
Parillo et al. (4)	Prednisone	102	Change in EF at 3 mo	Modest benefit (4 EF units vs. 2 EF units in the placebo)
Mason et al. (Myocarditis Treatment Trial) (5)	Prednisone and cyclosporine	111	Change in EF at 6 mo	No significant effect (increase of 10 EF units vs. 7 EF units with placebo)
McNamara et al. (IMAC Trial) (6)	Immune globulin	62	Change in EF at 6 mo	No treatment effect (increase of 14 EF units in both groups)

EF, ejection fraction.
From Feldman AM, McNamara D. Myocarditis. *N Engl J Med* 2000;343:1388–1398, with permission.

myocarditis on endomyocardial biopsy for only 214 of 2,233 screened patients. Of these individuals, 111 met the other entry criteria and were randomized. Overall, LV function improved significantly over time from a mean of 0.25 at baseline to 0.34 at 28 weeks. No treatment effect was evident with immunosuppressive therapy, as the improvement in LVEF was similar in the two groups (0.10 with immunosuppressive therapy vs. 0.07 in the control group) (Fig. 93.1). No long-term difference in survival was seen (*p* = .96), with an overall mortality of 20% at 1 year and 56% at 4.3 years (Fig. 93.2). In current practice, the absence of therapeutic benefit for immunosuppression in the MTT has all but eliminated its use in adults with suspected myocarditis.

Recent research has focused on the use of intravenous immunoglobulin (IVIG) as an immune modulating agent (115–117). High-dose IVIG has been used in a number of autoimmune disorders, including idiopathic thrombocytopenic purpura (118), Guillain-Barré syndrome (119), and dermatomyositis (120). Based on effectiveness in Kawasaki's disease (121), a coronary vasculitis in children, pediatricians began investigating its use in myocarditis and reported significant improvement in LV function compared to that of historical controls (122). Subse-

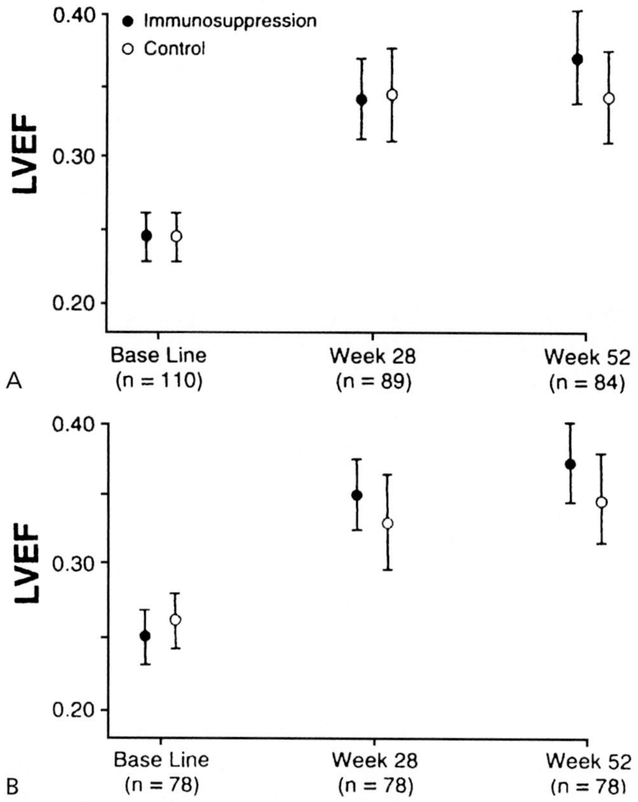

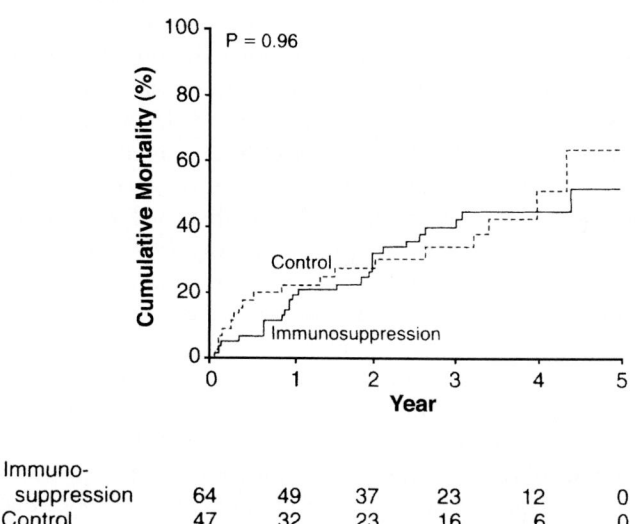

FIGURE 93.1 Serial change in left ventricular ejection fraction (LVEF) for all patients enrolled in the Myocarditis Treatment Trial **(A)** and only those who had paired studies **(B)**, showing comparable improvement in LVEF in the two groups. (From Mason JW, O'Connell JB, Herskowitz A, et al. A clinical trial of immunosuppressive therapy for myocarditis. *N Engl J Med* 1995;333:269–275, with permission. Copyright © 1995 Massachusetts Medical Society. All rights reserved.)

FIGURE 93.2 Cumulative mortality in subjects receiving immunosuppression and controls from the Myocarditis Treatment Trial, showing no difference between the groups. (From Mason JW, O'Connell JB, Herskowitz A, et al. A clinical trial of immunosuppressive therapy for myocarditis. *N Engl J Med* 1995;333:269–275, with permission. Copyright © 1995 Massachusetts Medical Society. All rights reserved.)

quently, two small series were reported in adults with new-onset dilated cardiomyopathy and myocarditis (123) and peripartum cardiomyopathy (124) that suggested enhanced improvement in LVEF compared to historical controls.

The therapeutic role of immunoglobulin for adults with recent-onset inflammatory cardiomyopathy was evaluated in the IMAC trial (6). This multicenter study randomized 62 patients to 2 g per kg IVIG or a placebo infusion at the time of initial presentation with new-onset heart failure. All enrolled patients had evaluation that was consistent with a primary dilated cardiomyopathy or myocarditis, had an LVEF of 0.40 or less, and were randomized within 6 months of their onset of cardiac symptoms. All underwent an endomyocardial biopsy; however, patients with and without cellular inflammation on biopsy were included. Overall, the clinical characteristics of the IMAC and MTT study populations were quite similar (*e*Table 93.3.1). The primary end point was the change in LVEF at 6 months after randomization. Overall, LVEF improved significantly from 0.25 at baseline to 0.42 at 12 months. No treatment effect was evident, as the improvement at 6 months was 14 EF units in both groups and at 12 months was 16 EF units with IVIG versus 15 with placebo (Fig. 93.3). Overall event-free survival [events defined as death, transplantation, or need for LV assist device (LVAD)] was 91% at 1 year and 88% at 2 years (Fig. 93.4), and there were no significant differences between treatment groups. ☙ p48

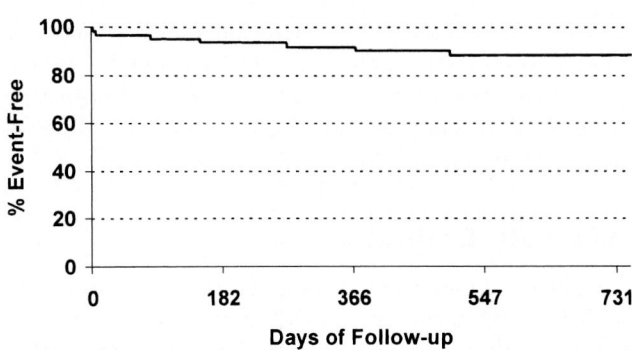

FIGURE 93.4 Event-free survival for patients with new-onset dilated cardiomyopathy and myocarditis enrolled in the IMAC trial (events defined as death, cardiac transplantation, or need for left ventricular assist device). Event-free survival 91% at 1 year and 88% at 2 years.

CLINICAL MANAGEMENT: EVALUATION

Presentation

The classic presentation for a patient with myocarditis is symptoms of chest pain or dyspnea in the setting of an acute febrile illness. However, subacute myocarditis (inflammation with mild or no LV dysfunction) may present without any cardiac symptoms. Occasionally, these cases are surreptitiously diagnosed in the setting of an acute viral syndrome by the incidental finding of electrocardiographic (ECG) abnormalities (131) or elevations of cardiac enzymes (132,133). Just as cardiac symptoms are not necessarily part of the presentation with myocarditis, neither is an acute febrile illness. Fever was present in only a minority of patients in the MTT (5) (*e*Table 93.3.1).

In patients who present with LV dysfunction, the most common cardiac symptoms are those of congestive heart failure (dyspnea, fatigue, and chest discomfort) (134). In general, heart failure symptoms are more left sided, although signs of right-sided failure, in particular peripheral edema, or symptoms of hepatic congestion (abdominal discomfort or nausea) can be seen. Palpitations are a common presenting complaint and may represent atrial or ventricular arrhythmias (135–137). Atrial arrhythmias generally reflect left atrial hypertension or irritation from associated pericarditis. Ventricular dysrhythmias, although usually associated with heart failure and significant LV dysfunction, are occasionally seen with relatively preserved LV function and presumably originate from an inflammatory focus within the ventricle (138).

Adult patients who present with symptoms of heart failure due to myocarditis typically do so with no signs of systemic inflammation (5,6) and come to medical attention months after the initial symptom complex began. In this regard, the presentation in young children is distinctly different from that of adults, perhaps reflecting differences in the pediatric viral milieu. Children are more likely to present within days of the onset of symptoms (122) and

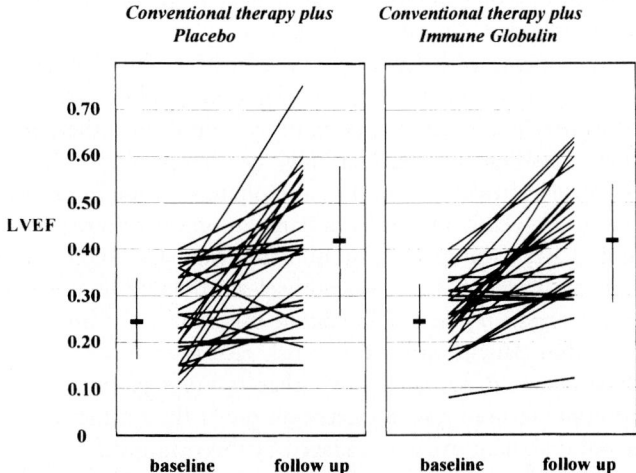

FIGURE 93.3 Left ventricular ejection fraction (LVEF) over time by treatment. LVEF by radionuclide scan at baseline and 12 months postrandomization in patients randomized to placebo and immunoglobulin. Overall, LVEF improved significantly over time (12 months LVEF significantly higher than baseline, *p* <.001). However, no differences by treatment group were evident (*p* = not significant for comparisons by treatment). (From McNamara DM, Holubkov R, Starling RC, et al., for the IMAC investigators. A controlled trial of intravenous immune globulin for recent onset dilated cardiomyopathy. *Circulation* 2001;103:2254–2259, with permission.)

have more systemic signs of an acute inflammatory state. As patients who present earlier generally have a higher probability of spontaneous recovery once systemic inflammation has resolved, this may lead to a higher probability of significant LV recovery in children.

Diagnostic Evaluation

The clinical examination of patients with suspected myocarditis should focus on signs of ventricular dysfunction. Although tachycardia and borderline hypotension may reflect an acute febrile syndrome, they may also be the first signs of significant hemodynamic compromise. In acute cases, rales on the pulmonary examination provide evidence of left-sided failure; however, in patients with a more insidious presentation a clear lung examination can be heard despite significant dyspnea and marked elevations in left-sided filling pressure. Elevated jugular venous pressure, hepatic tenderness, or peripheral edema is consistent with right-sided failure and suggests right ventricular involvement.

The ECG remains an important clinical tool in evaluating cases of suspected myocarditis (131). Common findings are diffuse and nonspecific ST- and T-wave abnormalities. In cases of fever and acute chest pain, PR depression and diffuse global ST elevation may allow a rapid diagnosis of pericarditis. Low voltage may be evident, particularly in those with an associated pericardial effusion. Occasionally, myocarditis presents with ECG findings suggestive of myocardial infarction in a specific vascular territory. Although this form of myocarditis that mimics the presentation of myocardial infarction has been well described (139–142), it remains important in such cases to rule out an acute ischemic event and to have a low threshold for proceeding with rapid coronary angiography.

Serum analysis for patients with a suspected myocarditis should include creatine phosphokinase (CPK) with appropriate fractionation or, alternatively, cardiac troponin. Elevations of CPK tend to be moderate, in the range of 200 to 1,000, even in cases of fulminant myocarditis. In young men who present with dilated cardiomyopathy with a persistent chronic elevation of CPK, a detailed family history should be obtained, as chronic elevations in CPK may reflect not persistent myocarditis but dystrophinopathy, a familial X-linked disorder (88).

For patients who present with an acute febrile illness, acute and convalescent sera against most common viral pathogens should be performed. Such a panel should include Coxsackie B, influenza A and B, cytomegalovirus, and appropriate adenoviral forms (59). A mild leukocytosis may be seen, particularly with a lymphocyte predominance. Marked leukocytosis should elicit a thorough evaluation for a systemic bacterial infection in which LV dysfunction may be secondary to septicemia. Peripheral eosinophilia should suggest the possibility of eosinophilic myocarditis, a syndrome that is frequently related to drug or other allergies. Serologic testing should include antinuclear antibody and rheumatoid factor, looking for occult connective tissue disease or other systemic autoimmune disease. Testing for other cardiac-specific autoantibodies, for example, those directed against cardiac myosin or the adrenergic beta-receptor, remains investigational and is not part of clinical screening.

In young patients with chronic cough or dyspnea, chest x-ray findings of cardiomegaly or interstitial edema often initiate the cardiac consultation. Usually, marked cardiomegaly is associated with a more insidious progressive course. In these patients, as in chronic dilated cardiomyopathy, findings on chest x-ray of pulmonary edema may be minimal despite markedly elevated left-sided filling pressures. In contrast, acute fulminant myocarditis can present with florid alveolar edema and acute respiratory failure, but, given the short time course of the illness, a relatively normal-sized cardiac silhouette.

In any patient with suspected myocarditis, an echocardiogram should be performed. This one test gives clinicians the maximum information about LV size and function and right ventricular involvement (143,144). The presence of a pericardial effusion, relatively small chamber size with decreased systolic function, and increased LV wall thickness are essentially diagnostic of an active process of myocardial inflammation. In general, decrease in LV systolic function is global, although marked segmental wall motion abnormalities can be seen. However, the echogenicity of the myocardium itself does not change with active inflammation, and therefore the echo images of the myocardium itself do not help in the specific diagnosis of cardiac inflammation. Despite this limitation, echocardiography remains clinically the most useful tool for clinical management and should be a part of any diagnostic evaluation.

In patients with LV systolic dysfunction and significant hemodynamic impairment, consideration should be given to invasive hemodynamic assessment by right heart catheterization. Persistent tachycardia may be compensatory for a decrease in stroke volume and a resultant decrease in cardiac output. As acute myocardial inflammation can affect systolic and diastolic properties, pulmonary capillary wedge and right atrial pressures are frequently elevated out of proportion to the apparent decrease in systolic function. In addition, in any adult patient with cardiac risk factors, coronary artery disease should be ruled out either by angiography or by appropriate noninvasive evaluation given the distinctly different treatment pathway engaged by this diagnosis.

Endomyocardial Biopsy

In the 1960s, the development of techniques for transvenous endomyocardial right ventricular biopsy made possible the antemortem diagnosis of myocardial inflammation (15,145). By the mid-1980s, its critical role in managing patients after cardiac transplant led to increased use in the evaluation of native myocardial disease (146). Infiltrates of inflammatory

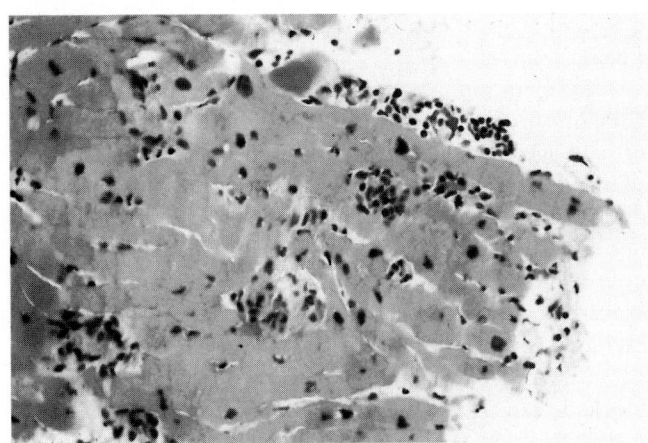
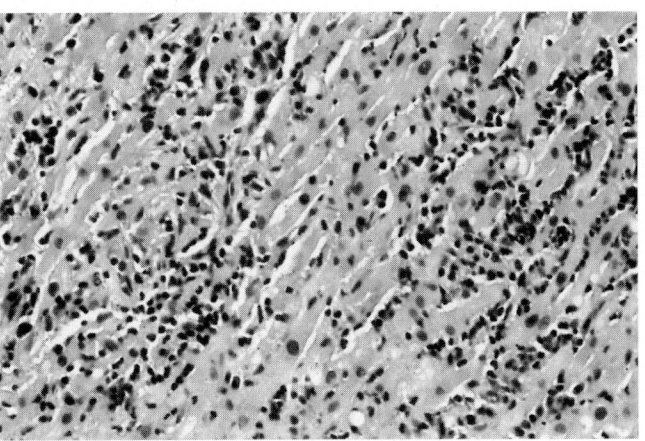

FIGURE 93.5 Histopathologic appearance of borderline myocarditis (lymphocytic infiltrates *without* myocyte necrosis) **(A)** and myocarditis (lymphocytic infiltrates *with* myocyte necrosis) **(B)**. **A:** ×350 magnification; **B:** ×300 magnification. (From Feldman AM, McNamara D. Myocarditis. *N Engl J Med* 2000;343:1388–1398, with permission. Copyright © 2000 Massachusetts Medical Society. All rights reserved.)

cells invading the myocardium on biopsy rapidly became the gold standard for the diagnosis of myocarditis, which previously had relied on more indirect clinical assessment. However, the sensitivity of endomyocardial biopsy has historically been limited by sampling error. Biopsy samples are taken from the apical portion of the right ventricular septum, as limiting sampling to this region lessens the risk of complications, namely, acute tricuspid regurgitation or cardiac perforation and tamponade. Autopsy studies of patients who are known to have myocarditis have estimated the sensitivity of endomyocardial biopsy at no better than 60% to 70% because of regional sampling error (147).

In addition, the finding of cellular inflammation as indicative of myocarditis is dependent on interpretation. In an effort to have more consistent pathologic guidelines, a group of leading cardiac pathologists met in Dallas in 1986 to establish a consensus for the definition of myocarditis (148). The Dallas criteria defined "borderline myocarditis" as the presence of mononuclear cell infiltrates without myocyte necrosis (Fig. 93.5A and *e*Fig. 93.5.1) and "myocarditis" as cellular infiltration with myocyte necrosis (Fig. 93.5B and *e*Fig. 93.5.2). Despite this widely accepted consensus, interpretation remains problematic and physician dependent (149). After review by the study pathology panel of the endomyocardial biopsies from patients enrolled in the MTT (all of whom were believed by their local pathologists to have histologic myocarditis), 36% were not thought to have Dallas criteria myocarditis or borderline myocarditis (5). Conversely, a "negative" biopsy does not rule out myocarditis, as patients without cellular inflammation on biopsy may still follow a clinical course that is suggestive of myocarditis. In the IMAC study, 16 of 20 patients who normalized their EF (greater than or equal to 0.50) during follow-up had biopsies that were interpreted as negative for cellular inflammation at entry. Most such cases of reversible LV dysfunction in retrospect had a clinical syndrome that was strongly suggestive of transient myocardial inflammation.

Two additional considerations are important in determining the role of endomyocardial biopsy in the workup of suspected myocarditis. First, for endomyocardial biopsy in native hearts the risk of a major complication, in particular cardiac tamponade, approaches 1% (150,151), significantly higher than in cardiac transplant patients. In addition, currently there are few histologically guided therapies; therefore, biopsy findings of cellular inflammation usually do not change therapeutic plans and are of minimal prognostic value (6,152). This absence of specific biopsy-guided therapy has led the American College of Cardiology to classify endomyocardial biopsy for the evaluation of heart failure due to unexplained myocardial dysfunction as a "class II procedure . . . acceptable but of uncertain efficacy and may be controversial" (7).

In patients with fulminant myocarditis, endomyocardial biopsy may have more clinical utility than in the compensated patient. Patients with fulminant disease and hemodynamic compromise are more likely to have giant-cell myocarditis (*e*Fig. 93.5.3). Although it remains investigational, data from the Giant Cell Registry (8,153) suggest that immunosuppression therapy may be appropriate in patients with giant-cell myocarditis. In addition, biopsy evidence of a dynamic destructive process may help guide the timing of therapeutic interventions such as LVAD placement or cardiac transplantation. Although in this very-high-risk subset biopsy may assist in these therapeutic decisions, it should be performed at a tertiary referral center where such end-stage supportive therapies are readily available.

MEDICAL MANAGEMENT OF MYOCARDITIS

In the absence of proven benefit in prospective clinical trials, immunosuppressive therapy is not recommended for adult patients with isolated myocarditis. For individuals with myocarditis as part of a systemic autoimmune disorder, such as sarcoid, systemic lupus erythematosus, or polymyositis, immunosuppressive therapy may be beneficial but is generally directed against the systemic disorder (e.g., prednisone for active sarcoid). The need for therapeutic intervention is determined by systemic markers of inflammation (serum CPK from skeletal muscle in polymyositis) and not on measures of myocardial function or findings on biopsy.

The medical therapy of patients with suspected myocarditis is therefore supportive and is dependent on the degree of LV dysfunction. In general, patients with myocarditis can be divided into three broad categories based on the severity of LV compromise: (a) myocarditis and preserved LV function; (b) myocarditis with LV dysfunction and class I–III heart failure; and (c) myocarditis with LV dysfunction and class IV heart failure, or fulminant myocarditis.

Patients with Myocarditis and Preserved Left Ventricular Function

This group of patients frequently present in a setting of an acute febrile illness with ECG abnormalities or chest pain due to associated pericarditis. Therapy in this case consists of observation and partial restriction of activities. Although chest pain due to isolated pericarditis can be treated with indomethacin or nonsteroidal antiinflammatory agents, these agents should be avoided in cases with myocarditis, as they potentiate myocyte necrosis in murine viral models (154–156). In the absence of LV dysfunction, there is no indication for beta-adrenergic receptor antagonists or angiotensin-converting enzyme (ACE) inhibitors. In general, it is recommended that aerobic activities or heavy lifting be avoided for at least 6 to 8 weeks (157). Cardiac assessment, generally ECG and echocardiography, should be repeated roughly 6 to 8 weeks after presentation to guard against progressive cardiac involvement. Endomyocardial biopsy is of limited clinical utility and is not recommended. In general, cases of myocarditis with either mild or no LV dysfunction are self-limited and carry an excellent prognosis.

Myocarditis Associated with Left Ventricular Dysfunction and Class I–III Heart Failure

Recommended therapy is similar to that for patients with LV dysfunction in the absence of myocarditis. ACE inhibitors or angiotensin-receptor blockers are recommended for all patients. Pulmonary congestion or symptoms of fluid overload should be treated with a loop diuretic, generally at the lowest effective dose. Digoxin should be added in patients with New York Heart Association class III heart failure; however, given potential proarrhythmic and proinflammatory (158) effects it should be maintained at a low

dose and avoided entirely in minimally symptomatic (class I or II) subjects.

Consideration should be given to beta-adrenergic antagonists. Caution should be used, however, in the use of such agents in individuals with relatively small chamber size and tachycardia. In such acute patients with systolic dysfunction without a compensatory increase in LV chamber size, tachycardia is compensatory for low stroke volume, and slowing of the heart rate precipitously can exacerbate a low-output state. Although caution must be exercised, given the potential beneficial effects of blocking adrenergic overstimulation in such patients, low-dose beta-blockade can still be considered.

In the absence of atrial fibrillation or a clinical embolic event, anticoagulation in patients with myocarditis and low EF remains controversial, as in noninflammatory dilated cardiomyopathy. Echocardiography is recommended, and if a mural thrombus (159) is detected, 6 to 12 months of low-dose warfarin with an international normalized ratio of 2 to 3 is recommended. In the absence of a mural thrombus or history of embolic event, warfarin is not universally recommended, and there exists much variation in standard practice.

In patients with myocarditis and LV dysfunction, ventricular arrhythmias are frequently seen. Although their management is similar to that of other patients with nonischemic cardiomyopathy, it should be noted that the potential stimulus for ventricular arrhythmias, myocardial inflammation, may resolve. In patients who present with cardiac arrest or aborted sudden death, an implantable defibrillator should be considered, given the potential risk of recurrence. However, in patients with symptomatic nonsustained ventricular tachycardia, amiodarone therapy can be considered an alternative. Multicenter studies in congestive heart failure (160,161) have shown that low-dose amiodarone therapy can be used without significant hazard and may actually improve survival in nonischemic cardiomyopathies. Therefore, amiodarone may offer some protection during the acute inflammatory period, with the potential benefit that it can be gradually withdrawn once the inflammatory period has resolved, particularly if systolic function improves. Amiodarone therapy should also be considered for treatment of symptomatic atrial dysrhythmias.

In general, in patients with LV dysfunction, strenuous physical activity is limited for a period of several months. Follow-up evaluation of LV dysfunction in 3 to 6 months and at 12 months after presentation is recommended. In patients with severe LV dysfunction and class II–III heart failure, we generally defer listing for cardiac transplantation for a period of at least 6 to 12 months, as a significant percentage of patients, from 30% to 50%, exhibit substantial improvement in LV dysfunction in the first year after presentation (6,21,22). In patients with persistent severe LV dysfunction at 12-month follow-up and significant functional limitations, metabolic stress testing should be performed to determine if further evaluation for transplant listing is indicated.

Fulminant Myocarditis: Myocarditis Associated with Hemodynamic Compromise and Class IV Heart Failure

Reports from the single-center registry at Johns Hopkins suggest that for patients with acute lymphocytic myocarditis and severe hemodynamic compromise, long-term prognosis (and the probability of LV recovery) may be better than for patients who present with more insidious chronic disease (162). In addition, dramatic recovery of LV function has been reported in patients with fulminant myocarditis that is maintained with LVAD support and has led to renewed interest in the use of assist devices as "bridges to recovery" rather than transplantation (163–168). Hemodynamic unloading should theoretically rest inflamed myocardium; however, the role of mechanical support in facilitating recovery is difficult to determine, and the use of LVADs is currently reserved for patients who are failing despite maximal inotropic therapy. For patients with cardiogenic shock and aggressive myocarditis, consideration should be given to referral to a tertiary center where both cardiac transplantation and device support are more accessible.

Giant-Cell Myocarditis

In patients with fulminant disease, evaluation for possible giant-cell myocarditis is the primary indication for endomyocardial biopsy. Patients with giant-cell myocarditis were excluded from the Johns Hopkins study, as their prognosis and potential for recovery are significantly worse than for those with lymphocytic myocarditis (8,28). Anecdotal reports (153,169) and the Giant Cell Registry (8) suggest that immunosuppressive therapy, in particular the combination of cyclosporine and the anti–T-lymphocyte antibody muromonab-CD3, may improve transplant-free survival. Given the grim prognosis of giant-cell myocarditis with conventional therapy, immunosuppression should be considered. This remains investigational as the subject of an ongoing multicenter trial.

Postrecovery

For patients whose LV size and systolic function completely normalize, ACE inhibitor therapy and beta-receptor antagonists can gradually be discontinued. In many such patients, subjective limitations in functional capacity and objective limitations in metabolic stress testing may persist, potentially because of a slower recovery of diastolic function (170). Overall prognosis of such patients remains excellent. Although a chance of recurrence of myocarditis

exists, most investigators believe that this is seen only in a minority of patients.

CONTROVERSIES AND PERSONAL PERSPECTIVES

Despite the absence of proven benefit in both the IMAC (6) and MTT trials (5), the search for an immune modulatory therapy which improves patient outcome remains the elusive "Holy Grail" of current myocarditis research. Interestingly, in both trials, patients with more active systemic inflammation actually appeared to have a better prognosis, leading some investigators to question whether suppression of inflammation is the appropriate goal of acute therapy. In the IMAC study, patients with higher initial plasma TNF-α levels tended to have more LV recovery and a higher LVEF at 12-month follow-up (107). In the MTT, patients with an active systemic inflammatory response at presentation (higher white-cell count or autoantibody titer) had less initial impairment of left ventricular function (5). Taken together, these data support the hypothesis that it is not the initial inflammatory event per se, but the myocardial response and subsequent transition to chronic disease that is the true culprit of this pathologic process. For many patients with acute myocarditis, supportive therapy is all that is needed. It is those patients with persistent inflammation who appear to progress toward cardiomyopathy, and identifying and targeting this subset should be the subject of future investigations. Indeed, recent trials in more chronic heart failure suggest a potentially more beneficial therapeutic role for immune modulation than has been seen in previous studies of acute new onset disease (174).

An additional point of controversy remains about whether newer molecular techniques will improve the clinical utility of endomyocardial biopsy and lead to a renaissance of its use in general practice. As important as investigations of gene expression are to the understanding of basic pathogenesis, the same factors which have limited the clinical utility of conventional histology, in particular sampling error, limited tissue availability, and the potential procedural morbidity, will remain significant obstacles despite molecular advances. It is likely that systemic markers of inflammation will be of increasing diagnostic importance, and that future innovations in noninvasive imaging techniques will continue to diminish the current clinical role of endomyocardial biopsy.

ACKNOWLEDGMENTS

I am indebted to Dr. Barry London and Dr. Srinivas Murali for their helpful comments, to Dr. Jake Demetris for providing the photomicrographs, and to Mrs. Marge Altvater for assistance in the preparation of the manuscript.

THE FUTURE

Primary dilated cardiomyopathy remains an important cause of morbidity. Although myocarditis and cardiac inflammation clearly play a role in its early pathogenesis, the clinical heterogeneity of its natural history remains an enigma. Two similar patients who present with LV dysfunction and myocarditis can embark on distinctly different courses, one to complete recovery and the other to chronic cardiomyopathy, cardiac transplantation, or death. The major challenge in the treatment of inflammatory heart disease is to distinguish at presentation those patients who are destined for recovery from those on the path to end-stage heart failure. In current clinical practice, most tools including endomyocardial biopsy are of limited use in this regard. Future investigations that focus on circulating cytokines or other inflammatory mediators, or on additional molecular techniques to enhance the role of biopsy, are needed to decipher these very distinct subsets.

One added untapped resource for the future will be provided by the ongoing research of the human genome project. Genetic background exerts a powerful influence on outcomes with myocarditis, but the genetic loci that are responsible for modulating recovery remain unknown. The human genome project will provide a wealth of information on human genetic variants for scores of genes of interest over the next decade. Studies of the impact of genetic background on the natural history of the disorder and on the efficacy of therapeutic intervention will be of critical importance. It is extremely likely that the current revolution in human genetics will have a significant impact on how we treat patients with inflammatory heart disease within the next decade.

REFERENCES

1. Lange LG, Schreiner GF. Immune mechanisms of cardiac disease. *N Engl J Med* 1994;330:1129–1135.
2. Feldman AM, McNamara D. Myocarditis. *N Engl J Med* 2000;343:1388–1398.
3. Dec GW, Fuster V. Idiopathic dilated cardiomyopathy. *N Engl J Med* 1994;331:1564–1575.
4. Parillo JE, Cunnion RE, Epstein SE, et al. A prospective, randomized, controlled trial of prednisone for dilated cardiomyopathy. *N Engl J Med* 1989;321:1061–1068.
5. Mason JW, O'Connell JB, Herskowitz A, et al., for the Myocarditis Treatment Trial investigators. A clinical trial of immunosuppressive therapy for myocarditis. *N Engl J Med* 1995;333:269–313.
6. McNamara DM, Holubkov R, Starling RC, et al., for the IMAC investigators. A controlled trial of intravenous immune globulin for recent onset dilated cardiomyopathy. *Circulation* 2001;103:2254–2259.
7. Williams JF, Bristow MR, Fowler MB, et al., for the ACC/AHA task force report. Guidelines for the evaluation and treatment of heart failure. *J Am Coll Cardiol* 1995;26:1376–1398.
8. Cooper LT, Berry GJ, Shabetai R, et al. Idiopathic giant-cell myocarditis—natural history and treatment. *N Engl J Med* 1997;336:1860–1866.
9. Hosenpud JD, Bennete LE, Keck BM, et al. The registry of the International Society for Heart and Lung Transplantation: sixteenth official report. 1999. *J Heart Lung Transplant* 1999;18:611–626.
10. Kawai C. From myocarditis to cardiomyopathy: mechanisms of inflammation and cell death. Learning from the past for the future. *Circulation* 1999;99:1091–1100.
11. Mattingly TW. Changing concepts of myocardial diseases. *JAMA* 1965;191:127–131.
12. Kibrick S, Benirschke K. Severe generalized disease (encephalohepato-myocarditis) occurring in newborn period and due to infection with Coxsackie virus group B: evidence of intra-uterine infection with this agent. *Pediatrics* 1958;22:857–874.
13. Lerner AM. Experimental approach to virus myocarditis. *Prog Med Virol* 1965;7:97–115.
14. Smith WG. Adult heart disease due to Coxsackie virus group B. *Br Heart J* 1966;28:204–220.
15. Sakakibara S, Konno S. Endomyocardial biopsy. *Jpn Heart J* 1962;3:537–543.
16. Jin O, Sole MJ, Butany JW, et al. Detection of enterovirus RNA in myocardial biopsies from patients with myocarditis and cardiomyopathy using gene amplification by polymerase chain reaction. *Circulation* 1990;82:8–16.
17. Aukrust P, Ueland T, Muller F, et al. Elevated circulating levels of C-C chemokines in patients with congestive heart failure. *Circulation* 1998;97:1136–1143.
18. Limas CJ, Goldenberg IF, Limas C. Autoantibodies against β-adrenoreceptors in human dilated cardiomyopathy. *Circ Res* 1989;64:97–103.
19. Richardson P, McKenna W, Bristow M et al. Report of the 1995 World Health Organization/International Society and Federation of Cardiology task force on the definition and classification of cardiomyopathies. *Circulation* 1996;93:841–842.
20. Davies MJ. The cardiomyopathies: a review of terminology, pathology and pathogenesis. *Histopathology* 1984;8:363–393.
21. Dec GW, Palacios IF, Fallon JT, et al. Active myocarditis in the spectrum of acute dilated cardiomyopathies: clinical features, histologic correlates, and clinical outcome. *N Engl J Med* 1985;312:885–890.
22. Steimle AE, Stevenson LW, Fonarow GC, et al. Prediction of improvement in recent onset cardiomyopathy after

referral for heart transplantation. *J Am Coll Cardiol* 1994;23:553–559.

23. Lieberman EB, Hutchins GM, Herskowitz A, et al. Clinicopathologic description of myocarditis. *J Am Coll Cardiol* 1991;18:1617–1626.

24. Burke AP, Saenger J, Mullick F, Virmani R. Hypersensitivity myocarditis. *Arch Pathol Lab Med* 1991;115:764–769.

25. Fenoglio JJ, McAllister HA, Mullick FG. Drug related myocarditis. I. Hypersensitivity myocarditis. *Hum Pathol* 1981;12:900–907.

26. Galiuto L, Enriquez-Sarano M, Reeder GS, et al. Eosinophilic myocarditis manifesting as myocardial infarction: early diagnosis and successful treatment. *Mayo Clinic Proc* 1997;72:603–610.

27. Beghetti M, Wilson GJ, Bohn D, et al. Hypersensitivity myocarditis caused by an allergic reaction to cefaclor. *J Pediatr* 1998;132:172–173.

28. Davidoff R, Palacios P, Southern J, et al. Giant cell versus lymphocytic myocarditis. A comparison of their clinical features and long term outcomes. *Circulation* 1991;83(3):953–961.

29. Lorell B, Alderman EL, Mason JW. Cardiac sarcoidosis. Diagnosis with endomyocardial biopsy and treatment with corticosteroids. *Am J Cardiol* 1978;42:143–146.

30. Jolles PR, Tatum JL. SLE myocarditis. Detection by Ga-67 citrate scintigraphy. *Clin Nucl Med* 1996;21:284–286.

31. Litovsky SH, Burke AP, Virmani R. Giant cell myocarditis: an entity distinct from sarcoidosis characterized by multiphasic myocyte destruction by cytotoxic T cells and histocytic giant cells. *Mod Pathol* 1996;9:1126–1134.

32. Melvin KR, Richardson PJ, Olson EG, et al. Peripartum cardiomyopathy due to myocarditis. *N Engl J Med* 1982;307:731–734.

33. Codd MB, Sugrue DD, Gersh BJ, et al. Epidemiology of idiopathic and hypertrophic cardiomyopathy. *Circulation* 1989;80(3):564–572.

34. Hufnagal G, Pankuweit S, Schonian U, Maisch B. The European Study of Epidemiology and Treatment of Cardiac Inflammatory Diseases (ESETCID). First epidemiology results. *Herz* 2000;25(3):279–285.

35. Saphir O. Myocarditis, a general review with an analysis of 240 cases. *Arch Pathol* 1951;32:1000.

36. Gore E, Saphir O. Myocarditis, a classification of 1402 cases. *Am Heart J* 1947;34:827–830.

37. Blankenhorn MA, Gall EA. Myocarditis and myocardosis: a clinicopathologic appraisal. *Circulation* 1956;X111:217–223.

38. Drory Y, Turetz Y, Hiss Y, et al. Sudden unexpected death in persons less than 40 years of age. *Am J Cardiol* 1991;68:1388–1392.

39. Huber SA. Animal models: immunological aspects. In: Banatvala JE, ed. *Viral infections of the heart.* London: Arnold, 1993:82–109.

40. Henke A, Huber SA, Stelzner A, et al. The role of CD8+ T lymphocytes in coxsackievirus B3-induced myocarditis. *J Virol* 1995;69:6720–6728.

41. Wilson FM, Miranda QR, Chason JL, Lerner M. Residual pathologic changes following murine Coxsackie A and B myocarditis. *Am J Pathol* 1969;55:253–265.

42. Matsumori A, Kawai C. An animal model of congestive (dilated) cardiomyopathy: dilatation and hypertrophy of the heart in the chronic stage in DBA/2 mice with myocarditis caused by encephalomyocarditis virus. *Circulation* 1982;66:355–360.

43. Godeny EK, Gauntt CJ. Interferon and natural killer cell activity in Coxsackie virus B3–induced myocarditis. *Eur Heart J* 1987;8:433–435.

44. Liu CC, Young LHY, Young JDE. Mechanisms of disease: lymphocyte-mediated cytolysis and disease. *N Engl J Med* 1996;335:1651–1659.

45. Gebhard JR, Perry CM, Harkins S, et al. Coxsackievirus B3–induced myocarditis. Perforin exacerbates disease, but plays no detectable role in virus clearance. *Am J Pathol* 1998;153:417–428.

46. Zaragoza C, Ocampo C, Saura M, et al. The role of inducible nitric oxide synthase in the host response to coxsackievirus myocarditis. *Proc Natl Acad Sci U S A* 1998; 95:2469–2474.

47. Seko Y, Tsuchimochi H, Nakamura T, et al. Expression of major histocompatibility complex class I antigen in murine ventricular myocytes infected with Coxsackie virus B3. *Circ Res* 1990;69:360–367.

48. Seko Y, Matsuda H, Kato K, et al. Expression of intercellular adhesion molecule-1 in murine hearts with acute myocarditis caused by coxsackievirus B3. *J Clin Invest* 1993;91:1327–1336.

49. Kishimoto C, Kuribayashi K, Masuda T, et al. Immunological behavior of lymphocytes in experimental viral myocarditis: significance of T-lympho in the severity of myocarditis and silent myocarditis in BALB/c-nu/nu mice. *Circulation* 1985;71:1247–1254.

50. Woodruff JF, Woodruff JJ. Involvement of T lymphocytes in the pathogenesis of Coxsackie B3 heart disease. *J Immunol* 19974;113:1726–1734.

51. Kishimoto C, Abelmann WH. Monoclonal antibody for the prevention of acute Coxsackie B3 myocarditis in mice. *Circulation* 1989;79:1300–1308.

52. Kyu B, Matsumori A, Sato Y, et al. Cardiac persistence of cardioviral RNA detected by polymerase chain reaction in a murine model of dilated cardiomyopathy. *Circulation* 1992;86:1605–1614.

53. Bowles NE, Archard LC, Olsen EGJ, Richardson PJ. Detection of Coxsackie-B-virus-specific RNA sequences in myocardial biopsy sample from patients with myocarditis and dilated cardiomyopathy. *Lancet* 1986;1:1120–1123.

54. Schwaiger A, Umlauft F, Weyrer K, et al. Detection of enteroviral ribonucleic acid in myocardial biopsies from patients with idiopathic dilated cardiomyopathy by polymerase chain reaction. *Am Heart J* 1993;126:406–410.

55. Fujioka S, Koide H, Kitaura Y, et al. Molecular detection and differentiation of enteroviruses in endomyocardial biopsies and pericardial effusions from dilated cardiomyopathy and myocarditis. *Am Heart J* 1996;131:760–765.

56. Kubota T, McTiernan CF, Frye CS, et al. Dilated cardiomyopathy in transgenic mice with cardiac-specific overexpression of tumor necrosis factor-alpha. *Circ Res* 1997;81:627–635.

57. Neu N, Rose NR, Beisel KW, et al. Cardiac myosin induces myocarditis in genetically predisposed mice. *J Immunol* 1987;139:3630–3636.

58. Fairweather D, Lawson CM, Chapman AJ, et al. Wild isolates of murine cytomegalovirus induce myocarditis and

antibodies that cross-react with virus and cardiac myosin. *Immunology* 1998;94:263–270.

59. Fairly CK, Ryan M, Wall PG, Weinberg J. The organisms reported to cause infective myocarditis and pericarditis in England and Wales. *J Infect Dis* 1996;32:223–225.

60. Grumbach IM, Heim A, Pring-Akerblom P, et al. Adenoviruses and enteroviruses as pathogens in myocarditis and dilated cardiomyopathy. *Acta Cardiol* 1999;54:83–88.

61. Matsumori A, Matoba Y, Sasayama S. Dilated cardiomyopathy associated with hepatitis C virus infection. *Circulation* 1995;92:2519–2525.

62. Okabe M, Fukuda K, Arakawa K, Kikuchi M. Chronic variant of myocarditis associated with hepatitis C virus infection. *Circulation* 1997;96:22–24.

63. Kao JH, Hwang JJ. Hepatitis C virus infection and chronic active myocarditis. *Circulation* 1998;98:1044–1045.

64. Cohen IS, Anderson DW, Virmani R, et al. Congestive cardiomyopathy in association with the acquired immunodeficiency syndrome. *N Engl J Med* 1986;315:628–630.

65. Lipshultz SE, Easley KA, Orav EJ, et al. Left ventricular structure and function in children infected with human immunodeficiency virus. Group for the Pediatric Pulmonary and Cardiac Complications of Vertically Transmitted HIV Infection (P2C2 HIV) study group. *Circulation* 1998;97:1246–1256.

66. Barbaro G, DiLorenzo G, Grisorio B, Barbarini G. Incidence of dilated cardiomyopathy and detection of HIV in myocardial cells of HIV-positive patients. Gruppo Italiano per lo Studio Cardiologico dei Pazienti Affetti da AIDS. *N Engl J Med* 1998;339:1093–1099.

67. Bowles NE, Kearney DL, Ni J, Perez-Atayde AR, et al. The detection of viral genomes by polymerase chain reaction in the myocardium of pediatric patients with advanced HIV disease. *J Am Coll Cardiol* 1999;34:857–865.

68. Dias JCP. Control of Chagas' disease in Brazil. *Parasitol Today* 1987;3:336–339.

69. World Health Organization. Sixth program report: Chapter 6: Chagas' disease. Special Program for Research and Training in Tropical Diseases. 1983;Document TDR, PR-6, 83.6-CHA, YNDP, World Bank, WHO.

70. Chadrasekar B, Melby PC, Troyer DA, Freeman GL. Induction of proinflammatory cytokines in experimental acute chagasic cardiomyopathy. *Biochem Biophys Res Comm* 1996;223:365–371.

71. Higuchi M, Reis MM, Aiello VD, et al. Association of an increase in CD8+ T cells with the presence of *Trypanosoma cruzi* antigens in chronic, human, chagasic myocarditis. *Am J Trop Med Hy* 1997;56:458–489.

72. Williams A. Aspergillus myocarditis. *Am J Pathol* 1974; 61:247–248.

73. Walsh TJ, Hutchins GM, Buckley BH, Mendelsohn G. Fungal infections of the heart. Analysis of 51 autopsy cases. *Am J Cardiol* 1980;45:357–366.

74. Duffield JS, Jacob AJ, Miller HC. Recurrent, life threatening atrioventricular dissociation associated with toxoplasma myocarditis. *Heart* 1996;76:453–454.

75. Montoya JG, Jordan R, Lingamneni S, et al. Toxoplasmic myocarditis and polymyositis in patients with acute acquired toxoplasmosis diagnosed during life. *Clin Infect Dis* 1997;24:676–683.

76. Lampert MB, Lang RM. Peripartum cardiomyopathy. *Am Heart J* 1995;130:860–870.

77. Huerta EM, Erice A, Espino RF, et al. Post-partum cardiomyopathy and acute myocarditis. *Am Heart J* 1985;110:1079–1081.

78. Rizeq MN, Rickenbacher PR, Fowler MB, Billingham ME. Incidents of myocarditis in peripartum cardiomyopathy. *Am Heart J* 1994;74:474–477.

79. Foelich CJ, Goodwin JS, Bankhurst AD, Williams RC. Pregnancy, a temporal fetal graft of suppressor cells in autoimmune disease. *Am J Med* 1980;69:329–331.

80. Kovithavongs T, Dossetor JB. Suppressor cells in human pregnancy. *Transplant Proc* 1978;10:911–913.

81. Damek DM, Shuster EA. Pregnancy and multiple sclerosis. *Mayo Clin Proc* 1997;72:977–989.

82. Midei MG, DeMent SH, Feldman AM, et al. Peripartum myocarditis and cardiomyopathy. *Circulation* 1990;81:922–928.

83. Demakis JG, Rahimtoola SH. Peripartum cardiomyopathy. *Circulation* 1971;44:964–968.

84. Billingham ME. Pharmacotoxic myocardial disease: an endomyocardial study. In: Sekiguchi C, Olsen EGJ, Goodwin JF, eds. *Myocarditis and related disorders.* Tokyo: Springer-Verlag, 1985:278–282.

85. Feenstra J, Grobbee DE, Remme WJ, Stricker BH. Drug-induced heart failure. *J Am Coll Cardiol* 1999;33:1152–1162.

86. Singal PK, Iliskovic N. Doxorubicin-induced cardiomyopathy. *N Engl J Med* 1998;339:900–905.

87. Michels VV, Moll PP, Miller FA, et al. The frequency of familial dilated cardiomyopathy in a series of patients with idiopathic dilated cardiomyopathy. *N Engl J Med* 1992;326:77–82.

88. Towbin JA, Hejtmancik, Brink P, et al. X-linked cardiomyopathy. Molecular evidence of linkage to the Duchenne muscular dystrophy gene at the Xp21 locus. *Circulation* 1993;87:1854–1865.

89. Olson TM, Michels VV, Thibodeau SN, et al. Actin mutations in dilated cardiomyopathy, a heritable form of heart failure. *Science* 1998;280:750–752.

90. Kamisago M, Sharma SD, DePalma SR, et al. Mutations in sarcomere protein genes as a cause of dilated cardiomyopathy. *N Engl J Med* 2000;343:1688–1696.

91. Mestroni L, Rocco C, Gregori D, et al. Familial dilated cardiomyopathy: evidence for genetic and phenotypic heterogeneity. *J Am Coll Cardiol* 1999;34:181–190.

92. Baig MK, Goldman JH, Caforio ALP, et al. Familial dilated cardiomyopathy: cardiac abnormalities are common in asymptomatic relative and may represent early disease. *J Am Coll Cardiol* 1998;31:195–201.

93. Michels VV, Moll PP, Rodeheffer RJ. Circulating heart autoantibodies in familial as compared to nonfamilial idiopathic dilated cardiomyopathy. *Mayo Clin Proc* 1994;69:24–27.

94. Caforio ALP, Keeling PJ, Zachara E. Evidence from family studies for autoimmunity in dilated cardiomyopathy. *Lancet* 1994;344:773–777.

95. Tazelaar HD, Billingham ME. Leukocytic infiltrates in idiopathic dilated cardiomyopathy. *Am J Surg Pathol* 1986;10:405–412.

96. Kuan AP, Chamberlain W, Malkiel S, et al. Genetic con-

trol of autoimmune myocarditis mediated by myosin-specific antibodies. *Immunogenetics* 1999;49:79–85.

97. McKenna CJ, Codd KA, McCann HA, Sugrue DD. Idiopathic dilated cardiomyopathy: familial prevalence and HLA distribution. *Heart* 1197;77:549–552.

98. Albert LJ, Inman RD. Molecular mimicry and autoimmunity. *N Engl J Med* 1999;341:2068–2074.

99. Limas C, Limas CJ, Boudoulas H. T-cell receptor gene polymorphisms in familial cardiomyopathy: correlation with anti–β-receptor autoantibodies. *Am Heart J* 1992;124:1258–1263.

100. Levine B, Kalman J, Mayer L, et al. Elevated circulating levels of tumor necrosis factor in severe chronic heart failure. *N Engl J Med* 1990;323:236–241.

101. Torre-Amione G, Kapadia S, Benedict C, et al. Proinflammatory cytokine levels in patients with depressed left ventricular ejection fraction: a report from the Studies of Left Ventricular Dysfunction (SOLVD). *J Am Coll Cardiol* 1996;27:1201–1206.

102. Kubota T, Alvarez RJ, Miyagishima M, et al. Expression of proinflammatory cytokines in the failing human heart: comparison of recent onset and endstage cardiomyopathy. *J Heart Lung Transplant* 2000;19:819–824.

103. MacGowan GA, Mann DL, Kormos RL, et al. Circulating interleukin-6 in severe heart failure. *Am J Cardiol* 1997;79:1128–1131.

104. Bozkurt B, Alvarez RJ Jr, McNamara DM, et al. Explant myocarditis: evidence for the role of inflammation in decompensation of advanced heart failure patients. *J Am Coll Cardiol* 1998;31[2 Suppl]:330A.

105. Deswal A, Bozkurt B, Seta Y, et al. Safety and efficacy of a soluble P75 tumor necrosis factor receptor (Enbrel, enteracept) in patients with advanced heart failure. *Circulation* 1999;99:3224–3226.

106. Felix SB, Staudt A, Dorffel WV, et al. Hemodynamic effects of immunoadsorption and subsequent immunoglobulin substitution in dilated cardiomyopathy. *J Am Coll Cardiol* 2000;35:1590–1598.

107. McNamara DM, Starling R, Dec GW, et al. Plasma cytokines in acute cardiomyopathy: evolution over time, correlations with functional studies, and potential role in recovery. *Circulation* 2000;102[Suppl]:2020A(abst).

108. Patel D, Haynes BF. New surrogate markers for autoimmune activity. *J Clin Invest* 1998;102:1075–1076.

109. Rose NR, Beisel KW, Herskowitz A, et al. Cardiac myosin and autoimmune myocarditis. *Ciba Found Symp* 1987;129:3–24.

110. Klein R, Maich B, Kochsiek K, Berg PA. Demonstration of organ-specific antibodies against heart mitochondria (anti-M7) in sera from patients with some forms of heart diseases. *Clin Exp Immunol* 1984;58:283–292.

111. Schultheiss HP, Bolte HD. Immunological analysis of autoantibodies against the adenine nucleotide translocator in dilated cardiomyopathy. *J Mol Cell Cardiol* 1985;17:603–617.

112. Fu LX, Magnusson Y, Bergh CH, et al. Localization of a functional autoimmune epitope on the second extracellular loop of the human muscarinic receptor in patients with idiopathic dilated cardiomyopathy. *J Clin Invest* 1993;91:1964–1968.

113. Maisch B, Wedeking U, Kochsiek K. Quantitative assessment of anti-laminin antibodies in myocarditis and perimyocarditis. *Eur Heart J* 1987;8:233–235.

114. Hahn EA, Hartz VL, Moon TE, et al. The Myocarditis Treatment Trial: design methods and patient enrollment. *Eur Heart J* 1995;16:162–167.

115. Geha RS. Regulation of the immune response by idiotype-anti-idiotype interactions. *N Engl J Med* 1981;305:25–28.

116. Dietrich G, Kaveri SV, Kazatchkine MD, et al. Modulation of autoimmunity by intravenous immune globulin through interaction with the function of the immune/idiotypic network. *Clin Immunol Immunopathol* 1992;62:S73–S81.

117. Oates JA, Woods AJ. Manipulating the immune system with immune globulin. *N Engl J Med* 1992;326:107–116.

118. Berchtold P, McMillian R. Intravenous immunoglobulin: new aspects of mechanism of action in chronic ITP. In: Imbach P, ed. *Immunotherapy with intravenous immunoglobulins.* London: Academic Press, 1991:245–252.

119. Thorton CA, Griggs RC. Plasma exchange and intravenous immunoglobulin treatment of neuromuscular disease. *Ann Neurol* 1994;35:260–268.

120. Dalakas MC, Illa I, Dambrosia JM, et al. A controlled trial of high-dose intravenous immune globulin infusions as treatment for dermatomyositis. *N Engl J Med* 1993;329(27):1993–2000.

121. Newberger JW, Takahashi M, Burns JC, et al. The treatment of Kawasaki syndrome with intravenous gamma globulin. *N Engl J Med* 1986;315:341–347.

122. Drucker MA, Colan SD, Lewis AB, et al. Gammaglobulin treatment of acute myocarditis in the pediatric population. *Circulation* 1994;89:252–257.

123. McNamara DM, Rosenblum WD, Janosko KM, et al. Intravenous immune globulin in the therapy of myocarditis and acute cardiomyopathy. *Circulation* 1997;95:2476–2478.

124. Bozkurt B, Villanueva FS, Holubkov R, et al. Intravenous immune globulin in the therapy of peripartum cardiomyopathy. *J Am Coll Cardiol* 1999;34:177–180.

125. Matsumori A, Tomioka N, Kawai C. Protective effect of recombinant alpha interferon on Coxsackievirus B3 myocarditis in mice. *Am Heart J* 1988;115:1229–1232.

126. Miric M, Miskovic A, Brkic S, et al. Long term follow up of patients with myocarditis and idiopathic dilated cardiomyopathy after immunomodulatory therapy. *FEMS Immunol Med Microbiol* 1994;10:65–74.

127. Miric M, Miskovic A, Vasiljevic JD, et al. Interferon and thymic hormones in the therapy of human myocarditis and idiopathic dilated cardiomyopathy. *Eur Heart J* 1995;16:150–152.

128. Doerffel WV, Felix SB, Wallukat G, et al. Short term hemodynamic effects of immunoadsorption in dilated cardiomyopathy. *Circulation* 1997;95:1994–1997.

129. Gullestad L, Aass H, Fjeld JG, et al. Immunomodulating therapy with intravenous immunoglobulin in patients with chronic heart failure. *Circulation* 2001;103:220–225.

130. Maisch B, Hufnagel G, Schonian U, et al., for the ESET-CID investigators. The European Study of Epidemiology and Treatment of Cardiac Inflammatory Disease (ESET-CID). *Eur Heart J* 1995;16:173–175.

131. Heikkila J, Karjalainen J. Evaluation of mild acute infectious myocarditis. *Br Heart J* 1982;47:381–391.

132. Smith SC, Ladenson JH, Mason JW, Jaffe AS. Elevations of cardiac troponin I associated with myocarditis. Experimental and clinical correlates. *Circulation* 1996;95:163–168.

133. Lauer B, Niederau C, Kuhl U, et al. Cardiac troponin T in patients with clinically suspected myocarditis. *J Am Coll Cardiol* 1997;30:1354–1359.

134. Dec GW, Palacios IF, Fallon JT, et al. Active myocarditis in the spectrum of acute dilated cardiomyopathies: clinical features, histologic correlates, and clinical outcome. *N Engl J Med* 1985;312:885–890.

135. Karjalainen J, Viitasalo M, Kala R, Heikkila J. 24-hour electrocardiographic recordings in mild acute infectious myocarditis. *Ann Clin Res* 1984;16:34–39.

136. Tai Y-T, Law C-P, Fong P-C, et al. Incessant automatic ventricular tachycardia complicating acute Coxsackie B myocarditis. *Cardiology* 1992;30:339–344.

137. Zeppilli P, Santini C, Palmieri V, et al. Role of myocarditis in athletes with minor arrhythmias and/or echocardiographic abnormalities. *Chest* 1994;106:373–380.

138. Vignola PA, Aonuma K, Swaye PS. Lymphocytic myocarditis presenting as unexplained ventricular arrhythmias: diagnosis with endomyocardial biopsy and response to immunosuppression. *J Am Coll Cardiol* 1984;4:812–819.

139. Frustaci A, Maseri A. Localized left ventricular aneurysms with normal global function caused by myocarditis. *Am J Cardiol* 1992;70:1221–1224.

140. Costanzo-Nordin MR, O'Connell JB, Subramanian R. Myocarditis confirmed by biopsy presenting as acute myocardial infarction. *Br Heart J* 1985;53:25–29.

141. Dec GW, Waldman H, Southern J, et al. Viral myocarditis mimicking acute myocardial infarction. *J Am Coll Cardiol* 1992;20:85–89.

142. Pasquini JA, Gottdiener JS, Cutler DJ, Fletcher RD. Myocarditis with transient left ventricular apical dyskinesis. *Am Heart J* 1985;109:371–373.

143. Gibson DG. Value and limitations of echocardiography in the diagnosis of myocarditis. *Eur Heart J* 1987;8:85–88.

144. Pinamonti B, Alberti E, Cigalotto A, et al. Echocardiographic findings in myocarditis. *Am J Cardiol* 1988;62:285–291.

145. Mason JW. Techniques for right and left ventricular endomyocardial biopsy. *Am J Cardiol* 1978;41:887–892.

146. Fowles RE, Mason JW. Role of cardiac biopsy in the diagnosis and management of cardiac disease. *Prog Cardiovasc Dis* 1984;27:153–172.

147. Hauk AJ, Kearney DL, Edwards WD. Evaluation of postmortem biopsy specimens from 38 patients with lymphocytic myocarditis: implications for role of sampling error. *Mayo Clin Proc* 1989;64:1235–1245.

148. Aretz HT, Billingham ME, Edwards WD. Myocarditis, a histopathologic definition and classification. *Am J Cardiovasc Pathol* 1987;1:3–14.

149. Shanes JG, Gahli J, Billingham ME, Edwards WD. Interobserver variability in the pathological interpretation of endomyocardial biopsy results. *Circulation* 1987;75:401–405.

150. Starling RC, Van Fossen DB, Hammer DF, Unverferth DV. Morbidity of endomyocardial biopsy in cardiomyopathy. *Am J Cardiol* 1991;68:133–136.

151. Deckers JW, Hare JM, Baughman KL. Complications of transvenous right ventricular endomyocardial biopsy in adult patients with cardiomyopathy: a seven year survey of 546 consecutive diagnostic procedures in a tertiary referral center. *J Am Coll Cardiol* 1992;19:43–47.

152. Grogan M, Redfield MM, Bailey KR, et al. Long-term outcome of patients with biopsy-proved myocarditis: comparison with idiopathic dilated cardiomyopathy. *J Am Coll Cardiol* 1995;26:80–84.

153. Menghini VV, Savcenko V, Olson LJ, et al. Combined immunosuppression for the treatment of idiopathic giant cell myocarditis. *Mayo Clin Proc* 1999;74:1221–1226.

154. Costanzo-Nordin MR, Reap EA, O'Connell JB, et al. A nonsteroid antiinflammatory drug exacerbates Coxsackie B3 murine myocarditis. *J Am Coll Cardiol* 1985;6:1078–1082.

155. Rezkalla S, Khatib G, Khatib R. Coxsackievirus B3 murine myocarditis: deleterious effects of nonsteroidal anti-inflammatory agents. *J Lab Clin Med* 1986;107:393–395.

156. Rezkalla S, Khatib R, Khatib G, et al. Effect of indomethacin in the late phase of Coxsackievirus myocarditis in a murine model. *J Lab Clin Med* 1988;112:118–121.

157. Friman G, Ilback NG. Acute infection: metabolic responses, effect on performance, interaction with exercise, and myocarditis. *Int J Sports Med* 1998;19:S172–S182.

158. Matsumori A, Igata H, Ono K, et al. High doses of digitalis increase the myocardial production of proinflammatory cytokines and worsen myocardial injury in viral myocarditis: a possible mechanism of digitalis toxicity. *Jpn Circ J* 1999;63:934–940.

159. Kojima J, Miyazaki S, Fujiwara H, et al. Recurrent left ventricular mural thrombi in a patient with acute myocarditis. *Heart Vessels* 1988;4:120–122.

160. Singh SN, Fletcher RD, Fisher S, et al. Amiodarone in patients with congestive heart failure and asymptomatic ventricular arrhythmia. *N Engl J Med* 1995;333:77–82.

161. Doval HC, Nul DR, Grancelli HO. Randomized trial of low-dose amiodarone in severe congestive failure. *Lancet* 1994;344:493–498.

162. McCarthy RE, Boehmer JP, Hruban RH, et al. Long-term outcome of fulminant myocarditis as compared with acute (nonfulminant) myocarditis. *N Engl J Med* 2000;342:690–695.

163. Reiss N, El-Banayosy A, Posival H, et al. Management of acute fulminant myocarditis using circulatory support systems. *Artif Organs* 1995;20:964–970.

164. Martin J, Sarai K, Schindler M, et al. MEDOS HIA-VAD biventricular assist device for bridge to recovery in fulminant myocarditis. *Ann Thorac Surg* 1997;63:1145–1146.

165. Marelli D, Laks H, Amsel B, et al. Temporary mechanical support with the BVS 5000 assist device during treatment of acute myocarditis. *J Cardiol Surg* 1997;12:55–59.

166. Kawahito K, Murata S, Yasu T, et al. Usefulness of extracorporeal membrane oxygenation for treatment of fulminant myocarditis and circulatory collapse. *Am J Cardiol* 1998;82:910–911.

167. Dipla K, Mattiello JA, Jeevanandam V, et al. Myocyte

recovery after mechanical circulatory support in humans with end-stage heart failure. *Circulation* 1998;97:2316–2322.

168. Zafeiridis A, Jeevanandam V, Houser SR, Margulies KB. Regression of cellular hypertrophy after left ventricular assist device support. *Circulation* 1998;98:656–662.

169. Levy NT, Olson LJ, Weyand C, et al. Histologic and cytokine response to immunosuppression in giant-cell myocarditis. *Ann Intern Med* 1998;128:648–650.

170. Semigran MJ, Thaik CM, Fifer MA, et al. Exercise capacity and systolic and diastolic ventricular function after recovery from acute dilated cardiomyopathy. *J Am Coll Cardiol* 1994;24:462–470.

171. Kleinert S, Weintraub RG, Wilkinson JL, Chow CW. Myocarditis in children with dilated cardiomyopathy: incidence and outcome after dual therapy immunosuppression. *J Heart Lung Transplant* 1997;16:1248–1254.

172. Lee KJ, McCrindle BW, Bohn DJ, et al. Clinical outcomes of acute myocarditis in childhood. *Heart* 1999;82:226–233.

173. Zales VR, Wright KL. Endocarditis, pericarditis, and myocarditis. *Pediatr Ann* 1997;26:116–121.

174. Bozkurt B, Torre-Amione G, Warren MS, et al. Results of targeted anti-tumor necrosis factor therapy with etanercept (ENBREL) in patients with advanced heart failure. *Circulation* 2001;103:1044–1047.

94

CARDIAC TRANSPLANTATION

DALE G. RENLUND
DAVID O. TAYLOR

▼▼ *ADDITIONAL ELECTRONIC TOPICS*

OVERVIEW

Despite major pharmacologic advances in the management of heart failure, cardiac transplantation is the most effective treatment for selected patients with end-stage heart failure. Sound, evidence-based immunosuppressive strategies have decreased morbidity and mortality, enabling the successful transplantation of even less than ideal candidates. Most infections and rejections are either preventable or treatable, and 1-year and 3-year survival rates exceed 85% and 80%, respectively. Cardiac allograft vasculopathy limits long-term survival and is the major cause of death after the first few years. Nonetheless, approximately 50% of recipients are alive 10 years after transplantation. Because of this success, the number of patients who could potentially benefit from cardiac transplantation is even greater than previously thought, which results in an ever-increasing donor to recipient dispar-

D. G. Renlund: Department of Internal Medicine, University of Utah School of Medicine, LDS Hospital, Salt Lake City, Utah

D. O. Taylor: Division of Cardiology, University of Utah School of Medicine, Salt Lake City, Utah

ity. Not only must every effort be made to increase the number of donors and use every appropriate donor heart, but care must be taken to ensure that individuals listed as candidates for cardiac transplantation are those who are likely to benefit the most. Potentially suitable candidates should be referred early in the course of their end-stage disease to heart failure and transplant specialists so that transplantation can be appropriately timed or alternative treatment options implemented. After transplantation, the care of recipients should be directed, at least in part, by transplant physicians.

HISTORICAL PERSPECTIVE

Although much progress has been made in pharmacologic therapy for heart failure, the most effective treatment for selected patients with end-stage heart disease is cardiac transplantation. Patients with severe heart failure have a 1- to 2-year mortality approaching 50% despite appropriate and advanced medical treatment (1). Heart transplantation alters the course of end-stage heart disease, with 1-year, 3-year, and 10-year survival rates exceeding 85%, 80%, and 50%, respectively (2) (eFig. 94.0.1). More than 55,000 procedures have been performed in over 330 centers worldwide, and nearly 3,000 additional procedures are performed each year (2). Although certain demographic variables influence the likelihood of survival after cardiac transplantation (e.g., retransplantation, older recipient and donor age, higher pulmonary vascular resistance, and longer duration of ischemia) (2) (eTable 94.0.1), survival and quality of life continue to improve (3–6). Heart transplantation is not experimental.

During the first month after cardiac transplantation, donor heart dysfunction predominates as a cause of death. The propensity to reject the transplanted heart decreases over time. Consequently, the first few months after transplantation present not only the highest risk of rejection but also the highest risk of infection because of the higher doses of immunosuppressive agents used. Between 1 and 12 months after transplantation, not surprisingly, infection and acute rejection predominate as causes of death. After the first few years, cardiac allograft vasculopathy (CAV) and malignancy become the leading causes of death, the former accounting for a quarter of the deaths in transplant recipients (2–4) (eFig. 94.0.2). ▼ p53

CLINICAL PROFILE

Recipient Selection

Indications

Cardiac transplantation is indicated for one of the many reasons listed in Table 94.1 (1,7–9). Cardiac transplantation is not indicated, however, simply because of an ejection fraction of less than 20%, a past history of functional class III or IV symptoms of heart failure, or a previous history of ven-

tricular arrhythmias. Also, before transplantation is considered, a thorough search for reversible or surgically amenable cardiac disease must be completed and optimal medical management implemented. Patients should either have failed to improve with a trial of beta-blocker therapy or have clear contraindications to beta-blocker use. Confidence that the medical therapy is optimal is increased when the therapy is directed or administered by heart failure specialists. ▼ p54

Assessment of Risk of Mortality and Morbidity after Transplantation

Patients meeting indications for cardiac transplantation are evaluated to determine whether they are at higher than

TABLE 94.1 INDICATIONS FOR CARDIAC TRANSPLANTATION CANDIDACY

Cardiogenic shock or low-output state requiring mechanical assistance (e.g., respirator, intraaortic balloon pump, ventricular assist device, total artificial heart) with, at worst, reversible end-organ damage

Refractory heart failure or low-output state requiring continuous inotropic support and invasive monitoring

NYHA class III or IV symptoms with objective documentation of marked functional limitation and poor 12-mo prognosis despite optimal medical therapy (peak oxygen consumption <14 mL/kg/min, documented progression of heart failure symptoms, clinical instability, or marked serial decline in peak oxygen consumption)

Recurrent or rapidly progressive heart failure symptoms unresponsive to optimal dosage of vasodilators and diuretics

Severe hypertrophic or restrictive cardiomyopathy with NYHA class IV symptoms

Refractory angina pectoris despite maximally tolerated dosage of beta-blockers, calcium channel blockers, and nitrates, not amenable to revascularization or transmyocardial laser revascularization due to distal vessel disease or severity of left ventricular dysfunction with severe ischemic symptoms consistently limiting day-to-day activities, accompanied by objective evidence of myocardial ischemia within the first two stages of a standard Bruce exercise protocol

Recurrent symptomatic, life-threatening ventricular arrhythmias despite maximal antiarrhythmic therapy by all appropriate conventional medical and surgical modalities (multiple firings from an ICD for documented VT and VF or prolonged periods of documented electromechanical dissociation after ICD conversion of VT or VF)

Cardiac tumors confined to the myocardium with a low likelihood of metastasis at time of transplantation

Hypoplastic left heart syndrome

Complex congenital heart disease with progressive ventricular failure that is not amenable to conventional surgical repair or palliation

In infants, children, and adolescents, progressive deterioration in left ventricular ejection fraction or functional status despite optimal medical therapy, failure to grow secondary to advanced heart failure symptoms, or a progressive rise in pulmonary vascular resistance that would be expected to preclude transplantation at a later date

ICD, implantable cardioverter-defibrillator; NYHA, New York Heart Association; VF, ventricular fibrillation; VT, ventricular tachycardia.

acceptable risk for a poor outcome after transplantation (7,10–14). Anecdotal experience of successfully overcoming isolated risk factors should not justify ignoring known risks in the majority of situations. Table 94.2 lists characteristics

that increase the risk of morbidity and mortality after cardiac transplantation. These risk factors do not necessarily represent absolute exclusionary criteria. For example, combined heart-liver or heart-kidney transplantation is feasible in

TABLE 94.2 CHARACTERISTICS INCREASING THE RISK OF MORBIDITY AND MORTALITY AFTER CARDIAC TRANSPLANTATION

Characteristic	Increase in risk
PVR >6 Wood units, unresponsive to vasodilators	Marked
PVR >6 Wood units, decreasing in response to vasodilators but not <3–4 Wood units	Moderate
PVR >3 Wood units, decreasing <3 Wood units in response to vasodilators	Minimal
Pulmonary artery systolic pressure >70 mm Hg, unresponsive to treatment	Marked
Transpulmonic gradient (mean PAP – PCWP) >15–20 mm Hg	Moderate
Transpulmonic gradient (mean PAP – PCWP) 10–15 mm Hg	Minimal
Active, untreated infection	Marked
Treated infection currently controlled on antibiotics	Moderate
Recent resolved infection	Minimal
Irreversible, severe hepatic disease	Marked
Moderate hepatic dysfunction not clearly related to cardiac congestion	Moderate
Mild hepatic enzyme elevations likely related to cardiac congestion	Minimal
Irreversible, severe renal disease	Marked
Moderate renal dysfunction not clearly related to low cardiac output	Moderate
Mild renal dysfunction likely related to low cardiac output	Minimal
Irreversible pulmonary disease with FEV_1 <1 L or FVC <50% predicted	Marked
Irreversible pulmonary disease with FEV_1 ≤1.5 L or FVC <65% predicted	Moderate
Mild/moderate pulmonary disease with FEV_1 >1.5 L or FVC >65% predicted	Minimal
Recent pulmonary infarction	Moderate
Age 50–60 yr	Minimal
Age 60–70 yr	Moderate
Age >70 yr	Marked
Age 1–5 yr	Minimal
Diabetes mellitus with significant end-organ damage	Moderate to marked
Diabetes mellitus without end-organ damage	Minimal
Cerebrovascular disease, severe, symptomatic	Marked
Cerebrovascular disease, mild to moderate, asymptomatic	Minimal
Peripheral vascular disease, severe, symptomatic	Marked
Peripheral vascular disease, mild to moderate, asymptomatic	Minimal
Gastrointestinal bleeding, active	Marked
Peptic ulcer disease, treated	Minimal
Diverticulitis, recent	Moderate
Chronic active hepatitis	Moderate to marked
Chronic hepatitis C infection with low viral load and benign liver biopsy results	Minimal
Human immunodeficiency virus positive	Marked
Malignancy, recent	Marked
Malignancy, remote	Minimal
Myocardial infiltrative disease	Marked
Myocardial inflammatory disease	Moderate
Major affective disorder or schizophrenia with poor control	Marked
Major affective disorder or schizophrenia with good control	Moderate
Personality disorders	Moderate
Cigarette abuse	Moderate
Substance abuse, active unresolved	Marked
Substance abuse, resolved albeit recent	Moderate
Medical noncompliance	Marked
Obesity, moderate (120–140% ideal body weight or BMI 30–35)	Minimal to moderate
Osteoporosis	Minimal to moderate
Lack of social support	Minimal to moderate

BMI, body mass index (weight in kg divided by height in m²); FEV_1, forced expiratory volume in 1 s; FVC, forced vital capacity; PAP, pulmonary artery pressure; PCWP, pulmonary capillary wedge pressure; PVR, pulmonary vascular resistance.

selected patients with both end-stage heart and liver disease or end-stage heart and kidney disease (12,13). ▼ p55

Management of the Patient while Awaiting Transplantation

While the patient awaits transplantation, his or her general health and hemodynamic compensation must not be allowed to deteriorate without intervention. A low threshold for hospitalization and more intensive heart failure treatment are mandated for any hemodynamic deterioration that may manifest as significant azotemia, refractory salt and water overload, persistent hypotension, altered mental status, or even gastrointestinal distress. Signs and symptoms of low cardiac output should prompt escalation in therapy from intravenous diuretics to intravenous inotropic agents, and from intravenous inotropic agents to intraaortic balloon pump or left ventricular assist devices (see Chapter 95). Heart transplant candidates who nonetheless develop irreversible end-organ failure in other organ systems or who are likely to die despite transplantation are not transplanted. Therapeutic approaches to the prevention of sudden death, including the use of an implantable cardioverter defibrillator, as appropriate, are considered. The routine placement of an implantable cardioverter defibrillator in heart transplant candidates in the absence of standard indications for use has not been proven. ▼ p56

Donor Selection

Donor selection is influenced by many factors, including ABO blood type compatibility, donor-recipient size disparity, presence of intrinsic cardiac disease, and presence of transmissible infectious or malignant diseases (15–18). The risk of using a specific donor heart is always balanced against the risk one is willing to take with regard to a particular recipient. A decision to use a marginal donor heart may sometimes be made if the condition of the potential recipient warrants the risk and the potential recipient consents. ▼ p57

To avoid intrinsic cardiac disease, electrocardiography, echocardiography, and (at times) coronary angiography are used. Electrocardiographic abnormalities that generally preclude the use of a donor heart include evidence of myocardial infarction and significant ventricular arrhythmias. Echocardiographic abnormalities that generally preclude the use of a donor heart include significant global hypokinesis, significant valvular abnormalities, and moderate to severe left ventricular hypertrophy. In addition, evidence of a significant cardiac contusion with a significantly elevated troponin level generally precludes use of the donor heart. Although older donor hearts are associated with a higher risk (*e*Table 94.0.1), many have been successfully used (2,19). Even in the absence of risk factors for coronary artery disease, coronary angiography is recommended in male donors older than 45 years and in female donors older than 50 years. The presence of risk factors for coronary

artery disease prompts coronary angiography in even younger donors. Some donor hearts with significant coronary artery or valvular disease have been transplanted successfully with simultaneous bypass surgery or valve replacement, but doing so is not yet standard care. Brain death can cause time-dependent changes in left ventricular function (20) that may be related to catecholamine release. Donor heart dysfunction may be reversible, and thyroid hormone is frequently administered to improve donor heart function. Clearly using an irreversibly damaged donor heart is to be avoided.

To avoid transmitting infectious disease with the donated heart, a series of tests are performed to determine the suitability for transplantation. A history of behaviors, especially recent, that predispose to human immunodeficiency virus (HIV) infection or viral hepatitis (e.g., intravenous drug use); positivity for HIV, hepatitis B surface antigen (HB$_S$Ag), or hepatitis C; and uncontrolled gram-negative sepsis generally preclude donor use. The use of a heart from an HB$_S$Ag-positive donor could be considered, however, if the recipient is also HB$_S$Ag positive. Due to the differences in virulence of various hepatitis C subtypes, the use of hepatitis C–positive donors' hearts in hepatitis C–positive recipients remains controversial. Generally, if the donor has a malignancy not confined to the cranium, the donor heart is not used (16–18,21). The final decision to transplant a particular heart is made at the time of visual inspection. ▼ p58

Donor Allocation

Given the increasing donor to recipient disparity, the procurement and methods of allocation of all solid organs are frequently debated. Of course, everything should be done to decrease candidate waiting time, increase the use of suitable donor hearts, and increase the willingness of the population at large to donate (16,21,22). Hearts are allocated based on mandated guidelines. In the United States, hearts are allocated to specific patients based on blood type, size, proximity of the donor to the candidate's transplant center, and the disease severity and waiting time of the candidate (23). ▼ p59

ANATOMIC CONSIDERATIONS

Donor Cardiectomy

In donor cardiectomy and transplant surgery, one key to successful transplantation is the minimization of donor heart ischemic time (24,25). Ischemic time (from the time of aortic cross-clamping in the donor to release of aortic cross-clamp in the recipient) of less than 4 hours is generally acceptable, although some risk is conferred by every hour of donor heart ischemia (risk = 1.0 + 0.26 per hour for each hour over 3 hours) (2) (*e*Table 94.0.1). ▼ p60

Implantation Techniques

Lower and Shumway Technique

Three implantation techniques are available: the traditional Lower and Shumway technique, the bicaval technique, and the rarely used heterotopic technique (24–28). Concern about the loss of normal atrial anatomy using the Lower and Shumway technique has led to the more frequent use of the bicaval technique. The bicaval technique may result in a longer donor heart ischemic time but is associated with lower right atrial pressure, lower incidence of atrial tachyarrhythmias, lower diuretic dose, less need for pacing, less tricuspid valve incompetence, and shorter hospital stay. An improved atrial kick contribution to cardiac output may also decrease the incidence of thrombus formation in the left atrium (29). Heterotopic cardiac transplantation can be performed with the donor heart placed in the right lower thorax in parallel to the recipient heart, which is left in place. ❦ p61

PATHOPHYSIOLOGY OF THE TRANSPLANTED HEART

Cardiac Allograft Function and Inotropic Support

The function of the newly transplanted cardiac allograft is influenced by preexplant variables (e.g., degree of inotropic support, cardiopulmonary resuscitation, and trauma), the ischemic insult during explant and implantation, effectiveness of cardioplegia, and total denervation. Inotropic support (using isoproterenol, dobutamine, or milrinone) is usually required for 2 to 5 days, depending on donor heart function. ❦ p62

If global ischemia is the cause of poor allograft function, recovery is likely. Even poorly functioning cardiac allografts can return to normal function after as little as 1 week. In most cardiac transplant recipients, measures of left ventricular function, such as ejection fraction, are normal within 1 to 2 weeks after transplantation. Resting hemodynamics tend to normalize over time as well.

Denervation and Reinnervation

Although the cardiac allograft is totally denervated at the time of transplantation, over a period of months to years it reinnervates at least partially in the majority of recipients (30–34). When totally denervated, the heart responds differently to many common cardiovascular medicines. The response to direct beta-adrenergic agonists (isoproterenol, dobutamine, epinephrine, norepinephrine) is qualitatively unchanged. The sympathomimetic amines that act indirectly by releasing catecholamines from nerve terminals (dopamine, ephedrine, metaraminol bitartrate, and mephentermine sulfate) are likely diminished, and supersensitivity to adenosine is occasionally seen. ❦ p63

Exercise Capacity

Despite demonstrably normal left ventricular function, most patients do not achieve a normal exercise capacity (32). Many patients are inadequately rehabilitated (33). In others, concomitant pulmonary or vascular disease limits exercise tolerance. Administered immunosuppressive agents, particularly corticosteroids, undoubtedly take their toll and likely affect even the structure of skeletal muscle in transplant recipients (34). Nonetheless, all recipients are encouraged to rehabilitate to the extent possible, preferably, at least early on, in organized cardiac rehabilitation programs.

Cardiac Arrhythmias

Sinus node dysfunction is common early after transplantation and appears to be more common when the traditional Lower and Shumway technique is used than when the bicaval technique is used. Transient bradycardia can be treated with temporary pacing or administration of theophylline. Permanent bradycardia, which can occur late after transplantation, eventually necessitates use of an electronic pacemaker in approximately 5% of patients.

As with many other types of cardiac surgery, postoperative atrial tachyarrhythmias may occur and are generally approached as usual. Cardiac allograft rejection, however, is considered in the differential diagnosis, and the pharmacologic interventions need to take into account the denervation (35). Late after transplantation, recipient remnant atrial to donor atrial conduction (across the suture line) has been observed (36). Early on, postoperative ventricular ectopy can be seen, but it usually resolves without the need for long-term treatment. After the postoperative period, electrophysiologic disease may become manifest or may develop. Generally, traditional approaches are appropriate, including the use of antiarrhythmic agents, devices, or interventions.

CARDIAC ALLOGRAFT REJECTION

Pathophysiology of Cardiac Allograft Rejection (the Immune System)

Transplantation of an organ between members of the same species is known as allotransplantation; hence, the use of the term *cardiac allograft*. Alloantigens are molecules recognized as foreign (or nonself) by the recipient immune system. In the absence of immunosuppression, destruction of the organ bearing alloantigens occurs (37–43).

HLA antigens are serologically identified alloantigens that have been shown to correspond to the human major histocompatibility complex (MHC). These cell surface antigens are subclassified as MHC class I (HLA-A, HLA-B, and HLA-C) or MHC class II (HLA-DP, HLA-DQ, and HLA-DR) and have distinctly different roles in the rejection process.

The sequence of events leading to cardiac allograft rejection encompasses antigen recognition (Fig. 94.1A), pri-

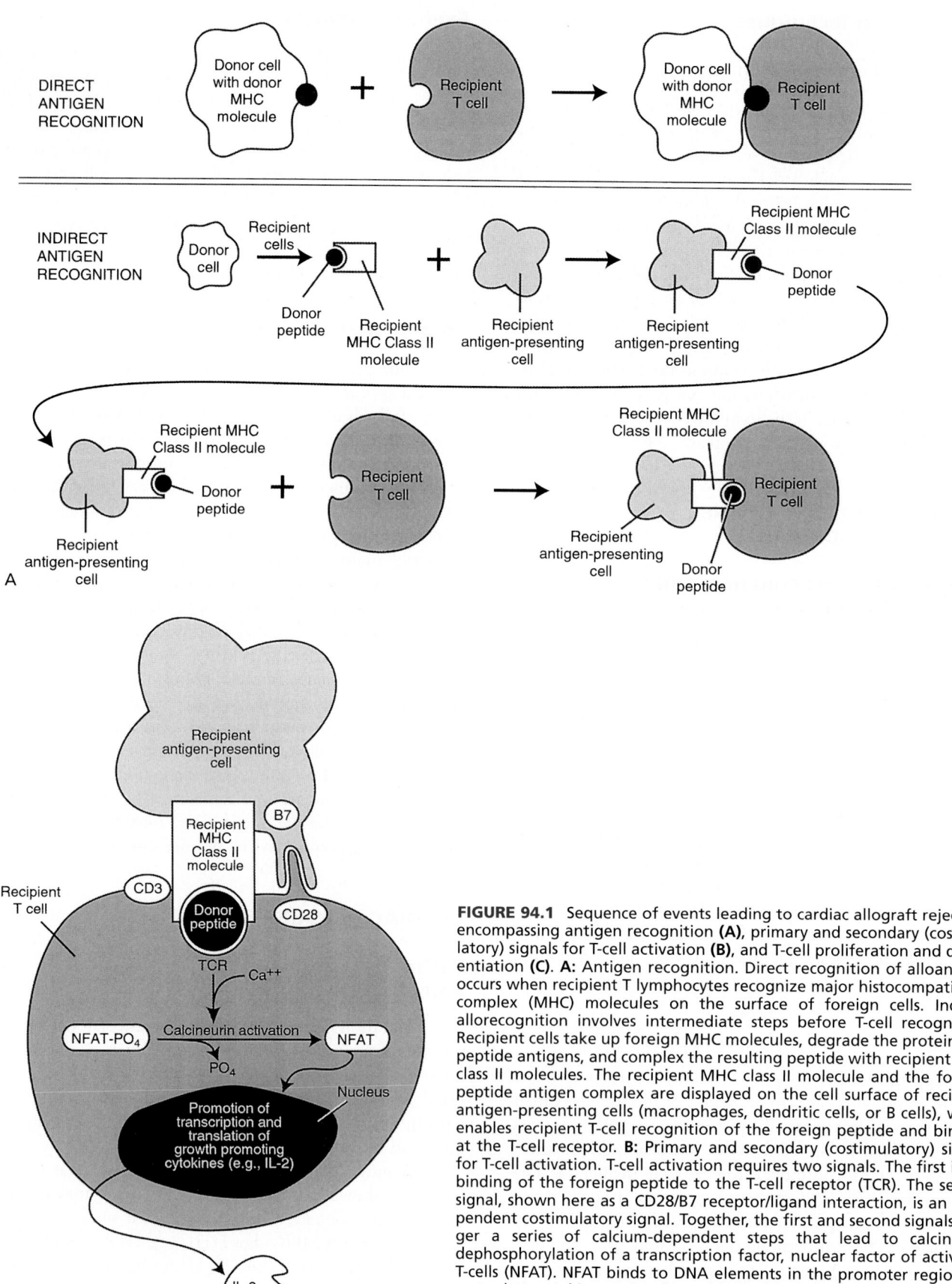

FIGURE 94.1 Sequence of events leading to cardiac allograft rejection, encompassing antigen recognition **(A)**, primary and secondary (costimulatory) signals for T-cell activation **(B)**, and T-cell proliferation and differentiation **(C)**. **A:** Antigen recognition. Direct recognition of alloantigen occurs when recipient T lymphocytes recognize major histocompatibility complex (MHC) molecules on the surface of foreign cells. Indirect allorecognition involves intermediate steps before T-cell recognition. Recipient cells take up foreign MHC molecules, degrade the protein into peptide antigens, and complex the resulting peptide with recipient MHC class II molecules. The recipient MHC class II molecule and the foreign peptide antigen complex are displayed on the cell surface of recipient antigen-presenting cells (macrophages, dendritic cells, or B cells), which enables recipient T-cell recognition of the foreign peptide and binding at the T-cell receptor. **B:** Primary and secondary (costimulatory) signals for T-cell activation. T-cell activation requires two signals. The first is the binding of the foreign peptide to the T-cell receptor (TCR). The second signal, shown here as a CD28/B7 receptor/ligand interaction, is an independent costimulatory signal. Together, the first and second signals trigger a series of calcium-dependent steps that lead to calcineurin dephosphorylation of a transcription factor, nuclear factor of activated T-cells (NFAT). NFAT binds to DNA elements in the promoter regions of many key cytokine genes [e.g., interleukin-2 (IL-2), interferon-γ, and tumor necrosis factor (TNF)-α], which leads to the transcription and translation of growth-promoting cytokines. (*continued*)

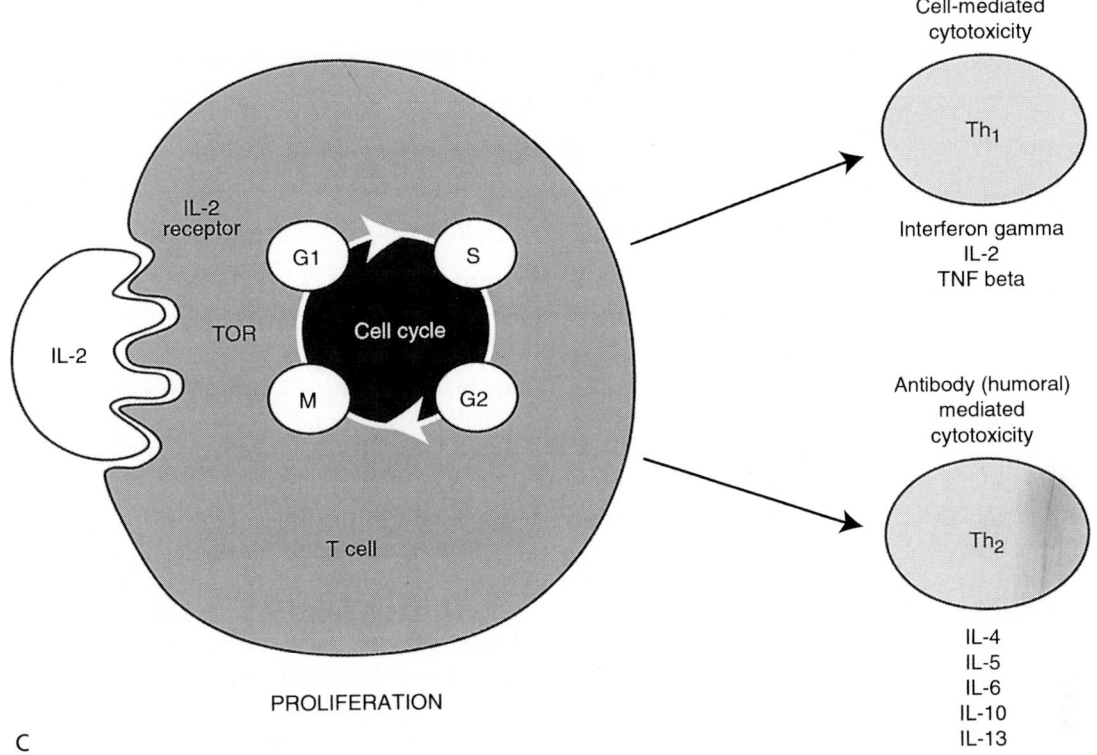

C

FIGURE 94.1 *Continued.* **C:** T-cell proliferation and differentiation. When growth-promoting cytokines (e.g., IL-2) bind to receptors on the surface of T lymphocytes, intracellular signaling occurs that allows the cell to enter the cell cycle and undergo mitosis (M) and clonal amplification. Undifferentiated T cells differentiate into Th$_1$ (cell-mediated cytotoxicity) or Th$_2$ [antibody (humorally)-mediated cytotoxicity] subsets depending on the influences of various cytokines. Both cell-mediated and humorally mediated cytotoxic immune responses may cause allograft destruction. G$_1$ and G$_2$, growth phases; S, synthesis phase; TOR, target of rapamycin.

mary and secondary (costimulatory) signals for T-cell activation (Fig. 94.1B), and T-cell proliferation and differentiation (Fig. 94.1C). ❦ p64

In brief, after the heart is transplanted, proinflammatory cytokines are elaborated and recipient inflammatory cells (e.g., macrophages) are recruited into the cardiac allograft. Donor passenger leukocytes migrate from the allograft into host lymphoid tissue, and recipient leukocytes enter the allograft. T-cell stimulation occurs via a T-cell receptor signal and a necessary costimulation signal. Cytokine production leads to the generation of effector cells for cell-mediated and antibody (humoral)-mediated immunity. Destruction of the allograft occurs via involvement of antibody, cytotoxic T lymphocytes, macrophages, and cytokines.

Types of Cardiac Allograft Rejection

Cardiac allograft rejection is an immunologic process that, left unchecked, leads to allograft destruction. Rejection has been variously classified but may be defined histologically, functionally, or clinically. The most generally recognized categories are hyperacute, acute cellular, and acute vascular (humoral) rejection. In cardiac transplantation, the term *chronic rejection* generally refers to CAV.

Although hyperacute rejection is due to preformed, donor-specific antibodies in the recipient, the presence of such antibodies does not always result in hyperacute rejection. When it occurs, hyperacute rejection is a vigorous immune response that takes place within minutes to hours. The outcome, without repeat transplantation or total artificial heart support, is uniformly fatal. The best method for avoiding hyperacute rejection is to avoid transplanting a donor heart into a patient who is sensitized to the donor (a positive donor-specific cross-match). Screening PRA is useful because prospective cross-matching is frequently impractical (44). PRA screening is performed by exposing recipient serum to lymphocytes from 50 or more random individuals. A normal result of 0% reactivity suggests a low risk that a retrospective cross-match would be positive. For PRA reactivity greater than 10%, prospective cross-matching is generally warranted (45,46). ❦ p65

Acute cellular rejection is the most common form of rejection and occurs at least once in approximately half of heart transplant recipients (47). Even though the propensity toward allograft rejection decreases over time and nearly half of the rejection episodes occur in the first 2 to 3 months, late rejection can and does occur. Rejection occurring early after transplantation tends to be more aggressive

TABLE 94.3 ENDOMYOCARDIAL BIOPSY GRADING SCALE USED BY THE INTERNATIONAL SOCIETY FOR HEART AND LUNG TRANSPLANTATION

Grade	Finding	Rejection severity
0	No infiltrates, normal myocytes	None
1A	Focal perivascular or interstitial infiltrates without necrosis	Borderline mild
1B	Diffuse but sparse infiltrates without necrosis	Mild
2	One focus only with aggressive infiltrate and/or myocyte damage	Mild or focal moderate
3A	Multifocal aggressive infiltrates and/or myocyte damage	Moderate
3B	Diffuse inflammatory infiltrates with necrosis	Borderline severe
4	Diffuse aggressive polymorphous infiltrate with edema, hemorrhage, and vasculitis, with necrosis	Severe

and life-threatening than late-occurring rejection. Acute cellular rejection is most frequently diagnosed by endomyocardial biopsy graded in accordance with the International Society for Heart and Lung Transplantation (ISHLT) criteria (48) (Table 94.3 and *e*Fig. 94.1.1). Certain factors increase the risk for rejection. For instance, both increasing age and male gender appear to be associated with decreased cardiac allograft rejection (49,50). All patients are at risk for rejection, however, and are carefully followed regardless of demographic variables.

Vascular rejection may be manifest by otherwise unexplained cardiac allograft dysfunction with or without histologic evidence. Histologic evidence is scant cellular infiltrate but abundant colocalized immunoglobulin and complement components in the allograft microvasculature seen on one or more biopsy specimens. In addition, vascular rejection may be manifest only histologically in the absence of allograft dysfunction (47). 🏴 p66

Diagnosis of Cardiac Allograft Rejection

Surveillance for allograft rejection generally centers on the routine use of endomyocardial biopsy (51). Endomyocardial biopsy is initially performed weekly (for the first 4 to 8 weeks) and then at gradually increasing intervals. Twelve to 24 months after transplant, biopsies are performed every 3 to 6 months. Over time, some patients are managed without routine endomyocardial biopsies (52). After the diagnosis of rejection, the endomyocardial biopsy interval is, of course, altered. 🏴 p67

Clinically, most rejection episodes are detected by surveillance endomyocardial biopsies and manifest no signs or symptoms. If the episode is symptomatic, the most frequent symptom is fatigue. Later in the rejection process, exercise intolerance or frank heart failure symptoms may occur. Physical findings, if present, may include relative hypotension (decrease in systolic blood pressure of more than 20 mm Hg from baseline), elevated jugular venous pressure, or a third heart sound gallop. Symptoms or signs such as those mentioned prompt an urgent endomyocardial biopsy. An enlarging pericardial effusion or worsened indices of systolic or diastolic function determined by echocardiography may herald rejection. Fever is

an infrequent manifestation of rejection. Atrial or ventricular arrhythmias are considered indicative of allograft rejection until proven otherwise. Clearly, if the patient has significant allograft dysfunction, signs of heart failure may be present.

Many noninvasive strategies for the early diagnosis of cardiac allograft rejection have been evaluated in an attempt to decrease the dependence on endomyocardial biopsy (53–57). Generally, sensitivities of 85% to 90% can be achieved with fair specificity. No technique has as yet eliminated the clinical practice of routine endomyocardial biopsy surveillance. 🏴 p68

Pharmacology of Immunosuppressive Agents

Suppression of the recipient immune system (Fig. 94.1) is necessary to prevent and treat cardiac allograft rejection. The pharmacology of currently available agents is summarized in Table 94.4. Polypharmacy is almost always used to minimize the toxicity of individual agents and to block the immune system in multiple locations (58–72). Immunosuppression is conveniently considered in three phases: early rejection prophylaxis (perioperatively and for the first several weeks after transplantation), long-term maintenance prophylaxis (immunosuppression in the absence of allograft rejection), and the augmentation in immunosuppression after the diagnosis of allograft rejection.

Prevention and Treatment of Cardiac Allograft Rejection

Early Rejection Prophylaxis

To prevent cardiac allograft rejection perioperatively and for the first several weeks after transplantation, multiple agents are administered. Generally, "triple therapy" is used, consisting of (a) cyclosporine or tacrolimus; (b) azathioprine, mycophenolate mofetil, or sirolimus; and (c) corticosteroids (61–72). Although not perfect, triple therapy has proven to be simple and effective for most patients. In some patients with marginal renal function, early administration of cyclosporine or tacrolimus can lead to

TABLE 94.4 PHARMACOLOGY OF IMMUNOSUPPRESSIVE AGENTS

Agent	Identification	Mechanism of action	Administration	Toxicity	Drug interactions and uses
Cyclosporine[a]	Cyclic undecapeptide produced by the fungus *Tolypocladium inflatum Gams*	Binds to cyclophilin, inhibits calcineurin-dependent transcription and translation of cytokine genes, particularly IL-2.	p.o. or i.v., oral to i.v. dose adjustment is 3:1, marked individual variation in bioavailability, oral dosage 6–8 mg/kg/d, targeted to level or toxicity.	Renal effects, hypertension, gingival hyperplasia, hirsutism, tremor, headache, paresthesias, flushing	Metabolism decreased by ketoconazole, diltiazem hydrochloride, verapamil hydrochloride, erythromycin, cimetidine, grapefruit; metabolism increased by phenytoin, phenobarbital, isoniazid, rifampin, carbamazepine; used in long-term maintenance immunosuppression.
Tacrolimus	Macrolide isolate of *Streptomyces tsukubaensis*	Binds to FK-binding protein, inhibits calcineurin-dependent transcription and translation of cytokine genes, particularly IL-2.	p.o. or i.v., oral to i.v. dose adjustment is 5:1, marked individual variation in bioavailability, oral dose 0.05–0.15 mg/kg/d, targeted to level or toxicity.	Renal effects, hypertension, tremor, headache, flushing, paresthesias, glucose intolerance	Metabolism decreased by ketoconazole, diltiazem, verapamil, erythromycin, cimetidine, grapefruit; metabolism increased by phenytoin, phenobarbital, isoniazid, rifampin, carbamazepine; used in long-term maintenance immunosuppression, may substitute for cyclosporine to treat rejection.
Azathioprine	Prodrug of 6-mercaptopurine	Inhibits purine ring biosynthesis, decreasing synthesis of DNA and RNA.	p.o. or i.v., no significant oral to i.v. adjustment, 1–2 mg/kg/d, WBC to remain >4,500/mm^3.	Macrocytic anemia, leukopenia, pancreatitis, cholestatic jaundice, hepatitis	Allopurinol slows metabolism by inhibiting xanthine oxidase; when used with allopurinol, azathioprine dosage is decrease by two-thirds and WBC monitored; used in long-term maintenance immunosuppression.
Mycophenolate mofetil	Morpholinoethylester of mycophenolic acid	Inhibits inosine monophosphate dehydrogenase, inhibiting the *de novo* pathway for guanine nucleotide biosynthesis.	p.o. or i.v., no significant oral to i.v. adjustment, 2,000–6,000 mg/d.	Gastrointestinal distress, leukopenia	No significant interactions; used in long-term maintenance immunosuppression, may substitute for azathioprine to treat rejection.
Sirolimus	Macrocyclic triene antibiotic produced by *Streptomyces hygroscopicus*	Binds to FK-binding protein, inhibits IL-2– and IL-6–driven events.	p.o., loading dose 6 mg, then 2 mg/d.	Hypertriglyceridemia, thrombocytopenia, leukopenia	Metabolism decreased by diltiazem and ketoconazole; metabolism increased by rifampin; interactions probably similar to those for cyclosporine; used in long-term maintenance and treatment of rejection.
Cyclophosphamide	Type of nitrogen mustard	Activated by a cytochrome P-450–catalyzed reaction in the liver to form alkylating species, cross-links DNA, preventing lymphocyte proliferation.	p.o. or i.v., oral to i.v. dose adjustment is 1.4:1; oral dose is 0.5–1.0 mg/kg/d, WBC to remain >4,500/mm^3.	Pancytopenia, hemorrhagic cystitis, alopecia	Additive effect with other inhibitors of lymphocyte proliferation, may substitute in the short term to treat vascular rejection.
Methotrexate sodium	Folic acid analogue	Inhibits dihydrofolate reductase, inhibiting purine biosynthesis.	p.o. or i.v., oral to i.v. dose adjustment is 1.4:1; oral dose is 7.5–15 mg/wk, WBC to remain >4,500/mm^3.	Pancytopenia, mucositis, alopecia, cirrhosis	Additive effect with other inhibitors of lymphocyte proliferation, may be used in recurring or refractory rejection.

(continued)

TABLE 94.4 *(Continued)*

Agent	Identification	Mechanism of action	Administration	Toxicity	Drug interactions and uses
Corticoster-oids	Synthetic or semisyn-thetic ana-logues of adrenocor-ticotropic hormones	Lymphocytolysis, inhibits release and action of vari-ous interleukins, interferes with antigen receptor interactions.	p.o. or i.v. with methylpredniso-lone and hydro-cortisone (no significant oral to i.v. dose adjust-ment), p.o. with prednisone, pred-nisone 1 mg = hydrocortisone 4 mg = methylpred-nisolone 0.8 mg; maintenance dos-age of prednisone is 0.0–0.1 mg/kg/d.	Pituitary-adrenal suppression, cushingoid habitus, glu-cose intoler-ance, hyperlipid-emia, hyper-tension, posterior sub-capsular cata-racts, myopathy, osteoporosis, skin fragility, PUD	Multiple drug interactions, none clinically significant; used in long-term maintenance immunosuppression and in the treatment of established rejection episodes.
Muromonab-CD3 anti-body (OKT3)	IgG$_{2A}$ murine mono-clonal immuno-globulin molecule	Binds to the CD3 sur-face antigen of lymphocytes, inhibits antigen recognition, opsonizes lym-phocytes.	i.v. only, 2.5–5.0 mg/d.	Fever, chills, gas-trointestinal distress, pul-monary edema, HAMA formation	No interactions; used in early rejection prophylaxis and in the treatment of rejection.
Antithy-mocyte globulin (ATG)	Equine poly-clonal anti-bodies to human thymocytes	Opsonizes lympho-cytes.	i.v. only, 10–20 mg/kg/d.	Fever, chills, serum sickness, leukopenia, thrombocy-topenia	No interactions; used in early rejection prophylaxis and in the treatment of rejection.
Thymoglobu-lin	Rabbit poly-clonal anti-bodies to human thymocytes	Opsonizes lympho-cytes.	i.v. only, 1.5 mg/kg/d.	Fever, chills, serum sickness, leukopenia, thrombocy-topenia	No interactions; used in early rejection prophylaxis and in the treatment of rejection.
Daclizumab	Chimeric mono-clonal IgG1 antibody	Blocks the IL-2 receptor α chain.	1 mg/kg i.v. once before transplant, repeated an addi-tional four times at 2-wk intervals.	Gastrointestinal distress	No interactions; used in early rejection prophylaxis.
Basiliximab	Chimeric mono-clonal IgG$_{1K}$ antibody	Blocks the IL-2 receptor α chain.	20 mg i.v. 2 h before transplant and repeated 4 d after.	Gastrointestinal distress	No interactions; used in early rejection prophylaxis.

HAMA, human antimouse antibody; IgG, immunoglobulin G; IL, interleukin; PUD, peptic ulcer disease; WBC, white blood cell count.
[a]Cyclosporine is available in two formulations, oil based and microemulsion based. The latter is associated with better bioavailability.

significant transient renal dysfunction and volume reten-tion. To avoid the early use of cyclosporine or tacrolimus in patients at high risk of renal dysfunction (serum creati-nine level higher than 2.0 mg per dL before transplant), OKT3, one of a variety of antilymphocyte globulins, or even IL-2 receptor blockers may be used perioperatively (67–69). Antilymphocyte antibody-based early rejection prophylaxis can safely delay cyclosporine or tacrolimus administration until after cardiac and renal function have stabilized. Disadvantages to using antilymphocyte anti-body-based early rejection prophylaxis include first-dose reactions, greater expense, more complicated immuno-

suppression, and potentially more immunosuppressive side effects. ❧ p69

Long-Term Maintenance Immunosuppression

The majority of patients is maintained long term on tri-ple therapy. Because the propensity to reject decreases over time, dosages of all three drugs may be decreased accordingly. Cyclosporine and tacrolimus are usually maintained long term at levels less than half of those used early after transplant. Similarly, although azathioprine may have been used early after transplant to target white blood cell counts in the 4,500 to 5,500 per mm^3 range, long-term doses larger than 2 mg per kg per day are generally not used. Long-term doses of mycophenolate mofetil generally decrease from 3,000 mg per day to 2,000 mg per day. Prednisone can safely be withdrawn in patients who demonstrate a low propensity to reject (73). Advantages of corticosteroid-free maintenance immunosuppression include reversal of most corticosteroid-induced side effects.

Treatment of Established Cardiac Allograft Rejection

The treatment of cardiac allograft rejection depends on several factors: severity of rejection (ISHLT grade of endomyocardial biopsy specimens), time since transplant, rejection and immunosuppressive history, and hemodynamic status of the patient. Even "mild" rejection (ISHLT grades IB and II) may warrant augmentation of immunosuppression in the setting of allograft dysfunction. In treating rejection, one generally optimizes or increases the dosages of maintenance immunosuppressors and markedly increases corticosteroid dosages. In corticosteroid-refractory rejection or in rejection episodes associated with hemodynamic instability, antilymphocyte antibodies such as OKT3 or one of a variety of antithymocyte globulins are added. Mild rejection in hemodynamically stable patients, those without evidence of allograft dysfunction, is not treated. Some data, however, suggest that occurrence of even mild rejection may increase the likelihood of CAV. Moderate rejection in the absence of hemodynamic instability is usually treated initially with a several-day course of either intravenous or high-dose oral corticosteroids. If a subsequent biopsy specimen shows resolution, the maintenance dosages are continued. If a subsequent biopsy specimen does not show resolution, however, then intravenous corticosteroids are used. Failure of a second course of corticosteroids to resolve the rejection episode generally leads to the use of antilymphocyte antibodies (*e*Fig. 94.1.2).

Rejection frequently may be treated by changing the maintenance immunosuppression. For instance, mycophenolate mofetil may be substituted for azathioprine, or tacrolimus for cyclosporine, or both substitutions may be made (74). Sirolimus may be added to or substituted into the regimen. The most vexing problem in immunosuppressive management is treating recurring or refractory rejection. Patients who require high dosages of maintenance immunosuppressive agents are at high risk of developing untoward, life-threatening immunosuppressive side effects. In difficult situations, one can add an agent to the treatment regimen (e.g., methotrexate sodium or sirolimus), consider the substitutions mentioned earlier, or even consider total lymphoid irradiation (75). An interesting new approach to dealing with rejection is photopheresis, which has been shown to decrease rejection

when given as early rejection prophylaxis and may be able to treat ongoing rejection (76).

CARDIAC ALLOGRAFT VASCULOPATHY

Pathophysiology of Cardiac Allograft Vasculopathy

After the first few years posttransplantation, CAV is the leading cause of death and the cause of significant morbidity (2,77,78). The prevalence of angiographically detectable disease approaches 50% to 60% at 5 years. The prevalence of disease detected by intravascular ultrasonography or at autopsy is greater. Thus far, the improvements in immunosuppression have not greatly affected the incidence and morbidity associated with CAV development. CAV is not a homogeneous disease; rather, it changes over time. Early, CAV is characterized by diffuse and distal involvement, whereas later-onset coronary artery disease is more proximal, focal, and eccentric. Because the vasculopathy is localized to the vascular bed of the transplanted heart, CAV cannot be totally explained by any property of the medications used after cardiac transplantation.

Histologically, CAV is characterized by proliferation and migration of smooth muscle cells, proliferation and migration of macrophages, intact elastic lamina, increased ground substance and foam cells, and macrophage-engulfed cholesterol (*e*Fig 94.1.3) (79). Angiographically, several types of lesions have been described, as shown in Figure 94.2 (80).

Various risk factors have been identified for the development of CAV diagnosed by angiography, intravascular ultrasonography, or angioscopy (2,78–95). Although older

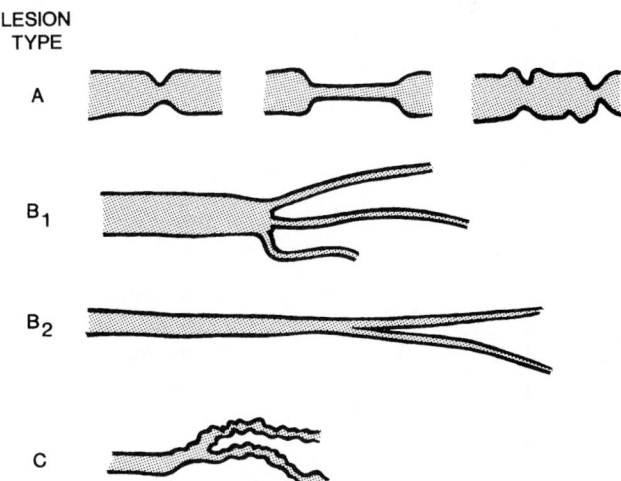

FIGURE 94.2 Types of lesion seen in cardiac allograft vasculopathy. Cardiac allograft vasculopathy can present with a variety of lesions, most of which are not amenable to revascularization. (From Gao SZ, Alderman EL, Schroeder JS, et al. Accelerated coronary vascular disease in the heart transplant patient: coronary arteriographic findings. *J Am Coll Cardiol* 1988;12:334–348, with permission.)

donor hearts are associated with an increased risk of the development of CAV at 3 years after transplantation [risk = 1.0 + 0.073 per year for each additional year of donor age above 30 years; *p* <.0001 (2)], given the significant and growing donor to recipient disparity, older donor hearts will likely continue to be used with even greater frequency. Not surprisingly, coronary artery disease leading to the need for cardiac transplantation is associated with a 33% increased risk of developing CAV at 3 years (2). The influence on CAV of the more common risk factors for native coronary artery disease (e.g., hypertension, diabetes, cigarette use, hyperlipidemia, hyperhomocysteinemia, low folate and vitamin B$_6$ concentrations) is likely greater later after transplantation (82,83). ▼ p70

Diagnosis of Cardiac Allograft Vasculopathy

The clinical presentation of CAV early after transplant may be silent, manifesting as acute myocardial infarction, congestive heart failure, arrhythmias, wall motion abnormalities, or sudden death. Later, typical angina pectoris may occur due to focal, albeit incomplete, reinnervation. Most CAV is diagnosed by routinely scheduled yearly surveillance angiography, although many noninvasive techniques have been evaluated in an attempt to decrease the need for invasive testing (96–98). ▼ p71

Regrettably, angiography is insensitive in detecting CAV (*e*Fig. 94.1.3). Compared with angiography, intravascular ultrasonography (or other techniques, see Chapter 85) is more sensitive, detecting disease in a much larger percentage of patients (99,100). Intravascular ultrasonography predicts the development of angiographic coronary artery disease and is predictive of morbidity and mortality (99). However, early diagnosis of CAV has not been shown to affect long-term outcomes.

Treatment of Cardiac Allograft Vasculopathy

The treatment of established disease appears to be limited to retransplantation and revascularization techniques, because augmented immunosuppression has not been conclusively shown to prevent progression. Retransplantation is the only option for patients with type B and C lesions, especially because transmyocardial laser revascularization is unlikely to be beneficial in the long term with current techniques (101). Retransplantation for CAV can, if performed years after the initial transplantation, result in survival rates of nearly 80% at 1 year after retransplantation (2). ▼ p72

COMPLICATIONS AFTER CARDIAC TRANSPLANTATION

The complications encountered after cardiac transplantation are legion. Recipients are at risk for cardiac, immunosuppression-related, and other complications. Although largely not preventable, most problems can be mitigated, at least in part. The cardiac complications have been addressed earlier in this chapter.

Immunosuppression-Related Complications

Infectious Complications

Infection is common in organ transplant recipients (102). The types of infections expected in cardiac transplant recipients vary depending on the time from transplantation. This is because the intensity of immunosuppression administered varies directly with the propensity for rejection, and the propensity to reject decreases over time. Figure 94.3 depicts the changing frequencies of bacterial, viral, protozoal, and fungal infections after transplantation (103).

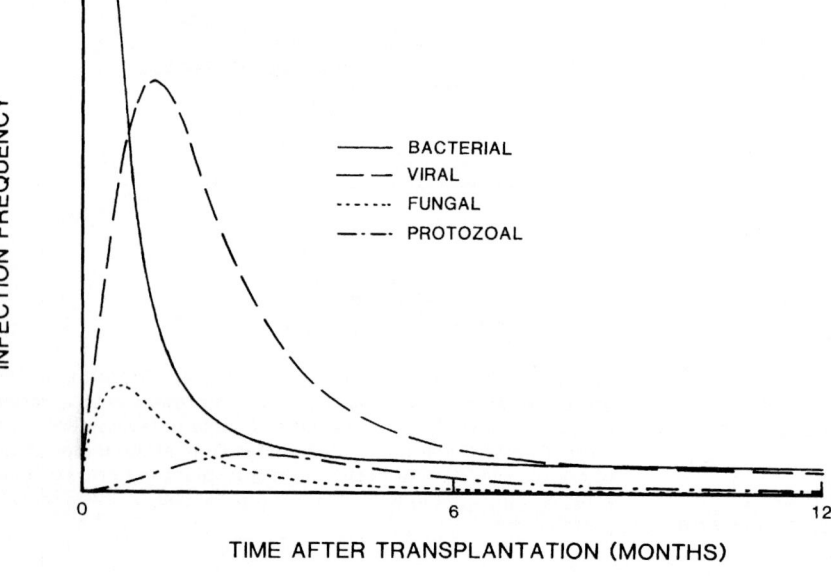

FIGURE 94.3 Risk of infection after cardiac transplantation. The risk of infection from various etiologic agents peaks at different times after cardiac transplantation. (Adapted from Miller LW, Naftel DC, Bourge RC, et al. Infection after heart transplantation: a multi-institutional study. *J Heart Lung Transplant* 1994;13:384, with permission.)

Bacteria and viruses account for more than 80% of infections after transplantation. The most common bacterial infections early after transplantation are nosocomial, due to infected intravascular catheters or lines, or gram-negative pneumonias. As can be seen in Figure 94.3, the risk decreases rapidly over time. The most common viral infections are caused by herpes viruses, CMV, and herpes simplex. Although CMV infection used to be associated with significant morbidity and mortality, the use of ganciclovir has significantly improved the prognosis (104,105). However, ganciclovir-resistant CMV is occasionally seen. Patients who are CMV seronegative who receive a heart from a seropositive donor are at greatest risk for aggressive disease. Attempts to prevent CMV disease in these patients have been less fruitful than in patients who are seropositive before transplantation. Although fungi and protozoa account for less than 15% of infections after transplantation, such infections can be associated with the worst prognosis (106). Fungal infections occur in patients who require intensive treatment over a prolonged period before transplantation or in whom significant rejection occurs in the setting of a bacterial infection that requires the use of broad-spectrum antibiotics. ▼ p73

Given the potential morbidity and mortality associated with infections during the first posttransplant year, infection prophylaxis is common. This has reduced the morbidity and mortality after cardiac transplantation for CMV infection, *Pneumocystis carinii* pneumonia, and toxoplasmosis (107,108). Prophylactic regimens are commonly used against CMV (if either recipient or donor is seropositive), toxoplasmosis (especially if the recipient tests negative and the donor tests positive), *P. carinii*, *Candida albicans*, and herpes simplex (*e*Table 94.4.1). Whether or not influenza vaccines should be given is not entirely clear. Concern exists about administering them early after transplantation; however, they are given to recipients who are at high risk (109).

Renal Insufficiency

Five years after heart transplantation, 8.5% of recipients have a serum creatinine level higher than 2.5 mg per dL, and 1.9% require long-term dialysis (2). Although some renal dysfunction is related to preexisting renal disease, most is acquired. Cyclosporine and tacrolimus are nephrotoxic and probably account for the majority of renal problems (110–113). Minimizing the dosages of these and other nephrotoxins, avoiding dehydration, and searching carefully for nonimmunosuppression-related reversible causes are warranted (111). ▼ p74

Hypertension

After transplantation, hypertension occurs in approximately two-thirds of recipients (2). Hypertension is more prevalent in cyclosporine-treated recipients (70% to 90%) than in tacrolimus-treated recipients (30% to 50%). In nontransplant patients, hypertension is a significant risk factor for vascular disease and to assume otherwise in transplant recipients is unwise. The role of hypertension in the development of renal dysfunction and CAV among long-term survivors is not known.

Even though most hypertensive cardiac transplant recipients require pharmacologic treatment, moderate limitation of salt intake, maintenance of ideal body weight, and moderate exercise are encouraged. Generally, blood pressures consistently greater than 140/90 mm Hg are treated. Either angiotensin-converting enzyme (ACE) inhibitors or calcium channel blockers in conventional dosages are effective monotherapy for many patients (114,115). Some patients are prone to hyperkalemia due to the combined effect of cyclosporine and ACE inhibition on the kidney. Due to decreased metabolism of cyclosporine and tacrolimus, the use of either diltiazem or verapamil necessitates lowering of the dosages of cyclosporine or tacrolimus and initially more frequent cyclosporine or tacrolimus level monitoring. Use of both an ACE inhibitor and a calcium channel blocker is effective in many patients in whom neither class of drugs alone is sufficient. Diuretics are effective in some patients, although rarely as monotherapy. Dehydration should, of course, be avoided with the concomitant use of cyclosporine or tacrolimus. ▼ p75

Osteoporosis

By the time most patients undergo cardiac transplantation, the risk of osteoporosis and other skeletal complications is high. Prolonged inactivity and, in some cases, prolonged heparin administration can demineralize bone and put the patient at risk for complications. Further bone loss occurs due to high-dose corticosteroid therapy. Bone loss is rapid in the first 6 months after transplantation and is most marked in the lumbar spine. Vertebral compression fractures and aseptic necrosis of the femoral head are among the most common skeletal problems after heart transplantation. Due to the morbidity associated with osteoporosis, patients at risk are treated (116–118). Postmenopausal women are generally prescribed estrogen replacement therapy. Postmenopausal women and all patients with evidence of pretransplant osteoporosis receive calcium salts (e.g., calcium carbonate 1,000 to 1,500 mg per day in divided doses) and upwardly titrated doses of calcitriol (beginning at 0.25 µg every other day) while awaiting transplantation and indefinitely thereafter (116). Alendronate sodium (10 mg per day) may effectively increase bone density and can be safely added to calcium salts and calcitriol (117). ▼ p76

Hyperlipidemia

After cardiac transplantation, hyperlipidemia is common (119) and requires treatment in as many as 50% of recipients (2). All patients are encouraged to limit intake of cholesterol and other fats, maintain ideal body weight, and exercise. Minimization of corticosteroid dosage, when possible, is also generally helpful. Serum cholesterol levels greater than 200 mg per dL (or levels of low-density lipoprotein cholesterol above 100 mg per dL) are treated. If levels are not successfully lowered with dietary and other behavior modification, pharmacologic treatment is instituted. Although use of gemfibrozil (in doses up to 600 mg twice daily) can be successful is some patients with mild to moderate hyperlipidemia, particularly in the setting of hypertriglyceridemia, moderate to severe hypercholesterolemia generally requires the use of a 3-hydroxy-3-methyl-glutaryl coenzyme A (HMG-CoA) reductase inhibitor (119,120). The combination of cyclosporine or tacrolimus and an HMG-CoA reductase inhibitor increases the risk of rhabdomyolysis over that for the HMG-CoA reductase inhibitor alone. When used, HMG-CoA reductase inhibitors should be started at low dosage and the dosage should be increased periodically while levels of creatine kinase and liver enzyme are monitored. Combining an HMG-CoA reductase inhibitor with gemfibrozil or nicotinic acid in lipid-lowering doses (1 g per day or more) can cause rhabdomyolysis, and these combinations are used cautiously in transplant patients. Bile acid sequestrants, probucol, and fish oil (omega-3 free fatty acids) are infrequently used to treat hyperlipidemia after transplantation. ▼ p77

Malignancy

After transplantation, cardiac allograft recipients have an increased risk of malignancy compared with the general population. The overall degree of immunosuppression may be more important than any intrinsic property associated with a particular drug. Care is taken to avoid overimmunosuppression. By 5 years after transplantation, nearly 10% of survivors have experienced a malignancy (2). Fortunately, nearly half are skin cancers, occurring predominantly in those who would otherwise be at risk (121). Because locally invasive skin cancer can be fatal if not treated promptly and adequately, routine screening is performed. Posttransplant lymphoproliferative disease (PTLD) occurs in less than 2% of patients (122). PTLD can be refractory to any treatment or relatively localized and benign, responding simply to reduction in immunosuppression (123). The Epstein-Barr virus (EBV), a lymphotropic virus that infects more than 90% of the population by adulthood, is thought to be the etiologic agent responsible for most cases of PTLD (123,124). ▼ p78

Although other malignancies occur in heart transplant recipients, the behavior of prostate, breast, and cervical cancer and of other solid tumors seems no different than in the general population.

Biliary Disease

The incidence of biliary disease is greater in cardiac transplant recipients than in nontransplant patients (125). The incidence

may be as high as 8%, which represents a 17-fold increase over the incidence in the general population. ▼ p79

Generally, presence of any abdominal symptoms coupled with cholelithiasis warrants surgical intervention. Laparoscopic cholecystectomy is the procedure of choice in uncomplicated situations (126).

Pregnancy

Successful pregnancies after heart transplantation have been reported (127). Maternal and fetal risk is undoubtedly higher than in the general population and transplant recipients are so counseled. Once the recipient is pregnant, close collaboration with an obstetrician knowledgeable with regard to high-risk cases is warranted to avoid teratogenic drugs and manage the pregnancy. Immunosuppressive drug levels are monitored frequently, as volume changes and metabolic changes occur during pregnancy. Radiation exposure can be minimized by using echocardiographically guided endomyocardial biopsies.

Management of the Cardiac Transplant Recipient Undergoing Surgery

Due to bone complications, biliary disease, and other surgically amenable problems, many cardiac transplant recipients undergo noncardiac surgery. In general, antibiotic prophylaxis is used for dental procedures and other procedures in which the risk of septicemia is high. The risk associated with noncardiac surgery depends on the status of the allograft. In patients without ongoing rejection, significant coronary disease, or left ventricular dysfunction, the risk is low. Before all elective procedures, an endomyocardial biopsy is performed, and the most recent angiogram is reviewed. Patients receiving corticosteroids within the preceding 9 months receive stress doses of corticosteroids. If intravenous immunosuppressants are to be needed due to prolonged ileus, appropriate dosage adjustments are made.

CONTROVERSIES AND PERSONAL PERSPECTIVES

Controversies in Recipient Selection

The impact of cardiac transplantation on the mortality of patients with end-stage heart failure should not obfuscate the fact that the need for transplantation generally represents a failure of heart muscle disease prevention or early detection and treatment. Viewed simplistically, decreasing the number of patients who could benefit from cardiac transplantation by preventive and early treatment measures is of greater importance than perfecting cardiac transplantation for those who need it.

Medical advances have made it possible to successfully transplant patients who were previously considered inap-

THE FUTURE

During the next decade, the induction of donor-specific tolerance will be furthered, which will decrease the need for pharmacologic immunosuppression. Because both xenotransplantation and permanent mechanical circulatory support systems will emerge as clinically appropriate, the donor to recipient disparity will stabilize as alternatives to allotransplantation are provided for selected patients with end-stage heart disease.

propriate candidates. Although individual patient advocacy is admirable, physicians bear a responsibility in their stewardship over donor hearts. Physicians must balance two competing interests—those of individual patient advocacy and societal responsibility—to ensure that appropriate candidates are given donor hearts.

Controversies in Transplant Center Restriction

The United States currently has over 150 heart transplant centers. Given that just over 2,000 heart transplants are performed in the United States each year, the average is a little over one transplant per center per month. Data suggest that centers performing a low number of transplants do so with increased risk to recipient survival. Therefore, reason suggests that the number of centers should be limited to improve overall patient survival, to ensure continued expertise, to further develop the science and art of transplantation, and to minimize cost.

Cost of Transplantation: Who Should Pay?

An unstated consideration in selecting a transplant candidate is the ability to pay. Many heart transplant centers will not list a patient unless funding for the procedure is secure. Patients from lower socioeconomic classes are not afforded the same opportunity for transplantation as others. The answer to the question of who should pay is not unique to transplantation but underlies much of the policy that governs health economics (128). The only resource scarcer than funding is donor hearts.

REFERENCES

1. Aaronson KD, Mancini DM. Mortality remains high for outpatient transplant candidates with prolonged (>6 months) waiting list time. *J Am Coll Cardiol* 1999;33:1189–1195.
2. Hosenpud JD, Bennett LE, Keck BM, et al. The Registry of the International Society for Heart and Lung Transplantation: seventeenth official report—2000. *J Heart Lung Transplant* 2000;19:909–931.
3. Ketheesan N, Tay GK, Witt CS, et al. The significance of HLA matching in cardiac transplantation. *J Heart Lung Transplant* 1999;18:226–230.
4. Hosenpud JD, Edwards EB, Lin H-M, et al. Influence of HLA matching on thoracic transplant outcomes: an analysis from the UNOS/ISHLT thoracic registry. *Circulation* 1996;94:170–174.
5. Grady KL, Jalowiec A, White-Williams C. Predictors of quality of life in patients at one year after heart transplantation. *J Heart Lung Transplant* 1999;18:202–210.
6. Kavanagh T, Yacoub MH, Kennedy J, et al. Return to work after heart transplantation: 12-year follow up. *J Heart Lung Transplant* 1999;18:846–851.
7. Miller LW. Criteria for selection of recipients and donors for cardiac transplantation. *Graft* 1999;2:S49–S53.
8. Metra M, Faggiano P, D'Aloia A, et al. Use of cardiopulmonary exercise testing with hemodynamic monitoring in the prognostic assessment of ambulatory patients with chronic heart failure. *J Am Coll Cardiol* 1999;33:943–950.
9. De Marco T, Goldman L. Predicting outcomes in severe heart failure. *Circulation* 1997;95:2597–2599.
10. Young JB. Redevelopment of disease in cardiac allografts. *Graft* 1999;2:S54–S59.
11. Grady KL, White-Williams C, Naftel D, et al. Are preoperative obesity and cachexia risk factors for post heart transplant morbidity and mortality: a multi-institutional study of preoperative weight-height indices. *J Heart Lung Transplant* 1999;18:750–763.
12. Narula J, Bennett LE, DiSalvo T, et al. Outcomes in recipients of combined heart-kidney transplantation. *Transplantation* 1997;63:861–867.
13. Befeler AS, Schiano TD, Lissoos TW, et al. Successful combined liver-heart transplantation in adults: report of three patients and review of the literature. *Transplantation* 1999;68:1423–1427.
14. Borkon AM, Muehlebach GF, Jones PG, et al. An analysis of the effect of age on survival after heart transplantation. *J Heart Lung Transplant* 1999;18:668–674.
15. Miller LW. Criteria for selection of recipients and donors for cardiac transplantation. *Graft* 1999;2:S49–S53.
16. Gridelli B, Remuzzi G. Strategies for making more organs available for transplantation. *N Engl J Med* 2000;343:404–410.
17. Delmonico FL, Snydman DR. Organ donor screening for infectious diseases: review of practice and implications for transplantation. *Transplantation* 1998;65:603–610.
18. Stephens JK, Everson GT, Elliott CL, et al. Fatal transfer

of malignant melanoma from multiorgan donor to four allograft recipients. *Transplantation* 2000;70:232–236.

19. Young JB. Age before beauty: the use of "older" donor hearts for cardiac transplantation. *J Heart Lung Transplant* 1999;18:488–491.

20. Pratschke J, Wilhelm MJ, Kusaka M, et al. Brain death and its influence on donor organ quality and outcome after transplantation. *Transplantation* 1999;67:343–348.

21. Kauffman HM, Bennett LE, McBride MA, et al. The expanded donor. *Transplant Rev* 1997;11:165–190.

22. Hauptman PJ, O'Connor KJ. Procurement and allocation of solid organs for transplantation. *N Engl J Med* 1997;336:422–431.

23. Renlund DG, Taylor DO, Kfoury AG, et al. New UNOS rules: historical background and implications for transplant management. *J Heart Lung Transplant* 1999;18:1065–1070.

24. Yacoub M, Mankad P, Ledingham S. Donor procurement and surgical techniques for cardiac transplantation. *Semin Thorac Cardiovasc Surg* 1990;2:153–161.

25. Adams DH. Surgical techniques in heart transplantation. *Graft* 1999;2:119–122.

26. Lower RR, Stofer RC, Shumway NE. Homovital transplantation of the heart. *J Thorac Cardiovasc Surg* 1961;41:196.

27. El-Gamel A, Yonan NA, Grant S, et al. Orthotopic cardiac transplantation: a comparison between the standard and the bicaval Wythenshawe technique. *J Thorac Cardiovasc Surg* 1995;109:721–730.

28. Morris-Thurgood J, Cowell R, Paul V, et al. Hemodynamic and metabolic effects of paced linkage following heterotopic cardiac transplantation. *Circulation* 1994;90:2342–2347.

29. Bainbridge AD, Cave M, Roberts M, et al. A prospective randomized trial of complete atrioventricular transplantation versus ventricular transplantation with atrioplasty. *J Heart Lung Transplant* 1999;18:407–413.

30. Bengel FM, Ueberfuhr P, Ziegler SI, et al. Serial assessment of sympathetic reinnervation after orthotopic heart transplantation: a longitudinal study using PET and C-11 hydroxyephedrine. *Circulation* 1999;99:1866–1871.

31. Schwaiblmair M, von Scheidt W, Uberfuhr P, et al. Functional significance of cardiac reinnervation in heart transplant recipients. *J Heart Lung Transplant* 1999;18:838–845.

32. Osada N, Chaitman BR, Donohue TJ, et al. Long-term cardiopulmonary exercise performance after heart transplantation. *Am J Cardiol* 1997;79:451–456.

33. Kobashigawa JA, Leaf DA, Lee N, et al. A controlled trial of exercise rehabilitation after heart transplantation. *N Engl J Med* 1999;340:272–277.

34. Bussierers LM, Pflugfelder PW, Taylor AW, et al. Changes in skeletal muscle morphology and biochemistry after cardiac transplantation. *Am J Cardiol* 1997;79:630–634.

35. Cui G, Kobashigawa J, Chung T, et al. Atrial conduction disturbance as an indicator of rejection after cardiac transplantation. *Transplantation* 2000;70:223–227.

36. Lefroy DC, Fang JC, Stevenson LW, et al. Recipient-to-donor atrioatrial conduction after orthotopic heart transplantation: surface electrocardiographic features and estimated prevalence. *Am J Cardiol* 1998;82:444–450.

37. Sayegh MH, Turka LA. The role of T-cell costimulatory activation pathways in transplant rejection. *N Engl J Med* 1998;338:1813–1821.

38. Delves PJ, Roitt IM. The immune system: first of two parts. *N Engl J Med* 2000;343:37–49.

39. Delves PJ, Roitt IM. The immune system: second of two parts. *N Engl J Med* 2000;343:108–117.

40. Klein J, Sato A. Advances in immunology: the HLA system (first of two parts). *N Engl J Med* 2000;343:702–709.

41. Klein J, Sato A. Advances in immunology: the HLA system (second of two parts). *N Engl J Med* 2000;343:782–786.

42. von Andrian UH, MacKay CR. Advances in immunology: T-cell function and migration—two sides of the same coin. *N Engl J Med* 2000;343:1020–1034.

43. Dallman MJ. Immunobiology of graft rejection. In: Ginns LC, Cosimi AB, Morris PJ, eds. *Transplantation.* Cambridge, MA: Blackwell Science, 1999:23–42.

44. Itescu S, Tung TC, Burke EM, et al. Preformed IgG antibodies against major histocompatibility complex class II antigens are major risk factors for high-grade cellular rejection in recipients of heart transplantation. *Circulation* 1998;98:786–793.

45. Tambur AR, Bray RA, Takemoto SK, et al. Flow cytometric detection of HLA-specific antibodies as a predictor of heart allograft rejection. *Transplantation* 2000;70:1055–1059.

46. John R, Lietz K, Burke E, et al. Intravenous immunoglobulin reduces anti-HLA alloreactivity and shortens waiting time to cardiac transplantation in highly sensitized left ventricular assist device recipients. *Circulation* 1999;100[Suppl II]:II-229–II-235.

47. Ma H, Hammond EH, Taylor DO, et al. The repetitive histologic pattern of vascular cardiac allograft rejection: increased incidence associated with longer exposure to prophylactic murine monoclonal anti-CD3 antibody (OKT3). *Transplantation* 1996;62:205–210.

48. Winters GL, Marboe CC, Billingham ME. The International Society for Heart and Lung Transplantation grading system for heart transplant biopsy specimens: clarification and commentary. *J Heart Lung Transplant* 1998;17:754–760.

49. Renlund DG, Gilbert EM, O'Connell JB, et al. Age-associated decline in cardiac allograft rejection. *Am J Med* 1987;83:391–398.

50. Johnson MR, Naftel DC, Hobbs RE, et al. The incremental risk of female sex in heart transplantation: a multiinstitutional study of peripartum cardiomyopathy and pregnancy. *J Heart Lung Transplant* 1997;16:801–812.

51. Baughman, KL. History and current techniques of endomyocardial biopsy. In: Baumgartner WA, Reitz BA, Achuff SA, eds. *Heart and heart-lung transplantation.* Philadelphia: WB Saunders, 1990.

52. Brunner-La Rocca HP, Kiowski W. Identification of patients not requiring endomyocardial biopsies late after cardiac transplantation. *Transplantation* 1998;65:533–538.

53. Harada K, Reller MD, Shiota T, et al. Echocardiographic indexes of rejection in pediatric cardiac transplant recipients managed without maintenance steroid immunosuppression. *Am J Cardiol* 1997;79:693–696.

54. Angermann CE, Nassau K, Stempfle H-U, et al. Recogni-

tion of acute cardiac allograft rejection from serial integrated backscatter analyses in human orthotopic heart transplant recipients: comparison with conventional echocardiography. *Circulation* 1997;95:140–150.

55. Aranda JM Jr, Weston MW, Puleo JA, et al. Effect of loading conditions on myocardial relaxation velocities determined by Doppler tissue imaging in heart transplant recipients. *J Heart Lung Transplant* 1998;17:693–697.

56. Moidl R, Chevtchik O, Simon P, et al. Noninvasive monitoring of peak filling rate with acoustic quantification echocardiography accurately detects acute cardiac allograft rejection. *J Heart Lung Transplant* 1999;18:194–201.

57. Rubin PJ, Hartman JJ, Hasapes JP, et al. Detection of cardiac transplant rejection with 111-In-labeled lymphocytes and gamma scintigraphy. *Circulation* 1996;94[Suppl II]:II-298–II-303.

58. Diasio RB, LoBuglio AF. Immunomodulators: immunosuppressive agents and immunostimulants. In: Hardman JG, Limbird LE, Molinoff PB, et al., eds. *Goodman and Gilman's the pharmacological basis of therapeutics*, 9th ed. New York: McGraw-Hill, 1996:1291–1308.

59. Chabner BA, Allegra CJ, Curt GA, et al. Antineoplastic agents. In: Hardman JG, Limbird LE, Molinoff PB, et al., eds. *Goodman and Gilman's the pharmacological basis of therapeutics*, 9th ed. New York: McGraw-Hill, 1996:1233–1287.

60. Schimmer BP, Parker KL. Adrenocorticotropic hormone; adrenocortical steroids and their synthetic analogs; inhibitors of the synthesis and actions of adrenocortical hormones. In: Hardman JG, Limbird LE, eds. *Goodman and Gilman's the pharmacological basis of therapeutics*, 10th ed. New York: McGraw-Hill, 2001:1649–1677.

61. Eisen HJ, Hobbs RE, Davis SF, et al. Safety, tolerability and efficacy of cyclosporine microemulsion in heart transplant recipients: a randomized, multicenter, double-blind comparison with the oil based formulation of cyclosporine—results at six months after transplantation. *Transplantation* 1999;68:663–671.

62. Taylor DO, Barr ML, Radovancevic B, et al. A randomized, multicenter comparison of tacrolimus and cyclosporine immunosuppressive regimens in cardiac transplantation: decreased hyperlipidemia and hypertension with tacrolimus. *J Heart Lung Transplant* 1999;18:336–345.

63. Meiser BM, Uberfuhr P, Fuchs A, et al. Single-center randomized trial comparing tacrolimus (FK506) and cyclosporine in the prevention of acute myocardial rejection. *J Heart Lung Transplant* 1998;17:782–788.

64. Kobashigawa J, Miller L, Renlund D, et al. A randomized active-controlled trial of mycophenolate mofetil in heart transplant recipients. *Transplantation* 1998;66:507–515.

65. Kelly PA, Kahan BD. Pharmacokinetics and pharmacodynamics of sirolimus. *Graft* 1999;2:189–192.

66. Ferron GM, Jusko WJ. Clinical pharmocokinetics and pharmacodynamics of glucocorticoids in transplant patients. *Graft* 1999;2:182–186.

67. Renlund DG. OKT3 for induction of immunosuppression and treatment of rejection in cardiac allograft recipients. *Clin Transplant* 1993;7:393–402.

68. Kovarik JM. Basiliximab: pharmacokinetics and immunodynamics in clinical transplantation. *Graft* 1999;2:193–195.

69. Vincenti F, Kirkman R, Light S, et al. Interleukin-2-receptor blockade with daclizumab to prevent acute rejection in renal transplantation. *N Engl J Med* 1998;338:161–165.

70. Watkins PB, Leichtman A. The molecular basis of cyclosporin A metabolism, pharmacokinetics and drug interactions. *Graft* 1999;2:177–181.

71. Meiser BM, Pfeiffer M, Schmidt D, et al. Combination therapy with tacrolimus and mycophenolate mofetil following cardiac transplantation: importance of mycophenolic acid therapeutic monitoring. *J Heart Lung Transplant* 1999;18:143–149.

72. Schuler W, Sedrani R, Cottens S, et al. SDZ RAD, a new rapamycin derivative: pharmacological properties in vitro and in vivo. *Transplantation* 1997;64:36–42.

73. Taylor DO, Bristow MR, O'Connell JB, et al. Improved long-term survival after heart transplantation predicted by successful early withdrawal from maintenance corticosteroid therapy. *J Heart Lung Transplant* 1996;15:1039–1046.

74. Onsager DR, Canver CC, Jahania MS, et al. Efficacy of tacrolimus in the treatment of refractory rejection in heart and lung transplant recipients. *J Heart Lung Transplant* 1999;18:448–455.

75. Ross HJ, Gullestad L, Pak J, et al. Methotrexate or total lymphoid radiation for treatment of persistent or recurrent allograft cellular rejection: a comparative study. *J Heart Lung Transplant* 1997;16:179–189.

76. Barr ML, Meiser BM, Eisen HJ, et al. Photopheresis for the prevention of acute rejection in cardiac transplantation. *N Engl J Med* 1998;339:1744–1751.

77. Weis M, von Scheidt W. Cardiac allograft vasculopathy: a review. *Circulation* 1997;96:2069–2077.

78. Costanzo MR, Naftel DC, Pritzker MR, et al. Heart transplant coronary artery disease detected by coronary angiography: a multiinstitutional study of preoperative donor and recipient risk factors. *J Heart Lung Transplant* 1998;17:744–753.

79. Gao S-Z, Hunt SA, Schroeder JS, et al. Early development of accelerated graft coronary artery disease: risk factors and course. *J Am Coll Cardiol* 1996;28:673–679.

80. Gao SZ, Alderman EL, Schroeder JS, et al. Accelerated coronary vascular disease in the heart transplant patient: coronary arteriographic findings. *J Am Coll Cardiol* 1988;12:334–348.

81. Mehra MR, Ventura HO, Jain SP, et al. Heterogeneity of cardiac allograft vasculopathy: clinical insights from coronary angioscopy. *J Am Coll Cardiol* 1997;29:1339–1344.

82. Gupta A, Moustapha A, Jacobsen DW, et al. High homocysteine, low folate, and low vitamin B_6 concentrations: prevalent risk factors for vascular disease in heart transplant recipients. *Transplantation* 1998;65:544–550.

83. Cooke GE, Eaton GM, Whitby G, et al. Plasma atherogenic markers in congestive heart failure and posttransplant (heart) patients. *J Am Coll Cardiol* 2000;36:509–516.

84. Brunner-La Rocca HP, Schneider J, Kunzli A, et al. Cardiac allograft rejection late after transplantation is a risk factor for graft coronary artery disease. *Transplantation* 1998;65:538–543.

85. Hornick P, Smith J, Pomerace A, et al. Influence of acute rejection episodes, HLA matching, and donor/recipient

phenotype on the development of "early" transplant-associated coronary artery disease. *Circulation* 1997;96[Suppl II]:II-148–II-153.

86. Weis M, Wildhirt SM, Schulze C, et al. Endothelin in coronary endothelial dysfunction early after human heart transplantation. *J Heart Lung Transplant* 1999;18:1071–1079.

87. Hosenpud JD, Morris TE, Shipley DG, et al. Cardiac allograft vasculopathy: preferential regulation of endothelial cell–derived mesenchymal growth factors in response to a donor-specific cell-mediated allogeneic response. *Transplantation* 1996;61:939–948.

88. Valantine HA, Gao S-Z, Menon SG, et al. Impact of prophylactic immediate post-transplant ganciclovir on development of transplant atherosclerosis: a post-hoc analysis of a randomized placebo-controlled trial. *Circulation* 1999;100:61–66.

89. Yun JJ, Fischbein MP, Laks H, et al. Early and late chemokine production correlates with cellular recruitment in cardiac allograft vasculopathy. *Transplantation* 2000;69:2515–2524.

90. Faulk WP, Labarrere CA, Torry RJ, et al. Serum cardiac troponin-T concentrations predict development of coronary artery disease in heart transplant patients. *Transplantation* 1998;66:1335–1339.

91. Lin H, Ignatescu M, Wilson JE, et al. Prominence of apolipoproteins B, (a), and E in the intimae of coronary arteries in transplanted human hearts: geographic relationship to vessel wall proteoglycans. *J Heart Lung Transplant* 1996;15:1223–1232.

92. Hosenpud JD, Mauck KA, Hogan KB. Cardiac allograft vasculopathy: IgM antibody responses to donor-specific vascular endothelium. *Transplantation* 1997;63:1602–1606.

93. Fredrich R, Toyoda M, Czer LSC, et al. The clinical significance of antibodies to human vascular endothelial cells after cardiac transplantation. *Transplantation* 1999;67:385–391.

94. Benza RL, Grenett HE, Bourge RC, et al. Gene polymorphisms for plasminogen activator inhibitor-1/tissue plasminogen activator and development of allograft coronary artery disease. *Circulation* 1998;98:2248–2254.

95. Labarrere CA. Anticoagulation factors as predictors of transplant-associated coronary artery disease. *J Heart Lung Transplant* 2000;19:623–633.

96. Spes CH, Klauss V, Mudra H, et al. Diagnostic and prognostic value of serial dobutamine stress echocardiography for noninvasive assessment of cardiac allograft vasculopathy: a comparison with coronary angiography and intravascular ultrasound. *Circulation* 1999;100:509–515.

97. Carlsen J, Toft JC, Mortensen SA, et al. Myocardial perfusion scintigraphy as a screening method for significant coronary artery stenosis in cardiac transplant recipients. *J Heart Lung Transplant* 2000;19:873–878.

98. Allen-Auerbach M, Schoder H, Johnson J, et al. Relationship between coronary function by positron emission tomography and temporal changes in morphology by intravascular ultrasound (IVUS) in transplant recipients. *J Heart Lung Transplant* 1999;18:211–219.

99. Liang DH, Gao S-Z, Botas J, et al. Prediction of angiographic disease by intracoronary ultrasonographic findings in heart transplant recipients. *J Heart Lung Transplant* 1996;15:980–987.

100. Wolford TL, Donohue TJ, Bach RG, et al. Heterogeneity of coronary flow reserve in the examination of multiple individual allograft coronary arteries. *Circulation* 1999;99:626–632.

101. Mehra MR, Uber PA, Prasad AK, et al. Long-term outcome of cardiac allograft vasculopathy treated by transmyocardial laser revascularization: early rewards, late losses. *J Heart Lung Transplant* 2000;19:801–804.

102. Fishman JA, Rubin RH. Infection in organ-transplant recipients. *N Engl J Med* 1998;338:1741–1751.

103. Miller LW, Naftel DC, Bourge RC, et al. Infection after heart transplantation: a multiinstitutional study. *J Heart Lung Transplant* 1994;13:381–393.

104. Rubin RH. Prevention and treatment of cytomegalovirus disease in heart transplant patients. *J Heart Lung Transplant* 2000;19:731–735.

105. Barber L, Egan JJ, Lomax J, et al. A prospective study of a quantitative PCR ELISA assay for the diagnosis of CMV pneumonia in lung and heart-transplant recipients. *J Heart Lung Transplant* 2000;19:771–780.

106. Grossi P, Farina C, Fiocchi R, et al. Prevalence and outcome of invasive fungal infections in 1,963 thoracic organ transplant recipients. *Transplantation* 2000;70:112–116.

107. Couchoud C, Cucherat M, Haugh M, et al. Cytomegalovirus prophylaxis with antiviral agents in solid organ transplantation: a meta-analysis. *Transplantation* 1998;65:641–647.

108. Olsen SL, Renlund DG, O'Connell JB, et al. Prevention of *Pneumocystis carinii* pneumonia in cardiac transplant recipients by trimethoprim/sulfamethoxazole. *Transplantation* 1993;56:359–362.

109. Fraund S, Wagner D, Pethig K, et al. Influenza vaccination in heart transplant recipients. *J Heart Lung Transplant* 1999;18:220–225.

110. Campistol JM, Sacks SH. Mechanisms of nephrotoxicity. *Transplantation* 2000;69:SS5–SS10.

111. MacDonald AS. Management strategies for nephrotoxicity. *Transplantation* 2000;69:SS31–SS36.

112. Baan CC, Balk AHMM, Holweg CTJ, et al. Renal failure after clinical heart transplantation is associated with TGF-β1 codon 10 gene polymorphism. *J Heart Lung Transplant* 2000;19:866–872.

113. Parry G, Meiser B, Rbago G. The clinical impact of cyclosporine nephrotoxicity in heart transplantation. *Transplantation* 2000;69:SS23–SS26.

114. Brozena SC, Johnson MR, Ventura H, et al. Effectiveness and safety of diltiazem or lisinopril in treatment of hypertension after heart transplantation. *J Am Coll Cardiol* 1996;27:1707–1712.

115. Schwitter J, DeMarco T, Globits S, et al. Influence of felodipine on left ventricular hypertrophy and systolic function in orthotopic heart transplant recipients: possible interaction with cyclosporine medication. *J Heart Lung Transplant* 1999;18:1003–1013.

116. Stempfle H-U, Werner C, Echtler S, et al. Prevention of osteoporosis after cardiac transplantation: a prospective, longitudinal, randomized, double-blind trial with calcitriol. *Transplantation* 1999;68:523–530.

117. Shane E, Rodino MA, McMahon DJ, et al. Prevention of bone loss after heart transplantation with antiresorptive therapy: a pilot study. *J Heart Lung Transplant* 1998;17:1089–1096.

118. Braith RW, Mills RM Jr, Welsch MA, et al. Resistance exercise training restores bone mineral density in heart transplant recipients. *J Am Coll Cardiol* 1996;28:1471–1477.

119. Kobashigawa JA, Kasiske BL. Hyperlipidemia in solid organ transplantation. *Transplantation* 1997;63:331–338.

120. Magnani G, Carinci V, Magelli C, et al. Role of statins in the management of dyslipidemia after cardiac transplant: randomized controlled trial comparing the efficacy and safety of atorvastatin with pravastatin. *J Heart Lung Transplant* 2000;19:710–715.

121. Lampros TD, Cobanoglu A, Parker F, et al. Squamous and basal cell carcinoma in heart transplant recipients. *J Heart Lung Transplant* 1998;17:586–591.

122. Mihalov ML, Gattuso P, Abraham K, et al. Incidence of post-transplant malignancy among 674 solid-organ-transplant recipients at a single center. *Clin Transplant* 1996;10:248–255.

123. Paya CV, Fung JJ, Nalesnik MA, et al. Epstein-Barr virus–induced posttransplant lymphoproliferative disorders. *Transplantation* 1999;68:1517–1525.

124. Darenkov IA, Marcarelli MA, Basadonna GP, et al. Reduced incidence of Epstein-Barr virus–associated posttransplant lymphoproliferative disorder using preemptive antiviral therapy. *Transplantation* 1997;64:848–852.

125. Vega KJ, Pina I, Krevsky B. Heart transplantation is associated with an increased risk for pancreaticobiliary disease. *Ann Intern Med* 1996;124:980–983.

126. Milas M, Ricketts RR, Amerson JR, et al. Management of biliary tract stones in heart transplant patients. *Ann Surg* 1996;223:747–753.

127. Branch KR, Wagoner LE, McGrory CH, et al. Risks of subsequent pregnancies on mother and newborn in female heart transplant recipients. *J Heart Lung Transplant* 1998;17:698–702.

128. Kasiske BL, Cohen D, Lucey MR, et al. Payment for immunosuppression after organ transplantation. *JAMA* 2000;283:2445–2450.

SURGICAL CONSIDERATIONS IN THE TREATMENT OF HEART FAILURE

NICHOLAS G. SMEDIRA

▼ ADDITIONAL ELECTRONIC TOPICS

INTRODUCTION

Heart failure is a major epidemic. Patients who would have otherwise died after acute coronary events or patients with chronic ventricular dysfunction are surviving, albeit with reduced left ventricular (LV) function and diminished quality of life. Medical therapies for these patients have improved dramatically, but survival in patients with advanced heart failure remains poor. Similar to medical therapies, great strides have been made in the surgical treatment of patients with cardiac disease. Currently, the mortality for primary and reoperative coronary artery bypass

grafting (CABG) at The Cleveland Clinic Foundation is less than 2%. Improvements in preoperative medical care, anesthetic management, perfusion technology, myocardial protection, inotropic agents, intensive care unit care, and postoperative medical therapy all have played important roles. These advances have encouraged the application of surgical techniques to patients with severe heart failure resulting in similarly low morbidity and mortality.

The goal of this chapter is to review the current state of surgical interventions for chronic heart failure. The focus is on surgical risk assessment, management of ischemic cardiomyopathy with revascularization and remodeling, mitral valve procedures, and LV assist devices (LVADs). Acute cardiogenic shock and mechanical complications of acute myocardial infarctions (MIs) are addressed in Chapter 19.

N. G. Smedira: Department of Thoracic and Cardiovascular Surgery, The Cleveland Clinic Foundation, Cleveland, Ohio

Because the field is rapidly changing, an effort was made to summarize information published in the last decade, and references are limited to important contributions in each area during this time period. Surgical videos and illustrations of the various procedures described are present on the CD-ROM that accompanies this textbook.

RISK ASSESSMENT

Patients at the highest risk for surgical morbidity and mortality are often the patients most likely to gain some improvement in quality of life or a survival benefit. Solid data are now available to estimate the risk of coronary revascularization and valvular intervention. What is often much more difficult is determining whether functional recovery of the ventricle will occur postoperatively and whether this is in fact a prerequisite for symptom resolution or has a survival advantage.

Series evaluating this early risk of coronary revascularization have concluded that the degree of LV dysfunction is no longer important. This is probably incorrect and reflects the practice of defining LV dysfunction at some arbitrary relatively high level of ejection fraction (EF). Rao et al. reviewed the Toronto General Experience in 4,558 CABG patients (1). The strongest predictor of mortality was LVEF less than 20%. When compared with patients with EFs between 20% and 40%, the mortality for patients with EF less than 20% increased from 3% to 11% (Table 95.1). The addition of advanced age, reoperation, and the need for emergency operation significantly increases the risk of revascularization. Using the equation generated by the analysis, an institution can input the variables and arrive at the patient's estimated risk (*e*Fig. 95.0.1).

Other risk factors in patients with ischemic cardiomyopathy include obesity, poor target vessels for revascularization, need for intraaortic balloon pump, and severity of congestive heart failure (CHF) symptoms or New York Heart Association (NYHA) functional class (2–6).

The presence of clinical heart failure deserves attention. In general, there is a poor correlation between EF and functional class. From the Duke database, approximately 20% of

TABLE 95.1 ODDS RATIO FOR MORTALITY AFTER CORONARY REVASCULARIZATION

Variable	Odds ratio	95% Confidence interval
Left ventricular ejection fraction		
40–60%	1.62	(0.93–2.83)
20–40%	2.02	(1.11–3.68)
<20%	8.10	(3.91–16.80)
Repeat operation	4.86	(2.97–7.95)
Age ≥70 yr	2.79	(1.85–4.19)
Emergency operation	2.69	(1.25–5.79)

TABLE 95.2 RELATIONSHIP BETWEEN EJECTION FRACTION AND CONGESTIVE HEART FAILURE CLASS

Ejection fraction (%)	Congestive heart failure class				
	0	I	II	III	IV
<0.25	1.1	10.8	5.0	6.0	18.2
0.25–0.35	6.5	14.9	15.0	26.5	29.5
0.36–0.45	15.8	29.7	21.7	22.9	22.8
0.46–0.55	28.0	20.3	25.8	26.5	22.8
>0.55	47.0	24.3	32.5	18.1	6.8

From Wechsler AS, Junod FL. Coronary bypass grafting in patients with chronic congestive heart failure. *Circulation* 1989;79[Suppl I]:I-92–I-96, with permission.

patients were in NYHA class IV in each quintile of EF below 55% (7) (Table 95.2). Olhshansky et al. reviewed data from the CABG Patch trial, which shows that when corrected for degree of CHF, EF failed to predict outcome across EF quartiles (*e*Table 95.2.1) (8). If they arbitrarily selected EFs above and below 0.27, then CHF predicted mortality in each group (*e*Table 95.2.2). These data support clinical experience that has found that the EF is at best a rough indicator of clinical well-being and that therapy to eliminate or reduce heart failure signs and symptoms before intervention may significantly affect early survival.

Some data are available to assess the risk of valve interventions in patients with reduced LV function. In 257 patients with a mixture of aortic and mitral interventions, predictors of hospital mortality mirrored those of coronary revascularization and included lower EF, reoperations, ischemic mitral disease, and emergency surgery (9). Predictors of decreased 10-year survival were age greater than 60 years, aortic regurgitation, and diuretic use. The authors suggest that the more advanced the heart failure, as reflected by the diuretic use, the worse the prognosis. For patients with severe aortic stenosis and low gradients secondary to severe LV dysfunction, surgery has a relatively high published mortality with few defined risk factors except older age (10,11).

At The Cleveland Clinic Foundation, we have used a severity scoring system that uses many of the variables identified as risk factors after coronary bypass surgery. Compared with the early 1980s, the patients undergoing surgery a decade later are in higher risk groups, yet have lower risk adjusted morbidity and mortality. It is noteworthy that stroke mortality has declined substantially. This reflects use of a single cross-clamp technique, frequent use of transesophageal echocardiography, and avoidance of aortic manipulation if ascending atheroslerosis is present (*e*Figs. 95.0.2 and 95.0.3, *e*Table 95.2.3) (12). Currently, isolated mitral valve operations at The Cleveland Clinic Foundation are now consistently performed with a less than 2% operative risk of death (Fig. 95.1).

There lies the quandary. Surgical risk has been reduced substantially for even the highest risk subgroups, a result

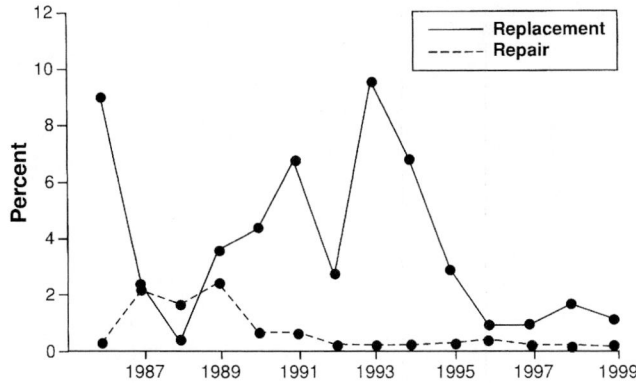

FIGURE 95.1 Operative mortality for isolated mitral valve operations at The Cleveland Clinic Foundation.

that is undoubtedly multifactorial and reflects improvements in preoperative preparation and management of heart failure, surgical techniques and myocardial protection, and intraoperative and postoperative care. Most patients survive the operation, but the real dilemma is identifying the patient most likely to benefit from the procedure.

ISCHEMIC CARDIOMYOPATHY: ROLE OF SURGICAL REVASCULARIZATION

The rationale behind revascularization is based on the concept that a chronically ischemic ventricle contains hibernating myocardium that will improve functionally with improvement of myocardial blood flow. This concept was first introduced by Rahimtoola (13,14). In a busy heart failure surgical section, the question of which patient with ischemic cardiomyopathy is a candidate for revascularization arises daily. The only randomized study to help with this decision is the Coronary Artery Surgery Study (CASS) study (15,16). It is important to note that the patients enrolled in this study had mild angina and were excluded if heart failure was present and if the EF was below 0.36. In the medically treated cohort excluded from surgery because of a low EF, survival was quite poor (17). It is true that these studies are nonrandomized, but it suggests that the subgroup of patients with the lowest EF have the poorest survival (*e*Fig. 95.1.1). Data supporting the value of surgical revascularization in this subgroup of patients was presented by Alderman and colleagues (18). They reviewed these patients who were evaluated for the CASS study but excluded because the EF was less than 36%. Surgically treated patients had more angina, more left main stenosis, and less heart failure (18). In addition to these differences, there was crossover into the surgical group. Medically treated patients with severely reduced LV function and three-vessel disease had dismal survival over 8 years. Overall they showed that surgically treated patients did better and

the greatest benefit was seen in the patients with the lowest EFs (Fig. 95.2).

Patient Selection

Patients with angina and severe LV dysfunction are candidates for surgical therapy assuming adequate targets for revascularization (19,20). Baker et al. concluded that this approach is favored by review of the literature, improves EF and angina by 30% to 50%, and reduces NYHA functional class by one (19). It must be noted, however, that these are nonrandomized trials, somewhat outdated, and with small numbers. However, clinical experience supports these findings (*e*Fig. 95.2.1). The more difficult question is when to intervene in patients without angina. It is primarily in this group of patients in which viability and functional studies have their greatest impact. It is beyond the scope of this chapter to detail the utility of functional studies. In general, the greater the number of viable myocardial segments, the greater the increase in postoperative EF and exercise capacity. However, improvement in quality of life and functional class has not correlated with the volume of hibernating myocardium (21).

To assess myocardial viability in patients with ischemic cardiomyopathy and heart failure, the author relies primarily on positron emission tomography (PET) and magnetic resonance imaging (MRI) scans. MRI has the advantage of assessing wall motion and perfusion, identifying scar distribution, and determining chamber volume and valve function. The study has its limitations, however. Approximately 10% of patients cannot tolerate the confined spaces of the MRI scanner and another 10% to 20% are excluded from the study because of the presence of pacemakers or internal

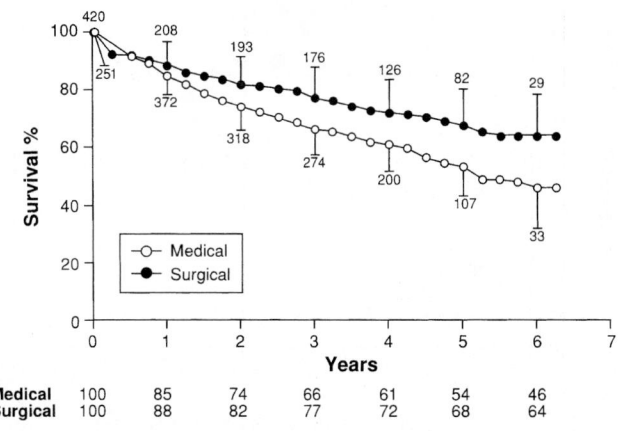

Medical	100	85	74	66	61	54	46
Surgical	100	88	82	77	72	68	64

P = 0.0007
Log Rank Stat = 11.522

FIGURE 95.2 Comparison of medically and surgically treated CASS registry patients excluded from the study because of an ejection fraction less than 36%. [Alderman EL, Fisher LD, Litwin P, et al. Results of coronary artery surgery in patients with poor left ventricular function (CASS). *Circulation* 1983;68:785–795, with permission.]

defibrillators. The patient receives intravenous gadolinium, which is taken up by myocardial scar (*e*Figs. 95.2.2 and 95.2.3). Kim et al. have shown that the absence of enhancement of the myocardium by gadolinium predicts improvement in wall motion after revascularization, whereas greater than 75% transmural uptake of gadolinium is indicative of scar and irreversible segmental dysfunction (22).

DiCarli and colleagues have evaluated the utility of PET scans in conjunction with clinical symptoms. Patients with PET mismatch (greater than 5% of myocardium, which is a low percentage), with and without angina, have a survival advantage over medical therapy. Sudden death was a common event in the medically treated patients, supporting the thesis that hibernating myocardium is a more unstable substrate than scar. In patients without angina, the use of PET matching of low perfusion and no metabolic activity predicts no survival benefit with revascularization (23). Other studies confirm this but suggest that quality of life and exercise capacity increase in this group. Because the number of patients assessed is small, further studies are necessary to define the role of revascularization in patients with heart failure and limited amounts of viable myocardium.

The size or volume of the ventricle is another important variable predicting outcome. Yamaguchi et al. showed that in patients with EFs less than 30%, if the LV end systolic volume index was greater than 100 mL per m², those patients did not have an increase in EF postrevascularization and had significantly worse 5-year survival and event-free survival (Figs. 95.3, 95.4, and 95.5) (24). It is likely

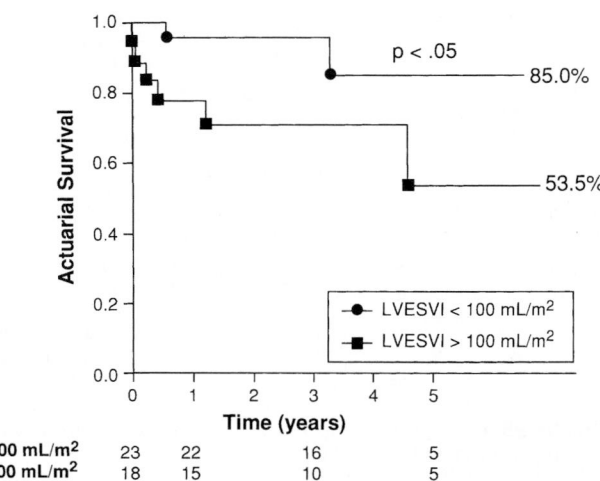

< 100 mL/m²	23	22	16	5
> 100 mL/m²	18	15	10	5

FIGURE 95.4 Ischemic cardiomyopathy and ventricular enlargement greater than 100 mL per m² is associated with reduced survival after revascularization. LVESVI, left ventricular end systolic volume index. (From Yamaguchi A, Takashi I, Adachi H. Left ventricular volume predicts postoperative course in patients with ischemic cardiomyopathy. *Ann Thorac Surg* 1998;65:434–438, with permission.)

that, in the future, some assessment of ventricular volume will be used to determine the likelihood of functional recovery of the revascularization.

Current Practice

Given the critical shortage of donor organs for transplantation, all patients with ischemic cardiomyopathy are assessed for nontransplant alternatives. For patients with angina, multivessel disease, and normal to mild chamber enlargement, revascularization can be expected to improve function and

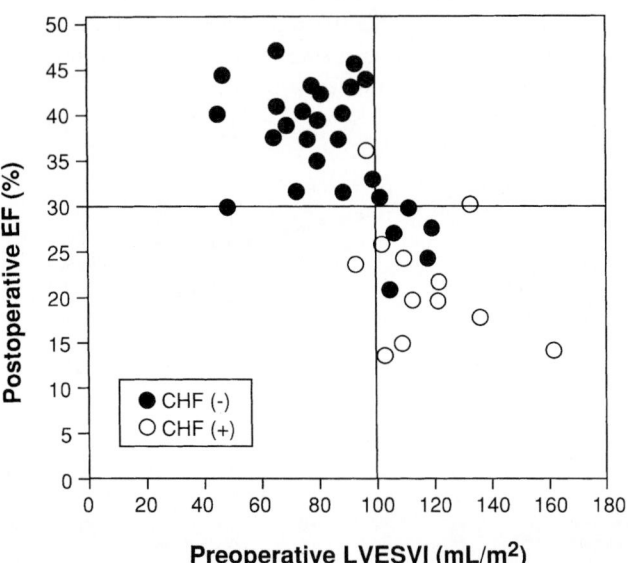

FIGURE 95.3 For patients with ischemic cardiomyopathy, ejection fraction (EF) less than 30% and left ventricular end systolic volume index (LVESVI) greater than 100 mL per m² functional recovery was unlikely after revascularization. CHF, congestive heart failure. (From Yamaguchi A, Takashi I, Adachi H. Left ventricular volume predicts postoperative course in patients with ischemic cardiomyopathy. *Ann Thorac Surg* 1998;65:434–438, with permission.)

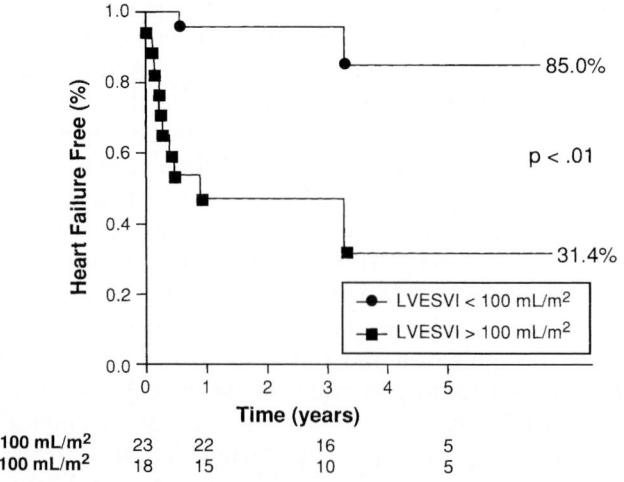

< 100 mL/m²	23	22	16	5
> 100 mL/m²	18	15	10	5

FIGURE 95.5 Event-free survival after revascularization is significantly reduced in the larger ventricle. LVESVI, left ventricular end systolic volume index. (From Yamaguchi A, Takashi I, Adachi H. Left ventricular volume predicts postoperative course in patients with ischemic cardiomyopathy. *Ann Thorac Surg* 1998;65:434–438, with permission.)

survival. A common clinical practice rarely described in the literature is to base revascularization decisions on target vessel quality. Langensburg et al. showed that in a small series of patients with ischemic cardiomyopathy, patients with vessels rated as poor had 100% mortality after revascularization (2). For patients with only heart failure symptoms, markedly enlarged ventricles, and previous operations (all predictors of increased operative risks), functional studies are obtained to help support surgical intervention. A PET scan showing mismatch of greater than 15% of the myocardial mass supports intervention. If PET corroborates extensive scarring, then isolated revascularization is not considered. A combination of anterior scar, ventricular enlargement, and lateral and inferior ischemia or hibernation directs the surgeon toward revascularization and a remodeling procedure.

Patients with a markedly enlarged ventricle, fair to poor targets, and limited viability, especially if the procedure is a reoperation, are at high risk for postcardiotomy pump failure and are assessed preoperatively for transplant candidacy. If postcardiotomy pump failure occurs, then an LVAD may be used to bridge the patient to transplantation.

SURGICAL TECHNIQUES

The goal of intervention is complete revascularization and meticulous myocardial protection. Because antegrade and retrograde blood cardioplegia provide outstanding protection of these marginal ventricles, an effort should be made to graft all bypassable targets. The approach of "get in and get out" is no longer supportable. The left internal thoracic artery should be used to bypass the left anterior descending artery and not avoided because it is a high-risk case. In fact, Leavitt et al. have shown in a large series of 21,873 consecutive patients that the use of the internal thoracic artery reduced in-hospital mortality and adverse events, especially in the higher risk patients (25). During reoperations the greatest risk is atheroembolization from diseased vein grafts. This would be potentially fatal in patients with marginal LV function. Gentle dissection, use of retrograde cardioplegia, and early ligation of diseased vein grafts all help minimize this problem.

For patients with more diffuse disease, coronary endarterectomy or laser transmyocardial revascularization have been employed. The efficacy and safety of these techniques are not known at this time.

DIRECT VENTRICULAR REMODELING

Partial Left Ventriculectomy

Randas Batista introduced partial left ventriculectomy (PLV) in late 1995 based on the law of LaPlace and the reduction of wall stress with a decrease in chamber radius. The procedure and its promoter drew a great deal of attention and interest

from heart failure physicians and patients with end-stage heart disease. This procedure offered an alternative to patients who were not candidates for transplant or LV assist devices or preferred to avoid or delay transplantation. More important, it encouraged physicians to look for more unconventional approaches to end-stage heart failure, and along with the contemporaneous success with mitral valve repair in patients with end-stage cardiomyopathy, surgeons were emboldened to attempt surgery in these high-risk patients.

Patient Selection and Technique

In most published series, patients undergoing PLV had idiopathic dilated cardiomyopathy with or without mitral regurgitation. LV dimensions needed to be greater than 7.0 cm; at The Cleveland Clinic Foundation, all patients were transplant candidates (33).

A wedge of ventricular myocardium weighing an average 96 g (range, 30 to 290 g) was resected in the coronary distribution of the lateral circumflex artery. This removed the muscle between the papillary muscles. If this was thought to be insufficient for radius reduction, the papillary muscles were detached, more myocardium was resected, and the papillary muscles reattached. Mitral valve repair or replacement was performed in most patients. An incremental but potentially significant advance in patient selection was described by Suma et al. (34). Early in The Cleveland Clinic experience, the preoperative MRI scans suggested that the lateral wall was functioning the best and the anterior wall and septum were akinetic and scarred. After lateral wall resection, the anterior and septal walls sometimes had improvement in function, but often they did not. Suma et al. intraoperatively looked at regional wall motion of the decompressed ventricles (on partial bypasses) with transesophageal echocardiography. If all walls show improved motion while decompressed on partial cardiopulmonary bypass, the patient is not a candidate for PLV and undergoes mitral valve surgery alone. If the anterior wall and septum are akinetic with good lateral wall function, a modified endoventricular circular patch plasty is performed even for idiopathic dilated ventricles. For lateral wall akinesis, the standard PLV is done (34).

Results

There were astonishing successes and dismal failures after PLV, with an inability to predict outcomes (35) (Table 95.3). In general, ventricular volume and wall stress were reduced,

TABLE 95.3 PARTIAL LEFT VENTRICULECTOMY RESULTS

Operative mortality	3–20%
Early left ventricular assist device (The Cleveland Clinic Foundation)	15%
2-year survival	50–60%
3-year event-free survival	30%

TABLE 95.4   RESULTS OF TARGETED VENTRICULAR REDUCTION[a]

| | EVCPP ± CABG/value | Group I | Group II | |
		LV reduction ± value	LV reduction ± value	Valve alone
No.	33	24	16	13
Mortality	7/33	12/24	1/16	2/33
Hospital + late (%)	21.2	50.0	6.3	15.4
IABP/LVAD	1/0	6/0	0/0	1/1
Return to heart failure	3	4	3	2
Follow-up (d)	377 ± 228	365 ± 323	272 ± 109	316 ± 156
Median (d)	362	278	262	368

CABG, coronary artery bypass grafting; EVCPP, endoventricular circular patch plasty; IABP, intraaortic balloon pumping; LV, left ventricular; LVAD, left ventricular assist device.

[a]Group I patients underwent standard partial left ventriculectomy. In Group II, ventricular remodeling was done after the dysfunctional walls were identified by partial decompression on cardiopulmonary bypass; otherwise they underwent valve repair alone if there was no evidence of regional dysfunction.

From Suma H, Isomura T, Horii T. Non-transplant cardiac surgery for end-stage cardiomyopathy. *J Thorac Cardiovasc Surg* 2000;119:1233–1245, with permission.

EF increased, but central hemodynamics were unchanged. Surgical mortality was high, and longer-term results were poor (36–41). The experience of Suma et al. suggests that a more selective approach to resection in elective patients can be done safely with good results (Table 95.4).

The reason for the unpredictability of PLV remains unclear. Computer analysis has shown that volume reduction by wall segment resection improves end systolic elastance but worsens diastolic compliance (Figs. 95.6 and 95.7) (42–44). The net effect is a decreased slope of the Starling relationship and worse cardiac pump function. Additional factors such as coronary artery injury in the resection closure further compromise cardiac function.

Currently, most centers have abandoned PLV as a therapy for idiopathic dilated cardiomyopathy. However, some European and Asian centers continue to pursue this approach in both ischemic and dilated cardiomyopathies.

In general, early operative mortality is high (approximately 20%), and long-term results are not known. New devices such as the Myosplint (Myocor, Inc., Plymouth, MN) may accomplish the same stress reduction without the high morbidity and mortality (see New Surgical Therapies for Congestive Heart Failure).

REMODELING THE ISCHEMIC VENTRICLE

Indications for Ventricular Remodeling

As mentioned previously [▼ p85], traditionally patients have presented with symptoms of cardiac failure and have

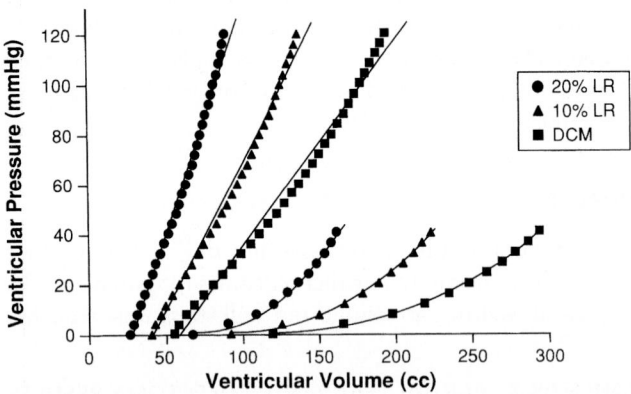

FIGURE 95.6 Finite element analysis predicting improvement in elastance with deterioration in compliance after lateral partial left ventriculectomy. DCM, dilated cardiomyopathy; LR, lateral resection. (From Ratcliffe MB, Hong J, Salahieh A, et al. The effect of ventricular volume reduction surgery in the dilated, poorly contractile left ventricle: a simple finite element analysis. *J Thorac Cardiovasc Surg* 1998;116:566–577, with permission.)

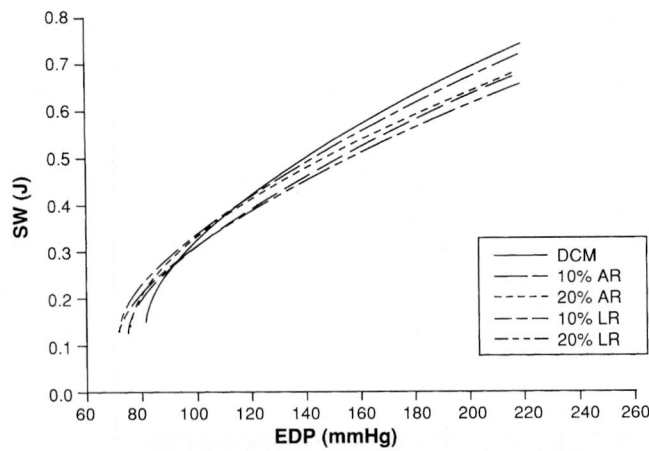

FIGURE 95.7 Overall result of partial left ventriculectomy with worsening of the Starling relationship. AR, apical resection; DCM, dilated cardiomyopathy; EDP, end diastolic pressure; LR, lateral resection; SW, stroke work. (From Ratcliffe MB, Hong J, Salahieh A, et al. The effect of ventricular volume reduction surgery in the dilated, poorly contractile left ventricle: a simple finite element analysis. *J Thorac Cardiovasc Surg* 1998;116:566–577, with permission.)

undergone aneurysm repair at this stage. Currently, asymptomatic patients with ventricular enlargement after an anterior MI should be considered for remodeling. Recommendations vary, but an end diastolic volume greater than 150 to 200 mL, end diastolic dimension of greater than 6.0 to 6.5 cm, or LV end systolic volume index of greater than 60 to 70 mL per m^2 are reasonable guidelines. In our ischemic remodeling group, the average end diastolic volume was 240 mL (end diastolic volume index = 97 mL per m^2) by three-dimensional echo or MRI, whereas Dor's patients had end diastolic volumes ranging from 205 to 246 mL by biplane cineangiography for akinetic and dyskinetic ventricles, respectively (47–49). We use MRI to assess regional wall motion abnormalities in conjunction with clinical status to exclude patients from remodeling. In patients with massively enlarged ventricles or those with extensive wall thinning with class IV symptoms and patients on inotropes, ventilators, or balloon pumps are considered for transplantation or LVAD.

MITRAL VALVE SURGERY IN REDUCED LEFT VENTRICULAR FUNCTION

Historically mitral valve surgery in the setting of reduced LV function was thought to be associated with prohibitive perioperative mortality. The oft quoted mortality of greater than 30% arose from papers published in the 1980s (50). Significant advances have been made since those series in the understanding of the mechanism of mitral insufficiency, the need to preserve papillary annular continuity, and improvements in myocardial protection and surgical techniques that have resulted in substantial improvement in survival. Currently, mitral valve interventions of all types including ischemic mitral regurgitation have an operative mortality of less than 10% (51–53).

Mechanism

Surgical dogma stated that replacement of the mitral valve in the setting of reduced ventricular function would eliminate the pop-off mechanism for the failing ventricle and result in deterioration in LV function (54). In fact, the mechanism for LV dysfunction was the common practice of excising both the anterior and posterior leaflets and chordal attachments. This loss of the papillary annular connection immediately worsened LV function and resulted in a more spherical ventricular shape with increased wall stress. As experience with mitral valve repair grew, it was demonstrated that when compared with mitral replacement LV function was maintained by repair. This led to the expansion of repair techniques in patients with LV dysfunction. It is worthwhile to note that mitral valve replacement that spares the subvalvular apparatus may be as useful as mitral replacement (55).

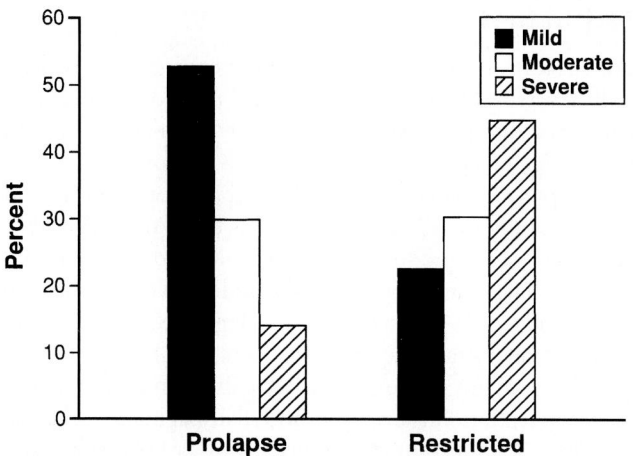

FIGURE 95.8 Relationship of valve pathology and ventricular function. *Mild, moderate,* and *severe* refer to ventricular dysfunction. (From Hendren WG, Nemec JJ, Lytle BW, et al. Mitral valve repair for ischemic mitral insufficiency. *Ann Thorac Surg* 1991;52:1246–1252, with permission.)

In patients with dilated cardiomyopathy, the mitral valve leaflets are usually normal and the mitral regurgitation is related to annular dilatation and apical displacement of the papillary muscles as the chamber enlarges. In ischemic cardiomyopathy, the pathology is much more varied (*e*Table 95.4.1) (56).

Ischemic injury to the papillary muscles results in regional wall motion abnormalities; muscle elongation and fibrosis lead to leaflet prolapse centrally and at the commissures. Postinfarction ventricular enlargement apically displaces the papillary muscles yet infrequently results in annular dilatation. Ischemic injury to the valve may cause morphologic changes similar to those seen with myxomatous valve disease. This results in reduced leaflet coaptation and restricted leaflet motion. These distinctions are important for determining repair techniques.

In general, patients with restricted leaflet motion have more severe reduction in LV function and significantly worse survival at 3 years (Fig. 95.8). ❦ p86

Indications for Mitral Valve Repair or Replacement with Reduced Left Ventricular Function

Clinically, there are no published data available to separate out patients with heart failure and mitral regurgitation so advanced that the patients would be better served by heart transplantation. In general, patients requiring continuous intravenous inotropes are not considered for mitral valve surgery. Patients weaned from inotropes have been successfully operated on. On the other side of the coin, the best approach for patients with 2 to 3+ mitral regurgitation remains unclear. In general, if preoperative echoes have shown 3+ mitral regurgitation and revascularization is unlikely to eliminate the regurgitation, valve repair should be considered.

Techniques

For successful surgical results when operating on ventricles with severe reduction in LV function, meticulous attention to myocardial protection, complete revascularization, and knowledge of valve repair techniques is paramount.

Chapter 21 focuses on valve repair techniques, and details can be found elsewhere in this text. Annuloplasty is the main technique for patients with dilated mitral annuli (*e*Figs. 95.8.3 and 95.8.4). The addition of a stitch to approximate the leaflets (Alfieri) (*e*Fig. 95.8.5) may help reduce late mitral regurgitation from apical displacement but this remains to be proven. Repair techniques such as leaflet resection for prolapse and flail segments, chordal transfer and shortening, papillary muscle plication, and commissural plication are used as necessary. In general, ischemic mitral regurgitation tends to be multifactorial and repairs more difficult. Chordal-sparing mitral valve replacement may be simpler, more effective, and result in similar short- and long-term outcomes.

MECHANICAL CIRCULATORY SUPPORT

A detailed discussion of mechanical circulatory support is beyond the scope of this chapter, but it is extremely important in the surgical management of patients with end-stage heart disease. Mechanical support can be categorized in multiple ways depending on the duration of support (acute or chronic), type of pump (pulsatile vs. continuous flow), completely implantable, implantable or external, total heart replacement, or ventricular assist devices (Table 95.5).

Currently, mechanical support is indicated for postcardiotomy pump failure, acute MI with cardiogenic shock, as a bridge to transplantation, and for patients with the potential for myocardial recovery. Permanent implant or destination therapy is the ultimate goal of mechanical support but has yet to be realized. The REMATCH trial may help define the role of implantable LVADs as an alternative for patients with end-stage cardiomyopathy (60).

Postcardiotomy Support

The need for postcardiotomy mechanical support is declining, despite increasing numbers of high-risk operations (61). To date, all short-term support devices have had equivalent outcomes with approximately 30% of patients surviving the hospitalization (62–65). Despite numerous advances in caring for these patients over the past 20 years, only the ability to convert these patients to an implantable LVAD has improved survival to nearly 50% (66,67). Samuels et al. have recommended that earlier initiation of mechanical support in the operating room to avoid the toxic effects of high doses of inotropes could improve outcome (68).

Bridge to Transplant

The largest collective experience worldwide with mechanical support has been in the group of patients bridged to transplant. The three most common devices are the TCI HeartMate (Fig. 95.9) (Thermo Cardiosystem, Woburn, MA), Novacor (WorldHeart Corp., Ottawa, Canada), and Thoratec VAD (Thoratec Laboratories, Berkeley, CA). A much smaller experience has accumulated with the Cardiowest (Cardiowest Technologies, Tucson, AZ) total artificial heart.

In general, these pumps have worked quite well, with 60% to 75% of patients surviving to transplant (66,69,70). Complications are frequent, including thromboemboli, pump-related infections, and mechanical and valve dysfunction. It is hoped that the smaller axial flow pumps will reduce or eliminate some of these problems as the implantation is much simpler and the pumps are smaller so infection may be less (Fig. 95.10). There are no valves, which may reduce the risk of thromboemboli and eliminates the problem of valve failure.

Ventricular Recovery

It was noticed early in the LVAD bridge to transplant that many hearts had decreased in size, remodeled, and improved in function. Some worked so well that the pump was removed and transplant avoided.

TABLE 95.5 CHARACTERISTICS OF MECHANICAL SUPPORT DEVICES

Device	Pulsatile	Short- and long-term	Internal
Extracorporeal membrane oxygenation	No	Short	No
ABIOMED	Yes	Short	No
AB-180	No	Short	Yes
HeartMate	Yes	Long	Yes
Novacor	Yes	Long	Yes
Thoratec	Yes	Short/long	Yes
LionHeart	Yes	Long	Completely
DeBakey	No	Long	Yes
Jarvik 2000	No	Long	Yes
ABIOCOR	Yes	Long	Completely

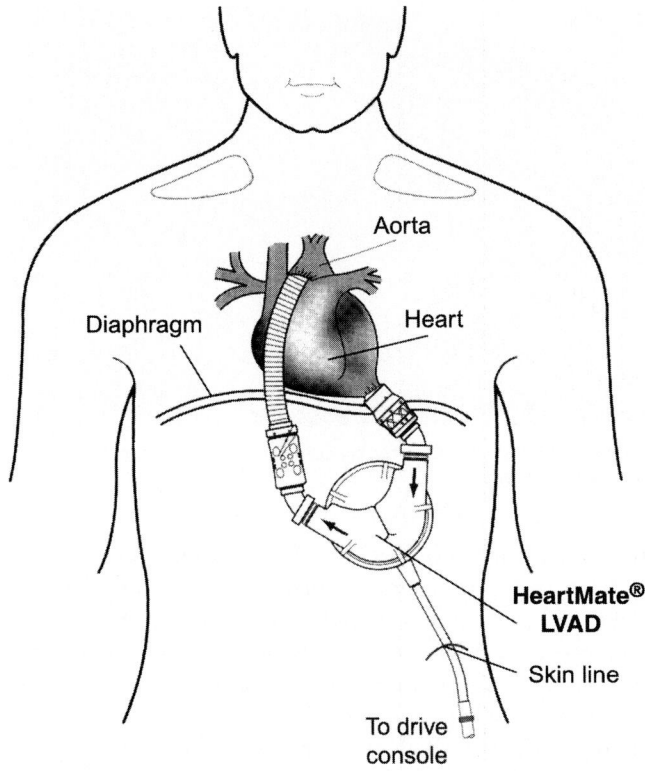

FIGURE 95.9 HeartMate left ventricular assist device (LVAD). (From Slaughter MS, Pappas PS, Tatooles AJ. Modified implant technique for the pneumatic HeartMate left ventricular assist system. *Journal of Congestive Heart Failure and Circulatory Support* 2000;1:123–125, with permission.)

In addition to macroscopic changes, neurohormonal and histologic changes supported the concept that unloading the ventricle may promote recovery. It has been more difficult to characterize ventricles and patients who may recover on support. Hetzer et al. reported the largest experience with 23 patients weaned from LVAD support (71). In general, only patients with idiopathic dilated cardiomyopathy, younger patients, those with shorter durations of heart failure symptoms, and those with greater and earlier remodeling while on support had lasting recovery. It is estimated that of the patients supported with LVADs for long-standing ischemic or dilated cardiomyopathies less than 10% will be recoverable. Given the declining number of donor hearts, identifying even a small group of potentially weanable patients is critical. Additionally, the best support parameters that rest the ventricle but also load it to promote recovery and avoid atrophy and fibrosis remain to be determined. Finally, adjuvant pharmacology, gene therapy, or myoblast transfer may be needed to increase the number of weanable patients.

Destination Therapy

The original purpose of mechanical support funding was to develop a permanent cardiac substitute. That dream remains elusive. Current LVADs work well as a temporary bridge to transplantation but are unlikely to provide the durability and quality of life necessary for more widespread application. The REMATCH trial will provide some insight into how close to the goal we are (60).

Future Devices

The next generation of devices will be the continuous flow pumps (72). These are either axial (straight) or centrifugal (right angle inflow and outflow relationship) miniature pumps that generate flow through high-speed revolution of an impeller blade (Fig. 95.10). The advantages of these pumps are they are much smaller and can be used in pediatric patients and small adults, limited dissection is needed to create a pump pocket, they are quiet, they work without valves, and they are technically easier to convert to a com-

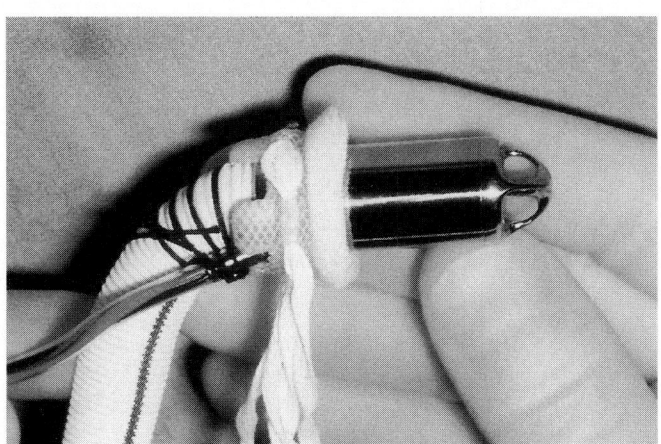

A

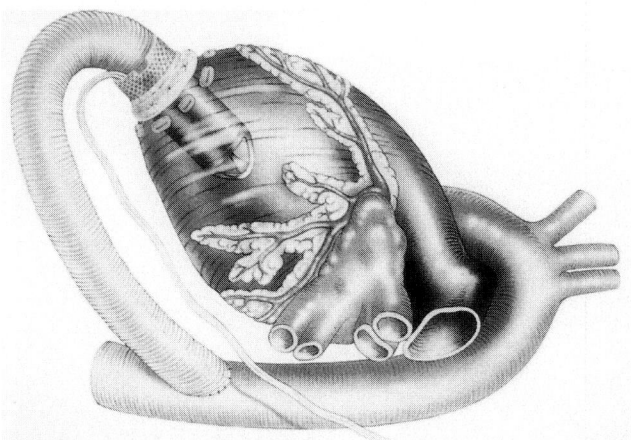

B

FIGURE 95.10 A,B: Jarvik axial flow pump. The metal portion is inserted into the apex of the ventricle with the graft anastomosed to the descending thoracic aorta. (From Katsumata T, Westaby S. Implantable axial flow impeller pumps. *J Circ Support* 1998;1:13–19, with permission.)

pletely implantable design. They currently are in trial in Europe, and trials will begin soon in the United States. It is hoped that the smaller continuous flow pumps will have fewer complications with greater durability and provide an alternative for nontransplant candidates.

NEW SURGICAL THERAPIES FOR CONGESTIVE HEART FAILURE

Acorn Cardiac Support Device

Cardiomyoplasty was developed with the idea that the trained muscle would augment systolic function of the ventricle. Research showed this augmentation was infrequent and the major advantage was a result of a passive girdling of the LV that reduced wall stress, decreased future LV enlargement, and occasionally reversed remodeled the ventricle. This led to the development of a simple mesh-like jacket (Figs. 95.11 and 95.12) that is slipped around the heart with the hopes of preserving or improving myocardial properties.

Animal studies are quite promising. In an ischemic heart failure model in dogs, the CSD after 3 to 6 months resulted in lower end systolic and end diastolic volumes, improved adrenergic reserve, and showed no evidence of constricting the myocardium. These investigators showed that the CSD attenuates cardiomyocyte stretch, limits cardiomyocyte hypertrophy, and improves sarcoplastic reticulum Ca^{2+} ATPase cycling (73).

In two small series published as abstracts, the Acorn CSD (Acorn Cardiovascular, St. Paul, MN) appears to reduce LV size and improve functional class. Currently, a randomized trial is under way that has two arms: CSD alone versus medical therapy, and CSD plus mitral valve surgery versus mitral valve surgery alone. The cardiomyoplasty experience has helped guide the selection of patients. This device will likely be most beneficial in retarding progression of chamber enlargement. This requires its applica-

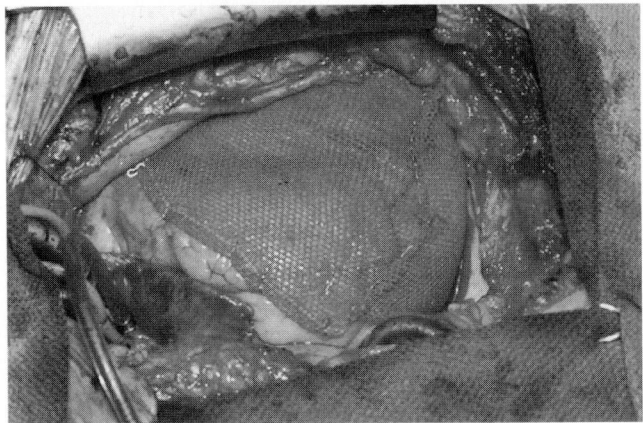

FIGURE 95.12 Acorn after placement around the left ventricle and right ventricle.

tion in patients with class II to III symptoms and moderate (6.0 to 7.5 cm) chamber enlargement. More advanced stages of heart failure are unlikely to benefit from the CSD and operative mortality will be substantially higher. An interesting application of this technology would be in patients after a large acute MI to prevent remodeling. Identifying patients at high risk for remodeling after an acute MI remains to be completely defined.

Myosplint

Unlike the Acorn CSD, which passively remodels the ventricle, the Myosplint (Myocor Inc., Plymouth, MN) actively and acutely reshapes the LV. Conceived after the Batista principle that geometric reduction in LV size should improve wall stress, the Myosplint is a transventricular splint with epicardial pads that reduce the LV radius by creating a bilobular or two-chamber LV (Figs. 95.13 and 95.14).

In early animal studies, LVEF increased from 19% to 38% with significant decreases in end systolic volume (75). It is anticipated that this device will be applied to patients

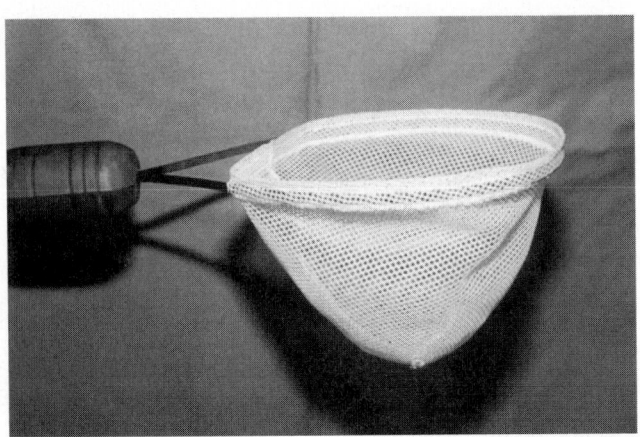

FIGURE 95.11 Acorn mesh.

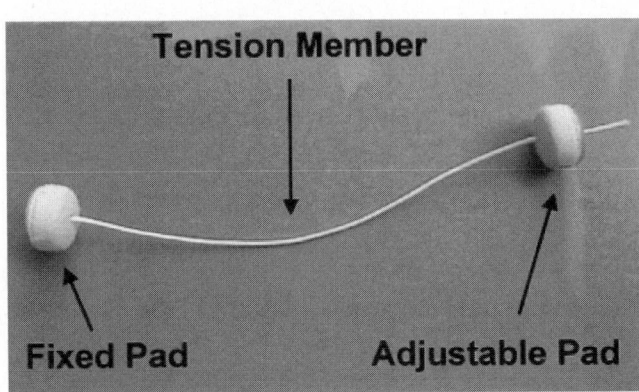

FIGURE 95.13 Myosplint tension member. This metal wire traverses the left ventricle in three spots from base to apex.

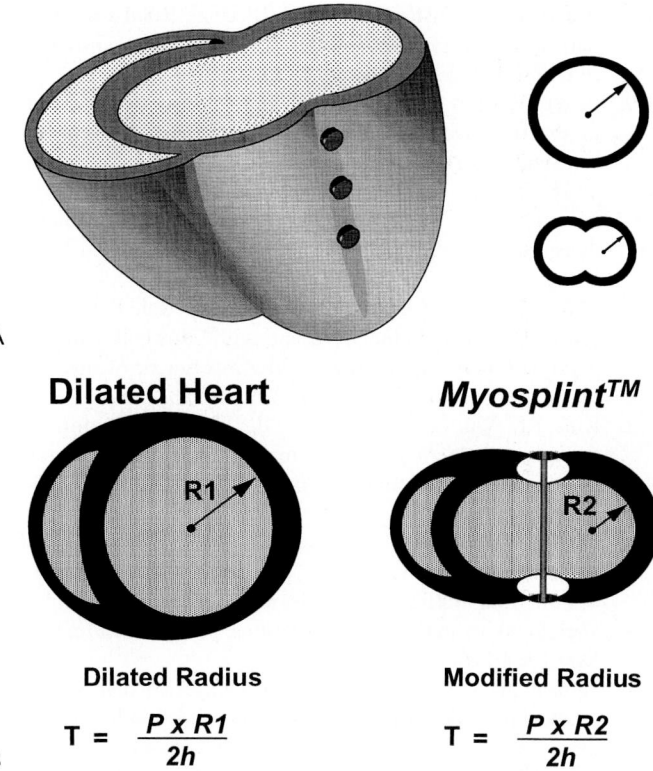

Dilated Heart   ***Myosplint*™**

Dilated Radius   **Modified Radius**

$$T = \frac{P \times R1}{2h}$$ $$T = \frac{P \times R2}{2h}$$

FIGURE 95.14 A,B: Myosplint concept. Stress reduction through ventricular shape change **(A).**

with more advanced heart failure symptoms and larger ventricular volumes.

CONTROVERSIES AND PERSONAL PERSPECTIVES

The statistics speak for themselves. An ever-growing pool of patients with heart failure, limited biologic replacement therapy, and an enlarging armamentarium of surgical therapies and devices suggest that surgery for heart failure will continue to play an important role in treating these patients.

The greatest difficulty in choosing a therapy is the rapidly changing landscape of heart failure medicine. In addition to angiotensin-converting enzyme inhibitors and beta-blockers, angiotensin-receptor blockers, anti–tumor necrosis factor, and other immunotherapy, biventricular pacing, automatic internal cardiodefibrillators, and gene and myoblast therapy are all being assessed in these patients and may affect ventricular remodeling, ischemia, arrhythmias, and mitral regurgitation such that they compete favorably with a surgical procedure. Conversely, waiting until the patient's disease is so far advanced before considering surgical therapy significantly increases the operative risk and most certainly diminishes the benefit. As this chapter outlines, operations for heart failure can be done with low mortality and the concerns that these are high-risk procedures and should be avoided are no longer true. The real question is, Do they provide an improvement in the quality of life of the patient and secondarily do they prolong survival at a reasonable cost?

Uncertainty remains as to the benefit of procedures with advanced heart failure. Patients with extensive myocardial ischemia or hibernation by functional studies should undergo revascularization. There is no justification to consider these patients for inclusion in a randomized trial. On the other hand, there is a great deal of uncertainty and conflicting information about the value of revascularization in patients with only heart failure symptoms, no ischemia or hibernation, and markedly enlarged ventricles. This group should and likely will be evaluated in a randomized trial that includes remodeling and revascularization versus medical therapy.

Other randomized trials are investigating the role of mitral valve repair in end-stage patients compared with medical therapy and the benefit of repair valves with lesser degrees of mitral regurgitation to prevent remodeling.

Assist devices are seen as the answer to end-stage heart disease. Some people say no one should die from heart failure without a trial on an assist device, probably with an AICD to reduce the risk of sudden death. It is hoped that the smaller rotary pumps will make the implant easier, be totally implantable, and run forever. The REMATCH trial may give us some insight into these issues. The profession and society as a whole will need to decide what cost we are willing to expend to improve the quality of and, it is hoped, extend the duration of life in these patients. This undoubtedly will assume greater urgency in the next few years.

THE FUTURE

The lines between heart failure medicine and surgery will grow less distinct. Operations will be performed earlier to prevent the deleterious effects of remodeling and long-standing valve insufficiency. Adjuvant gene or myoblast therapy along with tissue engineering may allow us to rebuild segments of damaged myocardium. Assist devices will get smaller, more durable, completely implantable, and less expensive, justifying a wider application of this technology.

REFERENCES

1. Rao V, Ivanov J, Weisel RD, et al. Predictors of low cardiac output syndrome after coronary artery bypass. *J Thorac Cardiovasc Surg* 1996;112:38–51.

2. Langenburg SE, Buchanan SA, Blackbourne LH, et al. Predicting survival after coronary revascularization for ischemic cardiomyopathy. *Ann Thorac Surg* 1995;58:1193–1197.

3. Kaul TK, Agnihotri AK, Fields BL, et al. Coronary artery bypass grafting in patients with an ejection fraction of twenty percent or less. *J Thorac Cardiovasc Surg* 1996;111:1001–1012.

4. Argenziano M, Spotnitz HM, Whang W, et al. Risk stratification for coronary bypass surgery in patients with left ventricular dysfunction. *Circulation* 1999;100[Suppl II]:II119–II124.

5. Yau TM, Fedak PW, Weisel RD, et al. Predictors of operative risk for coronary bypass operations in patients with left ventricular dysfunction. *J Thorac Cardiovasc Surg* 1999;118:1006–1013.

6. Milano CA, White WD, Smith R, et al. Coronary artery bypass in patients with severely depressed ventricular function. *Ann Thorac Surg* 1993;56:487–493.

7. Wechsler AS, Junod FL. Coronary bypass grafting in patients with chronic congestive heart failure. *Circulation* 1989;79[Suppl I]:I92–I96.

8. Olshansky B, Telfer EA, Curtis AB, et al. Predictive value of preoperative left ventricular ejection fraction and functional class for mortality and morbidity after high-risk coronary artery bypass grafting. *Am J Cardiol* 2000;85:1489–1491.

9. Duarte IG, O'Murphy CO, Kosinski AS, et al. Late survival after valve operation in patients with left ventricular dysfunction. *Ann Thorac Surg* 1997;64:1089–1095.

10. Connolly HM, Oh JK, Schaff HV, et al. Severe aortic stenosis with low transvalvular gradient and severe left ventricular dysfunction. *Circulation* 2000;101:1940–1946.

11. Powell DE, Tunick PA, Rozenzweig BP, et al. Aortic valve replacement in patients with aortic stenosis and severe left ventricular dysfunction. *Arch Intern Med* 2000;160:1337–1341.

12. Estafanous FG, Loop FD, Higgins TL, et al. Increased risk and decreased morbidity of coronary artery bypass grafting between 1986 and 1994. *Ann Thorac Surg* 1998;65:383–389.

13. Rahimtoola SH. A perspective on the three large multicenter randomized clinical trials of coronary bypass surgery for chronic stable angina *Circulation* 1985;72[Suppl V]:123.

14. Rahimtoola SH. The hibernating myocardium. *Am Heart J* 1989;117:211.

15. Kaiser GC, Davis KB, Fisher LD, et al. Survival following coronary artery bypass grafting in patients with severe angina pectoris (CASS). *J Thorac Cardiovasc Surg* 1989;89:513.

16. Myers WO, Schaff HV, Gersh BJ, et al. Improved survival of surgically treated patients with triple vessel coronary artery disease and severe angina pectoris. *J Thorac Cardiovasc Surg* 1989;97:487.

17. Emond M, Mock MB, Davis KB, et al. Long term survival of medically treated patients in the Coronary Artery Surgery Study (CASS) Registry. *Circulation* 1994;90:2645–2657.

18. Alderman EL, Fisher LD, Litwin P, et al. Results of coronary artery surgery in patients with poor left ventricular function (CASS). *Circulation* 1983;68:785–795.

19. Baker DW, Jones R, Hodges J. The role of revascularization in the treatment of patients with moderate or severe left ventricular systolic dysfunction. *JAMA* 1994;272:1528–1534.

20. Marwick TH. The viable myocardium: epidemiology, detection, and clinical implications. *Lancet* 1998;351:815–819.

21. Marwick TH, Zuchowski C, Lauer MS, et al. Functional status and quality of life in patients with heart failure undergoing coronary bypass surgery after assessment of myocardial viability. *J Am Coll Cardiol* 1999;33:750–758.

22. Kim RJ, Wu E, Rafael A, et al. The use of contrast-enhanced magnetic resonance imaging to identify reversible myocardial dysfunction. *N Engl J Med* 2000;343:1445–1453.

23. DiCarli MF, Maddahi J, Rohshar S. Long-term survival of patients with coronary artery disease and left ventricular dysfunction: implications for the role of myocardial viability assessment in management decisions. *J Thorac Cardiovasc Surg* 1998;116:997–1004.

24. Yamaguchi A, Takashi I, Adachi H. Left ventricular volume predicts postoperative course in patients with ischemic cardiomyopathy. *Ann Thorac Surg* 1998;65:434–438.

25. Leavitt BL, O'Connor GT, Ilmstead EM, et al. Use of the internal mammary artery graft and in-hospital mortality and other adverse outcomes associated with coronary artery bypass grafting. *Circulation* 2001;103:507–512.

26. Mickleborough LL, Maruyama H, Takagi Y, et al. Results of revascularization inpatients with severe left ventricular dysfunction. *Circulation* 1995;92[Suppl II]:II73–II79.

27. Elefteriades JA, Morales DLS, Gradel C, et al. Results of coronary artery bypass grafting by a single surgeon in patients with left ventricular ejection fraction <30%. *Am J Cardiol* 1997;79:1573–1578.

28. Elefteriades JA, Tolis G, Levi E, et al. Coronary artery bypass grafting in severe left ventricular dysfunction: excellent survival with improved ejection fraction and functional state. *J Am Coll Cardiol* 1993;22:1411–1417.

29. Anderson WA, Ilkowski DA, Mahan VL, et al. Coronary artery bypass grafting in patients with chronic congestive heart failure: a 10-year experience with 203 patients. *J Cardiol Surg* 1997;12:167–175.

30. Luciani GB, Montalbano G, Casali G, et al. Predicting long term functional results after myocardial revascularization in ischemic cardiomyopathy. *J Thorac Cardiovasc Surg* 2000;120:478–489.

31. Migrino RQ, Young JB, Ellis SG, et al. End-systolic index at 90 to 180 minutes into reperfusion therapy for acute myocardial infarction is a strong predictor of early and late mortality. *Circulation* 1997;96:116–121.

32. Lee TH, Hamilton MA, Stevenson LW. Impact of left ventricular cavity size on survival in advanced heart failure. *Am J Cardiol* 1993;72:672–676.

33. McCarthy PM, Starling RC, Wong J, et al. Early results with partial left ventriculectomy. *J Thorac Cardiovasc Surg* 1997;114:755–765.

34. Suma H, Isomura T, Horii T. Non-transplant cardiac sur-

gery for end-stage cardiomyopathy. *J Thorac Cardiovasc Surg* 2000;119:1233–1245.

35. Starling RC, McCarthy PM. Partial left ventriculectomy: sunrise or sunset? *Eur J Heart Failure* 1999;1:313–317.

36. Moreira LF, Stolf NAG, Bocchi EA, et al. Partial left ventriculectomy with mitral valve preservation in the treatment of patients with dilated cardiomyopathy. *J Thorac Cardiovasc Surg* 1998;115:800–807.

37. Schreuder JJ, Steendijk P, van der Veer FH, et al. Acute and short-term effects of partial left ventriculectomy in dilated cardiomyopathy. *J Am Coll Cardiol* 2000;36:2104–2114.

38. Popovic Z, Miric M, Gradinac S, et al. Effects of partial left ventriculectomy on left ventricular performance in patients with nonischemic dilated cardiomyopathy. *J Am Coll Cardiol* 1998;32:1801–1808.

39. Laks H, Marelli D. The current role of left ventricular reduction for treatment of heart failure. *J Am Coll Cardiol* 1998;32:1809–1810.

40. Katsumata T, Westaby S. An objective appraisal of partial left ventriculectomy for heart failure. *Journal of Congestive Heart Failure and Circulatory Support* 1999;1:97–106.

41. Etoch SW, Koenig SC, Laureano MA. Results after partial left ventriculectomy versus heart transplantation for idiopathic cardiomyopathy. *J Thorac Cardiovasc Surg* 1999;117:952–959.

42. Dickstein ML, Spotnitz HM, Rose EA, et al. Heart reduction surgery: an analysis of the impact on cardiac function. *J Thorac Cardiovasc Surg* 1997;113:1032–1040.

43. Ratcliffe MB, Hong J, Salahieh A, et al. The effect of ventricular volume reduction surgery in the dilated, poorly contractile left ventricle: a simple finite element analysis. *J Thorac Cardiovasc Surg* 1998;116:566–577.

44. Ratcliffe M. Batista's operation: what have we learned? *J Am Coll Cardiol* 2000;36:2115–2118.

45. Cox JI. Left ventricular aneurysms: pathophysiologic observations. *Semin Thorac Cardiovasc Surg* 1997;9:113–122.

46. Dor V, Sabatier M, Di Donato M. Efficacy of endoventricular patch plasty in large postinfarction akinetic scar and severe left ventricular dysfunction: comparison with a series of large dyskinetic scars. *J Thorac Cardiovasc Surg* 1998;116:50–59.

47. Dor V. Surgical management of left ventricular aneurysms by the endoventricular patch plasty technique. *Operative Techniques in Cardiac & Thoracic Surgery* 1997;2:139–150.

48. Dor V, Sabatier M, Didonato M. Late hemodynamic results after left ventricular patch repair associated with postinfarction akinetic or dyskinetic aneurysm of the left ventricle. *J Thorac Cardiovasc Surg* 1995;110:1291–1301.

49. Westaby S. Coronary artery surgery in heart failure patients. *Journal of Congestive Heart Failure and Circulatory Support* 2000;1:113–118.

50. Hendren WG, Nemec JJ, Lytle BW, et al. Mitral valve repair for ischemic mitral insufficiency. *Ann Thorac Surg* 1991;52:1246–1252.

51. Chen FY, Adams DH, Aranki SF, et al. Mitral valve repair in cardiomyopathy. *Circulation* 1998;98:II124–II127.

52. Bolling, SF, Deeb MG, Bach DS. Mitral valve reconstruction in elderly, ischemic patients. *Chest* 1996;109:35–40.

53. Cohn LWH, Couper GS, Kinchla NM, et al. Decreased operative risk of surgical treatment of mitral regurgitation with or without coronary artery disease. *J Am Coll Cardiol* 1990;16:1575–1578.

54. Kirklin JW. Replacement of the mitral valve for mitral incompetence. *Surgery* 1972;72:827–836.

55. Cohn LH, Rizzo RJ, Adams DH, et al. The effect of pathophysiology on the surgical treatment of ischemic mitral regurgitation: operative and late risks of repair versus replacement. *Eur J Cardiothorac Surg* 1995;9:568–574.

56. David TE. Techniques and results of mitral valve repair for ischemic mitral regurgitation. *J Cardiol Surg* 1994;9[Suppl]:274–277.

57. Gangemi JJ, Tribble CG, Ross SD, et al. Does the additive risk of mitral valve repair in patients with ischemic cardiomyopathy prohibit surgical intervention? *Ann Surg* 2000;231:710–714.

58. Bolling SF, Deeb GM, Brunsting LA, et al. Early outcome of mitral valve reconstruction in patients with end-stage cardiomyopathy. *J Thorac Cardiovasc Surg* 1995;109:676–683.

59. Bolling SF, Pagani FD, Deeb GM, et al. Intermediate-term outcome of mitral reconstruction in cardiomyopathy. *J Thorac Cardiovasc Surg* 1998;115:381–388.

60. Rose EA, Modskowitz AJ, Sollano PM, et al. REMATCH trial: rationale, design, and end points. Randomized evaluation of mechanical assistance for the treatment of congestive heart failure. *Ann Thorac Surg* 1999;67:723–730.

61. Smedira NG, Blackstone EH. Postcardiotomy ECMO support: risk factors and outcomes. *Ann Thorac Surg* 2001;71:S60–S66.

62. Smedira NG, Moazami N, Golding CM, et al. Clinical experience with 229 adults on ECMO: survival at 5 years. *J Thorac Cardiovasc Surg* 2001;122:92–102.

63. Magovern GJ Jr, Simpson KA. Extracorporeal membrane oxygenation for adult cardiac support: the Allegheny experience. *Ann Thorac Surg* 1999;68:655–661.

64. McBride LR, Naunheim KS, Fiore AC, et al. Clinical experience with 111 Thoratec ventricular assist devices. *Ann Thorac Surg* 1999;67:1233–1239.

65. Guyton RA, Schonberger JPAM, Everts PAM, et al. Postcardiotomy shock clinical evaluation of the BVS 5000 Biventricular System. *Ann Thorac Surg* 1993;56:346–356.

66. Körfer R, El-Banayosy A, Arusoglu L, et al. Temporary pulsatile ventricular assist devices and biventricular assist devices. *Ann Thorac Surg* 1999;68:678–683.

67. DeRose JJ, Umana JP, Argenziano M, et al. Improved results for postcardiotomy cardiogenic shock with the use of implantable left ventricular assist devices. *Ann Thorac Surg* 1997;64:1757–1763.

68. Samuels LE, Kaufman MS, Thomas MP, et al. Pharmacological criteria for ventricular assist device insertion following postcardiotomy shock: experience with the Abiomed BVS system. *J Card Surg* 1999;14:288–293.

69. Portner PM, Jansen PG, Oyer PE, et al. Improved outcomes with an implantable ventricular assist system: a multicenter study. *Ann Thorac Surg* 2001;70:205–209.

70. McCarthy PM, Smedira NG, Vargo RL, et al. One hundred patients with the HeartMate left ventricular assist device: evolving concepts and technology. *J Thorac Cardiovasc Surg* 1998;115:904–912.

71. Hetzer R, Muller JH, Weng YG, et al. Midterm follow-up of patients who underwent removal of a left ventricular assist device after cardiac recovery from end-stage dilated cardiomyopathy. *J Thorac Cardiovasc Surg* 2000;120:843–855.

72. Katsumata T, Westaby S. Implantable axial flow impeller pumps. *J Circ Support* 1998;1:13–19.

73. Saavedra FW, Tunn R, Mishima T, et al. Reverse remodeling and enhanced adrenergic reserve from a passive external ventricular support in experimental dilated heart failure. American Heart Association, November 13, 2000.

74. Slaughter MS, Pappas PS, Tatooles AJ. Modified implant technique for the pneumatic HeartMate left ventricular assist system. *Journal of Congestive Heart Failure and Circulatory Support* 2000;1:123–125.

75. Mueller XM, Tevaearai HT, Tucker O, et al. A new device for less invasive left ventricular volume reduction. STS, New Orleans, January 29–31, 2001:216.

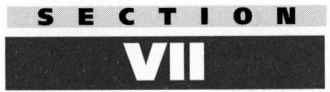

MOLECULAR CARDIOLOGY

JUDITH L. SWAIN

GENERAL TECHNIQUES IN MOLECULAR CARDIOLOGY

MARK E. LIEB
MARK B. TAUBMAN

▼▼ ADDITIONAL ELECTRONIC TOPICS

Smooth Muscle Cell Culture p87;   Coculture Techniques p88;   Other Cell Types p89;   RNA (Northern) Blot Analysis p90;   Promoter Analysis p91;   Constructing and Screening Complementary DNA Libraries p92;   Constructing and Screening Genomic Libraries p93; Functional (Expression) Cloning p94;   Subtraction Techniques p95;   Differential Display of Messenger RNA p96;   Yeast Two-Hybrid System p97

HISTORICAL PERSPECTIVE

A series of critical experiments in the 1950s and early 1960s established what has come to be known as the central dogma of molecular biology. These experiments demonstrated that deoxyribonucleic acid (DNA) is the genetic material responsible for transmitting heritable information, that DNA is "transcribed" into messenger ribonucleic acid (mRNA), and that mRNA is then "translated" into proteins. However, several crucial discoveries were required before detailed analyses of these processes could be routinely made. One of these was the identification of a series of DNA-processing enzymes

M. E. Lieb: Department of Medicine, Mount Sinai School of Medicine of the City University of New York, New York, New York
M. B. Taubman: Department of Medicine, The Cardiovascular Institute, Mount Sinai School of Medicine of the City University of New York, New York, New York

from bacteria and bacteriophages. These enzymes included restriction endonucleases, which cleave DNA at sequence-specific sites; polymerases, which synthesize new DNA from a DNA template; and ligases, which can join two pieces of DNA together. This technology ushered in the era of recombinant DNA, allowing small pieces of DNA to be isolated, sequenced, ligated to other pieces of DNA, radiolabeled, and used as molecular probes.

The discovery of the enzyme reverse transcriptase had a particularly great impact on the field of molecular biology. Reverse transcriptase synthesizes DNA from an RNA template, thus allowing one to make a strand of DNA that is complementary to the mRNA. The ability to synthesize complementary DNA (cDNA) from mRNA isolated from a specific tissue was critical to the development of cDNA libraries, ushering in the era of molecular cloning. Other important technical advances included the development of nucleic acid and protein gel electrophoresis to separate different species by size, systems for "blotting" nucleic acids and proteins on filters so that they can be subjected to a variety of analyses, the development of "hybridization" techniques to identify specific DNA and RNA molecules, and the advent of DNA sequencing. The development of viral and plasmid "vectors" that are designed to introduce DNA into a variety of cells where it can be transcribed into mRNA and then translated into proteins has provided powerful tools for the functional analysis of specific genes as well as the generation of recombinant proteins, a number of which are now routinely used in clinical medicine.

The development of appropriate experimental models was critical to the application of molecular techniques to basic investigation in cardiovascular disease. A critical breakthrough was the establishment of culture systems for studying the individual cellular components of the cardiovascular system. The ability to study each cell type as an essentially "pure" culture provided the initial stimulus for a vast array of studies that examined cell surface receptors, transmembrane signals, gene regulation, and the pathways involved in growth, migration, and control of shape. A variety of "coculture" models have been developed to examine interactions among cell types. The breakthroughs in tissue culture techniques have been paralleled by the development of a variety of animal models of cardiovascular disease. These include models of vessel injury, congestive heart failure, and dyslipidemia, as well as animals with genetic preponderance toward hypertension, atherosclerosis, and other cardiac diseases. These *in vivo* models have been complementary to cell culture and have allowed investigators to verify findings in culture using a more clinically relevant setting. The ability to generate "transgenic" animals—animals whose genetic makeup has been altered using recombinant DNA techniques—has allowed investigators to examine the functions of specific *in vivo* models and to develop small animal models that more closely mimic human pathology.

This chapter is designed as an overview of some of the major molecular and cellular techniques that are used in contemporary cardiovascular research. The revolution in molecular biology over the previous century has provided the tools to examine biologic processes at their most basic level. As is evident throughout this text, the application of molecular techniques to cardiovascular research has led to major advances in our understanding of the pathobiology of cardiovascular disease. Although the techniques described are widely used in many areas of biologic investigation, our focus is on their application to cardiovascular investigation; as such, we hope that it provides a frame of reference for understanding the experiments described in the other chapters of this book. The following sections of this chapter describe the cell culture and *in vivo* models that were developed to allow the application of basic molecular techniques to the study of cardiovascular diseases, the

major methods used in the study of gene expression, the techniques for molecular cloning, and the methods used to alter gene expression.

MODELS USED IN CARDIOVASCULAR RESEARCH

The development of appropriate experimental models was critical to the application of molecular techniques to cardiovascular research. Hundreds of models have been developed over the past few decades to help further our understanding of cardiovascular pathology. This section provides an overview of some of the models that are most commonly used.

Cell Culture

Cardiovascular diseases involve complex interaction among multiple cell types. As is discussed in later sections, state-of-the-art techniques are being increasingly refined to allow gene expression to be monitored in individual cells in their natural milieu. In spite of these advances, the ability to examine pure populations of cells in an environment that can be experimentally controlled has provided a wealth of information about the biologic properties of each cell type and continues to be a powerful approach. The relevance of data obtained from cell culture systems to the intact organism must be established experimentally. Hence, the ability to move rapidly from cell culture, to animal models, to clinical studies, and back is an important feature of contemporary molecular cardiology. The following paragraphs outline some of the procedures that are used to study cells in culture, the problems inherent in such cell culture systems, and more recent approaches to addressing cell-cell interactions.

Endothelial Cell Culture

Studies on vascular endothelium have also extensively availed themselves of cell culture. Unlike smooth muscle cells, endothelial cells are present as a single layer lining the intima. Therefore, smaller amounts of endothelial cells can be obtained from blood vessels. These cells also tend to develop senescence more quickly than smooth muscle and therefore provide a greater challenge in obtaining large numbers of cells. A favorite choice for endothelial cell culture has been the human umbilical vein endothelial cell. This cell can usually be passaged four to five times, and a large number of cells can be obtained from individual placentas (8). The ready availability of placentas has been instrumental in the popularity of these cells. Other sources include arterial endothelial cells from bovine, rat, and human sources. Unlike smooth muscle cells, endothelial cells grow poorly on plastic or glass and are usually grown on a matrix of gelatin, collagen, or fibronectin.

Two particularly important properties of cultured endothelial cells have received considerable attention. The first is the ability of endothelial cells to respond directly to shear or turbulence (9). This has led to the development of a variety of cell culture systems to study endothelial cell biology under various flow conditions. The second property is the ability of microvascular endothelial cells to form capillaries under appropriate cell culture conditions (10). This has allowed investigators to use cell culture to model capillary formation, such as that seen in tumor angiogenesis and in angiogenesis associated with ischemia.

Cardiac Myocyte Culture

Cardiac myocytes that are isolated by explant or enzymatic digestion of fetal and adult hearts maintain their contractile phenotype in culture on plastic and have been particularly useful for electrophysiologic as well as molecular biologic studies (reviewed in reference 11). Because they are at or near terminal differentiation, cardiac myocytes that are isolated from late stages of development do not divide in culture and, therefore, can only be used as primary cultures. Isolation of relatively pure populations of myocytes requires dissection to isolate the chamber of interest, mechanical and enzymatic disruption, and serial plating or density centrifugation to remove fibroblasts (which grow rapidly in culture and would quickly outnumber the myocytes). The passage of cardiac myocytes in serial culture has thus far been limited to transformed or cardiac tumor–derived cells that show varying degrees of differentiation in culture. The ability to expand large quantities of fetal cardiac myocytes in culture to repopulate damaged myocardium *in vivo* remains a major goal.

In Vivo Models

Despite the invaluable contribution of cell culture, the utility of molecular cardiology to improve the treatment of human disease is dependent on the development of animal models that accurately mimic these diseases. Although naturally occurring animal models of cardiovascular disease have been exploited, many of the common human diseases are rarely seen in animals. In recent years, the increasing application of transgenic technology to cardiovascular research has allowed the development of more sophisticated mouse models of cardiovascular pathology. Although the small size of the mouse presents challenges, a variety of diagnostic techniques have been adapted for its use, including echocardiography (14), micromanometry (15), and *in vivo* magnetic resonance imaging (16).

Atherosclerosis

One model that is commonly used to study atherosclerosis and arterial injury involves the use of balloon catheters to denude the endothelium and to injure the media (17). The

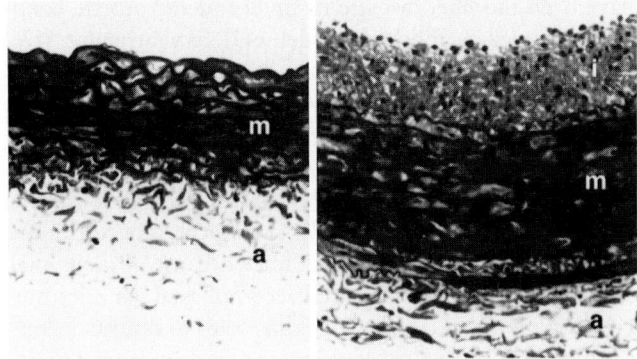

FIGURE 96.1 Intimal hyperplasia following balloon injury of the rat aorta. Cross section of a normal rat aorta **(left)** stained with hematoxylin and eosin and a rat aorta 2 weeks after balloon catheter injury **(right)** showing the development of a thickened intima (i). a, adventitia; m, media.

approach to catheterization is similar to that used in human angioplasties, involving cannulation of a distal artery and passage of a balloon-tipped catheter into the area to be injured. Injuries can range from gentle endothelial denudation to injuries that tear the internal elastic lamina and damage the media. Alternative approaches include external injury to the artery, for example, using a forceps to crush the artery (18,19), or internal injury using air (20) or electrical stimulation (21). Such models have been used in rats, rabbits, transgenic mice, dogs, pigs, and nonhuman primates. The hallmark of this model is the development of intimal hyperplasia, characterized by the migration and proliferation of smooth muscle cells in the intima. An example is shown in Figure 96.1. ▼ p98

In addition to acute arterial injury, a variety of *in vivo* systems have been used to model the more chronic development of atherosclerosis, such as that seen in human disease. These have included the use of high-fat/high-cholesterol diets in rabbits (reviewed in reference 23), pigeons (24), pigs (25), and nonhuman primates (26–28). Although these diets are often associated with the types of lesions that are seen in early atherosclerosis, they are not as severe as those seen in human disease (29). A variety of genetically engineered hyperlipidemic transgenic mice that more closely resemble the complex lesions of human atherosclerosis have been developed (30). The study of genetically altered mice has led to dramatic advances in the study of lipoprotein metabolism and atherosclerosis. (See reference 31 for an in-depth review.) In spite of these advances, challenges still remain. A critical feature of human unstable coronary syndromes is the rupture of atherosclerotic plaques, and the lack of plaque rupture is a shortcoming of the dyslipidemic animal models.

Congestive Heart Failure

A variety of large animal models that were developed to study the hemodynamic aspects of congestive heart failure have been modified for use in small rodents. Aortic banding is a well-established model of left ventricular (LV) hypertrophy due to pressure overload. The progression of LV hypertrophy to progressive LV dysfunction and overt heart failure has been documented in guinea pigs and rats. Similar effects have been observed following renal artery ligation (32) and after the administration of a high-salt diet to Dahl salt-sensitive rats (33). Surgical procedures are more technically challenging in mice because of their small size, but aortic banding can be accomplished via microsurgical techniques (34). Aortic banding leads to cardiac decompensation in mice that express specific transgenes (35,36) and in mice treated with cyclosporin (37). Coronary artery ligation as a model of myocardial infarction with subsequent LV failure has a long history in cardiovascular research and has been adapted to the mouse (38). Murine models of viral myocarditis with cardiac failure have been extensively studied (well reviewed in reference 39). A hereditary form of dilated cardiomyopathy occurs in a strain of Syrian hamsters (40); the underlying genetic defect has been identified (41,42). Although naturally occurring inherited cardiomyopathy models are lacking in the mouse, an array of transgenic models has been generated (see reference 43 for review). In addition to the models of dilated cardiomyopathy, an important model of hypertrophic cardiomyopathy has been developed by introduction of a missense mutation analogous to a mutation that causes familial hypertrophic cardiomyopathy into the murine alpha-cardiac myosin heavy-chain gene (44).

ANALYSIS OF GENE EXPRESSION

The central dogma in molecular biology is that the genetic information stored in DNA is transcribed to RNA and then translated to proteins. In strictest terms, *gene expression* refers to the process by which a gene is "turned on" to produce mRNA. However, it often is used to describe the entire process by which activation of a gene leads to an increase in its protein. This section describes approaches that are used to examine mRNA and protein.

Ribonuclease Protection Assays

Ribonuclease (RNAse) protection assay uses a sequence-specific labeled cRNA molecule as a probe to hybridize with RNA in solution (50,51). Base pairing between the labeled probe and the mRNA of interest results in double-stranded cRNA-RNA hybrids that are resistant to digestion by RNAse. Following hybridization, samples are digested with RNAse to destroy the unhybridized, single-stranded probe and mRNA. The products of digestion are then run on a polyacrylamide gel. The gel is dried, and the "protected" bands are detected by autoradiography (Fig. 96.2). One advantage of this technique is the extremely high degree of

base pairing that is needed to prevent RNAse from digesting the cRNA-RNA hybrids. Even two consecutive base pair mismatches are sufficient to allow the RNAse to digest the hybrid at the point of the mismatch. This technique thus allows for the identification of mRNA that is virtually 100% complementary to the cRNA probe. The area that corresponds to the alternative spliced exon is degraded by the RNAse. RNAse protection assays are usually more sensitive than RNA blot analysis and can therefore be used to detect lower levels of mRNA. Kits are commercially available to generate specific probes for the detection of multiple mRNAs in a single sample at one time.

Unlike RNA blot hybridization, RNAse protection assays do not usually identify highly related isoforms unless they are generated by the process of alternative splicing, in which identical exons, representing regions of 100% iden-

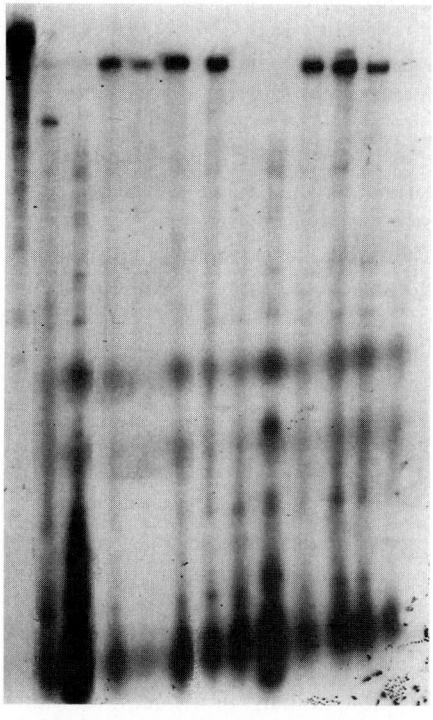

FIGURE 96.2 Ribonuclease (RNAse) protection. To examine the expression of the rat gene SM-20, an antisense P-32–labeled RNA probe was synthesized by *in vitro* transcription using a plasmid containing the rat SM-20 complementary DNA and the recognition site for T3 polymerase. The 420–base pair (bp) probe contained a 40-bp sequence from the plasmid vector and a 384-bp sequence complementary to SM-20 messenger RNA (mRNA). Total RNA, 10 µg per lane, from a variety of tissues was hybridized with the rat probe, incubated with RNAse, and then analyzed by polyacrylamide gel electrophoresis. Lane 1 of the autoradiogram shows the undigested probe. When the probe was hybridized to RNA from mouse heart (lane 2), part of the probe was protected from RNAse digestion, implying that there is partial sequence identity between the rat and mouse SM-20 mRNA. Rat tissues that express the SM-20 mRNA (lanes 4–7, 10–12) showed full protection of the complementary region of the probe. Yeast transfer RNA (lane 13) and RNA from tissues that do not express SM-20 (lanes 3, 8, 9) failed to protect the probe.

tity, are spliced to different exons. This results in partial protection of the cRNA probe, corresponding to the area that contains the shared exon.

Polymerase Chain Reaction

The most sensitive approach for identifying and amplifying specific DNA or mRNA sequences is polymerase chain reaction (PCR) (Fig. 96.3). Standard PCR involves the synthesis of a set of primers (sense and antisense) that correspond to the 5' and 3' ends of the segment of DNA to be amplified. DNA (genomic DNA, or plasmid DNA) is used as a template. To amplify sequences from mRNA, a cDNA copy of the mRNA is generated by reverse transcription and used as a template in the PCR reaction. To begin the PCR, template DNA is incubated in solution with the primers, all four deoxyribonucleotides, and a temperature-stable DNA polymerase. Three reactions are performed in a thermocycler that allows for very rapid changes of temperature. The initial step is the denaturation of the double-stranded DNA template by heating to approximately 95°C. The next step is annealing (performed between 37°C and 65°C) of the primers to the denatured template. This is followed by synthesis of complementary DNA strands by the heat-stable DNA polymerase (performed at ~72°C). At the beginning of the next cycle, the newly synthesized DNA is denatured (at ~95°C) to produce new single-stranded templates. This cycle is repeated 20 to 40 times to achieve greater than 1 million–fold amplification of the sequence of interest. The products are then resolved on agarose or poly-acrylamide gels. PCR can be used to identify and amplify a single molecule of viral DNA from a single cell. It can also be used to identify DNA that contains a specific mutation.

The sensitivity of reverse-transcription (RT)–PCR enables one to amplify from just a few molecules of mRNA. RT-PCR can therefore be used to examine mRNA from a single cell or from small tissue samples, such as those obtained from cardiac biopsies or coronary arthectomies. One disadvantage of RT-PCR is that it is difficult to use for quantitation. During the early cycles, there is exponential amplification and a direct relationship between the amount of original DNA template and the amount of product. As the number of cycles increases, the reagents in the reaction tube cannot sustain the continued exponential amplification. The rate of accumulation of PCR product falls off in an unpredictable way. Once this occurs, the final yield of product may have little relationship to the original amount of starting material. A variety of procedures involving the use of internal standards and varying cycle lengths have been used to allow "semiquantitation" of RT-PCR, but these techniques can be cumbersome. Real-time quantitative PCR is designed to circumvent these problems (reviewed in references 52 and 53). In this technique, the reaction is carried out in a thermocycler equipped with fluorescence detection and specialized software. The incorporation of dyes that are specific for double-

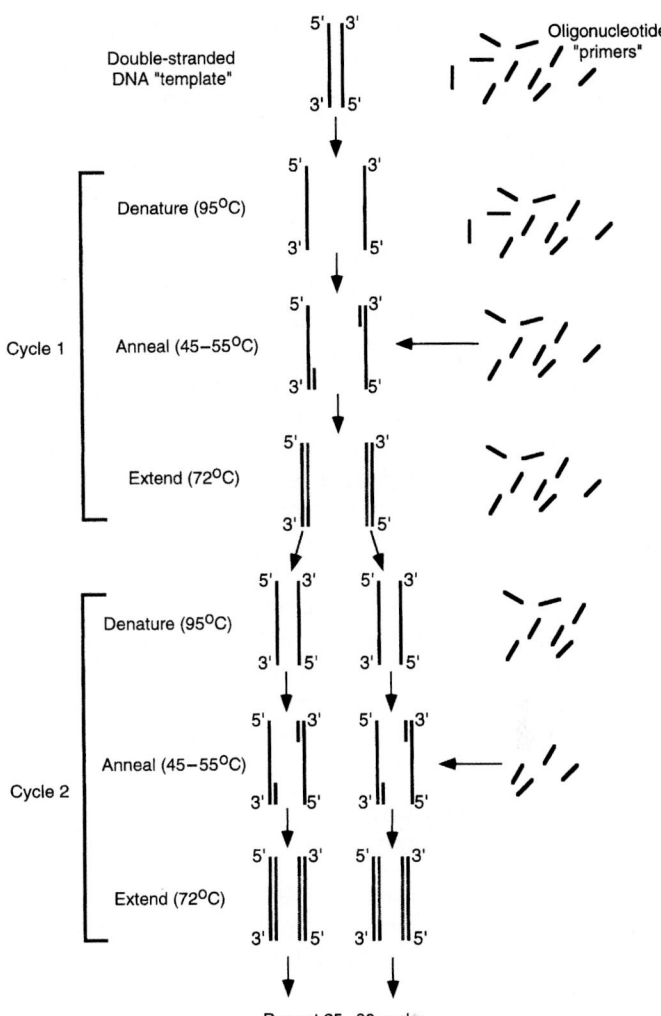

FIGURE 96.3 Polymerase chain reaction for amplification of DNA. The schematic shows two complete cycles of polymerase chain reaction. The procedure is repeated for a total of 25 to 30 cycles.

stranded DNA or the release of fluorescence from specially designed primers is continuously monitored. The numbers of cycles that are required to permit fluorescence detection are then correlated to the quantity of starting material.

In Situ Hybridization

The above techniques involve the identification and measurement of mRNA from samples extracted from cells or tissues. *In situ* hybridization provides a method for identifying mRNA in intact cells or tissue samples (54). The general strategy is similar to that used for RNAse protection assays and involves the generation of single-stranded, labeled cRNA probes. Rather than being hybridized in solution, the probes are incubated with cells or tissue sections fixed on slides or cover slips. After hybridization, the slides are washed at high stringency. In the case of radiolabeled probes, the slides are covered with photographic emulsion for several weeks and then developed. For digoxigenin-labeled probes, the slides are analyzed using antibodies to digoxigenin and colorimetric detection. They are then examined by light- or dark-field microscopy. After detection of radiolabeled probes, mRNA appears as grains associated with cell bodies. After detection with digoxigenin-labeled probes, it appears as colored staining. With either labeling technique, slides can be counterstained such that the normal cellular architecture can be determined. This procedure thus allows one to identify specific cells that express mRNA. In the early stages of murine development, embryos are small enough to allow penetration of cRNA probes without sectioning. This allows intact embryos to be examined by light microscopy to determine the expression of developmentally regulated genes. Although *in situ* hybridization is excellent for localizing sites of mRNA expression, it is not ideal for quantitation. Nevertheless, semiquantitative approaches have been used based on the number of grains seen. The availability of increasingly sophisticated imaging systems should allow for more reliable quantitation. An example of the use of *in situ* hybridization to examine gene expression in an animal model of balloon arterial injury is shown in *e*Figure 96.3.1.

New Directions: Laser Capture Microdissection

As discussed in the section Models Used in Cardiovascular Research, cardiovascular diseases involve complex interaction among multiple types of cells, and the ability to culture pure preparations of these cells has been critical to work in molecular cardiology. Still, each of the cell culture models has inherent limitations. It would be ideal to be able to study the individual cell types within pathologic lesions. *In situ* hybridization and immunostaining allow gene expression to be examined in tissue sections but are of limited sensitivity and do not permit comprehensive analysis of gene expression.

Laser capture microdissection (LCM) is a technique developed at the National Cancer Institute that allows pure cell populations to be microscopically dissected from tissue sections so that their DNA, RNA, and proteins can be analyzed (55). Briefly, a glass slide with a routine tissue section is overlain with a transparent thermal polymer film and placed on a microscope. Once the investigator visualizes the cells of interest, a brief burst of infrared laser light is directed at the area, causing the cells to adhere to the thermoplastic film. The cells can then be recovered from the film and subjected to molecular analysis, including RT-PCR followed by gene-array screening (56). The National Cancer Institute maintains a website devoted to LCM (http://dir.nichd.nih.gov/lcm/lcm.htm) to distribute information regarding the rapidly evolving uses of LCM. Figure 96.4 shows an application of LCM to isolate macrophages from an atherosclerotic plaque.

Analysis of Transcription

The above techniques measure steady-state levels of mRNA and can be used to assess the accumulation of mRNA in response to a particular stimulus, for example, arterial balloon injury or treatment with agonists. Steady-state mRNA levels represent a balance between transcription of new mRNA and changes in the stability of the transcribed message. It should be noted that the term *induction* has been most typically used to describe mRNA transcription. However, it is sometimes used to describe any increase in mRNA levels, whether it be due to changes in transcription, mRNA stability, or a combination of both. Several approaches have been used to examine specifically the transcriptional component.

Nuclear Run-On (or Run-Off) Analysis

Nuclear run-on (or run-off) analysis (57) has been the gold standard for examining mRNA transcription. This tech-

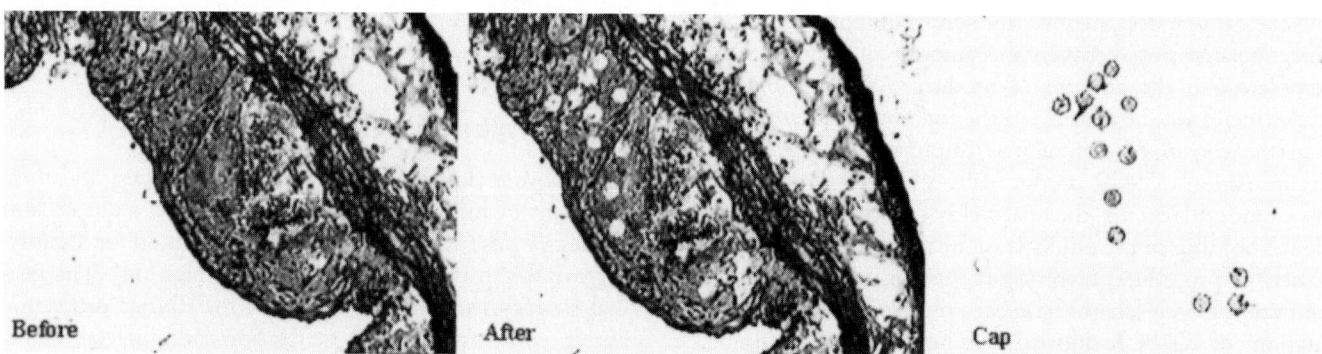

FIGURE 96.4 Laser capture microdissection (LCM) of atherosclerotic plaque. Sections of atherosclerotic plaque were immunostained to detect macrophage-derived foam cells and then covered with a thermoplastic film. Short bursts of infrared laser light were used to attach 15-μm circular fragments of macrophage-rich tissue to the film. Tissue section is shown before LCM **(left)** and after LCM **(middle)**. Thermoplastic film with adherent 15-μm specimens **(right)**. (Photo courtesy of Eugene Trogan, Hayes M. Dansky, and Edward A. Fisher, Mount Sinai School of Medicine.)

nique is based on the principle that isolated nuclei contain RNA that is in the process of being transcribed. One can complete this process (elongation) in a test tube by adding ribonucleotides. In contrast, transcription cannot be initiated in a test tube under the same conditions. By including a radiolabeled ribonucleotide in the reaction, one can measure the level of transcription that occurs at the moment that the nuclei were collected. ᷱ p99

Protein Identification

A variety of approaches are used to identify proteins. In some cases, functional assays can be used, particularly in the case of specific enzymes. More often, antibodies are used to identify specific proteins.

Immunoprecipitation

For immunoprecipitation, extracts that contain the desired protein are incubated with a specific antibody. An antibody-binding reagent, complexed to beads, is then used to precipitate the complex by centrifugation. Two approaches can be used for quantitation. In the first, the protein is labeled *in vivo* using radiolabeled amino acids. Most commonly, sulfate-35 (S-35)–methionine is used. The labeled material can then be counted using liquid scintillography. To provide maximum specificity, the precipitated complex can be run on a sodium dodecyl sulfate polyacrylamide gel that separates proteins by size in a fashion similar to that described for mRNA. The gel is then subjected to autoradiography. After this, the protein of interest can be verified by its position relative to known-sized markers and the amount of protein assayed either by densitometric analysis of the autoradiogram, by cutting out the band and measuring radioactivity in a scintillation counter, or by the use of a phosphoimager. An example of autoradiography is shown in Figure 96.5.

Western Blot Analysis

An alternative to immunoprecipitation is Western blot analysis (Fig. 96.6). In this technique, the protein extract is first run on a polyacrylamide gel. The proteins in the gel are then transferred to a membrane, and the membrane is incubated with an antibody that is specific for the protein in question. A variety of approaches can then be used to identify the antibody, most often involving the use of a secondary antibody, followed by enzymatic detection (see the section Enzyme-Linked Immunosorbent Assay). Western blot analysis has the same advantage as running immunoprecipitates on gels: It allows for confirmation of the desired protein by comparison with either size markers or by using purified protein as a control. In addition, it does not require prior labeling of the protein. Thus, Western blot analysis can be used to identify proteins in animal

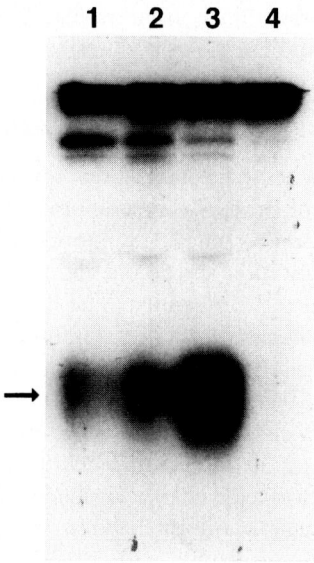

FIGURE 96.5 Immunoprecipitation. VSMC proteins were labeled *in vivo* by incubating cultured cells for 4 hours with sulfate-35–methionine. Protein lysates were isolated from cells that did not receive further treatment (lane 1) and cells labeled in the presence of 1 µM angiotensin II (lane 2) or 20 ng per mL platelet-derived growth factor (PDGF; lanes 3 and 4). Samples were precipitated with anti-JE antiserum (lanes 1–3) and preimmune serum (lane 4) and then analyzed by polyacrylamide gel electrophoresis followed by autoradiography. JE protein (*arrow*) was precipitated by the immune serum and showed elevated levels in cells exposed to angiotensin II or PDGF. [From Taubman M, Rollins B, Poon M, et al. JE mRNA accumulates rapidly after aortic injury and in platelet derived growth factor–stimulated vascular smooth muscle cells. *Circ Res* 1992;70(2),314–325, with permission.]

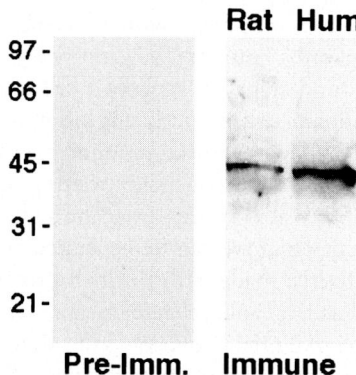

FIGURE 96.6 Western blot analysis. Protein lysates (25 µg per lane) of rat and human cultured vascular smooth muscle cells were loaded onto a 12% polyacrylamide gel. After electrophoresis and transfer to nitrocellulose, the blots were incubated with preimmune rabbit serum (Pre-Imm.) and antiserum against the rat protein SM-20. The blots were washed and then incubated with horseradish peroxidase–conjugated donkey antirabbit antibody. Detection of bound antibody was accomplished by exposing the blots to photographic film immediately after incubation with a chemiluminescent substrate for horseradish peroxidase. (From Wax SD, Tsao L, Lieb ME, et al. SM-20 is a novel 40-kd protein whose expression in the arterial wall is restricted to smooth muscle. *Lab Invest* 1996;74:797–808, with permission.)

models of arterial injury, from cardiac biopsies, or from atherectomy samples.

Enzyme-Linked Immunosorbent Assay

Several approaches have been used for rapid large-scale quantification of protein. These approaches have been of particular import in clinical laboratories, where large-scale and rapid quantitation is required and very small amounts of protein need to be measured. The most common techniques involve enzyme-linked immunosorbent assay (ELISA). In one approach, samples coat the bottom of 96-well immunosorbent plates. Nonspecific binding is blocked by incubating wells with normal horse serum and albumin. Wells are then rinsed and incubated with specific antibody. The wells are washed and the antibody detected using a variety of enzyme-based procedures. A commonly used method involves incubating with a biotinylated secondary antibody (e.g., horse antimouse or antirabbit immunoglobulin G) followed by avidin-conjugated horseradish peroxidase and then a developing solution that contains the chromogenic substrate *O*-phenylenediamine dihydrochloride. Protein concentrations are determined by comparison of light absorption of the samples to a standard curve that is generated using purified protein. A variety of kits are commercially available, as are automated ELISA readers.

Radioimmunoassay

Radioimmunoassay requires the availability of purified protein and a specific antibody. The purified protein is radiolabeled, usually with iodine-125, and the radiolabeled protein is immunoprecipitated with a specific antibody and counted in a gamma counter. To quantify levels of the target protein from a solution, such as a cell extract, culture medium, or human serum, increasing amounts of the solution are incubated with a fixed amount of iodinated protein. If the solution contains significant amounts of the target protein, it will compete away the radiolabeled protein. A competition curve can be generated and compared to a standard curve made with purified protein. This is a particularly sensitive and reliable means for quantifying protein. Its one potential drawback is the ability of a closely related but not identical protein to compete effectively with the target protein.

Immunohistochemistry

Immunohistochemistry uses antibodies in a fashion analogous to that described for *in situ* hybridization. Specific antibodies can be used to identify proteins in cell culture or in tissue sections. These techniques have been particularly useful for localizing proteins in tissue sections from experimental animal models or human specimens. Like *in situ* hybridization, they are less useful for quantitation. Immu-

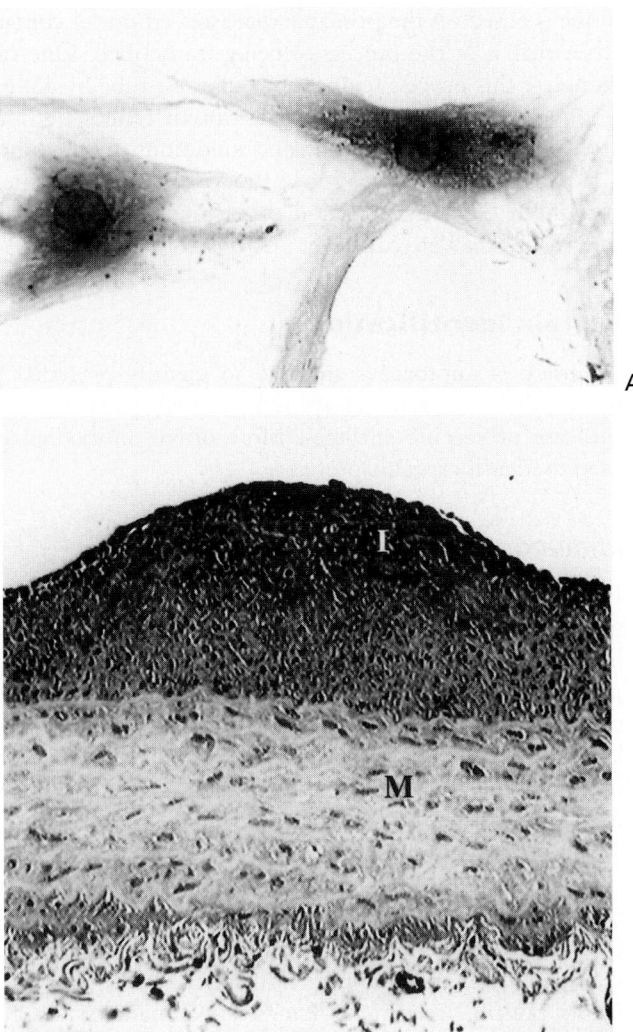

FIGURE 96.7 Immunohistochemistry. **A:** Immunohistochemical detection of tissue factor in cultured vascular smooth muscle cells. **B:** Immunohistochemical detection of the protein SM-20 in a section of an injured rat artery. Strongest immunostaining is seen in the intima (I) but is also seen in the media (M).

nohistochemistry can be used with light microscopy, confocal microscopy, or electron microscopy, the latter allowing for precise cellular localization of proteins. Double- and triple-labeling techniques are available to colocalize proteins. In addition, immunohistochemistry can be performed together with *in situ* hybridization. Examples of immunohistochemistry of cultured cells and tissue are shown in Figure 96.7.

MOLECULAR CLONING

In molecular cloning, genetic information from a species or cell type of interest is expanded in bacteria (or other simple hosts) to allow the isolation of DNA containing a single sequence of interest. Foreign DNA is introduced into bacteria most commonly in the form of plasmids (small pieces of circular DNA that replicate within bacteria) or bacteriophage (viruses that infect bacteria). The plasmids or phage that are used have been extensively engineered to facilitate the process of molecular cloning and are referred to as *cloning vectors*.

To begin the process of cloning, known quantities of DNA and of the cloning vector are digested with a restriction endonuclease and joined together by the enzyme DNA ligase. The result is a collection of millions of copies of the vector, each containing a single DNA fragment, referred to as the *insert*. This collection is called a *DNA library*; a high-quality library is one in which all of the DNA sequences that are present in the starting material are represented in the final pool of ligated vector.

If the starting material for the library is genomic DNA, the library is referred to as a *genomic library*. Because each somatic cell in an organism contains a complete copy of the genome, the tissue chosen for generating a genomic library is based on convenience. Genomic libraries contain exons and introns and thus may not provide direct information about the sequence of the mRNA or the protein. They are particularly valuable for isolating the promoter and associated regulatory sequences involved in gene transcription. Most of the information that has been obtained on the regulation of gene transcription has required cloning the regulatory regions from genomic libraries. Fragments that are isolated from genomic libraries are also necessary for generating transgenic animals.

Often, the sequence of interest is the mRNA that encodes a particular protein. In this case, the library is designed to represent the unique set of mRNA species that are expressed in a specific tissue or cell type at the moment of isolation. To allow mRNA sequences to be cloned using the same powerful techniques as genomic DNA, a DNA copy is made of the single-stranded mRNA using the enzymes reverse transcriptase and DNA polymerase. The resulting library is known as a *cDNA library*. The cDNA represents a faithful copy of the mRNA and therefore can be used to determine the sequence of the mRNA and to deduce the sequence of the protein encoded by the mRNA. A high-quality cDNA library contains copies of all of the mRNA transcripts that are present in the starting material; a high proportion of the copies will be full length, and the number of cDNA copies of a particular transcript will be directly proportional to the mRNA transcript's abundance.

Screening Libraries

Once an appropriate library has been constructed, the actual cloning process takes place. In its simplest form this involves "screening the library" with a radioactive probe that has a sequence similar to that of the clone of interest. Briefly, the phage or plasmid library is introduced into

bacteria and spread out on agar plates so that the individual clones are physically separated from each other. The bacteria are allowed to grow overnight, greatly amplifying the amount of plasmid or phage DNA that is present in each colony on the plates. The next day, sheets of nitrocellulose filter are briefly layered on top of the plates so that some of the DNA from each colony adheres to the nitrocellulose. The DNA that sticks to the filters is then denatured and "hybridized" by incubation with a solution that contains the radioactive probe. The nitrocellulose filters are washed and then subjected to autoradiography. Hybridizing clones are identified as spots on the autoradiogram and then recovered from the original agar plates by lining up the filters with the plates. The recovered clone is then amplified and spread onto agar plates, and the process is repeated until the clone is purified to homogeneity. The probe can be labeled to allow nonradioactive detection. Alternatively, the probe may be an antibody. In this case, the library can be introduced into bacteria that can express the protein sequences encoded by the cDNA. In cases in which no DNA or antibody probe exists, the cloning process is adapted to screen the library using a functional assay.

Use of DNA Libraries for Comparing Expression of Multiple Genes

The above strategies all involve screening libraries for "known" genes or genes that encode known proteins or specific functions. A number of strategies have been designed to find novel genes or to identify sets of genes that have been induced by specific circumstances, for example, genes activated by treatment with platelet-derived growth factor or genes induced during muscle differentiation. Technical innovations have made these types of comparisons increasingly robust.

The earliest approach to large-scale comparisons of gene expression was differential screening of cDNA libraries (*eFig. 96.7.1*). This was an extension of the standard methods described previously for screening libraries by hybridization. A cDNA library was generated from mRNA that was isolated from the cells or tissues of interest. After the library was plated, duplicate nitrocellulose lifts were made from the same bacterial lawn. The duplicate filters were then hybridized to labeled cDNA or cRNA probes made from RNA that was isolated under different conditions and subjected to autoradiography. If the duplicate membranes were nearly identical, a transcript present at high levels in one probe and at low levels in the other probe would be expected to show a corresponding difference of intensity after annealing to its corresponding clone on the two membranes. This somewhat crude technique has largely been supplanted by the use of arrayed libraries (discussed in the section Recent Advances in Molecular Cloning). Additional techniques for differential cloning including subtraction techniques and differential display of mRNA are discussed in the CD-ROM and the online version of this text.

Recent Advances in Molecular Cloning

Automation and new resources associated with the large-scale genome sequencing efforts have dramatically changed the common approach to molecular cloning. A limitation to the library screening approach is that each time the library is spread out onto agar plates, the identity of the millions of randomly dispersed clones is unknown. The only clones that are identified are those that are being specifically probed. In addition, the nitrocellulose filters can only be screened several times before new plates must be generated, creating a new array of millions of isolated colonies. Automation can improve this situation by arraying the library in a known configuration. Individual clones are picked off the plates and transferred to numbered wells on multiwell microtiter plates. The library is now "arrayed" and can be duplicated as many times as needed in this configuration. One way of screening an arrayed library is by having a robot "spot" an aliquot of each clone in an identifiable location on a membrane and then hybridizing the membrane with a labeled probe. Alternatively, the spots can be placed in a microscopic array for hybridization and detection using one of the microarray ("gene chip") technologies. In either case, the location of the hybridizing signal tells the investigator which well of the microtiter plate contains the clone of interest. Taking this one step further, the array can be constructed entirely of sequenced clones so that after identifying the location on the membrane by hybridization, the investigator can immediately have access to information about the clone's identity. When screening commercially available membranes (or microarrays), it is unnecessary for an investigator to actually possess the library—the individual clones of interest can be obtained from the vendor after their location is identified by screening.

In theory, hybridizing a gene array with a probe derived from the mRNA of a specific tissue identifies all of the arrayed genes that are actively expressed in the tissue. Thus, hybridizing duplicate arrays with probes derived from normal and diseased tissues can identify genes that are regulated in pathologic conditions. For example, a DNA array containing 6,000 genes was used to identify genes activated in a transgenic mouse model of lethal cardiomyopathy (67). Hybridization of identical arrays with probes derived from different tissues is essentially a modern version of the differential cloning strategy discussed previously except that now the identity of the clones has been established beforehand and there is no limit on the number of conditions that can be compared (other than the expense associated with acquiring the arrays).

Two types of resources generated through the publicly funded genome projects are particularly useful and, in many cases, can make the traditional techniques for molecular cloning unnecessary. The first applies to genomic cloning and the second to cDNA cloning. Each of the genome projects generates a library of overlapping, large genomic clones that are used in the sequencing process. In the early stages of a genome project, arrayed membranes produced from these libraries are usually available commercially. As the project progresses, vast amounts of sequence information from the individual clones is deposited in the public databases and is freely accessible via the Internet. By the time the genome project is completed, genomic library screening can be effectively accomplished "*in silico*" by searching the databases for the sequence of interest. If the actual genomic material is needed (e.g., for a promoter analysis or making a transgenic animal), a phone call or e-mail can replace the actual cloning process. The second resources are the expressed sequence tag libraries. These are cDNA libraries from a wide variety of tissues that are being systematically arrayed. Each clone is partially sequenced, and the sequence is deposited in the public databases. After an expressed sequence tag of interest is identified through a search of the public database, the actual clones can be obtained from a number of vendors. Certainly, these resources are evolving too rapidly for any printed source of information to be current. The National Center for Biotechnology Information maintains the public sequence databases in the United States, and its website is an excellent source of further information (http://www.ncbi.nlm.nih.gov).

MOLECULAR METHODS FOR ALTERING GENE EXPRESSION

A major approach for studying protein function is to either overexpress a protein that is normally not present at high levels in a particular cell type or to decrease the expression of the protein. Many of the techniques are similar to those described previously, and studies that use these techniques are described in detail in subsequent chapters.

Overexpression in Cell Culture

The basic strategies are similar to those described in expression cloning. Plasmid vectors are constructed containing promoters that are active in mammalian cells. The cDNA that encodes the protein to be overexpressed is then ligated into the vector, and the vector is transfected into the cells. Two types of promoters are used. Constitutive promoters, such as the cytomegalovirus promoter, are always active and thus continually generate large amounts of the target protein. Inducible promoters, such as the metallothionein or mouse mammary tumor virus promoter, are relatively inactive until the cells are treated with specific inducers, such as divalent cations or glucocorticoids, respectively. The plasmids are introduced into the cells using a variety of techniques, including transfection with calcium phosphate, DEAE-dextran, cationic liposomes, or electroporation. A second approach is to use viral vectors, such as retroviruses or adenoviruses. These "infections" have higher efficiencies of DNA transfer into cells than transfections. Expression can either be transient or stable. In the latter, transfections or infections are performed with vectors that contain a selectable marker, such as neomycin or hygromycin resistance, and stable clones are isolated in the presence of high levels of the appropriate antibiotic. Stable overexpressing lines can be used to generate high levels of recombinant proteins for a variety of studies.

Overexpression in Animals

Two general approaches have been used to overexpress proteins in animals. The first mimics cell culture and requires the introduction of expression vectors into animals. Like cell culture, these studies can use transfections with liposomes or, more typically, viral vectors. A particular target for such work has been the arterial wall, where DNA can be introduced locally using catheters. Plasmids have also been injected directly into cardiac muscle, to overexpress proteins and to perform *in vivo* promoter analyses.

The second approach to overexpression uses transgenic animals. In this technique, a gene that encodes a desired protein is injected into embryos at the earliest stages of development. Animals that incorporate the gene into their germline transmit it to their offspring. The gene's product is expressed by the "transgenic" animal during development and at maturation. For such studies, the choice of promoters is critical. Nonspecific promoters drive the expression of the gene in virtually all types of cells and tissues. However, many tissue-specific promoters exist that target expression to a particular organ. For example, the cardiac myosin heavy-chain promoter directs expression largely to the heart. In this way, one can overexpress a particular protein in heart muscle.

Underexpression in Cell Culture

The inhibition of specific protein expression is more problematic than overexpression, although many of the techniques are analogous. One approach is to transfect or infect cells with plasmids that contain cDNA in the antisense orientation. On transcription, antisense mRNA is produced that specifically binds to the normal ("sense") mRNA. The double-stranded RNA either remains as a stable complex, unable to be translated into protein, or is rapidly degraded. An example of this approach was the generation of smooth muscle cell lines with abnormal adhesion properties because of decreased expression of the matrix protein, osteopontin (68). The technique depends on generating levels of antisense mRNA that are significantly in excess of the normal sense mRNA. It often results in decreased levels of specific protein synthesis but does not completely inhibit synthesis of the target protein. Such studies usually require stable transfections to analyze the results of protein inhibition adequately and to provide an environment in which all of the cells display lower levels of the target protein.

The use of antisense oligonucleotides has provided an important alternative to transfection of antisense cDNAs. These small fragments can bind to the target mRNA, destabilizing the mRNA or preventing it from binding to the ribosome and being translated. Antisense oligonucleotides may also affect transcription by binding to nuclear DNA. The advantage of this approach is that oligonucleotides can be easily synthesized and are taken up by cells in culture with much higher efficiency than large plasmids. Therefore, they can be used in transient transfection studies. Oligonucleotides can also be used in animal models and have been used extensively in attempts to inhibit gene expression in the arterial wall, where they can be delivered by catheters or by absorption from the adventitial surface. One concern about the use of antisense oligonucleotides is nonspecific effects that are unrelated to their binding to mRNA and the potential for more than one species of mRNA to be inhibited. Nevertheless, the use of antisense oligonucleotides, particularly in cell culture, has provided many insights into the importance of specific proteins in a variety of cell processes.

Alternatives to antisense oligonucleotides are ribozymes, RNA molecules with enzymatic activity (see reference 69 for review). Like protein enzymes, ribozymes cleave RNA at specific sites. However, because of the ability of RNA to form complementary base pairs with other RNA, ribozymes can be synthesized to cleave a particular mRNA species. Ideally, this cleavage is catalytic, thereby allowing a small number of ribozyme molecules to cleave, and thus inactivate, a large number of mRNA molecules. In most cases, ribozymes are believed to act catalytically as well as like antisense oligonucleotides. Ribozymes are usually synthesized in the form of their corresponding cDNAs and introduced into cells via plasmids. Their uptake into cells thus follows the same rules as those of transfection or infection of vectors that contain sense or antisense cDNAs. Like other antisense strategies, ribozymes can often decrease levels of protein synthesis but do not fully "knock out" gene expression.

Underexpression in Animals

As noted previously, antisense oligonucleotides have been used to reduce gene expression in animal models. However, the most effective way to inhibit gene expression is to generate transgenic animals in which the gene of interest has been knocked out (reviewed in reference 70). In this approach, the gene is first isolated from a genomic library. It is then altered to produce a nonfunctioning gene, usually through the introduction of a premature stop codon, resulting in a truncated nonfunctioning protein. The gene, coupled to a selectable marker, is then introduced into embryonic stem (ES) cells; by the process of "homologous recombination," a small number of stem cells replace their native gene with the genetically altered one. This process of recombination is not significantly different from that which occurs in nature during meiosis, leading to genetic variation and sometimes serious abnormalities. By growing cells in the selection medium, the appropriate ES cells can be isolated. These are then used to generate mosaic animals whose germ cells contain one chromosome that lacks a functioning gene. After mating, these animals transmit the targeted allele to their offspring, who then are heterozygous for the targeted allele. By crossing these heterozygotes, one can generate mice that are homozygous for the nonfunctioning gene. The generation of knockout mice has produced a revolution in molecular biology, in that it has created hundreds of different animals that lack a specific gene product. Unlike all of the previously mentioned approaches, these animals can potentially be completely deficient in the target gene. In addition, one set of knockout mice can be bred with another to examine the interactions between two specific gene products. Although current work has used mice (because of the ease of generating mouse ES cells and of injecting mouse oocytes), knockout strategies are now being applied to other mammals as well and offer great promise for examining gene expression *in vivo*.

Disrupting a gene by homologous recombination in the manner described removes the gene from all tissues throughout the entire life of the organism. Knocking out a gene that is required at an early stage of development is likely to cause lethality at the earliest point in development that its protein product is required, eliminating the opportunity to determine the protein's function in tissues that appear at later points in development. To circumvent this problem and to allow the function of a gene to be examined in a specific tissue, conditional knockouts can be generated using the Cre/lox site-specific recombination system (reviewed in reference 71). In this technique, a gene encoding the site-specific recombinase "Cre" is attached to a promoter that drives expression in the tissue to be studied and is introduced into a mouse by transgenic techniques. Another mouse, in which the gene to be disrupted is flanked by specific recognition sequences for the recombinase ("lox" sites), is generated by homologous recombination in ES cells. The mice are crossed to produce offspring that carry the Cre recombinase transgene and the targeted gene (flanked by lox sites). When the tissue-specific promoter is turned on during development, the recombinase is expressed and causes the gene between the two lox sites to be efficiently removed. The resulting animal is a genetic mosaic in which the majority of cells that express the Cre recombinase are missing the targeted gene.

CONTROVERSIES AND PERSONAL PERSPECTIVES

Mouse Models of Cardiovascular Disease

The powerful techniques for targeted gene disruption that have been described are critical to contemporary biomedical research. Because knockout mice have phenotypes that closely resemble a number of human cardiovascular diseases, they are widely used as models. This is particularly true of mice with targeted disruptions of genes involved in lipoprotein metabolism that develop arterial lesions very similar to those seen in human arteriosclerosis. Despite the utility of these powerful models, there are several theoretical and practical considerations that should be kept in mind.

When targeting a gene by homologous recombination, there is an assumption that targeting will result in specific loss of the gene's product and will not directly affect the expression of other genes. Although the loss of the gene's product can be verified, the upregulation of another gene in the vicinity of the targeting can occur (72) and may readily escape detection. Such upregulation could have an important effect on the observed phenotype. In addition, the genetic background of the mice may have a profound effect on the observed phenotype. A particularly striking example is the vast difference in the extent of atherosclerosis observed in apolipoprotein E knockout mice based on their genetic background (73). To circumvent these concerns, one would ideally disrupt a gene using several different targeting strategies and then test the mutants to see if they are allelic (or use a transgene to "rescue" the mutant phenotype). The resultant knockouts could then be crossed onto several different genetic backgrounds. However, the time and expense of generating a mouse knockout are considerable, and seldom are different knockouts intentionally made for the same gene. Where they exist, subtle differences in the mutant phenotypes are not uncommon.

The standard approach to gene targeting by homologous recombination involves targeting the gene of interest in ES cells derived from one mouse strain and then transferring the targeted allele into a specific inbred strain by mating. Multiple rounds of backcrossing the targeted allele into the inbred strain are repeated until (after more than ten generations) the resulting mice are considered to be *congenic*, meaning identical to the inbred strain at all loci except for the targeted allele. Although the initial generations of targeted animals may be useful as experimental subjects, background genetic heterogeneity is high, and littermates must be used as controls. From a practical viewpoint, the investigator

THE FUTURE

The complete sequencing of the human genome is a critical milestone in the history of molecular biology, not only for the wealth of information that it provides but as a stunning example of how high-throughput techniques can be used to tackle basic problems in biology. As these technologies continue to evolve, the same trends toward miniaturization, increased speed, and decreased cost that are seen in other industries can be anticipated in molecular biology. The ability to characterize gene expression extensively in progressively smaller samples will permit wider application of these techniques to clinical medicine, further narrowing the gap between the clinical and basic sciences.

must be able to genotype the animals readily and to maintain a large enough colony of animals to ensure that adequate numbers with each genotype are available. In congenic strains the genetic background is uniform, but it is important to recognize that this "identity" is transient. Carrying a deleterious mutation in the homozygous state for multiple generations will favor the accumulation of new mutations over time that will tend to mitigate the severity of the mutant phenotype. Thus, even when using congenic strains, the "cleanest" experiment from a genetic perspective is one in which the homozygotes have had minimal opportunity for genetic drift from the control animals.

Gene Expression and Molecular Cloning

A major focus of cardiovascular research (and of this chapter) is the analysis of gene expression in normal and diseased tissues and the cloning of individual genes. Until recently, technical constraints limited most studies to the examination of only a few genes at a time. In the "postgenome era," there has been a shift toward performing far more comprehensive analysis of arrays that may include thousands of genes at one time. When studying such large sets of genes, each experiment produces a wealth of information that is then subjected to computational analysis. In previous investigations that focused on a single gene at a time, there was a natural tendency to study those genes that demonstrated the greatest difference in expression among conditions. In the large data sets generated by array screening, large numbers of genes with relatively modest degrees of regulation will be identified. If these robust analyses are to live up to their full promise, a major challenge for investigators will be to identify the underlying patterns and biologic significance of these more subtle forms of gene regulation. The rapidly developing field of proteomics should help provide rapid ways of determining whether subtle changes in mRNA are translated into important changes in protein levels and activity. Undoubtedly, exciting new approaches will be developed to combine experimental and computational biology.

REFERENCES

1. Campbell J, Campbell G. Methods of growing vascular smooth muscle in culture. In: Campbell J, Campbell G, eds. *Vascular smooth muscle in culture.* Boca Raton, FL: CRC Press, 1987:15–22.
2. Ross R. The smooth muscle cell. II. Growth of smooth muscle in culture and formation of elastic fibers. *J Cell Biol* 1971;50:172–186.
3. Thie M, Schlumberger W, Semich R, et al. Aortic smooth muscle cells in collagen lattice culture: effects on ultrastructure, proliferation and collagen synthesis. *Eur J Cell Biol* 1991;55:295–304.
4. Campbell J, Campbell G. Phenotypic modulation of smooth muscle cells in primary culture. In: Campbell J, Campbell G, eds. *Vascular smooth muscle in culture.* Boca Raton, FL: CRC Press, 1987:39–56.
5. Bowen-Pope D, Majesky M, Ross R. Growth factors for vascular smooth muscle cells. In: Campbell J, Campbell G, eds. *Vascular smooth muscle in culture.* Boca Raton, FL: CRC Press, 1987:71–92.
6. Owens G, Rovner A, Murphy R. Contractile protein expression and cytodifferentiation in cultured vascular smooth muscle cells. In: Campbell J, Campbell G, eds. *Vascular smooth muscle in culture.* Boca Raton, FL: CRC Press, 1987:57–70.
7. Campbell J, Campbell G, eds. *Vascular smooth muscle in culture.* Boca Raton, FL: CRC Press, 1987.
8. Jaffe E, Nachman R, Becker C, Minick C. Culture of human endothelial cells derived from umbilical veins. Identification by morphologic and immunologic criteria. *J Clin Invest* 1973;52(11):2745–2756.
9. Davies P, Remuzzi A, Gordon E, et al. Turbulent fluid shear stress induces vascular endothelial cell turnover in vitro. *Proc Natl Acad Sci U S A* 1986;83:2114–2117.
10. Folkman J, Haudenschild C. Angiogenesis in vitro. *Nature* 1980;288:551–556.
11. Kohtz SD. Studies of cardiac myocytes in culture: a developmental perspective. In: Marks A, Taubman M, eds. *Molecular biology of cardiovascular disease.* New York: Marcel Dekker, 1997:81–110.
12. O'Conner S, Davies P. Microcarrier culture of vascular smooth muscle cells. In: Campbell J, Campbell G, eds. *Vascular smooth muscle in culture.* Boca Raton, FL: CRC Press, 1987:23–38.

13. Luscinskas F, Gimbrone MJ. Endothelial-dependent mechanisms in chronic inflammatory leukocyte recruitment. *Annu Rev Med* 1996;47:413–421.

14. Tanaka N, Dalton N, Mao L, et al. Transthoracic echocardiography in models of cardiac disease in the mouse. *Circulation* 1996;94(5):1109–1117.

15. Palakodeti V, Oh S, Oh BH, et al. Force-frequency effect is a powerful determinant of myocardial contractility in the mouse. *Am J Physiol* 1997;273[3 Pt 2]:H1283–H1290.

16. Fayad ZA, Fallon JT, Shinnar M, et al. Noninvasive in vivo high-resolution magnetic resonance imaging of atherosclerotic lesions in genetically engineered mice. *Circulation* 1998;98(15):1541–1547.

17. Clowes A, Reidy M, Clowes M. Kinetics of cellular proliferation after arterial injury: I. Smooth muscle growth in the absence of endothelium. *Lab Invest* 1983;49(3):327–333.

18. Banai S, Shou M, Correa R, et al. Rabbit ear model of injury-induced arterial smooth muscle cell proliferation. Kinetics, reproducibility, and implications. *Circ Res* 1991;69:748–756.

19. Braam M, Cooley B, Gould J. Topical heparin enhances patency in a rat model of arterial thrombosis. *Ann Plast Surg* 1995;34:148–153.

20. Sarembock I, Gertz S, Thome L, et al. Effectiveness of hirulog in reducing restenosis after balloon angioplasty of atherosclerotic femoral arteries in rabbits. *J Vasc Res* 1996;33:308–314.

21. Romson J, Haack D, Lucchesi B. Electrical induction of coronary artery thrombosis in the ambulatory canine: a model for in vivo evaluation of thrombolytic agents. *Thromb Res* 1980;17:841–853.

22. Stemerman M. Thrombogenesis of the rabbit arterial plaque. *Am J Pathol* 1973;73:7–26.

23. Jayo J, Schwenke D, Clarkson T. Atherosclerosis research. In: Manning P, Ringler D, Newcomer C, eds. *The biology of the laboratory rabbit.* San Diego: Academic Press, 1994:367–380.

24. Jerome W, Lewis J. Early atherogenesis in White Carneau pigeons. I. Leukocyte margination and endothelial alterations at the celiac bifurcation. *Am J Pathol* 1984;116:56–68.

25. Lerman A, Webster M, Chesebro J, et al. Circulating and tissue endothelin immunoreactivity in hypercholesterolemic pigs. *Circulation* 1993;88:2923–2928.

26. Kaplan J, Manuck S, Adams M, et al. Plaque changes and arterial enlargement in atherosclerotic monkeys after manipulation of diet and social environment. *Arterioscler Thromb* 1993;13:254–263.

27. Geary R, Williams J, Golden D, et al. Time course of cellular proliferation, intimal hyperplasia, and remodeling following angioplasty in monkeys with established atherosclerosis. A nonhuman primate model of restenosis. *Arterioscler Thromb Vasc Biol* 1996;16:34–43.

28. Sasahara M, Raines E, Chait A, et al. Inhibition of hypercholesterolemia-induced atherosclerosis in the nonhuman primate by probucol. I. Is the extent of atherosclerosis related to resistance of LDL to oxidation? *J Clin Invest* 1994;94:155–164.

29. Watanabe Y. Serial inbreeding of rabbits with hereditary hyperlipidemia (WHHL-rabbit). *Atherosclerosis* 1980;36:261–268.

30. Breslow J. Mouse models of atherosclerosis. *Science* 1996;272:685–688.

31. Fazio S, Linton MF. Mouse models of hyperlipidemia and atherosclerosis. *Front Biosci* 2001;6:D515–D525.

32. Capasso JM, Palackal T, Olivetti G, et al. Left ventricular failure induced by long-term hypertension in rats. *Circ Res* 1990;66(5):1400–1412.

33. Inoko M, Kihara Y, Morii I, et al. Transition from compensatory hypertrophy to dilated, failing left ventricles in Dahl salt-sensitive rats. *Am J Physiol* 1994;267[6 Pt 2]:H2471–H2482.

34. Rockman HA, Ross RS, Harris AN, et al. Segregation of atrial-specific and inducible expression of an atrial natriuretic factor transgene in an in vivo murine model of cardiac hypertrophy. *Proc Natl Acad Sci U S A* 1991;88(18):8277–8281.

35. Hirota H, Chen J, Betz UA, et al. Loss of a gp130 cardiac muscle cell survival pathway is a critical event in the onset of heart failure during biomechanical stress. *Cell* 1999;97(2):189–198.

36. Zhang D, Gaussin V, Taffet GE, et al. TAK1 is activated in the myocardium after pressure overload and is sufficient to provoke heart failure in transgenic mice. *Natl Med* 2000;6(5):556–563.

37. Esposito G, Prasad SVN, Rapacciuolo A, et al. Cardiac overexpression of a Gq inhibitor blocks induction of extracellular signal-regulated kinase and c-Jun NH2-terminal kinase activity in in vivo pressure overload. *Circulation* 2001;103(10):1453–1458.

38. Patten RD, Aronovitz MJ, Deras-Mejia L, et al. Ventricular remodeling in a mouse model of myocardial infarction. *Am J Physiol* 1998;274[5 Pt 2]:H1812–H1820.

39. Kawai C. From myocarditis to cardiomyopathy: mechanisms of inflammation and cell death: learning from the past for the future. *Circulation* 1999;99(8):1091–1100.

40. Bajusz E, Baker JR, Nixon CW, Homburger F. Spontaneous, hereditary myocardial degeneration and congestive heart failure in a strain of Syrian hamsters. *Ann N Y Acad Sci* 1969;156(1):105–129.

41. Nigro V, Okazaki Y, Belsito A, et al. Identification of the Syrian hamster cardiomyopathy gene. *Hum Mol Genet* 1997;6(4):601–607.

42. Sakamoto A, Abe M, Masaki T. Delineation of genomic deletion in cardiomyopathic hamster. *FEBS Lett* 1999;447(1):124–128.

43. Ikeda Y, Ross J Jr. Models of dilated cardiomyopathy in the mouse and the hamster. *Curr Opin Cardiol* 2000;15(3):197–201.

44. Geisterfer-Lowrance AA, Christe M, Conner DA, et al. A mouse model of familial hypertrophic cardiomyopathy. *Science* 1996;272(5262):731–734.

45. Thomas P. Hybridization of denatured RNA and small DNA fragments transferred to nitrocellulose. *Proc Natl Acad Sci U S A* 1980;77:5201–5205.

46. Rost A-K, Köhler T, Heilman S, et al. A rapid and simple method to prepare digoxigenin-labeled DNA-probes by using PCR-generated DNA-fragments. *Eur J Clin Chem Clin Biochem* 1995;33(4):A59.

47. Sambrook J, Fritsch E, Maniatis T. *Molecular cloning: a laboratory manual,* 2nd ed. Cold Spring Harbor, NY: Cold Spring Harbor Laboratory Press, 1989.
48. Feinberg A, Vogelstein B. A technique for radiolabeling DNA restriction endonuclease fragments to high specific activity. *Anal Biochem* 1983;132:6–13.
49. Feinberg A, Vogelstein B. Addendum: a technique for radiolabeling DNA restriction endonuclease fragments to high specific activity. *Anal Biochem* 1984;137:266–267.
50. Zinn K, DiMaio D, Maniatis T. Identification of two distinct regulatory regions adjacent to the human beta-interferon gene. *Cell* 1983;34:865–879.
51. Melton D, Krieg P, Rebagliati M, et al. Efficient in vivo synthesis of biologically active RNA and RNA hybridization probes from plasmids containing a bacteriophage SP6 promoter. *Nucleic Acids Res* 1984;12:7035–7056.
52. Orlando C, Pinzani P, Pazzagli M. Developments in quantitative PCR. *Clin Chem Lab Med* 1998;36(5):255–269.
53. Bustin SA. Absolute quantification of mRNA using real-time reverse transcription polymerase chain reaction assays. *J Mol Endocrinol* 2000;25(2):169–193.
54. Awgulewtsch A, Utset M, Hart C, et al. Spatial restriction in expression of a mouse homeobox locus within the central nervous system. *Nature* 1986;320:328–335.
55. Emmert-Buck MR, Bonner RF, Smith PD, et al. Laser capture microdissection. *Science* 1996;274(5289):998–1001.
56. Simone NL, Bonner RF, Gillespie JW, et al. Laser-capture microdissection: opening the microscopic frontier to molecular analysis. *Trends Genet* 1998;14(7):272–276.
57. Groudine M, Peretz M, Weintraub H. Transcriptional regulation of hemoglobin switching in chicken embryos. *Mol Cell Biol* 1981;1:281–288.
58. Gorman C, Moffat L, Howard B. Recombinant genomes which express chloramphenicol acetyltransferase in mammalian cells. *Mol Cell Biol* 1982;2:1044–1051.
59. Nordeen S. Luciferase reporter gene vectors for analysis of promoters and enhancers. *BioTechniques* 1988;6:454–457.
60. Seed B, Sheen J. A simple phase-extraction assay for chloramphenicol acetyltransferase activity. *Gene* 1988;67:271–277.
61. Brasier A, Tate J, Habener J. Optimized use of the firefly luciferase as a reporter gene in mammalian cell lines. *BioTechniques* 1989;7:1116–1122.
62. Mack CP, Owens GK. Regulation of smooth muscle alpha-actin expression in vivo is dependent on CArG elements within the 5' and first intron promoter regions. *Circ Res* 1999;84(7):852–861.
63. Regan CP, Adam PJ, Madsen CS, et al. Molecular mechanisms of decreased smooth muscle differentiation marker expression after vascular injury. *J Clin Invest* 2000;106(9):1139–1147.
64. Murphy TJ, Alexander RW, Griendling KK, et al. Isolation of a cDNA encoding the vascular type-1 angiotensin II receptor. *Nature* 1991;351(6323):233–236.
65. Vu T, Hung D, Wheaton V, et al. Molecular cloning of a functional thrombin receptor reveals a novel proteolytic mechanism of receptor activation. *Cell* 1991;64:1057–1068.
66. Davis R, Weintraub H, Lassar A. Expression of a single transfected cDNA converts fibroblasts to myoblasts. *Cell* 1987;51:987–1000.
67. Redfern CH, Degtyarev MY, Kwa AT, et al. Conditional expression of a Gi-coupled receptor causes ventricular conduction delay and a lethal cardiomyopathy. *Proc Natl Acad Sci U S A* 2000;97(9):4826–4831.
68. Weintraub AS, Giachelli CM, Krauss RS, et al. Autocrine secretion of osteopontin by vascular smooth muscle cells regulates their adhesion to collagen gels. *Am J Pathol* 1996;149(1):259–272.
69. Doherty EA, Doudna JA. Ribozyme structures and mechanisms. *Annu Rev Biochem* 2000;69:597–615.
70. Muller U. Ten years of gene targeting: targeted mouse mutants, from vector design to phenotype analysis. *Mech Dev* 1999;82(1–2):3–21.
71. Sauer B. Inducible gene targeting in mice using the Cre/lox system. *Methods* 1998;14(4):381–392.
72. Moore RC, Lee IY, Silverman GL, et al. Ataxia in prion protein (PrP)-deficient mice is associated with upregulation of the novel PrP-like protein doppel. *J Mol Biol* 1999;292(4):797–817.
73. Dansky HM, Charlton SA, Sikes JL, et al. Genetic background determines the extent of atherosclerosis in ApoE-deficient mice. *Arterioscler Thromb Vasc Biol* 1999;19(8):1960–1968.

GENETIC STUDIES OF MYOCARDIAL AND VASCULAR DISEASE

QING WANG
REED E. PYERITZ
CHRISTINE E. SEIDMAN
CRAIG T. BASSON

▼▼ ADDITIONAL ELECTRONIC TOPICS

Atrial Fibrillation q01;   Conduction Defects q02;   Familial Atrioventricular Defects q03;   McKusick-Kaufman Syndrome q04;   Total Anomalous Pulmonary Venous Return q05;   Velocardiofacial Syndrome q06;   Velocardiofacial Syndrome: Clinical Features q07; Velocardiofacial Syndrome: Genetic Studies q08;   Tetralogy of Fallot q09;   Cardiac Looping Defects (Heterotaxy, or Left-Right Malformations) q10;   Bicuspid Aortic Valve q11;   Pulmonic Stenosis q12;   Familial Mitral Valve Prolapse q13;   Ebstein's Anomaly q14; Restrictive Cardiomyopathy q15;   Familial Aortic Aneurysm q16;   Ehlers-Danlos Syndrome q17;   Cutaneous Venous Malformations with Glomus Cells q18

OVERVIEW

Genetic factors contribute to the pathogenesis of a wide variety of disorders that affect cardiac and vascular structure

Q. Wang: Departments of Molecular Genetics and Molecular Cardiology, The Cleveland Clinic Foundation, Cleveland, Ohio
R. E. Pyeritz: Division of Medical Genetics, Department of Medicine, University of Pennsylvania School of Medicine, Philadelphia, Pennsylvania
C. E. Seidman: Department of Genetics, Harvard Medical School, Boston, Massachusetts
C. T. Basson: Cardiology Division, Weill Medical College of Cornell University, New York Presbyterian Hospital–Cornell Medical Center, New York, New York

and function. Advances in molecular genetics since the 1980s have provided remarkable insights into the genes responsible and pathogenic mechanisms of cardiovascular disease. Disease-causing genes have been identified for cardiac arrhythmic disorders [e.g., long QT syndrome (LQT), idiopathic ventricular fibrillation (IVF)], congenital heart disease [e.g., Holt-Oram syndrome, Ellis-van Creveld syndrome, atrial septal defect (ASD) with atrioventricular (AV) block, cardiac myxoma], hypertrophic cardiomyopathy, dilated cardiomyopathy, arrhythmogenic right ventricular dysplasia, and familial vascular anomalies [e.g., Marfan syndrome (MFS), patent ductus arteriosus, supravalvular aortic stenosis, lymphedema]. Genetic studies of human cardiovascular disorders continue to provide insight into molecular mechanisms underlying morphogenesis, development, and physiologic function of the cardiovascular system. Molecular genetic analysis of cardiovascular disease permits DNA-based diagnosis, which will promote new approaches to risk stratification and therapy. These exciting molecular discoveries have raised the hope of genetic testing, drug development, and gene-based therapies for a variety of cardiovascular disorders. In this chapter, we discuss major advances in the genetics of myocardial and vascular disease.

GLOSSARY

Allele: Alternative forms of a gene or a genetic locus.
Allelic: A condition in which two phenotypically different traits are the result of different mutations in the same gene.
Compound heterozygote: An individual with one mutation in one allele of a given gene and a different mutation in the other allele of the gene. Compound heterozygous mutations are usually associated with autosomal recessive disease.
Heterogeneity: *Allelic* or *intragenic heterogeneity* is different genotypes at the same genetic locus that cause a similar phenotype. *Locus heterogeneity* refers to a situation in which a disease is caused by defects at different genetic loci.
Heterozygote: An individual with a mutation in one copy of a given gene but without a mutation in the other copy. Heterozygous mutations are usually associated with autosomal dominant disease.
Homozygote: An individual with the identical sequence in both alleles of a given gene. Homozygous mutations are usually associated with autosomal recessive disease.
Linkage analysis: Analysis to determine whether two or more genetic traits (a marker locus and a disease trait) are cosegregating within a pedigree.
Positional cloning: A technique used to identify the underlying genetic cause of a disease based primarily on finding the location of the defective gene.

INTRODUCTION

Cardiovascular disease is the leading cause of death in developed countries. Genetic factors play an important role in the pathogenesis of cardiovascular disease. Each human being is variably estimated to have at least 30,000 to 40,000 different genes (1–3). Mutations in single or multiple genes can cause cardiovascular disease. The revolutionary advances in molecular genetics over the past 15 years have provided new insights into the responsible genes and pathogenic mechanisms of cardiovascular disease (*e*Fig.

100.0.1). Some of these diseases are individually quite prevalent. Many of the most common diagnoses, such as "stroke," "heart attack," "hypertension," or "heart failure," subsume several distinct disorders. Other cardiovascular conditions are quite rare but have proven instructive in terms of the etiology and pathogenesis of common disease processes, such as atherosclerosis, aneurysms, and dysrhythmia. Mendelian disorders may be rare and can be caused by mutations in a single gene with profound consequences. Many of the more common disorders are not simply inherited, yet have a few or perhaps many genes that stochastically interact with each other and the environment to produce pathology.

Monogenic cardiovascular disorders can be inherited as autosomal dominant, autosomal recessive, or X-linked traits. A rapidly increasing number of the genes responsible for such disorders have been mapped to specific chromosomal regions by linkage analysis and identified by candidate gene or positional cloning approaches (*e*Fig. 100.0.1) (4,5). The "working draft" of the human genome sequence will greatly facilitate identification of additional genes. A recent tabulation of genes that have been mapped and are associated with human phenotypes numbers just more than 1,000; just over one-fourth involve the cardiovascular system (5).

Analysis of the genetics of common disease is far more complicated, whether in terms of populations, families, or molecules, than that for simply inherited conditions. Nonetheless, considerable progress has been made, both in experimental animals and in humans, in identifying genes that contribute to the cause, pathogenesis, or both of common diseases such as coronary artery disease and hypertension. In many instances, specific genetic variations that confer an increased risk of developing a condition can now be identified before symptoms develop. The challenge is to devise approaches to modulating the risk in those so identified.

This chapter reviews the major advances in the molecular genetics of single gene disorders of the cardiovascular system. The genetics of complex diseases, such as coronary artery disease and hypertension, is covered in other chapters in this textbook.

DISORDERS OF CARDIAC RHYTHM AND CONDUCTION

Cardiac arrhythmias are a common cause of morbidity and mortality, accounting for 300,000 to 400,000 sudden deaths each year in the United States alone (6,7). A number of mendelian conditions account for an unknown but clearly underestimated fraction of this mortality.

Long QT Syndrome

LQT is characterized by prolongation of the QT interval and T-wave abnormalities on electrocardiograms (ECGs) and symptoms of syncope, seizures, and sudden death, usually from a specific ventricular arrhythmia, *torsades de pointes* (8–10). Two inherited forms of LQT have been reported: autosomal dominant LQT (Romano-Ward syndrome) with normal hearing (8,9) and the much rarer autosomal recessive LQT (Jervell-Lange-Nielsen syndrome) associated with congenital deafness (9,11). It appears that patients with Jervell-Lange-Nielsen syndrome have a more adverse course and higher rate of sudden death. The primary defect at the tissue level involves cardiac repolarization, and the prolonged QT interval, when corrected for heart rate, is usually (but not always) evident on standard 12-lead ECG (*e*Fig. 100.0.2). Autosomal dominant LQT has an incidence of approximately 1 per 10,000, without apparent ethnic or geographic predilection (12,13). A set of clinical criteria to assist in diagnosis has been developed (*e*Fig. 100.0.2) (14). Although most clinical events are "triggered" by excitement, exercise, emotional upset, and the like, sudden death can occur during sleep. Some have suggested LQT as a cause of sudden infant death syndrome (15–17).

Molecular Genetics

The first LQT gene was mapped to chromosome 11p15.5 (*LQT1*) in 1991 (18). Since then, at least five other genetic loci for LQT have been identified on chromosome 7q35–36 (*LQT2*) (19), 3p21–24 (*LQT3*) (19), 4q25–27 (*LQT4*) (20), 21q22 (*LQT5*) (21), and 21q22 (*LQT6*) (22), and further locus heterogeneity exists. Five disease genes have been cloned or identified, and mutations have been described in each gene. *KVLQT1* (*LQT1*), *HERG* (*LQT2*), *KCNE1* (*LQT5*), and *KCNE2* (*LQT6*) all encode potassium channel subunits. *SCN5A* (*LQT3*) encodes the cardiac sodium channel protein. Heterozygous mutations in these genes cause autosomal dominant LQT. Homozygous or compound heterozygous mutations in *KVLQT1* and *KCNE1* cause Jervell-Lange-Nielsen syndrome. The LQT gene on chromosome 4q25–27 has been mapped in one family, but it has not been cloned yet.

Cardiac Potassium Channel Gene KVLQT1

KVLQT1, the LQT1 gene on chromosome 11p15.5, is the first novel gene cloned for LQT (23). This gene encodes a potassium channel alpha-subunit with a conserved potassium-selective pore-signature sequence flanked by six transmembrane-spanning segments (S1 to S6). People who are heterozygous for mutations in *KVLQT1* are at risk for autosomal dominant LQT. However, people who have mutations in both of their *KVLQT1* alleles have the more severe disease, autosomal recessive LQT with congenital deafness (24,25). Mutations in *KVLQT1*, when heterozygous, cause loss of channel function, altered channel gating, and/or a dominant-negative effect (26) in which the mutant form of the channel subunit interferes with the function of the normal form. The KVLQT1 protein normally functions by interacting with MinK, a short potassium channel subunit with a mere 130 amino acids and only one transmembrane-spanning segment (27,28). The physical interaction between KVLQT1 and MinK produces the slowly activating potassium current (I_{Ks}) in cardiac myocytes.

Various ion currents such as I_{Ks} are responsible for the different phases of the cardiac action potential (CAP) (*e*Fig. 100.0.2). One CAP corresponds to one heart beat. The time course of one CAP can be divided into five phases: upstroke of rapid depolarization (phase 0); rapid repolarization following the peak (phase 1); a plateau (phase 2); rapid repolarization (phase 3); and the period between the maximum negativity (maximum diastolic potential) and the upstroke of the next action potential (phase 4) (*e*Fig. 100.0.2) (29,30). The I_{Ks} potassium current acts at the repolarization phase (phase 3). KVLQT1 mutations reduce the repolarizing cardiac I_{Ks} current, causing delayed repolarization and prolongation of the CAP duration, and prolongation of the QT interval on ECG.

Cardiac Potassium Channel Gene *HERG*

The *LQT2* gene on chromosome 7q35–36 was identified as *HERG*, which encodes a cardiac potassium channel core–forming subunit with six transmembrane segments (31). This channel ordinarily generates the rapidly activating delayed rectifier potassium current (I_{Kr}) in the heart. LQT-associated mutations in *HERG* act through either a loss-of-function or a dominant-negative mechanism (32). The I_{Kr} potassium current is a major current at the repolarization phase of CAP. HERG mutations reduce the repolarizing cardiac I_{Kr} current, thus causing prolongation of the CAP duration, leading to prolongation of the QT interval on ECG.

Cardiac Sodium Channel Gene *SCN5A*

The gene associated with LQT3 on chromosome 3p21–24 is the cardiac sodium channel gene, *SCN5A* (12,33). It encodes a large protein of 2,016 amino acids with a putative structure of four homologous domains (DI-DIV), each of which contains six membrane-spanning segments (S1 to S6) (34). The sodium current I_{Na} generated by this channel is responsible for the depolarization phase of the CAP and contributes some current at the plateau phase. LQT-causing mutations in *SCN5A* act through a gain-of-function mechanism, in which the mutant channel functions, but with altered properties. Four *SCN5A* mutations (ΔKPQ, N1325S, R1644H, E1784K) generate the persistent noninactivated sodium current in the plateau phase of the CAP (35–39). One *SCN5A* mutation (D1790G) shifts steady-state inactivation by −16 mV in the presence of the beta$_1$-subunit (40). The E1784K mutation shifts the voltage dependence of steady-state inactivation toward more negative potentials (5 mV), and coexpression with the beta$_1$-subunit exaggerates the negative shift. The mutation R1623Q increases the probability of long openings and causes early reopenings, producing a threefold prolongation of sodium current decay (41,42). Although the LQT-causing mutations in *SCN5A* produce variable degrees of altered channel function, they all lead to the increase of inward plateau sodium current, prolonging the action potential duration and the QT interval on ECG.

Cardiac Potassium Channel Gene *KCNE1* (*MinK*)

As in *KVLQT1*, heterozygous mutations in *MinK* cause autosomal dominant LQT, but homozygous or compound heterozygous mutations in *MinK* cause autosomal recessive LQT (21,43). MinK interacts with KVLQT1 and HERG, recapitulating I_{Ks} with KVLQT1 and augmenting the amplitude of I_{Kr} generated by HERG (44). Different MinK mutations appear to have different effects on KVLQT1 and HERG (44). Mutation V47F alters I_{Ks} currents, and increases the HERG current. W87R alters I_{Ks} currents only. D76N suppresses both KVLQT1 and HERG currents. Mutant L51H channels are processed improperly and interact with neither KVLQT1 nor HERG.

Cardiac Potassium Channel Gene *KCNE2*

This gene, also called *MiRP1*, for minK-related peptide 1, encodes an integral component of a potassium channel. This gene has high homology with KCNE1; their close linkage (70 kb apart on chromosome 21q22) suggests that one arose as a result of gene duplication of the other. Mutations in *KCNE2* cause LQT6 (22). MiRP1 is a small integral membrane subunit that assembles with HERG to form I_{Kr}. Recently, MiRP1 was shown to interact with KVLQT1, resulting in a great change of the amplitude and gating properties of the KVLQT1 current (45).

The KCNE family includes another member, *KCNE3* (46), but no mutations in *KCNE3* were reported in LQT patients.

Potassium Channel Gene *Kir2.1* and Andersen's Syndrome

Mutations in the Kir2.1 inward rectifier potassium channel were recently identified in patients with Andersen's syndrome, which is characterized by QTc prolongation, periodic skeletal muscle paralysis, and mild dysmorphic features (46a). Kir2.1 mutations act by either loss-of-function mechanism or a dominant negative mechanism. Kir2.1 consists of only two transmembrane segments, M1 and M2, flanking a pore region and may generate the I_{K1} potassium current at the terminal repolarization phase (phase 3) and for maintenance of the cardiac resting potential.

Genotype-Phenotype Correlation in Long QT Syndrome

Mutations in *KVLQT1* and *HERG* cause approximately 40% of LQT cases, respectively, whereas mutations in *SCN5A* are associated with 10% of cases (47). Mutations in *KCNE1* and *KCNE2* are rare. Patients with LQT1 tend to have frequent exercise-related cardiac events, whereas most with LQT3 experience cardiac events during sleep or at rest. Patients with LQT2 may experience cardiac events both at rest and during exercise. The risk of cardiac events is higher in LQT1 and LQT2 than in LQT3; however, the likelihood of dying during a cardiac event is significantly higher among LQT3 patients (48). LQT1, LQT2, and possibly LQT3 genotypes are associated with different but typical ST-T–wave patterns on ECG (49).

Diagnosis, Genetic Testing, and Treatment

LQT can be diagnosed with reasonable certainty if QTc is 0.47 second or longer for asymptomatic individuals or if QTc is 0.45 second or longer for symptomatic individuals (29,30). LQT is not likely if QTc is less than 0.41 second in males and less than 0.43 second in females. Many mutation carriers as well as normal people have QTc ranging from 0.41 second to 0.46 second, which significantly limits the power of ECG diagnosis of LQT patients. Sudden death occurs in 10% to 30% symptomatic LQT patients (13), and it may occur with the first syncope. These factors make genetic testing extremely important. Current genetic testing for LQT patients is carried out only in research laboratories. Only positive results—that is, identification of a mutation—confirm the diagnosis.

The identification of LQT genes has led to the development of gene-specific therapies for LQT patients (30). Sodium channel–blocking agents such as mexiletine and flecainide can shorten QTc for LQT3 patients (50,51). Raising the serum potassium concentration shortens QTc for LQT2 patients (52). Potassium channel–opening agents and verapamil may be beneficial to patients with potassium channel mutations (13). All these therapies are at the investigational stage, and it is not clear whether these therapies can eliminate life-threatening ventricular arrhythmias.

All symptomatic patients as well as all asymptomatic children require treatment (13). For most LQT patients, administration of a beta-blocker is the initial choice of therapy. Beta-blockers are effective in patients with KVLQT1 and HERG mutations. Other therapeutic options include pacing and implantation of a cardioverter-defibrillator in combination with beta-blockers.

Idiopathic Ventricular Tachycardia and Ventricular Fibrillation

Idiopathic Ventricular Fibrillation with Right Bundle Branch Block and ST-Segment Elevation ("Martini"-Brugada Syndrome)

IVF is ventricular fibrillation without underlying structural heart disease and other electrolyte disorders such as LQT. IVF can be classified into two types: IVF with normal ECG and IVF with an ECG feature of right bundle branch block and persistent ST-segment elevation (STE) in leads V1 to

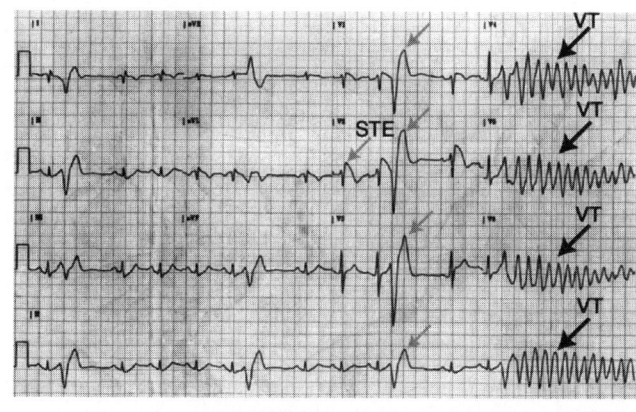
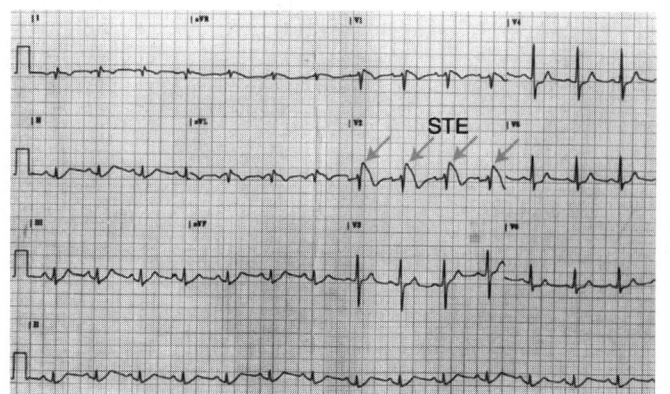

FIGURE 100.1 Twelve-lead electrocardiograms (ECGs) showing typical features of idiopathic ventricular fibrillation with right bundle branch block and ST-segment elevation (STE) ("Martini"-Brugada syndrome). **A:** ECG recorded immediately after the patient arrived at the emergency room because of an episode of syncope and seizures. The episode was triggered by cold-related fever. Note the presence of STE and development of polymorphic ventricular tachycardia (VT) after a ventricular premature contraction. **B:** ECG recorded 11 hours after the syncopal episode. The patient recovered after a cardioversion. Note the typical STE (mainly in lead V2). After the episode, a defibrillator was implanted in the patient. (Unpublished data, Carlos Oberti, Palmira Vanzini, Alvaro Rivara, and Qing Wang.)

V3 (IVF with STE) (Fig. 100.1), which was first described by Martini et al. and is now often referred to as *Brugada syndrome* (53–55). In a small percentage of patients with IVF, a family history of sudden death or even IVF can be found, with inheritance as an autosomal dominant pattern (56).

In 1998, the first gene for IVF with STE (Brugada syndrome) was identified as *SCN5A*, the cardiac sodium channel gene (56). *SCN5A* mutations were also identified in IVF patients without STE on ECG (56,57). The IVF mutations are functionally different from *SCN5A* mutations associated with LQT. The IVF mutations act by a loss-of-function mechanism (16,56,58,59). *SCN5A* mutations may account for 15% to 35% of IVF patients (56,60), and other genes are involved and remain to be identified.

Catecholaminergic Ventricular Tachycardia

Families with stress-induced ventricular tachycardia [catecholaminergic ventricular tachycardia (CVT)] occurring in the structurally intact heart have been reported (61). Clinical symptoms of CVT include a family history of juvenile sudden death and stress-induced syncope. The inheritance pattern appears to be autosomal dominant, and a genetic locus for CVT was mapped to 1q42–q43 (61). The gene for CVT has recently been identified as the cardiac ryanodine receptor gene (*RYR2*) (62,63). Mutations in *RYR2* (62,63) were identified in autosomal dominant families presenting with bidirectional ventricular tachycardia that was reproducibly induced by exercise stress testing and/or isoproterenol infusion without structural heart abnormalities. As discussed later, *RYR2* mutations also cause arrhythmogenic right ventricular dysplasia (ARVD).

Polymorphic ventricular tachycardia can segregate in families as an autosomal recessive trait, and an autosomal recessive polymorphic ventricular tachycardia gene was mapped to 1p13–21 (64); however, the gene remains to be cloned.

Right Ventricular Outflow Tract Tachycardia

Right ventricular outflow tract (RVOT) tachycardia is a paroxysmal IVT with the focal origin localized to the RVOT. A functional mutation of F200L in the guanosine triphosphate binding protein inhibitory subunit alpha-i2 gene (GNAI2) on chromosome 3p21 was identified in a patient with RVOT tachycardia (65). Mutation F200L is a somatic mutation because it was identified in a biopsy sample from the arrhythmogenic focus but not from peripheral lymphocytes or the sample distant from the arrhythmogenic focus. This finding raises the possibility that common RVOT tachycardia is a somatic cell genetic disorder caused by mutations in specific somatic cells.

Wolff-Parkinson-White Syndrome

The Wolff-Parkinson-White syndrome (WPW) is cardiac conduction defect characterized by a short PR interval, an increased duration of QRS complex, and a delta wave on ECG, and supraventricular tachyarrhythmias. A single mutation (R302Q) in the $gamma_2$-subunit of AMP-activated protein kinase was identified in two families with WPW, establishing a molecular basis for WPW (72a).

CONGENITAL STRUCTURAL HEART DISEASE

Many structural congenital cardiac anomalies have anatomic and physiologic manifestations that can be diagnosed at birth or even prenatally. Such anomalies occur in more than 5% of all live births and 10% of stillborns (73,74). Although some of these are sporadic events that result from somatic or *de novo* germline mutations, a significant portion represent familial transmission of disease. The increased risk of structural congenital heart disease in the first-degree relatives of patients with structural cardiac anomalies has long been recognized (75), and autosomal dominant, autosomal recessive, and X-linked modes of transmission have all been reported (5,75).

Mendelian patterns of inheritance can also vary in some disorders with a recognized heritable genetic basis. For instance, situs inversus can occur as an isolated heritable finding or as a component either of visceral heterotaxy syndromes (X-linked or autosomal recessive) or of autosomal recessive Kartagener syndrome. Molecular genetic analysis of such disorders has been limited by kindred size and low penetrance. Insights may be gleaned, however, from murine models (e.g., mutations in the *iv* and *inv* genes can produce murine *situs inversus*) (76,77). Macroscopic chromosomal aberrations and rearrangements (including trisomies of chromosomes 13, 18, and 21) have been associated with variable forms of congenital structural heart disease in the context of complex extracardiac abnormalities. Subtle mutations occur more often, however, and can cause discrete congenital cardiac malformations as well as syndromes with cardiac components. Recent advances in molecular biology have begun to elucidate the fundamental genetic mechanisms underlying such heritable cardiac disorders.

Septation Defects

Defects in the atrial and ventricular septa are the most commonly reported congenital cardiac anomalies. Studies have reported an incidence of greater than 5% of live births (74,78), and this is likely to be an underestimate given that both ventricular septal defects (VSDs) and ASDs may occur in isolation and may close spontaneously during infancy. Many VSDs as well as ASDs occur in the setting of other cardiac and extracardiac anomalies and can have grave physiologic consequences such as the development of Eisenmenger syndrome.

Holt-Oram Syndrome

Clinical Manifestations

Holt-Oram syndrome is characterized by cardiac septation defects in the setting of upper limb deformity (79). It is the most common form of "heart-hand syndrome" and occurs in at least 0.95 per 100,000 individuals (80). All individuals affected by Holt-Oram syndrome exhibit some degree of malformation of the arms or hands (*e*Fig. 100.1.1); such malformation is frequently asymmetric and may be unilateral. Although the initial descriptions of this syndrome focused on abnormalities of the thumb (typically triphalangism or aplasia) (*e*Fig. 100.1.1A), the most common

manifestations are carpal bone malformations or fusions (5,79,80). These may be evident only radiographically and in fact may be the only clinical evidence of Holt-Oram syndrome in a given patient. On the other hand, limb malformation may be sufficiently severe for individuals to present with phocomelia (*e*Fig. 100.1.1B), and the syndrome has been called a "pseudo-thalidomide syndrome."

Approximately 75% of Holt-Oram syndrome patients (81) have some cardiac abnormality (*e*Fig. 100.1.2). In most cases, these defects are ASD or VSD, which range in size, number, and location. Most ASDs are ostium secundum defects, and most VSDs are muscular. Severely affected individuals may present with multiple VSDs (sometimes termed "Swiss cheese septum") as well as ASDs, and rare individuals with AV canal defects have been reported. Many Holt-Oram syndrome patients will present with conduction disease (ranging from sinus bradycardia and first-degree AV block to AF and high-grade AV block). Conduction disease occurs independent of the presence or size of septation defects in a given patient. Other cardiac anomalies, including anomalous pulmonary venous drainage, abnormal isomerism, mitral valve prolapse, as well as persistent left superior vena cava and more rarely hypoplastic left heart syndrome and tetralogy of Fallot, have all been reported to occur in some patients with Holt-Oram syndrome (5).

Genetic Studies

Holt-Oram syndrome is an autosomal dominant disorder. Sporadic disease may represent a *de novo* germline mutation—that is, individuals who present with sporadic disease usually can transmit the disorder to their offspring. Despite its highly variable pattern of expression, Holt-Oram syndrome is highly penetrant in affected families.

Initial linkage analysis studies (82,83) revealed that the gene defect for Holt-Oram syndrome resides on the long arm of chromosome 12 (although this locus does not account for all other heart-hand syndromes). Recent studies (84,85) have demonstrated that Holt-Oram syndrome is caused by mutations on chromosome 12q24.1 that inactivate the *TBX5* gene. TBX5 is a member of the T-box family of transcription factors, and it is expressed in the embryonic human heart and forelimb (86,87). Atrial expression is much greater than ventricular expression in humans, mice, and chicks (86–90). It is currently unknown which genes are activated by this transcription factor, and the precise mechanism whereby *TBX5* haploinsufficiency causes cardiac and limb malformation is under active investigation. Studies correlating *TBX5* genotypes with Holt-Oram syndrome phenotypes suggest that mutations that produce truncation of the TBX5 protein have a higher incidence of both severe cardiac and severe limb malformation than less common missense mutations, which only alter a single amino acid (91). In the case of missense mutations, their location within the T-box appears to mediate the severity of cardiac versus limb malformations (91–93). The role of *TBX5* mutations in isolated septation defects and common atria syndromes also remains to be demonstrated. Detection of *TBX5* mutations in the families of Holt-Oram syndrome patients now permits accurate diagnosis of the syndrome even in subtly affected individuals (*e*Fig. 100.1.2). In the future, delineation of TBX5-mediated regulation of cardiac development may provide new approaches to gene therapy for septation defects.

Ellis-van Creveld Syndrome

Like Holt-Oram syndrome, Ellis-van Creveld syndrome represents an association of cardiac septation defects with skeletal abnormalities (94). Transmitted in an autosomal recessive pattern, Ellis-van Creveld syndrome is most obviously characterized by dwarfism with particularly evident shortening of the distal extremities. Other features include polydactyly, carpal bone abnormalities, nail dystrophy, upper lip deformity, and premature dental eruption. Cardiac abnormalities typically include ASDs and common atrium. Linkage analysis (95) of interrelated Amish families and unrelated Hispanic kindreds affected by Ellis-van Creveld mapped the genetic defect to a locus at chromosome 4p16. More recently, positional cloning studies have identified disease-causing mutations in the novel *EVC* gene, whose function remains unknown (96). Cytogenetic abnormalities of distal chromosome 4p have been associated with ostium secundum ASDs in the setting of craniofacial abnormalities in the Wolf-Hirschhorn syndrome (97). The relationship (if any) of the chromosome 4p Ellis-van Creveld locus to this syndrome is as yet unknown.

Familial Atrial Septal Defects with Atrioventricular Block

In the syndrome of familial ASD with AV block, ASDs occur without associated skeletal malformation, as seen in Holt-Oram or Ellis-van Creveld syndrome. Some individuals exhibit conduction delay manifest as progressive AV block. This condition is transmitted in families as an autosomal dominant trait. Schott et al. (98) used linkage analysis to study families with this disorder and demonstrated that the disease gene mapped to chromosome 5q35. They subsequently applied a candidate gene strategy to identify the disease gene as the *NKX2.5* gene at this locus. *NKX2.5* is a member of the large NK homeobox transcription factor gene family. The prototypical member of this family is the *Drosophila* tin man gene, without which the fly heart fails to develop.

Schott et al. (98) and Benson et al. (99) demonstrated a number of mutations in the *NKX2.5* gene that cause familial ASD with AV block. These mutations include not only nonsense and other mutations that are predicted to result

in *NKX2.5* haploinsufficiency but also a number of missense mutations. Recently, Kashahara et al. (100) studied a number of truncated forms of NKX2.5 as well as mutant NKX2.5 isoforms resulting from missense mutations observed in humans. They observed decreased NKX2.5 activity in all cases not only via NKX2.5 haploinsufficiency but also through impaired DNA binding or defective protein-protein interactions with essential cofactors.

Of note, although Lyons et al. (101) had initially noted that knockout mice who were homozygous null for *NKX2.5* died during embryogenesis with a failure of cardiac looping, subsequent analyses (101,102) have demonstrated both ASDs and conduction disease in mice heterozygous null for *NKX2.5*. Benson et al. (99) noted a number of protean manifestations of *NKX2.5* mutations in human patients. Not only do individuals with *NKX2.5* mutations exhibit ASDs, but also they may be affected by a number of other forms of congenital structural heart disease, including VSDs, tetralogy of Fallot, subvalvular aortic stenosis, pulmonary atresia, double-outlet right ventricle, and Ebstein's anomaly. However, no genotype-phenotype correlations have been observed (98,99,103) to allow the association of any particular form of congenital heart disease with any given single or group of *NKX2.5* mutations. Thus, the mechanism whereby *NKX2.5* mutations result in ASDs versus other forms of congenital heart disease remains unknown.

Conotruncal Abnormalities

Conotruncal abnormalities may account for more than 15% of congenital heart disease (112) and include malformation of the ventricular outflow tracts or the developing branchial arches. On the basis of animal studies in which neural crest cells have been experimentally ablated, defects in neural crest cell function/migration in the primitive contruncus are thought to be at the root of these abnormalities. Despite reports of autosomal dominant and recessive transmission (5), genetic investigation of many human conotruncal disorders has generally been limited by the impaired survival of affected individuals. With the advent of modern surgical repair of such disorders, however, improved survival of individuals affected by conotruncal malformations, including transposition of the great vessels, truncus arteriosus, and double-outlet right ventricle, has aided molecular genetic studies of these disorders, particularly velocardiofacial syndrome (VCFS) and tetralogy of Fallot.

Familial Valvular Disease

Abnormalities of the aortic, pulmonic, mitral, and pulmonic valves are common associations of a variety of complex cardiac malformation syndromes. These syndromes exhibit all modes of transmission. Examples of heritable

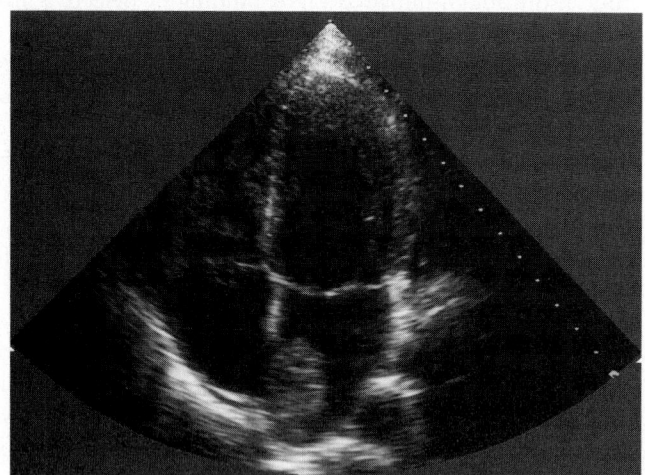

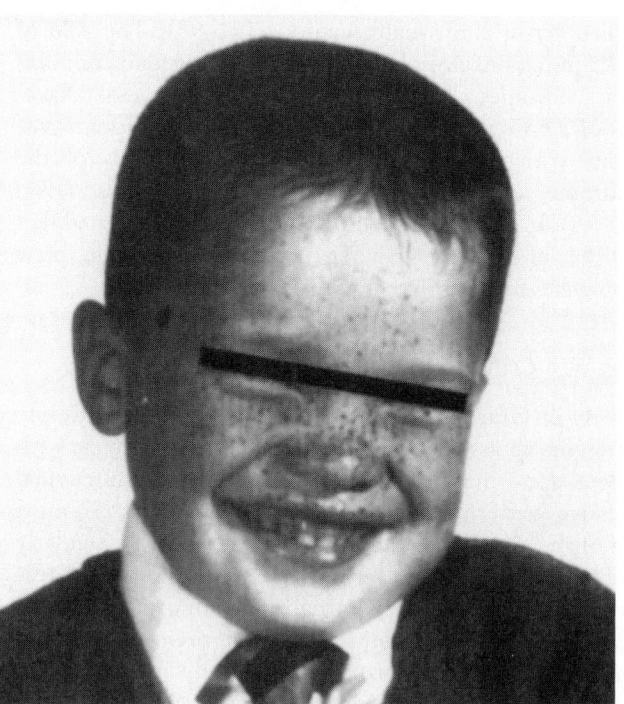

A

B

FIGURE 100.2 Cutaneous and cardiac involvement in the Carney complex. **A:** An apical four-chamber, two-dimensional echocardiographic view of the heart from an individual affected by Carney complex. Although the ventricular myocardium is structurally normal, a large mass arising from the interatrial septum can be seen in the left atrium. Histopathology of this mass after surgical removal demonstrated that it was an atrial myxoma. Cutaneous findings in this individual were similar to those seen in **B. B:** This child, a cousin of the individual illustrated in **A**, exhibits the typical cutaneous hyperpigmentation of the Carney complex. His face illustrates the excessive and atypical freckling pattern in this syndrome, including freckles on his lips. Note, as well, the large nevi on his right ear and between his right ear and right eye. In adulthood, he developed an atrial myxoma. Individuals in this family carry the haploinsufficient ΔFSterGly208 mutation in the PRKAR1α gene.

entities of which valvular abnormalities are major components are highlighted below.

Familial Cardiac Myxoma

Clinical Manifestations

Intracardiac tumors are themselves rarely evident at birth, although they may be features of complex syndromes whose signs and symptoms can be observed immediately postpartum. Intracardiac myxomas account for one-third to one-half of all primary cardiac tumors and are generally regarded as isolated benign tumors of the left atrium of middle-aged women; they are amenable to surgical resection and rarely recur or metastasize. Approximately 7% of individuals with intracardiac myxomas have a familial history of intracardiac myxoma (Fig. 100.2), and these individuals are often young and as likely to be male as female. Tumors in such individuals may occur in any cardiac chamber (although atrial involvement is more common than ventricular), may be multicentric, and frequently recur at intracardiac sites distant from the original tumor despite complete surgical resection (152,153). Moreover, familial atrial myxomas (Fig.

100.2A) usually occur as part of a complex syndrome. Previously referred to by acronyms such as *NAME* (*n*evi, *a*trial myxoma, *m*yxoid neurofibromata, *e*phelides) and *LAMB* (*l*entigines, *a*trial myxoma, *m*ucocutaneous myxoma, *b*lue nevi), these syndromes are encompassed by the eponym Carney complex. Carney complex is characterized by not only intracardiac myxomas, but also by extracardiac myxomas in the setting of lentiginosis (Fig. 100.2B) and endocrine dysfunction. This syndrome is transmitted in an autosomal dominant fashion, and although it is highly penetrant, disease manifestations are highly variable even among individuals within a given family (153). Although at least one-third of individuals will ultimately present with an intracardiac tumor, diagnosis is facilitated by the fact that almost all individuals will exhibit some abnormal form of hyperpigmentation even in infancy (154,155).

Genetic Studies

Linkage analyses (155) demonstrated that a gene defect at a locus on chromosome 17q caused Carney complex in several families. Subsequent candidate-positional cloning studies (156,157) demonstrated that mutations in the gene encoding the R1α regulatory subunit of cyclic adenosine monophosphate–dependent protein kinase A (*PRKAR1α*) cause Carney complex. All of the *PRKAR1α* mutations identified to date (156–159) result in haploinsufficiency. Although development of some tumors may be associated with loss of heterozygosity at the *PRKAR1α* locus (157), other tumors (156) maintain the wild-type allele and continue to synthesize the PRKAR1α subunit. Thus, *PRKAR1α* may function as a tumor suppressor gene in the heart, but tumorigenesis may be the result of a constitutional mutation in *PRKAR1α* along with acquired mutation of other tumor suppressor genes as has been demonstrated for the NF1 gene in neurofibromatosis (160,161).

Carney complex is likely genetically heterogeneous (158,162). A minority of families have been described in whom mutational analysis has failed to demonstrate *PRKAR1α* mutations and in which potential recombination exists between the Carney complex phenotype and the *PRKAR1α* gene. A second locus (154) has been described on chromosome 2p, but thus far, the statistical significance of this locus remains unclear. Ongoing investigation will likely identify at least one other Carney complex disease gene. In the interim, for those families in whom linkage can be demonstrated of Carney complex to chromosome 17, DNA-based testing may help identify individuals at risk for cardiac myxoma formation and who will benefit from annual surveillance echocardiography (156,163).

CARDIOMYOPATHIES: ADULT-ONSET DEFECTS OF CARDIAC STRUCTURE

Cardiomyopathies are a heterogeneous group of primary myocardial disorders characterized by impaired ventricular function. These are traditionally classified as dilated, hypertrophic, or restrictive, based on anatomic and hemodynamic features. With an estimated prevalence of 36.5 per 100,000 individuals, dilated cardiomyopathies occur most commonly (164,165) and are associated with cardiac chamber dilation and depressed ventricular contractility. Hypertrophic cardiomyopathies are defined by an increase in myocardial mass with myocyte and myofibrillar disarray and abnormalities of both diastolic and systolic function (164). Although the incidence of familial hypertrophic cardiomyopathy (FHC) is unknown, an echocardiographic survey demonstrated unexplained hypertrophy in 1 of 500 young adults (166). Restrictive cardiomyopathies are the least common of these disorders; these are characterized by normal cardiac dimensions and abnormal ventricular diastolic function with preserved systolic function.

Clinical and research efforts have demonstrated that both dilated and hypertrophic cardiomyopathies are often familial. By contrast, restrictive cardiomyopathies are rarely inherited. Familial cardiomyopathies have been reported to be inherited as autosomal (dominant or recessive), X-linked,

and matrilinear (presumably mitochondrial) disorders (167,168). Combined with recent advances in human molecular genetics, these observations have permitted significant progress toward identifying the genetic etiology of inherited cardiomyopathies. These endeavors will have a substantial impact on clinical medicine, including the immediate opportunity for accurate diagnosis. Such gene-based diagnosis also creates a scaffolding for ongoing analyses of clinical outcomes and therapies. In the future, understanding genetic mechanisms of cardiomyopathies may provide optimally targeted therapy instead of the currently available palliative therapy or cardiac transplantation. In this section, we explore in more detail current understanding of genetic etiologies of each form of cardiomyopathy and how they may relate to clinical presentation and management.

Familial Hypertrophic Cardiomyopathy

Clinical Features

FHC is an autosomal dominant disorder characterized by increased ventricular mass, hyperkinetic systolic function, and impaired diastolic relaxation. The cardiac hypertrophy found in this inherited disorder may affect either ventricle but usually involves the left ventricle and is often predominant in the interventricular septum (169,170). Histologic examination of affected myocardium reveals myocyte and myofibrillar disarray, which, if extensive, is pathognomonic (170). Symptoms of FHC are diverse and variable, including exertional dyspnea, angina pectoris, and sudden death, which can occur even in asymptomatic individuals (169). Hypertrophic cardiomyopathy is clinically significant because it is one of the most commonly recognized causes of sudden death in apparently healthy young adults (169,171,172). Hypertrophic cardiomyopathy can occur as a sporadic disease, but affected individuals can be shown to have familial disease with echocardiographic features of cardiac hypertrophy in first-degree relatives. Penetrance in familial disease is age-related, with the clinical manifestations of the disease typically developing in adolescence. In adults, penetrance may not be complete, although estimates of penetrance depend on the diagnostic criteria used. Although several studies of the natural history of FHC have demonstrated an annual mortality rate of 2% to 4% from sudden death (171), reports on ambulatory FHC patients suggest a more benign prognosis (169). The mechanism for sudden death is often unknown, and both primary arrhythmias and hemodynamic factors have been proposed. Atrial dysrhythmias, particularly fibrillation, are frequently problematic in FHC patients independent of their history of sudden death.

Physical findings (particularly a systolic murmur that increases with maneuvers that decrease preload) or ECG abnormalities (e.g., inferior Q waves and left ventricular hypertrophy) may suggest FHC. However, the mainstay of diagnosis in the adult is the observation by two-dimensional echocardiography of left ventricular hypertrophy (*e*Fig. 100.2.1) without obvious explanation (e.g., aortic stenosis or long-standing hypertension). Associated echocardiographic findings include asymmetric hypertrophy (particularly of the interventricular septum), a dynamic left ventricular outflow tract pressure gradient, and systolic anterior motion of the anterior mitral valve leaflet. With the discovery of genetic causes of hypertrophic cardiomyopathy, the natural history of disease has been expanded to include a preclinical stage. Most often this occurs in the young because hypertrophy may not develop until after adolescent growth has been completed (173). However in some adults, development of the morphologic features of disease may not be manifest until late in life. Although echocardiograms are, by definition normal throughout this preclinical stage, these individuals sometimes show ECG abnormalities.

Genetic Studies

Molecular genetic analyses have demonstrated that FHC is a disease of the sarcomere. Linkage analyses and positional cloning studies of kindreds with FHC have demonstrated that hypertrophic cardiomyopathy is a genetically heterogeneous disorder; a mutation in one of many sarcomeric genes can produce a clinically indistinguishable phenotype. To date, studies have demonstrated that mutations in genes for beta-myosin heavy chain (MHC) (chromosome 14q1) (174), cardiac troponin T (chromosome 1q31) (175), alpha-tropomyosin (chromosome 15q2) (175), myosin-binding protein C (chromosome 11p13–q13) (176), ventricular myosin regulatory light chain (chromosome 12q2) (177), ventricular myosin essential light chain (chromosome 3p) (177), cardiac actin (chromosome 15q14) (178), and titin (chromosome 2q31) (179) can all produce FHC.

Beta-cardiac MHC mutations are detected in approximately 35% to 40% of FHC patients, and extensive analyses of FHC patients have led to the identification of more than 50 mutations in the beta-cardiac MHC gene (180–182). The gene defects that cause FHC are typically family-specific—that is, unique mutations are found in different families (termed *allelic* or *intragenic heterogeneity*). All mutations are missense; the nucleotide change results in the replacement of the normally encoded amino acid with a different residue. Mutations are all localized to the globular head or head-rod junction in the molecule (183).

Different beta-cardiac MHC gene mutations appear to correlate with survival in patients with FHC (181,183,184). Several mutations have been identified that are associated with a significant risk of sudden and/or premature death (malignant mutations), whereas other mutations correlate with long-term survival (benign mutations). Kaplan-Meier curves for survival with FHC illustrate these different profiles (Fig. 100.3). For instance, near-normal survival is found in individuals with the Val606Met

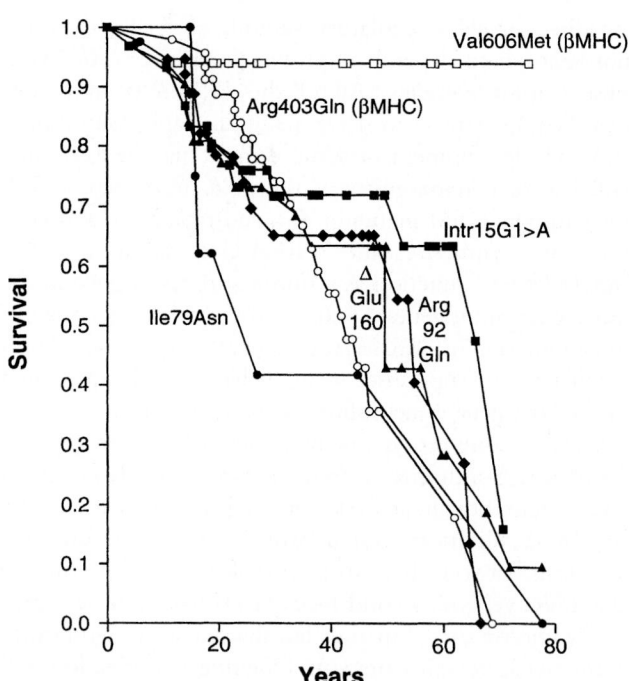

FIGURE 100.3 Kaplan-Meier product-limit curves for survival in patients with hypertrophic cardiomyopathy caused by different mutations. Survival data are plotted for all persons carrying a given mutation. The survival of individuals with hypertrophic cardiomyopathy caused by cardiac troponin T mutations [Intron 15 G₁→A (■), Ile79Asn (●), ΔGlu160 (▲), and Arg92Gln (◆)] is similar to that in persons with a malignant beta-cardiac myosin heavy chain mutation (Arg403Gln) but significantly shorter than that in persons with a benign myosin mutation (Val606Met). (*p* <.03 for the comparison with each troponin T mutation and *p* = .006 for the comparison with all troponin T mutations.) Myosin mutations are shown in ❑ and ❍. (From Watkins H, McKenna W, Thierfelder L, et al. Mutations in the genes for cardiac troponin T and alpha-tropomyosin in hypertrophic cardiomyopathy. *N Engl J Med* 1995;332:1058, with permission.)

(benign) beta-MHC mutation. In contrast, approximately half of individuals with the Arg403Gln (malignant) beta-MHC mutation are dead by age 50 years. Because there are no good clinical predictors of risk for premature death in hypertrophic cardiomyopathy, acquisition of more survival data from the full spectrum of sarcomere mutations may be extremely useful for stratifying patient risk and allowing appropriate intervention.

Despite this correlation between survival and alteration in charge of the mutated amino acid, considerable variation remains in the extent and distribution of hypertrophy even within a given family, all of whom have the same genetic basis for FHC. Recent analyses (185) of the anatomic features of FHC categorized according to different genetic etiologies have confirmed earlier work, thereby suggesting that other factors (genetic or environmental, or both) are important in modulating the hypertrophic phenotype. In addition, such factors undoubtedly also modulate the frequency of sudden death in FHC. Studies that correlate the clinical features of FHC in individuals with distinct genetic etiologies are an area of active research, and assessing various factors' impacts in light of the genetic background on which they occur will, it is hoped, improve risk stratification in patients.

In addition to beta-cardiac MHC mutations, mutations in other sarcomere components can also produce FHC (175,177,186). Defects in cardiac troponin T (175,187) and myosin-binding protein C (188,189) each account for approximately 15% of all cases of FHC. A wide range of different defects cause FHC in these genes, including missense mutations, insertions, deletions, and defects in splice signals. FHC caused by mutations in cardiac troponin T often has reduced penetrance, and the hypertrophic phenotype associated with these mutations can be subtle—that is, affected individuals appear to have modest increases in the maximum left ventricular hypertrophy (detected by echocardiography). Despite this, survival of individuals with FHC caused by cardiac troponin T mutations is often quite poor and comparable to that seen with malignant beta-cardiac MHC gene mutations. These findings suggest that genetic diagnosis may be particularly important in families with mutations in cardiac troponin T. A very different clinical profile is produced by cardiac myosin-binding protein C mutations (188,189). Hypertrophic cardiomyopathy caused by these defects can exhibit delayed expression, such that hypertrophy does not become manifest until middle age. Survival with myosin-binding protein C mutations is variable; some defects have near normal survival, whereas others have a poorer prognosis.

Other gene mutations are rarer causes of hypertrophic cardiomyopathy. Alpha-tropomyosin mutations account for approximately 5% (175), and a few mutations have been defined in the genes encoding the ventricular myosin regulatory and essential light chains (177), cardiac actin (178), and titin (179) in patients with FHC. Individuals with mutations in alpha-tropomyosin appear to have a variable presentation of FHC; severity of hypertrophy among families with unique mutations differs. Nonetheless, survival among such individuals is good, with only rare sudden death. Ongoing evaluations are needed to better assess the disease phenotype in individuals with mutations in ventricular myosin regulatory and essential light chains, cardiac actin, and titin.

Current research also centers on identification of other genetic causes of cardiac hypertrophy. For instance, clinicians have recognized an association between cardiac hypertrophy and electrical abnormalities, including Wolff-Parkinson-White syndrome and progressive atrioventricular block (190). Recent investigations (72a,190a) have established that defects in the gene encoding the gamma$_2$ regulatory subunit of AMP-activated protein kinase (*PRKAG2*) on chromosome 7q3 cause this phenotype. Although this disorder was initially felt to be a variant of hypertrophic cardiomyopathy, histopathology and biochemical features

of *PRKAG2* defects indicate this to be a novel glycogen storage disease of the heart (190b). Similarly, hypertrophic cardiomyopathy has been associated with the autosomal dominant Noonan's syndrome (craniofacial malformation, axial skeletal abnormalities, pulmonic stenosis, and hypertrophic cardiomyopathy) as well as the neuromuscular disorder Friedreich's ataxia (191). Mutations have recently been identified (192) in the novel frataxin gene on chromosome 9q from individuals with Friedreich's ataxia. At this time, however, no physiologic function has yet been ascribed to the frataxin gene, and the mechanism by which these mutations cause the cardiac manifestations of this syndrome are unclear. A hypertrophic cardiomyopathy occurs also in the context of multisystem neuromuscular disease. These disorders result from mutations in mitochondrial proteins encoded within the nuclear and mitochondrial genomes (reviewed in reference 172 and not discussed further in this chapter).

Strategies for understanding how sarcomere mutations result in cardiac hypertrophy are an avenue of active investigation. Mutated sarcomeric proteins are generally thought to produce disease via a dominant negative effect—that is, the mutated protein directly alters sarcomeric function. *In vitro* analysis of mutated myosins has suggested altered biochemical and biophysical properties of the protein. Although early data suggested that mutations in myosin caused a loss of function (193), more recent data indicate the opposite. *In vitro* analyses (194) of single molecule mechanics of Arg403Gln myosin showed supranormal actin-activated adenosine triphosphatase activity, increased generated force, and accelerated sliding with respect to actin filaments. These data indicate a gain in function resulting from this missense mutation. Ongoing evaluation of models (195–199) in which human mutations have been engineered into the mouse or rabbit genomes has helped define the physiologic and cellular consequences of FHC-causing mutations. These models also provide the opportunity to define intracellular signals and pathways that respond to perturbation in sarcomere structure or function, or both. Such data may provide a new framework for the rational design of therapeutic agents.

More immediately, the definition of distinct genetic etiologies for FHC permits gene-based diagnosis in some families. As noted, FHC is an autosomal dominant disorder that is equally inherited by men and women. Because only one mutated gene is sufficient to cause autosomal dominant diseases, 50% of the offspring of an affected individual will inherit the disease-causing mutation. In individuals for whom a sarcomere mutation has been identified, gene-based diagnosis of all family members is now possible. Gene-based diagnosis can be particularly beneficial to families with a high incidence of sudden death. Not only can this information target longitudinal evaluation to children who are genotype positive (200,201), but in addition these data can prevent unnecessary restrictions on children who are not at risk of developing FHC.

Familial Dilated Cardiomyopathies

Clinical Features

Dilated cardiomyopathy occurs as a primary disorder of the myocardium characterized by cardiac dilation (*e*Fig. 100.3.1) and impaired ventricular function or secondary to toxic, metabolic, or infectious agents (reviewed in reference 164). The incidence of dilated cardiomyopathies is approximately 37 per 100,000 individuals (164,202), and these prevalent disorders contribute substantially to overall incidence of heart failure in the United States (164,165,202). Indeed, dilated cardiomyopathy accounts for up to one-third of heart failure in individuals between the ages of 25 and 65 (164,202), and is the most common indication for heart transplantation. In addition to signs and symptoms of congestive heart failure, pericardial effusion and conduction disturbances are often observed. Thromboembolic events, syncopal episodes, and unexplained sudden death further contribute to substantial morbidity and mortality associated with dilated cardiomyopathy.

Pathologic findings also suggest that familial dilated cardiomyopathy is heterogeneous. Myocyte necrosis in the absence or presence of inflammation, fibrosis, and/or conduction system disease have all been noted (203). Cellular studies have identified a variety of physiologic defects (172,204) in dilated cardiomyopathy, including impaired sarcoplasmic reticulum calcium handling, atypical myocyte potassium currents, and autoantibodies to a variety of cardiomyocyte antigens, but have not provided a unified pathophysiologic or molecular mechanism (205). These data suggest that multiple gene defects individually or together may cause myocardial dysfunction that results in chamber dilation and dysfunction.

Genetic Studies

Primary dilated cardiomyopathy occurs as sporadic disease. Although elucidation of the initiating cause for idiopathic dilated cardiomyopathy in a single affected individual is often impossible, several studies have demonstrated that more than 25% of affected probands have an affected relative (202,206). Familial dilated cardiomyopathy can be inherited as a matrilinear, X-linked, autosomal recessive, or autosomal dominant trait (167,168). Dilated cardiomyopathy due to mitochondrial mutation is one component of multisystem disease (164); these disorders are not discussed further. Autosomal dominant transmission is the most prevalent mode of transmission that has fostered application of molecular genetic approaches to identify gene defects that cause dilated cardiomyopathy. Premature morbidity and mortality in familial dilated cardiomyopathy ini-

tially hindered genetic studies of this disorder but with advances in the genome project, issues such as small family size have become less significant obstacles. Increasingly genetic loci and disease genes have been defined. Identification of the full complement of mutations that cause familial dilated cardiomyopathy is also likely to provide insights into the causes of sporadic disease; in some instances these may be due to *de novo* mutations in genes that also cause heritable disease.

Familial dilated cardiomyopathy (5,204,206) can be associated with a variety of cardiac findings, including atrial cardiomyopathy, conduction system abnormalities (particularly AV block), valvular disease, and ventricular tachycardia. Extracardiac manifestations are sometimes present; the coexistence of subclinical or overt skeletal myopathy is particularly common (167).

Mutations in three X-linked genes cause dilated cardiomyopathy. In addition to cardiac disease, these defects cause muscular dystrophy (Duchenne's or Becker's muscular dystrophy and Emery-Dreifuss muscular dystrophy) or the complex phenotype of Barth's syndrome.

In Duchenne's/Becker's muscular dystrophy, proximal muscular atrophy is the most striking feature, but most patients will exhibit some degree of cardiac involvement (207). Ninety-five percent of Duchenne's patients will exhibit some manifestation of dilated cardiomyopathy by the end of their lives, and in many, signs and symptoms appear before the age of 6. Cardiomyopathy tends to present after puberty in Becker patients. In some Duchenne's/Becker's patients, dilated cardiomyopathy is the dominant clinical finding. These cardiomyopathies result from deletions of the 5' muscle promoter of the dystrophin gene (208). Such individuals exhibit pathologic findings of dystrophy on skeletal muscle biopsy, but may remain subclinical. A similar phenotype has been demonstrated in a recently described family with a premature stop codon and consequent dystrophin protein truncation (209). However, when the dystrophin promoter region in a large series of patients with idiopathic cardiomyopathy was examined, no mutations were identified (210). Thus, it is thought that this is a relatively rare etiology for adult-onset sporadic dilated cardiomyopathy.

Emery-Dreifuss muscular dystrophy often presents with dilated cardiomyopathy and AV conduction abnormalities in the setting of progressive skeletal muscle dysfunction and contractures. Although atrial dysrhythmias (paralysis, fibrillation, and flutter) are common, infranodal disease with slow junctional rhythms and AV block frequently causes symptoms. Mutations in the emerin gene cause this disorder (211), but the precise function of this protein as well as the contribution of emerin mutations to more common adult-onset cardiomyopathy remains unknown.

Barth's syndrome is a frequently lethal infantile disorder in which patients exhibit dilated cardiomyopathy associated with short stature and neutropenia. Although the genetic locus established by linkage analyses overlaps with the Emery-Dreifuss locus, recent positional cloning studies (212) have demonstrated that Barth's syndrome is caused by mutations in a distinct gene called *tafazzin*. Investigation of alternative splicing of tafazzin transcripts is an area of active research and may help explain the variable phenotypes in Barth's syndrome.

Autosomal dominant dilated cardiomyopathy is the most common form of hereditary primary dilated cardiomyopathy. To date, 17 distinct chromosomal loci have been reported (5) and more will likely be identified in the future. Disease genes that map to chromosomes 1q32, 2q31, 6q12–16, 9q13–q22, 14q11, and 15q14 cause isolated cardiac disease. Loci on chromosomes 1q21, 2q11–q22, 3q22–p25, 6q23, and 19q13.2 cause dilated cardiomyopathy in association with conduction system disease (5,70,213–217). Dilated cardiomyopathy that is caused by a mutated gene encoded on chromosome 10q21–q23 (216) is associated with mitral valve prolapse, whereas dilated cardiomyopathy due to mutation on chromosome 6q23–24 (218) is associated with sensorineural hearing loss. In several instances, these genomic locations have been defined by analyses of a single family, and in many instances specific gene defects have not yet been identified. In addition to the considerable variation in associated clinical manifestations, the age of onset of ventricular dilatation, systolic dysfunction, and frank heart failure can vary considerably. Early-onset disease that affects children and young adults characterizes some gene mutations, whereas others often present in middle-aged and older adults.

Conduction abnormalities are particularly prevalent in some families with autosomal dominant dilated cardiomyopathy. Individuals typically present early in life (before overt chamber dilatation) with sinoatrial node dysfunction, which may progress to supraventricular tachyarrhythmias and His-Purkinje system conduction delay. Pacemaker implantation is often required. Although mutations at three distinct loci are known to produce this phenotype, only one disease-causing gene has been identified. Mutations in the gene encoding lamin A and C isoforms (on chromosome 1q21) can cause this disease (219). Missense mutations that perturb the structure of the alpha-helical domain of these peptides usually cause dilated cardiomyopathy and conduction disease. Other mutations (missense and nonsense) in lamin can produce two different diseases, Emery-Dreifuss syndrome (220) or familial partial lipodystrophy (221). Emery-Dreifuss is a childhood-onset muscular dystrophy with contractures and adult-onset cardiac conduction abnormalities. Familial partial lipodystrophy (Dunnigan-type) is a metabolic disorder characterized by abnormal deposition of fat, insulin-resistant diabetes, and cardiac conduction system disease. The mechanisms by which distinct mutations in lamins cause these three different clinical phenotypes is unknown. Lamins are components of the nuclear envelope and may both contribute to the integrity of the nucleus; these may also participate in nuclear-cytoplasmic trafficking and in transcriptional regulation.

Dilated cardiomyopathy that occurs in isolation can be due to mutations in sarcomere protein genes. Although most mutations in these proteins cause hypertrophic cardiomyopathy, some missense mutations in cardiac actin (222) or the beta-cardiac MHC gene (223) and a deletion in cardiac troponin T (223) cause cardiac dilatation and dysfunction. Presumably these have distinct effects on the biophysical properties of the sarcomere than do mutations that result in cardiac hypertrophy. Although understanding the mechanisms by which different mutations produce these different cardiac morphologies is an area of active research, an important clinical observation came from this genetic research. The onset of cardiac failure occurs early in those individuals with dilated cardiomyopathy due to sarcomere gene mutations. Signs and symptoms of heart failure and even sudden death may present during childhood.

Arrhythmogenic Right Ventricular Dysplasia

Clinical Features

ARVD refers to a condition of progressive atrophy of the myocardium with fatty or fibrofatty tissue replacement (225–227). Although this primary myocardial disorder typically involves the right ventricle and pathologic findings are initially found there, left chamber involvement is not uncommon. The pathology can be segmental or diffuse and transmural. Right ventricular wall thickness can be normal or increased by fatty infiltration, but replacement of myocardium by fibrofatty tissue usually results in marked thinning of the right ventricular wall, often with aneurysmal dilatation. Histologic features include myocardial necrosis and focal inflammation (lymphocytic infiltrates). Pathologic specimens that demonstrate greater than 3% fat and greater than 40% fibrosis tissue have been considered pathognomonic for suggested ARVD.

Clinical recognition of the disease involves demonstration of perturbed structure and function. Endomyocardial biopsy should evidence the histopathology discussed above. Angiography and magnetic resonance imaging can be particularly helpful for defining right ventricular dilatation and/or aneurysm and diminished function (segmental or global dyskinesis/akinesis). Two-dimensional echocardiography has limited sensitivity in defining right ventricular abnormalities and may therefore be most helpful in longitudinal assessment rather than initial diagnosis. ECG findings of ARVD include right ventricular T-wave inversion, an epsilon wave, ventricular conduction delays, and ventricular tachycardia with left bundle branch block morphology (5).

Symptoms in ARVD can be absent during childhood and young adulthood, and in these ages the first manifestation of disease is often sudden death (228,229). Life-threatening arrhythmias characterize the disorder and appear to increase with disease duration. Affected adults can also develop symptoms of heart failure.

Genetics

Seven genetic loci have been mapped for autosomal dominant ARVD (230): *ARVD1* on chromosome 14q23–24 (231), *ARVD2* on 1q42–43 (232), *ARVD3* on 14q12–22 (233), *ARVD4* on 2q32.1–32.2 (234), *ARVD5* on 3p23 (235), *ARVD6* on 10p14–12 (236), and *ARVD7* on 10q22.3 (237). Recently, the ARVD2 gene has been identified as the cardiac ryanodine receptor gene (*RYR2*) (238). Tiso et al. (238) identified four missense mutations in *RYR2* in four ARVD families. The RYR2 protein induces the release of calcium from the sarcoplasmic reticulum into the cytosol and is involved in excitation-contraction coupling of myocardial cells. As discussed previously, mutations in RYR2 also cause catecholaminergic polymorphic ventricular tachycardia (62,63). Therefore, catecholaminergic polymorphic ventricular tachycardia and ARVD are allelic disorders. Other causative genes for autosomal dominant ARVD remain to be cloned or identified.

ARVD with an autosomal recessive inheritance pattern has also been reported in the setting of Naxos disease. Naxos disease was first reported in families on the Greek island of Naxos (239), and it is the triad of autosomal recessive ARVD, palmoplantar keratoderma, and woolly hair. The genetic locus for autosomal recessive ARVD (Naxos disease) was mapped to chromosome 17q21 (240). Recently, a homozygous 2-bp deletion in the plakoglobin gene was identified in patients with Naxos disease (241). The 2-bp deletion is located at the 3' end of the plakoglobin gene and causes a frameshift and creates a premature stop codon, leading to truncation of the plakoglobin protein by 56 amino acids. Plakoglobin is a major protein in the desmosomes and the intermediate junctions. Plakoglobin interacts with other desmosomal proteins, such as desmoglein I (242), and cell-cell adhesion proteins, such as E- and N-cadherin (243), linking it to the actin-based cytoskeleton. As discussed previously, mutations in the cardiac actin gene cause both dilated and hypertrophic cardiomyopathies. Thus, ARVD, dilated cardiomyopathy, and hypertrophic cardiomyopathy may share the same genetic pathogenic pathway—that is, mutations in a network of proteins in the cytoskeleton.

VASCULAR DISEASE

The vascular system is composed of four types of vessels based on anatomic and functional differences: arteries, capillaries, veins, and lymphatics. ▼▼ q19

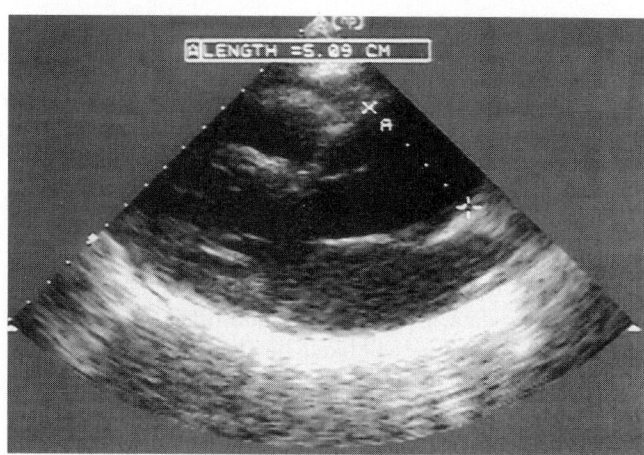

FIGURE 100.4 Aortic root dilatation in Marfan syndrome. A parasternal long-axis two-dimensional echocardiographic view of the heart from an individual affected by Marfan syndrome is shown. Note the marked dilatation of the aortic root, particularly at the sinuses of Valsalva (*dashed line*). The maximal measurement of the width of the aortic root at the sinuses in this individual was 5.09 cm.

Marfan Syndrome

MFS is an autosomal dominant disorder of fibrous connective tissue with manifestations in the cardiovascular, skeletal, and ocular systems (246). Cardiovascular features include mitral valve prolapse, mitral regurgitation, dilatation of the aortic root, and aortic regurgitation (Fig. 100.4). The major life-threatening cardiovascular complications are aneurysm of the aorta and aortic dissection (4). The gene for MFS was mapped to chromosome 15q21.1 and identified as *FBN1*, which encodes fibrillin-1, the principal component of the extracellular microfibrils (247–249). Microfibrils are present in extracellular matrices in early mammalian development and later throughout the body, which helps explain the extensive pleiotropic features of MFS. Life expectancy in MFS, which previously averaged in the third to fourth decades, has been considerably extended by a combination of advice against vigorous exertion, chronic beta-adrenergic blockade, and prophylactic aortic root repair when the diameter reaches 50 to 55 mm in the adult (250,251). More than 300 distinct mutations in *FBN1* have been found in MFS patients, but clinical utility of mutation searching is limited (252,253). Mutations in this gene also cause related conditions, such as MASS phenotype and familial aortic aneurysm (FAA) (4).

Mutations in the gene encoding fibrillin-2 (*FBN2*) on chromosome 5q23 have been identified to cause congenital contractural arachnodactyly, which shares skeletal abnormalities with MFS but is less commonly associated with cardiovascular abnormalities (254). Another gene has been mapped to chromosome 3p24.2–25 in a single family with marfanoid skeletal and vascular features (255,256).

Patent Ductus Arteriosus

Failure of the ductus arteriosus to close at birth occurs in approximately 0.05% of all full-term infants; patent ductus arteriosus comprises approximately 10% of all congenital heart defects (5). A small fraction of patent ductus arteriosus occurs in variable association with abnormal facial and hand development in the autosomal dominant Char syndrome. This condition was mapped to 6p12–p21, and the gene was recently shown to be a transcription factor, *TFAP2B*, that is expressed in neural crest cells (261).

Supravalvular Aortic Stenosis and Williams Syndrome

Supravalvular aortic stenosis is characterized by localized or diffuse congenital narrowing of the ascending aorta most pronounced just distal to the aortic valve (262). This is a common finding in Williams syndrome but can occur as an isolated autosomal dominant trait (263). In both instances, the supravalvular aortic stenosis is due to defects (often deletion) of one copy of the tropoelastin gene (*ELN*), which maps to chromosome 7q11.2 (262). Williams syndrome is characterized by infantile hypercalcemia, a face reminiscent of an elf, mental retardation but a gregarious personality, and dental abnormalities (264). The additional defects in Williams syndrome are due to deletion of genes surrounding *ELN*, making this condition a "contiguous gene deletion syndrome" (263). The cardiovascular defects in Williams syndrome, which include peripheral pulmonic stenosis, tend to be severer in males for unclear reasons (265). In both supravalvular aortic stenosis and Williams syndrome, the arterial constriction is not limited to the proximal aorta. Over time, a diffuse arteriopathy develops, which predisposes to stroke, myocardial infarction, and hypertension. The developmental impact of deletion of one *ELN* allele has been examined in mice made hemizygous at this locus. A loss of 50% of normal tropoelastin mRNA and protein was compensated by a 35% increase in the number of elastic lamellae and smooth muscle in arteries (266).

Mucocutaneous Venous Malformations

Mucocutaneous venous malformations is a vascular anomaly associated with gastrointestinal bleeding. A gene for mucocutaneous venous malformations was mapped to chromosome 9p21 and cloned (270). The mutated gene codes for the receptor kinase *TIE2*, which is expressed specifically in endothelial cells. The *TIE2* mutations caused a six- to tenfold increase in the phosphorylation activity or ligand-independent hyperphosphorylation of the receptor (270), suggesting a gain-of-function mechanism for development of venous malformations.

Lymphedema

Hereditary primary lymphedema is a developmental disorder of the lymphatic system that leads to a chronic tissue swelling resulting from deficient lymphatic drainage (5,272). A gene for hereditary lymphedema was mapped to chromosome 5q35.3 and identified (273,274). The mutated gene, the *FLT4* gene, encodes vascular endothelial growth factor receptor-3, a receptor for the vascular endothelial growth factor C (274).

An autosomal dominant condition of lymphedema of variable age of onset coupled with a double row of eyelashes (distichiasis) is due to mutations in a gene, *FOXC2*, that encodes a transcription factor (275).

Cerebral Cavernous Malformations

Cerebral cavernous malformations, or cavernous angiomas, are vascular malformations that may involve any part of the central nervous system and sometimes cause seizures, hemorrhage, or focal neurologic deficit (5). Three genetic loci for cerebral cavernous malformations have been identified: CCM1 on chromosome 7q11.2–21 (276,277), CCM2 on 7p15–13 (278), and CCM3 on 3q25.2–27 (278). The *CCM1* gene has been identified, and it encodes KRIT1, a protein that interacts with RAP1A (KREV1), which is a member of the RAS family of GTPases (279). The CCM2 and CCM3 genes remain to be identified.

Hereditary Hemorrhagic Telangiectasia

Hereditary hemorrhagic telangiectasia (HTT), or Rendu-Osler-Weber syndrome, is a vascular dysplasia leading to telangiectases and arteriovenous malformations of skin, mucosa, and viscera (the lung, liver, and brain) (5). The frequent complications of mucosal involvement are epistaxis and gastrointestinal bleeding. Two genes for HHT have been identified: the endoglin gene on chromosome 9q34.1 and the *ACVRL1* gene on 12q11–14 (280,281). The endoglin gene encodes a transforming growth factor-β binding protein, its mutations cause HHT1, which is associated with a high frequency of pulmonary arteriovenous malformations (280). The *ACVRL1* gene codes for an activin receptor–like kinase, also a transforming growth factor-β binding protein. The *ACVRL1* mutations cause HHT2, which rarely have pulmonary arteriovenous malformations (281).

CONTROVERSIES AND PERSONAL PERSPECTIVES

As increasing numbers of genes associated with cardiovascular diseases are identified, accurate adult and prenatal diagnoses of these conditions become technically feasible. Although few such tests are currently available on a routine

THE FUTURE

The genetic studies of cardiovascular disease will go through multiple phases, including disease gene identification, diagnostic genetic testing, pharmacogenomics, and therapy. We are currently at the peak of the gene discovery phase. Genes for many rare monogenic cardiovascular disorders have been identified. Study of common diseases is progressing, both in animals and in humans. Future studies will continue to identify new genes for the monogenic forms of cardiovascular diseases as well as the primary genetic causes for complex and polygenic disorders such as coronary artery disease, heart failure, and hypertension. Ultimately, genetic testing will benefit many patients by providing risk assessment and allowing implementation of medical surveillance and lifestyle planning programs to reduce risks. The novel field of pharmacogenomics has just started, and therapies based on disease gene discoveries may take an unpredictable length of time to reach and benefit patients. The completion of the sequencing of the human genome and the development of new bioinformatic tools promise rapid progress in all these four fields in the near future.

clinical basis, we can certainly anticipate commercial application of such testing in the future. In addition, although most research efforts have in the past focused on less common monogenic disorders, more recent studies have begun to identify genetic abnormalities that confer risk for common polygenic cardiovascular disorders such as hypertension and atherosclerosis. Clearly, definition of DNA-based diagnosis for both monogenic and polygenic disorders will be of great interest to patients and their physicians.

As with any clinical test, however, guidelines need to be developed for when to conduct and how to apply DNA testing. In some cases, preliminary genotype-phenotype studies have shown that certain mutations can predict an increased risk of mortality (e.g., sudden death in FHC and the beta-MHC Arg403Gln mutation) or morbidity (e.g., severe cardiac and limb malformation in Holt-Oram syndrome and *TBX5* mutations, which produce protein truncation). However, such DNA-based pre- and postnatal prognostication is limited by the variable expression of disease gene mutations; even within families that inherit "malignant" mutations, there are individuals who show minimal disease manifestations. Moreover, management options (including both currently available standard pharmacologic therapy and anticipated gene manipulation therapy) derived from DNA-based risk stratification have yet to be elucidated. Although studies (282) of at least one disease gene, huntingtin, have demonstrated that there are few significant negative psychological consequences to preclinical diagnosis, outcomes of studies demonstrating a universal benefit to such testing are not yet available.

Thus, we believe that at this time, DNA-based diagnosis should be selectively applied. Frequently, establishment of familial disease patterns by history is more than adequate for diagnosis and management when coupled with routine physical examination and imaging modalities. In fact, because a thorough family history and noninvasive evaluation may often be sufficient, they should always be carefully performed. Thorough consideration must be given to each patient's cultural, social, and financial situation, as well as his or her medical condition. In addition, before DNA-based testing, the physician should conduct a careful discussion with each patient regarding the reliability, medical risks, and clinical, social, and financial implications of both positive and negative test results and how they might have an impact on the patient's medical and personal decision making. To facilitate the appropriate application of DNA-based diagnoses, all candidate patients should be counseled both before and after testing by a physician with experience in both clinical genetics and the disease state in question.

In summary, genetic studies will have far-reaching effects on the diagnosis, treatment, and prevention of heart disease. They will lead to precise and definitive genetic diagnoses (including prenatal diagnosis), early detection of persons at high risk for disease development (even in the absence of symptoms), more rational and specific therapeutic intervention, and ultimately, prevention of many cardiovascular disorders.

ACKNOWLEDGMENTS

This work was partly supported by a Scientist Development grant from the American Heart Association National Center (QW), Grant-In-Aid from the American Heart Association Ohio-Affiliate (QW), a grant from CCF Lerner Research Institute (QW), the Fourjay Foundation Cardiovascular Research grant (QW), a Doris Duke Charitable Foundation Innovation in Clinical Research Award (QW), NIH grants HL65630 (QW), NHLBI ROI HL66214 (CTB), NHLBI ROI HL61785 (CTB), and P50HL52320 (CES), the Edward Mallinckrodt, Jr. Foundation (CTB), the March of Dimes Birth Defects Foundation (CTB), and Howard Hughes Medical Institute (CES). We apologize to those authors whose work is either not cited or is cited in review papers due to strict space limitation.

REFERENCES

1. Ewing B, Green P. Analysis of expressed sequence tags indicates 35,000 human genes. *Nat Genet* 2000;25:232–234.
2. Roest CH, Jaillon O, Bernot A, et al. Estimate of human gene number provided by genome-wide analysis using tetraodon nigroviridis DNA sequence. *Nat Genet* 2000;25:235–238.
3. Liang F, Holt I, Pertea G, et al. Gene index analysis of the human genome estimates approximately 120,000 genes. *Nat Genet* 2000;25:239–240.
4. Pyeritz RE. Marfan syndrome and other disorders. Fibrillin. In: Rimoin DL, Conner JM, Pyeritz RE, Korf B, eds. *Principles and practice of medical genetics*. New York: Churchill Livingstone, 2001 (*in press*).
5. *Online mendelian inheritance in man, OMIM TM*. Center for Medical Genetics, Johns Hopkins University (Baltimore) and National Center for Biotechnology Information, National Library of Medicine (Bethesda). 1996. URL: http://www.ncbi.nlm.nih.gov/omim.
6. Kannel WB, Cupples LA, D'Agostino RB. Sudden death risk in overt coronary heart disease: the Framingham Study. *Am Heart J* 1987;113:799–804.
7. Moodie DS. Adult congenital heart disease. *Curr Opin Cardiol* 1995;10:92–98.
8. Ward, OC. A new familial cardiac syndrome in children. *J Ir Med Assoc* 1964;54:103–106.
9. Romano C. Congenital cardiac arrhythmia. *Lancet* 1965; 1:658–659.
10. Wang Q, Bowles NE, Towbin JA. The molecular basis of long QT syndrome and prospects for therapy. *Mol Med Today* 1998;4:382–388.
11. Jervell A, Lange-Nielsen F. Congenital deafmutism, functional heart disease with prolongation of the QT interval, and sudden death. *Am Heart J* 1957;54:59–78.
12. Wang Q, Shen J, Li Z, et al. Cardiac sodium channel mutations in patients with long QT syndrome, an inherited cardiac arrhythmia. *Hum Mol Genet* 1995;4:1603–1607.
13. Vincent GM. The molecular genetics of the long QT syndrome: genes causing fainting and sudden death. *Annu Rev Med* 1998;49:263–274.
14. Schwartz PJ, Moss AJ, Vincent GM, et al. Diagnostic criteria for the long QT syndrome. An update. *Circulation* 1993;88:782–784.
15. Priori SG, Napolitano C, Giordano U, et al. Brugada syndrome and sudden cardiac death in children. *Lancet* 2000;355:808–809.
16. Wan X, Chen S, Sadeghpour A, et al. Accelerated inactivation in a mutant Na(+) channel associated with idiopathic ventricular fibrillation. *Am J Physiol* 2001;280:H354–H360.
17. Schwartz PJ, Priori SG, Dumaine R, et al. A molecular link between the sudden infant death syndrome and the long QT syndrome. *N Engl J Med* 2000;343:262–267.
18. Keating M, Atkinson D, Dunn C, et al. Linkage of a cardiac arrhythmia, the long QT syndrome, and the Harvey ras-1 gene. *Science* 1991;252:704–706.
19. Jiang C, Atkinson D, Towbin JA, et al. Two long QT syndrome loci map to chromosomes 3 and 7 with evidence for further heterogeneity. *Nat Genet* 1994;8:141–147.
20. Schott JJ, Charpentier F, Peltier S, et al. Mapping of a gene for long QT syndrome to chromosome 4q25–27. *Am J Hum Genet* 1995;57:1114–1122.
21. Schulze-Bahr E, Wang Q, Wedekind H, et al. KCNE1 mutations cause Jervell and Lange-Nielsen syndrome. *Nat Genet* 1997;17:267–268.
22. Abbott GW, Sesti F, Splawski I, et al. MiRP1 forms IKr potassium channels with HERG and is associated with cardiac arrhythmia. *Cell* 1999;97:175–187.
23. Wang Q, Curran ME, Splawski I, et al. Positional cloning of a novel potassium channel gene: KVLQT1 mutations cause cardiac arrhythmias. *Nat Genet* 1996;12:17–23.
24. Neyroud N, Tesson F, Denjoy I, et al. A novel mutation in the potassium channel gene KVLQT1 causes the Jervell and Lange-Nielsen cardioauditory syndrome. *Nat Genet* 1997;15:186–189.
25. Splawski I, Timothy KW, Vincent GM, et al. Molecular basis of the long-QT syndrome associated with deafness. *N Engl J Med* 1997;336:1562–1567.
26. Sanguinetti MC. Long QT syndrome: ionic basis and arrhythmia mechanism in long QT syndrome type 1. *J Cardiovasc Electrophysiol* 2000;11:710–712.
27. Barhanin J, Lesage F, Guillemare E, et al. K(V)LQT1 and IsK (minK) proteins associate to form the I(Ks) cardiac potassium current. *Nature* 1996;384:78–80.
28. Sanguinetti MC, Curran ME, Zou A, et al. Coassembly of K(V)LQT1 and minK (IsK) proteins to form cardiac I(Ks) potassium channel. *Nature* 1996;384:80–83.
29. Wang Q, Chen Q, Li H, et al. Molecular genetics of long QT syndrome from genes to patients. *Curr Opin Cardiol* 1997;12:310–320.
30. Wang Q, Chen Q, Towbin JA. Genetics, molecular mechanisms and management of long QT syndrome. *Ann Med* 1998;30:58–65.
31. Curran ME, Splawski I, Timothy KW, et al. A molecular basis for cardiac arrhythmia: HERG mutations cause long QT syndrome. *Cell* 1995;80:795–803.
32. Sanguinetti MC, Curran ME, Spector PS, et al. Spectrum of HERG K+-channel dysfunction in an inherited cardiac arrhythmia. *Proc Natl Acad Sci U S A* 1996;93:2208–2212.
33. Wang Q, Shen J, Splawski I, et al. SCN5A mutations associated with an inherited cardiac arrhythmia, long QT syndrome. *Cell* 1995;80:805–811.
34. Gellens ME, George AL Jr, Chen LQ, et al. Primary structure and functional expression of the human cardiac tetrodotoxin-insensitive voltage-dependent sodium channel. *Proc Natl Acad Sci U S A* 1992;89:554–558.
35. Bennett PB, Yazawa K, Makita N, et al. Molecular mechanism for an inherited cardiac arrhythmia. *Nature* 1995; 376:683–685.
36. Dumaine R, Wang Q, Keating MT, et al. Multiple mechanisms of Na+ channel–linked long-QT syndrome. *Circ Res* 1996;78:916–924.
37. Wang DW, Yazawa K, George AL, Jr., et al. Characterization of human cardiac Na+ channel mutations in the congenital long QT syndrome. *Proc Natl Acad Sci U S A* 1996;93:13200–13205.
38. Wei J, Wang DW, Alings M, et al. Congenital long-QT syndrome caused by a novel mutation in a conserved acidic domain of the cardiac Na+ channel. *Circulation* 1999;99:3165–3171.

39. Clancy CE, Rudy Y. Linking a genetic defect to its cellular phenotype in a cardiac arrhythmia. *Nature* 1999;400:566–569.

40. An RH, Wang XL, Kerem B, et al. Novel LQT-3 mutation affects Na+ channel activity through interactions between alpha- and beta1-subunits. *Circ Res* 1998;83:141–146.

41. Kambouris NG, Nuss HB, Johns DC, et al. Phenotypic characterization of a novel long-QT syndrome mutation (R1623Q) in the cardiac sodium channel. *Circulation* 1998;97:640–644.

42. Makita N, Shirai N, Nagashima M, et al. A de novo missense mutation of human cardiac Na+ channel exhibiting novel molecular mechanisms of long QT syndrome. *FEBS Lett* 1998;423:5–9.

43. Splawski I, Tristani-Firouzi M, Lehmann MH, et al. Mutations in the hminK gene cause long QT syndrome and suppress IKs function. *Nat Genet* 1997;17:338–340.

44. Bianchi L, Shen Z, Dennis AT, et al. Cellular dysfunction of LQT5-minK mutants: abnormalities of IKs, IKr and trafficking in long QT syndrome. *Hum Mol Genet* 1999;8:1499–1507.

45. Tinel N, Diochot S, Borsotto M, et al. KCNE2 confers background current characteristics to the cardiac KCNQ1 potassium channel. *EMBO J* 2000;19:6326–6330.

46. Schroeder BC, Waldegger S, Fehr S, et al. A constitutively open potassium channel formed by KCNQ1 and KCNE3. *Nature* 2000;403:196–199.

46a. Plaster NM, Tawil R, Tristani-Firouzi M, et al. Mutations in Kir2.1 cause the developmental and episodic electrical phenotypes of Anderson's syndrome. *Cell* 2001;105:511–519.

47. Splawski I, Shen J, Timothy KW, et al. Spectrum of mutations in long-QT syndrome genes. KVLQT1, HERG, SCN5A, KCNE1, and KCNE2. *Circulation* 2000;102:1178–1185.

48. Zareba W, Moss AJ, Schwartz PJ, et al. Influence of genotype on the clinical course of the long-QT syndrome. International Long-QT Syndrome Registry Research Group. *N Engl J Med* 1998;339:960–965.

49. Zhang L, Timothy KW, Vincent GM, et al. Spectrum of ST-T-wave patterns and repolarization parameters in congenital long-QT syndrome: ECG findings identify genotypes. *Circulation* 2000;102:2849–2855.

50. Schwartz PJ, Priori SG, Locati EH, et al. Long QT syndrome patients with mutations of the SCN5A and HERG genes have differential responses to Na+ channel blockade and to increases in heart rate. Implications for gene-specific therapy. *Circulation* 1995;92:3381–3386.

51. Benhorin J, Taub R, Goldmit M, et al. Effects of flecainide in patients with new SCN5A mutation: mutation-specific therapy for long-QT syndrome? *Circulation* 2000;101:1698–1706.

52. Compton SJ, Lux RL, Ramsey MR, et al. Genetically defined therapy of inherited long-QT syndrome. Correction of abnormal repolarization by potassium. *Circulation* 1996;94:1018–1022.

53. Viskin S, Belhassen B. Polymorphic ventricular tachyarrhythmias in the absence of organic heart disease: classification, differential diagnosis, and implications for therapy. *Prog Cardiovasc Dis* 1998;41:17–34.

54. Martini B, Nava A, Thiene G, et al. Ventricular fibrillation without apparent heart disease: description of six cases. *Am Heart J* 1989;118:1203–1209.

55. Brugada P, Brugada J. Right bundle branch block, persistent ST segment elevation and sudden cardiac death: a distinct clinical and electrocardiographic syndrome. A multicenter report. *J Am Coll Cardiol* 1992;20:1391–1396.

56. Chen Q, Kirsch GE, Zhang D, et al. Genetic basis and molecular mechanism for idiopathic ventricular fibrillation. *Nature* 1998;392:293–296.

57. Akai J, Makita N, Sakurada H, et al. A novel SCN5A mutation associated with idiopathic ventricular fibrillation without typical ECG findings of Brugada syndrome. *FEBS Lett* 2000;479:29–34.

58. Wan X, Wang Q, Kirsch GE. Functional suppression of sodium channels by beta(1)-subunits as a molecular mechanism of idiopathic ventricular fibrillation (in process citation). *J Mol Cell Cardiol* 2000;32:1873–1884.

59. Wang D, Makita N, Kitabatake A, et al. Enhanced Na+ channel intermediate inactivation in Brugada syndrome. *Circ Res* 2000;87:E37–E43.

60. Priori SG, Napolitano C, Gasparini M, et al. Clinical and genetic heterogeneity of right bundle branch block and ST-segment elevation syndrome: a prospective evaluation of 52 families. *Circulation* 2000;102:2509–2515.

61. Swan H, Piippo K, Viitasalo M, et al. Arrhythmic disorder mapped to chromosome 1q42–q43 causes malignant polymorphic ventricular tachycardia in structurally normal hearts. *J Am Coll Cardiol* 1999;34:2035–2042.

62. Priori SG, Napolitano C, Tiso N, et al. Mutations in the cardiac ryanodine receptor gene (hRyR2) underlie catecholaminergic polymorphic ventricular tachycardia. *Circulation* 2001;103:196–200.

63. Laitinen PJ, Brown KM, Piippo K, et al. Mutations of the cardiac ryanodine receptor (RyR2) gene in familial polymorphic ventricular tachycardia. *Circulation* 2001;103:485–490.

64. Lahat H, Eldar M, Levy-Nissenbaum E, et al. Autosomal recessive catecholamine- or exercise-induced polymorphic ventricular tachycardia: clinical features and assignment of the disease gene to chromosome 1p13-21. *Circulation* 2001;103:2822–2827.

65. Lerman BB, Dong B, Stein KM, et al. Right ventricular outflow tract tachycardia due to a somatic cell mutation in G protein subunit alpha i2. *J Clin Invest* 1998;101:2862–2868.

66. Feinberg WM, Blackshear JL, Laupacis A, et al. Prevalence, age distribution, and gender of patients with atrial fibrillation. Analysis and implications. *Arch Intern Med* 1995;155:469–473.

67. Wolf PA, Abbott RD, Kannel WB. Atrial fibrillation: a major contributor to stroke in the elderly. The Framingham Study. *Arch Intern Med* 1987;147:1561–1564.

68. Van Wagoner DR, Nerbonne JM. Molecular basis of electrical remodeling in atrial fibrillation (in process citation). *J Mol Cell Cardiol* 2000;32:1101–1117.

69. Brugada R, Tapscott T, Czernuszewicz GZ, et al. Identification of a genetic locus for familial atrial fibrillation. *N Engl J Med* 1997;336:905–911.

70. Brink PA, Ferreira A, Moolman JC, et al. Gene for progressive familial heart block type I maps to chromosome 19q13. *Circulation* 1995;91:1633–1640.

71. Kyndt F, Schott JJ, Probst V, et al. A new locus for isolated progressive cardiac conduction defect maps to 16q23–24 (abstract). *Circulation* 2001;102:II358.

72. Schott JJ, Alshinawi C, Kyndt F, et al. Cardiac conduction defects associate with mutations in SCN5A. *Nat Genet* 1999;23:20–21.

72a. Gollob MH, Green MS, Tang AS, et al. Identification of a gene responsible for familial Wolff-Parkinson-White syndrome. *N Engl J Med* 2001;344:1823–1831.

73. Olson EN, Srivastava D. Molecular pathways controlling heart development. *Science* 1996;272:671–676.

74. Roguin N, Du ZD, Barak M, et al. High prevalence of muscular ventricular septal defect in neonates. *J Am Coll Cardiol* 1995;26:1545–1548.

75. Lamy M, Dwgrouchy J, Schweisguth O. Genetic and nongenetic factors in the etiology of congenital heart disease: a study of 1188 cases. *Am J Hum Genet* 1957;9:17.

76. Brueckner M, D'Eustachio P, Horwich AL. Linkage mapping of a mouse gene, iv, that controls left-right asymmetry of the heart and viscera. *Proc Natl Acad Sci U S A* 1989;86:5035–5038.

77. Yokoyama T, Copeland NG, Jenkins NA, et al. Reversal of left-right asymmetry: a situs inversus mutation. *Science* 1993;260:679–682.

78. Moe DG, Guntheroth WG. Spontaneous closure of uncomplicated ventricular septal defect. *Am J Cardiol* 1987;60:674–678.

79. Holt M, Oram S. Familial heart disease with skeletal malformations. *Br Heart J* 1960;22:236.

80. Csaba E, Marta V, Czeizel E. Holt-Oram-syndrome. *Orvosi Hetilap* 1991;131:73.

81. Smith AT, Sack GH, Taylor GJ. Holt-Oram syndrome. *J Pediatr* 1979;95:538.

82. Basson CT, Cowley GS, Solomon SD, et al. The clinical and genetic spectrum of the Holt-Oram syndrome (heart-hand syndrome). *N Engl J Med* 1994;330:885–891.

83. Basson CT, Solomon SD, Weissman B, et al. Genetic heterogeneity of heart-hand syndromes. *Circulation* 1995;91:1326–1329.

84. Basson CT, Bachinsky DR, Lin RC, et al. Mutations in human TBX5 cause limb and cardiac malformation in Holt-Oram syndrome. *Nat Genet* 1997;15:30–35.

85. Li QY, Newbury-Ecob RA, Terrett JA, et al. Holt-Oram syndrome is caused by mutations in TBX5, a member of the Brachyury (T) gene family. *Nat Genet* 1997;15:21–29.

86. Hatcher CJ, Goldstein MM, Mah CS, et al. Identification and localization of TBX5 transcription factor during human cardiac morphogenesis. *Dev Dyn* 2000;219:90–95.

87. Hatcher CJ, Kim MS, Mah CS. TBX5 transcription factor regulates cell proliferation during cardiogenesis. *Dev Biol* 2001;230:177–188.

88. Bruneau BG, Logan M, Davis N, et al. Chamber-specific cardiac expression of Tbx5 and heart defects in Holt-Oram syndrome. *Dev Biol* 1999;211:100–108.

89. Liberatore CM, Searcy-Schrick RD, Yutzey KE. Ventricular expression of tbx5 inhibits normal heart chamber development. *Dev Biol* 2000;223:169–180.

90. Chapman DL, Garvey N, Hancock S, et al. Expression of the T-box family genes, Tbx1-Tbx5, during early mouse development. *Dev Dyn* 1996;206:379–390.

91. Basson CT, Huang T, Lin RC, et al. Different TBX5 interactions in heart and limb defined by Holt-Oram syndrome mutations. *Proc Natl Acad Sci U S A* 1999;96:2919–2924.

92. Yang J, Hu D, Xia J, et al. Three novel TBX5 mutations in Chinese patients with Holt-Oram syndrome. *Am J Med Genet* 2000;92:237–240.

93. Cross SJ, Ching YH, Li QY. The mutation spectrum in Holt-Oram syndrome. *J Med Genet* 2000;37:785.

94. Ellis RWB, van Creveld S. A syndrome characterized by ectodermal dysplasia, polydactyly, chondro-dysplasia and congenital morbus cordis: report of three cases. *Arch Dis Child* 1940;15:65.

95. Polymeropoulos MH, Ide SE, Wright M, et al. The gene for the Ellis-van Creveld syndrome is located on chromosome 4p16. *Genomics* 1996;35:1–5.

96. Ruiz-Perez VL, Ide SE, Strom TM, et al. Mutations in a new gene in Ellis-van Creveld syndrome and Weyers acrodental dysostosis. *Nat Genet* 2000;24:283–286.

97. Gandelman KY, Gibson L, Meyn MS, et al. Molecular definition of the smallest region of deletion overlap in the Wolf-Hirschhorn syndrome. *Am J Hum Genet* 1992;51:571–578.

98. Schott JJ, Benson DW, Basson CT, et al. Congenital heart disease caused by mutations in the transcription factor NKX2-5. *Science* 1998;281:108–111.

99. Benson DW, Silberbach GM, Kavanaugh-McHugh A, et al. Mutations in the cardiac transcription factor NKX2.5 affect diverse cardiac developmental pathways. *J Clin Invest* 1999;104:1567–1573.

100. Kasahara H, Lee B, Schott JJ, et al. Loss of function and inhibitory effects of human CSX/NKX2.5 homeoprotein mutations associated with congenital heart disease. *J Clin Invest* 2000;106:299–308.

101. Lyons I, Parsons LM, Hartley L, et al. Myogenic and morphogenetic defects in the heart tubes of murine embryos lacking the homeo box gene Nkx2-5. *Genes Dev* 1995;9:1654–1666.

102. Biben C, Weber R, Kesteven S, et al. Cardiac septal and valvular dysmorphogenesis in mice heterozygous for mutations in the homeobox gene Nkx2-5. *Circ Res* 2000;87:888–895.

103. Goldmuntz E, Hoes KB, Kenton ML, et al. NKX2.5 mutations in patients with tetralogy of Fallot. *Pediatr Res* 2000;47:43A.

104. Korenberg JR, Chen XN, Schipper R, et al. Down syndrome phenotypes: the consequences of chromosomal imbalance. *Proc Natl Acad Sci U S A* 1994;91:4997–5001.

105. Cousineau AJ, Lauer RM, Pierpont ME, et al. Linkage analysis of autosomal dominant atrioventricular canal defects: exclusion of chromosome 21. *Hum Genet* 1994;93:103–108.

106. Sheffield VC, Pierpont ME, Nishimura D, et al. Identification of a complex congenital heart defect susceptibility locus by using DNA pooling and shared segment analysis. *Hum Mol Genet* 1997;6:117–121.

107. Stone DL, Agarwala R, Schaffer AA, et al. Genetic and physical mapping of the McKusick-Kaufman syndrome. *Hum Mol Genet* 1998;7:475–481.

108. Stone DL, Slavotinek A, Bouffard GG, et al. Mutation of a gene encoding a putative chaperonin causes McKusick-Kaufman syndrome. *Nat Genet* 2000;25:79–82.

109. Correa-Villasenor A, Ferencz C, Boughman JA, et al. Total anomalous pulmonary venous return: familial and environmental factors. The Baltimore-Washington Infant Study Group. *Teratology* 1991;44:415–428.

110. Bleyl S, Nelson L, Odelberg SJ, et al. A gene for familial total anomalous pulmonary venous return maps to chromosome 4p13–q12. *Am J Hum Genet* 1995;56:408–415.

111. Ramer JC, Mowrey PN, Robins DB, et al. Five children with del (2)(q31q33) and one individual with dup (2)(q31q33) from a single family: review of brain, cardiac, and limb malformations. *Am J Med Genet* 1990;37:392–400.

112. Hoffman JE. Congenital heart disease: incidence and inheritance. *Pediatr Clin North Am* 1990;37:25.

113. Budarf ML, Collins J, Gong W, et al. Cloning a balanced translocation associated with DiGeorge syndrome and identification of a disrupted candidate gene. *Nat Genet* 1995;10:269–278.

114. Driscoll DA, Spinner NB, Budarf ML, et al. Deletions and microdeletions of 22q11.2 in velo-cardio-facial syndrome. *Am J Med Genet* 1992;44:261–268.

115. Driscoll DA, Salvin J, Sellinger B, et al. Prevalence of 22q11 microdeletions in DiGeorge and velocardiofacial syndromes: implications for genetic counseling and prenatal diagnosis. *J Med Genet* 1993;30:813–817.

116. Lindsay EA, Botta A, Jurecic V, et al. Congenital heart disease in mice deficient for the DiGeorge syndrome region. *Nature* 1999;401:379–383.

116a. Jerome AL, Papaioannou V. DiGeorge syndrome phenotype in mice mutant for the T-box gene, *Tbx1. Nat Genet* 2001;27:286.

116b. Lindsay EA, Vitelli F, Su H, et al. *Tbx1* haploinsufficiency in the DiGeorge syndrome region causes aortic arch defects in mice. *Nature* 2001;410:97.

116c. Merscher S, Funke B, Epstein JA, et al. *TBXl* is responsible for cardiovascular defects in Velo-Cardio-Facial/DiGeorge syndrome. *Cell* 2001;104:619.

117. Aranega A, Egea J, Alvarez L, et al. Tetralogy of Fallot produced in chick embryos by mechanical interference with cardiogenesis. *Anat Rec* 1985;213:560–565.

118. Fyler DC. Report of the New England regional infant cardiac program. *Pediatrics* 1980;65:375.

119. Takahasi K, Kido S, Hoshino K. Frequency of a 22q11 deletion in patients with conotruncal cardiac malformations: a prospective study. *Eur J Pediatr* 1995;154:878.

120. Goldmuntz E, Clark BJ, Mitchell LE, et al. Frequency of 22q11 deletions in patients with conotruncal defects. *J Am Coll Cardiol* 1998;32:492–498.

121. Schinzel A, Schmid W, Fraccaro M, et al. The "cat eye syndrome": dicentric small marker chromosome probably derived from a no. 22 (tetrasomy 22pter to q11) associated with a characteristic phenotype. Report of 11 patients and delineation of the clinical picture. *Hum Genet* 1981;57:148–158.

122. Mears AJ, Duncan AM, Budarf ML, et al. Molecular characterization of the marker chromosome associated with cat eye syndrome. *Am J Hum Genet* 1994;55:134–142.

123. Mears AJ, el Shanti H, Murray JC, et al. Minute supernumerary ring chromosome 22 associated with cat eye syndrome: further delineation of the critical region. *Am J Hum Genet* 1995;57:667–673.

124. Krantz ID, Smith R, Colliton RP, et al. Jagged1 mutations in patients ascertained with isolated congenital heart defects. *Am J Med Genet* 1999;84:56–60.

125. Eldadah ZA, Hamosh A, Biery NJ, et al. Familial tetralogy of Fallot caused by mutation in the jagged1 gene. *Hum Mol Genet* 2001;10:163–169.

126. Supp DM, Brueckner M, Potter SS. Handed asymmetry in the mouse: understanding how things go right (or left) by studying how they go wrong. *Semin Cell Dev Biol* 1998;9:77–87.

127. Supp DM, Witte DP, Potter SS, et al. Mutation of an axonemal dynein affects left-right asymmetry in inversus viscerum mice. *Nature* 1997;389:963–966.

128. Supp DM, Brueckner M, Kuehn MR, et al. Targeted deletion of the ATP binding domain of left-right dynein confirms its role in specifying development of left-right asymmetries. *Development* 1999;126:5495–5504.

129. Mochizuki T, Saijoh Y, Tsuchiya K, et al. Cloning of inv, a gene that controls left/right asymmetry and kidney development. *Nature* 1998;395:177–181.

130. Britz-Cunningham SH, Shah MM, Zuppan CW, et al. Mutations of the Connexin43 gap-junction gene in patients with heart malformations and defects of laterality. *N Engl J Med* 1995;332:1323–1329.

131. Kosaki K, Bassi MT, Kosaki R, et al. Characterization and mutation analysis of human LEFTY A and LEFTY B, homologues of murine genes implicated in left-right axis development. *Am J Hum Genet* 1999;64:712–721.

132. Kosaki R, Gebbia M, Kosaki K, et al. Left-right axis malformations associated with mutations in ACVR2B, the gene for human activin receptor type IIB. *Am J Med Genet* 1999;82:70–76.

133. Bamford RN, Roessler E, Burdine RD, et al. Loss-of-function mutations in the EGF-CFC gene CFC1 are associated with human left-right laterality defects. *Nat Genet* 2000;26:365–369.

134. Gebbia M, Ferrero GB, Pilia G, et al. X-linked situs abnormalities result from mutations in ZIC3. *Nat Genet* 1997;17:305–308.

135. Roberts WC. The congenitally bicuspid aortic valves: a study of 85 autopsy cases. *Am J Cardiol* 1970;26:72.

136. Emanuel R, Withers R, O'Brien K. Congenitally bicuspid aortic valves: clinicogenetic study of 41 families. *Br Heart J* 1978;40:1402.

137. Saenger P. Turner's syndrome. *N Engl J Med* 1996;335:1749–1754.

138. Jamieson CR, van dB, I, Brady AF, et al. Mapping a gene for Noonan syndrome to the long arm of chromosome 12. *Nat Genet* 1994;8:357–360.

138a. Tartaglia M, Mehler EL, Golberg R, et al. Mutations in *PTPNll*, encoding the protein tyrosine phosphatase SHP-2, cause Noonan syndrome. *Nat Genet* 2001 (*in press*).

139. Allanson JE, Upadhyaya M, Watson GH, et al. Watson syndrome: is it a subtype of type 1 neurofibromatosis? *J Med Genet* 1991;28:752–756.

140. Tassabehji M, Strachan T, Sharland M, et al. Tandem duplication within a neurofibromatosis type 1 (NF1) gene exon in a family with features of Watson syndrome and Noonan syndrome. *Am J Hum Genet* 1993;53:90–95.

141. Upadhyaya M, Shen M, Cherryson A, et al. Analysis of mutations at the neurofibromatosis 1 (NF1) locus. *Hum Mol Genet* 1992;1:735–740.

142. Spinner NB, Rand EB, Fortina P, et al. Cytologically balanced t(2;20) in a two-generation family with Alagille syn-

drome: cytogenetic and molecular studies. *Am J Hum Genet* 1994;55:238–243.

143. Rand EB, Spinner NB, Piccoli DA, et al. Molecular analysis of 24 Alagille syndrome families identifies a single submicroscopic deletion and further localizes the Alagille region within 20p12. *Am J Hum Genet* 1995;57:1068–1073.

144. Li L, Krantz ID, Deng Y, et al. Alagille syndrome is caused by mutations in human Jagged1, which encodes a ligand for Notch1. *Nat Genet* 1997;16:243–251.

145. Oda T, Elkahloun AG, Pike BL, et al. Mutations in the human Jagged1 gene are responsible for Alagille syndrome. *Nat Genet* 1997;16:235–242.

146. Cooper MJ, Abinader EG. Family history in assessing the risk for progression of mitral valve prolapse. Report of a kindred. *Am J Dis Child* 1981;135:647–649.

147. Strahan NV, Murphy EA, Fortuin NJ, et al. Inheritance of the mitral valve prolapse syndrome. Discussion of a three-dimensional penetrance model. *Am J Med* 1983;74:967–972.

148. Kyndt F, Schott JJ, Trochu JN, et al. Mapping of X-linked myxomatous valvular dystrophy to chromosome Xq28. *Am J Hum Genet* 1998;62:627–632.

149. Disse S, Abergel E, Berrebi A, et al. Mapping of a first locus for autosomal dominant myxomatous mitral-valve prolapse to chromosome 16p11.2–p12.1. *Am J Hum Genet* 1999;65:1242–1251.

150. Danielson GK, Maloney JD, Devloo RA. Surgical repair of Ebstein's anomaly. *Mayo Clin Proc* 1979;54:185–192.

151. Danielson GK, Driscoll DJ, Mair DD, et al. Operative treatment of Ebstein's anomaly. *J Thorac Cardiovasc Surg* 1992;104:1195–1202.

152. Carney JA, Gordon H, Carpenter PC, et al. The complex of myxomas, spotty pigmentation, and endocrine overactivity. *Medicine (Baltimore)* 1985;64:270–283.

153. McCarthy PM, Piehler JM, Schaff HV, et al. The significance of multiple, recurrent, and "complex" cardiac myxomas. *J Thorac Cardiovasc Surg* 1986;91:389–396.

154. Stratakis CA, Carney JA, Lin JP, et al. Carney complex, a familial multiple neoplasia and lentiginosis syndrome. Analysis of 11 kindreds and linkage to the short arm of chromosome 2. *J Clin Invest* 1996;97:699–705.

155. Casey M, Mah C, Merliss AD, et al. Identification of a novel genetic locus for familial cardiac myxomas and Carney complex. *Circulation* 1998;98:2560–2566.

156. Casey M, Vaughan CJ, He J, et al. Mutations in the protein kinase A R1alpha regulatory subunit cause familial cardiac myxomas and Carney complex. *J Clin Invest* 2000;106:R31–R38.

157. Kirschner LS, Carney JA, Pack SD, et al. Mutations of the gene encoding the protein kinase A type I-alpha regulatory subunit in patients with the Carney complex. *Nat Genet* 2000;26:89–92.

158. Kirschner LS, Sandrini F, Monbo J, et al. Genetic heterogeneity and spectrum of mutations of the PRKAR1A gene in patients with the Carney complex. *Hum Mol Genet* 2000;9:3037–3046.

159. Basson CT, Aretz HT. A 27 year old woman with syncope, TIA, and intracardiac masses. *N Engl J Med* 2001 (*in press*).

160. Cichowski K, Shih TS, Schmitt E, et al. Mouse models of tumor development in neurofibromatosis type 1. *Science* 1999;286:2172–2176.

161. Vogel KS, Klesse LJ, Velasco-Miguel S, et al. Mouse tumor model for neurofibromatosis type 1. *Science* 1999;286:2176–2179.

162. Basson CT, MacRae CA, Korf B, et al. Genetic heterogeneity of familial atrial myxoma syndromes (Carney complex). *Am J Cardiol* 1997;79:994–995.

163. Goldstein MM, Casey M, Carney JA, et al. Molecular genetic diagnosis of the familial myxoma syndrome (Carney complex). *Am J Med Genet* 1999;86:62–65.

164. Codd MB, Sugrue DD, Gersh BJ, et al. Epidemiology of idiopathic dilated and hypertrophic cardiomyopathy. A population-based study in Olmsted County, Minnesota, 1975–1984. *Circulation* 1989;80:564–572.

165. Cohn JN, Bristow MR, Chien KR, et al. Report of the National Heart, Lung, and Blood Institute Special Emphasis Panel on Heart Failure Research. *Circulation* 1997;95:766–770.

166. Maron BJ, Gardin JM, Flack JM, et al. Prevalence of hypertrophic cardiomyopathy in a general population of young adults. Echocardiographic analysis of 4111 subjects in the CARDIA Study. Coronary Artery Risk Development in (Young) Adults. *Circulation* 1995;92:785–789.

167. Mestroni L, Rocco C, Gregori D, et al. Familial dilated cardiomyopathy: evidence for genetic and phenotypic heterogeneity. Heart Muscle Disease Study Group. *J Am Coll Cardiol* 1999;34:181–190.

168. Grunig E, Tasman JA, Kucherer H, et al. Frequency and phenotypes of familial dilated cardiomyopathy. *J Am Coll Cardiol* 1998;31:186–194.

169. Spirito P, Chiarella F, Carratino L, et al. Clinical course and prognosis of hypertrophic cardiomyopathy in an outpatient population. *N Engl J Med* 1989;320:749–755.

170. Maron BJ, Gottdiener JS, Bonow RO, et al. Hypertrophic cardiomyopathy with unusual locations of left ventricular hypertrophy undetectable by M-mode echocardiography. Identification by wide-angle two-dimensional echocardiography. *Circulation* 1981;63:409–418.

171. McKenna W, Deanfield J, Faruqui A, et al. Prognosis in hypertrophic cardiomyopathy: role of age and clinical, electrocardiographic and hemodynamic features. *Am J Cardiol* 1981;47:532–538.

172. Kelly DP, Strauss AW. Inherited cardiomyopathies. *N Engl J Med* 1994;330:913–919.

173. Maron BJ, Spirito P, Wesley Y, et al. Development and progression of left ventricular hypertrophy in children with hypertrophic cardiomyopathy. *N Engl J Med* 1986;315:610–614.

174. Geisterfer-Lowrance AA, Kass S, Tanigawa G, et al. A molecular basis for familial hypertrophic cardiomyopathy: a beta cardiac myosin heavy chain gene missense mutation. *Cell* 1990;62:999–1006.

175. Thierfelder L, Watkins H, MacRae C, et al. Alpha-tropomyosin and cardiac troponin T mutations cause familial hypertrophic cardiomyopathy: a disease of the sarcomere. *Cell* 1994;77:701–712.

176. Watkins H, McKenna WJ, Thierfelder L, et al. Mutations in the genes for cardiac troponin T and alpha-tropomyosin in hypertrophic cardiomyopathy. *N Engl J Med* 1995;332:1058–1064.

177. Poetter K, Jiang H, Hassanzadeh S, et al. Mutations in

either the essential or regulatory light chains of myosin are associated with a rare myopathy in human heart and skeletal muscle. *Nat Genet* 1996;13:63–69.

178. Mogensen J, Klausen IC, Pedersen AK, et al. Alpha-cardiac actin is a novel disease gene in familial hypertrophic cardiomyopathy. *J Clin Invest* 1999;103:R39–R43.

179. Satoh M, Takahashi M, Sakamoto T, et al. Structural analysis of the titin gene in hypertrophic cardiomyopathy: identification of a novel disease gene. *Biochem Biophys Res Commun* 1999;262:411–417.

180. Anan R, Greve G, Thierfelder L, et al. Prognostic implications of novel beta cardiac myosin heavy chain gene mutations that cause familial hypertrophic cardiomyopathy. *J Clin Invest* 1994;93:280–285.

181. Fananapazir L, Epstein ND. Genotype-phenotype correlations in hypertrophic cardiomyopathy. Insights provided by comparisons of kindreds with distinct and identical beta-myosin heavy chain gene mutations. *Circulation* 1994;89:22–32.

182. Seidman CE, Seidman JG. Hypertrophic cardiomyopathy. In: Scriver CR, Beaudet A, Sly WS, Vogelstein B, eds. *The metabolic and molecular basis of inherited disease.* New York: McGraw-Hill, 2001.

183. Watkins H, Rosenzweig A, Hwang DS, et al. Characteristics and prognostic implications of myosin missense mutations in familial hypertrophic cardiomyopathy. *N Engl J Med* 1992;326:1108–1114.

184. Anan R, Greve G, Thierfelder L, et al. Prognostic implications of novel beta cardiac myosin heavy chain gene mutations that cause familial hypertrophic cardiomyopathy. *J Clin Invest* 1994;93:280–285.

185. Solomon SD, Wolff S, Watkins H, et al. Left ventricular hypertrophy and morphology in familial hypertrophic cardiomyopathy associated with mutations of the beta-myosin heavy chain gene. *J Am Coll Cardiol* 1993;22:498–505.

186. Roberts R, Sigwart U. New concepts in hypertrophic cardiomyopathies, part I. *Circulation* 2001;104:2113–2116.

187. Moolman JC, Corfield VA, Posen B, et al. Sudden death due to troponin T mutations. *J Am Coll Cardiol* 1997;29:549–555.

188. Niimura H, Bachinski LL, Sangwatanaroj S, et al. Mutations in the gene for cardiac myosin-binding protein C and late-onset familial hypertrophic cardiomyopathy. *N Engl J Med* 1998;338:1248–1257.

189. Yu B, French JA, Carrier L, et al. Molecular pathology of familial hypertrophic cardiomyopathy caused by mutations in the cardiac myosin binding protein C gene. *J Med Genet* 1998;35:205–210.

190. MacRae CA, Ghaisas N, Kass S, et al. Familial hypertrophic cardiomyopathy with Wolff-Parkinson-White syndrome maps to a locus on chromosome 7q3. *J Clin Invest* 1995;96:1216–1220.

190a. Blair E, Redwood C, Ashrafian H, et al. Mutations in the gamma(2) subunit of AMP-activated protein kinase cause familial hypertrophic cardiomyopathy: evidence for the central role of energy compromise in disease pathogenesis. *Hum Mol Genet* 2001;10:1215–1220.

190b. Arad M, Benson W, Perez-Atayde AR, et al. Kinase mutations cause glycogen storage disease mimicking hypertrophic cardiomyopathy. *J Clin Invest* 2001 (*in press*).

191. Casazza F, Morpurgo M. The varying evolution of Friedreich's ataxia cardiomyopathy. *Am J Cardiol* 1996;77:895–898.

192. Campuzano V, Montermini L, Molto MD, et al. Friedreich's ataxia: autosomal recessive disease caused by an intronic GAA triplet repeat expansion. *Science* 1996;271:1423–1427.

193. Cuda G, Pate E, Cooke R, et al. In vitro actin filament sliding velocities produced by mixtures of different types of myosin. *Biophys J* 1997;72:1767–1779.

194. Tyska MJ, Hayes E, Giewat M, et al. Single-molecule mechanics of R403Q cardiac myosin isolated from the mouse model of familial hypertrophic cardiomyopathy. *Circ Res* 2000;86:737–744.

195. Geisterfer-Lowrance AA, Christe M, Conner DA, et al. A mouse model of familial hypertrophic cardiomyopathy. *Science* 1996;272:731–734.

196. Yang Q, Sanbe A, Osinska H, et al. A mouse model of myosin binding protein C human familial hypertrophic cardiomyopathy. *J Clin Invest* 1998;102:1292–1300.

197. Oberst L, Zhao G, Park JT, et al. Dominant-negative effect of a mutant cardiac troponin T on cardiac structure and function in transgenic mice. *J Clin Invest* 1998;102:1498–1505.

198. Tardiff JC, Factor SM, Tompkins BD, et al. A truncated cardiac troponin T molecule in transgenic mice suggests multiple cellular mechanisms for familial hypertrophic cardiomyopathy. *J Clin Invest* 1998;101:2800–2811.

199. Marian AJ, Wu Y, Lim DS, et al. A transgenic rabbit model for human hypertrophic cardiomyopathy. *J Clin Invest* 1999;104:1683–1692.

200. Rosenzweig A, Watkins H, Hwang DS, et al. Preclinical diagnosis of familial hypertrophic cardiomyopathy by genetic analysis of blood lymphocytes. *N Engl J Med* 1991;325:1753–1760.

201. Ho CY, Lever HM, DeSanctis R, et al. Homozygous mutation in cardiac troponin T: implications for hypertrophic cardiomyopathy. *Circulation* 2000;102:1950–1955.

202. Michels VV, Moll PP, Miller FA, et al. The frequency of familial dilated cardiomyopathy in a series of patients with idiopathic dilated cardiomyopathy. *N Engl J Med* 1992;326:77–82.

203. Bharati S, Surawicz B, Vidaillet HJ Jr, et al. Familial congenital sinus rhythm anomalies: clinical and pathological correlations. *Pacing Clin Electrophysiol* 1992;15:1720–1729.

204. Dec GW, Fuster V. Idiopathic dilated cardiomyopathy. *N Engl J Med* 1994;331:1564–1575.

205. Chen J, Chien KR. Complexity in simplicity: monogenic disorders and complex cardiomyopathies. *J Clin Invest* 1999;103:1483–1485.

206. Miklos C. Familiaris dilatativ cardiomyopathia. *Orvosi Hetilap* 1990;134:507.

207. Nigro G, Comi LI, Limongelli FM, et al. Prospective study of X-linked progressive muscular dystrophy in Campania. *Muscle Nerve* 1983;6:253–262.

208. Muntoni F, Cau M, Ganau A, et al. Brief report: deletion of the dystrophin muscle-promoter region associated with X-linked dilated cardiomyopathy. *N Engl J Med* 1993;329:921–925.

209. Franz WM, Cremer M, Herrmann R, et al. X-linked dilated cardiomyopathy. Novel mutation of the dystrophin gene. *Ann N Y Acad Sci* 1995;752:470–491.

210. Michels VV, Pastores GM, Moll PP, et al. Dystrophin analysis in idiopathic dilated cardiomyopathy. *J Med Genet* 1993;30:955–957.

211. Bione S, Maestrini E, Rivella S, et al. Identification of a

novel X-linked gene responsible for Emery-Dreifuss muscular dystrophy. *Nat Genet* 1994;8:323–327.

212. Bione S, D'Adamo P, Maestrini E, et al. A novel X-linked gene, G4.5, is responsible for Barth syndrome. *Nat Genet* 1996;12:385–389.

213. Kass S, MacRae C, Graber HL, et al. A gene defect that causes conduction system disease and dilated cardiomyopathy maps to chromosome 1p1–1q1. *Nat Genet* 1994;7:546–551.

214. Durand JB, Bachinski LL, Bieling LC, et al. Localization of a gene responsible for familial dilated cardiomyopathy to chromosome 1q32. *Circulation* 1995;92:3387–3389.

215. Olson TM, Keating MT. Mapping a cardiomyopathy locus to chromosome 3p22–p25. *J Clin Invest* 1996;97:528–532.

216. Bowles KR, Gajarski R, Porter P, et al. Gene mapping of familial autosomal dominant dilated cardiomyopathy to chromosome 10q21–23. *J Clin Invest* 1996;98:1355–1360.

217. Krajinovic M, Pinamonti B, Sinagra G, et al. Linkage of familial dilated cardiomyopathy to chromosome 9. Heart Muscle Disease Study Group. *Am J Hum Genet* 1995;57:846–852.

218. Schonberger J, Levy H, Grunig E, et al. Dilated cardiomyopathy and sensorineural hearing loss: a heritable syndrome that maps to 6q23–24. *Circulation* 2000;101:1812–1818.

219. Fatkin D, MacRae C, Sasaki T, et al. Missense mutations in the rod domain of the lamin A/C gene as causes of dilated cardiomyopathy and conduction-system disease. *N Engl J Med* 1999;341:1715–1724.

220. Bonne G, Di Barletta MR, Varnous S, et al. Mutations in the gene encoding lamin A/C cause autosomal dominant Emery-Dreifuss muscular dystrophy. *Nat Genet* 1999;21:285–288.

221. Shackleton S, Lloyd DJ, Jackson SN, et al. LMNA, encoding lamin A/C, is mutated in partial lipodystrophy. *Nat Genet* 2000;24:153–156.

222. Olson TM, Michels VV, Thibodeau SN, et al. Actin mutations in dilated cardiomyopathy, a heritable form of heart failure. *Science* 1998;280:750–752.

223. Kamisago M, Sharma SD, DePalma SR, et al. Mutations in sarcomere protein genes as a cause of dilated cardiomyopathy. *N Engl J Med* 2000;343:1688–1696.

224. Aroney C, Bett N, Radford D. Familial restrictive cardiomyopathy. *Aust N Z J Med* 1988;18:877–878.

225. Angelini A, Thiene G, Boffa GM, et al. Endomyocardial biopsy in right ventricular cardiomyopathy. *Int J Cardiol* 1993;40:273–282.

226. Blake LM, Scheinman MM, Higgins CB. MR features of arrhythmogenic right ventricular dysplasia. *AJR Am J Roentgenol* 1994;162:809–812.

227. McKenna WJ, Thiene G, Nava A, et al. Diagnosis of arrhythmogenic right ventricular dysplasia/cardiomyopathy. Task Force of the Working Group Myocardial and Pericardial Disease of the European Society of Cardiology and of the Scientific Council on Cardiomyopathies of the International Society and Federation of Cardiology. *Br Heart J* 1994;71:215–218.

228. Marcus FI, Fontaine GH, Guiraudon G, et al. Right ventricular dysplasia: a report of 24 adult cases. *Circulation* 1982;65:384–398.

229. Thiene G, Nava A, Corrado D, et al. Right ventricular cardiomyopathy and sudden death in young people. *N Engl J Med* 1988;318:129–133.

230. Wang Q, Pyeritz RE. Molecular genetics of cardiovascular disease. In: Topol EJ, ed. *Textbook of cardiovascular medicine*, Vol. 3. New York: Lippincott Williams & Wilkins, 2000:1–12.

231. Rampazzo A, Nava A, Danieli GA, et al. The gene for arrhythmogenic right ventricular cardiomyopathy maps to chromosome 14q23–q24. *Hum Mol Genet* 1994;3:959–962.

232. Rampazzo A, Nava A, Erne P, et al. A new locus for arrhythmogenic right ventricular cardiomyopathy (ARVD2) maps to chromosome 1q42–q43. *Hum Mol Genet* 1995;4:2151–2154.

233. Severini GM, Krajinovic M, Pinamonti B, et al. A new locus for arrhythmogenic right ventricular dysplasia on the long arm of chromosome 14. *Genomics* 1996;31:193–200.

234. Rampazzo A, Nava A, Miorin M, et al. ARVD4, a new locus for arrhythmogenic right ventricular cardiomyopathy, maps to chromosome 2 long arm. *Genomics* 1997;45:259–263.

235. Ahmad F, Li D, Karibe A, et al. Localization of a gene responsible for arrhythmogenic right ventricular dysplasia to chromosome 3p23. *Circulation* 1998;98:2791–2795.

236. Li D, Ahmad F, Gardner MJ, et al. The locus of a novel gene responsible for arrhythmogenic right-ventricular dysplasia characterized by early onset and high penetrance maps to chromosome 10p12–p14. *Am J Hum Genet* 2000;66:148–156.

237. Melberg A, Oldfors A, Blomstrom-Lundqvist C, et al. Autosomal dominant myofibrillar myopathy with arrhythmogenic right ventricular cardiomyopathy linked to chromosome 10q. *Ann Neurol* 1999;46:684–692.

238. Tiso N, Stephan DA, Nava A, et al. Identification of mutations in the cardiac ryanodine receptor gene in families affected with arrhythmogenic right ventricular cardiomyopathy type 2 (ARVD2). *Hum Mol Genet* 2001;10:189–194.

239. Protonotarios N, Tsatsopoulou A, Patsourakos P, et al. Cardiac abnormalities in familial palmoplantar keratosis. *Br Heart J* 1986;56:321–326.

240. Coonar AS, Protonotarios N, Tsatsopoulou A, et al. Gene for arrhythmogenic right ventricular cardiomyopathy with diffuse nonepidermolytic palmoplantar keratoderma and woolly hair (Naxos disease) maps to 17q21. *Circulation* 1998;97:2049–2058.

241. McKoy G, Protonotarios N, Crosby A, et al. Identification of a deletion in plakoglobin in arrhythmogenic right ventricular cardiomyopathy with palmoplantar keratoderma and woolly hair (Naxos disease). *Lancet* 2000;355:2119–2124.

242. Mathur M, Goodwin L, Cowin P. Interactions of the cytoplasmic domain of the desmosomal cadherin Dsg1 with plakoglobin. *J Biol Chem* 1994;269:14075–14080.

243. Knudsen KA, Wheelock MJ. Plakoglobin, or an 83-kD homologue distinct from beta-catenin, interacts with E-cadherin and N-cadherin. *J Cell Biol* 1992;118:671–679.

244. Risau W. Mechanisms of angiogenesis. *Nature* 1997;386:671–674.

245. Griffioen AW, Molema G. Angiogenesis: potentials for pharmacologic intervention in the treatment of cancer, cardiovascular diseases, and chronic inflammation. *Pharmacol Rev* 2000;52:237–268.

246. De Paepe A, Devereux RB, Dietz HC, et al. Revised diagnostic criteria for the Marfan syndrome. *Am J Med Genet* 1996;62:417–426.

247. Dietz HC, Pyeritz RE. Mutations in the human gene for fibrillin-1 (FBN1) in the Marfan syndrome and related disorders. *Hum Mol Genet* 1995;4:1799–1809.

248. Pyeritz RE. The Marfan syndrome. *Annu Rev Med* 2000;51:481–510.

249. Schrijver I, Liu W, Brenn T, et al. Cysteine substitutions in epidermal growth factor-like domains of fibrillin-1: distinct effects on biochemical and clinical phenotypes. *Am J Hum Genet* 1999;65:1007–1020.

250. Shores J, Berger KR, Murphy EA, et al. Progression of aortic dilatation and the benefit of long-term beta-adrenergic blockade in Marfan's syndrome. *N Engl J Med* 1994;330:1335–1341.

251. Gott VL, Greene PS, Alejo DE, et al. Replacement of the aortic root in patients with Marfan's syndrome. *N Engl J Med* 1999;340:1307–1313.

252. Maron BJ. Cardiovascular risks to young persons on the athletic field. *Ann Intern Med* 1998;129:379–386.

253. Yuan ZR, Kohsaka T, Ikegaya T, et al. Mutational analysis of the Jagged 1 gene in Alagille syndrome families. *Hum Mol Genet* 1998;7:1363–1369.

254. Putnam EA, Zhang H, Ramirez F, et al. Fibrillin-2 (FBN2) mutations result in the Marfan-like disorder, congenital contractural arachnodactyly. *Nat Genet* 1995;11:456–458.

255. Collod G, Babron MC, Jondeau G, et al. A second locus for Marfan syndrome maps to chromosome 3p24.2–p25. *Nat Genet* 1994;8:264–268.

256. Dietz HC, Pyeritz RE. Marfan syndrome and related disorders. In: Scriver CR, Beaudet A, Sly WS, Valle D, eds. *The metabolic and molecular basis of inherited disease.* New York: McGraw-Hill, 2001.

257. Milewicz DM, Michael K, Fisher N, et al. Fibrillin-1 (FBN1) mutations in patients with thoracic aortic aneurysms. *Circulation* 1996;94:2708–2711.

258. Francke U, Berg MA, Tynan K, et al. A Gly1127Ser mutation in an EGF-like domain of the fibrillin-1 gene is a risk factor for ascending aortic aneurysm and dissection. *Am J Hum Genet* 1995;56:1287–1296.

259. Vaughan CJ, Casey M, He J, et al. Identification of a chromosome 11q23.2–q24 locus for familial aortic aneurysm disease, a genetically heterogeneous disorder. *Circulation* 2001;103:2469–2475.

260. Guo D, Hasham S, Kuang SQ, et al. Familial thoracic aortic aneurysms and dissections: genetic heterogeneity with a major locus mapping to 5q13–14. *Circulation* 2001;103:2461–2468.

261. Satoda M, Zhao F, Diaz GA, et al. Mutations in TFAP2B cause Char syndrome, a familial form of patent ductus arteriosus. *Nat Genet* 2000;25:42–46.

262. Curran ME, Atkinson DL, Ewart AK, et al. The elastin gene is disrupted by a translocation associated with supravalvular aortic stenosis. *Cell* 1993;73:159–168.

263. Ewart AK, Morris CA, Atkinson D, et al. Hemizygosity at the elastin locus in a developmental disorder, Williams syndrome. *Nat Genet* 1993;5:11–16.

264. Osborne LR. Williams-Beuren syndrome: unraveling the mysteries of a microdeletion disorder. *Mol Genet Metab* 1999;67:1–10.

265. Wessel A, Pankau R, Kececioglu D, et al. Three decades of follow-up of aortic and pulmonary vascular lesions in the Williams-Beuren syndrome. *Am J Med Genet* 1994;52:297–301.

266. Li DY, Faury G, Taylor DG, et al. Novel arterial pathology in mice and humans hemizygous for elastin. *J Clin Invest* 1998;102:1783–1787.

267. Schwatz A, Byers PH. The Ehlers-Danlos syndrome. In: Rimoin DL, Conner JM, Pyeritz RE, Korf B, eds. *Principles and practice of medical genetics.* New York: Churchill Livingston, 2001 (*in press*).

268. Pepin M, Schwarze U, Superti-Furga A, et al. Clinical and genetic features of Ehlers-Danlos syndrome type IV, the vascular type. *N Engl J Med* 2000;342:673–680.

269. Pyeritz RE. Ehlers-Danlos syndrome. *N Engl J Med* 2000;342:730–732.

270. Vikkula M, Boon LM, Carraway KL III, et al. Vascular dysmorphogenesis caused by an activating mutation in the receptor tyrosine kinase TIE2. *Cell* 1996;87:1181–1190.

271. Boon LM, Brouillard P, Irrthum A, et al. A gene for inherited cutaneous venous anomalies ("glomangiomas") localizes to chromosome 1p21–22. *Am J Hum Genet* 1999;65:125–133.

271a. Vikkula M, Brouillard P, Mulliken JB et al. Truncating mutations in the glomulin gene cause glomuvenous malformations (abstract). *Am J Hum Genet* 2001;69S:183.

272. Ferrell RE, Pyeritz RE. Hereditary disorders of the lymphatic and venous systems. In: Rimoin DL, Conner JM, Pyeritz RE, Korf B, eds. *Principles and practice of medical genetics.* New York: Churchill Livingston, 2001 (*in press*).

273. Ferrell RE, Levinson KL, Esman JH, et al. Hereditary lymphedema: evidence for linkage and genetic heterogeneity. *Hum Mol Genet* 1998;7:2073–2078.

274. Karkkainen MJ, Ferrell RE, Lawrence EC, et al. Missense mutations interfere with VEGFR-3 signalling in primary lymphoedema. *Nat Genet* 2000;25:153–159.

275. Fang J, Dagenais SL, Erickson RP, et al. Mutations in FOXC2 (MFH-1), a forkhead family transcription factor, are responsible for the hereditary lymphedema-distichiasis syndrome (in process citation). *Am J Hum Genet* 2000;67:1382–1388.

276. Dubovsky J, Zabramski JM, Kurth J, et al. A gene responsible for cavernous malformations of the brain maps to chromosome 7q. *Hum Mol Genet* 1995;4:453–458.

277. Gunel M, Awad IA, Finberg K, et al. A founder mutation as a cause of cerebral cavernous malformation in Hispanic Americans. *N Engl J Med* 1996;334:946–951.

278. Craig HD, Gunel M, Cepeda O, et al. Multilocus linkage identifies two new loci for a mendelian form of stroke, cerebral cavernous malformation, at 7p15–13 and 3q25.2–27. *Hum Mol Genet* 1998;7:1851–1858.

279. Laberge-le Couteulx S, Jung HH, Labauge P, et al. Truncating mutations in CCM1, encoding KRIT1, cause hereditary cavernous angiomas. *Nat Genet* 1999;23:189–193.

280. McAllister KA, Grogg KM, Johnson DW, et al. Endoglin, a TGF-beta binding protein of endothelial cells, is the gene for hereditary haemorrhagic telangiectasia type 1. *Nat Genet* 1994;8:345–351.

281. Johnson DW, Berg JN, Baldwin MA, et al. Mutations in the activin receptor-like kinase 1 gene in hereditary haemorrhagic telangiectasia type 2. *Nat Genet* 1996;13:189–195.

282. Wiggins S, Whyte P, Huggins M, et al. The psychological consequences of predictive testing for Huntington's disease. Canadian Collaborative Study of Predictive Testing. *N Engl J Med* 1992;327:1401–1405.

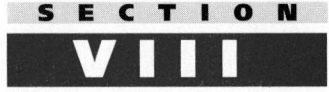

VASCULAR BIOLOGY AND MEDICINE

JEFFREY M. ISNER

THE BIOLOGY OF RESTENOSIS

ERIC VAN BELLE
CHRISTOPHE BAUTERS
JEFFREY M. ISNER

▾▾ *ADDITIONAL ELECTRONIC TOPICS*

The Early Phase: Smooth Muscle Cell Activation q20;   Hormonal Factors q21;   Mechanical Factors q22;   Proliferation and Restenosis q23;   Vessel Remodeling q24;   Effects on Vessel Remodeling q25;   Antithrombotic Effects q26;   Stent Reendothelialization q27; Brachytherapy and Thrombosis q28

OVERVIEW

Neointimal thickening, also referred to as *neointimal hyperplasia*, occurs in response to experimental arterial injury with a balloon catheter. This process, which is mainly the consequence of a growth response of the smooth muscle cells (SMCs), is maximal 1 to 4 weeks after the initial injury. It occurs in different vascular beds (coronary arteries, peripheral arteries) and in various animal species, including rats, rabbits, and pigs. A marked hyperplastic response can be observed after a single injury performed in normal vessels but also in animal models in

E. Van Belle: Department of Cardiology, Hôpital Cardiologique, Lille, France
C. Bauters: Department of Cardiology, CHRU de Lille, Lille, France
J. M. Isner: Department of Medicine/Vascular Medicine, Tufts University School of Medicine, St. Elizabeth's Medical Center, Boston, Massachusetts (Deceased)

which a first injury combined with a hypercholesterolemic diet has induced a stenosis that can then be dilated with an angioplasty balloon catheter. Neointimal formation involves the activation, proliferation, and migration of SMCs, and the production of extracellular matrix (ECM).

The factors that control neointimal thickening include growth factors, hormonal factors, and mechanical factors. Growth factors released at the site of injury play a major role in the response of SMCs to balloon injury and include platelet-derived growth factor (PDGF), basic fibroblastic growth factor (bFGF), transforming growth factor-β (TGF-β), and insulin-like growth factor-1 (IGF-1). Hormonal factors include angiotensin II, serotonin, and endothelin. Mechanical factors include trauma related to interventional devices and the mechanical events that comprise plaque rupture.

Experimental evidence is increasing that neointimal hyperplasia is not the sole mechanism leading to lumen renarrowing after angioplasty, namely, that arterial remodeling also plays a major role in this process. Studies performed in animals and human subjects have established the potential for "constrictive remodeling" to reduce vessel wall area after angioplasty, which indirectly narrows the vessel lumen and thus contributes to restenosis.

Delinquent reendothelialization has been shown to have a permissive, if not facilitatory, impact on SMC proliferation. This inverse relationship has been attributed to certain functions of the endothelium, including barrier regulation of permeability, thrombogenicity, and leukocyte adherence, as well as to growth-inhibitory molecules. More recent studies have confirmed this notion by demonstrating that administration of endothelial cell mitogens may facilitate endothelial cell regeneration, reduce neointimal thickening, and promote recovery of endothelial dysfunction after balloon injury.

Histologic findings after stent deployment in animal models and analyses of specimens retrieved from patients with in-stent restenosis have established that this complication of endovascular stents is due to intimal hyperplasia. Application of endothelial cell mitogens to promote endothelialization of the stent struts seems to reduce the thickness of the stent neointima in animal models.

Studies have also shown that endovascular brachytherapy might interfere with the various mechanisms involved in the restenosis process, and this new approach is currently under investigation in humans to treat or to prevent restenosis.

INTRODUCTION

Percutaneous transluminal coronary angioplasty (PTCA) has become a well-established technique for myocardial revascularization of patients with coronary artery disease (1–3). The use of PTCA remains limited by restenosis, however, which occurs in 30% to 60% of patients despite performance of a successful procedure (4–9). If one assumes that 500,000 PTCA procedures are performed per year in the United States (10), then more than 150,000 patients develop restenosis every year.

During the last decade, numerous agents have been used in an attempt to prevent restenosis (5,11–13). Despite positive results in animal models, no pharmacologic therapy has been found to significantly decrease the risk of restenosis in humans. These apparent discrepancies between animal models and the clinical situation were probably related mainly to an incomplete understanding of the mechanisms of restenosis in humans as well as in animal models. During the last few years, important experimental and clinical studies have allowed a better understanding of the various processes that occur after PTCA and that may lead to restenosis. The purpose of this chapter is to review the available information relevant to the response of the vascular wall to injury. The focus is on four major processes: neointimal hyperplasia, vessel remodeling, thrombosis, and endothelial regeneration. The mechanisms of these processes, as well as their relative contributions to lumen renarrowing in animals and humans, are reviewed in an attempt to reconcile results for animal models of restenosis with the clinical situation.

NEOINTIMAL HYPERPLASIA

Neointimal Hyperplasia after Experimental Arterial Injury

During the past 10 to 15 years, multiple studies have described the process of neointimal thickening—also known as *neointimal hyperplasia*—that occurs in response to experimental arterial injury with a balloon catheter (6,14–22) (Fig. 105.1). This process is due largely to growth of the SMCs and is maximal 1 to 4 weeks after the initial injury (Fig. 105.2). Neointimal thickening occurs both in coronary arteries and in peripheral arteries and is found in various animal species, including rats, rabbits, and pigs (14,22–26). A single injury performed in a normal vessel can produce a marked hyperplastic response (14,22,27). Neointimal hyperplasia is also observed in animal models fed a hypercholesterolemic diet after a first injury to induce a stenosis that can then be dilated with an angioplasty balloon catheter (double-injury model) (17,18). Neointimal formation involves several steps: SMC activation, proliferation, and migration, and the production of ECM.

Proliferation and Migration of Smooth Muscle Cells

Activation of SMCs is associated with a shift from a contractile to a synthetic phenotype (40–42) and leads to proliferation, migration, and synthesis of ECM. Proliferation of medial SMCs is evident 24 hours after experimental balloon injury and continues for at least 2 weeks (16). At least 20% to 40% of medial SMCs are activated and enter the cell cycle between 24 hours and 3 days after balloon denudation (43). *In vivo* animal studies have demonstrated the extent to which cell-cycle events are temporally coordinated after balloon injury (44). These cells then migrate to the intima through breaks in the internal elastic membrane. SMCs are observed on the luminal side of the internal elastic lamina 4 days after injury to rat arteries (14). Many of these neointimal cells continue to proliferate for several cycles, but nearly half of the migrating cells do not synthesize DNA (43). Proliferation and migration should thus be considered as two distinct mechanisms leading to neointimal thickening; as discussed later, some factors may affect

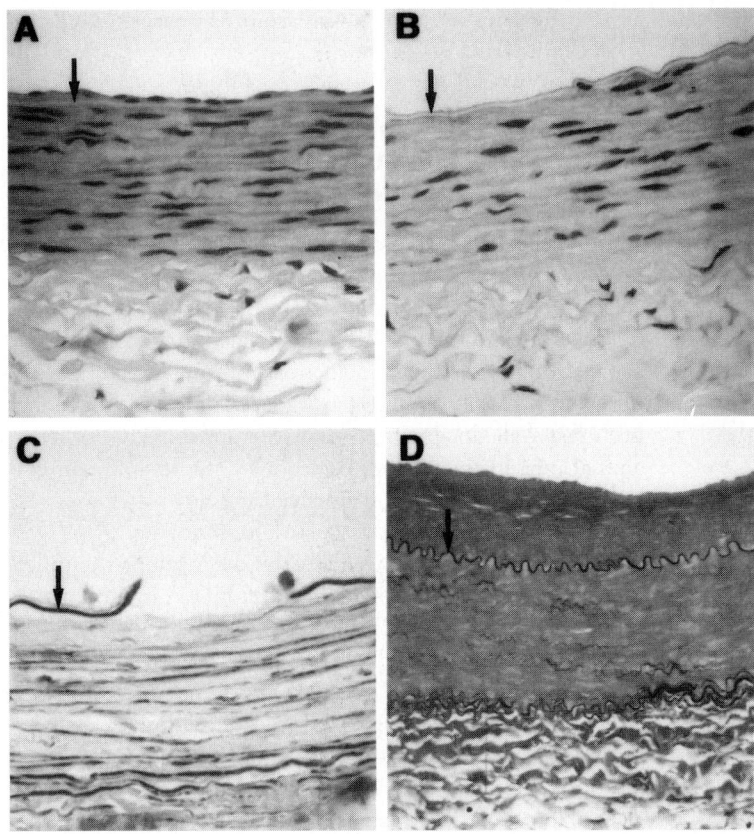

FIGURE 105.1 Experimental balloon denudation of rabbit aorta. **A:** Noninjured artery. **B:** Immediately after balloon denudation, complete deendothelialization is apparent. **C:** Immediately after balloon denudation, a break is also seen in the internal elastic membrane. **D:** Twenty-eight days after balloon denudation, neointimal thickening is observed. Arrow indicates the internal elastic lamina.

SMC migration but have no effect on SMC proliferation, and vice versa (15).

Synthesis of Extracellular Matrix

In animal models, the degree of intimal thickening is maximal after 3 months (14). The additional volume that accumulates after 2 to 4 weeks reflects the adjunctive synthesis of ECM by synthetic SMCs. Experimental balloon denudation is followed by a marked increase in expression of the genes that code for ECM proteins such as collagen and elastin in the arterial wall (45). Similarly, the reexpression of embryonic forms of fibronectin occurs in the media and adventitia of rabbit arteries 24 to 48 hours

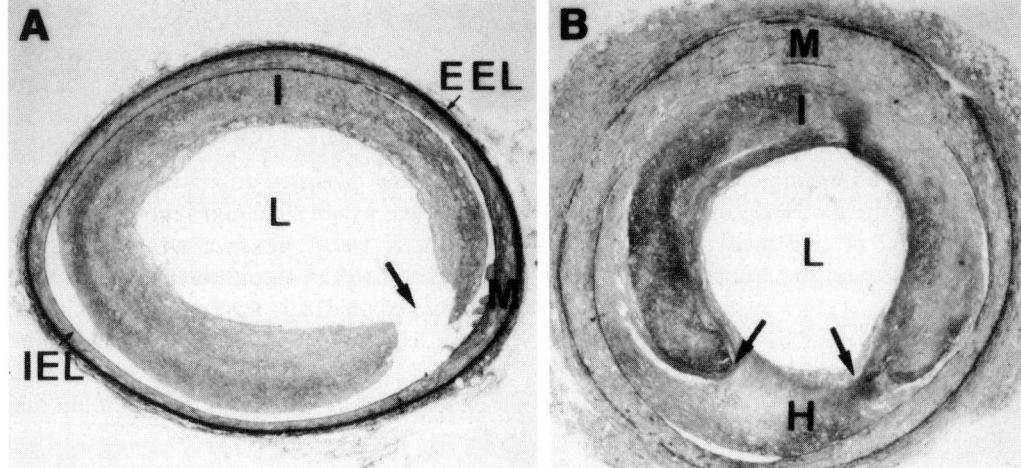

FIGURE 105.2 Experimental balloon angioplasty of an iliac artery in the hypercholesterolemic rabbit model. **A:** Immediately after balloon angioplasty, rupture (*arrow*) of the atherosclerotic lesion is seen. **B:** Twenty-eight days after balloon angioplasty, site of plaque rupture is "grouted in" by neointimal hyperplasia (H), maximal at the site of plaque rupture (elastic tissue stain). EEL, external elastic lamina; I, intima; IEL, internal elastic lamina; L, lumen; M, media.

after injury. Two weeks after balloon denudation, when the neointima is formed, fibronectin messenger RNAs (mRNAs) as well as the fibronectin protein accumulate in the luminal layers of the neointima (46). Fibronectin, as well as other matrix constituents characterized by the presence of an RGD amino acid sequence such as osteopontin (47) and vitronectin, is likely to facilitate SMC migration by interaction with certain integrins expressed by activated SMCs (48). As pointed out by Schwartz et al. (49), cellular components constitute only approximately 11% of neointimal volume, and the remainder is ECM. After 2 to 3 months, SMCs return to a contractile phenotype, and no further significant increase in intimal thickening occurs (50).

Potential Regulators of Neointimal Formation

Although the process of neointimal formation has been relatively well described, the factors that control it are still under intense investigation. The candidates for this regulation include growth factors, hormonal factors, and mechanical factors.

Growth Factors

Growth factors released at the site of injury play a major role in the response of SMCs to balloon injury. Platelets are an important source of PDGF, but endothelial cells, macrophages, and SMCs may themselves secrete PDGF after arterial injury (40,51–53). PDGF may be critical for SMC migration from media to intima; however, its absence does not limit SMC proliferation (23,54). Indeed, using an antibody to PDGF, Ferns et al. (54) were able to reduce neointimal SMC accumulation after experimental angioplasty without affecting mitogenic activity.

Basic fibroblast growth factor, an *in vivo* angiogenic factor (55) that is mitogenic for SMCs as well as endothelial cells through specific receptors (56,57), may also play a role in restenosis. SMCs within the tunica media, when damaged by an oversized balloon, may release bFGF due to stretch or crush injury. The liberated bFGF can then mediate the initial wave of cell division within this layer of the blood vessel. Infusion of an antibody that neutralizes bFGF reduces the first cycle of SMC replication by up to 80% in the arterial media after balloon denudation but has no effect on the resulting neointimal thickening (58).

Additional growth factors that have been implicated in the development of restenosis include TGF-β and IGF-1. TGF-β mRNA is increased in SMCs after arterial wall injury and reaches a maximum before the phase of ECM synthesis (59,60). TGF-β is known to modulate fibronectin expression (61) and may be important in the control of ECM synthesis (62,63). TGF-β is produced by SMCs, platelets, and endothelial cells (51,64). The main source of IGF-1 is SMCs, and its mRNA expres-

sion undergoes a tenfold increase in the weeks after balloon denudation (65).

Neointimal Formation after Percutaneous Transluminal Coronary Angioplasty in Humans

An important issue is to determine whether evidence for certain pathophysiologic mechanisms of restenosis demonstrated in experimental models can be supported by clinical observations in humans. Although angiographic studies have exhaustively detailed the incidence and time course of restenosis after PTCA, the arterial wall response in humans has been less well documented than responses in experimental animal models. Nevertheless, necropsy studies and contemporary diagnostic tools of invasive cardiology such as directional atherectomy, intravascular ultrasonography (IVUS), and angioscopy have allowed a better description and understanding of neointimal formation after PTCA in humans.

Apoptosis and Restenosis

Previous studies have suggested that development of restenosis represents the net outcome of SMC proliferation and programmed cell death, or apoptosis (103–105a), and that cellular proliferation is associated with apoptosis rates that are higher than those observed in primary lesions; this is true for coronary as well as peripheral vascular sites (104) (Fig. 105.3).

The possibility, if not the likelihood, exists that proliferation and apoptosis are temporally dissociated. Specifically, the contribution of SMC proliferation to the genesis of the restenotic lesion may peak relatively early after angioplasty, as has been repeatedly demonstrated in various animal models (106–112) studied at early time points seldom sampled in human subjects. Apoptosis, in contrast, may become more frequently recognizable at a later time. This latter concept is in fact consistent with previous animal studies reported by Clowes et al. (113) in the balloon-injured rat carotid artery. They found that proliferative activity of vascular SMCs, as determined by use of tritiated thymidine, persisted at relatively high levels (3.8%) for up to 12 weeks after balloon injury. Total arterial SMC content at 12 weeks, however, was unchanged from that measured at 2 weeks. In the absence of cell death, Clowes et al. calculated that this level of ongoing proliferation should have led to a 36% increase in cell number. Because this increase was not observed, they made the clairvoyant deduction that "cell death must account for our finding."

Extracellular Matrix and Restenosis

Although vascular SMC proliferation and the resulting hypercellular nature of the fibroproliferative tissue have been the focus of most studies of restenosis, it is the ECM

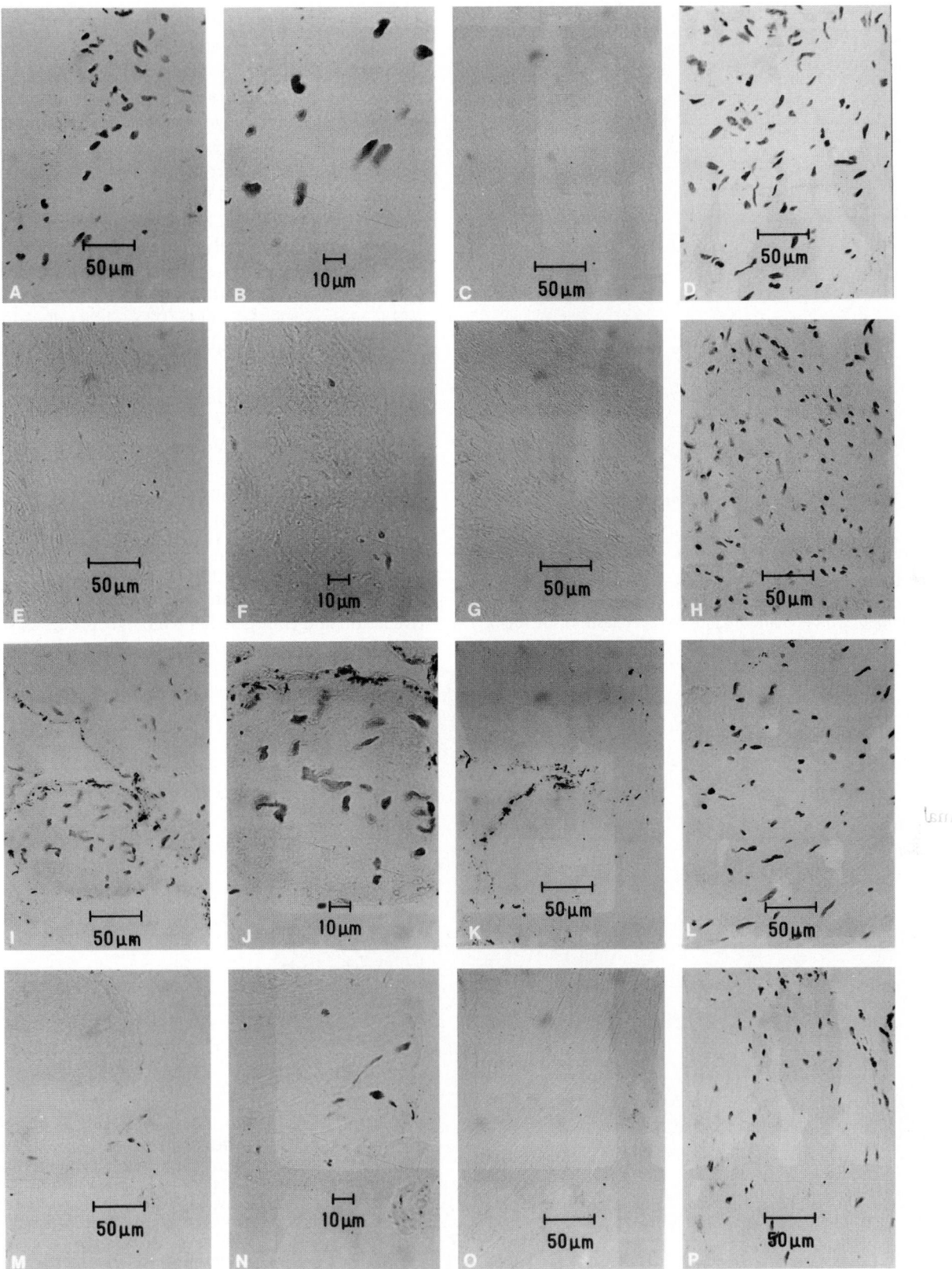

FIGURE 105.3 Apoptosis in human vascular lesions retrieved by directional atherectomy and identified by immunostaining of primary atherosclerosis. This composite photograph illustrates the use of terminal deoxytransferase (TdT)–mediated deoxyuridine 5-triphosphate–biotin nick end labeling to immunostain sections from specimens representative of the four groups of lesions studied: peripheral restenosis **(A–D)**, peripheral primary **(E–H)**, coronary restenosis **(I–L)**, and coronary primary **(M–P)**. Negative control was incubated in the absence of the TdT enzyme. One section of each tissue was processed as a positive control by pretreatment with deoxyribonuclease.

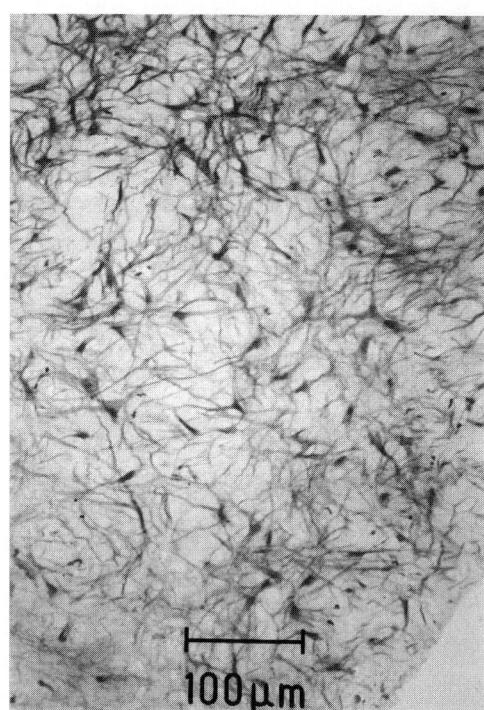

FIGURE 105.4 Restenosis specimen with abundant extracellular matrix. Note characteristic light-hued area in which are embedded stellate-shaped, synthetic smooth muscle cells (elastic tissue stain).

that in fact accounts for the bulk volume of these lesions (Fig. 105.4). Together with activated SMCs, ECM having a distinctively lighter hue on histochemical staining comprises the classic restenotic focus (114). Various collagen subtypes and proteoglycans have been demonstrated to comprise the ECM of atherectomy specimens (115), and certain constituents, particularly collagen, are derived from adventitial fibroblasts (116). The contribution of two proteoglycans in particular, biglycan and decorin (Fig. 105.5), known to be differentially modulated during ECM elaboration and differentially regulated by TGF-β_1 (Fig. 105.6), have been found to be differentially distributed in primary versus restenotic lesions (115). Extracellular deposits of biglycan were found to be characteristic of the loose, rich ECM typical of restenosis, whereas staining for decorin was limited to weak staining intensity in the more compact transition zone between loose ECM and dense connective tissue typical of advanced lesions composed of hypocellular fibrous plaque. More recently, the glycosaminoglycan hyaluronic acid (Fig. 105.7) has been shown to be a characteristic constituent of the loose myxoid ECM of human restenotic arteries (117). The presence of hyaluronic acid may be a marker for an initial phase of the ECM remodeling that occurs during the development of a fibroproliferative lesion and could facilitate biologic processes such as cell

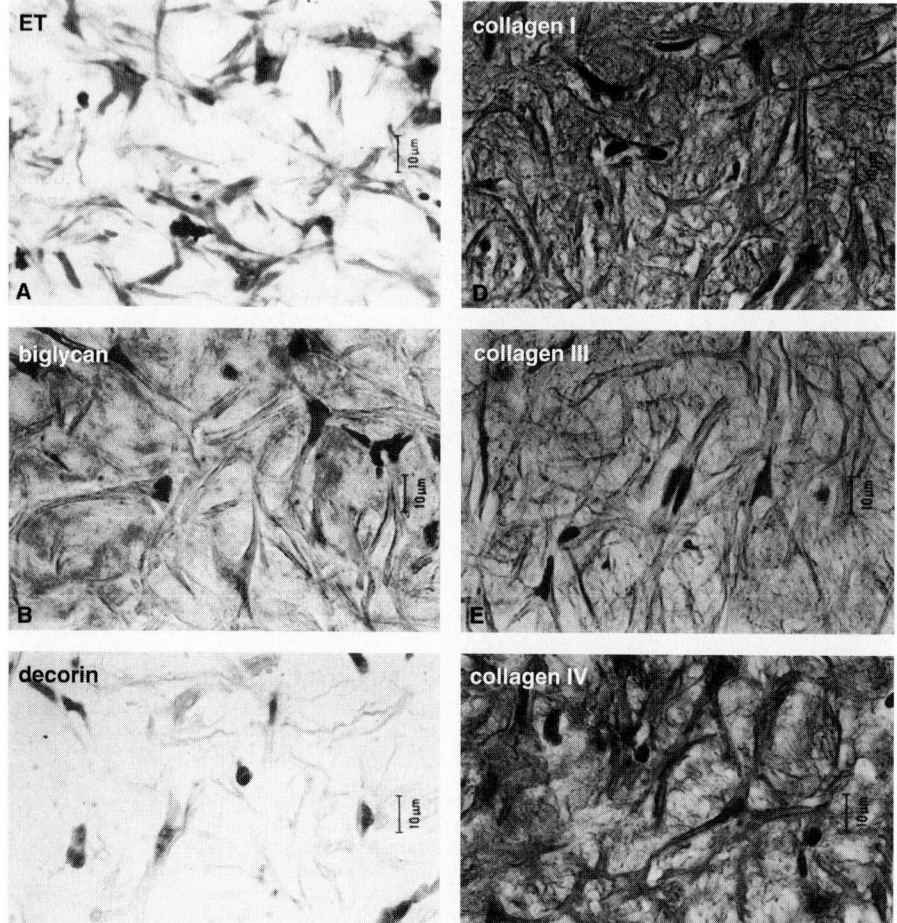

FIGURE 105.5 High-magnification photomicrographs taken from serial sections of a restenotic lesion (6 months after angioplasty) showing a fibroproliferative focus. Stellate-shaped α-actin–positive smooth muscle cells (not shown) are embedded in a loose extracellular matrix (elastic tissue trichrome stain) **(A)**. Immunostaining shows disseminated biglycan deposits **(B)**, no decorin **(C)**, and a loose network of collagen type I **(D)** and type III **(E)**. Staining for collagen type IV **(F)**, although also present in an interstitial distribution, is most intense around the perimeter of the cells.

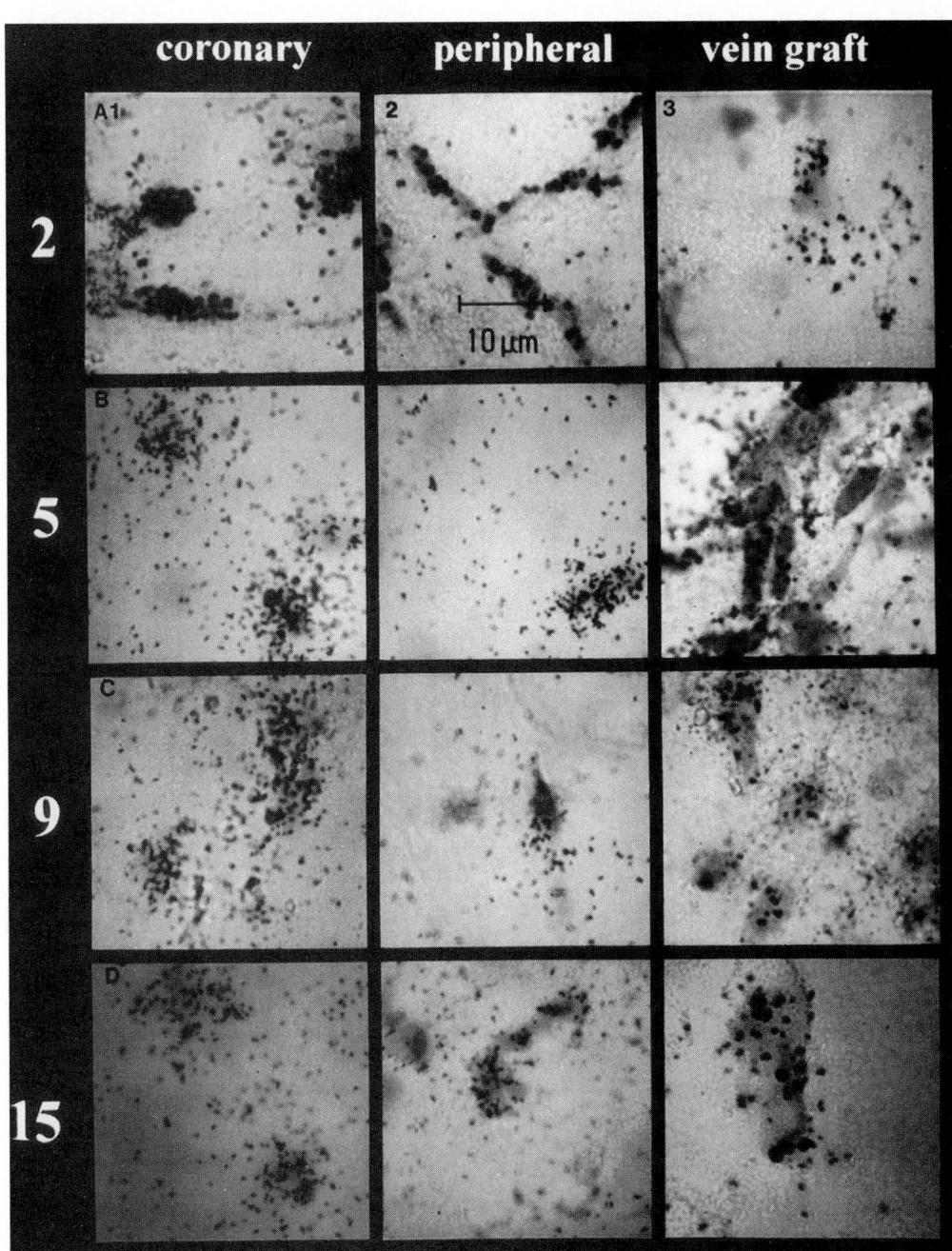

FIGURE 105.6 *In situ* hybridization performed on specimens retrieved by directional atherectomy from restenotic lesions in coronary and peripheral arteries and vein grafts. Numbers on the left refer to the time interval (months) between previous intervention and atherectomy procedure. Dark black silver grains overlying smooth muscle cells denote messenger RNA for transforming growth factor-β.

migration. Furthermore, because hyaluronic acid is heavily hydrated, the proposal has been made that (a) this hydrated feature of restenotic lesions may be responsible for the distinctive hue of the restenotic lesion; and (b) gradual loss of water or replacement of hyaluronan by collagen, or both, converts the restenotic lesion into a compact scar, with the resulting cicatrization then pulling in the arterial wall, which leads to constrictive remodeling (Fig. 105.8).

Angioscopic Findings

Evidence for neointimal formation after PTCA in humans can also be obtained from angioscopic studies (118,119) (Fig. 105.9). Although the angioscopic appearance of a pri-

mary lesion is extremely variable in terms of color, shape, and presence of superimposed thrombus, the angioscopic appearance of a lesion that was dilated a few months earlier is almost unvaryingly that of a stable smooth white plaque without thrombus (119). These differences reflect the magnitude of the changes occurring at the lesion site during the months after PTCA. The smooth concentric white aspect of the plaque is likely to be a consequence of neointimal hyperplasia that leads to a remodeling of the inner part of the vessel. Interestingly, this angioscopic aspect is not limited to restenotic lesions (greater than 50% stenosis by angiography) but is also observed in vessels that are widely patent at 6-month angiographic follow-up. This suggests that a significant healing process of the inner part of the

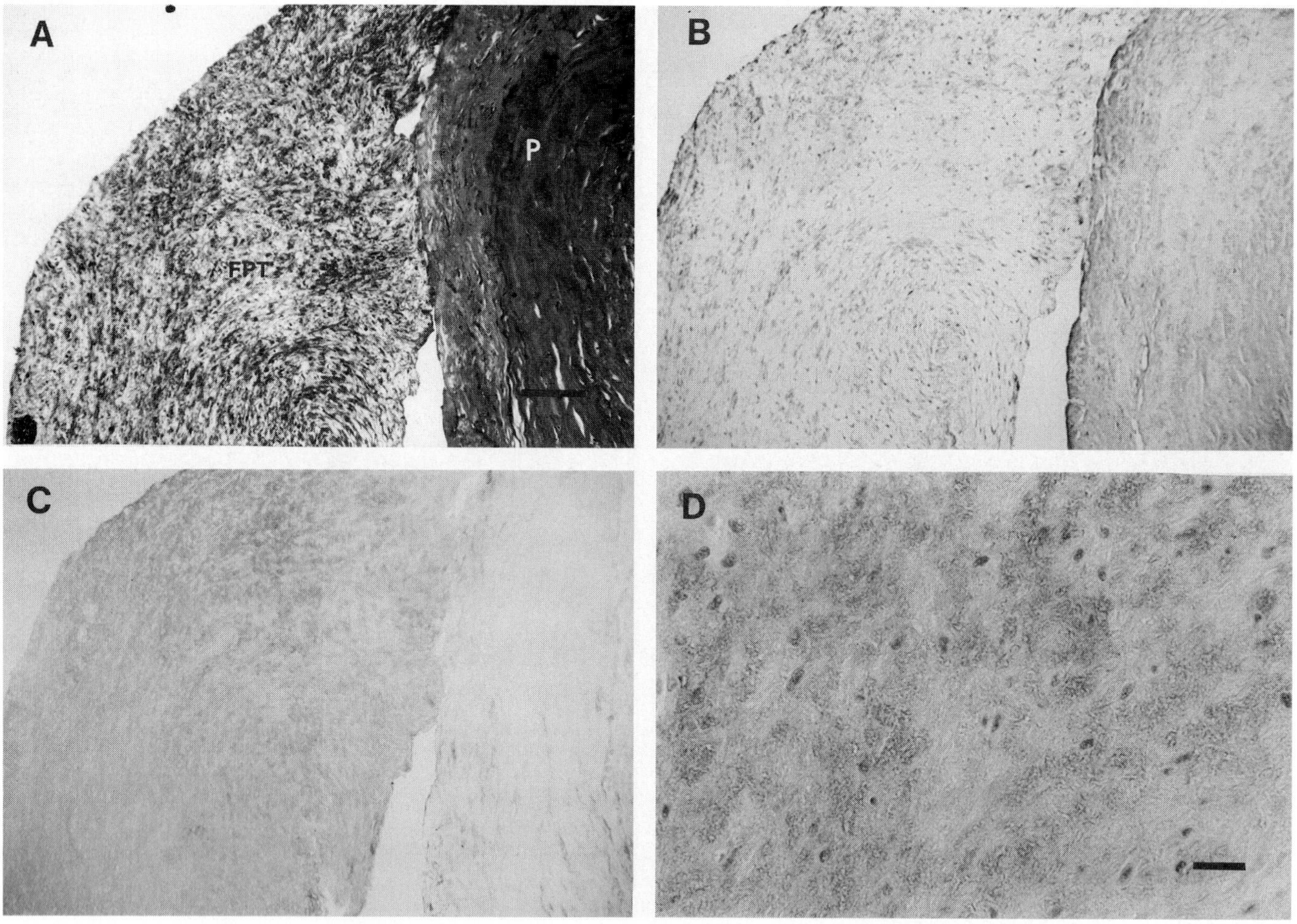

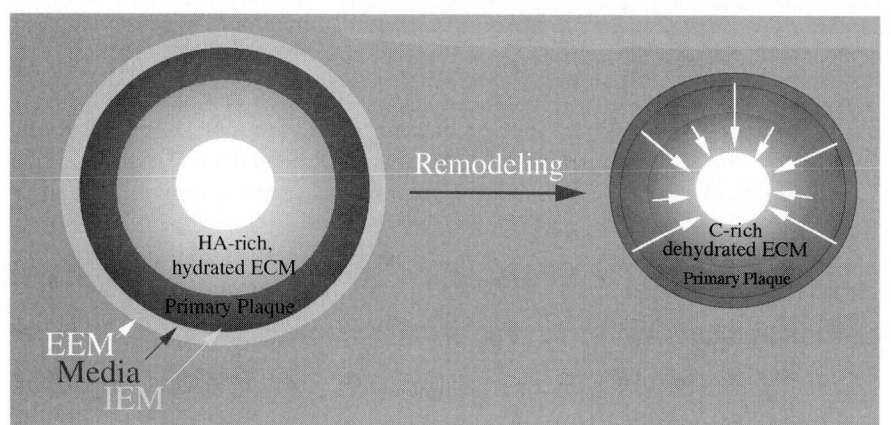

FIGURE 105.7   A: Low magnification of the elastic tissue trichrome staining of a restenotic lesion retrieved 7 months after angioplasty. A large restenotic focus (fibroproliferative tissue, FPT) is clearly demarcated from dense, compact matrix typical of primary plaque (*P*) (bar = 10 μm). **B:** In this adjacent section, the restenotic focus shows patchy staining for collagen type III, whereas collagen staining in areas of primary plaque is much more homogeneous. **C:** Staining for hyaluronic acid (HA) is inversely related to that for collagen, with dense, homogeneous staining for HA in the restenotic regions and only focal deposits of HA in primary plaque. **D:** High-power view of restenotic portion of previous specimen, double-stained for HA and proliferating-cell nuclear antigen (PCNA). The numerous PCNA-positive smooth muscle cells in this tissue are surrounded by an HA-rich matrix (bar = 10 μm).

FIGURE 105.8 As hyaluronic acid (HA), heavily hydrated, is replaced by collagen (C), resulting dehydration of the extracellular matrix (ECM) may exert a cicatrizing effect on the arterial wall, retracting the dimensions of the artery wall, much as a contracting scar pulls in skin. This process is proposed to contribute to constrictive remodeling of the vessel wall. EEM, external elastic membrane; IEM, internal elastic membrane.

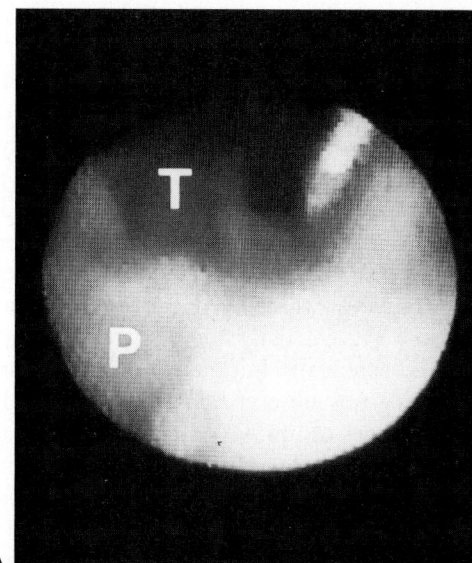

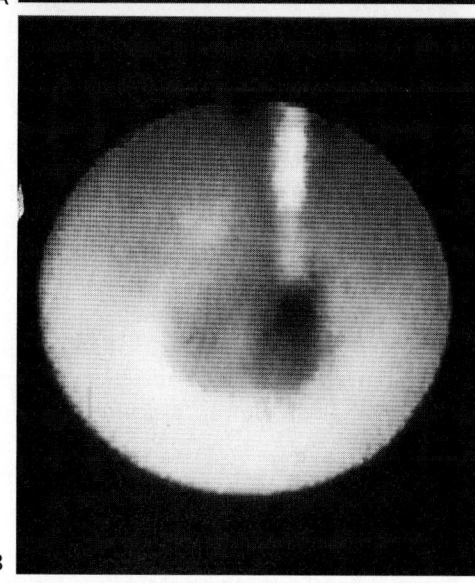

FIGURE 105.9 Serial images before angioplasty and 6 months after angioplasty. **A:** Angioscopic appearance of a lesion before angioplasty in a patient with unstable angina discloses a yellow plaque (*P*) with a superimposed red thrombus (*T*). **B:** Angioscopy of the same lesion 6 months after successful angioplasty; angioscopy now discloses a white, smooth, concentric lesion without thrombus.

vessel (probably related to neointimal hyperplasia) may occur without deleterious effects in terms of lumen size.

THROMBOSIS

Immediately after experimental balloon injury, endothelial denudation induces platelet adhesion and aggregation, which results in release of the constituents of their alpha granules within a few minutes (6,23). Numerous mitogenic substances, including PDGF, are thus released at the site of injury and may be involved in the process of SMC activation (130). Experiments performed in thrombocytopenic

animals have demonstrated the fundamental role of platelets in determining the extent of neointimal thickening after arterial injury (131). Experiments involving a canine model of endothelial injury have demonstrated that the intensity of cyclic flow variations related to platelet accumulation constitutes a major determinant of neointimal thickening (132). Thrombocytopenia has been shown to inhibit migration of activated SMCs from the media to the intima but to have no effect on the initial cycle of cell proliferation (23). Coagulation proteins such as thrombin may also be implicated in the response of SMCs (133). Thrombin has mitogenic properties for SMCs (134) and has been demonstrated to induce multiple growth-related signals in SMCs, including the expression of the c-*fos* protooncogenes (135). Finally, the volume of thrombus at the PTCA site may also play a role in the subsequent restenosis process; Schwartz et al. (49), based on observations made in the porcine coronary injury model, proposed that the volume of intracoronary thrombus resulting from PTCA may serve as a scaffold that determines the subsequent volume of neointima.

Clinical studies have suggested that thrombus formation may play a role in restenosis after PTCA in humans. The contribution of thrombosis to lumen renarrowing may be especially marked when PTCA is indicated for an unstable coronary syndrome. High restenosis rates have been observed, for example, in patients in whom angioplasty was performed at an infarct-related lesion (136,137) or in patients with severe unstable angina (138,139). The impact of local versus systemic factors on restenosis after PTCA of patients with unstable angina was studied (139). To assess these factors, a group of patients was identified who had unstable angina with a clearly defined culprit lesion and who underwent successful double-vessel angioplasty during a single catheterization session. Using quantitative angiography, the incidence of restenosis at culprit and nonculprit lesions was compared. The late loss at culprit lesions (0.87 ± 0.75 mm) was significantly greater than the equivalent value for nonculprit lesions (0.33 ± 0.69 mm; $p < .01$). Restenosis occurred at 67% of culprit lesions and at 32% of nonculprit lesions ($p < .01$). These results suggest that the increased rate of restenosis in patients with unstable angina predominantly reflects the influence of local lesion-related factors.

Because the pathophysiology of unstable angina or acute myocardial infarction, or both, involves episodes of plaque rupture associated with platelet aggregation and thrombus formation (140–142), studies have been designed to examine the relationship between thrombus and restenosis (118,143). Coronary angioscopy is to date the reference technique for the detection of intracoronary thrombus in humans. More than 50% of the thrombi detected by angioscopy are not detected by angiography (144,145). Ninety-nine consecutively treated patients who underwent coronary angioscopy before and immediately after a successful PTCA procedure and who had angiographic follow-up 6 months later were studied (118). To assess the role of an angioscopically visible thrombus at the PTCA site on the risk of restenosis, patients were classified into three groups: no thrombus, lining thrombus, and protruding thrombus. An angioscopic protruding thrombus at the PTCA site was associated with significantly greater loss in luminal diameter (late loss: no thrombus, 0.47 ± 0.52 mm; lining thrombus, 0.59 ± 0.67 mm; protruding thrombus, 1.07 ± 0.77 mm; p <.05). The restenosis rate (greater than 50% stenosis at follow-up) was also higher in the case of an angioscopic protruding thrombus (no thrombus, 38%; lining thrombus, 47%; protruding thrombus, 65%).

The mechanisms by which an intraluminal thrombus may increase the risk of restenosis after PTCA are not known specifically, but at least two hypotheses may be invoked. First, as discussed earlier, thrombosis may stimulate neointimal formation (49,131,132). However, a significant proportion of the restenoses observed after PTCA of lesions with superimposed thrombus are in fact due to total occlusion of the vessel at follow-up (118,143). These occlusions may occur as a final step in severely restenotic lesions but also may be the consequence of a thrombotic event occurring early after PTCA.

ENDOTHELIAL REGENERATION

Endothelial Regeneration after Experimental Arterial Injury

Endothelial Regrowth

In the hours after experimental angioplasty, endothelial cells rapidly enter the replication cycle to restore endothelial continuity. Proliferation and migration can be initiated either by loss of contact inhibition, stretch, or growth factors secreted by endothelial cells, SMCs, and circulating cells (15,56). Endothelial regeneration starts from the leading edge of the denuded area and from the ostia of collateral or branch arteries or both (146). Reendothelialization begins within the first 24 hours of arterial denudation and ceases 6 or 10 weeks later, depending on animal species (19). The rate and extent of endothelial regrowth are related to animal models and experimental conditions, but the most important factor seems to be the severity of the initial injury. Indeed, although complete reendothelialization can be achieved after small denuding injuries (147,148), endothelial cells have been found to be incapable of sustained regrowth after widespread denudation (19,20,149). Even if complete reendothelialization occurs, the regenerated endothelium often displays abnormal morphologic characteristics. In contrast to normal endothelial cells, regenerating endothelial cells grow as a sheet with close cell-to-cell contacts, no longer aligned with blood flow, and are both polygonal in shape and

irregular in size, with cytoplasm bulging toward the lumen (19,146,148–150).

Studies have emphasized the important role of endothelial cell growth factors in the reendothelialization process. Lindner et al. (56) have shown that systemic administration of bFGF (120 μg over an 8-hour period) after balloon catheter denudation of the rat carotid artery induces a highly significant increase in the replication rate of endothelial cells at the leading edge of the regrowth process. In this study, when bFGF was given over a longer period of time (12 μg daily for 12 days), a significant increase in the extent of endothelial outgrowth onto the denuded surface was observed. A study of the effect of much lower dosages of bFGF (systemic administration of 2.5 μg twice a week for 2 weeks) on the extent of endothelial regrowth after balloon denudation of rabbit iliac arteries found that animals in the bFGF group had a significantly greater degree of reendothelialization than did controls (151). Similar results have been observed with the use of acidic fibroblast growth factor in the same model (152). Stimulation of endothelial regrowth can also be achieved with vascular endothelial growth factor (VEGF). Asahara et al. (153) have demonstrated that a single local administration of VEGF (100 μg) immediately after balloon injury of the rat carotid artery is sufficient to significantly increase carotid artery reendothelialization at 2 and 4 weeks after injury. More recently, gene transfer of a plasmid encoding VEGF was associated with accelerated endothelial regrowth in a rabbit model (154) (Fig. 105.10). Taken together, these results demonstrate that both bFGF and VEGF are powerful stimuli of endothelial regrowth *in vivo* and suggest that they may participate in the spontaneous reendothelialization that occurs after injury.

Role of Progenitor Endothelial Cells in Reendothelialization

Work by Asahara et al. (155) has established that circulating mononuclear cells isolated from peripheral blood using antibodies to CD34 or Flk-1 can differentiate into endothelial cells *in vitro*. *In vivo*, such circulating endothelial cell progenitor cells were shown to incorporate into sites of angiogenesis, and more recent studies have indicated that such cells may contribute to reendothelialization at sites where balloon angioplasty has resulted in endothelial denudation. These findings thus suggest the need to reevaluate the conventional paradigm in which endothelial cells responsible for reendothelialization are considered to proliferate and migrate from intact endothelium at the proximal and distal boundaries of the balloon-injured segment, or from branch vessels. Some as-yet-undefined proportion of these endothelial cells may in fact be derived from circulating endothelial cell progenitor cells. Still to be determined is whether primary alterations in the proteoglycan "landing

LacZ-Tf   VEGF-Tf

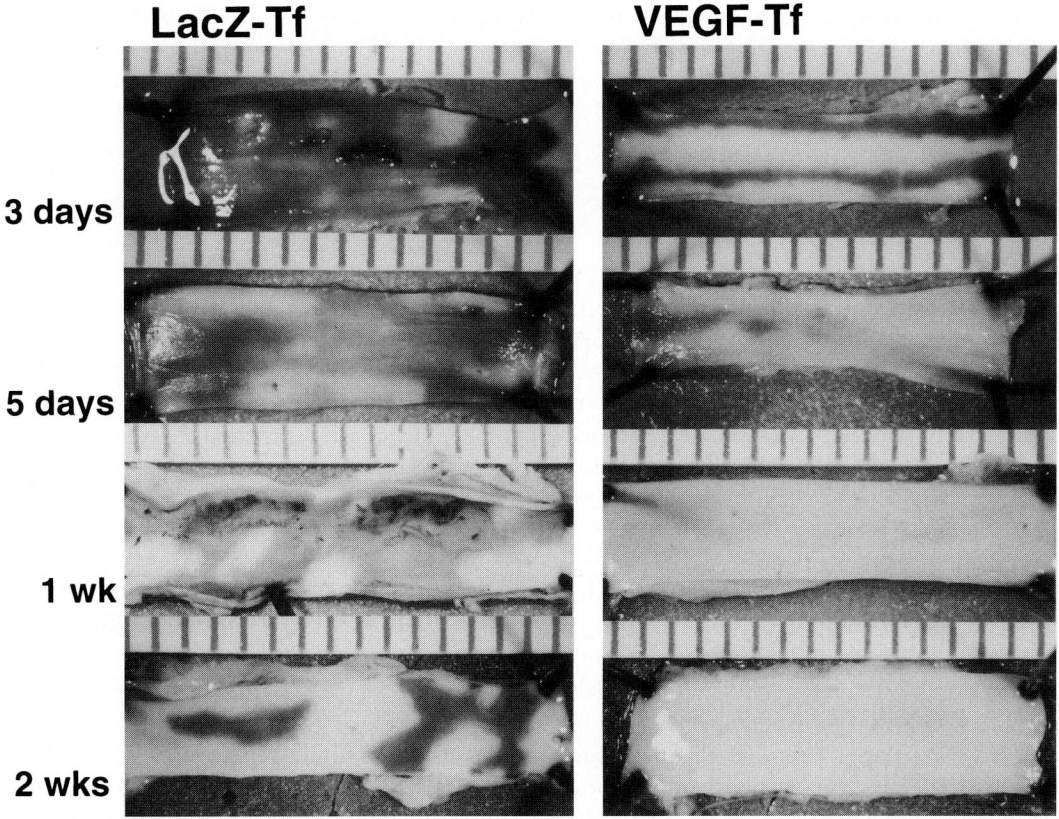

FIGURE 105.10 Representative macroscopic appearance of intimal surface of balloon-injured arteries transfected with control gene encoding β-galactosidase (LacZ-Tf) and gene encoding vascular endothelial growth factor (VEGF-Tf) at 3 days, 5 days, 1 week, and 2 weeks after gene transfer. Animals received systemic injection of Evans blue dye before sacrifice. Stained areas denote absent endothelium; reendothelialized areas, not stained by dye, appear white. Reendothelialization is accelerated in animals given VEGF-Tf.

pad" that constitutes the denuded segment—for example, expression of osteopontin or fibronectin beginning at the wound edges and progressing to the center of the denuded segment—determine the sequence in which such circulating progenitor cells may attach, differentiate, migrate, and proliferate.

Endothelial Dysfunction

The functional properties of regenerated endothelium have also been shown to be abnormal (27,148,156). After vascular injury, endothelium-dependent relaxation to vasodilator agonists is depressed in arteries with regenerated endothelium at a time when the ability of underlying vascular SMCs to relax or contract is unchanged. The severity of the endothelial dysfunction seems to be dependent on the nature of the initial injury. In a rabbit iliac artery model of angioplasty, impaired endothelium-dependent relaxation was found 4 weeks after the procedure only if animals experienced severe injury (148). Similarly, studies performed after coronary angioplasty in humans have demonstrated abnormal responses of previously dilated sites to endothe-

lium-dependent agonists such as serotonin (157) and acetylcholine (158).

Endothelial dysfunction may be related to a reduction in the ability of endothelial cells to produce endothelium-derived relaxing factors (159–161). Indeed, enhancing the production and release of NO may reverse endothelial dysfunction. In a rabbit model of balloon-injured iliac arteries, L-arginine, given in animal drinking water, restored acetylcholine-induced relaxations 4 weeks after vascular injury when these responses were depressed in the control group (27). This finding is in agreement with a reported study in which a constant intravenous infusion of the NO donor SPM-5185 significantly accelerated the functional recovery of the regenerating endothelium (162).

Importantly, the function of the endothelium that regenerates in response to exogenous administration of bFGF or VEGF seems to be normal (151,154). This demonstrates that endothelial cell growth factors are not only associated with a beneficial anatomic effect but also with an improvement in endothelial cell function. Similar results have been reported in other models of endothelial dysfunction. For example, the administration of angiogenic growth factors has been demonstrated to restore endothelium-dependent responses in arterial beds perfused via collaterals (163–165) and in hypercholesterolemic rabbits (166,167).

Impact of Endothelial Regeneration on Restenosis

Effects on Neointimal Hyperplasia

Previous investigations have underscored the principle of cross talk between endothelial cells and SMCs (149,168–170). Neointimal thickness is closely related to the presence of a regenerated endothelium. Indeed, intimal areas that are rapidly covered by continuous endothelium are protected from the accumulation of intimal SMCs, whereas typical intimal hyperplasia occurs in areas where reendothelialization is delayed.

Endothelium, in addition to its well-known role in regulating vessel tone and platelet aggregation, seems to modulate proliferative activity of the underlying SMCs. *In vitro* studies have emphasized a possible role for NO in controlling SMC growth (171,172). NO donors inhibit DNA synthesis in cultured SMCs, and similar effects achieved by administration of the analog 8-bromo-cyclic-guanosine monophosphate implicate the cyclic guanosine monophosphate pathway, physiologically activated by NO, in SMC growth regulation. Endothelial cells may maintain SMC quiescence through the growth-inhibitory effect of NO (172). Dysfunctional regenerating endothelium in which NO production is compromised may thus contribute to the development of a thickened intima due to reduced inhibition of platelet aggregation as well as SMC proliferation. Intriguingly, animal experiments have in fact documented that endothelial cell recovery is slower over damaged media than over normal media (173). On the basis that NO synthase catalyzes the synthesis of NO after oxidation of terminal guanidine-nitrogen atoms of L-arginine (174,175), several authors have administered this precursor locally or systemically and confirmed *in vivo* the efficacy of NO in preventing intimal hyperplasia (21,176,177).

Investigational experience with endothelial cell mitogens has yielded similar results. As discussed earlier, Asahara et al. demonstrated that a single local application of the endothelial cell–specific mitogen VEGF, either as a recombinant protein (153) or as naked DNA (154) (Fig. 105.10), is sufficient to facilitate endothelial repair after balloon injury (153). In these studies neointimal thickening was correspondingly attenuated to a statistically significant degree in VEGF-treated animals (Fig. 105.11). Somewhat different results have been observed in the case of FGF-induced reendothelialization. Lindner et al. (55), using high dosages of bFGF (12 µg daily for 12 days in a rat model), found a significant increase in neointimal thickening. By contrast, Bjornsson et al. (152), using low dosages

of acidic FGF [a mitogen for SMCs *in vitro* (178)] in the same model, observed an inhibition of neointimal thickening. The present authors found that administration of 2.5 µg of bFGF twice a week for 2 weeks in a rabbit model was associated with a very significant increase in endothelial regrowth but with no change in neointimal thickening (151). As bFGF is also a growth factor for SMCs, its final effect on neointimal thickening may be the consequence of a balance between stimulatory and inhibitory mechanisms on SMC growth. Factors such as the dosage used, the duration of the treatment, and the animal model studied may explain discrepancies between studies. On the other hand, the results obtained with VEGF are probably mainly the consequence of reendothelialization, without detrimental effect on SMC—that is, proliferation—because VEGF high-affinity binding sites are limited to endothelial cells.

IMPACT OF ENDOVASCULAR STENTS ON THE BIOLOGY OF RESTENOSIS

Coronary stenting is emerging as an effective treatment for patients with coronary artery disease (184–186). Changes in antithrombotic regimens and in the technique of implantation have allowed coronary stenting to be performed with excellent immediate outcome (187–189). As a result, the proportion of patients receiving a stent as an adjunct to conventional balloon angioplasty is increasing exponentially. Studies have shown that implantation of permanent metal prosthetic stents results in significantly lower rates of clinically and angiographically determined recurrence than with conventional balloon angioplasty (190,191). Even if restenosis is less frequent, however, it remains a significant problem after coronary stenting. Rates of angiographically identified restenosis varying between 13% and 32% have been reported after successful coronary stenting (190–192). Importantly, the mechanisms of restenosis within coronary stents differ very significantly from those of restenosis after conventional balloon angioplasty.

Stent and Vessel Remodeling

Serial intravascular ultrasonographic studies have indicated that stents do not recoil over the long term (193,194). Implantation of an intracoronary stent seems to eliminate any component of arterial remodeling, either enlargement or constriction. As vessel remodeling is the major mechanism of restenosis after conventional balloon angioplasty (125), its elimination is probably the main explanation for the decrease in restenosis rate after coronary stenting.

In-Stent Restenosis

Because stents are considered to neutralize geometric effects, including remodeling (121), development of rest-

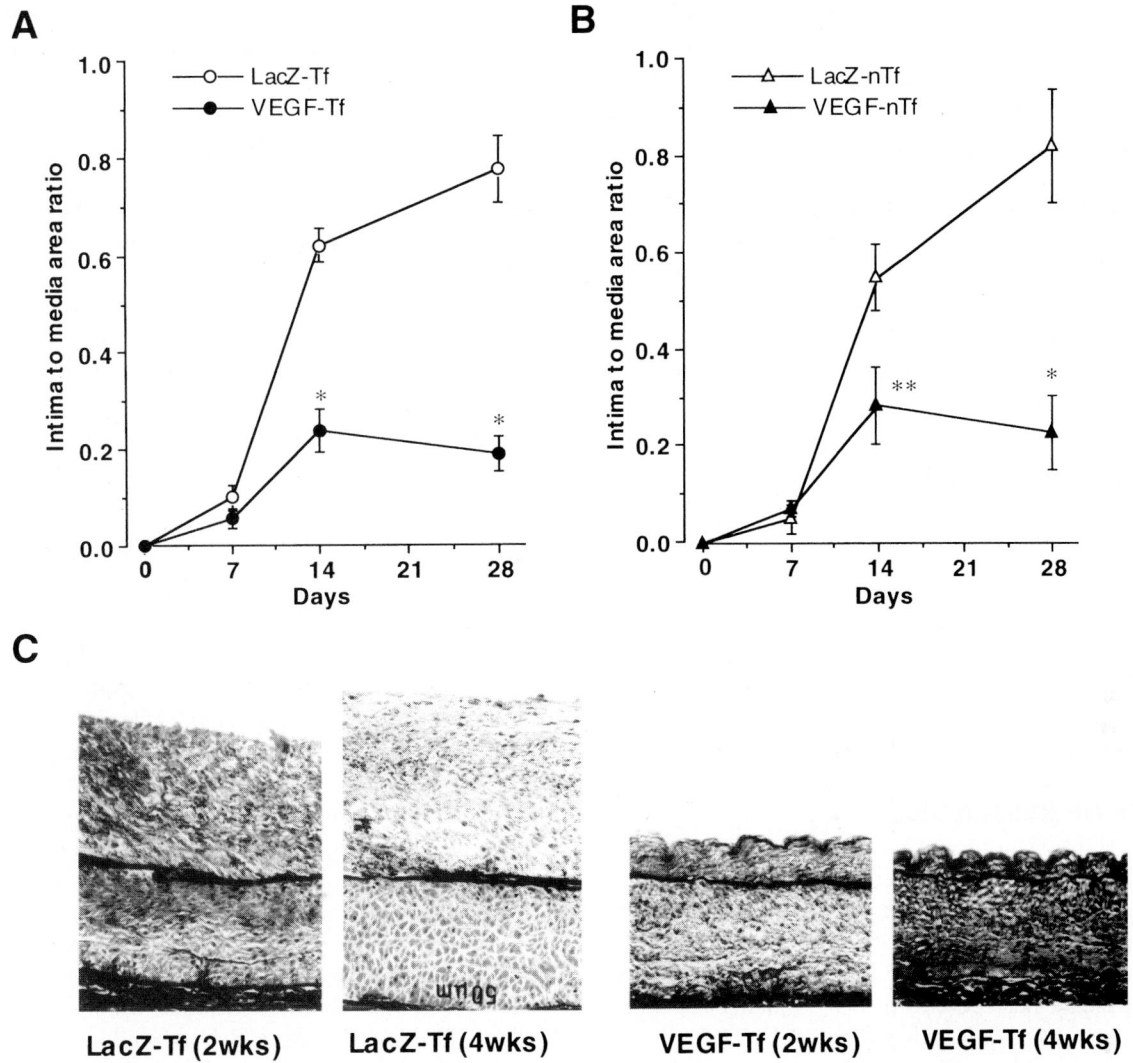

FIGURE 105.11 A: Arteries transfected with control gene encoding β-galactosidase (LacZ-Tf) showed progressive neointimal thickening through 4 weeks. Significantly less intimal thickening was observed among arteries transfected with gene encoding vascular endothelial growth factor (VEGF-Tf), including regression of intimal thickening between 2 and 4 weeks (*, $p < .01$ vs. LacZ-Tf). **B:** Contralateral balloon-injured, nontransfected arteries in VEGF group (VEGF-nTf) developed less intimal thickening and displayed no progression during weeks 2 to 4 compared with those in LacZ-nTf group (*, $p < .01$ vs. LacZ-nTf; **, $p < .05$). **C:** Representative effect of transfection on intimal thickening for LacZ-Tf and VEGF-Tf at 2 and 4 weeks posttransfection.

enosis after stent implantation has been attributed principally to SMC proliferation. Successful application of intravascular radiation to limit thickening of stent neointima in a variety of animal models (195–197), on the premise that proliferating cells display enhanced sensitivity to ionizing radiation, constitutes indirect support for this notion. Likewise, accelerated endothelialization of stents after catheter delivery of the gene encoding VEGF has been shown to markedly reduce SMC proliferation and thereby reduce luminal narrowing due to thickening of the stent neointima (198).

Histologic findings reported for a limited number of patients have suggested that in-stent restenosis is characterized by SMC hyperplasia. Pathologic analysis of graft seg-

ments surgically retrieved from two patients described by Anderson et al. (199) revealed "smooth muscle cells with abundant eosinophilic cytoplasm and minimal interstitial tissue" in the tissue overlying the stent wires. Among four patients with in-stent restenosis described by van Beusekom et al. (200), "tissue that narrowed the vessels always consisted of SMCs (often with a 'dendritic' appearance) within an extensive extracellular matrix." The extent of residual proliferative activity among these hypercellular foci was not specifically investigated in either series of patients. ▾ q29

Inflammatory cells, including foreign body granulomata formation, have been described in at least one previous animal study of endovascular stents (205). Although neither giant cells nor granulomata were observed in these specimens, occasional inflammatory cells were identified by CD45 immunostaining. A relatively small human alveolar macrophage-56 population was identified as well, but the contribution of both cell types to restenosis in these ten cases seems limited.

The role of thrombus in restenosis, including in-stent restenosis, is unclear. Schwartz et al. (206) have suggested that mural thrombus may constitute the primordial infrastructure that is subsequently colonized by activated SMCs. Thrombus was in fact observed in 60% of ten specimens in the cohort described and thus cannot be excluded as a factor contributing to the genesis of in-stent restenosis.

Stents and Thrombosis

As discussed earlier, thrombosis may contribute to restenosis. Stent implantation per se may increase the thrombotic response of the vessel wall. Thrombosis, however, may be significantly reduced by new antithrombotic regimens (189) and the use of heparin-coated stents (192).

IMPACT OF ENDOVASCULAR BRACHYTHERAPY ON THE BIOLOGY OF RESTENOSIS

Endovascular brachytherapy is currently under investigation in humans to treat or prevent coronary restenosis after standard balloon angioplasty or coronary stenting. Although preliminary results are encouraging and suggest that this strategy may be effective in reducing restenosis rates at 6 months in selected patients (212,213), several issues are still unresolved. For example, the optimal dosage, the nature of the source (beta vs. gamma), and the ideal mode of administration (external irradiation vs. catheter-based irradiation, stent-based vs. wire-based delivery) are unknown. In addition, although long-term results of radiation are still uncertain, the suggestion has been made that endovascular brachytherapy may be harmful and may increase the rate of restenosis at the edge of stents (214) or increase the rate of thrombotic events (215,216). The effects of radiation on the restenotic process and on the cellular components involved in vascular healing are discussed in the following sections.

Brachytherapy and Vessel Remodeling

Animal and IVUS studies have shown that brachytherapy may alter vessel remodeling. In porcine coronary arteries (217,218), administration of intravascular irradiation at the time of balloon injury was associated with a larger external diameter of coronary vessels at 14 days than in animals receiving balloon injury alone. Consistent with this observation, a serial IVUS study (219) involving patients treated

with balloon angioplasty and receiving beta irradiation found that 16 of 22 patients (76%) had vessel enlargement at 6 months. Similarly, Condado et al. (220) reported a negative late loss by angiography at 6 months in 10 of 22 patients (45%) treated with gamma radiation. This effect seems to be related to inhibition of adventitial fibrosis as suggested by the decrease in the number of adventitial cells expressing alpha-actin immunostaining after intravascular irradiation (218,221).

One must also point out, however, that animal experiments using external beam radiation have shown that irradiation may induce vessel constriction rather than vessel enlargement at 4 weeks (217). These effects were related to fibroblast proliferation and inflammation in the myocardium and to an increase in interstitial and perivascular fibrosis.

Brachytherapy and Intimal Hyperplasia

Studies have shown that intravascular radiation using a beta or gamma source may reduce intimal hyperplasia after balloon angioplasty at 14 days and 6 months in pigs (222–224) and at 6 weeks in rabbits (225). Similar results were found in animal models using beta-emitting stents (226–228). Results of preliminary trials showing that intravascular irradiation associated with stent implantation may reduce restenosis at 6 months suggest that this is also the case in humans (212). IVUS studies performed in humans are also consistent with a reduction of intimal hyperplasia at 6 months (229). Whether these results may last over the long term is not clear, however. Indeed, endovascular irradiation has also been associated with delayed arterial wound healing, including delayed endothelialization and persistent fibrin deposition in the intima 3 months after the implantation of beta-emitting stents in rabbits (230). In addition, smooth muscle cells with a synthetic rather than contractile phenotype produced large amounts of collagen 6 months after endovascular radiotherapy (217). Reports showing that intimal hyperplasia may continue to increase beyond the 6-month point in patients treated by endovascular brachytherapy are also consistent with these observations (231,232). Finally, some reports suggest that radiation may increase, rather than decrease, intimal hyperplasia. This has been observed with beta-emitting stents in animal models (233–235) as well as in humans at the stent edges (214).

Radiation inhibits proliferation and migration of endothelial and vascular smooth muscle cells and inhibits proliferation of myofibroblasts as demonstrated *in vitro* and *in vivo* (218,236,237). *In vitro*, the effects of radiation on endothelial cells and vascular SMCs relate to induction of G_0/G_1 arrest, without evidence of cell viability alteration, apoptosis, or ultrastructural changes (237,238). The absence of an effect of radiation on apoptosis was confirmed *in vivo* (218).

The apparently contradictory results observed in animal models and in humans seem to depend on the dosage, the method of delivery, and the timing of follow-up. The increase in intimal hyperplasia is thought to be secondary to insufficient direct inhibitory effect of radiation on proliferation and migration of vascular SMCs associated with stimulation of the production of collagen (6), a key component of ECM and intimal hyperplasia. The lack of the endothelial barrier may also indirectly stimulate the growth of vascular SMCs (239).

Brachytherapy and Reendothelialization

Balloon angioplasty and stent implantation induce disruption of the endothelial lining. Radiation, by inhibiting endothelial cell proliferation and migration (236), may delay the reendothelialization process. Endothelialization remains incomplete 2 to 3 months after implantation of beta-emitting stents in animals (230), and analysis of human coronary artery specimens also shows limited endothelialization at 2 months (230). Delayed reendothelialization may have some impact on endothelial function and may explain the impaired endothelium-dependent relaxation observed at 6 weeks after endovascular brachytherapy and balloon injury in animals (240). Endothelial function seems to have returned to normal at 6 months, however, as observed in patients treated with endovascular brachytherapy (241). Delayed endothelialization may also partly explain some of the side effects that have been reported in some circumstances with endovascular brachytherapy, such as increased thrombus formation (242,243) and increased intimal hyperplasia (243–245). A study showing that the combination of agents able to stimulate reendothelialization may reduce thrombus formation after endovascular brachytherapy provides additional support to this hypothesis (244).

CONTROVERSIES AND PERSONAL PERSPECTIVES

Certain issues pertaining to the biology of restenosis have generated some controversy. Four, in particular, merit comment. The first issue is the extent to which SMC proliferation contributes to restenosis. All animal studies, without exception, have shown that when tissue sampling can be performed at arbitrary, including early, times, evidence of SMC proliferation is abundant. Most, indeed nearly all, human studies of tissues obtained at necropsy or surgery (including atherectomy) have shown evidence of SMC hyperplasia. The controversy has been generated largely because of one study in which proliferative activity was observed (using PCNA staining) in 15% to 20% of atherectomy specimens, whereas in a subsequent study PCNA staining was infrequent. The difference between these two studies may be explained largely by differences in methodology: In the latter study, a PCNA stain was identified as positive only if the staining intensity corresponded to that of control tissues colabeled for PCNA and the S-phase–specific marker bromodeoxyuridine. Such an analysis tests SMCs in S phase, as opposed to proliferating SMCs stained by PCNA in G_1 and G_2 as well. Because proportionately far more cells are in G_1 and G_2 at any given time, this methodology severely underestimates proliferative activity. Furthermore, because animal studies indicate that peak proliferative activity occurs soon after the initial injury, the extent of cellular proliferation seen at the time of intervention represents a fraction of the proliferative activity responsible for generating hyperplastic lesions typical of restenosis.

A second issue is the role of constrictive remodeling in the pathogenesis of restenosis. No controversy exists that constrictive remodeling, first demonstrated by the laboratory of Cornelius Borst, contributes to restenosis. This has been inferentially confirmed by the clinical experience with endovascular stents, in which the reduction of restenosis is assumed to represent successful inhibition of remodeling. What is controversial is the extent to which remodeling contributes to restenosis in general. Clinical studies performed using high-resolution IVUS to follow patients treated by angioplasty without stents may clarify this issue; the authors' own personal perspective, however, is that remodeling accounts for proportionately fewer cases of restenosis than does SMC proliferation. Parenthetically, published data regarding stenosis that develops within a stent has unequivocally indicated that SMC proliferation is the culprit.

A third issue also relates to the pathogenesis of restenosis, namely, the role of postangioplasty mural thrombus. Some have held the view that such mural thrombus forms the infrastructure of the restenotic lesion; indeed, good data are available from animal models of stent restenosis to support this interpretation. Others have questioned this view, based on patients studied by angiography and particularly angioscopy postangioplasty, in whom evidence of such mural thrombus has been difficult to identify. Suffice it to say that even if mural thrombus does not itself comprise a precursor scaffold for neointimal thickening, the possibility remains that elements derived from transient thrombus formation—for example, thrombin—contribute to neointimal thickening via their mitogenic effect on SMCs.

Finally, what is perhaps the most controversial issue of all relates not to restenosis per se but instead to one principal means used to study its pathogenesis: the use of animal models. Species that have been used for this purpose include mouse, rat, rabbit, pig, and primate. Although certain of these models have gained favored status at one time or another, none has been shown to be uniquely predictive of what happens when a certain intervention is performed in human species. Each has certain advantages and liabili-

THE FUTURE

Subsequent studies may further disclose the extent to which SMC proliferation, vessel remodeling, and thrombosis proportionately contribute to restenosis. Much of this may come with investigation of stented arteries, because the remodeling component should be minimal and SMC is currently considered to represent the key pathogenetic mechanism of in-stent restenosis.

Current studies focusing on the interaction of key integrins and their respective ligands may also clarify the extent to which upregulation of specific integrins in SMCs contributes to restenosis and, correspondingly, whether this represents a suitable target for antirestenosis strategies.

The role played by progenitor endothelial cells in passivating the site of balloon injury should be clarified by ongoing studies. Resolution of this issue will determine the extent to which conventional concepts regarding the source of endothelial cells responsible for reendothelialization need to be modified. These studies may also offer insights into the potential for such precursor cells, with or without administration of endothelial cell mitogens, to constitute a novel therapy for expediting reendothelialization and thereby inhibiting restenosis.

Identification of genotypes that predispose to restenosis will receive increasing attention. Successful execution of such investigations will not only assist in management decisions regarding percutaneous revascularization but may also provide clues to restenosis prevention.

---

ties. No basis exists, however, for considering any one, two, or combination of these to be uniquely valid in a scientific sense. At best, each offers only the opportunity to establish proof of concept, and when considered in such context, each may be instructive.

SUMMARY

Restenosis is clearly a multifactorial entity. SMC proliferation, elaboration of ECM, thrombosis, and vascular remodeling all contribute to its pathogenesis. The contribution of these individual elements does not seem to be consistently proportional from one patient to another, or even from one lesion to another in the same patient. Similarly, the mechanisms of restenosis after coronary stent implantation are different from those of restenosis after conventional balloon angioplasty.

In the absence of a single therapy that effectively addresses all of these pathogenic elements, the capability to routinely preempt restenosis will likely require accurate clinical identification and understanding of the principal factor governing the biology of a given restenotic lesion.

REFERENCES

1. Gruentzig A, Senning A, Siegenthaler WE. Nonoperative dilatation of coronary artery stenosis: percutaneous transluminal coronary angioplasty. *N Engl J Med* 1979;301:61–68.
2. deFeyter PJ, Serruys PW. Percutaneous transluminal coronary angioplasty for unstable angina. In: Topol EJ, ed. *Textbook of interventional cardiology*, 2nd ed. Philadelphia: WB Saunders, 1994:274–291.
3. Holmes DR Jr, Berger PB. Complex and multivessel dilation. In: Topol EJ, ed. *Textbook of interventional cardiology*, 2nd ed. Philadelphia: WB Saunders, 1994:231–250.
4. Bauters C, Meurice T, Hamon M, et al. Mechanisms and prevention of restenosis: from experimental models to clinical practice. *Cardiovasc Res* 1996;31:835–846.
5. McBride W, Lange RA, Hillis LD. Restenosis after successful coronary angioplasty: pathophysiology and prevention. *N Engl J Med* 1988;318:1734–1737.
6. Liu MW, Roubin GS, King SB III. Restenosis after coronary angioplasty: potential biologic determinants and role of intimal hyperplasia. *Circulation* 1989;79:1374–1387.
7. Bauters C, Lablanche JM, McFadden EP, et al. Clinical characteristics and angiographic follow-up of patients undergoing early or late repeat dilation for a first restenosis. *J Am Coll Cardiol* 1992;20:845–848.
8. Bauters C, McFadden EP, Lablanche JM, et al. Restenosis rate after multiple percutaneous transluminal coronary angioplasty procedures at the same site: a quantitative angiographic study in consecutive patients undergoing a third angioplasty for a second restenosis. *Circulation* 1993;88:969–974.
9. Hillegass WB, Ohman EM, Califf RM. Restenosis: the clinical issues. In: Topol EJ, ed. *Textbook of interventional cardiology*, 2nd ed. Philadelphia: WB Saunders, 1994:415–435.
10. Califf RM. Restenosis: the cost to society. *Am Heart J* 1995;130:680–684.
11. Herrman JPR, Hermans WRM, Vos J, et al. Pharmacological approaches to the prevention of restenosis following angioplasty: the search for the holy grail? (Part I). *Drugs* 1993;46:18–52.
12. Franklin SM, Faxon DP. Pharmacologic prevention of restenosis after coronary angioplasty: review of the randomized clinical trials. *Coron Artery Dis* 1993;4:232–242.
13. Popma JJ, Califf RM, Topol EJ. Clinical trials of restenosis after coronary angioplasty. *Circulation* 1991;84:1426–1436.

14. Clowes AW, Reidy MA, Clowes MM. Kinetics of cellular proliferation after arterial injury: I. Smooth muscle growth in the absence of endothelium. *Lab Invest* 1983;49:327–333.

15. Casscells W. Migration of smooth muscle and endothelial cells: critical events in restenosis. *Circulation* 1992;86:723–729.

16. Majesky MW, Schwartz SM, Clowes MM, et al. Heparin regulates smooth muscle S phase entry in the injured-rat carotid artery. *Circ Res* 1987;61:296–300.

17. Lafont A, Guzman LA, Whitlow PL, et al. Restenosis after experimental angioplasty: intimal, medial, and adventitial changes associated with constrictive remodeling. *Circ Res* 1995;76:996–1002.

18. Kakuta T, Currier JW, Haudenschild CC, et al. Differences in compensatory vessel enlargement, not intimal formation, account for restenosis after angioplasty in the hypercholesterolemic rabbit model. *Circulation* 1994;89:2809–2815.

19. Reidy MA, Clowes AW, Schwartz SM. Endothelial regeneration: V. Inhibition of endothelial regrowth in arteries of rat and rabbit. *Lab Invest* 1983;49:569–575.

20. Reidy MA, Standaert D, Schwartz SM. Inhibition of endothelial cell regrowth: cessation of aortic endothelial cell replication after balloon catheter denudation. *Arteriosclerosis* 1982;2:216–220.

21. McNamara DB, Bedi B, Aurora H, et al. L-arginine inhibits balloon catheter-induced intimal hyperplasia. *Biochem Biophys Res Commun* 1993;193:291–296.

22. Bauters C, De Groote P, Adamantidis M, et al. Proto-oncogene expression in rabbit aorta after wall injury: first marker of the cellular process leading to restenosis after angioplasty? *Eur Heart J* 1992;13:556–559.

23. Fingerle J, Johnson R, Clowes AW, et al. Role of platelets in smooth muscle cell proliferation and migration after vascular injury in rat carotid artery. *Proc Natl Acad Sci U S A* 1989;86:8412–8416.

24. Steele PM, Chesebro JH, Stanton AW, et al. Balloon angioplasty: natural history of the pathophysiological response to injury in a pig model. *Circ Res* 1985;57:105–112.

25. Schwartz RS, Murphy JG, Edwards WD, et al. Restenosis after balloon angioplasty: a practical proliferative model in porcine coronary arteries. *Circulation* 1990;82:2190–2200.

26. Santoian EC, Schneider JE, Gravanis MB, et al. Angiopeptin inhibits intimal hyperplasia after angioplasty in porcine coronary arteries. *Circulation* 1993;88:11–14.

27. Hamon M, Vallet B, Bauters C, et al. Long-term oral administration of L-arginine reduces intimal thickening and enhances neoendothelium-dependent acetylcholine-induced relaxation after arterial injury. *Circulation* 1994;90:1357–1362.

28. Miano JM, Viasic N, Tota RR, et al. Localization of *fos* and *jun* proteins in rat aortic smooth muscle cells after vascular injury. *Am J Pathol* 1993;142:715–724.

29. Van Belle E, Bauters C, Wernert N, et al. Angiotensin converting enzyme inhibition prevents proto-oncogene expression in the vascular wall after injury. *J Hypertens* 1995;13:105–112.

30. Hamon M, Bauters C, Wernert N, et al. Heparin does not inhibit oncogene induction in rabbit aorta following balloon denudation. *Cardiovasc Res* 1993;27:1209–1213.

31. Bauters C, Van Belle E, Wernert N, et al. Angiopeptin inhibits oncogene induction in rabbit aorta after balloon denudation. *Circulation* 1994;89:2327–2331.

32. Pardee AB. G_1 events and regulation of cell proliferation. *Science* 1989;246:603–608.

33. Reed JC, Alpers JD, Nowell PC, et al. Sequential expression of protooncogenes during lectin-stimulated mitogenesis of normal human lymphocytes. *Proc Natl Acad Sci U S A* 1986;83:3982–3986.

34. Riabowol KT, Vosatka RJ, Ziff EB, et al. Microinjection of fos-specific antibodies blocks DNA synthesis in fibroblast cells. *Mol Cell Biol* 1988;8:1670–1676.

35. Heikkila R, Schwab G, Wickstrom E. A c-myc antisense oligodesoxynucleotide inhibits entry into S phase but not progress from G_0 to G_1. *Nature* 1987;328:445–449.

36. Simons M, Edelman ER, DeKeyser JL, et al. Antisense c-myb oligonucleotides inhibit arterial smooth muscle cell accumulation *in vivo*. *Nature* 1992;359:67–70.

37. Bennett MR, Anglin S, McEwan JR, et al. Inhibition of vascular smooth muscle cell proliferation in vitro and in vivo by c-myc antisense oligodeoxynucleotides. *J Clin Invest* 1994;93:820–828.

38. Gorski DH, LePage DF, Patel CV, et al. Molecular cloning of a diverged homeobox gene that is rapidly downregulated during the G_0/G_1 transition in vascular smooth muscle cells. *Mol Cell Biol* 1993;13:3722–3733.

39. Weir L, Chen D, Pastore C, et al. Expression of *GAX*, a growth-arrest homeobox gene, is rapidly downregulated in rat carotid artery during the proliferative response to balloon injury. *J Biol Chem* 1995;270:5457–5461.

40. Thyberg J, Hedin U, Sjölund M. Regulation of differentiated properties and proliferation of arterial smooth muscle cells. *Arteriosclerosis* 1990;10:966–990.

41. Schwartz SM, Campbell CR, Campbell JH. Replication of smooth muscle cells in vascular disease. *Circ Res* 1986;58:427–444.

42. Rubbia L, Gabbiani G. Phénotype des cellules musculaires lisses artérielles et athérosclérose. *Med/Sciences* 1989;53:389–395.

43. Clowes AW, Clowes MM. Kinetics of cellular proliferation after arterial injury: II. Inhibition of smooth muscle growth by heparin. *Lab Invest* 1985;52:611–616.

44. Wei GL, Krasinski K, Kearney M, et al. Temporally and spatially coordinated expression of cell cycle regulatory factors after angioplasty. *Circ Res* 1997;80:418–426.

45. Boyd CD, Kniep AC, Pierce RA, et al. Increased elastin mRNA levels associated with surgically induced intimal injury. *Connect Tissue Res* 1988;18:65–78.

46. Bauters C, Marotte F, Hamon M, et al. Accumulation of fetal fibronectin mRNAs after balloon denudation of rabbit arteries. *Circulation* 1995;92:904–911.

47. Weintraub AS, Giachelli CM, Krauss RS, et al. Autocrine secretion of osteopontin by vascular smooth muscle cells regulates their adhesion to collagen gels. *Am J Pathol* 1996;149:259–272.

48. Clark RAF, Tonnesen MG, Gailit J, et al. Transient functional expression of avb3 on vascular cells during wound repair. *Am J Pathol* 1996;148:1407–1421.

49. Schwartz RS, Holmes DR, Topol EJ. The restenosis paradigm revisited: an alternative proposal for cellular mechanisms. *J Am Coll Cardiol* 1992;20:1284–1293.

50. Clowes AW, Clowes MM, Kocher O, et al. Arterial smooth muscle cells in vivo: relationship between actin isoform expression and mitogenesis and their modulation by heparin. *J Cell Biol* 1988;107:1939–1945.

51. Assoian RK, Grotendorst GR, Miller DM, et al. Cellular transformation by coordinate action of three peptide growth factors from human platelets. *Nature* 1984;309:804–806.

52. Walker LN, Bowen-Pope DF, Ross R, et al. Production of platelet-derived growth factor-like molecules by cultured arterial smooth muscle cells accompanies proliferation after arterial injury. *Proc Natl Acad Sci U S A* 1986;83:7311–7315.

53. Wilcox JN, Smith KM, Williams LT, et al. Platelet-derived growth factor mRNA detection in human atherosclerotic plaques by in situ hybridization. *J Clin Invest* 1988;82:1134–1143.

54. Ferns GA, Raines EW, Sprugel KH, et al. Inhibition of neointimal smooth muscle accumulation after angioplasty by an antibody to PDGF. *Science* 1991;253:1129–1132.

55. Lindner V, Lappi DA, Baird A, et al. Role of basic fibroblast growth factor in vascular lesion formation. *Circ Res* 1991;68:106–113.

56. Lindner V, Majack RA, Reidy MA. Basic fibroblast growth factor stimulates endothelial regrowth and proliferation in denuded arteries. *J Clin Invest* 1990;85:2004–2008.

57. Lindner V, Majack RA, Reidy MA. Basic FGF induces the proliferation of vascular cells in injured arteries. *FASEB J* 1990;4:A625.

58. Lindner V, Reidy MA. Proliferation of smooth muscle cells after vascular injury is inhibited by an antibody against basic fibroblast growth factor. *Proc Natl Acad Sci U S A* 1991;88:3739–3743.

59. Bassols A, Massaque J. Transforming growth factor β regulates the expression and structure of extracellular matrix chondroitin/dermatan sulfate proteoglycans. *J Biol Chem* 1988;263:3039–3045.

60. Nikol S, Isner JM, Pickering JG, et al. Expression of transforming growth factor-β1 is increased in human vascular restenosis lesions. *J Clin Invest* 1992;90:1582–1592.

61. Border WA, Ruosslahti E. Transforming growth factor-β in disease: the dark side of tissue repair. *J Clin Invest* 1992;90:1–7.

62. Sporn MB, Roberts AB, Wakefield LM, et al. Some recent advances in the chemistry and biology of transforming growth factor-β. *J Cell Biol* 1987;105:1039–1045.

63. Roberts AB, Sporn MB, Assoian RK, et al. Transforming growth factor type β. Rapid induction of fibrosis and angiogenesis in vivo and stimulation of collagen formation in vitro. *Proc Natl Acad Sci U S A* 1986;83:4167–4170.

64. Antonelli-Orlidge A, Saunders KB, Smith SR, et al. An activated form of transforming growth factor-β is produced by cocultures of endothelial cells and pericytes. *Proc Natl Acad Sci U S A* 1989;86:4544–4548.

65. Cercek B, Fishbein MC, Forrester JS, et al. Induction of insulin-like growth factor I messenger RNA in rat aorta after balloon denudation. *Circ Res* 1990;66:1755–1760.

66. Dzau VJ. Vascular renin angiotensin: a possible autocrine or paracrine system in control of vascular function. *J Cardiovasc Pharmacol* 1984;6:S377–S382.

67. Rakugi H, Kim DK, Krieger JE, et al. Induction of angiotensin converting enzyme in the neointima after vascular injury: possible role in restenosis. *J Clin Invest* 1994;93:339–346.

68. Morishita R, Gibbons GH, Ellison KE, et al. Evidence for direct local effect of angiotensin in vascular hypertrophy: in vivo gene transfer of angiotensin converting enzyme. *J Clin Invest* 1994;94:978–984.

69. Pratt RE, Dzau VJ. Pharmacological strategies to prevent restenosis: lessons learned from blockade of the renin-angiotensin system. *Circulation* 1996;93:848–852.

70. Berk BC, Vekhstein V, Gordon HM, et al. Angiotensin II-stimulated protein synthesis in cultured vascular smooth muscle cells. *Hypertension* 1989;13:305–314.

71. Turla MB, Thompson MM, Corjay MH, et al. Mechanisms of angiotensin II- and arginine vasopressin-induced increases in protein synthesis and content in cultured rat aortic smooth muscle cells. *Circ Res* 1991;68:288–299.

72. Daemen MJAP, Lombardi DM, Bosman FT, et al. Angiotensin II induces smooth muscle cell proliferation in the normal and injured rat arterial wall. *Circ Res* 1991;68:450–456.

73. Powell JS, Clozel JP, Muller RKM, et al. Inhibitors of angiotensin-converting enzyme prevent myointimal proliferation after vascular injury. *Science* 1989;245:186–188.

74. Clozel JP, Hess P, Michael C, et al. Inhibition of converting enzyme and neointima formation after vascular injury in rabbits and guinea pigs. *Hypertension* 1991;18:I-155–I-159.

75. Osterrieder W, Muller RK, Powell JS, et al. Role of angiotensin II in injury-induced neointima formation in rats. *Hypertension* 1991;18[Suppl 4]:II-60–II-64.

76. Van Belle E, Vallet B, Auffray JL, et al. Chronic inhibition of nitric oxide synthesis reverses the effects of ACE inhibition on neo-endothelium-dependent relaxation and on intimal thickening after balloon injury. *Am J Physiol* 1996;270:H298–H305.

77. Farhy RD, Carretero OA, Ho KL, et al. Role of kinins and nitric oxide in the effects of angiotensin converting enzyme inhibitors on neointima formation. *Circ Res* 1993;72:1202–1210.

78. Vanhoutte PM, Houston D. Platelets, endothelium and vasospasm. *Circulation* 1985;72:728–734.

79. Nemecek GM, Coughlin SR, Handley DA, et al. Stimulation of aortic smooth muscle cell mitogenesis by serotonin. *Proc Natl Acad Sci U S A* 1986;83:674–678.

80. Moalic JM, Bauters C, Himbert D, et al. Phenylephrine, vasopressin and angiotensin II as determinants of proto-oncogene and heat-shock protein gene expression in adult rat heart and aorta. *J Hypertens* 1989;7:195–201.

81. Iwaki K, Sukhatme VP, Shubeita HE, et al. Alpha- and beta-adrenergic stimulation induces distinct patterns of immediate early gene expression in neonatal rat myocardial cells. *J Biol Chem* 1990;265:13809–13817.

82. Yanagisawa M, Kurihara H, Kimura S, et al. A novel potent vasoconstrictor peptide produced by vascular endothelial cells. *Nature* 1988;332:411–415.

83. Clozel M, Fischli W, Guilly C. Specific binding of endothelin on human vascular smooth muscle cells in culture. *J Clin Invest* 1989;83:1758–1761.

84. Komuro I, Kurihara H, Sugiyama T, et al. Endothelin stimulates c-fos and c-myc expression and proliferation of vascular smooth muscle cells. *FEBS Lett* 1988;238:249–259.

85. Hirata Y, Takagi Y, Fukuda Y, et al. Endothelin is a potent mitogen for rat vascular smooth muscle cells. *Arteriosclerosis* 1989;78:225–228.

86. Douglas SA, Louden C, Vickery-Clark LM, et al. A role for endogenous endothelin-1 in neointimal formation after rat carotid artery balloon angioplasty: protective effects of the novel nonpeptide endothelin receptor antagonist SB 209670. *Circ Res* 1994;75:190–197.

87. Azuma H, Hamasaki H, Niimi Y, et al. Role of endothelin-1 in neointima formation after endothelial removal in rabbit carotid arteries. *Am J Physiol* 1994;267:H2259–H2267.

88. Fingerle J, Tina AUYP, Clowes AW, et al. Intimal lesion formation in rat carotid arteries after endothelial denudation in absence of medial injury. *Arteriosclerosis* 1990;10:1082–1087.

89. Walker LN, Ramsay MM, Bowyer DE. Endothelial healing following defined injury to rabbit aorta: depth of injury and mode of repair. *Arteriosclerosis* 1983;47:123–130.

90. Kulik TJ, Rothman A, Glennon ET, et al. Stretching vascular smooth muscle causes inositol phosphates turnover. *Circulation* 1989;80[Suppl 11]:198(abst).

91. Clowes AW, Clowes MM, Reidy MA. Role of acute distension in the induction of smooth muscle proliferation after endothelial denudation. *Fed Proc* 1987;46:720(abst).

92. Kohler TR, Jawien A. Flow affects development of intimal hyperplasia after arterial injury in rats. *Arterioscler Thromb* 1992;12:963–971.

93. Kohler TR, Kirkman TR, Kraiss LW, et al. Increased blood flow inhibits neointimal hyperplasia in endothelialized vascular grafts. *Circ Res* 1991;69:1557–1565.

94. Johnson DE, Hinohara T, Selmon MR, et al. Primary peripheral arterial stenoses and restenoses excised by transluminal atherectomy: a histopathologic study. *J Am Coll Cardiol* 1990;15:419–425.

95. Garrat KN, Edwards WD, Kaufmann UP, et al. Differential histopathology of primary atherosclerotic and restenotic lesions in coronary arteries and saphenous vein bypass grafts: analysis of tissue obtained from 73 patients by directional atherectomy. *J Am Coll Cardiol* 1991;17:442–448.

96. Isner JM, Kearney M, Bauters C, et al. Use of human tissue specimens obtained in vivo by directional atherectomy to study restenosis and related human vascular disorders. *Trends Cardiovasc Med* 1994;4:213–221.

97. Austin GE, Norman NB, Hollman J, et al. Intimal proliferation of smooth muscle cells as an explanation for recurrent coronary artery stenosis after percutaneous transluminal coronary angioplasty. *J Am Coll Cardiol* 1985;6:369–375.

98. Gravanis MB, Roubin GS. Histopathologic phenomena at the site of percutaneous transluminal coronary angioplasty: the problem of restenosis. *Hum Pathol* 1989;20:477–485.

99. Isner JM, Kearney M, Berdan LG, et al. Core pathology lab findings in 425 patients undergoing directional atherectomy for a primary coronary artery stenosis and relationship to subsequent outcome: the CAVEAT study. *J Am Coll Cardiol* 1993;21:380A(abst).

100. Isner JM, Kearney M, Bortman S, et al. Sequential biopsy of human atheromata in vivo: longitudinal analysis of atheromatous coronary arterial wall in 11 patients treated for primary and restenosis lesions by directional atherectomy. *J Am Coll Cardiol* 1993;21:74A(abst).

101. Pickering JG, Weir L, Jekanowski J, et al. Proliferative activity in peripheral and coronary atherosclerotic plaque among patients undergoing percutaneous revascularization. *J Clin Invest* 1993;91:1469–1480.

102. Carter AJ, Laird JR, Farb A, et al. Morphologic characteristics of lesion formation and time course of smooth muscle cell proliferation in a porcine proliferative restenosis model. *J Am Coll Cardiol* 1994;24:1398–1405.

103. Bochaton-Piallat M-L, Gabbiani F, Redard M, et al. Apoptosis participates in cellularity regulation during rat aortic intimal thickening. *Am J Pathol* 1995;146:1059–1064.

104. Isner JM, Kearney M, Bortman S, et al. Apoptosis in human atherosclerosis and restenosis. *Circulation* 1995;91:2702–2711.

105. Nakamara T, Nishizawa T, Hagiya M, et al. Modular cloning and expression of human hepatocyte growth factor. *Nature* 1989;342:440–443.

105a. Davies MJ. Apoptosis in cardiovascular disease. *Heart* 1997;77:498–501.

106. Giraldi AA, Esposo OM, Meis JM. Intimal hyperplasia as a cause of restenosis after percutaneous transluminal coronary angioplasty. *Arch Pathol Lab Med* 1985;6:369–375.

107. Garratt KN, Edwards WD, Kaufmann UP, et al. Differential histopathology of primary atherosclerotic and restenotic lesions in coronary arteries and saphenous vein bypass grafts: analysis of tissue obtained from 73 patients by directional atherectomy. *J Am Coll Cardiol* 1991;17:442–448.

108. Isner JM, Kearney M, Berdan LG, et al. Core pathology lab findings in 425 patients undergoing directional atherectomy for a primary coronary artery stenosis and relationship to subsequent outcome: the CAVEAT study. *J Am Coll Cardiol* 1993;21:380A(abst).

109. Gordon D, Reidy MA, Benditt EP, et al. Cell proliferation in human coronary arteries. *Proc Natl Acad Sci U S A* 1990;87:4600–4604.

110. Hanke H, Strohschneider T, Oberhoff M, et al. Time course of smooth muscle cell proliferation in the intima and media of arteries following experimental angioplasty. *Circ Res* 1990;67:651–659.

111. Ohno T, Gordon D, San H, et al. Gene therapy for vascular smooth muscle cell proliferation after arterial injury. *Science* 1994;265:781–784.

112. Clowes AW, Clowes MM. Kinetics of cellular proliferation after arterial injury: II. Inhibition of smooth muscle growth by heparin. *Lab Invest* 1985;52:611–616.

113. Clowes AW, Reidy MA, Clowes MM. Kinetics of cellular proliferation after arterial injury: I. Smooth muscle growth in the absence of endothelium. *Lab Invest* 1983;49:327–333.

114. Tsujimoto Y, Croce CM. Analysis of the structure, transcripts, and protein products of bcl-2, the gene involved in human follicular lymphoma. *Proc Natl Acad Sci U S A* 1986;83:5214–5218.

115. Riessen R, Isner JM, Blessing E, et al. Regional differences in the distribution of the proteoglycans biglycan and decorin in the extracellular matrix of atherosclerotic and restenotic human coronary arteries. *Am J Pathol* 1994;144:962–974.

116. Shi Y, O'Brien JE, Ala-Kokko L, et al. Origin of extracellular matrix synthesis during coronary repair. *Circulation* 1997;95:997–1006.

117. Riessen R, Wight TN, Pastore C, et al. Distribution of hyaluronan during extracellular matrix remodeling in human restenotic arteries and balloon-injured rat carotid arteries. *Circulation* 1996;93:1141–1147.

118. Bauters C, Lablanche JM, McFadden EP, et al. Relation of coronary angioscopic findings at coronary angioplasty to angiographic restenosis. *Circulation* 1995;92:2473–2479.

119. Bauters C, Lablanche JM, Renaud N, et al. Morphologic changes after percutaneous transluminal coronary angioplasty of unstable plaques: insights from serial angioscopic follow-up. *Eur Heart J* 1996;17:1554–1559.

120. Post MJ, Borst C, Kuntz RE. The relative importance of arterial remodeling compared with intimal hyperplasia in lumen renarrowing after balloon angioplasty: a study in the normal rabbit and in the hypercholesterolemic Yucatan micropig. *Circulation* 1994;89:2816–2821.

121. Isner JM. Vascular remodeling: honey, I think I shrunk the artery. *Circulation* 1994;89:2937–2941.

122. Glagov S. Intimal hyperplasia, vascular remodeling, and the restenosis problem. *Circulation* 1994;89:2888–2891.

123. Glagov S, Weisenberg E, Zarins CK, et al. Compensatory enlargement of human atherosclerotic coronary arteries. *N Engl J Med* 1987;316:1371–1375.

124. Losordo DW, Rosenfield K, Kaufman J, et al. Focal compensatory enlargement of human arteries in response to progressive atherosclerosis: in vivo documentation using intravascular ultrasound. *Circulation* 1994;89:2570–2577.

125. Mintz GS, Popma JJ, Pichard AD, et al. Arterial remodeling after coronary angioplasty: a serial intravascular ultrasound study. *Circulation* 1996;94:35–43.

126. Kovach JA, Mintz GS, Kent KM, et al. Serial intravascular ultrasound studies indicate that chronic recoil is an important mechanism of restenosis following transcatheter therapy. *J Am Coll Cardiol* 1993;21:484A(abst).

127. Strauss BH, Chisholm RJ, Keeley FW, et al. Extracellular matrix remodeling after balloon angioplasty injury in a rabbit model of restenosis. *Circ Res* 1994;75:650–658.

127a. Mondy JS, Lindner V, Miyashiro JK, et al. Platelet-derived growth factor ligand and receptor expression in response to altered blood flow in vivo. *Circ Res* 1997;81:320–327.

127b. Smith JD, Bryant SR, Couper LL, et al. Soluble transforming growth factor–β type II receptor inhibits negative remodeling, fibroblast transdifferentiation, and intimal lesion formation but not endothelial growth. *Circ Res* 1999;84:1212–1222.

128. Shi Y, Pieniek M, Fard A, et al. Adventitial remodeling after coronary arterial injury. *Circulation* 1996;93:340–348.

129. Scott NA, Cipolla GD, Ross CE, et al. Identification of a potential role for the adventitia in vascular lesion formation after balloon overstretch injury of porcine coronary arteries. *Circulation* 1996;93:2178–2187.

130. Goldberb ID, Stemerman MB. Vascular permeation of platelet factor 4 after endothelial injury. *Science* 1980;209:611–612.

131. Friedman RJ, Stemerman MB, Wenz B, et al. The effect of thrombocytopenia on experimental arteriosclerotic lesion formation in rabbits. *J Clin Invest* 1977;60:1191–1201.

132. Willerson JT, Yao SK, McNatt J, et al. Frequency and severity of cyclic flow alternations and platelet aggregation predict the severity of neointimal proliferation following experimental coronary stenosis and endothelial injury. *Proc Natl Acad Sci U S A* 1991;88:10624–10628.

133. Fuster V, Badimon L, Badimon JJ, et al. The pathogenesis of coronary artery disease and the acute coronary syndromes. *N Engl J Med* 1992;326:242–250.

134. McNamara CA, Sarembock IJ, Gimple LW, et al. Thrombin stimulates proliferation of cultured rat aortic smooth muscle cells by a proteolytically activated receptor. *J Clin Invest* 1993;91:94–98.

135. Berk BC, Taubman MB, Gragoe EJ, et al. Thrombin stimulated events in cultured vascular smooth muscle cells. *J Biol Chem* 1990;265:1734–1740.

136. Bauters C, Khanoyan P, McFadden EP, Restenosis after delayed coronary angioplasty of the culprit vessel in patients with a recent myocardial infarction treated by thrombolysis. *Circulation* 1995;91:1410–1418.

137. Brodie BR, Grines CL, Ivanhoe R, et al. Six-month clinical and angiographic follow-up after direct angioplasty for acute myocardial infarction: final results from the primary angioplasty registry. *Circulation* 1994;25:156–162.

138. Leimgruber PP, Roubin GS, Hollman J, et al. Restenosis after successful coronary angioplasty in patients with single-vessel disease. *Circulation* 1986;73:710–717.

139. De Groote P, Bauters C, McFadden EP, et al. Local lesion-related factors and restenosis after coronary angioplasty: evidence from a quantitative angiographic study in patients with unstable angina undergoing double-vessel angioplasty. *Circulation* 1995;91:968–972.

140. Falk E. Unstable angina with fatal outcome: dynamic coronary thrombosis leading to infarction and/or sudden death. *Circulation* 1985;71:699–708.

141. Falk E. Plaque rupture with severe pre-existing precipitating coronary thrombosis: characteristics of coronary atherosclerotic plaques underlying fatal occlusive thrombi. *Br Heart J* 1983;50:127–134.

142. Davies MJ, Thomas AC. Plaque fissuring: the cause of acute myocardial infarction, sudden ischemia death, and crescendo angina. *Br Heart J* 1985;53:363–373.

143. Violaris AG, Melkert R, Herrman JPR, et al. Role of angiographically identifiable thrombus on long-term luminal renarrowing after coronary angioplasty. *Circulation* 1996;93:889–897.

144. Lablanche JM, Hamon M, McFadden EP, et al. Angiographically silent thrombus frequently persists after thrombolytic therapy for acute myocardial infarction: a prospective angioscopic study. *Circulation* 1993;88:3203(abst).

145. den Heijer P, Foley DP, Escaned J, et al. Angioscopic versus angiographic detection of intimal dissection and intracoronary thrombus. *J Am Coll Cardiol* 1994;24:649–654.

146. Clowes AW, Collazzo RE, Karnovsky MJ. A morphologic and permeability study of luminal smooth muscle cells after arterial injury in the rat. *Lab Invest* 1978;39:141–150.

147. Lindner V, Reidy MA, Fingerle J. Regrowth of arterial endothelium. Denudation with minimal trauma leads to complete endothelial cell regrowth. *Lab Invest* 1989;61:556–563.

148. Weidinger FF, McLenachan JM, Cybulski MI, et al. Persistent dysfunction of regenerated endothelium after bal-

loon angioplasty of rabbit iliac artery. *Circulation* 1990;81:1667–1679.

149. Haudenschild CC, Schwartz SM. Endothelial regeneration: II. Restitution of endothelial continuity. *Lab Invest* 1979;41:407–418.

150. Spagnoli LG, Pietra GG, Villaschi S, et al. Morphometric analysis of gap junctions in regenerating arterial endothelium. *Lab Invest* 1982;46:139–148.

151. Meurice T, Bauters C, Auffray JL, et al. Basic fibroblast growth factor restores endothelium-dependent responses after balloon injury of rabbit arteries. *Circulation* 1996;93:18–22.

152. Bjornsson TD, Dryjski M, Tluczek J, et al. Acidic fibroblast growth factor promotes vascular repair. *Proc Natl Acad Sci U S A* 1991;88:8651–8655.

153. Asahara T, Bauters C, Pastore C, et al. Local delivery of vascular endothelial growth factor accelerates reendothelialization and attenuates intimal hyperplasia in balloon-injured rat carotid artery. *Circulation* 1995;91:2793–2801.

154. Asahara T, Chen D, Kearney M, et al. Accelerated re-endothelialization and reduced neointimal thickening following catheter transfer of phVEGE$_{165}$. *Circulation* 1996;94:3291–3302.

155. Asahara T, Morohara T, Sullivan A, et al. Isolation of putative progenitor endothelial cells for angiogenesis. *Science* 1997;275:964–967.

156. Shimokawa H, Aarhus LL, Vanhoutte PM. Porcine coronary arteries with regenerated endothelium have a reduced endothelium-dependent responsiveness to aggregating platelets and serotonin. *Circ Res* 1987;61:256–270.

157. McFadden EP, Bauters C, Lablanche JM, et al. Response of human coronary arteries to serotonin after injury by coronary angioplasty. *Circulation* 1993;88:2076–2085.

158. Kirigaya H, Aisawa T, Ogasawara K, et al. Incidence of acetylcholine-induced spasm of coronary artery subjected to balloon angioplasty. *Jpn Circ J* 1993;57:883–890.

159. Furchgott RF, Zawadzki JV. The obligatory role of endothelial cells in the relaxation of arterial smooth muscle by acetylcholine. *Nature* 1980;288:373–376.

160. Palmer RMJ, Ferrige AG, Moncada S. Nitric oxide release accounts for the biological activity of endothelium-derived relaxing factor. *Nature* 1987;327:524–526.

161. Saroyan RM, Roberts MP, Light JT, et al. Differential recovery of prostacyclin and endothelium-derived relaxing factor after vascular injury. *Am J Physiol* 1992;262:H1449–H1457.

162. Guo J, Milhoan KA, Tuan RS, et al. Beneficial effect of SPM-5185, a cysteine-containing nitric oxide donor, in rat carotid artery intimal injury. *Circ Res* 1994;75:77–84.

163. Bauters C, Asahara T, Zheng LP, et al. Physiologic assessment of augmented vascularity induced by vascular endothelial growth factor in the rabbit ischemic hindlimb. *Am J Physiol* 1994;267:H1263–H1271.

164. Bauters C, Asahara T, Zheng LP, et al. Recovery of disturbed endothelium-dependent flow in the collateral-perfused rabbit ischemic hindlimb after administration of vascular endothelial growth factor. *Circulation* 1995;91:2802–2809.

165. Selke FW, Wang SY, Friedman M, et al. Basic FGF enhances endothelium-dependent relaxation of the collat-eral-perfused coronary microcirculation. *Am J Physiol* 1994;267:H1303–H1311.

166. Van Belle E, Rivard A, Chen D, et al. Hypercholesterolemia attenuates angiogenesis, but does not preclude augmentation by angiogenic cytokines. *Circulation* 1997;96:2667–2674.

167. Meurice T, Bauters C, Vallet B, et al. Basic fibroblast growth factor restores endothelium-dependent responses of hypercholesterolemic rabbit thoracic aorta. *Am J Physiol* 1996;272:H613–H617.

168. Stemerman MB, Spaet TH, Pitlick F, et al. The pattern of reendothelialization and intimal thickening. *Am J Pathol* 1977;87:125–142.

169. Fishman JA, Ryan GB, Karnovsky MJ. Endothelial regeneration in the rat carotid artery and the significance of endothelial denudation in the pathogenesis of myointimal thickening. *Lab Invest* 1975;32:339–351.

170. Reidy MA. Endothelial regeneration: VII. Interaction of smooth muscle cells with endothelial regrowth. *Lab Invest* 1988;59:36–43.

171. Scott-Burden T, Vanhoutte PM. The endothelium as a regulator of vascular smooth muscle proliferation. *Circulation* 1993;87[Suppl V]:V-51–V-55.

172. Garg UC, Hassid A. Nitric oxide-generating vasodilators and 8-bromo-cyclic guanosine monophosphate inhibit mitogenesis and proliferation of cultured rat vascular smooth muscle cells. *J Clin Invest* 1989;83:1774–1777.

173. Doornekamp FNG, Borts C, Post MJ. Endothelial cell recoverage and intimal hyperplasia after endothelium removal with or without smooth muscle cell necrosis in rabbit carotid artery. *J Vasc Res* 1996;33:146–155.

174. Palmer RMJ, Moncada DSA, Moncada S. Vascular endothelial cells synthesize nitric oxide from L-arginine. *Nature* 1988;333:664–666.

175. Moncada S, Higgs A. The L-arginine–nitric oxide pathway. *N Engl J Med* 1993;329:2002–2012.

176. von der Leyen HE, Leyen VD, Gibbons GH, et al. Gene therapy inhibiting neointimal vascular lesion: in vivo transfer of endothelial cell nitric oxide synthase gene. *Proc Natl Acad Sci U S A* 1995;92:1137–1141.

177. Taguchi J, Abe J, Okasaki H, et al. L-arginine inhibits neointimal formation following balloon injury. *Life Sci* 1993;53:387–392.

178. Winkles JA, Friesel R, Burgess WH, et al. Human vascular smooth muscle cells both express and respond to heparin-binding growth factor I (endothelial cell growth factor). *Proc Natl Acad Sci U S A* 1987;84:7124–7128.

179. Langille BL. Remodeling of developing and mature arteries: endothelium, smooth muscle, and matrix. *J Cardiovasc Pharmacol* 1993;21[Suppl 1]:S11–S17.

180. Langille BL, O'Donnell F. Reductions in arterial diameter produced by chronic decreases in blood flow are endothelium-dependent. *Science* 1986;231:405–407.

181. Gibbons GH, Dzau VJ. The emerging concept of vascular remodeling. *N Engl J Med* 1994;330:1431–1438.

182. Radomski MW, Palmer RMJ, Moncada S. The antiaggregating properties of vascular endothelium: interactions between prostacyclin and nitric oxide. *Br J Pharmacol* 1987;92:639–646.

183. Rubanyi GM. The role of endothelium in cardiovascular

homeostasis and diseases. *J Cardiovasc Pharmacol* 1993; 22[Suppl 4]:S1–S14.

184. Sigwart U, Puel J, Mirkovitch V, et al. Intravascular stents to prevent occlusion and restenosis after transluminal angioplasty. *N Engl J Med* 1987;316:701–706.

185. Serruys PW, Strauss BH, Beatt KJ, et al. Angiographic follow-up after placement of a self-expanding coronary artery stent. *N Engl J Med* 1991;324:13–17.

186. Kimura T, Yokoi H, Nakagawa Y, et al. Three-year follow-up after implantation of metallic coronary-artery stents. *N Engl J Med* 1996;334:561–566.

187. Van Belle E, McFadden EP, Lablanche JM, et al. Two-pronged antiplatelet therapy with aspirin and ticlopidine without systemic anticoagulation: an alternative therapeutic strategy after bailout stent implantation. *Coron Artery Dis* 1995;6:341–345.

188. Colombo A, Hall P, Nakamura S, et al. Intracoronary stenting without anticoagulation accomplished with intravascular ultrasound guidance. *Circulation* 1995;91:1676–1688.

189. Schomig A, Neumann FJ, Kastrati A, et al. A randomized comparison of antiplatelet and anticoagulant therapy after the placement of coronary-artery stents. *N Engl J Med* 1996;334:1084–1089.

190. Serruys PW, de Jaegere P, Kiemeneij F, et al. A comparison of balloon-expandable-stent implantation with balloon angioplasty in patients with coronary artery disease. *N Engl J Med* 1994;331:489–495.

191. Fischman DL, Leon MB, Baim DS, et al. A randomized comparison of coronary-stent placement and balloon angioplasty in the treatment of coronary artery disease. *N Engl J Med* 1994;331:496–501.

192. Serruys PW, Emanuelsson H, van der Giessen W, et al. Heparin-coated Palmatz-Schatz stents in human coronary arteries: early outcome of the Benestent-II pilot study. *Circulation* 1996;93:414–422.

193. Mintz GS, Popma JJ, Pichard AD, et al. Differing mechanisms of late arterial responses to transcatheter therapy: a serial quantitative angiographic and intravascular ultrasound study. *Eur Heart J* 1995;Suppl:385(abst).

194. Mintz GS, Pichard AD, Kent KM, et al. Endovascular stents reduce restenosis by eliminating geometric arterial remodeling: a serial intravascular ultrasound study. *J Am Coll Cardiol* 1995;25:36A(abst).

195. Hehrlein C, Gollan C, Donges BS, et al. Low-dose radioactive endovascular stents prevent smooth muscle cell proliferation and neointimal hyperplasia in rabbits. *Circulation* 1995;92:1570–1575.

196. Waksman R, Robinson KA, Crocker IR, et al. Intracoronary radiation before stent implantation inhibits neointima formation in stented porcine coronary arteries. *Circulation* 1995;92:1383–1386.

197. Laird JR, Carter AJ, Kufs WA, et al. Inhibition of neointimal proliferation with low-dose irradiation from a β-particle-emitting stent. *Circulation* 1996;93:529–536.

198. Gallino A, Mahler F, Probst P, et al. Percutaneous transluminal angioplasty of the arteries of the lower limbs: a 5-year follow-up. *Circulation* 1984;70:619–623.

199. Anderson PG, Bajaj RK, Baxley WA, Roubin GS. Vascular pathology of balloon-expandable flexible coil stents in humans. *J Am Coll Cardiol* 1992;19:372–381.

200. van Beusekom HMM, Van der Giessen WJ, van Suylen RJ, et al. Histology after stenting of human vein bypass grafts: observations from surgically excised grafts 3 to 320 days after stent implantation. *J Am Coll Cardiol* 1993; 21:45–54.

201. Strauss BH, Umans VA, van Suylen RJ, et al. Directional atherectomy for treatment of restenosis within coronary stents: clinical, angiographic and histologic results. *J Am Coll Cardiol* 1992;20:1465–1473.

202. Gelb AB, Kamel OW, LeBrun DP, et al. Estimation of tumor growth fractions in archival formalin-fixed, paraffin-embedded tissues using two anti-PCNA/cyclin monoclonal antibodies. *Am J Pathol* 1992;141:1453–1458.

203. Kearney M, Pieczek A, Haley L, et al. Histopathology of stent restenosis in patients with peripheral artery disease. *Circulation* 1997;95:1998-2002.

204. Wei GL, Krasinski K, Kearney M, et al. Temporally and spatially coordinated expression of cell cycle regulatory factors after angioplasty. *Circ Res* 1997;80:418–426.

205. Karas SP, Gravanis MB, Santoian EC, et al. Coronary intimal proliferation after balloon injury and stenting in swine: an animal model of restenosis. *J Am Coll Cardiol* 1992;20:467–474.

206. Schwartz RS, Holmes J, Topol EJ. The restenosis paradigm revisited: an alternative proposal for cellular mechanisms. *J Am Coll Cardiol* 1992;20:1284–1293.

207. Palmaz JC, Windeler SA, Garcia F, et al. Atherosclerotic rabbit aortas: expandable intraluminal grafting. *Radiology* 1986;160:723–726.

208. Schatz RA, Palmaz JC, Tio FO, et al. Balloon-expandable intracoronary stents in the adult dog. *Circulation* 1987;76:450–457.

209. Hardhammar PA, van Beukesom HMM, Emmanuelsson HU, et al. Reduction in thrombotic events with heparin-coated Palmaz-Schatz stents in normal porcine coronary arteries. *Circulation* 1996;93:423–430.

210. Van Belle E, Tio FO, Couffinhal T, et al. Stent endothelialization: time course, impact of local catheter delivery, feasibility of recombinant protein administration, and response to cytokine expedition. *Circulation* 1997;94:438–448.

211. Van Belle E, Tio FO, Chen D, et al. Passivation of metallic stents following arterial gene transfer of phVEGF$_{165}$ inhibits thrombus formation and intimal thickening. *J Am Coll Cardiol* 1997;29:1371–1379.

212. Teirstein PS, Massullo V, Jani S, et al. Catheter-based radiotherapy to inhibit restenosis after coronary stenting. *N Engl J Med* 1997;336:1697–1703.

213. King SB, Williams DO, Chougule P, et al. Endovascular beta-radiation to reduce restenosis after coronary balloon angioplasty: results of the beta energy restenosis trial (BERT). *Circulation* 1998;97:2025–2030.

214. Albiero R, Adamian M, Kobayashi N, et al. Short- and intermediate-term results of (32)P radioactive beta-emitting stent implantation in patients with coronary artery disease: the Milan Dose-Response Study. *Circulation* 2000;101:18–26.

215. Costa MA, Sabat M, van der Giessen WJ, et al. Late coronary occlusion after intracoronary brachytherapy. *Circulation* 1999;100:789–792.

216. Waksman R, Bhargava B, Mintz GS, et al. Late total

occlusion after intracoronary brachytherapy for patients with in-stent restenosis. *J Am Coll Cardiol* 2000;36:65–68.

217. Marijianowski MM, Crocker IR, Styles T, et al. Fibrocellular tissue responses to endovascular and external beam irradiation in the porcine model of restenosis. *Int J Radiat Oncol Biol Phys* 1999;44:633–641.

218. Waksman R, Rodriguez JC, Robinson KA, et al. Effect of intravascular irradiation on cell proliferation, apoptosis, and vascular remodeling after balloon overstretch injury of porcine coronary arteries. *Circulation* 1997;96:1944–1952.

219. Sabate M, Serruys PW, van der Giessen WJ, et al. Geometric vascular remodeling after balloon angioplasty and beta-radiation therapy: a three-dimensional intravascular ultrasound study. *Circulation* 1999;100:1182–1188.

220. Condado JA, Waksman R, Gurdiel O, et al. Long-term angiographic and clinical outcome after percutaneous transluminal coronary angioplasty and intracoronary radiation therapy in humans. *Circulation* 1997;96:727–732.

221. Wilcox JN, Waksman R, King SB, et al. The role of the adventitia in the arterial response to angioplasty: the effect of intravascular radiation. *Int J Radiat Oncol Biol Phys* 1996;36:789–796.

222. Waksman R, Robinson KA, Crocker IR, et al. Intracoronary low-dose beta-irradiation inhibits neointima formation after coronary artery balloon injury in the swine restenosis model. *Circulation* 1995;92:3025–3031.

223. Waksman R, Robinson KA, Crocker IR, et al. Endovascular low-dose irradiation inhibits neointima formation after coronary artery balloon injury in swine. A possible role for radiation therapy in restenosis prevention. *Circulation* 1995;91:1533–1539.

224. Mazur W, Ali MN, Khan MM, et al. High dose rate intracoronary radiation for inhibition of neointimal formation in the stented and balloon-injured porcine models of restenosis: angiographic, morphometric, and histopathologic analyses. *Int J Radiat Oncol Biol Phys* 1996;36:777–788.

225. Verin V, Popowski Y, Urban P, et al. Intra-arterial beta irradiation prevents neointimal hyperplasia in a hypercholesterolemic rabbit restenosis model. *Circulation* 1995;92:2284–2290.

226. Hehrlein C, Gollan C, Donges K, et al. Low-dose radioactive endovascular stents prevent smooth muscle cell proliferation and neointimal hyperplasia in rabbits. *Circulation* 1995;92:1570–1575.

227. Hehrlein C, Stintz M, Kinscherf R, et al. Pure beta-particle-emitting stents inhibit neointima formation in rabbits. *Circulation* 1996;93:641–645.

228. Carter AJ, Laird JR, Bailey LR, et al. Effects of endovascular radiation from a beta-particle-emitting stent in a porcine coronary restenosis model. A dose-response study. *Circulation* 1996;94:2364–2368.

229. Mintz GS, Weissman NJ, Teirstein PS, et al. Effect of intracoronary gamma-radiation therapy on in-stent restenosis: an intravascular ultrasound analysis from the gamma-1 study. *Circulation* 2000;102:2915–2918.

230. Farb A, Tang AL, Shroff S, et al. Neointimal responses 3 months after (32)P beta-emitting stent placement. *Int J Radiat Oncol Biol Phys* 2000;48:889–898.

231. Kay IP, Sabate M, Costa MA, et al. Positive geometric vascular remodeling is seen after catheter-based radiation followed by conventional stent implantation but not after radioactive stent implantation. *Circulation* 2000;102:1434–1439.

232. Teirstein PS, Massullo V, Jani S, et al. Three-year clinical and angiographic follow-up after intracoronary radiation: results of a randomized clinical trial. *Circulation* 2000;101:360–365.

233. Taylor AJ, Gorman PD, Farb A, et al. Long-term coronary vascular response to (32)P beta-particle-emitting stents in a canine model. *Circulation* 1999;100:2366–2372.

234. Taylor AJ, Gorman PD, Hudak C, et al. The 90-day coronary vascular response to (90)Y-beta particle-emitting stents in the canine model. *Int J Radiat Oncol Biol Phys* 2000;46:1019–1024.

235. Schulz C, Niederer C, Andres C, et al. Endovascular irradiation from beta-particle-emitting gold stents results in increased neointima formation in a porcine restenosis model. *Circulation* 2000;101:1970–1975.

236. Fischell TA, Kharma BK, Fischell DR, et al. Low-dose, beta-particle emission from "stent" wire results in complete, localized inhibition of smooth muscle cell proliferation. *Circulation* 1994;90:2956–2963.

237. Fareh J, Martel R, Kermani P, et al. Cellular effects of beta-particle delivery on vascular smooth muscle cells and endothelial cells: a dose-response study. *Circulation* 1999;99:1477–1484.

238. Gajdusek CM, Tian H, London S, et al. Gamma radiation effect on vascular smooth muscle cells in culture. *Int J Radiat Oncol Biol Phys* 1996;36:821–828.

239. Asahara T, Bauters C, Pastore C, et al. Local delivery of vascular endothelial growth factor accelerates reendothelialization and attenuates intimal hyperplasia in balloon-injured rat carotid artery. *Circulation* 1995;91:2793–2801.

240. Thorin E, Meerkin D, Bertrand OF, et al. Influence of postangioplasty beta-irradiation on endothelial function in porcine coronary arteries. *Circulation* 2000;101:1430–1435.

241. Sabate M, Kay IP, van Der Giessen WJ, et al. Preserved endothelium-dependent vasodilation in coronary segments previously treated with balloon angioplasty and intracoronary irradiation. *Circulation* 1999;100:1623–1629.

242. Vodovotz Y, Waksman R, Kim WH, et al. Effects of intracoronary radiation on thrombosis after balloon overstretch injury in the porcine model. *Circulation* 1999;100:2527–2533.

243. Cottin Y, Kollum M, Chan R, et al. Vascular repair after balloon overstretch injury in porcine model: effects of intracoronary radiation. *J Am Coll Cardiol* 2000;36:1389–1395.

244. Vodovotz Y, Waksman R, Cook JA, et al. *S*-Nitrosoglutathione reduces nonocclusive thrombosis rate following balloon overstretch injury and intracoronary irradiation of porcine coronary arteries. *Int J Radiat Oncol Biol Phys* 2000;48:1167–1174.

245. Waksman R. Late thrombosis after radiation. Sitting on a time bomb. *Circulation* 1999;100:780–482.

106

ANGIOGENESIS

JEFFREY M. ISNER

▼ ADDITIONAL ELECTRONIC TOPICS

Autocrine Loop as a Feature of Angiogenic Cytokines q30; Angiogenic Cytokines and Vascular Permeability q31; Direct versus Indirect Cytokines q32; Site-Specific Effects of Angiogenic Cytokines q33; Role of Nitric Oxide in Mediating Effects of Angiogenic Growth Factors q34; Experimental Studies in Animal Models of Myocardial Ischemia q35; Clinical Studies Using Gene Transfer q36; Transmyocardial Laser Revascularization q37

OVERVIEW

The development of blood vessels can be considered in several contexts. Vasculogenesis and angiogenesis are the processes that are responsible for the development of the circulatory system, the first functional unit in the developing embryo (1). Therapeutic angiogenesis includes the development of collateral blood vessels that supply ischemic tissues, either endogenously or in response to administered growth factors. Pathologic angiogenesis includes the role of postnatal neovascularization in the pathogenesis of arthritis, diabetic retinopathy, and, most notably, tumor growth and metastasis (2).

J. M. Isner: Department of Medicine/Vascular Medicine, Tufts University School of Medicine, St. Elizabeth's Medical Center, Boston, Massachusetts (Deceased)

Because recapitulation of the embryonic paradigm forms the basis for therapeutic, as well as pathologic, angiogenesis, this chapter addresses selected aspects of embryonic blood vessel development. Therapeutic angiogenesis represents a natural response to myocardial ischemia in particular and tissue ischemia in general, and, along with novel strategies that have been devised to augment this response, is discussed in detail. Although pathologic angiogenesis is beyond the scope of the current chapter, certain principles that have emerged from studies of pathologic neovascularization are considered for the implications that they may have for cardiovascular disease.

VASCULOGENESIS AND ANGIOGENESIS

Vasculogenesis refers to the *in situ* formation of blood vessels from progenitor endothelial cells (ECs), or angioblasts (3).

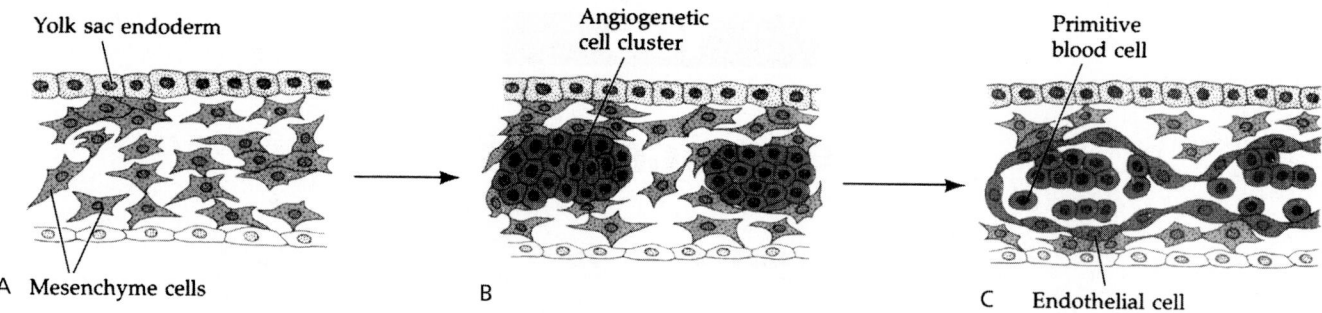

FIGURE 106.1 Blood islands. Blood vessel formation is first seen in the wall of the yolk sac, where **(A)** undifferentiated mesenchyme condenses to form **(B)** angiogenic cell clusters. **C:** The centers of these clusters form the blood cells, and the outside of the clusters develop into blood vessel endothelial cells. (From Gilbert SF. *Developmental biology*, 4th ed. Sunderland, MA: Sinauer Associates, 1997:342, with permission.)

It is necessary to distinguish between vascular development that takes place in the yolk sac of the embryo from that which occurs in the embryo proper. Extraembryonic vasculogenesis begins as a cluster formation, or blood island (Fig. 106.1). Growth and fusion of multiple blood islands in the yolk sac of the embryo ultimately give rise to the yolk sac capillary network (4); after the onset of blood circulation, this network differentiates into an arteriovenous vascular system (5). The integral relationship between the elements that circulate in the vascular system—the blood cells—and the cells that are principally responsible for the vessels themselves—ECs—is implied by the composition of the embryonic blood islands. The cells that are destined to generate hematopoietic cells are situated in the center of the blood island and are termed *hematopoietic stem cells* (*HSCs*). Endothelial progenitor cells (EPCs), or angioblasts, are located at the periphery of the blood islands. In addition to this spatial association, HSCs and angioblasts share certain antigenic determinants, including Flk-1, Tie-2, and CD34. These progenitor cells have consequently been considered to derive from a common precursor, putatively termed a *hemangioblast* (6–8).

Vasculogenesis that occurs within the embryo proper is currently considered to involve differentiation of so-called solitary angioblasts—that is, angioblasts that are not intimately associated with concomitantly differentiating HSCs (3). The sole exception to this is a small region in the aorta, termed *paraaortic clusters*. *In situ* differentiation of such solitary angioblasts occurs primarily from mesodermal cells in contact with endoderm. These angioblasts may migrate and fuse with other angioblasts and capillaries or form vessels *in situ*. Blood elements that circulate within the blood vessels of the embryo proper are believed to derive from the yolk sac or paraaortic clusters.

In contrast to *in situ* differentiation of progenitor cells that are required to establish the primordial vascular network, extension of the primitive vasculature involves angiogenesis—that is, sprouting of new capillaries from the preexisting network; by definition, this implicates dif-

ferentiated ECs as the responsible cellular element. Full development of the circulatory system involves recurrent remodeling, as some vessels regress, presumably by apoptosis, and others branch or are invested with a multilayer architecture characteristic of medium to large arteries and veins, or both. The extensive EC proliferative activity, which constitutes the basis for angiogenesis in the embryo, contrasts with extraordinary EC quiescence in the adult, in whom the interval for EC turnover is estimated to be more than 1,000 days (9).

Classic Paradigm for Angiogenesis

Until recently, vasculogenesis was considered to be restricted to the embryo, and new blood vessel formation in adult species was inferred to be the exclusive consequence of angiogenesis. The full paradigm for angiogenesis has been suggested to begin with "activation" of ECs within a parent vessel, followed by disruption of the basement membrane and subsequent migration of ECs into the interstitial space, possibly in the direction of an ischemic stimulus (10) (Fig. 106.2). Concomitant and/or subsequent EC proliferation, intracellular-vacuolar lumen formation, pericyte "capping," and production of a basement membrane complete the developmental sequence.

During angiogenesis, migration always precedes proliferation by approximately 24 hours (11). This principle was best demonstrated in classic experiments performed by Sholley et al. (12). Using a model of inflammation-induced angiogenesis of the rat cornea, initiation of vascular sprouting was shown to occur in the absence of EC proliferation. EC proliferation in this model was suppressed by X-irradiation with 2,000 or 8,000 rads before application of the inflammatory stimulus. In irradiated corneas displaying no cellular proliferation, vascular sprouting at 2 days was similar to that seen in contralateral shielded corneas. Although neovascular growth was subsequently blunted and ultimately ceased by 4 to 7 days, these experiments documented the critical if not exclusive roles of migration and

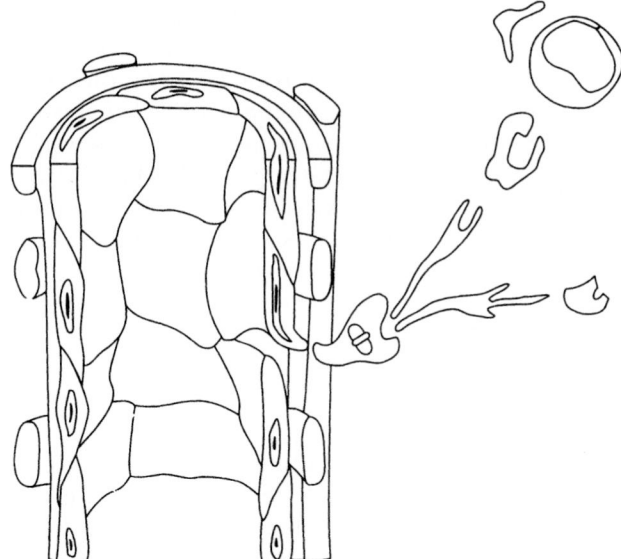

FIGURE 106.2 Classic paradigm for angiogenesis. Endothelial cells break free from their basement membrane and surrounding extracellular matrix, migrate, proliferate, and remodel (i.e., form a lumen), thus generating new blood vessels or "sprouts" from the parent vessel. (From D'Amore PA, Thompson RW. Mechanisms of angiogenesis. *Annu Rev Physiol* 1987;49:453–464, with permission.)

redistribution of preexisting ECs in the commencement of neovascularization. Similar implications resulted from work by Nicosia et al. (13): Fibronectin was shown to promote, in a dose-dependent fashion, the elongation of microvessels that sprout from explants of rat aorta placed in serum-free collagen gel—despite the fact that neither deoxyribonucleic acid (DNA) synthesis nor mitotic activity was increased in comparison to fibronectin-negative gels. Fibronectin was therefore inferred to promote angiogenesis *in vitro* by migratory recruitment of preexisting ECs. Subsequent studies have established the critical role played by plasmin and other proteases in promoting migration through preexisting matrix (14,15).

In contrast to these *in vivo* inflammatory and *in vitro* organ culture models, angiogenesis that develops in response to experimental vascular obstruction, that is, collateral vessel development, has been shown by several previous investigators to involve proliferation of not only ECs but smooth muscle cells (SMCs) as well. Several important principles were elucidated by these studies.

First, evidence of EC proliferation is nearly absent in normal arteries (16,17), a finding that is consistent with an estimated EC turnover time of "thousands of days" in quiescent microvasculature (9). Even a relatively low percentage of EC proliferation observed in response to arterial occlusion or exogenous growth factors may therefore represent considerable enhancement of EC proliferative activity and, when considered in relation to a denominator of thousands of ECs, is clearly sufficient to provide the

basis for new blood vessel formation. Second, peak EC proliferation that contributes to naturally occurring collateral development in the setting of vascular occlusion varies from 2.6% to 3.5% in the canine coronary circulation (16,18), from 5% to 6% in the rodent renal vasculature (19), and less than 1% in swine coronaries (20). The contrasting rates of EC proliferation between the canine and swine coronary circulations are indeed representative of the contrasting propensity for natural collateral artery development in these two species. Third, proliferation of SMCs, the additional requisite cell type for the formation of larger blood vessels, is an implicit component of angiogenesis, regardless of animal species or circulatory site. In fact, Schaper et al. (21) speculated more than 30 years ago that "it is tempting to assume that EC proliferation not only serves the purpose of forming the endothelium of a finally larger artery but rather actively participates in the development of the tunica media." Fourth, proliferative activity—for SMCs as well as ECs—is highest at the level of the smallest-diameter collateral vessels, the so-called midzone collateral segments (16,18,22,23). Fifth, although evidence of EC and SMC proliferation alone does not necessarily distinguish new vessel development from an increase in the size of preexisting vessels, adjunctive data regarding increased capillary density (24,25) support the notion that proliferative activity does in fact reflect true angiogenesis.

Ligand-Receptor Systems Modulate Vasculogenesis and Angiogenesis

A series of gene-targeting studies has elucidated the role of certain ligands or their receptors, or both, in vasculogenesis and angiogenesis. The phenotypic characteristics of these "knockout" mice are relevant to adult cardiovascular disease because of the implications they may have for the role played by these same ligand-receptor systems in promoting postnatal angiogenesis.

As indicated previously, KDR (the murine equivalent is known as *Flk-1* or *VEGFR-2*), the principal receptor for vascular endothelial growth factor (VEGF), is expressed by angioblasts and HSCs. It is perhaps not surprising, therefore, that mice deficient in this gene die *in utero* between 8.5 and 9.5 days postcoitum as the result of an early defect in the development of hematopoietic cells and ECs. Yolk sac blood islands were absent at 7.5 days, organized blood vessels could not be observed in the embryo and yolk sac at any stage, and hematopoietic progenitors were severely reduced (26). Markers of early endothelial precursors, such as Flt-1, Flt-4, and Tie-2, were expressed, but a marker of later endothelial development, Tie-2, could not be detected, indicating a deficiency of mature ECs (26). Expression of CD34, a marker of HSCs, was greatly reduced as well. The absence of blood islands and blood vessels in these mice established that the Flk-1 signaling pathway is required very early in the development of endothelial lineage and may be important for blood cell development as well.

Findings in the Flk-1 knockout mouse predicted what was to be found when the ligand, VEGF, was deficient. Mice that were deficient in even one of two VEGF alleles died *in utero* between days 10.5 and 12. Blood island formation (vasculogenesis) and vascular sprouting from pre-existing vessels (angiogenesis) were again impaired (27,28). The failure of blood vessel ingrowth was accompanied by apoptosis and disorganization of neuroepithelial cells. The heterozygous lethal phenotype was interpreted as evidence for tight dose-dependent regulation of embryonic vessel development by VEGF. Parenthetically, the aortas of VEGF-deficient mice have been noted to be hypoplastic, similar to those observed in mice deficient in endothelial nitric oxide (NO) synthase (P. Huang, *personal communication*, 2001). It is interesting to speculate that this may reflect the role of NO in VEGF-modulation of EC function.

The tyrosine kinase Flt-1 receptor (VEGF-R1) constitutes a second high-affinity binding receptor for VEGF. Mouse embryos that are homozygous for a targeted mutation in the Flt-1 locus formed fully differentiated ECs in embryonic and extraembryonic regions but assembled these cells into abnormal vascular channels and died *in utero* (29). Blood islands, for example, were disorganized, consisting of intermixed angioblasts and HSCs. In the head mesenchyme, instead of progressive development of individual small vessels, large fused vessels were seen that contained internally localized groups of ECs. These findings were interpreted as evidence that the Flt-1 signaling pathway may regulate normal EC cell-cell or cell-matrix interactions during vascular development.

Tie-1 and Tie-2 (30) comprise a second family of receptor tyrosine kinases, other than the VEGF family, in which expression is nearly specific for ECs. Mice embryos that are deficient in Tie-1 fail to establish structural integrity of otherwise differentiated ECs (31); consequently, erythrocytes extravasate through the blood-vessel EC (but not between ECs), leading to death immediately after birth with widespread hemorrhage. Embryos that are homozygous mutant for Tie-2 die earlier (day 10.5 *in utero*), with dilated vessels lacking distinction between small and large vessels; absence of ordered branching has been inferred as evidence of disordered angiogenesis. Vasculogenesis *per se* was not disrupted.

Successful disruption of the ligand for Tie-2, angiopoietin-1 (32,33), resulted in embryonic lethality by day 12.5, with defects similar to those seen in the Tie-2 receptor knockout. These included defects in organized branching, so that vessels remained dilated and almost syncytial. No change occurred in the total number of ECs, however.

The critical roles played by VEGF and its receptors in governing vasculogenesis and angiogenesis, and the Tie receptor/ligand family in maturation of the vascular network, have implications for the roles of these EC mitogens in promoting angiogenesis under circumstances of tissue ischemia in adults. In contrast to the lethal consequences of VEGF and Tie deficiencies, it is interesting to note that mice in which gene targeting has been used to disrupt the gene for basic fibroblast growth factor (bFGF) survive to maturity with no apparent phenotypic abnormalities of either the vascular or hematopoietic systems (G. Dorn and T. Deutschman, *personal communication*, 2001).

Remodeling

Remodeling in angiogenesis refers to the formation of a vascular lumen. Whereas multiple cell types, including ECs, grown *in vitro* on a collagen-matrix gel form cords, the presence of a lumen distinguishes vessels, or tubes, from solid cords. The presence of a lumen is clearly fundamental to the function of the circulatory system; however, the mechanisms that are responsible for tube formation are perhaps the least well understood aspect of angiogenesis (34). As Risau has pointed out, because isolated ECs may combine to form a lumen *in vitro* (35), lumen formation must represent an intrinsic feature or differentiation program of these cells (3). Mechanisms that have been discussed include the joining of polarized ends of capillary ECs in a ring-like fashion or, alternatively, simple deletion of a portion of the cell (vacuole formation) (36). Adding further to the complexity is the requirement to form qualitatively differing luminal and abluminal surfaces. Finally, it is inferred that remodeling comprises a coordinated process of lumen formation and vessel extension, with fusion of individual cells and their lumina via cell-cell adhesion molecules. The specific molecules that are responsible for vessel extension remain ambiguous. It is presumed that this aspect of vessel formation is subject to the regulatory factors that are responsible for vascular development in the embryo, as discussed above. In this respect, it is interesting to note that VEGF, for example, upregulates gap junction expression (specifically connexin 43) in ECs (37).

Nascent Vessels

Capillary growth rates (i.e., the velocity of neovascularization) range from 0.23 to 0.80 mm per day, depending on the experimental system used or the type of tumor, or both (38). The light microscopic features of newly formed vessels have been distinguished from those of native vessels (39). Whereas a histologic section of a capillary blood vessel in the normal brain reveals one or two ECs per lumen, in a brain tumor such as a glioblastoma, five to ten ECs may occupy one lumen. Tumor-induced vessels often appear dilated and saccular. Moreover, tumors may contain giant capillaries and arteriovenous shunts without intervening capillaries, so that blood may even flow from one venule to another.

Ultrastructural analysis of newly formed vessels has focused on features that are potentially responsible for augmented permeability. Dvorak et al. (40,41), for example, found that vascular leakage could not be attributed to passage of molecules through inter-EC junctions or injured tumor endothelium but instead involved transendothelial transport via a novel cytoplasmic organelle that they termed the *vesicular-vacuolar organelle*. Others (42) have reported VEGF-induced ultrastructural features that are consistent with endothelial fenestration.

Matrix-Integrin Interactions

Activated or proliferative ECs have been shown to express high levels of $\alpha v\beta_3$ (43,44). In nonhuman primates that were subjected to focal cerebral ischemia, for example, microvascular expression of $\alpha v\beta_3$ was noted in ischemic, but not nonischemic, tissues (45). Ligation of $\alpha v\beta_3$ on proliferating ECs promotes a critical adhesion-dependent cell survival signal, leading to inhibition of p53 activity, decreased expression of p21$^{WAF1/CIP1}$, and suppression of the bax cell death pathway (46). The intracellular molecular conflict that results from blocking $\alpha v\beta_3$ thus leads to unscheduled apoptosis and the abrogation of angiogenesis (44,46,47). Failure to ligate $\alpha v\beta_3$ may therefore inhibit the ability of actively cycling cells to ligate extracellular matrix proteins, including fibronectin, vitronectin, fibrinogen, and osteopontin, thereby influencing adhesion, migration, and, ultimately, survival of these cells (48).

Consistent with this notion, the integrin $\alpha v\beta_3$ has been shown to be required for angiogenesis *in vivo* (43), and antagonists of this integrin have been shown to inhibit angiogenesis by inducing apoptosis (44). Basic FGF, which has been shown to protect ECs from apoptosis (49), is known to modulate integrin expression by ECs (50–52). VEGF, by upregulation of the β_3 integrin and fibronectin, may similarly inhibit apoptosis by enhancing EC adhesion to matrix proteins (53). This notion is thus consistent with the concept that VEGF may exert a survival effect on ECs (43,44,54–56). These findings suggest that the net increase in EC viability after VEGF administration is not limited to the mitogenic effects of VEGF on ECs but is supplemented by the potential for VEGF to inhibit apoptosis.

Vasculogenesis in the Adult

Postnatal neovascularization was previously considered to result exclusively from the proliferation, migration, and remodeling of fully differentiated ECs derived from preexisting blood vessels, that is, angiogenesis (3,9,16). The formation of blood vessels from EC progenitors, or angioblasts (i.e., vasculogenesis), has been considered to be restricted to embryogenesis (5,57). However, the use of

HSCs derived from peripheral blood in lieu of bone marrow to provide sustained hematopoietic recovery can be reasoned to constitute inferential evidence for circulating stem cells (58). Given the common ancestry of HSCs and angioblasts, the hypothesis that stem cells circulating in peripheral blood might under selected circumstances differentiate into ECs was investigated (59,60). Flk-1 and a second antigen, CD34, shared by angioblasts and HSCs (26,61–71), were used to isolate putative angioblasts from the leukocyte fraction of peripheral blood. *In vitro*, these cells differentiated into ECs (Fig. 106.3). In animal models of ischemia, heterologous, homologous, and autologous EC progenitors are incorporated into sites of active angiogenesis (Fig. 106.4). These findings thus suggest that circulating EC progenitors may contribute to neoangiogenesis in adult species, consistent with vasculogenesis.

Parenthetically, these findings may have implications for augmenting collateral vessel growth to ischemic tissues (see Therapeutic Angiogenesis) and for delivery of anti- or proangiogenic agents, respectively, to sites of pathologic or utilitarian angiogenesis. A potentially limiting factor in strategies designed to promote neovascularization of ischemic tissues (72) is the resident population of ECs that is competent to respond to administered angiogenic cytokines (73). This issue can be successfully addressed with autologous EC transplants (74–76) (Fig. 106.5). The fact that progenitor ECs are home to foci of angiogenesis suggests potential utility as autologous vectors for gene therapy. For antineoplastic therapies, CD34+ mononuclear peripheral blood cells (MB^{CD34+}) could be transfected with or coupled to antitumor drugs or angiogenesis inhibitors. For treatment of regional ischemia, angiogenesis could be amplified by transfection of MB^{CD34+} to achieve constitutive expression of angiogenic cytokines or provisional matrix proteins, or both (77).

Angiogenesis within Blood Vessels: the Special Case of the Vasa Vasorum

The vasa vasorum consist of blood vessels that vary in size from vessels with single or multiple SMC layers to simple endothelial channels (78). In all but large or atherosclerotic vessels, the vasa vasorum are confined essentially to the adventitia of the blood vessel wall (79). This microcirculatory system presumably exists for the purpose of nourishing large and medium-sized blood vessels, including the aorta and epicardial coronary arteries. The vasa vasorum constitute a reservoir for postnatal angiogenesis that has been studied for its potential contribution to the growth and development of neointimal thickening.

Examination of human atherosclerotic specimens obtained by directional atherectomy (80–82) or at necropsy (83), together with studies performed in a variety of animal models (84–87), has clearly documented that extension of the vasa vasorum typically accompanies plaque growth and

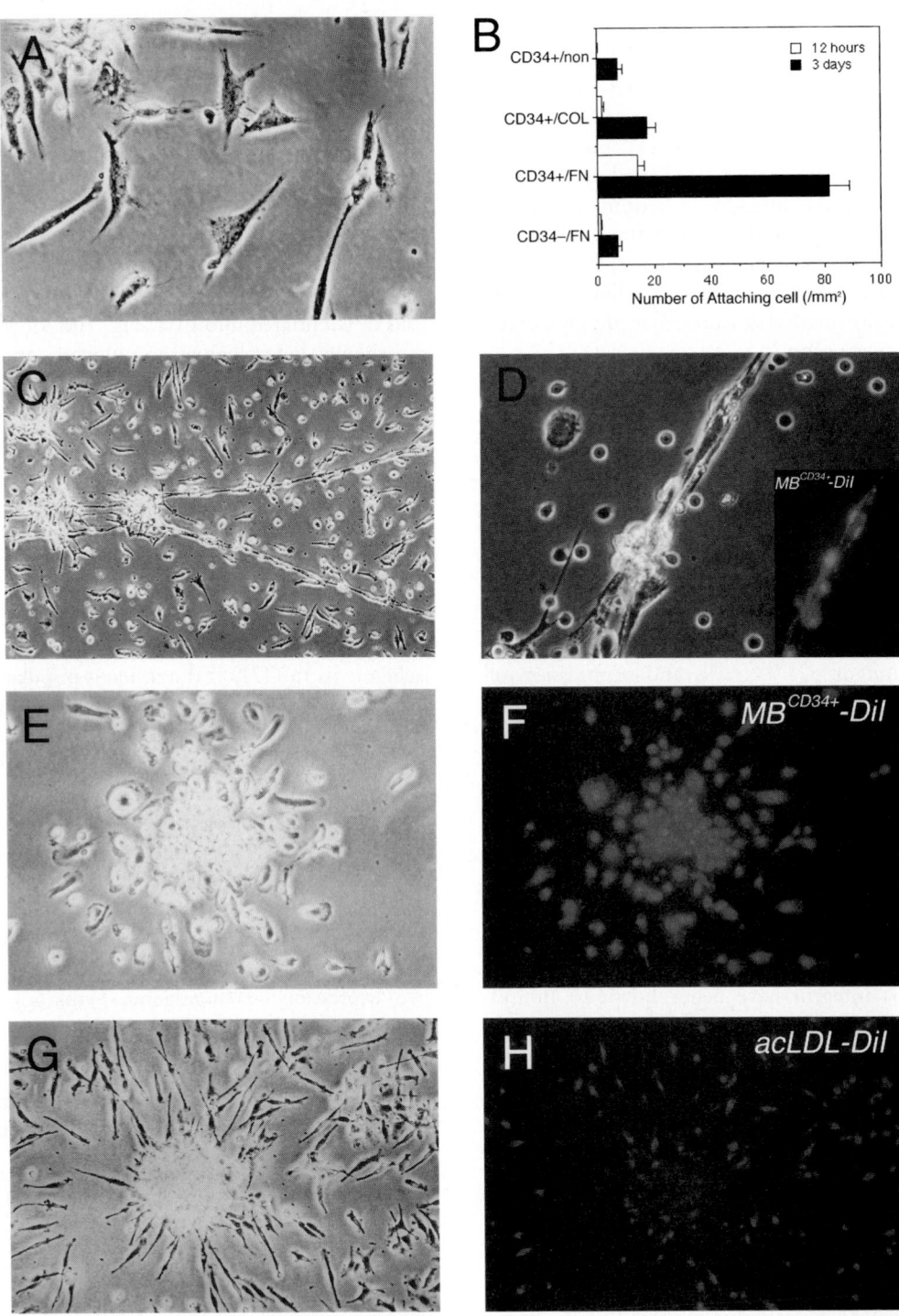

FIGURE 106.3 Attachment, cluster formation, and capillary network development by progenitor endothelial cells *in vitro*. **A:** Spindle-shaped attaching cells (AT^{CD34+}) 7 days after plating CD34+ mononuclear peripheral blood cells (MB^{CD34+}) (5 × 10 per mm^2) on fibronectin with standard medium. **B:** Number of AT^{CD34+} 12 hours and 3 days after single culture of MB^{CD34+} on plastic alone (CD34+/non), collagen coating (CD34+/COL), or fibronectin (CD34+/FN) and MB^{CD34-} on fibronectin (CD34–/FN). AT^{CD34+} yielded a significantly higher number of cells at 12 hours and 3 days when plated on fibronectin. Network formation **(C)** and cord-like structures **(D)** were observed 48 hours after plating coculture of MB^{CD34+}, labeled with DiI fluorescent dye, and unlabeled MB^{CD34-} (ratio of 1:100) on fibronectin-coated dish. These cords consisted principally of DiI-labeled MB^{CD34+}-derived cells (AT^{CD34+}). Beginning 12 hours after coculture, MB^{CD34+}-derived cells demonstrated multiple foci of cluster formation **(E,F)**. AT^{CD34+} sprout from the periphery, whereas round cells remain in the center and detach from the cluster several days later. After 5 days, uptake of DiI-labeled acLDL was seen in AT^{CD34+} at the periphery but not the center of the cluster **(G,H)**. (From Asahara T, Murohara T, Sullivan A, et al. Isolation of putative progenitor endothelial cells for angiogenesis. *Science* 1997;275:964–967, with permission.)

by inference "nourishes" the developing vascular lesion (Fig. 106.6). The ultimate extension of this principle is evidence suggesting that balloon injury to the arterial wall stimulates proliferation of vasa vasorum in conjunction with intimal thickening (88).

Experiments performed by Shweiki et al. (89) have identified hypoxia and glucose deprivation as the elements that are responsible for stimulating microangiogenesis in underperfused tissues. As indicated previously, EC mitogens, including VEGF (89), bFGF (90–92), and acidic fibroblast growth factor (aFGF) (93), have been implicated in mediating such neovascularization. In the case of aFGF, Nabel et al. (94) have reported that arterial gene transfer of complementary DNA encoding aFGF to the arterial wall may result in neointimal microangiogenesis. It is thus intriguing to consider the developing primary or restenotic lesion as relatively underperfused and, as is the model for tumor development (95), dependent for continued growth on triggering augmented vascularization. Given the established association between diabetes and restenosis, it is further intriguing to consider that neointimal or medial cells, or both, that are relatively deprived of intracellular glucose and capable of elaborating angiogenic cytokines may facilitate combinatorial growth of vessel and plaque.

These findings have begun to undergo reevaluation for possible implications that they may have in designing novel treatment strategies for atherosclerosis and restenosis. Conceptually, this is not unrealistic. More than two decades of research aimed at elucidating the role of angiogenesis in tumor growth and metastases have led to the identification of several classes of agents that are capable of interfering with angiogenesis (95). From the standpoint of drug delivery, even if the agent were not preferentially targeted to the neovessels of the plaque or wall, or both, a variety of interventional devices (96) are now clinically available to execute local delivery to selected segments of the human vasculature. q38

ANGIOGENIC CYTOKINES

Beginning a little over a decade ago (105), a series of polypeptide growth factors (Table 106.1) was purified, sequenced, and demonstrated to be responsible for natural as well as pathologic angiogenesis. These angiogenic cytokines all share in common the ability to act as mitogens for ECs.

Among the various growth factors that have been shown to promote angiogenesis, VEGF (106), also known as *vascular permeability factor* (107) and *vasculotropin* (108), is an EC-specific mitogen. Moreover, a plethora of studies have documented upregulation of VEGF in various cell types after exposure to other angiogenic cytokines. VEGF can thus be considered a prototypical angiogenic cytokine and for this reason is discussed here in further detail. Specific

aspects of the remaining angiogenic cytokines in Table 106.1 can be found in the accompanying lists of citations.

At least five VEGF genes have now been identified: VEGF-1 (or VEGF-A), VEGF-2 (or VEGF-C), VEGF-3 (or VEGF-B), VEGF-D, and VEGF-E. In turn, four homodimeric species of VEGF-1 have been identified, with each monomer having 121, 165, 189, or 206 amino acids, respectively (109). The secretion pattern of the four isoforms differs markedly. $VEGF_{121}$ is a weakly acidic polypeptide that does not bind to heparin and is freely soluble in the conditioned medium of transfected cells. The heparin-binding capabilities of the remaining three isoforms are progressively augmented as the result of a stepwise enrichment in basic residues. Thus, $VEGF_{165}$, the predominant form secreted by a variety of normal and transformed cells (40), is a basic heparin-binding glycoprotein with an isoelectric point of 8.5; while secreted, a significant portion remains bound to the cell surface or extracellular matrix. The $VEGF_{189}$ isoform includes 24 additional amino acids and has been shown not to be freely secreted but instead remains nearly completely bound to the cell surface or extracellular matrix, or both (110). $VEGF_{206}$ is a rare isoform that has so far been identified only in a human fetal liver complementary DNA library.

The teleologic basis for the 121, 165, and 189 isoforms that result from alternative splicing of the VEGF-1 transcript has remained enigmatic. It has been proposed (111) that the heparin-binding feature of angiogenic growth factors such as VEGF may explain in part their protracted efficacy due to binding of the growth factor by heparan sulfate proteoglycans present on the luminal surface of the vascular endothelium or within the extracellular matrix, or both. Although $VEGF_{121}$ lacks heparin-binding ability, all three isoforms bind to the Flk-1 receptor, which transduces the mitogenic signal (112), including $VEGF_{121}$, which binds exclusively to Flk-1 (113). Plate et al. (114) speculated that the three principal isoforms might mediate distinct EC functions. We considered that angiogenesis induced by VEGF may be differentially dependent on the extent to which each particular isoform used is freely secreted and soluble. The magnitude of freely secreted $VEGF_{121}$ isoform that reaches the ischemic focus from the site of synthesis, for example, might be superior to that achieved with the $VEGF_{165}$ isoform; alternatively, avid binding of the $VEGF_{189}$ isoform to the basement membrane or extracellular matrix, or both (115), might result in more protracted bioavailability and thereby yield an outcome superior to that of $VEGF_{165}$. q39

Synergism of Angiogenic Cytokines

Studies from several groups have disclosed evidence for a synergistic effect of growth factors on angiogenesis *in vitro*. Pepper et al. (174) demonstrated that, whereas EC migration and capillary lumen formation were inhibited by TGF-

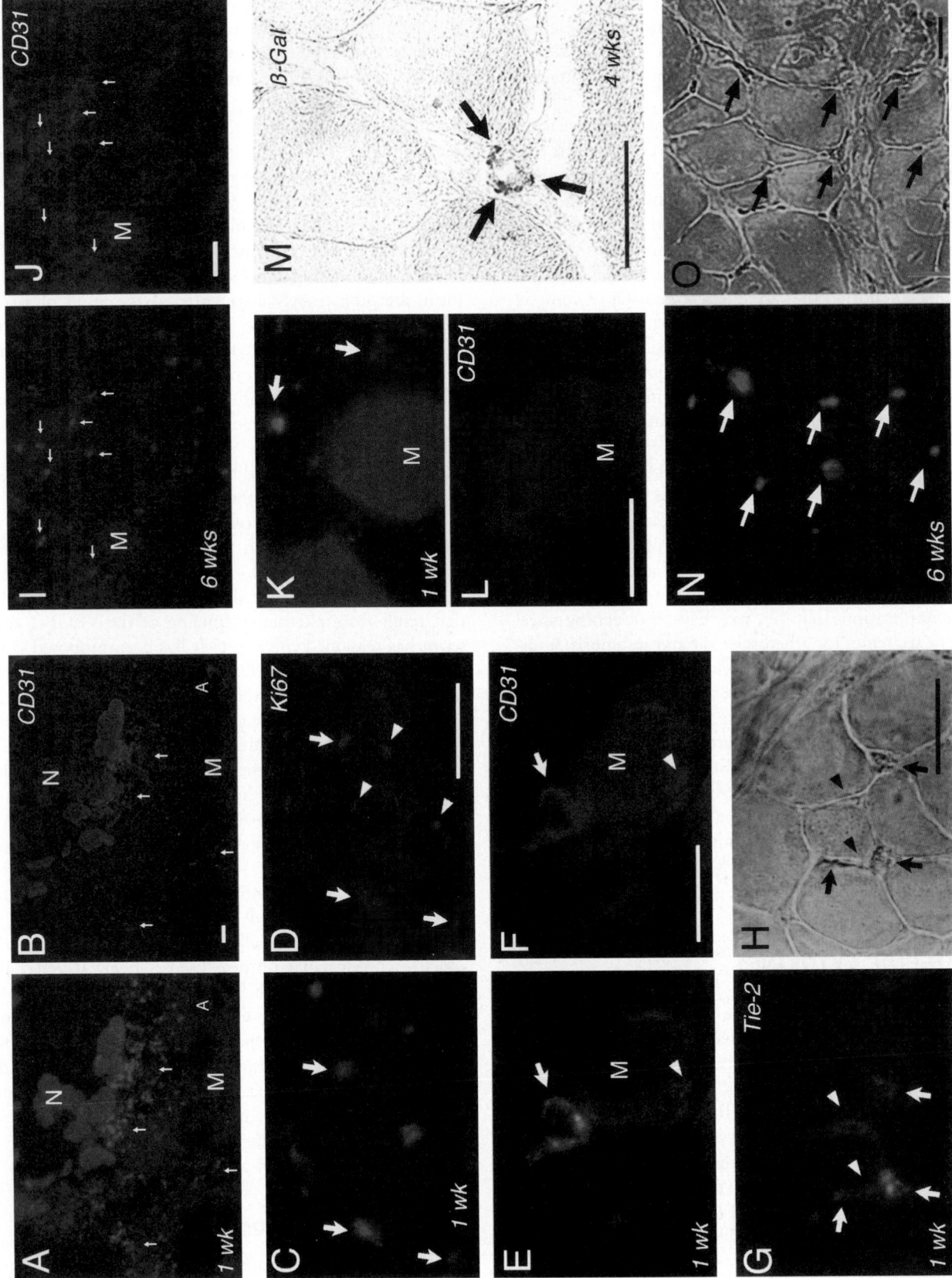

◄

FIGURE 106.4 Heterologous **(A–L)**, homologous **(M)**, or autologous **(N and O)** endothelial cell (EC) progenitors incorporate into sites of angiogenesis *in vivo*. **A,B:** CD34+ mononuclear peripheral blood cells (MB^CD34+^; *arrows*), labeled with the fluorescent dye Dil, between skeletal myocytes **(M)**, including necrotic **(N)** myocytes 1 week after injection; most are colabeled with CD31 (*arrows*). Note preexisting artery (a), identified as CD31 positive but Dil negative. **C,D:** Evidence of proliferative activity among several Dil-labeled MB^CD34+^-derived cells (*arrows*), indicated by coimmunostaining for Ki^67^ antibody. Proliferative activity is also seen among Dil-negative, Ki^67^-positive capillary ECs (*arrowheads*); both cell types comprise neovasculature. **E:** Dil and CD31 in capillary ECs (*arrows*) between skeletal myocytes, photographed through double filter 1 week after Dil-labeled MB^CD34+^ injection. **F:** Single green filter shows CD31 expression in Dil-labeled capillary ECs, integrated into capillary with native (Dil-negative, CD31-positive) ECs (*arrowheads*). **G:** Immunostaining 1 week after MB^CD34+^ injection showing capillaries comprised of Dil-labeled MB^CD34+^-derived cells expressing Tie-2 receptor. Several MB^CD34+^-derived cells (*arrows*) are Tie-2 positive and are integrated with some Tie-2–positive host capillary cells (*arrowheads*) identified by the absence of red fluorescence. **H:** Phase-contrast photomicrograph of same tissue section shown in **G** indicates corresponding Dil-labeled (*arrows*) and -unlabeled (*arrowheads*) capillary ECs. **I,J:** Six weeks after administration, MB^CD34+^-derived cells colabel for CD31 in capillaries between preserved skeletal myocytes. **K,L:** One week after injection of MB^CD34–^, isolated MB^CD34–^ derived cells (*arrows*) are observed between myocytes but do not express CD31. **M:** Immunostaining of β-galactosidase (β-gal) in tissue section harvested from ischemic muscle of B6,129 mice 4 weeks after administration of MB^Flk-1+^ isolated from transgenic mice constitutively expressing β-gal. (Flk-1 cell isolation was used for selection of EC progenitors due to lack of a suitable antimouse CD34 antibody.) Cells overexpressing β-gal (*arrows*) have been incorporated into capillaries and small arteries; these cells were identified as ECs by anti-CD31 and anti-BS-1 lectin. **N,O:** Sections of muscles harvested from rabbit ischemic hindlimb 4 weeks after administration of autologous MB^CD34+^. Red fluorescence indicates localization of MB^CD34+^-derived cells in capillaries, seen (*arrows*) in phase-contrast photomicrograph **(O)**. Each scale bar indicates 50 mm. (From Asahara T, Murohara T, Sullivan A, et al. Isolation of putative progenitor endothelial cells for angiogenesis. *Science* 1997;275:964–967, with permission.)

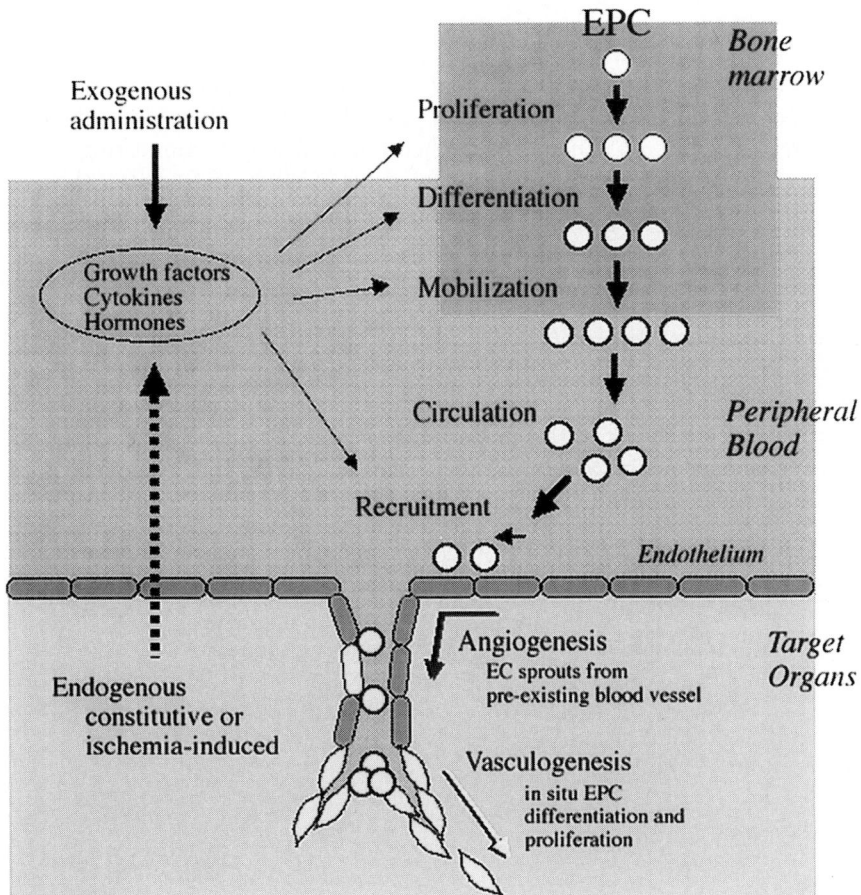

FIGURE 106.5 Neovascularization encompasses angiogenesis and vasculogenesis. Angiogenesis represents the classic paradigm for new vessel growth, as mature, differentiated endothelial cells (ECs) break free from their basement membrane and migrate as well as proliferate to form sprouts from parental vessels. Vasculogenesis involves participation of bone marrow–derived endothelial progenitor cells (EPCs), which circulate to sites of neovascularization, where they differentiate *in situ* into mature ECs. Growth factors, cytokines, or hormones released endogenously in response to tissue ischemia, or administered exogenously for therapeutic neovascularization, act to promote EPC proliferation, differentiation, and mobilization from bone marrow, via the peripheral circulation, to neovascular foci.

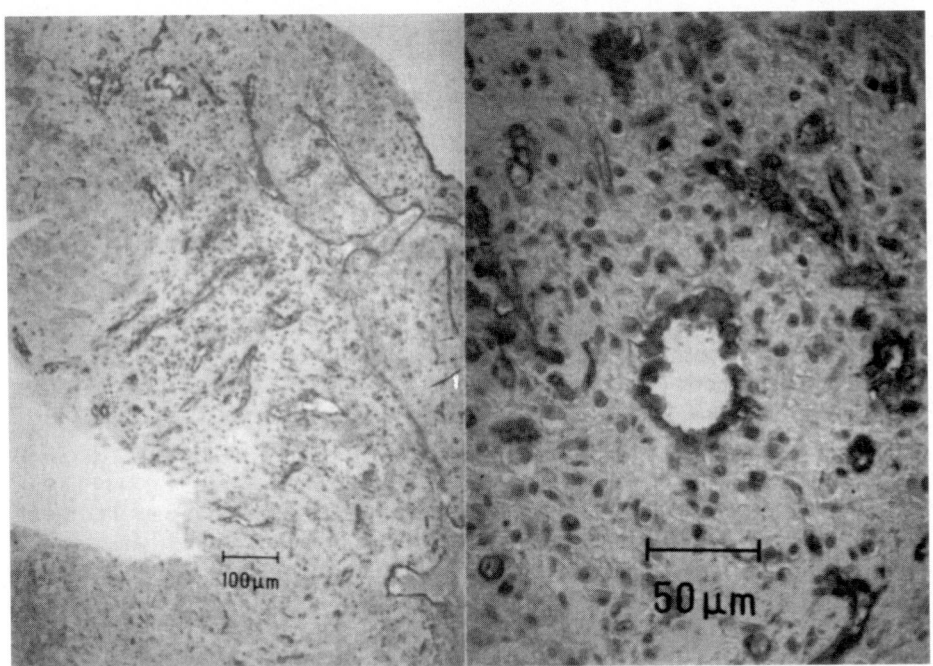

FIGURE 106.6 Identification of vasa vasorum in low-power **(left)** and higher-power **(right)** photomicrographs of atherosclerotic specimen obtained by directional atherectomy. Yellow-brown reaction product of Ulex immunostain identifies the endothelium of the vasa vasorum.

β1 alone, a lower concentration of TGF-β1 potentiated the effect of bFGF- and VEGF-induced migration. Furthermore, these same authors (186) showed that adding VEGF or bFGF to microvascular ECs grown on the surface of three-dimensional collagen gels induced the cells to invade the underlying matrix and form capillary-like tubules. When these same two mitogens were added simultaneously, however, they induced an angiogenic response that was far greater than additive and occurred with greater rapidity than the response to either cytokine alone. Goto et al. (187) measured the combined effect of VEGF and bFGF on the proliferative and morphologic changes exhibited by bovine capillary ECs cultured in a gel of type I collagen; when the two factors were added simultaneously, the number of cells and the number of cord-like structures were greater than the sum of those that were stimulated with either growth factor alone. Results of *in vivo* studies performed in the author's laboratory (188) are in agreement

with these previous *in vitro* experiments. Necropsy examination documented an increase in vascularity at the capillary level, consistent with the classic definition of angiogenesis that was formulated by Klagsbrun and Folkman (189). Moreover, the angiographic luminal diameter of the stem artery was significantly greater in the group treated with VEGF + bFGF than VEGF or bFGF alone.

The potential therapeutic benefit of stimulating formation of larger, more "mature" collaterals is suggested by the physiologic evidence of increased downstream perfusion that was documented on serial measurements of the lower limb blood pressure ratio. The dramatic increase in blood pressure ratio in rabbits treated with VEGF + bFGF between day 0 and day 10 compared with that seen after administration of either growth factor alone is likely to be a consequence of better arterial reconstitution in the combined therapy group. This conclusion is further supported by findings in the author's laboratory in which the combi-

TABLE 106.1 ANGIOGENIC CYTOKINES AND GENES USED IN CLINICAL ANGIOGENESIS TRIALS

Cytokine	Protein	Gene Ph	Gene Ad	EC specific	Pleiotropic	Secretory sequence
VEGF$_{165}$	✓	✓		✓		✓
VEGF$_{121}$			✓	✓		✓
VEGF-2 (VEGF-C)		✓		✓		✓
HIF-1a			✓			
FGF-1 (aFGF)	✓				✓	
FGF-1 modified		✓			✓	✓
FGF-2 (bFGF)	✓				✓	
FGF-4			✓		✓	✓

a, acidic; Ad, adenoviral vector; b, basic; EC, endothelial cell; FGF, fibroblast growth factor; HIF, hypoxia inducible factor; Ph, plasmid human; VEGF, vascular endothelial growth factor.

nation of VEGF and bFGF was found to have a synergistic effect on maximum flow reserve in this same animal model, compared to bFGF or VEGF alone (C. Bauters, *unpublished observations*, 2001).

The fundamental basis for the synergistic effect of VEGF and bFGF *in vivo* remains to be elucidated. Although VEGF is EC specific, bFGF is also a potent mitogen for a variety of other cell types, including SMCs. Direct stimulation of SMCs by bFGF might be responsible for certain of the *in vivo* effects that have been observed, such as the increase in the angiographic luminal diameter of the stem artery.

Conversely, the increase in capillary density and capillary-muscle fiber ratio in the ischemic muscles is more likely to be a consequence of a synergistic effect on ECs similar to that observed in the previously cited *in vitro* experiments. It is important in this regard to underscore the independent receptor systems that are responsible for signaling the mitogenic effects of VEGF and bFGF in ECs (67,190,191). Thus, amplification of the endothelial response to these mitogens is feasible based on their independent receptor systems alone. ▼ q40

THERAPEUTIC ANGIOGENESIS

The therapeutic implications of angiogenic growth factors were identified by the pioneering work of Folkman and colleagues more than two decades ago (206). Their work documented the extent to which tumor development was dependent on neovascularization and suggested that this relationship might involve angiogenic growth factors that were specific for neoplasms.

More recent investigations have established the feasibility of using recombinant formulations of such angiogenic growth factors to expedite and/or augment collateral artery development in animal models of myocardial and hindlimb ischemia. This novel strategy for the treatment of vascular insufficiency has been termed *therapeutic angiogenesis* (25).

Rationale for Therapeutic Angiogenesis in Patients with Occlusive Vascular Disease

Although ischemia from vascular occlusion upregulates expression of angiogenic growth factors, the fact that certain patients present with disabling angina indicates that such natural compensatory processes are not always sufficient. This can be explained in two possible ways: Either the production of angiogenic cytokines is inadequate or patients' response to them is attenuated. It has been shown that angiogenesis is impaired in older versus younger animals (207), secondary to reduced VEGF expression. Similar reductions in VEGF expression were observed in nonobese diabetic mice (208) and in hypercholesterolemic mice (209). These limitations in VEGF expression can be overcome in part by VEGF supplementation (208,209). Patients with advanced coronary disease are often older and may have diabetes, hypercholesterolemia, or other undetermined characteristics, limiting their capacity to upregulate angiogenic cytokines in response to ischemia, but may nevertheless respond to exogenous angiogenic cytokines. Significantly higher VEGF production in response to hypoxia was demonstrated in monocytes harvested from patients with angiographically visible collaterals, compared to those with reduced collaterals, suggesting that individual differences in cytokine expression may constitute yet another basis for variations in the magnitude of collateral development (210).

Reduced expression of angiogenic cytokines is not the only factor that contributes to the heterogeneous response to collateral vessel development. Marked genetic heterogeneity in the response to growth factor–stimulated angiogenesis has been observed in different strains of inbred mice (211). Age-related reduction in EC viability has also been demonstrated (207). Endothelial dysfunction accompanies many of the known coronary risk factors and may reduce endothelial responsiveness to angiogenic growth factors. Also, the responsiveness of EPCs to hypoxic stimuli may well be deficient and potentially limit therapeutic angiogenesis. Strategies to increase EC responsiveness and to enhance EPC production or availability are therefore reasonable targets for therapeutic angiogenesis (212–214).

Angiogenic Protein versus Gene Therapy

Angiogenic cytokines can be administered as the natural recombinant human protein or by gene transfer. Recombinant protein is a more conventional approach and typically displays a more precise dose-response relationship than gene transfer. Recombinant protein is usually administered systemically and is therefore limited by potential adverse effects of the high plasma concentrations that are required to achieve adequate myocardial uptake. These include hypotension and edema with VEGF (215,216) and anemia, thrombocytopenia, and renal toxicity for FGF (217,218). Data regarding the kinetics of recombinant protein circulation suggest that intravenous delivery is unlikely to result in sufficient myocardial uptake or residence time to achieve important biologic effects; intracoronary delivery constitutes an alternative route of parenteral administration (219).

The ideal regimen for therapeutic angiogenesis is a single administration that provides a sustained but transient (2–3 weeks) increase in local angiogenic protein concentration at foci of myocardial ischemia. A limited rise in systemic VEGF levels would be expected to reduce the potential for distant unwanted side effects. Currently available gene therapy strategies approach this ideal. Naked DNA and adenoviral vectors produce only transient transfection, ideal for the time scale that is required for angiogenesis. The principal challenge is that optimal transfection in the case of naked DNA is best achieved by intramyocardial injection, although intracoronary administration may be sufficient for adenoviral gene transfer (220). Unlike viral vectors, plasmid DNA does not induce inflammation. Although naked DNA gene transfer is less efficient than viral-mediated transduction, uptake of naked DNA is augmented in muscle (221), particularly ischemic or inflamed muscle (119,222).

Routes of Administration

Angiogenic cytokines and genes have been administered via a wide variety of routes. Injection sites include intravenous, selective pulmonary artery, left atrium, intracoronary, selective intracoronary, transepicardial intramyocardial at time of bypass surgery or via thoracotomy, transendocardial intramyocardial by electromechanical catheter, periadventitial at time of bypass surgery or by thoracotomy, and intrapericardial. Because local delivery of recombinant protein or gene can be considered ideal (223), trials in patients have favored the intracoronary (adenovirus) or intramyocardial (naked DNA or adenovirus) route. Although not an issue if performed as a part of a coronary bypass procedure, the attendant risk of surgery is otherwise a limitation of the transepicardial route; in the future, this may be averted by the catheter-based transendocardial approach (*e*Fig. 106.6.8).

Translation of Therapeutic Myocardial Angiogenesis from Bench to Bedside

The species differences in myocardial collateralization and the relatively small area of ischemia that is produced in the pig model underscore the difficulty in taking the results from animal models of myocardial ischemia directly to the clinical arena for myocardial angiogenesis. In addition, the heart is a difficult organ to access directly for either vascular or intramyocardial administration of angiogenic factors, and assessment of neovascularization and blood flow is not trivial. Consequently, to investigate therapeutic angiogenesis in

human subjects, a strategy was adopted of first studying patients with peripheral artery disease, specifically critical limb ischemia. The rationale for this included consideration of two issues. First, in patients with critical limb ischemia, the risk (limb loss)-benefit (limb salvage) ratio is appropriate for a novel therapeutic, due to the absence of any effective medical therapy (252). Second, access to ischemic skeletal muscle is straightforward, requiring only a superficial, nearly painless injection with a 27-gauge needle.

The effects of VEGF gene transfer were initially studied in patients with critical limb ischemia by delivering the gene to a patent arterial site in the ischemic limb upstream from the site of occlusion (72,253). Subsequently, however, this approach was replaced by direct intramuscular injection (198,254). Clinical benefit, including abolition of rest pain, limb salvage, and healing of ischemic ulcers, was associated with objective findings of improved perfusion (Figs. 106.7 through 106.10), including increase in ankle-brachial index, angiographic evidence of new collaterals, and improved leg blood flow on magnetic resonance angiography. Having established proof of the concept for therapeutic angiogenesis in human subjects, extrapolation of these findings to patients with myocardial ischemia were sought (255).

Evaluating Clinical Results of Myocardial Angiogenesis

No consensus has been reached regarding how best to evaluate the efficacy of therapeutic angiogenesis in patients with coronary heart disease. Most clinical studies have focused on the clinical end points that were used historically to evaluate new antianginal drugs, namely, angina class, exercise time, and quality of life. Each of these, however, is potentially subject to placebo and training effects, which cannot be eliminated in phase I trials and may limit the power of smaller phase II studies to detect a meaningful difference. Although these parameters may ultimately prove useful for establishing efficacy in larger phase II/III

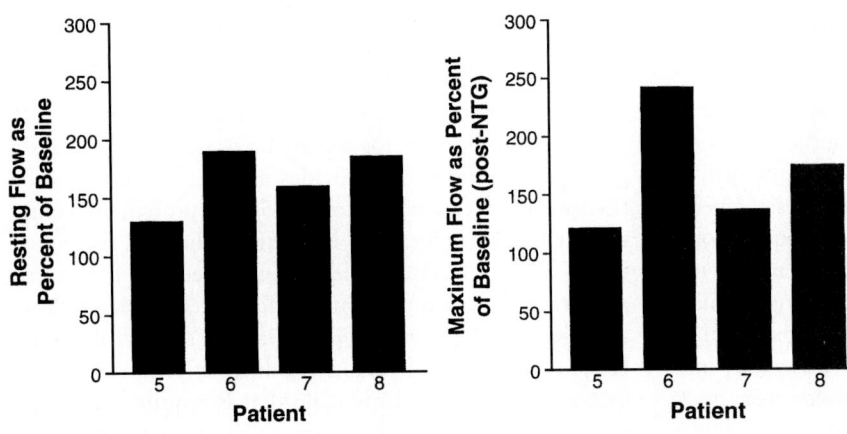

FIGURE 106.7 Resting flow **(left)** and maximum flow stimulated by intraarterial administration of nitroglycerin (NTG) **(right)** are augmented by 100% to 250% above baseline measurements in four patients undergoing gene therapy with 1,000 µg (patients 5, 6, 7) or 2,000 µg (patient 8) naked DNA encoding vascular endothelial growth factor. Blood flow was measured with intraarterial Doppler wire (FloMap, Cardiometrics).

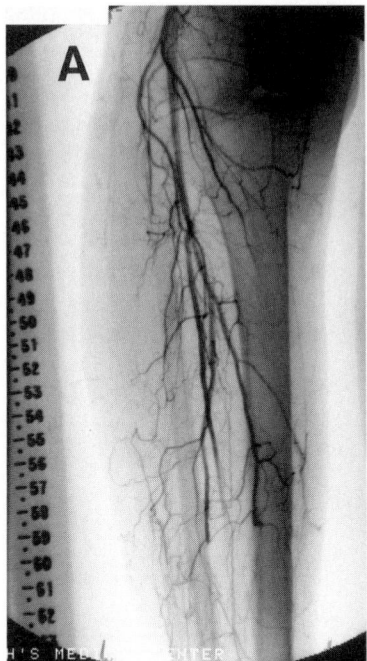
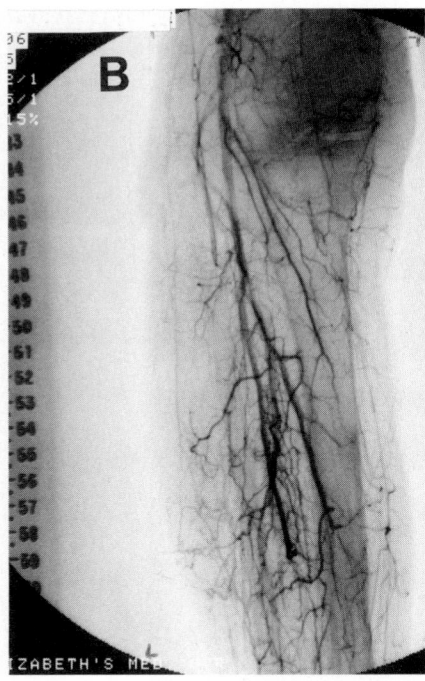

FIGURE 106.8 Selective digital subtraction angiograms performed in patient with critical limb ischemia due to occlusion of all three infrapopliteal vessels at midcalf level. Immediately before **(A)** and 1 month after gene therapy with 2,000 µg naked DNA encoding vascular endothelial growth factor **(B)**. The latter angiogram disclosed a plethora of new collateral vessels in the ischemic limb.

trials, additional objective evaluations may help to establish evidence of biologic effects that are attributable to therapeutic angiogenesis.

Rest and stress single-photon emission computed tomography (SPECT) perfusion imaging with thallium-201 or technetium-99m sestamibi provide objective estimates of relative myocardial blood flow and are used widely and routinely in clinical practice. As such, evidence of

improved relative myocardial perfusion on images recorded before and after gene transfer may constitute inferential evidence of angiogenesis.

Percutaneous catheter-based electromechanical mapping (256,257) is a novel technique that provides concurrent imaging of myocardial viability and endocardial wall motion (*e*Figs. 106.6.8 and 106.10.1); analysis of the two resulting maps can be used to identify foci of hibernating

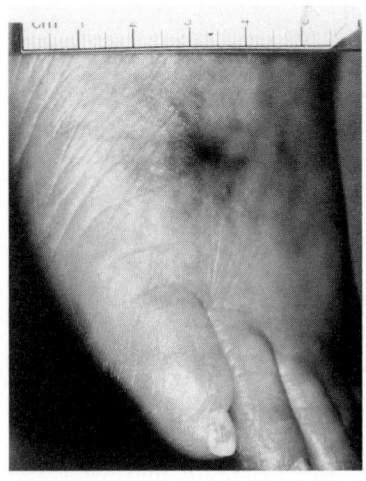
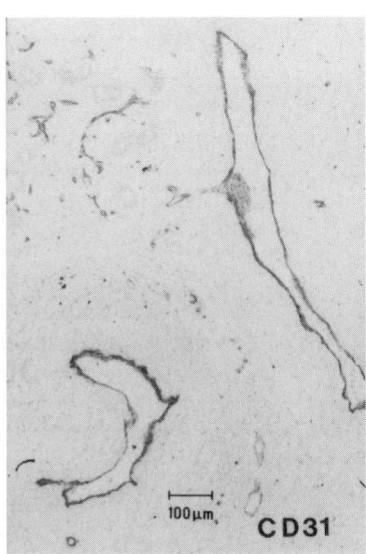
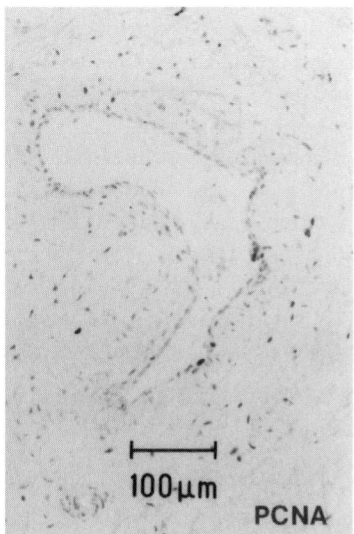

FIGURE 106.9 One of three spider angiomas that developed approximately 1 week after gene therapy in the distal portion of the ischemic limb of a patient whose angiograms are shown in Figure 106.8. Photomicrographs of tissue sections immunostained with antibody to endothelial antigen CD31 indicate the vascularity of the lesion, and immunostain of the adjacent section for proliferating cell nuclear antigen (PCNA) indicates the extent of proliferative activity among endothelial cells in the lesion.

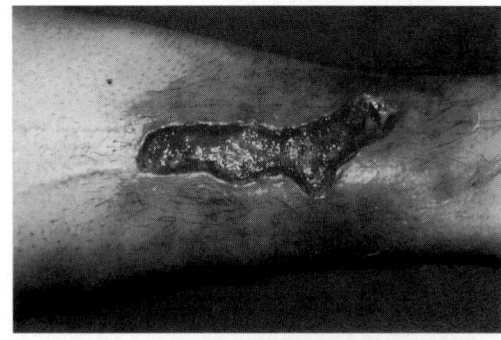

Before Skingraft Placement

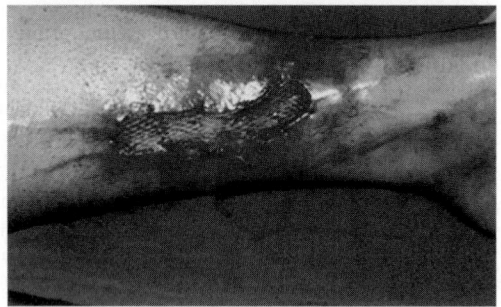

Directly after Skingraft Placement

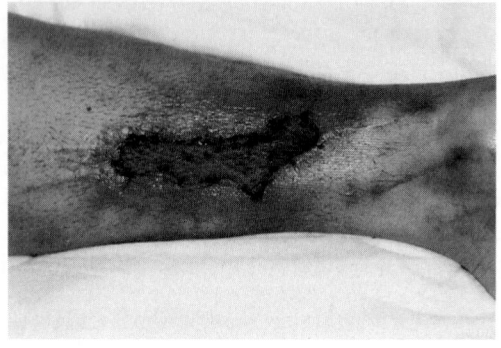

First Bandage Removal (Day 4)

FIGURE 106.10 Successful placement of split-thickness skin graft in first patient treated with intramuscular administration of naked DNA encoding plasmid human vascular endothelial growth factor ($phVEGF_{165}$). After two intramuscular injections of 2,000 μg $phVEGF_{165}$, the patient's ankle-brachial index increased from 0.28 to 0.55, angiography disclosed new collateral vessels in the ischemic limb, and a 9 × 3–cm wound at the site of vein harvest in the medial calf healed sufficiently to permit successful grafting.

myocardium, which can be serially evaluated before and after gene transfer (258).

Positron emission tomography using $^{13}NH_3$ or $H_2^{15}O$ can quantify regional coronary blood flow at rest and during vasodilation and has been used to demonstrate increased flow after a variety of interventions (259), but the technique is not widely available. Novel modifications of magnetic resonance perfusion imaging to detect foci of neovascularization (260,261) may prove useful for evaluation of angiogenesis after confirmation of reproducibility, sensitivity, and specificity by other centers.

Serial measures of left ventricular function have not proved consistently useful in animal or clinical studies to date. Angiographic studies have likewise failed to depict consistently reproducible evidence of neovascularization, even in animal or clinical studies with evidence of improved myocardial perfusion. This is likely due to the fact that the diameter of most collaterals formed in response to arterial occlusion or therapeutic angiogenesis, or both, is less than 200 μm (20)—that is, beyond the resolution of conventional angiography and certainly beyond

the spatial resolution of magnetic resonance angiography. Consistent with this notion is the fact that the increased resolution achieved by synchrotron radiation imaging has disclosed new collateral vessels in preclinical studies that could not be identified by conventional angiographic techniques (262).

Initial Results of Therapeutic Myocardial Angiogenesis in Patients with Coronary Disease

Tables 106.2 and 106.3 list completed and ongoing clinical trials of recombinant proteins and genes used for therapeutic angiogenesis, although data regarding the major end points have been published in only five, with two currently in press. Patients in these trials generally have severe angina that is unresponsive to medical therapy and are unsuitable for conventional revascularization. Many of the studies have been small phase I trials without control groups, designed primarily to establish safety or to evaluate dose-related effects, or both. Nevertheless, almost all have

TABLE 106.2 CLINICAL STUDIES OF RECOMBINANT PROTEINS FOR MYOCARDIAL ANGIOGENESIS—COMPLETED AND IN PROGRESS

Angiogen	Administration Route	Administration Dose	Population, phase	Active/placebo (n)	Follow-up	Outcome	PI/company	Reference(s)
FGF-1 + heparin + fibrin glue	Intramyo near LAD at CABG	0.01 mg/kg	3VD + distal LAD disease after LIMA insertion, phase I	20/20	12 wk, 3 yr	New vessels bypassing distal LAD, ↑ flow (angio gray scale) vs. placebo. ↓ angina, ↓ antianginal drugs, similar angio improvement at 3 yr	Stegmann	263–265
FGF-1 + heparin + fibrin glue	Intramyo at thoracotomy	0.01 mg/kg for each involved vascular bed	Severe angina, no option, phase I	20/0	6 and 12 wk	SPECT perfusion and exercise capacity reported significantly improved compared to baseline	Stegmann	266
FGF-2 + heparin alginate	Periadventitial implant at CABG	1 or 10 µg FGF-2 per implant, 10 implants/patient	Ungraftable artery, viable myocardium, phase I	8/0	3 mo	1 perioperative infarction in area of implant; all angina-free postop; variable changes in perfusion scan	Simons	323
FGF-2 + heparin alginate	Periadventitial implant at CABG	10 or 100 µg total dose FGF-2 or placebo divided into 10 implants	Ungraftable artery, undergoing CABG, viable myocardium, phase I	16/8	3 mo, longer clinical	2 operative deaths; 3 Q MI; less angina, reduced perfusion defect size with high dose	Simons	267
FGF-2	14 intravenous, 52 intracoronary	Incremental 0.33–48-µg/kg total dose, 2 × 10 min 10-mL infusions (2 distributions)	No option CAD, inducible ischemia, phase I	66/0	1, 2, 6 mo	↑ Exercise time, ↓ angina, ↑ QOL, ↑ LV function, ↑ nuclear perfusion, ↑ MRI flow	Simons/Chiron	268, 270, 271
FGF-2	Intracoronary	0.3-, 3.0-, or 30.0-µg/kg total dose, 2 × 10 min 10-mL infusions (2 distributions)	No option CAD, reversible perfusion defects, phase II, FIRST multicenter study	337 total 3:1 active/placebo	90 d, 6 mo	90-day exercise time (65 s vs. 45 s for placebo) and stress nuclear perfusion no different from placebo, less angina ($p = .057$), trend to improved overall result in older and more symptomatic patients	Simons/Chiron	277
VEGF$_{165}$	Intracoronary	5–167 ng/kg/min 10 min each artery	Angina + VUNE, phase I	15/0	30, 60 d	↓ angina 13/15; improved rest nuclear perfusion in high dose	Henry/Genentech	269, 272, 273
VEGF$_{165}$	Intravenous	17–100 ng/kg/min over 1–4 hr	Angina + VUNE, phase I	28/0	60 d	Perfusion scan improved 2 grades in 40% of rest, 20% of stress; ↑ angio collaterals in 38%	Henry/Genentech	272
VEGF$_{165}$	Intracoronary plus 3 × intravenous	17, 50 ng/kg/min IC 20 min, + IV 4 hr days 3, 6, 9	Angina + VUNE, phase II VIVA multicenter study	115/63	60 d, 120 d, 1 yr (part)	Day 60 similar ↑ exercise time for active and placebo, similar ↓ angina, QOL as placebo; nuclear perfusion, angiography, no change day 60; day 120 high dose ↓ angina vs. placebo, trend to ↑ exercise time; trend to ↑ angina class at 1 yr	Henry/Genentech	272, 274, 276

CABG, coronary artery bypass graft surgery; CAD, coronary artery disease; FGF, fibroblast growth factor; intramyo, intramyocardial injection; FIRST, FIolan International Randomized Survival Trial; IC, intracoronary; LAD, left anterior descending coronary artery; LIMA, left internal mammary artery; LV, left ventricle; MRI, magnetic resonance imaging; PI, principal investigator; Q MI, Q-wave myocardial infarction; QOL, quality of life; SPECT, single-photon emission computed tomography; 3VD, 3-vessel coronary artery disease; VEGF, vascular endothelial growth factor; VIVA, Vascular Endothelial Growth Factor in Ischemia for Vascular Angiogenesis; VUNE, viable underperfused myocardium in patients not eligible for revascularization.

TABLE 106.3 CLINICAL STUDIES OF GENE TRANSFER FOR MYOCARDIAL ANGIOGENESIS—COMPLETED AND IN PROGRESS

Angiogen	Administration		Population phase	Active/placebo (n)	Follow-up	Outcome	PI/company	Reference(s)
	Route	Dose						
PhVEGF$_{165}$	Intramyo: thoracotomy	125 μg (10), 250 μg (10), 500 μg (10)	No option CAD, refractory stable angina; phase I	30/0	2 and 6 mo, 1 yr, longer clinical	1 late postop death (4.5 mo) and 1 late death at 28.5 mo; less angina and NTG, ↑ ex time, improved rest/stress nuclear perfusion, ↑ function e.m. mapping	Isner Genentech	255, 258, 278, 279
AdVEGF$_{121}$	Intramyo: with CABG or at thoracotomy	4 × 10^8 to 4 × 10^{10} particle units	Ischemic nonby-passable region, phase I	21/0: CABG (15), thoracotomy (6)	30 d	2 perioperative, 1 late death with CABG, ↓ angina, ↑ function sestamibi, ↑ Rentrop and collateral score	Crystal Genvec	284
AdVEGF$_{121}$	Intramyo: video thoracotomy, thoracoscopy	4 × 10^{10} particle units	Severe angina, not ideal for revascularization, phase I	10/0: thoracotomy (6), thoracoscopy (4)	30 d	1 death at 40 d; in progress	Crystal Genvec	285
PhVEGF-2	Intramyo: thoracotomy	200 μg (10), 800 μg (10), 2,000 μg (10)	No option CAD, refractory stable angina; phase I	30/0	30, 60, 90 d; longer clinical	1 perioperative death; less angina and NTG, ↑ exercise time, improved nuclear perfusion, ↓ angina class ≥2 in 70%; ↑ function e.m. mapping	Isner VGI	286, 287
PhVEGF-2	Intramyo: via e.m. catheter in LV	200 μg	No option refractory stable angina; phase I multicenter	6 (including 3 single-blind control crossed over to active)	30, 60, 90 d; longer clinical	Less angina and NTG at 60 and 90 d; improved rest nuclear perfusion at 90 d; ↑ function e.m. mapping	Isner VGI	124
PhVEGF-2	Intramyo: via e.m. catheter in LV	200 μg (6/3), 800 μg (6/3), 2,000 μg (6/3)	No option refractory stable angina; phase I/II multicenter	19 (2:1 active vs. placebo); total of 27 proposed	60 and 90 d, longer clinical	In progress	Isner VGI	124
Ad FGF-4	Intracoronary AGENT study	3 × 10^8 to 10^{11} virus particles, incremental	Class 2–3 angina, 1 open vessel with other options; phase I/II	67 (3:1 active vs. placebo)	4 and 12 wk	Reported to show significant improvement in treadmill time at 4 and 12 wk vs. placebo	Hammond CTI, Berlex, Schering	Personal communication

Ad, adenoviral vector; AGENT, Adenovirus FGF Angiogenic Gene Therapy Agent Trial; CABG, coronary artery bypass graft surgery; CAD, coronary artery disease; e.m., electromechanical; FGF, fibroblast growth factor; intramyo, intramyocardial injection; LV, left ventricle; NTG, nitroglycerin; Ph, plasmid human; PI, principal investigator; VEGF, vascular endothelial growth factor.

reported encouraging reductions in angina and nitroglycerin consumption and, in certain cases, improvement in exercise time and/or improvement in objective measures of left ventricular perfusion or function, or both.

Clinical Studies Using Recombinant Proteins

The first clinical study of recombinant protein for myocardial ischemia used intramyocardial injections of FGF-1 (aFGF) with heparin in patients who were undergoing left internal mammary bypass of the left anterior descending coronary artery (263,264) (Table 106.2). Twenty patients received active drug, and 20 received heat-denatured protein as placebo. The authors used a novel form of imaging to suggest improved collateralization of the distal left anterior descending coronary artery in comparison to placebo. This effect was maintained at 3-year follow-up (265). At 3 years, 16 of 17 patients who were given FGF were in Canadian functional class I compared to 12 of 16 control subjects, and only 1 of 17 given FGF required nitrates compared to 12 of 16 controls ($p < .01$). In addition, fewer patients given FGF were on calcium channel blockers (1 of 17 vs. 10 of 16) or beta-blockers (5 of 17 vs. 10 of 16). The same group completed an uncontrolled study of FGF-1 injected transepicardially via minithoracotomy in patients with severe angina that was unsuitable for conventional revascularization (266). Compared to baseline preoperative values, SPECT perfusion and exercise capacity were reported to be improved at 6 and at 12 weeks.

Periadventitial implantation of FGF-2 (bFGF) administered intraoperatively in heparin alginate beads at the site of a nonbypassable artery has been evaluated in a placebo-controlled trial of patients who were undergoing concomitant bypass surgery (267). Despite a relatively high perioperative mortality and morbidity attributed to the advanced nature of coronary artery disease in the patient cohort, the investigators reported less angina in the active treatment group. Trends to less severe stress nuclear perfusion defects and less evidence of ischemia by magnetic resonance imaging were noted as well in the high-dose FGF-2 group.

Three uncontrolled phase I studies of intravenous or intracoronary FGF-2 or VEGF recombinant protein have been completed (Table 106.2). These studies overall reported less angina and improved exercise time and improvements in either nuclear or magnetic resonance imaging perfusion or left ventricular function (268–273).

Results of phase I studies, designed by definition to assess safety, must be interpreted with caution. Typically, the number of patients who are enrolled in such trials is relatively small, and for those lacking a control group, a placebo effect cannot be excluded. For studies in which recombinant protein or gene is administered in conjunction with conventional revascularization, it may be difficult to determine the relative contributions of the angiogenic agent versus bypass surgery to the symptomatic response.

Two larger placebo-controlled phase II studies of intracoronary ± intravenous recombinant protein have been completed. The Vascular Endothelial Growth Factor in Ischemia for Vascular Angiogenesis (VIVA) study compared two doses of VEGF-1 protein to placebo in 178 patients who were given a single intracoronary infusion followed by three separate intravenous infusions (274–276). The primary end point of exercise duration was not different from placebo in the VIVA study; in each of the three groups, the increase in exercise time at 60 days, approximately 45 seconds, was similar. At 120 days, the high-dose group maintained the improvement, with an increase of 47 seconds over baseline, whereas the placebo group showed only a 14-second improvement. Although this difference was not significant, given the relatively small numbers and the large placebo effect, the possibility of a type II error cannot be excluded. No significant differences from placebo were found in angina grade or quality-of-life measures at 60 days, although there was a significant reduction in angina grade at 120 days in the high-dose group. Angiographic and nuclear perfusion studies were interpreted to show no differences between active therapy and placebo at 60 days.

Perhaps the most striking finding in the VIVA trial was that, in spite of exclusion of patients with evidence of a malignancy, three patients were diagnosed and one died of cancer within the 120-day follow-up period, and worsening retinopathy developed in one patient. Remarkably, all of these individuals had been fortuitously randomized to the placebo group.

The Flolan International Randomized Survival Trial (FIRST) compared a single intracoronary dose of FGF-2 (bFGF) with placebo in 337 patients. The 90-day results (277) failed to show significant differences from placebo in the primary end point of exercise time (65 vs. 45 seconds' improvement, $p = .64$) or in rest or stress nuclear perfusion. Angina frequency determined by the Seattle Angina Questionnaire was less in the FGF group, although this did not achieve statistical significance. In a *post hoc* analysis, a significant improvement in exercise time was seen in patients who were older than 63 years (80 vs. 40 seconds, $p = .03$). The otherwise negative primary endpoint results of the VIVA and FIRST studies using intracoronary ± intravenous protein administration underscore the concern that the pharmacokinetics of recombinant protein administered into the vascular space may lead to inadequate local delivery of angiogenic growth factor within the ischemic myocardium, as suggested by studies reported previously using labeled ligand (219,223).

Potential Risks of Inducing Angiogenesis

The risks associated with therapeutic angiogenesis include those that are specific to the growth factor *per se* and those generic to strategies of promoting angiogenesis. With regard to the former, risks thus far recognized clinically in associa-

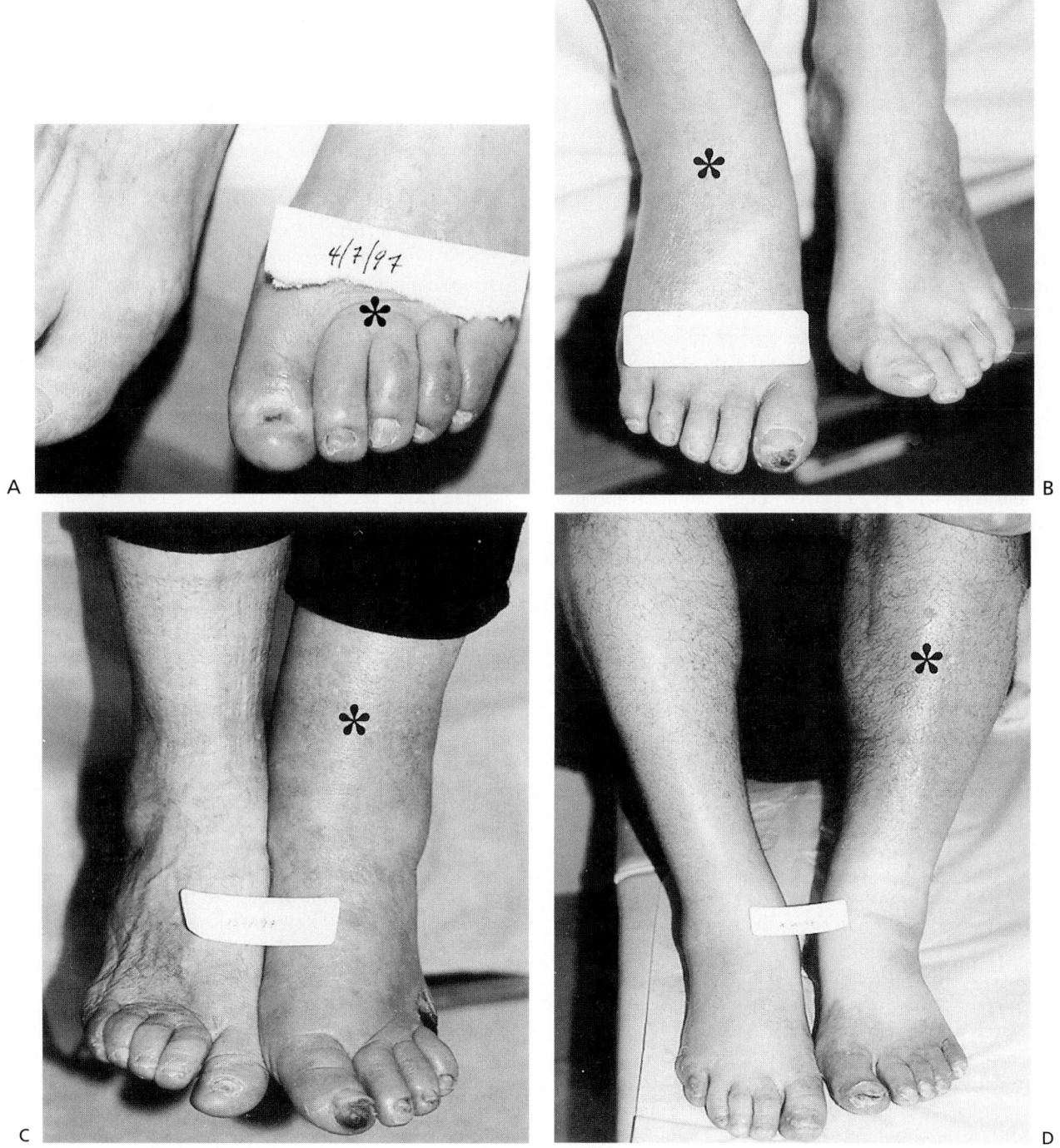

FIGURE 106.11 Representative examples of lower extremity edema (*asterisks*) according to clinical grade in four patients after intramuscular plasmid human vascular endothelial growth factor$_{165}$ gene transfer. **A:** Grade 1. **B:** Grade 2. **C:** Grade 3. **D:** Grade 4.

tion with VEGF depend on the mode of administration. Administration of recombinant protein can lead to hypotension (215,293), because VEGF upregulates NO synthesis (164,205); this complication, however, has never been described after gene transfer in either animals or humans. Although experiments performed in transgenic mice that were engineered to overexpress VEGF ± angiopoietin have

been interpreted to suggest lethal permeability-enhancing effects of VEGF (294), evidence of enhanced permeability in humans has been limited to transient lower extremity edema (Fig. 106.11) in patients with critical limb ischemia following VEGF gene transfer (216). A third issue concerns the development of angiomas in mice (295) or rats (247) that were treated with transduced myoblasts or supraphysiologic doses of plasmid DNA, respectively. Importantly, in the latter study, no angiomas were observed when the dose of administered plasmid DNA was reduced by 50% (R. A. Kloner et al., *unpublished data*, 2001). Except for these studies, no other preclinical or clinical reports, including those that used adenoviral vectors, have described this complication. With bFGF, hypotension may also result from the use of recombinant protein—again mediated via augmented NO release—but has not been described after gene transfer. Use of recombinant protein has also been associated with proteinuria (218).

More generic safety issues concern the potential to stimulate tumor vascularity and growth in the case of occult neoplasms, as well as the potential to exacerbate proliferative or hemorrhagic retinopathy, or both, in patients with diabetes, in view of the high VEGF levels that are demonstrated in the ocular fluid of patients with active proliferative retinopathy (296). With regard to carcinogenesis, there are neither *in vitro* nor *in vivo* data to date to suggest that VEGF increases the risk of neoplastic growth or metastases, or both, although longer-term follow-up will be required to address this issue in clinical trials. With regard to retinopathy, more than 100 patients who received VEGF-1 or -2 have now been treated at the author's institution and undergone serial funduscopic examinations before and after gene transfer by an independent group of retinal specialists; none to date (up to 4 years follow-up) has shown evidence of new retinopathy, despite the fact that nearly one-third had a history of diabetes or remote retinopathy, or both (297).

Another concern stems from the demonstration that inhibitors of angiogenesis tested in an apolipoprotein E–deficient mouse model of atherosclerosis inhibited plaque growth and intimal neovascularization (104). It is important to underscore the fact that these experiments were designed to test the hypothesis that inhibition of plaque angiogenesis would reduce the growth of atherosclerotic lesions; the experiments were not designed to test the hypothesis that administration of agents that promote angiogenesis would enhance atherosclerosis. To this end, several animal studies (103,298–300) and clinical studies of human subjects (301,302) (Table 106.4) fail to support the notion that accelerated atherosclerosis is a likely consequence of administering angiogenic cytokines; the outcome, in fact, is quite the opposite, in that administration of VEGF led to a statistically significant reduction in intimal thickening due to accelerated reendothelialization. The data available to date thus do not support the notion that acceleration of atherosclerosis is a consequence of VEGF-induced stimulation of angiogenesis.

TABLE 106.4 STUDIES REGARDING VASCULAR ENDOTHELIAL GROWTH FACTOR AND NEOINTIMAL THICKENING

First author (reference no.)	Year	Species	Target vessel	Trauma	VEGF Gene	VEGF Protein	Mode of delivery	Neointimal thickening Increased	Neointimal thickening Decreased	Neointimal thickening Unchanged
Asahara (103)	1995	Rat	Carotid artery	Balloon		✔	Dwell		✔	
Asahara (300)	1996	Rabbit	Femoral artery	Balloon	✔		Balloon catheter		✔	
Lazarous (227)	1996	Dog	Femoral artery	Balloon		✔	i.v.	✔		
Van Belle (298)	1997	Rabbit	Iliac artery	Balloon/stent		✔	Balloon catheter		✔	
Van Belle (299)	1997	Rabbit	Iliac artery	Balloon/stent	✔		Balloon catheter		✔	
Inoue (324)	1998	Human	Coronary	None			Autopsy specimens	✔[a]		
Luo (325)	1998	Rabbit	Vein graft	Surgery	✔		Topical		✔	
Isner (253)	1998	Human	SFA/profunda	Balloon	✔		Balloon catheter			✔
Vale (301)	1998	Human	SFA	PTA	✔		Balloon catheter		✔[b]	
Laitinen (302)	1998	Human	Coronary	PTCA	✔		Balloon catheter			✔
Henry (326)	1999	Human	Coronary	None	✔		i.c./i.v.			✔
Hiltunen (327)	2000	Rabbit	Aorta	Balloon/chol	✔		Balloon catheter		✔	
Celletti (328)	2001	Mouse, rabbit	Aorta	Chol		✔	i.p./i.m.	✔		

chol, cholesterol; i.c., intracoronary; i.p., intraperitoneal; PTA, percutaneous transluminal angioplasty; PTCA, percutaneous transluminal coronary angioplasty; SFA, superficial femoral artery; VEGF, vascular endothelial growth factor.
[a]Increased intimal thickening associated with increased VEGF immunostain.
[b]Versus historical controls.

CONCLUSIONS

The immediate goal of clinical research in therapeutic myocardial angiogenesis with either protein administration or gene transfer is to demonstrate efficacy in larger-scale, placebo-controlled trials. To be sure, the rate at which regulatory agencies have permitted clinical trials of gene therapy, as opposed to recombinant protein or TMR, to progress has delayed achieving this objective. In addition, it should be acknowledged that clinical evaluation of therapies designed to promote collateral development would benefit from improvements in imaging capabilities that permit routine, high-resolution imaging of vessels less than 200 μm in diameter, typical of synchrotron radiation (262) but not possible with current angiographic imaging suites. Given the goal of optimizing tissue exposure to growth factor, it remains to be demonstrated that this can be achieved with single or even multiple injections of recombinant protein; recognizing this, certain groups are currently investigating sustained-release formulations of recombinant protein (N. Ferrara, *personal communication*, 2001). In contrast, sustained release is an inherent feature of gene transfer, at least over a period of 2 to 4 weeks in the case of naked plasmid or adenoviral gene transfer (119,319), and thus constitutes a potential advantage for gene therapy. Subsequent studies will be required to confirm preliminary suggestions that the levels and duration of gene expression achieved with naked plasmid DNA are of sufficient magnitude to achieve therapeutic angiogenesis while avoiding adverse effects and to optimize the choice, dose, and route of administration of angiogenic growth factor. Similarly, clinical trials will ultimately be required to test combinations of growth factors (188,320) in an attempt to reproduce the cascade evolved by nature to elaborate vascular networks.

Finally, complementary strategies that are not limited to supplying the growth factor, but instead enrich the cellular population capable of responding to the ligand, may be required for optimally robust vascularity. A number of studies (207–209,212,214,321,322) have suggested that the viable population of ECs capable of responding to angiogenic cytokine replacement may represent a limiting factor in trials of angiogenesis. Preliminary attempts to address this by a strategy of "supply side" angiogenesis, administering expanded populations of endothelial progenitors harvested from the patient's own circulating blood volume, have successfully augmented hindlimb (74) and myocardial (75) angiogenesis. Clinical implementation of such a strategy will require further research into techniques for harvesting and separating cells and stimulation of their growth *ex vivo* before reinfusion at the time of cytokine stimulation. Implicit in this approach is the development of paradigms capable of identifying which patients are likely to have inadequate cytokine (21) or cellular responses to ischemia, so that therapy can be tailored and therapeutic angiogenesis targeted appropriately.

CONTROVERSIES AND PERSONAL PERSPECTIVES

The most daunting controversy in the clinical field of therapeutic angiogenesis is the task of executing a definitive clinical trial with regard to efficacy of either recombinant protein or gene transfer. Federal regulatory agencies have thus far been more permissive with regard to the more conventional of these two options, namely, recombinant protein. Unfortunately, the short half-life and greater difficulty of establishing site-preferential delivery have constituted recognized liabilities of this approach, and, not surprisingly, clinical trials to date have established limited evidence that recombinant proteins are efficacious for therapeutic angiogenesis.

Clinical trials of gene therapy for therapeutic angiogenesis have come under far greater scrutiny by federal regulatory agencies, and, thus, available clinical data regarding the efficacy of this delivery strategy to date are less robust than those for recombinant protein. The ability to extend the half-life of the angiogenic agent considerably as well as optimize local concentrations while minimizing systemic exposure is an inherent advantage of gene transfer; evidence of efficacy in the limited clinical investigations carried out thus far indeed suggests that these conceptual features translate into clinical advantages for therapeutic angiogenesis.

It is hoped that the clinical evidence to date that gene transfer for therapeutic angiogenesis is safe and well tolerated will now permit larger-scale, appropriately randomized trials to be performed at the more accelerated pace necessary to establish definitive evidence of therapeutic utility. In particular, it is noteworthy that many of the potential toxicities raised by experiments involving a variety of genetically engineered mice have not been borne out in clinical trials of either protein or gene therapy performed to date. Specifically, clinical trials to date do not suggest that the use of angiogenic cytokines accelerates atherosclerosis; indeed, the preclinical and more limited clinical data now available suggest that certain angiogenic cytokines, such as VEGF, may have utility for preventing restenosis; this strategy is parenthetically being tested clinically (using gene transfer) for patients with lower extremity vascular disease and will soon begin for patients with coronary artery disease, as catheter and as stent delivery of the transgene.

Finally, the potential to use cell therapy as an adjunct or even independent mode of therapeutic angiogenesis has now been established in preclinical studies and is about to be tested in human subjects. This therapeutic approach has great appeal, as it constitutes a "supply side" approach to replacing senescent ECs with robust precursors that may integrate into neovascular foci and at the same time delivers with each cell a "payload" of angiogenic cytokines that may facilitate neovascularization. It is likely that this approach will emerge as an effective option for promoting lower extremity and myocardial revascularization.

THE FUTURE

The identification of angiogenic growth factors has generated the opportunity for novel therapies in the treatment of a variety of diseases. This includes pathologic angiogenesis, such as diabetic retinopathy, rheumatoid arthritis, and cancer. In these cases, antibodies or naturally occurring angiogenesis inhibitors, or both, are being investigated clinically to antagonize key angiogenic factors. The strategy is designed to eliminate the vascular infrastructure and thereby minimize the extent of pathologic consequences to the patient.

A complementary strategy is now emerging for the treatment of cardiovascular diseases. Clinical trials of therapeutic angiogenesis have already been initiated in patients with myocardial ischemia and peripheral vascular disease and are imminent for patients with heart failure. These include trials of recombinant protein therapy as well as gene transfer. Protein and gene transfer have thus far been shown to be safe in human subjects. Preliminary trials of recombinant protein have shown limited evidence of efficacy. Preliminary applications of gene therapy have established proof of concept that angiogenic growth factors can augment myocardial perfusion. Subsequent clinical trials will determine the relative advantages of protein versus gene therapy, in terms of bioactivity and cost and safety; the maximum extent of clinical improvement that can be expected; and how the therapeutic outcome may be affected by certain features of the host.

It is also likely that future investigations may clarify the impact on established risk factors for vascular disease, such as lipid dyscrasias and diabetes, on native angiogenesis; thus, risk factor modifications may be useful for indirectly aiding natural angiogenesis in ischemic territories. It is intriguing to consider the possibility that one may be able to identify certain genotypic characteristics that may indicate why some patients form robust collateral networks whereas others fail to do so.

The role of EC progenitors in natural as well as therapeutic angiogenesis will be clarified by future studies. Recent studies have forced us to modify the classic concept that collateral development occurs solely by migration of fully differentiated ECs. It is now clear that circulating stem or progenitor cells, or both, contribute to such neovascularization. What remains to be determined is the proportion of new vessel growth that results from circulating stem cells versus parent vessel ECs. Finally, clinical trials will soon investigate the possibility that EC progenitors may be used in strategies of "supply side" therapeutic angiogenesis, specifically, whether administration of enriched or mixed populations of EC or less lineage-defined progenitors, including cells that are engineered to secrete proangiogenic agents, complement the impact of angiogenic cytokines on collateral vessel growth.

REFERENCES

1. Gilbert SF. *Developmental biology*, 4th ed. Sunderland, MA: Sinauer Associates, 1997:342.
2. Folkman J. Angiogenesis in cancer, vascular, rheumatoid and other disease. *Nature Med* 1995;1:27–30.
3. Risau W. Differentiation of endothelium. *FASEB J* 1995;9:926–933.
4. Risau W, Flamme I. Vasculogenesis. *Ann Rev Cell Dev Biol* 1995;11:73–91.
5. Risau W, Sariola H, Zerwes H-G, et al. Vasculogenesis and angiogenesis in embryonic stem cell–derived embryoid bodies. *Development* 1988;102:471–478.
6. Flamme I, Risau W. Induction of vasculogenesis and hematopoiesis in vitro. *Development* 1992;116:435–439.
7. His W. Leoithoblast und angioblast der wirbelthiere. *Abhandl K S Ges Wiss Math Phys* 1900;22:171–328.
8. Weiss M, Orkin SH. In vitro differentiation of murine embryonic stem cells: new approaches to old problems. *J Clin Invest* 1996;97:591–595.
9. Folkman J, Shing Y. Angiogenesis. *J Biol Chem* 1992;267:10931–10934.
10. D'Amore PA, Thompson RW. Mechanisms of angiogenesis. *Annu Rev Physiol* 1987;49:453–464.
11. Ausprunk DH, Folkman J. Migration and proliferation of endothelial cells in preformed and newly formed blood vessels during tumor angiogenesis. *Microvasc Res* 1977;14:53–65.
12. Sholley MM, Ferguson GP, Seibel HR, et al. Mechanisms of neovascularization: vascular sprouting can occur without proliferation of endothelial cells. *Lab Invest* 1984;51:624–634.
13. Nicosia RF, Bonanno E, Smith M. Fibronectin promotes the elongation of microvessels during angiogenesis in vitro. *J Cell Physiol* 1993;154:654–661.
14. Pepper MS, Montesano R. Proteolytic balance and capillary morphogenesis. *Cell Differ Dev* 1990;32:319–328.
15. Pepper MS, Ferrara N, Orci L, et al. Vascular endothelial growth factor (VEGF) induces plasminogen activators and plasminogen activator inhibitor-1 in microvascular endothelial cells. *Biochem Biophys Res Commun* 1991;181:902–906.
16. Schaper W, Brahander MD, Lewi P. DNA synthesis and mitoses in coronary collateral vessels of the dog. *Circ Res* 1971;28:671–679.
17. Cowan DF, Hollenberg NK, Connelly CM, et al. Increased collateral arterial and venous endothelial cell

turnover after renal artery stenosis in the dog. *Invest Radiol* 1978;13:143–149.

18. Pasyk S, Schaper W, Schaper J, et al. DNA synthesis in coronary collaterals after coronary artery occlusion in conscious dog. *Am J Physiol* 1982;242:H1031–H1037.

19. Ilich N, Hollenberg NK, Williams DH, et al. Time course of increased collateral arterial and venous endothelial cell turnover after renal artery stenosis in the rat. *Circ Res* 1979;45:579–582.

20. White FC, Carroll SM, Magnet A, et al. Coronary collateral development in swine after coronary artery occlusion. *Circ Res* 1992;71:1490–1500.

21. Schaper W, Schaper J, Xhonneux R, et al. The morphology of intercoronary anastomoses in chronic coronary artery occlusion. *Cardiovasc Res* 1969;3:315–323.

22. Cuevas P, Carceller F, Ortega S, et al. Hypotensive activity of fibroblast growth factor. *Science* 1991;254:1208–1210.

23. Bucay M, Nguy JH, Barrios R, et al. Impaired macro- and microvascular growth in hypercholesterolemic rabbits. *J Am Coll Cardiol* 1992;19:151A(abst).

24. Graham AM, Baffour R, Burdon T, et al. A demonstration of vascular proliferation in response to arteriovenous reversal in the ischemic canine hind limb. *J Surg Res* 1989;47:341–347.

25. Takeshita S, Zheng LP, Brogi E, et al. Therapeutic angiogenesis: a single intra-arterial bolus of vascular endothelial growth factor augments revascularization in a rabbit ischemic hindlimb model. *J Clin Invest* 1994;93:662–670.

26. Shalaby F, Rossant J, Yamaguchi TP, et al. Failure of blood-island formation and vasculogenesis in Flk-1 deficient mice. *Nature* 1995;376:62–66.

27. Carmeliet P, Ferreira V, Breier G, et al. Abnormal blood vessel development and lethality in embryos lacking a single VEGF allele. *Nature* 1996;380:435–439.

28. Ferrara N, Carver-Moore K, Chen H, et al. Heterozygous embryonic lethality induced by targeted inactivation of the VEGF gene. *Nature* 1996;380:439–442.

29. Fong GH, Rossant J, Gertsenstein M, et al. Role of flt-1 receptor tyrosine kinase in regulating the assembly of vascular endothelium. *Nature* 1995;376:66–70.

30. Sato TN, Qin Y, Kozak CA, et al. Tie-1 and Tie-2 define another class of putative receptor tyrosine kinase genes expressed in early embryonic vascular system. *Proc Natl Acad Sci U S A* 1993;90:9355–9358.

31. Sato TN, Tozawa Y, Deutsch U, et al. Distinct roles of the receptor tyrosine kinases Tie-1 and Tie-2 in blood vessel formation. *Nature* 1995;376:70–74.

32. Davis S, Aldrich TH, Jones PF, et al. Isolation of angiopoietin-1, a ligand for the TIE2 receptor by secretion-trap expression cloning. *Cell* 1996;87:1161–1169.

33. Suri C, Jones PF, Patan S, et al. Requisite role of angiopoietin-1, a ligand for the TIE2 receptor, during embryonic angiogenesis. *Cell* 1996;87:1171–1180.

34. Ingber DE, Folkman J. How does extracellular-matrix control capillary morphogenesis? *Cell* 1989;58:803–805.

35. Folkman J, Haudenschild C. Angiogenesis in vitro. *Nature* 1980;288:551–556.

36. Bar T, Guldner F-H, Wolff JR. "Seamless" endothelial cells of blood capillaries. *Cell Tissue Res* 1984;235:99–106.

37. Saffitz JE, Sullivan A, Isner JM. Regulation of endothelial cell connexin expression by vascular endothelial growth factor. *Circulation* 1996;94:I-238(abst).

38. Folkman J. Tumor angiogenesis. In: Becker FF (ed). *Cancer biology.* New York: Plenum Press, 1975:355–388.

39. Jain RK. Determinants of tumor blood flow. *Cancer Res* 1988;48:2641–2647.

40. Dvorak HF, Brown LF, Detmar M, et al. Vascular permeability factor/vascular endothelial growth factor, microvascular hyperpermeability, and angiogenesis. *Am J Pathol* 1995;146:1029–1039.

41. Kohn S, Nagy JA, Dvorak HF, et al. Pathways of macromolecular tracer transport across venules and small veins. Structural basis for the hyperpermeability of tumor blood vessels. *Lab Invest* 1992;67:596–607.

42. Roberts WG, Palade GE. Increased microvascular permeability and endothelial fenestration induced by vascular endothelial growth factor. *J Cell Sci* 1995;108:2369–2379.

43. Brooks PC, Clark RAF, Cheresh DA. Requirement of vascular integrin alpha-v-beta-3 for angiogenesis. *Science* 1994;264:569–571.

44. Brooks PC, Montgomery AMP, Rossenfeld M, et al. Integrin alpha-v-beta-3 antagonists promote tumor regression by inducing apoptosis of angiogenic blood vessels. *Cell* 1994;79:1157–1164.

45. Okada Y, Copeland BR, Hamann GF, et al. Integrin alpha-v-beta-3 is expressed in selected microvessels after focal cerebral ischemia. *Am J Pathol* 1996;149:37–44.

46. Stromblad S, Becker JC, Yebra M, et al. Suppression of p53 activity and p21^{WAF1CIP1} expression by vascular cell integrin alpha-v-beta-3 during angiogenesis. *J Clin Invest* 1996;98:426–433.

47. Breier G, Albrecht U, Sterrer S, et al. Expression of vascular endothelial growth factor during embryonic angiogenesis and endothelial cell differentiation. *Development* 1992;114:521–532.

48. Ruoslahti E, Reed JC. Anchorage dependence, integrins, and apoptosis. *Cell* 1994;77:477–478.

49. Fuks Z, Persaud RS, Alfieri A, et al. Basic fibroblast growth factor protects endothelial cells against radiation-induced programmed cell death in vitro and in vivo. *Cancer Res* 1994;54:2582–2590.

50. Defilippi P, Silengo L, Tarone G. Regulation of adhesion receptors expression in endothelial cells. *Microbiol Immunol* 1993;184:87–98.

51. Enenstein J, Walsh NS, Kramer RH. Basic FGF and TGF-β differentially modulate integrin expression of human microvascular endothelial cells. *Exp Cell Res* 1992;203:499–503.

52. Klein S, Giancotti FG, Presta M, et al. Basic fibroblast growth factor modulates integrin expression in microvascular endothelial cells. *Mol Biol Cell* 1993;4:973–982.

53. Spyridopoulos I, Brogi E, Kearney M, et al. Vascular endothelial growth factor inhibits endothelial cell apoptosis induced by tumor necrosis factor-alpha: balance between growth and death signals. *J Mol Cell Cardiol* 1997;29:1321–1330.

54. Friedlander M, Brooks PC, Shaffer RW, et al. Definition of two angiogenic pathways by distinct alpha v integrins. *Science* 1995;270:1500–1502.

55. Alon T, Hemo I, Itin A, et al. Vascular endothelial growth factor acts as a survival factor for newly formed retinal vessels and has implications for retinopathy of prematurity. *Nature Med* 1995;1:1024–1028.

56. Katoh O, Tauchi H, Kawaishi K, et al. Expression of the vascular endothelial growth factor (VEGF) receptor gene

KDR, in hematopoietic cells and inhibitory effect of VEGF on apoptotic cell death caused by ionizing radiation. *Cancer Res* 1995;55:5687–5692.

57. Pardanaud L, Altman C, Kitos P, et al. Relationship between vasculogenesis, angiogenesis and haemopoiesis during avian ontogeny. *Development* 1989;105:473–485.

58. Asahara T, Murohara T, Sullivan A, et al. Isolation of putative progenitor endothelial cells for angiogenesis. *Science* 1997;275:964–967.

59. Wu MH-D, Shi Q, Wechezak AR, et al. Definitive proof of endothelialization of a Dacron arterial prosthesis in a human being. *J Vasc Surg* 1995;21:862–867.

60. Shi Q, Wu MH, Hayashida N, et al. Proof of fallout endothelialization of impervious dacron grafts in the aorta and inferior vena cava of the dog. *J Vasc Surg* 1994;20:546–556.

61. Civin CI, Banquerigo ML, Strauss LC, et al. Antigen analysis of hematopoiesis. VI. Flow cytometric characterization of My-10-positive progenitor cells in normal human bone marrow. *Exp Hematol* 1987;15:10–17.

62. Katz F, Tindle RW, Sutherland DR, et al. Identification of a membrane glycoprotein associated with hemopoietic progenitor cells. *Leuk Res* 1985;9:191–198.

63. Andrews RG, Singer JW, Bernstein ID. Monoclonal antibody 12-8 recognizes a 115-kd molecule present on both unipotent and multipotent hematopoietic colony-forming cells and their precursors. *Blood* 1986;67:842–845.

64. Fina J, Molgard HV, Robertson D, et al. Expression of the CD34 gene in vascular endothelial cells. *Blood* 1990;75:2417–2426.

65. Soligo D, Delia D, Oriani A, et al. Identification of CD34⁺ cells in normal and pathological bone marrow biopsies by OBEND10 monoclonal antibody. *Leukemia* 1991;5:1026–1030.

66. Ito A, Nomura S, Hirota S, et al. Enhanced expression of CD34 messenger RNA by developing endothelial cells of mice. *Lab Invest* 1995;72:532–538.

67. deVries C, Escobedo JA, Ueno H, et al. The *fms*-like tyrosine kinase, a receptor for vascular endothelial growth factor. *Science* 1992;255:989–991.

68. Terman BI, Carrion ME, Kovacs E, et al. Identification of a new endothelial cell growth factor receptor tyrosine kinase. *Oncogene* 1991;6:1677–1683.

69. Matthews W, Jordan CT, Gavin M, et al. A receptor tyrosine kinase cDNA isolated from a population of enriched primitive hematopoietic cells and exhibiting close genetic linkage to c-kit. *Proc Natl Acad Sci U S A* 1991;88:9026–9030.

70. Millauer B, Wizigmann-Voos S, Schnurch H, et al. High affinity VEGF binding and developmental expression suggest *Flk-1* as a major regulator of vasculogenesis and angiogenesis. *Cell* 1993;72:835–846.

71. Yamaguchi TP, Dumont DJ, Conlon RA, et al. *flk-1*, an *flt*-related receptor tyrosine kinase is an early marker for endothelial cell precursors. *Development* 1993;118:489–498.

72. Isner JM, Pieczek A, Schainfeld R, et al. Clinical evidence of angiogenesis following arterial gene transfer of phVEGF$_{165}$. *Lancet* 1996;348:370–374.

73. Tschudi MR, Barton M, Bersinger NA, et al. Effect of age on kinetics of nitric oxide release in rat aorta and pulmonary artery. *J Clin Invest* 1996;98:899–905.

74. Kalka C, Masuda H, Takahashi T, et al. Transplantation of ex vivo expanded endothelial progenitor cells for therapeutic neovascularization. *Proc Natl Acad Sci U S A* 2000;97:3422–3427.

75. Kawamoto A, Gwon H-C, Iwaguro H, et al. Therapeutic potential of *ex vivo* expanded endothelial progenitor cells for myocardial ischemia. *Circulation* 2001;103:634–637.

76. Schatteman GC, Hanlon HD, Jiao C, et al. Blood-derived angioblasts accelerate blood-flow restoration in diabetic mice. *J Clin Invest* 2000;106:571–578.

77. Senger DR, Ledbetter SR, Claffey KP, et al. Stimulation of endothelial cell migration by vascular permeability factor/vascular endothelial growth factor through cooperative mechanisms involving the avb3 integrin, osteopontin, and thrombin. *Am J Pathol* 1996;149:293–305.

78. Williams JK, Heistad DD. Structure and function of vasa vasorum. *Trends Cardiovasc Med* 1996;6:53–57.

79. Heistad DD, Armstrong ML, Marcus ML. Hyperemia of the aortic wall in atherosclerotic monkeys. *Circ Res* 1981;48:669–675.

80. O'Brien ER, Garvin MR, Dev R, et al. Angiogenesis in human coronary atherosclerotic plaques. *Am J Pathol* 1994;145:883–894.

81. Isner JM, Kearney M, Bauters C, et al. Use of human tissue specimens obtained in vivo by directional atherectomy to study restenosis and related human vascular disorders. *Trends Cardiovasc Med* 1994;4:213–221.

82. Depre C, Havaux X, Wijns W. Neovascularization in human coronary atherosclerotic lesions. *Cathet Cardiovasc Diag* 1996;39:215–220.

83. Zhang Y, Cliff WJ, Schoefli GI, et al. Immunohistochemical study of intimal microvessels in coronary atherosclerosis. *Am J Pathol* 1993;143:164–172.

84. Geiringer E. Intimal vascularization and atherosclerosis. *J Pathol Bacteriol* 1951;63:201–211.

85. Wolinsky H, Glagov S. Nature of species differences in the medial distribution of aortic vasa vasorum in mammals. *Circ Res* 1967;20:409–421.

86. Heistad DD, Marcus ML, Law EG, et al. Regulation of blood flow to the aortic media in dogs. *J Clin Invest* 1978;62:133–140.

87. Barger AC, Beeuwkes R III, Lainey LL, et al. Hypothesis: vasa vasorum and neovascularization of human coronary arteries: a possible role in the pathophysiology of atherosclerosis. *N Engl J Med* 1984;310:175–177.

88. Williams JK, Armstrong ML, Heistad DD. Endothelial denudation stimulates proliferation of vasa vasorum. *J Vasc Med Biol* 1990;2:12–17.

89. Shweiki D, Neeman M, Itin A, et al. Induction of vascular endothelial growth factor expression by hypoxia and by glucose deficiency in multicell spheroids: implications for tumor angiogenesis. *Proc Natl Acad Sci U S A* 1995;92:768–772.

90. Flugelman MY, Virmani R, Correa R, et al. Smooth muscle cell abundance and fibroblast growth factors in coronary lesions of patients with nonfatal unstable angina: a clue to the mechanism of transformation from the stable to the unstable clinical state. *Circulation* 1993;88:2493–2500.

91. Cuevas P, Gonzalez AM, Carceller F, et al. Vascular response to basic fibroblast growth factor when infused onto the normal adventitia or into the injured media of the rat carotid artery. *Circ Res* 1991;69:360–369.

92. Edelman ER, Nugent MA, Smith LT, et al. Basic fibroblast growth factor enhances the coupling of intimal

hyperplasia and proliferation of vasa vasorum in injured rat arteries. *J Clin Invest* 1992;89:465–473.

93. Brogi E, Winkles JA, Underwood R, et al. Distinct patterns of expression of fibroblast growth factors and their receptors in human atheroma and nonatherosclerotic arteries: association of acidic FGF with plaque microvessels and macrophages. *J Clin Invest* 1993;92:2408–2418.

94. Nabel EG, Yang ZY, Plautz G, et al. Recombinant fibroblast growth factor-1 promotes intimal hyperplasia and angiogenesis in arteries *in vivo*. *Nature* 1993;362:844–846.

95. Folkman J. Clinical applications of research on angiogenesis. *N Engl J Med* 1995;333:1757–1763.

96. Riessen R, Isner JM. Prospects for site-specific delivery of pharmacologic and molecular therapies. *J Am Coll Cardiol* 1994;23:1234–1244.

97. Williams JK, Armstrong ML, Heistad DD. Vasa vasorum in atherosclerotic coronary arteries: responses to vasoactive stimuli and regression of atherosclerosis. *Circ Res* 1988;62:515–523.

98. Feldman LJ, Isner JM. Gene therapy for the vulnerable plaque. *J Am Coll Cardiol* 1995;26:826–835.

99. Barger AC, Beeuwks R III. Rupture of coronary vasa vasorum as a trigger of acute myocardial infarction. *Am J Cardiol* 1990;66:41G–43G.

100. Barker SGE, Cottam TS, Baskerville PA, et al. Arterial intimal hyperplasia after occlusion of the adventitial vasa vasorum in the pig. *Arterioscler Thromb* 1993;13:70–77.

101. Lindner V, Majack RA, Reidy MA. Basic fibroblast growth factor stimulates endothelial regrowth and proliferation in denuded arteries. *J Clin Invest* 1990;85:2004–2008.

102. Bjornsson TD, Dryjski M, Tluczek J, et al. Acidic fibroblast growth factor promotes vascular repair. *Proc Natl Acad Sci U S A* 1991;88:8651–8655.

103. Asahara T, Bauters C, Pastore CJ, et al. Local delivery of vascular endothelial growth factor accelerates reendothelialization and attenuates intimal hyperplasia in balloon-injured rat carotid artery. *Circulation* 1995;91:2793–2801.

104. Moulton KS, Heller E, Konerding MA, et al. Angiogenesis inhibitors endostatin and TNP-470 reduce intimal neovascularization and plaque growth in apolipoprotein E–deficient mice. *Circulation* 1999;99:1726–1732.

105. Shing Y, Folkman J, Sullivan J, et al. Heparin-affinity purification of a tumor-derived capillary endothelial cell growth factor. *Science* 1984;223:1296–1299.

106. Ferrara N, Henzel WJ. Pituitary follicular cells secrete a novel heparin-binding growth factor specific for vascular endothelial cells. *Biochem Biophys Res Commun* 1989;161:851–855.

107. Keck PJ, Hauser SD, Krivi G, et al. Vascular permeability factor, an endothelial cell mitogen related to PDGF. *Science* 1989;246:1309–1312.

108. Plouet J, Schilling J, Gospodarowicz D. Isolation and characterization of a newly identified endothelial cell mitogen produced by AtT-20 cells. *EMBO J* 1989;8:3801–3806.

109. Tischer E, Mitchell R, Hartmann T, et al. The human gene for vascular endothelial growth factor: multiple protein forms are encoded through alternative exon splicing. *J Biol Chem* 1991;266:11947–11954.

110. Houck KA, Leung DW, Rowland AM, et al. Dual regulation of vascular endothelial growth factor bioavailability by genetic and proteolytic mechanisms. *J Biol Chem* 1992;267:26031–26037.

111. Yanagisawa-Miwa A, Uchida Y, Nakamura F, et al. Salvage of infarcted myocardium by angiogenic action of basic fibroblast growth factor. *Science* 1992;257:1401–1403.

112. Keyt BA, Nguyen HV, Berleau LT, et al. Identification of vascular endothelial growth factor determinants for binding KDR and FLT-1 receptors. *J Biol Chem* 1996;271:5638–5646.

113. Gitay-Goren H, Cohen T, Tessler S, et al. Selective binding of $VEGF_{121}$ to one of the three vascular endothelial growth factor receptors of vascular endothelial cells. *J Biol Chem* 1996;271:5519–5523.

114. Plate KH, Breier G, Weich HA, et al. Vascular endothelial growth factor and glioma angiogenesis: coordinate induction of VEGF receptors. Distribution of VEGF protein and possible in vivo regulatory mechanisms. *Int J Cancer* 1994;59:520–529.

115. Park JE, Keller G-A, Ferrara N. The vascular endothelial growth factor (VEGF) isoforms: differential deposition into the subepithelial ECM and bioactivity of ECM-bound VEGF. *Mol Biol Cell* 1993;4:1317–1326.

116. Takeshita S, Tsurumi Y, Couffinhal T, et al. Gene transfer of naked DNA encoding for three isoforms of vascular endothelial growth factor stimulates collateral development in vivo. *Lab Invest* 1996;75:487–502.

117. Miles AA, Miles EM. Vascular reactions to histamine, histamine liberators or leukotoxins in the skin of the guinea pig. *J Physiol* 1952;118:228–257.

118. Carmeliet P, Ng Y-S, Nuyens D, et al. Impaired myocardial angiogenesis and ischemic cardiomyopathy in mice lacking the vascular endothelial growth factor isoforms $VEGF_{188}$. *Nature Med* 1999;5:495–502.

119. Tsurumi Y, Takeshita S, Chen D, et al. Direct intramuscular gene transfer of naked DNA encoding vascular endothelial growth factor augments collateral development and tissue perfusion. *Circulation* 1996;94:3281–3290.

120. Joukov V, Pajusola K, Kaipainen A, et al. A novel vascular endothelial growth factor, VEGF-C, is a ligand for the Flt4 (VEGFR-3) and KDR (VEGFR-2) receptor tyrosine kinases. *EMBO J* 1996;15:290–298.

121. Olofsson B, Pajusola K, Kaipainen A, et al. Vascular endothelial growth factor B, a novel growth factor for endothelial cells. *Proc Natl Acad Sci U S A* 1996;93:2576–2581.

122. Witzenbichler B, Asahara T, Murohara T, et al. Vascular endothelial growth factor-C (VEGF-C/VEGF-2) promotes angiogenesis in the setting of tissue ischemia. *Am J Pathol* 1998;153:381–394.

123. Cao Y, Linden P, Farnebo J, et al. Vascular endothelial growth factor C induces angiogenesis in vivo. *Proc Natl Acad Sci U S A* 1998;95:14389–14394.

124. Vale PR, Losordo DW, Milliken CE, et al. Randomized, placebo-controlled clinical study of percutaneous catheter-based left ventricular endocardial gene transfer of VEGF-2 for myocardial angiogenesis in patients with chronic myocardial ischemia. *Circulation* 2000;102:II-563(abst).

125. Maglione D, Guerriero V, Viglietto G, et al. Isolation of a human placenta cDNA coding for a protein related to the vascular permeability factor. *Proc Natl Acad Sci U S A* 1991;88:9267–9271.

126. Maglione D, Guerriero V, Viglietto G, et al. Two alternative mRNAs coding for the angiogenic factor, placenta

growth factor (PIGF), are transcribed from a single gene of chromosome 14. *Oncogene* 1993;8:925–931.

127. Hauser S, Weich HA. A heparin-binding form of placenta growth factor (PIGF-2) is expressed in human umbilical vein endothelial cells and in placenta. *Growth Factors* 1993;9:259–268.

128. DiSalvo J, Bayne ML, Conn G, et al. Purification and characterization of a naturally occurring vascular endothelial growth factor. Placenta growth factor heterodimer. *J Biol Chem* 1995;270:7717–7723.

129. Park JE, Chen HH, Winer J, et al. Placenta growth factor: potentiation of vascular endothelial growth factor bioactivity, in vitro and in vivo, and high affinity binding to *Flt*-1 but not to *Flk*-1/KDR. *J Biol Chem* 1994;269:25646–25654.

130. Cao Y, Linden P, Shima D, et al. In vivo angiogenic activity and hypoxia induction of heterodimer of placenta growth factor/vascular endothelial growth factor. *J Clin Invest* 1996;98:2507–2511.

131. Carmeliet P, Collen D. Molecular analysis of blood vessel formation and disease. *Am J Physiol* 1997;273:H2091–H2104.

132. Pajusola K, Aprelikova O, Pelicci G, et al. Signaling properties of FLT4, a proteolytically processed receptor tyrosine kinase related to two VEGF receptors. *Oncogene* 1994;9:3545–3555.

133. Lee J, Gray A, Yuan J, et al. Vascular endothelial growth factor–related protein: a ligand and specific activator of the tyrosine kinase receptor Flt4. *Proc Natl Acad Sci U S A* 1996;93:1988–1992.

134. Mignatti P, Morimoto T, Rifkin DB. Basic fibroblast growth factor released by single, isolated cells stimulates their migration in an autocrine manner. *Proc Natl Acad Sci U S A* 1991;88:11007–11011.

135. Jaye M, Lyall RM, Mudd R, et al. Expression of acidic fibroblast growth factor cDNA confers growth advantage and tumorigenesis to Swiss 3T3 cells. *EMBO J* 1988;7:963–969.

136. Myoken Y, Okamoto T, Kan M, et al. Release of fibroblast growth factor-1 by human squamous cell carcinoma correlates with autocrine cell growth. *In Vitro Cell Dev Biol* 1994;30A:790–795.

137. Schweigerer L, Neufeld G, Friedman J, et al. Capillary endothelial cells express basic fibroblast growth factor, a mitogen that promotes their own growth. *Nature* 1987;325:257–259.

138. Villaschi S, Nicosia RF. Angiogenic role of endogenous basic fibroblast growth factor released by rat aorta after injury. *Am J Pathol* 1993;143:181–190.

139. Bensaid M, Malecaze F, Prats H, et al. Autocrine regulation of bovine retinal capillary endothelial cell (BREC) proliferation by BREC-derived basic fibroblast growth factor. *Exp Eye Res* 1989;48:801–813.

140. Namiki A, Brogi E, Kearney M, et al. Hypoxia induces vascular endothelial growth factor in cultured human endothelial cells. *J Biol Chem* 1995;270:31189–31195.

141. Iizuki M, Yamauchi M, Ando K, et al. Quantitative RT-PCR assay detecting the transcriptional induction of vascular endothelial growth factor under hypoxia. *Biochem Biophys Res Commun* 1994;205:1474–1480.

142. Houck KA, Ferrara N, Winer J, et al. The vascular endothelial growth factor family: identification of a fourth molecular species and characterization of alternative splicing of RNA. *Mol Endocrinol* 1991;5:1806–1814.

143. Ladoux A, Frelin C. Expression of vascular endothelial growth factor by cultured endothelial cells from brain microvessels. *Biochem Biophys Res Commun* 1993;194:799–803.

144. Shweiki D, Itin A, Soffer D, et al. Vascular endothelial growth factor induced by hypoxia may mediate hypoxia-initiated angiogenesis. *Nature* 1992;359:843–845.

145. Goldberg MA, Dunning SP, Bunn HF. Regulation of the erythropoietin gene: evidence that the oxygen sensor is a heme protein. *Science* 1988;242:1412–1415.

146. Goldberg MA, Schneider TJ. Similarities between the oxygen-sensing mechanisms regulating the expression of vascular endothelial growth factor and erythropoietin. *J Biol Chem* 1994;269:4355–4359.

147. Schuler GD, Cole MD. GM-CSF and oncogene mRNA stabilities are independently regulated in trans in a mouse monocytic tumor cell. *Cell* 1988;55:1115–1122.

148. Linial M, Gunderson N, Groudine M. Enhanced transcription of c-myc in bursal lymphoma cells requires continuous protein synthesis. *Science* 1985;230:1126–1132.

149. Sporn MB, Roberts AB. Autocrine secretion—10 years later. *Ann Intern Med* 1992;117:408–414.

150. Dvorak HF. Tumors: wounds that do not heal. Similarities between tumor stroma generation and wound healing. *N Engl J Med* 1986;315:1650–1659.

151. Underwood JC, Carr I. The ultrastructure and permeability characteristics of the blood vessels of a transplantable rat sarcoma. *J Pathol* 1972;107:157–166.

152. Brogi E, Wu T, Namiki A, et al. Indirect angiogenic cytokines upregulate VEGF and bFGF gene expression in vascular smooth muscle cells, while hypoxia upregulates VEGF expression only. *Circulation* 1994;90:649–652.

153. Stavri GT, Zachary IC, Baskerville PA, et al. Basic fibroblast growth factor upregulates the expression of vascular endothelial growth factor in vascular smooth muscle cells: synergistic interaction with hypoxia. *Circulation* 1995;92:11–14.

154. Petrovaara L, Kaipainen A, Mustonen T, et al. Vascular endothelial growth factor is induced in response to transforming growth factor-beta in fibroblastic and epithelial cells. *J Biol Chem* 1994;269:6271–6274.

155. Cohen T, Nahari D, Cerem LW, et al. Interleukin 6 induces the expression of vascular endothelial growth factor. *J Biol Chem* 1996;271:736–741.

156. Witzenbichler B, Van Belle E, Chang L, et al. Scatter factor (SF) induces vascular endothelial growth factor (VEGF) expression in vascular smooth muscle cells (VSMC) and acts synergistic to VEGF on endothelial cell (EC) migration in vitro. *Circulation* 1996;94:I-593–I-594(abst).

157. Warren RS, Yuan H, Matli MR, et al. Induction of vascular endothelial growth factor by insulin-like growth factor 1 in colorectal carcinoma. *J Biol Chem* 1996;271:29483–29488.

158. Senger DR, Galli SJ, Dvorak AM, et al. Tumor cells secrete a vascular permeability factor that promotes accumulation of ascites fluid. *Science* 1983;219:983–985.

159. Kubes P, Granger DN. Nitric oxide modulates microvascular permeability. *Am J Physiol* 1992;262:H611–H615.

160. Nguyen LS, Villablanca AC, Rutledge JC. Substance P increases microvascular permeability via nitric oxide–mediated convective pathways. *Am J Physiol* 1995;268:R1060–R1068.

161. Laszlo F, Whittle BJR, Evans SM, et al. Association of microvascular leakage with induction of nitric oxide syn-

thase: effects of nitric oxide synthase inhibitors in various organs. *Eur J Pharmacol* 1995;283:47–53.

162. Bowerman RE, Pinkerton CA, Kirk B, et al. Disruption of a coronary stent during atherectomy for restenosis. *Cathet Cardiovasc Diag* 1993;71:364–366.

163. Fujii E, Irie K, Ogawa A, et al. Role of nitric oxide and prostaglandins in lipopolysaccharide-induced increase in vascular permeability in mouse skin. *Eur J Pharmacol* 1996;297:257–263.

164. van der Zee R, Murohara T, Luo Z, et al. Vascular endothelial growth factor (VEGF)/vascular permeability factor (VPF) augments nitric oxide release from quiescent rabbit and human vascular endothelium. *Circulation* 1997;95:1030–1037.

165. Klagsbrun M, D'Amore PA. Regulators of angiogenesis. *Annu Rev Physiol* 1991;53:217–239.

166. Sato N, Beitz JG, Kato J, et al. Platelet-derived growth factor indirectly stimulates angiogenesis in vitro. *Am J Pathol* 1993;142:1119–1130.

167. Pierce GF, Tarpley JE, Yanagihara D, et al. Platelet derived growth factor (BB homodimer), transforming growth factor-beta1, and basic fibroblast growth factor in dermal wound healing. *Am J Pathol* 1992;140:1375–1388.

168. Risau W, Drexler H, Mironov V, et al. Platelet-derived growth factor is angiogenic in vivo. *Growth Factors* 1992;7:261–266.

169. Beitz JG, Kim IS, Calabresi P, et al. Human microvascular endothelial cells express receptors for platelet-derived growth factor. *Proc Natl Acad Sci U S A* 1991;88:2021–2025.

170. Smits A, Hermansson M, Nister M, et al. Rat brain capillary endothelial cells express functional PDGF B-type receptors. *Growth Factors* 1989;2:1–8.

171. Bar RS, Boes M, Booth BA, et al. The effects of platelet-derived growth factor in cultured microvessel endothelial cells. *Endocrinology* 1989;124:2021–2025.

172. D'Amore P, Smith SR. Growth factor effects on cells of the vascular wall: a survey. *Growth Factors* 1993;8:61–75.

173. Roberts AB, Sporn MB, Assoian RK, et al. Transforming growth factor type-beta: rapid induction of fibrosis and angiogenesis in vivo and stimulation of collagen formation in vitro. *Proc Natl Acad Sci U S A* 1986;83:4167–4171.

174. Pepper MS, Vassalli JD, Orci L, et al. Biphasic effect of transforming growth factor-β1 on in vitro angiogenesis. *Exp Cell Res* 1993;204:356–363.

175. Chen JK, Hoshi H, McKeehan WL. Transforming growth factor type β specifically stimulates synthesis of proteoglycans in human adult arterial smooth muscle cells. *Proc Natl Acad Sci U S A* 1987;84:5287–5291.

176. Madri J, Pratt B, Tucker A. Phenotypic modulation of endothelial cells by transforming growth factor-beta depends upon the composition and organization of the extracellular matrix. *J Cell Biol* 1988;106:1375–1382.

177. Winkles JA, Gay CG. Serum, phorbol ester, and polypeptide mitogens increase class 1 and 2 heparin binding (acidic and basic fibroblast growth factor) gene expression in human vascular smooth muscle cells. *Cell Growth Differ* 1991;2:531–540.

178. Pola R, Ling LE, Silver M, et al. The morphogen sonic hedgehog is an indirect angiogenic agent upregulating two families of angiogenic growth factors. *Nature Med* 2001;7:706–711.

179. Wang GL, Semenza GL. Characterization of hypoxia-inducible factor 1 and regulation of DNA binding activity by hypoxia. *Blood* 1993;268:21513–21518.

180. Shima DT, Deutsch U, D'Amore PA. Hypoxic induction of vascular endothelial growth factor (VEGF) in human epithelial cells is mediated by increases in mRNA stability. *FEBS Lett* 1995;370:203–208.

181. Levy AP, Levy NS, Wegner S, et al. Transcriptional regulation of the rat vascular endothelial growth factor gene by hypoxia. *J Biol Chem* 1995;270:13333–13340.

182. Levy NS, Levy AP, Goldberg MA, et al. Regulation of vascular endothelial growth factor isoforms by hypoxia and identification of a novel truncated vascular endothelial growth factor isoform in cardiac myocytes. *Circulation* 1994;90:I-521(abst).

183. Vincent KA, Shyu K-G, Luo Y, et al. Angiogenesis is induced in a rabbit model of hindlimb ischemia by naked DNA encoding a HIF-1a/VP16 hybrid transcription factor. *Circulation* 2000;102:2255–2261.

184. Tsurumi Y, Murohara T, Krasinski K, et al. Reciprocal relationship between VEGF and NO in the regulation of endothelial integrity. *Nature Med* 1997;3:879–886.

185. Li J, Hampton T, Morgan JP, et al. Stretch-induced VEGF expression in the heart. *J Clin Invest* 1997;100:18–24.

186. Pepper MS, Ferrara N, Orci L, et al. Potent synergism between vascular endothelial growth factor and basic fibroblast growth factor in the induction of angiogenesis in vitro. *Biochem Biophys Res Commun* 1992;189:824–831.

187. Goto F, Goto K, Weindel K, et al. Synergistic effects of vascular endothelial growth factor and basic fibroblast growth factor on the proliferation and cord formation of bovine capillary endothelial cells within collagen gels. *Lab Invest* 1993;69:508–517.

188. Asahara T, Bauters C, Zheng LP, et al. Synergistic effect of vascular endothelial growth factor and basic fibroblast growth factor on angiogenesis in vivo. *Circulation* 1995;92:II-365–II-371.

189. Klagsbrun M, Folkman J. Angiogenesis. In: Sporn MB, Roberts AB, eds. *Peptide growth factors and their receptors II*. New York: Springer-Verlag, 1990:459–586.

190. Terman BI, Dougher-Vermazen M, Carrion ME, et al. Identification of the KDR tyrosine kinase as a receptor for vascular endothelial cell growth factor. *Biochem Biophys Res Commun* 1992;187:1579–1586.

191. Klagsbrun M, Baird A. A dual receptor system is required for basic fibroblast growth factor activity. *Cell* 1991;67:229–231.

192. Pu LQ, Sniderman AD, Brassard R, et al. Enhanced revascularization of the ischemic limb by means of angiogenic therapy. *Circulation* 1993;88:208–215.

193. Baffour R, Berman J, Garb JL, et al. Enhanced angiogenesis and growth of collaterals by in vivo administration of recombinant basic fibroblast growth factor in a rabbit model of acute lower limb ischemia: dose-response effect of basic fibroblast growth factor. *J Vasc Surg* 1992;16:181–191.

194. Takeshita S, Pu L-Q, Zheng L, et al. Vascular endothelial growth factor induces dose-dependent revascularization in a rabbit model of persistent limb ischemia. *Circulation* 1994;90:II-228–II-234.

195. Bauters C, Asahara T, Zheng LP, et al. Site-specific therapeutic angiogenesis following systemic administration of vascular endothelial growth factor. *J Vasc Surg* 1995;21:314–325.

196. Berkman RA, Merrill MJ, Reinhold WC, et al. Expression of the vascular permeability factor/vascular endothelial growth factor gene in central nervous system neoplasms. *J Clin Invest* 1993;91:153–159.

197. Rohovsky S, Kearney M, Pieczek A, et al. Elevated levels of basic fibroblast growth factor in patients with limb ischemia. *Am Heart J* 1996;132:1015–1019.

198. Baumgartner I, Pieczek A, Manor O, et al. Constitutive expression of phVEGF$_{165}$ following intramuscular gene transfer promotes collateral vessel development in patients with critical limb ischemia. *Circulation* 1998;97:1114–1123.

199. Bauters C, Asahara T, Zheng LP, et al. Physiologic assessment of augmented vascularity induced by VEGF in ischemic rabbit hindlimb. *Am J Physiol* 1994;267:H1263–H1271.

200. Thieme H, Aiello LP, Takagi H, et al. Comparative analysis of vascular endothelial growth factor receptors on retinal and aortic vascular endothelial cells. *Diabetes* 1995;44:98–103.

201. Brogi E, Schatteman G, Wu T, et al. Hypoxia-induced paracrine regulation of VEGF receptor expression. *J Clin Invest* 1996;97:469–476.

202. Brock TA, Dvorak HF, Senger DR. Tumor-secreted vascular permeability factor increases cytosolic Ca^{2+} and von Willebrand factor release in human endothelial cells. *Am J Pathol* 1991;138:213–221.

203. Ku DD, Zaleski JK, Liu S, et al. Vascular endothelial growth factor induces EDRF-dependent relaxation in coronary arteries. *Am J Physiol* 1993;265:H586–H592.

204. Leibovich SJ, Polverini PJ, Fong TW, et al. Production of angiogenic activity by human monocytes requires an L-arginine/nitric oxide-synthase–dependent effector mechanism. *Proc Natl Acad Sci U S A* 1994;91:4190–4194.

205. Murohara T, Asahara T, Silver M, et al. Nitric oxide synthase modulates angiogenesis in response to tissue ischemia. *J Clin Invest* 1998;101:2567–2578.

206. Folkman J. Tumor angiogenesis: therapeutic implications. *N Engl J Med* 1971;285:1182–1186.

207. Rivard A, Fabre J-E, Silver M, et al. Age-dependent impairment of angiogenesis. *Circulation* 1999;99:111–120.

208. Rivard A, Silver M, Chen D, et al. Rescue of diabetes related impairment of angiogenesis by intramuscular gene therapy with adeno-VEGF. *Am J Pathol* 1999;154:355–364.

209. Couffinhal T, Silver M, Kearney M, et al. Impaired collateral vessel development associated with reduced expression of vascular endothelial growth factor in ApoE –/– mice. *Circulation* 1999;99:3188–3198.

210. Schultz A, Lavie L, Hochberg I, et al. Interindividual heterogeneity in the hypoxic regulation of VEGF: significance for the development of the coronary artery collateral circulation. *Circulation* 1999;100:547–552.

211. Rohan RM, Fernandez A, Udagawa T, et al. Genetic heterogeneity of angiogenesis in mice. *FASEB J* 2000;14:871–876.

212. Isner JM, Asahara T. Angiogenesis and vasculogenesis as therapeutic strategies for postnatal neovascularization [Perspective]. *J Clin Invest* 1999;103:1231–1236.

213. Asahara T, Kalka C, Isner JM. Stem cell therapy and gene transfer for regeneration. *Gene Ther* 2000;7:451–457.

214. Isner JM. Tissue responses to ischemia: local and remote responses for preserving perfusion of ischemic muscle. *J Clin Invest* 2000;106:615–619.

215. Hariawala M, Horowitz JR, Esakof D, et al. VEGF improves myocardial blood flow but produces EDRF-mediated hypotension in porcine hearts. *J Surg Res* 1996;63:77–82.

216. Baumgartner I, Rauh G, Pieczek A, et al. Lower-extremity edema associated with gene transfer of naked DNA vascular endothelial growth factor. *Ann Intern Med* 2000;132:880–884.

217. Mazue G, Bertolero MG, Jacob F, et al. Preclinical and clinical studies with recombinant human basic fibroblast growth factor. *Ann NY Acad Sci* 1991;638:329–340.

218. Cooper LT, Hirsch AT, Regensteines JG, et al. A double-blind, placebo-controlled, phase II study of basic fibroblast growth factor in the treatment of intermittent claudication. *Circulation* 2000;102:II-373(abst).

219. Lazarous DF, Shou M, Stiber JA, et al. Pharmacodynamics of basic fibroblast growth factor: route of administration determines myocardial and systemic distribution. *Cardiovasc Res* 1997;36:78–85.

220. Giordano FJ, Ping P, McKirnan D, et al. Intracoronary gene transfer of fibroblast growth factor-5 increases blood flow and contractile function in an ischemic region of the heart. *Nature Med* 1996;2:534–539.

221. Wolff JA, Ludtke JJ, Acsadi G, et al. Long-term persistence of plasmid DNA and foreign gene expression in mouse muscle. *Hum Mol Genet* 1992;1:363–369.

222. Takeshita S, Isshiki T, Sato T. Increased expression of direct gene transfer into skeletal muscles observed after acute ischemic injury in rats. *Lab Invest* 1996;74:1061–1065.

223. Laham RJ, Rezaee M, Garcia L, et al. Tissue and myocardial distribution of intracoronary, intravenous, intrapericardial and intramyocardial ^{125}I-labeled basic fibroblast growth factor (bFGF) favor intramyocardial delivery. *J Am Coll Cardiol* 2000;35:10A(abst).

224. Schaper W, Munoz-Chapuli R, Wolf C, Ito W. Collateral circulation of the heart. In: Ware JA, Simons M, eds. *Angiogenesis and cardiovascular disease.* New York: Oxford University Press, 1999:159–198.

225. Unger EF, Banai S, Shou M, et al. Basic fibroblast growth factor enhances myocardial collateral flow in a canine model. *Am J Physiol* 1994;266:H1588–H1595.

226. Lazarous DF, Scheinowtiz M, Shou M, et al. Effects of chronic systemic administration of basic fibroblast growth factor on collateral development in the canine heart. *Circulation* 1995;91:145–153.

227. Lazarous DF, Shou M, Scheinowitz M, et al. Comparative effects of basic fibroblast growth factor and vascular endothelial growth factor on coronary collateral development and arterial response to injury. *Circulation* 1996;94:1074–1082.

228. Rajanayagam MA, Shou M, Thirumurti V, et al. Intracoronary basic fibroblast growth factor enhances myocardial collateral perfusion in dogs. *J Am Coll Cardiol* 2000;35:519–526.

229. Shou M, Thirumurti V, Rajanayagam S, et al. Effect of basic fibroblast growth factor on myocardial angiogenesis in dogs with mature collateral vessels. *J Am Coll Cardiol* 1997;29:1102–1106.

230. Harada K, Grossman W, Friedman M, et al. Basic fibroblast growth factor improves myocardial function in chronically ischemic porcine hearts. *J Clin Invest* 1994;94:623–630.

231. Lopez JJ, Edelman ER, Stamler A, et al. Basic fibroblast growth factor in a porcine model of chronic myocardial ischemia: a comparison of angiographic, echocardio-

graphic and coronary flow parameters. *J Pharmacol Exp Ther* 1997;282:385–390.

232. Laham RJ, Rezaee M, Post M, et al. Intrapericardial delivery of fibroblast growth factor-2 induces neovascularization in a porcine model of chronic myocardial ischemia. *J Pharmacol Exp Ther* 2000;292:795–802.

233. Banai S, Jaklitsch MT, Casscells W, et al. Effects of acidic fibroblast growth factor on normal and ischemic myocardium. *Circ Res* 1991;69:76–85.

234. Unger EF, Shou M, Sheffield CD, et al. Extracardiac to coronary anastomoses support regional left ventricular function in dogs. *Am J Physiol* 1993;264:H1567–H1574.

235. Lopez JJ, Edelman ER, Stamler A, et al. Angiogenic potential of perivascularly delivered aFGF in a porcine model of chronic myocardial ischemia. *Am J Physiol* 1998;274:H930–H936.

236. Tabata H, Silver M, Isner JM. Arterial gene transfer of acidic fibroblast growth factor for therapeutic angiogenesis in vivo: critical role of secretion signal in use of naked DNA. *Cardiovasc Res* 1997;35:470–479.

237. Lopez JJ, Laham RJ, Stamler A, et al. VEGF administration in chronic myocardial ischemia in pigs. *Cardiovasc Res* 1998;40:272–281.

238. Harada K, Friedman M, Lopez JJ, et al. Vascular endothelial growth factor in chronic myocardial ischemia. *Am J Physiol* 1996;270:H1791–H1802.

239. Hughes CG, Biswas SS, Yin B, et al. Intramyocardial but not intravenous vascular endothelial growth factor improves regional perfusion in hibernating porcine myocardium. *Circulation* 1999;100:I-476(abst).

240. Banai S, Jaklitsch MT, Shou M, et al. Angiogenic-induced enhancement of collateral blood flow to ischemic myocardium by vascular endothelial growth factor in dogs. *Circulation* 1994;89:2183–2189.

241. Tio RA, Tkebuchava T, Scheuermann TH, et al. Intramyocardial gene therapy with naked DNA encoding vascular endothelial growth factor improves collateral flow to ischemic myocardium. *Hum Gene Ther* 1999;10:2953–2960.

242. Vale PR, Milliken CE, Tkebuchava T, et al. Catheter-based gene transfer of VEGF utilizing electromechanical LV mapping accomplishes therapeutic angiogenesis: pre-clinical studies in swine. *Circulation* 1999;100:I-512(abst).

243. Vale PR, Tkebuchava T, Milliken CE, et al. Percutaneous electromechanical mapping demonstrates efficacy of pVGI.1 (VEGF2) in an animal model of chronic myocardial ischemia. *Circulation* 1999;100:I-22(abst).

244. Mack CA, Patel SR, Schwarz EA, et al. Biologic bypass with the use of adenovirus-mediated gene transfer of the complementary deoxyribonucleic acid for vascular endothelial growth factor 121 improves myocardial perfusion and function in the ischemic porcine heart. *J Thorac Cardiovasc Surg* 1998;115:168–176.

245. Lee LY, Patel SR, Hackett NR, et al. Focal angiogen therapy using intramyocardial delivery of an adenovirus vector coding for vascular endothelial growth factor 121. *Ann Thorac Surg* 2000;69:14–24.

246. Lazarous DF, Shou M, Stiber JA, et al. Adenoviral-mediated gene transfer induces sustained pericardial VEGF expression in dogs: effect on myocardial angiogenesis. *Cardiovasc Res* 1999;44:294–302.

247. Schwartz ER, Speakman MT, Patterson M, et al. Evaluation of the effects of intramyocardial injection of DNA expressing vascular endothelial growth factor (VEGF) in a myocardial infarction model in the rat—angiogenesis and angioma formation. *J Am Coll Cardiol* 2000;35:1323–1330.

248. Lee RJ, Springer ML, Blanco-Bose WE, et al. VEGF gene delivery to myocardium: deleterious effects of unregulated expression. *Circulation* 2000;102:898–901.

249. Vale PR, Losordo DW, Tkebuchava T, et al. Catheter-based myocardial gene transfer utilizing nonfluoroscopic electromechanical left ventricular mapping. *J Am Coll Cardiol* 1999;34:246–254.

250. Deutsch E, Tarazona N, Sanborn TA, et al. Percutaneous endocardial gene therapy: patterns of in-vivo gene expression related to regional myocardial delivery. *J Am Coll Cardiol* 2000;35:6A(abst).

251. Kornowski R, Fuchs S, Vodovotz Y, et al. Catheter-based transendocardial injection of adenoviral VEGF$_{121}$ offers equivalent gene delivery and protein expression compared to a surgical-based transepicardial injection approach. *J Am Coll Cardiol* 2000;35:73A(abst).

252. Schainfeld RM, Isner JM. Critical limb ischemia: nothing to give at the office? *Ann Intern Med* 1999;130:442–444.

253. Isner JM. Arterial gene transfer for naked DNA for therapeutic angiogenesis: early clinical results. *Adv Drug Deliv Rev* 1998;30:185–197.

254. Isner JM, Baumgartner I, Rauh G, et al. Treatment of thromboangiitis obliterans (Buerger's disease) by intramuscular gene transfer of vascular endothelial growth factor: preliminary clinical results. *J Vasc Surg* 1998;28:964–975.

255. Losordo DW, Vale PR, Symes J, et al. Gene therapy for myocardial angiogenesis: initial clinical results with direct myocardial injection of phVEGF$_{165}$ as sole therapy for myocardial ischemia. *Circulation* 1998;98:2800–2804.

256. Ben-Haim SA, Osadchy D, Schuster I, et al. Nonfluoroscopic, in vivo navigation and mapping technology. *Nature Med* 1996;2:1393–1395.

257. Gepstein L, Goldin A, Lessick J, et al. Electromechanical characterization of chronic myocardial infarction in the canine coronary occlusion model. *Circulation* 1998;98:2055–2064.

258. Vale PR, Losordo DW, Milliken CE, et al. Left ventricular electromechanical mapping to assess efficacy of phVEGF$_{165}$ gene transfer for therapeutic angiogenesis in chronic myocardial ischemia. *Circulation* 2000;102:965–974.

259. Huggins GS, Pasternak RC, Alpert NM, et al. Effects of short-term treatment of hyperlipidemia on coronary vasodilator function and myocardial perfusion in regions having substantial impairment of baseline dilator reserve. *Circulation* 1998;98:1291–1296.

260. Pearlman JD, Hibberd MG, Chuang ML, et al. Magnetic resonance mapping demonstrates benefits of VEGF-induced myocardial angiogenesis. *Nature Med* 1995;1:1085–1089.

261. Pearlman JD, Laham RJ, Simons M. Coronary angiogenesis: detection in vivo with MR imaging sensitive to collateral neocirculation—preliminary study in pigs. *Radiology* 2000;214:801–807.

262. Takeshita S, Isshiki T, Tanaka E, et al. Use of synchrotron radiation microangiography to assess development of small collateral arteries in a rat model of hindlimb ischemia. *Circulation* 1997;95:805–808.

263. Schumacher B, Pecher P, von Specht BU, et al. Induction of neoangiogenesis in ischemic myocardium by human growth factors: first clinical results of a new treatment of coronary heart disease. *Circulation* 1998;97:645–650.

264. Schumacher B, Stegmann T, Pecher P. The stimulation of neoangiogenesis in the ischemic human heart by the growth factor FGF: first clinical results. *J Cardiovasc Surg* 1998;39:783–789.

265. Stegmann TJ, Hoppert T, Schlurmann W, et al. First angiogenic treatment of coronary heart disease by FGF-1: long-term results after 3 years. *Cardiac Vasc Regeneration* 2000;1:5–10.

266. Stegmann TJ, Hoppert T, Schneider A, et al. Induction of myocardial neoangiogenesis by human growth factors. A new therapeutic option in coronary heart disease. *Herz* 2000;25:589–599.

267. Laham RJ, Sellke FW, Edelman ER, et al. Local perivascular delivery of basic fibroblast growth factor in patients undergoing coronary bypass surgery: results of a phase 1 randomized, double-blind, placebo-controlled trial. *Circulation* 1999;100:1865–1871.

268. Laham RJ, Chronos NA, Leimbach M, et al. Results of a phase 1 open label dose escalation study of intracoronary and intravenous basic fibroblast growth factor (rFGF-2) in patients (pts) with severe ischemic heart disease: 6 months follow-up. *J Am Coll Cardiol* 2000;35:73A(abst).

269. Henry TD, Rocha-Sing K, Isner JM, et al. Intracoronary administration of recombinant human vascular endothelial growth factor (rhVEGF) to patients with coronary artery disease. *Am Heart J* 2001;142:872–880.

270. Laham RJ, Chronos NA, Pike M, et al. Intracoronary basic fibroblast growth factor (FGF-2) in patients with severe ischemic heart disease: results of a phase 1 open-label dose escalation study. *J Am Coll Cardiol* 2000;36:2132–2139.

271. Udelson JE, Dilsizian V, Laham RJ, et al. Therapeutic angiogenesis with recombinant fibroblast growth factor-2 improves stress and rest myocardial perfusion abnormalities in patients with severe symptomatic chronic coronary artery disease. *Circulation* 2000;102:1605–1610.

272. Henry TD, Abraham JA. Review of preclinical and clinical results with vascular endothelial growth factors for therapeutic angiogenesis. *Curr Interv Cardiol Rep* 2000;2:228–241.

273. Hendel RC, Henry TD, Rocha-Singh K, et al. Effect of intracoronary recombinant human vascular endothelial growth factor on myocardial perfusion: evidence for a dose-dependent effect. *Circulation* 2000;101:118–121.

274. Henry TD, Annex BH, Azrin MA, et al. Final results of the VIVA trial of rhVEGF for human therapeutic angiogenesis. *Circulation* 1999;100:I-476(abst).

275. Ferguson JJ. Meeting highlights: highlights of the 48th scientific sessions of the American College of Cardiology. *Circulation* 1999;100:570–575.

276. Henry TD, McKendall GR, Azrin MA, et al. VIVA trial. One year follow up. *Circulation* 2000;102:II-309(abst).

277. Kleiman NS, Califf RM. Results from late-breaking clinical trials sessions at ACCIS 2000 and ACC 2000. *J Am Coll Cardiol* 2000;36:310–311.

278. Symes JF, Losordo DW, Vale PR, et al. Gene therapy with vascular endothelial growth factor for inoperable coronary artery disease: preliminary clinical results. *Ann Thorac Surg* 1999;68:830–837.

279. Vale PR, Losordo DW, Dunnington C, et al. Direct myocardial injection of phVEGF165: results of complete patient cohort in phase 1/2 clinical trial. *Circulation* 1999;100:I-477(abst).

280. Esakof DD, Maysky M, Losordo DW, et al. Intraoperative multiplane transesophageal echocardiography for guiding direct myocardial gene transfer of vascular endothelial growth factor in patients with refractory angina pectoris. *Hum Gene Ther* 1999;10:2315–2323.

281. Shen Y-T, Vatner SF. Mechanism of impaired myocardial function during progressive coronary stenosis in conscious pigs: hibernation versus stunning? *Circ Res* 1995;76:479–488.

282. Wijns W, Vatner SF, Camici PG. Hibernating myocardium. *N Engl J Med* 1998;3:173–181.

283. Dilsizian V, Bonow RO. Current diagnostic techniques of assessing myocardial viability in patients with hibernating and stunned myocardium. *Circulation* 1993;87:1–20.

284. Rosengart TK, Lee LY, Patel SR, et al. Angiogenesis gene therapy: phase I assessment of direct intramyocardial administration of an adenovirus vector expression VEGF121 cDNA to individuals with clinically significant severe coronary artery disease. *Circulation* 1999;100:468–474.

285. Rosengart TK, Lee LY, Port JL, et al. Video assisted epicardial delivery of angiogenic gene therapy to the human myocardium utilizing an adenovirus vector encoding for VEGF121. *Circulation* 1999;100:I-770(abst).

286. Vale PR, Milliken CE, Fortuin FD, et al. Effective gene transfer of phVEGF-2 for therapeutic angiogenesis in chronic myocardial ischemia as assessed by NOGA™ left ventricular electromechanical mapping. *Circulation* 2000;102:II-689(abst).

287. Hendel RC, Vale PR, Losordo DW, et al. The effects of VEGF-2 gene therapy on rest and stress myocardial perfusion: results of serial SPECT imaging. *Circulation* 2000;102:II-769(abst).

288. Schofield PM, Sharples LD, Caine N, et al. Transmyocardial laser revascularisation in patients with refractory angina: a randomised controlled trial. *Lancet* 1999;353:519–524.

289. Burkhoff D, Schmidt S, Schulman SP, et al. Transmyocardial laser revascularisation compared with continued medical therapy for treatment of refractory angina pectoris: a prospective randomised trial. *Lancet* 1999;354:885–890.

290. Allen KB, Dowling RD, Fudge TL, et al. Comparison of transmyocardial revascularization with medical therapy in patients with refractory angina. *N Engl J Med* 1999;341:1029–1036.

291. Frazier OH, March RJ, Horvath KA, et al. Transmyocardial revascularization with a carbon dioxide laser in patients with end-stage coronary artery disease. *N Engl J Med* 1999;341:1021–1028.

292. Aaberge L, Nordstrand K, Dragsund M, et al. Transmyocardial revascularization with CO_2 laser in patients with refractory angina pectoris: clinical results from the Norwegian randomized trial. *J Am Coll Cardiol* 2000;35:1170–1177.

293. Horowitz JR, Rivard A, van der Zee R, et al. Vascular endothelial growth factor/vascular permeability factor produces nitric oxide–dependent hypotension. *Arterioscler Thromb Vasc Biol* 1997;17:2793–2800.

294. Thurston G, Suri C, Smith K, et al. Leakage-resistant blood vessels in mice transgenically overexpressing angiopoietin-1. *Science* 1999;286:2511–2514.

295. Springer ML, Chen AS, Kraft PE, et al. VEGF gene delivery to muscle: potential role of vasculogenesis in adults. *Mol Cell* 1998;2:549–558.

296. Aiello LP, Avery RL, Arrigg PG, et al. Vascular endothelial growth factor in ocular fluids of patients with diabetic retinopathy and other retinal disorders. *N Engl J Med* 1994;331:1480–1487.

297. Vale PR, Rauh G, Wuensch DI, et al. Influence of vascular endothelial growth factor on diabetic retinopathy. *Circulation* 1998;17:I-353(abst).

298. Van Belle E, Tio FO, Couffinhal T, et al. Stent endothelialization: time course, impact of local catheter delivery, feasibility of recombinant protein administration, and response to cytokine expedition. *Circulation* 1997;95:438–448.

299. Van Belle E, Tio FO, Chen D, et al. Passivation of metallic stents following arterial gene transfer of phVEGF$_{165}$ inhibits thrombus formation and intimal thickening. *J Am Coll Cardiol* 1997;29:1371–1379.

300. Asahara T, Chen D, Tsurumi Y, et al. Accelerated restitution of endothelial integrity and endothelium-dependent function following phVEGF$_{165}$ gene transfer. *Circulation* 1996;94:3291–3302.

301. Vale PR, Wuensch DI, Rauh GF, et al. Arterial gene therapy for inhibiting restenosis in patients with claudication undergoing superficial femoral artery angioplasty. *Circulation* 1998;98:I-66(abst).

302. Laitinen M, Hartikainen J, Hiltunen MO, et al. Catheter-mediated vascular endothelial growth factor gene transfer to human coronary arteries after angioplasty. *Hum Gene Ther* 2000;11:263–270.

303. Mirhoseini M, Muckerheide M, Cayton MM. Transventricular revascularization by lasers. *Lasers Surg Med* 1982;2:187–198.

304. Yamamoto N, Kohmoto T, Gu A, et al. Angiogenesis is enhanced in ischemic canine myocardium by transmyocardial laser revascularization. *J Am Coll Cardiol* 1998;31:1426–1433.

305. Mack CA, Patel SR, Rosengart TK. Myocardial angiogenesis as a possible mechanism for TMLR efficacy. *J Clin Laser Med Surg* 1997;15:275–279.

306. Hughes GC, Lowe JE, Kypson AP, et al. Neovascularization after transmyocardial laser revascularization in a model of chronic ischemia. *Ann Thorac Surg* 1998;66:2029–2036.

307. Burkhoff D, Fisher PE, Apfelbaum M, et al. Histologic appearance of transmyocardial laser channels after 4 1/2 weeks. *Ann Thorac Surg* 1996;61:1532–1534.

308. Fisher PE, Khomoto T, DeRosa CM, et al. Histologic analysis of transmyocardial channels: comparison of CO$_2$ and holmium:YAG lasers. *Ann Thorac Surg* 1997;64:466–472.

309. Whittaker P, Kloner RA, Przyklenk K. Laser-mediated transmural myocardial channels do not salvage acutely ischemic myocardium. *J Am Coll Cardiol* 1993;22:302–309.

310. Isner JM. Pathology. In: Isner JM, Clarke RH, eds. *Cardiovascular laser therapy.* New York: Raven Press, 1989:63.

311. Malekan R, Reynolds C, Narula N, et al. Angiogenesis in transmyocardial laser revascularization: a nonspecific response to injury. *Circulation* 1998;98:II-62–II-66.

312. Rimoldi O, Burns SM, Rosen SD, et al. Measurement of myocardial blood flow with positron emission tomography before and after transmyocardial laser revascularization. *Circulation* 1999;100:II-134–II-138.

313. Al-Sheikh T, Allen KB, Straka SP, et al. Cardiac sympathetic denervation after transmyocardial laser revascularization. *Circulation* 1999;100:135–140.

314. Hughes GC, Landolfo KP, Lowe JE, et al. Diagnosis, incidence, and clinical significance of early postoperative ischemia after transmyocardial laser revascularization. *Am Heart J* 1999;137:1163–1168.

315. Kwong KF, Kanellopoulos GK, Nickols JC, et al. Transmyocardial laser treatment denervates canine myocardium. *J Thorac Cardiovasc Surg* 1997;114:883–890.

316. Kwong KF, Schuessler RB, Kanellopoulos GK, et al. Nontransmural laser treatment incompletely denervates canine myocardium. *Circulation* 1998;98:II-67–II-72.

317. Lauer B, Junghans U, Stahl F, et al. Catheter-based percutaneous myocardial laser revascularization in patients with end-stage coronary artery disease. *J Am Coll Cardiol* 1999;34:1663–1670.

318. Leon MB, Baim DS, Moses JW, et al. A randomized blinded clinical trial comparing percutaneous laser myocardial revascularization (using Biosense LV mapping) vs placebo in patients with refractory coronary ischemia. *Circulation* 2000;102:II-565(abst).

319. Lemarchand P, Jones M, Yamada I, et al. In vivo gene transfer and expression in normal uninjured blood vessels using replication-deficient recombinant adenovirus vectors. *Circ Res* 1993;72:1132–1138.

320. Asahara T, Chen D, Takahashi T, et al. Tie2 receptor ligands, angiopoietin-1 and angiopoietin-2 modulate VEGF-induced postnatal neovascularization. *Circ Res* 1998;83:233–240.

321. Van Belle E, Rivard A, Chen D, et al. Hypercholesterolemia attenuates angiogenesis but does not preclude augmentation by angiogenic cytokines. *Circulation* 1997;96:2667–2674.

322. Luscher TF, Noll G. Endothelium dysfunction in the coronary circulation. *J Cardiovasc Pharmacol* 1994;24:16S–26S.

323. Sellke FW, Laham RJ, Edelman ER, et al. Therapeutic angiogenesis with basic fibroblast growth factor: technique and early results. *Ann Thorac Surg* 1998;65:1540–1544.

324. Inoue M, Itoh H, Ueda M, et al. Vascular endothelial growth factor (VEGF) expression in human coronary atherosclerotic lesions. *Circulation* 1998;98:2108–2116.

325. Luo Z, Asahara T, Tsurumi Y, et al. Reduction of vein graft intimal hyperplasia and preservation of endothelium-dependent relaxation by topical vascular endothelial growth factor. *J Vasc Surg* 1998;27:167–173.

326. Henry TD, Annex BH, Azrin MA, et al. Double blind, placebo controlled trial of recombinant human vascular endothelial growth factor—the VIVA trial. *J Am Coll Cardiol* 1999;33:384A(abst).

327. Hiltunen MO, Laitinen M, Turunen MP, et al. Intravascular adenovirus-mediated VEGF-C gene transfer reduces neointima formation in balloon-denuded rabbit aorta. *Circulation* 2000;102:2262–2268.

328. Celletti FL, Waugh JM, Amabile PG, et al. Vascular endothelial growth factor enhances atherosclerotic plaque progression. *Nature Med* 2001;7:425–429.

DISEASES OF THE AORTA

PETER C. SPITTELL

▼▼ ADDITIONAL ELECTRONIC TOPICS
Aortic Dissection: Pathogenesis q41;   Aortic Dissection: Predisposing Factors q42;   Aortitis: Pathogenesis q43

OVERVIEW

Increased awareness of the clinical features of acquired diseases of the thoracic and abdominal aorta and familiarity with currently available diagnostic techniques are basic to their effective treatment. Acute dissection of the thoracic aorta, one of the most common fatal aortic conditions that is encountered clinically, is commonly misdiagnosed and has a markedly increased mortality during the first 48 hours after the onset of symptoms. Aortic dissection should always be included in the differential diagnosis of a patient with unexplained syncope, stroke, congestive heart failure, acute arterial occlusion, or an abnormal aortic contour on chest radiography, even in the absence of chest pain. In suspected acute aortic dissection, institution of beta-adrenergic blockade followed by rapid diagnosis with transesophageal echocardiography (TEE) is indicated. If ascending aortic dissection is present, emergent surgical therapy is indicated. Indications for surgical resection of a thoracic aortic aneurysm include symptomatic aneurysm and an aneurysm diameter of 6 cm or greater (>5.0 cm in diameter in patients with Marfan syndrome). Unless there are contraindications, elective surgical resection of thoracic aortic aneurysm that results from trauma, even when asymptomatic, is indicated

P. C. Spittell: Department of Medicine, Mayo Medical School; and Department of Internal Medicine, Division of Cardiovascular Disease, Mayo Medical Center, Rochester, Minnesota

TABLE 108.1 AORTIC DISEASE: ETIOLOGY

Aging
Atherosclerosis
Hypertension
Infection
Inflammatory disorders
Degenerative changes
Trauma
Neoplasia

because of the unpredictability of these aneurysms and the low risk of elective surgical repair. Surgical repair of an abdominal aortic aneurysm (AAA) is indicated when aneurysm diameter reaches 5 cm. In good-risk patients, selective repair of an AAA is indicated when the diameter reaches 4.5 cm. Surgical resection is the treatment of choice in patients with an inflammatory AAA, regardless of diameter. All patients with Marfan syndrome should be placed on a beta-adrenergic blocking agent if no contraindications exist. When an uncommon type of aortic disease is suspected (i.e., Takayasu's disease or giant-cell aortitis), invasive diagnosis should be pursued (angiography and/or arterial biopsy).

INTRODUCTION

Acquired diseases of the thoracic and abdominal aorta are encountered frequently in cardiologic practice. Their clinical presentation is highly variable, ranging from occult disease to classic clinical presentations. Numerous etiologic factors, acting singly and in combination, have been identified (Table 108.1). Diagnosis is possible by noninvasive means in most patients, but some types of aortic diseases require a high index of suspicion and invasive angiographic study or arterial biopsy. Awareness of the clinical features of acquired diseases of the thoracic and abdominal aorta and familiarity with currently available diagnostic techniques are basic to their effective treatment.

AORTIC DISSECTION

Acute dissection of the thoracic aorta is one of the most common catastrophic aortic conditions that is encountered in clinical practice. Its incidence has been reported to be approximately 2.9 in 100,000 per year (1). The variable manifestations of aortic dissection, in combination with a mortality in untreated cases of as high as 1% per hour during the first 48 hours after the onset of symptoms, underscore the importance of a high index of suspicion and prompt diagnosis and therapy (2–4). Noninvasive testing [TEE, computed tomography (CT), or magnetic resonance imaging (MRI)] allows an accurate diagnosis to be made in the majority of patients (5). Effective treatment

exists, so that future improvements in initial and long-term survival in acute aortic dissection depend on increased clinical awareness, rapid noninvasive diagnosis, and the early institution of appropriate medical or surgical therapy, or both.

Classification

The most widely used classification system for acute aortic dissection is that of DeBakey and associates (29), which recognizes three types of dissections (Fig. 108.1). Type I dissection arises in the ascending aorta and extends distally, type II dissection is limited to the ascending aorta, and type III dissection arises at or just distal to the origin of the left subclavian artery and extends distally or, rarely, retrogradely into the arch of the ascending aorta. ❦ q44

Clinical Features

Due to variable involvement of the aorta and its branches by the dissecting process, the patient with acute aortic dissection may have clinical manifestations of ischemia of various organ systems, singly or in combination, as well as symptoms and signs of cardiac disease. The diverse presentations of aortic dissection can provide for difficult diagnosis, and misdiagnosis commonly occurs (2,11). Despite major advances in the noninvasive diagnosis of aortic dissection and in medical and surgical therapy, up to 55% of patients in reported series die without a correct antemortem diagnosis (1,2,11,32,33). Therefore, a high index of clinical suspicion in any likely setting is imperative.

The classic presentation of a patient with acute aortic dissection, occurring in up to 94% of patients, is the sudden onset of severe pain, usually beginning in the anterior chest, radiating to the back, and moving distally as the dissection progresses (1,30). The pain is most commonly described as sudden in onset with a "ripping," "tearing," or "stabbing" quality; this is in contrast to the crescendo nature of the discomfort of acute myocardial infarction. ❦ q45

A cardiac murmur may be present, usually at the cardiac base, and may be systolic, diastolic, or both. A diastolic murmur of aortic regurgitation indicates involvement of the ascending aorta and is heard in up to 50% of patients with type I aortic dissection. Congestive heart failure, when present in association with proximal aortic dissection, is most often due to severe aortic regurgitation (9,30), but cases of congestive heart failure due to rupture of the dissecting process into the right or left atrium or right ventricle have also been reported (34–36). Myocardial infarction occurs in 1% to 2% of patients and is due to compromise of the coronary ostium by the hematoma or intimal flap. Peripheral pulse deficits are noted in approximately 40% of patients (3,30), more commonly with proximal aortic dissection. Pulse deficits may be transitory due to oscillation of the intimal flap or distal

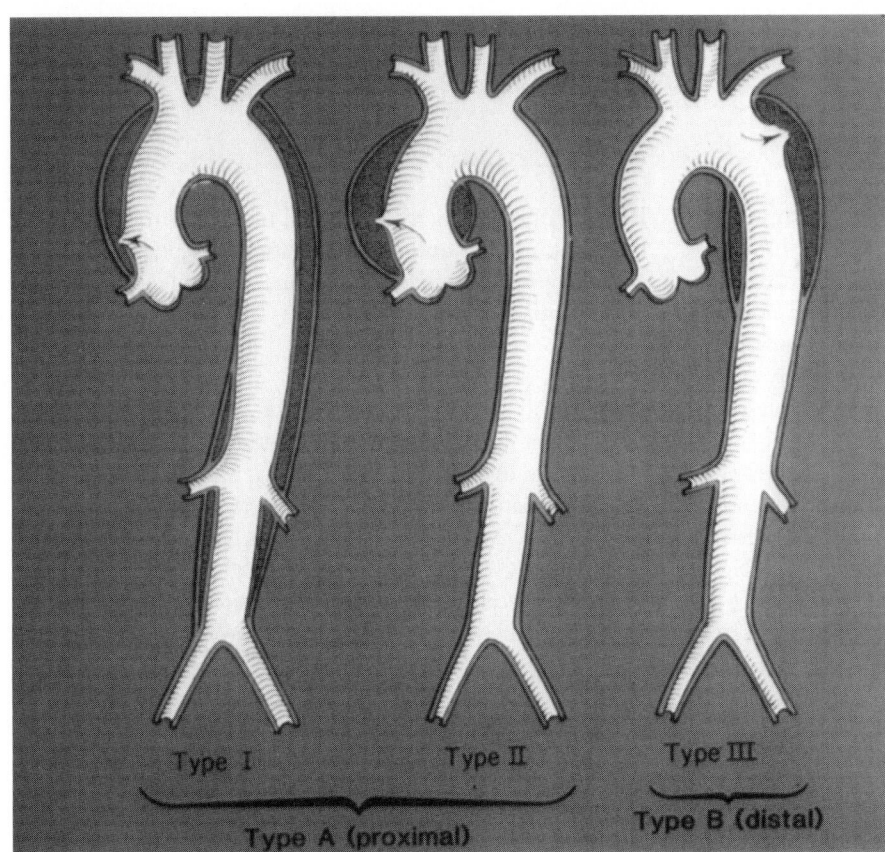

FIGURE 108.1 Classification of aortic dissection. Type I: primary tear in ascending aorta and dissection involving aortic arch and distal aorta for a variable distance. Type II: dissection involving only ascending aorta. Type III: primary tear distal to subclavian artery origin, extending distally for a variable distance. (Modified from DeBakey ME, Henly WS, Cooley DA, et al. Surgical management of dissecting aneurysms of the aorta. *J Thorac Cardiovasc Surg* 1965;49:130–149.)

reentry of the hematoma into the true lumen. Acute lower-extremity ischemia, with or without chest pain, as a result of dissection extending into the iliac arteries occurs in 6% to 12% of patients (3,37,38) and may provide an important clue to the diagnosis (37). Other cardiovascular findings include a difference in blood pressure between the arms, tachycardia, friction rubs, bruits, pulsus paradoxus, and cardiac tamponade.

Syncope in a patient with aortic dissection is an important event, as it usually results from rupture of the dissecting process into the pericardial space producing cardiac tamponade (11,30). Less commonly, rupture occurs into the left pleural space producing left hemothorax (11). Neurologic deficits, including cerebrovascular accident, disturbances of consciousness, ischemic paraparesis, and ischemic peripheral neuropathy, occur in more than 40% of patients, more commonly with proximal aortic dissection (1,39). Other, less-frequent findings include Horner's syndrome, a pulsatile sternoclavicular joint (40), vocal cord paralysis, hemoptysis (41), superior vena cava syndrome (42), upper airway obstruction (43), hematemesis (44), pleural effusion, unilateral pulmonary edema (45), signs of mesenteric or renal infarction, fever (46), and deep venous thrombosis (11).

As a general rule, aortic dissection should always be considered in the differential diagnosis of a patient with unexplained syncope, stroke, congestive heart failure, acute arterial occlusion, or an abnormal aortic contour on chest radiography, even in the absence of chest pain.

Diagnosis

MRI is an excellent noninvasive method for diagnosing aortic dissection [▼ q46] (63) (*e*Fig. 108.1.3). It is superior to TEE and CT in detecting arch vessel involvement and in identifying the anastomosis in patients who are managed with surgical therapy, and it may facilitate comparison of serial studies (5,59,64). Gated spin-echo MRI accurately demonstrates the entry site and intimal flap (65) and may be the optimal method for demonstrating thrombus formation and entry site location within all segments of the aorta (66). The ability to obtain oblique and longitudinal planes of section makes MRI especially valuable in demonstrating dissection without intimal tear (5,60,67). Disadvantages of MRI include cost, examination time, reduced availability, and standard contraindications to MRI. The most important limitation of MRI in acute aortic dissection is its nonportability, limiting its use in hemodynamically unstable patients.

Aortography, the traditional definitive diagnostic method in aortic dissection, is able to localize the site of origin of the dissection and delineate the extent of the dissection, as well as the circulation to vital organs. Diagnostic aortographic features include opacification of the false lumen, deformity of the true lumen by the false lumen, widening of the aorta, narrowing or occlusion of branches of the aorta, and the presence of an intimal flap (68). Disadvantages of aortography include nonportability, invasive technique, exposure to ionizing radiation, the use of i.v. contrast agents, and an inherent delay in diagnosis. False-negative aortogram results can occur if there is simultaneous and equal opacification of the true and false lumina or if the false channel is very faintly opacified (69). Intravascular ultrasound, in combination with standard aortographic technique, greatly improves the accuracy of aortography, can be performed rapidly and safely, and could serve as an accessory diagnostic procedure in selected patients with suspected aortic dissection (70,71).

In view of the increased early mortality of untreated acute aortic dissection, the screening test chosen depends on which test is most readily available at a particular institution and the patient's hemodynamic status (*e*Fig. 108.1.4). Noninvasive diagnosis of acute dissection by TEE, MRI, or CT, if readily available, is preferred, as it avoids the risks and delays that are inherent in invasive angiography (72).

Management

The initial treatment objectives in suspected aortic dissection are to control pain, reduce systemic blood pressure, and lower dP/dT to the lowest level that is compatible with maintenance of adequate visceral, renal, and cerebral perfusion (73). In hypertensive patients, treatment consists of an i.v. beta-adrenergic blocking agent, most commonly propranolol, in combination with i.v. sodium nitroprusside (*e*Table 108.1.2). ◥ q47

PENETRATING AORTIC ULCER

Penetrating aortic ulcer shares several clinical features with aortic dissection, especially type III aortic dissection, but the absence of certain clinical signs favors a diagnosis of penetrating aortic ulcer. Results of noninvasive imaging studies are usually distinctive, allowing differentiation of penetrating aortic ulcer from typical aortic dissection (96,97). Differentiation between the two disorders is important in view of the fact that the natural history of penetrating aortic ulcer is less well defined; therefore, treatment may differ from that currently used for classic aortic dissection (96,97).

Pathogenesis

Penetrating aortic ulcer refers to an atherosclerotic lesion of the thoracic aorta that undergoes ulceration that penetrates the internal elastic lamina of the thoracic aorta, resulting in formation of one of the following: intramural hematoma

within the media of the aortic wall, a true saccular aneurysm, a pseudoaneurysm, or transmural aortic rupture (98) (Fig. 108.2). ◥ q48

Risk Factors

Risk factors for penetrating aortic ulcer are similar to those for aortic dissection, the most common being advanced age, chronic systemic hypertension, and evidence of atherosclerotic disease (105). ◥ q49

Clinical Features

The clinical presentations of penetrating aortic ulcer and acute aortic dissection are similar, the most common being an elderly patient with systemic hypertension and the acute onset of severe pain in the chest, back, and, less commonly, epigastrium. Unlike aortic dissection, the pain is rarely migratory. Because the most common site of penetrating aortic ulcer is in the descending thoracic aorta, a murmur of aortic regurgitation, pericardial friction rub, and peripheral pulse deficits are not seen. In addition, visceral vessel involvement has not been reported. Neurologic deficits are very rare, but acute lower-extremity paraplegia has been reported (98). In a patient with a history that is compatible with aortic dissection, the *absence* of physical findings suggests the diagnosis of penetrating aortic ulcer. Asymptomatic penetrating aortic ulcer does occur and is usually incidentally discovered as enlargement of the descending thoracic aorta or a hilar mass on routine chest radiography (98,101).

Laboratory Findings

Routine laboratory studies are nonspecific with penetrating aortic ulcer. The chest radiograph is the most helpful of the routine laboratory tests because it is often abnormal. It may demonstrate mediastinal widening, focal or diffuse enlargement of the descending thoracic aorta, a hilar mass, left apical mass, bilateral pleural effusion, or isolated left pleural effusion (96,97). However, normal chest radiographic findings do not exclude penetrating aortic ulcer. The most common electrocardiographic abnormality is left ventricular hypertrophy from chronic systemic hypertension.

The findings on CT, MRI, TEE, and aortography in patients with penetrating aortic ulcer are characteristic, allowing differentiation of penetrating aortic ulcer from classic aortic dissection (*e*Fig. 108.2.1).

Management

Treatment is individualized, as the natural history of penetrating aortic ulcer and indications for surgery are not well defined. The natural history of an intramural hematoma has been shown by serial noninvasive imaging studies to follow a course of resorption of the hematoma and aortic

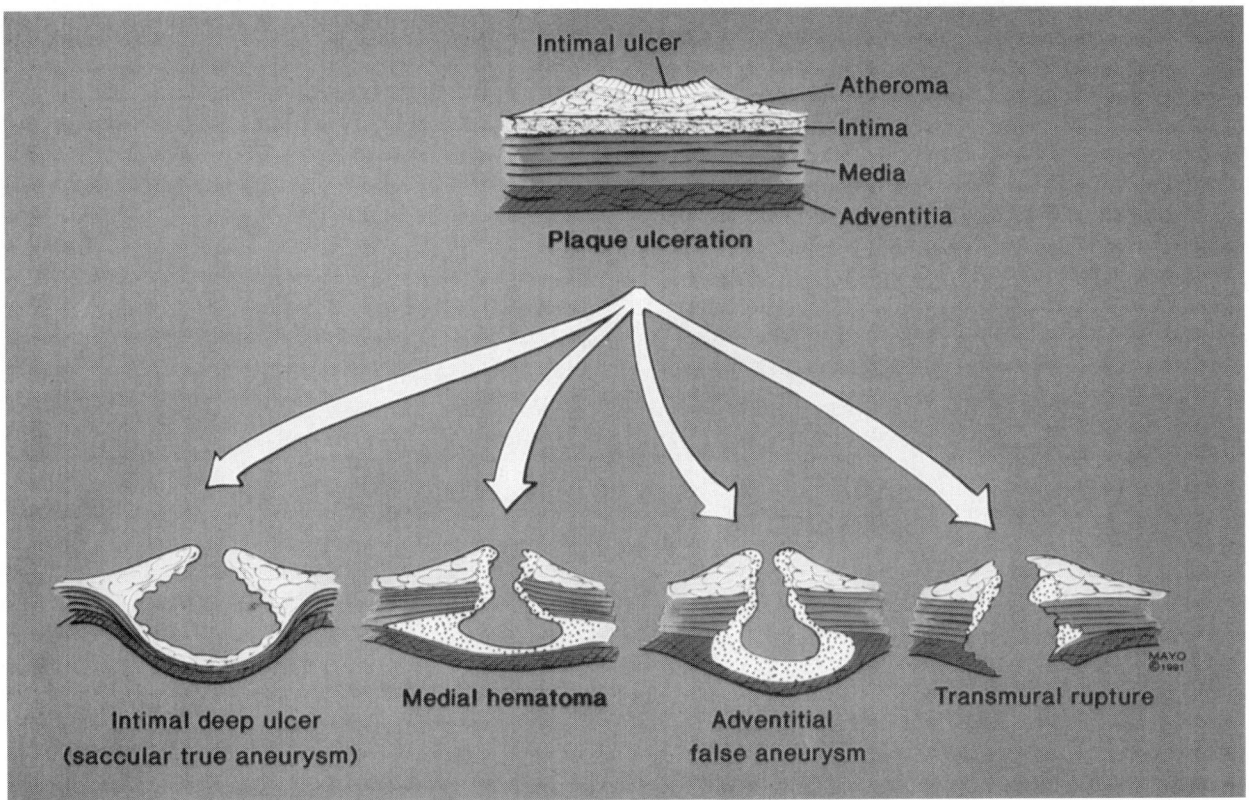

FIGURE 108.2 Pathologic consequences of penetrating atherosclerotic ulcer of the aorta. Atheromatous ulceration that burrows deeply into an atheroma can result in one of four potential outcomes (*from left to right*): a true saccular aneurysm, a medial hematoma, an adventitial false aneurysm, or transmural rupture. An intramural (medial) hematoma is the most commonly observed fate of a penetrating aortic ulcer.

dilation in the region of the involved aorta (97,98). Patients with an intramural hematoma should be treated medically, with special emphasis placed on control of blood pressure, preferably with a beta-adrenergic blocking agent. Ascending aortic involvement, progressive aortic dilation, persistent symptoms, or difficult-to-control hypertension is an indication for surgery. When saccular aneurysm or pseudoaneurysm is the result of a penetrating atherosclerotic ulcer of the aorta, surgery is recommended.

ANEURYSMAL DISEASE

An aneurysm can be defined as a permanent localized dilation of an artery. Because atherosclerosis is the most common cause of arterial aneurysm, aneurysmal disease and its complications are frequent clinical problems. Once initiated, an aneurysm tends to enlarge progressively. Although most aneurysms enlarge in an occult fashion, pressure of the aneurysm on surrounding structures or eventual rupture may occur. Furthermore, nonlaminar flow within the aneurysm leads to the formation of laminated thrombus, which may lead to distal embolization. Despite advances in noninvasive imaging and surgical techniques, the diverse

presentations of aortic aneurysm can challenge the best of clinicians at times, making the aphorism of Sir William Osler, "There is no disease more conducive to clinical humility than aneurysm of the aorta," (106) appropriate even today.

Thoracic Aortic Aneurysm

Atherosclerosis is the most common cause of aneurysmal disease of the aorta; thus, aneurysms are more common in men than in women (5:1) and are rare in patients who are younger than 50 years of age. Less common causes include congenital defects of the arterial wall, hypertension, tobacco use, familial tendency, inherited disorders of connective tissue, infections, arteritis, sudden deceleration, entrapment, and trauma. q50

Most aneurysms of the thoracic aorta are asymptomatic, being incidentally discovered on chest radiography (115,116). When symptoms develop, the aneurysm is usually large enough to encroach on surrounding structures and cause chest pain, back pain, dyspnea, dysphagia, cough, hoarseness, or stridor. When there is venous compression (*e*Fig. 108.2.2), compression of other structures (e.g., fixation of a vocal cord), or encroachment on the chest wall, corresponding findings may be noted. The symptoms and signs of congestive heart failure may predominate when there is significant aortic regurgitation. Atheroembolism is not an infrequent clinical presentation of aortic aneurysm. As a result of slowing of flow in the peripheral portions of the aneurysm, laminated mural thrombus develops and may subsequently embolize to the distal arterial circulation (68).

On a plain radiograph, an aneurysm appears as a rounded or smooth density in the central portion of the chest if it is not obscured by other structures (Fig. 108.3). Unless there is calcification in its wall, the aneurysm may be difficult to differentiate from intrathoracic tumor in the central chest or from simple elongation and torsion of the aorta. Aortography has been the classic method to diagnose thoracic aortic aneurysm, but CT, particularly with i.v. contrast enhancement; MRI; and combined TTE and TEE have become the noninvasive diagnostic tests of choice (117–121).

The prognosis of untreated thoracic aortic aneurysm is poor, with 3-year survival rates as low as 25% (122). Factors that seem to worsen the prognosis are female gender, diastolic hypertension, size greater than 6 cm, traumatic aneurysm, and associated coronary and cerebrovascular disease. The cumulative risk of rupture is 20% after 5 years (123). The 5-year risk of rupture as a function of aneurysm size at recognition is 0% for aneurysms less than 4 cm in diameter, 16% for those 4.0 to 5.9 cm, and 31% for aneurysms of 6 cm or more (123). Because of the poor prognosis for the untreated patient with a thoracic aortic aneurysm, surgical treatment is justified unless comorbid medical conditions contraindicate an operation. Based on previous natural history studies (115,116,123), the following seem to be reasonable indications for surgical treatment: (a) an aneurysm that is symptomatic, (b) an aneurysm with a diameter of 6 cm or greater, (c) an aneurysm that enlarges under observation, and (d) an aneurysm in a person with poorly controlled systemic hypertension.

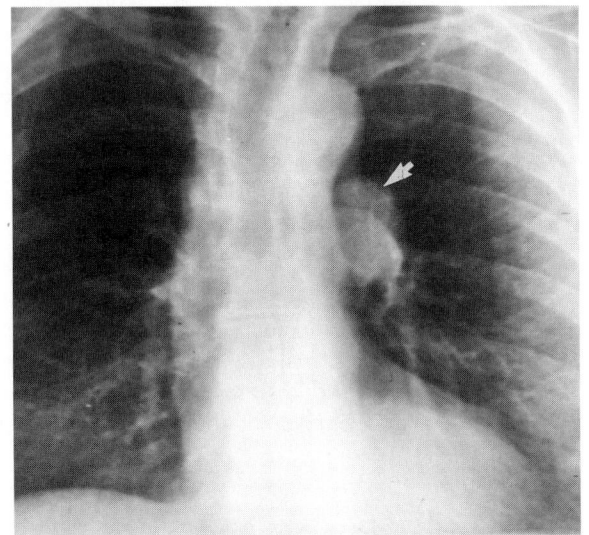

A

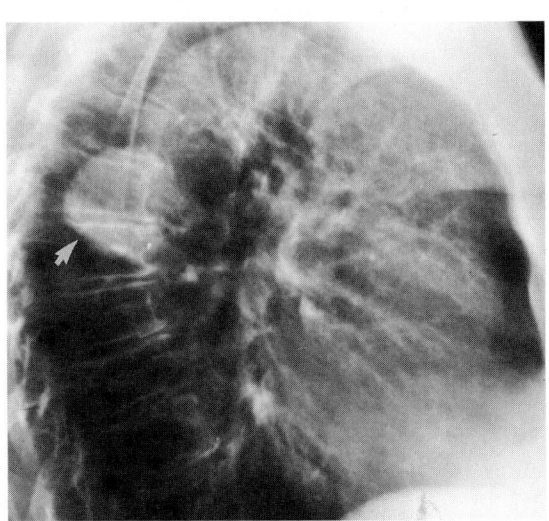

B

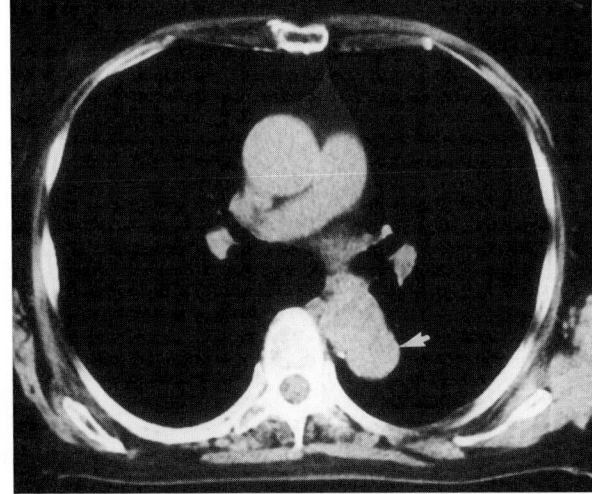

C

FIGURE 108.3 A: Posteroanterior chest radiograph demonstrates a left hilar mass (*arrow*). **B:** Lateral view demonstrates a mass adjacent to the proximal descending thoracic aorta (*arrow*). **C:** Computed tomographic scan demonstrates the mass to be a saccular aneurysm (*arrow*) of the proximal descending thoracic aorta.

Unless there are contraindications, elective surgical resection of thoracic aortic aneurysms that result from trauma, even when asymptomatic, is indicated because of the inability to predict rupture (124,125). Prophylactic surgical treatment of aortic root dilation greater than 5.0 cm in diameter in the person with Marfan syndrome is advisable to prevent the complications of aortic dissection and rupture (126,127). ▼ q51

Abdominal Aortic Aneurysm

Approximately three-fourths of all atherosclerotic aneurysms involve the abdominal aorta. Men are affected more frequently than women (9:1), and the majority of patients are older than 50 years. Hypertension often coexists and further contributes to aneurysm formation (7). Current smoking also increases the risk of aneurysm rupture and reduces long-term survival (131). A familial tendency for development of AAA is well established, with sex-linked and autosomal patterns of inheritance involved (132,133). ▼ q52

A less common cause of AAA that frequently goes unrecognized is trauma, usually blunt (i.e., seat belt injury), which can result in the formation of true aneurysm and pseudoaneurysm of the abdominal aorta in persons of any age.

The majority of patients with AAA are asymptomatic, emphasizing the importance of increased clinical awareness for the condition, especially when risk factors for aneurysmal disease are present. The most frequent and important physical finding in AAA is the presence of a pulsatile abdominal mass. The sensitivity of abdominal palpation for the detection of AAA is 43% overall (57% for aneurysms >4.0 cm in diameter, 29% for aneurysms <4.0 cm in diameter) (135). ▼ q53

When an AAA is symptomatic without rupture, the most common complaint is abdominal pain, intermittent or constant, over the preceding days or weeks. Recent-onset low back pain can occur and may be due to dissection within the aneurysm or retroperitoneal hematoma. Abdominal pain that radiates to the flank, groin, or testes may be a dominant or associated complaint. If atheroembolism from AAA has occurred, painful blue toes, livedo reticularis, hypertension, and renal insufficiency develop (*e*Fig. 108.3.1). Less commonly, intermittent claudication from embolization of the muscular branches of the lower extremity arteries can occur.

The most frequent complication of AAA is rupture, which occurs most often when aortic diameter exceeds 5 cm (140). Rupture of an AAA is characterized by the triad of severe pain, hypotension, and a tender abdominal mass. The pain is acute in onset, constant, and severe, most commonly located in the lumbar area or diffusely throughout the abdomen with radiation into the flanks, genitals, or legs. The abdominal aorta is usually tender to palpation, and there may be peritoneal signs if free rupture into the peritoneal cavity has occurred. Findings suggestive of a ruptured AAA or contained rupture represent a true surgical emergency, and prompt diagnosis and surgical therapy are crucial to improve survival. ▼ q54

AAA can be accurately diagnosed with ultrasonography, CT, or MRI and magnetic resonance angiography (MRA) (Fig. 108.4). Angiography is not needed to diagnose AAA, but it is useful when a juxtarenal aneurysm is suspected or when delineation of associated peripheral, renal, or visceral arterial occlusive disease is indicated before surgical repair.

Natural history studies of AAAs demonstrate an increase in risk of rupture when aneurysm diameter exceeds 5 cm (140,146). Elective resection and graft replacement have a surgical mortality of less than 5%, but emergent surgical treatment after the aneurysm has ruptured has a much higher mortality (145).

In the poor-risk patient with an aneurysm of less than 5 cm in diameter, observation of the aneurysm with serial ultrasound examinations every 3 to 6 months is appropriate. Some evidence has been found that long-term beta-adrenergic blockade may decrease the rate of expansion of AAA (147).

Endovascular repair of AAA, first reported in 1991 (148), is being used with increasing success (149–151). Advances in technology over the past 10 years and more well-defined indications have established endovascular repair of AAA as a safe and effective procedure in selected patients (151–153). With second-generation devices, the procedure is initially successful in greater than 95% of patients, with 2-year success rates that are comparable to those of standard surgical repair (151,152). ▼ q55

OCCLUSIVE DISEASE

Etiology

Occlusive disease of the aorta is most commonly due to advanced atherosclerosis. Additional causes include giant-cell arteritis and Takayasu's disease. Rarely, primary intimal sarcoma of the aorta can cause occlusive or embolic symptoms, or both (*e*Fig. 108.4.1).

Atherosclerosis

Atherosclerosis in the thoracic aorta usually involves the origin of the brachiocephalic arteries, principally the left subclavian and occasionally the innominate artery. Although atherosclerotic disease of the aortic arch branches is usually asymptomatic, stenosis of the origin of the left or right subclavian artery may cause intermittent claudication of the arm of sufficient degree to warrant surgical treatment. With complete occlusion of the origin of either subclavian artery, collateral blood flow to the arm may be derived principally from the cerebral circulation via

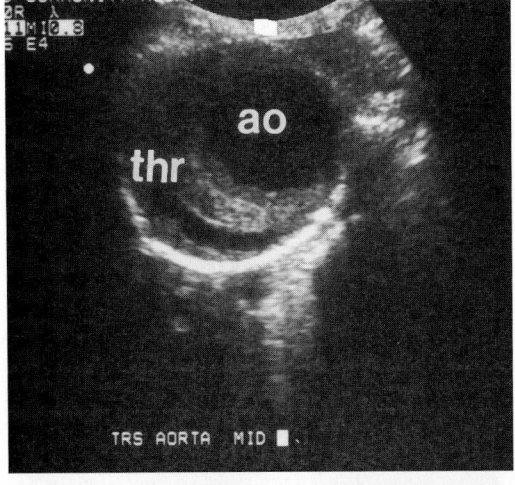

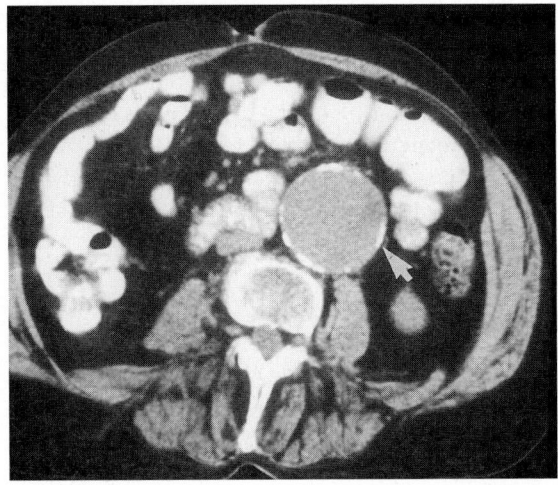

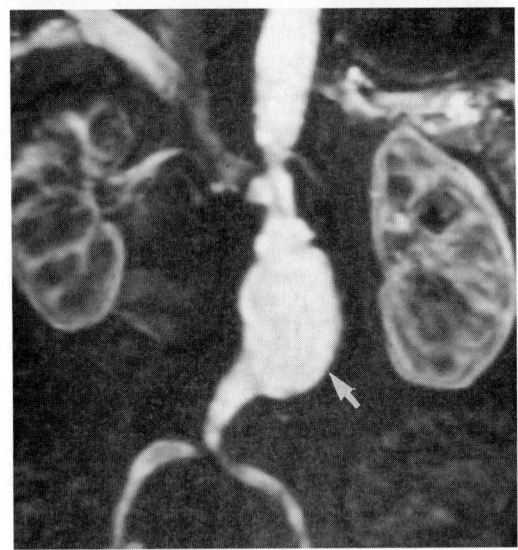

FIGURE 108.4 Noninvasive imaging in the diagnosis of abdominal aortic aneurysm. **A:** Ultrasound examination demonstrates large abdominal aortic aneurysm with large amount of laminated thrombus (thr). ao, aortic lumen. **B:** Computed tomographic study demonstrates large abdominal aortic aneurysm with calcification of the aortic wall (*arrow*). **C:** Magnetic resonance angiography demonstrates infrarenal abdominal aortic aneurysm (*arrow*).

reversed flow through the ipsilateral vertebral artery, so-called subclavian steal. This results in episodes of transient cerebral ischemia, especially when the ipsilateral arm is exercised. ⚓ q56

Acquired coarctation of the thoracic aorta due to focally obstructive calcific atherosclerotic disease is rare but has been reported (156). Symptomatic patients present with upper extremity hypertension and reduced blood pressure in the lower extremities, with or without intermittent claudication.

Micro- or macroemboli from atherosclerotic plaque and thrombus in the thoracic aorta are important causes of stroke and peripheral embolization. Aortic atheromas occur with a prevalence of approximately 27% in patients with previous embolic events, and aortic atheromas are also strong predictors of coronary artery disease (157,158). Assessment of thoracic aortic atherosclerotic plaque is most accurately obtained with TEE. Plaque thickness of greater than 4 mm and mobile thrombus (of any size) are associated with an increased risk of embolism (158). Embolism can occur spontaneously, in relation to invasive angiographic procedures, secondary to warfarin or thrombolytic

therapy, and secondary to cardiac surgical procedures that require cardiopulmonary bypass. Treatment is surgical resection if a focal source of embolism is present and the patient's general medical condition permits. Preliminary research suggests that warfarin may be beneficial in reducing subsequent embolic events, but further randomized trials are required (157).

Giant-Cell Arteritis

The cause of giant-cell arteritis (formerly called *temporal arteritis* or *cranial arteritis*) is unknown. The dominant clinical symptom is usually headache; the most frequent and dreaded complication is blindness. The classic physical finding is prominent, inflamed, or tender temporal arteries. Significant involvement of the aorta and large arteries is being recognized with increasing frequency.

Giant-cell arteritis is a subacute and chronic inflammatory process with local and systemic manifestations. It is generally seen in persons older than 55 years, and it is twice as common in women as in men. Involvement of the thoracic aorta and its branches may be minimal and asymptomatic, but when it is more extensive it can result in occlusion of one or more branches of the aortic arch (159), dilatation or saccular aneurysm of the aorta (160), or even aortic dissection (160).

The diagnosis is typically established by biopsy of the superficial temporal artery. However, MRI/MRA or standard contrast angiography is required to confirm the diagnosis of aortic and branch vessel involvement and to differentiate this disorder from atherosclerotic occlusion. The ascending aorta can be dilated, and there may be thickening of its wall; involvement of branches of the arch, when present, is often bilateral, with segmental areas of smooth, tapered arterial stenosis or occlusion, or both, in the absence of atherosclerotic changes.

Management of the patient with aortic or large-artery involvement by giant-cell arteritis is principally by administration of corticosteroids in adequate doses (beginning with 45–60 mg prednisone daily), often in combination with methotrexate (161). Arterial changes are reversible with adequate therapy, but when pharmacologic therapy has been insufficient to suppress the arteritis, there may be progressive involvement of the aorta and resultant dissection or rupture.

Takayasu's Disease

This disorder, also called *pulseless disease* and *idiopathic medial aortopathy and arteriopathy*, is another syndrome of arteritis that involves the aorta and its branches. In contrast to patients with giant-cell arteritis, most individuals with Takayasu's disease are younger than 40 years; it also occurs more commonly in women (>80% of cases).

The early subacute phase of fever, anorexia, malaise, weight loss, night sweats, and fatigue often go unrecognized, with the diagnosis first being suspected when symptoms and signs of the occlusive phase develop. The clinical manifestations of occlusion may include cerebrovascular insufficiency, arterial insufficiency of the upper or lower extremities, or mesenteric insufficiency, depending on the location of the aortitis and arteritis. Hypertension is very common; it occurs as a result of acquired aortic coarctation or involvement of the renal arteries by the arteritis.

MRA or standard contrast aortography is of great value in the diagnosis of Takayasu's disease. Segmental narrowing of a variable length of descending or abdominal aorta or narrowing of the origin of major branches of the aorta occurs as a result of thickening of the aorta or arterial wall (*e*Fig. 108.4.2). This usually allows distinction of Takayasu's disease from other causes of the aortic arch syndrome (162). Although aneurysmal dilatation of the thoracic aorta can occur in Takayasu's disease (163), it is not common or distinctive in this disorder.

Therapy with corticosteroids, sometimes combined with anticoagulant therapy, is effective for patients in the early phase of the disease in controlling systemic symptoms and allowing return of pulses. For the patient in the later occlu-

sive phase, surgical treatment to bypass the obstruction may be indicated to relieve hypertension caused by the acquired coarctation or renal artery stenosis (164). Similarly, other occlusive arterial lesions may require surgical treatment for relief of ischemic manifestations.

TRAUMATIC RUPTURE OF THE THORACIC AORTA

Pathogenesis

Trauma to the thoracic aorta may result from crushing injury and deceleration, as well as from penetrating injuries, or it may be iatrogenic from intraaortic procedures. Aortic rupture from sudden deceleration is the most common traumatic condition of the thoracic aorta that is encountered clinically. Rupture of the thoracic aorta as a result of sudden deceleration may vary in degree from incomplete laceration to complete transection. The injury occurs most often as a result of an automobile accident but may also occur in falls from heights or compression by heavy objects (165). With horizontal deceleration, as in automobile accidents, 80% of the aortic ruptures occur at the isthmus of the thoracic aorta just distal to the origin of the left subclavian artery and near the attachment of the ligamentum arteriosum, the point of aortic fixation where the shearing stress is maximal (166).

Clinical Features

Traumatic aortic rupture should be suspected whenever an injury involves sudden deceleration or chest trauma, either blunt or penetrating. The presence of chest contusions or penetrating wounds, rib or sternal fractures (167), hypertension in the arms (168), decreased or absent pulses in the legs (169), or evidence of fluid in the left side of the chest (170) is a clue to the possibility of aortic rupture.

Radiologic Features

The only finding on radiography of the chest may be widening of the mediastinum (170). The presence of left pleural fluid in association with mediastinal widening is an even stronger clue (170). Associated rib, clavicle, or sternal fractures may also be seen.

Diagnosis

In a patient with suspected traumatic rupture of the thoracic aorta, TEE, CT, or aortography should be performed emergently to confirm the diagnosis and localize the site of aortic rupture (171–173) (*e*Fig. 108.4.3). TEE is the initial test of choice, as it permits rapid diagnosis and effective triage of patients (173). The echocardiographic signs of aortic injury are complex and may be confined to a short section of the aorta. Therefore, examination by a physician who is highly trained in echocardiography is necessary in such cases.

Prognosis

Most patients with traumatic aortic rupture die before they reach a hospital, but as many as 20% may survive long enough to permit diagnosis and treatment (165). Some patients survive the aortic laceration and later present with so-called chronic traumatic thoracic aortic aneurysm; approximately half of these lesions become unstable and enlarge at some time in their course, but there are no criteria to predict which will do so (124).

Treatment

In the acute setting, extreme alertness, prompt diagnosis, and immediate surgical repair are necessary. Ordinarily, end-to-end anastomosis is not feasible, and therefore a prosthetic graft is interposed after resection of the lacerated area (174).

For chronic traumatic thoracic aortic aneurysm, we and others (124,125) favor surgical treatment, even though some of these patients may survive without surgery for long periods, because of the unpredictable course of this lesion and the low morbidity and mortality of elective surgical repair.

AORTITIS

Aortitis refers to a group of disorders with diverse etiologies. Although not a particularly common primary problem, aortitis, because of its role in aortic regurgitation, aortic dissection, and aneurysmal disease, is an important disorder of the thoracic and abdominal aorta.

Etiology

Inflammatory change can occur in the wall of the aorta in response to any type of injury. One way of classifying aortitis that involves a systematic approach to diagnosis is shown in *e*Table 108.1.3. Giant-cell arteritis and Takayasu's disease have already received attention in this chapter in the discussion of the arteritides in the section Occlusive Disease.

Clinical Features

Syphilitic aortitis, unless complicated, is usually asymptomatic. Other manifestations of tertiary lues may be seen in 10% to 30% of patients. With aneurysm formation, usually saccular in type, there may be signs of compression of other mediastinal structures; rarely, bony erosion occurs. When significant aortic regurgitation develops, a diastolic murmur and signs of a widened pulse pressure are noted.

In other types of infectious aortitis ("mycotic" aneurysm), the findings are those of infectious endocarditis.

Usually no specific signs of mycotic aneurysm are seen unless it encroaches on a surrounding structure or it ruptures. With other types of aortitis, the clinical signs are those of the underlying disease.

Radiographic Features

The diagnosis of aortitis is often first suspected from the findings on a chest radiograph (dilation of the ascending aorta or aneurysm). Linear calcification of the ascending aorta and not the arch is most suggestive of syphilitic aortitis. Calcification can also be seen with other types of aortitis and in atherosclerotic disease, but it does not usually involve the ascending aorta alone.

TEE, CT, MRI, and aortography are all accurate in demonstrating the extent of aortic dilatation and any aneurysmal change. Aortography or MRA is generally required to define any branch artery occlusion that may be present.

Diagnosis

The diagnosis of aortitis is usually inferred from any related clinical or chest radiographic findings, or both. Aortography can also demonstrate coronary ostial involvement in patients with syphilitic aortitis and Takayasu's disease. Further differentiation of the type of aortitis depends on associated findings of syphilis (serologic findings and characteristic calcification) or an associated systemic illness.

Prognosis

The prognosis for patients with syphilitic aortitis is about the same as that for the general population (178), and death from its complications, other than aneurysm, is unusual. The prognosis for syphilitic aortic aneurysm, on the other hand, is poor, particularly when it is large enough to cause symptoms (179).

Aortic rupture or dissection is a potential complication of giant-cell arteritis. Otherwise, the prognosis of aortitis is generally that of the underlying systemic disorder.

Treatment

The preventive value of adequate therapy of early syphilis is the most important therapeutic aspect of syphilitic aortitis. Therapy of other types of aortitis is basically that of the underlying disorder. Management of any aneurysm, aortic regurgitation, or arterial occlusive disease is the same as that for such a lesion when it is due to other causes.

MARFAN SYNDROME

Marfan syndrome is a generalized disorder of connective tissue and is relatively common, with an incidence of 1 per 20,000. The incidence of Marfan syndrome does not differ according to gender, race, or ethnicity. It is an autosomal dominant disorder with extremely variable expression (180–182). Sporadic mutations account for approximately 25% of cases. The cause of Marfan syndrome has been found to be a defect in fibrillin; the gene that encodes fibrillin is on chromosome 15q15–21 (183,184).

Clinical diagnostic criteria for Marfan syndrome depend on manifestations in the skeletal, cardiovascular, and ocular systems and the family history (185). A "marfanoid" body habitus is not diagnostic of Marfan syndrome in the absence of other characteristic features or a well-documented family history of Marfan syndrome. ▼ q57

Cardiovascular abnormalities are clinically apparent in 40% to 60% of patients with Marfan syndrome, whereas 80% to 95% of patients have cardiovascular findings by echocardiography or pathologic examination. The most common cardiovascular abnormalities are mitral valve prolapse with or without mitral regurgitation and dilation of the ascending aorta, which may result in aortic regurgitation, aortic dissection, or aortic rupture (180,185–189). Less commonly reported abnormalities are tricuspid valve prolapse and dilation of the main pulmonary artery. Cardiovascular complications, especially aortic root dilation with dissection or rupture, account for most of the early mortality in patients with Marfan syndrome. Before effective surgical techniques, most patients with Marfan syndrome died in the fourth and fifth decades of life (186,190).

Aortic abnormalities are found in 60% to 90% of patients (191). The prevalence of aortic root enlargement is greater in males than in females (192). Throughout life, the diameter of the aortic root is usually abnormal in proportion to body surface area in patients with Marfan syndrome; there is symmetric involvement of the sinuses of Valsalva and sinotubular ridge. Aortic dilation is usually progressive, likely due to abnormalities in aortic wall elastic properties such as increased wall stiffness (193,194). Aortic dilation may be limited to the sinuses of Valsalva or may involve the proximal and mid-ascending aorta. Generalized aortic dilation in patients with Marfan syndrome is a marker for increased risk of subsequent aortic complications (195). Dilation of the aorta is often accompanied by aortic regurgitation, and these patients often have a diastolic aortic regurgitation murmur (192). Aortic valve prolapse associated with a myxomatous aortic valve may also cause aortic regurgitation in patients without significant aortic dilation.

Aortic dissection in patients with Marfan syndrome is associated with aortic root dilatation (>6 cm) and a family history of dissection (196). Increased wall stress (Laplace's law) in the dilated aorta may contribute to the pathogenesis of aortic dissection in these patients. Dissection most commonly involves the ascending aorta, although isolated distal dissection may also occur. Pregnancy in patients with Marfan syndrome is associated with an increased risk of aortic dissec-

tion, especially during the third trimester, parturition, and the first month postpartum (197,198). ▼ q58

Treatment

Beta-adrenergic blockade to reduce the rate of dilation of the ascending aorta in Marfan syndrome has been shown to be beneficial (200–203). Progressive aortic root dilation occurs throughout life in patients with Marfan syndrome, the rate of dilation being greatest during early childhood and adolescent years. Although aortic root diameter increases over time in all patients, the rate of increase is significantly less in patients who are treated with beta-adrenergic blockade (202). Furthermore, beta-adrenergic blockade seems to improve survival without congestive heart failure, aortic regurgitation, aortic dissection, and aortic surgery (202). Therefore, patients with Marfan syndrome should begin beta-blockade therapy at the earliest age possible, and the dose should be adjusted to the largest dose that is tolerable. Atenolol has become the drug of choice for many physicians because of its relative cardioselectivity and the less frequent occurrence of adverse effects compared with lipid-soluble agents. Although no other drugs have been subjected to formal testing, verapamil, because of its negative inotropic action, is preferred in patients who cannot tolerate beta-adrenergic blocking agents (201).

Patients with aortic diameters greater than 5.0 cm have an increased risk of aortic dissection and should undergo prophylactic surgery (126). Patients with Marfan syndrome and ascending aortic aneurysm can undergo elective surgery with a low operative risk and excellent long-term survival with low morbidity. Aortic diameters less than 4 cm can be followed annually by echocardiography. Patients with aortic diameters between 4 and 5 cm should be observed more closely (every 6 to 12 months), especially if they have generalized aortic dilation and aortic regurgitation.

CONTROVERSIES AND PERSONAL PERSPECTIVES

Long-term management of type III aortic dissection continues to be an area of debate. Currently, most patients with type III aortic dissection are initially treated medically, with a beta-adrenergic blocking agent and adequate control of hypertension, and followed with noninvasive testing for the development of progressive aortic dilation and aneurysm formation, findings that might indicate the need for surgical intervention. Opinions differ about the indications for and timing of any surgical intervention in patients with "uncomplicated" type III aortic dissection. We and others currently advocate surgical therapy for patients with type III dissection after 2 to 3 weeks of pharmacologic therapy, if the patient's general condition does not contraindicate this approach (90,91). If pharmacologic therapy does not relieve pain and stabilize the dissection, prompt surgical therapy is also indi-

THE FUTURE

With regard to aortic dissection, continued efforts at earlier clinical recognition, allowing for more rapid diagnosis and treatment, are needed. Inclusion of aortic dissection in the differential diagnosis of patients presenting with acute chest pain is important, especially in view of the current widespread use of early i.v. thrombolytic therapy in patients with suspected acute myocardial infarction. Biochemical techniques will be integrated into the initial evaluation of patients with suspected aortic dissection. For example, elevated levels of smooth muscle myosin heavy-chain protein have been demonstrated to have a sensitivity and specificity of 91% and 98%, respectively, in patients with acute aortic dissection (206).

Based on the current size boundaries, the timing of surgical resection of aneurysms is less than perfect. For example, in patients with Marfan syndrome, an ascending aortic diameter of greater than 5 cm is associated with a small, although real, risk of rupture, and the risk increases significantly when aortic diameter exceeds 6 cm. Currently, surgery is indicated for patients with Marfan syndrome who have an ascending aortic diameter of greater than 5.5 cm, although surgery is less complicated and has less morbidity and mortality in patients with smaller aneurysms. The timing of surgical repair of AAA, in relation to aneurysm size, also requires further study. Currently, patients who are in otherwise good general health with an AAA diameter of greater than 4.5 cm are considered for *selective* surgical treatment. In the future, it is hoped that more emphasis will be placed on accurately determining aneurysm expansion rate to identify those patients with more rapid expansion rates who are at increased risk of rupture.

Increased efforts in identifying populations at risk for AAA are also clearly needed to allow more effective screening programs and identification of patients in the earlier stages of disease. Identification of less advanced aneurysmal disease may allow for earlier institution of pharmacologic therapy (i.e., beta-adrenergic blockade) and may lead to favorable alterations in the natural history of disease (i.e., decreased aneurysm expansion rate). Therapeutic agents that are targeted at the cellular level, for example, matrix metalloproteinases, may limit the growth of small AAAs. Personal ultrasound imagers will likely find increased utility in screening for aneurysmal

disease and become an integral portion of the physical examination in patients who are at increased risk for development of an AAA. Earlier detection of AAA at a smaller size and careful clinical follow-up may also allow for more appropriate timing of surgical intervention and a decrease in mortality from ruptured AAA. Furthermore, the role of medical therapy (i.e., corticosteroids) in inflammatory AAA, in addition to or in place of surgical therapy, warrants further study.

Clearly, the most exciting and promising advance in the treatment of aortic disease will involve the use of percutaneous endovascular techniques to place stents, bypass grafts, and other therapeutic agents. Percutaneous placement of an endovascular stent to treat AAA, as well as thoracic aortic aneurysm, and aortic dissection may become the optimal method of treatment in the future. Furthermore, percutaneous stent or stented graft placement may allow treatment of diffuse atherosclerotic disease of the aorta in patients with atheroembolic disease who would otherwise not tolerate extensive aortic reconstructive surgery. Indications for endovascular stent placement will clearly increase in patients who cannot tolerate aortic surgery but otherwise have an acceptable prognosis. With further improvements in catheter and stent technology and, therefore, fewer initial and long-term complications, endovascular stent therapy will certainly find increasing indications.

Future improvements in imaging techniques, in particular MRA and three-dimensional TEE, will allow for more accurate diagnosis and improved preoperative planning. The ability to provide the most accurate three-dimensional information about aortic intimal flaps, aneurysm anatomy, and atherosclerotic disease will be crucial to future advancements in medical and surgical treatment of these disorders.

Improvements in imaging techniques, in particular MRA and three-dimensional TEE, will allow for more accurate and earlier diagnosis of aortic aneurysms with an associated improvement in the timing of surgical treatment. Further improvements in percutaneous endovascular techniques to place stents and bypass grafts will lead to increasing indications. In addition, therapeutic agents will be developed to effectively retard the growth rate of AAAs.

cated. Transluminal placement of an endovascular stent-graft device in type III aortic dissection has been successfully performed and may provide an alternative to surgery in highly selected patients in the future (92,204).

Debate is ongoing regarding the best noninvasive test in suspected aortic dissection. CT, MRI, and TEE, using current-generation technology, all have an exceedingly high sensitivity and specificity (>95%) in the diagnosis of aortic dissection. Currently, the diagnostic test of choice in suspected acute aortic dissection is TEE because of its rapid availability, portability, ability to provide a comprehensive cardiovascular assessment, and intraoperative applications. If TEE is not immediately available and the patient is stable hemodynamically, CT and MRI can be used as a substitute for TEE. Coronary angiography is not required in patients with acute proximal aortic dissection due to the high early mortality that is associated with this disease and inherent delays that are present with angiography (78). MRI is the preferred test in patients with chronic aortic dissection.

Equally as controversial is the treatment of patients with certain types of penetrating aortic ulcers. Although the natural history of an intramural hematoma is generally benign (i.e., resorption of the hematoma and compensatory dilation of the involved aorta) (101), the natural history of saccular aneurysm and pseudoaneurysm (due to penetrating aortic ulcer) is presently not known. Further study in this area is needed. Equally important are improved surgical techniques to decrease the risk of perioperative spinal cord ischemia and resultant paraplegia in patients undergoing thoracic aortic surgery.

The utility of beta-adrenergic blockade therapy in patients who have aneurysmal disease but not Marfan syndrome is poorly understood. The rare reports of the utility of beta-adrenergic blockade in these patients show benefit in decreasing aneurysm expansion rate, but the number of studies and patients involved are exceedingly small. Presently, our practice has been to institute a beta-blocking agent in all patients with aneurysmal disease if no contraindications to such therapy exist. Furthermore, most of these patients have concomitant coronary artery disease and systemic hypertension, which are well-established indications for beta-adrenergic blockade therapy.

Another highly controversial topic in aortic disease, especially in view of the current emphasis on cost containment in medicine, is screening for AAA. Screening programs for the general population have not been clinically or economically effective. It has been demonstrated, however, that screening certain populations who are at risk for development of an AAA (i.e., older than 70 years, hypertension, tobacco use, family history of AAA, etc.) identifies a group of patients with a significantly increased incidence of AAA compared with the general population. Targeting "high-risk" patients in future aneurysm screening programs will be more clinically meaningful and cost effective (205).

REFERENCES

1. Meszaros I, Morocz J, Szlavi J, et al. Epidemiology and clinicopathology of aortic dissection. *Chest* 2000;117:1271.
2. Hirst AE Jr, Johns VJ, Kime SW Jr. Dissecting aneurysm of the aorta: a review of 505 cases. *Medicine* 1958;37:217.
3. Lindsay J Jr, Hurst JW. Clinical features and prognosis in dissecting aneurysm of the aorta: a re-appraisal. *Circulation* 1967;35:880.
4. McCloy RM, Spittell JA, McGoon DC. The prognosis in aortic dissection (dissecting aortic aneurysm or hematoma). *Circulation* 1965;31:665.
5. Nienaber CA, von Kodolitsch Y, Nicolas V, et al. The diagnosis of thoracic aortic dissection by noninvasive imaging procedures. *N Engl J Med* 1993;328:1.
6. Roberts WC. Aortic dissection: anatomy, consequences, and causes. *Am Heart J* 1981;101:195.
7. Spittell JA Jr. Hypertension and arterial aneurysm. *J Am Coll Cardiol* 1983;1:523.
8. Slater EE, DeSanctis RW. Diseases of the aorta. In: Braunwald E, ed. *Heart disease, a textbook of cardiovascular medicine.* Philadelphia: WB Saunders, 1980:1597–1632.
9. Larson EW, Edwards WD. Risk factors for aortic dissection: a necropsy study of 161 cases. *Am J Cardiol* 1984;53:849.
10. Wilson SK, Hutchins GM. Aortic dissecting aneurysms: causative factors in 204 subjects. *Arch Pathol Lab Med* 1982;106:175.
11. Spittell PC, Spittell JA, Joyce JW, et al. Clinical features and differential diagnosis of aortic dissection: experience with 236 cases (1980–1990). *Mayo Clin Proc* 1993;68:642.
12. Fukuda T, Tadavarthy SM, Edwards JE. Dissecting aneurysms of the aorta complicating aortic valvular stenosis. *Circulation* 1976;53:169.
13. Svensson LG, Crawford ES, Coselli JS, et al. Impact of cardiovascular operation on survival in the Marfan patient. *Circulation* 1989;80[Suppl I]:I-233.
14. Carter AJ, Brinker JA. Dissection of the ascending aorta associated with coronary angiography. *Am J Cardiol* 1994;73:922.
15. Sakamoto I, Hayashi K, Matsunaga N, et al. Aortic dissection caused by angiographic procedures. *Radiology* 1994;191:467.
16. Jacobs LE, Fraifeld M, Kotler MN, et al. Aortic dissection following intraaortic balloon insertion: recognition by transesophageal echocardiography. *Am Heart J* 1992;124:536.
17. Pieters FA, Widdershoven JW, Gerardy AC, et al. Risk of aortic dissection after aortic valve replacement. *Am J Cardiol* 1993;72:1043.
18. Still RJ, Hilgenberg AD, Akins CW, et al. Intraoperative aortic dissection. *Ann Thorac Surg* 1992;53:374.
19. Murphy DA, Craver JM, Jones EL, et al. Recognition and management of ascending aortic dissection complicating cardiac surgical operations. *J Thorac Cardiovasc Surg* 1983;85:247.
20. Nordt TK, Rauch B, Mattfeldt T, et al. Acute myocardial infarction due to proximal aortic dissection in giant cell aortitis. *Am Heart J* 1990;122:1151.
21. Walts AE, Dubois EL. Acute dissecting aneurysm of the aorta as the fatal event in systemic lupus erythematosus. *Am Heart J* 1977;93:378.
22. Schacter N, Perloff JK, Mulder DG. Aortic dissection in Noonan's syndrome (46XY Turner). *Am J Cardiol* 1984;54:464.
23. Price WH, Wilson J. Dissection of the aorta in Turner's syndrome. *J Med Genet* 1983;20:61.

24. McDermott JC, Schuster MR, Crummy AB, et al. Crack and aortic dissection. *Wis Med J* 1993;92:453.

25. Fisher A, Holroyd BR. Cocaine-associated dissection of the thoracic aorta. *J Emerg Med* 1992;10:723.

26. Biagini A, Maffei S, Baroni M, et al. Familial clustering of aortic dissection in polycystic disease. *Am J Cardiol* 1993;72:741.

27. Iino T, Eguchi K, Sakai M, et al. Polyarteritis nodosa with aortic dissection: a necrotizing vasculitis of the vasa vasorum. *J Rheumatol* 1992;19:1632.

28. Gates JD, Clair DG, Hechtman DH. Thoracic aortic dissection with renal artery involvement following blunt thoracic trauma: case report. *J Trauma* 1994;36:430.

29. DeBakey ME, Henly WS, Cooley DA, et al. Surgical management of dissecting aneurysms of the aorta. *J Thorac Cardiovasc Surg* 1965;49:130.

30. Slater EE, Desanctis RW. The clinical recognition of dissecting aortic aneurysm. *Am J Med* 1976;60:625.

31. Daily PO, Trueblood W, Stinson EB, et al. Management of acute aortic dissection. *Ann Thorac Surg* 1970;10:237.

32. Sullivan PR, Wolfson AB, Leckey RD, et al. Diagnosis of acute thoracic aortic dissection in the emergency department. *Am J Emerg Med* 2000;18:46.

33. Burchell HB. Aortic dissection (dissecting hematoma) of the aorta. *Circulation* 1955;12:1068.

34. Perryman RA, Gay WA. Rupture of dissecting thoracic aortic aneurysm into the right ventricle. *Am J Cardiol* 1972;30:277.

35. Nicod P, Firth BG, Peshock RM, et al. Rupture of dissecting aortic aneurysm into the right atrium: clinical and echocardiographic recognition. *Am Heart J* 1984;107:1276.

36. Oliveira JSM, Bestetti RB, Marin-Neto JA, et al. Ruptured aortic dissection into the left atrium: a rare cause of congestive heart failure. *Am Heart J* 1991;121:936.

37. Amer NC, Schaeffer HC, Domingo RT, et al. Aortic dissection presenting as iliac-artery occlusion: an aid to early diagnosis. *N Engl J Med* 1962;266:1040.

38. DeBakey ME, McCollum CH, Crawford ES, et al. Dissection and dissecting aneurysms of the aorta: twenty-year follow-up of five hundred twenty-seven patients treated surgically. *Surgery* 1982;92:1118.

39. Moersch FP, Sayre GP. Neurologic manifestations associated with dissecting aneurysm of the aorta. *JAMA* 1950;144:1141.

40. Logue RB, Sikes C. A new sign in dissecting aneurysm of the aorta: pulsation of a sternoclavicular joint. *JAMA* 1952;148:1209.

41. McCarthy C, Dickson GH, Besterman EMM, et al. Aortic dissection with rupture through ductus arteriosus into pulmonary artery. *Br Heart J* 1972;34:428.

42. Spitzer S, Blanco G, Adam A, et al. Superior vena cava obstruction and dissecting aortic aneurysm. *JAMA* 1975;233:164.

43. Giannoccaro PJ, Marquis J-F, Chan K-L, et al. Aortic dissection presenting as upper airway obstruction. *Chest* 1991;99:256.

44. Roth JA, Parekh MA. Dissecting aneurysm perforating the esophagus [Letter]. *N Engl J Med* 1978;299:776.

45. Kagele SF, Charan NB. Unilateral pulmonary edema: an unusual cause. *Chest* 1992;102:1279.

46. Giladi M, Pines A, Averbuch M, et al. Aortic dissection manifested as fever of unknown origin. *Cardiology* 1991;78:78.

47. Hirata K, Kyushima M, Asato H. Electrocardiographic abnormalities in patients with acute aortic dissection. *Am J Cardiol* 1995;76:1207.

48. Yacoub MH, Schottenfeld M, Kittle CF. Hematoma of the interatrial septum with heart block secondary to dissecting aneurysm of the aorta: a clinicopathologic entity. *Circulation* 1972;46:537.

49. Earnest F IV, Muhm JR, Sheedy PF. Roentgenographic findings in thoracic aortic dissection. *Mayo Clin Proc* 1979;54:43.

50. Hagan PG, Nienaber CA, Isselbacher EM, et al. The International Registry of Acute Aortic Dissection (IRAD): new insights into an old disease. *JAMA* 2000;283:897.

51. Enia F, Ledda G, Lo Mauro R, et al. Utility of echocardiography in the diagnosis of aortic dissection involving the ascending aorta. *Chest* 1989;95:124.

52. Khanderia BK, Tajik AJ, Taylor CL, et al. Aortic dissection: review of value and limitations of two-dimensional echocardiography in a six-year experience. *J Am Soc Echocardiogr* 1989;2:17.

53. Mathew T, Nanda NC. Two-dimensional and Doppler echocardiographic evaluation of aortic aneurysm and aortic dissection. *Am J Cardiol* 1984;54:379.

54. Isselbacher EM, Cigarroa JE, Eagle KA. Cardiac tamponade complicating proximal aortic dissection: is pericardiocentesis harmful? *Circulation* 1994;90:2375.

55. Erbel R, Engberding R, Daniel W, et al. Echocardiography in the diagnosis of aortic dissection. *Lancet* 1989;1:457.

56. Simon P, Owen AN, Havel M, et al. Transesophageal echocardiography in the emergency surgical management of patients with aortic dissection. *J Thorac Cardiovasc Surg* 1992;103:1113.

57. Armstrong WF, Bach DS, Carey L, et al. Spectrum of acute dissection of the ascending aorta: a transesophageal echocardiographic study. *J Am Soc Echocardiogr* 1996;9:646.

58. Wiet SP, Pearce WH, McCarthy, et al. Utility of transesophageal echocardiography in the diagnosis of disease of the thoracic aorta. *J Vasc Surg* 1994;20:613.

59. Deutsch HJ, Sechtem U, Meyer H, et al. Chronic aortic dissection: comparison of MR imaging and transesophageal echocardiography. *Radiology* 1994;192:645.

60. Nienaber CA, Spielmann RP, von Kodolitsch Y, et al. Diagnosis of thoracic aortic dissection: magnetic resonance imaging versus transesophageal echocardiography. *Circulation* 1992;85:434.

61. Chirilo F, Cavallini C, Longhini C, et al. Comparative diagnostic value of transesophageal echocardiography and retrograde aortography in the evaluation of thoracic aortic dissection. *Am J Cardiol* 1994;74:590.

62. Moncada R, Churchill R, Reynes C, et al. Diagnosis of dissecting aortic aneurysm by computed tomography. *Lancet* 1981;1:23867

63. Kersting-Sommerhoff BA, Higgins CB, White RD, et al. Aortic dissection: sensitivity and specificity of MR imaging. *Radiology* 1988;166:651.

64. Fattori R, Bacchi-Reggiani L, Bertaccini P, et al. Evolution of aortic dissection after surgical repair. *Am J Cardiol* 2000;86:868.

65. Chung JW, Park JH, Kim HC, et al. Entry tears of thoracic aortic dissections: MR appearance on gated SE imaging. *J Comput Assist Tomogr* 1994;18:250.

66. Nienaber CA, von Kodolitsch Y, Brockhoff CJ, et al. Comparison of conventional and transesophageal echocardiography with magnetic resonance imaging for anatomical mapping of thoracic aortic dissection: a dual noninvasive imaging study with anatomical and/or angiographic validation. *Int J Imaging* 1994;10:1.

67. Yamada T, Tada S, Harda J. Aortic dissection without intimal rupture: diagnosis with MR imaging and CT. *Radiology* 1988;168:347.

68. Spittell JA Jr. Clinical aspects of aneurysmal disease. *Curr Probl Cardiol* 1980;5:1.

69. Eagle KA, Quertermous T, Kritzer GA. Spectrum of conditions initially suggesting acute aortic dissection but with negative aortograms. *Am J Cardiol* 1986;57:322.

70. Weintraub AR, Erbel R, Gorge G, et al. Intravascular ultrasound imaging in acute aortic dissection. *J Am Coll Cardiol* 1994;24:495.

71. Yamada E, Matsumura M, Kyo S, et al. Usefulness of a prototype intravascular ultrasound imaging in evaluation of aortic dissection and comparison with angiographic study, transesophageal echocardiography, computed tomography, and magnetic resonance imaging. *Am J Cardiol* 1995;75:161.

72. Rizzo RJ, Aranki SF, Aklog L, et al. Rapid noninvasive diagnosis and surgical repair of acute ascending aortic dissection: improved survival with less angiography. *J Thorac Cardiovasc Surg* 1994;108:567.

73. Wheat MW Jr, Palmer RF, Bartley TD, et al. Treatment of dissecting aneurysms of the aorta without surgery. *J Thorac Cardiovasc Surg* 1965;50:364.

74. Palmer RF, Lasseter KC. Nitroprusside and aortic dissecting aneurysm [Letter]. *N Engl J Med* 1976;294:1403.

75. Grubb BP, Sirio C, Zehs R. Intravenous labetalol in acute aortic dissection. *JAMA* 1987;258:78.

76. Miller DC. Acute dissection of the aorta: continuing need for earlier diagnosis and treatment. *Mod Concepts Cardiovasc Dis* 1985;54:51.

77. Jex RK, Schaff HV, Piehler JM, et al. Repair of ascending aortic dissection. *J Thorac Cardiovasc Surg* 1987;93:375.

78. Penn MS, Smedira N, Lytle B, et al. Does coronary angiography before emergency aortic surgery affect in-hospital mortality? *J Am Coll Cardiol* 2000;35:889.

79. Movsowitz HD, Levine RA, Hilgenberg AD, et al. Transesophageal echocardiographic description of the mechanism of aortic regurgitation in acute type A aortic dissection: implications for aortic valve repair. *J Am Coll Cardiol* 2000;36:884.

80. Crawford ES, Svensson LG, Coselli JS, et al. Surgical treatment of aneurysm and/or dissection of the ascending aorta, transverse aortic arch, and ascending aorta and transverse aortic arch: factors influencing survival in 717 patients. *J Thorac Cardiovasc Surg* 1989;98:659.

81. Cosseli JS, Crawford ES. Composite valve-graft replacement of aortic root using separate Dacron tube for coronary artery reattachment. *Ann Thorac Surg* 1989;47:558.

82. Pannenton JM, The SH, Cherry KJ, et al. Aortic fenestration for acute or chronic aortic dissection: an uncommon but effective procedure. *J Vasc Surg* 2000;32:711.

83. Beregi JP, Prat A, Gaxotte V, et al. Endovascular treatment for dissection of the descending aorta. *Lancet* 2000;356:482.

84. Sabik JF, Lytle BW, Blackstone EH, et al. Long-term effectiveness of operations for ascending aortic dissection. *J Thorac Cardiovasc Surg* 2000;119:946.

85. Elefteriades JA, Lovoulos CJ, Coady MA, et al. Management of descending aortic dissection. *Ann Thorac Surg* 1999;67:2002.

86. Miller DC. The continuing dilemma concerning medical versus surgical management of patients with acute type B dissections [Review]. *Semin Thorac Cardiovasc Surg* 1993;5:33.

87. DeSanctis RW, Doroghazi MD, Austen WG, et al. Aortic dissection. *N Engl J Med* 1987;317:1060.

88. Glower DD, Fann JI, Speier RH, et al. Comparison of medical and surgical therapy or uncomplicated descending aortic dissection. *Circulation* 1990;82[Suppl IV]:IV-39.

89. Matsuda Y, Yamada Z, Morooka N, et al. Prognosis of patients with medically treated aortic dissections. *Circulation* 1991;84[Suppl III]:III-7.

90. Jex RK, Schaff HV, Piehler JM, et al. Early and late results following repair of dissections of the descending thoracic aorta. *J Vasc Surg* 1986;3:226.

91. Neya K, Omoto R, Kyo S, et al. Outcome of Stanford type B aortic dissection. *Circulation* 1992;86[Suppl 5]:II1.

92. Dake MD, Miller DC, Semba CP, et al. Transluminal placement of endovascular stent-grafts for the treatment of descending thoracic aortic aneurysms. *N Engl J Med* 1994;331:1729.

93. Walker PJ, Dake MD, Mitchell RS, et al. The use of endovascular techniques for the treatment of complications of aortic dissection. *J Vasc Surg* 1993;18:1042.

94. Glower DD, Fann JI, Speier RH, et al. Comparison of medical and surgical therapy or uncomplicated descending aortic dissection. *Circulation* 1990;82[Suppl IV]:IV-39.

95. Matsuda Y, Yamada Z, Morooka N, et al. Prognosis of patients with medically treated aortic dissections. *Circulation* 1991;84[Suppl III]:III-7.

96. Stanson AW, Kazmier FJ, Hollier LH, et al. Penetrating atherosclerotic ulcers of the thoracic aorta: natural history and clinicopathologic correlations. *Ann Vasc Surg* 1986;1:15.

97. Hussain A, Glover JL, Bree R, et al. Penetrating atherosclerotic ulcers of the thoracic aorta. *J Vasc Surg* 1989;9:710.

98. Spittell PC, Edwards WD, Stanson AW, et al. The clinical consequences of penetrating aortic ulcer (aortic intramural hematoma). *J Am Coll Cardiol* 1993;21:312A.

99. Shennan T. Dissecting aneurysms. Special report series nE 193. *Med Res Council (Great Britain)* 1933–1934;86.

100. Willius FA, Cragg RW. A talk on dissecting aneurysm of the aorta. *Cardiac Clin* 1941;16:41.

101. Kazerooni EA, Bree RL, Williams DM. Penetrating atherosclerotic ulcers of the descending thoracic aorta: evaluation with CT and distinction from aortic dissection. *Radiology* 1992;183:759.

102. Yucel EK, Steinberg FL, Egglin TK, et al. Penetrating aortic ulcers: diagnosis with MR imaging. *Radiology* 1990;177:779.

103. Willens HJ, et al. Transesophageal echocardiography in the diagnosis of diseases of the thoracic aorta (Pt 1). Aortic

dissection, aortic intramural hematoma, and penetrating atherosclerotic ulcer of the aorta. *Chest* 1999;116:1772.

104. Vilacosta I, San Roman JA, Aragoncillo P, et al. Penetrating atherosclerotic aortic ulcer: documentation by transesophageal echocardiography. *J Am Coll Cardiol* 1998;32:83.

105. Coady MA, Rizzo JA, Elefteriades JA. Pathologic variants of thoracic aortic dissections. Penetrating atherosclerotic ulcers and intramural hematomas. *Cardiol Clin* 1999;17:637.

106. Osler W, Bean WB, eds. *Sir William Osler aphorisms.* Springfield, IL: Charles Thomas Publisher, 1961.

107. Ellis PR, Cooley DA, DeBakey ME. Clinical considerations and surgical treatment of annulo-aortic ectasia: report of successful operation. *J Thorac Cardiovasc Surg* 1961;42:363.

108. Lemon DK, White CW. Annuloaortic ectasia: angiographic, hemodynamic and clinical comparison with aortic valve insufficiency. *Am J Cardiol* 1978;41:482.

109. Waller BF, Zoltick JM, Rosen JH, et al. Severe aortic regurgitation from systemic hypertension (without aortic dissection) requiring aortic valve replacement: Analysis of four patients. *Am J Cardiol* 1982;49:473.

110. Lande AM, Berkmen YM. Aortitis: pathologic, clinical and arteriographic review. *Radiol Clin North Am* 1976;14:219.

111. Fuster V, Kottke BA, Juergens JL. Atherosclerosis. In: Juergens JL, Spittell JA, Fairbairn JF II, eds. *Allen-Barker-Hines Peripheral Vascular Diseases*, 5th ed. Philadelphia: WB Saunders, 1980:219.

112. Johansen K. Aneurysms. *Sci Am* 1982;247:110.

113. Roberts WS. The hypertensive diseases: evidence that systemic hypertension is a greater risk factor to the development of other cardiovascular diseases than previously suspected. *Am J Med* 1975;59:523.

114. Greipp RB, Ergin MA, Lansman SL, et al. The natural history of thoracic aortic aneurysms. *Semin Thorac Cardiovasc Surg* 1991;3:258.

115. Joyce JW, Fairbairn JF II, Kincaid OW, et al. Aneurysms of the thoracic aorta: a clinical study with special reference to prognosis. *Circulation* 1964;29:176.

116. Pressler V, McNamara JJ. Thoracic aortic aneurysm: natural history and treatment. *J Thorac Cardiovasc Surg* 1980;79:489.

117. Posniak HV, Demos TC, Marsan RE. Computed tomography of the normal aorta and thoracic aneurysms. *Semin Roentgenol* 1989;24:7.

118. DeMaria AN, Bommer W, Neumann A, et al. Identification and localization of aneurysms of the ascending aorta by cross-sectional echocardiography. *Circulation* 1979;59:755.

119. Mintz GS, Kotler MN, Segal BL, et al. Two dimensional echocardiographic recognition of the descending thoracic aorta. *Am J Cardiol* 1979;44:232.

120. Lois JF, Gomes AS, Brown K, et al. Magnetic resonance imaging of the thoracic aorta. *Am J Cardiol* 1987;60:358.

121. Kamp O, van Rossum AC, Torenbeek R. Transesophageal echocardiography and magnetic resonance imaging for the assessment of saccular aneurysm of the transverse thoracic aorta. *Int J Cardiol* 1991;33:330.

122. Bickerstaff LK, Pairolero PC, Hollier LH, et al. Thoracic aortic aneurysm: a population based study. *Surgery* 1982; 92:1103.

123. Clouse WD, Hallett JW Jr, Schaff HV, et al. Improved prognosis of thoracic aortic aneurysms. A population-based study. *JAMA* 1998;280:1926.

124. Fleming AW, Green DC. Traumatic aneurysms of the thoracic aorta: report of 43 patients. *Ann Thorac Surg* 1974;18:91.

125. Quaini E, Colombo T, Donatelli F, et al. Chronic traumatic aneurysms of the descending thoracic aorta. *Tex Heart Inst J* 1985;12:143.

126. McDonald GR, Schaff HV, Pyeritz RE, et al. Surgical management of patients with the Marfan syndrome and dilatation of the ascending aorta. *J Thorac Cardiovasc Surg* 1981;81:180.

127. Baumgartner WA, Cameron DE, Redmond JM, et al. Operative management of Marfan syndrome: the Johns Hopkins experience. *Ann Thorac Surg* 1999;67:1859.

128. Lynch DR, Dawson TM, Raps EC, et al. Risk factors for the neurologic complications associated with aortic aneurysms. *Arch Neurol* 1992;49:284.

129. Singh MP, Bentall HH. Complete replacement of the ascending aorta and the aortic valve for the treatment of aortic aneurysm. *J Thorac Cardiovasc Surg* 1972;63:218.

130. Selle JG, Robicsek F, Daugherty HK, et al. Technical options in repairing the diseased ascending aorta with aortic valve involvement. *Ann Thorac Surg* 1981;32:578.

131. Smoking, lung function and the prognosis of abdominal aortic aneurysm. The UK small aneurysm trial participants. *Eur J Vasc Endovasc Surg* 2000;19:636.

132. Johansen K, Koepsell T. Familial tendency for abdominal aortic aneurysm. *JAMA* 1986;256:1934.

133. Tilson MD, Seashore M. Fifty families with abdominal aortic aneurysms in two or more first-order relatives. *Am J Surg* 1984;147:551.

134. Kearney RA, Eisen HJ, Wolf JE. Nonvalvular infections of the cardiovascular system. *Ann Intern Med* 1994;121:219.

135. Fowl RJ, Blebea J, Stallion A, et al. Prevalence of unsuspected abdominal aortic aneurysm in male veterans. *Ann Vasc Surg* 1993;7:117.

136. Sommerville RL, Allen EV, Edward JE. Bland and infected arteriosclerotic abdominal aortic aneurysms: a clinico-pathologic study. *Medicine* 1959;38:207.

137. Bruce CJ, Spittell PC, Montgomery SC, et al. Personal ultrasound imager: abdominal aortic aneurysm screening. *J Am Soc Echocardiogr* 2000;13:674.

138. Siepel T, Clifford DS, James PA, et al. The ultrasound-assisted physical examination in the periodic health evaluation of the elderly. *J Fam Pract* 2000;49:628.

139. Heather BP, Poskitt KR, Earnshaw JJ, et al. Population screening reduces mortality rate from aortic aneurysm in men. *Br J Surg* 2000;87:750.

140. Nevitt MP, Ballard DJ, Hallet JW. Prognosis of abdominal aortic aneurysms: a population based study. *N Engl J Med* 1989;321:1009.

141. Pennell RC, Hollier LH, Lie JT, et al. Inflammatory abdominal aortic aneurysms: a thirty-year review. *J Vasc Surg* 1985;2:859.

142. Sterpetti AV, Hunter WJ, Feldhaus RJ, et al. Inflammatory aneurysms of the abdominal aorta: incidence, pathologic, and etiologic considerations. *J Vasc Surg* 1989;9:643.

143. Nitecki SS, Hallett JW Jr, Stanson AW, et al. Inflamma-

tory abdominal aortic aneurysms: a case-control study. *J Vasc Surg* 1996;23:860.

144. Testart J, Plissonnier D, Peillon C, et al. Inflammatory abdominal aortic aneurysm. Role of corticosteroid therapy. *J Mal Vasc* 2000;25:201.

145. Hertzer NR, Beven EG, Young JR, et al. Coronary artery disease in peripheral vascular patients: a classification of 1000 coronary angiograms and results of surgical management. *Ann Surg* 1984;199:223.

146. Estes JE Jr. Abdominal aortic aneurysm: A study of one hundred and two cases. *Circulation* 1977;2:258.

147. Leach SD, Toole AL, Stern H, et al. Effect of β-adrenergic blockade on the growth rate of abdominal aortic aneurysms. *Arch Surg* 1988;123:606.

148. Parodi JC, Palmaz JC, Barone HD. Transfemoral intraluminal graft implantation for abdominal aortic aneurysms. *Ann Vasc Surg* 1991;5:491.

149. Parodi JC, Criado FJ, Barone HD, et al. Endoluminal aortic aneurysm repair using a balloon-expandable stent-graft device: a progress report. *Ann Vasc Surg* 1994;8:523.

150. Moore WS, Rutherford RB. Transfemoral endovascular repair of abdominal aortic aneurysm: results of the North American EVT phase I trial. *J Vasc Surg* 1996;23:543.

151. Zarins CK, Wolf YG, Lee WA, et al. Will endovascular repair replace open surgery for abdominal aortic aneurysm repair? *Ann Surg* 2000;232:501.

152. May J, White GH, Waugh R, et al. Comparison of first- and second-generation prostheses for endoluminal repair of abdominal aortic aneurysms: a 6-year study with life table analysis. *J Vasc Surg* 2000;32:124.

153. Buth J. Endovascular repair of abdominal aortic aneurysms. Results from the EUROSTAR registry. EUROpean collaborators on stent-graft techniques for abdominal aortic aneurysm repair. *Semin Interv Cardiol* 2000;5:29.

154. Zarins CK, White RA, Hodgson KJ, et al. Endoleak as a predictor of outcome after endovascular aneurysm repair: AneurRx multicenter clinical trial. *J Vasc Surg* 2000;32:90.

155. Patel A, Toole JF. Subclavian steal syndrome: Reversal of cephalic blood flow. *Medicine (Baltimore)* 1965;44:289.

156. Sadony V, Kayambo GH, Walz M, et al. Acquired coarctation due to calcified thrombus in atherosclerosis of the descending thoracic aorta: two cases and a review. *Eur J Cardiothorac Surg* 1989;3:464.

157. Ferrari E, Vidal R, Chevallier T, et al. Atherosclerosis of the thoracic aorta and aortic debris as a marker of poor prognosis: benefit of oral anticoagulation. *J Am Coll Cardiol* 1999;33:1317.

158. Tunick PA, Kronzon I. Atheromas of the thoracic aorta: clinical and therapeutic update. *J Am Coll Cardiol* 2000;35:545.

159. Hunder GG, Ward LE, Burbank MK. Giant-cell arteritis producing an aortic arch syndrome. *Ann Intern Med* 1967;66:578.

160. Evans JM, O'Fallon WM, Hunder GG. Increased incidence of aortic aneurysm and dissection in giant cell (temporal) arteritis: a population-based study. *Ann Intern Med* 1995;122:502.

161. Jover JA, Hernandez-Garcia C, Morado IC, et al. Combined treatment of giant-cell arteritis with methotrexate and prednisone. *Ann Intern Med* 2001;134:106.

162. Lande A, Berkmen YM. Aortitis: pathologic, clinical and arteriographic review. *Radiol Clin North Am* 1976;14:219.

163. Cull DL, Parent FN III, Wheeler JR, et al. Thoracic aortic ectasia in a patient with Takayasu's disease. *Ann Vasc Surg* 1991;5:470.

164. Ishikawa K. Survival and morbidity after diagnosis of occlusive thromboaortopathy (Takayasu's disease). *Am J Cardiol* 1981;47:1026.

165. Parmley RF, Mattingly TW, Manion WC. Penetrating wounds of the heart and aorta. *Circulation* 1958;17:953.

166. Cammack K, Rapport RL, Paul J, et al. Deceleration injuries of the thoracic aorta. *Arch Surg* 1959;79:244.

167. Greendyke RM. Traumatic rupture of aorta: special reference to automobile accidents. *JAMA* 1966;195:527.

168. Fox S, Pierce WS, Waldhausen JA. Acute hypertension: its significance in traumatic aortic rupture. *J Thorac Cardiovasc Surg* 1979;77:622.

169. Eiseman B, Rainer WG. Clinical management of post-traumatic rupture of the thoracic aorta. *J Thorac Surg* 1958;35:347.

170. Stoney RJ, Roe BB, Redington JV. Rupture of thoracic aorta due to closed-chest trauma. *Arch Surg* 1964;89:840.

171. Raptopoulos V, Sheiman RG, Phillips DA, et al. Traumatic aortic tear: screening with chest CT. *Radiology* 1992;182:667.

172. Berenfeld A, Barraud P, Lusson JR, et al. Traumatic aortic ruptures diagnosed by transesophageal echocardiography. *J Am Soc Echocardiogr* 1996;9:657.

173. Goarin JP, Catoire P, Jacquens Y, et al. Use of transesophageal echocardiography for diagnosis of traumatic aortic injury. *Chest* 1997;112:71.

174. Duhaylongsod FG, Glower DD, Wolfe WG. Acute traumatic aortic aneurysm: the Duke experience from 1970 to 1990. *J Vasc Surg* 1992;15:331.

175. Shahian DM, Javid H, Faber LP, et al. Lesions of the thoracic aorta and its arch branches simulating neoplasm. *J Thorac Cardiovasc Surg* 1981;81:251.

176. Mundth ED, Darling RC, Alvarado RH, et al. Surgical management of mycotic aneurysms and the complications of infection in vascular reconstructive surgery. *Am J Surg* 1969;117:460.

177. Heggtveit HA, Hennigar GR, Morrione TG. Panaortitis. *Am J Pathol* 1963;42:151.

178. Rich C Jr, Webster B. The natural history of uncomplicated syphilitic aortitis. *Am Heart J* 1952;43:321.

179. Kampmeier RH. Saccular aneurysm of the thoracic aorta: a clinical study of 633 cases. *Ann Intern Med* 1938;12:624.

180. McKusick VA. The cardiovascular aspects of Marfan syndrome: a heritable disorder of connective tissue. *Circulation* 1955;11:321.

181. Pyeritz RE. The Marfan syndrome. *Am Fam Physician* 1986;34:83.

182. Sun QB, Zhang KZ, Cheng TO, et al. Marfan syndrome in China: a collective review of 564 cases among 98 families. *Am Heart J* 1990;120:934.

183. Dietz HC, Cutting GR, Pyeritz RE, et al. Marfan syndrome caused by a recurrent de novo missense mutation in the fibrillin gene. *Nature* 1991;352:337.

184. Kainulainen K, Sakai LY, Child A, et al. Two mutations in Marfan syndrome resulting in truncated fibrillin polypeptides. *Proc Natl Acad Sci U S A* 1992;89:5917.

185. Beighton P, de Paepe A, Danks D, et al. International nosology of heritable disorders of connective tissue, Berlin 1986. *Am J Med Genet* 1988;29:581.

186. Murdoch JL, Walker BA, Halpern BL, et al. Life expectancy and causes of death in the Marfan syndrome. *N Engl J Med* 1972;286:804.

187. Hirata K, Triposkiadis F, Sparks E, et al. The Marfan syndrome: cardiovascular physical findings and diagnostic correlates. *Am Heart J* 1992;123:743.

188. Roberts WC, Honig HS. The spectrum of cardiovascular diseases in the Marfan syndrome: a clinicomorphic study of 18 necropsy patients and comparison to 151 previously reported necropsy patients. *Am Heart J* 1982;104:115.

189. Marsalese DL, Moodie DS, Vacante M, et al. Marfan syndrome: natural history and long-term follow-up of cardiovascular involvement. *J Am Coll Cardiol* 1989;14:422.

190. Silverman DI, Burton KJ, Gray J, et al. Life expectancy in the Marfan syndrome. *Am J Cardiol* 1995;75:157.

191. Brown OR, DeMots H, Kloster FE, et al. Aortic root dilatation and mitral valve prolapse in Marfan syndrome: an echocardiographic study. *Circulation* 1975;52:651.

192. Come PC, Fortuin NJ, White RI, et al. Echocardiographic assessment of cardiovascular abnormalities in the Marfan syndrome: comparison with clinical findings and with roentgenographic estimation of aortic root size. *Am J Med* 1983;74:465.

193. Hirata K, Triposkiadis F, Sparks E, et al. The Marfan syndrome: abnormal aortic elastic properties. *J Am Coll Cardiol* 1991;18:57.

194. Jeremy RW, Huang H, Hwa J, et al. Relation between age, arterial distensibility, and aortic dilatation in the Marfan syndrome. *Am J Cardiol* 1994;74:369.

195. Roman MJ, Rosen SE, Kramer-Fox R, et al. Prognostic significance of the pattern of aortic root dilation in the Marfan syndrome. *J Am Coll Cardiol* 1993;22:1470.

196. Gott VL, Pyeritz RE, Magovern GJ Jr, et al. Surgical treatment of aneurysms of the ascending aorta in the Marfan syndrome: results of composite-graft repair in 50 patients. *N Engl J Med* 1986;314:1070.

197. Pyeritz RE. Maternal and fetal complications of pregnancy in the Marfan syndrome. *Am J Med* 1981;71:784.

198. Elkayam U, Ostrzega E, Shotan A, et al. Cardiovascular problems in pregnant women with the Marfan syndrome. *Ann Intern Med* 1995;123:117.

199. Pyeritz RE, Wappel MA. Mitral valve dysfunction in the Marfan syndrome: clinical and echocardiographic study of prevalence and natural history. *Am J Med* 1983;74:797.

200. Ose L, McKusick VA. Prophylactic use of propranolol in the Marfan syndrome to prevent aortic dissection. *Birth Defects* 1977;13:163.

201. Rosen SE, Roman MJ, Kramer-Fox R, et al. The effect of chronic beta-blockade therapy on aortic root dilatation in patients with the Marfan syndrome. *Am J Genet* 1993;47:157.

202. Shores J, Berger KR, Pyeritz RE. Progression of aortic dilatation and the benefit of long-term b-adrenergic blockade in Marfan syndrome. *N Engl J Med* 1994;330:1335.

203. Salim MA, Alpert BS, Ward JC, et al. Effect of beta-adrenergic blockade on aortic root rate of dilation in the Marfan syndrome. *Am J Cardiol* 1994;74:629.

204. Czermak BV, Waldenberger P, Fraedrich G, et al. Treatment of Stanford type B aortic dissection with stent grafts: preliminary results. *Radiology* 2000;217:544.

205. Spittell PC, Ehrsam JE, Seward JB. Screening for abdominal aortic aneurysm during transthoracic echocardiography in a hypertensive patient population. *J Am Soc Echocardiogr* 1997;10:722.

206. Suzuki T, Katoh H, Tsuchio Y, et al. Diagnostic implications of elevated levels of smooth-muscle myosin heavy-chain protein in acute aortic dissection. *Ann Intern Med* 2000;133:537.

NONINVASIVE ASSESSMENT OF VASCULAR DISEASE

D. EUGENE STRANDNESS, JR.

OVERVIEW

This chapter reviews the application of the currently available indirect and direct methods of noninvasive testing that have been shown to be of value in the evaluation of peripheral vascular disease. The diseases considered include those most commonly seen in the practice of the cardiovascular specialist. The reader can determine which testing procedure(s) will best fit the patient population that he or she is addressing. It should also be evident how useful these testing procedures can be for evaluating the results of interventional therapy as well as the natural history of peripheral vascular disease without any form of intervention.

HISTORICAL PERSPECTIVE

Vascular diseases are broadly defined as afflictions of the arterial and venous system, the lymphatics, and the microcirculation. For the purpose of this chapter, those that involve the large- and medium-sized arteries are reviewed.

D. E. Strandness, Jr.: Department of Surgery, University of Washington Medical Center, Seattle, Washington (Deceased)

The objective evaluation of peripheral vascular disease is finally reaching a mature stage. Although indirect and direct noninvasive methods were slow to be accepted, they have now become a daily part of our practice. As is noted in this chapter, there is increasing evidence that angiographic methods can be bypassed for diagnostic reasons and before surgical intervention. This is a remarkable change in practice and is one that will continue into the future. It is also evident that the natural history of vascular disease as well as the outcome following any form of intervention can be done by noninvasive means. It is no longer acceptable to document outcome based on physician interpretation alone without confirmatory studies, which are the topic of this chapter.

One of the first methods of objectively assessing arterial perfusion to the limbs was to assess the ankle systolic blood pressure and relate it to the arm systolic blood pressure [ankle/brachial index (ABI)] (1,2). This very simple determination was slow to become accepted until it was realized that it could provide an immediate indication of success or failure of arterial reconstructions. It is now a standard method to document outcome and monitor disease progression. ❦ q69

Ultrasound

The introduction of ultrasound undoubtedly had the greatest impact on the field of noninvasive assessment. The first development of major importance was the observation by Satomura (6) that ultrasound could be transmitted through the skin to detect frequency shifts in flowing blood. He showed that moving blood would shift the frequency of the transmitted ultrasound in a manner that could be detected and recorded. This was a remarkable observation that changed the entire picture with regard to the investigation of blood flow. Our group very quickly picked up on this method and developed the first device that could be used to detect arterial and venous blood flow from all levels of the limb (7,8). However, it had several major problems and drawbacks. It was nondirectional, and the observer could not always be sure which vessel was being interrogated by the method. However, one of its major advantages in its simplest format was that it could also be used to measure ankle systolic blood pressure. Even today, this is one of its most common applications.

One of the greatest concerns with the earliest systems was that the observer had to train his or her ear to interpret arterial and venous blood flow patterns. Although the normal and abnormal velocity patterns could be recognized, it was not possible to present the earliest systems in an understandable analog format that could be made from any desired recording site. This greatly hampered the rapid acceptance of the method.

Progress was rapid in this field, going from the simple continuous wave (CW) Doppler to the pulsed system (9), which permitted selective sampling from many depths along the path of the sound beam. In addition, it became possible to develop systems that would permit an accurate determination of the direction of blood flow (10). This innovation was

quickly followed by the development of ultrasonic arteriography (11), which, by combining the pulsed Doppler with a position sensing arm, could be used to depict the anatomy of the flowing blood in any accessible arterial segment. This worked, but it was tedious to use and subject to numerous artifacts related to patient motion, depth, and anatomy of the underlying artery. It was quite clear that the best solution would be to combine the value of the ultrasonic B-mode image with a pulsed Doppler integrated into the system. This was accomplished in 1974 (12,13). Once this was done, the progress depended more on technology than anything else, and it was rapid. By the 1980s, the method was being widely applied to study disease in the large- and medium-sized vessels, wherever it was found. This was the most important development in this century, as it relates to the noninvasive study of diseases of the arterial and venous circulation. This fact will become evident as this chapter evolves.

INDIRECT NONINVASIVE TESTING

Beginning in the late 1960s, numerous indirect methods were introduced for the study of arterial and venous function (5,8,14–17). By definition, an indirect method is one that derives its value and information from physiologic sensors placed on a limb. These sensors can be used to obtain information on pressure and flow. From this information, it is possible to document important aspects of vascular function. All of these methods are used to measure systolic limb blood pressure, monitor digit/limb pulse volume changes, and assess (either qualitatively or quantitatively) limb blood flow.

Plethysmography

Systolic Blood Pressures

Systolic blood pressures are commonly expressed as absolute values or as a ratio to that recorded from the arm, often referred to as the *ABI* or *toe systolic/brachial index (TSPI)* [❦ q70].

1. *Ankle.* Normally, the systolic pressure at the ankle is higher than that recorded from the arm. This gives an ABI of greater than 1.0. For clinical purposes the value that is normally taken to indicate that peripheral arterial occlusive disease (PAOD) is present is less than 0.90. The variability in the measurement is ±0.15% (23,24).
2. *Toe.* Toe measurements are most commonly taken in diabetics, in whom medial calcification of the tibial and peroneal arteries is common. When this occurs, the ABI is falsely high. The normal TSPI is greater than 0.60. The variability in measurement is ±0.17%.
3. *Segmental pressures.* It is possible to measure pressures at the ankle, calf, above knee, and upper thigh. This is done by cuffs that are placed in these locations with the

sensor on the toe. The segmental pressures are used to define the level of occlusive involvement (*e*Fig. 109.0.1). This method has been replaced by ultrasonic duplex scanning in most laboratories (5).

4. *Absolute pressure levels.* It is important not only to assess the ABI and TSPI, but also to record the actual number, because it may have value from a clinical standpoint. For example, an absolute pressure of greater than 50 mm Hg is found with excellent collateral circulation. The absolute levels can also be useful in predicting when an open lesion might heal.

The ankle or toe pressures should also be measured from the arm using the same method. It is not advisable to use the stethoscopic measured arm pressure for calculation of either the ABI or the TSPI. It is now apparent that this simple measurement can be a good marker for atherosclerosis in other areas, such as the coronary/carotid artery.

Exercise Testing

The pressure recordings can be used to test the effect of exercise. Normally, the ankle systolic pressure does not decrease with moderate treadmill exercise. If occlusive disease and intermittent claudication occur, there is a drop in the ankle systolic pressure and a delayed recovery time (17,25–27). The time it takes for the ankle systolic pressure to recover is referred to as the *period of postexercise hyperemia.* It is not uncommon in cases of very severe claudication for the recovery to take more than 20 minutes.

Continuous Wave Doppler

With the development of Doppler systems, it became possible to generate information on the arterial and venous flow patterns in health and disease (8,14). The advantage of these simple systems is that they can be used at the bedside to measure ankle systolic blood pressure and assess the arterial flow patterns from the level of the tibial arteries to the external iliac artery in the leg and from the palmar circulation to the subclavian in the arm. The disadvantage of this method is that its use depends on a subjective interpretation of the audible velocity signals. However, the incorporation of this into imaging systems has produced a powerful diagnostic method that is now widely used.

COMMONLY PERFORMED TESTING PROCEDURES: ARTERIAL

Limb Blood Pressures

When a patient is first seen and suspected of having PAOD, it is necessary to measure the ABI, which provides confirmation of the presence of disease but also gives a rough index of its severity. Although presence or absence of peripheral pulses has been the major physical finding in documenting the presence of occlusive disease, this is not sufficiently sensitive or specific. That is why the simple measurement of ankle pressure and the ABI is so important. The criteria that are commonly used are as follows (28):

1. Abnormal levels are those less than 0.90.
2. An ABI of greater than 0.50 is most commonly seen with single-segment disease.
3. An ABI of less than 0.50 is commonly observed with multisegment disease.
4. For follow-up, a decrease of greater than 0.15 is consistent with disease progression. An ABI increase of greater than 0.15 is indicative of improvement in the collateral circulation.
5. If the ankle arteries are incompressible or the patient is a diabetic, the TSPI should be measured. As noted previously, this is normally greater than 0.60 (23).
6. In patients in whom it is not clear if the exercise-induced pain is due to arterial disease or some neurospinal cause, it is necessary to perform an exercise test (29). If an exercise test is performed, a normal ankle blood response is a drop of less than 20% from baseline, with recovery in less than 3 minutes. The treadmill walking time used is 2.0 mph on a 12% grade. For patients with suspected arterial disease, the maximal walking time used is 5 minutes, because this is sufficient to bring out any of the hemodynamic abnormalities. Most patients cannot walk this long even at this low workload. It is common practice to calculate the ABI after exercise, but this should not be done. The reason for this is that arm systolic pressure normally increases after exercise in proportion to the workload (17,25–27). Thus, it is only necessary to express the postexercise values in absolute units.

The most common error made by vascular laboratories is to calculate the ABI after exercise is completed. As has been noted, normally exercise induces an increase in arm systolic pressure, which, if used for the calculations, would lower the ABI, making the observer think that the testing is abnormal. After exercise, it is only necessary to measure the absolute levels of ankle systolic blood pressure.

Velocity Waveform Analysis

Because ultrasound can reach the major arteries of the upper and lower limbs, it is possible to use the CW Doppler to investigate the patterns at nearly all levels in which occlusive lesions are commonly found. Most use this method at the bedside and audibly interpret the back-scattered Doppler shift signals. It is also possible to obtain analog recordings that can provide hard copy verification. The most reliable method of analyzing the velocity patterns is by fast Fourier transform analysis. This method accurately presents the velocity information and the intensity of the back-scattered ultrasound. It is now the standard method used with Doppler ultrasound. The velocity patterns commonly observed follow.

Lower Limb

The normal velocity patterns exhibit a triphasic flow pattern from the level of the abdominal aorta to the tibial arteries at the ankle (Fig. 109.1). The three components are forward, reverse, and forward flow. If arterial occlusion is present, there will be no detectable signals from the site of involvement. Distal to the occlusion is damping of the arterial velocity patterns, with recordings showing a monophasic pattern (*e*Fig. 109.1.1). This is easily recognized by its audible characteristics.

Upper Limb

The only differences seen in the upper limb in normal subjects relate to the reverse flow component that is observed

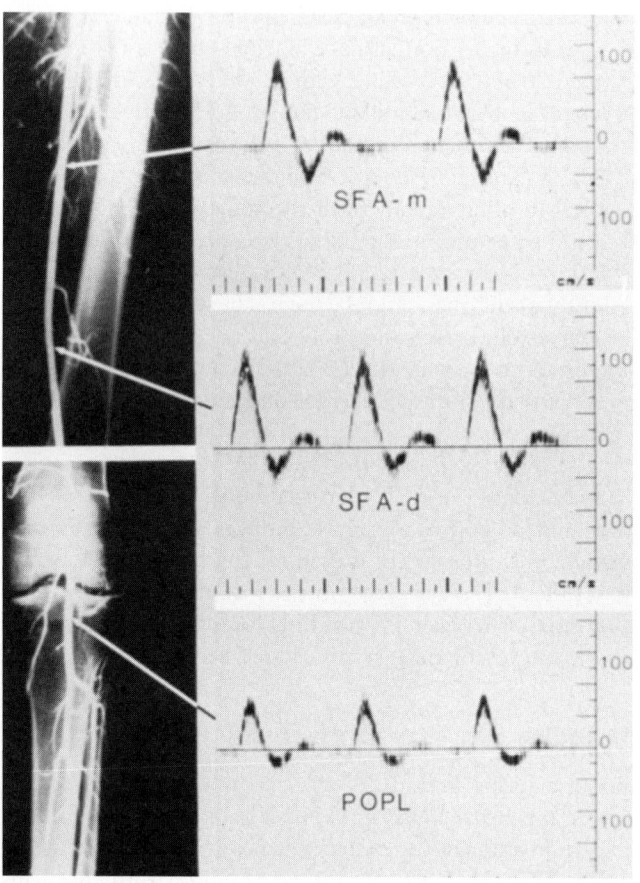

FIGURE 109.1 Hemodynamics of the normal arterial system. The normal arterial velocity patterns from the level of the abdominal aorta to the tibial arteries at the ankle are similar to those shown here. Flow is forward-reverse-forward, with a clear window beneath the systolic peak. POPL, popliteal artery; SFA-d, distal superficial femoral artery; SFA-m, medial superficial femoral artery. (From Strandness DE Jr. *Duplex scanning in vascular disorders,* 2nd ed. New York: Raven Press, 1993, with permission.)

in the radial and ulnar arteries. Up to 50% of normal subjects do not have a reverse flow component at this level. The end diastolic velocity is above zero, and the waveform itself is biphasic. This is due to the fact that resistance to flow is lower than in those with the triphasic waveform. With arterial occlusion are monophasic flow patterns, as observed in the lower limb.

DIRECT NONINVASIVE TESTING

Ultrasonic Duplex Scanning

The major advance in vascular testing was the development of ultrasonic duplex scanning (12,13,34,35). The method takes advantage of two ultrasonic methods, B-mode imaging and pulsed Doppler, by combining them into a single system. The major advantage of the method is that the imaging permits selective and accurate placement of the sample volume of the pulsed Doppler to sites of interest. The Doppler components of the system can now be expressed by color Doppler, power Doppler real-time fast Fourier transform spectral analysis that is used to document the velocity patterns at specific sites (36–40).

Carotid Artery Screening

One of the more common problems that needs evaluation is extracranial atherosclerosis. Although there are exceptions, its most common site of involvement is the carotid bifurcation. At this site, the plaque takes its origin in the posterolateral aspect of the bulb. As it evolves, it gradually enlarges to encompass the entire bulb and undergoes degeneration to become the complicated plaque. In this form, the lesion increasingly narrows the artery, and there is frequent loss of surface covering (ulceration). At these sites, the plaque can rupture to release emboli or provide the nidus for thrombosis of the internal carotid artery to occur. Both of these events are common causes of transient ischemic attacks (TIAs) and strokes (41–44).

Several aspects of carotid bifurcation disease are of great interest to all cardiovascular specialists.

1. It is a common cause of stroke.
2. The results of four large, randomized clinical trials have demonstrated that carotid endarterectomy is superior to conventional medical therapy in the prevention of stroke (45–49).
3. Evidence has been found that the stroke rate following arteriography is comparable to that secondary to carotid endarterectomy.
4. The incidence of carotid disease is high in patients with coronary artery disease and peripheral artery disease.
5. Ultrasonic duplex scanning is the preferred method of screening.

RESULTS OF CLINICAL TRIALS

During the 1980s, there was considerable skepticism about the role of carotid endarterectomy in the prevention of stroke. Many prominent neurologists essentially asked for a moratorium on the operation until its efficacy had been tested by prospective clinical trials (49–54). As a result of this skepticism, four major trials were undertaken—two in symptomatic patients and two in asymptomatic patients. These trials are now finished; therefore, it is possible to review the results and place their conclusions in proper perspective. The major issue has now been resolved, which is that carotid endarterectomy is superior to conventional medical therapy for certain categories of lesions. However, some problems remain that affect our practice in this area. A brief summary of the results details the issues involved.

Impact of Clinical Trials on Clinical Approach

Although the trials all suggest that endarterectomy is of benefit in the prevention of stroke, they have also created a great deal of confusion. The following questions have arisen.

1. Who should be screened? Some answers are known: (a) All patients who have symptoms that suggest carotid artery disease, (b) patients with bruits (57), and (c) individuals who are in a high-risk category for stroke should be screened. These include patients who are undergoing coronary artery bypass grafting, those with peripheral vascular disease, type 2 diabetics with a history of cardiovascular disease, and patients with renovascular hypertension (58,59). However, many questions also remain.

Considerable disagreement is found as to who should be screened. A consortium of Canadian neurologists addressed this issue and concluded that there was very little level 1 evidence to suggest screening even for patients who are normally considered to be at risk (60). This runs contrary to most specialists who deal with atherosclerotic disease in many different arterial circulations. It is clear that the presence of disease in one of the major vascular beds (coronary, peripheral, and carotid) is very likely to be associated with disease that is potentially serious in other areas. However, there is unlikely to be good evidence to suggest that screening of the general population is of value.

2. What screening procedure should be used? The NASCET investigators have suggested that ultrasound is not reliable enough to warrant its use. They maintain that contrast arteriography remains the best available method. Unfortunately, the ultrasound data from the NASCET study were seriously flawed, because there was no attempt at quality control (61).

3. When should arteriography be done? This is important because cerebral arteriography is not only costly but dangerous as well. In recent years, there has been a shift

away from its routine use even in symptomatic patients, with more reliance on duplex ultrasound. In addition, there is growing evidence that carotid endarterectomy can be safely done on the basis of ultrasound alone when it is properly performed and interpreted (62–65).

4. Which cases demand that an arteriogram be done? This occurs in approximately 10% of cases (62): (a) unusual anatomy (coils and kinks) in which interpretation of the ultrasound studies is difficult, (b) cases in which the disease is not confined to the bulb, and (c) instances in which so much calcium is in the bulb that it is difficult to estimate the degree of stenosis.

5. What type of arteriogram should be done, and how should it be read? Selective arteriography is the most commonly done, but it provides only limited views of the bulb. Which artery should be taken as the normal reference artery? At present, most still use the distal internal carotid artery, but one must recognize that it greatly underestimates the degree of involvement. The European group has suggested that the common carotid artery now be used as the normal reference artery, but this has been rejected by the NASCET group (66,67).

6. How can one use the conflicting data on degree of diameter reduction from the clinical trials? For example, how can a 50% or 60% diameter reduction found in the VAT (47) and ACAS (48) trials be reconciled against the higher degree of stenosis found in NASCET (45) and ECST (45)? As noted previously, this is largely related to the methodology used in terms of the ultrasound and the arteriography that was used. A fact of great importance is the intra- and interobserver variability found with all of these studies. It is not possible to define with great precision the exact degree of stenosis by any of the present means at hand. For arteriography, this can be comfortably assumed to be in the ±20% range (68). In the case of ultrasound, it has been long recognized that classification of disease into rather broad categories of clinical relevance made sense. This has proved to be true.

7. What impact is MRA going to have on this field? One must remember that it is also an arteriogram in the sense that interpretation of the presented images is very similar. In addition, the signal dropout problem remains an important issue that cannot be disregarded. This can make the estimate of the true degree of diameter reduction a very difficult problem.

Current Clinical Approach

It is obvious that the cutoff points for each of the clinical trials is very confusing, because they seem to disagree in many respects. For example, why should a 50% or 60% diameter reduction of the carotid artery be of surgical importance in an asymptomatic patient but not apply to a symptomatic patient? This makes no sense, but that is what we are forced to live with, given the results of the randomized trials. Although calipers were used in the trials to estimate the degree of narrowing, this is not a common procedure in clinical practice.

When we introduced the use of duplex ultrasound for the evaluation of carotid artery disease, it was necessary to adapt the velocity criteria for varying degrees of stenosis (35,39,57,65). In addition, it became apparent that the method could not be used to determine precisely the degree of narrowing but could be usefully applied to determine categories of narrowing that might have relevance to clinical practice. We went through several validation trials that compared our results with cut-film selective carotid arteriograms that also included views of the aortic arch, three views of the bulb, the carotid siphon, and intracranial views (39,69,70). The categories finally arrived at (39) have been modified slightly to make them more useful clinically. The current classification scheme is as follows:

1. *Normal.* No evidence has been found on B-mode imaging of a lesion in the posterolateral aspect of the bulb. In addition, boundary layer separation has to be present.
2. *Less than 50% stenosis.* Plaque is present (with or without acoustical shadowing), but the peak systolic velocity does not exceed 125 cm per second at the site of narrowing.
3. *Narrowing of 50% to 79%.* For this category of disease, the peak systolic velocity at the site of greatest narrowing is greater than 125 cm per second, with an end diastolic velocity of less than 140 cm per second (*e*Fig. 109.1.6).
4. *Stenosis of 80% to 99%.* The end diastolic velocity exceeds 140 cm per second.
5. *Occlusion.* No detectable flow in the internal carotid artery.

How did duplex ultrasound using these criteria compare with arteriography? The best way of comparing two diagnostic tests is to calculate the kappa statistic. If there is perfect agreement, the kappa value is 1.0. If there is random distribution of values, the kappa value is 0.0. For one neuroradiologist reading the films a second time, the kappa statistic is 0.711 ± 0.054. For two neuroradiologists reading the same films, the kappa statistic is 0.568 ± 0.058. For duplex scanning and one radiologist, the kappa statistic is 0.769 ± 0.039. For most diagnostic tests used in medicine, kappa values in the range of 0.5 to 0.8 are considered to be satisfactory.

How should the data be used clinically? After several years of experience, we came to the following conclusions based on natural history studies (57,71–74):

1. The less than 50% diameter reducing lesions are generally of little clinical relevance and can be followed by an annual examination to document progression versus stability.
2. The 50% to 79% stenosis in an asymptomatic patient is also a relatively benign lesion, but it warrants closer follow-up. We recommend that these patients have a study performed every 6 months to assess stability of the lesion. If it progresses, the patient should be considered for endarterectomy (*e*Fig. 109.1.7).
3. The 80% to 99% lesions are particularly dangerous and, in our view, should be considered candidates for operation.
4. The total occlusions cannot be opened surgically. However, even with an asymptomatic occlusion, the annual stroke rate on the side of the occlusion is in the range of 2% per year.

The clinical trials have posed new problems in terms of classification by ultrasound. However, it is possible to estimate the degree of stenosis defined by the trials without a major change in how the study is done. The method simply requires that the user divide the peak systolic velocity at the site of the stenosis by that found in the common carotid artery. Using this method, it has been possible to determine the 60% and 70% cutoff points defined by ACAS and NASCET.

Although one can use different cutoff points for the 60% cutoff, the author favors using a value of 3.2. This gives a positive predictive value of 85%, with a negative predictive value of 93% and overall accuracy of 89% (75).

For greater than 70% stenosis, the ratio is 4.0. This provides a positive predictive value of 76%, with a negative predictive value of 96% and overall accuracy of 88% (76).

It is obvious by using receiver operator curves that different ratios can be used depending on one's personal approach to patients who might be candidates for operation. With symptomatic patients, one would not want to miss the appropriate patient. In asymptomatic patients, it is important to limit the number of invasive studies whenever possible or reasonable (75,76).

What about plaque morphology as determined by ultrasound and arteriography (42,77–80)? Can this be used as a surrogate finding to tell the physician which direction to go (*e*Fig. 109.1.8)? Although it is agreed that loss of surface covering (ulceration) is a common cause for the accumulation of thrombotic debris and embolization, none of the current imaging methods is sufficiently sensitive to make them accurate enough to make this determination. Thus, one is forced at the present time to use the degree of narrowing as the sole determinant of when one should proceed with operation. Another common concept is that intraplaque hemorrhage precedes the sudden increase in size of a lesion rendering the patient symptomatic (81,82). This has also been discounted. Our own studies suggest that the most important factor to determine outcome of a stenotic lesion is the fibrous cap (83–88). If it remains intact, one has little to worry about. On the other hand, if it disrupts, the outcome depends on the material that is forced into the cerebral circulation. This could be thrombus, necrotic debris with cholesterol crystals, or lipid. The challenge over the next decade is to develop methods of studying the fibrous cap *in vivo*.

MRA is the latest method that is available for visualization of the carotid bifurcation. It is attractive because it is totally noninvasive and offers the opportunity of replacing conventional arteriography that will totally eliminate the risk and also lower the cost. The problem, however, is as shown in *e*Figure 109.1.9. As the degree of stenosis increases, there is often signal dropout, making it impossible to estimate the degree of diameter reduction. ❦ q71

UPPER AND LOWER EXTREMITY ARTERIAL DISEASE

Arm

At the outset, it can be stated with certainty that the upper extremity is largely spared the ravages of atherosclerosis, except for the involvement of the subclavian artery at its origin. Even when the subclavian artery is totally occluded, it is unusual for this to lead to any symptoms at all. Surprisingly, arm claudication is rare, probably due to the fact that the vertebral artery, which serves as an excellent collateral source of blood to the arm, is sufficient to maintain the arm pain free even with exercise. If there is an anomalous origin of the vertebral artery from the arch of the aorta, claudication is commonly seen. However, this is rare (89).

What about the role of reverse flow in the vertebral artery and its place in the development of vertebrobasilar insufficiency? Again, although reverse flow is common in the vertebral artery with subclavian artery disease, it is rarely the cause of posterior circulation symptoms.

How does one recognize or suspect the presence of a subclavian artery stenosis or occlusion? Several clues may be found, some of which are as follows:

1. The presence of a supraclavicular bruit.
2. A differential in arm systolic pressure of 15 mm Hg or greater on the side of the disease.
3. A monophasic brachial artery velocity pattern.
4. The demonstration of a stenosis or occlusion by duplex scanning. With this method, it is also possible to document the direction of blood flow in the ipsilateral vertebral artery.

Leg

PAOD is very common in the Western world. The atherosclerosis that is responsible affects specific arteries more frequently than others and is magnified in the presence of diabetes. Although specific problems are associated with this disease, it must be recognized that it can be present without producing any symptoms at all. When it is a clinical problem, it presents in one or two ways, or both. The most common is pain with walking (intermittent claudication) or with critical ischemia (90,91). The latter is simply

described as ischemia that is sufficient to warrant an amputation unless more blood can be brought to the limb.

It is important to emphasize the differences in the disease patterns between diabetics and nondiabetics. These are as follows:

1. A peripheral neuropathy is seen in up to 40% of patients with diabetes mellitus who also have PAOD (92).
2. In diabetics, there is a much higher incidence of medial calcification of the tibial and peroneal arteries (23).
3. The presence of medial calcification and the occlusive lesions of atherosclerosis are not related.
4. The occlusive lesions are much more common in the tibial and peroneal arteries of diabetics, with similar extent of involvement of the superficial femoral artery. Interestingly, less occlusive disease is found in the aorto-iliac segments in diabetic patients (92,93).

These factors are important to understand when considering the need for, or the understanding of, the noninvasive tests that are to be performed. It is necessary to realize that the indirect and direct testing procedures are of value here. It should be understood that patients with acute ischemia (due to emboli or thrombosis) demand immediate attention when compared to those with the chronic form of the disease.

Acute Limb Ischemia

When a patient has acute limb ischemia, the physician has to provide immediate action, because delays lead to progressive ischemia and tissue loss. In the past, the majority of cases of acute ischemia were secondary to emboli from the heart. Although this still occurs, acute thrombosis in the setting of atherosclerosis or from emboli that arise from an ulcerated plaque is much more common. The common complaints in this setting are pain, paresthesias, paralysis plus pallor, and pulselessness. If the acute ischemia is critical, the physician must realize that progressive tissue death will begin within the 4- to 6-hour time frame. It is also important to realize that the muscles begin to die first, with the skin coming later. ❦ q72

Chronic Limb Ischemia

Patients who present with either intermittent claudication or critical ischemia are first evaluated by the standard clinical evaluation and measurement of the ABI. If some form of intervention is going to be required, it has become a standard practice to carry out an ultrasonic duplex scan (94–98). With improvement in the technology and availability of a wide variety of transmitting frequencies and scan heads, it is now possible to assess the arterial flow from the level of the abdominal aorta to the tibial arteries at the ankle. From a clinical standpoint, the lesions that are of interest are total occlusions and stenoses that narrow the artery by more than

50% in terms of diameter reduction. The scans are done with the following guidelines in mind (94):

1. Isolated stenoses/short occlusions of the aorta/common iliac arteries are best treated by angioplasty.
2. Long occlusions of the aorto-iliac system are best treated by operative means.
3. Lesions that are distal to the inguinal ligament are best treated by surgical means.
4. Combined disease of the aorto-iliac and femoropopliteal segment can best be treated by angioplasty for the proximal lesions and bypass grafting for the below–inguinal ligament lesions.

The screening procedure used relies primarily on the following parameters for making a determination of the degree of involvement:

1. A triphasic velocity waveform is good evidence of a normal arterial system proximal to the recording site (89).
2. The degree of stenosis is estimated by noting the following changes.
3. For the stenoses that are less than 50% in terms of diameter reduction, the velocity pattern at the site of narrowing shows an increase of 30% to 100% in the peak systolic velocity with preservation of the reverse flow component (94,95,97).
4. For greater than 50% stenosis, the peak systolic velocity increases by more than 100% with loss of the reverse flow component (94,99) (Fig. 109.2).
5. With total occlusion, no flow is detected.

The prospective studies that have been done comparing the results with arteriography have given the results shown in Table 109.1. This scanning procedure has been useful not only in identifying the procedure that is most likely to succeed but in providing the necessary baseline data to assess the long-term outcome. Another major advantage of duplex scanning is that it is possible to carry out saphenous vein mapping. The most satisfactory method of treating lesions distal to the inguinal ligament is to use the saphenous vein. However, it is not possible to assess its suitability in terms of diameter and length without some imaging method. Duplex is ideal because it can provide both bits of

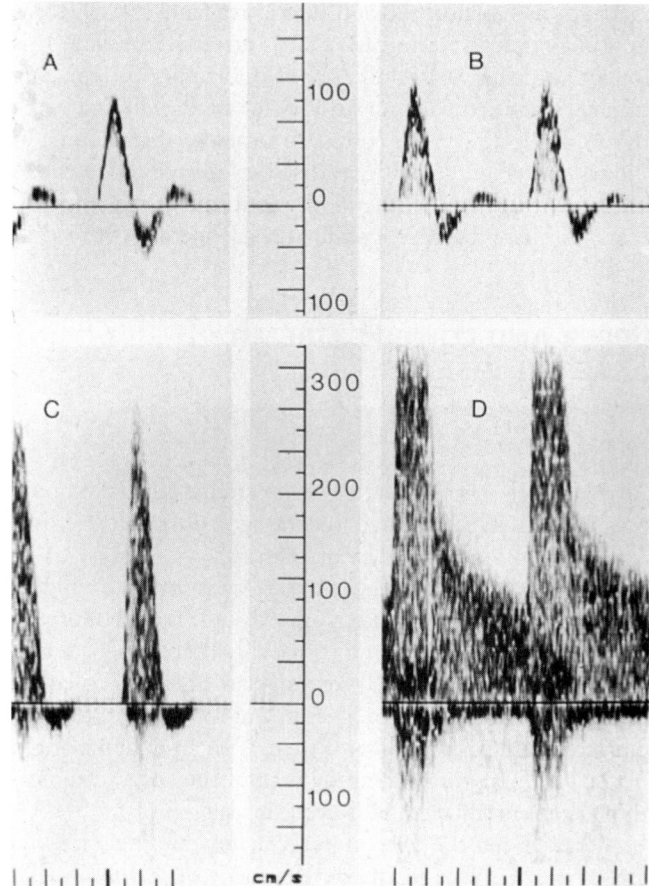

FIGURE 109.2 Velocity patterns recorded from peripheral arteries. In **A**, a normal triphasic waveform is shown. With a 1% to 19% narrowing (**B**), the only change observed is some slight spectral broadening. When the stenosis is in the 16% to 49% diameter reducing range (**C**), there is a peak systolic velocity change between 30% and 100% from the immediately adjacent proximal artery. Flow reversal is often preserved, but spectral broadening will be noted. With a greater than 50% stenosis (**D**), the peak systolic velocity increases by an amount greater than 100% from the adjacent proximal artery. The reverse flow is now gone, and there is marked spectral broadening. (From Strandness DE Jr. *Duplex scanning in vascular disorders*, 2nd ed. New York: Raven Press, 1993, with permission.)

information along with marking their course on the skin (100). In instances in which the leg veins may be inadequate, or if they had been previously stripped or used for other bypass procedures, it is also possible to scan the arms

TABLE 109.1 COMPARISON BETWEEN ULTRASONIC DUPLEX SCANNING AND ARTERIOGRAPHY IN DETECTING A LESS THAN OR GREATER THAN 50% DIAMETER REDUCING STENOSIS

Arterial segment	Sensitivity (%)	Specificity (%)	Positive predictive value (%)	Negative predictive value (%)
Iliac	94	96	94	96
Common femoral	66	100	100	91
Profunda	33	91	40	88
Superficial femoral—proximal	95	100	100	93
Superficial femoral—mid	100	84	82	100
Superficial femoral—distal	91	85	78	94
Popliteal	91	85	78	94
All segments	87	94	88	93

for suitable conduits. This procedure also is being used by cardiac surgeons, who may need to know the status of available veins for coronary bypass grafting. ❧ q73

VISCERAL ARTERIAL STUDIES

The two common areas in the abdomen that are frequently the sites of atherosclerotic narrowing and occlusion are the mesenteric arteries and the renal arteries.

Mesenteric Arteries

Involvement of the mesenteric arteries (celiac, superior, and inferior mesenteric arteries) is responsible for two major clinical problems: acute mesenteric ischemia and chronic mesenteric angina (fear of food syndrome) (101–106). Although involvement of these arteries is common, the clinical syndromes are uncommon due to the excellent collateral circulation that exists between the major inputs to the gut. In fact, it is now well appreciated that one must have involvement of all three major vessels for intestinal angina to occur. Acute mesenteric ischemia is most often secondary to embolic occlusion and results in a dramatic clinical presentation that demands immediate attention. The urgency of this situation does not lend itself to noninvasive studies.

Chronic mesenteric angina is represented by the fear of food syndrome. Patients find that cramping abdominal pain and diarrhea develop when they eat. This results in dramatic weight loss. Although the diagnosis may be quite clear in some instances, in many cases symptoms develop that suggest the diagnosis and some independent method of evaluation is demanded. The only established method of making this diagnosis is to perform lateral aortography with visualization of the origins and the first few centimeters of the celiac and superior mesenteric arteries (*e*Fig. 109.2.2). The advantage of duplex scanning is that the same arteries can be interrogated to assess their status. In the author's experience, if the syndrome is present, there must be very-high-grade stenoses or occlusions of both of these vessels (101–106). Recently, it has also been possible to assess the inferior mesenteric artery.

Renal Arteries

Although patients with renovascular hypertension constitute approximately 5% of the total population with hypertension, detection by noninvasive means has traditionally been difficult (107). In fact, it is agreed that the most certain method of establishing disease of the renal arteries has been arteriography. Most screening tests have not been very useful because of their poor predictive value. With the availability of lower-frequency scan heads (2.0 to 3.5 MHz) and color Doppler, it is not only possible to reach the renal arteries but to assess the presence of disease and its contribution to the parenchyma.

TABLE 109.2 RESULTS OF USING 180-CM-PER-SECOND PEAK SYSTOLIC VELOCITY FOR THE CUTOFF POINT OF DETECTING A RENAL ARTERY STENOSIS[a]

Duplex	Normal	Disease	Total
Velocity <180 cm/s	9	4	13
Velocity >180 cm/s	1	60	61
Total	10	64	74

[a]Sensitivity: 94%; specificity: 90%; accuracy: 93%.

The guidelines that have been worked out for detecting and grading the degree of stenosis are as follows:

1. The normal peak systolic velocity in the abdominal aorta at the level of the renal arteries is in the range of 100 cm per second. The variability is rather broad (±20%), making the absolute values less useful for quantitating the degree of stenosis.
2. To avoid unnecessary false-positive tests that might lead to arteriography, we elected to use a peak systolic velocity of 180 cm per second as the cutoff point for detecting narrowing. This value is 2.5 standard deviations above normal. If, at any point along the length of the renal artery, a value greater than 180 cm per second is found, the patient is classified as having renal artery stenosis (108) (Table 109.2).
3. Because the development of hypertension depends on the presence of a high-grade stenosis (greater than 60% diameter reduction), it is important to have criteria for detecting this degree of narrowing. It has been found that if the ratio of the peak systolic velocity at the site of the stenosis divided by that recorded from the aorta at the level of the renal artery (the renal-aortic ratio) exceeds 3.5, the stenosis is classified as being greater than 60% in terms of diameter reduction (Table 109.3, Fig. 109.3).
4. The inability to detect flow from the renal artery and finding a kidney less than 9.0 cm in length are taken as evidence of renal artery occlusion.
5. It is also important to measure the end diastolic ratio, which is the peak systolic velocity divided by the end diastolic velocity. The normal value is 0.34. This should be recorded from the distal renal artery and the parenchyma of the kidney itself. It reflects the parenchymal renal resistance and may be useful in predicting the response to revascularization. In patients with fibromuscular dysplasia, the end diastolic ratio is always normal, whereas in patients with renal atherosclerosis, it is often low.
6. For all follow-up studies, it is important to assess renal length. It has been shown that with greater than 60% diameter reducing lesions, there is often a loss of renal mass. This fact may well indicate the need for earlier intervention to preserve renal function (109).

Considerable progress has been made in identifying lesions in the renal artery and in predicting the long-term

TABLE 109.3 COMPARISON OF DUPLEX SCANNING VERSUS ARTERIOGRAPHY
FOR DETECTION OF A GREATER THAN 60% DIAMETER REDUCING STENOSIS[a]

Duplex	<60% diameter reduction	>60% diameter reduction	Occluded	Total
RAR <3.5	15	3	1	19
RAR >3.5	11	45	0	56
Occluded	0	0	10	10
Total	26	48	11	85

RAR, renal-aortic ratio.
[a]Sensitivity: 92%; specificity: 58%; accuracy: 81%.

outcome without intervention. It is clear that the high-grade lesions not only are very prone to progress but are frequently followed by loss of renal mass (110,111). We have also come to realize the effect of parenchymal disease on the entire process and the results of intervention, be it surgical or interventional. Patients with atherosclerotic renal artery disease very commonly have arteriolar nephrosclerosis as a complicating feature. This makes the outcome of any form of intervention unpredictable. In contrast, patients with fibromuscular hyperplasia have an entirely different course. Although high-grade lesions and hypertension develop, parenchymal disease does not occur, and patients usually receive an excellent result from renal angioplasty. In addition, individuals with fibromuscular dysplasia do not progress to renal artery occlusion and do not end up in renal failure. ❧ q74

Vein Graft Surveillance

It has been found that the longevity of saphenous vein grafts that are used to bypass occlusions in the leg can be increased by frequent duplex ultrasound surveillance, particularly dur-

ing the first year (112–115). It has also been shown that up to 80% of vein grafts develop a lesion within the first 6 months. Not all of these fibromuscular lesions go on to narrow the graft progressively and lead to thrombosis, but by correcting the higher-grade lesions, the assisted secondary patency at 3 years will be in the range of 90% (*e*Fig. 109.3.1). The criteria used to define the degree of stenosis depend on the ratio of the peak systolic velocity just proximal to a lesion divided into that found at the site of the lesion. We have found that a ratio of 3:5 is predictive of a high-grade (greater than 75% diameter reduction) stenosis that should be corrected by either transluminal angioplasty or direct surgical repair.

COMMONLY PERFORMED PROCEDURES: VENOUS

Screening for Acute Deep Vein Thrombosis

The introduction of duplex ultrasound with color Doppler has revolutionized our diagnostic approach to this very

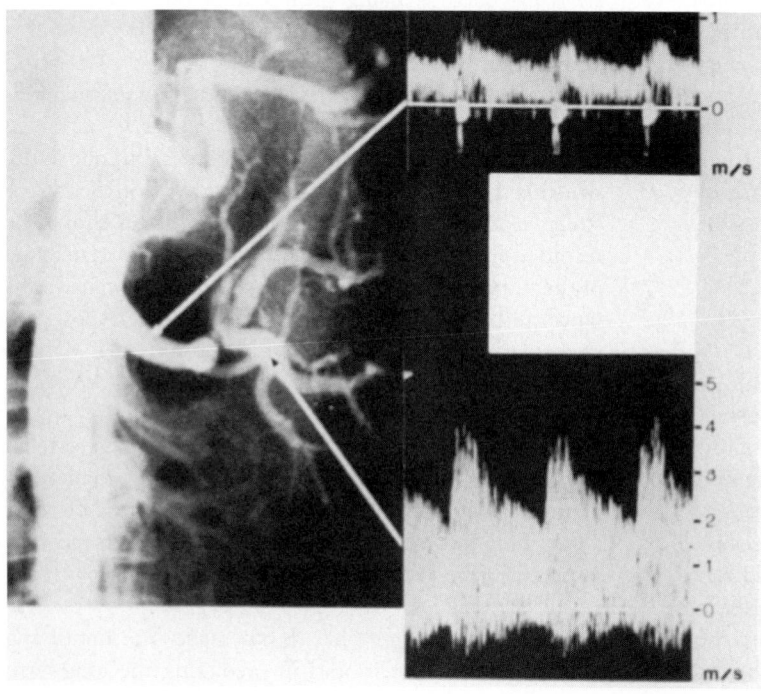

FIGURE 109.3 Velocity patterns recorded at the level of the renal hilus show a dramatic increase in peak systolic velocity (renal-aortic ratio less than 3.5). This is a case of fibromuscular hyperplasia (see text). (From Strandness DE Jr. *Duplex scanning in vascular disorders*, 2nd ed. New York: Raven Press; 1993, with permission.)

TABLE 109.4 ACCURACY OF THROMBUS VISUALIZATION AND INCOMPRESSIBILITY IN DETECTING ACUTE DEEP VEIN THROMBOSIS

	Contrast venography	Sensitivity (%)	Specificity (%)	Positive predictive value (%)	Negative predictive value (%)
Thrombus visualization	n = 38	19/38 (50)	11/12 (92)	19/20 (95)	11/30 (37)
Incompressibility	n = 38	30/38 (79)	8/12 (67)	30/34 (88)	8/16 (50)

important area of vascular disease (116,117). This method has, in fact, eliminated the need for contrast venography, which is a real advance in this field. To be successfully applied, the method takes advantage of two modalities, the B-mode image and the flow patterns. The criteria for each segment of the venous circulation are as follows:

1. Thrombus visualization. In 50% of cases of acute DVT, the thrombus itself can be visualized (*e*Fig. 109.3.2). Although it is tempting to try to age the thrombus on the basis of its echogenic characteristics, this must be done with care. It appears that the earlier thrombi are more uniformly echogenic, but this does not indicate the age of the thrombus or when it may have started.

2. Because not all thrombi can be seen on the image, the second maneuver that is carried out is to test the compressibility of the visualized segment. If the two walls of the vein can be completely coapted, it is assumed that no thrombi are present. In some areas, compression is not feasible. These include the superficial femoral vein in the adductor canal and the iliac veins and the inferior vena cava. One must depend on thrombus visualization and the flow patterns to establish the status of these segments.

3. As noted in the section Continuous Wave Doppler, the venous flow patterns are also very useful in establishing the presence of acute DVT (118). These, as noted, are related to the spontaneity of the flow and its relationship to respiration. The one area where flow cannot be used effectively is for the deep veins of the calf. Here, flow under resting conditions is so low that spontaneous venous flow signals may not be seen even in normal subjects. The criteria for occlusion depend on compressibility and the appearance of flow with augmentation that is performed by compressing the limb distal to the site of probe placement.

4. One area of concern at the time of the original appearance of this text was the problems related to studying the veins of the calf. These are small paired veins, and with imaging alone they are often difficult to visualize. However, with the availability of color Doppler, it is now feasible to study this area as well. It is also possible to document the status of the soleal sinuses and the gastrocnemial veins.

With the availability of this testing procedure, physicians are more willing to request the test. In our early experience with this method, the positive yield for the procedure was in the range of 25% (119). The overall accuracy of the method for the detection of acute venous thrombosis is shown in Table 109.4.

This is another area that is moving rapidly, in large part due to the availability of low-molecular-weight heparin, which permits some patients with DVT to be treated as outpatients. The sensitivity of the testing has led to the question of how to deal with isolated calf vein thrombosis. Is it necessary to treat and for how long? Opinion is divided on this subject due to the fact that thrombi below the knee rarely lead to serious and fatal pulmonary embolism. What is not known relates to the role of the veins in this location to the development of the postthrombotic syndrome. This question will be answered in the years to come.

Chronic Venous Disease

Patients who require some form of evaluation represent three major categories: those with primary varicose veins, those with secondary varicose veins, and those with the postthrombotic syndrome. Distinct ultrasonic features assist in proper classification of these patients. For each of these categories, it is necessary to establish the integrity of the venous valves at all levels of the limb (superficial and deep) (120). To do this, a variety of maneuvers can be used to establish valve competency. These are as follows:

1. Reflux with performance of Valsalva's maneuver. By suddenly increasing intraabdominal pressure, it is possible to detect reversal of flow in veins with incompetent valves. The problem with this maneuver is that one competent valve in the iliac veins may prevent the detection of incompetence in valves in the common femoral and superficial femoral vein. It is only reliable for the common and superficial femoral veins. This method does not permit quantification of the degree of reflux.

2. For the popliteal and distal vein valves, forceful limb compression is used. The principle is the same as for Valsalva's maneuver. The sudden creation of a reverse pressure gradient promotes reflux if the valves are unable to coapt completely.

3. To provide a quantitative method, a cuff method was developed that was performed in the upright position. The procedure is as follows (121,122): (a) Cuffs are placed at the thigh, below the knee, at the ankle, and on the foot, and (b) with the patient upright and the limb to be tested non-weight bearing, the cuffs are rapidly inflated to different pressures. For example, the 24-cm thigh cuff is inflated

to 80 mm Hg, the 12-cm calf and ankle cuff to 100 mm Hg, and the 7-cm foot cuff to 120 mm Hg. The key is rapid inflation and deflation. The inflation time is 3 seconds, with deflation taking only 0.3 second.

4. To document reflux, the duplex transducer is placed proximal to the cuff itself. With cuff deflation, there is a reversal of the pressure gradient, with reversal of flow attempting to replace the volume displaced by cuff inflation.

When this procedure was used on 30 normal legs, 95% of the times taken for venous valve closure were less than 0.5 second. The veins tested were the common femoral, superficial femoral, profunda femoris, popliteal, and posterior tibial at the calf and ankle level. This method has the advantage of examining the entire venous system segment by segment from the groin to the ankle. The greater and lesser saphenous veins can also be evaluated

These methods of study are used for the evaluation of the location and extent of valvular incompetence. This is particularly helpful for documenting the changes that occur with acute DVT, the effects of spontaneous thrombolysis, and the long-term sequelae of acute DVT (123–125).

Given the availability of duplex ultrasound for the sequential study of acute DVT, it became possible to follow patients on a regular basis from the time of the event to document the long-term outcome. One of the first things to be discovered was that spontaneous thrombolysis was much more common than was previously suspected and could have a dramatic effect on long-term outcome. Killewich et al. (123) found that among 21 patients followed sequentially, recanalization developed by 7 days in 44% and in 100% by 90 days. The percentage of initially involved segments that remained occluded decreased to a mean of 44% by 30 days and 14% by 90 days. This finding may well explain what Browse et al. had observed in 1981 (126). They noted that there did not appear to be any relationship between the extent of the original thrombosis and long-term outcome, namely, the development of the postthrombotic syndrome. Spontaneous lysis must play a large role in the long-term outcome.

In addition, repeat duplex ultrasound studies have permitted a look at venous valve function and its relationship to the timing of recanalization and the rate of spontaneous lysis. Markel et al. (127) and Meissner et al. (128) have clearly shown a relationship between the rate of thrombus lysis and retention of venous valve competence. Van Ramshorst et al. (124) noted a similar decrease in thrombus load in the first 6 months after the acute DVT. Recanalization with reestablishment of flow occurred in 87% of the 23 completely occluded segments.

Johnson et al. (125) examined the relationship between the dynamic changes that occur and the long-term outcome in 78 patients (83 legs) followed by sequential studies for a median of 3 years. At the time of the last visit, 49 limbs (59%) were free of symptoms. Interestingly, 12% of

the previously occluded limbs had no ultrasound evidence of chronic venous disease—they were entirely normal. The 41% of limbs that had evidence of the postthrombotic syndrome had more than three times the odds of having combined reflux and residual obstruction.

These studies clearly point out the need not only for the initial screening examination, but also for a repeat study at the time of completion of therapy. It is only then that one will be able to predict the long-term outcome and advise the patient as to the lifetime outcome. These studies are also important in those patients who may come back with recurrent symptoms that are suggestive of recurrent venous thrombosis. This occurs in up to 10% of patients who are given conventional anticoagulant therapy.

CONTROVERSIES AND PERSONAL PERSPECTIVES

Is Noninvasive Testing Necessary?

When noninvasive testing for peripheral vascular disease was introduced, there was an enormous amount of resistance to this whole effort. This was largely due to the fact that the medical community had come to depend on a careful history and physical examination followed by angiography to establish the diagnosis. This became the only accepted method for planning therapy, for all vascular beds on the arterial and venous side of the circulation. The ideas and techniques for documenting the role of noninvasive testing gradually took hold and, with the introduction of ultrasonic duplex scanning, the progress and its acceptance became accelerated, and this process is continuing even today. It is my view that now, with the widespread availability of these newer devices along with trained people to use them, they are and will become even more important fixtures in our armamentarium. I do not believe that I could practice high-quality medicine without these devices and techniques.

Noninvasive Testing Alone before Surgical Intervention

We are beginning to see a revolution in the area of noninvasive testing alone before surgical intervention. It is now clear that increasing numbers of centers are starting to perform procedures such as carotid endarterectomy without the benefit of arteriography. Even a few years ago, this would have been considered heresy, and today many critics of this approach are still to be found. Why has the scene begun to change and what might be its impact? Studies have shown that contrast arteriograms are unduly costly and potentially dangerous, a fact that we all knew but were willing to accept because there was little else available (62,63). Now, it is common in centers with good quality control to perform carotid endarterectomy without the benefit of arteriography. This is going to continue into the future and will be extended to other vascular beds as well. Another striking change is the acceptance of duplex imaging alone for patients in clinical trials randomized to the surgical arm of the trial. This represents a major change.

Role of the Technologist

One of the major problems with ultrasound methods is that they are very operator dependent. The outcome of any study is entirely dependent on the skill of the examiner. Traditionally, tests performed by technologists have been finally interpreted by a physician, who either reviews the study directly or reviews hard copy output from key parts of the study. For example, for most radiologic examinations, the technologist performs the x-ray in a standard method and then gives it to the radiologist for review. This is entirely different with vascular ultrasound.

The entire examination is performed by the technologist, who follows certain guidelines, but these must be used and often modified in the context of what is being observed. In addition, the technologist must have a good grasp of regional anatomy and physiology in health and disease. At the end of each examination, the technologist has to formulate an impression based on the findings. Although this information is given to the physician for final review and approval, it is rare for the physician to change the impression of the examining technologist. This level of responsibility has caused considerable concern, particularly on the part of the radiology community members, who feel very uncomfortable from a diagnostic standpoint with the inroads made by these non-MDs. It is this level of responsibility that makes these technologists so important. They recognize their duty and level of responsibility. They generally do it very well and form the backbone of every good vascular diagnostic laboratory.

A very important step in improving quality control in this area was the establishment of the Intersocietal Commission for the Voluntary Accreditation of Vascular Laboratories. This independent reviewing body has representatives of all of the major specialty groups on its board. Certification is a very difficult job, requiring a great deal of work on the part of the laboratory that is requesting certification. Certification is for 3 years only. This program is moving forward very rapidly and will, in my view, create a ripple effect in the medical community concerning standards of performance for diagnostic methods of this type.

Role of Long-Term Studies

In cardiovascular disease, the era of treating and then discharging a patient without objective evaluation of the results must become a thing of the past. Patients who have these chronic illnesses must be under constant surveillance,

and repeat studies must be performed whenever necessary to document outcome. Much of the confusion over certain forms of therapy has occurred because of the lack of objective follow-up. It now appears that we have made a major advance in attitude over the methods of follow-up. For example, in the stent trials that are currently under way, (carotid and renal) ultrasonic duplex scanning is accepted as the method. It is clear that one cannot resort to using blood pressure response alone as an index of technical and physiologic success.

The past 20 years have seen the rapid proliferation of diagnostic methods for the evaluation of vascular disease. The field has matured, and the poorer methods have been quickly replaced by more effective techniques such as ultrasonic duplex scanning. In addition, there has been a slow but deliberate movement to get away from the invasive angiographic approaches. This has been most successful in the field of acute DVT, for which venography is only rarely performed today in the United States. As noted earlier, there are other areas, such as carotid bifurcation, in which contrast studies are being done less and less.

From a diagnostic standpoint, the only new methods that might alter the way we do business in the future revolve around intravascular ultrasound, spiral CT scanning, and magnetic resonance imaging (MRI) and angiography. These are all imaging methods that, at present, provide anatomic information alone. One fact that is not often remembered about such methods is the difficulty in quantitating the images themselves. Each of these methods has an application that can be of assistance for specific applications, some of which are as follows:

1. Intravascular ultrasound. Although currently in limited use, it appears to have found a place for the immediate evaluation of transluminal angioplasty with or without stenting. For example, after an iliac artery percutaneous transluminal angioplasty, visualization by the use of intravascular ultrasound may permit the detection of a dissection that can be corrected by the placement of a stent. Another very controversial area in which this has been recommended is for carotid artery angioplasty and stenting. Here, as in the iliac arteries, the ultrasound could be used to determine to what extent the stent has been properly placed and seated with regard to the walls of the arteries themselves. However, it is not clear even now whether this type of study is essential. It is apparent that endovascular grafting of all types is proceeding without the use of this method.

2. Spiral computed tomography (CT) can produce elegant three-dimensional displays of discrete anatomic areas such as the abdominal aorta. Here, this method was touted as being necessary as the primary diagnostic test to be done before placement of endoluminal aortic stent grafts. It provides information as to the size, location, and extent of the aneurysm itself. It can provide information as to the feasibility of placing a stent graft and its relationship to the

THE FUTURE

The future will see a deliberate movement away from invasive angiographic approaches, which will be replaced by more effective methods, such as ultrasonic duplex scanning. Imaging methods such as intravascular ultra-sound, spiral CT scanning, MRI, and MRA will evolve to provide more than basic anatomic function. However, cost may be an inhibiting factor in the development of these technologies.

renal arteries but as yet has not replaced conventional CT scanning. CT scanning can be used to detect paraprosthetic leaks after endovascular grafting. At the present time this constitutes one of the major problems that can occur with this form of treatment. It does have limitations that must be recognized. It requires between 100 and 200 mL contrast material and provides only limited areas of interrogation. For example, it would not be possible at the moment to extend the studies distal to the inguinal ligament, which is a disadvantage. It is also clear that color duplex imaging may be superior for the detection of endoleaks. This will be determined in the next few years.

3. It is most likely that the future will find ultrasound as the initial diagnostic study, to be followed by MRA-MRI when further diagnostic confirmation is needed. Considerable savings will still result, with absolutely no morbidity or mortality from the diagnostic studies themselves. This will be a major advance for our society.

Potential problems can be seen on the horizon that will limit the development and application of new technology. For example, the cost of new devices such as MRA will greatly limit their implementation. In addition, once they are in place within a hospital, the demand for their services will be such that it will be necessary to limit their use severely. Not enough systems will be available to satisfy the needs of the medical community. As one knows, this is all related to the availability of money and the costs of delivering health care. For example, it is very unlikely that many of the needed postoperative or postangioplasty studies will be paid for in the future. However, one would hope that those institutions that can carry out such studies will provide the necessary information to determine which categories of cases need such follow-up.

From a technological standpoint, what are some areas that badly need better data? One very important area is the morphology of the carotid bifurcation plaque. We have learned that the outcome with regard to such lesions is related to the degree of narrowing: the tighter the lesion, the more likely an adverse outcome. However, even given these facts, it is clear that most patients with similar degrees of narrowing do not have an ischemic event. The difference must lie in the morphology of the lesion. The current evidence, which appears to be consistent, is that the problem most likely lies within the fibrous cap. If it remains intact,

there is little risk to the patient, but if fissuring occurs with rupture, an adverse outcome is more likely to occur. At present, there are no good methods of looking at the fibrous cap *in vivo*. Ultrasound can provide some information with regard to plaque morphology, but it is not specific enough to allow a detailed study of the fibrous cap. MRI may have some role here, but the work that needs to be done to prove its value will take a long time. The major problem will not only be a description of the lesion itself but its verification of the findings by *ex vivo* histologic confirmation. By necessity, this will have to be a method that allows three-dimensional reconstruction of the plaque.

REFERENCES

1. Winsor T, Payne JH, Rudy N, Beatty JO. Collateral circulation in health and disease. *Arch Surg* 1957;74:20.
2. Goetz RH. The diagnosis and treatment of vascular diseases. *Br J Surg* 1949;37:140.
3. Sumner DS, Strandness DE Jr. The relationship between calf blood flow and ankle pressure in patients with intermittent claudication. *Surgery* 1969;65:763–771.
4. Whitney RJ. The measurement of volume changes in human limbs. *J Physiol (Lond)* 1953;121:1.
5. Strandness DE Jr, Bell JW. Peripheral vascular disease: diagnosis and objective evaluation using a mercury strain gauge. *Ann Surg* 1965;161[Suppl]:1–35.
6. Satomura S. Study of flow patterns in peripheral arteries by ultrasonics. *J Acoust Soc Jpn* 1959;15:151–158.
7. Rushmer RF, Baker DW, Stegall HF. Transcutaneous Doppler flow detection as a nondestructive technique. *J Appl Physiol* 1966;21:554–566.
8. Strandness DE Jr, Schultz RA, Sumner DS, Rushmer RF. Ultrasonic flow detection: a useful technique in the evaluation of peripheral vascular disease. *Am J Surg* 1967;113:311–320.
9. Baker DW. Pulsed ultrasonic Doppler blood flow sensing. *IEEE Trans Biomed Eng* 1970;17:170–185.
10. McCleod FD Jr. *Progress report, directional Doppler blood flow meter.* NRG 33-010-074, Cornell University, 1969.
11. Hokanson DE, Mozersky DJ, Sumner DS, Strandness DE Jr. Ultrasonic arteriography: a new approach to arterial visualization. *Biomed Eng* 1971;6:420.
12. Barber FE, Baker DW, Nation AWC, et al. Ultrasonic duplex echo Doppler scanner. *IEEE Trans Biomed Eng* 1974;21:109–113.

13. Barber FE, Baker DW, Strandness DE Jr. Duplex scanner II for simultaneous imaging of artery tissues and flow. *Ultrasonics Symposium Proc IEEE* 1974;74CH0896-ISU.

14. Strandness DE Jr, McCutcheon EP, Rushmer RF. Application of a transcutaneous Doppler flowmeter in evaluation of occlusive arterial disease. *Surg Gynecol Obstet* 1966; 122:1039–1045.

15. Strandness DE Jr, Bell JW. Ankle blood pressure responses after reconstructive arterial surgery. *Surgery* 1966;59:514–516.

16. Carter SA. The relationship of distal systolic blood pressures to healing of skin lesions in limbs with arterial occlusive disease, with special reference to diabetes mellitus. *Scand J Clin Lab Invest* 1973;31[Suppl 128]:239–243.

17. Carter SA. Response of ankle systolic pressure to leg exercise in mild or questionable arterial disease. *N Engl J Med* 1972;287:578–582.

18. Gensler SW, Haimovici H, Hoffert P, et al. Study of vascular lesions in diabetic, non-diabetic patients. *Arch Surg* 1965;617–622.

19. Hull RD, Raskob GE, Ginsberg JS, et al. A noninvasive strategy for the treatment of patients with suspected pulmonary embolism. *Arch Intern Med* 1994;154:289–297.

20. Raines JK. The pulse volume recorder in peripheral arterial disease. In: Bernstein EF, ed. *Vascular diagnosis*, 4th ed. St. Louis: Mosby, 1993:534–543.

21. Wheeler HB, Pearson D, O'Connel D, Mullick SC. Impedance plethysmography: techniques, interpretation and results. *Arch Surg* 1972;104:164–169.

22. Wheeler HB, Hirsh J, Wells P, Anderson FA Jr. Diagnostic tests for deep vein thrombosis: clinical usefulness depends on probability of disease. *Arch Intern Med* 1994;154: 1921–1928.

23. Orchard TJ, Strandness DE Jr. Assessment of peripheral vascular disease in diabetes. *Circulation* 1993;88:819–828.

24. Baker JD, Dix D. Variability of Doppler ankle pressure with arterial occlusive disease: an evaluation of ankle index and brachial-ankle pressure gradient. *Surgery* 1981;89:134–137.

25. Stahler C, Strandness DE Jr. Ankle blood pressure response to graded treadmill exercise. *Angiology* 1967;18: 237–241.

26. Strandness DE Jr. Exercise testing in the evaluation of patients undergoing direct arterial surgery. *J Cardiovasc Surg* 1970;11:192–200.

27. Skinner JS, Strandness DE Jr. Exercise and intermittent claudication: I. Effect of repetition and intensity of exercise. *Circulation* 1967;36:15–22.

28. Marinelli MR, Beach KW, Glass MJ, et al. Noninvasive testing vs. clinical evaluation of arterial disease: a prospective study. *JAMA* 1979;241:2031–2034.

29. Goodreau JJ, Greasy JK. Rational approach to the differentiation of vascular and neurogenic claudication. *Surgery* 1978;84:749–757.

30. Strandness DE Jr, Langlois YE, Cramer MM, et al. Long-term sequelae of acute venous thrombosis. *JAMA* 1983;250:1289–1292.

31. Haeger K. Problems of acute venous thrombosis. I. The interpretation of symptoms and signs. *Angiology* 1969;20: 219–223.

32. Strandness DE Jr. Hemodynamics of the normal arterial and venous system. In: Strandness DE Jr, ed. *Duplex scanning in vascular disorders*, 2nd ed. New York: Raven Press, 1993:45–79.

33. Sumner DS, Baker DW, Strandness DE Jr. The ultrasonic velocity detector in a clinical study of venous disease. *Arch Surg* 1968;97:75–80.

34. Strandness DE Jr. *Duplex scanning in vascular disorders*, 2nd ed. New York: Raven Press, 1993.

35. Phillips DJ, Powers JE, Eyer MK, et al. Detection of peripheral vascular disease using duplex scanner III. *Ultrasound Med Biol* 1980;6:205–218.

36. Blackshear WM Jr, Phillips DA, Chikos PM, Strandness DE Jr. Carotid artery velocity patterns in normal and stenotic vessels. *Stroke* 1980;11:67–71.

37. Beach KW. Physics and instrumentation for ultrasonic duplex scanning. In: Strandness DE Jr, ed. *Duplex scanning in vascular disorders*, 2nd ed. New York: Raven Press, 1993:273–317.

38. Faught WE, Mattos MA, Van Bemmelen PS, et al. Color-flow duplex scanning of carotid arteries: new velocity criteria based on receiver operator characteristic analysis for threshold stenoses used in the symptomatic and asymptomatic carotid trials. *J Vasc Surg* 1994;19:818–828.

39. Langlois YE, Roederer GO, Chan ATW, et al. Evaluating carotid artery disease: the concordance between pulsed Doppler/spectrum analysis and angiography. *Ultrasound Med Biol* 1983;9:51–63.

40. Langlois YE, Roederer GO, Strandness DE Jr. Ultrasonic evaluation of the carotid bifurcation. *Echocardiography* 1987;4:141–149.

41. Davies MJ, Woolf N. Atherosclerosis: what is it and why does it occur? *Br Heart J* 1993;69[Suppl]:S3–S11.

42. Imparato AM, Riles TS, Gorstein F. The carotid bifurcation plaque: pathologic findings associated with cerebral ischemia. *Stroke* 1979;10:238–245.

43. Fisher M. Occlusion of the internal carotid artery. *Arch Neurol Psychiat* 1951;65:346–377.

44. Ricotta JJ, Schenk E. Angiographic and pathologic correlates in carotid artery disease. *Surgery* 1986;99:284–292.

45. Beneficial effect of carotid endarterectomy in symptomatic patients with high-grade carotid stenosis. North American Symptomatic Carotid Endarterectomy trial collaborators. *N Engl J Med* 1991;325:445–463.

46. European Carotid Surgery Trialists' Collaborative Group. MRC European carotid surgery trial. Interim results for symptomatic patients with severe (70–99%) or with mild (0–29%) stenosis. *Lancet* 1991;337:1235–1243.

47. Hobson RW, Weiss DG, Fields WS, et al. Efficacy of carotid endarterectomy for asymptomatic carotid stenosis. *N Engl J Med* 1993;328:221–227.

48. Executive Committee Asymptomatic Carotid Atherosclerosis Study. Endarterectomy for asymptomatic carotid artery stenosis. *JAMA* 1995;273:1421–1428.

49. European Carotid Surgery Trialists' Collaborative Group. MRC European carotid surgery trial: interim results for symptomatic patients with severe (70–99%) or with mild stenosis. *Lancet* 1991;337:1235–1243.

50. Easton JD, Sherman DG. Stroke and mortality rate in carotid endarterectomy: 228 consecutive operations. *Stroke* 1977;8:565–568.

51. Chambers BR, Norris JW. The case against surgery for asymptomatic carotid stenosis. *Stroke* 1984;15:964–967.

52. Barnett HJM, Plum F, Walton JN. Carotid endarterectomy: an expression of concern. *Stroke* 1984;15:941–943.

53. Brott T, Thallinger K. The practice of carotid endarterectomy in a large metropolitan area. *Stroke* 1984;15:950–955.

54. Easton JD, Wilterdink JL. Carotid endarterectomy: trials and tribulations. *Ann Neurol* 1994;35(1):5–17.

55. Barnett HJ, Taylor DW, Eliasziw M, et al. Benefit of carotid endarterectomy in patients with symptomatic moderate or severe stenosis. North American Symptomatic Carotid Endarterectomy Trial. *N Engl J Med* 1998;339:1415–1425.

56. Farrell B, Fraser A, Sandercock P, et al. European Carotid Surgery Trial Collaborator Group. Randomised trial of endarterectomy for recently symptomatic stenosis: final results of the MRC European carotid surgery trial (ECST). *Lancet* 1998;351;1379–1387.

57. Roederer GO, Langlois YE, Jager KA, et al. The natural history of carotid arterial disease in asymptomatic patients with cervical bruits. *Stroke* 1984;15:605–613.

58. Chan A, Beach KW, Martin DC, Strandness DE Jr. Carotid artery disease in NIDDM diabetes. *Diabetes Care* 1983;6:562–569.

59. Louie J, Isaacson JA, Zierler RE, et al. Prevalence of carotid and lower extremity arterial disease in patients with renal artery stenosis. *Am J Hypertens* 1994;7:436–439.

60. Perry JR, Szalai JP, Norris JW. Consensus against both endarterectomy and routine screening for asymptomatic carotid artery stenosis. *Arch Neurol* 1997;54:25–28.

61. Strandness DE Jr. What you didn't know about the North American Symptomatic Carotid Endarterectomy Trial (NASCET). *J Vasc Surg* 1995;21:163–165.

62. Dawson DL, Zierler RE, Strandness DE Jr, et al. The role of duplex scanning and arteriography before carotid endarterectomy: a prospective study. *J Vasc Surg* 1993;18:673–683.

63. Cartier QR, Cartier P, Fontaine A. Carotid endarterectomy without angiography. The reliability of Doppler ultrasonography and duplex assessment in preoperative assessment. *Can J Surg* 1993;36:411–416.

64. Ricotta JJ, Holen J, Schenk E, et al. Is routine arteriography necessary prior to carotid endarterectomy? *J Vasc Surg* 1984;1:96–102.

65. Strandness DE Jr. Angiography before carotid endarterectomy—no. *Arch Neurol* 1995;52:832–833.

66. Rothwell PM, Gibson RJ, Slattery J, et al. Equivalence of measurements of carotid stenosis: a comparison of three methods on 1001 angiograms. *Stroke* 1994;25:2435–2439.

67. Eliasziw M, Smith RF, Singh N, et al. Further comments on the measurement of carotid stenosis from angiograms. *Stroke* 1994;25:2445–2449.

68. Chikos PM, Fisher LD, Hirsch JH, et al. Observer variability in evaluating extracranial arterial stenosis. *Stroke* 1983;14:885–892.

69. Phillips DJ, Greene FM, Langlois YE, et al. Flow velocity patterns in the carotid bifurcations of young presumed normal subjects. *Ultrasound Med Biol* 1983;9:19–49.

70. Blackshear WM, Phillips DJ, Thiele BL, et al. Detection of carotid occlusive disease by ultrasonic imaging and pulsed Doppler spectral analysis. *Surgery* 1979;86:698–706.

71. Roederer GO, Langlois YE, Chan RTW, et al. Is siphon disease important in predicting the outcome of carotid endarterectomy? *Arch Surg* 1983;118:1177–1181.

72. Roederer GO, Langlois YE, Jager KS, et al. A simple parameter for accurate classification of severe carotid disease. *Bruit* 1989;3:174–178.

73. Roederer GO, Langlois YE. Postendarterectomy carotid ultrasonic duplex scanning concordance with arteriography. *Ultrasound Med Biol* 1983;9:73–78.

74. Johnson BF, Verlato F, Bergelin RO, et al. Clinical outcome in patients with mild and moderate carotid stenosis. *J Vasc Surg* 1995;21:120–126.

75. Moneta GL, Edwards JM, Papanicolaou G, et al. Screening for asymptomatic internal carotid artery stenosis: duplex criteria for discriminating 60% to 99% stenosis. *J Vasc Surg* 1995;21:989–994.

76. Moneta GL, Edwards JM, Chitwood RW, et al. Correlation of North American Symptomatic Carotid Endarterectomy Trial (NASCET) angiographic definition of 70% to 99% internal carotid artery stenosis with duplex scanning. *J Vasc Surg* 1993;17:152–160.

77. Lusby RJ, Ferrall LD, Ehrenfeld WF, et al. Carotid plaque hemorrhage: its role in production of cerebral ischemia. *Arch Surg* 1982;117:1479–1488.

78. Reilly LM, Lusby RJ, Hughes L, et al. Carotid plaque histology using real-time ultrasonography. *Am J Surg* 1983;146:188–193.

79. Hill SL, Donato AT. Ability of the carotid duplex scan to predict stenosis, symptoms, and plaque structure. *Surgery* 1994;116:914–920.

80. Edwards JH, Kricheff II, Riles T, Imparato A. Angiographically undetected ulceration of the carotid bifurcation as a cause of embolic stroke. *Radiology* 1979;132:369–373.

81. Imparato AM, Riles T, Mintzer R, Bauman F. The importance of hemorrhage in the relationship between gross morphological characteristics and cerebral symptoms in 376 carotid artery plaques. *Ann Surg* 1983;197:195–203.

82. Lusby RJ, Ferrell L, Ehrenfeld W, et al. Carotid plaque hemorrhage: its role in the production of cerebral ischemia. *Arch Surg* 1982;117:1429–1488.

83. Lennihan L, Kupsky WJ, Mohr JP, et al. Lack of association between carotid plaque hematoma and ischemic cerebral symptoms. *Stroke* 1993;18:879–881.

84. Thackray BD, Burns DH, Ferguson MS, et al. Three dimensional reconstruction of atherosclerotic plaque from the carotid bifurcation. *Am J Cardiol Imaging* 1994;9:149–156.

85. Lendon CL, Davies MJ, Born GVR, Richardson PD. Atherosclerotic plaque caps are locally weakened when macrophage density is increased. *Atherosclerosis* 1991;87:87–90.

86. Fuster V, Stein B, Ambrose JS, et al. Atherosclerotic plaque rupture and thrombosis: evolving concepts. *Circulation* 1990;82[Suppl]:II-47–II-59.

87. Hatsukami TS, Thackray BD, Primozich JP, et al. Echolucent regions in carotid plaque: preliminary analysis com-

paring three-dimensional histologic reconstructions to sonographic findings. *Ultrasound Med Biol* 1994;20:743–749.

88. Davies MJ, Richardson PD, Woolf N, et al. Risk of thrombosis in human atherosclerotic plaques: role of extracellular lipid, macrophage, and smooth muscle cell content. *Br Heart J* 1993;69:377–381.

89. Strandness DE Jr. Peripheral arterial system. In: Strandness DE Jr, ed. *Duplex scanning in vascular disorders*, 2nd ed. New York: Raven Press, 1994:159–195.

90. European Working Group on Critical Leg Ischemia: second European consensus document on chronic critical leg ischemia. *Circulation* 1991;84[Suppl IV]:IV-1–IV-26.

91. Strandness DE Jr. A perspective on critical ischemia. *Crit Ischaemia* 1993;3(2):34–38.

92. Strandness DE Jr., Priest RR, Gibbons GE. A combined clinical and pathological study of nondiabetic and diabetic vascular disease. *Diabetes* 1964;13:366–372.

93. Wheelock FC Jr. Transmetatarsal amputation and arterial surgery in diabetic patients. *N Engl J Med* 1961;264:316–320.

94. Jager KA, Phillips DJ, Martin RL, et al. Noninvasive mapping of lower limb arterial lesions. *Ultrasound Med Biol* 1985;11:515–521.

95 Kohler TR, Nance DR, Cramer MM, et al. Duplex scanning for diagnosis of aortoiliac and femoropopliteal disease: a prospective study. *Circulation* 1987;76:1074–1080.

96. Hatsukami TS, Primozich J, Zierler RE, Strandness DE Jr. Color Doppler characteristics in normal lower extremity arteries. *Ultrasound Med Biol* 1992;16:167–171.

97. Hatsukami TS, Primozich JP, Zierler RE, et al. Color Doppler imaging of lower extremity arterial disease: a prospective validation study. *J Vasc Surg* 1992;16:527–533.

98. Edwards JM, Coldwell DM, Goldman ML, Strandness DE Jr. The role of duplex scanning in the selection of patients for transluminal angioplasty. *J Vasc Surg* 1991;13:69–74.

99. Kohler TR, Andros G, Porter JM, et al. Can duplex scanning replace arteriography for lower extremity arterial disease? *Ann Vasc Surg* 1990;4:280–287.

100. Leather RP, Kupkinski AM. Preoperative evaluation of the saphenous vein as a suitable graft. *Semin Vasc Surg* 1988;1:51.

101. Strandness DE Jr. The mesenteric and portal circulation. In: Strandness DE Jr, ed. *Duplex scanning in vascular disorders*, 2nd ed. New York: Raven Press, 1993:217–229.

102. Moneta GL, Lee RW, Yeager RA, et al. Mesenteric duplex scanning: a blinded prospective study. *J Vasc Surg* 1993;17:79–86.

103. Moneta GL, Taylor DC, Helton WS. Duplex ultrasound measurement of postprandial intestinal blood flow: effect of meal composition. *Gastroenterology* 1988;95:1294–1301.

104. Jager KA, Fortner GS, Thiele BL, Strandness DE Jr. Noninvasive diagnosis of intestinal angina. *J Clin Ultrasound* 1984;12:588–591.

105. Jager KA, Bollinger A, Valli C, Ammann R. Measurement of mesenteric blood flow by duplex scanning. *J Vasc Surg* 1986;3:462–469.

106. Nicholls SC. Use of hemodynamic parameters in the diagnosis of mesenteric insufficiency. *J Vasc Surg* 1986;3:507–510.

107. Strandness DE Jr. The renal arteries. In: Strandness, DE Jr, ed. *Duplex scanning in vascular disorders*, 2nd ed. New York: Raven Press, 1993:197–215.

108. Hoffman U, Edwards JM, Carter S, et al. Role of duplex scanning for the detection of atherosclerotic renal artery disease. *Kidney Int* 1991;39:1232–1239.

109. Guzman RP, Zierler RE, Isaacson JA, et al. Renal atrophy and arterial stenosis: a prospective study with duplex ultrasound. *Hypertension* 1994;23:346–350.

110. Caps MT, Zierler RE, Polissar NL, et al. Risk of atrophy in kidneys with atherosclerotic renal artery stenosis. *Kidney Int* 1998;53:735–742.

111. Caps MT, Perissinotto C, Zierler RE, et al. Prospective study of atherosclerotic disease progression in the renal artery. *Circulation* 1998;98(25):2866–2872.

112. Mattos MA, Van Bemmelen PS, Hodgson KJ, et al. Does correction of stenoses identified with color duplex scanning improve infrainguinal graft patency? *J Vasc Surg* 1993;17:54–66.

113. Idu MM, Blankenstein JD, de Gier P, et al. Impact of color-flow duplex surveillance program on infrainguinal vein graft patency: a five year experience. *J Vasc Surg* 1993;17:42–53.

114. Mills JL, Harris J, Taylor LM, et al. The importance of routine surveillance of distal bypass grafts with duplex scanning: a study of 379 reversed vein grafts. *J Vasc Surg* 1990;12:379–389.

115. Caps MT, Bergelin RO, Primozich JP, Strandness DE Jr. Vein graft lesions: time of onset and rate of progression. *J Vasc Surg* 1995;22:466–475.

116. Killewich LA, Bedford GR, Beach KW, Strandness DE Jr. Diagnosis of deep venous thrombosis: a prospective study comparing duplex scanning to contrast venography. *Circulation* 1989;79:810–814.

117. Comerota AJ, Katz ML, Hashemi HA. Venous duplex imaging for the diagnosis of acute deep venous thrombosis. *Haemostasis* 1993;23[Suppl 1]:61–71.

118. Moneta GL, Bedford G, Beach KW, Strandness DE Jr. Duplex assessment of venous diameters, peak velocities and flow patterns. *J Vasc Surg* 1988;8:286–291.

119. Markel A, Manzo RA, Bergelin R, Strandness DE Jr. Acute deep vein thrombosis: diagnosis, localization, risk factors. *J Vasc Med Biol* 1992;3:432–439.

120. Van Bemmelen PS, Bedford G, Beach KW, Strandness DE Jr. Status of the valves in superficial and deep venous system in chronic venous disease. *Surgery* 1991;109:730–734.

121. Van Bemmelen PS, Bedford G, Strandness DE Jr. Quantitative segmental evaluation of venous valvular reflux with ultrasonic duplex scanning. *J Vasc Surg* 1989;10:425–431.

122. Van Bemmelen PS. Segmental evaluation of venous reflux. In: Bernstein EF, ed. *Vascular diagnosis*, 4th ed. St. Louis: Mosby, 1993.

123. Killewich LA, Bedford GR, Beach KW, Strandness DE Jr. Spontaneous lysis of deep venous thrombosis: rate and outcome. *J Vasc Surg* 1989;9:89–97.

124. Van Ramshorst B, Van Bemmelen PS, Hoeneveld H, et al.

Thrombus regression in deep venous thrombosis: quantification of spontaneous thrombolysis with duplex scanning. *Circulation* 1992;86:414–419.

125. Johnson BF, Manzo RA, Bergelin RO, Strandness DE Jr. Relationship between changes in the deep venous system and the development of the postthrombotic syndrome after an episode of lower limb deep vein thrombosis. *J Vasc Surg* 1994;21:307–313.

126. Browse NL, Clemenson G, Thomas ML. Is the postphlebitic leg always postphlebitic? Relation between phlebographic appearance and late sequelae. *BMJ* 1981;281: 1167–1170.

127. Markel A, Manzo RA, Bergelin RO, Strandness DE Jr. Valvular reflux after deep vein thrombosis: incidence and time of occurrence. *J Vasc Surg* 1992;15:377–384.

128. Meissner MH, Manzo RA, Bergelin RO, et al. Deep venous insufficiency: the relationship between lysis and subsequent reflux. *J Vasc Surg* 1993;18:596–608.

CEREBROVASCULAR DISEASE

CATHY A. SILA
ANTHONY J. FURLAN

OVERVIEW

The term *stroke* encompasses a heterogeneous group of cerebrovascular disorders, each with its own set of clinical presentations, etiologies, and management strategies. Hypertension

C. A. Sila: Cerebrovascular Center, Section of Stroke and Neurologic Intensive Care, The Cleveland Clinic Foundation, Cleveland, Ohio

A. J. Furlan: Cerebrovascular Center, Section of Stroke and Neurologic Intensive Care, Department of Neurology, The Cleveland Clinic Foundation, Cleveland, Ohio

is the single most important risk factor for stroke. Cerebral infarction accounts for 80% to 85% of all strokes, intracerebral hemorrhage for 10% to 15%, and subarachnoid hemorrhage for 5% to 6%. Of all cerebral infarctions, 20% to 30% are due to atherothrombosis or thromboembolism from the extracranial or intracranial vessels and can be managed by carotid revascularization or antithrombotic therapy. Lacunar infarcts make up another 20% to 25%, and their treatment focuses on risk-factor management. Cardioembolic sources account for 15% to 20% of cerebral infarctions; nearly half are associated with nonvalvular atrial fibrillation (NVAF), and many warrant anticoagulation. In at least 30% of cases of cerebral infarct, the cause remains unclear. Stroke prevention typically targets high-risk patients with a transient ischemic attack (TIA) or minor stroke and includes antithrombotic therapy with aspirin, clopidogrel bisulfate, ticlopidine hydrochloride, dipyridamole, or warfarin sodium. Intervention in acute ischemic stroke is modeled after therapeutic strategies in acute myocardial infarction (MI); however, the diversity of ischemic stroke mechanisms and the risk for brain hemorrhage have impeded the development of acute therapy protocols.

GLOSSARY

Angiographically occult: Vascular abnormality that is not delineated by cerebral angiography.

Complicated migraine (migraine stroke): A neurologic deficit that replicates the symptoms of prior migraine attacks but that is not transient, with other causes of stroke having been excluded.

Lacunar: Small, 3-mm to 2-cm infarcts of the deep subcortical structures resulting from vascular occlusion of penetrating branches of the larger cerebral arteries.

Penumbra: The border zone of ischemic, but not infarcted, tissue that surrounds the infarcted core of a cerebral infarct.

Stroke: A generic term for a group of cerebrovascular disorders in which part of the brain is transiently or permanently affected by ischemia or hemorrhage, or in which one or more blood vessels of the brain are primarily affected by a pathologic process, or both.

Transient ischemic attack: Sudden, focal, painless neurologic deficit of ischemic cause resolving within 24 hours but typically clearing within 15 minutes.

ANATOMIC CONSIDERATIONS

Epidemiology and Risk Factors

Stroke is one of the three leading causes of death in the United States and developed nations. Cerebrovascular mortality rates have been declining since the 1920s. Before the 1950s, the decline in mortality from stroke reflected changes in death certificate coding due to the recognition that most sudden deaths were related to cardiac disease rather than stroke. The rate of decline in cerebrovascular mortality was 1% per year in the 1950s and accelerated to 5% per year in the mid-1970s. The decline in cerebrovascular mortality was greater than that in cardiovascular disease in general and has been linked to declining rates of incidence of infarction and intracerebral hemorrhage, as well as to a decreased case fatality rate (43). The decline in mortality from stroke may have plateaued, however (44). A

TABLE 110.1 RISK FACTORS FOR STROKE

Nonmodifiable
Advanced age
Gender
Race
Family history of stroke
Modifiable
Hypertension
Transient ischemic attacks or prior stroke
Cardiac disease
Nonvalvular atrial fibrillation
Acute myocardial infarction
Valvular heart disease
Impaired myocardial function
Asymptomatic carotid artery stenosis
Hyperlipidemia
Diabetes mellitus
Cigarette smoking
Alcohol abuse
Hypercoagulable states

recent increase in stroke fatality rates may reflect improved case ascertainment and aging of the population. As stroke typically follows cardiovascular events by 5 to 10 years, the stroke rate may increase as survival after cardiovascular events improves.

Stroke risk factors, defined in populations at risk, provide a framework for individual patient management (45–47) (Table 110.1). Primary prevention in asymptomatic and presymptomatic individuals is the ultimate goal.

Hypertension

Hypertension is the single most important risk factor for both ischemic and hemorrhagic stroke. The risk of stroke is directly related to the magnitude of elevation of both the systolic and diastolic blood pressures for both genders and all age groups (48). Stroke risk is at least threefold higher in individuals with definite hypertension (higher than 160/95) and 1.5 times higher in those with borderline hypertension. Isolated systolic hypertension increases stroke risk two to four times, even after one controls for age and diastolic blood pressure. Improvements in detecting and managing hypertension have been linked to the observed decline in stroke mortality.

Cardiac Disease

The presence of cardiac disease, including coronary artery disease (CAD), congestive heart failure (CHF), left ventricular hypertrophy, and cardiac arrhythmias, doubles the risk of stroke. This powerful relationship between stroke and cardiac disease is attributable to a number of mechanisms. Atherothrombotic stroke shares the same risk factors as CAD, and MI is the most frequent cause of death in patients with ischemic stroke (49). Cardiogenic embolism accounts for 15% to 20% of all ischemic strokes, of which half are due to atrial fibrillation (AF). The major causes of cardiogenic cerebral embolism are NVAF, acute MI, ventricular aneurysm, rheumatic heart disease, and prosthetic cardiac valves (Table 110.2). Potential cardioembolic sources of stroke include mitral valve prolapse, patent foramen ovale, atrial septal aneurysm, spontaneous echo contrast, left atrial enlargement, aortic arch atheromatous disease, and mitral annular calcification.

Atrial Fibrillation

AF in patients with rheumatic mitral valve disease has long been recognized as a cause of stroke and systemic embolism. Epidemiologic studies identified the importance of chronic NVAF in the absence of rheumatic heart disease when stroke risk was increased fivefold after adjustment for other risk variables (50). The prevalence of NVAF increases with advancing age from 6.7% for those aged 50 to 59 years to 36.2% for those aged 80 to 89 years (51,52). More than one-third of ischemic strokes occurring in the elderly are in the setting of AF, and one-third of patients with AF will experience a stroke sometime during their lifetime. Clinically silent cerebral infarcts are also present on CT in more than one-third of patients with AF (53) (Fig. 110.1). The risk factors for stroke in patients with NVAF established by the Atrial Fibrillation investigators and Stroke Prevention and Atrial Fibrillation classification schemes have been combined into the CHADS$_2$ index to estimate stroke risk (54–57) (Table 110.3). This risk-stratification scheme assigns one point each for *C*ongestive heart failure, *H*ypertension, *A*dvanced age, and *D*iabetes and two points for prior *S*troke or TIA.

TABLE 110.2 CARDIAC RISK FACTORS FOR STROKE AND CORRESPONDING INCREASE IN RISK

Risk factor	Increase in risk
Cardioembolic stroke	2%–4% recurrent stroke within 30 days
Atrial fibrillation	1%/yr: <65 yr, no risk factors
	4.9%/yr: <65 yr, ≥1 risk factors
	4.3%/yr: 65–75 yr, no risk factors
	5.7%/yr: 65–75 yr, ≥1 risk factors
	3.5%/yr: >75 yr, no risk factors
	8.1%/yr: >75 yr, ≥1 risk factors
Acute MI	1%–3% all MI, 2%–6% anterior wall MI, 15% LV thrombus, clustered within 3 mo
LV hypertrophy on electro-cardiogram	Twofold increase
Dilated cardiomyopathy	1%–3%/yr
Rheumatic mitral stenosis	5%/yr, 18-fold increase with AF, three- to sixfold increase without AF
Bioprosthetic aortic valve	0.2%–2.9%/yr stroke + systemic embolism
Bioprosthetic mitral valve	0.4%–1.9%/yr stroke + systemic embolism
Mechanical aortic valve	12.3%/yr stroke + systemic embolism
Mechanical aortic valve, anticoagulated	1.4%–3.9%/yr stroke + systemic embolism
Mechanical mitral valve	22.2%/yr stroke + systemic embolism
Mechanical mitral valve, anticoagulated	1.1%–6.5%/yr stroke + systemic embolism
Patent foramen ovale	0%–4%/yr
Cardiac morbidity for patients with transient ischemic attack, stroke, or bruits	5%/yr absolute

AF, atrial fibrillation; LV, left ventricular; MI, myocardial infarction.

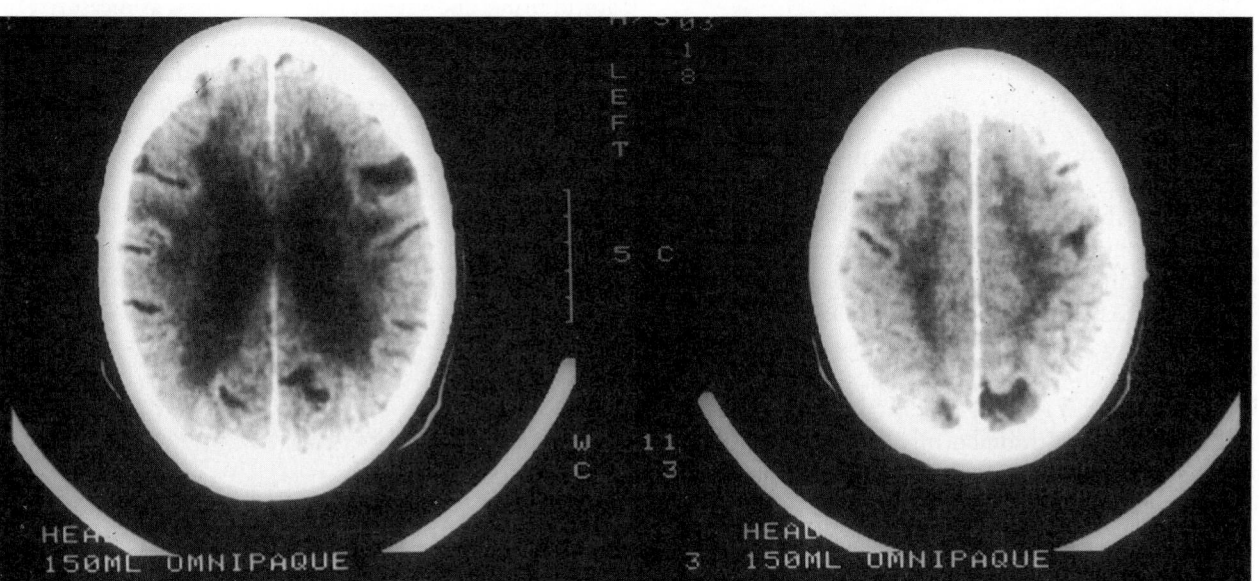

FIGURE 110.1 Small cortical infarcts and periventricular white matter disease in an octogenarian with hypertension and chronic atrial fibrillation.

TABLE 110.3 RISK FACTORS FOR STROKE WITH ATRIAL FIBRILLATION

Independent risk factors
Prior stroke or transient ischemic attack
Age ≥75 yr
Hypertension
Recent congestive heart failure
Diabetes mellitus
Factors posing increased risk
Female gender
Left ventricular dysfunction
Left atrial enlargement
Thrombus or "smoke" in left atrium, left atrial appendage
Mitral annular calcification
Cigarette smoking

Myocardial Infarction

Before the advent of thrombolytic therapy, stroke complicated 0.8% to 5.5% of acute MIs (58–60). An embolic mechanism is supported by pathologic studies demonstrating left ventricular mural thrombi in 38% to 67% of cases, typically in the apex in patients with anteroapical infarctions (61,62). Transthoracic echocardiography (TTE) detects mural thrombi or severe wall motion abnormalities, which place patients at increased risk for embolic stroke, although embolization may occur even in the absence of detectable thrombus on echocardiography (63,64). The distribution of cerebral emboli reflects cerebral blood flow patterns, with the majority affecting the anterior circulation, particularly the middle cerebral artery. Although 90% of cerebral embolic events occur within the first 2 weeks after MI, risk for stroke continues for 4 to 6 months, with a minority of patients having a lifelong risk. Risk factors for stroke include older age, history of stroke, paroxysmal AF, anterior or apical location, impaired left ventricular function, and severity of MI as measured by levels of creatine phosphokinase, CHF, or advanced Killip class (65–68).

Valvular Heart Disease

Rheumatic mitral stenosis alone increases stroke risk by sixfold, and when it is associated with AF, stroke risk by increases 18-fold. Embolism occurs with all degrees of rheumatic mitral valve disease but is less frequently a complication of pure mitral regurgitation (69).

The risk of prosthetic valve thromboembolism is higher for valves in the mitral than in the aortic position, higher for multiple prosthetic valves than for single, and higher for caged ball valves than for tilting disc or bileaflet valves. Additional risk factors for thromboembolism include prior thromboembolism, AF, CAD, an enlarged left atrium, and left atrial thrombus (70).

Impaired Myocardial Function

Clinical evidence of impaired cardiac function, including CAD and CHF, again doubles the risk for stroke. In hetero-geneous groups of patients with cerebrovascular disease, 86% have angiographic evidence of CAD, which is severe in 40% as determined by noninvasive studies or cardiac catheterization (71). The neurologic presentation does not predict severity of CAD.

Transient Ischemic Attack

A TIA is a sudden, painless, focal neurologic dysfunction from a vascular cause resolving within 24 hours. This clinical definition predated CT scanning, and the median duration of a TIA is now known to be only 12 minutes. Twenty-five percent of those fulfilling the traditional criteria have evidence of cerebral infarction on CT or MRI (72). From aggregate data, TIA is associated with a 4% to 12% annual risk of stroke and a 10% to 17% annual risk of death, two-thirds of which are vascular deaths (73–76). The highest risk for stroke is in the first year after onset of TIA, especially in the first few months.

The North American Symptomatic Carotid Endarterectomy Trial (NASCET) reported nine risk factors associated with an increased risk of stroke in patients with atherosclerosis-related TIA (77,78). The 2-year risk of stroke ranged from 17% to nearly 40%, depending on the number of risk factors present (Table 110.4).

Asymptomatic Carotid Artery Stenosis

The frequency of cervical bruits increases with age and is 7% to 10% in those patients older than 65 years. Cervical bruits correlate poorly with the degree of underlying carotid artery stenosis, however, as only half of arteries with bruits harbor significant internal carotid artery stenosis and only half of the relevant stenoses produce an audible bruit. Carotid bruits and carotid plaque thickness as measured by ultrasonography are markers of systemic atherosclerosis and increased risk of vascular events, although they are not a good predictor of ipsilateral cerebral infarction. Stroke risk

TABLE 110.4 REDUCTION IN RELATIVE RISK FOR IPSILATERAL STROKE AFTER ENDARTERECTOMY IN NASCET[a]

Stenosis (%)/no. of risk factors	Reduction in relative risk (%)
90–99	75
80–89	63
70–79	63
70–99	65
≥7 risk factors	78
6 risk factors	76
≤5 risk factors	38

NASCET, North American Symptomatic Carotid Endarterectomy Trial.
[a]Risk factors in NASCET: age >70 years; male gender; systolic blood pressure >160 mm Hg; diastolic blood pressure >90 mm Hg; symptoms within 31 days; history of stroke; stenosis >80%; plaque ulceration; history of smoking, hypertension, myocardial infarction, congestive heart failure, diabetes mellitus, claudication, or hyperlipidemia.

increases with the degree of carotid stenosis, from 1.3% per year for stenosis of less than 75% to 3.3% per year for stenosis greater than 75% (79,80). Even in the higher-risk group, however, the rate of ipsilateral cerebral infarction was only 2.5% per year, whereas the combined risk for myocardial ischemia and vascular death was 9.9% per year (81). Hence, asymptomatic carotid artery disease is a better indicator of MI and vascular death than stroke. The most important independent predictors of carotid artery stenosis are duration of cigarette smoking, hypertension, diabetes mellitus, and systolic blood pressure at the time of examination (82).

Diabetes Mellitus

Diabetes mellitus correlates strongly with hypertension, but it is an independent risk factor for cerebral infarction, especially in women, who have rates of intermittent claudication and cardiovascular complications similar to those for men. When adjusted for hypertension and diabetes, obesity is no longer an independent risk factor for stroke. The incidence of type 2 diabetes has increased dramatically, and it is a major contributor to small subcortical, or lacunar, strokes. Although aggressive treatment of hypertension among those with type 2 diabetes has been shown to reduce stroke risk, tight diabetic control has not (91). Hyperglycemia at the onset of cerebral infarction is a poor prognostic factor associated with increased infarct size (92).

Genetic Factors

The familial effect of stroke predominantly reflects genetic influences of known risk factors for stroke such as hypertension, diabetes, and hyperlipidemia as well as learned behaviors of cigarette smoking, diet, and physical activity (97). However, more than 50 monogenetic disorders account for uncommon causes of stroke, including amyloid angiopathy, coagulopathies, homocystinuria, familial cavernous malformations, saccular or berry aneurysms, and intracranial aneurysms associated with polycystic kidney disease, Ehlers-Danlos syndrome type IV, and Marfan syndrome.

CEREBRAL ISCHEMIA AND INFARCTION: CLINICAL PROFILE

The signs and symptoms of cerebral ischemia and infarction are related to the location and the volume of brain tissue injured as well as to the mechanism of injury. Symptoms of ischemia in the carotid territory include monocular blindness (amaurosis fugax), contralateral hemiparesis, and aphasia. These symptoms can be further divided into anterior cerebral and anterior/posterior or deep middle-cerebral artery territory symptoms (Table 110.5, Figs. 110.2 through 110.4). Vertebrobasilar

TABLE 110.5 CLINICAL MANIFESTATIONS OF CEREBRAL ARTERIAL OCCLUSIONS

Carotid occlusion	Manifestation
Ophthalmic artery	Amaurosis fugax (i.e., total or partial monocular blindness, usually altitudinal)
Anterior cerebral artery	Contralateral weakness involving leg more than proximal arm
Middle cerebral artery: Anterior branches	Contralateral motor and sensory loss, maximal for face, hand, and arm; if dominant hemisphere, nonfluent (Broca) aphasia
Posterior branches	Contralateral hemisensory loss and homonymous hemianopsia; if dominant hemisphere, fluent (Wernicke) aphasia
Deep perforating branches: lenticulostriate, anterior choroidal	Contralateral hemiparesis affecting face, arm, and leg about equally

Vertebrobasilar arterial occlusion	Manifestation
Bilateral symptoms	Binocular visual loss, quadriparesis, altered consciousness
Crossed symptoms	Ipsilateral cranial nerve/contralateral limbs
Combined symptoms	Dysarthria, diplopia, nausea, vomiting, vertigo, ataxia

ischemia is characterized by bilateral neurologic symptoms (e.g., quadriplegia) that are frequently accompanied by vertigo, dysarthria, or diplopia (106–108). Infarction related to arteriolar or penetrator arterial occlusive disease produces several lacunar syndromes (109,110). The most common are pure motor hemiparesis, pure sensory syndrome, and ataxic hemiparesis (Table 110.6, *e*Fig. 110.4.1, *e*Fig. 110.4.2). A stereotyped pattern of symptoms suggests a focal stenosis, whereas variable symptoms referable to multiple vascular territories suggest a proximal source of embolism (e.g., heart) or a multifocal arteriopathy (e.g., vasculitis) (111).

CEREBRAL ISCHEMIA AND INFARCTION: MANAGEMENT PRINCIPLES

Primary Prevention of Stroke: Strategies for Targeting High-Risk Patients

For most patients, appropriate screening consists of a thorough history and physical examination guided by knowledge of predisposing risk factors. The examination may provide important clues such as the presence of retinal Hollenhorst plaques, cervical bruits, an irregular pulse, or a cardiac murmur.

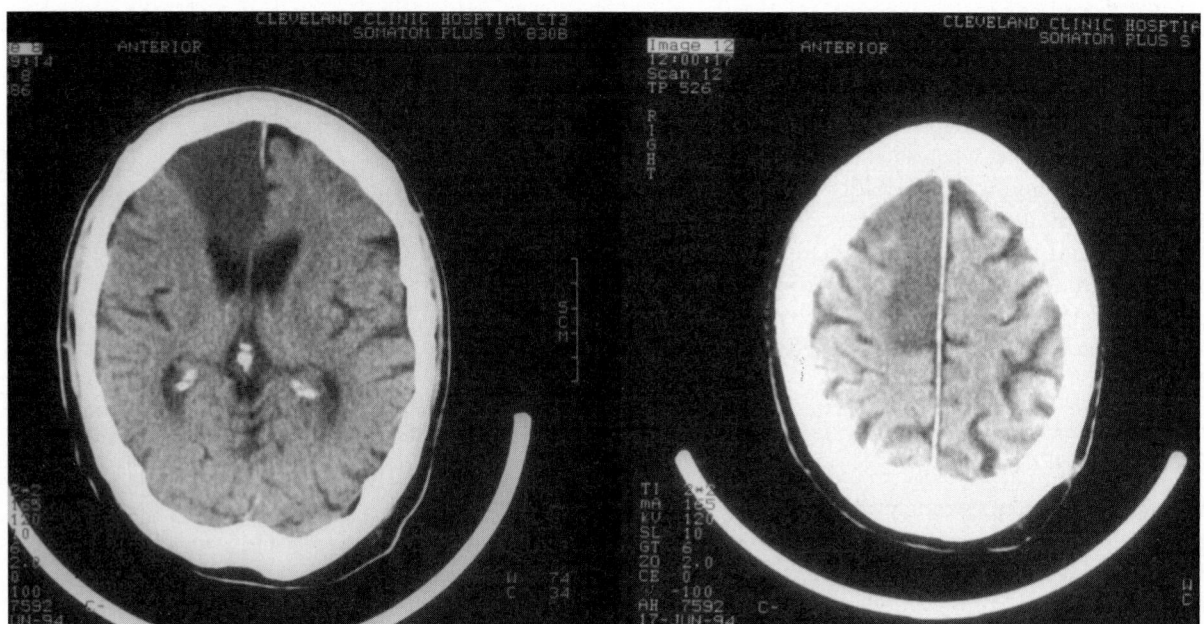

FIGURE 110.2 An anterior cerebral artery territory infarction at 7 days.

Patients with Hypertension

The efficacy of hypertension management for stroke prevention has been confirmed by a series of controlled clinical trials performed over the past 30 years. From a metaanalysis of 14 trials, a 35% to 40% reduction in stroke risk was obtained with a 5- to 6-mm Hg reduction in diastolic blood pressure over 5 years (112). Population studies have been less convincing, however, which possibly reflects less strict blood pressure control in a community setting. ❦ r05

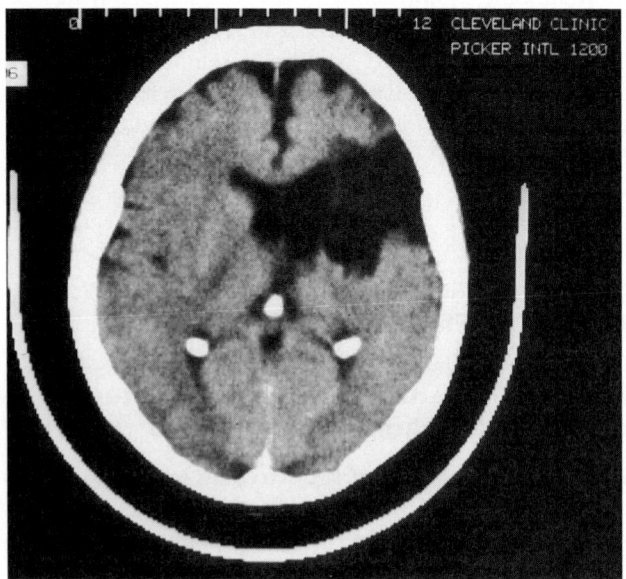

FIGURE 110.3 A chronic anterior division middle cerebral arterial infarction with encephalomalacia.

Patients with Acute Myocardial Infarction

Three large randomized clinical trials (126–128) demonstrated that short-term anticoagulant therapy reduced stroke incidence from a rate of 2.3% to 5.0% to a rate of 0.8% to 1.7% after MI. Studies (129–132) assessing longer-term anticoagulant therapy after acute MI have demonstrated a reduction in embolic stroke that needs to be balanced by the increased risk for ICH. Such therapy is recommended for patients at increased risk for embolic stroke, such as those with AF, prior systemic embolism, CHF, two-dimensional echo evidence of mural thrombus, or persistent left ventricular dysfunction.

Patients with Valvular Heart Disease

Mitral Stenosis
The use of oral anticoagulation with warfarin at an INR range of 2.0 to 3.0 is recommended to prevent cerebral and systemic emboli in patients with rheumatic mitral valve disease and either chronic or paroxysmal AF or prior systemic embolism, based primarily on nonrandomized studies with historical controls (level IV evidence) (133). Even in the absence of AF, long-term anticoagulant therapy is recommended for certain subgroups, such as those with mitral stenosis associated with enlargement of the left atrium greater than 5.5 cm, those for whom left atrial spontaneous echo contrast is present, and those about to undergo balloon valvuloplasty (134).

Prosthetic Cardiac Valves
Antithrombotic therapies to prevent thromboembolic complications from prosthetic valves vary by the type of valve,

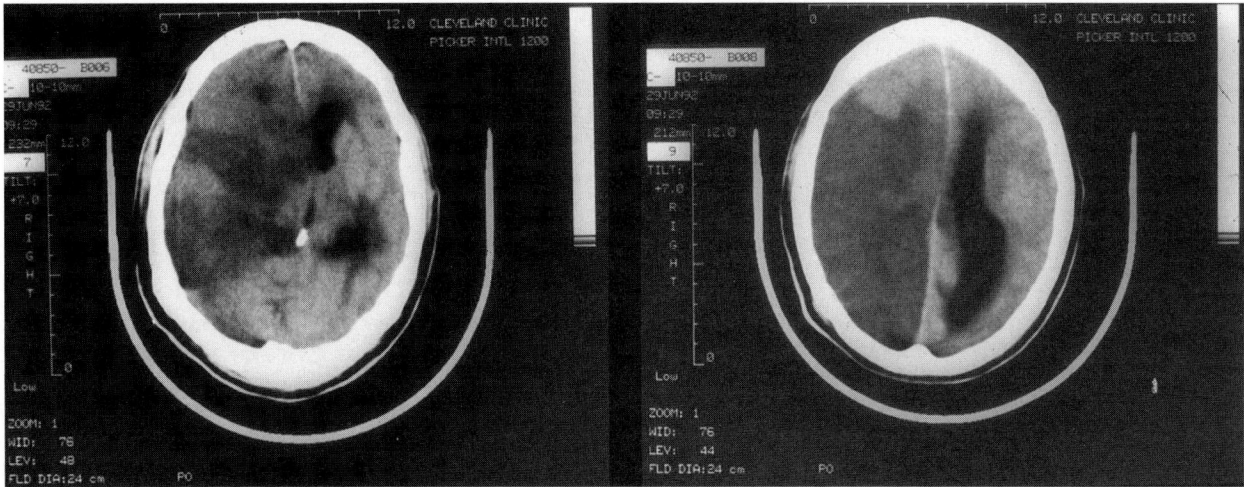

FIGURE 110.4 A carotid artery occlusion resulting in infarction of the middle and posterior cerebral artery territories that has spared the anterior cerebral artery. The midline shifts produced by the ischemic cerebral edema have resulted in hydrocephalus.

valve position, and other comorbidities. For mechanical prosthetic cardiac valves, permanent anticoagulation is strongly recommended, and the relationship between efficacy and intensity of anticoagulation is often described by U-shaped curves (level III and V evidence) (135). Thromboembolic risk is higher for caged-ball and caged-disc valves than for bileaflet valves, higher for mitral valves than for aortic valves, and higher with AF or after failure of oral anticoagulant therapy alone.

Mitral Valve Prolapse

Mitral valve prolapse is identified in 1% to 10% of echocardiographic studies, with a slightly higher incidence in those with symptoms of cerebral ischemia than in controls (138). Although pathologic studies have identified platelet-fibrin aggregates on the valvular surface, mitral valve prolapse is more likely to be the cause of stroke when other risk factors are present, such as an associated atrial septal abnormality or hypercoagulable state (139). Antiplatelet therapy with aspirin, 160 to 325 mg per day, is recommended for secondary stroke prevention; anticoagulation therapy is reserved for those for whom antiplatelet therapy is ineffective (level V evidence).

TABLE 110.6 LACUNAR SYNDROMES AND THEIR TYPICAL LOCATIONS

Pure motor hemiparesis: internal capsule, pons
    Pure motor hemiparesis with crossed III nerve palsy: midbrain
    Pure motor hemiparesis with crossed VI nerve palsy: pons
Ataxic hemiparesis: pons
    Dysarthria/clumsy hand: pons or capsule
Pure sensory syndrome: ventral thalamus
Lateral medullary syndrome (Wallenberg): medulla
Sensorimotor stroke: thalamus capsule
Thalamic dementia: anterior thalamus

Calcific Aortic Stenosis

Embolization of calcific debris can complicate valvuloplasty for calcific aortic stenosis (140). Although calcific emboli have been demonstrated, primarily in autopsy studies, the risk of stroke in the absence of AF remains uncertain. No evidence exists of any therapy that prevents embolization, but anticoagulation is not warranted (141).

Mitral Annular Calcification

Calcification of the mitral annulus can be identified in up to 30% of elderly patients with stroke, but it is also present in 20% of elderly patients without stroke and is associated with other risk factors such as hypertension, AF, CHF, and carotid stenosis. As with calcific aortic stenosis, its role as a cardioembolic cause of stroke and optimum therapy remains uncertain (142).

Patients Undergoing Cardiovascular Procedures

Stroke complicates 2% to 5% of coronary revascularizations and up to 15% of operations that require opening of the cardiac chambers. Much of the risk is related to the cardiopulmonary bypass circuit, which can contribute to cerebral injury through a number of mechanisms, including hypoperfusion, embolization, and a provoking of a systemic inflammatory response. Additional factors include prolongation of the cardiopulmonary bypass time related to the complexity of the case, potential for embolism of valve debris, and embolism of air and particulates during mechanical de-airing of the heart. "Off-pump" coronary artery bypass surgery or the use of emboli capture devices may become the superior alternative for those at increased risk of stroke. Stroke is related to aortic arch emboli in 32%, cardiogenic emboli in 12%, hypoperfusion in 12%, and concomitant cerebrovascular disease in 11%. Stroke risk factors include atherosclerosis of the proximal aorta, hypertension, diabetes, prior cerebrovascular disease, history of neurologic disease, age older than 70 years, history of pulmonary disease, and postoperative AF (157–159). Clinically recognizable encephalopathy persisting to the fourth postoperative day occurs in 3% to 12%, although 80% of these patients recover to be able to perform normally on a simple mental status test by the time of discharge. Prospective investigations using extensive neuropsychological test batteries, however, have found that 35% to 75% of patients have impairments in cognitive function, which is severe in 20% of cases, within the first 7 to 10 days, and 10% to 30% have persistent significant deficits at 3 to 6 months. Neuroimaging studies using MRI techniques suggest that the presence of preoperative cerebral atrophy and postoperative ischemic changes manifesting as lesions on diffusion-weighted or T2-weighted MRI brain scans correlate with cognitive dysfunction, findings which support a theory of multifocal microembolism (eFig. 110.4.4). Excessive alcohol consumption, postoperative AF, a history of peripheral vascular disease or prior coronary artery bypass graft, and cerebral atrophy by neuroimaging have also been reported as risk factors for cognitive decline. These identified risk factors for postoperative encephalopathy appear to reflect a patient's "cerebral reserve" for withstanding a diffuse or multifocal ischemic insult.

Paraplegia from spinal cord infarction is a rare complication of intraaortic balloon counterpulsation support (160) (eFig. 110.4.5).

Cerebral embolism complicates 0.1% to 1.0% of cardiac catheterizations and 0.2% to 0.3% of coronary interventions. Defects in the vertebrobasilar circulation account for 60% to 70% of cases presenting with combinations of confusional states, cortical blindness or hemianopic visual field defects, and intrinsic brainstem signs. The mechanism is generally felt to be embolic in nature, either from manipulation of the guidewire or during catheter flushing. Focal defects resolve within 48 hours in approximately half of patients; however, some strokes have been fatal. Rarely, a confusional state with headache and cortical blindness mimicking hypertensive encephalopathy or subarachnoid hemorrhage can occur. The cause is unknown, but the condition typically resolves within 48 hours with antihypertensive therapy (161–163) (eFig. 110.4.6).

The risk of embolic stroke ranges from 1.4% to 11% for aortic valvuloplasty and 3.2% to 4.2% for mitral valvuloplasty. In the presence of an atrial thrombus, systemic embolism can result during mitral valvuloplasty, which prompted the recommendations for 3 months of anticoagulation therapy and transesophageal echocardiography before each procedure. Embolic events during aortic valvuloplasty are often highly focal, small neurologic deficits suggesting small calcific emboli (134).

The frequency of hypoxic-ischemic encephalopathy or stroke due to hypotension before insertion of a left ventric-

ular assist device (LVAD) varies up to 25% in surgical series. Subsequent stroke from embolism of air or thrombus, or coagulopathy-related hemorrhage occurs in an additional 10% to 20% and is greater with longer durations of pump assist and during manipulation of the pump (164) (eFig. 110.4.7).

Secondary Prevention of Stroke: Prevention of Recurrent Ischemia in Patients Presenting with Transient Ischemic Attack or Major or Minor Cerebral Infarction

In patients with symptomatic retinal or cerebral ischemia, an evaluation is necessary to identify the underlying mechanism and to provide a rational basis for treatment. Depending on the clinical scenario, a complete history and physical and neurologic examination, some structural neuroimaging such as a CT scan of the brain, and basic systemic testing of blood as well as an electrocardiogram (ECG) may suffice; however, more typically, additional tests including noninvasive vascular studies, MRI, or TTE are performed (165). Additional levels of testing include cerebral angiography, transesophageal echocardiography, and assays of coagulation factors (165a).

Checking for a Cardiac Source of Embolism

Some clinical features can clue the clinician to a proximal source of embolism, including (a) nonlacunar involvement of the cortex or cerebellum in multiple vascular territories; (b) evidence of systemic embolism, syncope, palpitations, seizures at onset, or rapid resolution of a neurologic deficit; or (c) stroke in a young patient without risk factors for premature atherosclerosis. Because emboli are more likely to lodge in the middle cerebral artery or the posterior cerebral artery, certain clinical syndromes are overrepresented, such as Wernicke aphasia, ideomotor apraxia, isolated hemianopia, or top-of-the-basilar syndrome (168). Also, because cerebral emboli spontaneously lyse in at least 30% of patients, which leads to reperfusion of the ischemic area, rapid recovery or hemorrhagic infarction also suggests an embolic mechanism. Several misconceptions about cardioembolic symptoms also warrant mention. Although repetitive ischemic symptoms referable to the same arterial territory make a proximal source less likely, cerebral emboli may travel repeatedly to the same artery, typically the middle cerebral artery. Retinal ischemia manifesting as transient monocular blindness may be the only clue to cardiac embolization. The prototypical onset is in an awake, active patient, but cardiac embolization can occur at any time of the day or night regardless of the level of activity. Although 90% of embolic strokes are maximal at onset, the remainder have a stuttering onset that reflects initial embolization with superimposed thrombus formation in a vessel with stagnant flow caused by a partially occluding embolus. A cardioembolic mechanism cannot always be inferred by the presence of a potential cardioembolic source, because an estimated 30% of patients with a cardioembolic source have concomitant cerebrovascular atherosclerosis that may also be the cause.

Echocardiography

TTE is indicated in young patients with unexplained cerebrovascular symptoms and in all patients with symptoms or signs of heart disease. In elderly patients with no evidence of heart disease, however, TTE is of limited use and is not cost effective (169,170). Transesophageal echocardiography can disclose potential cardioembolic sources of embolism, including the aortic arch, patent foramen ovale, atrial septal defects, and atrial septal aneurysms. As these conditions can be detected in up to 30% of selected populations, however, their etiologic role requires additional study (171–175).

Electrocardiographic Monitoring

ECG monitoring may reveal a variety of dysrhythmias, particularly in patients with subarachnoid hemorrhage or ICH, and should otherwise be reserved for patients with syncope or palpitations at onset, unexplained stroke, and other cardiac symptoms or signs (176–179).

Cerebral Angiography

The presence of branch occlusion or delayed perfusion of distal arterial branches in the absence of a more proximal arterial source of embolism suggests a more proximal source of embolism, such as the heart. Because of spontaneous clot lysis, however, angiography performed more than 24 hours after symptom onset frequently proves normal. Angiography has been useful in clinical trials investigating intraarterial delivery of thrombolytic agents after cerebral embolism.

Therapeutic Options for Patients with Transient Ischemic Attack and Stroke

Most clinical trials for stroke prevention have involved patients with TIA or minor stroke. Major treatments include antiplatelet therapy, anticoagulant therapy, and carotid endarterectomy.

Antiplatelet Therapy

Aspirin

Aspirin remains the standard preventive therapy for patients at risk for stroke. Its indications have grown from the initial U.S. Food and Drug Administration (FDA) approval in 1980, which specified its use in men with TIAs "due to fibrin platelet emboli" based on a trial in which 1,300 mg was taken daily. In a metaanalysis of 31 trials encompassing over 29,000 patients with cerebrovascular disease, the risk reduction for the combined end point of stroke, MI, or vascular death was 25%, but the major effect

was from the 22% reduction in nonfatal stroke (33). Treatment was effective regardless of sex, middle or older age, or presence of hypertension or diabetes mellitus. Subgroup analyses (based on less than 400 events) in 25 trials showed no significant differences in reduction of vascular events for dosages of 75 to 150 mg (26%), 160 to 325 mg (28%), and 500 to 1,500 mg (21%), and documenting the optimum aspirin dosage would require a megatrial to avoid bias and random errors. ⚑ r06

Thienopyridines: Ticlopidine and Clopidogrel

Clopidogrel and ticlopidine are both thienopyridine derivatives that inhibit platelet aggregation by selectively and irreversibly inhibiting the adenosine diphosphate–dependent activation of fibrinogen binding via the glycoprotein IIb/IIIa complex. The Ticlopidine Aspirin Stroke Study (181) compared ticlopidine 250 mg twice daily with aspirin 650 mg twice daily in patients with TIAs or minor strokes. Ticlopidine reduced the overall risk for fatal or nonfatal stroke by 19% compared with aspirin, but in the first year of treatment the reduction in risk with ticlopidine proved 48% superior to that with aspirin. In the Canadian-American Ticlopidine Study (182), ticlopidine reduced recurrent stroke by 34% and reduced the combined risk for stroke, MI, or vascular death by 30% in patients with brain infarction. Ticlopidine proved effective in both men and women. Serious adverse events occurred in 2% of patients receiving both aspirin and ticlopidine, with gastrointestinal bleeding being the major side effect of aspirin. Significant neutropenia (i.e., absolute neutrophil count less than 450 per mm^3) occurred in less than 1% of ticlopidine-treated patients and almost exclusively within the first 3 months of therapy. Accordingly, a complete blood count with a differential count must be taken every 2 weeks for the first 3 months of ticlopidine therapy. Thrombotic thrombocytopenic purpura has been reported at an estimated rate of 200 to 625 cases per million ticlopidine-treated patients among those with cerebrovascular disease and after coronary interventions. As 80% of cases appeared within the first month of therapy, patients should be counseled to seek medical attention if fever, bruising, or neurologic symptoms develop (183). This safety and efficacy profile has limited the use of ticlopidine primarily to cases in which aspirin therapy has failed, although it remains under study in the African-American Antiplatelet Stroke Prevention Study.

A regimen of clopidogrel 75 mg once daily was compared to therapy with aspirin 325 mg daily in 19,185 patients with a recent stroke or MI or symptomatic peripheral vascular disease. The Clopidogrel versus Aspirin in Patients at Risk of Ischemic Events study demonstrated a 9% relative risk reduction in the combined end point of stroke, MI, or vascular death for clopidogrel over aspirin (5.32% vs. 5.83%) (39). Although subset analyses were not powered to look at cerebrovascular patients separately, the major benefit was seen for patients with peripheral arterial disease, and results were not statistically significant for those patients who entered with cerebrovascular events. The 75-mg dosage of clopidogrel was selected to achieve bleeding times comparable to those with ticlopidine 250 mg twice a day. Side effects of rash and diarrhea were more frequent, but gastrointestinal symptoms and gastrointestinal bleeding were lower with clopidogrel. As the incidence of severe neutropenia was similar to that of aspirin (0.04% vs. 0.02%), hematologic monitoring is not warranted. In postmarket surveys, the risk of thrombotic thrombocytopenic purpura has been found to be 3.7 cases per million clopidogrel-treated patients against a background rate of four cases per million person-years in the general population (184,185). Given the efficacy data and superior safety profile, clopidogrel has essentially replaced ticlopidine as an aspirin alternative.

Carotid Endarterectomy for Symptomatic Carotid Stenosis

In the 1980s the Rand report (190) suggested that one-third of carotid endarterectomies were performed for inappropriate indications and that indications for another one-third were questionable. Several randomized trials (77,143–146,191–193) have subsequently evaluated the safety and efficacy of carotid endarterectomy (*e*Tables 110.6.2–110.6.4). The best indication for carotid endarterectomy is for the prevention of ipsilateral carotid territory ischemic stroke in patients with a recent TIA or minor ischemic stroke due to severe carotid bifurcation atherosclerosis. This position is supported by the results of the NASCET and ECST studies (194).

North American Symptomatic Carotid Endarterectomy Trial
Starting in 1987, NASCET randomly assigned patients who had carotid territory TIA or nondisabling ischemic stroke within the past 3 months and who had ipsilateral 30% to 99% internal carotid stenosis to receive best medical management (including antiplatelet therapy) alone or with surgery. The degree of stenosis was determined by comparing the angiographic residual lumen diameter at the narrowest point to the normal vessel diameter just distal to the carotid bulb (*e*Fig. 110.5.2). The "NASCET method" has become a standard for describing carotid stenosis and differs importantly from other methods. Carotid stenosis was stratified by angiographically defined severity as moderate (30% to 69%) or severe (70% to 99%).

Perioperative Morbidity and Mortality in the North American Carotid Endarterectomy Trial. The perioperative stroke morbidity and mortality rate in all patients with severe carotid stenosis was 5.8%, which included a major stroke and death rate of 2% and a mortality rate of less than 1%. In comparison, during the 30-day perioperative period, stroke and death occurred in 3.3% of the group receiving medical treatment. The perioperative stroke morbidity and mortality rate in all patients with moderately severe carotid stenosis was 6.7%, which included a major stroke rate of 1.6% and a mortality rate of 1.2%. In comparison, stroke and death occurred in 2.4% of the group given medical treatment within 30 days. The net increase in 30-day risk with carotid endarterectomy for patients with moderate symptomatic stenosis was 4.3% for any stroke or death and 2% for disabling stroke or death. Characteristics that doubled the risk of perioperative stroke or death included contralateral carotid occlusion, evidence of an ipsilateral cerebral infarct on CT or MRI, left-sided carotid disease, diabetes, diastolic blood pressure above 90 mm Hg, absence of a history of MI or angina, and ingestion of less than 650 mg of aspirin per day, but not age or gender.

Among patients with symptomatic carotid stenosis of more than 50%, the risk of ipsilateral stroke was highest immediately after the initial ischemic event, declined gradually to 3% per year within 2 to 3 years with medical therapy alone, then dropped rapidly to 2% per year within 10 days of carotid endarterectomy. If patients with symptomatic carotid stenosis escaped recurrent symptoms for 2 or 3 years after the index ischemic event, they had little to gain from having subsequent surgery.

When Preventive Therapies Fail: Acute Ischemic Stroke Intervention

The American Heart Association (AHA) Stroke Council has published guidelines for the management of acute ischemic stroke, which have been updated for thrombolysis (195–197,270). A critical concept is time to treatment, because intravenous thrombolytic therapy must be initiated within 3 hours of stroke onset (Table 110.7).

Standard management includes respiratory support, aspiration precautions, and prevention of deep vein thrombosis. One of the most important issues in acute stroke is hemodynamic management (103,104). An algorithm for blood pressure management in patients with acute ischemic stroke has been published by the AHA (198). If the patient

TABLE 110.7   NINDS SYMPOSIUM: ACUTE STROKE TREATMENT GOALS[a]

Treatment goal	Time (min)
Door to doctor	10
Access to stroke expertise	15
Door to computed tomographic scan done	25
Door to computed tomographic scan read	45
Door to drug (intravenous t-PA)	60
Access to neurosurgical expertise	120
Door to monitored bed	180

NINDS, National Institute of Neurological Disorders and Stroke; t-PA, tissue-type plasminogen activator.
[a]NINDS Symposium on Rapid Identification and Treatment of Acute Stroke; December 1996; Arlington, VA.

has a history of hypertension, blood pressure should be kept in the mildly elevated range; some patients require higher blood pressure elevations to maintain cerebral perfusion, although this may increase the risk for cerebral edema or hemorrhage. Sustained hypertension (higher than 185/110) must be strictly avoided in patients undergoing thrombolysis. Pharmacologic agents used to decrease blood pressure should allow for minute-to-minute titration. Intravenous labetalol hydrochloride 5 to 10 mg is initially recommended when blood pressure must be lowered after acute stroke. Intravenous sodium nitroprusside is rarely required; such patients are not eligible for thrombolysis.

Aggravation of tissue acidosis from excessive anaerobic metabolism of glucose may exacerbate ischemic damage. Intravenous solutions therefore should not contain glucose, and blood glucose levels should be kept to less than 180 mg per dL and carefully monitored (92). Cerebral edema is usually maximal 3 to 7 days after cerebral infarction. Cerebral edema is best treated in an intensive care unit with ICP monitoring, osmotic dehydration, and sometimes hemicraniectomy.

Thrombolytic Therapy

Based on the National Institute of Neurological Disorders and Stroke (NINDS) trial, the FDA approved the use of intravenous tissue-type plasminogen activator (t-PA) for ischemic stroke within 3 hours of symptom onset in June 1996 (198). Intravenous t-PA within 3 hours of onset remains the only FDA-approved treatment of acute ischemic stroke. Virtually no experience has been gained with newer thrombolytic agents in acute stroke. The approval of intravenous t-PA has resulted in a much more aggressive approach to acute stroke therapy in many ways analogous to treatment of acute coronary syndromes (199). Because of the narrow therapeutic window and the risk of hemorrhage, thrombolysis in acute stroke is one of the most controversial issues in neurology today (200–205).

Intravenous Thrombolysis

Intravenous administration has the important advantages of time, ease of administration, and widespread availability. Many small series investigating intravenous thrombolysis have been performed. A metaanalysis (206) of 12 thrombolytic trials performed since 1980 found an absolute increase in symptomatic hemorrhages of 7% [odds ratio (OR), 3.62; 95% confidence interval (CI), 2.73 to 4.80] and a 3.7% increase in death (OR, 1.36; 95% CI, 1.14 to 1.62). A significant 6.5% absolute reduction in poor outcome was seen, however; 61.5% of patients (798 of 1,297) randomly assigned to receive thrombolysis were dead or dependent compared with 65.0% (864 of 1,270) who did not receive thrombolysis (OR, 0.75; 95% CI, 0.63 to 0.88). ♥ r07

Risks of Hemorrhagic Transformation

Several series have found no relationship between recanalization and hemorrhage risk, although these series usually refer to early as opposed to delayed recanalization (220,226,228–232). The amount of ischemic damage is a key factor in the development of hemorrhage after thrombolysis. Early CT changes and severity of initial deficit, both indicators of the extent of ischemic damage, are currently some of the best predictors of hemorrhagic transformation (199,207,233).

Several factors have been associated with hemorrhage after thrombolysis for both stroke and MI, including thrombolytic dose (230,234), blood pressure (19,230,235–237), advanced age, and prior head injury (199,230,234,235,238,239). Age was the most important identifiable risk factor in one of the largest series investigating thrombolysis-related ICH (238). Because of the increased risk in elderly patients, an upper age limit was initially placed on patients being considered for coronary thrombolysis. These patients were found still to benefit from treatment, and the generally accepted age limit has increased. The strong relationship between advanced age and hemorrhage was demonstrated again in the NINDS and ECASS trials. At this time, no strict age cutoff exists for administering thrombolytics for stroke. Physicians need to take into account the increased risk of hemorrhage in patients aged 75 and older when making the decision to initiate thrombolysis. ♥ r08

Thrombolysis in the Community Setting

Several phase IV series of t-PA use in experienced stroke centers have been published (241–243) that demonstrate similar rates of symptomatic ICH as seen in the NINDS trial. In the Cleveland metropolitan area, only 1.8% of all ischemic stroke patients admitted to hospitals and 10% arriving within 3 hours of symptom onset received intravenous t-PA (244). A systematic audit of t-PA use in Cleveland, performed in 1997 to 1998, found a higher symptomatic ICH rate (15.7%) (244), which suggests that the efficacy seen in clinical trials and experienced centers may not necessarily be replicated in communities. The presence of protocol deviations is associated with higher rates of symptomatic ICH (243). Major early signs of infarction on CT portend a worse prognosis and increased hemorrhage risk; such patients probably should not receive intravenous rt-PA. These signs can be missed (207,217,245). In a study of the accuracy of interpretation of head CT scans by emergency physicians, only 43% correctly recognized a remote infarction as being old. Their ability to detect early CT changes was 0% for scans rated as "difficult" and 46% for scans rated as "intermediate" in difficulty (245).

Use of Ancrod

The defibrinogenating agent ancrod, derived from Malayan pit viper venom, has been studied in acute stroke (246).

The positive results of the Stroke Treatment with Ancrod Trial were not replicated in a European study.

Anticoagulation and Antiplatelet Therapy

Use of Low-Molecular-Weight Heparin

Researchers have investigated the use of low-molecular-weight heparin in treating acute ischemic stroke (274). The Fraxiparine in Stroke Study (275) reported improved neurologic outcome at 6 months that was not present at 3 months in patients treated with low-molecular-weight heparin compared to those treated with placebo. Although this study has generated much interest, its methodologies have been criticized and its results must be interpreted with caution. The Trial of ORG 10172 in Acute Stroke Treatment (TOAST) evaluated the heparinoid Org 10172 in a randomized trial of the treatment of acute ischemic stroke. No overall benefit was found, and the rate of intracerebral hemorrhage in patients with more severe strokes was significant (NIHSS higher than 14). Subgroup analysis suggested a trend toward benefit for those patients with acute stroke due to large vessel atherosclerosis (276).

Glycoprotein IIb/IIIa Receptor Antagonism

The glycoprotein IIb/IIIa receptor is the final common pathway for platelet binding to fibrinogen and has demonstrated efficacy in prevention of thrombus formation in acute coronary syndromes and interventional procedures. In acute ischemic stroke, a dose-escalation study demonstrated that abciximab is safe when given as a 0.25-mg-per-kg bolus and 0.125-mg-per-kilogram-per-minute infusion (277). A phase II trial, Abciximab (ReoPro) in Acute Ischemic Stroke, is under way to test its use in treating acute ischemic stroke of less than 6 hours' duration. The role of IIb/IIa agents in stroke prevention is less clear, as several prevention trials with oral IIb/IIIa agents have been stopped early due to increased mortality rates and lack of apparent efficacy.

Controversies and Personal Perspectives

Choice of Antithrombotic Therapy

The optimum dosage of aspirin for preventing stroke has become less controversial. Dosages from 50 mg to 325 mg have their advocates and a few trials still are using 650 mg to 1,300 mg. The FDA has approved aspirin in doses of 50 mg to 325 mg for the prevention of stroke and TIAs. A metaanalysis found no significant effect of aspirin dose on stroke risk reduction (278).

Treatment of patients who remain symptomatic on aspirin is still controversial. An increasing number of alternatives to aspirin are available. Despite the lack of definitive evidence that clopidogrel specifically reduces the risk of stroke, it has replaced ticlopidine for most cerebrovascular indications. Combinations of antiplatelet agents likely will soon supplant single-agent therapy. Although the 50-mg aspirin plus 400-mg extended-release dipyridamole formulation has significant benefit for stroke risk reduction, the lack of demonstrated cardiovascular risk reduction is problematic in patients with multisystem atherosclerosis. The Clopidogrel in Unstable Angina to Prevent Recurrent Ischemic Events (CURE) trial (279) suggests that the combination of clopidogrel and aspirin is safe and effective for coronary risk reduction, and this combination is being specifically studied in the Management of Atherothrombosis with Clopidogrel in High-Risk Patients with Recent Transient Ischemic Attack or Ischemic Stroke (MATCH) trial. The Warfarin Aspirin Symptomatic Intracranial Disease study and the SPAF study demonstrated that antiplatelet or antithrombotic efficacy varies depending on the cause of the patient's cerebrovascular symptoms and on other poorly understood variables. These findings suggest that, in the future, therapy may well be determined by a number of selective factors.

Carotid Revascularization and Endovascular Therapies

Clinical trials have clarified the role of endarterectomy in symptomatic patients, but recommendations for asymptomatic patients remain controversial. The authors' conservative recommendations are based on (a) the particular cerebral event to be prevented (i.e., TIAs vs. all strokes vs. severe ipsilateral strokes), (b) the patient group in which such an event is to be prevented (e.g., men vs. women), and (c) the cost at which such prevention is to be achieved, both in terms of negative outcomes and economics. The lack of standard reporting of endarterectomy complication rates among surgeons and the performance of endarterectomy based on noninvasive testing alone are causes of concern. Carotid artery stenting has been proposed as an alternative to endarterectomy in cases of postradiation therapy carotid stenosis, restenosis after endarterectomy, and stenosis in high-risk patients with severe comorbidities, as well as in symptomatic, surgically inaccessible intracranial stenoses (280–282). Despite glowing case reports, however, the poor results with carotid angioplasty in the reported randomized trials should provoke a cautious advance of the technique, improved patient selection, then proof of equivalent efficacy in controlled clinical trials before it is widely embraced (283,284).

Endovascular techniques for aneurysm obliteration continue to carry substantial complication rates and uncertain longevity but are emerging as promising alternatives to aneurysm surgery ready for comparison in a clinical trial (285–287). Angioplasty is emerging as a promising treatment for vasospasm secondary to subarachnoid hemorrhage when standard medical therapy has failed (288–291).

CEREBRAL HEMORRHAGE: CLINICAL PROFILE

Nontraumatic ICHs are referred to as *primary* or *spontaneous* when no evidence is seen of an underlying cause, and as *secondary* when they occur because of a vascular malformation or aneurysm, coagulopathy, primary or metastatic tumor, or granuloma (292). Although time to diagnosis and overall mortality have improved with neuroimaging techniques and hypertension therapy, early mortality remains high at 30% to 40%. ⊽ r09

Hypertension

Arterial hypertension is blamed for 70% to 90% of primary ICHs related to rupture of small perforating arteries damaged by lipohyalinosis and microaneurysm formation (298,299).

Amyloid Angiopathy

Beta-amyloid protein deposits within the media and adventitia of small meningeal and cortical vessels produce vascular fragility, which leads to lobar hemorrhages that tend to be multiple or recurrent. The most common cause of nonhypertensive hemorrhage in the elderly, amyloid angiopathy is also implicated in ICH complicating thrombolysis (300–302) (Fig. 110.5).

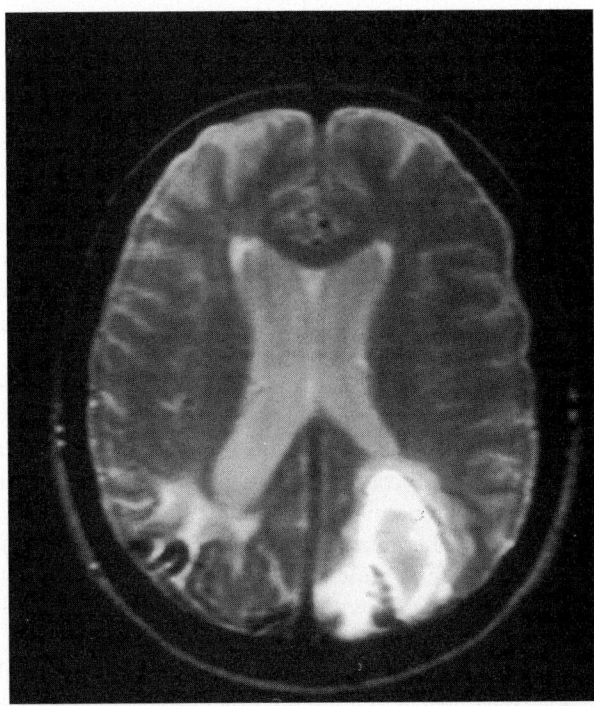

FIGURE 110.5 Residual hemosiderin in the right occipital lobe from a remote hemorrhage and subacute blood in the left occipital lobe in a patient with amyloid angiopathy.

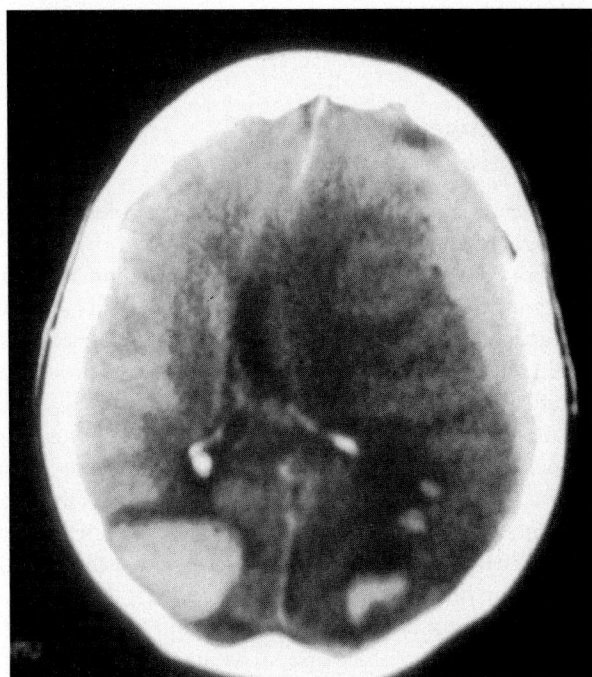

FIGURE 110.6 Complex multiple intracranial hemorrhages after coronary thrombolysis for acute myocardial infarction.

Coagulopathy-Induced Intracranial Hemorrhage

Anticoagulant-related ICHs account for 9% of all ICHs, and typically occur in patients on long-term or excessive oral anticoagulation. Other risk factors include increasing age, poorly controlled hypertension, and, probably, underlying cerebral amyloid angiopathy (306).

ICH is the most feared complication of thrombolytic therapy for acute ischemic stroke as well as a rare but serious complication of thrombolytic treatment of acute MI, peripheral vascular disease, and pulmonary embolism. Risk factors include advanced age, hypertension, low body weight, underlying hypertensive cerebrovascular disease, and amyloid angiopathy. Although hemorrhages are most commonly confluent, solitary, and lobar, the spectrum includes multiple, deep, or infratentorial hemorrhages, and associated subdural, intraventricular, and subarachnoid bleeding (235,238) (Fig. 110.6).

Drug-Related Intracranial Hemorrhage

Recreational drugs associated with ICH include the sympathomimetics, most commonly cocaine; amphetamines; and phencyclidine (307). Phenylpropanolamine has now been removed from appetite suppressants and cough and cold remedies, after it was associated with hemorrhagic stroke in women (308,309). An underlying structural cause, such as underlying arteriovenous malformation or aneurysm, is common, and rare cases of occlusive vasculopathy that mimics vasculitis have been described.

CEREBRAL HEMORRHAGE: MANAGEMENT PRINCIPLES

Surgical Evacuation for Intracranial Hemorrhage

Surgical evacuation for ICH should be considered before neurologic deterioration leads to coma and irreversible brainstem damage, although patient selection remains highly controversial. Symptomatic cerebellar ICHs are usually evacuated because of the unpredictable course and risk of rapid and progressive brainstem compression, producing respiratory arrest and death. Accessible subcortical ICHs, particularly those involving the nondominant hemisphere or noneloquent areas of the brain, are also amenable to surgical evacuation, and such evacuation should be considered in patients who present with relatively preserved neurologic function that subsequently begin to deteriorate (319). Surgical therapy does not improve outcome with ICHs affecting basal ganglia and the brainstem, and advanced age, large hematoma volume, and a depressed level of consciousness on evaluation are consistent predictors of poor neurologic outcome (320,321).

SUBARACHNOID HEMORRHAGE: CLINICAL PROFILE

Despite major advances in neurosurgical techniques over the past two decades, the acute mortality of approximately 10% continues to pose the major obstacle to treatment of subarachnoid hemorrhage. An additional 50% of patients die within 3 months, and of those who survive, more than half are left with a major neurologic or neurocognitive disability and a diminished quality of life (322,323).

The most common symptom of subarachnoid hemorrhage is a headache of noteworthy severity, ranging from the thunderclap prodromal headache with a minor leak to the sudden, severe, often exertional headache present in 45% of patients (324–326). Syncope at onset results from global cerebral hypoperfusion when the rupture causes a precipitous spike in ICP that approaches the mean arterial pressure and thus reduces cerebral perfusion pressure. Clinical grading of the patient based on headache and mental status is important in predicting prognosis and chance of recovery. The most commonly used scale is the Hunt and Hess classification scheme (eTable 110.7.2).

A CT scan of the brain without contrast performed within 24 hours shows positive findings in 92% but by 48 hours bears only a 75% chance of demonstrating cisternal or subarachnoid blood (Fig. 110.7). If no hemorrhage is seen, a lumbar puncture is recommended to establish the diagnosis. Selective intraarterial cerebral angiography remains the standard for diagnosis and planning of a therapeutic surgical or endovascular approach (327,328).

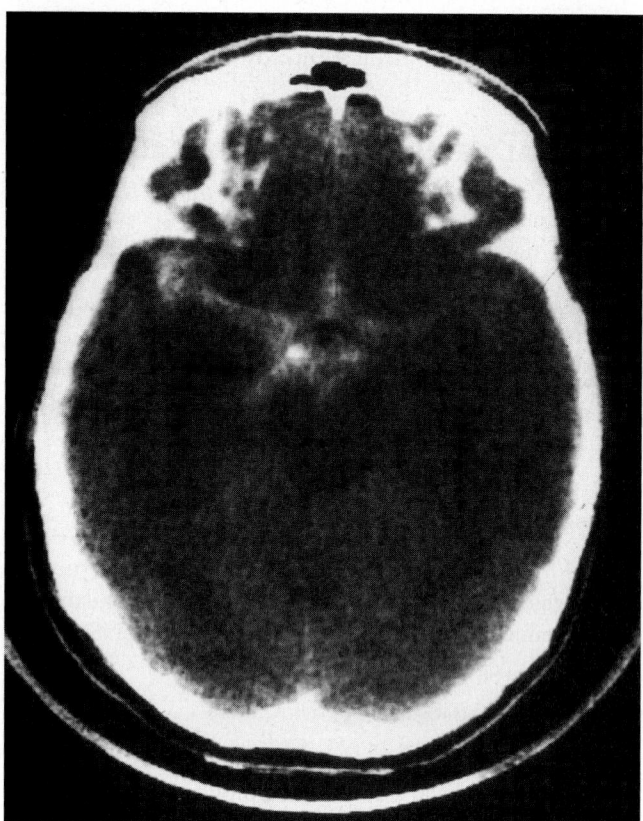

FIGURE 110.7 Computed tomographic scan showing cisternal blood in acute subarachnoid hemorrhage.

Aneurysms

Most intracranial aneurysms are *saccular* and are believed to be outpouchings of the arterial wall as a result of a congenital defect in the muscular layer, a degenerative process in the internal elastic membrane, or a combination of both processes. They most frequently occur at bifurcations, branch and bending points within the arterial tree, with the majority at the base of the brain on the circle of Willis. They are associated with polycystic kidney disease, coarctation of the aorta, Ehlers-Danlos syndrome, neurofibromatosis, fibromuscular dysplasia, and arteriovenous malformations (329,330).

Mycotic aneurysms are a complication of subacute bacterial endocarditis in which an infective embolus produces a local arteritis and septic degeneration of the vessel wall. The true incidence of mycotic aneurysms is unknown and would require cerebral angiography in a large series of patients with subacute bacterial endocarditis to ascertain. The location of such aneurysms at peripheral cerebral branch sites and their small size defy adequate visualization by any currently available noninvasive neuroimaging technique, including MRA (327). The neurologic profile most suggestive of a possible mycotic aneurysm is a focal neurologic deficit consistent with cerebral embolism. In patients who have successfully completed their full course of appropriate antibiotic therapy,

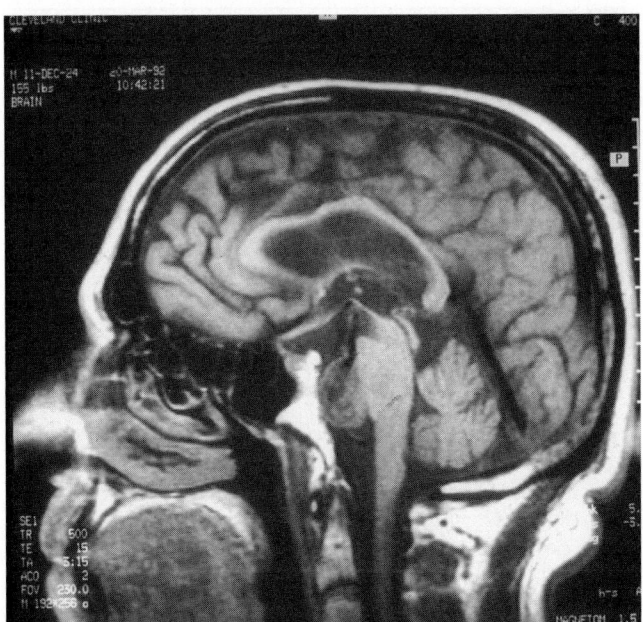

FIGURE 110.8 Magnetic resonance image demonstrating a large fusiform basilar arterial aneurysm producing brainstem compression and transient ischemic attacks.

the risk for late mycotic aneurysm rupture is estimated to be less than 3% (136,137).

Atherosclerotic aneurysms are tortuous vessels that are most frequently located in the vertebrobasilar system; however, they can affect the major intracranial internal carotid branches. Symptoms are produced by mass effect, ischemia from branch artery occlusions, and obstructive hydrocephalus but rarely from rupture (Fig. 110.8).

SUBARACHNOID HEMORRHAGE: MANAGEMENT PRINCIPLES

Subarachnoid hemorrhage carries the highest mortality of all stroke and warrants highly specialized management (337–339). The introduction of microsurgical techniques has substantially reduced operative morbidity and mortality, but nonoperative complications of rebleeding, vasospasm, and hydrocephalus continue to contribute to the poor outcome in many patients (339–342).

Rebleeding occurs in 30% of patients, is highest in the first 3 weeks, and carries a much higher morbidity and mortality risk (343). Transient episodes of hypertension have often been observed to precede and to perhaps precipitate rebleeding, but antihypertensive treatment per se has not been shown to improve outcome (344). Nevertheless, precautions for patients with aneurysm include a combination of bed rest, analgesia, stool softeners, dim lighting, and strict visitor limitations; in short, avoidance of any stimulus that may cause agitation or excitement and result in a rise in blood pressure. The optimal blood pressure range in the post–subarachnoid

hemorrhage period remains undefined but generally is within approximately 5% of the premorbid range.

Vasospasm

Vasospasm is clinically present in approximately 30% of patients, although angiographic evidence is present in approximately 70% (345,346). Symptoms of a focal neurologic deficit with a depression of consciousness usually begin between the third and fifth days after subarachnoid hemorrhage and peak between the fifth and fourteenth days, resolving over a period of weeks. Transcranial Doppler ultrasonography is useful in diagnosis and helps guide hypervolemic, hypertensive therapy (347,348). Hyponatremia often parallels the time course of vasospasm, is due to natriuresis or cerebral salt wasting and volume contraction mediated by atrial natriuretic factor, and is managed with intravascular administration of isotonic fluids (349,350). Oral nimodipine, 60 mg every 4 hours started within 4 days of the hemorrhage and continuing for 21 days, has been shown to reduce poor outcome due to vasospasm for patients of good neurologic condition after the ictus (i.e., Hunt and Hess grades I, II, and III) (351–356).

Medical Comorbidities

Subarachnoid hemorrhage is often accompanied by a massive rise in circulating levels of catecholamines that results in subendocardial ischemia, infarction, and arrhythmias. Premature ventricular complexes, bradyrhythmias, or supraventricular tachycardias occur in up to 90% of patients; however, potentially malignant arrhythmias such as atrioventricular dissociation, idioventricular arrhythmias, and ventricular tachycardia occur in 20% to 40% of patients. Arrhythmias are most frequent in the first 48 hours after subarachnoid hemorrhage, are often associated with QTc prolongation or hypokalemia, and may lead to sudden death.

Common pulmonary complications of subarachnoid hemorrhage include aspiration pneumonia and pulmonary edema. Pulmonary edema after subarachnoid hemorrhage may be due to elevated cardiac filling pressures or may be neurogenic, to which pulmonary capillary tight junction disruption is postulated as an important contributor.

Hydrocephalus complicates 20% of cases and when acute and untreated, carries a grave prognosis. Hydrocephalus more frequently develops insidiously, resulting in impaired consciousness, lower limb spasticity, and increased ICP. Ventricular drainage is recommended for symptomatic patients; however, catheterization carries a risk for rebleeding and infection, and catheter patency may be difficult to maintain (357–358a).

Seizure-like events are more common at the ictus but may also occur in a delayed fashion and carry a potential risk for rebleeding. Use of prophylactic anticonvulsants in the early posthemorrhage period is recommended; however, long-term continuation is not necessary if the patient has been seizure free (359).

THE FUTURE

A better understanding of the risk factors specific for each stroke subtype will advance preventive strategies. Endovascular interventions will evolve and mature, combined with thrombolysis for acute ischemic stroke, as an alternative to surgery for aneurysms and vascular malformations and in the treatment of inaccessible occlusive disease. Stroke health care delivery systems will continue to evolve to allow better patient access to care.

REFERENCES

1. Clarke E. Apoplexy in the Hippocratic writings. *Bull Hist Med* 1963;37:301–314.
2. Willis T. *Cerebri anatome: Cui accessit nervorum descriptio et usus.* Londini: J. Flesher, 1664.
3. Wepfer JJ. Observationes anatomicae, ex cadaveribus eorum, quos sustulit apoplexia cum exercitatione de ejus loco affecto. In: Schaffhausen JOH, ed. *Caspari Suteri.* 1658.
4. Rostan L. *Recherches sur le ramollissement du cerveau: ouvrage dans lequel on s'efforce de distinguer les diverses affections de ce viscere par des signes caracteristiques.* Paris: Bechet, 1823.
5. Fields WS, Lemak NA. *The history of stroke: its recognition and treatment.* New York: Oxford University Press, 1989:12–20.
6. Gowers WR. *Diagnosis of diseases of the brain and spinal cord.* New York: William Wood, 1885:164–165.
7. Chiari H. Über das verhalten des tielungswinkels der carotis communis bei der endarteris chronica deformans. *Verh Dtsch Ges Pathol* 1905;9:326–330.
8. Hunt JR. The role of the carotid arteries in the causation of vascular lesions of the brain with remarks on certain special features of the symptomatology. *Am J Med Sci* 1914;147:704–713.
9. Moniz E. L'encephalographic arterielle son importance dans la localisation des tumeurs cérébrales. *Rev Neurol* 1927;2:72–90.
10. Loman J, Myerson A. Visualization of the cerebral vessels by direct injection of thorium dioxide (Thorotrast). *AJR Am J Roentgenol* 1936;35:188–193.
11. Seldinger SI. Catheter replacement of the needle in percutaneous arteriography. *Acta Radiol* 1953;39:368–376.
12. Modic MT, Weinstein MA, Chilcote WA, et al. Digital subtraction angiography of the intracranial vascular system: comparative study in 55 patients. *AJR Am J Roentgenol* 1981;38:287–295.
13. Fisher CM. Occlusion of the internal carotid artery. *Arch Neurol Psychiatry* 1951;65:346–377.
14. Fields WS, North RR, Hass WK, et al. Joint study of extracranial arterial occlusion as a cause of stroke: organization of study and survey of patient population. *JAMA* 1968;203:955–960.
15. Hass WK, Fields WS, North RR, et al. Joint study of extracranial arterial occlusion: arteriography, techniques, sites and complications. *JAMA* 1968;203:961–968.
16. Bauer RB, Meyer JS, Fields WS, et al. Joint study of extracranial arterial occlusion: progress report of controlled study of long-term survival in patients with and without operation. *JAMA* 1969;208:509–518.
17. Blaisdell WF, Clauss RH, Galbraith JG, et al. Joint study of extracranial arterial occlusion: a review of surgical considerations. *JAMA* 1969;209:1889–1895.
18. Fields WS, Maslenikov V, Meyer JS, et al. Joint study of extracranial arterial occlusion: progress report of prognosis following surgery or nonsurgical treatment for transient cerebral ischemic attacks and cervical carotid artery lesions. *JAMA* 1970;211:1993–2003.
19. Fields WS, Lemak NA. Joint study of extracranial arterial occlusion: internal carotid artery occlusion. *JAMA* 1976;235:234–238.
20. Rose WM. Anticoagulant in management of cerebral infarction: record of poor result obtained. *Med J Aust* 1950;1:503–504.
21. Askey JM, Cherry CB. Thromboembolism associated with auricular fibrillation: continuous anticoagulant therapy. *JAMA* 1950;144:97–100.
22. Veterans Administration. An evaluation of anticoagulant therapy in the treatment of cerebral vascular disease. *Neurology* 1961;11:132–138.
23. Groch SN, McDevitt E, Wright IS. Long-term study of cerebral vascular disease. *Ann Intern Med* 1961;55:358–367.
24. Pearce JMS, Gubbay SS, Walton JN. Long-term anticoagulant therapy in transient cerebral ischemic attacks. *Lancet* 1965;1:6–9.
25. Craven LL. Prevention of coronary and cerebral thrombosis. *Miss Valley Med J* 1956;78:213–215.
26. Harrison MJG, Marshall J, Meadows JC, et al. Effect of aspirin in amaurosis fugax. *Lancet* 1971;2:743–744.
27. Mundall J, Quintero P, von Kaulla K, et al. Transient monocular blindness and increased platelet aggregability treated with aspirin: a case report. *Neurology* 1972;22(3):280–285.
28. Fields WS, Lemak NA, Frankowski, et al. Controlled trial of aspirin in cerebral ischemia. *Stroke* 1977;8:301–316.
29. Fields WS, Lemak NA, Frankowski, et al. Controlled trial of aspirin in cerebral ischemia. Part II: surgical group. *Stroke* 1978;9:309–319.
30. Canadian Cooperative Study Group. A randomized trial of aspirin and sulfinpyrazone in threatened stroke. *N Engl J Med* 1978;299:53–59.
31. Bousser MG, Eschwege E, Haguenau M, et al. AICLA controlled trial of aspirin and dipyridamole in the secondary prevention of atherothrombotic cerebral ischemia. *Stroke* 1983;14:5–14.

32. Sorensen PS, Pedersen H, Marquardsen J, et al. Acetylsalicylic acid in the prevention of stroke in patients with reversible cerebral ischemic attacks: a Danish study. *Stroke* 1983;14:15–22.

33. Antiplatelet Trialists' Collaboration. Secondary prevention of vascular disease by prolonged antiplatelet treatment. *BMJ* 1988;296:320–331.

34. UK-TIA Study Group. United Kingdom transient ischaemic attack (UK-TIA) aspirin trial: interim results. *BMJ* 1988;296:316–320.

35. ESPS Group. European Stroke Prevention Study. *Stroke* 1990;21:1122–1130.

36. The Dutch TIA Trial Study Group. A comparison of two doses of aspirin (30 mg versus 283 mg a day) in patients after a transient ischemic attack or minor ischemic stroke. *N Engl J Med* 1991;325:1261–1266.

37. The SALT collaborative group. Swedish Aspirin Low-dose Trial (SALT) of 75 mgm aspirin as secondary prophylaxis after cerebrovascular ischaemic events. *Lancet* 1991;338:1345–1349.

38. Diener HC, Cunha L, Forbes C, et al. European Stroke Prevention Study 2. Dipyridamole and acetylsalicylic acid in the secondary prevention of stroke. *J Neurol Sci* 1996;143:1–13.

39. CAPRIE Steering Committee. A randomized, blinded, trial of clopidogrel versus aspirin in patients at risk of ischemic events (CAPRIE). *Lancet* 1996;348:1329–1339.

40. Sandercock P, Molyneux A, Warlow C. Value of computed tomography in patients with stroke: Oxfordshire Community Stroke Project. *BMJ* 1985;290:193–197.

41. Kinkel WR, Jacobs L. Computerized axial transverse tomography in cerebrovascular disease. *Neurology* 1976;26:924–930.

42. Special report from the National Institute of Neurological Disorders and Stroke. Classification of cerebrovascular diseases III. *Stroke* 1990;21:637–676.

43. Garraway WM, Whisnant JP, Furlan AJ, et al. The declining incidence of stroke. *N Engl J Med* 1979;300:449–452.

44. Broderick J, Phillips SJ, Whisnant JP, et al. Incidence rates of stroke in the eighties: the end of the decline in stroke? *Stroke* 1989;20:577–582.

45. Kannel WB, Blaisdell FW, Gifford R, et al. Risk factors in stroke due to cerebral infarction. *Stroke* 1971;2:423–428.

46. Wolf PA, D'Agostino RB, Belanger AJ, et al. Probability of stroke: a risk profile from the Framingham study. *Stroke* 1992;22:312–318.

47. Sacco RL, Mohr JP, Tatemichi TK, et al. Infarction of undetermined cause: the NINCDS stroke data bank. *Ann Neurol* 1989;25:382–390.

48. Kannel WB, Wolf PA, Verter J, et al. Epidemiologic assessment of the role of blood pressure in stroke: the Framingham study. *JAMA* 1970;214:301–310.

49. Cerebral Embolism Task Force. Cardiogenic brain embolism. *Arch Neurol* 1986;43:71–84.

50. Wolf PA, Dawber TR, Thomas HE, et al. Epidemiologic assessment of chronic atrial fibrillation and the risk of stroke: the Framingham study. *Neurology* 1978;28:973–977.

51. Wolf PA, Abbott RD, Kannel WB. Atrial fibrillation: a major contributor to stroke in the elderly: the Framingham study. *Arch Intern Med* 1987;147:1561–1564.

52. Furberg CD, Psaty BM, Manolio TA, et al. Prevalence of atrial fibrillation in elderly subjects (the Cardiovascular Health Study). *Am J Cardiol* 1994;74:236–241.

53. Peterson P, Madsen EB, Brun B, et al. Silent cerebral infarction in atrial fibrillation. *Stroke* 1987;18:1098–1100.

54. European Atrial Fibrillation Trial Study Group. Secondary prevention in nonrheumatic atrial fibrillation after transient ischemic attack or minor stroke. *Lancet* 1993;324:1255–1262.

55. Atrial Fibrillation investigators. Risk factors for stroke and efficacy of antithrombotic therapies in atrial fibrillation: analysis of pooled data from five randomized controlled trials. *Arch Intern Med* 1994;154:1449–1457.

56. The Stroke Prevention in Atrial Fibrillation investigators. Predictors of thromboembolism in atrial fibrillation: clinical features in patients at risk. *Ann Intern Med* 1992;116:1–5.

57. Gage BF, Waterman AD, Shannon W, et al. Validation of clinical classification schemes for predicting stroke: results from the National Registry of Atrial Fibrillation. *JAMA* 2001;285:2864–2870.

58. Johannessen KA, Nordrehaug JE, von der Lippe G. Left ventricular thrombosis and cerebrovascular accident in acute myocardial infarction. *Br Heart J* 1984;51:553–556.

59. Komrad MS, Coffey CE, Coffey KS, et al. Myocardial infarction and stroke. *Neurology* 1984;34:1403–1409.

60. Behar S, Tanne D, Abinader E, et al. Cerebrovascular accident complicating acute myocardial infarction: incidence, clinical significance, and short- and long-term mortality rates. *Am J Med* 1991;91:45–50.

61. Weinreich DJ, Burke JF, Pauletto FJ. Left ventricular mural thrombi complicating acute myocardial infarction. *Ann Intern Med* 1984;100:789–794.

62. Meltzer RS, Visser CA, Fuster V. Intracardiac thrombi and systemic embolization. *Ann Intern Med* 1986;104:689–698.

63. Asinger RW, Mikell FL, Elsperger J, et al. Incidence of left ventricular thrombus after acute transmural myocardial infarction: serial evaluation by two-dimensional echocardiography. *N Engl J Med* 1981;305:297–302.

64. Schweizer P, Bardos P, Erbel R, et al. Detection of left atrial thrombi by echocardiography. *Br Heart J* 1984;51:553–556.

65. Maggiono AP, Franzosi MG, Santoro L, et al. The risk of stroke in patients with acute myocardial infarction after thrombolytic and antithrombotic treatment. *N Engl J Med* 1992;327:1–6.

66. Vaitkus P, Barnathan ES. Embolic potential, prevention, and management of mural thrombus complicating anterior myocardial infarction: a meta-analysis. *J Am Coll Cardiol* 1993;22:1004–1009.

67. Martin R, Bogousslavsky J. Mechanism of late stroke after myocardial infarct: the Lausanne Stroke Registry. *J Neurol Neurosurg Psychiatry* 1982;56:760–764.

68. Tanne D, Reicher-Reiss H, Boyko V, et al. Stroke risk after anterior wall acute myocardial infarction. *Am J Cardiol* 1995;76:825–826.

69. Coulshed N, Epstein EJ, McKendrick CS, et al. Systemic embolism in mitral valve disease. *Br Heart J* 1970;32:26–34.

70. Edmunds LH. Thromboembolic complications of current cardiac valvular prosthesis. *Ann Thorac Surg* 1982;34:96–106.

71. Hertzer NR, Young JR, Beven EG, et al. Coronary angiography in 506 patients with extracranial cerebrovascular disease. *Arch Intern Med* 1985;145:849–852.

72. Toole JF. The Willis Lecture: transient ischemic attacks, scientific method, and new realities. *Stroke* 1991;22:99–104.

73. Sandok BA, Furlan AJ, Whisnant JP, et al. Guidelines for the management of transient ischemic attacks. *Mayo Clin Proc* 1978;53:665–674.

74. Marzewski DJ, Furlan AJ, St. Louis P, et al. Intracranial internal carotid artery stenosis: long-term progress. *Stroke* 1982;13:821–824.

75. Bogousslavsky J, Regli F. Prognosis of symptomatic intracranial obstruction of internal carotid artery. *Eur Neurol* 1983;22:351–358.

76. Bogousslavsky J, Desplaud PA, Regli F. Prognosis of high-risk patients with nonoperated symptomatic extracranial carotid tight stenosis. *Stroke* 1988;19:108–111.

77. North American Symptomatic Carotid Endarterectomy Trial Collaborators. Beneficial effect of carotid endarterectomy in symptomatic patients with high-grade carotid stenosis. *N Engl J Med* 1991;325:445–453.

78. Easton JD, Wilterdink JL. Carotid endarterectomy: trials and tribulations. *Ann Neurol* 1994;35:5–17.

79. Roederer GO, Langlois YL, Jager KA, et al. The natural history of carotid arterial disease in asymptomatic patients with cervical bruits. *Stroke* 1984;15:605–613.

80. Chambers BR, Norris JW. Outcome in patients with asymptomatic neck bruits. *N Engl J Med* 1986;15:860–865.

81. Norris JW, Zhu CZ, Bornstein NM, et al. Vascular risks of asymptomatic carotid stenosis. *Stroke* 1991;22:1485–1490.

82. Ingall TJ, Homer D, Baker HL Jr, et al. Predictors of intracranial carotid artery atherosclerosis. *Arch Neurol* 1991;48:687–691.

83. Iso H, Jacobs DR, Wentworth D, et al. Serum cholesterol levels and six-year mortality from stroke in 350,977 men screened for the multiple risk factor intervention trial. *N Engl J Med* 1989;320:904–909.

84. Yano K, Reed DM, MacLean CJ. Serum cholesterol and hemorrhagic stroke in the Honolulu heart program. *Stroke* 1989;20:1460–1465.

85. Tell GS, Crouse JR, Furberg CD. Relation between blood lipids, lipoproteins, and cerebrovascular atherosclerosis. *Stroke* 1988;19:423–430.

86. Hachinski V, Graffagnino C, Beaudry M, et al. Lipids and stroke: a paradox resolved. *Arch Neurol* 1996;53:303–308.

87. Sacks F, Pfeiffer M, Moye L, et al. The effect of pravastatin on coronary events after myocardial infarction in patients with average cholesterol levels. *N Engl J Med* 1996;335:1001–1009.

88. White HD, Simes RJ, Anderson NE, et al. Pravastatin therapy and the risk of stroke. *N Engl J Med* 2000;343:317–326.

89. Shepherd J. The West of Scotland Coronary Prevention Study: a trial of cholesterol reduction in Scottish men. *Am J Cardiol* 1995;76:113C–117C.

90. Downs JF, Clearfield M, Weiss S, et al. for the AFCAPS/TexCAPS research group. Primary prevention in acute coronary events with lovastatin in men and women with average cholesterol levels. Results of AFCAPS/TexCAPS. *JAMA* 1998;279:1615–1622.

91. The Diabetes Control and Complications Trial Research Group. The effect of intensive treatment of diabetes on the development and progression of long-term complications in insulin-dependent diabetes mellitus. *N Engl J Med* 1993;329:977–986.

92. Toni D, De Michele M, Fiorelli M, et al. Influence of hyperglycemia on infarct size and clinical outcome of acute ischemic stroke patients with intracranial arterial occlusion. *J Neurol Sci* 1994;123:129–133.

93. Harris EN, Chan JKH, Asherson RA, et al. Thrombosis, recurrent fetal loss, thrombocytopenia: predictive value of IgG anticardiolipin antibodies. *Arch Intern Med* 1986;146:2153–2156.

94. Levine SR, Deegan MJ, Futrell N, et al. Cerebrovascular and neurological disease associated with antiphospholipid antibodies: 48 cases. *Neurology* 1990;40:1181–1189.

95. Mannoussakis MN, Tzioufas AG, Silis AG, et al. High prevalence of anticardiolipin antibody and other autoantibodies in a healthy population. *Clin Exp Immunol* 1987;69:557–565.

96. Gillum LA, Mamadipudi SK, Johnston SC. Ischemic stroke risk with oral contraceptives: a meta-analysis. *JAMA* 2000;284:72–78.

97. Alberts MJ. Genetic aspects of cerebrovascular disease. *Stroke* 1991;22:276–280.

98. Gorelick PB. Alcohol and stroke. *Stroke* 1987;18:268–270.

99. Abbott RD, Yin Y, Reed DM, et al. Risk of stroke in male cigarette smokers. *N Engl J Med* 1987;317:1237–1245.

100. Colditz GA, Bonita R, Stampfer MJ, et al. Cigarette smoking and risk of stroke in middle-aged women. *N Engl J Med* 1988;318:937–941.

101. Shinton R, Beevers G. Meta-analysis of relation between cigarette smoking and stroke. *BMJ* 1989;298:789–794.

102. Selman WR, Spetzler RF. Therapeutics for focal cerebral ischemia. *Neurosurgery* 1980;6:446–452.

103. Yatsu FM, Zivin J. Hypertension in acute ischemic strokes. *Arch Neurol* 1985;42:999–1000.

104. Powers WJ. Acute hypertension after stroke. *Neurology* 1993;43:461–467.

105. Ahmed SH, Hu CJ, Paczynski R, et al. Pathophysiology of ischemic injury. In: Fisher M, ed. *Stroke therapy*, 2nd ed. Woburn, MA: Butterworth–Heinemann, 2001:25–58.

106. Caplan LR. Top of the basilar syndrome. *Neurology* 1980;30:72–79.

107. Troost BT. Dizziness and vertigo in vertebrobasilar disease. Part I. Peripheral and systemic causes of dizziness. *Stroke* 1980;11:301–303.

108. Troost BT. Dizziness and vertigo in vertebrobasilar disease. Part II. Central causes and vertebrobasilar disease. *Stroke* 1980;11:413–415.

109. Fisher CM. Lacunar strokes and infarcts: a review. *Neurology* 1982;32:871–876.

110. Mohr JP. Lacunes. *Stroke* 1982;13:3–10.

111. Chimowitz MI, Furlan AJ, Sila CA, et al. Etiology of motor or sensory stroke: a prospective study of the predictive value of clinical and radiological features. *Ann Neurol* 1991;30:519–525.

112. Collins R, Peto R, MacMahon S, et al. Blood pressure, stroke, and coronary artery disease. *Lancet* 1990;335:827–838.

113. Veterans Administration Cooperative Study Group on Antihypertensive Agents. Effects of treatment on morbidity in hypertension. 1. Results in patients with diastolic blood pressures averaging 115 through 129 mm Hg. *JAMA* 1967;202:116–122.

114. Management Committee. The Australian therapeutic trial in mild hypertension. *Lancet* 1980;1:1261–1267.

115. Hypertension Detection and Follow-up Program Cooperative Group. The effect of treatment on mortality in "mild" hypertension. *N Engl J Med* 1982;307:976–980.

116. SHEP Cooperative Research Group. Prevention of stroke by antihypertensive drug treatment in older persons with isolated systolic hypertension. *JAMA* 1991;265:3255–3264.

117. Albers GW, Sherman DG, Gress DR, et al. Stroke prevention in nonvalvular atrial fibrillation: a review of prospective randomized trials. *Ann Neurol* 1991;30:511–518.

118. Peterson P, Godtfredsen J, Boysen G, et al. Placebo-controlled, randomized trial of warfarin and aspirin for prevention of thromboembolic complications in chronic atrial fibrillation: the Copenhagen AFASAK study. *Lancet* 1989;I:175–179.

119. The Stroke Prevention in Atrial Fibrillation investigators. Preliminary report of the Stroke Prevention in Atrial Fibrillation study. *N Engl J Med* 1990;322:863–868.

120. The Stroke Prevention in Atrial Fibrillation investigators. The Stroke Prevention in Atrial Fibrillation study: final results. *Circulation* 1991;84:527–539.

121. The Boston Area Anticoagulation Trial for Atrial Fibrillation investigators. The effect of low-dose warfarin on the risk of stroke in patients with nonrheumatic atrial fibrillation. *N Engl J Med* 1990;323:1505–1511.

122. Connally SJ, Laupacis A, Gent M, et al. Canadian Atrial Fibrillation Anticoagulation (CAFA) Study. *J Am Coll Cardiol* 1991;18:349–355.

123. Stroke Prevention in Atrial Fibrillation investigators. Warfarin versus aspirin for prevention of thromboembolism in atrial fibrillation: Stroke Prevention in Atrial Fibrillation II study. *Lancet* 1994;343:687–691.

124. Stroke Prevention in Atrial Fibrillation investigators. Adjusted-dose warfarin versus low-intensity, fixed-dose warfarin plus aspirin for high-risk patients with atrial fibrillation: Stroke Prevention in Atrial Fibrillation III randomised clinical trial. *Lancet* 1996;348:633–638.

125. Laupacis A, Albers G, Dalen J, et al. Antithrombotic therapy in atrial fibrillation. *Chest* 1998;114:579S–589S.

126. Medical Research Council. Assessment of short-term anticoagulant administration after myocardial infarction. *BMJ* 1969;1:335–342.

127. Veterans Administration Cooperative Study. Anticoagulants in acute myocardial infarction: results of a cooperative trial. *JAMA* 1973;225:724–729.

128. Drapkin A, Mersky C. Anticoagulant therapy after acute myocardial infarction: relation of therapeutic benefit to patient's age, sex, and severity of infarction. *JAMA* 1972;222:541–549.

129. Report of the 60+ Reinfarction Study Research Group. A double-blind trial to assess long-term anticoagulant therapy in elderly patients after myocardial infarction. *Lancet* 1980;2:989–994.

130. Smith P, Arnesen H, Holme I. The effect of warfarin on mortality and reinfarction after myocardial infarction. *N Engl J Med* 1990;323:147–152.

131. ASPECT research group. Effect of long-term oral anticoagulant treatment on mortality and cardiovascular morbidity after myocardial infarction. *Lancet* 1994;343:499–503.

132. Loh E, St. John-Sutton M, Wun CC, et al. Ventricular dysfunction and the risk of stroke after myocardial infarction. *N Engl J Med* 1997;336:251–257.

133. Salem DN, Levine HJ, Pauker SG, et al. Antithrombotic therapy in valvular heart disease. *Chest* 1998;114:590S–601S.

134. Nishimura RA, Holmes DR, Ruder GS. Percutaneous balloon valvuloplasty. *Mayo Clin Proc* 1990;65:198–220.

135. Stein PD, Alpert JS, Copeland J, et al. Antithrombotic therapy in patients with mechanical and bioprosthetic heart valves. *Chest* 1995;95[Suppl]:371S–379S.

136. Salgado AV, Furlan AJ, Keys TF, et al. Neurologic complications of endocarditis: a 12 year experience. *Neurology* 1989;39:173–178.

137. Hart RG, Foster JW, Luther MF, et al. Stroke in infective endocarditis. *Stroke* 1990;21:695–700.

138. Wolf PA, Sila CA. Cerebral ischemia with mitral valve prolapse. *Am Heart J* 1987;113:1308–1315.

139. Petty GW, Orencia AJ, Khandheria BK, et al. A population-based study of stroke in the setting of mitral valve prolapse: risk factors and infarct subtype classification. *Mayo Clin Proc* 1994;69:632–634.

140. Davidson CJ, Skelton TN, Kisslo KB, et al. The risk of systemic embolization associated with percutaneous balloon valvuloplasty in adults. *Ann Intern Med* 1988;108:557–560.

141. Mills P, Leech G, Davies M, et al. The natural history of non-stenotic bicuspid aortic valve. *Br Heart J* 1978;40:951–957.

142. Boon A, Lodder J, Cheriex E, et al. Mitral annulus calcification is not an independent risk factor for stroke: a cohort study of 657 patients. *J Neurol* 1997;244(9):535–541.

143. CASANOVA study group. Carotid surgery versus medical therapy in asymptomatic carotid stenosis. *Stroke* 1991;22:1229–1235.

144. Hobson RW, Weiss DG, Fields WS, et al. for the Veterans Cooperative Study Group. Efficacy of carotid endarterectomy for asymptomatic carotid stenosis. *N Engl J Med* 1993;328:221–227.

145. Mayo Asymptomatic Carotid Endarterectomy study group. Results of a randomized controlled trial of carotid endarterectomy for asymptomatic carotid stenosis. *Mayo Clin Proc* 1992;67:513–518.

146. Executive Committee for the Asymptomatic Carotid Atherosclerosis Study. Endarterectomy for asymptomatic carotid artery stenosis. *JAMA* 1995;273:1421–1428.

147. Howard G, Chambless LE, Baker WH, et al. A multi-center validation study of Doppler ultrasound versus angiogram. *J Stroke Cerebrovasc Dis* 1991;1:166–173.

148. Toole JF, Castaldo JE. Accurate measurement of carotid stenosis: chaos in methodology. *J Neuroimaging* 1994;4:222–230.

149. Chervu A, Moore WS. Carotid endarterectomy without arteriography. *Ann Vasc Surg* 1994;8:296–302.

150. Toole J. Quality-based medicine. *Arch Neurol* 1997;54:23–24.

151. Perry JR, Szalai JP, Norris JW, for the Canadian Stroke Consortium. Consensus against both endarterectomy and routine screening for asymptomatic carotid artery stenosis. *Arch Neurol* 1997;54:25–28.

152. Barnett HJM, Meldrum HE, Eliasizw M. The dilemma of surgical treatment for patients with asymptomatic carotid disease. *Ann Intern Med* 1995;123:723–725.

153. Barnett HJM, Meldrum DE, Eliasizw M. Do the facts and figures warrant a 10-fold increase in the performance of carotid endarterectomy on asymptomatic patients? *Neurology* 1996;46:603–608.

154. Brott T, Toole JF. Medical compared with surgical treatment of asymptomatic carotid artery stenosis. *Ann Intern Med* 1995;123:720–722.

155. Sila CA. Carotid stenosis: current management strategies in perspective. *Cleve Clin J Med* 2000;67:851–861.

156. Cote R, Battista RN, Abrahamowicz M, et al. Lack of effect of aspirin in asymptomatic patients with carotid bruits and substantial carotid narrowing. *Ann Intern Med* 1995;123:649–655.

157. Breuer AC, Furlan AJ, Hanson MR, et al. Central nervous system complications of coronary artery bypass graft surgery: prospective analysis of 421 patients. *Stroke* 1983;14:682–687.

158. Ricotta JJ, Faggioli GL, Castilone A, et al. Risk factors for stroke after cardiac surgery: Buffalo Cardiac-Cerebral Study Group. *J Vasc Surg* 1995;21:359–364.

159. Roach GW, Kanchuger M, Mangano CM, et al. Adverse cerebral outcomes after coronary bypass surgery. *N Engl J Med* 1996;335:1857–1863.

160. Harvey JC, Goldstein JE, McCabe JC, et al. Complications of percutaneous intra-aortic balloon pumping. *Circulation* 1981;64:1114–1117.

161. Dawson DM, Fischer EG. Neurologic complications of cardiac catheterization. *Neurology* 1977;27:496–497.

162. Kosmorsky G, Hanson MR, Tomsak RL. Neuro-ophthalmologic complications of cardiac catheterization. *Neurology* 1988;38:483–485.

163. Galbreath C, Salgado ED, Furlan AJ, et al. Central nervous system complications of percutaneous transluminal coronary angioplasty. *Stroke* 1986;17:616–619.

164. Goldstein DJ, Oz MC, Rose EA. Implantable left ventricular assist devices. *N Engl J Med* 1998;339:1522–1533.

165. Salerno SM, Landry FJ, Schick JD, et al. The effect of multiple neuroimaging studies on classification, treatment, and outcome in acute ischemic stroke. *Ann Intern Med* 1996;124:21–26.

165a. Bushnell CD, Goldstein LB. Diagnostic testing for coagulopathies in patients with ischemic stroke. *Stroke* 2000;31:3067–3078.

166. Bogdahn U, Becker G, Winkler J, et al. Transcranial color-coded real-time sonography in adults. *Stroke* 1990;21:1680–1688.

167. Masaryk TJ. Noninvasive carotid imaging: caveat emptor. *Radiology* 1993;186:325–331.

168. Caplan LR, Hier DB, D'Cruz I. Cerebral embolism in the Michael Reese Stroke Registry. *Stroke* 1983;14:530–536.

169. Tegeler CH, Downes TR. Cardiac imaging in stroke. *Stroke* 1991;22:1206–1211.

170. Sirna S, Biller J, Skorton DJ, et al. Cardiac evaluation of the patient with stroke. *Stroke* 1990;21:14–23.

171. Amerenco P, Cohen A, Tzourio C, et al. Atherosclerotic disease of the aortic arch and the risk of ischemic stroke. *N Engl J Med* 1994;331:1474–1479.

172. Toyoda K, Yasaka M, Nagata S, et al. Aortogenic embolic stroke: a transesophageal echocardiographic approach. *Stroke* 1992;23:1056–1061.

173. Pop G, Sutherland GR, Koudstaal, et al. Transesophageal echocardiography in the detection of intracardiac embolic sources in patients with transient ischemic attacks. *Stroke* 1990;21:560–565.

174. Cabanes L, Mas JL, Cohen A, et al. Atrial septal aneurysm and patent foramen ovale as risk factors for cryptogenic stroke in patients less than 55 years of age. *Stroke* 1993;24:1865–1873.

175. Hanna JP, Sun JP, Furlan AJ, et al. Patent foramen ovale and brain infarct, echocardiographic predictors, recurrence, and prevention. *Stroke* 1994;25:782–786.

176. Oppenheimer SM. The insular cortex and the pathophysiology of stroke-induced cardiac changes. *Can J Neurol Sci* 1992;19:208–211.

177. Oppenheimer SM, Hachinski VC. The cardiac consequences of stroke. *Neurol Clin* 1992;10:167–176.

178. Goldstein DS. The electrocardiogram in stroke: relationship to pathophysiological type and comparison from prior tracings. *Stroke* 1979;10:253–259.

179. Bell C, Kapral M. Use of ambulatory electrocardiography for the detection of paroxysmal atrial fibrillation in patients with stroke. Canadian Task Force on Preventive Health Care. *Can J Neurol Sci* 2000;27:25–31.

180. Steering Committee of the Physicians' Health Study Research Group. Final report on the aspirin component of the ongoing physicians health study. *N Engl J Med* 1989;321:129–135.

181. Hass WK, Easton JD, Adams HP, et al. for the Ticlopidine Aspirin Stroke Study group. A randomized trial comparing ticlopidine hydrochloride with aspirin for the prevention of stroke in high-risk patients. *N Engl J Med* 1989;321:501–507.

182. Gent M, Blakely JA, Easton JD, et al. for the CATS group. The Canadian-American Ticlopidine Study (CATS) in thromboembolic stroke. *Lancet* 1989;1:1215–1220.

183. Bennett CL, Davidson CJ, Raisch DW, et al. Thrombotic thrombocytopenic purpura associated with ticlopidine in the setting of coronary artery stents and stroke prevention. *Arch Intern Med* 1999;159(21):2524–2528.

184. Bennett CL, Connors JM, Carwile JM, et al. Thrombotic thrombocytopenic purpura associated with clopidogrel. *N Engl J Med* 2000;342(24):1773–1777.

185. Wood AJ. Thrombotic thrombocytopenic purpura and clopidogrel—a need for new approaches to drug safety. *N Engl J Med* 2000;342:1824–1826.

186. Jonas S. Anticoagulant therapy in cerebrovascular disease: review and meta-analysis. *Stroke* 1988;19:1043–1048.

187. Mohr JP, Thompson JLP, Lazar RM, et al. A comparison of warfarin and aspirin for the prevention of recurrent ischemic stroke. *N Engl J Med* 2001;345:1444–1451.

188. Chimowitz MI, Kokkinos J, Strong J, et al. The warfarin-aspirin symptomatic intracranial disease study. *Neurology* 1995;45:1488–1493.

189. Babikian VL, Levine SR. Therapeutic considerations for stroke patients with antiphospholipid antibodies. *Stroke* 1992;23[Suppl I]:I33–I37.

190. Khamashta MA, Cuadrado MJ, Mujic F, et al. The management of thrombosis in the antiphospholipid-antibody syndrome. *N Engl J Med* 1995;332:993–997.

191. Winslow CM, Solomon DH, Chassin MR, et al. The appropriateness of carotid endarterectomy. *N Engl J Med* 1988;318:721–727.

192. Barnett HJM, Taylor DW, Eliasziw M, et al. for the North American Symptomatic Carotid Endarterectomy Trial Collaborators. The benefit of carotid endarterectomy in symptomatic patients with moderate and severe stenosis. *N Engl J Med* 1988;339:1415–1425.

193. European Carotid Surgery Trialists' Collaborative Group. Randomized trial of endarterectomy for recently symptomatic carotid stenosis: final results of the MRC European Carotid Surgery Trial (ECST). *Lancet* 1998;351:1379–1387.

194. European Carotid Surgery Trialists' Collaborative Group. MRC European Carotid Surgery Trial: interim results for patients with severe (70% to 99%) or with mild (0% to 29%) carotid stenosis. *Lancet* 1991;337:1235–1243.

195. Moore WS, Barnett HJM, Beebe HG, et al. Guidelines for carotid endarterectomy. *Stroke* 1995;26:188–201.

196. A Working Group on Emergency Brain Resuscitation. Emergency brain resuscitation. *Ann Intern Med* 1995;122:622–627.

197. Adams HP, Brott TG, Furlan AJ, et al. Guidelines for thrombolytic therapy for acute stroke: a supplement to the guidelines for the management of patients with acute ischemic stroke. *Circulation* 1996;94:1167–1174.

198. Emergency Cardiac-Care Committee and Subcommittees, American Heart Association. Guidelines for cardiopulmonary resuscitation and emergency cardiac care. IV. Special resuscitation situations. *JAMA* 1992;268:2242–2250.

199. The National Institute of Neurological Disorders and Stroke rt-PA Stroke Study Group. Tissue plasminogen activator for acute ischemic stroke. *N Engl J Med* 1995;333:1581–1587.

200. Marler JR, Jones PW, Emr M, eds. Rapid identification and treatment of acute stroke. Proceedings of a national symposium. Bethesda, MD: National Institutes of Health, 1997. NIH publication no. 97–439.

201. Brott T. Thrombolysis for stroke. *Arch Neurol* 1996;53:1305–1306.

202. Riggs JE. Tissue-type plasminogen activator should not be used in acute ischemic stroke. *Arch Neurol* 1996;53:1306–1308.

203. Hachinski V. Thrombolysis in acute stroke. *Arch Neurol* 1996;53:1308.

204. Caplan LR, Mohr JP, Kistler JP, et al. Thrombolysis—not a panacea for ischemic stroke. *N Engl J Med* 1997;337:1309–1310.

205. Grotta J. t-PA—the best current option for most patients. *N Engl J Med* 1997;337:1310–1312.

206. Tognoni G, Roncaglioni MC. Dissent: an alternative interpretation of MAST-I. *Lancet* 1995;346:1515.

207. Wardlaw JM, Warlow CP, Counsell C. Systematic review of evidence on thrombolytic therapy for acute ischaemic stroke. *Lancet* 1997;350:607–614.

208. Hacke W, Kaste M, Fieschi C, et al. Intravenous thrombolysis with recombinant tissue plasminogen activator for acute hemispheric stroke. The European Cooperative Acute Stroke Study (ECASS). *JAMA* 1995;274:1017–1025.

209. Donnan GA, Davis SM, Chambers BR, et al. Streptokinase for acute ischemic stroke with relationship to time of administration. *JAMA* 1996;276:961–966.

210. The Multicenter Acute Stroke Trial—Europe study group. Thrombolytic therapy with streptokinase in acute ischemic stroke. *JAMA* 1996;335:145–150.

211. The Multicenter Acute Stroke Trial—Italy (MAST-I) group. Randomised controlled trial of streptokinase, aspirin and combination of both in treatment of acute ischaemic stroke. *Lancet* 1995;346:1509–1514.

212. The NINDS t-PA Stroke Study Group. Generalized efficacy of t-PA for acute stroke, subgroup analysis of the NINDS t-PA stroke trial. *Stroke* 1997;28:2119–2125.

213. The NINDS t-PA Stroke Study Group. Intracerebral hemorrhage after intravenous t-PA therapy for ischemic stroke. *Stroke* 1997;28:2109–2118.

214. Hacke W, Steiner T, Bluhmki E, et al. Dichotomized endpoints and combined global endpoint statistics applied to the ECASS intention to treat data set. *Stroke* 1998;29:303(abst).

215. Hacke W, Kaste M, Fieschi C, et al. Randomised double-blind placebo-controlled trial of thrombolytic therapy with intravenous alteplase in acute ischaemic stroke (ECASS II). *Lancet* 1998;352:1245–1251.

216. Clark WM, Wissman S, Albers GW, et al. Recombinant tissue-type plasminogen activator (alteplase) for ischemic stroke 3 to 5 hours after symptom onset—the ATLANTIS study: a randomized controlled trial. *JAMA* 1999;282:2019–2026.

217. Furlan A, Higashida R, Wechsler L, et al. Intra-arterial prourokinase for acute ischemic stroke—the PROACT II study: a randomized controlled trial. *JAMA* 1999;282:2003–2011.

218. del Zoppo GJ, Higashida RT, Furlan AJ, et al. PROACT: a phase II randomized trial of recombinant pro-urokinase by direct arterial delivery in acute middle cerebral artery stroke. *Stroke* 1998;29:4–11.

219. Lewandowski CA, Frankel M, Tomsick TA, et al. Combined intravenous and intra-arterial r-TPA versus intra-arterial therapy for acute ischemic stroke. Emergency Management of Stroke (EMS) bridging trial. *Stroke* 1999;30:2598–2605.

220. Brückmann H, Ferbert A, del Zoppo G, et al. Acute basilar thrombosis: angiologic-clinical comparison and therapeutic implications. *Acta Radiol* 1987;369[Suppl]:38–42.

221. Hacke W, Zeumer H, Ferbert A, et al. Intra-arterial thrombolytic therapy improves outcome in patients with acute vertebrobasilar occlusive disease. *Stroke* 1988;19: 1216–1222.

222. Brandt T, von Kummer R, Muller-Kuppers M, et al. Thrombolytic therapy of acute basilar artery occlusion, variables affecting recanalization and outcome. *Stroke* 1996;27:875–881.

223. Mitchell PJ, Gerraty RP, Donnan GA, et al. Thrombolysis in the vertebrobasilar circulation: the Australian Urokinase Stroke Trial. *Cerebrovasc Dis* 1997;7:94–99.

224. Cross DT, Moran CJ, Akins P, et al. Relationship between clot location and outcome after basilar artery thrombolysis. *AJNR Am J Neuroradiol* 1997;18:1221–1228.

225. Huemer M, Niederwieser V, Ladurner G. Thrombolytic treatment for acute occlusion of the basilar artery. *J Neurol Neurosurg Psychiatry* 1995;58:227–228.

226. Wijdicks EF, Nichols DA, Thielen KR, et al. Intra-arterial thrombolysis in acute basilar artery thromboembolisms: the Initial Mayo Clinic experience. *Mayo Clin Proc* 1997;72:1005–1013.

227. Herderscheê D, Limburg M, Hijdra A, et al. Recombinant tissue plasminogen activator in two patients with basilar artery occlusion. *J Neurol Neurosurg Psychiatry* 1991;54: 71–73.

228. Becker KJ, Purcell LL, Hacke W, et al. Vertebrobasilar thrombosis: diagnosis, management, and the use of intra-arterial thrombolytics. *Crit Care Med* 1996;24:1729–1742.

229. von Kummer R, Hacke W. Safety and efficacy of intravenous tissue plasminogen activator and heparin in acute middle cerebral artery stroke. *Stroke* 1992;23:646–652.

230. Mori E, Yoneda Y, Tabuchi M, et al. Intravenous recombinant tissue plasminogen activator in acute carotid artery territory stroke. *Neurology* 1992;42:976–982.

231. Levy DE, Brott TG, Haley EC, et al. Factors related to intracranial hematoma formation in patients receiving tissue-type plasminogen activator for acute ischemic stroke. *Stroke* 1994;25:291–297.

232. del Zoppo GJ, Poeck K, Pessin MS, et al. Recombinant tissue plasminogen activator in acute thrombotic and embolic stroke. *Ann Neurol* 1992;32:78–86.

233. Mori E, Tabuchi M, Yoshida T, et al. Intracarotid urokinase with thromboembolic occlusion of the middle cerebral artery. *Stroke* 1988;19:802–812.

234. Bozzao L, Angeloni U, Bastianello S, et al. Early angiographic and CT findings in patients with hemorrhagic infarction in the distribution of the middle cerebral artery. *AJNR Am J Neuroradiol* 1991;12:1115–1121.

235. Gore JM, Sloan M, Price TR, et al. Intracerebral hemorrhage, cerebral infarction, and subdural hematoma after acute myocardial infarction and thrombolytic therapy in the Thrombolysis in Myocardial Infarction Study. Thrombolysis in Myocardial Infarction, phase II, pilot and clinical trial. *Circulation* 1991;83:448–459.

236. Simoons ML, Maggioni AP, Knatterud G, et al. Individual risk assessment for intracranial haemorrhage during thrombolytic therapy. *Lancet* 1993;342:1523–1528.

237. Selker HP, Beshansky JR, Schmid CH, et al. Presenting pulse pressure predicts thrombolytic therapy-related intracranial hemorrhage, Thrombolytic Predictive Instrument (TPI) Project results. *Circulation* 1994;90:1657–1661.

238. Anderson JL, Karagounis L, Allen A, et al. Older age and elevated blood pressure are risk factors for intracerebral hemorrhage after thrombolysis. *Am J Cardiol* 1991;68: 166–170.

239. Gebel JM, Sila CA, Sloan MA, et al. Thrombolysis-related intracranial hemorrhage: a radiographic analysis of 244 cases from the GUSTO-1 trial with clinical correlation. *Stroke* 1998;29:563–569.

240. Larrue V, von Kummer R, del Zoppo G, et al. Hemorrhagic transformation in acute ischemic stroke, potential contributing factors in the European Cooperative Acute Stroke Study. *Stroke* 1997;28:957–960.

241. Sloan MA, Price TR, Petito CK, et al. Clinical features and pathogenesis of intracerebral hemorrhage after rt-PA and heparin therapy for acute myocardial infarction: the Thrombolysis in Myocardial Infarction (TIMI) II pilot and randomized clinical trial combined experience. *Neurology* 1995;45:649–658.

242. Chiu D, Krieger D, Villar-Cordova C, et al. Intravenous tissue plasminogen activator for acute ischemic stroke: feasibility, safety, and efficacy in the first year of clinical practice. *Stroke* 1998;29:18–22.

243. Albers GW, Bates VE, Clark WM, et al. Intravenous tissue-type plasminogen activator for treatment of acute stroke, the Standard Treatment with Alteplase to Reverse Stroke (STARS) study. *JAMA* 2000;283:1145–1150.

244. Buchan AM, Barber PA, Newcommon N, et al. Effectiveness of t-PA in acute ischemic stroke. Outcome relates to appropriateness. *Neurology* 2000;54:679–684.

245. Katzan IL, Furlan AJ, Lloyd LE, et al. Use of tissue-type plasminogen activator for acute ischemic stroke: the Cleveland area experience. *JAMA* 2000;283(9):1151–1158.

246. Schriger DL, Kalafut M, Starkman S, et al. Cranial computed tomography interpretation in acute stroke: physician accuracy in determining eligibility for thrombolytic therapy. *JAMA* 1998;279:1293–1297.

247. Sherman DG, Atkinson RP, Chippendale T, et al. Intravenous ancrod for treatment of acute ischemic stroke, the STAT Study: a randomized controlled trial. *JAMA* 2000;283:2395–2403.

248. Gentling E, Barnett HJM, Fields WS, et al. Cerebral ischemia: the role of thrombosis and antithrombotic therapy. *Stroke* 1977;8:150–175.

249. Millikan CH, McDowell FH. Treatment of progressing stroke. *Stroke* 1981;12:397–409.

250. Carter AB. Anticoagulation treatment ion–progressing stroke. *BMJ* 1961;2:70–73.

251. Fisher CM. Anticoagulant therapy in cerebral thrombosis and cerebral embolism. A national cooperative study, interim report. *Neurology* 1961;11:119–131.

252. Putnam SF, Adams HP. Usefulness of heparin in initial management of patients with recent transient ischemic attacks. *Arch Neurol* 1985;42:960–962.

253. Duke RJ, Bloch RF, Alexander GG, et al. Intravenous heparin for the prevention of stroke progression in acute

partial stable stroke: a randomized controlled trial. *Ann Intern Med* 1986;105:825–828.

254. Haley EC Jr, Kassell NF, Torner JC. Failure of heparin to prevent progression in progressing ischemic infarction. *Stroke* 1988;19:10–14.

255. Biller J, Bruno A, Adams HP Jr, et al. A randomized trial of aspirin or heparin in hospitalized patients with recent transient ischemic attacks: a pilot study. *Stroke* 1989;20:441–447.

256. Ramirez-Lassepas M, Quinones MR, Nino HH. Treatment of acute ischemic stroke open-trial with continuous intravenous heparinization. *Arch Neurol* 1986;42:386–390.

257. Keith DS. Heparin therapy for recent transient focal cerebral ischemia. *Mayo Clin Proc* 1987;62:1101–1106.

258. Estol CJ, Pessin MS. Anticoagulation: is there still a role in atherothrombotic stroke? *Stroke* 1990;21:820–824.

259. Sage JI. Stroke: the use and overuse of heparin in therapeutic trials. *Arch Neurol* 1985;42:315–317.

260. Phillips SJ. An alternative view of heparin anticoagulation in acute focal brain ischemia. *Stroke* 1989;20:295–298.

261. Chamorro A, Vila N, Saiz A, et al. Early anticoagulation after large cerebral embolic infarction: a safety study. *Neurology* 1995;45:861–865.

262. Marsh EE III, Adams HP Jr, Biller J, et al. Use of antithrombotic drugs in the treatment of acute ischemic stroke: a survey of neurologists in practice in the United States. *Neurology* 1989;39:1631–1634.

262a. Irino T, Watanabe M, Nishide M, et al. Angiographical analysis of acute cerebral infarction followed by "cascade"-like deterioration of minor neurological deficits. What is progressing stroke? *Stroke* 1983;14:363–368.

263. Cerebral Embolism Study Group. Immediate anticoagulation of embolic stroke: a randomized trial. *Stroke* 1983;14:668–676.

264. Gautier JC. Stroke in progression. *Stroke* 1985;16:729–733.

265. Cerebral Embolism Study Group. Immediate anticoagulation of embolic stroke: brain hemorrhage and management options. *Stroke* 1984;15:779–789.

266. Shields RW Jr, Laureno R, Lachman T, et al. Anticoagulant-related hemorrhage in acute cerebral embolism. *Stroke* 1984;15:426–437.

267. Petty GW, Tatemichi TK, Sacco RL, et al. Fatal or severely disabling cerebral infarction during hospitalization for stroke or transient ischemic attack. *J Neurol* 1990;237:306–309.

268. Dobkin BH. Heparin for lacunar stroke in progression. *Stroke* 1983;14:421–423.

269. Babikian VL, Kase CS, Pessin MS, et al. Intracerebral hemorrhage in stroke patients anticoagulated with heparin [Review]. *Stroke* 1989;20:1500–1503.

270. Adams HP, Brott TG, Crowell RM, et al. Guidelines for the management of patients with acute ischemic stroke. *Circulation* 1994;90:1588–1601.

271. International Stroke Trial collaborative group. The International Stroke Trial (IST): a randomized trial of aspirin, subcutaneous heparin, both or neither, among 19,435 patients with acute ischemic stroke. *Lancet* 1997;349:1569–1581.

272. CAST (Chinese Acute Stroke Trial) collaborative group. CAST: randomised placebo-controlled trial of early aspirin use in 20,000 patients with acute ischaemic stroke. *Lancet* 1997;349:1641–1649.

273. Granger C, Hirsh J, Califf R, et al. Activated partial thromboplastin time and outcome after thrombolytic therapy for acute myocardial infarction: results from GUSTO-I trial. *Circulation* 1996;93:870–878.

274. Hirsh J, Raschke R, Warkentin TE, et al. Heparin: mechanism of action, pharmacokinetics, dosing considerations, monitoring, efficacy, and safety. *Chest* 1995;108[Suppl]:258S–275S.

275. Kay R, Wong KA Sing, Yu YL, et al. Low–molecular weight heparin for the treatment of acute ischemic stroke. *N Engl J Med* 1995;333:1588–1593.

276. Biller J, Massey EW, Marler JR, et al. A dose escalation study of Org 10172 (low–molecular weight heparinoid) in the treatment of acute cerebral infarction. *Neurology* 1989;39:262–265.

277. The Abciximab in Ischemic Stroke investigators. Abciximab in acute ischemic stroke: a randomized, double-blind, placebo-controlled, dose-escalation study. *Stroke* 2000;31:601–609.

278. Algra A, van Gijn J. Aspirin at any dose above 30 mg offers only modest protection after cerebral ischaemia. *J Neurol Neurosurg Psychiatry* 1996;60(2):197–199.

279. The CURE Trial Investigators. CURE Trial. *N Engl J Med* 2001;345:494–502.

280. Tsai FY, Matovich V, Hieshima G, et al. Percutaneous transluminal angioplasty of the carotid artery. *AJNR Am J Neuroradiol* 1986;7:349–358.

281. Porta M, Munari LM, Belloni G. Percutaneous angioplasty of atherosclerotic carotid stenosis. *Cerebrovasc Dis* 1991;1:265–272.

282. Higashida RT, Hieshima GB, Tsai FY, et al. Transluminal angioplasty of the vertebral and basilar artery. *Am J Neurol Radiol* 1987;8:745–750.

283. Spence D, Eliasziw M. Endarterectomy or angioplasty for treatment of carotid stenosis? *Lancet* 2001;357:1722–1723.

284. Beebe HG, Archie JP, Baker WH, et al. Concern about safety of carotid angioplasty. *Stroke* 1996;27:197–198.

285. Guglielmi G, Vinuela F, Dion J, et al. Electrothrombosis of saccular aneurysms via endovascular approach. II. Preliminary clinical experience. *J Neurosurg* 1991;75:8–14.

286. Casasco AE, Aymard A, Gobin YP, et al. Selective endovascular treatment of 71 intracranial aneurysms with platinum coils. *J Neurosurg* 1993;79:3–10.

287. Higashida RT, Halbach VV, Barnwell SL, et al. Treatment of intracranial aneurysms with preservation of the parent vessel: results of percutaneous balloon embolization in 84 patients. *Am J Neuroradiol* 1990;11:633–640.

288. Eskridge JM, Newell DW, Pendelton GA. Transluminal angioplasty for treatment of vasospasm. *Neurosurg Clin North Am* 1990;1:387–399.

289. Higashida RT, Halbach VV, Cahan LD, et al. Transluminal angioplasty for treatment of intracranial arterial vasospasm. *J Neurosurg* 1989;71(pt 1):648–653.

290. Newell DW, Eskridge JM, Mayberg MR, et al. Angioplasty for the treatment of symptomatic vasospasm following subarachnoid hemorrhage. *J Neurosurg* 1989;71(pt 1):654–660.

291. Kassell NF, Helm G, Simmons N, et al. Treatment of cerebral vasospasm with intra-arterial papaverine. *J Neurosurg* 1992;77:848–852.

292. Ojemann RG, Heros RC. Spontaneous brain hemorrhage. *Stroke* 1983;14:468–475.

293. Kase CS, Mohr JP. Supratentorial intracerebral hemorrhage. In: Barnett HJM, Mohr JP, Stein BM, et al., eds. *Stroke: pathophysiology, diagnosis, and management.* New York: Churchill Livingstone, 1986:525–547.

294. Weisberg L. Multiple spontaneous intracerebral hematomas: clinical and computed tomographic correlations. *Neurology* 1981;31:897–900.

295. McCormick WF, Rosenfield DB. Massive brain hemorrhage: a review of 144 cases and an examination of their causes. *Stroke* 1973;4:946–954.

296. Ropper AH, Davis KR. Lobar cerebral hemorrhage: acute clinical syndromes in 26 cases. *Ann Neurol* 1980;8:141–147.

297. Kase C, Williams JP, Wyatt DA, et al. Lobar intracerebral hematomas: clinical and CT analysis of 22 cases. *Neurology* 1982;32:1146–1150.

298. Douglas MA, Haeror AF. Long-term prognosis of hypertensive intracerebral hemorrhage. *Stroke* 1982;13:88–91.

299. Kelley RE, Berger JR, Scheinberg P, et al. Active bleeding in hypertensive intracerebral hemorrhage: computed tomography. *Neurology* 1982;32:852–856.

300. Kase CS. Intracerebral hemorrhage: nonhypertensive causes. *Stroke* 1986;17:590–595.

301. Itoh Y, Yamada M, Hayakawa M, et al. Cerebral amyloid angiopathy: a significant cause of cerebellar as well as lobar cerebral hemorrhage in the elderly. *J Neurol Sci* 1993;116:135–141.

302. Vonsattel JPG, Myers R, Hedley-Whyte ET, et al. Cerebral amyloid angiopathy without and with cerebral hemorrhages: a comparative histological study. *Ann Neurol* 1991;30:637–649.

303. Toffol GJ, Biller J, Adams HP. Nontraumatic intracerebral hemorrhage in young adults. *Arch Neurol* 1987;44:483–485.

304. Norman D. Vascular disease: hemorrhage. In: Brant-Zawadzki M, Norman D, eds. *Magnetic resonance imaging of the central nervous system.* New York: Raven Press, 1987:209–220.

305. Brant-Zawadzki M, Kelly W. Brain tumors. In: Brant-Zawadzki M, Norman D, eds. *Magnetic resonance imaging of the central nervous system.* New York: Raven Press, 1987:159.

306. Wintzen AR, DeJonge H, Loeliger EA, et al. The risk of intracerebral hemorrhage during oral anticoagulant treatment. *Ann Neurol* 1984;16:533–558.

307. Levine S. Cocaine and stroke. *Stroke* 1989;20:841–843.

308. Kase CS, Foster TE, Reed JE, et al. Intracerebral hemorrhage and phenylpropanolamine use. *Neurology* 1987;37:399–404.

309. Kerna WN, Viscoli CM, Brass LM, et al. Phenylpropanolamine and the risk of hemorrhagic stroke. *N Engl J Med* 2000;343:1826–1832.

310. Chen ST, Chen SD, Hsu CY, et al. Progression of hypertensive intracerebral hemorrhage. *Neurology* 1989;39:1509–1514.

311. Hayashi M, Kobayashi H, Kawano H, et al. Treatment of systemic hypertension and intracranial hypertension in cases of brain hemorrhage. *Stroke* 1988;19:314–321.

312. Broderick J, Brott T, Tomsick T. Ultra-early evaluation of intracerebral hemorrhage (ICH). *Stroke* 1989;20:158.

313. Duff TA, Ayeni S, Levin AB, et al. Nonsurgical management of spontaneous intracerebral hematoma. *Neurosurgery* 1981;9:387–392.

314. Papo I, Janny P, Caruselli G, et al. Intracranial pressure time course in primary intracerebral hemorrhage. *Neurosurgery* 1979;4:504–511.

315. Ropper AH, King RB. Intracranial pressure monitoring in comatose patients with cerebral hemorrhage. *Arch Neurol* 1984;41:725–728.

316. Ropper AH, Rockoff MA. Treatment of intracranial hypertension. In: Ropper AH, Kennedy SF, eds. *Neurological and neurosurgical intensive care,* 2nd ed. Rockville, MD: Aspen Publishers, 1988:23–41.

317. Tellez H, Bauer RB. Dexamethasone as treatment in cerebrovascular disease. I. A controlled study in intracerebral hemorrhage. *Stroke* 1973;4:541–546.

318. Poungvarin N, Bhoopat W, Viriyavejakul A, et al. Effects of dexamethasone in primary supratentorial intracerebral hemorrhage. *N Engl J Med* 1987;316:1229–1233.

319. McKissock W, Richardson A, Taylor J. Primary intracerebral hemorrhage: a controlled trial of surgical and conservative treatment in 180 unselected cases. *Lancet* 1961;1:221–226.

320. Tuhrim S, Dambrosia JM, Price TR, et al. Prediction of intracerebral hemorrhage survival. *Ann Neurol* 1988;24:258–263.

321. Portenoy RK, Lipton RB, Berger AR, et al. Intracerebral hemorrhage: a model for the prediction of outcome. *J Neurol Neurosurg Psychiatry* 1987;50:976–979.

322. Torner JC. Epidemiology of subarachnoid hemorrhage. *Semin Neurol* 1984;4:354–369.

323. Longstreth WT Jr, Koepsell TD, Yerby MS, et al. Risk factors for subarachnoid hemorrhage. *Stroke* 1985;16:377–385.

324. Mayberg MR. Warning leaks and subarachnoid hemorrhage. *West J Med* 1990;153:549–550.

325. Leblanc R. The minor leak preceding subarachnoid hemorrhage. *J Neurosurg* 1987;66:35–39.

326. Vermeulen M, van Gijn J. The diagnosis of subarachnoid hemorrhage. *J Neurol Neurosurg Psychiatry* 1990;53:365–372.

327. Ross JS, Masaryk TJ, Modic MT, et al. Intracranial aneurysms: evaluation by MR angiography. *AJNR Am J Neuroradiol* 1990;11:449–455.

328. Forster DM, Steiner L, Hakanson S, et al. The value of repeat panangiography in cases of unexplained subarachnoid hemorrhage. *J Neurosurg* 1978;48:712–716.

329. Levey AS, Pauker SG, Kassirer JP. Occult intracranial aneurysms in polycystic kidney disease: when is cerebral arteriography indicated? *N Engl J Med* 1983;308:986–994.

330. Berg HW, Dippel DW, Limbrug M, et al. Familial intracranial aneurysms: a review. *Stroke* 1992;23:1024–1030.

331. Rosehorn J, Eskesen V, Schmidt K. Unruptured intracranial aneurysms. An assessment of the annual risk of rup-

ture based on epidemiological and clinical data. *Br J Neurosurg* 1988;2:369–377.

332. International Study of Unruptured Intracranial Aneurysms Investigators. Unruptured intracranial aneurysms—risk of rupture and risks of surgical intervention. *N Engl J Med* 1998;339:1725–1733.

333. Jane JA, Kassell NF, Torner JC, et al. The natural history of aneurysms and arteriovenous malformations. *J Neurosurg* 1985;62:321–323.

334. McCormick WF, Acosta-Rua GJ. The size of intracranial saccular aneurysms: an autopsy study. *J Neurosurg* 1970;33:422–427.

335. Wiebers DO, Whisnant JP, Sundt TM Jr, et al. The significance of unruptured intracranial saccular aneurysms. *J Neurosurg* 1987;66:23–29.

336. Crompton MR. Mechanism of growth and rupture in cerebral berry aneurysms. *BMJ* 1966;5496:1138–1142.

337. Mayberg MR, Batjer HH, Dacey R, et al. Guidelines for the management of aneurysmal subarachnoid hemorrhage. *Stroke* 1994;25:2315–2328.

338. Ojemann RG. Management of the ruptured intracranial aneurysm [Editorial]. *N Engl J Med* 1981;304:725–726.

339. Kassell NF, Torner JC, Haley EC Jr, et al. The International Cooperative Study on the Timing of Aneurysm Surgery. I. Overall management results. *J Neurosurg* 1990;73:18–36.

340. Graf CJ, Nibbelink DW. Cooperative aneurysm study of intracranial aneurysms and subarachnoid hemorrhage: report on a randomized treatment study. III. Intracranial surgery. *Stroke* 1974;5:559–601.

341. Kassell NF, Boarini DJ, Adams HP, et al. Overall management of ruptured aneurysm: comparison of early and late operation. *Neurosurgery* 1981;9:120–128.

342. Kassell NF, Torner JC, Jane JA, et al. The International Cooperative Study on the Timing of Aneurysm Surgery. II. Surgical results. *J Neurosurg* 1990;73:37–47.

343. Locksley HB. Natural history of subarachnoid hemorrhage, intracranial aneurysms, and arteriovenous malformation: based on 6368 cases in the cooperative study. *J Neurosurg* 1966;25:219–239.

344. Wijdicks EF, Vermeulen M, Murray GD, et al. The effects of treating hypertension following aneurysmal subarachnoid hemorrhage. *Clin Neurol Neurosurg* 1990;92:111–117.

345. Kassell NF, Sasaki T, Colohan AR, et al. Cerebral vasospasm following aneurysmal subarachnoid hemorrhage. *Stroke* 1985;16:562–572.

346. Adams HP Jr, Kassell NF, Torner JC, et al. Predicting cerebral ischemia after aneurysmal subarachnoid hemorrhage: influences of clinical condition, CT results, and antifibrinolytic therapy. A report of the Cooperative Aneurysm Study. *Neurology* 1987;37:1586–1591.

347. Aaslid R, Huber P, Nornes H. Evaluation of cerebrovascular spasm with transcranial Doppler ultrasound. *J Neurosurg* 1984;60:37–41.

348. Awad IA, Carter LP, Spetzler RF, et al. Clinical vasospasm after subarachnoid hemorrhage: response to hypervolemic hemodilution and arterial hypertension. *Stroke* 1987;18:365–372.

349. Wijdicks EF, Vermeulen H, Hijdra A, et al. Hyponatremia and cerebral infarction in patients with ruptured intracra-

nial aneurysms: is fluid restriction harmful? *Ann Neurol* 1985;17:137–140.

350. Rosenfeld JV, Barnett GH, Sila CA, et al. The effect of subarachnoid hemorrhage on blood and CSF atrial natriuretic factor. *J Neurosurg* 1989;71:32–37.

351. Allen G, Ahn H, Preziosi T, et al. Cerebral arterial spasm: a controlled trial of nimodipine in patients with subarachnoid hemorrhage. *N Engl J Med* 1983;308:619–624.

352. Petruk KC, West M, Mohr G, et al. Nimodipine treatment in poor-grade aneurysm patients: results of a multicenter double-blind placebo-controlled trial. *J Neurosurg* 1988;68:505–517.

353. Philippon J, Grob R, Dagreou F, et al. Prevention of vasospasm in subarachnoid haemorrhage: a controlled study with nimodipine. *Acta Neurochir (Wien)* 1986;82:110–114.

354. Pickard JD, Murray GD, Ilingworth R, et al. Effect of oral nimodipine on cerebral infarction and outcome after subarachnoid hemorrhage: British aneurysm nimodipine trial. *BMJ* 1989;298:636–642.

355. Gilsbach J, Reulen H, Ljunggren B, et al. Early aneurysm surgery and preventive therapy with intravenously administered nimodipine: a multicenter, double-blind, dose-comparison study. *Neurosurgery* 1990;26:458–464.

356. Gilsbach JM, Harders AG. Morbidity and mortality after early aneurysm surgery: a prospective study with nimodipine prevention. *Acta Neurochir (Wien)* 1989;96:1–7.

357. Pare L, Delfino R, Leblanc R. The relationship of ventricular drainage to aneurysmal rebleeding. *J Neurosurg* 1992;76:422–427.

358. Hasan D, Vermeulen M, Wijdicks EF, et al. Management problems in acute hydrocephalus after subarachnoid hemorrhage. *Stroke* 1989;20:747–753.

358a. Milhorat TH. Acute hydrocephalus after aneurysmal subarachnoid hemorrhage. *Neurosurgery* 1987;20:15–20.

359. Hart RG, Byer JA, Slaughter JR, et al. Occurrence and implications of seizures in subarachnoid hemorrhage due to ruptured intracranial aneurysms. *Neurosurgery* 1981;8:417–421.

360. Hacke W, Warach S. Diffusion-weighted MRI as an evolving standard of care in acute stroke. *Neurology* 2000;54:1548–1549.

361. Fisher M, Albers GW. Applications of diffusion-perfusion magnetic resonance imaging in acute ischemic stroke. *Neurology* 1999;52:1750–1756.

362. Wahlgren NG, Ranasinha KW, Rosolacci T, et al. Clomethiazole acute stroke study (CLASS): results of a randomized controlled trial of clomethiazole vs placebo in 1360 acute stroke patients. *Stroke* 1999;30:21–28.

363. Trust Study Group. Randomized, double-blind, placebo-controlled trial of nimodipine in acute stroke. *Lancet* 1990;336:1205–1209.

364. American Nimodipine Study Group. Clinical trial of nimodipine in acute ischemic stroke. *Stroke* 1992;23:3–8.

365. Diener HC, Hacke W, Hennerici M, et al. Lubezole in acute ischemic stroke: a double-blind, placebo-controlled phase II trial. *Stroke* 1996;27:76–81.

366. Albers GW, Atkinson RP, Kelley RE, et al. for the Dextrorphan Study Group. Safety, tolerability, and pharmacokinetics of the N-methyl-D-aspartate antagonist

dextrorphan in patients with acute stroke. *Stroke* 1995;26:254–258.

367. Grotta J, Clark W, Coull B, et al. Safety and tolerability of the glutamate antagonist CGS 19755 (Selfotel) in patients with acute ischemic stroke. *Stroke* 1995;26:602–605.

368. Muir KW, Lees KR. A randomized, double-blind, placebo-controlled pilot trial of intravenous magnesium sulfate in acute stroke. *Stroke* 1995;26:1183–1188.

369. Parkinson FE, Rudolphi KA, Fredholm BB. Propentofylline: a nucleoside transport inhibitor with neuroprotective effects in cerebral ischemia. *Gen Pharmacol* 1994;25:1053–1058.

370. The RANTTAS investigators. A randomized trial of tirilazad mesylate in patients with acute stroke (RANTTAS). *Stroke* 1996;27:1453–1458.

371. Clark WM, Warach S, Pettigrew LC, et al. for the Citicoline Stroke Study Group. A randomized dose-response trial of citicoline in acute ischemic stroke patients. *Neurology* 1997;49:671–678.

372. Clark WM, Raps EC, Tong DC, et al. Cervene (nalmefene) in acute ischemic stroke: final results of a phase III efficacy study. *Stroke* 2000;31:1234–1239.

373. North American Glycine Antagonist in Neuroprotection Investigators (GAIN). Phase II studies of the glycine antagonist GV 150526 in acute stroke. *Stroke* 2000;31:358–365.

374. Krieger DW, De Georgia MA, Abou-Chebl A, et al. Cooling for Acute Ischemic Brain Damage (COOL AID): feasibility and safety of induced hypothermia for severe acute ischemic stroke. *Stroke* 2001;32(8):1847–1854.

DISEASE OF PERIPHERAL VESSELS

KENNETH ROSENFIELD
PETER R. VALE
JEFFREY M. ISNER

▼▼ ADDITIONAL ELECTRONIC TOPICS

   K. Rosenfield: Department of Cardiovascular Medicine and Research, Tufts University School of Medicine, St. Elizabeth's Medical Center, Boston, Massachusetts
   P. R. Vale: Department of Vascular Medicine, University of New South Wales School of Medicine, St. Vincent's Hospital, St. Vincent's Clinic, Sydney, Australia
   J. M. Isner: Department of Medicine/Vascular Medicine, Tufts University School of Medicine, St. Elizabeth's Medical Center, Boston, Massachusetts (Deceased)

OVERVIEW

Although their primary focus remains in the diagnosis and treatment of cardiac disorders, many cardiovascular specialists are no longer limiting themselves to treatment of coronary artery disease (CAD) but instead are adopting a "global vascular management" strategy for their patients. This approach has been promulgated by institutions setting up divisions of vascular medicine under two premises. First, the peripheral vasculature makes up the largest single "organ system" in the body—one that is complex and fascinating in its biology and dynamic in its function. The peripheral vessels hold many biologic secrets that, when unlocked, will open doors for new therapies for both noncoronary and coronary diseases. Second, both patients and medical science could benefit from the perspective and knowledge gained from a medical (as opposed to surgical) subspecialty whose sole focus encompasses the evaluation and management of vascular disease.

Cardiovascular specialists can no longer realistically limit their focus to the coronary vasculature. The coronary and noncoronary circulations are interdependent; they commonly coexist and may each cause disabling or life-threatening symptoms. Furthermore, they are affected by the same disease processes and often require similar treatment modalities. The approaches to treatment of one often depend on the other. For example, patients requiring vascular surgery generally have higher cardiac risk than those undergoing nonvascular surgery because of the increased prevalence of CAD in this group. Likewise, many patients under treatment for CAD are disabled by symptomatic peripheral arterial disease (PAD); post–myocardial infarction patients with claudication may not be able to be appropriately rehabilitated without treatment of their PAD.

Toward that end, the ensuing chapter is designed to provide a brief overview of the major disease states that occur in the peripheral arteries, as well as a synopsis of current treatment for each condition. The principal focus of the chapter, however, is on the management of *atherosclerotic* PAD. By far the most common disorder of lower extremities encountered by North American physicians, it afflicts more than 20% of men and women combined older than the age of 75 years (1). An aging population guarantees that the prevalence will continue to increase. Significant technological advances, especially in percutaneous therapies, over the past 10 years now enable safer and more efficacious treatment of atherosclerotic PAD. Knowledge about the range of therapeutic options available, and in which patients to apply them, is critical to the optimal management of these patients.

DISEASE STATES OF THE PERIPHERAL ARTERIES

Atherosclerosis

PAD, or arteriosclerosis obliterans, is the most common cause of symptomatic obstruction in the peripheral arterial tree. The pathophysiologic basis of PAD is identical to that of coronary artery atherosclerosis; the same risk factors are also associated, including tobacco smoking, diabetes mellitus, hypertension, hyperlipidemia, a positive family history, and advanced age. The estimated prevalence of PAD in people age 65 years or older is 20%; this estimate may, in fact, be conservative due to the presence of a large number of patients who have either asymptomatic disease or in whom the symptoms

are not recognized as being due to arterial obstruction. The latter group, those in whom PVD symptoms are overlooked or falsely attributed to other etiologies (deconditioning, arthritis), make up an important subset who, if appropriately diagnosed, might benefit from available treatments.

The clinical presentation of patients with PAD is highly variable and depends on the involved vascular territory. Lower extremity symptoms range from mild discomfort during intense exercise to the presence of constant rest discomfort, painful ulceration, or frank gangrene. Claudication is described variably as pain, tightness, aching, soreness, hardness, or heaviness that occurs in the calf, buttocks, hips, or arch of the foot during ambulation and resolves with rest, similar to the pattern of exertional angina in CAD. Although intermittent claudication can be mild and nondisabling, it can become severely disabling. Pain at rest occurs if the impairment of blood flow is severe enough that oxygen and nutrient supply falls below the resting requirements of the distal tissue. Where the level of tissue ischemia is severe, cell injury and death will occur, leading to tissue breakdown, clinically manifested as ulceration or gangrene. Neither of these is likely to resolve without restoration of nutrient (usually pulsatile) flow to the affected extremity. Similar symptoms occur in the hand or forearm of patients with severe atherosclerosis of vessels supplying the upper extremities.

As is the case in CAD, symptoms related to PAD rarely occur until the atherosclerotic process has narrowed the vessel diameter by at least 50%. However, the presence of one or more lesions with 50% or more narrowing does not imply that the patient will be symptomatic. Indeed, a large number of patients with PAD remain asymptomatic, even in the presence of severe and extensive disease. Patients with complete occlusion of the major blood supply to a limb or organ may have no symptoms if an ample collateral supply is present. Rutherford et al., by defining the signs and symptoms according to their intensity and combining these with noninvasive data, developed a series of categories to describe the severity of chronic limb ischemia (Table 111.1) (2). Such standardization has greatly enhanced the ability of investigators to perform meaningful comparative analyses of treatment strategies. Furthermore, it has facilitated decision making for clinicians regarding optimal therapy for a given level of limb ischemia.

Natural History of Peripheral Arterial Disease

An important consideration in any treatment strategy of patients with PAD is the natural history of both symptomatic and asymptomatic disease. The uninterrupted clinical course of lower extremity arterial disease is usually one of slow progression of symptoms over time (3). Approximately 70% of patients will remain unchanged or even less symptomatic after 5 to 10 years; less than 30% will progress to require intervention; and less than 10% will need amputation. Patients with diabetes mellitus, who comprise a

TABLE 111.1 CLINICAL CATEGORIES OF CHRONIC LIMB ISCHEMIA

Grade	Category	Clinical description	Objective criteria
0	0	Asymptomatic	Normal treadmill/stress test
	1	Mild claudication	Completes treadmill exercise,[a] ankle pressure after exercise <50 mm Hg but >25 mm Hg less than brachial
I	2	Moderate claudication	Between categories 1 and 3
	3	Severe claudication	Cannot complete treadmill exercise and ankle pressure after exercise <50 mm Hg
II	4	Ischemic rest pain	Resting ankle pressure <60 mm Hg; ankle or metatarsal pulse volume recording flat or barely pulsatile; toe pressure <40 mm Hg
	5	Minor tissue loss—nonhealing ulcer, focal gangrene with diffuse pedal ischemia	Resting ankle pressure <40 mm Hg; flat or barely pulsatile ankle or metatarsal pulse volume recording; toe pressure <30 mm Hg
III	6	Major tissue loss—extending above transmetatarsal level, functional foot no longer salvageable	Same as category 5

[a]5 minutes at 2 mph on a 12% incline.
Adapted from Rutherford RB, Flanigan DP, Guptka SK. Suggested standards for reports dealing with lower extremity ischemia. *J Vasc Surg* 1986;4:80–94.

large percentage of patients with PAD, are a unique subgroup in terms of prognosis and natural history of the disease. Diabetics have a higher likelihood of developing critical limb ischemia; indeed, their amputation rate is seven times greater than in nondiabetic patients with PAD.

Therapy for Atherosclerotic Peripheral Arterial Disease

The goals of therapy are to maintain functional status, reduce or eliminate ischemic symptoms, and prevent progression of disease. Insofar as PAD is a marker for systemic atherosclerosis, a secondary goal is to reduce the incidence of coronary and cerebrovascular events. Therapeutic options include conservative measures, percutaneous intervention, and surgery. With respect to noninvasive measures, risk factor modification (cessation of smoking is paramount) should thus be an important part of any treatment plan and may reduce progression of disease. Because limb ischemia may stimulate collateral growth, formal exercise training in a supervised setting may increase claudication-free walking distance by approximately twofold in patients with mild or moderate symptoms. Those with severe claudication, rest pain, or tissue loss (e.g., Rutherford category of 3 or more) are less likely to benefit from exercise.

Patients with PAD should receive drug treatment for coexisting disease (e.g., hypertension), risk factor modification (e.g., hyperlipidemia), and prophylaxis against thrombotic events associated with atherosclerosis (e.g., antiplatelet drugs), predominantly to reduce associated cardiac and cerebrovascular morbidity and mortality. No pharmacologic agent has proved efficacious enough to produce significant improvement in symptoms of PAD to gain widespread acceptance or use. Two established drugs, however, have gained U.S. Food and Drug Administration

approval. Pentoxifylline (Trental), a rheolytic agent, has shown up to a 21% increase over placebo in walking distance; patients most likely to benefit were those with symptoms for longer than 1 year and an ankle-brachial index of less than 0.80. However, most investigators agree that Trental is of little overall value in the treatment of symptomatic PAD (4). Cilostazol (Pletal), a phosphodiesterase III inhibitor with vasodilator and antiplatelet activity, more recently gained approval and has demonstrated benefit in some patients. In randomized trials, cilostazol led to a 47% increase in walking distance compared with placebo (13%) and improved quality of life (5). Prostaglandins have been used in several studies of patients with critical limb ischemia with some success (6). A number of vasodilator (e.g., calcium channel blockers, alpha-adrenergic antagonists), antiplatelet (e.g., aspirin, ticlopidine, clopidogrel) (7), and metabolic agents (L-carnitine, L-arginine) (8) have been studied, but none has been conclusively demonstrated to improve symptoms related to PAD.

Another novel form of "medical" or "noninvasive" therapy currently under investigation in early phase I and II clinical trials is the use of growth factors to treat critical limb ischemia (9,10). The premise behind this treatment is that the obstructed main vessel may not require recanalization if flow can be augmented by the development of more collateral vessels, a process termed *therapeutic angiogenesis*. Angiogenic cytokines (e.g., vascular endothelial growth factor and basic fibroblast growth factor) can be administered as recombinant protein or as gene encoding for that protein, either by direct intravascular infusion or site-specific intramuscular injection.

Invasive therapy, including percutaneous revascularization and surgery, is the most effective therapy for immediate relief of symptoms related to PAD. Major advances in recent years have facilitated less invasive treatment modalities. The latter two-thirds of this chapter are devoted to the implementation of these new techniques and their results vis-à-vis surgical therapy.

Atheroembolism

Atheroembolism is a particularly malignant consequence of advanced atherosclerotic PAD. It is caused by embolization of micro- or macroscopic friable or ulcerated atherosclerotic plaque debris, liberated from the proximal arterial tree, either spontaneously or after provocation by direct surgical or catheter manipulation. Atheroembolism may result in ischemia or infarction of the tissue supplied by the small arteries and capillaries to which the debris travels. Atheroembolism to the lower extremities may be focal, in which one or more toes are involved (causing the so-called blue toe syndrome) or diffuse, causing bilateral livedo reticularis, cyanosis, and pain; ischemia may progress to painful ulceration and gangrene, depending on the embolic load and the status of the underlying vasculature. Involvement of the renovascular bed may result in deterioration of renal function.

The treatment strategy for atheroembolism includes conservative local measures for the affected tissue and, importantly, appropriate steps to avoid future embolic events. These steps might include antiplatelet therapy and avoidance of future surgical and catheter manipulation near the presumed source of embolization, such as the abdominal aorta. Occasionally, especially in the case of recurrent atheroembolism, exclusion of the embolic source, either via percutaneous or surgical means, is recommended.

Acute Limb Ischemia

Acute limb ischemia most commonly occurs as a result of embolic arterial occlusion; the embolic source is cardiac in more than three-fourths of cases, and atrial fibrillation is responsible for the vast majority. *In situ* thrombosis of diseased native extremity vessels occurs less frequently; when spontaneous thrombosis does occur, especially in the absence of an underlying high-grade stenosis, the possibility of a previously unrecognized hypercoagulable state must be entertained. Bypass graft thrombosis with or without underlying impediment to flow is another frequent cause of acute limb ischemia.

Diagnosis

The clinical presentation of acute limb ischemia is typically dramatic, with acute onset of severe pain followed shortly thereafter by paresthesia and, ultimately, motor dysfunction (e.g., paralysis). On examination the extremity is cool, pale, and pulseless. Rutherford and colleagues described a series of clinical categories of acute limb ischemia (Table 111.2), with well-defined diagnostic criteria that help determine whether the affected limb is viable, in imminent jeopardy (e.g., "threatened"), or already irreversibly damaged (15). Whether a given patient will present with one category or another depends on many factors, including the duration of occlusion, the level and etiology of the occlusion, the status of the underlying vessels, and general factors (blood pressure, cardiac output, presence/absence of diabetes, oxygen saturation). Paradoxically, it is often the patient with less underlying PAD who develops the most severe ischemia—for example, the patient with atrial fibrillation and normal peripheral vessels who embolizes to the common femoral or popliteal arteries. The presence of better-developed collaterals in the patient with preexisting PAD can be protective.

Therapy

Patients with acute limb ischemia, especially those with threatened limbs, require immediate attention and an accelerated effort to restore nutrient flow to the jeopardized limb. Treatment for each patient is individualized, as discussed later in this chapter. Options include surgical or catheter-based thrombectomy, bypass, thrombolytic therapy, or direct percutaneous recanalization.

CURRENT THERAPEUTIC APPROACH TO PERIPHERAL ARTERIAL DISEASE

Role of Catheter-Based Interventions

Since the pioneering work of Dotter, Judkins, Gruentzig, and others (16,17), technical innovations have resolved many of the limitations (large-profile balloons, stiff

TABLE 111.2 CLINICAL CATEGORIES OF ACUTE LIMB ISCHEMIA

Category	Description	Capillary return	Muscle weakness	Sensory loss	Doppler signals	
					Arterial	Venous
Viable	Not immediately threatened	Intact	None	None	Audible (ankle pressure >30 mm Hg)	Audible
Threatened	Salvageable if promptly treated	Intact, slow	Mild, partial	Mild, incomplete	Inaudible	Audible
Irreversible	Major tissue loss, amputation regardless of treatment	Absent (marbling)	Profound, paralysis	Profound, anesthetic	Inaudible	Inaudible

Adapted from Rutherford RB, Flanigan DP, Guptka SK. Suggested standards for reports dealing with lower extremity ischemia. *J Vasc Surg* 1986;4:80–94.

guidewires, and poor imaging equipment), and consequently reduced the hazards associated with the early years of percutaneous transluminal angioplasty (PTA). Catheter profiles have been streamlined, limiting complications related to vascular access. Novel materials for balloon and guidewire construction have facilitated passage through occluded vessels and permitted routine access to more remote vascular sites with less risk and greater efficacy. Directional and rotational atherectomy and laser irradiation now enable "debulking" of atheroma. Endovascular stents have dramatically improved both short-term and long-term outcomes of PTA (18–21). Foremost among improvements in imaging techniques has been the introduction of intravascular ultrasound (IVUS), digital enhancement of conventional contrast images, and magnetic resonance imaging. ❦ r27

The increasing popularity of percutaneous revascularization as first-line therapy for patients with PAD underscores the need for vascular specialists to have a comprehensive understanding of the mechanisms of angioplasty, indications for intervention, expected outcome, and potential complications of a given revascularization procedure.

Imaging in Percutaneous Angioplasty

Conventional contrast angiography remains the time-honored approach for lesion characterization. It is, however, limited by the fact that it depicts the vessel lumen only; plaque and vessel wall are viewed as a "negative imprint" on the contrast-filled lumen (23). Although this allows for characterization of lumen topography, irregularities within the vessel wall may only be inferred from the negative imprint. Furthermore, contrast angiography is limited to a single planar view per injection; as such, information regarding the circumferential nature of the plaque is not provided.

Pathologic evaluation of dilated vessels typically discloses plaque fractures and stretching of the arterial wall; the exact contribution of these, versus plaque compression and other factors that might augment lumen area, remains controversial. Most *in vivo* attempts to identify the mechanisms responsible for successful (or unsuccessful) PTA have been limited by the lack of ability to adequately assess the morphology and geometry of a lesion before and after treatment, and at the time of restenosis using standard angiographic imaging methods.

Intravascular Ultrasound

IVUS has become a very useful adjunctive imaging technique to contrast angiography by providing a cross-sectional view of the vessel similar to a histologic section, thereby addressing many of the angiographic limitations. IVUS is unequivocally superior to contrast angiography in its ability to demonstrate detailed characteristics at the interface of the lumen and vessel wall as well as within the plaque. Indeed, experimental and clinical experience indicates that IVUS images correlate remarkably well with histologic examination; IVUS is exquisitely sensitive in detecting details that are angiographically "silent" (Figs. 111.1 and 111.2) (24,25). For instance, angiographically normal sites that are adjacent to target lesions almost always demonstrate disease when imaged by IVUS. Similarly, calcified plaque, characterized by "acoustic shadowing," is detected by IVUS in a majority of vessels undergoing angioplasty, a feature grossly underappreciated by angiography (26). Similarly, angiographically normal-appearing vessels are often found by IVUS to have diffuse plaque deposition, indicating a much more advanced stage of atherosclerosis than would have been presumed otherwise.

ANATOMIC REGIONS OF INTEREST

Therapy for certain sites within the peripheral circulation, particularly those previously considered to be inaccessible by the percutaneous approach, is evolving rapidly. Likelihood of success and chances for clinical improvement vary in degree according to the region of interest and extent of disease. However, because the management of an individual lesion in a particular patient depends on a number of factors, any classification or categorizing of recommendations is difficult (30). Weighted consideration of these individual issues is therefore required to determine, for any given combination of lesions, the appropriateness of nonsurgical revascularization (Table 111.3).

AORTOILIAC OBSTRUCTIVE DISEASE

Most stenotic disease in the infrarenal abdominal aorta and iliac arteries is atherosclerotic in origin. The excellent procedural and long-term results of aortoiliac PTA, enhanced by stenting, are so predictable that the physical finding of a diminished femoral pulse is a useful sign for identifying patients who are likely to derive benefit. ❦ r28

Aortoiliac Stenosis

Percutaneous therapy represents the first line of therapy for aortoiliac stenoses. Acute technical and clinical success of PTA alone for iliac stenoses exceeds 90%, and 1- and 5-year patency rates range from 75% to 95% and 55% to 85%, respectively (30,37). Stents have been shown to rescue the flow-limiting complications, reduce the acute recoil, and improve on the immediate hemodynamic results of PTA for aortoiliac stenoses, with acute technical success rates of 90% to 100% (*e*Fig. 111.2.1 and Fig. 111.3) (30,38–45). Significant improvements in long-term patency have also been achieved in patients randomized to PTA and stent

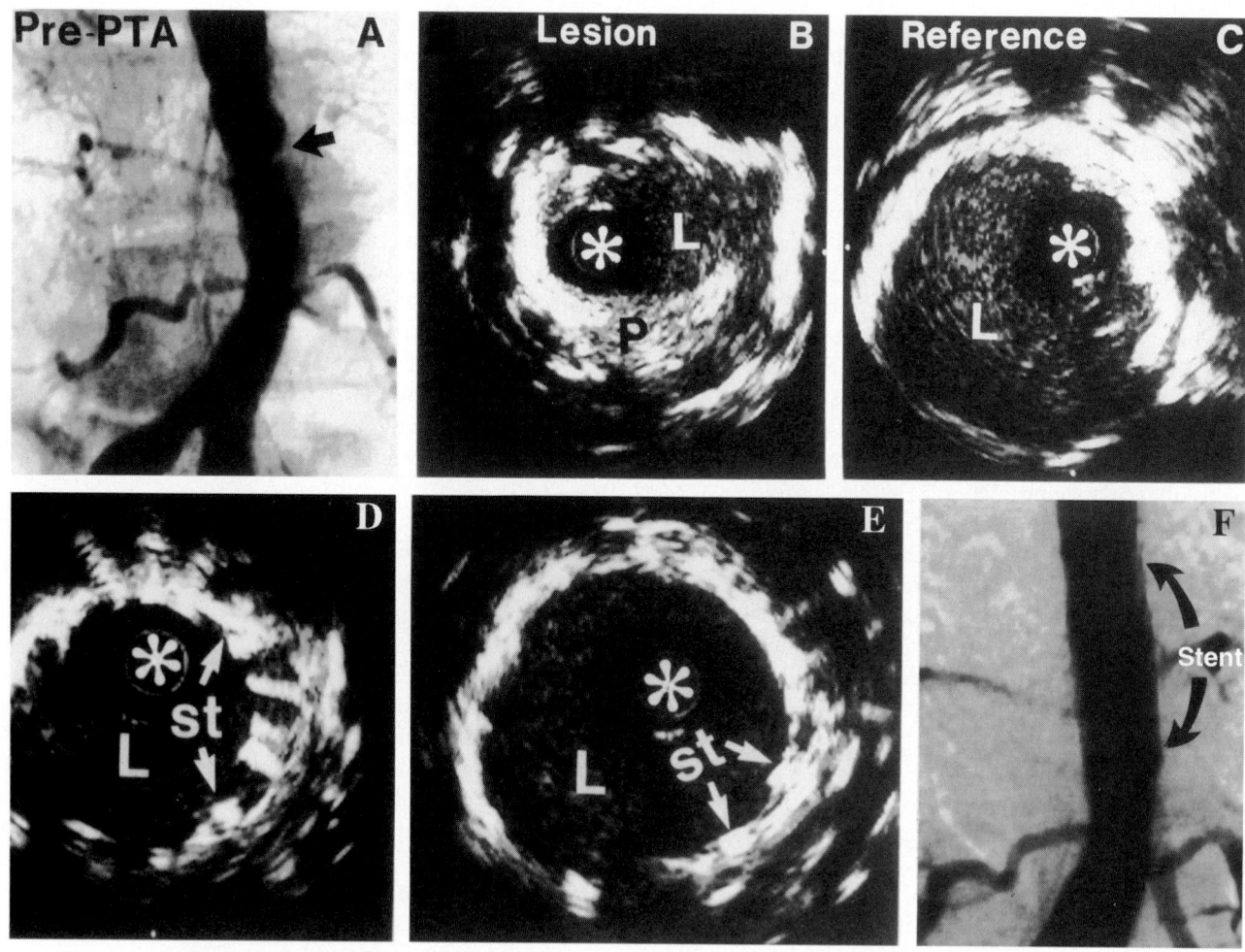

FIGURE 111.1 Superior imaging of eccentric aortic lesion by intravascular ultrasound (IVUS) compared with angiography. This 63-year-old woman presented with accelerated bilateral buttocks claudication, occurring at 1 to 2 blocks. **A:** Conventional anteroposterior angiography failed to disclose any significant stenosis; mild irregularity (*arrow*) was seen within the distal aorta. After discovering a large pressure gradient (see Fig. 111.4), IVUS examination was performed. **B:** IVUS image depicting focal eccentric plaque (P) narrowing the lumen (L) in distal aorta. **C:** IVUS from reference site distal to stenosis depicts normal lumen dimensions. **D:** Although lumen (L) is now enlarged compared with pre-percutaneous transluminal angioplasty (PTA), IVUS after 9-mm PTA/stent demonstrates stent underexpansion, with all struts (st) between 2 and 5 o'clock not in apposition to the arterial wall. **E:** IVUS after 12-mm PTA demonstrates complete expansion of stent, with all struts (st) now completely apposed to arterial wall and overall lumen (L) area further increased. **F:** Angiogram after 12-mm PTA shows slight decrease in luminal irregularity where stent has been redilated (*arrows*). *, IVUS catheter.

versus PTA alone: The angiographic patency (93%) in patients studied at 5-year follow-up rivals the best clinical patency reported at a similar time interval in patients undergoing operative revascularization (21,30).

Aortoiliac Occlusion

The approach to iliac occlusion is in evolution, moving from a predominantly surgically oriented therapy, to consideration of thrombolysis preceding PTA, and now toward a preference for primary PTA/stenting. There are two specific considerations in this regard. The first is the enhanced ability to traverse the segment of occluded artery (even

chronic occlusions) by advancements in guidewire (e.g., hydrophilic) and catheter technologies (46) and novel technical approaches, such as the so-called pull-through technique (Figs. 111.3 and 111.4) (47), a combination that has yielded an extremely high procedural success rate, especially in lengthy occlusions. The second issue concerns the specter of acute limb-threatening ischemia resulting from distal embolization in direct (nonlytic) recanalization of iliac occlusions, previously reported to occur with alarming frequency (48). The current incidence of embolization in this setting is exceedingly low, especially if a strategy of initial underdilation followed by stent deployment is used; the stent provides a scaffold, which, in theory, affixes the

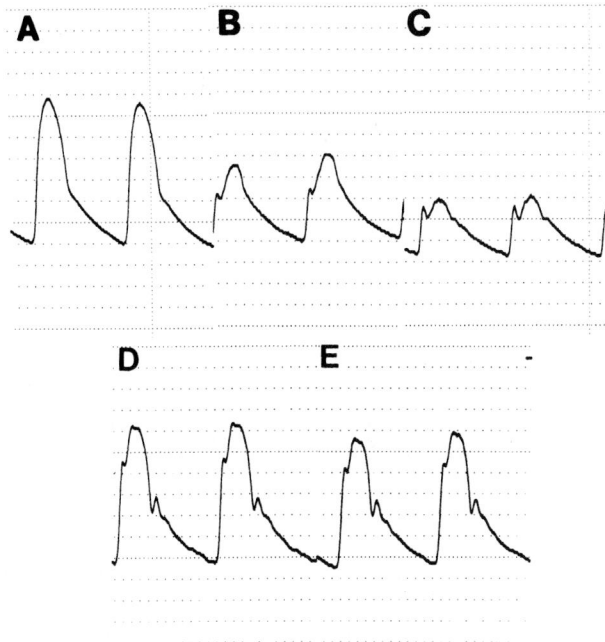

FIGURE 111.2 Intraarterial transstenotic pressure gradient before and after percutaneous transluminal angioplasty in the patient from Figure 111.3. **A:** Baseline blood pressure from aorta proximal to lesion. **B:** Pressure obtained simultaneously from aorta distal to lesion demonstrates 30-mm Hg peak gradient, which becomes exacerbated after administration of intraarterial nitroglycerin **(C)**. Proximal **(D)** and distal **(E)** aortic pressures after percutaneous transluminal angioplasty/stent are nearly identical, indicating hemodynamic improvement.

thrombus/plaque to the vessel wall, thus reducing the likelihood of distal embolization. The exception is the case of documented recent thrombosis, where use of thrombolytic therapy is unequivocally indicated (Fig. 111.4) (49–51). The extent to which lytic therapy may further optimize the treatment of less acute iliac occlusions by exposing an underlying lesion and converting an occlusion to a stenosis remains to be defined.

PTA alone for aortoiliac occlusions has less favorable results than for stenoses; the technical success rate of PTA of segmental (external or common) iliac occlusions is 80% to 85% (37,52) and long-term patency rates are close to 80% at 1 year and 55% at 5 years (53). Consequently, stenting is the preferred primary therapy for aortoiliac occlusions (40,44,53); indeed, a strategy of primary stent deployment for aortoiliac disease has been adopted by many investigators (43,45,54). A metaanalysis (55) of more than 2,100 patients showed greater immediate success rate (96% vs. 91%) and higher 4-year patency rates (61% vs. 54%) for stents than for PTA alone; stents also reduced the relative risk of 4-year failure by nearly 39% over PTA alone. Disease severity and relative proximal locations also have a positive influence on the outcome of revascularization by stenting (42). In patients with only focal aortoiliac or common iliac lesions, the rates for complete relief of symptoms

and 3-year persistent clinical benefit approach 90% and 95%, respectively, compared with 85% and 98% for patients with external iliac disease and 60% and 60% for patients with multilevel infrainguinal disease.

SUPERFICIAL FEMORAL AND POPLITEAL ARTERIES

Previous experience has failed to document any significant differences in either acute or long-term results for percutaneous revascularization of the SFA versus the popliteal artery; accordingly, both are herein considered together under the heading of SFA. r29

Occlusion of the Superficial Femoral Artery or Popliteal Artery

Among patients studied angiographically for consideration of revascularization, occlusions are more prevalent than stenoses. Two technical advances have facilitated treatment of SFA occlusions, even lengthy (more than 10 cm) or chronically occluded segments. The first is the use of hydrophilic wires. At our institution, the Glidewire was used to attempt percutaneous revascularization of 109 SFA total occlusions and was successfully advanced across the occluded segment in 107 (98%); PTA alone or in combination with DA and/or laser angioplasty was then used to complete percutaneous revascularization in all 107 patients (46). Improvements in ankle-brachial index (from 0.48 pre- to 0.82 postrevascularization) and in Rutherford class (one grade or more) were observed in 94% at 1-month follow-up. This experience was noteworthy for two reasons in particular. First, 50 lesions measured 5 to 10 cm in length and 21 were more than 20 cm long; consequently, mean occlusion length (9.8 cm) exceeded that reported in most previous series. Second, IVUS examination during these procedures demonstrated a subintimal route of recanalization in approximately one-third of patients (89).

The second advance is the use of thrombolytic therapy (Fig. 111.5), which has been proven effective, even for some patients with chronic total occlusions, because occlusion of the lower extremity arteries is typically characterized by a lengthy, gelatin-like thrombus superimposed on a high-grade atherosclerotic lesion. In such cases, lytic therapy can be effective in converting a long occlusion to one that is either shorter or no longer occlusive and thereby more amenable to mechanical revascularization. r30

Preliminary use of rheolytic thrombectomy devices (92,93) (Angiojet; Possis Medical Systems, Minneapolis, MN) either in lieu of or in conjunction with thrombolytic therapy has demonstrated encouraging results for treatment of acute and chronic thrombus in the SFA/popliteal (as well as other sites) and highlighted the potential for this device to reduce procedure time, hospital stay, and risks associated

TABLE 111.3 REVASCULARIZATION STRATEGY FOR VARIOUS LOCATIONS (AS OF 2001)

Arterial site and lesion type	Revascularization strategy					Clinical indication (e.g., Rutherford category/other)[a]	
	Percutaneous				Surgery	Percutaneous	Surgery
	Balloon angioplasty (PTA)	Adjunctive therapy					
		Stent	Thrombolysis	Other			
Iliac and infrarenal aorta							
Stenosis	Treatment of choice	Approved for suboptimal PTA result. Useful for unfavorable lesions. Primary stenting likely improves results and reduces restenosis.		Preliminary experience with early endografts not better than bare stent.	Reserved for cases of severe diffuse disease deemed inappropriate for PTA/stent.	2/3 or more	3 or more
Occlusion	Appropriate for short occlusion; lengthy occlusions also may respond, especially with adjunctive thrombolysis or primary stenting	Primary stenting indicated.	Essential for treatment of recent occlusion (<1 mo). Also may be used for chronic occlusions.	Preliminary experience with early endografts not better than bare stent.	Useful for lengthy occlusion, especially if distal aorta is stenosed or occluded.	2/3 or more	2/3 or more
Aneurysm		Stent-grafts (covered stents) approved in United States; first line of therapy for high-risk surgical candidates (due to comorbidity) who have anatomically suitable AAA.		Coils and occlusion devices required in some instances of AAA stent-grafting.	Remains current accepted gold standard for conventional-risk patients.	AAA 5-cm diameter or more and/or rapidly expanding in high-risk surgical patient; AAA causing thromboembolism	AAA 5-cm diameter or more and/or rapidly expanding; AAA causing thromboembolism
Common femoral	Reserved for patients with severe fibrosis due to previous surgery; some reports of PTA as first line of therapy in selected patients	Not approved; flexible stents may be used under certain "salvage" situations.			Preferred treatment, especially if in association with proximal/distal bypass.	2/3 or more	2/3 or more
Profunda femoris	Reserved for cases of severe or limb-threatening ischemia with no good surgical options; stakes high if SFA occluded already	Not approved; little experience reported thus far, but anecdotal acute success.			Preferred treatment for proximal disease (endarterectomy plus patch). Mid/distal vessel not easily accessed.	4 or more	3 or more

SFA/popliteal

Stenosis	Treatment of choice for short lesions; can be used in lengthy lesions as initial treatment; long-term results less favorable, but risk < surgery	Not approved; useful for "bail-out" indication; investigation under way using self-expanding device; initial trials with balloon-expandable stents show suboptimal results.	Useful only if non-occlusive thrombus present.	a) Directional atherectomy may be useful to debulk focal/eccentric stenoses but no clear-cut long-term improvement over PTA alone. b) Rotational atherectomy occasionally useful for calcified plaque. c) Trials under way using covered stents.	Reserved for cases of diffuse disease deemed inappropriate for PTA or DA.	2/3 or more
						3 or more
Occlusion	Treatment of choice for short (<7 cm) occlusion	Not approved; useful for bail-out indication; investigation under way for occlusion <10 cm.	Use highly recommended for recent (<1 mo) thrombosis/occlusion; some operators also prefer for chronic occlusion; may convert short or long occlusion into focal or segmental stenosis, facilitating treatment.	Treatment of choice for lengthy (e.g., >10 cm) occlusion.		
Infrapopliteal	Appropriate choice for treatment of discrete stenosis or focal occlusion	Not approved; useful to salvage failed PTA, especially in poor surgical patients.	Useful for recent thrombosis or thromboembolism.	a) Rotational atherectomy may be useful to debulk calcified lesions. b) Trials under way using excimer laser as adjunctive treatment.	Treatment of choice for lengthy diffuse disease/long occlusion(s), and not suitable or high-risk for percutaneous treatment.	3/4 or more
						4 or more
Subclavian stenosis/occlusion	Preferred treatment for stenosis; successful in most occlusions	Not approved; stents useful to optimize PTA results.	Indicated for recent occlusion (<1 mo). May facilitate PTA in chronic occlusion but little published experience.	Reserved for PTA non-candidates or failures who have severe symptoms.	Moderate arm claudication, subclavian steal syndrome, or coronary steal syndrome, or coronary steal via internal mammary artery	Severe arm claudication and/or subclavian steal syndrome

(continued)

TABLE 111.3 (Continued)

Arterial site and lesion type	Revascularization strategy					Clinical indication (e.g., Rutherford category/other)[a]	
	Percutaneous				Surgery	Percutaneous	Surgery
	Balloon angioplasty (PTA)	Stent	Adjunctive therapy				
			Thrombolysis	Other			
Vertebral	Preferred treatment for proximal stenosis	Not approved; useful for suboptimal PTA result, especially proximal vessel.	Useful and potentially life-saving in acute/subacute thrombosis.		Reserved for PTA failures and symptomatic occlusions.	Unequivocal symptoms of vertebral basilar insufficiency: visual/vestibular disturbance, posterior circulation TIA	Severe symptoms of vertebral basilar insufficiency; PTA impossible or unsuccessful
Basilar	Preferred treatment	Not approved; useful for flow-limiting dissection after PTA.	Life-saving in acute/subacute thrombosis with ongoing symptoms.		Reserved for cases of failed thrombolysis/PTA; may be primary therapy for occluded basilar with stable but persistent symptoms.	Acute/subacute/progressing symptoms of vertebral basilar insufficiency, posterior fossa or brainstem CVA/TIA	Same as for percutaneous but stable enough to undergo surgery
Carotid							
Innominate and common carotid (intrathoracic)	Preferred therapy for patients with symptoms or asymptomatic patients with critical stenosis	Not approved, but positive results; compelling reasons supporting primary (e.g., nonprovisional) stenting to prevent recoil, turbulence, thrombosis, and reduce stenosis.	No published data.		Reserved for symptomatic patients who are not PTA candidates.	Mild to severe symptoms or asymptomatic with stenosis >80% or 85%. Possible role preoperatively before coronary artery bypass graft	Moderate to severe symptoms
Bifurcation and proximal internal carotid artery	Experimental but favorable results in recent, nonrandomized clinical trials (if performed with stenting)	Investigational; appropriate for patients *not amenable* to CEA due to anatomic factors and/or comorbid conditions; some believe preferred for patients amenable to, but higher risk for, CEA.	Anecdotal reports of successful use in conjunction with PTA and stent for "active" or "acute" lesion.	a) Rheolytic thrombectomy—anecdotal reports of success in acute carotid thrombosis.	Accepted gold standard for lesions amenable to CEA.	Symptomatic or critical asymptomatic stenosis, if CEA not feasible; possibly for high-risk CEA patients	Fulfill North American Symptomatic Carotid Endarterectomy Trial or Asymptomatic Carotid Artery Study criteria

	PTA	Stent	Thrombolysis	Surgery	Indications for PTA/stent[a]	Indications for surgery[a]
	b) IIB/IIIA inhibitors—may be useful in carotid stent/PTA. Studies under way. c) Emboli protection devices—preliminary experience suggests benefit to capture emboli.					
Renal Fibromuscular disease	Treatment of choice	Not approved; anecdotal reports for lesions with recoil or restenosis.		Reserved for branch stenosis not amenable to PTRA.	Moderate HTN; accelerated or refractory HTN; renal insufficiency	Accelerated or refractory HTN; not amenable to PTA
Atherosclerotic (ostial or nonostial)	Preferred treatment for nonostial lesions; for ostial lesions, incidence of recoil and restenosis high with POBA	Not yet approved by the U.S. Food and Drug Administration, but large body of experience and several prospective trials demonstrating improved results over POBA for ostial lesions.	Reserved for acute thrombosis, an infrequent event.	Previously accepted standard for ostial disease, though PTA with stent likely equally effective with significantly less risk; preferred treatment for renal artery stenosis arising within aortic aneurysm or inaccessible for PTRA/stent.	HTN refractory or resistant to medical treatment; accelerated HTN; progressive renal dysfunction; CHF; angina. No benefit yet demonstrated when creatinine normal and HTN easily controlled by medical treatment	Same indications for PTRA when PTRA technically not feasible
Mesenteric	Reasonable first line of therapy but untested compared with surgery	Not approved, but anecdotal reports favorable; probable treatment of choice for ostial lesions.		Previously accepted standard but PTA plus stent may be equal with less risk.	Significant clinical evidence of mesenteric ischemia	Clear-cut evidence of mesenteric ischemia and PTA/stent not feasible

AAA, abdominal aortic aneurysm; CEA, carotid endarterectomy; CHF, congestive heart failure; CVA, cerebrovascular accident; DA, directional atherectomy; HTN, hypertension; med Rx, medical therapy; POBA, plain old balloon angioplasty; PTA, percutaneous transluminal angioplasty; PTRA, percutaneous transluminal renal artery angioplasty; SFA, superficial femoral artery; TIA, transient ischemic attack.

aIndications vary widely depending on risk-benefit ratio of a given procedure in a given patient. These are intended to be general guidelines only.

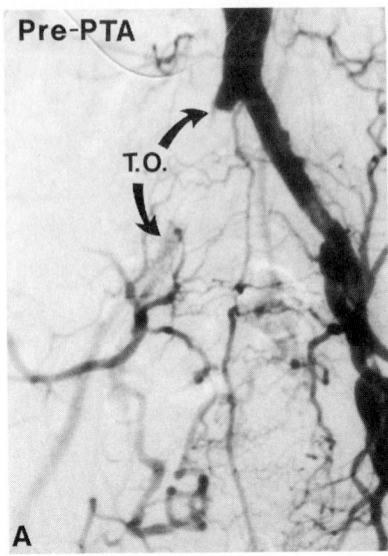
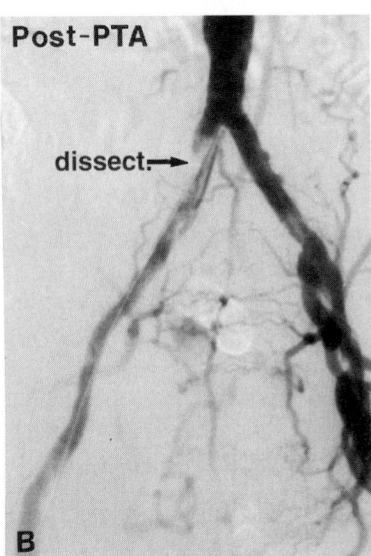
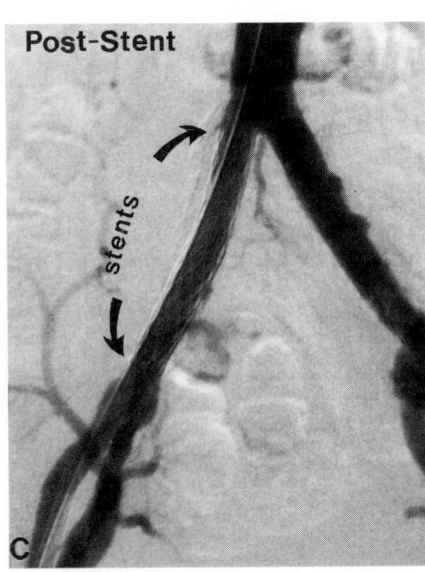

FIGURE 111.3 Percutaneous transluminal angioplasty (PTA) and stent deployment in chronically occluded right common iliac artery. **A:** Baseline angiogram demonstrates 5-cm total occlusion (T.O.) of right common iliac artery with reconstitution of external and internal iliac arteries. Occlusion was crossed using combination of angled and straight Glidewires, buttressed by a 4-Fr. catheter. **B:** Post-PTA angiogram demonstrating patent common iliac artery with extensive dissection (dissect.). **C:** Final angiogram after deployment of two Palmaz stents. Common iliac artery is widely patent. Baseline mean gradient of 37 mm Hg was reduced to 1 mm Hg. Patient is asymptomatic 4 years later.

with prolonged infusion of thrombolytic therapy (*e*Fig. 111.5.1).

The extent to which favorable acute procedural results in patients with chronic total occlusion will ultimately extend the role of percutaneous revascularization remains to be defined. Certainly for patients with nonhealing lesions or threatened limb loss in whom the risks of surgery are considered prohibitive, or in whom veins are unavailable for distal bypass, percutaneous revascularization of even lengthy occluded segments may facilitate healing. In similar types of patients with rest pain or severe claudication, PTA may be used to achieve pain relief at a lower risk than conventional surgical reconstruction. For patients with less severe symptoms, improved ability to revascularize does not in and of itself constitute a sufficient basis for routine invasive therapy. ⚓ r31

Current Recommendations for Superficial Femoral and Popliteal Disease

The acute technical success of balloon angioplasty for SFA/popliteal stenosis or occlusion is currently in the range of 90%. The principal factors in long-term patency are the status of the runoff vessels and the presence of occlusion. Long-term patency of 50% can be anticipated at 5 years; this is significantly less than that of iliac angioplasty. Thus, the threshold for intervention below the inguinal ligament should be higher. However, for patients with claudication severe enough to warrant intervention, PTA is the preferred initial treatment. This applies to both stenoses and occlusions that are amenable to revascularization. Lengthy, flush

occlusions of the SFA may not be approachable. Endovascular stents as a primary approach are not indicated. However, at present they have a limited role in salvage of acute PTA failures or complications (*e*Fig. 111.5.2). For chronic critical ischemia, or even acute limb-threatening ischemia, surgery is the preferred modality. However, one caveat to that is in the case of patients in whom the need for coronary bypass grafting is anticipated; in these patients, as long as instrumentation does not preclude future surgical intervention, PTA may be preferred to preserve the leg veins for future coronary bypass surgery.

INFRAPOPLITEAL ARTERIES

Published clinical experience involving percutaneous revascularization of the anterior tibial, tibioperoneal trunk, posterior tibial, and peroneal arteries, although dating to the time of Dotter and Judkins' original work (17), has nevertheless been far more limited than that described for aortoiliac and SFA sites. This is related to several issues, including the fact that claudication is rarely due to isolated disease of the infrapopliteal arteries; knee-to-foot patency of one of the three major branches is generally regarded as sufficient to prevent critical lower limb ischemia; restenosis rates in these vessels have typically been the highest of any of the lower extremity sites; and obstructive disease in these arteries is often occlusive or diffuse and complicated by heavy calcific deposits. Furthermore, diabetics have a high incidence of infrapopliteal disease, which is associated with diffusely atretic vessels that respond poorly to balloon dilation.

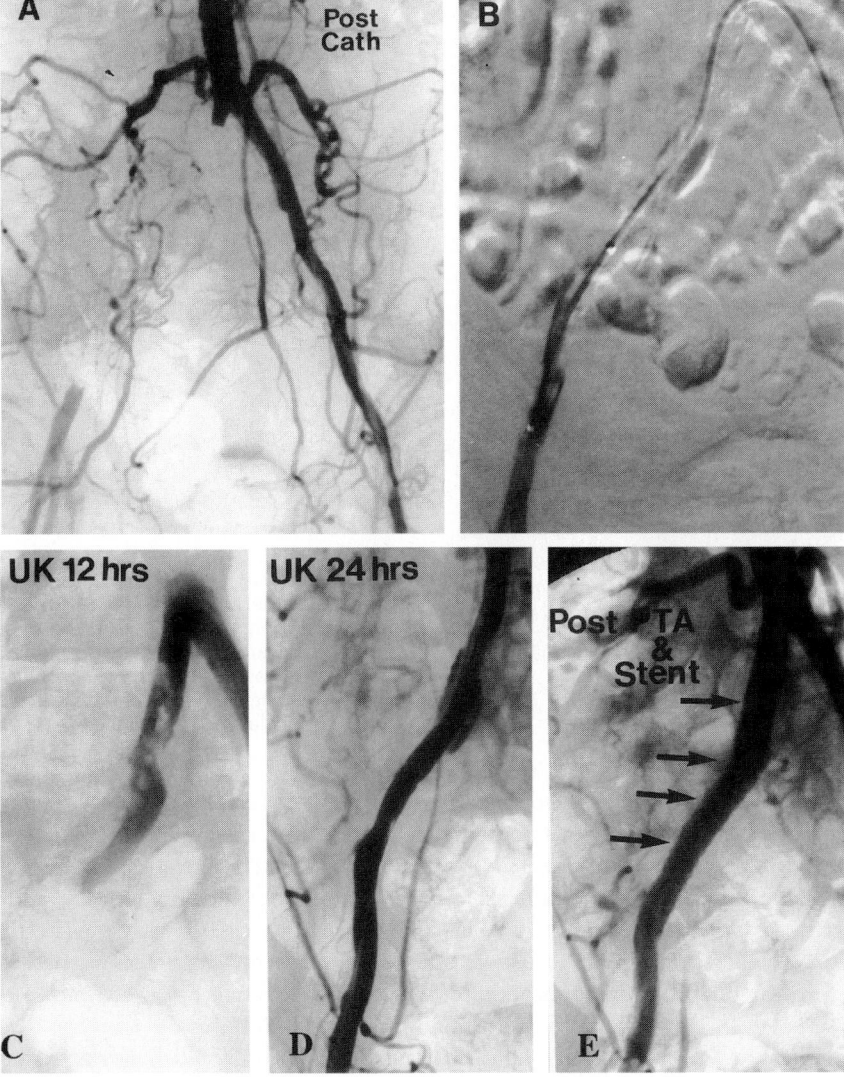

FIGURE 111.4 Thrombolysis, percutaneous transluminal angioplasty (PTA), and stent deployment in a patient with acute onset of right lower extremity ischemia after diagnostic cardiac catheterization (Cath). **A:** Baseline arteriogram demonstrates lengthy fresh occlusion of right common iliac artery, with reconstitution of common femoral artery by collaterals. **B:** Occlusion crossed in antegrade fashion from contralateral side and infusion of urokinase (UK) begun via Mewissen catheter and Katzen wire. **C:** After 12 hours of UK, common and external iliac arteries are now partially patent but have extensive dissection, residual thrombus, and blind cul-de-sac. Thrombolytic therapy therefore continued. **D:** After 24 hours of UK, vessel is now patent and thrombus resolved, but extensive dissection remains. **E:** After deployment of two Palmaz stents, the iliac artery is widely patent, with amelioration of dissection and elimination of the cul-de-sac. The patient remains asymptomatic 18 months later.

The ability to treat infrapopliteal disease has improved with technological advances, and the application of techniques used for coronary arterial revascularization has consequently resulted in a more widespread application of percutaneous revascularization for infrapopliteal disease (101). Despite this, many of the patients treated with infrapopliteal angioplasty to date have been those who were too high risk or otherwise unqualified for bypass surgery. The latter is still considered to be the standard of care for patients with critical limb ischemia due to infrapopliteal disease. Regardless of the conduit (reversed vein, *in situ* vein, or prosthetic material), patency rates are nonetheless inferior to those of more proximal reconstruction. It is conceivable that the long-term clinical outcome of percutaneous therapy may ultimately equal that of distal bypass grafting. Over the past decade, reports have documented that stenotic and even short occlusions of one or more infrapopliteal arteries can be revascularized percutaneously with a high degree of efficacy and at extraordinarily low risk

(102,103) both for critical limb ischemia and for claudication. These studies have demonstrated technical and clinical success rates in the range of 80% to 95% (the success rate in stenoses is superior to that in occlusions).

It must be emphasized that the goals of infrapopliteal revascularization often differ from those of above-the-knee therapy and vary with clinical presentation. In most patients with claudication, for example, below-knee angioplasty is not necessary, as treatment of coexisting proximal disease alone is often sufficient for symptomatic relief. There is a subset of patients who claudicate due solely to infrapopliteal disease for whom percutaneous therapy is becoming more popular. Such a strategy should be reserved, at least for the present, for patients who have severe symptoms (Rutherford category 3). Infrapopliteal PTA may also be justified in claudicants who undergo proximal revascularization (either with surgery or PTA), in whom the runoff is severely impaired, as outflow may be the principal determinant of long-term patency for femo-

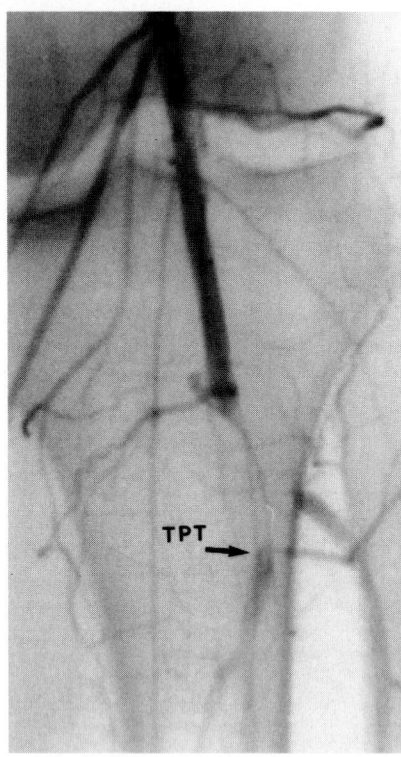
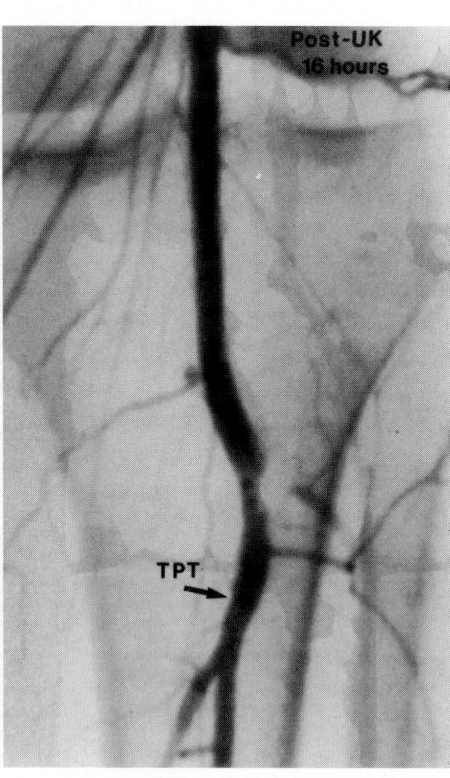

FIGURE 111.5 A: Acute embolic occlusion in an elderly woman with chronic atrial fibrillation. **B:** Rest pain resolved promptly after administration of urokinase (UK). Patency was restored to tibioperoneal trunk (TPT). The patient remains asymptomatic 4 years later.

A,B

ropopliteal revascularization. In patients with rest pain or ischemic ulceration, restoration of uninterrupted patency of at least one of the three major infrapopliteal arteries is generally required to obviate symptoms and/or heal a distal ischemic lesion. In this group of patients, aggressive application of percutaneous revascularization may achieve extremely gratifying results, even in patients with calcified and/or lengthy total occlusions (Fig. 111.6).

One point concerning percutaneous infrapopliteal revascularization requires special emphasis: the incidence of restenosis—which remains high—should not be a factor in the decision to use a percutaneous approach for what is, in many of these patients, a short-term problem. If uninterrupted patency of even one vessel can be achieved, the improvement in antegrade nutrient flow is typically adequate to facilitate limb salvage. Once healed, most patients will do satisfactorily, even in the face of documented reocclusion or restenosis. This strategy is further supported by the fact that both short- and long-term outcomes of distal surgical reconstruction for infrapopliteal disease are likewise imperfect (104). It is also conceivable that both of these revascularization strategies will be supplemented in many instances by the strategy of therapeutic angiogenesis (10,105,106). ⛛ r32

BYPASS GRAFTS

Percutaneous revascularization represents an alternative to operative reconstruction for failing or failed native or prosthetic conduits. Nonsurgical revascularization has several obvious advantages: It saves the patient the morbidity and additional hospitalization associated with a repeat surgical procedure; it does not require the availability or use of additional native veins; and in certain cases it may obviate the need to use prosthetic materials for distal reconstruction, an application for which such materials have been shown to confer lower patency rates (108,109).

The published results of PTA of *stenotic* lower extremity bypass grafts are extremely variable. [⛛ r33] Series in the surgical literature suggest that, although PTA can be acutely successful, the long-term patency is inferior to that associated with surgical revision (110,111). Our own approach to stenotic grafts is to make at least one attempt at percutaneous revascularization. This approach is derived from consideration of several issues. First, percutaneous revascularization of stenotic grafts is most often technically straightforward. Second, the risk of serious complications is low. Third, the contribution of adjunctive diagnostic and therapeutic techniques, including IVUS, DA, and endovascular stents, to preservation of graft patency remains essentially untested. Fourth, surgical revision itself is complicated by imperfect long-term patency (56,112,113). ⛛ r34

The approach to *occluded* lower extremity bypass conduits varies widely from institution to institution. Revascularization strategy should be based on consideration of numerous factors, including degree of ischemia present, type of graft material (e.g., prosthetic or autogenous vein), age of the graft, level of obstruction and accessibility for catheter-directed thrombolysis, presumed etiology of occlu-

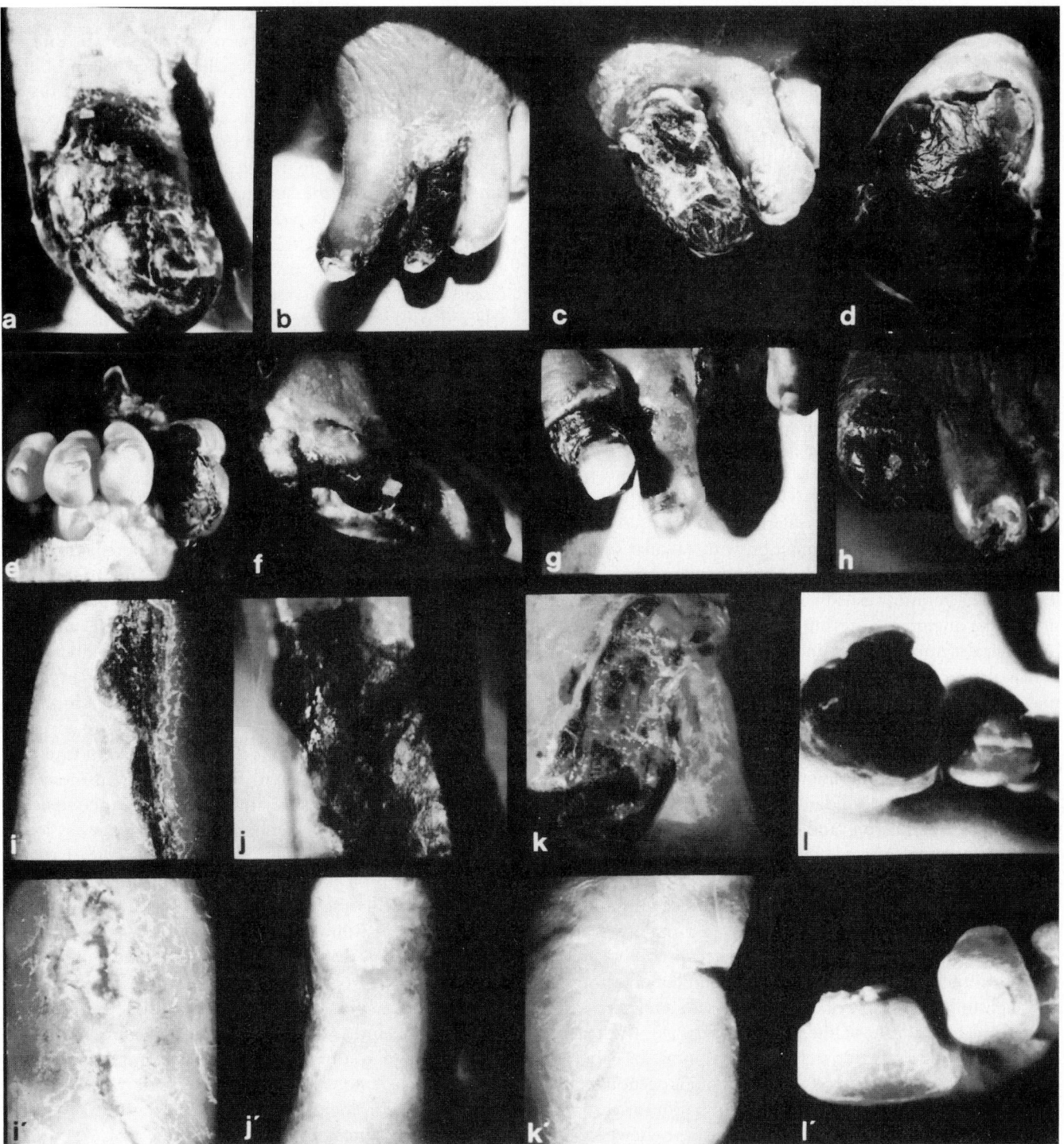

FIGURE 111.6 Composite figure showing the extent of severely ischemic alterations that typically develop before patients or their physicians seek medical consultation regarding the basis for these findings and possible treatment options. In most of these cases, amputation ultimately was required. For the patient whose limbs were photographed at the time of initial presentation in **i** through **l**, the corresponding photographs **i'** through **l'** demonstrate the appearance after percutaneous revascularization. These patients illustrate one of the most difficult groups of patients seen by specialists in vascular medicine. Earlier diagnosis and institution of therapy clearly are required to prevent the development of such extensive disease if the risk of amputation in these patients is to be reduced. It should be recognized, however, that when the extent of disease has reached even this degree, amputation and bypass surgery are not the only available treatment options. Percutaneous revascularization often may be successful in rescuing limbs of these patients; regardless of the subsequent incidence of restenosis, in the absence of recurrent foot, ankle, or lower leg trauma, such lesions will often remain clinically silent after satisfactory healing.

sion, and presence of comorbid conditions. Often, determination of the factor(s) responsible for graft failure is not possible before reestablishing enough flow to visualize the graft angiographically. Review of previous angiograms, including previous baseline (pregraft) and immediate post-grafting ("completion") studies, often provides a clue as to the factors that may have contributed to thrombosis. In cases of early graft failure (e.g., less than 3 months), reexamination of the angiograms for signs of technical or anatomic problems is crucial. Findings such as inadequate inflow to the graft due to proximal atherosclerosis, absence of adequate distal runoff vessels, mild residual narrowing at proximal or distal anastomotic sites, and presence of residual venous side branches are all potential sources of graft compromise that can have been underestimated or unrecognized altogether. Reevaluation of the patient's clinical and hematologic parameters is equally important: It is not unusual to detect an occult hypercoagulable state, such as protein C or S deficiency, which predisposed the patient to graft thrombosis.

Decisions regarding revascularization of an occluded graft should be made in conjunction with vascular surgical colleagues. Thrombosis of a very recently placed graft (e.g., less than 1 month) usually suggests the presence of an underlying anatomic or technical issue that is better treated by surgical thrombectomy and revision. The exception to that is the prosthetic graft (especially infrainguinal), which may thrombose spontaneously in the absence of obvious pathology, presumably because of the presence of thrombogenic foreign material. In these patients, even with recently placed grafts, prompt initiation of catheter-directed thrombolytic therapy may rapidly restore patency and enable angiographic evaluation and treatment of flow-limiting lesions. If none is detected, aggressive treatment with combined anticoagulation and antiplatelet agents is initiated in an attempt to prevent recurrent spontaneous thrombosis. Patients presenting with acute or subacute thromboses (less than 14 days) are best treated with catheter-directed thrombolysis (49,91). An alternative is balloon embolectomy, although this strategy may be associated with a higher morbidity and mortality over the ensuing year (91). Catheter-directed thrombolysis also remains an option for late or delayed (more than 3 months) occlusion of autogenous vein grafts. Angiography after successful elimination of thrombus often identifies a stenosis—anastomotic or elsewhere—that may have been primarily responsible for the graft occlusion. Treatment of the stenotic site with balloon angioplasty or DA can successfully restore long-term patency.

CAROTID ARTERIES

Atherosclerotic disease predominates at the common carotid bifurcation, a site easily accessible for surgical carotid endarterectomy (CEA). Indeed, revascularization of carotid arteries has, until recently, been considered to be exclusively within the purview of surgery. Since the first CEA more than 30 years ago, the associated morbidity, mortality, cost, and patient inconvenience associated with this procedure have been reduced considerably, such that CEA is currently recognized as the gold standard of therapy for patients deemed to require carotid revascularization. Supporting this are the landmark North American Symptomatic Carotid Endarterectomy Trial and Asymptomatic Carotid Artery Study trials demonstrating that surgical endarterectomy, when performed for carotid bifurcation disease by experienced vascular surgeons on appropriately selected patients, is effective in reducing the likelihood of stroke compared with medical therapy (130,131).

Carotid balloon angioplasty (CPTA) was performed as early as 1983, but due to the excellent results associated with CEA and concerns about the potential for distal embolization (132) and vessel recoil/thrombosis, the use of PTA for carotid disease (especially at the bifurcation) was limited to single-center anecdotal reports. Currently most institutions reserve percutaneous treatment of carotid arteries for those circumstances wherein the surgical risk is increased (133–136), such as in patients with either high cervical stenosis (i.e., under the angle of the mandible) or stenosis within the proximal common carotid artery near the aortic arch, which would require extensive intrathoracic surgery. In addition, patients with prior neck irradiation or radical neck dissection and those with restenosis at a previous endarterectomy site have also been considered appropriate for percutaneous intervention because of the increased risk of surgery in these subsets. Successful PTA, especially with the adjunctive use of endovascular stents, in these high-risk patients has led to consideration of the possibility that the less invasive, percutaneous approach might be applied more widely for carotid artery disease (Fig. 111.7).

The work of Roubin, Iyer, Yadav, Vitek (133,137,138), and others (139) demonstrated superior results of primary (as opposed to provisional) stenting (CPTA/stent) in carotid arteries, possibly due to more complete effacement of the plaque and associated ulcerations, reduction in elastic recoil, and restoration of laminar flow. Intermediate-term results demonstrate comparable safety (particularly the risk of neurologic events) and efficacy to CEA, especially when taking into account the selection of patients in higher-risk categories (lesion site, comorbid conditions) (140–143) (Fig. 111.8). Although technologic advances in stents, sheaths/guiding catheters, and diagnostic catheters may have contributed to the improved results, the reduction in events is principally due to increased operator experience and refinements in selection criteria.

Subsequently, prospective randomized trials have been initiated to compare the percutaneous versus surgical modalities to identify the role for CPTA/stenting. CAVA-

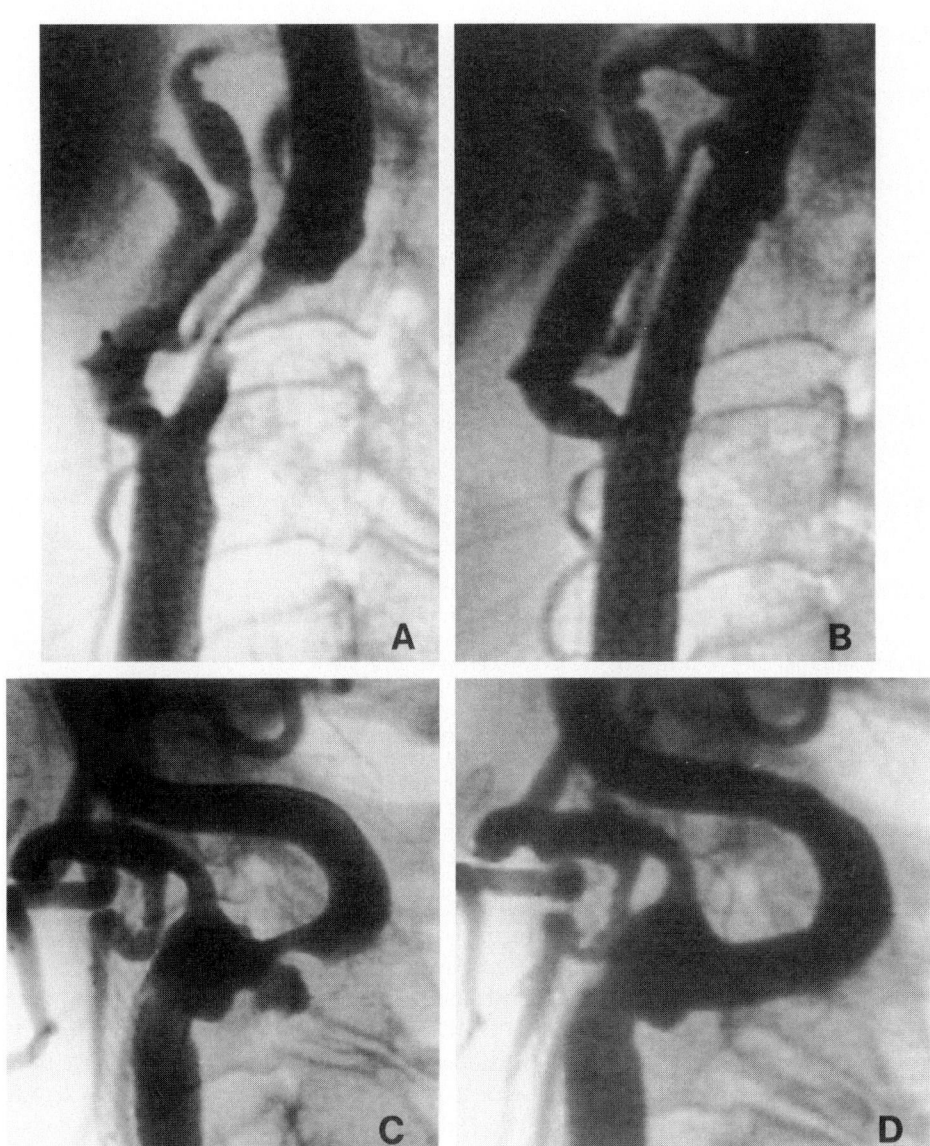

FIGURE 111.7 Bilateral carotid artery revascularization with balloon angioplasty and stent deployment in an 82-year-old asymptomatic male with "isolated hemispheres." **A:** High-grade stenosis of right internal carotid artery. **B:** Status post-percutaneous transluminal angioplasty and Wallstent deployment, with marked improvement and only mild residual narrowing. Wallstent extends into common carotid artery. No significant compromise in external carotid artery. **C:** High-grade, ulcerated stenosis in proximal left internal carotid artery, revascularized 4 weeks after percutaneous transluminal angioplasty of the right side. **D:** Status post percutaneous transluminal angioplasty and Palmaz stent deployment in proximal left internal carotid artery. Excellent result with no residual stenosis. Both procedures were uneventful, and the patient remains asymptomatic at 1-year follow-up.

TAS (144) enrolled 504 patients (253 CEA, 251 CPTA) and reported comparable 30-day major stroke and mortality rates between surgery and angioplasty. The Carotid Revascularization Endarterectomy Versus Stent Trial, a large National Institutes of Health–sponsored multicenter study, promises ultimately to provide more definitive information regarding the role of CPTA/stenting, at least in patients with symptomatic disease (145,146).

It remains to be determined what will be the best stent design for use in the carotid arteries. Despite initial excellent results with balloon-expandable Palmaz biliary stents (139,140), the infrequent but troublesome occurrence of stent compression (147) has led most investigators to favor the use of self-expanding stents that are lower profile, flexible, and able to be placed accurately. There are also tremendous enthusiasm and anticipation surrounding the development of distal protection devices to avoid embolization during carotid angioplasty (*e*Fig. 111.8.1). Clinical trials in Europe (148) and early investigational studies in the United States have shown promising results with devices involving the use of a distal trap, or umbrella, encasing a filter, which collects particulate debris. It is anticipated that these will significantly reduce the embolic complications associated with CPTA/stenting.

RENAL ARTERIES

The primary goals of renal artery revascularization are to improve control of hypertension; preserve or restore renal function; or treat the physiologic effects of severe RAS, which include congestive heart failure (CHF), recurrent flash pulmonary edema, and angina. Associated secondary benefits may include reduction in antihypertensive medications, ability to more safely administer angiotensin-converting enzyme inhibitors in patients with chronic CHF or

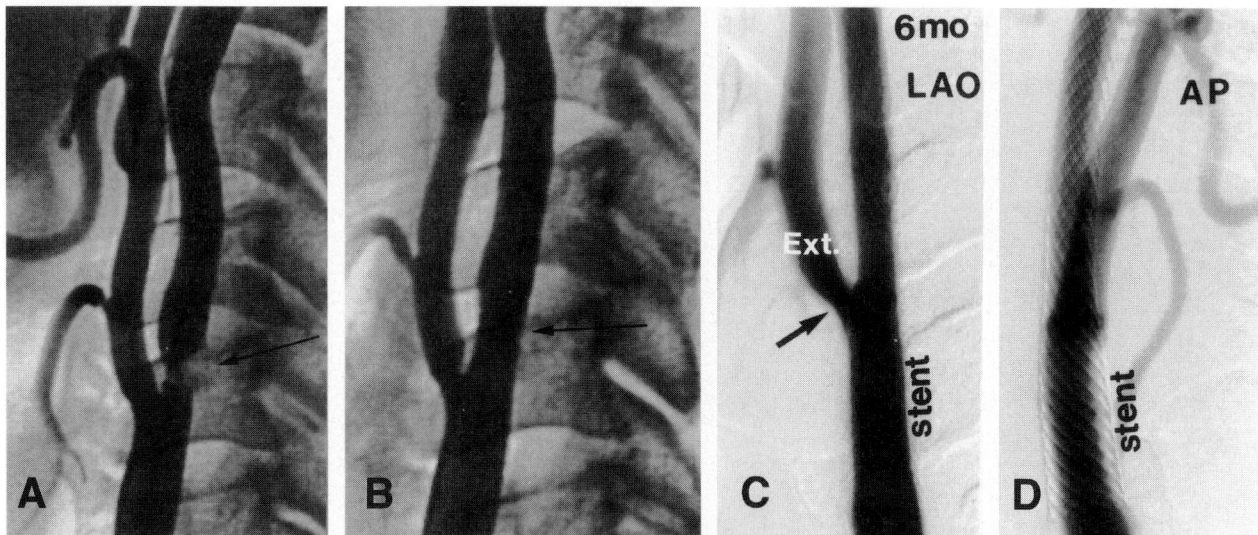

FIGURE 111.8 Carotid stent deployment in an 82-year-old patient with highly unstable angina on intravenous nitroglycerin, awaiting coronary artery bypass graft. Contralateral internal carotid artery is completely occluded, and both vertebral arteries are 95% narrowed. **A:** Before percutaneous transluminal angioplasty, internal carotid artery has severe, ulcerated, focal stenosis (*arrow*). **B:** After percutaneous transluminal angioplasty and deployment of Wallstent. Stenosis now ameliorated (*arrow*); flow improved into internal carotid artery. External carotid artery (Ext.) is minimally compromised. Patient subsequently underwent uneventful coronary artery bypass graft 1 day after percutaneous transluminal angioplasty. Left anterior oblique (LAO) **(C)** and anteroposterior (AP) **(D)** angiograms of right carotid artery 6-month status post Wallstent deployment demonstrate widely patent carotid artery. In **(C)**, Wallstent covers origin (*arrow*) of external carotid artery, which remains patent. Minimal neointimal growth within stent is seen in anteroposterior view. Patient remains free of neurologic and cardiac symptoms 14 months later.

cardiomyopathy, and, occasionally, elimination of the need for dialysis. ▼ r35

Fibromuscular Disease

Surgical revascularization for severe hypertension due to FMD is exemplary in the hands of surgeons with extensive experience (150), but the role of surgery has nonetheless declined for this entity, a reflection of the fact that PTA alone is quite effective. For lesions localized within the main renal artery or its primary branches, studies report acute technical success in excess of 90%, initial clinical success (elimination or significant reduction in hypertension at 6-month follow up) of 85% to 90%, 5-year recurrence rates of less than 10%, and long-term clinical benefit in 80% to 90% (151–153). Hence, the threshold for PTA in patients with FMD is relatively low; patients with persistent, even modest, hypertension on medications should be treated, especially if they are young, so as to avoid the long-term consequences of hypertension.

The experience with PTA for FMD involving branch vessels and/or aneurysmal disease is limited. Although surgical revascularization is still advocated using extracorporeal reconstruction of the branch vessels, reports of technical and clinical outcomes approaching 85% suggest that PTA may offer an effective alternative treatment (154); the decision to attempt PTA on smaller branch vessels, however,

must be weighed against the potential to cause dissection, thrombosis, and loss of the kidney.

The use of endovascular stents has not generally been advocated in FMD patients for two main reasons. First, the results with balloon angioplasty alone for FMD have been excellent, with lower recurrence rates than atherosclerotic disease. Second, the biologic effects and long-term consequences of placing stents in these lesions are unknown. Nonetheless, there have been anecdotal reports of stenting for refractory or recurrent FMD lesions.

Atherosclerotic Renal Artery Stenosis

Percutaneous treatment of atherosclerotic RAS has been less gratifying than that of FMD. However, balloon angioplasty can provide a safe and effective modality for renal revascularization, with a favorable risk-benefit ratio. In a pooled analysis of multiple early studies, percutaneous transluminal renal artery angioplasty (PTRA) resulted in improved renal function in 43% of patients, stabilization in 35%, and continued worsening (e.g., no beneficial effect of PTRA) in 22% (155) but was hampered by a high restenosis rate, which approached 70% at 6 to 12 months, primarily related to the predilection for immediate and delayed elastic recoil as a result of the high prevalence (approximately 80% to 90%) of thick, calcified aorto-ostial plaque. The mortality rate in most series is less than 1%; contrast-related and atheroembolic events are surprisingly infrequent; and the majority of reported complications is related to vascular access.

On the other hand, primary surgical revascularization in appropriately selected good surgical candidates has shown to be effective both with respect to restoration of patency and favorable clinical outcome (preservation of renal function and reduction of hypertension) (155,156), and although the associated mortality can be significant (between 2% and 17%) (155,157,158), progression of surgical experience and technique (using extraanatomic bypass techniques) has resulted in significant reduction in mortality rates (150,159). ◥ r36

The factor that is most predictive of initial failure or recurrence after PTRA alone is lesion location: Balloon dilation of stenoses located at the ostium are generally associated with an acute success rate of 50% or less and high restenosis rates (152,153,161). Although modifications in angioplasty technique, such as use of guiding catheters (162) and enhancement in imaging using IVUS (163), may facilitate PTRA, it is likely that the major limitation to successful dilation of ostial lesions will continue to be the elastic recoil of plaque, which is partially aortic in origin. Recent experiences using stents during PTRA to augment lumen size and reduce recoil, particularly for ostial stenoses, have clearly demonstrated much more complete amelioration of the stenosis and transstenotic pressure gradient compared with balloon angioplasty alone (Fig. 111.9) (164,165). Blum and colleagues, in a study of stent deployment for failed angioplasty of ostial lesions (166), reported 11% restenosis (more than 50% stenosis), 92% secondary patency at 60 months, 16% reversal of and 62% improvement in hypertension, and stability of renal function even in patients with baseline renal dysfunction. Palmaz (167) analyzed results from renal artery stenting in eight series (mean follow-up of 10.9 months); hypertension was improved in 56% or cured in 10%; renal function improved in 27% and stabilized (e.g., no further deterioration) in 38%; restenosis occurred in approximately 16% of patients; and major complications occurred in 4.9%. These results support the routine use of stents for renal ostial stenoses.

Complications related to balloon angioplasty and/or stenting of renal arteries occur in less than 10% of patients and commonly relate to access. The most feared complication, which probably occurs more frequently than is clinically appreciated, is that of atheroembolism into either renal vascular or peripheral vascular beds. Other complications of percutaneous renal revascularization include dissection of the renal artery or the wall of the aorta, acute or delayed thrombosis, and rupture of the renal artery.

Current Recommendations for the Treatment of Renal Artery Stenosis

The percutaneous approach is the initial choice of therapy for atherosclerotic renal artery stenosis. Furthermore, the evidence is overwhelming that stents, whether used prima-

rily or provisionally, greatly enhance the results of PTA. Surgery is reserved for patients in whom PTA is less suitable, such as those with branch vessel disease, total occlusions, and stenosis in a renal artery that arises from within an AAA. The question remains of when revascularization should be undertaken. In considering this issue, 40% of patients with atherosclerotic renal artery stenosis will progress over 5 to 10 years. Furthermore, a small subset of patients (10% to 20%) will demonstrate deterioration in renal function immediately after revascularization, presumably due to cholesterol embolization or contrast toxicity. Patients with progressive renovascular disease—in association with steady decline in renal function, hypertension that is accelerated or difficult to control, or CHF—will generally benefit from renal revascularization. Patients who have recently developed end-stage renal disease, partly or wholly due to RAS, may also benefit from revascularization (158,168); PTRA may enable such patients to discontinue or avoid imminent dialysis (Fig. 111.10). ◥ r37

HEMODIALYSIS CONDUITS

More than 120,000 patients are dependent on hemodialysis, and recent evidence shows an increase of 10% per year (178). Nowadays, with the expanding dialysis population enjoying an increased life expectancy, preservation of vascular access sites has become increasingly important. Repeated large-gauge needle punctures, increased sheer forces and intraluminal pressure during dialysis, and postdialysis compression of puncture sites are all factors that may contribute to the high incidence of stenosis and thrombosis in dialysis conduits, be they arteriovenous fistulas or Gore Tex grafts. Arteriovenous fistulas tend to develop fibrous strictures at, and proximal to, sites of repeated puncture. Gore Tex grafts develop stenoses principally localized to the venous and arterial anastomoses; accumulation of pseudointima within the body of the graft may also predispose to graft failure. Surgical revision typically involves several days of hospitalization and placement of temporary access. A more important consequence of surgical revision, however, is the use of proximal vein, which may limit options for future surgical management. PTA has played an increasingly important role in maintaining the functional status of hemodialysis access conduits. The use of PTA for dialysis conduits requires a different perspective from PTA at other sites: Because the patency of dialysis conduits is problematic, regardless of whether surgery or other approaches are used, restenosis is tolerated at a higher frequency than in nearly all other circumstances.

Percutaneous treatment of stenotic or occluded grafts or fistulae is usually technically straightforward (*e*Fig. 111.10.2). Acute success rates of 70% to 95% have been reported (178–180). However, primary restenosis rates are higher than for PTA in most other vascular beds, up to

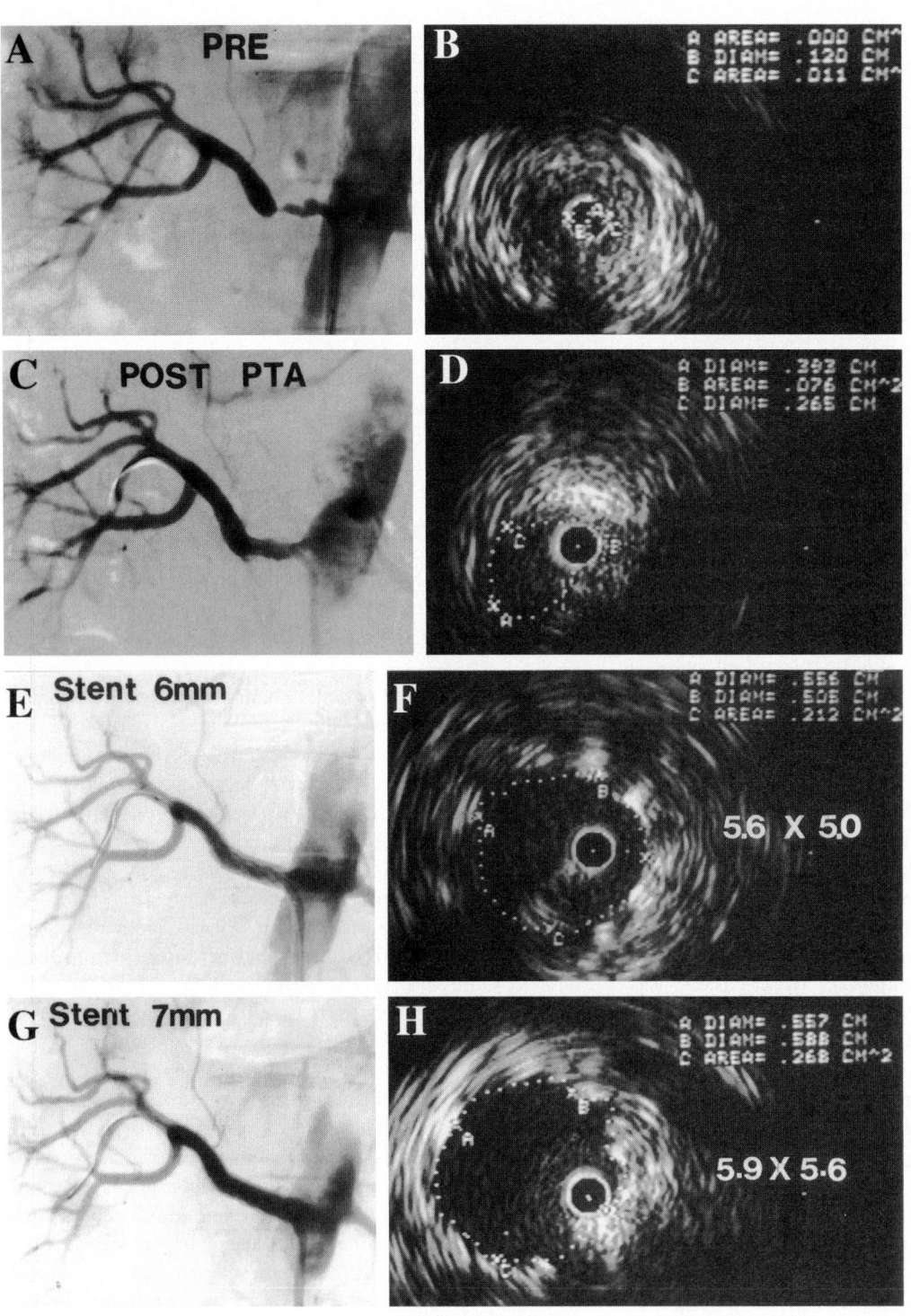

FIGURE 111.9 Percutaneous transluminal angioplasty (PTA) of the proximal renal artery lesion, guided by intravascular ultrasound (IVUS). **A:** Baseline angiogram depicts severe proximal renal artery stenosis. **B:** Corresponding IVUS image shows plaque abutting catheter circumferentially. **C:** Post-PTA, irregular lumen with plaque fracture and residual stenosis. **D:** IVUS post-PTA shows only modest enlargement of the lumen. **E:** Deployment and dilation of a Palmaz stent with a 6-mm balloon; angiographic result much improved over PTA alone. **F:** IVUS shows doubling in lumen diameter over PTA alone. However, in spite of excellent angiographic appearance, IVUS shows that the diameter of the treated segment is still less than the "reference segment." **G:** After inflation with a 7-mm balloon, the angiographic result is slightly better. **H:** IVUS now shows the size of stented vessel is equal to that of the reference segment. This case highlights the usefulness of IVUS in renal angioplasty.

60% and 80% at 1 and 2 years, respectively (180,181). *Secondary* patency, however, has been quite acceptable (more than 70% at 2 years) in series in which the investigators closely monitored graft function and performed early angiography and repeat PTA in cases of recurrent stenosis (180). Thus, although the average graft may remain functional only for 4 to 6 months after a single PTA, as opposed to 14 to 18 months after surgical revision (178), close monitoring of graft function and appropriately timed interven-

tion can enhance the results of the percutaneous strategy and delay the need for graft revision.

Angioplasty of offending lesions in dialysis conduits often requires use of high-pressure (up to 20 atmospheres) inflation because of the fibrotic nature of the strictures within the venous system and at the graft anastomosis. IVUS is particularly useful for determining the reference diameter and quantifying the extent of recoil (182). Even aggressive angioplasty using oversized balloons, however, is

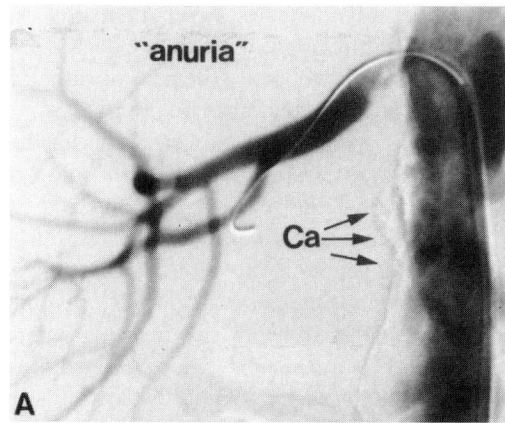

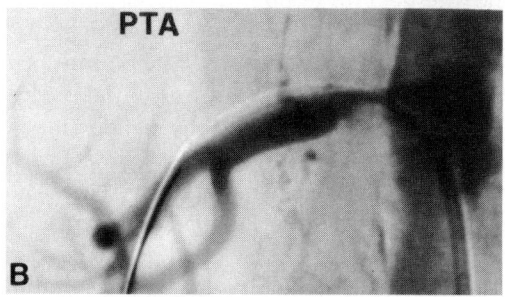

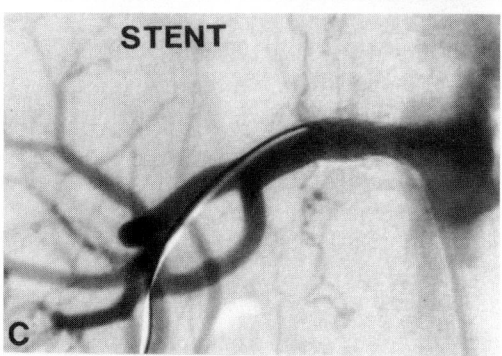

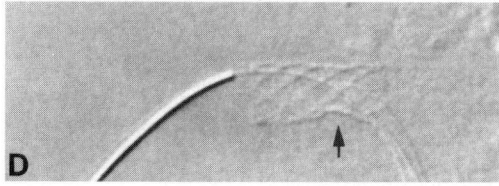

FIGURE 111.10 "Salvage" renal angioplasty and stent deployment in a woman with recent onset of renal failure, anuria, and severe, refractory congestive heart failure requiring intubation. **A:** Baseline angiogram obtained after traversing subtotal occlusion of right renal artery with guidewire. Aorta is very heavily calcified (Ca), and left renal artery is occluded; left kidney is nonfunctional. **B:** Status post balloon angioplasty alone [percutaneous transluminal angioplasty (PTA)] for this heavily calcified ostial stenosis; extensive recoil is evident. **C:** Vessel widely patent after stent deployment. Not significantly obstructive. **D:** Stent configuration without contrast demonstrates minor dimple (*arrow*) along inferior border caused by resistant aortic plaque. Patient began making urine immediately while on the angiographic table. Dialysis was discontinued immediately, and the patient left the hospital with a creatinine of 1.2 off dialysis 4 days after stent deployment. She remains off dialysis 1 year later.

often insufficient, in which case adjunctive treatment with DA may be useful to "cut" the fibrous band. Endovascular stents have also been investigated, but their role remains to be determined.

As suggested by several studies (178,179,183), management of dialysis conduits requires the cooperative efforts of a team consisting of nephrologists, vascular surgeons, and interventionalists. The nephrologists and dialysis nursing staff must pay close attention to the hemodynamic function of access sites during dialysis. Increase in venous pressure, decrease in arterial flow, increase in recirculation, and poor dialysis efficiency are all occurrences that should trigger the request for a diagnostic angiogram. Focal stenoses can be treated initially using PTA and, for resistant lesions, DA. Thereafter, patients should be monitored particularly closely, as one can expect a high incidence of restenosis. Repeated percutaneous interventions, in the interest of preserving the access site and avoiding the need to sacrifice additional vein, are appropriate. However, in cases of recurrent early failure and/or extensive graft degeneration, surgical revision becomes necessary.

CONTROVERSIES AND PERSONAL PERSPECTIVES

In general, the same rigorous standards that have been applied to studies evaluating management strategies in CAD have not thus far been applied to studies of peripheral artery revascularization (15). The development by Rutherford, Becker, and others of uniform standards for reporting results of interventions paves the way for the performance of prospective multicenter trials, which should enable more accurate comparison between various treatment strategies (2).

When Is It Appropriate to Revascularize?

The spectrum of thresholds for intervention is very broad, ranging from practitioners who will refer only PAD patients with advanced ischemia (Rutherford category 4) to those who consider lifestyle-limiting claudication grounds for considering revascularization. The former (conservative) approach is based on the premise that (a) this disease is not generally life-threatening and usually not limb-threatening; (b) any intervention uses up scarce health care dollars and limited resources; (c) the results of both PTA and surgery are imperfect; (d) complications can occur and are not entirely predictable; and (e) patients can occasionally be rendered worse off after (failed) intervention. However, an approach to patients solely based on these premises ignores the progress made in recent years treating PAD; the therapeutic armamentarium for and clinical experience with percutaneous revascularization has markedly improved the prospects of patients with PAD. In the bygone era, there was little reason to perform diagnostic angiography unless surgery was indicated, justifiably so given the risks of major reconstructive surgery in a high-risk population with coronary and cerebrovascular disease, thereby restricting surgery to patients with altogether disabling claudication or threatened limb loss.

In the current era, intervention at an earlier stage of symptomatic disability is possible due to the lower risks and lower costs of nonsurgical revascularization. As has been pointed out by Kumpe and Rutherford (184), "[T]he advantages to the patient able to undergo angioplasty rather than surgery . . . are lower initial morbidity and mortality, no need for general anesthesia, shorter hospital stay, [and] less trauma." This is true even when one adds to the morbidity of PTA that of diagnostic angiography. Complications of PTA are for the most part minor and typically do not require surgical treatment (185). Access-related events account for most complications [2% to 8% in most series (184–186)]; these range from the less serious and more common (e.g., groin hematoma) to the serious but rare (e.g., retroperitoneal hematoma) (187). The incidence of complications at the angioplasty site—1% to 7% in most series (185,186,188)—is similar to that in percutaneous transluminal coronary angioplasty, and consists principally of acute occlusion; as with PTA, many of these can be managed with lytic or adjunctive mechanical therapy, including stents, so that the need for emergent surgery due to a jeopardized limb is rare. Distal embolization has been reported in up to 5% of cases (186). Most, however, are clinically silent (185), and even those that might be potentially problematic can often be obviated pre-PTA or treated successfully post-PTA by judicious use of lytic therapy.

It is nevertheless true that both the risks and cost of percutaneous revascularization increase with the complexity and extent of anatomic involvement. The decision to revascularize the patient with claudication in 2001 must therefore take into account two principal considerations. The first is the patient's symptoms. Reduction in pulse amplitude or inability to palpate one or more pulses on physical examination altogether supports a vascular basis for the patient's complaints. Noninvasive testing (189–191) continues to represent an indispensable and necessary initial step in the evaluation of PAD; importantly, failure to detect an abnormal ankle-brachial index at rest does not exclude the presence of severe obstruction, particularly in diabetic or other patients with calcified, noncompressible arteries. Exercise or alternative stress testing may be required to elicit hemodynamic evidence of symptomatic vascular obstructions. Duplex (189), including color-flow (191), examinations may help to clarify such discrepancies. Angiographic examination, however, is still required to define the second consideration, namely the full extent and complexity of the anatomic basis for symptomatic disability, although current advancements in magnetic resonance imaging allow a noninvasive approach.

Once having clarified the anatomic basis for claudication, the recommendation to advise percutaneous revascularization is then individualized. Two patients, for example, may be similarly limited, and in both, the degree of limitation may be inadequate to justify the risks of vascular surgical reconstruction. Diagnostic angiography may suggest that percutaneous revascularization has a high likelihood of technical success in one patient who may thus be a suitable candidate for percutaneous revascularization. In the second patient, certain risks and a complex of anatomic factors suggesting a low likelihood of acute or long-term success may dictate that only surgical revascularization would constitute effective therapy, in which case it may be appropriate to defer the risk of surgery until the patient is more critically disabled. Angiography may thus critically raise or lower the threshold for recommending that an intervention be performed. In previous days, when higher-risk and higher-cost surgery represented the sole option to medical and exercise therapy, it could be reasonably argued that the decision to proceed with angiography could come down to consideration of symptomatic disability only. The option of performing lower-risk and lower-cost PTA, however, implies that the threshold for responding to a given level of symptomatic disability may be raised or lowered, depending on the extent and complexity of anatomic findings.

Should the patient treated by percutaneous revascularization return with clinical evidence of restenosis, repeat percutaneous intervention is probably indicated for the same reasons that led to the recommendation for the original procedure. A certain proportion of these patients—as has been clearly documented in certain patients undergoing one or more repeat coronary angioplasty procedures (192,193)—will achieve a satisfactory long-term result after the second intervention. In those who fail repeated percutaneous attempts to achieve long-term patency, the decision to undergo surgical revascularization may involve a reassessment of the patient's anatomy and clinical status.

Who Should Decide on the Revascularization Strategy, and Who Should Perform Percutaneous Interventions?

This controversy deserves but a few short lines. The concepts that are promulgated by some individuals within various specialties (vascular surgery: "our disease"; radiology: "our procedures"; cardiology: "our patients") have no place in the workup and management of patients with PAD. Justification for so-called turf wars is difficult to find and seems to be based mainly on issues only tangentially related to patient care, at best. Such "battles" preclude cross-fertilization and exchange of knowledge and ideas among specialties. As such, patient care stands to suffer from the underuse of resources that could have been helpful.

The ideal approach to management of PAD, a truly multidisciplinary disease, requires coordinated input from experts in cardiology, vascular surgery, radiology, and vascu-

THE FUTURE

As the population ages and patients are surviving with their heart disease, physicians are now grappling with the increased prevalence and disabling effects of vascular disease at other arterial sites, including carotids, renals, and lower extremities. Over the next 10 years, cardiologists will become much more aware and knowledgeable about PAD and involved in management issues related to this disease. Concurrently, detection and recognition of PAD will increase. The available treatment options, both conservative and invasive, will expand as well. Intensive efforts will be devoted to prevent the onset and halt the progression of vascular disease using powerful new lipid-lowering agents and aggressive risk factor modification. Similar resources will be used to prevent secondary recurrence after successful initial treatment. New innovative pharmaceutical agents currently under development may prove to be effective in treatment of intermittent claudication.

Invasive therapy for PAD will continue to shift toward a predominantly percutaneous, as opposed to surgical, approach. As interventions become more effective and safer, the threshold for treatment will be lowered and the number of percutaneous interventions will rise, probably dramatically. Restenosis, which remains the greatest enigma of percutaneous revascularization, will continue to complicate outcomes. However, the use of endovascular stents, which have already had a favorable impact on restenosis in coronary and iliac arteries, will be applied routinely to other vascular sites, including renal, carotid, vertebral mesenteric, aortic, and femoropopliteal vessels.

Meanwhile, additional promising strategies to reduce restenosis, including genetic and molecular manipulations and x-ray therapy, will be refined and will augment the beneficial impact of endovascular stents, further reducing the incidence of restenosis. The use of sophisticated imaging techniques, such as IVUS, MRA, and spinal computed tomography, will facilitate diagnosis and enhance the results of revascularization. These will also enable complex percutaneous procedures (e.g., exclusion of aneurysms by stent-grafting) to be performed with less risk and optimal results. Although novel treatment modalities will continue to be developed, third-party payors will require more rigorous documentation of outcomes using standardized measures that have not previously seen widespread application in PAD studies. There remains a concern that scrutiny by third-party payors and reduction in resources will stifle creative new research. As a consequence of the emphasis on risk factor modification, the aging of the population, and the shift toward catheter-based therapies, cardiologists will become increasingly involved with management of PAD. Finally, for patients who previously may have had to opt for amputation in the absence of viable options for conventional revascularization, the possibility of encouraging the formation of new vascular conduits by introducing angiogenic factors may offer these patients new hope for limb salvage. Indeed, if the angiogenesis trials and other molecular investigations currently under way produce favorable results, this could profoundly alter the way we approach both peripheral vascular and cardiovascular disease.

lar medicine. Formal or informal multidisciplinary vascular conferences provide an invaluable forum for exchange of knowledge and information, as well as an opportunity to develop management strategies for individual patients.

Regarding the performance of percutaneous interventions, such skills are not "specialty specific." Whoever has acquired a good fund of knowledge and has fulfilled the requirements set forth by their institution, requirements presumably that are based more or less on the published guidelines of American College of Cardiology/American Heart Association, should be capable of performing the procedures for which he or she is trained.

REFERENCES

1. Creager MA, Halperin JL, Coffman JD. Raynaud's phenomenon and other vascular disorders related to temperature. In: Loscalzo J, Creager MA, Dzau VJ, eds. *Vascular medicine: a textbook of vascular biology and diseases.* Boston: Little, Brown & Company, 1996:965–997.
2. Rutherford RB, Flanigan DP, Guptka SK. Suggested standards for reports dealing with lower extremity ischemia. *J Vasc Surg* 1986;4:80–94.
3. European Working Group on Critical Leg Ischemia. Second European consensus document on chronic critical leg ischemia. *Circulation* 1991;84[Suppl IV]:IV-1.
4. Creager MA. Can claudication be treated medically? *J Vasc Med Biol* 1989;1:269–271.
5. Money SR, Herd JA, Isaacsohn JL, et al. Effect of cilostazol on walking distances in patients with intermittent claudication caused by peripheral vascular disease. *J Vasc Surg* 1998;27:267–275.
6. Hiatt WR. Current and future drug therapies for claudication. *Vasc Med* 1997;2:257–262.
7. CAPRIE Steering Committee. A randomized, blinded trial of clopidogrel versus aspirin in patients at risk of ischemic events (CAPRIE). *Lancet* 1996;348:1329–1339.
8. Halperin JL, Creager MA. Arterial obstructive diseases of

the extremities. In: Loscalzo J, Creager MA, Dzau VJ, eds. *Vascular medicine: a textbook of vascular biology and diseases.* Boston: Little, Brown & Company, 1996:825–852.

9. Isner JM, Baumgartner I, Rauh G, et al. Treatment of thromboangiitis obliterans (Buerger's disease) by intramuscular gene transfer of vascular endothelial growth factor: preliminary clinical results. *J Vasc Surg* 1998;28:964–975.

10. Baumgartner I, Pieczek A, Manor O. Constitutive expression of phVEGF$_{165}$ following intramuscular gene transfer promotes collateral vessel development in patients with critical limb ischemia. *Circulation* 1998;97:1114–1123.

11. Wolff SM, Pariser KM. The clinical spectrum of vasculitis. In: Loscalzo J, Creager MA, Dzau VJ. *Vascular medicine: a textbook of biology and diseases.* Boston: Little, Brown & Company, 1996:999–1031.

12. Olin JW, Lie JT. Thromboangiitis obliterans (Buerger's disease). In: Loscalzo J, Creager MA, Dzau VJ. *Vascular medicine: a textbook of biology and diseases.* Boston: Little, Brown & Company, 1996:1033–1049.

13. Isner JM, Baumgartner I, Rauh G, et al. Treatment of thromboangiitis obliterans (Buerger's disease) by intramuscular gene transfer of vascular endothelial growth factor: preliminary clinical results. *J Vasc Surg* 1998;28:964–975.

14. Schafer AI. The hypercoagulable states. *Ann Intern Med* 1985;102:814–828.

15. Rutherford RB, Becker GJ. Standards for evaluating and reporting the results of surgical and percutaneous therapy for peripheral arterial disease. *Radiology* 1991;181:277–281.

16. Gruentzig AR. Transluminal dilatation of coronary artery stenosis (letter to editor). *Lancet* 1978;1:263.

17. Dotter CT, Judkins MP. Transluminal treatment of arteriosclerotic obstruction. Description of a new technic and a preliminary report of its application. *Circulation* 1964;30:654–670.

18. Dorros G, Jaff M, Jain A, et al. Follow-up of primary Palmaz-Schatz stent placement for atherosclerotic renal artery stenosis. *Am J Cardiol* 1995;75:1051–1055.

19. Isner JM, Rosenfield K. Redefining the treatment of peripheral artery disease. Role of percutaneous revascularization. *Circulation* 1993;88:1534–1557.

20. Long AL, Page PE, Raynaud AC, et al. Percutaneous iliac artery stent: angiographic long-term follow-up. *Radiology* 1991;180:771–778.

21. Richter GM, Roeren T, Brado M. Further update of the randomized trial: iliac stent placement versus PTA-morphology, clinical success rates, and failure analysis. *J Vasc Interv Radiol* 1993;4:30.

22. Isner JM, Pieczek A, Rosenfield K. Untreated gangrene in patients with peripheral artery disease. *Circulation* 1994;89:482–483.

23. Marcus ML, Skorton DJ, Johnson MR, et al. Visual estimates of percent diameter coronary stenosis: "a battered gold standard." *J Am Coll Cardiol* 1988;11:882–885.

24. Isner JM, Rosenfield K, Kelly K, et al. Percutaneous intravascular ultrasound examination as an adjunct to catheter-based interventions: preliminary experience in patients with peripheral vascular disease. *Radiology* 1990;175:61–70.

25. Rosenfield K, Isner JM. Intravascular ultrasound in patients undergoing coronary and peripheral arterial revascularization. In: Topol EJ, ed. *Textbook of interventional cardiology.* Philadelphia: WB Saunders, 1994:1153–1185.

26. Honye J, Mahon DJ, Nakamura S, et al. Enhanced diagnostic ability of intravascular ultrasound imaging compared with angiography (abstract). *Circulation* 1992;86:I-324–I-320.

27. Koelemay MJW, Lijmer JG, Stoker J, et al. Magnetic resonance angiography for the evaluation of lower extremity arterial disease: a meta-analysis. *JAMA* 2001;285:1338–1345.

28. Rosenfield K, Losordo DW, Ramaswamy K, et al. Qualitative assessment of peripheral vessels by intravascular ultrasound before and after interventions (abstract). *J Am Coll Cardiol* 1990;15:107A.

29. Nakamura S, Colombo A, Gaglione A, et al. Intracoronary ultrasound observations during stent implantation. *Circulation* 1994;89:2026–2034.

30. Dormandy JA, Rutherford RB. TASC Working Group: management of peripheral arterial disease. *J Vasc Surg* 2000;31:S1–S296.

31. O'Keeffe ST, Woods BO, Breslin DJ, Tsapatsaris NP. Blue toe syndrome: causes and management. *Arch Intern Med* 1992;152:2197–2202.

32. Lopez-Galarza LA, Ray LI, Rodriguez-Lopez J, Diethrich EB. Combined percutaneous transluminal angioplasty, iliac stent deployment, and femorofemoral bypass for bilateral aortoiliac occlusive disease. *J Am Coll Surg* 1997;184:249–258.

33. Schroder A, Muckner K, Riepe G, et al. Semiclosed iliac recanalisation by an inguinal approach—modified surgical techniques integrating interventional procedures. *Eur J Vasc Endovasc Surg* 1998;16:501–508.

34. Cooper CJ, Moore JA, Burket MW. Intraaortic balloon pump insertion after percutaneous revascularization in patients with aortoiliac stenosis. *Circulation* 1998;98:I-444.

35. Tadavarthy AK, Sullivan WA Jr, Nicoloff D, et al. Aorta balloon angioplasty: 9-year follow-up. *Radiology* 1989;170:1039–1041.

36. Audet P, Therasse E, Oliva VL, et al. Infrarenal aortic stenosis: long-term clinical and hemodynamic results of percutaneous transluminal angioplasty. *Radiology* 1998;209:357–363.

37. Johnston KW. Iliac arteries: reanalysis of results of balloon angioplasty. *Radiology* 1993;186:207–212.

38. Palmaz JC, Garcia O, Schatz RA, et al. Placement of balloon-expandable intraluminal stents in iliac arteries: first 171 procedures. *Radiology* 1990;174:969–975.

39. Martin EC, Katzen BT, Benenati JF, et al. Multicenter trial of the Wallstent in the iliac and femoral arteries. *J Vasc Interv Radiol* 1995;6:843–849.

40. Murphy TP, Webb MS, Lambiase RE, et al. Percutaneous revascularization of complex iliac artery stenoses and occlusions with use of Wallstents: three-year experience. *J Vasc Interv Radiol* 1996;7:21–27.

41. Onal B, Ilgit ET, Yucel C, et al. Primary stenting for complex atherosclerotic plaques in aortic and iliac stenoses. *Cardiovasc Intervent Radiol* 1998;21:386–392.

42. Laborde JC, Palmaz JL, Rivera FJ, et al. Influence of anatomic distribution of atherosclerosis on the outcome of revascularization with iliac stent placement. *J Vasc Intervent Radiol* 1995;6:513–521.

43. Sullivan TM, Childs MB, Bacharach JM, et al. Percutaneous transluminal angioplasty and primary stenting of the iliac arteries in 288 patients. *J Vasc Surg* 1997;25:829–838.

44. Treiman GS, Schneider PA, Lawrence PF, et al. Does stent placement improve the results of ineffective or complicated iliac artery angioplasty? *J Vasc Surg* 1998;28:104–112.

45. Tetteroo E, van Engelen AD, Spithoven JH, et al. Stent placement after iliac angioplasty: comparison of hemodynamic and angiographic criteria. Dutch Iliac Stent Trial Study Group. *Radiology* 1996;201:155–159.

46. Pieczek AM, Langevin RE Jr, Razvi S, Rosenfield K. Successful percutaneous revascularization of 180/190 (95%) consecutive peripheral arterial total occlusions using hydrophilic ("Glide") wire (abstract). *Circulation* 1992;86:I-704.

47. Ginsburg R, Thorpe P, Bowles CR, et al. Pull-through approach to percutaneous angioplasty of totally occluded common iliac arteries. *Radiology* 1989;172:111–113.

48. Ring E, Freiman D, McLean G, Schwartz W. Percutaneous recanalization of common iliac artery occlusions: an unacceptable complication rate? *AJR Am J Roentgenol* 1982;139:587–589.

49. The STILE Investigators. Results of a prospective randomized trial evaluating surgery versus thrombolysis for ischemia of the lower extremity. *Ann Surg* 1994;220:251–268.

50. Ouriel K, Veith FJ, Sasahara AA. A comparison of recombinant urokinase with vascular surgery as initial treatment for acute arterial occlusion of the legs. *N Engl J Med* 1998;338:1105–1111.

51. Working Party on Thrombolysis in the Management of Limb Ischemia. Thrombolysis in the management of lower limb peripheral arterial occlusion—a consensus document. *Am J Cardiol* 1998;81:207–218.

52. Blum U, Gabelmann A, Redecker M, et al. Percutaneous recanalization of iliac artery occlusions: results of a prospective study. *Radiology* 1993;189:536–540.

53. Henry M, Amor M, Ethevenot G, et al. Percutaneous endoluminal treatment of iliac occlusions: long-term follow-up in 105 patients. *J Endovasc Surg* 1998;5:228–235.

54. Tetteroo E, van der Graaf Y, Bosch JL, et al. Randomised comparison of primary stent placement versus primary angioplasty followed by selective stent placement in patients with iliac-artery occlusive disease. Dutch Iliac Stent Trial Study Group. *Lancet* 1998;351:1153–1159.

55. Bosch JL, Hunink MG. Meta-analysis of the results of percutaneous transluminal angioplasty and stent placement for aortoiliac occlusive disease. *Radiology* 1997;204:87–96.

56. Veith FJ, Gupta SK, Wengerter KR, et al. Changing arteriosclerotic disease patterns and management strategies in lower-limb-threatening ischemia. *Ann Surg* 1990;212:402–414.

57. Brewster DC, Cambria RP, Darling RC, et al. Long-term results of combined iliac balloon angioplasty and distal surgical revascularization. *Ann Surg* 1989;210:324–331.

58. Eagle KA, Coley CM, Newell JB, et al. Combining clinical and thallium data optimizes preoperative assessment of cardiac risk before major vascular surgery. *Ann Intern Med* 1989;110:859–866.

59. Blum U, Voshage G, Beyersdorf F, et al. Endoluminal stent-grafts for infrarenal abdominal aneurysms. *N Engl J Med* 1997;336:13–20.

60. Zarins CK, White RA, Schwarten D, et al. AneuRx stent graft versus open surgical repair of abdominal aortic aneurysms: multicenter prospective clinical trial. *J Vasc Surg* 1999;29:292–308.

61. D'Ayala, M, Hollier LH, Marin ML. Endovascular grafting for abdominal aortic aneurysms. *Cardiothorac Vasc Surg* 1998;78:491–500.

62. Perko MJ, Norgaard M, Herzog TM. Unoperated aortic aneurysms: a survey of 170 patients. *Ann Thorac Surg* 1995;59:1204–1209.

63. Ruebben A, Tettoni S, Muratore P, et al. Percutaneous endoluminal bypass of iliac aneurysms with a covered stent. *Cardiovasc Intervent Radiol* 1998;21:339–342.

64. Waibel PP, Wolf G. The collateral circulation in occlusions of the femoral artery. *Surgery* 1966;4:912–918.

65. Varty K, London NJM, Ratliff DA, et al. Percutaneous angioplasty of the profunda femoris artery: a safe and effective endovascular technique. *Eur J Vasc Surg* 1993;7:483–487.

66. Smith GD, Shipley MJ, Rose G. Intermittent claudication, heart disease risk factors, and mortality: the Whitehall Study. *Circulation* 1990;82:1925–1931.

67. Murray JG, Apthorp LA, Wilkins RA. Long-segment (>10 cm) femoropopliteal angioplasty: improved technical success and long-term patency. *Radiology* 1995;195:158–162.

68. Johnston KW. Femoral and popliteal arteries: reanalysis of results of balloon angioplasty. *Radiology* 1992;183:767–771.

69. Hunink MG, Donaldson MC, Meyerovitz MF, et al. Risks and benefits of femoropopliteal percutaneous balloon angioplasty. *J Vasc Surg* 1993;17:183–184.

70. Matsi PJ, Manninen JI, Vanninen RL, et al. Femoropopliteal angioplasty in patients with claudication: primary and secondary patency in 140 limbs with 1-2-year follow-up. *Radiology* 1994;191:727–733.

71. Capek P, McLean GK, Berkowitz HD. Femoropopliteal angioplasty. Factors influencing long-term success. *Circulation* 1991;83:I-70–I-80.

72. Pickering JG, Weir L, Jekanowski J, et al. Proliferative activity in peripheral and coronary atherosclerotic plaque among patients undergoing percutaneous revascularization. *J Clin Invest* 1993;91:1469–1480.

73. Simons M, Leclerc G, Safian RD, et al. Relation between activated smooth muscle cells in coronary artery lesions and restenosis after atherectomy. *N Engl J Med* 1993;328:608–613.

74. Dorros G, Lyer S, Lewin R, et al. Angiographic follow-up and clinical outcome of 126 patients after percutaneous directional atherectomy (Simpson AtheroCath) for occlusive peripheral vascular disease. *Cathet Cardiovasc Diagn* 1991;22:79–84.

75. Haji-Aghaii M, Fogarty TJ. Balloon angioplasty, stenting, and role of atherectomy. *Surg Clin North Am* 1998;78:593–616.

76. Vroegindeweij D, Tielbeek AV, Buth J, et al. Directional atherectomy versus balloon angioplasty in segmental femoropopliteal artery disease: two-year follow-up with color-flow duplex scanning. *J Vasc Surg* 1995;21:255–269.

77. Dorros G, Lyer S, Zaitoun R, et al. Acute angiographic and clinical outcome of high speed percutaneous rotational atherectomy (Rotablator). *Cathet Cardiovasc Diagn* 1991;22:157–166.

78. White CJ, Ramee SR, Escobar A, et al. High-speed rotational ablation (Rotablator) for unfavorable lesions in peripheral arteries. *Cathet Cardiovasc Diagn* 1993;30:115–119.

79. Sanborn TA, Cumerland DC, Greenfield AJ. Percutaneous laser thermal angioplasty: mitral results and 1-year follow-up in 129 femoropopliteal lesions. *Radiology* 1988;168:121–125.

80. White CJ, Ramee SR, Collins TJ, et al. Recanalization of arterial occlusions with a lensed fiber and a holmium:YAG laser. *Lasers Surg Med* 1991;11:250–256.

81. Isner JM, Donaldson RF, Deckelbaum LI, et al. The excimer laser: gross, light microscopic, and ultrastructural analysis of potential advantages for use in laser therapy of cardiovascular disease. *J Am Coll Cardiol* 1985;6:1102–1109.

82. Henry M, Amor M, Ethevenot G, et al. Palmaz stent placement in iliac and femoropopliteal arteries: primary and secondary patency in 310 patients with 2–4 year follow-up. *Radiology* 1995;197:167–174.

83. Cejna M, Illiasch H, Waldenberg P, et al. PTA vs Palmaz stent in femoropopliteal obstructions: a prospective randomised trial—long term results. *Radiology* 1998;209:492.

84. Damaraju S, Cuasay L, Le D, et al. Predictors of primary patency failure in Wallstent self-expanding endovascular prostheses for iliofemoral occlusive disease. *Tex Heart Inst J* 1997;24:173–178.

85. Sapoval MC, Long AL, Raynaud AC, et al. Femoropopliteal stent placement: long-term results. *Radiology* 1992;184:833–839.

86. Gray BH, Sullivan TM, Childs MB, et al. High incidence of restenosis/reocclusion of stents in the percutaneous treatment of long-segment superficial femoral artery disease after suboptimal angioplasty. *J Vasc Surg* 1997;25:74–83.

87. Strecker EP, Boos IB, Gottmann D. Femoropopliteal artery stent placement: evaluation of long-term success. *Radiology* 1997;205:375–383.

88. Rosenfield K, Schainfeld R, Pieczek A, et al. Restenosis of endovascular stents due to stent compression. *J Am Coll Cardiol* 1997;29:328–338.

89. Rosenfield K, Losordo DW, Ramaswamy K, et al. Three-dimensional reconstruction of intravascular ultrasound images recorded in 68 consecutive patients following percutaneous revascularization of totally occluded arteries: in vivo evidence that the neolumen frequently includes subintimal component (abstract). *Circulation* 1991;84:II-686.

90. Comerota AJ, Weaver FA, Graor RA, et al. Surgery versus thrombolysis for occluded lower extremity bypass grafts: results of a prospective randomized trial. *Ann Surg* 1994;220:251–268.

91. Ouriel K, Shortell CK, DeWeese JA, et al. A comparison of thrombolytic therapy with operative revascularization in the initial treatment of acute peripheral arterial ischemia. *J Vasc Surg* 1994;19:1021–1030.

92. Silva JA, Ramee SR, Collins TJ, et al. Rheolytic thrombectomy in the treatment of acute limb-threatening ischemia: immediate results and six-month follow-up of the multicenter Angiojet Registry. *Cathet Cardiovasc Diagn* 1998;45:386–393.

93. Mathie AG, Bell SD, Saibil EA. Mechanical thromboembolectomy in acute embolic peripheral arterial occlusions with use of the Angiojet rapid thrombectomy system. *J Vasc Interv Radiol* 1999;10:583–590.

94. Dolmatch B, Rholl KS, Moskowitz LB, et al. Blue toe syndrome: treatment with percutaneous atherectomy. *Radiology* 1989;172:799–804.

95. Brewer ML, Kinnison ML, Perler BA, White RI Jr. Blue toe syndrome: treatment with anticoagulants and delayed percutaneous transluminal angioplasty. *Radiology* 1988;166:31–36.

96. Kumpe DA, Zwerdinger S, Griffin K. Blue digit syndrome: treatment with percutaneous transluminal angioplasty. *Radiology* 1988;166:37–44.

97. Isner JM, Walsh K, Rosenfield K, et al. Arterial gene therapy for restenosis. *Hum Gene Ther* 1996;7:989–1011.

98. Isner JM, Asahara T. Angiogenesis and vasculogenesis as therapeutic strategies for postnatal neovascularization (perspective). *J Clin Invest* 1999;103:1231–1236.

99. Vale PR, Wuensch DI, Rauh GF, et al. Arterial gene therapy for inhibiting restenosis in patients with claudication undergoing superficial femoral artery angioplasty (abstract). *Circulation* 1998;17:I-66.

100. Waksman R. *Vascular brachytherapy*, 2nd ed. New York: Futura Publishing, 1998.

101. Bakal CW, Sprayregen S, Scheinbaum K, et al. Percutaneous transluminal angioplasty of the infrapopliteal arteries: results in 53 patients. *AJR Am J Roentgenol* 1990;154:171–174.

102. Dorros G, Jaff MR, Murphy KJ, Mathiak L. The acute outcome of tibioperoneal vessel angioplasty in 417 cases with claudication and critical limb ischemia. *Cathet Cardiovasc Diagn* 1998;45:251–256.

103. Hanna GP, Fujise K, Kjellgren O, et al. Infrapopliteal transcatheter interventions for limb salvage in diabetic patients: importance of aggressive interventional approach and role of transcutaneous oximetry. *J Am Coll Cardiol* 1997;30:664–669.

104. Parsons RE, Suggs WD, Lee JJ, et al. Percutaneous transluminal angioplasty for the treatment of limb threatening ischemia: do the results justify an attempt before bypass grafting? *J Vasc Surg* 1998;28:1066–1071.

105. Isner JM, Walsh K, Symes J, et al. Arterial gene transfer for therapeutic angiogenesis in patients with peripheral artery disease. *Hum Gene Ther* 1996;7:959–988.

106. Asahara T, Bauters C, Zheng LP, et al. Synergistic effect of vascular endothelial growth factor and basic fibroblast growth factor on angiogenesis in vivo. *Circulation* 1995;92:II-365–II-371.

107. Berkowitz HD, Fox AD, Deaton DH. Reversed vein graft stenosis: early diagnosis and management. *J Vasc Surg* 1992;15:130–142.

108. Hallet JW Jr, Brewster DC, Darling RC. The limitation of polytetrafluoroethylene in the reconstruction of femoropopliteal and tibial arteries. *Surg Gynecol Obstet* 1981;152:819–821.

109. Veith FJ, Gupta SK, Ascer E, et al. Six-year prospective multicenter randomized comparison of autologous saphenous vein and expanded polytetrafluoroethylene grafts in infrainguinal arterial reconstructions. *J Vasc Surg* 1986;3:104–114.

110. Perler BA, Osterman FA, Mitchell SE, et al. Balloon dilatation versus surgical revision of infra-inguinal autogenous vein graft stenoses: long-term follow-up. *J Cardiovasc Surg* 1990;31:656–661.

111. Whittemore AD, Donaldson MC, Polak JF, Mannick JA. Limitations of balloon angioplasty for vein graft stenosis. *J Vasc Surg* 1991;14:340–345.

112. Brewster DC, LaSalle AJ, Robison JG. Factors directing patency of femoropopliteal bypass grafts. *Surg Gynecol Obstet* 1983;157:437–442.

113. Whittemore AD, Clowes AW, Couch NP. Secondary femoropopliteal reconstruction. *Ann Surg* 1981;193:35–42.

114. Avino AJ, Bandyk DF, Gonsalves AJ, et al. Surgical and endovascular intervention for infrainguinal vein graft stenosis. *J Vasc Surg* 1999;29:60–71.

115. Porter DH, Rosen MP, Skillman JJ, et al. Mid-term and long-term results with directional atherectomy of vein graft stenosis. *J Vasc Surg* 1966;23:554–567.

116. Ozdil E, Krajcer Z, Angelini P. Percutaneous balloon angioplasty with adjunctive stent placement in the mesenteric vessels in a patient with Takayasu's arteritis. *Circulation* 1996;93:1940–1941.

117. Arend WP, Michel BA, Bloch DA, et al. The American College of Rheumatology 1990 criteria for the classification of Takayasu arteritis. *Arthritis Rheum* 1990;33:1129–1134.

118. Tanimoto A, Hiramatsu K. Percutaneous transluminal angioplasty for Takayasu's arteritis. *Semin Interv Radiol* 1993;10:1–7.

119. Millaire A, Trinca ZM, Marache P, et al. Subclavian angioplasty: immediate and late results in 50 patients. *Cathet Cardiovasc Diagn* 1993;29:8–17.

120. Henry M, Amor M, Henry I, et al. Percutaneous transluminal angioplasty of the subclavian arteries. *J Endovasc Surg* 1999;6:33–41.

121. Ansel GM, Barry SG, Yakubov JS. Primary stenting of symptomatic subclavian artery stenosis. *Circulation* 1996;94[Suppl I]:58.

122. Al-Mubarak N, Liu MW, Dean LS, et al. Immediate and late outcomes of subclavian artery stenting. *Catheter Cardiovasc Interv* 1999;46:169–172.

123. Sullivan TM, Gray BH, Bacharach M, et al. Angioplasty and primary stenting of the subclavian, innominate, and common carotid arteries in 83 patients. *J Vasc Surg* 1998;28:1059–1065.

124. Burke DR, Gordon RL, Mishkin JD, et al. Percutaneous transluminal angioplasty of subclavian arteries. *Radiology* 1987;164:699–704.

125. Hebrang A, Maskovic J, Tomac B. Percutaneous transluminal angioplasty of the subclavian arteries: long-term results in 52 patients. *AJR Am J Roentgenol* 1991;156:1091–1096.

126. Dorros G, Lewin RF, Jamnadas P, Mathiak LM. Peripheral transluminal angioplasty of the subclavian and innominate arteries utilizing the brachial approach: acute outcome and follow-up. *Cathet Cardiovasc Diagn* 1990;19:71–76.

127. Kumar K, Dorros G, Bates CM, et al. Primary stent deployment in occlusive subclavian artery disease. *Cathet Cardiovasc Diagn* 1995;34:281–285.

128. Hadjipetrou P, Cox S, Piemonte T, Eisenhauer A. Percutaneous revascularization of atherosclerotic obstruction of aortic arch vessels. *J Am Coll Cardiol* 1999;33:1238–1245.

129. Mufti SI, Young KR, Schulthesis T. Restenosis following subclavian artery angioplasty for treatment of coronary-subclavian steal syndrome: definitive treatment with Palmaz-stent placement. *Cathet Cardiovasc Diagn* 1994;33:172–174.

130. ACAS Study Group. Endarterectomy for asymptomatic carotid artery stenosis. *JAMA* 1995;273:1421–1428.

131. North American Symptomatic Carotid Endarterectomy Trial Collaborators. Beneficial effect of carotid endarterectomy in symptomatic patients with high-grade stenosis. *N Engl J Med* 1991;325:445–453.

132. Ohki T, Marin ML, Lyon RT, et al. Ex vivo human carotid artery bifurcation stenting: correlation of lesion characteristics with embolic potential. *J Vasc Surg* 1998;27:463–471.

133. Yadav JS, Roubin GS, King P, et al. Angioplasty and stenting for restenosis after carotid endarterectomy. *Stroke* 1996;27:2075–2079.

134. Hobson RW, Goldstein JE, Jamil Z. Carotid restenosis: operative and endovascular management. *J Vasc Surg* 1999;29:228–238.

135. Waigand J, Gross CM, Uhlich F, et al. Elective stenting of carotid artery stenosis in patients with severe coronary artery disease. *Eur Heart J* 1998;19:1365–1370.

136. Mathur A, Roubin GS, Gomez CR. Elective carotid artery stenting in the presence of contralateral occlusion. *Am J Cardiol* 1998;81:1315–1317.

137. Roubin GS, Yadav S, Iyer SS, Vitek J. Carotid stent-supported angioplasty: a neurovascular intervention to prevent stroke. *Am J Cardiol* 1996;78:8–12.

138. Iyer SS, Yadav S, Vitek J. Technical approaches to angioplasty and stenting of the extra-cranial carotid arteries (abstract). *Circulation* 1995;92:I-383.

139. Diethrich EB. Carotid angioplasty and stenting. Will they match the gold standard? *Tex Heart Inst J* 1998;25:1–9.

140. Satler LF, Hoffmann R, Lansky A, et al. Carotid stent-assisted angioplasty: preliminary technique, angiography, and intravascular ultrasound observations. *J Invasive Cardiol* 1996;8:23–30.

141. Yadav JS, Roubin GS, Iyer S, et al. Elective stenting of the extracranial carotid arteries. *Circulation* 1997;95:376–381.

142. Wholey MH, Wholey M, Bergeron P. Current global status of carotid artery stent placement. *Cathet Cardiovasc Diagn* 1998;44:1–6.

143. Henry M, Amor M, Masson I, et al. Angioplasty and stenting of the extracranial carotid arteries. *J Endovasc Surg* 1998;5:293–304.

144. Sivaguru A, Venables GS, Beard JD. European carotid angioplasty trial. *J Endovasc Surg* 1996;3:16–20.

145. Hobson RW. Status of carotid angioplasty and stenting trials. *J Vasc Surg* 1998;27:791.

146. Hobson RW, Brott T, Ferguson R. CREST: Carotid Revascularization Endarterectomy Versus Stent Trial. *Cardiovasc Surg* 1997;5:457–458.

147. Mathur A, Dorros G, Iyer SS, et al. Palmaz stent compression in patients following carotid artery stenting. *Cathet Cardiovasc Diagn* 1997;41:137–140.

148. Theron J. Protected carotid angioplasty and carotid stents. *J Mal Vasc* 1996;21:113–122.

149. Gruntzig A, Kuhlmann U, Lutolf U, et al. Treatment of renovascular hypertension with percutaneous transluminal dilation of a renal-artery stenosis. *Lancet* 1978;1:801–802.

150. Novick AC, Ziegelbaum M, Vidt DG, et al. Trends in surgical revascularization for renal artery disease: ten years' experience. *JAMA* 1987;257:498–501.

151. Klinge J, Mali WP, Puijlaert CB, et al. Percutaneous transluminal renal angioplasty: initial and long-term results. *Radiology* 1989;171:501–506.

152. Sos TA, Pickering TG, Phil D. Percutaneous transluminal renal angioplasty in renovascular hypertension due to atheroma or fibromuscular dysplasia. *N Engl J Med* 1983;309:274–279.

153. Tegtmeyer CJ, Dyer R, Teates CD, et al. Percutaneous transluminal dilatation of the renal arteries. *Radiology* 1980;135:589–599.

154. Cluzel P, Raynaud A, Beyssen B, et al. Stenoses of renal branch arteries in fibromuscular dysplasia: results of percutaneous transluminal angioplasty. *Radiology* 1994;193:227–232.

155. Rimmer JM, Gennari FJ. Atherosclerotic renovascular disease and progressive renal failure. *Ann Intern Med* 1993;118:712–719.

156. Libertino JA, Flam TA, Zinman LN, et al. Changing concepts in surgical management of renovascular hypertension. *Arch Intern Med* 1988;148:357–359.

157. Messina LM, Zelenock GB, Yao KA, Stanley JC. Renal revascularization for recurrent pulmonary edema in patients with poorly controlled hypertension and renal insufficiency. *J Vasc Surg* 1992;15:73–82.

158. Libertino JA, Bosco PJ, Ying CY, et al. Renal revascularization to preserve and restore renal function. *J Urol* 1992;147:1485–1487.

159. Hansen KJ, Starr SM, Sands E. Contemporary surgical management of renovascular disease. *J Vasc Surg* 1992;16:319–331.

160. Weibull H, Bergqvist D, Bergentz SE, et al. Percutaneous transluminal renal angioplasty versus surgical reconstruction of atherosclerotic renal artery stenosis: a prospective randomized study. *J Vasc Surg* 1993;18:841–852.

161. Sos TA. Angioplasty for the treatment of azotemia and renovascular hypertension in atherosclerotic renal artery disease. *Circulation* 1991;83[Suppl I]:I-162–I-166.

162. White CJ, Ramee SR, Collins TJ, et al. Guiding catheter-assisted renal artery angioplasty. *Cathet Cardiovasc Diagn* 1991;23:10–13.

163. Rosenfield K, Losordo DW, Harding M, et al. Intravascular ultrasound of renal arteries in patients undergoing percutaneous transluminal angioplasty: feasibility, safety, and initial findings, including 3-dimensional reconstruction of renal arteries (abstract). *J Am Coll Cardiol* 1991;17:204A.

164. Rees CR, Palmaz JC, Becker GJ, et al. Palmaz stent in atherosclerotic stenoses involving the ostia of the renal arteries: preliminary report of a multicenter study. *Radiology* 1991;181:507–514.

165. Dorros G, Prince C, Mathiak L. Stenting of a renal artery stenosis achieves better relief of the obstructive lesion than balloon angioplasty. *Cathet Cardiovasc Diagn* 1993;29:191–198.

166. Blum U, Krumme B, Flugel P, et al. Treatment of ostial renal artery stenoses with vascular endoprostheses after unsuccessful balloon angioplasty. *N Engl J Med* 1997;336:459–465.

167. Palmaz JC. The current status of vascular intervention in ischemic nephropathy. *J Vasc Interv Radiol* 1998;9:539–543.

168. Jamieson GG, Clarkson AR, Woodroff AJ, Faris I. Reconstructive renal vascular surgery for chronic renal failure. *Br J Surg* 1984;71:338–340.

169. Hansen KJ, Thomason RB, Craven TE, et al. Surgical management of dialysis-dependent ischemic nephropathy. *J Vasc Surg* 1995;21:197–211.

170. Rajachandran MS, Schainfeld R, Chaudhry GM, et al. Episodic pulmonary edema (CHF) in association with global renal ischemia from renal artery stenosis (RAS): successful treatment by renal artery stenting (PTRA). *J Am Coll Cardiol* 1997;29:486A.

171. Jaff MR, Olin JW. Atherosclerotic stenosis of the renal arteries. *Tex Heart Inst J* 1998;25:34–39.

172. Harden PN, Macleod MJ, Rodgers RS, et al. Effect of renal-artery stenting on progression of renovascular renal failure. *Lancet* 1997;349:1133–1136.

173. Shannon HM, Gillespie IM, Moss JG. Salvage of the solitary kidney by insertion of a renal artery stent. *AJR Am J Roentgenol* 1998;171:217–222.

174. Johnson KW, Lindsay TF, Walker PM. Early and late results and suggested surgical approach for chronic and acute mesenteric ischemia. *Surgery* 1995;118:1–7.

175. Cohn JM, Molavi B, Collar A. Stenting of a superior mesenteric artery lesion via the right arm approach. *J Invasive Cardiol* 1999;11:503–505.

176. Matsumoto AH, Angle JF, Tegtmeyer CJ. Mesenteric angioplasty and stenting for chronic mesenteric ischemia. In: Perler BA, Becker GI, eds. *Vascular intervention: a clinical approach*. New York: Thieme, 1998:545–556.

177. Khosla S, Zhang SY, Jenkins JS. Endovascular stent revascularization of mesenteric and celiac arteries for the management of chronic mesenteric ischemia. *Circulation* 1997;96:I-275.

178. Gaylord GM, Taber TE. Long-term hemodialysis access salvage: problems and challenges for nephrologists and interventional radiologists. *J Vasc Interv Radiol* 1993;4:103–107.

179. Kumpe DA, Cohen MA, Durham JD. Treatment of failing and failed hemodialysis access sites: comparison of surgical treatment with thrombolysis/angioplasty. *Semin Vasc Surg* 1992;5:118–127.

180. Turmel-Rodrigues L, Pengloan J, Blanchier D, et al. Insufficient dialysis shunts: improved long-term patency rates with close hemodynamic monitoring, repeated percutaneous balloon angioplasty, and stent placement. *Radiology* 1993;187:273–278.

181. Glantz S, Gordon DH, Lipkowitz GS, et al. Axillary and subclavian vein stenosis: percutaneous angioplasty. *Radiology* 1988;168:371–373.

182. Isner JM, Rosenfield K, Losordo DW, et al. Combination balloon-ultrasound imaging catheter for percutaneous transluminal angioplasty: validation of imaging, analysis

of recoil, and identification of plaque fracture. *Circulation* 1991;84:739–754.

183. Sullivan KL, Besarab A, Bonn J, et al. Hemodynamics of failing dialysis grafts. *Radiology* 1993;186:867–872.

184. Kumpe DA, Rutherford RB. Percutaneous transluminal angioplasty for lower extremity ischemia. In: Rutherford RB, ed. *Vascular surgery*, 3rd ed. Philadelphia: WB Saunders, 1992:759–761.

185. O'Keeffe ST, Woods BO, Beckmann CF. Percutaneous transluminal angioplasty of the peripheral arteries. In: Breslin DJ, ed. *Cardiology clinics. Peripheral vascular disease in the elderly.* Philadelphia: WB Saunders, 1991:519–521.

186. Gardiner GA Jr, Meyerovitz MF, Stokes KR, et al. Complications of transluminal angioplasty. *Radiology* 1986;159:201–208.

187. Trerotola SO, Kuhlman JE, Fishman EK. Bleeding complications of femoral catheterization: CT evaluation. *Radiology* 1990;174:37–40.

188. Orron DE, Kim DS. Percutaneous transluminal angioplasty. In: Kim DS, Orron DE, eds. *Peripheral vascular imaging and intervention.* Philadelphia: WB Saunders, 1990:393–408.

189. Kohler TR, Nance DR, Cramer MM, et al. Duplex scanning for diagnosis of aortoiliac and femoropopliteal disease: a prospective study. *Circulation* 1987;76:1074–1080.

190. Johnston KW, Hosang MY, Andrews DF. Reproducibility of noninvasive vascular laboratory measurements of the peripheral circulation. *J Vasc Surg* 1987;6:147–152.

191. Rosenfield K, Kelly SM, Fields CD, et al. Non-invasive assessment of peripheral vascular disease by color flow Doppler/two-dimensional ultrasound. *Am J Cardiol* 1989;64:247–251.

192. Teirstein PS, Hoover C, Ligon B, et al. Repeat restenosis: efficacy of the third and fourth coronary angioplasty (abstract). *J Am Coll Cardiol* 1987;9:63A.

193. Quigley PJ, Hlatky MA, Hinohara T, et al. Repeat percutaneous transluminal coronary angioplasty and predictors of recurrent restenosis. *J Am Coll Cardiol* 1989;63:409–413.

RENAL ARTERY DISEASE

JEFFREY W. OLIN
SUSAN M. BEGELMAN

OVERVIEW

Renal artery stenosis (RAS) is most commonly due to either fibromuscular dysplasia (FMD) or atherosclerosis. The former predominates in young women, whereas the latter is almost exclusively seen in individuals over the age of 55. Frequently, RAS is discovered incidentally during imaging studies for other reasons (atrophic or small kidney), or at autopsy. Incidental RAS is quite common (1,2), whereas renovascular hypertension occurs in only 1% to 5% of all patients with hypertension (3). The predominant

clinical manifestation of FMD is hypertension. The hypertension can frequently be cured or significantly improved with percutaneous transluminal angioplasty (PTA). The predominant clinical manifestations of atherosclerotic RAS include hypertension, renal failure (ischemic nephropathy), and recurrent episodes of congestive heart failure and flash pulmonary edema (4,5).

The presence of anatomic RAS does not necessarily establish that the hypertension or renal failure is caused by the RAS. Many patients have had essential (primary) hypertension for years and then develop atherosclerotic RAS later in life. In patients with long-standing hypertension, it is unlikely to achieve a cure of the hypertension with surgical or percutaneous intervention. However, 50% to 80% of patients do experience improvement in blood

---

J. W. Olin: The Heart and Vascular Institute, Morristown, New Jersey
S. M. Begelman: Department of Cardiovascular Medicine, Section of Vascular Medicine, The Cleveland Clinic Foundation, Cleveland, Ohio

pressure control (4,6–10). Ischemic nephropathy or flash pulmonary edema only occurs in the presence of bilateral renal artery disease or disease to a solitary functioning kidney. Percutaneous or surgical revascularization can lead to improvement or stabilization in renal function and improvement in congestive heart failure if the patients are selected carefully (8,11). Screening tests for RAS have improved considerably over the last decade. Although captopril renography was used almost exclusively in the past, duplex ultrasound of the renal arteries or magnetic resonance angiography (MRA) has replaced other modalities as the screening test of choice in many centers. Rarely does an arteriogram have to be performed for diagnostic purposes only.

Management of RAS consists of three possible strategies: medical management, surgical management, or percutaneous therapy with balloon angioplasty and stent implantation. The treatment of choice to control hypertension in patients with fibromuscular disease is percutaneous angioplasty. Renal artery stenting has replaced surgical revascularization for most patients with atherosclerotic disease who require an intervention.

PATHOPHYSIOLOGY

Experimental Models of Renovascular Hypertension

Pickering clarified the difference between renovascular hypertension and RAS: "The demonstration of a RAS in a hypertensive patient does not necessarily establish a diagnosis of renovascular hypertension, because essential hypertension may accelerate the development of atheromatous plaques, which do not necessarily have any functional significance. Ideally, it is necessary to demonstrate that there is also renal

ischemia, since this is thought to be the stimulus that raises the blood pressure, and leads to a decline of renal function" (19). Most investigators believe that there must be at least a 70% reduction in luminal diameter for a RAS to cause either hypertension or ischemic nephropathy (5,20,21).

Animal models for renovascular hypertension have helped to elucidate the pathophysiology of hypertension in patients with RAS (20,22–24). The renin-angiotensin-aldosterone system plays an important role, as shown in Figure 112.1 (10). In animals, the 2K-1C model is the classic model for renin-mediated hypertension and is analogous to unilateral RAS in humans. The one-kidney, one-clip model of renovascular hypertension is a model for volume-mediated hypertension and is analogous to bilateral RAS or RAS to a solitary functioning kidney in humans. Although the acute phases of both of these models are similar, different events occur in the chronic phase.

In the 2K-1C model (unilateral RAS), decreased renal blood flow stimulates the production of renin (Fig. 112.1A). Renin cleaves the proenzyme angiotensinogen to form angiotensin I and, in the presence of angiotensin-converting enzyme (ACE), is converted to angiotensin II. Angiotensin II has several important functions: (1) It elevates blood pressure directly by causing systemic vasoconstriction; (2) it stimulates aldosterone secretion, causing sodium reabsorption and potassium and hydrogen ion secretion in the cortical collecting duct; and (3) it changes the intrarenal hemodynamics, such as diminishing glomerular filtration, by decreasing glomerular capillary surface area and redistributing intrarenal blood flow. The salt and water retention (caused by excess aldosterone production) is rapidly excreted by the contralateral (normal) kidney by pressure natriuresis. This produces a cycle of renin-dependent hypertension (25–27). ▼ r53

In the one-kidney, one-clip model of renovascular hypertension, there is a similar decrease in blood flow to

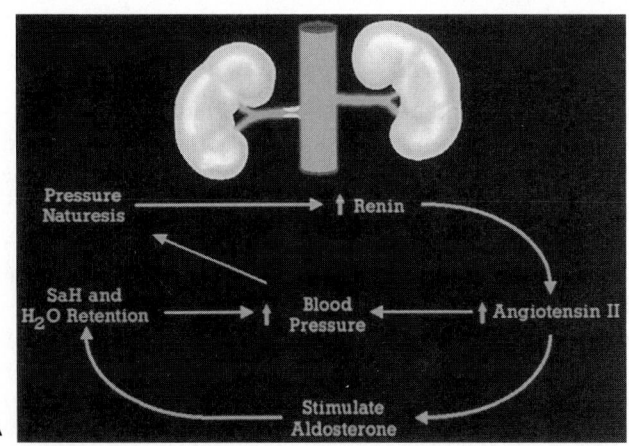

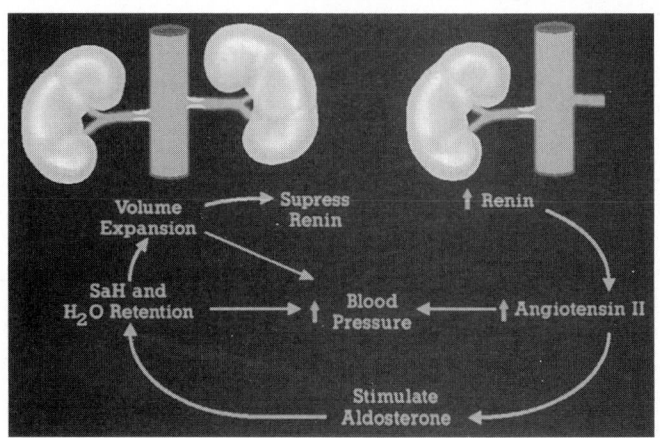

FIGURE 112.1 Pathogenesis of renovascular hypertension in unilateral **(A)** and bilateral **(B)** renal artery stenosis. (From Olin JW, Novick AC. Renovascular disease. In: Young JR, Olin JW, Bartholomew JR, eds. *Peripheral vascular diseases*, 2nd ed. St. Louis: Mosby, 1996:321–342, with permission.)

the affected kidney(s), acutely causing the secretion of renin and synthesis of angiotensin II and aldosterone (Fig. 112.1B) (10). Angiotensin II directly elevates blood pressure, and aldosterone causes salt and water retention. In this model there is not a normal kidney that can *sense* the elevated blood pressure; therefore, pressure natriuresis does not occur. The increased aldosterone causes sodium and water retention and volume expansion. The expanded plasma volume suppresses plasma renin activity, thus converting the animal from renin-mediated hypertension to volume-mediated hypertension (28,33). During this stage, administration of an ACE inhibitor or ARB does not decrease blood pressure or change renal blood flow (35). Dietary restriction of sodium or administration of diuretics returns the subject to a renin-mediated form of hypertension and restores sensitivity to an ACE inhibitor or ARB. Functional renal insufficiency may occur in humans when ACE inhibitors are administered to patients with bilateral RAS or RAS to a solitary kidney, especially in the volume-contracted state. ▼ r54

Pathophysiology of Ischemic Nephropathy

There are numerous reports suggesting that patients who develop azotemia while receiving ACE inhibitors have bilateral RAS, RAS to a solitary kidney, or decompensated congestive heart failure in the sodium-depleted state (44–49).

There are two mechanisms by which renal functional impairment may occur with the use of antihypertensive agents. The first may occur with any antihypertensive agent when a critical perfusion pressure is reached below which the kidney no longer receives adequate perfusion. This has been shown by the infusion of sodium nitroprusside in patients with high-grade bilateral RAS. When the critical perfusion pressure was reached, the urine output, renal blood flow, and glomerular filtration rate declined and later returned to normal when the blood pressure increased above this critical perfusion pressure (44). The exact pressure necessary to perfuse a kidney with RAS varies with the degree of stenosis and is different among different patients.

The second mechanism is confined to patients receiving ACE inhibitor or ARB agents and may occur despite no significant change in blood pressure (49). Patients with high-grade bilateral RAS or RAS to a solitary kidney may be highly dependent on angiotensin II for glomerular filtration. This is particularly common in patients who receive a combination of ACE inhibitor and diuretic (50) or in patients who are placed on a sodium-restricted diet (51). Under these circumstances, the constrictive effect of angiotensin II on the efferent arteriole allows for the maintenance of normal transglomerular capillary hydraulic pressure, thus allowing glomerular filtration to remain normal in the presence of markedly diminished blood flow (Fig. 112.2). In this instance, glomerular filtration is highly dependent on angiotensin II. When an ACE inhibitor is

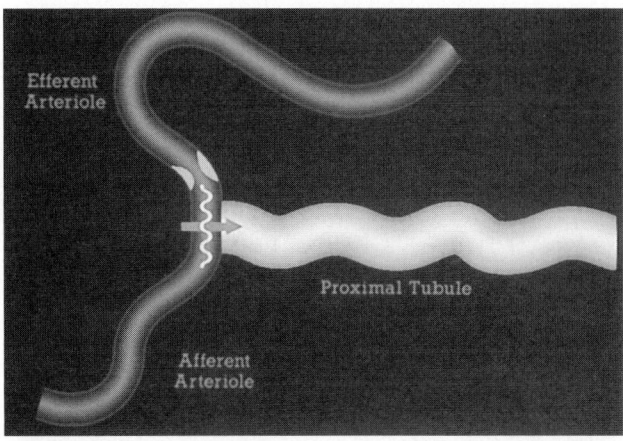

FIGURE 112.2 Patients with high-grade bilateral renal artery stenosis or renal artery stenosis to a solitary kidney may be highly dependent on the efferent arteriolar constriction caused by angiotensin II in preserving transglomerular capillary hydraulic pressure (*arrow*) and glomerular filtration rate. When an angiotensin-converting enzyme inhibitor is given, the efferent arteriole dilates, transglomerular capillary hydraulic pressure is not maintained, and blood is shunted from the afferent arteriole to the efferent arteriole, bypassing glomerular filtration.

administered, the efferent arteriolar tone is no longer maintained, and glomerular filtration is therefore decreased. A similar situation occurs in patients with decompensated congestive heart failure who are sodium depleted (47). Hricik and associates (51) demonstrated the important role that sodium balance plays in the azotemia associated with bilateral RAS or RAS to a solitary functioning kidney (*e*Table 112.0.1). When an ACE inhibitor alone was given, there was no change in renal function. However, if the patient was sodium depleted and then an ACE inhibitor was administered, the patient developed acute renal failure. This was rapidly reversed with the administration of intravenous fluids. ▼ r55

ANATOMIC CONSIDERATIONS

Atheromatous Lesions

Approximately 90% of all renovascular lesions are secondary to atherosclerosis (5). Although atherosclerotic RAS may occasionally be isolated to the renal artery alone, it is more commonly a manifestation of generalized atherosclerosis involving the aorta, coronary, cerebral, and peripheral vessels. Atherosclerotic RAS most often occurs at the ostium or the proximal 2 cm of the renal artery (Fig. 112.3). Distal arterial or branch involvement is distinctly uncommon (10).

Fibromuscular Dysplasia

FMD is a nonatherosclerotic, noninflammatory disease that most commonly affects the renal arteries and is the sec-

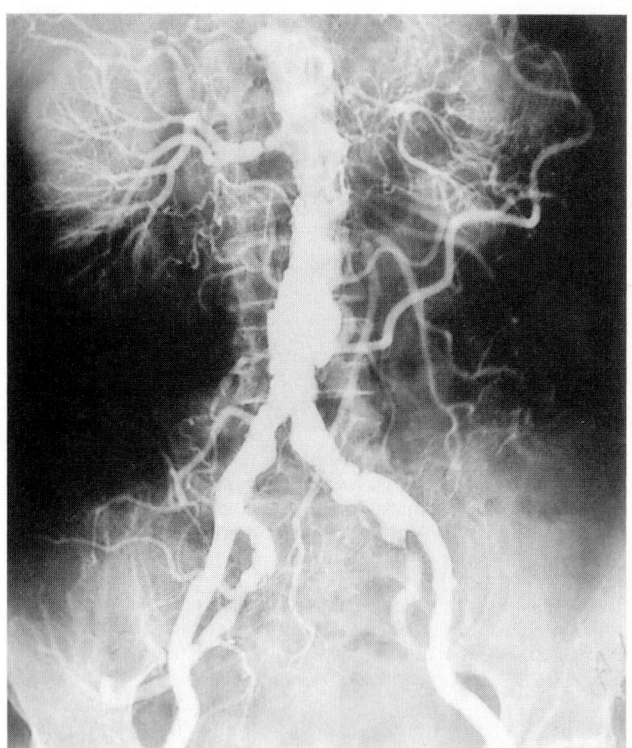

FIGURE 112.3 Aortogram showing severe proximal stenosis of the right renal artery. The left renal artery is occluded. Note the severe atherosclerosis in the aorta and iliac arteries. There is a large wandering artery of Drummond, indicating severe stenosis or occlusion of the superior mesenteric artery.

ond most common cause of RAS. The most common clinical presentation is that of hypertension in a young woman. FMD has been demonstrated in virtually every vascular bed. Renal artery involvement occurs in 60% to 75% of patients with FMD, followed by cervicocranial arteries in 25% to 30%, visceral arteries in 9%, and arteries of the extremities in approximately 5% of patients (68). It may present as a systemic disease (affecting a combination of the carotids, mesenteric, subclavian, and extremity vessels) in up to 28% of patients (69). The diagnosis is rarely made pathologically, but is usually determined by its typical angiographic appearance (Fig. 112.4). Although atherosclerosis involves the origin and proximal portion of the renal arteries, FMD characteristically involves the distal two-thirds of the artery and may involve the branches (70).

The lesions of FMD are thought to be congenital dysplasias with maldevelopment of the fibrous, muscular, and elastic tissues of the renal artery. They are subcategorized according to the layer of the arterial wall involved (71). This classification is important since each type of fibrous dysplasia has distinct histologic and angiographic features, and each type occurs in a different clinical setting (Table 112.1).

Medial FMD has been further divided into medial hyperplasia (the only type in which there is true smooth

muscle hyperplasia), perimedial dysplasia, and medial fibroplasia. Medial fibroplasia is the histologic finding in nearly 80% of all cases of FMD. It tends to occur in 25- to 50-year-old women and often involves both renal arteries. It has a "string of beads" appearance angiographically, with the "bead" diameter larger than the proximal, unaffected artery (Fig. 112.4). The areas of stenosis are often overshadowed by contrast medium in the microaneurysms, making the degree of actual stenosis difficult to assess. This beading is due to thickening of the media, interspersed by areas of aneurysmal dilatation. Microscopically, the internal elastic membrane is focally variably thinned and lost. Within the alternating thickened areas much of the muscle is replaced by collagen, hence the term *medial fibroplasia*. In other areas, thinning of the media occurs to the point of complete loss, and microaneurysms can be seen as saccules lined by only the external elastica. In extreme cases, giant aneurysms may be found in association with medial fibroplasia. Progression to total occlusion is rare in this subtype. Medial fibroplasia responds well to PTA. ❦ r56

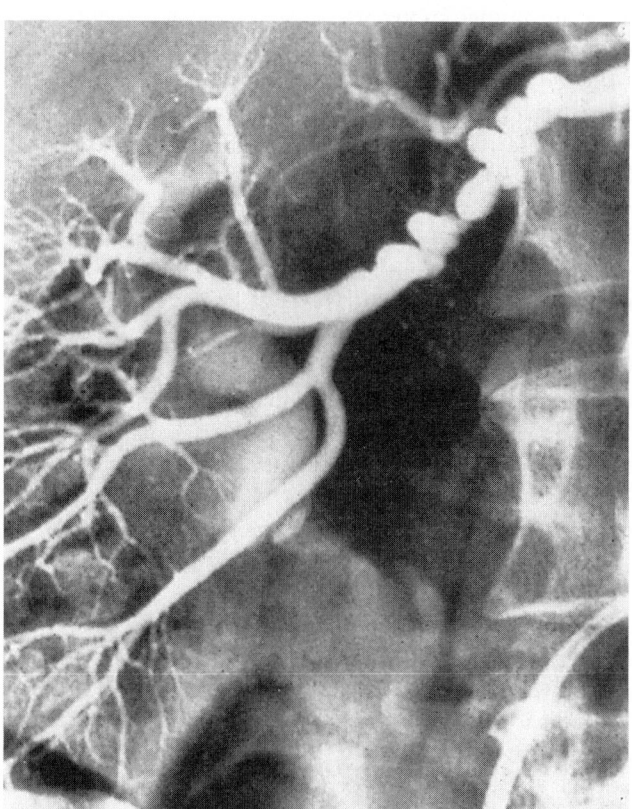

FIGURE 112.4 This renal arteriogram demonstrates typical medial fibroplasias of the renal artery. The "string of beads" appearance of the renal artery involves the distal portion of the main renal artery, and the "beads" are larger than the normal diameter of the artery. (From Olin JW, Novick AC. Renovascular disease. In: Young JR, Olin JW, Bartholomew JR, eds. *Peripheral vascular diseases,* 2nd ed. St. Louis: Mosby, 1996:321–342, with permission.)

TABLE 112.1 CLASSIFICATION OF FIBROMUSCULAR DYSPLASIA

Classification	Frequency	Pathology	Angiographic appearance
Medial dysplasia			
Medial fibroplasia	75–80%	Alternating areas of thinned media and thickened fibromuscular ridges containing collagen; internal elastic membrane may be lost in some areas.	"String of beads" appearance in which the diameter of the "beading" is larger than the diameter of the artery
Perimedial fibroplasia	10–15%	Extensive collagen deposition in the outer half of the media.	"Beading" in which the "beads" are smaller than the diameter of the artery
Medial hyperplasia	1–2%	True smooth muscle cell hyperplasia without fibrosis.	Concentric smooth stenosis (similar to intimal disease)
Intimal fibroplasia	<10%	Circumferential or eccentric deposition of collagen in the intima. No lipid or inflammatory component; internal elastic lamina fragmented or duplicated.	Concentric focal band; long smooth narrowing
Adventitial (periarterial) fibroplasia	<1%	Dense collagen replaces the fibrous tissue of the adventitia and may extend into surrounding tissue.	

From Begelman SM, Olin JW. Fibromuscular dysplasia. *Curr Opin Rheumatol* 2000;12:41–47, with permission.

CLINICAL ASPECTS OF RENAL ARTERY STENOSIS

Primary or essential hypertension is present in over 60 million Americans. Renovascular disease and renal parenchymal disease are the most common secondary causes of hypertension after obesity, excess alcohol ingestion, drug abuse, and oral contraceptives. Patients with atherosclerotic RAS have the usual risk factors for atherosclerosis. Past or present smoking is especially common in patients with renovascular disease (80,81). There is conflicting information on the prevalence of RAS in blacks. Although Keith et al. reported that renovascular disease was much more common in whites than it was in blacks (82), others (83) have shown that the prevalence of renovascular hypertension is similar in blacks and whites. Blacks with primary (essential) hypertension are more likely to have severe hypertension leading to vital organ damage [i.e., stroke, end-stage renal disease (ESRD)] than whites.

Although the effect of atherosclerosis on the coronary and carotid arteries is well recognized, involvement of the renal arteries is frequently overlooked. It is known that patients with atherosclerotic RAS succumb prematurely from myocardial infarction and stroke (8,84–86). Therefore, early diagnosis and treatment are of vital importance to avoid premature morbidity and mortality.

Natural History of Renal Artery Stenosis

Knowledge of the natural history of atherosclerotic renovascular disease is extremely important in the subsequent management of patients with RAS. Most natural history studies reported in the literature were retrospective studies. It is not only important to study anatomic end points (i.e., progression of stenosis), but also clinical end points (i.e., frequency of chronic renal failure and ESRD).

These clinical end points have been lacking in many reports.

Clinical End Points

Several studies have evaluated clinical end points (deterioration of renal function, loss of renal mass, survival) as they relate to patients with progressive RAS. Dean et al. (106) evaluated 41 patients with atherosclerotic renovascular disease and renovascular hypertension randomly selected for nonoperative management. Serial renal function studies were performed prospectively on these 41 patients with a mean follow-up of 28 months (range, 6 to 102 months). Nineteen of 41 patients (46%) experienced an increase in serum creatinine between 25% and 120%, and the glomerular filtration rates dropped 25% to 50% in 12 (29%) patients. Fourteen patients (37%) experienced a reduction in renal length of more than 10%. Although not a direct measure of renal function, loss of renal mass has been associated with a loss of renal function.

The effect of RAS on kidney size has been well studied (112,113). Using duplex ultrasound, Caps and colleagues (113) prospectively followed 204 kidneys in 122 patients with known RAS for a mean of 33 months. The 2-year cumulative incidence of renal atrophy was 5.5%, 11.7%, and 20.8% in kidneys with a baseline renal artery disease classification of normal, less than 60% stenosis, and greater than or equal to 60% stenosis ($p = .009$, log rank test).

However, a question that has really never been satisfactorily answered is how common is atherosclerotic RAS as a cause of ESRD? Scoble et al. (114) found that atherosclerotic renovascular disease was the cause of ESRD in 14% of patients starting dialysis therapy. Mailloux and colleagues (86) reviewed the causes of ESRD in 683 patients over a 20-year period. Eighty-three patients (12%) had documented RAS as a cause of ESRD. Because these investigators only performed arteriography in patients in whom they highly suspected RAS, it is entirely possible that the true incidence of RAS as a cause of ESRD was seriously underestimated. RAS should be searched for in every patient starting dialysis if a clear-cut etiology for the ESRD is not known.

Connolly et al. (84) showed that the 2-year actuarial *renal* survival (percent of patients remaining off dialysis) was 97.3% for patients with unilateral RAS, 82.4% in patients with bilateral RAS, and 44.7% in patients who have stenosis or occlusion to a solitary functioning kidney. Patients on dialysis have a shortened life expectancy. The average life expectancy in a patient with ESRD greater than age 65 is only 2.7 years (115,116). The survival estimates are even worse if the patient has atherosclerotic renovascular disease as the cause of ESRD. Mailloux and associates (86) have shown that median survival for patients with renovascular disease was 25 months compared with 55 months in patients with malignant hypertension and 133 months for patients with polycystic kidney disease. The 2-year survival on dialysis in patients with renovascular disease was 56%, 5-year survival 18%, and 10-year survival only 5%. These data underscore the fact that patients with atherosclerotic RAS who progress to ESRD and require dialysis have extremely high mortality.

In addition, the mere presence of RAS, even before developing ESRD, portends a poor prognosis. Patient survival decreases as the severity of RAS increases (117), with 2-year survival rates of 96% in patients with unilateral RAS, 74% in patients with bilateral RAS, and 47% in patients with stenosis or occlusion to a solitary functioning kidney. Dorros and associates (9) demonstrated that as the serum creatinine increases, the survival decreases in patients with atherosclerotic RAS. The 3-year probability of survival was 92 ± 4% for patients with a serum creatinine less than 1.4 mg per dL, 74 ± 8% for patients with a serum creatinine of 1.5 to 1.9 mg per dL, and 51 ± 8% for patients with a serum creatinine greater than or equal to 2.0 mg per dL.

Long-term survival was investigated at Duke University in a cohort of 1,235 patients who underwent abdominal aortography at the time of cardiac catheterization. The 4-year survival rate of subjects without RAS was 88% versus 67% for those with RAS (117).

Clinical Clues to the Diagnosis of Renal Artery Stenosis

A multicenter study was performed to determine a set of clinical characteristics that would identify individuals with a higher likelihood of having hypertension due to renal arterial disease (118). The clinical clues to suggest renal artery disease have changed considerably since that time (Table 112.2) (9).

TABLE 112.2   CLINICAL CLUES TO THE DIAGNOSIS OF RENAL ARTERY STENOSIS

Onset of hypertension after the age of 55
Exacerbation of previously well-controlled hypertension
Malignant hypertension
Resistant hypertension
Epigastric bruit (systolic/diastolic)
Unexplained azotemia
Azotemia while receiving angiotensin-converting enzyme inhibitors or angiotensin-receptor blocking agents
Atrophic kidney or discrepancy in size between the two kidneys
Recurrent congestive heart failure or "flash" pulmonary edema
Atherosclerosis elsewhere

Hypertension

- What was the age of onset?
- Has the hypertension suddenly become more difficult to control?
- Did the patient have malignant or accelerated hypertension?
- Does the patient have resistant hypertension?

Individuals who develop hypertension between the ages of 30 and 55 usually have primary (essential) hypertension. If the initial diagnosis of hypertension is made before the age of 30, it is usually due to FMD. Because atherosclerosis occurs in older individuals, it is usually the cause of RAS after the age of 55. It is not uncommon for patients to have years of primary hypertension and as they age, develop atherosclerotic RAS. This cohort of patients may have had well-controlled blood pressure that suddenly became more difficult to control. Accelerated or malignant hypertension has also been associated with a high prevalence of RAS. Davis and colleagues (103) demonstrated that renovascular hypertension was present in 32% of 76 white patients and 11% of 29 black patients studied with grade III or IV hypertensive retinopathy. *Resistant hypertension* is defined as failure to normalize blood pressure less than 140/90 mm Hg (119) after a good medical regimen consisting of at least three drugs with different mechanisms of action. The diagnosis of renovascular disease should be strongly considered in patients with resistant hypertension.

Physical Examination

- Does the patient have evidence of atherosclerosis elsewhere?
- Does the patient have an epigastric bruit?

In general, the physical examination is of limited help. Evidence of coronary, cerebral, or peripheral arterial disease is associated with a higher likelihood of renal artery disease due to the systemic nature of atherosclerosis. Although a systolic abdominal bruit is common and nonspecific, the presence of a systolic/diastolic bruit, especially over the epigastrium, may point to underlying renal artery disease (120). The presence of a diastolic component to the bruit indicates that the degree of narrowing of the artery is severe since there is continued flow during diastole (120). A systolic/diastolic bruit more often occurs in patients with fibromuscular disease (53%) than in patients who have atherosclerotic disease (12.5%) (121). Hunt et al. found a systolic/diastolic bruit in one-third of patients with atherosclerotic renovascular disease and in 75% of patients with fibromuscular disease (122). The presence of a bruit is helpful, but the absence does not exclude the diagnosis of either atherosclerotic renovascular disease or FMD.

Renal Function

- Are the kidneys of differing sizes?
- Has the patient ever developed azotemia associated with ACE inhibitors or angiotensin II receptor blocking agents?
- Does the patient have unexplained azotemia?
- Is the patient receiving dialysis without a clear cause for end-stage renal disease?

Gifford et al. (123) found that 71% of patients (53 of 75 patients) with an atrophic kidney had severe stenosis or complete occlusion of the renal artery ipsilateral to the small kidney. Three studies have shown that if there is a discrepancy in the size between the two kidneys or if one kidney is atrophic, there is a 60% chance that the contralateral renal artery (normal-sized kidney) is severely stenotic (10,124). Therefore, the presence of an atrophic kidney or a discrepancy in size between the two kidneys demands a thorough investigation for the presence of renovascular disease.

There are numerous reports suggesting that patients who develop azotemia while receiving ACE inhibitors have bilateral RAS, RAS to a solitary kidney, or decompensated congestive heart failure in the sodium-depleted state (44–48). The mechanisms have been discussed in detail earlier in this chapter.

Congestive Heart Failure and Pulmonary Edema

- Does the patient have unexplained congestive heart failure?
- Has the patient had recurrent episodes of "flash" pulmonary edema?

Recurrent congestive heart failure and flash pulmonary edema not related to ischemic heart disease can result from bilateral RAS (or unilateral RAS to a single functioning kidney). In our renal artery stent series, 39 patients (19% of all patients undergoing renal artery stent implantation from 1991 to 1997) had recurrent episodes of congestive heart failure or flash pulmonary edema as the primary indication for renal artery stenting (11). Although it is not completely understood, the mechanism of congestive heart failure may be related in part to the inability to use ACE inhibitors or ARBs, direct toxic effects of angiotensin II on myocardial function, or the inability to adequately control volume.

DIAGNOSIS OF RENOVASCULAR DISEASE

The ideal imaging procedure should (a) identify the main renal arteries as well as accessory or polar vessels; (b) localize the site of stenosis or disease; (c) provide evidence for the hemodynamic significance of the lesion; and (d) identify associated pathology (i.e., abdominal aortic aneurysm, renal mass, and so forth) that may have an effect on the treatment of the renal artery disease (124,125). The most sensitive and specific methods to identify RAS include the noninvasive imaging techniques such as duplex ultrasound, computed tomographic (CT) angiography, and MRA. Although intravenous digital subtraction angiography was used in the past, it no longer is used because of the large contrast loads required and poor image quality.

Arteriography

Angiography, the gold standard for arterial imaging, is rarely required to make the *diagnosis* of RAS. Usually one or more of the noninvasive modalities can accurately make the diagnosis. Exceptions to this general rule may occur in patients with FMD that primarily affects the branches of the renal arteries and patients with renal artery aneurysms. Angiography or intraarterial digital subtraction angiography has several distinct advantages as an imaging modality. All portions of the renal artery, including the intrarenal branches, can be well visualized. In addition, accessory renal arteries can be identified, and one can determine kidney size and gross function (the presence of a nephrogram). However, angiography is invasive and costly compared with other imaging modalities. Although not common, complications associated with angiography include access site complications such as a hematoma, pseudoaneurysm, arterial venous fistula, as well as acute renal failure from contrast-induced nephrotoxicity and atheromatous embolization to the kidneys, bowel, or lower extremities. Therefore, angiography is a poor *screening* test for RAS, but an excellent confirmatory test once it has been decided that revascularization (PTA, stent, surgery) is indicated.

It is important to recognize that the renal arteries often come off of the aorta posteriorly and, therefore, oblique views of the aorta may be needed to visualize the origins of the renal arteries well. Pressure gradients should also be obtained to confirm the physiologic significance of a given lesion. ♥ r57

Renal Arteriography at the Time of Cardiac Catheterization

Because RAS is so common in patients with coronary artery disease, some physicians recommend the routine performance of an aortogram on the "way out" after performing a cardiac catheterization (2,132). We are opposed to routine "drive-by angiography" at the time of cardiac catheterization. It adds additional time and contrast to the procedure. In addition, the quality of the images is often suboptimal. There may not be adequate views of the origin of the renal arteries, especially when they arise posteriorly from the aorta.

However, if the patient has a clear-cut indication for intervention (inability to control the blood pressure with a good antihypertensive regimen, jeopardy of renal function, or recurrent episodes of congestive heart failure), and the clinician is prepared to perform angioplasty and stenting should significant RAS be discovered, then an aortogram at the time of cardiac catheterization is not an unreasonable approach.

Knowing that the patient has RAS adds nothing to the patient's overall management other than to tempt the angiographer to stent this renal artery lesion in the absence of accepted clinical indications. This has been termed the *renal oculosten(t)otic reflex* (133).

Direct Screening Tests

Evaluation of the renal arteries is essential in acute or chronic renal failure, poorly controlled hypertension, or recurrent congestive heart failure that is not directly caused by myocardial ischemia (134). Imaging modalities are also useful to screen for restenosis after percutaneous or surgical revascularization of the renal arteries. Every patient who has undergone percutaneous intervention for RAS should be put in a surveillance program to detect restenosis. Technological advances in spiral CT angiography and MRA provide aortic and renal artery imaging that compares well with the quality and accuracy of angiography. In fact, MRA has virtually replaced diagnostic angiography for the evaluation of aortic and renal artery disease. Factors such as the patient's body habitus, the degree of renal impairment, and cost may help to determine which screening test is used. However, institutional experience and expertise are perhaps the most important factors determining which of the noninvasive imaging studies is used as a screening test for renovascular disease.

Duplex Ultrasonography

Duplex ultrasonography is an excellent test to detect RAS. It is the least expensive of the imaging modalities and pro-vides useful information about the degree of stenosis, the kidney size, and other associated disease processes, such as obstruction, and may even predict which patients can expect an improvement in blood pressure control or renal function after renal artery angioplasty and stenting (135). The location and degree of stenosis can accurately be determined by duplex ultrasound of the renal artery. Duplex ultrasound can be performed without altering the antihypertensive regimen and does not require contrast agents that may have an adverse effect on renal function. ♥ r58

A recent study used Doppler ultrasonography to predict the outcome of therapy in patients with RAS (136). One hundred thirty-eight patients with greater than 50% RAS underwent renal artery angioplasty or surgery for blood pressure control or preservation of renal function. A renal resistance index of at least 80 accurately identified patients in whom angioplasty or surgery was not associated with improved blood pressure, renal function, or kidney survival. Ninety-seven percent of patients with an increased renal resistance index demonstrated no improvement in blood pressure, and 80% had no improvement in renal function. The authors suggest that the increased resistive index identifies structural abnormalities in the small vessels of the kidney. Such small vessel disease has been seen with long-standing hypertension associated with nephrosclerosis or glomerulosclerosis (145). If this study is confirmed, it could provide a method for predicting which patients will improve after percutaneous intervention.

Renal artery duplex is an excellent test for the follow-up of RAS after percutaneous therapy or surgical bypass (*e*Fig. 112.4.4C) (7,146–148). Unlike MRA and CT angiography (which may be affected by artifact or scatter produced by the stent), ultrasound transmission through the stent is not a problem. Hudspeth et al. (147) compared angiography with duplex ultrasound for follow-up of RAS after angioplasty and demonstrated a sensitivity and specificity of 69% and 98%, respectively, for detecting stenosis greater than 60%. All patients who have undergone percutaneous intervention should be placed in a surveillance program in an attempt to identify restenosis and treat it before the artery occludes. After PTA and stent implantation, a renal artery duplex should be obtained at 6 months, 12 months, and yearly thereafter.

The sensitivity of identifying accessory renal arteries is approximately 67%. If there is a high index of suspicion for RAS and the duplex examination fails to reveal a significant stenosis, one may suspect an accessory vessel as the culprit.

Magnetic Resonance Angiography

Like CT angiography, MRA provides excellent imaging of the abdominal vasculature and associated anatomic structures (*e*Fig. 112.4.6). The examination does not require nephrotoxic contrast agents and therefore provides a good alternative to CT angiography in patients with renal insufficiency, congestive heart failure, or a contrast allergy. In general, the procedure is similar to CT angiography. The examination is performed with the patient supine. The patient must be able to cooperate and refrain from breathing during contrast-enhanced sequences or the quality of the study may be compromised.

Each examination should begin with acquisition of routine T1- and T2-weighted images to evaluate the kidneys, adrenal glands, and associated soft tissues. Time-of-flight and phase contrast are noncontrast techniques commonly used for vascular imaging. Software is available for both two-dimensional and three-dimensional imaging. The initial source images are completed in approximately 20 minutes. The reformatting process usually requires an additional 30 to 45 minutes. Maximum intensity projection and multiplanar reconstructions are the most commonly used postprocessing algorithms.

When compared with angiography, MRA has demonstrated a sensitivity of 90% to 100% and a specificity of 76% to 94% (155–159). However, MRA does not have the same sensitivity and specificity in patients with FMD.

Contrast-enhanced MRA provides a superior quality study when compared with noncontrast studies. Gadolinium chelate is the contrast agent of choice. Other contrast agents are under development and may improve the current imaging techniques. Unlike ionic and nonionic iodinated contrast agents, gadolinium is not nephrotoxic and can be used safely in patients with renal insufficiency. The imaging time is substantially shortened, and 20- to 40-second acquisition times are not uncommon. This eliminates some artifact created by gross patient movement (160). Signal strength is increased, providing for better visualization of distal small caliber vessels (161). Unlike flow-based techniques (time-of-flight, phase contrast), areas of slow flow or turbulence may be better visualized. The signal depends only on gadolinium concentration in the vessel. Thus, flow-related artifacts are almost entirely avoided. Thornton et al. (161) compared breath-hold MRA with conventional digital subtraction angiography in 42 patients. They demonstrated a sensitivity of 100% and a specificity of 98% for detecting greater than 50% stenosis. Overall MRA revealed 85 of 87 renal arteries, 20 of 20 stenoses, and 5 of 5 occlusions. The two arteries not identified were accessory vessels. Other studies have demonstrated a sensitivity and specificity between 91% and 100% and 79% and 98%, respectively (162,163,174). ✌ r59

PRINCIPLES OF MANAGEMENT

There has been a paradigm shift in management of atherosclerotic renal artery stenosis. Before 1990, if a patient met the criteria for intervention, surgical renal artery revascularization was almost always performed. However, since the introduction of stents, surgical revascularization is rarely performed solely for the treatment of renal artery disease. Despite advances in the technical aspects of angioplasty and stent implantation, there has been a paucity of controlled clinical trials assessing the role of renal artery angioplasty and stenting to control hypertension or preserve renal function. Because of a lack of controlled clinical trials, there remains some controversy as to the most appropriate treatment of atherosclerotic renal artery disease.

The four modalities currently available for the treatment of RAS are medical therapy, percutaneous balloon angioplasty, angioplasty with stent placement, and surgical revascularization. For the purpose of this discussion, *revascularization* is defined as restoration of blood flow to the kidney. This includes both percutaneous as well as surgical techniques. The etiology of the lesion, the patient's comorbidities, and the technical expertise of the treating physician must be taken into consideration when considering the type of treatment that will be employed.

The following items are the indications for revascularization:

- At least a 70% stenosis of one or both renal arteries *and*
- Inability to adequately control the blood pressure despite a good antihypertensive regimen *or*
- Chronic renal insufficiency not related to another clear-cut cause (disease should be bilateral or stenosis to a solitary functioning kidney). The treatment of an elevated serum creatinine with unilateral disease is controversial, and there are no good clinical trials to help guide the clinician (199).
- Dialysis-dependent renal failure in a patient without a definite cause of ESRD (200–202).
- Recurrent congestive heart failure or flash pulmonary edema not attributable to a cardiac cause (11,46,203).

In all patients, risk factor modification is important. Patients should be advised to stop smoking, lose weight, and exercise. Control of diabetes and appropriate management of hyperlipidemia are equally important. Because the majority of lesions is attributable to atherosclerosis or FMD, comments regarding therapy focus on these two diseases.

Medical Therapy

All patients with hypertension should be treated medically, even if they undergo intervention. Antiplatelet agents should be prescribed to help to lower the extremely high cardiovascular morbidity and mortality that occur in this patient population. Many patients have superimposed essential hypertension and will still require medications long term. Despite the etiology, the guidelines of the Sixth Joint National Committee on Prevention, Detection, Evaluation, and Treatment of High Blood Pressure should be followed (204). Patients with unilateral disease often have renin-mediated hypertension. They should be placed on an

ACE inhibitor or an ARB. Beta-blockers, which block renin secretion, and calcium channel blockers, which may counteract the direct effects of angiotensin II on the smooth muscle wall, are also first-line therapy. In individuals with bilateral disease or disease to a solitary functioning kidney, ACE inhibitors or ARBs should be used with caution, because this class of drugs can precipitate acute renal failure.

Patients with RAS who are treated solely with medical therapy should be carefully followed for progression of disease. This should include three important strategies:

- Follow the blood pressure closely and work to achieve a goal blood pressure within the guidelines of Sixth Joint National Committee.
- Follow the renal function every 3 months. If the serum creatinine begins to rise and there is no other explanation, consider revascularization.
- Place the patient into a surveillance program with serial duplex ultrasound imaging. The kidney size, volume, and severity of the stenosis can be closely followed. If the patient begins to lose volume to the affected kidney, consider revascularization.

Percutaneous Transluminal Angioplasty

PTA for RAS was first performed successfully by Gruntzig in 1978 (205). PTA has become widely used to treat individuals with renovascular disease. Technical success reflects the immediate outcome of the intervention (i.e., angiographic result and improvement in the pressure gradient), whereas long-term success is related to improvement in clinical parameters (i.e., blood pressure, renal function, and congestive heart failure).

PTA is the treatment of choice for FMD. Stenting is generally not indicated for patients with FMD because they respond so well to PTA alone. Sos et al. (206) performed PTA in 31 patients with FMD and demonstrated a technical success rate of 87.1%. Blood pressure was cured in 59.3% and improved in 33.3%. The cure or improvement in blood pressure was maintained in 93% of patients over an average follow-up of 16 months. Ramsay and Waller (207) reviewed ten published series of patients with FMD and reported that the hypertension was cured in 50% and improved in 42%. In a series of 85 lesions in 66 patients, PTA was technically successful in 100%. There was an 8% late recurrence rate at a mean of 15.7 months. Blood pressure was cured in 39% and improved in 59% of patients over a mean follow-up period of 39 months (208). Fourteen of these patients were treated for both hypertension and preservation of renal function. Before PTA, the mean serum creatinine was 2.4 mg per dL and after PTA the serum creatinine was 1.7 mg per dL (mean follow-up of 33 months). This represented an overall improvement of renal function in 86% of individuals.

Although the trend toward greater success for lesions due to FMD than atherosclerosis has been duplicated in many studies, the degree of overall cure has not been consistently demonstrated. A large retrospective series from the Mayo Clinic evaluated 105 patients with FMD who underwent PTA. While PTA resulted in blood pressure improvement in 85%, only 22% were classified as "cured" (mean follow-up of 42.7 months) (209). ⚐ r60

Comparison of Medical Therapy and Percutaneous Transluminal Angioplasty

There are three randomized prospective trials comparing medical management with angioplasty for blood pressure control in patients with atherosclerotic RAS. Each of the three studies has significant drawbacks precluding any definite conclusions. Plouin et al. (221) randomized 49 patients with unilateral RAS and found no significant difference in blood pressure control at 6 months (140/81 mm Hg in the PTA group vs. 141/84 mm Hg in the medical therapy–alone group). However, patients in the angioplasty group required less antihypertensive medication. In the medical group, 7 of 26 patients developed refractory hypertension and subsequently underwent PTA.

Webster et al. (222) randomized 55 of 135 eligible patients (44%) and followed them for 6 months. A significant fall in blood pressure from baseline occurred in the patients with bilateral RAS who were randomized to PTA (152/83 mm Hg in the PTA group vs. 171/91 mm Hg in the medical therapy group). This difference was not seen in patients with unilateral RAS.

The largest randomized, prospective study was published by van Jaarsveld et al. (223). One hundred six patients with angiographically documented RAS were randomly assigned to PTA or medical therapy and had blood pressure and renal function assessed at 3 and 12 months. Baseline blood pressure was 179/104 mm Hg and 180/103 mm Hg in the angioplasty and drug therapy groups, respectively. At 3 and 12 months, there was no significant difference in blood pressure control between the two groups, but the PTA group was on fewer antihypertensive medications. There were several rather serious problems with this study (224). Forty-four percent of patients randomized to medical therapy crossed over to the balloon angioplasty group, resulting in dilution of the long-term outcome differences. In spite of this, the initial angioplasty group required less antihypertensive therapy than the medical group ($p < .001$). There was a favorable trend to all primary outcome events, and with the small sample size we calculated that the chance of a type II error was substantial. Perhaps most importantly, the authors chose a 50% diameter reduction as the cut-off for "hemodynamically significant" renal artery lesions despite the fact that the evidence is clear that a lesion of at least 70% stenosis is required to cause significant hypertension or a decrement

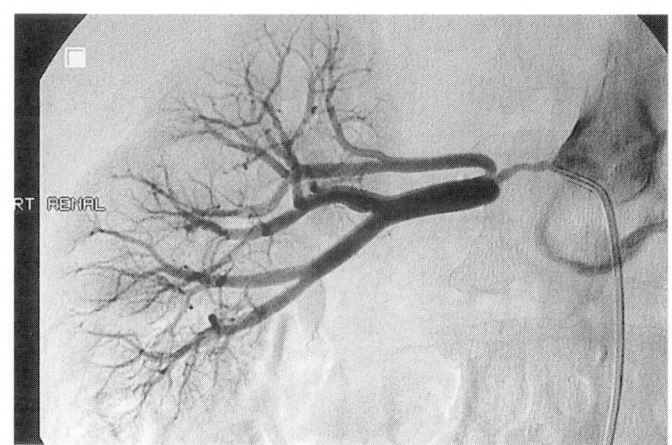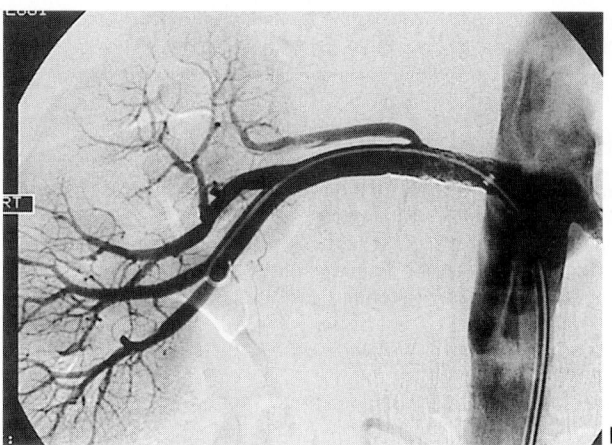

FIGURE 112.5   A: Severe stenosis to the right renal artery. **B:** Excellent angiographic result after stent placement.

in renal function (5). Only 57% of patients had stenosis of greater than 70%.

The primary problems with PTA alone are that a good technical result is virtually impossible with ostial lesions (221) and the restenosis rate is high (211,225).

Renal Artery Stents

Due to the high restenosis rate with angioplasty alone, endovascular stents offer a significant advantage over PTA in patients with atherosclerotic disease, especially those with ostial stenosis. The degree of stenosis poststenting approaches zero and most dissection flaps caused by PTA alone are successfully sealed with stents (Fig. 112.5). Despite the widespread use of stents in thousands of renal arteries since the late 1980s, there is still no U.S. Food and Drug Administration approval of these devices for the renal circulation.

There are a few important technical caveats when stenting the renal arteries:

- The shortest stent to adequately cover the lesion should be used.
- The stent must extend 1 to 2 mm into the aorta in patients with ostial disease.
- The stent must be fully expanded. A common problem encountered is to underdeploy the stent. It may be worthwhile to do the first 15 to 20 cases with intravascular ultrasound to be certain the stent is adequately expanded. It is also important to make sure that no postprocedure pressure gradient exists. ⚐ r61

Comparison of Percutaneous Transluminal Angioplasty and Endovascular Therapy with Stenting

The first randomized, prospective study comparing angioplasty alone with angioplasty and stenting was published (228): Eighty-five patients with ostial lesions were ran-

domized to receive PTA alone (42 patients, 51 arteries) or PTA and stent (42 patients, 52 arteries). Secondary stent implantation was allowed if the PTA failed immediately or during the first 6 months of therapy. The primary technical success rate (individual arteries) was 57% for PTA group and 88% for PTA with stent group. At 6 months, the primary patency was 29% for the PTA group and 75% for the stent group. Because this was an intention-to-treat analysis and 12 patients underwent stenting in the PTA group, there were no clinical differences between the two groups.

A publication of 163 patients (200 arteries) with atherosclerotic RAS evaluated the patency rates in patients undergoing PTA alone and those undergoing PTA and stent implantation. For ostial disease, the 12-month primary patency rate for PTA was 21 of 33 arteries (34%) and for PTA and stent was 4 of 21 arteries (80%) ($p = .002$) (229).

A metaanalysis of 14 studies compared the technical and clinical effect of renal artery PTA and stent implantation (Table 112.3) (7,8,228–239). The stent patients had a higher technical success rate and a lower restenosis rate when compared with patients only receiving PTA (98% vs. 77% and 17% vs. 26%; $p < .001$). The mean follow-up was 17 months for patients receiving a stent and 19 months for PTA patients. Complications of renal artery stent placement are shown in *e*Table 112.3.1. Hypertension was improved or cured in 69% of patients, and renal function improved or stabilized in 68% of patients. It should be noted that the complication rate varies considerably between centers, and high-volume centers generally can perform renal artery stenting with minimal morbidity and mortality. Although all studies reported use of an antithrombotic agent during the procedure and most patients were discharged on an antiplatelet agent, the regimens varied.

Two studies evaluated the effect that renal artery stent implantation had on preserving renal function (237,240). Both studies used the reciprocal of the serum creatinine to determine the rate of decline or improvement in renal func-

TABLE 112.3 CLINICAL AND ANGIOGRAPHIC FOLLOW-UP IN PATIENTS WHO UNDERWENT RENAL ARTERY STENT PLACEMENT

Study	No. of patients	Stent	Technical success (%)	Follow-up (mo)	Hypertension (%) Cure	Hypertension (%) Improved	Renal function (%) Improved	Renal function (%) Stable	Restenosis (%)	Complications
Wilms (231)	11	Wall-stent	83	7	30	40	0	0	29	3 (25%)
Kuhn (232)	10	Strecker	80	11	29	43	50	NM	25	4 (40%)
Rees (226)	28	Palmaz	96	7	11	54	36	36	39	5 (18%)
Hennequin (233)	21	Wall-stent	100	32	14	86	17	50	20	4 (19%)
van de Ven (228)	24	Palmaz	100	6	68	5	36	64	13	3 (11%)
Henry (234)	59	Palmaz	100	14	19	57	20	NM	9	2 (3%)
Iannone (235)	63	Palmaz	99	10	4	35	36	45	14	11 (13%)
Blum (7)	68	Palmaz	100	27	16	62	NM	NM	11	0 (0%)
Bosclair (236)	33	Palmaz	100	13	6	61	41	35	—	6 (17%)
Harden (237)	32	Palmaz	100	6	NM	NM	34	34	13	1 (3%)
White (227)	100	Palmaz	99	6	NM	NM	20	NM	19	2 (2%)
Rundback (238)	45	Palmaz	94	17	NM	NM	NM	NM	25	5 (9%)
Shannon (239)	21	Palmaz	100	9	NM	NM	43	29	0	2 (9%)
Dorros (8)	163	Palmaz	100	48	3	51	NM	NM	—	23 (11%)
Total	678	—	98[a]	16[a]	20[a]	49[a]	30	38	17	11[a]

NM, not mentioned.
[a]Mean based on random effects model.
From Leertouwer TC, Gussenhoven EJ, Bosch JL, et al. Stent placement for renal arterial stenosis: where do we stand? A meta-analysis. *Radiology* 2000;216:78–85, with permission.

tion. Harden et al. (237) placed renal artery stents in 32 patients (33 arteries) and reported that renal function improved or stabilized in 22 (69%) patients. In 25 patients with complete follow-up, Watson and associates (240) demonstrated that all exhibited a negative slope to the reciprocal of the serum creatinine. After stent placement, the slopes were positive in 18 patients and less negative in 7 patients.

Surgical Revascularization

Surgical revascularization has been used much less frequently than in the past. This is due in large part to the excellent technical results that can be achieved with angioplasty and stents. As previously noted, many patients can now undergo renal artery stent implantation as an outpatient procedure at a fraction of the cost of surgical revascularization.

Current indications for surgical revascularization include the following items:

■ Patients with branch disease from FMD that cannot be adequately treated with balloon angioplasty (241).
■ Patients with recurrent stenosis after stenting; however, this has been extremely rare in our experience (11).

■ Patients who require simultaneous aortic surgery (abdominal aortic aneurysm repair or symptomatic aortoiliac disease); even in this circumstance, it may be advisable to stent the renal artery first and then proceed with aortic reconstruction. The mortality of aortic replacement and renal artery revascularization is higher than either procedure alone (242). ▼ r62

Patient Selection for Intervention to Preserve Renal Function

One can often identify those patients in whom such disease poses a significant threat to overall renal function. Patients who are at a markedly increased risk are those with greater than 75% bilateral RAS or severe stenosis to a single functioning kidney. In this patient subgroup, the risk of total occlusion of the renal artery is significant, and if this occurs, the clinical outcome is a critical decrease in functioning renal mass with resulting renal failure (21,46,86,108,114,201,204).

The benefit of undertaking revascularization for preservation of renal function in patients with unilateral RAS and a normal contralateral renal artery is not established. If the contralateral kidney is anatomically and functionally normal, revascularization for this purpose is clearly not warranted. If the opposite kidney is functioning but involved with some type of parenchymal disorder, revascularization of the ischemic kidney may benefit some patients, but specific indications for this approach are not well defined.

Complete occlusion of the renal artery most often eventuates in irreversible ischemic damage of the involved kidney. However, in some patients with gradual arterial occlusion, the viability of the kidney can be maintained through the development of collateral arterial supply (262,263). There are certain clues that may help to predict renal salvageability in patients with an occluded renal artery:

- Angiographic demonstration of late filling of the distal renal arterial tree by collateral vessels on the side of total arterial occlusion (*e*Fig. 112.5.1) (264)
- Renal size of 8 to 9 cm
- Function of the involved kidney on a renal flow scan
- The presence of a nephrogram after a contrast arteriogram
- A renal biopsy showing well-preserved glomeruli and an absence of significant glomerulosclerosis

Revascularization to preserve renal function in patients with atherosclerotic RAS is most likely to be beneficial in patients with less severe renal impairment (serum creatinine less than 3.0 mg per dL) (265,266). When the serum creatinine is greater than 4.0 mg per dL, there is a greater chance that significant parenchymal renal disease exists along with main RAS. The most common underlying parenchymal renal disease in patients with RAS is severe nephrosclerosis or atheromatous embolization. ▼▼ r63

Revascularization for Control of Congestive Heart Failure or Flash Pulmonary Edema

There have been numerous reports demonstrating that surgical or endovascular revascularization is indicated for the treatment of congestive heart failure or flash pulmonary edema in some patients (11,41,42,201,205,270,271). This subgroup of patients most often has significant bilateral RAS or RAS to a single functioning kidney. The left ventricular systolic function may be normal or impaired (11). We reported 39 patients who underwent renal artery stent implantation for control of congestive heart failure (11). This represented 19% of our renal artery stent population. In this series, 18 (46%) patients had bilateral RAS and 21 (54%) patients had stenosis to a solitary functioning kidney. Renal artery stent implantation was technically successful in all 39 patients. The blood pressure was improved in 72% of patients. Renal function was improved in 51%, stable in 26%, and the renal function deteriorated in 23% of patients. The mean number of hospitalizations for congestive heart failure before stenting was 2.37 ± 1.42 (range,

1 to 6) and poststenting was 0.30 ± 0.65 (range, 0 to 3; p <.001). Seventy-seven percent of patients had no further hospitalizations after renal artery stenting over a mean follow-up period of 21.3 months. It was anecdotally noted that some patients were unable to be diuresed despite large doses of loop diuretics before stenting. Several patients began diuresing in the angiography suite immediately following stent placement.

The mechanism by which RAS causes congestive heart failure and pulmonary edema is not well defined. The improvement poststenting may in part be related to the ability to use ACE inhibitors, especially for those with impaired left ventricular function and the ability to better control volume.

CONTROVERSIES AND PERSONAL PERSPECTIVES

There have been many advances in the diagnosis of RAS in the last decade. In addition, catheter, balloon, and stent technology have revolutionized the treatment of renal artery disease. Whereas surgical revascularization was the treatment of choice a decade ago, endovascular stent implantation is now used to treat virtually all patients with RAS who require treatment. There is a large body of literature supporting the use of angioplasty and stent implantation for atherosclerotic RAS. However, there is a paucity of randomized prospective trials comparing renal artery stents with medical therapy and surgical revascularization. There will probably never be a randomized trial comparing stents with surgical bypass, because most clinicians now believe that that would not be ethical. Although there is compelling evidence to suggest that stent implantation can improve or at least stabilize renal function in many patients, there remain 15% to 20% of patients in whom renal function deteriorates after percutaneous intervention. Reasons for this deterioration include contrast injury, atheromatous embolization, or perhaps the renal failure was not caused by the RAS per se, but some other etiology (i.e., nephrosclerosis). It is often difficult to predict which patients will exhibit a decline in renal function after percutaneous intervention. The time has come for a prospective, controlled, randomized trial comparing renal artery stent implantation with medical therapy for preservation of renal function. This trial should randomize three distinct groups: bilateral RAS greater than 75%; RAS (greater than 75%) to a single functioning kidney; and unilateral RAS (greater than 75%) with an elevated serum creatinine level.

Just because the renal artery obstruction can be corrected safely does not mean that it should be corrected. Despite better balloons, catheters, and stents and better training in endovascular techniques, the temptation to dilate a RAS because it is there should be suppressed. Percutaneous renal intervention should be performed for one

THE FUTURE

Over the last decade, renal artery angioplasty and stenting have become much safer because of better equipment and more experienced operators. However, renal function does not improve or may even worsen in 15% to 20% of patients undergoing stent implantation, and blood pressure is not improved in 20% to 50% of patients after intervention. Two important advances will occur in the future: more accurate ways to predict response to therapy (i.e., identify the patient most likely to demonstrate improvement in blood pressure control and preservation of renal function), and protection of the kidneys during the procedure. The first will occur by measuring such parameters as the resistive index and functional flow reserve. The second will occur with emboli protection devices similar to those used in the carotid and coronary circulations.

of three indications: to better control the blood pressure in patients with suboptimal control despite a good antihypertensive regimen, preserve renal function, or treat congestive heart failure.

REFERENCES

1. Olin JW, Melia M, Young JR, et al. Prevalence of atherosclerotic renal artery stenosis in patients with atherosclerosis elsewhere. *Am J Med* 1990;88:46N–51N.
2. Harding MB, Smith LR, Himmelstein SI, et al. Renal artery stenosis: prevalence and associated risk factors in patients undergoing routine cardiac catheterization. *J Am Soc Nephrol* 1992;2:1608–1616.
3. Gifford RW Jr. Evaluation of the hypertensive patient with emphasis on detecting curable causes. *Milbank Mem Fund Q* 1969;47:170–186.
4. Novick AC, Scoble J, Hamilton G, eds. *Renal vascular disease.* London: WB Saunders, 1996.
5. Safian RD, Textor SC. Renal artery stenosis. *N Engl J Med* 2001;344:431–442.
6. Novick AC, Ziegelbaum M, Vidt DG, et al. Trends in surgical revascularization for renal artery disease. Ten years experience. *JAMA* 1987;257:498–501.
7. Blum U, Krumme B, Flugel P, et al. Treatment of ostial renal-artery stenosis with vascular endoprostheses after unsuccessful balloon angioplasty. *N Engl J Med* 1997;336:459–465.
8. Dorros G, Jaff M, Mathiak L, et al. Four-year follow-up of Palmaz-Schatz stent revascularization as treatment for atherosclerotic renal artery stenosis. *Circulation* 1998;98:642–647.
9. Rimmer J, Gennari FJ. Atherosclerotic renovascular disease and progressive renal failure. *Ann Intern Med* 1993;118:712–719.
10. Olin JW, Novick AC. Renovascular disease. In: Young JR, Olin JW, Bartholomew JR, eds. *Peripheral vascular diseases,* 2nd ed. St. Louis: Mosby, 1996:321–342.
11. Gray BH, Olin JW, Sullivan TM, et al. Clinical benefit of renal PTA/stent for CHF patients. *Circulation* 1998;98[Suppl]:I-485.
12. Goldblatt H, Lynch J, Hanzal RF, et al. Studies in experimental hypertension. I. The production of persistent elevation of systolic blood pressure by means of renal ischemia. *J Exp Med* 1934;59:347–379.
13. Houssay BA, Taquini AC. Accion vascoconstrictora de la sangre venosa del rinon isqeimiado. *Rev Soc Argent Biol* 1938;14:5–14.
14. Braun-Menendez E, Fasciolo JC. Mecansimo del accion hipertensora de la sangre venosa del rinon en isquemia incompleta aguda. *Rev Soc Argent Biol* 1939;15:401–411.
15. Braun-Menendez E, Fasciolo JC. Accion vascoconstrictora mecansimo e hipertensora de la sangre venosa del rinon en isquemia incompleta aguda. *Rev Soc Argent Biol* 1939;15:161–172.
16. Page IH, Helmer OM. Crystalline pressor substance (angiotonin) resulting from the reaction between renin and renin activator. *J Exp Med* 1940;71:29–42.
17. Skeggs LT, Marsh WH, Kahn JR, et al. The purification of hypertensin. I. *J Exp Med* 1954;100:363–370.
18. Elliott DF, Peart WS. Amino acid sequence in a hypertensin. *Nature* 1956;117:527–528.
19. Pickering TG, Topol EJ, Califf RM, eds. Renal artery disease. In: *Textbook of cardiovascular medicine.* Philadelphia: Lippincott-Raven, 1997:2623–2641.
20. Imanishi M, Akabane S, Takamiya M, et al. Critical degree of renal artery stenosis that causes hypertension in dogs. *Angiology* 1992;43:833–842.
21. Textor SC, Wilcox C. Ischemic nephropathy/azotemic renovascular disease. *Semin Nephrol* 2000;20:489–502.
22. Brunner HR, Kirshman JD, Sealey JE, et al. Hypertension of renal origin: evidence for two different mechanisms. *Science* 1971;174:1344–1346.
23. Gavras H, Brunner HR, Vaughan ED Jr, et al. Angiotensin-sodium interaction in blood pressure maintenance of renal hypertensive and normotensive rats. *Science* 1973;180:1369–1372.
24. Swales JD, Thurston H, Queiroz FP. Dual mechanism for experimental hypertension. *Lancet* 1971;2:1181–1183.
25. Gavras H, Brunner HR, Thurston H, et al. Reciprocation of renin dependency in renal hypertension. *Science* 1979;188:1316–1317.
26. Gross F. The renin-angiotensin system in hypertension. *Ann Intern Med* 1971;75:777–787.
27. Mohring J, Mohring B, Naumann H-J, et al. Salt and water balance and renin activity in renal hypertension of rats. *Am J Physiol* 1975;228:1847–1855.

28. Wilcox CS, Cardozo J, Welch WJ. AT1 receptors and TxA2/PGH2 receptors maintain hypertension throughout 2K, 1C Goldblatt hypertension in the rat. *Am J Physiol* 1996;271:R891–R896.

29. Bengis RG, Coleman TG. Antihypertensive effect of prolonged blockage of angiotensin formation in benign and malignant one- and two-kidney Goldblatt hypertensive rats. *Clin Sci* 1979;57:53–62.

30. Doyle AE, Duffy SG. Sodium balance and plasma renin activity during the development of two-kidney Goldblatt hypertension in rats. *Clin Exp Pharmacol Physiol* 1980;7: 293–304.

31. Phillips MI. Function of angiotensin in the central nervous system. *Annu Rev Physiol* 1987;49:413–435.

32. Harrison DG. Endothelial function and oxidant stress. *Clin Cardiol* 1997;20:II-11–II-17.

33. Vaughan ED Jr, Buhler FR, Laragh JH, et al. Renovascular hypertension; renin measurements to indicate hypersecretion and contralateral suppression, estimate renal plasma flow and score for surgical curability. *Am J Med* 1973;55: 402–414.

34. Dzau VJ, Siwek LG, Rosen S, et al. Sequential renal hemodynamics in experimental, benign and malignant hypertension. *Hypertension* 1981;3:[Suppl I]:63–68.

35. Rostand SG, Lewis D, Watkins JB, et al. Attenuated pressure natriuresis in hypertensive rats. *Kidney Int* 1982;21: 331–338.

36. Nakamoto H, Ferrario CM, Fuller SB, et al. Angiotensin-(1-7) and nitric oxide interaction in renovascular hypertension. *Hypertension* 1995;25:796–802.

37. Sigmon DH, Beierwlates WH. Endothelium-derived constricting factor in renovascular hypertension. *Hypertension* 1995;25:803–808.

38. Bianchi C, Bonadio M, Andriole VT. Influence of postural changes on the glomerular filtration rate in nephroptosis. *Nephron* 1976;16:161–172.

39. Pickering TG, Sos TA, James GD. Comparison of renal vein renin activity in hypertensive patients with stenosis of one or both renal arteries. *J Hypertens* 1985;3[Suppl 3]:S291–S293.

40. Vensel LA, Devereux RB, Pickering TG. Cardiac structure and function in renovascular hypertension produced by unilateral and bilateral renal artery stenosis. *Am J Cardiol* 1986;58:575–582.

41. Pickering TG, Herman L, Devereux RB, et al. Recurrent pulmonary edema as a manifestation of renovascular hypertension: treatment by angioplasty or surgical revascularization. *Lancet* 1988;II:551–552.

42. Bloch MJ, Trost DW, Pickering TG, et al. Prevention of recurrent pulmonary edema in patients with bilateral renovascular disease through renal artery stent placement. *Am J Hypertens* 1999;12:1–7.

43. Sutters M, Al-Kutoubi MA, Mathias CJ, et al. Diuresis and syncope after renal angioplasty in a patient with one functioning kidney. *BMJ* 1987;295:527–528.

44. Textor SC, Tarazi RC, Novick AC, et al. Regulation of renal hemodynamics and glomerular filtration rate in patients with renovascular hypertension during converting enzyme inhibition with captopril. *Am J Med* 1984;76:29–37.

45. Silas JH, Klenka Z, Solomon SA, et al. Captopril induced reversible renal failure: a marker for renal artery stenosis affecting a solitary kidney. *BMJ* 1983;286:1702–1703.

46. Jacobson HR. Ischemic renal disease: an overlooked clinical entity? *Kidney Int* 1988;34:729–743.

47. Packer M, Lee WH, Medina N, et al. Functional renal insufficiency during long-term therapy with captopril and enalapril in severe congestive heart failure. *Ann Intern Med* 1987;106:346–354.

48. Textor SC. Renal failure related to ACE inhibitors. *Semin Nephrol* 1997;17:67–76.

49. Textor SG. Pathophysiology of renal failure in renovascular disease. *Am J Kid Dis* 1994;24:642–645.

50. Watson ML, Bell GM, Muir AL, et al. Captopril/diuretic combinations in severe renovascular disease: a cautionary note. *Lancet* 1983;2:404–405.

51. Hricik D, Browning PJ, Kopelman R, et al. Captopril-induced functional renal insufficiency in patients with bilateral renal-artery stenosis or renal-artery stenosis to a solitary kidney. *N Engl J Med* 1983;308:373–376.

52. Grone H, Helmchen U. Impairment and recovery of the clipped kidney in two kidney, one clip hypertensive rats during and after anti-hypertensive therapy. *Lab Invest* 1986;54:645–655.

53. Jackson B, Franze L, Sumithran E, et al. Pharmacologic nephrectomy with chronic angiotensin converting enzyme inhibitor treatment in renovascular hypertension in the rat. *J Lab Clin Med* 1990;115:21–27.

54. Hricik DE, Dunn MJ. Angiotensin-converting enzyme inhibitor-induced renal failure: causes, consequences and diagnostic uses. *J Am Soc Nephrol* 1990;1:845–858.

55. Shanley PF. The pathology of chronic renal ischemia. *Semin Nephrol* 1996;16:21–32.

56. McManus JFA, Lupton CH. Ischemic obsolescence of renal glomeruli: the natural history of the lesions and their relation to hypertension. *Lab Invest* 1960;9:413–434.

57. Stoddard LD, Puchtler H. Human renal vascular lesions and hypertension. *Pathol Ann* 1996;4:253–268.

58. Vidt DG, Eisele G, Gephardt GN. Atheroembolic renal disease: association with renal artery stenosis. *Cleve Clin J Med* 1998;56:407–413.

59. Wilson C, Byrom FB. The vicious circle in Bright's disease. Experimental evidence from the hypertensive rat. *QJM* 1940;10:65–96.

60. Eng E, Veniant M, Floege J, et al. Renal proliferative and phenotypic changes in rats with two-kidney, one-clip Goldblatt hypertension. *Am J Hypertens* 1994;7:177–185.

61. Zimbler MS, Pickering TG, Sos TA, et al. Proteinuria in renovascular hypertension and the effects of renal angioplasty. *Am J Cardiol* 1987;59:406–408.

62. Ie EH, Karschner JK, Shapiro AP. Reversible nephrotic syndrome due to high renin state in renovascular hypertension. *Neth J Med* 1995;46:136–141.

63. Hariharan S, Pandey AP, Jacob CK, et al. Nephrotic-range proteinuria with renal artery stenosis: its reversal after transluminal angioplasty. *Nephron* 1987;47:77.

64. Chen R, Novick AC, Pohl M. Reversible renin mediated massive proteinuria successfully treated by nephrectomy. *J Urol* 1995;153:133–134.

65. Kumar A, Shapiro AP. Proteinuria and nephrotic syn-

drome induced by renin in patients with renal artery stenosis. *Arch Intern Med* 1980;140:1631–1634.

66. Thadhani R, Passcual M, Nickeleit V, et al. Preliminary description of focal segmental glomerulosclerosis in patients with renovascular disease. *Lancet* 1996;347:231–233.

67. Bartholomew JR, Olin JW. Atheromatous embolization. In: Young JR, Olin JW, Bartholomew JR, eds. *Peripheral vascular diseases*, 2nd ed. St. Louis: Mosby, 1996:261–270.

68. Gray BH, Young JR, Olin JW. Miscellaneous arterial diseases. In: Young JR, Olin JW, Bartholomew JR, eds. *Peripheral vascular diseases*, 2nd ed. St. Louis: Mosby, 1996:425–440.

69. Lüscher TF, Keller HM, Imhof HG, et al. Fibromuscular hyperplasia: extension of the disease and therapeutic outcome; results of the University Hospital Zurich Cooperative Study on Fibromuscular Hyperplasia. *Nephron* 1986;44[Suppl 1]:109–114.

70. Begelman S, Olin JW. Fibromuscular dysplasia. *Curr Opin Rheumatol* 2000;12:41–47.

71. Harrison EG, McCormack LJ. Pathologic classification of renal arterial disease in renovascular hypertension. *Mayo Clin Proc* 1971;46:161–167.

72. Stanley JC, Gewertz BL, Bove EL, et al. Arterial fibroplasia, histopathologic character and current etiologic concepts. *Arch Surg* 1975;110:561–566.

73. Stokes JB, Bonsib SM, McBride JW. Diffuse intimal fibromuscular dysplasia with multiorgan failure. *Arch Intern Med* 1996;156:2611–2614.

74. Halley SE, White WB, Ramsby GR, et al. Renovascular hypertension in Moyamoya syndrome. Therapeutic response to percutaneous transluminal angioplasty. *Am J Hypertens* 1988;1:348–352.

75. Shoskes DA, Novick AC. Surgical treatment of renovascular hypertension in Moyamoya disease: case report and review of the literature. *J Urol* 1995;153:450–452.

76. Yamada I, Himeno Y, Matsushima Y, et al. Renal artery lesions in patients with Moyamoya disease: angiographic findings. *Stroke* 2000;31:733–737.

77. Novick AC. Renal artery aneurysms and arteriovenous malformation. In: Novick AC, Straffon RA, eds. *Vascular problems in urologic surgery*. Philadelphia: WB Saunders, 1982:189–204.

78. Abud O, Chechile GE, Sole-Balcells F. Aneurysm and arteriovenous malformation. In: Novick AC, Scoble J, Hamilton G, eds. *Renal vascular disease*. London: WB Saunders, 1996:35–46.

79. Poutasse EF. Renal artery aneurysms. *J Urol* 1975;113:443–449.

80. Nicholson JP, Teichman SL, Alderman MH, et al. Cigarette smoking and renovascular hypertension. *Lancet* 1983;2:765–766.

81. Black HR, Cooper KA. Cigarette smoking and atherosclerotic renal artery stenosis. *J Clin Hyper* 1986;4:322–330.

82. Keith TA. Renovascular hypertension in black patients. *Hypertension* 1982;4:438–443.

83. Svetkey LP, Kadir S, Dunnick NR, et al. Similar prevalence of renovascular hypertension in selected blacks and whites. *Hypertension* 1991;17:678–683.

84. Connolly JO, Higgins RM, Walters HL, et al. Presentation, clinical features and outcome in different patterns of atherosclerotic renovascular disease. *QJM* 1994;87:413–421.

85. Mailloux LU, Bellucci AG, Mossey RT, et al. Predictors of survival in patients undergoing dialysis. *Am J Med* 1988;84:855–862.

86. Mailloux LU, Napolitano B, Bellucci AG, et al. Renal vascular disease causing end-stage renal disease, incidence, clinical correlates, and outcomes: a 20-year clinical experience. *Am J Kid Dis* 1994;24:622–629.

87. Dustan HP, Humphries AW, De Wolfe VG, et al. Normal arterial pressure in patients with renal arterial stenosis. *JAMA* 1964;187:1028–1029.

88. Holley KE, Hunt JC, Brown AL, et al. Renal artery stenosis: a clinical-pathological study in normotensive and hypertensive patients. *Am J Med* 1964;37:14–22.

89. Schwartz CJ, White TA. Stenosis of renal artery: an unselected necropsy study. *BMJ* 1964;2:1415–1421.

90. Uzu T, Inoue T, Fujii T, et al. Prevalence and predictors of renal artery stenosis in patients with myocardial infarction. *Am J Kidney Dis* 1997;29:733–738.

91. Wilms G, Marchal G. The angiographic incidence of renal artery stenosis in the arteriosclerotic population. *Eur J Radiol* 1990;10:195–197.

92. Choudrhi AH, Cleland JGF, Rowlands PC, et al. Unsuspected renal artery stenosis in peripheral vascular disease. *BMJ* 1990;301:1197–1198.

93. Swartbol P. Renal artery stenosis in patients with peripheral vascular disease and its correlation to hypertension. A retrospective study. *Int Angiol* 1992;11:195–199.

94. Missouris CG, Buckenham T, Cappucio FP, et al. Renal artery stenosis: a common and important problem in patients with peripheral vascular disease. *Am J Med* 1994;96:10–14.

95. Metcalfe W, Reid AW, Geddes CC. Prevalence of angiographic atherosclerotic renal artery disease and its relationship to the anatomical extent of peripheral vascular atherosclerosis. *Nephrol Dial Transplant* 1999;14:105–108.

96. Scoble JE. The epidemiology and clinical manifestations of atherosclerotic renal disease. In: Novick AC, Scoble J, Hamilton G, eds. *Renal vascular disease*. London: WB Saunders, 1996:303–314.

97. Gross CM, Kramer J, Waigand J, et al. Relation between arteriosclerosis in the coronary and renal arteries. *Am J Cardiol* 1997;80:1478–1481.

98. Jean WJ, Al-Bitar I, Zwicke D, et al. High incidence of renal artery stenosis in patients with coronary artery disease. *Cathet Cardiovasc Diagn* 1994;32:8–10.

99. Louie J, Issacson JA, Zierler RE, et al. Prevalence of carotid and lower extremity arterial disease in patients with renal artery stenosis. *Am J Hypertens* 1994;7:436–439.

100. Zierler RE, Bergelin RO, Polissar NL, et al. Carotid and lower extremity arterial disease in patients with renal artery atherosclerosis. *Arch Intern Med* 1998;158:761–767.

101. Rossi GP, Rossi A, Zanin L, et al. Excess prevalence of extracranial carotid artery lesions in renovascular hypertension. *Am J Hypertens* 1992;5:8–15.

102. Missouris CG, Papavassiliou MB, Khaw K, et al. High prevalence of carotid artery disease in patients with athero-

matous renal artery stenosis. *Nephrol Dial Transplant* 1998;13:945–948.

103. Davis BA, Crook JE, Vestal RE, et al. Prevalence of renovascular hypertension in patients with grade III or IV hypertensive retinopathy. *N Engl J Med* 1979;301:1273–1276.

104. Wollenweber J, Sheps SG, Davis GD. Clinical course of atherosclerotic renovascular disease. *Am J Cardiol* 1968; 21:60–71.

105. Meaney TF, Dustan HP, McCormack LJ. Natural history of renal arterial disease. *Radiology* 1968;91:881–887.

106. Dean RH, Kieffer RW, Smith BM, et al. Renovascular hypertension. *Arch Surg* 1981;116:1408–1415.

107. Schreiber MJ, Pohl MA, Novick AC. The natural history of atherosclerotic and fibrous renal artery disease. *Urol Clin North Am* 1984;11:383–392.

108. Tollefson DFJ, Ernst CB. Natural history of atherosclerotic renal artery stenosis associated with aortic disease. *J Vasc Surg* 1991;14:327–331.

109. Crowley JJ, Santos RM, Peter RH, et al. Progression of renal artery stenosis in patients undergoing cardiac catheterization. *Am Heart J* 1998;136:913–918.

110. Zierler RE, Bergelin RO, Isaacson JA, et al. Natural history of atherosclerotic renal artery stenosis: a prospective study with duplex ultrasonography. *J Vasc Surg* 1994;19:250–258.

111. Zierler RE, Bergelin RO, Davidson RC, et al. A prospective study of disease progression in patients with atherosclerotic renal artery stenosis. *Am J Hypertens* 1996;9:1055–1061.

112. Guzman RP, Zierler RE, Isaacson JA, et al. Renal atrophy and arterial stenosis: a prospective study with duplex ultrasound. *Hypertension* 1994;23:346–350.

113. Caps MT, Zierler RE, Polissar NL, et al. Risk of atrophy in kidneys with atherosclerotic renal artery stenosis. *Kidney Int* 1998;53:735–742.

114. Scoble JE, Maher ER, Hamilton G, et al. Atherosclerotic renovascular disease causing renal impairment—a case for treatment. *Clin Nephrol* 1989;31:119–122.

115. USRDS 1993 Annual Data Report. Bethesda, MD: The National Institutes of Health, National Institutes of Diabetes and Digestive Diseases, 1993.

116. Eggers PW, Connerton R, McMullan M. The Medicare experience with end stage renal disease: trends and incidence, prevalence and survival. *Health Care Finance Review* 1984;5:69–88.

117. Conlon PJ, O'Riordan E, Kalra P. New insights into the epidemiologic and clinical manifestations of atherosclerotic renovascular disease. *Am J Kid Dis* 2000;35:573–587.

118. Simon N, Franklin SS, Bleifer KH, et al. Clinical characteristics of renovascular hypertension. *JAMA* 1972;220:1209–1218.

119. The Sixth Report of the Joint National Committee on Prevention, Detection, Evaluation, and Treatment of High Blood Pressure. *Arch Intern Med* 1997;24:2413–2446.

120. Olin JW. Evaluation of the peripheral circulation. In: Izzo JL, Black HR, eds. *Hypertension primer*, 2nd ed. Dallas: American Heart Association, 1999:323–326.

121. Eipper DF, Gifford RW, Stewart B, et al. Abdominal bruits in renovascular hypertension. *Am J Cardiol* 1976; 37:48–52.

122. Hunt JC, Sheps SG, Harrison EG, et al. Renal and renovascular hypertension. A reasoned approach to diagnosis and management. *Arch Intern Med* 1974;133:988–999.

123. Gifford RW Jr, McCormack LJ, Poutasse EF. The atrophic kidney: its role in hypertension. *Mayo Clin Proc* 1965;40:834–852.

124. Carman T, Olin JW, Czum J. Noninvasive imaging of renal arteries. *Urol Clin North Am* 2000 (in press).

125. Prince MR. Renal MR angiography: a comprehensive approach. *J Magn Reson Imaging* 1998;8:511–516.

126. Schreier DZ, Weaver FA, Frankhouse J, et al. A prospective study of carbon dioxide-digital subtraction vs. standard contrast arteriography in the evaluation of the renal arteries. *Arch Surg* 1996;131:503–508.

127. Hawkins IF Jr, Wilcox CS, Kerns SR, et al. CO_2 digital angiography: a safer contrast agent for renal vascular imaging? *Am J Kid Dis* 1994;24:685–694.

128. Caridi JG, Hawkins IF Jr. CO_2 digital subtraction angiography: potential complications and their prevention. *J Vasc Interv Radiol* 1997;8:383–391.

129. Cardi JG, Stavropoulous SW, Hawkins IF Jr. CO_2 digital subtraction angiography for renal artery angioplasty in high-risk patients. *AJR Am J Roentgenol* 1999;173:1551–1556.

130. Caridi JG, Stavropoulos SW, Hawkins IF Jr. Carbon dioxide digital subtraction angiography for renal artery stent placement. *J Vasc Interv Radiol* 1999;10:635–640.

131. Spinosa DJ, Matsumoto AH, Angle JF, et al. Renal insufficiency: usefulness of gadolinamide-enhanced renal angiography to supplement CO_2-enhanced renal angiography for diagnosis and percutaneous treatment. *Radiology* 1999; 210:663–672.

132. Stack R. Renal artery stenosis—under-diagnosed and under-treated in the cardiac patient. *J Invasive Cardiol* 1999;11:103–106.

133. White CJ. The renal oculosten(t)otic reflex. *Cathet Cardiovasc Diagn* 1996;37:251.

134. Carman T, Olin JW. Diagnosis of renal artery stenosis: what is the optimal diagnostic test? *Curr Interv Cardiol Rep* 2000;2:111–118.

135. Radermacher J, Chavan A, Bleck J, et al. Use of Doppler ultrasonography to predict the outcome of therapy for renal artery stenosis. *N Engl J Med* 2001;344:410–417.

136. Olin JW. Role of duplex ultrasonography in screening for significant renal artery disease. *Urol Clin North Am* 1994;21:215–226.

137. Isaacson J, Neumyer MM. Direct and indirect renal arterial duplex and Doppler color flow evaluations. *J Vasc Technology* 1995;19:309–316.

138. Hanson KJ, Tribble RW, Reavis SW, et al. Renal duplex sonography: evaluation of clinical utility. *J Vasc Surg* 1990;12:227–236.

139. Hoffman U, Edwards JM, Carter S, et al. Role of duplex scanning for the detection of atherosclerotic renal artery disease. *Kidney Int* 1991;39:1232–1239.

140. Kohler TR, Zierler RE, Martin RL, et al. Noninvasive diagnosis of renal artery stenosis by ultrasonic duplex scanning. *J Vasc Surg* 1986;4:450–456.

141. Malatino LS, Polizzi G, Garozzo M, et al. Diagnosis of renovascular disease by extra- and intrarenal Doppler parameters. *Angiology* 1998;49:707–721.

142. Miralles M, Santiso A, Gimenez A, et al. Renal duplex scanning: correlation with angiography and isotopic renography. *Eur J Vasc Surg* 1993;7:188–194.

143. Olin JW, Piedmonte MR, Young JR, et al. The utility of duplex ultrasound scanning of the renal arteries for diagnosing significant renal artery stenosis. *Ann Intern Med* 1995;122:833–838.

144. Kim SH, Kim WH, Choi BI, et al. Duplex Doppler US in patients with medical renal disease: resistive index vs. serum creatinine level. *Clin Radiol* 1992;45:85–87.

145. Ruilope LM, Lahera V, Rodicio JL, et al. Are renal hemodynamics a key factor in the development of and maintenance of arterial hypertension in humans? *Hypertension* 1994;23:3–9.

146. Bakker J, Beutler JJ, Elgersma OEH, et al. Duplex ultrasonography in assessing restenosis of renal artery stents. *Cardiovasc Intervent Radiol* 1999;22:475–480.

147. Hudspeth DA, Hansen KJ, Reavis SW, et al. Renal duplex sonography after treatment of renovascular disease. *J Vasc Surg* 1993;18:381–390.

148. Taylor DC, Kettler MD, Moneta GL, et al. Duplex ultrasound scanning in the diagnosis of renal artery stenosis: a prospective evaluation. *J Vasc Surg* 1988;7:363–369.

149. Beregi JP, Elkohen M, Deklunder G, et al. Helical CT angiography compared with arteriography in the detection of renal artery stenosis. *AJR Am J Roentgenol* 1996;167:495–501.

150. Halpern EJ, Rutter CM, Gardiner Jr GA, et al. Comparison of Doppler US and CT angiography for evaluation of renal artery stenosis. *Acad Radiol* 1998;5:524–532.

151. Johnson PT, Halpern EJ, Kuszyk BS, et al. Renal artery stenosis: CT angiography—comparison of real-time volume-rendering and maximum intensity projection algorithms. *Radiology* 1999;211:337–343.

152. Kim TS, Chung JW, Park JH, et al. Renal artery evaluation: comparison of spiral CT angiography to intra-arterial DSA. *J Vasc Interv Radiol* 1998;9:553–559.

153. Rubin GD, Dake MD, Napel S, et al. Spiral CT of renal artery stenosis: comparison of three-dimensional rendering techniques. *Radiology* 1994;190:181–189.

154. Kawashima A, Sandler CM, Ernst RD, et al. CT evaluation of renovascular disease. *RadioGraphics* 2000;20:1321–1340.

155. Hertz SM, Holland GA, Baum RA, et al. Evaluation of renal artery stenosis by magnetic resonance angiography. *Am J Surg* 1994;168:140–143.

156. Kent KC, Edelman RR, Kim D, et al. Magnetic resonance imaging: a reliable test for the evaluation of proximal atherosclerotic renal artery stenosis. *J Vasc Surg* 1991;13:311–318.

157. Leung DA, Hoffman U, Pfammatter T, et al. Magnetic resonance angiography versus duplex sonography for diagnosing renovascular disease. *Hypertension* 1999;33:726–731.

158. Loubeyre P, Revel D, Garcia P, et al. Screening patients for renal artery stenosis: value of three-dimensional time-of-flight MR angiography. *AJR Am J Roentgenol* 1994;162:847–852.

159. Loubeyre P, Trolliet P, Cahen R, et al. MR angiography of renal artery stenosis: value of the combination of three-dimensional time-of flight and three-dimensional phase-contrast MR angiography sequences. *AJR Am J Roentgenol* 1996;167:489–494.

160. Saloner D. Determinants of image appearance in contrast-enhanced magnetic resonance angiography: a review. *Invest Radiol* 1998;33:488–495.

161. Thornton MJ, Thornton F, O'Callaghan J, et al. Evaluation of dynamic gadolinium-enhanced breath-hold MR angiography in the diagnosis of renal artery stenosis. *AJR Am J Roentgenol* 1999;173:1279–1283.

162. De Cobelli F, Venturini M, Vanzulli A, et al. Renal artery stenosis: prospective comparison of color Doppler US and breath-hold, three-dimensional, dynamic, gadolinium-enhanced MR angiography. *Radiology* 2000;214:373–380.

163. Hahn U, Miller S, Nägele T, et al. Renal MR angiography at 1.0T: three-dimensional (3D) phase-contrast techniques versus gadolinium-enhanced 3D fast low-angle shot breath-hold imaging. *AJR Am J Roentgenol* 1999;172:1501–1508.

164. Maxwell MH, Gonick, HC, Wiita R, et al. Use of the rapid sequence intravenous pyelogram: the diagnosis of renovascular hypertension. *N Engl J Med* 1964;270:213–220.

165. Bookstein JJ, Abrams HL, Buenger RE, et al. Radiologic aspects of renovascular hypertension. II. The role of urography and unilateral renovascular disease: cooperative study of renovascular hypertension. *JAMA* 1972;220:1225–1230.

166. Kaufman JJ. Renovascular hypertension: the UCLA experience. *J Urol* 1979;121:139–144.

167. Thornbury JR, Stanley JC, Fryback DG. Hypertensive urogram: a nondiscriminatory test for renovascular hypertension. *AJR Am J Roentgenol* 1982;138:43–49.

168. Maxwell MH, Rudnick M, Waks AU. New approaches to the diagnosis of renovascular hypertension. *Adv Nephrol* 1985;14:285–304.

169. Müller FB, Sealey JE, Case CB, et al. The captopril test for identifying renovascular disease in hypertensive patients. *Am J Med* 1986;80:633–644.

170. Blaufox MD, Middleton ML, Bongiovanni J, et al. Cost efficacy of the diagnosis and therapy of renovascular hypertension. *J Nucl Med* 1996;37:171–177.

171. Emovon OE, Klotman PE, Dunnick NR, et al. Renovascular hypertension in blacks. *Am J Hypertens* 1995;9:18–23.

172. Wilcox CS, Williams CM, Smith TB, et al. Diagnostic uses of angiotensin-converting enzyme inhibitors in renovascular hypertension. *Am J Hypertens* 1988;1:344S–349S.

173. Hughes JS, Dove HG, Gifford RW Jr, et al. Duration of blood pressure elevation in acutely predicting surgical cure of renovascular hypertension. *Am Heart J* 1981;101:408–413.

174. Vaughan ED Jr, Bühler FR, Laragh JH, et al. Renovascular hypertension: renin measurements to indicate hypersecretion and contralateral suppression, estimate renal plasma flow, and score for surgical curability. *Am J Med* 1973;55:402–414.

175. Pickering TG, Sos TA, James GD, et al. Comparison of renal vein renin activity in hypertensive patients with

stenosis of one or both renal arteries. *J Hypertens* 1985; 3[Suppl 3]:S291–S293.

176. Maxwell MH, Marks LS, Lupu AN, et al. Predictive value of renin determinations in renal artery stenosis. *JAMA* 1977;238:2617–2620.

177. Marks LS, Maxwell MH, Varady PD, et al. Renovascular hypertension: does the renal vein renin ratio predict operative results? *J Urol* 1976;115:365–368.

178. Novick AC, Straffon RA, Stewart BH, et al. Diminished operative morbidity and mortality in renal revascularization. *JAMA* 1981;246:749–753.

179. Olin JW, Vidt DG, Gifford RW Jr, et al. Renovascular disease in the elderly: an analysis of 50 patients. *J Am Coll Cardiol* 1985;5:1232–1238.

180. Maxwell MH, Lupu AN, Taplin GV. Radioisotope renogram in renal arterial hypertension. *J Urol* 1968;100:376–383.

181. Nally JV, Clarke HS Jr, Grecos GP, et al. Effect of captopril on ^{99m}Tc-diethylenetriaminepentaacetic acid renograms in two-kidney, one clip hypertension. *Hypertension* 1986;8:685–693.

182. Ploth DW. Angiotensin-dependent renal mechanisms in two-kidney, one-clip renal vascular hypertension. *Am J Physiol* 1983;245:F131–F141.

183. Nally JV, Barton DP. Contemporary approach to the diagnosis and evaluation of renovascular hypertension. *Urol Clin N Am*, 2001 (in press).

184. Black HR, Bourgoignie JJ, Pickering T, et al. Report of the working party group for patient selection and preparation. *Am J Hypertens* 1991;4:745S–746S.

185. Setaro JF, Saddler MC, Chen CC, et al. Simplified captopril renography in diagnosis and treatment of renal artery stenosis. *Hypertension* 1991;18:289–298.

186. Derkx FHM, Tan-Tjiong HL, Wenting GJ, et al. Captopril test for the diagnosis of renal artery stenosis. In: Glorioso N, Laragh JH, Rapelli A, eds. *Renovascular hypertension.* New York: Raven Press, 1987:295–305.

187. Prigent A, Cosgriff P, Gates GF, et al. Consensus report on quality control of quantitative measurements of renal function obtained from the renogram: International Consensus Committee from the Scientific Committee of Radionuclides in Nephrourology. *Semin Nucl Med* 1991;29:146–159.

188. Dondi M. Captopril renal scintigraphy with ^{99m}Tc-mercaptoacetyltriglycine (^{99m}Tc-MAG$_3$) for detecting renal artery stenosis. *Am J Hypertens* 1991;4:737S–740S.

189. Fommei E, Ghione S, Hilson AJW, et al. Captopril radionuclide test in renovascular hypertension: a European multicentre study. *Eur J Nucl Med* 1994;20:617–623.

190. Geyskes GG, Oei HY, Puylaert CBAJ, et al. Renography with captopril. Changes in a patient with hypertension and unilateral renal artery stenosis. *Arch Intern Med* 1986;146:1705–1708.

191. Sfakianakis GN, Bourgoignie JJ, Daffe D, et al. Single dose captopril scintigraphy in the diagnosis of renovascular hypertension. *J Nucl Med* 1987;28:1383–1392.

192. Erbsloh-Moller B, Dumas A, Roth E, et al. Furosemide ^{131}I-hippuran renography after angiotensin-converting enzyme inhibition for the diagnosis of renovascular hypertension. *Am J Med* 1991;90:23–40.

193. Mann SJ, Pickering RG, Sos TA, et al. Captopril renography in the diagnosis of renal artery stenosis: accuracy and limitations. *Am J Med* 1991;90:30–40.

194. Elliott WJ, Martin WB, Murphy MB. Comparison of two noninvasive screening tests for renovascular hypertension. *Arch Intern Med* 1993;153:755–764.

195. van Jaarsveld BC, Krijnen P, Derkx FH, et al. The place of renal scintigraphy in the diagnosis of renal artery stenosis. Fifteen years of clinical experience. *Arch Intern Med* 1997;157:1226–1234.

196. Mittal BR, Kumar P, Arora P, et al. Role of captopril renography in the diagnosis of renovascular hypertension. *Am J Kidney Dis* 1996;28:209–213.

197. Miralles M, Covas MI, Martinez ME, et al. Captopril test and renal duplex scanning for the primary screening of renovascular disease. *Am J Hypertens* 1997;10:1290–1296.

198. Johansson M, Jensen G, Aurell M, et al. Evaluation of duplex ultrasound and captopril renography for detection of renovascular hypertension. *Kidney Int* 2000;58:774–782.

199. Jaff MR, Olin JW. Revascularization of atherosclerotic renal artery stenosis—indications for intervention. *Texas Heart J* 1998;25:34–39.

200. Novick AC, Textor SC, Bodie B, et al. Revascularization to preserve renal function in patients with atherosclerotic renovascular disease. *Urol Clin North Am* 1984;11:477–490.

201. Kaylor WM, Novick AC, Ziegelbaum M, et al. Reversal of end stage renal failure with surgical revascularization in patients with atherosclerotic renal artery occlusion. *J Urol* 1989;141:486–488.

202. Hansen KJ, Thomason RB, Craven TE, et al. Surgical management of dialysis-dependent ischemic nephropathy. *J Vasc Surg* 1995;21:197–209.

203. Olin JW, Harjai K, Graor RA. Recurrent pulmonary edema in a patient with atherosclerotic renal artery stenosis. *J Vasc Med Biol* 1993;4:216–220.

204. The sixth report of the Joint National Committee on prevention, detection, evaluation, and treatment of high blood pressure. *Arch Intern Med* 1997;24:2413–2446.

205. Gruntzig A, Kuhlmann U, Vetter W, et al. Treatment of renovascular hypertension with percutaneous transluminal dilatation of a renal-artery stenosis. *Lancet* 1978;1:801–802.

206. Sos TA, Pickering TT, Sniderman K, et al. Percutaneous transluminal renal angioplasty in renovascular hypertension due to atheroma or fibromuscular dysplasia. *N Engl J Med* 1983;309:274–279.

207. Ramsay LE, Waller PC. Blood pressure response to percutaneous transluminal angioplasty for renovascular hypertension: an overview of published series. *BMJ* 1990;300:569–572.

208. Tegtmeyer CJ, Hartwell GD, Selby JB, et al. Results and complications of angioplasty in aortoiliac disease. *Circulation* 1991;83:153–160.

209. Bonelli FS, McKusick MA, Textor SC, et al. Renal artery angioplasty: technical results and clinical outcome in 320 patients. *Mayo Clin Proc* 1995;70:1041–1052.

210. Cluzel P, Raynaud A, Beyssen B, et al. Stenoses of renal branch arteries in fibromuscular dysplasia: results of per-

cutaneous transluminal angioplasty. *Radiology* 1994;193:227–232.

211. Klow NE, Paulsen D, Vatne K, et al. Percutaneous transluminal renal artery angioplasty using the coaxial technique. Ten years experience from 591 procedures in 419 patients. *Acta Radiol* 1998;39:594–603.

212. Luft FC, Grim CE, Weinberger MH. Intervention in patients with renovascular hypertension and renal insufficiency. *J Urol* 1983;130:654–656.

213. Pickering TG, Sos TA, Saddekni S, et al. Renal angioplasty in patients with azotemia and renovascular hypertension. *J Hypertens* 1986;4[Suppl 6]:S667–S669.

214. Bell GM, Reid J, Buist TA. Percutaneous transluminal angioplasty improves blood pressure and renal function in renovascular hypertension. *QJM* 1987;63:393–403.

215. O'Donovan RM, Gutierrez OH, Izzo JL Jr. Preservation of renal function by percutaneous renal angioplasty in high-risk elderly patients: short-term outcome. *Nephron* 1993;60:187–92.

216. Canzanello VJ, Millan VG, Spiegel JE, et al. Percutaneous transluminal renal angioplasty in management of atherosclerotic renovascular hypertension: results in 100 patients. *Hypertension* 1989;13:163–172.

217. Martin LG, Casarella WJ, Gaylord GM. Azotemia caused by renal artery stenosis: treatment by percutaneous angioplasty. *Am J Radiol* 1988;150:839–844.

218. Cicuto KP, McLean GK, Oleaga JA, et al. Renal artery stenosis: anatomic classification for percutaneous transluminal angioplasty. *AJR Am J Roentgenol* 1981;137:599–601.

219. Hayes JM, Risius B, Novick AC, et al. Experience with percutaneous transluminal angioplasty for renal artery stenosis at the Cleveland Clinic. *J Urol* 1988;139:488–492.

220. Peterson RA, Baldauf CG, Millward SF, et al. Outpatient percutaneous transluminal angioplasty: a Canadian experience. *J Vasc Interv Radiol* 2000;11:327–332.

221. Plouin PF, Chatellier G, Darne B, et al. Blood pressure outcome of angioplasty in atherosclerotic renal artery stenosis. Essai Multicentrique Medicaments vs Angioplastie (EMMA) Study Group. *Hypertension* 1998;31:823–829.

222. Webster J, Marshall F, Abdalla M, et al. Randomised comparison of percutaneous angioplasty vs. continued medical therapy for hypertensive patients with atheromatous renal artery stenosis. Scottish and Newcastle Renal Artery Stenosis Collaborative Group. *J Hum Hypertens* 1998;12:329–335.

223. van Jaarsveld BC, Krijnen P, Pieterman H, et al. The effect of balloon angioplasty on hypertension in atherosclerotic renal-artery stenosis. Dutch Renal Artery Stenosis Intervention Cooperative Study Group. *N Engl J Med* 2000;342:1007–1014.

224. Tan WA, Wholey MH, Olin JW. Renal angioplasty and hypertension [letter]. *N Engl J Med* 2000;343:438.

225. Plouin P-F, Darne B, Chatellier G, et al. Restenosis after a first percutaneous transluminal renal angioplasty. *Hypertension* 1993;21:89–96.

226. Rees CR, Palmaz JC, Becker GJ, et al. Palmaz stent in atherosclerotic stenoses involving the ostia of the renal arter-

ies: preliminary report of a multicenter study. *Radiology* 1991;181:507–514.

227. White CJ, Ramee SR, Collins TJ, et al. Renal artery stent placement: utility in lesions difficult to treat with balloon angioplasty. *J Am Coll Cardiol* 1997;30:1445–1450.

228. Van de Ven PJ, Kaatee R, Beutler JJ, et al. Arterial stenting and balloon angioplasty in ostial atherosclerotic renovascular disease. A randomised trial. *Lancet* 1999;353:282–286.

229. Baumgartner I, von Aesch K, Do DD, et al. Stent placement in ostial and nonostial atherosclerotic renal arterial stenosis: a prospective follow-up study. *Radiology* 2000;216:498–505.

230. Leertouwer TC, Gussenhoven EJ, Bosch JL, et al. Stent placement for renal arterial stenosis: where do we stand? A meta-analysis. *Radiology* 2000;216:78–85.

231. Wilms GE, Peene PT, Baert AL, et al. Renal artery stent placement with the use of the Wallstent endoprosthesis. *Radiology* 1991;179:457–462.

232. Kuhn FP, Kutkuhn B, Torsello G, et al. Renal artery stenosis: preliminary results of treatment with the Strecher stent. *Radiology* 1991;180:367–372.

233. Hennequin LM, Joffre FG, Rousseau HP, et al. Renal artery stent placement: long-term results with the Wallstent endoprosthesis. *Radiology* 1994;191:713–719.

234. Henry M, Amor M, Henry I, et al. Stent placement in the renal artery: three-year experience with the Palmaz stent. *J Vasc Interv Radiol* 1996;7:343–350.

235. Iannone LA, Underwood PL, Nath A, et al. Effect of primary balloon expandable renal artery stents on long-term patency, renal function and blood pressure in hypertensive and renal insufficient patients with renal artery stenosis. *Cathet Cardiovasc Diagn* 1996;37:243–250.

236. Boisclair C, Therasse E, Oliva VL, et al. Treatment of renal angioplasty failure by percutaneous renal artery stenting with Palmaz stents: midterm technical and clinical results. *AJR Am J Roentgenol* 1997;168:245–251.

237. Harden PN, MacLeod MJ, Rodger RS, et al. Effect of renal-artery stenting on progression of renovascular renal failure. *Lancet* 1997;349:1113–1136.

238. Rundback JH, Gray RJ, Rozenblit G, et al. Renal artery stent placement for the management of ischemic nephropathy. *J Vasc Interv Radiol* 1998;9:413–420.

239. Shannon HM, Gillespie IN, Moss JG. Salvage of the solitary kidney by insertion of a renal artery stent. *AJR Am J Roentgenol* 1998;171:217–222.

240. Watson PS, Hadjipetrou P, Cox SV, et al. Effect of renal artery stenting on renal function and size in patients with atherosclerotic renovascular disease. *Circulation* 2000;102:1671–1677.

241. Novick AC, Ziegelbaum M, Vidt DG, et al. Trends in surgical revascularization for renal artery disease. *JAMA* 1987;257:498–501.

242. Tarazi RY, Hertzer NR, Beven EG, et al. Simultaneous aortic reconstruction and renal revascularization: risk factors and late results in eighty-nine patients. *J Vasc Surg* 1987;5:707–714.

243. Ernst CB, Stanley JC, Marshall FF, et al. Autogenous saphenous vein aortorenal autografts: a ten-year experience. *Arch Surg* 1972;105:855–864.

244. Stoney RJ, Olofsson PA. Aortorenal arterial autografts: the last two decades. *Ann Vasc Surg* 1988;2:169–173.

245. Cormier JM, Fichelle JM, Laurian C, et al. Renal artery revascularization with polytetrafluoroethylene bypass graft. *Ann Vasc Surg* 1990;4:471–478.

246. Novick AC, Jackson CL, Straffon RA. The role of renal autotransplantation in complex urologic reconstruction. *J Urol* 1990;143:452–457.

247. Van Bockel JH, Van Den Akker PJ, Chang PC, et al. Extracorporeal renal artery reconstruction for renovascular hypertension. *J Vasc Surg* 1991;13:101–110.

248. Brewster DC, Darling RC. Splenorenal arterial anastomosis for renovascular hypertension. *Ann Surg* 1979;189: 353–358.

249. Khauli R, Novick AC, Ziegelbaum W. Splenorenal bypass in the treatment of renal artery stenosis: experience with 69 cases. *J Vasc Surg* 1985;2:547–551.

250. Chibaro EA, Libertino JA, Novick AC. Use of the hepatic circulation for renal revascularization. *Ann Surg* 1984;199:406–411.

251. Valentine RJ, Martin JD, Myers SI, et al. Asymptomatic celiac and superior mesenteric artery stenoses are more prevalent among patients with unsuspected renal artery stenoses. *J Vasc Surg* 1991;14:195–199.

252. Fry RE, Fry WJ. Supraceliac aortorenal bypass with saphenous vein for renovascular hypertension. *Surg Gynecol Obstet* 1989;168:180–182.

253. Novick AC, Stewart R, Hodge E, et al. Use of the thoracic aorta for renal arterial reconstruction. *J Vasc Surg* 1994;19:605–609.

254. Hansen KJ, Starr SM, Sands E, et al. Contemporary surgical management of renovascular disease. *J Vasc Surg* 1992;16:319–330.

255. Bredenberg CE, Sampson LN, Ray FS, et al. Changing patterns in surgery for chronic renal artery occlusive diseases. *J Vasc Surg* 1992;15:1018–1023.

256. Libertino JA, Bosco PJ, Ying CY, et al. Renal revascularization to preserve and restore renal function. *J Urol* 1992;147:1485–1487.

257. Lawrie GM, Morris GC, Claeser DH, et al. Renovascular reconstruction: factors affecting long-term prognosis in 919 patients followed up in 31 years. *Am J Cardiol* 1989;63:1085–1092.

258. Hallett JW, Fowl R, O'Brien PC, et al. Renovascular operations in patients with chronic renal insufficiency: do the benefits justify the risks? *J Vasc Surg* 1987;4:622–627.

259. Van Bockel JH, Van Schilfgaarde R, Felthuis W, et al. Surgical treatment of renovascular hypertension caused by arteriosclerosis: I. influence of preoperative factors on blood pressure control early and late after reconstructive surgery. *Surgery* 1987;101:698–705.

260. Libertino JA, Flam TA, Zinman LN, et al. Changing concepts in surgical management of renovascular hypertension. *Arch Intern Med* 1988;148:357–359.

261. Weibull H, Bergqvist D, Bergentz S-E, et al. Percutaneous transluminal renal angioplasty versus surgical reconstruction of atherosclerotic renal artery stenosis: a prospective randomized study. *J Vasc Surg* 1993;18:841–852.

262. Zinman L, Libertino JA. Revascularization of the chronic totally occluded renal artery with restoration of renal function. *J Urol* 1977;18:517–521.

263. Schefft P, Novick AC, Stewart BH, et al. Renal revascularization in patients with total occlusion of the renal artery. *J Urol* 1980;124:184–186.

264. Olin JW, Young JR, Graor RA. Thrombolytic therapy for renal artery occlusions. *Cleve Clin J Med* 1989;56:432–438.

265. Bedoya L, Ziegelbaum M, Vidt DG, et al. The effect of baseline renal function on the outcome following renal revascularization. *Cleve Clin J Med* 1989;56:415–421.

266. Mercier C, Piquet P, Alimi Y, et al. Occlusive disease of the renal arteries and chronic renal failure: the limits of reconstructive surgery. *Ann Vasc Surg* 1990;4:166–170.

267. Textor SC, Novick AC, Steinmuller DR, et al. Renal failure limiting antihypertensive therapy as an indication for renal revascularization. *Arch Intern Med* 1983;143:2208–2211.

268. Dean RH, Tribble RW, Hansen KJ, et al. Evolution of renal insufficiency in ischemic nephropathy. *Ann Surg* 1991;213:446–455.

269. Olin JW. Is survival different for renal artery stenosis patients on dialysis compared with other patients with end-stage renal disease? *J Invasive Cardiol* 1998;10:105–108.

270. Diamond JR. Flash pulmonary edema and the diagnostic suspicion of occult renal artery stenosis. *Am J Kid Dis* 1993;21:328–330.

271. Messina LM, Zelenock GB, Yao KA, et al. Renal revascularization for recurrent pulmonary edema in patients with poorly controlled hypertension and renal insufficiency: a distinct subgroup of patients with atherosclerotic renal artery occlusive disease. *J Vasc Surg* 1992;15:73–80.

INDEX

Page numbers followed by the letter *f* refer to figures; those followed by the letter *t* refer to tables.